Critical Care

Provided through an Educational Grant from

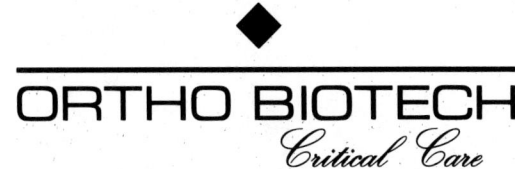

ORTHO BIOTECH
Critical Care

Critical Care

THIRD EDITION

JOSEPH M. CIVETTA, MD

Professor and Chief
Division of Surgical Critical Care
Department of Surgery
University of Miami School of Medicine
Miami, Florida

ROBERT W. TAYLOR, MD

Clinical Associate Professor of Medicine
Director, Critical Care Training Program
St. John's Mercy Medical Center
St. Louis University
St. Louis, Missouri

ROBERT R. KIRBY, MD

Professor of Anesthesiology
University of Florida College of Medicine
Gainesville, Florida

With 203 additional contributors

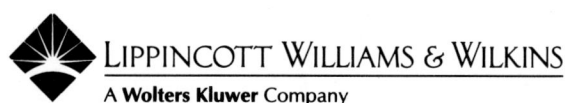

LIPPINCOTT WILLIAMS & WILKINS
A **Wolters Kluwer** Company
Philadelphia · Baltimore · New York · London
Buenos Aires · Hong Kong · Sydney · Tokyo

Acquisitions Editor: Lisa McAllister
Developmental Editor: Emilie Linkins
Project Editor: Ellen M. Campbell
Production Manager: Caren Erlichman
Production Coordinator: MaryClare Malady
Design Coordinator: Melissa Olson
Indexer: Alexandra Nickerson
Compositor: Compset Inc.
Printer: Courier Book Company/Westford

Third Edition

Library of Congress Cataloging-in-Publication Data

Critical care / [edited by] Joseph M. Civetta, Robert W. Taylor,
  Robert R. Kirby ; with 203 additional contributors.—3rd ed.
     p.   cm.
  Includes bibliographical references and index.
  ISBN 0-397-51527-8 (alk. paper)
  1. Critical care medicine. I. Civetta, Joseph M. II. Taylor,
Robert W. (Robert Wesley), 1949–   . III. Kirby, Robert R.
  [DNLM: 1. Critical Care. 2. Intensive Care Units. WX 218
C9334 1996]
  RC86.7.C69   1996
  616'.028—dc20
  DNLM/DLC
  for Library of Congress   96-15571
                                                          CIP

Care has been taken to confirm the accuracy of the information presented
and to describe generally accepted practices. However, the authors, editors,
and publisher are not responsible for errors or omissions or for any consequences from application of the information in this book and make no
warranty, express or implied, with respect to the contents of the publication.

The authors, editors, and publisher have exerted every effort to ensure
that drug selection and dosage set forth in this text are in accordance with
current recommendations and practice at the time of publication. However,
in view of ongoing research, changes in government regulations, and the
constant flow of information relating to drug therapy and drug reactions,
the reader is urged to check the package insert for each drug for any
change in indications and dosage and for added warnings and precautions.
This is particularly important when the recommended agent is a new or
infrequently employed drug.

Some drugs and medical devices presented in this publication have Food
and Drug Administration (FDA) clearance for limited use in restricted
research settings. It is the responsibility of the health care provider to
ascertain the FDA status of each drug or device planned for use in their
clinical practice.

9 8 7 6 5 4 3

To the memory of my parents, Rose and Mike Civetta,
and my dear friend, Clare McGuire.

For my wife, Judy, who provides the love
that makes it all possible.

To my children, Nancy, Betsy, Peter, Jenny, and Katy—
they add spice to my life—and to Kayla of the next generation.

Joseph M. Civetta, MD

My efforts for this edition are dedicated to my wife, Pat,
and children, Lindsey, Matthew, and Jon,
each of whom helped me over the rough spots.

Robert W. Taylor, MD

Dedicated to Margie and Robbie
to acknowledge the many family nights and weekends given up
so that I could work on this book.

Robert R. Kirby, MD

With our heartfelt thanks to Sandy Saunders, Hope Olivo,
Gail C. Frazer, Carolyn S. Linenbroker and Ramona Kilby:
no one but another editor knows how much they do to make a book a reality.
There are so many details, tasks, and drudgery that would stop the editors
but, thank goodness, not our assistants.

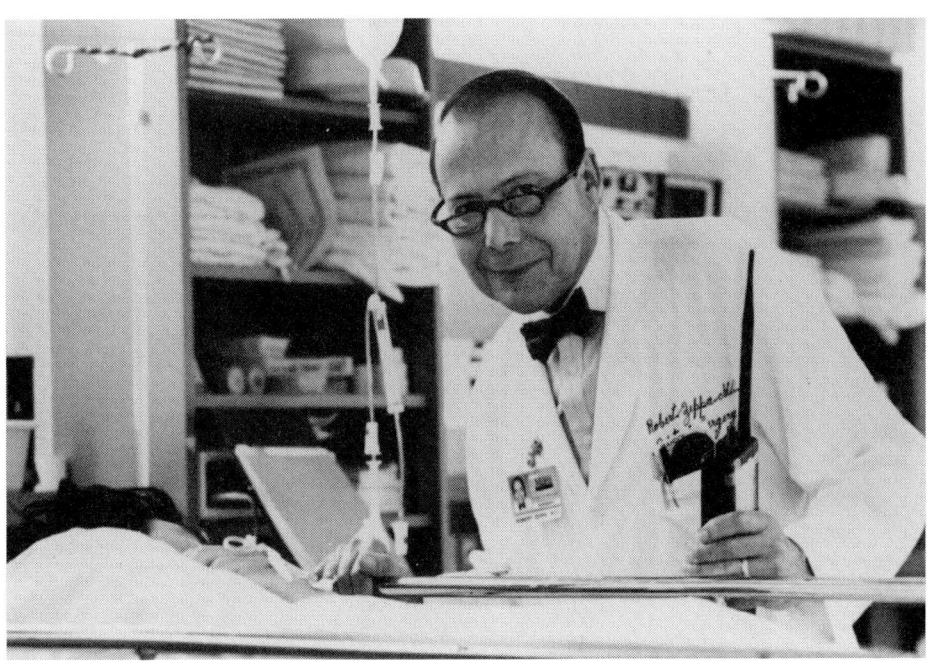

Special Dedication

DR. ROBERT ZEPPA died in 1993 while at work at the University of Miami/Jackson Memorial Medical Center, which he had loved and to which he had devoted the last twenty-five years of his life. The accompanying photograph captures him best, at the bedside of a patient in the Ryder Trauma Center, carrying the "brick." This is the nickname for the two-way radio, used by the physicians to control triage and care of trauma patients, which was chosen by the surgery residents assigned to trauma resuscitation. It was so named because this is a heavy responsibility even with faculty backup as provided by Dr. Zeppa in the picture. He was Chairman of the Department of Surgery of the University of Miami, Surgeon in Chief at Jackson Memorial Medical Center, Chief of the Trauma Service, and the Chief of the Ryder Trauma Center, but still took his 24-hour trauma in-house call until his untimely death. He was an extraordinary man, both in vision and in practical matters. He believed in the collaborative, multidisciplinary practice of critical care in the "living physiology laboratory," as he termed the intensive care unit. As a Professor of Surgery and Physiology, he was one of the first not to just see the link between these two disciplines but, as he described in the Foreword to the first edition of this book, to ensure that this vision became reality in his own department. Two of us (JMC and RRK) had the special good fortune to work with him in developing the concepts and the realities of the "living physiology laboratory."

He was extraordinary, too, for his vision of medicine. He was chosen a number of times by the students to be the commencement speaker at the University of Miami School of Medicine. We chose to include his vision from one of the addresses as the opening statement of the first chapter of this book. He taught that the practice of medicine is a responsibility and a joy for the same reasons: it is a responsibility to stay up-to-date and a joy to do so because it keeps one vital and aware of the dedication necessary to be a physician.

Not only was he a man of vision but again a practical one, for no one demonstrated these two goals on a daily basis more than he. Some believe that his greatest monument is the Ryder Trauma Center. Dade County, Florida had a tumultuous history in the battle to develop a trauma network, its subsequent failure, and the inevitable pressure on the university teaching–county hospital to care for critically injured patients. In his vision, given an adequate facility, the problem would be solved by clustering all of the patients at the institution which was dedicated to provide the care, the teaching, and the research so necessary in this field. As a practical man, he was behind the incredible community effort that resulted in the construction of the $27 million facility, and was deeply involved in the process that resulted in the special sales tax voted by the population of Dade County to support the missions of Jackson Memorial Hospital, including trauma care. The Ryder Trauma Center is now the only trauma center for adult trauma patients in Dade County, with its population of 2 million souls.

Yet even such a substantial "concrete" monument is not a truly fitting memorial for Dr. Zeppa. His visions and his love for patients, students, and residents will live on in the minds and memories of his disciples and associates. This was his essence and this we will endeavor to keep alive for succeeding generations.

JOSEPH M. CIVETTA
ROBERT W. TAYLOR
ROBERT R. KIRBY

Contributors

THOMAS E. AHLERING, MD

Associate Professor of Surgery
Chief, Division of Urology
University of California at Irvine
Orange, California

JAMES A. ALEXANDER, MD

Professor and Division Chief
Thoracic and Cardiovascular Surgery
University of Florida College of Medicine
Gainesville, Florida

OSCAR A. ALVAREZ, MD

Division of Gastroenterology
University of Texas Health Science Center at San Antonio
San Antonio, Texas

JUDITH R. ANDERSON, MD

Clinical Assistant Professor of Medicine
Division of Infectious Diseases
University of Colorado Health Sciences Center
Denver, Colorado
Consultant, Infectious Diseases
North Colorado Medical Center
Greeley, Colorado

MARK E. APPLEMAN, MD

Chief, Infectious Diseases
Newport Hospital
Newport, Rhode Island

CHRISTOPHER J. ARMSTRONG

Justice, Appeals Court
Commonwealth of Massachusetts
Boston, Massachusetts

RAMON A. ARROYO, MD

Assistant Professor of Medicine
F. Edward Hebert College of Medicine
Bethesda, Maryland
Wilford Hall Medical Center
Lackland Air Force Base, Texas

MICHAEL J. BANNER, PhD, RRT

Associate Professor of Anesthesiology and Physiology
Director, Anesthesiology Research Laboratories
University of Florida College of Medicine
Gainesville, Florida

TINA E. BANNER, RN, MN

Director, Cardiovascular Center
*   and Cardiac Catheterization Laboratory*
Shands Hospital at the University of Florida
Gainesville, Florida

ROGER R. BARRETTE, MD, FACS, FCCM

Director, Surgical Progressive Care Unit
Associate Director, Trauma Life-Support Center
The Mercy Hospital of Pittsburgh
Clinical Assistant Professor of Anesthesiology/Critical Care
University of Pittsburgh School of Medicine
Pittsburgh, Pennsylvania

RICHARD J. BARTH, MD

Clinical Assistant Professor of Medicine
University of South Dakota
Central Plains Clinic, Ltd.
Sioux Falls, South Dakota

ROBERT H. BARTLETT, MD

Professor of Surgery
Section of General Therapy
University of Michigan Medical Center
Ann Arbor, Michigan

LAWRENCE S. BERMAN, MD
Associate Professor of Anesthesiology and Pediatrics
University of Florida College of Medicine
Gainesville, Florida

WALTER C. BERNARDS, MD
Associate Clinical Professor of Anesthesiology
Oregon Health Sciences Center
Staff Anesthesiologist
St. Vincent Hospital
Portland, Oregon

PALMER Q. BESSEY, MD
Professor of Surgery
Director of Trauma, Burns, and Surgical Critical Care
Department of Surgery
University of Rochester Medical Center
Rochester, New York

WILLIAM H. BICKELL, MD
Assistant Professor of Surgery
Section of Emergency Medicine
Oklahoma University
Associate Director
Department of Emergency Service
St. Francis Hospital
Tulsa, Oklahoma

PAUL B. BLANCH, BA, RRT
Equipment Manager
Respiratory Care Services
Shands Hospital at the University of Florida
Gainesville, Florida

FREDERICK R. BODE, MD
Associate Professor of Clinical Medicine
Division of Pulmonary and Critical Care Medicine
University of Missouri—Columbia
Columbia, Missouri

EDWARD H. BOYLE, JR., MD
Senior Surgical Research Fellow
University of Washington Medical Center
Seattle, Washington

PHILIP G. BOYSEN, MD, FACP, FCCP
Professor and Chair
Department of Anesthesiology
University of North Carolina
School of Medicine
Chapel Hill, North Carolina

CHARLES E. BRADY, III, MD
Division of Gastroenterology
University of Texas Health Science Center at San Antonio
San Antonio, Texas

BARUCH A. BRODY, PhD
Center for Ethics
Baylor College of Medicine
Houston, Texas

DAVID L. BROWN, MD
Professor of Anesthesiology
Mayo Medical School
Department of Anesthesiology
The Mayo Clinic and Foundation
Rochester, Minnesota

BRIAN A. BROZNICK, MD, CPTC
Executive Director
Center for Organ Recovery and Education
Pittsburgh, Pennsylvania

MATHEW E. BRUNSON, MD
Assistant Professor of Surgery
University of Florida College of Medicine
Gainesville, Florida

CHARLES L. BRYAN, MD
Associate Professor of Medicine
Division of Pulmonary Diseases & Critical Care Medicine
University of Texas Health Science Center at San Antonio
San Antonio, Texas

GEORGE W. BURKE, III, MD
Associate Professor of Surgery
Division of Transplantation
Department of Surgery
University of Miami School of Medicine
Miami, Florida

RICHARD K. BURT, MD
Director
Allogeneic Bone Marrow Transplantation
Northwestern University
Northwestern Memorial Hospital
Chicago, Illinois

PATRICIA M. BYERS, MD, FACS
Associate Professor of Clinical Surgery
Division of Trauma Services
Department of Surgery
University of Miami School of Medicine
Miami, Florida

MATTHEW T. CARPENTER, MD
Assistant Professor of Medicine
F. Edward Hebert College of Medicine
Bethesda, Maryland
Wilford Hall Medical Center
Lackland Air Force Base, Texas

C. JAMES CARRICO, MD
Professor and Chairman
Department of Surgery
University of Texas Southwestern Medical Center
Dallas, Texas

EDDY H. CARRILLO, MD
Assistant Professor
Department of Surgery
University of Louisville
Louisville, Kentucky

NED H. CASSEM, MD
Associate Professor of Psychiatry
Harvard Medical School
Chief of Psychiatry
Massachusetts General Hospital
Boston, Massachusetts

DONALD CATON, MD
Professor of Anesthesiology, Obstetrics, and Gynecology
University of Florida College of Medicine
Gainesville, Florida

GAETANO CIANCIO, MD
Division of Transplantation
Department of Surgery
University of Miami School of Medicine
Miami, Florida

MICHAEL J. CICALE, MD
Associate Professor of Medicine
Pulmonary Division
University of Florida College of Medicine
Gainesville, Florida

JOSEPH M. CIVETTA, MD
Professor and Chief
Division of Surgical Critical Care
Department of Surgery
University of Miami School of Medicine
Miami, Florida

DAVID CLAS, MD
Assistant Professor of Surgery
Université de Montréal
Hopital Maisonneuve-Rosemont
Montréal, Quebec
Canada

THEODORE COLTON, ScD
Professor and Chair
Department of Epidemiology and Biostatistics
Boston University School of Public Health
Boston, Massachusetts

ROBERT B. CONSTANT, MD
Clinical Endocrinologist
Diabetes & Endocrine Center of Orlando
Orlando, Florida

VICENTE CORTES, MD
Assistant Professor of Surgery
University of Connecticut School of Medicine
Assistant Director, EMS/Trauma Service
Hartford Hospital
Hartford, Connecticut

GEORGE E. CRAWFORD, MD
Program Director and Chief
Division of Medicine
Wilford Hall Medical Center
Lackland Air Force Base, Texas

JOSEPH M. DARBY, MD
Associate Professor of Anesthesiology/Critical Care Medicine
University of Pittsburgh School of Medicine
Director, Trauma and Neurosurgical ICU
Presbyterian University Hospital
Pittsburgh, Pennsylvania

LAURIE K. DAVIES, MD
Associate Professor of Anesthesiology
Chief, Cardiothoracic Division
University of Florida College of Medicine
Gainesville, Florida

RICHARD F. DAVIS, MD
Professor of Anesthesiology
Oregon Health Sciences University
Chief, Anesthesiology Service
Veterans Affairs Medical Center
Portland, Oregon

W. ROSS DAVIS, MD
East Alabama Cardiovascular Associates
Opelika, Alabama

R. PHILLIP DELLINGER, MD
Professor and Chief
Pulmonary and Critical Care Medicine
University of Missouri—Columbia
Harry S. Truman Memorial Veterans' Hospital
Columbia, Missouri

RICHARD C. DENNIS, MD, FACS
Associate Professor of Surgery and Anesthesiology
Boston University School of Medicine
Chief, Section on Critical Care Medicine
Boston Medical Center Hospital
Boston City Hospital
Boston, Massachusetts

SCOTT A. DEPPE, MD, FACP, FCCM, FCCP
Consultant in Critical Care Medicine and Hyperbaric Oxygen
Augusta Regional Medical Center
Clinical Associate Professor of Medicine
Medical College of Georgia
Augusta, Georgia

STEPHEN DERDAK, DO, Lt. Col.
Chief, Pulmonary Critical Care
United States Air Force
Wilford Hall Medical Center
Lackland Air Force Base, Texas

KENNETH F. DES ROSIER, MD
Assistant Professor of Medicine
F. Edward Hebert College of Medicine
Bethesda, Maryland
Wilford Hall Medical Center
Lackland Air Force Base, Texas

JACK A. DIPALMA, MD
Division of Gastroenterology
University of South Alabama
Mobile, Alabama

RICHARD S. DOWNEY, MD
Emory University Medical School
Augusta, Georgia

ROBERT J. DOWNEY, MD
Divisions of Thoracic Surgery and Critical Care
Memorial Sloan-Kettering Cancer Center
New York, New York

MIMI EMIG, MD
Assistant Professor of Medicine
Uniformed Services University of the Health Sciences
Bethesda, Maryland
Chief, Infectious Diseases
Scott Air Force Base, Illinois

F. KAYSER ENNEKING, MD

Assistant Professor of Anesthesiology
University of Florida College of Medicine
Gainesville, Florida

FERRIC C. FANG, MD

Assistant Professor of Medicine, Pathology, and Microbiology
Director, Clinical Microbiology Laboratory
Division of Infectious Diseases
University of Colorado Health Sciences Center
Denver, Colorado

J. CHRISTOPHER FARMER, MD, FACP, FCCP

Associate Professor of Clinical Medicine and Surgery
Uniformed Services University of the Health Sciences
Bethesda, Maryland
Director, Critical Care
Wilford Hall Medical Center
Lackland Air Force Base, Texas

JOHN A. FARMER, MD

Division of Cardiology
Ben Taub General Hospital
Houston, Texas

STEPHEN F. FLAHERTY, MD, Maj., USMC

Critical Care Trauma Fellow
Section on Critical Care Medicine
Boston University Medical Center and Boston City Hospital
Boston, Massachusetts
Clinical Assistant Professor of Surgery
Uniformed Services University of the Health Sciences
Bethesda, Maryland

ORLANDO G. FLORETE, JR., MD

Clinical Assistant Professor
Departments of Anesthesiology and Medicine
University of Florida College of Medicine
Health Science Center/Jacksonville
Jacksonville, Florida

JAMES F. FLYNN, MD, FRCPC

Clinical Assistant Professor
Memorial University of Newfoundland
Health Sciences Centre
St. John's, Newfoundland
Canada

BARBARA J. FONER, MD

Department of Critical Care Medicine
St. John's Mercy Medical Center
St. Louis University
St. Louis, Missouri

RICHARD J. FOWL, MD

Section of Vascular Surgery
Mayo Clinic Scottsdale
Scottsdale, Arizona

JILL I. FREEDMAN, MD

Special Fellow in Anesthesiology
University of Florida College of Medicine
Gainesville, Florida

ROBERT E. FROMM, JR., MD, MPH

Associate Professor of Medicine
Baylor College of Medicine
Department of Emergency Services
The Methodist Hospital
Houston, Texas

REED M. GARDNER, PhD

Medical Informatics
LDS Hospital/University of Utah
Salt Lake City, Utah

ENRIQUE GINZBURG, MD

Assistant Professor of Clinical Surgery
Division of Trauma, Vascular Surgery, & Critical Care
Department of Surgery
University of Miami School of Medicine
Miami, Florida

MICHAEL L. GOOD, MD

Chief, Anesthesiology Service
Veterans Affairs Medical Center, Gainesville
Associate Professor of Anesthesiology
University of Florida College of Medicine
Gainesville, Florida

SALVATORE R. GOODWIN, MD

Professor of Anesthesiology and Pediatrics
Medical Director
Pediatric Intensive Care Unit
University of Florida College of Medicine
Gainesville, Florida

NIKOLAUS GRAVENSTEIN, MD

Professor of Anesthesiology and Neurosurgery
University of Florida College of Medicine
Gainesville, Florida

JONATHAN GREENBERG, MD, JD, FACS

Teaching Faculty
Orlando Regional Medical Center
Orlando, Florida

STEPHEN B. GREENBERG, MD

Professor of Medicine
Baylor College of Medicine
Chief, Medical Service
Ben Taub General Hospital
Houston, Texas

MICHAEL A. GREENE, MD

Assistant Professor of Pediatric Cardiovascular Surgery
Division of Thoracic & Cardiovascular Surgery
University of Florida College of Medicine
Gainesville, Florida

DAVID H. GREMILLION, MD, FACP

University of North Carolina
School of Medicine
Wake Medical Center, AHEC
Raleigh, North Carolina

AKE N. A. GRENVIK, MD, PhD

Distinguished Service Professor of Critical Care Medicine
Director, Multidisciplinary Critical Care Training Program
University of Pittsburgh School of Medicine
Pittsburgh, Pennsylvania

JOYCE GRISSOM, MD
Director, Movement Disorders Clinic
Department of Neurology
Wilford Hall Medical Center
San Antonio, Texas

THOMAS GRISSOM, MD
Assistant Professor of Anesthesiology
Uniformed Services University of the Health Sciences
Bethesda, Maryland
Program Director
Anesthesia Critical Care Fellowship
Wilford Hall Medical Center
San Antonio, Texas

JEFFREY S. GROEGER, MD
Medical Director, Special Care Unit
Memorial Sloan-Kettering Cancer Center
Associate Professor of Medicine
Cornell University Medical College
New York, New York

RICHARD L. GROTZ, MD
Fellow, Colon and Rectal Surgery
Mayo Medical School and Mayo Clinic
Rochester, Minnesota

GREGORY GULLAHORN, MD
Residency Director
Co-Director, Critical Care Anesthesia
Department of Anesthesiology
Naval Medical Center—San Diego
San Diego, California

RONALD A. HARTMANN, Pharm D, BCPS
Director of Pharmacy
St. John's Mercy Medical Center
St. Louis, Missouri

J. STEVEN HATA, MD
Assistant Professor
Pulmonary, Critical Care, and Environmental Medicine
University of Missouri—Columbia
School of Medicine
Columbia, Missouri

STEPHEN O. HEARD, MD
Associate Professor of Anesthesiology and Surgery
Co-Director, Surgical Intensive Care Units
University of Massachusetts Medical Center
Worcester, Massachusetts

SUDARSHAN HEBBAR, MD
Associate
Kidney Associates of Kansas City, P.C.
Kansas City, Missouri

JAY B. HIGGS, MD
Associate Professor of Clinical Medicine
F. Edward Hebert College of Medicine
Bethesda, Maryland
Wilford Hall Medical Center
Lackland Air Force Base, Texas

RICHARD J. HOWARD, MD
Professor of Surgery
University of Florida College of Medicine
Gainesville, Florida

JUDITH A. HUDSON-CIVETTA, RN, MSN
Research Associate
Division of Surgical Critical Care
Department of Surgery
University of Miami School of Medicine
Miami, Florida

JAMES M. HURST, MD
Professor of Surgery
Vice Chair, Clinical Department of Surgery
University of Cincinnati Medical Center
Cincinnati, Ohio

WILLIAM L. ISLEY, MD
Associate Professor of Medicine
Chief, Division of Endocrinology, Diabetes, & Metabolism
University of Missouri—Kansas City
School of Medicine
Kansas City, Missouri

CHRISTOPHER F. JAMES, MD
Associate Professor of Anesthesiology
University of Florida College of Medicine
J. Hillis Miller Health Science Center
Gainesville, Florida

K. N. JEEJEEBHOY, MD, BS, FRCP(C)
Professor of Medicine
University of Toronto Faculty of Medicine
Director, Nutrition and Digestive Disease Program
St. Michael's Hospital
Toronto, Ontario
Canada

EDGAR J. JIMENEZ, MD
Fellow, Department of Critical Care Medicine
St. John's Mercy Medical Center
St. Louis, Missouri

JAY A. JOHANNIGMAN, MD
Assistant Professor of Surgery
Division of Trauma and Critical Care
Department of Surgery
University of Cincinnati Medical Center
Cincinnati, Ohio

CESAR A. KELLER, MD
Professor of Internal Medicine
Division of Pulmonology and Pulmonary Occupational Medicine
St. Louis University Health Sciences Center
St. Louis, Missouri

ROBERT R. KIRBY, MD
Professor of Anesthesiology
University of Florida College of Medicine
Gainesville, Florida

ORLANDO C. KIRTON, MD, FACS
Assistant Professor of Clinical Surgery
Division of Trauma & Surgical Critical Care
Department of Surgery
University of Miami School of Medicine
Miami, Florida

STEPHEN M. KOCH, MD
Assistant Professor of Anesthesia and Internal Medicine
University of Texas Medical School at Houston
Houston, Texas

ERIC T. KUNICHIKA, MD
Department of Anesthesiology
Florida Hospital
Orlando, Florida

ANTHONY LAI, MD
South Florida Perinatal Associates
Miami, Florida

SAMSUN LAMPOTANG, PhD
Assistant Professor of Anesthesiology and Mechanical Engineering
University of Florida College of Medicine
Gainesville, Florida

DENNIS P. LAWLOR, MD
Pulmonary/Critical Care Medicine
Wilford Hall Medical Center
Lackland Air Force Base, Texas

A. JOSEPH LAYON, MD
Associate Professor of Anesthesiology, Surgery, and Medicine
Associate Director of Critical Care and Emergency Medicine
Associate Director, UF/Shands Burn Center
Chief, Emergency Medical Services
University of Florida College of Medicine
Gainesville, Florida

DOUGLAS R. LEIGH, MD
Chief, Department of Infectious Diseases
Keesler Medical Center
Keesler Air Force Base, Mississippi

KIMBERLY A. LENTZ, MD
Assistant Professor of Clinical Radiology
University of Miami School of Medicine
Miami, Florida

JOE U. LEVI, MD
Professor of Surgery
Division of General Surgery
Department of Surgery
University of Miami School of Medicine
Miami, Florida

STEWART J. LEVINE, MD
Staff Physician
Critical Care Medicine Department
Clinical Center
National Institutes of Health
Bethesda, Maryland

DAVID H. LINDNER, DO
Fellow, Critical Care Medicine
St. John's Mercy Medical Center
St. Louis University
St. Louis, Missouri

ALAN S. LIVINGSTONE, MD
Professor and Vice Chairman of Surgery
Chief, Division of Surgical Oncology
University of Miami School of Medicine
Miami, Florida

LAURIE A. LOIACONO, MD
Fellow, Division of Critical Care Medicine
Department of Surgery
Hartford Hospital
Hartford, Connecticut

SALVATORE LOPALO, CRNA, MS Ed, MA
Associate in Anesthesiology
University of Florida College of Medicine
J. Hillis Miller Health Science Center
Gainesville, Florida

KEN P. MADDEN, MD, PhD
Department of Neurosciences
Marshfield Clinic
Marshfield, Wisconsin

LARRY C. MARTIN, MD
Associate Professor of Surgery
Director of Trauma Services
Department of Surgery
Ohio State University
Columbus, Ohio

LUIS S. MATOS, MD, MPH
Associate Professor of Clinical Surgery
Chief, Division of Hyperbaric Medicine
Department of Surgery
University of Miami School of Medicine
Miami, Florida

GEORGE M. MATUSCHAK, MD
Professor of Internal Medicine and Pharmacological Science
Division of Pulmonology
Department of Internal Medicine
St. Louis University Health Science Center
St. Louis, Missouri

SUSAN MCCAFFREY, RN
Associate Director
Quality Management
Hartford Hospital
Hartford, Connecticut

LAURENCE MCCULLOUGH, MD
Professor of Medicine and Medical Ethics
Center for Medical Ethics and Health Policy
Baylor College of Medicine
Houston, Texas

MARK G. MCKENNEY, MD, FACS

Assistant Professor of Clinical Surgery
Division of Trauma
Department of Surgery
University of Miami School of Medicine
Miami, Florida

THOMAS L. MCKIERNAN, MD, FACC, FSCAI

Associate Professor of Clinical Medicine
Director, Division of Cardiology
Loyola University of Chicago
Stritch School of Medicine
Maywood, Illinois

PATRICK C. MCKILLION, MD

Assistant Professor
Division of Pulmonary, Critical Care, and Environmental Medicine
Department of Internal Medicine
University of Missouri—Columbia
School of Medicine
Columbia, Missouri

ROGER S. MECCA, MD

Chairman, Department of Anesthesiology
Danbury Hospital
Danbury, Connecticut

MANDEEP R. MEHRA, MD

Clinical Assistant Professor of Medicine
Louisiana State University
School of Medicine
Director of Ambulatory Services
Advanced Heart Failure and Cardiac Transplantation
Ochsner Medical Institutions
New Orleans, Louisiana

GREGORY P. MELCHER, MD, FACP

Associate Professor of Medicine
Uniformed Services University of the Health Sciences
Chairman and Program Director
Department of Infectious Diseases
Wilford Hall Medical Center
Lackland Air Force Base, Texas

RICHARD J. MELKER, MD, PhD

Associate Professor of Anesthesiology and Pediatrics
University of Florida College of Medicine
Gainesville, Florida

LESLIE W. MILLER, MD, FACC

Professor of Medicine and Surgery
Division of Cardiology
St. Louis University Health Sciences Center
St. Louis, Missouri

WILLIAM W. MONAFO, MD

Professor of Surgery
Washington University School of Medicine
Active Staff, Barnes Hospital
Chief of Surgery
St. Louis Regional Medical Center
St. Louis, Missouri

GARY L. MUELLER, MD, FACP

Consulting Endocrinologist
Summit Endocrinology
Summit Medical Center
Nashville, Tennessee

RICHARD S. MUTHER, MD, FACP

Clinical Professor of Medicine
University of Missouri—Kansas City
School of Medicine
Director of Hemodialysis
Research Medical Center
Kansas City, Missouri

ANTONI M. NEJMAN, DDS, MD

Director, Surgical Intensive Care Unit
Department of Veterans Affairs Medical Center
Department of Anesthesiology
University of Miami School of Medicine
Miami, Florida

LOREN D. NELSON, MD

Director, Surgical Trauma Intensive Care Unit
Orlando Regional Medical Center
Orlando, Florida
Clinical Associate Professor
Department of Surgery
University of Florida College of Medicine
Gainesville, Florida

JOAN M. NIEHOFF, MD

Resident, Anesthesia Program
University of Michigan Medical Center
Ann Arbor, Michigan

SCOTT H. NORWOOD, MD

Director, Trauma Service
East Texas Medical Center
Tyler, Texas

DIEGO NUNEZ, JR., MD

Professor and Director
Emergency-Trauma Radiology
Department of Radiology
University of Miami School of Medicine
Miami, Florida

DANIEL J. O'BRIEN, PhD, RN

Associate Professor of Critical Care Nursing
Thoracic and Cardiovascular Surgery
University of Florida College of Medicine
Gainesville, Florida

LORETTA M. O'BRIEN, Major, USAF

Staff Clinician
Department of Infectious Disease
David Grand United States Air Force Medical Center
Travis Air Force Base, California

MARC D. PALTER, MD

Assistant Professor of Surgery
University of Connecticut
School of Medicine
Medical Director, Neurosurgical ICU
Attending Staff, Trauma Service
Hartford Hospital
Hartford, Connecticut

ROBERT I. PARKER, MD

Vice Chairman for Academic Affairs
Associate Professor of Pediatrics
Director, Pediatric Hematology—Oncology
Department of Pediatrics
State University of New York—Stony Brook
Stony Brook, New York

MICHAEL D. PECK, MD

Associate Professor of Surgery
Department of Surgery
University of Miami School of Medicine
Assistant Director
University of Miami
Jackson Memorial Medical Center
Miami, Florida

KENNETH A. PERRET, MD

University of Texas Health Science Center at San Antonio
San Antonio, Texas

WILLIAM T. PERUZZI, MD

Associate Professor of Anesthesiology
Associate Chair of Perioperative Services
Chief, Section of Critical Care Medicine
Department of Anesthesiology
Northwestern University Medical School
Chicago, Illinois

WILLIAM W. PFAFF, MD

Professor Emeritus
Department of Surgery
University of Florida College of Medicine
J. Hillis Miller Health Science Center
Gainesville, Florida

TIMOTHY H. POHLMAN, MD

Department of Surgery
University of Washington
School of Medicine
Seattle, Washington

NORMAND RACINE, MD, FRCP(C)

Assistant Professor of Medicine
Cardiology Division
Université de Montréal
Hopital Notre Dame
Montréal, Québec
Canada

CARL E. RAVIN, MD

Professor and Chairman
Department of Radiology
Duke University Medical Center
Durham, North Carolina

CHARLES A. REASNER, MD, FACP, FACE

Associate Professor of Medicine
Chief of Clinical Endocrinology
University of Texas Health Sciences Center at San Antonio
San Antonio, Texas

GERALD M. REID, MD

Clinical Assistant Professor of Medicine
University of Missouri—Kansas City
School of Medicine
Director of Hemodialysis
Dialysis Clinics Inc. Dialysis Unit
Kansas City, Missouri

H. DAVID REINES, MD, FACS, FCCM

Chief of Surgery
Newton Wellesley Hospital
Professor of Surgery
Tufts University Medical School
Newton, Massachusetts

MATTHEW M. RICE, MD, JD

Assistant Clinical Professor of Emergency Medicine
Uniformed Services University of the Health Sciences
Assistant Clinical Professor of Medicine
University of Washington School of Medicine
Chair, Department of Emergency Medicine
Madigan Army Medical Center
Tacoma, Washington

R. DWAINE RIEVES, MD

Medical Officer
Food and Drug Administration
Center for Biologics Research and Evaluation
Rockville, Maryland

JAMIE ROCHE, MD

Director
Quality Management
Hartford Hospital
Hartford, Connecticut

LOREN A. ROLAK, MD

Department of Neurosciences
Marshfield Clinic
Marshfield, Wisconsin
Associate Clinical Professor of Neurology
University of Wisconsin Medical School
Madison, Wisconsin

BRADLEY H. RUBEN, DO, FCCP, FACA

Anesthesiology, Critical Care
Seven Rivers Hospital
Family Practice, Meadowcrest Family Practice
Crystal River, Florida

PAUL A. RUTECKI, MD

Associate Professor of Neurology & Neurosurgery
University of Wisconsin Medical School at Madison
Director, Francis M. Forster and University of Wisconsin
  Epilepsy Center
William S. Middleton Veterans Affairs Hospital
Madison, Wisconsin

RICHARD RYSKAMP, MD

Department of Critical Care Medicine
St. John's Mercy Medical Center
St. Louis University
St. Louis, Missouri

JEFFREY A. SADOWSKY, MD
Department of Critical Care Medicine
St. John's Mercy Medical Center
St. Louis University
St. Louis, Missouri

SHARON M. SALAMAT, MD, PhD
Assistant Professor of Clinical Obstetrics & Gynecology
Division of Perinatology
Department of Obstetrics and Gynecology
University of Miami School of Medicine
Miami, Florida

ARAVIND B. SANKAR, MD
Division of Cardiothoracic Surgery
Department of Surgery
University of Texas Medical Branch
Galveston, Texas

PAUL SATISH, MD
Associate Director of Critical Care Center
Columbia Memorial Hospital
Jacksonville, Florida

DAVID A. SCHENK
Assistant Clinical Professor of Medicine
University of Texas Medical School at San Antonio
Associate Professor
Uniformed Services University of the Health Sciences
Chief, Pulmonary/Critical Care Medicine
Wilford Hall Medical Center
Lackland Air Force Base, Texas

ROBERT SCHLICHTIG, MD
Department of Anesthesia
Oakland VA Medical Center
Pittsburgh, Pennsylvania

DAVID A. SEARS, MD
Professor of Medicine
Baylor College of Medicine
Houston, Texas

ERAN SEGAL, MD
Instructor in Anesthesiology
Sackler School of Medicine
Tel Aviv University
Department of Anesthesiology
Sheba Medical Center
Tes-Hashomer, Israel

JOAN SHAFFER, MD
Department of Critical Care Medicine
St. John's Mercy Medical Center
St. Louis University
St. Louis, Missouri

BARRY A. SHAPIRO, MD
Professor and Chairman
Department of Anesthesiology
Northwestern University Medical School
Chicago, Illinois

DAVID V. SHATZ, MD, FACS
Assistant Professor of Clinical Surgery
Division of Trauma and Surgical Critical Care
Department of Surgery
University of Miami School of Medicine
Miami, Florida

JAMES H. SHELHAMER, MD
Department of Critical Care Medicine
National Institutes of Health
Bethesda, Maryland

SCOTT A. SHIKORA, MD, FACS
Assistant Professor of Surgery
Tufts University School of Medicine
Director, Surgical Intensive Care Units
Faulkner Hospital
Boston, Massachusetts

AVNER SIDI, MD
Associate Professor of Anesthesiology
University of Florida College of Medicine
Gainesville, Florida

DANNY SLEEMAN, MD
Associate Professor of Clinical Surgery
Division of Surgical Critical Care
Department of Surgery
University of Miami School of Medicine
Miami, Florida

ROBERT A. SMITH, MS, RRT
Assistant Professor
Department of Anesthesiology
University of South Florida
College of Medicine
Tampa, Florida

JORGE LUIS SOSA, MD
Director
Laparoscopic Institute of South Florida
Miami, Florida

RICHARD L. SPIELVOGEL, MD
Professor and Chair
Department of Dermatology
Medical College of Pennsylvania
*   and Hahnemann University Medical School*
Philadelphia, Pennsylvania

DONALD S. STEVENS, MD
Assistant Professor
Department of Anesthesiology
Director, Pain Management Services
University of Massachusetts Medical Center
Worcester, Massachusetts

DAVID A. STRIKER, MD
Department of Critical Care Medicine
St. John's Mercy Medical Center
St. Louis University
St. Louis, Missouri

WARREN J. STRITTMATTER, MD
Division of Neurology
Duke University Medical Center
Durham, North Carolina

CONNIE E. TAYLOR, MD
Department of Anesthesiology
Tulane Medical Center
New Orleans, Louisiana

ROBERT W. TAYLOR, MD
Clinical Associate Professor of Medicine
Director, Critical Care Training Program
St. John's Mercy Medical Center
St. Louis University
St. Louis, Missouri

STEPHEN P. TAYLOR, MD
Department of Critical Care Medicine
St. John's Mercy Medical Center
St. Louis University
St. Louis, Missouri

DAN R. THOMPSON, MD, FACP, FCCM
Medical Director, Trauma/Intensive Care Unit
The Mercy Hospital of Pittsburgh
Clinical Assistant Professor of Anesthesiology and Critical Care
The University of Pittsburgh
School of Medicine
Pittsburgh, Pennsylvania

SUBHASH TODI, MD
Clinical Research Fellow
Assistant Clinical Professor
Department of Critical Care Medicine
St. John's Mercy Medical Center
St. Louis University
St. Louis, Missouri

FREDERICK L. TRENT, MD
Clinical Assistant Professor
Departments of Anesthesia and Medicine
University of Florida College of Medicine
Gainesville, Florida

STEVEN J. TROTTIER, MD
Assistant Clinical Professor
Department of Critical Care Medicine
St. John's Mercy Medical Center
St. Louis University
St. Louis, Missouri

ANDREAS G. TZAKIS, MD
Professor of Surgery
Chief, Division of Liver and GI Transplantation
Department of Surgery
University of Miami School of Medicine
Miami, Florida

ALBERT J. VARON, MD
Professor of Clinical Anesthesiology and Surgery
Director, Division of Trauma Anesthesia and Critical Care
Department of Anesthesia
University of Miami School of Medicine
Miami, Florida

CARLOS A. VAZ FRAGOSO, MD
Pulmonary Division
Danbury Hospital
Danbury, Connecticut

HECTOR O. VENTURA, MD
The Advanced Heart Failure and Cardiac Transplant Program
Ochsner Medical Institutions
New Orleans, Louisiana

BAHMAN VENUS, MD, FCCM, FCCP
Chair, Department of Critical Care Medicine
Columbia Memorial Hospital
Jacksonville, Florida

CHRISTOPHER VEREMAKIS, MD
Chairman, Critical Care Medicine
Chairman, Graduate Medical Education
St. John's Mercy Medical Center
St. Louis University
St. Louis, Missouri

PHILIP A. VILLANUEVA, MD
Associate Professor of Clinical Neurological Surgery
Department of Neurological Surgery
University of Miami School of Medicine
Miami, Florida

GEORGE WALLACE-BARNHILL, PhD
Professional Therapy Associates
Hollywood, Florida
The Retreat Psychiatric Hospital
Clinical Director
Resolutions Partial Hospitalization Program
*   for Women with Trauma*
Sunrise, Florida

C. GILLON WARD, MD
Professor of Surgery
Department of Surgery
University of Miami School of Medicine
Director, Burn Center
University of Miami
Jackson Memorial Medical Center
Miami, Florida

MARC G. WEBB, MD
Assistant Professor of Clinical Surgery
Division of Liver and GI Transplantation
Department of Surgery
University of Miami School of Medicine
Miami, Florida

CHARLES A. WEBER, MD
Assistant Clinical Professor of Internal Medicine
University of Wisconsin Medical School
Meriter Park Hospital
Madison, Wisconsin

WILLIAM WEHRMACHER, MD, FACC, FACP
Clinical Professor of Medicine
Adjunct Professor of Physiology
Loyola University Medical Center
Maywood, Illinois

VALERIE WELLS, RN

Clinical Educator
Surgical Intensive Care Unit/Cardiovascular Intensive Care Unit
Surgical Hospital Center
Jackson Memorial Medical Center
Miami, Florida

DEBORAH WEPPLER, RN, MSN

Clinical Specialist
Division of Liver/Gastrointestinal Transplantation
Jackson Memorial Medical Center
Miami, Florida

M. JACK WILLIAMS, MD

Clinical Professor of Surgery
University of Texas
Health Science Center
Houston, Texas

RICHARD E. WINN, MD

Professor of Internal Medicine
Texas A&M College of Medicine
Director, Division of Pulmonary Medicine
Scott & White Clinic and Hospitals
Temple, Texas

MICHAEL G. WISE, MD

Clinical Professor of Psychiatry
Louisiana State University
School of Medicine
Tulane University School of Medicine
New Orleans, Louisiana
Uniformed Services University of the Health Sciences
F. Edward Hebert School of Medicine
Bethesda, Maryland

NEIL S. YESTON, MD

Professor of Surgery
University of Connecticut
School of Medicine
Director, Division of Critical Care Medicine
Department of Surgery
Hartford Hospital
Hartford, Connecticut

ERNLÉ YOUNG, PhD

Clinical Professor of Medicine (Ethics)
Stanford University Center for Biomedical Ethics
Palo Alto, California

GARY PAUL ZALOGA, MA, MD, FCCM, FCCP

Professor of Anesthesia/Critical Care Medicine
Bowman Gray School of Medicine
Head, Section of Critical Care
Wake Forest University Medical Center
Winston-Salem, North Carolina

JANICE L. ZIMMERMAN, MD, FCCM, FCCP

Associate Professor of Medicine
Baylor College of Medicine
Houston, Texas

ALEJANDRO ZULUAGA, MD

Clinical Associate Professor of Radiology
University of Antioquia
Medellin, Colombia

JOSEPH B. ZWISCHENBERGER, MD

Professor of Surgery and Medicine
Division of Cardiothoracic Surgery
University of Texas Medical Branch
Galveston, Texas

GREGORY A. ZYCH, MD

Associate Professor of Orthopedics and Rehabilitation
Chief, Division of Orthopedic Trauma
Department of Orthopedics and Rehabilitation
University of Miami School of Medicine
Miami, Florida

Foreword to the First Edition

I am honored to have been asked to write the foreword for this comprehensive new textbook entitled *Critical Care*, edited by Drs. Civetta, Taylor, and Kirby. My perspective during this endeavor stems from the early attempts in the 1950s to segregate the sickest patients into appropriate nursing units at the North Carolina Memorial Hospital. In 1971 when I was offered the Chair in Surgery at the University of Miami School of Medicine, the then-young surgical intensive care unit was not administered by the Department of Surgery. I asked for the SICU to be placed administratively within the Department of Surgery as a condition for accepting this position. The reason for such a request was to provide a classroom for the teaching of applied pharmacology and abnormal physiology to house officers. To this end it became imperative to recruit a surgeon who had the strongest interest in this area. The Department of Surgery and I were fortunate that Dr. Civetta was available, and the rest, in terms of development of this unit, is history.

It has been a most satisfying experience to have watched young people of all three basic disciplines come through the training program in our SICU under the directorship of Dr. Civetta. I am especially gratified that our surgical residents, at the end of their 5 years, demonstrate competence in the care of the multi-injured patient, the severe diabetic, and the patient with myocardial compromise. Insofar as such medical conditions affect diagnoses of surgical patients, then surgeons must have the ability to cope successfully with these problems. The converse is equally true today: other specialists such as internists and anesthesiologists must understand the problems of surgical patients. It has been my strong belief that only by direct participation in a critical care unit would such skills be acquired.

It is especially heartwarming for me to provide this foreword for the most comprehensive book on critical care I have ever imagined. It should serve readers in all disciplines, thus conceptually and practically advancing the cause of multidisciplinary critical care.

My fond regards and congratulations to the editors for their editorial skills.

ROBERT ZEPPA, MD

Preface to the Third Edition

A Third Edition poses new and perhaps more difficult challenges for the editors. The first edition has an immediate goal to create a book de novo. We, in common with most editors, tried to organize structure and content to help the reader during his or her first experience in the intensive care unit and so to create a book that would be read and useful. This concept, of course, introduces a problem, because one would like to have mastered some body of knowledge before beginning the experience designed to teach it. Arthur Block, in the anthology *Murphy's Law and Other Reasons Why Things Go Wrong*, lists Finagle's first rule: "to study a subject best, understand it thoroughly before you start."

We created the "Immediate Concerns" at the beginning of clinical chapters and tried to organize the book into sections that would provide not only the medical knowledge but also the growing knowledge of other disciplines necessary to practice intensive care. These included legal, ethical, psychological, and societal viewpoints. We also chose specialists and sub-specialists, such as thoracic surgeons, urologists, hematologists, and oncologists, as authors and asked them to express their viewpoints to those specializing in critical care. This approach represented an attempt to give value and insight into daily bedside care to the clinical chapters. We tried to accomplish this goal by instructing the authors to write down all the things they considered important to transmit to the intensivists who, in many institutions, would be charged with the minute-to-minute responsibility for the care of the primary operating surgeon's or a medical specialist's patients. We hope that this would lead to true synergy of care and collaborative practice.

The second edition had obvious new objectives for us. Once we saw the actual book, we realized that despite our attempts, both redundancies and vacuums occurred in the choice of chapters and the materials contained therein. We gained different perspectives through the eyes of various reviewers and we tried to take to heart their well-intentioned criticisms. And finally, we needed to include the important developments that had occurred since the original manuscripts were submitted. This meant new material in some chapters as well as the addition of totally new chapters. Thus, the second edition contained 40 new or newly authored chapters, 22 rewritten chapters, and 50 other chapters with extensive revisions. This effort eventually culminated in 2,000 pages, which made the book less than ideal for helping to solve bedside crises, the concept behind the "Immediate Concerns" sections. Therefore, a year later, we extracted information from many chapters in which immediate knowledge would be essential and published it in the *Handbook of Critical Care*. This effort was pocket-sized and contained in outline form material we thought would be useful at the bedside. Each outline in the handbook referred back to the master chapter in the textbook so that the reader could learn relevant background, physiology, and pathophysiology, and obtain references for further study.

Then came this Third Edition. While we were tempted to polish and update the format and content, we felt that since ten years had passed from the time we started the first edition, readers would best be served if we "started over." Also, in all of medicine but especially in critical care, an increased emphasis on decision-making has evolved, together with many changes in the delivery of health care. Changes in the scientific basis of critical care were also numerous, not just in physiology as represented in our chapters titled "Essential Physiologic Concerns," but also in a new perspective which we termed "Modulating the Response to Injury." Therefore, we decided to "re-engineer" the entire textbook.

Decision-making in all its dimensions is the basis for the 13 chapters in Section I. The individual chapters on physiologic concerns, which led the sections on organ system problems in the second edition, were grouped together in

Section II. The third section, consisting of 10 chapters, discusses modulating the response to injury. Our hope was to summarize current knowledge, but more importantly, to provide a foundation for interpreting new developments which surely would be forthcoming after publication. More than 20 chapters in Section IV deal with techniques, procedures, and treatment. Section V, "Monitoring: Practical Applications," contains an additional 8 chapters. In all, 63 chapters precede discussion of specific patients, illnesses, or organ systems.

New chapters deal with splanchnic flow and resuscitation, interventional radiology, feeding tube placement, work of breathing and respiratory muscle fatigue, continuous ST segment monitoring, and protecting the practitioner. Recruitment of experts for the first edition was relatively easy. However, conceptually and practically, it was sometimes difficult to ask the same author ten years later to bring the same enthusiasm and perspective to the task of another revision for the Third Edition. Interests and responsibilities change over a decade; thus we chose to ask many original authors to allow a new author to do the initial revision. In this way we hoped to add enthusiasm and a new perspective, yet maintain the senior author's experience, prior contributions, and editing skills. We believe this combination revitalizes and *retains* time-tested material. As a result, this edition presents 32 new chapters and 36 more with new first authors (roughly one-half of the book).

We also listened to what our readers told us. We were glad to find that many thought the book was useful; when faced with a clinical problem, they found valuable, applicable information. This fact encouraged us to try and make the book more concrete and specific. The Immediate Concerns sections, in most chapters, were subdivided into Major Problems, Stress Points, Essential Diagnostic Tests and Procedures, and Initial Therapy. Each author was urged to devise chapters to guide clinical practice: what to think of first, what should be done in daily practice, and what to do when initial interventions are insufficient.

"New and improved" is probably the most overused phrase in advertising, yet our challenge was to validate this concept. Critical care medicine has changed since the first edition; we have tried to create a Third Edition that reflects current practice, yet will remain relevant at least a few years. If we have done so, it is due to the efforts of the authors, both old and new, and especially the staff at Lippincott–Raven. They devised a continuous, intensive production schedule that permitted simultaneous submission of manuscripts, our editing, their copy-editing, shipment of galleys to the editors, and production of page proofs. They even held out page proofs to the last minute so that references "in press" at the time of submission could be updated.

Finally, the Second Edition of the *Handbook of Critical Care* has been prepared simultaneously, and we hope this package will help provide information at the bedside and material to establish a firm foundation of critical care knowledge.

The complete revision of the format, new goals, and new production schedule had one final result for us, the editors: this was no longer a re-revision, which would have been a tedious task, but the realization of a new vision. For us that was as exciting as the creation of the first edition itself.

JOSEPH M. CIVETTA
ROBERT W. TAYLOR
ROBERT R. KIRBY

Contents

SECTION I   1

DECISION-MAKING

Chapter 1   3

How to Read a Medical Article and Understand Basic Statistics

Joseph M. Civetta
Theodore Colton

Critical Reading of the Medical Literature   4
Fundamentals of Biostatistics in Medical Research   9
Interpretation of Study Results   14
Coda   20

Chapter 2   21

Setting Objectives: Perspectives for Care

Orlando C. Kirton
Joseph M. Civetta

The Economic Issues: Is Economics King?   22
Selection of "Appropriate" Patients   22
Generic Goals of Intensive Care   23
Beneficence, Nonmaleficence, and Distributive Justice   24
Patient Autonomy   25
"Futility of Care"   25

The Family: Compassion and Avoiding Conflict   26
Immediate Objective: Examine Societal Values   27
Immediate Objective: Examine Bedside Care   29
Appendix 2-1: Advance Directive: Living Will   29
Appendix 2-2: Health Care Proxy Designation and
   Acceptance Form   31
Appendix 2-3: Durable Power of Attorney for Health Care
   and Health Care Surrogate Designation Form   32
Appendix 2-4: Affidavit   33

Chapter 3   35

Collaborative Care: Physician and Nursing Interactions

Danny Sleeman
Judith A. Hudson-Civetta
Joseph M. Civetta

The Surgeon Before the ICU   35
Members of the Team   35
Communications   36
Problems With Communication   37
Special Situations   37
Fellows' Function and Interrelationships   37
Functioning as a Team   39
Factors Contributing to Collaboration   40
Allocating Nursing Care   40
Nursing Care Functions   41
Allocation of Nursing Resources   41

Chapter 4   49

Clinical Decision-Making

David V. Shatz
Joseph M. Civetta

Clinical Data as Scientific Variables   50
Cardiopulmonary Resuscitation and Do-Not-Resuscitate
   Orders   50
Elements of Clinical Care   52
The Influence of Time   55
First Vantage Point: Source of Admissions   55
Second Vantage Point: On ICU Admission   56
Third Vantage Point: Short-Term ICU Outcome   56
Fourth Vantage Point: Continued ICU Care   57
Fifth Vantage Point: Long-Term ICU Patients   58
Last Vantage Point: Discharge From Intensive
   Care   59

Chapter 5   63

Life and Death in the ICU: Ethical Considerations

Ernlé W. D. Young

Medical Ethics   63
The "Futility" Debate   73
Factors Compelling Treatment Even in the Likelihood
   of a Negative Outcome   74
Physician Aid-in-Dying   77

Chapter 6   81

Informed Consent and Refusal

Laurence B. McCullough

Key Considerations to Practice Informed Consent   81
When Patients Refuse Critical Care Intervention   84
Ethical Foundations of Informed Consent   85
Special Considerations   86

Chapter 7   89

Understanding Reactions of Patient and Family

George L. Wallace-Barnhill

Psychological Concepts   89
Staff Involvement With Families   91
The Patient in the ICU   92

Chapter 8   95

Iatrogenesis

Mark G. McKenney
Joseph M. Civetta

Type 1 Iatrogenesis: Incorrect Diagnosis   96
Type 2 Iatrogenesis: Therapy-Related   96
Type 3 Iatrogenesis: Procedure-Related   97
Type 4 Iatrogenesis: Laboratory Error   99
Type 5 Iatrogenesis: Decubitus Ulcer   100
Type 6 Iatrogenesis: Falls   101
Discussion and Legal Aspects   101

Chapter 9   105

Judicial Involvement in Treatment Decisions

Christopher Armstrong

The Beginnings of Court Involvement   106
A Consensus Emerges   107
Points on Which There Is No Consensus   114

Chapter 10   117

Important Legal Concepts in Critical Care

Baruch A. Brody

Informed Consent and the Refusal of Treatment   117
Levels of Care for Terminal Patients   119
Brain Death   122
Organ Transplantation   124

Chapter 11   127

Prediction and Definition of Outcome

Joseph M. Civetta

Cost Considerations   127
Definition of Outcome   128
Goals for Intensive Care   131
Descriptions of Quantitative Indices   134

Chapter 12   149

Resuscitation Outcomes

William H. Bickell
Matthew M. Rice

Immediate Concerns   149
Outcomes of Resuscitation   150

Outcome After Out-of-Hospital Cardiac Arrest 150
Hospital Course of Patients Successfully Resuscitated From
  Out-of-Hospital Cardiac Arrest 154
Outcome After In-Hospital Cardiac Arrest 155
Neurologic Outcome After CPR 157
Termination of Resuscitation 157
On What Should the Decision to Terminate CPR Be
  Based? 158
Is Age a Factor to Be Considered in the Decision to Stop
  CPR? 159
Can the End-Tidal Carbon Dioxide Concentration or
  Coronary Perfusion Pressure Help Determine When to
  Stop CPR? 159
Should the Cost of Patient Care or the Postresuscitation
  Quality of Life Be Considered in the Decision to Stop
  CPR? 159
Who Should Decide to Terminate CPR? 159
Terminating Resuscitative Efforts Out-of-Hospital 160
Legal Implications of Terminating CPR 160
How Is It Possible to Determine Whether the Physician Is
  on Solid Legal Ground When Terminating CPR? 160
What Are the Considerations of Advance Directives and
  Family Interests in the Decision to Stop CPR? 161

Chapter 13   163

Quality Assessment and Improvement in the Adult Intensive Care Unit

Neil S. Yeston
Jamie Roche
Susan McCaffrey

Establishing a Program 164
A Quality Improvement Model for Surgical Critical
  Care 165
Risk Management 175
Critical Paths 175
The JCAHO Survey 176

SECTION II   187

ESSENTIAL PHYSIOLOGIC CONCERNS

Chapter 14   189

The Lungs and Their Function

Roger S. Mecca
Carlos A. Vaz Fragoso

Static Lung Volumes: Anatomic Considerations 189
Pulmonary Compliance 193
Airway Resistance 196
Gas Exchange 198
Ventilation-Perfusion Matching 199
Fluid and Protein Homeostasis 202
Central Control of Ventilation 204
Protective Functions 205
Metabolic Activity 205

Chapter 15   209

Respiratory Muscle Function and the Work of Breathing

Michael J. Banner

Immediate Concerns 209
Respiratory Muscles 210
Clinical Implications of Respiratory Muscle Loading 216
Decreasing Respiratory Muscle Afterload 219

Chapter 16   227

Cardiovascular System

Avner Sidi
Richard F. Davis

Cardiac Electrical Activity 227
Cardiac Contraction 231
Intrinsic Regulation of Cardiac Function 233
Characteristics of the Heart as a Pump 236
Ventricular Interaction 241
Ventricular Vascular Coupling 241
Neurogenic Control of the Cardiovascular System 242
Passive and Active Control of Systemic and Coronary Artery
  Size and Vasomotion 246
Metabolic Demand and Oxygen Supply of the
  Heart 247

Chapter 17   255

Acid–Base Chemistry and Physiology

Robert R. Kirby
Walter C. Bernards

Chemistry of Acids and Bases 255
Respiratory Derangements 257
Metabolic Derangements 257
Metabolic Compensation for Primary Respiratory
  Disturbances 258
Respiratory Compensation for Primary Metabolic
  Disturbances 259
Problem Solving 259
Metabolic Acidosis and Alkalosis 260
Respiratory Acidosis and Alkalosis 263

Chapter 18   265

Coagulation

Robert I. Parker

Immediate Concerns   265
Physiology and Biochemistry of Primary Hemostasis   265
Physiology and Biochemistry of Secondary Hemostasis   267
Physiology and Biochemistry of Fibrinolysis   270
Coagulation as an Integrated System   272

Chapter 19   273

Central Nervous System Physiology

Christopher Veremakis
David H. Lindner

Immediate Concerns   273
Mechanisms of Brain Injury   274
Therapeutic Considerations During Brain
    Resuscitation   278
Specific Therapeutic Options in Brain Resuscitation   283

Chapter 20   291

The Host Response to Injury
and Infection

Timothy H. Pohlman
Edward M. Boyle, Jr.

Reticuloendothelial System   292
Plasma Protein Defenses   296
Immunity   299

Chapter 21   303

Allergy and Immunology

R. Dwaine Rieves
Stewart J. Levine
James H. Shelhamer

Immediate Concerns   303
Overview   304
Antigen Recognition and Processing   304
Antigen Clearance   306
Antigen Clearance and Inflammation   308
Immune Defects and Critical Illness   308
Immunotherapy   311
Complications of Immunotherapy   313

Chapter 22   315

Pregnancy

Donald Caton

Pregnancy-Imposed Stress   315
Changes at Term   316
Coordination   318

SECTION III   323

MODULATING THE RESPONSE
TO INJURY

Chapter 23   325

Metabolic Response to Injury
and Critical Illness

Palmer Q. Bessey
Richard S. Downey
William W. Monafo

Immediate Concerns   325
General Features of the Response to Injury   326
Intermediary Metabolism in Critical Illness   327
Regulation of the Metabolic Responses to Critical
    Illness   331
Clinical Care and Metabolic Responses to Critical
    Illness   333

Chapter 24   337

Oxygen Delivery and Consumption
in Critical Illness

Robert Schlichtig

Immediate Concerns   337

Chapter 25   343

Progression to Multiple Organ
System Failure

George M. Matuschak

Immediate Concerns   343
Definitions   345
Epidemiology   346
Pathogenesis   347
Organ System Interactions   351

Clinical Features 352
Prevention and Treatment 353

Chapter 26 359

Shock

Edgar J. Jimenez

Immediate Concerns 359
Overview 364
Definition 365
Classification and Clinical Recognition 365
Pathophysiologic Mechanisms of Shock 368
Management 373
Prognosis 381

Chapter 27 389

Cardiogenic Shock

John A. Farmer

Immediate Concerns 389
Classification 390
Etiology 390
Clinical Manifestations 395
Therapy 395

Chapter 28 405

Sepsis and Septic Shock

Janice L. Zimmerman
Robert W. Taylor

Immediate Concerns 405
Epidemiology and Etiology 406
Pathophysiology 407
Organ System Dysfunction in Sepsis 407
Clinical Manifestations 408
Diagnostic Considerations 409
Management of Sepsis 409

Chapter 29 413

Fluid and Electrolytes

Gary P. Zaloga
Robert R. Kirby
Walter C. Bernards
A. Joseph Layon

Immediate Concerns 413
Fluid Compartments 414

Electrolytes 415
Intraoperative and Postoperative Fluid Therapy 433
Hypoosmolar States 437

Chapter 30 443

Splanchnic Flow and Resuscitation

Orlando C. Kirton
Joseph M. Civetta

The Intestinal Microcirculation 443
Cellular Energy Metabolism 444
Intestinal Ischemia 445
Reperfusion Injury 445
Dysoxic Versus Normoxic State 446
Global Parameters of Delivery and Utilization:
   The Controversy 446
The Gastrointestinal Tract and Multiple Organ System
   Failure 447
Relevant Clinical Studies 448
The Monitoring Plan 450
Who Should Be Monitored? 451
Approach to Therapy 452
Future Investigations 452

Chapter 31 457

Enteral and Parenteral Nutrition

Patricia M. Byers
K. N. Jeejeebhoy

Immediate Concerns 457
Introduction 458
The Importance of a Nutritional Support Service 459
Nutritional Assessment and Patient Selection 459
Nutritional Requirements 460
Routes and Techniques of Administration 464
Nutritional Therapy of Patients with Organ System
   Dysfunction 468
Complications 468

Chapter 32 475

Pharmacologic Principles

Subhash K. Todi
Ronald A. Hartmann

Pharmacokinetics and Pharmacodynamics 475
Pharmacotherapy in Renal Diseases 478
Pharmacotherapy in Liver Disease 481
Adverse Drug Reactions 482

SECTION IV   489

TECHNIQUES, PROCEDURES, AND TREATMENT

Chapter 33   491

Fundamentals of Cardiopulmonary Resuscitation

Robert R. Kirby
Richard S. Melker

Immediate Concerns   491
Initial Considerations   492
Airway Patency   492
Breathing   495
Circulation   496
Defibrillation and Cardioversion   497
Pulseless Electrical Activity, Bradycardia, and Asystole   499
Pharmacologic Therapy   499

Chapter 34   507

Clean and Aseptic Technique at the Bedside

Judith A. Hudson-Civetta
Joseph M. Civetta

Questions Regarding Handwashing   507
Importance of Nosocomial Blood Stream Infection   510
Sources of Bacteria   510
Insertion Protocols   511
A Practical Bedside Approach   511
Preparation of Site and Dressing   511
Technique of Skin Preparation   512
Maintenance of Intravascular Catheters   514
Semiquantitative Culture Specimens Using Guidewire Exchange   515
Guidelines for the Use of Guidewires   517

Chapter 35   521

Vascular Cannulation

Bahman Venus
Paul Satish

Immediate Concerns   521
Venous Cannulation   522
Pulmonary Artery Cannulation   538
Peripheral Arterial Cannulation   539

Chapter 36   545

Temporary Cardiac Pacemakers

W. Ross Davis

Immediate Concerns   545
Indications for Temporary Pacing   545
Electrode Catheters and External Pacemaker Units   546
Procedures for Establishing Temporary Pacing   548

Chapter 37   553

Important Intensive Care Procedures

Neil S. Yeston
Richard L. Grotz
Laurie A. Loiacono

Thoracentesis   553
Tube Thoracostomy   556
Heimlich Catheter Insertion   560
Chest Tube Bottles   561
Paracentesis   562
Diagnostic Peritoneal Lavage   563
Intraabdominal Pressure Measurement   568
Venous Cutdown   569
Defibrillation   573
Cardioversion   575
Pericardiocentesis   577
Transtracheal Aspiration   580

Chapter 38   587

Interventional Radiology

Diego Nunez
Kimberly A. Lentz
Alejandro Zuluaga

Vascular Procedures   587
Nonvascular Procedures   590

Chapter 39   599

Feeding Tube Placement

Scott A. Shikora

Immediate Concerns   599
Overview   600
Determining the Most Appropriate Tube Type, Site, and Placement Technique   600
Tube Options   601
Placement Technique Options   602

Chapter 40   609

Mechanical Cardiac Assist Devices

Thomas L. McKiernan
William H. Wehrmacher

Purpose   609
Synchronized Coronary Venous Retroperfusion   611
Ventricular Assist Devices   611

Chapter 41   613

Antithrombotic and Thrombolytic Therapy

Steven J. Trottier

Immediate Concerns   613
Antiplatelet Therapy   613
Antithrombotic Therapy   615
Thrombolytic Therapy   622

Chapter 42   631

Renal Replacement Therapies

Sudarshan Hebbar
Richard S. Muther

Immediate Concerns   631
Physiology   632
Extracorporeal Therapies   632
Peritoneal Dialysis   636
Choice of Therapy   636

Chapter 43   639

Transfusion Therapy

Richard C. Dennis
David Clas
Joan M. Niehoff
Neil S. Yeston

Immediate Concerns   639
Acute Massive Hemorrhage   640
Subacute Blood Volume Deficiency   643
Chronic Anemia   644
History of Blood Transfusion   644
Red Blood Cell Transfusion   645
Fresh Frozen Plasma   648
Cryoprecipitate   649

Platelets   649
DDAVP   651
Technical Aspects of Blood Product Administration   651
Transfusion Complications   652
Refusal of Transfusion   656

Chapter 44   661

Decreasing the Need for Homologous Blood Transfusion

Stephen F. Flaherty
Richard C. Dennis

Immediate Concerns   661
Optimization of Red Cell Production   663
Autotransfusion   663
Passive Blood Loss in the ICU   665
Blood Substitutes   666

Chapter 45   669

Extracorporeal Circulation for Respiratory or Cardiac Failure

Joseph B. Zwischenberger
Aravind B. Sankar
Robert H. Bartlett

Immediate Concerns   669
Background   670
Pathophysiology   671
Patient Selection   671
Techniques and Management   672
Venovenous ECMO   675
The ECMO Team   676
Complications   677
Results   678
Laboratory Investigation   679
Cardiac Support   679

Chapter 46   683

Fiberoptic Bronchoscopy

J. Steven Hata
David A. Schenk
R. Phillip Dellinger

Immediate Concerns   683
Complications   684
Fiberoptic Bronchoscopy in Airway Management   686

Chapter 47   703

Oxygen Therapy

Robert A. Smith

Immediate Concerns   703
Therapeutic Considerations   704
Potential Complications   704

Chapter 48   711

Mechanical Ventilation

Michael J. Banner
Samsun Lampotang
Paul B. Blanch
Robert R. Kirby

Immediate Concerns   711
Peak Inflation Pressure   712
Ventilator Classification   712
Microprocessor-Controlled Ventilators   715
Conventional Mechanical Ventilatory Techniques   719
New or Experimental Techniques   727
Spontaneous Breathing   729
The Work of Breathing   734
Special Techniques   737
Transport Ventilation   738
Side Effects and Complications   739

Chapter 49   745

Ventilatory Support Modes

Orlando C. Kirton

Noninvasive Techniques   745
Truly Assisted Ventilation   747
Near-Total Ventilatory Support   750
Minimal Excursionary Ventilation   753
Spontaneous Augmented Low-Volume Ventilation   754

Chapter 50   757

Airway Management

Orlando G. Florete
Robert R. Kirby

Immediate Concerns   757
General Principles   758
Anatomic Considerations   759
Drugs   762
Esophageal, Pharyngeal, and Laryngeal Tubes   763
Tracheal Intubation   764

Tracheotomy   769
Cricothyroidotomy   770
Cuff Inflation   770

Chapter 51   777

Hyperbaric Medicine

Luis A. Matos

Immediate Concerns   777
Clinical Application   779
Indications   780
Care Before HBO Therapy   781

Chapter 52   787

Intrahospital Transport

Gregory M. Gullahorn

Immediate Concerns   787
Overview   788
Transport Scenarios   789
Planning: Preparatory Phase   792
On the Road Again: Transport Phase   794
Home at Last: Posttransport Stabilization   794
Individualizing Approaches   795

Chapter 53   803

Interhospital Transport of the Critically Ill

Robert E. Fromm

Immediate Concerns   803
Overview   803
Prehospital Practitioners   804
Air Medical Transport   805
Approach to the Transport of the Critically Ill   807

Chapter 54   809

Pain Control

David L. Brown
James F. Flynn

Immediate Concerns   809
Patient Selection   811
Analgesic Technique   811
Clinical Management   816
Problems and Related Complications   817
Special Considerations   819

Chapter 55   821

Sedation and Paralysis

Antoni M. Nejman

Immediate Concerns   821
Sedation   822
Paralysis   828

SECTION V   837

MONITORING: PRACTICAL APPLICATIONS

Chapter 56   839

Invasive Pressure Monitoring

Reed M. Gardner

Equipment   839
Equipment Setup   841
Complications of Invasive Pressure Monitoring   844
Signal Amplification, Processing, and Display   844

Chapter 57   847

Arterial, Central Venous, and Pulmonary Artery Catheters

Albert J. Varon

Immediate Concerns   847
Introduction   848
Arterial Catheters   850
Central Venous Catheters   852
Pulmonary Artery Catheters   853
Derived Cardiopulmonary Parameters   861

Chapter 58   867

Assessment of Cardiopulmonary Function

Nikolaus Gravenstein
Michael L. Good
Tina E. Banner

Relative Attributes   867
Clinical Assessment of Cardiopulmonary Function   868
Noninvasive Blood Pressure Measurement   870
Electrocardiography   873
Pulse Oximetry   875
Capnometry   877

Noninvasive Assessment of Cardiac Output   883
Echocardiography   884
Invasive Cardiac Output Determinations   886

Chapter 59   899

Continuous ST Segment Monitoring

David V. Shatz
Valerie R. Wells

Prevalence of Silent Ischemia   899
Significance of Perioperative Ischemia   900
Pathophysiologic Basis of Electrocardiographic Changes   901
Advantages of ST Segment Monitoring   901
Limitations of ST Segment Monitoring   902
Indications for Monitoring   902
Lead Placement   902
Monitor Setup   903
Troubleshooting Alarm Conditions   905
Definition of Ischemic Events   906
Therapeutic Options   906

Chapter 60   909

Venous Saturation Monitoring and Usage

Joseph M. Civetta
Loren D. Nelson

Immediate Concerns   909
Physiology of Oxygen Transport   910
Assessment of Oxygen Transport Balance   911
Monitoring Oxygen Transport   912
Clinical Usefulness of Continuous $S\bar{v}O_2$ Monitoring   912
Combined Venous and Pulse Oximetry   916
Arterial Venous Oxygen Content Difference   916
Intrapulmonary Shunt   916
Applicability   917
Appendix 1: Normal Range, Units, and Derivation for Common Oxygen Transport Terms   917
Appendix 2: Clinical Examples   918

Chapter 61   921

Blood Gas Analysis

Barry A. Shapiro
William T. Peruzzi

Interpretive Guidelines   922
Arterial Oxygenation   923
Ventilation   924
Acute Respiratory Alkalosis   926
Metabolic Acid–Base Imbalances   926
Clinical Assessment of Oxygenation   928

Hypoxemia and Oxygen Therapy   929
Tissue Oxygenation   930
Noninvasive Monitoring   931
Carbon Dioxide Stores   932
Carbon Monoxide Poisoning   933
Aberrant Intracellular Metabolism   934
Cardiopulmonary Resuscitation and Low Flow States   934
Temperature Correction   936
Point of Care Analyzers and Blood Gas Monitors   938

Chapter 62   941

Neurologic Monitoring

Thomas Grissom
Joyce Grissom
J. Christopher Farmer

Cerebral Function   941
Cerebral Perfusion   946
Cerebral Metabolism   951
Neurologic Imaging   952

Chapter 63   957

Radiographic Imaging

Carl E. Ravin

Plain Chest Radiograph   957
Evaluation of Life-Support and Monitoring Devices   965
Abdominal Radiography   969
Newer Imaging Technology   971
Magnetic Resonance Imaging   978

SECTION VI   985

THE SURGICAL PATIENT

Chapter 64   987

Perioperative Pulmonary Function Testing and Consultation

Philip G. Boysen
Robert R. Kirby

Immediate Concerns   987
General Considerations   988
Assessment for Lung Resection   989
Assessment for Abdominal Surgery   992
Specific Therapeutic Measures   994

Postoperative Care   995
Mechanical Ventilation and the Work of Breathing   996

Chapter 65   999

Preoperative Evaluation of High-Risk Surgical Patients

David L. Brown
Stephen O. Heard
Donald S. Stevens
Robert R. Kirby

Immediate Concerns   999
Overview   1000
Concurrent Disease   1001
Management   1004
Prevention of Complications   1006
Special Considerations   1007

Chapter 66   1013

Anesthesia: Physiology and Postanesthesia Problems

Eran Segal
A. Joseph Layon

Immediate Concerns   1013
Uptake and Distribution of Inhalational Agents   1015
Inhalation Agents and Organ System Function   1017
Intravenous Agents   1021
Preferred Anesthetic Techniques for Critically Ill
    Patients   1026
Postanesthetic Problems   1026

Chapter 67   1037

Initial Triage of the Trauma Patient

Larry C. Martin

Immediate Concerns   1037

Chapter 68   1045

Secondary Triage of the Trauma Patient

Marc D. Palter
Vicente Cortes

Immediate Concerns   1045
Obtaining the Patient's History and History of Injury   1047

Reassessing the ABCs While Maintaining Vital
    Functions   1047
Persistent Shock   1050
Blunt Cardiac Injury   1052
Compartment Syndrome   1052
Intraabdominal Hypertension (Intraabdominal
    Compartment Syndrome)   1053
Delayed Diagnosis   1054
Pelvic Fractures   1058

Chapter 69   1065

Evaluation of Bleeding in the Surgical Patient

Timothy H. Pohlman
C. James Carrico

Immediate Concerns   1065
Evaluation of Bleeding   1067
Etiologies of Postoperative Bleeding   1067
Complex Postoperative Bleeding Problems   1071

Chapter 70   1075

Abdominal Trauma: Diagnostic Steps and Postoperative Considerations

Vicente Cortes
Marc D. Palter
Mark McKenney

Immediate Concerns   1075
General Considerations in Abdominal Injury   1077
Penetrating Injuries   1079
Blunt Injuries   1080
Mortality and Morbidity in Abdominal Trauma   1082
Specific Injuries   1083

Chapter 71   1099

Evaluating the Acute Abdomen

Jorge Luis Sosa
H. David Reines

Immediate Concerns   1099
Introduction   1100
Anatomy   1100
History   1101
Physical Examination   1102
Adjunctive Procedures   1102
Therapy   1103
Special Conditions   1104

Chapter 72   1109

The Complicated Postoperative Abdomen

Danny Sleeman
Scott Norwood

Immediate Concerns   1109
Evaluating the Elective Postoperative Patient   1110
Normal Postoperative Course   1111
Evaluating the Postoperative Abdomen for Sepsis   1112
Specific Surgical Problems   1113
Tube Technology   1116

Chapter 73   1121

Surgical Aspects of Hepatobiliary Disease

Alan S. Livingstone
Jorge Luis Sosa

Immediate Concerns   1121
Management of the Cirrhotic Patient   1122
Early Postshunt Complications   1123
Surgical Management of Ascites   1125
Major Hepatic Resections   1126
Budd-Chiari Syndrome   1127
Hemobilia   1127
Postoperative Cholecystitis   1127
Cholangitis   1128
Biliary Fistula After Cholecystectomy   1128

Chapter 74   1131

Thoracic Surgery

Eddy H. Carrillo
M. Jack Williams

Immediate Concerns   1131
Thoracic Surgery   1133
Preoperative Considerations   1133
Management of the Postthoracotomy Patient   1133
Thoracic Trauma   1137
Special Situations and Procedures   1143

Chapter 75   1147

Postoperative Management of the Adult Cardiac Surgical Patient

Daniel J. O'Brien
James A. Alexander

Immediate Concerns   1147
The First 8 Postcardiopulmonary Bypass Hours   1148

The Next 16 Post-CPB Hours   1148
The Second 24 Post-CPB Hours   1149
The Third 24 Post-CPB Hours   1149
Monitoring and Managing Cardiovascular
    Performance   1150
Special Concerns   1155

Chapter 76   1161

Postoperative Management of the Pediatric Cardiac Surgical Patient

Laurie K. Davies
Michael A. Greene

Immediate Concerns   1161
Hemodynamic Issues   1162
Respiratory Management   1169
Laboratory Values   1170
Cardiac Rhythm and Pacing   1170
Temperature   1171
Sedation and Paralysis   1171
Infections and Antibiotics   1171
Renal Failure and Diuretics   1172
Limb Ischemia   1172
Bleeding   1173
Later Concerns   1173
Transplantation   1175

Chapter 77   1177

Vascular Surgery and Trauma

Enrique Ginzburg
James M. Hurst
Richard J. Fowl

Immediate Concerns   1177
Principles of Intensive Care for the Vascular Patient   1178
Problems Common to All Vascular Reconstructions   1180
Management of Specific Reconstructions   1182
Vascular Trauma   1187
Management of Specific Vascular Injuries   1187
Thrombolytic Therapy   1189
Aortic Dissection   1191

Chapter 78   1195

Neurologic Injury: Prevention and Initial Care

Philip A. Villanueva
Bradley H. Ruben
Jonathan Greenberg

Immediate Concerns: Head Injury   1195
Immediate Concerns: Spinal Injury   1197

Head Injury   1198
Spinal Cord Injury   1208

Chapter 79   1219

Multiple Fractures

Gregory A. Zych

Immediate Concerns   1219
Diagnosis of Fractures and Dislocations   1220
Specific Treatment Methods   1221
Special Problems   1226
Complications   1227

Chapter 80   1231

Orthopedic Complications

Jill I. Freedman
F. Kayser Enneking

Immediate Concerns   1231
Spinal Surgery   1232
Joint Replacement   1234
Pathologic Processes Common to Orthopedic
    Patients   1235
Miscellaneous Problems   1245

Chapter 81   1253

Urologic Surgery and Trauma

Thomas E. Ahlering

Immediate Concerns   1253
Major Urologic Postoperative Management   1254
Urogenital Trauma   1256

Chapter 82   1265

Burn Injury

Michael D. Peck
C. Gillon Ward

Immediate Concerns   1265
Management of Respiratory Problems   1266
Management of Cardiovascular Problems   1267
Complications of Resuscitation   1268
Maintenance of Electrolyte Homeostasis and Acid–Base
    Balance   1269
Management of Renal Failure   1270
Management of Bleeding Disorders   1270
Provision of Nutritional Support   1271
Diagnosis and Treatment of Serious Infections   1272
Care of the Burn Wound   1273

The Importance of Physiotherapy   1274
The Psychosocial Needs of the Patient and Family   1274
The Team Approach to Burn Care   1274

Chapter 83   1277

The Obese Surgical Patient

Scott A. Shikora
Jay A. Johannigman

Immediate Concerns   1277
Overview   1278
Cardiovascular Disease   1278
Pulmonary Disease   1279
Thromboembolic Disease   1280
Soft Tissue Problems   1281
Sepsis   1281
Drug Dosing   1282
Nutritional Support   1282

SECTION VII   1287

ORGAN TRANSPLANTATION

Chapter 84   1289

Organ Transplantation: An Overview of Problems and Concerns

Ake Grenvik
Joseph M. Darby
Brian A. Broznick

Immediate Concerns   1289
Current Transplantation Activities   1290
Organ Need Versus Supply   1291
Evolution of the Brain Death Concept   1291
Procedural Considerations   1292
Organ Procurement, Recovery, and Preservation   1295
Transplantation Organizations and Allocation of
   Organs   1296

Chapter 85   1301

Renal Transplantation

Matthew E. Brunson
William W. Pfaff
George W. Burke, III
Gaetano Ciancio

Immediate Concerns   1301
Immunosuppressants and Their Complications   1303
Minimizing Infections in the Immunocompromised
   Host   1305
Other Problems   1305

"Stable" Allograft Recipients Readmitted to the ICU   1306
Other Conditions   1308

Chapter 86   1311

The Renal and Pancreatic Allograft Recipient

George W. Burke, III
Gaetano Ciancio

Immediate Concerns   1311
Overview   1312
Initial ICU Admission   1312
Immunosuppression   1314
Secondary ICU Admissions   1315

Chapter 87   1317

Heart-Lung, Double-Lung, and Single-Lung Transplantation

Cesar A. Keller

Indications   1317
Initial Management   1317
Postoperative Management   1320

Chapter 88   1333

Heart Transplantation

Leslie W. Miller

Indications   1333
Candidate Selection: Hemodynamic Assessment   1333
Initial Postoperative Management   1334
Immediate Concerns   1335

Chapter 89   1341

Orthotopic Liver Transplantation

Mathew E. Brunson
Richard J. Howard

Immediate Concerns   1341
Early Graft Function and Primary Nonfunction   1342
Coagulation Abnormalities   1343
Hemodynamic Function and Fluid Therapy   1343
Immunosuppression   1344
Hypertension   1345
Other Early Problems   1345
Assessing and Optimizing Graft Function   1346
Complications   1347
Late Readmissions to the ICU   1350
Consultation   1350

Chapter 90   1353

Intestinal and Multivisceral Transplantation

Marc G. Webb
Andreas G. Tzakis

Immediate Concerns: Preoperative Care   1353
Immediate Concerns: Postoperative Care   1354
Overview   1354
Preoperative and Operative Care   1355
Postoperative Care   1360

Chapter 91   1367

Bone Marrow Transplantation

Richard K. Burt

Immediate Concerns (First 30 Days)   1367
Intermediate Concerns (Days 30 to 100)   1377
Late Concerns (Beyond Day 100)   1377

SECTION VIII   1387

THE OBSTETRIC PATIENT

Chapter 92   1389

Cardiac Disease and Hypertensive Disorders in Pregnancy

Christopher F. James

Immediate Concerns   1389
Hypertensive Disorders   1392
Cardiac Disease   1393
Cardiac Surgery During Pregnancy   1397
Pregnancy After Cardiac Surgery   1398
Cardiopulmonary Resuscitation   1398

Chapter 93   1401

Hemorrhagic Disorders

Connie E. Taylor

Immediate Concerns   1401
Cardiovascular Changes With Obstetric Drugs   1402
Coagulation Changes   1403
Hemorrhagic Complications   1403
Coagulopathies   1406

Chapter 94   1409

Pulmonary Abnormalities

Robert R. Kirby

Immediate Concerns   1409
Physiologic Considerations   1410
Ventilation and Perfusion   1411
Diagnosis and Treatment of Respiratory Failure   1412

Chapter 95   1419

Trauma and the Acute Abdomen

Sharon Salamat
Anthony Lai

Immediate Concerns   1419
Initial Assessment and Management   1420
Diagnostic Studies   1421
Specific Management   1423
Postoperative Period   1424
Delivery Concerns   1425
Maternal Brain Death   1425

Chapter 96   1429

Fetal Monitoring Concerns

Donald Caton

Immediate Concerns   1429
Special Considerations   1430
Fetal Oxygenation   1431
Monitoring   1432
Chronic Adaptations   1433
Acute Adaptations   1434

SECTION IX   1437

ENVIRONMENTAL HAZARDS

Chapter 97   1439

Protecting the Practitioner: Acquired Immunodeficiency Syndrome and Hepatitis

Salvatore Lopalo
A. Joseph Layon

Acquired Immunodeficiency Syndrome   1439
Health Care Workers and HIV Transmission   1440

Testing of Health Care Workers After Possible
  Exposure 1441
Prevention 1442
The Hepatitides 1444
Protective and Therapeutic Measures 1447

Chapter 98   1451

Temperature-Related Injuries

J. Christopher Farmer

Immediate Concerns 1451
Hypothermia 1451
Hyperthermia 1454
Malignant Hyperthermia and the Neuroleptic Malignant
  Syndrome 1457

Chapter 99   1463

Toxicology: General Approach

Jeffrey A. Sadowsky

Immediate Concerns 1463
History 1464
Diagnosis and the General Approach to the Poisoned
  Patient 1467
Pregnancy 1475
Treatment Refusal: The Uncooperative Patient 1475
Appendix 99-1: Toxicology Information 1475

Chapter 100   1483

Toxicology: Specific Drugs
and Poisons

Richard P. Ryskamp
Robert W. Taylor

Acetaminophen 1483
Salicylates 1486
Cyclic Antidepressants 1489
Lithium 1493
Antipsychotic Drugs 1494
Benzodiazepines 1495
Beta-Blockers 1496
Calcium Channel Blockers 1497
Digitalis 1498
Theophylline 1499
Alcohols 1501
Insecticides: Cholinergic Agents 1504

Chapter 101   1511

Substance Abuse and
Withdrawal: Alcohol, Cocaine,
and Opioids

Joan Shaffer

Immediate Concerns 1511
Ethanol 1512
Cocaine 1514
Opioids 1517

Chapter 102   1523

Envenomation

Charles L. Bryan
Charles A. Weber
Kenneth A. Perret

Immediate Concerns 1523
Venomous Snake Bites 1524
Black Widow Spider Bites 1528
Brown Recluse Spider Bites 1530
Scorpion Envenomation 1532
Marine Envenomations 1533

Chapter 103   1537

Electrical Injuries

Kenneth A. Perret
Charles A. Weber
Charles L. Bryan

Immediate Concerns 1537
Classification 1538
Basic Mechanisms in Electrical Injury 1538
Clinical Manifestations and Management 1539

Chapter 104   1543

Anaphylaxis

Stewart J. Levine
R. Dwaine Rieves
James H. Shelhamer

Immediate Concerns 1543
Clinical Manifestations 1544
Management 1546
Prevention 1549
Pathogenesis 1550
Implications and Outcome 1550

SECTION X   1553

INFECTIOUS DISEASE

Chapter 105   1555

An Approach to the Use of Antimicrobial Agents

George E. Crawford
Mimi Emig

Immediate Concerns   1555
Principles of Antibiotic Selection   1556
Antibiotic Therapy   1561
Prophylactic Antibiotics   1565
Antimicrobials Useful in the Critical Care Unit   1566

Chapter 106   1573

The Prevalence and Importance of Nosocomial Infections in the Intensive Care Unit

Mark G. McKenney
Scott Norwood

Immediate Concerns   1573
Risk Factors and Scope of Nosocomial Infections in Critical Illness   1575
Hospital-Acquired Respiratory Infections   1575
Catheter-Related Nosocomial Infections   1577
Surgical Wound Infections   1581
Hospital-Acquired Urinary Tract Infections   1582
Fungal Infections   1583
Sinusitis   1583
Antibiotic-Associated Pseudomembranous Colitis   1583
Hospital-Acquired Ventriculitis and Meningitis   1584

Chapter 107   1589

An Approach to the Febrile ICU Patient

David V. Shatz
Scott Norwood

Immediate Concerns   1589
Definition, Pathophysiology, and Purpose   1591
Common Causes of Fever   1592
Fever as a Predictor of Infection   1592
Recommended Approach to Fever Evaluation   1593

Chapter 108   1603

Infections in the Immunocompromised Host

Gregory P. Melcher
Douglas R. Leigh

Immediate Concerns   1603
Approach to the Immunocompromised Host   1604
The Granulocytopenic Patient   1605
The Corticosteroid-treated Patient   1606
The Renal Transplant Recipient   1609
Bone Marrow Transplant Recipient   1613

Chapter 109   1617

Human Immunodeficiency Virus in the Intensive Care Unit

Loretta M. O'Brien
Richard E. Winn

Immediate Concerns   1617
Pulmonary Manifestations of HIV   1618
Neurologic Manifestations of HIV Infection   1626
Sepsis and Bacteremia   1627
Gastrointestinal Manifestations of HIV   1629
Fever of Unknown Origin   1630
ICU Utilization in HIV Infection   1630
Control of HIV Infection in the ICU   1630

Chapter 110   1635

Neurologic Infections

David H. Gremillion

Immediate Concerns   1635
Clinical Presentation and Initial Diagnostic Measures   1635
Establishing the Diagnosis   1639
Management   1641
Prevention of Bacterial Meningitis   1642
Complications of Bacterial Meningitis   1643
Special Clinical Considerations   1644

Chapter 111   1649

Urinary Tract Infections

Mark E. Appleman
Richard E. Winn

Immediate Concerns   1649
Cystitis   1650

Pyelonephritis   1650
Prostatitis   1654
Nosocomial Infections   1654
Fungal Infections   1655

Chapter 112   1657

Bacterial Infections

Judith R. Anderson
Ferric C. Fang

Staphylococcus aureus   1657
Coagulase-Negative Staphylococci (Including
   Staphylococcus epidermidis)   1661
Streptococcal and Enterococcal Infections   1663
Streptotoccus pyogenes (Group A Streptococcus)   1663
Streptococcus agalactiae (Group B Streptococcus)   1664
Streptococcus pneumoniae   1664
Viridans Streptococci   1665
Streptococcus milleri/intermedius Group   1665
Enterococci   1666
Moraxella (Branhamella) catarrhalis   1666
Neisseria meningitidis   1666
Neisseria gonorrhoeae   1667
Bacillus Infections   1668
Corynebacteria (Diphtheroids)   1668
Listeria monocytogenes   1668
Nocardia   1668
Acinetobacter   1669
Campylobacter and *Helicobacter*   1669
Enterobacteriaceae   1669
Enterobacter   1669
Escherichia   1670
Klebsiella   1670
Proteus   1670
Salmonella   1670
Serratia   1671
Shigella   1671
Yersinia   1671
Other Enterobacteriaceae   1672
Flavobacterium   1672
Francisella   1672
Haemophilus influenzae   1672
Other HACEK Organisms   1673
Legionella   1673
Pasteurella   1673
Pseudomonas aeruginosa   1673
Pseudomonas (burkholderia) cepacia   1674
Stenotrophomonas (xanthomonas) maltophilia   1675
Vibrios and Related Organisms   1675
Anaerobic Cocci   1675
Actinomycosis   1675
Clostridial Infections   1676
Propionibacterium acnes   1678
Anaerobic Gram-Negative Bacilli   1678
Bartonella (Rochalimaea) Infections   1679
Capnocytophaga   1679

Chlamydia   1680
Mycobacterium avium-intracellulare   1680
Mycobacterium kansasii   1680
Mycobacterium tuberculosis   1680
Mycoplasmal Infections   1681
Rickettsial Infections   1682
Borrelia   1682
Leptospirosis   1682
Syphylis   1682

Chapter 113   1685

Fungal and Viral Infections

Stephen B. Greenberg

Fungal Infections   1685
Viral Infections   1691

Chapter 114   1703

Unusual Infections

Richard E. Winn

Rickettsial Diseases   1703
Ehrlichia   1706
Brucellosis   1706
Tularemia   1707
Plague   1708
Borreliosis   1708
Hantavirus Pulmonary Syndrome   1709
Hemorrhagic Fever   1709
Head and Neck Infections   1710
Cerebral Malaria   1711

SECTION XI   1715

CARDIOVASCULAR DISEASE AND DYSFUNCTION

Chapter 115   1717

Evaluation of Chest Pain in the ICU

Stephen P. Taylor

Immediate Concerns   1717
Differentiation of Chest Pain Syndromes   1719
Differential Diagnosis of Life-Threatening Causes of
   Chest Pain   1720
Differential Diagnosis of Non–Life-Threatening Causes of
   Chest Pain   1724

Chapter 116   1727

Acute Myocardial Infarction: Contemporary Management Strategies

Normand Racine

Immediate Concerns   1727
Role of Aspirin in Acute Myocardial Infarction   1727
Thrombolysis   1728
Percutaneous Transluminal Coronary Angioplasty   1733
Role of Heparin in Acute Myocardial Infarction   1733
Role of Intravenous β-Adrenergic Blocking Agents   1734
Role of Intravenous Nitroglycerin   1735
Role of Calcium Channel Blockers   1735
Lidocaine   1736
Angiotensine-Converting Enzyme Inhibitors (ACE-i)   1736
Heart Failure and Cardiogenic Shock   1737
Differentiation From Chronic Heart Failure   1737
Mechanical Complications   1737
Right Ventricular Infarction Diagnosis and Therapy   1738
Cardiogenic Shock   1738
Clinical Guidelines for Hemodynamic Monitoring   1738
Recommended Approach to Congestive Heart
   Failure   1739
Noninvasive Imaging Techniques   1740
Q Wave and Non-Q Wave Myocardial Infarctions   1742

Chapter 117   1749

Heart Failure

Mandeep R. Mehra
Hector O. Ventura

Immediate Concerns   1749
Introduction   1750
Epidemiology of Heart Failure   1751
Etiopathogenesis   1752
Neurohormonal Activation in Advanced Heart
   Failure   1752
Neurohormonal Activation: Adaptation or
   Maladaption?   1753
Prognostic Factors in Advanced Heart Failure   1753
Clinical Trials in the Medical Management of Heart
   Failure   1755
Pooled Studies of ACE Inhibitors   1756
Clinical Use of ACE Inhibitors   1756
Oral Inotropic Therapy–Hopeless or a Glimmer of
   Hope?   1756
A Summary of Clinical Trials in Advanced Heart
   Failure   1757
The Unique Management of Refractory Advanced Systolic
   Heart Failure   1758
Tailored Medical Therapy   1759
Practical Aspects of Intravenous Inotropic Therapy   1760
Fluid Removal in Refractory Heart Failure   1761
Non-pharmacological Cardiac Assistance   1762

Selection Criteria for Implantable Ventricular Assist
   Devices   1763
Emerging Pharmacologic Therapeutics in Heart
   Failure   1763
Diastolic Dysfunction: The Other Side of the Coin   1764

Chapter 118   1769

Valvular Heart Disease

W. Ross Davis

Immediate Concerns   1769
Critical Illness Caused by Valvular Heart Disease   1769
Complicating Cardiac Valvular Disease in Critically Ill
   Patients   1770
Considerations in Specific Valvular Abnormalities   1770

Chapter 119   1781

Cardiac Arrhythmias

W. Ross Davis

Immediate Concerns   1781
Diagnostic Maneuvers   1781
Supraventricular Arrhythmias   1783
Ventricular Arrhythmias   1783
Wide Complex Tachycardia   1784
Atrioventricular Block   1784
Management   1784

Chapter 120   1787

Infective Endocarditis

Stephen B. Greenberg

Immediate Concerns   1787
Overview   1787
Epidemiology   1788
Pathology and Pathogenesis   1788
Diagnostic Criteria   1789
Clinical Manifestations   1790
Laboratory Tests   1790
Microbiology   1791
Therapy   1793

Chapter 121   1803

The Pericardium

Thomas L. McKiernan

Acute Pericarditis   1803
Cardiac Tamponade   1805
Constrictive Pericarditis   1808
Postpericardiotomy Syndrome   1809

Chapter 122   1811

Hypertensive Emergencies and Urgencies

Patrick C. McKillion
R. Phillip Dellinger

Immediate Concerns   1811
Specific Considerations   1816
Hypertensive Urgencies   1819

SECTION XII   1823

PULMONARY DISEASE AND DYSFUNCTION

Chapter 123   1825

The Acute Respiratory Distress Syndrome

Barbara J. Foner
Scott H. Norwood
Robert W. Taylor

Immediate Concerns   1825
Overview   1826
Etiology   1826
Pathophysiology   1828
Clinical Presentation   1830
Treatment   1831
Novel Forms of Mechanical Ventilation   1835
Monitoring   1836
Complications   1836
Outcome   1836

Chapter 124   1841

Community Acquired Pneumonia

Dennis P. Lawlor
Mimi Emig

Immediate Concerns   1841
Characterization of Pneumonia   1842
Pathogens in Community Acquired Pneumonia   1842
New Pathogens   1843
Old Pathogens, New Problems   1843
Host Defense and Susceptibility   1844
Initial Diagnostic Evaluation   1846
Evaluation and Treatment of Pleural Effusions   1848
Lung Abscess   1849
Empiric Antibiotics   1850
Duration of Therapy   1852
Adjunctive Treatment   1852
Clinical Response to Therapy   1852
Invasive Testing   1852

Chronic Lung Infections   1854
Radiographic Resolution   1855
Prophylaxis   1855
Evaluation of Recurrence   1856
Future Directions   1856

Chapter 125   1861

Aspiration Syndromes

Salvatore R. Goodwin

Immediate Concerns   1861
Classification   1862
Further Diagnostic Concerns   1864
Subsequent Management   1865
Prevention   1868

Chapter 126   1875

Drowning and Near-Drowning

Eric T. Kunichika
Lawrence S. Berman

Immediate Concerns   1875
Presentation   1877
Pathophysiology   1877
Treatment   1878
Neurologic Sequelae   1880
Fluids and Electrolytes   1880
Renal Failure   1880
Hematologic Changes   1881
Sequelae   1881
Ice Water Submersion   1882
Prognosis and Outcome   1882
Other Concerns   1883

Chapter 127   1887

Venous Thrombosis and Pulmonary Embolism

Mandeep R. Mehra
Frederick R. Bode

Immediate Concerns   1887
Venous Thromboembolism: Ubiquitous Yet Undiagnosed   1888
The Medical ICU and Deep Venous Thrombosis: The Case for Routine Prophylaxis   1889
Natural History of Venous Thromboembolism   1891
Clinical Features and Diagnosis of Venous Thromboembolism   1891
Therapy of Venous Thromboembolism   1897
Future Directions   1901

Chapter 128   1905

Other Embolic Syndromes

Scott A. Deppe
Dan R. Thompson
Roger R. Barrette

Immediate Concerns   1905
Arterial Embolism of Gas, Cholesterol, or Fat   1905
Venous Air Embolism   1907
Fat Embolism Syndrome   1908
Amniotic Fluid Embolism   1910

Chapter 129   1917

Acute Respiratory Failure in Chronic Obstructive Lung Disease

Michael J. Cicale
Frederick L. Trent

Immediate Concerns   1917
Definitions   1918
Etiology   1919
Pathophysiology   1919
Management   1919
Complications   1927
Prognosis   1929

Chapter 130   1931

Life-Threatening Bronchospasm in the Asthmatic Patient

R. Phillip Dellinger

Immediate Concerns   1931
Pathophysiology and Pulmonary Function in Severe
   Asthma   1932
Diagnosis   1934
Admission Decisions   1936
Therapy   1936
Indications for Tracheal Intubation   1939
Summary of Treatment Priorities   1942
Nontraditional Therapy of Severe Bronchospasm   1943

Chapter 131   1947

Inhalation Injury

David A. Striker

Immediate Concerns   1947
Fire and Smoke   1948

Thermal Injury   1949
Pathogenesis   1950
Histopathology   1950
Clinical Presentation and Diagnosis   1950
Treatment   1951
Classification   1952

Chapter 132   1959

Pulmonary Barotrauma

David L. Brown
Robert R. Kirby

Immediate Concerns   1959
Pneumothorax   1960
Other Extra-Alveolar Air Conditions   1964
Prevention of Barotrauma and Related
   Complications   1965
Surveillance for Pulmonary Barotrauma   1966

SECTION XIII   1969

NEUROLOGIC DISEASE AND DYSFUNCTION

Chapter 133   1971

Altered Mental Status and Coma

Warren J. Strittmatter

Immediate Concerns   1971
Emergency Evaluation   1971
Bedside Evaluation of Coma   1972
Additional Studies   1975
Bilateral Hemispheric Lesions   1975
Brain Stem Lesions   1976
Metabolic–Toxic Etiologies   1977

Chapter 134   1981

Seizures and Status Epilepticus

Paul A. Rutecki

Immediate Concerns   1981
Definitions and Classification   1982
Etiology   1982
Pathophysiology   1983
Initial Therapy and Management   1983
Pharmacologic Therapy   1984
Laboratory Evaluation   1986
Prognosis   1986
Special Cases   1986

Chapter 135   1989

Cerebrovascular Disease

Ken P. Madden
Loren A. Rolak

Immediate Concerns   1989
Stroke   1990
Other Cerebrovascular Diseases   1999

Chapter 136   2005

Neuromuscular Disorders

Stephen Derdak

Immediate Concerns   2005
Guillain-Barré Syndrome (Acute Autoimmune
    Inflammatory Demyelinating
    Polyneuropathology)   2005
Myasthenia Gravis   2011

Chapter 137   2017

Behavioral Disturbances in the Intensive Care Unit

Michael G. Wise
Ned H. Cassem

Immediate Concerns   2017
Diagnosis and Clinical Features of a Delirium   2018
Behavioral Disorders Without Cognitive
    Dysfunction   2024

SECTION XIV   2031

GASTROINTESTINAL DISEASE AND DYSFUNCTION

Chapter 138   2033

Gastrointestinal Bleeding

Jack A. DiPalma

Immediate Concerns   2033
Overview   2033
Approach to Diagnosis and Management of Upper
    Gastrointestinal Bleeding   2034
Treatment for Gastrointestinal Bleeding   2035

Critical Assessment of Available Interventions   2037
Stress Ulceration   2037
Approach to Lower Gastrointestinal Bleeding   2040

Chapter 139   2045

Fulminant Hepatic Failure

Marc G. Webb
Andreas G. Tzakis

Immediate Concerns   2045
Etiology and Prognosis   2046
Complications and Treatment   2047

Chapter 140   2055

Pancreatic Disease

Danny Sleeman
Joe U. Levi

Immediate Concerns   2055
Overview   2056
Diagnosis of the Disease Process   2056
Classification   2057
Treatment of Acute Pancreatitis   2057
Surgical Management   2059

Chapter 141   2065

Inflammatory Bowel Disease

Charles E. Brady
Oscar A. Alvarez

Immediate Concerns   2065
Fulminant Colitis and Toxic Megacolon   2066
Colonic Perforation and Massive Hemorrhage   2069

Chapter 142   2071

Esophageal Disorders

Jack A. DiPalma

Immediate Concerns   2071
Esophageal Obstruction   2071
Foreign Bodies   2073
Corrosive Injury   2073
Esophageal Perforation   2075
Medication Injury   2076

SECTION XV   2079
RENAL AND ENDOCRINE DISEASE AND DYSFUNCTION

Chapter 143   2081
Acute Renal Failure

Richard S. Muther

Immediate Concerns   2081
Differential Diagnosis of Acute Azotemia   2081
Differential Diagnosis of Acute Renal Failure   2084
Pathophysiology   2086
Prevention of ARF   2088
Treatment and Supportive Care   2088
Prognosis and Recovery   2090

Chapter 144   2093
Impact of Chronic Renal Failure

Gerald M. Reid
Richard S. Muther

Immediate Concerns   2093
Hypotension   2094
Chest Pain   2096
Cardiac Arrhythmias   2096
Respiratory Failure   2097
Disordered Consciousness   2098

Chapter 145   2101
Disordered Glucose Metabolism

Dan R. Thompson

Immediate Concerns   2101
Disordered Glucose Metabolism   2102
Diabetic Ketoacidosis   2102
Hyperosmolar Hyperglycemic Nonketotic Disease   2106
Decompensated Diabetes Mellitus in Patients With
    Coexistent Medical or Surgical Problems   2107

Chapter 146   2111
Hypothalamic and Pituitary Disease

Charles A. Reasner II
Gary L. Mueller

Immediate Concerns   2111
Overview   2112
Hypothalamic–Anterior Pituitary Unit   2112
Neurohypophysis   2116

Chapter 147   2121
Adrenal Disease

Robert B. Constant
Richard J. Barth

Immediate Concerns   2121
Physiology of the Adrenal Gland   2122
Adrenal Hormone Insufficiency   2123
Adrenal Hormone Excess (Cushing's Syndrome)   2125
Clinical Use of Glucocorticoid Medications   2125
Adrenal Function Tests   2126

Chapter 148   2129
Pheochromocytoma

Gary L. Mueller
Charles A. Reasner II

Immediate Concerns   2129
Presenting Symptoms and Signs   2130
Pathology   2130
Diagnosis   2131
Management   2133
Prevention of Complications   2133
Special Considerations   2133

Chapter 149   2137
Thyroid Disease

William L. Isley

Immediate Concerns   2137
Thyrotoxicosis   2137
Hypothyroidism   2142
Drugs, Thyroid Disease, and Thyroid Function   2146
Thyroid Function in Nonthyroidal Illness and Aging   2146
Airway Obstruction   2147

SECTION XVI   2151
SKIN AND MUSCLE DISEASE AND DYSFUNCTION

Chapter 150   2153
Critical Care of Rheumatic Disease

Jay B. Higgs
Ramon A. Arroyo
Kenneth F. Des Rosier
Matthew T. Carpenter

Immediate Concerns   2153
Overview   2155
Principles and Pitfalls in the Critical Care of Rheumatic
   Disease   2155
Vasculitis   2159
Critical Care of Systemic Lupus Erythematosus   2164
Systemic Sclerosis   2171

Chapter 151 2175

Dermatologic Conditions

Richard L. Spielvogel

Immediate Concerns   2175
Erythema Multiforme   2175
Toxic Epidermal Necrolysis   2177
Staphylococcal Scalded Skin Syndrome   2178
Generalized Pustular Psoriasis (Von Zumbusch)   2179
Erythroderma and Exfoliative Dermatitis   2181
Pemphigus   2182
Bullous Pemphigoid   2183
Eczema Herpeticum (Kaposi's Varicelliform
   Eruption)   2184
Varicella-Zoster Infections   2185
Drug Eruptions   2186
Purpura   2188
Acquired Immunodeficiency Syndrome   2191
Contact Dermatitis   2191
Necrotizing Fasciitis   2192

Chapter 152 2195

Rhabdomyolysis

J. Christopher Farmer

Immediate Concerns   2195
Complications   2196
The Clinical Syndrome of Rhabdomyolysis   2198

Chapter 153 2203

Preventive Care

Deborah Weppler
Joseph M. Civetta

Skin and Subcutaneous Tissues   2203
Musculoskeletal System Considerations   2207
Subtle Infectious Processes   2209
Miscellaneous Conditions   2211
Types of ICU Beds   2212

SECTION XVII 2215

HEMATOLOGIC AND ONCOLOGIC DISEASE AND DYSFUNCTION

Chapter 154 2217

Coagulation Disorders

Robert I. Parker

Immediate Concerns   2217
Overview   2218
An Approach to the Patient With an Actual or Suspected
   Coagulation Disorder   2218
Conditions Associated With Serious Bleeding or a High
   Probability of Bleeding   2220
Thrombotic Syndromes   2229
Laboratory Abnormalities Not Associated With
   Bleeding   2229
Selected Disorders   2230

Chapter 155 2231

Hematologic Diseases

David A. Sears

Reduced Blood Counts   2231
Increased Blood Counts   2239
Altered Blood Rheology   2241

Chapter 156 2245

Oncologic Emergencies

Robert J. Downey
Jeffrey S. Groeger

Cancer Hypercalcemia   2245
Acute Tumor Lysis Syndrome   2247
Obstructive Syndromes   2248
Neurologic Syndromes   2249
Cardiac Tamponade   2250
Gastrointestinal Emergencies: Neutropenic
   Enterocolitis   2250
Toxicity of Chemotherapy   2251

Appendix   2255

Critical Care Catalog

Stephen M. Koch

Appendix A: Prefixes and Conversions   2255
Appendix B: Dubois Body Surface Area
   Nomogram   2256
Appendix C: Fluids and Electrolytes   2257

Appendix D: Acid-Base   2259
Appendix E: Formulas   2261
Appendix F: Pharmacology   2266
Appendix G: Dermatomes   2273
Appendix H: Organ Injury Scaling   2273

Index   2283

Critical Care

Decision-Making

Critical Care, Third Edition, edited by Joseph M. Civetta,
Robert W. Taylor, and Robert R. Kirby.
Lippincott-Raven Publishers, Philadelphia, PA © 1997.

CHAPTER 1

How to Read a Medical Article and Understand Basic Statistics

Joseph M. Civetta
Theodore Colton

Continuing self-education and appraisal of the medical literature are simultaneously a responsibility and a joy for the physician who intends to keep abreast of new developments and incorporate new research findings into clinical practice. It is a responsibility, given the tremendous accrual of new knowledge. It is a joy because this stimulus keeps the mind alive and renews the original feelings that prompted the study of medicine.[1] Feinstein[2] notes, "The statistician brings a long tradition of intellectual neglect of the significance of management of clinical data. He finds as his collaborators, clinicians who have a long tradition of intellectual fear of statistics." He also observed that the numerical method was introduced into clinical medicine in 1836 by Pierre Louis, who helped end the popularity of blood-letting by counting and comparing the results of patients treated in various ways. Louis was both attacked and vilified according to Feinstein who refers to Louis' experience as, "A caveat for any clinician who questions an accepted therapy of his era and who urges his colleagues to make better use of their senses and statistics in evaluating therapy." He also quotes Louis, "Let those, who engage hereafter in the study of therapeutics, pursue an opposite course to that of their predecessors. Let them labor to demonstrate rigorously the influence and the degree of influence of any therapeutic agent, on the duration, progress, and termination of a particular disease." Thus, the reader faces strong positive and negative stimuli to pursue the goals of this chapter.

The medical literature contains reports of well-conceived, well-conducted, and well-analyzed studies in addition to reports of ill-conceived, poorly conducted, and inadequately analyzed studies. How is it possible to tell the good from the bad? Although this remains a continuing and perplexing problem for the clinician, we hope to provide some assistance in separating the wheat from the chaff. Although the reader may make some inferences, guided by prior knowledge of the quality of a journal, for instance, we should approach the evaluation of an existing medical report and the creation of our own research in a more formal and structured manner. Although it is tempting to read the title, abstract, and conclusions and then rush to apply the new methodology or treatment, we should spend the time to evaluate the entire article. This has the dual advantages of training our often capricious minds and also avoiding errors caused by our precipitous acceptance of the new finding. Remember, "jumping to conclusions seldom leads to happy landings."[3] The high-quality journal that uses vigorous peer review and meticulous editorial appraisal is likely to publish good, solid, and sound reports of medical studies. But even with such journals, the occasional poor paper can slip through the peer review editorial process and achieve the "importance" of publication. With the proliferation of journals, it is also true that articles that fail to pass the stringent peer review of prestigious journals may also achieve publication in another journal that is struggling to fill its allotted pages. Hence, it is important that the clinician, in assessing medical reports in areas of particular interest, has the ability to assess critically and formulate judgments concerning the strengths and weaknesses of published medical reports.

CRITICAL READING
OF THE MEDICAL LITERATURE ∎

A formalized process aids particularly in evaluating a medical report to ensure that the conclusions are well supported and to further the development of the reader's own critical acumen. The steps in the process are outlined in Table 1-1. These are general questions that apply to virtually any research report involving the collection and analysis of data.

OBJECTIVE AND HYPOTHESIS

Obviously, the most pertinent starting point is an understanding of the investigator's objective. The investigator has the obligation to state clearly and specifically the purpose of the study conducted, but this may be difficult to discern. In such cases, we may question whether the author had, indeed, a clear objective. "Fishing expeditions," that is, extensive data collection projects with the intention of exploring and identifying important relationships, achieve success when the captain knows where the fish are. In other words, the so-called gold mine of data does not guarantee that statistical search will lead to pay dirt and reveal important new relationships. The author, or we as researchers, must formulate specific objectives and a clear-cut hypothesis for testing. Lack of an understanding of objectives handicaps the reader and the author in any assessment or interpretation of the results.

A more specific and somewhat more subtle question in assessing objectives is classification of a study as descriptive and exploratory versus analytic. Using epidemiologic terminology, descriptive studies are those that "describe" diseases, characterize disease patterns, and explore relationships, particularly in regard to person, place, and time. Such studies mainly serve the purpose of "hypothesis generation." The specific hypothesis can then be tested by an analytic study, one whose primary objective involves the test of a specific hypothesis.

To illustrate this distinction, a descriptive study reported the use of high-level positive end-expiratory pressure (PEEP) in acute respiratory insufficiency in patients who developed severe, progressive, acute respiratory insufficiency despite aggressive application of conventional respiratory therapy.[4] Later, the term *optimal PEEP,* introduced in the first study, was updated in another descriptive study of 421 patients reported in 1978.[5] The second study entailed treatment of a large group with respiratory failure using

TABLE 1-1. Focal Points When Reading Medical Reports

(1) Objective and hypothesis
(2) Study design
(3) Methodology and observations
(4) Presentation of findings and results
(5) Data analysis
(6) Discussion and conclusions
(7) Abstract or summary

titration of PEEP in conjunction with intermittent mandatory ventilation but using cardiovascular interventions to support cardiac function until a preselected end point of 15% shunt could be achieved. The first study represented a description of the development of a treatment regimen; in the second study, refinements in this treatment regimen were applied to a broader population. Later, a hypothesis was constructed to test whether, in moderate arterial hypoxemia, there was any improvement in patient outcome or resource utilization using "optimal PEEP" compared with similar modalities of therapy, with an end point defined as achievement of nearly complete arterial oxygen saturation at nontoxic inspired oxygen fractions.

The hypothesis that PEEP titration to achieve an intrapulmonary shunt of less than 20% would have a better outcome or would achieve faster resolution of the disease process could not be substantiated in the analytic study.[6] The two descriptive studies[4,5] identified a specific hypothesis that the third or analytic study tested.

STUDY DESIGN

The reader should consider carefully the definitions of the groups studied and the population to which the investigators intend to refer their findings. For instance, in the three studies quoted, the reader might assume that the failure to prove the hypothesis in the third study invalidated the findings of the two earlier descriptive studies. The third, an analytic study, however, involved only patients with early and moderate arterial hypoxemia. The original group of patients who were studied specifically excluded these patients and concentrated on developing therapy for those who had persistent hypoxemia despite aggressive application of conventional respiratory therapy. Thus, a technique that reversed hypoxemia in patients who were refractory to the then "conventional therapy" of acute respiratory insufficiency was found not to be useful in another population that had only moderate hypoxemia and did not have true adult respiratory distress syndrome. If the authors do not state clearly the populations with which they are dealing, the readers can easily lose this important distinction. This has even greater importance in review articles that may omit the important qualifiers or modifiers found in the original reports. The fact that a particular form of therapy useful in advanced disease has no particular advantage in patients with mild disease indicates that therapy should be restricted to patients who can benefit from treatment, rather than arrive at some alternative conclusion that titration of PEEP to preselected end points has no advantage.

The reader should examine carefully the Materials and Methods section for a description of the study design. Epidemiologically, there are two major classifications of study design: experimental and observational. Loosely defined, an experimental study is one in which the investigator has control over or can manipulate the major factor under study. The epitome of the experimental study is the randomized controlled trial in which the investigator demonstrates "control" over the factor under study by randomizing patients to various regimens. Many prophylactic and therapeutic studies tend to be experimental in design. It cannot be assumed that just because a study was experimental and the investigator may have randomized patients that the study was well done and its conclusions are valid. Experimental studies are prone to various sources of bias and to poor execution. The label *randomized* is not equivalent to assurance of high quality, nor does it alone add validity to the study. Thus, randomized studies also need careful assessment of their design, methods, analyses, and conclusions. One other factor, *blinding*, is often viewed as an attribute of the highest quality studies. If subjective elements are used to judge the effectiveness of treatment, there is a compelling rationale to blind the investigators. If there are subjective assessments of the patients' response, there is a compelling rationale to blind the subjects. If all of the outcome variables are objective, blinding, strictly speaking, is unnecessary. Thus, in the assessment of a new medication to relieve pain, double blinding (both subjects and investigators) is necessary.

When the investigators cannot manipulate the major factor under study, they must rely on what has been observed; this study is an observational study. We should not view observational studies as being inferior to experimental studies. Clearly, a tight, well-designed, well-executed experimental study carries the greatest strength of evidence, but observational studies can also provide substantial, sound medical evidence. In fact, a well-planned and well-executed observational study can be much more informative than a weakly designed and poorly executed randomized study. There are various approaches to the design of observational studies, such as cross-sectional, case control, prospective cohort, and retrospective cohort. The interested reader should consult basic epidemiology or statistics textbooks for further descriptions of these various design strategies and for the relative strengths and weaknesses of each design format.[7,8]

With respect to observational studies, the reader should determine whether the data collection was prospective or retrospective. The principal advantage of prospective data collection is that the researchers, having clearly identified the objectives, can ensure collection of this relevant information in a manner that they can determine. Retrospective analysis of medical records depends on what happens to appear in the record, often with no indication of the manner in which the information was obtained. For example, sex, age, and hospital outcome (survival or death) are key data elements that may not appear for *every patient* in a retrospective chart review. Clearly, without a specified protocol, the researcher cannot anticipate that a daily blood gas, serum creatinine, or any other intermittent measurement dependent on a specific order will appear in the chart. Everyone should attempt a retrospective study (at least once) to learn the pitfalls and the impossibility of obtaining a complete data base. This would enable each of the then-frustrated researchers to read other retrospective studies both with a great deal of deserved skepticism and with empathy for the difficulties with such research.

Selection of the study group is another important step. The researcher should look for possible sources of selection that would make the sample atypical or nonrepresentative. Even such seemingly "random" allocation of cases such as alternate days may introduce an unappreciated bias. For instance, the Trauma Service at the University of Miami/Jackson Memorial Medical Center had two separate teams that alternated coverage every 24 hours. Patients admitted on alternate days, therefore, are cared for by different teams of physicians. A study that entailed alternate-day assignment to treatment groups would entail, as well, the factor of differences in physician practice style, a factor that could not be disentangled in analysis of study results.

We must also consider the nature of the control group or standard of comparison. We frequently encounter the "historical control" group that usually has a "poorer" result than the contemporary group. The problem, of course, is that the basic assumption that the modality of treatment under investigation is the only cause for the difference in results is clearly erroneous. It has been tempting to ascribe the remarkable reduction in wartime mortality from World War II to Korea to Vietnam to the marked diminution in delay between injury and treatment. However, the entire surgical training experience changed during that time, an almost completely new pharmacopoeia was available in Vietnam, and, most assuredly, many other variables are yet unaccounted for between the two eras. In fact, the principal reason for randomization in a study is to attempt to distribute the unknown and potentially important variables equally among groups to avoid selection bias. We may also see this effect if subjects accrue slowly and the study thus runs over many years. Other aspects of therapy may change and have a greater impact on outcome than the original variable selected for study.

Two aspects of clinical research that sometimes perplex beginning researchers and inexperienced readers are validity and generalizability. *Validity* deals with the ability of a study to give a scientifically sound answer to the question posed. Insofar as possible, this answer should be free from bias, uninfluenced by the effects of other related or confounding variables and with good statistical precision. Only then is there a basis for a *valid* study result.

Generalizability deals with extrapolation of study findings to a larger population or to other groups. Assessment of generalizability depends on the degree to which the study subjects are representative of some larger target population and how well the selection of study subjects simulates the process of drawing a random sample from a population.

The ideal is for studies to be both valid and generalizable. In practice, this is rarely the case. In the design of clinical research, investigators face many situations in which they must choose between validity and generalizability. When faced with a choice, undoubtedly they should opt for validity. Without a valid study, an investigator has little or nothing of scientific merit. The investigator may have actually drawn a random sample from a larger population and have virtually ideal generalizability. But, if in the process, validity was threatened or compromised, the findings are worthless. With findings of questionable or doubtful validity, there is nothing of value to generalize. Generalizability plays a subordinate role and, in fact, should not surface until validity has been firmly established. Often the reader must assume the onus of assessment of generalizability and of whether findings can be extrapolated to other populations.

METHODOLOGY AND OBSERVATIONS

In the reporting of research results, clarity in the definitions of the terms and measurements made has great importance. The more clearly the authors (or we as potential researchers) define the terms, including diagnostic criteria, measurements made, and the criteria of outcome, the more likely it is that we, the readers, can interpret the findings correctly and gain a proper perspective. For instance, in the field of invasive catheter-related infection, terms such as "colonization," "contamination," and "infection of the catheter" abound. Authors often use these terms differently, leading to great difficulty in interpretation and synthesis of results from different studies. Furthermore, a "positive culture" may represent different bacteriologic methodologies: some authors use a semiquantitative culture of an intracutaneous catheter segment,[9] whereas others use blood cultures aspirated through the catheter.[10] Clearly, results from one methodology may not be comparable to another, and interpretations based on differing methodologies may lead to different conclusions.

We must also try to evaluate the methods of classification or of measurement. The essential question is to assess whether inconsistencies in observation or evaluation could have sufficient impact to influence materially the results of the study. We also must evaluate the reliability and reproducibility of the observations. This is more difficult to assess. Frequently, some clues inform the reader of the author's concern with and awareness of reproducibility and reliability. When a subjective element enters into an assessment, an author often refers to and sometimes provides data on the results of evaluations by independent observers and their degree of agreement. *Interrater reliability* refers to the ability of two or more independent raters to make the same observations. *Intrarater reliability* refers to an observation made by the same rater over two or more different times. With respect to abstracting information from charts, interrater and intrarater reliability is usually in the range of only 80% to 90%. An author who devotes some attention to issues concerning measurement or laboratory error seemingly would be cognizant of the importance of reproducibility and reliability. It is well to be suspicious of results from a study that seems entirely devoid of concern with these elements, especially if some subjective element is clearly involved in either diagnosis, observation, or assessment of outcome.

PRESENTATION OF FINDINGS OR RESULTS

Authors must walk the fine line of clear and concise data presentation in the Results section without editorializing or drawing conclusions from the data they presented. Remember, the facts should speak for themselves. The author must still detour into enough necessary detail for the reader to judge the importance of the data. Important findings require proper documentation. If a small number of subjects are presented, a table listing the important demographic characteristics is useful so that the reader has a clear understanding of the population studied.

It is surprising how often numerical inconsistencies are contained within reports published in even the most reputable medical journals. This may be partly caused by the many drafts and revisions compounded by textual proofreading, computational and tabular proofreading, and other processes. Because of the frequency of these errors, the reader may wish to use some quick checks: columns and rows should add up to their indicated totals; percentages of mutually exclusive categories should add up to 100%; numbers in tables and figures should agree with those in the text; and totals in various tables describing the same population should agree. With the ubiquitous presence of hand-held calculators and personal computers, we can even run some of our own statistical tests, especially when the reported results appear incompatible with our quick mental assessment or even personal bias!

Clarity and precision are important criteria to judge the overall scientific validity of an article. Assessments, comparisons, and judgments belong in the Discussion section. However, when these are enthusiastically included in the Results section, they strongly suggest bias in the author's approach. Strictly speaking, investigators should undertake an analytic study when they can wholeheartedly support affirmation or rejection of the hypothesis under test. Thus, inclusion of subjective opinions (e.g., "markedly improved outcome") in the Results section may be a subtle indication that the investigators performed the study to confirm their preexisting personal views.

DATA ANALYSIS

In reality, the first question we, as readers, should ask is "Are the data worthy of statistical analysis?" We must then examine the methods of statistical analysis to determine whether they were appropriate to the source and nature of the data and whether the analysis was correctly performed and interpreted. These questions are difficult to answer. However, we recognize that this is an entire field to itself for which this chapter should stimulate the reader to pursue more vigorous study.

One of the first issues that should cross the reader's mind is to ask whether the observed and reported finding could result simply from chance, the luck of the draw, or sampling variation. An arsenal of statistical methodology is available ranging from simple (e.g., t-test, chi-square test) to sophisticated (multiple logistic regression, Cox proportional hazards model) to examine the role of chance in the analysis of study results. Each medical reader may not have sufficient expertise to assess whether the investigators have chosen their methodology appropriately and have correctly performed the statistical analyses. We hope that the journal's peer review process has included some form of assessment of the statistical aspects of the report. Until we, the readers, learn enough, we must solicit expert biostatistical assistance. However, three points should be remembered. First, it is the author's responsibility to provide the reader with information on the specific statistical analysis used in assessing the role of chance. Second, whatever the level of significance reported, no matter how small the *p* value, we can never rule out chance with certainty. An exceedingly small *p* value (1 instance in 1000) denotes that chance is an unlikely explanation of the result, but the possibility remains, although unlikely, that this is indeed that one instance in 1000. The third point is that a statistically significant result is not necessarily important or indicative of a real effect, only that an effect of chance has been ruled out with some reasonable certainty. Often we must apply context or perspective to the author's work. We have discussed the importance of reliability and reproducibility.

As clinicians, we know that measurements of pulmonary artery occlusion pressure (PAOP) differ among observers. For instance, estimation of PAOP from a visual inspection of the oscilloscope tracing may be 3 to 4 mm Hg different from the results calculated electronically and displayed in digital form on the monitor. In reviewing the effects of a drug, however, some investigators may interpret a change of the same magnitude (3 to 4 mm Hg) as an "effect" of the therapy. Thus, in addition to deciding whether a particular result is "statistically significant," that is, if it represents a real event (or results from chance), we must decide whether it has any real clinical, biologic meaning.

Furthermore, in our interpretation of study results we must, with reasonable certainty, rule out the possibility of *bias* and *confounding*. A result may be highly significant statistically but the study design and conduct could lead to a substantially biased result, or there may be some other related variable that also explains statistically significant results.

Confounding refers to effects of one or more related variables. In its strict epidemiologic definition, a confounding variable is one that is associated with both the "exposure" (or independent variable), and with the "outcome" (or dependent variable) under study. For example, in an observational study comparing the mortality experience of two modalities of treatment for head injuries, an obvious "confounding" variable would be the severity of the injury. Clearly, the severity of the injury relates to the dependent variable under study: mortality. The injury severity, however, may also have an association with the independent variable: the choice of the particular modality of treatment. Thus, any finding of a difference in mortality between modalities of treatment, no matter how statistically significant the difference, might be explained by the confounding effects of the severity of injury.

The important point is to judge whether the authors have considered all of the pertinent known confounding variables in their analyses and have taken proper steps to account for their effects. The reader, without substantive knowledge of the particular field of study, may be unable to delineate what pertinent potential confounding variables should have been considered. We (authors and readers) must cautiously proceed with forming conclusions.

Bias refers to a systematic departure from the truth. Bias may exist in many forms, and many statistical and epidemiologic adjectives can precede the word "bias" to denote some specific hazard or snag that can lead to a departure from the truth. Sackett[11] provides a useful compendium of the various biases that lurk to ensnare the unwary investigator,

and the unwary reader, in the conduct of biomedical research. We shall use the three adjectives: selection, observation, and analysis.

Selection bias refers to how subjects were entered into the study. Is the manner of selection of persons for study such that the study will result in substantial distortion of the truth? As a simple example, consider a study comparing outcome of surgery in patients who agree and volunteer to undergo the operation with those who refuse. Those who choose surgery may be better operative risks (at least from their own perception) probably with less comorbid disease than that found in the nonsurgical group. Of course, other factors may have influenced the other group to refuse surgery. Still, the difference in the outcome of surgery might be more likely to result from the selective nature of the groups rather than from any real effect of the surgical procedure.

Observation bias refers to the methodology for handling and evaluating subjects during the course of the study. If a therapeutic intervention group receives more attention, more supportive therapy, and more intense scrutiny than a control group, an observed difference in outcome might more likely be explained by observation bias rather than by any real effects of the intervention. Retrospective studies are particularly prone to observation bias.

Analysis bias refers to fallacies that exist in the choice of statistical methods to analyze data. An example is the "average age at death" fallacy. Calculation of average-age-at-death among decedents does *not* measure longevity; it reflects mainly the age composition of the total members of the groups, mostly those who are alive. For example, consider a newspaper report of a study that compared the average age at death of U.S. professional football players with professional baseball players.[12] The report stated that football players died, on average, 7 years earlier than baseball players. It would be erroneous to conclude that this differential reflects the more hazardous and traumatic aspects of professional football compared with professional baseball. In fact, professional football is a much newer sport (dating from the mid-1920s) than professional baseball (dating from the 1860s). Consequently, the total group of professional baseball players is considerably older than the total group of professional football players. As an extreme example of this average-age-at-death bias, consider the result anticipated in a comparison of the average-age-at-death in a children's hospital with that in a retirement community hospital.

When, in the assessment of a study, we can rule out with reasonable certainty that the finding does *not* result from chance, bias, or confounding, we are well on the road to determining a real and meaningful effect.

Finally, it is important to emphasize that the interpretation of *statistical significance* does not in and of itself connote medical or biologic importance. Correlation and regression illustrate this distinction and the misinterpretation that often occurs. Correlations are used to describe the degree of association between independent variables, such as blood pressure and age. With regression, this implies that we can choose one variable as dependent and one (or more) as independent. Our concern with regression is the relationship between an independent and dependent variable, namely, what happens to the dependent variable as we alter the independent variable. We use the linear regression equation, $Y = a + bX$, to predict values of the dependent variable Y from the independent variable, X, where b is the slope of the regression line and a is the intercept. Both correlation and regression may be presented familiarly as a scatter diagram and usually involve some analysis of the "statistical significance" of this relationship. The relation of a correlation coefficient in the case of a perfect linear relationship would yield a value of 1. Correlation coefficients of 0.5 or less might achieve "statistical significance" at a p value of less than 0.001, particularly when the sample size is large, (i.e., there are a large number of data points). The square of the correlation coefficient (and multiplication by 100) indicates the percentage of the variance of the dependent variable explained by the variance in the independent variable. Given a regression coefficient of 0.5, 25% of the dependent variable's variance would be explained by changes in the independent variable, although 75% remains unexplained. This may be a highly statistically significant relationship, with, say, $p < 0.001$; that is, there is a likelihood of less than 1 in 1000 that this has occurred by chance. Many authors and readers do not understand clearly the separation of the statistical reliability of the relationship and the *importance* of the statistical relationship. They often place a high weight of importance on relationships of minor causal significance (low r value) only because it is highly unlikely to result from chance (low p value). To illustrate this point, some years ago the hemodynamic and respiratory data for numerous disparate patients were combined and subjected to regression analysis.[13]

Venous oxygen content and intrapulmonary shunt had a statistically significant relation ($p < 0.01$) with an r value of 0.46. A glance at individual data points in the scatter diagram (Fig. 1-1) reveals that there are sufficient departures from the line depicting the regression equation such that it would be valueless to attempt to predict shunt from venous oxygen content for a new patient even within the observed range of values. Therefore, other factors must have an even greater weight to explain the other 79% percentage of variance ($r = 0.46$, $r^2 = 0.21$, or 21% of variance). Obviously, the degree of pulmonary disease in this instance would have the greatest effect in determining the intrapulmonary shunt. Thus, there is a *weak* although causal link between the two variables (low r value) and a *strong* likelihood that a relationship exists, that is, that the result was not due to chance (low p value). The problem occurs when we or other authors are searching for a relationship and infer an important causal physiologic relationship based on "statistical significance." Thus, we must remember that the p value, the significance of the statistical result, reflects merely the likelihood of chance at the level specified rather than the precision of the result; a lower p value, then, does not make the result more biologically important or clinically significant.

DISCUSSION AND CONCLUSIONS

In the Discussion section, the author provides an interpretation of findings. Here the author can attach clinical relevance to the reported statistically significant findings. The findings

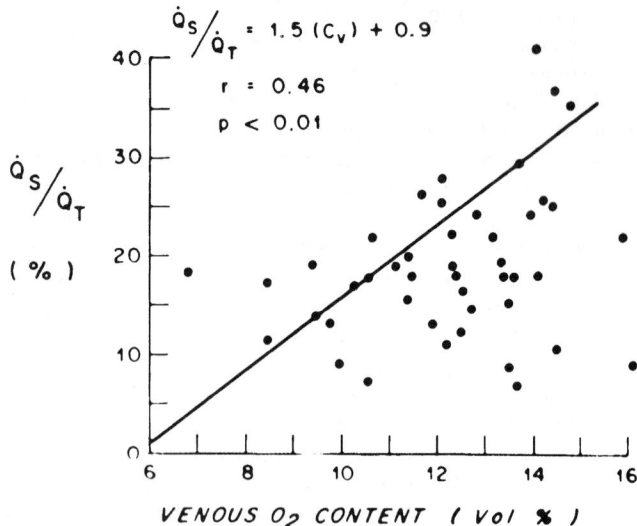

FIGURE 1-1. Scattergram plotting venous oxygen content and intrapulmonary shunt. Regression coefficient of 0.46 indicates that 21% of the variance in shunt is explained by variance in venous oxygen content. This relation is "statistically significant" ($p < 0.01$); it is unlikely to result from chance. Notice that this would not be a clinically important relationship to predict shunt from venous oxygen content. The relationship partly derives from the calculation of shunt. The denominator of the shunt equation is as follows: capillary oxygen content minus venous oxygen content; thus venous oxygen content numerically appears as both "independent" and part of the "dependent" variable.

may be compared with those of other studies and interpretations. Possible explanations for results can be postulated and differences from other reports in the literature explained. Hopefully the author bases the conclusions on the findings. This is not always the case. When we discuss the results, we should consider whether they have any meaning in the real world of bedside practice. A "significant" but relatively small difference in cardiac performance discovered only in carefully controlled circumstances has little resemblance to the constantly changing status of the critically ill patient in whom such a finding may not have any real import. We must ask ourselves whether the demonstrated result is important in influencing or directing bedside practice. We must retain our skepticism and use it to balance enthusiasm.

Later we discuss the concept of power relating to the necessary size of the sample. Authors who conclude that results would have been statistically significant if only a larger sample had been available display their lack of foresight and preparation; clearly, the time to discover the proper sample size is at the outset, the study-planning phase. Rather, it would be refreshing to encounter conclusions that forthrightly admitted that the hypothesis was incorrect, that the study showed that therapy did not lead to improvement, or that the investigator headed off on the wrong track. Negative reports of this sort will prevent other investigators from pursuing ideas that turn out to be flawed and can also direct investigators, including themselves, along more fruitful pathways.

The reporting of negative studies has been addressed from an editorial standpoint.[14] Angell states, ". . . it is widely believed that reports of negative studies are less likely to be published than those of positive studies and some data have been put forth to support this belief . . . it is assumed that editors and reviewers are biased against negative studies, considering them less inherently interesting than positive studies. However, a bias against publishing negative studies would distort the scientific literature."[14] Although she believes that the *New England Journal of Medicine* publishes fewer negative reports than positive ones, it is not a matter of policy. She asks, "Does it deal with an important question? Is the information new and interesting? Was the study well done? . . . We feel a particular obligation to publish a negative study when it contradicts an earlier study we have published and is of a similar or superior quality. When a good study addresses an important question, the answer is interesting and the work deserves publication whether the result is positive or negative."[14]

Finally, we should consider whether the conclusions are relevant to the questions posed by the investigators. Far too many reports begin with "unwarranted assumptions" in the introduction, end with "foregone conclusions" in the discussion, and contain in between a mass of barely relevant data. If we care to spend the time necessary to review published reports and, in particular, to do the preparation necessary before we embark on our own clinical investigations, such discouraging assessments will occur much less frequently.

ABSTRACT OR SUMMARY

Although we know that we should spend time in analyzing the medical literature, it is clear that, given the pressures of everyday life and the journals that appear with seemingly increasing frequency on our desks each month, we are often tempted to read only the title and the abstract. One final caveat: there may be important disparities among the results, discussion, and abstract. One memorable report compared two forms of fluid resuscitation. Three patients in one group had been given from two to three times the amount specified in the protocol. With exclusion of these patients properly in the data analysis, *as noted* in the results section, there were *no* differences between the two groups. With inclusion of patients with protocol violations, there was a "statistically significant" difference. The abstract cited the "statistically significant" analysis without any reference to the patients who should have been excluded. The authors' conclusion of a statistically significant difference in treatment modalities was, in fact, denied by their own results. If you are in a hurry, do not just read the abstract and move on; come back and read the article properly when you have enough time.

FUNDAMENTALS OF BIOSTATISTICS IN MEDICAL RESEARCH ■

This section presents some of the fundamentals of descriptive statistics and is an introduction to inferential statistics, primarily to alert the readers to certain important caveats in the interpretation of results of statistical analyses. We readily acknowledge the limitations of the fundamentals presented here. However, we hope that we will stimulate the reader both to seek expert assistance initially and to pursue further study.

Two distinctive components to statistical methods are

Descriptive statistics: methods that deal with the organization, summarization, and presentation of data
Inferential statistics: methods that deal with the drawing of inferences about populations from results obtained in study samples.

The main contemporary interest in statistics for clinical research is inferential statistics. This leads to the tests of significance, p values, and confidence limits that pervade the medical literature.

DESCRIPTIVE STATISTICS

(1) Types of Data

We encounter two major classes of data: quantitative and categorical. *Quantitative* data deal with measured quantities such as age, blood pressure, or arterial or oxygen tension. Quantitative data may be subdivided into *discrete* when only certain values are possible, such as the number of patients currently in the intensive care unit, or *continuous* when any value is possible. An example is serum sodium values, which could be reported as whole numbers such as 140 mEq/L or in decimals, 140.6 mEq/L, depending on the accuracy of the measuring instrument. *Categorical* data deal with attributes such as living or dead, hypertensive or not, and blood type. Similarly, categorical or qualitative variables may be subdivided into *ordinal* and *nominal* categories. The forgoing examples, such as living or dead or blood type, are nominal or named variables. Yes and no categories, such as the presence or absence of hypertension, may be called *dichotomous*. Ordinal variables consist of numbers, such as a ranking scale for pain. Because these are subjective assessments rather than objective measurements, they are not considered continuous quantitative variables.

(2) Fourfold Table for Quantal Data

Many medical investigations involve the comparison of two groups: a *study group* and a *comparison group*. When the data are categorical, the *fourfold* or *2 × 2 table* is a convenient device for summarizing the results. The fourfold table has two columns, corresponding to the study and comparison groups, and two rows, corresponding to the dichotomous data collected (e.g., success or failure, live or die, respond or do not respond). The four cells in the body of the table provide the study results.

The obvious descriptive measure with quantal data is the *percentage* with the attribute. From a fourfold table, the clinician compares the percentages with the attribute in the study and comparison groups. For simplicity, we choose examples from one study to illustrate various points.[6] The study design consisted of randomizing patients into groups with two different end points for the titration of PEEP. In group I, the authors used 5 cm H_2O PEEP to maintain the partial arterial pressure of oxygen (PaO_2) greater than 65 mm Hg at an inspired oxygen fraction (FIO_2) of 0.45. If PaO_2 fell below this level, PEEP was titrated until PaO_2 rose to the treatment goal, 65 mm Hg. In group II, the authors increased PEEP until physiologic shunt was reduced to less than 0.2. The authors compared the two groups for outcome and resources used: 6 (33%) of 18 patients in group I died; and 5 (25%) of 20 patients in group II died. This can be displayed as a fourfold table (Table 1-2).

As we shall see later, depending on the situation, the clinician can compare the percentages by examining their *difference,* their *ratio,* or, in epidemiology, their *odds ratio.* Authors should always report the numbers used to calculate percentages. In fact, many journals and abstract rules require that the basic data be reported.

(3) Descriptive Measures for Quantitative Data

The two descriptive characteristics of prime importance are *location* and *spread.*

For location, the most common measures used are the *mean* (arithmetic average), *median* (middlemost value), and *mode* (most frequently occurring). For purposes of statistical inference, the *mean* and *median* are most frequently used. The *mode* is rarely used in clinical research.

For spread, the most obvious is the *range* (highest minus lowest), but it has limited use for inference. The measure of spread ubiquitous in research is the *standard deviation* (SD), defined as

$$SD = \sqrt{\frac{\sum (x - \bar{x})^2}{n - 1}}$$

A convention many investigators follow with studies involving quantitative data is to summarize results as mean ± SD.

WARNING: Another convention involves expression of results as mean ± standard error (SE), where SE is some other quantity (discussed later). The author's onus in a medical article is to indicate whether the number following the ± is SD or SE.

(4) Normal or Gaussian Distribution

The normal or Gaussian distribution is a theoretic mathematic curve (i.e., an equation can be written for it) that has particular importance in statistical work. It has the familiar bell-shaped appearance. The distribution can be described entirely by its mean and SD.

TABLE 1-2.   Titrating PEEP in Early, Moderate, and Arterial Hypoxemia

	GROUP I	GROUP II
Died	6	5
Did not die	12	15
Total patients studied	18	20
% Died	33.3	25.0

PEEP, positive end-expiratory pressure.

Empirically, the distribution of many quantitative measurements tends to approximate a normal distribution in shape (e.g., weight, examination scores, IQs).

Particular properties of the normal distribution are that its

Mean ± 1 SD encompasses about 65% of the measurements;

Mean ± 2 SD encompasses about 95% of the measurements;

Mean ± 3 SD encompasses almost all measurements.

Unfortunately, many populations in critical care are not normal in the sense that the distribution of many quantitative measurements does not approximate a Gaussian distribution. For instance, in any clinical series, a few patients tend to remain in the hospital far longer and tend to skew the distribution to the right on a scale of increasing duration of hospital stay. Because hospital charges are proportional to the time spent in the hospital, the reader might anticipate that the distribution of hospital charges would not be normal. In the PEEP study, the hospital charges in group I patients were $32,000 ± $18,000 (mean ± SD).[6] Clearly, hospital charges do *not* approximate a normal distribution. If we had naively calculated mean ± 2 to encompass 95% of the patients, we would see that the lowest value is an impossible negative charge, $−4000. Whether data under study follow an approximately normal distribution can influence the choice of method for analysis. In the above example, to compare charges in the two study groups—rather than use the t-test, which has an implicit assumption that the data follow an approximately normal distribution—the Mann-Whitney U test was used, which does not entail any assumption regarding the shape of the distribution of the data. With the wide availability of statistical computer packages, it is possible to readily calculate means and standard deviations, regardless of whether the data are normally distributed (even with ordinal data such as ranking scales). If all of the data are of similar sign (that is all positive or all negative) and the standard deviation is greater than half of the mean, the data clearly will *not* be normally distributed. The median and range can be used as descriptive statistics and, in addition to the Mann-Whitney U test for testing differences between two unpaired treatments, other nonparametric tests of significance are available. These include the following: the Wilcoxon signed rank test, which tests for differences between two paired treatments; the Kruskal-Wallis analysis of variance (see later) for testing differences between more than two treatments; and the Spearman rank correlation, which can be used to test the strength of association between two variables.

The more important use of the normal distribution in statistics is in the process of statistical inference, which we are now ready to discuss.

STATISTICAL INFERENCE

(1) Background and Objectives

The ultimate result of statistical tests of significance is presentation in a report of a "*p* value" and a claim that findings were "statistically significant" or "not statistically significant." These claims result from a series of numerical calculations. In today's world of electronic aids, we can deemphasize the calculation ritual and emphasize the underlying rationale for the statistical test of significance and the proper interpretation of its result.

We focus here on the comparison of two groups of observations: a study group and a comparison group. The data under consideration could be categorical or quantitative. In fact, the nature of the data involved in the comparison dictates the statistical methods for analysis. Categorical data lead to chi-square tests (sometimes cited with Yates' correction), whereas quantitative data lead to t-tests (or, as occur alternatively, nonparametric Wilcoxon rank tests or the Mann-Whitney test).

(2) Concept of Sampling Variations and Definition of SE

Basic to statistical inference is the underlying concept of *sampling variation,* namely, that any quantity calculated in a sample (e.g., proportion, mean, median, and SD) will differ with different samples (of the same size) from an underlying population. The variation in this quantity from sample to sample is sampling variation.

For example, consider quantal data and calculation in a sample of the proportion of persons who have the attribute under study. Think of many repeat samples of the same size from this population with, in each sample, determination of the proportion with the attribute. The variation among the proportions in the various repeat samples is the *sampling variation of a proportion.*

As a second example, consider quantitative data and the calculation of a mean for the sample. Think of many repeat samples of the same size from this population and, with each sample, determination of the mean. The variation among means in the repeat samples is the *sampling variation of a mean.*

If we consider using the SD to describe variation, we come to the definition of *SE,* the SD for sampling variation of some quantity (e.g., proportion or mean) calculated in each of the repeat samples. For our first example, the SD among proportions for repeat samples of the same size is the *SE of a proportion.* For our second example, the SD among means for repeat samples of the same size is the *SE of a mean.*

Finally, without going through the laborious process of empirically obtaining repeat samples, statistical theory indicates that [a] for proportions, the SE of a proportion (SE_p) is

$$SE_p = \sqrt{P(1-P)/n}$$

where n = sample size and P = proportion in the population with the attribute; and [b] for means, the SE of a mean ($SE_{\bar{x}}$) is

$$SE_{\bar{x}} = \sigma/n$$

where n = sample size and σ = SD in the population.

NOTES.   When the SD (σ) in the entire population is unknown, which is almost always the case, the SD in the sample, s, should be used as an estimate of σ. Thus,

$$est\ SE_{\bar{x}} = s/\sqrt{n}.$$

The choice of mean $\pm$ SD or mean $\pm$ SE depends on the purported use of the data. If the intention is to indicate variation of individual values about a mean, the choice is mean $\pm$ SD. If the intention is to indicate sampling variation in many different samples or stability of the mean and to conduct a statistical inference regarding the mean, then the choice is mean $\pm$ SE.

The calculation of $SE_{\bar{x}}$ results in a smaller number than SD because it is SD divided by the square root of the sample size. Sometimes, however, we will find mean $\pm$ SE used to indicate variation of individual values about a mean in a single sample, although the choice should be mean $\pm$ SD. This could be a mistake in transforming or selecting the data, but another inference is that the authors believe this somehow "tightens" the data by appearing to mask the actual variation of individual values in the sample.

An amazing but mathematically provable feature is that if a distribution of the means or proportions from repeat samples of the same size is plotted, the distribution tends to follow a normal or Gaussian curve. The mathematical derivation of this is called the Central Limit Theorem. The fact that sampling distributions of a mean and a proportion are normal is the reason why the normal distribution is the basis for many of the methods of statistical inference we encounter in research.

(3) Specifications for a Test of Significance

Three specifications are necessary to perform a test of significance. The clinician must specify a *null hypothesis,* set a *significance level,* and determine whether to conduct a *one- or two-sided* test.

NULL HYPOTHESIS.   The null hypothesis generally states that there is no difference between two groups or no effect of treatment. When comparing two groups with categorical data, the null hypothesis concerns the proportions with the attributes in the two larger "study" and "comparison" populations from which the study data came. The obvious null hypothesis is that the proportions with the attribute are the same in the study and comparison populations. The PEEP study compared mortality rates in the two groups.[6] The null hypothesis states that, in the underlying populations from which these study samples come, there is no difference in mortality rates.

For the comparison of two groups with the quantitative data, the null hypothesis is that the means in the underlying study and comparison populations are identical, or, alternatively, that the difference in population means is zero.

SIGNIFICANCE LEVEL.   As is seen later, the test of significance involves making a decision under uncertainty and based on chance. Setting a significance level is the *arbitrary* selection of a small enough chance for making a choice. Convention in both medical and nonmedical research dictates 0.05 or 5% and 0.01 or 1% as the typical levels of significance. Choice of 5% indicates that an event occurring only 1 time in 20 or less is sufficiently rare to risk drawing a conclusion that excludes chance as a likely explanation of what was observed. Choice of 1% is more conservative and indicates that an event occurring only 1 time in 100 or less is sufficiently rare to risk drawing a conclusion that excludes chance as a likely explanation of what was observed.

How should we determine whether 5% or 1% or some other value is a proper level of significance? Because this is an arbitrary selection, several factors bear on this selection process. For instance, if a particular form of treatment carries a high risk of serious side effects, we might choose a level of 1%. On the other hand, if the disease has an extremely high mortality rate, we might raise the level of significance to 5%, allowing a greater possibility for chance to have produced the results but not discarding a real result based on too strict a criterion. If the problem addressed is widespread and the proposed remedy simple and inexpensive, we might elect a higher level of significance, whereas an expensive, complicated, difficult-to-effect modality of therapy might more properly be judged by a lower significance level.

To refer again to the PEEP study, the chosen level of significance was 0.05. The level of significance was chosen because the mortality rate may have been considered high (favoring a higher level), the therapy was simple, and neither arm entailed higher charges or more complicated interventions.

ONE- OR TWO-SIDED TEST. A one- or two-sided test pertains to the nature of the alternatives entertained in contrast to the null hypothesis. More specifically, if in the comparison of two groups the clinician considers as alternatives to the null hypothesis only that the population mean or proportion in the study group may be higher than that in the comparison group, this is a *one-sided test*. If, however, the possibility is considered that the population mean or proportion in the study group may be either higher or lower than that in the comparison group, this is a *two-sided test*. In general, the two-sided test is the more conservative. In trials, although the clinician may have every anticipation that the new therapy will perform better than the standard, the possibility often exists that it may perform worse. Hence, the more conservative two-sided test would be adapted in such a situation.

If we are increasing PEEP to attempt to increase PaO_2, we might analyze our results with a one-sided test. If we chose a two-sided test, we entertain the possibility that PEEP lowers the partial pressure of oxygen (PO_2). In practice, we chose the more conservative two-sided test to compare mortality rates in the two groups of the PEEP study.

(4) Rationale for the Test of Significance

Central to the application of statistical methods is the notion that a study consists of a random sample from some underlying population. One calculates a descriptive statistic in the sample, a proportion (or rate or percentage) for quantal data, and a mean for quantitative data. The inference to be drawn concerns the respective statistic in the underlying population, that is, the population proportion or the population mean.

The situation we have prescribed then concerns two populations: a "study" and "comparison" as well as two samples, one from the study and one from the comparison population. We further presume that with quantal data we have calculated the sample proportion in each of our study and comparison samples. In the PEEP example, the sample proportions are 33.3% and 25.0%, respectively, in groups I and II. With quantitative data, we presume calculation of the sample mean in each of our study and comparison samples.

The rationale for the test of significance is that we presume that the null hypothesis we have specified regarding the populations is true. We then determine, using methods based on the mathematic theory of probability, the chance that we would obtain results in our samples that were as extreme as or more extreme than what we have actually observed. If this chance is sufficiently small, then we claim that the results obtained with our samples are not compatible with the specified null hypothesis, and our study has provided us evidence to refute the null hypothesis. This is the meaning of *statistically significant*.

If the chance we determine is *not* sufficiently small, then we claim that the results obtained with our samples are, indeed, compatible with the specified null hypothesis, and our study provides no evidence to refute the null hypothesis. This is the meaning of *not statistically significant*.

By "sufficiently small," we mean the chance we had selected with our significance level specification, namely, the conventional 5% or 1%.

Finally, if we determine the chance of extremities in only one direction from the null hypothesis specification, we are performing a one-sided test. If we determine the chance of extremities in either direction from the null hypothesis specification, we are performing a two-sided test.

Stated simply, the test of significance is an indication of whether chance is a likely (not statistically significant) or an unlikely (statistically significant) explanation of the discrepancy between the stated null hypothesis and the observed results in the study samples.

(5) Distinction Between Paired and Independent Samples for the Comparison of Two Groups

We need to distinguish between two different forms of comparative studies: paired samples and independent samples. *Paired samples* occur when each observation in the study sample has, by the nature of the investigation, a matching or paired observation in the comparison sample. The most obvious paired situation is a "before–after" study, or one in which the patient serves as his or her own control. Sometimes investigators individually match subjects on various characteristics (e.g., age, sex, race, socioeconomic status) and conduct a paired sample study.

When, as described in the study methodology, there is no evident individual matching of study with comparison sample observations, the design is obviously *independent samples*.

(6) Four Situations for the Comparison of Two Groups

With two types of data (quantal and quantitative) and two study designs (paired samples and independent samples), we have four situations for the comparison of two groups. Table 1-3 indicates some pertinent statistical tests of significance for each situation.

(7) Example

To illustrate the above points, consider the PEEP study discussed previously. Patients were randomized to one of two study groups, with 18 assigned to group I and 20 to group II. Among the various study outcomes investigated, Table 1-2 presents the relevant fourfold table for mortality. Consider a test of significance comparing mortality rates in the two groups. A perusal of the Methods section of the report indicates no individual matching or pairing of patients in the two groups; hence, we are dealing with independent samples. The data for this particular comparison, Died or Did Not Die, are clearly categorical. Hence, our interest is in comparison of proportions in independent samples, which, according to Table 1-3, indicates chi-square as an appropriate method of statistical analysis.

Recall that we have stated previously that we are testing the null hypothesis of no difference in mortality in the underlying populations for the two interventions under study. When we perform our test of significance we are asking: if the null hypothesis is correct and there is no real difference, how often by chance alone would we obtain a mortality difference in samples of n = 18 in group I and n = 20 in group II of 33.3% − 25.0% = 8.3% or something more extreme? When we specified a two-tailed test, we stated our interest in considering deviations as extreme or more extreme in *both* directions from the null hypothesis value of zero.

Following the calculation ritual for chi-square in independent samples, we obtain a chi-square value (with use of Yates' correction and 1 df) of 0.04. From a table of the chi-square distribution, this yields a probability (p value) of 0.84 or 84%. Having chosen a significance level of 5%—that is, we considered 5% or 1 chance in 20 as sufficiently infrequent—clearly 84% far exceeds 5%. Hence, the test of significance concludes "not statistically significant." In other

words, chance or sampling variation does, indeed, constitute a plausible explanation for the observed difference in mortality rates for the two study groups. Thus, on the basis of the results of this study, we have no reason to doubt the null hypothesis. The observed difference in mortality rates between the two study groups is well within the possibility of chance variation.

The McNemar test is another type of chi-square analysis that can be used to compare proportions in a before and after determination on the same group of subjects, namely, a paired sample of categorical data.

In addition to mortality rate, the PEEP study examined other variables, some of which are shown in Table 1-4. These include number of days in the surgical intensive care unit, number of days intubated, number of arterial and venous blood gas determinations, number of inotropic or vasoactive drugs administered, and frequency with which more than 5 cm H_2O PEEP was required to achieve the desired end points. The first five variables involve quantitative data, and, for each variable, Table 1-4 shows the respective means and SDs for the 18 patients in group I and the 20 patients in group II. In each instance, a test of significance was conducted to compare the two group means. Because this is a comparison of two means in independent samples, a relevant calculation ritual according to Table 1-3 is the independent samples t-test.

In each instance, the null hypothesis under test is that, in the underlying population from which these study data came, there is no difference in the means. Each test involved choice of a 5% significance level and use of a two-sided test. In each instance, the outcome of the test of significance was "not significant" ($p > 0.05$).

Interpretation of these results is that in each of the five tests comparing means, the results observed in the study samples are, indeed, compatible with the null hypothesis statement that, in the respective populations, no difference exists between means for each of these variables. In other words, if each of the null hypotheses of no difference in means is true, the results observed in the study sample, or something more extreme in either direction from the null, could have occurred by chance or by sampling variation. Thus, on the basis of these study results, the two interventions do not differ with respect to mean effects for each of these variables.

TABLE 1-3. Study Design and Data Type Comparisons

DATA	DESIGN	COMPARISON	NAME OF TEST
Quantal	Paired	Proportions (by means of untied pairs)	McNemar's chi-square (exact binomial when sample size is small)
Quantal	Independent samples	Proportions	Chi-square (with Yates' correction) (Fisher's exact test when sample size is small)
Quantitative	Paired samples	Means Medians?	Paired samples t-test Wilcoxon signed rank test
Quantitative	Independent samples	Means Medians	Independent samples t-test Wilcoxon rank sum test of Mann-Whitney U-test

TABLE 1-4.   Titrating PEEP Study: Resources Used°

	GROUP I (n = 18)	GROUP II (n = 20)	p VALUE
SICU days	5.3 ± 3	6.6 ± 5	NS†
Days intubated	3.4 ± 3	5.3 ± 5	NS
No. of arterial blood gas determinations	25.0 ± 16	32.0 ± 19	NS
No. of venous blood gas determinations	11.0 ± 3	15.0 ± 4	NS
No. of inotropic/vasoactive drugs	1.7 ± 1.5	2.2 ± 1.8	NS
Required > 5 cm H_2O PEEP to achieve end-points, % of patients	27.8	95.0	0.00008

PEEP, positive end-expiratory pressure; SICU, surgical intensive care unit.
°Data are mean ± SD
†NS, not significant, $p > 0.05$.

The final data item in Table 1-4 gives the percentage of patients who required more than 5 cm H_2O of PEEP to achieve the desired end points. As with the mortality data, comparison of the two groups on this variable entails a comparison of two proportions in independent samples and entails the chi-square test. Performing the same calculation ritual as with the mortality data leads to a chi-square (with use of Yates' correction and 1 df) of 15.6. This yields a p value of 0.00008, or, more roughly, $p < 0.0001$ (i.e., less than a 1 in 10,000 chance). Here, too, the null hypothesis is equal population frequency for the two interventions. The chosen significance level is 5% (or 1 chance in 20), and a two-tailed test was selected. Clearly, the p value we calculated, 1 in 10,000, is far below our chosen significance level, 1 in 20. Hence, our results are "statistically significant" ($p < 0.05$). In other words, the sample results in this study are *not* compatible with the null hypothesis of no difference in the two interventions for this variable. The results we observed are unlikely to have occurred by chance or sampling variation alone. Thus, our study *does* provide sufficient evidence to doubt or refute the null hypothesis that these two interventions require the same frequency of use of more than 5 cm H_2O of PEEP. We could state, "Significantly more patients in the group II intervention compared with group I required more than 5 cm H_2O of PEEP to achieve the desired end points ($p < 0.05$)." Alternatively, the previous statement could appear with a parenthetical "$p < 0.0001$," as shown in Table 1-4, or with the actual p value calculated, "$p = 0.00008$." In other words, this difference in sample rates, 27.8% in group I and 95% in group II, is unlikely to have occurred purely by chance, and we can construe this as substantial evidence in this study to refute the null hypothesis.

INTERPRETATION OF STUDY RESULTS ■

CAUTIONS AND CAVEATS

As we proceed from statistical analysis of data to the field of statistical inference, we must be aware of cautions and caveats in the use, abuse, interpretation, and misinterpretation of the tests of significance.

(1) "Statistically Significant" and "Not Statistically Significant"

Many terms used are used, correctly and incorrectly, to express the concepts *statistically significant* and *not statistically significant*. However, these terms should be used only in accordance with the equivalency outlined in Table 1-5.

(2) Implying or Stating the Null Hypothesis

The null hypothesis must be clearly implied or specifically stated. The results of a test of significance always refer to some null hypothesis regarding unknown population values. The investigator's responsibility is either to state the null hypothesis specifically or to have it clearly implied in the description of the investigation. In studies involving the comparison of two groups, the implicit null hypothesis is that no difference exists (in proportions or means) between the "study" and "comparison" populations. A "statistically significant" or "not statistically significant" result without clear indication of the null hypothesis is uninterpretable.

(3) Significance Level

The chosen significance level or citation of a p value must always appear. The citation of a p value occurs commonly in medical research. The investigator, from the calculation ritual in performing the selected test of significance, obtains a probability value from reference to a statistical table. The exact probability determined may be cited (e.g., $p = 0.047$ or $p = 0.00008$), or the smallest commonly used level for which results can be significant may be chosen (e.g., $p < 0.05$ or $p < 0.0001$). Today, when statistics are usually calculated by computer programs, the exact values are usually calculated.

Statements that "results were statistically significant" or "results were not statistically significant" without indication somewhere of a significance level or citation of a p value are meaningless.

(4) "Proving the Null Hypothesis"

The null hypothesis can never be proved to be true. Results that are "not statistically significant" mean only that evidence

TABLE 1-5. Equivalency of Terms Commonly Used

Statistically significant	=	Rejected null hypothesis	=	Sample value not compatible with null hypothesis value	=	Sampling variation is an unlikely explanation of discrepancy between null hypothesis and sample values
Not statistically significant	=	Do not reject null hypothesis	=	Sample value compatible with null hypothesis value	=	Sampling variation is a likely explanation of discrepancy between null hypothesis and sample values

is insufficient to disprove the null hypothesis. It may be that the null hypothesis, in reality, is *not* true but that the conducted study was too small and lacked the precision to detect differences from the null hypothesis. A result of "not statistically significant" means that the clinician must live with the null hypothesis until such time that further evidence arises that might disprove it.

To avoid any connotation of proving the null hypothesis true when results are not statistically significant, we use the convoluted wording "failure to reject the null hypothesis" rather than the simpler and more direct "accept the null hypothesis."

(5) Specific and General Use of "Significance"

Be cautious in the use of the word "significance" in its specific, statistical context and its vague, general usage to denote importance. Basically, statistical significance does not mean importance. A result may be "statistically significant," but clinically it may be totally unimportant. Some medical journals discourage use of the word significant in anything other than its technical statistical context.

(6) Interpreting Tests of Significance

Interpretation of the outcome of a test of significance presupposes that determination of the study samples simulates random sampling from underlying populations. The calculation ritual for tests of significance can be applied to any set of numbers. The interpretation of the results of a test of significance depends on the assumption that the study samples were obtained by a process that reasonably simulates random selection of a sample from a larger population. A useful point to keep in mind is to ask, before examination of the results of a test of significance, whether the investigator had the *right* to perform a test of significance with the data. If the study is prone to strong effects of bias and uncontrolled confounding, the test of significance becomes irrelevant (see section on Data Analysis).

(7) "Multiple Peeks" Problem: Repeat Analyses of Accumulating Data

Worshipping at the shrine of the 5% significance level, an interesting suggestion is to analyze accumulating data in a study after every few observations and to stop the study as soon as the cumulative data achieve statistical significance at the 5% level. Statistically, this is an entirely fallacious

procedure. The actual significance level with this procedure will not be 5% but something *much higher*, thus increasing the likelihood that chance alone is responsible for the "difference" observed. Using conventional statistical tests such as t-tests and chi-square, the actual significance level depends on the number of peeks or analyses performed with the accumulating data. In fact, it can be shown mathematically that even if the null hypothesis is exactly true, the investigators will ultimately find a statistically significant result although they may have to continue obtaining observations and analyzing the cumulative results for a long time.

If the clinician wishes to take multiple peeks with repeat analyses of data as they accumulate, special statistical techniques[15] must be used that were devised for this situation, namely, *sequential methods* (see Chap. 8 in *Statistics in Medicine*[7]).

(8) "Multiple Comparisons" Problem: Many Tests of Significance Within a Single Study

With the ability to collect many measurements on a wide variety of variables in a single study, and the availability of computers to grind out the calculation rituals for tests of significance, a study may involve a large number of tests of significance and the reporting of their respective *p* values.

With many variables tested, their corresponding *p* values require cautious interpretation. As we shall indicate later, one way to view the chosen significance level is to consider it as the chance to make an incorrect decision and reject a null hypothesis that is true. Thus, specification of a 5% significance level means that we are willing to risk a 5% or 1 in 20 chance of coming to the wrong conclusion in our analysis and rejecting the null hypothesis when it is true. What this means is that among every 100 tests of significance we encounter in which the null hypothesis actually is true, five have resulted in the erroneous conclusion of statistical significance.

Thus, if a study involves 100 tests of significance with various data items, we would anticipate that 5% or five tests would produce statistically significant results by chance alone. The extreme in multiple statistical testing is to let the statistical analysis drive the investigation. Investigators may decide that rather than specify particular hypotheses for testing, they will conduct a study collecting information on as many variables as possible and then, from the tests of significance for each variable, choose and report those variables that turn out statistically significant at the 5% level. Not only is this improper use of statistical methods, but also it is poor science. It is often termed a "fishing expedition," but in reality it would be a poor study design for a fishing trip as well: too much ocean and too few fish!

When a study does involve several statistical comparisons, specific techniques are available for dealing with this situation, namely, *multiple comparisons procedures*, which can preserve the predetermined significance level for the statistical testing.[16,17] Although, for illustrative purposes, we did *not* use any multiple comparisons procedure, certainly the PEEP study results (see Table 1-4) lend themselves to consideration of a multiple comparisons procedure.

Thus far we have limited discussion to comparison of two groups by means of t tests for *quantitative* data. If more than two groups exist, the appropriate test would be the analysis of variance, often abbreviated ANOVA. To determine statistical significance, this test analyzes the variance between groups and within groups. The null hypothesis in this instance states that there are no differences among any of the group means. However, if the null hypothesis is rejected, and analysis reveals that a difference is unlikely to result from chance, ANOVA does not identify which group or groups are different. The researcher must perform additional analysis. Again, most common statistical programs print the subsequent multiple comparisons procedures as part of the statistical results in the ANOVA package. Which test is appropriate for your study or determining whether the authors have used the appropriate test requires consultation with a statistician or further study.

Often, clinical studies entail measurements of response of the variable under study over time in two or more different groups. Here, repeated measures ANOVA is the appropriate statistical test. For instance, we could use repeated measures ANOVA to compare the effect of PEEP on the first, second, and third days of the study between the "adequate oxygenation" and "minimal shunt" groups.

(9) *Playing by the Rules of the Game*

We realize that the structure of statistical tests of significance involves some arbitrary choices (such as choice of a significance level) and some unrealistic oversimplification in its dichotomization of the world (such as significant or not significant). If this hypothesis-testing framework is chosen for drawing inferences from study findings, results should be reported properly, with correct terminology, according to the rules of the game and without editorializing. Thus, within the framework, after choosing a significance level, results are either "significant" or "not significant" at that chosen level. It is customary to indicate the smallest significance level at which that result would have been significant. For example, although the 5% significance level was chosen for the test, the calculated p value for comparison of percentage of patients requiring more than 5 cm H_2O of PEEP was 0.0008. Hence, the results could be reported with one of the following three notations: $p < 0.05$, $p < 0.0001$, or $p = 0.0008$. What is irksome is when results are *not* significant at the chosen level, but authors often write, "There was a clear trend toward significance," or "The findings suggest a difference, but they did not achieve statistical significance." Clearly, results are or are not significant. The

qualifications of "a clear trend" or "suggest a difference" constitute unnecessary editorializing. If comments such as these are made, they should appear in the Discussion section of an article and not in the Results section. The astute reader is, indeed, wary of the arbitrariness and limitations of the process of statistical testing and does not need additional editorializing by the authors while assessing a study's findings.

Another perspective on this is that deployment of tests of significance according to the rules does mean that, say at a chosen 5% significance level, a calculated p value of 0.047 is "significant," whereas nearly the same sample result that leads to a calculated p value of 0.053 is "not significant." The experienced researcher and reader are well aware of this limitation and apparent paradox with tests of significance. But, if we have chosen to play the game, we must play by the rules and not hedge or qualify the reporting of the findings.

The limitations and arbitrariness surrounding tests of significance are reasons why many investigators, and many biostatisticians, are shifting toward confidence limits for reporting research results. Although the same principles of statistical inference are involved in calculation and interpretation of a confidence interval, it provides more information than the mere reporting of a p value from a test of significance.

TYPE I AND TYPE II ERRORS

With the use of statistical tests of significance to test hypotheses, it is important to understand the two errors that arise in the conclusions drawn:

(1) *Type I or α Error*

When we choose the 5% significance, we, alternatively, have stated that we are willing to risk 5% chance of erroneously rejecting a true null hypothesis (i.e., claiming statistical significance when, in fact, the null hypothesis is true). This incorrect decision or error is called the *type I error, α error, or error of the first kind.*

(2) *Type II or β Error*

Obviously, the above definition implies that there is a corresponding *type II error, β error, or error of the second kind.* In this situation, the null hypothesis is false, and some alternative hypothesis regarding the population values prevails. The incorrect conclusion we make is to fail to reject the null hypothesis when, in fact, the null hypothesis is false. In other words, β or type II error is coming to the erroneous conclusion of "not statistically significant" when, in fact, the null hypothesis is false and there really *is* a difference between the study and comparison groups.

We, as readers and authors, must make some decisions with respect to the possibility of introducing either type I or type II errors. For instance, if a particular form of treatment is hazardous and has life-threatening side effects, we want to be sure that a true difference exists before rejecting the null hypothesis. We may, therefore, choose a lower level of significance (p value = 0.01 rather than p value = 0.05) to make it less likely that the difference is a result of chance alone. We have diminished the likelihood of introducing a hazardous form of therapy based on results that, indeed, were the outcome of chance. On the other hand, if a safe form of treatment has a small therapeutic effect, we might not wish to fall into a type II error, in other words, coming to the erroneous conclusion that there was not a statistically significant difference between the two groups when, in fact, there was a true difference.

(3) Power

Power of a statistical test is defined simply as the complement of the β or type II error, that is,

$$\text{Power} = 1 - \beta$$

Thus, the power of a statistical test refers to the chance of correctly rejecting the null hypothesis when, in fact, the null hypothesis is false.

PLANNING THE SAMPLE SIZE OF A STUDY

With these definitions we have three important quantities involved in a statistical test of significance:

(i) the sample size, *n*
(ii) α error associated with the null hypothesis
(iii) β error associated with an alternative hypothesis

Providing any two of the above items allows us to determine the value of the third. For example, with specification of (i) the sample size of the study and (ii) the α error chosen for the null hypothesis, we can determine, for any specific alternative hypothesis, the β error, that is, the chance of making an erroneous conclusion of "not statistically significant" when, in fact, that specific alternative hypothesis is true.

Of more use, perhaps, is that with specification of (ii) the α error associated with the null hypothesis and (iii) the β error for some specific alternative hypothesis, we can then determine *n*, the sample size needed for the study. For comparative investigations, this means that an investigator must provide an α error and a β error for a specific difference (usually called a clinically meaningful difference). (Alternatively, rather than β error, the researcher could just as well frame the specification in terms of power, that is, the study is planned to have a certain specified power for a specific difference.)

The above is the rationale for the answer the statistician provides to the question, "How big a sample do I need?" The investigator must specify the α and β errors, have some idea of the underlying variability in the measurements under consideration (expected SD), and select a value to represent a true difference between the experimental and control groups.

The equation to calculate the size of the sample contains the SD and the terms for the percentage point of a normal distribution for α and β errors in the numerator and the true difference in the denominator. A *higher* specified level

of significance for each results in a lower numerator and a lower quotient or sample number. Thus, if we select an α or β error of 0.05 compared with 0.01, we need a smaller sample. On the other hand, if a greater variability occurs in the measurements, a large sample size is necessary. The sample size also depends on the value selected for a true difference. Determining whether mortality rate is reduced from 25% to 10% takes a smaller sample than an anticipated reduction from 25% to 20%. If the existing mortality rate is low (4%), therapy that would truly result in halving the rate to 2% would require a study involving a large number of patients (further details and methods of calculation are provided in *Statistics in Medicine*,[7] pp 142-146).

Consider the PEEP study we used earlier as an example to illustrate tests of significance. Consider the mortality data as shown in Table 1-2 in which the mortality rate in both groups combined is roughly 30%. Suppose we plan some new intervention that we anticipate will reduce mortality. How large a comparative study do we need to test this new intervention (study group) against conventional therapy (comparison group)?

Clearly, the null hypothesis is that mortality in the study and that in the comparison groups are identical. When confronted with the statistical question regarding type I error, suppose we indicate that we plan to perform a two-sided test at the 5% level. We chose a two-sided test because although we have every anticipation that our new intervention will reduce mortality, some possibility exists that it might result in an increase in mortality. If such an adverse consequence did occur, we would want to be able to detect such a possibility in our analysis. Hence, we have opted for the more conservative two-sided test. When we chose the 5% significance level or α = 0.05, we have specified our type I error; that is, we have indicated that we wish a 5% or 1 in 20 chance of erroneously rejecting the null hypothesis, namely, erroneously claiming a statistically significant difference in our study when, in fact, no real difference in mortality exists.

We now have to specify our type II error. As a first step, we must choose what difference in mortality we consider clinically important. Suppose we choose a difference of 10%. This means that if, in fact, our new intervention reduces mortality by 10%, say, from 30% to 20%, we deem this as a clinically important effect that we wish to detect. In fact, when pressed, we might state that we wish to have a 10% type II error for this effect. In other words, we wish to have only a 10% or one in ten chance of erroneously failing to reject the null hypothesis when this magnitude of effect exists, that is, if there is, in reality, an effect of reduction of mortality by 10% (i.e., absolute 10% difference), we wish our study to have only one chance in ten of arriving at the erroneous conclusion of "no significant difference" in mortality.

We could, alternatively, have made the above specification in terms of statistical power rather than type II error. We would then say that if the real reduction in mortality is 10% (i.e., absolute 10% difference), we wish our study to have 90% power to detect such a difference. In other words, we wish to have a study such that there are nine chances in ten that our results will lead to the correct conclusion of "statistically significant difference" when, in fact, a true difference in mortality of this magnitude exists.

With these specifications, calculations reveal that we need a sample size of 420 patients in each of the study and comparison groups or a total of 840 patients in the investigation. If this number is beyond the resources available to us, we would have to relinquish something in our error specifications. Our sample size determination would yield a smaller number if we were to increase α error (e.g., from 5% to 10%) or increase our β error (e.g., from 10% to 20%) or choose a larger clinically meaningful minimum difference in mortality rate (e.g., 15% instead of 10%).

Another approach to the collective bargaining between biostatistician and clinical investigator in determination of sample size is for the investigator to indicate to the biostatistician the maximum number of patients that can be anticipated for the study. The biostatistician can then determine, for various alternative choices of clinically meaningful differences, just what statistical power the study would have to determine such differences.

ANALYZING DIAGNOSTIC TESTS

Contempory medical literature abounds with descriptions of attributes of new diagnostic tests such as sensitivity and specificity. The definitions and calculation of these terms can be derived from a 2 × 2 table (Fig. 1-2). Sensitivity is the ability of a test to detect a disease and is calculated by dividing the true positives, the number of times the test is positive when the attribute is present, (a), by the same number plus the false negatives, the number of times the test is negative when the condition is present, (c). The formula then is a/(a + c). Specificity refers to the test being negative when the disease is not present. It can be calculated by

taking the true negatives, the number of times that the test is negative in the absence of disease, (d), and dividing it by the same quantity plus b or false positives, the test is positive although the attribute is absent. The formula for specificity thus is d/(d + b). Two other commonly used terms are positive and negative predictive values. The positive predictive value is the chance of having the attribute if the test is positive. This is calculated as the ratio of the true positives (a) in which the test is positive when the attribute is present and the sum of all situations in which the test is positive, which includes true positives (a) and false positives (b). The formula for positive predictive value then is a/(a + b). Negative predictive value states the accuracy of the test to exclude the attribute if the test is negative. It is calculated from the ratio of true negatives (d) and all negative test results, (d + c), both true and false negatives. The formula for negative predictive value is d/(d + c).

CONFIDENCE INTERVALS (LIMITS)

Confidence intervals are alternatives to tests of significance for drawing inferences regarding populations from observations in a sample. They are based on the same considerations of sampling variation as discussed with tests of significance. From results in a sample, a calculation ritual leads to determination of confidence limits and the confidence interval. The interval gives a range of values within which the true underlying population value lies. If a 95% confidence interval is calculated, the chance is 95% or 19 in 20 that the limits calculated embrace the true population value; the smaller the sample size, the wider the confidence interval.

For the comparison of two groups, we can calculate confidence intervals on the difference in percentages or in means. These, as indicated earlier, provide an interval within which the true difference in population proportions or means lies.

Again, consider the PEEP study as an illustration. With regard to mortality, the difference observed in the study was 33.3% − 25.0% = 8.3%. Calculation of 95% confidence limits on this difference yields −20.6% to 37.2%. Thus, based on our sample results, we state with 95% confidence that in the population from which the study samples came, the difference in mortality rates is somewhere between −21% (i.e., an absolute difference in mortality rate 21% higher in group II than in group I) and +37% (i.e., an absolute difference in mortality rate 37% higher in group I than in group II). The term "95% confidence" means that when we state that the true population difference is somewhere between −21% to +37%, there is a 95% or 19 in 20 chance that these limits *do* embrace the true population difference; there is a 5% or 1 in 20 chance that the true population difference is outside these limits.

Clearly, the limits calculated above are wide because of the small sample sizes involved, namely, about 20 patients per group. Confidence limits are sensitive to sample size and shrink as sample size increases. For example, if these same sample results, namely, 33.3% and 25%, had arisen from a study quintupled in size, that is, with 100 patients in each of groups I and II, 95% confidence limits on the

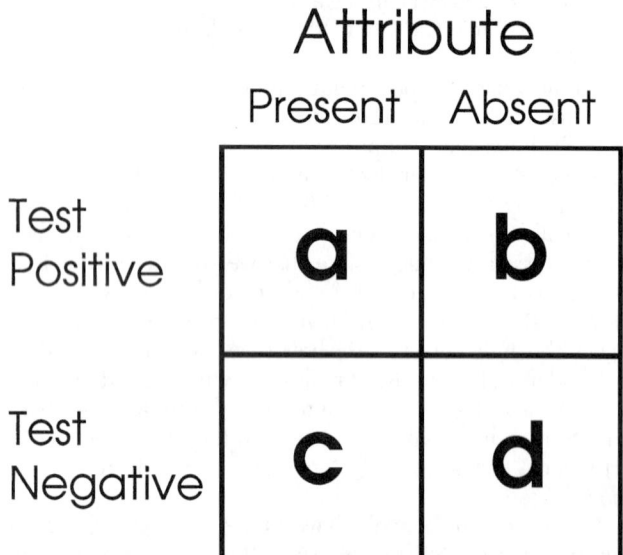

Attribute

Present   Absent

Test Positive	**a**	**b**
Test Negative	**c**	**d**

FIGURE 1-2. A 2 × 2 contingency table for diagnostic tests. Sensitivity, specificity, positive predictive value, negative predictive value, and accuracy can be calculated according to formulae. a, true positives; b, false positives; c, false negatives; d, true negatives.

Determination of the Odds Ratio

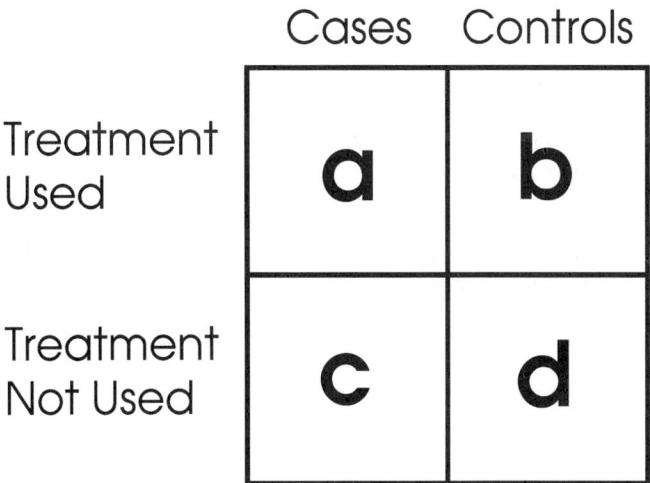

FIGURE 1-3. The 2 × 2 contingency table also can be used to calculate odds ratios. In this situation, cases and controls are in the columns whereas treatment and no treatment are in the rows.

true population difference in percentage mortality would be −4.2% to +20.9%.

Confidence limits are compatible with the results of tests of significance. For example, if 95% confidence limits on the difference in two proportions or means include zero, then a two-tailed test at the 5% level would yield the result of "not statistically significant." If the 95% confidence limits does *not* include zero, then the two-tailed test at the 5% level would yield the result of "statistically significant." In the PEEP study just mentioned, the 95% confidence intervals (−21% to +37%) included zero, which is compatible with the test result of "no significant difference" in mortality rates.

If, in a comparative study of proportions, the clinician is interested in the *ratio* of the two proportions (i.e., relative risk), the confidence interval on the ratio can be calculated. If, for example, a 95% confidence interval of the ratio of two rates includes 1, there is no significant increase in relative risk, tested by a two-tailed test at the 5% level. If 1 is outside the 95% confidence interval, a significant increase in relative risk occurs, with a two-tailed test at the 5% level.

The clinician often encounters calculation of the odds ratio to give an estimate of relative risk, particularly in case-control studies. It can be calculated from a 2 × 2 contingency table (Fig. 1-3). The ratio is calculated from the product of a (treatment used in cases) and d (treatment not used in controls) divided by b (treatment not used in cases) times c (treatment used in controls). The formula then is ad/bc.

Confidence intervals are gaining in popularity in clinical research. Particularly for epidemiologic studies, they provide more useful information than corresponding tests of significance.

However, often authors do not calculate confidence intervals. This is especially important when no occurrences of a particular outcome have occurred in a relatively small study group. It is erroneous to extrapolate this finding of zero responses to the general population. It has been shown that with sample sizes greater than 30, at a $p = 0.05$, "... if none of n patients shows the event about which we are concerned, we can be 95% confident that the chance of this event is at most 3 in n."[18] For instance, in a study of in-hospital cardiopulmonary resuscitation, Taffet and colleagues[19] reported that none of the $n = 68$ patients older than 70 years of age who received cardiopulmonary resuscitation (CPR) survived until discharge. Although the authors did not recommend setting age limits for CPR, the clinician fears an inference of "hopelessness" from the study of CPR in patients older than 70 years of age. Using the rule of 3/n, a one-sided upper 95% confidence limit is that we might reasonably expect up to 4.4% of patients older than the age of 70 years to survive. We should then discuss futility as a condition for withholding CPR with this latter figure in mind as a reasonable upper limit. Some might judge that, indeed, a less than 5% chance of survival justifies withholding CPR. However, this issue needs direct discussion, and clearly we should not draw the inference that that study *proved* that no patient older than 70 years of age could possibly survive CPR.

WARNING: With confidence limits on a mean, notice that these provide an interval within which the population mean likely lies. The confidence interval does *not* provide limits within which individual observations lie. It is entirely incorrect to interpret, for example, a 95% confidence interval on a mean as limits that encompass the values for 95% of individual subjects.

OTHER COMMON REGRESSION ANALYSES

In addition to linear regression, described previously (Y = a + bX), there are other mathematic relationships linking two variables, including curvilinear (e.g., quadratic, cubic) or logarithmic functions. Once again, all of the commonly used statistical packages provide these functions (perhaps too) easily and conveniently. Also, multiple regression techniques can be used when there are several independent variables. The Harris-Benedict equation to predict energy expenditure is a commonly used multiple regression equation. The dependent variable predicted must be quantitative, although qualitative and quantitative variables can be used as predictors. Qualitative variables are described as present (using a coefficient of one) or absent (zero as coefficient which cancels the term when multiplied). When the predicted or dependent variable is categorical, such as living or dead, the appropriate regression technique is logistic regression. The many severity of illness indices, such as the Acute Physiology and Chronic Health Evaluation (APACHE) and the Mortality Prediction Model, exemplify the use of logistic regression to calculate the risk of mortality.

CODA ■

In a way, we can compare our current medical journals with daily newspapers and television news programs. They report the most "up-to-the-minute" information; the reports may be incomplete, certain important details may be missing, and it may be difficult to fit the results reported into the existing framework of previous information. Sometimes this may indicate that the existing framework needs to be changed sharply; at other times, subsequent reports reveal flaws in the methodology or in the interpretation of the "newest" report.

Inertia may be interpreted in terms of the difficulty in moving a stationary object. Remember, too, inertia also refers to the difficulty in moving an object from the direction in which it is moving. When the preponderance of data points in one direction, we should not be too hasty in changing directions based on a single study that shows the opposite result. On the other hand, the purpose of this entire exercise, reading and contributing to the medical literature, is to add to existing knowledge or sharpen the focus and to change directions when necessary. A sense of proportion or balance is necessary: to choose a level of significance; to determine and accommodate types I and II errors; to distinguish chance from real effects; to separate statistical likelihood of difference from the importance of that difference; to give clinical dimensions to real experimental differences; to weigh costs and detrimental effects of therapy against the beneficial effects of improving outcome in devastating illness; or to improve the quality of life or diminish the costs of care when survival is not the only important determinant of outcome.

If the medical literature bears any resemblance to the news media in general, our tasks can only become more difficult in the future. While more and more information

becomes more easily available with less and less validation, we may pass to a future that goes beyond Andy Warhol's dictum that everyone will be famous for 15 minutes. We may likely be heading for a future in which *everything* is true for only 15 minutes. Unfortunately, it will always take more than 15 minutes to analyze a medical report correctly. We will be faced with an overwhelming input of information. We must learn to reject quickly the flighty, flimsy, and faulty, and to concentrate on science with substance.

REFERENCES ■

1. Zeppa R: Commencement address, University of Miami School of Medicine, June 1987 (unpublished)
2. Feinstein AR: Biologic and statistical implications of clinical taxonomy. In: *Clinical Judgment*. Baltimore, Williams & Wilkins, 1967:209
3. Peter LJ, Dana B: *The Laughter Prescription*. New York, Ballantine Books, 1982:131
4. Kirby RR, Downs JB, Civetta JM, et al: High level positive end-expiratory pressure (PEEP) in acute respiratory insufficiency. *Chest* 1975;67:156
5. Gallagher TJ, Civetta JM, Kirby RR: Terminology update: optimal PEEP. *Crit Care Med* 1978;6:323
6. Nelson LD, Civetta JM, Hudson-Civetta JA: Titrating positive end-expiratory pressure therapy in patients with early, moderate arterial hypoxemia. *Crit Care Med* 1987;15:14
7. Colton T: *Statistics in Medicine*. Boston, Little, Brown, 1974
8. Hennekeus CH, Buring, J: *Epidemiology in Medicine*. Boston, Little, Brown, 1987
9. Hudson-Civetta JA, Civetta JM, Martinez OV, et al: Risk and detection of pulmonary catheter–related infection in septic surgical patients. *Crit Care Med* 1987;15:29
10. Applefeld JJ, Caruthers TE, Reno DJ, et al: Assessment of the sterility of the long term cardiac catheterization using the thermodilution Swan-Ganz catheter. *Chest* 1978;74:377
11. Sackett DL: Biases in analytic research. *J Chronic Dis* 1979;32:51
12. *Real Paper*, Boston, Massachusetts, 1978
13. Civetta JM: Critical illness: the non-steady state. *Surg Forum* 1972;23:153
14. Angell M: Negative studies. *N Engl J Med* 1989;321:464
15. Armitage P: *Sequential Medical Trials*. Springfield, IL, Charles C Thomas, 1960
16. Bliss CI: *Statistics in Biology*, vol 1. New York, McGraw-Hill, 1967
17. Dixon WJ, Massey FJ Jr: *Introduction to Statistical Analysis*, 3rd ed. New York, McGraw-Hill, 1969
18. Hanley JA, Lippman-Hand A: If nothing goes wrong, is everything all right? *JAMA* 1983;249:1743
19. Taffet GE, Teasdale TA, Luchi RJ: In-hospital cardiopulmonary resuscitation. *JAMA* 1988;260:2069

Critical Care, Third Edition, edited by Joseph M. Civetta,
Robert W. Taylor, and Robert R. Kirby.
Lippincott-Raven Publishers, Philadelphia, PA © 1997.

CHAPTER 2

■

Setting Objectives: Perspectives for Care

Orlando C. Kirton
Joseph M. Civetta

The first objective of critical care might be to decide which patients should be treated. Once this seemed simple: choose the sickest patients. The concept that stimulated the formation of intensive care units (ICUs) seemed to be an effective guideline for selecting appropriate candidates for these units. Younger[1] suggests several goals that may be achieved by medical interventions:

Goal 1: Returning the patient to an independent state that improves the quality of life
Goal 2: Lengthening life for some purposeful period, such as continuing treatment to enable the patient to accomplish certain goals before death
Goal 3: Postponing death because of the sanctity of life
Goal 4: Achieving strictly physiologic goals, such as the raising of blood pressure by vasoactive agents or preventing death from ventilatory failure by using mechanical ventilation.

ICUs were created to concentrate three critical components: (1) the sickest patients, (2) the highly technical and expensive equipment, and (3) the staff with the knowledge and experience to treat the patients and use the equipment with the goals of improving efficiency, efficacy, and reducing costs. By omitting terminal patients and those who would fare well enough in routine care areas, practitioners should have been able to select appropriate patients for intensive care *based on these medical and organizational factors.*

Currently, however, there are financial, legal, ethical, moral, and religious aspects to the delivery of care, termina-

tion of life support, utilization of scarce resources, malpractice, and rising medical costs, all of which impact and, perhaps, have greater weight than "mere" patient–physician–disease interactions.

The Edwin Smith Surgical Papyrus is, perhaps, the oldest existing medical document.[2] It was scribe-copied around 1600 B.C.E. from a document possibly written 5000 years ago. It is a collection of 48 case descriptions, classified by three different verdicts, the term used to describe the diagnosis: (1) "an ailment which I will treat"; (2) "an ailment with which I will contend"; or (3) "an ailment not to be treated." Thus, in the earliest of medical documents, physicians were cautioned to recognize the ailments that were beyond their curative powers, ailments not to be treated. We believe that one of the current problems is that we have stopped identifying these ailments and separating them from the ones we should treat. We have substituted what Ronald Preston calls *aspirational heroism*—a belief that science and technology should defeat disease and death.[3] This is not true. Bulkin and Lukashok[4] succinctly express the result of this belief:

> . . . viewing death as unnatural causes us to confuse our inability to cure with failure. If we could recognize an ailment that "ought not be treated" because it cannot be treated successfully, we would realize that the term *life support* in such a case is inaccurate—continued intervention can only prolong dying, not support life.

This distinction is not always clear; however, the issues and need for open discussion are gradually becoming more widely recognized by the medical profession and society in general.

Cessation of vital signs (cardiac activity and breathing) was always considered a sign of death. Now it is often termed *cardiac arrest* and after prompt resuscitation, indeed, these patients are not dead but are functioning, active members of society. On the other hand, cardiac and respiratory activity no longer necessarily signify life. The concept of brain death, stimulated by successful human organ transplantation, has evolved and achieved medical and legal status.

We face these situational incompatibilities most acutely in the ICU where we have learned that terms such as "sicker" and "alive longer" carry implications unknown in human history. Patients may enter an unprecedented state of prolonged dying, a period lasting from days to weeks to months and even years, if we maintain careful attention to numerous details of bedside care and continue measures often termed *life support*. The transition from life to death, especially when artificially lengthened and almost "frozen in time," make it difficult to decide when a patient is just sick enough to be in the ICU with a potential to survive after treatment or so sick that the natural progression to death occurs even if delayed or prolonged by our perhaps poorly termed life-support techniques.

As ICU practitioners, we must delineate goals for intensive care, understand the limitations of current care, examine the process of bedside care, adjust our functioning to conform with the hospital's goals and resources, and finally, remain congruent with overall societal values. Therefore, a simple list of admission and discharge requirements likely would be both impossible to construct and untenable, even if created.

THE ECONOMIC ISSUES: IS ECONOMICS KING? ■

All eyes focus on the fact that medical costs generally are increasing. At the same time, all eyes focus on the spectacular successes achieved in transplantation, although costs for an individual liver transplant patient in our hospital actually exceeded $1 million for the hospitalization and the procedure. George Orwell's major error in *1984* was not in predicting the *type* of future but in attributing the *cause* of the changes to direct governmental intervention.[5] Many of the changes have occurred without obvious "Big Brother" control. Many "Newspeak" concepts, if not the words, are with us today. For instance, the term *doublethink* referred to the developed ability to hold two contradictory ideas in the mind at the same time and not to notice that they were diametrically opposed. Thus, it does not seem contradictory today to expect to lower costs and introduce better and more expensive forms of effective therapy at the same time. We must await society's realization that this is a problem that must be addressed humanistically, not politically, and, if medical science is to continue to discover, refine, and improve therapy, the conflict between the desire to lower costs and the need to improve care will actually become more acute.

As we attempt to select admission criteria for the proper use of the ICU, we must depreciate the current focus on money and medicolegal considerations, notwithstanding their considerable visibility and impact. We must remember Fein's[6] important observation, "we live in a society, not an economy." Unfortunately, continually rising costs for medical care have been cited as the reason to institute major changes in health care financing; these changes have an impact on the delivery of care. Moreover, there is a growing tendency to try to exclude patients from the ICU based on what we believe to be an incomplete appraisal of the role of intensive care in today's hospital environment.[7-9] There is also an ominous specter to this emphasis on rising costs: cost containment, if poorly conceived and implemented, will reduce the access to care as well as the quality of care, yet fail to achieve true savings. Opinions are divergent with respect to the directions that should be taken. Proponents of prospective payment systems, such as diagnosis related groups (DRGs) used by Medicare, believed that it would solve many of the ills attributed to cost-based reimbursement. We should notice that the DRG system was not designed as a tool for reimbursement. Siegel and colleagues[10] conclusively showed that a reimbursement system based on DRGs would result in gross inequities for level 1 trauma centers because of the nonnormal distribution of the complications associated with severe injury. Moreover, no one has outcome criteria to assess the effects of this system with regard to intensive care.

Critical care medicine practiced in the ICU consumes a disproportionately large fraction of U.S. health care resources. The bed capacity of the roughly 7400 nationwide ICUs comprise less than 10% of all hospital beds, yet ICUs consume approximately 20% of total hospital costs. Increases in the U.S. health care delivery costs continue to exceed the gross national product. Whereas total hospital beds are decreasing nationwide, paralleling a decrease in hospital occupancy, the actual number and percentage of ICU beds have increased, paralleling the increase in occupancy. From 1986 to 1992, however, the increases in ICU cost per day were less than the increases in overall health care costs. The percent of gross domestic product occupied by nationwide ICU costs was 0.7% in 1986, and 1988 and 0.9% in 1992.[11]

The focus on cost containment has not been confined to the ICU. In fact, ICU staffing levels and equipment generally have been affected far less than in many other areas of the hospital. The reality is even worse; with a nationwide nursing shortage and crisis, both ICUs and routine care areas often have fewer nurses working than the number of positions allocated or the planned staffing level.

SELECTION OF "APPROPRIATE" PATIENTS ■

The set of moral principles governing the generic goals of the health care provider, as elucidated by Beauchamp and Childress,[12] include (1) *beneficence*, our efforts to do good for the patient; (2) *nonmaleficence*, avoidance of intentional harm; (3) *distributive justice*, the equitable and appropriate allocation of resources; and (4) *autonomy*, respect for the patient's right of self-determination.

Life was simpler when we believed that we could characterize patients as too well, too sick, and just right for intensive care. In this conception, a patient was an appropriate candidate for intensive care if the illness was deemed too severe for care in a routine hospital area (death could be predicted) and *the illness was likely to respond to treatment in the ICU.* Unfortunately, few disease states and even fewer patients meet those criteria such that there is unequivocal evidence of the efficacy of intensive care.[13] This classification system fails to recognize that these distinctions are not always possible and not necessarily desirable. Although "terminal" patients would experience little benefit from the ICU, neither clinicians nor patients and their families usually want ICU admission. Although 80% or more of patients in the United States currently die in hospitals, and many patients with terminal illnesses are readmitted to the hospital primarily to die, the motivating force is not one last-ditch effort to avoid death but rather comfort for the patient and relief of stress on the family. One third of patients with terminal illnesses using hospice techniques of home care, who had planned to die at home, have been readmitted to acute care hospitals because of an inability to manage these problems at the end.[14] Patients with acute devastating illness, even if admitted to the ICU, usually have a prompt fatal outcome. Exclusion of the patient who is "too sick" has little salutary effect in terms of treatment goals and essentially no impact on resources—less than 1% of patient-days.[15] In fact, to choose all of the appropriate patients, we must, by design, broaden the admission criteria, thus including patients who ultimately might be deemed "too sick" because of our inability to select only the appropriate patients. In like manner, we often extend our selection process to include patients who may be considered "too well" for intensive care. Some have proposed that patients be excluded if the risk of mortality or morbidity is low or if the need for treatment is low.[8–10] Given the current hypersensitive medicolegal scrutiny, particularly blurring the distinction between bad outcome and negligence, it seems hard to believe that the negligible financial saving of a single day's observation in the ICU is likely to be considered a justifiable defense for the refusal to admit such patients, should a complication needing treatment develop in an excluded patient.

When we studied elective admissions to our ICU, about 30% of requested patients were considered so stable at the end of the operation that ICU admission was deferred and the patients were sent to the recovery room for routine postoperative care.[16] There was no difference in the total hospital bills, that is, the elimination of the 1-day admission did not result in savings. Although unnecessary admissions are clearly wasteful, an analysis of the risk of complications proposed by the Consensus Development Conference weighted two distinct factors: the risk of complication and the likelihood of successful treatment.[13] Clearly, patients at a markedly increased risk deserve the observation currently available only in ICUs. If equivalent treatment of a developed complication can be reasonably expected in routine care areas and the ICU, no advantage to ICU admission can be postulated. However, when delay in diagnosis or

treatment can be predicted from the staffing and equipment levels currently available in a given hospital's routine care areas, ICU admission would seem warranted.

The development of adverse cardiac events has been a major cause of morbidity and mortality after noncardiac surgery. Mangano and associates[17] report that myocardial ischemia occurred postoperatively in 41% of monitored patients and was associated with a 2.8-fold increase in the odds of all adverse cardiac outcomes and a 9.2-fold increase in the odds of an ischemic event.

Varon and colleagues'[18] descriptive study reviewed the accuracy and effectiveness of preoperative ICU consultations and found that physician judgment was able to decide who would potentially benefit from preoperative ICU admission for invasive monitoring based on identifiable risk factors. Patients who were admitted preoperatively were, indeed, at higher risk for cardiovascular complications. The patients identified as low risk and who were not admitted had essentially no perioperative myocardial infarctions. The physician's judgment seemed capable of identifying the proper patients for ICU admission.

An analogous study examined the prognostic significance of using dipyridamole-thallium single-photon emission scanning in identifying patients at risk of perioperative cardiovascular morbidity and mortality who were undergoing aortic surgery.[19] All patients were screened preoperatively (i.e., patients were selected with both low and high *risk factors*). The authors found 54% of all patients to have abnormal scan results, even among patients who had no risk factors. In patients with one of two multivariant-derived risk factors (age older than 65 years, definite coronary artery disease), the complication rate was 24%; in individuals with both risk factors, the cumulative cardiac complication rate was 39%. Of greatest interest was that the number of perioperative cardiac events were the *same* in patients who had positive scan results and those who had negative scan results. The authors conclude that dipyridamole-thallium scanning was not an accurate screening test, but more importantly, clinical judgment was useful.

GENERIC GOALS OF INTENSIVE CARE

We need a different perspective, a qualitative basis for categorizing patients depending on the generic goals of intensive care.[20] Three categories have been identified that distinguish surgical ICU patients from routine postoperative surgical patients but generally apply to all specialty ICU patients as well: (1) monitoring/observation, (2) extensive nursing requirements, and (3) constant physician supervision. Patients are considered appropriate candidates for ICU admission for "just" *monitoring and observation* even if they are physiologically stable. Examples of this include patients with stable pelvic fractures, liver or splenic lacerations, or those who have had major vascular reconstruction (graft patency and perioperative ischemia). These patients must have a recognized risk of complications and should be admitted when the likelihood of recognition and successful treatment is higher in the intensive care setting. Intensive monitoring and observation were never particularly easy or effective in routine care areas; after all, one of the earliest forms of intensive care in this country, the coronary care unit, was created to correct this deficiency. Monitoring and observation with early institution of effective treatment for simple, premonitory arrhythmias have been well documented to reduce mortality. However, the issue of monitoring and observation must be addressed quantitatively as well as qualitatively. The patient:nurse ratio is 12:1 during the night shift in our regular hospital care areas. Allowing time for necessary administrative functions and their physiologic needs, the nurses have less than 30 minutes per shift available for any individual patient. This may be accomplished by establishing intermediate care areas or "overnight recovery rooms"[21]; in practice, the same patients must be provided with increased nursing surveillance outside of the ICU. The particular "solution" is not the issue. Increased staffing and more equipment will be necessary to create the monitoring/observation environment, no matter where it is located or what name is used. Monitoring/observation patients belong in today's ICU.

Examples of *extensive nursing requirement* include pulmonary toilet, major wound care, and mechanical ventilation. The same limitations apply to patients who need extensive nursing requirements. Frequent position changes, complex dressings, intake and output measurements, laboratory testing, and myriad additional nursing tasks are beyond the capabilities of the small nursing contingent assigned to floor care areas. The measures designed to improve efficiency that have been enacted over recent years clearly eliminated the type and number of personnel necessary to accomplish these tasks; this was reasonable because these capabilities were included in the ICU as a part of the overall design. These patients make up approximately 60% of our patient population but are a most important focus for more than mere numbers.[22] These patients are generally physiologically stable; using most indices of severity, they are neither very sick nor very well. They constitute a large percentage of the daily ICU population for the following reasons. Patients in the monitoring/observation class, if they remained stable, are discharged within 1 or 2 days and no longer are counted in the ICU population. If they develop complications, they enter the extensive nursing requirement category. Although the extensive care group may be physiologically stable, careful monitoring and observation are always necessary. The complexity and frequency of nursing tasks that exceed the reasonable expectations of time available in general nursing units are the motivating force behind ICU admission. These patients remain in the ICU for extended periods and are subjected to many complications related to the primary admitting diagnosis and to subsequent failure of initially functioning organ systems, especially related to the interrelationships among sepsis, immune function, and nutritional state, all of which create demands on nursing resources. Patients who need extensive nursing care must also be admitted to the ICU.

The third group is characterized as the patients requiring *constant physician care*. They are physiologically unstable, and physicians and nurses must remain at the bedside, re-

acting to changes and implementing, validating, and refining further therapy. Patients requiring constant physician care—10% to 20% of our population—can stay in this category only for a short period of time; thereafter, the acute abnormalities are resolved successfully, in which case they commonly enter the extensive nursing care category or, if therapy has been unsuccessful, they die. They conform to the popular image of intensive care because of the elements of high technology, rapid but efficient activity, crises, and perhaps, dramatic successes. There is no problem in the selection of these patients for ICU admission. Yet, even in these circumstances, once this acute stage passes, as it must, the reality includes other elements as well, such as the nearness of death and illnesses lasting months, because it is rare that the devastating illness resulting in their initial classification can resolve rapidly. It is this form of intensive care, prototypical in initial concept, that must evolve beyond crisis orientation in medical and nonmedical areas to develop consonance with evolving societal values.

BENEFICENCE, NONMALEFICENCE, AND DISTRIBUTIVE JUSTICE ■

Critical care today requires a focus beyond the needs of a specific patient and must encompass the total number of patients who could be considered eligible for care, given the number of available beds. Because the beds are so expensive, the hospital clearly cannot afford to maintain an excess of beds with available staffing to accommodate emergency admissions.

At the outset, however, it is important to remember that although the *problem* needs a solution, the *solution* may be effected step by step so that, in most cases, no patient is deprived of necessary care. This process, however, usually requires creativity, cooperation, and a great deal of work to bring to a successful conclusion. In fact, much of the day in many ICUs (ours included) is spent in this fashion. The physical process of discharge can be accelerated (often hours elapse waiting for the "recipient" bed to be emptied, for a family member to pick up the patient, or medications to be ready). The bed must be changed, and the room must be cleaned, creating delays in waiting for housekeeping; actual transfer may be dependent on transport personnel; the personnel on the floor may wish to wait until after shift report; and so on. To expedite discharge (especially at night), we have the responsible service write contingency orders on stable patients who are about ready for transfer. These orders are activated if an ICU bed is required in an emergency. In addition, all patients deemed ready for discharge are discussed at the beginning of ICU rounds to enable administrative routines to be set in motion as quickly as possible. Other possible solutions include the provision of special duty nurses for patients who might require extra monitoring outside the unit; another ICU may temporarily "loan" a vacant bed; overnight care may be provided in a recovery room in place of ICU admission; extra nursing personnel may be enticed to work overtime or give up a day off; nursing personnel may be added to the unit's staff temporarily from another ICU, supervisory personnel, or an agency; and even physicians have been recruited to provide independent and dependent nursing role functions. Using overtime or "day off" personnel, although sometimes necessary and possible, is a major factor in increasing the stress of daily ICU life because these crises, that is, more patients than can be cared for by the available assigned nursing staff, occur regularly: staffing cannot be predicated on peak requirements. Continuously asking the staff to work double shifts or to work on days off have been mentioned as factors leading to "burn-out," an inner pressure to resign from a position previously highly desired.

Unfortunately, no matter how creatively and diligently the participants work, new patients arrive when all beds are full and all temporizing measures have been exhausted. This serious problem has existed for the last 20 years despite the incredible expansion of the number of ICU beds during that era. In terms of the ethical principle of distributive justice, one method commonly and effectively used is "first come, first served." Care is apportioned to appropriate candidates seeking admission; these patients may continue to receive care until their outcome is determined. This seemingly simple principle was confounded during the evolution of critical care through the creation of the unprecedented prolonged dying state. The difficulty in making such choices was examined by the National Institutes of Health Consensus Development Conference on Critical Care Medicine in 1983[13]:

> It is not medically appropriate to devote limited ICU resources to patients without reasonable prospect of significant recovery when patients who need those services and who have a significant prospect of recovery from acutely life-threatening disease or injury are being turned away due to lack of capacity. It is inappropriate to maintain ICU management of a patient whose prognosis has resolved to one of persistent vegetative state, and it is similarly inappropriate to employ ICU resources where no purpose will be served but a prolongation of the natural process of death.

PATIENT AUTONOMY ■

Decision-making based on self-determination is the definition of autonomy. However, this translates not only into the right to choose, but also the right to *refuse* life-sustaining treatments. The competent patient has the right to choose or *refuse* based on the concepts of *informed consent, and informed refusal,* the components of which include the following: (1) the provision of sufficient and accurate information from the health care provider; (2) patient comprehension; and (3) the exercise of free choice (Chap. 6). We, as physicians, have an obligation to our patients to allow them to choose a peaceful and dignified death. Thomlinson and Brody[23] argue that futility judgments can be endorsed on nonpaternalistic grounds and that failure to make such judgments truly undermine the autonomous choice of patients or their legally appointed guardian or surrogate. For the sake of patient autonomy, physicians must be able to restrict the alternatives for treatment that are made available in consideration of their patient's welfare.

The same elements necessary for informed consent are, thus, necessary for informed refusal of continued care. However, physicians often feel impelled to initiate and to continue "everything" to prolong the lives of critically ill patients. Weir and Gostin[24] point out that a tragic consequence is that patients who lack decision-making capacity are sometimes given life-sustaining treatment that is not consistent with their previous preferences, not in the their best interest, and not wanted by their families.

"FUTILITY OF CARE" ■

Throughout history, the absence of vital signs (heart rate and respiratory rate) was considered a sure sign of death until brain death was defined for transplantation purposes. Some families refuse to accept brain death today whereas others define death as a persistent vegetative state or other state in which the "personhood" of the patient would no longer be present. According to these concepts, life is life when it possesses dignity, value, and meaning to the person, and in the absence of these qualities defines a state of dying, which ends in death (Chap. 5).

The definition of futility includes those situations in which (1) further therapy seems useless and unreasonable and (2) the treatment is likely to do more harm than good. The word futility is derived from the Latin word *futilis*—that which easily pours out or is considered of no value, incapable of producing the wanted or desired result.[25]

It is derived from the Greek myth when the daughters of the king Argos murdered their husbands under his instructions, and were then condemned for this act by the gods to collect water for eternity using leaky sieves.

Schneiderman and coworkers[26] attempted to quantify futility. To them, futility can be defined as useless care if there have been no survivors in a physician's last 100 cases, or if the literature supports uniformly fatal outcome. They also considered care to be futile if it only preserves a vegetative state or requires continued dependence on intensive care.

From another perspective, the Society of Critical Care Medicine's task force on ethics[27] states that interventions are justified by the scientific evidence of benefit. When benefit cannot be achieved or can no longer be reasonably expected, interventions loose their justifications and may be withdrawn.

Luce[25] articulates the physician's societal obligations to provide futile care:

> Physician refusal to provide futile or unreasonable care is supported by the ethical principles of non-maleficence, beneficence, and distributed justice. Physicians are not ethically required to provide futile or unreasonable care, especially to patients who are brain dead, vegetative, critically or terminally ill, with little chance of recovering and are unlikely to benefit from cardiopulmonary resuscitation.

From an ethical standpoint, the health care team is not obligated to provide care because of demands by the family or the patient. The celebrated Barber,[28] Baby L,[29] Baby K,[30] and Helen Wanglie[31] court cases addressed physicians' rights and liabilities concerning the withholding and withdrawing of futile care but not conclusively (Chaps. 9 and 10).

In April, 1995, a superior court jury in Suffolk, Massachusetts exonerated physicians and a hospital from civil liability in discontinuing a ventilator and failing to resuscitate despite objections of a family member.[32] After the patient's death, a suit was filed by the patient's daughter who had been hostile to the providers and refused to participate in discussions to stop treatment. The court asked the jury to decide whether the patient, Katherine Gilgunn, a 72-year-old comatose woman with irreversible brain damage and multiple comorbid and chronic health problems would have wanted to be kept on life support if she could have made the decision herself. The jury was instructed by the judge to balance her preference against the medical judgment to withdraw such treatment in the content of not whether, but for how long, and at what cost, her life might be extended. The jury found in favor of the physicians that resuscitation would have been futile and that the failure to resuscitate was not negligent. If this is upheld on appeal, the physicians' right to withdraw futile therapy would have a legal precedent. As pointed out by Brett and McCullough,[33] futile care should not be provided if it deprives others of necessary care. This would be consistent with the ethical principle of distributive justice, the fair equitable and appropriate distribution of medical resources in society. Do not resuscitate (DNR) orders may be based on the wishes of competent patients or information about the patient's wishes pronounced by an appropriate patient's surrogate to provide a mechanism for withholding resuscitation in the event of a cardiopulmonary arrest (or perhaps, more accurately, when the patient dies).[34] Health care institutions must develop policies to deal with DNR orders in the setting of anesthesia in surgery because it is estimated that 15% of patients with DNR orders undergo a surgical procedure.[35] The patient's wishes are best served through an open discussion of options, therapy, and expectations between the patient, family or proxy, and the health care team.

THE FAMILY: COMPASSION AND AVOIDING CONFLICT

The best method of avoiding confrontation, in regards to discontinuing futile treatment, is to establish trust with the family through communication. This communication must be established early and it must be honest and open.[36] One must emphasize the real prognosis and the limitations of medical care; the articulation of these realities must be consistent among all care providers. The communication should set limits with respect to the future medical plans and also with respect to who will communicate with the family. The family must not be allowed to pit one member of the team against another in the quest to find inconsistencies. For some reason, they believe that differing opinions among care givers gives them a wedge to force the provider to do something that will make the patient better. Unreasonable

expectations are common and are usually based on irrational premises. Daily conferences with an individual member or the entire family can be set up so that the same participants from the providers and family have a chance to develop trust through communication. The family should never be positioned to believe that they are being asked to decide whether or not to continue treatment, or as specifically stated by many families, to "pull the plug." Physicians must never ask for permission to stop treatment. It is wrong ethically and medically. The role of the family is to provide information concerning the patient's wishes. The role of the physician is to describe the future course and what can be achieved by medical care. The death of the patient depends entirely on the untreatable disease, not on the physician's wishes, nor on the family's wishes. The question should never be, "What do you want us to do?" nor should you ever accept the answer, "I don't want him [or her] to suffer." The proper question is, "If your loved one could speak to us, what would he [or she] say in this situation?" The proper answer is, "I know that he [or she] would not want to continue with the treatment if the outcome is hopeless." Most problems result from inadequate insight into the patient–family chemistry and lack of understanding of the differences between the proper questions and answers.

At patient care conferences, the physician must instruct the family that everything (reasonable and effective) has been done and that there are no alternatives, thus removing the burden from the family. Make it clear that further therapy or attempts at resuscitation would increase the patient's suffering before inevitable death and that continuation of therapy is not in the best interest of the patient. Families who are in denial or have unrealistic beliefs do not listen to logic, especially discussions of withdrawing treatment based on distributive justice. Distributive justice should not be used in these discussions, because it always fails and often becomes a focus for the family to express anger. When confrontation or irrational expectations persist, communication should be intensified, not avoided; it should be enriched with patience and compassion for the family who persists in demanding that "everything be done," understandably torn by anguish, guilt, and anger.

Document in the chart (as a minimal standard of acceptable care) all discussions and anticipated problems as well as the rationale behind all current and future plans, that is, what has been achieved through group consensus of the care providers and also what limits have been placed on care, including initiating new treatments and DNR orders. Whereas decisions may be made by team consensus, the actions must be communicated to the family, and the family members told that certain treatments will be withheld and that DNR orders have been written.

We treat approximately 1500 ICU patients a year with a 10% mortality rate. Of the 150 deaths, the forgoing measures were successful in approximately 98% of those cases. In situations where confrontation is unavoidable, early consultation with the institutional bioethics committee may provide an appropriate forum, allowing both the family and care givers to voice their views and interpretations. They may be able to overcome the stalemate that exists between the bedside provider and the increasingly resistant family. They can also provide an outside reality check by confirming the actions of the team and the predicted course of the patients. Ultimately, however, legal intervention may be necessary. Courts should be considered to be the last resort.

IMMEDIATE OBJECTIVE: EXAMINE SOCIETAL VALUES ■

The medical goal of the preservation of life is associated with the societal value of the sanctity of life whereas a second goal, the alleviation of suffering, is associated with the quality of life. These two principles may become incompatible, in which case one or the other must predominate. If they become incompatible at the beginning of life, one might chose preservation of life associated with the sanctity of life as more important than the alleviation of suffering (for example, placing a chest tube for a tension pneumothorax with less than ideal local anesthesia). However, as the end of life is reached, alleviation of suffering should be chosen as more important than the preservation of life because the quality of life is the ascendant societal value, in line with the principal of nonmaleficence (see Chap. 5 for an in-depth discussion).

A theoretic point of utility represents a transition beyond which life cannot be extended with value, dignity, and meaning as defined by the patient's wishes. This transition point has two characteristics: (1) objective medical evidence that death is inevitable, and (2) subjective information that the patient would not accept this quality of life. From the beginning of life until this point is reached, we direct our care and efforts toward cure, associating the sanctity of life with preservation of life (principle of beneficence). However, once that point is passed, efforts should be directed to caring for the patient and caring for the family adjusting to dying (principle of nonmaleficence). We elevate the quality of life associated with the alleviation of suffering above prolongation of life.[37]

Physicians are often uncertain about the legality of abating life-sustaining treatment and may often be given conservative legal advice by attorneys working for the hospital. Also, physicians may be troubled by the prospect of civil or even criminal liability if they do not continue to use everything within their power—although all of the states that have considered the question of liability have adopted the view that a physician acting in good faith and within established professional standards of care cannot incur civil or criminal liability.[24] This topic received increased public attention after the *Cruzan* case, which was the first "right to die" case considered by the U.S. Supreme Court. Nancy Cruzan was in a persistent vegetative state, maintained by tube feedings and hydration. Her parents wished to withdraw artificial nutrition. Although the parents stated that the patient had said that she would not want to continue living should she have to live as a "vegetable," the Missouri Supreme Court held that the family cannot assume the choice to abate treatment for an incompetent person in the absence of "clear and convincing evidence" of her wishes. The U.S. Supreme Court upheld the Missouri decision.

Later, additional evidence from Miss Cruzan's coworkers was presented in a Missouri court; the trial judge considered that this did represent clear and convincing evidence and authorized withdrawal of tube feedings. She died December 26, 1990. The Supreme Court did recognize that a competent patient had a constitutionally protected "liberty" in refusing unwanted medical treatment. It also implicitly recognized that this right to refuse treatment could be exercised by a surrogate. The right to refuse treatment is also based on the common law right of self-determination and the constitutionally derived right of privacy, which can be traced back to an 1891 U.S. Supreme Court decision. Furthermore, in a technical sense, most of the court recognized the constitutional right to refuse life-sustaining treatment. In addition to the four dissenting justices, Justice Sandra Day O'Connor in her concurring opinion concluded that such a right exists. Orentlicher[38] drew some inferences from the Supreme Court decision: (1) the right to refuse medical treatment is not limited to patients who are terminally ill, a common phrase used in state statutes; (2) the right to refuse treatment includes the right to refuse artificially supplied nutrition and hydration; (3) the right to refuse treatment may be exercised through living wills, durable powers of attorney, or other advance directives, even in the absence of a state advance-directive statute. Implicit in the Supreme Court's holding that a state can require clear and convincing evidence of a patient's wishes before permitting withdrawal of treatment is the principle that a state must *permit* withdrawal when there is clear and convincing evidence that the patient would want the treatment withdrawn.[38] As a corollary, the instructions in an advance directive would be valid whether or not they exceed the kind of instructions covered by the state's advance-directive statute. Every person should have a written advance directive. Because it is difficult to anticipate all of the decisions that will have to be made or to write instructions with enough specificity to avoid uncertainty in their interpretation, appointment of a surrogate decision-maker ensures that a person chosen by the patient will be able to decide on behalf of the patient, even when unforeseen circumstances arise. The use of a surrogate can avoid the possibility of ambiguous instructions. Based on this growing understanding that patients have a right to choose a surrogate as well as the conditions that they would or would not wish for themselves, our Bioethics Committee created an advance directive ("living will") containing descriptions of various situations that might be considered acceptable or not acceptable to individual patients. It also lets patients appoint a surrogate decision-maker to avoid the ambiguities mentioned earlier.[38] The "Advance Directive," "Durable Power of Attorney for Health Care and Health Care Surrogate Form," the "Affidavit" designating a health care surrogate proxy, and the "Health Care Proxy Designation and Acceptance Form" are shown in Appendices 2-1 through 2-4 at the end of this chapter.

The legal liability issue is still mentioned frequently by physicians when confronted with decisions to withdraw or withhold therapy. "Every court in every jurisdiction that has addressed the question of physician liability—including the Barber court—has found physicians participating in the case to be free from civil or criminal sanctions."[24] Weir and Gostin also point out that a few cases indicate the physicians in health care institutions providing treatment for autonomous or non-autonomous patients are at risk of liability when *treatment is continued* against the wishes of a patient or a patient's surrogate. Physicians who do not honor reasonable decisions to abate life-sustaining treatment may face charges of malpractice, battery, intentional infliction of emotional distress, and violation of the common law and constitutionally based right to refuse medical treatment.[39]

Orentlicher[38] is equally emphatic:

Physicians should initiate discussions about life-sustaining treatment and the advisability of advance directives with their patients. Physicians should also document the patient's preferences in the patient's medical record thereby insuring that there is sufficient evidence of the patient's preferences even if the patient does not write an advance directive. Such documentation would almost certainly satisfy even the strictest procedural safeguards. Documentation of an individual's wishes need not be a cumbersome process.

In this regard, the words of Wanzer and colleagues[14] are both inspiring and powerful:

The care of the dying is an art that should have its fullest expression in helping patients cope with the technologically complicated medical environment that often surrounds them at the end of life. The concept of a good death does not

mean simply the withholding of technological treatments that serve only to prolong the act of dying. It also requires the art of deliberately creating a medical environment that allows a peaceful death. . . . The hopelessly ill patient must have whatever is necessary to control pain. In the patient whose dying process is irreversible, the balance between minimizing pain and suffering and potentially hastening death should be struck clearly in favor of pain relief. It is morally correct to increase the dose of narcotics to whatever dose is needed even though the medication may contribute to the depression of respiration or blood pressure, the dulling of consciousness, or even death, provided the primary goal of the physician is to relieve suffering. The proper dose of pain medication is a dose that is sufficient to relieve pain and suffering, even to the point of unconsciousness. . . . Dying patients may require palliative care of an intensity that rivals even that of curative efforts. Even though aggressive curative techniques are no longer indicated, professionals and families are still called upon to use intensive measures—extreme responsibility, extraordinary sensitivity, and heroic compassion.

Cook and colleagues[40] analyzed a survey instrument polling 149 ICU attending staff, 142 house staff, and 1070 ICU nurses in the Canadian Health Care System, concerning their decision to discontinue or withdraw care based on 12 detailed clinical scenarios in which the patient was declared incompetent and no family or friends were available for

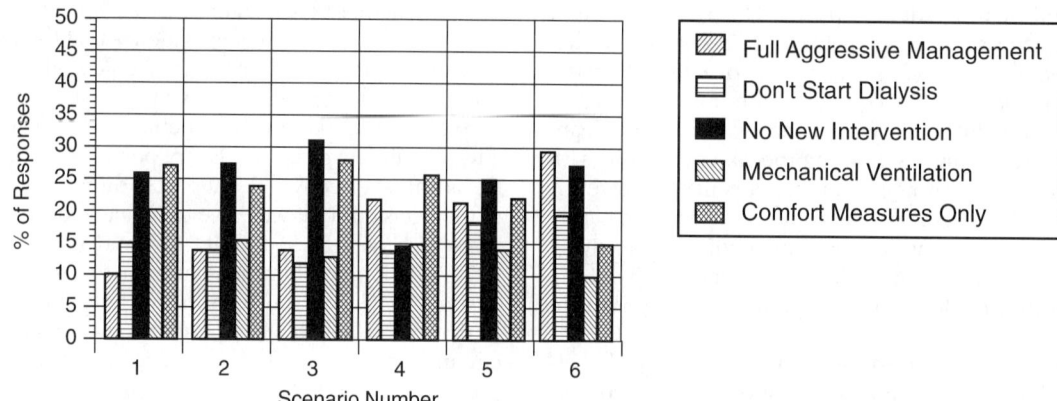

FIGURE 2-1. Distribution of responses to each scenario. The height of each column represents the portion of respondents who chose the particular response options, from full aggressive management to comfort measures only. Each scenario is characterized by whether the patient was 75 years of age (+) or 45 years of age (−); whether the Acute Physiology and Chronic Health Evaluation II score indicated at 10% chance of survival (+) or 50% chance of survival (−); whether the patient had prior breast cancer (+) or did not have prior breast cancer (−); or whether the patient had prior cognitive impairment (+) or did not have prior cognitive impairment (−). The scenarios are labeled as 1 to 6 by the numbers along the x axis. For example, the first scenario describes a 75-year-old patient with urosepsis and a 10% probability of survival with prior breast cancer and prior cognitive impairment; the second scenario describes a 75-year-old patient with urosepsis and a 50% probability of survival with prior breast cancer and no prior cognitive impairment.

surrogate judgment. The respondents consistently identified the following as important to their decision: likelihood of surviving the immediate episode, likelihood of long-term survival, premorbid cognitive function, and age of the patient. In only 1 of 12 scenarios did more than 30% of the respondents make the same therapeutic decision (Fig. 2-1). In 8 of 12 scenarios, more than 10% of the respondents chose the opposite extreme, that is, patient management resonated between full aggressive intensive care to comfort measures only. It is amazing that about the same percentage of people wanted to continue everything (up to dialysis) (summation of the first two bars in scenario 1) as those respondents who were willing to withdraw all support (comfort measures only). The variability of respondent choice of the level of care likely reflected the individual's ethical, moral, and religious values that inextricably impacted on their medical decision making. The ultimate goal must be to develop guidelines for use of scarce resources that reflect the values of our society, and that what is implemented will minimize the input of individual idiosyncratic values of health care workers on life and death decisions. Until accurate predictors are available and until there is a consensus concerning "reasonable prospect," the problem will continue. Society seems to be wrestling with this problem today, having only reached reasonable consensus on a much simpler problem: the definition of brain death (most states have statutes).

IMMEDIATE OBJECTIVE: EXAMINE BEDSIDE CARE

The improved efficiency of the utilization of resources and a better focus for the care of patients who are dying are attainable objectives. Diminishing unnecessary activity will decrease complications and have salutary effects. Having more time to be with patients and their families will decrease our sense of failure and fulfill the important goal of caring. Physicians and nurses can return to thinking, assessing, and decision-making instead of frenetically ordering, reacting, and intervening which, we believe, accurately describes informational overload created by undue emphasis on high technology. In this way, we can respond to Fuchs' exhortation that physicians consider the possibility of contributing more by doing less.[41] In responding, however, we must never forget that the societal, not merely economic, impact of medical care is our principal consideration. We must first contribute more by achieving a greater understanding of the medical care process. Only then can we know how to do less at the beside. We *can* and must distinguish between costly and high-quality care—they are not necessarily synonymous.

CONCLUSION

It is a common axiom that to learn about the future we must often return to a study of the past. Instead of a restricted focus on technology in intensive care, we must reemphasize the marvelous therapeutic quality of the physician–patient relationship, the principle tool possessed by our predecessors. Medical "success" needs human dimensions to achieve fulfillment and be sustaining for both patient and staff. For the patient who survives, we can make the experience less fearful. Indeed, we must remember that patients often completely "forget" their stay in the ICU, although we can remember many seemingly rational conversations. Denial, the mind's defense against memories that cannot be tolerated, is most powerful. We need to remember how helpless the patients must feel. A sympathetic approach will help, but we should strive to diminish their dependency when possible by giving them some control. For the dying patient, we will supply the only needs that matter and can be met: an easing of the lonely, frightening, and often painful transition to death. For society, we will preserve the scarce resources. Health care professionals have an obligation to educate the public about the limitations of our art, that "doing everything" is not always best for the patient or the grieving family. "Physicians should do every thing they believe may be of benefit for their patients unless society or the institution establishes guidelines that limit interventions they desire."[42] For ourselves, as professionals, we will better understand and practice the art and science of medicine at the bedside, and for ourselves, just those members of the human race who happen to have chosen medicine as a profession, we can more confidently approach the future, secure in the knowledge that our human qualities are society's greatest medical resource.

APPENDIX 2-1

ADVANCE DIRECTIVE (LIVING WILL)

YOU MAY ADD, CHANGE OR CROSS OUT ANY WORDS ON THIS FORM

I, _____ , have a right to life-prolonging procedures including food and water (nutrition and hydration), and I also have a right to have life-prolonging procedures stopped or no new ones started. I can choose someone to do this for me if I am unconscious, in a coma, incompetent, or otherwise mentally or physically incapable of making my wishes known.

I understand that treatments or medications which take away pain, suffering, anxiety, or other forms of distress will not be withheld or withdrawn (even if they hasten my death).

By signing below, I hereby choose _____ , whose telephone numbers are _____ (work) and _____ (home), and whose address is _____ as my designee.

By signing below, I hereby choose _____ , whose telephone numbers are _____ (work) and _____ (home), and whose address is _____ as my alternate designee.

I would like my designee (if I have named one), my health care or residential facility, physician, or other health care provider, to read my answers to the following questions and use my answers to help them carry out my wishes if I am unable to do that myself.

1. If I have a terminal condition, from which I will probably not recover or survive and my death will likely occur within weeks,
   a. I would want life-prolonging procedures to be:
   _____ withheld/withdrawn _____ continued
   b. I would want artificially administered food and water such as tube or intravenous feedings to be:
   _____ withheld/withdrawn _____ continued
   c. If my heart or breathing stopped, I would want my doctor to try to restart it through CPR or other means: _____ YES _____ NO

2. If I have a medical condition that is steadily getting worse and my doctor has told me that there is no reasonable possibility of recovery, but I could survive in this condition for weeks or even months,
   a. I would want life-prolonging procedures to be:
   _____ withheld/withdrawn _____ continued
   b. I would want artificially administered food and water such as tube or intravenous feedings to be:
   _____ withheld/withdrawn _____ continued
   c. If my heart or breathing stopped, I would want my doctor to try to restart it through CPR or other means: _____ YES _____ NO

3. If I am in an irreversible coma, persistent vegetative state, or other condition where my doctor has determined that there is no reasonable medical likelihood I will ever be awake or able to make medical decisions for myself again,
   a. I would want life-prolonging procedures to be:
   _____ withheld/withdrawn _____ continued
   b. I would want artificially administered food and water such as tube or intravenous feedings to be:
   _____ withheld/withdrawn _____ continued
   c. If my heart or breathing stopped, I would want my doctor to try to restart it through CPR or other means: _____ YES _____ NO

4. If I must live in a hospital or nursing home for the rest of my life because I am unable to feed or groom myself or take care of my other bodily functions such as responding to my toilet needs,
   a. I would want life-prolonging procedures to be:
   _____ withheld/withdrawn _____ continued
   b. I would want artificially administered food and water such as tube or intravenous feedings to be:
   _____ withheld/withdrawn _____ continued
   c. If my heart or breathing stopped, I would want my doctor to try to restart it through CPR or other means: _____ YES _____ NO

5. If I have progressive or permanent memory loss such that I am no longer able to recognize my family and friends or communicate my thoughts to others,
   a. I would want life-prolonging procedures to be:
   _____ withheld/withdrawn _____ continued
   b. I would want artificially administered food and water such as tube or intravenous feedings to be:
   _____ withheld/withdrawn _____ continued
   c. If my heart or breathing stopped, I would want my doctor to try to restart it through CPR or other means: _____ YES _____ NO

6. If I am in the hospital with a serious condition and my doctor and I have decided to continue treatment because we believe it may be effective and treatment seems to be

going well, if my heart or breathing unexpectedly stopped, I would want my doctor to try to restart it through CPR or other means:

_____ YES   _____ NO

7. In my current state of health, if my heart or breathing unexpectedly stopped, I would want my doctor to try to restart it through CPR or other means:

    _____ YES   _____ NO

8. If I am pregnant I want the instructions I have given above to be followed, prior to the time that my fetus is determined to be viable:

    _____ YES   _____ NO

If not, please give any alternative instructions here:

_____

_____

_____

_____

I understand that I can make quality of life choices. I am not asking anyone else to make quality of life choices for me. This document merely directs others to carry out the quality of life choices I have made. If, in the course of making decisions for me, my designee is dissatisfied with any determination of my attending physician, my designee may substitute another attending physician.

If I cannot make medical decisions for myself, I want the directions in this Declaration to be accepted and fulfilled as the final expression of my legal right to accept or refuse medical or surgical treatment and to accept the consequences of my decisions.

I understand the fulll import of this Declaration, and I am emotionally and mentally competent to make this Declaration.

By executing this Declaration, I am revoking all prior Declarations.

_____   _____

Date   Patient

In signing this Declaration on the date noted above, I state that the declarant is known to me and I believe him/her to be of sound mind. I certify that I am not the declarant's designee named in this document.

_____

Witness

In signing this Declaration on the date noted above, I state that the declarant is known to me and I believe him/her to be of sound mind. I certify that I am not the declarant's spouse, blood relative or designee as named in this document.

_____

Witness

APPENDIX 2-2   ■

HEALTH CARE PROXY DESIGNATION AND ACCEPTANCE FORM

I, _____ , hereby agree to serve as the health care proxy for _____ ("the patient"), with the authority to make health care decisions for the patient if she/he is unable to do so her/himself. I bear the following relationship to the patient:

_____ .

I understand that my authority as the patient's health care proxy begins when two doctors determine that the patient is unable to make health care decisions for her/himself and ends as soon as the patient regains the ability to make necessary medical decisions.

In making health care decisions for the patient, I agree to make the decisions which I reasonably believe the patient would have made under the circumstances. I understand that if asked to make a decision regarding the withholding or withdrawal of life-prolonging procedures, my decision must be supported by clear and convincing evidence that the decision would have been the one the patient would have chosen had she/he been competent. Also, before making decisions regarding life-prolonging procedures, I must determine that the patient does not have a reasonable probability of recovering competency and being able to decide for her/himself and that the patient has a terminal condition.

If the patient has executed a living will or other form of advance directive, I agree to obtain a copy of the directive and consider it evidence of the patient's wishes with regard to medical and treatment decisions.

I understand that as the patient's health care proxy, I have the following responsibilities:

1. To act for the patient and to make all health care decisions for the patient in matters regarding the patient's health care during the patient's incapacity. In accordance with the patient's instructions, unless such authority has been expressly limited by the patient.
2. To consult expeditiously with appropriate health care providers to provide informed consent in the best interest of the patient, and make only health care decisions for the patient which she or he believes the patient would have made under the circumstances if the patient were capable of making such decisions.
3. To provide written consent using an appropriate form whenever consent is necessary.
4. To be provided access to the appropriate clinical records of the patient.
5. To apply for public benefits, such as Medicare and Medicaid, for the patient and have access to information regarding the patient's income and assets and banking and financial records for to the extent required to make application.
6. To authorize the release of information and clinical records to appropriate persons to ensure the continuity of the patient's health care and, if appropriate, to authorize the transfer and admission of the patient to or from a health care facility.

_____   _____

Date   Signature of Health Care Proxy

_____

Address

_____

_____

Phone

APPENDIX 2-3   ■

DURABLE POWER OF ATTORNEY FOR HEALTH CARE AND HEALTH CARE SURROGATE DESIGNATION FORM

I, _____ , have the right to choose someone to make health care decisions for me if I cannot make such decisions myself or if I cannot make my wishes known or provide informed consent. That person would be known as my health care surrogate.

By signing below, I hereby select _____ , whose address is _____ , and whose phone numbers are _____ (work) and _____ (home), and whose relationship to me is as follows, _____ , as my alternate surrogate.

I fully understand that this document allows the surrogate I have named above to make health care decisions for me. My surrogate will be able to provide, withhold or withdraw consent for me, will be able to apply for public benefits to help pay for my health care expenses and will be able to arrange for my admission to or transfer from a health care facility.

I would like to give the following instructions to my surrogate:

I _____ (do) _____ (do not) want my surrogate to be able to provide consent for the withholding or withdrawal of life-prolonging procedures.

If I am pregnant, I _____ (do) _____ (do not) want my surrogate to be able to provide consent for the withholding or withdrawal of life-prolonging procedures prior to the viability of my fetus.

Additional instructions:

_____

_____

_____

I have executed this form voluntarily and not as a condition of treatment or admission to a health care facility.

It is my intent that this durable power of attorney for health care shall not be affected by my disability except as provided by statute.

I have sent copies of this document to the following people in addition to my surrogate:

_____

_____

_____

_____   _____
Date   Patient

In signing this document on the date noted above, I state that the declarant is known to me and I believe her/him to be of sound mind. I am not the surrogate or alternate surrogate named in this document.

_____
Witness

In signing this document on the date noted above, I state that the declarant is known to me and I believe her/him to be of sound mind. I am not the surrogate or alternative surrogate named in this document or the declarant's spouse or blood relative.

_____
Witness

APPENDIX 2-4 ■

AFFIDAVIT

BEFORE ME, the undersigned authority, personally appeared
_____ who after being duly sworn on oath deposes and says:
    (FRIEND)

1. I am of full age, I am competent and under no legal disability.
2. I have personal knowledge of the facts contained in this affidavit.
3. My address is _____
                        (ADDRESS)

    My phone numbers are _____   _____
                          (HOME PHONE)   (WORK PHONE)
4. I am a close friend of _____
                                 (PATIENT)
    I have known him/her for approximately _____ years.
5. I am willing and able to become involved in his/her health care.
6. I have maintained such regular contact with him/her so as to be familiar with his/her activities, health and religious beliefs, and his/her wishes regarding medical care.

FURTHER AFFIANT SAYETH NAUGHT

_____
          (SIGNATURE OF FRIEND)

State of Florida, County of Dade

The foregoing instrument was acknowledged before me this _____ day of _____ , 199__ by _____

_____ who is personally known to me or who has produced _____ as identification and who did (did not) take an oath.

_____

REFERENCES

1. Younger SJ: Who defines futility? *JAMA* 1988;260:2094
2. Hook D: The Edwin Smith surgical papyrus. *Bull Cleveland Med Library Assoc* 1973;20:23.
3. Preston RP: *The Dilemmas of Care: Social and Nursing Adaptations to the Deformed, the Disabled and the Aged.* New York, Elsevier, 1979
4. Bulkin W, Lukashok H: Rx for dying: the case for hospice. *N Engl J Med* 1988;318:376
5. Orwell G: *1984.* New York, Harcourt Brace Jovanovich, 1949
6. Fein R: On measuring economic benefits of health programs. In: McLachlan G, McKeown T (eds). *Medical History and Medical Care: A Symposium of Perspectives.* London, Oxford University Press, 1971:179
7. Fogel R: Medicare: past overuse of intensive care services inflates hospital payment. In: *Report to the Secretary of Health and Human Services,* United States General Accounting Office. GAO/HRD-86-25, March 1986
8. Knaus WA: When is intensive care inappropriate? New "prognostic" measures provide answers. *Hosp Med Q* 1986:14
9. Henning RJ, McClish D, Daly B, et al: Clinical characteristics and resource utilization of ICU patients: implications for organization of intensive care. *Crit Care Med* 1987;15:264
10. Siegel JH, Shafi S, Goodarz S, et al: A quantitative method for cost reimbursement and length of stay quality assurance in multiple trauma patients. *J Trauma* 1994;37:928
11. Halpern NA, Bettes L, Greenstein R: Federal and nationwide intensive care units and health care costs: 1986–1992. *Crit Care Med* 1994;22:2001
12. Beauchamp TL, Childress JF: *Principles of Biomedical Eithics,* 4th ed. New York, Oxford University Press, 1994
13. Critical Care Medicine, Consensus Development Conference Summary. Bethesda, MD, National Institutes of Health, 1983;4(6)
14. Wanzer SH, Federman DD, Adelstein SJ, et al: The physicians' responsibility toward hopelessly ill patients. *N Engl J Med* 1989;320:844
15. Civetta JM, Hudson-Civetta JA, Nelson LD: Evaluation of APACHE II for cost containment and quality assurance. *Ann Surg* 1990;212:266
16. Civetta JM, Varon AJ, Yu M, et al: Accuracy of structured ICU consultations. *Crit Care Med* 1989;17:S87
17. Mangano DT, Browner WS, Hollenberg M, et al: Association of perioperative myocardial ischemia with cardiac morbidity and mortality in men undergoing noncardiac surgery. *N Engl J Med* 1990;323:1782
18. Varon AJ, Hudson-Civetta JA, Civetta JM, et al: Preoperative intensive care unit consultations: accurate and effective. *Crit Care Med* 1993;21:234
19. Baron JF, Mundler O, Bertrand M, et al: Dipyridamole-thallium scintigraphy and gated radionuclide angiography to assess cardiac risk before abdominal aortic surgery. *N Engl J Med* 1994;330:663
20. Civetta JM: The inverse relationship between cost and survival. *J Surg Res* 1973;14:265
21. Teres D, Steingrub J: Can intermediate care substitute for intensive care? *Crit Care Med* 1987;15:280
22. Civetta JM, Hudson-Civetta J, Nelson LD: Costly care: data problems and proposing remedies [abstract]. *Crit Care Med* 1985;202:524
23. Tomlinson T, Brody H: Futility and the ethics of resuscitation. *JAMA* 1990;264:1276
24. Weir RF, Gostin L: Decisions to abate life-sustaining treatment for nonautonomous patients: ethical standards and legal liability for physicians after Cruzan. *JAMA* 1990;264:1846
25. Luce JM: Physicians do not have a responsibility to provide futile or unreasonable care if a patient or family insists. *Crit Care Med* 1995;23:760
26. Schneiderman LJ, Jecker NS, Jonsen AR: Medical futility: its meaning and ethical implications. *Ann Intern Med* 1990;112:949
27. Task force on ethics of the Society of Critical Care Medicine: Consensus report on the ethics of foregoing life-sustaining treatments in the critically ill. *Crit Care Med* 1990;18:1435
28. *Barber v Superior Court,* 147 Cal App 3d 1006, 195 Cal Rptr 484 (Ct App 1983)
29. Paris JJ, Crone RK, Reardon F: Physicians' refusal of requested treatment: the case of Baby L. *N Engl J Med* 1990;322:1012
30. *In re Baby K,* 16F. 3d590, petition for rehearing en banc denied, no. 93-1899(L), CA-93-G8-A, 28 March (4th Cir. 1994)
31. *In re Helen Wanglie.* Fourth Judicial District (Dist. Ct. Probate Ct. Div.) Px-91-283. Minnesota, Hennepin County
32. Ellemont J: Jury sides with doctors on elderly woman's life support. *Boston Globe,* April 22, 1995
33. Brett AS, McCullough LB: Defining the limits of the physician's obligation. *N Engl J Med* 1986;315:1347
34. Bedell SE, Pelle P, Maher PL, et al: Do-not-resuscitate orders for critically patients in the hospital. *JAMA* 1986;256:233
35. Margolis JO, McGrath BJ, Kussin PS, et al: Do not resuscitate (DNR) orders during surgery: ethical foundations for institutional policies in the United States. *Anesth Analg* 1995;80:806
36. Elpern EH, Silver MR, Burton LA: When families force life-support decisions: what should the medical team do? *J Crit Illness* 1991;6:1131
37. Civetta JM: Critical care: how should we evaluate our progress. *Crit Care Med* 1992;20:1714
38. Orentlicher D: The right to die after *Cruzan. JAMA* 1990;264:2444
39. *Estate of Leach v Shapiro,* 13 Ohio App 3d, 469 NE2d 1047 (1984)
40. Cook DJ, Guyatt GH, Jaeschke R, et al: Determinants in Canadian health care workers of the decision to withdraw life support from the critically ill. *JAMA* 1995;273:703
41. Fuchs VR: A more effective, efficient, and equitable system. *West J Med* 1976;125:3
42. Sprung CL, Eidelman LA, Steinberg A: Is the physician's duty to the individual patient or to society? *Crit Care Med* 1995;23:618

Critical Care, Third Edition, edited by Joseph M. Civetta,
Robert W. Taylor, and Robert R. Kirby.
Lippincott-Raven Publishers, Philadelphia, PA © 1997.

CHAPTER 3

Collaborative Care: Physician and Nursing Interactions

Danny Sleeman
Judith A. Hudson-Civetta
Joseph M. Civetta

As medical knowledge increases, the patient population grows older, technology advances, and the need for intensive care grows, the interrelationships among physicians—and other medical personnel—become more complex. The success of an intensive care unit (ICU) hinges on these interrelationships, which are examined in this chapter according to four major areas. The first examines physicians within and outside the ICU who must interact smoothly. The fellow's role and responsibilities and a guide to planning the day forms the second section. The concept of the ICU team and how the physician's orders affect nursing practice and unit efficiency are described in the last two sections.

THE SURGEON BEFORE THE ICU

Before the development of ICUs and intensivists, surgeons directed the entire postoperative course of their patients. Because surgeons pioneered the development of physiologic perioperative care, they were also intimately involved in the care of their patients during the ICU portion of a patient's hospital admission. This practice has recently changed. Patients are sicker with more physiologic changes occurring with increased frequency. At the same time, surgeons are less available, are doing more extensive operations and patient consultations, or are performing often-lengthy ambulatory surgical procedures. They are also spending more time on documentation and paperwork. Full-time ICU personnel,

with specialized training in critical care, often care for the patients in the surgeon's absence. The operating surgeon and the ICU team must interact to maintain optimal patient management.

MEMBERS OF THE TEAM

The identification of various members on the surgical and ICU teams is important before further discussion of their roles can be undertaken (Fig. 3-1).

The ICU fellow should communicate the patient's status to the attendings on both the surgical and ICU teams. The interaction between the ICU fellow and the senior residents of the surgical team is the level on which many decisions reflecting changes in management occur. The fellows and team senior residents must discuss which decisions need confirmation by their respective attendings. The consulting services may be brought into the patient's management at the agreed-on request of either the ICU or surgical team. The nurses in the ICU are vital for nursing care of the patient and also for keeping the ICU fellow abreast of the patient's condition. The same holds true for the respiratory therapists and the ICU fellow in terms of the goals for respiratory management. The junior members of the surgical and ICU teams are in the early stages of their careers and training and should not have independent decision-making responsibility.

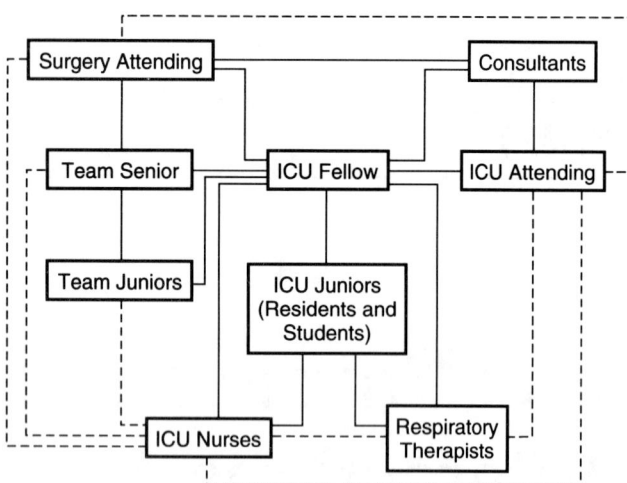

FIGURE 3-1. Diagram illustrating the interrelations among ICU personnel. Communication is centralized in the Fellow. Solid lines indicate commonly used routes; dotted lines signify available avenues that are used less frequently.

THE SURGICAL ATTENDING

The surgeon provides the patient with the most continual care and information so that the patient and family can understand what to expect during the course of the illness. For the attending's patients, the surgical attending is ultimately responsible for a patient's prehospital, intrahospital, and posthospital care, as well as the long-term follow-up. For the "staff" patients, the surgical attending also is ultimately responsible to guarantee the best management of the patients cared for through the hospital clinics. These responsibilities should not be dismissed once the patient enters an ICU, especially in today's litigious society. The attending should make daily rounds on these patients and have regular communication with the ICU team. But recently critical care has progressed rapidly, and some aspects of a patient's management should be left to the ICU team, whose knowledge of critical care equipment, techniques, and pharmacology is usually more detailed and current. They also have to make the many adjustments in daily patient intensive care.

THE SURGERY TEAM SENIORS

The surgery team seniors are the agents through which the surgical attendings can maintain minute-to-minute management of the patients without being physically present. They provide an essential link between the ICU team and the surgery attending. They are also able to provide assistance in managing the many minor surgical problems as they arise (e.g., opening an infected wound, changing the initial dressing). They usually write ICU admission or discharge orders, communicate needs for admissions and scheduling of surgical procedures (both in main operating rooms or at the ICU bedside), and coordinate with the nurses the timing of complex dressing changes.

THE ICU ATTENDING

An ICU attending has a diversified role. The attending should understand physiology and pathophysiology, manage critical care patients, know technical aspects of the monitors and equipment, be a stimulating researcher and an effective educator, be a diplomatic manager and politician, and have the empathy required to deal with dying patients and their families. The attending must always be ready to discuss management with the non-ICU team, nurses, respiratory therapists, and patient or families. Usually the attending is ultimately responsible for decisions relating to admissions or discharges to the ICU. The ICU attending may be involved in specific management decisions of the extremely ill patients and should be able to settle any disputes among the various teams or ICU members.

ICU attendings should have the final say but effect this position diplomatically through accessing and processing information and forming judgments; otherwise they will be deemed ineffective managers.

THE CONSULTANTS

The consultant of a particular service provides an important educational role to the critical care team. They provide further knowledge in certain specific areas that might not be known by the critical care team, despite excellent training. A consultant's role should be to answer the specific questions that are asked by the ICU or surgical teams. This expectation can be realized only if specific questions are formulated *and* communicated directly. Relying on a hastily written consult form in the chart may result in unnecessary and unwanted or unwarranted opinions about other aspects of management and no answer to the problem. The consultants should not expect suggestions to be implemented without discussing the pertinent aspects with the ICU team. It is preferable to have the discussion orally before committing remarks to the legal record (the patient's chart).

THE ICU JUNIOR RESIDENTS

The junior residents on rotation through an ICU are in the ICU to learn the basics of caring for a critically ill patient and to recognize the physiologic abnormalities. During on-call periods, they are assigned patients; they are then responsible for collecting data, analyzing it, and formulating an assessment and management plan. Although their management plan may not be implemented in its entirety, the junior residents are able to develop some of the cognitive skills required in managing critically ill patients. They should give formal presentations of their patients during the teaching rounds and receive immediate feedback on their understanding, assessment, and skills. The nursing interrelationships are discussed later.

COMItUNICATIONS ■

The smooth functioning of any system is dependent on effective communication. *When* to communicate may lead to problems unless all major deteriorations in a patient's condition are made known to all involved, regardless of the time of day. Communication is not a courtesy but a necessity because of patient responsibility. It also forces an orderly presentation of the problem and solution. It helps refine decision-making yet avoids errors and misdirections that occur when one acts independently.

PROBLEMS WITH COMMUNICATION ■

Having invested much time and effort in a patient's surgery and care, the surgeon may focus only on the positive aspects of a patient's status and seem to ignore the negative data. They may feel that the ICU team is pestering them with unwanted details if more negative than positive parameters are identified. Because many long-term ICU patients die after similar courses of progressive multiple system failure and sepsis, the ICU team, on the other hand, may have a *pessimistic* outlook on a patient's course. They may seem anxious to withdraw support on some patients. Specially scheduled conferences among the surgical and ICU teams with the four key personnel—the ICU team, the surgical team, nursing staff, and the family—may be required to develop a unified, mutually agreeable approach to the patient's management. This enhances the patient's care and provides uniformity in the information given to the patients and families. Perhaps the desire to create the numerous illness severity scoring systems rested on the hope that objective data might help in the management of these conflicts. Unfortunately, such help is not available despite the vigorous ongoing efforts in the long-term patients for whom it is most difficult to differentiate, on clinical grounds, potential survivors from those who will die.

SPECIAL SITUATIONS ■

The subspecialty teams usually have a more restricted focus and less experience with overall patient management necessary in the ICU; therefore, they tend to "give over" the care of the patient to the ICU team. The ICU team may be uncomfortable with the specific problems related to the subspecialties (e.g, balanced orthopedic traction or plugged, special-drainage catheters). The growth of the specialties in medicine has led to the development of specialized ICUs. While each ICU concentrates on a particular type of patient with a specialized knowledge base, their knowledge of other areas may not be as current. Mutual exchange, part of the philosophy of the founders of the Society of Critical Care Medicine, may be considered even more important because knowledge and technology have expanded.

FELLOWS' FUNCTION AND INTERRELATIONSHIPS ■

In addition to structure, daily function is important. Every institution has different responsibilities for fellows, residents, or medical students and different hours and arrange-

ments for coverage. However, several functions of the fellow seem to be universal and can be assessed by observing in detail a day in the life of an ICU fellow.

TEACHING ROUNDS

Morning rounds are the most important activity for gaining knowledge, communicating, and planning the day's treatment goals. Rounds should be multidisciplinary, including the charge nurse, each patient's bedside nurse in turn, the respiratory therapist, and others who might want to participate, such as the pharmacist and dietitian. Either the fellow or attending must also make rounds at the bedside with the team, because patient observation is the key to detecting problems (e.g., incorrectly positioned endotracheal tube, inappropriate ventilator settings, abdominal distention, abnormal breathing patterns, wound infection, and incorrect pulmonary artery waveform analysis).

Like the opening paragraph of a newspaper article, the first few sentences of the presentation should capture the essence of the problem and direct the listener to the appropriate areas of focus. A long, roundabout history starting with numerous superfluous details about why the patient was admitted and dwelling on unrelated medical history bores the listeners and distracts them from hearing important data.

Present the who, why, when, where, and what: (1) briefly state the patient's name, age, sex, and attending; (2) explain why the patient was admitted; (3) explain when and where the events happened; and (4) describe the sequence of events and the medical interventions. The report is not complete without an assessment of the problems and, finally, discussion of the plans for the day and expectations for the patient and disease process (prognosis).

Be ready to explain and defend each therapeutic maneuver, but be willing to change the treatment plans if better ideas are expressed by the other team members.

PRIORITIZATION, ORGANIZATION, AND DAILY CHORES

Despite emergencies, having routines and a sense of control over a hectic unit is important. For example, having a routine reassures the team members and nurses that formal work rounds are indeed done, and when the care plan is discussed daily, questions can be asked, allowing problems to be discussed and dealt with promptly and efficiently.

The fellow ensures that all chores are done in a timely fashion. The nurse and resident must understand clearly the goals for their patient for that day; the fellow checks the patient at regular intervals to ensure that therapeutic maneuvers are done properly and various results are obtained, and to decide on further treatment modalities. The fellow's place is at the bedside of critically unstable patients. This responsibility cannot be delegated to junior residents. When second-to-second decisions, such as titration of drugs, are being made, only physical presence ensures that therapy is given properly, that ineffective drugs or dosages are changed quickly until the desired result is obtained. The residents learn by watching the fellow in action and helping with the minute-to-minute details of crisis care.

Communicating with family is also an important part of being in charge. Family members quickly recognize the fellow as having authority and knowledge. One of the most crucial lessons is not to give conflicting messages to the family—nothing confuses, distresses, and angers the family more than to hear one physician say their loved one has no chance and another physician, perhaps from a wish to spare their feelings, give the opposite message. It is mandatory that prognosis be discussed on rounds with the entire team present, that all understand the situation, and that all involved give the same message.

NEW ADMISSIONS

If the fellow is asked to see a patient whose condition is deteriorating in a routine care area, assess the patient as soon as possible in person and make plans for a safe transfer to the ICU. If the patient is in severe respiratory distress, intubate the patient electively before transfer—do not be forced to do so inside the elevator. Make sure all appropriate devices for a safe transfer (such as oxygen, electrocardiograph monitor, and pulse oximeter) are available. If possible, take time to explain to the patient and family why the transfer is necessary, what to expect in the ICU, and, especially, that the family will be allowed to visit their loved one in the ICU. A short, clear explanation has a beneficial and calming effect on both the patient and family.

Before a definite decision is made to admit the patient to the ICU, discuss the "numbers" with the ICU charge nurse. If beds or nursing staff are not available, special arrangements will be necessary.

If special items such as ventilators, transducers, and other equipment are needed in the ICU, give the information ahead of time so that it will be ready on patient arrival. Admissions, which can occur any time of day, range from patients who are in or about to experience cardiac arrest to stable patients who need to be monitored for potential life-threatening problems.

If the patient arrives in critical and unstable condition, the fellow should direct therapeutic maneuvers and urgent diagnostic testing simultaneously by dividing tasks and allocating them to the appropriate personnel.

Initial resuscitation of a severely hypotensive unfamiliar patient is analogous to resuscitation of a trauma victim, and the following priorities should apply:

1. Immediately call for supportive personnel, if the available level is not adequate.
2. Get immediate control of the patients's airway. The most experienced person should perform the intubation—this is not the time for teaching.
3. Obtain immediate venous access for fluids, pressors, or both.
4. When blood pressure is acceptable, procedures such as arterial line or pulmonary artery catheter insertion that help in the diagnosis and management of the patient can be performed—do not delay therapy to perform these procedures. Deaths have occurred while the physician was engrossed in trying to gain central access.

5. Send the necessary immediate laboratory work and adjust initial therapy according to the results.

Fortunately, because most patients are not this critically ill, the nursing staff usually has time to "hook up" the patient to various monitors. The fellow and receiving team should be at the patient's bedside because this is the best time to gather information from the transporting physician, whether it is the anesthesiologist, emergency room doctor, surgeon, or house officer.

After the busy work of settling the patient has been completed and while laboratory results are pending, a more orderly and complete history, physical examination, and chart review can be done. The fellow should make sure that a team member takes the time to review the patient's chart and past medical records, if available. Skill is required to pull out the pertinent facts from a distressingly thick chart, but it pays to start at the beginning of the record with the emergency room admission sheet or initial history and physical examination to get a perspective of the patient's hospital course.

After the history and physical examination are completed, the next phase of patient assessment is formulating follow-up plans, both short and long term, to tidy up current problems.

If information is inadequate, other sources are sought: (1) old charts (including telephone calls to other hospitals); (2) family members and other physicians; and (3) additional laboratory and diagnostic studies and procedures.

Short-term follow-up consists of frequent checks, treating immediate problems, and reevaluating the situation until a coherent picture of the patient, the diagnosis, and the treatment has evolved. Do not rely on nursing staff and junior residents to call with subtle signs that might be harbingers of major problems. No news is *not* good news!

SIGNING OUT/AFTERNOON ROUNDS

A second daily round serves the following purposes:

1. Daily chores and therapeutic maneuvers discussed in morning rounds can be followed up.
2. Further treatment modalities necessary for the evening can be planned.
3. Information on new admissions can be shared with the team.

TEACHING, SUPERVISION, AND ORIENTATION

To be able to teach a topic, one has to understand and organize the material for accurate presentation. Although most teaching occurs during work rounds, it is helpful for the fellow in preparation for the future after training to have didactic sessions with residents, nurses, or other personnel who request it. Everyone learns if certain problems and pathophysiology are explained using patients in the ICU as examples.

Orienting new residents is another function of the fellow. It is important to explain clearly the routines and policies of the ICU, what is expected of their performance, and to answer any questions. The supervising of junior residents, all of whom are at different levels of training and have varying talents and interests, is another responsibility of the fellow. All medical students should be closely supervised. A fine line exists between being overly protective and being negligent.

EVALUATION OF ELECTIVE CONSULTATIONS

For surgical patients undergoing major procedures or with significant medical illnesses, ICU care is often desirable. Patients can be considered for postoperative care or preoperative admission for invasive monitoring and cardiovascular "fine tuning." Try to see patients as early as possible so that the necessary testing and transfer can be accomplished before nightfall!

GROWTH AND RESEARCH

At first, everyone has a sense of insecurity in a new role and environment, and the days are filled with learning routines, getting to know different and eccentric personalities (both in and outside the ICU), reviewing previously learned information, and mastering new material. The fellow, while gaining experience and becoming more skilled at coordination and supervision, begins to function more autonomously. Many fellows, especially those with academic interests, get involved in research. Research in critical care medicine is a wide-open field. Endless topics need to be investigated. The fellow can elect to take an extra year solely for research if there is no time during the clinical rotation.

FUNCTIONING AS A TEAM

To write orders effectively, physicians must understand more than medical concepts. The ICU is a unique environment, which often seems to be fiercely protected by the permanent ICU staff—nurses, physicians and others. Understanding the motivations of the regular personnel and the problems faced by newcomers can facilitate joining the team.

One pragmatic approach to this difficult issue is collaborative practice: the interaction between nurses and physicians that uses the knowledge and skills of both professions to enhance patient care. First, a relationship based on mutual trust and respect must be developed. Other key features include active and assertive contributions from both parties, a negotiating process that builds on these contributions, and clarification of the goals and expectations of both parties.[1] Collaborative practice requires tact and diplomacy, considering that many different personalities are involved. Remembering that people who work in an ICU are functioning under considerable stress helps one to better accept another's idiosyncrasies. Only then can we accomplish our goal in caring for the critically ill.

Greenburg and associates[2] describe an ICU as a high-tension environment because of the random appearance of catastrophic events or unpredictable clinical crises. "Uncer-tainty produces anxiety and anxiety readily translates into stress."[3] Because of the stress, defenses are set up to protect new physicians—at least while they enter the established ICU for the first time—and nurses, who may need to express the proprietary "rights" of the establishment—the "permanent" ICU staff. Physicians may, justifiably, be fearful because they are unfamiliar with procedures and with the environment, independent of the recognized gaps in their medical knowledge about the care of critically ill.

Nurses, too, feel protective, ostensibly for the patients and to ensure that protocols are followed. But, again, the order and structure can greatly help them to cope with the activity, acuteness of illness, and interpersonal stressors. Thus, the protection also has great value for the nurse.

Lack of adherence by new physicians to the protocols and to the traditions of the unit has a profound impact on the morale of the nursing and other permanent staff. Coping mechanisms for even the smallest stressors, whether patient or environmentally related, can be abandoned because of anger, frustration, and apathy. The development of important team relationships become bogged down, if not halted.

Motivation to encourage an existing team to incorporate new members is difficult to initiate. This lack of motivation in all parties to address this issue is caused by the immature or nonexistent relationships within the group. The ability to negotiate and communicate effectively is important to the morale and cohesiveness of the unit as well as care of the critically ill patient.

When the development of the team fails, cliques begin to form within the unit, all attempting to find ways to maintain their morale, some constructive and others destructive. The main components of professional collaboration—development of the relationship, mutual trust and respect, effective communication with negotiation, and clarification of goals and expectations—are endangered.

There must be consistent evidence that the administrative staff (medical director, other attending physicians, head nurse, and associate head nurses) are working toward protecting the order and structure of the unit. A new physician who is not willing to participate or acknowledge the existence of the team can cause a disturbance powerful enough to reverberate through the framework of even a well-established unit. This results in many long-term consequences for team members, such as mistrust in the leadership's ability to command, unit stress, and depression.

Knowing how we handle stress and how it handles us can benefit the new ICU physician and all members of the ICU team. We must understand that we handle stress differently. Some laugh and joke, others are solemn, others shout, and some become quiet and withdrawn. Initially, new ICU physicians are unaware of everyone's stress-releasing mechanisms, just as their coworkers are unaware of theirs. Recognition and respect for the human elements in this equation underlie all attempts at collaborative practice. The emphasis of teamwork should be on *what is right*, not necessarily *who is right*. Caring for patients is a team effort. The team includes nurses, respiratory therapists, junior residents, and other ancillary personnel.

A system of checks and balances is used. Fellows, junior residents, nurses, and respiratory therapists must be aware of the daily plan of care. Each member is responsible for individual tasks but continually monitors the entire patient care process to ensure that daily goals are being achieved. Therefore, inquiries about therapy are not meant to question an individual's judgment but to ensure that the rationale is understood and the plan of care is consistent—by the questioner as well as the questioned. However, new team members (physicians) are almost always tested by members who perceive themselves as constants (nurses). Team membership has to be "earned." This requires recognition of the importance of the other team members, decision-making skills, judgment, and honesty—all demonstrated by adhering to group-approved behavior. This behavior—the unwritten rules of the game—is based on the desires of the organizational hierarchy. Initially, it is easiest to accept the unit's correct way to earn a spot on the team roster. Later, new ideas can be introduced using a collaborative approach. If this approach is not used, and a new physician starts by correcting "errors" or by introducing new (and better?) ways, the reaction is often defensiveness, isolation, and hostility instead of trust and acceptance. Deviation from established protocols is considered an unwillingness to be part of the team, not evidence of a superior way of doing a task, and it is disruptive to morale, can heighten organizational stress, and ultimately can obstruct the delivery of optimum health care. The fellow or resident must make decisions and plans for therapy and may be asked, at times, to explain the rationale. This should not be viewed as a criticism of judgment but as an opportunity for teaching new ideas and reinforcing old information. This ensures that all team members have the same plan of therapy in mind.

The *nurses* may be the most informed members of the team in terms of the actual status of the patient. The information needed to make an assessment should be on the flow sheet. If it is not, the nurses are the best resource. They may also be helpful by guiding the new ICU fellow or resident through the various systems of a particular institution. Nurses may be able to assist in expediting test results or in identifying whom to call to schedule a test. If a team member is unsure about how to complete a task, checking with the nurse will save time and energy.

Different family members must receive the same messages concerning the patient's progress. Family members are also dealing with stress and generally hear what they want to hear, or are capable of hearing. Therefore, simple and clear language should be used. Family members who cannot accept a poor prognosis often confront team members separately in desperate attempts to alter outcome through manipulation. All of the physicians and nurses involved should discuss the patient's case to provide consistent information to deal with this problem.

FACTORS CONTRIBUTING TO COLLABORATION ■

Physicians become acutely aware of the demands placed on them to be active team members, in fact, to be one of the leaders within the team. Yet, personal goals are a major factor in determining whether the physician chooses to become a team member. Unfortunately, some choose not to tolerate the trials of earning team membership and reject the concept of the team approach. New physicians on the unit often speak of continually being questioned about their particular plan of therapy or thought process in providing interventions. In the best of circumstances, the questioners are attempting to understand the rationale for therapy and to learn from the physician's previous experiences. They are also looking for pleasure and stimulation in working as part of the team. This is not to say that, at times, judgments are not questioned; although this is a delicate situation, such questioning may be necessary. An ability to be open in conveying perceptions and to validate them is vitally important. (Example: "I feel as if you think I have not made the correct decision.") The real issue—which only you can decide for yourself—is, do you want to do your work as part of a team, or do you want to be an independent practitioner explaining your actions only if you wish? If the latter, it will be extremely difficult to mobilize the best efforts from the necessary members to provide optimal health care for your patients, because this attitude often is perceived as defensive, condescending, supercilious, or outright antagonistic—none of which encourages whole-hearted cooperation. Collaborative practice is a method of goal setting that allows team members to devise a means of achieving those goals by relying on individual member's strengths and resources.[3] Contributions from each team member, trust and respect for those contributions, negotiations that lead to new ways of conceptualizing the issues, communication, and clarification of roles and expectations all lead to the development of a working relationship,[1] the kind of relationship necessary for working effectively in a high-stress environment.

ALLOCATING NURSING CARE ■

In this cost-sensitive era, nurse and physician members of the ICU team are confronted daily with the mandate to deliver an increasing number of patient days (PDs) of intensive care to older and sicker patients with decreased total health care resources. This mandate is felt most acutely in medical centers that are categorized as both tertiary care referral centers and level I regional trauma centers. Patient populations demonstrate the following: (1) a significant increase in the average length of patient stay; (2) an increase in the acuteness of patient illness, age, and number of comorbidities; (3) an increase in the number of patients for whom outcome is uncertain (patient population with greater than a 13-day ICU stay with mortality rates from 40% to 50%); and (4) a reduction in the number of elective surgical patients and a simultaneous increase in the number of blunt- or penetrating-trauma victims. Our hospital (University of Miami/Jackson Memorial Medical Center, Miami, Fla) has undergone changes, and the effects are delineated in Tables 3-1 and 3-2. Unfortunately, no magic cost-containment formula has been issued by the bureaucrats to be used at the bedside by the ICU practitioner. Because the costs of nursing personnel are known to be one of the highest in an

TABLE 3-1. Comparison of Demographics

VARIABLE	1984	1989
Total no. patients	374	309
Survivors	294	215
Deaths	80	94
% Mortality	21%	30%
% Trauma	35%	63%
% Elective	65%	37%
Stay ≥2 wk	28	61
% Population	7.5%	20%
% Mortality	57%	39%

TABLE 3-2. Comparison of Utilization

	1984		1989	
VARIABLE	ICU Stay (d)	APACHE II	ICU Stay (d)	APACHE II
Total no. patients	4.2 ± 5.5	11.8 ± 7.4	9 ± 13.2	15.3 ± 9
Stay ≥ 2 wk	20.7 ± 5.9	15.4 ± 7.4	29.5 ± 17.7	17 ± 7.1

institution[4-6] and because the availability of experienced ICU nurses is limited,[7] we must evaluate and, when possible, change our practice so that we may provide efficient, productive nursing care for the ICU patient while maintaining the quality of care. This section reviews the allocation of nursing care in the ICU through discussion of the following areas: a brief description of the different roles and care functions of the ICU nurse; the evolution of the study of nursing resource allocation in the ICU, developing categories of nursing care, quantifying delivered nursing care, and improving nursing efficiency and productivity in equivalent illness; correlations between the severity of patient illness, the amount and type of nursing care required, and the role of the physician's preferences expressed through written orders; and descriptions of our nursing care classified according to the severity of illness and level of physician interventions.[8,9]

NURSING CARE FUNCTIONS ■

In most ICUs in this country, nursing *care* is not limited to nursing *tasks* (measure and record). Appropriate ICU nursing addresses the whole patient and all disease processes: systematic determination of a patient's problems and needs, establishing the priority of those problems, making a plan to solve them, implementing that plan, and evaluating the extent to which the plan was effective in resolving the problems identified.[10] Given the limited number of residency positions and fellowships to train ICU physicians, it seems reasonable for physicians to learn about ICU nursing care during their ICU training because it is safe to predict that in the absence of physicians physically present in most ICUs, this description of nursing care will portray actual bedside ICU care for patients in the physician's future practice. Certainly, in the ideal ICU environment in which the nurse manager and the medical director direct by collaborative practice, a mutual understanding and support of role function is essential.

Within a PD of 24 *possible* hours, the hours of nursing care *delivered* to each patient are dependent on the nurse–patient ratio. If this ratio is 1:2, then only 12 hours of nursing care are available. Mostly, the nurse staffing allocations to

an ICU, although idealized to be 1:1 in the past, are based on an overall 1:2 ratio.[7,11]

Nursing care in the ICU is composed of dependent role functions, independent role functions, and a mixture of the two. The dependent role encompasses the tasks necessary to complete and document the orders written by the physician, for example, the administration and documentation of an ordered medication. In the independent role, the nurse performs functions such as preventive skin care for a long-term immobile patient (turning, massage of reddened areas, range-of-motion exercises, careful skin hygiene). A mixture of independent and dependent roles is most common. For example, a physician writes an order for wet-to-dry abdominal wound dressing every 8 hours. First, the order is transcribed and included in the patient's care plan (dependent). Each nurse assesses the status of wound healing, looks for evidence of infection, and evaluates the condition of the skin surrounding the wound (independent). The dressing is changed as prescribed (dependent). Finally, if excoriation is noticed, the nurse will start the use of skin-protective measures such as the application of Karaya powder and an absorbable gelatin sponge to absorb pressure. From one perspective, the major goal of ICU medical therapy is to promote patient wellness. Physician's orders are the most common method to outline and transmit the specific medical therapies to reach the goal of wellness. Yet, to prevent compromise of the quality of patient care, physician's orders also should have the following nonmedical goals: to increase efficiency and productivity of patient care; to support the independence of nursing assessment regarding the patient's physiologic stability; and to control the costs of intensive care and thus impact on total hospital costs. The most important way to accomplish these ends is to think carefully to avoid the unnecessary.

ALLOCATION OF NURSING RESOURCES ■

In the past, we have confused activity with productivity and have allocated nursing resources with little regard for determining the patient's need for the tasks performed. A good example of this activity is the nearly universal "requirement" for hourly measurement and recording of vital signs and intake and output for the first, if not all, ICU days in all patients. This activity does not fulfill the physiologic need of every patient and only wastes valuable nursing resources.

To provide some scientific basis for nursing allocations in the ICU, we conducted staffing studies first in 1976 through 1977[12] and again in 1984[13] to quantify the nursing care delivered in our own general surgical/trauma adult ICU. The first study, conducted prospectively, evaluated 61 PDs in 14 different patients. *Nursing time* was defined as the total hours actually delivered by the nurses to accomplish the necessary and ordered patient care. According to this methodology, if the sum of nursing time exceeded 24 hours, even a 1:1 nurse–patient ratio would be insufficient. Nursing care was divided into major categories and further subdivided into specific tasks and activities. Procedures by different people were observed to determine the time required to perform each activity properly; the time required by less experienced nurses was combined with more proficient nurses to derive "average values." Supervisory nursing personnel then independently observed and confirmed the validity of the time quantification. The results demonstrated that the average nursing care required per patient was 19.6 hours. We divided the patients into three classifications (Table 3-3): class 1, patients requiring 12 hours or less of nursing care; class 2, requiring 13 to 24 hours; and class 3, requiring more than 24 hours of nursing care in a 24-hour PD to simulate nurse–patient ratios of 1:2, 1:1, and more than 1:1, respectively. Table 3-3 also contains the results of the 1984 study, as well as scores of the Therapeutic Intervention Scoring System (TISS) and Acute Physiology and Chronic Health Evaluation (APACHE) II[14].

In 1976, according to our calculations, a nurse patient ratio of 1:2 was inadequate for 89% of the PDs sampled. A 1:1 ratio was, indeed, "necessary," and the charge nurse had to have been free of a direct patient assignment to assist with the class 3 patients (those who required more than 24 hours of care per PD, which is more than one nurse could provide). After the study, we attempted to increase our nursing staffing to achieve a level of sufficient coverage to deliver the "required and ordered" care; no attempt was made to evaluate whether the *patient* actually physiologically *required* all of the nursing care delivered. Parenthetically, we learned that we, among others, often use the phrase

"The patient required . . ." when we really mean "We choose to use. . . ." The importance of this distinction rests in the awareness that if we realize that the latter is actually true, changes may then be made.

By 1984, two related problems had arisen that forced us to evaluate our nursing practice. First, our hospital had a shortage of *nurses* applying for positions in any of the 12 ICUs; and second, a shortage of nursing *positions* (full-time equivalents [FTEs] in the surgical ICU table of organization) also existed, resulting from the nationwide and hospital-wide cost–reimbursement focus. We began, at first haphazardly and then systematically, to evaluate our nursing care practice and protocols. We asked if hourly *recorded* vital signs were really necessary for 24 hours after admission, that is, did the recording of observed stable numbers add anything to the patient's care or improve outcome? This systematic evaluation was spurred by our realization that laboratory testing could be markedly decreased without affecting outcome or quality of care.[8] Also, we had observed a tremendous difference in the frequency of vital signs performed in an international study of APACHE: patients with the same score had the same outcome regardless of vital sign recording frequency.[15] The surgical ICU nursing management and medical directors collaboratively changed our practice style and effected these changes by changing or eliminating set frequencies defined in standing orders: substituting *observation* of continuously monitored vital signs for *recording* in all stable patients; simplifying intake and output recording; eliminating previously routine tasks that were of unproven value, such as daily prophylactic chest physiotherapy on all ventilated patients; diminishing laboratory work; and deleting repetition of other tasks or discarding tasks we redefined as unnecessary. The patient care protocols that evolved are discussed according to the simple patient classification (Chap. 2) derived from earlier studies,[9,16] with implications for the types of orders the physician should write. Although our personal preferences are used as examples, we propose only that the general principles and approach are worthy of investigation in other institutions. Finally, from April to June 1984, we repeated the staffing study with an updated list of categories, activities, and average times. Newly added activities that could not be abstracted from the flow sheet, such as time spent with the family, were recorded directly.

TABLE 3-3. Classification of Patients by Nursing Care Hours

		CLASS 1 ≤12 h	CLASS 2 13–24 h	CLASS 3 >24 h	TOTAL
% of total PDs	1976	11%	69%	20%	61 PDs
	1984	66%	34%		148 PDs
Nursing h/patient	1976	11.71 ± 0.6	19.1 ± 3.3	26.0 ± 1.4	19.6 ± 4.8
	1984	10.2 ± 1.4	14.9 ± 2.4		11.9 ± 3.0
TISS	1976	16.1 ± 2.9	26.8 ± 6.5	36.6 ± 3.3	27.6 ± 7.9
	1984	19.0 ± 6.7	32.6 ± 9.6		23.9 ± 10.2
APACHE II	1976	12.4 ± 4.9	12.5 ± 4.9	16.0 ± 2.7	11.9 ± 5.2
	1984	11.5 ± 5.96	18.3 ± 8.7		13.7 ± 8.3

PDs, patient days.

We had been able to effect a major reduction in the average number of nursing hours per patient per class and a redistribution of patients from the classes consuming a large number of nursing hours to the lowest category (see Table 3-3). The effect on overall ICU function was to increase the number of PDs provided by 30% at a 10% increase in costs and an 8% increase in FTEs (Table 3-4). The major shifts in the distribution of patients according to class are most dramatically illustrated by the increase from 11% to 66% of patients now in class 1, requiring less than 12 hours of nursing care per PD, and the complete elimination of the patients requiring more than 24 hours of nursing care. No difference occurred in mean APACHE II or TISS scores between the 2 years, nor was there a significant difference in mortality. We infer that our overall patient population remained the same, at least as judged by the physician's perception of the degree of illness and therapy, physiologic status on admission, and outcome. Thus, we have achieved an increased productivity and efficiency of nursing care by collaborative practice change, which directed the elimination of nonessential but previously "required" tasks. Most of the eliminations were outgrowths of our unit's parochialism or arbitrary (often published) standards, also based on opinion rather than data, which had become cemented into our daily practice, enforced unfailingly on each entering new physician or nurse but clearly amenable to study and modification.

Before physicians write orders for a patient in the ICU, they must first determine the patient's general and unique needs. An efficient method to determine needs is to classify the patient according to the primary objectives of ICU care: monitoring/observation; extensive nursing requirements; and constant medical care (Chap. 2).

We must restrict the allocation of nursing care in the monitoring/observation patients so that these patients can continue to receive this necessary quantum of care in the ICU but not waste resources by too many routine orders. Patients who need extensive ICU nursing care are stable physiologically, and physicians need to curtail their enthusiasm for long lists of orders for completeness or other perceived reasons; because they are stable physiologically, their needs will be met by independent nursing functions. In the case of the patient who is physiologically unstable and requires constant physician attention, the nursing care engendered will be voluminous and contain both dependent

(orders and interventions) as well as independent nursing interventions.

ORDERS FOR PATIENT MONITORING AND OBSERVATION

The monitoring/observation class generally consists of patients who are admitted to the ICU usually for 1 day and ultimately survive. In our ICU, these patients typically need less than 12 hours of care in a 24-hour period and, therefore, can easily be "doubled" with a more demanding patient for the nursing assignment.[10] These patients are primarily elderly patients undergoing major elective surgery with a known risk of postoperative complications and often have many risk factors such as preexisting cardiovascular disease, chronic obstructive lung disease, or diabetes mellitus.[17] These high-risk patients are at risk to develop potentially devastating complications that cannot be cared for on a general ward.[17–19] They are often admitted to the ICU preoperatively, primarily for invasive hemodynamic monitoring and then, postoperatively, for observation and anticipatory care. If we remember this need and restrict other activity and laboratory testing, these patients can be cared for properly and efficiently. They represented about 30% of the patients but consume only 6% of the total PDs in our study.[16] Our nursing protocol covers assessment of physiologic stability: vital signs, measurements from invasive monitoring devices, temperatures, and surveillance measures. Values are obtained on admission but then *the interval between measurements is rapidly and progressively lengthened.* Table 3-5 outlines our current vital signs/measurements protocol. We quickly realized that observation *alone* of these physiologic parameters, mostly displayed continuously, was adequate *unless* changes occurred, at which time *recording* would be performed as well. Recording can usually be advanced to every 4 hours within 4 to 8 hours. Orders can specify the alarms for whatever monitoring devices are in use (see Table 3-5). Limits should be chosen by combining knowledge of the individual patient's physiologic status with the range for normal values. Thus, they serve as early warning systems or surveillance devices to signal change to the nurse and physician. No orders need to be written for calibration in most ICUs because the procedures are part of nursing standards.

Fluid intake in parenteral or enteral form also is recorded in a manner designed to reduce repetitive, inefficient—and potentially inaccurate—charting. Each individual site of infusion is assigned a column and the rate as well as total solution infused are recorded once per nursing shift (every 12 hours) unless the rate or type of solution changes (Fig. 3-2). To indicate when a new container of infusate is begun, an arrow is placed in that column, and the initial volume is entered. The total for each fluid infused is calculated by multiplying the hours of infusion times the rate (usual products for common rates are quickly learned), and the grand total is calculated by cross-adding all column totals. This is recorded once a shift. The amount of urine output is *observed* while in the collection chamber of a urometer or on the display of an electronic device every 1 to 2 hours but measured and recorded hourly only if the amount is near

TABLE 3-4. Comparison of Patient Populations and Nursing Care

	1976	1984
Total nursing h/patient	19.6 ± 4.8	11.9 ± 3*
TISS	27.6 ± 7.9	23.9 ± 10.2
APACHE II	11.9 ± 5.2	13.7 ± 8.3
Deaths	6(46%)	17(26%)
Labor costs ($)	994,358	1,102,642
Patient days	2431	3152

*Significant difference $p < 0.05$.

TABLE 3-5. Vital Sign/Measurement Protocol°

VARIABLE	FREQUENCY
NONINVASIVE	
Apical heart rate/rhythm	q 15 min × 4 → q 30
Respiratory rate/quality	min × 2 →
Peripheral pulse oximetry (arterial oxygen saturation)	→ q 1 hr × 1–2 h → q 4 h
Temperature: rectal, rectal probe, PA, or bladder	q 1–2 h if abnormal; otherwise q 4 h
Cuff blood pressure	On admission or when questioned or when arterial catheter questioned
INVASIVE	
Mean arterial pressure	
Systolic/diastolic arterial pressure	
PA mean pressure	As above: rapidly
PA occlusion pressure	advance if patient
Central venous pressure	stable
Intracranial pressure	
PA mixed venous O_2 saturation	

PA, pulmonary artery; q, every.

°Alarms for each patient's predicted and acceptable variability can be set to provide constant surveillance with the exception of the following intermittent measurements: cuff blood pressure, rectal and PA temperature, and PA occlusion pressure.

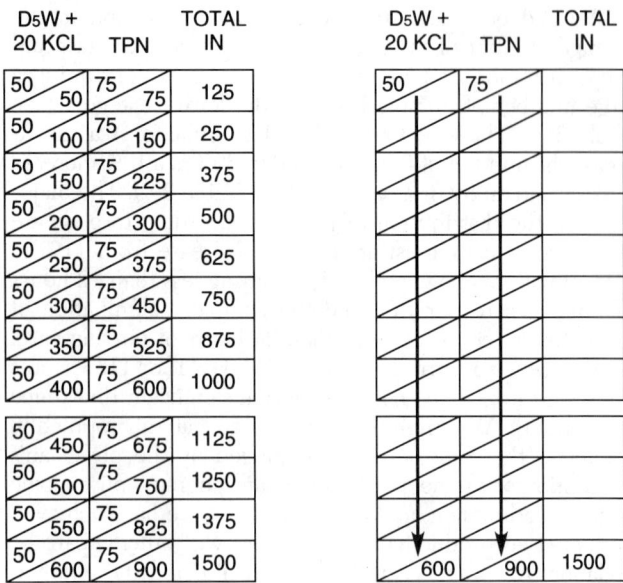

FIGURE 3-2. Comparison of the recording of IV intake. We previously kept hourly linear and cumulative totals, never used by either nurses or physicians in stable patients. We agreed to record the rate and use an arrow to indicate the hours at that rate. In these examples, 60 entries and 34 calculations were replaced by 5 entries and 1 calculation. The information contained is the same. The hour-by-hour totals can be calculated, if need be (although need never seems to be). The 55 omitted entries and 33 unnecessary calculations were only possibilities for error. D_5W, 5% dextrose in water; KCL, potassium chloride; TPN, total parenteral nutrition; TOTAL IN, total intake.

or below the unit's "worry" limit (e.g., 50 mL/hour or 0.5 mL/kg). Urine volume is *recorded* every 4 hours for most patients to even once per shift when there are no actual or anticipated problems. All other fluid outputs such as gastric secretions and fluid from surgically placed drains are measured and recorded every 12 hours, although observation alone is more frequent (Fig. 3-3). The nurses cross-check each other's intake and output *totals* at the end of each shift and initial the flow sheet to prevent errors.

Routine respiratory care of the monitoring/observation patient should include auscultation and recording of breath sounds. Suction of the endotracheal tube may be done on admission but is usually done only when necessary because of accumulated or excessive secretions. If the patient appears hypoxemic or hyercapnic, the chest is auscultated. Incentive spirometry and coughing are taught to the patient and provided every 4 hours. We no longer use prophylactic chest physiotherapy or routine suctioning, again, shortening the list of older standing orders.

Most ICUs have defined protocols for the dressings used for invasive monitoring devices, other apparatus, and wounds. These protocols, although differing to some degree, are usually formulated from general published guidelines or the policies of the hospital infection control and ICU committees. Needless to say, each new fellow or resident need not waste time or ink in writing his or her own preferences. Hygienic measures, which include a bath, mouth care,

Foley catheter care, back or skin care, comfort measures, and cleaning the incontinent patient are all, we believe, independent nursing functions and do not require written orders. Mobilization or activity is begun by turning and positioning the patient from side to side every 2 hours and performing range of motion exercises every 12 hours. Ambulation is usually done in collaboration with the physician as soon as possible (both in terms of orders and help!).

In summary, then, the physician's orders for the monitoring/observation patient should include the following: each—and only—specific laboratory test used to detect an expected complication, for example, a hematocrit to detect suspected hemorrhage; orders to wean ventilatory support and extubate as well as for any arterial blood gas required; alarm limits for continuous monitoring devices and ranges for clinically monitored parameters; intravenous fluid therapy; changes in the basic regimen while the patient's physiologic condition changes (e.g., an order for a fluid bolus if the physician suspects hypovolemia); and medications.

ORDERS FOR PATIENTS WITH EXTENSIVE NURSING REQUIREMENTS

These patients are stable physiologically but consume more nursing care hours than those in the monitoring/observation class. Interventions for specific problems related to length of stay have become an important priority. In this group of

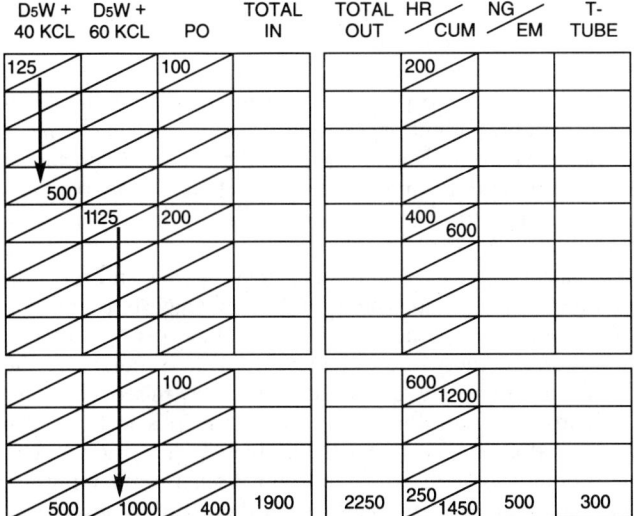

FIGURE 3-3. Intake and output according to the described simplifications. Only the essential information is included. In stable patients, urine volumes are measured only intermittently, although hourly observation is continued. Tube drainages are measured only once each shift unless volumes are large or unless total intake and output figures should be calculated more frequently in the rare patient with clinical instability justifying more detail. D₅W, 5% dextrose in water; KCL, potassium chloride; PO, oral intake; TOTAL IN, total intake; TOTAL OUT, total output; HR/CUM, hourly/cumulative output; NG/EM, nasogastric emesis output.

patients with extensive nursing requirements, these interventions are focused on the following major areas: (1) general skin integrity, (2) muscle and joint mobility, (3) patient hygiene, (4) decreased patient resistance to infection, and (5) patient safety. Problems may occur in each of these areas that prolong general hospital stay, for example, a nosocomial pneumonia or a decubitus ulcer, which places even more economic stress on the health care system. The uncertainty of patient outcome or survival has also generated another area for nursing assessment and intervention.

Clinical examples of patients in this class include a former monitoring/observation patient who has developed complications such as infection or failure of one or more organ systems; the long-term patient with multitrauma; or a readmission to the ICU for treatment of complications. The role of physician orders is primarily anticipatory. Some clinical examples include assessment and treatment of the malnourished state; detection and treatment of the sources of infection; detection and treatment of organ systems failure; and ventilatory support. Specific orders could include adjustments in the composition or rate of parenteral nutrition infusion; a directed evaluation for fever; chest physiotherapy every 6 hours for a specific abnormality (i.e., an atelectatic right upper lobe); an order for a 2-hour urine creatinine clearance to evaluate suspected renal dysfunction; and an order for an increase in the level of positive end-expiratory pressure with subsequent physiologic evaluation in a patient with respiratory failure.

The nursing role in this class is more than extensive in just a temporal sense; it is independent, involving the active

treatment of current problems and active prevention of further complications. Because these patients are reasonably stable physiologically, vital signs and measurements need only be recorded every 2 to 4 hours, using observation and the assistance from the monitoring alarms as in the monitoring/observation group. Sudden elevation in temperature is a common occurrence. Continuous core temperature can be measured by pulmonary artery catheter or special Foley catheters to eliminate the frequent manual measurement of rectal temperatures to detect elevations or while cooling the patient.

Respiratory care of these patients is essentially the same, although because of a higher prevalence of moderate respiratory failure and pulmonary secretions, auscultation of breath sounds because of suspected hypoxemia, indicated endotracheal suctioning for secretions, and the assessment of the effectiveness of bronchodilator therapy are more frequent. Intake and output procedures are also handled in a similar manner to the monitoring/observation patient. More infusions or more complicated drainage systems, generating some of the increased nursing care, result in the patient's classification in extensive nursing care.

Hygiene and daily care activities such as the dressing changes are the same as those previously described; however, these interventions become of higher priority and are time consuming. Mobilization and ambulation may be especially difficult in the patient with complicated wounds and many tubes, and especially if the patient is weakened by a long illness, this category is a high priority for care and consumes considerable time.

In the area of general skin care, preventive assessment as well as active early intervention into specific problems are the keys (Chap. 154). Full range of active and passive motion exercises should be begun as soon as a patient is physiologically stable and subsequently performed every 12 hours. The patient and family should be involved whenever possible. ICU patients have generalized as well as specific loss of muscle tone progressing to muscle atrophy, especially those who are long term (greater than 1 week). A physical therapy consult may be of particular value when long-term care is anticipated or exists. The patient can be systematically evaluated for mobility deficits and muscle and joint deterioration, and suggestions can be made for treatment; all of these can be incorporated into the nursing care plan, but the therapist will add to limited nursing care resources by actually performing a complete set of exercises each day and will also reinforce proper exercise technique for the staff. Problems that might require further hospital stay in a rehabilitation center may be avoided or ameliorated.

Decreased resistance to infection is the third area that requires increased attention to prevent, ameliorate, or decrease the incidence of nosocomial infection. An urgent need exists for strict adherence to the Centers for Disease Control guidelines for handwashing and asepsis in the ICU, for example, sterile dressing changes (Chap. 34). Nurses must be especially careful when handling invasive devices such as urinary catheters, intravenous and intraarterial catheters, endotracheal or tracheostomy tubes, and intracranial pressure tubes and while providing scrupulous wound care. The nurse must also monitor the patient for the signs and symptoms of the following nosocomial infections: pneumonia, tracheobronchitis, intravascular device–related bacteremia, urinary tract infection, sinusitis, and wound infection. Surveillance for infection should include assessment for the following: fever and fever patterns when present; increase in the white blood cell count; increase in amount or change in color or odor of pulmonary secretions; a regional decrease in breath sounds or the appearance of adventitious sounds; appearance of sediment in the urine or complaint of bladder spasms; erythema or purulence at a site of intravascular catheterization; a wound, or a site of skin breakdown; and the results of any cultures sent to the laboratory. When infection is diagnosed by the ICU team and treatment is instituted, the nurse must administer much of the treatment (antibiotics), monitor the patient's response to treatment (improvement in wound healing or serum antibiotic levels), and alleviate or reduce symptoms such as fever.

Proper infusion protocols should be developed for parenteral and enteral nutrition as well as guidelines for monitoring the side effects of therapy. Both types should be delivered by pump to ensure accurate delivery rates, save nursing time, and decrease infusion rate–related side effects. Complications of parenteral therapy may include hypoglycemia, hyperglycemia, glycosuria, and intravascular device–related infection. Aspiration and diarrhea are the most frequent problems associated with enteral alimentation and are more prevalent in patients with a decreased level of consciousness or who are restricted to bedrest. The team should first ascertain correct feeding tube placement. The nurse can place a small amount of food coloring in the tube feeding (5 mL of coloring per 500 mL of feeding) to differentiate it from pulmonary secretions; measure residual volumes every 4 hours; elevate the patient's back; assess for bowel sounds and abdominal distention; maintain the correct and a constant infusion rate; and provide management and treatment of diarrhea or fecal impaction.

Patient safety is related to the following factors: alcohol or drug abuse and the attendant potential for substance withdrawal; an increasingly elderly ICU population with a propensity for falls; and the increase in the prevalence of serious head injury with improved patient transport and resuscitation. A neurologic assessment should be performed routinely every 12 hours on all patients and, with evidence of head injury, the frequency should increase to match the frequency of vital sign assessment. Patient history should be obtained from the family if the patient is unable to cooperate. This assessment should include reorientation to current surroundings and status as necessary. Promotion of patient safety should include the following measures: elevated side rails; low bed height when the nurse is away from the bedside; adequate sedation for pain or substance withdrawal; and limb restraints as necessary in the presence of patient agitation, disorientation, or hallucinations to prevent self-injury. All aberrant patient behavior, nursing intervention, and patient response to treatment should be documented. JCAHO regulations necessitate a physician's order for restraints. In addition, a note must be written in the progress note listing what measures had been used unsuccessfully and the reason for the restraints. The order must specify the type of restraints and a time limit, no more than 72

hours. Nurses must document the use of restraints and assessments of patient safety.

Uncertain patient outcome or survival is the final area of focus in this group of patients. Particularly for the long-term patient, patient and family teaching and involvement in patient care and planning is of the utmost importance. Consistent and frequent communication of the patient's plan of care and the patient's response to therapy must be undertaken. *Early* referral to available support services (e.g., religious, language interpreters, social service, and rehabilitation counselors) and incorporation of suggested interventions into the nursing plan of care alleviates patient and family stress. Increasing the amount of time spent with the family in answering questions, dispelling misconceptions, and providing comfort and caring functions is time well spent and is beneficial to the family as well as the nurse.

Although patient education and discharge planning are a part of the routine nursing care of the monitoring/observation patient, this category assumes much more importance in the extensive nursing requirement patient because of the longer ICU stay. Particular emphasis is placed on procedures in which the patient can be an active participant. Discharge planning that involves people from other services, such as the nutritional support team or the social worker, are begun as soon as possible.

In general, the need for nursing care in this category still is less than 12 hours per PD, but more than needed for the monitoring/observation patient. A 1:2 nurse:patient ratio can be used; this assignment, however, may approach the limit of 24 hours of care per PD, and the nurse may need support as well as assistance from the physician, the charge nurse, and ancillary personnel.

ORDERS FOR PATIENTS NEEDING CONSTANT PHYSICIAN CARE

The constant physician care group requires intensive intervention from the physician and the nurse. Examples of these patients include a multisystem trauma victim with multiple physiologic abnormalities, or an emergency admission for liver transplant or the adult respiratory distress syndrome. The nursing hours required by these patients range from 13 to 24 hours. Although the nurse–patient ratio generally remains 1:2, for this to succeed, an attempt must be made to pair this patient with one requiring minimal care. If this is not possible, if there is no "light" or stable patient, a 1:1 ratio is necessary.

The vital signs and measurements for these patients may be done hourly or more often if changes are occurring rapidly; however, the frequency may be decreased when physiologic stability is achieved. Again, this assessment of stability and observation in place of continued rote recording can reduce the total number of nursing hours expended.

Although the remaining nursing protocols for the constant physician care patients are similar to those already described, the instability of the patient, resulting in more and different interventions, increases the frequency and complexity of nursing care. While the need for dependent role functions increases (response to orders for medications), so, too, does the independent nursing function. The unstable patient requires a multiperspective assessment to avoid critical oversights. These patients generate the most written orders by the physician, most of which are related to changing interventions necessary to achieve physiologic stability, such as the type and rate of vasoactive infusions and testing necessary to evaluate the cause of the patient's problems, such as a chest radiograph to rule out pneumothorax.

To summarize, the physician must create general orders as in the previous categories. The physiologic instability that results in constant attention creates specific orders. Although these patients receive the largest number of nursing care hours, careful clinical decision-making and information processing resulting in excellent chart documentation brings order to potential chaos and improves the likelihood of successful outcome. Harmonious interaction within the ICU team is a decidedly positive side effect. The physician, instead of believing that the length of the order sheet is a good reflection of the thoroughness and ultimate value of medical care, can learn that writing orders may confuse activity with productivity.

REFERENCES ■

1. Weiss SJ, Davis HP: Validity and reliability of the collaborative practice scales. *Nurs Res* 1985;34:299
2. Greenburg AG, Civetta JM, Barnhill GW: Neglected components of intensive care. *J Surg Res* 1979;26:494
3. Gottlieb L, Rowat K: The McGill model of nursing: a practice-derived model. *Adv Nurs Sci* 1987;9:51
4. Morgan A, Daly C, Murawski B: Dollar and human costs of intensive care. *J Surg Res* 1973;14:441
5. McKibbin RC, Brimmer PF, Galliher JM, et al: Nursing costs and DRG payments. *Am J Nursing* 1985;12:1353
6. Schroeder RE, Rhodes AM, Shields RE: Nurse acuity systems: cash vs. grasp (a determination of nurse staff requirements). *Nurs Forum* 1984;21:72
7. Cullen DJ: Surgical intensive care: current perceptions and problems. *Crit Care Med* 1981;9:2905
8. Civetta JM, Hudson-Civetta JA: Maintaining quality of care while reducing charges in the ICU: 10 ways. *Ann Surg* 1985;202:524
9. Cullen DJ, Civetta JM, Briggs BA, et al: Therapeutic intervention scoring system: a method for quantitative comparison of patient care. *Crit Care Med* 1974;2:57
10. Dossey BM: The nursing process. In: Kenner CV, Guzzetta CE, Dossey BM (eds). *Critical Care Nursing: Body–Mind–Spirit*. Boston, Little, Brown, 1981
11. Sullivan S, Breu C: Survey of critical care nursing practice. IV. Staffing and training of intensive care unit personnel. *Heart Lung* 1982;11:237
12. Hudson J, Caruthers T, Lantiegne K: Intensive care nursing requirements: resource allocation according to patient status. *Crit Care Med* 1979;7:69
13. Hudson-Civetta JA, Civetta JM, Weppler D, et al: Improved nursing efficiency and productivity. *Crit Care Med* 1987;15:351
14. Knaus WA, Draper EA, Wagner DP, et al: APACHE II: a severity of disease classification system. *Crit Care Med* 1985;13:818
15. Knaus WA, Wagner DP, Loirat P, et al: A comparison of intensive care in the U.S.A and France. *Lancet* 1982;ii:642
16. Civetta JM: The inverse relationship between cost and survival. *J Surg Res* 1973;14:265
17. Civetta JM, Hudson-Civetta JA: Cost effective use of the ICU. In: Eiseman B (ed). *Cost Effectiveness in Surgery*. Philadelphia, WB Saunders, 1987:13
18. Critical Care Medicine, Consensus Development Conference Summary. Washington, DC, National Institutes of Health, 1983;4(6)
19. Civetta JM, Hudson-Civetta J, Nelson LD: Costly care: data, problems, and proposing remedies. *Crit Care Med* 1986;14:357

Critical Care, Third Edition, edited by Joseph M. Civetta,
Robert W. Taylor, and Robert R. Kirby.
Lippincott-Raven Publishers, Philadelphia, PA © 1997.

CHAPTER 4

Clinical Decision-Making

David V. Shatz
Joseph M. Civetta

Our earliest exposure to clinical decision-making probably occurs when we are taught as medical students to construct a differential diagnosis at the end of the initial history and physical examination. At that time, the quality of our efforts was often judged by the length of the list—a superficial, quantitative index. Thereafter, learning the prevalence of disease states, we might have prioritized our list in terms of the frequency of occurrence. Although frequency is important, in certain "crisis" situations in the intensive care unit (ICU), reversibility (especially with mechanical problems) must be placed at the top of the list. For example, hypoxemia caused by a disconnected ventilator can—and must be—rapidly reversed if detected; the disconnected ventilator will be detected in time only if it heads the list of possibilities.

Clinical decision-making must be a process of many steps based on elements gathered over time. Some of the information must be gleaned from the past, providing the basis of decisions made in the present and forming the framework for plans for the future. The process can be viewed from separate vantage points during the passage of time to assess the objectives of therapy and the results attained. Reevaluations are necessary and desirable as the perception of the patient's illness evolves, resulting in realistic appraisals at each succeeding stage. These two determinants of decision-making coalesce to form a continuously changing perception in the mind of the clinician. Elements are added and deleted, augmented and subtracted, weighted or discounted, appreciated or unrecognized, or incorrectly assessed. No wonder, in this ever-changing and poorly delineated process, we consider clinical decision-making to be a part of the art of medicine, which seems to relieve it (and us) of the necessity to be scientific.

This viewpoint has been examined elegantly by Alvin Feinstein in his monograph *Clinical Judgment*.[1] It is proba-

bly the most comprehensive examination of the subject and extraordinarily revealing in terms of the description of the problem and solutions. Feinstein has painstakingly examined many myths, dispelled them unerringly, and replaced them with logical scientific alternatives, over 100 years old but largely unknown in clinical medicine. He begins by pointing out that the method of clinical judgment is not reproducible and so, "we have been taught to call it 'art' and to consign its intellectual aspects to some mystic realm of intuition that was 'unworthy' of scientific attention because it was used for the practical every day work of clinical care." Modern clinicians concerned with laboratory investigations of pathogenesis or mechanisms of cellular biology believe that the problems of clinical therapy are a mere application of basic science to clinical care. Behind this dismissal, according to Feinstein, is the traditional belief that the therapeutic aspects of medicine can never be "a science" and that clinical judgment can never be "scientific": "The personal environmental management of the patient is a challenge to the clinician's judgment as a humanistic healer. Treatment of the patient is a challenge to the clinician's judgment as an experimental scientist."

The argument about whether clinical medicine is an art or a science is often ended by partitioning the whole into two parts: one, called *art*, is the clinical portion done at the bedside; the other, called *science*, is done in the laboratory. We have seemed to accept the current fashion of making the words *research* and *science* synonymous with laboratory activity, whereas the words *healing* and *art* are reserved for bedside care.[2] There is nothing scientifically shameful in the label of art. There is science in art, such as the combination of selected colors to make specific shade, the angles of spatial perspective, and the timing of each measure in music or selection of proper notes to fit the range of specific instruments. There is also art in science: the intuition that converts serendipity into insight and the aesthetic taste that brings elegance to creation, execution, evaluation, and communication of experiments. Art and science may differ, not in perception, wisdom, imagination, and discipline, but in the type, verification, arrangement, preservation, and reproducibility of the raw material. Without intuition, imagination, or aesthetics, the scientist is a dullard. Without rationality, discipline, or logic, the artist is a doodler, concludes Feinstein.[2]

CLINICAL DATA AS SCIENTIFIC VARIABLES ■

We must remember that to obtain the data and preserve the humanistic tradition of clinical medicine, the patient must be examined artfully while, simultaneously, to satisfy the exacting requirements that data and therapy must fulfill in modern science, the patient must be examined scientifically. Clinical medicine is more than analysis, dissection, and division; rather, the clinician deals with a synthesis of the whole organism and all of its properties and variations. "Of all man's activities, clinical medicine is the most scientific art and the most humanistic science. The art and science are intermingled, symbiotic, and inseparable. Without the art there can be no data for the science. Without the science there can be no reason for the art."[3]

CARDIOPULMONARY RESUSCITATION AND DO-NOT-RESUSCITATE ORDERS ■

In 1960, Kouwenhoven and associates[4] reported the use of closed chest cardiac massage in patients who had cardiac arrest. The overall survival rate was 70% (Fig. 4-1). By negation, cardiopulmonary resuscitation (CPR) and nonsurvival represents 30%. Recently, the survival rate for CPR prac-

RECENT REPORTS:

ALL CARDIAC ARRESTS REPORTED

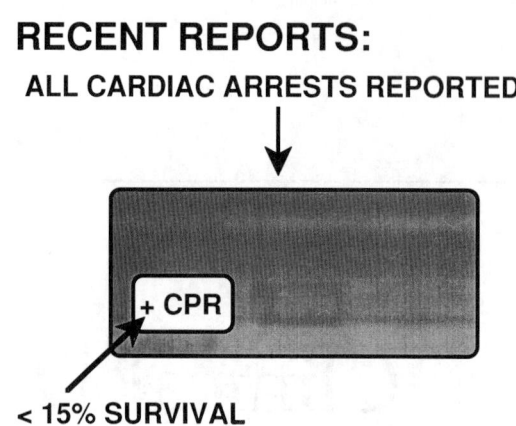

< 15% SURVIVAL

FIGURE 4-2. Using the same definitions, the set of patients who survived CPR reported in many recent series is seen to be much smaller and corresponds to the rectangle labeled less than 15% survival.

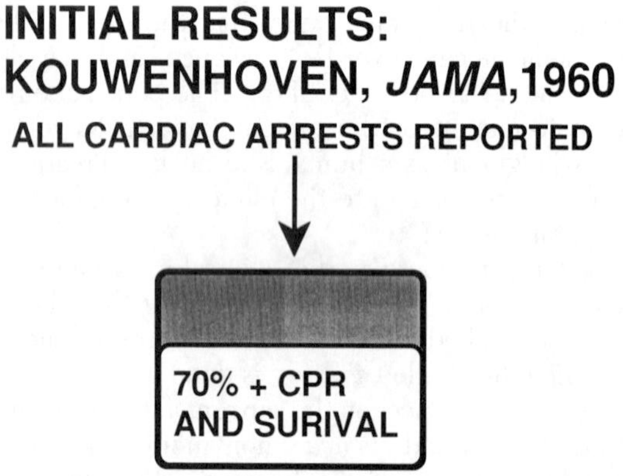

ticed on any hospitalized patient is more likely to be less than 15%[5] (Fig. 4-2). Kouwenhoven's initial results appeared to be far better at first glance. However, this may not be the case, because the universe of patients to be considered for CPR may have been defined differently.

If we try to classify the successes in Kouwenhoven's initial study, we can divide them (for this discussion) into three subsets or groups (Fig. 4-3). Group 1 had an acute electrical event such as ventricular fibrillation that occurred after a myocardial infarction. Group 2 had an electrical event without myocardial infarction. In many of the studies of CPR performed outside of the hospital by emergency medical services, up to 50% of patients with ventricular fibrillation who are subsequently resuscitated have no evidence of a myocardial infarction. One may postulate a third group with some other disease or event initiating the cardiac arrest. Using Venn diagrams, we can analyze patients with myocardial infarctions (Fig. 4-4). Subset 1 represents patients who

INITIAL RESULTS: KOUWENHOVEN, *JAMA*,1960

ALL CARDIAC ARRESTS REPORTED

70% + CPR AND SURIVAL

FIGURE 4-1. Venn diagram of the initial results reported by Kouwenhoven and associates[4] of all the patients considered to have a cardiac arrest and in whom cardiopulmonary resuscitation (CPR) was rendered: 70% survived. Thus, the outside rectangle represents the set of all patients who were given CPR, and the white smaller rectangle represents the 70% who survived.

ALL CARDIAC ARRESTS REPORTED

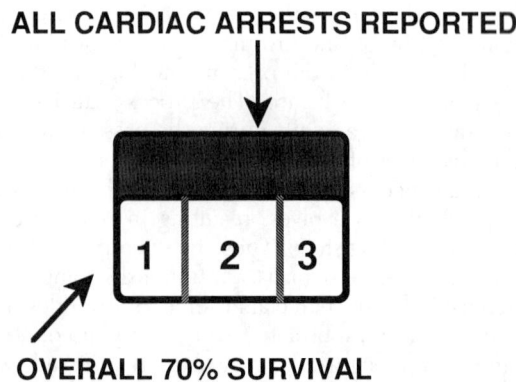

OVERALL 70% SURVIVAL

FIGURE 4-3. In this Venn diagram, the 70% of the patients who were subjected to CPR and survived is divided into three smaller subsets: subset 1 represents patients who had cardiac arrest and myocardial infarction; subset 2 represents patients who had an electrical event precipitating cardiac arrest; and subset 3 represents all other patients who had a cardiac arrest, CPR, and survived.

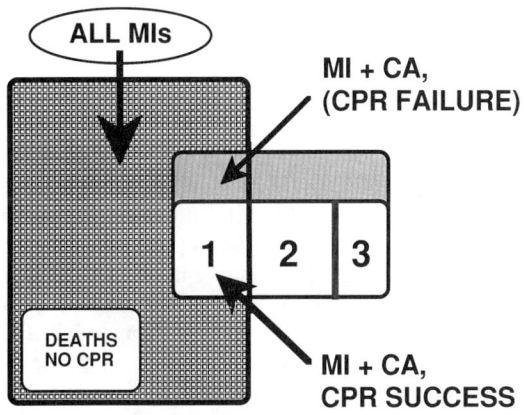

FIGURE 4-4. A Venn diagram of all patients with myocardial infarctions (MIs), depicted as the rectangle in squares. Some patients had a cardiac arrest (CA) and received CPR. The light stippled area represents patients who were not resuscitated, whereas the white subset 1 represents patients with a myocardial infarction and cardiac arrest who survived after CPR. Other patients who had myocardial infarctions died and did not receive CPR. They are depicted in the white subset in the left lower corner.

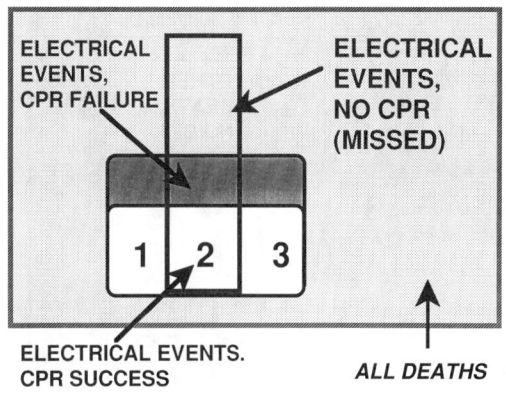

FIGURE 4-5. A description of the patients who had electrical events. Subset 2 represents patients who had CPR and survived. The dark stippled area depicts patients who had an electrical event not associated with a myocardial infarction and then received CPR but were not resuscitated. The group of patients who had electrical events but were not diagnosed is represented as the light stippled area. Because they were not diagnosed and CPR was not administered, several patients might have been saved. They are now a subset of the large stippled area representing all patients who died.

had a cardiac arrest associated with an electrical event, who received CPR and were successfully resuscitated. Another group, represented by the lightly stippled area, also had a myocardial infarction and cardiac arrest and received CPR, but were not resuscitated. These two groups make up only a small percentage of all patients with myocardial infarctions seen by the set marked in squares. In addition, another group of patients exists who died without CPR, seen in the lower left corner. One could make this more complicated by identifying subsets of patients with hypotension, pulmonary edema, cardiogenic shock, and so forth. Continuing our description of the process that resulted in the concern that CPR currently is less successful than when initially described, we examine group 2, which contains patients who were successfully resuscitated after electrical events (Fig. 4-5). In addition to these patients are patients who also had electrical events and CPR but were not successfully resuscitated, seen in the lightly stippled area. Finally, there is another group of patients who had a cardiac arrest resulting from an undiagnosed electrical event, so that the patients did not receive CPR. These patients became a subset of all deaths but not of patients who received CPR and would not be reported in the outcome of any study of the effectiveness of CPR. In a similar fashion, we can examine the other sets to which patients in group 3 belong. These patients are defined as those who were successfully resuscitated after cardiac arrest but did not have either an isolated electrical event or a myocardial infarction. Another group of patients satisfied the conditions of other causes and received CPR but were not successfully resuscitated; this is seen in the striped area. In addition are many patients (wavy areas) who died without having received CPR. Even among hospitalized patients, CPR is not universally performed[5] (Fig. 4-6).

However, the crucial logical failing that has resulted in the low success rate can be seen in Figure 4-7. Patients with

cardiac arrest are depicted in the center in the white set labeled *CPR success* (subdivided into groups 1, 2, and 3, as discussed earlier) and the three striped sets linearly displayed above the CPR success group. These represent the 30% of patients described in Kouwenhoven's original article who had a cardiac arrest, had CPR, but were not resuscitated. If we accept, for the sake of argument, that these six subsets, three of success and three of failure, represent all of the patients who *should be considered to have had a cardiac arrest and should be considered for CPR, the "problem" of only a 15% success rate today becomes revealed as a nonproblem.* For instance, in many ICUs, many patients have multiple organ system failure (MOSF), the conjoined set of the sets labeled 1 and 2 in Figure 4-7. Subset 1 represents patients with MOSF who die, whereas subset 2 represents patients who survive (remember, the size of a set depicted in the Venn diagram does not refer to a quantity but only to a specific quality). What has been depicted is that patients with MOSF who die represent a subset of other deaths who do not receive CPR (appropriately). Subset 1 does not intersect with the striped area and the clear area, which represent patients who truly had a cardiac arrest, some of whom were successfully resuscitated and the others who were not. Had we recognized that CPR is a technique to be applied only to patients who have had a cardiac arrest, we, as clinicians, could have forestalled all of the problems that have arisen from the indiscriminate application of a technique to a group of patients who did not have the necessary antecedent (true cardiac arrest). Thus, CPR should not be applied to all patients whose heart has stopped, because many of those patients are appropriately classified as patients who *die* rather than having had a *cardiac arrest.* Our failure to use the therapy for the specific group of patients with the appropriate antecedent has resulted in significant suffering for patients and families, wasted resources, supposed

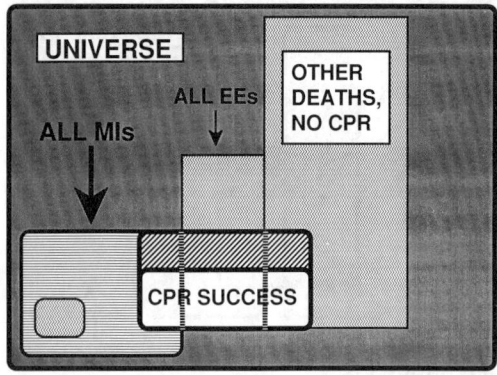

FIGURE 4-6. The Venn diagrams get increasingly complicated, but this level of complexity is necessary to understand the current dilemma in applying CPR to the wrong patients. The wavy areas represent patients who die without receiving CPR. Notice that the central area labeled *CPR success* and the banded area immediately above it (*CPR failures*) encompass only a small percentage of the patients who died. Particularly important is the large rectangle to the right showing other deaths that did not receive CPR. Should CPR be given to patients who did not have an antecedent for successful resuscitation (subsets 1, 2, and 3), one would expect that the success rate would be extremely low. Indeed, CPR should be given only to patients who had a cardiac arrest. MIs, myocardial infarctions; EEs, electrical events.

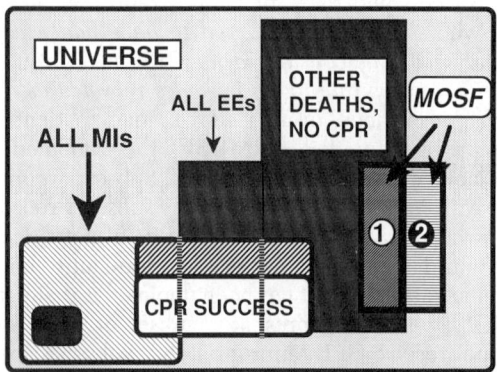

FIGURE 4-7. A Venn diagram placing patients with multiple organ system failure (MOSF) in the perspective that they should not be subjected to CPR. In doing so, subsets 1 and 2 represent all patients with MOSF. Patients in subset 1 died and patients in subset 2 survived. Notice there is no intersection of subset 1 with the striped and clear areas representing patients who had a cardiac arrest. Because no intersection occurs, patients who have MOSF die rather than have a cardiac arrest. Had this distinction been recognized, no patient in this situation would have been subjected to CPR. By restricting CPR to patients who have a cardiac arrest and are appropriate candidates for CPR, the success rate will rise once again. In reality, this means that the therapeutic modality of CPR will not be used in patients who die. In this way, more societal goals will be satisfied, resources will be saved, and the results of CPR will be "improved." MIs, myocardial infarctions; EEs, electrical events.

"ethical dilemmas," and unnecessary legislation. Appropriate application of the technique might have substantiated Kouwenhoven's results.

Unfortunately, Kouwenhoven's 35-year-old data, coupled with the seemingly universal success of CPR in television drama, has adversely affected the lay public's perception of the success of CPR. Hence, the consensus of medical futility and the decision to withhold further life-support measures, including CPR, is frequently a difficult process for the physician and family members. Maintaining in one's mind the distinction of a dying heart versus one sustaining a arrhythmic cardiac arrest eases the decision process somewhat. Familiarity with survival probabilities nationally and at one's own institution further relieves the physician of the sense of guilt stemming from the concern of premature withdrawal or withholding of support. Ultimately, knowing the patients' desires for "heroic" efforts, or lack thereof, can further guide the physician's hand during the patient's terminal processes of life.[6,7] False perception of the true outcome prospects after CPR probably has led to the fact that upward of 90% of elderly patients in geriatric units favor CPR for themselves[8–11]; 20% to 45% of patients with such serious disabilities as coma or terminal illness similarly opt for CPR.[6,8–10,12–14] However, statistics show that elderly patients undergoing out-of-hospital CPR in cities with good emergency medical systems survive to hospital discharge in only 10% of cases.[15,16] Chronically ill patients have even less chance of survival to hospital discharge after CPR (less than 5%)[17–19] When properly educated as to the true outcome probabilities after CPR, half of elderly patients will opt to forgo CPR should they be faced with that situation.[20] In fact, of those older than 65 years of age, few want CPR if faced with an acute or chronic disease process.

The emotional and ethical concerns of a do-not-resuscitate order can be further relieved if a patient has a properly executed advance directive. To qualify for Medicare funds, hospitals must provide information to all patients on admission concerning advance directives and the hospital's policy toward them under Health Care Financing Administration regulations. Advance directives posing several different scenarios with variable outcome possibilities are often the best understood format (see Appendix in Chapter 2). And in the unfortunate event that no advance directive is available when the patient becomes incompetent to make decisions regarding future care, family members may be able to provide information under the principle of substituted judgment. However, it is not what the family member desires, but what the *patient* would want. Once again, this relieves the family of the guilt or burden of making the decision regarding withdrawal or withholding of life support.

ELEMENTS OF CLINICAL CARE

Analysis of clinical care distinguishes the following elements: the health care status of the patient; newly acquired diseases and complications; selection and sequencing of the diagnostic evaluation; an assessment of the likely effects of therapy; a clinical decision (identification of the problem and selection of therapy); short-term and long-term objectives; changes in the diagnosis and therapy influenced by acquisition of new information; and definition of outcome.

HEALTH CARE STATUS OF THE PATIENT

General demographic information such as sex, age, and other socioeconomic variables are available but have failed to provide insight into the management of a unique, individual patient. Usable knowledge concerning the impact of preexisting chronic disease states is at a rudimentary stage in intensive care. Although we know that an elderly patient with diabetes, hypertension, and arteriosclerosis may tolerate surgery poorly, we have not quantitated either the degree of functional impairment or the subsequent effect on total health status.[21,22] The qualitative assessments that are available may help in selecting patients for preoperative invasive monitoring.[23,24]

NEWLY ACQUIRED DISEASES AND COMPLICATIONS

The numerous scoring systems that have been devised and are discussed in Chapter 11 generally fail because of the undue reliance on mensuration. We must learn to describe symptoms, signs, diseases, and complications verbally rather than by measurement and to identify functional clusters of patients. Clinical manifestations and functions can be specific, distinct, and independent evidence of the total state of a patient. The reliance on statistical analyses based on mensuration, unfortunately, will continue to fail because the wrong yardsticks have been used. Only when the specific classifications, both pretherapeutically and posttherapeutically, have been created can we analyze these effects in such a way that we can predict outcome. Doing so is important because identifying the severity of disease is less important than identifying patients who will be the most challenging. Patients with the least severe disease will use few ICU resources, will survive, and cause no particular problems in identification, utilization of resources, or bioethical considerations. Patients who are most severely ill may be identified to test new forms of therapy to affect the high mortality rates inevitably present but, again, have little impact on overall ICU utilization, costs, or even bioethical considerations because the severity of the disease determines outcome in a relatively short period of time. The most difficult group to characterize comprises those who will ultimately spend long periods of time in the ICU, require careful identification of the disease and appropriate forms of therapy, and have an outcome that is in doubt for weeks to months at a time, thus creating problems in all of the spheres previously mentioned. Currently, we have identified these patients only retrospectively, and the challenge for predictive indices to describe diseases and complications is a formidable one.

SELECTION AND SEQUENCING OF THE DIAGNOSTIC EVALUATION

The number of potentially useful diagnostic tests is vast and ever-increasing. Particularly in intensive care, many of these tests may be used repetitively. Often the explosion of utilization has been glibly attributed to a better awareness of physi-

cians and nurses to use these tests of proven superiority to traditional history-taking and physical examination; however, the proper timing, sequence, and repetition of diagnostic testing have not been assessed by outcome criteria. Given the absence of scientific knowledge for selection of initial and subsequent laboratory testing, methods have been devised and tested to control laboratory testing.[25] Interestingly, more than half the tests could be eliminated in patients with the same severity of illness in the same proportions without affecting the time spent in the ICU or survival. These guidelines (Chap. 11) should encourage further scrutiny in the selection and sequencing of subsequent testing. In terms of efficiency, many tests are often selected initially. This removes the possibility of omission and may be justified to speed both diagnosis and management. It may be far cheaper and certainly faster to order a $50 specific laboratory test for all patients at the same time or in place of a cheaper screening test, even if half of the group would be eliminated by the screening test, *if* simultaneous testing could eliminate an extra day of ICU care in the other half. Thinking rather than behaving automatically is the key to eliminating unnecessary testing without creating unnecessary delays.

AN ASSESSMENT OF THE LIKELY EFFECTS OF THERAPY

We must constantly evaluate the possible forms of therapy in terms of the projected benefits and risks inherent in the therapy itself and as influenced by the patient's current health status and disease state. Perhaps of greater importance in the ICU is the distinction between "therapeutic" interventions and "manipulation." Therapy implies a chance for cure, which means evidence must link an improved outcome to the application of this remedy. For this reason, prospective randomized trials are considered to be a proper method of evaluating new forms of therapy. On the other hand, we might consider manipulation as the minute-to-minute response to abnormalities in physiologic variables based on a constant stated or unstated desire to return as many to the normal range in as short a period of time as possible (at least in time for morning rounds). Many of these unwritten orders are discernible as bedside habits that have no effect on outcome and result only in increased costs and poor utilization of nursing and laboratory personnel.

A CLINICAL DECISION

After assessing the patient's health status, recognizing newly acquired diseases or complications, selecting the proper diagnostic tests and their sequencing, and evaluating the potential forms of therapy, a discrete clinical decision is necessary. In fact, this decision, seemingly central and fundamental to care, is rarely evident in the medical record. Progress notes contain observations and data; rarely are impressions and judgments delineated clearly.[26] If the preceding four elements are analyzed and synthesized, the art of clinical decision-making will have been replaced, at least in part, by science. To the degree that this process has not been completed in the minds of the clinician, we may expect that the medical record lacks evidence of the decision-making. Conversely, we can view the current emphasis on adequate documentation as an additional force stimulating clinical decision-making.

SHORT- AND LONG-TERM OBJECTIVES

Identifying our expectations for treatment is important. We must also recognize that immediate objectives may be attained without the desired long-term effect. For instance, a patient in shock may be profoundly hypovolemic. Volume expansion is selected and implemented. The hypovolemia may be corrected and, indeed, cardiac function may improve. Much later, the patient may develop sepsis and die. The short-term objectives were correctly identified and attained through the process of clinical decision-making. The failure to achieve long-term success should not necessarily be construed as evidence of improper decision-making. Invasive monitoring has been criticized[27] because these important limiting interrelationships were not perceived. The failure to obtain a long-term objective should not be used as criticism of a technique that may only be directed at short-term objectives, such as improvement in cardiac function. The evolution of objectives is also part of the temporal framework of clinical decision-making.

ACQUISITION OF NEW INFORMATION

The changing nature of the decision-making process reflects the effects of diseases during evolution, changes created by the introduction of therapy, and the subsequent development of other complications. Thus, it is necessary to acquire new information and reassess the choice of diagnosis and the effects of therapy. The continually updated decision is also influenced by the passage of time and the selection of objectives appropriate to the evolved state of illness and response.

DEFINITION OF OUTCOME

Immediate results are gratifying but infrequent. Crises commonly reflect acute cardiorespiratory and oxygen transport problems. Clearly, initial success may not be sustained, and death may occur in the ICU or after discharge. An evaluation of long-term outcome, however, must form part of the process of initiating therapy, even in cases characterized as crises. In cases of cessation of cardiac activity, two immediate diagnoses are possible: cardiac arrest or death of the patient. If a judgment is made that the patient died, clearly, CPR would be inappropriate. We must incorporate long-term objectives into early decision-making.

Comprehending or formalizing the "benefits" of critical care is difficult at times. Survival in patients who otherwise would die is one, and a limited, criterion of evaluation. Patients may have improved quality of life, referenced to the state of acute illness and *not necessarily* the prior state of health. Life may be extended, but it may not be the same life expectancy as before the onset of the catastrophic illness. The benefit depends largely on the patient's perception of the value of the resulting quality and duration of life relative to that which was associated with the worst state in the ICU, not life before the onset of the illness.

We cannot delay current clinical decisions awaiting future improvements reflecting advances in the science of clinical judgment. Neither can we delay our own education in the foundations of the process, or the application of the knowledge so well developed in principle yet so poorly applied. Too often, under pressure to move forward to the next urgent case, we neglect to evaluate clinical judgment. Even mortality and morbidity conferences tend to focus on specifics rather than process. Clarity of understanding, improved communication, and better documentation in the medical record are immediate, obtainable objectives.

The decision-making can be summarized in terms of the stages of data collection involved in the processes of clinical judgment and informed consent (Fig. 4-8). Defining the iatrotrophic stimulus (the actual reason a patient seeks initial medical attention) is important because many patient values and variables result in patients seeking help at a particular time. Not all patients with a similar stage of a disease present at the same moment; as a result, information becomes available that is useful in dealing with the patient. The physician must then properly characterize these symptoms and signs with the emphasis on a careful, qualitative analysis that may then more clearly delineate the disease process. A second history is necessary to provide other needed details and to ascertain that features omitted are truly absent. The diagnosis may then be made and conveyed to the patient. The impact of this diagnosis should be carefully observed by the physician. An assessment of the reaction may help in judging how to proceed with presentation of further information and to help the patient comply with recommendations in the future. This information is then synthesized into a treatment plan. At this point, the patient's values should be explicitly explored and discussed because they reflect not only on a disease-oriented approach to therapy, but what is important to the patient. Subsequently, alternatives in therapy can be proposed and index variables selected for those particular targets of therapy of importance to the patient and physician. Having this information, the patient can, with our help, make

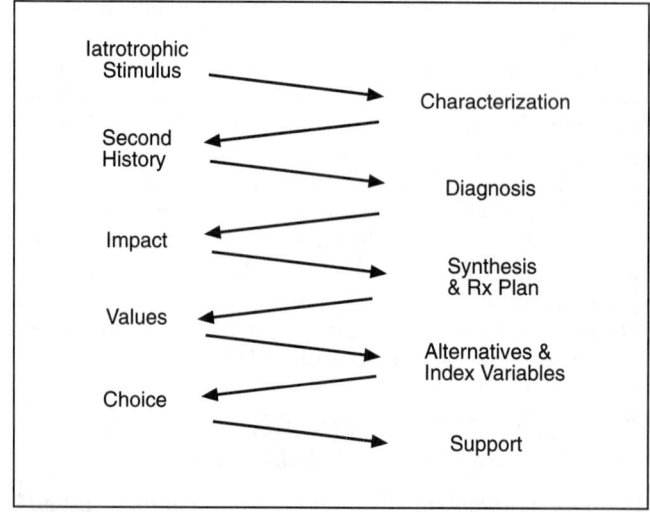

FIGURE 4-8. Stages of data collection involved in the processes of clinical judgment and informed consent. Rx, treatment.

a free, informed choice; and, finally, if we understand the iatrotrophic stimulus, have observed the impact of the diagnosis, have discussed the patient's values, and have heard the reasons for free choice, then we should be able to support the patient in all dimensions affected by the disease–patient interrelationships.

THE INFLUENCE OF TIME ■

Many methods have been proposed to assess severity of illness and risk of death or outcome variables such as sepsis or other complications. The groups studied include trauma patients, all ICU admissions, elective surgical candidates, patients scheduled for cancer surgery, and patients given a preoperative nutritional assessment. Parameters were found to be effective in prediction for each specific group of patients. Although it had been hoped that the vast mass of data, when subjected to proper statistical techniques in sufficient quantities, would quantify the degree of illness and predict the likelihood of recovery prospectively, these expectations have not been realized.[28] Many authors hoped that precise mathematical models could replace the uncertainties of clinical judgment; however, this prior uncertainty reflected that outcome is often determined by the unpredictable occurrence of catastrophic events, development of new illnesses or complications, iatrogenic events, and, especially, ultimate failure of organ systems functioning early in the patient's course. These same events must affect the reliability of all mathematical predictive systems. Refinements based on mensuration systems will only perpetuate the errors of the past and, by so doing, will inhibit new development using appropriate techniques.[29]

However, the predictive indices or scoring systems to extract the important elements can still examined at each temporal vantage point. Combined with the elements of the clinical care process, we can focus our attention on the relevant physiologic processes that have the greatest effect on survival at that vantage point (Fig. 4-9). In this way, clinical decision-making is concerned with appropriateness of therapy, given the existing circumstances for *this* patient at *this* point in the illness. We must consider decision-making in the context of creating a balance between the probable effects of disease and the wishes and values of the patient. Algorithms describing the disease apart from the patient give only an incomplete picture.

FIRST VANTAGE POINT: SOURCE OF ADMISSIONS ■

Patients admitted from emergency and elective sources should be considered separately. Emergency patients have a higher mortality rate and draw our special attention because of their initial acuity; thus, the important parameters to help decision-making are usually related to cardiorespiratory integrity. Further, little may be known, or there may be little time to amass other relevant information. In contrast, elective (usually surgical preoperative) patients are in a sta-

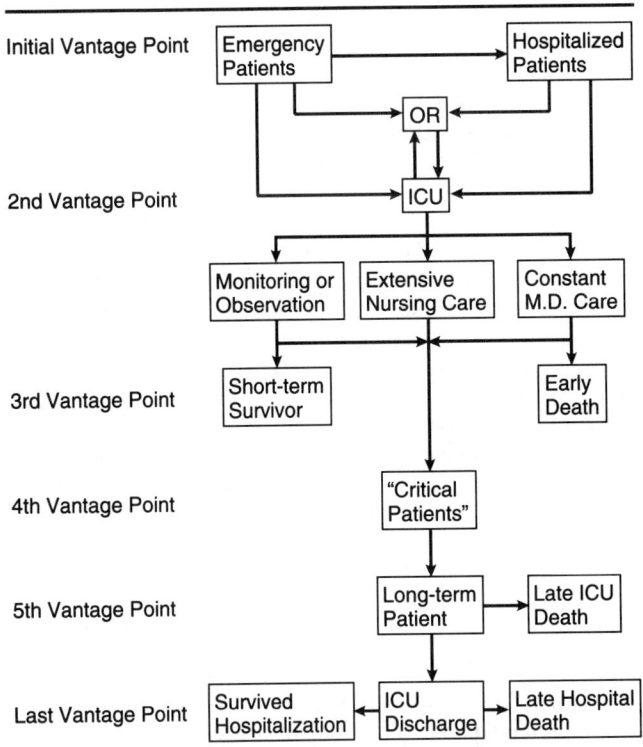

FIGURE 4-9. Clinical decision-making: the influence of time. OR, operating room; ICU, intensive care unit; M.D., physician's.

ble state, even if chronic illness is present; further, their course is based on the capacity to withstand future physiologic stress (physiologic reserve) rather than the capacity to respond to the existing stress that characterizes the emergency patients.

The greatest wealth of analyzed data exists for the multi-trauma patient. Many scales have been developed primarily for triage within trauma systems. They usually rely on simple measurements to be performed by paramedics or other non-physicians. Commencing in 1982, the Major Trauma Outcome Study[30] data base has been the basis for the Trauma and Injury Severity Score (TRISS) and, subsequently, A Severity Characterization of Trauma (ASCOT), which are models for predicting probability of death from trauma. The TRISS method[31] combined patient age, Injury Severity Score, and Revised Trauma Score (RTS) to predict survival to hospital discharge after injury. Although a better method than previous ones, several limitations were demonstrated.[32–34] Champion and his associates[33] addressed the limitations related to age, anatomic profile of the patient, and weighted values of the RTS components, in developing the ASCOT. However, recent studies[35] have demonstrated further limitations of these scoring systems. Scoring systems currently in use focus only on mortality and are fairly crude; using them to predict major outcomes other than survival requires substantial revision. However, these systems are not without value because they allow for more meaningful epidemiologic studies, comparison of interventions, provide a basis for injury control, and have potential application in estimating resource needs.

With respect to other types of emergencies such as gastrointestinal inflammation, obstruction, or perforation, distribution of patients within a community has not been seen as a problem; no similar triaging instruments exist. Similar types of abnormalities in cardiorespiratory integrity and end-organ function exist, however. For instance, the decision for urgent operation in patients with bowel obstruction and metabolic acidosis is made because of the derangement in cellular oxygen utilization suggestive of ischemic or infarcted bowel.

Patients considered to have compromised hemodynamic function are often admitted to the ICU preoperatively for invasive hemodynamic monitoring and assessment of the physiologic reserve of the cardiovascular system. The data base also includes other parameters of cardiorespiratory function that require invasive monitoring. These are also used to calculate oxygen transport and utilization parameters, which together form the basis of the decisions at the first vantage point (Table 4-1).

In addition to this assessment of baseline function, a stepwise approach to analysis of physiologic reserve, as follows, also has been used[16]:

Step 1. If patients are considered to have compromised hemodynamic function, invasive monitoring is used preoperatively.
Step 2. If there is evidence of inadequate baseline function such as decreased cardiac output or left ventricular stroke work, increased oxygen extraction, or inadequate oxygen delivery, then augmentation of ventricular function using preload, manipulation of afterload by vasodilators, and augmentation of contractility may be attempted.
Step 3. If none of the above measures improve function and oxygen delivery remains diminished, the risk of

TABLE 4-1. Physiologic Profile: Measured Parameters°

CARDIOVASCULAR
Cardiac output
Systematic arterial pressure
Heart rate
Pulmonary arterial pressure
Left ventricular filling pressure
Right ventricular filling pressure
Height and weight

RESPIRATORY
Hemoglobin
Inspired O_2 tension
Arterial O_2 tension
Arterial CO_2 tension
Arterial O_2 saturation
Venous O_2 tension
Venous O_2 saturation

°Parameters obtained by direct measurements including intravascular pressures and blood gases (require pulmonary artery catheterization).

developing cardiac complications and potential mortality is considered to be high. However, 95% of patients can be rendered suitable candidates for the intended surgery using this approach.[23,24]

Deterioration in clinical status may occur in the hospitalized patient. The parameters of sudden clinical deterioration necessitating emergency ICU admission usually are related to similar cardiorespiratory and oxygen transport values in other emergency patients.

SECOND VANTAGE POINT: ON ICU ADMISSION

Patients admitted to the ICU have one factor in common: a presumed increased risk of mortality or morbidity. In our process of clinical decision-making, we must examine the factors correlated with mortality. We will find that most predictors based on mortality use measurements are common to critically ill patients. Although the specific disease, the patient's physiologic reserve, and the presence of chronic diseases may all complicate the evaluation of the overall degree of illness in an individual patient, the most important components that influence immediate survival again reflect cardiorespiratory function and oxygen transport. On the other hand, in patients without major acute physiologic derangements, parameters reflecting the immune system, liver, kidneys, and nutritional state are more useful in the clinical decision.

THIRD VANTAGE POINT: SHORT-TERM ICU OUTCOME

The relationships among mortality rate, duration of ICU stay, and severity of illness are complex. In surgical ICUs, many patients are admitted for monitoring/observation and have short ICU stays. Few patients are so critically ill that they die despite all efforts within the same brief time. The *mortality rate* for short-term ICU admissions is low because it reflects the relatively few patients who die and the large number of the monitoring/observation patients who live. Clinical decision-making is relatively easy for both groups: little needs to be done for the monitoring/observation group and everything must be done for the most critical group, but usually intervention is possible only for a short time.[36] The mortality rate for patients who have long ICU admissions is much higher, commonly approaching 50%.[37] One might mistakenly conclude that long ICU admissions correlate with a higher severity of illness. This is not true because the short-term ICU admission group actually contains the patients with the most severe illness. The long-term group is the most problematic, especially to differentiate between what we want to do to achieve success, and what we should or must do, which may be much less or even, at times, nothing. Our sense of urgency to affect outcome may not be satisfied, but our actions will be appropriate.

We must distinguish between the aphorism of our training that focuses on crisis orientation: "Don't just stand there, do something"; instead, when we realize that death is inevitable, "Don't just do something, stand there." Decision-making becomes all the more difficult when dealing with patients in the middle of the severity of disease spectrum. Collection of information from both medical and patient-related sources must continue to allow reassessment and reappraisal of both risks and benefits. The longer the illness and the graver the prognosis, the less medicine has to offer and the greater the weight should be given to the patient's choice based on personal values (Chap. 6).

Most patients admitted for monitoring/observation do not and should not develop complications; therefore, the following day they are safely discharged to routine care areas. This decision is usually easy. In several cases, however, problems will develop; these patients may then require an increased level of nursing and physician care as well as an increased duration, which also correlates with higher costs.[38] Patients with the highest degree of abnormal cardiac, respiratory, and oxygen transport function will not only have a high mortality rate but also a short duration of intensive care before death occurs. Clinically, these patients clearly are the most severely ill and, not surprisingly, are so judged by predictive instruments. Therefore, we must determine the basis of the indices that can distinguish short-term survivors from early deaths. We can then focus on the identified components to direct our decision-making.

The Acute Physiology Score and Chronic Health Evaluation (APACHE) was introduced in 1981.[22] Initially, 34 physiologic measurements were obtained from the patient's clinical records; additionally a four-category designation of preadmission health status was made. Later, the APACHE II was developed, which was compressed to 12 routine physiologic measurements plus age and previous health status.[39] APACHE III has since been introduced to correct deficiencies in the previous versions.[40] Although APACHE III relates the score to mortality,[41] no qualitative changes have been made that would correct for the demonstrated deficiencies in APACHE II.[38,42–44] The Therapeutic Intervention Scoring System (TISS) assigned point values to interventions rather than physiologic abnormalities, as in APACHE.[45] Patterns of evolving cardiorespiratory function in surviving and nonsurviving patients were the basis of a third instrument.[46] Although the two previous indices had subjective weights assigned to the variables, actual measurements form the basis of the third predictive system. Finally, simple variables available at the time of admission were analyzed mathematically to form the basis of a fourth instrument.[47] Except for the complete listing of therapeutic interventions in TISS, the other three instruments contain approximately 12 individual components; 7 of them appear in at least two, and 4 of them appear in all three instruments (Table 4-2). This similarity underscores the fundamental biologic necessity for delivery of oxygen and cellular utilization. The fact that these parameters are few and have important statistical value supports the need for early and intense monitoring of cardiorespiratory function as well as oxygen transport. These parameters, then, are included in the diagnostic testing; the values form the basis of the selection of interventions. Reassessment in terms of short-term objectives is based on the demonstrated response to the chosen intervention.

TABLE 4-2. Common Elements in Acute Severity Indices

ELEMENT	INDICES*
Cardiovascular	
Blood pressure	APACHE II, TISS, CRV, MLR
Heart rate	APACHE II, TISS, CRV, MLR
Cardiac output	TISS, CRV
Respiratory	
Arterial oxygenation	APACHE II, TISS, CRV, MLR
Neurologic function	APACHE II, TISS, MLR
Oxygen transport	
Hemoglobin	APACHE II, CRV
Bicarbonate/pH	APACHE II, TISS, CRV, MLR
Renal function	APACHE II, TISS, MLR

APACHE II, Acute Physiology Score and Chronic Health Evaluation, Knaus et al[39]; TISS, Therapeutic Intervention Scoring System, Cullen et al[45]; CRV, cardiorespiratory variables, Shoemaker et al[46]; MLR, multiple logistic regression, Lemeshow et al.[47]

*Notice that TISS reflects therapeutic interventions chosen to affect listed variables.

FOURTH VANTAGE POINT: CONTINUED ICU CARE

Because outcome has already been decided for patients with the least and most degree of severity, the ICU contains patients midway along the severity spectrum.[38] Mortality rates will be higher, and halfway along the severity spectrum the mortality rate should be 50%, because the severity spectrum starts with patients with the least degree of illness (the mortality rate approaches 0%) and as a continuum extends to the most severe, those with lethal illnesses (with mortality rates approaching 100%).

These patients are the most important focus in terms of difficulty in achieving success, intensity of effort, resource utilization, legal issues, and bioethical problems. The distinction between those patients who will live and those who will ultimately die is impossible to achieve on admission; time and intervention are necessary to achieve resolution and to separate these groups. Decision-making is more difficult and more necessary. In this context, clinical judgment recognizes the need for effective intervention and the realization that such intervention does not produce immediate results; rather, a successful outcome can only be determined after a considerable investment of time. In a study of long-term patients, the average duration of stay was approximately 3 weeks in patients who ultimately lived or who died.[48] If resolution took this length of time, clearly the initial physiologic state must have been similar in both groups. When APACHE II and TISS were calculated repetitively, statistical separation of those who ultimately survived from those who died was only possible after 2 weeks of applied interventions. Because these patients are midway along the severity spectrum and because outcome was not determined for weeks, the indices designed to assess patients early in their course and heavily weighted to cardiorespiratory and oxygen transport parameters clearly cannot characterize the events that ultimately determine outcome in this small subgroup (7% of total) of patients. On the other hand, these patients used 35% of the total patient days of care.

Decision-making is a long and arduous problem balancing benefits and resource utilization. A predictive index must be based on data available at the time it is calculated. The events that actually determine outcome, evolution of the illness, unforeseen illnesses or complications, and especially, failure of organs functioning earlier, have not yet been "predicted"; decision-making depends on constant data gathering and reappraisal. The ICU patient is not like a train with both destination and direction fixed by the tracks. Rather, the patient's course must be "driven" by clinical judgment, much as a car is guided through traffic and around obstacles. Our next goal is to identify the clinical characteristics of the long-term patients at the time of their ICU admission. We can then recognize their probable course, which should focus on preventive aspects such as nutrition and avoidance of nosocomial infections while preparing the patient and family for the long and difficult road ahead.

FIFTH VANTAGE POINT: LONG-TERM ICU PATIENTS ■

Resource utilization is an important focus, but we must remember that our decision must include what *not* to do as well as what to do. The long-term patients are midway along the severity spectrum, and survival rates approximate 50%. We must continue to treat these patients because we recognize that the degree of physiologic abnormality, using our best quantitative methods, is not particularly high, nor can outcome be predicted accurately. The uncertainty of outcome affects the patients, their families, and the ICU staff. Because oxygen transport and cardiorespiratory parameters are not grossly deranged, it should be clear that usual ICU interventions, such as cardiovascular monitoring/interventions and ventilatory support, have little to offer these patients in terms of immediate improvement at this time. We have little true treatment to offer when renal, hepatic, and immune functions deteriorate, despite maintenance of cardiorespiratory function and nutritional support. In fact, patients who are at high risk of developing MOSF have had mortality rates of 50% even with minimal abnormalities demonstrated by acute scoring systems (APACHE II scores less than 10).[44]

We must temper our desire to use the "technological imperative," that is, to use everything in the therapeutic armamentarium until the moment of death. We must also recognize the impact of the uncertainty of outcome on the patient and family as well. Our desire to restore health to all of our patients must face the reality that nearly 50% of these patients ultimately die. Rather than view this as failure, we must include a new factor in our decisions, a perspective based on always achieving good from our medical interventions.

There are two principles or goals of medical care (Chap. 5). The first, which is consonant with the primary goal of intensive care, is the preservation of life. The second, more important in these patients, is the alleviation of suffering. As prognosis worsens, we must make decisions to strive for the alleviation of suffering and, again, depart from the illness-based algorithm approach, which concentrates only on diagnosis and treatment.

Based on the realization that death is an increasingly likely possibility in the long-term patients, and recognizing the limitation of early physiologic assessors for differentiating between patients who ultimately live or die, others have investigated more basic and fundamental biologic processes, such as methods of quantitating protein metabolism and immune function. These can reflect the ability of the host to heal and resist sepsis as well as reveal vital organ system function; these are often the capabilities that differentiate success from failure in prolonged and critical illness. The multiple organ failure syndrome is seen to have a metabolic basis in substrate–energy failure.[49] Many of these long-term patients have primarily or secondarily developed the sepsis syndrome. Analysis of long-term patients who survived and died showed significant differences[50]: patients who later died could be identified more than a week before death with a high degree of certainty (Table 4-3). Notice that many of these variables occur as a result of the failures in substrate metabolism, including increased urea, lactate, and glucose. However, the differences currently only underscore the fundamental defects in metabolic pathways that are beyond our capacity to influence. Most of the parameters that have been found to be discriminatory in these patients are related neither to acute cardiorespiratory dysfunction nor to the types of bedside assessment that were so prevalent in the

TABLE 4-3. Surviving and Dying Septic Patients: Discriminators and Nondiscriminators

---

DIFFERENCES

    Urea
    Lactate
    Z° nonessential amino acids
    α-Aminobutyrate
    Glucagon
    Z valine
    Z aspartate
    Z glutamine
    Glucose

NO DIFFERENCES

    pH
    P_{AO_2}
    Systematic blood pressure
    Heart rate
    Respiratory rate

° Z, fractional concentration of total group of amino acids rather than absolute amount of particular listed component. Notice that common components used in early predictors were of no value in these patients.

(Adapted from Moyer E, Cerra F, Chenier R, et al: Multiple systems organ failure. VI. Death predictors in the trauma–septic state: the most critical determinants. *J Trauma* 1981;21:862.)

early predictors and are deemed so responsive to active early ICU treatment. Our decision-making must achieve a different tone, direction, and even destination, at times.

It is unlikely that we will ever be able to predict with certainty all patients who will die or those who will not, despite any intervention we may provide. For the relatively few patients whose disease process is so severe that death is inevitable, we must provide comfort measures for both the patient and the family as an initial goal. For the not-so-obvious, we must focus our efforts on both the technological ICU procedures and on measures to alleviate the patient's suffering while we support the patient and await resolution based on the patient's ability to restore normal metabolic processes or, if this is impossible, to die ultimately. We must maintain efforts. We must continue our support. But we also have an equal imperative to avoid unnecessary manipulations that cannot influence the outcome and can only prolong dying, increasing stress to patients and families and draining already limited ICU resources.

LAST VANTAGE POINT: DISCHARGE FROM INTENSIVE CARE ▪

Our last, important clinical decision is made to effect discharge from the ICU. One might believe that if discharge were delayed until all major physiologic abnormalities had been resolved, patients would continue their recuperation in a routine hospital area and be discharged. However, mortality does not cease at ICU discharge, because a significant percentage of total hospital mortality occurs in the period between discharge from the ICU and hospital discharge. Because we rarely discharge dying patients to the floor, these deaths occur in patients considered well enough to be discharged with an expectation of survival, yet they die during their subsequent hospitalization. Thus, the decision for discharge is not easy, even given resolution of the acute physiologic abnormalities prompting admission. Certain problems, such as late arrhythmia or pulmonary embolism, may develop de novo. Respiratory arrest soon after ICU discharge in a patient treated for respiratory failure, however, may represent a poorly formulated decision. Our decisions must incorporate more than an appraisal of the risk of death. Many patients survive hospitalization only to be permanently placed in nursing homes or to undergo chronic hospitalization for severe physical and mental impairments. Thus, social parameters must enter our decision-making process and, at this stage, are more important than physiologic measurements. This has important implications for our care. Once again, high technology and repeated measurements, which are often important when significant physiologic abnormalities are the immediate determinants of outcome, must be restrained. Our decisions must be guided by an understanding that our role in caring for the patient may have to focus on a process of educating the patient and family with respect to short- and long-term prognosis. This direction varies according to the stage of the illness and the likelihood of successful outcome (see Chap. 6). In general, the higher the expected mortality rate or the greater the change in

quality of life, the more important it is to provide this information in a sympathetic and understanding way so that patients, or in the case of incompetent patients, the family, can properly exercise autonomy to choose the course most consistent with the patient's values. Preserving the patient's desires with regard to quality of life is important, but because the chain of events can rarely be foreseen, we should explore these issues before hospitalization or operation whenever possible. This is especially relevant when we are dealing with elderly patients with chronic diseases and specific diagnoses that have low success rates, such as carcinoma of the stomach or lung. We should recognize that information concerning quality of life that would be vital to know during prolonged illness is often unobtainable at that time. We must, therefore, include such deliberations in our preoperative evaluation, giving these patients the opportunity to consider their feelings about quality of life. In this manner, when patients pass on to the long-term ICU stage and reach the point of consideration of discontinuation of interventions to shorten the dying process, consensus will already be present among the patient, family, and physicians. The burden of decision will not be placed on distressed family members, quasi-incompetent patients, or well-meaning but, perhaps, poorly informed physicians.

CONCLUSION ▪

We can chose to take a passive role and treat problems as they arise, or we can aggressively monitor and seek potential problems long before they may otherwise manifest themselves. Continuous mixed venous oxygen saturation monitoring may alert one to an otherwise unsuspected alteration in cardiac output or oxygen consumption. Cardiac ischemia that might be missed on a once-daily electrocardiograph may become evident with continuous ST segment monitoring, during what may be otherwise considered benign routine ICU procedures (e.g., tracheal suctioning). Indeed, silent ischemia has been detected in 41% of high-risk vascular patients by this technique.[51] Detection of these ischemic events would, therefore, prompt aggressive therapy, thereby possibly averting a more permanent and catastrophic event (Chap. 59). "Hemodynamically compensated shock," as described by Fiddian-Green and coworkers,[52] otherwise undetectable by conventional parameters (hemodynamics, lactic acidosis, base deficit), but nonetheless a potential harbinger of MOSF, may be detected by an abnormally low gastric intramucosal pH and may be treated effectively by increasing global oxygen delivery, increasing splanchnic blood flow, or with agents designed to block ischemia-reperfusion injury[53-55] (Chap 30). Duration of mechanical ventilation may be unnecessarily prolonged if patients are weaned either too rapidly or not rapidly enough. Bedside monitoring of patient work of breathing not only gives an indication of excessive mechanical support or of work expended by the patient, but may also detect mechanical failures of the ventilator or circuitry, leading to iatrogenic respiratory failure (Chap. 15). Reversal of the persistently high mortality of ICU patients, therefore, may come not only as a result of new high-visiblity modalities such as endotoxin binding by monoclonal antibodies and blockade of production and end-organ effects of cytokines, but from active and anticipatory patient monitoring and therapy of common and fundamental processes such as resuscitation, ventilation, and cardiac function.

We often feel uncomfortable with the uncertainties of clinical judgment, long described as one of the arts of medicine. In our highly technological society and the environment in today's ICU, we perhaps vainly hope that this uncertainty can be dispelled by analyzing the massive data base accumulated. We should not dismiss clinical judgment by categorizing it as part of the art of medicine, but rather we should adopt Feinstein's perspective that it is scientific art and artful science, if only we can learn the proper scientific approach and apply the appropriate methodology rather than to continue to develop "new and improved" scoring systems using the same mathematical bases and the same faulty premises.[56] We should recognize that the expression of the art is as dependent on education and experience, as are music, theater, and painting. We must concentrate on learning the fundamentals, contained in the elements of the clinical care process and the components of the predictive indices, to improve our technique. The important determinants, when viewed from different vantage points during the ICU stay, are few in number and remarkably consistent among different instruments. Therefore, we can learn to focus on these elements as we try to characterize particular subgroups.

When the possibility of death increases, however, we must learn to restrict useless interventions and focus on caring for the patient and family. Our time should be spent in communication, explanation, and clarification rather than ordering new drugs, tests, or procedures. Patients seek medical *care*, not necessarily expecting *cure*. Technology, including intensive care, can then be seen as a method to enhance our clinical judgment when appropriate, but we should not look to technological solutions for social and societal issues, which are especially important in prolonged ICU care. Effective clinical decision-making still depends primarily on the processor: a knowledgeable and caring physician.

REFERENCES

1. Feinstein AR: Prologue. In: Feinstein AR (ed). *Clinical Judgment*. Baltimore, Williams & Wilkins, 1967:1
2. Feinstein AR: Art, science, and clinical observation. In: Feinstein AR (ed). *Clinical Judgment*. Baltimore, Williams & Wilkins, 1967:291
3. Feinstein AR: Science in clinical examination: standardization. In: Feinstein AR (ed). *Clinical Judgment*. Baltimore, Williams & Wilkins, 1967:328
4. Kouwenhoven WB, Jude JR, Knickerbocker GG: Closed chest massage. *JAMA* 1960;173:1064
5. Bedell SE, Delbanco TL, Cook EF, et al: Survival after cardiopulmonary resuscitation in the hospital. *N Engl J Med* 1983;309:569
6. Everhart MA, Pearlman RA: Stability of patient preferences regarding life-sustaining treatments. *Chest* 1990;97:159
7. Emanuel LL, Barry MJ, Stoeckle JD, et al: Advance directives for medical care: a case for greater use. *N Engl J Med* 1991;324:889
8. Schonwetter RS, Teasdale TA, Taffet G, et al: Educating the elderly: cardiopulmonary resuscitation decisions before and after intervention. *J Am Geriatr Soc* 1991;39:372
9. Uhlmann RF, Pearlman RA, Cain KC: Understanding of elderly patients' resuscitation preferences by physicians and nurses. *West J Med* 1989;150:705
10. Finucane TE, Shumway JM, Powers RL, et al: Planning with elderly patients for contingencies of severe illness: a survey and clinical trial. *J Gen Intern Med* 1988;3:322
11. Torian LV, Davidson EJ, Fillit HM, et al: Decisions for and against resuscitation in an acute geriatric medicine unit serving the frail elderly. *Arch Intern Med* 1992;152:561
12. Shmerling RH, Bedell SE, Lilienfeld A, et al: Discussing cardiopulmonary resuscitation: a study of elderly patients. *J Gen Intern Med* 1988;3:317
13. Danis M, Southerland LI, Garrett JM, et al: A prospective study of advance directives for life-sustaining care. *N Engl J Med* 1991;324:882
14. Frankl D, Oye RK, Bellamy PE: Attitudes of hospitalized patients toward life support: a survey of 200 medical inpatients. *Am J Med* 1989;86:645
15. Longstreth WT Jr, Cobb LA, Fahrenbruch CE, et al: Does age affect outcomes of out-of-hospital cardiopulmonary resuscitation? *JAMA* 1990;264:2109
16. Tresch DD, Thakur RK, Hoffman RG, et al: Comparison of outcome of paramedic-witnessed cardiac arrest in patients younger and older than 70 years. *Am J Cardiol* 1990;65:453
17. Appelbaum GE, King JE, Finucane TE: The outcome of CPR initiated in nursing homes. *J Am Geriatr Soc* 1990;38:197
18. Awoke S, Mouton CP, Parrott M: Outcomes of skilled cardiopulmonary resuscitation in a long-term-care facility: futile therapy? *J Am Geriatr Soc* 1992;40:593
19. Murphy DJ, Murray AM, Robinson BE, et al: Outcomes of cardiopulmonary resuscitation in the elderly. *Ann Intern Med* 1989;111.199
20. Murphy DJ, Burrows D, Santilli S, et al: The influence of the probability of survival on patients' preferences regarding cardioplumonary resuscitation. *N Engl J Med* 1994;330:545
21. DelGuercio L, Cohn JD: Monitoring operating risk in the elderly. *JAMA* 1980;243:1350
22. Knaus WA, Zimmerman JE, Wagner DP, et al: APACHE—acute physiology and chronic health evaluation: a physiologically based classification system. *Crit Care Med* 1981;9:591
23. Orlando R, Nelson LD, Civetta JM: Invasive preoperative evaluation of high risk patients. *Crit Care Med* 1985;13:263
24. Shibutani K, Del Guercio LRM: Preoperative hemodynamic assessment of the high-risk patient. *Semin Anesth* 1983;1:231
25. Civetta JM, Hudson-Civetta JA: Maintaining quality of care while reducing charges in the ICU: 10 ways. *Ann Surg* 1985;202:524
26. Weed LW: *Medical Records, Medical Education, and Patient Care: The Problem-Oriented Record as a Basic Tool*. Chicago, Year Book Medical Publishers, 1970
27. Robin ED: Death by pulmonary artery flow-directed catheter: time for a moratorium? *Chest* 1988;92:727
28. Kirby RR, Civetta JM: Critical care outcome. In: Brown DL (ed). *Risk and Outcome in Anesthesia*, 2nd ed. Philadelphia, JB Lippincott, 1991
29. Feinstein AR: Retrospection, experience and medical records. In: Feinstein AR (ed). *Clinical Judgment*. Baltimore, Williams & Wilkins, 1967:263
30. Champion HR, Copes WS, Sacco WJ, et al: The major trauma outcome study: establishing national norms for trauma care. *J Trauma* 1990;30:1356
31. Boyd CR, Tolson MA, Copes WS: Evaluating trauma care: the TRISS method. *J Trauma* 1987;27:370

32. Cayten CG, Stahl WM, Murphy JG, et al: Limitations of the TRISS method for interhospital comparisons: a multihospital study. *J Trauma* 1991;31:471

33. Copes WS, Champion HR, Sacco WJ: The Injury Severity Score revisited. *J Trauma* 1988;28:69

34. Markle J, Cayten CG, Byrne DW, et al: Comparison between TRISS and ASCOT methods in controlling for injury severity. *J Trauma* 1992;33:326

35. Hannan EL, Mendeloff J, Farrell LS, et al: Validation of TRISS and ASCOT using a non-MTOS trauma registry. *J Trauma* 1995;38:83

36. Civetta JM, Hudson-Civetta J: Costly care: data, problems and proposing remedies. *Crit Care Med* 1986;14:357

37. Civetta JM: The inverse relationship between cost and survival. *J Surg Res* 1973;14:265

38. Civetta JM, Hudson-Civetta JA, Nelson LD: Evaluation of APACHE II for cost containment and quality assurance. *Ann Surg* 1990;212:266

39. Knaus WA, Draper EA, Wagner DP, et al: APACHE II: a severity of disease classification system. *Crit Care Med* 1985;13:818

40. Wagner D, Draper E, Knaus W: Development of APACHE III. *Crit Care Med* 1989;17(Suppl):S199

41. Knaus WA, Wagner DP, Draper EA, et al: The APACHE III prognostic system: risk prediction of hospital mortality for critically ill hospitalized adults. *Crit Care Med* 1991;19 (Suppl):583

42. Kirton OC, Aragon C, Salas C, et al: Can APACHE II meaningfully stratify a surgical ICU sub-group? *Crit Care Med* 1991;19(Suppl):531

43. Civetta JM, Nelson LD, Hudson-Civetta JA, et al: Individual outcome prediction by APACHE II scores in a surgical ICU. *Crit Care Med* 1991;19(Suppl):536

44. Cerra FB, Negro F, Abrams J: APACHE II score does not predict multiple organ failure or mortality in postoperative surgical patients. *Arch Surg* 1990;125:519

45. Cullen DJ, Civetta JM, Briggs BA, et al: Therapeutic intervention scoring systems: a method for quantitative comparison of patient care. *Crit Care Med* 1974;2:57

46. Shoemaker WC, Pierchala BS, Chang P, et al: Prediction of outcome and severity of illness by analysis of the frequency distribution of cardiorespiratory variables. *Crit Care Med* 1977;5:82

47. Lemeshow S, Teres D, Pastides H, et al: A method for predicting survival and mortality of ICU patients using objectively derived weights. *Crit Care Med* 1985;13:519

48. Civetta JM: The clinical implications of ICU scoring systems. *Probl Crit Care* 1989;3:681

49. Siegel JH: Cardiorespiratory manifestations of metabolic failure in sepsis and the multiple organ failure syndrome. *Surg Clin North Am* 1983;63:379

50. Moyer E, Cerra F, Chenier R, et al: Multiple systems organ failure. VI. Death predictors in the trauma-septic state: the most critical determinants. *J Trauma* 1981;21:862

51. Mangano DT, Browner WS, Hollenberg M, et al: Association of perioperative myocardial ischemia with cardiac morbidity and mortality in men undergoing noncardiac surgery. *N Engl J Med* 1990;323:1781

52. Fiddian-Green RG, Haglund U, Gutierrez G, et al: Goals for the resuscitation of shock. *Crit Care Med* 1993;21:S25

53. Doglio GR, Pusajo JF, Egurrola MA, et al: Gastric mucosal pH as a prognostic index of mortality in critically ill patients. *Crit Care Med* 1991;19:1037

54. Gutierrez G, Bismar H, Dantzker DR, et al: Comparison of gastric intramucosal pH with measures of oxygen transport and consumption in critically ill patients. *Crit Care Med* 1992;20:451

55. Maynard N, Bihari D, Beale R, et al: Assessment of splanchnic oxygenation by gastric tonometry in patients with acute circulatory failure. *JAMA* 1993;270:1203

56. Civetta JM: New and improved scoring systems [editorial]. *Crit Care Med* 1990;18;1487

Critical Care, Third Edition, edited by Joseph M. Civetta,
Robert W. Taylor, and Robert R. Kirby.
Lippincott-Raven Publishers, Philadelphia, PA © 1997.

CHAPTER 5

Life and Death in the ICU: Ethical Considerations

Ernlé W. D. Young

Our contemporary technological ability to preserve and extend life in the intensive care unit (ICU) is impressive, to say the least. But for a few patients—those whose living can no longer be extended but whose dying can only be prolonged—the technology of the ICU has come to have sinister, even frightening, connotations. What most of us dread, more than death itself, is an inevitable process of dying that is meaninglessly and agonizingly protracted by artificial means. There are times when the instruments of healing become the tools of torture. There are situations in which the benefits of intensive care medicine are far outweighed by the harms inflicted in attempting to realize them. There are moments when death ought no longer to be resisted and fought back as an enemy, by any and all means possible, but is rather to be welcomed and embraced as a friend. And people generally are concerned that these times will not be discerned, these situations will remain unrecognized, these moments will be missed.

There are good grounds for this uneasiness. Sometimes it seems that there is an overwhelming fascination—even infatuation—with the toys of technology that prompts intensivists unconcernedly to play with them, in circumstances of life and death too momentous for mere games. And often intensivists are genuinely concerned that if they do not do everything possible for their patients, unquestioningly and unremittingly, they will later be sued. The defensive practice of medicine is an inevitable corollary to the litigious nature of American society.

Fortunately, some of the court cases discussed later have substantially alleviated physicians' legitimate concerns about possible malpractice litigation. There are now some good legal precedents for at times *not* doing everything it is possible to do. Also, the American Medical Association (AMA) and American Bar Association are beginning to look for alternatives to malpractice litigation to compensate and redress aggrieved consumers. However, these investigations are in their early stages, and the problem has yet to be resolved.

In addition to the technological imperative and the fear of malpractice litigation, a third factor motivates intensivists to cross the line between extending life and prolonging death in a sometimes inappropriate fashion: a lack of skill in ethical decision-making, especially when those involved in the decision-making process are many and speak with various voices. In the ICU of a modern medical center, ethical decision-making may involve not only the patient and the primary (community) physician, but also the family, the director of the ICU, various consultants, the house staff, the nurses, the respiratory therapists, the social worker, the chaplain, the ethics consultant or committee, and the hospital's legal counsel! This complicates issues to an extraordinary degree. It is far simpler not to make a decision at all. Yet, not making a decision is, itself, a decision. And in the circumstances that we are considering, it is one that can have dire consequences for the patient.

MEDICAL ETHICS ∎

Courses in medical ethics, which are offered in most medical schools, and ethics seminars for house staff attempt to redress this lack of skill. To describe the function of medical ethics in this regard, it is useful to begin by briefly considering the meaning of three other related terms: *morality,* *ethics,* and *law. Morality* comprises those attitudes, actions, or behaviors of an individual or of a group that reflect that individual's or group's vision of the highest good. *Ethics* is the discipline that has, as one of its functions, to study moral attitudes, actions, and behaviors analytically or descriptively, looking for consistency and coherency between them and the highest good they purport to reflect. The other function of ethics is prescriptive, or normative. It is to move from a description of what *is* happening in a situation fraught with moral ambiguity to suggest what *ought* to be going on if the vision of the highest good is to be translated accurately into what is said and done. This is the more difficult task of ethics, and it invites analytical criticism from others (which is one of the ways the cause of truth is furthered). The law may be considered to be the societal requirement or allowance, on the one hand, or prohibition, on the other, of attitudes, actions, and behaviors, which, in a given culture and at a certain time in history, are considered to be either moral or immoral. Just as morality changes from one cultural milieu to another and from one generation to the next, so the law reflects these differing perceptions. Fifty years ago, racial discrimination was well-entrenched in the United States. Its immorality was unquestioned; it was legally sanctioned and enforced in countless ways. The civil rights movement began to challenge racism as immoral. As the movement gathered momentum, racist laws came under attack as being unconstitutional. Eventually, both the moral perception of Americans as well as discriminatory laws were changed. Ethics functions with respect to the law much in the same way as it does in regard to morality. It analyzes what is going on in particular laws, assessing whether they accurately express a society's moral vision. And it makes normative proposals which, if adopted, would render the law less immoral or more moral than before.

Medical ethics, therefore, is that discipline concerned with moral issues arising in the contemporary practice of medicine. With respect to these proliferating problems, various positions begin to be formulated and adopted, either in practice or theoretically. Some of these positions become entrenched in the law, either legislatively or through case precedents. In its analytical or descriptive mode, medical ethics is interested in the facts adduced in support of a particular position—how accurate, extensive, or pertinent they are; in the implicit or explicit values of the various parties involved—how well or how poorly they are being respected and upheld, and whether consciously or unconsciously; and in the logical and rational consistency (or otherwise) of the arguments brought forward to bolster claims or to undergird conclusions. In its normative or prescriptive mode, medical ethics goes beyond analysis to suggest what ought to be happening, with reference either to particular cases or laws.

DEONTOLOGY AND UTILITARIANISM

At the rational level, medicine has traditionally responded to moral quandaries by appeal to evolving basic principles, rather than in ad hoc fashion. This is to say, medical ethics, to use the language of philosophers, has functioned either deontologically or in terms of rule-utilitarianism. For those who are not familiar with this terminology, it may be useful to explain it. The word *deontological* derives from the Greek, *deon*, meaning "it is necessary" or "it is required." A deontological ethics is one in which certain actions are declared obligatory, ab initio, at the outset, no matter what the circumstances or the consequences may be. For example, deontological norms require that we be truthful, that we maintain confidentiality, that we seek to benefit patients rather than ourselves, that we engage not to harm those in our care. The consequences of truth-telling, or preserving confidentiality, or acting beneficently or nonmaleficently, are not accorded primary significance in the process of deciding what to do in a given situation. *Utilitarianism* weighs the imagined results of various possible courses of action and decides what to do on the basis of the set of consequences thought to be most beneficial (or least detrimental) to the largest number of relevant parties. *Rule-utilitarianism* seeks to apply the rules, principles, or guidelines that experience has taught will produce the maximum amount of good (or the minimum amount of harm) for the greatest possible number. Beauchamp and Childress[1] effectively demonstrate how medical ethicists with a deontological approach and a rule-utilitarian orientation, starting from different premises, can agree on fundamental principles. (Act-utilitarianism, the other major form of consequentialist ethics, enjoins those *actions* which, in each new situation, it is thought will maximize the good or minimize the harm for the greatest number.)

MEDICOMORAL PRINCIPLES

Two primary medicomoral principles have traditionally informed the practice of medicine: preserving life and alleviating suffering. For the most part, these two principles can be applied concurrently, without conflict, to guide the physician's decisions and actions. However, in circumstances of critical or terminal illness, they sometimes come into conflict. Then it becomes possible to apply one principle only at the expense of the other. To continue, willy-nilly, to attempt to preserve life may, in fact, inflict rather than alleviate suffering. And consciously to strive to alleviate suffering may require abandoning the intention to continue to preserve life. In such situations where principles are in opposition to one another, the questions arise: Which principle ought to take precedence over the other, and when, and why? To these questions we must turn.

Some resolve a potential conflict between these two traditional medicomoral principles by insisting that preserving life always ought to take precedence over the concern to alleviate suffering. In terms of Figure 5-1, if X equals birth, Y equals death, and the curve equals the human life span, they insist that CARE ought to take the form of an unyielding

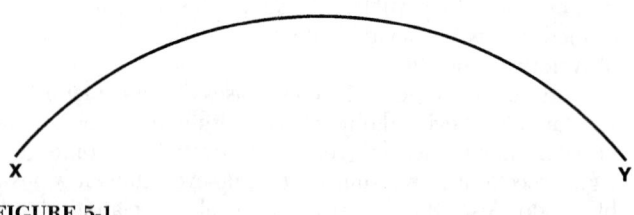

FIGURE 5-1.

Chapter 5. Life and Death in the ICU: Ethical Considerations **65**

and unremitting attempt to CURE, from X through Y. That is to say, the sanctity of the patient's life is valued above considerations of its quality, and death is perceived as an enemy to be fought back and kept at bay by all means, for as long as possible.

A segment of both patients and physicians espouse this philosophy of care. Their putative motives warrant consideration. Some patients have urgent, unfinished business to attend to before they die: a book to complete, a project to finalize, a legacy of one kind or another to wrap up. Understandably, they are willing to purchase as much time as they possibly can, without regard for the quality of their lives, by insisting that everything feasible be done to maintain their physical existence. Others, such as Helga Wanglie and her husband, Oliver, are avowed pro-lifers or "vitalists," holding that biologic existence alone is a sufficient good. Yet others are unable to come to terms with their own mortality and finiteness. The threat of nonbeing is so intense that they are willing to endure all kinds of harms—iatrogenic or disease-related—to hold off the inevitable, to remain in being, for as long as possible.

With respect to physicians, various motives prompt the adoption of a CARE = CURE philosophy from X to Y. One has to do with research. If a breakthrough can occur in treating a patient with what is generally thought to be an incurable and terminal condition, this may benefit a whole population of future patients. Another reason is to be discerned in the case of children afflicted with terminal illnesses: if unremitting, aggressive treatment can purchase an extra year or two of life for a child, no matter what the cost, that cost is worth paying because a year or two in the life of a 5- or 7-year old represents a considerable proportion of the total life span. Thirdly, just as some patients are temperamentally unable to come to terms with their inevitable mortality, so too are some physicians incapable of accepting "defeat;" to stop treating a terminal disease aggressively is unfortunately equated with failure.

There is, however, another way of looking at this whole conundrum. It revolves around point Z (Fig. 5-2). Point Z may be defined as the moment when the difference between attempting to extend life (with meaning, as defined by the patient) and merely prolonging death (in mindless and meaningless fashion) is discerned. Recognizing point Z, admittedly, is difficult. At least three factors enter into its determination. One is the accumulation of *objective* clinical data:

radiograph findings, computed tomographic scan results, or magnetic resonance imaging evidence that the disease is gaining the upper hand; further findings of untreatable metastases; or disastrous results of blood counts. A second is the *subjective* assessment of the patient who has determined that, having fought the good fight, the battle is no longer worth the candle: the deleterious effects of fighting on outweigh the benefits of sheer survival, without discernible quality. And, thirdly, there is *intuition*: the intuition of the clinician, the patient, or both, that the time has come to switch from a mode in which attempting to extend life ought to be the primary concern to a philosophy in which the quality of life is seen as more important; where death may be regarded no longer as an enemy to be resisted, but rather as a friend to be afforded hospitality.

If it is conceded that it is possible to discern point Z (and doing this requires more in terms of the art of medicine, perhaps, than its science, although they can be complementary, as in the case of APACHE III scores), then another philosophy of care emerges. From X through Z, the principle of preserving life ought to take precedence over that of alleviating suffering; the value of the sanctity of life ought to predominate over quality of life valuations; death ought to be seen more as a foe to be attacked and defended against than as a colleague to be embraced; and CARE should take the form of a resolute attempt to CURE. But from Z through Y, these principles and values are reversed. Now, alleviating suffering ought to take precedence over the principle of attempting to preserve life. Now, the quality of life requires more attention than the mere prolongation of physical existence. Now, death may appropriately be recognized and embraced as a welcome visitant. And now, CARE will take the form of ensuring *comfort* in the face of pain, *companying with* the dying person (rather than abandoning or segregating him), and facilitating a *creative completion* of the patient's inner journey (which will move spiritual counselors and companions from the sidelines to center field). Now, it will also be possible to view the withdrawal or withholding of aggressive life-sustaining technologies *as an appropriate expression of the concern to care.*

Accordingly, this chapter is devoted initially to describing some principles that I have found helpful in the ICU in facilitating ethical decision-making about the withdrawal or withholding of aggressive, heroic, life-sustaining technologies, and to identifying those who might be party to the decision-making process, along with their appropriate roles. At relevant points, reference is made to major court decisions on withdrawing or withholding life-sustaining interventions. Legislation and policy statements that have a bearing on the topic are also considered. Later, I turn to two recent developments that are likely to dominate the ethical landscape throughout the remainder of this decade: the so-called *futility debate* and physician aid-in-dying (or physician-assisted suicide).

Whether what follows is termed deontological or rule-utilitarian does not matter. What matters is that there *are* some rational guiding principles to help the intensivist in making difficult ethical decisions. Five may be delineated. From my perspective, they serve as broad guidelines rather than as rigid and inflexible, context-invariant rules.

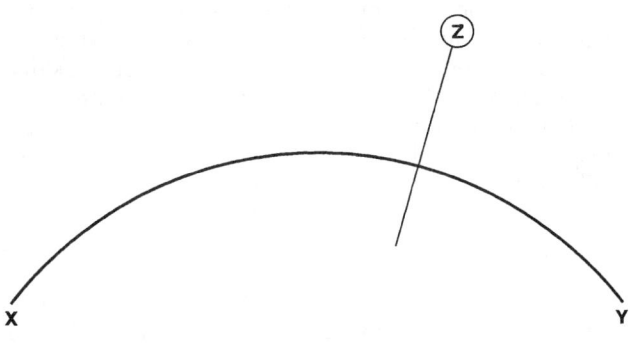

FIGURE 5-2.

Potential for Salvageability

The first is a common-sense principle, first enunciated (to my knowledge) by Cynthia B. Cohen,[2] that the criterion for admission to and continuance in an ICU is *the potential for salvageability*. As expressed by Cohen:

> All who are critically ill should not automatically be admitted to the ICU. A necessary condition for admission is that the patient be potentially salvageable, by which it is meant that the patient has a chance for returning to a state in which his or her life is not threatened. Patients who are immediately and irreversibly dying, and for whom it has been carefully determined that there is no known therapy, are not salvageable. They deserve comfort and support within the hospital but cannot benefit from intensive care.[2]

With respect to this first guideline, two qualifying comments are in order. One is that it is easier to apply at the time of admission to an ICU than when the discontinuance of intensive care is being contemplated because a patient is no longer deemed to be "salvageable." When admission to an ICU is being considered, it is usually sufficient that the patient be thought to have a 50/50 chance of recovery for the attempt to be made aggressively to preserve life. (This may change dramatically under the influence of "managed care.") But when it is becoming apparent that the patient is no longer salvageable and that, therefore, comfort and support rather than intensive care is more appropriate, a far higher level of certainty is mandated. Before agreeing to the discontinuance of life-sustaining therapies (because point Z is thought to have been reached), the intensivist wishes for a degree of certainty approaching 100%, rather than the 50% that may have sufficed at the outset.

A second qualifying remark is that the definition of salvageability is greatly determined by the resources that are available. A simple analogy clarifies this point. If a person were fortunate enough to inherit a Model T Ford (which had been locked in a garage for the last half century) and wanted it restored to its original, pristine, showroom condition, craftspeople are available who can accomplish such feats. Their work is beautiful to behold. If no limit exists to the funds allotted to such a project, the Ford could be totally restored, with genuine parts, or with parts handmade to the original specifications. However, if the budget was restricted to, let us say, $5000, it is highly unlikely that the same goal could be reached. For $5000 it might be possible to restore the upholstery, the chassis, the motor, or even the body to mint condition, but it is too much to expect that the whole car could be renovated; labor and parts together would cost more than the $5000 available.

In the same way, if resources are infinite (or are thought to be infinite, as was the case when intensive care had its genesis in the 1960s), the definition of salvageability can be loose, and the threshold for admittance to and continuance in an ICU can be low. But once resources are recognized as finite, and limits on expenditures have to be set (as is increasingly the case in the context of managed care), the definition of salvageability may have to be tightened and the threshold of eligibility for initial and continued intensive care raised commensurately.

These two disclaimers notwithstanding, Cohen's principle is helpful. It reminds us that caring can encompass several different activities. At times, caring means furnishing a patient with a respirator or with renal dialysis. At other times, it requires no more than palliation for pain and the discomfort, for example, of constipation. Hopefully, caring will never cease. However, the *form* caring takes is determined by medical and other factors, which are considered later in this chapter.

Cohen's principle accords well with the findings of a Consensus Development Conference held at the National Institutes of Health on March 7 through 9, 1983, to discuss issues related to the practice of critical care medicine. The conference identified three categories of patients:

1. Patients "with acute reversible disease for whom the probability of survival without ICU intervention is low, but the survival probability with such intervention is high"
2. Patients "with a low probability of survival without intensive care whose probability of survival with intensive care may be higher, but the potential benefit is not as clear"
3. Patients "admitted to the ICU, not because they are critically ill, but because they are at *risk* of becoming critically ill. The purposes of intensive care in these instances are to prevent a serious complication or to allow a prompt response to any complication that may occur."[3]

The conference went on to state that

> It is not medically appropriate to devote limited ICU resources to patients without reasonable prospect of significant recovery when patients who need those services, and who have a significant prospect of recovery from acutely life-threatening disease or injury are being turned away because of a lack of capacity. It is inappropriate to maintain ICU management of a patient whose prognosis has resolved to one of persistent vegetative state, and it is similarly inappropriate to employ ICU resources where no purpose will be served but a prolongation of the processes of death.[3]

Preserving Life

A second principle, mentioned earlier, is that of *preserving life*. This goes back to the Judaic element in the Judaeo-Christian heritage. The governing principle in Jewish medical ethics is the preservation of life. So fundamental is this principle in the tradition that things otherwise prohibited by Jewish law must be set aside to preserve life. "Thus even though it is forbidden to mutilate a corpse, heart and kidney transplants as well as corneal grafting are permitted, provided of course that the utmost care is taken to be sure that the person whose body is being used for the purpose is really dead."[4]

Nonmaleficence

A third principle is that of *nonmaleficence*. A duty not to harm is recognized in most deontological and rule-utilitarian ethical theories. The concept of nonmalificence is associated with the maxim *primum non nocere*: above all, or first of all, do no harm. According to Beauchamp and Childress:

> This maxim is frequently invoked by health care professionals, yet its origins are obscure and its implications unclear. Often proclaimed the fundamental principle in the Hippocratic tradition of medical ethics, it is not found in the Hippocratic corpus, and a venerable statement sometimes confused with it—"at least, do no harm"—is a strained translation of a single Hippocratic passage.[5]

Of course, as these authors point out, harm can be variously defined: in terms of death, disability, distress, or deprivation of freedom and pleasure. Further, harms—however defined—have to be weighed against hoped-for, compensatory benefits: all medical interventions inflict *some* harm. Usually, the harm inflicted is minimal and the ensuing benefits are many. In the ICU, however, this may not always be the case. Where someone has been determined to be no longer salvageable, there will not be any hoped-for, compensatory benefit to offset the iatrogenic harms being inflicted by aggressive life-sustaining measures. Applying this principle in such situations then becomes fairly straightforward.

Allied closely to the negative principle of nonmaleficence is the positive concept of *alleviating suffering*, which goes back to the Hippocratic corpus. We have already alluded to this principle. Not to harm entails, as a corollary, a concern to alleviate suffering, whether physical or psychological. For the most part, in medicine, it is possible to apply the second principle (that of attempting to preserve life) and this third principle (doing no harm or alleviating suffering) simultaneously and without conflict. As has been remarked, however, in circumstances of terminal illness, the one principle can usually be upheld only at the expense of the other. Then a decision has to be made about which should predominate over the other, and when, and why. We have suggested how this ranking of principles might take place, and this point is discussed in more detail later.

Autonomy

Fourth is the principle of *autonomy*. The origins of this norm can be traced back to the emphasis in the Judaeo-Christian tradition on respect for persons. Respecting the personhood of others requires that we allow and enable them, so far as possible, to be self-determining agents. Immanuel Kant, in insisting that every human being always be treated as an end and never as a means to an end, embedded this principle more deeply in the Western tradition.

However, as Candace Cummins Gauthier points out in a careful examination of the nature of autonomy in Kant and in John Stuart Mill, "it becomes apparent that personal autonomy is best understood not as a positive freedom, a freedom to receive or be given something, but rather a negative freedom, a freedom from interference."[6] What began as a negative right to noninterference in matters of private choice, with the strict proviso that a person's choices ought not to harm or endanger others, is believed (in American popular culture) to be a positive entitlement to have whatever a person wants, especially if someone else is paying for it. We shall return to this development in our discussion of "futility."

Justice

Last is the principle of *justice*. Understood in its most basic terms, justice may be thought of as fairness. Fairness, when it comes to distributing scarce resources equitably, requires that we do not do for some what we are unwilling or unable to do for all. To expend more than a million dollars on a single patient, who in the end dies in the ICU 14 months and 16 surgical procedures after admission, is one issue. To expend such colossal amounts of money on *all* potential ICU patients is another. Manifestly, it is impossible. The principle of justice, much to the fore in an era of cost containment, poses the question: How can we fairly allocate ICU resources? How can we equitably distribute among the many claimants for our services those limited benefits we have to offer?

Let one thing be stated now, most emphatically: decisions *within the ICU* ought not be made on economic, rather than on medical, grounds. It is not acceptable, from an ethical point of view, once having begun to offer a patient intensive care, to decide to discontinue aggressive therapy because it is costing too much. Doing this would violate the moral contract entered into with the patient at the time of admission. This point of view is endorsed by the 1983 National Institutes of Health Consensus Development Conference on Critical Care Medicine.[3]

Nevertheless, it is morally licit for considerations of distributive justice to enter into the decision-making process *before the patient is admitted to the ICU*, in terms of a raised threshold of eligibility for costly, technological life-sustaining services. Given the finiteness of our resources, it is morally acceptable for a hospital to decide not to offer intensive care, for example, to a patient with a metastatic, terminal disease process. If this policy is publicly stated, ahead of time, to everyone concerned—staff members as well as patients and their family members—no objection can be made to this attempt to raise the threshold of eligibility for what the ICU is able to provide.

APPLICATION OF MEDICOMORAL PRINCIPLES

Having enunciated five basic ethical principles pertinent to decision-making in the ICU, they must be ranked in order of priority, identifying their points of applicability. Concerning the first three, the following can be said. While the patient is considered to be salvageable (as defined both medically and by the resources available) and is therefore on the X–Z segment of the curve in Figure 5-2, preserving life ought to take precedence over the principle of doing no harm or alleviating suffering. However, once it is decided that a patient is no longer salvageable, that is, is on the Z-Y segment of the curve, intensive care is no longer the most appropriate form of care, and the principle of nonmaleficence or alleviating suffering assumes priority over preserving life. Defining salvageability—both medically and in terms of the resources available (and thus deciding that the Z-point has been reached)—is the key to reranking principles and accordingly reordering priorities from attempting to cure to comforting.

The fourth principle, autonomy, ought to have its place throughout the decision-making process. So far as possible, medical decisions ought not to be made by physicians acting unilaterally. (The emergency room setting provides one obvious exception to this general norm.) Usually, this is unproblematic as long as the patient continues to be conscious and competent. Difficulties in the continued exercise of autonomy arise when patients become unconscious or incompetent. Various measures have been devised to meet these difficulties. These are mentioned later. Furthermore, as has been indicated, autonomy is often construed to be an entitlement to services that are medically inappropriate or useless, especially when a third party is paying for them rather than the patient or family.

As has already been suggested, the fifth principle, distributive justice, ought to have its place outside the ICU, in the arena of institutional and public policy, rather than within the ICU itself. Once having initiated treatment for medical reasons, it is unacceptable to terminate treatment for economic reasons. Economic considerations should have their place in deciding which patients not to treat intensively in the first place.

In situations where aggressive therapy has been initiated, but it has become apparent that the patient is no longer salvageable, doing no harm (or alleviating suffering) becomes more important than continuing with the (futile and potentially harmful) attempt to preserve life. If intensive care is no longer the most appropriate form of care, and palliative or supportive care is indicated, who can and who ought to decide to limit treatment? A summary answer to this question is provided in Table 5-1. In what follows, the summary points made in the table are further explicated, with reference to pertinent court decisions, legislation, and policy statements.

The principle of autonomy requires that patients assume the primary role in all decisions to limit therapy, wherever this is possible. Usually, the interest patients have in deciding to limit therapy is that of not wanting the process of dying in a meaninglessly and painfully prolonged manner when life can no longer be extended with "quality"—according to patients' own definitions. I say "usually," because occasionally some patients are so afraid of death that they will do anything and endure all manner of hardship to prolong the inevitable. Patients in this category present a different ethical problem: To what extent does an "unsalvageable" patient have the right to demand costly and possibly scarce ICU resources in a futile attempt to keep death at a distance? In this case, the principles of autonomy and justice are in conflict. Because autonomy is never an absolute, even in societies like ours (none of us is free not to pay taxes, or not to obey the highway code, or not to have our children immunized, or not to educate our children), this may be an area in which concern for the common good (represented by the principle of justice) ought to take precedence over the principle of autonomy (inadequately construed as unbridled freedom).

Limitation or Refusal of Treatment

If the patient is conscious and competent, no insurmountable obstacles are in the way of exercising the right to refuse treatment. This right has been recognized by the AMA and the American Hospital Association, and is included in the commonly accepted Patient's Bill of Rights. However, the case of *Bartling v Superior Court*[7] is a reminder that this "right" cannot be taken for granted and of the fact that it has been upheld by court action in a single jurisdiction. Mr. Bartling, 70 years old, had multiple medical problems. His condition had become compromised after a pneumothorax sustained during a biopsy of a lung mass. He had a chest tube inserted, was given a tracheostomy, and was placed on a ventilator. Throughout, Mr. Bartling remained conscious and competent and on several occasions attempted to remove the ventilator tubing. Mr. Bartling repeatedly requested that ventilatory support be discontinued. The treating physicians and the hospital refused to comply with his request and continued to restrain Mr. Bartling so that he could not extubate himself. Richard S. Scott, a doctor and lawyer active in the right-to-die movement, took up this case on Mr. Bartling's behalf. The lower court denied the request for an injunction restraining the hospital and the physicians from administering medical care to which the patient had not given consent. The case was appealed. Before the appeal court could rule, Mr. Bartling died, still connected to his ventilator. So important was this case deemed to be, however, that the Court of Appeal ruled posthumously, holding that ". . . competent adult patients, with serious illnesses which are probably incurable, but have not been diagnosed as terminal, have the right, over the objection of their physicians and the hospital, to have life-support equipment disconnected despite the fact that withdrawal of such devices will surely hasten death." Typically, obstacles in the way of the patient limiting intensive care therapy have arisen only when the patient has become either unconscious or incompetent. From the patient's point of view, the prior concern was, How can I continue to exercise my autonomy beyond the point of unconsciousness and incompetence? And from the physician's perspective, the consideration was, How does the clinician do what the patient seemingly would have wanted, without becoming overly vulnerable to malpractice litigation?

Early attempts to surmount these obstacles included the so-called Living Will (now recognized as a legally valid document) and the California Natural Death Act, or its equivalent. The Natural Death Act had several deficiencies. One major problem was that, according to the provisions of the Act, the Directive to Physicians could only be executed by persons who were at the time and had been for at least 14 days previously, terminally ill, as defined in the Act. (Mr. Bartling was not terminally ill, as defined in the Act, when he asked to be allowed to exercise his right to refuse treatment.) This prevented the Natural Death Act from being of assistance to persons who, not being terminally ill beforehand, had later sustained massive, irreversible neurologic or physiologic insults, or both, whether iatrogenically or through accidents.

These problems have since been recognized, and the Natural Death Act was amended in 1991 to allow all compe-

TABLE 5-1. Principles Potentially Party to the Decision-Making Process

	INTEREST IN THE DECISION-MAKING PROCESS	OBSTACLES IN THE WAY OF DOING THIS	HOW THESE OBSTACLES MAY BE OVERCOME	REMAINING PROBLEMS
THE PATIENT				
Should, ideally, play the *primary* and *central* role in limiting therapy	Not wanting death prolonged when life cannot be further extended with meaning and quality according to the patient's own definition *Principle:* Autonomy	None, so long as the patient is conscious and competent *and* "unsalvageable" (irreversibly terminal)	Appeal to the "right to refuse treatment," recognized by the AMA and the AHA	The case of *Mr. Bartling*
		Unconsciousness or incompetence	Natural Death Act (or its equivalent), Durable Power of Attorney for Health Care	Ignorance or neglect of these measures; patient not legally "qualified"; patient not identified as having executed such a document
		The patient not yet seen as unsalvageable, the disease process not yet seen as irreversible and terminal	Either: The Bartling precedent Or: The team continuing to treat. For how long? The case of *Elizabeth Bouvia*	Risk of litigation for assault and battery
THE FAMILY				
Should, ideally, play a role *secondary* to the patient and *advisory* to the team in decisions to limit therapy	Same as the patient's, expressed above *Principle:* As above	The family's guilt over "ending the patient's life" by their decision: defining "quality" of life for someone else	Prior unambiguous, regularly updated written statements of patient's wishes; verbal testimony	Absence of any such statement, written or verbal; the famliy divided in its opinions
	Wanting to end their own suffering, rather than the patient's.	The team's contract is always with the patient first and foremost; the family is secondary	The team continuing to act in accordance with the *patient's* expressed wishes (if known), or according to the *patient's* best interest, medically perceived	The possibility of legal repercussions from disgruntled family members
	Ulterior motivation: wanting to save further expense, or the desire to inherit	Again, the patient's interests take precedence over those of the family; decisions must be made on medical, not economic grounds		Documenting all decisions and collaborative decision-making important
THE CRITICAL CARE TEAM				
Should, ideally, play a role *secondary* to the patient, but more *assertive* than the family in limiting therapy	Medical judgment about "unsalvageability" with the patient who is perceived as terminal Medical judgment about the irreversibility of the patient's condition (vegetative state)	Unrealistic attitudes in the family; family members with unfinished business to complete; legal hazards of withdrawing ventilatory, then intravenous, support The case of *Clarence Herbert*	Continuing treatment *and* initiating emotional and spiritual support of family until family ready to let go; AMA guidelines following the *Barber* case	The possibility of civil, but not criminal, legal repercussions

(continued)

TABLE 5-1.   *(continued)*

	INTEREST IN THE DECISION-MAKING PROCESS	OBSTACLES IN THE WAY OF DOING THIS	HOW THESE OBSTACLES MAY BE OVERCOME	REMAINING PROBLEMS
THE HOSPITAL AS AN INSTITUTION	Fear of malpractice litigation may cause dying to be prolonged; concern to conserve shrinking fiscal resources may cause living not to be extended	Institutional intrusion into the privacy of the physician–patient relationship, now an inevitability; conflict with patient autonomy	New Jersey Supreme Court ruling in the cases of *Hilda Peter, Nancy Jobes,* and *Kathleen Farrell* (June 1987)	The need for more legislative guidelines
SOCIETY				
Economically: Society should *not* make decisions within the ICU itself	*Principles:* Nonmaleficence, alleviating suffering Conservation of scarce resources *Principle:* Distributive Justice	Policy decisions are typically made in ad hoc fashion, not in rational, principled manner	Institutional guidelines for eligibility for ICU services, publicly proclaimed; societal involvement in policy decisions	The increased bureaucratization of medicine; policies applicable across the board do not sufficiently allow for the uniqueness of individuals
Legally: Court decisions affect what happens in the ICU, as do state and federal legislation	Autonomy of the patient	Varies from state to state	Lobbying for national standards	What is ethical is being reduced to what is legal
	Assisted suicide	Right-to-Life lobby	Education, lobbying	Slippery slope

AHA, American Hospital Association; AMA, American Medical Association; ICU, intensive care unit.

tent adults, at any time, to specify their preferences regarding both treatment and nontreatment. The only difference between the Directive to Physicians in terms of the Natural Death Act and the Durable Power of Attorney for Health Care (discussed next), is that the latter (as the name implies) allows patients to designate a proxy to act as decision-maker on their behalf in the event of their becoming incompetent or incapacitated.

California legislated its "proxy directive," commonly known as the Durable Power of Attorney for Health Care, in January 1985. This document empowers another person, selected by the patient, to make decisions regarding health care on the patient's behalf and in accordance with the patient's expressed wishes, if the patient should later become unconscious or incompetent. Ordinary powers of attorney do not survive the makers' incompetence. This one remains in effect; hence its appellation, "durable." Several other states have since emulated California in this respect. All follow the recommendation of a presidential commission that durable powers of attorney be preferred to living wills, "since they are more generally applicable and provide a better vehicle for patients to exercise self-determination."[8]

In the United States Supreme Court case of Nancy Beth Cruzan,[9] it was recognized, if only hypothetically, that a state has no right to keep a comatose patient alive against the patient's previously expressed wish to be allowed to die in circumstances had been reached.

In 1990, the Federal government enacted that Patient Self-Determination Act as part of the Omnibus Budget Reconciliation Act. The Patient Self-Determination Act became effective in January 1991. As a condition for participation in Medicare or Medicaid programs, the Act requires hospitals, skilled nursing facilities, home health agencies, hospice programs, and prepaid health care organizations to furnish patients with information about advance directives. In spite of this legislation, it is estimated that only 15% to 17% of eligible Americans have executed advance directives.

Typically, one obstacle in the way of attending physicians simply acceding to a patient's request to terminate life-sustaining treatment is that the patient may not be considered unsalvageable or terminal on medical grounds. For a salvageable or nonterminal patient to decline treatment that could possibly restore the patient to functionality—at least for the foreseeable future—seems tantamount to a suicidal death wish or evidence of insanity. The (benignly paternalistic) instinct in such cases is to continue treating, hoping that either the suicidal impulse or the insanity will prove temporary and will later give way to retroactive consent. Yet there are people like Mr. Bartling in ICUs who are neither terminal, nor crazy, nor irrationally suicidal. Entirely rationally, they wish to exercise their right to refuse further aggressive treatment. The treating physician is then faced with a dilemma: either to presume that the patient being treated is in the category that Mr. Bartling has compelled the court to recognize, or that the patient is somehow "incompetent" and that, therefore, the patient's expressed wishes need to be overruled, at least until such time as competency can be established. An informed refusal of potentially beneficial treatment is the other side of the coin of informed consent. The only moral stipulation is that the refusal should be an informed one: the probable consequences of the refusal should have been made clear, and the patient should be competent to comprehend these.

The Family's Role

The role of the family in decisions to limit therapy should be secondary to the patient (on the strength of the principle of autonomy) and should be advisory to the critical care team rather than assertive. The distinction between advisory and assertive is important. To allow the initiative for decision-making to pass from the critical care team to the family (where the patient is no longer available to actively participate in the decision-making process, either directly or indirectly with a Durable Power of Attorney for Health Care) is the same as assigning responsibility for making the decision to the family. This means that later the family could come to feel guilty for decisions made that resulted in the patient's death. Because the underlying disease process usually is the cause of death, not the withdrawal or withholding of life-sustaining measures, it seems unnecessarily cruel to saddle the family with an additional burden of guilt for the decision to limit (futile) aggressive therapy. The critical care team should consult closely with the family to act in accordance with their interpretation of the patient's wishes, yet themselves assume responsibility for the decision eventually made.

Ideally, the family's interest in desiring to limit therapy would be identical to that of the patient: not wanting dying to be protracted when life cannot any longer be extended with qualities consistent with the patient's own self-understanding. This presupposes that the family knows what capacities the patient would have considered indispensable for a meaningful life. Where there is good evidence that the family does represent the patient's wishes and interests (either because of a prior written statement by the patient or reiterated verbal statements to which all members of the family could attest), there are no foreseeable problems. But where there was no prior written or verbal statement by the patient, and where the family is divided in its opinions about what the patient would have wanted if able to verbalize this, the critical care team has no alternative but to play it safe, that is, to be conservative and to continue to treat.

Occasionally, the critical care team may have reason to suspect that the family is not representing the patient's best interests but rather, their own: either in seeking to alleviate their own suffering or, worse, in wanting to hasten the patient's demise (e.g., to inherit an estate). Wherever such suspicions surface, the team has no alternative, morally speaking, but to remind itself that its primary obligation is to the patient, not to the family, although a family member may be the legal surrogate decision-maker. The burden of proof is on the medical caregiver. In such circumstances, the team must continue to act either in accordance with the patient's expressed wishes or in what is thought to be the patient's best interests, medically perceived. The reasons for doing so should be carefully documented in the patient's chart, because in such situations the possibility always exists that disgruntled family members will later sue the treating team for malpractice.

Occasionally, it will be necessary to seek a court-appointed guardian to resolve the problem. However, this usually takes so much time (approximately 3 months) as to make taking this route impractical when acute medical decisions must be made.

The Critical Care Team

The term *critical care team* has been used in this discussion. The reasons for a team approach in critical care and the dynamics within the team need to be addressed, however briefly. Apart from the technology, what makes modern intensive care possible is the sophistication and concentration of intensive care nurses in such units. Because of their extensive technical, pharmacologic, psychological, and nursing competence, registered nurses have developed and are steadily asserting their own distinct professional identity. No longer are they willing to be subservient to physicians; they are acknowledged caregivers in their own right, and seek to be recognized as such. Moreover, because of the nature of their training and the strategic position they occupy within ICUs (registered nurses are the one group of professionals in ICUs who are with the patient 24 hours a day), nurses have a pivotal role to play in the communication process: between other members of the team, between the team and the patient or family, and between various family members.

For these reasons, nurses in ICUs must be regarded as the partners of physicians, not as their handmaidens, and be accorded their due place in the team, especially with respect to the process of making decisions about withholding or withdrawing intensive care therapies. (Incidentally, the *Barber* case [discussed later] illustrates the potentially devastating consequences of not according intensive care nurses an equal place as partners in the team. It was the supervisory ICU nurse, who had long been disgruntled with what she considered to be unilateral decision-making by the intensive care physicians, who initiated a report to the district attorney whose assistant later charged Drs. Leonard Barber and Robert Nejdl with murder.)

Other members of the team may include community physicians, who often admit patients to ICUs, consulting physicians, house officers (in teaching hospitals), respiratory therapists, social workers, chaplains, and, more and more, an ethics consultant or hospital ethics committee representative. A recent article in the *Journal of the American Medical Association* draws attention to the way residents at the bedside frequently believe that their attending physicians are out of touch with current problems and ethical approaches.

They experience considerable stress when attending physicians make decisions without discussing them with the residents beforehand, yet expect the residents to comply with these decisions, unquestioningly, after the fact. As the author points out:

> Little attention has been paid to the issue of whether residents are always bound to the decisions of their attending physicians, and whether it may ever be appropriate for residents to decline to participate in the life-sustaining care of patients on the basis of ethical grounds.[10,11]

Although the attending ICU physicians ultimately take responsibility for decisions made in the ICU, those that are difficult or complex should always be decided in collaborative, rather than unilateral, fashion. This makes good sense in terms of human interactions and relationships within the unit. It also makes good sense from a legal perspective. A decision, however controversial, that has been thoroughly discussed among the members of the team, carefully concluded, and meticulously documented is the best defense against litigation.

LIMITATION OF THERAPY. The team's role in limiting therapy should be secondary to that of the patient (on the basis of the principle of autonomy), but assertive, not merely advisory, vis-a-vis the family. It is physicians who are licensed to practice medicine, not family members per se. And, as discussed earlier, assertiveness on the part of the team (after careful consultation with the family) can substantially alleviate the family's guilt over deciding to end the patient's life. After all, it is the disease process or the accident itself that ultimately ends the patient's life, not the decision to avoid prolonging meaningless suffering. The interest of the team in deciding to limit therapy ought to be primarily medical. On *medical* grounds, judgments ought to be made about a patient's unsalvageability or the irreversible chronicity of the patient's condition (e.g., a persistent vegetative state). Such determinations trigger the reranking of principles discussed earlier and the switching from one form of care (intensive) to another (palliative), with the attempt to cure replaced by the concern to assure the patient's comfort. Such determinations will cause death to be resisted no longer, but to be hailed as a welcome guest. The principle of alleviating suffering and nonmaleficence will predominate over the principle of preserving life.

HUMANITARIAN REASONS. The team may hesitate to implement decisions reached in this way, both for humanitarian reasons and for fear of legal repercussions. The humanitarian concerns could include allowing a family with an unrealistic view of the patient's condition the time necessary to adjust to the reality of the situation, or allowing members of the family time to complete unfinished business with the patient.

An anecdote illustrates this last point. After a 51-year-old patient in our ICU had been determined to be legally dead by the brain death criterion, she was placed on mechanical ventilation for another week to allow her 18-year-old son time to complete his own unfinished business with her. He had left home in anger a year earlier and had not seen his mother after that. His siblings were present with her before her surgery (from which she never recovered), but he was not. When he finally arrived at the hospital, his mother was unresponsive. Nevertheless, he was encouraged to talk to her *as if she could hear and understand what he was saying to her*. During the week before ventilatory support was discontinued, he told her that he was sorry about his earlier behavior and that he loved her. Finally, when he had expressed what he had not previously verbalized and had begun to forgive himself for what had been amiss in his relationship with his mother, the respirator was disconnected. The patient died immediately. In this new era of managed care, it is unlikely that such humanitarian treatment of the family is still possible.

LEGAL REPERCUSSIONS. Fear of legal repercussions has been the motivation for the team hesitating to implement a decision based on good medical grounds. Initially, this fear was exacerbated by the case of *Barber v People*,[12] in which two physicians, Leonard Barber and Robert Nejdl, were charged with murder and conspiracy to commit murder after life-support measures were withdrawn from Clarence Herbert, a patient in a deeply comatose state, in accordance with the wishes of the family. However, the court's eventual ruling and subsequent developments have relieved these anxieties considerably. Physicians are *more* secure than they were before while proceeding to implement decisions about the withdrawal of life-sustaining procedures on medical grounds in accordance with family desires. The facts of the case are as follows.

Clarence Herbert, a 55-year-old security guard, had come into the hospital for an ileostomy closure. The operation had been completed successfully. While in the recovery room, Mr. Herbert went into cardiopulmonary arrest. He was resuscitated, intubated, and transported to the ICU where he was placed on a respirator. He did not regain consciousness. He went into what the physicians described as an irreversible coma secondary to extensive brain damage. The electroencephalogram showed minimal brain activity. Mrs. Herbert and her eight children unanimously asked that ventilatory support be withdrawn from Clarence Herbert, and that he be allowed to die naturally. They went so far as to express this in writing: "We, the immediate family of Clarence LeRoy Herbert, would like all machines taken off that are sustaining life. We release all liability to Hosp. Dr. & Staff." Three days after his cardiopulmonary arrest, Mr. Herbert was taken off the respirator. To the dismay of all concerned, Mr. Herbert did not die; he began breathing spontaneously. Two days later, on the family's insistence that intravenous (IV) feeding lines be withdrawn and that the nasogastric (NG) feeding tube be removed in compliance with their written request that *"all machines [be] taken off that are sustaining life,"* Mr. Herbert ceased to receive hydration and nourishment. Six days after that he died. Sandra Bardenilla, an ICU nurse, called the county's Health Services Department to file a formal complaint; the department referred the case to the district attorney. The deputy district attorney, Nikola M. Mikulicich, initiated the prosecution of Drs. Barber and Nejdl for murder. The physicians petitioned the Court of Appeal to issue a writ of prohibition against the trial court, restraining it from taking further action against them. The court of appeal did so, with Justice Fleming observing that "a murder prosecution is a poor way to design an ethical and moral code for doctors who are faced with decisions concerning the use of costly and extraordinary 'life support' equipment."[13]

Based on the decision in *Barber v Superior Court*, the Board of the Los Angeles County Bar Association (LACBA) approved, on December 11, 1985, and the Board of the Los Angeles County Medical Association (LACMA) ratified, on January 6, 1986, a document entitled *Principles and Guidelines Concerning the Forgoing of Life-Sustaining Treatment for Adult Patients*. In this document, it is expressly stated that

> All life-sustaining interventions, including nutrition and hydration, are legally equivalent. It is legally acceptable for the caregiver to withhold or withdraw any or all of them. It is recognized, however, that nutrition and hydration have a powerful symbolic significance to both the members of the general public and to many caregivers.

That is to say, the insertion of IV lines and NG feeding tubes are regarded as *medical interventions* (which, like all medical interventions, may be withheld or withdrawn in appropriate circumstances), not basic requirements like food and drink.

In March 1986, the AMA's judicial council approved a new policy on withdrawing medical treatment. In this far-reaching policy statement, the AMA proclaims that it would be ethical for doctors to withhold "all means of life prolonging medical treatment, including food and water, from patients in irreversible comas." The court decision in *Barber v People*, these two policy statements by the joint LACBA-LACMA Committee on Biomedical Ethics, and the position now taken by the AMA should go a long way toward alleviating intensivists' fears that the withdrawal or withholding of life-sustaining interventions, *including hydration and nutrition with of IV and NG feeding tubes,* could result in criminal action against them. However, the possibility of *civil* action remains; this is what Drs. Leonard Barber and Robert Nejdl faced next.

Society's Impact

The last row in Table 5-1 concerns society. Society impinges in many ways on those involved in decisions to limit therapy in the ICU; however, society's primary impact is in terms of economic and legal constraints. From the economic perspective, society's interest in limiting therapy is based on the principle of distributive justice: the need to allocate fairly among the many claimants for them the limited resources available for intensive care. Public policy decisions in the United States are made in ad hoc fashion rather than in a principled way, for example, according to the proposals of John Rawls.[14] As has already been asserted, if economic considerations are to enter into decisions made about intensive care (as inevitably they must), they need to take effect at the policy level *beforehand*, rather than in the clinical

situation *after the fact*. This is true in terms of institutional and societal budgetary constraints. Inevitably, this will lead to increased bureaucratization in the practice of medicine, with the concomitant danger that policies applicable across the board will not prove flexible enough to meet the unique needs of individuals. Only those with strong convictions about the respect that is due to persons will be able to temper justice with mercy, and thus make "the system" work in a more—rather than less—humane fashion.

Society is having an increasing impact on decisions to limit therapy in the ICU in terms of court decisions and legislation. At this level, hopefully the guiding principle will be that of patient autonomy. At the same time, physicians acting out of respect for patient autonomy require to be exonerated from all possible legal repercussions. If this does not happen, self-interest on the part of the caregivers is bound to outweigh concerns about upholding the right of individual patients to be self-determining, so far as possible, in matters related to their medical care. Further court precedents are to be expected. One such precedent is the verdict in the case of Elizabeth Bouvia, the quadriplegic who, in 1983, unsuccessfully sought court permission to starve herself to death at Riverside General Hospital–University Medical Center (Riverside, CA). Subsequently, she was again admitted to a southern California hospital. Again, the physicians treating her refused her request for removal of a life-sustaining feeding tube. Again, she petitioned the court to order it removed. Her motive in wanting the feeding tube removed, she claimed, was not to starve herself to death. Rather, it was to be able to choose her own treatment. She believed that her caloric intake was sufficient, without IV hydration or NG nutrition, to sustain life. Her physicians disagreed. Her "continued refusal to eat adequate food was viewed by the staff as an attempt at suicide starvation," county attorneys for the hospital stated in their court papers. This time, the court ruled in Ms. Bouvia's favor, and the NG tube was withdrawn. Subsequently, when her physicians sought to deny her IV morphine for control of her constant pain, Ms. Bouvia again petitioned the court. The court ruled in her favor.[15]

THE "FUTILITY" DEBATE ◼

From the strictly rational perspective of guiding biomedical ethical principles, it could be argued that expensive aggressive treatments can and should be limited when (1) little hope exists of *benefiting* the patient, (2) negative outcomes are almost certain and the treatment is likely to be disproportionately *harmful* to the patient, and (3) continuing to treat deprives others of resources that would clearly benefit them (thus subverting the principle of *distributive justice*). In practice, however, there may be insurmountable difficulties present in the way of taking this rational course, as the following case makes clear.

"Judith Pierce" was a 26-year-old African-American woman, unmarried, with two children aged 11 and 9 years, respectively. The three of them lived with her father and his two other daughters. She had a long history of drug abuse and had been on welfare for all of her adult life. In 1989, she developed end-stage renal disease and had been on hemodialysis, 3 days a week, since that time. In April 1993, while on hemodialysis, she went into cardiopulmonary arrest. The initial attempt at resuscitation in the dialysis unit was unsuccessful, and she was transferred by ambulance to the emergency department of the medical center, where the attempt continued. It took 45 minutes to restore cardiac function. She was intubated, taken to the ICU, and placed on a ventilator.

On admission to the ICU, the attending nephrologist, who had been treating Judith since 1989 and knew her well, attempted to explain to her father and sisters what had happened and to prepare them for a bleak prognosis, which was dependent on the results, over the next few days, of several clinical neurologic tests. After 3 weeks in the ICU, the neurology service unequivocally pronounced Judith to be in a persistent vegetative state, having lost irretrievably all neocortical function. There was, however, residual brain stem function, which encouraged the hope that she could be weaned from the ventilator.

The nephrologist, neurologist, ICU fellow, and ethicist met with Judith's father and sisters to discuss continued hemodialysis for a patient in a persistent vegetative state. The father, who always had his Bible in his hand, reacted angrily to the recommendation that the patient ought not to continue to receive hemodialysis and be allowed to have a natural and peaceful death. He accused the physicians (who, like myself, were all white) of being "racists," "murderers," and "atheists." He believed in God and was confidently expecting a miracle. The patient, he insisted, should continue to undergo dialysis. The attending nephrologist was so frustrated (and insulted) by this response that he withdrew from the case after giving the family the names of other nephrologists with whom they could consult. We also gave the family names of other neurologists, so that they could have the benefit of a second opinion. Subsequently, a second neurologic team confirmed the initial diagnosis, and the nephrologist who had taken on the case supported the original recommendation that hemodialysis be discontinued. At this point, the family threatened to sue the hospital if that recommendation were carried out, insisting again on continued aggressive treatments while they awaited a miracle. They were joined in this discussion by two pastors from their church, one of whom stated that he had known a woman in a persistent vegetative state who had recovered completely after the church had begun praying for her.

The patient was weaned from the ventilator 4 months later and was discharged to a skilled nursing facility where she continued to receive hemodialysis three times a week. After 10 months, she died in this facility. The cost of treating her was borne by MediCal and amounted to approximately one million dollars.

This case suggests that when a negative outcome is almost—but not absolutely—certain, one or more of several factors may compel the team to treat rather than limit treatment.

FACTORS COMPELLING TREATMENT EVEN IN THE LIKELIHOOD OF A NEGATIVE OUTCOME ■

PROBABILITY, NOT CERTAINTY

First, in cases like this, those advocating that continued aggressive treatment is inappropriate are inevitably in a realm of probability rather than absolute certainty. At most, this patient's neurologists could say that the probability that she would survive with any meaningful quality of life was exceedingly small; they could not say with absolute certainty that she would die sooner rather than later, or that she would not recover any cognitive function.

The extraordinary case of Carrie A. Coons makes this evident.[16] Carrie Coons, an 86-year-old New York woman, was diagnosed as being in a persistent vegetative state. On April 9, 1989, after being unresponsive for 5 months, Mrs. Coons regained consciousness, took small amounts of food by mouth, and engaged the next day in conversation. Only days before, a judge had granted her family's request that the feeding tube keeping her alive be removed. Her unexpected recovery left her doctor and her family baffled. Medically, her case raises questions about the reliability of a diagnosis of *irreversible* unconsciousness.

The question, then, is: How high a degree of probability is needed to approach certainty? 95%? 99%? 99.9%? We have neither a medical nor a societal consensus about this. Individual physicians and family members are thus equally at liberty to play the odds. *Nevertheless, while the probability of a negative outcome approaches certainty, it is reasonable to insist that the burden of proof shift from those wishing to limit to those wanting to continue with aggressive treatments.*

DESCRIBING THE SITUATION AS FUTILE DOES NOT SOLVE THE PROBLEM

A second difficulty concerns the definition of futility. Futility could be defined in terms of *statistical probability*. Schneiderman and coworkers[17] hold that if a treatment has not worked in 99 previous cases, it may be considered futile in the 100th case. That is to say, they consider odds of 1 in a 100 to be so poor as to represent futility. However, to those who play the lottery, odds of 1 in a 100 may seem excellent! A second way of looking at futility is in terms of *physiologic inefficacy*: in the case of Judith Pierce, the fact that hemodialysis will not reverse the damage done to Judith's brain during the time she was anoxic. However, from the family's perspective, continued hemodialysis buys time for the miracle for which they are praying to occur. Futility could also be defined as *the inability to postpone death*. This definition is not helpful in this case; by continuing to dialyze Judith, death can be postponed, albeit not indefinitely. Fourth, futility could be defined as *the inability to maintain a quality of life acceptable to the patient*. Most of us would not want our existence to be prolonged when the quality of our lives was unacceptably low—and this is how we would categorize being in a persistent vegetative state. The family, however, clearly believes that Judith's quality of life is acceptable. All four ways of looking at futility should converge before a conclusion is drawn. In this case, there is no convergence. This leaves us with a weakened argument for declaring continued aggressive treatment to be medically futile.[18]

DEFINING HARMS

A third problem has to do with deciding what is harmful to the patient. When the benefits of continued treatment are outweighed by the harms, or, to put it another way, when the harms of continued treatment are disproportionately massive relative to the meager benefits, then both the medical and the moral imperative is to stop aggressive treatments and to make the patient as comfortable as possible until death occurs. But in this case, how are harms to be defined? It is not possible to fall back on the notion of harms associated with Judith Pierce's neurologic status, because the family considered her life to be worthwhile even in her vegetative condition and confidently expected God to reverse the neurologic damage. Only future possible harms may be invoked: the burdens of prolonged and repeated medical and surgical procedures and possible complications, including pain, infection, and cardiac arrest. Until these have occurred, it is difficult to argue that the harms of continued treatment are disproportional to the benefits. Besides, from the family's perspective, death is a harm worse than all other possible harms mentioned.

CONFRONTING POWERFUL BELIEF SYSTEMS

Fourthly, in situations of medical futility, powerful belief systems often undergird the position of those insisting on the continued provision of treatments that others deem futile. These beliefs may be religious, or they may be entirely secular. They could be the beliefs of the family, or they could be those of the nurse or physician. Ethnic and cultural beliefs and values further complicate the picture.

These beliefs may not be amenable to rational persuasion: beliefs are typically held with passion. We not only live by our beliefs, on occasion we are also ready to die for them.

In this case, the religious beliefs of the family were reinforced by the pastor who claimed to have seen a woman in a persistent vegetative state restored to cognitive awareness in answer to prayer. And, additionally, it seemed that the family believed the treating team's recommendation to withdraw hemodialysis to have been racially motivated. They suspected the "white" establishment of genocidal tendencies. Hence, they characterized the treating team as "racists" and "murderers." There was no rational way of circumventing beliefs as powerful as these.

THE TECHNOLOGICAL IMPERATIVE

This case illustrates a fifth difficulty: the way in which our society generally subscribes to the "technological imperative." This means that if something can be done, we, too, readily assume that it should be done. Clearly, this was the family's view in the Judith Pierce case. It was possible

technologically to sustain Judith's existence (I shall not call it life); therefore, this must be done.

Most of us have at least three objections to this. One is that it fails to distinguish between an effect and a benefit. Continuing to dialyze this patient has the effect of keeping her alive. But many would question whether this is benefiting her as a person. The things that are being done *to* her are not necessarily doing anything *for* her. Those who succumb to the technological imperative seem not to be aware of this distinction. A second objection is that once a society subscribes to the technological imperative, it allows technology to become its master instead of its servant. The reverse surely ought to be the case: the technology is present only to serve human ends. Third, buying into the technological imperative is symptomatic of our societal unwillingness to confront the inescapable fact of our own mortality. To deny our finiteness, the fact that death is part of life, we tend to grasp at any technological straw. This leads directly into a sixth difficulty.

THE AMERICAN MYTH OF MEDICAL IMMORTALITY

In many ways, medicine is the victim of its own success. Our successes foster the illusion that medicine is able to keep even death at bay—indefinitely. This feeds into our cultural denial of death, a phenomenon that Ernest Becker[19] wrote about 20 years ago. Together, the successes of medicine and our cultural denial of death lead to a situation well described by Daniel Callahan:

> What might be called the death fallacy—the notion that our mortality should be wholly under our control—has two components, one moral, the other medical. The moral part is the belief that we have an unlimited obligation to combat death and lethal disease.... The medical part is the potent assumption that death is essentially an accident, correctable with enough money, will, and scientific ingenuity.... In other industrial countries [someone in a PVS] is not likely to be subjected to aggressive treatment. They have made the judgment that in certain cases the price of continued treatment is simply too burdensome to the patient and to society.[20]

As a society, we have failed to make that judgment. Therefore, the nephrologist and neurologist who want to limit treatment are out on a limb.

"LIFE-SUPPORT": A MISNOMER

A seventh difficulty comes to light in situations of so-called medical futility: the technologies that make possible modern intensive care are frequently referred to as *life-support* systems. This is a misnomer. It suggests that aggressive treatment unambiguously supports life. Whereas this is often the case, it is also true that frequently these same technologies merely prolong dying and inflict suffering. Intensive care is not an unmixed blessing. Failure to appreciate this, on the part of the public at large and of physicians, leads to the erroneous conclusion that withholding or withdrawing these technologies is to deprive someone of "life." It may be more accurate to say that in many cases, especially those of medical futility, the life of the patient as a person has already ended; withholding or withdrawing aggressive care merely prevents further harm being done to the patient or prevents the prolongation of an inevitable and now meaningless process of dying. For this reason, use of the term *life-support* is to be discouraged. It is preferable to speak of *mechanical* or *artificial* support systems.

TRANSFERRING SAVINGS

An eighth problem arising in situations of seeming futility is that it is unpersuasive to appeal to the principle of distributive justice as a reason for no longer continuing with apparently futile treatment when there is no effective mechanism for transferring the savings effected to where they might do more good. In cases where the medical expenses are being met in full by third-party payers or insurers, financial concerns may not necessarily be in the foreground. In other cases, where MediCal is paying only a small proportion of a hospital's charges, they may be of more immediate concern.

The question *must* be asked: Wouldn't this money be better spent taking care of people whose problems are reversible with appropriate medical treatment? The difficulty is that no ready mechanism exists for transferring the savings that would result from not providing futile care to pay for the care of others for whom it would clearly do more good. Only in a centralized system can transfers like this be effected. Ours is a complicated mix of privately and publicly funded medical care in which the left hand seldom knows what the right is doing. This considerably weakens the appeal to the principle of distributive justice as a reason for no longer providing medically futile treatments.

LACK OF PHYSICIAN ASSERTIVENESS

Although it was not an issue in this particular case, a ninth often-encountered difficulty may be mentioned: the marked tentativeness of younger physicians, generally, and of the house staff, particularly, in deference to patient and family preferences and assertions of patient autonomy. Many house officers have a discernible reluctance to make a strong recommendation after discussing the medical options. Instead, and too often, they set out the options and then ask, "What would you like us to do?" The predictable response of many families to this question is, "Everything." Those who abdicate their professional authority in this way prepare for themselves the trap into which they then fall. Once having been ensnared, extricating themselves becomes a daunting and formidable challenge.

We need to remind ourselves that respect for the autonomy of patients means that they or their proxies have the right to *negotiate* treatment (or nontreatment) decisions with those whose responsibility it is to practice medicine.

THE THREAT OF LITIGATION

In the Judith Pierce case, the family threatened that if Judith's hemodialysis were discontinued, they would sue the hospital.

Logic suggests that where there is a *medical consensus* about the uselessness of continued aggressive treatment, where there has been *consultation* with other relevant specialists and with the bioethics consultant or committee, and all this has been carefully *documented*, the team is on reasonably safe legal ground. Of course, people can sue for any reason. But, logically, the kind of process I am suggesting should make it extremely unlikely that a suit could succeed. Not so. Health maintenance organizations that have sought to deny patients expensive treatments not considered to be established therapy have been sued—and have lost.

And in this case, the adverse publicity associated with legal action was probably enough to cow the hospital into submission. Rather than face litigation, it continued to provide Judith with hemodialysis, three times a week, until she was discharged to the skilled nursing facility.

These ten factors at times make it difficult to take a rational, ethical approach to problem-solving in cases of seeming medical futility.

- Inevitably, this is an area of probability, not certainty
- Defining futility is problematic
- Deciding what is harmful to the patient is also fraught with complexity
- Powerful, deeply held, belief systems are often operative
- The technological imperative is extremely potent in our society
- We are up against the American myth of medical immortality
- The term *life-support* is a dangerous misnomer
- No good mechanism exists for transferring savings resulting from limiting treatment thought to be futile to the care of others for whom treatment would result in obvious benefits
- Difficulties are often invited because of an overly tentative and insufficiently assertive posture on the part of the treating physicians
- The threat of litigation, or of adverse publicity associated with litigation, is often enough to scare a hospital into submission.

So, is there a way forward? And if there is, what is it? These are the *real* ethical issues when negative outcomes are almost, but not absolutely, certain. In closing, let me suggest briefly that there may be three options, only one of which, in my view, is desirable.

One would be to refer cases like this to the courts, and have judges decide what ought to be done. I, for one, do not believe that judges are qualified to make medical decisions—nor do the judges I have spoken to want to be put in the position of having to do this. In any case, as has been mentioned, the courts have upheld the plaintiffs more consistently than the defendants in cases where health maintenance organizations have sought to limit unproved or marginally beneficial treatments.

Secondly, we might wait for the state to decide which treatments it will and will not pay for. If the approach Oregon has adopted to the use of its Medicaid funds is more widely emulated, it is possible that treatments for patients in various categories would be ranked in order of priority, and that the budget would determine how far down that list the state could go. Also, in Oregon, in situations of apparent futility the burden of proof is shifted from those who want to limit treatment to those wanting to continue with an aggressive course. At the moment, there is no sign that other states are moving in the direction Oregon has taken.

This leaves us with a third option: that of physicians themselves beginning at the county, state, and national levels to define the standard of care for patients in various categories. In a unique experiment, hospitals in Denver are seeking to define a standard of care for conditions they jointly and publicly determine to be futile, starting with what they call Guidelines for the Use of Intensive Care in Denver, or GUIDE. Continued resuscitation efforts in the emergency department for victims of cardiopulmonary arrest in whom prehospital resuscitation attempts have failed also have been deemed not worthwhile.[21] This process needs to be extended to conditions such as persistent vegetative state.

This is the option I favor. Professionals must take up this medical and ethical challenge of beginning to define a standard of care for various conditions commonly encountered. As a community and then a national consensus begins to emerge, this will strengthen the hand of the isolated clinician, or even the isolated clinical team, attempting to make tough decisions in accordance with these standards.

PHYSICIAN AID-IN-DYING ■

Before turning to the subject of physician-assisted suicide, we must briefly consider the physician's use of powerful narcotics such as morphine in alleviating suffering and also in hastening death.

The moral issue is clear. It is permissible to hasten death by using morphine when the physician's *intention* is to alleviate suffering, and death is the unintended, secondary consequence of this. In such cases, the prescribed dosage must be commensurate with the patient's pain and drug tolerance. It is impermissible to administer morphine with the *intention* of hastening death, with the dosage level incommensurate with either the patient's pain or drug-tolerance. Turning specifically to physician-assisted suicide, during the last decade this issue has come to the forefront of the national biomedical ethics agenda as a result, inter alia, of the following practices, cases, personalities, and legislation (defeated in Washington and California, but approved by the voters in the state of Oregon):

1983: The Netherlands experiment began; it allows physicians to respond to repeated requests from competent, terminally ill patients with intractable pain for help in dying. It was legally recognized in 1993.
1986: Roswell and Emily Gilbert were married for 51 years. Emily had been diagnosed with Alzheimer's disease in 1973 and also had osteoporosis; her spinal column was collapsing. Roswell (76 years old), shot her through the head while she sat on their couch. He was the first American to be convicted and sent to jail for "mercy killing." He was later released after expressing remorse for what he had done.
1988: The unnamed medical resident in "It's Over, Debbie,"[22] purportedly gave a terminally ill cancer patient

in intractable pain a fatal injection 5 minutes after meeting her.
1990: Dr. Jack Kevorkian helped Janet Adkins die. Kevorkian has since assisted more than 20 others to die.
1991: Dr. Timothy Quill publicly confessed to helping his terminally ill patient, "Diane," die by writing a prescription for barbiturates that she subsequently used in an overdose.[23]
1991: Derek Humphry's *Final Exit* was published. This do-it-yourself suicide manual remained on the *New York Times* best seller list for more than 12 weeks.
1991: Proposition 119, which would have legalized physician-assisted suicide in the state of Washington, was defeated.
1992: Proposition 161, which would have legalized physician-assisted suicide in the state of California, was defeated.
1994: Measure 16, which made it legal for physicians in the state of Oregon to prescribe medication so that terminally ill patients in intractable pain could end their own lives, was passed. Measure 16 is being challenged in the courts.

As in any debate, predictably, more than one side exists. Those who are in favor of physicians helping competent, terminally ill patients with intractable pain to die typically make two arguments: one based on the ethical principle of respect for *autonomy*, and the other on the principle of *beneficence*.

The argument based on autonomy is that choosing to die with the direct aid of a physician when life (and suffering) no longer have meaning is the ultimate act of self-determination, the logical next step in the so-called right-to-die movement. The right-to-die movement (so called because, strictly speaking, death is not so much a right as a destiny) has sought to give patients control over the manner and circumstances of their death. In the decades since the case of Karen Ann Quinlan came before the court, this movement has steadily asserted the right of the competent adult to forgo life-sustaining treatments—usually focusing on withholding and withdrawing treatment. Proponents of physician aid-in-dying hold that the culminating point of this movement is the next step from passively forgoing treatments to actively helping patients who request this to die.

What is unclear in this argument is why physicians ought to be compelled to take the step from respecting patients' autonomy to themselves intervening to end patients' lives. Autonomy is not an absolute principle, automatically overriding all others. This is where the second argument comes in.

The other line of reasoning appeals to the principle of *beneficence*. This requires physicians to benefit their patients. For patients who are imminently dying and who have terrible pain, death may be viewed as the greatest imaginable benefit. If a competent patient so deems it, then the physician is bound by the principle of beneficence to provide what the patient wants. The possible flaw in this argument is latent in the question it begs: Is death a benefit or a harm? The patient may consider it a benefit. Society generally holds death to be a harm: Roswell Gilbert harmed his wife when he took her life—at least this was the view of the courts that found him guilty of homicide and sentenced him to jail. The burden of proof rests on proponents of physician aid-in-dying to show that life for the terminally ill with unrelievable suffering is a greater harm than death itself.

Those opposed to physician aid-in-dying make several different arguments, which, when taken together, are compelling. Some assert that medicine is an intrinsically ethical profession, which is why killing patients has been prohibited from the time the Hippocratic corpus came into being: doing this goes beyond what has traditionally been considered to be the morally legitimate role of the physician, which is to heal.

Others appeal to the "slippery slope" argument: if we permit competent terminally ill patients in unmitigable pain to request and receive physician aid-in-dying, it will be difficult to hold the line here; inexorably, the next step will be ending the lives of the no longer competent. This argument has more to commend it than an emotive harking back to the horrors of the Third Reich. Several legal scholars are concerned that the 14th amendment to the U.S. Constitution, the "equal rights" amendment, would make it difficult not to extend to the incompetent the same rights accorded to the competent.

Other lines of argument against physician aid-in-dying are that professionals' advocacy for life would be weakened by it, that the emphasis would shift away from sophisticated techniques for pain management and control to the "quick fix," that society's interest in preventing suicide generally would be severely compromised, that informed consent would not be a limiting condition for physician-assisted suicide, and that the social sanction of physician-assisted suicide presumes a responsibility to monitor the process to keep it within agreed-upon limits—killing, then, would become bureaucratized and standardized.

I, personally, had major moral reservations about the proposed legislation that was submitted to the voters in the state of Washington in 1991 and to Californians in 1992. It contained no requirement to question the management of the terminally ill person's pain. Aggressive pain management has become commonplace in major medical centers, which usually offer a specialized pain service to patients. Physicians have to wonder what those in rural medical practice know about the most modern and sophisticated techniques for managing pain. Before simply acceding to a terminally ill patient's request to die because of unbearable pain, alternative methods of dealing with the pain ought at least to be explored. Similarly, there was no requirement that patients requesting aid-in-dying be examined for *treatable* depression, or that family members (or significant others) concur that the request to be helped to die is not inconsistent with the patient's previously expressed values and is not out of character. Neither was there any required waiting period. Nor was the quality of the relationship between the patient and the physician willing to provide aid-in-dying subject to scrutiny. These, in my view, were all serious flaws in these pieces of proposed legislation.

Measure 16, the Oregon initiative, which was passed by the voters in 1994 but is being challenged in the courts, is more modest than either Proposition 161 or Proposition 191. It merely allows the physician to write a prescription

for terminally ill patients with intractable pain which they themselves must fill and use when they finally decide that death is preferable to life. Yet, the same questions about pain management, treatable depression, and the concurrence of family members or significant others, and the quality of the physician–patient relationship need to be asked, and answered satisfactorily, before even this more limited measure can be regarded as ethical. Besides, even the writing of a prescription involves physicians in the process of enabling patients to die; the arguments against physician-assisted suicide summarized earlier are no less relevant here.

There is an enormous leap from ethics in the clinical relationship to the arena of public policy. Seen within the context of the clinical relationship Dr. Quill had with his patient, a relationship going back for at least 8 years, what he did for Diane seems both compassionate and morally appropriate. In this respect, Quill's action was vastly different from that of the unnamed medical resident in "It's Over, Debbie" who ended his patient's life after an acquaintance of a few minutes, or from those of Dr. Kevorkian who seems not to have had any clinical relationship at all with those he has helped to die. But even if aid-in-dying can sometimes be justified within the context of the clinical relationship, how can physicians move from this to the arena of public policy?

There are three possibilities.

One is to attempt to allow in the United States what physicians in the Netherlands have been doing for more than a decade. The Royal Dutch Society for the Promotion of Medicine carefully drew up guidelines for physician aid-in-dying, which in 1993 were recognized by the Dutch Parliament. Physicians who help their patients to die in accordance with these guidelines are not prosecuted.

I do not believe this approach could work in our own country. Holland is a small nation, its population is highly homogeneous, and, in the classic sense of the word, it is a universally liberal society. Ours is vastly larger and more heterogeneous country and, overall, far less liberal. In Holland, review of the documentation concerning the nature of the illness, the patient's competence, the family's concurrence, and the repeated nature of the request, is conducted *after-the-fact*. Retrospective review, it seems to me, is like closing the barn door after the horse has fled. Besides, there are disquieting reports that in the Netherlands the line allowing only competent terminally ill adult patients in dreadful pain to seek aid in dying is frequently crossed: reports indicate that incompetent patients and children are being helped to die as well.

A second option is to legalize, prospectively, some form of physician-assisted suicide as Oregon has attempted to do. I am opposed to across-the-board or blanket permission to enable people in this special category to die. Although I am generally opposed to slippery slope arguments (why there is a slope to begin with, and why it is so slippery is seldom explained), they do have weight with respect to the present topic. Fourteenth Amendment concerns are well founded, as are concerns about what adding aid-in-dying to their repertoire will do to physicians' professional norms and to the physician–patient relationship.

As a third way forward, I propose an alternative public policy to that of blanket legalization of physician aid-in-dying. I suggest that there should be committees, perhaps at the county level, legally empowered to review concurrently and either approve or decline requests for physician aid-in-dying on a case-by-case basis. Every committee would be comprised of a psychiatrist, an expert in pain management, someone skilled in counseling the dying, and representatives of the general community. To assure consistency between counties, these committees would be required to ask exactly the same questions about diagnosis and prognosis, competence, treatable depression, pain management, the concurrence of family members or significant others, the patient's wish over time (which requires that there be a waiting period), the quality of the physician–patient relationship, and the method a physician willing to comply with a request proposes to use to help end a patients' life. Satisfactory answers to these questions would allow approval of the request and the exemption of the physician from legal consequences or repercussions in that one case only.

Committees have served us well, both in research involving animals and human subjects and in clinical ethics. Far from impeding progress, committee review has helped assure the integrity of research and facilitate clinical ethical decision-making. I see no reason why committees at the county level should not provide an invaluable function and safeguard against abuse in this controversial area as well.

CONCLUSION　■

At least five driving forces, together, continually create fresh ethical quandaries in the contemporary practice of medicine: the discovery of new diseases (like AIDS); the advent of new technologies (such as the Jarvick VII implantable heart); fresh legal judgments and legislative measures; powerful economic pressures such as capitation; and sociologic phenomena such as nurses developing and asserting their own distinctive professional identity. Interestingly, all five factors conjoin and are focussed in the modern ICU. Here the ethical issues are presented most acutely and with the utmost poignancy. It is possible, however, to approach these problems in a principled way, such as that outlined in this chapter. It is also possible to identify those who are potentially able to participate in decisions to limit therapy, and to suggest what weight their respective contributions ought to have, and why. This, too, has been discussed in this chapter. My hope is that the material presented here at the reflective level will be helpful to those existentially bound up in the decision-making process in the clinical situation.

REFERENCES　■

1. Beauchamp TL, Childress JF: *Principles of Biomedical Ethics*, 4th ed. New York, Oxford University Press, 1994
2. Cohen CB: Ethical problems of intensive care. *Anesthesiology* 1977;17:217
3. National Institutes of Health: *National Institutes of Health Consensus Development Conference Summary, vol 4, no 6.* Washington, DC, Department of Health and Human Services, 1983
4. *Dictionary of Medical Ethics*. New York, Crossroad, 1981:263
5. Beauchamp TL, Childress JF: *op. cit.*, p 189
6. Gauthier CC: Philosophical foundations of respect for autonomy. *Kennedy Inst Ethics J* 1993;1:21
7. 163 Cal. App. 3d 190, 209 Cal. Rptr. 220
8. Deciding to forego life-sustaining treatment: ethical, medical, and legal issues in treatment decisions. In: *The President's Commmission for the Study of Ethical Problems in Medicine and Biomedical and Behavioral Research*. Washington, DC, Government Printing Office, 1983
9. US Supreme Court, *Cruzan v Director*, Missouri Dept. of Health, U.S. 580 SLW 4916, June 25, 1990
10. Winkenwerder W: Ethical dilemmas for house staff physicians. *JAMA* 1985;254:3454
11. Moral disagreements during residency training and doctor's orders [editorial]. *JAMA* 1985;254:3467
12. 147 Cal. App. 3d 1006, 195 Cal. Reptr. 484
13. *Barber and Nejdl v. Superior Court,* 147 Cal. App. 3d 1006, at 1011
14. Rawls J: *A Theory of Justice*. Cambridge, MA, Harvard University Press, 1971
15. *Bouvia v Superior Court* (Glenchur), 179 Cal. App. 3d 1127, 225 Cal. Rptr. 297 (1986)
16. Steinbock B: Recovery from persistent vegetative state? The case of Carrie Coons. *Hastings Center Report* 1989;19:4:14
17. Schneiderman LJ, Jecker NS, Jonsen AR: Medical futility: its meaning and ethical implications. *Ann Intern Med* 1990;112:12:949
18. Truog RD, Brett AS: The problem with futility. *N Engl J Med* 1992;326:1560
19. Becker E: *The Denial of Death*. New York, The Free Press, 1973
20. Callahan D: Our fear of dying. *Newsweek*, October 4, 1993:20
21. Gray WA, Capone RJ, Most AS: Unsuccessful emergency department resuscitation: are continued efforts in the emergency department justified? *N Engl J Med* 1991;325:1393
22. It's over, Debbie. *JAMA* 1988;259:2:272
23. Quill TE: A case of individualized decision making. *N Engl J Med* 1991;324:691

Critical Care, Third Edition, edited by Joseph M. Civetta,
Robert W. Taylor, and Robert R. Kirby.
Lippincott-Raven Publishers, Philadelphia, PA © 1997.

CHAPTER 6

■

Informed Consent and Refusal

Laurence B. McCullough

KEY CONSIDERATIONS TO PRACTICE INFORMED CONSENT ■

There are five key considerations in applying a practice of informed consent in critical care medicine: (1) the elements of informed consent, (2) degrees of disclosure, (3) four strategies for obtaining informed consent, (4) informed consent in the care of incompetent patients, and (5) preventive ethics.

ELEMENTS OF INFORMED CONSENT

Informed consent has two main features. First, it is a *process* involving the physician and the patient; it is not simply the signature of the patient on a hospital form or a nod of the patient's head. These are only indications that the process has taken place and should not be regarded as informed consent. Second, as a process, informed consent has three elements:

Patients must be provided with an adequate amount of information about their condition: the ways in which it might be treated (including diagnostic interventions, not just therapies); the risks and benefits of alternative treatments; the prognoses of various treatments; and the risks, benefits, and prognosis of nontreatment.

Patients must understand this information. They must interpret this information in terms of their values and beliefs to determine what, in their own view, is the best course of intervention.

Patients must choose a course of intervention or nonintervention that is free of controlling constraints.

DEGREES OF DISCLOSURE

One central problematic feature of informed consent is the degree of disclosure required of the physician to satisfy the first condition of informed consent. The key word in the above formulation is *adequate.* What is an adequate amount of information? Three standards have emerged, and all are relevant to critical care medicine. Each requires progressively more disclosure.

The first standard is the *professional community standard,* in which adequate disclosure is defined by the customary rules or traditional practices of the professional community of relevantly trained and experienced physicians. Increasingly, in a specialty like critical care medicine, the benchmark will be a national standard, not a regional or local one (e.g., the risks of complications of arterial catheterization to monitor arterial blood pressure and gases). This is a physician-centered standard; the next two are patient centered.

The second standard of disclosure is the *reasonable person standard,* in which the physician discloses what a hypothetical reasonable person would want to know. *Reasonable* means that the patient is free of unreasoning fears and other coercive psychological problems, can think clearly, and should participate in the decision. A helpful benchmark for disclosure under this standard is that the physician should share with the patient any information that has entered into the clinical judgment about diagnosis and about diagnostic and therapeutic interventions. The patient can then assess the risks and benefits of available alternatives and, indeed, whether to accept or refuse the physician's determination that a particular procedure be initiated.

The third standard of disclosure is the *subjective standard.* This is the most demanding standard. It requires that the physician aim for the ideal of providing for the patient all of the information that this patient, here and now, needs to know. This standard makes the physician vulnerable to being second guessed. Nonetheless, in some circumstances in critical care medicine, it is the appropriate standard.

STRATEGIES FOR OBTAINING INFORMED CONSENT

There are four ethically distinct situations in critical care, which do not always occur in a temporal sequence. These four situations, regardless of the temporal sequence, are ethically different, with different requirements for disclosure and communication. This heterogeneity requires a heterogenous approach to informed consent in critical care.

Situation One

The patient is in crisis and is at grave risk of loss of life or of serious disease, injury, or handicapping condition. There is usually little time to act, if action is to benefit the patient. In these circumstances, the appropriate standard of disclosure is the professional community standard. The patient should be told of the condition, how it can be most effectively addressed, the most common risks and benefits of treatment, and the risks of nontreatment. The second and third elements sometimes, perhaps frequently, will be not fully satisfied. The operating assumption is that most reasonable persons want to avoid unnecessary death, disease, injury, or handicap if reasonably safe and effective treatment is available. This assumption would be invalid in instances when the patient has made a prior determination of what would be wanted in certain situations (e.g., a living will or some other form of advance directive), as might occur in a patient admitted in situation three (described later) who experiences a cardiac arrest and has a living will that explicitly rules out cardiopulmonary resuscitation because it is against the patient's wishes.

Situation Two

The patient has been stabilized, and further diagnosis and treatment remain to be done. In instances when situation one temporarily precedes situation two, it is not justified to assume that the patient's initial consent to intervention amounts to consent for continuing intervention. This is because the patient's condition must be addressed in the long term. The kind of information the patient must consider in the first situation—what intervention will prove to be of *immediate* benefit—is different from the kind of information that must be considered and evaluated in the second situation—what diagnostic and therapeutic interventions will be of *continuing* benefit, and of how great a benefit. The reasonable person standard emerges in situation two as the appropriate standard of treatment, because the patient has the time to assess his or her condition and its prognosis under alternative interventions. The critical care patient's needs in situation two can rarely best be met through a single course of therapy. In addition, some diagnostic and therapeutic

interventions may carry considerable risk of failure and be accompanied by what most reasonable persons would regard as significant, long-term pain and suffering. These are important matters in the life of any person and are best decided by that person. For example, in situation two, code status should be discussed with the patient, and the patient's autonomous decision (i.e., one that satisfies the three elements of informed consent) should be implemented.

Situation Three

The patient's prognosis seems to be worsening, and it is not clear whether the patient will recover. Conversely, it is not clear whether the patient will not recover. This situation in critical care is distinctly different from the first two. In the first and second situations, the physician has reason to believe that the patient will directly benefit from intervention; the patient is expected to recover and leave the hospital to resume his or her life. Interventions are undertaken with this goal as justification. In the third situation, the physician cannot proceed with such confidence toward a beneficial outcome. The justification for continuing interventions becomes that of exploring whether it is fully justified to continue, that is, to determine whether recovery to some reasonable degree is possible. Consent should be sought to a trial of continuing intervention, observing that it might fail to benefit the patient.

In a trial of intervention, the physician's clinical judgment becomes more subjective; therefore, the subjective standard of disclosure becomes relevant. Further diagnostic or therapeutic interventions usually involve significant levels of pain and suffering, as well as iatrogenic risks from invasive or painful monitoring techniques. Respect for the patient's autonomy requires that the patient know why the physician believes that such risks be considered, so that the patient can decide whether it is worth going on, that is, whether the patient can possibly change to situation two of critical care or whether to change to situation four. The standard for disclosure in this situation should be a blend of the reasonable person and subjective standards.

Situation Four

The patient's prognosis turns grim, and reasonable and well-founded clinical judgment indicates that the patient is not expected to recover. The patient is judged either to be dying in such a way that further intervention cannot prevent death (intervention is futile in preventing a physiologic outcome, death) or to be in a permanent "vegetative" state from which recovery is not expected (intervention is futile in terms of overall benefit). The decisions to be made in these kinds of critical care cases reach to the heart of the human experience: whether someone will be allowed to die; how someone will die; and how someone will be remembered by loved ones, friends, and care-givers. The subjective standard should therefore guide disclosure. Given the deep human significance of the issues to be decided, primary—indeed overriding—consideration should be given to the patient's decisions.

INFORMED CONSENT IN THE CARE OF INCOMPETENT PATIENTS

The above guidelines apply to competent patients: those who are able to think and communicate (by speaking, writing, or nodding) for themselves. Informed consent in the care of incompetent patients poses special challenges. Traditionally, physicians turned to family members for guidance. Physicians still do so, but other factors must be considered, including living wills and other advance directives, durable power of attorney, hospital ethics committees, and court review.

The main emphasis of informed consent is on the *patient's* values and beliefs and respect for them in the patient's life and decisions about medical treatment and care. Can this priority be sustained in caring for incompetent patients? The answer is a qualified *yes*.

Adult critical care patients have already lived their lives according to values and beliefs that they have found significant and meaningful. Many of these values and beliefs have to do with medical care and being treated with dignity and respect by physicians, nurses, and hospitals. This is especially true of elderly patients, many of whom have given a good deal of thought to such matters as whether they want to be on a respirator or undergo resuscitation should they experience cardiac arrest. This dimension of aging in our society is too frequently overlooked in critical care.

When previously competent patients become incompetent, the following strategy is ethically justified. First, the physician should attempt to restore the patient to a condition of competence. When this result is achieved, the above four strategies can be followed. When the patient cannot recover to a condition of competence, previous values and beliefs—the patient's values history—should guide intervention.[1] This values history may be given specific, even detailed, expression in a living will or other form of advance directive. The values history also can be reconstructed with the aid of family members, loved ones, and the patient's primary physician. Family members should not first be asked (as they often are), "What do you want us to do?" Rather, the questions are, "What was important to your spouse/parent/relative?" "On the basis of that, what do you think he or she would want us to do?" "Did your spouse/parent/relative say anything directly about the sorts of interventions we are considering, like resuscitation or respirators?"

Patients and families most likely will not have thought as much about specific diagnostic interventions when they are first proposed or if they have not been experienced earlier. However, they will have values and beliefs about pain and suffering and how much pain and suffering are worth enduring to undergo medical interventions. This dimension of values and beliefs about medical care is especially important in developing a values history relevant to assessing the worth of diagnostic interventions that involve significant levels of risks of complications and of pain and suffering.

Values histories are relevant to all four situations in critical care. Hence, they should be obtained by critical care physicians routinely for incompetent patients. If a reliable values history cannot be determined, the physician should be guided by judgment of what is in the patient's interest, taking into account the values and wishes of family members. In such circumstances, hospital ethics committees can play a useful role because they can provide a forum for careful and critical evaluation of the physician's judgment.

Some patients have never been competent (e.g., infants, young children, and adults with severe or profound mental retardation). In these circumstances, the physician should be guided by judgment of the patient's interest, again in consultation with an ethics committee, if available.

The role of the family in cases of incompetent and never-competent patients has two parts. On the one hand, they are the moral fiduciaries of the patient. They are expected to authorize interventions that are in the patient's interest, on the basis of respect for the patient's values history (in the case of formerly competent patients) and on the basis of values and beliefs that are important to them (in the case of never-competent patients). In this respect, the family's moral relationship with the patient parallels that of the physician, who is also expected to act in a way that protects and promotes the interest of the patient. On the other hand, the results of medical interventions sometimes have an adverse effect on the interests of family members. In this respect, the family is a third party to the physician–patient relationship, and their interests as third parties can be harmed by what the physician does. This is especially pertinent if critical care will result in long-term care for the patient, which in our society is usually provided by the family. Families should be assisted in distinguishing these two legitimate roles and in focusing primarily on what is in the interest of the patient.

Increasingly, the critical care of no-longer-competent and never-competent patients is influenced by the law. Courts in several states have made landmark rulings that may influence the courts in other states. Legislatures have enacted statutes to sanction living wills and other forms of advance directives. Two responses to this potentially stressful situation seem appropriate. First, if the physician is uncertain about the legal dimensions of a case, an attorney should be consulted. Physicians are not trained to be experts in the law and are often erroneous in their legal judgments. Such consultations should be obtained and considered in clinical judgment. Beware of the attorney who assures the physician that a particular intervention is always the safe course for the physician—it may not be in the patient's interest. Rather, ask for an assessment of benefits and risks for the patient of appropriate alternatives. Second, court review of deeply conflicting cases is an option, but one that should be exercised after careful and thorough consideration. Courts in different, and even in the same, jurisdictions have handed down conflicting opinions regarding similar case situations. In addition, court hearings may introduce factors such as an excessively strong desire on the part of the hospital to protect itself, which turns the primary focus away from the patient's interest to those of third parties.

PREVENTIVE ETHICS

One unfortunate development in recent years has been to focus all of the attention on informed consent and decision-making on critical care itself. Should this patient be on full code status? Should we keep this patient on the respirator, or should we turn it off? Should we monitor blood gases on patients with increasingly poor prognoses or on patients who are dying? These are important questions, but they can be anticipated for many patients before they enter the critical care setting.

Many of the patients in critical care units in our hospitals have chronic diseases and disabilities. The reason that they are in the critical care unit is that they have experienced an acute episode requiring intensive care. In many of these cases, such an event was predictable, given the patient's underlying chronic condition. This is especially true with elderly patients whose chronic condition worsens, resulting in hospitalization.

A major role exists for primary care physicians, surgeons, and critical care physicians in the application of *preventive ethics* to critical care. Recall the previous discussion of basing decisions regarding incompetent patients on the patient's values history. Probably, the least advantageous time to obtain such a history is when the patient is in the critical care unit. Compared with the patient, the family is the less advantageous source of such a history. The best source is the patient. The primary care physician working with chronically ill patients can obtain a values history during regular visits with the patient.[1] The future of the patient's chronic condition can be explained (it should have been already) and the possibility of hospitalization raised, including details about the sorts of interventions available. The surgeon can explain postoperative risks of various diagnostic or therapeutic interventions that might be indicated if the patient needs to be admitted to the critical care unit or if such admission is a standard postoperative strategy. There should be frank discussion of the possibility of future intervention, recommendation against such intervention, and discussion of this recommendation with the patient.

The patient should consider these matters, and values and preferences should be discussed with the physician. This information should be recorded in the patient's chart. If necessary and if the patient consents, the physician or surgeon should arrange sessions with the patient and the patient's family so that they have the opportunity to learn what the patient wants if critical care hospitalization should occur, either as a part of the natural history of a chronic condition or as a result of complications of surgery.

The physician or surgeon should then ensure that the contents of the values history are communicated accurately to the patient's critical care physicians. Managed care that is well managed provides an opportunity to implement guidelines that require gathering such information well in advance of critical events. The role for critical care physicians is threefold: (1) to encourage their referring physicians to obtain values histories in advance, (2) to act on those values histories when they provide adequate guidance about diagnostic and therapeutic interventions, and (3) to insist on development of institutional policies that sanction these two clinical strategies.

WHEN PATIENTS REFUSE CRITICAL CARE INTERVENTION ■

Sometimes, as an outcome of the informed-consent process, patients refuse critical care intervention. A refusal, by itself, is not evidence of incompetence on the part of the patient. Indeed, the patient should be presumed to be competent unless there is reliable clinical evidence—not an untested, subjective clinical impression—to the contrary. Patients should also be presumed to have good reasons, by their lights, for refusing. Part of respect for the autonomy of the patient is respect for those reasons, even if they are not embraced by the physician.

If patients refuse critical care interventions in situation four, their refusal should be respected, whether it is directly expressed or, for the no-longer-competent patient, expressed in advance through a living will or durable power of attorney. The refusal of interventions in situation three also should be respected. For both situations three and four, from the point of view of the beneficence model, there is no *compelling* justification for continued critical care.

Advance directives should also be respected in situation one. In their absence, when a patient refuses intervention and when the situation is immediately life-threatening and there is no time to discuss the patient's refusal with the patient, it is justified to initiate intervention, with a view to removing the life-threatening factors, so that the patient's refusal can be discussed.

This brings us to a refusal in situation two–type cases. The first response should be to elicit the patient's reasons for the refusal. If patients are discovered to hold factually mistaken beliefs about their condition, this should be pointed out to them; the factually correct information should be provided; and they should be invited to reconsider their refusal. If patients hold factually correct beliefs about their condition and have, by their own lights, a good reason to refuse, it is consistent with respect for the autonomy of the patients to ask if they would be willing to discuss alternatives and hear the physician's case for them. This opens the door to respectful persuasion—pointing out how those alternatives are consistent with the patient's reasons—and negotiation. Respectful persuasion and negotiation should not be undertaken with the goal of imposing a decision on patients against their refusal, for that would constitute unwarranted paternalism in almost all cases. Rather, the goals should be to give the patients the opportunity to reconsider and to provide the physician the opportunity to learn why the patients' refusal makes sense to them. Both goals enhance respect for the autonomy of the patient by the physician and respect for the integrity of clinical judgment by the patient—two worthy aims. This preventive ethics strategy should be the main response of physicians to possible requests for physician-assisted suicide, especially those based on fear of uncontrolled pain. A physician's unwillingness to participate should be clearly explained to the patient and supported by institutional policy.

In the end, the decision about whether to live or die is not a decision that is controlled by the beneficence model, because medicine possesses no competence to decide such matters, only whether a death is unnecessary vis-à-vis risks of morbidity. The decision about whether to live or die is controlled by the autonomy model, and this is why, ethically, that decision finally belongs to the patient.

ETHICAL FOUNDATIONS OF INFORMED CONSENT ■

The concept and practice of informed consent entered the history of medicine in the 20th century. The roots of this historical change were in the law at first, and later (in the last 30 years) in ethics. Informed consent cannot be found in the writings of medical ethics before the beginning of our century. As Faden and Beauchamp[2] have shown, before our century, matters of disclosure or "truth telling" were handled in one of two ways. One view was that physician discretion should be the guiding principle, with patients being told little or nothing about their condition and treatment. This approach would lead to minimal disclosure. Patients were to accept what was offered to them, which was usually little more than comfort and support, given the extremely limited therapeutic power of medicine in previous centuries. A second view was that the physician should be forthcoming with the patient, including dying patients. The justification for this approach was twofold: (1) such an approach benefits the patient by alleviating fears based on ignorance or uncertainty, and (2) this approach respects the dignity of patients.

The contemporary understanding of the ethics of informed consent derives mainly from the second of these two approaches. The fundamental ethical principle on medical practice in the West, from its beginnings in ancient Greece, has been that the physician should protect and promote the interest of the patient, as these are understood from a rigorous clinical perspective. Medicine, until the beginning of the 20th century, assumed for itself the task of defining for patients what was in their interest.

In ethical theory, the principle of beneficence directs us to seek for others in our dealings with them the greater balance of goods over harms. To apply this principle, the clinician must have some sense of the goods to be sought and the harms to be avoided. Western medicine, drawing on pervasive values in our culture, claims to have such a sense when it comes to medical care, based on its competencies. Medicine is competent to seek for patients the goods of avoiding unnecessary death (death that can be prevented at reasonable risks of morbidity) and preventing, curing, or at least ameliorating morbidity in the form of disease, injury, handicap, and unnecessary pain and suffering (pain and suffering that are not achieving the other goods). Given this understanding of beneficence in medicine, we can say that there is a beneficence model of moral responsibility in medicine that directs the physician to those interventions that are beneficial to patients from medicine's perspective.[3]

The hallmark of the beneficence model is that its balancing of goods and harms is objective in character. By this I mean that the model requires the physician to avoid, as much as possible, idiosyncratic balancing among the goods and harms of the model. Thus, a worry that sharing uncertainties with situation three critical care patients would be harmful must be based on more than the physician's own intuitions or experience. Rather, such judgments should have a firm empirical foundation in the overall experience of critical care physicians and patients. Objectivity in the application of the beneficence model, speaking more generally, thus means that the physician can give reasons and provide a justification for a clinical judgment about what is and is not in the interest of the patient.

As a result of the influence of law (with its principle of respect for the self-determination of individuals) and of ethics (with its principle of respect for the autonomy of individuals), another perspective on the interest of the patient must be acknowledged: that of the patient for the patient. Human beings have values and beliefs by which they live their lives and that do not desert them when they become ill and find themselves in a critical care unit under a physician's care. Because these values and beliefs shape individuals and their lives, they are to be accorded respect. Otherwise, we treat each other as things, as "means" merely to our own ends, as the 18th century philosopher Immanuel Kant would put it. The ethical principle of respect for autonomy directs us to acknowledge and implement the autonomous decisions of others, those decisions that reflect or express their values and beliefs—even if, and especially if, those values and beliefs happen to differ from our own. This ethical principle is at the heart of the autonomy model of moral responsibility in medicine.[3]

The distinctive feature of medical ethics is that both of these models must be taken into account by physicians. Each directs the physician to important but incomplete views on what counts as the interest of the patient. No account of the ethics of medicine is adequate unless reference is made to both models.

This is certainly the case for informed consent. The beneficence model justifies the practice of informed consent on the grounds that it promotes important goods in patient care, chiefly trust and cooperation. In the absence of these two attitudes on the part of the patient, it is usually difficult, if not impossible, to seek for the patient the goods of the beneficence model. The beneficence model is also the primary ethical foundation of the professional community standard of disclosure, presumably because professional practice is based on a shared judgment of what level of disclosure promotes trust and cooperation. This matter, however, is open to empirical investigation and dispute. This is the reason why the professional community standard, although the legal standard in most states, is being criticized in the medical ethics literature.

The autonomy model plays an obvious role in justifying the practice of informed consent, because the entire thrust of this model is to make the patient's perspective on the patient's own interest the primary consideration. The autonomy model justifies both the reasonable person and subjective standards of disclosure. The autonomy model is also the primary justification for both the second and third elements of informed consent. The second element emphasizes respect for and attention to the values and beliefs of the patient by the physician. The third element emphasizes the importance of voluntary decisions on the part of the patient. Most accounts of autonomy in the literature acknowledge that full autonomy, in the sense of making decisions that are totally *unconstrained,* is an ideal not open to achievement by humans. Rather, it is acknowledged that we act under a variety of internal influences (physical and psychological factors) and external influences (other persons and institutions). The goal of an autonomous decision, therefore, is a decision that is not *controlled* by such influences and thus is to this extent the person's own.[2]

Temptation exists with the autonomy model to shift all responsibility to the patient along with decisional authority. This practice would represent a misunderstanding of both informed consent and the ethical principle of respect for autonomy. With respect to the latter, we must recognize that informed consent is a two-party process. And, in critical care, given its four ethically distinct situations, a constant give and take occurs between the physician's and patient's perspectives on the patient's interest. For example, situation one care relies more heavily on a beneficence model–based approach to informed consent, whereas situation four care relies more on an autonomy model–based approach. The clinical realities of critical care medicine make impossible, and thus impractical, a single-model approach to understanding the ethical dimensions and thus the practice of informed consent.

Shifting the full burden of decision-making to patients, under the guise of respecting their autonomy, usually amounts to just the opposite. This move is often made in frustration or even anger with the decisions patients make or with their general personality type (e.g., the "demanding" patient). What it amounts to is an attempt to isolate or even psychologically to abandon the patient. "Here, you decide!" is not an offer to help a patient think through an often difficult and perhaps tragic situation—as it should be under any reasonable interpretation of respect for autonomy—but is a power play that results in alienating patients even further. In short, the introduction of the ethical principle of respect for autonomy into medical ethics, along with the changes that this brings for such matters as informed consent, should be seen as enriching the moral life in medicine.

SPECIAL CONSIDERATIONS ■

Although a great deal has been written about the ethical and legal dimensions of informed consent, less work has been done on its psychological dimensions. Important questions remain to be investigated if informed consent in its three elements, as described earlier, is to become a more common practice in critical care medicine and medicine in general.[4]

These questions concern the psychological "markers" for the three elements themselves. The first element is fairly easy to measure, to the extent that it depends on what the physician discloses. To the extent that achieving a standard of disclosure depends on the patient's cognitive and affective capacities to absorb the information that is being disclosed, the first element of informed consent is more difficult to measure. Mental status examinations may provide some indication of the level of such capacities but not as much as we need. These examinations attempt to measure such capacities as short-term memory, logical functioning, and the like, but do so with varying degrees of reliability, especially in the critical care patient.

The second element requires that patients evaluate the disclosed information on their own terms. This involves the patient considering the risks and benefits of alternative interventions and their prognoses and rank-ordering them from most preferable (or best) to least preferable (or worst). We need further study of the psychological markers that will indicate with some reliability when this process is occurring, how it can be facilitated and strengthened, and when it is completed.[5]

The third element poses similar difficulties. Critical care patients are under a great deal of stress, as in the situation one patient in the early hours of care. However, we must recognize that a patient's diminished ability to make choices in the first hours of care, or at any other time during the course of hospitalization, does not necessarily imply that that capacity has been lost altogether. The point of distinguishing situations in critical care is to call attention to the changing capacity of patients for autonomous decision-making and to encourage the assumption that patients in situations two, three, and four, especially, possess a greater capacity for autonomous decision-making than commonly assumed. The main goal here is for the physician to identify and alleviate internal influences that threaten to control a patient's decision-making capacity. Psychiatric involvement with and support of critical care patients may be of considerable use in striving for this ethically significant goal.

"To what extent is the patient making a decision to satisfy someone else?" is a question that is appropriately raised regarding the third element of informed consent. In this situation the "someone else" may be a family member or a member of the health care team, including the physician. Again, the goal should be to prevent such influences from becoming controlling factors, even if we still have difficulty in identifying when an external factor has, indeed, become controlling. This is an especially important consideration for elderly patients who have absorbed the ageism of our society and thus suffer from reduced self-esteem. Ageism can also be exhibited by members of the health care team, an attitude that is without justification.

CONCLUSION ■

Informed consent as a practice is founded in the two main models of moral responsibility in medicine generally and in critical care medicine particularly. It has three elements and involves three standards of disclosure, all of which are relevant to critical care medicine. I have proposed four strategies for informed consent in critical care medicine and have addressed matters of informed consent and incompetent patients, along with the important role of the physician in preventive ethics. Patients' refusals of intervention also have been discussed. More study and full appreciation of the psychological markers of informed consent are needed. Medical ethics has created for clinical medicine an important new area for investigating and improving the quality of patient care.

REFERENCES

1. Doukas DJ, McCullough LB: The values history: the evaluation of the patient's values and advance directives. *J Fam Pract* 1991;32:145
2. Faden RR, Beauchamp TL: *A History and Theory of Informed Consent*. New York, Oxford University Press, 1986
3. Beauchamp TL, McCullough LB: *Medical Ethics: The Moral Responsibilities of Physicians*. Englewood Cliffs, NJ, Prentice-Hall, 1984
4. McCullough LB: An ethical model for improving the patient–physician relationship. *Inquiry* 1988;25:454
5. White BC: *Competence to Consent*. Washington, DC, Georgetown University Press, 1994

Critical Care, Third Edition, edited by Joseph M. Civetta,
Robert W. Taylor, and Robert R. Kirby.
Lippincott-Raven Publishers, Philadelphia, PA © 1997.

CHAPTER 7

■

Understanding Reactions of Patient and Family

George L. Wallace-Barnhill

For a more compassionate and effective physician–patient relationship, the medical profession must recognize and accept the psychological dynamics that permeate the intensive care unit (ICU) environment. Physicians need to acknowledge that all injury, regardless of severity—but certainly critical injury—is more than a physiological event.

When patients and families are faced with the crisis of an ICU experience, few are prepared for the physical trauma, or the often devastating psychological repercussions they must face.

Advances in medical technology, particularly with invasive monitoring equipment, have changed the process of dying in America. It is estimated that of the people who will die within the next year, 80% will die in hospitals or nursing homes. Therefore, physicians must understand and communicate with patients and families, particularly during times of extended crises and uncertainty.

There is a great need to *humanize* the ICU and provide honest communication with patients and families. Our task is to provide an environment in which families can learn to cope with their emotions during these crises. Understanding these psychological factors leads to more productive medical interventions, in the broad sense, by not restricting our point of view to procedures and medications.

PSYCHOLOGICAL CONCEPTS ■

Most people are familiar enough with psychological terminology to recognize the term *defense mechanisms*. Most nonprofessional personnel, however, do not comprehend the concepts of defense mechanisms or, more importantly, what purposes they serve and why they are implemented.

Few experiences in life force us to recognize our humanness and vulnerability more than those that place us out of control of our lives or the life of someone we love. There is no better example of this than that of a family facing the crisis of having a loved one in an ICU.

The impact of complex psychological and emotional factors on families can be devastating. Fully comprehending the physical injury that has befallen a loved one can be enough to render even a well-adjusted family unstable, at least temporarily.

ACUTE STRESS DISORDER

Depending on the emotional dynamics of the relationship to the patient, loved ones may experience *acute stress disorder*.[1] Knowledge and awareness of the symptoms related to this disorder may help health care professionals deal more effectively with traumatized family members.

The following characteristics distinguish acute stress disorder from less severe reactions:

1. The person's response to knowing about the threat of death or serious injury to a loved one involves intense fear, helplessness, or horror
2. The person must experience at least three of the following dissociative symptoms:
   a. a sense of numbing, detachment or absence of emotional responsiveness
   b. a reduction in awareness of the surroundings (e.g., being in a daze)
   c. derealization (feelings of unreality)
   d. depersonalization (being detached from oneself)
   e. dissociative amnesia (inability to recall important aspects about the traumatic event).

In addition, the person may experience exaggerated symptoms of anxiety or increased arousal (e.g., difficulty sleeping, irritability, poor concentration, hypervigilence, exaggerated startle response, motor restlessness).

This disturbance may also cause significant distress or impairment of the individual's ability to pursue some necessary tasks such as mobilizing personal resources to inform family members about the trauma. These symptoms usually last a minimum of 2 days to a maximum of 4 weeks.

DENIAL

Denial is a common term used to define a personal mechanism of defense against the reality of a given situation. This deception (denial) is an attempt to disavow the existence of unpleasant reality. Among adults, it is probably more accurately described as a resistance.

Denial aids a person's efforts to filter information. Because of its use in limiting awareness to only positive information, people using this defense frequently make poor judgments. At best, this mechanism is only a temporary reprieve from the realities of the circumstances that stimulated the denial response. Therefore, denial serves a useful, albeit temporary, purpose by allowing time to accept the reality of a given situation at a pace that is more tolerable to a person's senses.

It is crucial for physicians to establish open lines of two-way communication with families. The early interactions during this crisis are vitally important and determine the pattern and degree of communication through the ordeal. Family members' initial reactions, including shock and denial, may interfere with the effective communication and clarity of understanding. Although patients and families have difficulty totally comprehending bad news, it is *no* news that is the most difficult to assess. Therefore, even disheartening news *should* be presented. The manner in which it is presented is important, as is the attitude of the presenter. The attending physician primarily responsible for the ICU treatment should relay the initial information to the family and, therefore, set the tone for all subsequent family contacts. Families are usually most receptive if medical information is presented in a straightforward manner with carefully chosen, simple words.

FEAR

Regardless of how family members present themselves, whether stoic, seemingly unemotional and in control, or out of control and behaving hysterically, the most overriding concern is fear of death for their loved one.

The fear is related to accepting the reality of a loved one's near-death condition and is awesome. Verbalization of fears by family members, however, should be viewed as an improvement over their use of denial. Their confrontation of these fears and anxieties should be supported by the ICU team. Families should be encouraged to openly discuss their feelings regarding the uncertainty of the circumstances.

Determining how each family will respond to this stressful circumstance is impossible. Most families are aware of their psychological dynamics and are cognizant of the extent to which these forces are in play, even if they are not aware of terminology. An emotionally threatened family usually can be reassured if ICU personnel can accept their sometimes dramatic emotional shifts rather than rushing in to provide a resolution. The willingness of families to express their thoughts and feelings is directly related to how they perceive their acceptance by the ICU staff. In other words, family members will usually withdraw if they sense that it is unsafe for them to express their emotions openly. Often families control their feelings and behavior in such a manner as to protect the staff from being uncomfortable. If this situation continues, it may have a negative effect on the physician–family relationship throughout the course of treatment. Therefore, a personal exchange of honest information and emotions is recommended to reduce the level of fear inherent in every family during crisis.

Although certain emotional or psychological responses are expected, the actual process of dealing with these powerful feelings is unique to each family. Therefore, ICU personnel and physicians, in particular, should become involved with families as soon as possible and establish a supportive relationship of communication and care. With the exception of the knowledge that their loved one is receiving the best medical treatment, the physician's attitude is the second most important factor for families.

Physicians should become aware of their own personal feelings of discomfort and uncertainty in dealing with families. When families are offered the physician's human side with the physician's doubts, fears, and, frequently, the inability to predict the outcome for loved ones, families' tensions are reduced. Effective management of their own discomfort is a first step for ICU personnel in supporting their patients' and families' emotional responses.

LOSS OF CONTROL

In addition to the initial shock, the need for temporary denial, and the fear engendered in a crisis, families feel *immobilized* by their inability to control the outcome of the patient's life. These feelings of helplessness exaggerate the alteration in the family homeostasis. A period of family disintegration ensues until a meaningful role or sense of worth can be established for each family member. Many factors affect the time required for this family adjustment. They include the following:

1. Age and importance of the patient to the family
2. Number of family members directly involved
3. Individual relationships within the family
4. Amount of interpersonal stress at the time of the crisis
5. General psychological stability of the family unit.

Other less tangible familial factors include feelings of guilt or responsibility for things said or done, petty jealousy, competitiveness, hostilities, and interpersonal differences.

The ICU staff should learn to recognize and accept the onset of these dynamics among family members. Physicians and nurses should be concerned if family members display an absence of emotion. Emotional response varies among individual families and cultures with different ethnic and religious backgrounds. These differences make it impossible to prescribe an acceptable set of responses appropriate for all situations. Anger and rage are common emotional responses among patients' families during acute periods of crisis. If unresolved, these feelings may cause further disintegration within a family struggling to stabilize itself. In extreme circumstances, these feelings may lead to the destruction of some relationships within the family structure. Although most people seem to believe that emergency or family crisis situations have a tendency to pull family members together and to bring out the best in everyone involved, in actuality, this assumption is usually valid only for families who already have strong, healthy relationships. For less-stable families, the crisis situation tends to exacerbate their problems and drive them further apart.

STAFF INVOLVEMENT WITH FAMILIES

Staff response to family members is crucial to the establishment of emotional and behavioral stability for all concerned. While family members gain access to more and more information about what is going on, their anxieties and fears are reduced rather than increased. Knowing what is happening to the patient, even if negative, is less frightening than not knowing. This direct involvement with families helps them cope more effectively with feelings of helplessness and addresses their sense of immobilization regarding the patient. This acceptance and involvement of the family by the ICU staff permits the family to focus their fears and concerns more constructively. In addition, it provides a psychological sense of communal spirit of purpose, and it gives the family a feeling of worth and of much-needed hope.

Physicians and patients or their families should talk with each other honestly on a daily basis. Decisions should be made through meaningful dialogue and compromise. This patient–physician interchange is based on the concept that patients are the recipients of medical decision-making as well as active participants. Further, this decision-making approach is a process among the primary people involved and based on the premise that the best decisions and treatment for a particular patient are most likely to emerge from this process.

Although patients and families are encouraged to participate in and take serious responsibilities for critical care decisions, it is the physician's obligation to initiate and guide the decision-making process.

The task of effectively representing the ICU's or hospital's position regarding what are often life-threatening circumstances should not be left to the least experienced personnel. The perceptions and impressions, real and imagined, that families glean from these meetings have a powerful and lasting impact on all concerned.

Physicians need to accept families as a part of their treatment responsibility. Working with families for the benefit of the patient decreases the probabilities that disgruntled family members may react out of fear, threat, or ignorance and seek recourse by personal or legal means.

ICU physicians and nurses are experts who dedicate themselves to work in critical care. They are expected to provide answers when the questions are about death. Tragically, health professionals are not specifically trained or experienced in the affect-laden circumstances of helping others face death. When called on to buffer the powerful impact of grief or to make sense out of death to family members, they are often unsuccessful. When medical treatment has failed, only these relatively unskilled people are available to help families adjust to the death of a loved one, a time when even a highly trained and skilled person might have difficulty in handling this most complex human drama.

Too often, physicians, who may be competent in medical complexities of patient care, are lost when it comes to human sensitivity and emotional understanding during the devastating events that occur from the time of an ICU admission until the final outcome.

Although some medical school curricula provide training in these areas, most physicians are not truly prepared to deal with grieving, threatening, hysterical, stubborn, blaming, dependent, time-consuming, arrogant patients or their family members.

The responsibilities of competent critical care physicians are enormous, because they must make medical treatment decisions that affect other peoples' lives forever. Physicians mostly focus on decision-making from the perspective of medical recovery as the only goal. Often this expectation is unrealistic; physicians then experience stress because their only goal is beyond what can be provided for a patient. Physicians need to learn how to help patients and their families during the dying process. This can be accomplished only if physicians permit themselves to look at their own humanness and vulnerability and accept their own mortality.

The unexpressed but powerfully motivating expectation of medicine and society to defeat death is unrealistic. The process of decreasing pressure on health care professionals that is exhibited as physical, psychological, or emotional stress could begin with providing an ICU environment where medical competence is expected, but the acceptance of medical personal humanness is demanded.

HOW TO INVOLVE FAMILIES

Dealing with families will become easier if the following suggestions are considered. Physicians must honestly assess their personal reactions and feelings about a given family. If the personal feelings are positive, the family members will recognize that the physician likes them and conclude that the physician *cares* about the patient. This initial receptiveness will reduce family members' initial fears and uncertainties substantially. A physician's personal response to a given family may sometimes be negative, however. The more physicians permit themselves to experience these negative feelings without guilt or judgment, the more accepting they will become of themselves. This process further reduces any tension or hesitation on the part of the physicians and allows them to interact with the family with a more relaxed attitude. Often physicians inadvertently deal directly with families without regard to or identification of these inner feelings. When this occurs, families respond to the negativism that is being displayed unwittingly by the physician. This type of interchange creates tension and mistrust between family members and the ICU physician. These initial impressions are real and tend to be long lasting. Therefore, close attention and some mental preparation can go far in promoting a healthier and more effective treatment approach for all concerned. The establishment of a positive interchange with family members will directly improve their cooperation throughout the patient's course of treatment.

For a family with which *positive* rapport has been established, flexible visiting hours may be permitted. For ICU patients, loss of physical and psychological contact with familiar surroundings and loved ones is stressful. Therefore, additional visiting time with family members may decrease emotional as well as physical stress and positively contribute to the recovery process. These family members will create fewer problems regarding interactions with other ICU personnel. In addition, this positive arrangement between physician and family permits the establishment of meeting times between a designated family representative and a staff person. This process saves staff time and effort trying to cope with many members of the same family.

Meetings with a family representative should be scheduled on a regular basis. A private office or room should be designated for this purpose; this reinforces trust and confidentiality and also provides a meeting place where other family members can be told the content of the meeting. Finally, it provides a haven for family members to share emotions and console each other in times of grief.

Families who are provided this attention and personal as well as professional response are usually better prepared to handle decisions regarding medical, legal, or ethical considerations such as termination of life support, discontinuing aggressive treatment, or do-not-resuscitate orders. In dealing with families, it is crucial to remember that hope for survival of the family's loved one is the most important factor in their ability to cope, regardless of the medical odds. Most people eventually accept and deal with even the gravest of situations if they are given some hope. However, at times it is extremely difficult for staff members to assess accurately the psychological needs of each family member. Some families are not prepared for or capable of accepting, hearing, or interpreting the truth. In this situation, emotional tension between the family and the staff may develop. However, the ICU staff should recognize that a family's negative behavioral reactions usually reflect feelings of uncertainty and dread and should not be taken personally. Remember, for families, each hour of each day may be filled with hopes and expectations that often are unrealistic. The dreaded feeling that the disease or injury may ultimately prove fatal is constantly present, although rarely expressed. Tolerating the constant pressure of seeing a loved one near death is difficult without having some degree of optimism. Family members must focus so much energy on maintaining a positive, hopeful attitude that often discouraging news is either not heard or is denied so that a false sense of optimism may prevail.

Some families are not receptive to even the most appropriate of staff responses. The staff needs to determine what factors are precipitating the negative responses. For example, family members realize that their loved one is not "getting well," and they cannot or will not accept the reality that the patient is dying. Because the patient is not getting better,

then the patient *must not* be receiving the best treatment, and as a result of this "psychological rationalization" and factual distortion, the family becomes verbally and behaviorally dissatisfied with the ICU staff. In other words, staff must deal directly with the underlying problem (fear of their loved one's death) rather than focusing on the behavioral symptoms presented by the family. When necessary, however, a mental health professional may need to evaluate the family. A consultant could evaluate the psychological dynamics of the family as a unit and assess their psychological strengths and weaknesses. A consultant could also provide appropriate alternative approaches to dealing more effectively with the family. Finally, if the family unit or any individual member of the family is seriously disturbed, appropriate recommendations and referral for treatment can be offered at this time.

THE PATIENT IN THE ICU ■

With few exceptions, there is probably no more terrifying situation than being a patient in an ICU. A constant fear of death is present, although some patients have a temporary feeling of omnipotence for having survived the disease or injury that caused them to be admitted.

The modern ICU surrounds patients with a massive array of equipment that spouts forth a mountain of data in various shapes, sights, and sounds. The ICU environment requires *major* adjustments, both mentally and emotionally. Having been thrust into an unknown environment for which they have no frame of reference requires a Herculean adjustment. Patients must struggle to gain any sense of stability and self-control. The reality is that they have become almost totally dependent, that is, lost control over their environment and personal well-being. They are no longer in charge of even the simplest body functions, including respiration, urination, and defecation. The need for a constant stream of medical data requires constant subjugation to physical examinations and probing into even the most private parts. The patient's routine functions like bathing, hair washing, and brushing teeth become someone else's assignment on the morning shift. This sudden and absolute state of total dependence on others for survival is usually devastating to ICU patients.

COMMON REACTIONS

Almost every ICU patient experiences severe sleep deprivation. Often the members of the health care team are responsible for disrupting patients' sleep patterns. Although the importance of sleep is generally recognized by health professionals, priorities are dictated by life-threatening physiologic needs that outweigh the need for sleep. The conditions in an ICU are inadvertently conducive to mental alterations as well as critical illness itself. The environment is self-contained, with little outside stimulation; body movement is minimal; the temperature is usually constant; and the noise level, although initially abrasive, becomes essentially "white noise," providing little alternative stimulation. Personnel come and go; they, of course, must pay attention to individual body parts or specific machinery, and this may be perceived as not being aware of the whole patient. Staff must, therefore, make special efforts to react to, talk to, and reassure patients in an attempt to ameliorate rather than contribute to the subtle but real slippage toward psychosis.

Intensive care psychosis is a diagnosis often applied to patients exhibiting acute agitation varying from mild confusion to advanced delirium. Patients' feelings may follow a pattern varying from intense fear and anxiety to denial and depression. If this sequence of spiraling emotions is not halted, it is followed by increased dependency, leading to a state of paranoia with patients fearing for their life and being temporarily disconnected from reality.

This state of psychosis has been referred to as an *acute organic brain syndrome*, involving impaired intellectual functioning. Some form of mental aberration begins to appear in patients who spend more than 5 to 7 days in an ICU, and the longer the stay the greater the risk.[2] The reported percentage of occurrence of this syndrome ranges from 2% to 70%.[3] Some of the inconsistency may result from the terminology, which ranges from mental aberration, perceptual distortion, illusions, and hallucinations to delirium.

Patients who have sustained severe trauma, prolonged surgical procedures, and lengthy anesthesia have a greater tendency to develop this diagnosis. The common features of this ICU syndrome consist of clouding of the consciousness, decreased ability to maintain attention, orientation difficulties, memory problems, and labile affect. Patients may display symptoms of altered time perception, lack of emotion, feelings of surrealism, a sense of detachment, loss of control, and revival of memories.

ICU patients face constant concern about death as well as fears for loved ones and concerns for those dependent on them financially or emotionally. This stress, in addition to the reality of their physical state, can cause extreme despondency or depression. The accumulation of environmental and situational factors affects all ICU patients to varying degrees, depending on their personality characteristics, physical state, extent of physical trauma, degree and severity of any surgery performed and subsequent responses, and length of stay in the ICU.

The problem of communication for ICU patients is extraordinary. The patient's inability to express thoughts verbally to ICU staff or to convey feelings to loved ones creates severe emotional distress. In addition, the experience of being attached to monitoring machines and, particularly, to the respirator for ventilatory support produces a real sense of personal paranoia. The ICU staff members and families must be aware that these reactions may occur. They should be prepared to deal with them appropriately. For example, occasionally patients may feign drowsiness or other symptoms to avoid frustration or embarrassment because of the inability to communicate in a conventional fashion. Family members may respond defensively to this dilemma by shortening their visits, *observing* the patient rather than talking to the patient, and behaviorally withdrawing from the patient. If these or other manifestations by families or patient are recognized by the ICU staff, it may be helpful to present the staff's assessment openly to the family. If given in a concerned, helpful manner, the family may use this time to respond with their feelings of frustration and fear related to the situation, thereby providing an opportunity directly to reduce some degree of familial tension. Hopefully, together with the staff, a more effective, personal approach can be suggested to help the patient.

The ICU physician may wish to respond to a patient's symptoms of depression or psychosis with medications. Although the symptoms are relieved, the patient usually is rendered inaccessible to family members. This act of emotionally immobilizing a patient negates what time may remain for the patient and family. It bars them from precious time to discuss and relate those most intimate of feelings and decisions. If patients are not in pain, they should not be medicated. If pain is present, it should be relieved with small medication doses, titrated to achieve success without oversedation, if possible. An alternative is to offer increased human contact and physical touching with a family member. Many ICU survivors do not recall their experiences, no matter how bad, after they have recovered. Most pertinent to this discussion, however, is the importance of the lucid time spent with loved ones, especially for the patient who does not survive.

From my own personal experience living through months of a surgical ICU stay with my brother, I can attest to the powerful importance of time and opportunity for communication. Robert survived with severe, multiple injuries for $2\frac{1}{2}$ months after a car accident. The normal visiting policy of 5 minutes each hour was suspended, and I was permitted to stay with him throughout the day. Until the last week before he died, Robert was mentally alert and awake for much of the time. There were days when he suffered from depression, and there were days that he suffered visual hallucinations. Robert often had to ask me to confirm if monsters were floating above his bed. We would talk about his visions, and then he would laugh as if realizing the absurdity of his thoughts. When Robert suffered from severe depression, his hands would grasp my arm as I leaned next to him, and we would cry. Invariably, however, before I left for the night, he would turn his face to look at me and then, with his hand, give me the "thumbs up" signal. Robert survived two additional surgical procedures before his last operation, which revealed widespread peritonitis. He suffered from septic shock, complete renal failure, worsening respiratory failure, and coma. Shortly before his death, Robert's wife Kathe and I agreed to discontinue therapy.

If Robert had been chemically treated for his depression and periodic psychotic states, we would never have experienced the last $2\frac{1}{2}$ months of his life with him.

WHEN DEATH IS IMMINENT

Families may respond with despair and disbelief on hearing from their loved one's physician that nothing more can be done. Some families wish to continue treatment at any cost despite overwhelming odds against survival or continued life with dignity. Therefore, families and physicians frequently disagree over the appropriateness of specific therapy. Fortunately, such disagreements are usually resolved within the patient–physician–family triad. Physicians should not feel threatened when patients or families assume a greater role in decision-making regarding medical treatment. In a moral, ethical, and legal sense, families should be and are empowered to participate in this decision-making. Although there will certainly continue to be situations that can be resolved only through the legal processes, many such problems can be prevented by more effective communication by ICU physicians involved. When the inevitability of impending death is apparent, the medical staff must recognize and provide for family needs to allow the acceptance of death. Civetta[4] believes that "providing an environment in which families can learn to cope with this unpleasant reality should, indeed, be one of the physician's most important goals." When confronted with the reality that their loved one will not survive, however, families may not respond as expected. They are forced to give up the hopes and beliefs that have kept them together and helped them to tolerate this ordeal. Thus, regardless of prior discussion and counseling, physicians should expect reactions of denial and disbelief. Usually time is the main requirement for family members to adjust to and accept the reality of the death of their loved one. Most adjustments occur within 24 to 48 hours. If not, it is wise to secure the service of an experienced mental health professional before life-sustaining treatment is withdrawn. Unless all ICU beds are occupied and a critically ill or injured but potentially viable patient is waiting for a bed, any urgency to act quickly is ill advised. During this time, physicians should shift their efforts and attend to the needs of the family. This realignment of treatment objectives may allay feelings of antagonism and resistance that arise in the family in response to the imminent death of their loved one.

In circumstances when the death of the patient follows prolonged ICU treatment, the family may initially feel relieved. They may respond this way not because their loved one has died but because the *ordeal* is finally over. Expressions of relief may be unspoken, inhibited by restrictions imposed by feelings of guilt. Nonetheless, the need for some sense of closure is greater than our ability to endure uncertainty.

Immediately after the death of a patient, ICU staff interactions with the family are needed and appropriate. Therefore, the responsibility of the physicians and other ICU personnel should not terminate with the patient's death. In addition to responses to family members on an individual basis, more formal meetings should be arranged for all interested staff plus family members.

The meetings need not be strictly formal, although some responsibility for comments and responses, both personally and professionally, should be presented by significant staff involved. These meetings provide a dual purpose for staff and family. Family members may want to know the exact manner in which the patient died. Was their loved one alone at the time of death? Was the death peaceful?

These meetings also provide an opportunity for families to communicate and share deep feelings of gratitude to the medical staff. Physicians and other ICU personnel often are left in doubt about the thoughts of family members. For example, the staff may wonder what the family thought about the quality of treatment and patient care. Is the family angry? Does the family blame the staff? Do they think their loved one was tortured, or do they think treatment was discontinued too soon or prolonged unnecessarily? Does the family understand that the ICU staff really cared and did their best? Answers to such questions may help foster acceptance of death for families as well as staff.

REFERENCES ■

1. American Psychiatric Association: *Diagnostic and Statistical Manual of Mental Disorders*, 4th ed. Washington, DC, American Psychiatric Association, 1994
2. Kleck JL: Means to forestall ICU syndrome explored. *Anesth News* 1984;10:10
3. Hackett TP, Cassem NH: *Handbook of General Psychiatry.* Boston, Massachusetts General Hospital, 1978
4. Civetta JM: Beyond technology: intensive care in the 1980s. *Crit Care Med* 1981;9:763

Critical Care, Third Edition, edited by Joseph M. Civetta,
Robert W. Taylor, and Robert R. Kirby.
Lippincott-Raven Publishers, Philadelphia, PA © 1997.

CHAPTER 8

▼

Iatrogenesis

Mark G. McKenney
Joseph M. Civetta

Iatrogenesis, or as Kane titled a 1980 paper, "Just What the Doctor Ordered,"[1] must have originated soon after one person undertook to provide some form of medical care for another. However, its recognition in print awaited the evolution of high-technology medical care. In 1955, Barr titled an article "The Hazards of Modern Diagnosis and Therapy: The Price We Pay."[2] He stated, "Although incalculable benefits have come to mankind with the introduction of . . . newer diagnostic and therapeutic procedures, hazards of medical management have at the same time enormously increased. Not one of the occasionally indispensable diagnostic tests may be undertaken without risk." Moser, in 1956, titled an article "Diseases of Medical Progress."[3] He defined the problem as "diseases that would not have occurred if sound therapeutic principles had not been employed." He aptly pointed out that "progress in every sphere of human endeavor creates new problems at each turn." The magnitude of the problem on a general medical service at a university hospital became startlingly clear in a report by Steel and coworkers.[4] They found that 36% of 815 patients had an iatrogenic illness. In 9% of all persons admitted, the illness was considered major because it threatened life or produced considerable disability. In 2%, the iatrogenic illness contributed to the patient's death. In all, 497 iatrogenic occurrences were discovered in these 815 patients. Iatrogenic illness significantly increased the risk of death during that hospitalization. Robin[5] described four particular types of iatrogenesis that were related to critical care. Combining the definitions used by Steel and Robin, we can divide iatrogenesis into six groups:

Type 1: Illness or injury secondary to an incorrect diagnosis
Type 2: Illness secondary to therapy
Type 3: Illness secondary to a procedure

Type 4: Illness or injury secondary to a laboratory error
Type 5: Decubitus ulcer occurring in the hospital
Type 6: Injury secondary to a fall in the hospital

Despite the implications that iatrogenic occurrences necessarily accompany modern medicine and medical progress, and despite the disclaimer that "iatrogenic" should not be construed to imply culpability—both concepts espoused by physician authors—the emphasis has changed markedly in the last few years. Through the process initially titled *quality assurance* and now in its current iteration as *continuous quality improvement*, the Joint Commission on Accreditation of Health Care Organizations has taken major steps to change this almost complacent attitude linking medical progress, technology, and iatrogenic occurrences. The current focus is to link process to outcome, demonstration of total quality improvement, selection of important aspects of care and, ultimately, comparison of performance through a national data bank[6] (Chap. 13). Furthermore, the era of auditing and control within the medical profession also has ended. No longer will iatrogenic occurrences be discussed only at the bedside or in mortality and morbidity conferences. Professional review organizations already monitor many demographic aspects of care and identify discrepancies in the quality of care. These changes may result in loss of reimbursement for the hospital and individual sanctions against physicians who have accumulated too many points assessed for quality-of-care problems.[7]

It is immaterial whether the lackadaisical approach to these problems justified government intervention; an organized and demonstrable monitoring and evaluation process is mandated. Given the pervasive nature of iatrogenic occurrences, even if an outside stimulus has been added, this stimulus should intensify efforts by the medical profession to minimize all aspects of iatrogenic problems.

TYPE 1 IATROGENESIS: INCORRECT DIAGNOSIS ■

Type 1 iatrogenic injury are those illnesses or injuries resulting from an incorrect diagnosis or interpretation. Many specific diagnoses have similar clinical presentations, and individual cases rarely present in a classic fashion. This is a fertile field for type 1 iatrogenic injuries. Of course, we are always at risk for missing the subtle presentation of an uncommon problem, and, indeed, our delight in the clinical pathologic conference reflects our fascination with the obscure or unlikely diagnosis, which furthers our exaltation of the clinician-detective. Another problem is incorrectly attaching a name to a particular clinical presentation. We might consider that a *differential diagnosis* is a cautious method of hedging one's bets. Type 1 iatrogenesis can also lead to inappropriate therapy and procedures, thus increasing the incidence of types 2 and 3 iatrogenesis.

An interesting approach to examining the problems of iatrogenesis was developed by Meador[8] in his article, "The Art and Science of Nondisease" (clearly tongue in cheek). If clinicians are unaware of his perspective on nondisease, they could fall into frequent errors of misdiagnosis (type 1 iatrogenesis). This can also lead to overuse of laboratory testing, with a subsequent increase in type 4 iatrogenesis. Meador[8] reasons that because disease is an abnormal state that can be classified, we think of nondisease or health as all-encompassing and nonspecific. However, because patients are frequently thought to have a specific disease, which is not substantiated on further investigation, Meador asks, "What, then, does the patient have? He must have something. The argument will be presented that he or she has a particular nondisease." He describes a middle-aged, slightly obese woman with facial rounding, a ruddy complexion, and prominent hair on the upper lip. Cushing's disease was excluded by the appropriate laboratory tests. This patient, he believes, has *non-Cushing's disease*. His classification of nondisease is pertinent to the intensive care unit (ICU) population. For example, non-Cushing's disease would be classified as a *mimicking syndrome,* which is probably most common in endocrine disorders.

Two other important classes of nondisease are *radiographic over-interpretation syndromes* and the *over-interpretation of physical finding syndrome.* Unless these entities are readily identified, multiple nondiseases can be combined, such as the over-interpretation of physical signs leading to the radiographic over-interpretation syndrome, together with a touch of the laboratory error syndrome. This becomes a nondisease that often requires 14 days to run its diagnostic course.

In short, recognition of nondisease as a clinical entity can avert the pitfalls of misdiagnosis and overuse of laboratory testing and establish that a patient is free from a disease that may be suspected but is then not confirmed on further diagnostic testing. This label, which is applied after the true disease has been excluded, can prevent the next eager clinician from repeating the unnecessary diagnostic workup.

Iatrogenesis can occur from over-diagnosis and also from misdiagnosis. As soon as an incorrect diagnostic "label" is attached to a specific patient, the thinking and investigation expended on uncovering unknown factors usually cease. Thus, the real illness eludes identification and continues to exert its effects unabated, undiagnosed, and untreated. This effect is further perpetuated when each succeeding group of practitioners accepts the erroneous label and fails to re-evaluate the situation. One case history should suffice.

A quasiritualistic workup of a fever in a critically ill postoperative patient included the search for pulmonary complications such as atelectasis or pneumonia, urinary tract infection, wound infections, bacteremia secondary to invasive monitoring catheters, and so on. This patient had an increased white blood cell count, a tracheal culture positive for pathogens, infiltrates visible on chest radiograph, and purulent tracheal secretions. The label of pneumonitis was affixed to this patient; however, the true source of the fever and signs of inflammation was a septic antecubital vein, which would have been amenable to simple excision. Unfortunately, this procedure was not performed for almost 1 week. Ultimately, 3 months later, the patient died of sepsis and multiple organ system failure. At postmortem examination, multiple abscesses throughout the kidneys and lungs were found; cultures contained the same organisms that were identified in the septic vein.

Teaching and research must reflect a new perspective: gaining understanding of the decision-making process does not demean the role or ability of the experienced expert clinician. It emphasizes the necessity to identify the data collected and the reasoning used, which leads the individual clinician to conclusions missed by the rest of us.

TYPE 2 IATROGENESIS: THERAPY-RELATED ■

Type 2 iatrogenesis is an illness or injury secondary to therapy. Medications produced the highest number of iatrogenic complications; not surprisingly, a greater exposure produced a greater incidence of complications and a greater number of major complications. Steel and associates observed[4] exposure to drugs as a particularly important factor in iatrogenic illness. They showed that in the patients with no complications, an average of seven drugs were used, whereas those with major complications were subjected to 17 different medications. In fact, 42% of the total occurrences were drug related, compared with 35% related to diagnostic and therapeutic procedures (type 3 iatrogenesis) and 23% classified as miscellaneous. Of the drug-related complications, 19% were considered major.

The list of the most commonly associated drugs included nitrates, digoxin, aminophylline, antiarrhythmics, anticoagulants, penicillins, antihypertensives, propranolol, and benzodiazepines. Major complications occurred in one third or more of patients who had complications caused by digoxin, anticoagulants, antihypertensives, or propranolol. Drug-related iatrogenic occurrences must be prevalent in our ICU patients, given the degree of illness and frequency of use. Goals and outcomes should be identified when using medication. "Therapeutic interventions" should be distinguished from "manipulations." Therapy implies a chance for cure; that is, scientific evidence links outcome to the application of a particular remedy. For this reason, prospective randomized trials are considered proper for evaluating new forms of therapy. Manipulations can be considered as the minute-to-minute responses to abnormalities in physiologic variables based on a constant stated or unstated desire to return as many of these abnormalities to normal in as short a period as possible. Because these efforts do not seem to affect outcome, the only possible results are deleterious. If many drugs can be presumed to represent manipulations, we may be able to decrease the major complication rates significantly.

Hospitalization itself has been associated with increasing nosocomial infections. Britt and Deackoff[9] studied nosocomial infection rates as a function of age and length of hospitalization. The average daily rate per 1000 patient days increased from 2.2 days in the 21- to 45-year-old population to approximately 7 days in patients aged 75 years and older. Rates of nosocomial infection increased from approximately 1 per 1000 patient days for stays of 3 days or less to approximately 10 times that number if the hospital stay was prolonged beyond 1 week. The increases were similar for all age groups studied; the higher rates in the elderly population resulted from the continued accumulation of nosocomial infections during extended hospitalization while patients awaited nursing home placement.

Because iatrogenic occurrences require the interaction of a patient and the medical care system, the length of stay predicted the likelihood of a complication and the likelihood of a major complication. Thus, patients who escaped complications stayed about 1 week, those with minor complications were under care for about 2 weeks, and those with severe complications were hospitalized for nearly 3 weeks. Although these predisposing conditions and temporal relationships clearly must increase the risk of iatrogenic complications, they also determine the patients who are in most need of our care.

TYPE 3 IATROGENESIS: PROCEDURE-RELATED ▪

Type 3 iatrogenesis is illness secondary to a procedure. Each time a procedure is performed, the risks and benefits must be considered. The iatrogenic result after a nonindicated subclavian venipuncture, the pneumothorax, in fact represents only a small subset of all iatrogenic aspects of inappropriate evaluation and diagnosis (type 1 iatrogenesis), testing (possible type 4 iatrogenesis), and interventions (possible type 3 iatrogenesis).

We must also consider the serious morbidity and mortality associated with invasive devices caused by nosocomial infections in ICU patients. The National Nosocomial Infection Surveillance System[10] reports that the median nosocomial infection rate associated with Foley catheters was 8.7 per 1000 catheter days. The ventilator-associated pneumonia rate was 14.0 per 1000 catheter days, and the intravascular line–associated bloodstream infection rate was 5.4. Nosocomial infection rates vary according to the type of ICU: rates

were 3.5 times higher in burn ICUs (54.4 per 1000) than in coronary care units (14.9 per 1000).

Devices and interventions transform immunocompromised and critically ill patients into hosts for nosocomial infections. From 1986 to 1990, the National Nosocomial Infection Surveillance System[11] analyzed 1621 months of data from 66 hospitals. The most common sites of infection were those associated with intrusions: pneumonia, 30.7% (endotracheal tubes and ventilators); urinary tract infections, 24.4% (Foley catheters); and bloodstream infections, 15.9% (intravascular devices). The most frequently reported pathogens again reflect the iatrogenic aspect of these illnesses because the organisms are not commonly associated with infections occurring outside ICUs. The most prevalent infections were caused by *Pseudomonas aeruginosa* (13.2%), *Staphylococcus aureus* (11.8%), *Candida* (10.2%), coagulase-negative *Staphylococcus* (9.6%), enterococci (8.6%), and *Enterobacter* sp. (8.4%).

Although using an unnecessary monitoring device clearly offers the patient no advantage and increases the risk of harm,[5] this has been translated into a relatively noncritical appraisal of current invasive monitoring practice. Patients who experienced hypotension or pulmonary edema after acute myocardial infarction were studied retrospectively by Gore and colleagues[12] in a large metropolitan area. No management protocol was used. Clinicians, acting independently, chose to use or not to use pulmonary artery (PA) catheterization to aid in managing these patients. No criteria for selection were established either beforehand or retrospectively. Mortality rates in the invasively monitored group were higher (Table 8-1).

As the authors observed:

> [G]iven the retrospective observational nature of the present study, and its reliance on the use of the medical record as its primary source of data, we could not determine if patients with specified hemodynamic complications of acute MI who received a PA catheter were indeed sicker than patients with these complications who did not have a PA catheter inserted. The decisions to place these catheters were made by scores of physicians, with varying levels of skills in the use of the PA catheter, at 16 different hospitals over a 10-year period. It is unlikely that there was a uniform or even a consistent pattern of practice with regard to the use of PA catheterization throughout the periods studied.

The authors also stated that, "appropriate reservation must be exercised in the interpretation of data from non-randomized/observational studies." Some objective data seem to support the bias toward using PA catheters in the sicker patients (Table 8-2). However, they concluded that these results should be used to promote a randomized prospective study.

However, an accompanying editorial, "Death by Pulmonary Artery Catheter,"[13] dismisses the authors' concerns and concludes that perhaps over 100,000 patients had died since 1975 as a result of the "excess mortality" induced by unnecessary PA catheterization. Robin[13] recommended an immediate moratorium until the question could be resolved. Because a diagnosis does not uniformly result in agreed-on diagnostic and therapeutic interventions, this controversy has received an unfortunate amount of attention even in

TABLE 8-1. Case Fatality Rates

COMPLICATION	WITH PULMONARY ARTERY CATHETER (%)	WITHOUT PULMONARY ARTERY CATHETER (%)	DIFFER-ENCE (%)	p
Congestive heart failure	45	25	+20	<0.001
Hypotension	48	32	+16	<0.001
Shock	74	79	−5	ns
Any	44	23	+21	<0.001

ns, not significant.
Adapted from Gore JM, Goldberg RJ, Spodick DH, et al: A community-wide assessment of the use of pulmonary artery catheters in patients with acute myocardial infarction. *Chest* 1987;92:721.

daily newspapers, as can be seen in the newspaper headline, "Diagnostic Tool May Be Fatal."[14]

Gore and colleagues[12] incorrectly identify a possible source of selection bias in choosing patients who may or may not have been initially more critically ill. The physicians involved were treating their own patients, and it seems reasonable to suppose that there was intentional selection of sicker patients for invasive monitoring. Selection bias implies that an unknown factor was operative: in this series, severity of illness that is not quantitated in the report was immediately assessed by the clinicians. In general, the amount of infarcted myocardium is expressed initially as the degree of "pump failure" and later as an ascending mortality rate. This, in fact, was demonstrated in the study. Thus, an alternative inference is that patients with the more severe initial clinical manifestations secondary to a larger myocardial infarction were appropriately selected for invasive monitoring. Invasive monitoring may aid in delineation of abnormal hemodynamics, and this information may assist clinicians in selecting interventions. Possibly the group that had PA catheters would have had an even higher mortality without the intervention.

The previously mentioned study[12] then might be interpreted as validation of clinical judgment; in fact, a worst-case scenario would be that the mortality rate in nonmonitored patients would have been higher than that in those selected for monitoring because the sickest patients would not have been identified. Criticism then might have been leveled justifiably against clinicians who had been unable to assess the severity of initial presentation. The primary problem

TABLE 8-2. Possible Confounding Variables*

Large infarct (peak CK > 5× normal)
Men
Q wave infarct
Length of stay

CK, creatine kinase.
*Variables noted by Gore and coworkers[12] to be associated with more severe myocardial infarction and occurring in a significantly higher percentage of patients who received pulmonary artery catheter.

with the study and the editorial is that the clinical decision-making process was never outlined. This did not prevent interpreting disparate outcomes as a function of the use or misuse of a monitoring tool.

The ultimate result may be that undue caution and fear of litigation will deprive patients of useful monitoring instead of saving them from increased risk. Thus, the improper focus on the tool rather than the process again highlights that iatrogenesis has many aspects.

Again, if the PA catheter is just a "tool," it is appropriate to consider the knowledge and experience of the "worker." A multiple-choice examination dealing with the PA catheter was given to nearly 500 physicians.[15] The examination consisted of 31 questions. The mean unscaled score of correct responses was 20.7 (67% correct). The authors report that the mean score was significantly associated ($p < 0.01$) with level of training, frequency of insertion, frequency of PA catheter data and treatment, specialty area, and primary or secondary medical school affiliation by one factor analysis of variance. Indeed, the data support the concept of a structured and hierarchical residency training system (Table 8-3). A small set of selected, experienced, and skilled clinicians achieved high scores (27 to 31 correct). However, PGY (postgraduate year) 1 average was 16.4, with a consistent increase with the level of training and experience. Clearly, therefore, the lower-level residents need supervision for insertion and also for interpreting and applying the information that is obtained. It is also gratifying to see that fellows in critical care training approached the level of attending scores. Therefore, exposure and education in the use of PA catheters occurs in a satisfactory fashion. What is also clear (but perhaps should go without saying) is that junior residents should not be permitted either to insert or to use the data obtained independently, any more than PGY 1 surgical residents should be allowed to perform aortic aneurysm resections independently. Thus, this study documents that the training process "works" and that a significant degree of supervision and evaluation is necessary in critical care and in other medical disciplines. Establishing critical care training programs and special certification in critical care by various member boards of the American Board of Medical Specialties seems to be an appropriate step in achieving these ends.

TABLE 8-3. Correct Responses (Primary Medical School Affiliate Hospitals)°

Total items on test	31.0
Skilled, effective clinicians	28.8
Attending physicians	23.3
Fellow or PGY-4	23.1
PGY 2–3	20.8
PGY 1	16.4

°Results extracted from 31-item questionnaire. A clear relation exists between level of training and experience and the no. of correct responses.
PGY, postgraduate year of training.
Adapted from Iberti TJ, Fischer EP, Leibowitz AB, et al: A multicenter study of physicians' knowledge of the pulmonary artery catheter. *JAMA* 1990; 264:2928.

Robin[13] sets criteria for judging medical tests (although he uses them specifically for evaluating PA catheters):

The use of the catheter is a form of medical test. By its use alone, no one ever cured pulmonary edema or any other pathophysiologic disturbance. Its effectiveness can only be judged in terms of improved patient outcome. The only benefit (to patients) that would be acceptable would be firm evidence that its use improved decision-making and that as a result of improved decision-making, patient outcomes were improved. This means that the only justification for the use of a test depends on demonstrating a better outcome for patients. No such data have been provided for the use of pulmonary flow catheters.

Notice that no current test or monitoring modality used for hemodynamic monitoring satisfies Robin's criteria. No data support the use of arterial or central venous pressure monitoring, cardiac output, arterial and mixed venous oximetry, and even inspection, palpation, percussion, and auscultation.

The incorporation of new technology is not limited to the ICU. Feinstein[16] discusses this elegantly:

Nor has any era of man been spared the occupational disruption of new technology. Whenever introduced, a new technological advance has been initially rejected and feared: rejected, because of the belief it could not work as well as existing devices; feared, because of the suspicion that it might. A constant source of wry amusement in any era is to read the deprecations of the initial reception given to technology developed in a previous era. For example, Laennec's introduction of the stethoscope was not greeted as a universal symbol of the clinician that it has become. Said the *London Times* in 1834, ". . . that it will ever come into general use notwithstanding its value . . . [is] extremely doubtful; because its beneficial application requires much time and gives a good bit of trouble both to the patient and the practitioner, because its hue and character are foreign and opposed to all of our habits and associations. . . . There is something even ludicrous in the picture of a great physician proudly listening through a long tube applied to the patient's thorax."[17]

Clearly, we have much to do in validating our interventions and, until that occurs, an unknown risk of iatrogenesis persists. However, moratoria on all forms of nonvalidated medical tests (choosing a single one seems presumptuous and ill advised) are neither feasible nor in the patient's interest. Clear decision-making, identifying indications, goals, risks, and benefits for each person, limits possible iatrogenic interventions while we learn to collect and interpret validating data correctly.

The specific aspects of technical complications, especially those associated with invasive monitoring procedures, are covered in detail in the chapters describing the specific techniques and procedures.

TYPE 4 IATROGENESIS: LABORATORY ERROR ■

Type 4 iatrogenesis is illness or injury secondary to laboratory error. An array of potentially useful laboratory tests face the clinician. Many of these tests, particularly in the ICU, are performed repeatedly. Often, the explosion of test use has been glibly attributed to better awareness of the proven superiority of these diagnostic tests to the traditional methods of history taking and physical examination. However, the proper timing, sequence, and repetition of laboratory testing have not been studied in relation to outcome; this would make it possible for us to understand how many and how often laboratory tests should be used.

We examined ten ways (Table 8-4) to improve the efficiency of care by decreasing unnecessary laboratory testing.[18] This approach could make a favorable impact on total patient care by diminishing the incidence of laboratory error, thus lessening type 4 iatrogenesis. In addition, this approach might help to control costs while maintaining the quality of care. Hospital laboratory charges and the frequency of use of 28 commonly performed tests were abstracted from the itemized patient bills of 50 patients treated in April 1983 and, 8 months after the interventions, in a second group of 50 patients treated in February 1984. The total number of tests (Table 8-5) decreased by 2803 (42%), or 56 per patient per admission. In 1983, 2254 blood gas tests were performed, or 45 per patient. In 1984, the number was 1313, or 26 per patient. We were astounded at the average of 23 tests per patient per day. As a result of the interventions planned and implemented, this number was reduced to 13 in February 1984 and decreased to approximately 8 per patient per day in 1987. Since then, the use of both pulse and mixed venous

TABLE 8-4. Ten Ways to Diminish Laboratory Charges

1. Principles of management
2. Elimination of standing orders
3. Classification of patients
4. Written guidelines for laboratory testing
5. Mandatory communication among care givers
6. No repetitive orders
7. Single order for a single test
8. Removal of monitoring catheters
9. Constant administrative attention
10. Feedback

TABLE 8-5. Overall Utilization

	1983	1984	COMMENT
ICU days (% hospitalization)	15%	19%	Not different
Total tests	6703	3900	↓ 2803; $p <0.05$
Tests/patient	134	78	↓ 56 (42%)
Total blood gases	2254	1313	↓ 941
Blood gases/patient	45	26	↓ 19; $p <0.025$
Total tests/patient/d	23	13	↓ 10

ICU, intensive care unit.
Mean values per patient are reported.
T-test for two means used for statistical comparisons.

oximetry has reduced the number to just two to three per day for most patients. No change in the severity of illness, distribution of patients, duration of ICU stay, length of hospitalization, or hospital mortality rate was observed. For our then 12-bed unit, this could be extrapolated to diminish the total number of tests by more than 40,000 per year. Now that we supervise 40 beds, this may be extrapolated to more than 130,000 unnecessary tests.

Our changes in what Stern and Epstein[19] identify as *physician practice style*—how and why tests were generated—reduced costs in the ICU with the attendant necessary reduction of type 4 iatrogenesis and thus had an impact on patient care. Insecurity, inexperience, habit, training patterns, tradition, and fatigue seem to be responsible for the proliferation of testing. This model of decreasing laboratory testing demonstrated that the quality of care was not dependent on our practice style and that *costly* and *high quality* were not necessarily synonymous. Similar thinking has led to similar findings at other institutions (Chap. 11). We must learn to distinguish the necessary yet costly elements from those that are unnecessary and that contain only the potential for harm.

Another common occurrence that can increase type 4 iatrogenesis in the ICU is the *upper/lower limit syndromes*. Whenever the upper or lower limit of normal variation is reached, repetitive testing almost always follows until we recognize that this patient's values are in the normal range. The most common ICU occurrence is repetitive testing of potassium levels. We continually reestablish that the patient has the upper/lower limit syndrome, and to ensure that the patient remains in this desirable classification, we often institute therapy for this nondisease (i.e., supplementing potassium for near lower-limit values and discarding all potassium-containing infusions as the level approaches the upper limit).

Meador also explores *laboratory error syndromes*. In these cases, the repetitive testing that automatically follows seems to achieve a salutary end. This group of nondiseases is the most responsive to treatment, merely repeating the test cures the patient. Meador[8] states, "In what other nondisease or disease can one see a rise in the hemoglobin level from 6 to 14 g/100 mL in 2 hours with only one iron tablet?" He also mentions a specific variant of the nondiseases, *paroxysmal nocturnal errors*, because many of them occur during the night shift.

Another manifestation may be a subcategory of Robin's *informational overload*, to which Meador applies the term *any laboratory test available syndrome*. This may lead to what has been called *serendipitomania*, the common habit of ordering all laboratory tests in hopes of falling onto a disease.[20] Unfortunately, the clinician usually falls onto a nondisease or into type 4 iatrogenesis. Fuchs'[21] exhortation that we "consider the possibility of contributing more by doing less" is important. The immense amount of data usually collected in the ICU must be organized to determine its use and relevance. We must learn what is the necessary and sufficient data base. However, we must not forget that the societal, not merely the economic, impact of medical care must remain our principal consideration. When we first contribute more by achieving a greater understanding of the medical care process, we can knowledgeably do less at the bedside.

TYPE 5 IATROGENESIS: DECUBITUS ULCER ■

Type 5 iatrogenesis is decubitus ulcer occurring in the hospital. Decubitus ulcers are a common, life-threatening, expensive problem for patients. Pressure ulcers have been estimated to be responsible for 60,000 deaths per year in the United States.[22] Four percent to 14% of hospitalized patients develop pressure sores.[23-25] They occur even more commonly in extended care facilities and are especially common in the elderly. The average cost of treating a decubitus ulcer in 1987 was estimated at over $1000 (range, $47 to over $10,000).[26] With the increase in morbidity and mortality from loss of skin integrity and the increased costs, prevention of decubitus ulcers must be the goal. In addition, prevention has been shown to be more cost effective than treatment.[27] Risk factors for developing dreaded "bed sores" are common in ICUs; these include immobility, inactivity, increased age, malnutrition, and incontinence.[28-32] Supine patients develop increased pressure over bony prominences; the most common sites are over the sacrum, heels, spine, hip, knees, costal margins, and the occiput.[33-35] Patients in the sitting position are at risk for developing pressure ulcers over the ischial tuberosities. Pressure ulcers also have been linked to poor nutrition, especially vitamin C deficiency and hypoalbuminemia.[36-39] Vitamin C aids in iron absorption and is required for protein collagen absorption. Adequate caloric intake also is needed to avoid negative nitrogen balance and tissue breakdown. Another risk factor common in critically ill patients is incontinence. Urinary and fecal incontinence increase the probability of developing skin breakdown. Maceration and excoriation are increased when the skin is subjected to excess moisture and bacteria from stool and urine.

Prevention of decubitus ulcers (Chap. 154) is aimed at optimizing nutrition and patient positioning. Patients in the ICU should be repositioned every 2 hours. Positioning should be scheduled to accommodate the day's activities (dressing changes, line changes, gastrostomy feedings).[40] Competent patients must be encouraged to "weight shift" to reduce the number of pressure ulcers. These patients also may benefit from an overhead trapeze bar. Foam and air mattresses can be used to decrease pressure in patients who are immobile. Patients who are incontinent of urine should have either a condom Foley or disposable briefs. If the patient is incontinent of feces, regular toileting, disposable briefs, and possibly a rectal tube should be considered to minimize the length of time that stool is left in contact with the skin. Also, the cause of the incontinence must be investigated.

Iatrogenic decubitus ulcers occurring in the ICU cannot be regarded as inevitable. Many of these patients have multiple risk factors, but this should increase our use of preventive measures, which are cost effective, and should decrease the morbidity and mortality of iatrogenic decubitus ulcers.

TYPE 6 IATROGENESIS: FALLS

Type 6 iatrogenesis is a fall in the hospital. A patient fall is easily dismissed as an unavoidable accident, but with this attitude, no responsibility is assumed and nothing is done to prevent further falls. Falls frequently occur under similar situations, thus making them predictable and avoidable. Falls constitute a common source of mortality and morbidity in elderly patients. Octogenarians have a mortality from falls that is eight times that of patients in their sixth decade of life or younger.[41] In addition, there is an increased disability for the elderly if they sustain a fall.[42] Elderly persons who fracture their hip in a fall have a 20% mortality rate, and only 25% achieve a full preinjury recovery.[43]

The first step to reduce the number of in-hospital falls is to identify those at risk. Janken and colleagues[44] retrospectively reviewed the hospital chart of patients who fell and compared it with patients aged 60 years and older who were hospitalized during the same period of time but did not fall. She found that seven variables were significantly related to fall status both on the admission and on the fall day: (1) general weakness, (2) decreased mobility of the lower extremities, (3) sleeplessness, (4) incontinence, (5) confusion, (6) depression, and (7) substance abuse. This lends further support that patients at high risk for a fall can be identified. Many of these patients can be identified at hospital admission. Interestingly, this study found that patients taking narcotics (assumed to be a high risk group) were not at an increased risk of falling.

Once high-risk patients are identified, limited resources can be specifically channeled to reduce type 6 iatrogenesis. These patients should be in a safe environment where preventive measures have been taken.[45] The walkways should be free of clutter and well lit. Wet floors should be clearly marked and traffic rerouted. Steps should be clearly marked at the top and bottom. All floors should be nonglare and nonskid. Grab bars should be strategically placed and easy to access. Wheelchairs, walkers, and crutches should be maintained in good condition, and clients should be instructed on safe use. Patients who have already fallen comprise an especially high-risk group. One of ten patients who have fallen once in the hospital will fall again.[46] Some patients

are at high risk from their medical illnesses. Several devices can signal when the high-risk patient is getting out of bed or out of a chair.[45-48] A sensing pad can be placed on the patient's bed or chair that activates an alarm when the patient gets up (Bed Check, Bed Check Corporation, Tulsa, OK). Ambularm (Alert Care Incorporated, Mill Valley, CA) is placed on the thigh and senses when the patient stands up. Using these devices on the highest risk patients alerts the health care workers when a patient is standing up.

Falls cannot be viewed as unavoidable accidents. The number of falls at an institution can be reduced and is related to the patient's environment. Health care workers must take responsibility to ensure safe surroundings for the patients. To paraphrase Ross,[45] "Does a fall in a nontherapeutic or nonsupportive environment represent malpractice?" Further research is required to identify the accuracy of picking out high-risk patients and to assess the effectiveness of therapy. The onus of responsibility rests on the institutions where patients are treated to follow the pattern of falls, identify the high-risk groups, and follow the results of treatment. Only then will we be able to decrease type 6 iatrogenesis.

DISCUSSION AND LEGAL ASPECTS

Steel and associates[4] conclude that it may be logically sound to speculate that the benefit of hospitalization far exceeds the risk. However, they state that because of the severity of illness of the population in hospitals, the natural progression of disease, and the value of alternative modes of therapy, mechanisms must be developed to assess the hazards of hospitalization in an ongoing manner. Technological, educational, and administrative means can then be sought to reduce the number and severity of untoward events, and the efficacy of such efforts can be ascertained.

Thus far we have considered iatrogenesis solely from the viewpoint of the medical practitioner. Another perspective has been investigated as part of an interdisciplinary study of medical injury and malpractice litigation. Brennan and associates[49] reviewed over 30,000 randomly selected records from acute care hospitals in New York State in 1984. Adverse events occurred in 3.7% of the hospitalizations, and 28% of these events were judged to result from negligence. Although 70% of the adverse events gave rise to disability lasting less than 6 months, 14% led to death. The authors estimated that nearly 100,000 adverse events occurred in New York State hospitals, and over 27,000 involved negligence.

In a second analysis, the nature of these adverse events was investigated.[50] Nearly 48% were linked to operative procedures. However, only 17% were thought to be related to negligence. Interestingly, the authors point out that operations involve many technical steps and, therefore, offer many opportunities for errors. Not all errors can be considered negligent, but it is because of the complicated nature of surgical procedures that adverse events occur so frequently. In addition, the incidence of adverse events was associated with increasing patient age. Again, elderly patients who have less physiologic reserve and more severe illnesses seem to develop more adverse reactions. However, only 3% of the adverse events occurred in ICUs—also the site of many technical procedures and also a location used by many elderly patients. Even if the distinction between error and negligence is important in tort law, wherein medical negligence is defined as failure to meet the standard practice of an average qualified physician, the types of errors are important from a quality assurance standpoint and from our own desire to improve medical practice. Performance errors were most frequent, and of these, 75% were related to technique. Inadequate preparation of the patient before the procedure and inadequate monitoring afterward accounted for another 10% each (multiple errors could be present). Errors of prevention included failure to take precautions to prevent accidental injury, failure to use indicated tests, failure to act on the results of tests or findings, and avoidable delay in treatment. The latter three errors were also the most frequent types in the classification of diagnostic errors.

Many of the adverse events identified were neither preventable nor predictable, given the current state of medical knowledge; for example, idiosyncratic drug reactions in patients who had never taken the drug or postoperative myocardial infarction in young patients with no previous evidence of heart disease. Other unpreventable adverse events occur with predictable frequency, such as wound infections after clean elective surgery. If a high rate is encountered, however, this may be a problem for an individual physician, quality assurance, and risk management.

Everyone acknowledges that some degree of error is inherent in all human activity, and medicine is no exception. Accordingly, standards of practice must include an acceptance of this fact. Leape and coworkers[50] conclude the following:

> [A]dverse events result from the interaction of the patient, the patient's disease, and the complicated, highly technical system of medical care provided not only by a diverse group of doctors, other caregivers, and support personnel, but also by a medical-industrial system that supplies drugs and equipment. Reducing the risk of adverse events requires an examination of all these factors as well as their relation with each other.

These studies are notable for two important reasons: (1) nearly 1 of 25 patients will have an adverse event; (2) of these, nearly 30% will be caused by negligence. Because negligence is defined as substandard performance, its incidence can be reduced. Although it is interesting to speculate on a lawyer's reaction to the estimate of over 27,000 adverse events involving negligence occurring in New York State in a single year, we must be careful not to characterize our own iatrogenic occurrences as inevitable or unpredictable. Careful self-scrutiny and unit-wide quality assurance programs must examine details of care to reduce the proportion of negligent adverse events as much as possible.

CONCLUSION

Medical knowledge and our professional skills may not be able to treat each devastating critical illness, but we must not view this with a sense of failure. Rather, it is an opportunity for the expression of those unique human resources that aid the family and patient in coping with the dying process. The opposite course, persisting in hopeless situations, completely blocks the achievement of these important objectives.

We must accept the responsibility to investigate, quantify, and delineate our clinical care so that the subtle effects introduced by bias and lack of understanding (i.e., iatrogenesis in its broadest sense) can be minimized. The ultimate effect of purifying, clarifying, distilling, and delineating bedside intensive care will be in eliminating misinterpretations, misdirections, and misadventures—iatrogenesis.

Medicine has been described as an art and a science. The frequency with which the imprecise term "art" is used reflects the clinician's inability to identify the necessary data base used to form decisions or to relate this decision to subsequent diagnostic evaluation, therapeutic interventions, or clinical expectations for survival. Feinstein[16] has clarified the issue elegantly. Current "science" relies on continuous measurement techniques. Clinical judgment must rely on a different form of mathematics, Boolean algebra for its logic and group and set theory as its measurement tool (Chap. 4). The result is that the clinical decision-making process rarely is documented in the medical record, which prevents subsequent analysis of the total process of care. The particular diagnosis does not uniformly result in specific diagnostic and therapeutic interventions, and we can consider this one of the most important iatrogenic aspects of our care.

REFERENCES ■

1. Kane RL: Iatrogenesis: just what the doctor ordered. *J Community Health* 1980;5:149
2. Barr DP: Hazards of modern diagnosis and therapy: the price we pay. *JAMA* 1956;159:1452
3. Moser RH: Diseases of medical progress. *N Engl J Med* 1956;255:606
4. Steel K, Gertman PM, Crescenzi C, et al: Iatrogenic illness on a general medical service at a university hospital. *N Engl J Med* 1981;304:638
5. Robin ED: A critical look at critical care. *Crit Care Med* 1983;11:144
6. Joint Commission on Accreditation of Health Care Organizations: *Accreditation Manual for Hospitals.* Chicago, JCAHO, 1990
7. Joint Commission on Accreditation of Health Care Organizations: New scoring guidelines adapted from hospital QA activities. In: *The Joint Commission Perspectives Newsletter.* Chicago, JCAHO, 1990;10:1
8. Meador CK: The art and science of nondisease. *N Engl J Med* 1965;272:92
9. Britt M, Deackoff K: Nosocomial infections in the "old." [abstract B/48]. Third International Conference on Nosocomial Infections, Atlanta, Georgia, 1990:56
10. Edwards JR, Jarvis W, The National Nosocomial Infection Surveillance System (NNIS): Nosocomial infection rates in adult and pediatric intensive care units (ICU) in the United States, 1986–90 [abstract 52]. American Society of Microbiology, Conference on Chemical Germicides, Atlanta, Georgia, July 1990:28
11. Edwards J, Jarvis W, The National Nosocomial Infections Surveillance System (NNIS): The distribution of nosocomial infec-

tions by site and pathogen in adult and pediatric intensive care units in the United States, 1986–1990 [abstract B/19]. American Society of Microbiology, Conference on Chemical Germicides, Atlanta, Georgia, July 1990

12. Gore JM, Goldberg RJ, Spodick DH, et al: A community-wide assessment of the use of pulmonary artery catheters in patients with acute myocardial infarction. *Chest* 1987;92:721

13. Robin ED: Death by pulmonary artery flow-directed catheter: time for a moratorium [editorial]? *Chest* 1987;92:727

14. Krieger LM: Diagnostic tool may be fatal. *San Francisco Examiner*, October 17, 1987

15. Iberti TJ, Fischer EP, Leibowitz AB, et al: A multicenter study of physicians' knowledge of the pulmonary artery catheter. *JAMA* 1990;264:2928

16. Feinstein AR: *Clinical Judgment*. Baltimore, Williams & Wilkins, 1967

17. McKosick VA: *A Cardiovascular Sound in Health and Disease*. Baltimore, Williams & Wilkins, 1958:12

18. Civetta JM, Hudson-Civetta JA: Maintaining quality of care while reducing charges in the ICU: 10 ways. *Ann Surg* 1985;202:524

19. Stern RS, Epstein AM: Institutional responses to prospective payment based on diagnosis-related groups: implications for cost, quality, and access. *N Engl J Med* 1985;312:621

20. Pittman JA Jr: Personal communication with Clifton Meador. In Meador CK: The art and science of nondisease. *N Engl J Med* 1965;272:92

21. Fuchs VR: A more effective, efficient and equitable system. *West J Med* 1976;125:3

22. Kynes P: A new perspective on pressure sore prevention. *J Enterostomal Ther* 1986;13:42

23. Brandeis B, Morris JN, Nash DJ, et al: Incidence and healing rates of pressure ulcers in the nursing home. *Decubitus* 1989;2:60

24. Ek AC, Bowman G: A descriptive study of pressure sores: the prevalence of pressure sores and the characteristics of patients. *J Adv Nurs* 1982;7:51

25. Langemo DK, Olson B, Hunter S, et al: Incidence of pressure sores in acute care, rehabilitation, extended care, home health, and hospice in one locale. *Decubitus* 1989;2:42

26. Alterescu V: The financial costs of inpatient pressure ulcers to an acute care facility. *Decubitus* 1989;2:14

27. Oot-Giromini B, Bidwell FC, Heller NB, et al: Pressure ulcer prevention versus treatment: comparative product cost study. *Decubitus* 1989;2:52

28. Andersen KE, Jensen O, Kvorning SA, et al: Decubitus prophylaxis: a prospective trial of the efficiency of alternating-pressure, air mattresses and water-mattresses. *Acta Derm Venereol (Stockh)* 1982;63:227

29. Bergstrom N, Braden BJ, Laguzza A, et al: The Braden scale for predicting pressure sore risk. *Nurs Res* 1987;36:205

30. Gosnell D: An assessment tool to identify pressure sores. *Nurs Res* 1973;22:55

31. Norton D, McLaren R, Exton-Smith AN: *An Investigation of Geriatric Nursing Problems in Hospitals*. Edinburgh, Churchill Livingstone, 1962

32. Taylor KN: Assessment tools for the identification of patients at risk for the development of pressure sores: a review. *J Enterostomal Ther* 1988;15:201

33. Kosiak M: Etiology and pathology of ischemic ulcers. *Arch Phys Med Rehabil* 1959;40:62

34. Lindan O, Greenway RN, Piazza JM: Pressure distribution on the surface of the human body. *Arch Phys Med Rehabil* 1965;46:378

35. Seiler WO, Stahlein HB: Recent findings on decubitus ulcer pathology: implications for care. *Geriatrics* 1986;41:47

36. Husain T: An experimental study of some pressure effects on tissues with reference to the bedsore problem. *J Pathol Bacteriol* 1953;66:347

37. Allman RM, Laprade CA, Noel LB, et al: Pressure sores among hospitalized patients. *Ann Intern Med* 1986;105:337

38. Bergstrom N, Norvell K, Braden B: Instant nutritional assessment, serum albumin, and total lymphocyte count as predictors of pressure sore risk. *Gerontologist* 1988;28(Suppl):76A

39. Taylor TV, Rimmer S, Day B, et al: Ascorbic acid supplementation in the treatment of pressure sores. *Lancet* 1974;ii:544

40. Kelley LS, Mobily PR: Iatrogenesis in the elderly: impaired skin integrity. *J Gerontol Nurs* 1991;17:24

41. Louia M: Falls and their causes. *J Gerontol Nurs* 1983;3:142

42. Jensen JS, Tondevold E: Mortality after hip fractures. *Acta Orthop Scan* 1979;50:161

43. Hofeldt F: Proximal femoral fractures. *Clin Orthop* 1987;218:12

44. Janken JK, Reynolds BA, Swiech K: Patient falls in the acute care setting: identifying risk factors. *Nurs Res* 1986;35:215

45. Ross JR: Iatrogenesis in the elderly: contributors to falls. *J Gerontol Nurs* 1991;17:19

46. Lynn FH: Incidents: need they be accidents? *Am J Nurs* 1980;80:1098

47. Meissner BA: Patient fall prediction. *Nurs Management* 1988;16:78

48. Hendrich AL: An effective unit-based fall prevention plan. *J Nurs Qual Assur* 1988;3:28

49. Brennan TA, Leape LL, Laird NM, et al: Incidence of adverse events and negligence in hospitalized patients: results of the Harvard Medical Practice Study I. *N Engl J Med* 1991;324:370

50. Leape LL, Brennan TA, Laird NM, et al: The nature of adverse events in hospitalized patients: results of the Harvard Medical Practice Study II. *N Engl J Med* 1991;324:377

Critical Care, Third Edition, edited by Joseph M. Civetta, Robert W. Taylor, and Robert R. Kirby. Lippincott-Raven Publishers, Philadelphia, PA © 1997.

CHAPTER 9

∎

Judicial Involvement in Treatment Decisions

Christopher J. Armstrong

In the years between the Karen Ann Quinlan decision (1976)[1] and the decision of the United States Supreme Court in the Nancy Cruzan case (1990),[2] appellate courts throughout the United States were required to address a problem that might be called the downside of modern medical advances: the growing ability of medicine to stave off death almost indefinitely, holding the patient in a kind of technological limbo, midway between life and death, without hope of cure, usually at great emotional cost to the family or friends and financial cost to them or to society. Common sense suggested that there came a point where medical intervention did more harm than good and nature should be allowed to take its course. As early as 1955, Pope Pius XII cautioned medical practitioners against "a technological attitude that threatens to become an abuse,"[3] and other observers depicted "[t]he ultimate horror [not as] death but the possibility of being maintained in limbo, in a sterile room, by machines controlled by strangers."[4] Although common sense could identify technological abuse in extreme cases, no one had articulated practical and generally ac-

cepted guidelines for determining when the line had been crossed from the appropriate to the excessive.

The concept of withholding life-sustaining treatment was not new. The public generally assumed that medical practitioners did everything in their power to sustain the lives of the critically ill patients; however, those in the profession knew that the truth was not so simple. They knew of instances in which, by written or verbal orders, available resuscitation was intentionally withheld in the aftermath of cardiac arrest,[5] in which severely defective newborns were permitted to die from treatable conditions,[6] and in which hospitalization and antibiotic therapy were withheld from severely debilitated patients in nursing homes,[7] pneumonia, for example, being treated (paraphrasing Osler) as "the old man's friend." Doctors as a group were not eager to discuss these matters openly.

Destroying the public misconception might impair confidence in the profession. Knowledge of the fact of choice would trouble many families unnecessarily. The wise family physician was treating the family as well as the patient, a family whose concerns and troubles he understood. Where difficult decisions had to be made, he would not hesitate to spare the family and take the burden on himself.

Three factors conspired to destroy the myth. One was the gradual breakdown of the once-intimate relationship

---

1. *Matter of Quinlan,* 70 N.J. 10 (1976)

2. *Cruzan v Director, Missouri Dept. of Health,* 110 S. Ct. 2841 (1990)

3. Quoted in the Vatican Declaration on Euthanasia, May 5, 1980, appearing in Appendix C of the Report of the President's Commission of the Study of Ethical Problems in Medicine and Biomedical and Behavioral Research, Deciding to Forego Life Sustaining Treatment (1983)

4. Steel, "The Right to Die: New Options in California," 93 Christian Century (July–Dec. 1976), quoted in *In re Torres,* 357 N.W. 2d 332, 340 (Minn.1984)

---

5. Rabkin, Gillerman, Rice: Orders not to resuscitate. *N Engl J Med* 1976;295:364

6. Duff, Campbell: Moral and ethical dilemmas in the special care nursery. *N Engl J Med* 1973;289:90

7. Brown, Thompson: Nontreatment of fever in extended care facilities. *N Engl J Med* 1979;300:1246

between the doctor and the family. In an age of group practices and hospital-based or clinic-based practices and ever more rarefied specialization, treating physicians were often relative strangers to the patient and his family. The second factor, to a large extent related to the first, was the growth of malpractice litigation, which made the doctor, knowing little of the family with whom he was dealing, chary of potential legal liability, and ever more cognizant of the dangers of acting in the absence of documented informed consent. The third factor, certainly the most dramatic and pervasive, was the revolution in drugs and technology. No longer was medical care "both cheap and useless."[8] New discoveries, at first gradually and then exponentially, increased the range of treatment options and their potential impact. By the 1970s, it had become possible to extend life in some form for indeterminate periods if the technology could be brought to bear while the patient was still alive or, indeed, within a few minutes after his death (by traditional tests). The doctor's decision, which took the form of benign neglect in earlier, more discrete times, now took stark and unambiguous forms, such as whether to "pull the plug" on a mechanical ventilator. No longer could the fact of *choice* be submerged. It had to come, in Fried's words, "out of the closet"[9] and into the public domain.

THE BEGINNINGS OF COURT INVOLVEMENT

The debut of the problem in the public realm was tumultuous. The occasion was the trial concerning the fate of Karen Ann Quinlan, a 21-year-old in a persistent vegetative state (PVS) whose parents sought removal of a respirator. The trial caught the public imagination. Pundits wrote of euthanasia and mercy killings. Public prosecutors spoke threateningly of suicide and, worse, murder. It is interesting to reflect (in light of the later support of right-to-life opposition by many prominent voices within the Roman Catholic Church) that the Quinlan parents' request for termination of ventilator support was supported by their parish priest and the New Jersey Catholic Bishops' Conference. The opposition came from public prosecutors, the hospital, the treating physicians, and the State of New Jersey.

The Quinlan decision was unanimous and spoke for humanistic values above technology. The result of the first public exposure seemed reassuring to doctors. The problem had been aired; the court had sanctioned a decision to withdraw life-sustaining treatment; and the contention that such a withdrawal could be indictable as homicide was seemingly put to rest. The court had suggested a viable decision-making process, involving consultation and consensus among the treating physician, the patient (if competent) or family, and a hospital ethics committee. It had exonerated medical practitioners from civil liability, and it had rejected the idea—

anathema to most physicians—that courts should normally have to become involved in such decisions. Comfortingly, it had characterized court involvement as a "gratuitous encroachment upon the medical profession's field of competence."[10]

The *Quinlan* decision was followed within 1 year, however, by the influential *Saikewicz* decision in Massachusetts,[11] which rejected the *Quinlan* view and called (as the *Saikewicz* case was understood at the time) for judicial resolution of decisions to terminate treatment.[12] Within a short time thereafter, the New York Court of Appeals, in *Matter of Storar*,[13] emphatically rejected the developing substituted judgment doctrine that had played a role in the *Quinlan* decision and had been the cornerstone of the analysis of the *Saikewicz* opinion. The celebrated *Earle Spring* case brought "right to life" groups into the debate, charging euthanasia,[14] and in New York and some other states district attorneys were threatening prosecution of doctors who terminated life-sustaining treatment. Frustrated groups advocating "natural death" options sought relief from state legislatures, some of which passed natural death acts over often vocal "right to life" opposition that treated the question of natural death as indistinguishable from abortion. The resulting "living will" legislation was often so narrow in scope as to be almost useless in the view of the advocates and so couched with legal conditions as to be intimidating to medical practitioners. What doctors most feared seemed to be happening. Far from providing understanding and guidance, the legal community—courts, legislatures, lawyers—seemed hopelessly enmeshed in conflict and confusion.

Physicians, in this early period, were understandably dismayed. They, along with nurses and hospitals, were on the firing line where treatment decisions had to be made. But the initial confusion was predictable. In a democratic country, the process of hammering out significant policy is not orderly. Democracy encourages dissent; the federal system encourages a diversity of approaches. The process looks chaotic, but, when it works well, it can forge a societal consensus that derives its durability from the fact that alternatives have been examined, tried, and found wanting.

10. 170 N.J. at 50

11. *Superintendent of Belchertown State School v. Saikewicz,* 373 Mass. 728 (1977)

12. *Saikewicz,* 373 Mass. at 758–759: "We reject the approach adopted by the New Jersey Supreme Court in the *Quinlan* case of entrusting the decision whether to continue artificial life support to the patient's guardian, family, attending doctors, and hospital 'ethics committee' ... [s]uch questions of life and death seem to us to require the process of detached but passionate investigation and decision that forms the ideal on which the judicial branch of government was created. Achieving this ideal is our responsibility and that of the lower court, and is not to be entrusted to any other group purporting to represent the 'morality and conscience of our society,' no matter how highly motivated or impressively constituted."

13. *Matter of Storar,* 52 N.Y. 2d 363 (1981)

14. *Matter of Spring,* 380 Mass. 629 (1980). The story of the involvement of right to life groups is recounted in Paris' "Death, Dying, and the Courts: The Travesty and Tragedy of the Earle Spring Case." *Linacre Quarterly,* Feb. 1972

8. Avorn: Benefit and cost analysis in geriatric care: turning age discrimination into health policy. *N Engl J Med* 1984;310:1294

9. Fried: Terminating life support: out of the closet! *N Engl J Med* 1976;295:390

Physicians who were critical of the confusion in the aftermath of the *Quinlan* and *Saikewicz* cases would do well to reflect on the conflicts within their own profession in the early stages of the debate. Many of the major court cases were marked by sharp divisions of opinion among doctors concerning the dictates of medical ethics.[15] Articles surveying physicians' attitudes in these matters displayed similar, deep-seated divisions.[16] The medical profession seemed as much in need of standards as the larger society.

A CONSENSUS EMERGES

After the initial period of deep doctrinal division, the courts within a decade had reached a substantial consensus in many aspects of termination of treatment decisions. In achieving this consensus, they were strongly influenced by a landmark document, *Deciding to Forego Life-Sustaining Treatments*, published in 1983 by the President's Commission for the Study of Ethical Problems in Biomedical and Behavioral Research, and by thoughtful position papers and consensus statements of several professional groups. It must be emphasized that the judicial consensus does not imply unanimity; significant procedural variations exist from state to state, and on particular points one or two states may diverge from substantive principles recognized by the majority. The point, however, is that the consensus is now sufficiently developed that for several years it has been meaningful to speak in terms of "rules" and "exceptions to the rules." What follows is a discussion of the "rules" or principles that the courts have adopted for dealing with decisions to withhold or withdraw life-sustaining treatments.

It should also be noted that not all appellate courts have addressed these issues; indeed, the substantive decisions have arisen in only about 25 jurisdictions. The consensus, however, is more significant than the numbers would indicate, because courts, when faced with new problems, traditionally look for guidance to the manner in which other courts have dealt with the same problems.[17] Moreover, the

several principles that comprise the consensus should derive stability from the fact that they are in harmony with the traditional and accepted roles of physicians, patients, and families in determining courses of medical treatment.

The largely settled principles are presented below, together with a brief discussion of the application of each.

(1) *A competent adult has the right to refuse medical treatment, a right that is not absolute but is subject to qualification by certain state interests.* Prior to the Supreme Court's decision in the *Cruzan* case, most courts assumed that the right of an individual to refuse medical treatment was supported not only by the common law but also by the right of privacy protected by the Due Process Clause of the United States Constitution. The *Cruzan* decision seems to have confirmed that view.[18] The law definitely rejects the vitalist principle that underlies the thinking of many in the "right to life" movement: that human life must be preserved at all costs. Cases applying the principle have often involved elderly patients refusing major surgery, such as leg amputations,[19] Jehovah's Witnesses refusing blood transfusions,[20] or lucid patients with devastating conditions—Lou Gehrig's disease or quadriplegia—seeking removal of life support.[21] These amputation and transfusion cases illustrate that the state does not always insist "that human life be saved where the affliction is curable."[22]

The state interests that sometimes justify overriding the wishes of the competent patient have been identified as "(1) the preservation of life, (2) the protection of the interests of innocent third parties, (3) the prevention of suicide, and (4) maintaining the ethical integrity of the medical profession."[23] The first of these is often said to be "the most significant"[24] of the four state interests. Taken literally, however, it could destroy the free choice principle. Recent cases have tended to sidestep it as a factor in cases of terminal or incurable illness.[25] "The general state interest in the preservation of life—most weighty where the patient, properly

---

15. The *Quinlan* case was an example. Another was *Brophy v New Eng. Sinai Hosp.*, 398 Mass. 417 (1986)

16. See Shaw, Randolph, Maynard: Ethical issues in pediatric surgery: a natural survey of pediatricians and pediatric surgeons. *Pediatrics* 1977;60:588; Todres, Krane, Howell: Pediatricians' attitudes affecting decision making in defective newborns. *Pediatrics* 1977;60:197

17. The 4–3 decision of the Missouri Supreme Court in *Cruzan v Harmon*, 760 S.W. 2d 408 (Mo. 1988), however, was a striking example of the power of a court to reject out-of-state authority. The *Cruzan* decision explicitly recognized the existence of a consensus in favor of termination, citing roughly fifty decisions contrary to the position it elected to take. See 760 S.W. 2d at 412–413, fn. 4. The result was a major constitutional issue whether Federal due process permitted a state to take so divergent a position in an area fraught with considerations of personal liberty and privacy. The 5–4 decision of the United States Supreme Court, on narrow reasoning, ruled that Missouri's position was not forbidden by the United States Constitution. See *Cruzan v Director, Missouri Department of Health*, 110 S. Ct. 2841 (1990)

18. This is the generally accepted reading of a sentence in the majority decision that reads: "The principle that a competent person has a constitutionally protected liberty interest in refusing unwanted medical treatment may be inferred from our prior decisions." 110 S. Ct. at 2851. The four dissenters also accepted this proposition. Only one member (Scalia, J.) questioned it.

19. Examples are *Lane v Candura*, 6 Mass. App. Ct. 377 (1978), and *Matter of Quackenbush*, 156 N.J. Super. 282 (1978)

20. E.g., *Matter of Osborne*, 294 A. 2d 372 (D.C. 1972); *Matter of Melideo*, 88 Misc. 2d 974 (N.Y. Sup. Ct. 1976)

21. E.g., *Staz v Perlmutter*, 362 So. 2d 160 (Fla. App. 1978); aff'd. 379 So. 2d 359 (Fla. 1980); *Matter of Farrell*, 108 N.J. 335 (1987); *Bouvia v Superior Court*, 225 Cal. Rptr. 297 (Ct. App. 1986); *Tune v Walter Reg Army Medical Hospital*, 602 F. Supp. 1452 (1985); *State v McAfee*, 259 Ga. 579 (1989)

22. *Saikewicz*, 373 Mass. at 742

23. *Saikewicz*, 373 Mass. at 741

24. *Id.*

25. The state interest in the preservation of life may play a decisive role in states that do not utilize substituted judgment analysis in cases of incompetent patients, because it can be invoked as a reason for continuing life support to patients who derive no benefit from treatment, such as those in a permanent vegetative state.

treated, can return to reasonable health, without great suffering, and a decision to avoid treatment would be aberrational—carries far less weight where the patient is approaching the end of a normal life span, where the afflictions are incapacitating, and where the best that medicine can offer is an extension of suffering."[26] Cases involving the second state interest—protection of the rights of innocent third parties—have usually involved refusals of needed blood transfusions by healthy pregnant women[27] or by basically healthy treatable adults with young children to support.[28] The trend of decisions has been increasingly to emphasize patient autonomy over the interests of third parties.[29] Prevention of suicide—the third countervailing state interest—has not led to overriding a competent patient's refusal of treatment in any reported appellate case.[30] Courts have universally accepted a distinction between suicide and allowing a life-threatening condition to take its natural course, without treatment or artificial life support.[31]

The fourth state interest—maintaining the ethical integrity of the medical profession—has carried different connotations in different decisions. To the *Quinlan* and *Saikewicz* courts, it meant a consensus of medical practitioners, where one could be shown to exist, that withholding treatment would be ethically unjustified in particular circumstances. Other courts have used the concept in which a particular patient seeks institutional treatment but seeks also to limit the course of that treatment in a manner violative of sound medical practice, for example, consenting to surgery while

denying consent for any necessary blood transfusions.[32] To some courts the concept has meant that a physician or hospital may not be required to act in a way in which the physician or hospital views as immoral, as long as the patient may be transferred to the care of others who do not share that view.[33] The last application is one on which courts are divided. It is discussed below in the section on unresolved questions.

Earlier decisions tended to emphasize the countervailing state interests and to be skeptical of a decision to forego life-sustaining treatment. The trend in recent cases has been to emphasize that patient autonomy governs except in those situations in which the countervailing state interest is for some reason "compelling."[34] Often quoted in this respect are the words of Justice Letts in *Satz v. Perlmutter*:

> It is all very convenient to insist on continuing Mr. Perlmutter's life so that there can be no question of foul play, no resulting civil liability, and no possible trespass in medical ethics. However, it is quite another matter to do so at the patient's sole expense and against his competent will, thus inflicting never ending physical torture on his body until the inevitable, but artificially suspended moment of his death. Such a course of conduct invades the patient's constitutional right of privacy, removes his freedom of choice and invades his right to self-determination.[35]

(2) An incompetent patient has the same right as a competent patient to avoid treatment, and the right may be asserted in his behalf by an appropriate surrogate. Most courts accept this general principle, but there is some underlying disagreement as to the basis of the right and as to the manner in which it may be asserted. The *Saikewicz* court, using the term "substituted judgment," conceptualized the right as precisely analogous to the right of a competent patient to withhold consent. It envisions the surrogate's role as one of determining as nearly as possible what the incompetent patient would choose of he were competent to make a choice. The standard is said to be subjective; the surrogate will give or withhold consent based on the incompetent's choice, whether wise or foolish.[36] Other courts tend to view the role of the surrogate as himself or herself making the necessary decision for the incompetent patient,[37] at least where the patient has not left specific instructions, which

26. *Brophy v New Eng. Sinai Hosp.*, 398 Mass. 417, 433, fn.8 (1986), quoting from *Matter of Spring*, 8 Mass. App. Ct. 831, 845–846 (1979), rev'd in part 380 Mass. 629 (1980)

27. *Raleigh Fitkin–Paul Mem. Hosp. v Anderson*, 42 N.J. 421 (1964); *Crouse–Irving Hosp. v Paddock*, 127 Misc. 2d 101 (N.Y. Sup. Ct. 1985); *Matter of Jamaica Hosp.*, 128 Misc. 2d 1006 (1985); *Jefferson v Griffin Spaulding County Hosp.*, 247 Ga. 86 (1985)

28. *Holmes v Silver Cross Hosp.*, 340 F. Supp. 125 (D, 111, 1972); *Application of President & Directors of Georgetown College*, 331 F. 2d 1000 (D.C. Cir.), cert. den. 377 U.S. 978 (1964); *Winthrop Univ. Hosp. v Hess*, 128 Misc. 2d 804 (N.Y. Sup. Ct. 1985)

29. See *Norwood Hosp. v Munoz*, 409 Mass. 116, 127–130 (1991; 38-year-old mother with husband, child, and elderly father in household allowed to refuse blood transfusions); *Wons v Public Health Trust of Dade County*, 500 So. 2d 679 (Fla. D.C. App. 1987), aff'd. 541 So. 2d 96 (Fla. 1989) (mother of two children refusing blood transfusions); *Fosmire v Nicoleau*, 75, N.Y. 2d 218, 229–230 (1990; patient's right to refuse treatment "not conditional on patient being without minor children or dependents")

30. *Matter of Gannett*, 547 A. 2d 609 (Del.Ch. 1988), involving a prison immate's hunger strike, was analyzed as a case of mental illness rather than as an attempted suicide of a competent person. Force-feeding was authorized.

31. *Saikewicz*, 373 Mass. at 743, fn. 11; *Matter of Conroy*, 98 N.J. 321, 350–351 (1985); *Bouvia v Superior Court*, 170 Cal. App. 3d. 1127, 1144–1145 (1986); *Delia v Westchester County Med. Center*, 516 N.Y.S.2d 677, 692 (App. Div. 1987); *In re Colyer*, 660 P. 2d 738, 743 (Wash. 1983); *Rasmussen by Mitchell v Fleming*, 741 P. 2d 667, 671 (Ariz. 1986); *Satz v Perlmutter*, 362 So. 2d at 162 (Fla. 1978); *In re Gardner*, 534 A. 2d. 947, 955–956 (Me. 1987); *McConnell v Beverly Enterprises—Conn.*, 553, A. 2d. 596, 605 (Conn. 1989)

32. *Application of President & Directors of Georgetown College*, 331 F. 2d at 1009; *United States v George*, 239 F. Supp. 752, 754 (d. Conn. 1965); *John F. Kennedy Memorial Hosp. v Hesston*, 58 N.J. 576, 582–583 (1971)

33. An example is the *Brophy* case, 398 Mass. at 440–441, where the court agreed that the patient (who was in a permanent vegtative state) was legally entitled to the removal of a gastrostomy, but declined to require that the removal take place at the chronic care hospital where he was a patient. The decision noted that other nearby hospitals were available and willing to assume care of the patient during the removal and thereafter.

34. See *In re Torres*, 357 N.W. 2d 332, 339 (Minn. 1984)

35. *Satz v Perlmutter*, 362 So. 2d at 164

36. *Lane v Candura*, 6 Mass. App. Ct. 377, 383 (1978); *Brophy v New Eng. Sinai Hosp., Inc.*, 398 Mass. 417, 430 (1986)

37. Examples include *Matter of Jobes*, 108 N.J. 394, 415–416 (1987); *In re Hamlin*, 689 P. 2d 1372, 1377–1378 (Wash. 1984)

normally will control.[38] Surrogates can be of two types: first, the family, friend, or person named by the patient in a durable power of attorney, who presumably knows in detail the patient's situation in life and his or her moral values and attitudes toward death and dependency on life support; and, second, a professional surrogate, such as an attorney appointed by a court as guardian for an elderly person with no family or close friends. The latter as a practical matter, can often do little other than evaluate the patient's interests in the traditionally objective sense: balancing the burdens of treatment against the potential benefits to the patient. The substituted judgment and surrogate decision-making approaches differ analytically but in most cases reach identical results in consideration of much the same reasons. The substituted judgment approach ascertains what the patient would have wanted by considering his expressed views on mechanical life support, his moral and religious predilections, and the objective situation in which he finds himself (i.e., the expected benefits of treatment versus its burdens). The surrogate decision-making approach, as least as to family or friend type surrogates, reflects the patient's value system because the surrogate presumably knows how the patient would react to his medical dilemma. The differences, in other words, are generally more theoretical than real; and many courts simply and sensibly blend the two approaches, indicating that great weight should attach to the patient's expressions of views while competent or, if his views are unknown, to the views of his family or designated surrogate.[39]

The substituted judgment approach, most plausible where the views of the patient were expressed at some time before the lapse into incompetency, has been criticized as meaningless when applied to infants or to mentally retarded patients who have never been competent to have or express a meaningful choice.[40] Its advantage may be that it tends to facilitate consideration of intangible factors—those related to personal dignity, concern for loved ones, concern even for cost—that the surrogate knows, but cannot demonstrate, would enter into the thinking of most competent persons similarly situated. The objective "patient's interests" test, if narrowly applied, can become bureaucratic, resulting in mechanical decisions to continue life support in situations where it is of no benefit to the patient, and is both exorbitantly costly and a source of anguish to the patient's loved ones, simply because it cannot be shown by reference to objective criteria, such as pain, that it is better for the patient not to prolong the ordeal.[41]

Fortunately, most courts have resisted the temptation to approach these cases mechanically. When the patient's actual views are not known but it is clear that continued treatment is of no benefit, most courts have not imposed technical legal barriers to humane decision-making. Courts have been influenced by the thought of religious leaders that a decision not to treat can be justified "as an acceptance of the human condition, or a wish to avoid the application of a medical procedure disproportionate to the results that can be expected, or a desire not to impose excessive expense on the family or the community."[42]

Three highest state courts have declined to permit surrogate decision-making or substituted judgment. New York is the clearest exception. Its decisional law is that a termination of medical life support can be based only on the patient's clearly and deliberately stated wishes, expressed while the patient was competent.[43] Those wishes must be shown by clear and convincing evidence, not by idle and casual comments.[44] Treatment must be continued, it seems, where the patient has never been competent to make his own decision,[45] or where the patient neglected to set down his wishes when competent. Human nature being what it is, the latter group is and will doubtless continue to make up a strong majority. In the famous *Cruzan* case, the Supreme Court of Missouri, on a four to three vote, refused to allow the parents of a young woman in a permanent vegetative state to terminate artificial feeding.[46] Recognizing the consensus to the contrary among other state courts, it elected to follow the New York approach of requiring clear and convincing

---

38. Examples include *Guardianship of Browning*, 568 So. 2d 4, 13 (Fla. 1990); *Matter of Peter by Johanning*, 108 N.J. 365, 377 (1987). Some courts use the terms "substituted judgment" and "surrogate decision-making" interchangeably. The confusion is understandable, because the surrogate is, in effect, substituting his judgment for that of the incompetent patient.

39. See, e.g., *In re Torres*, 357 N.W. 2d at 338–339; *Matter of Hamlin*, 689 P. 2d 1372, 1375–1376 (Wash. 1984); *Rasmussen by Mitchell v Fleming*, 154 Ariz. 207, 221–222 (1987); *Guardianship of L.W.*, 167 Wis. 2d 53, 77–81 (1992); *In re Rosebush*, 195 Mich. App. 675 (1992)

40. See *Matter of Storar*, 52, N.Y. 2d at 380

41. In New Jersey, for example, the *Conroy* case seems to require (where the incompetent patient's actual views are not known) that life support must be continued except where "the recurring, unavoidable and severe pain of the patient's life with the treatment [is] such that the effect of administering life-sustaining treatment would be inhumane." 987 N.J. at 366. See the moving protest against this restrictive standard by Judge Stanton in *Matter of Visbeck*, 510 A. 2d 125, 130–133 (N.J. Super. Ct. 1986). The *Storar* case indicates that New York law is similarly restrictive. See discussion in *Matter of Hier*, 18 Mass. App. Ct. 200, 206–207 (1984)

42. Vatican Declaration on Euthanasia, May 5, 1980. See fn. 3, supra

43. *In re Eichner*, 52 N.Y. 2d 363 (1981)

44. *Westchester County Med. Center v O'Connor*, 72 N.Y. 2d 517 (1980)

45. *Matter of Storar*, 52 N.Y. 2d 363 (1981) (mandating continuation of blood transfusions to retarded adult with terminal cancer). See discussion of New York cases in *Matter of Hier*, 18 Mass. App. Ct. 200, 206–207 (1984). As a practical matter, decisions to terminate pointless, death-prolonging treatments are probably not infrequent, even in New York, due to two other features of the New York decisions: first, the parties are not required to obtain court approval of decisions to terminate treatment, and, second, the formal expression of wishes by the patient while competent need not be written. Thus physicians doubtless rely in some cases on the family's assurance that the patient while competent decisively made his wishes known.

46. *Cruzan v Harmon*, 760 S.W. 2d 408 (Mo. 1988)

evidence that the patient while competent had expressed his or her wishes with some solemnity. A third state, Maryland, appears to have joined New York in precluding surrogate decision-making.[47] Missouri, on the other hand, appears to have narrowed the *Cruzan* holding so that it applies only to termination of artificial feeding.[48]

Missouri's *Cruzan* decision was narrowly upheld by the United States Supreme Court, the first "right to die" case to reach that court.[49] It is important to understand the precise holding in *Cruzan*. The Supreme Court was not endorsing the view of the Missouri Supreme Court. It merely held that the Federal Constitution did not *forbid* states from structuring their law as Missouri did. A state may thus preclude surrogate decision-making or substituted judgment, insisting instead on clear and convincing expressions of intent by the incompetent patient while competent. Thus, the Federal Constitutional right of privacy, previously assumed by many courts to preclude most state intervention in private (i.e., family and doctor) decision-making process in this area, is not quite so broad. The *Cruzan* decision *did* affirm that the Federal Constitution protected the right of a competent patient to refuse treatment, and it implied that the patient's wishes expressed while competent must be honored in the event of later incompetency. Thus, the *Cruzan* decision has given a strong boost to the living wills or other formal statements of intent, and to durable power of attorney, whereby a competent person designates another to make health care decisions for him should he later become incompetent.[50] In the majority of states, however, the *Cruzan* decision should make little or no difference. In most states the extension of autonomy to the incompetent patient, acting through another, is firmly grounded in the state's common law, the state statutory law or, in some cases, the state's constitution.[51] It does not depend on a federal right of privacy. The consensus in this regard is unimpaired by *Cruzan*.

(3) *The family of an incompetent patient is presumptively an appropriate surrogate to act in his behalf.* Although there has been little discussion of the principle in court decisions prior to *Quinlan*, it has long been taken for granted by physicians and hospitals that they may look to parents, spouses, and children to give valid consent to treatment when the patient is incompetent to make the choice. "Almost invariably," the *Jobes* court wrote, "the patient's family has an intimate understanding of the patient's medical attitudes and general world view and therefore is in the best position to know the motives and considerations that would control the patient's medical decisions."[52] In deciding that the family is presumed also to be the appropriate surrogate to participate in decisions not to continue treatment,[53] courts have confirmed the traditional view of the family's role.

The presumption may be rebutted. Circumstances may come to the attention of physicians or hospital staff indicating that the family is not an appropriate participant in the treatment decision. Obviously, the presumption is strongest when applied to the immediate family of the patient who lives with him, and weakest in the case of distant relatives who have to be searched out; strong when their view seems like the normal view of a loving and emotionally involved family, weaker when their view seems unconcerned or aberrational. As one court has stated, "[in] individual cases, health care providers and courts have to be wary about idiosyncratic decisions made by surrogates."[54] An important and long-standing example is that courts have regularly overridden idiosyncratic choices of parents to refuse needed medical treatment for children.[55] Here, physicians and hospital staff must necessarily rely on experience and common sense, knowing there is little likelihood that they will be held accountable if they act in good faith.[56] Serious doubts about the role of the family in treatment decisions may sometimes necessitate the assistance of a court.

(4) *Court proceedings are generally unnecessary to secure approval of a decision to withhold or withdraw life-sustaining medical treatment, except in cases of dispute or where the incompetent patient lacks an appropriate surrogate to act on his behalf.* The *Quinlan* decision in 1976 rejected the notion that the courts should decide termination of treatment cases on a case-by-case basis. Later cases, including

47. *Mack v Mack*, 329 Md. 188 (1993), rejecting petition of wife to withdraw artificial feeding from husband who, 9 years earlier, had been injured in automobile accident and was in a persistent vegetative state, on ground that there was no clear and convincing evidence that husband, before the accident, had left instructions to that effect.

48. *In re Warren*, 858 S.W. 2d 263 (Mo. Ct. App. 1993) (DNR order allowed by substituted judgment. *Cruzan* limited to decisions to terminate artificial feeding; otherwise, evidence not required of patient's expression of intent while competent).

49. *Cruzan v Director, Missouri Dept. of Health*, 110 S. Ct. 2841 (1990)

50. The states that at the time of *Cruzan* had formal living will or durable power of attorney laws were listed in Justice O'Connor's concurring opinion, 110 S. Ct. 2857–2858, 1), 385 Mass. 697, 707–710 (1982)

51. Examples of state constitutional protection for decisions to refuse treatment are found in *Guardianship of Browning*, 568 So. 2d 4, 10 (Fla. 1990) and *Rasmussen by Mitchell v Fleming*, 741 P. 2d at 682 (Ariz. 1987)

52. *Matter of Jobes*, 108 N.J. 394, 415 (1987)

53. *Rasmussen by Mitchell v Fleming*, 741 P. 2d 667, 672 (Ariz. App. 1986); *In re L.H.R.*, 253 Ga. 439, 446–447 (1984); *John F. Kennedy Hosp. v Bludworth*, 452 So. 2d 921 (Fla. 1984); *Matter of Hamlin*, 689 P. 2d 1372, 1377 (Wash. 1984); *Matter of J.N.*, 406 A. 2d 1275 (D.C. Ct. App. 1979); *In re L.H.R.*, 253 Ga. 439 (1984); *Barber v Superior Court*, 147 Cal. App. 3d 1006 (Ct. App. 1983). See also *Matter of Spring*, 8 Mass. App. Ct. 831, 840 and fn. 9 (1979), rev'd in part, 380 Mass. 629, 638 (1980), *Custody of a Minor* (No. 1), 385 Mass. 697, 707–710 (1982); *In re Rosebush*, 195 Mich. App. 675, 686–7 (1992); *Estate of Longeway*, 133 Ill. 2d 33, 49–50 (1989); *Matter of Lawrance*, 579 N.E. 2d 32, 41–42 (Ind. 1991); *Matter of Fiori*, 652 A. 2d 1350, 1355–1358 (Pa. Super. 1995)

54. *Matter of Visbeck*, 510 A. 2d 125, 132 (N.J. Super. Ct. 1986)

55. *Custody of a Minor*, 375 Mass. 733 (1978) (parent choosing vitamin treatment over chemotherapy for child with leukemia). *Jehovah's Witnesses v Kings County Hosp.*, 390 U.S. 598 (1966), and *Matter of Sampson*, 29 N.Y. 2d 900 (1972; parents refusing blood transfusions for children)

56. See *infra*, consensus point 8.

the *Saikewicz* case in Massachusetts and *Leach v Akron General Medical Center* in Ohio,[57] cast doubt on the *Quinlan* view, but it is now clear that all courts that have addressed the point, with the possible exception of Ohio's, have adopted the view that prior court approval is not legally required.[58] This is true even in Massachusetts, where the Supreme Judicial Court has clarified or amended its statement in the *Saikewicz* case, so as to make it clear that

> . . . our opinions should not be taken to establish any requirements of prior judicial approval that would not otherwise exist. . . . [T]he standard for determining whether the treatment was called for is the same after the event as before; negligence cannot be based solely on failure to obtain prior court approval, if the approval would have been given. . . . Thus absence of court approval does not result in automatic civil liability for withholding treatment; court approval may serve the useful purpose of resolving a doubtful or disputed question of law or fact. . . .[59]

Some courts require that the decision of a family (or guardian) and attending physicians to terminate life-sustaining treatment be reviewed and approved by a third party, such as a hospital ethics committee,[60] other physicians,[61] or a prognosis committee.[62] If the incompetent patient does not have a family or guardian, ordinarily resort must be had to a court to obtain either the appointment of a guardian with the authority to act for the patient or a substituted judgment decision by the court.[63] New Jersey has adopted a unique procedure, applicable to sapient (i.e., non-PVS) patients in nursing homes, that requires the appointment of a guardian (whether or not the patient has a family) and

involvement of the State's ombudsman.[64] Illinois had established a requirement of court approval prior to a surrogate decision to terminate artificial nutrition and hydration, so that the court can ferret out improper motives of family members.[65] Most states rely on physicians and nurses to sense such motives. When there is irreconcilable disagreement between physicians and family members, resort should be had to a court.

Courts appreciate the logistical impossibility of deciding all termination-of-treatment questions on a case-by-case basis. In the *Torres* case, for example, the Minnesota Supreme Court noted that "an average of about ten life support systems are disconnected weekly in Minnesota."[66]

(5) *The entry of a no-code (or DNR) order on a patient's chart does not require prior judicial approval.* The principal case on this subject is *Matter of Dinnerstein*, which held prior judicial approval unnecessary.[67] Most deaths in our time occur in hospitals; most are signalled by cardiac arrest.

> As it cannot be assumed that legal proceedings . . . will be initiated in respect of more than a small fraction of all terminally ill or dying elderly patients, [a requirement of prior judicial approval of no-code orders] would require attempts to resuscitate dying patients in most cases, without exercise of medical judgment, even when that course of action could aptly be characterized as a pointless, even cruel, prolongation of the act of dying.[68]

When cardiac arrest is anticipated immediately as part of the terminal stage of incurable illness, resuscitation is

57. 68 Ohio Misc. 1 (1980)

58. *Rasmussen by Mitchell v Flemming*, 741 P. 2d 674, 690) Ariz. 1987); *John F. Kennedy Hosp. v Bludworth*, 452 So. 2d 921, 925 (Fla. 1984); *Barber v Superior Court*, 147 Cal. App. 3d 1006, 1021 (1983); *Parker v United States*, 406 A. 2d 1275, 1282 (D.C. Ct. App. 1979); *In re L.H.R.*, 253 Ga. 439, 446–447 (1984); *In re Torres*, 357 N.W. 2d 332, 341, fn. 4 (Minn. 1984); *Matter of Hamlin*, 689 P. 2d 1372, 1378 (Wash. 1984); *Matter of Spring*, 380 Mass. 629, 636 (1980); *Matter of Storar*, 52 N.Y. 2d 363 (1981); *Matter of Jobes*, 108 N.J. 394, 423 (1987); *Matter of Drabick*, 245 Cal. Rptr. 840, 844–849 (Cal. App. 1988); *Matter of Lawrance*, 579 N.E. 2d 32, 41–42 (Ind. 1991); *Guardianship of L.W.*, 167 Wis. 2d 53, 92–93 (1992); *In re Rosebush*, 195 Mich. App. 675, 686–687 (1992); *DiGrella by Parrent v Elston*, 858 S.W. 2d 698, 709–710 (Ky. 1993); *Matter of Fiori*, 652 A. 2d 1350, 1356–1357 (Pa. Super. 1995). Illinois appears to follow the rule except as to withdrawal of artificial feeding, where prior court approval *was* required by *Estate of Longeway*, 133 Ill. 2d 33, 51 (1989). But see fn. 65.

59. *Matter of Spring*, 380 Mass. at 636, 639. The earlier statement in the *Saikewicz* case (see fn. 12, *supra*) was explained to mean only that, "when a court is properly presented with the legal question, whether treatment may be withheld, it must decide that question and not delegate it to some private person or group." 380 Mass. at 639

60. *Matter of Quinlan*, 70 N.J. at 54

61. *John F. Kennedy Hosp. v Bludworth*, 452 So. 2d at 926

62. *Matter of Hamlin*, 689 P. 2d at 1377–1378

63. *Matter of Conroy*, 98 N.J. at 381–382 (guardian); *Matter of Hamlin*, 689 P. 2d at 1378 (guardian); *Custody of a Minor (No. 1)*, 385 Mass. at 708–710 (substituted judgment determination)

64. See *Matter of Conroy*, 98 N.J. at 381–385, as modified by *Matter of Peter by Johanning*, 108 N.J. at 374

65. *Estate of Longeway*, 133 Ill. 33, 51 (1989). The Illinois requirements for prior court approval of withdrawal has been superseded by the Illinois Surrogacy Act (Ill. Pub. Act 87–749, N.B. 2334, 87th Gen. Assembly, 91st Sess., 1991)

66. 357 N.W. 2d at 341, see fn. 4

67. *Matter of Dinnerstein*, 6 Mass. App. Ct. 466 (1978). Five other appellate decisions have touched on no-code orders. Two were dismissed as moot, the patient having died. *Strickland v Deaconess Hospital*, 735 P. 2d 74 (Wash. App. 1987); *In re Riddlemoser*, 317 Md. 496 (1989). An Indiana decision, *Payne v Marion General Hospital*, 549 N.E. 2d 1043 (Ind. App. 1990), held that a physician could be civilly liable for entering a no-code order at the behest of the patient's sister, without consulting the patient. The case was remanded for trial to determine if the patient had been, as alleged, competent and not terminally ill. In *In re Warren*, 858 S.W. 2d 263 (Mo. Ct. App. 1993), a DNR order was held properly entered with consent of patient's guardian, despite lack of evidence of patient's wishes; *Cruzan* was held to apply only to withdrawal of artificial feeding. In *Morgan v Olds*, 417 N.W. 2d 232 (Iowa App. 1987), the court affirmed a jury verdict for a hospital and doctor who intentionally did not resuscitate plaintiff's husband; he had been weaned from respirator several hours earlier. (The plaintiff disputed hospital's contention that she had approved course of treatment.) A Massachusetts jury in 1995 rejected a daughter's claim for damages based on entry of no-code order for her mother without the daughter's consent. *Gilgunn v Massachusetts General Hospital*, Suffolk Superior civil no. 92-4820. An appeal has been entered in the Appeals Court.

68. *Matter of Dinnerstein*, 6 Mass. App. Ct. at 471

manifestly inappropriate,[69] whether or not the patient's family has been consulted or approved.[70] In such cases, there is no real treatment decision to be made; rather, the situation "presents a question peculiarly within the competence of the medical profession of what measures are appropriate to ease the imminent passing of an irreversibly, terminally ill patient in light of the patient's history and condition and the wishes of the family."[71] When the death is not expected immediately but the patient is suffering from an untreatable, debilitating illness or is greatly enfeebled by the afflictions of age, the entry of a no-code order should normally be discussed with and determined by the patient (if appropriate) or the family.

There may be cases in which a "family, through ignorance, misunderstanding, fear, or guilt," demands resuscitation of an irreversibly dying patient or, conversely, insists "on a DNR order for a patient the physician believes has a good chance of recovering."[72] In such cases, after education or persuasion fail, the physician or hospital, whose first duty is to the patient, may find it appropriate to seek the assistance of a court.

(6) *A decision to terminate treatment is subject to the same legal standards as a decision not to begin the treatment.* Each court that has considered the question has agreed that no distinction should be drawn between withdrawing and withholding treatment. Leading decisions have been the *Barber* case in California, the *Conroy* case in New Jersey, and the *Brophy* case in Massachusetts.[73] A person who "has a right to refuse treatment in the first instance has a concomitant right to discontinue it."[74] This position accords with that taken by the influential President's Commission for the Study of Ethical Problems in Medicine and Biomedical and Behavioral Research in 1983.[75]

A contrary view was, until recently, prevalent among physicians, who doubtless reasoned from the principle that a physician, having undertaken care of a patient, should not abandon him or her.[76] But terminating a treatment is not abandonment if the treatment turns out to be pointless. Respirator support may be required to give time for evaluation, but if the evaluation shows that nothing can be done to benefit the patient, the reason for respirator support is gone. "From a policy standpoint, it might well be unwise to forbid persons from discontinuing a treatment under circumstances in which the treatment could be permissibly withheld. Such a rule could discourage families and doctors from even attempting certain types of care and could thereby force them into hasty and premature decisions to allow a patient to die."[77] Thus, in 1983, the National Institutes of Health Consensus Development Conference on Critical Care Medicine concluded that "[i]t is inappropriate to maintain ICU management of a patient whose prognosis has resolved to one of persistent vegetative state, and it is similarly inappropriate to employ ICU resources where no purpose will be served but a prolongation of the natural process of death." That view is fully consistent with the decisions of all courts that have spoken to the point.

(7) *Rules concerning withdrawal of treatment apply equally to withdrawal of nutrition and hydration by artificial means.* Artificial means include intravenous feeding, nasogastric tubes, gastrostomies, central hyperalimentation, and the like.[78] The first and leading case of withdrawal of feeding was the *Barber* case in California, in which physicians, at the family's request, withdrew a nasogastric tube from a patient in a permanent vegetative state.[79] The physicians were charged with murder. The court quashed the charges, holding that withdrawal of artificial feeding was no different from withdrawing any other medical treatment not benefiting the patient. "Medical procedures to provide nutrition and hydration are more similar to other medical procedures than to typical human ways of providing nutrition and hydration. Their benefits and burdens ought to be evaluated in the same manner as any other medical procedure."[80] The court adopted, in effect, the conclusion by the President's Commission Report the same year,[81] and since that time the

69. "The purpose of cardiopulmonary resuscitation is the prevention of sudden, unexpected death. Cardiopulmonary resuscitation is not indicated in certain situations, such as in cases of terminal irreversible illness where death is not unexpected or where prolonged cardiac arrest dictates the futility of resuscitation efforts. Resuscitation in these circumstances may represent a positive violation of an individual's right to die with dignity." AMA standards for cardiopulmonary resuscitation (CPR) and emergency cardiac care (EEC). *JAMA* 1974;227:837,864

70. New York, atypical in this respect also, has enacted legislation mandating, except in unusual cases, that consent be obtained from the patient or, if the patient is incompetent, from his family or guardian, prior to the entry of a no-code order. N.Y. Pub. Health Law art. 29-B. Physicians report that the result is numerous resuscitation attempts that are medically contraindicated, simply because the necessary consents have not been obtained. K. Prager, M.D., Columbia College of Physicians & Surgeons, letter to *Wall Street Journal*, May 3, 1990

71. *Matter of Dinnerstein*, 6 Mass. App. Ct. at 475

72. Paris, Reardon: Dilemmas in intensive care medicine: an ethical and legal analysis. *J Intensive Care Med* 1986;1:75,79

73. Respectively, 147 Cal. App. 3d at 1016;98 N.J. at 370;398 Mass. at 438

74. *Satz v Perlmutter*, 362 So. 2d at 163

75. Deciding to Forego Life-Sustaining Treatment at 181–183

76. *Ascher v Gutierrez*, 533 F. 2d 1235 (D.C. Cir. 1976)

77. *Matter of Conroy*, 98 N.J. at 370

78. "Life-prolonging medical treatment includes medication and artificially or technologically supplied respiration, nutrition or hydration." Statement of American Medical Assn. Council on Ethical and Judicial Affairs (1986), also stating: "Even if death is not imminent but a patient's care is beyond doubt irreversible and there are adequate safeguards to confirm the diagnosis and with the concurrence of those who have the responsibility for the care of the patient, it is not unethical to discontinue all means of life-prolonging medical treatment."

79. *Barber v California*, 147 Cal. App. 3d 1006 (1983)

80. *Id.*, at 1016–1017. The language was adapted from Lynn, Childress: Must patients always be given food and water? *Hastings Ctr Rep* 1983;13:17,20.

81. Deciding to Forego Life-Sustaining Treatment, at 90, 288

position taken in *Barber* has in turn been adopted by virtually all courts that have spoken on the point.[82]

No high court decision is directly contrary. The Missouri Supreme Court's decision in the *Cruzan* case seemed to differentiate between artificial nutrition and hydration and other life-sustaining medical treatments,[83] but the decision was made to turn on other factors, that is, the absence of clear and convincing evidence of the comatose patient's wishes. When the parents, in a subsequent proceeding, marshaled clear and convincing evidence of their daughter's wishes, a lower court saw no obstacle to ordering the feeding tube halted. The *Longeway* decision in Illinois established a procedural requirement of prior court approval for a withdrawal of artificial feeding but otherwise treated artificial feeding as indistinguishable from other medical treatments.[84] In 1988, the Washington Supreme Court, unable to assemble a majority, in effect deferred the question of termination of artificial feeding to the legislature.[85]

(8) *A physician or hospital acting in good faith will not be held civilly or criminally liable for acquiescing in the wish of the patient's family that artificial life-support measures be terminated.* This is a corollary of the principle that a court decision is normally not required or desirable except in cases of dispute or cases without an appropriate surrogate. Because decision-making within the physician–patient–family triad is authorized by the law, such a decision cannot in itself be a source of liability. Here the courts recognize that determinations when to continue and when to terminate treatment require a sophisticated exercise of judgment, and the law will not inhibit the physician's exercise of his best judgment by second-guessing it at a later date. Rather, the courts have indicated that the highest standard to which a

physician will be held is that he must act without negligence and in good faith.[86]

The unusual action of the California courts in quashing the criminal prosecution in the *Barber* case should serve as an example to physicians that, in this sensitive area, the courts will not countenance the misuse of the criminal process for political reasons. Massachusetts' highest court has stated, "Little need be said about criminal liability: there is precious little precedent, and what there is suggests that the doctor will be protected if he acts on a good faith judgment that is not grievously unreasonable by medical standards."[87] The Florida Supreme Court has stated, "To be relieved of the potential civil and criminal liability, guardians, consenting family members, physicians, hospitals, or their administrators need only act in good faith. For them to be held civilly or criminally liable, there must be a showing that their actions were not in good faith but intended to harm the patient."[88] The New Jersey Supreme Court stated that "if the [health care] professional has made a good faith determination in this regard, he or she will not be subject to any criminal or civil liability."[89] There is no reason to think that other courts, should the question come before them, will not act similarly to protect physicians and hospital staff who honestly exercise their best professional judgment in this complex and sensitive area. Fifteen years after the *Quinlan* decision, the author has found no reported case that has imposed civil or criminal liability on a physician or hospital for a decision to terminate life support.[90] Fears of physicians in this respect seem seriously overblown.

(9) *The right of a patient to have life-sustaining treatment withdrawn does not imply a right to commit suicide, and one who knowingly assists a patient to commit suicide is*

---

82. *Matter of Conroy*, 98 N.J. at 372–374; *Brophy v New Eng. Sinai Hosp.*, 398 Mass. at 435–440; *Bouvia v Superior Court*, 179 Cal. App. 3d at 1141; *Corbett v D'Iessandro*, 487 So. 2d 368, 371 (Fla. Dist. Ct. App. 1986); *Matter of Hier*, 18 Mass. App. Ct. 207–208, *Gray by Gray v Romeo*, 657 F. Supp. 580, 586–587 (D.R.I. 1988); *In re Gardner*, 534 A. 2d 947, 954 (Me. 1987); *Matter of Peter by Johanning*, 108 N.J. 365, 379–383 (1987); *Rasmussen by Mitchell v Fleming*, 741 P. 2d 674, 684 (1987); *McConnell v Beverly Enterprises-Conn.*, 553 A. 2d 596, 602–603 (Conn. 1989); *In re Severns*, 425 A. 2d 156, 160 (Del. Ch. 1987); *Delio v Westchester County Medical Center*, 516 N.Y. S. 2d 677, 688–689 (1987); *Guardianship of L.W.*, 167 Wis. 2d 53, 70–71 (1992); *Guardianship of Myers*, 62 Ohio Misc. 2d 763, 769 (1993); *Matter of Fiori*, 652 A. 2d 1350, 1351 (Pa. Super. 1995); *DiGrella by Parrent v Elston*, 858 S.W. 2d 698, 707, and fn. 5 (Ky. 1993); *Matter of Lawrance*, 579 N.E. 2d 32, 39–40 (Ind. 1991)

83. *Cruzan v Harman*, 760 S.W. 2d at 423–424

84. *Estate of Longeway*, 133 Ill. 2d 33, 45, 51 (1989)

85. *Guardianship of Grant*, 747 P. 2d 445, as amended by 757 P. 2d 534 (Wash. 1987 and 1988). Four justices thought artificial nutrition and hydration indistinguishable from other medical treatments; three drew a distinction, declining to authorize termination of artificial feeding without explicit legislative authorization; and two opposed any withdrawal of life-sustaining treatment from one who had not, while competent, declared that to be his wish.

86. *Matter of Spring*, 380 Mass. at 639

87. *Id.* at 637

88. *John F. Kennedy Hosp. v Bludworth*, 452 So. 2d at 926

89. *Matter of Jobes*, 108 N.J. 394, 419 (1987)

90. Two courts have suggested the possibility of civil or criminal liability for erroneous decisions to withhold or withdraw treatment. In *Payne v Marion General Hosp.*, 549 N.E. 2d 1043, 1046, 1050 (Ind. App. 1990), a physician was charged with negligence for acquiescing in the request of the patient's sister in entering a no-code order without consulting the patient, who, it was alleged, was competent and not terminally ill. The case was remanded for trial to determine if those allegations were true. In *Matter of P.V.W.*, 424 So. 2d 1015 (La. 1982), it was said that there could be civil or criminal liability if life support of a child were terminated in violation of the provision of a Louisiana statue mandating medical treatment for children (subject to exceptions) regardless of disabilities. A jury verdict exonerating a physician and a hospital from civil liability for failing to resuscitate was upheld in *Morgan v Olds*, 417 N.W. 2d 232 (Iowa App. 1987). In a 1995 Massachusetts case that has not yet been considered on appeal, a jury exonerated a physician and hospital from civil liability for entering a DNR order and failing to resuscitate despite finding that the patient would have opted for resuscitation; the jury, in answers to special questions, found that resuscitation would have been futile and that the failure to resuscitate was not negligent. *Gilgunn v Massachusetts General Hospital*, Suffolk Superior civil no. 92-4280

criminally liable. The secure establishment, in the post-*Quinlan* period, of the ethical and legal bases for termination-of-life-support decisions has led to discussion in professional journals and elsewhere of physician-assisted suicide; that is, where a physician, at the request of, or with the concurrence of, the patient, administers a poison or other agent adapted to and intended to cause death, or, alternatively, supplies the poison or other agent to the patient knowing of the patient's intention to use it to kill himself. Whatever the status of the ethical debate, the law is clear that physician-assisted suicide will expose the physician to criminal liability. Some states have adopted statutes specifically to that effect[91] other jurisdictions have treated assistance to a suicide as murder[92] or manslaughter.[93] Recent decisions of trial courts holding unconstitutional statutes forbidding physician-assisted suicide have in turn been reversed on appeal.[94] There is no doubt that the common law and statutory constraints prohibiting physician-assisted suicide are constitutionally valid and are in effect in most states. In any event, it is universally true that the law distinguishes sharply between a patient refusing life support and a patient seeking medical help to bring about death. In every state but Oregon (see footnote 91), the latter involves potential criminal exposure for the physician or other medical assistor.

POINTS ON WHICH THERE IS NO CONSENSUS

Two questions of major significance to medical providers have been discussed in court decisions but cannot be said to be the subject of consensus as of 1995. On the first, futile care, decisional law is too sparse. On the second, implementation of court ordered termination despite ethical objections, the decisional law is too closely divided.

(1) *Must a hospital or physician furnish futile care at the insistence of the patient's family?* The sparsity of decisional law on this question probably reflects the reluctance of health care providers—particularly hospitals—to take a public position facially at odds with their underlying mission to provide health care. A hospital's readiness to acquiesce in a family's insistence on futile care may ultimately be tested by increasing cost pressures on the health care system.

A clear distinction must be drawn between the question discussed above—that is, the patient's or surrogate's right to *refuse* treatment—and the question discussed here—the patient's or his family's right to *insist on* a treatment that the health care provider deems medically inappropriate or futile. Logically, decisions upholding the patient's right to refuse treatment offer little support for an asserted right to force others to provide treatment. The constitutionally and statutorily recognized right to privacy, to be let alone, has nothing in common with an asserted right to demand medical treatment from an unwilling physician.

Three cases have surfaced in the courts. A case filed in Massachusetts, reported as "Baby L,"[95] involved physicians who regarded further pediatric ICU care of a 2-year-old with massive neurologic deficits as inhumane. The mother sought a court order, but the case was mooted when a physician at another pediatric ICU agreed to assume care. The widely reported Helga Wanglie case in Minnesota[96] involved an elderly PVS patient whose family insisted on indefinite life support that was deemed wasteful and pointless by the physicians and the hospital. The latter sought a court order naming a disinterested conservator to evaluate treatment. The Probate Court declined to do so, naming Helga Wanglie's husband as her conservator. Helga Wanglie died 3 days later, before an appeal could be taken. The Probate Court decision,[97] not having been tested on appeal, lacks precedential value, even in Minnesota. The third case, however, that of "Baby K," was decided in a Federal Circuit Court of Appeals and does have precedential value.

Baby K was born in 1992 with anencephaly. She was placed on a respirator and physicians then explained to the parents that normally such babies die soon after birth and that it was impossible for her ever to attain consciousness. The mother refused to approve a DNR order. The baby was finally transferred to a nursing home but was required periodically to return to the hospital in respiratory distress. When the hospital indicated that it would further refuse admissions for treatment it deemed inappropriate, the mother, over the objections of the father and a guardian ad litem, obtained from a Federal court an order that the hospital accept Baby K and undertake treatment.[98] Refusal, the court held, would violate the Emergency Medical Treatment and Active Labor Act (EMTALA, the so-called antidumping law),[99] the Rehabilitation Act of 1973,[100] and the American with Disabilities Act.[101] The decision was upheld by the Court of Appeals under EMTALA, it being unnecessary to

91. See, e.g., Wash. Rev. Code 9A 36.060; Mich. C L 752.1027. A collection of state statutes on assisted suicide can be found in *People v Kevorkian*, 447 Mich. 436, 478, fn. 51 (1994). Oregon has a statute that forbids assisted suicide, Or. Rev. St. 163.125 (1)(b); but in November 1994, the voters passed, by ballot initiative, the Death with Dignity Act, permitting physicians, under certain circumstances, to prescribe lethal medication for terminally ill persons.

92. *People v Roberts*, 211 Mich. 187 (1920)

93. *Persampieri v Commonwealth*, 343 Mass. 19 (1961)

94. See *People v Kevorkian*, 447 Mass. 436 (1994), reversing decisions of Michigan Circuit Court and Court of Appeals; *Compassion in Dying v Washington*, 49 F. 3d 586 (1995), reversing decision of U.S. District Court judge reported at 850 F. Supp. 1454 (W.D. Wash. 1994)

95. Paris, Crone, Reardon: Physicians' refusal of requested treatment: the case of Baby L. *N Engl J Med* 1990;322:1012

96. *New York Times*, January 10, 1991

97. *In re Helga Wanglie*, Fourth Judicial District (Dist. Ct., Probate Ct. Div.) PX-91-283 Minnesota, Hennepin County. At that point Helga Wanglie had been in the ICU on ventilator support for seventeen months at a cost reported to be in excess of $700,000. See Miles SH: Informed demand for "nonbeneficial" medical treatment. *N Engl J Med* 1991;325:512

98. *In the Matter of Baby K*, 832 F. Supp. 1022 (E.D. Va. 1993)

99. 42 U.S.C. *st* 1395 dd

100. 29 U.S.C. *st* 794

101. 42 U.S.C. *st* 1201 et seq

rule on the other asserted bases.[102] The act applies to any hospital with an emergency department, which must stabilize the condition of any patient presenting with an emergency medical condition.[103] Whereas the *Baby K* decision is binding precedent only in the Fourth Circuit, the antidumping law applies in all states, so the ruling is of concern in all states.

(2) *Must a physician or hospital comply with a termination order over his or its ethical objections?* Courts have divided on the question whether a health care provider who has connected a life-support system may be required to withdraw it, notwithstanding his or its ethical objections. The *Brophy* court in Massachusetts declined to so order, deferring to the ethical integrity of the provider, a chronic care hospital, which was willing to assist the family with a transfer to another hospital.[104] Its view was followed by a New York court in the *Delio* case.[105] More jurisdictions have reached a contrary result with respect to hospitals, usually premised on the failure of the hospital to make its policy known to the patient or his family at the outset.[106] The *Barber* case and the President's Commission rejected the distinction between initiating and withdrawing mechanical life support, analogizing artificial feeding, for example, to continuous manual feeding. The same distinction could afford a broader rationale for requiring the medical providers who initiate life support to effect the termination when such support is reasonably deemed no longer appropriate by the patient or his surrogate.

CONCLUSION ◼

It is difficult to appreciate how far the debate has moved in 20 years without recalling the contentions made to courts in *Quinlan* and other cases and comparing those contentions with where we are today. In the early stages of the debate, the focus was on the applicability of criminal concepts, like murder and abetting suicide, and on the need to establish legal mechanisms—the most comprehensive being full court review in every case—to protect patients from possibly unscrupulous or uncaring decisions by doctors and families. The very language of the debate seemed to promise an unavoidable involvement of lawyers and courts in every case in which doctors and patients or their families decided to withhold or withdraw an available life-sustaining treatment. The norm implicit in the debate seemed to be that all available technologies should be applied and that any deviation from that norm was fraught with serious legal consequences.

Two decades later, in contrast, those fears have been very largely put to rest. Despite some unanswered questions, courts across the country have reached something approaching consensus on principles that comprehensively protect private decision-making within the traditional physician–patient–family triad and insulate the decision-makers from criminal and civil liability for decisions, not manifestly unreasonable, made in good faith.[107] At the beginning of the decade, medical providers lay vulnerable to criticism because the public had little understanding of the life-and-death decisions being made daily in health care institutions. The glare of publicity was inevitable and profoundly uncomfortable for physicians and families alike. The debate was at times intemperate and vehement, but today medical providers are in a more tenable position because a significant part of the public has come to understand, if only in a general way, a truth long hidden within the medical profession; that an important part of the physician's role is knowing when the time has come to terminate medical intervention and to permit the passage to death.

102. *Matter of Baby K*, 16 F. 3d 590 (4th Cir. 1994), cert. denied, 115 S. Ct. 91

103. The act alternatively authorizes transfer to another hospital prior to stabilization, but the consent of the receiving hospital is required, as well as either (1) a written request for transfer by the patient or surrogate, or (2) a certification that the medical benefits expected outweigh the risks of transfer.

104. *Brophy v New Eng. Sinai Hosp.*, 398 Mass. 417, 440–441 (1986)

105. *Delio v Westchester County Medical Center*, 516 N.Y. S. 2d 677, 693 (App. Div. 1987)

106. *Gray by Gray v Romeo*, 697 F. Supp. 580, 590–591 (1988); *Tune v Walter Reed Army Medical Hosp.*, 602 F. Supp. at 1455 (Dist. Col.); *Matter of Jobes*, 108 N.J. 394 (1987); *In re Requena*, 213 N.J. Super. 443 (App. Div.), aff'g 213 N.J. Super. 475 (Ch. Div. 1986)

107. A significant (although controversial) illustration of the protective attitude of courts toward private decision-making was the response of both the New York and Federal courts to attempts by outside agencies (both private and governmental) to intrude into the physician–family decision-making process in the much-publicized Baby Jane Doe case. See *Weber v Stony Brook Hosp.*, 95 App. Div. 2d 587 (1983), aff'd. 60 N.Y. 2d 208 (1983); *United States v Univ. Hosp. of New York*, 575 F. Supp. 607 (E.D.N.Y. 1983), aff'd. 729 F. 2d 144 (2nd Cir. 1984)

Critical Care, Third Edition, edited by Joseph M. Civetta,
Robert W. Taylor, and Robert R. Kirby.
Lippincott-Raven Publishers, Philadelphia, PA © 1997.

CHAPTER 10

■

Important Legal Concepts in Critical Care

Baruch A. Brody

This chapter surveys the major values and themes that have shaped the legal treatment of four issues of vital concern to all intensivists: informed consent and the refusal of treatment, levels of care for terminal patients, brain death, and organ transplantation. Its purpose is neither to change physicians into attorneys nor to offer advice about specific cases. Rather, it provides the background information that clinicians need to understand the legal issues raised by specific cases and to fruitfully interact with the legal system to resolve the issues in question.

INFORMED CONSENT AND THE REFUSAL OF TREATMENT

■

One of the fundamental principles of contemporary medical ethics and medical jurisprudence is that a physician must obtain the free and informed consent of a patient, or a patient's surrogate if the patient is incompetent, before medical care is provided. Providing treatment without that consent—unless certain conditions (discussed later) are met—has been treated by the courts either as a battery or as a form of medical negligence, even if the treatment is indicated and is performed in a competent fashion.[1,2] This principle emerged clearly in the United States in a series of cases at the beginning of this century.[3] The basic rationale for this

principle is embodied in the following famous quote from Justice Cardozo in *Schloendorff v. Society of New York Hospitals*, a case in which a surgeon removed a fibroid tumor after the patient consented only to an abdominal examination under anesthesia[4]:

> Every human being of adult years and sound mind has a right to determine what shall be done with his own body; and a surgeon who performs an operation without his patient's consent commits an assault, for which he is liable in damages.

Whether interpreted as a constitutional right to privacy or as a common law right to self-determination, the basic theme is clear.

Whereas the early cases emphasized the need for consent, the post–World War II cases emphasized the requirement that the consent be informed. In the 1957 case of *Salgo v. Leland Stanford Jr. University Board of Trustees*,[5] involving a patient who became paralyzed after a translumbar aortography, the court found that physicians have a duty to disclose "any facts which are necessary to form the basis of an intelligent consent by the patient to proposed treatment."

Clinicians confront many questions as they attempt to implement this principle in daily practice. Among them are the following: (1) What level of information should be supplied to the patient? (2) Are there cases in which informed consent is not required? (3) Which interventions require explicit consent and for which interventions can consent be implied? (4) From whom should consent be obtained if the

---

1. 70 C.J.S 90–96 (1987)
2. 61 *Am Jur* 2nd 174–200 (1981)
3. Faden R, Beauchamp T: *A History and Theory of Informed Consent*. New York, Oxford University Press, 1986

4. 211 N.Y. 125 105 N.E. 92 (1914)
5. 317 P.2d 170 (1957)

patient is a minor or an incompetent adult? and (5) How should refusals of consent be treated? This chapter provides an overview of the legal responses to these questions, but state law on each of them varies according to different responses by courts and legislatures, so appropriate counsel should always be consulted in complex situations.

LEVEL OF INFORMATION

It is not the rule of law in any jurisdiction that patients must be informed of all the information that the physician knows before the consent is informed. Such a requirement would be impossible to fulfill (because the patient lacks the background information) and unhelpful (because the patient would be swamped under a mass of information). Different requirements have been developed in different states; the latest detailed summary and analysis is from 1981.[6] In general, however, two major approaches have been adopted:

1. *The professional standard rule.*[7] The duty of a physician is limited "to those disclosures which a reasonable medical practitioner would make under the same or similar circumstances."
2. *The reasonable patient rule.* The duty of a physician is to disclose[8] "all those facts, risks, and alternatives that a reasonable man in the situation which the physician knows or should have known to be the plaintiff's would deem significant in making a decision to undergo the recommended treatment."

This latter rule has found favor with most commentators, partly because the first approach presupposes a professional standard that may not exist, and partly because the second approach fits better with the concept of self-determination, which grounds the whole requirement of informed consent. In applying the reasonable patient rule, physicians should indicate the patient's condition, the proposed treatment, its benefits (with the likelihood of their occurring), its risks (with the likelihood of their occurring), and any feasible alternatives. In some contexts, other information (e.g., cost) is also appropriate. At least one study[9] indicates that most of this information is usually supplied, so the two approaches may not be as different as is sometimes supposed.

One major ambiguity in applying the reasonable patient rule is defining the alternatives that should be mentioned. Should they be limited to the alternatives that the physician thinks is reasonable, or must they also include those thought to be reasonable by some other physician or group of physicians? Should they be limited to those that are reasonably available, or must they also include those available somewhere? These important ambiguities need to be clarified.

EXCEPTIONS

Two major exceptions have traditionally been recognized to the requirement of informed consent.[10] The first is the emergency exception, which allows a physician to treat a patient when significant harm is imminent, when the patient is incapable of consenting, and when no surrogate is available in a timely fashion to give consent. Not allowing physicians to treat in these circumstances would be harmful to the patient, and we are entitled to assume that the patient would consent if possible. This emergency exception applies to recognized therapies. There is considerable controversy about the use without consent of experimental therapies as part of research protocols in emergency settings. One restrictive view allows this only when there are no more than minimal risks to the patients or subjects. A different view is that this is permissible when the potential benefits outweigh the potential risks. Various in-between positions also have been proposed. Hopefully this important issue will soon be clarified.[11] The second exception is the therapeutic privilege exception, which allows physicians to withhold information when its disclosure poses a sufficient threat of harm to the patient. The courts, which have recognized the second exception, have warned against its overuse and have urged, as an alternative, disclosures to and obtaining consent from available surrogates.

IMPLIED CONSENT

Are these cases in which consent can be assumed? This issue is particularly important for intensivists who order numerous interventions for each patient. It seems impossible and unnecessary to require consent for each intervention after a full process of disclosure, but it seems equally incorrect to take the patient's consent to the initial hospitalization as consent to every ordered intervention. Some institutions have adopted policies as to which procedures require separate written consent, but such policies do not fully resolve this issue. Little has been explicitly said about this issue in the ICU setting, although there is some relevant material from surgical cases discussing implied consent and extended consent. Perhaps the best that can be said is that, absent an emergency, a general consent to ICU care should be obtained by the ICU physician at the time of admission to the unit, and that additional specific consents should be obtained for major interventions and major changes in strategy.

PEDIATRIC AND INCOMPETENT PATIENTS

Consent is normally obtained from competent adult patients. From whom does one obtain consent when dealing with minor patients? The general rule is that parents or legal guardians provide the required consent in nonemergency

6. Rosoff AJ: *Informed Consent.* Rockville, Aspen Systems, 1981

7. *Natanson v. Kline,* 186 Kan 393, 350 P.2d 1093 (1960)

8. *Cooper v. Roberts,* 220 Pa Super 260, 286 A.2d 647 (1971)

9. Greenberg LW et al: Giving information for a life-threatening diagnosis. *AJDC* 1984;138:649

10. *Canterbury v. Spence,* U.S. Court of Appeals, District of Columbia Circuit 464 Fed 2d 772 (1972)

11. Brody BA: *Ethical Issues in Drug Testing, Approval, and Pricing.* New York, Oxford University Press, 1994

situations for patients younger than 18 years of age. Statutory schemes (which have been reviewed as of 1990)[12] allow for other family members to provide consent when the parents are unavailable. Two special problem areas should be noted, and advice of counsel should be sought in such cases: (1) when the parents refuse consent for needed therapy—counsel should advise on whether and how to obtain the necessary court orders to provide the needed care; and (2) when the patient is an older minor who is married, is pregnant or is a parent, is no longer living at home, is mature of judgment, or is seeking help for substance abuse, venereal disease, or acute psychological problems—counsel should advise on the specific rules of the state as to whose consent is required.[12,13] What does one do when the patient is not a competent adult, and how is competency determined? These are harder questions, and not enough attention has been paid to them except in the context of refusing life-threatening therapy. An extreme position would be to insist that patients must be declared incompetent by a court and that consent must be obtained from a court-appointed guardian. Although such a process may be necessary in controversial cases or where no surrogate is available, the many cases involving incompetent patients make such a policy unrealistic, and the availability of close family members to serve as surrogates makes such a policy unnecessary. What has emerged as an alternative to this extreme position is the practice of clinicians making informal judgments that a patient is incompetent and then seeking consent from the available family members. A recent Texas statute that has endorsed this practice deserves to be followed elsewhere.[14] Recent commentators[15] observe that this process needs to be studied to formulate standards for its future use. In the interim, physicians can assess competency by seeing whether the patient can receive information, remember it, use it in making decisions, make a decision and give reasons for it, and appropriately assess the information in their reasoning.[16] If the patient is judged to be sufficiently incompetent, consent should be sought from the closest available family member. Family disputes, especially when the patient is marginally incompetent or the intervention is controversial, often require outside adjudication.

REFUSALS

A clear implication of the principle of informed consent is that interventions should not be provided to competent adult patients who refuse to give consent to their provision. A cautionary note has to be kept in mind. It is always important to probe the basis of the refusal. Studies[17] have shown that such refusals often result from communication failures and other breakdowns in the patient–physician relationship and can be resolved by communications that frankly address lingering doubts and confusions. Refusals of consent should be respected, but one must first be sure that one is facing a real and an informed refusal. For many, the most troubling cases involve competent nonterminally ill patients who refuse treatment that will reverse life-threatening conditions. A type of case that has attracted some attention involves elderly patients of marginal competence with gangrenous feet refusing amputations, preferring to die rather than to live without their feet. In at least one such case,[18] such a refusal was respected although the patient was not fully competent. Several recent cases have involved courts allowing discontinuation of respiratory support for quadriplegic patients who refused further support.[19] Finally, many (but by no means all) courts have respected the right of competent adult Jehovah's Witnesses to refuse blood transfusions although this refusal would result in their death.[20] Clinicians and courts will, no doubt, continue to struggle with these implications of the principle of informed consent in the future.

LEVELS OF CARE FOR TERMINAL PATIENTS

The increased capacity of medicine to sustain the life of patients who would otherwise have died has given rise to substantial clinical questions with important ethical and legal dimensions. Since the mid-1970s,[21,22] a consensus has emerged that life-sustaining therapy can be withheld or withdrawn from the appropriate patients after the appropriate decisional processes. Disagreement exists, however, about the precise definition of the patients and processes, and this disagreement is reflected in differences in the laws of the various states. This chapter highlights the main points of agreement and disagreement, looking at three classes of patients: competent adult patients, adult patients who are no longer competent, and pediatric patients.

12. Morrisey JM et al: *Consent and Confidentiality in the Health Care of Children and Adolescents*, 2nd ed. New York, Free Press, 1990

13. Holder A: *Legal Issues in Pediatric and Adolescent Medicine*. New Haven, Yale University Press, 1985

14. Texas 1993 H.B. 2545 and S.B. 332

15. Buchanan AG, Brock DK: *Deciding for Others*. New York, Cambridge University Press, 1989

16. Brody BA: *Life and Death Decision-Making*. New York, Oxford University Press, 1988:100

17. Applebaum R, Roth L: Patients who refuse treatment in medical hospital. *JAMA* 1983;250:1296

18. *Matter of Quackenbush*, 156 N.J. Super 282, 383 A.2d 785 (1978)

19. Kolata G: Saying life is not enough: the disabled demand rights and choices. *New York Times*, Jan. 31, 1991:B6

20. Obade CC: Legal aspects of critical care decision-making. In: Gosfield A (ed). *1989 Health Law Handbook*. New York, Clark Boardman, 1989:321

21. *In re Quinlan*. 70 N.J. 10 355 A.2d 647 (1976)

22. Critical Care Committee of the Massachusetts General Hospital: Optimum care for hopelessly ill patients. *N Engl J Med* 1976;295:362

COMPETENT ADULT PATIENTS

Competent adult patients with terminal illnesses facing acute life-threatening medical problems present the easiest case for analysis. As explained in a recent Supreme Court decision,[23] the right of such patients to refuse physician-recommended life-extending therapy is grounded both in the common law doctrine of informed consent, with its implication that informed competent patients can refuse therapy, and in the constitutional rights of privacy and liberty. Given the strong bases for this right of refusal, it is not surprising that many courts (as noted earlier) have extended their recognition of that right to patients who are not necessarily terminally ill and to patients who are refusing artificial nutrition or hydration.[24] An issue that has not been adequately litigated, and which is discussed later, is whether such patients have a right to receive wanted treatment for such life-threatening problems when their physicians judge that the provision of such treatment is unlikely to be successful and is, therefore, futile.

NO LONGER COMPETENT ADULT PATIENTS

Greater controversy exists when the patient is no longer competent. In such cases, we cannot be guided by the contemporaneous wishes of the patient. To provide for a mechanism whereby competent adults can plan in advance for decision-making under these circumstances, most states have passed statutes recognizing living wills or natural death act declarations, whereby patients direct in advance that life-sustaining therapy be withheld when they are terminally ill. The differing provisions of these statutes recently have been carefully analyzed and summarized.[25] Such statutes often restrict their validity to patients who are terminally ill in a narrowly defined sense, limit the forms of therapy that may be withheld or withdrawn (e.g., so that artificial nutrition and hydration is not covered), and are unclear as to whether they remain in effect if the no-longer competent patient evidences a wish for further life-sustaining therapy. Because of all these problems, living wills may not be as helpful as originally envisioned. Interest has, therefore, turned to another mechanism, durable powers of attorney, whereby patients direct in advance who is authorized to make decisions about their medical care, including refusing life-sustaining therapy, when they are no longer competent to make such decisions. Congress[26] has required that all Medicare-participating institutions inform individuals of their rights under state law to accept or refuse therapy and to formulate advance directives (such as living wills or durable powers of attorney) relating to the provision of such care. The congressional view is that this will limit the number of controversial cases involving no-longer competent adults whose wishes about life-sustaining therapy are unknown.

It is likely that there will still be many no-longer competent adult patients who will not have implemented any advance directive. Three options exist for decision-making in such cases. One is to have a court-approved guardian act as a surrogate decision-maker or to have the court itself play that role. The second is to allow decisions to be made by the patient's family. The third is to have the decision made (or at least reviewed) by a hospital ethics committee. Each of these positions has its adherents. The first view's primary (although by no means exclusive) advocate has been the Supreme Judicial Council of Massachusetts since its 1977 decision in the *Saikewicz*[27] case, although its 1980 decision in the *Spring* case[28] made it clear that even it will allow informal family decision-making in at least some cases. The second view has been adopted by many courts. Among the most prominent decisions advocating it are two 1984 cases: the Florida case of *J.F.K. Memorial Hospital v. Bludworth*,[29] and the Washington case of *In re Hamlin*,[30] which also alluded to a possible consultative role of a hospital ethics committee. Of particular interest is the reasoning in the latter decision, which explained why the court moved away from formal guardianship hearings:

> In *Colyer*, we stated that guardianship hearings would not be overly burdensome, but upon reflection, the approach that best accommodates these most fundamental societal decisions is to allow the surrogate decision-maker, the family, to make the decision free of the cumbersomeness and costs of legal guardianship proceedings.

Although no firm data exist, it is reasonable to speculate that these considerations of practicality and of trust in the family have resulted in most decision-making to forgo life-sustaining therapy for adult incompetent patients with no advance directives being made by families and physicians, with the advice of hospital ethics committees when there is disagreement or uncertainty.

This solution is not available when the patient has no known family, and less has been written about such cases. In 1992, a New York State Task Force proposed[31] a reasonable approach: life-prolonging interventions can be withheld from such patients when the attending physician and another physician chosen by the hospital agree that the patient will die in a short time, despite the provision of such interventions; they also may be withheld in other cases with the concurrence of a bioethics committee. It remains to be seen whether this approach will be adopted more widely or whether physicians will need to obtain the concurrence of a court-appointed guardian.

Whoever is the surrogate decision-maker in such cases, the question remains: What standard should be used in

23. *Cruzan v. Director, Missouri Dept. of Health*, 58 LW 4916 (June 25, 1990)

24. *Bouvia v. Superior Court*, 255 Cal Reptr. 297 (1986)

25. Meisel A: *The Right to Die*. New York, John Wiley, 1989

26. 1990 Omnibus Budget Reconciliation Act, Section 4206

27. *Superintendent of Belchertown State School v. Saikewicz*, 373 Mass. 728, 370 N.E. 2d 417 (1977)

28. *In re Spring*, 380 Mass. 629, 405 N.E. 2d 115 (1980)

29. *J.F.K. Memorial Hospital v. Bludworth*, 452 So. 2d 921 (1984)

30. *In re Hamlin*, 102 Wash 2d 810, 689 P.2d 1372 (1984)

31. New York State Task Force on Life and the Law: *When Others Must Choose*. New York, The Task Force, 1992

making the decision to forgo life-sustaining therapy? Several recently reviewed standards[32] have been advocated:

1. *The clear and convincing evidence standard.* Adopted by courts in New York[33] and Missouri,[34] this standard requires clear and convincing evidence of the patient's expressed intent that they not receive the therapy in question. Although not requiring that the evidence be in writing in the form of an advance directive, this standard will often be hard to satisfy without such written evidence.

2. *The substituted judgment (or subjective) standard.* Adopted by most courts, this standard requires that the surrogate, in light of the available evidence, make the judgment that the patient would most likely have made.

3. *The best interest (or objective) standard.* Exclusively adopted in only a few cases but advocated by commentators,[35] this standard requires that the surrogate make an objective assessment of what would be in the patient's best interest in light of the extent of life preserved, the preservation of functioning during that life, and the available relief from pain and indignity.

These standards have been usefully combined by the Supreme Court of New Jersey in a influential triad of cases from 1985 to 1987[36]; priority should be given to the former standards when the evidence they require is available, but the objective standard should increasingly be used as the evidence of the patient's wishes is less and less available.

Clinicians need to be informed of the approach adopted in their state regarding the identity of the surrogate decision-maker and the standard to be applied. A recent Supreme Court decision[23] makes it clear that states are allowed to continue to adopt different approaches. All of these complexities provide clinicians with an additional motive to encourage still-competent adult patients to implement advance directives that will help avoid these ambiguities. The recent federal legislation (noted earlier), which requires that patients be informed about these matters, is clearly a step in the right direction.

Before turning to pediatric patients, two points of controversy should be observed. The first has to do with withholding artificial nutrition or hydration from incompetent patients (whether terminal or merely severely disabled, such as persistent vegetative patients). Whereas controversy continues among commentators,[37] the courts are increasingly accepting the decision to discontinue that form of support,[38] although several living will statutes exclude food and fluids from their provisions.[39]

The second has to do with providing "futile" forms of therapy. Until now, the focus have been on the right of patients and their surrogates to forgo life-sustaining therapy when they judge it to be inappropriate. What, however, should happen if they insist on the provision of such therapy, but the physicians believe that it is futile in light of the low probability of it making a real difference? May the physician refuse to provide such therapies? Does the patient have a right to receive them? Increasingly, major medical groups have insisted that the physician has no obligation to provide such therapies, although a recent survey of these opinions[40] has revealed that these groups are employing different concepts of futility. Moreover, in the first major appellate case to deal directly with this issue,[41] the court ruled that at the request of the parents, physicians must continue to provide an anencephalic infant (Baby K) with life-prolonging interventions judged to be futile by the providers. The question of the obligation to provide futile interventions is, therefore, far from settled.

PEDIATRIC PATIENTS

Pediatric patients raise an additional set of issues. As minors, they are usually not capable of making binding decisions about their health care, although some exceptions are noted later. Moreover, in the case of pediatric patients, unlike the case of formerly competent adult patients, little sense can be made of any substituted judgment approach. In general, then, parents must be entrusted with the authority to make binding decisions about their children's care. They are expected to make them in light of a best interest standard, and courts have been willing to interpose their judgment (especially when the child's condition is life threatening and the treatment likely to be efficacious) when they believe that the parental decision is not in the child's best interest. This is true even when the parental decision (e.g., the refusal of transfusions by parents who are Jehovah's Witnesses) is based on religious beliefs. But does the right of parents extend to refusing life-prolonging therapy for their dying children? That is the additional issue that must be considered.

Four states (Arkansas, Louisiana, New Mexico, and Texas) have answered the questions by specific provisions in their natural death acts, which authorize parents to implement such directives on behalf of their dying children. The use of such directives is apparently helpful.[42] There exist, moreover, several court decisions affirming that parental

32. Developments: Medical technology and the law. *Harvard Law Rev* 1990;103:1519

33. *In re Westchester County Medical Center on Behalf of O'Connor*, 531NE.2d 607 (1988)

34. *Cruzan v. Harman*, 760 S.W. 2d 408 (1988)

35. Dresser R, Robertson J: Quality of life and non-treatment decisions for incompetent patients: a critique of the orthodox approach. *Law Med Health Care* 1989;17:234

36. *In re Conroy*, 98N.J. 321, 486 A.2d 1209 (1985); *In re Jobes*, 108 N.J. 394, 529 A.2d 434 (1987); and *In re Peter*, 108 N.J. 365, 529 A.2d 419 (1987)

37. Cranford R, Brody B, Armstrong P, et al: The persistent problem of PVS. *Hastings Center Report* 1988;18:26

38. Cruzan *Supra* note 23, footnote 6

39. Meisel, *Supra* note 25, Section 11.15

40. Brody B, Halevy A: Is futility a futile concept? *J Med Philos* 1995;2:123

41. *Matter of Baby K*, 1994 WL 38674 (Fourth Circuit) Feb. 10, 1994

42. Jefferson L et al: The use of the Natural Death Act in pediatric patients. *Crit Care Med* 1991;19:901

right independent of any legislation.[43] In general, then, the answer to our question is affirmative. There are, however, two further complicating factors that must be considered, one having to do with newborns and the other with adolescents.

The Child Abuse Amendment of 1984[44] (the second version of the Baby Doe laws) requires that each state receiving federal funds must have in place a program for dealing with child abuse that consists of withholding medically indicated treatment from infants facing life-threatening conditions. Most jurisdictions have such a program in place, and such programs limit the discretion of parents (even with physician concurrence) to decide to withhold life-sustaining therapy from infants (children younger than 1 year of age or those whose problems date back to when they were younger than that age). In general, all medically indicated treatment must be provided unless the infant falls into one of three classes: (1) the infant is chronically and irreversibly comatose; (2) the provision of the treatment would be futile in terms of survival and would merely prolong dying; (3) the provision of the treatment would be virtually futile in terms of survival and inhumane under such circumstances. Even in such cases, appropriate nutrition, hydration, and medication must be provided. Studies[45] have shown that practicing neonatal intensivists find the provisions of this legislation unclear and unhelpful. Not surprisingly, many refer such cases to infant care review committees, whose formation was encouraged by the legislation to help clarify ambiguities before terminating life-sustaining therapy.

As children grow into adolescence, they acquire greater decisional capacities. Adolescence also marks that period of time at which they increasingly receive decisional authority. These facts raise an important question for intensivists dealing with the issue of continuing life-sustaining therapy for adolescent patients: What are the roles of the patient and of the parents in that decision? Clinicians[46,47] have increasingly advocated a greater role for such patients, although the exact role at different ages is still a matter of controversy. The law[48] also has given increasing decisional authority to mature minors, to married minors, to minors who are parents, and to emancipated minors. Should adolescents then have the final decisional authority over life-preserving therapy, or should that authority continue in the hands of their parents? Texas, as part of its natural death act,[49] has said that such patients, if competent, can supersede the parental decision to forgo further life-sustaining therapy. It does not state, however, the age of the patient who is covered, nor does it

address the issue of the adolescent who wishes, with or against parental wishes, to forgo life-sustaining treatment. The legal literature has not resolved these issues. Moreover, several 1994 cases were decided in opposite directions.[50] A Florida court allowed 15-year-old Benito Agrelo to stop taking antirejection medications because of painful side effects, and he died. However, a California court ordered compulsory chemotherapy for Lee Lor, a 15-year-old Hmong girl who, together with her family, rejected it on cultural grounds. The best strategy for clinicians is surely to strive to build a consensus in the family, but the Lor case demonstrates remaining legal ambiguities.

BRAIN DEATH

The classic definition of death refers to the irreversible cessation of spontaneous cardiac and respiratory function. Despite occasional fears about the premature diagnosis of death and a resulting premature burial, this definition served society well until two medical developments raised problems for its continued use. First, the ability of physicians to artificially support respiration and circulation often makes it difficult to determine whether spontaneous functioning has ceased. Moreover, the development of organ transplantation requires the determination of death as soon as possible in supported patients before organs deteriorate.

Both of these concerns motivated a 1968 report by an ad hoc committee of the Harvard Medical School.[51] That report offered a new definition of death: the condition of a permanently nonfunctioning brain (confusingly called "irreversible coma"). Such patients are unreceptive and unresponsive to stimuli, neither move spontaneously nor breathe on their own, and exhibit no central reflexes. An isoelectric electroencephalogram (EEG), although not required, was viewed in the report as being of great confirmatory value.

This report led to many clinical and legal responses in the years that followed. These many responses have, unfortunately, led to much confusion, so we need to follow them carefully, beginning with the legal responses. The simplest response, the adoption of brain death as the primary if not the sole definition of death, was advocated in 1978 by the National Conference of Commissioners on Uniform State Laws in their Uniform Brain Death Act, which reads as follows[52]:

> For legal and medical purposes, an individual who has sustained irreversible cessation of all functioning of the brain, including the brain stem, is dead. A determination under this section must be made in accordance with reasonable medical standards.

43. *In re L.H.R.*, 253Ga 439, 321 SE 2d 716 (1984); *In re P.V.W.*, 424 SO 2d 1015 (1982)

44. PL 98–457

45. Kopelman L et al: Neonatologists judge the "Baby Doe" regulations. *N Engl J Med* 1988;318:677

46. Nitschke R et al: Therapeutic choices made by patients with end-stage cancer. *J Pediatr* 1982;101:471

47. Leikin S: A proposal concerning decisions to forgo life-sustaining treatment for young people. *J Pediatr* 1989;115:17

48. Holder A: Minors' rights to consent to medical care. *JAMA* 1987;257:3400

49. Texas Health and Safety Code Title 8, Section 672.007

50. Slap G, Jablow M: When young patients refuse treatment. *New York Times*, Nov. 10, 1994:B3; and Slap G, Jablow M: Girl flees after clash of cultures on illness. *New York Times*, November 12, 1994:6

51. Ad Hoc Committee of the Harvard Medical School to Examine the Definition of Brain Death: A definition of irreversible coma. *JAMA* 1968;205:337

52. Uniform Brain Death Act 12 *U.L.A.* 16 (1990 Suppl.)

Although adopted at one time or another by six state legislatures and several state courts, this approach has mostly been abandoned. It has been replaced by statutes that offer alternative definitions of death. The most common is the Uniform Determination of Death Act, recommended by the same National Conference in 1980 and adopted by legislation in 26 states and the District of Columbia, and by some state courts; it reads as follows[53]:

An individual who has sustained either (1) irreversible cessation of circulatory and respiratory functions, or (2) irreversible cessation of all functions of the entire brain, including the brainstem, is dead. A determination of death must be made in accordance with accepted medical standards.

This approach, although preserving continuity with the past as well as making the changes required by modern technology, does not clarify when each of these definitions is to be employed. A third approach, originally advocated by Professors Capron and Kass[54] and adopted by legislation or by court decisions in several states, stipulates that the brain death definition should be used when artificial means of support preclude use of the traditional cardiopulmonary definition.

Although the resulting legal variations make it advisable that practicing physicians know what approach has been adopted in their state either by the legislature or by the courts, intensivists can avoid many of these legal niceties, because most of their dying patients are on life support and their death is defined by all three approaches in terms of brain death.

Two crucial points should be noted. First, although eminent philosophers,[55,56] lawyers,[57] and clinicians[58] have argued for a neocortical approach to brain death according to which a patient is dead if their cortex (but not necessarily the rest of their brain) has irreversibly ceased functioning, no jurisdiction has adopted that approach. This means that clinicians must ascertain that all parts of the brain, including the stem, have irreversibly ceased functioning. Second, all of the legal definitions refer to reasonable and accepted medical standards for determining brain death, but none indicate what are those standards. For these two reasons, the legal definitions have generated significant clinical literature as to what are the reasonable and accepted standards for determining that the entire brain has irreversibly ceased functioning.

The Harvard committee's emphasis on the use of such tests as an EEG has been criticized as unnecessary if clinical findings are carefully reviewed, and as unhelpful because the test environment often produces a misleading nonisoelectric EEG. Recently, the most influential clinical attempt to provide criteria for brain death was the recommendation of the medical consultants to the President's Commission,[59] whose criteria are as follows:

1. Cerebral function has ceased (as evidenced by cerebral unreceptivity and unresponsivity) and brain stem function is absent (as evidenced by an absence of stem reflexes—pupillary, corneal, oculocephalic, oculovestibular, and oropharyngeal—and an absence of respiratory effort even after an adequate challenge such as the extended apnea test[60]).
2. This cessation is irreversible because the cause of the coma is established and is not reversible (not from sedation, hypothermia, neuromuscular blockage, or shock), and because it has been absent for an adequate period of time (6 hours if there is a confirmatory EEG, 12 hours otherwise).

Whereas EEG testing is referred to on several occasions in the committee's report, the major impact of an EEG is to lessen the amount of time required before the cessation is judged to be irreversible.

These medical consultants believed that irreversibility of cessation of functioning is harder to determine in younger children whose brains were thought to have greater resistance to damage and greater capacity to recover functioning. A joint task force of neurologists and pediatricians[61] called for more extensive testing of children younger than 1 year of age. From 7 days of age to 2 months, two full clinical examinations and two EEGs separated by 48 hours are recommended. From 2 months to 1 year of age, two examinations and two EEGs separated by 24 hours are recommended.

Although none of these criteria have the force of law, they help define what are reasonable and accepted medical standards for determining brain death. In many hospitals in which this author consults, the medical staff has formally adopted these standards to provide guidance and protection to the clinicians called on to determine brain death. It has recently been demonstrated, however, that the satisfaction of these standards does not mean a total cessation of brain functioning, especially neurohormonal functioning.[62] It remains to be seen whether this will lead to new standards or to a different understanding of brain death.

53. Uniform Determination of Death Act 12 *U.L.A.* 320 (1990 Suppl.)

54. Capron A, Kass L: A statutory definition of the standards for determining brain death. *Univ Penna Law Rev* 1972;121

55. Veatch RM: The whole-brain oriented concept of death: an outmoded philosophical formulation. *J Thanatol* 1975;3:13

56. Engelhardt HT: *The Foundations of Bioethics*. New York, Oxford, 1986

57. Smith DR: Legal recognition of neocortical death. *Cornell Law Rev* 1986;71:850

58. Youngner SJ, Barlett ET: Human death and high technology. *Ann Intern Med* 1983;99:252

59. Report of the Medical Consultants on the Diagnosis of Death: guidelines for the determination of death. *JAMA* 1981; 246:2184

60. Belsh JM, Blatt R, Schiffman PL: Apnea testing in brain death. *Arch Intern Med* 1986;146:2385

61. Report of Special Task Force: Guidelines for the determination of brain death. *Pediatrics* 1987;80:298

62. Halevy A, Brody B: Brain death: reconciling definitions, criteria, and tests. *Ann Intern Med* 1993;119:519

ORGAN TRANSPLANTATION ■

Organ transplantation raises an extensive set of legal issues concerning procurement, distribution, and financing. These issues have been addressed to varying degrees, and the resulting legal principles are complex. This section provides an overview of what has been accomplished, emphasizing the aspects that are most relevant from a clinical perspective.

The basic legal framework for the procurement of cadaver organs is provided by the Uniform Anatomical Gift Act (UAGA), endorsed by the National Conference of Commissioners on Uniform State Laws in 1968 and adopted by all state legislatures in the early 1970s.[63] The basic policy of that act is to provide individuals with an opportunity in advance of their death to donate their organs for use in transplantation. Families may donate organs after the death of the patient if the patient has made no advance provisions, but the UAGA makes it clear that donor advance donations take precedence over family objections. Only two states (Florida and New York) have given certain family members the right to veto the donation, and the recent revision of the UAGA has made this point even clearer. Nevertheless, standard practice[64] has been to accept donations only if the family concurs, partly because one often doesn't know about advance donations in a timely manner and partly because transplant programs want to avoid the stresses that would arise if they attempted to harvest organs against family wishes.

Because of this standard practice and because most people have not make an advance donation, the procurement effort is directed toward families. After considerable evidence that many clinicians failed to even approach families of potential donors, congress amended the Social Security Act in 1986[65] to establish a requirement that any hospital receiving funds from Medicare or Medicaid must develop a protocol for identifying potential donors and for approaching families with the option of organ donation. This national "required request" approach supplemented a variety of state laws that required the same thing. However, some have criticized this approach on the grounds that it inappropriately shifts the locus of decision-making to families rather than reinforcing the original policy of respecting the views of the patient, and the American Medical Association has called for a policy of mandated choice where individuals are required to state their preferences when renewing their driver's license.[66]

National policy, since the National Organ Transplant Act of 1984,[67] specifically prohibits the purchasing of organs from the family. Some clinicians have attempted to argue for such a policy—using data from third-world countries where organs are being purchased—because of the poor results obtained when using such organs.[68] That analysis has been challenged, and the best defense[69] of the policy seems to be that our social values reject the idea of treating the body or its parts as a commodity.

Two special cases of organ procurement have attracted considerable attention. The first is procuring organs from anencephalics. In 1994, the Council on Ethical and Judicial Affairs of the American Medical Association[70] concluded that it should be permissible to procure organs from living anencephalic infants because "the infant has never experienced, and will never experience, consciousness." Currently, however, such procurements would be illegal in all states. It remains to be seen whether this new approach will be adopted. The second is a protocol developed by the University of Pittsburgh in 1992.[71] According to it, dying patients who are going to have life support removed anyway can have this done in the operating room so that organs can be procured. Central to this protocol is the determination of death after 2 minutes of cardiopulmonary death without any attempts at resuscitation. Whether this satisfies the current legal requirement of irreversibility is unclear.

The discussion turns from organ procurement to organ distribution. The fundamental legal structure for distribution was created by the above-mentioned National Organ Transplant Act of 1984. Among its major provisions was the creation of a national organ procurement and transplantation network. A contract for such network was formulated and awarded to a nonprofit corporation in Virginia, the United Network for Organ Sharing (UNOS). Because of reimbursement restrictions, all active centers participate in this network.

From the clinical perspective, the crucial functions of UNOS are to maintain a list of individuals awaiting transplantation, to promulgate criteria for allocating organs to such individuals, and to match harvested organs with recipients. Extensive UNOS policies cover these issues,[72] which involve elements of local sharing and national sharing and compromises between medical need and medical benefit. All of these issues were given an extensive analysis by an important task force[73] created by Congress in 1984, whose recommendations form the basis of many UNOS policies.

Finally, the question of third-party reimbursement is addressed; this is an extremely important issue because transplants are procedures for which few patients could pay with-

63. Uniform Anatomical Gift Act 8ULA 15 (1983)

64. Task Force on Organ Transplantation: *Organ Transplantation: Issues and Recommendations*. Washington, D.C., Dept. of Health and Human Services, April 1986

65. PL 99–509 Section 9318

66. Developments: Medical technology and the law. *Harvard Law Rev* 1990:103:1519; Council on Ethical and Judicial Affairs: Strategies for cadaveric organ procurement. *JAMA* 1994;272:809

67. 42 U.S.C. §274e

68. Salahudeen AK et al: High Mortality among recipients of bought living unrelated donor kidneys. *Lancet* 1990;ii:725

69. Al-Khader AA: Living non-related kidney transplantation in Bombay. *Lancet* 1990ₓ:1002

70. Council on Ethical and Judicial Affairs: *Code of Medical Ethics: Current Opinions With Annotations*. Chicago, AMA, 1994

71. Arnold RM, Youngner SJ (eds): Ethical, psychosocial, and public policy implications of procuring organs from non-heart-beating cadavers. *Kennedy Inst Ethics J* 1993;3:A1

72. *Policies of United Network for Organ Sharing*. Virginia, UNOS, March 1990, Section 3

73. Task Force, *Supra* Note 64

out such reimbursement. The Social Security Amendments of 1972 covered the cost of treating end-stage renal disease, including dialysis and transplantation, under the Medicare program.[74] Heart transplantation was originally covered by Medicare in November 1979. That coverage was suspended in June 1980 but was reinstated in April 1987, and liver transplantation was covered in 1991.[75] A 1993 survey[76] showed that although Medicare did not cover pancreatic transplantation, it was paying for much of the costs because of the association with kidney transplantation. Medicaid coverage varied among the states and among the procedures.

Private insurers have found it difficult to deny covering transplantation when it is the patient's best hope. This is evident from a 1994 survey[77] of insurance reimbursement for bone marrow transplantation for breast cancer—still an experimental procedure—that showed tremendous variation among insurers, but also showed that attempts to deny coverage when challenged usually have failed. Clearly, then, the legal framework for financing transplantation is not fully developed at this point, no doubt reflecting the fact that the financing of health care in the United States involves many different third-party payers.

74. PL 92–603

75. Organ transplants: deciding who lives, who dies, and who pays. *Medical Benefits*, August 15, 1991:6

76. Evans RW et al: An economic analysis of pancreas transplantation. *Clin Transplant* 1993;7:166

77. Peters WB, Rogers Mark C: Variation in approval by insurance companies of coverage for autologous bone marrow transplantation for breast cancer. *N Engl J Med* 1994;330:473

Critical Care, Third Edition, edited by Joseph M. Civetta,
Robert W. Taylor, and Robert R. Kirby.
Lippincott-Raven Publishers, Philadelphia, PA © 1997.

CHAPTER 11

Prediction and Definition
of Outcome

Joseph M. Civetta

The definition of outcome was a relatively simple matter before the current era in which costs have become such a central issue. In an evaluation of the outcome of intensive care, survival from intensive care, although easy to measure and of fundamental importance, is not the only determinant. Some patients improve enough to be discharged from the intensive care unit (ICU) only to die before discharge from the hospital. Other patients survive hospitalization to be permanently placed in nursing homes or undergo chronic hospitalization for severe physical and mental impairments. Today, however, the *outcomes movement* and managed care have additional goals, born of cost containment and the fears of health care rationing. These include understanding the effectiveness of interventions, better decision-making, developing guidelines and "critical pathways," and optimizing use of resources. Life or death, in fact, are not the only important outcomes considered by patients; rational choices among treatments depend on how patients view their predicament, a personalized assessment of specific risks and benefits.

Quantitative indices have been developed to provide a more precise and accurate tool to evaluate the degree of illness and the likelihood of recovery. Outcome can be accurately predicted in approximately 85% to 90% of cases. The failure rate should not be construed as representing a shortcoming of methodology, but rather, that the necessary data are not and will never be available in all cases. Because most systems collect information at the time of ICU admission or during the first 24-hour period, unique determinants of outcome, such as catastrophic new illnesses or iatrogenic events, cannot be predicted. Of greater importance are the patients who develop multiple organ system failure (MOSF) and sepsis, ultimately dying of failure of organ systems that

were functioning at ICU admission. Finally, most predictive indices are weighted for acute physiologic changes, predominantly of cardiorespiratory and oxygen transport functions. In MOSF, these indicators usually may be close to normal even moments before death.

Goals for predictive indices include evaluation of the performance of an individual unit, interunit comparisons, and a method to control the populations in prospective studies. These goals are reasonable for most patients; it is important to develop indices that can also identify resource use (i.e., proper selection of diagnostic and therapeutic interventions) and to measure outcomes, beyond the limitations incurred if survival alone is selected, that are relevant to patients' values and desires.

COST CONSIDERATIONS ∎

When costs for medical care exceeded 10% of the gross national product (GNP) a few years ago, responses varied and included changes in medical care financing,[1] high visibility of costly technology,[2] and the introduction of cost effectiveness as a perspective for viewing medical care.[3] Intensive care deserves special scrutiny because it generates approximately 2% of the GNP. Three potential methods exist for achieving control of costs: (1) reevaluating criteria for admission, (2) diminishing charges generated during the ICU admission, and (3) attempting to hasten discharge. Evaluation of criteria for admission is covered in Chapter 2.

The "appropriate" patient must be considered to be the one who could not survive without intensive care but who actually does survive given such care. This patient is difficult

127

to define accurately, and patients admitted to most ICUs include those who might otherwise be considered too sick or too well. Patients who are "too well," that is, those who could survive without intensive care, often are given observation and intensive nursing care and consume a small portion of ICU bed days. These patients, if excluded, may paradoxically cause increased costs and resource utilization if complications develop in routine care areas where therapy in response to developed complications (in contrast to preventive care) is neither as effective nor as rapid. If terminally ill patients are excluded, patients who are severely ill usually die rapidly and, again, use few bed days. Some patients, however, may respond favorably to intensive treatment and survive, an outcome not possible if all of these patients are excluded. Control can be achieved by evaluating—and diminishing—expenditures while patients are in the ICU.

Restriction of unnecessary diagnostic testing preserves patients from harms associated with incorrect test results and interpretations, technical errors from inappropriate procedures, and the confusion resulting from too much data. Limitation of the ICU stay is, actually, most important for patients who ultimately die. We must recognize the distinction between living and dying. When our efforts cannot have a salutary outcome in terms of survival, we must change directions and accept the inevitability of death. (This subject is covered in greater detail in Chapter 5). Earlier recognition will alleviate suffering and stress for patient, family, and ICU staff and will conserve limited resources.

We can now proceed to a more detailed evaluation of outcomes and predictive indices, define various goals for intensive care independent of the emphasis on mortality, and evaluate measures for cost control based on these deliberations.

DEFINITION OF OUTCOME ■

The relationship between severity of illness and survival or death is important, but does not account for some of the most important societal factors at this time: evaluation of the process of care, effective use of resources, cost containment, and, most important, understanding the patients' values—when care is considered necessary, what patients think of various risks and benefits, and how they obtain and use information in making these choices.

Patients clearly view their predicaments in different ways. Some patients with severe symptoms may not choose surgery, whereas others find limitation of lifestyle a sufficient reason to undergo hazardous operations. Investigations into these factors has been termed *outcome research*.[4] It holds out hope that full entitlement to effective health care is attainable within the limits of our national willingness to fund medical care. Current levels of use of expensive procedures, many of which incorporate intensive care, may not reflect the level of demand if patients were fully informed of their options and if they understood the probabilities of various outcomes. If demand fell, then rationing based on the assumption that demand cannot be met because of financial restraints might not be considered. Proponents believe that we will gain increased understanding of the effectiveness of

different interventions, allow patients and physicians to make better decisions using this information, aid in the development of guidelines for physicians, and optimize the use of resources by third-party payers.[5] The technology to do so has been labeled *outcomes management*[6] and is described as the technology of patients' experience designed to help patients, payers, and providers make rational, medical care–related choices based on better insight into the effect that these choices have on the patients' life.

In contrast to the predictive systems and indices that have been developed and are discussed in this chapter, the data necessary for outcomes management consist of information and analysis of clinical, financial, and health outcomes that best estimate the relationship between medical interventions and health outcomes as well as the relationship between health outcomes and money. Instead of attempting greater precision or incorporating more physiologic measurements, outcomes management would place greater reliance on standards and guidelines to aid physicians in selecting appropriate interventions, to systematically measure the functioning and well-being of patients and clinical outcomes, and to analyze results most appropriate to the concerns of each decision maker.[7]

These goals and terminology are not new but need to be newly applied. In contrasting laboratory and clinical medicine, Feinstein[6] pointed out that two important differences occur in the design of experiments: repetition and variation. In the laboratory, both are under the control of the investigator. However, in a clinical therapeutic experiment, the clinician cannot reproduce the same patient and must, instead, obtain a population whose diverse illnesses constitute the various subgroups that form the clinical spectrum of that disease. In addition, Feinstein listed many factors that now might be considered part of outcomes research: vocational incapacitation, scholastic requirements, pain, familial problems, psychological reactions, financial burdens, and "many other features of the panorama of human life."[6]

Therefore, we must be concerned with citing the objectives of each therapeutic situation.[8] Possible targets for treatment include basic abnormalities of the disease itself, associated arrangements manifested in tests, and clinical symptoms and signs. The criteria include the following: whether a particular manifestation or target is present or absent; the quantity, severity, or degree of manifestation; a significant change in the manifestation; and, finally, cluster designations that represent a total effect, such as "improved" or "deteriorated." The major problem with all existing indices is that neither the goals of outcomes management nor the targets and criteria of clinical judgment have been used. By concentrating on the severity of illness—which bears little relationship to the goals and targets outlined—and its relationship to survival or death, we have been led away from the perplexing problems facing society in an analysis of outcome and costs. No index has yet achieved the goals set out by their developers. In the words of the National Institutes of Health Consensus Development Conference on Critical Care Medicine,

> The combination of life-threatening diseases, finite resources, invasive therapeutic and monitoring techniques and high costs makes the need for adequate data on which to

base decision a high priority. Such research is aimed at determining how ICUs can be used for the maximum benefit of the ICU population. This research should include procedures for "triaging" patients so that admission is not denied to patients who can most benefit from an ICU as well as excluding patients who have no reasonable chance to benefit. Research aimed at developing accurate outcome predictors as a function of initial presenting condition, diagnoses, and other on-going prognostic variables should be encouraged.[9]

Even the newest indices do not attain these goals for individual patients.

COST AND COST EFFECTIVENESS

The element of resource allocation, although not fundamental to medical care, is fundamental to reimbursement for that care. We must therefore examine some of the problems associated with this approach.

The relation between cost and charge has been difficult to unravel for many reasons. Certain areas of the hospital, such as the laundry and utilities, create costs without generating any revenue. These costs may be apportioned in different ways to various charges, such as medications and laboratory tests. Furthermore, over the years, charges have been raised according to formulas applied under the auspices of government or third-party payers. For instance, if a charge were "too high," the excess might be apportioned to another charge that was below the limit or ceiling (Fig. 11-1). Accordingly, to trace an individual charge backward to the fundamental costs often is impossible. "Best guess" estimates in our hospital range from a cost of 35% of charge for laboratory determinations to 70% for the daily bed charge. Perhaps as a result of the inability to trace charges back to costs or because costs of health insurance have affected the prices of consumer goods while being available to fewer and fewer people, changes have occurred in health care financing. Independent of legislative action and governmental policy, managed care has penetrated most markets, reaching 40% to 50% in California and Minnesota. The first step involves negotiations at discounted prices for professional and hospital services. "Bundled" prices for hospitalization for such operations as coronary artery bypass transfer the risk to the provider. While the amount to be given to both the physician and the hospital diminishes, efficiency must increase and needless expenditures be curtailed. After all of the fat in the system has been trimmed, additional diminution in the reimbursement may limit access or result in inferior care. Before that point is reached, however, an individual outlier, which is the patient who experiences complications and has a prolonged stay, can end up wiping out the meager remaining profit from the other patients treated. Thus, the phrase "risk is assumed by the providers" means that physicians can lose money by providing expensive services. Finally, under capitation systems, the health care providers agree to accept a certain amount for all lives covered in the plan but in return have to provide all the services *required* by the population. This leads to a reversal of the prior medical system that rewarded productivity: the more one did, the more one made. Now a surgeon makes more money by not operating while the managed care company, the hospital and the physician group usually split the capitation income. Thus, if no operations are performed, hospital costs are saved and these monies are distributed among the three participants. Clearly, expert care performed with no complications will enable services to be provided at a minimal cost without provider risk. Excesses and inefficiencies must be identified and curtailed, but the specter of limiting, withholding, or withdrawing care based on economic necessities looms larger and larger.

It seems sensible to examine the reasons for these costs to understand how we might approach the problem of control from within the medical profession. The number of patients admitted is not as indicative of resource utilization as are the patient days consumed (product of the number of patients each day and the number of days considered). The 375 patients studied in our surgical ICU (SICU) consumed 1664 days of intensive care.[10] Of these 375, 110 patients were admitted for 1 day and ultimately survived. These patients were mostly elderly patients undergoing major elective surgery with a known risk of postoperative complications. Additionally, 14 patients were admitted and died during the first 24 hours. Together, these 124 patients represented 34% of admissions yet used only 5% of the patient days and generated 8% of the total charges. Thus, elimination of these patients as too well or too sick by developing restrictive admission policies would not result in a major reduction in charges.

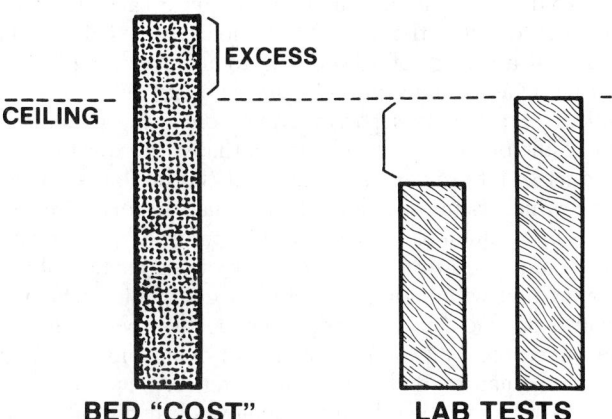

FIGURE 11-1. Apportionment of excess hospital charges from bed "cost" to laboratory tests.

SEVERITY OF ILLNESS

These two groups represent the opposite ends of the severity spectrum: the least severe (too well) are discharged quickly because little care is needed, and the most severely ill die rapidly despite maximum therapeutic efforts. The patients whose ICU stay lasted more than 2 weeks, however, should be an important focus. Twenty-eight patients (7%) used 583 (35%) of the ICU days and generated 36% of the total charges, yet 12 (44%) survived (Table 11-1). Because survival was nearly 50%, such patients must be considered appropriate for ICU care; because they consume so many ICU days, they create many problems in terms of ethics, law, and resource allocation, among other societal concerns.

TABLE 11-1.   Spectrum of Severity of Illness

	LEAST						MOST					
	Living						*Deaths*					
ICU stay (days)	1	2	3–4	5–6	7–13	>13	>13	13–7	6–5	4–3	2	1
Patients	110	71	52	27	21	12	16	20	9	10	13	14
ICU days used	110	142	170	146	184	258	325	182	49	35	26	14
Charge/patient ($K)	20	20	28	30	60	113	71	55	36	23	18	23

Both rapid recovery (least severe = little care needed) and rapid death (most severe = little time for/success of intervention) are relatively low in charges. The patients who stayed longer than 2 wks were 7% of the sample, yet generated the highest resource utilization.
ICU stay (days) = length of ICU admission until discharge as hospital survivor for living or, in deaths, length of ICU admission for those who died in ICU or before hospital discharge.
Charge/patient ($K) in thousands of dollars.

PREDICTION AND RESOURCE UTILIZATION

Our inability to predict survival or death accurately on admission presents society with an unclear picture concerning the desirability of continuing therapeutic efforts. If we could define accurately whether a patient had a 10%, 1%, or 0.1% chance of survival, society could decide if it wished to pay for treatment of 9, 99, or 999 patients with fatal illnesses for medical care to achieve one survivor. Given an average ICU charge of $50,000 per patient in our hospital in 1994, this would represent the investment of $500,000, $5,000,000, or $50,000,000 per survivor. One problem is that no current prognostic indicator can give us this level of resolution; a second problem is that society (the people, the government, and the insurance carriers) gives no clear directive as to how much should be expended in a single case. A recent case in Florida made headlines: an indigent infant under the care of Health and Rehabilitative Services (HRS) was being considered for small bowel transplantation. Given the limited overall HRS budget, the question was raised whether distributive justice would be well served by devoting the anticipated resources to a single individual or whether they would be better spent providing immunizations and basic health care to a larger number of other patients under HRS jurisdiction. The courts ruled that the infant should receive the transplantation; after many months of care for many complications, the child died. The total hospital bill was in excess of $800,000.

COST-CONTAINMENT EFFORTS

We must address our cost-containment efforts toward the other two areas of control: expenditures while patients are in the unit and the decision for discharge. In general, it is well recognized that ICU deaths are often associated with MOSF and sepsis.[11,12] Our true therapeutic efforts, that is, interventions that cure disease, are limited in these patients. MOSF is characterized by involvement of the central nervous system, the liver, immune system or host response, renal function, and coagulation, among others. We do not have effective therapeutic modalities in these states. Our two control measures, then, can be to restrict unnecessary

diagnostic testing and to recognize that the variations in the patient cause a desire to influence outcome by minute-to-minute manipulations and repetitive laboratory testing in the hopes that these will change outcome. In reality, the converse is true: excessive efforts carry no chance for improvement, thus leaving only the possibility for errors, iatrodemics, and iatrogenic occurrences.[13]

Instead of devoting our energies to manipulations and useless testing, we should focus our attention on assessment and evaluation to determine when the patient has no chance for survival: living has ceased and dying has begun (Chap. 5). This is important because it is an equally valid goal for medical care to alleviate suffering and to avoid prolongation of dying when death is inevitable.

In our 375-patient sample, 82 patients (22%) died after being treated in the ICU for an average of 7.7 days per patient. These patients used 632 ICU days, which represents 38% of the total expended for all 375 patients. We might set a goal, therefore, to bring the percentage of days expended on dying patients into a reasonable proportion to the percentage of dying patients. If this were possible—by this I mean that we could identify more accurately the point at which living ceases and dying begins—we could hope to equalize the duration of stay for survivors and patients who died. Because the average duration of those who survived was 3.5 days per patient, this would imply a "savings" of 3.2 days per dying patient, or 262 patient days. This would represent a savings of 16% of the total ICU days *without* restricting admissions and *without* changing outcome. The difficulty we face to separate living from dying patients is the result of an unwanted and, perhaps, unexpected by-product of intensive care: creation of the prolonged dying state, which is unprecedented in human history. Current terms in common use reflect our discomfort in dealing with these concepts. Most often, we speak of termination of life support and withholding or withdrawing of life-sustaining treatment, when, from another perspective, we could say the same process is the termination of dying and accepting death, the natural end of human existence.

Clearly, it may be difficult to achieve clear distinction or resolution from the perspectives of the patient, the family, the medical profession, and society in all cases, but that should not diminish the strong sense of need to make these decisions as early as possible in the truly "critical" patient.

GOALS FOR INTENSIVE CARE ■

All ICU patients are not similar in terms of the goals of ICU admission, the dimensions for care used, or the resources necessary. They can be separated by goals into three groups: patients admitted for intensive observation or "monitoring only," patients who are stable physiologically but need extensive nursing care, and patients given essentially full-time medical and nursing care. Intensive observation is a necessary goal for ICU care because it represents a quantum of care impossible to achieve on a routine nursing unit. As an important corollary, however, we must be certain that observation is the only necessity: excessive ordering just because the patient is in the ICU must be avoided, and routine or "automatic" laboratory testing should be avoided.

In the second group, nursing care beyond that which is available on general nursing units is needed. Because these patients are physiologically stable, little moment-to-moment need exists for medical intervention; the physician's role is primarily anticipatory. Unnecessary manipulations and tests should be avoided because they cannot improve outcome and only increase costs.

The physiologically unstable patients constitute the third group. Physicians at the bedside generate a proliferation of orders, testing, and manipulations, which seem to be proportional to the perceived degree of the illness. However, even in these patients, utilization can be reviewed, perceptions changed, and use curtailed in many ways without compromising the quality of care.

The plethora of information generated by unrestrained laboratory testing and uncontrolled utilization of nursing time results in the creation of an array of data to be digested on a day-to-day basis. Robin termed this *informational overload*.[13] It can potentially harm the patient as a result of the physician's or nurse's inability to detect important abnormalities and to prioritize an approach because of the overwhelming amount of data to be evaluated. Curtailing unnecessary testing and unnecessary nursing activity diminishes frenetic yet unproductive activity. When the hubbub abates, the necessity for clear thinking and assessment on the part of the physician stands out.

The proliferation of tests mandates the development of scientific criteria and judgment for choosing the proper tests, frequency, and sequence. In Feinstein's words,

> If (the physician) orders too many tests indiscriminately, he wastes every one's time, effort, and money. The costs may bankrupt the patient (or the health insurance program), and the multitude of tests may overwhelm the laboratory's capacity for accurate results. If the clinician orders too few tests believing that his purely clinical reasoning needs no supplementation or confirmation by precise para-clinical aids, he runs the risk of making major diagnostic and therapeutic blunders.[14]

In the ICU, therefore, testing and technology should be considered in three steps of increasing utilization. The "observation only" patients must have few tests ordered. By definition, repetitive testing is not the quantum of care necessary; rather, it is the continuous observation not possible outside the ICU. Patients admitted for intensive nursing care often have associated physiologic derangements such as acute respiratory failure and cardiovascular dysfunction. They therefore tend to be fitted into parochial methods of treatment or clinical "protocols," including the laboratory testing to be used. At other times, extensive testing is considered necessary to avoid risk exposure. Most often, however, it is not the absence of a test result in the chart that results in a malpractice suit. The real issue is the difficulty in clinical decision-making, committing a judgment to the medical record, and communicating it to the patient and family.

We must remain committed to treatment of the patient with a poor but possible salutary outcome. Although we recognize that a 1% or 10% chance of survival clearly translates into a preponderance of similar patients who will die, we—the medical profession and society—wish to achieve success when possible. This desire must recognize that over-utilization of resources, including materials, personnel, and time, does not help to attain the successful outcome in the low-probability case.

At the University of Miami/Jackson Memorial Medical Center, laboratory testing was used as a model to determine whether modification in existing patterns of care could be accomplished without affecting the quality of care because the frequency of laboratory tests can be quantified; thus, assessment before and after interventions was feasible.[10] Although increased efficiency was one goal, it was hoped that the process would also lead to better teaching methods based on improved decision-making in the care of patients. In 1983, laboratory charges were $10,000, and the calculated ICU laboratory charges (calculated from the frequency of 28 identified tests abstracted from the patient's bills) were $6160 per patient. The patients spent 15% of their total hospitalization but generated 61% of their total laboratory charges in the ICU. The staff was astonished to find that 134 tests were ordered per patient, or 23 tests per patient per ICU day. In 1984, after the interventions had been made, laboratory charges were $6300, and the calculated ICU laboratory charges were $2894, representing a decrease of $3226 or 53%. Total number of ICU tests per patient decreased by 56 (42%).

Six months later, the frequency was again assessed and had diminished even further to approximately eight tests per patient per ICU day. The introduction of arterial pulse and mixed venous oximetry has permitted elimination of more blood gas analyses and, as a result, total laboratory utilization has continued to decrease. Initially, laboratory testing was diminished by 67%, or more than 60,000 tests per year. Total charges have diminished more than $3,000,000 and, using the 35% cost-basis, represents a $1,000,000 savings to the hospital. Notice that the mortality, distribution of patients by Therapeutic Intervention Scoring System (TISS) class, and average TISS score remained the same throughout the period of study (Table 11-2). I consider that the eliminated testing was unnecessary.

We can now examine ways to control testing that were implemented and the effect on specific laboratory tests.

TABLE 11-2. Description of Population

	BEFORE	AFTER
CLASS IV		
No. of patients	10	12
TISS (24 h)	39	40
Deaths	2	4
CLASS III		
No. of patients	32	30
TISS (24 h)	27	25
Deaths	3	4
CLASS II		
No. of patients	8	8
TISS (24 h)	12	15
Deaths	0	0
TOTAL		
No. of patients	50	50
TISS (24 h)	28	27
Deaths	5	8

TISS, Therapeutic Intervention Scoring System; Before, 1983 samples; After, 1984 samples.
No. in each class and TISS were compared by T-tests for two means. Mortality between groups was compared by chi-square test. No differences occurred. TISS scores were calculated 24 h after admission.

PRINCIPLES OF MANAGEMENT

Much of our behavior is automatic and is not based on scientific data. Therefore, as a management principle, it was believed that change was permissible whenever the existing policy was based only on tradition or parochialism. For instance, at the University of Miami/Jackson Memorial Medical Center, a program for the calculation of various parameters of renal function had been incorporated into the ICU programmable calculator. Unnecessary widespread usage in normal patients was identified and mentioned daily. A significant decrease occurred in the number of ordered tests for urinary creatinine, osmolarity, and electrolytes as a result of the "spotlight" approach: identifying the patient and discussing indications and need.

We suspected, in contrast to the thinking of others,[2] that a lot of "little ticket" items would make a significant impact; therefore, we resolved to examine each detail of care to uncover areas for potential small savings. Our pathology department had acquired an automated cell counter (ACC) to perform what had traditionally been called a complete blood count (CBC). We had not been aware that the terminology had changed so that CBC included a differential white blood count (WBC) with an extra $10 charge. Accordingly, we emphasized the substitution of ACC for CBC in routine circumstances. The augmented numbers of ACCs and diminished CBCs translate into diminished charges of approximately $25,000 per year.

Finally, we promulgated the phrase that "thinking, not screening, detects rare abnormalities." Calculation of the amylase:creatinine clearance ratio had been proposed to help detect subtle cases of pancreatitis. However, the indications for this screening technique were gradually broadened in our unit to many stable, postoperative patients, which increased the number of tests without finding unsuspected cases of pancreatitis. Once recognized, this practice was spotlighted and the screening eliminated. The effects of these principles are shown in Table 11-3.

DELETION OF STANDING ORDERS FOR TESTING

Standing orders were designed to eliminate several problems. An inexperienced person, responsible for writing orders, might overlook an important test. A busy practitioner, performing the same procedure frequently, might save a great deal of time by having preprinted orders to cover the usual postoperative situations. Preprinted orders would also increase the likelihood that they could be deciphered. On the other hand, imprecise thinking in the past might become codified as "tradition," and laboratory testing might proliferate. Arterial blood gas analyses (ABGs) are the most frequently ordered test in intensive care.[11] Our unit was no exception, resulting in an incidence of 9.3 tests for ABGs per patient per day, or 45 during the average ICU stay.[10] This frequency reflected our standing order to obtain blood gas values for every change in the patient's condition and after each change in ventilatory support. In practice, blood gas values also were obtained at the end of each nursing shift and before the morning and evening medical reports. All could be justified under our standing orders. Blood gas values were then ordered individually with an initial decrease of 19 blood gas tests per patient. Encouraged by these early results, we continued to stress test-by-test evaluation; the current incidence is less than two blood gas measurements per patient per day.

In our investigation of factors leading to the high frequency of ABG analyses, we observed that the presence of an arterial line seemed to correlate with the incidence of blood gas analyses. Accordingly, we reviewed the indications for an arterial line. Often it was maintained for "convenience" and, in those instances, contributed to the total number of blood gas analyses. This observation has been confirmed more recently[15] and, again, points to the subtle determinants of human behavior, which can have major effects on resource utilization and costs, only discoverable if these factors are considered important on the "micro" level.

STRUCTURED DECISION TREES TO SELECT TESTS

One intention of standing laboratory orders was to decrease the likelihood that a fatigued or inexperienced staff member might overlook a clinically relevant test. Because our gross overutilization was an unanticipated result, standing orders for testing were deleted. We substituted structured decision trees to help select appropriate tests in commonly encountered situations such as the "fever workup" and nutritional support monitoring. These decision trees were also created to aid in the initial selection of laboratory testing, depending

TABLE 11-3. Tests Related to Management Principles

	BEFORE	AFTER	CHARGE ($)	SAVINGS ($)
CHANGE WHEN NO SCIENTIFIC SUPPORTING DATA				
Creat (U)	4.7	0.7	22	88.00
Osm (U)	2.2	0.9	18	23.40
Elec (U)	3.0	1.2	44	79.20
EACH DETAIL OF CARE EXAMINED				
ACC	5.2	7.5	23	−52.90
CBC with diff	5.5	2.3	33	105.60
THINKING, NOT SCREENING, DETECTS ABNORMALITIES				
Amylase (S)	3.7	1.2	27	67.50
Amylase (U)	2.5	0.1	27	65.80
K^+	7.0	2.6	21	92.40

Creat, creatinine; osm, osmolarity; Elec, electrolytes; U, urinary; S, serum; ACC, automated cell count; CBC with diff, complete blood count with differential; K^+, potassium.
Mean no. of tests/intensive care unit admission/patient in 1983 (before) and 1984 (after). Groups compared using t-test for two means. All values were significant.
Savings in dollar charges to patient.

on the source of admission: elective preoperative admissions for invasive hemodynamic monitoring, routine postoperative admissions, and emergency admissions. For instance, elective preoperative admissions usually have all of the necessary testing completed before admission to the ICU. No useful purpose had been served by the routine repetition of these tests just because the patient's *location* in the hospital had changed (i.e., routine nursing care area to ICU) rather than the patient's physiologic status.

Testing of routine postoperative patients was a slightly more complex issue. These patients often remained intubated, had new catheters inserted into the central circula-

tion, may have had hypotension or arrhythmias during the operation and received many blood transfusions, or had had oliguria. "Blanket testing" had been ordered in our unit for nearly all postoperative patients because at least one or more of these conditions usually applied. In Table 11-4, however, these conditions are separated with my "suggestions" for appropriate ordering. This separation into specific clinical indications results in a decreased overall incidence of individual tests because they were no longer grouped (Table 11-5).

With respect to emergency admission, the decision tree included an admonition to check for prior laboratory orders

TABLE 11-4. Schematic for Selecting Laboratory Tests

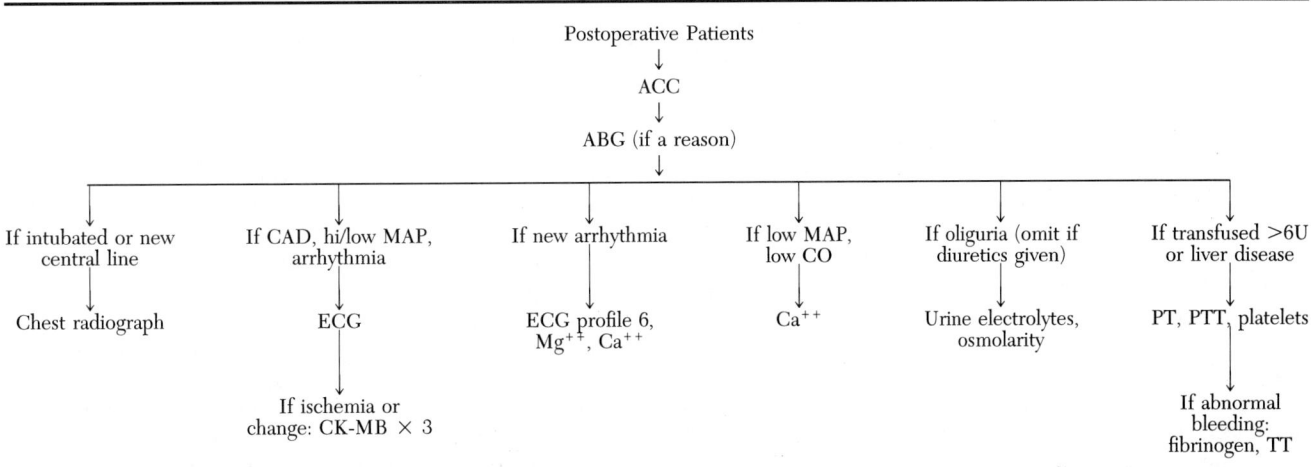

ACC, automated cell count (hematocrit, hemoglobin, white blood cell count); Ca^{++}, calcium; CAD, coronary artery disease; CK-MB, creatine kinase (main band); MAP, mean arterial pressure; Mg^{++}, magnesium; ABG, arterial blood gas; TT, thrombin time; CO, cardiac output; ECG, electrocardiogram; PTT, partial thromboplastin time; PT, prothrombin time.

TABLE 11-5. Structured Decision Trees to Select Test

	BEFORE	AFTER	CHARGE ($)	SAVINGS ($)
Cardiac enzymes	2.3	1.2	30	33.00
CK-MB	2.2	1.4	30	24.00
Liver enzymes	2.2	1.5	48	33.60
Ca^{++}	3.5	2.8	24	16.80
Mg^{++}	3.3	1.3	23	46.00

Ca^{++}, calcium; CK-MB, creatine kinase (main band); Mg^{++}, magnesium.
Average no. of tests/patient during ICU admission in 1983 (before) and 1984 (after). Groups compared using t-test for two means. All values were significant.

TABLE 11-6. No Orders for Repeated Testing

	BEFORE	AFTER	CHARGE ($)	SAVINGS ($)
Profile 8	2.8	1.1	45	76.50
PT/PTT	5.4	2.4	54	162.00
Platelets	5.5	1.7	23	87.40
Fibrinogen	1.0	0.4	28	16.80
Osmolarity	2.9	0.4	20	50.00

PT, prothrombin time; PTT, partial thromboplastin time.
Average no. of tests/patient during ICU admission in 1983 (before) and 1984 (after). Group comparisons performed using t-test for two means. All values were significant.

because most available tests often are ordered during the initial assessment of the multiple-injury or severely ill patient in the emergency room. Repetition of the same tests is not necessary after ICU admission (usually only 1 hour later) but was common practice.

NO ORDERS FOR REPEATED TESTING

When efforts are designed to avoid omissions, initial orders are often repeated at specified time intervals. Even if necessary initially, it is unlikely that all such repetitions are necessary; in this case, we "encouraged" a new order to be entered after reassessment and review of available information. Combinations provided by the laboratory, such as our profile 8, fell into this class, as did repetitive testing of coagulation parameters in many patients who had no evidence of a coagulation disorder (Table 11-6).

I believe that control of laboratory testing is a convenient model to examine bedside practice. Many habits and traditions were discovered that could be eliminated with even a moment's thought. Perhaps the intensity of our prior activity precluded any chance or need for close scrutiny. Our experience led to the hope that the diminished activity could have salutary effects. Physicians and nurses can return to decision-making and thinking instead of frenetic ordering, reacting, and intervening—Robin's informational overload.[13] Laboratory testing has been examined in other centers. Roberts and associates[15] "hypothesized that a cost effective, practical management approach could be applied in adult medical and surgical ICUs to reduce the frequency of diagnostic testing in a sustainable manner, and that this would result in cost savings." Instead of emulating our manual approach, they used computer-based information systems to create monthly reports. In addition, they monitored utilization for 2 years after the interventions had been applied. They also discovered details in the units that resulted in wasted ordering and designed practical solutions. They, too, attacked blood gas analyses as the most common ICU laboratory test by devising a detailed algorithm to cut down the observed practice that arterial and mixed venous ABG samples were routinely sent even in stable patients. They concluded, "an information based multi-disciplinary management team can produce marked and sustained reductions in unnecessary

testing in a cost effective manner."[15] Whereas experts grab headlines in the debates about health care financing, "money is wasted in dribs and drabs at the bedside."[16] Necessary, even if costly, elements can be preserved so that quality is maintained. Our task is to recognize overutilization resulting in overload so that efficiency can be improved while charges are diminished.

In a different environment, the outpatient clinic, merely placing the charges for tests and total charge for an individual patient on the computer screen that is used to order tests resulted in a significant decrease in laboratory utilization in one institution.[17] No differences occurred in three chosen measures of possible adverse outcomes (number of hospitalizations, emergency room visits, and outpatient visits). However, after the charges were removed from the computer screen, the difference in ordering patterns also vanished. This study is revealing for two different reasons: even minor interventions can have important effects, and administrative attention must be ongoing to sustain the desired result.

Next, the quantitative methods to assess severity and predict survival are examined.

DESCRIPTIONS OF QUANTITATIVE INDICES

Shoemaker and coworkers[18] have concentrated on cardiorespiratory patterns and oxygen transport variables. Rather than focusing therapy on normalizing values, their perspective reflected Claude Bernard's observation that the bodily responses to injury and illness are compensatory and have survival value. They believed that the values of patients who survived life-threatening cardiorespiratory problems were appropriate to be applied prospectively to the critically ill patient, and they devoted their efforts to an analysis of the cardiorespiratory patterns of patients who survived and died.

By analyzing the number of right and wrong predictions and combining the results for all variables, Shoemaker and colleagues achieved an average correct prediction of 85%.

An advantage of this method is that the data are readily available, given a decision to use invasive monitoring and laboratory testing. The disadvantages, however, recognized by the authors, reflect the fact that cardiorespiratory causes are not the only determinants of outcome. Also, their later automated system would be expensive to initiate. The ability to predict survivors after elective surgery should be high because mortality rates for most elective surgery are low. An error rate of 15% in the group of patients who ultimately were predicted to die is excessive in terms of serving as a basis for decisions for continuing or discontinuing therapy.

Phillips and coworkers[19] tried to establish whether outcome could be predicted at an early stage to determine why patients died and to concentrate diagnostic and management resources in those areas and establish criteria for withdrawal of therapy in patients who did not meet established criteria for brain death. In contrast to the optimistic outlook expressed by Shoemaker's group, Phillips and coworkers did not find any absolute predictors of outcome. Low-prevalence, high-impact factors such as renal failure and coma were identified, but variables that would support the exclusion of certain patients before ICU admission were not identified. With respect to discontinuing life support in the absence of brain death, they ultimately outlined a process based on comprehension of the nature of the illness, an adequate time interval for care, and a hopeless prognosis accepted by all nurses, physicians, and the patient's relatives, rather than a predictive model.

Much controversy exists and many articles have been written about prospective utilization of supernormal values of oxygen delivery in the last few years. It has been difficult to study these populations for several reasons. Patients in the control groups, in which no interventions are specifically intended to increase oxygen delivery, often have a spontaneous increase in oxygen delivery that meets or exceeds the treatment group specification. Also, patients in the treatment group do not respond to interventions and have values similar to the control groups. Finally, oxygen consumption often is measured indirectly through the application of the Fick Principle and thus is subject to mathematical coupling as described by Archie.[20] A prospective, randomized study of driving oxygen delivery with dobutamine after ensuring adequate volume resuscitation has shown an increased mortality in the treatment group.[21] The popularity of using supernormal values has been diminishing in the last few years while clinicians have recognized the problems of crossover and mathematic coupling. Because more articles and editorials have criticized this approach, the balance has shifted away from using cardiorespiratory variables as either therapeutic goals or prognostic indices.

Lemeshow and colleagues[22] described another method for predicting survival and mortality rate of ICU patients using a multiple logistic regression model. They collected a few and easily obtained variables (Table 11-7). The result was expressed as a probability rather than a score. Using 0.5 as a cutoff for predicting mortality rate, 87% and 85% of the patients were correctly classified at admission and at 24 hours, respectively. More recently they have extended the mortality probability model to 48 and 72 hours after finding that the 24-hour model demonstrated poor calibration and discrimination at 48 and 72 hours.[23] The new models contain the same 13 variables and coefficients but differ in their constant terms, which increase in a manner that reflects the increasing probability of mortality with increasing length of stay in the ICU. Their study population has always included many patients who had a short duration of ICU stay and were discharged alive, thus leaving a group with increased likelihood of mortality. In fact they conclude, "the increasing constant terms and associated increase in the probability of hospital mortality exemplify a common clinical adage that if a patient's clinical profile stays the same, he or she is actually getting worse."[23] They suggested "a low probability of mortality based on the 72 hour model, in combination with clinical judgment and evidence that ICU care is not being administered, could help to identify a patient who is a candidate for discharge to a less intensive care environment."[23] They do not advocate using probabilities to justify limiting ICU care, especially for points beyond 72 hours. The authors believe that this technique is superior because it is based on statistically derived weights for its variables rather than subjectively determined values common to the Acute Physiology Score and Chronic Health Evaluation (APACHE) and TISS (see text that follows). The data were easy to gather, and the variables were few in number, which would make it easier to use as a general predictive index. The variables included at admission: age, cirrhosis, intracranial mass effect, metastatic neoplasm, and nonelective surgery. At 24 hours, interval assessments are coma or deep stupor, creatinine level greater than 2 mg/dL, infection, mechanical ventilation, partial pressure of arterial oxygen (PaO_2) less than 60 mm Hg, prothrombin time more than 3 seconds above standard, urine output less than 150 mL per 8 hours, and infusion of vasoactive drip for longer than 1 hour. Again, similar to all other systems, the very well and the very sick were easily distinguished; also, approximately 15% to 20% of the patients were misclassified.

In 1973, I[24] described the three groups of intensive care patients used at the beginning of this chapter by subjectively estimating the amount of care. Later, Cullen and associates[25] presented TISS as a method for quantitating categories of ICU patients. This was an outgrowth of the anecdotal "tube sign" in use among the surgical resident staff at the Massachusetts General Hospital in the 1960s: the higher the number of "tubes" used, the less likely was survival. The basic premise of TISS was that the more seriously ill patient received more therapeutic interventions independent of a specific diagnosis, and the severity of illness could be quantified by the interventions used. The interventions were weighted from 1 to 4 points. However, this presumed that physicians seeing a similarly ill patient would prescribe the same therapy which, empirically, is not the case. However, TISS separated the four classes of patients, with class I representing a patient receiving routine postanesthesia care. Classes II, III, and IV represented observation only, extensive nursing care, and intensive physician care groups, respectively.

Nearly 10 years later, the TISS system was updated because of changing perspectives regarding therapeutic interventions[26] (Table 11-8). No difference occurred in overall point score using the updated system.

Whereas the original TISS score concentrated on the three ICU classes, an intermediate TISS has been introduced for non-ICU patients.[27] It was developed to better identify medical patients who may not require intensive

TABLE 11-7. Demographic and Discrete Variables at Time of ICU Admission

VARIABLE	VITAL STATUS AT HOSPITAL DISCHARGE	NO.	%	MEAN	SD	p VALUE°
Age	Alive	592	(79.8)	56.9	(19.10)	
	Dead	150	(20.2)	68.6	(16.28)	<0.001
Systolic blood pressure	Alive	593	(79.9)	139.2	(29.83)	
	Dead	149	(20.1)	118.1	(38.13)	<0.001†
Heart rate	Alive	574	(80.6)	95.7	(24.15)	
	Dead	138	(19.4)	106.2	(30.50)	<0.001†
No. of organ failures	Alive	593	(79.8)	1.4	(0.71)	
	Dead	150	(20.2)	2.3	(1.19)	<0.001†

VARIABLE CODING	ALIVE		DEAD		p VALUE‡
	No.	%	No.	%	
Service at admission (medical/sugical)	207	(69.7)	90	(30.3)	
	386	(86.5)	60	(13.5)	<0.001
Infection at admission (no/probable)	400	(88.1)	54	(11.9)	
	193	(66.8)	96	(33.2)	<0.001
CPR before admission	580	(83.0)	119	(17.0)	
	13	(29.5)	31	(70.5)	<0.001
Type of admission (elective/emergency)	215	(95.1)	11	(4.9)	
	378	(73.1)	139	(26.9)	<0.001
Po₂ (mm Hg) (>60/≤60)	555	(81.3)	128	(18.7)	
	38	(63.3)	22	(36.7)	0.002
Bicarbonate (mEq/L) (≥18/<18)	569	(80.7)	136	(19.3)	
	24	(63.2)	14	(36.8)	0.13
Creatinine (mg/dL) (≤2.0/>2.0)	573	(80.8)	136	(19.2)	
	20	(58.8)	14	(41.2)	0.004
Level of consciousness (coma or deep stupor/not)	584	(84.6)	106	(15.4)	
	9	(18.4)	40	(81.6)	<0.001

CPR, cardiopulmonary resuscitation; Po₂, partial pressure of oxygen.
°Based on Student's t-test.
†Because homogeneity of variances was significant at the α <0.01 level, a separate variance estimate was used.
‡Derived using chi-square tests for dichotomous variables.
Lemeshow S, Teres D, Pastides H, et al: A method for predicting survival and mortality of ICU patients using objectively derived weights. *Crit Care Med* 1985;13:519.

therapy but need cardiopulmonary monitoring which is available through flexible monitoring systems in the regular hospital units. Also, it can be used to determine the need for additional hospital facilities such as more ICU beds or intermediate care areas. In these cost-conscious times, it is increasingly necessary to develop objective measures to help support decision making in "marginal" cases. Managed care will not provide extra dollars for low-risk monitoring patients, yet the costs of a developed complication in an excluded patient wipes out any remaining profit.

One advantage of TISS is its simplicity to perform because it lists interventions easily recognized at the patient's bedside. It also quantitates the physician's perception of the illness, which translates into requirements for nursing care and other aspects of total patient care. Its basic, fundamental, and most important limitation is that the physician's perception of illness can change over time, and there is no current method of guaranteeing that different physicians faced with

the same patient and the same illness would agree on the same intervention.

First introduced in 1981, APACHE has been described as a physiologically based classification system consisting of two parts: the acute physiology score (APS) and the chronic health evaluation.[28] The APS was a weighted sum of each of 34 physiologic measurements obtained from the patient's clinical record within the first 24 hours of ICU admission. If a physiologic variable was not measured, it was assumed to be normal or not necessary to estimate the severity of illness. The second portion was a four-category designation of preadmission health status. The physiologic variables collected in APACHE were weighted from 0 to 4 according to a group consensus as to the perceived significance of abnormality, similar to the a priori judgments contained in TISS. Thereafter, the data were subjected to logistic multiple regression adding age, sex, operative status, and indication for admission. A risk of death was calculated and used to

TABLE 11-8. Therapeutic Intervention Scoring System–1983

4 POINTS

    (a) Cardiac arrest or countershock within 48 h°
    (b) Controlled ventilation with or without PEEP°
    (c) Controlled ventilation with intermittent or continuous muscle relaxants°
    (d) Balloon tamponade of varices°
    (e) Continuous arterial infusion°
    (f) Pulmonary artery catheter
    (g) Atrial or ventricular pacing°
    (h) Hemodialysis in unstable patient°
    (i) Peritoneal dialysis
    (j) Induced hypothermia°
    (k) Pressure-activated blood infusion°
    (l) G-suit
    (m) Intracranial pressure monitoring
    (n) Platelet transfusion
    (o) IABA (intraaortic balloon assist)
    (p) Emergency operative procedures (within past 24 h)°
    (q) Lavage of acute gastrointestinal bleeding
    (r) Emergency endoscopy or bronchoscopy
    (s) Vasoactive drug infusion (>1 drug)

3 POINTS

    (a) Central IV hyperalimentation (includes renal, cardiac, hepatic failure fluid)
    (b) Pacemaker on standby
    (c) Chest tubes
    (d) Intermittent mandatory ventilation (IMV)° or
    (e) Continuous positive airway pressure (CPAP)
    (f) Concentrated K^+ infusion by central catheter
    (g) Nasotracheal or orotracheal intubation°
    (h) Blind intratracheal suctioning
    (i) Complex metabolic balance (frequent intake and output)°
    (j) Multiple ABG, bleeding or stat studies (>4/shift)
    (k) Frequent infusions of blood products (>5 U/24 h)
    (l) Bolus IV medication (nonscheduled)
    (m) Vasoactive drug infusion (1 drug)
    (n) Continuous antidysrhythmia infusions
    (o) Cardioversion for dysrhythmia (not defibrillation)
    (p) Hypothermia blanket
    (q) Arterial line
    (r) Acute digitalization—within 48 h
    (s) Measurement of cardiac output by any method
    (t) Active diuresis for fluid overload or cerebral edema

    (u) Active Rx for metabolic alkalosis
    (v) Active Rx for metabolic acidosis
    (w) Emergency thora-, para-, and pericardiocenteses
    (x) Active anticoagulation (initial 48 h)°
    (y) Phlebotomy for volume overload
    (z) Coverage with more than 2 IV antibiotics
    (aa) Rx of seizures or metabolic encephalopathy (within 48 h of onset)
    (bb) Complicated orthopedic traction°

2 POINTS

    (a) CVP
    (b) 2 peripheral IV catheters
    (c) Hemodialysis—stable patient
    (d) Fresh tracheostomy (less than 48 h)
    (e) Spontaneous respiration by endotracheal tube or tracheostomy (T piece or trach mask)
    (f) Gastrointestinal feedings
    (g) Replacement of excess fluid loss°
    (h) Parenteral chemotherapy
    (i) Hourly neuro vital signs
    (j) Multiple dressing changes
    (k) Pitressin infusion IV

1 POINT

    (a) ECG monitoring
    (b) Hourly vital signs
    (c) 1 peripheral IV catheter
    (d) Chronic anticoagulation
    (e) Standard intake and output (q 24 h)
    (f) Stat blood tests
    (g) Intermittent scheduled IV medications
    (h) Routine dressing changes
    (i) Standard orthopedic traction
    (j) Tracheostomy care
    (k) Decubitus ulcer°
    (l) Urinary catheter
    (m) Supplemental oxygen (nasal or mask)
    (n) Antibiotics IV (2 or less)
    (o) Chest physiotherapy
    (p) Extensive irrigations, packings, or debridement of wound, fistula, or colostomy
    (q) Gastrointestinal decompression
    (r) Peripheral hyperalimentation/intralipid therapy

ABG, arterial blood gas readings; CVP, central venous pyelogram; ECG, electrocardiogram; IV, intravenous; K^+, potassium; neuro, neurologic; q, every; PEEP, positive end-expiratory pressure; Rx, therapy; stat, immediate.
°Therapeutic Intervention Scoring System explanation code.
4-Point Interventions: (a) Point score for 2 d after most recent cardiac arrest. (b) This does not mean intermittent mandatory ventilation which is a 3-point intervention. It does mean that regardless of the internal plumbing of the ventilator, the patient's full ventilatory needs are being supplied by the machine. Whether or not the patient is ineffectively breathing around the ventilator is irrelevant if the ventilator is providing all the patient's needed minute ventilation. (c) For example, D-tuborcurarine chloride, pancuronium (Pavulon), metocurine (Metubine). (d) Use Sengstaken-Blakemore or Linton tube for esophageal or gastric bleeding. (e) Pitressin infusion via inferior mesenteric artery (IMA), superior mesenteric artery (SMA), or gastric artery catheters for control of gastrointestinal bleeding, or other intraarterial infusion. This does not include

(continued)

TABLE 11-8.   *(continued)*

standard 3 mL/h heparin flush to maintain catheter patency. (g) Active pacing even if a chronic pacemaker. (h) Include first 2 runs of an acute dialysis. Include chronic dialysis in patient whose medical situation now renders dialysis unstable. (j) Continuous or intermittent cooling to achieve body temperature less than 33°C. (k) Use of a blood pump or manual pumping of blood in the patient who requires rapid blood replacement. (p) May even be the initial emergency operative procedure—precludes diagnostic test, (i.e., angiography, computed tomographic scan).
3-Point Interventions: (d) The patient is supplying some of his own ventilatory needs. (g) Not a daily point score. Patient must have been intubated in the ICU (elective or emergency) within 24 h. (i) Measurement of intake/output above and beyond the normal 24-h routine. Frequent adjustment of intake according to total output. (x) Includes Rheomacrodex. (bb) For example, Stryker frame, Circ-Olectric.
2-Point Interventions: (g) Replacement of clear fluids over and above the ordered maintenance level.
1-Point Interventions: (k) Must have a decubitus ulcer. Does not include preventive therapy.
Keene AR, Cullen DJ: Therapeutic Intervention Scoring System: update 1983. *Crit Care Med* 1983;11:1.

determine the number of expected deaths in an attempt to relate outcome to the initial severity of illness as assessed by APACHE. When this method was applied in different hospitals, the authors found substantial differences in the severity of acute illness among the hospitals, but projected death rates were similar to the observed deaths in each hospital.[29] Their studies then compared intensive care in the United States and France.[30]

Patients admitted to French ICUs were significantly younger, remained in the ICU twice as long, and had hourly vital sign monitoring and invasive hemodynamic monitoring at half the rate of U.S. patients. The probability of hospital death at any given APS score was the same in both countries.

In 1985, APACHE II was described, which compressed the APS from 34 to 12 routine physiologic measurements plus age and previous health status[31] (Table 11-9). Again, mortality rate was closely correlated to increasing APACHE II score. The number of patients correctly classified was 85.5%. In the validation study performed in 13 tertiary care hospitals, the authors used the same methodology that was used previously to validate APACHE.[32] In the first studies, APACHE was considered validated because observed death rates were similar to expected rates provided by the predictive APACHE model. In the validation of APACHE II, actual and predicted death rates were compared using group results as a standard. When one hospital had significantly better results and another had significantly inferior results, failure of validation was not mentioned.[32] In its place, the differences were interpreted: the authors concluded that these were related more to the interaction and coordination of each hospital's intensive care staff than to the unit's administrative structures, amount of specialized treatment used, or the hospital teaching status. Unfortunately, the interpretations have been widely quoted in both the medical and lay press. That APACHE II did not meet the authors' previous validation standard[29,30] has generally escaped notice.

Two additional limitations are not inherent in the system itself but seemed to depend on the interpretations of the authors. First, APACHE II has been promulgated as a useful tool in clinical trials or in nonrandomized or multi-institutional studies of therapeutic efficacy. The authors believe that APACHE II scores will help investigators determine whether control and treatment groups are similar. They also

plan to compare the expected death rate with the actual death rate as a test of therapeutic efficacy; however, an incorrect overall classification rate of 15% but, unfortunately, misclassification of 50% of the deaths makes this unlikely. The "strength" of calculating APACHE II in the first 24 hours—to eliminate the effects of treatment—also ignores that subsequently developed complications and illnesses determine outcome of the patients who use the most resources and who have a 50% mortality rate, but the system does not identify which patients live or die. The author of APACHE II believes it should be used to answer questions concerning restriction of intensive care services from patients who are too healthy or too sick to benefit from aggressive care, despite the fact that APACHE previously demonstrated that neither group consumes significant resources.[33]

More recently, APACHE III has been developed. Its goal is "to provide physicians, hospitals, and patients, with nationally representative information that will improve the quality and use of adult medical/surgical ICU services."[34] It includes seven chronic health items (AIDS, hepatic failure, lymphoma, solid tumor with metastases, leukemia or multiple myeloma, immunocompromise, and cirrhosis). Physiologic variables have been increased to include five new variables (blood urea nitrogen, urine output, serum albumin, bilirubin, and glucose). In addition, creatinine level is scored differently in the presence or absence of acute renal failure. The Glasgow Coma Score is included with new weights. Finally, a combined variable including serum pH and partial pressure of carbon dioxide (Pco_2) was developed to establish weights for common acid–base disorders. The weighting of vital signs in laboratory abnormalities is distinctly different from the zero to four scoring in APACHE and APACHE II (Fig. 11-2). The patient's treatment location immediately before ICU admission was also added because it was believed to hold important prognostic significance. Notice that an automated version has been produced to capture physiologic and clinical data automatically "without primary data collection costs" (although automated equipment and software must be purchased from a private corporation).[34] The authors observe, "when patient volume precluded data collection on consecutive admissions, we used an alternating data collection scheme (e.g., every second or third patient)."[35] Overall correct classification on the first day was

TABLE 11-9. The APACHE II Severity of Disease Classification System

	HIGH ABNORMAL RANGE			
PHYSIOLOGIC VARIABLE	+4	+3	+2	+1
(1) Temperature—rectal (°C)	≥41°	39–40.9°		38.5–38.9°
(2) MAP mm Hg	≥160	130–159	110–129	
(3) Heart rate ventricular response	≥180	140–179	110–139	
(4) Respiratory rate (nonventilated or ventilated)	≥50	35–49		25–34
(5) Oxygenation: $(A - a)DO_2$, or PaO_2 (mm Hg)				
(a) FIO_2 0.5 record $(A - a)DO_2$	≥500	350–499	200–349	
(b) FIO_2 0.5 record only PaO_2				
(6) Arterial pH	≥7.7	7.6–7.69		7.5–7.59
(7) Serum sodium (mm/L)	≥180	160–179	155–159	150–154
(8) Serum potassium (mm/L)	≥7	6.6–9		5.5—5.9
(9) Serum creatinine (mg/100 mL) (Double point score for acute renal failure	≥3.5	2–3.4	1.5–19	
(10) Hematocrit (%)	≥60		50–59.0	46–49.9
(11) WBC (Total/mm³) (in 1.000 s)	≥40		20–39.9	15–19.9
(12) Glasgow Coma Score (GCS) Score = 15 minus actual GCS				

APACHE, Acute Physiology Score and Chronic Health Evaluation; DO_2, oxygen delivery; FIO_2, fraction of inspired oxygen; MAP, mean arterial pressure; PaO_2, partial arterial pressure of oxygen; WBC, white blood cell count.
Adapted from Knaus WA, Draper EA, Wagner DP, et al: APACHE II: a severity of disease classification system. *Crit Care Med* 1985;13:818.

88.2% compared with 85.5% for APACHE II. The five-point increase in the APACHE III score (range, 0 to 299) is independently associated with a statistically significant increase in the relative risk of hospital death within each of 78 major medical and surgical disease categories compressed from an initial list of 212 such categories. However, inspection of data for 1467 trauma admissions showed a decrease in mortality from a score of 50 to 60 and a jump from a less than 50% mortality rate to a more than 80% mortality rate associated with an increased APACHE score of 90 to 100. Interestingly, weighting for the variables in APACHE and APACHE II were assigned by group consensus. In APACHE III, computer-derived weights were initially calculated but, "where discrepancies existed (e.g., a mean blood pressure of 60 mm Hg assigned a lower coefficient indicating a lower risk of death than a mean pressure of 70 mm Hg) we adjusted the ranges.... [I]n a few cases where the results of the analyses remained incompatible with established physiologic patterns, we adjusted the estimated weights by using clinical judgment."[35] Later, however, the authors state that objective prognostic estimates derived from APACHE III have at least three potential advantages compared with clinical judgment.

Similar to the extension of the Mortality Prediction Model (MPM), APACHE III authors have derived equations to determine the daily risk of hospital deaths during each of the first 7 days of ICU care.[36] One thousand thirty-three patients who had a daily risk estimate of more than 90% during any of their initial 7 ICU days had a 90% mortality rate but represented only 47% of all ICU deaths and 31%

of the total hospital deaths. Only one third of the patients remained in the ICU for longer than 3 days. Mortality for the entire sample was 17% but was 40% for those remaining in the ICU for 7 days or longer. The implications for the APS were different: the same score on day 6 is associated with greater than a twofold increase in mortality (25% to 55% for a score of 50). The receiver operating curve (ROC) area actually decreased from day 1 through day 7 (0.9 to 0.84), as did the r^2 value (0.4 to 0.35). The confidence limits for predicted risk of hospital death ranged from 2% to 20%. The authors observe that a patient with a 93% probability of hospital death has 95% confidence limits on the prediction of 96% to 89%. Although they state that confidence limits are sufficiently narrowed to be potentially useful for making probability estimates for an individual patient, this is precisely the area in which individuals, patients, families, and care givers differ in expectations for continued treatment versus withdrawal of support. In my personal experience, families, nurses and physicians alike have expressed differing opinions with regard to 10%, 5%, or 1% likelihood of survival, however estimated. This has been reported in the study of more than 1300 ICU attending staff, house staff, and nurses in Canada.[37] Given a scenario of a 75-year-old patient with urosepsis, a 10% probability of survival (based on APACHE II score), breast cancer with vertebral metastases, and prior cognitive impairment, nearly 28% chose to discontinue inotropes and mechanical ventilation but continue comfort measures, 22% would stop inotropes but continue mechanical ventilation and comfort measures, 25%

					0					
			8 ≤39	5 40–49	**Pulse** 50–99 beats/min	1 100–109	5 110–119	7 120–139	13 140–154	17 ≥155
	23 ≤39	15 40–49	7 60–69	6 70–79	**Mean BP** 80–99 mm Hg	4 100–119	7 120–129	9 130–139	10 ≥140	
20 ≤32.9	16 33–33.4	13 33.5–33.9	8 34–34.9	2 35–35.9	**Temperature** 36–39.9°C	4 ≥40				
		17 ≤5	8 6–11*	7 12–13	***Respiratory rate** 14–24 b/min	6 25–34	9 35–39	11 40–49	18 ≥50	
		15 ≤49	5 50–69	2 70–79	**Pao₂** ≥80 mm Hg					
					†A-aDO₂ ≥80 mm Hg	7 100–249	9 250–349	11 350–499	14 ≥500	
				3 ≤40.9	**Hematocrit** 41–49%	3 ≥50				
			19 <1.0	5 1.0–2.9	**WBC** 3.0–19.9 mm³	1 20–24.9	5 ≥25			
				3 <43 / ≤0.4	**‡Creatine s̄ ARF** 44–132 μmol/dL / 0.5–1.4 mg/dL	4 133–171 / 1.5–1.94	7 ≥172 / ≥1.95			
					‡Creatine c̄ ARF 0–132 mol/dL / 0–1.4 mg/dL	10 ≥133 / ≥1.5				
15 ≤399	8 400–599	7 600–899	5 900–1499	4 1500–1999	**Urine Output** 2000–3999 mL/day	1 ≥4000				
					BUN ≤6.1 mmol/L / ≤16.9 mg/dL	2 6.2–7.1 / 17–19	7 7.2–14.3 / 20–39	11 14.4–28.5 / 40–79	12 ≥28.6 / ≥80	
			3 ≤119	2 120–134	**Sodium** 135–155 mEq/L	4 ≥155				
			11 ≤19 / ≤1.9	6 20–24 / 2.0–2.4	**Albumin** 25–44 g/L / 2.5–4.4 g/dL	4 ≥45 / ≥4.5				
					Bilirubin ≤34 μmol/L / ≤1.9 mg/dL	5 35–51 / 2.0–2.9	6 52–85 / 3.0–4.9	8 **86–135** / **5.0–8.0**	16 ≥136 / ≥8.0	
			§8 ≤2.1 / ≤39	§9 2.2–3.3 / 40–59	**Glucose** 3.4–11.1 mmol/L / 60–199 mg/dL	3 11.2–19.3 / 200–349	5 ≥19.4 / ≥350			

FIGURE 11-2. APACHE III physiologic scoring for vital signs and laboratory tests. Top number in each box represents point score for abnormality. BP, blood pressure; BUN, blood urea nitrogen; Pao₂, partial arterial pressure of oxygen; WBC, white blood count; b, breaths; c̄, without; s̄, with.

°For patients on mechanical ventilation, no points are given for respiratory rates between 6 and 11.

†Only use alveolar to arterial oxygen tension difference (A-aDO₂) for intubated patients with fraction of inspired oxygen (FIO₂) ≤ 0.5.

‡Acute renal failure (ARF) is defined as creatinine ≥ 1.5 mg/day and urine output < 410 mg/day, with no chronic dialysis.

§Glucose ≤ 39 mg/dL is lower weight than 40 to 59.

(Redrawn from Knaus W, Wagner D, Draper E, et al: The APACHE III prognostic system risk prediction of hospital mortality for critically ill hospitalized adults. *Chest* 1991;100:1619.)

would continue all current management but not add new therapy, 15% would continue aggressive management but withhold dialysis if it became necessary, and the final 10% would continue full aggressive management including dialysis.

The difficulty in predicting survival and death in the long term ICU patient is even more disheartening. Despite nearly 15 years of additions and refinements, no predictive index provides sufficient discrimination to enable it to be used to help in decision-making for individual patients. It is especially discouraging because this particular area, prolonged resource utilization and uncertain outcome, is the most important problem in this era of limited resources. Furthermore, repetitive calculations of APACHE III equations require extensive daily laboratory testing, which may not be justified in this cost-sensitive environment. If values are missing, then they are assumed to be normal, which would then rob the predictive equation of its accuracy because this assumption is not justified in long-term ICU patients. We also live in a litigious society. Whereas patients and families accept the uncertainties of human judgments in most cases, it is not clear whether a higher standard might be expected for computer-derived predictions. It might be too expensive, then to calculate such a prediction (1) the purchase of software and hardware may be beyond the ICU budget, (2) the increased testing necessary to construct daily predictions may not be possible for capitated patients or those covered under bundled pricing, and (3) a plaintiff's lawyer may derive the opposite interpretation of the reported statistics, that is, about 12% of the patients were misclassified and the predictions lost reliability over time. It is not surprising that both the ROC area and r^2 diminished. The two thirds of the patients who left the units on days 1 through 3 were either very well and had low scores or very sick and died within that 3-day period and had very high scores. Those who remained for long periods of time have already been shown to have had indistinguishable initial scores and that the average score of all patients remaining in the ICU whether they ultimately lived or died, remained statistically indistinguishable for the first 2 weeks.[38]

VALUES AND LIMITATION OF PREDICTIVE INDICES

Prediction of the potential usefulness of intensive care for an individual patient is a lofty objective. Most indices easily separate patients at the ends of the severity spectrum. It is unlikely that any index completed at the time of the patient's admission can do this for the problematic long-term patient. When sequential APACHE II calculations were made in long-term ICU patients, separation of the scores of the patients who actually died from those who actually survived occurred after 1 week of ICU care (Table 11-10). Further, calculations of APACHE II made 24 hours before actual death revealed a score associated with a predicted 35% mortality rate. TISS scores decreased over time even in patients who died. This underscores the basic premise that TISS represents a physician's perspective of the patient's illness reflected in the choice of interventions. The patients die of MOSF and not of acute catastrophic cardiorespiratory failure; the latter alone is highly weighted in TISS and APACHE.

If a vital factor is not included in the calculation of the index, its effect cannot be predicted. The *sepsis syndrome* is difficult to define yet is often the cause of death in ICU patients. If an organ system is functioning normally on admission and is so measured by the included variables, the ultimate effect of later dysfunction cannot be predicted.

In addition, because prediction is an imperfect science, most authors discuss the false classification rate, which approximates 10% to 15% for all predictive indices.[39] Practically speaking, the known false classification rates will be expressed in ways that are detrimental to present standards of care. One type of false classification is that patients who are predicted to live may die even with ICU care. In fact, the policy of the exclusion of "low-risk monitor" patients does not address the issue of later development of significant complications. The Consensus Development Conference[9] discussed the potential for the development of complications in excluded patients citing that, if these patients were to be excluded safely, care in routine care areas should be no less effective than care in the ICU. However, because ICUs cluster the sickest patients and because skilled nursing care is limited both within and outside the ICU, this premise is not justified. The increase in mortality rates with long-term ICU admissions and the lack of consistent correlation of survival, low admission APACHE score, and short ICU duration of care all suggest that this exclusion of patients based on low APACHE scores would not be safe.[38] In fact, this policy would recreate conditions identical with those that led to the development of SICUs over 20 years ago.

The second expression of a false classification rate is that patients who are predicted to die actually live with ICU care. This is substantiated by the fact that patients with a high initial APACHE score have a higher survival rate with

TABLE 11-10. Repetitive APACHE II Calculations in Patients With Prolonged ICU Stay

	SURVIVORS—AFTER PROLONGED ICU STAY (>13 d)								DIED—AFTER PROLONGED ICU STAY (>13 d)						
Day	1	2	3	5	7	14	F	Day	1	2	3	5	7	14	F
APACHE II°	12	10.8	9.9	12.9	11.4	9.4	7.6	APACHE II	16.5	14.7	16	14.6	16.4	20.9	21.6
% Mortality predicted	12	12	12	12	12	6	6	% Mortality predicted	20	20	20	20	20	35	35

F, day before ICU discharge.
Knaus WA, Draper EA, Wagner DP, et al: APACHE II: a severity of disease classification system. *Crit Care Med* 1985;13:818.

PATIENTS WITH SAME INITIAL APACHE 2 DIVIDED INTO ABOVE AND BELOW MEAN STAY

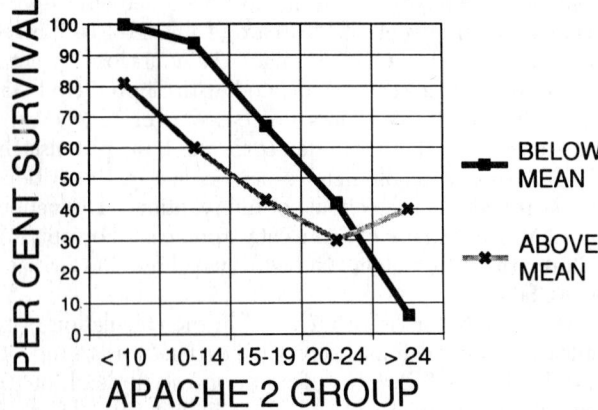

FIGURE 11-3. Patients were subdivided into five groups according to their admission APACHE II scores. For groups with APACHE II scores < 10 and 10 to 14, a statistically significant increase in mortality rate occurred with increased duration of ICU stay. Conversely, for patients whose APACHE II scores were more than 24, the mortality rate was significantly higher if the duration of ICU stay was more than 5 days. Thus, there were opposite and statistically significant differences in mortality rates for the patients with the highest and lowest APACHE scores, depending on the duration of ICU stay.

increased duration of ICU stay (Fig. 11-3). However, if this care is not provided immediately (patients are excluded as too sick), it seems highly likely that an early death will result. In terms of the actual number of patient days and percentage of total ICU days expended, little savings can be achieved. The increased survival rate associated with a longer duration of ICU stay suggests that the resolution of even a severe degree of physiologic abnormality is possible only if patients are given continued care; if ICU admission is denied, it is likely that these patients will die.

In addition to these general limitations, there are specific considerations with respect to surgical patients. The original APACHE system[28] was intended to assess the patient independent of therapy. Although the artifacts of using 24 hours of data has been addressed regarding both quality of care and pre-ICU stabilization times, APACHE scores in surgical patients may be artifactually raised or lowered, depending on chosen therapeutic objectives. In elective surgical patients, one might view the anesthesiologists' physiologic objective as maintaining the lowest possible APACHE score by anticipating and preventing abnormalities so that no acute physiology points are accrued. Well-cared-for patients will be penalized because they have not accumulated enough points from physiologic abnormalities to qualify for ICU admission. These patients will be relegated to lesser care facilities, which will be viewed as appropriate yet less expensive for the measured degree of their "noncritical" illness. This premise can only be disproven by the development of serious complications that lead to markedly increased costs, longer subsequent ICU stays for developed complications, and preventable deaths.

Over 10 years ago, Zook and Moore[40] recognized that the opposite was true and stated that "considerable cost saving and reduction in human suffering would be possible if the frequency of adverse events could be reduced, even by a small percentage." Thus, the potential for increased costs and suffering seems to be greater than any possible savings that might result from a policy of exclusion on the basis of current predictive indices.

The authors of APACHE III have attempted to improve the discharge decisions by using a quantitative estimation of risk of next-day therapy using the APACHE III data base of 17,440 ICU admissions.[41] Predictive equations were constructed for each of the first 3 days. After considerable study, they chose to evaluate patients predicted at less than 10% risk for active treatment. The subsequent number and type of therapy received, ICU readmission rate, and survival were calculated to see if these criteria could be applied to permit safe discharge to an intermediate care area or hospital ward and thus reduce ICU bed demand without compromising patient safety. On day 1, 6080 patients were predicted at greater than 10% risk of needing active treatment and actually received treatment. An additional 2809 were predicted to be at high risk but did not actually receive active treatment. A total of 4648 were not actively treated and were correctly predicted to be at low risk, whereas there was a 5% false-negative rate (250 patients were actively treated although they were predicted to be at low risk). Similar false-negative rates of 5.1% were seen on day 2 and day 3 (5.4%). Of the patients predicted to be at less than 10% risk of needing active treatment, 3.4% received endotracheal intubation and mechanical ventilation, and 0.5% of patients had a cardiac arrest. The authors believe that this degree of accuracy is comparable with clinical judgment, as suggested by the strong association between the predicted risk of active treatment and the actual discharge rates observed. Again, the issue of whether mathematic predictions will be afforded the same latitude in terms of error making as clinical judgment may be relevant. A 1-day "snapshot" of ICU practice in the United States was described by Groeger and associates.[42] Data were obtained regarding 25,871 patients in 2876 separate ICUs, representing 38.7% of the nation's ICUs. By extrapolation, approximately 67,000 patients would reside in the nation's ICUs on a given day. From the data presented in the Zimmerman article, then on a daily basis, approximately 2278 patients would be intubated and receive mechanical ventilation, 335 would experience a cardiac arrest, and, if patients had been discharged according to the criterion of less than 10% risk of requiring actual treatment, 10,300 patients would have been discharged and received treatment. Reintubations, cardiac arrests, and active treatment do occur among patients who are discharged according to clinical judgment; however, further study is needed to evaluate whether the risks can be lowered and whether adverse occurrences after discharge decisions based on statistical predictions will be palatable to patients (and their lawyers) or helpful in resolving the ethical and financial problems that prompted this investigation.

With respect to artifacts in scores, the opposite may also occur: the use of intentional hypotension, hypothermia, muscle paralysis, and mechanical ventilation may result in a high score, supposedly measuring severe physiologic abnormalities, yet may be associated with a low mortality rate. Patients who have undergone cardiac surgery have been excluded from APACHE II analysis, perhaps because the effect of these often-selected therapeutic interventions render incorrect mortality predictions. Patients who experience trauma in urban areas with well-developed emergency medical systems, which have short response times, may never develop abnormalities in APACHE II components because of the rapid initiation of therapeutic support. The extent that this counteracts and obviates effects that would have occurred if treatment had been unavailable is immeasurable.

In most hospitals, admission and duration of ICU stay are carefully scrutinized and further exclusionary tactics, particularly in surgical patients, must be followed by an increase in morbidity, hospital costs, and mortality. Given the scarcity of available ICU beds in the ICU at my institution, we have been using a clinical triage system, attempting to add to the validity of ICU-exclusion decision by incorporating additional opinions and additional data into the decision-making process.[43] In our hospital, only 5% of elective surgical patients were considered by their surgeons for postoperative intensive care. If, at the end of the operation, in the opinion of the surgeon and anesthesiologist, the patient was considered to be stable, to have tolerated the procedure well, and to be at low risk for developing problems requiring ICU care, the patient was transferred to the recovery room. Twenty-nine percent of the patients satisfied these criteria. Mortality rate in this group of patients was significantly lower than in patients actually admitted to the ICU.

A second specific surgical consideration is that the severity of physiologic abnormality, as judged by APACHE II, does not seem to be an appropriate measure of resource utilization. Hospital charges and ICU bed days are not correlated with APACHE II scores. Indeed, the patients who die within 1 day and have the highest APACHE scores have bed days that are identical with those of survivors given 1 day of ICU care who have the lowest APACHE scores and are at the opposite end of the spectrum (Fig. 11-4). The same nonlinear relationship between severity of illness and charges that we found (Fig. 11-5) has been confirmed for another predictive index (MPM) as well.

From a quality assurance standpoint, if individual unit mortality rates were higher than overall rates in the national data base, unit performance could be judged as inferior. Remember that this problem is not just a question of scientific validity, because interpretations are already made by the government and the public, often incorrectly based on presently available overall hospital mortality information.[44]

The unfortunate implication that hospitals with high death rates deliver poor quality of care has been made in numerous newspaper articles after the release of this information. Higher observed mortality rates, whenever caused by specific problems inherent in determining the severity of illness in carefully attended patients during surgery, then create extensive and unnecessary review to determine whether performance was inferior. The increased time, effort, and expense used for these nonmedical functions must unavoidably increase the costs and decrease the efficiency of dollar resources by reducing the amount of time and number of personnel available to provide true medical care functions. To the extent that this occurs, the application of current predictive indices to surgical patients will not attain

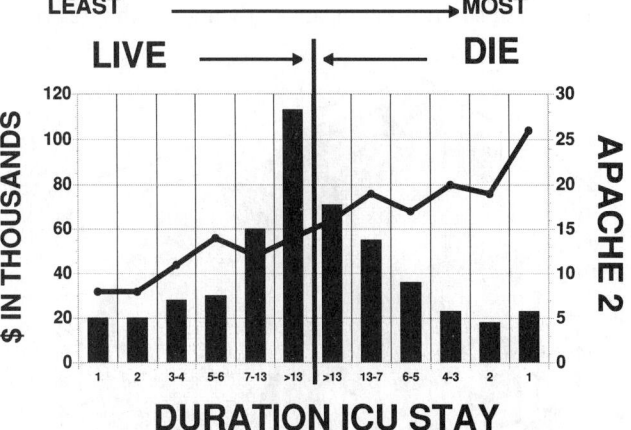

FIGURE 11-5. A severity-of-illness spectrum was again created on the premise that patients who stayed in the unit for 1 day and survived were the least sick, whereas patients who died during their first ICU day were the sickest. This spectrum, based on the duration of ICU stay, increases to a midway point for patients who stayed for more than 2 weeks and lived, with the next sickest group representing patients who stayed for more than 2 weeks and died. APACHE II scores show a pattern of generally increasing values from the least to the most sick. However, total hospital charges (in thousands of dollars) bear no relationship to the APACHE II scores. Thus, increasing severity of illness is not accompanied by increasing charges. In fact, the patients with the highest APACHE scores (1-day patients who died) had identical hospital bills to those with the lowest APACHE scores (1-day patients who lived).

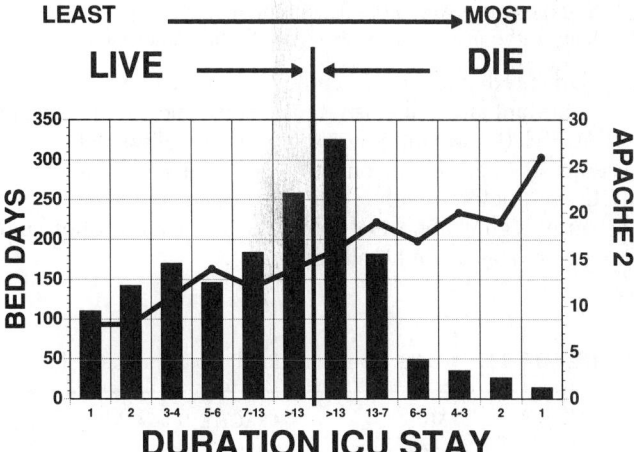

FIGURE 11-4. The severity-of-illness spectrum is based on the premise that the least–sick patient spent 1 day in the ICU and lived, and the sickest patient spent 1 day in the ICU and died. Total use of bed days (*bars*) and APACHE II scores (*line overlay*) are graphically represented. There is no overall correlation, and, in fact, patients with the highest APACHE scores (*right*) used the least bed days. There would be little savings from their exclusion.

the objectives of quality assurance and cost containment but contribute to producing the opposite effect.

Any methodology that hopes to attain the objectives of cost containment and quality assurance must describe the population in a uniform manner, especially if this description is said to be independent of treatment.[28] However, when patients are considered from the standpoint of initial APACHE II scores and duration of illness, neither symmetry nor uniformity is present (Fig. 11-6). The marked difference in survival within an APACHE II group, depending on the duration of ICU stay, indicates that therapy must have an effect and that other important variables affect outcome.

Because MOSF is of such importance in terms of resource utilization and mortality and because its long duration makes clinical predictions difficult, APACHE II score (A2S) was evaluated in surgical patients to predict the onset of MOSF and morality.[45] However, A2S significantly underestimated the potential for development of MOSF. Patients were grouped by A2S: with an A2S score of 5, the mortality rate was 50%, rising to 60% at A2S 10, and 75% at 15. Expected mortality rates were 0%, 4%, and 8%, respectively. The authors observed that the segment of the SICU population studied had the highest ICU resource use. Yet, because it is characteristic of the MOSF process that the extent of organ injury does not become manifest until several days after ICU admission, A2S both theoretically and practically cannot contribute to prediction or mortality of MOSF. Outcome predictive models also have been evaluated for individual patients in a medical ICU.[46] Three indices were evaluated: the MPM, APACHE II, and the Simplified Acute Physiology Score.[47] There were differences among the various scores in terms of correct predictions (Table 11-11). Prediction of survival was, again, fairly high, with rates vary-

ing from 85% to 95%. Well patients are usually easy to identify by clinicians, and confirmation by indices is not really helpful, although it may be expensive if laboratory testing—either manual or automated data collection—and processing costs are considered. Prediction of death was problematic, with no more than 50% of deaths identified. The authors[46] also observed that application of A2S to diagnostic subgroups, using disease-adapted risk calculations, revealed marked inconsistencies between the estimated risk and the observed mortality rate.

Although overall classification rates were slightly lower (approximately 75%) than most other reported series (in which 85% are usually correctly identified),[39] the authors concluded that the inaccuracy of the methods made them ineffective for predicting individual outcome and that they provide little advantage over clinical decision-making. In another medical ICU population, an inverse relationship existed between APACHE II score and mortality in respiratory failure resulting from cardiogenic pulmonary edema.[48] This report was considered remarkable by the authors of APACHE II. In fact, they stated,

> . . . [T]herefore, in a search for possible explanations behind the results of Fedullo et al, we respectfully ask the authors to consider the following. One explanation for these findings would be that the computer codes identifying surviving and deceased patients were reversed at some point during the analysis. We wonder whether the authors have checked back to original medical records for those cases to be sure that they are accurate.[49]

Feinstein[50] has a different perspective:

> When medical records have been used in the past to note severity of illness, the main difficulty has not been the absence of suitable data, but the absence of the investigators' attention to the suitable data. Investigators, who considered only the demographic data and the para-clinical data of "disease" while ignoring the clinical data of illness, were unable to classify severity effectively—but then often concluded that the defect was in the data of the medical records rather than in the investigators' concept of what data to analyze.

Early prediction of the death of a specific patient remains an important and still elusive goal. The principle underlying APACHE (to weight physiologic abnormality) defeats its usefulness in predicting outcome in patients with prolonged ICU stays before death, even when calculated repetitively, because highly abnormal physiologic characteristics and long-term stay are mutually exclusive.

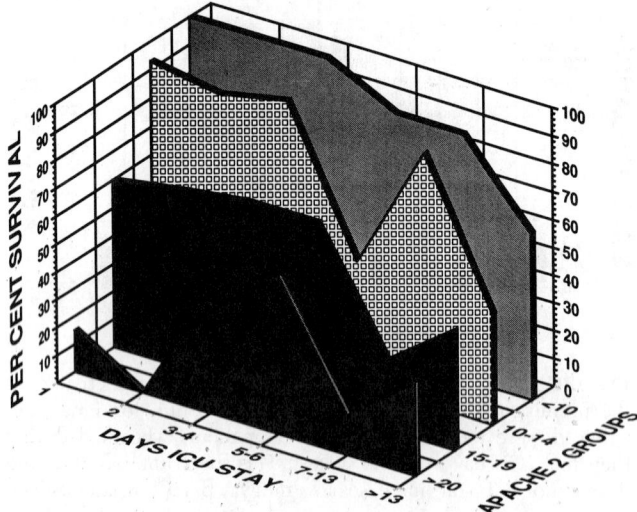

FIGURE 11-6. Three-dimensional representation of survival rates as a function of APACHE II score and duration of ICU stay. For a given APACHE II group, markedly different mortality rates occur, depending on duration of stay. Neither symmetry nor uniformity on any axis is present. Therefore, factors other than admission APACHE II scores must affect mortality rates, and these factors would not be evaluated if APACHE II alone were used as an assessment tool.

TABLE 11-11. Correct Outcome Prediction in a Medical ICU[46]

	MPM (%)	APACHE II (%)	SAPS (%)
Death	45	51	21
Survival	85	85	97
Overall	73	76	76

MPM, Mortality Prediction Model; SAPS, Simplified Acute Physiology Score.[47]

TABLE 11-12. ANOVA Intergroup Comparisons

	TOTAL POINTS	DAYS PAC	DAY 1 CVFn	LAST CVFn
# Diff	0/20	0/20	3/20	0/20
p Value	0.33	0.61	0.003	0.24

ANOVA, analysis of variance; CVFn, cardiovascular function; # Diff, no. of intergroup comparisons with a significant difference by Scheffe test; PAC, post–acute care.

Finally, risk stratification is a desirable attribute claimed for A2S. We wondered if this were possible for hemodynamically unstable patients.[51] If this were so, patients grouped by A2S should not only have different mortality rates but different needs for monitoring, interventions, and resulting cardiovascular function (CVFn). A2S was significantly correlated with mortality rates. However, virtually no stratification of total intervention points, days of monitoring, nor initial or final CVFn was encountered (Table 11-12). Of 80 intergroup comparisons, 77 were not statistically significant. When the total number of interventions was regressed with the APACHE II first day score, the coefficient of determination (r^2) was 0.001 and the slope of the regression line was 0.1. Thus, over 99% of the variance was not explained. A regression analysis performed between initial CVFn and the APACHE II score showed an r^2 of 0.00006 and the slope of the regression line of 0.0001. Both regression lines were therefore nearly horizontal, showing no stratification of either CVFn or the number of interventions used according to the patients' APACHE II score. Even when patients were further divided into those who lived and died, first CVFn was different only in an unexpected way (patients with low A2S who died had hyperdynamic function and those with high A2S who lived had hypodynamic function: basically the opposite of the usually reported favorable association of hyperdynamic function with survival).

CONCLUSION

Outcome, prediction, cost containment, and clinical judgment must be linked together in current medical practice. Clarification and refinements to existing systems do not seem to be appropriate solutions. First, we need to investigate new methodology to judge therapeutic interventions and to achieve outcomes desired by patients and by society. Second, we must investigate the factors that truly determine patients' values. Third, we must spend these immense resources wisely. Perhaps Feinstein[50] provided the correct answer even before the questions were asked. New mathematic approaches must be investigated. Considering the tremendous time and financial investment in both the developing and daily use of APACHE III, a 2.5% improvement in prediction compared with a remaining 12% misclassification rate was disappointing. An additional theoretic limitation related to transforming multidimensional variables into a one-dimensional score such as APACHE, the Apgar score, or the Glasgow Coma Score has been described by Antonio Boba (personal communication, March, 1991). These scales take various dimensions and transform them into a single, numerical, one-dimensional sequence. Boba states, ". . . a word of caution should be said about the implicit assumption that because the values in question can be arranged along an axis isomorphic to the axis of ordered integers that whatever manipulation is automatically permissible with a positive integer is also automatically permissible for the values themselves." In other words, combining rates, sizes, concentrations, and percents and forming a single linear scale leads to discontinuity and repetition of values, and does not create a linear relationship among all of the variables. By stripping the units from each variable and combining the integers that remain, an assumption is made that a linear scale has been created. It has never been clear that the same point total for hypertension and bradycardia has the same clinical implication as for hypotension and tachycardia.

An alternative to the use of multiple logistic regression, common to the indices thus far described, are connectionist models such as neural networks. In cases where input variables are interrelated similar to the hypertension–bradycardia (which might indicate increased intracranial pressure) and hypotension–tachycardia (which would be associated with hypovolemia), connectionist models may outperform classic predictive methods. Neural nets have been used in predicting outcome from gram-negative sepsis,[52] predicting chronicity in the SICU,[53] making the diagnosis of acute pulmonary embolism,[54] predicting length of stay in an ICU after cardiac surgery,[55] and predicting weaning from respiratory support.[56] Whereas current studies have performed as well or better than traditional statistical methodology, many problems still exits, as described by Buchman and associates.[53] A practical ceiling to the number of variables that can be handled by a neural network exists. Diagnoses need to be coded to prevent interpretation of numerical labels such as the ICD-9 codes as continuous variables. Omissions degrade the neural network, and effective data replacement strategy is necessary. If many laboratory tests are required, then our cost-sensitive environment will be in the same predicament using neural networks as conventional statistical methods. Validation errors from automatic data collection from bedside devices have replaced transcriptional and calculation errors. This problem will be common to APACHE III, which also relies on automated bedside data collection. Finally, the connectionist approach does not permit the user to understand the relationships among the relevant variables. A neural network provides the predictions with perhaps greater power but at the expense of insight into the model itself. Despite these limitations, given the "wall" seemingly hit by all of the newest iterations of the surviving predictive indices, alternative methodologies should be investigated.

Finally, we have been forced to evaluate outcome in terms of resource allocation and cost. Is intensive care worth the price? A study of nearly 11,000 patients in Finland[57] provides heartening data. Patients were followed for 5 years after their discharge from intensive care. Although nearly 15% died within the first 6 months, after this time period, the survival curve of ICU patients became parallel to that of the general population for the rest of the period of observation. The excess mortality was greatest in patients who had experienced cardiac arrest: only 30% were alive at 6 months after ICU discharge. Thus, patients who survive the ICU, survive hospitalization, and survive for 6 months thereafter can expect a mortality rate equivalent to the general population. The long-term outcome of intensive care thus seems to be worth the cost.

REFERENCES ■

1. Stern RS, Epstein AM: Institutional responses to prospective payment based on diagnosis-related groups: implications of cost, quality, and access. *N Engl J Med* 1985;312:621
2. Showstack JA, Stone MH, Schroeder SA: The role of changing clinical practices in the rising costs of hospital care. *N Engl J Med* 1985;313:1201
3. Klarman HE: Application of cost-benefit analysis to health systems technology. *J Occup Med* 1974;16:172
4. Wenneberg JE: Sounding board: outcomes research, cost containment, and the fear of health care rationing. *N Engl J Med* 1990;323:1202
5. McClung JA, Kamer RS: Sounding board: the outcomes movement. Will it get us where we want to go? *N Engl J Med* 1990;323:266
6. Feinstein AR: The objectives of treatment. In: *Clinical Judgment*. Baltimore, Williams & Wilkins, 1967:231
7. Ellwood PM: Special report: Shattuck lecture. Outcome management: a technology of patient experience. *N Engl J Med* 1988;318:1549
8. Feinstein AR: Indexes and criteria of therapeutic response. In: *Clinical Judgment*. Baltimore, Williams & Wilkins, 1967:247
9. National Institutes of Health. Consensus Development Conference Summary. Washington, DC, Department of Health and Human Services, 1983;4(6).
10. Civetta JM, Hudson-Civetta JA: Maintaining quality of care while reducing charges in the ICU: 10 ways. *Ann Surg* 1985;202:524
11. Drucker WR, Gavett JW, et al: Toward strategies for cost containment in surgical patients. *Ann Surg* 1983;198:284
12. Campion EW, Mulley AG, Goldstein MA, et al: Medical intensive care for the elderly: a study of current use, costs, and outcomes. *JAMA* 1981;246:2052
13. Robin ED: A critical look at critical care. *Crit Care Med* 1983;11:144
14. Feinstein AR: The diagnostic taxonomy of disease: problems in therapy. In: *Clinical Judgment*. Baltimore, Williams & Wilkins, 1967:103
15. Roberts DE, Bell DD, Ostryzniuk T, et al: Eliminating needless testing in intensive care: an information-based team management approach. *Crit Care Med* 1993;21:1452
16. Civetta JM: No headlines, just headway [editorial]. *Crit Care Med* 1993;21:1416
17. Tierney WM, Miller ME, McDonald CJ: Special article: the effect on test ordering of informing physicians of the charges for outpatient diagnostic tests. *N Engl J Med* 1990;322:1499
18. Shoemaker WC, Pierchala BS, Potter Chang, et al: Prediction of outcome and severity of illness by analysis of the frequency distribution of cardiorespiratory variables. *Crit Care Med* 1977;5:82
19. Phillips GD, Austin KL, Runciman WB: Deaths in intensive care. *Med J Aust* 1980;424
20. Archie JP: Mathematic coupling of data: *Ann Surg* 1981;193:296
21. Hayes M, Timmins A, Yau E, et al: Elevation of systemic oxygen delivery in the treatment of critically ill patients. *N Engl J Med* 1994;330:1717
22. Lemeshow S, Teres D, Pastides H, et al: A method for predicting survival and mortality of ICU patients using objectively derived weights. *Crit Care Med* 1985;13:519
23. Lemeshow S, Klar J, Teres D, et al: Mortality probability models for patients in the intensive care unit for 48 or 72 hours: a prospective, multicenter study. *Crit Care Med* 1994;22:1351
24. Civetta JM: The inverse relationship between cost and survival. *J Surg Res* 1973;14:265
25. Cullen DJ, Civetta JM, Briggs BA, et al: Therapeutic intervention scoring system: a method for quantitative comparison of patient care. *Crit Care Med* 1974;2:57
26. Keene AR, Cullen DJ: Therapeutic intervention scoring system: update 1983. *Crit Care Med* 1983;11:1
27. Cullen D, Nemeskal R, Zaslavsky A: Intermediate TISS: a new therapeutic intervention scoring system for non-ICU patients. *Crit Care Med* 1994;22:1406
28. Knaus WA, Zimmerman JE, Wagner DP, et al: APACHE—acute physiology and chronic health evaluation: a physiologically based classification system. *Crit Care Med* 1981;9:591
29. Knaus WA, Draper EA, Wagner DP, et al: Evaluating outcome from intensive care: a preliminary multihospital comparison. *Crit Care Med* 1982;10:491
30. Knaus WA, Wagner DP, Loirat P, et al: A comparison of intensive care in the U.S.A. and France. *Lancet* 1982;62:642
31. Knaus WA, Draper EA, Wagner DP, et al: APACHE II: a severity of disease classification system. *Crit Care Med* 1985;13:818
32. Knaus WA, Draper EA, Wagner DP, et al: An evaluation of outcome from intensive care in major medical center. *Ann Intern Med* 1986;104:410
33. Knaus WA: When is intensive care inappropriate: new "prognostic" measures provide answers. *Hosp Med Q* 1986;14
34. Zimmerman JE (ed): APACHE III study design: analytic plan for evaluation of severity and outcome. Summary and Acknowledgments. *Crit Care Med* 1989;17:S174
35. Knaus W, Wagner D, Draper E, et al: The APACHE III prognostic system risk prediction of hospital mortality for critically ill hospitalized adults. *Chest* 1991;100:1619
36. Wagner D, Knaus W, Harrell F, et al: Daily prognostic estimates for critically ill adults in intensive care units: results from a prospective, multicenter, inception cohort analysis. *Crit Care Med* 1994;22:1359
37. Cook DJ, Guyatt GH, Jaeschke R, et al: Determinants in Canadian health care workers of the decision to withdraw life support in the critically ill. *JAMA* 1995;273:703
38. Civetta JM, Hudson-Civetta J, Nelson LD: Evaluation of APACHE II for cost containment and quality assurance. *Ann Surg* 1990;212:266
39. Kirby RR, Civetta JM: Critical care. In: Brown DL (ed): *Risk and Outcome in Anesthesia*, 2nd ed. Philadelphia, JB Lippincott, 1991
40. Zook CJ, Moore FD: High-cost users of medical care. *N Engl J Med* 1980;302:996
41. Zimmerman J, Wagner D, Draper E, et al: Improving intensive care unit discharge decisions: supplementing physician judgement with predictions of next day risk for life support. *Crit Care Med* 1994;22:1373
42. Groeger J, Guntupalli K, Strosberg M, et al: Descriptive analysis of critical care units in the United States: patient characteristics and intensive care unit utilization. *Crit Care Med* 1993;21:279

43. Civetta JM, Varon AJ, Yu M, Hudson-Civetta JA: Accuracy of structured ICU consultations. *Crit Care Med* 1989;17:S87

44. 1986 Hospital Mortality Information. *Federal Register* 1987;52: 30,741

45. Cerra FB, Negro F, Abrams J: APACHE II score does not predict multiple organ failure or mortality in postoperative surgical patients. *Arch Surg* 1990;125:219

46. Schafer JH, Maurer A, Jochimsen F: Outcome prediction models on admission in a medical intensive care unit: do they predict individual outcome? *Crit Care Med* 1990;18:111

47. LeGall JR, Loirat P, Alperovitch A, et al: A simplified acute physiology score for ICU patients. *Crit Care Med* 1984;12: 975

48. Fedullo AJ, Swinburne AJ, Wah GW, et al: APACHE II score and mortality in respiratory failure due to cardiogenic pulmonary edema. *Crit Care Med* 1988;16:1218

49. Knaus WA, Wagner DP: Selection bias and the relationship between APACHE II and mortality. *Crit Care Med* 1990;18: 793

50. Feinstein AR: Retrospection, experience, and medical records. In: *Clinical Judgment*. Baltimore, Williams & Wilkins, 1967: 264

51. Kirton OC, Aragon C, Salas C, et al: Can APACHE II fully stratify a surgical ICU sub-group? *Crit Care* 1991;19:S36

52. Chalfin D, Flaster E, Fein A: The use of neural networks (NN'S) to predict outcome for critically ill patients with gram-negative sepsis. *Crit Care Med* 1995;23(Suppl):A51

53. Buchman T, Kubos K, Seidler A, et al: A comparison of statistical and connectionist models for the prediction of chronicity in a surgical intensive care unit. *Crit Care Med* 1994;22:750

54. Patil S, Henry JW, Rubenfire M, et al: Neural netwwork in the clinical diagnosis of acute pulmonary embolism. *Chest* 1993;104:1685

55. Tu JV, Guerriere MRJ: Use of a neural network predictive instrument for length of stay in the intensive care unit following cardiac surgery. *Comput Biomed Res* 1993;26:220

56. Ashutosh K, Lee H, Mohan C, et al: Prediction criteria for successful weaning from respiratory support: statistical and connectionist analyses. *Crit Care Med* 1992;20:1295

57. Niskanen M, Kari A: Five-year survival after intensive care: comparison of 10,976 patients with general population. *Crit Care Med* 1995;23(Suppl A):A20

Critical Care, Third Edition, edited by Joseph M. Civetta,
Robert W. Taylor, and Robert R. Kirby.
Lippincott-Raven Publishers, Philadelphia, PA © 1997.

CHAPTER 12

■

Resuscitation Outcomes

William H. Bickell
Matthew M. Rice

IMMEDIATE CONCERNS ■

MAJOR PROBLEMS

Cardiac arrest outcome is heavily influenced by the patients' prearrest medical condition and the events of the resuscitation. The prognosis for long-term survival in those successfully resuscitated can be predicted by the level of consciousness and hemodynamic stability. Resuscitation is successful in only one of three attempts. Therefore, in most patients who have had a cardiac arrest, a decision must be made to terminate cardiopulmonary resuscitation (CPR).

STRESS POINTS

1. Prearrest medical conditions that predict an unsuccessful resuscitation effort include:
   A. Homebound lifestyle
   B. Metastatic cancer
   C. Cerebrovascular accidents with residual neurologic deficit
   D. Renal failure
   E. Left ventricular dysfunction
   F. Hypotension or metabolic acidosis before the arrest
   G. Recurrent cardiac arrest during the same hospital stay
   H. Sepsis
2. Factors during the resuscitation effort predicting increased mortality include:
   A. Unwitnessed collapse
   B. CPR delayed longer than 4 minutes; advanced cardiac life support (ACLS) delayed more than 10 minutes

   C. Bradyasystolic arrest rhythms
   D. Fine ventricular fibrillation (ventricular fibrillation amplitude less than 0.2 mV)
   E. CPR for longer than 15 minutes
   F. Dilated pupils despite adequate ventilation and external chest compression
3. In patients who respond to resuscitation, in-hospital mortality from cardiogenic shock or hypoxic encephalopathy can be predicted in the comatose patient or in those who require adrenergic agonists for blood pressure stabilization. Patients who are alert and hemodynamically stable after resuscitation have a 97% chance of full recovery.

ESSENTIAL PROCEDURES

Successful outcomes in cardiac arrest depend on what has been termed by the American Heart Association as the "the chain of survival" (i.e., early access to care, early CPR, early defibrillation, and early advanced life support). The failure to optimize all links in the chain of survival results in poor resuscitation rates and neurologic disabilities.

TERMINATION OF RESUSCITATION (NORMOTHERMIC ADULTS)

1. CPR should be terminated if inappropriately initiated in patients exhibiting rigor, dependent lividity, or when a do-not-resuscitate (DNR) order is in effect.
2. CPR should be terminated when it is determined that the cardiovascular system is unresponsive. Cardiovascular unresponsiveness is generally indicated by 30 minutes of CPR or advanced life support without resumption of intrinsic cardiac output, or bradyasystolic

arrest rhythms that persist despite attempted myocardial pacing and appropriate pharmacologic therapy.

3. Resuscitation efforts can be terminated out-of-hospital by the on-line medical control physician when the following conditions have been met: (1) endotracheal intubation has been accomplished; (2) intravenous (IV) access has been achieved; (3) appropriate IV medications have been administered; (4) appropriate countershocks for ventricular fibrillation have been delivered; (5) attempted external pacing for bradyasystolic rhythms has been accomplished; and (6) persistent asystole or agonal electrocardiographic patterns are present, with no reversible causes having been identified (e.g., hypothermia).

OUTCOMES OF RESUSCITATION   ■

The resuscitation of cardiopulmonary arrest victims has been practiced for more than 6000 years. Rescue breathing using the mouth-to-mouth technique was described in the Bible (II Kings 4:34). In 1892, Maass[1] described the use of external chest compression for the resuscitation of cardiac arrest induced by chloroform. In 1899, Prevost and Batelli[2] demonstrated that ventricular fibrillation could be reversed and regular cardiac activity restored by applying alternating current to the heart. It was not until 1960, however, that all of these elements (ventilation, external chest compression, and defibrillation) were combined in a coordinated effort for the successful resuscitation of a 45-year-old patient with ventricular fibrillation.[3] This monumental effort heralded the beginning of modern resuscitation. Since that time, the American Heart Association, in conjunction with the National Research Council, promoted and developed training standards for CPR and emergency cardiac care. As a result, training in emergency cardiac care has been provided to physicians and to allied health personnel involved in emergency and critical care. In addition, nearly 20 million Americans have been trained in CPR.

In caring for cardiac arrest victims, physicians are inevitably confronted with questions about prognosis. Family, friends, or possibly, the patients themselves, want to know the chances of surviving until hospital discharge and the functional status after discharge. The prognosis is also of value to the medical care team for determining the patients' future needs and in allocating medical resources. Answering these questions requires a thorough knowledge of the outcome of CPR.

Data on the outcome of CPR are not readily available. The studies that have been published on this subject focus primarily on out-of-hospital arrest and report a remarkably wide range of success. Attempting to draw conclusions based on the available data is difficult because the results are limited by the lack of standard terminology, definitional inconsistencies, and the variety of formats for reporting outcome. It is difficult to gain information from the studies that report cardiac arrest from all causes (trauma, medical, environmental) because of the vast differences in outcome of the different causes. This chapter, therefore, focuses on cardiac arrest resulting from heart disease. This population is not only more homogeneous but also represents most of the patients for whom CPR is initiated.

OUTCOME AFTER OUT-OF-HOSPITAL CARDIAC ARREST   ■

In 1992, cardiovascular disease accounted for 913,908 deaths (half of the deaths from all causes).[4] Nearly 600,000 of these deaths were from coronary artery disease, most of which were sudden deaths secondary to cardiac arrhythmias. More than two thirds of the sudden deaths take place outside the hospital within 2 hours after the onset of symptoms.[5,6] Ventricular fibrillation is the cause of cardiac arrest in most sudden deaths. In more than 50% of these patients, there is no evidence of myocardial infarction on the electrocardiogram or in cardiac enzyme studies, which accounts for the large number of patients who do not experience premonitory symptoms before the actual arrest.[7]

Survival rate after out-of-hospital cardiac arrest ranges from 2% to nearly 80% in selected patient populations.[8,9] Several identifiable factors result in profound changes in survival.

FACTORS AFFECTING SURVIVAL

Community Emergency Medical Services System

Before 1960, the prehospital management of cardiac arrest victims consisted of transport only. Survival for such patients was essentially nonexistent. With the introduction of the external chest compression technique, CPR was delivered in selected communities. In 1969, Adgey and others[10] introduced the concept of definitive field management for out-of-hospital cardiac arrest with the implementation of a mobile coronary care unit. This concept provided mobile medical services that previously had been limited to a fixed facility.

Currently, mobile units are staffed with EMTs who provide three levels of care: basic life support (EMT-A), EMTs certified in the use of a defibrillator (EMT-D), and EMTs certified in advanced life support (EMT-paramedic). Basic life support consists primarily of CPR, whereas advanced life support includes endotracheal intubation, defibrillation, and intravenous pharmacologic therapy. Community EMS systems provide mobile units staffed at the level of EMT-A, EMT-D, or EMT-paramedic. The level of EMS care relies primarily on available resources and community funding. The clinical course of cardiac arrest patients managed by EMT-A, EMT-D, and EMT-paramedic EMS systems is shown in Figure 12-1. The predicted effects of prehospital paramedic care over that provided by EMT-A are a twofold increase in the success of resuscitation and a threefold increase in the rate of survival to hospital discharge. The effect of adding the capability of prehospital defibrillation to a basic life support system (EMT-D) is a twofold increase in survival to hospital discharge. The direct comparison of adjacent communities and the prospective evaluation of communities that upgrade their EMS system to either EMT-D or paramedic level of care substantiates these data.[12,13,17,18]

FIGURE 12-1. Comparison of the clinical course of out-of-hospital cardiac arrest victims managed by emergency medical technicians providing basic life support or cardiopulmonary resuscitation (EMT-A); emergency medical technicians providing basic life support and defibrillation (EMT-D); and emergency medical technicians providing cardiopulmonary resuscitation, defibrillation, endotracheal intubation, and intravenous pharmacologic therapy (EMT-paramedic). (Derived from the combined data of Adgey et al,[10] Cobb et al,[11] Eisenberg et al,[12] Vertesi et al,[13] Stueven et al,[14] Roth et al,[15] and Stults et al.[16])

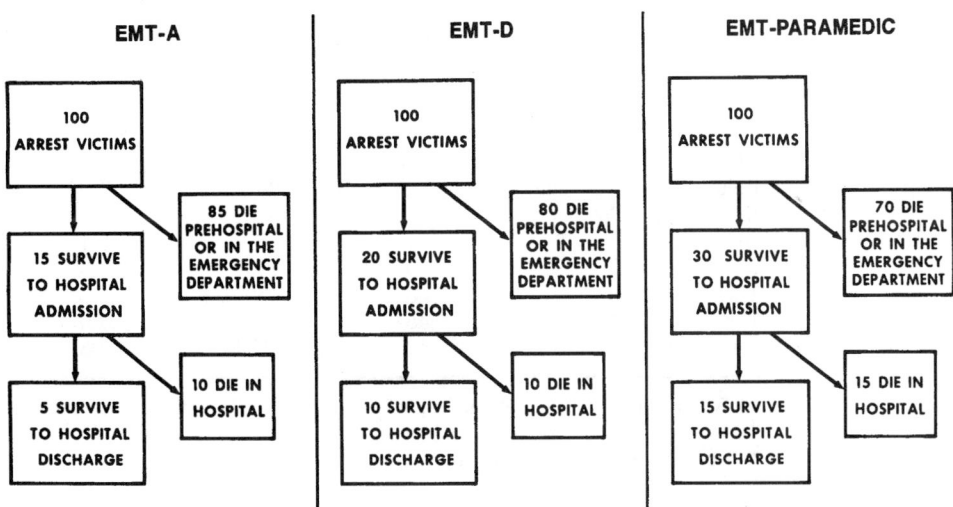

Recently, Eisenberg and associates[19] have shown that a tiered system in which the first responder is an EMT-A or EMT-D followed shortly thereafter by a paramedic-level second responder is a further enhancement over what would be achieved by a single-tier system of paramedic first responders. This improvement in survival results from a reduction in the time to initiation of basic life support and defibrillation.

Cardiac Rhythm

The cardiac rhythm as determined at the time of initial patient evaluation is shown in Figure 12-2. The most predominant rhythm is ventricular fibrillation, occurring in 63%, followed by asystole and pulseless electrical activity (PEA; electromechanical dissociation [EMD], pseudo-EMD, idioventricular escape rhythms, and bradyasystolic rhythms) in 31% and ventricular tachycardia in 6%.[9] The rhythm discovered at the time of initial patient evaluation is not necessarily the rhythm at the onset of cardiac arrest. Over time, ventricular fibrillation, if untreated, will eventually convert to asys-

tole. Similarly, ventricular tachycardia in the arrested heart is unstable and rapidly converts to ventricular fibrillation. Thus, the incidence of ventricular fibrillation and ventricular tachycardia may be greater than that currently reported if the rhythm at the onset of arrest could be determined. Cardiac rhythm is a strong predictor of the cardiac arrest victim's outcome. Survival rate in cardiac arrest patients presenting with ventricular fibrillation is reported in the range of 11% to 52%, with an overall survival rate of 22% (Table 12-1). For the subgroup of patients with ventricular tachycardia, survival to hospital discharge is reportedly 67%.[9] Both asystole and PEA carry a dismal prognosis with an overall mortality rate of 97% (see Table 12-1). The reason for this discrepancy in outcome can be understood from the etiology of the arrhythmias. Bradyasystolic rhythms are generally secondary to global ischemia, massive myocardial infarction, or cardiac chamber rupture, or they simply represent the terminal rhythm in untreated ventricular fibrillation. On the other hand, ventricular fibrillation frequently results from the transient instability of myocardial conduction, which is potentially reversible.

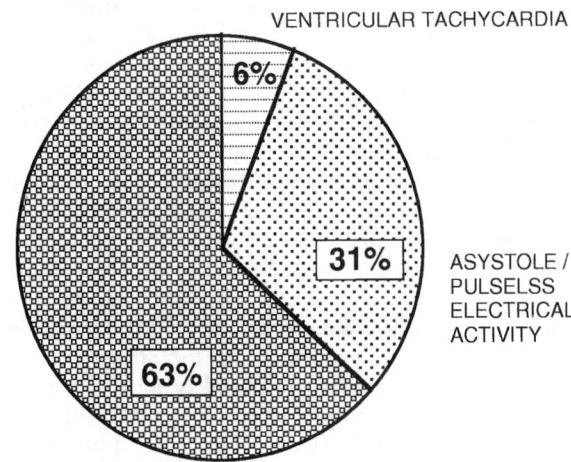

FIGURE 12-2. Incidence of cardiac arrhythmias discovered at the time of initial patient evaluation after out-of-hospital cardiac arrest.

TABLE 12-1. Controlled Studies in Advanced Life Support (Paramedic) Systems That Report Rhythm and Survival[*]

COMMUNITY	VF/VT	SURVIVORS	ASYSTOLE/PEA	SURVIVORS
Charlottesville, VA[20]	23	5	3	3
Belfast, Northern Ireland[10]	48	25	65	0
King County, WA[21]	442	131	179	9
Irvine, CA[22]	14	6	12	0
Pittsburgh, PA[15]	98	15	89	3
Torrance, CA[23]	50	15	40	0
York County, PA[24]	454	51	593	14
Overall	1129	248 (22%)	981	29 (3%)

VF/VT, the reported no. of patients with ventricular fibrillation/ventricular tachycardia; PEA, pulseless electrical activity.
[*]Discharge from the hospital alive.

Witnessed Versus Unwitnessed Cardiac Arrest

Unwitnessed cardiac arrest (collapse not witnessed by the EMS system or bystanders) usually indicates a prolonged anoxia time and is, therefore, associated with a decreased survival. Studies in King County, Washington, have specifically examined this variable and demonstrate a 75% reduction in survival for unwitnessed cardiac arrest.[25] The presenting cardiac rhythm in unwitnessed arrest is more frequently asystole. This fails to explain the poor results completely, however, because patients found in ventricular fibrillation after an unwitnessed collapse have a significantly reduced survival.[25]

Amplitude of the Ventricular Fibrillatory Waveform and Postcountershock Rhythm

The amplitude of ventricular fibrillation (as measured by the greatest peak-to-peak sinusoidal wave occurring before attempted defibrillation) is a powerful predictor of the subsequent clinical course. Fine ventricular fibrillation (0.2 mV or less) is as readily converted as coarse ventricular fibrillation (more than 0.2 mV); however, the resulting postcountershock rhythms are significantly different.[26] Patients exhibiting fine ventricular fibrillation are more likely to convert to asystole or a pulseless idioventricular rhythm and are, therefore, less likely to survive. Weaver and colleagues[26] showed that the survival rate in patients with fine ventricular fibrillation was a dismal 6% compared with 36% in patients with coarse ventricular fibrillation. Survival in fine ventricular fibrillation approaches that of primary bradyasystolic arrest and may represent the bridge between viability and death. Some cases of fine ventricular fibrillation possibly may represent atrial fibrillation with ventricular asystole. The occasional observation of isolated P waves after countershock supports this contention and helps to explain the poor survival. The initial resulting heart rate and rhythm after countershock also correlate well with the subsequent hospital course and survival. Liberthson and associates[27] have demonstrated progressive improvement in survival with increasing heart rate after defibrillation (Fig. 12-3). Further, survival is greater in those with postcountershock supraventricular

rhythms than in those with junctional or idioventricular rhythms (Fig. 12-4). The poor prognosis in patients with postcountershock bradyarrhythmias is probably related to the anoxic metabolic derangement of prolonged arrest, thus accounting for the inability of the heart to support supraventricular rhythms. In addition, bradyarrhythmias may enhance ventricular irritability, thereby predisposing these patients to recurrent arrest.

Out-of-Hospital Bystander CPR

In 1960, Kouwenhoven and coworkers[3] reported on the effectiveness of external chest compression in the experimental management of ventricular fibrillation and in the clinical management of cardiac arrest. Widespread acceptance of the concept and practice of CPR ensued. As a result, complications from this procedure rapidly surfaced. The combination of positive-pressure ventilation and external chest com-

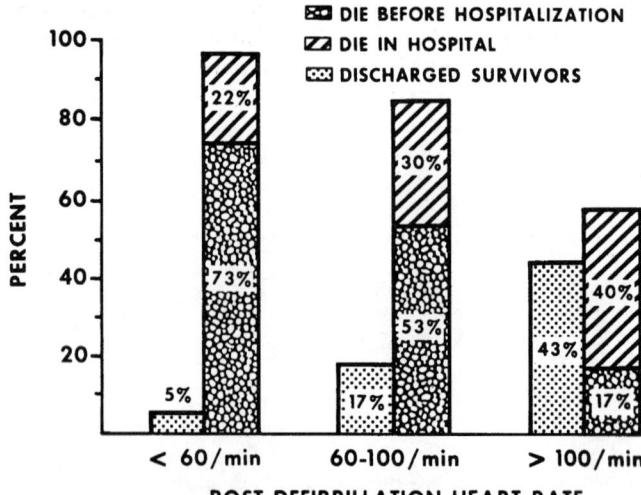

FIGURE 12-3. Prognostic implications of the initial heart rate after out-of-hospital defibrillation. (Liberthson RR, Nagel EL, Hirschman JC, et al: Prehospital ventricular fibrillation: prognosis and follow-up course. 1974;291:317.)

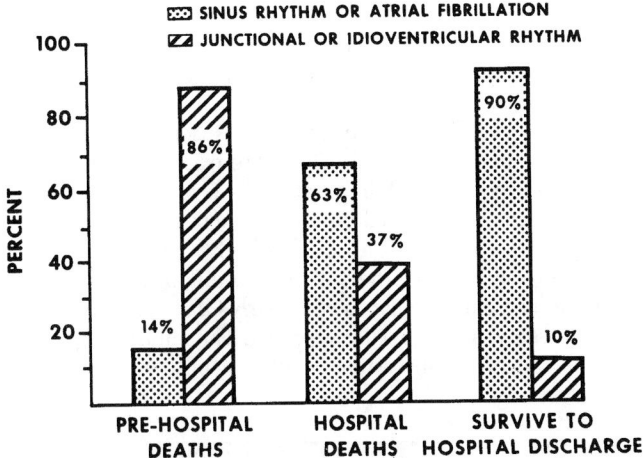

FIGURE 12-4. Prognostic implications of the initial cardiac rhythm after out-of-hospital defibrillation. (Liberthson RR, Nagel EL, Hirschman JC, et al: Prehospital ventricular fibrillation: prognosis and follow-up course. 1974;291:317.)

pression resulted in the following complications: fractures of the ribs and sternum; pneumothoraces; lacerations of the myocardium, liver, spleen, and kidney; cerebral and pulmonary edema; and bone marrow and fat embolism. Further, research into the hemodynamic effects of external chest compression demonstrates a strikingly low blood flow that is far below the levels necessary for cerebral or myocardial viability.[28]

The high rate of complications combined with the low critical organ perfusion has led many investigators to question whether conventional CPR contributes to human resuscitation. CPR as a modality by itself has been shown clinically and experimentally to be incapable of halting or reversing the process of anoxic cellular necrosis, although its independent efficacy has been demonstrated in hypothermia, respiratory arrest, and drug overdose.[29] However, the concept behind

the clinical practice of CPR is not that the procedure stops or reverses the process of death; rather, it extends the window of possible resuscitation. Despite the surprisingly low rates of critical organ perfusion, CPR has been shown experimentally to maintain ventricular fibrillation and extend the time over which defibrillation will produce a supraventricular rhythm and an adequate cardiac output.

The controlled clinical evaluation of the theory that CPR improves outcome is difficult. For most patients, the rhythm at the onset of arrest is not known; thus, it is not possible to determine clinically whether CPR maintains the heart in fibrillation. Further, one cannot randomly allocate CPR versus no CPR or control the factors that influence outcome such as arrest location, rhythm, and time to definitive care. Nonetheless, information on survival in bystander versus delayed CPR is available. Over the last decade, at least nine EMS systems have demonstrated that survival is increased when CPR is bystander initiated versus delayed until arrival of EMS personnel (Table 12-2). The Milwaukee paramedic system, however, reported that bystander CPR was of no benefit in coarse ventricular fibrillation.[36]

Caution must be exercised in extrapolating these results to the general issue of early CPR. First, the rhythm selected for study has been shown to reflect arrest conditions that uniformly result in a favorable outcome. Coarse ventricular fibrillation, as discussed earlier, is associated with a witnessed arrest and a brief time to definitive care. Thus, for the subgroup of patients presenting to paramedic level personnel with coarse ventricular fibrillation, the beneficial effects of early (bystander) CPR may not begin to surface. Second, the fundamental question of whether CPR maintains ventricular fibrillation for a longer time was not addressed. In the Pittsburgh EMS system when CPR was bystander initiated, the initial rhythm recorded by paramedics was ventricular fibrillation or ventricular tachycardia in 71%.[15] When CPR was delayed until arrival of the field team, the initial rhythm was ventricular tachycardia or ventricular fibrillation in only 46%. This finding supports the contention

TABLE 12-2. Controlled Studies of Survival* From Out-of-Hospital Cardiac Arrest: Bystander CPR Versus Delayed CPR

			% DISCHARGED FROM HOSPITAL	
COMMUNITY	SYSTEM	RHYTHM	*Bystander CPR (%)*	*Delayed CPR (%)*
Oslo, Norway[30]	BLS	Not reported	36	8
Birmingham, AL[31]	ALS	VF/VT	86	50
Seattle, WA[32]	ALS	VF	43	21
Winnipeg, Canada[33]	BLS	VF/VT	25	5
Iceland[9]	BLS	All rhythms	42	6
Vancouver, Canada[13]	ALS	All rhythms	21	6
Los Angeles, CA[35]	ALS	All rhythms	22	5
King County, WA[35]	ALS	All rhythms	23	12
Pittsburgh, PA[16]	ALS	VF/VT	24	7

CPR, cardiopulmonary resuscitation; BLS, basic life support (i.e., CPR only); ALS, advanced life support (i.e., BLS, defibrillation, endotracheal intubation, and intravenous drug therapy); VF/VT, ventricular fibrillation/ventricular tachycardia; VF; ventricular fibrillation.
*Discharged from the hospital alive.

that CPR maintains the heart in ventricular fibrillation or ventricular tachycardia and delays the anoxic progression to asystole.

Location of Cardiac Arrest

Survival after cardiac arrest has been observed to be higher when collapse occurs outside the home.[37] This has been attributed to the fact that arrest outside the home is more often witnessed, a bystander is more likely to initiate CPR, and the patient is more likely to present with ventricular fibrillation at the time of evaluation by the EMS system. These factors, as previously discussed, strongly correlate with an improved survival. However, these variables fail to explain completely the observed decrease in mortality after cardiac arrest outside the home. Although other factors such as the sedentary lifestyle of home arrest victims have been proposed, the precise cause has not been ascertained.

Time to Definitive Care and Resuscitation

The time from collapse to definitive care (defibrillation, intubation, and intravenous drug therapy) correlates well with the response time (time from dispatch to scene arrival) of the mobile advanced life support unit. The relation between response time and survival is shown in Figure 12-5. Each minute of increase in response time results in a reduction in survival of approximately 5%.[14,25] The duration of the resuscitation effort also has an inverse correlation with survival. Because of the inevitable relationship between the time to cardiac stabilization and the duration of cellular anoxia, prolonged resuscitation results in an increase in mor-

tality. Resuscitation time may be predetermined by the viability of the myocardium. Nevertheless, the time to cardiac stabilization partly reflects the treatment delivered in the field. Thus, an emphasis on immediate (quick-look) defibrillation and an efficient, coordinated resuscitation effort will yield an improved survival. The mere existence of an EMS system staffed with EMT-paramedic–level personnel does not guarantee an optimal outcome. Successful outcomes in cardiac arrest depend on how well all of the resuscitation efforts are linked together in the aforementioned chain of survival (i.e., early access to care, early CPR, early defibrillation, and early advanced life support). The failure to optimize all links in the chain results in inferior outcomes.

HOSPITAL COURSE OF PATIENTS SUCCESSFULLY RESUSCITATED FROM OUT-OF-HOSPITAL CARDIAC ARREST ∎

The most immediate concern for patients resuscitated from out-of-hospital cardiac arrest is recurrent ventricular fibrillation. This problem occurs in 25% to 60% of the patients surviving to hospital admission (generally within the first 24 hours).[27] The greatest risk is in those with atrioventricular or intraventricular conduction defects. Warning arrhythmias (i.e., ventricular premature contractions) are not reliable indicators of recurrent ventricular fibrillation.

The cause of in-hospital mortality after out-of-hospital resuscitation is not commonly reported. Arrhythmias are a relatively infrequent cause of death, despite the observation of electrophysiologic instability in up to 90% during the early phase of hospitalization.[9] Cardiac causes of death (i.e., ventricular fibrillation and cardiogenic shock) account for 41% to 50% of the in-hospital mortality (Table 12-3). Most patients die directly or indirectly from the central nervous system consequences of cardiac arrest.

SURVIVAL AFTER HOSPITAL DISCHARGE

Ventricular fibrillation is the arrhythmia from which 96% of the survivors of out-of-hospital cardiac arrest are resuscitated and subsequently discharged from the hospital. Any discus-

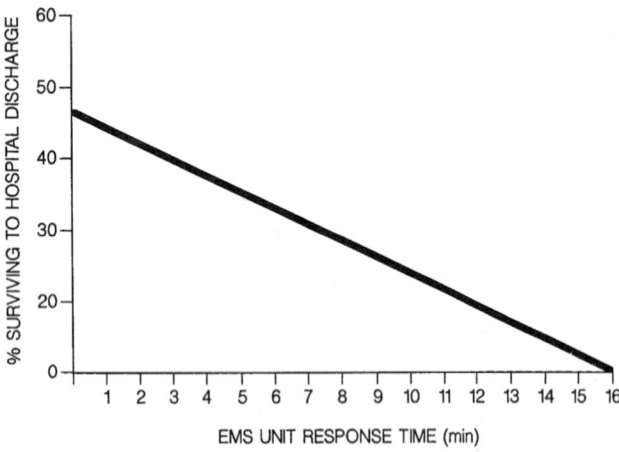

FIGURE 12-5. Relation between response time (i.e., time from dispatch to scene arrival) of the mobile emergency medical services system unit and survival in patients with out-of-hospital ventricular fibrillation. (Derived from Stueven H, Troiano P, Thompson B, et al: Bystander/first responder CPR: ten years' experience in a paramedic system. *Ann Emerg Med* 1986;15:707; and Eisenberg M, Hallstrom A, Bergner L, et al: The ACLS score: predicting survival from out-of-hospital cardiac arrest. *JAMA* 1981;246:50.)

TABLE 12-3. Etiology of In-Hospital Mortality in Patients Resuscitated From Out-of-Hospital Cardiac Arrest

	JACKSON MEMORIAL HOSPITAL, MIAMI[9] (%)	ROYAL VICTORIA HOSPITAL, BELFAST[10] (%)
Ventricular fibrillation	10	8
Cardiogenic shock	31	42
Anoxic encephalopathy	38	50
Sepsis°	21	Not reported

°Occurred in comatose patients on mechanical ventilation.

sion about survival after hospital discharge, therefore, must focus primarily on this subgroup of cardiac arrest victims. Because ventricular fibrillation is a well-recognized complication of myocardial infarction, cardiac arrest is attributed to this mechanism, particularly in cases in which atherosclerotic heart disease is discovered at autopsy. Evidence of myocardial infarction is found in only 40%,[7] however, which indicates that many episodes of cardiac arrest result from primary ventricular fibrillation (i.e., ventricular fibrillation without associated acute myocardial infarction). Hence, two basic categories make up most of the survivors from out-of-hospital cardiac arrest: (1) ventricular fibrillation secondary to acute myocardial infarction, and (2) primary ventricular fibrillation. The separation of these two patient groups is more than just an epidemiologic exercise, because their subsequent survival after hospital discharge is markedly different. In patients with ventricular fibrillation secondary to acute myocardial infarction, survival after hospital discharge is significantly greater than that of patients with primary ventricular fibrillation.[11] The reason for this disparity in survival can be understood from the underlying causes of electrophysiologic instability. In patients with acute myocardial infarction, the propensity for developing ventricular fibrillation is of brief duration, whereas ventricular fibrillation without acute myocardial infarction is generally related to chronic disease processes and, therefore, is likely to recur.

From the observations of recurrent out-of-hospital cardiac arrest, the cause of mortality is most often sudden death from ventricular fibrillation. This generally occurs within 4 months of hospital discharge.[11] Most of these recurrent episodes of cardiac arrest occur without prodromal symptoms, thus reducing the likelihood that acute preventive measures (e.g., self-administration of lidocaine) would be effective, as some have suggested. For most of these patients, hope for survival rests with bystander CPR and the rapid delivery of advanced life support. More recent technologic advances, such as implanted defibrillators and automatic defibrillators in the home, may be important adjuncts in selected patients.

From the forgoing discussion, it is evident that several factors improve the chance of surviving out-of-hospital cardiac arrest. Location of arrest, witnessed versus nonwitnessed collapse, and cardiac rhythm are obviously the given conditions that cannot be altered. However, several factors—time to the initiation of CPR, EMS system response time, and resuscitation time—can be favorably changed. For example, community programs for training citizens in basic life support will reduce the time to the initiation of CPR and facilitate access into the EMS system; improvements in the logistics of mobile EMS unit dispatch will reduce response time; and an emphasis on early defibrillation with efficient, well-coordinated resuscitation efforts will reduce resuscitation time. For the nearly 2000 victims with out-of-hospital cardiac arrest daily, overall long-term survival rates of nearly 40% are within the realm of possibility. Achieving this goal may be the greatest challenge for critical care medicine.

OUTCOME AFTER IN-HOSPITAL CARDIAC ARREST

Before 1974, standards for the performance of CPR and emergency cardiac care were nonexistent.[38] Cardiac arrest therapeutics varied substantially from one medical center to the next. Now-abandoned modalities such as alternating-current defibrillation and intramuscular drug administration were routinely used. Often, nurses were not trained in CPR, and arrest management teams were organized only during daytime hours. As a result, mortality was markedly increased when physicians were not immediately available to begin CPR and during the evening hours when there was no functional team for cardiac arrest management. Further, our limited knowledge of resuscitation physiology during the early practice of CPR resulted in some unusual therapeutic interventions. This is exemplified in the following excerpt: "In some patients, external cardiac massage was effective to the point at which the patient regained consciousness, and required intravenous sodium amylobarbitone sedation to allow external cardiac massage to continue."[39]

Although numerous manuscripts have been published on the subject of in-hospital cardiac arrest, few yield meaningful data because of the aforementioned problems. Further, many authors include in their arrest results patients with simple syncope, seizures, Stokes-Adams attack, or those with primary respiratory arrest. Although these conditions may result in loss of consciousness, they are not conditions with true cardiac arrest (i.e., unresponsive, apneic, pulseless) and hence carry a better prognosis. This section focuses on the outcome in cardiac arrest secondary to heart disease, thus dealing with the patients who require defibrillation or the full sequelae of CPR and emergency cardiac care.

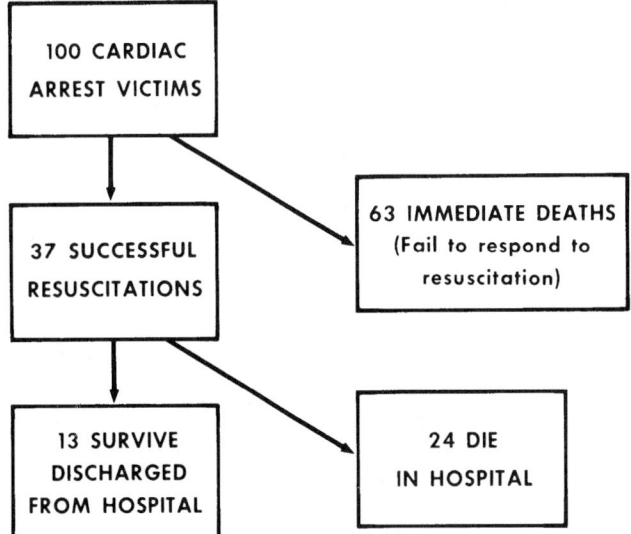

FIGURE 12-6. Clinical course after in-hospital cardiac arrest and attempted cardiopulmonary resuscitation. (Derived from the data of Bedell et al,[40] Peatfield et al,[41] Messert and Quglieri,[42] Jeresaty et al,[43] Hollingsworth,[44] Gregory and Grace,[45] Hofkin,[46] Johnson et al,[47] and Grace and Minogue.[48]

The overall clinical course of in-hospital cardiac arrest victims is shown in Figure 12-6. The factors that negatively influence survival are divided into prearrest, arrest, and post-resuscitation variables.

PREARREST MEDICAL CONDITIONS PREDICTING INCREASED MORTALITY

For patients with cancer, renal failure, or homebound life-style, the mortality rate after cardiac arrest and attempted resuscitation exceeds 95%.[40] In addition, survival is essentially nonexistent in patients with sepsis, in those with preexisting neurologic deficit resulting from a cerebral vascular accident, or in those who have had a previous cardiac arrest during the same hospital stay. In addition, prearrest conditions such as hypotension and metabolic acidosis portend a poor outcome. In contrast, the mortality rate in patients with none of the above characteristics is reportedly 34%.[40]

FACTORS DURING THE RESUSCITATION EFFORT PREDICTING INCREASED MORTALITY

As in the prehospital environment, survival is more favorable in patients with ventricular fibrillation as opposed to asystole and PEA (EMD, pseudo-EMD, idioventricular escape rhythms, and bradyasystolic rhythms; Table 12-4). The subgroup of arrest secondary to torsade de pointes has demonstrated a remarkable survival rate of 88%.[40] The need for endotracheal intubation during resuscitation is associated with increased mortality. In general, patients who require intubation are those who fail to respond to immediate resuscitative efforts such as precordial thump or "quick-look" defibrillation and, therefore, require a longer resuscitation. Consequently, mortality increases when intubation is required. The time required for cardiac stabilization (i.e., re-

suscitation time) directly reflects the time of cellular anoxia. As a result, the chances for survival decrease with increasing resuscitation time. The mortality rate in patients whose resuscitation effort is less than 15 minutes is approximately 40% and leaps to 95% with resuscitation efforts greater than 15 minutes. Interestingly, numerous authors have failed to report any survivors after resuscitation efforts of greater than 30 minutes.[40,43]

FACTORS PREDICTING MORTALITY AFTER SUCCESSFUL RESUSCITATION

The prognosis for survival until hospital discharge in patients successfully resuscitated is determined primarily by the level of consciousness and hemodynamic stability. Mortality from cardiogenic shock or hypoxic encephalopathy can be predicted in those who require adrenergic agonists for blood pressure stabilization or in the comatose patient. Conversely, patients who are alert and hemodynamically stable after resuscitation have a 97% chance for full recovery.[40]

Predicting Mortality: Cause and Effects

In the forgoing discussion, several factors that predict increased mortality have been presented. Some of these factors are *not* the primary cause of mortality; rather, they are merely the manifestation of an underlying condition. For example, the functional status of the left ventricle determines both survival and the arrest rhythm. Increasing left ventricular dysfunction increases the incidence of asystole. In cardiogenic shock, the arrest rhythm is mostly asystole or EMD. In the absence of left ventricular dysfunction, the arrest rhythm is generally ventricular fibrillation. An increased incidence of bradyasystolic arrest also is found in patients with cancer, renal failure, and homebound lifestyles. Ventricular fibrillation, therefore, apparently occurs in the

TABLE 12-4. Controlled Studies of In-Hospital Cardiac Arrest That Report Rhythm and Survival to Hospital Discharge

HOSPITAL	VF/VT	SURVIVORS	ASYSTOLE/ PEA	SURVIVORS
Royal Melbourne Hospital, Australia[39]	24	8	14	0
Hospital of the University of Pennsylvania, Philadelphia[49]	33	3	45	2
Sinai Hospital of Baltimore[46]	16	7	12	0
St. Francis Hospital, Hartford, CT[43]	148	41	81	9
University of Virginia Hospital, Charlottesville, VA[44]	105	15	108	2
Hollywood Presbyterian Hospital[50]	63	14	60	0
Beth Israel Hospital, Boston[40]	97	26	Not reported	Not reported
Overall	486	114 (23%)	320	13 (4%)

VF/VT, the reported no. of patients with ventricular fibrillation/ventricular tachycardia; PEA, pulseless electrical activity.

less severely compromised host, whereas asystolic rhythms occur with increasing frequency as the severity of illness increases. Furthermore, a prospective study of cardiac arrest victims has shown that mortality is primarily determined by the underlying medical condition.[40] Factors such as arrest rhythm or metabolic status merely reflect the underlying disease. This explains why aggressive resuscitation efforts such as attempted cardiac pacing have mostly been unsuccessful in patients with bradyasystolic arrest rhythms. The primary problem is not the cardiac rhythm but the underlying disease.

IS AGE A FACTOR PREDICTING THE OUTCOME OF CPR?

The physiologic reserve of a given organ system would be expected to decline over time; hence, age may be considered a contributing factor influencing the outcome of CPR. Although elderly patients can be initially resuscitated and hospitalized as successfully as younger patients, the elderly are less likely to survive to hospital discharge.[51] Moreover, it has been demonstrated that, in selected populations, survival is essentially nonexistent. For example, Taffet and coworkers,[52] in a study of cardiac arrest occurring at a veterans administration hospital, found that survival to hospital discharge is essentially nonexistent in patients older than 70 years of age. In a similar vein, it has been shown that CPR in residents of nursing homes results in no long-term survivors.[53] However, not all authors concur that the outcome of CPR in the elderly is dismal. Several clinical studies examining this issue have found that although survival from cardiac arrest is lower in the elderly, age alone is a weak predictor of survival after resuscitation attempts.[40,51,54] The most important factors influencing survival relate to the physical condition of the patient before cardiac arrest, the circumstances of the arrest (e.g., witnessed versus nonwitnessed), and the time required to achieve intrinsic cardiac activity. The poor outcomes for the elderly are, therefore, more related to the concomitant disease and the events of the arrest itself than to age.

DOES THE IN-HOSPITAL LOCATION OF THE CARDIAC ARREST INFLUENCE SURVIVAL?

Before the functional organization of cardiac arrest teams, the location in which the cardiac arrest occurred had a significant influence on survival. The chances for survival were greatest in the operating room or the intensive care unit and least in the general wards. Since the institution of standards for emergency cardiac care and the organization of cardiac arrest teams, no difference has been reported in survival between the emergency center, general wards, operating room, or the intensive care unit. However, it cannot be concluded from the standpoint of cardiac arrest management that an intensive care setting is unnecessary. The underlying medical condition of the arrest population must be considered. The achievement of similar survival rates in patients with a greater severity of illness may partly justify the resources expended in the intensive care environment.

CLINICAL COURSE AFTER HOSPITAL DISCHARGE: SURVIVAL AND FUNCTIONAL STATUS

For patients who survive CPR and who are ultimately discharged from the hospital, there is a steady annual death rate of 10% for the first 5 years, but thereafter the death rate levels off and approaches that of the general population. The rate functional status of the survivors (based on the New York Heart Association's classification of functional capacity before and after arrest) is, for the most part, unchanged.[55] In addition, 60% of the survivors return to work, thus reflecting the potentially reversible mechanisms of cardiac arrest. The major residual disability for the survivors of CPR is the limitation in activity and confinement to home. This limitation results primarily from the fear of recurrent arrest and not from any change in physical capability.

NEUROLOGIC OUTCOME AFTER CPR ■

In an 18-month prospective review of 294 consecutive cardiac arrest patients, Bedell and coworkers[40] reported that new-onset neurologic dysfunction occurs in 2% of the long-term survivors. All other patients surviving to hospital discharge were alert, oriented, and had a normal memory as determined by the Wechsler memory scale. Other investigators reporting on the outcome of cardiac arrest have confirmed this remarkably low incidence of neurologic complications after in-hospital CPR.[43,48,55-57] In contrast, patients surviving to hospital discharge after out-of-hospital cardiac arrest have a 30% incidence rate of new-onset neurologic dysfunction, which ranges from a loss of short-term memory to chronic vegetative states.[29,58] The increased incidence of neurologic complications after out-of-hospital cardiac arrest reflects the prolonged anoxia time and occurs predominately when CPR is delayed greater than 4 minutes.

About 90% of patients who are comatose after resuscitation either regain consciousness or die within 36 hours.[59] Only 10% never improve beyond the vegetative state and require institutional care. Although immediately after resuscitation it is difficult to determine which comatose patients will functionally recover, neurologic death or a chronic vegetative state can be accurately predicted in the patients lacking any two of the following brain stem reflexes: corneal, pupillary, or oculovestibular.

TERMINATION OF RESUSCITATION ■

Despite an unprecedented array of therapeutic interventions, resuscitation is successful in only one of three attempts. Therefore, in most cardiac arrest cases, a decision must be made to terminate CPR and declare the patient dead. At what point during the resuscitation should this decision be made? This is possibly the most difficult and final decision a physician can make. Information on the patient's medical history, metabolic and cardiopulmonary condition, and response to resuscitation combined with probabilities of survival and ethical, legal, and emotional considerations are distilled into a yes-or-no decision. Since the early practice of emergency cardiac care, the difficulty of predicting which patients will survive the resuscitative effort has been well appreciated. Consequently, it was recommended that CPR be continued until evidence of brain and cardiac death persists throughout 1 hour of adequate basic and advanced life support.[60] It was soon realized that maximum effort on all patients is unnecessary and impractical. The observation that survival is highly unlikely after 30 minutes of CPR or in patients with bradyasystolic arrest led to the recommendation that resuscitation be terminated if unsuccessful after 30 minutes or after 10 minutes of advanced life support if bradyasystolic rhythms persist.[61] Although these guidelines are useful in predicting the patients for whom continued resuscitation will not be successful, the possibility of survival can never completely be excluded. For example, resuscitation efforts of greater than 60 minutes have resulted in long-term survival, even in patients with bradyasystolic arrest. This is not to say that as a result of these reports all patients should be resuscitated for more than 1 hour before the effort is deemed futile. These patients who seemingly defy the odds and survive illustrate that this issue cannot be resolved by a rigid set of criteria. There is a need for flexibility in caring for individual patients.

ON WHAT SHOULD THE DECISION TO TERMINATE CPR BE BASED?   ■

Cardiopulmonary resuscitation should be terminated if inappropriately initiated. CPR should not be initiated on those who are obviously dead. The determination of death can be made definitively in patients exhibiting rigor mortis, dependent lividity, or generalized body decomposition.[62] Occasionally, CPR is initiated on the obviously dead by well-meaning EMTs or bystanders. When this is realized by the physician responsible for cardiac arrest management, CPR should be stopped. However, care should be taken to explain why resuscitation was terminated to the people who initiated the procedure. Another situation in which it would be inappropriate to initiate CPR is when a DNR order, which has been instituted in accordance with appropriate hospital policy, is in effect.[63] If CPR has been initiated, it should be terminated immediately when the information of the DNR order is confirmed.

Cardiopulmonary resuscitation should be terminated when it is determined that the cardiovascular system is unresponsive and hence further efforts are futile. We cannot determine with certainty which patients will not respond to continued resuscitation efforts. Nonetheless, it can be determined that under certain circumstances the probability of survival is exceedingly low. These clearly identifiable circumstances are (1) 30 minutes of CPR or emergency cardiac care without resumption of intrinsic cardiac output; and (2) bradyasystolic arrest rhythms that persist despite attempted myocardial pacing (i.e., external, transvenous, or transthoracic), intravenous pharmacologic therapy (i.e., atropine or

epinephrine), or both. With few notable exceptions, if intrinsic cardiac output is not achieved within 30 minutes, further efforts are futile.[40] Additionally, it is generally understood that the chances for survival after bradyasystolic arrest are slim.[64] Moreover, the failure to respond to appropriate therapeutic measures overwhelmingly indicates that the cardiac arrest was a terminal event and not a transient complication of cardiac impulse formation or conduction. These conditions do not dictate that survival is impossible. Nevertheless, if the decision is made to continue with further resuscitative efforts, it should be based on the consideration that the underlying factors precipitating cardiac arrest (i.e., hypothermia, drug overdose, or electrolyte disturbance) are treatable or have been reversed; hence, continued resuscitation may be successful. Beyond the two aforesaid conditions, determining when resuscitation is futile becomes more difficult. A consideration of the medical history in addition to the other prearrest and arrest factors that have a negative influence on survival is helpful in formulating this decision (Table 12-5). For example, mortality in patients with fine ventricular fibrillation (amplitude less than 0.2 mV) is similar to that in patients with bradyasystolic arrest.[26] If the patient with fine ventricular fibrillation fails to respond to multiple countershocks and appropriate pharmacologic interventions, it would be a rational decision to terminate resuscitation despite the observation of continued fibrillation. On the other hand, in the patient with no significant medical problems and favorable circumstances surrounding the arrest (i.e., torsade de pointes or coarse ventricular fibrillation), the clinician may opt for a more prolonged resuscitation,

TABLE 12-5. Predictors of Mortality After Cardiac Arrest and Attempted CPR

PREARREST

Homebound lifestyle
Cancer
Cerebrovascular accident with residual neurologic deficit
Renal failure
Sepsis
Left ventricular dysfunction
Hypotension (systolic blood pressure <100 mm Hg)
Metabolic acidosis
Recurrent cardiac arrest during the same hospital stay

ARREST

Unwitnessed collapse
CPR delayed >4 min; advanced cardiac life support delayed >10 min
Bradyasystolic arrest rhythms (asystole electromechanical dissociation/pulseless idioventricular rhythm)
Fine ventricular fibrillation (ventricular fibrillation amplitude <0.2 mV)
CPR for more than 15 min
Dilated pupils despite adequate ventilation and external chest compression
Endotracheal intubation

CPR, cardiopulmonary resuscitation.

possibly beyond 30 minutes if the patient has shown transient intrinsic cardiac activity.

IS AGE A FACTOR TO BE CONSIDERED IN THE DECISION TO STOP CPR?

Age as a factor that influences outcome in cardiac arrest is often discussed but infrequently researched. It has been suggested that patients older than 65 years of age be subjected to only brief resuscitation efforts because of the poor outcome and the possibility that a chronic vegetative state may occur with more extensive efforts; however, the data supporting this concept are either incomplete or nonexistent. Numerous clinical studies specifically examining this issue have determined that age as an independent factor is a weak predictor of either survival or the level of function after hospital discharge.[40,41,44,49,65–67] What most influences the prognosis in cardiac arrest is the underlying disease, not the date of birth.

CAN THE END-TIDAL CARBON DIOXIDE CONCENTRATION OR CORONARY PERFUSION PRESSURE HELP DETERMINE WHEN TO STOP CPR?

End-tidal carbon dioxide concentration ($PETCO_2$) is a measure of the partial pressure of carbon dioxide present at the end of an exhaled breath. Because carbon dioxide is the end metabolic product of aerobic metabolism, it is not surprising that $PETCO_2$ has been shown to correlate with cardiac output and, hence, oxygen delivery to tissues. Clinical studies have demonstrated that a sudden rise in $PETCO_2$ is often the first notification of restoration of a pulse and the return of spontaneous circulation.[68] Likewise, an initially low $PETCO_2$ that fails to elevate in response to resuscitative efforts is a harbinger of unsuccessful resuscitation. Coronary perfusion pressure is defined as the aortic pressure minus the right atrial pressure. This pressure represents the perfusion gradient of blood traveling through the coronary arteries to the myocardium. Similar to $PETCO_2$, progressive increases in coronary perfusion pressure have been shown to correlate with an improved chance of achieving a return of spontaneous circulation.[69]

Despite the encouraging reports of the predicted value of both $PETCO_2$ and coronary perfusion pressure, a return of spontaneous circulation by no means guarantees survival to hospital discharge. Studies examining $PETCO_2$ and coronary perfusion pressure in human CPR have focused predominantly on patients who have failed out-of-hospital resuscitative efforts. This group has been shown to have a uniformly poor outcome. It is, therefore, not surprising that although resuscitation may have been initially successful in selected patients, none survived to hospital discharge. There are no conclusive data to determine how either $PETCO_2$ or coronary perfusion pressure predicts survival to hospital discharge. Furthermore, the measurement of coronary perfusion pressure is impractical during resuscitative efforts because it involves invasive venous and arterial catheter placement and radiographic confirmation of position. As a result of the aforementioned difficulties of measurement and lack of data on long-term survival, we believe that neither $PETCO_2$ nor coronary perfusion pressure are useful in deciding when to stop CPR.

SHOULD THE COST OF PATIENT CARE OR THE POSTRESUSCITATION QUALITY OF LIFE BE CONSIDERED IN THE DECISION TO STOP CPR?

In this era of increasing fiscal restraint, cost is a frequently discussed reason for terminating or limiting care. The dramatization of the rising cost of medical care has contributed to the concern that prolonged resuscitation may result in a drawn-out death in the intensive care unit. Most patients who die, however, do so within 24 hours of the resuscitation effort.[49] The long, lingering death is the publicized exception rather than the common occurrence.

Frequent reference is made to the fact that coma, vegetative states, or severe cardiac disability may occur in survivors of CPR. In the judgment of some clinicians, these complications represent an unacceptable reduction in the quality of life, and, therefore, resuscitation should be terminated early in selected patient populations. Two problems arise when using postresuscitation quality of life in the decision to stop CPR: (1) it is impossible to predict which patients will have these complications; and (2) the termination of treatment based on the quality of life is a special judgment reserved for informed patients. Even if it were possible to predict postresuscitation complications accurately, the arrested patient could not evaluate this information to make the appropriate decision. In conclusion, it is our opinion that cost and the postresuscitation quality of life have no bearing on the judgment of when to stop CPR.

WHO SHOULD DECIDE TO TERMINATE CPR?

The decision of who should decide to terminate CPR rests with the physician who has the primary medicolegal responsibility for the patient during the cardiac arrest. This person is generally the leader of the cardiac arrest management team. What should be done if there is disagreement among the team members with regard to this decision? For example, if the nurse or EMT demands further efforts after resuscitation has been terminated, can the physician ethically disregard these requests? We suggest that he or she can if resuscitation was inappropriately initiated or the resuscitation effort is determined to be futile. Although the observations and suggestions of the other team members should be considered, the final decision of when to stop CPR must be made by the physician bearing primary responsibility for the patient's management during the arrest.

TERMINATING RESUSCITATIVE EFFORTS OUT-OF-HOSPITAL   ∎

Several investigators have demonstrated that hospital transport of adult cardiac arrest victims who have failed to respond to an adequate trial of out-of-hospital ACLS does not result in meaningful rates of survival. Moreover, the costs and risks associated with high-speed transport may outweigh the extremely small likelihood of benefits. The American Heart Association has, therefore, recommended that resuscitation may be discontinued out-of-hospital when the cardiovascular system is unresponsive after an adequate trial of ACLS.[62] The determination that the patient is nonresuscitatable should be made by the EMS medical director or an appropriately licensed on-line medical control physician who has reasonable assurances that the following conditions have been met: (1) endotracheal intubation has been accomplished; (2) IV access has been achieved; (3) appropriate medications have been administered according to ACLS protocol; (4) appropriate countershocks for ventricular fibrillation have been delivered; (5) attempted external pacing for bradyasystolic rhythms has been accomplished; and (6) persistent asystole or agonal electrocardiographic patterns are present, with no reversible causes having been identified (e.g., hypothermia). In EMS systems where resuscitation is terminated out-of-hospital, mechanisms must be established for the determination of cardiovascular unresponsiveness and appropriate disposition of the body by means other than the EMS vehicles. Furthermore, the care providers should be trained to deal in a caring and compassionate manner with the family and others that may be present.

LEGAL IMPLICATIONS OF TERMINATING CPR   ∎

Medicolegal liability in resuscitation is based primarily on the quality of care and the decision to provide, withhold, or withdraw care.[70] Legal difficulties inherent in medical practice generally arise when outcomes are in contrast to patient or family expectations. There has been surprisingly little litigation involving CPR because of the low expectations and the lack of precedent-setting cases in decisions involving the termination of CPR.

Traditionally, the attorney for the party filing a legal claim (plaintiff's attorney) attempts to prove that certain events occurred or failed to occur and hence resulted in harm or suffering to the patient. One of the key elements in medical malpractice is to prove a proximate cause between an adverse outcome and alleged action or inaction by a care provider. Under the principle of proximate cause, it is nearly impossible to demonstrate that terminating CPR resulted in the death of a patient who has already had a cardiac arrest. As a result, successful litigation specifically implicating this decision is essentially nonexistent. However, a recent legal concept is emerging that will impact the decision to stop CPR. This concept, loss-of-chance, refers to the ability of a party to recover damages when, because of inaction, the chance to avoid an adverse outcome was missed.[71] For example, Mr. H has a cardiac arrest at home and is brought to the hospital while CPR is ongoing. At the hospital, he is pronounced dead on arrival and thus no further resuscitative efforts are attempted. Under the principle of proximate cause, the attorney representing Mr. H's estate would have to prove that the failure to continue resuscitative efforts was the proximate cause of death. Again, this would be almost impossible to prove in the patient who had a cardiac arrest before the decision to stop CPR was made. Under the loss-of-chance doctrine, it would be necessary only to demonstrate that some identifiable percentage of people who are given appropriate emergency cardiac care survive under the same circumstances as Mr. H's. Because of the lack of such care, Mr. H was, therefore, denied a chance to survive. With the current medicolegal climate in the United States, loss-of-chance decisions are worrisome.

HOW IS IT POSSIBLE TO DETERMINE WHETHER THE PHYSICIAN IS ON SOLID LEGAL GROUND WHEN TERMINATING CPR?   ∎

The decisions and standards for terminating CPR in the out-of-hospital setting are clearly outlined and generally create little controversy; termination is permitted when effective spontaneous ventilation and circulation are restored, responsibility is passed to an equal or higher level of care, or resuscitation is physically impossible (i.e., exhaustion of resuscitators, environmental hazards).[62] Beyond these well-defined areas, there tends to be confusion about when to terminate CPR. Although these unclear areas make legal interpretation more complicated, the legal determination of death offers some guiding principles. All medical care should be stopped when the patient is determined to be legally dead. A legal pronouncement of death is made when a person has sustained either (1) irreversible cessation of all functions of the entire brain, including the brain stem; or (2) irreversible cessation of cardiopulmonary functions.[72] During CPR, the determination that irreversible cessation of all brain functions has occurred is not possible; hence, the responsiveness of the cardiovascular system is used to determine death. The finding of cardiovascular unresponsiveness (as determined using acceptable medical standards) indicates that the heart has died, and there is no legal purpose in continuing with further procedures or therapeutic interventions. It is to such accepted medical practice that a physician will be held in determining whether the basic standards of medical care were met. Thus, it rests with the medical community to adopt standards of cardiovascular unresponsiveness and for the practitioner to follow them to be best protected from successful litigation.

The concept of medical futility with regard to CPR is an often-debated issue. Physicians are not ethically obligated to provide or continue therapeutic procedures if their use would be futile. Therefore, an argument based on the futility of resuscitation, especially with regard to cardiovascular unresponsiveness, is a powerful argument for discontinuing CPR.

WHAT ARE THE CONSIDERATIONS OF ADVANCE DIRECTIVES AND FAMILY INTERESTS IN THE DECISION TO STOP CPR? ■

A prime consideration in withholding or terminating treatment is the refusal of such treatment by a competent individual. An adult with the capacity to make an informed decision is generally permitted to make decisions about the medical care offered, including refusal of treatment. Frequently, such decisions may be evidenced through advance directives. These directives are particularly useful when patients are incapable of expressing their consent. Advance directives are more frequently being recognized as documents reflecting the desires of the patient and may guide physicians in providing or withholding health care. Advance directives include the "living will" and the "durable power of attorney."[73] Although the living will is a document providing information on a patient's desires for treatment, a durable power of attorney is a document authorizing someone other than the patient to make medically related decisions when the patient becomes incapacitated.[73,74] The presence of valid advance directives provides adequate documentation for the individual's expression of desire to avoid unwanted medical care and procedures. Physicians may then feel more comfortable in not beginning, restricting, or terminating resuscitation. However, advanced directives may fail to describe what artificial means are acceptable and to consider legal limitations imposed by the state (i.e., pregnancy, dependent children). Therefore, a resuscitation, once begun, should aggressively be continued until these details are clarified.

DNR orders also may be considered an advance directive in reflecting the decision made by the patient, through the physician, on what types of medical care are desired.[75] They should, therefore, be honored when appropriately implemented and documented. Preferably a resuscitation would never begin on such a patient, but if begun before the DNR orders are discovered and verified, it should be stopped expeditiously once this is realized. Whenever possible, family members should be consulted in all resuscitation decisions. Such consultation assists in informed decision-making, prepares the family to accept death should it occur, and hence is less likely to result in a litigious outcome.

REFERENCES ■

1. Maass: Die Methode der Weiderbelebung bei Herztod nach Chloroformein Athmung. *Klin Wochenschr* 1892;9:265
2. Prevost JL, Batelli F: Sur quelques effects des descharges electriques sur le coeur des manniferers. *C R Acad Sci* 1899; 29:1267
3. Kouwenhoven WB, Jude JR, Knickerbocker GG: Closed-chest cardiac massage. *JAMA* 1960;173:1064
4. National Center for Health Statistics: Births, marriages, divorces, and deaths for March 1992. *Month Vital Stat Rep* 1992;39:3
5. Kuller L, Cooper M, Perper J, et al: Epidemiology of sudden death. *Arch Intern Med* 1972;129:714
6. *Heart Facts.* Dallas, American Heart Association, 1985:2
7. Baum RS, Alvarez H, Cobb LA: Survival after resuscitation from out-of-hospital ventricular fibrillation. *Circulation* 1974; 50:1231
8. Gudjonsson H, Baldvinsson E, Oddsson G, et al: Results of attempted cardiopulmonary resuscitation of patients dying suddenly outside the hospital in Reykjavik and the surrounding area, 1976–1979. *Acta Med Scand* 1982;212:247
9. Myerburg RJ, Conde CA, Sung RJ, et al: Clinical, electrophysiologic and hemodynamic profile of patients resuscitated from prehospital cardiac arrest. *Am J Med* 1980;68:568
10. Adgey AJ, Scott ME, Allen JD, et al: Management of ventricular fibrillation outside hospital. *Lancet* 1969;i:1169
11. Cobb LA, Baum RS, Alvarez H, et al: Resuscitation from out-of-hospital ventricular fibrillation: 4 years' follow-up. *Circulation* 1975;52(Suppl 3):223
12. Eisenberg MS, Copass MK, Hallstrom A, et al: Management of out-of-hospital cardiac arrest: failure of basic emergency medical technician services. *JAMA* 1980;243:1049
13. Vertesi L, Wilson L, Glick N: Cardiac arrest: comparison of paramedic and conventional ambulance services. *Can Med Assoc J* 1983;128:809
14. Stueven H, Troiano P, Thompson B, et al: Bystander/first responder CPR: 10 years' experience in a paramedic system. *Ann Emerg Med* 1986;15:707
15. Roth R, Stewart RD, Rogers K, et al: Out-of-hospital cardiac arrest: factors associated with survival. *Ann Emerg Med* 1984; 13:237
16. Stults KR, Brown DD, Schug VL, et al: Prehospital defibrillation performed by emergency medical technicians in rural communities. *N Engl J Med* 1984;301:219
17. Eisenberg MS, Bergner L, Hallstrom A: Out-of-hospital cardiac arrest: improved survival with paramedic services. *Lancet* 1980;i:812
18. Sherman MA: Mobile intensive care units: an evaluation of effectiveness. *JAMA* 1979;241:1899
19. Eisenberg MS, Horwood BT, Cummins RO, et al: Cardiac arrest and resuscitation: a tale of 29 cities. *Ann Emerg Med* 1990;19:179
20. Crampton RS, Aldrich RF, Gascho JA, et al: Reduction of prehospital ambulance and community coronary death rates by the community-wide emergency cardiac care system. *Am J Med* 1975;58:151
21. Bergner L, Eisenberg M, Hallstrom A, et al: *Evaluation of Paramedic Services for Cardiac Arrest*, DHHS publication no. (PHS)82-3310 (December 1981). Hyattsville, MD, National Center for Health Services Research Report Series. Springfield, VA, US Department of Health and Human Services, Public Health Services, Office of Health Research, Statistics and Technology, National Center for Health Services Research (Available from National Technical Information Services, 1982)
22. Iseri LT, Siner EJ, Humphrey SB, et al: Prehospital cardiac arrest after arrival of the paramedic unit. *J Am Coll Emerg Phys* 1977;6:530
23. Diamond NJ, Schofferman J, Elliott JW: Factors in successful resuscitation by paramedics. *J Am Coll Emerg Phys* 1977;6:42
24. Eitel DR, Walton SL, Guerci AD, et al: Out-of-hospital cardiac arrest: a 6-year experience in a suburban–rural system. *Ann Emerg Med* 1988;17:808
25. Eisenberg M, Hallstrom A, Bergner L: The ACLS score: predicting survival from out-of-hospital cardiac arrest. *JAMA* 1981;246:50
26. Weaver WD, Cobb LA, Dennis D, et al: Amplitude of ventricular fibrillation waveform and outcome after cardiac arrest. *Ann Intern Med* 1985;102:53
27. Liberthson RR, Nagel EL, Hirschman JC, et al: Prehospital

ventricular fibrillation: prognosis and a follow-up course. *N Engl J Med* 1974;291:317

28. Niemann JT: Differences in cerebral and myocardial perfusion during closed-chest resuscitation. *Ann Emerg Med* 1984;13:849
29. Cummins RO, Eisenberg MS: Prehospital cardiopulmonary resuscitation: is it effective? *JAMA* 1985;253:2408
30. Lund I, Skulberg A: Cardiopulmonary resuscitation by lay people. *Lancet* 1976x:702
31. Copley DP, Mantle JA, Rogers WJ, et al: Improved outcome for prehospital cardiopulmonary collapse with resuscitation by bystanders. *Circulation* 1977;56:901
32. Thompson RG, Hallstrom AP, Cobb LA: Bystander initiated cardiopulmonary resuscitation in the management of ventricular fibrillation. *Ann Intern Med* 1979;90:737
33. Tweed WA, Bristow G, Donen N: Resuscitation from cardiac arrest: assessment of a system providing only basic life support outside of hospital. *Can Med Assoc J* 1980;122:297
34. Guzy PM, Pearce ML, Greenfield S: The survival benefit of bystander cardiopulmonary resuscitation in a paramedic-served metropolitan area. *Am J Public Health* 1983;73:766
35. Eisenberg M, Bergner L, Hallstrom A: Paramedic programs and out-of-hospital cardiac arrest. I. Factors associated with successful resuscitation. *Am J Public Health* 1979;69:30
36. Kowalski R, Thompson BM, Horwitz L, et al: Bystander CPR in prehospital coarse ventricular fibrillation. *Ann Emerg Med* 1984;13:1016
37. Litwin PE, Eisenberg MS, Hallstrom AP, et al: The location of collapse and its effect on survival from cardiac arrest. *Ann Emerg Med* 1987;16:787
38. Standards for cardiopulmonary resuscitation (CPR) and emergency cardiac care (ECC). *JAMA* 1974;227(Suppl):833
39. Robinson JS, Sloman G, Matthew TH, et al: Survival after resuscitation from cardiac arrest in acute myocardial infarction. *Am Heart J* 1965;69:740
40. Bedell SE, Delbanco TL, Cook EF, et al: Survival after cardiopulmonary resuscitation in the hospital. *N Engl J Med* 1983;309:569
41. Peatfield RC, Sillet RW, Taylor D, et al: Survival after cardiac arrest in hospital. *Lancet* 1977;i:1223
42. Messert B, Quglieri CE: Cardiopulmonary resuscitation: perspectives and problems. *Lancet* 1976x:410
43. Jeresaty RM, Godar TJ, Liss JP: External cardiac compression in a community hospital: a 3-year experience. *Arch Intern Med* 1969;124:588
44. Hollingsworth JH: The results of cardiopulmonary resuscitation: a 3-year university hospital experience. *Ann Intern Med* 1969;71:459
45. Gregory JJ, Grace WJ: Resuscitation of the severely ill patient with acute myocardial infarction. *Am J Cardiol* 1967;20:836
46. Hofkin GA: Survival after cardiopulmonary resuscitation. *JAMA* 1967;202:653
47. Johnson AL, Tanser PH, Ulan RA, et al: Results of cardiac resuscitation in 552 patients. *Am J Cardiol* 1967;20:831
48. Grace WJ, Minogue WF: Resuscitation for cardiac arrest due to myocardial infarction. *Dis Chest* 1966;50:173
49. Stemmler EJ: Cardiac resuscitation: a 1-year study of patients resuscitated within a university hospital. *Ann Intern Med* 1965;63:613
50. Castagna J, Well MH, Shubin H: Factors determining survival with cardiac arrest. *Chest* 1974;65:527
51. Tresch DD, Ranjun KT, Raymond GH, et al: Comparison of outcome of paramedic-witnessed cardiac arrest in patients younger and older than 70 years. *Am J Cardiol* 1990;65:453
52. Taffet GE, Teasdale TA, Luchi RJ: In-hospital cardiopulmonary resuscitation. *JAMA* 1988;260:2069
53. Applebaum GE, King SE, Finucane TE: The outcome of CPR initiated in nursing homes. *J Am Geriatr Soc* 1990;38:197
54. Bonnin MJ, Pepe PE, Clark PS: Survival in the elderly after out-of-hospital cardiac arrest. *Crit Care Med* 1993;21:1645
55. Lemire JG, Johnson AL: Is cardiac resuscitation worthwhile?: a decade of experience. *N Engl J Med* 1972;286:970
56. Roser LA: Cardiopulmonary resuscitation experience in a general hospital: review of 116 consecutive resuscitation attempts during a two and one-half year period. *Arch Surg* 1967;95:658
57. Sandoval RG: Survival rate after cardiac arrest in a community hospital. *JAMA* 1965;194:675
58. Risto OR, Kajaste S, Kaste M: Neuropsychological sequelae of cardiac arrest. *JAMA* 1993;269:237
59. Levy DE, Bates D, Caronna JJ, et al: Prognosis in nontraumatic coma. *Ann Intern Med* 1981;94:293
60. Goldberg AH: Cardiopulmonary arrest. *N Engl J Med* 1974;290:381
61. Eliastam M: When to stop CPR. In: Auerbach PS, Budossi SA (eds). *Cardiac Arrest and CPR*. Rockville, MD, Aspen Publishing, 1983:215
62. *Textbook of Advanced Cardiac Life Support*. New York, American Heart Association, 1994
63. Miles SH, Cranford R, Schultz AL: The do-not-resuscitate order in a teaching hospital: considerations and a suggested policy. *Ann Intern Med* 1982;96:660
64. Smith JP, Bodai BI: Guidelines for discontinuing prehospital CPR in the emergency department: a review. *Ann Emerg Med* 1985;14:1093
65. Nachlas MM, Miller DI: Closed-chest cardiac resuscitation in patients with acute myocardial infarction. *Am Heart J* 1965;69:448
66. Mackintosh AF, Crabb ME, Grainer R, et al: The Brighton resuscitation ambulances: review of 40 consecutive survivors of out-of-hospital cardiac arrest. *Br Med J* 1978;1:1115
67. Eisenberg MS, Bergner L, Hallstrom A: Cardiac arrest in the community: importance of rapid provision and implications for program planning. *JAMA* 1979;241:1905
68. Callaham ML, Barton CW: Prediction of outcome of cardiopulmonary resuscitation from end-tidal carbon dioxide concentration. *Crit Care Med* 1990;18:358
69. Paradis NA, Martin GB, Rivers EP, et al: Coronary perfusion pressure and the return of spontaneous circulation in human cardiopulmonary resuscitation. *JAMA* 1990;263:1106
70. McIntyre KM: Medicolegal aspects of decision-making in resuscitation and life support. *Cardiovasc Rev Rep* 1983;4:46
71. *Herskovits v. Group Health*, 99 Wn. 2d 609, 664 P.2d 474 (1983)
72. Guidelines for the determination of death. *JAMA* 1981;246:2184
73. Eisendrath SJ, Jonsen AR: The living will: help or hindrance? *JAMA* 1983;249:2054
74. Peters DA: Advance medical directives: the case for the durable power of attorney in for health care. *J Legal Med* 1987;8:3
75. Mooney C: Deciding not to resuscitate hospital patients: medical and legal perspectives, Univ. 111. *Law Rev* 1986;4:1025

Critical Care, Third Edition, edited by Joseph M. Civetta,
Robert W. Taylor, and Robert R. Kirby.
Lippincott-Raven Publishers, Philadelphia, PA © 1997.

CHAPTER 13

Quality Assessment and Improvement in the Adult Intensive Care Unit

Neil S. Yeston
Jamie Roche
Susan McCaffrey

Before embarking on the creation of a truly effective quality assurance (improvement) program, one must appreciate that *everyone* involved in the treatment of critically ill patients is responsible for the quality of care delivered. Intensivists deal with a diverse group of patients hosting a variety of problems, all of which must be included in the evaluation and improvement in quality of care. This chapter presents a blueprint of a quality improvement program in a large university-affiliated surgical intensive care unit (ICU) and the impact of that program on patient care. In addition, we discuss the current use of critical paths and practice guidelines and conclude with a primer on the Joint Committee on Accreditation of Healthcare Organizations (JCAHO) survey.

The principals of total quality management and continuous quality improvement (CQI) underlie a new way of thinking about quality in health care. These principles have been employed effectively in the industrial world for over 40 years. Their use in health care requires that everyone involved in the process, whether directly or indirectly, must participate in the quality improvement program. This essential principle effectively shifts the power for solving problems from the top administrative level to caregivers and auxiliary personnel who are closest to the patient.

In the past, the Hartford Hospital (Hartford, CN) surgical ICUs were the source of major systems problems that adversely affected the operating room schedule for patients undergoing cardiothoracic surgery. Frequently, patients who required ICU postoperative care were delayed in the operating room or recovery room because "no beds were available in the ICU." Many of the beds that could have been available were occupied by patients ready to be transferred for whom no beds were available on the ward.

Not until an ad hoc group was organized that consisted of staff nurses, ward secretaries, transportation personnel, and members of the housekeeping force did the answer to this problem become apparent. They discovered that although the ICU team was prepared to transfer patients from the ICU in ample time to receive the first operating room cases of the day (i.e., by 11:00 AM), the housekeeping personnel were taking their lunch breaks at precisely the time they were needed to prepare rooms to receive the patients from the ICU. Once the problem had been identified, by including the housekeeping personnel in its evolution, it was resolved within 24 hours.

This is an example of improvement in patient care resulting from a paradigm shift away from the assumption that only the "leadership" can make effective problem-solving policy decisions to a realization that individuals closest to the problems can solve them.

ESTABLISHING A PROGRAM ◼

THE START-UP

When one embarks on a program to establish the principles of quality improvement, the goals appear almost insurmountable. This finding is especially true in the ICU where so many events occur at once that contemplation of the first move is intimidating. Hospital administrators may not be willing to provide support for this JCAHO-mandated activity. Low-cost self-help may be the only realistic solution. Given ownership of the problems, many intelligent, committed, industrious members of the health care team can function more effectively than anyone hired specifically to improve quality in the ICU. The previous example illustrates this point. The key words, ownership and authority, however, must not just be semantic but must be real and palpable for this "voluntary force" to be effective.

SELECTING A STEERING COMMITTEE

If you announce on Monday that, effective immediately, every member of the health care team will be responsible for the identification, evaluation, and resolution of problems, by Tuesday you will have created chaos. A steering committee or *quality council* should be organized to convert a centralized system (leadership making all of the decisions) into an efficient body of problem-solvers and continuous improvers of quality. The quality council should be composed of representatives from all of the vertically related departments that impact patient care: nursing, respiratory therapy, postanesthesia care unit, laboratory, and cardiothoracic surgery. The creation of such a system affords the opportunity to establish horizontal relationships between departments that, by tradition, have been vertically isolated.

Individuals representing departments that relate vertically should be invited on an ad hoc basis to address specific issues. In essence, the quality council sets policies, identifies major areas of concern to be evaluated, reviews those evaluations, and officially effects change. The process of tearing down vertical walls and making inroads into heretofore fairly autonomous fiefdoms can be accomplished only if the concept that the *patient* is central to the process of improving quality becomes paramount. This concept may seem overly simplistic or even trite, yet much can be accomplished when individuals, who previously were concerned only with their unique responsibilities, learn to respond as a group to problems. This focus can produce an ideal system that will create the best possible outcome for the ICU patient.

LEARNING TO SKI

Given the enormity of the activities in any ICU, one could spend endless hours contemplating which problems to tackle while accomplishing nothing. Solving problems one element at a time is essential. The strategy used by Olympic slalom skiers in negotiating a complicated and perilous course demonstrates a concept that we have found helpful in getting quality improvement programs off the ground. Slalom racers, too, face a formidable problem: a steep, precarious descent interrupted by an incessant number of obstacles. Any of these competitors, however, will tell you that if you look at the finish line, other than when the final gate has been passed, you are doomed to failure. Rather, each races from gate to gate, never looking past the one directly ahead, rapidly and methodically overcoming each obstacle, solving each problem and ultimately, successfully completing the course.

Using this strategy, one may also achieve a successful outcome in the ICU. Do not be paralyzed by the enormity or complexity of the problems. Selecting and resolving a few at a time leads to a better outcome at the bottom (or top) of the hill. Moreover, all participants will feel good about themselves because they have had a role in the process. And, most importantly, patient care will have been improved.

DEFINING THE SCOPE OF PRACTICE

Again, using the slalom racer example, "walk the course" before racing it. That is, know your obstacles and problems. Define the scope of your practice (Table 13-1). Who are you treating? What are their problems? Physically and therapeutically, what do you do to them and for them? This exercise allows you to identify more effectively the areas that require the greatest concentration of activity. Having surveyed the course in general, you will be ready to identify problem areas that may be amenable to improvement strategies.

INDICATOR SELECTION

Indicators are the clinical events in the ICU that occur at an observable *frequency* and expose the patient to a definable *risk*. They include logistical problems that may impact negatively on patient care or resources utilization. Select the indicators that seem essential to the quality of patient care. Do not be overly ambitious. The finish line will come soon enough! Remember, however, the main point. No matter what the results of your evaluation, you must never be satisfied that you have done enough. CQI principles dictate that room for improvement always exists. Only zero-based deficit defines true quality. Indicators identified in our ICU that are routinely monitored for improvement are listed in Table 13-2.

ESTABLISHING THRESHOLDS

A threshold is a level of occurrence above which a quality problem exists. It may be a complication rate or a systems problem. The goal is to keep the indicator frequency below the established thresholds. Some of these thresholds can be obtained from published outcome data. For example, the mortality and complication rates for major esophageal surgery have been reported; therefore, they may be used as "benchmarks" for comparison of like patients in your ICU.

Many ICU activity areas have no established outcome data. Here comparisons must be made locally or regionally. Regardless of the threshold established, an opportunity is always present to effect improvement. The following exam-

TABLE 13-1. Quality Assurance for Surgical Intensive Care Unit: Scope of Care

A. Type of patient
   1. Trauma: operative and nonoperative
   2. Emergency nontrauma: operative and nonoperative
   3. Cardiothoracic: operative and nonoperative
   4. General surgical
   5. Specialty surgical
B. Diagnoses and conditions
   1. Compromised cardiovascular function and arrhythmias
   2. Acute respiratory failure and airway management
   3. Acute and chronic renal failure
   4. Metabolic abnormalities
   5. Electrolyte abnormalities
   6. Neurologic injury and dysfunction
   7. Musculoskeletal injuries and problems
   8. Primarily and nosocomial infections
   9. Gastrointestinal problems and operations
   10. Disorders of pregnancy and gynecologic problems
C. Treatment/therapies
   1. Vasoactive central venous catheter insertion
   2. Arterial catheter insertion
   3. PA catheter insertion
   4. Transvenous pacemakers
   5. Total parenteral nutrition
   6. Enteral nutrition
   7. Hemodynamic calculations
   8. Ventilatory support (ventilators, CPAP)
   9. Antibiotic therapy
   10. Antiarrhythmic therapy
   11. Continuous sedation
   12. Muscle relaxants
   13. ICP monitoring
   14. Oximetry, arterial and mixed venous
D. Clinical activities: measurements of cardiac output and calculation of cardiopulmonary variables
   1. Detailed intake and output
   2. Monitoring vital signs
   3. Problem-oriented system evaluation
   4. Surgical wound care
   5. Care of open injuries
   6. Family support and counseling
E. Protocols
   1. PA catheter insertion
   2. Central venous catheter insertion
   3. Weaning
   4. Potassium
   5. Initial orders
F. Admission criteria
G. Discharge criteria

PA, pulmonary artery; CPAP, continuous positive airway pressure; ICP, intracranial pressure.

TABLE 13-2. SICU Indicators for Continuous Quality Improvement

   1. Admission/discharge criteria met
   2. ICU readmission rate
   3. Reintubation rate
   4. Self-extubation rate
   5. Pneumothorax rate
   6. Catheter infection rate
   7. Decubitus ulcer rate
   8. Stroke rate
   9. Cardiac arrest rate
   10. Blood conservation volume
   11. Weaning time
   12. Mortality rate
   13. Autopsy correlation

ples illustrate how these principles were put into practice in our ICU and how improvement in quality of practice was confirmed.

A QUALITY IMPROVEMENT MODEL FOR SURGICAL CRITICAL CARE ■

SETTING

The surgical ICU at Hartford Hospital, University of Connecticut, consists of 24 acute care and 8 intermediate critical care beds for the treatment of all general surgery and specialty surgery patients, including heart and liver transplantation, but excluding burn wounds in excess of 30% body surface area. The unit admits over 1700 patients per year. Administratively, it is run by a full-time, hospital-employed director who is assisted by eight associate directors, all of whom are board certified in surgery or anesthesiology, and all of whom have added qualifications in critical care medicine.

Nursing leadership consists of nurse managers, clinical specialists, and nurse educators. In addition, a member of the Pharmacy department consults daily in the unit. Formal ICU rotations are available to surgery, anesthesia, oromaxillofacial, and obstetrics and gynecology residents. Fellowship training in critical care is approved by the American Boards of Surgery and Anesthesiology.

ORGANIZATIONAL FRAMEWORK

In 1987, an Intensive Care Unit Collaborative Practice Committee (Quality Council) was established, the main function of which was to serve as a steering committee for quality of care issues in the surgical ICU. The committee was comprised of ICU leadership members in addition to individuals representing postanesthesia care, cardiothoracic surgery, respiratory therapy, pharmacology, staff nursing, and critical care residents. It identifies and receives all quality improvement issues from the various reporting sources. Occasionally, ad hoc teams are charged with the responsibility for monitoring, evaluating, and recommending improvements to resolve quality issues. Ultimately, the Council establishes, where appropriate, policy from the information received.

DATA COLLECTION

Voluntary personnel assisted in the data collection process because full-time personnel were not available. Staff nurses collected data on admission and discharge criteria, decubitus ulcer rate, and blood product usage. Respiratory therapists monitored reintubation and self-extubation. The remainder of the data were collected by the ICU fellows.

Currently, data are collected using an ICU registry tool (Fig. 13-1). The registry includes indicator data and is designed to be a scannable document (OpScan 5 Optical Mark Reader, National Computer Systems, Minneapolis, MN). This instrument scans at a rate of 2000 sheets per hour, eliminating the need for data entry personnel. In addition, the ICU registry is part of a relational data base that is related to data obtained from our ICU morbidity/mortality data base, also a scannable document (Fig. 13-2). All relevant quality-of-care data are captured, collated, and reported to the Council on a quarterly basis.

The following examples illustrate the impact of such a quality improvement program on the critical care environment (Table 13-3).

INDICATOR: ADMISSION AND DISCHARGE CRITERIA

As mandated by the JCAHO, we monitored our compliance with admission and discharge criteria as defined in our policy and procedure manual. Even before collecting the data, we

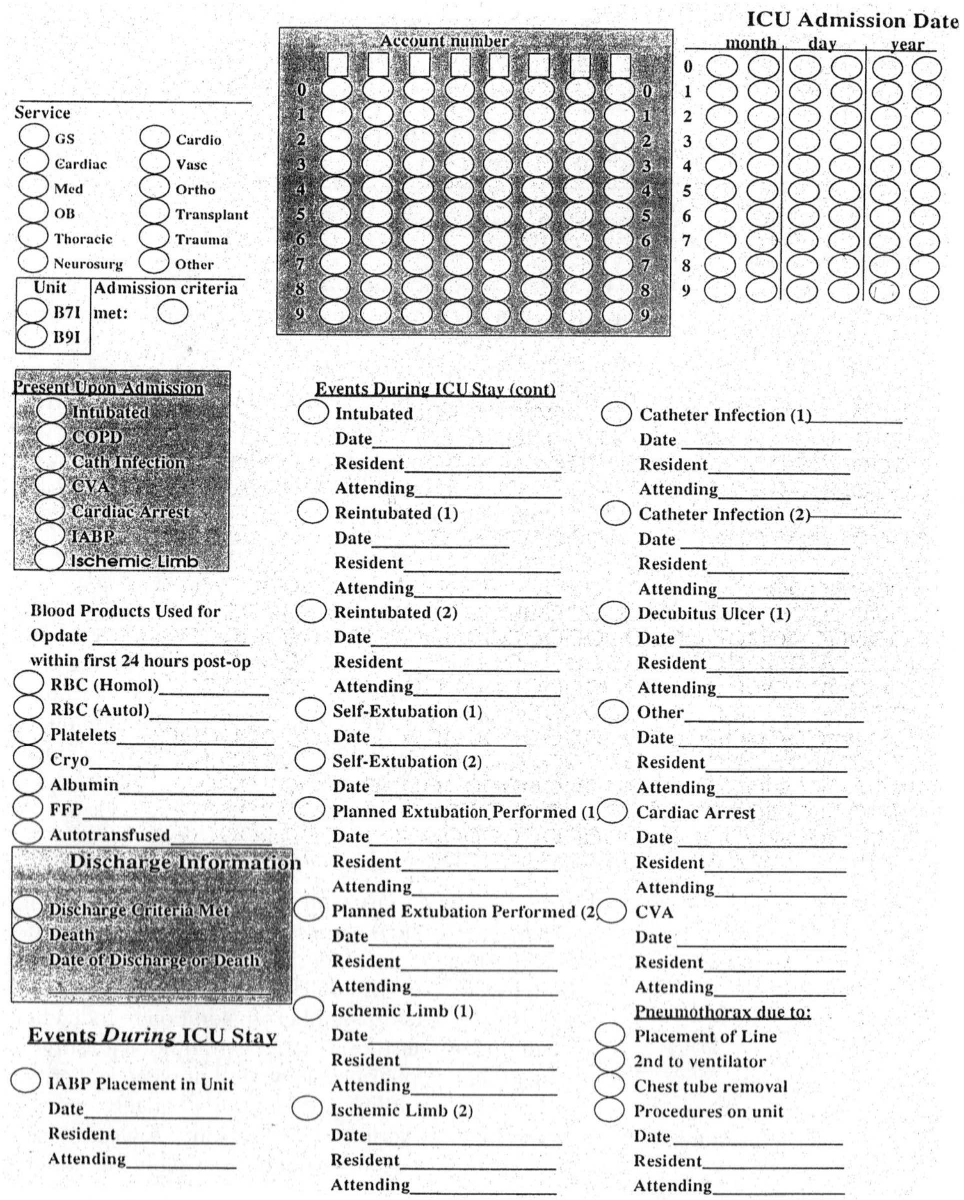
Account number
0 1 2 3 4 5 6 7 8 9

ICU Admission Date
month day year
0 1 2 3 4 5 6 7 8 9

Service
GS
Cardiac
Med
OB
Thoracic
Neurosurg
Cardio
Vasc
Ortho
Transplant
Trauma
Other

Unit
B7I
B9I

Admission criteria met:

Present Upon Admission
Intubated
COPD
Cath Infection
CVA
Cardiac Arrest
IABP
Ischemic Limb

Blood Products Used for
Opdate
within first 24 hours post-op
RBC (Homol)
RBC (Autol)
Platelets
Cryo
Albumin
FFP
Autotransfused

Discharge Information
Discharge Criteria Met
Death
Date of Discharge or Death

Events *During* ICU Stay
IABP Placement in Unit
Date
Resident
Attending

Events During ICU Stay (cont)
Intubated
Date
Resident
Attending
Reintubated (1)
Date
Resident
Attending
Reintubated (2)
Date
Resident
Attending
Self-Extubation (1)
Date
Self-Extubation (2)
Date
Planned Extubation Performed (1)
Date
Resident
Attending
Planned Extubation Performed (2)
Date
Resident
Attending
Ischemic Limb (1)
Date
Resident
Attending
Ischemic Limb (2)
Date
Resident
Attending

Catheter Infection (1)
Date
Resident
Attending
Catheter Infection (2)
Date
Resident
Attending
Decubitus Ulcer (1)
Date
Resident
Attending
Other
Date
Resident
Attending
Cardiac Arrest
Date
Resident
Attending
CVA
Date
Resident
Attending
Pneumothorax due to:
Placement of Line
2nd to ventilator
Chest tube removal
Procedures on unit
Date
Resident
Attending

FIGURE 13-1. Hartford Hospital ICU Registry data collection form.

SICU Morbidity and Mortality

Name _____   Account # _____

Date of conference _____   Age _____   Sex M ___ F ___

B71 ___   B7SD ___   B91 ___   B9SD ___   ICU attending _____

Service: C Surg ___   Trauma ___   Trans ___   Other ___
                G Surg ___   PVS ___   Thor ___

Cause of death: Cardiac ___   Resp ___
                        MSOF ___   Withdraw ___
                        Neuro ___   Hemorrhage ___
                        Sepsis ___

Complications:

ICU complication _____

☐ Cardiac   ☐ Respiratory
  ___ Arrhythmia   ___ Resp failure
  ___ Myocardial infarction   ___ PE
  ___ CHF   ___ ARDS
  ___ Cardiac arrest   ___ Reintubation
  ___ Low output state   ___ PTX
  ___ Other   ___ Self-extubation
                                           ___ Other

☐ Technical   ☐ Infections
  ___ PA cath complication   ___ Pneumonia
  ___ CVP complication   ___ Bacteremia
  ___ Heimlich complication   ___ UTI
  ___ Other   ___ Septic shock
                                           ___ Other

☐ Miscellaneous   ☐ Neurologic
  ___ DIC   ___ CVA
  ___ Readmission   ___ Coma
  ___ Liver failure   ___ Other
  ___ Renal failure
  ___ Other
  ___ Readmission to ICU

                            ☐ Error in judgment
                            ☐ Error in diagnosis
                            ☐ Error in technique
                            ☐ Delay—prehospital
                            ☐ Delay—preconsult
                            ☐ Delay—preoperative
                            ☐ Extradepartmental (specify) _____

Refer to quality assurance department
      ___ Yes   ___ No

Signature to verify information and review

_____ MD

FIGURE 13-2. Hartford Hospital morbidity and mortality data collection form.

knew that we were not universally in compliance with our own existing discharge criteria. The validity of these criteria was questionable, but the criteria had a long history of "that's how we've always done it." The criteria required that to be transferred from the ICU to the ward, a patient had to have achieved a room air PaO$_2$ in excess of 55 mm Hg. Although this practice was probably "safest" for patients who went to less monitored settings, it was systematically violated without apparent adverse outcome.

We evaluated the frequency of "breaking the rule" and the impact on patient care of the rule having been broken. After evaluating 101 consecutive discharges from the ICU, we discovered that 16% of patients were discharged with a room air PaO$_2$ of less than 55 mm Hg. However, the readmission rate for that group was identical (6%) to the other 84% of patients who had a PaO$_2$ greater than 55 mm Hg. Notwithstanding these data, nursing personnel were concerned about the possibility that the number of hours per patient per day required to care for those "sicker" patients (room air PaO$_2$ less than 55 mm Hg) would require disproportionately more nursing care. This possibility could have a negative impact on the care given to less sick patients.

Accordingly, we examined this hypothesis and failed to confirm either a difference in readmission rate or hours per patient day for either group. Consequently, the Quality Council voted to rescind the "Room Air" rule while continuing to carefully evaluate readmissions to the ICU that may have occurred as a result of hypoxemia. To date, we have not observed any increase in readmissions as a result of this action. Table 13-3A describes our current compliance with the published admission and discharge criteria in our unit.

INDICATOR: READMISSION RATE

A measure of appropriateness of one's discharge criteria is the rate of ICU readmission. This figure may differ from unit to unit and may be significantly different if a stepdown unit is available to serve as a buffer between the acute care ICU and the more convalescent ward environment. Our readmission rate for fiscal year 1993 to 1994 was 50 of 1898 patients (2.6%) (see Table 13-3B). Other institutions have reported readmission rates as high as 9.4%.[1] Regardless of the exact rate, we must refine our ICU registry to capture the data that might identify the exact reasons for readmission. The resulting identification of a "pattern of care" can then form the basis for the correction of problems that should ultimately reduce the rate of readmission even further.

INDICATOR: SELF-EXTUBATION

All ICU personnel who care for numerous, mechanically ventilated patients have experienced the often unpleasant experience of the inadvertently extubated patient. Such patients have the potential to sustain significant morbidity.[2] Data gleaned from our ICU morbidity/mortality conference indicate that this complication occurred often enough to be worthy of study. A systematic, prospective evaluation of the problem revealed that of 133 intubated patients, 8 extubated themselves. This "self-extubation rate" of 7.5% was well

TABLE 13-3. SICU Quality Improvement (6 months)

A. ADMISSION AND DISCHARGE CRITERIA MET

Criteria	No.	%
Admission criteria met	1892	99.7
Discharge criteria met	1873	98.7

B. READMISSION RATE

Patients (no.)	Readmits (no.)	Readmits (%)
1898	50	2.63

C. SELF-EXTUBATION RATE

Intubated patients (no.)	Self-extubations (no.)	Self-extubations (%)
1646	42	2.55

D. REINTUBATION RATE

Intubated patients (no.)	Reintubations (no.)	Reintubations (%)
16461	95	5.77

E. REINTUBATION RATE

Intubated	Reintubated	Rate (%)
154 (COLD)	11	7.14
1492 (No COLD)	61	4.1

% of reintubated patients without COLD: 61/72 (85%)
% of reintubated patients with COLD: 11/72 (15%)

F. PNEUMOTHORAX

Central catheters (no.)	Pneumothoraces (no.)	Pneumothoraces (%)
521	8	1.5

G. DECUBITUS ULCER RATE

Patients (no.)	Decubitus ulcers (no.)	Decubitus ulcers (%)
1898	10	0.53

H. CEREBROVASCULAR ACCIDENT RATE

Patients (no.)	CVA (no.)	CVA (%)
1898	17	0.9

I. CARDIAC ARREST RATE

Patients (no.)	Cardiac arrests (no.)	Cardiac arrests (%)
1898	29	1.53

COLD, chronic obstructive lung disease.

below the published rate of 11%, indicating in theory that the complication was not a "problem" in our ICU.

Using the principle of CQI, we chose to analyze and improve the system. The original protocol to protect against self-extubation and the restraint technology were both primitive. Accordingly, after reassessing our protocol in addition to evaluating new, potentially more effective temporary restraint technologies, we prospectively remonitored this indicator for improvement and identified that only 13 of 522 intubated patients had extubated themselves, a rate of

2.49%. Thus, we significantly reduced the threshold for self-extubation and monitored compliance (see Table 13-3C). Although only 42 of 1646 intubated patients in the 1993 to 1994 period self-extubated, we continue to strive for better outcomes. We have observed that most self-extubations occur in the immediate postoperative period by agitated patients emerging from anesthesia. Accordingly, a "Sedation Task Force" has been formed and charged to seek solutions.

INDICATOR: REINTUBATION RATE

A prime indicator of clinical judgment in the critical care environment is the ability to predict accurately those individuals who can be weaned from mechanical ventilation and successfully extubated. The literature is replete with measurements, formulas, and algorithms, too numerous to be reviewed in this chapter, that attempt to define the perfect predictor for extubation. We do not rely on a rigid protocol to determine who should be extubated and when. In general, patients are extubated who have an adequate PaO_2 (greater than 60 mm Hg), a fraction of inspired oxygen less than 0.5, a $PaCO_2$ of 35 to 45 mm Hg (or greater if premorbid arterial blood gas analysis revealed carbon dioxide retention), and a normal pH that is not associated with rapid shallow breathing or copious secretions. Table 13-3D depicts the resulting reintubation rate experienced in our ICU.

Establishment of meaningful thresholds for this complication requires the identification of three distinct patient groups: those who are expected to be weaned and extubated soon after intubation (24 to 48 hours), those with premorbid chronic obstructive lung disease (COLD), and those who require prolonged mechanical ventilation resulting from a variety of problems (e.g., pneumonia, acute respiratory distress syndrome [ARDS], and respiratory muscle weakness). Demling and associates identified thresholds for patients expected to be weaned and extubated shortly after being mechanically ventilated (4%),[3] but the threshold for patients who have significant COLD or advanced ARDS may be as high as 20%.[4]

The data presented in Table 13-3E allow us to differentiate our patient population into the groups described earlier. Although we are clearly at or below our threshold (i.e., reintubation rate of 4% non-COLD and 7.1% COLD), we seek to further improve our results. We currently are evaluating new technology (Bicore CP100, Riverside, CA) specifically designed to measure the patient and ventilator circuitry work of breathing to improve our ability to accurately predict the patients who can successfully sustain extubation.

INDICATOR: PNEUMOTHORAX RATE

Pneumothorax secondary to attempted central venous access is well known but poorly tolerated (patient, perpetrator, and chief-of-service alike). The incidence of this complication ranges from 0% to 5% with an average of 1% to 2%.[5] Even in the most able hands, this complication is sometimes unavoidable. However, logic and experience suggest that when the least experienced individual participates unsupervised in placing central catheters, the complication may be expected to exceed acceptable thresholds.

We developed a process of certifying house staff rotating through the ICU in the insertion of central venous catheters (single lumen, triple lumen, and pulmonary artery; Figs. 13-3 through 13-5). Once we have satisfactory evidence that the house officer is secure in the anatomy and technique of this procedure, the certification process is complete. A minimum of five successful insertions certifies that the house officers may perform the procedure unsupervised (except pulmonary artery catheters for which either an ICU fellow or attending is required to be in attendance).

Figure 13-6 represents the form used for collecting these and other data. Documentation of the certification process by individuals is kept in a three-ring binder. In addition, the house officer receives at the conclusion of the rotation, a summary of the procedures performed. A recent audit of the impact of this certification process evaluating 521 catheters inserted revealed a pneumothorax rate of 1.5% (see Table 13-3F).

INDICATOR: CATHETER INFECTION RATE

Initial surveillance of our catheter-related infections suggested a catheter-colonization incidence rate (greater than 15 colony-forming units) of 8.5% and an associated bacteremia incidence rate of 3.4%. Although the latter is within recognized acceptable thresholds,[6,7] any catheter-related infection potentially may result in significant morbidity or mortality. We modified the insertion and care protocol in collaboration with our infection control personnel. Subsequently, we demonstrated a reduction in catheter-related bacteremia to 1.3%. This change not only improved patient care, but also preempted the need for a more expensive solution, the use of silver-impregnated catheters. As a result of our improvement, quality of care standards were increased and resources were effectively conserved.

INDICATOR: DECUBITUS ULCER

The presence of a decubitus ulcer in the ICU is almost always related to poor nursing care. When we prospectively monitored the incidence of decubitus ulcers in our unit, only 33 of 562 patients (5.9%) developed this untoward event, compared with 8% reported previously.[8]

The ICU Quality Council appointed an ad hoc group to study the problem systematically. Sidarenko and coworkers[9] measured sacral and heel pressure (Fig. 13-7) on patients in recumbent and 45-degree sitting positions on three different mattresses, one of which was the standard mattress used in our ICU. Figures 13-8 and 13-9 depict the distinct benefit of two of the mattresses over the third. These data were used to justify the trial of one of the mattresses that transmitted less pressure.

Prospective monitoring of the next 734 consecutive patients admitted to the ICU demonstrated that the incidence rate of decubitus ulcers was reduced to 0.2%.[9] Of the last 1898 admissions to our ICU, only 10 patients (0.5%) had this complication (see Table 13-3G). This example represents another improvement in quality when the prior incidence of the problem was already below a satisfactory threshold.

Subclavian Vein Catheterization   Resident's name _____

Observed
Yes   No

1. Place the patient in supine position, with the head at least 15 degrees down to distend the neck veins and to prevent air embolism. Turn the patient's head away from the venipuncture side.   ___ ___

2. Clean the skin around the venipuncture site well and drape the area. Wear sterile gloves when performing this procedure   ___ ___

3. If the patient is awake, use a local anesthetic at the venipuncture site.   ___ ___

4. Introduce a large-bore needle, attached to a 6-mL syringe with 0.5 to 1 mL of saline, 1 cm below the junction of the middle and medial thirds of the clavicle.   ___ ___

5. After the skin has been punctured and with the bevel of the needle upward, expel the skin plug that may occlude the needle.   ___ ___

6. Hold the needle and syringe parallel to the frontal plane.   ___ ___

7. Direct the needle medially, slightly cephalad, and posteriorly behind the clavicle toward the posterior superior angle of the sternal end of the clavicle (toward a finger placed in the suprasternal notch).   ___ ___

8. Slowly advance the needle while gently withdrawing the plunger syringe.   ___ ___

9. When a free flow of blood appears in the syringe, rotate the bevel of the needle caudally; remove the syringe and occlude the needle with a finger to prevent air embolism.   ___ ___

10. Quickly insert the guide wire to a predetermined depth (the tip of the wire should be above the right atrium for fluid administration).   ___ ___

11. Remove the needle and advance the catheter over the wire.   ___ ___

12. Remove the wire.   ___ ___

13. Affix the catheter in place (i.e., with suture), apply antibiotic ointment, and dress the area.   ___ ___

14. Tape the intravenous tubing in place.   ___ ___

15. Attach the CVP to transducer (level at zero) with the level of the patient's right atrium.   ___ ___

16. Obtain a chest film to ascertain the position of the intravenous line and determine whether there exists a possible pneumothorax.   ___ ___

Preceptor's comments:

Patient assessed in proper sequence? Yes _____   No _____

Preceptor's name: _____

FIGURE 13-3. Hartford Hospital certification process of invasive catheter insertion—subclavian vein.

INDICATOR: CEREBROVASCULAR ACCIDENT

This indicator represents our ability to maintain effective cerebral blood flow while avoiding extremes of blood pressure. It also relates to the effectiveness of anticoagulation strategies when appropriate (e.g., atrial fibrillation, bioprosthesis). Continuous surveillance of this indicator is depicted in Table 13-3*H*. We are unaware of any published rates for this indicator and have arbitrarily selected a threshold of 2%.

INDICATOR: CARDIAC ARREST

Similarly, we selected the frequency of cardiac arrest as an indicator of our ability to maximize myocardial blood flow, avoid coronary artery ischemia, reduce myocardial oxygen demands, and prevent or treat malignant arrhythmias. Table 13-3*I* illustrates our ability to prevent this untoward event. Again, we are unaware of any published reports of these data for a surgical ICU and have arbitrarily selected a threshold of 3% as accepted frequency. Strategies for further reducing the incidence of this complication can be developed as a result of ongoing analysis of care.

INDICATOR: BLOOD PRODUCT CONSERVATION

In the ICU, hemoglobin and hematocrit frequently drift downward over time in a predictable fashion, often necessitating transfusion. This phenomenon often occurs without an identifiable source of blood loss except routine, and sometimes excessive, phlebotomy. Smoller and Kruskal[10] report

Central Venous Catheterization   Resident's name _____
Internal Jugular

		Observed
		Yes No

1. Place the patient in supine position, with the head at least 15 degrees down to distend the neck veins and to prevent air embolism. Turn the patient's head away from the venipuncture side.   ___ ___

2. Clean the skin around the venipuncture site well and drape the area. Wear sterile gloves when performing this procedure.   ___ ___

3. If the patient is awake, use a local anesthetic at the venipuncture site.   ___ ___

4. a) Introduce a needle, attached to a 6-mL syringe with 0.5 to 1 mL of saline, in the center of the triangle formed by the two lower heads of the sternocleidomastoid and the clavicle (central approach).   ___ ___

   b) Introduce the needle at the posterior edge of the sternocleidomastoid muscle 2 fingerbreaths above the clavicle.   ___ ___

5. After the skin has been punctured and with the bevel of the needle upward, expel the skin plug that may occlude the needle.   ___ ___

6. a) Direct the needle toward the ipsilateral nipple or hip and at a 30- to 45-degree angle to the skin (central approach).   ___ ___

   b) Direct the needle toward the medial clavicular head of the sternocleido-mastoid and parallel to the horizontal plane.   ___ ___

7. Slowly advance the needle while gently withdrawing the plunger of the syringe.   ___ ___

8. When a free flow of blood appears in the syringe, remove the syringe and occlude the needle with a finger to prevent air embolism.   ___ ___

9. Quickly insert the guide wire to a predetermined depth (the tip of the wire should be above the right atrium for fluid administration).   ___ ___

10. Remove the needle and advance the catheter over the wire.   ___ ___

11. Remove the wire.   ___ ___

12. Affix the catheter in place (i.e., with suture), and apply antibiotic ointment, and dress the area.   ___ ___

13. Tape the intravenous tubing in place.   ___ ___

14. Obtain a chest film to ascertain the position of the intravenous line and to determine whether there exists a possible pneumothorax.   ___ ___

Preceptor's comments:

Patient assessed in proper sequence? Yes _____   No _____

Preceptor's name: _____

FIGURE 13-4. Hartford Hospital certification process of invasive catheter insertion—internal jugular.

Insertion of a Pulmonary Artery Catheter   Resident's name _____

                                                                          Observed
                                                                          Yes   No

1. Follow the same procedure as for a CVP catheter, up to and including insertion of the   __   __
    guide wire.

2. Insert the dilator and introducer over the guide wire; remove the wire.   __   __

3. Remove the dilator, and suture the introducer in place.   __   __

4. Test the PA catheter balloon, and irrigate the CVP and PA port with D_5W.   __   __

5. Insert the PA catheter through the diaphragm and advance to 20 cm; inflate the balloon.   __   __

6. Advance slowly until the RV trace is seen (approximately 35 to 40 cm).   __   __

7. Advance until the PA trace is seen (approximately 35 to 40 cm). Stop.   __   __

8. With the balloon inflated, advance millimeter by millimeter until the wedge trace position   __   __
    is identified.

9. Deflate the balloon.   __   __

10. Reinflate the balloon slowly. If the wedge pressure is below 0.75 mL, deflate the balloon,   __   __
    withdraw it slightly, and reinflate it. The catheter should wedge with approximately 1 mL
    of air.

11. The PA catheter would be in wedge tract position (between 45 and 50 cm).   __   __

12. If the proper waver forms are not seen, deflate the balloon.   __   __

13. Apply a sterile dressing.   __   __

14. Rebalance and calibrate the transducer.

Preceptor's comments:

Patient assessed in proper sequence? Yes _____   No _____

Preceptor's name: _____

FIGURE 13-5. Hartford Hospital certification process of invasive catheter insertion—pulmonary artery.

that an average of 65 mL per day of blood is lost by the ICU patient to the phlebotomist.

The problem was brought to the attention of the ICU Quality Council by members of the nursing staff who had developed a closed reinfusion system designed to conserve blood lost to the ICU patient. This system reduced the obligatory amount of blood that was discarded to clear the line before the sample was drawn for laboratory evaluation. This volume previously lost for lab tests averaged 69 mL per patient per day. The closed system (Fig. 13-10) permitted the previously discarded blood volume to be retained and then reinfused after the sample was collected. This technique resulted in an average blood loss of only 35 mL per patient per day,[11] and a reduction in the incidence of transfusion in a stable, nonbleeding patient population from 51% to 40%.

INDICATOR: WEANING TIME, POSTCARDIOPULMONARY BYPASS PROCEDURES

Members of our cardiothoracic surgery department expressed concern that routine weaning of postoperative cardiopulmonary bypass patients was prolonged. We discovered that 33% of patients required in excess of 24 hours to be weaned from mechanical ventilation and successfully extubated. This period seemed to our cardiothoracic surgeons (and us) to be prolonged.

When the system was evaluated by an ad hoc group assigned by the ICU Quality Council, several inefficiencies were identified. Principal among them was the lack of a "weaning protocol." In addition, a required arterial blood gas analysis order for each reduction in intermittent mandatory ventilation also slowed extubation.

Consequently, a protocol was instituted that resulted in a reduction in mean time to extubation from 18 hours to 14 hours. Successful extubation of 98% of our patients after routine cardiopulmonary bypass occurred within 24 hours of their ICU admission. This modification, in addition to other refinements, helped to reduce almost immediately the ICU average length of stay from 4.4 days to 2.4 days and the total hospital length of stay from 17.9 days to 12.2 days. Further refinement of the process (e.g., critical paths, change in anesthetic technique) has enabled us to reduce the extubation time to 6 hours and to reduce our ICU length of stay to 1.6 days including step down. Quality improvement at its best!!

HARTFORD HOSPITAL PROCEDURES DEPT: SURGERY CCM

HISTORY NUMBER

DATE: _____
TIME: _____ AM
_____ PM

RESIDENT/PA FELLOW: _____
ATTENDING: _____

PERMIT SIGNED?: (Y) (N)
○ EMERGENT

ICU LOCATION: _____

ICU DIAGNOSIS
- ① CHF
- ② MYO INS.
- ③ MYO INF.
- ④ PNEU B,V,F
- ⑤ RESP. INS.
- ⑥ RESP. FAIL
- ⑦ CVA
- ⑧ CARD ARR.
- ⑨ SEP
- ⑩ SEP SH
- ⑪ CARDIO SH
- ⑫ HEMM _____
- ⑬ RENAL INSUFF
- ⑭ OLIG
- ⑮ NUTR DIFF
- ⑯ COMA
- ⑰ PE
- ⑱ ABN LYTES
- ⑲ ACID BASE
- ⑳ OTHER_____

PROCEDURE   (MARK MAX OF 1)
VASC
- ① CVP
- ② SWAN-GANZ
- ③ ARTERIAL LINE
- ④ FEM CATH
- ⑤ PACEMAKER
ASP
- ⑥ THORACENTESIS
- ⑦ PARACENTESIS
- ⑧ LP
- ⑨ JOINT ASPIRATION
- ⑮ DIALYSIS CATHETER
GI
- ⑯ TUBE THORACOSTOMY
BX
- ⑰ HEIMLICH CATHETER
- ⑱ TRACHEAL INTUBATION
- ⑲ CVP OVER WIRE
RX
- ⑳ PERITONEAL LAVAGE

ACCESS SITE
SIDE
- (R) RIGHT
- (L) LEFT
- (C) CENTER/MIDLINE
VEIN
- ① INTERNAL JUGULAR
- ② SUBCLAVIAN
- ③ FEMORAL
ART
- ④ AXILLARY
- ⑤ RADIAL
- ⑥ FEMORAL
SP
- ⑦ _____ INTERCOSTAL SPACE
- ⑧ _____ DISC SPACE
ABD
- ⑨ LOWER QUADRANT

INDICATION   (MARK MAX OF 3)
DX
- ① INFECTION
- ② NEOPLASM
- ③ BLEED
- ⑧ OTHER

CARD
- ⑨ HYPOTENSION
- ⑩ CHF
- ⑪ ASSESS VOLUME STATUS
- ⑫ BRADY/TACHY ARRYTHMIA

RESP
- ⑬ PULMONARY INFILTRATES
- ⑭ HYPOXEMIA
- ⑮ PLEURAL EFFUSION
- ⑯ RESPIRATORY FAILURE

REN
- ⑰ RENAL INSUFFICIENCY

OI
- ⑱ ASCITES
- ⑲ GI BLEED

RTC
- ㉓ BLOOD SAMPLE
- ㉔ ACCESS
- ㉕ INFUSION - MEDICINE
- ㉖ INFUSION - FLUID
- ㉗ INFUSION - NUTRITION
- ㉘ MONITOR

HEMODYNAMIC INFORMATION
- ① PAS _____
- ② PAD _____
- ③ PAM _____
- ④ PCWP _____
- ⑤ CO _____
- ⑥ CI _____
- ⑦ SVR _____
- ⑧ SVRI _____
- ⑨ O_2 DEL _____
- ⑩ O_2 CON _____
- ⑪ PV O_2 _____
- ⑫ MV SAT _____

COMPLICATION   (Y) (N)
CARD
- ① ARRYTHMIA
- ② CARDIAC ARREST
- ③ CARDIAC PERFORATION
- ④ HYPOTENSION
VASC
- ⑤ ARTERIAL CANNULATION
- ⑥ ARTERIAL INSUFFICIENCY
- ⑦ BALLOON RUPTURE
- ⑧ CATH/WIRE MIGRATION
- ⑨ CATH/WIRE TANGLE
- ⑩ THROMBOSIS
- ⑪ EMBOLISM
- ⑫ VENOUS INSUFFICIENCY
HEM
- ⑬ HEMORRHAGE - MAJOR
- ⑭ HEMORRHAGE - MINOR
- ⑮ HEMATOMA
RESP
ID
- ⑯ PNEUMOTHORAX
- ⑰ FEVER
- ⑱ INFECTION - LOCAL
- ⑲ INFECTION - SYSTEMIC
CNS
- ⑳ CNS SX
- ㉑ CEREBRAL HERNIATION
- ㉒ CSF LEAK
- ㉓ PARAPLEGIA
- ㉔ PERSISTENT HEADACHE
GI
GEN
- ㉕ BOWEL PERFORATION
- ㉖ DEATH
- ㉗ PAIN
- ㉘ DRUG REACTION
- ㉙ PERFORATION
- ㉚ PERSISTENT FLUID LEAK
- ㉛ OTHER
- ㉜ INADEQUATE SPECIMEN

FINDINGS
_____
_____
_____

FIGURE 13-6. Hartford Hospital Procedures Department data collection form.

INDICATOR: MORTALITY

To attribute a mortality reduction to directly measurable improvements in quality of care is difficult. Nevertheless, most ICUs are committed to comparing their "report cards" with those of like units as a benchmark of the quality of care that is being delivered in their institutions. Although no consensus exists for a system to compare the results from one ICU to another, we assessed our outcomes with others using Acute Physiology Score and Chronic Health Evaluation (APACHE) II scoring.[12] Figure 13-11 depicts our observed mortality compared with predicted rates.

INDICATOR: AUTOPSY CORRELATION

We attempted to correlate results of the postmortem examination with the care delivered to patients who have died in our ICU. Goldman and researchers[13] suggest a system of classification of postmortem findings that were related to diagnoses not recognized in the premorbid state (Table 13-4).

We evaluated 89 patients who died in our unit from 1986 through 1991. The ICU autopsy rate during that period was 22% to 26% per year, whereas the hospital autopsy rate was 13% to 16% per year. During that period, 47% of autopsies

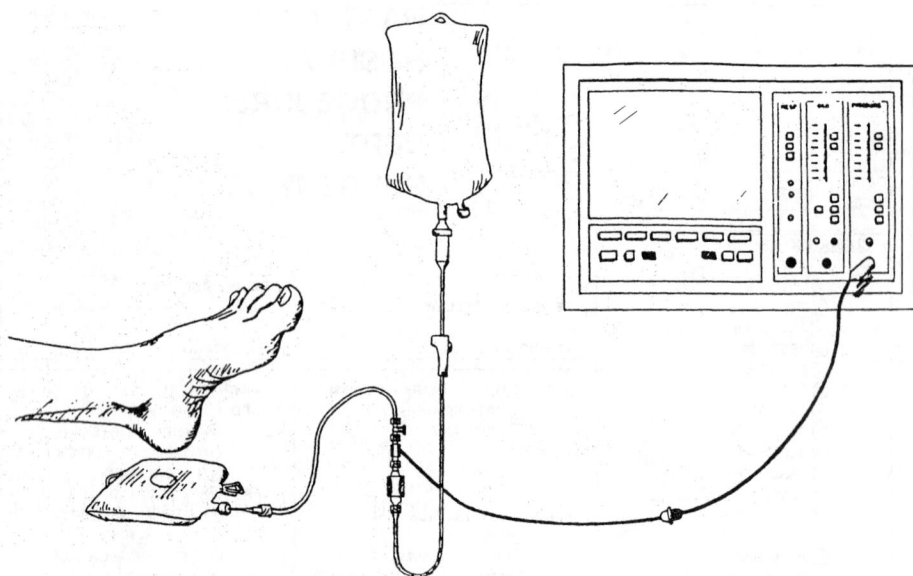

FIGURE 13-7. Instruments to measure sacral and heel pressure. (From Sideranko S, Quinn A, Burns K, et al: Effects of position and mattress overlay on sacral and heel pressures in a clinical population. *Res Nurs Health* 1992;15:245.)

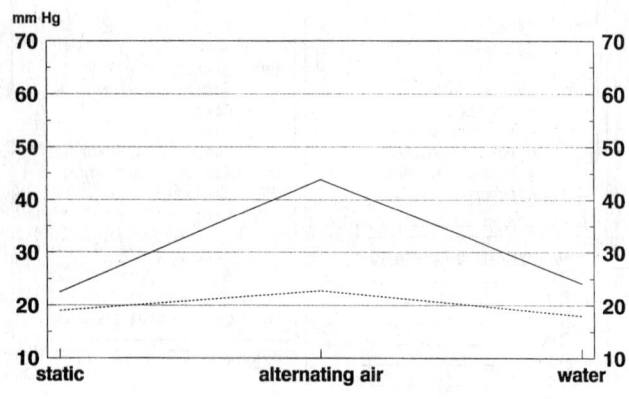

FIGURE 13-8. Recumbent sacrum (*solid line*) heel (*dashed line*). $P < .05$ for three-way interaction. (From Sideranko S, Quinn A, Burns K, et al: Effects of position and mattress overlay on sacral and heel pressures in a clinical population. *Res Nurs Health* 1992;15:245.)

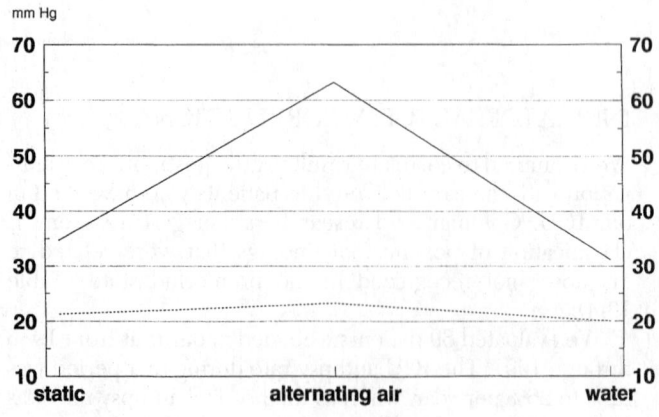

FIGURE 13-9. Sacrum (*solid line*) heel (*dashed line*) 45 degrees. Heel and sacral pressures measured in the 45-degree supine position with three different mattress types. $P < .05$ for three-way interaction. (From Sideranko S, Quinn A, Burns K, et al: Effects of position and mattress overlay on sacral and heel pressures in a clinical population. *Res Nurs Health* 1992;15:245.)

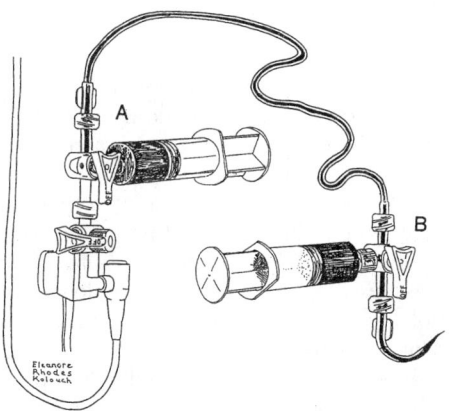

FIGURE 13-10. Blood conservation technology. (From Gleason, Grossman S, Campbell C: Minimizing diagnostic blood loss in critically ill patients. *Am J Crit Care* 1992;1:85.)

TABLE 13-4. Postmortem Findings Not Recognized Premortem

Class 1 A missed diagnosis, the detection of which would probably have altered management and would probably have resulted in a longer survival or possible cure

Class 2 A missed major diagnosis, the detection of which would not have altered therapy or outcome

Class 3 A missed minor diagnosis that would have changed outcome if detected premortem

Class 4 A missed minor diagnosis that may have contributed to the patient's death

Class 5 No unexpected findings

failed to reveal any major unexpected findings before death (class 5). Conversely, major unexpected autopsy findings were identified in 29% of cases. Further analysis revealed that undiagnosed fungal infections accounted for 54% of class I findings. This value rose to 80% in patients who underwent organ transplantation. Recognition of this outcome led us to conduct more rigorous surveillance of fungal infections in the ICU population. Hopefully, earlier identification and treatment of that disease process has the potential to reduce mortality.

RISK MANAGEMENT ■

The risk management program in our ICU includes reporting medication errors, patient falls, laboratory sample errors, major complications, and the identification of untoward events documented in incident reports. We strongly believe that the most effective risk management program is the presence of a highly organized, effective, quality improvement program. Failure of our ICU personnel to be implicated in risk management claims is impressive testimony of this tenet.

CRITICAL PATHS ■

CONCEPT

Critical paths are tools adopted by many health care institutions over the last decade to improve patient care. They exist in various formats and have been popularized principally through the efforts of Karen Zander.[14] A critical path is a plan that shows the critical or key events that must occur in a predictable and timely fashion to achieve collaboratively agreed-on patient outcomes based on patient needs. The goals of critical paths include lower cost, higher quality care; shifting the focus of care to better meet patient and family needs; opening lines of communication among caregivers; providing a mechanism for data collection and analysis for CQI; and education of patients and caregivers.

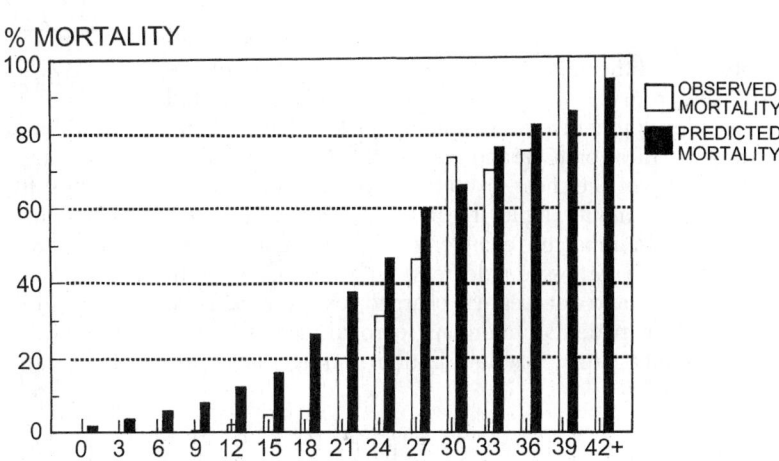

FIGURE 13-11. Predicted versus observed mortality, APACHE II score. (Based on intensive care unit registry, 10/1/93 to 9/30/94.)

IMPLEMENTATION

In most institutions, critical paths are paper documents that share similar characteristics. The format is generally grid-like (Fig. 13-12) with a time line on one axis and a menu on the other. The time line may be divided into units of time (hours, days, weeks) or phases of illness or development (e.g., trimesters of pregnancy). The menu includes expected outcomes, consults, patient activity, mobility, education, and discharge management elements, among others.

Critical paths are created through the combined efforts of the health care team after careful selection of the target population (usually on the basis of high volume or high cost). This step is followed by a review of the literature and published practice guidelines, benchmarking with other institutions, and an analysis of local clinical experience. The review leads to discussion aimed at developing consensus regarding what the most appropriate diagnostic interventions are for the typical patient in that population, as well as how best to coordinate and deliver those interventions. These activities, aimed at guiding the development of critical paths, often lead to new protocols and standing orders, with immediate impact on efficiency.

DOCUMENTATION

The path in its most complete form covers the entire episode of illness, incorporates patient and family issues, and is used by all members of the multidisciplinary team. It contains elements of documentation by all members, such that duplication is avoided and overall documentation time is decreased. Documentation, which is part of the legal record, is accompanied by a tool used for data collection regarding patient, caregiver, or system variance. From an analysis of these data, quality assurance and improvement activities are stimulated.

Many institutions include a third document, the patient path. It is written in simpler language, often with pictorials, and is given to the patient to provide a general orientation to the rhythm and coordination of the care that should be expected. Hartford Hospital has over 70 critical paths in various stages of implementation.

In analyzing the impact of critical paths on cost and quality, it is difficult to ferret out the contribution of the path itself from the many other epiphenomena associated with the development and maturation of a health care team. However, critical path creation at Hartford Hospital often has been one of the most pivotal activities nurturing team development. In this light, it can be viewed as having a primary role in impacting change derived from team effort. In one year, we witnessed a decrease in length of stay from 10.3 to 8.2 days and a decrease in charged costs from $26,300 to $22,650 for patients undergoing coronary artery bypass graft without cardiac catheterization during the same admission.[15]

PHYSICIAN PARTICIPATION

As with any new methodology, issues with implementation arise. Physician participation and buy-in, a critical success factor, is often cited as a major issue in institutions where physicians are primarily in the private practice arena. This problem is changing with managed care and package-pricing and will likely become less of an issue with time. However, it is one factor to consider in selecting patient populations for the first critical paths in a unit or an institution.

Liability issues are often raised by physicians. However, paths do not lock a patient into a particular plan of care. Physician's orders can always tailor the plan described in the path to meet the needs of the individual patient. The liability is thus not on the physician, unless the care ultimately prescribed is substandard and is the proximate cause of harm to the patient.

To avoid liability, the team creating a path should follow developmental guidelines, document the developmental process, clarify the purpose of the path, avoid singling out specific products, review and update the path regularly, and add a disclaimer to the path regarding how individual variation is handled with critical path methodology. Data ownership and confidentiality issues must be dealt with regarding variance analysis. Most institutions have chosen to incorporate the path into the record, leaving variance data in the realm of quality assurance.

BENEFITS

If these issues are addressed and the appropriate administrative support is given to the effort, critical paths can yield significant benefits to patients individually and at the level of patient populations. For individual patients, caregivers can view the updated snapshot provided by the path and adjust the delivery of care to best meet their needs in a manner that reinforces communication, coordination, and cost-effectiveness. With the analysis of variance data, teams of caregivers can identify opportunities for improvement and monitor the impact of new strategies on populations of patients.

THE JCAHO SURVEY ■

GENERAL CONCEPT

A multidisciplinary approach to care has long been an integral part of many critical care unit microsystems. These microsystems will be asked about their role in the hospital mission, and their interdepartmental relationships and interfaces with the organization as a whole. A sample survey question a critical care staff member might be asked is, "How do you collaborate with other clinical and nonclinical services throughout the organization to achieve better patient care or a better environment in which to provide that care?"

(text continues on page 184)

ADMISSION DATE:_____

DISCHARGE DATE:_____

ADMISSION UNIT:_____

LOS:_____   ACTUAL:_____

WAS PATIENT SEEN IN PATC?_____ DATE: _____

TX NEW PATHWAY: NAME: _____
CP010501
```

| PREADMISSION/ PRE-OP | A | V | PERIOPERATIVE/ INTRAOPERATIVE | A | V | 1ST POST-OP HOUR | A | V | 2ND-24TH POST-OP HOUR/ DAY 1 | A | V |
|---|---|---|---|---|---|---|---|---|---|---|---|
| DATE:_____ | | | DATE:_____ | | | DATE:_____ | | | DATE:_____ | | |
| **OUTCOMES** | | | **OUTCOMES** | | | **OUTCOMES** | | | **OUTCOMES** | | |
| 1 Patient demonstrates understanding of hospital course and post-operative care | | | 121 Hemodynamic Stability | | | 241 Adequate oxygenation/ventilation | | | 361 Adequate oxygenation/ventilation | | |
| 2 Preadmission testing completed | | | 122 Graft patency | | | 242 Hemodynamics within normal parameters | | | 362 Hemodynamically stable | | |
| 3 Plan for discharge established | | | 123 | | | 243 Patient seen by family | | | 363 Patient and family verbalize understanding of situation and surroundings | | |
| 4 | | | 124 | | | 244 Occlusive dressing intact | | | 364 Occlusive dressing intact | | |
| 5 | | | 125 | | | 245 No evidence of pneumothorax or significant pleural effusion | | | 365 No evidence of pneumothorax or significant pleural effusion | | |
| 6 | | | 126 | | | 246 | | | 366 Extubation | | |
| 7 | | | 127 | | | 247 | | | 367 No neuro or sensory deficits | | |
| 8 | | | 128 | | | 248 | | | 368 CT output less than 30cc/hour | | |
| 9 | | | 129 | | | 249 | | | 369 No nausea and/or vomiting | | |
| 10 | | | 130 | | | 250 | | | 370 Taking clear liquids by 24th hour | | |
| 11 | | | 131 | | | 251 Pain is controlled | | | 371 Pain is controlled | | |
| 12 | | | 132 | | | 252 Anxiety is controlled | | | 372 Anxiety is controlled | | |
| 13 | | | 133 | | | 253 | | | 373 Transfer to B9E by 24th post-op hour | | |
| **CONSULT** | | | **CONSULT** | | | **CONSULT** | | | **CONSULT** | | |
| 14 Anesthesia | | | 134 | | | 254 | | | 374 | | |
| 15 Cardiothoracic Surgeon | | | 135 | | | 255 | | | 375 | | |
| 16 Cardiologist | | | 136 | | | 256 | | | 376 | | |
| 17 Social Service | | | 137 | | | 257 | | | 377 | | |
| 18 Dietician | | | 138 | | | 258 | | | 378 | | |
| 19 | | | 139 | | | 259 | | | 379 | | |

**FIGURE 13-12.** Hartford Hospital critical pathway for coronary artery bypass graft. (*continued*)
```

NAME: _____   MEDICAL RECORD #: _____

PREADMISSION/ PRE-OP	A	V	PERIOPERATIVE/ INTRAOPERATIVE	A	V	1ST POST-OP HOUR	A	V	2ND-24TH POST-OP HOUR/DAY 1	A	V
DATE:_____			DATE:_____			DATE:_____			DATE:_____		
ASSESSMENT			**ASSESSMENT**			**ASSESSMENT**			**ASSESSMENT**		
20 History and Physical completed			140 Continuous monitoring of Cardiopulmonary hemodynamics pre, intra and post cardiopulmonary bypass			260 Continuous monitoring of EKG, hemodynamic lines, SAO2/SVO2, temperature, chest tube drainage			380 Continuous monitoring of EKG, hemodynamic lines, SAO2/SVO2, temperature, chest tube drainage		
21 Old Records			141 Nursing Assessment			261			381		
22 Cath report			142			262			382		
23 Cardiology nuclear studies			143			263			383		
24 Nursing Data Base			144			264			384		
25 Informed consent			145			265			385		
26			146			266			386		
TESTS			**TESTS**			**TESTS**			**TESTS**		
27 As per Standard Orders			147			267 As per Standard Orders			387 As per Standard Orders		
28			148 Blood sugar Q5-20 minutes after going on bypass if diabetic			268			388		
29			149 ABG's, Hgb, HCT Q30"			269			389		
30			150 Potassium, BS and platelets after warming			270			390		
31			151			271			391		
NUTRITION			**NUTRITION**			**NUTRITION**			**NUTRITION**		
32			152			272 NPO			392 Post extubation clear liquids		
33			153			273			393		
MEDICATIONS			**MEDICATIONS**			**MEDICATIONS**			**MEDICATIONS**		
34 Continue pre-operative medications			154 Anticoagulants per protocol			274 As per Standard Orders			394 As per standard orders		
35			155 Antibiotics per protocol			275			395		
36			156 Vasoactive medications as indicated			276			396		
37			157			277			397		
38			158			278			398		

FIGURE 13-12. *(continued)*

NAME: _____ MEDICAL RECORD #: _____

PREADMISSION/ PRE-OP	A	V	PERIOPERATIVE/ INTRAOPERATIVE	A	V	1ST POST-OP HOUR	A	V	2ND-24TH POST-OP HOUR/DAY 1	A	V
DATE: _____			DATE: _____			DATE: _____			DATE: _____		
TREATMENT/ INTERVENTION			**TREATMENT/ INTERVENTION**			**TREATMENT/ INTERVENTION**			**TREATMENT/ INTERVENTION**		
39			159 Surgical prep			279 Hemodynamic/cardiac monitoring as per Standards of Care			399 Hemodynamic/cardiac monitoring as per Standards of Care		
40			160 Continuous monitoring of Cardiopulmonary hemodynamics pre, intra, and post cardiopulmonary bypass			280 Autotransfuse until chest tube output is less than 50cc/hour			400 Autotransfuse until chest tube output is less than 50cc/hour		
41			161 Transfusion therapy per protocol			281			401 D/C LA line		
42			162			282			402 Vasoactive drips DC'd		
43			163			283			403 D/C PA cath within 24 hours		
44			164			284 Rewarm to temp 95-98 degrees F.			404 Rewarm to temp 95-98 degrees F.		
45			165			285 Ace wraps			405 Ace wraps		
46			166			286 Check CMS			406 Check CMS		
47			167			287 Temporary pacing if indicated			407 Temporary pacing if indicated		
48			168			288 Foley			408 Foley		
49			169			289 NG tube			409 D/C NG tube		
50			170			290 Respiratory Therapy: -Initial ventilation settings per anesthesia -Wean per ICU protocol			410 Respiratory Therapy: Wean and extubate per ICU protocol		
51			171			291			411 I.S. Q1H and prn after extubation		
52			172			292			412		
MOBILITY/ ACTIVITIES			**MOBILITY/ ACTIVITIES**			**MOBILITY/ ACTIVITIES**			**MOBILITY/ ACTIVITIES**		
53			173			293 Bedrest			413 OOB to chair by 24th hour		
54			174			294			414		
PSYCHOSOCIAL MANAGEMENT			**PSYCHOSOCIAL MANAGEMENT**			**PSYCHOSOCIAL MANAGEMENT**			**PSYCHOSOCIAL MANAGEMENT**		
55 Patient will have knowledge of their Bill of Rights			175			295 Assist family to identify coping			415		
56 Advance Directives			176			296			416 Offer spiritual/chaplain support		
57			177			297			417		

NAME: _____ MEDICAL RECORD #: _____

PREADMISSION/ PRE-OP	A	V	PERIOPERATIVE/ INTRAOPERATIVE	A	V	1ST POST-OP HOUR	A	V	2ND-24TH POST-OP HOUR/DAY 1	A	V
DATE: _____			DATE: _____			DATE: _____			DATE: _____		
EDUCATION			**EDUCATION**			**EDUCATION**			**EDUCATION**		
58 Visitation guidelines			178			298 Family support and updates on clinical condition			418 Patient/family support		
59 Cardiac surgery booklet			179			299 Orient family to the ICU			419		
60 Cardiac surgery classes			180			300			420		
61 Unit visit			181			301			421		
62			182			302			422		
DISCHARGE MANAGEMENT			**DISCHARGE MANAGEMENT**			**DISCHARGE MANAGEMENT**			**DISCHARGE MANAGEMENT**		
63 Initiate discharge plan			183			303			423		
64 Assess home environment			184			304			424		
65 Assess family support			185			305			425		
66			186			306			426		
PATIENT SPECIFIC NEEDS			**PATIENT SPECIFIC NEEDS**			**PATIENT SPECIFIC NEEDS**			**PATIENT SPECIFIC NEEDS**		
67			187			307			427		

FIGURE 13-12. *(continued)*

NAME: _____   MEDICAL RECORD #: _____

POST-OP DAY 2	A	V	POST-OP DAY 3	A	V	POST-OP DAY 4	A	V	POST-OP DAY 5	A	V	POST-OP DAY 6		
DATE:_____			DATE:_____			DATE:_____			DATE:_____			DATE:_____		
OUTCOMES			**OUTCOMES**			**OUTCOMES**			**OUTCOMES**			**OUTCOMES**		
68 Hemodynamically stable			188 Tolerating full diet			308 Adequate bowel function			428 Verbalizes understanding of discharge teaching			481 Verbalizes understanding of discharge instructions as per "Going Home After Your Open Heart Surgery"		
69 Awake and alert			189			309 Tolerating increased level of activity			429 Compliant with increased activity			482 Discharge to home		
70 No neuro or sensory deficits			190 No neuro or sensory deficits			310 No neuro or sensory deficits			430 No neuro or sensory deficits			483		
71 Pain is controlled			191 Pain is controlled			311 Pain is controlled			431 Pain is controlled			484		
72 Free of arrhythmias			192 Free of arrhythmias			312 Free of arrhythmias			432 Free of arrhythmias			485		
73 Peripheral pulses same as pre-op			193 Peripheral pulses same as pre-op			313 Peripheral pulses same as pre-op			433 Peripheral pulses same as pre-op			486		
74 Minimal pedal edema			194 Minimal pedal edema			314 Minimal pedal edema			434 Minimal pedal edema			487		
75 Adequate urine output			195 Adequate urine output			315 Adequate urine output			435 Adequate urine output			488		
76 Minimal anxiety			196 Minimal anxiety			316 Minimal anxiety			436 Minimal anxiety			489		
77 No evidence of pneumothorax or significant pleural effusion			197			317			437 Weight at or below preop weight			490		
78 Compliance with incentive spirometry			198 Compliance with incentive spirometry			318 Compliance with incentive spirometry			438 Compliance with incentive spirometry			491		
79 Exhibits no signs of infection			199 Exhibits no signs of infection			319 Exhibits no signs of infection			439 Exhibits no signs of infection			492		
80 Afebrile			200 Afebrile			320 Afebrile			440 Afebrile			493		
81			201			321			441 Wounds healed			494		
CONSULT			**CONSULT**			**CONSULT**			**CONSULT**			**CONSULT**		
82 Pastoral services			202			322			442			495		
83 PT/OT referral upon diagnosis of motor function neuropathy			203			323			443			496		
84 Social Service			204			324			444			497		
85			205			325			445			498		

FIGURE 13-12. *(continued)*

NAME: _____ MEDICAL RECORD #: _____

POST-OP DAY 2	A	V	POST-OP DAY 3	A	V	POST-OP DAY 4	A	V	POST-OP DAY 5	A	V	POST-DAY 6	A	V
DATE: _____			DATE: _____			DATE: _____			DATE: _____			DATE: _____		
ASSESSMENT			**ASSESSMENT**			**ASSESSMENT**			**ASSESSMENT**			**ASSESSMENT**		
86 As per standards of care			206 As per standards of care			326 As per standards of care			446 As per standards of care			499 As per standards of care		
87			207			327			447			500		
TESTS			**TESTS**			**TESTS**			**TESTS**			**TESTS**		
88 Chest X-Ray after CT removal			208 As per Standard Orders			328			448			501		
89			209			329			449			502		
90			210			330			450			503		
NUTRITION			**NUTRITION**			**NUTRITION**			**NUTRITION**			**NUTRITION**		
91 Advance to no added salt, low total fat diet if bowel sounds present			211			331			451			504		
92			212			332			452			505		
MEDICATIONS			**MEDICATIONS**			**MEDICATIONS**			**MEDICATIONS**			**MEDICATIONS**		
93 As per standing orders			213 As per standing orders			333 As per standing orders			453 As per standing orders			506 As ordered for discharge		
94			214			334			454			507		
TREATMENT/ INTERVENTION			**TREATMENT/ INTERVENTION**			**TREATMENT/ INTERVENTION**			**TREATMENT/ INTERVENTION**			**TREATMENT/ INTERVENTION**		
95 Discontinue pacer wires			215 D/C IV site (24 hour post D/Cing pacer wires)			335			455 Discuss available cardiac rehab programs			508 Daily weight		
96 Discontinue telemetry			216			336			456			509 Incentive spirometry 4-5 times a day		
97 Discontinue chest tubes			217			337			457			510		
98 Routine incisional care			218 Routine incisional care			338 Routine incisional care			458 Routine incisional care			511		
99 D/C foley			219			339			459			512		
100 Daily weight			220 Daily weight			340 Daily weight			460 Daily weight			513		
101 Incentive spirometry Q1-2 hours			221 Incentive spirometry Q1-2 hours			341 Incentive spirometry Q4 hours			461 Incentive spirometry 4-5 times per day			514		
102 O2 per B9E protocol			222 O2 per B9E protocol			342			462			515		
103			223			343			463			516		

FIGURE 13-12. *(continued)*

NAME: _____   MEDICAL RECORD #: _____

POST-OP DAY 2	A	V	POST-OP DAY 3	A	V	POST-OP DAY 4	A	V	POST-OP DAY 5	A	V	POST-OP DAY 6	A	V
DATE: _____			DATE: _____			DATE: _____			DATE: _____			DATE: _____		
MOBILITY/ ACTIVITIES			**MOBILITY/ ACTIVITIES**			**MOBILITY/ ACTIVITIES**			**MOBILITY/ ACTIVITIES**			**MOBILITY/ ACTIVITIES**		
104 Encourage to flex and extend feet, legs, thighs Q20"			224			344			464			517 Walk 5-6 minutes X2		
105 OOB to chair TID			225 OOB to chair for all meals			345 OOB to chair for all meals			465			518 Stairs for identified patients only		
106 Bathroom privileges with assistance			226 Walk for 2 minutes X2			346 Walk for 3-4 minutes X2			466 Walk 4-5 minutes X2			519		
107 Assist with ADL's			227 Minimal assistance with ADL's			347			467 Stairs for identified patients only			520		
108			228			348			468			521		
PSYCHOSOCIAL MANAGEMENT			**PSYCHOSOCIAL MANAGEMENT**			**PSYCHOSOCIAL MANAGEMENT**			**PSYCHOSOCIAL MANAGEMENT**			**PSYCHOSOCIAL MANAGEMENT**		
109 Assist patient and family with identifying coping mechanisms to reduce anxiety			229 Assist patient and family with identifying coping mechanisms to reduce anxiety			349			469			522		
110			230			350			470			523		
EDUCATION			**EDUCATION**			**EDUCATION**			**EDUCATION**			**EDUCATION**		
111 Pulmonary care			231 Incision care			351 Diet			471			524 Review discharge medications with patient and family		
112 Incentive spirometry			232 Signs and symptoms of infection			352 Activity and exercise			472			525		
113 Pain management			233 Bathing			353 Lifting instructions			473			526		
114			234 Weights			354			474			527		
115			235			355 Read "Going Home After Open Heart Surgery" pamphlet			475 Read "Going Home After Open Heart Surgery" pamphlet			528		
116			236			356 Pain management			476			529		
117			237			357			477			530		

FIGURE 13-12. *(continued)*

NAME: _____   MEDICAL RECORD #: _____

POST-OP DAY 2	A	V	POST-OP DAY 3	A	V	POST-OP DAY 4	A	V	POST-OP DAY 5	A	V	POST-OP DAY 6	A	V
DATE: _____			DATE: _____			DATE: _____			DATE: _____			DATE: _____		
DISCHARGE MANAGEMENT			**DISCHARGE MANAGEMENT**			**DISCHARGE MANAGEMENT**			**DISCHARGE MANAGEMENT**			**DISCHARGE MANAGEMENT**		
118 Reassess discharge plan			238 Reassess discharge plan			358 Reassess discharge plan			478 Formalize discharge plan			531		
119			239			359			479			532		
PATIENT SPECIFIC NEEDS			**PATIENT SPECIFIC NEEDS**			**PATIENT SPECIFIC NEEDS**			**PATIENT SPECIFIC NEEDS**			**PATIENT SPECIFIC NEEDS**		
120			240			360			480			533		

FIGURE 13-12. *(continued)*

NAME:

MEDICAL RECORD #:

LEGEND:

A=Accomplished: intervention/outcome reached

V=Variance: intervention/outcome not reached

NA=Non-applicable: intervention/outcome deemed not clinically applicable

X=indicates no intervention/outcome for that day

NAME:(Please Print) _____ INITIALS: _____ SIGNATURE: _____ TITLE: _____

NAME:(Please Print) _____ INITIALS: _____ SIGNATURE: _____ TITLE: _____

NAME:(Please Print) _____ INITIALS: _____ SIGNATURE: _____ TITLE: _____

NAME:(Please Print) _____ INITIALS: _____ SIGNATURE: _____ TITLE: _____

NAME:(Please Print) _____ INITIALS: _____ SIGNATURE: _____ TITLE: _____

NAME:(Please Print) _____ INITIALS: _____ SIGNATURE: _____ TITLE: _____

NAME:(Please Print) _____ INITIALS: _____ SIGNATURE: _____ TITLE: _____

NAME:(Please Print) _____ INITIALS: _____ SIGNATURE: _____ TITLE: _____

This critical path was developed through the concensus of a multidisciplinary group and depicts the sequence and timing of those critical events which drive the achievement of progressive patient outcomes during an episode of illness. This is not meant to represent the only acceptable way to design the care for a given patient nor would all patients' needs necessarily be met by such a path, therefore the content may be tailored to meet the needs of the individual patient.

The contents of this document incorporate the Standards of Patient Care.

CRITICAL PATHWAY APPROVED BY _____ ON _____

cp_cahg2.doc

FIGURE 13-12. *(continued)*

This kind of thinking is based on the premise that care is not delivered in a vacuum or in separate, discrete interventions but, rather, occurs along a continuum. The more coordinated the care is along the continuum, the better the outcome will be for the patient. Recently surveyed hospital ICUs reported that "in the ICU, the emphasis was on the multidisciplinary assessment and periodic reassessment of ventilated patients and the consistency of intravenous sedation given to patients transferred from the ER to the ICU."[16] Yet another comment indicated that "the surveyor also wanted staff nurses to assess the psychosocial (emotional and spiritual) needs of dying patients."[16]

PERSONNEL INVOLVEMENT

In addition to understanding the processes of patient assessment and care in their organizations, caregivers should be familiar with the mechanisms used to determine the level of appropriate care to be delivered and the setting in which the care is to be rendered. Comprehensive policies for admission must address a level of care and the specific goals for patient care, treatment, and rehabilitation. This format is in keeping with dimensions of performance, believed by JCAHO to be essential to a successful organization. These dimensions of performance speak to appropriate and respectful care available to meet patients' needs, provided in an effective and coordinated manner at the right time, using the appropriate resources to achieve the best possible patient outcome.

The survey process itself will be interactive to a greater degree than in the past and will include random and scheduled interviews with managers and staff as well as the customary document and medical record review. Employees will be approached throughout the survey process with the goal of assessing their organizational and role-specific knowledge. Questions evaluating the extent of employee understanding about patient rights, the mission of the hospital, life safety, organizational systems, and their role in the organization are fair game for surveyors. The interview process also includes patients and families to assess their understanding of reasons for hospitalization and the education provided to teach them about their illness, plan of treatment, and discharge plan.

The JCAHO views the Human Resource function as a critical aspect of organizational leadership and within that framework places heavy emphasis on personnel competency. (During an accreditation survey, competency reviews are conducted using selected staff records to assess documented orientation and training, continuing education, and specialty training (e.g., fire and disaster, cardiopulmonary resuscitation, and advanced cardiac life support).

SPECIFIC ANALYSES

Surveyed hospitals stated that a "major theme . . . was the need to link job descriptions, competency evaluations, education and performance appraisals to the age-specific needs of patient served."[17] Age groupings identified as having unique care needs are neonatal, pediatric, adolescent, and geriatric. Ancillary services such as Respiratory Therapy, Pulmonary Function Laboratory, Radiology, Pharmacy, and others need to identify their involvement with these age populations. Job descriptions, educational activities, and performance appraisals must address this involvement and support the competency to do so.

Finally, the performance improvement standard focuses on the organization's ability to design processes well and evaluates how these processes are continuously and systematically assessed to identify opportunities and implement strategies for improving patient care outcomes. On interview, employees may be asked to describe their role in performance improvement activities and to articulate how the processes and outcomes of care are evaluated, beginning with the mechanisms for selection of indicators for measurement, through the data collection and analysis process, to the impact on patient care and actions taken as a result.

The JCAHO is clearly aggressive in its quest to press health care institutions into a CQI environment. For many of us, these changes will not come easily or overnight. Changing the culture of the way work is accomplished can be a long, tedious process. Standards written by the JCAHO and the questions they ask are appropriate. If any one of us was in the role of patient or family member, the answers to these questions would be important to us. The JCAHO has written their intention to make the survey an educational process as well. Most of us welcome that approach and most decidedly could benefit from it. It's also good to know, whether or not we agree with all the details, that someone "out there" is as concerned about quality of care as we are.

REFERENCES ■

1. Snow N, Bergin KT, Horrigan TP: Re-admission of patients to the surgical intensive care unit: patient profiles and possibilities for prevention. *Crit Care Med* 1985;13:961
2. Coppolo D, May JJ: Self-extubation: a 12 month experience. *Chest* 1990;98:165
3. Demling RH, Truman R, Lind LJ, et al: Incidence and morbidity of extubation failure in surgical intensive care patients. *Crit Care Med* 1980;16:573
4. Rifkin M: Quality assessment and improvement in the ICU: its influence on bedside practice. In: Civetta JM, Taylor RW, Kirby RR (eds). *Critical Care*, 2nd ed. Philadelphia, JB Lippincott, 1992:1912
5. Seneff MG: Central venous catheterization: a comprehensive review. Part III. *J Intens Care Med* 1987;2:218
6. Norwood S, Ruby A, Civetta J, et al: Catheter-related infections and associated septicemia. *Chest* 1991;99:968
7. Samsoondar W, Freeman JB: Colonization of intravascular monitoring devices. *Crit Care Med* 1985;13:753
8. National Pressure Ulcer Advisory Panel: Pressure ulcers: prevalence, cost and risk assessment. Consensus Development Conference Statement. *Decubitus* 1989;2:24
9. Sideranko S, Quinn A, Burns K, et al: Effects of position and mattress overlay on sacral and heel pressures in a clinical population. *Res Nurs Health* 1992;15:245
10. Smoller BR, Kruskal MS: Phlebotomy for diagnostic laboratory tests in adults. *N Engl J Med* 1986;314:1233

11. Gleason E, Grossman S, Campbell C: Minimizing diagnostic blood loss in critically ill patients. *Am J Crit Care* 1992;1:85

12. Knaus WA, Draper EA, Wagner DP, et al: An evaluation of outcome from intensive care in major medical center. *Am Intern Med* 1986;104:410

13. Goldman L, Sayson R, Robbins S, et al: The value of the autopsy in three medical eras. *N Engl J Med* 1983;308:1000

14. Melum MM, Sinoris MK: Total Quality Management: The Health Care Pioneers. American Hospital Publishing, 1992

15. Allen L, Leggit M, Hartford Hospital. Personal communication

16. Survey Monitor Rounds the Corner in Briefings on JCAHO, October 1994

17. Type I of the month-age Specific Competency in Briefings on JCAHO, October 1994

Essential Physiologic Concerns

Critical Care, Third Edition, edited by Joseph M. Civetta,
Robert W. Taylor, and Robert R. Kirby.
Lippincott-Raven Publishers, Philadelphia, PA © 1997.

CHAPTER 14

■

The Lungs and Their Function

Roger S. Mecca
Carlos A. Vaz Fragoso

STATIC LUNG VOLUMES: ANATOMIC CONSIDERATIONS ■

The human lungs contain an intricate three-dimensional matrix of thin-walled alveoli supplied by small airways. Alveoli are in intimate approximation to a rich network of sinusoidal capillaries that originate in pulmonary arterioles and terminate in pulmonary venules. Alveoli, small airways, and capillaries are suspended in a net of collagen and elastin fibers that radiates outward from hilum to periphery. Radial orientation of suspensory fibers and surface tension in alveolar air–fluid interfaces promote reduction of lung volume. Lung distention increases this *elastic* force, so the lungs behave like three-dimensional springs. Distention also generates traction in suspensory fibers, which helps to keep alveoli and small airways expanded. The lungs are bordered by the rib cage, mediastinum, and diaphragm, forming a thoracic cavity. The diaphragm, a dome-shaped muscle that forms the thoracic cavity *floor*, curves upward into the thorax, whereas the ribs curve downward and forward from the thoracic vertebrae to the sternum. Diaphragmatic contraction and movement of the ribs upward and outward increase thoracic cavity volume.

PLEURAL PRESSURE

The outer surface of the lungs and inner surface of the chest cavity are lined by visceral and parietal pleura, respectively. These serous membranes are in close contact, with only a potential space between. The lungs are held expanded by the thoracic cavity, which resists their tendency to collapse. Simultaneously, the lungs pull the diaphragm and ribs upward and inward, respectively, opposing thoracic expansion. This three-dimensional dynamic equilibrium generates a subatmospheric (negative) intrapleural pressure (Ppl), maintaining uninterrupted contact between the pleural surfaces.

A break in pleural integrity permits lung collapse, diaphragmatic descent, and rib cage expansion, generating a pneumothorax. Ppl varies with location.[1] In dependent regions, lung weight opposes lung recoil, decreasing the net force tending to separate the pleura. In contrast, pleura covering nondependent lung must resist retractile lung forces and support the weight of lung tissue and fluid that "hang" beneath it. These gravitational effects generate a vertical Ppl gradient, with the least negative Ppl around dependent lung and the most negative pressure around nondependent lung (Fig. 14-1).

FUNCTIONAL RESIDUAL CAPACITY

At end-expiration, lung recoil and thoracic cavity expansion forces are at resting equilibrium. Lung volume at end-expiratory equilibrium is called the functional residual capacity (FRC). During normal tidal ventilation at any point in the thorax, Ppl reaches its least negative value at FRC. Radial forces that hold airspaces open are also weakest at FRC because elastin and collagen fiber stretch varies directly with lung volume (Fig. 14-2). The FRC remains relatively constant in healthy people throughout adult life.[2] If lung volume is reduced below normal FRC, radial traction becomes insufficient to hold some small airways open, so airspaces will collapse.

The lung volume at which airways first collapse can be defined as the closing capacity, although its clinical relevance is questionable. Normally, airway closure occurs only if lung volume falls far below normal FRC, so small airways remain patent throughout tidal ventilation. Chronic degenerative diseases and perhaps normal aging progressively reduce lung

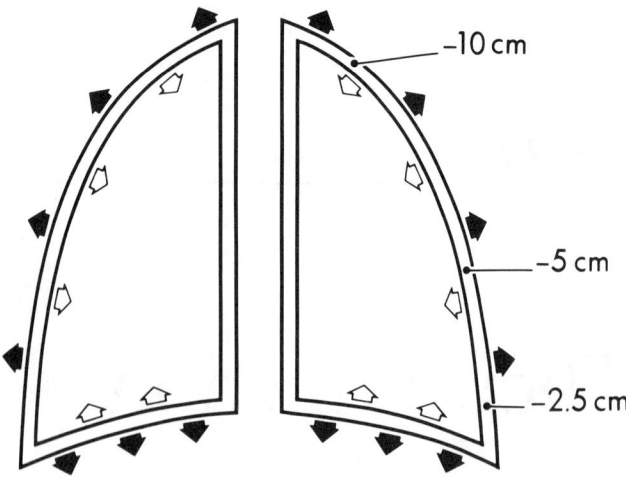

FIGURE 14-1. Pleural pressure gradient (erect position). (Mecca RS: Pulmonary physiology. In: Kirby RR, Taylor RW [eds]: *Respiratory Failure*. Chicago, Year Book Medical Publishers, 1986.)

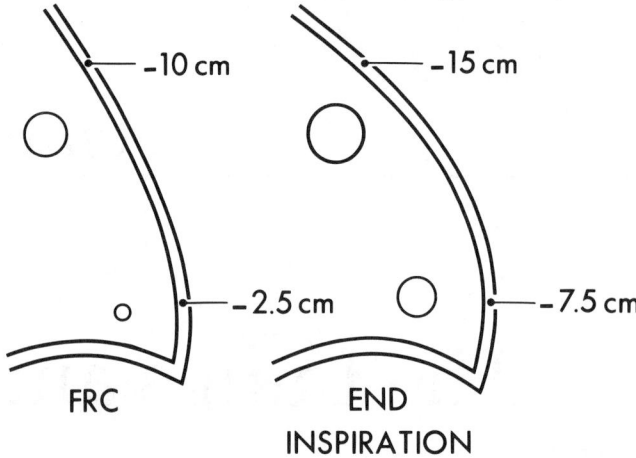

FIGURE 14-2. Variation of pleural pressure and alveolar size with lung volume. (Mecca RS: Pulmonary physiology. In: Kirby RR, Taylor RW [eds]: *Respiratory Failure*. Chicago, Year Book Medical Publishers, 1986.)

recoil and radial airway traction at a given lung volume, so that eventually airway closure appears at end-expiration. In a healthy supine man, this change occurs around 44 years of age.[3]

Increased lung volume during inspiration reopens airways, allowing fresh gas flow to distal airspaces. With more severe degenerative changes (e.g., closing capacity exceeds end-inspiratory lung volume), some small airways remain closed during inspiration, and distal airspaces collapse.

Acute pathologic conditions can transiently decrease FRC and promote airway closure, as can changes in position or increases of intraabdominal pressure. When FRC is reduced, airway collapse and loss of lung volume appears first in dependent regions of the lung where Ppl is least negative and radial traction is weakest.

Two broad categories of lung disease affect static lung volumes. Obstructive diseases such as status asthmaticus or chronic obstructive lung disease are characterized by obstruction to airflow through airways, prolonged expiration, and gas trapping. Resulting hyperinflation increases the FRC and the total lung capacity (TLC), the maximum achievable end-inspiratory lung volume. Restrictive diseases impede thoracic cavity and lung expansion, as occurs with chest wall abnormalities (e.g., scoliosis), neuromuscular problems (e.g., phrenic nerve injury), parenchymal diseases (e.g., interstitial lung disease, pulmonary edema), and pleural effusions, pneumothorax, or extrathoracic problems (e.g., increased intraabdominal pressure). Restrictive conditions reduce FRC and TLC. In both categories, pulmonary compliance is reduced and the potential for ventilation-perfusion ($\dot{V}/\dot{Q}$) mismatch or hypoventilation is increased.

Serial lung volume measurements assess disease severity and manage mechanical ventilation (MV) and weaning. Several techniques are available to measure specific lung volumes in intubated patients.[4] Unfortunately, they are clinically impractical. A cumbersome gas dilution technique for measuring FRC (e.g., open or closed circuit) can affect the inspired fraction of oxygen (F_{IO_2}) or interrupt MV. Radio-

graphic measurement of the TLC and FRC has yet to be validated during MV. Noninvasive respiratory impedance plethysmograph only approximates changes in the FRC. Other noninvasive bedside measurements can indirectly reflect FRC and TLC, negating the need for direct measurement (Table 14-1).

MECHANICS OF VENTILATION

Spontaneous ventilation involves repetitive creation of pressure gradients between ambient (mouth) pressure and alveolar pressure. These gradients overcome flow resistance in airways and generate gas movement in and out of the lungs. At end-expiration, pressure within the alveoli equals atmospheric pressure (assuming airway patency), so gas flow does not occur. During inspiration, inspiratory muscles actively expand the thoracic cavity, increasing the volume of the parenchymal airspaces. Because volume and pressure vary inversely, alveolar pressure must decrease below atmospheric, creating a pressure gradient that causes inward gas flow. When active expansion ceases, alveolar pressure quickly equalizes with ambient, the gradient disappears, and gas flow stops (Fig. 14-3). At end-inspiration, lung and chest wall forces are unbalanced because expansion has increased the tendency for the lungs to collapse and decreased the tendency for the chest cavity to spring outward. When inspiratory muscles relax, this disequilibrium allows lung retractile forces to reduce lung volume. Alveolar pressure increases above ambient pressure, forcing gas to flow outward until FRC is reached. This sequence describes one spontaneous tidal volume (VT) exchange.[5]

Routine bedside measurement of airway pressure gradients is usually done only during MV, using ventilator pressures. The *resistive pressure* (reflecting obstructive disease) is the difference between the peak inspiratory pressure (PIP) and the static or plateau inspiratory pressure (Pplat). PIP is measured after an unassisted machine inflation, whereas Pplat is measured 1 to 2 seconds later during an end-inspira-

TABLE 14-1. Critical Care Bedside Physiology: Obstructive (COLD) Versus Restrictive (ARDS)

PARAMETER	COLD	ARDS	COMMENTS
LEVEL 1: ROUTINE			
History, physical, chest radiograph	See text	See text	Define the clinical context
PaCO₂	Increased	Decreased	See text
PaO₂/FIO₂	Decreased	Decreased	Worse in ARDS (<150 mm Hg)
V̇E needs	Increased	Increased	Worse in ARDS (>20 L/min)
Cdyn	Decreased	Decreased	Worse in ARDS (<25 mL/cm H₂O)
Ces	Preserved	Decreased	Worse in ARDS (<25 mL/cm H₂O)
PIP–Pplat	Increased	~Normal	Worse in COLD (>5–10 cm H₂O)
Pplat–PEEP	~Normal	Increased	Worse in ARDS
auto PEEP	Increased	Increased	Worse in COLD and at a lower Ve
Raw	Increased	~Normal	Worse in COLD (>15)
VD/VT	Increased	Increased	Dependent on many factors
LEVEL 2: WHEN INDICATED			
REE (V̇CO₂, V̇O₂)	Increased	Increased	Ventilator–dependent or hypermetabolic
VD/VT	Increased	Increased	V̇E >10 L/min without an obvious cause
Pulmonary artery catheter	See text	See text	Shock with ? intravascular volume
LEVEL 3: RESEARCH			WEANABLE FROM MV IF . . .
P0.1	Increased	Increased	<6.0 cm H₂O
WOB	Increased	Increased	<0.75 J/L
TTIdi	Increased	Increased	<0.15
Static lung volumes	Increased	Decreased	See text
Impedance plethysmography	See text	See text	See text

ARDS, acute respiratory distress syndrome; COLD, chronic obstructive lung disease; Cdyn, dynamic compliance; Ces, static compliance; PaCO₂, arterial partial pressure of carbon dioxide; PIP, peak inspiratory pressure; MV, mechanical ventilation; FIO₂, fraction of inspired oxygen; Pplat, plateau inspiratory pressure; PEEP, positive end-expiratory pressure; Raw, airway resistance; REE, resting energy expenditure in Kcal/d; VD/VT, dead space ratio; P0.1, change in airway pressure at 0.1 second; WOB, work of breathing; PaO₂, arterial partial pressure of oxygen; TTIdi, tension time index diaphragm; V̇E, expired volume per minute; V̇CO₂, carbon dioxide production per minute; V̇O₂, oxygen consumption per minute.

tory hold. The greater the gradient (PIP − Pplat), the more pronounced the resistive work of breathing (WOB). Ventilator pressures also help to evaluate the resistive pressure relative to the machine's peak inspiratory flow rate (V̇I) during an unassisted mechanical tidal volume. This reflects the total airway resistance to gas flow, including resistance in the endotracheal tube and the ventilatory circuitry.[6] The *elastic pressure* (reflecting restrictive disease) is the gradient between the Pplat and the positive end-expiratory pressure (PEEP), which includes both applied PEEP and auto PEEP. Increased elastic pressure indicates a greater elastic WOB.

RESPIRATORY MUSCLES

During inspiration, chest cavity expansion is primarily achieved by contraction of the diaphragm, which inserts on the upper margins of the lower six ribs, the anterolateral aspects of the first three lumbar vertebrae, and the xiphoid. Motor innervation is supplied by the phrenic nerves, originating from spinal roots C3, C4, and C5. Contraction moves

the diaphragmatic dome downward like a piston, forcing the abdominal contents caudad and the ventral abdominal wall outward. Vertical chest cavity dimension increases 1 to 4 cm during quiet tidal ventilation, although excursion can exceed 8 cm during maximal inspiration. Contraction of the external intercostals pulls the ribs upward and outward, increasing the anteroposterior chest cavity diameter. The external intercostal muscles run from the lower, outer rib margins downward and forward to insert on the upper, outer margins of the ribs below.[7]

Tidal Ventilation

Quiet tidal inspiration is achieved by coordinated contraction of the diaphragm, the external intercostal muscles, the interchondral portions of the internal intercostals (parasternals), and the scalenes,[8] generating a subambient alveolar pressure of −2 to −3 cm H₂O (see Fig. 14-3). In vivo, these muscles operate at different points in their length tension curves, optimizing efficiency of inspiration across a wide range of

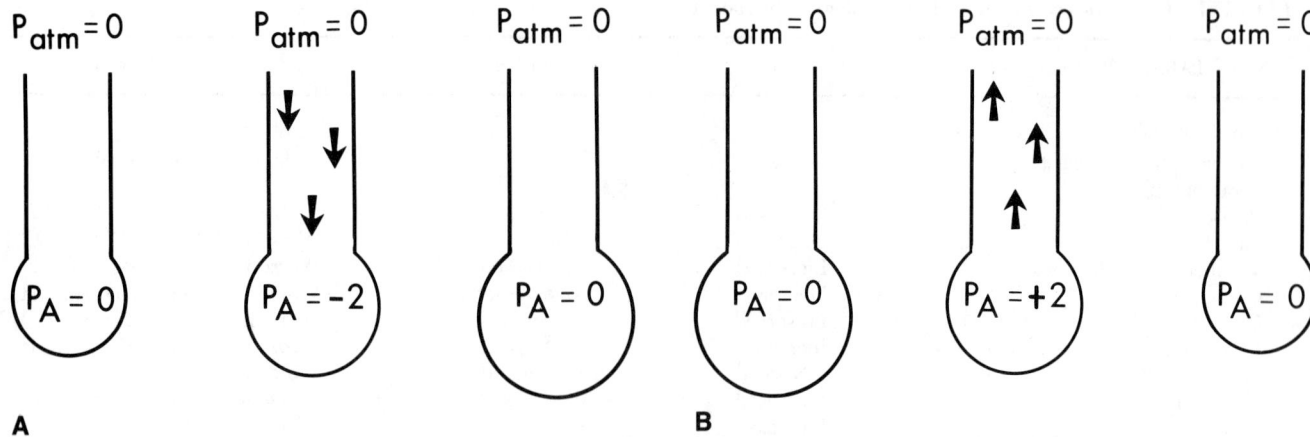

FIGURE 14-3. Alveolar pressure during spontaneous ventilation. (**A**) Inspiration. (**B**) Expiration. (Mecca RS: Pulmonary physiology. In: Kirby RR, Taylor RW [eds]: *Respiratory Failure*. Chicago, Year Book Medical Publishers, 1986.)

lung volumes. Effectiveness of diaphragmatic contraction depends on diaphragmatic stretch at end-expiration, lung compliance, intraabdominal pressure, and coordination with intercostal contraction. Quiet expiration usually occurs passively by recoil of the expanded lungs.

Extremes of Ventilation

Extremes of ventilation (greater than 40 to 50 L/minute) or marked increases in resistance to gas flow necessitate recruitment of accessory muscles to assist inspiration and to achieve active expiration. The sternocleidomastoid muscles are the major inspiratory accessory muscles that can significantly augment chest cavity expansion in normal humans.[9] Reduction of chest cavity volume during active expiration is achieved by contraction of internal interosseous intercostal muscles, which run upward and forward between the inner margins of adjacent ribs and pull the ribs downward and inward. Contraction of the rectus and transversus abdominis and the internal and external abdominal oblique muscles force the abdominal contents inward and the diaphragm upward. Various laryngeal and pharyngeal muscles, which modulate upper airway resistance, flow dynamics, and airway patency, are synchronized with muscles of ventilation through neural control from centers in the medulla.[10-12] Sensory feedback about pressure or positional changes from the larynx to the medulla is a key element of this control loop.

With otherwise normal physiologic features, adequate tidal ventilation usually can be maintained by one hemidiaphragm, or the intercostal muscles.[13-15] However, an increase in ventilatory requirements—or WOB—can precipitate ventilatory insufficiency. Neuromuscular disease, phrenic nerve trauma, hypocalcemia, malnutrition, and metabolic derangements reduce diaphragmatic and intercostal contractile strength, decrease ventilatory reserve, and interfere with weaning from MV.[16,17]

Vital Capacity

Monitoring ventilatory muscle function is important during management of respiratory failure and MV. Several noninva-

sive approaches yield relatively accurate information.[18,19] In nonintubated patients, visual evaluation of spontaneous ventilation and vital capacity (VC) measurements allow qualitative assessment of respiratory muscle strength. Tachypnea, small tidal volumes, accessory muscle recruitment, respiratory alternans, or abdominal paradox may imply respiratory muscle weakness or fatigue. Visual observations can be graphically quantitated with respiratory impedance plethysmography.[20] Whether routine use of plethysmography is cost effective when compared with physical examination and clinical judgment remains to be seen. VC can be measured in a cooperative patient with a portable spirometer. A reduction in the VC secondary to neuromuscular disease occurs before abnormalities in gas exchange arise. Carbon dioxide (CO_2) retention does not usually begin until the VC falls below 50% of the predicted value. If VC falls below 30 mL/kg, secretion clearance is impaired. A VC below 10 mL/kg warns of progressive CO_2 retention requiring ventilatory support.

Peak Pressures

During an occluded spontaneous breath, the maximal inspiratory pressure at residual volume (PI_{max}) and the maximal expiratory pressure at TLC (PE_{max}) reflect the maximal output of inspiratory and expiratory muscles, respectively. A PI_{max} less negative than -20 cm H_2O often predicts progressive CO_2 retention, whereas a PE_{max} less than 40 cm H_2O impairs coughing.[18]

Clinical Applications

For intubated, spontaneously ventilating patients, evaluation of breathing patterns, VC, and PI_{max} are useful to assess ventilatory muscle strength. Additional data on V_T, rate, and minute ventilation ($\dot{V}E$) is available from the ventilator. A shallow breathing index of less than 100 (rate/V_T = breaths/minute/L) with a $\dot{V}E$ less than 10 L/minute predicts respiratory muscle output adequate to sustain spontaneous ventilation.[6,21] Profiling PI_{max}, VC, breathing pattern, and ventilatory muscle load can help to accurately assess ventilatory muscle compromise and likelihood of continued ventilator dependence. However, measurement of VC and PI_{max} is less reliable in an intubated patient, given the impact of critical illness on patient cooperation and the problems associated with correct test performance. Alternative methods for more accurate assessment of ventilatory muscle strength, such as phrenic nerve stimulation with measurement of transdiaphragmatic pressures, have not been validated for impact on outcome or cost effectiveness.

FATIGUE

A decrease in the force-generating capacity of respiratory muscles (Table 14-2) contributes to ventilatory failure. When assessing decreased force-generating capacity, weakness must be distinguished from fatigue.[22] Weakness often reflects an irreversible, intrinsic muscle abnormality, whereas fatigue is reversible with rest. Approximately 75% of muscle fibers in respiratory muscles are oxidative types I and IIA, which are resistant to fatigue. Each individual exhibits a threshold respiratory load, below which fatigue should never occur. If decreased pulmonary compliance, increased airway resistance, or increased ventilatory demand expose the respiratory muscles to loads beyond the threshold, a gradual decline of force-generating capacity occurs until the muscles are unable to maintain adequate minute ventilation. The clinical sensation of dyspnea is most likely caused by perception of respiratory muscle fatigue rather than hypoxemia, hypercapnia, or low lung compliance.[23]

Central Component

Respiratory muscle fatigue may have a central component involving a decrease in motor outflow, which might protect against exhaustion, muscle injury, and complete ventilatory failure. Fatigued respiratory muscles may send afferent inhibitory impulses along the phrenic nerve, causing a decrease in the frequency of efferent motor firing.[24,25] Cortical influences or increased levels of endorphins also may play a role.

TABLE 14-2. Respiratory Muscle Fatigue

Central
  Decrease in CNS motor outflow
  Cortical influences
  Possibly modulated by endogenous opioids
Transmission
  Decrement of impulse generation at myoneural junction
    Neurotransmitter depletion
    Decreased postsynaptic excitability
Contractile
  High frequency
    Lactic acid accumulation
    Decreased Ca^{2+}, ATP
    Electrolyte disturbances
    Reduced muscle blood flow
  Low frequency
    Physical damage to muscle fibers

Impulse Generation and Contractile Response

A second element of respiratory muscle fatigue involves transmission fatigue, reflecting a decrement in impulse generation at the neuromuscular junction. This problem may be caused by neurotransmitter depletion or from decreased excitability of the muscle membranes. Contractile fatigue also occurs, reflecting a reversible impairment of contractile response, which is independent of drug effects or length tension relationships. Contractile fatigue has high-frequency and low-frequency elements.[26] High-frequency contractile fatigue resolves within minutes and is likely caused by lactic acid accumulation, depletion of calcium from the sarcoplasmic reticulum, electrolyte disturbances, or ATP depletion, any of which cause decrements in impulse propagation and excitation/contraction coupling. Reduction of muscle blood flow might also play a role. Low-frequency fatigue takes 24 hours to resolve and is probably caused by physical damage to muscle fibers during exertion.[27]

Miscellaneous Factors

Nutritional support, decreased muscle loading through optimization of airway resistance and pulmonary compliance, and specific training of respiratory muscles can decrease respiratory muscle fatigue and improve ventilatory function. Other interventions such as aminophylline infusion or external diaphragmatic pacing might be useful in patients with critical illness or minimal ventilatory reserve.[27–29]

In critically ill patients, both weakness and fatigue compromise muscle function. Diaphragmatic weakness can be caused by chronic steroid use, malnutrition, metabolic derangements, acute or chronic polyneuropathy, neuromuscular blockade, and mechanical disadvantage caused by chronic hyperinflation or trauma. In contrast, diaphragmatic fatigue often is caused by an increased WOB, by a decrease in diaphragmatic perfusion secondary to cardiovascular problems, or by inappropriate management of MV and weaning.

Clinically, it is difficult to separate the contributions of respiratory muscle weakness and fatigue, especially when baseline muscle status is unknown or adequate respiratory muscle rest has not been provided. Respiratory muscle load and performance should be evaluated frequently during MV or weaning, and potential reversibility of inadequate respiratory muscle performance should be estimated. Iatrogenic factors and elements of the underlying lung disease that contribute to weakness or fatigue should be minimized, and interventions should be chosen to optimize respiratory muscle performance.

PULMONARY COMPLIANCE ■

ELASTIC FORCES AND SURFACE TENSION

When deformed by an external force, an elastic object tends to restore its original resting dimensions by generating an equal and opposite internal force. When a hollow elastic object is inflated with positive pressure, the relationship between inflation pressure and volume is:

$$dV/dP = K \qquad (1)$$

in which dV is change in volume (deformation) and dP is the pressure difference between the inside and outside of the object (transmural pressure gradient). The constant, K, representing change in volume per unit change in transmural pressure gradient, is the compliance.

A human lung resists expansion, mimicking elastic behavior over a narrow range of lung volumes. However, stretch and reorientation of elastic tissues only partially explain lung retraction. Surface tension on the large air–fluid interface in alveoli and airways also contributes to lung recoil. Surface tension is a force generated in a fluid surface that tends to minimize the area of an air–fluid interface. If a surface is spherical, as in a bubble, surface tension generates pressure within the sphere, according to the law of Laplace:

$$P = 2T/r \qquad (2)$$

in which P is pressure between the inside and outside of the sphere, T is surface tension, and r is radius of the sphere.

Modeling alveoli as numerous interconnected bubbles exhibiting a tendency to minimize surface area would seem to account for overall lung recoil. However, if water surface tension were responsible for lung recoil, lung compliance would be much lower than observed in vivo. Also, the Laplace equation indicates that overall lung recoil should decrease as lung volume is increased. Finally, assuming all alveoli communicate, water surface tension would generate high internal pressures in small alveoli, forcing them to empty into larger, lower pressure alveoli. Such emptying would ultimately create one large air chamber.

The unique properties of pulmonary surfactant (surface active material) explain why alveolar pressure–volume relationships deviate from those predicted by surface tension equations.[30] Surfactant is a highly insoluble substance containing phospholipids, including lecithin, sphingomyelin, phosphatidylglycerol, and phosphatidylinositol. Some components are secreted by type II alveolar lining cells. A thin

layer of surfactant floats on the alveolar fluid lining, reducing the surface tension of the air–fluid interface. While alveolar radius increases, surface tension in the surfactant layer increases more than the surface tension decreases in the underlying fluid, causing a net increase in alveolar surface forces. Total lung recoil increases with increased lung volume, and large alveoli theoretically tend to empty into smaller ones, stabilizing alveolar size (Fig. 14-4). Surfactant also may help to prevent alveolar fluid accumulation and inhibit resorption of gas in obstructed airspaces. Instillation of natural or artificial surfactants can be useful in treating respiratory distress syndromes characterized by low pulmonary compliance caused by loss of endogenous surfactant and high alveolar surface tension.[31]

TIME, FREQUENCY, AND VOLUME DEPENDENCE

Lung compliance exhibits complex deviations from linear elastic behavior. If a lung is rapidly inflated and held at a given volume, pressure decreases exponentially from the initial value required to achieve inflation to a value 20% to 30% lower several seconds later, as if the lung parenchyma were relaxing. Inflation volume divided by the initial high pressure yields dynamic compliance (Cdyn), whereas division by the final holding pressure yields a greater effective static compliance (Ces)[32] (Fig. 14-5). Time dependence of compliance also implies a frequency dependence. Increasing the number of inflations per unit time results in a lower average compliance, because less time is available for "relaxation" between inflations.[33]

Sequentially inflating and deflating a lung reveals that the pressure required to maintain a given volume is greater on inflation than on deflation. This hysteresis is proportionally greater at large lung volumes. A plot of volume versus pressure yields a loop-shaped graph, or hysteresis curve, rather

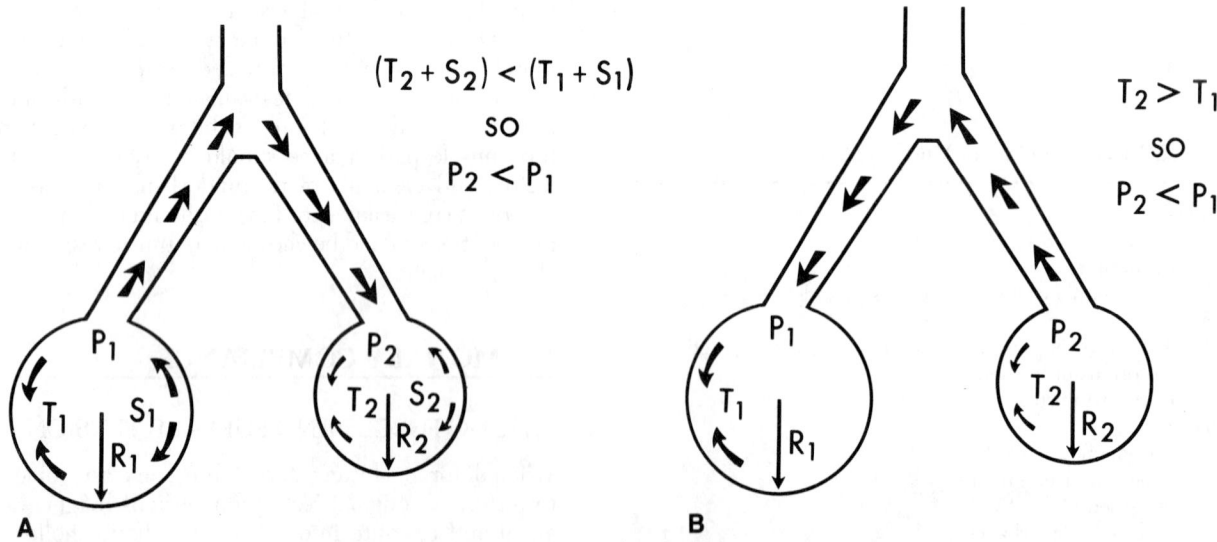

FIGURE 14-4. Alveolar surface force. (**A**) With surfactant. (**B**) Without surfactant. When surfactant is present, surface tension is directly related to alveolar volume. (Mecca RS: Pulmonary physiology. In: Kirby RR, Taylor RW [eds]: *Respiratory Failure.* Chicago, Year Book Medical Publishers, 1986.)

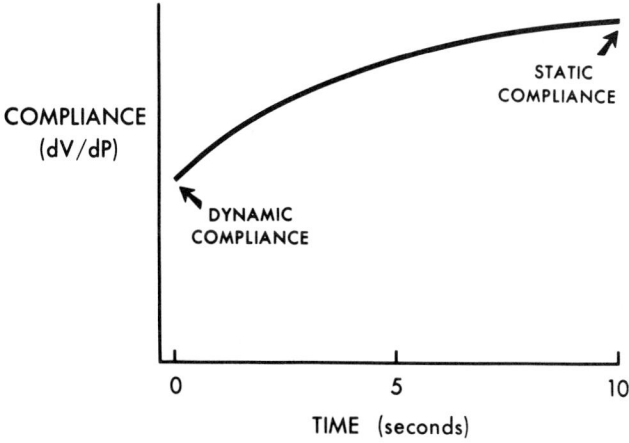

FIGURE 14-5. Time dependence of lung compliance. For a given lung inflation volume, initial high pressure determines *dynamic compliance.* Pressure decrease over time yields higher *static compliance.*

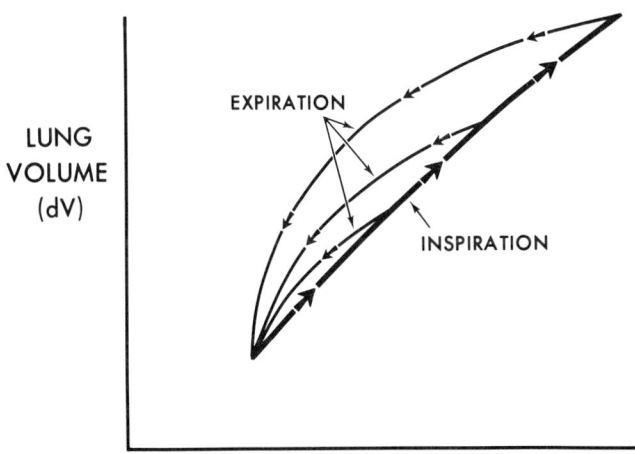

TRANSMURAL PRESSURE GRADIENT (dP)

FIGURE 14-6. Hysteresis. Pressure required for a given change in volume is greater during inflation (inspiration) than during deflation (expiration). (Mecca RS: Pulmonary physiology. In: Kirby RR, Taylor RW [eds]: *Respiratory Failure.* Chicago, Year Book Medical Publishers, 1986.)

than the straight line expected with an ideal elastic body (Fig. 14-6).

If a lung is repeatedly inflated and deflated with low tidal volumes, compliance gradually decreases during subsequent cycles. This volume dependence implies that periodic large inflations may be necessary for the maintenance of normal lung compliance. Although volume dependence of compliance is seldom of clinical importance, inflation volumes below 250 mL may cause a decrease in lung compliance if intercurrent larger inflations do not occur. Physiologic explanations of time dependence, hysteresis, and volume dependence remain obscure. Variation of surfactant activity may be a major determinant, although other mechanisms may be important.[1]

LUNG AND CHEST WALL INTERACTION

Chest cavity compliance is affected by diaphragmatic and intercostal muscle tone, and by factors that impede rib cage expansion or diaphragmatic descent into the abdomen. Factors that decrease chest cavity compliance contribute to a reduction of overall lung–thorax compliance and should be considered in any clinical setting of abnormal pressure–volume behavior.

Pulmonary Compliance

In vivo, change in volume of the intact lungs and thoracic cavity per unit change in transmural pressure is defined as pulmonary compliance:

1/pulmonary compliance
   = 1/lung compliance + 1/chest cavity compliance   (3)

Pulmonary compliance varies with lung–thorax volume in a complex fashion (Fig. 14-7). Within the usual range of lung volume, inspiration from FRC is assisted by spontaneous chest wall expansion, whereas expiration is achieved by passive lung recoil. These assist mechanisms allow a large

volume change with minimal pressure change. Pulmonary compliance is, therefore, highest when end-expiratory lung volume is at normal FRC. Lung volume below normal FRC promotes airway closure and atelectasis. A higher transmural pressure gradient is then required to reopen collapsed airspaces. Reduced lung volume often is caused by the diaphragm being forced upward into the chest, so outward chest cavity recoil does not increase proportionally. Pulmonary compliance is decreased at low lung volumes because more pressure is required to achieve expansion.[34,35]

Marked increases in lung volume also cause significant decreases in pulmonary compliance. A chest wall that is stretched to its equilibrium position offers little elastic assistance for further expansion. Expansion beyond the chest cavity equilibrium point impedes rather than assists inspiration. Similarly, at high lung volumes, the mechanical advantage and force of diaphragmatic contraction are reduced, decreasing the diaphragm's ability effectively to increase thoracic volume.

Pulmonary compliance is important clinically. A reduction of pulmonary compliance necessitates an increase in WOB (the energy expenditure required for spontaneous ventilation) to a point that respiratory muscle fatigue, exhaustion, and respiratory failure may supervene. Decreased pulmonary compliance also makes maintenance of FRC difficult. Reduced FRC, in turn, decreases radial traction on small airways, promoting airway closure and increased airway resistance, further increasing WOB. Decreased lung volume also interferes with $\dot{V}/\dot{Q}$ matching, predisposing to arterial hypoxemia. Low pulmonary compliance increases the positive pressure required to generate a given tidal volume with a mechanical ventilator. Excessive positive intrathoracic pressure increases the risk of barotrauma (pneumothorax, subcutaneous emphysema, air embolism) and impedes venous return to the heart, reducing cardiac output or increasing intracranial pressure.[36,37]

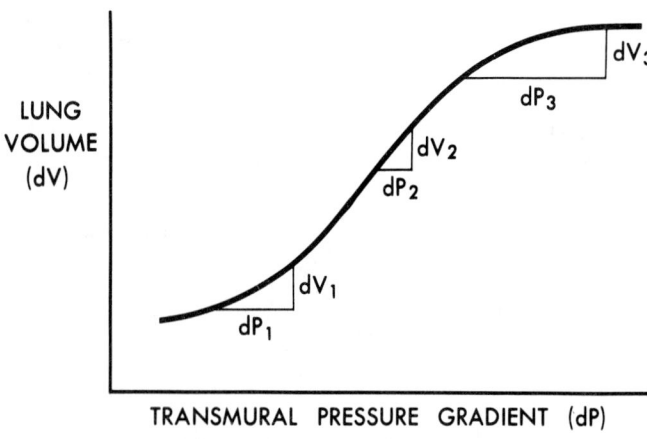

FIGURE 14-7. Pulmonary compliance versus lung volume. Relatively large pressure changes are required to achieve a given volume change at lung volumes far above or below normal functional residual capacity (FRC). (Mecca RS: Pulmonary physiology. In: Kirby RR, Taylor RW [eds]: *Respiratory Failure.* Chicago, Year Book Medical Publishers, 1986.)

In mechanically ventilated patients, ventilator airway pressures (PIP, Pplat) are used to estimate compliance, which in turn helps assess WOB.[4,6] The inflation volume is corrected for volume loss from compression in the ventilator circuit (3 to 5 mL/cm H_2O in adult circuits). A compliance above 50 mL/cm H_2O is considered normal, whereas a compliance below 25 mL/cm H_2O indicates an excessive WOB, which may interfere with weaning. Cdyn reflects elastic and resistive WOB, whereas the effective Ces reflects only the elastic WOB. When both compliances are proportionately reduced, the primary abnormality in the WOB is elastic. When compliance values are reduced disproportionately (e.g., Cdyn = 15, Ces = 30), it implies an increase in both elastic and resistive WOB. In contrast, if Cdyn is reduced but Ces is normal (Ces<<Cdyn), the primary WOB problem is resistive.

Measurement of esophageal pressures (Pes) during MV approximates pleural pressures and allows estimation of the pressure time index and the WOB. A change in Pes to less than 15 cm H_2O, a PTI less than 0.15, and a WOB less than 0.75 J/L during a spontaneous Vt indicate a nonlimiting WOB and predict successful weaning from MV. This assessment requires a computerized monitoring system and placement of an esophageal balloon catheter. The cost effectiveness of this technology is uncertain.[38]

AIRWAY RESISTANCE ■

LAMINAR AND TURBULENT FLOW

Flowing gas generates friction as gas molecules move past airway walls and one another. Overcoming this resistance to flow dissipates energy while pressure is reduced along the airway. For a given flow rate, the pressure gradient required to overcome resistance is expressed as follows:

$$P_p - P_d = \dot{Q} \times R \qquad (4)$$

in which $P_p - P_d$ represents the difference between proximal and distal pressures, $\dot{Q}$ is flow in volume per unit time, and R is resistance. An increase of resistance requires a greater pressure gradient to achieve constant flow or reduces flow if the pressure gradient remains constant.

Resistance to gas flow is influenced by flow velocity, airway geometry, and flow character. At low flow velocities through smooth straight tubes, gas molecules move in uniform, parallel streamlines characteristic of laminar flow. Resistance to laminar flow is calculated as:

$$R = \frac{8 \times \text{tube length} \times \text{gas viscosity}}{\pi \times (\text{radius})^4} \qquad (5)$$

At high flow rates or when airways are irregular or branching, streamlined laminar flow degenerates into a chaotic, unpredictable, turbulent pattern. Resistance to turbulent flow varies inversely with the fifth power of airway radius[39] and requires pressure gradients that vary directly with the square of flow rate.

ANATOMIC CONSIDERATIONS

Determinants

Airway resistance is determined primarily by airway radius, because other variables are essentially constant. Small changes in airway caliber markedly accentuate the impact of resistance on pulmonary gas flow.[40] For example, if airway effective radius is halved, resistance to laminar flow increases 16-fold, and the pressure gradient must also increase by 16-fold to maintain constant flow. Although the radii of individual airways decrease with each of 23 successive branchings, the total number of airways increases to a greater extent, resulting in an increase of total airway cross-sectional area with each successive generation. Therefore, overall resistance to gas flow is normally highest in the larger airways and decreases as the total cross-sectional area of smaller airways increases. Gas flow velocity also decreases in smaller airways because the same volume of gas flows through a progressively larger total cross-sectional area. Relatively high flow rates in large airways promote turbulence. While velocities decrease, the transition from turbulent to laminar flow also contributes to lower resistance in smaller airways.

Structure

Airways can be divided into three categories based on structure and size. The trachea and bronchi (generations 1 to 11) are large conduits encased in fibrous sheaths. These sheaths are not directly attached to the lung parenchyma, so large airways are not held open by retractile forces caused by lung expansion. Patency and support are provided by strong cartilaginous rings and smooth muscle within the airway walls. Positive intrathoracic pressure can compress the large airways, increasing airway resistance and limiting maximum forced expiratory flow rates. Bronchioles (generations 12 to

19) are small airways that have dense layers of smooth muscle in their walls but no significant cartilaginous wall support. They are attached to the lung parenchyma and rely on radial traction to maintain patency. Although these airways usually are not compressed by positive intrathoracic pressure, they undergo loss of support and closure when disease attenuates lung recoil. Alveolar ducts and alveoli (generations 20 to 23) are the smallest terminal airways. Their cross-sectional area is so large that gas movement and resistance to flow are negligible. Diffusion is the primary mechanism of gas exchange in alveolar ducts and alveoli.

CHANGES IN RESISTANCE

Mechanics

In view of its helical arrangement, contraction of airway smooth muscle decreases luminal cross-sectional area and increases resistance to gas flow. Localized constriction can selectively divert ventilation away from poorly perfused lung tissue and improve $\dot{V}/\dot{Q}$ matching. Smooth muscle tone is affected by many factors. Stimulation of beta-2 sympathetic nervous system (SNS) receptors in small airway walls by endogenous catecholamines or exogenous sympathomimetic medications activates adenyl cyclase, which increases the concentration of cyclic AMP and promotes relaxation by decreasing free intracellular calcium. Parasympathetic stimulation of muscarinic airway receptors causes smooth muscle contraction in larger airways.[41] Exposure to histamine promotes airway smooth muscle contraction, as might extremes of carbon dioxide partial pressures or alpha-adrenergic stimulation.

Peptides

A variety of neuropeptides originating in *peptidergic* neural structures in the lung also can affect airway smooth muscle tone.[42,43] Important among these are gastrin-releasing peptide, activated complement fragment C5A, leukotrienes C4 and D4, bradykinin, and a variety of neurokinins, including substance P and neurokinin A. Several other peptides induce bronchodilation, including peptide histidine methionine, vasopressin, oxytocin, atrial natriuretic peptide, and vasoactive intestinal peptide. Vasoactive intestinal peptide may be an important transmitter. In a poorly defined nonadrenergic, noncholinergic component of autonomic innervation of the lungs,[44] it possibly modulates release of inflammatory mediators from mast cells. In addition to direct effects, these peptides also interact with cholinergic and adrenergic mechanisms to affect smooth muscle tone.

Airway Pressure Changes

An increase in total airway resistance requires a compensatory increase in the pressure gradient to maintain a given level of ventilation. During spontaneous inspiration, a more negative intraalveolar pressure must be created, because ambient (mouth) pressure is unchanged. During expiration, greater positive alveolar pressure must be generated using muscles of expiration. Generation of excessive alveolar pres-

sure to overcome airway resistance significantly increases WOB, oxygen consumption, and CO_2 production.

Gas Trapping and Auto PEEP

Increased airway resistance often prolongs the time required for complete exhalation. If reduced expiratory flow precludes emptying of distal airspaces before the next breath is initiated, midexpiratory gas will be "trapped" in the alveoli and airways. Gas trapping forces subsequent inspirations to begin from a larger lung volume, increasing the energy required for expansion. Trapping dilutes inspired gas, causing hypercapnia and even hypoxemia by decreasing effective alveolar ventilation and alveolar Po_2.[39] Gas trapping also occurs if poorly supported airways in dependent lung regions close during tidal expiration.

In mechanically ventilated patients, increased expiratory resistance can cause auto PEEP, a positive pressure in the airways at end exhalation secondary to an inadequate expiratory time. Factors that favor development of auto PEEP include obstructive airway disease, $\dot{V}E$ requirements in excess of 10 L/minute, high ventilator rates with lower V_T, or low inspiratory flow rates. As with other forms of positive airway pressure, auto PEEP can contribute to barotrauma, reduce cardiac output, and interfere with interpretation of pulmonary arterial occlusion pressure. Auto PEEP will not be detected by the ventilator manometer, because positive pressure in the distal airways is not reflected on the manometer at end-exhalation.

Auto PEEP is more reliably identified using graphic waveform displays. On a flow-time curve, an expiratory flow rate that does not return to zero before the next machine-delivered breath suggests its presence. In general, the degree of auto PEEP varies directly with end-expiratory flow rate. Auto PEEP can also be estimated by reading the ventilator manometer pressure when the expiratory port is occluded during a passive exhalation just before the onset of inspiratory flow. If auto PEEP is present, ventilator settings should be changed to maximize expiratory time and minimize minute ventilation. Application of PEEP up to 10 to 15 cm H_2O, but not exceeding 80% to 85% of the auto PEEP, can act as a pneumatic splint to minimize dynamic airways' collapse. Bronchodilator therapy should be optimized.[45,46]

Complicating Factors

Compensatory physiologic adjustments sometimes worsen airway resistance. Positive intrathoracic pressure generated to overcome expiratory resistance compresses the large ensheathed airways. Increased inflow velocities through airways with reduced cross-sectional area promote turbulent flow, with a consequent increase in resistance. High flow velocities and turbulence are worsened if minute ventilatory requirements are augmented by hypercapnia, hypoxemia, or air hunger. High flow velocities also can push the smooth mucus lining the airways into a wavy, irregular configuration, reducing the cross-sectional area still further. Finally, high negative Ppl generated during labored inspiration promotes fluid accumulation around airways and can decrease their cross-sectional area. In the extreme, forced inspiration against an obstructed airway results in transient, occasionally severe hydrostatic pulmonary edema.[47]

Clinical Correlates

Increased airway resistance is caused by conditions that increase airway smooth muscle tone (asthma, reactive airway disease, chronic obstructive lung disease, potent airway stimulation) or by factors that interfere with airway smooth muscle regulation (beta-receptor blocking drugs, parasympathomimetic or alpha-agonistic medications, histamine release).[48,49] Inflammation and edema of the airways or accumulation of luminal secretions reduce cross-sectional area and increase resistance. Decreased lung recoil from chronic disease or loss of lung volume reduces radial traction and increases resistance. Obstruction caused by external compression (tumors, hematoma) or upper airway narrowing (croup, epiglottitis, laryngospasm) produces severe, life-threatening resistance changes.

GAS EXCHANGE   ■

PULMONARY CAPILLARIES

Carbon dioxide excretion and arterial oxygenation require a large interface that permits gas molecules to cross freely and rapidly between alveolar gas and pulmonary blood. Two populations of pulmonary capillaries exist within the alveolar matrix (Fig. 14-8). The first courses through corner junctions where adjacent alveoli merge at a "triple point." These junctional capillaries probably do not participate in gas exchange but instead are important for pulmonary fluid homeostasis. Other capillaries run in a sheet-like configuration within the alveolar septa dividing adjacent airspaces. Suspensory collagen fibers attach to septal capillaries, predominantly on the side facing the septal midplane. An increase in lung volume exerts traction on the suspensory fibers, bulging the septal capillary outward into the airspace on one side of the septum. (Roughly half the capillaries in a septum protrude

into each contiguous airspace, maximizing alveolar–capillary contact area).

Septal capillaries exhibit a thick vessel wall on the midplane side, with significant thinning where the capillary bulges into the airspace. The thin portion, composed of capillary endothelium, a fused basement membrane, and alveolar epithelium is involved in gas transfer. In contrast, the thick portion seems predominantly concerned with fluid and protein transfer between blood and the pulmonary interstitium. In some areas of the lung, alveolar septa exhibit pleats with capillary tufts inside.[50] These tufts are arteriovenous channels that bypass the capillary network and are sheltered from high intraalveolar pressures. Alveolar perfusion may originate in these vessels.

ALVEOLAR GAS COMPOSITION

Within a mixture of gases, each individual gas exerts a "partial" pressure in proportion to its fractional concentration. The sum of partial pressures of all gases and vapors equals total barometric pressure. To estimate the partial pressures of individual gases in alveoli, alveolar gas is assumed to be 100% saturated with water vapor at body temperature, and partial pressures of trace gases are ignored. Oxygen, CO_2, water vapor, and nitrogen are key components of alveolar gas, unless nitrogen has been replaced by nitrous oxide during anesthesia. In most instances, the alveolar partial pressure of carbon dioxide (P_{ACO_2}) approximates the systemic arterial partial pressure of carbon dioxide (P_{aCO_2}), a readily measured value.[51] Given ambient atmospheric pressure (P_B), the alveolar partial pressure of oxygen (P_{AO_2}) can be estimated using a simplified alveolar air equation[52]:

$$P_{AO_2} = [F_{IO_2} \times (P_B - P_{H_2O})] - P_{aCO_2}/R \qquad (6)$$

in which F_{IO_2} is the inspired concentration of oxygen expressed as a decimal, P_{H_2O} is saturated vapor pressure of water (47 mm Hg at 37°C), and R is the respiratory quotient (usually assumed to be 0.8). The F_{IO_2} should be held constant for 10 minutes to allow equilibration with FRC gas. Unless a patient is breathing ambient air (21% oxygen) or

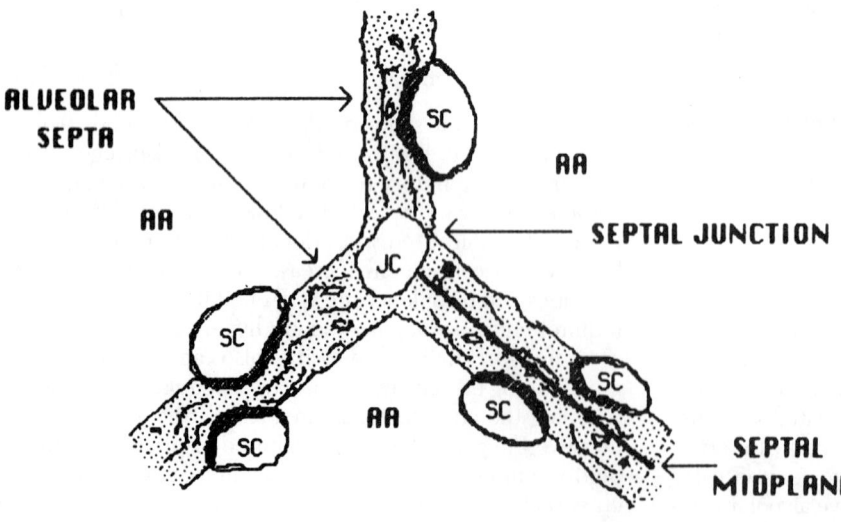

FIGURE 14-8. Schematic representations of the gas and fluid exchange areas within the lungs. SC, septal capillary; JC, junctional capillary; AA, alveolar airspace. (Mecca RS: Pulmonary physiology. In: Kirby RR, Taylor RW [eds]: *Respiratory Failure.* Chicago, Year Book Medical Publishers, 1986.)

a known percentage of oxygen in a closed system (endotracheal tube or tight-fitting mask with reservoir), the exact FIO_2 is often difficult to determine. Most devices used to deliver supplemental oxygen allow entrainment of room air during inspiration, reducing the actual percentage of oxygen in the trachea.

Once PAO_2 has been determined, an alveolar gas profile can be completed by using the equation:

$$PN_2 \text{ (or } PN_2O) = PB - (PH_2O + PAO_2 + PACO_2) \quad (7)$$

Estimation of alveolar partial pressures is important clinically, because they define one end of the diffusion gradient between blood and alveolar gas. Knowledge of PAO_2 is especially useful when evaluating the overall efficiency of pulmonary oxygen transfer.

BLOOD GAS COMPOSITION

Blood gas partial pressure is affected by the plasma solubility of each gas, which is constant if temperature is unchanged. In vivo, blood gas partial pressures vary directly with the number of free gas molecules dissolved. Because oxygen molecules bound to hemoglobin are in instantaneous equilibrium with "free" dissolved oxygen molecules, blood partial pressure reflects both dissolved and hemoglobin-bound fractions. Whole blood oxygen content is calculated as follows:

Blood O_2 content (mL/dL)
$$= 1.39 \times Hgb \times \% \text{ saturation} + (0.003 \times PaO_2) \quad (8)$$

in which Hgb is hemoglobin concentration (in grams per deciliter) and %saturation is percent saturation.

CO_2 molecules in blood are either dissolved, reversibly bound in red blood cells as carboxyhemoglobin, or involved in a carbonic acid–bicarbonate equilibrium:

$$CO_2 + H_2O \rightleftarrows H_2CO_3 \rightleftarrows H^+ + HCO_3^- \quad (9)$$

This equilibrium explains how increased $PaCO_2$ (reflecting dissolved molecules) decreases blood pH (a logarithmic expression of "free" hydrogen ion concentration). Dissolved CO_2 molecules are in instantaneous equilibrium with carboxyhemoglobin and carbonic acid–bicarbonate, so that the $PaCO_2$ reflects all three reservoirs.

GAS TRANSFER

Gas transfer between blood and alveoli occurs by passive molecular diffusion down partial pressure gradients. Diffusion distance across the thin side of septal capillaries is small, allowing rapid transfer of gas molecules. Exposure of pulmonary arterial blood to alveolar gas generates a rapid flux of oxygen and CO_2 molecules along their respective partial pressure gradients until new partial pressure equilibriums are reached. Oxygen molecules diffuse from a relatively high partial pressure in alveolar gas to a lower partial pressure in pulmonary arterial blood. Equilibration with alveolar PAO_2 is usually achieved before blood has traversed one third the length of an exchanging capillary. CO_2 molecules diffuse in an opposite direction along a gradient from pulmonary arterial blood to alveolar gas. Because of its in-

creased water solubility, CO_2 exchanges more rapidly across biologic barriers than does oxygen. Equilibration is almost instantaneous and is essentially unaffected by conditions that impede oxygen transfer.[53,54]

Partial pressures of nitrogen, nitrous oxide, and other inert gases are almost equal in alveoli and pulmonary blood unless the inspired concentration changes and a diffusion gradient is established. If an inert gas such as nitrogen is suddenly eliminated from the inspired mixture (as when a patient inhales 100% oxygen), much of the inert gas stored in FRC, blood, and tissue is quickly "washed out" by expiration. Depending on blood solubility, large volumes of inert gas can move into the alveoli, changing alveolar gas composition dramatically for short periods.

VENTILATION-PERFUSION MATCHING ■

Efficient gas exchange requires pulmonary arterial blood to flow through capillaries contiguous to alveoli containing fresh gas. Gas exchange is affected by the distribution of alveolar ventilation in proportion to pulmonary blood flow. If fresh gas delivery ceases, the partial pressures of alveolar gases quickly approach those in pulmonary arterial blood. Pulmonary and arterial blood passing unventilated or collapsed alveoli can neither gain oxygen nor unload CO_2, because the gradients necessary for diffusion are abolished. Instead, it is *shunted* through the lungs. In the pulmonary veins and left atrium, shunted blood extracts oxygen from the hemoglobin and plasma of oxygenated blood, resulting in a lowering of the PaO_2 in systemic arterial blood. Normally, 1% to 2% of right ventricular output is shunted physiologically through bronchial vessels, thebesian veins, and pulmonary arteriovenous anastomoses. Physiologic shunting partially explains the normal gradient between alveolar and arterial PO_2. A transient elevation of arterial CO_2 also occurs, but this change elicits a compensatory increase in ventilation that minimizes the impact of shunting on $PaCO_2$.

If blood flow to an alveolus is interrupted, ventilation to that airspace cannot contribute to gas exchange; this airspace is designated as *dead space*. The nasopharynx, oropharynx, trachea, and airways to the respiratory bronchiolar level comprise the normal anatomic dead space (approximately 2 mL/kg or 30% of a normal tidal volume). Interference with perfusion to the ventilated lung parenchyma creates additional *pathologic* dead space.[55] With constant total minute ventilation, an increase in dead space must decrease effective alveolar ventilation. Because the elimination of CO_2 varies linearly and directly with effective alveolar ventilation, increased dead space ventilation reduces CO_2 removal and leads to hypercapnia and respiratory acidemia, as described by the relationship for CO_2 homeostasis:

$$PaCO_2 = k \dot{V}CO_2/\dot{V}A \quad (10)$$

in which $\dot{V}CO_2$ is CO_2 production in milliliters per minute, and $\dot{V}A$ is alveolar ventilation in liters per minute. Alveolar ventilation can be expressed as follows:

$$\dot{V}A = \dot{V}E (1 - VD/VT) \quad (11)$$

in which $\dot{V}E$ is total minute ventilation in liters per minute and VD/VT is dead space ratio (percentage of VT not participating in gas exchange). Combining and substituting (equations 10 and 11) yields:

$$PaCO_2 = k\,\dot{V}CO_2/[\dot{V}E\,(1 - VD/VT)] \qquad (12)$$

For $PaCO_2$ to remain constant with increased VD/VT, a disproportionate increase in minute ventilation must occur. If total ventilatory requirement exceeds a patient's maximum ventilatory capability, progressive CO_2 retention occurs. Clinically, a VD/VT exceeding 0.6 at 10 L/minute usually indicates that a patient will not be able to maintain adequate CO_2 excretion during spontaneous ventilation, or will present significant problems with hypercapnia during weaning from MV. Measurement of $\dot{V}E$ often makes determination of VD/VT unnecessary. If the $\dot{V}E$ is less than 10 L/minute, VD/VT is almost always less than 60% and should not affect the patient's capacity to sustain spontaneous ventilation. Dead space does not affect PaO_2 significantly, because all pulmonary blood flow is still exposed to oxygen-rich fresh gas.

The lungs can be viewed as numerous $\dot{V}/\dot{Q}$ units with ratios ranging from 0 (shunt) through 1 (optimal) to infinity (dead space). Overall efficiency of gas exchange depends on a statistical distribution of $\dot{V}/\dot{Q}$ matching in millions of contributing units.[56] The concept of $\dot{V}/\dot{Q}$ matching has qualitative clinical applicability. Significant changes in gas exchange often are caused by subtle changes in $\dot{V}/\dot{Q}$ matching rather than by a complete cessation of blood flow or ventilation to one area of the lungs, especially when mechanisms that regulate the distribution of ventilation or perfusion are rendered ineffective.

DISTRIBUTION OF PULMONARY BLOOD FLOW

Both perfusion pressure and vascular resistance are important determinants of blood flow distribution within the pulmonary circulation. Blood flow through a vascular bed varies directly with the pressure gradient and inversely with resistance. Systolic pulmonary artery (PA) pressure is determined by preejection diastolic pressure, ventricular contractility, stroke volume, and compliance of large pulmonary vessels. Diastolic pressure is affected by the diastolic time interval (i.e., heart rate), pulmonary vascular resistance, and degree of left ventricular filling. Pressures within the PA are much lower than those in systemic vessels (e.g., approximately 25/10 mm Hg compared with 120/80 mm Hg) because PA wall compliance is high whereas pulmonary vascular resistance is relatively low.

Modifying Effects

As blood flows into smaller pulmonary vessels, gravity exerts a greater influence on intravascular pressure. Pressure in arteries located below the heart increases by an amount equal to the "weight" of a fluid column between the right atrium (taken as zero elevation) and the artery. Conversely, arteries located above the heart manifest a decreased intra-vascular pressure because upward blood flow is opposed by gravitational force. In smaller vessels, pressure is dissipated in overcoming resistance to flow caused by friction of cells, protein, and fluid against vessel walls and branch points. Most pressure reduction occurs by the time the blood passes the small muscular arterioles. Flow distal to arterioles is determined by capillary resistance, alveolar pressure, and pulmonary venous pressure. Relative distensibility and collapsibility of the small pulmonary vessels make pulmonary capillary resistance more significant in determining blood flow distribution than systemic capillary resistance.[57,58]

Lung Zones

The interaction between alveolar pressure and microvascular blood flow delineates three theoretical *zones*. In zone 1, alveolar pressure exceeds PA pressure, collapsing septal capillaries and precluding blood flow. Most zone 1 flow occurs through capillaries located in triple points and pleats (see Fig. 14-8). During spontaneous, ambient pressure ventilation, zone 1 should exist only in the most nondependent lung tissue, because maximum alveolar pressure is normally 2 to 4 cm H_2O. In zone 2, alveolar pressure is less than PA pressure but greater than pulmonary venous pressure. Zone 2 capillary flow should be intermittent and patchy, ceasing in septal vessels when microvascular pressure (P_{mv}) falls below alveolar pressure during expiration or diastole. In zone 3, PA and pulmonary venous pressures exceed alveolar pressure, and blood flow occurs throughout the cardiac cycle. Most healthy lung tissue falls within zone 3 unless alveolar pressure is elevated significantly above atmospheric. Zone 1 represents dead space (ventilation without perfusion); zone 2 contains high $\dot{V}/\dot{Q}$ units (ventilation in excess of perfusion); and zone 3 contains well-matched $\dot{V}/\dot{Q}$ units.[50,59]

Miscellaneous Factors

Capillary cross-sectional area and resistance are affected by pulmonary venous pressure, pleural and alveolar pressure, and lung volume. The effects of lung volume on septal and junctional capillary resistance are complex. Microvascular resistance probably is minimal at normal FRC but increases with a change in lung volume above or below FRC. Increased microvascular resistance in poorly expanded or collapsed lung may divert flow to better expanded regions, thereby improving $\dot{V}/\dot{Q}$ matching. This effect probably is minor because poor expansion or collapse usually occurs in dependent areas where P_{mv} and blood flow are highest. Negative alveolar pressure during inspiration tends to increase cross-sectional area. Extremes of negative or positive alveolar pressure can cause marked changes in regional blood flow distribution.

Regional blood flow also varies with PA pressure. Reduction of pressure decreases perfusion to nondependent lung regions. A decrease in PA pressure also blunts the impact of resistance differences among vascular beds. Increased PA pressure forces blood flow to nondependent areas, "recruits" previously underperfused vessels with high vascular resistance, and increases flow through physiologic and pathologic right-to-left shunts.

PULMONARY VASCULAR RESISTANCE

Hypoxic Pulmonary Vasoconstriction

Contraction of the circumferential wall muscle in individual arterioles or venules allows precise distribution of blood flow. Hypoxic pulmonary vasoconstriction (HPV) causes localized contraction of arterioles 200 to 300 μm in diameter, increased vascular resistance, and diversion of blood to better oxygenated airspaces in response to regional reduction of PaO_2. More global constriction in response to hypoxemia in PA blood increases PA pressure and redistributes blood flow to nondependent lung, recruiting poorly perfused capillaries and increasing surface area available for gas exchange.[60] HPV is attenuated by mediators, drugs, or increased PA pressure.[61-64]

Pathologic Factors

Many pathologic factors can influence pulmonary vascular tone.[65] Pulmonary arterioles are richly innervated with adrenergic receptors, so SNS activity or circulating catecholamines cause changes in resistance to flow. Generally, alpha-adrenergic stimulation causes vasoconstriction, whereas beta-adrenergic stimulation causes vasodilation. Numerous endogenous mediators (angiotensin, histamine, acetylcholine, bradykinin, serotonin, and vasopressin) and various neuropeptides cause vasoconstriction or vasodilation, depending on resting vascular tone. Individual effects and contributions of these substances to pulmonary vascular tone, HPV, pulmonary hypertension, and vasoconstriction with microembolism are controversial. Acidemia secondary to elevated arterial or alveolar PCO_2 causes pulmonary vasoconstriction, augmenting the effects of hypoxemia on pulmonary vascular resistance.[66] Nitric oxide exerts a potent, short-lived, vasodilatory effect on the pulmonary vasculature, and may play a role as a mediator in physiologic regulation of vascular tone.[67]

Vascular resistance between the pulmonary capillaries and the left atrium is usually minimal. However, pulmonary venules and small veins exhibit SNS innervation and can constrict in response to central nervous system (CNS) sympathetic outflow, reducing flow in upstream capillaries and arterioles. Poorly regulated SNS outflow associated with trauma, hypoxemia, or other pathologic conditions is sometimes associated with large increases in postcapillary resistance. The resulting increase of capillary pressure promotes accelerated fluid egress into the pulmonary interstitium, causing *neurogenic* pulmonary edema.[68] Compression or narrowing of pulmonary veins caused by positive intrathoracic pressure, increased interstitial fluid, tumor masses, or intimal thickening causes similar but less dramatic changes.

DISTRIBUTION OF VENTILATION

Pressure Gradients and Compliance

Distribution of ventilation is partially determined by pressure gradient differences within the airways. During spontaneous breathing, mouth pressure is constant and the effect of gravity on alveolar gas pressures is negligible. Therefore, only variations of alveolar pressures account for differences in airway pressure gradients during inspiration and expiration. These variations are related to differences in airspace compliances.

In contrast to unidirectional vascular flow, pulmonary gas flow is to and fro. During inspiration, gas flow through an airway fills distal airspaces and progressively reduces the airway pressure gradient. In a short time, alveolar pressure equals mouth pressure, and inspiratory flow ceases. Similarly, expiratory flow rapidly drains volume from expanded distal airspaces, again reducing the pressure gradient. Neglecting resistance, distribution of gas flow around airways is related to how quickly gradients in each individual airway or region of lung change with time. The pressure change occurring in a given airspace while it fills determines how much flow it will receive in comparison with others.

During inspiration, negative Ppl generated by chest cavity expansion is transmitted to the alveoli. In highly compliant airspaces, this transmitted negative pressure causes a substantial change in alveolar volume. In low-compliance airspaces, transmission of Ppl is attenuated by factors responsible for the poor compliance, and a smaller volume change results. The net result is a preferential distribution of gas flow to highly compliant areas within the lung. Airspace compliance also is affected by the surrounding tissues' distensibility, lung volume, interstitial hydration, intravascular volume, and body position.[69]

While alveolar volume increases, tension within the airspace wall and the surfactant–air–fluid interface increases, necessitating greater pressure changes to achieve additional expansion. Compliance, therefore, decreases as alveoli expand during inspiration. Distribution of ventilation is, in turn, affected by the different rates of change of compliance among alveoli and differences in their initial compliance. Alveoli that initially are highly compliant receive disproportionately greater ventilation during early inspiration. A rapid increase in volume decreases compliance of these alveoli below that of other airspaces that initially exhibited lower compliance. Gas flow is then diverted to these relatively underventilated alveoli at a later phase of inspiration.

Airway Resistance

Airways with low resistance receive more flow than those with higher resistance at comparable pressure gradients. Airway resistance, therefore, exerts a major effect on the distribution of ventilation.[70] Resistance in airways supplying poorly perfused distal airspaces may increase, diverting fresh gas to better perfused airspaces. PaO_2 probably is a primary stimulus regulating such bronchoconstriction. Pathologic increases in airway resistance can seriously derange $\dot{V}/\dot{Q}$ matching. In the extreme, airway closure denies fresh gas flow to respiratory bronchioles and alveoli, promoting shunt. Intermittent occlusion of small airways during tidal ventilation has more subtle effects. Ventilation will usually be sufficient to maintain alveolar patency but often will not match perfusion. Low $\dot{V}/\dot{Q}$ units are created, causing incomplete saturation of hemoglobin and reduction of PaO_2. Even after lung expansion pulls such airways open, their cross-sectional area is small compared with other airways. Intermittent closure is particularly damaging to $\dot{V}/\dot{Q}$ matching in dependent lung regions because the increased resistance diverts fresh gas away from well-perfused alveoli.

Although accurate assessment of in vivo gas distribution is difficult, clinical effects of compliance and resistance changes on flow can be described qualitatively. For example, in an erect position, apical alveoli exhibit high compliance and are supplied by small airways that are maintained patent by strong pleural retractile forces. During early inspiration, gas flow is preferentially distributed to the apical airways. This gas is predominantly dead space gas remaining in the large airways from the previous expiration. Because the apical airspaces also contain high $\dot{V}/\dot{Q}$ units, their initial high compliance diverts "stale" gas into poorly perfused alveoli. When these apical alveoli fill and their compliance falls, fresher gas is diverted to more compliant dependent alveoli with better perfusion. Storage of dead space gas in poorly perfused alveoli is an example of passive $\dot{V}/\dot{Q}$ matching.[55]

Pulmonary disease greatly influences airspace compliance and resistance and thus the distribution of ventilation. Atelectasis or consolidation eliminates ventilation to involved areas. Pulmonary edema, gas trapping, or retention of secretions reduces regional compliance, whereas destruction of lung tissue by emphysema increases compliance to abnormally high levels. Therapeutic application of positive-pressure ventilation alters regional compliance, especially if positive end-expiratory pressure or continuous positive airway pressure is used. Severe bronchospasm may increase airway resistance in a nonuniform fashion across the lung. Interstitial fluid accumulation and airway wall edema from obstructed lymphatics also change resistance. Pathologically increased resistance impedes gas flow through airways, negating more subtle diverting effects of selective bronchoconstriction. Increased airways resistance necessitates more time to complete expiration, which, in turn, reduces the time available for inspiration. A resulting rapid inspiration may not allow sufficient time for alveolar expansion, upsetting a balance between compliance changes and distribution of ventilation. If expiratory flow is so impeded that gas trapping occurs, adverse impact on alveolar compliance and distribution of blood flow can be profound.[71]

FLUID AND PROTEIN HOMEOSTASIS   ◼

Fluid and protein continuously pass across the microvascular endothelium of the pulmonary capillaries into lung tissue. Two separate influences promote fluid and protein movement: transmural hydrostatic pressure and transmural oncotic pressure.

ANATOMIC CONSIDERATIONS

Intravascular and airspace compartments (bounded by uninterrupted endothelial and epithelial cell layers, respectively) are separated by an interstitial compartment that is continuous from the hila through alveolar septa and suspensory tissue outward to the pleura. Intravascular fluid must move across the interstitial compartment to reach an airspace, assuming integrity of natural anatomic barriers. Pulmonary lymphatics originate in the interstitial space.

Sites of Exchange

Most pulmonary fluid and protein exchange occurs at a microvascular level, with both septal and junctional vessels participating (see Fig. 14-8). On the thin side of septal capillaries, fused basement membranes and tight junctions between alveolar epithelial cells impede movement of fluid and protein molecules. However, on the thick side facing the midplane of the alveolar septum, the basal lamina of capillary endothelium is widely separated from that of alveolar epithelium. This interstitial space contains connective tissue fibers, cellular constituents, mucopolysaccharide gel substance, contractile fibroblasts, and neural elements. Fluid exchange in septal capillaries probably occurs predominantly into the thick portion of the capillary–alveolar septal interface. Septal capillaries are directly affected by intraalveolar pressure because they are sandwiched between contiguous alveolar airspaces. Positive alveolar pressure compresses septal capillaries, reducing the transmural pressure gradient; negative alveolar pressure increases this gradient.

Junctional capillaries run in the intersections of alveolar septa and are completely surrounded by the interstitial space. Like the thick side of septal capillaries, these vessels probably do not participate in significant gas exchange. They are relatively unaffected by alveolar pressure, given their position in the alveolar matrix. However, increases of alveolar volume with spontaneous inspiration exert radial traction on these capillary walls, causing negative extravascular pressure and increased transmural pressure. Deflation alleviates this traction.[72]

Endothelial Permeability

Endothelial permeability to protein and cells varies in different portions of the pulmonary vasculature. Fluid and protein transfer seem to occur predominantly in capillary and proximal venular segments. Junctional gaps between endothelial cells usually allow passage of molecules smaller than 60 Å in diameter. Vasoactive substances or significant increases in P_{mv} may promote separation of loose intercellular junctions, causing an increase in permeability to fluid and protein. Increased permeability to protein results in higher interstitial protein concentration and a reduction of the transmural oncotic pressure.

Pressure Gradients

A low-magnitude negative-pressure gradient probably exists along the interstitial space, ranging from -3.3 mm Hg in the alveolar septa to approximately -9 to -10 mm Hg at the septal junctions and terminal lymphatics.[72] Increased surface tension caused by curvature differences between planar septal walls and rounded alveolar junctions may account for the greater negativity in junctional tissue. Also, radial stretch on junctional vessels during lung expansion may open intercellular junctions, promoting greater protein egress and creating an oncotic pressure gradient from septal to junctional tissue. After fluid and protein enter the terminal lymphatics, flow occurs through larger lymphatics against progressively less negative pressures, with eventual entry into the venous system. Fluid movement through valved lymphatics probably is assisted by a pumping action related to ventilation.

FLUID FLUX

Movement of fluid and solutes across microvascular endothelial barriers is described by the Starling equation:

$$\dot{Q}_f = [K_f(P_{mv} - P_{is})] - \sigma(\pi_{mv} - \pi_{is})] \quad (13)$$

in which $\dot{Q}_f$ is rate of filtration (volume/time), P is hydrostatic pressure, and π is oncotic pressure of microvascular (mv) and interstitial (is) compartments. Fluid conductance (Kf) is assumed to be large, indicating that microvascular walls are freely permeable to water. Similarly, σ (reflection coefficient) is assumed to be equal to 0 for small molecules but equal to 1 for large proteins, indicating that microvascular walls are freely permeable to electrolytes but impermeable to most large plasma proteins.

Hydrostatic Forces

Pulmonary microvascular pressure forces fluid across the capillary endothelium into the interstitial space. Usually, P_{mv} is approximately 7 mm Hg and is relatively unaffected by changes in PA pressure because the capillaries are distal to the primary resistance vessels, the pulmonary arterioles. However, an increase in left atrial or left ventricular enddiastolic pressure causes a corresponding increase in P_{mv}. The P_{mv} also is affected by gravity in that dependent capillaries have higher intravascular pressures than nondependent ones.

Normally, P_{is} is subambient, with an estimated value of approximately -8 to -9 mm Hg in a well-perfused lung. Negative interstitial pressure probably results from alveolar surface tension and perhaps from high plasma oncotic pressure as well. A negative P_{is} promotes fluid egress from capillaries by increasing the transmural pressure gradient.[73] Interstitial pressure varies with location in the lung and with changes in lung volume at a given location.

Osmotic-Oncotic Forces

Osmotic pressure varies directly with the number of free particles in a solution. Particle size is irrelevant. Water flows from an area of low osmotic pressure to one of higher osmotic pressure. In so doing, it dilutes the higher concentration of free molecules and equalizes osmotic pressure.

Differences between plasma and interstitial osmotic pressures are related to differing molecular concentrations across the endothelium. Because capillaries are freely permeable to electrolytes ($\sigma = 0$), intravascular and interstitial electrolyte concentrations are equal. However, significant protein concentration differences create a sizable *oncotic* gradient. Larger plasma proteins such as globulins are completely contained by endothelium ($\sigma = 1$), whereas smaller proteins such as albumin pass to a limited extent.

Although endothelium is slightly permeable to albumin, this protein accounts for most of the oncotic gradient because the number of molecules is far greater than other plasma proteins. Intravascular albumin concentration is always higher than that in the interstitium, assuming that the capillary endothelium is intact. Normal intravascular protein concentration yields a plasma oncotic pressure of approximately 28 mm Hg, which opposes fluid egress. Estimates of interstitial protein concentration (often based on lung lymph measurements) yield an approximate interstitial oncotic pressure of 13 mm Hg, which draws fluid out of the vessels. Acute changes in the transmural oncotic pressure gradient are predominantly caused by variation of interstitial albumin concentration, because serum concentration is relatively constant.

The estimated *net* transmural pressure is small, normally ranging from 0.2 to 0.5 mm Hg.[74] Change of one pressure in the transmural equilibrium often causes a compensatory change in an opposing pressure that attenuates the impact of the first change on overall fluid-solute flow into the interstitium. For example, increased P_{mv} or decreased π_{mv} should accelerate fluid and solute flux out of capillaries. However, fluid leakage increases P_{is} and decreases π_{is}, tending to maintain a normal gradient.[75] At steady state, a minor flux of fluid occurs from the intravascular space into the interstitial space that is continually removed by lymphatic drainage. The lymphatic system has a reserve capacity to absorb increased fluid flux to a point beyond which fluid accumulates and interstitial edema occurs.[76]

PULMONARY EDEMA

Several factors probably act in concert to prevent alveolar fluid accumulation. Alveolar epithelial cells have uniform, tight intercellular junctions that create a formidable barrier to solutes and water to a degree. Interstitial hydrostatic pressure beneath the epithelium is probably negative (-3.3 mm Hg), whereas interstitial oncotic pressure is undoubtedly higher than alveolar, because the alveoli normally do not contain significant amounts of free protein. Hydrostatic and oncotic pressure gradients, in conjunction with barrier characteristics of alveolar epithelium, strongly favor retention of fluid within the interstitial space. Rapid resorption of fluid, solutes, and protein from alveoli does occur.[77] Small radii of curvature in alveolar junctions may generate excessive surface tension, creating negative pressure "sumps" that draw fluid into the junctional interstitium. Alveolar fluid might interfere with surfactant activity, increasing surface tension and facilitating resorption. Intraalveolar protein is less easily absorbed than fluid. Clearance of large amounts probably involves phagocytotic activity.

Oncotic Pressure

Alterations of oncotic pressure alone seldom cause significant aberrations of pulmonary fluid homeostasis. Reduction of π_{mv} by severe hypoalbuminemia does not usually increase fluid transfer above the lymphatic drainage capability. Leakage of protein-poor fluid into the interstitium probably reduces interstitial protein concentration, tending to normalize the transmural oncotic gradient.

Pulmonary Microvascular Pressure

Increase in P_{mv} has a far greater impact on fluid homeostasis. Hydrostatic pulmonary edema is almost always related to increased P_{mv}. A compensatory increase of P_{is} is limited, because an elevation of 8 to 9 mm Hg would probably generate positive interstitial pressure, separation of alveolar epithelial cells, and alveolar flooding. Large increases of P_{mv} are possible, especially with left ventricular or mitral valve dysfunction. When P_{mv} reaches approximately 20 mm Hg, fluid flux approaches the drainage capacity of interstitial lymphatics. Accumulation occurs first in loose connective tissue near lymphatic origins and around small vessels and bronchioles. If P_{mv} rises above approximately 25 mm Hg, transudation across terminal airway epithelium and flooding of distal alveoli can occur (hydrostatic pulmonary edema).[78] Fluid flux might generate positive pressure in the alveolar septa as well, causing epithelial separation and direct alveolar flooding. Hydrostatic pulmonary edema can also be caused by extremes of negative pressure within the airspaces that generate a net filtration gradient similar to an increase in P_{mv}. This mechanism is responsible for pulmonary edema seen after forceful inspiratory efforts against an acute upper airway obstruction.[47]

Capillary Integrity

If capillary endothelial integrity is compromised, interstitial accumulation of fluid, protein, and even blood cells occurs, rapidly exceeding lymphatic drainage. The same pathophysiologic changes may disrupt alveolar epithelium.[79] Such increased permeability edema is much less dependent on intravascular pressure and is much more difficult to treat.

Mixed Pathology

Often, pulmonary edema is caused by a combination of increased intravascular pressure and increased capillary permeability. Each pathologic condition exhibits a mix of pressure and permeability characteristics. For example, pulmonary edema secondary to acute left ventricular dysfunction predominantly results from increased P_{mv}. However, some widening of capillary and venular intercellular gaps may occur, causing a capillary leak as well. Pulmonary edema resulting from systemic sepsis or the acute respiratory distress syndrome is predominantly caused by major increases in vascular permeability. However, elevations in P_{mv} generated by increased SNS activity or poor ventricular performance can also increase fluid flux.

CENTRAL CONTROL OF VENTILATION ▪

CARBON DIOXIDE

The CNS uses negative feedback mechanisms to monitor and regulate ventilation. A major component of ventilatory control is mediated by $PaCO_2$. CO_2 rapidly diffuses across the blood–brain barrier, so that elevation of $PaCO_2$ in arterial blood causes an immediate increase of CNS PCO_2 and pericellular free hydrogen ion concentration.[80,81] The reduced pH stimulates H^+-sensitive cells in the anterolateral cerebral medulla, increasing somatic outflow to ventilatory muscles. Ventilatory rate or depth increases, augmenting alveolar ventilation and CO_2 elimination. Subsequently, arterial blood with reduced $PaCO_2$ quickly reaches the brain, promoting diffusion of CO_2 out of the cerebrospinal fluid, reduction of respiratory center activity, and a decrease in alveolar ventilation. Elevation of CNS CO_2 does not cause a significant change in minute ventilation without a decrease in pH. In fact, a compensatory elevation of $PaCO_2$ usually occurs to compensate for chronic metabolic alkalosis. On the other hand, a reduction of cerebrospinal fluid pH increases ventilation despite a reduced $PaCO_2$. Respiratory compensation for chronic metabolic acidosis requires reduction of $PaCO_2$ below normal. At high partial pressure, CO_2 induces peripheral vascular dilation and myocardial depression. If $PaCO_2$ exceeds 150 to 250 mm Hg, cerebral function is affected in much the same fashion as by an anesthetic.[82]

OXYGEN

Chemoreceptor cells located in the carotid bodies (small, highly vascular organs near the carotid bifurcation) generate neural input to the respiratory center in response to reduced PaO_2. An increase in minute ventilation follows until elevation of PaO_2 reduces hypoxic feedback. Anemia, carbon monoxide poisoning, methemoglobinemia, or shifts in oxyhemoglobin dissociation characteristics alter the amount of oxygen available from each milliliter of blood. Although these abnormalities cause significant tissue hypoxia, an increase in minute ventilation does not occur if carotid PaO_2 remains normal. Therefore, the carotid body hypoxic drive mechanism monitors the efficacy of pulmonary oxygenation rather than systemic oxygen availability. Conversely, carotid body hypoperfusion related to hypotension or acute carotid occlusion can cause chemoreceptor hypoxia and an increase in minute ventilation, although pulmonary oxygenation and PaO_2 are normal. Carotid bodies also exhibit some sensitivity to $PaCO_2$/pH, contributing 10% to 20% of the total CNS ventilatory response to acidemia.[83,84]

NEURAL RECEPTORS

Lung volume and expansion are monitored and regulated, presumably to optimize compliance and $\dot{V}/\dot{Q}$ matching and to avoid respiratory muscle fatigue. Mechanoreceptors in the chest wall and diaphragm and slow adapting stretch receptors in the pulmonary parenchyma provide feedback on lung tissue deformation and chest cavity volume to pontine and medullary centers, which then alter the depth or pattern of inspiration.[85,86] This feedback is probably responsible for occasional large expansions (sighs or yawns) useful to maintain lung volume and compliance and might explain the air hunger encountered when lung expansion is limited by restrictive bandages, low pulmonary compliance, or inadequate ventilator volumes. These receptors probably also sense tissue deformation caused by vascular engorgement or interstitial fluid accumulation, contributing to the ventilatory changes associated with increased lung water. "J" receptors in the parenchyma seem to be activated by parenchymal inflammation, whereas rapidly adapting airway receptors generate afferent signals when exposed to noxious inhalants.

MISCELLANEOUS FACTORS

Ventilatory control is influenced by other CNS functions. Anxiety, agitation, or pain induce hyperventilation and respiratory alkalemia, as does increased autonomic activity.[87,88] Volitional or emotional input from cerebral cortical centers can override other drives, changing minute ventilation until extremes of pH and $PaCO_2$ are reached.[89-91] CNS reflexes regulating cough, swallowing, and phonation interact with central control of ventilation in a complex fashion. Motor output from ventilatory centers is also modulated by afferent input from laryngeal receptors along the superior laryngeal nerve. Various laryngeal receptors seem to monitor pressure and temperature as an index of flow and play a key role in coordination of pulmonary ventilatory cycling with upper airway patency.[92] Normal sleep has some inhibitory influence on ventilatory drive, causing a 4 to 8 mm Hg increase in $PaCO_2$ and a 3 to 10 mm Hg decrease in PaO_2, as well as significant changes in ventilatory patterns. WOB also exerts an inhibitory ventilatory influence mediated by afferent impulses from fatigued muscles of respiration or by the brain stem itself.[93]

A combination of ventilatory drives and inhibitory mechanisms determine motor output to muscles of respiration and minute ventilation. A change in one monitored variable will dominate control of ventilation until the adverse condition is alleviated. If severe $\dot{V}/\dot{Q}$ mismatching reduces PaO_2, hypoxic drive will override $PaCO_2$/pH drive and increase minute ventilation despite respiratory alkalemia. Conversely, if respiratory muscle fatigue is serious, inhibitory input will reduce ventilation in spite of CO_2 retention. If one drive is rendered ineffective by a disease or trauma, others will maintain ventilation. When chronic ventilatory insufficiency causes chronic elevation of $PaCO_2$, CNS sensitivity to pH diminishes and hypoxic drive dominates. Elevation of PaO_2 during administration of supplemental oxygen theoretically can produce severe hypoventilation and life-threatening acidemia in such patients. Conversely, bilateral carotid surgery can damage the carotid bodies, eliminating effective hypoxic drive.[94]

Many other factors influence the control of ventilation. Progesterone, doxapram, or aminophylline elicit increased minute ventilation by CNS stimulation. Systemic sepsis, paradoxical cerebrospinal fluid acidosis, or intracerebral trauma cause similar central hyperventilation and respiratory alkalemia. Narcotics or inhalation anesthetics depress sensitivity to both $PaCO_2$ and PaO_2.[95-97] The effectiveness of CNS control in maintaining adequate ventilation is altered in several disease states, including sleep apnea syndromes, apnea of prematurity, neuromuscular disorders (Guillain-Barré syndrome, poliomyelitis), spinal cord or brain stem trauma, increased intracranial pressure, and congenital heart disease.[16]

PROTECTIVE FUNCTIONS ■

REFLEX ACTIVITY

Laryngeal reflexes elicit a variety of protective responses that guard against aspiration of secretions or foreign matter into the lower airways. Cough reflexes that forcefully expel matter from the airway originate at both laryngeal and tra-

cheal levels and are probably mediated by intraepithelial, rapidly adapting receptors. A similar "expiration reflex" generates less forceful expiration accompanied by laryngeal constriction in response to vocal cord stimulation. This reflex is a common problem in lightly anesthetized patients.

Laryngospasm in response to mechanical airway stimulation also protects against aspiration. Reflex swallowing channels solid or liquid matter away from the tracheal inlet. Even reflex bronchospasm triggered by stimulation of laryngeal or tracheal mucosa probably has a protective function. Bronchospasm decreases airway cross-sectional area, thereby increasing velocity of expulsive air flow. Airway rigidity also increases, making airways less susceptible to collapse from positive intrathoracic pressure during expulsion. Finally, narrowed airways facilitate impaction of inhaled particles, protecting more distal airways from contamination during aspiration.

MUCOCILIARY TRANSPORT

Mucociliary transport along airways constitutes another important defense mechanism. Ciliated columnar epithelial cells line most of the airway lumenal surface, covered by a periciliary fluid layer that is probably formed through active chloride secretion across tracheal epithelium. The density of ciliated epithelium falls with increasing airway generations. Each cell projects approximately 200 to 250 cilia up into a second, 5 to 10 μm thick mucus layer lying over the periciliary fluid layer. The mucus layer is probably secreted by a variety of secretory cells interspersed in the epithelium and might be patchy rather than continuous. The fluid bilayer also has a significant pH buffering capability.

Volume and composition of mucus secretion are strongly influenced by a rich plexus of adrenergic, cholinergic, and peptidergic innervation.[98] ATP-dependent beating of the cilia propels the mucus layer with trapped particulate matter or bacterial debris toward the pharynx where it is cleared and swallowed. Mucus velocity varies between 2 mm/minute in small airways to 20 mm/minute in the trachea, with a total clearance between 10 and 100 mL/day. Ciliary clearance is greatly impeded by drying, cooling, aspiration or inhalation of caustic substances, and mechanical trauma.[99]

METABOLIC ACTIVITY ■

Pulmonary vascular endothelial cells are an ideal site for metabolic activity, because they constitute a large-surface monolayer that is exposed to the entire cardiac output. Several important endogenous substances are absorbed and metabolized by pulmonary endothelial cells, including serotonin, norepinephrine, and prostaglandins E and F. Other substances such as bradykinin, angiotensin, and adenine nucleotides are metabolized on endothelial cell surfaces. Lung injury can seriously interfere with these metabolic processes, causing significant physiologic aberrations. Changes in metabolism of these substances might prove useful as a severity index for pulmonary disease.[100] Several therapeutic compounds interact with pulmonary metabolic processes and can generate toxic metabolites that directly damage the pulmonary vasculature.[101]

REFERENCES   ■

1. Nunn JF: Elastic forces and lung volumes. In: *Applied Respiratory Physiology.* Oxford, Butterworth-Heinemann, 1993:36
2. Rehder K, Rah HM, Rodarte JR, et al: Airway closure. *Anesthesiology* 1977;47:40
3. Leblanc P, Ruff F, Milic-Emili J: Effects of age and body position on "airway closure" in man. *J Appl Physiol* 1970;28:448
4. Marini JJ: Lung mechanics determinations at the bedside: instrumentation and clinical application. *Respir Care* 1990;35: 669
5. Nunn JF: Pulmonary ventilation: mechanisms and the work of breating. In: *Applied Respiratory Physiology.* Oxford, Butterworth-Heinemann, 1993:117
6. Kacmarek RM: Noninvasive monitoring techniques in the ventilated patient. In: Kacmarek RM, Stoller JK (eds): *Current Respiratory Care.* St Louis, Mosby–Year Book, 1988:182
7. Roussos C, Macklem PT: Respiratory muscles. *N Engl J Med* 1982;307:786
8. De Troyer A, Estenne M: Functional anatomy of the respiratory muscles. *Clin Chest Med* 1988;9:175
9. De Troyer A, Estenne M, Vincken W: Rib cage motion and muscle use in high tetraplegics. *Am Rev Respir Dis* 1986; 133:1115
10. Von Euler C: Brain stem mechanisms for generation and control of breathing pattern. In: Cherniak NS, Widdicombe JG (eds). *The Respiratory System.* Bethesda, American Physiological Society, 1986:1
11. Van Lunteren E, Strohl KP: The muscles of the upper airways. *Clin Chest Med* 1986;7:171
12. Sant'Ambrogio FB, Mathew OP, Clark WD, et al: Laryngeal influences on breathing pattern and posterior cricoarytenoid muscle activity. *J Appl Physiol* 1985;58:1298
13. Arbonelius M, Lija B, Senyk J: Regional and total lung function in patients with hemidiaphragmatic paralysis. *Respiration* 1975;32:253
14. Eisele JH, Noble MIM, Katz J, et al: Bilateral phrenic nerve block in man. *Anesthesiology* 1972;37:64
15. Laroche CM, Carroll M, Moxham J, et al: Clinical significance of severe isolated diaphragm weakness. *Am Rev Respir Dis* 1988;138:962
16. Colice GL, Bernat JL: Neurologic disorders and respiration. *Clin Chest Med* 1989;10:521
17. Macklem PT: Normal and abnormal functions of the diaphragm. *Thorax* 1981;36:161
18. Kelly BJ, Luce JM: The diagnosis and management of neuromuscular diseases causing respiratory failure. *Chest* 1991;99: 1485
19. Vaz Fragoso CA: Monitoring in adult critical care. In: Kacmarek RM, Hess D, Stoller JK (eds): *Monitoring in Respiratory Care.* St Louis, CV Mosby, 1993:649
20. Krieger BP, Ershowsky P: Noninvasive detection of respiratory failure in the intensive care unit. *Chest* 1988;94:254
21. Yang KL, Tobin MJ: A prospective study of indices predicting the outcome of trials of weaning from mechanical ventilation. *N Engl J Med* 1991;324:1445
22. NHLBI Workshop Summary. Respiratory muscle fatigue. *Am Rev Respir Dis* 1990;142:474
23. Killian KJ, Jones NL: Respiratory muscles and dyspnea. *Clin Chest Med* 1988;9:237
24. Collett PW, Buchler B, Graham R, et al: The effect of small fiber phrenic afferents on respiratory motoneuron control. In: Sieck G, Gandevia SC, Cameron WE (eds). *Respiratory Muscles and Their Neuromotor Control,* vol 26. New York, Alan R Liss, 1987:205
25. Road J, Vahi R, Del Rio P, et al: In vivo contractile properties of fatigued diaphragm. *J Appl Physiol* 1987;63:471
26. Aubier M, Farkas G, Troyer A, et al: Detection of diaphragmatic fatigue in man by phrenic stimulation. *J Appl Physiol* 1981;50:538
27. Aldrich TK: Respiratory muscle fatigue. *Clin Chest Med* 1988; 9:225
28. Aubier M, Banzett RB, Bellamare F, et al: Respiratory muscle fatigue: report of the respiratory muscle fatigue workshop group. *Am Rev Respir Dis* 1990;142:474
29. Moxham J: Respiratory muscle fatigue: mechanisms, evaluation, and therapy. *Br J Anaesth* 1990;65:43
30. Van Golde IM, Battenburg JJ, Robertson B: The pulmonary surfactant system: biochemical aspects and functional significance. *Physiol Rev* 1988;68:374
31. Jobe A, Ikegami M: Surfactant for the treatment of respiratory distress syndrome. *Am Rev Respir Dis* 1987;136:1256
32. Marshall R, Widdicombe JG: Stress relaxation in the human being. *Clin Sci* 1961;20:19
33. Mills RJ, Cumming G, Harris P: Frequency dependent compliance at different levels of inspiration in normal adults. *J Appl Physiol* 1963;18:1061
34. Rehder K, Sender AD, Marsh HM: General anesthesia and the lung. *Am Rev Respir Dis* 1975;112:541
35. Caro CG, Butler J, Bubois AB: Some effects of restriction of chest cage expansion on pulmonary function in man. *J Clin Invest* 1960;39:573
36. Kumar A, Pontoppidan H, Falke KJ, et al: Pulmonary barotrauma during mechanical ventilation. *Crit Care Med* 1973;1:181
37. Qvist J, Pontoppidan H, Wilson R: Hemodynamic responses to PEEP. *Anesthesiology* 1975;42:45
38. Kaczmarek RM, Hess D: Routine measurement of work of breathing: is it necessary? *Respir Care* 1994;39;881
39. Nunn JF: Non-elastic resistance to gas flow. In: *Applied Respiratory Physiology.* Oxford, Butterworth-Heinemann, 1993:61
40. Ingram RA, Wellman JS, McFadden ER, et al: Relative contributions of large and small airways to flow limitation in normal subjects before and after atropine and isoproterenol. *J Clin Invest* 1977;59:696
41. Nadel JA, Barnes PJ: Autonomic regulation of the airways. *Annu Rev Med* 1984;35:451
42. Said SI: Effector actions: influence of neuropeptides of airway smooth muscle. *Am Rev Respir Dis* 1987;136:S52
43. Russell JA: Tracheal smooth muscle. *Clin Chest Med* 1986;7: 189
44. Diamond L, Altiere RJ, Thompson DC: The airway nonadrenergic, noncholinergic inhibitory nervous system. *Chest* 1988;93:1283
45. Ranieri VM, Giuliani R, Cinnella G, et al: Physiologic effects of positive end-expiratory pressure in patients with chronic obstructive pulmonary disease during acute ventilatory failure and controlled mechanical ventilation. *Am Rev Respir Dis* 1993;147:5
46. Pepe PE, Marini JJ: Occult positive end-expiratory pressure in mechanically ventilated patients with airflow obstruction: the auto-PEEP effect. *Am Rev Respir Dis* 1982;126:166

47. Wilms D, Shure D: Pulmonary edema due to upper airway obstruction in adults. *Chest* 1988;94:1090
48. Nodel JA: Autonomic regulation of airway smooth muscle. In: Nodel JA (ed). *Physiology and Pharmacology of the Airways*. New York, Marcel Decker, 1980:215
49. Hirschman CA: Airway reactivity in humans. *Anesthesiology* 1983;58:170
50. Gil J: The normal lung circulation: state of the art. *Chest* 1988;93:80S
51. West JB: Ventilation-perfusion relationships. *Am Rev Respir Dis* 1977;116:919
52. Riley RL, Lilienthal JL, Proemmel DD, et al: On the determination of the physiologically effective pressure of oxygen and carbon dioxide in alveolar air. *Am J Physiol* 1946;147:191
53. Piiper J: Pulmonary diffusion capacity and alveolar capillary equilibration. *Adv Exp Med Biol* 1988;227:19
54. Chang HK: Convection, diffusion and interactions in the bronchial tree. *Adv Exp Med Biol* 1988;227:39
55. Nunn JF: Distribution of pulmonary ventilation and perfusion. In: *Applied Respiratory Physiology*. Oxford, Butterworth-Heinemann, 1993:156
56. West JB: Ventilation/perfusion ratio inequality and overall gas exchange. In: *Ventilation/Blood Flow and Gas Exchange*. Oxford, Blackwell Scientific Publications, 1977:53
57. Sykes MK: The distribution of pulmonary blood flow. In: Prys-Roberts C (ed). *The Circulation in Anesthesia*. Oxford, Blackwell Scientific Publications, 1980:265.
58. West JB: Blood flow to the lung and gas exchange. *Anesthesiology* 1974;41:124
59. West JB, Dollery CT, Naimar A: Distribution of blood flow in isolated lung: relation to vascular and alveolar pressures. *J Appl Physiol* 1964;19:713
60. Marshall BE, Marchall C, Frasch F, et al: Role of hypoxic pulmonary vasoconstriction in pulmonary gas exchange and blood flow distribution. I. Physiologic concepts. *Intensive Care Med* 1994;20:379
61. Fishman AP: Hypoxia on the pulmonary circulation: how and where it acts. *Circ Res* 1986;38:221
62. Mathers J, Benumof JL, Wahrenbrock EA: General anesthetics and regional hypoxic pulmonary vasoconstriction. *Anesthesiology* 1977;46:111
63. Benumof JL: Hypoxic pulmonary vasoconstriction and sodium nitroprusside perfusion. *Anesthesiology* 1979;50:481
64. Benumof JL, Wahrenbrock EH: Blunted hypoxic pulmonary vasoconstriction by increasing lung vascular pressure. *J Appl Physiol* 1975;38:846
65. Marshall BE, Marchall C, Frasch F, et al: Role of hypoxic pulmonary vasoconstriction in pulmonary gas exchange and blood flow distribution. II. Pathophysiology. *Intensive Care Med* 1994;20:379
66. Malik AB, Kidd BSL: Independent effects of changes in H+ and CO_2 concentrations on hypoxic pulmonary vasoconstriction. *J Appl Physiol* 1973;34:318
67. Frostell C, Fratacci MD, Waiin JC, et al: Inhaled nitric oxide: a selective pulmonary vasodilator reversing hypoxic pulmonary vasoconstriction. *Circulation* 1991;83:2038
68. Theodore J, Robin ED: Speculations on neurogenic pulmonary edema. *Am Rev Resp Dis* 1976;113:405
69. Rehder K, Sessler AD, Rodante JR: Regional intrapulmonary gas distribution in awake and anesthetized-paralyzed man. *J Appl Physiol* 1977;42:391
70. Engel LA, Landau L, Tausing L, et al: Influence of bronchomotor tone on regional ventilation distribution at residual volume. *J Appl Physiol* 1976;40:411

71. West JB: Obstructive diseases. In: *Pulmonary Pathophysiology*. Baltimore, Williams & Wilkins, 1977:59
72. Weibel ER, Backofen H: Structural design of the alveolar septum and fluid exchange. In: Fishman AP, Renkin EM (eds). *Pulmonary Edema*. Bethesda, American Physiological Society, 1979:1
73. Taylor AE: Capillary fluid filtration: Starling force and lymph flow. *Circ Res* 1981;49:557
74. Guyton AC, Parker JC, Taylor AE, et al: Forces governing water movement in the lung. In: Fishman AP, Renkin EM (eds). *Pulmonary Edema*. Bethesda, American Physiological Society, 1979:65
75. Staub NC: Pulmonary edema. *Physiol Rev* 1974;54:678
76. Oppenheimer L: Lung fluid movement and its relevance to the management of patients with increased lung water. *Clin Intensive Care* 1990;1:103
77. Gee MH, Staub NC: Role of bulk fluid flow in protein permeability of the dog lung alveolar membrane. *J Appl Physiol* 1977;42:144
78. Staub NC: Pathways for fluid and solute fluxes. In: Fishman AP, Renkin EM (eds). *Pulmonary Edema*. Bethesda, American Physiological Society, 1979:113
79. Staub NC: Pulmonary edema due to increased microvascular permeability to fluid and protein. *Circ Res* 1978;43:145
80. Fleetham JA, Clarke H, Dhingra S, et al: Endogenous opiates and chemical control of breathing in humans. *Am Rev Respir Dis* 1980;121:1045
81. Bruce EN, Cherniak NS: Central chemoreceptors. *J Appl Physiol* 1987;62:389
82. Pavlin EG, Hornbein TF: Distribution of H+ and HCO3− between CSF and blood during respiratory acidosis in dogs. *J Physiol* 1975;228:1145
83. Ezaguirre C, Zapata P: Perspectives in carotid body research. *J Appl Physiol* 1984;57:931
84. Cunningham DJC: The control system regulating breathing in man. *Q Rev Biophys* 1974;6:433
85. Paintal AS: The mechanisms of excitation of type J receptors and the J reflex. In: Porter R (ed). *Breathing: Hering-Breuer Centenary Symposium*. Edinburgh, Churchill Livingstone, 1970:59
86. Katz S, Horres AD: Medullary respiratory neuron response to pulmonary emboli and pneumothorax. *J Appl Physiol* 1972;33:390
87. Burton MD, Johnson DC, Kazemi H: Adrenergic and cholinergic interaction in central ventilatory control. *J Appl Physiol* 1990;68:2092
88. Eger EI, Dolan WM, Stevens WC, et al: Surgical stimulation antagonizes the respiratory depression produced by forane. *Anesthesiology* 1972;36:544
89. Fink BR: Influence of cerebral activity in wakefulness on regulation of breathing. *J Appl Physiol* 1961;16:15
90. Phillipson EA: Control of breathing during sleep. *Am Rev Respir Dis* 1978;118:909
91. Shea SA, Walter J, Pelley K, et al: The effect of visual and auditory stimuli upon resting ventilation in man. *Respir Physiol* 1987;68:345
92. Sant'Ambrogio G, Mathew OP: Laryngeal receptors and their reflex responses. *Clin Chest Med* 1986;7:211
93. Poon CS: Optimal control of ventilation in hypoxia, hypercapnia, and exercise. In: Whipp BJ, Widberg DM (eds). *Modeling and Control of Breathing*. New York, Elsevier Biomedical, 1983:189
94. Wade JG, Larson CP, Hickey RF, et al: Effect of carotid endarterectomy on carotid chemoreceptor and baroreceptor function in man. *N Engl J Med* 1970;282:823

95. Weil JV, McCullough RE, Kline JS, et al: Diminished ventilatory response to hypoxia and hypercapnia after morphine. *N Engl J Med* 1975;292:1103

96. Knill RL, Gelb AW: Ventilatory responses to hypoxia and hypercarbia during halothane sedation and anesthesia in man. *Anesthesiology* 1978;49:244

97. Hirshman CA, McCullough RE, Cohen PJ, et al: Hypoxia ventilatory drive in dogs during thiopental, ketamine, or pentobarbital anesthesia. *Anesthesiology* 1975;43:628

98. Basbaum CB: Regulation of airway secretory cells. *Clin Chest Med* 1986;7:231

99. Wanner A: Mucociliary clearance in the trachea. *Clin Chest Med* 1986;7:247

100. Hart CM, Block ER: Lung serotonin metabolism. *Clin Chest Med* 1989;10:59

101. Duncan CA: Lung metabolism of xenobiotic compounds. *Clin Chest Med* 1989;10:49

Critical Care, Third Edition, edited by Joseph M. Civetta,
Robert W. Taylor, and Robert R. Kirby.
Lippincott-Raven Publishers, Philadelphia, PA © 1997.

CHAPTER 15

■

Respiratory Muscle Function and the Work of Breathing

Michael J. Banner

IMMEDIATE CONCERNS ■

MAJOR PROBLEMS

Work of breathing (WOB) assesses *afterload* on the respiratory muscles, that is, the load opposing respiratory muscle contraction. Increases in respiratory muscle afterloading and, thus, WOB result primarily from increased elastance and resistance. Because compliance is the reciprocal of elastance, as total compliance (lungs and chest wall) decreases, elastic loading of the respiratory muscles increases. The total resistive load is affected by airways and breathing apparatus resistances. Elastance, resistance, or both can significantly increase the afterload on the respiratory muscles, predisposing to muscle fatigue (loss of the force-generating capacity of the muscles), carbon dioxide retention, and hypoxemia.

Ventilatory support may be applied to partially or totally unload respiratory muscles. High levels of ventilatory support totally unload the muscles and, if applied for too long a period, may lead to atrophy. Conversely, too little support risks muscle fatigue. Unfortunately, in either case, the duration of mechanical ventilation may be needlessly prolonged for reconditioning/training if respiratory muscle atrophy is present or to provide needed rest if the muscles are fatigued. Optimization of ventilatory support to each patient's unique needs requires information of the afterload on the respiratory muscles as well as gas exchange. WOB measurements represent one approach to assess the afterload on the muscles and may provide a quantitative and goal-oriented method for appropriately setting the ventilator.

STRESS POINTS

1. Respiratory muscles are force generators, and the diaphragm accounts for 70% of normal tidal volume (V_T).
2. The diaphragm has high endurance capability well suited to low-tension, high-repetition activity (breathing). However, it can be readily fatigued by high resistive flow or increased duration of contraction.
3. Imposed WOB against a highly resistant ventilator circuit and endotracheal tube leads to fatigue. Patients with an already increased physiologic WOB because of respiratory disease tolerate such increases poorly.
4. Bedside measurement of WOB, including breath-by-breath analysis, and separation into its component parts is possible with a commercially available bedside monitor.
5. Previous estimates of WOB usually underestimated the actual value because of failure to assess chest wall compliance and its contributions.
6. Factors that load the respiratory muscles include increases of inspiratory flow rate and minute ventilation (alveolar and dead space), intrinsic positive end-expiratory pressure (PEEP), breathing apparatus resistance, and the ventilator response time. Many of these factors can be altered favorably by careful adjustment and replacement of highly resistant elements of the circuit (particularly the endotracheal tube).
7. Respiratory muscle fatigue results from an imbalance of energy supply and demand. It varies inversely with the removal of metabolites such as lactic acid.
8. Inferences as to WOB, such as increased respiratory

rate above 25 to 30 breaths per minute, can be misleading.

9. Successful weaning from mechanical ventilation often requires only a decrease in the imposed WOB. Pressure support ventilation (PSV) is uniquely capable of this goal when titrated in accordance with measured WOB.

ESSENTIAL DIAGNOSTIC TESTS AND PROCEDURES

1. Most patients can be followed by conventional assessment. However, when weaning, extubation, or both are difficult or seemingly impossible, direct measurement of airway and esophageal pressures and VT and calculation of WOB and its components using a bedside computer provide objective data not otherwise available.

2. Respiratory rate and breathing patterns should be continuously monitored, but their limitations for predicting fatigue, as detailed in this chapter, should be well understood.

INITIAL THERAPY

1. Decrease the imposed WOB to zero using PSV as the first step. This workload is of no value for muscle conditioning and predisposes to fatigue.

2. Add additional PSV as necessary to reduce the physiologic workload (elastance and resistance) to a normal level of 0.3 to 0.6 J/L.

3. Use the largest endotracheal tube that is unlikely to result in airway damage. A 1.0-mm increase of the inside diameter is associated with significantly less resistance work (parenthetically to be noted is that less air is needed for cuff inflation with larger tubes, thereby decreasing the risk of cuff-induced tracheal damage).

4. Do not reduce PSV below the level that eliminates imposed work. To do so reloads the respiratory muscles, predisposing to fatigue.

5. In difficult cases, use clinical parameters to supplement but not to replace direct WOB measurement.

RESPIRATORY MUSCLES ■

Respiratory muscles are the *force generators* that drive the respiratory system.[1] Regarded as the primary inspiratory muscle, the diaphragm accounts for approximately 70% of normal VT exchange. Other inspiratory muscles that account for the balance of tidal ventilation are the external intercostals, parasternals, and scalenes.[2] The sternocleidomastoid muscles are major *accessory* inspiratory muscles that have a predominantly pump-handle action on the rib cage, elevating the first ribs and sternum (Fig. 15-1). During quiet breathing, they are usually inactive but are always active during exercise and conditions of respiratory muscle loading.

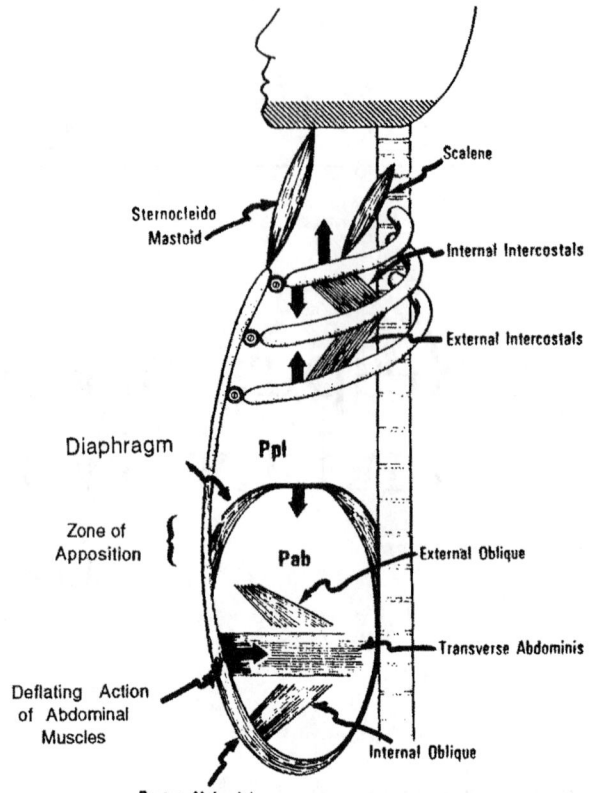

FIGURE 15-1. Diagrammatic representation of inspiratory and expiratory muscles; arrows indicate direction of action. Pab, abdominal pressure; Pp1, intrapleural pressure. (Modified from Roussos C: Function and fatigue of respiratory muscles. *Chest* 1985;88:S125.)

The internal intercostal and abdominal muscles are involved with exhalation. On contraction, the internal intercostal muscles lower the ribs, thus deflating the lungs. The external abdominal oblique, internal abdominal oblique, transverse abdominis, and rectus abdominis[1,2] (see Fig. 15-1) are the most important and powerful expiratory muscles. When these muscles contract, the abdominal wall is pulled inward, causing increased intraabdominal pressure that forces the diaphragm cephalad into the thoracic cavity.[3] Concomitantly, the lower ribs are pulled downward and medially. The net effect of these actions is deflation of the rib cage. Normally, exhalation is a passive process and the abdominal muscles are inactive. With increased muscle loads (e.g., increased airway resistance), however, the abdominal muscles are recruited and exhalation becomes an active, energy-consuming process.

THE DIAPHRAGM

Because the diaphragm is the primary muscle of inspiration, the physiologic characteristics and responses of this muscle during conditions of loaded and unloaded breathing are described.

Muscle Fiber Types

The adult diaphragm is composed of three types of skeletal muscle fibers: type 1 ($\leq$60%), type 2A ($\leq$20%), and type 2B ($\leq$20%)[4] (Table 15-1). Skeletal muscle fibers are differentiated on the basis of (1) velocity of shortening (fast and slow fibers), and (2) the major pathway to form ATP (oxidative and glycolytic fibers).[5] In general, muscle fibers are composed of two contractile protein filaments: myosin (thick filament) and actin (thin filament). Fibers containing myosin with high ATPase activity (enzyme that catalyzes the hydrolysis of ATP to ADP, releasing chemical energy stored in ATP) are classified as fast fibers; those containing myosin with lower ATPase activity are slow fibers. In general, the more energy that is available for contraction, the greater is the velocity of muscle fiber shortening.

OXIDATIVE PROPERTIES. Fibers containing high concentrations of mitochondria and oxidative enzymes (succinic dehydrogenase) have a high capacity for oxidative phosphorylation and are thus classified as oxidative. These fibers also have numerous capillaries and high myoglobin content. The large amounts of myoglobin give the muscle a dark red color; thus oxidative fibers are also referred to as "red muscle." In contrast, glycolytic fibers have few mitochondria but possess a high concentration of glycolytic enzymes and a large store of glycogen. These fibers have few blood vessels and contain little myoglobin. Because of the lack of myoglobin, glycolytic fibers are referred to as "white muscle." On the basis of these characteristics, type 1 fibers are referred to as slow oxidative fibers; type 2A are fast oxidative fibers; and type 2B, fast glycolytic fibers.[6]

FORCE GENERATION AND FATIGUE. Muscle fibers differ in terms of size and force development. Glycolytic fibers are larger in diameter than oxidative fibers. A greater force or tension can be developed by a large diameter muscle fiber. Consequently, a type 2B fiber (strength-oriented) can generate more force than a type 1 fiber during contraction.[4,5]

Fibers also differ in their ability to resist fatigue. Type 2B fibers fatigue rapidly, whereas type 1 fibers are resistant to fatigue (endurance oriented), a characteristic that allows them to maintain contractile activity for long periods. Type 2A fibers have an intermediate capacity to resist fatigue.[4,7]

RECRUITMENT. The muscle fiber types differ in terms of motor unit (all the muscle fibers innervated by a single motor nerve) recruitment order.[6] Motor units are recruited according to Henneman's size principle with type 1, type 2A, and then type 2B units added sequentially.[8,9] For heterogeneous muscle like the diaphragm, the earliest recruited motor units are the type 1, slow oxidative fibers with a rich capillary supply adapted to sustain aerobic work. At intermediate levels of force with moderate respiratory muscle loading, the type 2A motor units are also active; at higher levels of force with significant muscle loading, the type 2B motor unit fibers (the largest and most fatigable units) subsequently are recruited. The size principal ensures recruitment of motor units in order of increasing fatigability (or decreasing endurance)[6] (see Table 15-1).

ENDURANCE AND STRENGTH. In general, the diaphragm is an endurance-oriented (low-tension, high-repetition activity), not strength-oriented (high-tension, low-repetition activity) muscle because most of the muscle mass is composed of type 1, slow oxidative fibers. In fact, it is capable of impressive feats of endurance. An Olympic marathon runner can maintain high minute ventilation of approximately 50 L/minute several hours per day for many days in succession. Despite this endurance performance, the diaphragm can be fatigued in a matter of minutes by an increased resistance to flow rate or increased duration of muscle contraction.[4]

Actions

The diaphragm may be considered a piston with two parts (or two muscles). The *costal* section forms the sides of the "piston" with a zone of apposition to the ribs; the *crural*

TABLE 15-1. Characteristics of Diaphragmatic Muscle Fibers

	1	2A	2B
SHORTENING VELOCITY	Slow	Fast	Fast
ATPase activity	Low	High	High
Oxidative enzymes	High	High	Low
Mitochondrial content	High	High	Low
Capillary density	High	Intermediate	Low
Myoglobin content	High	High	Low
PRIMARY SOURCE OF ATP	Oxidative	Oxidative	Glycolytic
Glycogen content and enzymes	Low	Intermediate	High
Force	Lowest	Intermediate	Highest
Fiber diameter	Small	Intermediate	Large
Recruitment order	First	Second	Third
Resistance to fatigue	High	Intermediate	Low
Endurance	High	Intermediate	Low

section, or dome, forms the top.[1] After phrenic nerve stimulation, the costal diaphragmatic muscle fibers shorten in the zone of apposition, the diaphragm contracts and descends, the thoracic cavity expands, and the abdominal viscera are displaced caudally. Thus, the most important change in diaphragmatic shape is the piston-like axial displacement of the diaphragmatic dome as a result of shortening of the apposed muscle fibers. Simultaneously, intrapleural pressure decreases and abdominal pressure increases.[1,10] In addition to being an intrathoracic negative-pressure generator, the diaphragm is an intraabdominal positive-pressure generator for such functions as micturition, parturition, and defecation.

The *force* and *duration* of diaphragmatic contraction, useful for assessing muscle energy demands, can be measured.[1,3,7] Force generated during contraction is assessed by measuring the transdiaphragmatic pressure (Pdi), which is the difference between abdominal pressure (Pab) measured with a gastric balloon catheter and intrapleural pressure (Ppl) measured indirectly with an intraesophageal balloon catheter:

$$Pdi = Pab - Ppl$$

Normally, transdiaphragmatic pressure increases by approximately 10 cm H_2O during spontaneous inhalation. Healthy adults can generate maximal transdiaphragmatic pressures of approximately 100 to 150 cm H_2O.[11]

The duration of diaphragmatic contraction is the duty cycle of the breath taken as the ratio of inspiratory time to total respiratory cycle time (T_I/T_{tot}). Normally, the T_I/T_{tot} ratio is approximately 0.33.[10] The diaphragm, although contracting rhythmically from minute to minute, requires time to recover before contraction resumes. Impingement on this recovery time by an increase in respiratory rate, duration of contraction, or both, predisposes to respiratory muscle fatigue. An increase in respiratory rate, as in acute respiratory failure, causes a greater reduction in expiratory time than inspiratory time, thus increasing T_I/T_{tot} and contributing to the development of fatigue.[7,10] In patients with severe respiratory muscle loading, T_I/T_{tot} ratios as high as 0.50 to 0.60 have been measured.

By altering the excitation or stimulation frequency to the respiratory muscles, the CNS respiratory controllers affect the breathing pattern, that is, the force and duration of diaphragmatic contraction and respiratory rate.[2] On phrenic nerve stimulation, the neuromuscular junction is stimulated and the diaphragmatic muscle fiber membrane depolarizes and then repolarizes. These membrane potential changes are measured by an electromyogram (EMG) of the diaphragm. Muscle fiber shortening below relaxation length then ensues, resulting in increased transdiaphragmatic pressure. The greater the central discharge firing frequency and time of excitation from the central respiratory controllers, the greater the force and duration of diaphragmatic contraction, respectively. After a change in transdiaphragmatic pressure, a change in lung volume (VT) results.

MEASUREMENT OF WORK OF BREATHING

The load or afterload on the respiratory muscles is a reverse force that opposes the contractile force of the muscles and may be assessed by measuring the WOB, that is, by integrating the change in pressure (P) and the change in volume (dV)[12,13]:

$$\text{Work of breathing} = \int P \, dV$$

The total respiratory muscle work performed by a spontaneously breathing, intubated patient connected to a mechanical ventilator includes *imposed* and *physiologic* components (Table 15-2). The imposed WOB (work performed by the patient to breathe spontaneously through the endotracheal tube, ventilator breathing circuit, and demand-flow system) is an additional flow-resistive workload superimposed on the physiologic work.[14–16] Imposed work may equal or exceed the physiologic work under some conditions.[17–19]

Imposed work of the breathing apparatus is assessed by integrating the change in pressure measured at the carinal end of the endotracheal tube and VT.[20] Pressure at the carinal or tracheal end of the tube is measured by inserting a narrow (1-mm outside diameter), air-filled catheter through the tube and positioning it at the carinal end. VT is measured by integrating the flow signal from a miniature flow sensor (pneumotachograph) positioned between the "Y" piece of the breathing circuit and the endotracheal tube. These data are, in turn, directed to a commercially available, computerized, bedside monitor (Bicore, CP-100, Bicore Monitoring Systems, Allied Healthcare Products, Inc., Riverside, CA) that provides real time calculation and display of the imposed WOB[14] (Fig. 15-2).

Physiologic work includes elastic (work required to overcome the elastic forces of the respiratory system during inflation) and flow-resistive (work required to overcome the resistance of the airways and tissues to the flow of gas) components and is approximately 0.5 J/L of ventilation in normal adults[21] (clinically acceptable range is approximately 0.3 to 0.6 J/L).[22,23]

WOB performed by the patient on the respiratory system (physiologic work) and breathing apparatus (imposed work) during spontaneous ventilation is calculated by integrating the changes in esophageal pressure (indirect measurement of intrapleural pressure) and volume. Intraesophageal pressure is measured with a balloon catheter positioned in the middle to lower third of the esophagus. Correct position is confirmed using an occlusion test as described by Baydur and others[24] (i.e., after occlusion of the airway opening, the *change* in pressure at the airway opening and in the esophagus are nearly the same during spontaneous inspiratory efforts). VT is measured as described previously. Data from these measurements and measurement of chest wall compli-

TABLE 15-2. Work of Breathing Performed by a Spontaneously Breathing, Intubated Patient

TOTAL WORK OF BREATHING
PHYSIOLOGIC WORK
Elastic and flow resistive
IMPOSED WORK
Resistive work imposed by breathing apparatus (endotracheal tube, breathing circuit, demand-flow system, exhalation valves)

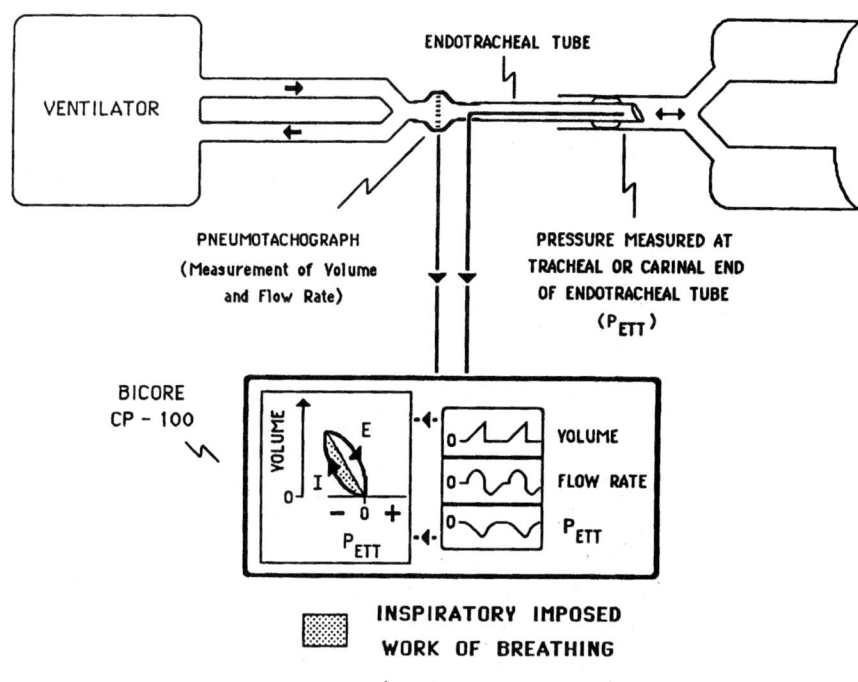

FIGURE 15-2. Imposed resistance work of the breathing apparatus is determined during spontaneous breathing by measuring change in pressure at the tracheal or carinal end of the endotracheal tube (PETT) and change in volume between the "Y" piece of the ventilator breathing circuit and the endotracheal tube. PETT and the change in volume are directed to a portable, bedside respiratory monitor (Bicore Monitoring Systems, Allied Healthcare Products, Inc., Riverside, CA) and are integrated to display a pressure–volume (work) loop and provide real time calculations of the inspiratory imposed work of breathing (i.e., the shaded area of the loop). I, inhalation; E, exhalation.

ance are processed and the WOB calculated using the Campbell diagram[13,25,26] (Fig. 15-3).

The Campbell Diagram

To compute WOB using the Campbell diagram, chest wall compliance must first be measured. Accuracy in measuring chest wall compliance requires a relaxed and mechanically ventilated patient. To measure chest wall compliance, a dose of 1 to 2 mg of midazolam is administered to induce relaxation, and then the mechanical ventilator rate is increased transiently to approximately 12 breaths/minute. Under conditions of mechanical inflation with a preselected VT and a relaxed patient, esophageal pressure increases. The monitor integrates the changes in esophageal pressure and volume to produce a pressure–volume loop, that moves in a counterclockwise direction. The slope of this pressure–volume loop is interpreted as chest wall compliance. This compliance value is stored in the monitor's computer memory. Measured chest wall compliance values for adult patients who were diagnosed with acute respiratory failure averaged 109 ± 37 mL/cm H_2O.

Next, 0.2 mg of flumazenil is given to reverse the effects of midazolam HCl so that the patient can resume spontaneous breathing. If complete reversal of the sedation is not achieved within 10 minutes, the dose is repeated. Total work during spontaneous breathing can then be computed using the Campbell diagram software.[27]

A validation study performed to assess the accuracy of the calculated work values displayed on the Bicore monitor compared with conventional measurement revealed a WOB correlation between the two sets of measurements that was nearly perfect ($r^2 = 0.99$, $p < 0.001$).[28] Bias was minimal (−0.05 J/L) and precision was excellent (±0.03 J/L).[29]

Alternative Measurements

The method described by Campbell has been applied to assess the WOB for adolescents[30] with compromised pulmonary mechanics and for adults receiving ventilatory support.[31–34] Use of the Campbell diagram, however, is tedious when conventional monitoring equipment is available; for these reasons, it has not been applied at the bedside. Other methods, all of which are less accurate, have been used.

Measurement of the area enclosed within an esophageal pressure—volume loop during spontaneous breathing *underestimates* WOB, because the area of the loop includes only the resistive work (physiologic plus imposed) and a small portion of the elastic work (see Fig. 15-3). Some investigators fitted a right triangle to the esophageal pressure—volume loop to infer elastic work; however, this approach also underestimates elastic WOB.[30] Measurement of the pressure change at the Y piece of the ventilator breathing circuit tubing or at the carinal end of the endotracheal tube and the change in volume during spontaneous breathing allows calculation *only* of the work imposed by the breathing circuit and the total breathing apparatus, respectively.[15,20] Thus, accurate measurement of the WOB (physiologic plus imposed) requires monitoring equipment with appropriate hardware and software to use the Campbell diagram.

LOADING FACTORS

For healthy, asymptomatic individuals, the afterload on the respiratory muscles results from normal impedance (compliance and resistance) and ventilation loads.[35] Increases in respiratory muscle loading result from a variety of physiologic and breathing apparatus factors. Physiologic factors include decreases in lung or chest wall compliance, or both,

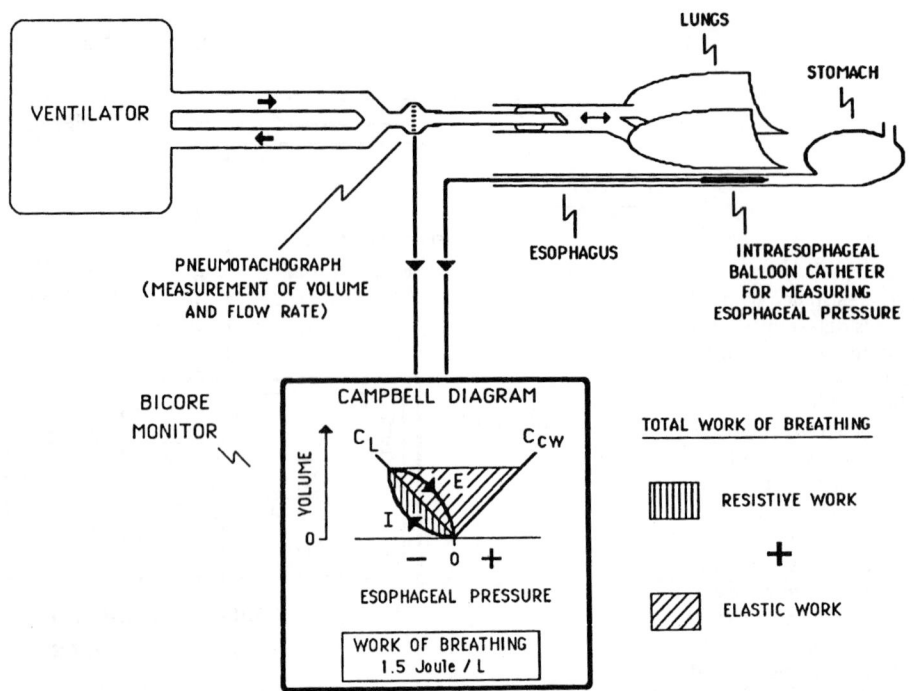

FIGURE 15-3. Clinical method of measuring the patient's work of breathing (WOB) (physiologic plus imposed work). Work is computed using the Campbell diagram, which relates the change in volume plotted over the change in esophageal pressure (inference of intrapleural pressure) during spontaneous inhalation (I) and exhalation (E). The change in volume is measured at the connection between the "Y" piece of the breathing circuit and the endotracheal tube with a miniature pneumotachograph (flow sensor). Esophageal pressure (Pes) is measured with an intraesophageal balloon positioned in the middle to lower third of the esophagus. These data are directed to a computerized, portable monitor (Bicore Monitoring System, Riverside, CA). The Pes–volume loop moves in a clockwise direction; the slope of the loop is lung compliance (CL). Chest wall compliance (Ccw) is obtained previously by mechanically ventilating a relaxed patient. Under these conditions the Pes–volume loop moves in a counterclockwise direction (not shown); the slope of the loop is Ccw. (This compliance value is stored in the monitor's computer memory and is used to construct the Campbell diagram). Inspiratory resistance WOB includes the physiologic resistive work on the airways and the resistive work on the breathing apparatus (vertical lines). Elastic WOB is the triangular shaped area subtended by the lung and chest wall compliance curves (diagonal lines). Total measured WOB, the sum of resistive and elastic work, is 1.5 J/L in this example. (Banner MJ, Gabrielli A, Layon AJ: Partially and totally unloading respiratory muscles based on real time measurements of work of breathing: clinical approach. *Chest* 1994;106:1835.)

secondary to pulmonary abnormalities, or to bronchoconstriction leading to peripheral, widespread narrowing of the airways that increase elastic and resistive loading, respectively (Figs. 15-4 and 15-5).

Spontaneous inspiratory flow rate demand affects resistive WOB directly. This relationship can be explained by an analogy of Ohm's Law of electricity, that is, change in pressure equals inspiratory flow rate demand multiplied by airway resistance. Assuming a fairly constant airway resistance over a range of flow rates, increases in the patient's peak inspiratory flow rate demand result in greater changes in pressure. Because work = ∫ P dV, a greater change in pressure with the same change in volume produces greater WOB.[20]

Minute Ventilation

Increases in alveolar and physiologic dead space minute ventilation also are forms of respiratory muscle loading that lead to increased WOB.[35] Under both conditions, the respiratory muscle pump is forced to work harder per minute (power) to meet the metabolic demands and maintain appropriate oxygen and carbon dioxide exchange. Assuming no change in oxygen consumption and carbon dioxide minute production, an increase in physiologic dead space ventilation from 1.5 to 3.0 L/minute requires the respiratory muscle pump to work proportionately harder to maintain the same alveolar minute ventilation.

Intrinsic PEEP

Increased levels of intrinsic positive end-expiratory pressure (PEEPi), or auto PEEP, as a result of increased expiratory airway resistance, inadequate exhalation time, or both, is another form of respiratory muscle loading. PEEPi must be counterbalanced by an equivalent change in alveolar pressure before air can flow into the lungs.[36] Consider a patient with dynamic hyperinflation and a PEEPi level of 5

FIGURE 15-4. Elastic work of breathing (WOB) varies inversely with lung compliance (CL). Functional residual capacity (FRC) is defined as the intersection of the lung and chest wall compliance (CCW) curves. Under conditions of normal lung compliance (*left*), a change in intrapleural pressure occurs accompanied by a change in tidal volume (VT) during spontaneous inhalation (I) and exhalation (E). The pressure–volume loop moves in a *clockwise* direction. Elastic WOB is the area indicated by the diagonal lines. Decreases in CL result in increased elastic WOB; notice flattened CL curve and increased elastic work area (diagonal lines) (*right*). In addition to decreased lung volume (decreased FRC), a greater change in intrapleural pressure is required to exchange a smaller tidal volume, a characteristic of acute respiratory failure.

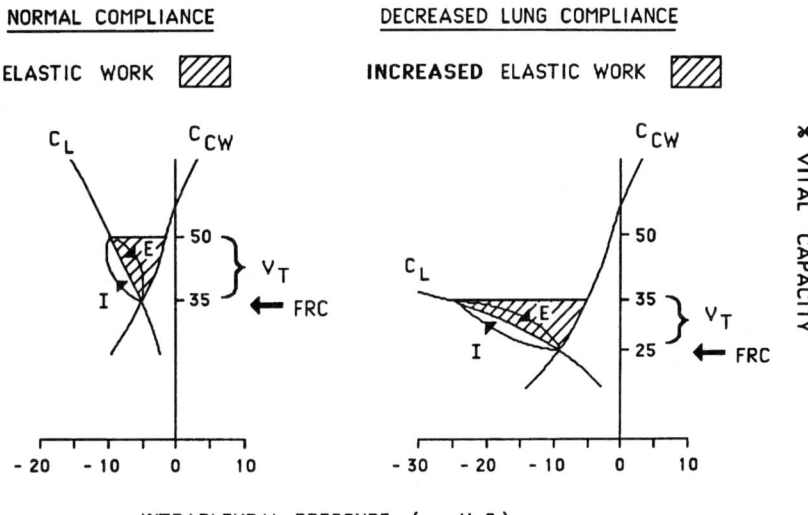

cm H_2O breathing room air spontaneously. Intraalveolar pressure must decrease by at least 6 cm H_2O (instead of 1 cm H_2O under normal conditions) so that alveolar pressure falls below ambient pressure. A pressure gradient between the mouth and alveoli must occur for air to flow into the lungs. Under these conditions, a greater decrease in pleural pressure is required than normal, and a greater WOB results.

Breathing Apparatus

Several breathing apparatus factors affect imposed WOB. *The endotracheal tube is probably the most significant resistor in the breathing apparatus.*[15,16,37–39] Breathing through a narrow internal diameter endotracheal tube attached to a highly resistive demand-flow continuous positive airway pressure (CPAP) system requires a large change in pressure

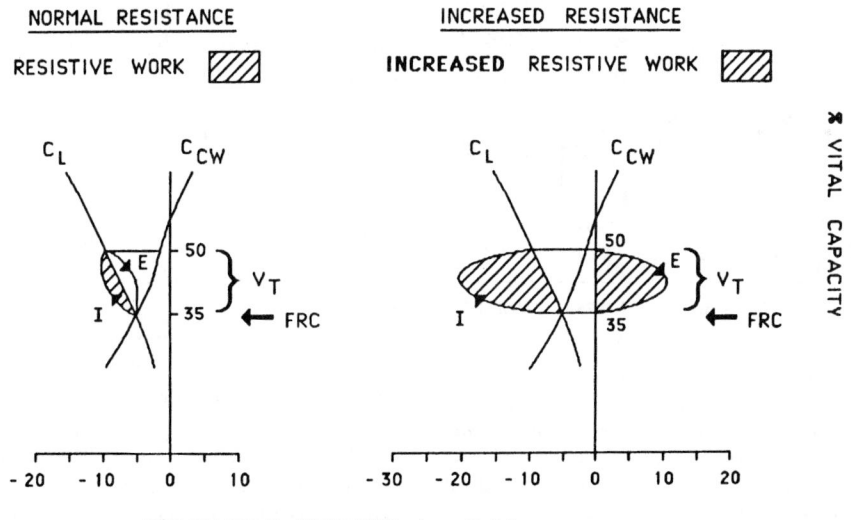

FIGURE 15-5. Increased resistance from airways resistance or imposed resistance of the breathing apparatus results in increased resistive work of breathing. Under conditions of normal resistance (*left*), a change in intrapleural pressure occurs accompanied by a change in tidal volume (VT) during spontaneous inhalation (I) and exhalation (E). Inspiratory resistive work of breathing is defined as the lower half of the intrapleural pressure–volume loop (area indicated by diagonal lines). Normally, exhalation is a passive process, and no resistive work is performed by the expiratory respiratory muscles. With increased resistance, the inspiratory muscles are loaded, resulting in a greater decrease in intrapleural pressure during inhalation and increased inspiratory resistive work (*right*). Expiratory resistance also may be present, causing expiratory muscle loading (abdominal muscles) and additional resistive workloads. FRC, Functional residual capacity; CL, lung compliance; CCW, chest wall compliance.

to move a specific volume. An increased resistive workload is imposed by the apparatus[39,40] (Fig. 15-6).

Ventilator Response Time

The response time of the ventilator (time delay from the initiation of spontaneous inhalation to the onset of flow in the airway) directly affects the imposed WOB. It is partly affected by the method of triggering the system "ON," and partly by the ventilator's sensitivity/trigger setting. The response characteristics of a ventilator's demand-flow CPAP system is improved by moving the pressure measuring/triggering site physically closer to the respiratory muscles, that is, at the tracheal or carinal end of the endotracheal tube.[41] Significantly less imposed work results from pressure-triggering the system ON at the carinal end of the endotracheal tube compared with the conventional method of pressure-triggering from inside the ventilator or using flow-by (flow triggered) initiation.[42,43] With pressure-triggering from inside the ventilator or with flow-by triggering, an initial *pressure* drop across the endotracheal tube must be generated by

the patient before *flow* is initiated. This effort results in significant increases in imposed work. By contrast, pressure triggering at the carinal end of the endotracheal tube effectively decreases the resistance by the endotracheal tube during spontaneous inhalation, thus decreasing the imposed WOB.

The sensitivity/trigger setting on the ventilator directly affects the imposed WOB. At a higher setting, a greater change in pressure is required to trigger the system ON, thereby increasing the WOB.[44]

CLINICAL IMPLICATIONS OF RESPIRATORY MUSCLE LOADING ■

FATIGUE

Increased respiratory muscle loading results in increases in the force and duration of diaphragmatic contraction and leads to an increased tension-time index of the diaphragm (TTdi).[3,7,10] TTdi is the product of transdiaphragmatic pressure over the maximum transdiaphragmatic pressure (Pdi_{max}) and the ratio of inspiratory time to total cycle time (TTdi = $Pdi/Pdi_{max} \times T_I/T_{tot}$). The TTdi is similar to the tension-time index for the heart and gives a useful approximation of muscle energy demands.[7,10] During spontaneous breathing, the change in transdiaphragmatic pressure is normally about 10 cm H_2O and the T_I/T_{tot} ratio is 0.33, effecting a TTdi of 0.03 (TTdi = 10 cm H_2O/100 cm $H_2O \times 0.33$). With increased respiratory muscle loading, Pdi may increase to 30 cm H_2O and T_I/T_{tot} to about 0.5, resulting in a TTdi of 0.15. Breathing patterns with a TTdi of about 0.15 to 0.20 are called *fatiguing* to indicate that the diaphragm will, in time, fail.[7,10] Presumably, when the *demand* of the diaphragm exceeds 0.15 to 0.20, sufficient energy supplies are not available.[7,10,44] This threshold TTdi is related to the limitation of blood perfusion and oxygen delivery to the muscle (Fig. 15-7).

ENERGY SUPPLY AND DEMAND

Respiratory muscle fatigue develops for the same reasons that one develops angina pectoris: *demand for energy exceeds the supply of energy.*[7,45] Energy supply refers to the proportion of cardiac output, blood perfusion, oxygen, and nutrients to the respiratory muscles that directly affect the synthesis of ATP. Respiratory muscle fatigue develops when ATP hydrolysis exceeds ATP synthesis as a result of an imbalance between energy supply and demand. Under conditions of increased muscle loading, respiratory muscle energy demands increase. Increases in muscle blood flow demand and oxygen consumption predispose to the development of muscle ischemia, fatigue, and respiratory failure.[45,46] VT decreases and increases in dead space to VT ratio and arterial carbon dioxide levels result when the respiratory muscles fail as force generators.

Respiratory muscle fatigue varies inversely with the removal of muscle metabolites.[7] A decreased rate of lactate removal results in increased intracellular hydrogen ion con-

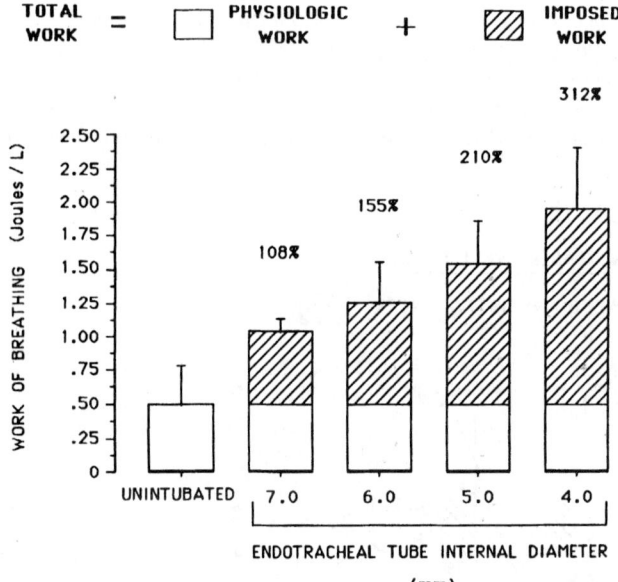

FIGURE 15-6. Influence of endotracheal tube size on imposed and total work of breathing (WOB). Before intubating a group of piglets (n = 8; weight, approximately 10 kg), the mean physiologic work, as measured using the method described by Campbell, was 0.5 J/L. Subsequently, all animals breathed through endotracheal tubes of 7-, 6-, 5-, and then 4-mm internal diameter, which were sequentially inserted into their tracheas. Imposed work of the endotracheal tube (diagonally striped columns) is superimposed on the physiologic work (open columns), yielding the total WOB or afterload on the respiratory muscles. The narrower the endotracheal tube, the greater the imposed and total WOB. Total work increased by 312% with the narrowest internal diameter endotracheal tube, predisposing to respiratory muscle fatigue. (Widner L, Banner MJ: A method of decreasing the imposed work of breathing associated with pediatric endotracheal tubes [abstract]. *Crit Care Med* 1992;20;S82.)

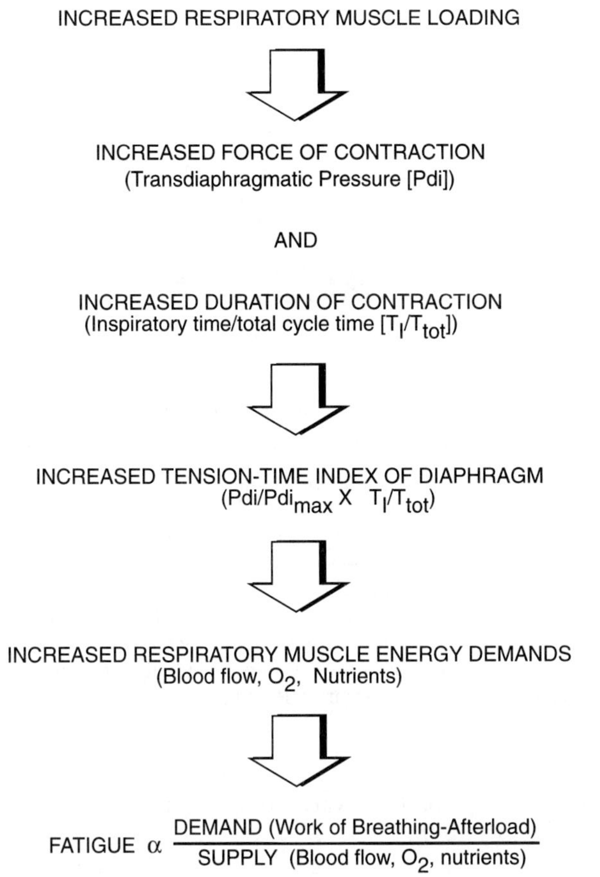

INCREASED RESPIRATORY MUSCLE LOADING

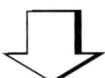

INCREASED FORCE OF CONTRACTION
(Transdiaphragmatic Pressure [Pdi])

AND

INCREASED DURATION OF CONTRACTION
(Inspiratory time/total cycle time [T_I/T_{tot}])

INCREASED TENSION-TIME INDEX OF DIAPHRAGM
(Pdi/Pdi_{max} X T_I/T_{tot})

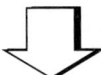

INCREASED RESPIRATORY MUSCLE ENERGY DEMANDS
(Blood flow, O_2, Nutrients)

$$\text{FATIGUE} \;\alpha\; \frac{\text{DEMAND (Work of Breathing-Afterload)}}{\text{SUPPLY (Blood flow, } O_2 \text{, nutrients)}}$$

FIGURE 15-7. Increased respiratory muscle loading and the subsequent effects leading to fatigue. Fatigue is defined as loss of the *force-generating* capacity of the respiratory muscles.

centration which, in turn, leads to decreases in muscle pH (normally about 7.0). When muscle pH decreases to about 6.4, glycolytic enzymes (phosphorylase and phosphofructokinase) are almost completely inactive.[7] Thus, the decrease in pH results in a slowing of the rate of ATP resynthesis. In addition, the fall in muscle fiber pH impairs calcium release from the sarcoplasmic reticulum.[7] Inhibition of ATP synthesis and the release of calcium compromises muscle contractile protein function and results in a decrease in the force-generating capacity of the respiratory muscles.

BREATHING PATTERN

Frequency

When pulmonary mechanics deteriorate, the respiratory muscles are loaded and WOB increases. As a result, the breathing pattern changes (Table 15-3). These changes are vagally mediated by afferent or sensory fibers (load sensors) in the lungs and respiratory tract. Three types of afferent fibers modulate the breathing pattern: (1) slowly adapting receptors (SARs); (2) rapidly adapting receptors (RARs) (also termed *deflation, cough,* or *irritant* receptors), both of

which are pulmonary stretch or mechanoreceptors; and (3) chemosensitive or C-fiber endings.[47] SARs are found in the bronchial smooth muscle fibers, RARs are situated in the superficial layers of the respiratory tract mucosa, and C-fibers are found in the airway epithelium.[47]

CNS MODULATION. The mechanoreceptors monitor changes in pulmonary mechanics and thoracic gas volume (functional residual capacity).[48,49] After a decrease in lung compliance (increase in respiratory muscle load), an increase in discharge activity occurs. Similar responses result after increases in total resistance.[48,49] C-fiber endings are activated by many substances produced in the lungs such as histamine, bradykinin, and some prostaglandins.[48,49] Some sympathetic afferents also may be activated in response to increases in mechanical loads.[48] Afferent discharge signals from the sensory fibers are directed by the vagus nerve to the central respiratory controllers in the CNS, modifying their output signals, which, in turn, modify the breathing pattern.[3]

Stimulation of these receptors produces patterns of rapid, shallow breathing and an optimal breathing frequency to minimize large changes in intrapleural pressure.[50] Patients with loaded respiratory muscles breathe at a faster rate and a smaller Vt to minimize the WOB, the so-called "minimal WOB" or "least average force" concept, producing the most energy-efficient combination of breathing frequency and Vt.[21,50,51] When the frequency is too low, much elastic work is required to produce large Vts; when the frequency is too high, much resistive work is required (as well as useless work to ventilate the dead space with each breath[50]) (Fig. 15-8). This mechanism also functions to protect the respiratory muscles from exhaustive, fatiguing contractions that can lead to muscle fiber splitting, hemorrhage, and self-destruction.[3]

LOCAL LOAD COMPENSATION. A local load-compensator mechanism has been described that involves muscle spindle receptors and motorneurons in the intercostal muscles and diaphragm.[48] This mechanism regulates muscle contraction to obtain the desired change in length (i.e., Vt). The demand for a given length change is transmitted from the muscle receptors to the motorneurons. As a result, a change in

TABLE 15-3. Manifestations of Loaded Respiratory Muscles and Fatigue*

Increased breathing frequency
Discoordinate respiratory movements, i.e., abdominal paradox (abnormal *inward* abdominal displacement during spontaneous inhalation, characteristic of a fatigued diaphragm) and respiratory alternans (alternating between abdominal paradox and normal breathing, which is characterized by an outward displacement of the abdominal wall during inhalation)
Hypercapnia and respiratory acidemia
Terminal fall in breathing frequency and minute ventilation

---

*Fatigue is defined as loss of the force-generating capacity of the muscles.

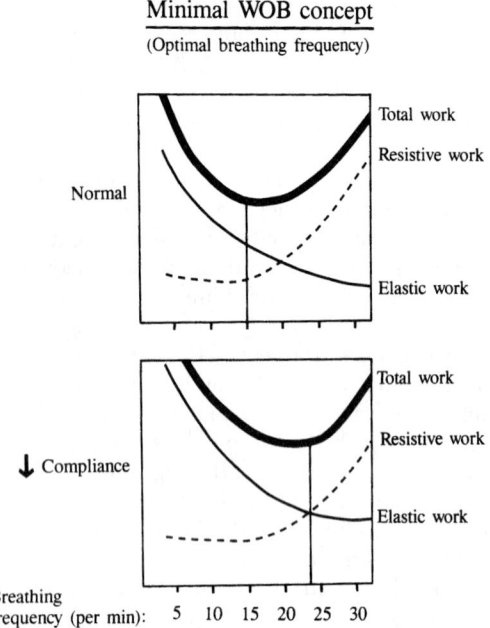

Minimal WOB concept

(Optimal breathing frequency)

FIGURE 15-8. Minimal work of breathing (WOB): optimal breathing frequency concept as described by Otis[21] and Sant' Ambrogio.[49] Total WOB (*thick line*) consists of resistive (*dashed line*) and elastic work (*thin line*). Under normal conditions (*top*), patients adopt a breathing frequency and tidal volume combination which corresponds to minimal total WOB, that is, for adults, an optimal breathing frequency and tidal volume are approximately of 12 to 15/ minute and 500 mL, respectively. Elastic work is excessive at lower breathing frequencies and higher tidal volumes. Conversely, resistive work increases at higher breathing frequencies and lower tidal volumes. The body adopts a motion that strains it the least. Under conditions of decreased compliance (increased elastance) the respiratory muscles are loaded (*bottom*), and a breathing frequency of 12/minute and tidal volume of 500 mL are no longer optimal because elastic work, and thus total WOB, are increased. The optimal breathing frequency and tidal volume combination corresponding to minimal total WOB are a frequency of approximately 25/minute and a tidal volume of about 250 mL. Thus, a rapid, shallow breathing pattern is a compensatory, energy-efficient breathing strategy to minimize WOB.

mechanical load (e.g., increased airway resistance) to the contracting muscle leads to compensatory adjustments in the activity of the motorneurons.

INFERRED WORK OF BREATHING. Clinicians use respiratory rate as an *inference* of the WOB.[52] An abnormal adult respiratory muscle workload is inferred when the spontaneous respiratory rate is greater than 25 to 30 breaths/minute; a breathing rate of 15 to 25 breaths/minute is inferred to mean that workload is tolerable and in a more normal range. These inferences, however, seem to be inaccurate and misleading with regard to the WOB.[31,53–55] Although patients breathing between 15 to 25 breaths/minute often demonstrate an apparently acceptable breathing pattern, the respi-

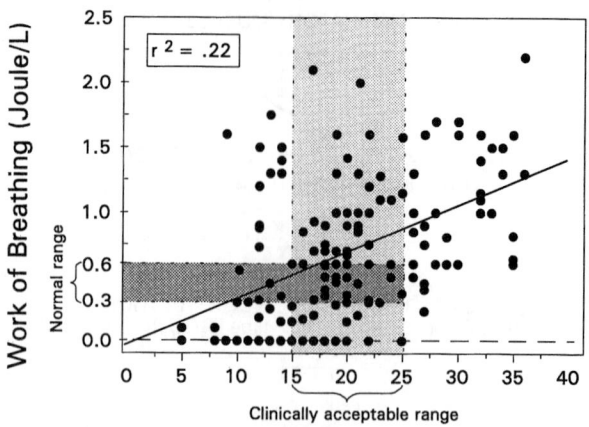

FIGURE 15-9. Relationship between WOB and spontaneous breathing rate. Although a positive and significant correlation was found ($r = 0.47$, $p < 0.001$), spontaneous breathing rate predicted or explained only 22% of the variance in work of breathing. Within a clinically acceptable breathing rate range of 15 to 25 breaths/ minute, some adults performed no work (predisposing to disuse respiratory muscle atrophy), others performed work in a normal range, and some performed work in a potentially fatiguing range (predisposing to respiratory muscle fatigue).

ratory muscle workloads vary from fatiguing, to normal, to zero[53,54] (Fig. 15-9).

ASSISTED SPONTANEOUS BREATHING. Unquestionably, the aforementioned physiologic, load-sensing and load-compensating mechanism functions during spontaneous breathing. Whether it functions in the same manner during assisted spontaneous breathing (i.e., PSV) is unknown. However, some altered role of the pulmonary stretch receptors in mediating the response seems likely, particularly when ventilatory support results in larger-than-normal VT (as is often the case during PSV) and restoration of functional residual capacity with CPAP. The focal point or question of this argument is, "Can the above physiologic, load-sensing and load-compensating mechanism be relied on to predict or infer respiratory muscle workloads *accurately* for all patients in respiratory failure treated with PSV?"

My data and that of others[53–56] reveal that the breathing pattern is not an accurate predictor of WOB and may provide preliminary evidence that this physiologic mechanism is, indeed, affected during positive-pressure ventilatory support. I believe that the breathing pattern should *not* be used as the primary guideline for selecting levels of PSV to unload the respiratory muscles. To infer a value for WOB by counting the breathing frequency and observing the breathing pattern seems as spurious as inferring a value for cardiac output by counting heart rate and observing urine output. Data also suggest that the perceived inspiratory effort sensation during spontaneous breathing (how the patient feels, degree of comfort) is not related to the presence of fatiguing or nonfatiguing diaphragmatic contractions.[57] A logical deduction is that WOB should be measured directly.

DECREASING RESPIRATORY MUSCLE AFTERLOAD

THERAPEUTIC OBJECTIVES

Objectives of therapy for loaded or fatigued muscles include the following: (1) decrease energy demand (WOB), and (2) increase energy supply (oxygen, blood flow, and nutrient delivery) to the respiratory muscles. PSV is advocated to unload the respiratory muscles, decrease the WOB, and decrease the energy demands of patients with decreased compliance and increased resistance.[22,52,58,59] It also augments spontaneous breathing by potentially decreasing the work imposed by the resistance of the breathing apparatus to zero.[14,37]

In the PSV mode, the ventilator is patient-triggered ON, and an abrupt rise in airway pressure to a preselected positive-pressure limit results from a variable flow rate of gas from the ventilator. As long as the patient maintains an inspiratory effort, airway pressure is held constant at the preselected level. Gas flow rate from the ventilator ceases when the patient's inspiratory flow rate demand decreases to a predetermined percentage of the initial peak mechanical inspiratory flow rate (e.g., 25%). The ventilator is thus flow-cycled "OFF" in the PSV mode.

Once the preselected inspiratory pressure limit is set, the patient *interacts* with the pressure-assisted breath and retains control over inspiratory time and flow rate, expiratory time, breathing rate, VT, and minute volume (Fig. 15-10). Patient work decreases, and ventilator work increases at incremental levels of PSV.[27,31,32]

Decreasing the afterload on a muscle to an appropriate level decreases the force and duration of muscle contraction (tension-time index),[7] energy demand, muscle ischemia, and fatigue. For a patient with an increased systemic vascular resistance of 2400 dyne·second·cm^{-5}, clinicians may choose

to unload the left heart by means of vasodilators. The response is a decreased afterload (systemic vascular resistance) to a more "normal" range and an increased velocity of myocardial muscle shortening and stroke volume (assuming no change in the energy supply, force-length [preload], and force-frequency [contractility] relationships of the muscle). In analogous fashion for a patient with increased respiratory muscle afterload/WOB, for example, 1.5 J/L, a clinician may also unload the respiratory muscles to a more normal range using PSV. The response is similar: a decrease in afterload (WOB) and energy demand and an increase in the velocity of muscle shortening and VT. Thus, *PSV is to the diaphragm as sodium nitroprusside is to the left ventricle* (Fig. 15-11).

PARTIAL AND TOTAL RESPIRATORY MUSCLE UNLOADING

The level of PSV may be set to partially or totally unload the respiratory muscles.[27,58-60] During partial unloading, PSV is increased until the patient's WOB is decreased to a tolerable range. My goal usually is 0.3 to 0.6 J/L, the normal range for physiologic WOB.[22,23] During inhalation with PSV, positive pressure actively assists lung inflation. A portion of the WOB is provided, relieving and unloading the respiratory muscles of the increased workload, and decreasing the force and duration of muscle contraction. Work is performed in part by the patient and in part by the ventilator, that is, a work-sharing approach. Partial respiratory muscle unloading is appropriate to provide a nonfatiguing workload and promote muscle conditioning (Fig. 15-12).

Titration of PSV

The level of PSV may be set to provide appropriate, or *optimal* respiratory muscle loads. The exact level of this load is not known, but some authorities suggest that near-normal

FIGURE 15-10. Airway pressure and flow waveforms are depicted for pressure support ventilation (PSV). After the ventilator is patient-triggered "ON," an abrupt rise in pressure ensues to a preselected limit, and a decelerating inspiratory flow waveform results. When the inspiratory flow rate decreases to a predetermined percentage of the initial peak inspiratory flow rate (e.g., 25%), the ventilator flow cycles "OFF." On the right, a greater inspiratory effort, a longer inspiratory time (T$_I$) and higher peak inspiratory flow rate demand are illustrated at the same level of PSV. The clinician sets the level of PSV, while the patient *interacts* with the pressure-supported breath and retains control over breathing rate, T$_I$, flow rate, and tidal volume.

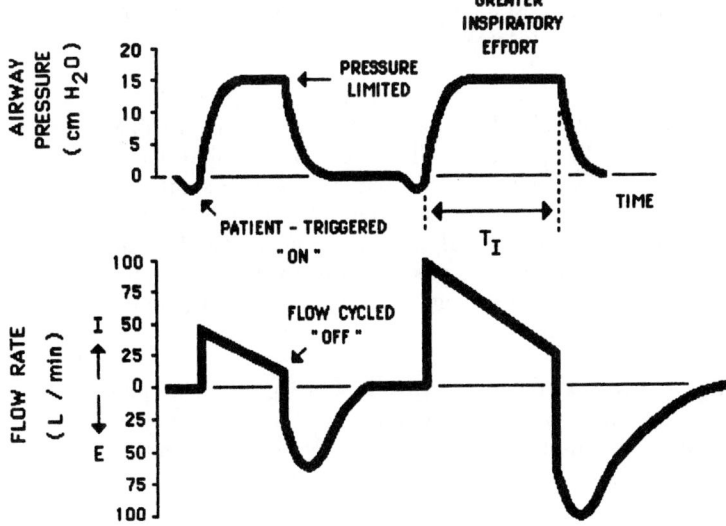

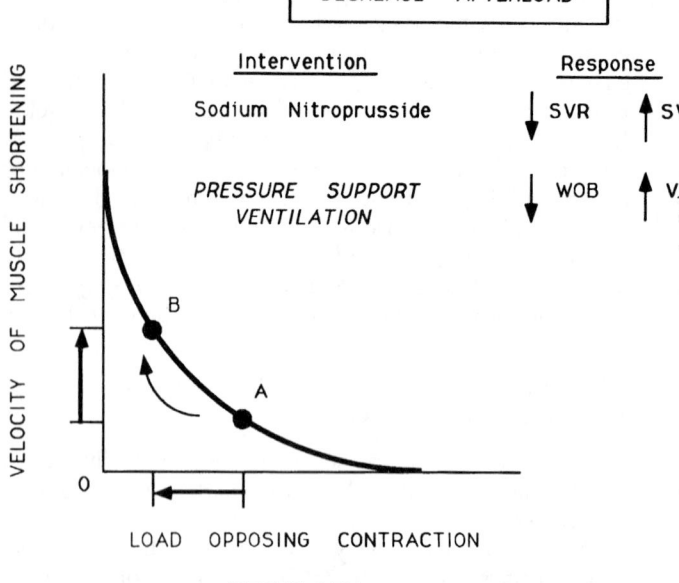

DECREASE AFTERLOAD

Intervention		Response
Sodium Nitroprusside	↓ SVR	↑ SV
PRESSURE SUPPORT VENTILATION	↓ WOB	↑ V_T

FIGURE 15-11. Relationship between the load or force opposing muscle contraction (afterload) and the velocity of muscle shortening. The afterload on the cardiac and respiratory muscles is a reverse force that opposes muscle contraction. The force-velocity relationship describes the ability of a muscle to move loads, that is, the speed of shortening is inversely related to the initial load on the muscle. With increased left ventricular afterload (increased systemic vascular resistance [SVR], *point A*), the velocity of muscle shortening is decreased, that is, decreased stroke volume (SV). Sodium nitroprusside decreases left ventricular afterload, causing a shift from point A to B and resulting in decreased SVR and increased SV. Pressure support ventilation is to the diaphragm as sodium nitroprusside is to the left ventricle. Application of pressure support ventilation decreases afterload on the respiratory muscles, causing a shift from point A to B and resulting in decreased WOB and increased tidal volume (V_T). (Banner MJ, Gabrielli A, Layon AJ: Partially and totally unloading respiratory muscles based on real time measurements of work of breathing: a clinical approach. *Chest* 1994;106:1835.)

workloads are well tolerated.[32,56] In a carefully done study, Brochard and coworkers[32] report that at PSV of approximately 15 cm H_2O, an optimal muscle load corresponded to a patient WOB 0.52 ± 0.12 J/L. An optimal load was defined as that which maintained maximal diaphragmatic electrical activity without fatigue (specifically, the lowest level of PSV at which no reduction in the ratio of high to low frequency components of the diaphragm's electromyographic signal occurred). A reduction of 80% or less of the initial high:low ratio is defined as incipient diaphragmatic fatigue.[61,62]

When the respiratory muscles were partially unloaded, we found that PSV of approximately 18 cm H_2O was required, corresponding to a patient WOB of 0.50 ± 0.12 J/L.[27] Combining these observations, my definition of partial respiratory muscle unloading (WOB in a normal range) correlates well with the optimal respiratory muscle load as defined by Brochard and associates.[32]

PATIENT CHARACTERISTICS. Physiologic patient characteristics should also be considered. Weak, malnourished, and chronically ill patients will not tolerate normal workloads as well as physically powerful individuals with short-term illness. The latter patients may be able to generate twice the normal work range without developing fatigue. Because the *load tolerance* may vary, setting the level of PSV so that the WOB is in a normal range is a reasonable initial guideline for many patients.[27]

ELASTANCE AND RESISTANCE. During normal, unassisted, spontaneous inspiration, pressure is generated by the respiratory muscles (Pmus) to overcome the elastic and resistive pressures of the respiratory system. Elastic pressure

(Pel) is the product of respiratory system elastance (E_{RS}) (reciprocal of compliance) and volume (V):

$$Pel = E_{RS} \text{ (cm } H_2O/L) \times V \text{ (L)}$$

Resistive pressure (Pres) is the product of total resistance (respiratory system plus breathing apparatus resistance) (R_{tot}) and inspiratory flow rate ($\dot{V}$):

$$Pres = R_{tot} \text{ (cm } H_2O/L/second) \times \dot{V} \text{ (L/second)}$$

During spontaneous breathing under normal conditions, the change in respiratory muscle pressure is approximately 5 cm H_2O. When the respiratory muscles are loaded under conditions of increased elastance (e.g., decreased lung compliance), resistance, or both, respiratory muscle pressure and WOB increase. For example,

$$Pmus = Pel + Pres$$
$$= 10 \text{ cm } H_2O + 10 \text{ cm } H_2O$$
$$= 20 \text{ cm } H_2O$$

Respiratory muscle pressure decreases to more normal levels when an appropriate amount of PSV is applied (e.g., 15 cm H_2O) to partially unload the respiratory muscles. For example,

$$Pmus = (Pel + Pres) - PSV$$
$$= (10 \text{ cm } H_2O + 10 \text{ cm } H_2O) - 15 \text{ cm } H_2O$$
$$= 5 \text{ cm } H_2O$$

During partial unloading, the ventilator acts as an extension of the patient's respiratory muscles. The pressure output of the muscles, and thus the WOB, is lessened because the

A. LOADED RESPIRATORY MUSCLES
(HIGH PRESSURE, LOW VOLUME WORK)

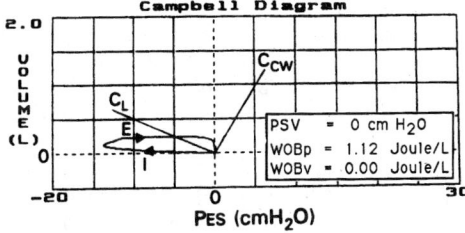

B. PARTIALLY UNLOADED RESPIRATORY MUSCLES
(LOW PRESSURE, HIGH VOLUME WORK)

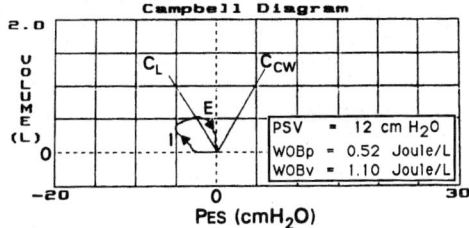

C. TOTALLY UNLOADED RESPIRATORY MUSCLES

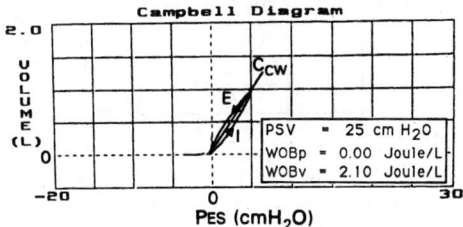

FIGURE 15-12. The work of breathing performed by the patient (WOBp) during three conditions: loaded, partially unloaded, and totally unloaded respiratory muscles. Work of breathing during spontaenous inhalation (I) and exhalation (E) is shown using the Campbell diagram display from a computerized, respiratory monitor (Bicore Monitoring Systems, Riverside, CA). (**A**) The level of pressure support volume (PSV) is zero, and the respiratory muscles are *loaded*, as indicated by the increased value for WOBp (normal, approximately 0.3 to 0.6 J/L). The esophageal pressure (Pes)–volume loop is abnormal and characterized by a *large* change in pressure and a *small* change in volume. The work of breathing performed by the ventilator (WOBv) to inflate the respiratory system is zero because the level of PSV is zero (WOBv is calculated by integrating the changes in airway pressure and volume). (**B**) A PSV of 12 cm H_2O is applied, the respiratory muscles are partially unloaded, and WOBp is in a normal, nonfatiguing range. Work is performed in part by the patient and in part by the ventilator. Notice that the esophageal pressure–volume loop is more normal in configuration, characterized by a *smaller* change in pressure and a *larger* change in volume. (**C**) PSV of 25 cm H_2O is applied, the respiratory muscles are totally unloaded, and virtually all of the work of breathing is provided by the ventilator. Notice also that the pressure–volume loop moves in a counterclockwise direction. (Banner MJ, Gabrielli A, Layon AJ: Partially and totally unloading respiratory muscles based on real time measurements of work of breathing: a clinical approach. *Chest* 1994;106:1835.)

workload is shared between the muscles and the ventilator (Fig. 15-13).

Available evidence suggests that total unloading, allowing fatigued respiratory muscles to rest and recover, is appropriate.[4,7,63] The time for respiratory muscle recovery after chronic fatigue is estimated to be at least 24 hours.[7] A reasonable approach is to totally unload the respiratory muscles of such patients for approximately 24 hours by using high levels of PSV (e.g., >30 cm H_2O). Subsequently, when appropriate, PSV may be decreased so that the patient WOB is in a normal, tolerable range and the respiratory muscles are partially unloaded[27] (see Fig. 15-13).

COMPONENTS OF PATIENT WORK OF BREATHING

As previously stated, WOB performed by a spontaneously breathing, intubated patient equals the sum of the imposed resistive work of the breathing apparatus, physiologic elastic work, and physiologic resistive work. The clinical importance of differentiating WOB into its component parts may be useful in shortening the duration of intubation and ventilatory support for some patients. A study was performed to determine whether adults recovering from respiratory failure, who were candidates for extubation, could be extubated *sooner* using the zero imposed WOB approach rather than a more conventional method employing low-level CPAP.[64]

Imposed work of the breathing apparatus was decreased to zero by applying PSV[14] (Fig. 15-14). In this crossover study design, the decision to extubate was made first while the patients received CPAP of 5 cm H_2O, then with the zero imposed WOB approach. With CPAP of 5 cm H_2O as the only test, the decision *not* to extubate was made for 70% of the patients based on increased total WOB, breathing frequency, and accessory muscle use (Table 15-4). A PSV level of 13 ± 3 cm H_2O was required to achieve zero imposed WOB. Under these conditions, because all indices were in an acceptable range, all patients were extubated with an 80% success rate (see Table 15-4). Blood gas exchange was comparable between the two test conditions.

Increases in total WOB with accessory muscle use, as a result of increased imposed work, may seem to represent an indication that intubation should be prolonged. Indeed, this was the interpretation with the conventional approach. In this study, most patients were extubated sooner (at least 1 day) by using zero imposed WOB as an extubation test.

My experience and that of others[18] suggests that all intubated, spontaneously breathing patients in respiratory failure should receive a *minimal* level PSV that reduces imposed WOB to zero.[14] Additional PSV may be required to decrease the abnormally high physiologic work associated with the disease process to a normal level.[27] Subsequently, as the patient's respiratory status improves, PSV may be decreased while ensuring that the WOB is in a nonfatiguing range (Fig. 15-15). PSV should not be decreased to zero or below the level required to decrease imposed work to zero. To do so functionally reloads the respiratory muscles and risks fatigue. Extubation at the level of PSV results in zero

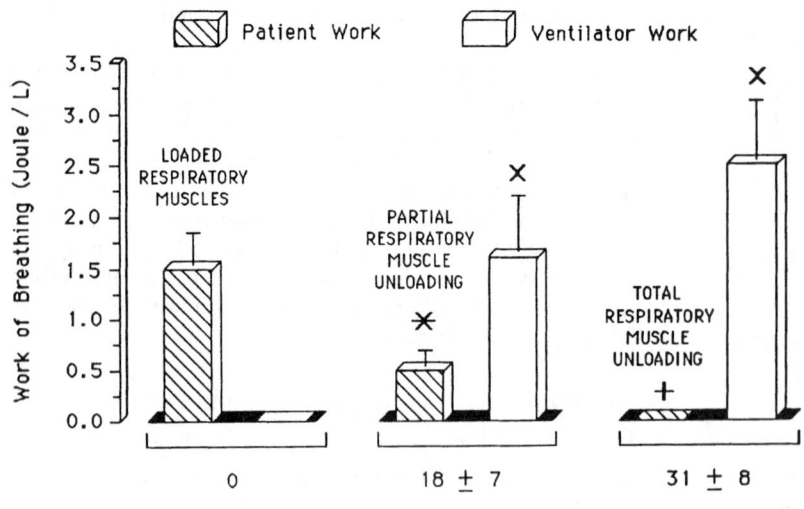

FIGURE 15-13. Work of breathing performed by the patient decreased to a normal range (asterisk) and work performed by the ventilator (X) increased significantly ($p < 0.05$) when the respiratory muscles were partially unloaded as the level of pressure support ventilation was raised from 0 to 18 ± 7 cm H_2O; work was performed in part by the patient and in part by the ventilator. A nonfatiguing workload was performed by the patient under these conditions. Patient work decreased further to zero (+) ($p < 0.05$) and ventilator work increased when the muscles were totally unloaded at a pressure support ventilation level of 31 ± 8 cm H_2O. Data are mean ± SD. (Banner MJ, Gabrielli A, Layon AJ: Partially and totally unloading respiratory muscles based on real time measurements of work of breathing: a clinical approach. *Chest* 1994;106:1835.)

A

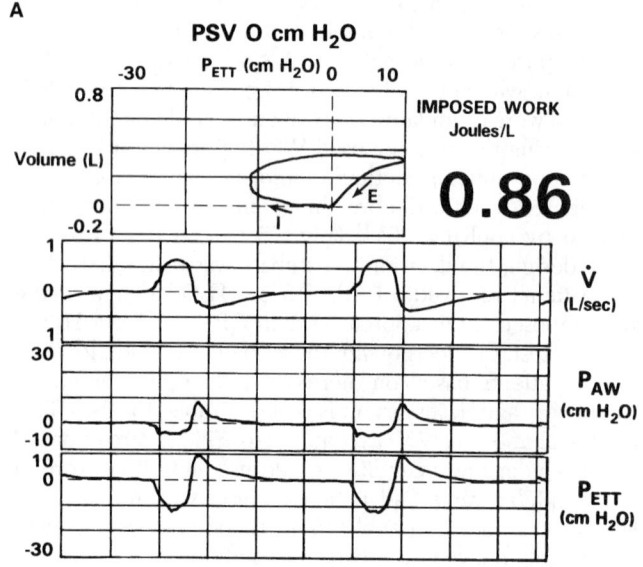

B

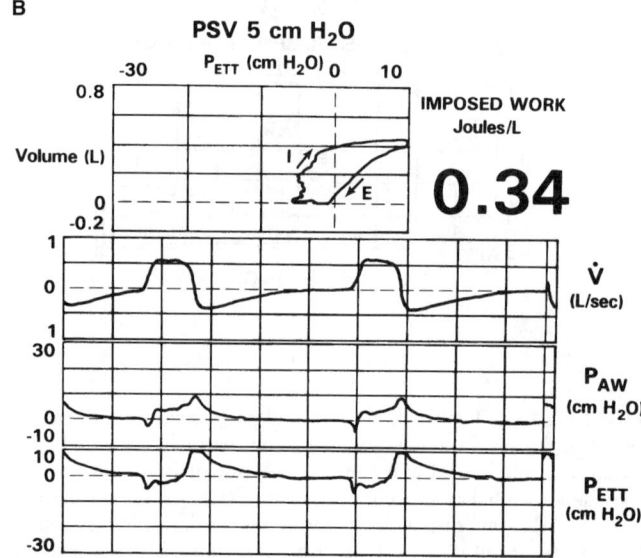

C

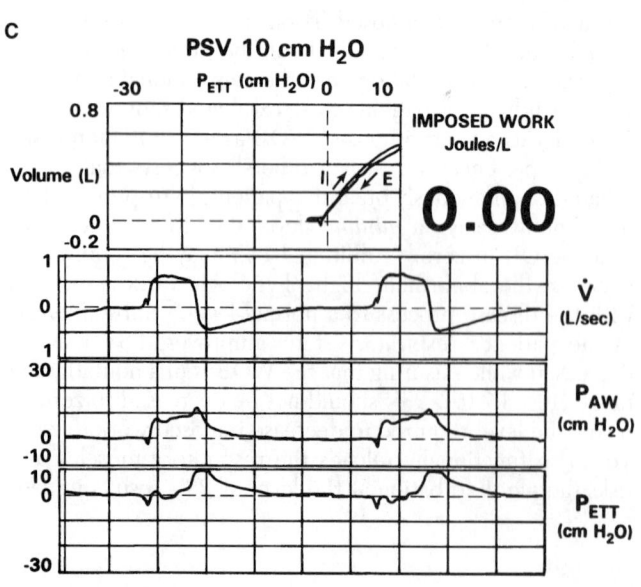

FIGURE 15-14. Recordings of imposed work of breathing obtained by integrating the changes in pressure at the tracheal or carinal end of the endotracheal tube (P_{ETT}) and volume at the "Y" piece of the ventilatory breathing circuit for a patient intubated with a 7.5-mm internal diameter endotracheal tube and connected to a ventilator (7200a, Puritan-Bennett) while breathing spontaneously with zero end-expiratory pressure. Inspiratory flow rate ($\dot{V}$) and airway pressure (P_{AW}) are measured at the Y piece of the breathing circuit (see fig. 15-2). The pressure–volume loop moves in a clockwise direction during inhalatin (I) and exhalation (E), and the area circumscribed within the loop is imposed work. (**A**) No PSV is applied. Notice the value of imposed work and that P_{ETT} decreases by a greater amount than P_{AW} during spontaneous inhalation because of the resistance of the endotracheal tube. (**B**) PSV of 5 cm H_2O is applied and imposed work decreases. P_{AW} increases after the initial decrease required to trigger the ventilator "ON," and P_{ETT} decreases by a lesser amount during inhalation compared with **A**. (**C**) PSV of 10 cm H_2O is applied, and imposed work decreases to zero. P_{AW} increases to a greater level, and P_{ETT} does not decrease during inhalation compared with **B**. Notice that volume increases from approximately 0.35 L in **A** to 0.50 L in **C** as a result of PSV. A *minimal* level of PSV is that which corresponds to *zero* imposed WOB.

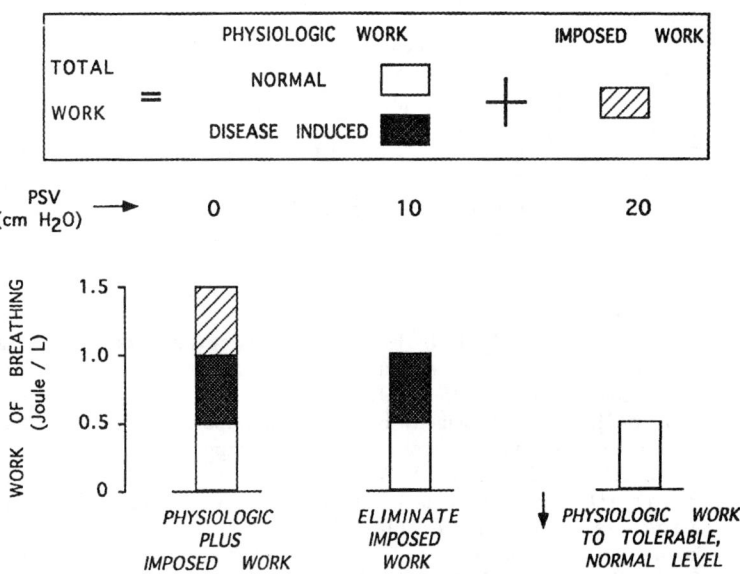

FIGURE 15-15. Model for partitioning the components of the work of breathing (WOB) and a rationale for applying pressure support ventilation (PSV) is depicted. In this example, at zero PSV, the total WOB performed by a spontaneously breathing, intubated patient is the physiologic work, which may be represented as an amount equivalent to a normal range (approximately 0.3 to 0.6 J/L); the increased elastic or resistive work induced by the pulmonary disease process; and the additional resistive workload imposed by the breathing apparatus. Total WOB is 1.5 J/L. Accordingly, 10 cm H_2O PSV is determined as the *minimal* level required to eliminate or decrease the imposed WOB to zero. However, the respiratory muscles are still afterloaded as evidenced by the increased physiologic WOB. Thus, the level of PSV is increased further to 20 cm H_2O to decrease the work to a tolerable level, which may correspond to a normal WOB.

TABLE 15-4. Readiness for Extubation Evaluated During Continuous Positive Airway Pressure and Zero Imposed Work of Breathing

	CPAP	ZERO IMPOSED WOB
Total WOB (J/L)	1.4 ± 0.3	$0.48 \pm 0.2°$
Physiologic WOB (J/L)	0.54 ± 0.25	0.48 ± 0.23
Imposed WOB (J/L)	0.86 ± 0.3	$0°$
Breathing frequency (breaths/min)	$27 \sim 4$	$20 \pm 3°$
Tidal volume (mL)	312 ± 90	$482 \pm 20°$
Breathing frequency/tidal volume	96 ± 38	$45 \pm 15°$
Accessory muscle use (yes/no)	7/3	0/10
Extubate? (yes/no)	3/7	10/0
Extubation successful (%)	—	80

WOB, work of breathing; CPAP, continuous positive airway pressure.

Values are means ± SD.

°p <0.05 compared with CPAP (N = 10).

imposed WOB; that is, about 10 cm H_2O for most adults seems reasonable.

SUMMARY AND CONCLUSIONS ■

Respiratory muscle WOB of intubated patients receiving ventilatory support may be visualized as a continuum; muscles at one end are highly loaded and at the other end are totally unloaded, predisposing to fatigue and atrophy, respectively. The terms "nosocomial respiratory failure" and "iatrogenic ventilator dependency"[18] describe the inappropriate prolongation of ventilatory support. This problem may result from respiratory muscle fatigue (caused by increased muscle loading from breathing through a highly resistive apparatus, increased physiologic work, or insufficient ventilatory support) or muscle atrophy (as a result of total unloading of respiratory muscles by too high levels of PSV).[18]

With either fatigue or atrophy, the respiratory muscles become weak, failing as force generators. Hypoventilation, hypercapnia, and failure to wean often result, thus prolonging the need for ventilatory support. Fatigue or atrophy can occur, in part, from lack of assessing and adjusting respiratory muscle afterload, thereby failing to perceive their often subtle onset. Measurement of the WOB provides objective and tested data that can be used to set ventilator modes such as PSV to prevent either occurrence and to expedite eventual weaning and extubation.

REFERENCES ■

1. Roussos C, Macklem P: The respiratory muscles. *N Engl J Med* 1982;307:786
2. De Troyer A: Respiratory muscles. In: Crystal RG, West JB (eds). *The Lung: Scientific Foundations*. New York, Raven Press, 1991:869
3. Roussos C: Function and fatigue of respiratory muscles. *Chest* 1985;88:S124
4. Braun NMT, Faulkner J, Hughes RL: When should respiratory muscles be exercised? *Chest* 1983;84:76
5. Vander AJ, Sherman JH, Luciano DS: *Human Physiology*, 5th ed. New York, McGraw-Hill, 1992:283
6. McKenzie DK, Gandevia SC: Skeletal muscle properties: diaphragm and chest wall. In: Crystal RG, West JB (eds). *The Lung: Scientific Foundations*. New York, Raven Press, 1991:649
7. Grassino A, Macklem PT: Respiratory muscle fatigue and ventilatory failure. *Ann Rev Med* 1984;35:625
8. Brooks VB: Motor control (part 1). In:*Handbook of Physiology*. Vol 11, *Motor Control*, section 1: *The nervous system*. Bethesda, MD: American Physiological Society, 1982:43, 345

9. Thomas CK, Ross BH, Stein RB: Motor-unit recruitment in human first dorsal interosseous muscle for static contractions in three different directions. *J Neurophysiol* 1986;55:1017

10. Jenkins FH, Olsen GN: Chronic obstructive lung disease and acute respiratory failure. In: Klein EF (ed). *Acute Respiratory Failure: Problems in Critical Care*, vol 1, no 3. Philadelphia, JB Lippincott, 1987:466

11. Laporta D, Grassino A: Assessment of transdiaphragmatic pressure in humans. *J Appl Physiol* 1985;58:1469

12. Milic-Emili J: Work of breathing. In: Crystal RG, West JB (eds). *The Lung: Scientific Foundations*. New York, Raven Press, 1991:1065

13. Banner MJ, Jaeger MJ, Kirby RR: Components of the work of breathing and implications for monitoring ventilator-dependent patients. *Crit Care Med* 1994;22:515

14. Banner MJ, Kirby RR, Blanch PB: Decreasing imposed work of the breathing apparatus to zero using pressure support ventilation. *Crit Care Med* 1993;21:1333

15. Bersten AD, Rutten AJ, Vedig AE: Additional work of breathing imposed by endotracheal tubes, breathing circuits, and intensive care ventilators. *Crit Care Med* 1989;17:671

16. Bolder PM, Healy EJ, Bolder AR: The extra work of breathing through adult endotracheal tubes. *Anesth Analg* 1986;65:853

17. Kirton O, Banner MJ, Axelrod A: Detection of unsuspected imposed work of breathing: case reports. *Crit Care Med* 1993;21:790

18. Civetta JM: Nosocomial respiratory failure or iatrogenic ventilator dependency. *Crit Care Med* 1993;21:171

19. Kirton OC, DeHaven B, Morgan J, et al: Endotracheal tube flow resistance and elevated imposed work of breathing masquerading as ventilator weaning intolerance [Abstract]. *Chest* 1993;104S:133S

20. Banner MJ, Kirby RR, Blanch PB: Site of pressure measurement during spontaneous breathing with continuous positive airway pressure: effect on calculating imposed work of breathing. *Crit Care Med* 1992;20:528

21. Otis AB: The work of breathing. In: Fenn WO, Rahn H (eds). *Handbook of Physiology: A Critical, Comprehensive Presentation of Physiological Knowledge and Concepts.* Section 3: Respiration. Washington, DC: American Physiological Society, 1964:463

22. Kacmarek RM: The role of pressure support ventilation in reducing work of breathing. *Respir Care* 1988;88:99

23. Amato MBP, Barbas CSV, Bonassa J: Volume assured pressure support ventilation (VASPV): a new approach for reducing muscle workload during acute respiratory failure. *Chest* 1992;102:1225

24. Baydur A, Behrakis P, Zin WA: A simple method for assessing the validity of the esophageal balloon technique. *Am Rev Respir Dis* 1982;126:788

25. Campbell EJM: *The Respiratory Muscles and the Mechanics of Breathing*. Chicago, Year Book Medical Publishers, 1958

26. Agostoni E, Campbell EJM, Freedman S: Energetics. In: Campbell EJM, Agostoni E, Davis JN, (eds). *The Respiratory Muscles: Mechanics and Neural Control*. Philadelphia, WB Saunders, 1970:115

27. Banner MJ, Kirby RR, Gabrielli A, et al: Partially and totally unloading the respiratory muscles based on real time measurements of work of breathing: a clinical approach. *Chest* 1994;106:1835

28. Blanch PB, Banner MJ: A new respiratory monitor that enables accurate measurement of work of breathing: a validation study. *Respir Care* 1994;39:897

29. Bland JM, Altman DG: Statistical methods for assessing agreement between two methods of clinical measurement. *Lancet* 1986;1:307

30. Zapletal A, Samanek M, Paul T: *Lung Function in Children and Adolescents*. New York, S Karger Publishers, 1987

31. Brochard L, Rua F, Lorino H: Inspiratory pressure support compensates for the additional work of breathing caused by the endotracheal tube. *Anesthesiology* 1991;75:739

32. Brochard L, Harf A, Lorino H: Inspiratory pressure support prevents diaphragmatic fatigue during weaning from mechanical ventilation. *Am Rev Respir Dis* 1989;139:513

33. Sassoon CS, Giron AE, Ely EA: Inspiratory work of breathing on flow-by and demand-flow continuous positive airway pressure. *Crit Care Med* 1989;17:1108

34. Van de Graff WB, Gordey K, Dornseif SE: Pressure support: changes in ventilatory pattern and components of the work of breathing. *Chest* 1991;100:1082

35. MacIntyre NR, Leatherman NE: Mechanical loads on the ventilatory muscles. *Am Rev Respir Dis* 1989;139:968

36. Marini JJ: Breathing effort and work of breathing during mechanical ventilation. In: Banner MJ (ed). *Positive-Pressure Ventilation: Problems in Critical Care*, vol 4, no 2. Philadelphia, JB Lippincott, 1990:184

37. Fiastro JF, Habib MP, Quan SF: Pressure support compensates for inspiratory work due to endotracheal tubes and demand continuous positive airway pressure. *Chest* 1988;93:499

38. Shapiro M, Wilson RK, Casar G: Work of breathing though different sized endotracheal tubes. *Crit Care Med* 1986;14:1028

39. LeSouef PN, England SJ, Bryan AC: Total resistance of the respiratory system in preterm infants with and without an endotracheal tube. *J Pediatr* 1984;104

40. Widner L, Banner MJ: A method of decreasing the imposed work of breathing associated with pediatric endotracheal tubes [abstract]. *Crit Care Med* 1992;20:S82

41. Kacmarek RM, Shimada Y, Ohmura A: Optimizing mechanical ventilatory assist. tube. *J Pediatr* 1984;104:108

42. Banner MJ, Blanch PB, Kirby RR: Imposed work of breathing and methods of triggering a demand-flow, continuous positive airway pressure system. *Crit Care Med* 1993;21:183

43. Messinger G, Banner MJ, Gabrielli A, et al: Tracheal pressure triggering a demand-flow CPAP system decreases work of breathing [abstract]. *Anesthesiology* 1994;81:A272

44. Tobin MJ, Skorodin M, Alexis CG: Weaning from mechanical ventilation. In: Taylor RW, Shoemaker WC (eds). *Critical Care: State of the Art*, vol 12. Fullerton, CA: Society of Critical Care Medicine, 1991:373

45. Bellemare F, Wight D, Lavigne CM, et al: Effect of tension and timing of contraction on blood flow of the diaphragm. *J Appl Physiol* 1983;54:1597

46. Cohen CA, Zagelbaumm G, Gross D, et al: Clinical manifestations of inspiratory muscle fatigue. *Am J Med* 1982;73:308

47. Barnes PJ: Neural control of airway smooth muscle. In: Crystal RG, West JB (eds). *The Lung: Scientific Foundations*. New York, Raven Press, 1991:903

48. Sant' Ambrogio G, Sant' Ambrogio FB: Reflexes from the airway, lung, chest wall, and limbs. In: Crystal RG, West JB (eds). *The Lung: Scientific Foundations*. New York, Raven Press, 1991:1383

49. Sant' Ambrogio G: Information arising from the tracheobronchial tree of mammals. *Physiol Rev* 1982;62:531

50. Otis AB, Fenn WO, Rahn HL: Mechanics of breathing in man. *J Appl Physiol* 1950;2:592

51. Kacmarek RM, Venegas J: Mechanical ventilatory rates and tidal volumes. *Respir Care* 1987;32:466

52. MacIntyre NR: Weaning from mechanical ventilatory support: volume-assisting intermittent breaths versus pressure-assisting every breath. *Respir Care* 1988;33:121

53. Banner MJ, Kirby RR, Kirton OC, et al: Breathing frequency and pattern are poor predictors of work of breathing in patients receiving pressure support ventilation. *Chest* 1995;108:1338.

54. Kirton O, Banner MJ, DeHaven CB, et al: Respiratory rate and related assessments are poor inferences of patient work of breathing [abstract]. *Crit Care Med* 1993:S242

55. Nathan SD, Ishaaya AM, Koerner SK, et al: Prediction of minimal pressure support during weaning from mechanical ventilation. *Chest* 1993;103:1215

56. Silas SL, Simpson SQ, Levy H: Rapid shallow breathing index does not correlate with airway occlusion pressure or work of breathing [abstract]. *Chest* 1993;104:130S

57. Bradley TD, Chartrand DA, Fitting JW, et al: The relation of inspiratory effort sensation to fatiguing patterns of the diaphragm. *Am Rev Respir Dis* 1986;134:1119

58. MacIntyre NR: Respiratory function during pressure support ventilation. *Chest* 1986;89:677

59. MacIntyre NR, Nishimura M, Usada Y: The Nogoya conference on system design and patient-ventilator interactions during pressure support ventilation. *Chest* 1990;97:1463

60. Banner MJ, Kirby RR, MacIntyre NR: Patient and ventilator work of breathing and ventilatory muscle loads at different levels of pressure support ventilation. *Chest* 1991;100:531

61. Gross D, Grassino A, Ross WRD, et al: Electromyogram pattern of diaphragmatic fatigue. *J Appl Physiol* 1979;46:1

62. Murciano D, Aubier M, Lecoguie Y, et al: Effects of theophylline on diaphragmatic strength and fatigue in patients with chronic obstructive pulmonary disease. *N Engl J Med* 1984; 311:349

63. Stoller JK: Physiologic rationale for resting the ventilatory muscles. *Respir Care* 1991;36:290

64. Banner MJ, Gabrielli A, Kirby RR, et al: Extubating at a pressure support ventilation level corresponding to zero imposed work of breathing [abstract]. *Anesthesiology* 1994;81:A271

Critical Care, Third Edition, edited by Joseph M. Civetta,
Robert W. Taylor, and Robert R. Kirby.
Lippincott-Raven Publishers, Philadelphia, PA © 1997.

CHAPTER 16

Cardiovascular System

Avner Sidi
Richard F. Davis

The primary physiologic roles of the heart and vascular system are to supply cellular oxygen and nutrients and to remove metabolic waste products to their excretory sites. In dealing with critically ill patients, regardless of the cause of their illness, one must have a firm grasp of the principles of normal cardiovascular physiology so that abnormalities can be readily detected, understood, and corrected. Abnormal cardiovascular function is a major predictor of adverse outcome in critical care and plays a key role in the pathophysiology of other major organ system failure. This chapter reviews the essential features of normal cardiovascular physiology.

CARDIAC ELECTRICAL ACTIVITY

Cardiac arrhythmias are a major source of cardiovascular morbidity and mortality in the critically ill patient population. A knowledge of cardiac electrophysiology is important in understanding and treating cardiac arrhythmias. The myocardium is composed of two predominant cell types: "working" muscle and the conduction system. Myocardial muscle fibers have the specialized ability to shorten against a load when electrically stimulated; this property forms the basis of cardiac contraction.

Electrical excitation, or depolarization, changes the physical properties of the myocardial cell membrane to allow calcium (Ca^{2+}) to enter the cell and activate the contractile apparatus. However, contractile efforts of individual working myocardial cells must be coordinated to produce effective contraction. The process is orchestrated by cells of the cardiac conduction system, which spontaneously depolarize and transmit electrical activity to the working cells in a specific time sequence. Any disturbance of these functions (forma-

tion and conduction of the impulse and the depolarization and repolarization of working myocardial cells) potentiates cardiac arrhythmias.

ACTION POTENTIAL

Depolarization and Repolarization

The electrical events during depolarization and repolarization can be demonstrated for single myocardial cells by microelectrodes that record the electrical potential difference across the surface membrane.[1] In working myocardial cells at rest, the transmembrane potential is stable, and the cell interior is negative by approximately 90 mV relative to the exterior; that is, the resting potential is −90 mV. This potential difference is determined primarily by the distribution of sodium (Na^+) and potassium (K^+). The Na^+ concentration is higher outside cells than inside, whereas K^+ is higher inside than outside.[2] The potential varies inversely with extracellular K^+ concentration. Hypokalemia produces hyperpolarization, whereas hyperkalemia tends to lower the measured value.

In contrast, extracellular Na^+ concentration has little influence on resting potential but critically influences the action potential (AP) amplitude. An electrical impulse markedly increases membrane permeability for Na^+. As a result, the cell interior becomes transiently positive by approximately 20 mV relative to the exterior. Depolarization and repolarization, when recorded from microelectrodes and displayed on an oscilloscope, produce the characteristic AP waveform. An external stimulus, which reduces resting membrane potential to the threshold level (normally about −65 mV), produces the AP. Once initiated, the AP is propagated by the sequential flow of electrical current from depolarized areas into adjacent, nondepolarized areas of the membrane. At each point, the local membrane potential is lowered to the threshold level, producing further depolarization.

Depolarization is initiated by a short-duration increase in the permeability of the cell membrane to Na^+ and Ca^{2+}. Two specific transmembrane channels for ion movement have been described.[3,4] The fast channel permits rapid entry of Na^+ into the cell and has a threshold of approximately -60 mV. The slow channel has a threshold of -20 mV and allows cellular entry of Ca^{2+}. That these channels are actual physical structures in the cell membrane is indicated by several lines of evidence. Conductance of Na^+ but not Ca^{2+} is blocked by tetrodotoxin, whereas Ca^{2+} conductance is inhibited by other divalent ions, such as manganese, lanthanum, and cobalt, and by calcium channel blocking drugs, such as verapamil, diltiazem, and nifedipine.[5] Also, the myocardial contractile response to membrane depolarization, which requires extracellular Ca^{2+}, is slight until the threshold of Ca^{2+} conductance is reached at about -30 mV, despite a large increase in Na^+ conductance at the more negative (-60 mV) membrane potential.

Depolarization opens fast Na^+ channels briefly, and Na^+ flows down its concentration gradient into the cell. This influx produces rapid depolarization and is termed phase 0 of the AP. It coincides with the QRS complex of the surface electrocardiogram (Fig. 16-1). Closure of the fast Na^+ channels results in a brief period, phase 1 of the AP, when the membrane potential rapidly returns toward zero, and initiates repolarization. Calcium entry by the slow channel keeps the cell isoelectric but still depolarized during phase 2 of the AP, corresponding in time to the ST segment of the surface electrocardiogram. During phase 3, K^+ efflux from the cell returns the membrane potential to the resting level of -90 mV. Although repolarization is complete at this point, the normal ionic gradient across the membrane is not yet reestablished. During phase 4, specialized membrane-bound enzyme systems (the sodium-potassium pump) effectively remove Na^+ from the cell interior and return K^+ to the cell. This pumping action involves ionic transport against the Na^+ and K^+ concentration gradients and is, therefore, a highly energy-dependent process that requires an abundant supply of adenosine triphosphate (ATP).

Automaticity

The AP recorded from cells in the conduction system, especially in the sinoatrial (SA) and atrioventricular (AV) nodes, differs from that of the working cells. In these cells, the resting potential (phase 4) is not isoelectric; rather, a slow, spontaneous depolarization of the membrane occurs, a property termed *automaticity*. This spontaneous diastolic depolarization is caused by a low membrane permeability to K^+ and a high resting permeability to Ca^{2+}. When the threshold potential is reached, an AP is propagated. Phase 0 of the AP recorded from cells in the SA and AV nodes results primarily from the entry of Ca^{2+} through the slow channels and has a lesser slope than that in the working cells.

The rate at which spontaneous diastolic depolarization produces a conducted AP is influenced by several factors. The slope of depolarization in SA nodal cells is closely controlled by autonomic nervous system activity.[6] Sympathetic activity (circulating catecholamines through beta$_1$-adrenergic activity) initiated predominantly by the right sympathetic chain increases the depolarization slope and thereby decreases the time required to reach threshold potential. Hence, the overall frequency of depolarization is increased. Vagal activity, in contrast, decreases this frequency through the action of acetylcholine, which increases K^+ conductance, producing hyperpolarization of the membrane; decreases the slope of phase 4; and increases threshold potential. Typically, cells of the SA node exhibit the highest frequency of spontaneous depolarization; therefore, the SA node is the dominant pacemaker for the heart, with resting frequencies ranging from 60 to 100/minute. Spontaneous depolarization in the AV node and the Purkinje system is masked by the conducted impulse from the SA node. However, the AV node and Purkinje system area may be conceptualized as "escape" or back-up pacemakers with intrinsic depolarization rates of 40 to 60/minute and 20 to 40/minute, respectively.

Refractoriness and Excitability

Two concepts are important in understanding the development of arrhythmias: excitability and refractoriness. Excitability is the property by which cardiac tissue depolarizes in

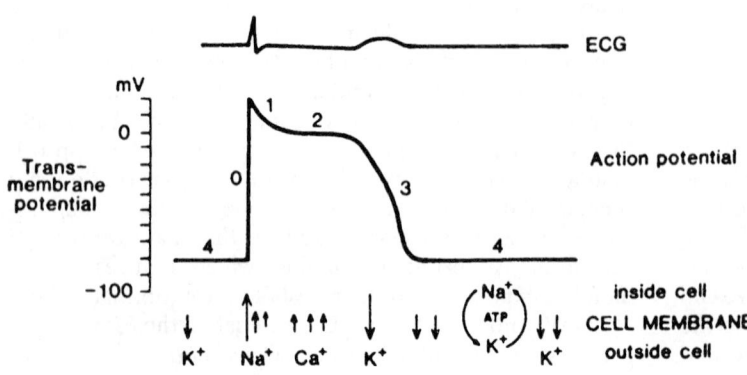

FIGURE 16-1. Schematic illustration of the action potential in a ventricular myocardial cell showing the relation of the action potential to the surface electrocardiogram (ECG) and the directional changes of the electrolytes across the cell membrane. K^+, potassium; Na^+, sodium; Ca^+, calcium; ATP, adenosine triphosphate. (Lewis AJ: Monitoring and dysrhythmia recognition in advanced cardiac life support. In: McIntyre KM, Lewis AJ [eds]: *Textbook of Advanced Cardiac Life Support.* Dallas, American Heart Association, 1983:59.)

response to a given stimulation. Increased excitability, which indicates responsiveness to a lesser stimulus or greater response to a baseline stimulus, is an important cause of arrhythmias. During depolarization and the early part of repolarization (i.e., phases 0, 1, 2, and the initial part of phase 3 of the AP), the cell cannot depolarize and produce another AP. This time interval is the *absolute refractory period*. For the latter portion of phase 3, a stronger than usual impulse can produce a propagated AP (i.e., excitability is decreased); this interval is the *relative refractory period*. The sum of these two periods is termed the *effective refractory period*. The relative refractory period is also referred to as the *vulnerable period*. An impulse occurring at this time reaches areas of the heart in various stages of repolarization, increasing the likelihood of repetitive but dysynchronous depolarization, as seen in ventricular fibrillation.

IMPULSE CONDUCTION

An AP is conducted from its origin in the SA node to its endpoint in the ventricular myocardium by discrete, specialized tissue pathways. From the SA node to the AV node, at least three pathways are involved, with velocities of 800 to 1000 mm/second. Conduction to the left atrium is mediated by the anterior interatrial myocardial band (Bachmann's bundle). Conduction velocity through the AV node is 20% to 25% of that through the atria (200 mm/second). This conduction delay is analogous to a capacitor in an electrical circuit and allows completion of both atrial activation and contraction before ventricular activation.

At its inferior margin, the AV node merges into the AV or His bundle, which divides into the left and right bundle branches. The left bundle divides early in its course into several components, which are commonly grouped into the left anterior and left posterior fascicles. The right bundle supplies the interventricular system near the cardiac apex and the right ventricle. Conduction velocity through the bundles and the Purkinje system is the most rapid in the conduction system—4000 mm/second. This feature ensures rapid, synchronous activation of the ventricle and preserves the activation sequence necessary for optimal efficiency.

The interventricular septum and papillary muscles are the first portions of the ventricular myocardium to contract, providing a framework for subsequent ventricular contraction and preventing prolapse of the AV valves. Sequential ventricular activation occurs first at the apical endocardium and last at the basal epicardium. This sequence produces an apical-to-basal, spiraling contraction pattern by which the heart "wrings out" its stroke volume.

EXCITATION–CONTRACTION COUPLING

Despite its complexity, cardiac electrical activity (membrane depolarization and impulse conduction) is a secondary system that functions meaningfully only when it produces myocardial contraction. Coupling of membrane excitation to mechanical contraction of myocardial muscle is mediated by transmembrane and transcellular flux of Ca^{2+} (Table 16-1). Unlike skeletal muscle, myocardial muscle requires at least

TABLE 16-1. Myocardial Excitation–Contraction Coupling

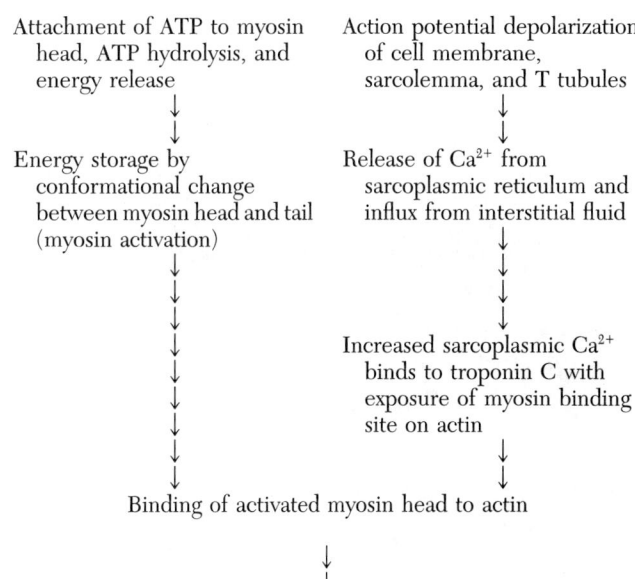

Release of potential energy, return to inactive myosin head and tail conformation; sliding of actin relative to myosin, with sarcomere shortening

some extracellular Ca^{2+} to initiate effective contraction. One substantial difference in the configuration of the conduction system cell AP and the myocardial cell AP is the duration of phase 2, which is caused by transmembrane (outside to inside) Ca^{2+} flux. During this phase, Ca^{2+} from intracellular (sarcoplasmic reticulum) and extracellular (interstitial) sources increases perhaps 100-fold in the myocardial cytosol.

The extracellular contribution is facilitated by the transverse (T) tubular system of myocardial cells. These T tubules are invaginations of the sarcolemma, an extension of the cell membrane, which are concentrated near Z bands (see later) and come into close contact, but not actual continuity, with the intracellular sarcoplasmic reticulum. The T tubule system vastly increases cell membrane surface area for ion transport and provides a mechanism for transmission of ATP to intracellular membranes.

Ultrastructural Changes

A brief consideration of myocardial cell ultrastructure is important. Working myocardial cells are large, 10 to 20 μm in diameter and 50 μm to 100 μm in length, containing hundreds of longitudinally arranged myofibrils that run the length of the cell (Fig. 16-2). Functionally, the myocardium is a syncytium of such cells. Myofibrils are composed of sarcomeres, which in turn contain the contractile proteins actin and myosin. Myosin (thick) filaments are interposed between actin (thin) filaments, which are attached at each end to a fibrous Z band. Other bands characterized by light microscopic study are the overlapping actin and myosin fil-

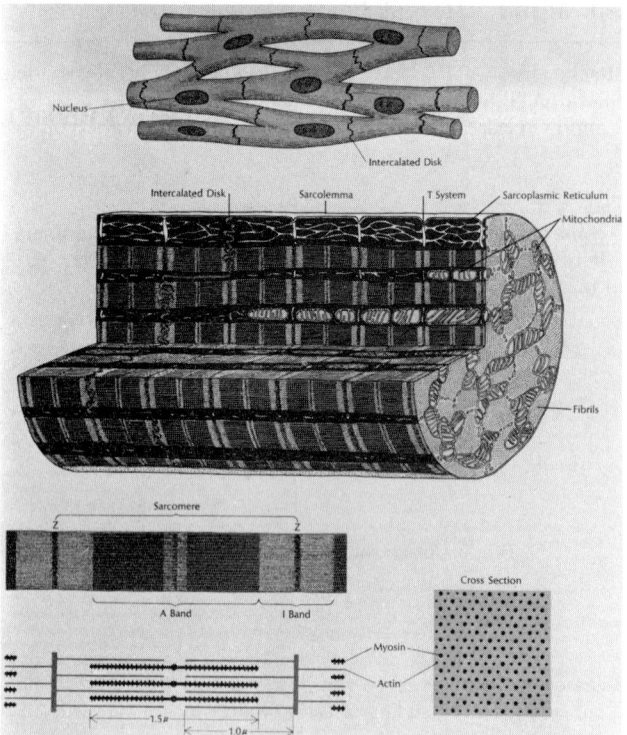

FIGURE 16-2. Diagrammatic representation of the ultrastructure of a segment of a ventricular myocardial cell. (Braunwald E: *The Myocardium: Failure and Infarction.* New York, H. P. Publishing, 1974:4.)

aments (A band) and the free actin filaments extending from each side of the Z band (I band).

At the molecular level, contraction is produced by interaction of actin and myosin such that the filaments appear to slide across one another, producing an increased length of overlap and a shortening of the sarcomere. Myosin molecules are composed of a globular "head," which is the center of ATPase activity and the site of attachment to actin, and an

elongated "tail," which winds around other myosin tails in a double-helical arrangement to provide strength to the fibril (Fig. 16-3).

The thin filament is actually a double helix composed of two chains of globular actin monomers. A third molecule, tropomyosin, consists of two elongated polypeptide chains that align with the grooves of the actin double helix. The fourth element is troponin, actually a composite of three subunits, which binds to tropomyosin in association with a chain of seven actin monomer units (see Fig. 16-3). Troponin subunits include troponin C, which contains the Ca^{2+} binding site; troponin I, which inhibits the formation of crossbridges between the thin filament and myosin; and troponin T, which physically holds troponin to tropomyosin.

With arrival of the AP, depolarization of the sarcolemma and T tubule system (and probably the sarcoplasmic reticulum membranes) occurs. This depolarization produces an approximate 100-fold increase in sarcoplasmic Ca^{2+}, although a lesser increase (5×10^{-7} to 6×10^{-6} mol/L) results in 90% of the maximum force of contraction.[7] Increased sarcoplasmic Ca^{2+} enhances the binding of Ca^{2+} to the troponin C component, producing a conformational change in troponin, and exposes the site on the actin monomer for binding to the myosin head.[8] Hydrolysis of ATP by actomyosin ATPase produces a conformational change between the myosin head and tail, which has the effect of storing potential energy. Attachment of the myosin head to the now-exposed binding site on the actin thin filament is followed by a return to the resting relation between the myosin head and tail. This latter step releases the stored potential (chemical) energy, and the myosin head attachment to the actin binding site produces mechanical movement of actin relative to myosin. Because actin is attached to the Z band area, and myosin overlaps actin through filamentous attachments to opposite ends of the sarcomere, sliding of the thick and thin filaments produces mechanical shortening of the sarcomere.

Myocardial relaxation during diastole can be thought of as a reversal of the above process. Triggered by a yet undefined

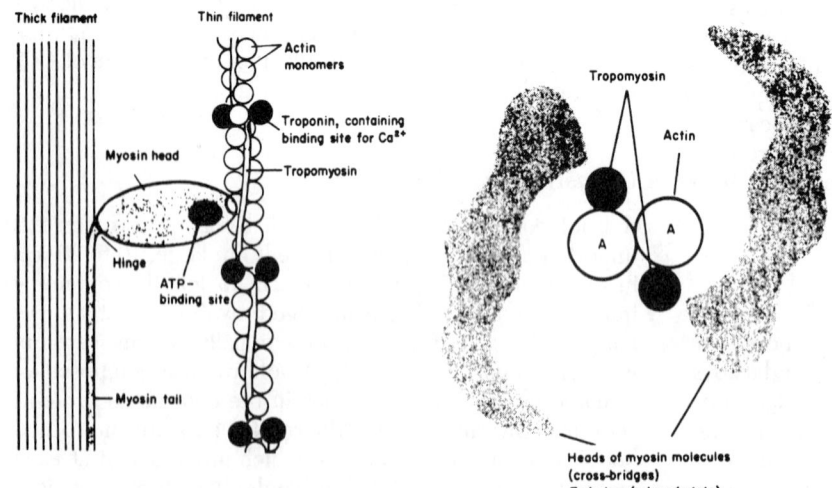

FIGURE 16-3. Diagrammatic representation of the interaction between actin and myosin. (Lehninger AL: *Biochemistry,* 2nd ed. New York, Worth Publishers, 1975.)

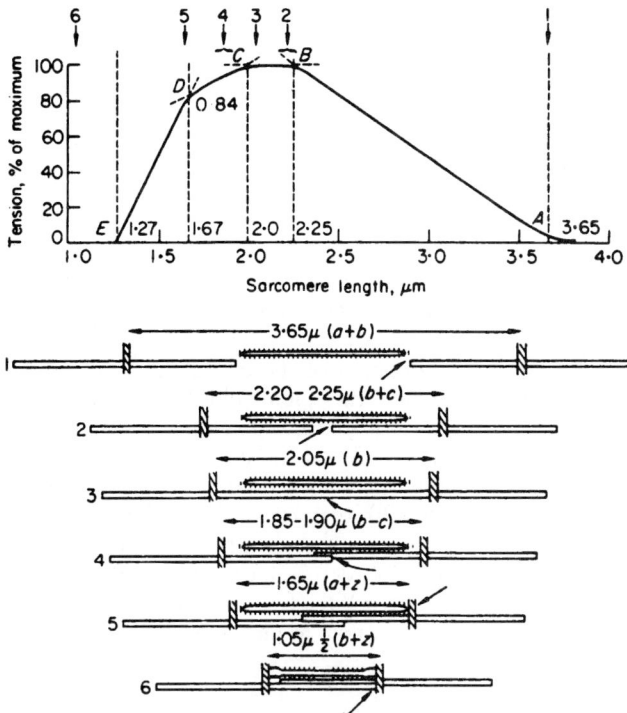

FIGURE 16-4. The relation between the resting sarcomere length and the tension developed by isolated papillary muscle fiber. At approximately 2.2 μm the fiber length is optimal and tension development is maximal. (Wilke DR: *Muscle.* London, Edward Arnold Publishers, 1968.)

CARDIAC CONTRACTION ■

ISOLATED MUSCLE PREPARATIONS

Although a complete discussion of cardiac muscle mechanics is beyond the scope of this chapter, a solid understanding of the fundamental concepts is important because much of the knowledge of cardiac muscle function stems from isolated muscle studies. In 1938, A.V. Hill[10] described studies of frog skeletal muscle and developed a conceptual model with two main components: the contractile element (CE) and the series elastic element (SE; Fig. 16-5). A major difference between skeletal and cardiac muscle is the resting tension found in cardiac muscle. Hence, the Hill model is often modified to include a parallel elastic element (PE) in addition to the SE.

Although these concepts have been accorded wide acceptance, the anatomic correlates of the elastic elements are obscure. The contractile apparatus itself resides in the actin and myosin filaments, but the elastic constituents may be in membrane structures, valves, and connective tissue or even in the elastic properties of the contractile filaments.

Initial shortening of the CE produces a stretch of the SE that transmits the force to the fixed ends of the isolated muscle preparation or to the cardiac skeleton in the intact heart. During this initial phase, much of the energy of contraction is expended by the contractile elements, but actual external work is not done because overall shortening does not occur; hence the term *isometric contraction* (*isovolemic* in the intact heart). When the force generated by the CE and transmitted by the SE is greater than the external restraining force, shortening of the whole muscle can occur. The PE

stimulus, sarcoplasmic Ca^{2+} concentration declines because of binding or reuptake by sarcoplasmic reticulum membrane with subsequent movement (diffusion or transport) to terminal cisternae of the sarcoplasmic reticulum or to the interstitial fluid. These processes are outlined in Table 16-1.

Of importance is the differentiation between the overall strength of the shortening process (i.e., the maximum force that is generated) and the intensity of the actin–myosin interaction (release of the stored potential energy during the change to resting configuration of the myosin molecule, which is contractility). The total force generated by a contraction can be augmented by an increase in force per actin–myosin interaction (contractility) or by increasing the number of actin–myosin interaction sites. Increasing the resting sarcomere length up to approximately 2.2 μm increases the number of actin and myosin sites involved in a given contraction, enhancing tension development[9] (Fig. 16-4). From that point, any increase or decrease of sarcomere length decreases tension development by decreasing the number of active sites involved in the contraction. At the subcellular level, this relation explains the Starling effect, in which increased preload enhances tension development. Contractility changes, in contrast, result from a change in the force developed by each active site and therefore alter the force of contraction independently of any change in the number of active sites.

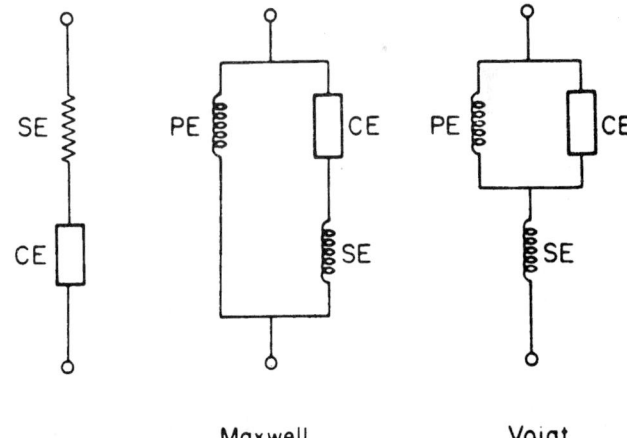

FIGURE 16-5. The original Hill two-element model for skeletal muscle is composed of a contractile element (CE) and a series elastic element (SE). Because cardiac muscle has a significant resting tension and the CE is assumed to be freely extensible at rest, a parallel elastic element (PE) is often added to the Hill model to account for the resting tension. The PE may be placed parallel with the SE (Maxwell model) or in series with the SE (Voigt model). (Prys-Roberts C: *The Circulation in Anaesthesia.* London, Blackwell Scientific Publications, 1980:69.)

functions to support resting tension and has relatively less influence on contraction.

By using a tension transducer, a lever arm with a stop, and a series of variable weights, one can make the papillary muscle contract from a controllable, initial length (preload) against a controllable resistive force (afterload)[11] (Fig. 16-6). Typically, the magnitude of shortening and the developed tension are plotted as a function of time. The slope of the length-time curve is the velocity of shortening, the maximum value of which is reached early for a given contraction.

In an isotonic contraction (muscle contraction against a fixed afterload), tension developed in the muscle reaches a plateau when shortening begins, and the tension remains constant despite further shortening until contraction ceases and relaxation begins. If one progressively increases the afterload for contractions that have the same preload, a series of length-time and tension-time curves are generated in which the maximum velocity of shortening declines until none occurs (i.e., velocity is zero).[12] At this point, the tension-time curve loses the plateau effect, and the maximum tension the muscle is capable of generating can be interpreted as the peak of the tension-time curve with zero shortening.

A common presentation of these relations is the force-velocity curve, in which the initial velocity of shortening is plotted against the afterload (force generated during isotonic contraction; Fig. 16-7). When the curve is extrapolated to the horizontal and vertical axes, both the theoretical maximum force possible (P_0), or force at zero velocity, and the maximum velocity (Vmax), or contraction velocity when afterload equals zero, are determined. Neither P_0 nor Vmax is a measurable quantity. Of the two, Vmax is most commonly used because it can be taken as an index of the myocardial contractile state.

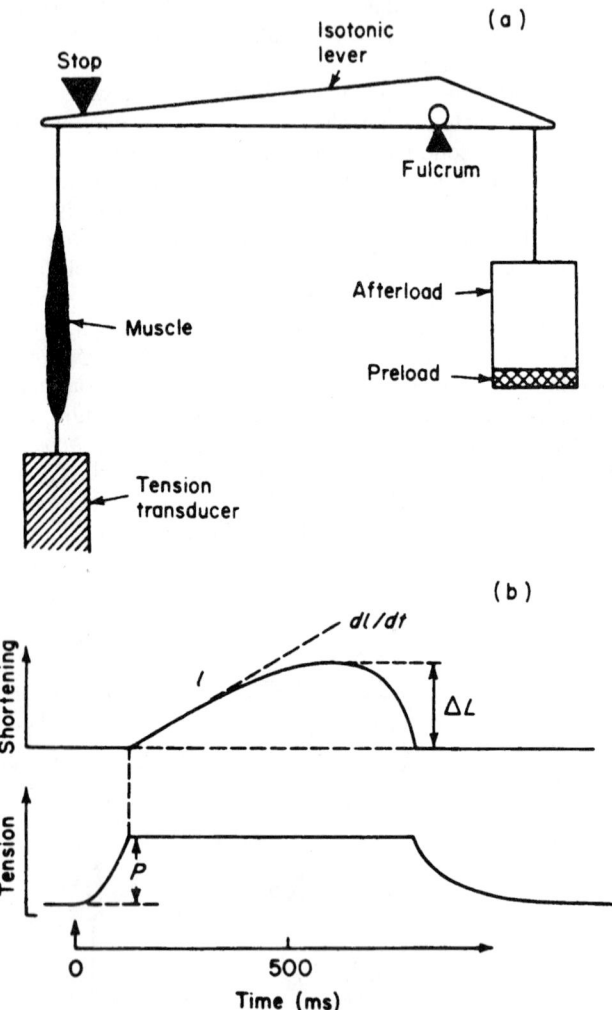

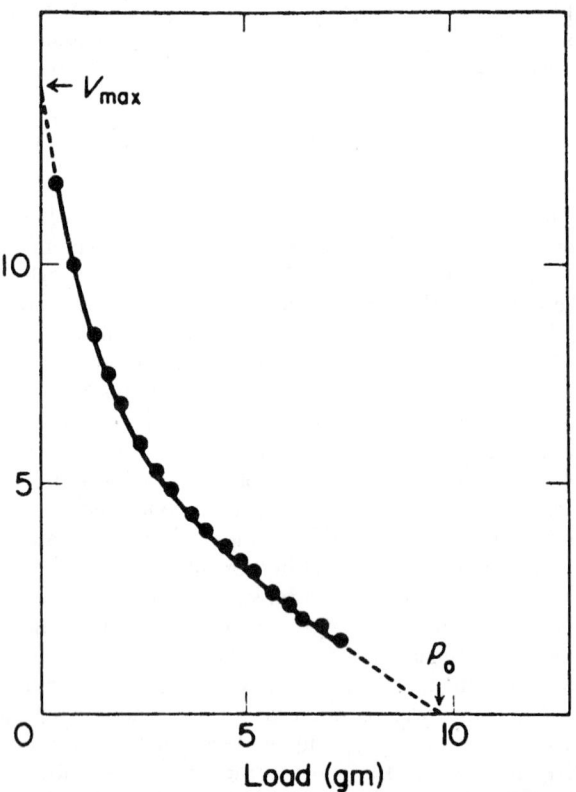

FIGURE 16-6. Recording of isometric and isotonic contractions from a papillary muscle. The muscle is attached to a tension transducer, and the initial length of the muscle is determined by a preload. A stop set on the tension arm keeps the initial muscle length constant before the onset of contraction. Additional load is added to the preload to produce an effective afterload, which is encountered only after the onset of contraction. The lower panel illustrates the plot of the degree of shortening and the tension developed over time during a contraction. The figure (*upper panel*) shows the inverse relation between the initial velocity of isotonic shortening and the resistive load encountered by the muscle. (Sonnenblick EH: Implications of muscle mechanics in heart. *Fed Proc* 1962;21:975.)

FIGURE 16-7. Relation between the initial velocity of shortening and afterload (force): the force-velocity relation. Vmax is the hypothetical maximum shortening velocity at zero afterload; P_0 is the hypothetical maximum possible force developed by the muscle at a zero contraction velocity. (Braunwald E, Ross J, Sonnenblick EH: *Mechanisms of Contraction of the Normal and Failing Heart.* Boston, Little, Brown, 1968.)

Consider the force-velocity curves in Figure 16-8. Increasing the preload of the isolated muscle (increasing the number of actin and myosin active sites that interact during contraction) increases the force-generating capability. Maximum force increases, but the intensity of each individual active site is not changed. Thus, Vmax is unchanged. In contrast, increasing the contractility of the actin–myosin interaction increases both Vmax and P_0 without a change of preload.

Because initial sarcomere length (preload), force generated, and velocity are clearly interactive, a three-dimensional representation is sometimes used[13] (Fig. 16-9). Work (force times distance) is shown on the horizontal plane, and power (force times velocity) is shown on the vertical plane. A single contraction begins at zero velocity, zero developed tension, and an initial length or preload (point A, see Fig. 16-9). During the initial phase of isometric contraction, the velocity of CE shortening rapidly reaches a maximum value (Vmax). However, when force is generated by the contraction, CE velocity decreases until a point (point C, see Fig. 16-9) is reached where developed tension equals the load; shortening of the entire muscle occurs isotonically (C → E) until velocity is again zero when contraction is completed. The area ABCD in Figure 16-9 represents power of the contraction (force times velocity during isotonic shortening), and the area ADEF is the actual work done (force times distance) during that period.

INTACT HEART

Information derived from the study of isolated papillary muscle preparations contributes substantially to our understanding of cardiac contraction, but important differences

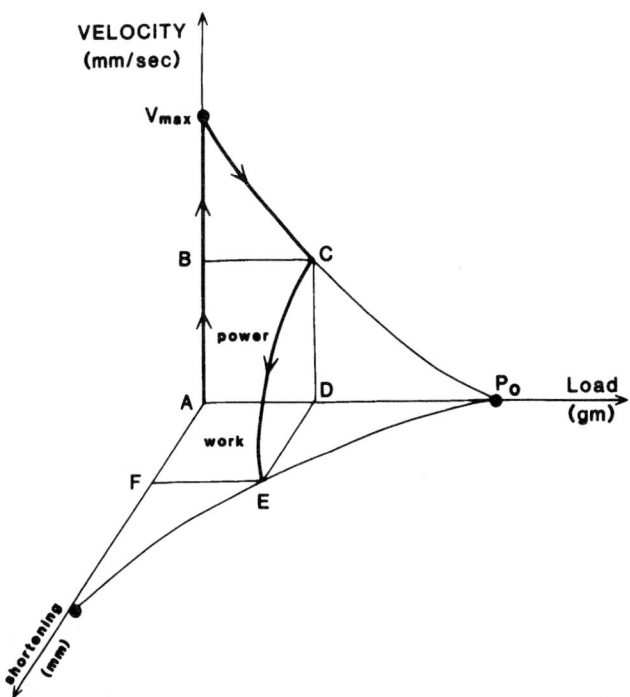

FIGURE 16-9. Schematic three-dimensional representation of the relation between contraction velocity load and degree of shortening. A single hypothetical contraction is shown by the heavy line through the power generated during that contraction (force × velocity is illustrated by the rectangle ABCD). The actual work done (force × distance) is shown by the rectangle ADEF.

between such preparations and the intact heart must be recognized. The geometric configuration of the ventricle, which is vaguely ellipsoid with a relatively thick wall and complex spiral arrangement of muscle fibers, is different from the thin, solid cylinder of papillary muscle with longitudinally oriented fibers.[14] Also, the pattern of ventricular contraction—with shortening from apex to base, increase of wall thickness and circumference, and variable contraction velocity between anterior and posterior sections—is markedly different from the simple linear shortening of the isolated muscle. Finally, although tension placed on the isolated muscle directly influences sarcomere length, in the intact heart, because of variations of compliance (both from one time to the next and from one ventricular location to another), no predictable relation exists between intraventricular pressure and ventricular end-diastolic volume. Clearly, one must be cautious in applying concepts derived from the study of isolated muscle.

INTRINSIC REGULATION OF CARDIAC FUNCTION ■

CONTRACTILITY

The primary difficulty in providing a useful measure of *contractility* is determination of a parameter of ventricular function that is independent of the two other variables that

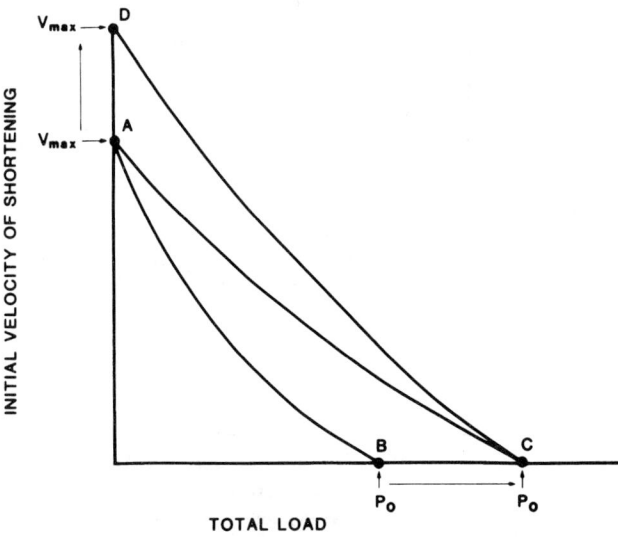

FIGURE 16-8. Differing force velocity curves. Curve AB represents the baseline state. Curve AC is produced by increasing preload, and curve DC is produced by increasing contractility. Notice that the increase in contractility produces an increase both in Vmax and P_0, whereas increased preload augments P_0 without significant change in Vmax.

control performance of the heart as a pump, that is, diastolic volume (preload) and aortic pressure (afterload). Ventricular contractility can be described by three variables and their interrelations: (1) velocity of shortening; (2) force of contraction; and (3) length of displacement. All of the functional indices that are ultimately derived reflect one or more of these variables and their interdependence. Thus, contractility, or the inotropic state, although conceptualized as the speed of the actin–myosin interaction and reasonably approximated by the Vmax of an isolated muscle preparation, remains an elusive concept in the intact circulation. Sympathetic stimulation, circulating catecholamines, and cardiac glycosides all enhance contractility, but no single common hemodynamic variable, measured or derived, indicates a change in contractility independent of changes in loading conditions (preload or afterload) or heart rate.

The heart rate influence on contractility has been appreciated as the treppe or Bowditch phenomenon. An increase in heart rate produces increased contractility. This effect is probably mediated by cardiac sympathetic innervation and is obtunded, but not abolished, during general anesthesia.[15] An increase in afterload (aortic pressure) also produces an increase in contractility by activation of aortic stretch receptors. This phenomenon has been termed the *Anrep effect* after its originator.[16]

The first-time derivative of ventricular pressure (dP/dt), or any of its derivatives (length, diameter, force, and velocity), is often used as an indicator of contractility. However, dP/dt and all of the associated derivations are subject to change by heart rate or loading conditions and, therefore, do not represent contractility alone. Of the many isovolemic indices, the dP/dt at a specific developed pressure (dp/dt/P) offers the least sensitivity to left ventricular (LV) end-diastolic pressure changes while retaining sensitivity to acutely induced changes in inotropic states. Despite these shortcomings, dP/dt (or one of its derivatives) is the best common hemodynamic indicator of the contractile state when afterload, preload, and heart rate are held constant (which rarely happens clinically).

PRELOAD: THE FRANK-STARLING PRINCIPLE

In 1895, Frank[17] described the increased pressure generated by the frog heart when the filling pressure was increased just before contraction. The presystolic or end-diastolic volume and filling pressure determine the magnitude of the all-or-none response. Frank's studies emphasized the dependence of the cardiac response on hemodynamic events immediately preceding excitation. But uncertainty remained whether the responsiveness of the heart was fundamentally related to changes in presystolic pressure (initial tension) or in presystolic volume (initial length).

Ernest Starling[18] in 1914 described the increased stroke volume produced when diastolic ventricular volume was increased or when venous return was augmented. The conclusion by Starling that cardiac responsiveness was primarily related to presystolic fiber length has been validated by nearly all investigators. Although it is common knowledge that fiber length and resting tension are closely related, Sarnoff and Berglund[19] demonstrated that other factors can

affect the responsiveness of the myocardium by showing that a "family" of curves (Fig. 16-10) relating stroke work and left atrial pressure exists for each ventricle, and that many other factors (humoral agents, neural influence, metabolic conditions) determine on which particular curve the ventricle operates at any given time. In the intact circulation, the volume of the venous return, loading conditions, Frank-Starling effect, and contractility are all interactive. Thus, the concept of a ventricular function curve relating preload to stroke work must be modified to include a family of such curves in which the ventricle moves along a single curve with changes in preload and also among the curves with changes in contractile states (see Fig. 16-10).

In any given circulatory state, a consistent relation exists between atrial pressure and stroke work of the ipsilateral ventricle. At high filling pressures, the curve flattens to a plateau. A descending limb (decrease of ventricular work with increased effective filling pressure) does not occur in the normal heart but may occur with a compromised myocardium. Such a relation was not consistently found between right atrial pressure and LV stroke work, between atrial pressure and stroke volume, or between atrial pressure and cardiac output.[19] The stroke volume is a function of the extent of shortening of myocardial fiber. Studies of isolated cardiac muscle seem to show that the extent of shortening during each contraction is dependent on three separate factors: (1) the preload (initial volume), which partly determines the myocardial sarcomere end-diastolic length; (2) the resistance to ventricular emptying, or afterload, which is closely related to the peak systolic tension developed by the myocardium and the aortic input impedance; and (3) the contractile or inotropic state of the myocardium.[20]

The interaction between these three variables and the extension of myocardial fiber shortening is illustrated in

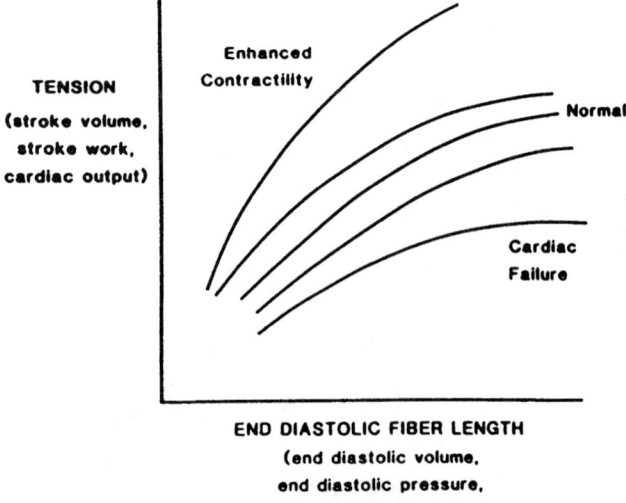

FIGURE 16-10. A "family" of ventricular function curves shows the relation between ventricular wall tension and diastolic fiber length (and their physiologically measurable analogs). (Cohn JN, Franciosa JA: Vasodilator therapy of cardiac failure. *N Engl J Med* 1977;297:27.)

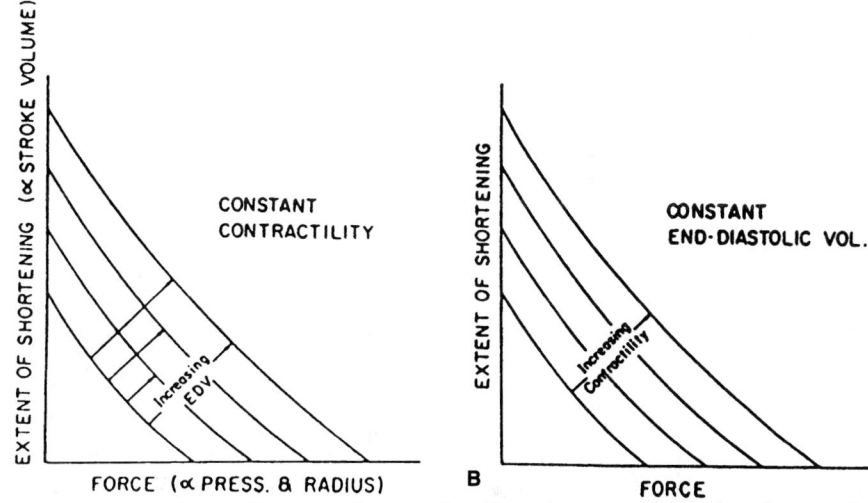

FIGURE 16-11. Dependence of extent of myocardial fiber shortening (and, therefore, in the intact ventricle, the stroke volume) on ventricular force, end-diastolic volume, and contractility. (**A**) Reciprocal relation between ventricular force (which is a function of intraventricular pressure, and according to Laplace's law, ventricular radius) and extent of myocardial fiber shortening. The contractile state of the ventricle is constant, and the extent of shortening is seen, at any level of intraventricular force, to be a function of ventricular end-diastolic volume. (**B**) The same reciprocal relation between force and extent of shortening but at a constant end-diastolic volume. The extent of shortening is seen, at any level of intraventricular force, to be a function of the level of the contractile state. (Braunwald E: Mechanics and energetics of the normal and failing heart. *Trans Assoc Am Physicians* 1971;84:63.)

Figure 16-11. A reciprocal relation exists between afterload (or force) and the extent of shortening. The force itself is a function of intraventricular pressure and, according to Laplace's law, the ventricular radius (the law of Laplace substitutes pressure multiplied by half the radius for wall tension [T]: T = radius / 2 × pressure). Each curve in Figure 16-11 represents this relation at a constant level of contractility (see Fig. 11*A*) or a constant end-diastolic volume (see Fig. 11*B*). While one of those variables (preload volume or contractility) is increased, that is, movement from inner to an outer curve, the extent of myocardial fiber shortening is increased at any given level of developed force or afterload.[21]

This mechanism, commonly termed the *Frank-Starling effect*, is primarily responsible for the matching of cardiac output and venous return and also, ultimately, the matching of right and LV output. The basis for the effect is the increasing fiber length stretches the sarcomere toward the optimal 2.2-μm length mentioned previously, providing a better "fit" between the actin and myosin contractile protein. This optimum overlapping provides the greatest number of force-generating sites, independent of the contractility effects. Typically, the heart operates well below this point on a steeply ascending curve where small fiber-length increments produce relatively large increments in developed tension.

The length–tension relation of a papillary muscle is shown in Figure 16-12. When the sarcomere is stretched beyond about 2.2 μm, the developed force decreases while the myofilaments become partially disengaged and fewer contractile are brought into play.[9] While the papillary muscle is increasingly stretched, the resting tension increases, first slowly and then more markedly. The stiffness of the muscle can be

defined as the slope of the curve relating the change in resting tension to the change in length. Relative to skeletal muscle, cardiac muscle is stiff, with resting tension rising exponentially as the sarcomeres approach 2.2 μm. Without resting tension, diastolic sacromere length is about 1.95 μm. Compressive forces in systole are necessary for shorter lengths, creating elastic recoil on relaxation. It was also shown that interaction exists between Starling effects (end-diastolic length) and contractile effects (Vmax). Increasing end-diastolic length also increases the contractility component, that is, more sites and higher performance per site. Experiments indicate that factors that govern the effectiveness of the excitation contraction cycle are length dependent, that is, this coupling is more effective at longer than shorter muscle lengths.[22] Thus, resting fiber length (or preload) and the contractile or inotropic state of the myocardium can no longer be considered theoretically as independent determinants of myocardial performance. The level of coupling is length dependent, and myofilament activation varies with length at the onset of cardiac contraction and continues to vary as length changes during contraction, as the fiber shortens.

AFTERLOAD: AORTIC IMPEDANCE

Ventricular ejection and performance are influenced by the sum of forces against which the ventricles contract[17] (Fig. 16-13). For the left ventricle, this sum of opposing forces (afterload or aortic input impedance) is composed of peripheral vascular resistance (friction), arterial capacitance (stiffness), mass of the aortic column of blood, and the blood viscosity.[7] Similar corresponding factors exist for the right

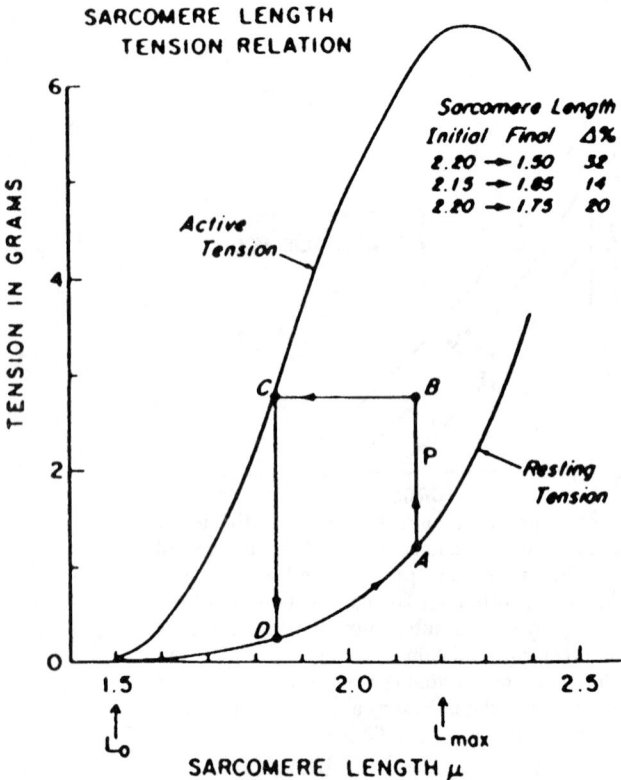

FIGURE 16-12. The relation between papillary sarcomere length, resting tension, and developed or active tension. Notice that active tension increases up to a sarcomere length of 2.2 μm (Lmax) and then decreases. The resting tension increases markedly above a sarcomere length of 2 to 2.2 μm, which corresponds to an end-diastolic pressure of about 10 to 12 mm Hg. The course of a normal contraction is shown in ABCD. Contraction starts at point A and develops a force equal to an imposed load P, reaching point B. The fiber then shortens until the active tension curve is reached at C, when relaxation occurs and returns the course to D at the end of systole. Normally, the ventricle functions on the ascending limb of the active tension curve at length below Lmax, where greatest active tension develops, with sarcomere lengths between 1.8 and 2.2 μm. The descending limb of the length-active tension curve occurs at sarcomere lengths greater than Lmax. (Sonnenblick EH, Spotnitz HM, Spiro D: Role of sarcomere in ventricular function and the mechanism of heart failure. *Circ Res* 1964; 15[Suppl 2]:70.)

ventricle. Thus, afterload is the sum of forces against which the left ventricle must act to eject blood into the aorta. The term *aortic input impedance* implies the instantaneous sum of these forces.[7] LV wall tension is thus an indicator of afterload (i.e., the tension is the result of the myocardium acting against this total opposing force), but it is not the same as afterload. In addition, preload has some relation to ventricular afterload, because end-diastolic volume directly determines ventricular radius at the onset of systole and thereby (by the Laplace relation) the amount of wall tension during the onset of the next contraction, which is related, but not identical, to afterload. For any given aortic input impedance, wall tension is higher with larger left ventricle

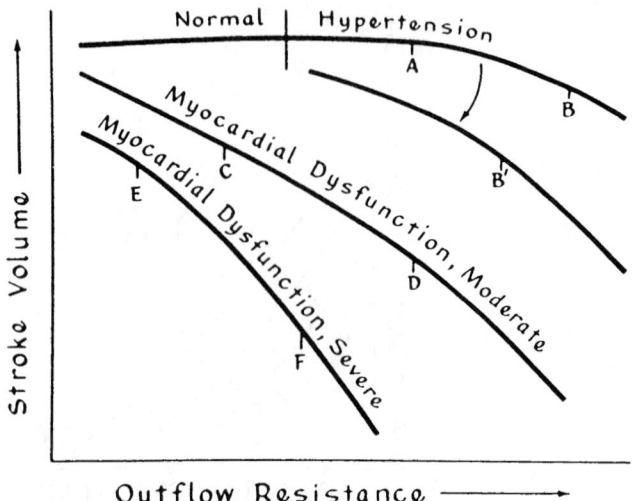

FIGURE 16-13. Ventricular function curves plotting stroke volume as a function of outflow resistance. (Cohn JN, Franciosa JA: Vasodilator therapy of cardiac failure. *N Engl J Med* 1977;297:27.)

volumes, provided that wall thickness is also constant. Increased thickness means less tension for any given LV pressure or volume, or aortic impedance, provided that the increased thickness does not alter the intrinsic elastic properties of the myocardium, a condition that is rarely present.

In conditions in which LV blood volume decreases rapidly after the onset of systole (e.g., mitral regurgitation), total impedance to LV emptying rapidly decreases during systole, as does the load on the ventricle. In general, afterload continuously but variably influences the force–velocity–time relations throughout the course of myocardial shortening. Because afterload influences the rate and extent of systolic emptying of the ventricle, it also directly influences ventricular end-systolic volume and, therefore, indirectly influences the diastolic characteristics of the next beat. A larger increase in end-systolic LV volume acutely increases the end-diastolic volume and, hence, the generated force of the subsequent beats. This effect combines with an augmentation of contractility, from the sympathomimetic effects of LV (and aortic) stretch receptor activation produced by the increased LV wall tension, to produce the Anrep effect or hemodynamic autoregulation.[16]

CHARACTERISTICS OF THE HEART AS A PUMP

PRESSURE–VOLUME RELATIONS

A clear understanding of the interaction between pressure and volume over time during cardiac contraction is key to an overall understanding of cardiac function (Fig. 16-14). Nearly a century ago, Frank represented the cycle of ventricular contraction as a loop in a plane defined by pressure (p) in the vertical direction and volume (v) in the horizontal direction[23] (Fig. 16-15). Thus, the pressure–volume loop

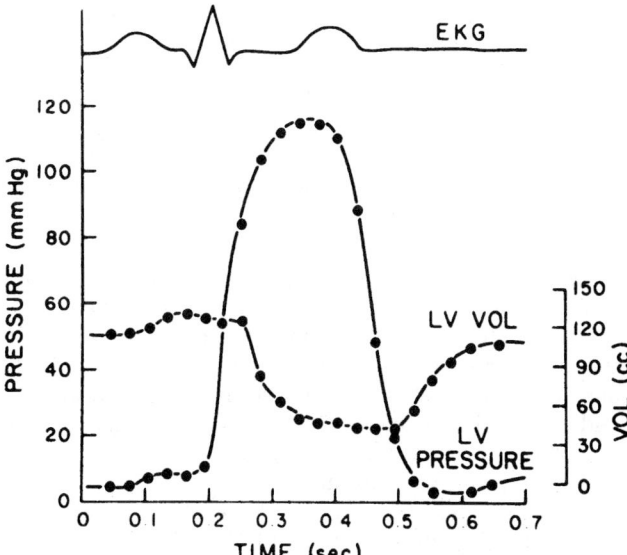

FIGURE 16-14. Simultaneous measurements of left ventricular pressure (LV) and volume plotted over time during a cardiac cycle. (Suga H: Left ventricular time-emptying pressure/volume ratio in systole as an index of myocardial inotropin. *Jpn Heart J* 1971;12:153; and Barash PG, Kopriva CJ: Cardiac pump function and how to monitor it. In: Thomas SJ [ed]: *Manual of Cardiac Anesthesia.* New York, Churchill Livingstone, 1984:1.)

representing a single contraction consists of a vertical ascending segment for the isovolemic contraction phase (A to B, Fig. 16-16), a curved horizontal segment for the ejection phase (B to C, see Fig. 16-16), a vertical descending segment for the isovolemic relaxation phase (C to D, see Fig. 16-16), and a horizontal curved segment that represents a filling phase (D to A, see Fig. 16-16).

The pressure–volume loop illustrates the external work of the ventricle (see Fig. 16-15), represented by the area circumscribed by the loop, and demonstrates the change in peak developed pressure obtained when the ventricle contracts isovolemically, beginning from various end-diastolic volumes (Fig. 16-17). The end-ejection (end-systolic) points of a series of pressure–volume loops obtained at varying diastolic volumes form a straight line for any given contractile state. The slope of this end-systolic pressure–volume relation is the best indicator of the contractile state in the intact heart.[24] An increase in the contractile state produces an upward and leftward shift (increased slope of the end-systolic pressure–volume line, whereas a decreased contractility decreases the slope). Likewise, when contractility is held constant, stroke volume from any given end-diastolic volume decreases while end-systolic pressure decreases[24] (see Fig. 16-17A). The end-systolic pressure–volume relation, therefore, predicts that either an increase or a decrease of end-diastolic volume will cause a shift of the end-systolic pressure–stroke volume relation along a single line, whereas an inotropic intervention, positive or negative, will cause a corresponding change in the slope of the end-systolic pressure–stroke volume relation (see Fig. 16-17B).

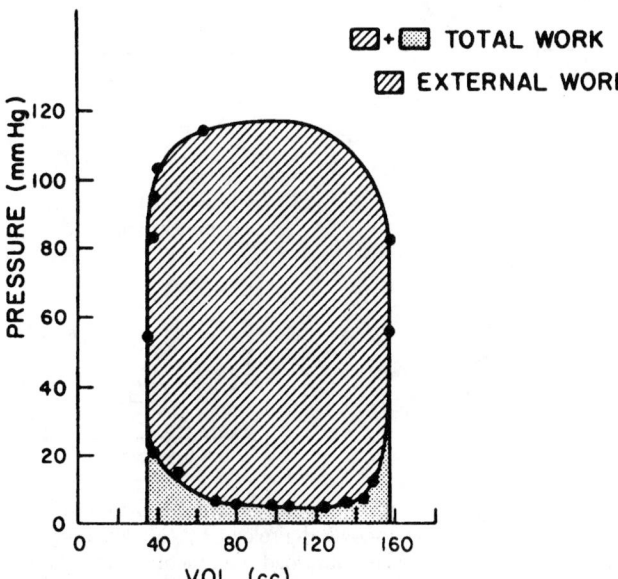

FIGURE 16-15. Plot of simultaneously measured left ventricular pressure and volume, the pressure–volume loop. (Adapted from Englar RL, Covell JW: Influence of the venous system on ventricular/arterial coupling. In: Yin FCP [ed]. *Ventricular/Vascular Coupling: Clinical, Physiological and Engineering Aspects.* New York, Springer-Verlag, 1987:20.)

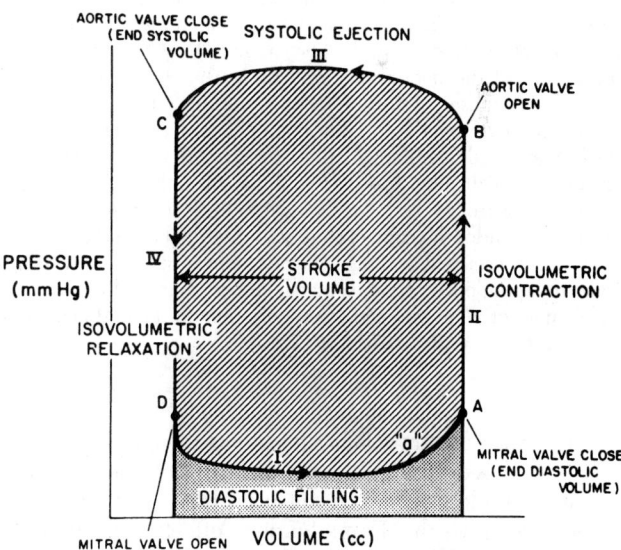

FIGURE 16-16. An idealized pressure–volume loop labeled to indicate corresponding events of the cardiac cycle. The stroke volume is the difference between ventricular volume at end-diastole and that at end-systole. (Barash PG, Kopriva CJ: Cardiac pump function and how to monitor it. In: Thomas SJ [ed]: *Manual of Cardiac Anesthesia.* New York, Churchill Livingstone, 1984:1.)

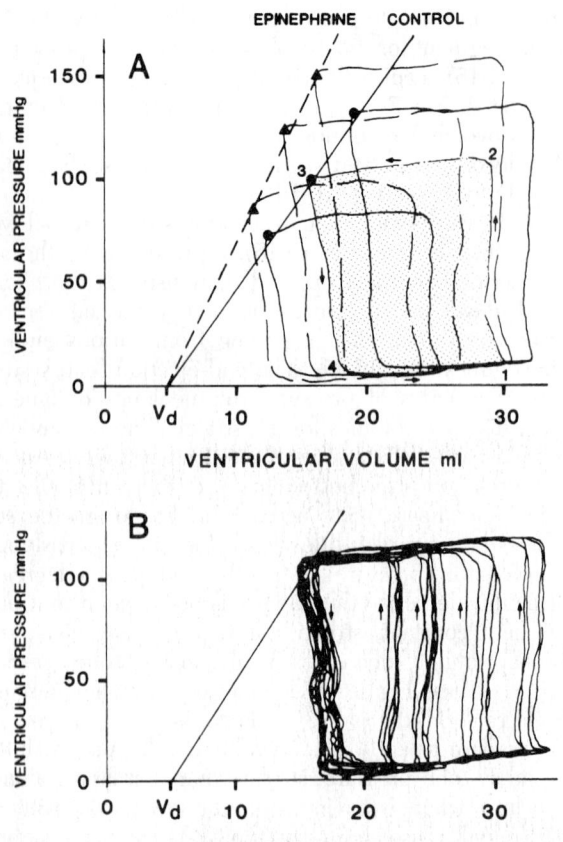

FIGURE 16-17. (**A**) Left ventricular pressure–volume loops of a denervated heart. Mean arterial pressure was fixed at three different levels while cardiac output was kept constant during both the control (*solid loops*) and the enhanced (2 μg/kg/min epinephrine infusion; *broken loops*) contractile states. The pressure–volume loop indicated by the shaded area is the data under load 1 during the control contractile state. The arrows show the direction of movement of the data points with time from 1 to 2 (isovolumic contraction phase), 2 to 3 (ejection phase), 3 to 4 (isovolumic relaxation phase), and 4 to 1 (diastolic filling phase). The solid and the broken rectilinear lines are the end-systolic data points gathered around a straight lilne (pressure–volume relation line). (**B**) Mean arterial pressure was kept constant while cardiac output was varied extensively under the control contractile state. The solid rectilinear line was transcribed from *A*. (Suga H, Sagawa K, Shoukas AA: Load independence of the instantaneous pressure-volume ratio of the canine left ventricle and effects of epinephrine and heart-rate on the ratio. *Circ Res* 1973;32:317.)

Thus, the left ventricle has the ability to generate a stroke volume that is dependent on preload, afterload, and contractile state. Preload effects result from the end-diastolic sarcomere length—the Frank-Starling effect (Fig. 16-18*A*). Sarcomere length is related to LV diastolic pressure by LV diastolic compliance (e.g., aortic stenosis, systemic hypertension, hypertrophic cardiomyopathy; see Fig. 16-18*B*), and small volume changes are associated with striking increases in filling pressures. When preload and contractility are held constant (see Fig. 16-18*C*), an inverse relation exists between afterload and stroke volume. When contractility is un-

changed, all end-systolic pressure–volume points fall on the same line. When preload and afterload are held constant, however, changes in stroke volume are directly proportional to changes in contractility (slope of end-systolic pressure–volume relation) (see Fig. 16-18*D*). Under these conditions, ejection fraction (i.e., stroke volume divided by end-systolic volume) is directly proportional to myocardial contractility.

The relation of stroke volume to end-diastolic volume has also been described in terms of stroke work (the product of stroke volume and the aortic pressure) and plotted relative to end-diastolic pressure (used as an index of end-diastolic volume). This derived relation, the common ventricular function curve, is flawed, as just discussed; stroke work at any given end-diastolic pressure is also altered by afterload and contractility changes.[25,26] Furthermore, wall thickness changes decrease LV compliance and, therefore, increase end-diastolic pressure for any volume.[27] Thus, an increased end-diastolic predictability was demonstrated for end-diastolic volume from measured end-diastolic pressure.[28]

These properties of the heart as a pump can be expressed in terms of segments of muscle in the ventricular wall. The end-diastolic volume, established by end-diastolic pressure, is reflected in initial fiber length, which is determined in turn by the resting tension or preload. The pressure developed by the ventricle, which leads to aortic valve opening and blood

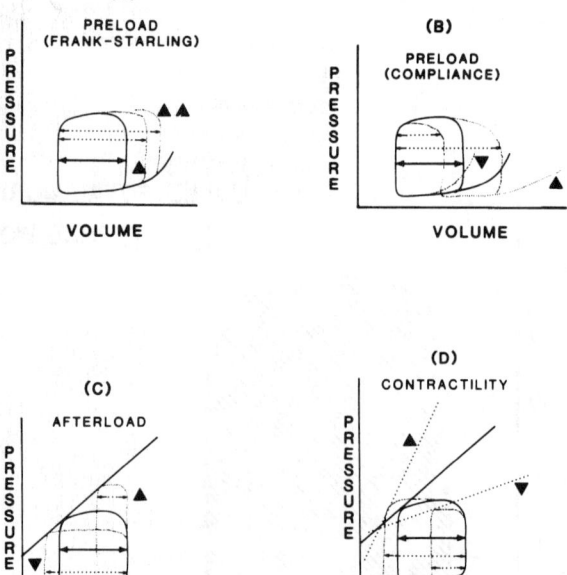

FIGURE 16-18. Changes in pressure–volume loop caused by the conditions shown. (**A**) Increased preload by the Frank-Starling mechanism (*arrows*), when afterload, contractility, and diastolic compliance remain constant. (**B**) Changes in diastolic compliance (*arrows*), when afterload and contractility remain constant. (**C**) Changes in afterload (*arrows*) when preload and contractility are constant. (**D**) Changes in contractility (*arrows*) when preload and afterload are constant. (Thomas S: Anesthetic management of the patient with valve disease and other unusual cardiac problems. In: *American Society of Anesthesiologists Refresher Course Lectures,* no. 276. Chicago, ASA, 1990:2.)

ejection, is related directly to afterload. Of course, afterload is not the pressure itself, but it is related directly to the pressure and the size of the ventricle. Thus, the tension in the wall (T) is a function of pressure (P) and radius (r) and is inversely related to wall thickness (h). Hence, a smaller heart generates less wall tension at the same pressure (modification of the Law of Laplace, or $T \cong P \times r \div h$). Moreover, the wall force tension declines during normal ejection while volume (or r) is reduced, although pressure (P) may continue to rise.

Thus, the LV pressure–volume curve is not fixed. Interventions shift the curve within a few beats, and long-term changes in the heart's operating environment produce chronic shifts.[28] Five potential mechanisms have been suggested to explain those changes: (1) changes in the LV geometry; (2) changes in myocardial passive mechanical properties; (3) incomplete relaxation from previous systole; (4) engorgement of the coronary circulation (the so-called erectile effect); and (5) interaction between the two ventricles. Geometric changes (e.g., hypertrophy or dilatation) tend to influence the pressure–volume curve as chronic responses to long-term changes. Changes in muscle elasticity are important in mediating some chronic shifts. Incomplete relaxation and coronary circulation engorgement are not significant determinants.[28] Strong evidence supports the role for right ventricular interaction and for an influence of the pericardium on ventricular function, especially for the right ventricle (see Ventricular Interaction).

Diastolic pressure contributes to the relation between LV pressure and volume (pressure–volume relationship): the LV systolic-pressure volume relation is not linear but concave to the volume axis. The true slope is, therefore, variable and not an index of contractility. Apparently, linearity or convexity results from inappropriate addition of the diastolic pressure–volume properties.[29]

Diastolic LV pressure–volume relation can change, showing a striking upward shift that signifies a marked decrease in the LV chamber distensibility.[20] Such diastolic dysfunction may result from extrinsic compression (i.e., by pericardial constriction or tamponade) and right ventricular overload, or other physiologic or anatomic abnormality that leads to increased resistance to diastolic filling of one or both ventricles. (Fig. 16-19).

Limitations

One potential limitation of pressure–volume relation stems from the fact that pressure may not be an accurate measure of end-systolic afterload. Afterload is the force that opposes ejection. In physical terms, force = pressure $\times$ area and accounts for the distribution of pressure over the surface to which the force is applied. When the force is applied to a thick-chambered sphere (e.g., the LV), it is described by the Laplace relation: stress = pressure $\times$ radius + 2 height-thickness. When the LV radius or thickness changes, end-systolic stress is more useful in demonstrating reduced afterload.[31]

Changes in the x-intercept of the force-volume or stress-volume line may occur with changes in the inotropic state instead of a change in slope.[31,32] A parallel shift in the stress-volume line results rather than a change in slope (Fig. 16-20). Such a shift is likely to occur when the inotropic state, and loading conditions are changed in a small ventricle. Because slope = change in Y (pressure or stress) + change in X (volume), the slope changes relatively less in a small ventricle when stress is used instead of pressure.

Finally, an additional limitation may occur because reflex changes in heart rate and the ionotropic state can occur during load-altering maneuvers. However, the linearity of stress–volume relations reported in most studies suggests

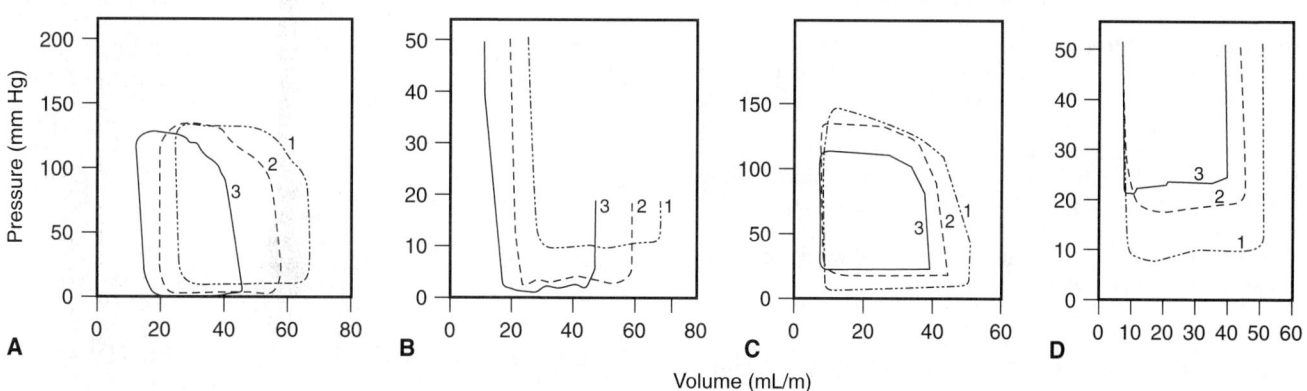

FIGURE 16-19. Left ventricular (LV) pressure–volume relation at increasing heart rate (atrial pacing) in a patient with normal coronary arteries (**A** and **B**) and a patient with multivessel coronary artery disease (**C** and **D**). The LV diastolic pressure–volume relation shifted downward with tachycardia in the patient without coronary disease, possibly resulting from relief of pericardial restraint and ventricular interaction. In contrast, the patient with coronary artery disease developed angina pectoris with pacing tachycardia, and this was associated with an upward shift in the LV diastolic pressure–volume relation. Pressures were measured with micromanometer catheters and volumes with radionuclide ventriculography. (Reproduced from Aroesty JM, McKay RG, Heller GV, et al: Simultaneous assessment of left ventricular systolic and diastolic dysfunction during pacing–induced ischemia. *Circulation* 1985;71:889.) A and B: ····· = 85 beats/min, --- = 100 beats/min, —— = 125 beats/min. C and D: ····· = 84 beats/min, --- = 110 beats/min, —— = 135 beats/min.

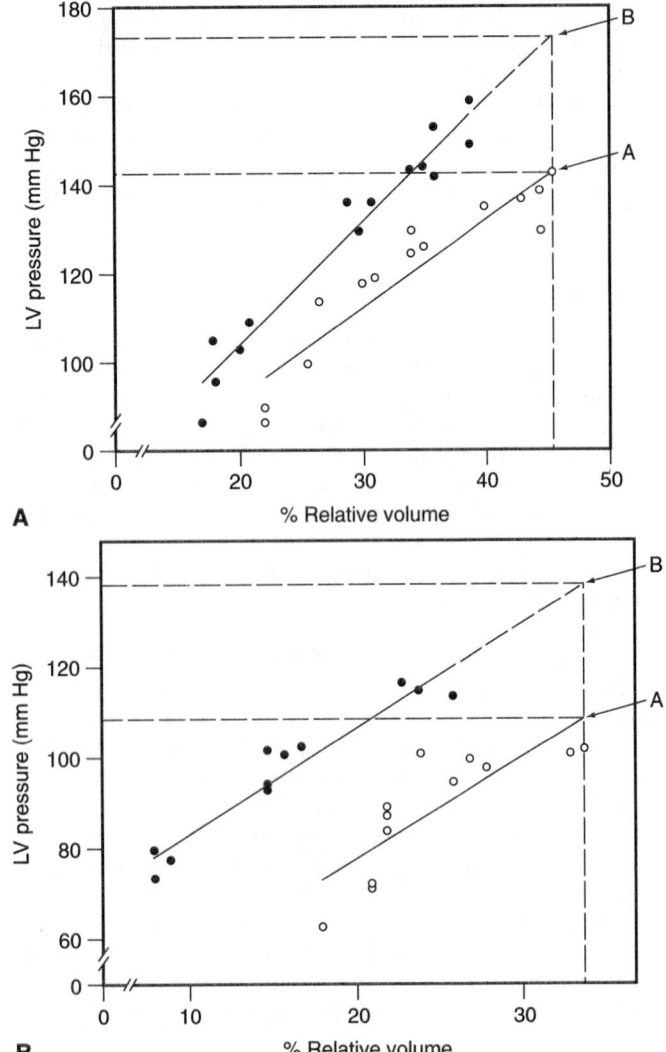

A

B

FIGURE 16-20. Effect of dobutamine on the end-systolic pressure–volume relation during nitroprusside washout in two representative patients (○, control; ●, dobutamine). Point A is the left ventricular pressure and relative volume at control end-systolic volume. Point B is left ventricular pressure and relative volume at control end-systolic volume during dobutamine infusion, extrapolated from linear regression of the end-systolic pressure–volume relationship. (**A**) Patient in whom there was an increase in slope. (**B**) Patient in whom there was an upward and leftward shift without an apparent change in slope.

that contractile function does not change much during loading.

PRESSURE–FLOW RELATIONS

In addition to ejecting the stroke volume from a given end-diastolic volume, the ventricle delivers the stroke volume with a velocity determined by its instantaneous volume and the resistance to ejection, that is, pressure (Fig. 16-21). Thus, when the end-diastolic volume is augmented (see Fig. 16-21, panel 2), stroke volume increases (b′ to c′), as does the ejection velocity. When arterial pressure is increased (see

Fig. 16-21, panel 3), the velocity of ejection and stroke volume are reduced. An inotropic intervention increases both (see Fig. 16-21, panel 4). The stroke power (product of stroke volume and aortic pressure divided by ejection duration, i.e., stroke work per unit time) is also increased at any end-diastolic volume, but, as with stroke work, it remains pressure dependent.

The Frank-Starling law of the heart does not play a major role in mediating increased LV performance, because LV end-diastolic volume does not increase during exercise. However, the increase in LV peak rapid filling rate is correlated with decreased end-systolic volume, suggesting that enhancement of LV filling during the shortened diastolic interval, is, at least in part, caused by LV suction.[33]

Simplification Attempts

Substitution of peak-systolic for end-diastolic pressure is an attractive feature of the pressure–volume relation because of its potential for being determined noninvasively. However, the close relation found between peak and end-systolic pressure[34] may not be constant, especially when large stroke volumes and pulse pressures are present (i.e., in aortic regurgitation). Then, the relation of peak-systolic to end-systolic pressure may be different.

The end-systolic pressure–volume ratio has been used as a measure of contractile function. Because the Y intercept of the pressure–volume line varies from patient to patient, this assumption is usually not justified, and this pressure–volume ratio does not truly represent the slope. However, it can be used in a single patient.

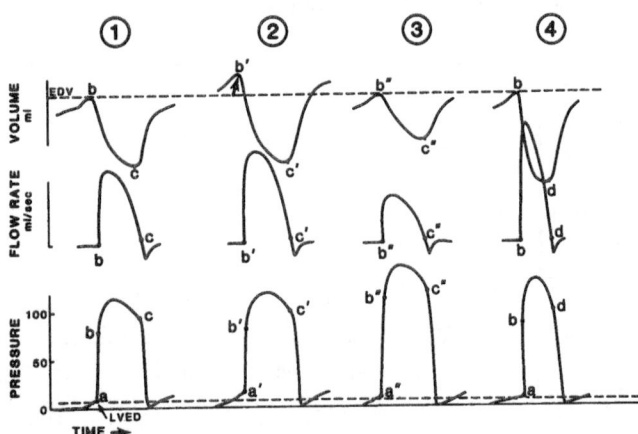

FIGURE 16-21. Effects of altered ventricular volume, pressure, and contractility. Intraventricular volume, aortic flow rate, and intraventricular pressure have been illustrated relative to time. (**Panel 1**) Control state. (**Panel 2**) Effects of an augmented end-diastolic volume. (**Panel 3**) Effects of increased intraventricular pressure. Diastolic volume has been maintained constant. (**Panel 4**) Effects of administering isoproterenol. Diastolic volume has been held constant. (Brutsaert DL, Sonnenblick EH: Cardiac muscle mechanics in the evaluation of myocardial contractility and pump function: Problems, concepts and directions. *Progr Cardiovasc Dis* 1973;16:342.)

The end-systolic stress–volume ratio, as mentioned previously, may be useful because stress data often have advantages over pressure in quantifying afterload when the ventricular size and thickness are abnormal. However, this ratio, like the pressure–volume ratio, is not a substitute for the slope. It may be particularly limited in small ventricles where volume value on X-intercept (V_D) is larger in relation to end-systolic volume.

VENTRICULAR INTERACTION

The right and left ventricles are joined by the common interventricular septum, and both are closely surrounded by fibrous, relatively inelastic pericardium. That the pericardium plays a significant role in controlling the compliance of the heart is shown by the increase in right ventricular distensibility that occurs after pericardiotomy.[35] Normally, the interventricular septum is slightly convex toward the right ventricle, largely because of the higher pressure and lower compliance of the left ventricle. Overdistension of the left ventricle or markedly decreased LV compliance can produce sufficient shift of the septum to compromise right ventricular filling, leading to reduced cardiac output. This example is one form of ventricular interaction.

The opposite effect, the so-called paradoxical septal shift, also can occur.[36] A marked decrease in right ventricular compliance caused, for example, by right ventricular infarction or significant pulmonary thromboembolism, shifts the septum leftward and effectively decreases compliance of the left ventricle, also reducing cardiac output. Additive factors include the varying impact of pulmonary vascular hypertension, the respiratory cycle, and, especially, mechanical positive-pressure ventilation, which increases right ventricular afterload and may actually decrease LV afterload.[37] Hence, on a beat-to-beat basis, left and right ventricular output often differ, despite the fact that over time they must be equal. The factor of intrathoracic pressure (ventilation mode) is an important influence on the performance of the left *versus* the right ventricle.[38] Positive-pressure ventilation can be a form of LV afterload reduction and right ventricular afterload augmentation. Negative intrathoracic pressure is the opposite. These effects add to the beat-to-beat disparity of right and LV stroke volume that is also caused (primarily) by phasic differences in venous return volume.

VENTRICULAR VASCULAR COUPLING

Although a primary focus of attention in cardiovascular physiology has been myocardial function, the heart is not an isolated pump. Rather, it provides the initial power to produce blood flow through the systemic and pulmonary vasculature. The overall efficacy of the circulation depends on the interactions of the pump and the vascular conduits. The venous system cannot be thought of as a passive conduit, because venous capacitance is subject to reflex and pharmacologic control to increase or decrease the volume of venous return.[39] Certainly the venous system is key to overall cardio-

vascular function, and venous return is the key regulator of cardiac output.[40]

The interaction of the arterial system and LV function is often misunderstood, but it is of fundamental importance to an understanding of the cardiovascular system.[41] Whereas flow in the distal arterioles and capillaries is nearly continuous, both pressure and flow are distinctly pulsatile proximal to the muscular arterioles, where maximum resistance to blood flow occurs. The phasic pumping function of the left ventricle produces this pressure and flow pulsatility, but the elastic properties of the arterial system greatly influence the energy expenditure required to produce the stroke volume and perfusion of the left ventricle. Under normal circumstances, a progressive increase in pressure and decrease in blood flow velocity occur as the pulse wave is transmitted from the central aorta to the periphery. Thus, systolic blood pressure in the radial or dorsalis pedis arteries is approximately 15% greater than central aortic pressure, whereas the mean value is nearly constant (Fig. 16-22).

This amplification of the pressure pulse illustrates the importance of elasticity of the arterial system. It is erroneous to consider peripheral resistance as equal to LV afterload. The calculation, by convention, is the quotient of mean arterial pressure and mean blood flow, which totally ignores arterial elasticity and the pulsatile pressure wave. Moreover, peripheral resistance considers the entire cardiac cycle, whereas the left ventricle "sees" arterial pressure only during systolic ejection (approximately one third of the cycle) in terms of its work output. As stated by Bramwell and Hill,[42] "The amount of energy which the heart has to expend per beat, other things being equal, varies inversely with the elasticity of the arterial system."

The arterial system primarily is a conduit, providing nutrient flow to peripheral tissues, and as an energy buffer to absorb the pulsatility of ventricular ejection and to deliver continuous flow to the periphery. This conduit function is efficient, because essentially no pressure drop occurs in the major arteries. However, resistance abruptly increases at the level of the arterioles, and this abrupt change results in a strong reflection of the pressure wave from the peripheral site toward the central vessels. This reflection is largely responsible for the amplification of the pressure pulse.

In a healthy circulatory system, the steady-state pressure and flow components (i.e., mean pressure and mean flow, classic vascular resistance) of ventricular load predominate. Only about 10% of the energy expended to produce flow is related to the pulsatile components. Under these optimal conditions, aortic mean systolic pressure is only 5 to 10 mm Hg greater than mean aortic pressure averaged throughout the cardiac cycle. The ideal aortic pressure wave form has a low-amplitude systolic peak, followed by an incisura caused by aortic valve closure, and by a second peak during diastole that is caused by elastic recoil of the great vessels and by the peripherally reflected pressure wave. Atherosclerotic arterial disease, hypertension, and aging all result in decreased distensibility of the arterial system and increased pulse wave velocity. Normal ventricular vascular coupling is functionally altered. The decreased distensibility has two primary effects: (1) a given arterial volume increment (stroke volume) requires a greater pressure increment; and (2) more rapid

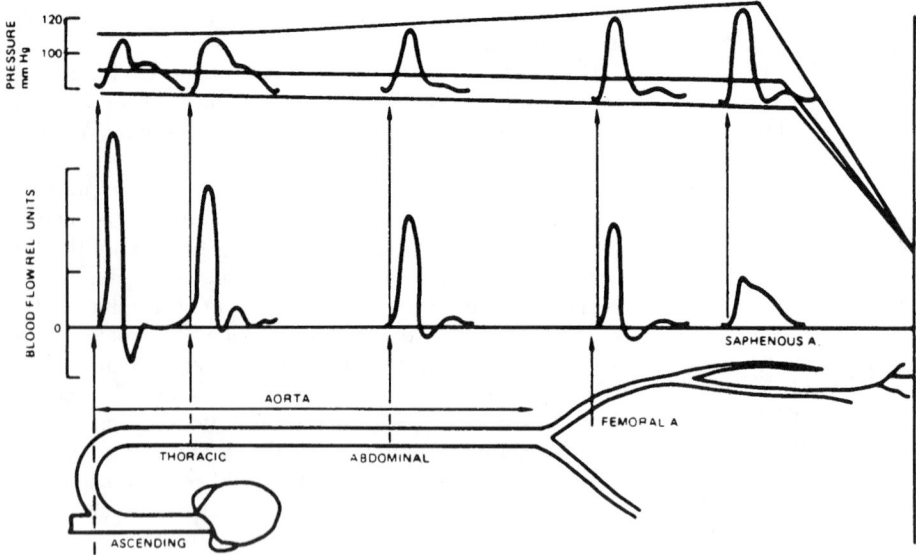

FIGURE 16-22. Schematic representation of the intrinsic amplification of the pressure pulse at progressively more distal arterial measurement sites. Notice that the actual flow pulse decreases while the pressure pulse increases. (McDonald DA: *Blood Flow in the Arteries,* 2nd ed. London, Edward Arnold Publishers, 1974.)

pressure wave propagation produces a more rapid return of reflected waves that can lead to summation with systolic pressure to increase further the systolic pressure load of the left ventricle. This increased pressure load increases energy expenditure of the left ventricle (increased wall tension), leading in chronic states to compensatory LV hypertrophy, and can compromise coronary blood flow.

Improved ventricular vascular coupling requires increased elasticity of the great vessels and delayed pressure wave reflection from the periphery. Mechanically, these effects are accomplished with intraaortic balloon counterpulsation. Specific pharmacologic improvement of ventricular vascular coupling is not available, although vasodilator therapy may have a beneficial influence on peripheral pressure wave reflection. Further study of the impact of critical illness on ventricular vascular coupling should produce improvements in cardiovascular management.

NEUROGENIC CONTROL OF THE CARDIOVASCULAR SYSTEM ∎

REGULATION OF THE HEARTBEAT

A discussion of the neurogenic control of cardiac activity may be subdivided into consideration of the regulation of pacemaker activity as well as myocardial performance. However, in the intact organism, a change in one almost invariably produces an alteration in the other. At a constant stroke volume, cardiac output is a linear function of the heart rate. Heart rate, in turn, is determined primarily by the rhythmicity of the SA node. The SA node is under the tonic influence of both divisions of the autonomic nervous system: sympathetic stimulation, in general, enhances automaticity, whereas parasympathetic stimulation inhibits it. Changes in heart rate usually involve reciprocal actions of the two divisions of the autonomic nervous system, but under certain conditions heart rate may change because of selective action

of one division. Ordinarily, in healthy resting adults, parasympathetic tone is predominant.

Parasympathetic Control

The cardiac parasympathetic fibers originate in the medulla oblongata. Vagal fibers pass inferiorly through the neck, in close proximity to the common carotid arteries, and then through the mediastinum to synapse with postganglionic cells located within the heart itself. Most of the cardiac ganglion cells are located near the SA node and AV conduction tissue. The right and left vagi are distributed differently to the various cardiac structures. (The left vagus mainly influences AV conduction tissue, and the right affects the SA node predominantly, but a considerable overlap exists between the two vagal trunks.) The SA and AV nodes are rich in cholinesterase; thus, the effect of a vagal impulse is short because the acetylcholine released in nerve terminals is rapidly hydrolyzed. Parasympathetic influences dominate over sympathetic effects at the SA node.[43]

Sympathetic Control

The cardiac sympathetic fibers originate in the intermediolateral columns of the upper five or six thoracic segments and lower one or two cervical segments of the spinal cord. They emerge from the spinal column through the white communicating branches and enter the paravertebral chain of ganglia. In many species, preganglionic and postganglionic neurons synapse mainly in the stellate ganglia. In humans, sympathetic neural impulses also travel through the cervical (superior, middle, and inferior) ganglia and the thoracic cardiac accelerator nerves (T1-4); sympathetic stimulation affects the SA and AV nodes, ventricular muscle and the conduction system.

The postganglionic cardiac sympathetic fibers approach the base of the heart along the adventitial surface of the great vessels, are distributed into an extensive epicardial plexus, and penetrate the myocardium accompanying branches of the coronary vessels. The adrenergic receptors in the nodal regions and myocardium are predominantly the beta subtype. As with the vagus, there is a differential distribution of the left and right sympathetic fibers: the left sympathetic chain has a greater distribution to LV myocardium, whereas the right is preferentially distributed to the conduction system. In general, increased sympathetic tone produces an increase on the chronotropic, dromotropic, and inotropic state of the heart. The effects of sympathetic stimulation decay gradually after cessation of stimulation, in contrast to vagal activity. Most norepinephrine released during stimulation is taken up again by nerve terminals, much of the remainder is carried away by the bloodstream, and relatively little is degraded in the tissues.

Neural centers regulating cardiac function are located mostly in the anterior half of the brain (frontal lobe, orbital motor and premotor cortex, temporal lobe, insula, and cingulate gyrus). Tachycardia can be induced by thalamic stimulation, and the variations in heart rate can be evoked by stimulating the hypothalamus. Cortical and diencephalic centers are responsible for initiating cardiac reactions during anxiety. Also, environmental alterations (e.g., temperature) may stimulate hypothalamic centers involved in cardiac response.

Reflex Control

Numerous investigators have confirmed observations made by Bainbridge in 1915 regarding the acceleration of the heart rate in response to intravenous administration of fluid.[44] Receptors that influence heart rate exist in both atria and are located principally in the caval–atrial junctions. Distension of these receptors sends afferent impulses centripetally in the vagi. Efferent impulses are carried down by fibers from both autonomic divisions to the SA node. The cardiac response is selective—changes in contractility are negligible. The Bainbridge reflex is prepotent over baroreceptor activity when blood volume is rising, but not under hypovolemic conditions (Fig. 16-23A).

Numerous studies have investigated the conflicting effects of left atrial and LV receptor stimulation on heart rate and mean arterial pressure. When left atrial receptors are stimulated, a reflex increase in heart rate is described as the *Bainbridge reflex.*[45,46] Conversely, LV receptor stimulation causes a bradycardia, and is described as the *Bezold-Janish reflex.*[47,48] Because these receptor populations are proximate anatomically, they likely can be activated simultaneously. Studies have shown a complex modulation of one reflex by the other.[47,49] Stimulation of left atrial receptors with simultaneous LV receptor activation alters the increase in heart rate (Fig. 16-24). Apparently, cardiovascular reflexes

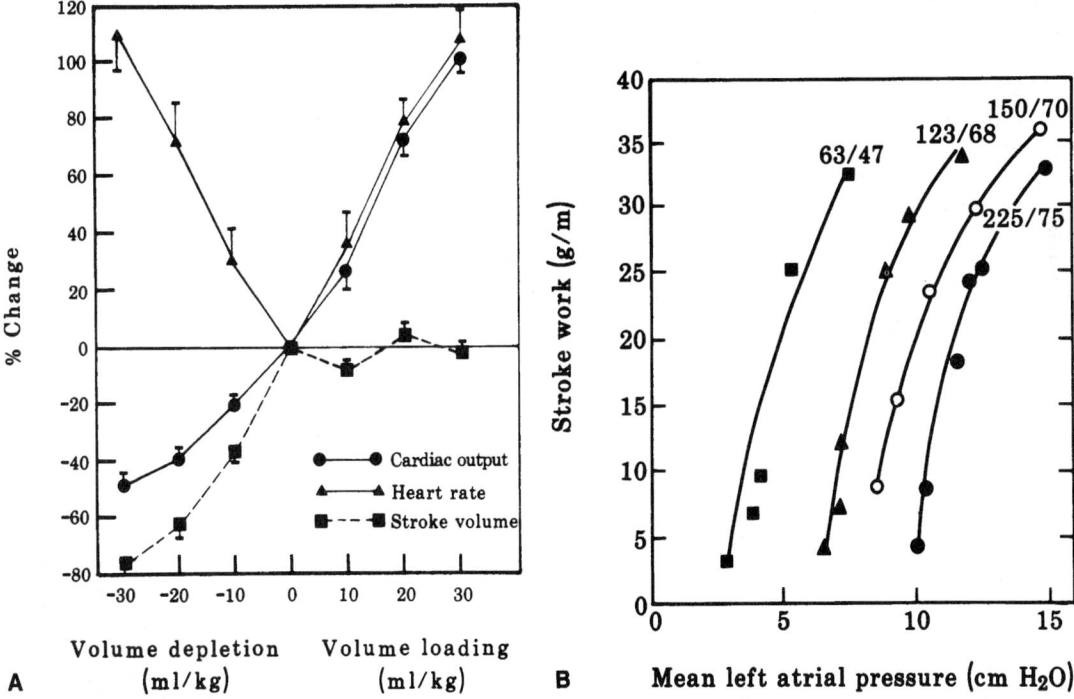

FIGURE 16-23. (**A**) Effects of blood transfusion and bleeding on cardiac output, heart rate, and stroke volume in unanesthetized dogs. (**B**) While the pressure in the isolated carotid sinus is progressively raised, the ventricular function curves shift to the right. The numbers at the tops of each curve represent the systolic/diastolic perfusion pressures (in mm Hg) in the carotid sinus regions of the dog. (Vanter SF, Boettcher DH: Regulation of cardiac output by stroke volume and heart rate in conscious dogs. *Circ Res* 1978;42:557; and Berne RM, Levy MN: Regulation of the heartbeat. In: Carson D [ed]. *Cardiovascular Physiology,* 5th ed. St Louis, CV Mosby, 1986:99.)

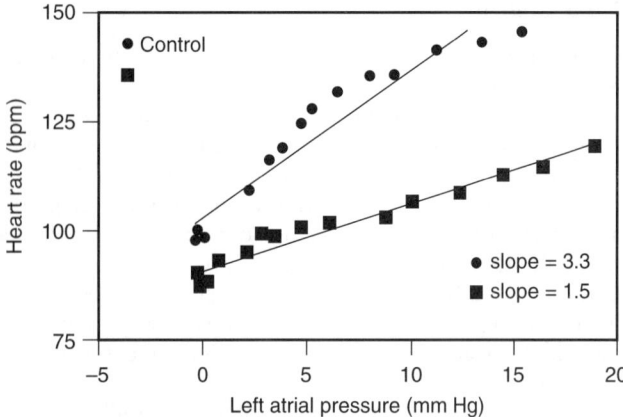

FIGURE 16-24. A graph of the heart rate versus left atrial pressure relationship from a typical veratridine experiment. The filled circles represent a control left atrial balloon inflation, whereas the filled squares represent a left atrial balloon inflation during an intracoronary infusion of veratridine (0.2 µg/kg/min). The lines through the data points show the calculated linear regressions used to determine the slopes of these responses.

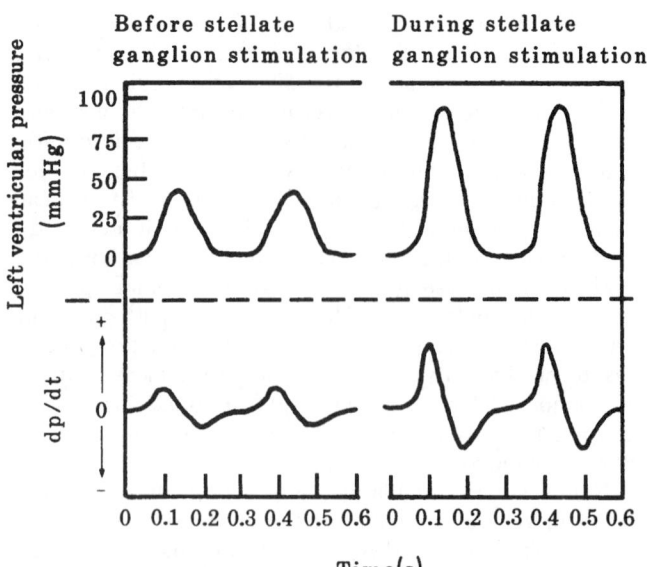

FIGURE 16-25. In an isovolumic left ventricle preparation, stimulation of cardiac sympathetic nerves evokes a substantial rise in peak left ventricular pressure and in the maximum rates of intraventricular pressure rise and fall (dp/dt). (Berne RM, Levy MN: Regulation of heartbeat. In: Carson D [ed]. *Cardiovascular Physiology*, 5th ed. St Louis, CV Mosby, 1986:96.)

are not discrete entities, but form part of an integrated network.[50] Also, the afferent arm of the Bainbridge reflex include sympathetic activation and vagal withdrawal.[50] However, the cardiac vagal neurons are more sensitive to baroreceptor input than are the sympathetic neurons.[51] That complex innervation and reflex modulation may explain why during hypovolemic states with sympathectomy (i.e., epidural block), the unopposed vagal response will cause bradycardia, rather than reflex tachycardia. Also, baroreceptor unloading (i.e., with nitroglycerin) is largely manifested by a decrease in sympathetic activation in heart failure.[52]

The inverse relation between arterial pressure and heart rate is dependent on baroreceptors located in the aortic arch and carotid sinuses. Reciprocal reflex changes in sympathetic and vagal activity occur even for small deviations in blood pressure within the normal range of pressures. Just as the stimulation of the baroreceptors affects heart rate, it also affects myocardial performance (see Fig. 16-23B). Stimulation of the sympathetic division of the autonomic nervous system increases atrial and ventricular contractility (Fig. 16-25), decreases the duration of systole, and increases the rate of ventricular relaxation during early phases of diastole. The shortening of systole and rapid relaxation assist ventricular filling. Neurally released norepinephrine interacts with beta-adrenergic receptors on the cardiac cell membranes to activate adenylate cyclase. This activation increases intracellular cyclic AMP concentration and activates protein kinases, consequently promoting protein phosphorylation, which augments opening of Ca^{+2} channels in myocardial cell membranes. The negative inotropic effect of vagal stimulation is less pronounced (Fig. 16-26).

Acetylcholine increases the intracellular concentration of cyclic guanosine monophosphate (cGMP), which may depress contractility. The increased concentration of cGMP and subsequent activation of guanylate cyclase in cell membrane activates K^+ channels and produces hyperpolarization of SA node cells or an increase in outward current in atrial cells.[53]

NEURAL CONTROL OF PERIPHERAL BLOOD FLOW

Several regions in the medulla influence cardiovascular activity. Stimulation of the dorsal lateral medulla causes vasoconstriction, enhanced heart rate, and increased contractility. Caudal and ventromedial to the pressor region is a zone that, when stimulated, decreases blood pressure. These areas comprise a physiologic, not an anatomic center. From the vasoconstrictor regions, fibers descend in the spinal cord and synapse at different thoracolumbar region levels (T1-L3). Fibers from the intermediolateral gray matter of the

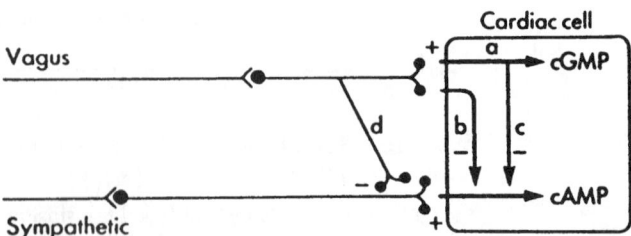

FIGURE 16-26. The interneuronal and intracellular mechanisms responsible for the vagal–sympathetic interactions. (Berne RM, Levy MN: Regulation of the heartbeat. In: Carson D [ed]. *Cardiovascular Physiology*, 5th ed. St Louis, CV Mosby, 1986:98.)

cord emerge with ventral roots and join the paravertebral sympathetic chains through the white communicating branches. Postganglionic gray (unmyelinated) branches join the corresponding segmental spinal nerves and are distributed peripherally to innervate the arteries and veins. The medullary vasoconstrictor regions are tonically active, and impulses originating in these regions reach the terminal branches, where a constrictor neurotransmitter (norepinephrine) is released. Vasoconstriction is elicited by interaction of norepinephrine with alpha₁-adrenergic receptors in the vascular smooth muscle. Such vasoconstriction shows cyclic variation, some of which occurs at the frequency of respiration (Traube-Hering waves), resulting from increases in efferent sympathetic impulses coincident with inspiration. Others are independent of and at a lower frequency than respiration (Mayer waves).[43]

Neural influence on the larger vessels is far less effective than it is on the microcirculation. Capacitance vessels are apparently less responsive to sympathetic nerve stimulation than are the muscular (resistance) vessels, because they reach maximum constriction at a lower frequency of stimulation than do the resistance vessels.[54] Furthermore, capacitance vessels do not possess beta-adrenergic receptors, nor do they respond to vasodilator metabolites.[43] Sympathetic cholinergic fibers also innervate the resistance vessels in skeletal muscle and skin. Their stimulation results in active dilation, which can be blocked by atropine. They arise in the motor cortex of the cerebrum and pass through the hypothalamus and ventral medulla before joining the other sympathetic outflow the spinal cord. Evidence does not support any tonic activity of these fibers.

Only small proportions of the resistance vessels of the body receive parasympathetic fibers. The efferent fibers of the cranial division of the parasympathetic system supply the vasculature of the head and most viscera, whereas fibers of the sacral divisions supply the vasculature of the genitalia, bladder and large bowel. The effect of this cholinergic innervation total vascular resistance is small.

The Vasovagal Response

The vasovagal response reflects arteriolar dilation (vaso-) and inappropriate cardiac slowing (-vagal), leading to arterial hypotension with loss of consciousness. Simultaneous vagal activation and sympathetic inhibition during this response are considered to be neural mechanisms that can be activated along two different pathways[55] (Fig. 16-27). One descends from corticohypothalamic centers to medullary cardiovascular centers (central type); the second pathway probably originates in the heart (peripheral type). The main determinants of neural activity in the peripheral type seems to be wall deformation and the inotropic state of the cardiac muscle. The combination of an increased inotropic stimulus to the heart and decreased LV volume is thought to give rise to contractions around an "empty" chamber, leading to deformation and activation of ventricular-mechanoreceptors.[56]

Hypovolemic hypotension may set in motion two opposing reflexes as previously described: the arterial baroreceptor

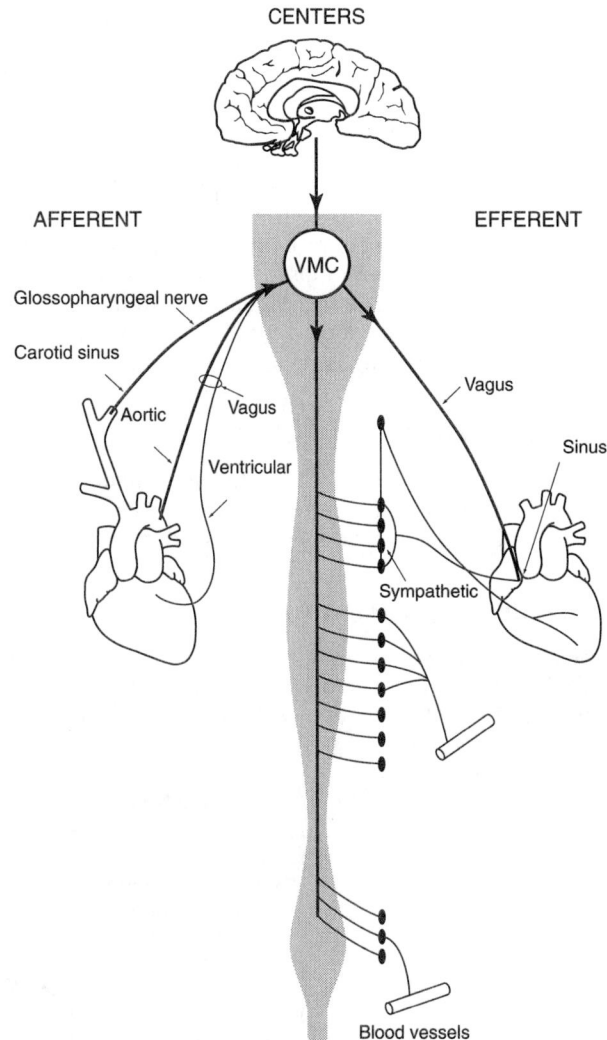

FIGURE 16-27. Cardiovascular part of the autonomic nervous system. Schematic representation of the two different pathways that may elicit the depressor response: the baroreceptor and depressor reflex arcs and the "central command" to the vasomotor centres (VMC). (Reproduced from Van Lieshout JJ: *Cardiovascular Reflexes in Orthostatic Disorders.* Amsterdam: Rodopi, 1989.)

and depressor reflex. The former is activated by a fall in arterial blood pressure and the latter by a decrease in ventricular filling volume (see Fig. 16-27). Antagonism between the control of filling pressure and volume of the heart, and the control system of systemic arterial pressure can cause imbalance. Thus, when syncope ensues, the depressor reflex overrides the baroreflex. This shift from presyncopal tachycardia to bradycardia (with or without hypotension) has been referred to as the *biphasic response.*[57] It is reflected by an initial noradrenaline elevation just before syncope, followed by a stable or declined level during the vasovagal response.[58]

PASSIVE AND ACTIVE CONTROL OF SYSTEMIC AND CORONARY ARTERY SIZE AND VASOMOTION

PASSIVE CONTROL

The factors that control coronary and peripheral artery size are passive and active. Passive factors (e.g., stenosis, lesion geometry, distal arteriolar resistance, and perfusion pressure) interact with smooth muscle tone and modulate flow. Small variations in tone, acting in concert with the hemodynamic factors noted previously, can limit flow when severe atherosclerotic narrowing is present.

ACTIVE CONTROL

The possible active factors that influence smooth muscle tone to alter the size of an artery can be divided into those that are endothelial dependent or independent (Fig. 16-28).

Endothelium-Dependent Mechanisms

Normal vascular endothelium releases one or more potent muscular autocoids termed *endothelium-derived relaxing factors* (EDRF). At least one of these appears to be nitric oxide (NO), and it mediates local arterial smooth muscle relaxation through activation of guanyl-cyclase to increase cGMP. This substance induces phosphorylation of intracellular proteins and initiates hydrolysis of phosphatidyl inositol, leading to reduction of cytosolic Ca^{+2} with resultant smooth muscle relaxation and vasodilation. When flow-rate increases in a large artery, shear stress in the endothelial surface is increased and sensed by endothelial cells, which in turn release EDRF.[59] Release is also triggered by acetylcholine, serotonin, and other agents acting at the endothelial receptors. EDRF also has a potent local antiaggregation effect on platelets. Endothelial dysfunction resulting from atherosclerosis, hypoxia, ischemia, and drugs may play a role in the genesis of arterial spasm, reduced flow, and reduced stimulus for release of EDRF in the functional adjacent endothelium.

Vascular endothelial cells reportedly produce a novel potent vasoconstrictor called *endothelin*.[60] The role of EDRF and endothelin in regulation of vascular tone indicates that they also modulate sympathetic transmitter release. Both seem to affect norepinephrine efflux indirectly by changing arterial flow, but not directly by interference with the release process itself.[61]

To conclude, endothelial functions or factors may affect vascular tone[62]: indirectly, by enzyme hydrolysis of vasoactive

Factors Involved in Coronary Vasomotion

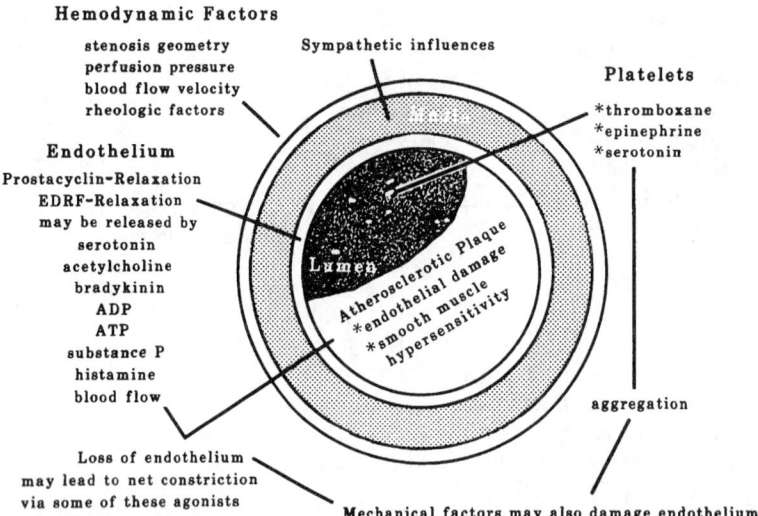

FIGURE 16-28. Role of passive and active factors involved in coronary vasomotion. Passive hemodynamic factors, such as stenosis geometry, perfusion pressure, blood flow velocity, and blood rheologic factors, which are determined mostly by large molecules like fibrinogen, interact to determine functional importance of a coronary stenosis. Active factors include the sympathetic nervous system, platelets, ecosinoids, and endothelium. Specific agonists (serotonin, acetylcholine, and bradykinin) act at receptor sites in endothelium, along with increases in blood flow to stimulate release of endothelial-derived relaxation factor (EDRF) and produce relaxation of vascular smooth muscle in the media. Mechanical factors, such as atherosclerotic plaque or even spasm, may result in loss of endothelial function and reduce EDRF to produce constriction by agonists that previously had caused dilatation. The factors determine the size of the lumen, particularly at the site of eccentric plaque. (Pepine CJ, Lambert CR: Coronary artery spasm: Pathophysiology, natural history, recognition, and treatment. In: Hurst JW [ed]. *The Heart, Arteries, and Veins,* 7th ed. New York, McGraw-Hill, 1990:1120.)

compounds (e.g., angiotensin-converting enzyme), producing a cascade of ectonucleodidases (e.g., ATP-ase) and sequentially degrading ATP to adenosine; and directly, by binding vasoactive compounds to receptors at the endothelial surface and including release of intracellular Ca^{2+}, which is a necessary signal for synthesis of different autocoids (e.g., PGI_2, EDRF) (Fig. 16-29).

Coronary vascular tone also might be affected by EDRF and endothelin, but its significance in coronary blood flow control is not fully evaluated.[61-63] EDRF formation in the coronaries may result from the high shear stress imposed on the endothelial lining by periodic diameter reduction and from direct deformation of the endothelium.[64] Some findings suggest that NO reduces baseline venous tone similarly to arterial tone.[65]

Impaired endothelium-dependent vasomotor control has been documented during ischemia,[66] hypercholesterolemia, atheromatosis, diabetes, hypertension, and reperfusion damage.[67] Because NO is an effective regulator of vascular tone and is produced in endothelial cells from L-arginine by NO synthase, L-arginine therapy may be effective.

Endothelium-Independent Mechanisms

Adrenergic nervous system stimulation by alpha-adrenergic receptor activation increases vascular smooth muscle tone. Modulation of sympathetic outflow by the endogenous central opiate system also may play a role in regulating arterial tone.[68] Although histamine may stimulate endothelium-dependent dilation, coronary spasm has been reported with histamine. Serotonin released from platelets has been proposed as a mechanism for arterial spasm, although its role in coronary spasm is minimal.

METABOLIC DEMAND AND OXYGEN SUPPLY OF THE HEART

PHYSIOLOGIC CONSIDERATIONS

The interrelation between oxygen requirements and availability, synonymous with the concept of metabolic demand and supply, is fundamental for any consideration of the

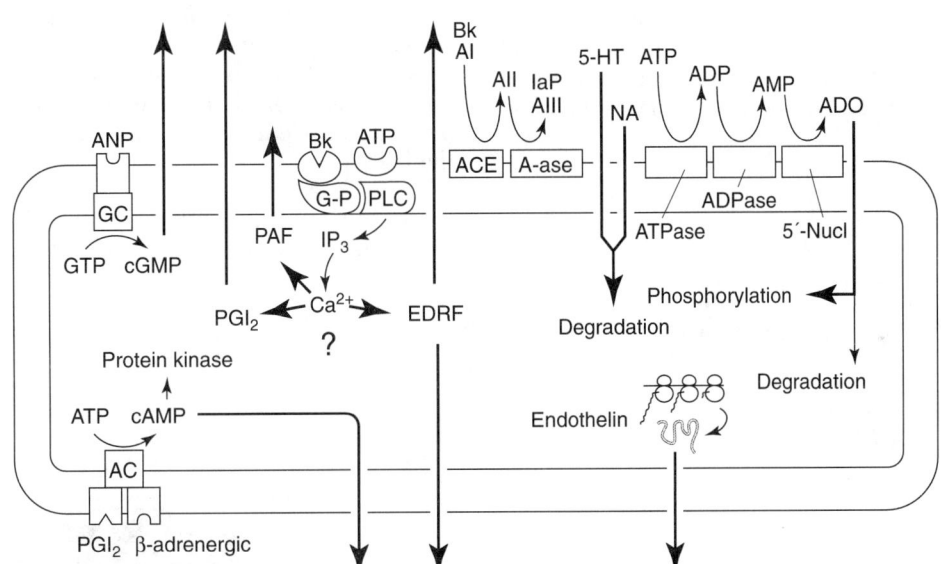

FIGURE 16-29. Schematic diagram of endothelial functions which directly or indirectly affect vascular tone. Indirect effects: Ectoenzymes at the luminal endothelial surface hydrolyse a number of vasoactive compounds (angiotensin-converting enzyme [ACE], which cleaves bradykinin [Bk] and converts angiotensin I [AI] to AII). A cascade of ectonucleotidases (ATPase, ADPase, 5'nucleotidase) sequentially degrades ATP to adenosine (ADO), which is taken up by the endothelium and further degraded or rephosphorylated to ATP. Circulating biogenic amines like serotonin (5-HT) or norepinephrine (NA) are also taken up and degraded. Direct effects: Vasoactive compounds bind to receptors at the endothelial surface which leads to an activation of phospholipase C (PLC) probably by mediation of G-proteins (G–P). The formation of inositol-1,4,5-trisphosphate (IP_3) induces the release of Ca^{2+} from intracellular stores. An elevation of intracellular Ca^{2+} is a necessary signal for the synthesis of the autocoids prostacyclin (PGI_2), platelet-activating factor (PAF) and EDRF (for the role of Ca^{2+} in the formation of EDRF, see text. Stimulation of adenylate cyclase (AC) or particulate guanylate cyclase (GC) (by atrial natriuretic peptide [ANP]) elicits the release of the second messengers cAMP and cGMP, whose potential role in the extracellular space is unknown. (Pohl U, Busse R: Endothelium-dependent modulation of vascular tone and platelet function. *Eur Heart J* 1990;11(Suppl B):35.)

heart's capacity to work. This is particularly the case for the ischemic heart, where this balance is compromised, and where an oxygen debt leads to a decline in ventricular performance, because the heart is an obligate aerobic organ.

Metabolic Demand

The major determinants of myocardial oxygen consumption ($M\dot{V}O_2$; Fig. 16-30) include systolic wall tension (determined by chamber pressure and geometry [volume plus wall thickening]), myocardial contractile state, and heart rate. Contributions of each are interdependent. The components of wall tension (Fig. 16-31) include the following: (1) the magnitude of developed force; (2) the interval during which force is generated and maintained (integral of systolic force); (3) rate of development; and (4) frequency (per unit of time). Alterations in the myocardial contractile state exert a predominant influence on the rate of force development and also may influence the magnitude of force development. Any increment in ventricular pressure or volume would be expected to raise all components except the frequency. Increments in the frequency of contraction result in augmentation of the contractile state and the rate of force development. Elevated heart rate decreases $M\dot{V}O_2$ per beat or contraction but not per minute. The interrelation between $M\dot{V}O_2$, the integral of force per minute (reflecting magnitude and duration of force plus the influence of heart rate), and the rate of force development (role of contractile state) is shown in Figure 16-32. An increment of any of these

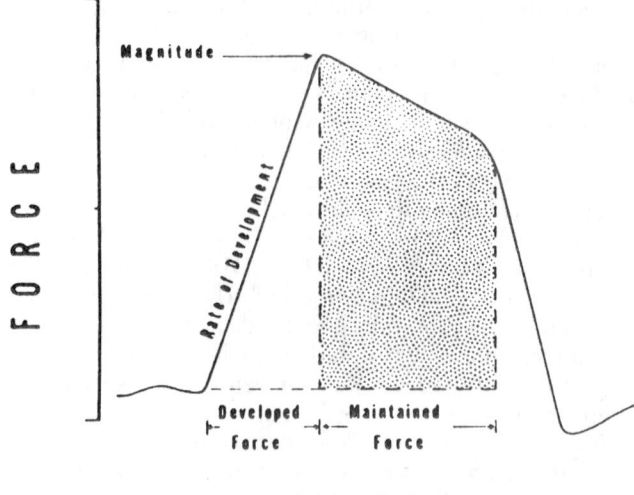

FIGURE 16-31. The major determinants of myocardial oxygen consumption expressed in relation to their influence on the components of systolic wall force. (Weber KT, Janicki JS: The metabolic demand and oxygen supply of the heart: physiologic and clinical considerations. *Am J Physiol* 1979;44:723.)

components of force requires an almost equivalent elevation in energy consumption.

A practical way to describe the energy requirements of the heart is to divide them into two groups, extrinsic and intrinsic, according to the interaction of the heart with the body.

EXTRINSIC REQUIREMENTS.   Extrinsic work of the heart is the work performed in pumping blood (force multiplied

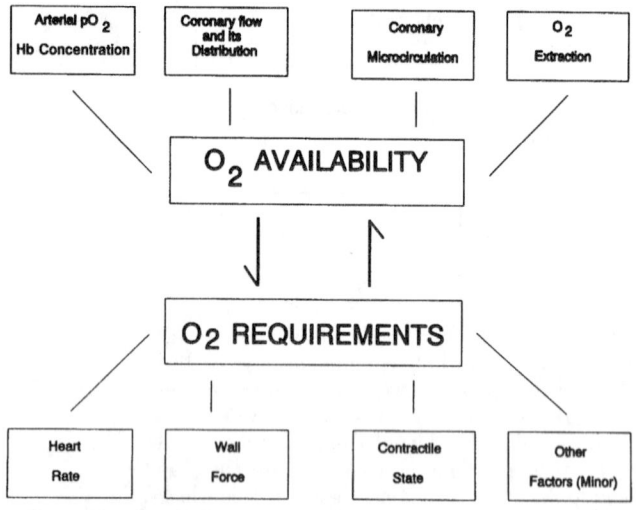

FIGURE 16-30. Schematic representation of the factors that regulate the demand and supply of oxygen in the heart cells and thereby reflect the heart's requirements for oxygen and its availability. Hb, hemoglobin. (Weber KT, Janicki JS: The metabolic demand and oxygen supply of the heart: physiologic and clinical considerations. *Am J Physiol* 1979;44:723.)

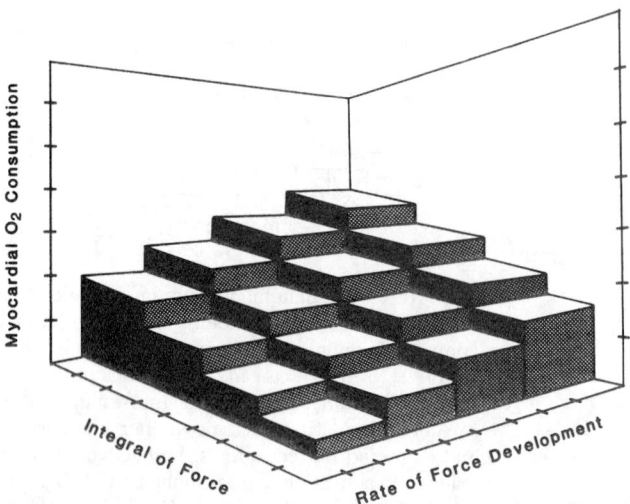

FIGURE 16-32. Three-dimensional representation of the interrelations among myocardial oxygen consumption (mL/min/100 g), the integral of systolic wall force per minute, and the peak of force development. (Weber KT, Janicki JS: The metabolic demand and oxygen supply of the heart: physiologic and clinical considerations. *Am J Physiol* 1979;44:724.)

by distance, or pressure × flow × time). The efficiency of the heart is the ratio of energy supplied to mechanical energy produced. However, $M\dot{V}O_2$ does not vary in a simple way with the work done—the efficiency varies depending on how its mechanical work is performed (e.g., by changing resistance or venous return). Sarnoff and colleagues[69] quantified this concept in 1958 (Fig. 16-33). They demonstrated that doubling cardiac work, by increasing the aortic pressure, doubled $M\dot{V}O_2$, but doubling work by doubling cardiac output increased $M\dot{V}O_2$ by less than one tenth. Sarnoff proposed that a clinical measure (referred to as the *tension-time index* [TTI]) be used for clinical estimation of oxygen consumption by the heart, which is the product of mean pressure during systole and the duration of systole as measured in the left ventricle. The most common clinical definition of TTI is the average pressure during ejection in the aortic root, multiplied by the duration of systole (in seconds per minute) in the aorta (when the aortic valve is open). The relation of TTI to a well-known index, the rate-pressure product, is not a good one, because $M\dot{V}O_2$ does not correlate just with peak systolic pressure during ejection but is a product of rate, peak systolic pressure, and duration of ejection.

INTRINSIC REQUIREMENTS. Intrinsic factors that determine $M\dot{V}O_2$ are influenced by the function of the myocardium itself. *Contractility* describes most intrinsic factors affecting $M\dot{V}O_2$ beyond basal requirements. The data in Figure 16-34 clearly demonstrate that a correlation exists between $M\dot{V}O_2$ and increased inotropic state. Increasing heart rate elevates $M\dot{V}O_2$ by increasing TTI, contractility, or

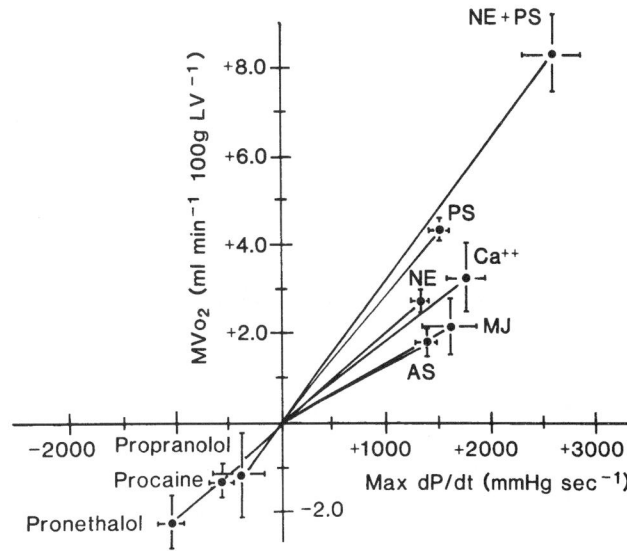

FIGURE 16-34. Relation between maximal intraventricular dP/dt and $M\dot{V}O_2$. Each point represents the average of a series of experiments with the associated standard error. AS, acetylstrophanthidin; Ca, calcium; NE, norepinephrine; PS, paired electrical stimulation. (Braunwald E: Mechanisms and energetics of the normal and failing heart. *Trans Assoc Am Physicians* 1971;84:63.)

both. Increasing the heart rate shortens the duration of ejection per beat (increased contractility per beat) and duration of ejection per minute (increased systolic wall tension per minute). Therefore, increased heart rate increases $M\dot{V}O_2$ by both intrinsic and extrinsic mechanisms.

Metabolic Supply

The amount of oxygen available to the myocardium (see Fig. 16-30) and its mitochondria is determined by (1) arterial oxygen content, which is directly related to hemoglobin concentration and hemoglobin oxygen saturation; (2) coronary flow and its distribution (oxygen delivery); (3) anatomic characteristics of the coronary microcirculation; and (4) PaO_2, which drives oxygen from capillaries into intracellular compartments. At the level of the myocardium, blood flow through the coronary vasculature is regulated almost entirely by the intrinsic localized vascular response in the myocardium. This mechanism is independent from neural control and is regulated by (1) oxygen demand—it is thought that decreased PaO_2 in the myocardium causes relaxation of coronary arterioles or that hypoxia causes vasodilator substances, such as adenosine, to be released; (2) carbon dioxide, which is released from metabolizing muscle; (3) lactate and pyruvate ions, which are released from muscle; (4) K^+ released during muscle activity; and (5) adenosine (discussed earlier).[70]

The increased coronary blood flow produced by increased cardiac work has been attributed to two possible mechanisms that reflect adaptation of the microcirculation to variations of metabolic demand: (1) redistribution of flow from nonex-

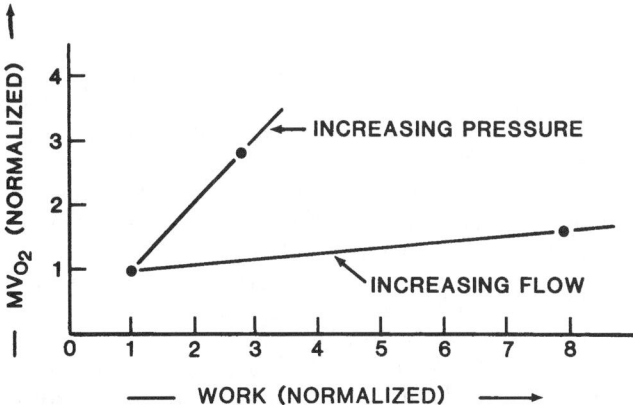

FIGURE 16-33. $M\dot{V}O_2$ versus pressure and flow. Isolated dog hearts were studied in preparation in which contractility presumably did not change. The change in myocardial oxygen consumption is presented (1) with a change in the rate of work by increasing mean aortic pressure while flow is held constant; doubling the rate of work in this way almost exactly doubles oxygen consumption; and (2) with a change in the rate of work by increasing flow while mean aortic pressure is held constant. The increase in oxygen consumption is minimal, and preload almost certainly increases. (Modified from Sarnoff SJ, Braunwald E, Welch GH Jr, et al: Hemodynamic determinations of oxygen consumption of the heart with special reference to the time-tension index. *Am J Physiol* 1958;192:148.)

METABOLIC RESERVE

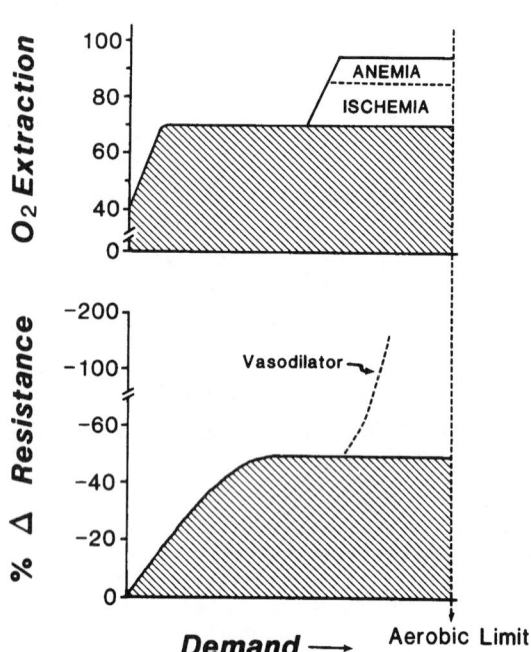

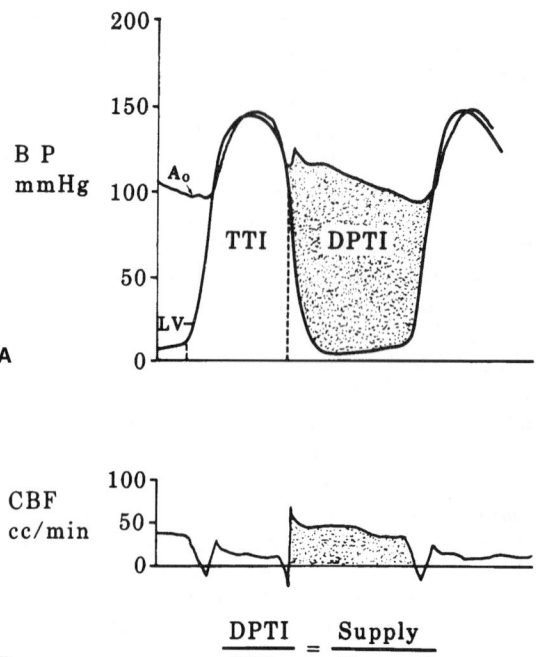

FIGURE 16-35. The metabolic reserve of the heart may be described by the changes in oxygen extraction (percent) and the percent decrease in coronary vascular resistance that occur in response to a progressive elevation in metabolic demand. Notice that oxygen extraction reaches a plateau early and does not increase again until the coronary vascular reserve has reached its optimal level. Myocardial ischemia or anemia promotes a greater extraction of oxygen. Coronary vasodilators, such as dipyridamole, may increase coronary flow are maximal, additional increments in demand result in cell hypoxia and, thus, the aerobic limit of the heart is exceeded. (Weber KT, Janicki JS: The metabolic demand and oxygen supply of the heart: physiologic and clinical considerations. *Am J Physiol* 1979;44:726.)

changing to exchanging vessels, and (2) recruitment in the number of perfused channels or density of open capillaries. The relative contribution of either mechanism, however, remains uncertain. Oxygen extraction may also increase but to a lesser extent than the flow elevation. These compensating adjustments in blood flow and oxygen extraction, which occur during acute or chronic elevation of work, constitute the metabolic reserve of the heart (Fig. 16-35).

Supply–Demand Ratio

Measurements of oxygen delivery (coronary flow × arterial oxygen content) and oxygen consumption (coronary flow × arteriovenous oxygen difference) do not establish the adequacy of delivered oxygen relative to mitochondrial oxygen consumption. Concentration of lactate and pyruvate, or the ratio of reduced to oxidized nicotinamide-adenine-dinucleotide (NADH/NAD), reflects the proportions of reduced to oxidized substrate and, hence, the adequacy of oxygen delivery to the intracellular compartment.

FIGURE 16-36. (**A**) Superimposed left ventricular and aortic pressure tracings. The stippled area is the difference between the two pressures in diastole—the diastolic pressure–time index (DPTI). The vertical dashed lines indicate the systolic area chosen to measure the systolic pressure time index—here labeled TTI. (**B**) Tracing of the phasic flow velocity in the left circumflex coronary artery. The stippled area indicates diastolic flow. (Hoffman JIE, Buckberg GD: Regional myocardial ischemia causes, prediction and prevention. *Vasc Surg* 1974;8:117.)

Clinical assessment of coronary artery supply by pressure measurement was tested by Beckberg and associates.[71] They defined the diastolic pressure–time index (DPTI) as the integral of the difference between aortic root and LV pressure during diastole. They then determined the ratio of supply to demand (DPTI/TTI or endocardial viability ratio) during steady-state condition and when either oxygen supply or demand was changed (Fig. 16-36). They also measured the change in ratio of endocardial to epicardial regional myocardial blood flow (RMBF) and found that it remained above 0.8 until the endocardial viability ratio fell below 0.8; at lower endocardial viability ratios, the endocardial–epicardial RMBF ratio also fell. The data suggest that endocardial viability is a reasonable predictor of endocardial to epicardial blood flow distribution and the overall adequacy of coronary blood flow, but its clinical usefulness is limited.

Coronary Autoregulation and Myocardial Oxygen Balance

A new variable has been introduced to express myocardial resistance to oxygen flow (Ro_2). This variable was defined as the ratio of coronary driving pressure to LV oxygen uptake.[72] Higher values indicate small consumption relative to generated aortic pressure and higher coronary reserve. Conditions that produce the highest obtainable value for RO_2 are considered optimal. An expression relating RO_2 to ventricular hemodynamic variables was developed and studied using a mathematical model of the cardiovascular system; and this model predicts that for each state of circulation, an optimal level of cardiac contractility exists for which coronary reserve is maximized (Fig. 16-37).

EFFECT OF ISCHEMIA ON MYOCARDIAL METABOLISM

Under normal aerobic conditions, myocardium derives its energy primarily from oxidative phosphorylation, a process localized in the mitochondria. Although many substrates can be used, oxidation of free fatty acids (FFA) predominates. Under aerobic conditions, carbohydrate metabolism proceeds by oxidation through the Krebs (tricarboxylic acid) cycle. During hypoxia, glycolytic flux initially increases because of enhanced uptake of glucose and increased phosphorylation. Glycogenolysis accelerates because of the transformation of phosphorylase b (Fig. 16-38). However, when anoxia supervenes, the lack of oxygen inhibits Krebs cycle activity, and glucose metabolism can proceed only by anaerobic glycolysis. Acidosis and accumulation of lactate and other metabolites then contribute directly to a marked inhibition of the glycolytic flux; the decline of high-energy phosphate stores is, therefore, faster compared with aerobic conditions.

The preferential myocardial use of FFA appears to depend on high activity of several enzyme systems, including acetyl-coenzyme A-carnitine transferase, which facilitates continuing transport of aCyl-coenzyme A to the mitochondria (see Fig. 16-38). The limited supply of oxygen inhibits oxidation of FFA, as does the increased ratio of NADH/NAD and reduced concentration of flavoproteins. Accumulation of aCyl-coenzyme A inhibits further formation of acetyl coenzyme A and creates an accumulation of acetyl-coenzyme A esters, which inhibit effective exchange of ADP and ATP to the mitochondria (see Fig. 16-38).

Under normal aerobic conditions, the myocardium extracts lactate from the arterial blood; the extraction fraction (percent change of arteriovenous difference) is in the range of 0.2 (20%). Decreased lactate extraction occurs during myocardial ischemia, and the usual positive ratio may be replaced by a negative ratio that means a net lactate production. This is also accompanied by an increase in coronary lactate–pyruvate ratio. Calculation of lactate extraction (LE) ratio is commonly reported as a means of quantifying the magnitude of ischemia. However, conventional LE calculation (arteriovenous lactate difference ÷ arterial lactate) ignores blood flow. Lactate flux (lactate arteriovenous difference) times blood flow in the ischemic area quantifies the actual amount of lactate consumed or produced in the myocardium. This latter calculation has a closer relation to measured changes in coronary blood flow than does LE.[73]

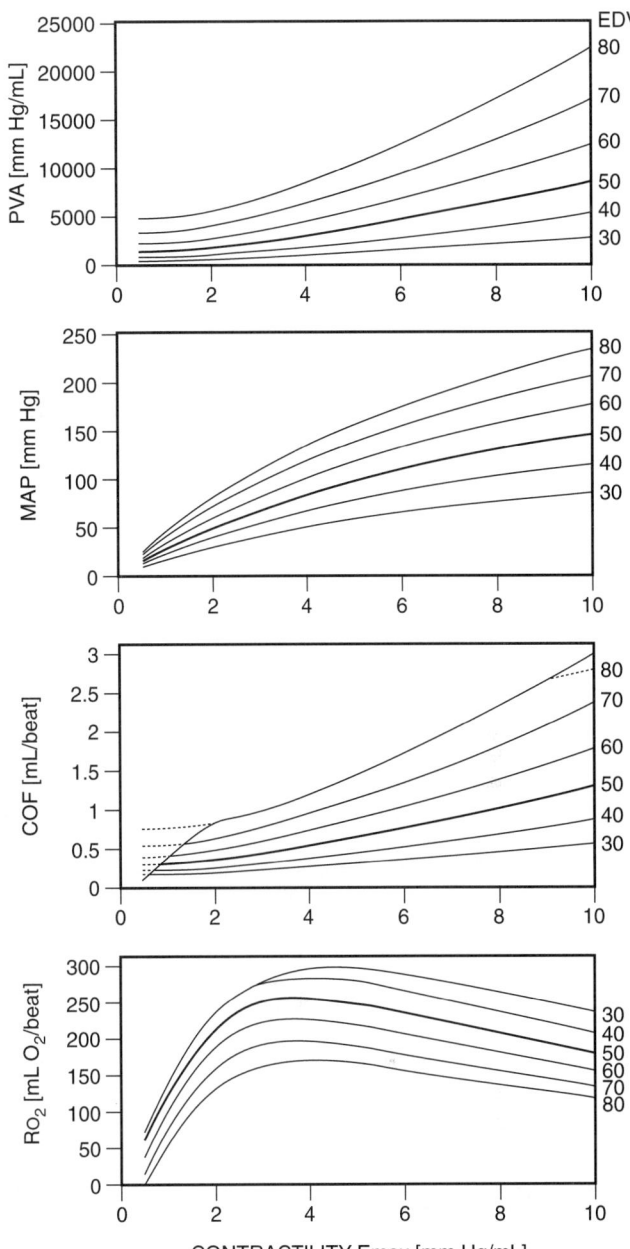

FIGURE 16-37. Pressure-volume area (PVA), mean aortic pressure (MAP), coronary flow (COF), and $\hat{R}O_2$ as functions of contractility (Emax), for different values of end-diastolic volume (HR = 120 bpm, peripheral resistance [Rps] = 3.0 mm Hg/mL). (Barnea O, Santamore WP: Coronary autoregulation and optional myocardial oxygen utilization. *Basic Res Cardiol* 1992;81:295.)

However, a problem with both calculations with regard to quantifying ischemia is that the magnitude of lactate production is not directly proportional to the severity of ischemia. Rather, lactate production sharply declines as blood flow falls to severely ischemic levels.

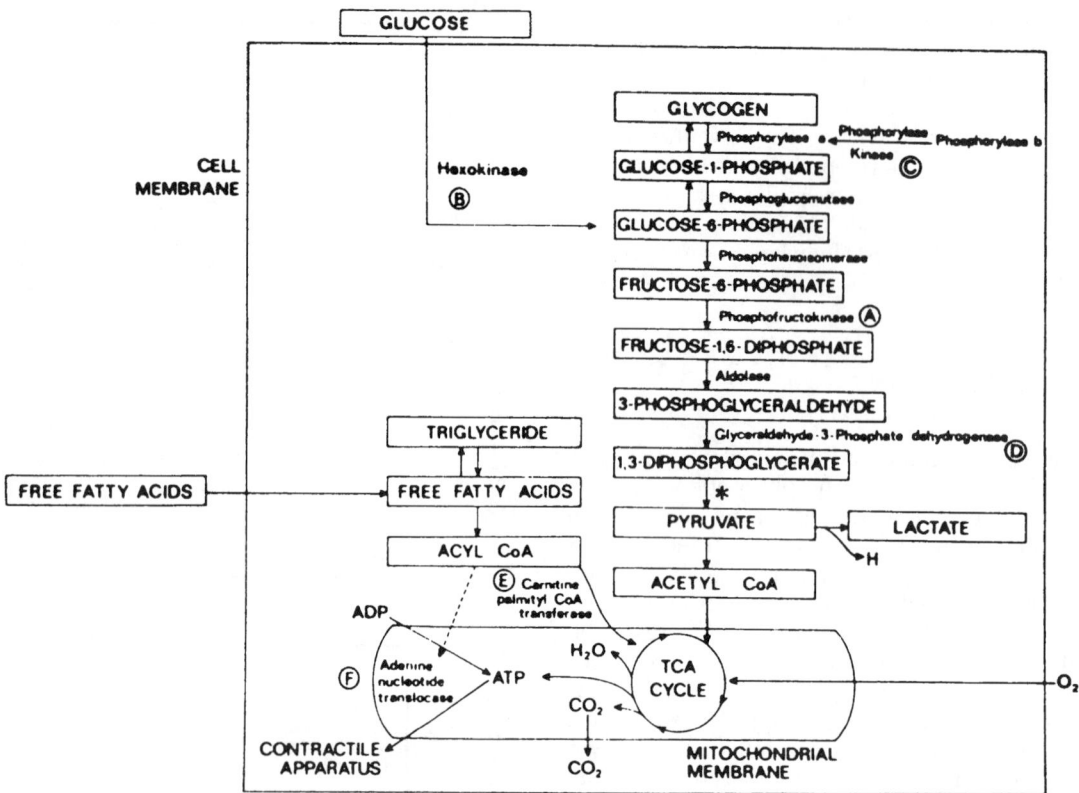

FIGURE 16-38. Effects of ischemia on glycolysis and free fatty acid metabolism. Ischemia increases intracellular lactate concentration; this accumulation inhibits several enzymes in the glycolytic pathway: Phosphofructokinase (**A**); hexokinase (**B**); and phosphorylase kinase (**C**), which prevents activation of phosphorylase b to phosphorylase a and therefore suppresses conversion of glycogen to glucose-1-phosphate. Glyceraldehyde-3-phosphate dehydrogenase (**D**) is suppressed by an elevation of intracellular lactate (° denotes that the glycolytic pathway has been condensed at this point). Ischemia increases the intracellular concentration of acyl CoA esters, in part because the intracellular accumulation of lactate inhibits carnitine palmityl coenzyme A transferase (**E**), the enzyme that catalyzes the transfer of acyl CoA from the cell cytoplasm to the mitochondria. Acyl CoA esters inhibit the effective exchange of ADP and ATP between the cytoplasm of the cell and the mitochondria by suppressing the activity of adenine nucleotide translocase (**F**). TCA, tricarboxylic acid. (Hillis LD, Braunwald E: Myocardial ischemia: parts I, II, and III. *N Engl J Med* 1977;971, 1034, and 1093.)

REFERENCES ■

1. Hoffman BF, Cranefield TF, Wallace AG: Physiological basis of cardiac arrhythmias. Parts I and II. *Mod Concepts Cardiovasc Dis* 1966;35:103

2. Wallace AG: Electrical activity of the heart. In: Hurst JW (ed). *The Heart, Arteries and Veins*, 6th ed. New York, McGraw-Hill, 1986:73

3. Zipes DP: Recent observations supporting the role of slow currents in cardiac electrical physiology. In: Wellens HJJ, Lie KI, Ganse MJ (eds). *The Conduction System of the Heart: Structure, Function, and Clinical Implications.* Philadelphia, Lea & Febiger, 1976:85

4. Cahalan M: Molecular properties of sodium channels in excitable membranes. In: Cotman CW, Post G, Nicholson GL (eds). *The Cell Surface and Neuronal Function.* Amsterdam, Elsevier, 1980

5. Prys-Roberts C: Electrophysiology: the origin of the heartbeat. In: Prys-Roberts C (ed). *The Circulation in Anaesthesia: Applied Physiology and Pharmacology.* Oxford, Blackwell Scientific Publications, 1980:29

6. Nobel D. *The Initiation of the Heartbeat.* Oxford, Oxford University Press, 1975

7. Schlant RC, Sonneblick EH: Normal physiology of the cardiovascular system. In: Hurst JW (ed). *The Heart, Arteries, and Veins*, 6th ed. New York, McGraw-Hill, 1986:37

8. Noble MI, Pollack GH: Molecular mechanisms of contraction. *Circ Res* 1977;40:333

9. Sonnenblick H, Spotnitz HM, Spiro D: The role of the sarcomere in ventricular function and the mechanism of heart failure. *Circ Res* 1964;14:17

10. Hill AV: The heat of shortening and the dynamic contents of muscle. *Proc R Soc Lond [Biol]* 1938;126:136

11. Sonnenblick H: Implications of muscle mechanics in heart. *Fed Proc* 1962;21:974

12. Braunwald E, Ross J, Sonnenblick EH: *Mechanisms of Contraction of the Normal and Failing Heart.* Boston, Little, Brown, 1968

13. Sonnenblick EH: The mechanics of myocardial contraction. In: Briller SA, Conn HL Jr (eds). *The Myocardial Cell: Structure, Function, and the Modification of Cardiac Drugs.* Philadelphia, University of Pennsylvania Press, 1966:173

14. Smith NT: Myocardial function in anesthesia. In: Prys-Roberts C (ed). *The Circulation in Anaesthesia: Applied Physiology and Pharmacology.* Oxford, Blackwell Scientific Publications, 1980:57

15. Higgins CB, Batner SF, Franklin D, et al: Extent of regulation of the heart's contractile state in conscious dog by alteration in the frequency of contraction. *J Clin Invest* 1973;52:1187

16. Von Anrep G: On the part played by suprarenals in the normal vascular reactions of the body. *J Physiol*,1912;45:307

17. Frank O: Zur dynamik des herzmuskels. *Z Biol* 1985;33:370 (Following Chatman CB, Vasserman E [translators]). *Am Heart J* 1959;58:282)

18. Patterson SW, Starling EH: On the mechanical factors which determine the output of the ventricle. *J Physiol* 1914;48:357

19. Sarnoff SJ, Berglund E: Ventricular function. I. Starling's law of the heart studied by means of simultaneous right and left ventricular function curves in the dog. *Circulation* 1954;9:706

20. Braunwald E, Ross J, Sonnenblick EH: Mechanism of contractions of the normal and failing heart. In: *Mechanisms of Contraction*, 2nd ed. Boston, Little, Brown, 1976:39

21. Braunwald E: Mechanisms and energetics of the normal and failing heart. *Trans Assoc Am Physicians* 1971;84:63

22. Lakatta EG: Length modulation of muscle performance: Frank-Starling law of the heart. In: Fozzard HA (ed). *The Heart and Cardiovascular System.* New York, Raven Press, 1986:819

23. Frank O: Die Grundform des arteriellen pulses. *Z Biol* 1898; 37:483

24. Sagawa K: The ventricular pressure–volume diagram revisited. *Circ Res* 1978;43:677

25. Sonnenblick EH, Downing SE: Afterload as a primary determinant of ventricular performance. *Am J Physiol* 1963:204:604

26. Sarnoff SJ, Mitchell JH: The control of the function of the heart. In: Dow P (ed). *Handbook of Physiology*, vol 1. Washington DC, American Physiological Society, 1962:489

27. Braunwald E, Ross J Jr: The ventricular end-diastolic pressure: appraisal of its value in the recognition of ventricular failure in man. *Am J Med* 1963;34:147

28. Glantz SA, Parmley WW: Factors which affect the diastolic pressure–volume curve. *Circ Res* 1978;42:171

29. Santamore WP, Peterson JT, Johnston WE, et al: Variable non-linearity in end systolic pressure–volume relationships results from interaction between end diastolic and developed pressure–volume relations. *Cardiovasc Res* 1991;25:36

30. Grossman W: Diastolic function and heart failure: an overview. *Eur Heart J* 1990 11(Suppl C):2

31. Carabello BA, Spann JF: The uses and limitations of end-systolic indexes of left ventricular function. *Circulation* 1984;69:1058

32. Leatherman GF, Shook TL, Leatherman SM, et al: Use of a conductance catheter to detect increased left ventricular inotropic state by end-systolic pressure–volume analysis. *Basic Res Cardiol* 1989; 84(Suppl 4):247

33. Tomai F, Ciavolella M, Gaspardone A, et al: Peak exercise left ventricular performance in normal subjects and in athletes assessed by first-pass radionuclide angiography. *Am J Cardiol* 1992;70:531

34. Marsh JD, Green LH, Wynne J, et al: Left ventricular end-systolic pressure-dimension and stress-length relations in normal human subjects. *Am J Cardiol* 1979;44:1311

35. Jenicki JS, Weber KT: The pericardium and ventricular in action, distensibility and function. *Am J Physiol* 1980;238:H4

36. Laver MB, Strauss HW, Pohost GM: Right and left geometry: adjustments during acute respiratory failure. *Crit Care Med* 1979;7:509

37. Robotham JL, Lixfield W, Holland L, et al: Effects of respiration on cardiac performance. *J Appl Physiol* 1978;44:703

38. Robotham JL, Lixfield W, Holland L, et al: The effects of positive end-expiratory pressure on right and left ventricular performance. *Am Rev Respir Dis* 1980;121:677

39. Engler RL, Covell JW: Influence of the venous system on ventricular/arterial coupling. In: Yin FCP (ed). *Ventricular/Vascular Coupling: Clinical, Physiological and Engineering Aspects.* New York, Springer-Verlag, 1987:20

40. Guyton AC: Cardiac output, venous return, and their regulation. In: Guyton AC (ed). *Textbook of Medical Physiology*, 4th ed. Philadelphia, WB Saunders, 1971:311

41. O'Rourke MF, Avolio AP, Nichols WW: Left ventricular–systemic arterial coupling in humans and strategies to improve coupling in diseased states. In: Yin FCP (ed). *Ventricular/Vascular Coupling: Clinical, Physiological and Engineering Aspects.* New York, Springer-Verlag, 1987:1

42. Bramwell JV, Hill AV: Velocity of transmission of pulse and elasticity of the arteries. *Lancet* 1922;1:891

43. Berne RM, Levy MN: Regulation of the heartbeat. In: Carson D (ed). *Cardiovascular Physiology*, 5th ed. St Louis, CV Mosby, 1986:76

44. Vanter SF, Boettcher DH: Regulation of cardiac output by stroke volume and heart rate in conscious dogs. *Circ Res* 1978; 42

45. Bainbridge FA: The influence of venous filling upon the rate of the heart. *J Physiol (Lond)* 1915;50:65

46. Kappagoda CT, Linden RJ, Snow HM: A reflex increase in heart rate from distension of the junction between the superior vena cava and the right atrium. *J Physiol (Lond)* 1972;220:177

47. Holmberg MJ, Gorman AJ, Cornish KG, et al: Attenuation of arterial baroreflex control of heart rate by left ventricular receptor stimulation in the conscious dog. *Circ Res* 1983;52:597

48. Mark AL: The Bezold-Jarisch reflex revisited: clinical implications of inhibitory reflexes originating in the heart. *J Am Coll Cardiol* 1983;1:90

49. Panzenbeck MJ, Tan W, Hajdu MA, et al: Intracoronary infusion of prostaglandin 12 attenuates arterial baroreflex control of heart rate in conscious dogs. *Cir Res* 1988;63:860

50. Hajdu MA, Cornish KG, Tan W, et al: The interaction of the Bainbridge and Bezold-Jarisch reflexes in the conscious dog. *Basic Res Cardiol* 1991;86:175

51. Kollai M, Koizumi K: Cardiac vagal and sympathetic nerve responses to baroreceptor stimulation in the dog. *Eur J Physiol (Plügere Arch)* 1989;413:365

52. Chen J-S, Wang W, Bartholet T, et al: Analysis of baroreflex control of heart rate in conscious dogs with pacing-induced heart failure. *Circulation* 1991;83:260

53. Ptattinger PJ, Martin JM, Hunter DD, et al: GTP-binding protein couple cardiac muscarinic receptors to a K channel. *Nature* 1985;317:536

54. Mellander S: Comparative studies on the adrenergic neuromoral control of the resistance and capacitance blood vessel cats. *Acta Physiol Scand* 1960;50(Suppl 176):1

55. van Lieshout JJ, Wieling W, Karemaker JM, et al: The vasovagal response. *Clin Sci* 1991;81:575

56. Abboud FM: Ventricular syncope: is the heart a sensory organ? *N Engl J Med* 1989;320:390

57. Henry JP: On the triggering mechanism of vasovagal syncope. *Psychosom Med* 1984;46:91

58. Goldstein DS, Spanarkel M, Pitterman A, et al: Circulatory control mechanisms in vasodepressor syncope. *Am Heart J* 1982;104:1071

59. Rubanyi GM, Romero CJ, Vanhoutte PM: Flow-induced release of endothelium-derived relaxing factor. *Am J Physiol* 1986;250:H1145

60. Yanagisawa M, Kurihara H, Kimura S, et al: A novel potent

vasoconstrictor peptide produced by vascular endothelial cells. *Nature* 1988;322:411

61. Wennmalm A, Karwatowska-Prokopczuk E, Wennmalm M: Role of the coronary endothelium in the regulation of sympathetic transmitter release in isolated rabbit hearts. *Acta Physiol Scand* 1980;136:81
62. Pohl U, Busse R: Endothelium-dependent modulation of vascular tone and platelet function. *Eur Heart J* 1990;11(Suppl B):35
63. Stewart DJ: Role of EDRF and endothelin in coronary vasomotor control. *Basic Res Cardiol* 1991;86(Suppl 2):77
64. Lamontagne D, Pohl U, Busse R: Mechanical deformation of vessel wall and shear stress determine the basal release of endothelium-derived relaxing factor in the intact rabbit coronary vascular bed. *Circ Res* 1992;70:123
65. Glick MR, Gehman D, Gascho JA: Endothelium-derived nitric oxide reduces baseline venous tone in awake instrumented rats. *Am J Physiol* 1993;265 (*Heart Circ Physiol* 34:H47–H51)
66. Winn MJ, Ku DD: Effects of regional ischaemia, with or without reperfusion, on endothelium dependent coronary relaxation in the dog. *Cardiovasc Res* 1992;26:250
67. Bassenge E: Clinical relevance of endothelium-derived relaxing factor (EDRF). *Br J Clin Pharmacol* 1992;34:37S
68. Pasyk S, Pitt B: Central opiate induced ventricular arrhythmias in the conscious dog. *Circulation* 1983;68:III-249
69. Sarnoff SJ, Braunwald E, Welch GH Jr, et al: Hemodynamic terminations of oxygen consumption of the heart with special reference to the time-tension index. *Am J Physiol* 1958;192:148
70. Feigl EO: Local control of coronary blood flow. *Coron Physiol Rev* 1983;63:54
71. Beckberg GD, Fixler DE, Archie JP, et al: Experimental subendocardial ischemia in dogs with normal coronary arteries. *Circ Res* 1972;30:67
72. Barnea O, Santamore WP: Coronary autoregulation and optional myocardial oxygen utilization. *Basic Res Cardiol* 1992;87:290
73. Sidi A, Davis RF: Lactate extraction fails to accurately reflect regional lactate production in the ischemic myocardium. *J Cardiothorac Vasc Anesth* 1989;3:321

Critical Care, Third Edition, edited by Joseph M. Civetta,
Robert W. Taylor, and Robert R. Kirby.
Lippincott-Raven Publishers, Philadelphia, PA © 1997.

CHAPTER 17

Acid–Base Chemistry and Physiology

Robert R. Kirby
Walter C. Bernards

Disturbances in acid–base homeostasis are common. Available technology, specifically pH and P_{CO_2} electrodes, make the measurement of these disturbances a simple matter. Nevertheless, the proper diagnosis and treatment of acid–base disorders remains one of the more difficult and poorly performed tasks in critical care medicine.

The fault, we believe, lies in large measure with the diverse terminology and the confusing mathematics used to present this subject. Physicians who experience little difficulty in handling far more complex problems involving other fluid and electrolyte imbalances are often bewildered by a subject in which concentrations are expressed as logarithms of inverted fractions. The rote use of derived or artificial parameters such as standard bicarbonate,[1] buffer base,[2] or base excess[3] has done little to increase understanding; when they are applied in the clinical setting without an appreciation of their limitations, serious errors in therapy may result.

This degree of confusion is unfortunate and unnecessary. An understanding of the chemistry of acids and bases sufficient to allow interpretation of the type of acid–base disturbance (i.e., respiratory, metabolic, or mixed) and to quantify the degree of disturbance is within the easy reach of every interested clinician.

CHEMISTRY OF ACIDS AND BASES

DEFINITIONS

The Brönsted-Lowry definition of acids and bases is generally accepted in the biological sciences. According to this definition, an acid is a substance that tends to dissociate or release hydrogen ions (H^+), and a base is a substance that tends to associate or bind H^+. Acids and bases, then, exist as conjugate pairs, examples of which are listed in Table 17-1. This table demonstrates that the charge on a molecule or ion, per se, has nothing to do directly with its acid property, that is, Table 17-1 includes acids that are positively charged, negatively charged, and neutral. The practice of defining most cations (positively charged ions) as bases and most anions (negatively charged ions) as acids, which arose before H^+ concentration ($[H^+]$) could be measured in a clinical setting, is not compatible with current concepts of acid–base chemistry.

Actual Concentrations and pH

In most biological fluids, the $[H^+]$ is extremely small, averaging 0.000,000,04 Mol/L of extracellular fluid (ECF). With severe acidosis, this value can increase to 0.00000016 Mol/L, and with severe alkalosis, it could decrease to 0.000000016 Mol/L. These are small numbers and are cumbersome to transcribe. Hence, Sorenson in 1909 suggested the expression of $[H^+]$ as the negative logarithm to the base 10, for which he introduced the symbol pH. Thus, a $[H^+]$ of 0.00000004 Mol/L may be expressed simply as pH 7.4; one of 0.00000016 Mol/L is pH 6.8; and one of 0.000000016 Mol/L is pH 7.8.

Although pH simplified the expression of $[H^+]$ and proved to be a help to chemists, it has presented difficulties to clinicians' understanding of acid–base chemistry.[4-6] To circumvent this difficulty and return $[H^+]$ to arithmetic rather than logarithmic expressions, Campbell[5] in 1962 introduced

TABLE 17-1. Examples of Acids° and Bases
That Exist as Conjugate Bases

ACID		CONJUGATE BASE
CH_3COOH	$\rightleftarrows$	$CH_3COO^- + H^+$
H_2PO_4	$\rightleftarrows$	$HPO_4 + H^+$
H_2CO_3	$\rightleftarrows$	$HCO_3 + H^+$
NH^{4+}	$\rightleftarrows$	$NH_3 + H^+$
HCO_3^-	$\rightleftarrows$	$CO_3 + H^+$
H_2SO_4	$\rightleftarrows$	$HSO_4 + H^+$

°Notice that an acid may have a positive, negative, or neutral charge.

the term *nanoequivalent*, a unit equal to 10^{-9} equivalent or one millimicroequivalent. In this chapter, we equate nanoequivalent to nanomole (nMol). The normal $[H^+]$ of blood and ECF is simply expressed as 40 nMol/L. The range of $[H^+]$ compatible with life is approximately 16 to 160 nMol/L (pH 7.8 to 6.8). Table 17-2 compares values for $[H^+]$ expressed as pH and nMol/L.

Many of the conceptual and quantitative difficulties experienced by the clinician when pH notations are employed can be avoided by the direct expression of $[H^+]$ in nanomoles. For example, the nonlinearity of the pH scale is immediately obvious from Table 17-2. A change of 0.2 pH unit in the range of moderate acidosis, from 7.2 to 7.0, denotes *four times* as large a change in actual hydrogen ion activity, as does an identical pH change in the range of moderate alkalosis—from pH 7.8 to 7.6. This nonlinearity of the pH scale has been the source of many clinical errors. Furthermore, the large changes in $[H^+]$, which normally can be tolerated (approximately 16 to 160 nMol/L), are obscured by the corresponding small absolute changes in pH. A similar tenfold alteration in sodium (Na^+) or potassium (K^+) concentration is incompatible with life.

Table 17-3 lists normal acid–base values. The following definitions are useful:

Acidemia: a hydrogen ion concentration above the normal range of 36 to 44 nMol/L (pH less than 7.36)
Alkalemia: a hydrogen ion concentration below the normal range of 36 to 44 nMol/L (pH greater than 7.44)

TABLE 17-2. Comparison of pH Values and H^+ (nMol/L)

pH	nMol/L
6.0	1000
6.8	160
7.0	100
7.2	63
7.4	40
7.6	25
7.8	16
8.0	10
9.0	1

TABLE 17-3. Normal Acid–Base Values

pH	7.40 ± 0.04
H^+	40.0 ± 4.0 nMol/L
Pco_2	40.0 ± 4.0 mm Hg
Actual bicarbonate	24.0 ± 2.0 mMol/L

Acidosis: a physiologic condition that would cause acidemia if uncompensated
Alkalosis: a physiologic condition that would cause alkalemia if uncompensated.

Processes causing acidosis or alkalosis are themselves conveniently subdivided into respiratory and metabolic categories. Respiratory acidosis denotes a primary (noncompensatory) rise in $Paco_2$ to above the normal range of 36 to 44 mm Hg. All other primary processes tending to cause acidemia are, by definition, metabolic. Similarly, respiratory alkalosis denotes a primary lowering of Pco_2 to below the normal range of 36 to 44 mm Hg. All other primary processes tending to cause alkalemia are, by definition, metabolic.

These definitions of acidosis and alkalosis have been a source of unnecessary confusion. The following example clarifies their current usage. A patient with chronic obstructive lung disease (COLD) leading to hypoventilation and a Pco_2 of 60 mm Hg can achieve a bicarbonate concentration ($[HCO_3^-]$) of 34 mMol/L and a normal pH of 7.38 because of renal production and conservation of HCO_3^-. It is not helpful to say that he has a normal acid–base status because his pH value is normal. He definitely has pulmonary disease causing a primary elevation in $Paco_2$. The potential semantic dilemma is avoided by reserving the terms *acidosis* and *alkalosis* to refer to the primary pathologic process and then to describe the degree and type of compensation. In this instance, it is correct to say that this patient has chronic respiratory acidosis but has full renal compensation. In previous years this renal response was referred to as *compensatory renal metabolic alkalosis*, but restriction of the terms acidosis and alkalosis to the primary processes, although referring to the secondary ones as compensatory, makes more sense.[7]

The presence of an acid–base disturbance is commonly ascertained through an analysis of arterial blood pH (pHa) and Pco_2 ($Paco_2$). With the exception of iatrogenic complications resulting from inappropriate mechanical ventilation, prolonged nasogastric suctioning, or the administration of sodium bicarbonate ($NaHCO_3$), most acid–base abnormalities originate intracellularly and are only secondarily manifested by extracellular composition changes measured in arterial blood. Thus, although we precisely define the abnormality of $[H^+]$ in the ECF compartment, often we can only guess at what disturbance is taking place intracellularly. Even if we are reasonably certain of the latter process, no specific therapy can be directed toward this intracellular component.

RESPIRATORY DERANGEMENTS ■

Carbon dioxide (CO_2) alters [H^+] according to the following reversible reaction:

$$CO_2 + H_2O \rightleftharpoons H_2CO_3 \rightleftharpoons H^+ + HCO_3^- \qquad (1)$$

Respiratory derangements, by virtue of their effect on the $PaCO_2$, may cause major changes in [H^+] within the body. For each acute 10-mm Hg deviation of $PaCO_2$ above or below 40 mm Hg, the pH changes by approximately 0.07 units. In actuality, this change is not entirely linear, but with small acute changes in $PaCO_2$, the accuracy of the arterial blood gas values can be checked by knowing the approximate magnitude of change in pH that *should* occur (providing a superimposed metabolic abnormality is not also present) for a given change in $PaCO_2$.

Because the relation between $PaCO_2$ and alveolar ventilation is straightforward, correction of the respiratory component in acid–base derangements is easy (at least in theory). If the pH is decreased and the $PaCO_2$ levels are increased, an increase in alveolar ventilation lowers $PaCO_2$ and returns pH toward normal. The opposite is also true. Remember that if *alveolar* ventilation is halved, $PaCO_2$ is approximately doubled. Similarly, if alveolar ventilation is doubled, $PaCO_2$ decreases by half. Respiratory disturbances and [H^+] can be assessed and corrected if this relation is appreciated:

$$\uparrow \dot{V}_A \rightarrow \downarrow CO_2 \rightarrow \uparrow pH \qquad (2)$$

METABOLIC DERANGEMENTS ■

Hydrogen ion concentration also is affected by metabolic processes. Syndromes of metabolic acidosis fall into two patterns that can be separated by calculating the anion gap.

$$\text{Anion gap} = Na^+ - (Cl^- + HCO_3^-) \qquad (3)$$

This gap represents unmeasured anions, most of which are offset by [H^+]. Thus, an increased anion gap often implies the presence of a metabolic acidosis. Alternatively, chloride (Cl^-) may increase as [H^+] rises (Table 17-4). Causes of metabolic acidosis can be categorized according to a pattern of anion (Cl^-) depletion into Cl^--responsive or Cl^--resistant types.

BUFFERS

Just as the change in $PaCO_2$ from a normal value of 40 mm Hg is the prime indicator of respiratory acid–base disturbance, a change in HCO_3^- generally reflects disturbances that are metabolic in origin. Quantification of a metabolic acid–base derangement, and separation of the respiratory and metabolic components of a mixed disturbance, are the major problems facing clinicians caring for patients with such disorders. The following example illustrates the difficulty.

A 70-kg patient has a pH of 7.0. Table 17-2 shows that the [H^+] of his ECF is 100 nMol/L. Normal ECF [H^+] is only 40 nMol/L; therefore, the patient has an excess of 60 nMol of H^+ in each liter of ECF. Because the ECF represents

TABLE 17-4. Types of Metabolic Acidosis

ANION GAP

   Renal failure
   Diabetic ketoacidosis
   Salicylism
   Lactic acidosis (and starvation)
   Toxins: methanol, paraldehyde, ethylene glycol

HYPERCHLOREMIC

   Renal tubular acidosis
   Acetazolamide therapy
   Diarrhea
   Ureteral diversions
   Addition of HCl (NH_4Cl, HCl, arginine, lysine)
   Early renal failure

sents approximately 20% of body weight, the 14 L of ECF in this patient contains a total of 840 nMol of excess H^+. (All calculations of acid–base disturbances are based on the assumption that the disturbance exists only in the ECF. This is a practical necessity, because ECF acid–base changes do not necessarily reflect intracellular changes, and intracellular changes, as noted previously, cannot be measured in the clinical setting.)

One HCO_3^- anion neutralizes one H^+ cation (equation 1). Will the administration of 840 nMol of $NaHCO_3$ neutralize all of the excess acidity in this hypothetical patient and convert the pH from 7.0 to a normal 7.4?

Even with the assumption that this patient's acidosis is strictly extracellular and that ventilation will be maintained at a level guaranteeing adequate elimination of all CO_2 formed by the reaction depicted in equation 1, the answer is no, because 840 nMol of $NaHCO_3$ is less than 0.001 mL of the usual clinical preparation (1 mMol/mL). Such a volume will have no measurable effect, even if it could be drawn into a syringe. But if not, wherein lies the error in these assumptions or calculations?

The answer is central and crucial to an understanding of the chemistry of acid–base balance disorders. All biological systems are characterized by the presence of buffers (i.e., weak acids and their salts) that bind reversibly with H^+ and effectively neutralize them. The major buffers consist of HCO_3^-, which represents 75% to 80% of the ECF buffering capacity against metabolically produced or exogenously administered acids, phosphate, protein, and hemoglobin. On the addition of H^+ (i.e., strong acids), the buffer anions tend to bind part of the added H^+ according to the following reversible reactions:

$$HCO_3^- + H^+ \rightleftharpoons H_2CO_3 \qquad (4)$$

$$HPO_4^{-2} + H^+ \rightleftharpoons H_2PO_4^- \qquad (5)$$

$$Prot^- + H^+ \rightleftharpoons HProt \qquad (6)$$

$$Hb^- + H^+ \rightleftharpoons HHb \qquad (7)$$

If the added H^+ remain bound as H_2CO_3, $H_2PO_4^-$, HProt, or HHb, they do not contribute to the acidity of the blood and are not measured by the pH electrode. But what part of added H⁺ is so bound?

A study by Pitts[8] provides the answer. He infused approximately 14 million nMol of dilute hydrochloric acid into each liter of a normal dog's ECF. Before the infusion, the [H⁺] was 36 nMol/L (pH 7.44); after the infusion, it rose to only 72 nMol/L (pH 7.14). Thus, of the added 14 million nMol of [H⁺], 13,999,964 were buffered, leaving only 36 in solution as free H⁺. These 36 nMol of free H⁺ are analogous to the 60 nMol/L of excess [H⁺] measured in the hypothetical patient under discussion. This small proportion of the excess acid load is all that can be actually measured (as pH) and, therefore, gives little direct assistance in quantifying the total acidosis. Any direct treatment aimed at the 36 nMol/L of excess free H⁺ would cause the reversible buffer reactions (equations 5 to 8) to move to the left and free an additional 36 nMol/L of bound H⁺. The pH could not return to normal until the entire 14 million nMol/L had been neutralized.

The clinical problem, then, is to determine the quantity of H⁺ that has been buffered. Whereas this *hidden* H⁺ cannot be measured directly, it can be calculated, because the total quantity of the buffer anions (i.e., HCO_3^-, HPO_4^-, Prot⁻, and Hb⁻) must have decreased by the same amount as did the H⁺: in this example, by 13,999,964 nMol. If the decrease in the buffer anions is determined, an exact quantification of the added H⁺ can be made.

The only buffer that can be measured accurately *and* separated into its prime components is HCO_3^-/H_2CO_3 (equation 4). If the decrease in [HCO_3^-] is calculated after a metabolic acid challenge, it will correspond to approximately 80% of the total buffer decrease caused by the added H⁺ within the blood and ECF. Accordingly, the total buffer change can be derived by the following equation:

$$\Delta \text{ Total buffers (mMol/L)} = \frac{[HCO_3^-]}{0.8} \qquad (8)$$

METABOLIC COMPENSATION FOR PRIMARY RESPIRATORY DISTURBANCES

If a rise or fall in [HCO_3^-] is used to reflect metabolic alkalosis or acidosis, we must first determine if any of the change has resulted from an alteration of ventilation (equation 1). Many methods have been proposed for making this correction, including determinations of standard HCO_3^-,[1] buffer base,[2] base excess,[3] and CO_2 combining power.[9] All of these methods are based on in vitro titrations of blood or plasma with CO_2; this titration varies from that which occurs in vivo. As a result, unless these methods are well understood and their limitations appreciated by the clinician using them, a marked hypercapnia or hypocapnia may be misdiagnosed as representing a primary metabolic disturbance and inappropriate therapy given.[10,11]

The most direct method for separating the respiratory and metabolic effects on the serum [HCO_3^-] is that provided by studies in the 1960s.[12-14] Changes in pHa and [HCO_3^-] were measured in experimental animals and human volunteers exposed to graded degrees of acute hypocapnia or hypercapnia, or in patients with uncomplicated chronic hypercapnia. The results, with calculated 95% confidence limits, are presented in Table 17-5. Any [HCO_3^-] excess or deficit from these values must be the result of a nonrespiratory cause, that is, metabolic alkalosis or acidosis. For example, a patient with acute uncomplicated respiratory acidosis and a $PaCO_2$ of 60 mm Hg should have a [HCO_3^-] between 25 and 28 mMol/L (see Table 17-5). If his [HCO_3^-] is less than 25 mMol/L, the patient also has an associated metabolic acidosis; if the [HCO_3^-] is more than 28 mMol/L, a metabolic alkalosis is present.

Table 17-5 is too extensive to be committed to memory. Fortunately, the alteration in [HCO_3^-] with changing $PaCO_2$

TABLE 17-5. Acute and Chronic Changes in $PaCO_2$, pHa, and [HCO_3^-]

$PaCO_2$ (mm Hg)	ARTERIAL pH		[HCO_3^-] (mMol/L)	
	Acute	*Chronic*	*Acute*	*Chronic*
15	7.61–7.74	—	15–21	—
20	7.55–7.66	—	18–23	10–14
25	7.49–7.59	—	20–24	13–16
30	7.45–7.53	7.38–7.51	21–26	17–23
35	7.40–7.48	—	22–27	—
40	7.37–7.44	7.37–7.51	23–27	22–31
45	7.33–7.39	—	24–28	—
50	7.31–7.36	7.35–7.47	24–28	27–35
60	7.24–7.29	7.33–7.44	25–28	31–40
70	7.19–7.23	7.30–7.42	26–29	33–44
80	7.14–7.18	7.28–7.39	26–29	—
90	7.09–7.13	—	27–29	—
100	—	7.24–7.35	—	42–54

is reasonably linear, which means it is predictable. This relationship allows the use of four rules-of-thumb for clinical application, making it unnecessary to have the table immediately at hand. Notice that the following holds true, in general:

1. During acute hypercapnia, $[HCO_3^-]$ increases 1 mMol/L for each 10 mm Hg increase in $PaCO_2$ above 40 mm Hg.
2. During chronic hypercapnia, $[HCO_3^-]$ increases 4 mMol/L for each 10 mm Hg increase in $PaCO_2$ above 40 mm Hg.
3. During acute hypocapnia, $[HCO_3^-]$ decreases 2 mMol/L for every 10 mm Hg decrease in $PaCO_2$ below 40 mm Hg.
4. During chronic hypocapnia, $[HCO_3^-]$ decreases 5 to 7 mMol/L for every 10 mm Hg decrease in $PaCO_2$ below 40 mm Hg.

RESPIRATORY COMPENSATION FOR PRIMARY METABOLIC DISTURBANCES ■

We have considered the metabolic changes (i.e., changes in $[HCO_3^-]$) that are expected as compensation for primary respiratory derangements. Here we briefly consider the respiratory compensations to be expected from primary metabolic derangements.

METABOLIC ACIDOSIS

Hyperventilation is a normal response to a metabolically induced decrease in pH. Albert and associates[15] quantified this response in patients with uncomplicated metabolic acidosis. They observed that $PaCO_2$ was equal to $1.54 [HCO_3^-] + 8.36$, with a standard error of ±1.11 mm Hg, (i.e., in metabolic acidosis with an actual $[HCO_3^-]$ of 12 mMol/L, the $PaCO_2$, with normal ventilation, should average $(1.54 \times 12) + 8.36 = 27$ mm Hg. The normal range for 95% of the population is 25 to 29 mm Hg. A $PaCO_2$ greater than 29 mm Hg, in the face of this severe acidosis, would represent an associated respiratory acidosis.

Alternatively, these data can be used to predict the normal $PaCO_2$ with a varying pH. Their calculated regression equation, relating PCO_2 to pH, is $PaCO_2 = -484.64 + 70.26$ pH with a standard error of 2.72. A more easily remembered form (the rule of sevens) is presented in Table 17-6. With each decrease in pH of 0.1 unit, the normal $PaCO_2$ decreases by 7 mm Hg.

This respiratory response is prompt, but if the metabolic acidosis persists, ventilatory compensation becomes less effective, perhaps resulting from muscle fatigue. Maximum compensation occurs at pH 7.1; if blood pH decreases below that level, it does not increase further (and may decrease). This response may be caused by the deleterious effects of the progressive acidosis on the respiratory center itself.

METABOLIC ALKALOSIS

Unlike the prompt and predictable respiratory response to metabolic acidosis, the ventilatory response to metabolic

TABLE 17-6. Rule of Sevens

pH	$PaCO_2$ WITH NORMAL RESPIRATORY COMPENSATION (mm Hg)
7.3	28 ± 5
7.2	21 ± 5
7.1	14 ± 5

alkalosis is variable and often small. Usually, the $PaCO_2$ does not rise above 45 mm Hg in response to a primary metabolic alkalosis. However, we have seen patients with a compensatory increase of $PaCO_2$ as high as 60 mm Hg.

PROBLEM SOLVING ■

Use of the foregoing rules-of-thumb makes the solution to acid–base disorders relatively simple, as demonstrated by the following clinical examples:

Case 1: An otherwise healthy, 70-kg man sustains acute airway obstruction during induction of anesthesia. He then regurgitates and aspirates liquid stomach contents. An endotracheal tube is inserted, and an arterial blood sample is sent to the clinical laboratory. The following values are reported: $PaCO_2 = 70$ mm Hg, pHa = 7.10, and $[HCO_3^-] = 21$ mMol/L.

Stepwise analysis proceeds in the following manner. A pHa below 7.36 represents acidosis. Thus, the patient is acidotic, and, because the $PaCO_2$ is 70 mm Hg, at least a portion of the abnormality is respiratory in origin. Is there also a component of metabolic acidosis? Application of rule-of-thumb (1) suggests that $[HCO_3^-]$ should be at least 3 mMol above the normal values of 24 mMol/L if only $PaCO_2$ is changed. The predicted $[HCO_3^-]$ is 27 mMol/L, but the actual $[HCO_3^-]$ in this patient is only 21 mMol/L, a deficit of 6 mMol/L. A combined respiratory and metabolic acidosis is present.

Case 2: A 56-year-old, 70-kg man with COLD and a resting $PaCO_2$ of 70 mm Hg sustains an acute perioperative myocardial infarction. The blood pressure is 80/50 mm Hg, and he is diaphoretic, cool, and clammy. Arterial blood gas analysis shows the following: $PaCO_2 = 70$ mm Hg, pHa = 7.10, and $[HCO_3^-] = 21$ mMol/L.

Here, the laboratory values are identical to the first case but the clinical setting is considerably different. The pHa of 7.10 confirms acidosis and the $PaCO_2$ of 70 mm Hg reveals that a respiratory abnormality is present. However, in this instance, one is dealing with chronic hypercapnia and the application of rule-of-thumb (3) predicts a $[HCO_3^-]$ of 36 mMol/L. Actual $[HCO_3^-]$ is only 21 mMol/L, a deficit of 15 mMol/L. The metabolic component of acidosis is much greater in this case than in the first, despite the identical blood gas/pH measurements and $[HCO_3^-]$.

Case 3: A 70-kg man with neither clinical findings nor history of chronic pulmonary disease is seen in the intensive care unit 8 hours after an emergency gastrectomy. He is intubated and mechanically ventilated with a tidal volume of 1000 mL and a minute ventilation of 8 L. Blood gas and pH values are as follows: pHa = 7.08, $PaCO_2$ = 80 mm Hg, and $[HCO_3^-]$ = 23 mMol/L.

The patient has a respiratory acidosis, whereas the $[HCO_3^-]$, which is only slightly altered from normal, suggests a minimal metabolic component. To more adequately quantify the latter, consider any alteration in $[HCO_3^-]$ caused by the respiratory acidosis. Rule-of-thumb (1) says that the acute 40-mm Hg elevation of $PaCO_2$ should cause the $[HCO_3^-]$ to increase by 4 mMol/L. If the $PaCO_2$ is reduced to 40 mm Hg, the $[HCO_3^-]$ will decrease by the same 4 mMol/L to 19 mMol/L. The decrease in $[HCO_3^-]$ is, therefore, 24 to 19, or 5 mMol/L. This patient's major problem is maladjustment of the ventilator. He needs twice the alveolar ventilation he is receiving, probably because of a significant increase in dead space.

Case 4: A patient without known pulmonary disease is seen in the intensive care unit in septic shock. His blood gas and pH values are as follows: pH = 7.10, $PaCO_2$ = 18, and $[HCO_3^-]$ = 5.5 mMol/L.

A severe metabolic acidosis is apparent from the patient's extremely low $[HCO_3^-]$. To begin rational treatment, we need to know his respiratory status and to quantify his acid excess. The work of Albert and coworkers[15] shows that his $PaCO_2$ is well within the range predicted for normal ventilatory response to this severe an acidosis. The low $PaCO_2$ does not reflect a respiratory alkalosis but a normal value under these circumstances. Indeed, a $PaCO_2$ higher than 20 mm Hg would be abnormal.

In evaluating acid–base data, it is important to have knowledge of any chronic elevation of PCO_2 and to be aware of any acute treatment, either in the form of alkali administration or ventilatory manipulations.

Case 5: A patient with uncomplicated COLD, pHa of 7.36, PCO_2 of 70 mm Hg, and $[HCO_3^-]$ of 38 mMol/L is intubated and treated with controlled mechanical ventilation. After 1 hour, his arterial values are pH = 7.62, $PaCO_2$ = 35 mm Hg, and $[HCO_3^-]$ = 35 mMol/L.

Without knowledge of the institution of mechanical ventilation in the face of COLD, the second set of blood gas values could be erroneously interpreted as indicating severe metabolic alkalosis resulting from improper therapy. Appreciation of the immediate past events in this patient's medical management makes proper evaluation possible.

In Case 1, ventilatory support is indicated to correct the respiratory acidosis, whereas in Case 2 it may be indicated to prevent a further increase in $PaCO_2$. If correction of the metabolic component is indicated, the following formula may be employed:

$$\text{Total } [HCO_3^-] \text{ deficit} = \text{weight (kg)}$$
$$\times \, 0.2 \text{ (percent body weight as ECF)}$$
$$\times \text{ deficit } [HCO^{3-}] \text{ (mMol/L)} \qquad (9)$$

Because the aforementioned patients weigh 70 kg, the amount of $NaHCO_3$ to be administered if correction is desired is as follows:

Case 1: $70 \times 0.2 \times 6 = 84$ mMol
Case 2: $70 \times 0.2 \times 15 = 210$ mMol
Case 3: $70 \times 0.2 \times 5 = 80$ mMol

METABOLIC ACIDOSIS AND ALKALOSIS ■

A thorough discourse of the causes, physiologic effects, and the therapy of acid–base disturbances is beyond the scope of this chapter. This section discusses these matters succinctly.

ACIDOSIS

Causes

Normal metabolism results in the formation of 40 to 60 mMol of metabolic acids per day in the average adult, most from the metabolism of protein. This amount may be compared with the daily production of 20,000 mMol of CO_2 (respiratory acid). The metabolic acid load normally presents little challenge to the body, and the clearance of metabolic acids can cease entirely for several days without major ill effects. Under abnormal conditions, however, the production of metabolic acids from the incomplete combustion of carbohydrates and lipids can be considerable. In diabetic acidosis, 500 to 1000 mMol of β-hydroxybutyric acid may be formed per day, and during cardiac arrest, lactic acid may be formed at a rate as high as 20 mMol/minute. These extremes require intervention.

Iatrogenic hyperchloremic metabolic acidosis has been a concern to some clinicians after resuscitation with hypertonic saline solutions, with or without a hyperoncotic colloid such as 10% dextran 60. The additional acid load might exacerbate an already existing lactic acidosis in a low-flow state or shock.[16] Substitution of acetate for Cl^- has been suggested to reduce this acid load by provision of a HCO_3^- precursor.[17] However, a study by Frey and associates[18] did not show improved efficacy of such a substitution. They compared equiosmolal solutions of sodium chloride–dextran 60 and sodium acetate–dextran 60 (2400 mOsm/kg)[19] for the resuscitation of dogs subjected to hemorrhagic shock. Mean arterial pressure was lower in the acetate-treated animals. Arterial pH was significantly lower in the Cl^--treated animals at 5, 30, and 60 minutes, as was plasma HCO_3^-. However, the acetate-treated animals had persistently elevated lactate concentration. The authors concluded that no significant advantages resulted from substitution of acetate for Cl^-, although acid–base status seemed to be improved.

Treatment

Primary therapy must always be directed toward reestablishing normal metabolic pathways, such as insulin for the diabetic and improved cardiac output in low flow states. Alkali therapy is reserved for situations where it is needed to regain or maintain a $[H^+]$ (pH) compatible with adequate cellular function. Even in these circumstances, treatment must be tempered with the realization that lactic acid and the ketone bodies represent only a temporary acid load. With the reestablishment of normal metabolism, those substances are catabolized to CO_2 and water, leaving no fixed acid residue. Any alkali given as therapy during the acute stage of the disease remains as an excess alkali load to be excreted by the body.

At what point therapy is necessary for preservation of function is unclear. Earlier work with isolated heart preparations suggests severe myocardial depression with minimal decrease in pH. Other evidence with the intact organism reveals, at least in some circumstances, that maintenance of good cardiovascular function and normal responsiveness to catecholamines persists at pH values as low as 7.1.[20]

BUFFER ADMINISTRATION.   Our practice is to be less aggressive with alkali therapy than in the past. We rarely intervene at pH values higher than 7.20 unless the patient is in a precarious clinical state, in which case attempts are made to correct all treatable abnormalities. Below pH 7.20, treatment is determined by an evaluation of both the pH and the actual [HCO_3^-]. In general, we treat a patient with a [HCO_3^-] of less than 15 mMol/L, although some authors advocate withholding HCO_3^- therapy until the pH falls below 7.1 or the [HCO_3^-] falls below 5 to 8 mMol/L.[21,22]

Dosage of alkali is based on a calculation of total ECF [HCO_3^-] deficit, as outlined earlier. In practice, about three quarters of the calculated amount would be given initially in case patient variability or errors in measurement are present. More can always be given; however, once $NaCHO_3^-$ is administered, it cannot be taken out. One might question whether the first and third patients discussed earlier need treatment. This decision must be based on clinical judgment, not rules-of-thumb. The latter allow quantification of the abnormality and represent the "science" of acid–base problems; the "art" is up to the physician.

In some circumstances, however, the calculated dose of HCO_3^- will be grossly inadequate, particularly with continuing acid production (or base loss) in acidosis of long standing, or in instances of extreme acidosis. In the latter two instances, the degree of intracellular involvement can be significant. Indeed, in the case of diabetic acidosis, the volume of distribution of HCO_3^- is commonly assumed to be 50% of body weight,[21,22] and in instances of severe acidosis (i.e., [HCO_3^-] of 1 to 4 mMol/L), Garella and associates[23] reported an apparent volume of distribution of as much as 200% of body weight. This extra buffer capacity may partly reside in bone. In most patients, however, the assumption that the HCO_3^- deficit is limited to the ECF (i.e., 20% of body weight) has proven clinically appropriate. Repeat blood gas and pH measurements after treatment points out the cases with a significant intracellular contribution.

This general plan of treatment is altered in the following circumstances:

1. *Mixed metabolic acidosis and respiratory alkalosis*: With such a mixed disorder, a patient can have a significant calculated HCO_3^- deficit with a near-normal pH. Treatment of the metabolic acidosis without concomitant correction of the hyperventilation leads to increasing pH. In the absence of information to the contrary, we assume that pH is the more important parameter to maintain, and will, therefore, withhold $NaHCO_3$ unless the hyperventilation can be simultaneously curtailed.

2. *Metabolic acidosis in the neonate*: Neonates run a high risk of intracranial hemorrhage from sudden marked changes in serum osmolality. The commonly used clinical solution of $NaHCO_3$ is highly hyperosmolar, containing a concentration of over 2000 mOsm/L. Simmons and associates[24] report a decrease from 13.4% to 2.6% in the incidence of intracranial hemorrhage in their neonatal intensive care unit following a policy of decreased amount and concentration of $NaHCO_3$ administration. They suggest diluting $NaHCO_3$ at least 1:2 with water before administration and limiting the total dose to no more than 8 mMol/kg/day. Although this study was questioned because of a lack of suitable controls, there seems little to lose in following these recommendations.

3. *Idiopathic lactic acidosis*: This rare, mostly fatal, clinical entity of uncertain origin and pathogenesis was first described by Huckabee.[25] It is characterized by the production of large amounts of lactic acid in the absence of clinical shock. The suggested site of lactic acid production may be regionally ischemic tissues. In a case report by Taradash and Jacobson,[26] vasodilator therapy with sodium nitroprusside led to a dramatic and permanent resolution. They believed that nitroprusside caused redistribution of the cardiac output so that lactic acid metabolism and acid–base equilibrium returned to normal.

Major revisions concerning the role of HCO_3^- therapy are taking place. The American Heart Association urges restraint in the use of $NaHCO_3$ during cardiopulmonary resuscitation.[27,28] Experimentally, HCO_3^- administered to correct severe, hypoxic lactic acidosis actually increases lactate production.[29] Part of the difficulty is related to the fact that CO_2, elaborated by the reaction of H^+ and HCO_3^- (equation 1), rapidly diffuses across cell membranes, creating intracellular acidosis even though the extracellular acidosis is decreased.[30-33] Substitutes for HCO_3^- have been suggested to offset this problem,[34,35] but they have not been documented to improve outcome.

ALKALOSIS

Causes

Metabolic alkalosis is a common finding in the seriously ill or injured patient. This is not always a benign condition, as suggested by reports describing a correlation between increasing pH and increasing mortality.[36,37] The exact physiologic or pathologic effects of metabolic alkalosis responsible for the increasing mortality are unknown, but the frequently associated hypokalemia is not causal. The causes of metabolic alkalosis are better known than their effects, and, as seen in Table 17-7, they are frequently iatrogenic. There are few

TABLE 17-7. Conditions Causing a Metabolic Alkalosis

Loss of acid gastric juice
Volume depletion, especially associated with low K^+ or Cl^-
Diuretic therapy
Adrenal cortical hormone excess
Hepatic coma
Administration of exogenous base
  Lactate, acetate, etc (intravenous fluids)
  Citrate (bank blood)
  Bicarbonate

alkalotic end products of metabolism, so alkalosis usually results from an excessive loss of acid, either from the stomach or kidney, or from alkali administration.

ACID LOSS.   Gastric acid loss from vomiting or continuous suction is easily appreciated, but renal acid excretion by perfectly normal kidneys in the face of marked body alkalosis is more difficult to understand. The explanation lies in the primacy of the renal function of maintaining ECF volume over the maintenance of factors such as acid–base balance and osmolality. In other words, when given a "choice" between maintaining ECF volume or sacrificing volume to maintain acid–base balance or osmolality, the kidney chooses the former. Accordingly, the excretion of H^+ by the kidney often is not determined by the body's acid–base state but by the body's need for Na^+ retention.

Sodium reabsorption occurs in the proximal tubules by active transport, with Cl^- following passively to maintain electrical balance. In the distal nephrons, sodium reabsorption occurs, at least in part, by a cation exchange mechanism where electrical balance is maintained by exchange of Na^+ for either K^+ or H^+. With a Na^+-avid kidney (e.g., hypovolemia, increased aldosterone), deficiency of either K^+ or Cl^- can lead to increasing renal loss of K^+ by the cation exchange mechanism and therefore to metabolic alkalosis. K^+ deficit has been held chiefly responsible for inappropriate aciduria, but evidence suggests that hypochloremia is more important.[38-40] For example, in patients with hypochloremic, hypokalemic metabolic alkalosis (with body K^+ deficits as large as 500 mMol), the alkalosis and aciduria are correctable with Cl^- administration, but not with K^+.

Hypokalemia is usually associated with the alkalosis, either as a contributing cause because increasing amounts of H^+ must be lost by the cation exchange mechanism, or as an effect because the relative scarcity of H^+ during alkalosis causes increasing amounts of K^+ to be lost by the cation exchange mechanism. The first five causes listed in Table 17-7 result from this basic mechanism. It is frequently seen in the geriatric surgical candidate treated with digitalis, diuretics, and a low sodium diet.

ALKALI ADMINISTRATION.   A significant amount of alkali is administered to sick patients, often without the physician's recognition. Organic anions, such as lactate, acetate, pyruvate, gluconate, and citrate, when metabolized, result in an increase of HCO_3^-. A liter of lactated Ringer's solution contains 25 mMol of HCO_3^- precursor, and Normosol con-

tains a full 50 mMol. An aneurysmectomy patient, who often receives 8 L or more of intravenous fluids during surgery and the first 2 postoperative days, accumulates a significant base load if the fluids are *balanced electrolyte solutions* (BES). Add to this the several hundred millimoles of HCO_3^- precursor as citrate in bank blood (1 Mol citrate = 3 Mols HCO_3^-),[41] and the acid and Cl^- loss secondary to nasogastric suction, and one can understand why so many of these patients develop significant alkalosis.

HCO_3^- administration is another cause of iatrogenic alkalosis. Its use in treating acidosis, especially during cardiac arrest, is commonly excessive, and has led to the previously mentioned revisions of the American Heart Association resuscitation protocol.[28] Most "routine" uses of HCO_3^-, such as with blood transfusions, after aortic cross-clamping, or during cardiopulmonary bypass, without measurement of acid–base parameters, are to be condemned.

Treatment

Most cases of metabolic alkalosis are iatrogenic and preventable. Acidic gastric losses should be replaced with a high Cl^--containing solution (half- or full-strength saline) and not with BES. Patients already alkalotic and in need of continuing replacement of ongoing ECF losses should be given saline solution rather than BES with its hidden alkali load. This simple step, that is, the administration of Cl^--rich saline solution, will prevent or correct most cases of metabolic alkalosis.

POTASSIUM SUPPLEMENTATION.   Hypokalemia is an almost inevitable partner of alkalosis and can reach staggering levels. Body K^+ deficits of 1000 mMol have been reported[38] and losses of 300 to 500 mMol are common. Whereas metabolic alkalosis can be corrected with Cl^- alone, the accompanying hypokalemia can itself be life-threatening and requires correction. The usual practice of administering 40 mMol of K^+ in 1 L of 5% dextrose can lead to acute exacerbation of hypokalemia, because the glucose causes an intracellular movement of K^+. With significant hypokalemia, K^+ should be administered at a rate of 10 to 40 mMol/hour, with frequent determinations of serum levels.

Not every case of metabolic alkalosis is correctable with Cl^- alone. The syndrome of saline-resistant metabolic alkalosis or *chloride-wasting nephropathy*[42] is characterized by the finding of persistent urinary excretion of Cl^- in the presence of metabolic alkalosis. This situation probably occurs when body K^+ depletion becomes severe, in excess of 500 mMol. Severe K^+ depletion of this magnitude by itself may alter the renal tubular handling of Cl^-, leading to Cl^- wasting and metabolic alkalosis. It is reversible with K^+ replacement.

ACID ADMINISTRATION.   Several cases of alkalosis resistant to K^+ and saline administration have been reported. These have responded to the administration of 0.1 to 0.2 Mol/L hydrochloric acid in either saline, 5% dextrose, or distilled water.[43,44] Ammonium chloride has been used for this same purpose, but it runs the risk, especially in the face of liver impairment, of causing a severe encephalopathy with coma.

THERAPY IN CHRONIC LUNG DISEASE. Metabolic alkalosis is a common finding in patients with COLD. In one series, fully 26% of such patients had a pH in excess of 7.45.[45] Diuretics and sodium restriction seem to be the prime causes. The depression of these patients' respiratory drives by the alkalosis can have a significantly deleterious effect on minute ventilation, and blood gas values can be improved by correcting the acid–base abnormality.[38,44] Saline and K^+ administration commonly are required.

RESPIRATORY ACIDOSIS AND ALKALOSIS

ACIDOSIS

The causes, effects, and therapy of respiratory acidosis are beyond the scope of this chapter. However, therapy consists first of defining and treating the underlying cause (i.e., narcotic or other drug overdose, paralysis, sepsis, shock, and COLD), and secondly in the judicious use of mechanical ventilation. Rarely should buffers be employed because the CO_2 formed (in the case of HCO_3^- buffer) cannot be exhaled.[45]

ALKALOSIS

Because of its frequency, the fact that it is commonly iatrogenic in origin, and its serious but poorly appreciated effects, respiratory alkalosis is an important problem. Table 17-8 lists the commonly associated conditions. The last listed cause, iatrogenic hyperventilation, is the most common in our experience and is easily prevented. Minute ventilation needs to be individualized to the level that results in a normal

TABLE 17-8. Clinical States in Which Respiratory Alkalosis May Occur

Drugs
  Salicylates
  Analeptics
  Doxapram
Hormones
  Progesterone
  Epinephrine
Hypermetabolic states
  Fever
  Exercise
  Thyrotoxicosis
Anoxia
CNS lesions
  Meningitis
  Encephalitis
  Hemorrhage
  Trauma
Hepatic failure
Shock
Gram-negative bacteremia (without fever or shock)
Any interstitial pulmonary disease
Iatrogenic hyperventilation

CNS, central nervous system.

TABLE 17-9. Effects of Acute Respiratory Alkalosis

Decreased cardiac output
Shift of the oxyhemoglobin dissociation curve to the left
Bronchoconstriction with increased V̇/Q̇ imbalance
Hypotension
Hypokalemia
Decreased cerebral blood flow
Decreased cerebral spinal fluid pressure
Posthyperventilation hypoxia
Resetting of central chemoreceptors

$PaCO_2$ and pHa. The appropriate range may be as little as 4 L/minute up to more than 30 L/minute in adults.

Patients with central nervous system lesions who hyperventilate are more difficult to manage. Trimble and coworkers[46] demonstrated a decrease in $P(A - a)O_2$ and increased cardiac output in five such patients after paralysis and 3% CO_2 supplementation to bring PCO_2 and pH to near normal levels. Evidence is lacking that this maneuver will improve ultimate mortality figures. Muscle paralysis may be indicated so that ventilation can be effectively controlled.

Table 17-9 lists the effects of acute respiratory alkalosis, some of which are life-threatening.

CONCLUSION

Many systems of acid–base analysis other than the ones discussed in this chapter have been used. Indeed, some are slightly more accurate than the recommendation given here of evaluating only the change in $[HCO_3^-]$ (after correction for the effect of altered PCO_2) when quantifying a metabolic disturbance. We believe, however, that the slight increase in accuracy of these alternative methods does not compensate for their significantly increased complexity.

Arterial blood generally is used to assess acid–base disturbances. However, in low-flow states and cardiac arrest, analysis of central mixed venous (and peripheral venous) blood may provide a better view of what is happening at the cellular level.[47] Arterial and venous discrepancies in measured and derived parameters can be significant.[30,31,48]

REFERENCES

1. Jörgenson K, Astrup P: Standard bicarbonate: its clinical significance and a new method for its determination. *Scand J Clin Lab Invest* 1957;2:122
2. Singer RB, Hastings AB: An improved clinical method for the estimation of disturbances of the acid–base balance of human blood. *Medicine* 1948;27:233
3. Astrup P, Siggaard-Andersen O, Jörgenson K, et al: The acid–base metabolism: a new approach. *Lancet* 1960;i:1035
4. Editor's choice: Henderson vs. Hasselbalch. *Anesth Analg* 1966;45:491
5. Campbell EJM: RI pH. *Lancet* 1962;i:681
6. Campbell EJM: RI pH. *Lancet* 1962;ii:154

7. Winters RW: Terminology of acid–base disorders. *Ann NY Acad Sci* 1965;133:211
8. Pitts RF: Mechanisms for stabilizing the alkaline reserves of the body. *Harvey Lect* 1952–43;48:172
9. Van Slyke DD, Cullen GD: Studies of acidosis. I. The bicarbonate concentration of the blood plasma: its significance and its determination as a measure of acidosis. *J Biol Chem* 1917;30:289.
10. Roos A, Thomas IJ: The *in vivo* and *in vitro* carbon dioxide dissociation curves of true plasma. *Anesthesiology* 1967;28:1048
11. Bunker J: The great transatlantic acid–base debate. *Anesthesiology* 1965;26:591
12. Arbus G, Hebert L, Levesque P, et al: Application of "significant band" for acute respiratory alkalosis. *N Engl J Med* 1969;280:117
13. Brackett NC, Cohen JJ, Schwartz WB: Carbon dioxide titration curve of normal man: effect of increasing degrees of acute hypercapnia on acid–base equilibrium. *N Engl J Med* 1965;272:6
14. Brackett NC, Wingo CF, Muren O, et al: Acid–base response to chronic hypercapnia in man. *N Engl J Med* 1969;280:124
15. Albert M, Dell R, Winters R: Quantitative displacement of acid–base equilibrium in metabolic acidosis. *Ann Intern Med* 1967;66:312
16. Rocha e Silva M, Braga GA, Prist R, et al: Physical and physiological characteristics of pressure-driven hemorrhage. *Am J Physiol* 1992;263:H1402
17. Smith GJ, Kramer GC, Peron P, et al: A comparison of several hypertonic solutions for resuscitation of bled sheep. *J Surg Res* 1985;39:517
18. Frey L, Kesel K, Prückner S, et al: Is sodium acetate dextran superior to sodium chloride dextran for small volume resuscitation from traumatic hemorrhagic shock? *Anesth Analg* 1994;79:517
19. Vassar MJ, Holcroft JW: Use of hypertonic-hyperoncotic fluids for resuscitation of trauma patients. *J Intens Care Med* 1992;7:189
20. Andersen M, Border J, Mouritzen C: Acidosis, catecholamines and cardiovascular dynamics: when does acidosis require correction? *Ann Surg* 1967;166:344
21. Felig P: Current concepts: diabetic ketoacidosis. *N Engl J Med* 1974;290:1360
22. Kassirer JP: Current concepts: serious acid–base disorders. *N Engl J Med* 1974;291:773
23. Garella S, Dana CL, Chazan JA: Severity of metabolic acidosis as a determinant of bicarbonate requirements. *N Engl J Med* 1973;289:121
24. Simmons M, Adcock E, Bard H, et al: Hypernatremia and intracranial hemorrhage in neonates. *N Engl J Med* 1974;291:6
25. Huckabee W: Abnormal resting blood lactate. II. Lactic acidosis. *Am J Med* 1961;30:840
26. Taradash MR, Jacobson LB: Vasodilator therapy of idiopathic lactic acidosis. *N Engl J Med* 1975;293:468
27. Emergency Cardiac Care Committee and Subcommittees, American Heart Association. Guidelines for cardiopulmonary resuscitation and emergency cardiac care. *JAMA* 1992;268:2210
28. Cummins RO (ed): *Textbook of Advanced Cardiac Life Support*, vol 7. Dallas, American Heart Association, 1994:14
29. Graf H, Leach W, Arieff A: Evidence for a detrimental effect of bicarbonate therapy in hypoxic lactic acidosis. *Science* 1986;227:754
30. Weil MH, Rackow EC, Trevino R, et al: Differences in acid–base state between venous and arterial blood during cardiopulmonary resuscitation. *N Engl J Med* 1986;315:153
31. Grundler W, Weil MH, Rackow EC: Arteriovenous carbon dioxide and pH gradients during cardiac arrest. *Circulation* 1986;74:1071
32. Young GP: Reservations and recommendations regarding sodium bicarbonate administered during cardiac arrest. *J Emerg Med* 1988;6:321
33. von Planta M, Weil MH, Gazmuri RJ, et al: Myocardial acidosis associated with CO_2 production during cardiac arrest and resuscitation. *Circulation* 1989;80:684
34. Sun JH, Filley GF, Hord K, et al: Carbicarb: an effective substitute for $NaHCO_3$ for the treatment of acidosis. *Surgery* 1987;102:834
35. Bersin RM, Arieff AI: Improved hemodynamic function during hypoxemia with carbicarb, a new agent for the management of acidosis. *Circulation* 1988;77:227
36. Wilson R, Gibson D, Percinel A, et al: Severe alkalosis in critically ill surgical patients. *Arch Surg* 1972;105:197
37. Steer M, Cloeren S, Bushness L, et al: Metabolic alkalosis and respiratory failure in critically ill patients. *Surgery* 1972;72:408
38. Schwartz W, Van Ypersele de Strihau C, Kassirer J: Role of anions in metabolic alkalosis and potassium deficiency. *N Engl J Med* 1968;279:630
39. Kassirer JP, Berkman PM, Laurenz DR, et al: The critical role of chloride in the correction of hypokalemic alkalosis in man. *Am J Med* 1965;38:172
40. Kassirer J, Schwartz W: The response of normal man to selective depletion of hydrochloric acid. *Am J Med* 1966;40:10
41. Barcenas C, Fuller T, Knochel J: Metabolic alkalosis after massive blood transfusion. *JAMA* 1976;236:953
42. Garella S, Chazan J, Cohen J: Saline resistant metabolic alkalosis: a "chloride-wasting" nephropathy. *Ann Intern Med* 1970;73:31
43. Abouna GM, Veazey PR, Terry DB Jr: Intravenous infusion of hydrochloric acid for treatment of severe metabolic alkalosis. *Surgery* 1974;75:194
44. Harken AH, Gabel RA, Fence V, et al: Hydrochloric acid in the correction of metabolic alkalosis. *Arch Surg* 1975;110:819
45. Vassallo CL, Gee JBL, Robin ED, et al: The failure of potassium salts to repair diuretic-induced hypokalemia and alkalosis in chronic hypercapnia. *Am Rev Resp Dis* 1968;97:804
46. Trimble C, Smith DE, Rosenthal MH, et al: Pathophysiologic role of hypocarbia in post-traumatic pulmonary insufficiency. *Am J Surg* 1971;122:633
47. Arieff AI: Indications for use of bicarbonate in patients with metabolic acidosis. *Br J Anesth* 1991;67:165
48. Androgue HJ, Rashad MN, Gorin AB, et al: Assessing acid–base status in circulatory failure. *N Engl J Med* 1989;320:1312

Critical Care, Third Edition, edited by Joseph M. Civetta,
Robert W. Taylor, and Robert R. Kirby.
Lippincott-Raven Publishers, Philadelphia, PA © 1997.

CHAPTER 18

Coagulation

Robert I. Parker

IMMEDIATE CONCERNS

MAJOR PROBLEMS

Normal coagulation represents a balance between intact local hemostatic mechanisms in response to vascular injury and the reactions that prevent systemic catalysis of coagulation. Disorders of coagulation result when local coagulation pathways are impaired, the protective mechanisms to prevent systemic spread of coagulation are inadequate, or these protective measures overrespond and interfere with local hemostasis. Several interactive factors are involved in normal coagulation (Table 18-1). These diverse components of coagulation may in turn be divided into the processes involved in primary and secondary hemostasis, as well as fibrinolysis.

STRESS POINTS

1. Primary hemostasis refers to the cascade of interactions between circulating platelets and a blood vessel (particularly the subendothelium) in the area of its injury. In many instances, primary hemostatic function provides a sufficient barrier against any further extrusion of blood and plasma, at least from small-caliber vessels.

2. Secondary hemostasis involves the activation of plasma coagulation proteins, ultimately leading to fibrin cross-linkage, platelet plug stabilization, and clot retraction.

3. The role of fibrinolysis and other related regulatory mechanisms is to "turn off" the various coagulation pathways and to cleave fibrin polymers to smaller degradation forms.

4. These events are physiologically important for recanalization and reestablishment of blood flow through an injured vessel. Fibrinolysis is also important in containing thrombosis as a local event.

PHYSIOLOGY AND BIOCHEMISTRY OF PRIMARY HEMOSTASIS

COMPONENTS

Primary hemostasis comprises several important activities: reflex vasoconstriction after vascular injury; platelet adhesion to vascular subendothelial structures; platelet activation and secretion; and platelet aggregation, plug formation, and clot retraction. These are modulated by biochemical and physiologic stimuli. Therefore, when any agents interfere with any of these steps, increased bleeding results.

The platelet is a complex structure, our understanding of which is primarily limited to observed phenomena. It is derived from megakaryocytes, which are found in the bone marrow, the lungs, and, rarely, in the peripheral circulation. The life span of the platelet is 8 to 9 days. The anatomic structure of the platelet seems to be closely related to its function. Its plasma membrane is rich in phospholipids, providing a ready availability of substrate (arachidonic acid) for the synthesis of prostaglandins and thromboxanes—compounds that modulate many of the functions of platelets. Platelet aggregation, granule release, and reflex vasoconstriction all are influenced by the presence of prostaglandins and thromboxanes.[1-4] Membrane receptors for collagen and other subendothelial proteins, several coagulation factors (including fibrinogen and von Willebrand factor), the adenine nucleotides (particularly adenosine diphosphate [ADP]), epinephrine, and serotonin also are found on the platelet surface. The binding of these agonists to their respective receptors is partly responsible for platelet adherence and aggregation. Dense and alpha-granules, located in the platelet cytoplasm, contain numerous proteins such as coagulation factors V, VIII, and XIII, fibrinogen, and von Willebrand factor; protease inhibitors; chemotactic factors; and platelet agonists (ADP, epinephrine, serotonin). Secretion of these

TABLE 18-1. Overview of the Factors Involved in Normal Hemostasis

PRIMARY HEMOSTASIS
Vessel wall
Platelets
Fibrogen
von Willebrand factor
Calcium ion

SECONDARY HEMOSTASIS
Coagulation proteins
Protease inhibitors
Phospholipids
Calcium ion

FIBRINOLYSIS
Fibrinolytic factors

platelet agonists further enhances platelet activation and hemostasis. These secreted proteins also play a role in the inflammatory response. Finally, the cytoplasm contains the microtubular apparatus, which is necessary for normal clot retraction (by altering platelet morphologic features). It also plays a role in platelet granule secretion.

The vascular endothelial cell is the other important cellular component of primary hemostasis. In a noninjured state, one of the most critical physiologic functions of the endothelial cell is to provide a nonthrombogenic interface to circulating blood. On injury, however, the exposed subendothelial structures provide a surface for platelet adhesion and subsequent aggregation. This typically occurs in conjunction with reflex vasoconstriction and the release of tissue factors and collagen, which in turn stimulate coagulation (secondary hemostasis). Tissue plasminogen activator (tPA) is also released from endothelial cells after injury. This activates the fibrinolytic system, thereby limiting excess thrombus formation and helping to maintain vascular patency. In addition, the activated endothelial cell presents a surface on which coagulation can proceed to take place; it also produces or secretes into the local environment various substances that function to modulate hemostasis, fibrinolysis, and local blood flow.

FUNCTION IN NORMAL COAGULATION

When the integrity of a blood vessel is disrupted, the subendothelial structures are exposed and various tissue factors are released. These tissue factors initiate coagulation but also include plasminogen activator, a stimulator of fibrinolysis. Production of the vasoconstrictor peptide endothelin by activated endothelial cells may reduce local blood flow, thereby contributing to platelet deposition. Within seconds, platelets begin to adhere to the exposed subendothelial structures (primarily collagen and, to a lesser extent, basement membrane proteins). Fibrinogen and, in particular, von Willebrand factor, also are required for normal platelet adherence. Their effects are mediated through specific membrane glycoprotein receptors to which these substances bind.

In a series of subsequent events, which are poorly understood, platelets are "activated," resulting in release of the alpha-granule and dense granule contents and the production of prostaglandins and thromboxanes. These events occur within seconds after vascular injury. The initial release of granule contents causes further platelet granule secretion, particularly ADP release, leading to additional platelet aggregation at the site of injury. Platelet activation also results in the development of platelet procoagulant activity, which is primarily mediated through surface expression of special coagulation factors (e.g., factors Va and VIIIa). Amplification of these actions and interactions leads to platelet plug formation within minutes. Prostaglandin and thromboxane synthesis and the subsequent influence of these substances on intraplatelet cyclic adenosine monophosphate (cAMP) levels and cytoplasmic ionic calcium concentrations play important modulatory roles in many of these activities.[1,3]

The platelet is also important to hemostasis through its provision of a phospholipid surface on which the intrinsic pathway of primary hemostasis may be initiated. These include, but are not limited to, the expression of coagulation factor Va on the platelet membrane surface. It is here that several coagulation factors interact and undergo zymogen activation (discussed later). As these processes proceed, thrombin is formed on the platelet membrane surface, which in turn directly stimulates further platelet granule release and aggregation, leading to platelet coalescence into a stable hemostatic plug. This plug is ultimately stabilized by fibrin polymer deposition and integration into its structure as secondary hemostasis proceeds. The activated platelets then cause retraction of the interlaced fibrin strands and a reduction in clot size, with the expulsion of its remaining liquid contents. This typically occurs within 3 to 10 minutes.

As one would suspect, these processes can quickly exceed regional hemostatic requirements, leading to excessive clot and platelet plug formation. Locally, the endothelial cell provides some capability to limit such action through the production of prostaglandin I_2 (often referred to as prostacyclin). Prostaglandin I_2 activates the adenyl cyclase of platelets, raising intraplatelet cAMP levels. By regulating cytoplasmic ionic calcium concentrations, cAMP prevents further platelet aggregation and granule release. Prostaglandin I_2 also impedes hemostasis by its action as a potent vasodilator.

LABORATORY ASSESSMENT

Abnormal function of primary hemostasis results from an impairment of platelet adherence to subendothelium. This can be caused by abnormalities in either the platelets or vascular structures. Platelet defects can be classified as quantitative or qualitative. The microscopic review of a peripheral blood smear allows one to estimate circulating numbers of platelets: each platelet visualized per high-power oil-immersion field approximates 15,000 platelets per microliter of whole blood. A normal count is roughly 150,000 to 400,000/ μL. The cause of a derangement in circulating platelet numbers cannot be ascertained from such a smear review, and bone marrow aspiration and biopsy are typically required to address the possibility of decreased platelet production. An assessment of platelet morphologic features from the peripheral smear, however, may provide clues as to the etiology of the thrombocytopenia. Specifically, platelet size and homogeneity suggest rates of platelet turnover. Experimental data (not universally accepted) indicate that, as a population, younger platelets are larger and denser than older platelets. Using this information, one can infer an increased platelet turnover rate if mean platelet size or density is increased. The finding of an increased mean platelet size in a thrombocytopenic patient suggests that peripheral destruction of platelets is involved in the etiology of the thrombocytopenia. However, the reader must be cautioned that some constitutional thrombocytopenias are characterized by the production of unusually large platelets.

Measurement of the template bleeding time provides a sensitive but nonspecific overall assessment of primary hemostasis. The modified Ivy technique is probably the most sensitive and standardized of those available.[5] A standardized incision is made on a relatively avascular area of the forearm, and the time required for bleeding to stop under standardized conditions is measured. Qualitative defects in platelet function, von Willebrand factor deficiency, afibrinogenemia, marked thrombocytopenia, and abnormalities in vascular collagen all can result in an abnormally prolonged bleeding time (normal is less than 10 minutes). Disorders of coagulation (secondary hemostasis) do *not* generally affect the bleeding time. A specific discussion of each of these important disorders is found in Chapter 154.

Platelet aggregation can be measured and assessed in vitro to further delineate the etiology of an apparent qualitative defect. Platelet-rich plasma is incubated with a platelet agonist, such as ADP, collagen, epinephrine, or thrombin, resulting in platelet activation and consequent aggregation. Platelet aggregation is measured by light transmission and absorbance, and analysis of the aggregation curves often allows deductions on the nature of the platelet defect to be made. There is also an assay for functional von Willebrand factor that uses platelet agglutination in the presence of the antibiotic ristocetin (ristocetin cofactor assay). Finally, clot retraction can be grossly quantitated.

PHYSIOLOGY AND BIOCHEMISTRY OF SECONDARY HEMOSTASIS ■

COMPONENTS

Secondary hemostasis represents a unique physiologic arrangement whereby the inactive components of coagulation (the zymogen forms of the enzymes) continuously circulate through the bloodstream but can be quickly activated in an area where bleeding occurs, thereby facilitating the regional conversion of blood from a liquid to a gel state. This is based on the ultimate conversion of fibrinogen to insoluble fibrin polymers. An ever-growing number of coagulation factors, as well as stimuli and inhibitors of coagulation, have been added to the structural scheme for coagulation. Secondary hemostasis has classically been divided into the intrinsic and extrinsic pathways, or cascades. Recently, however, it has become apparent that the interrelationships among these pathways are many, and that such an arbitrary division is not always consistent with their in vivo functional activity. Such a conceptual framework does, however, provide a means for understanding and interpreting the various laboratory studies used to identify a particular cause for an observed coagulopathy.

A simplified overview of the currently accepted coagulation pathways is illustrated in Figure 18-1. As can be seen, activation of factor XII along the intrinsic pathway ultimately leads to thrombin production and fibrin polymerization. The extrinsic pathway, on the other hand, is initiated by the interaction of a tissue factor and calcium ion with factor VII, leading to its activation from the zymogen form. The final common pathway to thrombin production proceeds from factor X activation, the point at which the two pathways converge. Again, the division of these pathways is relative, and several crossover points exist.

From a biochemical standpoint, the individual components of secondary hemostasis are better classified according to the functional requirements of each of the coagulation factors. In this regard, procoagulant factors can be divided into three groups: the contact factors, the vitamin K–dependent factors, and the thrombin-sensitive factors.[3] Table 18-2 lists each of these groups and their respective factors. Proteins C and S are included in the vitamin K–dependent list for completeness; however, they function as anticoagulant rather than procoagulant proteins. Protein M

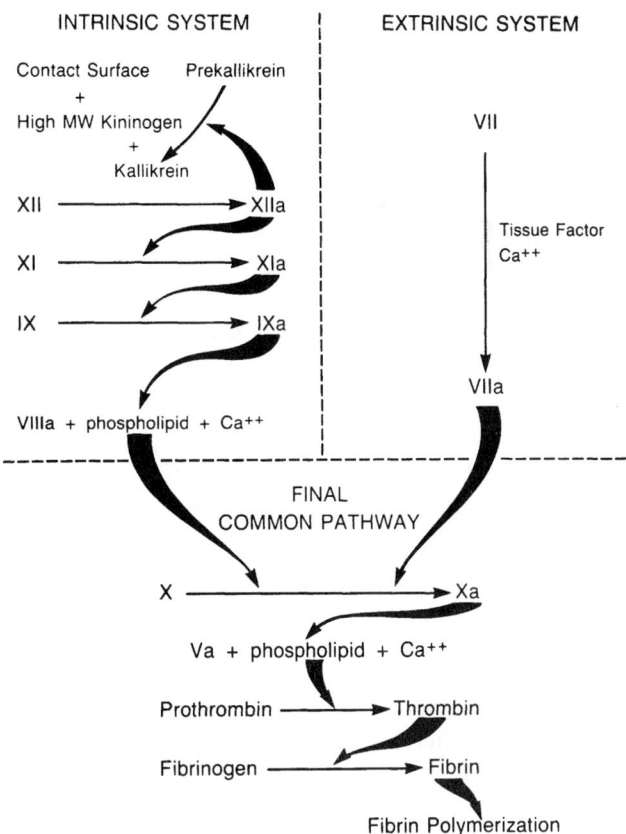

FIGURE 18-1. An overview of secondary hemostasis.

TABLE 18-2. Components of Secondary Hemostasis

VITAMIN K–DEPENDENT FACTORS

Factor II (prothrombin)
Factor VII (proconvertin)
Factor IX (Christmas factor)
Factor X (Stuart-Prower factor)
Protein C
Protein M
Protein S
Protein Z

CONTACT FACTORS

Factor XII (Hageman factor)
Factor XI
Prekallikrein (Fletcher factor)
High molecular weight kininogen (Fitzgerald factor)

THROMBIN-SENSITIVE FACTORS

Factor I (fibrinogen)
Factor V (proaccelerin)
Factor VIII (antihemophilic factor)
Factor XIII (Laki-Lorand factor)

and, perhaps, protein Z are procoagulant, although their specific functions are currently unknown.

Contact Factors

As noted in Table 18-2, the contact factors include factors XII and XI, along with high molecular weight kininogen and prekallikrein. These are referred to as contact factors because of their mode of activation. When factor XII contacts a negatively charged surface, such as platelet membrane phospholipid or subendothelial collagen, its activation from a zymogen form begins. Factor XI, high molecular weight kininogen, and prekallikrein all depend on their subsequent activation from factor XII; thus, all are considered contact (dependent) factors.

Factor XII exists in its native form as a single-chain glycoprotein. On surface contact and binding, it undergoes a conformational change that provides partial activation and, more importantly, renders it susceptible to further activation by prekallikrein, another single-chain glycoprotein of similar molecular weight. High molecular weight kininogen, a precursor of bradykinin, is also involved in the factor XII activation process.[4] In a reciprocal action, the now-activated factor XIIa in turn cleaves and activates prekallikrein to kallikrein, which activates still more factor XII. Kallikrein has additional effects on the activation of plasminogen (discussed in the section on fibrinolysis). Finally, factor XI, which is also bound to the negatively charged surface, is activated by factor XIIa. Unlike many of the other reactions in the coagulation cascade, calcium ion is not required as a cofactor for any contact factor activation steps.

Vitamin K–Dependent Factors

The vitamin K–dependent coagulation factors include prothrombin (factor II) and factors VII, IX, and X. In addition, four other vitamin K–dependent plasma proteins that are involved in normal coagulation have been identified: proteins C, S, Z, and M. All of these proteins share the unique biochemical feature of having γ-carboxyglutamic acid in their amino acid sequences as a result of vitamin K–dependent postribosomal modification. The γ-carboxyglutamic acid residues in turn facilitate the binding of these proteins to calcium ions. Calcium ion is a required cofactor for the normal function of these enzymes. In the absence of vitamin K, these proteins do not undergo γ-carboxylation and cannot function normally in the coagulation process.

Protein C and protein S have interrelated and codependent functions as anticoagulants. Protein C inactivates the activated cofactors Va and VIIIa. In addition, it stimulates fibrinolysis, possibly through activated protein C–mediated production of tPA. Protein S is a cofactor for the protein C–mediated inactivation of factors Va and VIIIa, functioning as an accelerator of this process.[4] Curiously, protein C activation is initiated by thrombin, an activated vitamin K–dependent factor that is responsible for fibrin formation. Thus, thrombin has a role in both primary and secondary hemostasis, as well as fibrinolysis. Protein M seems to be a procoagulant enzyme and may be involved in the activation of prothrombin to thrombin. The exact function of protein Z is unknown, but it is hypothesized to be procoagulant by virtue of its effect on qualitative platelet function.[3]

Prothrombin is proteolytically cleaved to thrombin through the combined actions of factors Va and Xa, along with calcium ion and a phospholipid surface, which is usually supplied by the platelet. Calcium bridges are reversibly formed from the phospholipid surface to the γ-carboxyglutamic acid residues during these reactions. Factor VII, like prothrombin, exists as a zymogen that can be activated by the other activated vitamin K–dependent factors (thrombin, IXa, and Xa). Factor XIIa and plasmin are also capable of factor VII activation. Factor VII has physiologic activity in both the intrinsic and extrinsic pathways. It also has the unique capability among the vitamin K–dependent factors of initiating coagulation in its nonactivated form as its single-chain form retains some degree of inherent biologic activity, even before proteolytic zymogen activation.[4] Factor IX may be activated by either factor VIIa or factor XIa and is likewise dependent on the presence of calcium ion. Thus, we see that a reciprocal, amplifying relationship exists between factors VII and IX because activation of one results in activation of the other, and so on.

This reciprocal activation of factors VII and IX by each other represents the major "cross talk" circuit between the intrinsic and extrinsic pathways.

Factor X has been called "the crossroads of the coagulation system." Macromolecular complexes formed along either the intrinsic or extrinsic coagulation pathway are capable of activating factor X. This γ-carboxyglutamic acid residue–laden double-chain protein is also activated by proteolytic cleavage. This process occurs while factor X is tightly bound by calcium ion to a negatively charged surface.

In summary, the activation steps of the vitamin K–dependent coagulation proteins occur through proteolytic cleavage; are calcium dependent; are generally "positive feedback loop" reactions; affect both intrinsic and extrinsic coagulation pathways, as well as fibrinolysis in the case of proteins C and S; and probably occur in vivo while bound to the platelet membrane surface.

Thrombin-Sensitive Factors

The thrombin-sensitive factors are so named because of their susceptibility to proteolysis by thrombin, which in most cases leads to their enzymatically active forms. These include fibrinogen and factors V, VIII, and XIII. The central importance of thrombin formation to normal coagulation and its regulation is again emphasized by these interactions, along with others discussed previously. As with the contact factors—but not the vitamin K–dependent coagulation proteins—there is no unifying or characteristic structure common to this group, although all of these factors can be identified on or within platelets.

Conversion of fibrinogen to fibrin, and its subsequent polymerization and incorporation into the matrix of a platelet plug, represents the endpoint for secondary hemostasis. Fibrinogen is a comparatively large, complex coagulation protein. Conversion to fibrin occurs when thrombin symmetrically cleaves two pairs of short polypeptides, fibrinopeptides A and B, from its amino terminal ends. The biochemical cause for the resulting activation is not known; however, spontaneous polymerization of fibrin monomer quickly follows. As fibrin is polymerized and becomes insoluble, it is also stabilized by the action of activated factor XIII. It is, however, susceptible to serial proteolysis and degradation by plasmin, yielding multiple forms of fibrin degradation products.

Factor V is also proteolytically activated by thrombin. Recall, too, that factor V is also present in platelet alpha-granules and can be secreted and expressed on the platelet membrane surface, where many of the coagulation reactions occur. In fact, the platelet as a source of factor Va for initial in vivo coagulation may be more important than the factor Va provided by serum activation.[1] Factor Va is inactivated by protein C and is a pivotal inhibitory point in preventing the continued coagulation of whole blood in vivo.

The factor VIII complex is composed of two separate glycoprotein moieties that have different structures and functions. The smaller of the two components is the factor VIII procoagulant glycoprotein. This is the protein that is deficient in hemophilia A and is acted on by thrombin to produce the activated clotting factor VIIIa. The presence of this clotting factor is critical for normal secondary hemostasis because of its function as a cofactor in the factor IXa–mediated conversion of factor X to Xa. Activated factor VIII (VIIIa) is subsequently inactivated by activated protein C or by prolonged exposure to thrombin. The procoagulant portion of the factor VIII complex (Table 18-3) is synthesized in the liver and complexes with von Willebrand factor in circulation. Because von Willebrand factor is essential for normal platelet adhesion to subendothelial structures, a deficiency of this glycoprotein results in a hemorrhagic diathesis.

Factor XIII is activated by the action of thrombin as well. Activated factor XIII (XIIIa) is in turn responsible for covalent bond formation between fibrin monomers as spontaneous polymerization occurs. In the absence of factor

TABLE 18-3. Functional Components of Factor VIII

FACTOR VIII:C, AHF

Synthesized in the liver(?), source of factor VIII procoagulant activity, has antigenic properties that allow radioimmunoassay quantitation of plasma samples

FACTOR VIII R:WF

von Willebrand factor, synthesized by endothelial cells and megakaryocytes, necessary for normal in vivo platelet function; also called bleeding time factor (factor VIII R:WF [BT]) or factor VIII–related antigen (factor VIII R:Ag)

XIIIa, the fibrin polymers that are formed are unstable and cannot provide sufficient matrix rigidity to the primary platelet plug. Deficiency of this factor results in delayed bleeding as a consequence of early clot breakdown.

FUNCTION IN NORMAL COAGULATION

Although the arbitrary division of coagulation pathways into intrinsic and extrinsic cascades does not always accurately reflect function in a patient, it does provide a means of "mapping out" the sequence of events that occur during coagulation. This approach also provides a framework for understanding the laboratory diagnostic assessment of a coagulation disorder.

The Intrinsic Pathway

It is assumed that disruption of endothelial integrity is the stimulus that triggers the intrinsic pathway. Factor XII first binds to the exposed negatively charged surface and undergoes a conformational change that results in its partial activation. More importantly, this conformational change allows the interaction of factor XII with prekallikrein and high molecular weight kininogen, resulting in more complete activation of factor XII. Activated factor XII (XIIa) reciprocally cleaves prekallikrein to kallikrein, which then becomes a more potent activator of factor XII. Factor XIIa then activates factor XI, which in turn activates factor IX in the mandatory presence of calcium ion. Finally, activated factor IX (IXa) complexes with factor VIIIa, calcium ion, and a phospholipid structure, forming a macromolecular unit capable of activating factor X.

Although factor VII is considered part of the extrinsic pathway, it also plays a role in the intrinsic pathway. In its single-chain, uncleaved zymogen form, factor VII has some degree of inherent enzymatic activity, through which it can activate factor IX. In addition, it is rapidly activated by factor XIIa, and in this form can activate factor IX more expeditiously.

There are two major points of amplification in the intrinsic pathway. The first is the factor XII–prekallikrein activation loop, which rapidly accelerates the initial coagulation series. The second is the positive feedback of factor VIIa on factor IX. In this feedback loop, factor IXa activates factor VII, which in turn greatly increases the reaction speed of factor

IX activation. Of these two amplification steps, only the loop involving factors IX and VII is of clinical importance because persons totally deficient in factor XII manifest no bleeding abnormalities.

The Extrinsic Pathway

The disruption of an endothelial surface, and the subsequent activation of the coagulation cascade, is not necessarily dependent on the initial binding of factor XII to a negatively charged surface. When such an injury occurs, a tissue factor is released from the damaged cells into the circulation. This tissue factor, the nature of which is not well understood, complexes with factor VII and calcium ion, resulting in factor VII activation. This macromolecular structure then activates factor X. This is the so-called extrinsic pathway. Activated factor VII (VIIa) can also activate the intrinsic pathway by activating factor IX, essentially bypassing the contact activation steps of the intrinsic cascade. Such crossover reactions between pathways are apparent, whereas amplification loops are not.

The Final Common Pathway to Coagulation

Factor X activation can be achieved by either the intrinsic or extrinsic pathway. Factor Xa complexes with factor Va, phospholipid, and calcium to form a large complex capable of converting prothrombin to thrombin. As thrombin is formed, it reciprocally activates factor V and thus greatly accelerates the reaction of thrombin activation. Thrombin now cleaves two pairs of short polypeptides from fibrinogen, and the resulting fibrin monomer rapidly and spontaneously polymerizes. In the final step of coagulation, thrombin further activates factor XIII, and factor XIIIa in turn causes noncovalent linkages to form between fibrin monomers, vastly increasing the tensile strength of the fibrin mesh within the platelet plug.

LABORATORY EVALUATION

Although the first step in identifying and classifying disorders of secondary hemostasis is *always* a careful history and physical examination, the focus here is on the laboratory evaluation of clotting disorders. The most commonly ordered screening test of clotting is the prothrombin time (PT). In this test, plasma is incubated with a lipoprotein thromboplastin that acts as a tissue factor for the extrinsic pathway. Factor VII is in turn activated, and so forth, down the coagulation schema. Thus, this test gives a sensitive measurement of factor VII availability and activity. Factor VII is usually the first of the coagulation factors to be depleted when oral anticoagulant therapy is begun (i.e., warfarin drugs); therefore, this test provides a good measure of the effects of the drug. Any acquired or congenital deficiencies of factors VII, X, or V, thrombin, or fibrinogen potentially may be reflected in a prolonged PT. Acquired deficiency of factor VII frequently accompanies significant liver disease.

The activated partial thromboplastin time (aPTT) is another commonly measured parameter of coagulation. Plasma is incubated with any of numerous substances, in effect providing a negatively charged surface for activation of the contact factors of coagulation. A phospholipid (which acts as a partial thromboplastin) is also added serially, along with calcium ion, so that the vitamin K–dependent factors down through the final common pathway of coagulation can be stimulated. Like the PT, the aPTT assesses factor X activation through fibrin formation. However, the aPTT measures coagulation through the intrinsic pathway and therefore is not sensitive to deficiencies or inhibitors of factor VII.

The thrombin time assesses both the quantitative and qualitative aspects of the conversion of fibrinogen to fibrin. Thrombin is incubated with plasma, and the time until appearance of a fibrin clot is measured. The myriad disorders associated with either availability or function of fibrinogen are assessed with this test. It is exquisitely sensitive to the presence of heparin and inhibitors of fibrin monomer polymerization (i.e., fibrin degradation products, dysfibrinogens). The reptilase time also provides an assessment of fibrinogen and its function. Like thrombin, the reptilase enzyme (derived from snake venom) cleaves polypeptides from fibrinogen, leading to activation and fibrin monomer formation. Unlike the thrombin time, however, the reptilase time is not affected by heparin.

Factor assays are also available for most of the important coagulation proteins involved in the clotting of blood. The general concept behind these assays involves providing the specific substrate for the factor that is suspected to be deficient. Subsequent time to clotting is then measured and clotting factor activity is reported as a percentage of normal activity.

PHYSIOLOGY AND BIOCHEMISTRY OF FIBRINOLYSIS

COMPONENTS

As discussed, normal hemostasis includes the regulation and inhibition of blood coagulation and fibrin clot formation in such a manner that regional blood loss from a damaged vessel is controlled without diffuse clot formation. For example, in the absence of a regulatory system, sufficient thrombin could locally be generated in 1 mL of whole blood to activate and coagulate all the fibrinogen in roughly 3 L of blood.[2] Inhibition of such a rapidly amplified system is essential.

The maintenance of blood fluidity is accomplished through multiple physiologic interactions (Table 18-4). This

TABLE 18-4. Factors That Maintain Blood Fluidity

CELLULAR COMPONENT
  (Phagocytic clearance of activated factors)
  Hepatocytes
  Reticuloendothelial system

HUMORAL COMPONENT
  (Direct inactivation of activated factors)
  Protein C
  Antithrombin III
  Plasmin (fibrinolysis)

initial discussion, however, is limited to the fibrinolytic system. The major enzyme component of the fibrinolytic system is plasminogen, the zymogen form of plasmin. It is primarily synthesized in the liver and circulates in the plasma at 10- to 20-mg/dL concentrations under basal conditions. Plasminogen concentrations, however, can greatly increase in response to inflammatory states, paralleling changes seen in fibrinogen levels. Consumption or decreased liver production accounts for subnormal serum concentrations. Interestingly, plasminogen is similar in size and structure to the contact activation factors. These same contact factors can in turn activate plasminogen, as is discussed in the following section.

FUNCTION IN NORMAL COAGULATION

Plasminogen activation occurs extrinsically, intrinsically, or exogenously. Intrinsic activation involves the contact factors of coagulation. As mentioned earlier, factor XIIa converts prekallikrein to kallikrein, which can then convert plasminogen to plasmin. Kallikrein also activates additional factor XII, so that amplification of the intrinsic pathway of coagulation also leads to simultaneous amplification of fibrinolysis. The involvement of the other contact factors seems necessary, but their role is not yet well understood.

The extrinsic activation of fibrinolysis, like the extrinsic pathway of coagulation, involves the presence of a tissue factor, in this case tPA. Although tPA is present in many tissues, it seems that its synthesis by vascular endothelial cells is key in the extrinsic activation of fibrinolysis. Several drugs, including vasopressin, 1-desamino-8-D-arginine vasopressin (DDAVP), and epinephrine, have the ability to enhance vessel wall production of tPA.[3] Pathophysiologic stimuli such as tissue anoxia or endothelial trauma also result in enhanced synthesis and secretion of tPA. tPA does not activate plasminogen in the absence of fibrin.

Finally, streptokinase and urokinase have been used clinically as exogenous activators of the fibrinolytic system. Streptokinase is a biologic product of certain Lancefield strains of beta-hemolytic streptococci and is antigenic in nature. Its mechanism of plasminogen activation seems related to a nonenzymatic, nonproteolytic reaction, through an alteration of the plasminogen active site that occurs on binding of the two molecules (streptokinase and plasminogen). The resultant complex directly cleaves a second molecule of plasminogen to its active form, plasmin. Urokinase was initially isolated from urine and fetal kidney cells but is now produced using recombinant DNA technology. In contrast to streptokinase, urokinase activates plasminogen through direct proteolytic action and is not antigenic. Recombinant human tPA (rh-tPA) also can be infused intravenously to activate fibrinolysis. Exogenously administered rh-tPA has identical actions as endogenously produced tPA.

Plasmin has the ability to digest fibrinogen and fibrin. Multiple sites of proteolysis have been described for both molecules, resulting in various by-products, known clinically as fibrin–fibrinogen degradation products. After spontaneous polymerization of fibrin monomers, factor XIIIa reacts with fibrin so that stabilizing covalent cross-linkages are formed between fibrin strands, which greatly improves the tensile strength of the fibrin structure. When plasmin digests

fibrin that has been cross-linked, a unique cleavage product, called the *D-dimer*, is formed. This can be measured and quantitated (discussed later).

After activation by any of the above described methods, fibrinolysis has the potential to interfere with normal hemostatic mechanisms. As stated, tPA does not activate plasminogen in the absence of fibrin, thus limiting fibrinolytic activity to the site of fibrin formation and thereby avoiding the systemic depletion of fibrinogen. (However, when used therapeutically, rh-tPA produces a systemic lytic state with dose-dependent depletion of plasma fibrinogen.) Further, several circulating plasma proteins exist that can inactivate plasmin. The most important of these are α_2-antiplasmin and α_2-macroglobulin. These efficient proteins have potent proteolytic activity, ensuring that any excess plasmin that finds its way into the general circulation is rapidly inactivated. Finally, C1 esterase inhibitor, an inhibitor of the complement system, also impedes the intrinsic activation of plasminogen by kallikrein. The activity of tPa is inhibited by PAI–1 (plasminogen activator inhibitor type 1) and to a lesser extent by PAI–2.

Several stimulators of fibrinolysis also exist. Thrombin stimulates the production and release of protein C, which in turn accelerates the production and local release of tPA. Platelet plug retraction is also a direct stimulus to fibrinolysis. Polymorphonuclear neutrophils, and perhaps monocytes, also may have the ability to stimulate or initiate fibrinolysis (possibly through interaction with platelets or platelet products), although the mechanism is unknown.[4]

LABORATORY EVALUATION

Tests that directly measure fibrinolytic function or activity are not as readily available as those that measure secondary hemostasis. In general, the PT, aPTT, and thrombin time are relatively insensitive to changes in fibrinolytic activity (including those induced by streptokinase or urokinase). Therefore, these tests are not useful in the diagnosis of increased fibrinolysis. An assay of plasma fibrinogen and fibrin degradation product levels provides some useful information concerning fibrinolysis or fibrinogenolysis, if basal levels are known. These quantitations clearly are not the tests of choice for either diagnosing or monitoring hyperfibrinolysis.

The most common test used to diagnose fibrinolysis is the euglobulin clot lysis time. However, it is not quantitative and is at best only a gross indicator of increased fibrinolytic activity. The test involves the precipitation of fibrinogen, plasminogen, and plasminogen activators by mixing a plasma sample with an acidic solution of low ionic strength. These precipitated proteins are then redissolved and allowed to clot, and the time to clot lysis is measured. A shortened time to clot lysis (less than 3 hours) indicates a state of increased fibrinolysis. Unfortunately, the degree of shortening of the euglobulin clot lysis time does not correlate with the extent of increased fibrinolysis. Further, difficulties in test interpretation can occur if the level of fibrinogen is low or if amounts of fibrin degradation products sufficient to impede clot formation are present.

Recently, assays for the D-dimer fibrin degradation product have been developed. The presence of increased amounts of D-dimer in plasma or serum indicates thrombin generation and active fibrinolysis. This test is theoretically negative in instances of primary fibrinolysis, where fibrinogen—not cross-linked fibrin—is being degraded (unless secondary bleeding with subsequent thrombin generation and clotting has already occurred). The absolute specificity of the commercially available D-dimer assays is directly related to the specificity of the anti–D-dimer antibody employed in the assay. Consequently, many of the assays may still recognize some amount of fibrinogen degradation products. Interpretation of a D-dimer assay result must accordingly be tempered by this realization. In cases of increased fibrinolysis, plasma levels of plasminogen will be low, and those of plasmin will be elevated.

COAGULATION AS AN INTEGRATED SYSTEM ■

The compartmentalization of the various aspects of coagulation, as presented here, is intended to ease the burden of conceptualization for the reader. In vivo coagulation physiology, however, can be understood only as an integrated system. Although many of these interactions have been discussed throughout this chapter, the central role of thrombin deserves final emphasis.

Within seconds after the vascular endothelium is denuded or injured, measurable levels of thrombin are present. This has several effects. Platelet aggregation and platelet granule release are strongly stimulated by thrombin while it is formed on the platelet surface. Thrombin also can modify circulating factor V so that its binding affinity is greatly increased, resulting in an increased rate of factor X activa-tion. Ultimately, this increases the rate of additional thrombin formation, all of which lead to an explosive potentiation of both primary and secondary hemostasis.[1] Finally, thrombin-mediated factor XIII activation is important in platelet plug–fibrin mesh stabilization.

Thrombin also controls its fate, to a certain extent, through a series of inhibitory events that it initiates simultaneously. While thrombin is released into the circulation, binding with the thrombomodulin receptor of intact endothelium occurs. Activated protein C is generated as a result of this binding. Protein C, in turn, in the presence of protein S, inactivates factors Va and VIIIa and stimulates plasminogen activation. Thrombin also binds with antithrombin III at the endothelial surface, effectively removing activated thrombin from the circulation. In addition to this interaction, other serum proteases, such as α_1-antitrypsin and α_2-macroglobulin, have some degree of activity against thrombin in a nonspecific fashion.

REFERENCES ■

1. Thompson AR, Harker LA: *Manual of Hemostasis and Thrombosis*. Philadelphia, FA Davis, 1983
2. Rifkind RA, Bank A, Marks PA, et al: Hemostasis: normal mechanisms. In: *Fundamentals of Hematology*. Chicago, Year Book Medical Publishers, 1986
3. Triplett DA: *Hemostasis: A Case Oriented Approach*. New York, Igaku-Shoin, 1985
4. Lammle B, Griffin JH: Formation of the fibrin clot: the balance of procoagulant and inhibitory factors. *Clin Lab Haematol* 1985; 14:281
5. Sultan C, Gouault-Heilmann M, Imbert M: *Manual of Hematology*. New York, John Wiley & Sons, 1985

Critical Care, Third Edition, edited by Joseph M. Civetta,
Robert W. Taylor, and Robert R. Kirby.
Lippincott-Raven Publishers, Philadelphia, PA © 1997.

CHAPTER 19

■

Central Nervous System Injury: Essential Physiologic and Therapeutic Concerns

Christopher Veremakis
David H. Lindner

IMMEDIATE CONCERNS ■

MAJOR PROBLEMS

Acute central nervous system injury occurs with head trauma, focal ischemia, global anoxia, metabolic derangements, or infection. The ultimate neurologic sequelae are the result of this primary injury and any secondary neuronal injury that may develop in the minutes to days after the initial insult. The emphasis of the critical care team should be on the prevention and treatment of this secondary injury. On initial contact, the evaluating physician should assume that the patient has ongoing secondary injury and act accordingly. Time is critical. All appropriate resuscitative efforts should be instituted without delay. Aggressive critical care can improve survival and functional neurologic recovery. The optimal care of patients with neurologic injury requires that the physician and staff recognize and understand the factors that lead to secondary injury and are able to focus therapy on preventing or ameliorating this process.

This chapter reviews (1) the physiologic principles governing the intracranial contents, (2) the mechanisms of secondary brain injury, and (3) a rational therapeutic approach to the neurologically injured patient. Emphasis is placed on the common pathophysiologic processes of secondary injury and the impact and interaction between the neurologic injury and systemic physiology. General recommendations and specific therapeutic options for brain resuscitation are discussed in the context of this altered physiologic makeup.

STRESS POINTS

1. Significant secondary ischemic injury complicates the primary central nervous system (CNS) insult in most forms of brain injury.
2. The secondary injury may comprise a large portion of the ultimate neurologic deficit.
3. Preventing secondary injury is the focus of neurologic critical care.
4. Secondary injury is most often the result of hypotension, hypoxemia, surgically correctable expanding mass lesions, elevated intracranial pressure (ICP), or intracranial oxygen supply–demand imbalance.
5. Tissue salvage is the therapeutic goal. Specific treatment (if available) must be instituted as rapidly as possible.
6. Surgically correctable lesions must be delineated rapidly.

ESSENTIAL DIAGNOSTIC TESTS AND PROCEDURES

1. Rapid general history and physical to define non-CNS disease

273

2. Rapid modified neurologic examination to define level of consciousness, motor function, and cranial nerve involvement
3. Noncontrast computed tomography (CT) to exclude surgical lesions, hemorrhage, or both
4. Electrolytes, glucose, calcium, prothrombin time, and partial thromboplastin time
5. ICP monitoring (if indicated)

INITIAL TREATMENT

1. Stabilize cardiopulmonary function.
2. Supplement with oxygen.
3. Intervene surgically (if applicable).
4. Correct hematologic and metabolic abnormalities.
5. Control ICP (if applicable).
6. Improve cerebral blood flow (CBF) (if applicable).
7. Control cerebral metabolic activity.
8. Institute cytoprotective therapy (if applicable).

MECHANISMS OF BRAIN INJURY

Central nervous system injury can be classified as primary or secondary, although the causes of secondary injury may follow the primary injury within seconds. Secondary damage is conceptually a part of the primary disease state but may be viewed as a complication and therefore is potentially preventable.

Recently, ischemia has been identified as the central mechanism of secondary cell injury in most forms of CNS insult. Interestingly, the injured brain seems to be more vulnerable to additional ischemic injuries because of impaired regulation of blood flow and chemical mediator–induced "sensitization" to further ischemic insults. Cerebral ischemia ultimately results from a mismatch of tissue oxygen supply to oxygen demand; oxygen delivery is inadequate for the metabolic requirements of the tissue. As in systemic tissue, this imbalance may occur as a consequence of impaired oxygen delivery, increased oxygen demand, or impaired tissue oxygen utilization. Global cerebral oxygen delivery ($C\dot{D}o_2$) is the product of CBF and arterial oxygen content (Cao_2). Consequently, decreased $C\dot{D}o_2$ may result from a generalized or focal decrease of CBF, a deficiency in hemoglobin concentration, or hypoxemia (Table 19-1). Cerebral metabolic consumption of oxygen ($CMRo_2$) is reduced in coma but may be increased by seizures, hyperthermia, or injury-induced release of excitatory amino acid neurotransmitters. The resulting oxygen debt rapidly causes the depletion of high-energy substrates and initiates anaerobic glycolysis and the failure of phosphocreatine and ATP production. Cerebral tissue oxygen uptake and utilization also may be impaired. Compared with other organs, the brain is especially vulnerable to ischemia because of its high resting energy requirement and the lack of oxygen stores.[1-4]

At the cellular level, the imbalance of oxygen supply and demand impairs the ATP-dependent sodium-potassium pump. Consequently, the cells lose ionic homeostasis. Potassium leaks out of the cell, and calcium, sodium, and water diffuse into the cells from the extracellular space. Oxidative phosphorylation is uncoupled, and cellular respiration is impaired as a result of the mitochondrial sequestration of calcium ion. Intracellular pH declines in direct relation to lactate production, and the damaged cells release excitatory neurotransmitters. This may further worsen ionic disequilibrium, perpetuate cellular injury, alter energy production, and promote iron-mediated free radical production. Cytoplasmic free calcium enhances the intracellular breakdown of lipids and proteins, promoting cell membrane degradation. With prolonged ischemia, oxygen stores are exhausted and cellular death ensues.[1-4]

Critical thresholds of cerebral oxygen delivery and consumption have been characterized for neuronal function and viability (Fig 19-1). A normal human adult has a CBF ranging from 30 to 70 mL/100 g/minute. Diminished CBF leads to progressive loss of electrical activity. Neuronal dysfunction develops below a flow of 20 mL/100 g/minute, the electroencephalogram becomes isoelectric, and synaptic transmission ceases at flows below 15 mL/100 g/minute. This level of flow has been described as the threshold of electrical failure. With further reduction of CBF below 10 mL/100 g/minute, there is failure of the ionic pump mechanisms and ATP depletion. This level has been described as the threshold of membrane failure.[1-4]

Brain tissue with blood flow between the upper limit of the threshold for electrical failure and the lower limit of the threshold for membrane failure illustrates the clinical

TABLE 19-1.   Cerebral Oxygen Delivery and Consumption

	APPROXIMATE VALUE
Cerebral blood flow (CBF)	50 mL/100 g/min
Systemic arterial oxygen content (Cao_2)	14–20 mL/100 mL
Jugular venous oxygen content ($Cjvo_2$)	8–13 mL/100 mL
Jugular venous oxygen saturation ($Sjvo_2$)	65%
Cerebral arterial–venous oxygen content difference [$C(a-v)o_2 = Cao_2 - Cjvo_2$]	6.3 mL/100 mL
Cerebral oxygen delivery ($C\dot{D}o_2 = CBF \times Cao_2$)	10 mL/100 g/min
Cerebral metabolic rate of oxygen consumption [$CMRo_2 = CBF \times C(a-v)o_2$]	3.5 mL/100 g/min

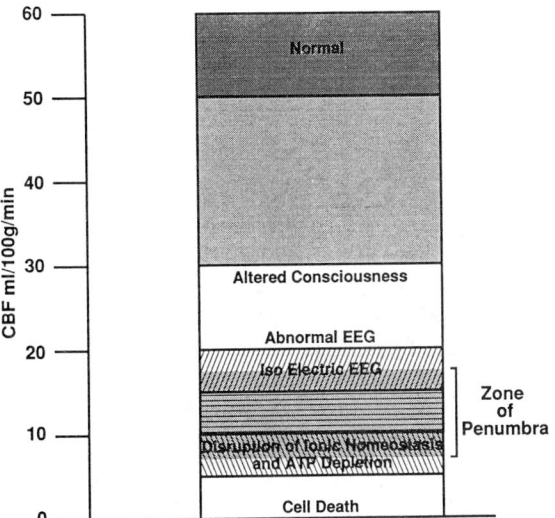

FIGURE 19-1. Flow thresholds for cerebral function and metabolism. As cerebral blood flow (CBF) is diminished, electroencephalographic silence occurs, followed by energy failure and disruption of ionic homeostasis. The zone of penumbra describes brain tissue with flows between the upper limit of the threshold of electrical failure and the lower limit of the threshold of membrane failure. EEG, electroencephalogram. (Modified with permission of the American Heart Association, Inc. From Astrup J, Symon L, Branston N, et al: Cortical evoked potential and extracellular K^+ and H^+ at critical levels of brain ischemia. *Stroke* 1977;8:51.)

concept of the ischemic penumbra introduced by Astrup.[2] Ischemic tissue in this zone is electrically silent and nonfunctional but marginally viable. Such tissue may recover if adequate flow is restored or may become irreversibly damaged with sustained ischemia. The duration and severity of ischemia as well as several metabolic factors (e.g. temperature, hyperglycemia) influence the extent of residual brain damage. The time window for reversibility and salvage of the penumbra in humans is unknown but in animal models is 4 hours or less. Incomplete ischemia may be tolerated for hours before irreversible damage occurs. Variations in regional vulnerability also play a role; gray matter is more sensitive to ischemia than white matter. Inhomogeneous vulnerability is the result of regional differences in collateral blood flow, capillary density, and basal metabolic activity.[2,5–7]

The injured brain is particularly vulnerable to secondary global hypoxic injury. Seemingly insignificant transient episodes of hypotension or hypoxemia may cause additional neuronal damage. Consequently, aggressive supportive care to stabilize oxygen transport and avoid even mild episodes of hypotension and hypoxemia is mandatory. Scrupulous monitoring and meticulous nursing care cannot be overemphasized. Nevertheless, despite successful optimization of the systemic circulation, further ischemic injuries frequently result from intracranial aberrations of CBF. The basic pathophysiologic mechanisms responsible for this damage include (1) ICP-induced injury, (2) loss of normal vasoregulatory control, (3) excessive cerebral metabolic demand, and (4) reperfusion injury.[8,9] Therefore, neurologic intensive care is directed toward preventing or reversing the pathophysio-

logic events that impair regional or global CBF or perpetuate the imbalance between CDo_2 and $CMRo_2$.

INTRACRANIAL PRESSURE

Under normal circumstances, the intracranial contents consist of the brain (80%), the cerebrospinal fluid (CBF, 10%), and blood (10%). Because the intracranial contents are enclosed in a nondistensible protective compartment (i.e., skull), any increase in the volume of one component causes a decrease in the volume of the other components, an increase in the pressure within the intracranial cavity, or a combination of the two. This principle is known as the Monro-Kellie doctrine. The pressure–volume relationship of the intracranial cavity is depicted in Figure 19-2. Because the brain is essentially noncompressible, any increase in intracranial volume initially decreases the CSF or the cerebral blood volume (CBV). Primary compensation results from the displacement of CSF into the distensible spinal subarachnoid space. A decrease of CBV through venoconstriction of CNS capacitance vessels provides additional compensatory volume displacement into the jugular venous system. (points 1 to 2, see Fig. 19-2). After these mechanisms are exhausted, additional small increases in intracranial volume result in marked elevations of ICP (points 2 to 3, see Fig. 19-2). Generalized increases of ICP decrease cerebral perfusion pressure, which may compromise CBF, especially if vasoregulation is impaired.

When elevated ICP is unevenly distributed throughout the cranium, pressure gradients may compress tissue altering capillary blood flow. Under extreme conditions, rapid changes in pressure may displace brain tissue into other cranial compartments, resulting in massive neuronal destruction termed a herniation syndrome. Under other circumstances, slow progressive volume encroachment, as occurs with tumors, may be well tolerated despite structural distortion because compensatory mechanisms maintain a low ICP. In this setting, however, minimal acute increases of

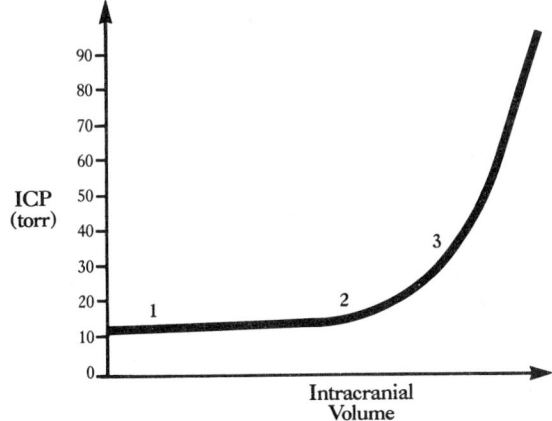

FIGURE 19-2. The curve describes the compliance characteristics of the intracranial compartment. The flat portion of the curve ($1 \rightarrow 2$) reflects the existing compensatory mechanisms as intracranial volume rises. ICP, intracranial pressure. (From Shapiro HM: Intracranial hypertension: therapeutic and anesthetic considerations. *Anesthesiology* 1975;43:445.)

intracranial volume may precipitously elevate ICP because intracranial compliance is decreased. If an elevated ICP is equally distributed throughout the brain and normal vaso-regulation of CBF is intact, high pressures may not be associated with functional neurologic impairment. Therefore, the deleterious effect of an elevated ICP is a function of the failure of normal compensatory mechanisms and the rate of change rather than the absolute ICP. Acute brain injury usually produces rapid elevations in ICP and impairment of normal vasoregulation. This characteristic pathophysiology provides the practical basis for clinical ICP monitoring. The most common clinical entities associated with pathologic increases of ICP include all forms of traumatic brain injury, intracranial bleeding, and any process that induces generalized edema.[10,11]

A normal ICP is 0 to 10 mm Hg; pathologic intracranial hypertension is defined as an ICP of 20 mm Hg or higher. Clinically significant ICP elevations develop in as many 55% of patients with traumatic head injury within the first 72 hours after injury and are associated with increased neurologic morbidity and mortality.[10,11] Persistent and uncontrollable ICP elevations occur in approximately 15% of head-injured patients and are usually fatal. Pathologic elevations are seen most frequently in association with intracranial hematomas and contusions, but significant elevations also may develop in the absence of focal lesions or midline shift on CT. Hyperemic CBF after traumatic head injury also is associated with increased ICP.[12] After cardiac arrest, sustained elevations of ICP are uncommon in the absence of underlying cranial disease or seizures. Raised ICP also plays a pathophysiologic role in toxic encephalopathies such as Reye's syndrome and fulminant hepatic failure, in large hemispheric strokes associated with cerebral edema, and in encephalitis and is adversely related to outcome in these syndromes.[13–15]

REGULATION OF CEREBRAL BLOOD FLOW

The brain receives 15% of the cardiac output. Global CBF is approximately 50 to 55 mL/100 g/minute but varies regionally from 20 to 80 mL according to metabolic activity. The CBV occupies 10% of the intracranial space, and most of this volume is stored within the venous capacitance vessels. The most common technique used clinically to measure CBF employs parenteral or inhaled radioactive xenon. The major determinants of CBF and cerebral vascular resistance are PaO_2, $PaCO_2$, pressure autoregulation, and the level of neuronal stimulation.

Under normal circumstances, CBF is closely regulated and matched to metabolic needs. The level of neural activity impacts CBF secondarily by flow-metabolism coupling in response to changes in $CMRo_2$. A more direct neuronal effect on CBF may exist, although there is no evidence of tonic autonomic regulation.[16–18]

Hypoxia and hypercapnia produce cerebral vasodilation and increase CBF (Fig. 19-3). Hypoxia does not have a significant impact unless the Po_2 drops below 50 torr. However, CBF and CBV are exquisitely sensitive to changes in the partial pressure of carbon dioxide. Within the physiologic range, a 1-mm Hg change in $PaCO_2$ results in a 3% to 4%

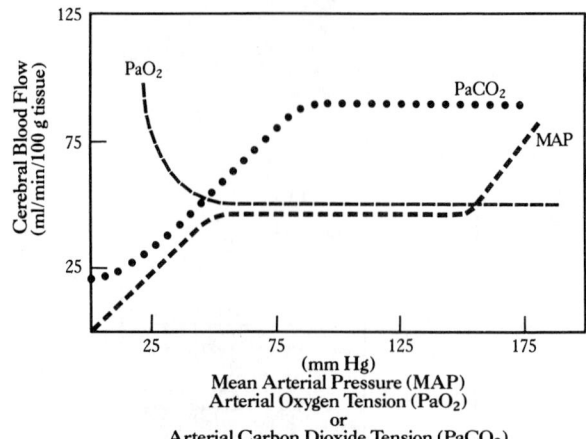

FIGURE 19-3. Changes in cerebral blood flow in response to changes in mean arterial pressure (MAP), arterial oxygen tension (PaO_2), or arterial carbon dioxide tension ($PaCO_2$). If autoregulation is intact, cerebral blood flow remains constant as MAP varies between 50 and 150 mm Hg.

change in CBF and a 0.04-mL/100 g change in CBV. These effects are mediated by alterations in extracellular fluid pH, which influences vascular smooth muscle. The marked dependence of CBF and CBV on $PaCO_2$ has important clinical implications, especially if intracranial pressure–volume compensatory mechanisms have reached their limits. Clinically, hypoventilation (hypercapnia) may precipitate a herniation syndrome in a patient with cerebral edema or mass effect. Conversely, induced hyperventilation (hypocapnia) may therapeutically lower or control an elevated ICP.[16–18]

The principle of autoregulation describes the mechanism by which a constant CBF is maintained over the normal range of mean arterial pressure (MAP), that is, between 50 and 100 mm Hg. Below 50 mm Hg or above 150 mm Hg, CBF becomes linearly related to blood pressure. These set points may be elevated in chronic hypertension because of hypertrophic and fibrotic changes in the resistance vessels. The true driving force of CBF is the cerebral perfusion pressure (CPP), which is defined as the difference between the MAP and the cerebral venous pressure. Arterial vasodilation compensates for a falling CPP, maintaining CBF until the lower autoregulatory limit is reached, after which CBF declines. Normally, CBF becomes compromised below a CPP of 50 mm Hg. Under pathologic conditions, however, pressure autoregulation is completely or partially disrupted and CBF is linearly related to CPP. In addition, CBF may be compromised at normal blood pressures. When ICP is elevated, CPP equals MAP minus ICP. Therefore, the ICP becomes the limiting downstream pressure. Because the interaction between ICP, cerebral vasoreactivity, blood volume, and dysfunctional autoregulation are complex, poorly understood, and variable within different regions of the brain, it is impossible to delineate the best set of cerebral hemodynamic/ventilatory parameters for each patient. As an example, in a patient with impaired autoregulation, raising MAP may either improve blood flow to an ischemic area or increase edema, CBV, and ICP, thus impairing perfusion further. As a general rule, ICP should be maintained below

20 to 25 mm Hg and cerebral perfusion pressure maintained at approximately 70 mm Hg.[16-19]

Many pathophysiologic events may operate to impair regional CBF in the injured brain, even if CPP or global CBF are adequate. Delineation of the importance of regional flow impairment awaits the refinement of techniques that allow quantification of regional flow variations in specific diseases and in response to specific therapeutic maneuvers.

PATHOLOGIC ALTERATIONS OF CEREBRAL BLOOD FLOW

Hypoperfusion After Brain Injury

Generalized and regional decreases in CBF have been reported after head injury, subarachnoid hemorrhage, stroke, and cardiac arrest. With restoration of circulation after cardiac arrest, four subsequent stages of cerebral reperfusion abnormalities have been described. In the first stage, a multifocal absence of cerebral perfusion (no reflow phenomenon) is seen immediately after the ischemic episode. The extent of no reflow depends on the duration and severity of the insult. This phenomenon has been attributed to microcirculatory obstruction at the capillary level and provides a pathophysiologic basis for irreversible damage resulting from the primary ischemic injury. No reflow may resolve spontaneously or persist in multiple areas of the brain. In the second stage, transient global hyperemia occurs during the first 10 to 20 minutes after circulation is restored and lasts for approximately 15 to 30 minutes. During the third stage, delayed global hypoperfusion develops at approximately 90 minutes after systemic reperfusion and persists for longer than 6 hours. Postischemic hypoperfusion is attributed to vasoconstriction and is an important cause of secondary brain injury. Finally, in the fourth stage, aberrant flow resolves or the abnormalities persist with complete cessation of blood flow and brain death.[3,16,20-22]

Hyperemia and Vasospasm

The luxury perfusion syndrome describes areas of injured brain with CBF in excess of cerebral metabolic needs. This loss of normal flow-metabolism coupling is presumably a result of impaired vasomotor regulation. Hyperemia may promote secondary brain injury by increasing intravascular hydrostatic pressure, producing edema and increasing ICP. Absolute and relative hyperemia have been observed after acute stroke, traumatic head injury, or after successful resuscitation in cardiac arrest. Bilateral diffuse brain swelling after traumatic injury in children results directly from hyperemia and increased CBV rather than primary brain edema. Although hyperemia is more common in pediatric patients, it may occur in comatose head-injured adults.[17,12,20,23]

Severe arterial vasospasm may result in significant ischemic injury and is the major source of postadmission morbidity after subarachnoid hemorrhage. Angiographic vasospasm may be present with or without clinical symptoms of cerebral ischemia. Vasospasm develops in as many as 35% of patients with severe head injury, although its relevance in this setting has not been clearly defined. The mechanisms responsible for vasospasm are poorly understood, but blood within the subarachnoid space is a necessary prerequisite. The activation or lysis of clot (i.e., platelets, mast cells, neutrophils, erythrocytes) may initiate an inflammatory response in blood vessels or may promote the release of endogenous vasoactive mediators. Vasospasm commonly develops within 3 to 10 days after subarachnoid bleeding, often involves multiple arteries near the area of hemorrhage, and may persist for up to 10 to 14 days.[16,21,24]

CEREBRAL METABOLISM

The brain uses approximately 20% of the body's total oxygen consumption. Global cerebral oxygen consumption ($CMRo_2$) averages 3.5 mL/100 g/minute and may be divided into two components: (1) basal metabolic energy, and (2) electrical work or "activation energy." Forty-five percent of the total brain energy consumption results from basal energy requirements. $CMRo_2$ is decreased by one third to one half in patients with severe brain injuries. Evidence suggests that this decrease results from the diminution of electrical work and is directly proportional to the depth of coma as reflected by the score on the Glasgow Coma Scale. Insertion of a percutaneous catheter through the jugular vein to the level of the jugular bulb allows sampling of venous blood and measurement of jugular venous saturation. Near-infrared spectrophotometry (niroscopy) provides a noninvasive method of monitoring cerebral venous oxygen saturation. $CMRo_2$ can be calculated as the product of the arterial–jugular venous oxygen content difference [$C(a - v)O_2$] and CBF. Simultaneous sampling of systemic arterial and jugular venous blood allows calculation of the $C(a - v)O_2$. Positron emission tomography, primarily available as a research tool, is capable of determining global and regional $CMRo_2$, oxygen extraction, and glucose metabolism. $CMRo_2$ increases with neuronal activity, seizures, and fever. A 1°C increase in temperature can raise $CMRo_2$ by as much as 10% to 15%. Hypothermia, the volatile anesthetics, barbiturates, and benzodiazepines decrease $CMRo_2$.[25-30]

Normally CBF is closely coupled to $CMRo_2$ and changes in parallel to match alterations in brain oxygen consumption, so that $C(a - v)O_2$ remains constant. A low CBF must be interpreted in terms of flow-metabolism coupling. For example, during general anesthesia, $CMRo_2$ decreases and CBF consequently decreases, and $C(a - v)O_2$ remains in the normal range (Table 19-2). If CBF is compromised, a constant $CMRo_2$ is maintained by increased oxygen extraction and, therefore, $C(a - v)O_2$ widens. Investigation of brain metabolism with positron emission tomography scanning has demonstrated that increased oxygen extraction maintains a normal $CMRo_2$ in the face of dropping CBF until compensatory mechanisms are exhausted. Thereafter, $CMRo_2$ decreases and cerebral lactate production increases in association with cellular disruption and infarction. Normal flow-metabolism coupling may be disrupted in some forms of brain injury. Tracking jugular venous desaturation may provide a mechanism of identifying early cerebral ischemia. The interrelationships of CBF, $CMRo_2$, and $C(a - v)O_2$ in normal and injured brain are summarized in Table 19-2. Because the major etiology of secondary injury involves

TABLE 19-2. Interrelationships of CBF, $CMRo_2$, and $C(a - v)o_2$ in Brain Injury

CIRCULATORY STATUS	CBF	$CMRo_2$	$C(a - v)o_2$
Normal	N	N	N
Compensatory flow-metabolism coupline	↓	↓	N
Compensatory flow-metabolism coupling	↑	↑	N
Ischemia	↓	N	↑
Infarction	↓	↓	↓
Hyperemia	↑/N	↓	↓

CBF, cerebral blood flow; $CMRo_2$, cerebral metabolic rate of oxygen consumption; $C(a - v)o_2$, cerebral arterial–venous oxygen content difference; N, normal.

an ischemic process, therapeutic maneuvers to decrease $CMRo_2$ may improve oxygen supply demand imbalance and therefore salvage neuronal tissue.[20,21,25]

BRAIN EDEMA

Injured brain, like other tissues, swells when it is damaged. Brain edema, defined as the abnormal accumulation of fluid within brain parenchyma associated with a volumetric enlargement of brain tissue, develops in response to many forms of intracranial disease, but also may complicate systemic disorders such as diabetic ketoacidosis and hepatic failure. Edema per se is not necessarily deleterious, but it may promote secondary injury by impairing regional (focal brain compression) or global CBF (ICP elevation). Herniation of the brain is the most devastating consequence of severe brain edema.

Three types of cerebral edema have been described: cytotoxic, vasogenic, and interstitial. Cytotoxic edema develops with cell membrane damage and failure of the ATP-dependent mechanisms that maintain ionic homeostasis and osmolar gradients. This form of edema is precipitated by systemic hypotension and hypoxia, hypoosmolar states, purulent meningitis, and by toxins that impair oxidative phosphorylation or cellular respiration.

Vasogenic edema occurs with the extravasation of protein-rich fluid from the intravascular to the extracellular space as a consequence of capillary endothelial damage. The pathophysiologic mechanism involves compromise of endothelial tight junctions, which are thought to comprise the blood–brain barrier. Hyperemia, hypertension above the upper autoregulatory limit, or CPP elevations with impaired autoregulation may exacerbate vasogenic edema. The severity of vasogenic edema depends on the pressure-dependent leakage of protein into the interstitium. This form of edema is found with brain tumor or abscess, contusion, hemorrhage, infarction, lead intoxication, and purulent meningitis.

Interstitial edema as occurs with obstructive hydrocephalus results from the shift of fluid from the ventricles into the periventricular interstitium. The volume of periventricular white matter is reduced, and extracellular fluid volume is increased.

Ischemic brain edema contains elements of vasogenic and cytotoxic edema. The magnitude of edema depends on the extent and duration of the insult. Cytotoxic swelling develops initially when CBF is decreased to less than 20 mL/100 g/minute. Vasogenic edema develops several hours later, with the breakdown the blood–brain barrier. Ischemic brain edema becomes maximal after several days as the extracellular space enlarges from continued protein leakage and necrotic changes. As edema evolves, ICP rises. Local increases in tissue pressure may further diminish flow below the ischemic threshold, advancing the perimeter of irreversible damage. Ischemic brain edema peaks 48 to 72 hours after the initial insult, and then resolves if additional mechanisms of secondary injury do not intervene.[31,32]

SUMMARY

Primary brain injury destroys neural tissue. Systemic cardiopulmonary instability often aggravates the brain insult. Ischemic cellular dysfunction initiates mechanisms that produce further injury at the cellular level, including calcium-mediated cell damage, intracellular acidosis, and the formation of free radicals and other toxic mediators. On the tissue level, primary injury can trigger a chain of events that impair cerebral perfusion, vascular reactivity, and regulation of intracranial volume, overwhelming normal compensatory mechanisms. As these mechanisms fail, regional or global decreases in CBF or increases in ICP diminish CPP and worsen tissue ischemia. These concepts are generally applicable to all forms of neurologic injury, although certain processes assume more or less prominence, depending on the initiating disease or condition. Table 19-3 lists the most frequent causes of primary brain injury and the characteristics of associated secondary injury.

THERAPEUTIC CONSIDERATIONS DURING BRAIN RESUSCITATION ■

INITIAL STABILIZATION

The most comprehensive goal of brain resuscitation is to restore the balance between cerebral oxygen supply and demand by resuscitation from the primary injury and prevention or amelioration of secondary neurologic injury. General and specific therapeutic strategies are directed toward im-

TABLE 19-3. Pathophysiologic Mechanisms of Secondary Ischemic Injury

PRIMARY DISEASE OR TRAUMA	PATHOPHYSIOLOIC MECHANISMS OF SECONDARY INJURY
Traumatic head injury	Hypotension, hypoxemia, mass lesions, edema, increased ICP, hyperemia, vasospasm, seizures
Subarachnoid hemorrhage	Rebleed, vasospasm, increased ICP, seizures
Ischemic stroke	Regional hypoperfusion, hyperemia, edema and increased ICP in massive strokes, reperfusion injury, seizures
Cardiac arrest	Hyperemia, reperfusion injury, delayed global hypoperfusion, seizures
Brain tumor	Compressive effect of mass lesion, vasogenic edema, elevated ICP, seizures
Metabolic encephalopathy, Reye's syndrome, fulminant hepatic failure	Toxins, edema, elevated ICP, seizures

ICP, intracranial pressure.

proving $C\dot{D}O_2$ by maximizing arterial oxygen content (CaO_2) and CBF or reducing $CMRO_2$.

Management of neurologic injury begins with the establishment of adequate cardiopulmonary function. Secondary brain insults are frequently caused by unrecognized or untreated episodes of hypoxemia and hypotension. The "ABCs" of basic life support (i.e., airway, breathing, circulation) must be addressed, followed by correction of shock, severe anemia, and hypoxemia. Stabilization of cardiopulmonary function may be the most powerful means of improving morbidity and mortality after severe brain injury. If systemic oxygen delivery is acceptable, general and specific therapies directed at brain resuscitation can be instituted simultaneously (Tables 19-4 and 19-5).[33,34]

A patient who presents as unconscious or uncommunicative, with focal neurologic defects or with a deteriorating neurologic examination, has ongoing secondary brain injury. Initial neurologic assessment involves evaluating the level of consciousness; breathing pattern; pupillary size, shape, and reactivity; eye movements (i.e., testing with calorics or doll's head maneuvers in the comatose patient); and delineation of purposeful or reflex motor activity. In the first 24 hours after brain injury, the standard "q 1 hr neuro check" is generally inadequate, and serial examination may be necessary every 15 to 30 minutes. Deterioration of the neurologic examination implies new ongoing secondary injury. The frequency of assessment should be guided by knowledge of the pathophysiologic features of the specific disease and the potential for rapid deterioration.

CT SCAN AND THE DIAGNOSIS OF EMERGENT SURGICAL LESIONS

The initial diagnostic evaluation must differentiate hemorrhagic from nonhemorrhagic brain insults and identify lesions that require surgical intervention. CT scan, the diag-

TABLE 19-4. Treatment Goals of Brain Resuscitation

GOAL	ACTION
Increased cerebral oxygen delivery	
Improve CaO_2	Avoid hypoxemia, O_2 Sat $\geq 93\%$
	Control airway
	Correct anemia, Hgb 9–10 g
Improve CBF	Stabilize BP
	Establish normovolemia
	Reduce ICP by minimizing cerebral venous pressure and intrathoracic pressure; avoid agitation
Reduce cerebral metabolic rate	Control hyperthermia
	Control seizures
	Control pain
	Avoid agitation, excessive stimulation, shivering

CaO_2, arterial oxygen content; CBF, cerebral blood flow; ICP, intracranial pressure; O_2 Sat, oxygen saturation; BP, blood pressure; Hgb, hemoglobin.

TABLE 19-5. Specific Treatment Options During Brain Resuscitation

CONDITION	ESTABLISHED TREATMENT	ADJUNCTIVE TREATMENT	INVESTIGATIONAL/ PROMISING	NOT BENEFICIAL
ICP elevation	Osmotic agents, CSF drainage	Hyperventilation, furosemide, barbiturates for refractory ↑ICP	Hypothermia	Steroids
Edema Ischemic Peritumor Interstitial	Osmotic diuretics Steroids	Furosemide Acetazolamide, steroids(?) for inflammatory etiology		Steroids
Vasospasm	Normovolemia, calcium channel blockers	Hemodilution-induced hypertension	Perfluorocarbons	
Focal ischemia	Supportive care	Hemodilution, anticoagulation(?) in some cases; glucose control	Calcium channel blockers, excitatory neurotransmitters, free radical scavengers Calcium channel blockers, excitatory neurotransmitters, free radical scavengers, hypothermia	Barbiturates

ICP, intracranial pressure; CSF, cerebrospinal fluid.

nostic procedure of choice, characterizes the extent of primary injury and the necessity for emergent surgical intervention. A mass lesion (e.g. epidural, subdural, intracerebral, or cerebellar hematoma) accompanied by significant brain shift is an indication for surgical removal. The importance of rapid identification and definitive treatment of expanding mass lesions cannot be overemphasized. Morbidity and mortality with subdural hematoma are significantly improved if evacuation occurs within 4 hours of presentation.[35] A high incidence of surgically correctable lesions is associated with a history of head trauma, recent neurologic surgery, anticoagulant therapy, ethanol abuse, and chronic hypertension. If an expanding mass lesion is strongly suspected, medical therapy to control ICP and prevent herniation should be instituted before and during CT scanning. Patients should be attended by a physician at all times. Temporizing measures pending surgical intervention include intubation, hyperventilation, and the intravenous administration of osmotic agents.

CT scan also generates important information concerning nonsurgical brain lesions. After traumatic head injury, the initial CT scan indicates the probability of significant ICP elevation. Sustained ICP elevations are relatively infrequent (15% to 30%) with a normal admission CT scan. Contusions or hematomas, with or without midline shift, are associated with ICP elevations in more than 50% of patients. However, the absence of a contusion or hematoma does not absolutely exclude later development of increased ICP. In one clinical series, abnormal ventricles (i.e., small, absent, or enlarged) reliably predicted the development of sustained ICP greater than 30 mm Hg during the first 72 hours after trauma. In

other series, only 33% of patients with "diffuse injury" (i.e. normal, reduced, or absent ventricles without midline shift) developed intracranial hypertension as opposed to 53% of patients with low-density CT lesions. In head-injured patients with normal results on CT scan, the risk of significant ICP elevation is increased if two or more factors are present: systolic blood pressure less than 90 mm Hg, abnormal motor posturing, or age older than 40 years. Because approximately one third of patients with normal admission CT scans develop new abnormalities (e.g., generalized brain swelling, delayed hematoma) during the first week after trauma, a follow-up CT scan should be obtained in a few days or at the first sign of clinical deterioration.[11,12,35-37] CT scan remains the best diagnostic test for identification of intracranial blood. On the other hand, cerebral infarction is poorly identified within the first 24 hours of an ischemic stroke.[38]

PHARMACOLOGIC AGENTS AND INTRACRANIAL PRESSURE

A variety of pharmacologic agents used in the intensive care setting may have profound effects on CBF and CBV. The volatile anesthetics are potent cerebral vasodilators, increasing CBF and decreasing $CMRo_2$. The dissociative anesthetic ketamine increases CBF without the "protective" effect of decreased $CMRo_2$; its use is not recommended in patients at risk for secondary neurologic injury. Haldol lowers the seizure threshold and also is not a preferred agent. Propofol has no direct effect on CBF and lowers $CMRo_2$ and ICP. However, it also uniformly lowers blood pressure and CPP by approximately 20% and therefore should be employed with caution. Barbiturates decrease $CMRO_2$ and CBF. The narcotic agents usually do not affect or decrease CBF and $CMRO_2$. The benzodiazepines decrease CBF and $CMRO_2$.[27,28,39]

The neuromuscular blocking agent succinylcholine has the advantage of rapid onset and short duration of action, but it has been reported to increase ICP during laryngoscopy and intubation. This agent also may cause hyperkalemia. Its use is not recommended in patients with brain injury. The nondepolarizing muscle relaxants and vecuronium have no direct effects on the cerebral circulation.[27,28,39]

Most evidence suggests that dopamine and other adrenergic agonists (e.g., epinephrine, norepinephrine, isoproterenol) do not directly affect cerebral vessels or CBF. If MAP is increased above the upper autoregulatory limit, CBF may increase in response to these agents. Many antihypertensive agents (e.g., nitroglycerin, nitroprusside, hydralazine) are cerebral vasodilators that increase CBV and may increase ICP while decreasing MAP. In patients with noncompliant intracranial dynamics, these agents can precipitate herniation syndromes. The treatment of hypertension in brain-injured patients is controversial. This topic and the pharmacologic effect of the commonly used antihypertensive agents is discussed in more detail in the section "Cardiovascular Concerns During Brain Resuscitation." Among the cerebral vasodilators, the calcium antagonists may be the least deleterious because their action is most pronounced on vasoconstricted vessels. The ganglionic blocker trimethaphan does not appear to directly increase ICP. Captopril shifts the lower autoregulatory limit down, preserving CBF at a lower MAP. Alpha- and beta-adrenergic blockers do not directly alter CBF and therefore may be the preferred agents for control of blood pressure in the brain-injured patient.[40,41]

PULMONARY CONCERNS DURING BRAIN RESUSCITATION

A variety of gas exchange abnormalities, ranging from mild hypoxemia to neurogenic pulmonary edema, are associated with brain injury. Abnormal ventilatory patterns, including Cheyne-Stokes respiration, central neurogenic hyperventilation, and apneustic and ataxic respiration, have been characterized, but association with the anatomic location of brain damage is not precise. Gas exchange abnormalities may occur with isolated CNS injury, but concomitant chest trauma often adds to the respiratory compromise. Pneumonia is a major cause of delayed morbidity and mortality in the brain-injured patient. Although aspiration and nosocomial infections are frequent late complications, prophylactic antibiotics should be avoided. Pulmonary embolism is an additional cause of delayed morbidity. Pneumatic leg compression is the recommended prophylaxis against deep vein thrombosis in the setting of trauma, tumor, or hemorrhage; nonhemorrhagic stroke may be treated with low-dose heparin.[42,43]

Hypoxemia and Abnormal Ventilation

Arterial hypoxemia has been observed in 20% to 45% of spontaneously breathing patients with severe head injury.

Increased venous admixture and shunt without apparent pulmonary damage occur early after isolated head trauma. Venous admixture greater than 13% strongly correlates with poor neurologic outcome and increased mortality. Abnormalities in venous admixture may develop for several reasons, including transient apnea at time of initial injury, microatelectasis, and subclinical or frank neurogenic pulmonary edema. Regardless of etiology, hypoxemia should be treated promptly. Supplemental oxygen is a minimal requirement.[10,42,43]

Neurogenic pulmonary edema, a form of noncardiogenic pulmonary edema, may occur after severe brain injury. This relatively infrequent complication is probably caused by transient massive sympathetic discharge consequent to cerebral ischemia. Systemic vasoconstriction redistributes blood to the pulmonary circuit, while pulmonary vasoconstriction exacerbates pulmonary vascular pressures. Pulmonary microvasculature is injured for unclear reasons. Moderate to severe increases in extravascular lung water with normal pulmonary artery occlusion pressure have been observed in 50% of patients with isolated head trauma or subarachnoid hemorrhage. The incidence of clinical neurogenic pulmonary edema is much less common, suggesting that subclinical pulmonary edema may be a common etiologic factor in pulmonary dysfunction after brain injury.[41,44]

Hypocapnia from spontaneous hyperventilation is a frequent early response to brain injury. Hypercapnia may develop and is associated with a poor outcome. Both hypercapnia and hypoxia produce cerebral vasodilation, which may worsen ICP. Standard precautions should be taken to ensure that the stuporous or comatose patient is able to maintain the upper airway without assistance. Impaired ventilation may result from aspiration as a result of depressed cough and gag reflexes, or from glossal-pharyngeal obstruction. Intubation may be necessary to protect the airway and, in conjunction with mechanical ventilation, may be required to provide therapeutic hyperventilation or to correct abnormalities in pulmonary gas exchange.

Intubation and Mechanical Ventilation

Intubation should be accomplished as smoothly as possible. Pharyngeal and laryngeal stimulation initiate a tremendous catecholamine surge that in turn may generate dangerously high ICPs. Even with normal ICP, sudden episodes of systemic hypertension may have adverse effects on the injured brain. Pretreatment with rapidly acting agents such as fentanyl (1–3 μg/kg), etomidate (0.1 to 0.3 mg/kg), propofol (0.5 to 1.0 mg/kg), or thiopental (0.5 to 2.0 mg/kg) may prevent these complications but may also cause hypotension. Intravenous lidocaine (1.5 mg/kg) prevents ICP elevation during intubation. Beta-adrenergic blockade also may be useful because it effectively blunts tachycardiac and hypertensive responses during laryngeal instrumentation. If paralysis is necessary, vercuronium or pancuronium are preferred to succinylcholine. When intubation can be delayed for 15 to 20 minutes, an intravenous bolus of mannitol may lessen the risk of ICP elevation during laryngeal stimulation.[39,45–47]

Positive-pressure ventilation increases intrathoracic pressure and impedes cerebral venous return, which may elevate

ICP. Additionally, increases in intrathoracic and intraabdominal pressure transmitted to the epidural veins produce venous engorgement with compression of the spinal subarachnoid space, causing translocation of CSF into the intracranial space. Suctioning, coughing, straining, nasogastric tube placement, and routine nursing measures may increase ICP by these mechanisms. Severe impairment of cerebral venous drainage may occur in patients "fighting" the ventilator, and sedation or muscle relaxants may be necessary to prevent elevating ICP. Raising the head 30 degrees and maintaining the head in the midline position maximize cerebral venous drainage and may help to blunt ICP responses during positive-pressure ventilation and routine pulmonary care. However, elevation of the head does not improve ICP in all patients and may actually increase ICP in some.[48-50]

The use of positive end-expiratory pressure (PEEP) for treatment of concomitant pulmonary dysfunction in brain-injured patients may also elevate ICP. PEEP increases intrathoracic pressure and decreases venous return, which may lower blood pressure, thus reducing CPP by two mechanisms. The extent to which moderate use of PEEP worsens ICP has been questioned. When pulmonary compliance is decreased, only a small fraction of the PEEP is transmitted to the mediastinum, minimizing the effect on cerebral venous pressure and ICP.[46] In one study in which head elevation was maintained, PEEP of up to 20 cm H_2O did not increase ICP even in patients with low intracranial compliance. In another series, PEEP of 5 to 15 cm H_2O did not produce clinically significant ICP elevations, affect CPP, or induce neurologic deterioration in any patient, even when ICP was 20 mm Hg or greater. Nevertheless, because the effect of PEEP on ICP is not easily estimated, PEEP should be applied only when absolutely necessary to improve oxygenation and only after euvolemia has been established. PEEP should be increase and decreased slowly, and ICP monitoring is essential if levels above 10 cm H_2O are employed.[43,48-50]

CARDIOVASCULAR CONCERNS DURING BRAIN RESUSCITATION

Electrocardiographic abnormalities and arrhythmias may be present after primary brain injury, alone or in combination with myocardial ischemia. CNS injury can be associated with histologic myocardial damage in the absence of coronary artery disease and probably results from sustained sympathetic hyperactivity. A hyperdynamic hemodynamic pattern with high cardiac output and normal or decreased systemic vascular resistance has been observed after head injury and attributed to this hyperadrenergic state.[51,52]

Hypotension and Fluid Resuscitation

Although it is a common complication of brain death and spinal cord injury, hypotension is not a usual early consequence of primary brain injury unless there is medullary damage. However, traumatic brain injury is frequently associated with systemic trauma that produces hypotension from hypovolemia or occasionally from cardiac dysfunction. Hypotension and anemia may have devastating effects on an already injured brain and should be vigorously corrected to maximize CPP and $C\dot{D}o_2$. In severe head injury, concurrent systolic blood pressure less than 90 mm Hg is associated with worsened morbidity and mortality.[10] In addition, hypotension in the first 24 hours is a significant risk factor for the later development of elevated ICP.[37]

The usual principles employed in shock resuscitation are applicable to the brain-injured patient. Pressor agents should not be administered until hypovolemia and severe anemia are corrected. Alpha- and beta-agonists and moderate doses of dopamine do not directly influence CBF but modify CPP through effect on MAP.[20] The administration of fluids for shock resuscitation of the brain-injured patient has been intensively studied in experimental brain injury. Colloid solutions offer no benefit over isotonic crystalloid solutions and are more expensive. Hypotonic solutions increase cerebral edema and ICP and should be avoided. There is no evidence that fluid restriction has a beneficial effect on cerebral edema, ICP, or mortality. Furthermore, volume depletion may precipitate hypotension or exacerbate reductions in CPP secondary to PEEP or head elevation.[53-56]

Patients should not be placed in the Trendelenburg position for the insertion of central venous lines. Lowering the head below the heart impedes cerebral venous return and may raise intracranial venous pressure. In patients with intracranial hypertension, CPP is maximal in the horizontal position. The head should be maintained in the midline position during catheter insertion because head and neck rotation occlude unilateral jugular venous flow. Internal jugular line placement carries some risk for venous occlusion, although jugular bulb catheterization has been accomplished without significant adverse sequelae.[12,25]

Hypertension

Hypertension is common after brain injury. The sympathetic discharge that accompanies primary injury may elicit hypertension de novo or exacerbate preexisting essential hypertension. Cushing's response is the hypertensive response that may accompany significant ICP elevations. It is attributed to brain stem ischemia or increased pressure on the vasomotor centers in the floor of the fourth ventricle. If ICP exceeds perfusion pressure, a sympathetically mediated systemic vasoconstriction causes a rise in MAP to restore CPP.[20] Vagally mediated bradycardia may precede or accompany the hypertension. Cushing's triad of bradypnea, bradycardia, and hypertension is often a preterminal event associated with herniation. Transient hypertensive responses of a lesser magnitude can occur in some patients with increased ICP. Essential hypertension frequently coexists with cerebrovascular disease and may complicate ischemic stroke and intracranial hemorrhage.

With the exception of intracranial bleeding or hypertensive encephalopathy, the treatment of hypertension after brain injury is controversial. An elevated perfusion pressure may benefit areas of segmental ischemia, and a lowered blood pressure may aggravate ischemic lesions.[20] With chronic hypertension, the autoregulatory limits are shifted upward because of increased cerebrovascular resistance, and the brain's tolerance to acute MAP elevations is improved, but tolerance to acute hypotension is impaired. Therefore, rapid control of blood pressure may precipitate global cerebral ischemia at a "normal" MAP. Conversely, if intracranial compliance is decreased, even a moderate rise in MAP may increase CBV and ICP. Additionally, with impaired autoregulation or a damaged blood–brain barrier, a rise in MAP produces vascular fluid extravasation, worsening intracranial bleeding or vasogenic edema and aggravating ICP and ischemia.[18,20]

Transient hypertension resulting from a hyperadrenergic state often responds to sedation or adequate analgesia. If antihypertensive therapy is indicated, the most appropriate choice of agent is problematic. Cerebral vasodilators may increase CBV, promote vasogenic edema, and increase ICP while decreasing MAP (and CPP). ICP elevation and neurologic deterioration have been reported with nitroglycerin, nitroprusside, and nifedipine.[40,41,57–59]

Adrenergic blockade does not directly alter CBF or ICP except through effects on MAP, and may provide an additional benefit by attenuating the hyperadrenergic response. Propranolol has been used successfully to treat hypertension after head injury. In a group of neurosurgical patients with hypertension poorly controlled by nitroprusside, intravenous labetalol in low to moderate doses adequately controlled blood pressure without adverse effects on CPP or ICP.[52,60]

It is difficult to ascertain the ideal blood pressure in the brain-injured patient. Therapy should be individualized, control of ICP optimized, and CPP maintained above 70 mm Hg. Iatrogenic hypotension is invariably worse than persistent mild or moderate hypertension. In general, a systolic blood pressure less than 200 mm Hg does not require treatment. Control of hypertension should be achieved in a conservative, nonprecipitous fashion. If ICP is elevated, pharmacologic cerebral vasodilation may produce neurologic deterioration; adrenergic blockade is the best option for controlling hypertension in this setting. ICP monitoring may facilitate treatment of significant hypertension.

METABOLIC CONCERNS DURING BRAIN RESUSCITATION

Several endocrinologic and metabolic abnormalities may develop after primary brain injury. Hyponatremia from the syndrome of inappropriate antidiuretic hormone or cerebral salt wasting increases cytotoxic edema and should be corrected. The former condition is treated with fluid restriction and the latter with salt and water replacement. Central diabetes insipidus also may occur, exacerbating hyperosmolality that may already be present as a consequence of diuretic therapy.[61]

Neurologic injury triggers a cascade of metabolic responses that result in a hypermetabolic, hypercatabolic, and hyperglycemic state. Immunocompetence is also compromised. Clinical evidence suggests that appropriate nutritional supplementation improves outcome. As with most critically ill patients, the enteral route is preferred, is less expensive, and is associated with a decreased incidence of sepsis. Because gastric paresis is common, early placement of a duodenal or jejunal feeding tube optimizes caloric and protein delivery. The advantage of special formulations in the care of brain-injured patients has not been established.[62]

Lactate accumulated during anaerobic glycolysis is the major cause of ischemic brain acidosis, and an increase in cerebral lactate after brain injury has been linked to worsened neurologic morbidity and outcome. Studies in experimental animals provide evidence suggesting that hyperglycemia worsens intracerebral lactate accumulation and acidosis during brain ischemia, presumably because of increased availability of substrate for anaerobic glycolysis. Hyperglycemia is associated with more pronounced brain edema and poorer neurologic outcome after experimental brain injury. Clinical investigations support the concept that hyperglycemia accentuates ischemic brain damage in humans. Pending further clarification of this issue, glucose-containing infusions should not be used during resuscitation from neurologic injury unless concurrent hypoglycemia exists, and hyperglycemia should be corrected with administration of short-acting insulin.[63]

SPECIFIC THERAPEUTIC OPTIONS IN BRAIN RESUSCITATION

MANEUVERS TO DECREASE INTRACRANIAL VOLUME AND PRESSURE

Elevated ICP is frequently a final common pathway in the production of secondary injury and is associated with worsened prognosis in brain injury.[10,14,15] In traumatic head injury, survival is greater than 80% in patients whose ICP remains less than 20 mm Hg but is greater than 90% in those with persistent uncontrollable elevations. Aggressive therapy to lower ICP improves survival in head injury and Reye's syndrome. Evidence that treatment of ICP reduces the mortality in global cerebral injury and massive stroke is less conclusive.[10,11,64]

Nonsurgical treatment of intracranial hypertension is directed at decreasing intracranial volume through manipulation of CSF or CBV or reduction of edema. ICP monitor–directed therapy is usually initiated at sustained pressures of 20 to 25 mm Hg. Although general treatment for elevated ICP is associated with improved outcome in traumatic brain injury, the efficacy of therapy specifically titrated by invasive measurement of ICP remains poorly delineated.[65,66] The available data are conflicting. In one study, treatment to decrease ICP was administered to severely head-injured patients without implementation of ICP monitoring; mortality was comparable with other clinical series using ICP monitor–guided therapy.[67] In another study, treatment of ICP based on invasive measurements offered no improvement in neurologic outcome or mortality over empiric therapy administered without consideration of actual measured ICP.[68] Clearly, aggressive therapy to reduce ICP can be instituted effectively without ICP monitoring. Nonetheless, advocates of ICP monitoring argue that because raised ICP strongly correlates with worsened morbidity and mortality and because monitoring permits early recognition of intracranial hypertension and precise titration of therapy, ICP monitoring is necessary in patients with severe traumatic injury.[19] The benefits of therapy guided by invasive ICP measurements must be weighed against the risk of complications (e.g., infection, hemorrhage) that occur in as many as 8% of patients. ICP monitoring should be considered if there is a strong probability of significantly increased ICP and if measures to lower ICP are likely to improve outcome.

Hyperventilation

Iatrogenic hyperventilation has traditionally been a mainstay in the treatment of elevated ICP. Hypocapnia induces cerebral vasoconstriction, reducing both CBV and CBF. Between a $PaCO_2$ of 40 and 25 mm Hg, each 1-mm Hg change mitigates a 3% decrease in blood flow and volume. ICP responds within minutes. The effectiveness of hyperventilation is more pronounced when CBF is hyperemic but is also maintained if CBF is normal or low. For many years, both prophylactic and therapeutic hyperventilation were employed as first-line therapy in patients with traumatic brain injuries.[12,69] Recent evidence, however, suggests that hyperventilation can, in fact, exacerbate secondary brain injury by decreasing CBF in a setting already characterized by pathologic vasomotor regulation and patchy ischemia. One single, prospective, randomized study of prophylactic hyperventilation after traumatic brain injury reveals a better 6-month outcome in patients kept normocapnic during the first 5 days of their hospitalization.[70] Hyperventilation seems to have a much greater and direct effect on CBF than on ICP. Consequently, it is no longer recommended as subacute or prophylactic therapy in the treatment of brain edema or elevated ICP. Nevertheless, acute hyperventilation remains the treatment of choice to rapidly control ICP (while awaiting more definitive therapy) in patients with precipitous neurologic deterioration. After stabilization of neurologic function, appropriate chronic therapy for control of ICP should be initiated and $PaCO_2$ returned to 30 mm Hg or higher.[70,71]

Osmotic Agents

The use of osmotic diuretics is a standard measure employed in the control of ICP. These agents create an osmotic gradient between the brain and the bloodstream and draw fluid from brain tissue. An intact blood–brain barrier is necessary to maintain this gradient. Dehydration occurs primarily in normal brain tissue rather than in injured, edematous tissue. Osmotic diuretics improve intracranial compliance by providing compensatory volume for edema, minimizing ICP elevations and focal vascular encroachment.[31]

Mannitol (20% solution) is the most commonly used osmotic agent. Intravenous doses of 0.25 to 1.0 g/kg reduce ICP within 20 to 30 minutes. The higher doses may be useful for acute decompression or severe ICP elevations, but the lower doses are also efficacious and may allow repeated treatments with fewer adverse effects. Mannitol is not thought to cross an intact blood–brain barrier, but it may penetrate the endothelium in injured tissue. In addition to its osmotic effect, mannitol is also a plasma expander that reduces hematocrit, decreases blood viscosity, and increases CBF.

The effects of osmotic diuretics last only 4 to 6 hours because the osmotic gradient narrows as blood concentrations diminish. Repeat dosing may be required as ICP rises and the neurologic condition deteriorates. Chronic osmotherapy beyond 48 to 72 hours is not advisable, because brain tissue tends to adapt to sustained serum hyperosmolality with increased intracellular osmolality. In addition, osmotic diuretics are not excluded from edematous tissue. As the plasma concentration of the hypertonic agent decreases, fluid may shift into injured tissue where the osmotic gradient is relatively high. Consequently, rebound ICP elevation may occur after repeated use of these agents.

The major complication of osmotic diuresis is hyperosmolality with hypernatremia. Serum osmolality should not exceed 310 to 320 mOsm or neuronal injury, rebound edema, metabolic injury, and renal failure may ensue. Because hyperosmotic agents can produce transient hypervolemia, they should be administered cautiously in the presence of congestive heart failure or ventricular dysfunction.

There is no defined role for the routine use of osmotic agents in obstructive hydrocephalus or cerebral edema unassociated with ICP elevations.[72]

Nonosmotic Diuresis and Cerebrospinal Fluid Drainage

The rate of CSF formation is approximately 500 mL/day. CSF production is decreased by the administration of furosemide (40 to 80 mg) or acetazolamide (250 mg two to four times daily). Acetazolamide may be beneficial in the treatment of interstitial edema, but it is of limited value in the treatment of vasogenic or cytotoxic edema, although it will counteract the hypochloremic metabolic alkalosis produced by furosemide. In brain-injured patients, intravenous furosemide (20 mg) decreases ICP without affecting CPP. In experimental and clinical brain injury, the combination of furosemide and mannitol produces greater brain shrinkage and more sustained ICP reductions than either agent alone.[73,74]

A catheter placed in the lateral ventricle allows both CSF drainage and continuous ICP monitoring. Removal of only a few milliliters of CSF may lower ICP. Fluid should be drained against a positive pressure to avoid ventricular collapse. Although this is a rapid method for acute ICP reduction, the invasive nature of the technique and the risk of infection make it a less than ideal alternative.

Corticosteroids

Although few drugs have been administered with as much fervor as steroids, the therapeutic indications for the use of these agents in brain injury are limited. The theoretic rationale for steroid administration is reduction of vasogenic edema through membrane stabilization, preservation of blood–brain barrier integrity, and inhibition of arachidonic acid release from cell membranes. A theoretic rationale also exists for the use of steroids in obstructive hydrocephalus resulting from inflammatory changes in the subarachnoid space or arachnoid villi, but this has not been well studied. There is no basis for a steroid influence on cytotoxic edema.

Several prospective, randomized clinical investigations have consistently demonstrated that steroids are not beneficial in the treatment of ischemic or traumatic edema. Steroid treatment does not reduce the mean ICP or improve neurologic outcome or mortality after severe head injury, intracerebral hemorrhage, or ischemic cerebral infarction.[75-78] Corticosteroid administration during brain resuscitation causes additional morbidity form systemic complications such as infection, sepsis, and hyperglycemia.[79]

Steroids have been employed in the treatment of peritumor edema associated with primary and metastatic brain tumors for more than 25 years, and their efficacy in this setting is established. Dexamethasone has decreased the hearing loss that complicates bacterial meningitis in pediatric patients, although no other beneficial effect on long-term neurologic outcome was apparent.[80]

Early treatment with high-dose methylprednisolone has recently been reported to improve neurologic outcome after spinal cord injury. This improvement has been attributed to the antioxidant free radical scavenging properties of high-dose steroids.[81]

MANEUVERS TO INCREASE CEREBRAL BLOOD FLOW

Iatrogenic Hypertension

In pathologic conditions (e.g., stroke, subarachnoid hemorrhage) in which global and regional ischemia exist without significant ICP elevation, manipulation of MAP to increase CPP has theoretic merit. Maintenance of CPP above 50 mm Hg is mandatory, but if autoregulation is impaired, further increases of CPP (70 to 80 mm Hg) may improve CBF. However, if ICP is increased, induced hypertension can worsen ICP and precipitate additional ischemia. Iatrogenic hypertension in conjunction with maximization of intravascular volume is useful in the management of vasospasm after subarachnoid hemorrhage.[82] Phenylephrine, dopamine, and other vasopressors have been successfully employed to increase CBF and reverse neurologic deficits.[83,84] Phenylephrine may be preferred if cardiac output is sufficient because it does not cause tachycardia. Currently, there is no role for iatrogenic hypertension in management of ischemic stroke, and the role of induced hypertension in traumatic head injury has not been defined.

Alterations of Blood Viscosity and Intravascular Volume

The principle that blood flow increases as blood viscosity decreases has been applied clinically with the use of hemodilution to treat focal ischemia and vasospasm. Hematocrit is a major determinant of blood viscosity, especially in the microcirculation or during low-flow states. A hematocrit of approximately 30% to 33% is optimal for maintaining a balance between improved blood flow from reduced viscosity and preserving oxygen transport as hematocrit decreases. Because blood viscosity is increased in stroke and because viscosity reductions may increase global and regional CBF, it is reasoned that hemodilution during an ischemic event may salvage tissue with marginal oxygen delivery and prevent further ischemic damage.

Hypervolemic hemodilution is produced by volume expansion with asanguineous fluids and may precipitate ICP increases or cardiac overload. Isovolemic hemodilution—accomplished by phlebotomy plus volume replacement—may be optimal in patients with impaired cardiovascular reserves or those at risk for ICP elevation. Both crystalloid and colloid may be used in hemodilution.

Initial clinical studies reported a therapeutic benefit with isovolemic and hypervolemic hemodilution in acute focal cerebral ischemia. However, several large, prospective, randomized multicenter trials of isovolemic hemodilution in the management of acute stroke demonstrate little or no improvement in neurologic outcome or survival. Hemodilution may be beneficial during crescendo transient ischemic attacks and as a prophylactic measure before carotid surgery. Further investigation is required.

Hypervolemic hemodilution, alone or in combination with iatrogenic hypertension, has been successfully employed in the treatment of ischemic complications from vasospasm associated with subarachnoid hemorrhage. Morbidity and mortality from vasospasm are reduced in most patients, although cardiopulmonary complications occur in as many as 19%. Hypervolemic hemodilution should be employed only if invasive hemodynamic monitoring guides therapy.[85-88]

MANEUVERS TO DECREASE METABOLIC DEMAND

Increased cerebral metabolic demand may precipitate tissue ischemia if CDo_2 is compromised or flow is uncoupled to metabolism. Mechanical obstruction to flow may prevent elevation of regional CBF to match increased metabolic needs, even if global CBF is adequate. $CMRo_2$ is often decreased after primary brain injury, but seizures, hyperthermia, a hypermetabolic state, excess motor activity, and pain raise oxygen demand and can exacerbate the oxygen debt. General measures to prevent $CMRo_2$ elevation include providing adequate analgesia and sedation and preventing postoperative shivering.

Regulation of Temperature

Fever often occurs in brain-injured patients without an infectious cause, and the consequent rise in $CMRo_2$ may produce ischemia if CDo_2 does not increase. Even if CBF increases to match a higher $CMRo_2$, the resulting elevation of CBV may produce compromise if intracranial compliance is reduced. Temperature elevations should be aggressively controlled with antipyretics and cooling blankets, if necessary.

Induced hypothermia has been shown to improve neurologic outcome in animal models of brain injury. Clinical studies have documented the feasibility and safety of moderate hypothermia in human patients. A multicenter randomized prospective trial in patients with severe traumatic head injury studying the effect of moderate hypothermia (32°C) is currently underway.[89]

Barbiturate Coma

Barbiturates depress neuronal function, decrease $CMRo_2$, and suppress seizure activity. CBF is reduced concurrently because flow-metabolism coupling results in vasoconstriction, and CBV and ICP are consequently lowered. Barbiturates have been used clinically to decrease ICP and provide cerebral protection by reducing $CMRo_2$. However, clinical investigations suggest that the indications for barbiturate coma and the overall benefits achieved are limited. A prospective, randomized, multicenter trial of intravenous thiopental administration (30 mg/kg) immediately after resuscitation from cardiac arrest demonstrates no difference in long-term mortality or neurologic outcome.[90] Two prospective, randomized clinical trials do not demonstrate a beneficial effect for barbiturates given as initial, rather than second-line, treatment in severe head injury. Similarly, barbiturate treatment of elevated ICP in association with stroke has not improved outcome.[91-93]

Barbiturates may have some value as an adjunctive, last-line measure in treating uncontrollable ICP elevations, which are associated with exorbitant mortality. Several clinical trials have employed barbiturate loading after standard measures failed to reduce ICP in patients with head injury and nontraumatic brain injury. Barbiturate coma produces sustained ICP reductions in as many as 50% of these patients with improvement in mortality, but not necessarily functional recovery. Pentobarbital coma for reduction of ICP is produced by a loading dose of 3 to 10 mg/kg, followed by a maintenance infusion of 1 to 3 mg/kg/hour to maintain serum barbiturate levels of 2.5 to 4 mg%. Barbiturate coma should not be considered a benign therapeutic maneuver. Because of respiratory depression, mechanical support of ventilation is mandatory. Hypotension occurs frequently secondary to vasodilation and myocardial depression. Hemodynamic monitoring for titration of volume administration and inotropic agents is mandatory.[90-94]

Seizures

Seizures greatly increase $CMRo_2$ and precipitate secondary brain injury. Ischemic brain damage is a recognized sequel of prolonged seizure activity, although CBF may increase in response to flow-metabolism coupling and seizure-induced hypertension. If focal or generalized seizures occur in the brain-injured patient, immediate treatment is mandatory. Intravenous benzodiazepine should be administered in incremental doses (e.g., 5 to 40 mg of diazepam or 2 to 8 mg of lorazepam) sufficient to terminate all seizure activity. Subsequently, a full loading dose of intravenous phenytoin (20 mg/kg) should be administered and followed by maintenance therapy (300 mg/day) to prevent seizure recurrence.

Anticonvulsant prophylaxis is recommended in head injury, subarachnoid hemorrhage, brain tumor, and cerebral abscess. The indication for anticonvulsant prophylaxis after ischemic brain injury is not as certain. Early seizures may develop after successful resuscitation in as many as 20% of cardiac arrest patients, but thiopental loading does not significantly lower the incidence of seizures. The benefit of prophylactic phenytoin therapy must always be weighed against the risk of serious adverse reactions (e.g. rash, anaphylaxis), which occur in as many as 15% of these patients.[95,96]

CYTOPROTECTION

As a consequence of primary injury, a cascade of cellular, metabolic, and chemical events increase the cell's vulnerability to secondary injury. Because this process evolves over time, a window of opportunity exists during which these chemical cascades may be potentially modulated to improve neuronal survival. Current research efforts emphasize three main areas of interest:

1. Exitatory amino acid (EAA) neurotransmitters (modulation)
2. Free radical scavengers (antioxidant therapy)
3. Calcium channel blockade

The injured brain releases increased quantities of excitatory amino acid neurotransmitters (e.g. glutamate, aspirate), which results in pathologic stimulation of neuronal and glial EAA receptors (e.g., N-methyl-D-aspartate receptor. Stimulation of these receptors produces chemically mediated transmembrane ionic shifts of calcium, resulting in intracellular calcium accumulation. Free cytoplasmic and mitochondrial calcium promotes irreversible cell injury through activation of proteases and phospholipases, cell membrane degradation, and inhibition of cellular respiration. A variety of EAA receptor antagonists and modulators have shown substantial promise in animal models of brain injury. Currently, clinical trials are underway evaluating the efficacy of these agents in traumatic brain injury and stroke.[38,97]

An additional mechanism of secondary cellular injury involves the formation or release of oxygen free radicals as a by-product of ischemia-reperfusion. Free radicals hasten cellular destruction by enhancing lipid peroxidation of cell membranes. Lipid peroxidation is also accelerated in the presence of free reactive iron. Two free radical scavengers, tirilazad and polyethylene-bound super oxide dismutase, are presently being studied in Phase III trials for the treatment of traumatic brain injury and subarachnoid hemorrhage.[98]

Calcium channel blockers inhibit voltage-sensitive calcium entry into cells and relax smooth muscle, causing vasodilation. The cerebroselective calcium antagonists cross the blood–brain barrier and act preferentially on cerebral vessels rather than on the peripheral vasculature or myocardium. These agents include the dihydropyridines (e.g., nimodipine, nicardipine, nilvadipine) and the diphenylalkylamines (e.g., flunarizine, cinnarizine).

The utility of calcium channel blockade in brain resuscitation is based on (1) the potential amelioration of adverse sequelae resulting from ischemic intracellular calcium overload, and (2) the potential increase in CBF secondary to cerebral vasodilation. As mentioned earlier, excessive calcium entry into cells initiates the final processes associated with cellular dissolution. In smooth muscle cells, increased calcium availability may mediate ischemic vasoconstriction or vasospasm. In experimental brain injury, administration of calcium antagonists counteracts vasoconstriction, reduces histologic damage, and improves CBF and neurologic recovery.

Several prospective, randomized, placebo-controlled clinical trials demonstrate that prophylactic oral nimodipine (60 to 90 mg every 4 hours) improved functional outcome in patients who have had ischemia-related neurologic deficits after subarachnoid hemorrhage. However, the incidence of symptomatic vasospasm, the incidence and severity of angiographic vasospasm, and overall mortality were not altered by nimodipine. The beneficial effects of nimodipine are possibly related to vasodilation of small arteries, with improvement of collateral flow, rather than reversal of vasospasm per se. Alternatively, the drug may protect neuronal metabolism during ischemia. Oral nimodipine therapy initiated *after* the onset of symptomatic vasospasm has no proven efficacy. Continuous intravenous nicardipine has been shown to reverse angiographic vasospasm but has not been shown to alter outcome. Further studies are pending.[99–105]

Current data regarding the efficacy of calcium antagonists in global ischemia do not support their administration. Prospective, randomized, multicenter trials of nimodipine in severe head injury and stroke fail to reveal any definite benefits. The potential therapeutic effects of magnesium, a competitive antagonist of calcium, have not been thoroughly studied in brain ischemia.[38,98,106]

CONCLUSION

Successful brain resuscitation limits damage from primary brain injury and prevents secondary injury. Cellular and tissue ischemia consequent to the initiating insult precipitates a cascade of events that promote injury. Systemic factors and extracranial organ dysfunction frequently complicate neurologic injury and may worsen an already complex pathophysiologic interaction. Intensive care management minimizes secondary damage and promotes healing. The primary therapeutic objective is to reestablish a favorable balance between cerebral oxygen supply and demand. General therapeutic measures (see Table 19-4) are directed toward improving $C\dot{D}o_2$ and CBF and minimizing $CMRo_2$ elevations.

Attention to pulmonary, cardiovascular, and metabolic disturbances associated with primary brain injury is necessary to avoid further cerebral ischemia. Several specific measures (see Table 19-5) have established efficacy in the treatment of ICP elevation, edema, and vasospasm. Various adjunctive and investigational therapeutic modalities may prevent or ameliorate secondary injury. Treatments that directly address cellular ischemia are currently being studied. The application of these therapies is dictated by the specific cause of primary brain injury. The ultimate goal of brain resuscitation is improvement of neurologic outcome with an enhanced quality of survival.

ACKNOWLEDGMENT

The authors gratefully acknowledge the assistance of Mrs. Carolyn Linenbroker in the preparation of this manuscript.

REFERENCES

1. Siesjo BK: Mechanisms of ischemic brain damage. *Crit Care Med* 1988;16:954
2. Astrup J: Energy-requiring cell functions in the ischemic brain. *J Neurosurg* 1982;56:482
3. Powers WJ: Hemodynamics and metabolism in ischemic cerebrovascular disease. *Neurol Clin* 1992;10:31
4. Sundt TM Jr, Sharbrough FW, Piepgras DG, et al: Correlation of cerebral blood flow and electroencephalographic changes during carotid endarterectomy. *Mayo Clin Proc* 1981;56:533
5. Abramson NS, Safar P, Detre KM, et al: Neurologic recovery after cardiac arrest: effect of duration of ischemia. *Crit Care Med* 1985;13:930
6. Sundt TM Jr, Grant WC, Garcia JH: Restoration of middle cerebral artery flow in experimental infarction. *J Neurosurg* 1969;31:311
7. Crowell RM, Olsson Y, Klatzo I, et al: Temporary occlusion of the middle cerebral artery in the monkey: clinical and pathological observations. *Stroke* 1970;1:439
8. Schmidley JW: Free radicals in central nervous system ischemia. *Stroke* 1990;21:1086
9. Hallenbeck JM, Dutka AJ: Background review and current concepts of reperfusion injury. *Arch Neurol* 1990;47:1245
10. Miller JD, Butterworth JF, Gudeman SK, et al: Further experience in the management of severe head injury. *J Neurosurg* 1981;54:289
11. Narayan RK, Kishore PR, Becker DP, et al: Intracranial pressure: to monitor or not to monitor? *J Neurosurg* 1982;56:650
12. Obrist WD, Langfitt TW, Jaggi JL, et al: Cerebral blood flow and metabolism in comatose patients with acute head injury. *J Neurosurg* 1984;61:241
13. Sakabe T, Tateishi A, Miyauchi Y, et al: Intracranial pressure following cardiopulmonary resuscitation. *Intensive Care Med* 1987;13:256
14. Shaywitz BA, Rothstein P, Venes JL: Monitoring and management of increased intracranial pressure in Reye syndrome: results in 29 children. *Pediatrics* 1980;66:198
15. Ropper AH, Shafran BL: Brain edema after stroke: clinical syndrome and intracranial pressure. *Arch Neurol* 1984;41:26
16. Bouma GJ, Muizelaar PJ: Cerebral blood flow in severe clinical head injury. *New Horizons* 1995;3:384
17. Lassen NA, Astrup J: Cerebral blood flow: normal regulation and ischemic thresholds. In: Weinstein PR, Faden AI (eds). *Protection of the Brain From Ischemia*. Baltimore, Williams & Wilkins, 1990:7
18. Paulson OB, Waldemar G, Schmidt JF, et al: Cerebral circulation under normal and pathological conditions. *Am J Cardiol* 1989;63:2C
19. Lang EW, Chesnut RM: Intracranial pressure and cerebral perfusion pressure in severe head injury. *New Horizons* 1995;3:400
20. Powers WJ: Hemodynamics and metabolism in ischemic cerebrovascular disease. *Neurol Clin* 1992;10:31
21. Voldby B, Enevoldsen EM, Jensen, FT: Regional CBF, intraventricular pressure, and cerebral metabolism in patients with ruptured intracranial aneurysms. *J Neurosurg* 1985;62:48
22. Hossman KA: Hemodynamics of postischemic reperfusion of the brain. In: Weinstein PR, Faden AI (eds). *Protection of the Brain From Ischemia*. Baltimore, Williams & Wilkins 1990:21
23. Bruce DA, Alavi A, Bilaniuk L, et al: Diffuse cerebral swelling following head injuries in children: the syndrome of "malignant brain edema." *J Neurosurg* 1981;54:170
24. Adams HP, Kassell NF, Torner JC, et al: Predicting cerebral ischemia after aneurysmal subarachnoid hemorrhage: influ-

ence of clinical condition, CT results, and antifibrinolytic therapy. *Neurology* 1987;37:1586

25. Robertson CS, Cormio M: Cerebral metabolic management. *New Horizons* 1995;3:410
26. McCormick PW, Stewart M, Goetting MG, et al: Noninvasive cerebral optical spectroscopy for monitoring cerebral oxygen delivery and hemodynamics. *Crit Care Med* 1991;19:89
27. McPherson RW, Kirsch JR, Traystman RJ: Optimal anesthetic techniques for patients at risk of cerebral ischemia. In: Weinstein PR, Faden AI (eds). *Protection of the Brain From Ischemia.* Baltimore, Williams & Wilkins, 1990:237
28. Messick JM, Newberg LA, Nugent M, et al: Principles of neuroanesthesia for the nonneurosurgical patient with CNS pathophysiology. *Anesth Analg* 1985;64:143
29. Powers WJ: Positron emission tomography, In: Weinstein PR, Faden AI (eds). *Protection of the Brain From Ischemia.* Baltimore, Williams & Wilkins, 1990:99
30. Olesen WD: Cerebral function, metabolism, and blood flow. *Acta Neurol Scand* 1974;57:38
31. Fishman RA: Brain edema. *N Engl J Med* 1975;14:706
32. Klatzo I: Brain edema following brain ischaemia and the influence of therapy. *Br J Anaesth* 1985;57:18
33. Tonnesen AS: Hemodynamic management of brain-injured patients. *New Horizons* 1995;3:499
34. Chesnut RM: Secondary brain insults after head injury: clinical perspectives. *New Horizons* 1995;3:366
35. Seelig JM, Marshall LF, Toutant SM, et al: Traumatic acute subdural hematoma: major mortality reduction in comatose patients treated within 4 hours. *N Engl J Med* 1981;304:1511
36. Lobato RD, Sarabia R, Rivas JJ: Normal computerized tomography scans in severe head injury. *J Neurosurg* 1986;65:784
37. Klauber MR, Toutant SM, Marshall LF: A model for predicting delayed intracranial hypertension following severe head injury. *J Neurosurg* 1984;61:695
38. Fisher M, Bogousslavsky J: Evolving toward effective therapy for acute ischemic stroke. *JAMA* 1993;270:360
39. Prielipp RC, Coursin DB: Sedative and neuromuscular blocking drug use in critically ill patients with head injuries. *New Horizons* 1995;3:456
40. Van Aken H, Cottrell JE, Anger C, et al: Treatment of intraoperative hypertensive emergencies in patients with intracranial disease. *Am J Cardiol* 1989;63:43C
41. Barry DI: Cerebrovascular aspects of antihypertensive treatment. *Am J Cardiol* 1989;63:14C
42. Demling R, Riessen R: Pulmonary dysfunction after cerebral injury. *Crit Care Med* 1990;18:768
43. Gildenberg PL, Frost EA: Respiratory care in head trauma. In: Becker DP, Povlishock JT (eds). *Central Nervous System Trauma Status Report.* Bethesda, National Institutes of Health, 1985:161
44. Mackersie RC, Christensen JM, Pitts LH, et al: Pulmonary extravascular fluid accumulation following intracranial injury. *J Trauma* 1983;23:968
45. Hamill JF, Bedford RF, Weaner DC, et al: Lidocaine before endotracheal intubation: intravenous or laryngotracheal? *Anesthesiology* 1981;55:578
46. Cucchiara RF, Benefiel DJ, Matteo RS, et al: Evaluation of esmolol in controlling increases in heart rate and blood pressure during endotracheal intubation in patients undergoing carotid endarterectomy. *Anesthesiology* 1986;65:528
47. Shapiro HM: Intracranial hypertension: therapeutic and anesthetic considerations. *Anesthesiology* 1975;43:445
48. Cooper KR, Boswell PA, Choi SC: Safe use of PEEP in patients with severe head injury. *J Neurosurg* 1985;63:552
49. Ropper AH, O'Rourke DO, Kennedy SK: Head position,

50. Burchiel KJ, Steege TD, Wylar AR: Intracranial pressure changes in brain-injured patients requiring positive end-expiratory pressure ventilation. *Neurosurgery* 1981;8:443
51. Talman WT: Cardiovascular regulation and lesions of the central nervous system. *Ann Neurol* 1985;18:1
52. Clifton GL, Robertson CS, Grossman RG: Management of the cardiovascular and metabolic responses to severe head injury. In: Becker DP, Povlishock JT (eds). *Central Nervous System Trauma Status Report.* Bethesda, National Institutes of Health, 1985:139
53. Shackford SR: Fluid resuscitation in head injury. *J Intensive Care Med* 1990;5:59
54. Wisner D, Busche F, Sturm J, et al: Traumatic shock and head injury: effects of fluid resuscitation on the brain. *J Surg Res* 1989;46:49
55. Ducey JP, Mozingo DW, Lamiell JM, et al: A comparison of the cerebral and cardiovascular effects of complete resuscitation with isotonic and hypertonic saline, hetastarch, and whole blood following hemorrhage. *J Trauma* 1989;29:1510
56. Morse ML, Milstein JM, Haas JE, et al: Effect of hydration on experimentally induced cerebral edema. *Crit Care Med* 1985;13:563
57. Gagnon RL, Marsh ML, Smith RW, et al: Intracranial hypertension caused by nitroglycerin. *Anesthesiology* 1979;51:86
58. Marsh ML, Shapiro HM, Smith RW, et al: Changes in neurologic status and intracranial pressure associated with sodium nitroprusside administration. *Anesthesiology* 1979;51:336
59. Hayashi M, Kobayashi H, Kawano H, et al: Treatment of systemic hypertension and intracranial hypertension in cases of brain hemorrhage. *Stroke* 1988;19:314
60. Orlowski JP, Shiesley D, Vidt DG, et al: Labetalol to control blood pressure after cerebrovascular surgery. *Crit Care Med* 1988;16:765
61. Wijdicks EF, Vermeulen M, ten Haaf JA, et al: Volume depletion and natriuresis in patients with a ruptured intracranial aneurysm. *Ann Neurol* 1985;18:211
62. Roberts PR: Nutrition in the head-injured patient. *New Horizons* 1995;3:506-517
63. Yatsu FM: Cardiopulmonary arrest and intravenous glucose. *J Crit Care* 1987;2:1
64. Eisenberg HM, Frankowski RF, Contant CF, et al: High dose barbiturate control of elevated intracranial pressure in patients with severe head injury. *J Neurosurg* 1988;69:15
65. Saul TG, Ducker TB: Effect of intracranial pressure monitoring and aggressive treatment on mortality in severe head injury. *J Neurosurg* 1982;56:498
66. Rockoff MA, Marshall LF, Shapiro HM: High dose barbiturate therapy in humans: a clinical review of 60 patients. *Ann Neurol* 1979;6:194
67. Stuart GG, Merry GS, Smith JA, et al: Severe head injury managed wihtout intracranial pressure monitoring. *J Neurosurg* 1983;59:601
68. Smith HP, Kelly DL, McWhorter JM, et al: Comparison of mannitol regimens in patients with severe head injury undergoing intracranial monitoring. *J Neurosurg* 1986;65:820
69. Havill JH: Prolonged hyperventilation and intracranial pressure. *Crit Care Med* 1984;12:72
70. Cold GE: Does acute hyperventilation provoke cerebral oligaemia in comatose patients after acute head injury? *Acta Neurochir (Wein)* 1989;96:100
71. Marion DW, Firlik A, McLaughlin MR: Hyperventilation therapy for severe traumatic brain injury. *New Horizons* 1995;3:439

72. Bullock R: Mannitol and other diuretics in severe neuro-trauma. *New Horizons* 1995;3:448

73. Pollay M, Fullenwider C, Roberts A, et al: Effect of mannitol and furosemide on blood–brain osmotic gradient and intra-cranial pressure. *J Neurosurg* 1983;59:945

74. Schettini A, Stahurski B, Young H: Osmotic and osmotic-loop diuresis in brain surgery. *J Neurosurg* 1982;56:679

75. Saul TG, Ducker TB, Salcman M, et al: Steroids in severe head injury: a prospective randomized clinical trial. *J Neurosurg* 1981;54:596

76. Kelly DF: Steroids in head injury. *New Horizons* 1995; 3:453-455

77. Poungvarin N, Bhoopat W, Viriyavejakul A, et al: Effects of dexamethasone in primary supratentorial intracerebral hemorrhage. *N Engl J Med* 1987;316:1229

78. Norris JW, Hachinski VC: High dose steroid treatment in cerebral infarction. *Br Med J* 1986;292:21

79. De Maria EF, Reichman W, Kenney PR, et al: Septic complications of corticosteriod administration after central nervous system trauma. *Ann Surg* 1985;202:248

80. Lebel MH, Freij BJ, Syrogiannopoulos GA: Dexamethasone therapy for bacterial meningitis: results of two double-blind, placebo-controlled trials. *N Engl J Med* 1988;319:964

81. Bracken MB, Shepard MJ, Collins WF, et al: A randomized, controlled trial of methylprednisolone or naloxone in the treatment of acute spinal-cord injury: results of the second national acute spinal cord injury study. *N Engl J Med* 1990; 322:1405

82. Kassell NF, Peerless SJ, Durward QJ, et al: Treatment of ischemic deficits from vasospasm with intravascular volume expansion and induced arterial hypertension. *Neurosurgery* 1982;11:337

83. Muizelaar JP, Becker DP: Induced hypertension for the treatment of cerebral ischemia after subarachnoid hemorrhage: direct effect on cerebral blood flow. *Surg Neurol* 1986;25: 317

84. Adams HP: Prevention of brain ischemia after aneurysmal subarachnoid hemorrhage. *Neurol Clin* 1992;10:251

85. Heros RC, Korosue K: Hemodilution for cerebral ischemia. *Stroke* 1989;20:423

86. Wood J, Fleischer A: Observations during hypervolemic hemodilution of patients with acute focal cerebral ischemia. *JAMA* 1982;248:2999

87. Scandinavian Stroke Study Group: Multicenter trial of hemodilution in acute ischemic stroke. I. Results in the total patient population. *Stroke* 1987;18:691

88. Hemodilution in Stroke Study Group: Hypervolemic hemodilution treatment of acute stroke: results of a randomized multicenter trial using pentastarch. *Stroke* 1989;20:317

89. Clifton GL: Hypothermia and hyperbaric oxygen as treatment modalities for severe head injury. *New Horizons* 1995; 3:474-478

90. Brain Resuscitation Clinical Trial I Study Group: Randomized clinical study of thiopental loading in comatose survivors of cardiac arrest. *N Engl J Med* 1986;314:397

91. Ward JD, Becker DP, Miller JD, et al: Failure of prophylactic barbiturate coma in the treatment of severe head injury. *J Neurosurg* 1985;62:383

92. Schwartz ML, Tator CH, Rowed DW, et al: The University of Toronto Head Injury Treatment Study: a prospective, randomized comparison of pentobarbital and mannitol. *Can J Neurol Sci* 1984;11:434

93. Woodcock J, Ropper A, Kennedy SK: High dose barbiturates in non-traumatic brain swelling: ICP reduction and effect on outcome. *Stroke* 1982;13:785

94. Wilberger JE, Cantella D: High-dose barbiturates for intracranial pressure control. *New Horizons* 1995;3:469

95. Deutschman CS, Haines SJ: Anticonvulsnat prophylaxis in neurological surgery. *Neurosurgery* 1985;17:510

96. Temkin NR, Dikmen SS, Wilensky AJ, et al: A randomized, double-blind study of phenytoin for the prevention of post-traumatic seizures. *N Engl J Med* 1990;323:497

97. Buchan A: Advances in cerebral ischemia: experimental approaches. *Neurol Clin* 1992;10:49

98. Smith DH, Casey K, McIntosh TK: Pharmacologic therapy for traumatic brain injury: experimental approaches. *New Horizons* 1995;3:562

99. Wong MC, Haley EC Jr: Calcium antagonists: stroke therapy coming of age. *Stroke* 1990;21:494

100. Allen GS: Role of calcium antagonists in cerebral arterial spasm. *Am J Cardiol* 1985;55:149B

101. Allen GS, Ahn HS, Preziosi TJ, et al: Cerebral arterial spasm: a controlled trial of nimodipine in patients with subarachnoid hemorrhage. *N Engl J Med* 1983;308:619

102. Philippon J, Grob R, Dagreou F, et al: Prevention of vasospasm in subarachnoid hemorrhage: a controlled study with nimodipine. *Acta Neurochir (Wein)* 1986;82:110

103. Petruk KC, West M, Mohr G, et al: Nimodipine treatment in poor grade aneurysm patients: results of a multicenter double-blind placebo-controlled trial. *J Neurosurg* 1988; 68:505

104. Pickard JD, Murray GD, Illingworth R, et al: Effect of oral nimodipine on cerebral infarction and outcome after subarachnoid hemorrhage: British Aneurysm Nimodipine Trial. *Br Med J* 1989;298:636

105. Kassell NF, Haley EC, Torner JC, et al: Nicardipine and angiographic vasospasm [abstract]. *J Neurosurg* 1991;74:341A

106. Gelmers HJ, Gorter K, De Weedt CJ, et al: A controlled trial of nimodipine in acute ischemic stroke. *N Engl J Med* 1988; 318:203

Critical Care, Third Edition, edited by Joseph M. Civetta,
Robert W. Taylor, and Robert R. Kirby.
Lippincott-Raven Publishers, Philadelphia, PA © 1997.

CHAPTER 20

The Host Response to Injury and Infection

Timothy H. Pohlman
Edward M. Boyle, Jr.

Humans possess an extensive repertoire of responses to infection and injury (Fig. 20-1). These highly complex defenses may be deployed concurrently or sequentially; many require precise regulation to prevent collateral damage to normal tissue. Four major homeostatic systems mediate host defense: the immune system, the reticuloendothelial system (RES), a system of four cross-reacting plasma protein cascades, and a complex system of neuroendocrine reactions. The neuroendocrine response to injury is described in Chapter 23, and this topic is not discussed further in this chapter. The principal functions of the immune system are to recognize self from non-self and to effect death or destruction of the latter. In contrast to the immune system, the RES is completely indiscriminate in defense of the host and, to function normally, it must be precisely regulated, generally by the immune system. The plasma protein defense system includes contact activation proteins, complement proteins, coagulation factors, and proteins of fibrinolysis that, similar to the RES system, also are indiscriminate in action. Therefore, these plasma protein cascades, like the RES, have distinct potential to induce collateral tissue damage. Another important feature of host defense is that the immune system and RES "talk" to one another through a vast network of cytokines and a smaller number of lipid-based mediators (e.g., platelet activating factor). Although the structure and function of the immune system and RES have been under investigation for over a century, the molecular biology of the cytokine network is a relatively recent topic of biomedical research. These components of host defense are operative to some degree in every critical ill patient. One or all of the systems described may still be active in the absence of

infection or acute injury, profoundly distorting the meaning of clinical data in the ICU.

Several experiments of nature demonstrate with supreme directness the importance of the immune system, RES, and the plasma protein defense system to host survival. The acquired immunodeficiency syndrome is caused by human immunodeficiency virus–induced destruction of CD4-bearing T lymphocytes ("helper" T cells). Gradual failure of cellular immunity (that together with humoral immunity constitutes the immune system of host defense) inevitably leads to death secondary to infection or neoplastic transformation. X-linked severe combined immunodeficiency syndrome is characterized by impairment of both cell-mediated and humoral immunity. Affected individuals die early from recurrent, severe infections. In several cases in this heterogeneous group of disorders, the disease occurs secondary to mutations in the common gamma-chain (g-c gene), which encodes a portion of the receptor heterodimer for interleukin (IL)-2, IL-4, IL-7, IL-9, and IL-15. Communication between immune cells, mediated by these cytokines, therefore fails to occur. Thus, severe combined immunodeficiency syndromes clearly demonstrate the importance of cytokine function in host defense. Within the RES, a congenital absence of CD11b/CD18 (leukocyte adherence deficiency [LAD] type 1), a glycoprotein expressed on most types of leukocytes, causes a profound susceptibility to life-threatening infection because leukocyte adherence to endothelium and leukocyte aggregation, both mediated by CD11b/CD18, does not occur. Although neutrophils from LAD-1 patients function normally in every other respect, failure of neutrophils in affected patients to adhere to the endothelial surface

291

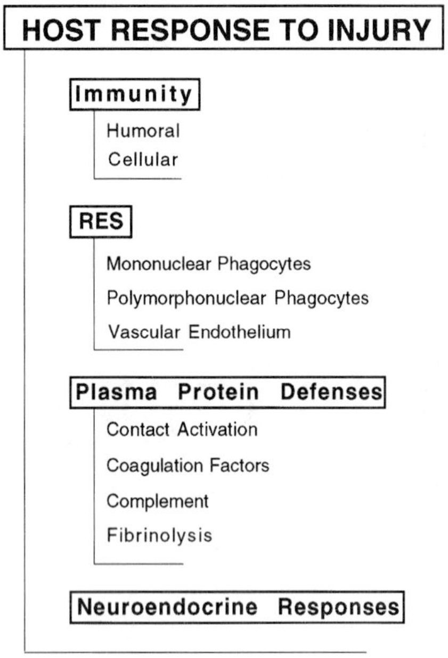

HOST RESPONSE TO INJURY

Immunity
Humoral
Cellular

RES
Mononuclear Phagocytes
Polymorphonuclear Phagocytes
Vascular Endothelium

Plasma Protein Defenses
Contact Activation
Coagulation Factors
Complement
Fibrinolysis

Neuroendocrine Responses

FIGURE 20-1. Host systems that defend against infection and injury: To some degree, all four host defense systems are operative in every critically ill patient. Principal features of the host response to injury are (1) all four systems are inextricably connected; (2) any or all host defense systems, or any of the component elements of each system, may be operative in the absence of infection or injury; and (3) each host response defense system is precisely regulated to prevent damage to normal tissue outside of an area of infection or injury. Neuroendocrine responses are discussed in Chapter 23. RES, reticuloendothelial system.

prevents migration to sites of infection and tissue damage. Dysfunction of the plasma protein cascade system occurs in patients with an inherited deficiency of one or more proteins of coagulation, fibrinolysis, complement, or contact activation. For example, a single coagulation factor deficiency such as hemophilia A produces profound abnormalities in host defense. Also, deficiencies of regulatory proteins of the plasma protein defense system can be equally deleterious to the host. For example, a deficiency of C1-inhibitor (C1-Inh), which regulates function of proteins in all four defense cascades, produces profound clinical abnormalities.

Life-threatening disease states develop when the immune system fails to discriminate self from non-self (autoimmunity), or when the RES or plasma protein defense system exceed regulatory boundaries. RES-mediated host injury occurs after RES-based inflammatory reactions, when this system, designed to function optimally at a local level, extends systemically. Thus, if an inflammatory response remains localized to the site of infection, this response, although destructive to tissue, benefits the host by containing and eliminating infecting microbes. If, however, the inflammatory response exceeds local boundaries and spreads to engulf one or more organ systems, the destructive nature of inflammation, manifested systemically, may compromise the homeostatic integrity of the host. The concept of a malignant spread of inflammation, even in the absence of a defin-

able infectious process, was first recognized by Carrico and coworkers[1] and was subsequently defined and designated the systemic inflammatory response syndrome (SIRS).[2-4] Furthermore, a second category of RES-mediated systemic inflammatory reactions, involving an entirely different spectrum of pathophysiologic events, recently has been recognized and designated ischemia-reperfusion injury. In various levels of severity, RES-mediated host injuries (either SIRS or ischemia-reperfusion injury) are, arguably, the most common cause of critical illness in the ICU (Fig. 20-2).

RETICULOENDOTHELIAL SYSTEM

MONONUCLEAR PHAGOCYTES

The host response to infection begins with activation of mononuclear phagocytes (Mϕ), in the form of either fixed tissue macrophages or circulating mononuclear cells. The principal functions of Mϕ are to present Mϕ-processed foreign antigen to the immune system and to secrete an initial wave of cytokines that initiate the inflammatory response. Although antigen processing and presentation by Mϕ have been studied extensively, less is known about the mechanisms mediating Mϕ activation and Mϕ cytokine expression. Recently, CD14, a glycosyl-phosphatidylinositol–anchored glycoprotein, was identified as a Mϕ surface receptor for bacterial lipopolysaccharide (LPS; endotoxin), a major virulence factor of gram-negative bacteria.[5-8] Patients with paroxysmal nocturnal hemoglobinuria lack glycosyl-phosphatidylinositol anchors on many of their cell types.[9] Phagocytes from patients with paroxysmal nocturnal hemoglobinuria respond weakly to LPS with minimal release of inflammatory cytokines, confirming the requirement of CD14 for normal Mϕ function.[10] LPS activation of Mϕ also requires an acute-phase reactant, LPS-binding protein, which presents LPS to CD14 on the Mϕ plasma membrane. Once CD14 acquires LPS, a transmembrane signal is generated, which activates a distinct 38-kd protein kinase of the MAPK family of protein kinases.[11] This pathway then ultimately results in new gene transcription and Mϕ activation.

Gram-negative sepsis, caused largely by the effect of LPS on the host, is a common complication in the ICU. Infections with gram-positive organisms, however, also are associated with substantial morbidity and mortality in critically ill patients and are etiologic agents of SIRS.[12] Although, gram-positive bacteria do not contain LPS, gram-positive bacterial cell walls do contain several LPS-like amphiphilic lipolymers[13] including lipoteichoic acid, lipomannan, lipopeptidoglycan, lipopoly-(N-acetyl-glucosamine), and lipoteichuronic acid. Recent studies suggest that amphiphilic, LPS-like molecules also may activate Mϕ through a CD14-dependent mechanism.[5]

Early response cytokines from Mϕ, including tumor necrosis factor (TNF), IL-1, and IL-6, are observed experimentally within minutes after an injection of either *Escherichia coli* or purified LPS. TNF levels rise and peak at approximately 90 minutes, after which they return to baseline levels by 4 to 6 hours post-LPS infusion. IL-1 in contrast, has a

A. ISCHEMIA-REPERFUSION

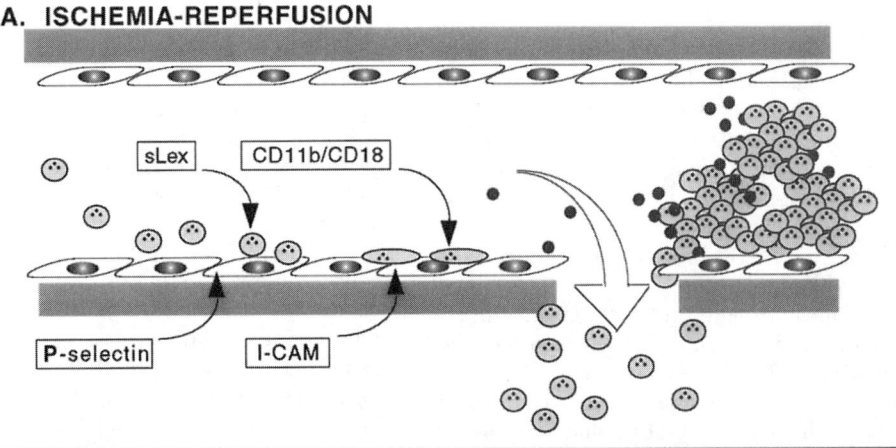

B. SEPSIS (SIRS)

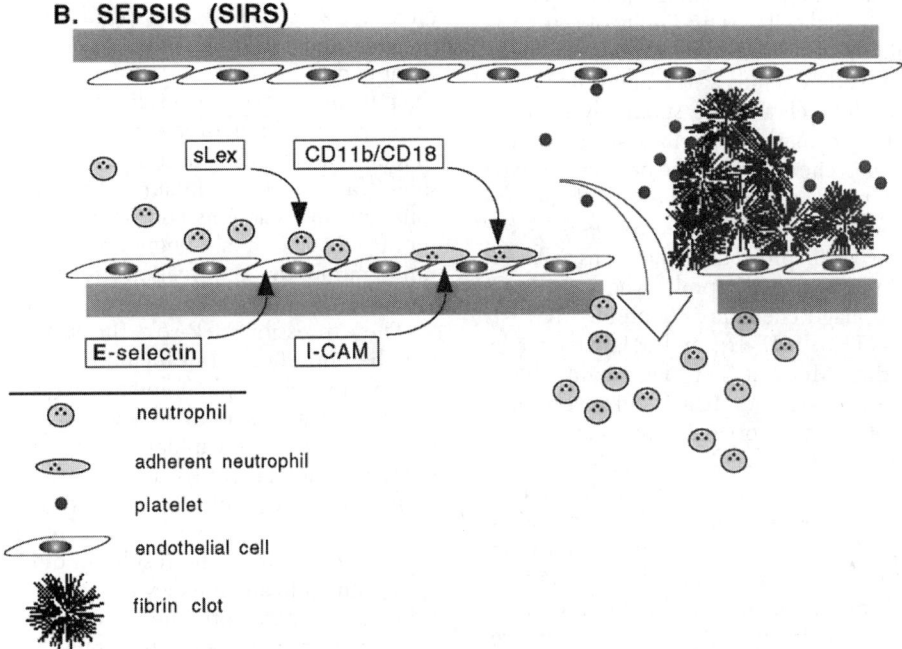

FIGURE 20-2. Systemic inflammatory response paradigms: The two types of systemic inflammatory responses that may occur are based on the nature of the injury to the patient. (**A**) Reperfusion of ischemic tissue generates oxygen-derived reactive molecules such as superoxide anion, hydroxyl radical, hydrogen peroxide, or hypochloric acid. Also, local mediators, such as nitric oxide and fixed-tissue mononuclear phagocytes expressing chemokines (not depicted in this figure), also may be involved. In this scheme, P-selectin is expressed after stimulation of endothelial cells with reactive oxygen species or complement fragments, in particular, C5a. Neutrophils then begin to roll along the endothelial cell surface and become activated by chemokine signals from juxtaposed endothelial cells, leading to firm adherence of the neutrophil to the endothelial cell surface. Under the influence of chemotactic cytokines (e.g., IL-8), neutrophils migrate across the vessel wall. Release of toxic neutrophil substances at any time during this sequence of events may lead to damage of the vessel or adjacent tissue. Furthermore, activated platelets and neutrophils may aggregate during reperfusion, producing "no-reflow" phenomena and aggrevating tissue injury. (**B**) Infection with gram-negative or gram-positive bacteria leads to the activation of fixed tissue and circulating mononuclear phagocytes. Macrophage-derived cytokines (tumor necrosis factor, IL-1, and IL-6) activate endothelial cells, with the conversion of endothelial cells into a specific phenotype. This endothelial cell activation phenotype includes expression of surface molecules that promote inflammation and coagulation. In a similar four-step sequence shown in **A** (tethering, signaling, adherence, and migration), neutrophils infiltrate through the vessel wall into surrounding tissue. Activation of platelets and intravascular tissue factor expression lead to intravascular coagulation. This systemic inflammatory response syndrome (SIRS) also has been referred to as disseminated intravascular inflammation to emphasize the parallel of this process with disseminated intravascular coagulation.

broader peak extending over 3 to 4 hours, whereas interferon-gamma and IL-6 levels rise continuously throughout the initial 8-hour period after the infusion of LPS. Cells that respond to TNF possess between 1000 and 10,000 cytokine receptors per cell, but only as little as 10% of these receptors need to be occupied at any one time for a maximum biological response.[14] TNF and IL-1 are found in invertebrates and thus have appeared early in evolution. Moreover, the most primitive invertebrates and, possibly, unicellular protozoa, may possess cytokine-like molecules. The early appearance in evolution of cytokines strongly underscores the fundamental importance of these molecules to the defense of the organism from environmental challenges.

In addition to cytokines, Mϕ secrete several smaller sized peptides, classified as chemokines, that mediate important inflammatory and immunoregulatory activities. Chemokines are expressed in several cell types including fibroblasts, endothelial cells, and epithelial cells.[15] This family of cytokines is divided into two subfamilies based on the orientation of the first two of four conserved cysteines at the amino-terminus of each peptide. The alpha-chemokine subfamily includes peptides in which the two marker cysteines are separated by one amino acid (C-X-C chemokines); the beta-chemokine subfamily consist of peptides containing the identifying cysteines adjacent to one another (C-C chemokines). C-X-C chemokines, including IL-8 (previously known as NAF or NAP-1), preferentially attract neutrophils, whereas the C-C chemokines (macrophage chemotaxis protein [MCP]-1, MCP-2, MCP-3, RANTES, MIP-1α, and MIP-1β) act by preferentially recruiting Mϕ but not neutrophils. Both groups of chemokines activate and attract leukocytes, and, therefore, this group of inflammatory mediators may exacerbate or extend an inflammatory reaction through a positive feedback mechanism. For example, MCP-1 induces IL-1 and IL-6 release from monocytes. Thus, MCP-1–recruited Mϕ also could release IL-1 after MCP-1 stimulation in an inflammatory site, which may further stimulate MCP-1 release from adjacent fibroblasts or endothelial cells, recruiting more leukocytes and amplifying the inflammatory response. These small peptides likely are the major mediators of leukocyte recruitment to and activation in inflammatory sites, although this has not been firmly established. Using monoclonal anti–IL-8 antibodies in rabbit models of septic and ischemia-reperfusion injuries, neutrophil accumulation is reduced up to 80%, demonstrating the potential clinical importance of this group of inflammatory mediators. IL-4, IL-10, and interferon-gamma seem to regulate expression of both cytokines and chemokines during endotoxemia.[16] Failure of the antiinflammatory effects of IL-4, IL-10, and interferon-gamma is an appealing but unsubstantiated explanation for systemic extension of a local homeostatic mechanism.

ENDOTHELIUM

Endothelial Cell Activation

Because of a strategic position between tissue and the vascular space bearing many circulatory inflammatory mediators, the endothelium of the vascular tree is ideally positioned to regulate the inflammatory response. Endothelial cells, considered for over a century as only a passive, nonthrombogenic inner lining of blood vessels, are known to transiently express an extensive array of surface membrane proteins. Activation of endothelial cells results in a profound change to a phenotype that promotes inflammation and thrombosis. Endothelial cell activation in inflammatory states is divided into early and late phases, determined by the nature of the stimulus inducing activation. Thrombin, histamine, complement fragment C5a, hypoxia, and oxygen-derived free radicals are agonists of early-phase endothelial cell activation. Within minutes of binding to cognate receptors on the endothelial cell surface, thrombin, histamine, or complement fragment C5a induce the rapid release of P-selectin (CD62P; Fig. 20-3), von Willebrand factor, and other constituents from endothelial cell Weibel-Palade bodies. P-selectin functions as an initiator of leukocyte adhesion to platelets and endothelial cells. The corresponding glycoprotein ligand on the activated neutrophil necessary for this adhesion has been identified.[17] The most prominent function of P-selectin in the inflammatory process is linked most directly to leukocyte adhesion in ischemia-reperfusion injuries. In several in vivo models, monoclonal antibody to P-selectin was found to inhibit a reperfusion inflammatory response.[18-26] However, inflammatory reactions associated with infection do not seem require P-selectin, although a reduction in white blood cell immigration to an infectious focus after treatment with monoclonal antibody to P-selectin has been reported.[27]

The expression of P-selectin on the surface of platelets may be important in an inflammatory process contributing to the "no reflow" phenomenon. This theory proposes that activated platelets and leukocytes together aggregate in the circulation, causing capillary obstruction.[28] This leads to increased ischemia and tissue injury because of the impaired delivery of energy substrate and oxygen to peripheral vascular bed. It is likely that what is recognized as ischemia-reperfusion injury is the result of both leukocyte adherence to endothelium and leukocyte aggregation. In that leukocyte integrins mediate both phenomena, it is difficult to separate these two processes experimentally.

Late-response endothelial cell functions are induced by Mϕ cytokines TNF and IL-1. (Highly purified bacterial lipopolysaccharides also induce every known endothelial cell function induced by TNF and IL-1.[29] The clinical relevance of this in vitro observation is uncertain, because any LPS that dissociates from blood-borne gram-negative bacteria is likely cleared extremely rapidly by Mϕ in vivo.) The endothelial cell response induced by TNF and IL-1 (and LPS) requires new protein synthesis, and thus the peak activity of these functions appears within 3 to 4 hours after stimulation with either cytokine. Responses induced by TNF and IL-1 in endothelial cells in vitro include the expression of leukocyte adherence molecules (E-selectin [CD62E; see Fig. 20-3], intracellular adhesion molecule [ICAM-1, ICAM-2], and vascular cell adhesion molecule [VCAM] and the conversion of the endothelial cell to a procoagulant phenotype. Like P-selectin, E-selectin has been determined to be a mediator in the initial transient adhesion phenomenon between neutrophils and endothelial cells; however, the adhesive bond between E-selectin and the leukocyte counter-structure rec-

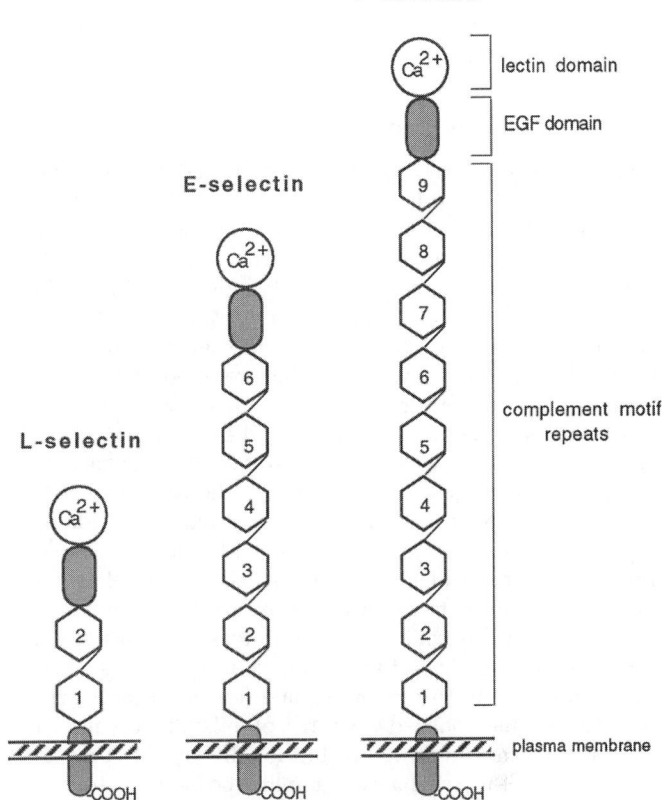

FIGURE 20-3. The general structures of selectin adherence molecules: Selectins are designated CD62L (L-selectin), CD62E (E-selectin), and CD62P (P-selectin), and all three have the same structural motif. Each selectin has a transmembrane hydrophobic domain joining the extracellular portion of the selectin molecule to an intracellular signalling domain at the carboxy-terminus of each selectin. Selectin intracellular domains are highly functional and may be responsible for generating activation signals that target adjacent neutrophils. At the amino-terminus, each selectin has a calcium-dependent, carbohydrate-binding lectin domain. Adjacent to the lectin domain is an epidermal grown factor (EGF)–like domain, and adjacent to the EGF-like domain are a variable number of repeats that are homologous with complement regulatory proteins. It has been suggested that the different number of repeating complement motifs among selectin family members has evolved to maintain a molecular distance between cells that is specific for each selectin. Preformed P-selectin is expressed on endothelial cells and platelets after storage in Weibel-Palade bodies and in alpha-granules, respectively. E-selectin is expressed only on endothelial cells, and before it is expressed, E-selectin must be synthesized after transcriptional activation of the E-selectin gene. L-selectin is expressed on all leukocytes except for one category of lymphocytes. Sialyl-Lewis x (sLe^x) and sialyl-Lewis a (sLe^a), or the sulfated forms of these fucose-containing tetrasaccharides, are recognized by the lectin domains of all three selectins, and several selectin ligands are characterized by the presence of sLe^x, sLe^a, or their sulfated derivatives. (Imhof BA, Dunon D: Leukocyte migration and adhesion. *Adv Immunol* 1995;58:345.)

ognized by E-selectin seems slightly stronger than is the bond created by a P-selectin–receptor interaction.[17] The counter-structure on the neutrophil surface associated with E-selectin binding includes a carbohydrate ligand (sLe^x and Le^x) and L-selectin. E-selectin is found exclusively on endothelial cells and is not constitutively expressed. In vivo, E-selectin expression can be detected in patients with both bacteremia and sustained hypotension but is not detected in bacteremic patients who are not in septic shock. Markedly elevated endothelial cell surface expression of E-selectin is detectable in baboons in experimental septic shock[30]; however, in baboons subjected to hypovolemic shock (ischemia-reperfusion injury), an increased expression of E-selectin over baseline is not observed.[31]

The immunoglobulin gene superfamily is composed of several adhesion molecules expressed on, but not exclusive to, endothelium. These adhesion molecules include ICAM-1, ICAM-2, and VCAM. ICAM-1 expression is inducible after stimulation of both endothelial cells and myocytes with inflammatory stimuli. Expression of ICAM-1 is maximal within 4 to 6 hours after stimulation of endothelial cells or cardiac myocytes with TNF or IL-1 in vitro, and, once expressed, persists up to 48 hours. ICAM-1 binds the leukocyte integrin CD11b/CD18 (also known as [MAC]-1), mediating the firm adherence stage of leukocyte transendothelial cell migration ICAM-2, which weakly binds leukocyte inte-

grins (particularly CD11/CD18), is constitutively expressed on endothelial cells, and whose expression is not increased during endothelial cell activation. Therefore, ICAM-1 seems to regulate high-volume, transendothelial leukocyte inflammatory traffic, whereas ICAM-2 regulates low-level constitutive leukocyte migration. The leukocyte ligand for VCAM-1 is another integrin, VLA-4, expressed on lymphocytes, monocytes, eosinophils, basophils, and natural killer cells, but not on neutrophils.[17] This interaction explains the role of VCAM-1 in cell-mediated immune reactions to injury such as transplant rejection. Monoclonal antibodies to VCAM-1 reduce rejection after cardiac transplantation[32] and attenuate certain autoimmune disorders,[33] demonstrating the clinical relevance of this endothelial cell adhesion molecule.

Tissue factor expressed on endothelial cells binds coagulation factor of VII, thereby activating the extrinsic pathway of coagulation. A factor VII–tissue factor interaction results in a transmembrane signal in endothelial cells, leading to a transient increase in intracellular Ca^{2+}. These Ca^{2+} transient alterations may lead to further Weibel-Palade discharge, thus reinitiating early response endothelial cell activation. Furthermore, expression of endothelial cell tissue factor promotes the formation of intravascular thrombin and subsequent intravascular coagulation. In addition to extending intravascular coagulation, intravascular thrombin also may propagate the activation of endothelial cell early inflammatory responses (e.g., P-selectin expression) in an autocrine or paracrine fashion.

Leukocyte Effector Functions

Once the endothelial cell has been activated and adhesion molecules have recruited neutrophils from the circulation to the activated endothelium, the neutrophil confers an enormous amount of nonspecific tissue damage. The main mechanism producing neutrophil-mediated tissue injury is the elaboration of cytotoxic by-products released from adherent, activated neutrophils stimulated by the inflammatory cascade. Although normally neutrophils are important scavengers, primed and activated to contain and eliminate foreign, infectious, and necrotic material, in the systemic host response to injury, the widespread leukocyte–endothelial margination causes tissue damage through the release of toxic substances such as oxygen-derived free radicals, oxidants, proteolytic enzymes, and lipid autocoids such as platelet activating factor and leukotriene B_4. Exocytosis of stored cytoplasmic contents results in an extracellular release of secretory products such as serine proteases, elastases, and myleoperoxidase. Secretory products include prostaglandins, prostacyclin, thromboxane, and leukotrienes. Arachidonic acid is metabolized to a series of inflammatory mediators by activated neutrophils, further driving this process. These stimulatory mechanisms amplify the inflammatory response and thus the tissue damage. Additionally, neutrophil activation results in an oxidative burst. The oxygen used in the oxidative burst produces hydrogen peroxide, hydroxyl radicals, and other destructive oxygen free radicals, which disrupt cellular functions and increase the degree of endothelial cell activation. Normally proteolytic enzymes, arachidonic acid metabolites, and free radicals, in combination with neutrophil phagocytic activity, respond to by neutralizing foreign invaders and clearing cellular debris and necrotic tissue. However, when neutrophils are called in to respond to injured cells, adjacent tissue with potentially reversible injury may be permanently damaged. When neutrophils adhere to large areas of endothelium as a result of massive systemic stress, multiple organ dysfunction can follow.

Leukocyte–Endothelial Cell Interactions

Recent studies, both in vitro and in vivo, demonstrate the fundamental importance of leukocyte interactions with the endothelium of the vascular tree and the subsequent emigration of leukocytes to the extravascular space. These basic cellular processes are postulated to occur in a coordinated four-step sequence: (1) tethering, (2) signaling, (3) adherence, and (4) migration.[34] Tethering, or rolling, refers to a transient, weak attachment of leukocytes to endothelium in the postcapillary venule where sheer forces are minimal. Also, other vessels in inflammatory sites dilate under the influence of nitric oxide (NO), prostaglandins, and other mediators, which reduces flow and sheer stresses, allowing more leukocytes to engage the vessel wall. Once leukocytes are at the vessel wall, endothelial cell selectins (P-selectin and E-selectin) mediate leukocyte "rolling" along the activated endothelium. Although selectin-mediated leukocyte adherence is transient, it is sufficient to permit transmission of signals by chemokines from endothelial cells or adjacent cells such as fibroblasts that activate leukocyte integrins. Activated leukocyte integrins then firmly bind to counter-structures on the endothelial cell surface. Lastly, adherent leukocytes begin diapedesis to endothelial cell junctions through which migration occurs. At any time in this sequence, early discharge of phagocyte lysosomal enzymes and oxygen radicals can produce substantial tissue damage out of proportion to the injury that produced the response.

The LAD syndromes illustrate the importance of these mechanisms to normal host defense. LAD-1 patients are unable to express integrins (CD11/CD18) on the leukocyte surface. Leukocytes fail to bind to the corresponding counter-structure on the endothelial cell surface, and as a result, LAD-1 patients exhibit neutrophilia and recurrent, life-threatening infections. The second subset of patients, LAD type 2, fail in production of the carbohydrate ligand on the leukocyte surface. These leukocytes fail to bind to endothelial cell selectins; thus, the initial weak neutrophil–endothelial cell interaction is blocked, and leukocyte adherence is only possible under conditions of extremely low shear stress. LAD-2 patients so far identified are also at an increased risk for infection, yet the severity of these infectious complications is less than that of the LAD-1 patients. These two experiments of nature suggest potential strategies with antiadherence therapy in systemic inflammatory responses. For example, administration of a monoclonal antibody that blocks leukocyte CD11/CD18 (producing a LAD-1–like defect), will completely inhibit ischemia-reperfusion syndromes, including that syndrome that follows shock and resuscitation. This antibody, however, predictably exacerbates infections in experimental animals, thus reducing a potential therapeutic window for future therapies based on this antibody. Alternatively, blocking P-selectin expression (a LAD-2–like defect) in experimental models of ischemia-reperfusion injury seems to be nearly as effective as CD11/CD18 blockade in amelioration of the injury, but without causing the same degree of susceptibility to infection.

PLASMA PROTEIN DEFENSES ■

COMPLEMENT

Complement (C') is a host defense mechanism primarily integrating specific humoral (antibody) and nonspecific cellular (phagocyte) components of an inflammatory response. However, because of redundant pathways of C' activation, and because of a membrane attack complex (MAC) that forms after complement activation, neither specificity nor phagocytosis is necessarily observed during C'-mediated events. Moreover, by-products of complement activation have the properties of inflammatory mediators inasmuch as these circulating peptide fragments from proteolytic cleavage of C' protein precursors have potent inflammatory properties. Thus, of any host defense mechanism, C' harbors the most potential for injuring the host.

Two pathways are recognized as initiators of complement activation, the classic pathway and the alternate pathway (Fig. 20-4). These converge at complement component C3, which is activated by either pathway. The alternate pathways differs functionally from the classic pathway in that the alternate pathway is always "primed" by a low level of spontaneous activation; furthermore, the alternate pathway has a positive feedback mechanism, which can rapidly amplify a C′-mediated response. The complement cascade is regulated by several inhibitors that have critical functions, as demonstrated by the presence of severe symptoms in patients who congenitally lack one or more complement regulatory proteins. An important factor that protects host cells from inadvertent injury by activated components of complement is decay-accelerating factor (DAF; CD55). DAF is expressed on all cell types and functions by accelerating the proteolytic activity of a C′ inhibitor in the fluid phase, factor I, on C3b. Manipulation of cellular DAF expression on endothelium of a donor organ has been considered as potential immunosuppression for xenotransplantation. This strategy involves stable transfection of DAF into xenograft endothelium before transplantation. Increased expression of DAF on the donor organ endothelium protects the graft from complement-mediated hyperacute rejection by the recipient.

Complement activation ultimately leads to the formation of the membrane attack complex (MAC) consisting of complement proteins C5b-C9. This complex creates an opening in the target cell (e.g., bacteria, virus, tumor cell) membrane and causes hypotonic lysis of cells susceptible to lysis, such as bacteria. The mechanism of action on nucleated cells is less clear. Endothelial cells unprotected from autologous complement fixation are activated by MAC insertion, causing vesiculation of membrane particles that express binding sites for coagulation factor V and promote prothrombinase activity. Complement-induced prothrombinase activity on endothelium may, therefore, contribute to microvascular thrombin deposition systemically during systemic complement activation or at local sites of inflammation cell. Complement activation also results in the formation of potential inflammatory mediators, C3a and C5a, classically referred to as anaphylatoxins.

C5a is a potent neutrophil chemotaxin and stimulus of leukoaggregation, which may contribute to ischemia-reperfusion injury. C5a also has been shown to activate endothelial cells in vitro, causing release of von Willebrand factor and P-selectin, simultaneously promoting coagulation and inflammation, respectively.[35]

CONTACT ACTIVATION PROTEINS

The major protein components of the plasma contact activation system are as follows: (1) prekallikrein; (2) high molecular weight kininogen; (3) Hageman factor, which is coagulation factor XII; and (4) coagulation factor XI. The recognition of coagulation factors XII and XI as major protein components of both the coagulation system and contact activation system demonstrates the essentially inseparable pathways of the plasma protein host defense systems. In addition to kinin release by contact activation, plasma kallikrein and Hageman factor also convert plasminogen to plasmin and activate the first component of complement, C1. Factor XII–deficient patients (Hageman factor), for example, have increased thromboembolic phenomenon because factor XII partly contributes to the initiation of fibrinolysis.[36] Thus, coagulation, fibrinolysis, and complement all may be activated by initiation of contact activation. Furthermore, plasmin, in a reciprocal fashion, catalyzes the formation of kinins, creating a positive feedback loop with a potential for rapid amplification of inflammatory reactions in plasma (Fig. 20-5).

Bradykinin generation by contact activation requires autoactivation of Hageman factor on foreign surfaces (e.g., bacterial outer membranes bearing lipopolysaccharides[37] or extravascular protein surfaces such as basement membrane). Extracorporeal membrane oxygenation circuits also represent a potential initiator of contact activation. Although contact activation is classically initiated by foreign surfaces, cells of the RES initiate contact activation with kinin formation and secondary activation of coagulation, complement, and

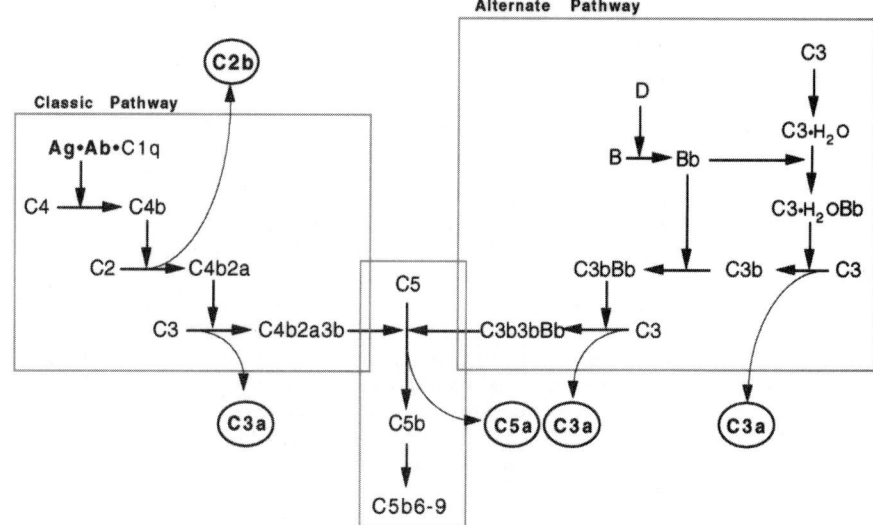

FIGURE 20-4. Molecular pathways of complement activation: The complement membrane attack complex may be generated by either activation of the *classic pathway* or *alternate pathway*. During the activation of either pathway, several inflammatory peptides are generated (*enclosed by ovals*). These complement fragments, also known as anaphylatoxins, have several biological activities through activation of cells of the reticuloendothelial system (RES). The prototype reaction of complement fragment–RES interactions is C5a receptor–mediated activation of endothelial cells leading to, in part, the expression of P-selectin.

fibrinolysis. Contact activation initially involves the interaction of the contact activation proteins with a negatively charged molecule such as heparin (or heparin-like molecules on RES cell surfaces), collagen, vascular basement membrane glycosaminoglycans, or dextran, resulting in the activation of Hageman factor (factor XII). In addition, endothelial cells express a high-affinity receptor that binds Hageman factor, which may accelerate activation. Prekallikrein is then converted to kallikrein by activated Hageman factor, and kallikrein subsequently converts high molecular weight kininogen to bradykinin. Bradykinin, released by this reaction (which is accelerated by tissue injury and exposure of proteoglycans), binds to specific receptors on adjacent cells to increase vasodilation and to increase capillary permeability. Vasodilation induced by bradykinin is likely mediated by NO.[8] Kinins also stimulate prostacyclin release, another potent vasodilator. Kinin-mediated hypotension in septic shock then may lead to cardiovascular dysfunction and end-organ injury. Injection of kallikrein into pigs produces a rapid increase in cardiac output, a marked decrease in mean arterial pressure, and a fall in pulmonary systemic resistance.[39] Within hours of administration of endotoxin to humans, a systemic inflammatory response evolves, characterized by hemodynamic instability, ventricular contraction abnormalities, and changes in pulmonary gas exchange and permeability. These deleterious changes are related to activation of the kallikrein–kinin system and of the fibrinolytic system.[40] However, bradykinin has been shown to have a cardioprotective effect after experimental myocardial ischemia through a mechanism involving the effects of hypoxia on endothelial cells. These observations suggest that blockade of kinin activity to reduce vasodilation and vascular permeability in such states as sepsis may possess untoward effects that are not anticipated.[41,42]

Kinin-mediated vasomotor activity is regulated by kinin degradation enzymes on endothelial cells, particularly angiotensinogen converting enzyme (ACE). Pharmacologic inhibition of ACE increases NO production in cultured endothelial cells by a kinin-dependent mechanism, suggesting that ACE inhibitors could produce kinin-generated, NO-mediated abnormalities in vasomotor tone. Prolongation of the half-life of bradykinin by ACE inhibitors may explain the antiischemic and cardioprotective effect of this class of drugs.[41]

The contact activation cascade is inhibited predominately by C1-Inh, a serine protease inhibitor that also regulates initial reactions in the classic pathway of complement activation. The inhibitory actions of C1-Inh on contact activation are through blockade of Hageman factor and kallikrein activities. A deficiency of C1-Inh can be inherited as an autosomal dominate trait known as hereditary angioedema. This syndrome is characterized by abdominal pain caused by acute edema of the bowel wall and acute edema of mucosa and subcutaneous tissues, particularly involving the face and neck. Notably, certain patients who have sustained massive blood loss and are then subjected to massive transfusion and

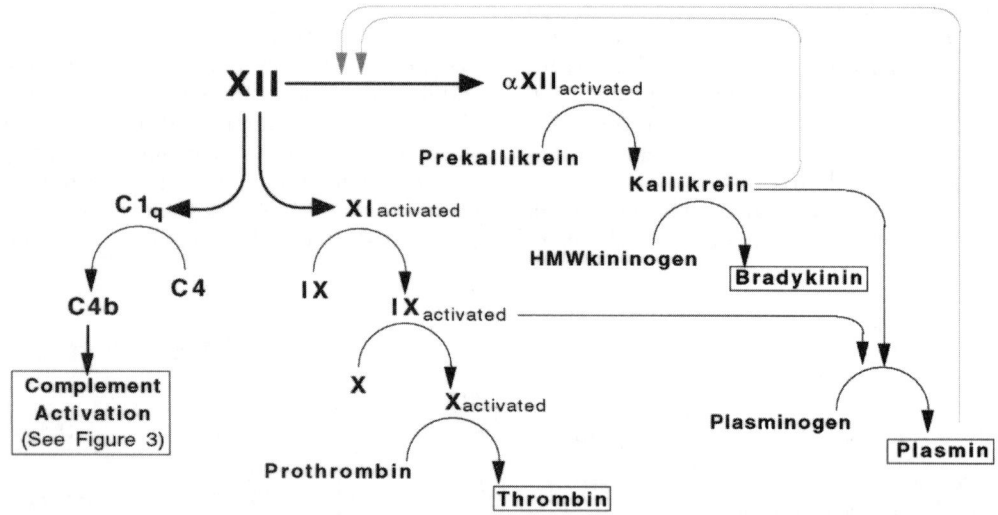

FIGURE 20-5. Molecular pathways of the plasma protein defense cascades: Factor XII, also called Hageman factor (for the individual in whom an inherited deficiency of factor XII was first recognized by Ratnoff and coworkers), is directly involved in complement activation, the formation of thrombin, and the generation of kinins. Factor XII is indirectly involved in the formation of plasmin from plasminogen through factor IX activation in the coagulation cascade, or through kallikrein during contact activation. Moreover, factor XII–mediated activation of the fibrinolytic pathway may lead to the activation of factor XII in a positive feedback loop, thus providing a mechanism for amplification of inflammation. Dysregulation of these four interrelated pathways on a systemic level causes a diffuse capillary leak syndrome. Massive tissue edema is frequently the cause of major organ dysfunction in the critically ill patient and is prominent after massive trauma and resuscitation. Angiotensin converting enzyme inhibitors block kinase II activity (not shown), a major regulator of kinin generation, and may cause clinically significant accumulations of bradykinin.

resuscitation (a systemic ischemia-reperfusion injury) are observed immediately after resuscitation to be markedly edematous, resembling patients with hereditary angio-edema. An angioedema-like syndrome after hypovolemic shock and resuscitation has been referred to previously as a diffuse capillary leak syndrome. The similarity between systemic ischemia-reperfusion syndrome and hereditary angioedema is also evident during celiotomy when massive bowel edema is occasionally encountered, precluding closure of the abdomen, or, if the abdomen is closed, causing abdominal compartment syndrome postoperatively. Fulminate respiratory failure during the first 12 to 24 hours in the ICU is also associated with some patients with this clinical course. These observations suggest that the clinical manifestations of systemic ischemia-reperfusion injury may partly be caused by a failure of C1-Inh–mediated inhibition of contact activation. Consistent with a potential role of C1-Inh in modulating systemic inflammatory reactions is the observation that infusion of C1-Inh during experimental gram-negative bacteremia prevents the development of shock.[43]

C1-Inh is a member of the serpin family of proteinase inhibitors. Serpin proteinase inhibitors have evolved substrate specificity by subtle alterations of the conformation of the reactive center loop motif common to all serpins. This necessarily makes these proteins unusually susceptible to phenotypic variation in inhibitory activity because of minor genetic changes in center loop codons.[44,45] These molecular observations may explain why an inflammatory response may exceed C1-Inh regulation in some individuals, resulting in a systemic ischemia-reperfusion injury after trauma, whereas other individuals do not develop this syndrome after similar or greater trauma.

COAGULATION

The coagulation system functions predominately in response to tissue injury. Similar to complement activation, two protein cascades converge on a common pathway to form clot. The extrinsic pathway, activated by tissue factor, initiates coagulation. Tissue factor is expressed constitutively on several cell types within and immediately outside the vessel wall, but under normal conditions is not expressed on vascular endothelium. Therefore, at the initiation phase, coagulation is localized to blood exposed only to cells outside the vascular space. The intrinsic pathway is thought to function in normal hemostasis as an amplifier of factor X activation and an accelerator of the conversion of prothrombin to thrombin. Hemophilia A and B clearly demonstrate the importance of the intrinsic pathway to normal hemostasis. Pathologically, the intrinsic pathway may promote abnormal intravascular clot formation that is remote from the site of an injury that initiates coagulation. Diffuse microvascular clot formation possibly contributes to clinical abnormalities in several pathologic states. The hemolytic-uremia syndrome and thrombotic thrombocytopenia purpura are characterized by hemolytic anemia resulting from passage of erythrocytes through microvascular thrombi consisting of platelets and fibrin strands with hyaline formation along the endothelial

cell surface; the hallmark of this microangiopathy is the appearance of fragmented erythrocytes (schistocytes) on the peripheral smear. Microangiopathy is not seen in all cases of disseminated intravascular coagulation, but it occurs in disseminated intravascular inflammation that is associated with a stimulus for coagulation.

An important relationship exists between the complement and coagulation systems by the interaction of protein S of the coagulation system with C4b-binding protein that regulates complement activity. Protein S is a cofactor for the endogenous anticoagulant, protein C. Protein S is bound by C4b-binding protein in serum. An elevation of the plasma concentration of free protein S, because of a decrease in the plasma concentration of C4b-binding protein, increases the amount of protein S that can interact with protein C and thereby enhances protein C–mediated anticoagulation. Protein C has a protective effect in experimental models of SIRS. Infusion of C4b-binding protein into primates with *E. coli* bacteremia markedly enhances the deleterious effects of this systemic inflammatory condition, causing a lethal injury with intravascular coagulation and organ dysfunction.[46] C4b-binding protein is an acute-phase reactant, and the level of C4b-binding protein can be expected to increase as a general response to injury. In cases of septic injury, a prominent acute-phase response with C4b-binding protein, therefore, may be harmful. These observations illustrate the complexity of the mechanisms that have evolved for localized injuries and infections. A maladaptive response is possible when such complex mechanisms are challenged by the more virulent, systemic illnesses of modern intensive care medicine.

FIBRINOLYSIS

During a normal hemostatic response to injury, fibrin clot formation is regulated by plasmin generated from plasminogen by the action of tissue plasminogen activator derived principally from endothelial cells. Both plasminogen and tissue plasminogen activator have a high affinity for fibrin on the surface of a clot, which localizes the action of plasmin, a powerful serine proteinase to the clot. Systemic intravascular fibrinolysis away from the site of injury is further regulated by the two other members of the serpin superfamily of serine protease inhibitor: plasminogen activator inhibitor and α_2-antiplasmin. Plasminogen activator inhibitor, also secreted by endothelial cells, is subject to rapid deactivation in plasma α_2-antiplasmin; in contrast is a plasma constituent and an extremely powerful inhibitor of plasmin in the circulation. α_2-Antiplasmin, however, is an inefficient inhibitor of plasmin at or near the clot surface. These redundant regulatory mechanisms may be partly the reason for the low incidence of primary fibrinolysis; the appearance of fibrin degradation products usually represents a compensatory response to disseminated intravascular coagulation.

IMMUNITY

Recognition of foreign antigen and discrimination from self is, arguably, the most complex component of the host response to injury. Mɸ engulf foreign antigen, process it by proteolytic breakdown, and then present this processed material to lymphocytes. Recognition of foreign antigens subsequently results in T-cell and B-cell activation. Lymphocyte activation generally requires two signals from the environment. The first signal consists of the foreign antigen binding to antigen-specific recognition receptors (the "T-cell receptor" for T cells, and surface-expressed IgM antibodies for B cells). Equally important is a co-stimulatory signal delivered by specific cytokines synthesized and secreted by the Mɸ during presentation of antigen. These cytokines include, among others, IL-1 and IL-2, which are T-cell stimulators, and IL-4, which co-stimulates the activation of B cells. Subsets of T cells, in turn, release several cytokines' signals that amplify an immune response. Activated lymphocytes then proceed through a complex process of differentiation into mature antibody-producing B cells and cytolytic T cells.

Helper T cells have an essential role in the orchestration of various immune responses. Helper T cells are divided into two T-cell clones, designated T_{H1} and T_{H2}, that secrete different patterns of cytokines. T_{H1} clones secrete primarily IL-2, interferon-gamma, and lymphotoxin. These cytokines mediate delayed-type hypersensitivity reactions. T_{H2} clones secrete IL-4, IL-5, IL-6, IL-10, IL-13, and granulocyte-macrophage colony-stimulating factor in addition to other immune regulatory cytokines and growth factors. This latter group of T cells and cytokines are associated with the elaboration of a specific antibody response.

Just as malfunction of the RES or the plasma protein defense system can produce severe collateral damage of normal tissue, deregulation of the immune system may have an equally detrimental effect on the host. Within the ICU, examples of immune-mediated host injury are the vasculitis syndromes, including, in particular, necrotizing vasculitis. A common pathologic mechanism in this spectrum of systemic disorders is immune complex deposition in the vessel wall. Two major groups of systemic vasculitis include the polyarteritis nodosa group of systemic necrotizing vasculitis and a subgroup characterized by hypersensitivity that also involves effector T cells: Henoch-Schönlein purpura, essential mixed cryoglobulinemia with vasculitis, and nonspecific vasculitis associated with other primary disorders. Other categories include Wegner's granulomatosis and giant cell arteritis. Moreover, in many critically ill patients, their derangements mimic those of known syndromes. In particular, the hemolytic-uremic syndrome and thrombotic thrombocytopenia purpura consist of abnormalities that overlap with common findings in critically ill patients. These include microangiopathic processes with anemia and microvascular clot formation. This may be accompanied by vessel thrombosis and occlusion, hemorrhage, and ischemic changes in surrounding tissue.

SUMMARY ■

A variety of clinical events initiate systemic inflammatory responses, including sepsis, trauma, thermal-injury, pancreatitis, extracorporeal circulation, or ischemia. Oxygen-derived free radicals, cytokines, complement, or the kallikrein–kinin contact activation system function as either mediators or effector molecules to respond immediately to injury or infection, and to activate the RES. These processes are extended by coagulation and fibrinolysis. The RES represents, in essence, an endothelial cell—-mononuclear phagocyte axis that simultaneously coordinates and mediates the host response to injury. Moreover, a major prerequisite event to injury is a neutrophil–endothelial interaction because inhibition of this event experimentally either completely inhibits or ameliorates these injuries. Immune reactions focus the host response to injury and infection. Host defense systems likely have evolved to respond to localized, well-defined injuries and infections. Modern intensive care, however, presents unprecedented physiologic challenges to the human host. For example, for all of mammalian evolution, a host response to acute blood loss after trauma was selected in the absence of fluid resuscitation. And, although fluid resuscitation is considered intuitively beneficial in the treatment of hemorrhage, and certainly, such therapy clearly reliably reverses hypovolemic shock, recent evidence indicates that such therapy also may allow "deregulation" of host defense systems that is detrimental to the host. This example illustrates that complex defense mechanisms, designed through several million years of natural selection to function at a local level, become maladaptive when manifest systemically.

REFERENCES ■

1. Carrico CJ, Meakins JL, Marshall JC, et al: Multiple organ failure syndrome. *Arch Surg* 1986;121:196
2. Bone RC, Balk RA, Cerra FB, et al: Definitions for sepsis and organ failure and guidelines for the use of innovative therapies in sepsis: The ACCP/SCCM Consensus Conference Committee, American College of Chest Physicians/Society of Critical Care Medicine. *Chest* 1992;101:1644
3. Bone RC: Toward an epidemiology and natural history of SIRS (systemic inflammatory response syndrome). *JAMA* 1992; 268:3452
4. Bone RC, Sibbald WJ, Sprung CL: The ACCP SCCM consensus conference on sepsis and organ failure. *Chest* 1992; 101:1481
5. Pugin J, Heumann ID, Tomasz A, et al: CD14 is a pattern recognition receptor. *Immunity* 1994;1:509
6. Tobias PS, Gegner J, Han J, et al: LPS binding protein and CD14 in the LPS dependent activation of cells. *Prog Clin Biol Res* 1994;388:31
7. Tobias PS, Ulevitch RJ: Lipopolysaccharide binding protein and CD14 in the lipopolysaccharide dependent activation of cells. *Chest* 1994;105(Suppl 3):48S
8. Ulevitch RJ, Tobias PS: Recognition of endotoxin by cells leading to transmembrane signaling. *Curr Opin Immunol* 1994; 6:125
9. Yeh ET, Rosse WF: Paroxysmal nocturnal hemoglobinuria and the glycosylphosphatidylinositol anchor. *J Clin Invest* 1994;93:2305
10. Duchow J, Marchant A, Crusiaux A, et al: Impaired phagocyte responses to lipopolysaccharide in paroxysmal nocturnal hemoglobinuria. *Infect Immunol* 1993;61:4280

11. Han J, Lee JD, Bibbs L, et al: A MAP kinase targeted by endotoxin and hyperosmolarity in mammalian cells. *Science* 1994;265:808

12. Bone RC: Gram positive organisms and sepsis. *Arch Intern Med* 1994;154:26

13. Reusch VM Jr: Lipopolymers, isoprenoids, and the assembly of the gram positive cell wall. *Crit Rev Microbiol* 1984;11:129

14. Tracey KJ, Cerami A: Tumor necrosis factor, other cytokines and disease. *Annu Rev Cell Biol* 1993;9:317

15. Lukacs NW, Kunkel SL, Allen R, et al: Stimulus and cell specific expression of C X C and CC chemokines by pulmonary stromal cell populations. *Am J Physiol* 1995;268(5 Pt 1):L856

16. Standiford TJ, Strieter RM, Lukacs NW, et al: Neutralization of IL-10 increases lethality in endotoxemia: cooperative effects of macrophage inflammatory protein 2 and tumor necrosis factor. *J Immunol* 1995;155:2222

17. Carlos TM, Harlan JM: Leukocyte endothelial adhesion molecules. *Blood* 1994;84:2068

18. Davenpeck KL, Gauthier TW, Albertine KH, et al: Role of P-selectin in microvascular leukocyte endothelial interaction in splanchnic ischemia reperfusion. *Am J Physiol* 1994;267(2 Pt 2):H622

19. Kubes P, Jutila M, Payne D: Therapeutic potential of inhibiting leukocyte rolling in ischemia/reperfusion. *J Clin Invest* 1995;95:2510

20. Lee WP, Gribling P, De Guzman L, et al: A P selectin immunoglobulin G chimera is protective in a rabbit ear model of ischemia reperfusion. *Surgery* 1995;117:458

21. Okada Y, Copeland BR, Mori E, et al: P selectin and intercellular adhesion molecule 1 expression after focal brain ischemia and reperfusion. *Stroke* 1994;25:202

22. Seekamp A, Till GO, Mulligan MS, et al: Role of selectins in local and remote tissue injury following ischemia and reperfusion. *Am J Pathol* 1994;144:592

23. Winn RK, Mihelicic D, Vedder NB, et al: Monoclonal antibodies to leukocyte and endothelial adhesion molecules attenuate ischemia reperfusion injury. *Behring Inst Mitt* 1993;92:229

24. Winn RK, Liggitt D, Vedder NB, et al: Anti P selectin monoclonal antibody attenuates reperfusion injury to the rabbit ear. *J Clin Invest* 1993;92:2042

25. Winn RK, Vedder NB, Mihelcic D, et al: The role of adhesion molecules in reperfusion injury. *Agents Actions* 1993;41(Suppl):113

26. Winn RK, Paulson JC, Harlan JM: A monoclonal antibody to P selectin ameliorates injury associated with hemorrhagic shock in rabbits. *Am J Physiol* 1994;267(6 Pt 2):H2391

27. Sharar SR, Sasaki SS, Flaherty LC, et al: P selectin blockade does not impair leukocyte host defense against bacterial peritonitis and soft tissue infection in rabbits. *J Immunol* 1993;151:4982

28. Jerome SN, Dor'e M, Paulson JC, et al: P selectin and ICAM 1 dependent adherence reactions: role in the genesis of postischemic no reflow. *Am J Physiol* 1994;266(4 Pt 2):H1316

29. Pohlman TH, Harlan JM: Endotoxin endothelial cell interactions. In: Morrison DC, Ryan J (eds). *Bacterial Endotoxic Lipopolysaccharides.* Boca Raton, CRC Press, 1992:459

30. Drake TA, Cheng J, Chang A, et al: Expression of tissue factor, thrombomodulin, and E selectin in baboons with lethal *Escherichia coli* sepsis. *Am J Pathol* 1993;142:1458

31. Redl H, Dinges HP, Buurman WA, et al: Expression of endothelial leukocyte adhesion molecule 1 in septic but not traumatic/hypovolemic shock in the baboon. *Am J Pathol* 1991;139:461

32. Orosz CG, Ohye RG, Pelletier RP, et al: Treatment with anti vascular cell adhesion molecule 1 monoclonal antibody induces long term murine cardiac allograft acceptance. *Transplantation* 1993;56:453

33. Yednock TA, Cannon C, Fritz LC, et al: Prevention of experimental autoimmune encephalomyelitis by antibodies against α_4, β_1 integrin. *Nature* 1992;356:63

34. Imhof BA, Dunon D: Leukocyte migration and adhesion. *Adv Immunol* 1995;58:345

35. Foreman KE, Vaporciyan AA, Bonish BK, et al: C5a induced expression of P selectin in endothelial cells. *J Clin Invest* 1994;94:1147

36. Levi M, Hack CE, de Boer JP, et al: Reduction of contact activation related fibrinolytic activity in factor XII deficient patients: further evidence for the role of the contact system in fibrinolysis in vivo. *J Clin Invest* 1991;88:1155

37. Reddigari S, Silverberg M, Kaplan AP: Assembly of the human plasma kinin forming cascade along the surface of vascular endothelial cells. *Int Arch Allergy Appl Immunol* 1995;107:93

38. Mombouli JV, Vanhoutte PM: Kinins and endothelial control of vascular smooth muscle. *Annu Rev Pharmacol Toxicol* 1995;35:679

39. Naess F, Roeise O, Johansen HT, et al: Hemodynamic and proteolytic effects of intravenous injection of purified human plasma kallikrein. *Am J Physiol* 1992;263(2 Pt 2):H405

40. Martich GD, Boujoukos AJ, Suffredini AF: Response of man to endotoxin. *Immunobiology* 1993;187:403

41. Linz W, Wiemer G, Gohlke P, Unger T, et al: Contribution of kinins to the cardiovascular actions of angiotensin converting enzyme inhibitors. *Pharmacol Rev* 1995;47:25

42. Linz W, Wiemer G, Scholkens BA: Cardioprotective actions of bradykinin in myocardial ischemia and left ventricular hypertrophy. *Braz J Med Biol Res* 1994;27:1949

43. Dickneite G: Influence of C1 inhibitor on inflammation, edema and shock. *Behring Inst Mitt* 1993;93:299

44. Stein PE, Carrell RW: What do dysfunctional serpins tell us about molecular mobility and disease? *Nat Struct Biol* 1995;2:96

45. Davis AE III, Bissler JJ, Cicardi M: Mutations in the C1 inhibitor gene that result in hereditary angioneurotic edema. *Behring Inst Mitt* 1993;93:313

46. Taylor FB Jr, Dahlback B, Chang AC, et al: Role of free protein S and C4b binding protein in regulating the coagulant response to *Escherichia coli.* *Blood* 1995;86:2642

Critical Care, Third Edition, edited by Joseph M. Civetta,
Robert W. Taylor, and Robert R. Kirby.
Lippincott-Raven Publishers, Philadelphia, PA © 1997.

CHAPTER 21

∎

Allergy and Immunology

R. Dwaine Rieves
Stewart J. Levine
James H. Shelhamer

IMMEDIATE CONCERNS ∎

MAJOR PROBLEMS

The various components of normal immune system function are tightly interwoven but may be grouped into a predominantly humoral response, a cell-mediated immune response, or a phagocytic cell response. The humoral response includes the production of antigen-specific immunoglobulins and the use of antigen-nonspecific complement proteins to augment antigen clearance. The cell-mediated immune response includes cytotoxic and antigen processing functions mediated by lymphocytes, macrophages, and other antigen presenting cells (APCs). The humoral response and cell-mediated immune response contribute to phagocytosis of certain antigens by neutrophils. In general, defects in the humoral immune response or phagocytic cell function result in a predisposition to bacterial and fungal infections. Defects in the cell-mediated response are associated with infections from viruses and more unusual bacterial and mycobacterial pathogens, many of which are opportunistic organisms.

Immunotherapies are used in treating many diseases. These immunotherapies include immunosuppressive drugs, cytokines, hematologic growth factors, antibodies, and plasmapheresis. Side effects of these immunotherapies are common and range from a predisposition to infection to a systemic inflammatory response resembling septic shock.

STRESS POINTS

1. B-lymphocyte production of antibody in response to an antigen does not require the antigen to be broken down into its composite peptide fragments by an APC.

2. The T-lymphocyte secretion of cytokines and activation of natural killer T lymphocytes in response to an antigen occurs only after processing of the antigen by certain APCs. These APCs, such as macrophages and dendritic cells, degrade the antigen into small fragments, which are subsequently exposed on their cell surface.

3. Certain cytokines are signaling molecules between the humoral immune system, cell-mediated immune system, and nonimmune cells. When produced in large quantities, certain cytokines, such as interleukin (IL)-1 and tumor necrosis factor (TNF), may produce fever, hypotension, and myalgia.

4. Immunoglobulin deficiencies may be associated with recurrent infections and have been implicated as a primary cause for bronchiectasis. Replacement therapy with intravenous immunoglobulin (IVIG) is effective in preventing infections.

5. The Fab fragment of an anti-digoxin antibody is an effective and rapid treatment for severe digoxin intoxication.

6. Plasmapheresis is a component of the therapy for several diseases including thrombotic thrombocytopenia purpura (TTP), Goodpasture's syndrome, and Guillain-Barré syndrome. Complications such as infection and protein depletion are common.

ESSENTIAL DIAGNOSTIC TESTS AND PROCEDURES

1. Quantitative serum immunoglobulins should be obtained if an immunoglobulin deficiency is suspected. Recurrent infections in association with normal serum

303

immunoglobulin levels should prompt consideration of referral for specialized examinations of phagocytic cell function.

2. Hereditary angioedema is characterized by a decreased serum C4 level and may be associated with a decrease in the level of total hemolytic complement.

3. Systemic inflammatory syndromes induced by cytokines used in cancer immunotherapies may mimic sepsis. The syndrome should not arbitrarily be attributed to a cytokine side effect. A search for a potential septic source usually should be pursued in these patients.

4. The amount of anti-digoxin Fab to be used in treating digoxin intoxication should be based on the suspected amount ingested. If the amount ingested is unknown and enough time has elapsed after ingestion to allow for near-equilibration of the absorbed dose, then the amount ingested can be estimated from the following formula:

Body burden of digoxin (mg) =

$$\frac{\text{serum digoxin level (ng/mL)} \times 5.6 \text{ (L/kg, distribution volume)} \times \text{weight (kg)}}{1000}$$

5. Placement of venous access for plasmapheresis should be made with consideration of the potential septic and hemorrhagic complications encountered with the procedures. Venous catheters should not be placed where hematoma formation may compromise the airway or where laceration of a vessel, should it occur, would not be amenable to digital compression.

INITIAL THERAPY

1. If treated patients with IgA deficiencies should be screened for the presence of IgA antibodies or receive IgA-depleted immunoglobulin. Infusion of pooled immunoglobulin into IgA-deficient patients has been associated with severe reactions because of the presence of anti-IgA antibodies in these patients.

2. Treatment of C1 inhibitor deficiency and its associated acute angioedema includes the use of subcutaneous or inhaled racemic epinephrine and C1 inhibitor preparations (if available). Chronic therapy includes the use of danazol or stanozolol to increase the body's C1 inhibitor production.

3. The dose of anti-digoxin Fab to be administered in the treatment of digoxin intoxication is based on the manufacturer's stated neutralization capability of each vial. Currently, 40 mg of Fab will neutralize 0.6 mg digoxin.

4. The replacement fluid to be used in plasmapheresis depends on the disease being treated and the patient's protein and fibrinogen stores. Fresh frozen plasma is recommended as replacement therapy for TTP, whereas combinations of saline and 5% albumin are used for most other diseases. Fibrinogen depletion may occur with frequent sessions, and cryoprecipitate may be needed for profound depletion or hypofibrinogenemia accompanied by hemorrhage.

5. The capillary leak syndrome associated with IL-2 administration is generally responsive to lowering of the IL-2 dose, use of corticosteroids, or both. Abrupt development of the syndrome may require the use of vasopressors and cautious volume replacement.

OVERVIEW ■

Immunity may be defined as the ability to recognize and respond to an antigen. An allergic response usually implies an immediate hypersensitivity response in which the response is initiated by mast cells coated with IgE. All facets of immunity are tightly integrated such that cell-mediated immune responses and humoral responses do not function as independently of each other as was once thought. Likewise, almost all nonimmune cellular and organ functions, such as those responsible for hemodynamic stability and body metabolism, have been shown to be partially modulated by networking cytokine messages from the multiple immune system cells.

ANTIGEN RECOGNITION AND PROCESSING ■

Cytokine signals from multiple immune system cells tightly regulate antigen processing and clearance responses (Fig. 21-1). Antigen binding to immunoglobulin receptors coating the B-lymphocyte membrane surface stimulates the cell to differentiate into an antibody-secreting plasma cell. This differentiation proceeds along two pathways: one requiring cytokine stimulation by T lymphocytes, the T-cell–dependent pathway; or a T-cell–independent pathway. The antigens recognized by B cells may be in their native, nondegraded form and do not require prior processing of the antigen by other immune system cells. In contrast, almost all T-cell responses require the new antigen to be first degraded into fragments by the various APCs of the body.[1] APCs include certain types of macrophages, dendritic cells of the spleen and lymph nodes, B lymphocytes, and Langerhans' cells of the skin and mucosa.

Multiple membrane receptors are used in APC interactions with T lymphocytes. These membrane proteins generally function as either antigen capture receptors or as scaffolds for antigen presentation to other cells. The most notable membrane proteins include the cluster of differentiation (CD) series, which also serve as markers by which certain cell populations and the major histocompatibility series (MHC) are classified. CD markers are characteristic of specific immune system cells, whereas MHC molecules are found on immune and nonimmune cells. MHC molecules, the scaffolds for antigen presentation, are genetically determined histocompatibility markers that are classified into two major groups on the basis of their glycoprotein cell surface structures. MHC class I molecules consist of a single glycoprotein chain penetrating the cell membrane and are present on virtually all nucleated cells. One component of the MHC class I complex, β2 microglobulin, may be present in a liberated form in serum and urine and has been found

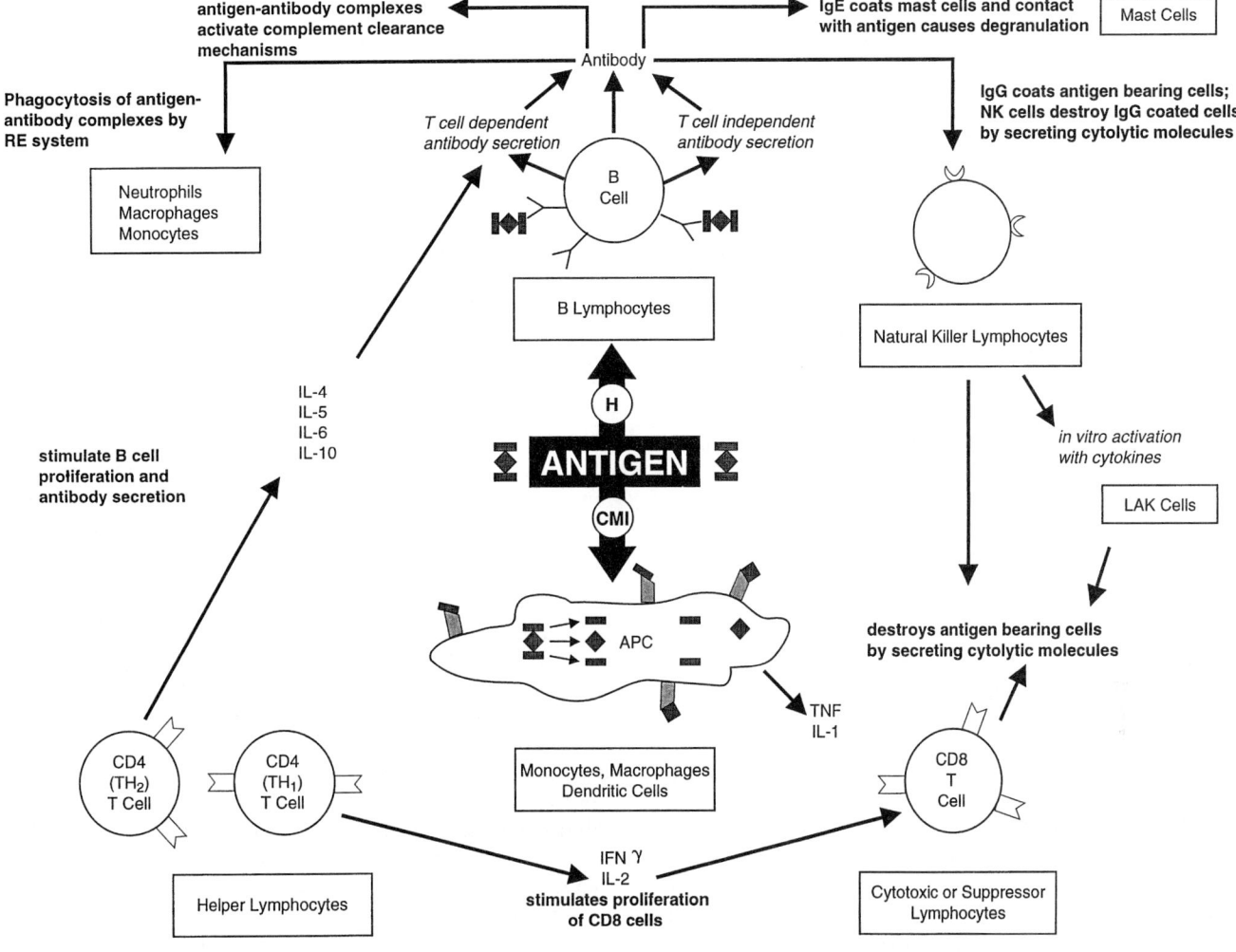

FIGURE 21-1. The major intersections of the humoral immune response (H) and the cell-mediated immune response (CMI) to an antigen. APC, antigen presenting cell; LAK, lymphokine-activated killer cells; NK, natural killer; RE, reticuloendothelial; IFN-γ, interferon-gamma; TNF, tumor necrosis factor; IL, interleukin; MHC, major histocompatibility complex.

⬓ = MHC molecules

⊓ = T cell receptors

⋃ = immunoglobulin receptors

Y = immunoglobulin

in increased concentrations in certain immune disorders. MHC class II molecules consist of two glycoprotein chains and are found primarily on APC. MHC class I molecules are involved in antigen presentation to the CD8 subpopulation of T lymphocytes. The CD8 population of T lymphocytes, which includes suppressor and cytotoxic lymphocytes (CTLs), functions to destroy a cell sheltering an antigen. MHC class II molecules are involved in antigen presentation to the CD4 subpopulation of T lymphocytes. The CD4 population of T lymphocytes, the helper lymphocytes, enhance antibody production by the B-lymphocyte population and may regulate the function of CD8 lymphocytes. CD4 lymphocytes are subdivided into two major classes, TH$_1$ or TH$_2$,

on the basis of the pattern of cytokines secreted.[2] The TH$_2$ group of CD4 cells secrete cytokines that partially suppress the cellular immune response, such as IL-10 and IL-4, but stimulate B-cell secretion of antibodies. The cytokines secreted by the TH$_1$ group of CD4 cells include IL-2 and interferon-gamma (IFN-γ), stimulants of the cell-mediated immune response. The systemic predominance of CD4 cells with either the TH$_1$ or TH$_2$ cytokine pattern has been associated with altered resistance to certain infections.

Once an antigen enters an APC, it is degraded to its peptide fragments. These antigen fragments are transported to the cell membrane, where they are exposed to neighboring cells within a complex that includes either MHC class I or MHC class II molecules. T lymphocytes and certain B lymphocytes subsequently recognize the MHC–Ag complex and initiate their antigenic response. All T lymphocytes recognize an antigen by specific T-cell receptor (TCR) molecules in their cell membrane. These TCR molecules function similar to a lock and key with the MHC–antigen complex. This tightly regulated interaction of APC with T lymphocytes may be bypassed in the presence of certain unique "superantigens." Superantigens are microbial antigens, such as the staphylococcal enterotoxins, which localize to the MHC scaffolds of APC without first undergoing endocytosis and degradation. Consequently, many more superantigen molecules may be displayed on the APC surface membrane than the molecules of processed antigens. This enhanced exposure of the superantigen results in widespread T-cell stimulation and the extensive systemic release of cytokines. The toxic shock syndrome has been attributed primarily to the function of the staphylococcal enterotoxin superantigens.[3]

ANTIGEN CLEARANCE

IMMUNOGLOBULIN AND COMPLEMENT

Once the immune system recognizes an antigen, clearance processes are used to destroy the extracellular antigen or the cells sheltering the antigen. The predominant mechanism for rapid clearance of extracellular antigen involves antibodies and complement. Antibodies circulating in the bloodstream or interstitial fluid may inactivate an antigen by stimulating phagocytic cell function, neutralization of toxic portions of the antigen, or inducing complement-mediated lysis of cells bearing the antigen–immunoglobulin complex. Immunoglobulins possess unique antigen specificity, thereby narrowing the inflammatory response to the antigenic target. The more generalized action of the complement system amplifies the inflammatory response. Complement components and immunoglobulins are strategic to optimal phagocytic cell function and modulation of mononuclear cell function.

Among the most notable functions of immunoglobulins are opsonization and the capacity to activate complement. IgG, IgM, and IgA are crucial to normal opsonization functions. Opsonization by IgG and IgM expedites clearance of circulating antigens, whereas the secretion of IgA onto mucosal surfaces facilitates clearance of invaders by mucosal surface macrophages and neutrophils. Because of its larger size, the function of IgM is confined primarily to intravascular clearance of antigens, whereas IgG readily diffuses into the extravascular space. IgA, secreted onto mucosal surfaces, may be degraded by certain bacterial proteases and the proteases released by the body during critical illnesses, predisposing to bacterial colonization and infections.[4] After being coupled with an antigen, immune complexes are normally cleared by phagocytic and red blood cells, although in certain disease states, antigen–antibody complexes may freely circulate, stimulating inflammatory reactions throughout the body.

The complement system is capable of generating a broad series of inflammatory actions associated with antigen clearance. These actions include lysis of cells bearing antigen–antibody complexes, chemotaxis of inflammatory cells, opsonization of antigens, and generation of anaphylactoid reactions. Complement activation may be accomplished by either the classic pathway or the alternate route. Antigen–antibody complexes initiate the classic pathway whereas the alternate route is initiated by antigenic protein aggregates, endotoxin or insoluble compounds with certain surface characteristics. With sequential proteolysis of complement substrates, various complement fragments with neutrophil and eosinophil chemotactic properties as well as vasodilatory effects are generated.

EFFECTOR CELL FUNCTION

The major cells involved in antigen clearance include APC and lymphocytes, neutrophils, and various organ-specific structural cells. Although many antigens may be destroyed within mononuclear or phagocytic cells by intracellular enzymes, some antigens may become sheltered within the cells. Clearance of these intracellular antigens requires lysis of the infected cell. T-lymphocyte function is the best-characterized cell lysis system for clearance of antigens sequestered within cells or on their surface. This T-lymphocyte–dependent clearance mechanism is crucial to clearance of tumor cells, transplanted tissue, and intracellular microbial pathogens. Coincident with presentation of processed antigen by APC, multiple cytokines and inflammatory mediators are secreted. Notable among the cytokines produced by APCs are IL-1 and TNF. In high systemic concentrations, both IL-1 and TNF have profound effects on body metabolism and are capable of inducing hypotension, fever, and cachexia and have been implicated in the manifestations of septic shock.[5]

Just as APCs release cytokines on antigen processing and exposure, T cells increase the secretion of lymphokines after TCR coupling to the presented antigen. These cytokines are crucial to regulation of the immune response (Table 21-1).

The cytolytic response of T lymphocytes has been best characterized by analysis of three major cell populations: CD8 suppressor and CTLs, natural killer cells, and killer lymphocytes. The CTL response refers primarily to cell killing by CD8 lymphocytes. After exposure to processed antigen, CD8 cells proliferate under the influence of the lymphokines IL-2 and IFN-γ. The activated CD8 cells synthesize and secrete membrane attack molecules, which results in lysis of the antigen-bearing cell. A second type of immune effector cell, the natural killer cell, has not been well characterized by either lineage or function; both a macrophage and lymphocyte lineage have been proposed. Similar to the cell lysis by CTL, natural killer cells lyse neighboring cells by secreting membrane attack molecules. Unlike the CTL response, natural killer cell lysis of antigen-bearing cells does not seem to be antigen specific. Killer lymphocytes, the third major cytolytic cell population, are coated with surface receptors for antibodies. Killer lymphocytes may localize to antigen-antibody–coated cells and release their cytotoxic granules. Antibody recognition is crucial to

TABLE 21-1. Selected Mediators of Inflammation and Immunity

MEDIATOR	FUNCTIONS
IL-1	Promotes neutrophil adherence and phagocytic function, promotes IL-2 production, stimulates fibroblast and endothelial cell proliferation, induces fever, stimulates hepatocyte acute-phase protein synthesis
IL-1 receptor antagonist	Blocks IL-1 receptor
IL-2	Stimulates T-lymphocyte proliferation and activation
IL-3	Stimulates proliferation of multilineage hematopoietic cells
IL-4	Stimulates B-lymphocyte proliferation and antibody secretion; inhibits macrophage production of IL-1, IL-6 and TNF; stimulates TH_2 subset proliferation
IL-5	Stimulates eosinophil proliferation and differentiation
IL-6	Stimulates B-lymphocyte proliferation and differentiation, stimulates epithelial and fibroblast proliferation in vitro, induces fever, inhibits TNF production
IL-7	Stimulates B- and T-lymphocyte precursor proliferation in bone marrow
IL-8	Neutrophil chemotactic factor, stimulates neutrophil degranulation, inhibits neutrophil adherence to endothelium
IL-9	Stimulates T-lymphocyte proliferation
IL-10	Stimulates B-lymphocyte proliferation and differentiation, inhibits TH_1 subset cytokine secretion
IL-11	Stimulates proliferation of hematopoietic stem cells
IL-12	Stimulates proliferation of TH_1 subset and cytokine secretion
IL-13	Stimulates T-lymphocyte proliferation and B-lymphocyte differentiation, suppresses macrophage cytokine secretion
TNF-α	Promotes release of multiple cytokines from mononuclear cells, produces effects similar to IL-1
IFN-γ	Promotes monocyte differentiation, enhances macrophage and dendritic cell MHC expression
Transforming growth factor β	Inhibits IL-2 stimulated lymphocyte proliferation, inhibits neutrophil adherence, multiple immunomodulatory functions
Platelet-derived growth factor	Stimulates macrophage cytokine production, stimulates fibroblast and smooth muscle cell proliferation, inhibits natural killer cell function
Transforming growth factor α	Stimulates proliferation of epithelial cells, fibroblasts, and endothelial cells
Platelet activating factor	Enhances neutrophil adherence to endothelial cells, chemoattractant for eosinophils, activates neutrophils, promotes platelet degranulation
Fibroblast growth factor	Stimulates endothelial cell proliferation and angiogenesis

IL, interleukin; TNF, tumor necrosis factor; TNF-α, tumor necrosis factor alpha; MHC, major histocompatibility complex; IFN-γ; interferon gamma.

this system, and killer lymphocyte function seems to be a component of antibody-dependent cytotoxicity. Natural killer cell and killer lymphocytes can be activated and made to proliferate in vitro under the influence of cytokines. These lymphokine-activated killer cells may be reinfused into the body and have been investigated as cancer immunotherapy.[6]

Unlike lymphocytes, neutrophils are capable of directly phagocytosing circulating antigens without processing by macrophages. After neutrophil phagocytosis, enzyme-laden lysosomes fuse with the antigen-containing phagosome, digesting and destroying the antigen. Neutrophils possess receptors for the Fc portion of immunoglobulins as well as receptors for complement components. Opsonization of antigens by immunoglobulins and complement markedly enhances phagocytic capability.

In addition to the primary immune effector cells, structural cells, such as those of the endothelium, epithelium, and connective tissue, are also important in an effective immune response. Not only are these cells capable of secreting cytokines and inflammatory mediators, they also possess MHC molecules and may function in antigen presentation to T lymphocytes. After stimulation, structural cells release proinflammatory and antiinflammatory mediators. The activation of structural cells by immune system cytokines may underlie the organ dysfunction associated with chronic septic states and multisystem organ failure.[7]

ANTIGEN CLEARANCE
AND INFLAMMATION ■

The antigen clearance process is enhanced within tissues by increased vascular flow, altered vascular permeability, and the recruitment of phagocytic and cytotoxic cells. Several physiologic mechanisms involved in circulating inflammatory cell adhesion to vascular endothelium and subsequent diapedesis have been described. Multiple adhesion molecules are present on both circulating inflammatory cells and endothelial cells. Adhesion molecules expressed on circulating leukocytes include the L-selectin molecules (most notably, LAM-1) and β2 integrin family of molecules (LFA-1 and MAC-1), which recognize specific endothelial cell ligands. These endothelial cell adhesion ligands include the P-selectin (GMP 140), E-selectin (ELAM-1) family of molecules and ICAM-1 and ICAM-2 molecules. Expression and function of these molecules is modulated by certain cytokines.

From both in vitro and in vivo studies, a paradigm for circulating leukocyte accumulation at inflammatory sites has evolved. The activation of tissue macrophages and other APC after exposure to an antigen results in the local release of TNF and IL-1. TNF and IL-1 stimulate endothelial cell expression of selectins and ICAM-1. Coupling of the endothelial selectin molecules with the leukocyte L-selectin molecules results in leukocyte "rolling." The subsequent interaction of leukocyte β2 integrin adhesion molecules with the ICAM-1 and ICAM-2 endothelial cell molecules correlates with leukocyte adhesion to the endothelium. In this model, TNF and IL-1 function as "early response cytokines" and stimulate the production of a second wave of cytokines by both structural and immune system cells.[8] Notable among this second wave of cytokines is IL-8, a potent leukocyte chemotaxin. IL-8 production by endothelial cells and tissue fibroblasts is a major component of the chemotactic gradient facilitating leukocyte migration across the endothelial surface. The release of multiple inflammatory mediators from migrating leukocytes (proteases, oxygen radicals, leukotrienes, platelet activating factor) expand the local inflammatory process. Conversely, several cytokines and soluble cytokine receptors are normally present to down-regulate or limit the inflammatory response. Among these "antiinflammatory" factors are soluble forms of the IL-1 and TNF receptors, IL-4, IL-10, IL-13, transforming growth factor-β, and IL-1 receptor antagonist.

Cytokines released into the systemic circulation as a consequence of either localized or systemic inflammation have been directly implicated in the pathophysiologic mechanisms of the organ dysfunction associated with major trauma, sepsis, and burns. Plasma concentration of IL-1, TNF, and IL-6 have been shown to correlate with mortality in septic shock.[9] In response to TNF, nitric oxide is produced by endothelial cells and, along with the other mediators, promotes smooth muscle relaxation and vasodilation. Whether these cytokines and mediators are the primary pathogenetic mediators for the shock syndrome or are markers for systemic inflammation is unclear.

IMMUNE DEFECTS AND
CRITICAL ILLNESS ■

Many life-threatening diseases represent the consequences of immune system defects.

Recurrent or unusual infections, increased susceptibility to neoplasia, and delayed healing characterize patients with immune system disorders. Although many immune system diseases overlap in immunopathogenesis, most immune system diseases may be classified on the basis of the predominant immune defect, be it congenital or acquired (Table 21-2). Additionally, many other chronic illnesses such as malnutrition, alcoholism, and diabetes mellitus are associated with subtle immunologic abnormalities potentially contributing to clinical disease. Immune system disorders may be grouped into disorders of humoral immunity, cell-mediated immunity, and phagocytic cell function.

COMPLEMENT

Defects of the complement system include deficiencies of individual complement component proteins, regulatory proteins, or complement receptors. Complement component deficiencies may be broadly grouped into early (C1–C4) or late component (C5–C8) deficiencies. A predisposition to *Streptococcus pneumoniae* and *Haemophilus influenzae* infections has been observed in patients deficient in early complement components. *Neisseria meningitidis* infections have been recognized as a sequelae of late component deficiencies. In contrast to patients with late component deficiencies, patients with early complement component deficiencies possess a uniquely higher incidence of autoimmune disease, especially systemic lupus erythematosus. In these patients, it has been suggested that the complement deficiency impairs effective clearance of circulating immune complexes, predisposing to autoimmune diseases. The consumption of complement in sepsis and septic shock has been clearly demonstrated. Whether complement activation is pathogenic or physiologic in septic shock remains unclear. Both the alternate and classic pathways of complement activation have been shown to be activated in septic shock, potentially related to a sepsis-induced inactivation of C1 inhibitor.[10]

The most clinically significant complement regulatory protein deficiency is loss of C1 inhibitor activity. This nonspecific esterase inhibitor is strategic in controlling the classic complement cascade and in inhibiting the action of several clotting factors. Although acquired forms of C1 inhibitor deficiency have been described, the autosomally dominant genetic defect is the most common. In patients with hereditary angioedema, a trauma or stress may precipitate uncontrolled activation of the complement system, culminating in systemic angioedema—nonpruritic limb edema, gastrointestinal disturbances, and upper airway obstruction. Unlike the angioedema associated with anaphylaxis, the angioedema associated with C1 inhibitor deficiency is much less responsive to epinephrine and glucocorticoids.[11] In addition to subcutaneous or inhaled epinephrine, the management of acute angioedema may include the use of fresh frozen plasma

TABLE 21-2.   Major Immunodeficiency Syndromes

DEFECT OR DISEASE	ETIOLOGY	CONSEQUENCE
IgG deficiency	In adults, usually acquired as a form of common variable hypogammaglobulinemia; the most severe form is congenital, X-linked hypogammaglobulinemia; Associated with ataxia telangiectasia, chronic lymphocytic leukemia and multiple myeloma	Recurrent infections, especially with *Streptococcus pneumoniae, Haemophilus* sp.
IgA deficiency	Thought to occur primarily as a congenital abnormality	Recurrent sinopulmonary infections, especially with *S. pneumoniae*
Early complement component (C2–C4) deficiencies	Congenital	Predisposition to autoimmune disease, e.g., systemic lupus erythematosus; increased risk for infections, especially with *S. pneumoniae*
Late complement component (C5–C8) deficiencies	Congenital	Increased risk for infections, especially with *Neisseria meningitidis* and *Neisseria gonorrhea*
C1 inhibitor deficiency	Primarily congenital, rarely acquired	Angioedema, abdominal distress, upper airway obstruction
Complement receptor deficiency	Congenital or acquired	Predisposition to autoimmune disease
Alternate complement pathway defects	Associated with sickle cell disease	Increased risk for infections, especially with *S. pneumoniae*
T-lymphocyte defects	AIDS, lymphoma, iatrogenic (especially glucocorticoid therapy and immunosuppressants used in solid organ transplantation)	Infection with opportunistic pathogens, especially *Pneumocystis carinii,* cytomegalovirus, herpes simplex, *Cryptococcus neoformans, Legionella*
Chronic granulomatous disease	Abnormal neutrophil oxidative metabolism, ineffective microbicidal activity, congenital	Recurrent bacterial and fungal infections, especially pyogenic infection of the skin, lymph nodes, liver, and lungs
Neutropenia	Most commonly iatrogenic (cytotoxic chemotherapy)	Bacterial and fungal infections
Leukocyte adhesion deficiency	Congenital absence of leukocyte adhesion molecules (LFA, MAC-1, selectins)	Recurrent skin, soft tissue, and lung infections; persistently elevated peripheral leukocyte counts
Chediak-Higashi syndrome	Congenitally abnormal neutrophil chemotaxis and degranulation, decreased microbicidal capacity	Associated with albinism and photophobia; recurrent infections
Job's syndrome	Congenitally abnormal neutrophil chemotaxis, delayed catabolism of IgE	Elevated serum IgE; sinusitis; otitis media; eczema; recurrent skin and soft tissue infections, especially with *Staphyloccus aureus*

AIDS, acquired immunodeficiency syndrome.

or, when available, purified C1 inhibitor replacement. As maintenance therapy, androgens such as danazol or stanozolol offer effective therapy and are usually effective in increasing the levels of serum C1 inhibitor. C1 inhibitor deficiency is characterized by deficient C1 functional activity in serum, along with low levels of C2 and C4, especially during acute episodes. Notably, the serum level of C3 or total hemolytic complement activity is commonly normal.

Few patients deficient in complement receptors have been described. The lack of cell surface complement receptors results in poor clearance of immune complexes. The elevated level of circulating immune complexes is thought to underlie the high prevalence of systemic lupus erythematosus in these patients.

IMMUNOGLOBULIN

Abnormalities of immunoglobulin production manifest most commonly as deficiencies, although the excessive production of immunoglobulins occasionally results in severe sequelae, as may occur in Waldenström's macroglobulinemia.

Infectious consequences of immunoglobulin deficiency result from most forms of immunoglobulin deficiency. The most common adult type of primary immunoglobulin deficiency is a selective deficiency of IgA. Although IgA deficiency has been associated with recurrent sinopulmonary infections and with *Giardia* intestinal infections, many of these patients remain asymptomatic. The clinical consequences of hypogammaglobulinemia are more frequent in patients with the heterogeneous disorders composing common variable hypogammaglobulinemia. Common variable hypogammaglobulinemia includes a group of disorders characterized by low or absent serum immunoglobulin levels and an enhanced risk for bacterial infections, especially sinopulmonary infections. Because the infections are usually recurrent and generally responsive to treatment, these patients may present in adulthood with bronchiectasis and lung destruction. Infections with encapsulated bacteria such as *Haemophilus* and *Streptococcus* are especially prevalent. The most frequently diagnosed immunoglobulin deficiency pattern in these patients is a decrease in all classes of immunoglobulins.[12] Prophylactic therapy with γ-globulin has proven to be effective in preventing infections.

Among the many disorders associated with elevated serum concentrations of immunoglobulins, diseases associated with excessive IgM production are especially notable for acute clinical sequelae. Because of their size and structure, IgM globulins possess unique properties, including cold insolubility (cryoglobulins) and the potential to greatly increase blood viscosity. Excessive IgM production may result from a clearly benign response to mycoplasma and viral infections or a neoplastic-like B-lymphocyte response (Waldenström's macroglobulinemia). The cold agglutinin response to infections rarely results in more than a mild hemolytic anemia, but the IgM levels associated with Waldenström's macroglobulinemia may produce life-threatening consequences. Viscosity-related sequelae include confusion, coma, visual impairment, and congestive heart failure. Plasmapheresis to lower the serum IgM level is effective therapy for these acute complications.

A normal antibody immune response to foreign material may occasionally result in dramatic clinical symptomatology. Especially notable examples are serum sickness and leukoagglutinin reactions. Serum sickness is characterized by the formation of circulating antigen–antibody complexes 7 to 10 days after injection of an antigenic protein into the body. With systemic deposition of the immune complexes, complement is activated and edema, rash, arthralgia, and fever result. The most common cases of serum sickness follow treatment with antithymocyte globulin (equine or rabbit origin) or snake antivenom (equine origin). Glucocorticoid therapy is usually indicated for severe serum sickness symptoms. The leukoagglutinin reaction results from the incidental transfusion of antibodies with red blood cells or plasma. Leukoagglutinin reactions result from the interaction of transfused antibodies with recipient neutrophils, prompting neutrophil sequestration in the lungs. Cough, dyspnea, and respiratory failure may follow the transfusion. Treatment is supportive, there being no specific therapy for the reactions.[13]

DISORDERS OF CELL-MEDIATED IMMUNITY

Acquired defects in lymphocyte and macrophage-regulated immunity are the most common immunodeficiencies encountered in adults. Three major groups of disorders account for most of these disorders: the acquired immunodeficiency syndrome (AIDS), various lymphohematologic ma-

lignancies, and iatrogenic immunosuppression. These diseases are associated with enhanced susceptibility to infections with common pathogens as well as a unique predisposition to infections with opportunistic microorganisms. The pathogenesis of one of the most devastating immune disorders, AIDS, involves selective depletion of the CD4 subset of T lymphocytes by retroviral infection. In these patients, lymphocyte depletion, combined with abnormal macrophage function and certain B-lymphocyte malfunctions, culminates in a plethora of potentially life-threatening infections. As with other patients with profound defects in lymphocyte-regulated immunity, patients with AIDS may commonly present with fulminant respiratory failure in association with diffuse pulmonary infiltrates.

Notable opportunistic respiratory pathogens in patients with defects in lymphocyte-regulated immunity include *Pneumocystis carinii*, *Listeria monocytogenes*, *Nocardia* sp., *Mycobacteria* sp., *Cryptococcus neoformans*, and cytomegalovirus. Before the AIDS epidemic, most cases of *Pneumocystis* pneumonia in adults occurred among iatrogenically immunosuppressed patients or patients with lymphoma, especially Hodgkin's lymphoma. Immunosuppressants primarily affecting lymphocyte function include those used in organ transplantation: glucocorticoids, antithymocyte globulin, OKT3 antilymphocyte globulin, azathioprine, and cyclosporine.

PHAGOCYTIC CELL FUNCTION

The most common abnormalities of phagocytic function are related to either an abnormal number or function of circulating neutrophils. The consequence of almost all neutrophil defects is infection, primarily bacterial and fungal, and, less commonly, viral. The incidence of infection among neutropenic patients correlates with the depression of the circulating neutrophil count and the duration of neutropenia. The risk of infection increases proportionally as the circulating neutrophil count falls below 1000 cells/mm^3 and is greater when the neutropenia persists over several days. This risk forms the basis for empiric antimicrobial therapy in neutropenic patients before pathogen identification.

The pathogenesis of neutrophil functional abnormalities has been most extensively studied among patients with congenital neutrophil defects. A history of recurrent lymphocutaneous or pulmonary infections with staphylococci or gram-negative bacilli, especially *Pseudomonas* sp. or *Serratia* sp., provides a clue to a potential underlying neutrophil function disorder. Notably, infections with obligate anaerobic bacilli are exceedingly rare among patients with neutrophil defects. Multiple congenital functional defects of neutrophils have been identified and are outlined in Table 21-2. Specific therapy exists for only one of these congenital disorders. Among certain patients with chronic granulomatous disease, the administration of IFN-γ has been shown to partially correct the neutrophil abnormality and dramatically lessen the incidence of infections.[14] Neutrophil dysfunction also has been implicated in the pathogenesis of infections complicating several chronic diseases, including diabetes mellitus, malnutrition, sickle cell disease, cirrhosis, and chronic alcoholism. Multiple in vitro neutrophil abnormalities have been demonstrated in these patients, especially abnormalities of chemotaxis and phagocytosis. Therapy for these neutrophil defects is nonspecific, including antimicrobial agents for infections and treatment of the underlying disease.

IMMUNOTHERAPY

A broad spectrum of immunotherapies has evolved over the last several years (Table 21-3). Immunotherapies may be broadly classified as either immune system stimulants or suppressants, but there is much mechanistic overlap. For example, the therapeutic effect of IVIG administration in the treatment of idiopathic thrombocytopenia purpura has been partially attributed to the immunosuppressive properties of the transfused immunoglobulin complexes.[15] Likewise, the actions of most immunosuppressive drugs are relatively global, with alterations in both cell-mediated immunity and humoral immunity.

IMMUNOTHERAPIES AND CRITICAL ILLNESS

Although the complications of immunosuppression commonly result in serious illnesses, only a few specific immunotherapies are used in caring for critically ill patients. These immunotherapies include the use of certain antibodies, antibody fragments, and plasmapheresis. Multiple other forms of immunotherapy for critically ill patients have been used with less consistent or no success. The use of immunosuppressives and antibodies in the management of septic shock has failed to demonstrate any clinical benefit.[16,17]

The administration of antibodies, either as pooled γ-globulin fractions or antigen-specific immunoglobulins, has demonstrable efficacy in many chronic medical illnesses. Certain antibodies and antibody fragments occupy a novel therapeutic role in the management of the critically ill patient.

A unique detoxifying mechanism for digoxin intoxication involves the use of the Fab fragment of an anti-digoxin antibody.[18] These fragments, produced in sheep, facilitate digoxin clearance with minimal side effects. Within minutes of infusion, serum free digoxin levels are usually undetectable, whereas immunoreactive digoxin levels (detecting the inactive digoxin–Fab complexes) are usually elevated. Digoxin–Fab complexes are excreted by the kidneys without the latent release of digoxin.

In general, anti-digoxin Fab therapy is indicated for digoxin-intoxicated patients presenting with life-threatening arrhythmias or digoxin intoxication accompanied by hyperkalemia. In addition to correcting the cardiac toxicity, the occasional hyperkalemia induced by digoxin poisoning commonly resolves with the Fab therapy. The commercially available anti-digoxin Fab product contains 40 mg of the Fab fragment, which is capable of binding 0.6 mg digoxin. The amount of Fab to be administered may be calculated either from knowledge of the amount ingested or by the formula (assuming that the drug has reached equilibrium levels):

$$\text{Body burden of digoxin (mg)} = \frac{\text{serum digoxin level (ng/mL)} \times 5.6 \text{ (L/kg, distribution volume)} \times \text{weight (kg)}}{1000}$$

The body burden of digoxin should be calculated and the appropriate number of anti-digoxin Fab vials administered. Clinical experience suggests that it is better to deliver the correct number or a slight excess of Fab vials rather than underdose the patient. Side effects, even in the presence of moderate renal insufficiency, have been mild. Rarely is there a need to readminister an Fab dose. After the Fab administration, serum potassium levels should be monitored because the most common side effect is hypokalemia, and cautious potassium supplementation may be necessary. Once the anti-digoxin Fab has been administered, serum digoxin levels are uninterpretable. With normal renal function, the digoxin–Fab complex is excreted with a half-life of 10 to 20 hours.

Multiple immunomodulatory agents, including antibodies to cytokines and soluble cytokine receptors, are under active investigation in the management of critical illnesses and their complications. Whereas initial clinical trials suggested some efficacy of certain anti-endotoxin antibodies, studies in larger patient populations clearly demonstrated no benefit and perhaps a harmful effect. Considering the complexity of the immune system regulatory mechanisms in critical illnesses, the interpretation of preliminary immunomodulatory studies should be done with caution.[19]

Plasmapheresis, the removal of plasma from blood with the reinfusion of cells and replacement fluids, has been used in many illnesses with variable success.[20] Plasmapheresis has been shown to be effective in several illnesses that commonly require management in the intensive care unit, including TTP, Guillain-Barré syndrome, myasthenia gravis, Waldenström's macroglobulinemia, and Goodpasture's syndrome. In general, plasmapheresis requires placement of either large-bore peripheral venous catheters or a temporary hemodialysis catheter. Most of the severe complications associated with plasmapheresis have been related to placement and maintenance of the venous access catheter. Hemorrhagic and septic complications are major concerns with respect to the choice of vascular access because of catheter manipulation during the pheresis sessions, the predisposition to hemorrhage associated with plasma extraction, and underlying renal and hemostatic derangements. Either peripheral venous catheters or femoral catheters are probably preferable to subclavian or internal jugular sites for patients with hemostatic derangements. Similarly, the appropriate replacement fluid varies with the clinical condition and disease. In general, fresh frozen plasma is the most appropriate replacement fluid in treating TTP, whereas 5% albumin with isotonic saline is usually used for most neurologic indications. The volume of replacement fluid is estimated by approximating the amount of plasma removed. Considering that one plasma volume is commonly removed with each session, the replacement volume can be estimated from the following equation:

TABLE 21-3. Major Immunotherapies

AGENTS	INDICATIONS	MAJOR SIDE EFFECTS/ COMPLICATIONS
IMMUNOSUPPRESSIVE DRUGS		
Corticosteroids	Multiple diseases associated with inflammation, graft rejection	Adrenal suppression, infection, altered glucose metabolism, cataracts, osteoporosis
Cytotoxic chemotherapies	Cancer therapy	Neutropenia, infection, mucosal ulceration
Methotrexate	Multiple diseases associated with inflammation, cancer therapy	Pneumonitis, hepatitis, neutropenia, infection
Cyclosporine	Graft rejection	Nephrotoxicity, hypertension
Azathioprine	Graft rejection, rheumatoid arthritis	Leukopenia, thrombocytopenia, infection
IMMUNOMODULATORY DRUGS		
Levamisole	Cancer therapy	Diarrhea, nausea, stomatitis, neurotoxicity, leukopenia, rash
ANTIBODIES		
Immunoglobulin (pooled human)	Immunoglobulin deficiency diseases, idiopathic thrombocytopenia purpura, myasthenia gravis, Guillain-Barré syndrome, CMV pneumonia in immunosuppressed patients	Myalgia, arthralgia, fever (especially on rapid infusion), aseptic meningitis, occasionally severe reactions in IgA-deficient patients, rarely anaphylaxis
Hyperimmune human immunoglobulins (hepatitis B, rabies, tetanus, Rho globulin, pooled globulin for hepatitis A, measles)	Passive prophylaxis for specific diseases	Myalgia and injection site inflammation when administered intramuscularly
Hyperimmune animal sera (spider antivenin, polyvalent snake antivenin)	Antidotes for envenomization	Anaphylaxis, serum sickness
Antithymocyte globulin	Graft rejection, aplastic anemia	Fever, chills, thrombocytopenia, serum sickness, anaphylaxis
OKT3 (murine monoclonal antibody to T lymphocytes)	Graft rejection	Cytokine syndrome (especially with first injection, infection)
Antidigoxin Fab fragment	Digoxin intoxication with arrhythmias	Hypokalemia, exacerbation of heart failure
Antiplatelet integrin receptor (ReoPro, 7E3 Fab)	Prevention of acute reocclusion after coronary angioplasty	Hemorrhage
CYTOKINES AND GROWTH FACTORS		
IL-2	Cancer therapy	Capillary leak syndrome, hypotension, pulmonary edema
IFN-α	Cancer therapy, certain forms of hepatitis	Flu-like syndrome: fever, headache, chills, myalgia
IFN-γ	Chronic granulomatous disease with recurrent infections	Flu-like syndrome: fever, myalgia, chills, headache
IFN-β	Multiple sclerosis	Flu-like syndrome: myalgia, fever; injection site inflammation
GCSF	Prevention of infections and episodes of febrile neutropenia after chemotherapy	Bone pain
GMCSF	Myeloid reconstitution after bone marrow transplantation	Capillary leak syndrome; pulmonary edema; pericardial effusion; flu-like syndrome: fever, myalgia, chills

CMV, cytomegalovirus; IL-2, interleukin-2; IFN, interferon; GCSF, granulocyte colony stimulating factor; GMCSF, granulocyte-macrophage colony stimulating factor.

$$Blood\ volume = weight\ (kg) \times 70\ mL$$

Replacement volume =

$$blood\ volume \times (1 - hematocrit,\ as\ a\ decimal)$$

Hence, for a 70-kg adult with a hematocrit of 40%, the replacement volume would be 2940 mL. The plasma volume to be removed, replacement volume, and type of replacement fluid must be individualized based on the patient's clinical condition. Almost 50% of patients undergoing plasmapheresis experience some complication. Most of the complications, such as muscle cramps, are mild and have been related to the citrate used in the circuit. Less commonly, hypofibrinogenemia, electrolyte deficiencies, and total protein deficiencies may develop. Patients undergoing frequent sessions should be monitored regularly for electrolyte levels, blood counts, and fibrinogen levels. Fibrinogen depletion, especially in patients with clinical conditions predisposing to hemorrhage, may be treated with cryoprecipitate.

COMPLICATIONS OF IMMUNOTHERAPY ■

The side effects of many immunotherapies include several severe illnesses. Infectious complications of immunosuppressive therapy account for the most common severe consequences of immunotherapies. However, several other severe, noninfectious clinical syndromes have been attributed to certain immunotherapies. These systemic reactions have been described most commonly with certain immunoglobulin or cytokine therapies. The infusion of γ-globulin (IVIG) may result in myalgia, low-grade fever, and back pain.[21] These relatively minor symptoms have been partially attributed to complement activation by immunoglobulin complexes and are usually effectively managed by slowing the rate of infusion or prophylaxis with antihistamines. Occasionally, IVIG infusions may result in systemic hypotension or anaphylaxis. These severe reactions, although rare, have been described most commonly among patients with IgA deficiencies who have preexisting antibodies to IgA. The IgA in the IVIG infusate is thought to initiate the subsequent antigen–antibody reaction. Immunoglobulins produced in animals, such as antithymocyte globulin and the antivenins, are among the most common causes of anaphylaxis or serum sickness. The immunosuppressive monoclonal antibody OKT3 is occasionally associated with a "cytokine release syndrome" shortly after infusion.[22] OKT3 is a murine monoclonal antibody that selectively depletes T lymphocytes and has proven useful in solid organ transplantation. The cytokine release syndrome manifests as fever, myalgia, dyspnea, and hypotension. This reaction is most common after the initial OKT3 infusion and has been attributed to the systemic release of IFN-γ and TNF. This syndrome may be prevented by prophylaxis with corticosteroids. Another cytokine-mediated syndrome is the capillary leak syndrome associated with IL-2 administration.[23] IL-2 is used in certain cancer therapies and multiple other investigational studies. The capillary leak syndrome, although apparently dose related, is common, and

in certain patient populations the incidence rate approaches 50%. The sepsis-like syndrome consists of hypotension, extravascular fluid sequestration, and occasionally pulmonary edema. Treatment includes vasopressor cardiovascular support and corticosteroids. Development of the syndrome may require a decrease in the interleukin dose or cessation of therapy.

CONCLUSION ■

Appropriate immunologic responses are crucial to recovery from most critical illnesses. The complex intercommunication among immune and nonimmune system cells manifests itself as many of the systemic symptoms commonly associated with acute illness, such as fever, hypotension, and protein depletion. Perturbation of the immune defense systems, whether on a congenital or acquired basis, complicates the recovery process and commonly prolongs otherwise curable illnesses. The expanding use of immunotherapies has been accompanied with the recognition of several severe systemic side effects and infectious consequences that, in themselves, result in serious illnesses.

REFERENCES ■

1. Nossal GJ: The basic components of the immune system. *N Engl J Med* 1987;316:1320
2. Romagnani S: Lymphokine production by human T cells in disease states. *Annu Rev Immunol* 1994;12:227
3. Marrack P: The staphylococcal enterotoxins and their relatives. *Science* 1990;248:705
4. Woods DE, Straus DC, Johanson WG, et al: Role of salivary protease activity in adherence of gram-negative bacilli to mammalian buccal epithelial cells in vivo. *J Clin Invest* 1981;68:1435
5. Dinarello CA, Wolff SM: The role of interleukin-1 in disease. *N Engl J Med* 1993;328:106
6. Rosenberg SA: Adoptive immunotherapy for cancer. *Sci Am* 1990;262:62
7. Bone RC: Sepsis and its complications: the clinical problem. *Clin Exp Immunol* 1994;22(Suppl):8
8. Strieter RM, Kunkel SL: Acute lung injury: the role of cytokines in the elicitation of neutrophils. *J Invest Med* 1994;42:640
9. Casey LC, Balk RA, Bone RC: Plasma cytokine and endotoxin levels correlate with survival in patients with the sepsis syndrome. *Ann Intern Med* 1993;119:771
10. Kalter ES, Daha MR, ten Cate JW, et al: Activation and inhibition of hagemean factor-dependent pathways and the complement system in uncomplicated bacteremia or bacterial shock. *J Infect Dis* 1985;151:1019
11. Frank MM: Complement in the pathophysiology of human disease. *N Engl J Med* 1987;316:1525
12. Rosen FS, Cooper MD, Wedgwood RJP: The primary immunodeficiencies. *N Engl J Med* 1984;311:300
13. Welborn JL, Hersch J: Blood transfusion reactions. *Postgrad Med* 1991;90:125
14. Ezekowitz RAB, Dinauer MC, Jaffe HS, et al: Partial correction of the phagocytic defect in patients with X-linked chronic granulomatous disease by subcutaneous interferon gamma. *N Engl J Med* 1988;319:146

15. Abe Y, Horiuchi A, Miyake M, et al: Anti-cytokine nature of natural human immunoglobulin: one possible mechanism of the clinical effect of intravenous immunoglobulin therapy. *Immunol Rev* 1994;139:5

16. The Veterans Administration Systemic Sepsis Cooperative Study Group: Effect of high-dose glucocorticoid therapy on mortality in patients with clinical signs of systemic sepsis. *N Engl J Med* 1987;317:659

17. Suffredini AF: Current prospects for the treatment of clinical sepsis. *Clin Exp Immunol* 1994;22:(Suppl):12

18. Taboulet P, Baud FJ, Bismuth C: Clinical features and management of digitalis poisoning: rationale for immunotherapy. *Clin Toxicol* 1993;31:247

19. Luce JM: Introduction of new technology into critical care practice: a history of HA-1A human monoclonal antibody against endotoxin. *Crit Care Med* 1993;21:1233

20. Strauss RG, Ciavarella D, Gilcher RO, et al: An overview of current management. *J Clin Apheresis* 1993;8:189

21. Duhem C, Dicato MA, Ries F: Side-effects of intravenous immune globulins. *Clin Exp Immunol* 1994;97(Suppl1):79

22. Suthanthiran M, Fotino M, Riggio RR, et al: OKT3-associated adverse reactions: mechanistic basis and therapeutic options. *Am J Kidney Dis* 1989;14(Suppl 2):39

23. Ognibene FP, Rosenberg SA, Lotze M, et al: Interleukin-2 administration causes reversible hemodynamic changes and left ventricular dysfunction similar to those seen in septic shock. *Chest* 1988;94:750

Critical Care, Third Edition, edited by Joseph M. Civetta,
Robert W. Taylor, and Robert R. Kirby.
Lippincott-Raven Publishers, Philadelphia, PA © 1997.

CHAPTER 22

Pregnancy

Donald Caton

Critically ill obstetric patients alarm many clinicians. The welfare of two patients—mother and child—hangs in the balance, and therein lies the challenge. Moreover, in realizing that pregnancy alters body processes, including the response to many drugs, clinicians fear that customary methods of treatment may be deleterious.

Insecurity surrounding the obstetric patient has been fostered by decades of clinical teaching and practice that emphasize singular aspects of pregnancy—those characteristics that distinguish pregnancy from a normal condition. Equating different with abnormal, physicians assume that principles of medical physiology no longer apply and look for new rules with which to manage these patients. In fact, pregnancy is simply a condition in which normal physiologic processes maintain maternal body homeostasis in the face of stress. When the character of the stress is identified, the response appears logical, orderly, and clinically manageable.

PREGNANCY-IMPOSED STRESS

CHARACTERISTICS

The major stress imposed by pregnancy is metabolic. At any stage of pregnancy, the metabolic rate of the mother is the arithmetic sum of her normal (nonpregnant) rate, the metabolic rate of the products of conception, and the slight increase caused by the physical work of carrying the extra tissue.[1] At term, maternal metabolism normally has increased by 20% to 30%, an amount greater than the increase of either maternal surface area or weight. The high metabolic activity of the products of conception causes the disproportion.[2] The metabolic rate of the fetus, placenta, and uterus exceeds that of the mother by a factor of two to four. Thus, a 60-kg woman who consumes 240 mL oxygen/minute (4 mL/kg) before pregnancy may consume as much as 320 mL

oxygen/minute by term, provided that her fetus, placenta, and uterus all are of average weight.[3,4]

Although oxygen consumption of fetus, placenta, and uterus can be as high as 20 mL/kg/minute, it varies in relation to fetal growth, a situation that applies to extrauterine and intrauterine growth. Highest rates occur in the fastest-growing fetuses and lowest in fetuses in whom growth is suspended. Thus, the metabolic stress imposed on the woman carrying a large, rapidly growing fetus is high for two reasons: first, because the total mass of fetal tissue is greater; second, because each unit mass of that tissue consumes oxygen at a higher rate. Recall that glucose and other metabolic substrates are consumed and that heat and other metabolic byproducts are produced in proportion to oxygen consumption. Therefore, measurements of oxygen consumption accurately reflect the total metabolic stress imposed on the mother.

RESPONSE

Women respond to metabolic stress with functional and structural changes in most tissue and organ systems. Collectively, these changes comprise the signs and symptoms of normal pregnancy. If carried to excess, however, they become pathologic and are called *diseases of pregnancy*. For example, when protracted, the nausea and vomiting of the first trimester become hyperemesis gravidarum. The normal increase of mean arterial pressure between the second and third trimesters becomes eclampsia. Physicians must know the normal patterns of change so that they can recognize when the boundaries have been surpassed, plan their response, and manage the underlying problems.

Ventilation

Maternal minute ventilation increases as a direct reaction to the metabolic challenge. This pulmonary response differs

315

from that which occurs with a simple increase of metabolic rate during exercise or hyperthermia. Upward displacement of the diaphragm and the rib cage by the enlarging uterus alters the mechanics of ventilation, causing decreased functional residual capacity. This change facilitates nitrogen washout, enhances inhalation anesthetic agent uptake, and limits the oxygen supply. The last factor, together with the increased metabolic rate, contributes to the rapid desaturation observed in pregnant women during periods of apnea.[5,6]

Pervasive change also occurs in the regulation of ventilation. Increased sensitivity of the respiratory nuclei in the brain stem causes a decrease in $PaCO_2$ to 30 to 35 mm Hg as early as the sixth week of pregnancy. The kidneys respond to the low $PaCO_2$ by proportionally decreasing plasma bicarbonate. Because the carbon dioxide–bicarbonate ratio remains almost constant, pH is only slightly increased; however, the decreased buffering capacity contributes to the mild feeling of dyspnea that many women experience during pregnancy, a phenomenon that also occurs during the luteal phase of the menstrual cycle.[7,8]

Cardiovascular

Increased blood flow to the skin and kidneys increases heat dissipation and the excretion of fixed acids (derived from increased metabolism) and contributes to increased cardiac output. Most of the additional cardiac output, however, goes to the placenta and uterus in direct support of the growing fetus.[9] Arteries, veins, and capillaries of many organs, especially the uterus, grow and dilate, and blood volume increases by as much as 50%. Plasma volume expansion exceeds that of the circulating red blood cell mass, contributing to the drop in hematocrit.[10–12]

While metabolic demands of the fetus increase throughout pregnancy, so, in theory, should cardiac output. In fact, it peaks at or about the sixth month, coinciding with the time cardiac patients often develop problems. From 6 months until term, the pattern varies; output increases in some patients but decreases or remains constant in others. Early in pregnancy, stroke volume causes most of the increment of cardiac output. Later, increases follow heart rate, a point of clinical significance when one deals with patients with mitral valve lesions in whom diastolic filling time limits performance.

Renal

Changes in renal function also satisfy the increased metabolic needs.[13] Renal blood flow, glomerular filtration rate, and renal tubular reabsorption increase. These changes are readily understood in terms of the mother's need to excrete surplus amounts of fixed acids and to accumulate water and salt needed for the additional 1 to 2 L of maternal blood, the amniotic fluid, and new fetal tissue. Water accumulation is an important part of the growth process. The water content of the conceptus exceeds 90%, although near term it falls toward normal newborn concentrations. Increased capillary permeability facilitates the movement of water from the vasculature into interstitial tissues. It also contributes to the appearance of dependent edema, particularly in the last weeks of pregnancy.

Hepatic

Enhanced protein synthesis by the liver may represent a vestigial response, important in egg-laying animals, in which the protein deposited in eggs is synthesized in the liver and then transported to the oviduct for deposition around the yolk. In patients, the extra proteins are important for blood volume expansion. Altered liver metabolism and excretion, blood volume, serum protein concentrations, and cardiodynamics contribute to the increased sensitivity of pregnant women to the effects of many drugs.

Miscellaneous

Several other changes in pregnancy support the increased need for metabolic substrates. In the central nervous system (CNS), a change in the set point of the appetite-regulating center, increased olfactory acuity, and greater affinity for certain foods with specific tastes all foster increased caloric intake and a tendency for weight gain. Concomitantly, diminished maternal neuromotor activity from hormonal depression of the CNS lessens caloric expenditure on activities not directly supportive of fetal growth and development.

Medical conditions that limit the cardiac response to pregnancy restrict fetal growth. As a result, estimates of fetal weight, determined reasonably accurately by ultrasound, can be used to measure the physiologic stress imposed on the mother and her capacity to respond. Increments of cardiac output during pregnancy are diminished in relation to the severity of disease in cardiac patients, as in the birth weight of their offspring. Similarly, when the weight of the fetus is appropriate for gestational age, it suggests the ability of the mother's cardiovascular system to support at least that level of growth.

CHANGES AT TERM ■

CARDIOPULMONARY

Labor imposes an additional metabolic stress. Oxygen consumption and carbon dioxide production increase from the physical work of labor and the response to pain. Cardiac output and minute ventilation increase proportionately, a significant stress in the cardiac or pulmonary patient with limited reserves.[14] Respiratory and vascular responses caused by labor cannot be blocked with appropriate anesthetic management, but pain can. Effective pain therapy, therefore, becomes an important part of management of the high-risk patient.

Not all components of the vascular response at term are metabolically derived. In the last days of pregnancy, uterine and mammary blood flow increase. Cardiac output increases during labor, although the highest rates occur in the immediate postpartum period, rapidly subsiding over the ensuing 6 to 24 hours. These patterns of change are important to those managing high-risk patients during the peripartum period. Nonmetabolic hormonal mechanisms cause some of the prepartum and most of the postpartum vascular responses. At delivery, the maternal metabolic rate drops abruptly by an amount equal to the intrauterine metabolic rate of the fetus and placenta.

UTERINE

Any tissue or cell capable of becoming more active does so during the peripartum period. The myometrium, quiescent for almost 9 months, begins spontaneous contractions that progress from weak and ineffectual to strong, regular, and coordinated. Changes related to cellular membrane phenomena include decreased membrane potential, increased rate of spontaneous discharge, increased responsiveness to external stimuli, such as oxytocin, and greater propensity to propagate electrical activity from one cell to the next. A "pacemaker" develops near the fundus that drives and coordinates contractions, culminating in dilatation of the cervix and expulsion of the fetus.

SMOOTH MUSCLE

Parallel changes occur in other smooth muscle (Table 22-1). Bronchioles become reactive, and the risk of intrinsic or induced (as with an endotracheal tube) asthma increases tremendously during the peripartum period. In addition, venous tone and smooth muscle irritability increase, changes apparent to anyone drawing blood from a postpartum patient. Spontaneous constriction of the capacitance circulation is an important defense against blood loss during vaginal delivery or delivery by cesarean section. However, it also contributes to the increased cardiac output and risk of postpartum congestive heart failure in the cardiac patient. Arrhythmias increase during the peripartum period, presumably influenced by the same agents that stimulate the myometrium. Estrogen concentrations, which rise abruptly before delivery, interact with and affect the cardiac muscle similarly to digitalis.

CENTRAL NERVOUS SYSTEM

The CNS also increases its activity during the last days of pregnancy.[15-17] Normally, most women notice a return of energy, less drowsiness, and increased neuromotor activity, a complex characterized as nesting behavior in many species. Reflexes releasing oxytocin, from stimulation of the nipple or dilatation of the cervix (Ferguson's reflex), become active and contribute to uterine activation. In its most extreme form, the increased neuromotor activity is manifested as the convulsions of eclampsia. Notice that estrogens, which are important in activating the myometrium at term, also are capable of causing convulsions in primates.

CONNECTIVE TISSUE

Connective tissue changes also occur in pregnancy. Water moves from the fetus and from the interstitial space of the mother into the maternal vasculature from whence it is excreted by the kidney, appearing as a diuresis during the last days of pregnancy. Commonly, but incorrectly, this phenomenon is attributed solely to extrinsic pressure of the uterus on the bladder. In response to rising concentrations of relaxin, a protein hormone produced in the ovary and possibly the placenta, the cervix softens and then dilates as the uterus begins to contract. Relaxin probably causes softening of other ligaments, detected by anesthesiologists as loss of the characteristic resistance of the ligamentum flavum during an epidural needle insertion.

TABLE 22-1. Smooth Muscle Response to Pregnancy

ORGAN SYSTEM	RESPONSE	CLINICAL EFFECT
UROGENITAL		
Uterus	Hyperplasia and hypertrophy; alterations in tone and irritability	Enlargement; relaxation until term, then contractions
Ureter	Same as above	Dilatation; decreased peristalsis, urinary retention, and infection
GASTROINTESTINAL		
Gastroesophageal sphincter	Decreased tone with some incompetence	Esophagitis
Stomach	Decreased peristalsis	Prolonged emptying
Bowel	Decreased peristalsis, increased transit time	Constipation
Gallbladder, bile ducts	Decreased tone, dilatation	Stasis, stone formation, infection
CARDIOVASCULAR		
Heart	Altered irritability peripartum	Dysrhythmias
Arterioles, venules	Growth of new vessels, enlargement of existing cells, alterations of tone and irritability	Engorgement of mucous membranes, epistaxis, spider angiomata, palmar erythema
RESPIRATORY		
Vasculature	Growth and enlargement of mucous membrane blood vessels	"Stuffy nose"
Bronchioles	Increased irritability, particularly peripartum	Asthma

COORDINATION ■

Despite its complexity, the maternal response to pregnancy is orderly in terms of the timing and pattern of physiologic and structural change. Conception and parturition exemplify coordination of events in time. Successful mating requires appropriate behavior (male attraction, female reception), a ripe follicle, a biochemical environment of the reproductive tract favorable for migration and activation of sperm, and a uterine mucosa prepared to receive the fertilized egg. Events at term are perhaps more intricate because they involve integration of complex events in the mother and fetus. Premature labor, a common clinical problem, represents an abnormality of timing, a situation in which the maturation of the child and the activation of the myometrium are out of synchrony.

Less dramatic than timing, but no less important, is regulating the amount of change. Successful pregnancy requires a balance between maternal and fetal needs. The fetus requires sufficient quantities of nutrients to be available at appropriate times. The mother, however, needs to accomplish this goal with the least possible expenditure of energy. At best, an imbalance can be biologically inefficient. At worst, it may be disastrous to the mother, child, or both. Without means to control the process, a woman whose reserves are limited by cardiac or pulmonary disease can be thrown into life-threatening heart failure trying to meet the metabolic demands of a fetus. On the other hand, consider twins or triplets: without mechanisms to signal the existence of a multiple pregnancy, the supply of nutrients might be wholly inadequate to support normal growth and development.

The uterine circulation exemplifies the balance achieved between mother and fetus, as well as the regulatory patterns of the variables involved in metabolic substrate delivery.[18-20] During pregnancy, uterine blood flow increases in proportion to the weight and metabolic activity of the fetus, placenta, and uterus. This response ensures an economy of effort, adequate but not greater than required to satisfy fetal needs at any given time. Blood flow, however, constitutes only one part of the delivery system. Where oxygen is concerned, other factors include maternal oxygen-carrying capacity and saturation, the diffusion capacity of the placenta, fetal oxygen-carrying capacity, and umbilical blood flow. Disruption of any one factor, if not too severe, rarely terminates the pregnancy but does induce compensatory changes in other components of the system. Higher than normal rates of uterine blood flow occur in a variety of conditions that impair oxygen delivery, including maternal anemia, chronic hypoxemia (residents at high altitude), and disruption of normal placental growth.

MECHANISMS OF INTEGRATION

In normal circumstances, various neural and endocrine mechanisms regulate and integrate physiologic and anatomic changes. Although their function continues during pregnancy, they must adjust to a whole new set of activities and demands emanating from the uterus. To an extent, existing control mechanisms become subordinate to new ones whose primary function is balancing maternal and fetal needs. This role is assumed by estrogens and progestogens.

Estrogens and progestogens regulate reproductive functions in most animal species. In most higher species, they are produced and released by the mother and the fetoplacental unit. Hormones produced by the latter affect the mother throughout pregnancy. Estrogens released by the blastocyst signal the onset of pregnancy; conversely, maternal estrogen and progesterone changes at term promote a complex series of events that culminate in parturition.

Between conception and term, the fetoplacental unit and maternal ovary produce hormones in proportion to the rate of fetal growth. Moreover, the magnitude of the maternal response to pregnancy seems to be directly related to the concentration or rate of hormonal synthesis. In the event of stress or unusual demands, with multiple gestation, for example, hormonal metabolic patterns adjust appropriately.

In short, estrogens and progesterone are important mechanisms of physiologic communication during pregnancy, and their capacity to induce alterations in structure and function is protean and pervasive. They coordinate change by direct effects on targeted organs and by inducing change in other hormonal systems (Tables 22-2 and 22-3).

Direct Effects

Direct effects of estrogens and progestogens on targeted tissues fall into three major categories: smooth muscle, CNS, and glandular.

SMOOTH MUSCLE
Structure. The most dramatic and best recognized effect of estrogens and progestogens is their influence on smooth muscle anatomy. Conjointly, they stimulate growth, causing hyperplasia and hypertrophy, particularly of the myometrium, which increases its weight fivefold to sixfold. In most species, the weight of the term uterus is proportional to the weight of its fetus. Similar, although less dramatic, changes occur in ureteral, gastrointestinal, bile duct, and vascular smooth muscle. Clinical manifestations of small vessel hyperplasia consist of telangiectasia of the head and neck, palmar erythema, stuffy nose, and gingival bleeding.

TABLE 22-2. Hormone Systems That Interact With Estrogens and Progesterone

CENTRAL NERVOUS SYSTEM
Catecholamines
Prolactin
Oxytocin
Endorphins
ACTH

ADRENAL
Glucocorticoids
Mineralocorticoids

ACTH, corticotropin.

TABLE 22-3. Effects of Estrogen and Progesterone on Membrane Phenomena

	ESTROGEN	PROGESTERONE
Polarization	↓	↑
Frequency of spontaneous discharge	↑	↓
Propagation of electrical activity	↑	↓
Response to other stimuli		
Oxytocin	↑	↓
Epinephrine	↑	↓
Mechanical stimulation	↑	↓
Uterine contractions	↑	↓
Cardiac dysrhythmias	↑	↓
CNS		
Drowsiness	↓	↑
Seizures	↑ ↓	?
Reflex response	↑	↓

CNS, central nervous system.

Function.   Large, equally important changes transpire in smooth muscle physiology. During most of pregnancy, smooth muscle tone and irritability are depressed. Spontaneous activity of and sensitivity to oxytocin and epinephrine are altered. Manifestations of diminished activity and their clinical correlates include dilation of peripheral veins, appearing as varicosities and hemorrhoids; decreased ureteral function, predisposing patients to urinary tract infections; decreased bowel activity, resulting in increased transit time and constipation; increased gastric emptying time and decreased gastroesophageal sphincter tone, causing symptoms of esophagitis; and decreased activity of the gallbladder and bile ducts, causing stasis and a tendency to stone formation. Clinical problems caused by smooth muscle relaxation during pregnancy include varicosities and urinary and bile stasis, which often continue to bother women later in life.

In response to endocrine changes at term, the intrinsic tone, irritability, and sensitivity of smooth muscle to extrinsic stimuli increase.[21] The most striking clinical manifestation is Braxton Hicks contractions, which later become contractions of true labor. Similar, although less dramatic, alterations in vascular smooth muscle occur. Capacitance vessels constrict, blood shifts centrally, and cardiac output increases when patients go into labor. Concomitant changes in smooth muscle tone and irritability affect the pulmonary circulation and may account for the increased pulmonary artery pressures normally measured during labor. The high incidence of asthma in parturients suggests similar involvement of bronchiolar smooth muscle. (The incidence of asthma also increases in the premenstrual period.)

CENTRAL NERVOUS SYSTEM.   "Depression" best characterizes the CNS response to pregnancy. Clinically, this alteration appears as diminished neuromotor activity and drowsiness (despite increased sleep requirements). A measurable difference in the proportion of time spent in rapid eye movement sleep is observed. Cerebellar function changes; women who normally excel at tasks requiring fine hand-eye coordination may experience difficulty. Depression of the cyclical activity of the hypothalamic–pituitary–gonadal axis occurs, causing the clinically apparent cessation of ovulation and menstruation. Generalized CNS depression, probably a direct response to progesterone, interacts synergistically with an altered pharmacodynamic state to increase the sensitivity of pregnant women to sedatives, narcotics, tranquilizers, and inhalation anesthetics.[22]

On the surface, other CNS functions seem to be stimulated. Notable examples are appetite, respiration, and vomiting. Sensitivity of the respiratory center increases as early as the sixth week of pregnancy, causing a decrease in arterial and alveolar P_{CO_2}, a change that persists through the remainder of the pregnancy. The drive is strong, summating with hypoxemia to lower the Pa_{CO_2} of pregnant women living at high altitude to 20 to 25 mm Hg. As mentioned previously, little change of pH occurs because the kidneys compensate with a proportional increase of bicarbonate excretion. Familiarity with these variables is important for anyone measuring the blood gas partial pressures and pH of pregnant women. A Pa_{CO_2} value greater than 35 mm Hg is abnormal until proven otherwise.

Vomiting occurs in many women during the first trimester of pregnancy, partly because of increased sensitivity of the vomiting center in the medulla, and partly because of increased sensitivity to odors. If vomiting is severe or continues past the first 3 months, it can cause serious metabolic derangements that are life-threatening to mother and child. Increased pigmentation of the face, areolae, and linea negra result from elevated concentrations of melanocyte-stimulating hormone. The systematic decrease of mean arterial pressure during the second trimester and its increase during the third trimester stem from a change of the blood pressure regulatory center in the brain stem. The hypertensive component of preeclampsia may reflect an inappropriate response of this mechanism.

Many other examples of altered CNS activity occur. Pregnancy induces change in most CNS functions. Depression is the character of the overall response, but examples of increased activity also occur, many of which are medically important. Change may reflect direct stimulation in some cases or inhibitory center depression in others.

GLANDS.   Many glands enlarge during pregnancy and their secretory activity is altered. Most conspicuous are changes in the mammary glands. Lactation at term concludes a sequence of steps that occurs throughout pregnancy and consists of duct proliferation, acinar development, colostrum production, and, finally, lactation. Salivary glands also secrete more, as is apparent in the copious secretions that often interfere with visualization during a tracheal intubation. Gastric gland hyperactivity contributes to symptoms of esophagitis and to increased risk of pulmonary damage from regurgitation and aspiration.

Indirect Effects

Generally, the more important a physiologic regulatory mechanism, the more it interacts with other regulatory mechanisms. This truism applies to estrogens and progestogens (see Table 22-2). In most instances, effects are reciprocal; changes in one hormone system induce appropriate change in others. Hormone regulatory mechanisms, including those peculiar to pregnancy, also interact reciprocally with the CNS, extending their capacity to respond to stress.

HORMONAL INTERACTIONS. The sequence of events at term illustrates the importance of hormonal interactions.[21,23–25] Normally, a spontaneous rise of fetal glucocorticoid concentrations triggers the events that culminate in labor and delivery. Placental metabolism of progesterone declines over a period of days, and estrogens rise precipitously during the last hours. Changes in estrogens and progesterone in turn produce CNS changes, including increased oxytocin concentration in the pituitary gland. An increase of maternal prolactin contributes to the onset of lactation and initiates instinctual changes, which are collectively termed *nesting behavior.* Coincidentally, changes in the fetus, partly induced by the altered hormonal milieu, prepare it for parturition and independent life.

STRESS. Some types of stress may initiate the same sequence of endocrine events that normally culminate in labor.[26–31] For example, hypoxia, hyperthermia or hypothermia, and psychological stress cause a premature rise in maternal or fetal glucocorticoids sufficient in selected cases to induce labor. In many species, the administration of glucocorticoids to the mother induces delivery within 24 hours.

The medical significance of such change depends on the circumstances. On the one hand, it affords the fetus, if not too young, a means to hasten the process of physiologic maturation, preparing it for survival after premature birth by inducing the biochemical changes necessary for surfactant production. On the other hand, it provides the mother a means to rid herself of pregnancy when her own survival is threatened. For an animal in the wild, threatened by predators or adverse environmental conditions, such a response may spell the difference between survival and death.

PREMATURE LABOR AND ABORTION. Originally, the capacity to abort a pregnancy in time of stress may have had similar survival value for humans. Trauma, surgery (particularly abdominal surgery), hyperpyrexia, and even psychological stress may induce premature labor. It is not difficult to imagine circumstances when such a response might be lifesaving for a woman. In this regard, it is noteworthy that the incidence and timing of premature labor among patients with certain types of congenital cardiac lesions seem to vary with the severity of the disease. Presumably, the physical limitations imposed by the cardiac problem induce a reaction that allows the mother to survive even at the cost of her pregnancy.

Abortion or premature labor is a drastic stress response, however. In other circumstances, a more moderate response, occurring in less-threatening circumstances, fosters an adaptive reaction that allows the fetus to survive and the pregnancy to continue. Disruption of normal placental growth initiates a change of progesterone metabolism, important

because it stimulates an overgrowth of existing placental tissue and higher-than-normal rates of uterine blood flow. This adaptive response is of sufficient magnitude to sustain normal rates of fetal growth to term.

DRUGS AND ANESTHESIA. Abortion after injury or stress has other implications. We have the medical tools to deal successfully with many problems that once were lethal to the mother, and we assume that we can manage her disease, using survival of the fetus and continuation of the pregnancy as the measure of success. In this regard, drugs and techniques already in use offer promise, and several affect maternal or fetal endocrinology. Regional anesthesia (spinal or epidural) modifies or delays the increase of corticotropin and glucocorticoid concentrations that normally occurs during surgery and physical stress. They even depress this response during labor.

Other drugs have similar effects. Etomidate seems to suppress adrenocortical activity, an undesirable effect in some intensive care unit patients, perhaps, but one with potential for the management of acutely stressed, pregnant patients. Althesin, a short-acting hypnotic, has a steroid configuration that closely resembles progesterone, although its effects on clinical endocrinology have not been studied. Considering the key role of glucocorticoids and other steroid hormones in the regulation and integration of events in pregnancy, these agents represent a significant potential medical control. Remember that the physiologic changes associated with pregnancy and parturition alter the maternal responses to administered drugs from those of the nonpregnant patient (Table 22-4).

Although drugs and regional anesthesia offer new opportunities for medical management, they also create a clinical dilemma. Currently, we have no means to differentiate stress that is severe enough to initiate labor or fetal death from that which stimulates an adaptive response. Neither do we know how to evaluate stress response. Both points are important if we expect to intervene and to regulate the endocrine patterns of the acutely ill or severely injured pregnant patient.

TABLE 22-4. Physiologic Changes That Alter the Response to Drugs

---

1. Increased blood volume and interstitial water content that change volume of distribution
2. Increased total plasma protein affecting binding of drugs
3. Increased glomerular filtration rate affecting excretion of drugs by the kidney
4. Change in the distribution of cardiac output—a smaller fraction goes to the heart and brain
5. Altered liver metabolism and excretion causing retention of some drugs to their more active forms
6. Increased drug sensitivity of some end organs, such as the brain and heart, from interaction with steroid hormones

CONCLUSION ■

Pregnancy involves extensive change in the function and structure of most tissue and organ systems in the body.[32] The amount and character of change are goal directed. Integration is accomplished through intricate hormonal interactions that affect many of the pharmacologic and physiologic activities important to physicians in critical care medicine. Currently, we do not know how to regulate this activity, although some techniques and drugs that are available seem to have potential usefulness in this area.

REFERENCES ■

1. Carpenter TM, Murlin JR: The energy metabolism of mother and child just before and just after birth. *Arch Intern Med* 1911;7:184
2. Morriss FH, Rosenreid CR, Resnik R, et al: Growth of uterine oxygen and glucose uptakes during pregnancy in sheep. *Gynecol Invest* 1974;5:230
3. Clapp JF, Abrams RM, Caton D, et al: The oxygen consumption of the uterus and its tissue contents in late gestation: a comparison of simultaneous measurements using two different techniques. *Q J Exp Physiol* 1972;57:24
4. Caton D, Henderson J, Wilcox CJ, et al: Oxygen consumption of the uterus and its contents and weight at birth of lambs. In: Longo LD, Reneau DD (eds). *Fetal and Newborn Cardiovascular Physiology*. New York, London, Garland STPM Press, 1976:123
5. Alaily AB, Carrol KB: Pulmonary ventilation in pregnancy. *Br J Obstet Gynaecol* 1978;85:518
6. Weinberger SE, Weiss ST, Cohen WR, et al: State of the art: pregnancy and the lung. *Am Rev Respir Dis* 1980;121:559
7. Mathida H: Influence of progesterone on arterial blood and CSF acid–base balance in women. *J Appl Physiol* 1981;51:1433
8. Blechner JN, Cotter JR, Stenger VG, et al: Oxygen, carbon dioxide, and hydrogen ion concentrations in arterial blood during pregnancy. *Am J Obstet Gynecol* 1968;100:1
9. Parry HJ: The vascular structure of the extraplacental uterine mucosa of the rabbit. *J Endocrinol* 1950;7:88
10. Hytten FE, Paintin DB: Increase in plasma volume during normal pregnancy. *J Obstet Gynaecol* 1963;70:402
11. Duffus GM, MacGillivray I, Denis KJ: The relationship between baby weight and changes in maternal weight, total body water, plasma volume, electrolytes and proteins and urinary oestriol excretion. *J Obstet Gynaecol Br Commonw* 1971;78:97
12. Caton WL, Roby CC, Reid DE, et al: The circulating red cell volume and body hematocrit in normal pregnancy and the puerperium. *Am J Obstet Gynecol* 1951;61:1207
13. Gibson HM: Plasma volume and glomerular filtration rate in pregnancy and their relation to differences in fetal growth. *J Obstet Gynaecol* 1973;80:1967
14. Ueland K, Novy M J, Peterson EN, et al: Maternal cardiovascular dynamics. *Am J Obstet Gynecol* 1969;104:856
15. Holzbauer M: Physiological aspects of steroids with anaesthetic properties. *Med Biol* 1976;54:227
16. Conney AH: Hormonal regulation of drug metabolism. In: Conney AH (ed). *Pharmacological Implications of Microsomal Enzyme Induction*. New York, Williams & Wilkins, 1967:344
17. Crawford JS, Rudofsky S: Some alterations in the pattern of drug metabolism associated with pregnancy, oral contraceptives, and the newly born. *Br J Anaesth* 1966;38:446
18. Caton D, Crenshaw C, Wilcox CJ: O₂ delivery to the pregnant uterus: its relationship to O₂ consumption. *Am J Physiol* 1979;237:R52
19. Caton D, Kalra PS: Endogenous hormones and regulation of uterine blood flow during pregnancy. *Am J Physiol* 1986;250:R265
20. Caton D, Kalra PS, Wilcox CJ: Relationships between maternal hormones and weight of newborn sheep. *Am J Physiol* 1983;244:R31
21. Nathanielsz PW: Endocrine mechanisms of parturition. *Annu Rev Physiol* 1978;40:411
22. Pfaff DW, McEwen BS: Actions of estrogens and progestins on nerve cells. *Science* 1983;219:808
23. Rawlings NC, Ward WR: Changes in steroid hormones in plasma and myometrium and uterine activity in ewes during late pregnancy and parturition. *J Reprod Fertil* 1976;48:355
24. Eguchi Y, Arishima K, Morikawa Y, et al: Rise of plasma corticosterone concentrations in rats immediately before and after birth and in fetal rats after the ligation of maternal uterine blood vessels or of the umbilical cord. *Endocrinology* 1977;100:1443
25. Turnbull AC, Fint APF, Jeremy JY, et al: Significant fall in progesterone and rise in oestradiol levels in human peripheral plasma before onset of labour. *Lancet* 1974;1:101
26. Price DB, Thaler M, Mason JW: Preoperative emotional states and adrenal cortical activity. *AMA Arch Neurol Psychiatr* 1957;77:646
27. Black S, Friedman M: Effects of emotion and pain on adrenocortical function investigated by hypnosis. *Br Med J* 1968;1:477
28. Lederman RP, Lederman E, Work BA, et al: The relationship of maternal anxiety, plasma catecholamines, and plasma cortisol to progress in labor. *Am J Obstet Gynecol* 1978;132:495
29. Wagner RL, White PF, Kan PB, et al: Inhibition of adrenal steroidogenesis by the anesthetic etomidate. *Lancet* 1983;310:1415
30. Gordon NH, Scott DB, Percy Robb IWP: Modification of plasma corticosteroid concentrations during and after surgery by epidural blockade. *Br Med J* 1973;1:581
31. Buchan PC, Milne MK, Browning MCK: The effect of continuous epidural blockade on plasma II-hydroxycorticosteroid concentrations in labour. *J Obstet Gynaecol Br Commonw* 1973;80:974
32. Bonica JS: Maternal anatomic and physiologic alterations during pregnancy and parturition. In: Bonica JS, McDonald JS (eds). *Principles and Practice of Obstetric Analgesia and Anesthesia*. Baltimore, Williams and Wilkins, 1995:45

Modulating the Response to Injury

Critical Care, Third Edition, edited by Joseph M. Civetta,
Robert W. Taylor, and Robert R. Kirby.
Lippincott-Raven Publishers, Philadelphia, PA © 1997.

CHAPTER 23

Metabolic Response to Injury and Critical Illness

Palmer Q. Bessey
Richard S. Downey
William W. Monafo

IMMEDIATE CONCERNS

MAJOR PROBLEMS

The metabolic response to injury and critical illness is characterized by an acceleration of whole body metabolism. This "hypermetabolism" is a generalized phenomenon that is initiated and sustained by a combination of humoral, neural, and environmental stimuli, and is proportional in intensity to the severity of injury. Nutritional reserves are mobilized from a variety of sites to provide glucose, amino acids, and fat substrate as required to meet the accelerated metabolic demands. These accelerated demands may be superimposed on a significant degree of premorbid starvation, with its attendant metabolic implications. With prolonged post-traumatic hypermetabolism, mobilization of metabolic reserves leads to a depletion of essential protein, fat, and carbohydrate stores. Major organ system dysfunction may occur with impairment of immune, skeletal muscle, cardiac, pulmonary, gastrointestinal, and renal function. Superimposed infection frequently develops. If unchecked, these events are associated with a significant increase in morbidity and mortality. Recognition of potentially reversible metabolic derangements is essential so that these untoward effects can be minimized or reversed.

This chapter addresses alterations in both energy metabolism and intermediary metabolism of the major tissue fuels known to occur with injury, sepsis, and other critical illnesses. A meaningful assessment of most metabolic derangements requires carefully controlled, steady-state measurements—data that are typically difficult if not impossible to obtain in the critical care setting, particularly in the presence of failure of one or more organ systems. Conventional laboratory tests that report the blood or tissue concentration of a particular substrate or metabolite may not afford insight into the underlying dynamic state. Moreover, changes in both the magnitude and the distribution of body water occur which affect the interpretation of these laboratory studies. Since changes in body water are difficult to measure, particularly in the critically ill, such data are usually unavailable.

STRESS POINTS

1. Immediately following injury and persisting for 24 to 48 hours is a period of "diminished circulatory vitality" termed the "ebb phase, which is usually associated with shock and resuscitation."
2. Oxygen consumption is typically decreased during the ebb phase because of inadequate oxygen delivery to the tissues.

3. Activation of the sympathetic nervous system and the hypothalamic–pituitary axis occurs during the ebb phase and gradually diminishes during convalescence.
4. The "flow phase" begins after stabilization and resuscitation and usually is fully developed 5 to 7 days after injury.
5. Body temperature, heart rate, cardiac output, oxygen consumption, respiratory rate, and minute ventilation all increase during the flow phase.
6. Changes in the flow phase gradually return toward normal as the patient recovers.
7. Increased protein synthesis occurs in the bone marrow and liver after injury, resulting in elevated acute phase reactants. In skeletal muscles, protein catabolism predominates, so that nitrogen excretion and muscle wasting are dramatically increased.
8. Blood glucose is typically elevated and intolerance to exogenous glucose is common.
9. Lipid stores are mobilized by the lipolysis of triglycerides to glycerol and free fatty acids. These are used in the liver and peripheral tissues as an energy source.
10. The metabolic responses to injury are regulated by complex neurohumoral mechanisms.
11. Catabolic counterregulatory hormones (cortisol, glucagon, epinephrine and norepinephrine) are increased. Insulin and growth hormone are variable.
12. Cytokines are elaborated during inflammation and also participate in the metabolic responses to injury and critical illness.

GENERAL FEATURES OF THE RESPONSE TO INJURY

EBB PHASE

In a series of observations first made more than 50 years ago and repeatedly confirmed in the essential details, Cuthbertson noted that patients with uncomplicated trauma, such

TABLE 23-1. Metabolic Responses to Critical Illness—Time Course

	EBB PHASE	FLOW PHASE
Oxygen consumption	↓	↑
Cardiac output	↓	↑
Body temperature	↓	↑
Nitrogen loss	—	↑
Blood glucose	↑	↑
Glucose production	—	↑
Lactate	↑	—
Free fatty acids	↑	↑
Catecholamines, glucagon, cortisol	↑	↑
Insulin	↓	↑
Insulin resistance	↑	↑
Cytokine production	—	↑

as long bone fractures, demonstrate characteristic clinical and laboratory findings during recovery (Table 23-1).[1-4] Immediately after injury and persisting for 24 to 48 hours is a period of "diminished circulatory vitality," termed by Cuthbertson the *ebb phase*.[4] It is now well recognized that these early systemic changes following trauma result primarily from a decreased cardiac output that attends hypovolemia from blood loss or extracellular fluid sequestration. Oxygen consumption is typically decreased during the ebb phase, in most instances owing to inadequate oxygen transport to the tissues. Body temperature tends to be subnormal. There is both clinical and laboratory evidence of intense activation of the sympathetic nervous system and of the hypothalamic–pituitary–adrenal axis. Serum glucose concentrations tend to be elevated (except in infants, whose small hepatic glycogen stores are rapidly depleted), and serum insulin levels are subnormal. Circulating catecholamines, lactate, and free fatty acids are typically elevated. As noted in detail elsewhere in this volume, treatment during the ebb phase is, of necessity, directed toward rapid resuscitation and correction of the acute physiologic derangements that attend hypovolemia and tissue hypoxia.

FLOW PHASE

As Cuthbertson originally noted, elevations of body temperature, respiratory rate, and pulse are consistently observed by the latter part of the first week after injury. Cardiac output by then has returned to the normal range and is accompanied by normovolemia or hypervolemia. The cardiac output characteristically continues to increase, reaching a plateau in the supernormal range by the end of the second week. Barring specific complications, regional blood flow to viscera, particularly the kidneys and liver, is also characteristically elevated, as is flow to the region of the wound. Weight loss begins to become apparent, although it may be masked—particularly in elderly patients—by delayed excretion of sodium and water loads (often of massive proportions) initially administered during resuscitation. Whole body resting oxygen consumption tends to rise to a plateau during the first 2 weeks after injury. Nitrogen excretion is also increased to a far greater extent than can reasonably be attributed to local tissue breakdown at the injury site. Cuthbertson correctly deduced that increased urinary nitrogen, sulfur, and phosphorus losses were manifestations of a generalized increase in muscle protein catabolism and not simply a consequence of resorption of injured or necrotic tissue. The increase in resting metabolic rate, which occurs in the presence of minimal or decreased caloric intake, necessitates the utilization and oxidation of the body's own fuel reserves.

During the flow phase, blood glucose is normal or elevated and tolerance to exogenous carbohydrate is decreased—"diabetes of injury."[5] Enhanced peripheral uptake of glucose is seen.[6] As discussed below, the rate of gluconeogenesis is accelerated; glucogenic amino acids (released primarily from skeletal muscle) are utilized as substrate for the formation of the new glucose. Serum insulin levels become normal or are elevated and insulin resistance is seen.[7] Circulating glucagon is dramatically increased. Superimposed stresses, such as surgical procedures or infection, frequently exacerbate the already increased metabolic demands. Adipose tissue, the major fuel reserve, is mobilized and oxidized after injury, but less preferentially than in starvation.

STARVATION: AN ADAPTIVE RESPONSE

Although patients often develop critical illness early after trauma and shock, noninjured or minimally injured patients may also become critically ill. In these cases especially the acute metabolic effects of critical illness are frequently superimposed on a preexisting state of either short-term or long-term starvation, an often unrecognized phenomenon that occurs in a high proportion of hospitalized patients.[8,9] In contrast to the hypermetabolism of critical illness, starvation is an adaptive mechanism designed to maintain euglycemia in the absence of caloric intake while meeting the metabolic requirements of functioning tissues and conserving protein stores.[10,11] These effects are readily reversible with simple refeeding.

The metabolic changes of starvation serve to meet the continued energy demands of the brain, renal medulla, hematopoietic tissue, and other metabolically active organs. The production of glucose from liver and muscle glycogen stores depletes those stores rapidly—typically within 12 to 24 hours—and alternative sources of energy must be used. Protein stores are next broken down, at rates of up to 120 to 140 g/day, to meet the large glucose requirements of such tissues as the brain. If this high rate of protein breakdown continued, it would result in overdepletion and death. However, during periods of fasting longer than 5 to 7 days, the primary fuel source shifts from protein to fat (the major fuel reserve). The ketone bodies acetoacetate and β-hydroxybutyrate replace glucose as the primary metabolic substrate for the brain. Influx of ketone bodies into the brain is largely determined by the ketone concentration in the blood.[12] Brain glucose use is markedly diminished with partial recycling of glucose through the Cori cycle.

Gluconeogenesis may develop in the kidneys, with a direct effect on the maintenance of acid–base status by the generation of ammonia. Insulin levels remain low to facilitate the mobilization of fat and protein reserves. Free fatty acids become the primary fuel source, whereas amino acids are used for protein synthesis. Markedly increased serum levels of free fatty acids and ketones are measured, with normal levels of glucose, glycerol, amino acids, lactate, and pyruvate. Animal studies suggest that starvation induces characteristic alterations in amino acid transport in gastrointestinal tract brush border membrane vesicles.[13] The gut nutritive transporters for glutamine and arginine are decreased. However, the gluconeogenic transporters for alanine, MeAIB and leucine, are maintained. Simple starvation can usually be tolerated without appreciable morbidity for 4 to 6 days postoperatively in previously well-nourished patients. However, the increase in catecholamine concentrations after surgery or following injury inhibits the metabolic adaptation to starvation. Consequently, the patient who is stressed and is unable to adapt to the additional stresses of starvation often requires early and aggressive exogenous nutritional support.

INTERMEDIARY METABOLISM IN CRITICAL ILLNESS

PROTEIN

Although proteins within the body cell mass are constant in amount, a dynamic flux exists for individual proteins, which results in an equilibrium between ongoing synthesis and breakdown.[14] Enterally or parenterally acquired amino acids, as well as endogenous amino acids derived from protein breakdown, contribute to protein synthesis. In normal healthy adults about 350 g of protein is synthesized daily, which usually matches protein breakdown, so that lean body mass remains constant within fairly narrow limits. Since dietary protein is normally only about 75 g/day, it is obvious that endogenous amino acids derived from protein catabolism are re-utilized for protein synthesis to a significant extent. Net protein losses can therefore result from either net reduction in rate of synthesis or acceleration of proteolysis.

An abrupt increase in protein synthesis occurs after injury, especially in the liver and bone marrow. Increased concentrations of several circulating acute phase reactants and related compounds can be measured. For example, C-reactive protein and α-acid glycoprotein levels may increase 20-fold. Fibrinogen, haptoglobin, and the other molecules have an increased rate of synthesis and a presumed survival benefit following injury. Thus, from a teleologic viewpoint, fibrinogen improves clotting efficiency; haptoglobins prevent renal injury by binding hemoglobin; complement is important in the immune response; increased synthesis of a variety of white blood cells presumably aids immunoreactivity; and increased rates of cell proliferation in the wound are necessary for wound healing. Liver alanine content acutely increases by as much as three times that before injury and serves as substrate for both acute phase reactant synthesis and gluconeogenesis.

In skeletal muscle, protein catabolism predominates. Increased net release of amino acids from muscle results in increased urinary urea nitrogen loss. These amino acids are subsequently used in part by the viscera for protein synthesis and gluconeogenesis. Uptake by the viscera of the amino acids released from skeletal muscle exceeds their production rate from muscle, so that the plasma levels of many amino acids are typically reduced. This graded and complex metabolic adaptation in muscle leads to muscle atrophy and weakness and would seem to be deleterious, whereas the protein metabolic response in liver appears to be beneficial.

There is considerable evidence that the response of muscle is not homogeneous. Many differences have been observed in the metabolism of muscles from animals subjected to different types of trauma, and individual muscles from the same animal may react differently.[15,16] In other words, it appears likely that the biochemical composition and physiologic function of individual muscles are significant determinants of their response to injury.

For example, we measured protein dynamics in incubated, intact rat epitrochlearis and soleus muscles following graded injuries.[15] (The epitrochlearis muscle is the fast-twitch, white-fiber muscle that functions intermittently to change limb position; the predominantly red-fiber soleus is

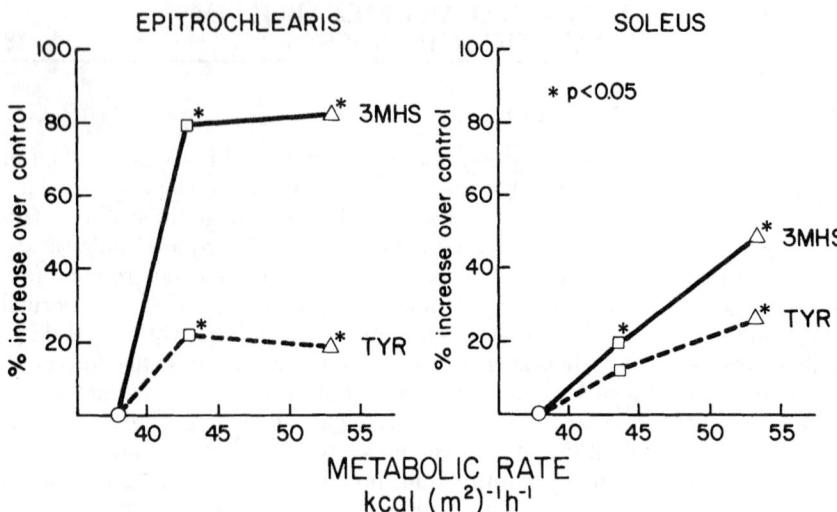

FIGURE 23-1. *Left.* Release from the epitrochlearis muscle of 3-methylhistidine (3MHS; *solid line*) and tyrosine (TYR: *broken line*) as a function of the metabolic rate on study day 5 for control (○), scalded (□), and excised (△) rats. *Right.* Release from the soleus muscle of 3MHS and TYR as a function of the metabolic rate on study day 5 for each animal group.

important in posture maintenance.) These injuries resulted in an increase in metabolic rate of about 15% in the least severely injured animals and approximately 40% in the more severely stressed animals. Protein synthesis was measured isotopically by phenylalanine incorporation. Breakdown rates of the mixed protein pool were determined by measurement of the rate of tyrosine release. The release rate of 3-methylhistidine was used to quantitate breakdown of myofibrillar protein (actin and myosin) in these muscles.

Protein synthesis rates were not significantly altered, except for increases in directly injured muscles. The relationship between catabolism in both the general protein pool and the myofibrillar protein is complex. Figure 23-1 demonstrates that the protein populations of the white-fiber epitrochlearis were considerably more labile in response to post-traumatic catabolic stimuli than were the same protein populations in the predominantly red-fiber soleus. Both the contractile proteins and to a lesser extent the mixed protein pool of the epitrochlearis evidenced this property. However, tyrosine release was not significantly elevated in the soleus, unlike the epitrochlearis. The proteolytic rate of contractile proteins in the soleus was significantly elevated, but to a lesser extent than in the epitrochlearis. Thus the protein constituents of a given muscle do not necessarily respond similarly. The lability of myofibrillar proteins in the white-fiber epitrochlearis exceeded that measured in the red-fiber soleus at both levels of injury severity tested. Other investigators have also observed protein lability in fast-twitch muscles and an accentuated response of myofibrillar protein breakdown in response to other catabolic stimuli such as starvation and sepsis.[17] Thus, muscles involved in intermittent activity and the contractile proteins—actin and myosin—appear to be the most severely affected by critical illness in these models. Similar phenomena may play a role in the development of the weakness and debility in patients who have recovered from critical illness.

Cuthbertson was one of the first investigators to conclude that the increased nitrogen loss following injury reflects not only a generalized increase in the breakdown rate of skeletal muscle[2] but also in other factors, especially inactivity. He estimated that as much as 40% of the increased nitrogen loss was due to disuse atrophy.[18] The classic studies of Deitrick and associates[19] demonstrated that normal subjects receiving an otherwise weight-maintaining diet developed negative nitrogen balance when immobilized in spica casts. Active muscle contraction (and even passive manipulation[18]) can reduce this source of nitrogen loss during critical illness. Thus, exercise and physical therapy even on a limited scale in critically ill patients may lessen debility.

AMINO ACIDS

Free amino acids are found in both the intracellular and the extracellular fluid compartments. Skeletal muscle is the largest protein mass in the body. The intracellular concentrations of free amino acids in muscle are approximately three times greater than those in the plasma. The total intracellular concentration of free amino acids typically decreases during critical illness. This is due in large part to a fall in the concentration of glutamine,[20] a nonessential amino acid, which accounts for 60% of the total intracellular pool.[21] Intracellular concentrations of some other amino acids such as phenylalanine, tyrosine, and alanine, and the branched-chain amino acids leucine, isoleucine, and valine usually increase during critical illness.[20] Following convalescence, amino acid levels return toward normal. The concentrations of free amino acids in plasma demonstrate similar alterations to those in the intracellular compartment and hypoaminoacidemia is generally observed in critical illness reflecting the fall primarily in the concentration of nonessential amino acids.

The intracellular amino acid pool is quantitatively the most important, but the extracellular compartment is principally involved in amino acid transport between several regional microvascular beds, such as those in the gastrointestinal (GI) tract, skeletal muscle, and liver. Therefore, net release or storage of amino acids is often determined from analysis of the extracellular compartment. During critical illness the net release of amino acids from peripheral tissue is increased. In a study of burn patients the net release of amino acid nitrogen was five times greater in the patients than in control subjects.[22] Furthermore, the rate of amino acid release was related to total burn size (injury severity) and appeared to represent a generalized metabolic response to critical illness. The accelerated peripheral release was matched by an increased amino acid uptake across the splanchnic bed.[23] The amino acids, glutamine and alanine, together account for a large portion of the total amino acid nitrogen exchanged between regional tissues.[24] These appear to be the major nitrogen carriers in the circulation, although all amino acids are required for protein synthesis. Glutamine and alanine both appear to have specific physiologic roles as well. Alanine is a major precursor for the hepatic production of glucose. In that conversion the nitrogen is incorporated into urea, which is subsequently excreted by the kidneys. Urea is the final step in the breakdown of body protein and usually represents an irreversible loss of nitrogen.

Glutamine is a nonessential amino acid, which has long been recognized to serve as a precursor for the production of ammonia in the kidney. This can be an important buffering mechanism for excreted acid. In addition, glutamine has a gluconeogenic potential through its conversion to Krebs cycle intermediates. However, in the last several years other key roles for glutamine have been discovered. It appears to be an important determinant of net skeletal muscle protein breakdown.[25] A variety of studies of intact animals, ex vivo preparations, and cell culture all document a relationship between intracellular glutamine concentration and either the protein synthetic rate or the net rate of protein degradation.[25,26] Furthermore, glutamine is an important respiratory fuel for the GI tract,[27] and probably other cell types as well, especially those that rapidly proliferate, such as bone marrow, fixed immunologic cells, and proliferative cells in wounds, and other foci of inflammation.

In summation, accelerated dissolution of muscle protein during critical illness provides a ready supply of amino acids to support protein synthesis in the wound, the liver, and other remote sites. Alanine and certain other amino acids may also be utilized for glucose production by the liver and to a lesser extent the kidney. Glutamine appears to be a specific fuel for the GI tract where it is converted to alanine. Unfortunately, this enhanced mobilization of amino acids from muscle protein leads to an irretrievable loss of nitrogen in the form of urea, ammonia, creatinine, uric acid, and other compounds that are excreted. The net effect on the patient is rapid erosion of muscle mass and worsening debility. Preliminary evidence suggests that a diet enhanced with glutamine and its precursor alpha-ketoglutarate may have a positive effect on protein synthesis in a trauma model.[28]

CARBOHYDRATES

Injury and critical illness result in major perturbations in glucose metabolism. Hyperglycemia, glycosuria, and impaired glucose tolerance are common findings in critically

TABLE 23-2. Fasting Glucose and Insulin Concentrations

SUBJECTS	GLUCOSE (mg/dL)	INSULIN (μU/mL)
Normals (n = 49)	78 ± 1	12 ± 1
Trauma patients (n = 19)	104 ± 2°	17 ± 2°

°$P < 0.02$

ill patients, and have led to the term *diabetes of injury.* These signs appear promptly during the ebb phase and persist until convalescence is largely completed. Initially, insulin output appears to be decreased, but normal or slightly elevated fasting insulin concentrations are usually found during the hyperdynamic flow phase (Table 23-2).[29] In response to a glucose load, insulin concentration may be supranormal.[5]

During the flow phase of convalescence, hepatic glucose production is stimulated and glucose flow throughout the extracellular fluid compartment is increased. The rate of glucose oxidation may be more than doubled during the flow phase.[30] Glucogenic amino acids released by muscle catabolism at the periphery provide substrate for the increase in hepatic gluconeogenesis. Not only is hepatic glucose output increased, but inhibition by exogenous glucose infusion is blunted.[31] Kinney has speculated that the increased glucose production is adaptive, as it may provide a substrate for the synthesis of acute phase glycoproteins and for connective tissue requirements of glucosoaminoglycans and fibroblasts.[32]

Glucose also serves as a fuel for the many cell types in a healing wound.[33] In studies of burn patients,[34] blood flow to a burned leg was greater than that to an uninjured extremity. The oxygen consumption of both injured and uninjured limbs was comparable but glucose uptake by the injured leg was significantly elevated. This was associated with an increased release of lactate produced by an aerobic glucose oxidation.

The increase in total glucose production and flow appears to correlate with the increase in oxygen consumption (injury severity) in patients with burns or other injuries. However, the respiratory quotient is typically in the range of 0.7 to 0.8, indicating that fat is the principal substrate being oxidized. The increased glucose production by splanchnic tissue is associated with an increased uptake of both lactate and glucogenic amino acids, especially alanine. Thus, the enhanced glucose production seen in critical illness reflects both synthesis of new glucose from amino acids and recycled glucose from lactate. Wolfe has documented increased glucose cycling in patients with burns.[35] The increased mass flow of glucose, while serving as a fuel for healing wounds and inflammatory tissue, also reflects inefficient "futile" cycling that serves mainly to produce heat.

Despite the increased mass flow of glucose during critical illness, patients are usually intolerant to exogenous glucose administration. Black and coworkers[5] induced and maintained fixed hyperglycemia in both patients recovering satis-

TABLE 23-3. Limits of Glucose Oxidation or Disposal

| SEVERITY OF ILLNESS | DISPOSAL RATES | | | STUDY |
	mg/kg × min	g/kg × day	kcal/day (70 kg)	
Postoperative	7	10.1	2400	Wolfe[32]
Moderate injury	6	8.6	2050	Black[5]
Severe burn	5	7.2	1710	Wolfe[31]

factorily from multiple trauma and age-matched controls. In the control subjects, glucose disposal continually increased in association with a steady rise in serum insulin concentrations. However, in the patients recovering from trauma, glucose disposal in response to fixed hyperglycemia was relatively steady despite insulin concentrations that were consistently greater than those achieved in the normal subjects. In the injured patients, no association between glucose disposal and insulin concentration was found. Glucose disposal was generally in the range of 6 to 7 mg/kg/min, even though the insulin concentrations were high.

In other studies, insulin was infused to maintain fixed hyperinsulinemia, and sufficient glucose was administered to maintain euglycemia. Glucose disposal was lower in patients than in controls at all doses and concentrations of insulin achieved. These studies provided quantitative evidence of insulin resistance in patients recovering from injury. This apparent limitation in the ability to utilize glucose during critical illness has been demonstrated in other studies as well.[36,37] This limitation seems to be related to the severity of injury (Table 23-3). Therefore, in the ICU the most seriously ill patients are progressively less able to utilize glucose to meet their total energy requirements.

LIPID

Fat oxidation tends to maximize between 8 and 14 days after injury. In contrast to stores of protein (6–7 kg) and carbohydrate (a few hundred grams), fat stores are large, normally accounting for about 14 kg of body weight in a healthy 70-kg man (Table 23-4). Fat reserves are mobilized by the lipolysis of triglycerides to glycerol and free fatty acids. The fatty acids are used both in the liver and in peripheral tissues as a source of energy. The increased lipolysis following injury is presumably regulated by the amount of 3′,5′-cyclic adenosine monophosphate, which in turn regulates the enzyme triglyceride lipase.[38] In the postinjury state, patients continue to burn fat even when given large amounts of glucose. The failure of exogenous glucose to limit fat oxidation is characteristic of hyperemetabolic critically ill or injured patients.

The triacylglycerol in adipose tissues is the primary lipid fuel reserve. After hepatic synthesis, triacylglycerol is incorporated into very low-density lipoproteins and transported in blood. In the peripheral tissues, hydrolysis precedes tissue uptake of fatty acids, which constitute a major fuel source for all tissues except red blood cells and brain. Free fatty acids are normally the major source of energy for resting skeletal muscle.

Plasma free fatty acids are elevated after injury; elevations are greatest with more severe injury. Normally the free fatty acid content of plasma and the metabolic turnover of fatty acids are directly related. The rate of lipolysis is typically sensitive to circulating levels of catecholamines, although glucagon and adrenocorticotropic hormones also modulate the response under some conditions.[39] Insulin stimulates both glucose and free fatty acid uptake in adipose tissue. In short, the balance between fat mobilization and storage is the result of complex neurohormonal interactions to which, in the setting of injury and acute illness, must be added the

TABLE 23-4. Average Adult Body Composition

COMPONENT	% BODY WEIGHT	kg	CALORIC VALUE
Carbohydrate (glucose, glycogen)	1	<1	1,000
Fat (adipose, triglyceride)	20 (variable)	14	130,200
Protein (muscle, plasma proteins)°	20	14	(56,000)
Water	55	38.5	0
Minerals	3–5	2–3.5	0
Total	100	70	

°Approximately one half of body protein is relatively metabolically inert and exists as structural protein in connective tissue, skin, cartilage, and bone. The remainder (6–7 kg) consists of visceral, plasma, and skeletal muscle protein, which is in a dynamic state. These proteins, which exist in the hydrated state, constitute the body cell mass. The readily available body caloric reserve of protein is therefore about 28,000 calories.

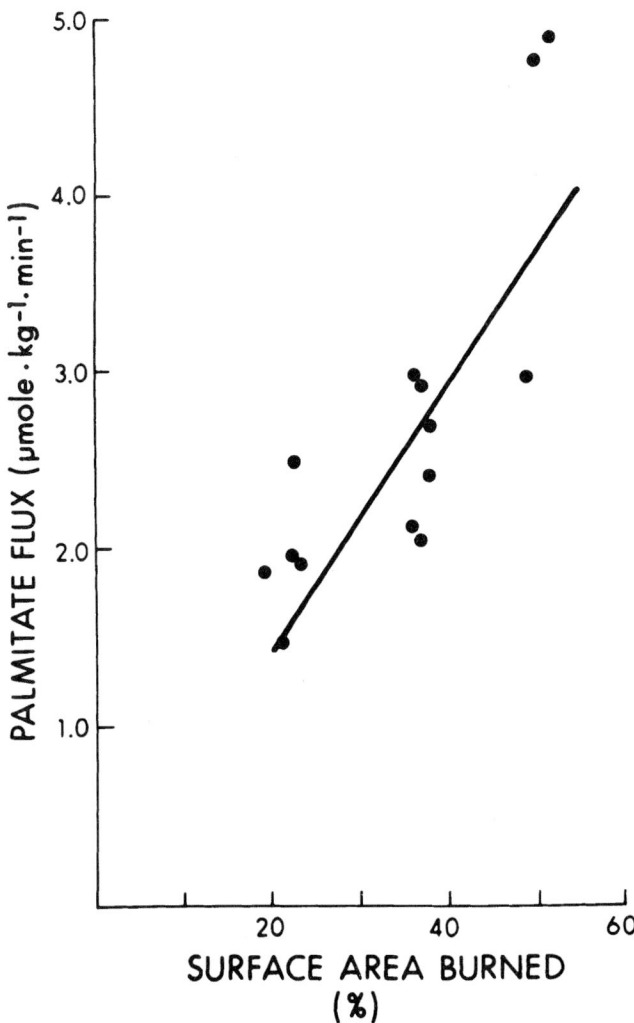

FIGURE 23-2. Relation between percent body surface area burned and plasma palmitate turnover. The equation Y = 0.074 × −0.115 describes this relation (r = 0.81; P < 0.01).

effects of major perturbations in blood flow to the adipose tissue, muscle, and liver, which depend on the postinjury interval and other uncontrollable variables.[40]

Galster and associates[41] used stable isotope measurement techniques to quantitate plasma palmitate turnover in patients with uncomplicated thermal burns of moderate severity. Although there was considerable variability, fatty acid flux and plasma fatty acid concentration in burn patients were directly related as they are in healthy subjects. We also found that palmitate flux was directly related to injury severity, as illustrated in Figure 23-2. Fatty acid turnover measurements reflect the net lipolytic rate, since fatty acids liberated from adipose tissue by hydrolysis can be re-esterified locally. Glycerol, however, cannot be re-esterified, and plasma glycerol turnover therefore represents the absolute lipolytic rate.

Glycerol turnover was measured in injured and infected patients by Carpentier and associates[42] and was found to be about twice normal, in contrast to the more modest 20% to 30% increase observed by Galster.[41] Several methodologic differences may explain this disparity. In Carpentier's study plasma glycerol was elevated, whereas in Galster's patients, plasma glycerol was decreased.

Recent studies in burn patients by Wolfe and associates[35] indicate that this increased rate of fatty acid turnover is because of increased cycling of fatty acids and glycerol, that is, the hydrolysis of triglycerides and re-esterification of the fatty acids with glycerol, a cyclical process resulting in no net quantitative change of substrate. The purpose of this and other so-called futile cycles is not clear, but since they usually involve the net generation of heat they may contribute to the increased heat production or hypermetabolism of critical illness.

REGULATION OF THE METABOLIC RESPONSES TO CRITICAL ILLNESS

It has been useful to consider the regulatory mechanisms of the responses to critical illness as a component of a neurohumoral reflex arc.[43] Afferent signals alert the body to the presence of an injury, invading bacteria, hypoxia, acidosis, and even to the presence of potential danger. Afferent input also indicates the presence, extent, and resolution of the inflammatory tissue or wound. The brain and central nervous system, and perhaps other organ systems, presumably process and interpret the afferent input and generate efferent signals that control the regional and systemic metabolic alterations observed clinically.

ENDOCRINE MEDIATORS

One of the most familiar neurohumoral reflex arcs is the endocrine system. During critical illness, the concentrations of the catabolic counterregulatory hormones—cortisol, glucagon, and the catecholamines, epinephrine and norepinephrine—are typically increased. These hormones serve as effector signals in the response to critical illness. Increases in concentration correlate with the severity of illness.[44–47] The catecholamines appear to play a role in the development of hypermetabolism.[48,49] Catecholamine turnover is proportional to burn size and hypermetabolism may be significantly decreased by α- and β-blockade. The catecholamines also influence normal glucose and insulin relationships. Porte and associates demonstrated the influence of the sympathoadrenal axis on the insulin response to glucose.[50] Insulin concentrations were substantially reduced with α-stimulation but they were enhanced by β-agonists. The catecholamines may also affect peripheral insulin action. Epinephrine infused into normal persons at doses associated with β-effects resulted in significantly reduced insulin-stimulated whole body glucose disposal and glucose uptake by forearm tissue.[51] The metabolic effects of cortisol include muscle wasting, glucose intolerance, and sodium retention. Glucagon stimulates hepatic glucose production.

Shamoon and coworkers[52] observed a synergistic effect of the three counterregulatory hormones—cortisol, glucagon, and epinephrine—on glucose production in humans, suggesting that combined hormonal effects were more complex than the addition of individual hormonal actions. Based on that observation, Bessey and associates[53] infused a mixture of hydrocortisone, glucagon, and epinephrine into normal persons continuously for 3 days. This hormonal infusion achieved concentrations of counterregulatory hormones similar to those observed in patients with mild to moderate injury. In addition, the hormonal infusion resulted in increased resting heart and respiratory rates, widened pulse pressure, and slightly elevated rectal temperature when compared with those of the same subjects during a control saline infusion. Hypermetabolism, negative potassium balance, increased endogenous glucose production, insulin resistance, sodium retention, and leukocytosis were also observed.

During the control studies, the subjects were maintained in nitrogen equilibrium by consuming a standard constant diet. During the hormonal infusion the subjects were in persistently negative nitrogen balance even though nutritional intake was identical to control. Whole body protein turnover was increased with hormonal infusion and this was due largely to an increase in protein catabolism. Thus, simple alteration of the hormone environment simulated many of the metabolic responses to injury even in the absence of a wound or inflammatory focus. The hormonal interactions were complex. For example, the increased metabolic rate appeared to represent additive effects of the hormones whereas negative nitrogen balance demonstrated synergistic interactions.

The development of insulin resistance appeared entirely because of the action of cortisol. Additional studies demonstrated a fall in skeletal muscle intracellular amino acid concentration following triple hormone infusion.[54] This was largely because of a decrease in intracellular glutamine. In view of the potential regulatory role of glutamine in muscle, these observations suggested that the hormonal environment might play a causative role in increasing net skeletal muscle proteolysis. However, other findings did not support that conclusion. The triple hormone infusion did not alter whole blood amino acid concentrations or amino acid efflux from the forearm. Although hormonal blockade has resulted in the reduction of net skeletal muscle proteolysis following injury,[55] alteration of the hormonal environment alone was not a sufficient stimulus to accelerate net skeletal muscle proteolysis. Thus, the stress hormones appear to be necessary but not completely responsible for the proteolytic response to critical illness. Other factors, therefore, must be involved in the determination of these clinical phenomena.

CYTOKINES

In the last several years, investigators have identified an ever increasing number of substances elaborated by inflammatory cells that influence the recruitment, proliferation, or function of other cells (Table 23-5; see Chap. 20). As a group these substances are known as *peptide regulatory factors* or *cytokines*. Some of these factors have primarily immuno-

TABLE 23-5.   Peptide Regulatory Factors—Cytokines

FAMILY	SOURCES	TARGET CELLS
Interleukins (IL 1-11)	Monocytes/macrophages, fibroblasts, epithelial cells	Hematopoietic cells, fibroblasts, lymphocytes, hepatocytes, brain
Tumor necrosis factors (TFN α, β)	Monocytes/ macrophages, lymphocytes	Endothelial cells; monocytes/ macrophages, neutrophils, fibroblasts; liver, muscle, lung, gut, kidney
Interferons (IFN α, β, γ)	Monocytes/macrophages, fibroblasts, epithelial cells	Multiple immune cells, phagocytes
Colony stimulating factors (Granulocyte CSF, Macrophage CSF, GM-CSF, erythropoietin)	Granulocytes, macrophages juxtaglomerular cells	Granulocyte precursors, erythroid precursors, monocytes/ macrophages
Growth factors (Epidermal GF; fibroblast GF; insulin-like GF 1, 2; nerve GF; platelet-derived GF; transforming GF α, β)	Multiple cell types	Multiple cells

modulatory effects and others affect cellular proliferation, growth, and differentiation. Some of the factors influence neighboring cells (paracrine action), some affect the cell from which they were secreted (autocrine action), and a few of the substances also appear to be able to affect cells in remote sites and thus exert systemic (endocrine) effects. Cytokines affect whole body nutrition and metabolism and are responsible for many of the clinically observed nutritional effects in critical illness and injury.[56]

Interleukin-1 (IL-1) was one of the first substances to be recognized as part of a more generalized class of peptides. Prior to its reclassification as an interleukin, this substance was variously referred to as endogenous pyrogen, leukocyte endogenous mediator, and lymphocyte activating factor. These different terms reflected studies on different components of the acute phase response. IL-1 is now recognized to be a protein or a family of proteins which appears to play a major role in the acute phase response to infection. A small amount of IL-1 injected intrathecally produces the same increase in body temperature as a much larger dose administered intravenously,[57] suggesting that IL-1 may act centrally and therefore function as an afferent signal in the metabolic responses to critical illness. Furthermore, IL-1 immunoreactivity has been demonstrated in the hypothalamus of humans,[58] indicating that IL-1 may be an intrinsic neuromodulator in central nervous system pathways that mediate the acute phase response. Baracos and associates[59] reported increased muscle proteolysis in vitro when tissues were incubated with a monocyte supernatant of IL-1. They further proposed that IL-1 induced elevated concentrations of the prostaglandin PGE_2, which was responsible for the increased proteolysis.

Other studies in intact animals suggested that IL-1 or one of its breakdown products could produce hypermetabolism, increase amino acid oxidation, and increase myofibrillar protein breakdown.[60] However, Moldawer and colleagues,[61] investigating the effects of IL-1 and skeletal muscle protein synthesis in vitro and in vivo, found that IL-1 alone had no effect on protein balance even though production of PGE_2 was increased. Antibody to IL-1 blocked the lymphoproliferative response to a monocyte preparation but did not alter protein degradation. Neither IL-1 nor PGE_2 appeared to affect skeletal muscle protein balance. Watters and coworkers[62] stimulated the production of IL-1 in normal humans with daily injections of the steroidal compound etiocholanolone, which resulted in sterile inflammation. Although the subjects manifested an acute phase response, they were not hypermetabolic and they remained in nitrogen equilibrium on a standard diet. Furthermore, the concentrations of catabolic hormones were not affected by the etiocholanolone injections. However, when these were administered to subjects receiving an infusion of the catabolic hormones, both inflammatory and metabolic responses were observed.[63] These findings suggest that both specific inflammatory and metabolic mediators determine the clinical responses to critical illness.

Tumor necrosis factor (TNF) is elaborated by activated macrophages and other inflammatory cell types.[64] It was originally discovered by investigators interested in the mech-

anisms by which some malignant tumors spontaneously regressed. Other investigators identified it as a serum factor that could induce anorexia and cachexia. Thus, TNF is also referred to as *cachectin*. The physiologic effects of TNF are dose related. Low concentrations can affect wound remodeling and other inflammatory cell functions, whereas high doses can produce shock and death. Michie and coworkers[65] administered recombinant human TNF to patients. TNF infusion led to a dose-dependent rise in the TNF concentration and to symptoms of headache, myalgia, and chills. In addition, the patients demonstrated fever, tachycardia, and an increase in adrenocorticotropic hormone (ACTH), indicating activation of the adrenal pituitary axis. Symptoms developed 30 to 60 minutes after the start of the infusion.

When these observations were compared with those of normal subjects who received endotoxin, it was apparent that the symptoms produced by endotoxin were similar to those following TNF. Furthermore, following endotoxin there was a sharp rise in TNF concentration similar to that observed with TNF infusion. The increase in TNF concentration preceded all clinical symptoms. Although the clinical responses persisted for several hours, TNF could only be detected in the circulation for a brief period of time and appeared to be cleared rapidly.

The importance of TNF in mediating the responses to endotoxin was dramatically demonstrated in studies by Tracey and associates.[66] When lethal doses of endotoxin were administered to baboons, death could be completely prevented by prior administration of TNF antibody. In human subjects when the cyclooxygenase inhibitor ibuprofen was given prior to endotoxin, the systemic symptoms and endocrine responses were attenuated even though the rise in TNF concentration and subsequent leukocytosis were still present.[67] Thus, TNF seems to be an important mediator in the responses to endotoxin, and it appears also to activate cyclooxygenase pathways.

Interleukin-2 (IL-2) is elaborated by activated helper (OKT-4) T cells and has important immunomodulatory functions. When administered alone or in combination with lymphokine activated killer cells, IL-2 has marked tumoricidal activity both in vitro and in vivo. However, IL-2 also is associated with toxic effects, including fever, tachycardia, flu-like symptoms, and elevations of the counterregulatory hormones. These responses are similar to those observed after endotoxin. However, following administration of IL-2, circulating TNF does not appear. Rather, the level of interferon-γ (IFN-Γ) increases following IL-2 administration, and this precedes the onset of host responses.[68] As in the case with endotoxin, ibuprofen attenuates the symptoms and endocrine changes induced by IL-2.

Interleukin-6 (IL-6), also elaborated by inflammatory cells, can stimulate myeloid cell growth as well as T-cell proliferation and differentiation often in association with IL-2 or IFN-Γ. IL-6 also appears to have a dominant stimulatory effect on the hepatocyte synthesis of acute phase proteins.[69] IL-1, TNF, and IFN-Γ appear to be accessory signals. Given the central importance of the liver in the metabolic responses to critical illness, IL-6 may prove to be an important systemic mediator as well.

CLINICAL CARE AND METABOLIC RESPONSES TO CRITICAL ILLNESS ■

Our understanding of the metabolic responses to critical illness serves as the basis for many current approaches to care for the critically ill. Often this includes care of an inflammatory mass or wound. The wound has a dominant, controlling effect on all of the responses associated with critical illness—both beneficial and detrimental. The control of the wound or control of the processes perpetuating or extending the inflammatory mass is essential to diminishing the metabolic responses to critical illness. Debridement of dead tissue, drainage of pus, coverage of wounds, reduction of fractures, and control of infection, as well as control of hemorrhage and appropriate resuscitation, all have a high priority in the care of the critically ill. Inadequate oxygen delivery may lead to ischemia, cellular dysfunction, and further extension of the inflammatory mass.

EPILOGUE

Enhancement of anabolic processes is also now feasible. Growth hormone is most notable in this regard. Recombinant human growth hormone may be administered safely without the side effects that were commonly observed formerly with crude preparations. Manson and Wilmore[70] found that daily administration of growth hormone could maintain positive nitrogen balance in normal subjects given hypocaloric diets. These observations were extended clinically by Jiang and coworkers in China.[71] They administered low-dose growth hormone to patients undergoing major abdominal surgery and maintained on hypocaloric intravenous feedings for 1 week postoperatively. The subjects receiving growth hormone had a markedly shortened period of negative nitrogen balance and lost less weight. In addition, growth hormone appeared to preserve both muscle mass and function as gauged by grip strength. Recently Herndon and associates[72] administered growth hormone to burned children. Those receiving the treatment had more rapid epithelialization of their donor sites and a shorter hospital stay following grafting. Further studies are required to define the appropriate circumstances in which growth hormone administration might be indicated in the critically ill.

REFERENCES ■

1. Cuthbertson DP: The influence of prolonged muscular rest on metabolism. *Biochem J* 1929;23:1328
2. Cuthbertson DP: The disturbance of metabolism produced by bony and non-bony injury with notes on certain abnormal conditions of bone. *Biochem J* 1930;24:1244
3. Cuthbertson DP: Observations on the disturbances of metabolism produced by injury to the limbs. *Q J Med* 1932;1:233
4. Cuthbertson DP: Post-shock metabolic response. *Lancet* 1942;1:433
5. Black PR, Brooks DC, Bessey PQ, et al: Mechanisms of insulin resistance following injury. *Ann Surg* 1982;196:420
6. Mizock BA: Alterations in carbohydrate metabolism during stress: a review of the literature. *Am J Med* 1995;98:75
7. Bessey PQ, Lowe KA: Early hormonal changes affect the catabolic response to trauma. *Ann Surg* 1993;218:476
8. Mullen JL, Gertner MH, Buzby GP, et al: Implications of malnutrition in the surgical patient. *Arch Surg* 1979;114:121
9. Steffee WP: Malnutrition in hospitalized patients. *JAMA* 1980;244:2630
10. Cahill GF: Starvation in man. *N Engl J Med* 1970;282:668
11. Levenson SM, Seifer E: Starvation: metabolic and physiologic responses. In: Burke JF (ed). *Surgical Physiology*. Philadelphia, WB Saunders, 1983:121
12. Hasselbalch SG, Knudsen GM, Jakobsen J, et al: Blood-brain barrier permeability of glucose and ketone bodies during short-term starvation in humans. *Am J Physiol* 1995;268:E1161
13. Sarac TP, Souba WW, Miller JH, et al: Starvation induces differential aminoacid transport. *Surgery* 1994;116:679
14. Kinney JM, Elwyn DH: Protein metabolism and injury. *Ann Rev Nutr* 1983;3:433
15. Downey RS, Monafo WW, Karl IE, et al: Protein dynamics in skeletal muscle after trauma: local and systemic effects. *Surgery* 1986;99:265
16. Tischler ME, Fagan JM: Response to trauma of protein, amino acid and carbohydrate metabolism in injured and uninjured rat skeletal muscle. *Metabolism* 1983;32:853
17. Hasselgren PO, James JH, Benson DW, et al: Total and myofibrillar protein breakdown in different types of rat skeletal muscle: effects of sepsis and regulation by insulin. *Metabolism* 1989;38:634
18. Cuthbertson DP: The physiology of convalescence after injury. *Br Med Bull* 1945;3:96
19. Deitrick JE, Wheldon GD, Shorr E: Effects of immobilization upon various metabolic and physiologic functions of normal men. *Am J Med* 1948;4:3
20. Askanazi J, Carpentier YA, Michelson CB, et al: Muscle and plasma amino acids following injury: influence of intercurrent infection. *Ann Surg* 1980;792:78
21. Bergstrom J, Fuerst P, Noree L-O, et al: Intracellular free amino acid concentration in human muscle tissue. *J Appl Physiol* 1974;36:693
22. Aulick LH, Wilmore DW: Increased peripheral amino acid release following burn injury. *Surgery* 1979;85:560
23. Wilmore DW, Goodwin CW, Aulick AH, et al: Effect of injury and infection on visceral metabolism and circulation. *Ann Surg* 1980;192:491
24. Garber AJ, Karl IE, Kipnis DM: Alanine and glutamine synthesis and release from skeletal muscle. I. Glycolysis and amino acid release. *J Biol Chem* 1976;251:826
25. Johnson DJ, Jiang ZM, Colpoys M, et al: Branched chain amino acid uptake and muscle free amino acid concentrations predict postoperative muscle nitrogen balance. *Ann Surg* 1986;204:513
26. Smith RJ: The role of skeletal muscle in interorgan amino acid exchange. *Fed Proc* 1986;45:2172
27. Souba WW, Wilmore DW: Postoperative alterations of arteriovenous exchange of amino acids across the gastrointestinal tract. *Surgery* 1983;94:342
28. Blomqvist BI, Hammarqvist F, von der Decken A, et al: Glutamine and alpha-ketoglutarate prevent the decrease in muscle free glutamine concentration and influence protein synthesis after total hip replacement. *Metabolism* 1995;44:1215
29. Allison SP, Hinton P, Chamberlain MJ: Intravenous glucosetolerance, insulin, and free fatty acid levels in burned patients. *Lancet* 1968;2:1113
30. Gump FE, Long CL, Killian P: Studies of glucose intolerance in septic injured patients. *J Trauma* 1974;14:378

31. Long, CL, Kinney JM, Geiger JW: Nonsuppressibility of gluco-neogenesis in septic patients. *Metabolism* 1976;25:193
32. Kinney JM: Injury. In: Richards JR, Kinney JM (eds). *Nutritional Aspects of Care in the Critically Ill.* Edinburgh, Churchill Livingstone, 1977:95
33. Im MJC, Hoopes JE: Energy metabolism in healing skin wounds. *J Surg Res* 1970;10:459
34. Wilmore DW, Aulick LH, Mason AD, et al: Influence of the burn wound on local and systematic responses to injury. *Ann Surg* 1977;186:444
35. Wolfe RR, Herndon DN, Jahoor F, et al: Effect of severe burn injury on substrate cycling by glucose and fatty acids. *N Engl J Med* 1987;317:403
36. Wolfe RR, Durkot MJ, Allsop JR, et al: Glucose metabolism in severely burned patients. *Metabolism* 1979;28:1031
37. Wolfe RR, O'Donnell TF Jr, Stone MD, et al: Investigation of factors determining optimal glucose infusion rate in total parenteral nutrition. *Metabolism* 1980;29:892
38. Carlson LA: Mobilization and utilization of lipids after trauma: relation to caloric homeostasis. In: Knight PR (ed). *Symposium on Energy Metabolism in Trauma.* London, J & A Churchill, 1970:155
39. Birke G, Carlson LA, von Euler US, et al: Studies on burns. XII. Lipid metabolism, catecholamine excretion, basal metabolic rate and water loss during treatment of burns with warm dry air. *Acta Chir Scand* 1972;138:321
40. Kinney JM: Surgical hyper-metabolism and nitrogen metabolism. In: Wilkinson AW, Cuthbertson D (eds). *Metabolism and the Response to Injury.* Tunbridge Wells, Pitman Medical, 1976:237
41. Galster AD, Bier DM, Cryer PE: Plasma palmitate turnover in subjects with thermal injury. *J Trauma* 1984;24:938
42. Carpentier YA, Askanazi J, Elwyn DH, et al: Effects of hypercaloric glucose infusion on lipid metabolism in injury and sepsis. *J Trauma* 1979;19:649
43. Wilmore DW, Long JM, Mason AD, et al: Stress in surgical patients as a neurophysiologic reflex response. *Surg Gynecol Obstet* 1976;142:257
44. Davies CL, Newman RJ, Molyneux SG, et al: The relationship between plasma catecholamines and severity of injury in man. *J Trauma* 1984;24:99
45. Rolih CA, Ober KP: The endocrine response to critical illness. *Med Clin N Am* 1995;79:211
46. Vaughan GM, Becker RA, Allen JP, et al: Cortisol and cortitrophin in burned patients. *J Trauma* 1982;22:263
47. Wilmore DW, Lindsey CA, Moylan JA, et al: Hyperglucagonaemia after burns. *Lancet* 1974;1:73
48. Wilmore DW, Long JM, Mason AD Jr, et al: Catecholamines: mediator of the hypermetabolic responses to thermal injury. *Ann Surg* 1974;180:653
49. Harrison TS, Seaton JF, Feller I: Relationship of increased oxygen consumption to catecholamine excretion in thermal burns. *Ann Surg* 1967;165:169
50. Porte D Jr, Robertson RP: Control of insulin secretion by catecholamines, stress, and the sympathetic nervous system. *Fed Proc* 1973;32:1792
51. Bessey PQ, Brooks DC, Black PR, et al: Epinephrine acutely mediates skeletal muscle insulin resistance. *Surgery* 1983;94:172
52. Shamoon HM, Hendler R, Sherwin RS: Synergistic interactions among anti-insulin hormones in the pathogenesis of stress hypoglycemia in humans. *J Clin Endocrinol Metab* 1981;52:1235
53. Bessey PQ, Watters JM, Aoki TT, et al: Combined hormonal infusion simulates the metabolic response to injury. *Ann Surg* 1984;200:264
54. Bessey PQ, Jiang Z-M, Johnson DJ, et al: Post-traumatic skeletal muscle proteolysis: the role of the hormonal environment. *World J Surg* 1989;13:465
55. Hulton N, Johnson DJ, Smith RJ, et al: Hormonal blockade modifies post-traumatic protein catabolism. *J Surg Res* 1985;39:310
56. Souba WW: Cytokine control of nutrition and metabolism in critical illness. *Curr Prob Surg* 1994;31:577
57. Turchik JB, Bornstein OL: Role of the central nervous system in acute-phase responses to leukocyte progress. *Infect Immun* 1980;30:439
58. Breder CD, Dinarello CA, Saper CB: Interleukin-1 immunoreactive innervation of the human hypothalamus. *Science* 1988;240:321
59. Baracos V, Rodeman HP, Dinarello CA, et al: Stimulation of muscle protein degradation and prostaglandin E_2 release by leukocytic pyrogen (Interleukin-1): a mechanism for increased degradation of muscle proteins during fever. *N Engl J Med* 1983;308:553
60. Clowes GHA, George BC, Villee CA, et al: Muscle proteolysis induced by a circulating peptide in patients with sepsis or trauma. *N Engl J Med* 1983;308:545
61. Moldawer LL, Svaninger G, Gelin J, et al: Interleukin-1 and tumor necrosis factor do not regulate protein balance in skeletal muscle. *Am J Physiol* 1987;253:766
62. Watters JM, Bessey PQ, Dinarello CA, et al: The induction of interleukin-1 in humans and its metabolic effects. *Surgery* 1985;98:298
63. Watters JM, Bessey PQ, Dinarello CA, et al: Both inflammatory and endocrine mediators stimulate host responses to sepsis. *Arch Surg* 1985;121:179
64. Old LJ: Tumor necrosis factor (TNF). *Science* 1985;230:630
65. Michie HR, Spriggs DR, Manogue KR, et al: Tumor necrosis factor and endotoxin induce similar metabolic responses in human beings. *Surgery* 1988;104:280
66. Tracey KJ, Fong Y, Hesse DG, et al: Anti-cachectin/TNF monoclonal antibodies prevent septic shock during lethal bacteremia. *Nature* 1987;330:662
67. Revhaug A, Michie HR, Manson JM, et al: Inhibition of cyclooxygenase attenuates the metabolic response to endotoxin in humans. *Arch Surg* 1988;123:162
68. Michie HR, Eberlein TJ, Spriggs DR, et al: Interleukin-2 initiates metabolic responses associated with critical illness in humans. *Ann Surg* 1988;208:493
69. Koj A: The role of interleukin-6 as the hepatocyte stimulating factor in the network of inflammatory cytokines. *Ann NY Acad Sci* 1989;557:1
70. Manson JM, Wilmore DW: Positive nitrogen balance with human growth hormone and hypocaloric intravenous feeding. *Surgery* 1986;100:188
71. Jiang, Z-M, He G-Z, Zhang S-Y, et al: Low-dose growth hormone and hypocaloric nutrition attenuate the protein-catabolic response after major operation. *Ann Surg* 1989;210:513
72. Herndon DN, Barrow RE, Kunkel KR, et al: Effects of recombinant human growth hormone on donor-site healing in severely burned children. *Ann Surg* 1990;212:424

Critical Care, Third Edition, edited by Joseph M. Civetta,
Robert W. Taylor, and Robert R. Kirby.
Lippincott-Raven Publishers, Philadelphia, PA © 1997.

CHAPTER 24

∎

Oxygen Delivery and Consumption in Critical Illness

Robert Schlichtig

IMMEDIATE CONCERNS ∎

MAJOR PROBLEMS

Each organ and each cell of each organ must have sufficient oxygen (O_2) to support its energy demand or it will die. The guiding principle is *dysoxia*, which is a generic name for insufficient O_2 delivery ($\dot{D}O_2$) to support O_2 demand. Dysoxia causes cell damage or death if not corrected quickly.[1] $\dot{D}O_2$ is the bulk quantity of O_2 delivered to a given tissue and is defined by the following equation:

$$\dot{D}O_2 \approx \dot{Q} \times SaO_2 \times [Hb]$$

where ($\dot{Q}$) is flow, SaO_2 is arterial O_2 saturation, and [Hb] is hemoglobin concentration. O_2 consumption ($\dot{V}O_2$) is the quantity of O_2 taken up by a given tissue, and is approximated by the following equation:

$$\dot{V}O_2 \approx \dot{Q} \times (SaO_2 - SvO_2) \times [Hb]$$

where SvO_2 is venous O_2 saturation. Units for $\dot{V}O_2$ and $\dot{D}O_2$ usually are not helpful in clinical management because O_2 demand varies so greatly among various clinical conditions. Nevertheless, the concepts are certainly essential. In this regard, the biphasic $\dot{V}O_2 - \dot{D}O_2$ model (Fig. 24-1) perhaps represents the most exciting and useful new concept in critical care medicine in recent years.[2] Although this model should rarely be taken literally in patient care (i.e., it is seldom worthwhile to construct an $\dot{V}O_2$ versus $\dot{D}O_2$ relationship for a patient), it is essential to recognize its most important point, namely, that there is a critical $\dot{D}O_2$ below which dysoxia commences. Attempts to show that $\dot{V}O_2$ is diffusion limited—as opposed to convection limited—have,

for all practical purposes, been unsuccessful, and clinicians should generally assume that an increase in $\dot{D}O_2$ by any method (increased SaO_2, increased Hb concentration, or increased $\dot{Q}$) is just as helpful.[3]

The first, and often most perplexing, clinical problem is to determine whether dysoxia exists. Unfortunately, we really don't have good ways of detecting dysoxia, with the exception of heart and brain. Consequently, a good deal of guess work is often needed. Making the best guess, in turn, requires scrupulous attention to many different parameters because no single parameter is sufficiently sensitive and specific to make the diagnosis.

The second problem is to determine how best to improve $\dot{D}O_2$ or to decrease O_2 demand. In this regard, equation 1 does not "say it all." For example, it is easy to forget that dysoxia can sometimes be treated by decreasing the O_2 demand. Imagination, constant attention, and experience also are often needed. For example, the best way to improve $\dot{D}O_2$, in some instances, is to check for auto PEEP and administer a bronchodilator.

The third problem is to direct the $\dot{D}O_2$ to the tissue regions that are dysoxic. In many instances, this simply can't be done, and we can only hope that the patient will respond favorably to our interventions. However, the clinician who worries about it seems more likely to improve regional $\dot{D}O_2$ than the clinician who doesn't. This can be done by choosing the therapeutic intervention that seems least likely to produce regional ischemia. For example, norepinephrine should probably be reserved for instances where other interventions fail or where a rapid and fail-safe response is needed.

This is scary and serious business where brave hearts, iron wills, and nerves of steel are desirable. The best way

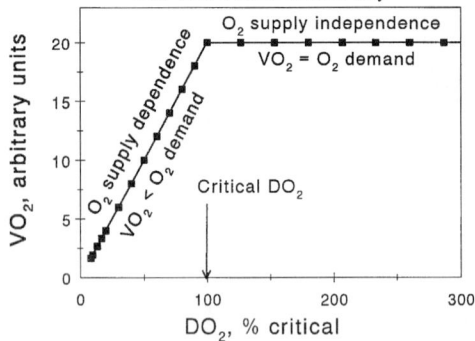

FIGURE 24-1. The biphasic $\dot{V}O_2 - \dot{D}O_2$ model. $\dot{V}O_2$ is a reasonable estimate of ATP turnover in the cells. If ATP turnover is adequate, then there is enough energy available to perform the work needed. If not, the cells become damaged, as shown by several elegant investigations.[1] One of several reasons that this model should not be taken literally is that $\dot{V}O_2$ is typically highly variable in any given patient.[1] Consequently, in an awake patient, covariation of $\dot{V}O_2$ and $\dot{D}O_2$ is much more likely to represent $\dot{D}O_2$ increasing to meet an increased oxygen (O_2) demand than it is to represent "O_2 supply dependence." Remember that there is always a critical $\dot{D}O_2$.

to acquire these attributes is to make a serious effort to thoroughly understand what is known about detection and treatment of dysoxia and to gain guided experience.

STRESS POINTS

1. *Expediency, expediency, expediency*: This cannot be over-stressed. Two given clinicians might perform exactly the same diagnostic tests and provide exactly the same treatment to two identical patients. However, the clinician who accomplishes these goals faster is the one who is more likely to have a surviving and undamaged patient (Fig. 24-2). Occasionally, this may mean physically running to the blood bank for units of blood. Although not strictly necessary, it often pays the clinician to stay healthy and physically fit.

2. *Irreversibility*: Once a tissue is dead, it is dead, and you can't bring it back. If your patient's systolic blood pressure is 40 mm Hg, the patient is almost certainly dysoxic in one or more tissue regions. In this instance, it is not acceptable to give 250 mL of normal saline over an hour or to wait until the dopamine infusion is prepared. A small bolus of epinephrine is usually more appropriate, but then it is necessary to watch closely for the cardiac arrhythmias, which sometimes follow. Pressors alone are rarely adequate and should be weaned as quickly as possible, usually as intravascular volume is increased.

   In addition, for goodness' sake, if your patient clearly has acute myocardial ischemia and if the blood pressure is significantly lower than the premorbid condition, add a pressor agent. Pressor agents are a sort of "poor man's balloon pump." The coronary arteries

fill only during diastole. They won't fill well with a lower-than-normal diastolic blood pressure because the arteriolar sphincters distal to the coronary obstruction are presumably already maximally vasodilated. Give a pressor, and *then* try to think of a a more benign way to treat the cardiac ischemia.

3. *Suspicion*: Coronary artery disease is an excellent example of the value of suspicion. A normal admission electrocardiogram (ECG) reading and absence of coronary history does not mean that your patient does not have coronary artery disease.[4] The more damaged the heart becomes, the less well it pumps, and the more difficult it is to maintain an adequate whole-body $\dot{Q}$ (i.e., cardiac output). Always be suspicions of coronary artery disease, or you may discover it too late.

4. *Resolve*: Once you have determined what diagnostic tests or treatments are needed, don't take "no" for an answer. For example, your patient is profoundly hypotensive from a new onset of atrial fibrillation and serum potassium concentration is 2 mMol, but the hospital rules are that potassium chloride may never be infused more rapidly than 10 mMol per hour. These concepts simply do not go together. Give the potassium chloride yourself if you have to. Change the rules later.

5. *Individuality*: Each patient is an individual, different from every other human being. There is no single cook book recipe that is appropriate for every patient with any given disease process. It is essential that you learn as much as you can about the ways that your patient differs from others. For example, a "dopaminergic" dose of dopamine does absolutely nothing for some

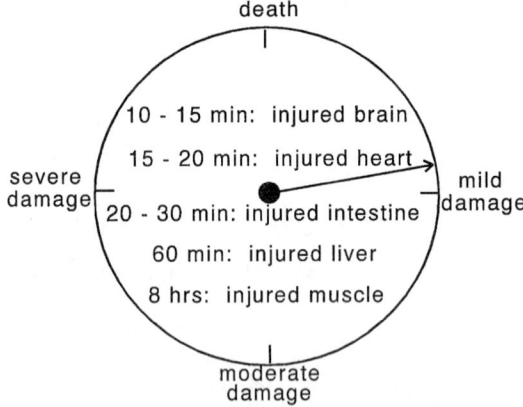

FIGURE 24-2. The dysoxia clock. It is often difficult to tell whether dysoxia exists. However, if the patient has acute encephalographic changes, if there is an acute unanticipated loss of neurologic function, or if there is profound hypotension, there is no excuse for providing anything less than your best and fastest work. Often, you need to "pitch in" manually because not enough nurses, respiratory therapists, and transporters are immediately available.

individuals, whereas it is a pressor for others. We academicians do our best to be accurate, but sometimes our statements are wrong or misinterpreted.

6. *Cooperation*: Patient treatment is most likely to flow smoothly and quickly when all of the clinicians like each other and feel free to offer suggestions. The nurse is commonly the only clinician in a crowded room who understands the problem exactly. But if nobody listens to the nurse, diagnosis and treatment will probably be delayed. The day of the Renaissance physician is long gone. We all have to work together.

7. *Prevention*: In general, in a well-run ICU, cardiac arrests should be relatively uncommon. Perhaps the most common mistake made by truly gifted clinicians is to forget to order antianginal medications for the patient with known stable angina, who depended on high doses of antianginal medication preoperatively, and who has just had an abdominal operative procedure. The patient is "NPO," and nobody remembers to administer nitroglycerin paste or intravenous beta-blocker.

8. *Discretion*: Some patients really don't appreciate our efforts to keep them alive because they really don't want to live. In the absence of information, it is usually wise to "do everything" until the long-term outcome seems clear. However, there are times when a quick telephone call to the patient's spouse or closest friend is at least as important as the urgent intubation. With a little imagination, reasonable temporizing measures often can be found.

ESSENTIAL DIAGNOSTIC TESTS AND PROCEDURES

1. *Pulse oximeter*: There should be a pulse oximeter for every patient in your ICU. The idea is this: it is so fast that the pulse oximeter is there even before before you think to order a blood gas. Sometimes the fastest and easiest way to increase $\dot{D}o_2$ is to increase the fraction of inspired O_2 (FIo_2). This is one reason why patients with acute myocardial ischemia and other shock states are always given supplemental O_2.

2. *Continuous ECG*: Tachycardia does not seem to be harmful in itself, provided that it does not produce myocardial ischemia or hypotension. However, if the patient is consistently tachycardiac, it is essential to be sure that it does not represent underlying disease (e.g., infection). Reasons to watch for tachyarrhythmias and bradyarrhythmias are not reviewed here.

3. *Arterial catheter*: Although uncommon, dysoxia can be present with a normal blood pressure. Conversely, dysoxia can seemingly be absent with a decreased blood pressure. However, continuous blood pressure monitoring is, at the least, a valuable trend monitor and "stays on the job" continuously, provided that the arterial catheter is inserted and maintained properly. In addition, the arterial catheter provides a quick and painless way to obtain frequent blood samples.

Be certain that the alarms are properly set in accordance with the patient's usual blood pressure.

4. *Blood gas measurement with standard base excess (SBE) concentration*: Not only does blood gas measurement provide a Po_2 value, permitting you to fine-tune the FIo_2, but it also provides a SBE concentration, an extraordinarily valuable and unnecessarily neglected clinical tool. Obtaining a SBE concentration is simple, accurate, and fast. Trauma surgeons have known this all along from clinical experience. Normal SBE concentration is 0 mMol. SBE concentration greater than zero means alkalosis. SBE concentration less than zero means acidosis. If you don't believe it, read about it[5] and discover that there is really no defense for not using it.

5. *Hb concentration*: Every ICU should have access to a cooximeter. It is unacceptable to wait 2 hours for a Hb concentration. A cooximeter provides an accurate Hb concentration within minutes.

6. *Twelve-lead ECG*: If your patient is hypotensive, don't forget to perform an ECG. Do it yourself if you have to. Often, we are surprised at what we find. On the other hand, don't be gullible. Myocardial ischemia is often the *result*—as opposed to the *cause*—of hypotension. For example, any patient with severe coronary artery disease will develop ECG changes if the blood pressure becomes low enough for any reason. Commonly, the primary problem is sepsis as opposed to myocardial ischemia. Both need to be treated. Never stop being suspicious.

7. *Lactate level*: An elevated lactate level does not necessarily indicate dysoxia, particularly during sepsis, and a normal lactate level does not necessarily indicate the absence of dysoxia.[3] Nevertheless, it is among the best tools that we have. If a lactate measurement cannot be obtained quickly, compare the current SBE concentration to the most recent SBE concentration. The numerical difference between them should be a good approximation of the change in the lactate level.

8. *Venous O_2 saturation* ($S\bar{v}o_2$): Mixed venous blood gases, obtained from a pulmonary artery catheter, are preferable. However, if the patient does not yet have a pulmonary artery catheter, blood from any central vein will do.[6] Think of $S\bar{v}o_2$ as the concentration of O_2 left in the blood after it has passed through the tissues (equation 2). If $S\bar{v}o_2$ is decreased (less than 70%), then O_2 demand is a large fraction of O_2 delivery.

Unfortunately, $S\bar{v}o_2$ is only a trend monitor because there really is no single critical value that applies to everybody.[1] However, it can be exceedingly useful in many situations. For example, if the systolic blood pressure of your cardiac surgical patient suddenly decreases to 30 mm Hg immediately postoperatively, should you immediately open the chest and look for tamponade? Or wait for a transesophageal echocardiogram? No. The patient might simply be vasodilated. This common, largely unexplained phenomenon is poorly documented in the literature but is real. The quickest way to diagnose it is to obtain a $S\bar{v}o_2$. If the $S\bar{v}o_2$ is 80%, then it is extremely unlikely that the $\dot{D}o_2$ is low. Phenylephrine hydrochloride (Neo-Synephrine) or norepinephrine bitartrate (Levophed) is all that is needed initially, followed by intravascular volume repletion, if indicated.

9. *Tests to investigate the etiology of decreased $S\bar{v}o_2$*: If your hospital cannot provide rapid access to a ventilation-perfusion scan or a pulmonary angiogram, then it probably should not have an ICU. "Stat" chest radiographs truly need to be immediate. Page the technician yourself if necessary to reinforce the sense of urgency. Sometimes our expertise as critical care clinicians is absolutely useless unless we can obtain the needed tests expediently. Your hypoxemic patient may just need some antibiotics to treat a pneumonia, but, then again, a chest tube or urgent therapeutic bronchoscopy may be needed.

10. *Tests to investigate the etiology of decreased blood pressure*: As noted, a central venous O_2 saturation can provide absolutely the quickest clue to the diagnosis of hypotension, provided that the cooximeter is nearby. In fact, sometimes it is all that is needed. Not all patients with sepsis-induced hypotension need pulmonary artery catheters. They usually have a normal or increased central venous O_2 saturation, and the cardiac output is usually elevated. Hence, often the only additional unexpected piece of information that can be obtained with a pulmonary artery catheter is the pulmonary artery occlusion pressure. If the central venous O_2 saturation is normal or elevated, if the blood pressure can be raised quickly with several liters of fluid, if the 12-lead ECG reading is unchanged, if urine output is adequate, and if neurologic status is reasonable, the patient often can be managed without a pulmonary artery catheter.

On the other hand, contrary to several publicized but truly ridiculous statements, pulmonary artery catheters are often absolutely essential, not only for diagnosis, but also for clinical management. If the cause of hypotension or metabolic acidosis cannot be immediately determined from the clinical history or test results, there simply is no better way to proceed. A seasoned intensivist dealing with normal anatomy and seasoned ICU nurses should be able to safely insert a pulmonary artery catheter and obtain a thermodilution cardiac output within 5 minutes, including sterile procedure. If the cardiac output is high, you are probably dealing with sepsis or liver failure or, occasionally, with adrenal insufficiency. If the cardiac output is low, you could be dealing with anything from myocardial ischemia, to cardiac tamponade, to a tension pneumothorax that was missed on chest radiographic examination, to massive pulmonary embolus, to severe auto PEEP. Proper treatment of each of these diagnostic entities is radically different, and the clock is ticking (see Fig. 24-2).

11. *Transesophageal echocardiogram*: Rapid availability of a transesophageal echocardiogram is nearly essential in the acute management of patients immediately after open heart surgery. It is not necessary for the clinician to be in the position of deciding whether to open a patient's chest in the ICU when the actual problem is stunned myocardium after inadequate cardioplegia (as opposed to cardiac tamponade). In the hands of a skilled diagnostician, transesophageal echocardiogram also can be used to diagnose anything from acute myocardial infarction, to dissecting aortic aneurysm, to mural thrombus.

12. *Consultants*: None of us is an expert at everything. Know your consultants and know who to call. For example, rapid diagnosis of a severe intracranial hemorrhage isn't much use if a neurosurgeon is not already standing by.

13. *Urinary drainage catheter*: Low urinary output does not necessarily mean inadequate renal perfusion. However, normal to increased urine output usually means that the kidneys are adequately perfused. Whether the remaining organs are also well perfused can be difficult to determine, but adequate urinary output is at least comforting for the clinician.

14. *Neurologic examination*: Is the CNS adequately perfused? Perform a cursory neurologic examination. It costs nothing and is easy to do.

15. *Arterial–gastric Pco_2 difference*: This certainly has not achieved the role of common clinical practice. However, it doesn't really fall into the category of a research tool and is entirely innocuous. Intramucosal pH should never be calculated.[5] A normal arterial–gastric Pco_2 difference is approximately 10 mm Hg, and a critical value will probably turn out to be 25 to 30 mm Hg, provided that the stomach contains no appreciable HCO_3^-, together with strong acid. Values greater than 100 mm Hg represent unequivocal ischemia. Although sensitivity is unknown, specificity seems highly likely.[5] Examples of good candidates for this test include patients on high-dose pressors, patients with new and unexpected hepatic transaminase levels, and patients who are struggling to breathe.

INITIAL THERAPY

1. *Airway*: $\dot{D}o_2$ to the tissues requires open communication of air and the trachea. It is usually not sufficient, but it is absolutely essential. Intubation sometimes isn't needed but is a safe and painless procedure in the hands of a skilled operator. If the endotracheal tube isn't needed or wanted, it can always be removed.

Sight is not your only useful sense during an intubation; the value of sound is little appreciated. If one can't see the vocal cords and if the patient is still breathing, one can usually still perform an intubation by (a) bending the tip of the endotracheal tube into a "hockey stick" shape; (b) fishing around in the general location of the (unseen) vocal cords; and (c) placing the proximal tip of the endotracheal tube next to your ear. If you can hear air movement, you must be near the vocal cords. Try it.

2. *Venous access*: In general, the lower the blood pressure, the larger the catheter. It is often wise to insert an 8.5-French pulmonary artery introducer because blood and fluids run fastest through these immediately available devices. If the patient's condition fails to improve quickly, you can later use it to float a pulmonary artery catheter.

3. *Intravascular volume administration*: Generally, intravascular volume administration is considered the most innocuous means of raising blood pressure, at least initially. I prefer colloids for acute emergencies but lactated Ringer's may work just as well. And don't be stingy. I was taught that patients seldom die (in the ICU) from drowning and have found this teaching to be correct, provided that the clinician knows how to finesse a mechanical ventilator. Unless the patient has renal insufficiency, excess volume administered usually can be rapidly removed using diuretics.

The convenience and importance of gravity is little appreciated. In the absence of a fluid pump (or fluid pumper, i.e., person with a large syringe), the fastest infusion rates are achieved when the fluid is nearest the ceiling. If you aren't tall enough, find a step stool.

4. *Blood*: Nobody seems to truly know what is the optimal hematocrit. However, 30% usually seems to be a reasonable target value.

5. *Pressors and inotropes*: As noted, arteriolar sphincters distal to a fixed obstruction should usually be considered to be maximally vasodilated. The only way to improve flow past a fixed arterial obstruction with maximally vasodilated arteriolar sphincters is to increase blood pressure. Excellent examples are myocardial ischemia and cerebral vasospasm after a subarachnoid hemorrhage.

In this regard, notice that the idea to create intraaortic balloon pumps arose from the observation that coronary sinus O_2 saturation and lactate levels improved during cardiogenic shock when pressors were administered.[7] Pressors first; intraaortic balloon pump later.

In the absence of a known fixed arterial obstruction, it is generally believed that a mean arterial blood pressure (MAP) greater than 60 mm Hg must be maintained to ensure adequate perfusion to all the organs. Let's suppose, for example, that pulmonary artery occlusion pressure is 30 mm Hg and MAP is 50 mm Hg. This leaves little coronary perfusion pressure. Alternatively, let's suppose that the vertical distance from the aortic valve to the frontal cerebral cortex is 5 cm. This translates to a hydrostatic pressure difference of roughly 10 mm Hg. If MAP is 50 mm Hg, mean pressure at the tip of the frontal cortex should be about 10 mm Hg less. Is this perfusion pressure within the limits of cerebral autoregulation? I prefer not to take the chance.

During profound hypotension, pressors are absolutely essential for initial management. You could wait for intravascular volume expansion alone to raise the patient's blood pressure, just as you could also routinely ignore stop signs. Regarding the latter, you would survive in most instances; sooner or later, however, you would find yourself in a fatal automobile accident—why take chances? Pressors first; wean them as soon as you are able. If arrhythmias are of concern, use Neo-Synephrine, preferably as a judicious bolus. Ever used it as a nasal spray during a cold? It works quickly.

6. *Vasodilators*: Nitroglycerin can improve flow past a partially reversible coronary obstruction or to tissue near the "border zone" of an ischemic area of myocardium. In high doses, nitroglycerin can be as effective as nitroprusside, thereby reducing myocardial work and improving forward flow.

7. *Treatment of auto PEEP*: As noted, severe auto PEEP alone can cause profound hypotension, particularly during intravascular volume depletion. In extreme instances, it can even masquerade as electrical–mechanical dissociation, unresponsive to therapy.[8] In addition to bronchodilators, decreased ratio of inspiratory time to expiratory time (I:E) must be tried, and there seems to be little wrong with permissive hypercapnia (i.e., maintaining SaO_2 at the minimum possible ventilatory rate).

8. *Reduction of O_2 demand*: In the instance of myocardial ischemia, beta-blockers are often helpful, provided that MAP can be maintained. In the instance of suspected renal injury, O_2 demand can be reduced using furosemide because about 70% of renal work is involved with reabsorbing sodium chloride. This is analogous to cardioplegia, where depolarization of cardiac myocytes with high-concentration potassium solution and cold (ice) permits minimal myocardial injury for up to 3 hours or so of zero myocardial blood flow.

9. *Hydrocortisone*: It is easy to forget or entirely miss the fact that your patient has been on steroids recently. Also, adrenal injury is probably more common than generally believed. For treating simple adrenal insufficiency, methylprednisolone is much too immunosuppressive and often doesn't work. Same for dexamethasone (Decadron). When in doubt, perform a quick corticotropin stimulation test and then immediately give 50 to 100 mg hydrocortisone every 8 hours.[9]

REFERENCES ∎

1. Schlichtig R, Tonnessen T, Nemoto EM: Detecting dysoxia in silent organs. In Prough DS, Traystman RJ (eds). *Critical Care State of the Art* Anaheim, CA, Society of Critical Care Medicine, 1993;14:239

2. Cain SM: Peripheral oxygen uptake and delivery in health and disease. *Clin Chest Med* 1983;4:139

3. Schlichtig R: O_2 uptake, O_2 delivery, and tissue wellness. In: Pinsky MR, Dhainaut JF (eds). *Pathophysiologic Foundations of Critical Care*. Baltimore, Williams & Wilkins, 1993

4. Hertzer NR, Beven EG, Young JR, et al: Coronary artery disease in peripheral vascular patients: a classification of 1000 coronary

angiograms and results of surgical management. *Ann Surg* 1984; 199:223

5. Schlichtig R: Base excess: a powerful clinical tool in the ICU. *Critical Care Symposium—1996.* Anaheim, CA, Society of Critical Care Medicine, 1996;1

6. Scheinman MM, Brown MA, Rapaport E: Critical assessment of use of central venous oxygen saturation as a mirror of mixed venous oxygen in severely ill cardiac patients. *Circulation* 1969; 40:165

7. Mueller HS, Ayres SM, Giannelli S, et al: Effect of isoproterenol, L-norepinephrine, and intraaortic counterpulsation on hemodynamics and myocardial infarction. *Circulation* 1972;45:335

8. Rogers P, Schlichtig R, Miro A, et al: Auto-PEEP: an occult cause of electromechanical dissociation. *Chest* 1991;2:492

9. Singh N, Gayowski T, Marino IR, et al: Acute adrenal insufficiency in critically ill liver transplant recipients. *Transplantation* 1995;59:1744

Critical Care, Third Edition, edited by Joseph M. Civetta,
Robert W. Taylor, and Robert R. Kirby.
Lippincott-Raven Publishers, Philadelphia, PA © 1997.

CHAPTER 25

∎

Progression to Multiple Organ System Failure

George M. Matuschak

IMMEDIATE CONCERNS ∎

MAJOR PROBLEMS

Progressive dysfunction of multiple organ systems, culminating in the syndrome of multiple organ system failure (MOSF), has become the leading cause of death in critically ill and injured patients. MOSF is a disease of medical progress. Broader use of ICU resources combined with improvements in single organ–directed therapy such as mechanical ventilation and dialytic techniques have reduced early mortality after major physiologic insults. This has permitted a more extensive ICU course for increasing numbers of patients after sepsis and trauma, during which basic pathogenetic mechanisms of inflammatory tissue injury proceed unchecked.

MOSF represents a systemic disorder of immunoregulation, endothelial dysfunction, and hypermetabolism with varying manifestations in individual organs. Mortality in MOSF is consistently augmented as the number of failing organ systems increases. This implies that changes in the function of all organs have equal pathogenetic significance; however, organs differ in their host defense functions and sensitivity to host-derived inflammatory mediators or reductions in oxygen delivery ($\dot{D}o_2$). Diagnosis and therapy therefore focus whenever possible on preventive measures. Changes in the cellular oxygen (O_2) supply both cause and complicate MOSF. Consequences include direct hypoxic organ damage, secondary ischemia-reperfusion (I/R) injury mediated by neutrophils and reactive O_2 species (ROS), and enhanced injury by activation of cytokines including tumor necrosis factor-alpha (TNF-α). Initial and subsequent ther-

apy follows a two-tiered approach, targeting systemic factors that contribute to ongoing inflammation and single organ–related problems. Efforts are first directed at stabilizing $\dot{D}o_2$ while addressing life-threatening derangements in acid-base balance and gas exchange. Prompt resuscitation of hemodynamic instability to defined endpoints that correlate with resolution of tissue O_2 debt minimize ischemia-related organ damage. The element of time is a critical factor. Delays in completing initial resuscitation, eliminating foci of infection or devitalized tissue, or treating de novo organ-specific problems such as oliguria all worsen outcome. Late-phase (e.g., over 72 hours) problems involve acquired immunosuppression, predisposition to secondary infection, and hypermetabolism, which impairs wound healing and host defense. Although numerous, the pathogenetic mechanisms of MOSF furnish opportunities to therapeutically intervene at multiple points.

STRESS POINTS

1. MOSF develops in up to 15% of critically ill medical or surgical patients who require ICU admission. Survival from MOSF is reduced in proportion to the number of failing organ systems irrespective of their identity; mortality rates in patients with one, two, or three failing organs average 30%, 50%, and greater than 70%, respectively.
2. Population-based but not individual risks of mortality can be predicted with high degrees of precision by several severity-of-illness scoring systems and models.

343

3. MOSF may result from "single-hit" insults such as severe infection or trauma or may evolve through several stages, each having characteristic clinical features.

4. An uncontrolled focus of infection, ongoing perfusion deficits resulting in diminished tissue $\dot{D}o_2$, injured or devitalized tissue, and persistent nonseptic inflammation commonly initiate and sustain MOSF.

5. Sepsis is not the only cause of fever or hypothermia and leukocytosis; these represent nonspecific manifestations of inflammation typified by the systemic inflammatory response syndrome (SIRS).

6. TNF-α, interleukin (IL)-1, IL-6, IL-8, platelet-activating factor, ROS, and nitric oxide (NO) are pivotal early mediators in the host response to infection and have multiple pathophysiologic effects relevant to MOSF.

7. Inappropriate regulation of the production of cytokines, eicosanoids, ROS, and NO is thought to be of causal significance in MOSF, as are pathologic neutrophil–endothelial interactions and crosstalk among elements of the coagulation, complement, and kinin cascades.

8. Tissue injury is augmented by synergism between cytokine-mediated inflammatory responses and shock-related physiologic changes caused by reductions in the cellular O_2 supply. Cell damage from imbalances in O_2 supply–demand can be exacerbated during reestablishment of perfusion and oxygenation by I/R and hypoxia-reoxygenation (H/R) injuries.

9. Clinically occult dysfunction of the gastrointestinal (GI) mucosal barrier in the ICU is common because of splanchnic ischemia from shock and its treatment by alpha-adrenoceptor agonists.

10. Neutrophil- and ROS-mediated intestinal I/R injury in the postresuscitation period is a potential mechanism of remote organ damage. This may lead to a domino-like sequence of organ failures.

11. Derangement of organ interactions in the gut–liver axis may result in endogenous endotoxemia and bacterial translocation. However, trials of selective decontamination of the GI tract by antibiotic protocols have not consistently prevented organ dysfunction or improved outcome.

12. The liver plays a pivotal but clinically inapparent role in systemic host defense through four mechanisms. First, mononuclear phagocytic (Kupffer) cell uptake processes control the magnitude and circulating half-life of endotoxin, bacteria, and vasoactive by-products. Second, production and export of TNF-α with other mediators directly modulate lung function and cardiovascular stability. Third, hepatobiliary clearance is important in the metabolic inactivation and detoxification of such mediators. And fourth, synthesis of acute-phase reactants regulate several key aspects of metabolism and inflammation.

13. Reductions in total hepatic blood flow ($\dot{Q}L$) and $\dot{D}o_2$, or its partitioning between portal venous and hepatic arterial flows, may alter the above mechanisms, thereby influencing systemic immunoregulation.

14. Acquired dysfunction of single organs may reflect worsening of preexisting limitations of functional reserve, or progression of organ-specific dysfunction from inadequate therapy or postoperative complications. Dysfunction also may reflect functional deterioration from ongoing damage in a single organ despite adequate therapy. Signs of established MOSF are manifested differently in each organ (e.g., acute respiratory distress syndrome [ARDS], acute renal failure [ARF]), yet such changes reflect generalized endothelial injury and inflammation.

15. Diverse medical conditions may mimic sepsis-related MOSF and should be excluded when appropriate. These include connective tissue diseases, intoxications, and neoplasms.

16. Typical metabolic responses in MOSF include hyperglycemia from insulin resistance, accelerated Cori cycle activity, and hepatic glucose release from gluconeogenesis and glycogenolysis. Hypertriglyceridemia results from TNF-α–related reductions in lipoprotein lipase activity. Hepatic lipogenesis is enhanced, increasing the respiratory quotient and minute ventilation. Marked protein catabolism from cytokine-mediated muscle proteolysis and urinary nitrogen wasting is typical.

17. Early rapid resuscitation from shock, irrespective of its etiology, attenuates I/R injury to regional organs and may decrease the incidence of MOSF.

18. Goal-oriented hemodynamic therapy to achieve supranormal values of $\dot{D}o_2$ and O_2 consumption ($\dot{V}o_2$) has improved organ dysfunction and outcome in some studies. If considered in high-risk patients, goal-oriented hemodynamic therapy should be initiated early after presentation and target values achieved within 12 to 24 hours.

ESSENTIAL DIAGNOSTIC TESTS AND PROCEDURES

Hemodynamic and Metabolic Monitoring

1. Begin assessing the adequacy of initial resuscitation efforts by noninvasive measures including skin color and temperature, arterial blood pressure, pulse rate, respiratory rate, mental status, and urine output; determine if metabolic acidosis is present from arterial blood gas and plasma bicarbonate ($NaHCO_3$) determinations. If acidosis is present, establish whether the anion gap and plasma lactate concentrations are increased.

2. Initiate invasive hemodynamic monitoring by arterial and central vascular catheterization. Central venous pressure estimates right heart filling but may not accurately gauge left ventricular preload with tricuspid insufficiency, preexisting heart disease, pulmonary hypertension, or ARDS. Exclude myocardial infarction as a cause of hemodynamic instability by electrocardiography and creatine kinase isoenzyme levels.

3. Perform pulmonary artery catheterization and continuously monitor mixed venous O_2 saturation ($S\bar{v}o_2$;

evaluate cardiac index (CI), $\dot{D}o_2$, $\dot{V}o_2$, and, if initially elevated, lactate concentrations to determine the adequacy of resuscitation and titrate therapy further.
4. After initiating crystalloid or colloid infusions to control hemodynamic instability, stabilize the blood hemoglobin level at 10 to 12 g/dL to optimize $\dot{D}o_2$.

Evaluation for Infection

1. For suspected sepsis on ICU admission, blood cultures (including fungal cultures where appropriate) should be immediately obtained, as should Gram stains and cultures of urine, an adequate sputum specimen (25 or more leukocytes per low-power field) or tracheobronchial washings, and wound discharges before antimicrobial therapy. Suspicious skin lesions should undergo culture by aspiration and biopsy. On discovery of fluid collections, perform thoracentesis and paracentesis within 12 hours or less; determine pH; and perform a Gram stain, culture, cell count, cytologic studies, glucose level, and other chemistries.
2. Evaluate the patient thoroughly for all infectious and potential noninfectious etiologies of MOSF.
3. For suspected nosocomial sepsis, reculture blood, urine, and sputum; evaluate all sites of vascular cannulation and remove catheters, if possible; consider fiberoptic bronchoscopy to obtain protected brush or bronchoalveolar lavage (BAL) samples in patients with pneumonia. Exclude infective endocarditis or endovascular infection by cardiac echography and scintigraphic scanning for high-grade or recurrent bacteremia.
4. Serially monitor renal, pancreatic, and hepatic function; exclude acalculous cholecystitis or pancreatitis by abdominal ultrasound; perform computed tomography of the sinuses, chest, abdomen, and pelvis when appropriate to define fluid collections; these should be drained and cultures performed.
5. Maintain a high index of suspicion for opportunistic fungal infection with *Candida* sp. despite negative results on blood culture.

INITIAL THERAPY

1. Resuscitation of hemodynamic instability should be rapidly initiated with crystalloid and colloid infusions followed by replenishment of the red cell mass. Crystalloid infusions should be limited when the patient already requires a high fraction of inspired O_2 (FIO_2) to treat severe permeability pulmonary edema (e.g., ARDS).
2. Vasopressors (dopamine, norepinephrine) are titrated to a systolic pressure of 90 to 100 mm Hg or a mean arterial pressure of 70 mm Hg or higher.
3. Evaluate and treat ionized hypocalcemia and severe metabolic acidosis if the response to catecholamine therapy is inadequate. $NaHCO_3$ is given to raise arterial pH to 7.1 or more; complications of $NaHCO_3$ therapy include hypernatremia, hyperosmolality, fluid overload, and ionized hypocalcemia.

4. If shock persists despite rapid and aggressive fluid resuscitation, consider endotracheal intubation and mechanical ventilation, irrespective of arterial blood gas values. With proper titration of ventilatory therapy, this averts respiratory muscle fatigue and arrest by reducing shock-related increases in the O_2 cost of breathing.
5. Evaluate and treat oliguria with the same urgency used in approaching chest pain. Differentiate prerenal causes by obtaining serum and urine osmolalities, Na^+, and creatinine before diuretic use; mannitol (25 g intravenously) or loop diuretics given early may attenuate incipient renal failure by increasing excretion of tubular casts, sloughed epithelial cells, or toxins such as myoglobin, thereby maintaining tubular patency. Low-dose dopamine infusions (3 μg/kg/minute or less) to stimulate renal dopaminergic receptors has been used without clear demonstration of benefit.
6. Stabilize long bone fractures early.
7. Initiate broad-spectrum antimicrobial therapy, including coverage against methicillin-resistant *Staphylococcus aureus* and *Staphylococcus epidermidis*; add coverage for suspected anaerobic intraabdominal sepsis.
8. Begin therapy with fluconazole or amphotericin B in patients at high risk for fungal sepsis despite negative results on blood culture when clinical findings are suggestive (e.g., extensive colonization by *Candida*, nonintertriginous skin rash, myositis, or retinitis).
9. Perform prompt reexploration for suspected intraabdominal sepsis and abscess formation.

DEFINITIONS

Central to the pathophysiologic mechanisms and clinical expression of MOSF is a pattern of immunophysiologic responses by the host of variable severity, known as SIRS.[1–3] SIRS is associated with numerous infectious, noninfectious, and inflammatory conditions. These include sepsis, major trauma, burns, pancreatitis, and immunologic disorders. By consensus,[1] SIRS has been defined to include one or more of the following clinical manifestations that represent acute, unexpected alterations: (1) body temperature above 38°C or below 36°C; (2) heart rate over 90 beats per minute; (3) tachypnea with a respiratory rate above 20 breaths per minute or hyperventilation with a $Paco_2$ less than 32 mm Hg; and (4) a white blood cell count above 12,000/μL or less than 4000/μL, or the presence of more than 10% immature band neutrophils. Although these criteria have been thought to be indicative of sepsis, at least 15% of patients enrolled in recent sepsis trials who met these criteria were subsequently found to have no evidence of infection.[4]

MOSF has been variably defined because of the spectrum of dysfunction occurring in single organ systems. One widely used classification scheme is the Acute Physiology Assessment and Chronic Health Evaluation II (APACHE II) scoring system[5] (Table 25-1). MOSF defined by this and other systems usually specifies severe dysfunction in at least two organ systems lasting a minimum of 24 to 48 hours. Recently,

TABLE 25-1. Definitions of Multiple Organ System Failure (MOSF)

CARDIOVASCULAR FAILURE
(PRESENCE OF ONE OR MORE OF THE FOLLOWING)

Heart rate ≤54/min
Mean arterial pressure ≤49 mm Hg
Ventricular tachycardia, ventricular fibrillation, or both
Serum pH ≤7.24 with Pco_2 ≤40 mm Hg

RESPIRATORY FAILURE
(PRESENCE OF ONE OR MORE OF THE FOLLOWING)

Respiratory rate ≤5/min or ≥49/min
$Paco_2$ ≥50 mm Hg
$P(A-a)O_2$ ≥350 mm Hg: $P(A-a)O_2 = 713 (Fio_2) - Paco_2 - Pao_2$
Ventilator or CPAP-dependent on day 4 of MOSF

RENAL FAILURE
(PRESENCE OF ONE OR MORE OF THE FOLLOWING)

Urine output ≤479 mL/24 h or ≤159 mL/8 h
Serum BUN ≥100 mg/dL
Serum creatinine ≥3.5 mg/dL

HEPATIC FAILURE

Serum bilirubin ≥6 mg/dL
Prothrombin time > 4 s over control (in the absence of systemic anticoagulation)

HEMATOLOGIC FAILURE

WBC ≤1000/μL
Platelets ≤20,000/μL
Hematocrit ≤20%

CENTRAL NERVOUS SYSTEM FAILURE

Glasgow Coma Scale score ≤6 (in the absence of sedation at any one point in the day)

$P(A-a)O_2$, alveolar-to-arteriole oxygen gradient; MOSF, multiple organ system failure; Fio_2, fraction of inspired oxygen; CPAP, continuous positive airway pressure; BUN, blood urea nitrogen; WBC, white blood cell count.

From Knaus WA, Wagner DP: Multiple systems organ failure: epidemiology and prognosis. *Crit Care Clin* 1989;5:221.

the term *multiple organ dysfunction syndrome* (MODS) has been proposed to better describe the constellation of severe dysfunction in multiple organ systems,[1] because "failure" implies a dichotomous event, which may not describe functional abnormalities that vary over a spectrum. The terms MOSF and MODS are currently used interchangeably by many investigators, although further refinement of definitions is likely.

EPIDEMIOLOGY

The incidence and mortality of MODS progressing to MOSF have been studied extensively in patients with acute medical illnesses and in those sustaining severe trauma or undergoing major operations.[6-12] Collectively, the data indicate that

MOSF is the principal cause of death in ICU patients. Information concerning the epidemiology of MOSF comes from three sources: (1) analyses of the outcome of single-organ dysfunction such as ARF or ARDS after supervening MOSF[6,7,11]; (2) prospective and retrospective surveys of the incidence of MOSF in medical, surgical, or mixed ICU populations[8-10,12]; and (3) comparative studies examining the prognostic utility of severity-of-illness scoring systems such as APACHE II or III,[5,13] Simplified Acute Physiology Score (SAPS) II,[14] and Mortality Probability Model (MPM) II.[15] Despite differences in ICU populations, study design, inclusion criteria, and methods of analysis among reports, several important findings have been consistently observed.

First, the incidence rate of MOSF is approximately 15% in unselected medical and surgical patients requiring ICU admission. In a large cohort of prospectively followed ICU admissions reported by Knaus and coworkers,[16] 891 of 5815 (15.3%) developed MOSF, defined as severe acquired dysfunction in two or more organ systems (by APACHE II scoring) that lasted at least 24 hours during critical medical illness or after trauma or major operation. Forty-nine percent of these patients met at least one definition for organ failure lasting at least 1 day. Similarly, 74 of 490 patients (15.1%) developed MOSF in the earlier prospective trial of extracorporeal membrane oxygenator support for acute respiratory failure.[6] Incidence figures for MOSF vary among other studies, reflecting in part variable definitions for organ failure. Notice that the incidence of MOSF is considerably higher in subsets of patients having any of three risk factors: (1) age older than 65 years[6] (older than 55 years in trauma patients[17]); (2) increased severity of illness as assessed by APACHE II scores, especially scores of 20 or more[17]; and (3) diagnosis of infection, established sepsis, or acute lung injury at the time of ICU admission. Goris and colleagues[9] report a 100% incidence rate of MOSF in 92 surgical patients prospectively followed after developing intraabdominal sepsis. In prospectively identified medical and surgical patients at risk for ARDS or with established ARDS, there was a 48% incidence rate of MOSF,[7] although in another study of similar patients, only 22 of 207 (10.6%) progressed to MOSF.[8] Recently, progression to lethal MOSF has been tracked among the 17,440 unselected medical-surgical ICU admissions of the APACHE III data base,[13] the 12,977 patients in the SAPS II data base,[14] and the 10,357 subjects in the MPM II 24-hour model.[15] Because each of these systems is an integrative model encompassing preadmission variables and comorbid conditions as well as indices of single-organ dysfunction, epidemiologic data regarding the impact of MOF per se on ICU mortality have not been completely defined. Marshall and others[18] report that a daily composite MODS score of impairment in six organ systems (cardiovascular, respiratory, renal, hepatic, hematologic, and central nervous system) reliably predicted ICU and hospital mortality of surgical patients.

A second, consistent finding across studies is that ICU mortality increases in direct relation to the number of acquired severe organ system failures.[6,7,10,13,18] Development of severe dysfunction in any single-organ system is associated with an incremental rate of mortality risk of 30% to 40%. Mortality rate generally rises to 50% to 60% when two organ systems are impaired, and to 80% to 100% when three or more organ systems are severely dysfunctional. These relations are independent of the identity of individual dysfunctional organ systems.[6,7,13,18] Rather, they may reflect host factors including age and comorbid conditions associated with preexisting functional organ impairment (e.g., chronic obstructive lung disease, renal insufficiency), immunosuppression, or acquired systemic sepsis. Thus, physiologic derangements accompanying severe single-organ dysfunction such as pneumonia predispose to MOSF.[19] Despite the reproducibility of these population statistics and their prognostic utility, direct extrapolation to predict outcome in individuals with MOSF remains imperfect.

PATHOGENESIS ◼

Diverse pathogenetic mechanisms have been proposed to account for the development of multiple organ dysfunction and failure. Most can be grouped under six main processes that involve molecular, cellular, and organ-specific events (Table 25-2). When the host inadequately controls the stimuli that promote inflammation, such as endotoxemia, cellular ischemia, or presence of injured tissue,[1,2,9,20,21] these mechanisms interact in vivo to culminate in MOSF. Although the final clinical expression of MOSF is similar regardless of these varied etiologies, there may be important cause-specific differences in pathogenesis, particularly in early stages more amenable to therapeutic intervention.

MOSF is a systemic disorder of immunoregulation, endothelial dysfunction, inflammatory organ damage, and hypermetabolism.[1,2,9,22–24] During progression of SIRS to MOSF, a key initiating mechanism is stimulation of mononuclear phagocytes, polymorphonuclear neutrophils (PMNs), and endothelial cells by microorganisms and their products.[25–27] A complex programmed sequence of molecular and cellular events follows, which, if inappropriately regulated at any of several steps, results in a self-amplifying process of inflammatory organ injury (Fig. 25-1). Most knowledge in this regard derives from studies of experimental gram-negative endotoxemia or human gram-negative sepsis.[28] Endotoxin may have modest direct endothelial toxicity. However, most of its deleterious effects are caused by host-derived protein and lipid mediators. Early after entry of endotoxin into the bloodstream, its cellular uptake may be prevented by binding of its toxic constituent lipid A to circulating and membrane-associated bactericidal permeability-increasing protein, a component of PMN azurophilic granules.[29,30] Alternatively, endotoxin's inflammatory effects can be facilitated by its association with the circulating acute-phase reactant lipopolysaccharide-binding protein (LBP), which competes with bactericidal permeability-increasing protein for endotoxin binding.[31,32] LBP–endotoxin interaction is followed by cellular internalization of the biologically active endotoxin–LBP complex through the cell differentiation surface receptor CD14.[33] These receptors are particularly abundant on mononuclear phagocytes, including tissue-based macrophages (e.g., alveolar macrophages, Kupffer cells). Within minutes, successive nuclear events involving tyrosine phosphoryla-

TABLE 25-2. Pathogenetic Mechanisms in Progression of SIRS to Multiple Organ Dysfunction and Failure

---

INAPPROPRIATE HOST REGULATION OF ENDOGENOUS INFLAMMATORY MEDIATORS

  Cytokines (TNF-α, IL-1, IL-6, IL-8)
  Chemokines (macrophage activation peptide, ENA-78)
  Platelet-activating factor
  Eicosanoids (prostaglandins, thromboxanes, leukotrienes)
  Nitric oxide
  Complement peptides

CYTOKINE-INDUCED CROSS TALK AMONG INFLAMMATORY MEDIATOR CASCADES

  Coagulation
  Complement
  Kinin/kininogen

GENERALIZED ENDOTHELIAL CELL ACTIVATION AND INJURY

  "Malignant" intravascular inflammation
  Microvascular thrombosis
  Paradoxic vasoconstriction

REDUCTIONS IN THE TISSUE O₂ SUPPLY

  Endothelial and parenchymal cell oxidative stress

ISCHEMIA-REPERFUSION, HYPOXIA-REOXYGENATION INJURY

  Activation of neutrophils and tissue-based macrophages
    Generation of reactive O₂ species
    Cytokine induction

PATHOLOGIC ORGAN SYSTEM INTERACTIONS

  Gut–liver axis
    Endogenous endotoxemia
    Bacterial translocation
  Liver–lung interactions

SIRS, systemic inflammatory response syndrome; TNF-α, tumor necrosis factor-alpha; IL, interleukin; ENA-78 epithelial neutrophil activating protein–78 (ENA–78).

tion, kinase activation, and proteolytic reactions linked to the cell's redox status activate transcription factors such as nuclear factor (NF)-κB.[34] These factors in turn bind to specific DNA sequences of multiple cytokine genes located within the major histocompatibility complex on chromosome 6. There follows increased production in the blood and tissues of the multifunctional cytokines' TNF-α, IL-1, IL-6, IL-8,[34,35–38] and other elements, including colony-stimulating factors.

The mechanisms by which these otherwise homeostatic events escape regulatory control to initiate inflammatory organ damage are not fully understood. Overexpression of cytokine production is prominent in models of sepsis[39,40] and experimental human endotoxemia,[41] or in patients with sepsis- and trauma-related MOSF.[21,35,42–44] However, TNF-α, IL-1, and other cytokines have dual beneficial and adverse effects, depending on the amount, timing, and anatomic locus of cytokine production,[45–47] as well as pathogen-specific and host factors. Earlier emphasis on the shock-inducing aspects of TNF-α or IL-1 overexpression has been balanced

Temporal Sequence of Progression vs Recovery of MOSF

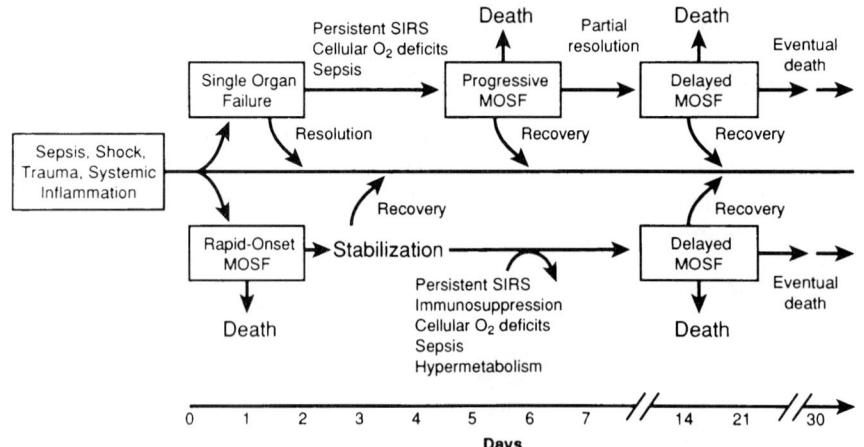

FIGURE 25-1. Temporal sequence of progression vs. recovery from multiple organ system failure (MOSF) after sepsis, trauma, shock, or systemic inflammation (e.g., acute pancreatitis) showing diverse possible outcomes. Rapid-onset MOSF follows such single-hit insults; progressive and delayed MOSF result from multiple-hit insults including ongoing inflammation, immunosuppression, cellular O_2 deficits, and secondary sepsis.

by recognition of their roles in host defense. These include upregulation of PMN microbicidal functions and antibody production, promotion of wound healing by fibroblast collagen synthesis, and coordination of appropriate changes in intermediary metabolism.[34,48] In addition, anticytokine strategies targeting TNF-α have not demonstrated improvement in 28-day survival in septic ICU patients. Moreover, cytokine antagonism has adversely affected survival in experimental bacterial peritonitis or abscesses.[45,49] The margin between promotion of host defense by compensatory cytokine responses versus cytokine-dependent progression to MOSF thus can be difficult to distinguish.[28] Moreover, in severe acute *Candida* sepsis, TNF-α and IL-1 are not pivotal mediators of the fungal septic shock syndrome, either in normal or neutropenic hosts.[50,51] As for sepsis, cytokine induction after trauma should be viewed as an expected part of the systemic response that, in itself, is not solely responsible for MOSF. Circulating levels of IL-6 and IL-8 were increased as early as 2 hours after severe traumatic injury (Injury Severity Score of 25 or more) in one study[38]; although levels remain elevated over 24 hours, they were not predictive of ARDS or MOSF.

Given the consequences of dysregulated cytokine production, multiple host strategies exist to limit excessive generation. Those involved after sepsis or trauma-associated endotoxemia are shown in Table 25-3. Nonendotoxemic stimuli associated with SIRS also lead to continued cytokine overexpression in blood and tissues if rates of synthesis are elevated or those of elimination are protracted. Figure 25-2 depicts synthetic pathways and coinduced regulatory mechanisms that modulate the production or action of TNF-α and IL-1. Antiinflammatory cytokines (IL-4, IL-10, and granulocyte colony-stimulating factor) are important,[52,53] as are activation of genes and enzymes regulating critical eicosanoid second messengers. Features of this network include bidirectional pathways, signal redundancy, and feedback inhibition or amplification. For example, TNF-α elevations after endotoxemia generate ROS that cause lipid peroxidation of cell membranes and organ damage.[54] However, ROS also stimulate further TNF-α expression by NF-κB activation during

reductions in tissue $\dot{D}o_2$ when oxidant production outstrips cellular antioxidant defense.[55] Likewise, TNF-α and IL-1 generate 20-carbon eicosanoids for entry into the cyclooxygenase pathway by activating the enzyme phospholipase A_2 (PLA_2). In a study of septic and posttraumatic ICU patients, increases in circulating PLA_2 were found to be strongly predictive of lethal MOSF in patients with peritonitis but not for those with multiple injuries.[56] Such increases result in production of an array of vasoactive prostaglandin and thromboxanes, or entry of arachidonate into the lipoxygenase pathway, generating leukotrienes (LTs) whose concentrations are elevated in patients with ongoing SIRS and ARDS.[57] Cyclooxygenase products, including prostacyclin and throm-

TABLE 25-3. Host Strategies Limiting Excessive Cytokine Generation After Endotoxemia

---

INTRAVASCULAR

   Increased circulating levels of BPI vs LBP
   Expression and shedding of soluble CD14 receptors
   Synthesis of other endotoxin-binding proteins

INTRACELLULAR

   Control of half-life of cytokine-specific mRNAs
   Modulation of translational efficiency of cytokine transcripts
   Production of antiinflammatory cytokines (e.g., IL-4, IL-6, IL-10)
   Production of cytokine receptor antagonists
      IL-1 receptor antagonist
   Feedback inhibition by cytokine 2nd messengers
      E series prostaglandins
   Downregulation of cytokine receptors
   Shedding of soluble TNF-α and IL-1 receptors
   Cytokine binding by acute-phase reactants
      α₂-macroglobulins
      High-density lipoproteins

BPI, bactericidal permeability-increasing protein; LBP, lipopolysaccharide-binding protein; IL, interleukin; TNF-α, tumor necrosis factor-alpha.

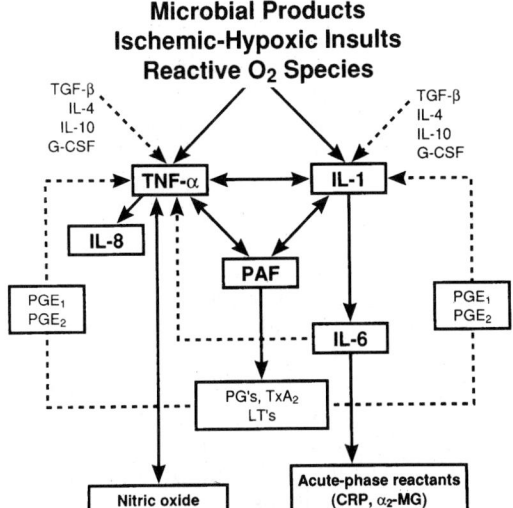

**Microbial Products
Ischemic-Hypoxic Insults
Reactive O₂ Species**

FIGURE 25-2. Schematic representation of key cytokine–eicosanoid interactions within a network of inflammatory mediators activated early after exposure to microbial products or noninfectious ischemic-hypoxic insults. Both stimulatory effects (solid arrows) and inhibitory effects (broken arrows) are shown. Microbial products and reactive O₂ species independently increase TNF-α and IL-1 gene expression, which coinduce PAF, IL-6, and IL-8, along with production of second messengers, including eicosanoids and nitric oxide. Antiinflammatory cytokines (TGF-β, IL-4, IL-10, and G-CSF), HSPs, and feedback inhibitory effects of E series PGs may attenuate biosynthesis of TNF-α and IL-1; α₂-receptors and receptor antagonists may neutralize or stabilize cytokine actions in the vasculature. TNF-α, tumor necrosis factor-alpha; TGF-β, transforming growth factor-beta; G-CSF, granulocyte colony-stimulating factor; HSPs, heat shock proteins; PAF, platelet-activating factor; PGs, prostaglandins; TxA₂, thromboxane A₂; LTs, leukotrienes; CRP, C-reactive protein; α₂-MG, α₂-macroglobulin; IL, interleukin.

boxane A₂, partly mediate cytokine-induced shock and multiple organ injury, events attenuated by prior pharmacologic inhibition of the cyclooxygenase pathway.[58] In contrast, E series prostaglandins and other agonists, which elevate intracellular cyclic AMP, dose-dependently downregulate cytokine gene expression.[59] Cytokine or oxidant-induced production of platelet-activating factor from cell membrane lipid bilayers further sustains TNF-α and IL-1 biosynthesis because of bidirectional stimulatory effects.[60] In conjunction with endotoxin, TNF-α and IL-1 synergistically amplify production of the potent vasodilatory and immunomodulatory autacoid NO to cause biphasic hypotension.[61-63] Early (60 to 120 minutes after endotoxemia) NO production is chiefly from the constitutive isoform of NO synthase in models of sepsis; subsequent (6 to 48 hours) sustained increases in NO production are caused by a molecular switching process whereby inducible NO synthase is preferentially activated by cytokines. The exact role of NO in human sepsis and, particularly, in septic shock, remains unclear. Like cytokines, NO mediates several beneficial host responses to sepsis, including preservation of microcirculatory perfusion within the liver[64] and antiaggregatory effects on PMNs.[65] Further, human phagocytes seem to produce scant amounts of NO

in contrast to experimental animals. For these reasons, NO synthase inhibition with currently available nonselective blockers has not convincingly improved survival in models of sepsis.[28]

The concept of crosstalk among inflammatory networks and noninflammatory protein cascades also is important in the pathogenesis of MOSF, and offers insights into potential therapeutic interventions. Such reciprocal interactions among the cytokine, coagulation, and complement systems occur in several phases (Fig. 25-3). Early after gram-negative bacteremia, cytokine-induced inflammatory activation of the extrinsic coagulation pathway causes binding of factor VIIa to tissue factor (TF). The factor VIIa–TF complex so formed activates factors IX and X, resulting in thrombin generation, fibrin formation within microvessels and alveolar spaces, and generalized endothelial dysfunction with respect to fluid transport and capillary leak.[66] A procoagulant endothelial phenotype is further induced by TNF-α and other cytokines by downregulation of thrombomodulin on endothelial cells. This impairs the activation of vitamin K–dependent protein C. Normally, activated protein C inactivates factors Va and VIIIa, thereby blocking thrombin formation, as well as platelet and PMN activation.[67] This may explain why the level of circulating protein C is strongly predictive of outcome in septic patients,[68] and why administering activated protein C to animal models of bacteremic shock improves both organ failure and survival.[69] Excessive generation of TF or depletion of bioactive protein C ushers in a coagulopathic phase characterized by disseminated intravascular coagulation (DIC) and consumption of fibrinogen and platelets; fibrin degradation products are formed by activation of plasminogen. Plugging of capillaries by fibrin, activated platelets, and PMNs decreases nutritive tissue perfusion, further deranging microvascular perfusion by ischemic swelling of endothelial cells and altered red cell deformability. DIC, as a manifestation of failure of the hematologic system, is attenuated

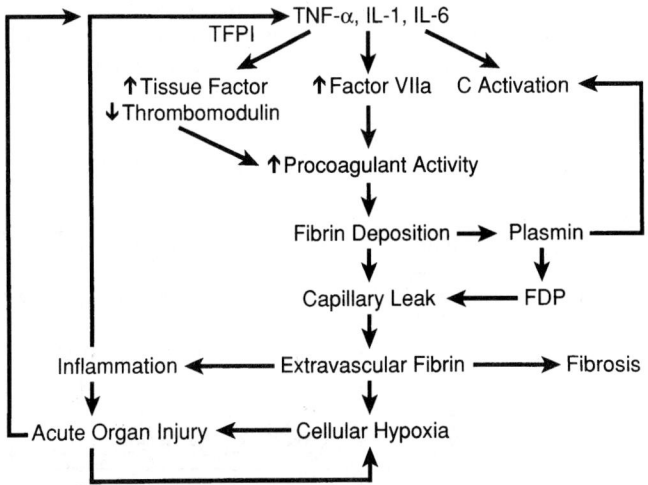

FIGURE 25-3. Crosstalk among elements of cytokine, coagulation, and complement (C) systems that predispose to progressive multiple organ injury during severe systemic inflammatory response syndrome accompanying sepsis, trauma, or inflammatory disorders.

by anti-TF antibodies or plasma-derived activated protein C in otherwise lethal *Escherichia coli* bacteremia in primates, in conjunction with improved organ function, survival, and cross-protective reductions in circulating TNF-α.[70] In contrast, pretreatment with anti–TNF-α antibodies improves survival but not postbacteremic DIC.[71] To hold this cytokine-activated inflammatory–coagulation axis in check, the regulatory anticoagulant tissue factor pathway inhibitor (TFPI) serves as a major physiologic inhibitor of TF.[71] Synthesized by the endothelium, TFPI binds to and neutralizes factor Xa. Plasma TFPI levels increase after severe injury, and their concentrations are elevated in BAL fluid from patients at risk for ARDS or who have established ARDS after sepsis or trauma.[66] TFPI administration also improves outcome from otherwise lethal experimental gram-negative bacteremia.[72]

In addition to the above interactions, C3a and C5a are involved in other sequences implicated in the pathogenesis of MOSF.[73] C peptides mediate local and remote organ injury after trauma or experimental I/R injury.[74] In particular, C5a primes PMNs for enhanced oxidant production while upregulating TNF-α production by mononuclear cells.[75] Both events contribute to time-dependent expression on PMNs and endothelial cells of specific adhesion molecules and ligands (Fig. 25-4). Such PMN–endothelial interactions support host defense by facilitating PMN efflux from the circulation and recruitment to foci of infection or injured tissue. However, interactions between PMNs and the endothelium become pathologic when PMN priming by endotoxin or C fragments are further upregulated for adhesion molecule expression and oxidant damage. In this regard, circulating concentrations of intercellular adhesion molecule-1 are increased on ICU admission in patients with sepsis, SIRS, and after trauma,[76,77] and correlate with vasopressor-dependent shock and MOSF. When pathologic PMN–endothelial interactions are accompanied by cytokine overexpression and intravascular fibrin, the stage is set for a self-amplifying process of "malignant" intravascular inflammation and organ injury, even after resolution of the initiating septic, traumatic, or inflammatory insult.

Synergism of physiologic with inflammatory changes occurs within each level of the host defense hierarchy during shock. Ultimately, this synergism is caused by changes in the cellular O_2 supply. The level of tissue O_2 availability and its dynamic fluctuation should be viewed as regulatory factors of inflammation in their own right that, when detected, are amenable to intervention. Overt and occult reductions in tissue $\dot{D}o_2$ contribute to MOSF by two mechanisms. First, endothelial and parenchymal cell oxidative stress from low intracellular Po_2 impairs aerobic metabolism and causes progressive cell swelling and irreversible mitochondrial dysfunction.[78] Second, such hypoxic cell damage can be paradoxically exacerbated by reestablishment of the O_2 supply to result in I/R and H/R organ injuries.[79,80] These are mediated by O_2-linked generation of ROS from xanthine oxidase (Fig. 25-5), mitochondria, resident tissue phagocytes, and infiltrating PMNs.[25] Irrespective of the cause of shock, I/R and H/R injury can amplify inflammatory organ by induction of TNF-α, IL-1, and other cytokines.[81] Both mechanisms of tissue injury usually occur simultaneously or in a sequence-dependent manner in acutely ill patients. Even so, data are limited with respect to the exact role of these processes in initiating or perpetuating MOSF. Most studies of severe SIRS have focused on dysregulation of cytokine biosynthesis[82] *or* on PMN-mediated reperfusion and reoxygenation injuries.[25,79,80] However, I/R and H/R occur in the presence of microbial products during cytokine-induced septic shock and its resuscitation; primary reductions in regional $\dot{O}_2$ during hypovolemic shock from trauma precede secondary endotoxemia or bacteremia. Postbacteremic induction of TNF-α from the liver and, possibly, other organs is significantly downregulated by a 30-minute secondary oxidative stress during global low-flow I/R or H/R.[83,84] Such downregulation was not observed in perfused rat liver when similarly timed hepatic I/R preceded intraportal *E. coli* bacteremia.[84] Persisting deficits in tissue $\dot{O}_2$ delivery therefore may modify inflammation in a complex manner in ICU patients. Inflammation can be perpetuated by increased cytokine transcription when ROS production outstrips intracellular reduced glutathione.[55] Administration of precursors with antioxidant effects similar to glutathione (e.g., *N*-acetyl-L-cysteine) reduce TNF-α levels by suppression of ROS-induced NF-κB activation, among other mechanisms.[85] Alternatively, inappropriate decreases in cytokine production by

Neutrophil Adhesion Cascade

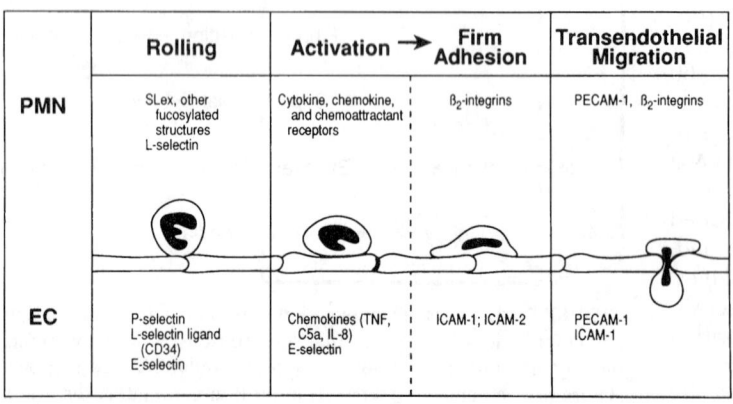

	Rolling	Activation →	Firm Adhesion	Transendothelial Migration
PMN	SLex, other fucosylated structures L-selectin	Cytokine, chemokine, and chemoattractant receptors	β$_2$-integrins	PECAM-1, β$_2$-integrins
EC	P-selectin L-selectin ligand (CD34) E-selectin	Chemokines (TNF, C5a, IL-8) E-selectin	ICAM-1; ICAM-2	PECAM-1 ICAM-1

FIGURE 25-4. Sequence of neutrophil (polymorphonuclear neutrophil [PMN]) and endothelial cell (EC)-specific expression of adhesion molecules during inflammatory mediator-induced cellular activation. SLex, sialyl Lewis carbohydrate tetrasaccharide; ICAM, intercellular adhesion molecule; PECAM, platelet-endothelial cell adhesion molecule. (From Talbott GA, Sharar SR, Harlan JM, *et al*: Leukocyte-endothelial interactions and organ injury: the role of adhesion molecules. *New Horizons* 1994;2:545.)

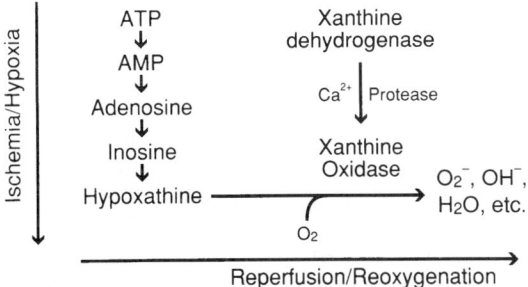

FIGURE 25-5. Xanthine oxidase–mediated generation of reactive O_2 species (ROS) causing ischemia-reperfusion or hypoxia-reoxygenation injury by lipid peroxidation and cytokine induction when ROS production exceeds antioxidant defenses. TFPI, tissue factor pathway inhibitor; FDP, fibrin degredation products; TNF-α, tumor necrosis factor-alpha. (Modified from McCord JM: Oxygen-derived free radicals in postischemic tissue injury. *N Engl J Med* 1989;312:159.)

less severe oxidative stress may be immunosuppressive and promote secondary infection.

ORGAN SYSTEM INTERACTIONS

Although outcome from MOSF is related to the number and not to the identity of severely dysfunctional organs, interactions among organ systems modulate progression of SIRS to MOSF by several mechanisms. Two examples are those within the gut–liver axis[86] and liver–lung interactions.[87] Recognition of these has been delayed because of practical difficulties in their assessment at the bedside. Within the gut–liver axis, anatomic, physiologic, and cellular factors functionally link these organs, as does their in-series vascular supply. The splanchnic circulation normally contains 20% to 25% of the systemic blood volume and receives 25% of the cardiac output.[88] Portal venous flow ($\dot{Q}$pv), representing mesenteric venous drainage, comprises nearly 75% of $\dot{Q}$L. Pressure-flow autoregulation is minimal in the portal circuit. Hepatic perfusion by $\dot{Q}$pv therefore is controlled by upstream hemodynamic events that modulate mesenteric arterial inflow or venous capacitance.[87] These factors predispose the gut to being both a target organ and a "motor" of early MOSF in two ways. First, the mesenteric circulation is sensitive to increases in alpha-adrenoceptor tone during circulatory stresses associated with shock and its treatment by alpha-adrenergic agonists.[88] These circumstances increase mesenteric arteriolar tone, thereby diminishing splanchnic arterial inflow. Second, the critical $\dot{D}o_2$ to maintain enterocyte integrity is higher than in other organs of the body during endotoxemia, such that intestinal $\dot{V}o_2$ becomes flow dependent despite minimal alterations in systemic hemodynamics.[89] Splanchnic venous pooling from endotoxemia further limits mesenteric and hepatic arterial flows.[90] Sustained but clinically occult mesenteric arteriolar vasoconstriction from inadequate fluid resuscitation or sympathoadrenal activation compromises the gut mucosal barrier by ROS-mediated injury because of high $\dot{V}o_2$ requirements of enterocytes.[91,92] There are four potential consequences:

1. Endogenous portal and systemic endotoxemia, which, by mediator activation, amplifies SIRS even without a focus of infection[2,93,94]: This mechanism was previously invoked to explain delayed hemodynamic instability that complicates initially successful resuscitation from hemorrhagic shock.[95]
2. Microbial overgrowth and translocation across intact gut epithelia, especially when associated with altered digestive tract microflora from prolonged use of broad-spectrum antibiotics or trauma[96]: Consistent with the sensitivity of the gut mucosal barrier to ischemic injury, bacterial translocation is enhanced in models of hemorrhagic shock as described by Deitch[86] (calcium and PLA$_2$ activation as well as ROS mediate these).[97] Translocation also has been reported in models of nutritional depletion, burns, and intraabdominal abscesses and in endotoxemia itself.[86]
3. Gut I/R injury and PMN-dependent remote organ damage, including ARDS[94,98]
4. Enhanced cytokine generation by the gut during ischemic intestinal injury, followed by export into portal venous blood and activation of the liver[99]

The significance of these mechanisms in ICU patients is incompletely defined because translocation of endotoxin, bacteria, and MOSF have not been consistently observed in other reports after trauma or hemorrhagic shock.[100–102]

Liver–lung interactions are increasingly recognized to modulate predisposition to and resolution of ARDS with MOSF.[87] They exemplify how dysfunction of a single organ can adversely affect remote organ performance by defined molecular and cellular pathways. Hepatic performance influences four interrelated elements of the systemic inflammatory response after sepsis or trauma to alter lung function:

1. *Control of endotoxemia, bacteremia, and vasoactive by-products of sepsis by mononuclear phagocytic (Kupffer cell) clearance:* This uptake of gram-negative endotoxin and microorganisms limits their magnitude and intravascular half-life. Kupffer cells, comprising nearly 80% of the body's mononuclear phagocytic system cell mass, are critical in this regard, although other determinants may affect their efficiency (e.g., characteristics of $\dot{Q}$L, preexisting liver disease). Several observations suggest that "spillover" of microbial products past mononuclear phagocytic system elements in the liver impairs pulmonary function: (1) ARDS is more frequent and lethal in patients with end-stage liver disease awaiting hepatic transplantation[103]; (2) ARDS resolution in such patients is enhanced by liver transplantation or retransplantation[104]; and (3) cholestatic liver injury and biliary cirrhosis amplify mortality and lung inflammation during endotoxemia.[105] High-grade portal endotoxemia may itself detrimentally affect $\dot{Q}$L. Halvorsen and others[106] showed that a 1 μg/hour intraportal infusion of endotoxin increased portal resistance by 160% and hepatic arterial resistance by 350% in a porcine model; endotoxin spillover to the lungs increased pulmonary vascular resistance.

2. *Hepatic cytokine production and export* is a second mechanism influencing lung function. The capacity for hepatic cytokine efflux is considerable: peak splanchnic TNF efflux 90 minutes after endotoxemia in human volunteers averaged 7 µg.[41] Because concentrations of free circulating TNF-α in established sepsis are in the picogram-per-milliliter range,[28] the liver may produce a large fraction of circulating TNF-α in early sepsis. Nonseptic stimuli such as hypoperfusion of the liver after trauma and experimental I/R injury also induce hepatic efflux of TNF-α and chemokines that increase lung microvascular permeability and inflammation.[81] Because decreases in $\dot{Q}L$ in the critically ill are common resulting from the above factors plus the effects of positive-pressure ventilation,[107] several components of the inflammatory response may amplify lung injury under these circumstances[108] (Fig. 25-6).

3. *Metabolic inactivation of inflammatory mediators by hepatobiliary elimination* is an important but incompletely understood process because there may be poor correlation with standard liver function tests. By analogy to the altered pharmacokinetics of drugs preferentially metabolized in the liver when hepatic dysfunction supervenes, the half-lives of endogenous mediators can be prolonged by impaired hepatobiliary function. Blood and BAL fluid concentrations of TNF-α and LTs are increased during ARDS with MOSF,[37,109] and both mediators are metabolized in the liver.[87] In sepsis models, impaired hepatocytic performance reproducibly enhances TNF-α– and LT-dependent mortality and lung inflammation.[110]

4. *Modulation of metabolic and inflammatory responses by hepatic acute-phase reactants* is connected with the other three elements of host defense. Kupffer cell–hepatocyte interactions after stress balance stimulatory effects of endotoxin, TNF-α, IL-1, and IL-6 against inhibitory effects of NO on hepatic protein synthesis.[111]

Cytokine-induced reprioritization of protein synthesis in ICU patients predictably decreases albumin and transferrin synthesis while increasing that of acute-phase reactants such as α₂-macroglobulin, C-reactive protein (CRP), fibrinogen, haptoglobin, and the proteinase inhibitor α₁-antitrypsin.[112]

Multiple proinflammatory and antiinflammatory cytokines bind to acute-phase reactants, especially α₂-macroglobulin,[113] although the significance of this during critical illness is still unclear. Neutralization of cytokine bioactivity, prolongation of bioactivity from preemptive binding by soluble cytokine receptors, and extension of bioactivity by interorgan transport and deposition are all possible consequences (Table 25-3). Acute-phase reactants also may be proinflammatory—as is the case for LBP[32,33]—or protective by dampening PMN-mediated inflammation. Blood levels of CRP are increased in ARDS patients, and these elevations correspond with decreased PMN chemotaxis.[114] Dietary or transgenic increases in serum CRP decrease experimental C-induced pulmonary leukosequestration and vascular permeability.[115] Collectively, these aspects of the hepatic acute-phase response should be viewed as part of a homeostatic repertoire that can be modified by liver dysfunction during progression of SIRS to MOSF.

CLINICAL FEATURES ■

MOSF can develop at any time during a patient's ICU course (see Fig. 25-1). There is much variation in its clinical expression, especially concerning the temporal pattern of sequential organ dysfunctions and their severity. It is unlikely that all organs have equal pathogenetic significance or severity of dysfunction despite meeting organ-specific criteria for failure. This is most true for splanchnic organs; neither gut mucosal barrier function nor hepatic immunoregulation are accurately assessed by standard clinical measures. Organ systems also are differentially susceptible to cellular damage, have differing substrate requirements for energy production, and show evidence of dysfunction at different times after sepsis or trauma. New-onset single-organ dysfunction in an ICU patient therefore should be approached from the perspective that it may have one or more of four causes: (1) illness-related worsening of intrinsically compromised organ-specific function (e.g., congestive heart failure, chronic renal insufficiency); (2) progression of organ-specific dysfunction from inadequate response to initial therapy or postoperative complications (e.g., pneumonia with resistant pathogens, intestinal anastomotic leak); (3) organ-specific

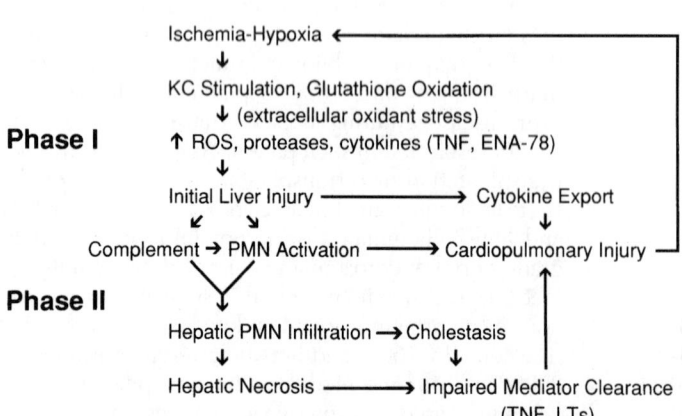

FIGURE 25-6. Pathologic organ interactions in the liver–lung axis. Dual-phase hepatic ischemia-reperfusion injury elicits production and export of reactive oxygen species (ROS), cytokines, and nitric oxide (not shown) in Phase I. Polymorphonuclear neutrophil (PMN)–dependent liver injury in Phase II causes progressive hepatocytic damage, cholestasis, and impaired hepatobiliary clearance of inflammatory mediators. TNF, tumor necrosis factor; ENA-78, epithelial neutrophil activating protein–78; LTs, leukotrienes; KC, Kupffer cells. (Modified from Jaeschke H, Farhood A, Bautista AP, *et al:* Complement activates Kupffer cells and neutrophils during reperfusion after hepatic ischemia. *Am J Physiol* 1993;264:G801.)

deterioration despite otherwise adequate therapy; and (4) a manifestation of systemic endothelial injury and inflammation that is simultaneously affecting multiple organs (e.g., MOSF-related ARDS with ARF and DIC).

Whereas the sequence of sequential organ system dysfunction is variable in MOSF, it is useful to think of SIRS progressing to MOSF in three stages, each associated with typical clinical features. In *Stage 1*, increases in microvascular permeability from inflammatory mediator activation result in respiratory alkalosis with modestly increased venous admixture. Increased volume requirements to maintain biventricular filling pressures and arterial pressure are common. Altered renal tubular function increases the fractional excretion of Na^+; tubular obstruction by ischemic cell swelling or cast formation contribute to oliguria, as do persistent reductions in the glomerular filtration rate. Collectively, these cause a need for diuretics to maintain urine output above 0.5 mL/kg/hour. Intestinal distention and normal or mildly cholestatic liver function indices are common, as are hyperglycemia from stress hormone release and insulin resistance,[24] confusion, and mild thrombocytopenia with a variable leukocyte count. Progression to *Stage 2* within hours or days (see Fig. 25-1) results in tachypnea, hypoxemia, and an increased O_2 cost of breathing from increased extravascular lung H_2O, despite a pulmonary artery occlusion pressure less than 18 mm Hg; elevated minute ventilatory requirements from sepsis or fever mandate intubation and mechanical ventilation. When preexisting cardiac reserve is not severely impaired, a hyperdynamic cardiovascular state evolves, typified by increases in the CI to 4.5 L/minute/m^2 or more and reductions in the systemic vascular resistance index to 800 dynes/second/cm^{-5} or less; parallel reductions occur in arterial vasomotor tone, requiring modest vasopressor dependency (e.g., dopamine, 10/μg/kg/minute or less). Mild generalized edema resulting from capillary leak, azotemia with or without oliguria, conjugated hyperbilirubinemia and hypoalbuminemia, lethargy, protein catabolism with urinary nitrogen wasting,[23] and intolerance to enteral feeding are all common. In *Stage 3*, the patient is edematous and overtly unstable from shock resistant to fluid administration that requires vasopressors (dopamine, more than 10/μg/kg/minute; norepinephrine; or epinephrine). ARDS, with a PaO_2 divided by FIO_2 value of 200 or less and diffuse bilateral pulmonary infiltrates requiring high levels of positive end-expiratory pressure, is complicated by barotrauma, hypercapnia, and nosocomial pneumonia. Renal deterioration occurs, including progressive azotemia, uremic metabolic acidosis, hyperkalemia, and volume overload requiring dialysis. Ileus is frequent, as is enzymatic evidence of pancreatitis; ischemic colitis or stress ulceration with GI bleeding is exacerbated by vitamin K–resistant prolongation of the prothrombin time and thrombocytopenia accompanying DIC. Clinical jaundice follows, with transaminase elevations, stupor or coma, muscle wasting, and lactic acidosis. Recurrent hemodynamic instability from catheter-related sepsis, postoperative abscess formation, devitalized tissue, or blood culture–negative opportunistic infection by *Candida* sp. often signal a final phase of variable length in which irreversible clinical deterioration occurs.

PREVENTION AND TREATMENT ■

Because our understanding of the pathogenesis of MOSF is incomplete, a proactive approach to prevent single-organ dysfunction should be central to the treatment plan of every ICU patient. Systemic factors that stimulate ongoing activation of inflammatory mediator pathways must be corrected whenever possible to minimize organ-specific dysfunction. This entails finding and treating sources of sepsis or injured tissue, correcting persisting deficits in $\dot{D}O_2$, and minimizing pathologic organ interactions (see Table 25-2). Successful management of MOSF encompasses three goals:

1. Analysis of all potential causes of new-onset single-organ dysfunction during titration of organ-specific support: Thus, stabilization of ARDS-related derangements in gas exchange by mechanical ventilation must be accompanied by simultaneous efforts to determine an etiologic diagnosis.
2. Balancing such support with potential cross-reacting organ interactions that adversely affect remote organ function: For example, increases in intrathoracic pressure during support of impaired lung function may be associated with adverse effects on the liver, kidney, and other organ systems.[107,116]
3. Frequent reassessment of the presumed cause of unresolved MOSF: Initiating and sustaining factors of inflammatory organ damage may differ over time (Table 25-4).

Key aspects of prevention and treatment of MOSF are shown in Table 25-5. Aggressive volume resuscitation from shock, irrespective of its cause, prevents or ameliorates MOSF. Overconservative fluid administration is the single biggest error. Conventional endpoints include the following: a systolic arterial pressure at or above 90 to 100 mm Hg or a mean arterial pressure of 70 mm Hg or higher; CI greater than 3.5 L/minute/m^2; pulmonary artery occlusion pressure of 12 mm Hg or higher; $S\bar{v}O_2$ of 70% or more; blood hemoglobin concentration of 10 to 12 g/dL in high-risk patients; urine output of 0.5 to 1 mL/kg/hour; resolution of lactic acidosis; and normal skin color or temperature. Even if met, these endpoints do not assure the adequacy of regional organ $\dot{D}O_2$ and tissue oxygenation.[117] CI represents total-body flow, and increases are not proportionately distributed among and within regional organs. In contrast, $\dot{D}O_2$ represents the bulk flow of O_2 to the tissues. Compared with nonsurvivors of critical illness, survivors have earlier restoration and higher values for $\dot{D}O_2$ and $\dot{V}O_2$.[118] The finding of pathologic, supply-dependent $\dot{V}O_2$ in patients with sepsis, ARDS, and other conditions[119,120] has been taken to indicate a tissue O_2 debt, even in the absence of lactic acidosis. Other studies have not confirmed supply-dependent $\dot{V}O_2$,[121,122] possibly because of mathematical coupling of the indices used to calculate $\dot{V}O_2$.[123] Because empirically supranormal $\dot{D}O_2$ values are associated with enhanced survival, goal-oriented hemodynamic therapy to achieve such supranormal values as a first approximation to optimize the physiologic response to stress has been evaluated to decrease organ dysfunction and mortality. These goals are mean or median values in the first 12 to 24

TABLE 25-4. Common and Uncommon Causes of Progression to MOSF

COMMON

Sepsis (bacteremic, nonbacteremic, nonbacterial)
Trauma
Aspiration of gastric contents
Acute pancreatitis
Infective endocarditis
Heat stroke
Systemic vasculitides
   Polyarteritis nodosa
   Wegener's granulomatosis
Connective tissue disease
   Systemic lupus erythematosis

UNCOMMON

Disseminated tuberculosis
Antiphospholipid antibody syndrome
Thrombotic thrombocytopenic purpura
Unusual microbial infections
   Erlichiosis
   Rocky Mountain spotted fever
   Plasmodium falciparum malaria
   Vibrio vulnificus sepsis
Intoxications/toxins
   Arsenic
   Ethylene glycol
   Organophosphates
   Mercury
   Methanol
   Amanita mushroom ingestion
   Scorpion, snake envenomation
Atrial myxoma
Pheochromocytoma

MOSF, multiple organ system failure.

hours after presentation of individual survivors and thus reflect wide ranges.[120,125] Data from randomized studies are conflicting,[124–127] possibly related to different timing of intervention across studies and because supranormal values differ somewhat among survivors of high-risk surgical operations, trauma, and septic and cardiogenic shock; the highest values observed in septic shock are CI greater than 5.5 L/minute/m^2, $\dot{D}o_2$ greater than 1000 mL/minute/m^2, and $\dot{V}o_2$ greater than 190 mL/minute/m^2.[128] Benefits in surgical patients, including reduced mortality, fewer days on mechanical ventilation, fewer ICU days, and decreased costs, have been reported,[124] but not consistently in septic patients or in mixed ICU populations. In a recent multicenter trial, Gattinoni and associates[129] strove for supranormal values of CI (4.5 L/minute/m^2 or more) or $\dot{S}\bar{v}o_2$ (70% or more) in a heterogeneous population of ICU patients using volume expansion, inotropic infusions, or both. Neither the number of dysfunctional organs, length of ICU stay, nor mortality were reduced. However, hemodynamic targets were able to reached in only 45% of the CI group and 67% of the $\dot{S}\bar{v}o_2$ group. If considered in patients at high risk for MOSF, then hemodynamic therapy targeting supranormal values of $\dot{D}o_2$ or $\dot{V}o_2$

as must be accomplished early (e.g., in less than 24 hours); otherwise, benefits may be marginal.[128]

Because the adequacy of splanchnic $\dot{D}o_2$ is difficult to infer from systemic hemodynamic parameters, more direct measures have been sought. Tonometrically measured intramucosal gastric pH (pHi), a metabolic index of splanchnic oxygenation, has been used to track gastric mucosal pH, and by extension, intestinal ischemia.[130–132] In one prospective study, only pHi and mixed venous pH values discriminated between survivors and nonsurvivors[133]; in another, therapy guided by pHi measurements to maintain values over 7.35 improved survival, even in patients whose pHi on admission to the ICU was normal.[134] Although these results are encouraging, further prospective studies of pHi monitoring are needed to define which patients derive benefit and the optimum timing of such intervention.

Table 25-5 indicates specific measures that should be undertaken in managing patients with MOSF. Of these, control of sepsis is critical although difficult, because all SIRS-related criteria, including fever and white blood cell elevations, reflect mediator-driven inflammatory responses and not infection per se. Because of the hypercatabolism associated with MOSF[24] and the imprecision of mathematical formulas in assessing true caloric and protein requirements, confirmatory studies should be performed. Measurement of $\dot{V}o_2$ and nitrogen balance by quantitating urinary excretion of urea are particularly important in guiding nutritional support.

Because of the multifactorial pathogenesis and the continuing high mortality of MOSF, a variety of novel mechanism-oriented approaches have been evaluated, primarily in patients with severe SIRS, sepsis, or septic shock. These

TABLE 25-5. Prevention and Therapeutic Management of MOSF

Prompt volume resuscitation to limit extent, duration of shock
   Pulmonary artery catheter-guided assessment of ventricular filling and O_2 transport
   Preemptive diuresis by mannitol, loop diuretics

Early fracture stabilization

Debridement of devitalized tissue

Control of sepsis
   Early empiric broad-spectrum antibiotics after cultures
   Pathogen-specific antibiotic coverage
   Drainage of all localized fluid collections
      Operative
      Nonoperative
   Reculture appropriate anatomic sites if response is inadequate
   Limit duration of intubation, intravascular catheters

Enteral, parenteral nutritional support
   $\dot{V}o_2$-directed caloric intake
   Confirmation of positive nitrogen balance

Consider alternative infectious, noninfectious causes of severe SIRS and MOSF

Titrate drug dosages to changes in end-organ function

MOSF, multiple organ system failure; SIRS, systemic inflammatory response syndrome; $\dot{V}o_2$, oxygen consumption per minute.

include antiendotoxin antibodies, monoclonal antibodies to TNF-α, TNF-α soluble receptor fusion proteins, receptor antagonists of IL-1 and bradykinin, and activated protein C.[135-137] None has conclusively improved 28-day survival,[28] although studies are ongoing. In view of the concept of the gut as the "undrained abscess" of MOSF,[138] selective decontamination of the GI tract has been proposed to reduce enteric aerobic gram-negative bacilli and other pathogens causing nosocomial pneumonia and MOSF. Although the incidence of nosocomial pneumonia has been reduced in certain studies of selective decontamination, no investigations of this modality have demonstrated improved ICU survival.[139-142] Future developments in the treatment of MOSF will include multiagent combinations of immunomodulatory agents, protocol-driven ICU management, and "first-strike" enhancement of host defense in high-risk patients with recombinant cytokines or other agents.[24] Such multimodality therapy combined with meticulous single-organ support hopefully will improve the outcome of this complex disorder.

REFERENCES

1. American College of Chest Physicians/Society of Critical Care Medicine Consensus Conference: Definitions for sepsis and organ failure and guidelines for the use of innovative therapies in sepsis. *Crit Care Med* 1992;20:864
2. Beal AL, Cerra FB: Multiple organ failure syndrome in the 1990s: systemic inflammatory response and organ dysfunction. *JAMA* 1994;271:226
3. Rangel-Frausto MS, Pittet D, Costigan M, et al: The natural history of the systemic inflammatory response syndrome (SIRS). *JAMA* 1995;273:155
4. Bone RC: Toward an epidemiology and natural history of SIRS (systemic inflammatory response syndrome. *JAMA* 1993; 25:270
5. Knaus WA, Wagner DP: Multiple systems organ failure: epidemiology and prognosis. *Crit Care Clin* 1989;5:221
6. National Heart, Lung, and Blood Institute, Division of Lung Diseases: *Extracorporeal Support for Respiratory Insufficiency: A Collaborative Study*. Bethesda, NIH, 1979
7. Bell RC, Coalson JJ, Smith JD, et al: Multiple organ system failure and infection in adult respiratory distress syndrome. *Ann Intern Med* 1983;99:293
8. Montgomery AB, Stager MA, Carrico CJ, et al: Causes of mortality in patients with the ARDS. *Am Rev Respir Dis* 1985;132:485
9. Goris RJA, te Boekhorst TP, Nuytinck JK, et al: Multiple organ failure: generalized autodestructive inflammation? *Arch Surg* 1985;120:1109
10. Barie PS, Hydo LJ, Fischer E: A prospective comparison of two multiple organ dysfunction/failure scoring systems for prediction of mortality in critical surgical illness. *J Trauma* 1994;37:660
11. Alexopoulos E, Vakianis P, Kokolina E, et al: Acute renal failure in a medical setting: changing patterns and prognostic factors. *Ren Fail* 1994;16:273
12. Kollef MH, Wragge T, Pasque C: Determinants of mortality and multiorgan dysfunction in cardiac surgery patients requiring prolonged mechanical ventilation. *Chest* 1995;107:1395
13. Knaus WA, Wagner DP, Draper EA, et al: The APACHE III prognostic system: risk prediction of hospital mortality for critically ill hospitalized adults. *Chest* 1993;100:1619
14. Le Gall JR, Lemeshow S, Saulnier F: A new simplified acute physiology score (SAPS II) based on a European–North American multicenter study. *JAMA* 1993;270:2957
15. Lemeshow S, Teres D, Avrunin JS, et al: MPM II: Mortality probability models based on an international cohort of intensive care unit patients. *JAMA* 1993;270:2478
16. Knaus WA, Draper EA, Wagner DP, et al: Prognosis in acute organ-system failure. *Ann Surg* 1985;202:685
17. Sauaia A, Moore FA, Moore EE, et al: Early predictors of postinjury multiple organ failure. *Arch Surg* 1994;129:39
18. Marshall JC, Cook DJ, Christou NV, et al: Multiple organ dysfunction score: a reliable descriptor of a complex clinical syndrome. *Crit Care* Med 1995;23:1638
19. Sauaia A, Moore FA, Moore EE, et al: Pneumonia: cause or symptom of postinjury multiple organ failure? *Am J Surg* 1993;166:606
20. Abello PA, Buchman TG, Bulkley GB: Shock and multiple organ failure. *Adv Exp Med Biol* 1994;366:253
21. Roumen RM, Redl H, Schlag G, et al: Inflammatory mediators in relation to the development of multiple organ failure in patients after severe blunt trauma. *Crit Care Med* 1995;23:474
22. Baue AE: Multiple organ failure, multiple organ dysfunction syndrome, and the systemic inflammatory response syndrome: where do we stand? *Shock* 1994;2:385
23. Cerra FB, Siegal JH, Coleman B, et al: Septic auto-cannibalism: a failure of exogenous nutritional support. *Ann Surg* 1980;192:570
24. Cerra FB: Hypermetabolism-organ failure syndrome: a metabolic response to injury. *Crit Care Clin* 1989;5:289
25. Fujishima S, Aikawa N: Neutrophil-mediated tissue injury and its modulation. *Intensive Care Med* 1995;21:277
26. Talbott GA, Sharar SR, Harlan JM, et al: Leukocyte-endothelial interactions and organ injury: the role of adhesion molecules. *New Horizons* 1994;2:545
27. Rosenbloom AJ, Pinsky MR, Bryant JL, et al: Leukocyte activation in the peripheral blood of patients with cirrhosis of the liver and SIRS: correlation with serum interleukin-6 levels and organ dysfunction. *JAMA* 1995;274:58
28. Natanson C, Hoffman WD, Suffredini AF, et al: Selected treatment strategies for septic shock based on proposed mechanisms of pathogenesis. *Ann Intern Med* 1994;120:771
29. Marra MN, Wilde CG, Griffith J, et al: Bactericidal/permeability-increasing protein has endotoxin-neutralizing activity. *J Immunol* 1990;144:662
30. Weiss J, Ellsbach P, Shu C, et al: Human bactericidal/permeability-increasing protein and a recombinant NH_2-terminal fragment cause killing of serum-resistant gram-negative bacteria in whole blood and inhibit tumor necrosis factor release induced by the bacteria. *J Clin Invest* 1992;90:1122
31. Heumann D, Gallay P, Betz-Corradin S, et al: Competition between bactericidal/permeability-increasing protein and lipopolysaccharide-binding protein for lipopolysaccharide binding to monocytes. *J Infect Dis* 1993;167:1351
32. Mezaros K, Aberle SD, Dedrick R, et al: Monocyte tissue factor induction by LPS: dependence on LPS-binding protein and CD14, and inhibition by a recombinant fragment of bactericidal/permeability-increasing protein. *Blood* 1994;83:2516
33. Wright SD, Ramos RA, Tobias PS, et al: CD14: a receptor for complexes of lipopolysaccharide (LPS and LPS-binding protein). *Science* 1990;249:1431
34. Giroir BP: Mediators of septic shock: new approaches for interrupting the endogenous inflammatory cascade. *Crit Care Med* 1993;21:780
35. Casey LC, Bone RC: Plasma cytokine and endotoxin levels correlate with survival in patients with the sepsis syndrome. *Ann Intern Med* 1993;119:771

36. Pruitt JH, Copeland EM III, Moldawer LL: Interleukin-1 and interleukin-1 antagonism in sepsis, systemic inflammatory response syndrome, and septic shock. *Shock* 1995;3:235

37. Suter PM, Suter S, Girardin E, et al: High bronchoalveolar levels of tumor necrosis factor and its inhibitors, interleukin-1, interferon, and elastase, in patients with adult respiratory distress syndrome after trauma, shock, or sepsis. *Am Rev Respir Dis* 1992;145:1016

38. Hoch RC, Rodriguez R, Manning T, et al: Effects of accidental trauma on cytokine and endotoxin production. *Crit Care Med* 1993;21:839

39. Tracey KJ, Lowry SF, Fahey TJ III, et al: Cachectin/tumor necrosis factor induces lethal shock and stress hormone responses in the dog. *Surg Gynecol Obstet* 1987;164:415

40. Creasey AA, Stevens P, Kenney J, et al: Endotoxin and cytokine profile in plasma of baboons challenged with lethal and sublethal *Escherichia coli*. *Circ Shock* 1991;33:84

41. Fong Y, Marano MA, Moldawer LL, et al: The acute splanchnic and peripheral tissue metabolic responses to endotoxin in humans. *J Clin Invest* 1990;85:1896

42. Marks JD, Marks CB, Luce JM, et al: Plasma tumor necrosis factor in patients with septic shock. *Am Rev Respir Dis* 1990;141:94

43. Pinsky MR, Vincent JL, Deviere J, et al: Serum cytokine levels in human septic shock: relation to multiple organ failure and mortality. *Chest* 1993;103:565

44. Roumen RM, Hendriks T, van der Jongekrijg J, et al: Cytokine patterns in patients after major vascular surgery, hemorrhagic shock, and severe blunt trauma: relation with subsequent adult respiratory distress syndrome and multiple organ failure. *Ann Surg* 1993;218:769

45. Echtenacher B, Falk W, Mannel DN, et al: Requirement of endogenous tumor necrosis factor/cachectin for recovery from experimental peritonitis. *J Immunol* 1990;145:3762

46. Munoz C, Carlet J, Fitting C, et al: Dysregulation of in vitro cytokine production by monocytes during sepsis. *J Clin Invest* 1991;88:1747

47. Boujoukos AJ, Martich GD, Spunski E, et al: Compartmentalization of the acute cytokine response in humans after intravenous endotoxin administration. *J Appl Physiol* 1993;74:3027

48. Van Deuren M, Dofferhoff ASM, van der Meer JWM: Cytokines and the response to infections. *J Pathol* 1992;168:349

49. Alexander HR, Sheppard BC, Jensen JC, et al: Treatment with recombinant human tumor necrosis factor-alpha protects rats against the lethality, hypotension, and hypothermia of gram-negative sepsis. *J Clin Invest* 1991;88:34

50. Matuschak GM, Klein CA, Tredway TL, et al: TNFα and cyclooxygenase metabolites do not modulate *C. albicans* septic shock with disseminated candidiasis. *J Appl Physiol* 1993;74:2432

51. Lechner AJ, Tredway TL, Brink D, et al: Differential systemic and intrapulmonary TNF-α production in *Candida* sepsis during immunosuppression. *Am J Physiol* 1993;263:L526

52. Vannier E, Miller LC, Dinarello CA: Coordinated antiinflammatory effects of interleukin-4. *Proc Natl Acad Sci USA* 1992;89:4076

53. Marchant A, Deviere J, Byl B, et al: Interleukin-10 production during septicaemia. *Lancet* 1994;343:707

54. Bautista AP, Meszaros K, Bojta J, et al: Superoxide anion generation in the liver during the early stage of endotoxemia in rats. *J Leukoc Biol* 1990;48:123

55. Shreck R, Rieber P, Baeuerle PA: Reactive oxygen metabolites as apparently widely used messengers in the activation of the NF-MB transcription factor and HIV-1. *EMBO J* 1991;10:2247

56. Uhl W, Beger HG, Hoffmann G, et al: A multicenter study of phospholipase A_2 in patients in intensive care units. *J Am Coll Surg* 1995;180:323

57. Bernard GR, Korley V, Swindell B, et al: Persistent generation of peptide leukotrienes in bronchoalveolar lavage fluid of patients with the adult respiratory distress syndrome. *Am Rev Respir Dis* 1991;144:263

58. Okusawa S, Gelfand JA, Ikejima T, et al: Interleukin-1 induces a shock-like state in rabbits: synergism with tumor necrosis factor and the effect of cyclooxygenase inhibition. *J Clin Invest* 1988;81:1162

59. Kunkel SL, Spengler M, May MA, et al: Prostaglandin E_2 regulates macrophage-derived tumor necrosis factor gene expression. *J Biol Chem* 1988;11:5380

60. Braquet P, Paubert-Braquet M, Bourgain R, et al: PAF/cytokine auto-generated feedback networks in microvascular immune injury: consequences in shock, ischemia, and graft rejection. *J Lipid Mediat* 1989;1:75

61. Szabo C: Alterations in nitric oxide production in various forms of circulatory shock. *New Horizons* 1995;3:2

62. Evans T, Carpenter A, Kinderman H, et al: Evidence of increased nitric oxide production in patients with the sepsis syndrome. *Circ Shock* 1993;41:77

63. Ochoa JB, Udekwu AO, Billiar TR, et al: Nitrogen oxide levels in patients after trauma and during sepsis. *Ann Surg* 1991;214:621

64. Harbrecht BG, Stadler J, Demetris AJ, et al: Nitric oxide and prostaglandins interact to prevent hepatic damage during murine endotoxemia. *Am J Physiol* 1994;266:G1004

65. Kanwar S, Kubes P: Nitric oxide is an antiadhesive molecule for leukocytes. *New Horizons* 1995;3:93

66. Sabharwal AK, Bajaj SP, Ameri A, et al: Tissue factor pathway inhibitor and von Willebrand factor antigen levels in adult respiratory distress syndrome and in a primate model of sepsis. *Am J Resp Crit Care Med* 1995;151:758

67. Esmon CT, Taylor FB, Snow TR: Inflammation and coagulation: linked processes potentially regulated through a common pathway mediated by protein C. *Thromb Haemost* 1991;66:160

68. Fourrier F, Chopin C, Goudemand J, et al: Septic shock, multiple organ failure, and disseminated intravascular coagulation: compared patterns of antithrombin III, protein C and protein S deficiencies. *Chest* 1992;101:816

69. Taylor FB, Chang A, Esmon CT, et al: Protein C prevents the coagulopathic and lethal effects of *E. coli* infusion in the baboon. *J Clin Invest* 1987;79:918

70. Taylor FB, Chang A, Ruf W, et al: Lethal *E. coli* septic shock is prevented by blocking tissue factor with monoclonal antibody. *Circ Shock* 1991;33:127

71. Taylor FB: Inflammatory-coagulation axis in the host response to gram-negative sepsis: regulatory roles of proteins and inhibitors to tissue factor. *New Horizons* 1994;2:555

72. Creasey AA, Chang AC, Feigen L, et al: Tissue factor pathway inhibitor reduces mortality from *Escherichia coli* septic shock. *J Clin Invest* 1993;91:2850

73. Goya T, Morisaki T, Torisu M: Immunologic assessment of host defense impairment in patients with septic multiple organ failure: relationship between complement activation and changes in neutrophil function. *Surgery* 1994;115:145

74. Hechtman HB: Mediators of local and remote injury following gut ischemia. *J Vasc Surg* 1993;18:134

75. Okusawa S, Yancey KB, van der Meer JWM, et al: C5a stimulates secretion of tumor necrosis factor from human mononuclear cells in vitro. *J Exp Med* 1988;168:443

76. Sessler CN, Windsor AC, Schwartz M, et al: Circulating ICAM-1 is increased in septic shock. *Am J Respir Crit Care Med* 1995;151:1420

77. Law MM, Cryer HG, Abraham E: Elevated levels of soluble ICAM-1 correlate with the development of multiple organ failure in severely injured trauma patients. *J Trauma* 1994; 37:100

78. Gutierrez G: Cellular energy metabolism during hypoxia. *Crit Care Med* 1991;19:619

79. McCord JM: Oxygen-derived free radicals in postischemic tissue injury. *N Engl J Med* 1985;312:159

80. Weiss SJ: Tissue destruction by neutrophils. *N Engl J Med* 1989;230:365

81. Colletti LM, Kunkel SL, Walz A, et al: Chemokine expression during hepatic ischemia/reperfusion-induced lung injury in the rat. *J Clin Invest* 1995;95:143

82. Goldie AS, Fearon KC, Ross JA, et al: Natural cytokine antagonists and endogenous antiendotoxin core antibodies in sepsis syndrome. *JAMA* 1995;274:274:172

83. Wibbenmeyer LW, Lechner AJ, Munoz CF, et al: Downregulation of E. coli–induced TNFα expression in perfused liver by hypoxia-reoxygenation. *Am J Physiol* 1995;268:G311

84. Epperly NA, Lechner AJ, Johanns CA, et al: Bidirectional effects of hepatic ischemia/reperfusion on E. coli–induced TNF-α gene expression. *Am J Physiol* 1996;270:R289

85. Zhang H, Spapen H, Nguyen DN, et al: Protective effects of N-acetyl-L-cysteine in endotoxemia. *Am J Physiol* 1994; 266:H1746

86. Deitch EA: Gut-liver axis in multiple systems organ failure: role of bacterial translocation and endotoxemia. In: Matuschak GM (ed). *Multiple Systems Organ Failure: Hepatic Regulation of Systemic Host Defense*. New York, Marcel Dekker, 1993:39

87. Matuschak GM: Liver-lung interactions in critical illness. *New Horizons* 1994;2:488

88. Parks DA, Jacobson ED: Physiology of the splanchnic circulation. *Arch Intern Med* 1985;145:1278

89. Nelson DB, Samsel RW, Wood LDH, et al: Pathological supply dependence of systemic and intestinal oxygen uptake during endotoxemia. *J Appl Physiol* 1988;64:2410

90. Pinsky MR, Matuschak GM: Cardiovascular determinants of the hemodynamic response to acute endotoxemia in the dog. *J Crit Care* 1986;1:18

91. Steffes CP, Dahn MS, Lange MP: Oxygen transport-dependent splanchnic metabolism in the sepsis syndrome. *Arch Surg* 1994;129:46

92. Landow L, Andersen LW: Splanchnic ischaemia and its role in multiple organ failure. *Acta Anaesthesiol Scand* 1994;38:626

93. Moore FA, Moore EE: Evolving concepts in the pathogenesis of postinjury multiple organ failure. *Surg Clin North Am* 1995;75:257

94. Turnage RH, Guice KS, Oldham KT: Endotoxemia and remote organ injury following intestinal reperfusion. *J Surg Res* 1994;56:571

95. Sori AJ, Rush BF, Lysz TW, et al: The gut as a source of sepsis after hemorrhagic shock. *Am J Surg* 1988;155:187

96. Moore FA, Moore EE, Poggetti R, et al: Gut bacterial translocation via the portal vein: a clinical perspective with major torso trauma. *J Trauma* 1991;31:629

97. Koike K, Moore EE, Moore FA, et al: Phospholipase A$_2$ inhibition decouples lung injury from gut ischemia-reperfusion. *Surgery* 1992;112:173

98. Turnage RH, Guice KS, Oldham KT: Pulmonary microvascular injury following intestinal reperfusion. *New Horizons* 1994;2:463

99. Deitch EA, Xu D, Ayala A, et al: Evidence favoring the role of the gut as a cytokine-generating organ in rats subjected to hemorrhagic shock. *Shock* 1994;1:141

100. Roumen RM, Hendriks T, Wevers RA, et al: Intestinal permeability after severe trauma and hemorrhagic shock is increased without relation to septic complications. *Arch Surg* 1993; 128:453

101. Schlichtig E, Grotmol T, Kahler H, et al: Alterations in mucosal morphology and permeability, but no bacterial or endotoxin translocation takes place after intestinal ischemia and early reperfusion in pigs. *Shock* 1995;3:116

102. Endo S, Inada K, Yamada Y, et al: Plasma endotoxin and cytokine concentrations in patients with hemorrhagic shock. *Crit Care Med* 1994;22:949

103. Matuschak GM, Rinaldo JE, Pinsky MR, et al: Effect of end-stage liver failure on the incidence and resolution of the adult respiratory distress syndrome. *J Crit Care* 1987;2:162

104. Matuschak GM, Shaw BW Jr: Adult respiratory distress syndrome associated with acute liver allograft rejection: resolution following hepatic retransplantation. *Crit Care Med* 1987; 15:878

105. Chang SW, Ohara N: Chronic biliary obstruction induces pulmonary intravascular phagocytosis and endotoxin sensitivity in rats. *J Clin Invest* 1994;94:2009

106. Halvorsen L, Roth R, Gunther RA, et al: Liver hemodynamics during portal venous endotoxemia in swine. *Circ Shock* 1993;41:166

107. Matuschak GM, Pinsky MR, Rogers RM: Effects of positive end-expiratory pressure on hepatic blood flow and performance. *J Appl Physiol* 1987;62:1377

108. Jaeschke H, Farhood A, Bautista AP, et al: Complement activates Kupffer cells and neutrophils during reperfusion after hepatic ischemia. *Am J Physiol* 1993;264:G801

109. Stephenson AH, Lonigro AJ, Hyers TM, et al: Increased concentrations of leukotrienes in bronchoalveolar lavage fluid of patients with ARDS or at risk of ARDS. *Am Rev Respir Dis* 1985;138:714

110. Matuschak GM, Mattingly M, Tredway TL, et al: Liver-lung interactions during E. coli endotoxemia: TNFα-leukotriene axis. *Am J Respir Crit Care Med* 1994;149:41

111. Harbrecht BG, Billiar TR: The role of nitric oxide in Kupffer cell–hepatocyte interactions. *Shock* 1995;3:79

112. Scanga G, Siegal JH, Brown G, et al: Reprioritization of hepatic plasma protein release in trauma and sepsis. *Arch Surg* 1985;120:18

113. Wollenberg GK, LaMarre J, Hayes MA: Cytokine interactions with α$_2$-macroglobulin. In: Matuschak GM (ed). *Multiple Systems Organ Failure: Hepatic Regulation of Systemic Host Defense*. New York, Marcel Dekker, 1993:293

114. Kew RR, Hyers TM, Webster RO, et al: Human C–reactive protein inhibits neutrophil chemotaxis *in vitro*: possible implications for the adult respiratory distress syndrome. *J Lab Clin Med* 1990;115:339

115. Heuertz RM, Xia D, Samols D, et al: Inhibition of C5a des arg–induced neutrophil alveolitis in transgenic mice expressing C-reactive protein. *Am J Physiol* 1994;266:L649

116. Rossaint R, Jorres D, Nienhaus M, et al: Positive end-expiratory pressure reduces renal excretion without hormonal activation after volume expansion in dogs. *Anesthesiology* 1992; 77:700

117. Wang P, Ba,ZF, Burkhardt J, et al: Measurement of hepatic blood flow after severe hemorrhage: lack of restoration despite adequate resuscitation. *Am J Physiol* 1992;G92

118. Shoemaker WC, Appel PL, Kram HB: Tissue oxygen debt as a determinant of lethal and nonlethal postoperative organ failure. *Crit Care Med* 1988;16:1117

119. Vincent JL, Roman A, DeBacker D, et al: Oxygen uptake/supply dependency: effects of short-term dobutamine infusion. *Am Rev Respir Dis* 1990;142:2

120. Shoemaker WC, Appel PL, Kram HB: Role of oxygen debt in the development of organ failure, sepsis, and death in high-risk surgical patients. *Chest* 1992;102:208

121. Ronco JJ, Phang PT, Walley KR, et al: Oxygen consumption is independent of changes in oxygen delivery in severe ARDS. *Am Rev Respir Dis* 1991;143:1267

122. Ronco JJ, Fenwick JC, Wiggs BR, et al: Oxygen consumption is independent of oxygen delivery by dobutamine in septic patients who have normal or increased plasma lactate. *Am Rev Respir Dis* 1993;147:25

123. Hanique G, Dugernier T, Laterra PF, et al: Significance of pathologic oxygen supply dependency in critically ill patients: comparison between measured and calculated methods. *Intensive Care Med* 1994;20:12

124. Tuchschmidt J, Fried J, Astiz M, et al: Elevation of cardiac output and oxygen delivery improves outcome in septic shock. *Chest* 1992;102:216

125. Bishop MH, Shoemaker WC, Appel PL, et al: Relationship between supranormal circulatory values, time delays, and outcome in severely traumatized patients. *Crit Care Med* 1993; 21:56

126. Boyd O, Grounds M, Bennett ED: A randomized clinical trial of the effect of deliberate perioperative increase of oxygen delivery on mortality in high-risk surgical patients. *JAMA* 1993;270:2699

127. Hayes MA, Timmins AC, Yau EHS, et al: Elevation of systemic oxygen delivery in the treatment of critically ill patients. *N Engl J Med* 1994;330:1717

128. Shoemaker WC: Temporal patterns of $\dot{D}o_2$ and $\dot{V}o_2$: predictions of outcome and therapeutic goals. In: Vincent JL (ed). *Yearbook of Intensive Care and Emergency Medicine*. Berlin, Springer-Verlag, 1994:132

129. Gattinoni L, Brazzi L, Pelosi P, et al: A trial of goal-oriented hemodynamic therapy in critically ill patients. *N Engl J Med* 1995;333:1025

130. Mythen MG, Webb AR: Intra-operative gut mucosal hypoperfusion is associated with increased post-operative complications and cost. *Intensive Care Med* 1994;20:99

131. Ivatury RR, Simon RJ, Havriliak D, et al: Gastric mucosal pH and oxygen delivery and oxygen consumption indices in the assessment of adequacy of resuscitation after trauma: a prospective, randomized study. *J Trauma* 1995;39:128

132. Marik PE: Gastric intramucosal pH: a better predictor of multiorgan dysfunction syndrome and death than oxygen-derived variables in patients with sepsis. *Chest* 1993;104:225

133. Gutierrez G, Bismar H, Dantzker DR, et al: Comparison of gastric intramucosal pH with measures of oxygen transport and consumption in critically ill patients. *Crit Care Med* 1992;20:451

134. Gutierrez G, Palizas F, Doglio G, et al: Gastric intramucosal pH as a therapeutic index of tissue oxygenation in critically ill patients. *Lancet* 1992;339:195

135. McCloskey RV, Straube RC, Sanders C, et al: Treatment of septic shock with human monoclonal antibody HA-1A: a randomized, double-blind, placebo-controlled trial. *Ann Intern Med* 1994;120:1

136. Fisher JC, Dhainaut JF, Opal SM, et al: Recombinant human interleukin-1 receptor antagonist in the treatment of patients with the sepsis syndrome: results from a randomized, double-blind, placebo-controlled trial. *JAMA* 1994;271:1836

137. Fein AM, Bernard GR, Criner GJ, et al: Treatment of severe systemic inflammatory response syndrome (SIRS) and sepsis with a novel bradykinin antagonist CP-0127: results of a randomized, double-blind, placebo-controlled trial. *JAMA* 1996 (in press)

138. Marshall JC, Christou NV, Meakins JL: The gastrointestinal tract: the undrained "abscess" of multiple organ failure. *Ann Surg* 1993;218:111

139. Gastinne H, Wolff M, Delatour F, et al: A controlled trial in intensive care units of selective decontamination of the digestive tract with nonabsorbable antibiotics. *N Engl J Med* 1992;326:594

140. Rocha LA, Martin MJ, Pita S, et al: Prevention of nosocomial infection in critically ill patients by selective decontamination of the digestive tract: a randomized, double blind, placebo-controlled study. *Intensive Care Med* 1992;18:398

141. Hammond JMJ, Saunders GL, Potgieter PD, et al: A double blind study of selective decontamination in intensive care. *Lancet* 1992;340:5

142. Cerra FB, Moddaus MA, Dunn DL, et al: Selective gut decontamination reduces nosocomial infections and length of stay, but not mortality or organ failure in SICU patients. *Arch Surg* 1992;127:163

Critical Care, Third Edition, edited by Joseph M. Civetta,
Robert W. Taylor, and Robert R. Kirby.
Lippincott-Raven Publishers, Philadelphia, PA © 1997.

CHAPTER 26

Shock

Edgar J. Jimenez

IMMEDIATE CONCERNS

MAJOR PROBLEMS

Shock may be difficult to define, but translating any definition into measurable parameters that can aid clinical recognition is more difficult still. How severe is severe? What actually constitutes organ dysfunction? These are questions that plague the literature on shock and the clinician faced with a patient exhibiting less than the full shock syndrome (Table 26-1). In this section, essential guidelines are presented to confront this condition.

Two common systemic manifestations of shock are metabolic acidosis and arterial hypotension; nevertheless, they are not prerequisites for recognition of the syndrome. Metabolic (lactic) acidosis results from tissue hypoxia and anaerobic metabolism, often complicated by hepatic function inadequate to metabolize the increased lactate. The severity of acidosis varies greatly and is correlated with a poor outcome.[1,2] A fall in arterial pressure can be a harbinger of potential shock and a common manifestation of shock itself. Marked decreases in systemic blood pressure inevitably lead to hypoperfusion and vital organ dysfunction. However, changes in regional vascular resistance can compensate for modest decreases in perfusion pressure, thereby maintaining perfusion to vital organs. Arterial hypotension often can be treated before vital organ dysfunction is clinically obvious, preventing irreversible organ dysfunction or ameliorating its severity.

The brain, heart, and kidneys are usually affected by shock. The severity of organ dysfunction and clinical presentation, however, vary with previous levels of organ function, compensatory mechanisms, and the cause of the shock syndrome. Although other organ systems are affected, they are not as helpful initially for clinical recognition and management.

The brain is able to autoregulate its perfusion despite moderate changes in perfusion pressure (in this case, mean systemic arterial pressure minus intracerebral pressure). Eventually, cerebral perfusion decreases if mean arterial pressure (MAP) falls below 60 to 70 mm Hg.[3,4] Cerebral perfusion falls at even higher levels of arterial pressure in previously hypertensive patients.[5] Although the decrease in cerebral perfusion affects all levels of brain function, the most common clinical manifestation is an acute change in mental state, varying from mild changes in mental acuity to frank coma.

The heart is particularly important because cardiac dysfunction from shock can perpetuate shock, leading to further coronary hypoperfusion and a cycle of ever-worsening cardiac dysfunction. This type of adverse feedback is common in the pathophysiologic mechanism of shock; breaking the cycle is a key aspect of management.

Cardiac dysfunction manifests itself in several ways. The most common presentation, tachycardia, is primarily caused by a reflex neurohumoral response to decreased myocardial performance. The pulse is frequently thready, indicating a low cardiac stroke volume. With coronary ischemia, more complex rhythm disturbances may occur, and these also can impair cardiac function. Systemic arterial hypotension increases coronary ischemia and worsens cardiac dysfunction. As the heart fails, left ventricular end-diastolic pressure rises, ultimately causing pulmonary edema and respiratory failure. The impairment in gas exchange causes hypoxemia, exaggerating tissue hypoxia. The most common clinical symptoms of coronary hypoperfusion are chest pain and dyspnea; physical signs include the appearance of a dyskinetic apical cardiac impulse, a new third or fourth heart

TABLE 26-1.   Clinical Recognition of Shock

ORGAN SYSTEM	SYMPTOM OR SIGN	CAUSES
CNS	Mental status changes	↓ Cerebral perfusion
	Pinpoint pupils	Narcotic overdose
Circulatory		
Heart	Tachycardia	Adrenergic stimulation, depressed contractility
	Other dysrhythmias	Coronary ischemia
	Hypotension	Depressed contractility secondary to ischemia or MDFs, right ventricular failure
	New murmurs	Valvular dysfunction, VSD
Systemic	Hypotension	↓ SVR, ↓ venous return
	↓ JVP	Hypovolemia, ↓ venous return
	↑ JVP	Right heart failure
	Disparate peripheral pulses	Aortic dissection
Respiratory	Tachypnea	Pulmonary edema, respiratory muscle fatigue, sepsis, acidosis
	Cyanosis	Hypoxemia
Renal	Oliguria	↓ Perfusion, afferent arteriolar vasoconstriction
Skin	Cool, clammy	Vasoconstriction, sympathetic stimulation
Other	Lactic acidosis	Anaerobic metabolism, hepatic dysfunction
	Fever	Infection

MDFs, myocardial depressant factors; VSD, ventricular septal defect; SVR, systemic vascular resistance; JVP, jugular venous pulsations.

sound, a new murmur of mitral regurgitation (representing papillary muscle dysfunction), and pulmonary crackles. Electrocardiographic signs (e.g., ST or T wave changes) of myocardial ischemia also can be expected.

Renal function depends critically on perfusion. The kidney, like the brain and heart, autoregulates its perfusion over a moderate range of arterial pressures. When hypoperfusion occurs, the glomerular filtration rate falls. Oliguria is a common manifestation of shock. As with other organs, the perfusion deficit may be absolute or relative; it may reflect an overall decrease of blood flow or an unfavorable redistribution. In the kidney, redistribution of blood flow from the renal cortex toward the renal medulla occurs as perfusion decreases.

When the skin is poorly perfused, its temperature falls and its color changes. It is often pale and dusky, representing oligemia and venous pooling of blood desaturated of oxygen. With concomitant hypoxemia, frank cyanosis can exist. Sympathetic nervous system stimulation, a compensation for hypotension, causes sweat gland hypersecretion. The result is the frequently observed cool, clammy skin of shock. However, shock can occur without these features. Activation of the coagulation system is common, although disseminated intravascular coagulation (DIC) is not often clinically evident at initial presentation. Liver failure is occasionally prominent. If shock is caused by infection, hyperglycemia and fever are usually present; paradoxically, hypothermia also can occur.

Shock may be classified into four groups—*hypovolemic (oligemic), cardiogenic, extracardiac obstructive,* and *distributive*—that may overlap synergistically (Table 26-2, Fig.

26-1). The recognition of these hemodynamic patterns (Table 26-3) may help elucidate the etiology and guide the management in complicated cases. The multiple organ dysfunction syndrome (MODS), observed in advanced cases, results as a "final common pathway" of these categories and has been associated with the initial or postreperfusion "triggering" of cytokine and other humoral and cell-mediated inflammatory responses.

STRESS POINTS

1. Shock is a syndrome characterized by an acute generalized disturbance in the normal circulatory pattern, resulting in ineffective perfusion and severe dysfunction of critical organs (Table 26-4).
2. Confusion, tachycardia, arterial hypotension, and oliguria are the most common early manifestations of brain, cardiac, and kidney dysfunction, respectively. More severe degrees of shock produce coma, myocardial ischemia, and pulmonary edema.
3. The possibility of a successful recovery increases with a rapid reversal of the precipitating factors and maintenance of the vital functions. Treatment must start *immediately* when the condition is suspected.
4. Although the syndrome is divided into four basic hemodynamic patterns, the pathophysiologic mechanisms overlap and may act synergistically. Septic shock (in essence, distributive shock) is the major cause of intensive care unit (ICU) mortality.[6-8]
5. The appearance of MODS with refractory hypotension and persistent lactic acidosis heralds a poor outcome.

TABLE 26-2.   Classification of Shock

HYPOVOLEMIC (OLIGEMIC)

Hemorrhagic
  Trauma (external, internal, retroperitoneal, or
    intraperitoneal bleed)
  Gastrointestinal
Nonhemorrhagic
  Dehydration
  Vomiting
  Diarrhea
  Fistulas
  Burns
  Polyuric (DKA, DI, adrenocortical insufficiency)
  "Third spacing" (peritonitis, pancreatitis, ascitis)

CARDIOGENIC

Myocardial
  Infarction (including stunning and hibernation)
  Contusion
  Myocarditis (viral, autoimmune, parasitic)
  Cardiomyopathies (e.g., hypertrophic, amyloid)
  Pharmacologic/toxic depression (beta-blockers, calcium
    channel blockers, TCA, anthracycline)
  Intrinsic depression (SIRS-related, i.e., "depressants,"
    acidosis, hypoxia)
Mechanical
  Valvular or dynamic stenosis
  Valvular regurgitation
  Ventricular septal defects
  Ventricular wall defects and aneurysms
Arrhythmias (tachycardias, bradycardias, atrioventricular
  blocks)

EXTRACARDIAC OBSTRUCTIVE

Extrinsic vascular compression
  Mediastinal tumors
Increased intrathoracic pressure
  Tension pneumothorax
  Positive-pressure ventilation
Intrinsic vascular flow obstruction
  Pulmonary embolism
  Air embolism
  Tumors
  Aortic dissection
  Aortic coarctation
  Acute pulmonary hypertension
Pericardic
  Tamponade (trauma, myocardial rupture, Dressler's
    syndrome, inflammatory, autoimmune, infectious,
    malignancy, uremia, or anticoagulation)
  Pericarditis (constrictive)
Miscellaneous (hyperviscosity syndrome, sickle cell crysis,
  polycytemia vera)

DISTRIBUTIVE

SIRS-related
  Sepsis (bacterial, fungal, viral, rickettsial)
  Pancreatitis
  Trauma
  Burns
Anaphylactic/anaphylactoid (Hymenoptera venoms,
  medications)
Neurogenic (spinal trauma)
Toxic/pharmacologic (vasodilators, benzodiazepines)
Endocrine (thyroid, myxedema, adrenal insufficiency)

DI, diabetes insipidus; DKA, diabetic ketoacidosis; TCA, tricyclic antidepressants; SIRS, systemic inflammatory response syndrome.

TABLE 26-3.   Common Hemodynamic Patterns in Shock

TYPE	CO	SVR	PAOP	CVP	S$\bar{\text{v}}$O$_2$
Hypovolemic (oligemic)	↓	↑	↓	↓	↓
Cardiogenic					
Left Ventricular MI	↓	↑	↑	Nl–↑	↓
Right Ventricular MI	↓	↑	Nl–↓°	↑°	↓
Extracardiac Obstructive					
Pericardial tamponade	↓	↑	↑†	↑†	↓
Massive pulmonary embolism	↓	↑	Nl–↓‡	↑	↓
Distributive					
Early	↓–Nl–↑	↑–Nl–↓	Nl	Nl–↑	Nl–↓
Early after fluid administration	↑	↓	Nl–↑	Nl–↑	↓–Nl–↑
Late	↓	↑	Nl	Nl	↓ (Rarely ↑)

CO, cardiac output; SVR, systemic vascular resistance; PAOP, pulmonary artery occlusion pressure; CVP, central venous pressure; S$\bar{\text{v}}$O$_2$, mixed venous oxygen saturation; MI, myocardial infarction.

°Occasionally, equalization of pressures suggesting periocardial tamponade may exist.
†Equalization (±3 mm Hg) of pressures is characteristic, including pulmonary artery diastolic and right ventricular end-diastolic pressure.
‡May be clinically unobtainable or uninterpretable.

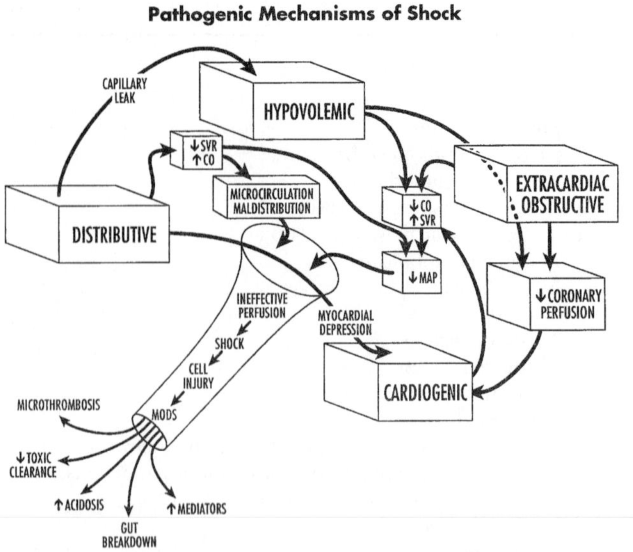

Pathogenic Mechanisms of Shock

FIGURE 26-1. Pathogenic mechanisms of shock. CO, cardiac output; MAP, mean arterial pressure; MODS, multiple organ dysfunction syndrome; SVR, systemic vascular resistance.

ESSENTIAL DIAGNOSTIC TESTS AND PROCEDURES

1. Consider as serious a systemic systolic blood pressure of less than 90 mm Hg or a drop of 40 mm Hg or more from the usual systolic pressure in patients with prior hypertension. An accurate blood pressure measurement is necessary to avoid falsely low readings, especially when treatment is initiated. Doppler devices or direct measurement by an indwelling catheter may be required during early assessment and management.

2. Obtain a series of baseline tests that include the following: complete blood cell count and differential; platelet count; complete serum chemistry profile; prothrombin and activated partial thromboplastin times; serum lactate; a urinalysis with microscopic sediment analysis; serum amylase; and arterial blood gases. A pregnancy test should be obtained in all female patients of childbearing age. A 12-lead electrocardiogram (ECG) and chest radiograph should be performed.

3. Blood, sputum, and urine Gram stains and cultures always should be ordered in cases of suspected sepsis. Consider other tests depending on other possible etiologies, like computed tomography scans, abdominal radiographs, or ultrasound; echocardiogram; ventilation-perfusion scan; angiograms; and cardiac isoenzymes or right-sided ECG.

4. In cases where a significant blood loss is observed, anticipated, or suspected, type and cross match for several units of packed red blood cells (RBCs) and fresh frozen plasma.

5. Keep in mind that certain etiologies, like tension pneumothorax or cardiac tamponade, can present with precipitous drops in blood pressure that may require immediate decompression before any initial tests.

INITIAL THERAPY

1. The airway should remain patent and the ventilation and oxygenation effective, or endotracheal intubation and mechanical ventilation should be implemented *at once.*

2. Secure at least two peripheral large-bore intravenous lines. Consider early catheterization of central veins with a pulmonary artery catheter *introducer* (8.5

TABLE 26-4.   Multiple Organ System Failure

ORGAN	PRESENTATION	SYNDROME
Lung	Hypoxemia + diffuse infiltrates	ARDS
Kidney	Creatinine >2 mg/dL or 2 × admission	
	Urine output <500 mL/24 h	Oliguric ARF
	Urine output >500 mL/24 h	Nonoliguric ARF
Liver	Bilirubin 2 mg/dL, AST and LDH 2 × admission	Cholestatic jaundice
	Intractable hyperglycemia or hypoglycemia	Hepatocyte failure
	Cholecystitis with nonlithogenic bile	Acalculous choleystitis
Gut	Upper GI bleeding, 2 U/24 h	Stress ulceration
	Endoscopically confirmed superficial ulceration	
Coagulation	Thrombocytopenia, prolonged PT and PTT with FDP	DIC, hypofibrinogenemia
Heart	Hypotension, CI <1.5 L/min/m², no MI	Myocardial failure
Central nervous system	Response only to painful stimuli	Obtundation of sepsis
Peripheral nervous system	Peripheral neuropathy	Generalized muscle weakness

ARDS, acute respiratory distress syndrome; ARF, acute renal failure; PT, prothrombin time; PTT, partial thromboplastin time; FDP, fibrin degradation products; CI, cardiac index; AST, aspartate aminotransferase; LDH, lactate dehydrogenase; DIC, disseminated intravascular coagulation; GI, gastrointestinal; 2 × admission, twice the level on admission.

French) if the peripheral access is difficult to obtain, when rapid or large volume replacements are anticipated, and to facilitate further hemodynamic monitoring in refractory or complicated cases.

3. Any hemodynamically relevant bradyarrhythmias or tachyarrhythmias should be managed (Chap. 118).

4. If congestive heart failure is not detected initially by physical examination or chest radiograph, blood pressure may be improved by a cautious trial of fluid administration (500 to 750 mL of a colloid or 1000 to 2000 mL of a crystalloid solution during the first hour).

5. When blood is required immediately, O-negative units may be used until type-specific uncrossmatched or the more time-consuming fully crossmatched units are available.

6. With moderate and severe decreases of systemic blood pressure, catecholamine infusions (Table 26-5) may be started as the fluid administration continues.

Dopamine is often used initially. In nonresponsive cases or with severe hypotension, adding or starting a norepinephrine infusion should be an *early* consideration (Fig. 26-2).

7. If hypotension does not improve or if signs of congestive heart failure are evident or emerge, hemodynamic monitoring with a thermistor-tipped pulmonary artery catheter[9] should be undertaken rapidly. These measurements can be useful in resolving conflicts between radiographic interpretations of pulmonary infiltrates and the clinical evaluation; in defining the prognosis associated with severe pulmonary edema; and in guiding fluid, vasopressor, and inotropic therapies.

8. In cases of suspected sepsis or if distributive shock of undetermined etiology ensues, empiric broad-spectrum antibiotic coverage should be started while a more specific evaluation is performed.

9. Patients with potential for adrenal insufficiency—

TABLE 26-5. Sympathomimetic Drugs

DRUG	USUAL IV DOSE	ADRENERGIC EFFECTS			ARRHYTHMOGENIC POTENTIAL	SETTING
		α	β	*Dopamine*		
Dopamine	1–2 μg/kg/min°	1+	1+	3+	1+	Oliguria despite "normal" blood pressure
	2–10 μg/kg/min	2+	2+	3+	2+	
	10–30 μg/kg/min	3+	2+	3+	3+	Initial emergency treatment of hypotension (any cause) and alternative treatment for bradycardia
Dobutamine	2–30 μg/kg/min	1+	3+	0	2+	Cardiac shock, cardiac pulmonary edema with marginal blood pressure
Norepinephrine	0.5–80 μg/min	3+	2+	0	2+	Initial emergency treatment of hypotension (any cause, especially sepsis)
Epinephrine	0.5–1 **mg**[§] (1:10,000)	1+	2+	0	3+	Cardiac arrest
	1–200 μg/min	2+	3+	0	3+	Severe hypotension and bradycardia
	0.3–0.5 **mg** SQ (1:1,000)[‡]					Anaphylaxis
Phenylephrine	20–200 μg/min	3+	0	0	0	Distributive shock when no cardiac effect desired
Isoproterenol	2–10 μg/min	0	3+	0	3+	Refractory bradycardia; denervated hearts; refractory torsade de pointes
Amrinone[†]	Load: 0.75 **mg**/kg over 3 min Then: 2–15 μg/kg/min	0	0	0	2+	Cardiogenic shock; usually as synergistic agent with dobutamine
Milrinone[†]	Load: 50 μg/kg over 10 min Then: 0.375–0.75 μg/kg/min	0	0	0	2+	Cardiogenic shock; usually as synergistic agent with dobutamine

IV, intravenous.
°Increases renal and splanchnic blood flow.
[†]Phosphodiesterase inhibitors; require loading dose.
[‡]SQ: Subcutaneous dosing, may be repeated every 15–20 min.
[§]Milligram doses are in bold to differentiate from micrograms.

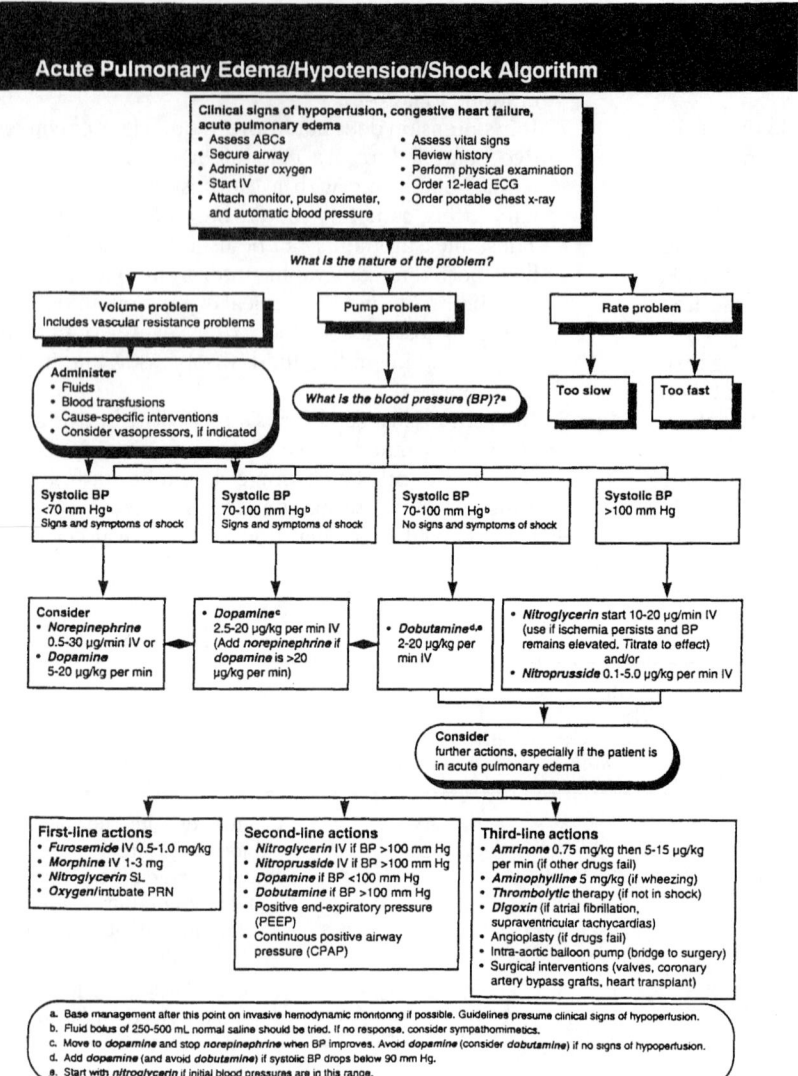

FIGURE 26-2. Acute pulmonary edema/hypotension/shock algorithm. IV, intravenous; ECG, electrocardiogram; BP, blood pressure. (With permission from *Textbook of Advanced Cardiac Life Support.* Dallas, American Heart Association, 1994: 1.)

another form of distributive shock—may present with refractory hypotension despite adequate fluid replacement and vasopressors. Dexamethasone therapy may be started before a corticotropin (ACTH) stimulation test (Chap. 146).

10. Patients presenting with cardiogenic ischemic events should be expeditiously screened for thrombolysis, should the blood pressure improve,[10] or prepared for emergent cardiac catheterization.[11] Similarly, the suspicion of a massive pulmonary embolus requires a rapid implementation of a perfusion scan or an angiogram for possible embolectomy or thrombolysis.[12]

11. Depending on the case, other interventions that to be considered are as follows: use of morphine sulfate, loop diuretics, and sublingual or intravenous nitroglycerin; or nitroprusside and intraaortic balloon pumping to manipulate preload and afterload, re-

spectively, when cardiogenic events with myocardial or valvular failure occur. In selected cases, where the blood pressure allows, cautious trials of dobutamine or milrinone infusions may improve contractility and decrease afterload.

OVERVIEW ■

The devastating effects of severe trauma have been part of clinical descriptions throughout the history of medicine since the times of Hippocrates. Nevertheless, the relationship of these descriptions with the French term *choc* and its English translation did not occur until the mid-18th century. It seems that the first evidence of an attempt to separate the initial insult from the posttraumatic disorders did not occur until the mid-19th century by Morris.[13]

Virtually every aspect of shock, from definition to treatment, remains controversial, and it has changed in time as we have continued to learn about this entity. This uncertainty is understandably frustrating, and the frustration is compounded by the knowledge that untreated shock inevitably leads to death. As a result, the physician in the ICU often must initiate management immediately, before an adequate database has been collected or a cause has been determined.

Unfortunately, despite decades of research, the mortality remains high.[8] The clear understanding of the interaction of different pathways leading to the physiologic derangements has eluded us until recently, when we have begun to identify the essentials of biomolecular phenomena involved in its pathophysiologic mechanisms. These include the release of cytokines, the cleavage of organelle and cell membranes, the formation of eicosanoid-based compounds, the activation of humoral- and cell-mediated inflammatory responses, the abnormalities in coagulation and cell adhesion, the formation of free radicals, the enhanced synthesis of nitric oxide,[14] and many others that initially or, as a reperfusion effect, alter the homeostasis. These issues are covered in detail in other chapters.

Following certain well-founded principles of therapy, we can improve the outcome of shock. This chapter emphasizes these principles and explains their physiologic basis following well-recognized hemodynamic profiles. Most successful outcomes ultimately depend on the prompt and effective treatment of the underlying disorder; therefore, general management issues discussed here must be accompanied by a simultaneous effort to diagnose and reverse the specific etiology.

DEFINITION ■

Although some researchers define shock as a metabolic defect, we prefer a more traditional definition that incorporates a perfusion abnormality as central to the pathophysiologic mechanism. *Shock is an acute clinical syndrome initiated by ineffective perfusion, resulting in severe dysfunction of organs vital to survival.*

Ineffective perfusion is a key concept for understanding and recognizing the shock state. Organ dysfunction initiated by other causes *is not* shock. Organ perfusion can be compromised by an overall decrease or maldistribution in cardiac output. Abnormalities in the distribution of blood flow within the organ can further aggravate organ dysfunction. Also, at different stages depending on the mechanism, the tissues themselves may be incapable of using what substrate is supplied, mimicking or worsening the effects of hypoperfusion.

Notice the emphasis on shock as a syndrome, that is, a relatively constant set of signs and symptoms that predictably result from well-described pathophysiologic events. Shock *is* a systemic disorder; the clinical presentation varies because each organ system is affected differently, depending

on the severity of the perfusion defect, the underlying cause, and prior organ dysfunction.

CLASSIFICATION AND CLINICAL RECOGNITION ■

Several well-recognized basic hemodynamic profiles have been described. For didactic reasons and to facilitate early intervention and etiologic diagnosis, we refer to the most widely accepted classification of shock proposed by Weil and Shubin in 1972,[15] which divides the syndrome into four major categories: hypovolemic, cardiogenic, extracardiac obstructive, and distributive (see Table 26-2). However, notice that this is an artificial separation and that there is frequent, considerable initial mixing and overlap within these categories because patients may present simultaneously with different precipitating and synergistic factors (see Fig. 26-1).

In septic shock, the systemic vascular resistance and the distribution of cardiac output are abnormal, but cardiomyopathic and hypovolemic features can play important roles as well, either as part of the primary mechanism (i.e., myocardial depression and capillary leakage) or as a concomitant illnesses (i.e., a myocardial infarction or a gastrointestinal hemorrhage). Similarly, although severe trauma is often associated to hypovolemic shock, neurologic and postanesthetic components may compound the clinical picture with distributive shock features, manifested by hypotension to a degree that is out of proportion to blood loss or other signs of hypovolemia.[16–18]

These categories converge also in the activation of shared, cascading pathophysiologic disturbances that are activated initially or as a reperfusion effect during resuscitation. In some cases, despite our most sophisticated monitoring and current therapeutic interventions, they continue to progress to the well-recognized multiorgan dysfunction and mortality associated with this syndrome.

HYPOVOLEMIC SHOCK (OLIGEMIC)

Hypovolemic shock occurs with various mechanisms that decrease the intravascular volume, including severe external or internal bleeds, marked fluid losses from a gastrointestinal (diarrhea, vomiting) or urinary (hyperosmolar states, diuretics) source. Also, fluid loss can occur from malnutrition; from "capillary leakage" into the interstitium or corporal cavities (the so-called "third spacing" that occurs after trauma, surgery, sepsis, and cardiac, liver, and kidney failure); or it can be compounded by added losses through damaged skin, as in the case of burns[19] and other epidermolytic or scalded conditions.

Hypovolemic shock produces the prototypic hemodynamic picture of the shock syndrome (see Table 26-3). It is characterized by marked decreases in cardiac diastolic filling pressures and volumes with the resulting decrease in stroke volume. Cardiac output is partially maintained by a compensatory tachycardia. Reflex increases in peripheral vascular resistance and myocardial contractility, mediated by neurohumoral mechanisms and associated with intrinsic autoregulation, maintain perfusion to the brain and heart. However, as the blood loss exceeds 20% to 25% of the intravascular volume, these compensatory mechanisms are no longer effective; arterial hypotension and decreasing cardiac output result. The normal blood volume of an adult is approximately 70 mL/kg, and hypotension is usually evident after an acute blood volume loss of 1500 mL or more. Classic clinical manifestations become evident, such as tachycardia with thready pulses, tachypnea, flat peripheral and neck veins, as well as some initial indicators of compromised end-organ perfusion like a pale, cool, and clammy skin with an increased capillary refill time above 2 seconds, decreased urinary output, and altered mental status.

The decrease in cardiac output diminishes oxygen transport to peripheral tissues. Tissues that can maintain their oxygen consumption by increasing oxygen extraction do so, leading to a widening of the arteriovenous oxygen content difference $[C(a - v)O_2]$. Eventually, this compensatory mechanism also fails, and tissue hypoxia and lactic acidosis supervene, usually heralding a poor outcome.[20-22] Cerebral and cardiac function are maintained by the diversion of blood flow from skin, muscle, and kidneys by neurohumoral mechanisms. When these compensatory mechanisms are no longer effective, cardiac function deteriorates further, worsening tissue oxygen delivery. It is recognized that sustained insults, like blood losses in excess of 40% for over 2 hours,[23-26] may result in disengaging inflammatory–mediator responses at a systemic level, which further compound and worsen the initial dysfunction, rendering any resuscitative effort as insufficient.

CARDIOGENIC SHOCK

The hemodynamic picture of cardiogenic shock from myocardial failure and that of hypovolemic shock are virtually identical, with an important exception: cardiogenic shock generates elevated cardiac chamber filling pressures that produce the characteristic clinical findings of pulmonary edema and increased jugular venous pulsations. In fact, shock should not be diagnosed as cardiogenic unless the cardiac index is below 2 L/minute/m² and the pulmonary artery occlusion pressure (PAOP) is greater than 17 to 20 mm Hg. In some cases, a trial of fluid administration is required to achieve these filling pressures. A low cardiac output in a patient with myocardial infarction and a low PAOP may reflect hypovolemia (e.g., excessive diuretic administration).

Many cardiac disorders can cause hypotension and shock (see Table 26-2), but all invariably decrease cardiac output. A primary failure of the contractile apparatus caused by ischemia, infarction, or cardiomyopathy is not always the responsible mechanism. Other causes of cardiogenic shock include bradyarrhythmia and tachyarrhythmia, conduction system disturbances, cardiac valvular lesions, mechanical complications of acute myocardial infarction (e.g., acute mitral valvular regurgitation, ventricular septal rupture), cardiac contusion, myocarditis, and end-stage cardiomyopathies of different etiology.

Cardiogenic shock from an acute left ventricular myocardial infarction occurs when more than 40% of the left ventricle is involved and may occur in 10% to 20% of Q wave infarcts.[27-29] Also, in this type of shock, a correlation between the degree of lactic acidosis and the predicted mortality has been described[30]; however, in general, the mortality exceeds 75% unless a surgically correctable lesion, such as a ventricular aneurysm or valvular dysfunction, is found.

Signs of peripheral vasoconstriction and distended neck veins may be prominent, pulmonary edema is frequent, and oliguria is virtually always present. Cardiac signs depend on the underlying cause, varying from an S_3 gallop to loud murmurs when valvular mechanisms are compromised or ruptures occur. Hemodynamic findings consist of decreased cardiac output, arterial hypotension, elevated PAOP, and a widened $C(a - v)O_2$ (see Table 26-3). Echocardiography or radionuclide ventriculography confirms poor left ventricular function.

Some complicating features—like myocardial wall or septal rupture, usually occurring between the third to seventh day after infarction—may change the hemodynamic pattern, showing, respectively, the equalization of diastolic pulmonary vascular and right ventricular pressures of cardiac tamponade (extracardiac obstructive), or right-sided failure (pulmonary embolus or right ventricular infarct). If any of these entities are suspected, *emergency* surface or transesophageal echocardiography or angiography should be obtained.

Remember that hypotension from other causes in patients with coronary artery disease can rapidly produce myocardial ischemia, infarction, shock, and death.[31,32]

Right Ventricular Infarct

An important variant of cardiogenic shock results from right ventricular dysfunction.[33,34] Right ventricular infarcts may be seen in as much as 50% of all inferior wall infarcts. However, cardiogenic shock only occurs in 10% to 20% of patients with right ventricular infarct.[35,36] The lungs are clear despite the presence of jugular venous distention. Occasionally, a prominent cervical venous pulse or distention during inspiration (Kussmaul's sign) may be observed. Hemodynamic findings vary, but they frequently include elevated right atrial pressure compared with the PAOP, elevated right ventricular diastolic pressure, and decreased pulmonary artery pressure. The cardiac output is decreased, and equalization of atrial and ventricular end-diastolic pressures commonly occurs. In this case, cardiac tamponade must be excluded (see Table 26-3). Echocardiography and radionuclide ventriculograms can help with this determination and demonstrate decreased right ventricular function. Left ventricular contractility may be normal or abnormal, depending on whether it is affected by ischemia. In the presence of right ventricular dysfunction, a pulmonary perfusion or ventilation-perfusion scan may be necessary to exclude pulmonary embolization, although in this case, pulmonary hypertension usually accompanies shock. Pulmonary hypertension can be diagnosed with Doppler echocardiography or hemodynamic monitoring. This type of myocardial infarction treatment differs markedly from that indicated for those affecting mainly the left ventricle and is discussed later.

EXTRACARDIAC OBSTRUCTIVE SHOCK

Extracardiac obstructive shock is associated with a physical impairment to adequate forward circulatory flow involving mechanisms different than primary myocardial or valvular apparatus dysfunction. Its etiology includes many diverse entities that either (1) impair the diastolic filling, like cardiac tamponade, tension pneumothorax, constrictive pericarditis, and compression of the great veins by mediastinal masses; or, (2) increase the right or left ventricular afterload, as is the case of massive pulmonary embolization,[37] acute pulmonary hypertension, or aortic dissection and systemic embolization, respectively.

The varied clinical presentation of this form easily overlaps with hypovolemic and cardiogenic shock, with the usual evidence of low output and compromised end-organ perfusion; and the presence or absence of distended neck veins, depending on the mechanism. Other signs, sometimes subtle, may be present, such as muffled heart sounds or pulsus paradoxus in the case of cardiac tamponade, or more dramatic ones like tearing and transfixing pain in the case of an aortic dissection.

Several hemodynamic patterns may be observed, depending on the cause (see Table 26-3), from frank decrease in filling pressures (as is the case of mediastinal compressions of great veins); to trends toward equalization of pressures in the case of cardiac tamponade and constrictive pericarditis; or to markedly increased right ventricular filling pressures with low PAOP in the case of a massive pulmonary embolization (when more than 50% to 60% of the vascular bed is affected).[38,39] As is the case with the previously discussed patterns of shock, cardiac output in this setting is usually decreased, the systemic vascular resistance is increased, and there is marked widening of the $C(a - v)O_2$.

DISTRIBUTIVE SHOCK

Distributive shock is often described, in its initial phases, as a hyperdynamic state with a high cardiac output, normal to low cardiac filling pressures, and the defining decreased systemic vascular resistance.[40-42] The mixed venous oxygen tension ($P\bar{v}O_2$) may be normal or increased, and the calculated oxygen consumption varies. This typical hyperdynamic pattern is most commonly associated with the *systemic inflammatory response syndrome* (SIRS),[43] triggered classically by sepsis.[44] SIRS also may be associated with other noninfectious insults like pancreatitis, multitrauma and tissue injury,[45] burns, immune-mediated organ injury, and in the late stages of hemorrhagic and other types of shock.

This hyperdynamic pattern with low systemic vascular resistance also is seen in some other entities such as adrenal insufficiency, hyperthyroidism, anaphylaxis, severe hepatic dysfunction, and neurogenic dysfunction (e.g., postanesthesia or spinal cord injuries).

The detailed description of SIRS and its complicated homeostatic disturbances is beyond the scope of this chapter and is found elsewhere in this book (Chaps. 20, 25, and 28). An understanding of SIRS is, however, vital for the critical care clinician because it is a leading cause of ICU mortality.[8,46]

Septic Shock

Septic shock is caused by infectious agents or their products in the bloodstream.[47] Gram-negative organisms are responsible for most cases. Also, with emerging importance, gram-positive bacteria,[48,49] fungi, and viruses[40,50,51] are capable of producing a syndrome indistinguishable from that caused by gram-negative bacteria as the generalized inflammatory response is mounted. Mortality overall can be in the order of 50% and probably higher for gram-negative–associated shock, even with aggressive treatment[52] and seems to correlate with the level of some cytokines.[53] Most of the deaths occur during the first week as a result of circulatory failure; only 25% occur at a later stage and usually present as overwhelming *MODS* (see Table 26-4).[54]

The initial host response to *SIRS* or *sepsis*, by definition,[44] is characterized by two or more of the following: (1) temperature above 38C or below 36C; (2) tachycardia (heart rate higher than 90 beats per minute); (3) tachypnea (respiratory rate above 20 breaths per minute) or respiratory alkalosis (PaCO$_2$ less than 32 mm Hg); and (4) abnormal leukocyte count (white blood cell count greater than 12,000 cells/mm^3 or less than 4000 cells/mm^3 or more than 10% bands). In *severe sepsis*, the clinical picture is compounded by hypotension or hypoperfusion with organ dysfunction manifested but not limited to lactic acidosis, decreased urinary output, and altered mental status. If, despite adequate fluid resuscitation, the above condition persists, *septic shock* ensues with the requirement of inotropes, vasopressors, or both to achieve acceptable vital parameters. As a result of these interventions, hypotension may not be apparent despite the persistent organ dysfunction seen on this complicated clinical picture.[55]

Although cardiac output is often elevated during septic shock, cardiac function and peripheral perfusion are abnormal.[41,56,57] Abnormalities in systolic function are characterized by decreases in stroke volume and depression of the ejection fraction.[58,59] Abnormalities in myocardial contractility have been demonstrated experimentally and may be caused by "myocardial depressant factors" that enhance the synthesis of myocardial nitric oxide[60-63] or coronary ischemia. Because contractility may be abnormal, increasing preload (e.g., with intravascular volume expansion) may not increase stroke volume and may instead exacerbate pulmonary edema.

Abnormalities in ventricular compliance (diastolic dysfunction) also occur in septic shock. An abnormal ventricular compliance means that the relationship between the PAOP and left ventricular end-diastolic volume is no longer normal. The interpretation of PAOP measurements in patients with sepsis is difficult and must be made with caution.

A significant decrease in systemic vascular resistance, often out of proportion to any increase in cardiac output, is common in septic shock and may be responsible for refractory hypotension in many patients. The pathogenesis of decreased peripheral vascular tone seems to be associated with systemic or locally produced mediators that induce the formation of nitric oxide.[64]

The classic hemodynamic picture of early sepsis (i.e., high cardiac output, low systemic vascular resistance, hypotension) is not always present. Experimental models of sepsis using nonhuman primates often demonstrate an early decrease in venous return as a result of intravascular volume loss and splanchnic redistribution of cardiac output.[65] The initial hemodynamic picture in this model resembles hypovolemic shock; the hyperdynamic picture in this model does not become evident *until* fluid resuscitation is accomplished. Whether a similar phenomenon occurs in humans is not clear because, in many instances, some degree of fluid resuscitation has already taken place before hemodynamic measurements are obtained. Other factors, such as the host response to sepsis and preexisting abnormalities of cardiac function, further confuse the hemodynamic picture. In the terminal stages of septic shock, cardiac function deteriorates, and the hemodynamic pattern often resembles that of cardiogenic shock.[66]

In septic shock, the mixed venous oxygen tension and saturation may be normal despite profound shock. The reasons for this apparently inappropriate increase are not clear, but decreased peripheral use, abnormal distribution of perfusion, and arteriovenous shunting all have been invoked. Sepsis may impose a cellular defect early in the course of shock, decreasing peripheral use of oxygen. Interpretation of mixed venous oxygen data should be undertaken with caution in patients with septic shock.

Several studies indicate that oxygen consumption may depend on oxygen delivery in sepsis.[17,67,68] In other forms of shock and under normal conditions, oxygen consumption is independent of delivery until a marked impairment in transport occurs. This threshold occurs at an oxygen delivery of approximately 7 mL/kg, about half the normal value. In sepsis, however, oxygen consumption seems to be linearly related to oxygen delivery, even beyond normal values for oxygen transport, although there is some concern that this finding is an artifact of measurement caused by "mathematical coupling."[69]

Neurogenic Shock

Shock after trauma of the spinal cord may occur without hypovolemia.[16,18] The condition also may be seen in association with general or spinal anesthesia. Hypotension occurs despite an increased cardiac output from marked loss of venous tone and pooling of blood peripherally, with the subsequent decrease in venous return and ventricular filling pressures. The arterial tone may be decreased, also manifested by a low peripheral vascular resistance; oxygen transport is increased; and the $C(a - v)O_2$ is narrowed. Oxygen consumption is usually unchanged. This hemodynamic picture is consistent with stress and with an inadequate, albeit increased, cardiac output attempting to maintain "normal" blood pressure. Whether it represents relative intrinsic myocardial depression (e.g., after surgery, caused by anesthetics) or release of breakdown products from tissue injury causing vasodilation is uncertain. When hypovolemia does not accompany trauma, hypotension is usually easily treated.

Anaphylactic Shock

The degranulation of mast cells and basophils can be precipitated by different mechanisms. *Anaphylactic* reactions consist of a hypersensitivity reaction after immunoglobulin-E (IgE) interaction with an antigen; in the cases when the mediator release occurs without this IgE-mediated mechanism, the term *anaphylactoid* is preferred (Chap. 21). The basophilic granules in these cells contain compounds like histamine, serotonin, proteolytic enzymes, and chemotactic factors that have "cascading" effects with other reactions, like the synthesis of eicosanoid-based compounds (platelet activating factor [PAF], leukotrienes, prostaglandins).[70]

Clinically, either reaction presents identically and follows a distributive pattern similar to that of septic shock, with a characteristic capillary leakage resulting in hypovolemia, the loss of systemic vascular resistance, and the hyperdynamic cardiac output with elements of myocardial depression.[71-73]

Adrenal Shock

The clinical and hemodynamic patterns of distributive shock can be precipitated by a sudden loss in the biosynthesis of mineralocorticoids and glucocorticoids, by the inability of the adrenal glands to mount a higher response in the presence of stressors, or after the abrupt cessation of replacement therapy. The former situation may be seen in cases of adrenal hemorrhage associated with sepsis (from bacterial, fungal, or human immunodeficiency virus), anticoagulation, malignant infiltration, or in the postoperative setting.[74-76] The other conditions may be seen in patients with chronic adrenal insufficiency or when concomitant illnesses (chronic obstructive lung disease, rheumatic diseases) require prolonged corticosteroid intake.

Not only is adrenal failure an uncommon presentation for this type of shock, but it may be more difficult to diagnose because it is usually masked by other coexisting illnesses. The clinical presentation in most instances is nonspecific; however, any clinical suspicion, anamnestic or physical—like a history of chronic steroid intake, the appearance of disproportionate fever and hypotension with minor infections, or shock refractory to fluids and vasopressors[77]—should warrant an immediate evaluation to determine a cortisol level and its response to ACTH stimulation. Stress doses of steroids should be started at once to rapidly revert this serious condition. The initial use of dexamethasone in these cases does not interfere if the ACTH stimulation and cortisol levels need to be delayed (Chap. 146).

PATHOPHYSIOLOGIC MECHANISMS OF SHOCK

The mechanisms controlling regional organ blood flow are of central importance to the pathophysiology of shock. Blood flow to an organ is a function of the perfusion pressure and the vascular resistance of the vessels supplying the organ. Hypoperfusion and dysfunction occur if vascular resistance cannot compensate for low systemic perfusion pressure or if systemic pressures cannot overcome high levels of resistance within the vessels supplying an organ. The former cause of organ hypoperfusion occurs in the brain and heart with severe systemic hypotension, and it is often important in kidney dysfunction. With marked changes in interregional blood flow distribution, as may occur in sepsis, multiple organ dysfunction can occur despite normal levels of systemic pressure. Factors affecting the microcirculation (i.e., perfusion at a cellular level) also may contribute to organ dysfunction. These factors include microvascular compression from cellular edema or abnormal vasoregulation from the release of vasoactive substances. The initial common denominator is perfusion that is not adequate to meet tissue metabolic needs.

CELLULAR INJURY

Shock affects specific organs by altering the functional integrity of their constituent cells. Cells require energy to function properly. Cell failure is caused by a deficiency in delivered substrate, an inability to use the nutrients that are delivered, or an inability to produce enough energy from them. Hypoperfusion decreases delivery of nutrients. The inability to use what is delivered results from the secondary consequences of hypoperfusion (cell injury), the direct toxic effects of an injurious agent, and cytokine-mediated or metabolic changes at the cellular level that are counterproductive to effective energy production.

Ineffective perfusion is the initiating event. With decreased delivery of oxygen and other needed nutrients, adenosine triphosphate (ATP) production diminishes. Maintenance and repair of cellular membranes are attenuated. Endoplasmic reticulum swelling is the first ultrastructural evidence of hypoxic damage. Mitochondria are affected next, with condensation of the inner compartment followed by progressive mitochondrial swelling. With continued cellular hypoxia, lysosome rupture releases degradative enzymes that contribute to intracellular digestion and intracellular calcium deposition. Lysosomal disruption may be the point of irreparable cell damage, analogous to clinical irreversibility. Restoration of normal substrate delivery after this point no longer prevents eventual cell death.

Another mechanism that has recently acquired great attention is the formation of free radicals in association with a reperfusion effect or the activation of neutrophils.[78–81] The accumulation of ATP degradation products (hypoxanthine)[82] during hypoperfusion potentiates the activity of the enzyme xanthine oxidase as the reperfusion process takes place and oxygen becomes available again in the affected tissues. By participating in this step, oxygen is converted to the active radical superoxide (O_2^-), which in turn generates other reactive species like hydrogen peroxide (H_2O_2) and hydroxyl (OH^-), contributing to ultrastructural membrane damage and potential irreversibility. As part of their in situ response, activated neutrophils also generate large amounts of superoxide and proteolytic enzymes that further contribute to cellular injury.[83] These reactions in turn facilitate the cleavage of cell membranes, increasing phospholipid substrates that enter the arachidonic acid pathway with the subsequent formation of leukotrienes, prostaglandins, and thromboxanes, among others.[84,85]

NEUROHUMORAL RESPONSES

Because trauma and hypovolemia are the most common threats to survival in animals, protective reflex responses have evolved. The key signal seems to be a fall in systemic blood pressure, indicating apparent hypovolemia (decreased effective arterial blood volume).[86] If hypotension results from causes other than hypovolemia, these same responses may be inappropriate or ineffective.

The response to hypovolemia in the otherwise healthy person is reproducible (Fig. 26-3). Any fall in blood volume initiates increased activity from carotid and aortic arch baroreceptors and from mechanoreceptors within the right atrium. The result is a neurohumoral response that includes increased sympathetic nervous system activity with direct cardiac stimulation and peripheral vasoconstriction, increased pituitary release of ACTH and antidiuretic hormone, and increased adrenocortical release of epinephrine and cortisol. Receptors in the afferent arterioles and macula densa of the kidneys are also affected, leading to stimulation of the renin–angiotensin–aldosterone system. The net effect is an integrated response to maintain blood pressure and to retain sodium and water. Because cerebral and cardiac perfusion are largely independent of pressure above a minimal level of pressure (autoregulation), blood flow (and therefore function) is initially preserved in these organs. In severe hypovolemia, these compensatory mechanisms are ineffective, and organ function deteriorates.

Other mediators besides catecholamines have vasoactive properties and are released into the circulation during shock, following complicated pathways and interrelations that are currently being studied.[41] These include prostaglandins, histamine, bradykinin, serotonin, beta-endorphins, and circulating myocardial depressant factors. The activation of macrophages and other monocytes results in the release of potent cytokines such as tumor necrosis factor-alpha (TNFα),[87–90] the interleukins (e.g., IL-1, IL-2), PAF,[91] interferon, and many others. These mediators, principally TNFα and IL-

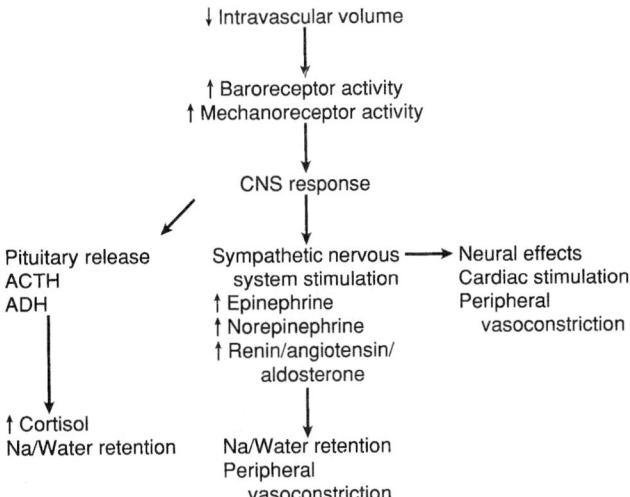

FIGURE 26-3. Expected neurohumoral response to hypovolemia. CNS, central nervous system; ACTH, corticotropin; ADH, antidiuretic hormone; Na, sodium.

1,[92] are capable of initiating all of the pathophysiologic and clinical manifestations associated with SIRS in general (i.e., septic shock).[93] The extent to which any of these substances contributes to the clinical picture of shock is still not completely elucidated. The number of substances involved, each with its own set of effects, as well as their response level (probably determined genetically and by previous exposures to precipitating factors), are some of the reasons why the clinical presentation and the effect of different therapeutic options varies so greatly (Chaps. 20, 25, and 28). This "cascade" affects intraorgan blood flow distribution; causes or promotes increased vascular permeability; alters neutrophil chemotaxis; generates intercellular adhesion molecules,[94] integrins, and selectins; contributes to noncardiogenic pulmonary edema; and alters myocardial and platelet function, leading to microvascular obstruction and dysregulation of the microcirculation.

As previously mentioned, the cleavage of the cytoplasmic and organelle membranes[95-98] by activated phospholipases not only generates eicosanoid-based compounds, but also contributes by altering the permeability to ions (calcium, potassium, sodium, chloride)[99,100] with the subsequent dysfunction associated with the loss of electrochemical gradients, particularly in conductive and contractile functions.

When shock results from other causes, the response described previously may change significantly. For example, infarcted myocardium is largely unresponsive to adrenergic stimulation, eliminating cardiac stimulation as an early compensatory mechanism during shock. Alternatively, peripheral vasoconstriction represents an increase in cardiac afterload; thus, it can be counterproductive, creating a cycle of worsening cardiac function and more intense peripheral vasoconstriction. In contrast, peripheral vasoconstriction is often absent or ineffective during the early stages of septic shock, and the observed myocardial dysfunction in this case may be related to the presence of circulating depressant factors or the overwhelming of autoregulation with resultant coronary hypoperfusion.

METABOLIC RESPONSES

The neurohumoral reflexes that occur during hypovolemic shock also elicit predictable metabolic responses. Catecholamine release causes insulin secretion to decrease, promoting glycogenolysis and lipolysis. Glucocorticoid release promotes gluconeogenesis; with decreased insulin availability, hyperglycemia occurs. Because cellular oxygen availability decreases, hyperglycemia contributes to lactic acid production,[101] which eventually inhibits gluconeogenesis, limiting substrate for needed cellular energy production. Without energy for glycolysis, the cell depends on lipolysis and the autodigestion of intracellular protein for energy. Initially, ketone bodies and the branched-chain amino acids are used as alternative fuel sources. Without oxygen, these sources become inefficient, leading to hypertriglyceridemia, increased beta-hydroxybutyric acid and acetoacetate levels, and changes in the amino acid concentration pattern. As these metabolic changes occur, set in motion by cellular hypoxia and promoted by systemic hormonal changes, structural changes continue within individual cells.

The metabolic response is apparently different in septic shock.[102] Hyperglycemia, hyperinsulinemia, and a decreased insulin–glucagon ratio occur if cardiac output is normal or supranormal. In contrast to hypovolemic shock, lipolysis in septic shock is relatively inhibited and earlier proteolysis occurs. Lactic acidemia is not prominent initially if cardiac output is elevated. If cardiac output is depressed, hypoglycemia, hypoinsulinemia, and lactic acidemia occur. Changes in hepatic gluconeogenesis may be involved in this transition. Simultaneously, there is a transition in plasma in which aromatic amino acids become more prominent than branched-chain amino acids. The clinical consequences of the increase in protein catabolism include hypoalbuminemia, anergy to skin test antigens, gastrointestinal ulceration, muscle wasting, and failure of wound healing. The patterns of carbohydrate, lipid, and amino acid composition in plasma have led some to speculate that nutritional support during sepsis can be specific for the metabolic abnormalities involved. Evidence to support this contention is still inconclusive.

EFFECT OF SHOCK ON SPECIFIC ORGANS

Heart

The heart is a critical organ in the pathophysiology of shock.[31] Because myocardial oxygen extraction is almost maximal under normal conditions, increased cardiac work (imposed by reflex sympathetic stimulation and peripheral vasoconstriction) must be met by increased coronary blood flow. When coronary perfusion is compromised, as it is during systemic hypotension, cardiac function suffers. Myocardial depressant factors that increase the biosynthesis of myocardial nitric oxide and impair the availability of calcium also may play a role in some forms of shock.[61,62,103] Underlying coronary disease adds to cardiac dysfunction. The redistribution of blood flow from endocardium toward epicardium (because of sympathetic stimulation) may impair cardiac performance, especially if overall coronary perfusion is compromised by systemic hypotension or atheromatous coronary disease. Cardiac output also can be compromised by arrhythmias caused by underlying coronary disease, adrenergic stimulation, drug administration, hypoxemia, or acidosis.

Fatty acids are the preferred substrate for cardiac metabolism under normal aerobic conditions. During anaerobic conditions imposed by hypoxemia or ischemia, the myocardium shifts to glycolysis. Anaerobic glycolysis, however, is insufficient to meet cardiac work demands for any length of time because the myocardial glycogen stores, as an alternative fuel source, are minimal and rapidly depleted.

In the absence of coronary stenosis, myocardial necrosis, as evidenced by the release of creatine kinase or electrocardiographic ST segment elevation and Q wave development, is unusual in shock. Unless shock is of cardiac origin, the heart usually plays a participatory role in which it is unable to compensate fully for arterial hypotension caused by hypovolemia, vasodilation, or other factors.

Brain

Like the heart, the brain almost exclusively depends on perfusion, rather than changes in extraction, to meet its oxidative metabolic needs. Protective mechanisms, collectively referred to as autoregulation, have evolved to guard perfusion. As with the heart, brain function also can be affected significantly by regional decreases in perfusion imposed by underlying cerebrovascular disease. Nevertheless, in uncompromised neural vasculature, the cerebral function seems to be maintained until the MAP reaches 50 to 60 mm Hg.[104] The factors that control cerebral autoregulation are incompletely understood but seem to include local carbon dioxide and oxygen tensions and the so-called Bayliss effect (i.e., contraction or dilation of arteriolar smooth muscle in the presence of increased or decreased intravascular pressure).

Cell death in the brain seems to occur by mechanisms similar to those elsewhere in the body, such as progressive cell swelling and autolysis caused by membrane dysfunction. Compared with the cytochrome aa$_3$ in oxidative phosphorylation, the hydroxylases involved in the synthesis of neurotransmitters from tyrosine and tryptophan show a lower affinity for oxygen. This may explain why some patients show significant changes in their mental status, despite what is considered as "adequate" overall oxygen delivery and in the absence of lactic acidosis. The encephalopathic processes that occur during septic shock are associated with an increased mortality.[105] However, just how vulnerable the brain is to anoxic injury is uncertain. In monkeys, significant neurologic recovery can occur despite complete and prolonged (16 minutes) lack of perfusion.[106] The adequacy and the method of resuscitation can critically influence postischemic recovery. Factors like the no-reflow phenomenon may be important. These observations have motivated investigation of specific brain resuscitation regimes. Despite interest and efforts in this area, specific modalities cannot be recommended at this time.

Other elements of the central and peripheral nervous system do not seem to be particularly vulnerable to the effects of shock, because irreversible dysfunction is rarely seen, especially if the brain recovers.

Lungs

Respiratory failure is common in shock. Despite early receptor stimulation that increases the respiratory drive, with augmentation of the minute volume and the resulting primary respiratory alkalosis, the sustained hypoperfusion results in the eventual dysfunction of respiratory muscles (e.g. diaphragm),[107] as well as the central driving mechanism itself. Pulmonary edema also may ensue as an early or late manifestation, depending on the etiology of shock. This can result from increased hydrostatic pressures observed in cardiogenic and some types of obstructive shock, or by increased capillary permeability seen in distributive shock and in the late phases of all other types, caused by injury of the alveolocapillary layers. Whether the therapy of shock contributes to pulmonary edema (in the absence of gross volume overload) is still an unsettled question.

With the release of inflammatory mediators and free radicals, the pulmonary circulation is severely impaired.[108] Diffuse alveolocapillary damage,[109] pulmonary hypertension, and abnormalities of normal hypoxic vasoconstriction all are associated with the appearance of the *acute respiratory distress syndrome* (ARDS) (Chap. 123). Pulmonary hypertension may be caused by hypoxemia, microthromboembolism, biochemical mediator release, or obliteration of the vascular bed. If severe, pulmonary hypertension limits cardiac output. However, other evidence indicates that endotoxin interferes with hypoxic vasoconstriction.[110] Losing this important compensatory mechanism can contribute to defects in oxygenation that are commonly observed in septic shock (increased shunt fraction).

Kidneys

Oliguria, as defined by a urinary output less than 0.5 mL/kg/hour, is a cardinal manifestation of shock. The pathogenesis of shock-related oliguria is more complex than mere renal hypoperfusion.[111-113]

Blood flow to the kidney is rarely reduced below 40% to 50% of normal levels, even in the face of more severe reductions in overall cardiac output. The decreased glomerular filtration rate results from additional mechanisms. Sympathetic stimulation, circulating catecholamines, angiotensin, and locally produced prostaglandins contribute to afferent arteriolar vasoconstriction and the redistribution of blood flow away from cortical glomeruli toward the renal medulla. The net effect is a decreased glomerular filtration rate. This change may be amplified by vasodilation of the efferent arteriole, but it is unlikely that this is a major independent factor. Additional fluid (and salt) conservation is promoted by the effects of aldosterone and antidiuretic hormone.

The reflex responses that cause oliguria can be further altered by therapy, primarily the use of vasoconstricting catecholamines, and by injury to the nephron caused by ischemia. Three pathologic changes are observed: (1) tubular necrosis with back-diffusion of glomerular infiltrate; (2) tubular obstruction by casts or other cellular debris; and (3) tubular epithelial damage with consequent interstitial edema and tubular collapse. Because acute renal failure (i.e., oliguria and azotemia) also can occur without these disorders, the pathologic changes may be secondary events that can amplify but rarely initiate acute renal failure. The appearance of microthrombi or an overt DIC can further decrease the glomerular filtration rate. These pathologic changes partially explain why restoration of normal hemodynamic function does not often lead to an immediate improvement in renal function. Although irreversible renal failure from shock alone is rare, fluid and electrolyte balance are often supported temporally by dialysis although the actual cause of shock has been reversed.

This mixture of reflex responses and primary ischemic damage to the kidney mirrors the variability in responses to therapy for oliguria. If afferent arteriolar vasoconstriction predominates, low-dose dopamine may help to preserve urine output by opposing the vasoconstriction. As pathologic changes occur, a loop diuretic or mannitol may diminish tubular obstruction by maintaining urine flow as long as overall intravascular volume remains constant. After there is obstruction or tubular necrosis, treatment is conservative, supported by dialysis while cellular repair and recovery take place.

Urine that is produced during shock often reflects the pathophysiologic changes occurring in the kidney. If reflex vasoconstricting mechanisms predominate (i.e., hypovolemic and cardiogenic shock), the urine is largely free of salt and is highly concentrated, showing a sodium concentration of less than 20 mMol/L, an osmolality in excess of 450 mOsm/L, a fractional excretion of sodium of less than 1%, a urine–to–plasma creatinine ratio of over 40, and an unremarkable sediment. However, with the effects of ischemic damage on tubular function and the development of acute tubular necrosis, salt retention and urine osmolality decrease, manifested by a sodium concentration of over 40 mMol/L, an osmolality less than 350 mOsm/L, a fractional excretion of sodium of over 2%, a urine–to–plasma creatinine ratio of less than 20, and an active sediment showing all ranges of RBC involvement, from simple hematuria to marked RBC dysmorphism and variable RBC cast formation. Even so, urine sediment and chemistries are not highly specific, and caution must be used to avoid overinterpretation.

Liver

Clinical manifestations of ischemic liver injury are not usually apparent in the early stages of shock as the organ participates in the release of acute phase reactants. As hepatic cells die, they release characteristic enzymes (i.e., aspartate aminotransferase, alanine aminotransferase).[114] Occasionally, an obstructive picture with elevated bilirubin and alkaline phosphatase predominates. Later, the synthesis of coagulation factors, albumin, and prealbumin may deteriorate.[115,116] Less clinically obvious is the impairment in the reticuloendothelial system function. Impaired hepatic clearance functions and reticuloendothelial system failure contribute to continued circulation of vasoactive substances that can perpetuate shock. The appearance of "shock liver" with massive hepatocytic necrosis is unusual and presents mainly in patients with preexisting liver conditions.[117,118]

Gastrointestinal Tract

Ischemic injury to the gut is manifested primarily by interstitial fluid sequestration and hemorrhage or necrosis of the mucosal lining. Ulcer formation[119] with exsanguinating hemorrhage can occur several days after normal hemodynamic function has been restored.[120] The ischemic lesions that develop in the gut usually can be prominent in the stomach,[121] with the rest of the gastrointestinal tract less frequently affected. Ischemic damage to the gut mucosa is especially likely in patients with underlying atherosclerotic disease involving the mesenteric arteries. A pseudomembranous enterocolitis can occur in patients who recover hemodynamically from shock, and it is probably associated with free radical injury during reperfusion.[122] Breakdown of the gut epithelium creates a port of entry for translocation of bacteria or deleterious bacterial products (endotoxin),[123–125] which

may be important in the pathogenesis of irreversible shock[126,127] by releasing mediators to the systemic circulation. The determination of the mucosal pH is described as a potential indicator of the therapeutic response and a marker of MODS.[128]

Pancreas

The importance of the pancreas in contributing to the clinical picture of shock is not established. A myocardial depressant factor is thought to be released from the pancreas, but its role in human disease has not been confirmed. The endocrine and exocrine functions of the pancreas seem rarely to be affected after normal cardiovascular function returns. The special effects of endotoxic or cardiogenic shock on pancreatic function have not been elucidated. However, pancreatitis is a well recognized etiology of SIRS.[44]

Blood

Rheologic alterations and changes in circulating cells may be important during shock. Blood viscosity increases dramatically, especially during burn-induced shock,[129] significantly impairing microcirculation. Although frank DIC is uncommon—except in cases of septic shock[130] and MODS—changes in platelet function associated with PAF, the expression of selectins, and the release of other vasoactive prostaglandins may contribute extensively to the clinical picture of shock, with significant microcirculatory hypoperfusion. Coagulation deficits in hemorrhagic shock may be associated with a dilutional thrombocytopenia after volume replacement, associated with an increased peripheral utilization.[131]

Because shock interferes with tissue oxygen delivery, its effect on the hemoglobin-oxygen dissociation curve has received considerable attention. In most shock states, the curve shifts slightly to the right, probably reflecting changes in 2,3-diphosphoglycerate and metabolic acidosis. This effect enhances the unloading of oxygen at the tissue level, all other factors being equal. However, this small change in affinity usually is trivial compared with the more important influence on oxygen delivery on overall decreased cardiac output or hypoxemia from pulmonary edema.

Multiple Organ Dysfunction Syndrome

If shock is recognized quickly and treated promptly and if the underlying cause is reversible, recovery is usually rapid, with few chronic sequelae. If treatment is excessively delayed for any reason or if the underlying cause cannot be effectively treated or reversed, death is usually inevitable.

In some cases, however, patients enter a chronic state in which blood pressure can be controlled with vasoactive agents but organ system function remains abnormal despite careful attention to intravascular volume and other hemodynamic parameters (see Table 26-4). This state, known as multiple organ dysfunction syndrome (MODS), represents the ultimate manifestation of SIRS and its potential etiologies (sepsis); it can be seen late in other types of shock. As we previously mentioned, the mortality rate in these patients exceeds 60%.

Our ignorance about MODS has generated several controversies about management. In the most conservative view, treatment should focus on managing problems caused by failure of individual organ systems, after circulation has been restored to normal values. This view, however, has been challenged. In analyzing hemodynamic data from large sets of surgical ICU patients, Shoemaker and colleagues[17,132,133] found that, compared with nonsurvivors and normal controls, survivors of shock had a higher oxygen consumption, blood volume, and cardiac output. These data indicate that oxygen consumption and oxygen delivery are linearly related in some shock syndromes such as septic shock. Based on these findings, the hemodynamic values achieved by the survivors of shock have been recommended as appropriate endpoints for resuscitation. Some reports suggest that this approach may improve outcome, and although contradicting data exist,[134-136] recent studies have shown improvement when the hemodynamic support begins early in the phase of "compensated shock" (detected by sophisticated noninvasive hemodynamic monitoring).[8] Verification is needed before broad application of this approach. The target parameters usually followed have been summarized by Parrillo[41] and are presented in Table 26-6.

Shock also has been viewed as a metabolic problem rather than a problem of perfusion deficits. Two schools of thought regarding the metabolic defects in shock have been identified: (1) the hormonal school, in which hormonal abnormalities induced by shock are thought to create the abnormal metabolic patterns observed; and (2) the energy-deficit school, in which a cellular deficit in metabolizing substrate is postulated.

Although there have been many observations of the hormonal and metabolic changes that accompany shock and sepsis, their etiologic importance and relationship to outcome remain uncertain. The liver and gut continue to be emphasized as initiators of metabolic derangements and in the development of MODS.[137,138] Advocates of the energy-deficit school believe that outcome may be improved by circumventing the metabolic disturbances. This view has led to controversy regarding nutritional support for patients in shock.[139,140] Because hemodynamic instability and changing fluid requirements characterize the first few days of most patients who survive the onset of shock, MODS is the rule by the time nutritional support is possible in these patients. The amount of calories required, the sources from which these calories should be obtained, and the amino acid composition of the solutions all have been debated. In general, while the patient remains dependent on vasoactive drugs, full nutritional support of any type is often limited by fluid requirements and renal function.

MANAGEMENT ■

Shock results from pathophysiologic disturbances associated with various disorders; management must be directed toward interrupting the downward spiral of events that perpetuate and amplify shock and toward treating the specific initiating cause.[141]

Regardless of the underlying cause, the initial management of shock must quickly address the following questions:

TABLE 26-6. Guidelines for the Care of Patients in Shock

ABNORMALITY	INTERVENTION	THERAPEUTIC GOAL
Hypotension	ICU monitoring, volume expansion, vasopressors	MAP ≥60 mm Hg PAOP 14–18 mm Hg
Tissue hypoperfusion	ICU monitoring, volume expansion, inotropic agents, vasopressors	Hemoglobin ≥10 g/dL Oxygen saturation ≥92% CI ≥2.2 L/min·m² in nondistributive shock CI ≥4.0 L/min·m² in distributive shock Serum lactate ≤2.2 mMol/L P$\bar{v}$o$_2$ >30 mm Hg or S$\bar{v}$o$_2$ > 55%

MODS	ICU monitoring, volume expansion, inotropic agents, vasopressors	Normalization or reversal of:
		  CNS: mental status
		  Renal: blood urea nitrogen, serum
		    creatinine, urinary output >0.5 mL/kg/h
		  Hepatic: serum bilirubin
		  Pulmonary: A–a gradient

Infection	Appropriate antibiotics/surgical drainage	Eradication
Inflammatory response	Mediator inhibition or modulation°	Reversal of effect

A–a, alveoloarterial; CNS, central nervous system; ICU, intensive care unit; MAP, mean arterial pressure; MODS, multiple orgasm dysfunction syndrome; PAOP, pulmonary artery occlusion pressure; P$\bar{v}$o$_2$, mixed venous oxygen partial pressure; S$\bar{v}$o$_2$, mixed venous oxygen saturation; CI, cardiac index.
°Experimental therapies.
Modified from Parrillo JE; Pathogenetic mechanisms of septic shock. *N Engl J Med* 1993; 328:1471.

Does the patient require tracheal intubation for airway protection and ventilatory support? Is the arterial hypotension severe enough to require immediate resuscitation? Is there an obvious or likely etiology identified, warranting the immediate implementation of confirmatory procedures in an *early* attempt to block, modify, or reverse the associated mechanisms?

These questions often must be answered before a satisfactory history, physical examination, and laboratory database are available. However, the consequence of failing to proceed aggressively can be irreversible organ failure instead of full recovery.

AIRWAY MANAGEMENT AND MECHANICAL VENTILATION

Most patients with the fully developed shock syndrome require tracheal intubation and mechanical ventilatory support, even if acute respiratory failure has not yet occurred. Clinical benefits are especially likely in patients with cardiogenic or septic shock; unlike hemorrhagic shock, these conditions are seldom rapidly reversible. Improvement may occur for several reasons. Recent data demonstrate that the respiratory muscles require a disproportionate share of the total cardiac output during shock.[142,143] Because other organs are deprived of needed nutrient blood flow, lactic acidosis is potentiated. Mechanical ventilation allows blood flow to be redistributed, tends to reverse lactic acidosis, and supports the patient until other therapeutic measures can be effective. Tracheal intubation also is indicated if mental status changes make adequate protection of the airway uncertain. Hypoxemia or inadequate respiratory compensation for a metabolic acidosis makes mechanical ventilatory support absolutely necessary.[144]

In the absence of the full shock picture, intubation and mechanical ventilation should be instituted after an assessment of gas exchange, work of breathing, and the ability to maintain a patent airway. Important signs that ventilatory support is necessary include cyanosis, severe tachypnea or bradypnea, use of accessory muscles during breathing, and mental obtundation. Auscultation of the chest may reveal crackles or wheezing, either of which can indicate pulmonary edema, ARDS, pneumonia, or anaphylaxis. Although acute respiratory failure is usually defined in terms of the arterial blood gas partial pressures, the presence of any of these clinical signs—especially in combination—requires immediate consideration of intubation and ventilatory support, even before the arterial blood gas results are known. We recommend using endotracheal tubes with the largest internal diameter tolerated by the patient (usually 7.5 or 8.0 mm) to facilitate suctioning or eventual bronchoscopic procedures. Issues regarding precise ventilator settings and management are controversial and are discussed elsewhere in this book; however, some of our initial guidelines include using calculated tidal volumes in the order of 7 to 10 mL/kg of lean body mass, initial limitation in the use of positive end-expiratory pressure,[145] an oxygen concentration that results in arterial saturations not less than 92%, and adequate ventilator rate and sedation to minimize the work of breathing. There are multiple variations to these parameters that ultimately depend on the etiology and the constant reevaluation of the interventions.

INITIAL THERAPY FOR HYPOTENSION

Aggressive resuscitative measures for arterial hypotension should be undertaken whenever the systolic blood pressure is unacceptably low (e.g., less than 90 mm Hg or a decrease of more than 40 mm Hg from usual values) and there are signs of vital organ dysfunction, including obtundation, oliguria, obvious pulmonary edema, and angina. Other important signs include tachycardia or bradycardia (an important primary cause of hypotension) and cool, clammy skin. The absence of these signs, especially with a normal mental status, may indicate that the arterial blood pressure has been underestimated. If this is a possibility, direct measurement of blood pressure by an arterial catheter should be obtained.

Initially, the placement of at least two large-bore (14 to 16 gauge), well-secured peripheral venous catheters should be performed. Prompt consideration should be given to early access of central veins with severe cases or when peripheral access is difficult or impossible to obtain. The placement of a pulmonary artery catheter *introducer* in this situation may offer a large-bore (usually 8.5 French) access with low resistance to flow for rapid fluid administration, and may facilitate further hemodynamic monitoring in complicated cases.

If blood pressure is truly low or accompanied by signs of organ dysfunction, the physician must choose a vasopressor agent (e.g., norepinephrine, dopamine) or intravascular volume expansion (e.g., blood, colloids, or isotonic crystalloid solutions). Often, a combination of a trial of volume expansion with a vasopressor is appropriate. In our view, the consequences of inadequate cerebral and coronary perfusion are potentially so disastrous that every effort must be made to rapidly restore arterial pressure to at least 90 mm Hg systolic or 60 mm Hg mean systemic level. This goal can be achieved most rapidly with a vasopressor, even if shock is caused by hemorrhage, while fluids are given simultaneously. Although vasoactive agents are least effective when intravascular volume is depleted, their use can be justified by the lethal consequences of prolonged systemic arterial hypotension: irreversible cerebral and cardiac injury. Because dopamine is not always successful, even at high infusion rates, because it depends on the release of the endogenous reserves of norepinephrine, *in severe cases* we believe that the direct agonist norepinephrine is the best initial choice (see Fig. 26-2). Some studies indicate that, especially in septic shock, norepinephrine may improve blood pressure and increase urine flow, but volume infusions often do little to cardiac performance.[146–148] Every attempt must be made to rapidly decrease the infusion rate of the vasopressor, to switch to a lower (and less vasoconstrictive) effective dose of dopamine, or to discontinue vasoactive agents altogether.

Theoretically, tilting a patient into the head-down position (i.e., Trendelenburg position) diverts blood volume into the central circulation, increasing cardiac filling and augmenting stroke volume. Studies, however, do not demonstrate any significant redistribution of blood volume centrally.[149] For this reason, and because the head-down position can worsen gas exchange and cardiac function, we *no longer recommend the Trendelenburg position* for the emergency management of shock. If this type of measure is desirable, it is sufficient to raise the legs above the level of the heart.

The choice of fluid for resuscitation is a matter of considerable controversy,[150-158] but several points should be kept in mind. Evidence of pulmonary edema at the outset is a strong contraindication to further fluid administration. Some patients with noncardiogenic forms of pulmonary edema and septic shock may respond to intravascular volume expansion without further exacerbation of their pulmonary edema, but this response is difficult to predict, especially at the time of initial presentation. Therefore, fluid administration should be minimized under these circumstances. Likewise, evidence of myocardial dysfunction (e.g., angina or significant ST segment elevation on the ECG)—even without obvious pulmonary edema—provides sufficient reason to avoid aggressive fluid administration during the initial management of shock. After additional information is obtained (especially hemodynamic data), a trial of volume expansion may be indicated.

With all other noncardiogenic forms of shock, intravascular volume expansion should be attempted. The actual choice of fluid frequently represents a compromise between what is readily available, what is required based on estimated or observed losses, and the kind of fluid being lost. Blood and colloid-containing solutions are more efficient and often more effective in rapidly expanding intravascular volume than are isotonic crystalloid solutions.

Fully crossmatched blood is the ideal and obvious choice for hemorrhage and the severely anemic patient with a compromised oxygen carrying capacity, but its preparation takes time; colloid or isotonic crystalloid solutions are usually given initially. Many experimental solutions and blood substitutes have been undergoing evaluation, but none can be recommended yet for routine use.[159,160] O-negative units of blood can be used in severe hemorrhage initially until more specific units are available. In most cases, the outcome of shock is probably not affected by the type of solution given during the first hours of resuscitation, but by the rate of administration. If administration is too slow, arterial hypotension or vasopressor use is unnecessarily prolonged; if too fast, the risk of pulmonary edema increases rapidly. No arbitrary formula should be adhered to dogmatically, but a reasonable approach is to administer 500 to 750 mL of a colloid or 1000 to 2000 mL of an isotonic crystalloid solution (i.e., normal saline or Ringer's lactate) during the first hour; this guideline *does not count* ongoing losses. In hemorrhagic shock, even more rapid administration may be necessary. Keep in mind that blood losses can be occult (e.g., internal bleeding after trauma, leaking aortic aneurysm, fractured femur shaft). At all times, the rate of administration should be adjusted frequently, using changes in blood pressure, urine output, or evidence of emerging pulmonary edema as important clinical endpoints. Additional fluid administration is dictated by the clinical response to this initial fluid challenge or by new information from hemodynamic and laboratory monitoring and may require combinations of crystalloids or colloidal solutions with blood products. A new and interesting concept in the management of penetrating injuries to the trunk utilizes delaying the fluid resuscitation until the operative intervention is initiated, with favorable results.[161,162] More studies are required before a change of this nature is widely accepted.

After this initial period, during which maintenance of a minimally acceptable mean systemic blood pressure, organ perfusion, and a trial of intravascular volume expansion are emphasized, attention must be directed toward acquiring additional data, defining the cause of the shock syndrome, and implementing appropriate further specific management.

LABORATORY AND BASIC STUDIES

Initial laboratory tests should include a complete chemistry profile with serum electrolytes, creatinine, blood urea nitrogen, liver function tests, calcium, magnesium and phosphate levels; a complete blood count and differential; a platelet count; prothrombin and activated partial thromboplastin times; a serum lactate level; a urinalysis with a detailed sediment analysis; a serum amylase level; and arterial blood gases. A pregnancy test should be performed in all female patients of childbearing age. A 12-lead ECG and chest radiograph are always indicated.

Other studies should be considered in specific conditions and may include blood, sputum, and urine Gram stains and cultures in all cases of suspected sepsis; more detailed imaging studies like computed tomography scans,[163] abdominal radiographs, or ultrasound; surface or transesophageal echocardiograms[164]; ventilation/perfusion scan; angiograms; cardiac isoenzymes or right-sided ECG in inferior wall infarcts[165]; and many others that are discussed in detail in specific chapters.

Typing and crossmatching for several units of packed RBCs and fresh frozen plasma should be ordered in when a significant blood loss is observed, anticipated, or suspected.

ENDPOINTS FOR RESUSCITATION

Because organ system dysfunction is a sine qua non for the diagnosis of shock, a return to normal function seems to be an appropriate endpoint for therapy. If shock is recognized quickly, resuscitative measures are initiated rapidly, and treatment of the underlying cause is instituted, restoration of normal organ system function is expected. Improvement in mental acuity, restoration of urine flow, and diminishing signs of myocardial ischemia all are useful signs that the treatment of shock has been effective. However, especially after prolonged ischemia, an extended period of time may be required before organ function fully returns to normal. It is often appropriate to adjust therapy before the actual return of normal organ function to avoid common side effects or complications.

An alternative approach is to titrate therapy according to relevant physiologic variables. Numerous parameters have been proposed, including measurements of arterial blood pressure, PAOP, cardiac output, lung water, mixed venous oxygen saturation, and oxygen consumption. None is specifically and universally accepted, and in most instances, *all* of these factors are frequently measured or calculated (see Table 26-6).[166]

Basic Hemodynamic Monitoring

Initial monitoring of the patient in shock includes noninvasively determining vital signs, cardiac rhythm, and urinary output. An accurate blood pressure measurement is necessary when treatment is initiated, especially to avoid falsely low readings.[167] Normally, blood pressure can be measured by cuff and stethoscope because Korotkoff sounds arise from turbulent blood flow distal to the point of vessel occlusion by the blood pressure cuff. Pressure may be underestimated by conditions that decrease the turbulence, including peripheral vascular disease, tachycardia with a small pulse pressure, and irregular rhythms like atrial fibrillation.[168] Doppler devices improve detection of pressure but do not always reliably resolve the problem.[169] When noninvasive methods are erratic, hypotension is profound, the patient is unresponsive to initial resuscitative measures, or clinical shock is present, invasive hemodynamic monitoring, including arterial and pulmonary arterial catheterization, is indicated.

Because central venous catheters often are placed early in the management of shock, it is usually possible to obtain a central venous pressure (CVP) measurement. If the patient is in the ICU, the CVP should be measured with the usual pressure tubing, transducers, and monitoring equipment. Water manometry is often inaccurate and therefore is usually inappropriate. It should be clear though, that *CVP is not an accurate means of monitoring volume resuscitation*, and should be used as a rough guideline. It is rarely necessary to push volume resuscitation beyond a CVP of 10 to 15 mm Hg unless obstructive shock or right ventricular infarction is involved. An initially low CVP (i.e., less than 5 mm Hg) may indicate hypovolemia. A CVP greater than 15 mm Hg, with an absent y-descent on the CVP tracing, suggests cardiac tamponade in the appropriate clinical setting.

Advanced Hemodynamic Monitoring

As previously discussed, the various shock syndromes clinically differ with respect to their hemodynamic profiles (see Table 26-3), and their patterns may be anticipated when we have identified possible etiologies; or, vice versa, a specific profile of a shock of unknown etiology can point us in the direction of other tests that may elucidate the diagnosis and guide more specific management issues.[170] Therefore, meticulous attention to hemodynamics is important in developing therapeutic strategies.[166,171,172] However, keep in mind that with time and therapy, hemodynamic profiles often change.

Most hemodynamic measurements used as physiologic parameters to guide therapy during shock are obtained with catheters, transducers, amplifiers, and bedside recorders. Careful recording and calibration are important because clinicians clearly alter therapy of shock based on the results of these measurements.[173,174] The results of hemodynamic measurements should be evaluated with respect to the total clinical picture, and the clinician should understand the sensitivity and specificity of these parameters and be aware that intrapatient variation is frequently observed. All of the hemodynamic measurements that are commonly used as endpoints are plagued by numerous potential artifacts (Table 26-7). Appropriate quality control in the ICU minimizes but does not eliminate these errors. It is important to know what, how, and when to monitor and how to interpret trends

TABLE 26-7. Common Artifacts in Hemodynamic Measurements

VARIABLE	ARTIFACT	CAUSES	COMMENTS/CORRECTIVE ACTION
Vascular pressures (including PAOP)	Overestimation of preload	Technical	Avoid with rigid nursing protocols
		Improper leveling of transducer	
		Improper calibration	
		Improper system frequency response	
		Respiratory:	Avoid digital readouts; use analogue tracings
		Not recording pressures at end-expiration during mechanical ventilation	
		Active expiratory effort	Suspect with respiratory distress; consider muscle paralysis, usually not significant with <10 cm H₂O PEEP
		PEEP	
		Improper positioning of catheter tip	Suspect if tip in upper lobes on chest radiograph or PAD < PAOP
		Cardiac:	
		Mitral regurgitation	Read PAOP as post–A wave
		Mitral stenosis	Interpret with caution as preload estimate
		Acute changes in LV compliance	Suspect in presence of myocardial ischemia

(continued)

TABLE 26-7. *(continued)*

VARIABLE	ARTIFACT	CAUSES	COMMENTS/CORRECTIVE ACTION
	Underestimation of preload	Technical (see above) Respiratory: Not recording pressures at end-expiration during spontaneous breathing	
Cardiac output	Inaccuracies	Technical: Incorrect injectable volume; thermistor contact with vessel wall; incorrect computational constant	Inspect temperature curves; suspect if PA waveform is dampened; follow rigid nursing protocol
		Cardiac: TR	Do not use in presence of significant TR
	Wide variation	Technical (as above)	Delete measurements with >20% variation from mean
		Respiratory: Variable respiratory rate during mechanical ventilation	Average measurements throughout respiratory cycle
Mixed venous oxygen saturation	Inaccuracies	Technical: Light reflecting against vessel wall, catheter kinking	Note computer error messages
		Presence of significant HgbCO	Measure HgbCO directly at least once
	Misinterpretation	Shifts in oxygen dissociation curve	Correlate with $P\bar{v}O_2$ measurements
		Dependence on oxygen delivery	Correlate with oxygen delivery measurements
Extravascular lung water	Inaccuracies	Inaccurate measurement of cardiac output (see above)	Correlate cardiac output with regular thermodilution measurements
	Underestimation	Presence of significant areas of nonperfused lung	Measurements suspect in presence of significant regional disease (e.g., lobar pneumonia) or known vascular obstruction
Systemic vascular resistance	Inaccuracies	Inaccurate measurement of cardiac output (see above)	
		Inaccurate measurement of blood pressure	Measure directly (see above)

PAD, pulmonary artery diastolic; LV, left ventricle; PA, pulmonary artery; TR, tricuspid regurgitation; PAOP, pulmonary artery occlusion pressure; PEEP, positive end-expiratory pressure; HgbCO, carboxyhemoglobin; $P\bar{v}O_2$, mixed venous oxygen partial pressure.

in the collected data. Because hemodynamic measurements are physiologic, they can be used most profitably to answer specific physiologic questions and to follow trends, rather than to be endpoints themselves.

Hemodynamic monitoring is most useful when the pathophysiologic mechanism of a shock syndrome is reasonably well understood, as in the case of cardiogenic or hypovolemic shock; in septic shock, the usefulness of hemodynamic monitoring is less clear because appropriate endpoints are not established. For instance, thermodilution cardiac output measurements usually are obtained with other hemodynamic measurements. A less than normal cardiac output (or index) is inadequate for a patient in shock and requires treatment, but it is not clear that the endpoint of treatment is simply a normal cardiac output, nor is it clear by what means the cardiac output should be raised.[132,133,175,176] This problem is especially apparent when septic shock is contrasted with cardiogenic or hypovolemic shock. In the latter conditions, a normal cardiac output is a reasonable endpoint. However, in septic shock, it is not clear whether the goal should be normal cardiac output or a supranormal cardiac output that maximizes oxygen delivery. A Belgian group recommends following the relationship between cardiac index and oxygen extraction ratio, instead of the traditional oxygen delivery and uptake, as a more reliable source to guide management.[177] On the other hand, some studies suggest that increasing oxygen delivery does not alone alter outcome; the debate continues.[136] In septic shock, we attempt to increase the *cardiac index* to approximately 4 L/minute/m² only if there is evidence of impaired tissue oxygenation, such as lactic acidosis or a mixed venous less than 30 mm Hg (SvO_2 less than 55%), and only if this can be accomplished without causing serious cardiac arrhythmias or worsening pulmonary edema.

Our approach to employing vasoactive drugs or fluid administration is based on the clinical situation. In patients with hypovolemic shock, fluid administration is the treatment of choice; in patients with cardiogenic shock (but with adequate filling pressures), vasoactive or inotropic drugs are preferred. In mixed forms of shock or if the cause of circulatory disturbance is poorly understood, the appropriate strategy for maximizing cardiac output is unclear, and actual practice differs widely. In such situations, we generally emphasize volume expansion if it can be accomplished without exacerbating pulmonary edema.

Volume expansion, although important, is difficult to monitor effectively. The PAOP, which is the most commonly used endpoint for volume resuscitation, may not accurately reflect end-diastolic volume or intravascular volume. Because of numerous sources of artifact in critically ill patients, a single measurement can be extremely difficult to interpret. The most reliable solution to this problem is to initiate a "therapeutic fluid challenge." The PAOP is used to make a "best guess" about what therapy is appropriate, and a regimen is initiated to test this clinical hypothesis. As new information is obtained, including changes in the PAOP or other responses to therapy, the validity of the original assumptions and their interpretation is reevaluated.

Assuming appropriate calibration and leveling of transducer equipment, the most common artifacts in PAOP measurement cause overestimation of the true value. Therefore, recordings of less than 10 mm Hg are rarely spuriously low, and fluid resuscitation can be used with relatively little risk. If pressures are between 20 and 25 mm Hg, errors in measurement are seldom so large; consequently, fluid restriction is usually appropriate. In the many instances of intermediate pressure, a fluid challenge is particularly useful.

A sensible approach to performing the challenge is to give fluid at a rate of 500 to 2000 mL/hour. If shock is caused by hypovolemia, 2 to 4 L of isotonic crystalloid or its equivalent usually reestablishes normal vital signs if there are no continued intravascular volume losses. Failure to reestablish vital signs suggests that other mechanisms are responsible (e.g., internal bleeding, myocardial depression, SIRS). The actual rate chosen for the infusion depends on the severity of shock, the choice of fluid, and the potential for causing or exacerbating pulmonary edema. Vital signs and the PAOP are checked every 10 to 15 minutes. When clinical signs of organ function change or the PAOP changes by more than 3 mm Hg, the patient is reevaluated. We recommend correlating changes in PAOP with changes in cardiac output or stroke volume. This relationship is especially important in patients with abnormalities in ventricular diastolic compliance. The rate of fluid administration should be adjusted to reflect these changes. We cannot overemphasize the superiority of this approach to the usual order to give fluids until the PAOP reaches some arbitrary value (e.g., 16 to 18 mm Hg).[174]

Data from several studies have reawakened the controversy about fluid resuscitation if septic shock and pulmonary edema simultaneously occur.[177-182] These studies indicate that a positive fluid balance may not be beneficial and may even be harmful in cases of pulmonary edema. None of these studies, however, address the problem of whether the preferred treatment of shock should then be vasopressors or volume expansion. Such uncertainty emphasizes even more the need to show that intravascular volume expansion improves cardiac output or oxygen delivery with hemodynamic monitoring. In the absence of decreased left ventricular compliance, optimal cardiac output can usually be accomplished with a PAOP of 8 to 12 mm Hg. Otherwise, cardiovascular function should be maintained with inotropic agents or vasoconstrictors, and fluid balance should be kept even or negative unless hemodynamic monitoring clearly demonstrates that additional volume expansion improves cardiovascular function. As hemodynamics improve, the sympathomimetics are weaned and the patient is maintained with the lowest tolerated filling pressures, as is also the case for noncardiogenic pulmonary edema (ARDS).

Using PAOP measurements as a guide to fluid management implies that the chance of causing or exacerbating pulmonary edema can be minimized in this way.

Another endpoint for judging successful resuscitation is the oximetric determination of SvO_2, especially during vasoactive drug infusions. This approach assumes that total-body oxygen consumption remains constant during the therapy. If cardiac output improves and oxygen consumption is stable, SvO_2 increases as oxygen extraction decreases. However, data suggest that oxygen consumption remains dependent on oxygen delivery in many critically ill patients, particularly those with ARDS or sepsis.[68,108] Interpretation of venous oximetry measurements in this group of patients is considerably less certain. Continuous venous oximetry can be recommended only for the titration of vasoactive agents in patients whose predominant problem is heart failure or cardiogenic shock. Its usefulness is problematic in hypovolemic and septic shock. For these reasons, in general, we prefer placement of the standard thermodilution pulmonary artery catheter instead of the more expensive varieties, like the oximetric or the right ventricular ejection fraction catheters, reserving use of the more expensive catheters for specific cases or research.

There has been considerable recent interest in what seems to be several promising *noninvasive* monitoring devices, like near-infrared spectroscopy to detect oxygen availability and utilization at tissular level, or thoracic electrical bioimpedance for continuous cardiac output measurements. These could be used with high-risk patients to detect "compensated states," before clinical hemodynamic instability is evident. Currently, more studies and refinement are necessary before the "golden standard" (pulmonary artery catheter with a thermistor tip) can be challenged.[8,183-187]

Pharmacologic Support of Blood Pressure

Pharmacologic agents—pressors in particular—may be required immediately to support blood pressure in the early stages of shock.[188,189] If these agents cannot be discontinued after intravascular volume expansion, continued pharmacologic support is necessary. Most drugs have combined effects. Table 26-5 compares the most currently used agents and gives their recommended doses.

Dopamine and dobutamine are the most commonly used inotropic agents in the treatment of shock.[190] Dopamine, an endogenous precursor of norepinephrine, has multiple dose-related effects. At low doses, beta-2 and dopaminergic effects are evident, and enhanced blood flow to renal and splanchnic beds is prominent. At higher doses, cardiac inotropy is seen; at still higher doses, vasoconstriction predominates. Dobutamine is a synthetic congener of isoproterenol with primarily beta-1 (cardiac) but also beta-2 (vasodilatory) stimulating properties. It has few insignificant vasoconstrictive or renal vasodilating effects.

If shock involves heart failure, dobutamine often can be used to advantage. Cardiac output usually is increased without marked increases in heart rate. A concomitant advantage is that the systemic vascular resistance and the PAOP usually fall during dobutamine infusions. These features make the use of dobutamine desirable, even in patients with ischemic coronary disease, as long as heart rate is not unduly increased and blood pressure holds. In cardiac failure, a simultaneous infusion of low-dose dopamine (less than 5 μg/kg/minute) enhances renal perfusion and urine output.[180]

If shock results from causes other than heart failure, a vasopressor agent is usually needed if volume replacement does not correct hypotension. High-dose dopamine is often used, although in our experience, it has frequently been ineffective. Norepinephrine, a catecholamine with primarily alpha-receptor agonist activity, is often then the drug of choice. When norepinephrine is required to maintain blood pressure, a simultaneous infusion of dopamine usually does not ameliorate its deleterious vasoconstrictive properties, although some physicians favor using low-dose dopamine to potentially enhance renal perfusion. Similarly, if dopamine is used in high doses to support blood pressure, simultaneous infusion of dobutamine does not make it possible to lower the dopamine infusion rate and thereby minimize its vasoconstrictive properties. When using dopamine or norepinephrine for blood pressure support, the most important factors to evaluate are the adequacy of intravascular volume resuscitation and the accuracy of blood pressure measurements. Both problems often require evaluation by invasive hemodynamic monitoring.

The "renal dosing" of dopamine has been challenged in recent articles[191] because the associated increase in urinary output observed may be more related to a diuretic mechanism involving ATPase at the distal tubular level rather than an actual increase in renal perfusion. Dobutamine at low doses has been associated with higher creatinine clearances than comparable doses of dopamine.[192]

Vasoactive drugs may alter the relationship between PAOP, left atrial pressure, and left ventricular end-diastolic pressure and volume through their effects on the pulmonary vascular bed and on cardiac tissue. Thus, a "high" PAOP does not necessarily mean that the patient cannot respond to volume infusion. Only a carefully executed and evaluated fluid challenge can determine this information.

The phosphodiesterase inhibitors amrinone and milrinone have potent inotropic properties that may be useful if dopamine or dobutamine are not effective.[193] Amrinone and milrinone also are vasodilators, which may contraindicate their use in shock. They have been used mainly as synergistic agents in refractory cardiogenic shock.

Reducing the systemic vascular resistance (afterload reduction) with direct-acting vasodilators can be a effective means of improving cardiac output in heart failure if systemic pressures are otherwise normal or even elevated. This approach, however, is extremely dangerous during shock if systemic pressures or cardiac filling pressures are low. We do not recommend it unless shock is caused by severe aortic or mitral valvular regurgitation or a dissecting aortic aneurysm.

The American Heart Association[194] has incorporated a revised algorithm for the management of acute pulmonary edema, hypotension, and shock into its guidelines of advanced cardiac life support (see Fig. 26-2).

Lactic Acidosis

Lactic acidosis is common during shock.[195] Metabolic acidosis itself is a known, although not potent, myocardial depressant, and it may interfere with the effectiveness of exogenously administered catecholamines. These and similar factors often are used as the rationale to aggressively treat lactic acidosis.[196]

The best treatment of lactic acidosis is unquestionably reversal of the underlying cause. Because this goal is usually not immediately attainable, intravenous sodium bicarbonate administration is occasionally given. The wisdom of this form of treatment has been questioned.[197] Experimental data indicate that exogenous sodium bicarbonate can actually worsen intracellular acidosis.[198] Perhaps for this reason, prospective clinical studies do not show any benefit from administering intravenous sodium bicarbonate.[199]

The emphasis should be prioritized toward correcting the underlying hemodynamic problem by restricting the use of sodium bicarbonate when the pH is below 7.1. In such cases, 100 to 150 mMol of intravenous sodium bicarbonate can be infused slowly and the effect on serum bicarbonate, arterial pH, and hemodynamics evaluated. If no effect is seen, the chance that additional sodium bicarbonate will change the course or outcome is slim.

New agents like a mixture of bicarbonate and sodium carbonate (Carbicarb) and dichloroacetate have shown promising results.[101,200]

ADJUNCTIVE SPECIFIC MANAGEMENT AND EXPERIMENTAL TECHNIQUES

Besides the general approach to management described in the earlier segments, some shock states warrant more specific interventions.

Cardiogenic Shock

In cardiogenic shock (Chap. 27) associated with myocardial infarction, a rapid screening should be performed to determine if the patient is a candidate for thrombolysis, should the pressure be increased and stabilized,[10] or, if the location allows, to undergo emergent cardiac catheterization and eventual revascularization of the main stenosis.[11,201,202] Depending on the circumstances, other agents (e.g., aspirin) might be considered at this early stage (see Chap. 116).

The administration of morphine, in doses of 2 to 4 mg intravenously (IV), as an analgesic and sedative, may contribute to the overall condition by decreasing the sympathoadrenergic discharge, decreasing the myocardial stress and oxygen requirements. It helps also by causing mild to moderate venodilation, therefore assisting in decreasing the preload. The specific use for this later effect is less justified in the presence of more effective and titratable preload reducers such as nitroglycerin (if the systolic blood pressure is 95 to 100 mm Hg or higher).

Recognizing other complications is essential to ensuring appropriate treatment. Shock from mitral valvular dysfunction is usually accompanied by congestive heart failure and implies severe papillary muscle dysfunction or rupture. Mitral regurgitation occurring as a result of ischemia may respond to standard antianginal therapy. Vasodilators such as sodium nitroprusside also may be useful by reducing the impedance to cardiac ejection and diminishing the effects of mitral regurgitation. Vasopressors should be avoided in acute mitral regurgitation because the increase in afterload increases the severity of the regurgitation. If shock persists, intraaortic balloon counterpulsation and mitral valve replacement often are required (Chap. 117).[203]

Right Ventricular Infarct

The main focus in the treatment of hypotension accompanying right ventricular infarction is maintenance of right ventricular filling pressure with intravascular volume expansion to maintain right ventricular preload (Chap. 115).[165] Left ventricular filling pressure should be used with measurements of cardiac output as an endpoint for further fluid administration. However, because the dilated right ventricle may cause the septum to bulge into the left ventricle and change left ventricular diastolic compliance (i.e., ventricular interdependence), little change in cardiac output may occur despite an increase in the PAOP.[33] If volume infusion is not sufficient to restore hemodynamic function to normal, inotropic therapy should be used. The inotropic agents of choice, such as dobutamine or dopamine, do not increase pulmonary vascular resistance.

Prognosis for the patient with right ventricular infarction and hypotension or shock is considerably better than that for the patient with the same findings as a result of left ventricular infarction.

Septic Shock

A hyperdynamic circulation in a patient with shock is sufficiently characteristic of sepsis that if the mechanism is not clear, empiric antibiotic therapy should be initiated and occult, specific sources of infection excluded (Chap. 28). The antibiotic coverage should be broad and usually should include an aminoglycoside (e.g., gentamicin, tobramycin, amikacin) and a semisynthetic penicillin combined with a β-lactamase inhibitor (e.g., piperacillin/tazobactam, ampicillin/sulbactam, ticarcillin/clavulinic acid). An alternative to the semisynthetic penicillins is a third-generation cephalosporin like cefotaxime or ceftriaxone; the latter is particularly important in suspected CNS infection or when there is increased incidence of penicillin-resistant *Streptococci*. Ceftazidime, cefoperazone, or imipenem are often specifically recommended for neutropenic patients or for infections possibly involving *Pseudomonas*. If anaerobic infection is suspected (e.g., a potential intraabdominal source), the combination penicillins previously mentioned can be used; clindamycin, metronidazole, cefoxitin, or chloramphenicol also can be added if imipenem is not part of the regimen. If *Staphylococcus aureus* may be involved (e.g., central venous catheter infection), a penicillinase-resistant antibiotic like oxacillin or nafcillin should be used; vancomycin should be substituted if a methicilin/oxacillin--resistant *S. aureus* infection is possible. Antibiotic therapy can be further refined if the specific clinical circumstance is taken into account. Surgical incision, drainage, or debridement should be undertaken for a closed-space infection (e.g., empyema, abdominal abscess).

Whether survival is improved when oxygen delivery and oxygen consumption are maximized in septic shock[197] (i.e., delivery should be increased until consumption no longer increases) is a matter of debate and ongoing research.[67,132,133,147] Several lines of evidence indicate that this approach may be reasonable. Most patients with sepsis have an elevated cardiac output, suggesting a physiologic attempt to maximize oxygen delivery.[66] The level of the cardiac output on presentation is inversely related to survival during sepsis, also suggesting that oxygen delivery is an important factor in determining outcome. However, increased oxygen delivery has not been associated with improved outcome in other studies and continues to be a matter of great controversy.[136]

Anaphylaxis

Hypotension associated with anaphylaxis (Chap. 104) can usually be treated effectively by volume expansion and the administration of 0.3 to 0.5 mL of 1:1000 aqueous epinephrine, given subcutaneously or intramuscularly. Epinephrine also usually improves urticaria and bronchospasm. The dose may be repeated in 15 to 20 minutes, or earlier if necessary. Local absorption of antigen (e.g., bee venom) may be retarded by application of a tourniquet and ice cold compresses and local infiltration with epinephrine. Bronchospasm also may be relieved by nebulizations with beta-agonists (albuterol), anticholinergics (ipratroprium bromide), and aminophylline. Oxygen should be administered and the airway maintained by cricothyrotomy, if necessary. Antihistamines (usually 50 mg of diphenhydramine hydrochloride, administered intramuscularly or IV) should be given early in the course. Vasopressors should be administered if hypotension persists despite the use of epinephrine and adequate volume replacement. A short course of corticosteroids is often prescribed, but because the effects of corticosteroids are delayed, it should not supplant any of the other measures described. Rarely, with severe myocardial depression associated with anaphylaxis, we have found intraaortic balloon pumping to be a life-saving support technique until myocardial recovery.

Other Methods of Supporting Blood Pressure

The military antishock trouser is an inflatable trouser and abdominal binder, providing circumferential external pressure. Its use is controversial because no improved survival has been observed[205]; we no longer recommend it in the management of shock.

The intraaortic balloon pump has frequently been used to treat cardiogenic shock. Although cardiac output increases regularly with this support, long-term outcome is not affected unless a surgically correctable lesion is the cause of shock or the patient overcomes the myocardial stunning. In such cases, the intraaortic balloon pump may allow hemodynamic stability to be achieved during preparation for surgery or for a short period postoperatively.

Other methods like ventricular assist devices, the artificial heart, and myoplastic surgery (with latissimus dorsi muscle) have been used as "bridging" alternatives before cardiac transplantation.

Extracorporeal membrane oxygenation has shown encouraging results in younger patients.[203,206]

Corticosteroids

Glucocorticoids have not been effective in treating sepsis or septic shock. The results of two multicenter studies showed that early administration of high-dose corticosteroids neither improved patient survival nor prevented nor reversed shock in septic patients.[207–209] Both studies were double-blinded, randomized, and placebo-controlled prospective trials. Although the protocols differed in minor ways, both studies treated septic patients with high-dose corticosteroids within 2 or 3 hours of the diagnosis, in addition to employing other appropriate supportive measures. Because both studies were well designed and corticosteroids were administered early in the clinical course but neither study demonstrated improved patient survival, we do not recommend the use of corticosteroids in septic shock.

Stress doses of glucocorticoids (100 mg of hydrocortisone IV every 6 or 8 hours or its equivalent) are appropriate for treating shock when it is associated with adrenal insufficiency, hypothyroidism, in patients with an impaired adrenal–pituitary axis, or in those who require steroids for treatment of an underlying immunologic diseases (e.g., vasculitis). Conversely, steroids are relatively contraindicated in patients with cardiogenic shock because they alter the healing process of the myocardium and may predispose the patient to myocardial rupture.[209]

High-dose steroid administration was advocated for cardiogenic and hypovolemic shock and for ARDS associated with septic shock. Neither animal nor clinical studies support the use of steroids in these patients.

Miscellaneous Investigational Agents

Dozens of therapeutic agents have been used experimentally in shock[50,210] including naloxone[211,212]; dichloroacetate[101,200]; magnesium chloride–ATP complex[213]; pentoxifylline; free radical scavengers and antioxidants[214,215]; cyclooxygenase,[216] lypooxygenase, and thromboxane synthase inhibitors[217]; calcium channel blockers[218]; different antibodies[219–223]; soluble receptors or receptor antagonists[224]; vaccines[225]; gene therapy[226]; and many more that look promising but require additional studies before their routine use and specific indications can be recommended.

PROGNOSIS

Outcome after the onset of shock depends on at least five variables: severity, temporal duration, underlying cause, preexisting vital organ dysfunction, and reversibility. Several index of severity scoring systems are still under evaluation.[227,228] In general, MAP of 60 to 70 mm Hg and a systolic pressure of 80 to 90 mm Hg are benchmarks often used to signify severity; below these levels, autoregulation of brain and coronary perfusion fails in the nonhypertensive individual. Lactate measurement is another means of estimating the severity of shock. The response to therapy also assesses severity. If shock is readily reversed by moderate intravascular volume expansion, it is less severe than if maintenance of systemic pressure requires large doses of vasopressor agents, even though initial blood pressure is the same in both cases. The severity of shock may reflect only the magnitude of the underlying cause (e.g., the amount of myocardium involved by infarction, the amount of blood lost from hemorrhage). However, other factors can affect severity, including preexisting disease (e.g., chronic congestive heart failure), inadequacy of compensatory mechanisms (e.g., beta-adrenergic blocking agents that interfere with a normal neurohumoral response), or counterproductive systemic responses (e.g., SIRS).

Reversibility represents a return to normal vital organ function as a result of treatment, and irreversibility is a failure to reestablish normal function despite correction of the underlying cause. The duration of shock before treatment and the response to treatment usually determine whether shock is reversible. Unfortunately, factors that control the temporal onset of irreversibility are incompletely understood, although severity, the duration of shock before treatment, and the response to treatment undoubtedly are important.

Irreversibility implies continued circulatory insufficiency and organ dysfunction. Prolonged shock can cause brain death or irreversible renal failure, but shock itself may still be reversible. Irreversibility is signaled clinically by the continued need for vasopressor agents to maintain an arbitrarily selected level of MAP (which is itself not always possible). Because systemic pressure is the product of cardiac output and systemic vascular resistance, the heart and the peripheral vasculature are always involved in determining reversibility.

Factors that contribute to depressed myocardial function during shock include myocardial damage from prolonged ischemia, metabolic acidosis, inadequate sympathetic stimulation or depleted tissue catecholamines, circulating myocardial "depressant factors" that may enhance the synthesis of nitric oxide, and lack of available metabolic substrate for myocardial contractile function.

Vasodilating factors, including prostaglandins, bradykinin, histamine, nitric oxide, and endorphins, may be released with prolonged shock. Locally, these substances can interfere with the ability of the peripheral vasculature to maintain systemic pressure. Exogenous substances like endotoxin may interfere with vasoconstriction. It is likely that more than one of these factors plays some role. After shock begins, a vicious cycle is created in which continued hypoperfusion produces further tissue ischemia, release of more vasodilating substances, more myocardial dysfunction, and continued systemic hypoperfusion. At this point, shock is usually irreversible.

Prognosis is improved if the duration of shock is kept to a minimum by early recognition and aggressive correction of the perfusion disturbances, even in "compensated states," and if the underlying cause is discovered and corrected.

REFERENCES ■

1. Henning RJ, Weil MH, Weiner F: Blood lactate as a prognostic indicator of survival in patients with acute myocardial infarction. *Circ Shock* 1982;9:307
2. Bakker J, Coffernils M, Leon M, et al: Blood lactate levels are superior to oxygen derived variables in predicting outcome in human septic shock. *Chest* 1992;99:956
3. Lassen NA: Cerebral blood flow and oxygen consumption in man. *Physiol Rev* 1959;39:183
4. Bond RF: Peripheral macro- and microcirculation. In: Schlag G, Redl H (eds). *Pathophysiology of Shock, Sepsis and Organ Failure*. Berlin, Springer-Verlag, 1993:893
5. Strandgaard S, Olesen J, Skinhoj E, et al: Autoregulation of brain circulation in severe arterial hypertension. *Br Med J* 1973;1:507
6. U.S. Bureau of the Census: *Statistical abstrct of the United States: 1994*, ed 114, sections 2 & 3. Washington, DC, 1994
7. National Center for Health Statistics: *Health, United States, 1986*, DHHS publ no (PHS) 87-1232. Washington, DC, Government Printing Office, 1986
8. Shoemaker WC: Invasive and noninvasive cardiopulmonary monitoring of acute circulatory dysfunction and shock. *Curr Opin Critical Care* 1995;1:189
9. Bishop MH: Invasive monitoring in trauma and other critical illness. *Curr Opin Critical Care* 1995;1:204
10. Garber PJ, Mathieson AL, Ducas J, et al: Thrombolytic therapy in cardiogenic shock: effect of increased aortic pressure and rapid tPA administration. *Can J Cardiol* 1995;11:30
11. Hibbard MD, Holmes DR Jr, Bailey KR, et al: Percutaneous transluminal coronary angioplasty in patients with cardiogenic shock. *J Am Coll Cardiol* 1992;19:639
12. Gulba DC, Schmid C, Borst HG, et al: Medical compared with surgical treatment for massive pulmonary embolism. *Lancet* 1994;343:576
13. Morris EA: *A Practical Treatise on Shock After Operations and Injuries*. London, Hardwicke, 1867
14. Anggard E: Nitric oxide: mediator, murderer, and medicine. *Lancet* 1994;343:1199
15. Weil MH, Shubin H: Proposed reclassification of shock states with special reference to distributive effects. In: Hinshaw LB, Cox BG (eds). *The Fundamental Mechanisms of Shock*. New York, Plenum Press, 1972:13
16. Moss GS, Saletta JD: Traumatic shock in man. *N Engl J Med* 1974;290:724
17. Shoemaker WC, Montgomery ES, Kaplan E, et al: Physiologic patterns in surviving and nonsurviving shock patients. *Arch Surg* 1973;106:630
18. Zipnick RI, Scalea TM, Trooskin SZ, et al: Hemodynamic responses to penetrating spinal cord injuries. *J Trauma* 1993;35:578, 582 [discussion]
19. Warden GD: Burn shock resuscitation. *World J Surg* 1992; 16:16
20. Dunham C, Siegel J, Weireter L: Oxygen debt and metabolic acidemia as quantitative predictors of mortality and the severty of the ischemia insult in hemorrhagic shock. *Crit Care Med* 1991;19:231
21. Viteck V, Cowley R: Blood lactate in the prognosis of various forms of shock. *Ann Surg* 1971;173:308
22. Schlag G, Redl H, Hallström S: The cell in shock: the origin of multiple organ failure. *Resuscitation* 1991;21:137
23. Bond RF, Johnson G III: Vascular adrenergic interactions during hemorrhagic shock. *Fed Proc* 1985;44:281
24. Rush BF: Irreversibility in posttransfusion phase of hemorrhagic shock. *Adv Exp Med Biol* 1971;23:215
25. Falk JL, O'Brien JF, Kerr R: Fluid resuscitation in traumatic hemorrhagic shock. *Crit Care Clin* 1992;8:323
26. Astiz ME, Rackow EC, Weil MH: Pathophysiology and treatment of circulatory shock. *Crit Care Clin* 1993;9:183
27. Goldberg RJ, Gore JM, Alpert JS, et al: Cardiogenic shock after acute myocardial infarction: incidence and mortality from a community-wide perspective. *N Engl J Med* 1991; 325:1117
28. Leor J, et al: Cardiogenic shock complicating acute myocardial infarction in patients without heart failure on admission: incidence, risk factors, and outcome. *Am J Med* 1993;94:265
29. Moritz A, Wolner E: Circulatory support with shock due to acute myocardial infarction. *Ann Thorac Surg* 1993;55:238
30. Afifi AA, Chang PC, Liu VY, et al: Prognostic indexes in acute myocardial infarction complicated by shock. *Am J Cardiol* 1974;33:826
31. Braunwald E, Sobel BE: Coronary blood flow and myocardial ischemia. In: Braunwald E (ed). *Heart Disease*. Philadelphia, WB Saunders, 1992:1175
32. Califf RM, Bengtson JR: Cardiogenic shock. *N Engl J Med* 1994;330:1724
33. Dell'Italia LJ: Right ventricular infarction. *J Intensive Care Med* 1986;1:246
34. Zehender M, Kasper W, Kauder E, et al: Right ventricular infarction as an independent predictor of prognosis after acute inferior myocardial infarction. *N Engl J Med* 1993;328:981
35. Cohn JN, Guiha NH, Broder Ml, et al: Right ventricular infarction: clinical and hemodynamic features. *Am J Cardiol* 1974;33:209
36. Roberts N, Harrison DG, Reimer KA, et al: Right ventricular infarction with shock but without significant left ventricular infarction: a new clinical syndrome. *Am Heart J* 1985;110: 1047
37. Stein PD: Pulmonary embolism. *Curr Opin Critical Care* 1995;1:23
38. Sharma GVRK, McIntyre KM, Sharma S, et al: Clinical and hemodynamic correlates in pulmonary embolism. *Clin Chest Med* 1984;5:421

39. McIntyre KM, Sasahara AA: The hemodynamic response to pulmonary embolism in patients without prior cardiopulmonary disease. *Am J Cardiol* 1971;28:288

40. Bamberger DM, Gurley MB: Microbial etiology and clinical characteristics of distributive shock. *Clin Infect Dis* 1994; 18:726

41. Parrillo JE: Pathogenetic mechanisms of septic shock. *N Engl J Med* 1993;328:1471

42. Glauser MP, Heumann D, Baumgartner JD, et al: Pathogenesis and potential strategies for prevention and treatment of septic shock: an update. *Clin Infect Dis* 1994;18:S205

43. Rangel-Frausto MS, Pittet D, Costigan M, et al: The natural history of the systemic inflammatory response syndrome (SIRS). A prospective study. *JAMA* 1995;273:117

44. Bone RC, Balk RA, Cerra FB, et al: Definitions for sepsis and organ failure and guidelines for the use of innovative therapies in sepsis: The ACCP/SCCM Consensus Conference Committee, American College of Chest Physicians/Society of Critical Care Medicine. *Chest* 1992;101:1644

45. Ahmed NA, Christou NV, Meakins JL: The systemic inflammatory response syndrome and the critically ill surgical patient. *Curr Opin Critical Care* 1995;1:290

46. The problem of sepsis: an expert report of the European Society of Intensive Care Medicine. *Intensive Care Med* 1994;20:300

47. Hoffman WD, Natanson C: Endotoxin in septic shock. *Anesth Analg* 1993;77:613

48. Wolf JE, Rabinowitz LG: Streptococcal toxic shock–like syndrome. *Arch Dermatol* 1995;131:73

49. Bone RC: Gram-positive organisms and sepsis. *Arch Intern Med* 1994;154:26

50. Natanson C, Hoffman WD, Suffredini AF, et al: Selected treatment strategies for septic shock based on proposed mechanisms of pathogenesis. *Ann Intern Med* 1994;120:771

51. Welbourn CR, Young Y: Endotoxin, septic shock and acute lung injury: neutrophils, macrophages and inflammatory mediators. *Br J Surg* 1992;79:998

52. Edwards JD: Management of septic shock. *Br Med J* 1993; 306:1661

53. Casey LC, Balk RA, Bone RC: Plasma cytokine and endotoxin levels correlate with survival in patients with sepsis syndrome. *Ann Intern Med* 1993;119:771

54. Parker SM, Shelhamer JH, Natanson C, et al: Serial cardiovascular variables in survivors and nonsurvivors of human septic shock: heart rate as an early predictor of prognosis. *Crit Care Med* 1987;15:923

55. Bone RC: Sepsis and its complications: the clinical problem. *Crit Care Med* 1994;22:S8

56. Carmona RH, Tsao T, Dae M, et al: Myocardial dysfunction in septic shock. *Arch Surg* 1985;120:30

57. Lefer AM, Jartin J: Origin of myocardial depressant factor in shock. *Am J Physiol* 1970;218:1423

58. Parker MM, Shelhammer JH, Bacharach SL, et al: Profound but reversible myocardial depression in patients with septic shock. *Ann Intern Med* 1984;100:483

59. Werdan K, Muller U, Reithmann C: "Negative inotropic cascades" in cardiomyocytes triggered by substances relevant to sepsis. In: Schlag G, Redl H (eds). *Pathophysiology of Shock, sepsis and Organ Failure.* Berlin, Springer-Verlag, 1993: 787

60. Moncada S, Higgs A: The L-arginine–nitric oxide pathway. *N Engl J Med* 1993;329:2002

61. Kumar A, Kosuri R, Thota V, et al: Nitric oxide and cyclic GMP generation mediates human septic serum–induced in vitro cardiomyocyte depression [abstract]. *Chest* 1993;104: 12S

62. Kumar A, Kosuri R, Kandula P, et al: Tumor necrosis factor–induced myocardial cell depression in-vitro is mediated by nitric oxide generation [abstract]. *Crit Care Med* 1993;21: S278

63. Parker MM, Parrillo JE: Myocardial function in septic shock. *J Crit Care* 1990;4:47

64. Thiemermann C, Szabö C, Mitchell JA, et al: Vascular hyporeactivity to vasoconstrictor agents and hemodynamic decompensation in hemorrhagic shock is mediated by nitric oxide. *Proc Natl Acad Sci USA* 1993;90:267

65. Carroll GC, Snyder JV: Hyperdynamic severe intravascular sepsis depends on fluid administration in cynomologous monkey. *Am J Physiol* 1982;243:R131

66. Hess ML, Hastillo MA, Greenfield LJ: Spectrum of cardiovascular function during gram-negative sepsis. *Prog Cardiovasc Dis* 1981;23:279

67. Abraham E, Bland RD, Cobo JC, et al: Sequential cardiorespiratory patterns associated with outcome in septic shock. *Chest* 1984;85:75

68. Haupt MT, Gilbert EM, Carlson RW: Fluid loading increases oxygen consumption in septic patients with lactic acidosis. *Am Rev Respir Dis* 1985;131:912

69. Ensinger H, Weichel T, Lindner KH, et al: Effects of norepinephrine, epinephrine, and dopamine on oxygen consumption in volunteers. *Crit Care Med* 1993;21:1502

70. Bochner BS, Lichtenstein LM: Anaphylaxis. *N Engl J Med* 1991;324:1785

71. Cooper DJ, Thompson CR, Walley KR, et al: Histamine decreases left ventricular contractility in normal human subjects. *J Appl Physiol* 1992;73:2530

72. Otero E, Onufer JR, Reiss CK, et al: Anaphylaxis-induced myocardial depression treated with amrinone. *Lancet* 1991; 337:682

73. Raper RF, Fisher MMD: Profound reversible myocardial depression after anaphylaxis. *Lancet* 1988;i:386

74. Claussen MS, Landercasper J, Cogbill TH: Acute adrenal insufficiency presenting as shock after trauma and surgery: three cases and review of the literature. *J Trauma* 1992;32: 94

75. Rao RH, Vagnucci AH, Amico JH: Bilateral massive adrenal hemorrhage: early recognition and treatment. *Ann Intern Med* 1989;110:227

76. Chin R: Adrenal crisis. *Crit Care Clin* 1991;7:23

77. Dorin Rl, Keams PJ: High output circulatory failure in acute adrenal insufficiency. *Crit Care Med* 1988;16:296

78. Redl H, Schlag G, Kneidinger R, et al: Activation/adherence phenomena of leukocytes and endothelial cells in trauma and sepsis. In: Redl H, Schlag G (eds). *Pathophysiology of Shock, Sepsis and Organ Failure.* Berlin, Springer-Verlag, 1993: 549

79. McCord JM: Oxygen-derived free radicals. *New Horizons* 1993;1:70

80. Brigham KL: Oxygen radicals: an important mediator of sepsis and septic shock. *Klin Wochenschr* 1991;69:1004

81. Haglund U, Gerdin B: Oxygen-free radicals (OFR) and circulatory shock. *Circ Shock* 1991;34:405

82. Saugstad OD, Ostrem T: Hypoxanthine and urate levels of plasma during and after hemorrhagic hypotension in dogs. *Eur Surg Res* 1977;9:48

83. Yokoyama Y, Parks DA: Circulating xanthine oxidase: release of xanthine oxidase from isolated rat liver. *Gastroenterology* 1988;94:607

84. Vadas P, Pruzanski W: Induction of group II phospholipase A_2 expression and pathogenesis of the sepsis syndrome. *Circ Shock* 1993;39:160

85. Anderson BO, Moore EE, Banerjee A: Phospholipase A_2 regu-

lates critical inflammatory mediators of multiple organ failure. *J Surg Res* 1994;56:199

86. Gutierrez G, Brown SD: Response of the macrocirculation. In: Schlag G, Redl H (eds). *Pathophysiology of Shock, Sepsis and Organ Failure*. Berlin, Speinger-Verlag, 1993:215

87. Tracey KJ, Cerami A: Tumor necrosis factor: an updated review of its biology. *Crit Care Med* 1993;21:S415

88. Beutler B, Grau GE: Tumor necrosis factor in the pathogenesis of infectious diseases. *Crit Care Med* 1993;21:S423

89. Tracey KJ, Cerami A: Tumor necrosis factor and regulation of metabolism in infection: role of systemic versus tissue levels. *Proc Soc Exp Biol Med* 1992;200:233

90. Moldawer LL: Biology of proinflammatory cytokines and their antagonists. *Crit Care Med* 1994;22:S3

91. Hosford D, Braquet P: The potential role of platelet-activating factor in shock and ischemia. *J Crit Care* 1990;5:115

92. Dinarello CA, Wolff SM: The role of interleukin-1 in disease. *N Engl J Med* 1993;328:106 [published erratum: *N Engl J Med* 1993;328:744]

93. Bellomo R: The cytokine network in the critically ill. *Anaesth Intensive Care* 1992;20:288

94. Korthuis RJ, Anderson DC, Granger DN: Role of neutrophil-endothelial cell adhesion in inflammatory disorders. *J Crit Care* 1994;9:47

95. Shires GT, Cunningham JN, Barker CRF: Alterations in cellular membrane function during hemorrhagic shock in primates. *Ann Surg* 1972;176:288

96. Campion SD, Lynch LJ, Rector FC, et al: Effect of hemorrhagic shock on transmembrane potential. *Surgery* 1969;66:1051

97. Trunkey DD, Illner H, Wagner IY, et al: The effect of septic shock on skeletal muscle action potentials in the primate. *Surgery* 1979;85:638

98. Minei IP, Fantini GA, Hesse DG, et al: Endotoxin infusion in human volunteers: assessment of the early cellular membrane response. *Surg Forum* 1987;38:102

99. Bergstrom J, Furst F, Holmstrom B, et al: Influence of injury and nutrition on muscle water and electrolytes: effect of elective operations. *Ann Surg* 1981;193:810

100. Sayeed MM: Membrane sodium-potassium transport and ancillary phenomenon in circulatory shock. In: Cowley R, Trump B (eds). *Pathophysiology of Shock, Anoxia and Ischemia*. Baltimore, Williams & Wilkins, 1982:112

101. Matthews JG, Lisbon A: Lactate metabolism in the critically ill patient. *Curr Opin Critical Care* 1995;1:267

102. Mizock B: Septic shock: a metabolic perspective. *Arch Intern Med* 1984;144:579

103. Gulick T, Chung MK, Pieper SJ, et al: Interleukin-1 and tumor necrosis factor inhibit cardiac myocyte adrenergic responsiveness. *Proc Natl Acad Sci USA* 1989;86:6753

104. Harper AM: Autoregulation of cerebral blood flow: influence of the arterial blood pressure on the blood flow though the cerebral cortex. *J Neurol Neurosurg Psychiatry* 1966;29:398

105. Sprung CL, Peduzzi PN, Shatney CH, et al: Impact of encephalopathy on mortality in the sepsis syndrome. *Crit Care Med* 1990;18:801

106. Gisvold SE, Safar P, Rao G, et al: Prolonged immobolization and controlled ventilation do not improve outcome after global brain ischemia in monkeys. *Crit Care Med* 1984;12:171

107. Johnson G, Henderson D, Bond RF: Morphological differences in cutaneous and skeletal muscle vasculature during compensatory and decompensatory hemorrhagic hypotension. *Circ Shock* 1985;15:111

108. Newman JH: Sepsis and pulmonary edema. *Clin Chest Med* 1985;6:371

109. Matthay MA: Function of the alveolar epithelial barrier under pathologic conditions. *Chest* 1994;105:67S

110. Weir K, Mlczoch J, Reeves J, et al: Endotoxin and prevention of hypoxic pulmonary vasoconstriction. *J Lab Clin Med* 1976;88:975

111. Wardle EN: Acute renal failure and multiorgan failure. *Nephron* 1994;66:380

112. Myer B, Moran S: Hemodinamically mediated acute renal failure. *N Engl J Med* 1986;314:97

113. Badr KF, Ichikawa I: Prerenal failure: a deleterious shift from renal compensation to decompensation. *N Engl J Med* 1988;319:623

114. Kitai T, Tanaka A, Tokuka A, et al: Changes in the hepatic oxygenation state during hemorrhage and following epinephrine or dextran infusion as assessed by near-infrared spectroscopy. *Circ Shock* 1993;41:197

115. Bor NM, Alvur M, Ercan MT, et al: Liver blood flow rate and glucose metabolism in hemorrhagic hypotension and shock. *J Trauma* 1982;22:753

116. Hawker F: Liver dysfunction in critical illness. *Anaesth Intensive Care* 1991;19:165

117. Champion HR, Jones RT, Trump BF, et al: A clinicopathologic study of hepatic dysfunction following shock. *Surg Gynecol Obstet* 1976;142:657

118. Moreau R, Hadengue A, Soupison T, et al: Septic shock in patients with cirrhosis: hemodynamic and metabolic characteristics and intensive care unit outcome. *Crit Care Med* 1992;20:746

119. Fusamoto H, Hagiwara H, Meren H, et al: clinical study of acute gastrointestinal hemorrhage associated with various shock states. *Am J Gastroenterol* 1991;86:429

120. Schuster DP, Rowley H, Feinstein S, et al: Prospective evaluation of the risk of upper gastrointestinal bleeding after admission to a medical intensive care unit. *Am J Med* 1984;76:623

121. DiPalma JA: Gastrointestinal complications in the critically ill and the role of the gut in multiple organ dysfunction syndrome. *Curr Opin Critical Care* 1995;1:121

122. Mainous MR, Deitch EA: Bacterial translocation. In: Schlag G, Redl H (eds). *Pathophysiology of Shock, Sepsis and Organ Failure*. Berlin, Springer-Verlag, 1993:265

123. Van Leeuwen PA, Boermeester MA, Houdijk AP, et al: Clinical significance of translocation. *Gut* 1994;35:S28

124. Fink MP: Adequacy of gut oxygenation in endotoxemia and sepsis. *Crit Care Med* 1993;21:S4

125. Berg RD: Bacterial translocation from the gastrointestinal tract. *J Med* 1992;23:217

126. Meakins JL, Marshall JC: The gut as the motor of multiple organ failure. In: Marston A, Bulkley GB, Fiddian-Green RG, et al (eds). *Splanchnic Ischemia and Multiple Organ Failure*. St Louis, Mosby, 1989:339

127. Haglund U: Systemic mediators released from the gut in critical illness. *Crit Care Med* 1993;21:S15

128. Fiddian-Green RG: Associations between intramucosal acidosis in the gut and organ failure. *Crit Care Med* 1993;21:S103

129. Muller MJ, Herndon DN: The challenge of burns. *Lancet* 1994;343:216

130. Thijs LG, de Boer JP, de Groot MC, et al: Coagulation disorders in septic shock. *Intensive Care Med* 1993;19:S8

131. Counts HB, Haisch C, Simon TL, et al: Hemostasis in massively transfused trauma patients. *Ann Surg* 1979;190:91

132. Shoemaker WC, Bland RD, Appel PL: Therapy of critically ill postoperative patients based on outcome prediction and prospective clinical trials. *Surg Clin North Am* 1985;65:811

133. Bishop MH, Shoemaker WC, Appel PL, et al: Prospective, randomized trial of survivor values of cardiac index, oxygen delivery, and oxygen consumtion as resuscitation endpoints in severe trauma. *J Trauma* 1995;38:780

134. Silance PG, Simon C, Vincent JL: The relation between cardiac index and oxygen extraction in acutely ill patients. *Chest* 1994;105:1190

135. Hayes MA, Timmins AC, Yau EHS, et al: Elevation of systemic oxygen delivery in the treatment of critically ill patients. *N Engl J Med* 1994;330:1717

136. Hinds C, Watson D: Manipulating hemodynamics and oxygen transport in critically ill patients. *N Engl J Med* 1995;333:1074

137. Pinsky MR, Matuschak G: A unifying hypothesis of multiple systems organ failure: failure of host defense homeostasis. *J Crit Care* 1990;5:108

138. Barton R, Cerra FB: The hypermetabolism multiple organ failure syndrome. *Chest* 1989;96:1153

139. Kudsk KA, Minard G: Enteral versus parenteral nutrition in the critically ill and injured. *Curr Opin Critical Care* 1995; 1:255

140. Barton RG: Nutrition support in critical illness. *Nutr Clin Pract* 1994;9:127

141. Giroir BP: Mediators of septic shock: new approaches for interrupting the endogenous inflammatory cascade. *Crit Care Med* 1993;21:780

142. Aubier MT, Trippenbach T, Roussos C: Respiratory muscle fatigue during cardiogenic shock. *J Appl Physiol* 1981;51:499

143. Hussain SNA, Graham R, Rutledge F, et al: Respiratory muscle energetics during endotoxin shock in dogs. *J Appl Physiol* 1986;60:486

144. Johnson TJ, Stothert JC: Respiratory evaluation and support in the ICU. *Curr Opin Critical Care* 1995;1:306

145. Idris AH, Staples ED, O' Brien DJ, et al: Effect of ventilation on acid-base balance and oxygenation in low blood-flow states. *Crit Care Med* 1994;22:1827

146. Desjars P, Pinaud M, Potel G, et al: A reappraisal of norepinephrine therapy in human septic shock. *Crit Care Med* 1987;15:134

147. Meadows D, Edwards JD, Wilkins RG, et al: Reversal of intractable septic shock with norepinephrine therapy. *Crit Care Med* 1988;16:663

148. Ognibene FP, Parker MM, Natanson C, et al: Depressed left ventricular performance: response to volume infusion in patients with sepsis and septic shock. *Chest* 1988;93:903

149. Reich DL, Konstadt SN, Raissi S, et al: Trendelenburg position and passive leg raising do not significantly improve cardiopulmonary performance in the anesthetized patient with coronary artery disease. *Crit Care Med* 1989;17:313

150. Rackow EC, Falk JL, Fein A, et al: Fluid resuscitation in circulatory shock: a comparison of the cardiorespiratory effects of albumin, hetastarch, and saline solutions in patients with hypovolemic and septic shock. *Crit Care Med* 1983;11:839

151. Shoemaker WC, Hauser CJ: Critique of crystalloid versus colloid therapy in shock and shock lung. *Crit Care Med* 1979;7:117

152. Puri V, Howard M, Paidipaty BB, et al: Resuscitation in hypovolemic shock: a prospective study of hydroxyethyl starch and albumin. *Crit Care Med* 1983;11:518

153. Tullis JL: Albumin. I. Background and use. *JAMA* 1977;237:355

154. Tullis JL: Albumin. II. Guidelines for clinical use. *JAMA* 1977;237:460

155. Monafo WW: Volume replacement in hemorrhage, shock and burns. *Adv Shock Res* 1980;3:47

156. Velanovich V: Crystalloid versus colloid fluid resuscitation: a meta-analysis of mortality. *Surgery* 1989;105:65

157. Napolitano LM: Resuscitation following trauma and hemorrhagic shock: is hydroxyethyl starch safe? *Crit Care Med* 1995;23:795

158. Goodin TH, Grossbard EB, Kaufman RJ, et al: A perfluorochemical emulsion for prehospital resuscitation of experimental hemorrhagic shock: a prospective, randomized, controlled study. *Crit Care Med* 1994;22:680

159. Rabinovici R, Neville LF, Rudolph AS, et al: Hemoglobin-based oxygen-carrying resuscitation fluids. *Crit Care Med* 1995;23:801

160. Dubick MA, Wade CE: A review of the efficacy and safety of 7.5% NaCl/6% dextran 70 in experimental animals and in humans. *J Trauma* 1994;36:323

161. Bickell WH, Wall MJ Jr, Pepe PE, et al: Immediate versus delayed fluid resuscitation for hypotensive patients with penetrating torso injuries. *N Engl J Med* 1994;331:1105

162. Owens TM, Watson WC, Prough DS, et al: Limiting initial resuscitation of uncontrolled hemorrhage reduces internal bleeding and subsequent volume requirements. *Trauma* 1995;39:200, 208 [discussion]

163. Milne ENC: Impact of imaging in the intensive care unit. *Curr Opin Critical Care* 1995;1:43

164. Khoury AF, Afridi I, Quinones MA, et al: Transesophageal echocardiography in critically ill patients: feasibility, safety, and impact on management. *Am Heart J* 1994;127:1363

165. Kinch JW, Ryan TJ: Right ventricular infarction. *N Engl J Med* 1994;330:1211

166. Fiddian-Green RG, Haglund U, Gutierrez G, et al: Goals for the resuscitation of shock. *Crit Care Med* 1993;21:S25

167. Eisenberg PR, Schuster DP: Clinical evaluation compared with invasive hemodynamic assessment. In: Snyder JV (ed). *Oxygen Transport in the Critically Ill.* Chicago, Year Book Medical Publishers, 1987:199

168. Bruner JMR, Krenis LJ, Krunsman JM, et al: Comparison of direct and indirect methods of measuring blood pressure. Parts I–III. *Med Instrum* 1981;15:11, 97, 182

169. Aaslid R, Brubakk AO: Accuracy of an ultrasound Doppler servo method for noninvasive determination of instantaneous and mean blood pressure. *Circulation* 1981;64:753

170. Foëx BA, Little RA: Hemodynamic evaluation of the critically ill surgical patient. *Curr Opin Critical Care* 1995;1:281

171. Mimoz O, Rauss A, Rekik N, et al: Pulmonary artery catheterization in critically ill patients: a prospective analysis of outcome changes associated with catheter-prompted changes in therapy. *Crit Care Med* 1994;22:573

172. Abou-Khalil B, Scalea TM, Trooskin SZ, et al: Hemodynamic responses to shock in young trauma patients: need for invasive monitoring. *Crit Care Med* 1994;22:633

173. Eisenberg PR, Jaffe AS, Schuster DP: Clinical evaluation compared to pulmonary artery catheterization in the hemodynamic assessment of critically ill patients. *Crit Care Med* 1984;12:349

174. Connors AF Jr, McCafree DR, Gray BA: Evaluation of right heart catheterization in the critically ill patient without acute myocardial infarction. *N Engl J Med* 1983;308:263

175. Pinsky MR: Beyond global oxygen supply-demand relations: in search of measures of dysoxia. *Intensive Care Med* 1994;20:1

176. Shoemaker WC, Appel PL, Kram HB: Hemodynamic and oxygen transport responses in survivors and nonsurvivors of high-risk surgery. *Crit Care Med* 1993;21:977

177. Schuller D, Mitchell JP, Calandrino FS, et al: Fluid balance

of patients in pulmonary edema has an important impact on outcome. *Am Rev Respir Dis* 1990;141:A141

178. Mitchell JP, Schuller D, Calandrino FS, et al: Prospective randomized trial of effect of fluid balance on the resolution of pulmonary edema. *Am Rev Respir Dis* 1990;141:A141.

179. Schuller D, Mitchell JP, Calandrino FS, et al: Early extravascular lung water reduction is associated with better outcome in non-cardiogenic pulmonary edema. *Chest* 1990;98:86S.

180. Simmons RS, Berdine GG, Seidenbeld JJ, et al: Fluid balance and the adult respiratory distress syndrome. *Am Rev Respir Dis* 1987;135:924

181. Humphrey H, Hall J, Sznajder I, et al: Improved survival in ARDS patients associated with a reduction in pulmonary capillary wedge pressure. *Chest* 1990;97:1176

182. Lowell JA, Schifferdecker C, Driscoll DF, et al: Postoperative fluid overload: not a benign problem. *Crit Care Med* 1990;18:728

183. Simonson SG, Piantadosi CA: Near-infrared spectroscopy for monitoring tissue oxygenation in the critical care setting. *Curr Opin Critical Care* 1995;1:197

184. Wo CC, Shoemaker WC, Bishop MH, et al: Noninvasive estimations of cardiac output and circulatory dynamics in critically ill patients. *Curr Opin Critical Care* 1995;1:211

185. Shoemaker WC, Wo CC, Bishop MH, et al: Multicenter trial of a new thoracic electrical bioimpedance device for cardiac output estimation. *Crit Care Med* 1994;22:1907

186. Groeneveld AB, Kolkman JJ: Splanchnic tonometry: a review of physiology, methodology, and clinical applications. *J Crit Care* 1994;9:198

187. Arnold J, Hendriks J, Ince C, et al: Tonometry to assess the adequacy of splanchnic oxygenation in the critically ill patient. *Intensive Care Med* 1994;20:452

188. Mueller HS: Inotropic agents in the treatment of cardiogenic shock. *World J Surg* 1985;9:3

189. Chernow B, Rainey TG, Lake CR: Endogenous and exogenous catecholamines. *Crit Care Med* 1982;10:409

190. McGhie AI, Golstein RA: Pathogenesis and management of acute heart failure and cardiogenic shock: role of inotropic therapy. *Chest* 1992;102:626S

191. McArthur CJ: Some recent controversies in intensive care. *Asian Cardiovasc Thorac Ann* 1995;3:4

192. Duke GJ, Breidis JH, Weaver RA: Renal support in critically ill patients: low-dose dopamine or low-dose dobutamine? *Crit Care Med* 1994;22:1919

193. Frishman WH, Dollery CT, Cruickshank JM: *Current Cardiovascular Drugs.* Philadelphia, Current Medicine, 1994:195

194. *Texbook of Advanced Cardiac Life Support.* Dallas, American Heart Association, 1994:1

195. Mizock BA, Falk JL: Lactic acidosis in critical illness. *Crit Care Med* 1992;20:80

196. Narins RG, Cohen J: Bicarbonate therapy for organic acidosis: the case for its continued use. *Ann Intern Med* 1987;106:615

197. Douglas ME, Downs JB, Mantini EL, et al: Alterations of oxygen tension and oxyhemoglobin saturation: a hazard of sodium bicarbonate administration. *Arch Surg* 1979;114:326

198. Ritter JM, Doktor HS, Benjamin N: Paradoxical effect of bicarbonate on cytoplasmic pH. *Lancet* 1990;335:1243

199. Cooper DJ, Walley KR, Wiggs RB, et al: Bicarbonate does not improve hemodynamics in critically ill patients who have lactic acidosis. *Ann Intern Med* 1990;112:492

200. Stacpoole PW, Wright EC, Baumgartner TG, et al: A controlled clinical trial of dichloroacetate for the treatment of lactic acidosis in adults: the Dichloroacetate Lactic Acidosis Study Group. *N Engl J Med* 1992;327:1564

201. Bedotto JB, Kahn JK, Rutherford BD, et al: Failed direct coronary angioplasty for acute myocardial infarction: in-hospital outcome and predictors of death. *J Am Coll Cardiol* 1993;22:690

202. Eckman MH, Wong JB, Salem DN, et al: Direct angioplasty for acute myocardial infarction: a review of outcomes in clinical subsets. *Ann Intern Med* 1992;117:667

203. Goldenberg IF: Nonpharmacologic management of cardiac arrest and cardiogenic shock. *Chest* 1992;102:596S

204. Russell JA, Phang PT: The oxygen delivery/consumption controversy: approaches to management of the critically ill. *Am J Respir Crit Care Med* 1994;149:533

205. Mattox KL, Bickell W, Pepe PE, et al: Prospective MAST study in 911 patients. *J Trauma* 1989;29:1104

206. Zwischenberger JB, Cox CS Jr: ECMO in the management of cardiac failure. *ASAIO J* 1992;38:751

207. Bone RC, Fisher CJ, Clemmer TP, et al: A controlled clinical trial of high-dose methylprednisolone in the treatment of severe sepsis and septic shock. *N Engl J Med* 1987;317:653

208. Veteran's Administration Systemic Sepsis Cooperative Study Group: Effect of high-dose glucocorticoid therapy on mortality in patients with clinical signs of systemic sepsis. *N Engl J Med* 1987;317:659

209. Roberto R, DeMillo V, Sobel BE: Deleterious effects of methylprednisolone in patients with myocardial infarction. *Circulation* 1976;53:204

210. Suffredini AF: Current prospects for the treatment of clinical sepsis. *Crit Care Med* 1994;22:S12

211. Curtis MT, Lefer AM: Protective actions of naloxone in hemorrhagic shock. *Am J Physiol* 1980;239:H416

212. Faden AI, Holaday JW: Experimental endotoxin shock: the pathophysiologic function of endorphins and treatment with opiate antagonists. *J Infect Dis* 1980;142:229

213. Harkema JM, Chaudry IH: Magnesium-adenosine triphosphate in the treatment of shock, ischemia, and sepsis. *Crit Care Med* 1992;20:263

214. Schiller HJ, Reilly PM, Bulkley GB: Tissue perfusion in critical illnesses: antioxidant therapy. *Crit Care Med* 1993;21:S92

215. Goode HF, Webster NR: Free radicals and antioxidants in sepsis. *Crit Care Med* 1993;21:1770

216. Jacobs ER, Soulsby ME, Bone RC, et al: Ibuprofen in canine endotoxin shock. *J Clin Invest* 1983;70:536

217. Bone RC: Phospholipids and their inhibitors: a critical evaluation of their role in the treatment of sepsis. *Crit Care Med* 1992;20:884

218. Maitra SR, Krikhely M, Dulchavsky SA, et al: Beneficial effects of diltiazem in hemorrhagic shock. *Circ Shock* 1991;33:121

219. Ziegler EJ, McCuthchan JA, Fierer J, et al: Treatment of gram-negative bacteremia and shock with human antiserum to a mutant *Escherichia coli. N Engl J Med* 1982;307:1225

220. Peake S: Monoclonal antibodies: immunotherapy for the critically ill. *Anaesth Intensive Care* 1993;21:739

221. The French National Registry of HA-1A (Centoxin) in Septic Shock: A cohort study of 600 patients. The National Committee for the Evaluation of Centoxin. *Arch Intern Med* 1994;154:2484

222. Bodmer M, Fournel MA, Hinshaw LB: Preclinical review of anti-tumor necrosis factor monoclonal antibodies. *Crit Care Med* 1993;21:S441

223. Pennington JE: Therapy with antibody to tumor necrosis factor in sepsis. *Clin Infect Dis* 1993;17:S515

224. Fisher CJ Jr, Dhainaut JF, Opal SM, et al: Recombinant human interleukin-1 receptor antagonist in the treatment of

patients with sepsis syndrome: results from a randomized, double-blind, placebo-controlled trial. Phase III rhIL-1ra Sepsis Syndrome Study Group. *JAMA* 1994;271:1836

225. St. John RC, Dorinsky PM: Immunologic therapy for ARDS, septic shock, and multiple organ failure. *Chest* 1993;103:932

226. Buchman TG: Manipulation of stress gene expression: a novel therapy for the treatment of sepsis? *Crit Care Med* 1994;22:901

227. Meade MO, Cook DJ: A critical appraisal and systematic review of illness severity scoring systems in the intensive care unit. *Curr Opin Critical Care* 1995;1:221

228. Carlet J, Nicolas F: Specific severity of illness scoring systems. *Curr Opin Critical Care* 1995;1:233

Critical Care, Third Edition, edited by Joseph M. Civetta,
Robert W. Taylor, and Robert R. Kirby.
Lippincott-Raven Publishers, Philadelphia, PA © 1997.

CHAPTER 27

Cardiogenic Shock

John A. Farmer

IMMEDIATE CONCERNS

MAJOR PROBLEMS

Cardiogenic shock is a major and frequently fatal complication of a variety of acute and chronic disorders that results in a primary impairment of the ability of the heart to maintain adequate tissue perfusion.

STRESS POINTS

1. Clinical criteria used to establish the diagnosis of cardiogenic shock include absolute or relative hypotension, which is defined as a systolic blood pressure less than 90 mm Hg or a blood pressure that has fallen to at least 30 mm Hg less than the individual's baseline blood pressure.
2. Cardiogenic shock thus may be a complication in patients with chronic hypertension who have an acute cardiac event that results in a decrease in blood pressure, but not to the 90-mm Hg systolic level.
3. However, if signs of organ dysfunction and tissue hypoperfusion accompany this condition, the individual thus qualifies for the diagnosis of cardiogenic shock.
4. The exact incidence of cardiogenic shock is difficult to definitely ascertain because of variability in diagnostic criteria and survival rates in the early phase of acute myocardial infarction. The Multicenter Investigation of Limitation of Infarct Size trial[1] documents an incidence rate of cardiogenic shock in 7% of subjects who were admitted to the hospital after having an acute myocardial infarction. Using multivariate analysis, the Worcester Heart Attack Study demonstrated that the incidence of acute myocardial infarction complicated by cardiogenic shock is increasing, which presumably

results from improved recognition and treatment of myocardial infarction in the early hours after formation of the acute occlusive thrombus.[2]

ESSENTIAL DIAGNOSTIC TESTS AND PROCEDURES

1. Bedside clinical criteria that provide evidence of reduced organ perfusion include oliguria, confusion, peripheral cyanosis, and evidence of peripheral vasoconstriction.
2. An accurate definition of cardiogenic shock also requires persistence of the shock state after correction of extracardiac conditions, such as hypovolemia or a variety of metabolic abnormalities including significant disturbances in acid-base metabolism, electrolyte abnormalities, or arrhythmias.
3. The pulmonary artery occlusion pressure is frequently in excess of 18 mm Hg, and the cardiac index is usually less than 2.2 L/minute/m^2.

INITIAL THERAPY

1. Cardiogenic shock in the setting of acute myocardial infarction warrants pharmacologic intervention to limit infarct size and includes using thrombolytic therapy, heparin, aspirin, nitrates, calcium channel blockers, beta-blockers, or a combination thereof.
2. Hemodynamic management includes optimization of preload and afterload and augmentation of contractility, when appropriate, with agents such as dobutamine, dopamine, norepinephrine, digitalis preparations, or phosphodiesterase inhibitors.
3. Surgical intervention in myocardial infarction has been used to limit infarct size by direct revascularization or

correction of mechanical defects of an acute ischemic event such as ventricular septal defects (VSDs), acute mitral insufficiency, free wall rupture, or left ventricular aneurysm.

4. Mechanical assist devices such as the intraaortic balloon pump are used as temporizing measures to optimize blood pressure, cardiac output, and tissue perfusion in patients with cardiogenic shock while further diagnostic procedures and disease staging are performed.

CLASSIFICATION

A variety of classification schemes have been proposed for the division of circulatory shock according to etiology and underlying hemodynamic mechanisms. Circulatory shock can be subdivided into four distinct classes on the basis of underlying mechanism plus hemodynamics; these classes should be considered and excluded before establishing a definite diagnosis of cardiogenic shock.

HYPOVOLEMIC SHOCK

Hypovolemic shock results from volume loss caused by conditions such as gastrointestinal bleeding or extravasation of plasma.

OBSTRUCTIVE SHOCK

Obstructive shock results from impedance of the circulatory channels by an intrinsic or extrinsic obstruction. Pulmonary embolism, dissecting aneurysm, and pericardial tamponade result in obstructive shock.

DISTRIBUTIVE SHOCK

Distributive shock is caused by conditions such as direct arteriovenous shunting and is characterized by decreased resistance or increased venous capacity from the vasomotor dysfunction that is associated with a normal or high resistance.

CARDIOGENIC SHOCK

Cardiogenic shock is characterized by primary myocardial dysfunction resulting in the inability of the heart to maintain an adequate cardiac output with subsequent compromising of metabolic requirements (Fig. 27-1). The most common etiologies are myocardial infarction or cardiomyopathy with a superimposed hemodynamic stress.

ETIOLOGY

The most common etiology of cardiogenic shock is acute myocardial infarction with a resultant loss of approximately 40% of functioning myocardium. Loss of myocardial function may occur in one massive myocardial infarction or may

result in a cumulative loss of pump function caused by serial smaller infarcts. Predominant involvement of the left ventricle is the form of myocardial infarction most commonly associated with cardiogenic shock, although recent clarification of the potential role of the right ventricle in the precipitation of the shock state has been recognized. Additionally, acute mechanical complications of myocardial infarction such as mitral insufficiency, free wall rupture, and acute VSD may result in the periinfarction occurrence of cardiogenic shock, as does the late development of left ventricular aneurysm (Table 27-1).

LEFT VENTRICULAR ACUTE MYOCARDIAL INFARCTION

Reduction in left ventricular performance is one of the major complications of ischemic heart disease. Several classifications that attempt to standardize the clinical and hemodynamic presentation of myocardial infarction have been proposed to aid in determining prognosis and the therapeutic approaches in patients with established cardiogenic shock or those who have the potential to progress to the shock state.

The Killip classification uses pure clinical bedside evaluation of the patient to establish prognostic indicators to predict the mortality associated with an acute myocardial infarction using the physical findings of congestive heart failure.[3]

Class I patients developed no overt signs of congestive heart failure, and these individuals had a low in-hospital mortality rate. This subgroup represented approximately 40% to 50% of all patients who presented with an acute myocardial infarction, and the in-hospital fatality rate was approximately 6%.

Class II patients demonstrated evidence of impaired ventricular function as manifest by persistent bibasilar rales and an audible third heart sound. This subset of patients accounted for approximately 30% to 40% of patients with acute myocardial infarction and resulted in a significant increase in in-hospital mortality rate, with an approximate tripling of the mortality rate relative to Class I, with a level of 17% being documented.

Class III patients were characterized by the development of acute pulmonary edema, which was seen in approximately 10% to 15% of patients admitted to the hospital. A significant mortality rate of 38% was seen in this group, who were treated in a conservative manner before the thrombolytic era.

Class IV patients had established cardiogenic shock with hypotension and signs of organ hypoperfusion. Cardiogenic shock occurred in approximately 5% to 10% of infarct patients in this series but was associated with a markedly increased in-hospital mortality rate of 80%, which was a function of both severity of the underlying illness plus the limited availability of definitive treatment at the time this classification was proposed.

The group at Cedars Sinai Medical Center Los Angeles, also developed a clinical classification of heart failure associated with acute myocardial infarction, which was subsequently refined by the availability of invasive hemodynamic monitoring using pulmonary artery catheters[4] (Table 27-2).

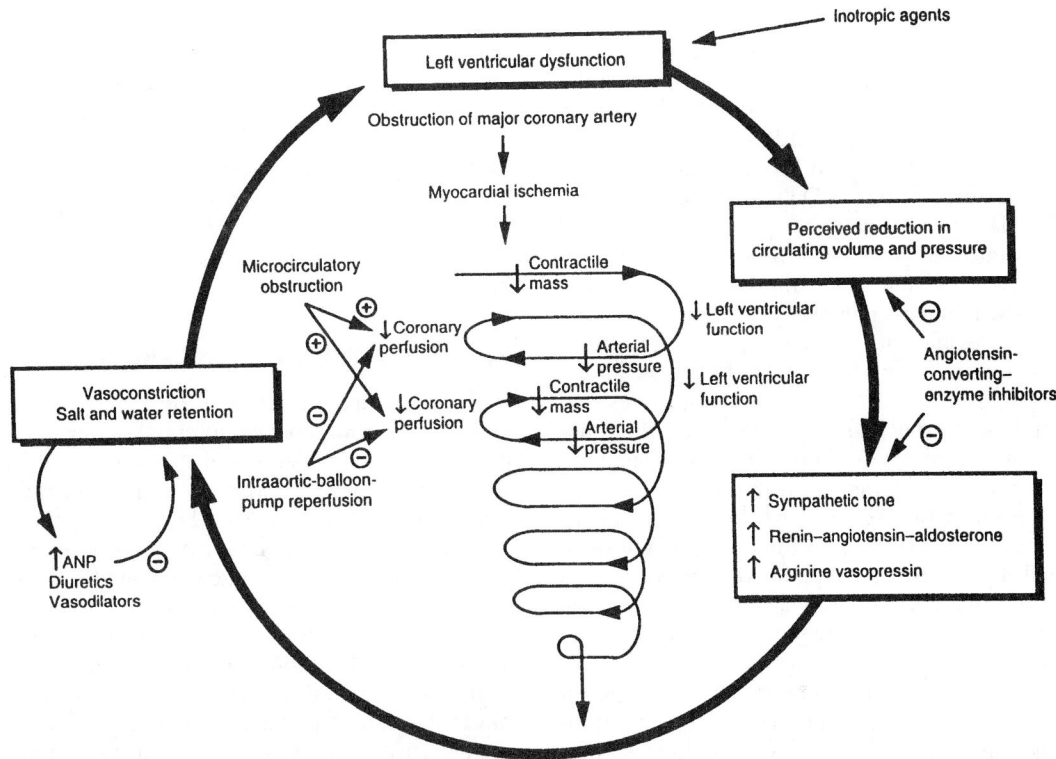

FIGURE 27-1. Neurohumoral and mechanical events that lead to death in patients with cardiogenic shock. ANP, atrial natriuretic peptide. (Used with permission from Califf RM, Bengston JR: Cardiogenic shock. *N Engl J Med* 1994;300:1724.)

The Cedars Sinai classification also subdivided patients with acute myocardial into four subsets based on the measurement of the pulmonary artery occlusion pressure, cardiac index, and clinical assessment.

Class I patients had no clinical evidence of pulmonary congestion or tissue hypoperfusion. Hemodynamic parameters measured in these subjects revealed the pulmonary artery occlusion pressure to be less than 18 mm Hg and the cardiac index to be in excess of 2.2 mm Hg. The advent and widespread use of pulmonary artery catheters clarified the concept of the ideal wedge that established the impact of diastolic dysfunction secondary to acute ischemia, with resul-

tant impaired relaxation and elevated filling pressures being required to maintain adequate cardiac output.

Class I patients accounted for 25% of subjects admitted to the coronary care unit, and there was an extraordinarily low in-hospital mortality rate of 1%. Patients who on clinical grounds demonstrated no evidence of hypoperfusion or pulmonary congestion would not be expected to benefit from invasive cardiac monitoring and frequent clinical reassessments; close attention paid to blood pressure and evidence of organ perfusion would represent adequate care.

Class II patients demonstrated pulmonary congestion as manifest by only an elevated pulmonary artery occlusion

TABLE 27-1. Contributing Factors to the Development of Cardiogenic Shock in Myocardial Infarction

1. Loss of left ventricular function
   Cumulative loss of myocardial tissue exceeding 40% of ventricular mass
   Myocardial infarction associated with bradyarrhythmias or tachyarrhythmias
   Hypovolemia or hypervolemia
2. Right ventricular infarction
3. Mechanical defects
   Papillary muscle dysfunction or rupture
   Ventricular septal defect
   Ventricular pseudoaneurysm
   Free wall rupture

TABLE 27-2. Hemodynamic Subsets and Mortality in Myocardial Infarction

SWAN-FORRESTER CLASS	MORTALITY RATE (%)
I CI >2.2 PAOP <18	<3
II CI >2.2 PAOP >18	9
III CI <2.2 PAOP <18	23
IV CI <2.2 PAOP >18	51

PAOP, pulmonary artery occlusion pressure; CI, cardiac index in liters per minute per square meter.

pressure greater than 18 mm Hg with an associated normal cardiac index. Class II patients also accounted for approximately 25% of patients admitted to the coronary care unit, but an 11% mortality rate was associated with this group. Mild pulmonary congestion is transiently seen in a significant percentage of patients admitted to the coronary care unit and has a multifactorial etiology. Diastolic dysfunction induced by ischemia with retrograde transmission of elevated filling pressures into the pulmonary venous circuit results in extravasation of fluid into the pulmonary bed because of Starling forces. Papillary muscle dysfunction with mild degrees of mitral insufficiency also are a potential cause of pulmonary congestion in this subgroup. Physical examination of these patients reveals mild to moderate rales and potentially a audible third heart sound associated with radiographic evidence of pulmonary venous hypertension. Dyspnea and orthopnea are the main symptoms superimposed on the clinical presentation of myocardial ischemia. Treatment in this group is centered on reduction of filling pressures to a level that relieves pulmonary venous congestion but does not result in an overzealous reduction of filling pressures below the ideal wedge. Excessive diuresis should be assiduously avoided, especially in patients who were euvolemic before the onset of their infarct. Despite signs of pulmonary congestion, these patients frequently are not intravascularly volume overloaded, and diuretic therapy may reduce filling pressures to a level that would impair cardiac output. Oxygenation should be maintained with adequate arterial saturation that may be monitored by oximetry. Vasodilator therapy in the form of nitroglycerin or inotropic agents with vasodilating capacity such as dobutamine are effective to return the hemodynamic parameters to normal. The usefulness and risk–benefit ratio of invasive hemodynamic monitoring in this subgroup of patients are controversial, although these patients frequently may be managed on clinical grounds.

Class III patients are characterized predominantly by clinical evidence of hypoperfusion. Hemodynamic monitoring reveals a pulmonary artery occlusion pressure less than 18 mm Hg and a cardiac index of less than 2.2 L/minute/m². The Class III subgroup accounts for approximately 15% of patients with acute myocardial infarction and is associated with a 23% mortality rate. Patients in this subgroup may be extremely difficult to manage on clinical grounds, and treatment can be facilitated by invasive hemodynamic monitoring to establish the volume status. Relative hypovolemia is determined by measuring the pulmonary artery occlusion pressure, which falls below that of the ideal wedge as predicted in ischemic states. Excessive diuresis is extremely problematic in this group of patients and may excessively decrease cardiac output because of the preexistent relative hypovolemia. Class III patients require restoration of intravascular volume to increase filling pressures to a degree that ensures adequate cardiac output and organ perfusion.

Class IV patients demonstrated elevated pulmonary artery occlusion pressures in excess of 18 mm Hg and a depressed cardiac index of less than 2.2 L/minute/m² and frequently qualify for the diagnosis of cardiogenic shock, which additionally requires clinical evidence of organ hypoperfu-

sion and dysfunction. This subgroup currently accounts for approximately 35% of patients with myocardial infarction and is associated with an in-hospital mortality rate of approximately 50%. Class IV patients may have a mechanical defect such as acute mitral insufficiency, free wall rupture, or VSD underlying the acute myocardial infarction; these are discussed separately. Oxygenation with the potential assisted ventilation in addition to inotropic and judicious use of vasodilator support is the recommended therapy in these subgroups.

RIGHT VENTRICULAR INFARCTION

Right ventricular infarction as the cause of cardiogenic shock had been discounted as a potential etiologic factor because prior experimental studies had demonstrated minimal impairment of cardiac output after induced right ventricular infarction in canine hearts.[5] The clinical diagnosis of right ventricular infarction should be considered when elevated jugular venous pressure is accompanied by hypotension, but the diagnosis may be difficult to establish clinically unless hemodynamic measurements, special electrocardiographic leads, echocardiography, or nuclear imaging are performed.[6] Right-sided precordial leads obtained by electrocardiography that demonstrates at least 1-mm ST elevation is approximately 70% sensitive in the diagnosis of right ventricular infarction. Echocardiography is an easily obtainable noninvasive study that demonstrates right ventricular dilation and impairment of wall motion of the right ventricle. Radionuclide angiography currently is considered to be the most sensitive means to diagnose right ventricular infarction.[7] A decrease in right ventricular ejection fraction that is associated with wall motion abnormalities is more than 90% sensitive in the diagnosis of a right ventricular infarction. Hemodynamic studies, which are also supportive of significant ischemic involvement of the right ventricle, are manifest by increases in right atrial pressures plus demonstration of resistance to diastolic filling, as shown by blunting of the y-descent that follows tricuspid valve opening. A square root sign or dip and plateau pattern in the diastolic pressure curve is commonly demonstrated in right ventricular infarctions but is not specific, and also may be associated with pericardial tamponade or restrictive cardiomyopathy.[8]

Cardiogenic shock in patients with right ventricular infarction frequently represents a substantial loss of functioning myocardium and carries a poor prognosis. Right ventricular infarction accompanied by cardiogenic shock is frequently associated with a variety of conduction abnormalities, including a high-grade atrioventricular block or significant rhythm disturbances. The treatment of right ventricular infarction complicated by cardiogenic shock centers around maintaining right ventricular filling pressures and assurance of adequate volume. Hemodynamic measurements may facilitate the estimate of volume loading required. Nitrates, diuretics, and other predominantly venodilating compounds should be avoided. Atrial fibrillation is frequently poorly tolerated by these patients and may require immediate electrical cardioversion. The use of digitalis in acute right ventricular infarction, even in the presence of atrial fibrillation, is controversial. Adequate inotropic support with vasodilating inotropic agents such as dobutamine are used if cardiac output fails to optimize after adequate volume loading.

MECHANICAL DEFECTS

A variety of mechanical defects may be associated with cardiogenic shock in the periinfarction stage (Table 27-3). Myocardial infarction resulting in cardiogenic shock from the appearance of mechanical defects such as acute mitral insufficiency, VSD, or free wall rupture represents a major complication and requires aggressive diagnostic and therapeutic interventions if the patient is expected to survive. Despite improvements in imaging techniques plus mechanical assist devices and emergency surgery, the mortality from these complications remains extremely high.

Acute Mitral Insufficiency

The mitral valve is a complicated apparatus and consists of the valvular annulus, leaflets, chorda tendineae, and papillary muscles plus potential functional alterations from involvement of the adjacent myocardium. Abnormalities affecting any of the components of the mitral valve may result in acute or chronic mitral insufficiency. The mitral valve annulus may be dilated and contribute to mitral insufficiency, although this complication is primarily associated with cardiomyopathies or connective tissue diseases such as Marfan's syndrome rather than an acute myocardial infarction. Calcification of the mitral valve annulus is common in the elderly and may alter coaptation of the mitral valve leaflets and result in mitral incompetence.

Acute mitral insufficiency caused by involvement of the valvular leaflets is associated with infective endocarditis from necrotizing organisms such as *Staphylococcus aureus* or *Enterococcus*, resulting in destruction of the valvular apparatus or traumatic penetrating injuries that involve the valve itself. Rupture of the chorda tendineae may also be seen in endocarditis or a variety of connective tissue diseases, including myxomatous degeneration or Marfan's syndrome.

Chordal rupture that results in severe impairment of left ventricular function depends on the number of involved structures and the rapidity with which the rupture occurs. Mitral insufficiency in the periinfarction state also may result from involvement of the surrounding myocardium or papillary muscles. Papillary muscles located adjacent to the infarction zone may simply become dysfunctional because of alteration of synchrony of contraction related to ischemia or progress to frank rupture from ischemic necrosis.

The degree of mitral insufficiency is a function of the degree of involvement and anatomic competence. The two papillary muscles (posteromedial and anterolateral papillary muscles) have different ischemic vulnerabilities because of the blood supply from the coronary arteries. The anatomic vascular supply represents end arteries that are solely supplied by terminal portions of the coronaries, thus rendering the papillary muscles vulnerable to ischemic involvement during an acute myocardial infarction. Papillary muscle dysfunction may result from intermittent ischemia during unstable angina or myocardial infarction with involvement of the adjacent myocardium.[9] Papillary muscle dysfunction is frequently characterized only by mild flow murmurs, which may be only grade I or grade II by auscultation. The anterolateral papillary muscle has a dual blood supply, which provides partial protection during ischemia. The diagonal branches of the left anterior descending and marginal branches from the circumflex supply blood to the anterolateral papillary muscle. The posteromedial papillary muscle is generally supplied solely from the posterior descending branch of the right coronary artery, thus increasing its vulnerability to ischemic-related dysfunction.

Significant ischemia involving the papillary muscle that results in complete rupture with fulminant mitral insufficiency is generally fatal because of the marked volume load ejected retrograde into the left atria and pulmonary venous bed.[10] However, if the major ischemic-related necrosis is distal and only involves rupture of the head of the papillary muscle, the resultant mitral insufficiency may be tolerated hemodynamically long enough to allow recognition, proper diagnosis, and surgical intervention. Mild ischemic involve-

TABLE 27-3. Complications of Myocardial Infarction

CHARACTERISTIC	VENTRICULAR SEPTAL RUPTURE	PAPILLARY MUSCLE RUPTURE	PAPILLARY MUSCLE DYSFUNCTION
Incidence	Unusual	Rare	Common
Murmur			
Type	Pansystolic	Early to pansystolic	Variable
Location	Left sternal border (95%)	Apex → axilla (50%)	Apex
Thrill	>50%	Rare	No
Clinical presentation	Left & right ventricular failure	Profound pulmonary edema	None to moderate left ventricular failure
Catheterization	O₂ step-up in right ventricle	Large left atrial V wave	Mild to moderate elevation of left atrial pressure

With permission from Crawford MH, O'Rourke RA: The bedside diagnosis of the complications of myocardial infarction. In: Eliot RS (ed). *Cardiac Emergencies.* Mount Kisco, NY, Futura, 1962.

ment of the papillary muscle may be increased in hemodynamic significance in the presence of preexisting left ventricular dilation, which alters the ability of the mitral leaflets to coapt. Right ventricular papillary muscle rupture may occur but is clinically uncommon. Involvement of papillary muscles in the right ventricle results in tricuspid insufficiency, which, if marked in severity, may result in subsequent right ventricular failure.

Papillary muscle rupture is a relatively uncommon complication of acute myocardial infarction and occurs in approximately 1% of patients having an acute ischemic event; the incidence rate has decreased in the thrombolytic era.[11] The peak incidence of papillary muscle rupture is within the first week after the onset of infarction, with most occurring between days 3 and 5. The diagnosis of papillary muscle rupture may be suspected on physical examination and has been facilitated with the advent of hemodynamic monitoring and echocardiography.

The physical examination in acute mitral insufficiency secondary to papillary muscle rupture differs from the findings associated with chronic valvular regurgitation because of the normal preinfarction left atrial compliance and resultant acute hyperdynamic state. A palpable thrill is an extremely uncommon finding in acute mitral insufficiency, and the radiation of the murmur also differs from the auscultatory findings in chronic conditions. The systolic murmur is soft, decrescendo, generally ends before the second heart sound, and is frequently best audible at the base of the heart as opposed to the apex, with radiation to the neck or the top of the head.

Echocardiography and Doppler ultrasound has been a major advance in the diagnosis of acute mitral insufficiency and its clinical separation from other mechanical lesions associated with a new murmur.[12] The left atrium and left ventricle are generally of normal size, and the ejection fraction is increased and frequently hyperdynamic. The mitral leaflet is flail and may frequently be demonstrated to prolapse into the left atrium. Doppler ultrasound with color flow study determines the presence and severity of mitral insufficiency and exclusion of an intracardiac shunt. The degree of mitral regurgitation may be quantitated using this readily available noninvasive tool.

Hemodynamic monitoring, including placement of a pulmonary artery catheter into the pulmonary artery with measurement of pulmonary artery and artery occlusion pressures, also is useful in mitral insufficiency, although the necessity of this intervention as a diagnostic tool has decreased with the advent of echocardiography. Placing a pulmonary artery catheter allows direct measurement of filling pressures and cardiac output. Additionally, the presence of a regurgitant wave in the pulmonary artery occlusive pressure tracing may be documented, which is strong evidence in favor of the presence of an acute mitral regurgitant lesion, especially when there is no evidence of a step-up in oxygen concentration in the right atria or right ventricle. Pulmonary artery catheterization is not necessary for diagnosis, but the use of invasive monitoring allows optimization of cardiac output, filling pressures, and adjustment of inotropic vasodilator and diuretic therapy on the basis of induced changes in pressures.

Ventricular Septal Defect

Rupture of the interventricular septum may present in a similar clinical manner as mitral insufficiency with the abrupt onset of congestive heart failure plus a new murmur, making the two conditions difficult to separate on clinical grounds. Rupture of the interventricular septum also occurs in the first week after the acute ischemic event with a peak incidence occurring between days 3 and 5. The prevalence rate of acute VSDs after an infarction is difficult to accurately determine but occurs within the range of 0.5% to 2.0%. The blood supply to the septum is supplied by septal perforating branches of the left anterior descending vessel, and thus acute VSD is more common in anterior myocardial infarctions, although the patients frequently have multivessel disease.

The diagnosis of acute VSD may be inferred on clinical grounds but frequently requires more sophisticated evaluation to accurately diagnose and quantify the defect, which is located in the muscular septum and may be multiple. The physical examination in acute VSD depends on the magnitude of the shunt, which is, in turn, a function of the size of the ventricular defect, right ventricular compliance, pulmonary artery pressures, and the inotropic state. A significant VSD is associated with the characteristic findings of the shock syndrome in addition to a new holosystolic murmur associated with a precordial thrill. A precordial thrill may be palpated in approximately 50% of patients with an acute VSD and is predominantly a function of the magnitude pressure gradient between the two chambers. The exact prevalence rate of rupture of the ventricular septum is unknown but may occur in up to 2% of myocardial infarctions and is the cause of death in approximately 5% of all fatal myocardial infarctions.

The diagnosis of VSD and its separation from acute mitral insufficiency has been facilitated by the advent of noninvasive and invasive diagnostic procedures. Two-dimensional echocardiography combined with Doppler flow study generally identifies a significant defect.[13] Contrast echocardiography using microbubble techniques also may aid in the diagnosis of acute VSD and establish the presence of an intracardiac shunt. Pulmonary artery catheterization demonstrates the absence of a V wave in the pulmonary wedge tracing plus an increase in oxygen saturation in the right ventricle compared with the right atrium. Generally, a step-up of approximately 10% in oxygen levels is required for the diagnosis. The mortality rate for septal defects is significant, with approximately 25% of patients dying within the first 24 hours, which increases to a 50% mortality at 1 week. Less than 10% survive 1 year when treated solely with medical therapy.[14]

Free Wall Rupture and Tamponade

Free wall rupture is a major complication of myocardial infarction and is difficult to diagnose premortem. The prevalence of this complication is unknown but may occur in up to 8% of all myocardial infarctions with approximately one third occurring in the first 24 hours after the onset of the ischemic event.[15] However, the peak incidence seems to be between days 5 and 7 after infarction. Rupture of the free wall is a major cause of mortality in acute ischemic events and is frequently associated with large transmural infarcts in the presence of an inadequately collateralized circulation. A variety of clinical characteristics predispose to free wall rupture, with this serious complication occurring more commonly in elderly hypertensive patients. Involvement of the left ventricle is the rule, although free wall rupture involving the right ventricle has been reported. Rupture of the free wall is frequently associated with the ventricular remodeling process in which a segmental infarction results in elevated left ventricular and diastolic pressure with expansion of the infarcted area. Expansion involves thinning of the affected area with regional hypertrophy in the adjacent region surrounding the infarct. A disproportionate dilatation occurs in the infarcted area, and the risk of free wall rupture is enhanced with high shearing forces and elevated pressures. Free wall rupture generally occurs in the border zone between the infarcted area and the normal surrounding myocardium. The advent of thrombolytic therapy has been postulated to potentially increase the risk of free wall rupture. However, this therapy has not been definitely associated with increased incidence of perforation of the ventricle. Thrombolytic therapy may actually minimize the extent of myocardial necrosis and thus decrease free wall rupture. The use of agents such as corticosteroids, which had been previously used as a potential intervention to limit infarct size by blunting the inflammatory response to tissue necrosis, has been associated with increased risk of free wall rupture.

Cardiac rupture presents clinically as a catastrophic syndrome that is frequently associated with sudden cardiac death unless a pseudoaneurysm forms. Hemopericardium with cardiac tamponade is difficult to diagnose acutely within a time frame that is adequate to institute definitive therapy. Cardiac tamponade after acute myocardial infarction also may be secondary to hemorrhagic pericarditis. However, massive hemopericardium generally is secondary to cardiac rupture and is frequently associated with the rapid development of electromechanical dissociation and a high mortality. The diagnosis of free wall rupture is difficult but should be suspected with sudden hypotension, elevated jugular venous pressures, muffled heart sounds, and a pulsus paradoxus. Echocardiography can document the presence of pericardial fluid and occasionally demonstrates the perforated free wall.[16,17] The classic signs of tamponade are present on echocardiography and are caused by the rising intrapericardial pressure compressing the right atrium and right ventricle, resulting in equalization of pressures plus right ventricular diastolic collapse. Definitive therapy involves pericardiocentesis plus volume and pressure support with early surgical intervention being necessary for salvage. Untreated free wall rupture is universally fatal, although isolated instances of successful aggressive intervention with surgical therapy have been reported.[18]

Left Ventricular Aneurysm

Left ventricular aneurysm is a relatively common complication of acute myocardial infarction and may occur in up to 15% of survivors.[19] A true aneurysm has a wide base with the ventricular walls composed entirely of myocardium, compared with a pseudoaneurysm, which generally has a narrow base with the walls consisting of pericardium and thrombotic debris. True aneurysms have a relatively low risk of free wall rupture but are associated with increased mortality because of several serious complications, including sudden death from ventricular arrhythmias, emboli from mural thrombus, and progressive loss of left ventricular function.[20] Aneurysms may develop early in the postinfarction period and can be asymptomatic or present with significant deterioration of left ventricular function. The presence of left ventricular aneurysm may be inferred by persistent ST elevation in the absence of chest pain or enzyme leakage.[21]

Echocardiography demonstrating dyskinesis is a valuable tool in diagnosing aneurysms, as is left ventricular angiography. Left ventricular angiography demonstrates paradoxic systolic distention during ventricular contraction. Successful treatment of the aneurysm may be achieved with resection of the involved myocardium, frequently in combination with saphenous vein or mammary artery bypass grafting because of the high associated prevalence of multivessel coronary artery disease. Surgical resection has been advocated in the presence of arrhythmias to eliminate the substrate for ventricular tachycardia, but electrophysiologic mapping techniques are necessary to demonstrate that the origin of the arrhythmia arises from the left ventricular aneurysm.

CLINICAL MANIFESTATIONS

The clinical manifestations of cardiogenic shock are a function of the underlying cause, and mechanical defects must be aggressively sought because of the need for definitive therapy. However, clinical recognition of the shock syndrome frequently requires prompt and aggressive stabilization procedures to be instituted before the definitive diagnosis of the underlying etiology. Hence, an early clinical diagnosis of cardiogenic shock must be made and stabilization procedures undertaken. A brief history and physical examination should be obtained with special attention to mental status, jugular venous pulsations, quality and intensity of heart sounds, presence and localization of a murmur, and presence of oliguria; readily obtainable laboratory tests such as electrocardiogram, portable chest radiograph, arterial blood gases and, if available, echocardiography frequently provide adequate clinical information to initiate stabilization therapy while a definitive diagnosis may be obtained.

THERAPY

PHARMACOLOGIC LIMITATION OF INFARCT SIZE

Several pharmacologic interventions have been used during acute myocardial infarction to minimize the extent of irreversible ischemic damage and decrease the likelihood of subsequent development of cardiogenic shock. Quantitative measurements of the extent of myocardial damage by electrocardiographic mapping and creatine kinase (CK) release are imprecise and frequently limit quantitative assessment of the potential therapeutic impact of pharmacologic interventions. Calcium channel blockers, beta-blockers, and nitrates have been the main agents that have undergone clinical analysis to minimize myocardial damage, whereas a variety of experimental or uncommonly used therapies have been evaluated in small-scale clinical trials. Nitrates are complex pharmacologic agents with arterial and venodilating activity in addition to other potential beneficial effects, such as alteration of prostacyclin metabolism. Nitrates, when administered as topical, oral, or sublingual agents, are predominately venodilators with subsequent venous pooling, decreased venous return, and lowering of pulmonary artery occlusion pressures. Reduction in venous return and optimization of occlusion pressures decrease left ventricular volume and improve subendocardial perfusion, thus reducing wall stress with the potential for minimizing infarct extent. Nitrates also have effects on systemic vascular resistance and epicardial coronary arteries, with resultant reduction of impedance to left ventricular ejection and increase in coronary blood flow.

Intravenously administered nitroglycerin has a more balanced arterial and venodilating effect. Clinical trials demonstrate that intravenous nitroglycerin administered at a level to decrease mean aortic pressure by 10%[22] result in a decrease in extension of a myocardial infarction and subsequent incidence of congestive heart failure. Intravenous nitroglycerin regimens have been shown to improve left ventricular ejection fraction and survival.[23] Nitrates administered intravenously also have been demonstrated to minimize the magnitude of infarct size, as monitored by CK, and alter infarct expansion with reduction in the subsequent remodeling process, which has been demonstrated to be associated with progression to congestive heart failure. Nitrates, when given by the intravenous route, are potent vasodilators and require careful blood pressure monitoring to prevent significant hypotension and bradycardia, which may paradoxically occur. Nitrates also may result in a beneficial redistribution of coronary flow to the subendocardium and do not result in coronary steals, which have been a major potential complicating factor in other potent intravenous vasodilators such as nitroprusside.

Calcium channel blockers are important agents in managing patients with classic and vasospastic angina. The calcium channel blocking agent acts by improving oxygen supply and demand relationships as a class effect. The significant decrease in systemic vascular resistance associated with these agents decreases oxygen demand and increase coronary flow, improving the balance between supply and demand. At pharmacologic doses, these agents also may have several other potentially beneficial effects, including antiplatelet activity.

Despite the documented beneficial effect of these agents in hypertension and angina, calcium channel blockers have not been proven to be beneficial in the treatment of acute myocardial infarction and do not definitely limit infarct size. Studies using nifedipine have been unable to demonstrate benefit with the administration of this agent in acute myocardial infarction. Diltiazem has been proven to be of benefit in non–Q wave infarction in the Diltiazem Reinfarction Study.[24] However, the Multicenter Diltiazem Postinfarction

Trial was not able to document a benefit to the administration of diltiazem in the postinfarction state when compared with placebo.[25] Subgroup analysis that was subsequently carried out showed a mortality benefit with diltiazem therapy when no pulmonary congestion was present. However, mortality was increased when diltiazem was administered to subjects whose infarction was complicated by pulmonary congestion, implying that this agent should not be used in patients who would be prone to developing cardiogenic shock. Studies performed in Denmark using intravenous verapamil followed by oral administration of this agent do not demonstrate a clear-cut benefit. Later studies using only oral verapamil do show the potential for benefit in mortality reduction, although these trials have not been reconfirmed.[26] Currently, the evidence for using calcium channel blockers for the treatment of acute myocardial infarction to limit infarct size and progression to cardiogenic shock is limited, and this mode of therapy cannot be recommended.

Beta-adrenergic blocking agents have been used in treating hypertension, atrial fibrillation, and a variety of ischemic conditions. Beta-blockers act predominantly by decreasing myocardial oxygen demand caused by the negative chronotropic and inotropic activities of these agents. Beta-blockers may have several other potentially beneficial effects, including antiplatelet activity, regression of left ventricular hypertrophy, and reduction in sudden cardiac death. Clinical trials using beta-blockade in acute myocardial infarction have yielded conflicting results. The Goteborg Trial administered metoprolol or placebo to subjects having an acute myocardial infarction and demonstrated a significant reduction in mortality at 90 days in the group randomly assigned to beta-blocker therapy.[27] Early administration of metoprolol was associated with a reduction in estimated infarct size, which presumably has an effect on early and long-term survival. Additionally, despite the fact that beta-blockers are not commonly used as antiarrhythmic agents, there was a documented decrease in sudden cardiac death in the beta-blocker group, which has been shown to be secondary to an increase in ventricular fibrillatory threshold.

The Metoprolol in Acute Myocardial Infarction Trial was able to demonstrate that the early administration of intravenous metoprolol in acute myocardial infarction was associated with a decrease in mortality in a high-risk subgroup of infarct patients, which was characterized by individuals with three or more of classic risk factors. Propranolol, which is a noncardioselective beta-blocker as opposed to the cardioselective activity of metoprolol, has not uniformly been demonstrated to decrease mortality or limit infarct size when administered early in acute myocardial infarction. However, the Beta-Blocker Heart Attack Trial did reduce mortality when propranolol was administered after the acute phase of the infarction had subsided.[28] Intravenous atenolol was studied in the First International Study of Infarct Survival Trial and demonstrated a 15% reduction in the early mortality of infarct patients who were given oral atenolol after the intravenous loading doses.[29] Beta-blockers also have been combined with thrombolytic therapy to limit infarct size. The Thrombolysis in Myocardial Infarction Trial (TIMI II-B) studied the impact of three 5-mg boluses of metoprolol administered at 5-minute intervals followed by oral metoprolol compared with thrombolysis plus oral metoprolol alone. The TIMI II-B trial demonstrated a decrease in nonfatal reinfarctions and recurrent ischemic episodes in the group who received immediate intravenous metoprolol followed by oral therapy compared with the delayed subgroup.

Use of beta-blockers in acute myocardial infarction must be undertaken with caution because of the potential of pre-cipitating atrioventricular block, reactive airways disease, or hypotension. Beta-blockers are best suited for administration in individuals with evidence of sympathetic overactivity or recurring chest pain combined with other indices of in-farct extension.[30]

Several agents have been used in small studies as ad-junctive therapy in acute myocardial infarction but have not reached widespread clinical use. Myocardial damage may be potentiated by the presence of reactive oxygen radicals, and interest has been generated concerning the potential benefit of free radical scavengers such as superoxide dismu-tase or catalase to potentially blunt the toxic effects of these compounds on viable myocardium. Free radical scavengers have been shown to be effective when administered before the onset of experimental infarcts; definitive clinical studies are currently ongoing.

Glucose insulin potassium infusions (polarizing solution) have been used for several years to reduce infarct size by altering free fatty acid metabolism.[31] Polarizing solution con-sists of 300 g of glucose, 50 U of regular insulin, and 80 mMol of potassium in 1 L of water delivered at 1.5 mL/kg/ hour. Ejection fraction and wall motion abnormalities have been documented to be improved after administering this solution and may be associated with decreased mortality. However, polarizing solution has not been studied exten-sively in the classic double-blind, placebo-controlled trials, and routine administration of this solution has not reached clinical acceptance.

Hyaluronidase may have antiinflammatory activity and modulate the immune response associated with acute myo-cardial infarction, which has been postulated to play at least a partial role in the extent of infarct size. Hyaluronidase has been administered in small clinical studies and was associ-ated with improvement of mortality and decreased develop-ment of Q waves, implying myocardial salvage, but it has not been thoroughly evaluated in large-scale clinical trials.[32]

Converting enzyme inhibitors have been administered orally and intravenously in clinical trials to halt progression to congestive heart failure in the Survival and Ventricular Enlargement and Consensus-II trials. The Survival and Ven-tricular Enlargement study used captopril in over 2000 pa-tients who had an acute anterior myocardial infarction when enrolled during the period from 3 to 16 days after the acute myocardial event.[33] These patients, who all had ejection frac-tions less than 40%, were randomized to receive captopril or a placebo and were demonstrated to have less progression to congestive heart failure and improved mortality when followed over a 42-month period. In addition to the mortality decrease, recurrent myocardial infarctions and hospitaliza-tions for heart failure were also altered by captopril. The Consensus-II trial used intravenous enalapril in the early phase of infarction followed by oral enalapril, but this trial was unable to demonstrate a mortality benefit when com-pared with placebo.[34] Converting enzyme inhibitors are at-tractive agents because of their effects on hemodynamics, microcirculation, and angiotensin-mediated vasoconstriction and should be considered especially in anterior infarcts with significant reductions in ejection fraction.

THROMBOLYSIS

Thrombolysis induced by pharmacologic agents or direct angioplasty is an attractive treatment for reestablishing coro-nary perfusion to minimize the extent of myocardial in-farction and progression to cardiogenic shock. The open artery hypothesis postulates that clinical outcome is depen-dent on maintaining adequate coronary perfusion to mini-mize ischemic damage mediated by vascular occlusion sec-ondary to an intravascular thrombus. Recent trials of coronary thrombolysis (GISSI, ISIS, GUSTO) demonstrate the prevalence rate of cardiogenic shock of approximately 3% on arrival to the hospital with a subsequent increase in the early time period of an acute myocardial infarction.[35] Early progression to cardiogenic shock is characterized de-mographically by a high prevalence of elderly patients, ante-rior infarctions, low ejection fractions, diabetes, and known prior myocardial infarction. Despite the theoretic attrac-tiveness of administration of recombinant tissue plasmino-gen activators or streptokinase in patients with established or impending cardiogenic shock, the mortality associated with established cardiogenic shock remains high despite thrombolytic therapy. GISSI-I and GISSI-II document ex-ceedingly high mortality rates in patients with established cardiogenic shock who received thrombolytic therapy, with the survival rate approximating 35%.[36] Prompt administra-tion of thrombolytic agents within the first hour of acute myocardial infarction may result in improved survival rates if reperfusion of the infarct-related artery can be sustained. Low coronary perfusion pressures in cardiogenic shock may play a potential role in the poor clinical outcome of these patients after thrombolytic therapy.

In vitro experimental infarct studies with reduced perfu-sion pressure have shown decreased diffusion of thrombo-lytic agents into clots with resultant impaired fibrinolysis.[37] Enhanced pressure increases the rate of dissolution of an intravascular thrombus, implying that in cardiogenic shock with systemic hypotension and a reduced transcoronary pres-sure gradient may result in blunted efficacy of thrombolytic agents. The metabolic abnormalities associated with cardio-genic shock including lactic acidosis also may alter the con-version of plasminogen to plasmin and limit the efficacy of these drugs in clot lysis. Failure from lytic agents to sustain vascular patency in patients with cardiogenic shock is an indication for consideration of early cardiac catheterization and direct angioplasty if no contraindications exist. Persistent hypotension, nonevolving ST elevation, continuing clinical evidence of myocardial ischemia, CK elevations, and clinical instability are potential indications for rescue coronary an-gioplasty, and this may result in increased survival.[38] Rescue angioplasty has not been systematically studied in random-ized, controlled trials to compare efficacy of thrombolytic therapy versus percutaneous transluminal coronary angio-plasty (PTCA) in shock. However, failure to maintain vessel patency seems to be a major indicator of decreased clinical success, and if thrombolytic therapy does not result in establishment of coronary perfusion, angioplasty should be considered as a therapeutic option. Cardiogenic shock secondary to mechanical defects such as papillary muscle dysfunction also has been treated successfully with PTCA, resulting in a decreased severity of mitral regurgitation with resolution of cardiogenic shock.[39] Failure of angioplasty with vascular collapse may be treated with stent placement, and anecdotal reports have demonstrated benefit with intravascular stent placement.

Thrombolytic agents should be administered to all patients with acute myocardial infarction who demonstrate evidence of the shock state if there are no contraindications to administering these drugs. Failure of evidence of reperfusion is a potential indicator for direct rescue angioplasty, although definitive clinical trials currently have not been performed.

PHARMACOLOGIC AGENTS

Inotropic Agents

The effectiveness of various inotropic agents in cardiogenic shock depends on the cause and underlying pathophysiologic mechanism of the shock state. With systemic hypotension, adequate perfusion of the coronary arteries must be maintained (Fig. 27-2).

DOPAMINE.   Dopamine is an endogenous catecholamine with positive inotropic properties secondary to stimulation of alpha- and beta-receptors plus dopamine receptors, which have been divided into two subtypes: DA_1 and DA_2.[40,41] DA_1 receptors are postsynaptic and induce dilation of the coronary, renal, and mesenteric vasculature. DA_2 receptors are located in autonomic ganglia and in the postganglionic sympathetic nervous system. Stimulation of DA_2 receptors blocks the release of endogenous catecholamines from intraneuronal storage sites. The effect of dopamine on alpha and beta activity is dose related. Low infusion dosages of dopamine

(2 to 5 μg/kg/minute) result in positive inotropic activity secondary to stimulation of the beta$_1$-receptors. Alpha-receptor stimulation occurs at dosages above 10 μg/kg/minute and results in a secondary increase in systemic vascular resistance caused by peripheral vasoconstriction. In addition to the inotropic effect, dopamine results in increased atrioventricular conduction from adrenergic stimulation. The effects of dopamine are thus dose dependent, and pharmacologic activity is a function of the amount of dopamine infused corrected for body weight. Initial pharmacologic responsiveness may be predicted by dose level. However, the individual response may be variable, and unless the clinical situation warrants large pressor doses to maintain blood pressure, dopamine infusion should begin at a low rate (1 μg/kg/minute) and gradually be increased while adjusting for clinical responsiveness. Cardiogenic shock with low tissue perfusion accompanied by hypotension may be treated in a more aggressive manner with progressively increasing doses of dopamine at 5-minute intervals.

Low-dose dopamine infusion results in stimulation of DA_2 receptors and minimal or no changes in heart rate, cardiac output, or blood pressure. Stimulation of DA_2 receptors results in renal vasodilation and increases glomerular filtration rate, renal blood flow, and sodium excretion. Reduction in cardiac output in shock frequently results in shunting of blood away from the renal vasculature and induction of a prerenal state with elevated blood urea nitrogen–to–creatinine ratios plus sodium retention. Dopamine is a useful agent to reverse the adverse redistribution of cardiac output, with a beneficial secondary effect on volume and sodium loss resulting from the increased amount of sodium presented to the loop of Henle, which allows increased efficacy of diuretics such as furosemide or bumetanide that predominantly act in this area of the kidney.

Medium dosing ranges of dopamine (5 to 10 μg/kg/min) result in an increase in cardiac output, which may also improve volume status by increasing renal blood flow. The cardiac effects of dopamine in this dosing range are secondary to stimulation of the β$_1$-adrenergic receptors caused by a secondary release of norepinephrine. The effect of dopamine is thus indirect and depends on a preexistent adequate storage level of endogenous catecholamines to induce its beneficial effect. Longstanding congestive heart failure is frequently associated with reduction in sympathetic receptors in the myocardium, and thus the efficacy of dopamine may be limited if prolonged congestive heart failure was present before the shock syndrome. Dopamine infusion at this dose range generally does not result in alterations of venous return secondary to venodilation. Thus, right atrial and pulmonary artery occlusion pressures may not be decreased by this level of infusion. Dopamine may be combined with either direct vasodilating compounds or other inotropic agents such as dobutamine, which combine inotropism with vasodilation. Medium dosing range infusions of dopamine are generally safe and effective in maintaining blood pressure; however, care must be instituted to ensure that acid-base status and electrolyte levels are optimized to avoid potential induction of arrhythmias with resultant malignant ventricular arrhythmias or marked sinus or supraventricular tachycardias, which would increase myocardial oxygen demand.

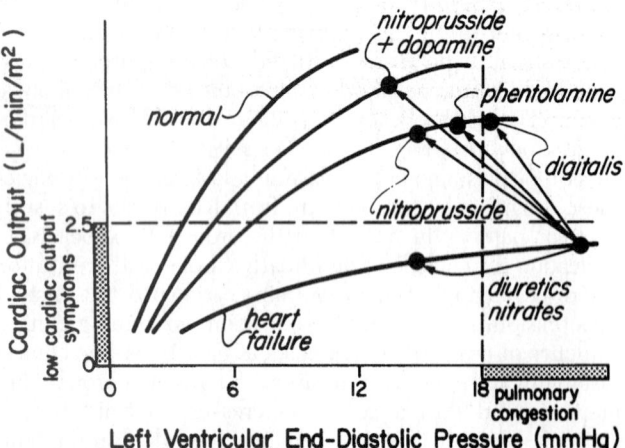

FIGURE 27-2. Inotropic and vasodilator therapy of cardiogenic shock. (Adapted from Mason DT: *Congestive Heart Failure.* New York, Yale Medical Books, 1976.)

High-range dopamine infusions (greater than 10 μg/kg/minute) result in activation of alpha-adrenergic receptors and a secondary norepinephrine release with secondary vasoconstriction and increased levels of systemic vascular resistance. Patients in frank cardiogenic shock may need markedly elevated levels of dopamine, and ranges up to 50 μg/kg/min have been used, which requires strict attention to volume status and repeated examinations to observe for excessive vasoconstriction or extravasation of the agent, or tissue necrosis results. Additionally, dopamine may interact with coadministered drugs with the potentiation of its pressor effects. Tricyclic antidepressants seem to increase the pressor response of direct-acting sympathomimetics and to decrease the sensitivity to indirect agents. Because dopamine has direct and indirect effects on the vasculature, this agent should be used with caution, especially with overdoses of the tricyclic drugs.[42] Although not commonly used, the rauwolfia alkaloids also may potentiate the pressor response of direct-acting sympathomimetics, resulting in hypertension. Monoamine oxidase inhibitors may result in an increased pressor response of dopamine, and the administered levels should be adjusted downward to compensate for this potential adverse effect.[43] Dopamine is an endogenous catechol that is degraded by catechol-o-methyltransferase and thus is not effective when administered in oral doses. Orally administered prodrugs have been used but have no role in the treatment of cardiogenic shock.

DOBUTAMINE. As opposed to dopamine, which is an endogenous catechol and immediate precursor of norepinephrine and epinephrine, dobutamine is a synthetic agent that stimulates predominantly β_1-adrenoreceptors[44] (Table 27-4). Mild activation of β_2- and alpha-receptors also may be seen with this agent, but the degree of stimulation is significantly decreased when compared with β_1-receptors. Administration of dobutamine results in a direct inotropic stimulation plus a secondary reflex vasodilation, which results in reduction of systemic vascular resistance and an increase in cardiac output. Dobutamine is a direct-acting agent, unlike dopa-

mine, and does not require the presence or release of intramyocardial norepinephrine to modulate its effects.

The pharmacologic mechanism of dobutamine is complicated because of its asymmetric structure and the drug is administered as a racemic mixture. The positive and negative isomers have been evaluated as to their relative activities in in vitro studies, but it is believed that in clinical situations, the positive isomer is predominantly responsible for the activation of the beta-receptor and determines the potential beneficial effects. The administration of dobutamine alters stimulation of beta-receptors in a differential manner, with an increased binding affinity for the predominantly cardiac β_1-adrenergic receptors, with direct inotropic effects being obtained from this finding. The inotropic effects of this agent are not coupled with an increased rate of arrhythmias when compared with epinephrine and norepinephrine, and there seems to be less adverse electrophysiologic effects when compared with dopamine. Because of the vasodilating effect of dobutamine, there are no major effects on arterial blood pressure, which is basically altered only minimally because of the decrease in systemic vascular resistance. The resultant hemodynamic effects result in an increase in cardiac output and stroke volume with dobutamine administration. The secondary increase in cardiac output results in improved renal blood flow and enhanced ability to excrete sodium and water. Dobutamine is effective in cardiogenic shock, assuming that the underlying etiology is not caused by valvular or subvalvular stenosis and the pharmacologic infusion does not result in significant hypotension, although this agent may be combined with dopamine to maintain blood pressure.

NOREPINEPHRINE. Norepinephrine is a powerful alpha-adrenergic agonist that results in significant peripheral vasoconstriction when administered within the usual dosage range of 2 to 8 μg/minute. Norepinephrine is generally instituted in the treatment of cardiogenic shock after failure of volume correction and dopamine to maintain adequate cardiac output and blood pressure.[45] Norepinephrine is a

TABLE 27-4. Dobutamine

ADRENERGIC RECEPTOR	SITE	ACTION
β_1	Myocardium	Increase atrial and ventricular contractility
	Sinoatrial node	Increase heart rate
	Atrioventricular conduction system	Enhance atrioventricular conductions
β_2	Arterioles	Vasodilation
	Lungs	Bronchodilation
α	Peripheral arterioles	Vasoconstriction
DA_1	Postsynaptic	Dilation of coronary, renal, and mesenteric vasculature
DA_2	Autonomic ganglia and postganglionic sympathetic nervous system	Decreased release of endogenous catechols

naturally occurring catecholamine that has both alpha- and β_1-adrenergic activity. Administration of this agent is generally associated with an increase in cardiac output. However, because of the increases in systemic vascular resistance and mean aortic blood pressure that occur after its infusion, cardiac output may be minimally affected. In addition to the effects on systemic vascular resistance, the pressure work of the left ventricle and oxygen consumption are increased after administration of norepinephrine. Norepinephrine also may result in shunting of blood away from various organ beds because of volume redistribution secondary to catecholamine sensitivity. Oliguria and azotemia from impaired renal blood flow may be worsened secondary to the norepinephrine-mediated vasoconstriction. Norepinephrine also has been associated with increased irritability of the ventricle with an increased electrical instability and potential adverse rhythm disorders.

DIGITALIS PREPARATIONS.   The use of digitalis in general and cardiogenic shock specifically has been controversial because of theoretic objections involving the use of this agent and the lack of controlled clinical trials documenting a beneficial impact on mortality.[46] Digitalis glycosides have complex mechanisms of action whose inotropic activity is modulated by increasing the availability of intracellular calcium secondary to inhibition of sodium-potassium ATPase. Inhibition of this ubiquitous enzyme, which is found not only in cardiac tissue but also in the central nervous system, gastrointestinal tract, and kidney, results in calcium influx by the activation of the sodium-calcium exchange mechanism. The level of free cytosolic calcium regulates the activity of tropomyosin in a such a way that increases in levels of calcium are associated with an increased force developed by interactions between actin and myosin filaments. Alterations in contraction are caused by variations in levels of cytosolic calcium, which can be moved in and out of the sarcoplasmic reticulum.

Digitalis has established inotropic effects, although the increase in cardiac output after administration of this drug is modest when compared with the more powerful intravenous inotropes such as dobutamine, dopamine, and norepinephrine. In addition to inotropic effects, digitalis increases the refractory period at the atrioventricular node and decreases conduction velocity in this tissue, which results in a negative chronotropic effect in patients with atrial fibrillation that may be associated with congestive heart failure and cardiogenic shock. Digitalis lacks the negative inotropic activity of other agents that have been used to slow the rate in atrial fibrillation, including beta-blockers and calcium channel blockers such as diltiazem and verapamil.[47] Digitalis increases vagal tone and has been shown to decrease levels of norepinephrine in chronic heart failure, which also may be secondary to decreased activity of the peripheral sympathetic nervous system. Digitalis also resets baroreceptor sensitivity and may have renal effects, although natriuresis is most likely secondary to increased renal blood flow from enhanced cardiac output.

Digitalis withdrawal has been demonstrated to result in worsening of heart failure in the randomized, double-blind, placebo-controlled study of digitalis withdrawal in patients who were also treated with converting enzyme inhibition. However, the role of digitalis in cardiogenic shock is limited as far as maintenance of cardiac output, although the autonomic effects of this agent with secondary decreases in the heart rate in atrial fibrillation would be of benefit.

ISOPROTERENOL.   Isoproterenol has both β_1- and β_2-adrenergic properties, and its administration is not associated with vasoconstriction. The administration of isoproterenol results in increased myocardial contractility, heart rate, and cardiac output. However, the powerful chronotropic and inotropic activities of this agent associated with decreased vascular resistance result in myocardial work and oxygen consumption being increased, and the net energy balance shifts to a detrimental relationship with respect to the myocardium. Isoproterenol thus is infrequently used in heart failure or cardiogenic shock unless the shock state is associated with bradyarrhythmias that do not respond to other therapies, but it is believed that the patient would clinically benefit from an increase in cardiac output secondary to chronotropic activity. Cardiogenic shock associated with acute valvular insufficiency also may be benefitted by isoproterenol if blood pressure and volume status are maintained. Isoproterenol thus has a limited role in the acute management of cardiogenic shock and has decreased in its clinical application.

PHOSPHODIESTERASE INHIBITORS.   Amrinone and milrinone are bipyridine derivatives that inhibit cellular levels of phosphodiesterase.[48] Inhibition of this key enzyme results in increased levels of cyclic AMP in cardiac muscle with resultant enhancement of protein phosphorylation by protein kinase. Increased levels of cyclic AMP in cardiac muscle result in increased inotropic and chronotropic activities. The methylxanthines were known to nonspecifically inhibit phosphodiesterase activity and result in mild enhancement of the inotropic state. Both amrinone and milrinone have been shown in experimental and clinical studies to increase cardiac output in patients with severe congestive heart failure or cardiogenic shock.[49]

Administering these agents results in reduction of filling pressures and increases in stroke volume and cardiac output. The chronotropic effects of amrinone and milrinone are modest, but a mild increase in heart rate may be documented unless inordinately large doses are used, which may result in severe peripheral vasodilation, hypotension, and tachycardia. The phosphodiesterase inhibitors have been studied in patients with pump failure after myocardial infarctions and, at a dosage level of 200 µg/kg/hour, have been shown to improve cardiac function. Comparison in clinical trials of amrinone to other vasodilating inotropes such as dobutamine documented a greater decrease in systemic and pulmonary venous pressures in the group that received amrinone.[50] The vasodilating activity of the phosphodiesterase inhibitors, while increasing cardiac output, may result in significant hypotension, requiring concomitant administration of sympathomimetic amines with at least partial alpha-activity such as norepinephrine to control pressure. The side effect profile of the phosphodiesterase inhibitors relates mainly to potential hematologic and gastrointestinal side effects. Nausea, vomiting, and diarrhea occur in many patients. Thrombocytopenia is common with amrinone, although the marked decreases in platelet counts to levels under 50,000 seems to be relatively rare and may be treated by dose reduction. Milrinone is more potent on a milligram basis when compared with amrinone and also has effects on the inotropic state and ventricular relaxation. Enoximone is an imidazole derivative that also results in phosphodiesterase inhibition.[51] Administration of this compound results in increased levels of cyclic AMP and contractile force in isolated muscle preparations. Intravenous enoximone results in an increase in cardiac index with a decrease in right-sided filling pressures, with only minimal impacts on systemic vascular resistance and heart rate. Enoximone seems to have a relatively mild side effect profile, and thrombocytopenia is uncommon with the use of this agent, which is currently undergoing a variety of controlled trials.

GLUCAGON.   Glucagon is uncommonly used in cardiogenic shock but has a potential advantage in that it has a different mechanism of action from other sympathomimetic amines and does not require beta-receptor stimulation to exert its inotropic effects.[52,53] Glucagon is administered in a dosing range of 4 to 6 mg intravenously, which may be followed by a constant infusion of 4 to 12 mg/hour. Glucagon administration increases cardiac output by approximately 20%, which is associated with a decrease in peripheral vascular resistance and less of an adverse negative effect on myocardial oxygen demand when compared with norepinephrine. The indications for glucagon have not been delineated, although it seems justifiable to administer this agent to patients with cardiogenic shock who do not respond to conventional therapy or cannot tolerate other agents because of the development of significant arrhythmias or hematologic toxicity.

SURGICAL INTERVENTION

Surgical intervention in myocardial infarction has been used to limit infarct size by direct revascularization or to correct the mechanical defects of an acute ischemic event such as VSDs, acute mitral insufficiency, free wall rupture, or left ventricular aneurysm. Surgical intervention for revascularization in acute myocardial infarction had been contraindicated on theoretic grounds because of the presumed high morbidity and mortality rates from cardiac catheterization and operative interventions during the unstable period of acute myocardial infarction. A variety of clinical studies subsequently determined that with available resources and personnel, coronary bypass surgery could be performed in an expeditious manner with an attendant low mortality. Bypass surgery has been used as primary therapy in acute myocardial infarction with an overall operative rate of approximately 5% for transmural infarctions plus a highly acceptable long-term mortality rate.[54,55] Evidence is accumulating that early revascularization by direct PTCA, intravenous or intracoronary thrombolytic agents, or bypass surgery in selected patients represents the treatment of choice in early myocardial infarction (less than 6 hours) to decrease myocardial necrosis and complication rates. Congestive heart failure, which occurs in the postmyocardial state, may be amenable to revascularization by surgical interventions, although large-scale, controlled, randomized studies are lacking. However, several surgical series have been reported documenting the effects of coronary bypass surgery in patients with an acute myocardial infarction complicated by cardiogenic shock with data available on early and long-term survival. Additionally, a registry for the impact of early revascularization of cardiogenic shock has been established by a multinational consortium. Surgical intervention in cardiogenic shock is fraught with considerable clinical problems and requires the presence of surgically accessible jeopardized but potentially viable myocardium, which has the potential to regain contractility after reestablishment of flow. Surgical intervention has the advantage of reestablishing flow not only in the infarct-related artery but in vessels not involved in the acute ischemic process but significantly obstructed. Viability of the myocardium in the periinfarction state may be difficult to determine secondary to problems with the acute delineation of stunned, hibernating, or irreversibly damaged myocardium. Nitroglycerin or dobutamine enhancement of ejection fraction is an indirect method of determining viability but is time consuming in a period where early revascularization is of prime importance.

Indications for surgical intervention in cardiogenic shock have not been completely delineated but should be considered in patients who fail to respond to volume correction and inotropic therapy. Failure of conventional medical interventions for cardiogenic shock should result in consideration of intraaortic balloon counterpulsation, which has been used as a temporizing measure to improve prognosis for revascularization. Emergent coronary artery bypass surgery, which has been preceded by placement of intraaortic balloon, demonstrates improved survival rates in cardiogenic shock to approximately 75%. Surgery for acute mitral insufficiency associated with cardiogenic shock in the postinfarction state is the only available definitive therapy for severe mitral regurgitation. The impact of acute mitral insufficiency on left ventricular performance may be underestimated by using ejection fraction as the index of function because the left ventricle ejects retrograde into the low compliance left atrial and pulmonary venous system. Medical therapy with inotropic support and systemic peripheral vasodilation improves regurgitant flow as calculated by the regurgitant fraction. Severe mitral insufficiency is associated with a variety of adverse pathophysiologic changes that result in a poor survival after surgical intervention, but the results are significantly better than medical treatment that results in essentially 100% mortality if marked mitral insufficiency is associated with cardiogenic shock.

Surgical intervention is generally required for acute VSDs, which occur in the muscular portion of the interventricular septum and may be multiple. However, two general anatomic types of acute VSDs have been described. A VSD resulting from occlusion of a posterior descending coronary artery that arises from the right coronary is associated with a defect located in the inferobasilar region of the septum. Anteroseptal myocardial infarctions, which are associated with thrombotic occlusion of the left anterior descending, are associated with mid-apical to anterior defects in the septum. The physiologic impact of a left-to-right shunt is a function of the quantitative amount of involved myocardium plus associated left ventricular dysfunction, pulmonary artery pressures, and right ventricular compliance. A significant left-to-right shunt markedly decreases forward flow with poor peripheral perfusion and the clinical characteristics of cardiogenic shock. If the left ventricular end-diastolic pressure is markedly elevated, left-to-right shunting will also occur during diastole and is associated with an extremely high 24-hour mortality rate of approximately 25%.[56,57] Medical treatment alone allows only a 20% survival beyond 60 days, and 1-year survival is less than 10%.

Surgical intervention in acute VSDs requires early and aggressive diagnostic and therapeutic interventions. Despite intraaortic balloon pumping and optimization of medical management, refinements in surgical technique have improved 1-year survival to 32% without coronary artery bypass. Evaluation of clinical trials that attempt to postpone therapy to improve the healing process have been questioned because this eliminates the most severely ill patients from definitive therapy and introduces a selection bias into the implications of therapy. Early surgical intervention with direct patch grafts plus coronary artery bypass has been employed in the early stage of acute myocardial infarction with severe VSDs and may result in survival rates of up to 75%.

Free wall rupture of the left ventricle has no acceptable nonsurgical therapy, even with a clotted hemopericardium, which may result in decreased further extravasation of blood into the pericardial space. The diagnosis of free wall rupture may be extraordinarily difficult on clinical grounds, and signs of pericardial tamponade should be actively sought. Pericardiocentesis with decompression of the pericardial space may be lifesaving in the short term but represents only a temporizing procedure. Cardiac rupture is essentially universally fatal, and surgical intervention may be successful with direct oversewing of the defect if recognized and managed in a timely fashion.[58,59]

Left ventricular aneurysm as a cause of cardiogenic shock may require surgical intervention as a definitive therapy. The remodeling process, which begins after an acute ischemic event with regional thinning and expansion of the infarct zone, may result in progressive decrease in left ventricular performance and the onset of clinical cardiogenic shock. If the aneurysmal dilation of the left ventricle involves more than 20% of the left ventricular mass, severe impairment of pumping ability ensues and potentially requires surgical intervention if no response to routine medical management, including intraaortic balloon pumping, is documented. Surgical intervention for aneurysms should be optimized in timing with adequate healing and fibrosis.

ASSIST DEVICES

The intraaortic balloon pump has been in clinical use for over 20 years to increase diastolic coronary arterial perfusion and to decrease left ventricular afterload.[60] The intraaortic balloon pump is a temporizing measure that does not increase myocardial oxygen demand and results in reduction of ventricular diastolic volume and reduces pulmonary congestion with an increase in cardiac output. The intraaortic

balloon pump is the most widely used circulatory assist device in patients with cardiogenic shock because of the ease of insertion, which may be accomplished either percutaneously or surgically. Effective counterpulsation results in stabilization and potential reversal of the shock state with improvement in peripheral perfusion but does require an adequate systemic pressure and left ventricular performance to maximize its use.

Profoundly hypotensive patients respond poorly to intraaortic counterpulsation, and the balloon pump has limited efficacy. Balloon pumping in selected patients allows optimization of blood pressure, cardiac output, and tissue perfusion in patients with cardiogenic shock while further diagnostic procedures and staging of the patient are performed. Intraaortic balloon pumping may be used prophylactically in patients with mechanical defects such as acute mitral insufficiency or VSD to increase coronary perfusion, allow time for healing, and restore cardiac output toward normal. The impact of intraaortic balloon pumping on long-term survival is controversial and depends on the indications for insertion, hemodynamic status, and etiology of the cardiogenic shock. Patient selection is a key issue, and early insertion of the intraaortic balloon may result in increased clinical benefit rather than procrastination until full-blown cardiogenic shock has developed.

Patients who are not expected to significantly benefit from intraaortic balloon pumping are elderly patients, patients with severe peripheral vascular disease, and patients with large myocardial infarctions exceeding 40% of left ventricular myocardium. The overall survival rate of patients with cardiogenic shock treated with the intraaortic balloon pump is approximately 40%. For subjects who required balloon insertion for large myocardial infarctions without a significant mechanical obstruction, the survival rate was only 27%. Complications may be documented in up to 30% of patients who undergo intraaortic balloon pumping and relate mainly to local vascular problems, including surgical trauma, emboli, infection, and hemolysis.

Left ventricular assist devices function as prosthetic ventricles but require a sternotomy for insertion. Assist devices may be used to support left ventricular performance, right ventricular performance, or a combination, depending on the underlying condition. The Pierce-Donachy left ventricular assist device (Thoratec, Berkeley, CA) has been used a bridge to transplantation and has been documented to improve cardiac output and filling pressures. Insertion of the Thortec device in patients with severe left ventricular dysfunction allowed survival to transplant in approximately 75% of 29 patients.[61] The indications for insertion of a left ventricular assist device are controversial, and this aggressive approach to support of the circulatory system may be used after failure of medical and intraaortic balloon pumping and in the presence of the potentially reversible component to the disease.

The Nimbus hemopump (Nimbus Medical, Inc., Rancho Cordova, CA) circumvents the problem associated with median sternotomy and allows a percutaneous placement of a cannula across the aortic valve, which is coupled to an extracorporeal power source. The Nimbus hemopump uses an Archimedes' spiral screw valve that rotates at approximately 25,000 revolutions per minute without significant hemolysis. The major complications associated with the Nimbus hemopump insertion include the initiation of ventricular arrhythmias and embolic phenomenon.[62]

CONCLUSIONS ■

Despite rapid advancement in pharmacologic thrombolytic therapy, mechanical revascularization techniques, and development of mechanical ventricular assist devices, cardiogenic shock remains a major clinical challenge with an associated high mortality. Improved survival in cardiogenic shock may be seen with an aggressive approach to diagnosis and management of the problem, with emphasis on early recognition and treatment of mechanical defects such as VSD, acute mitral insufficiency, and free wall rupture. Limitation of infarct size by minimizing the extent of infarcted tissue is the key component in all therapeutic strategies with the goal to maximize perfusion, limit irreversible cell death, and decrease potential for a secondary mechanical event.

REFERENCES ■

1. Hands ME, Rutherford JD, Muller JE: The in-hospital development of cardiogenic shock after myocardial infarction. *J Am Coll Cardiol* 1989;14:40
2. Goldberg RJ, Gore JM, Alpert JS: Cardiogenic shock after acute myocardial infarction. *N Engl J Med* 1991;325:1117
3. Killip T, Kimball JT: Treatment of myocardial infarction in a coronary care unit. *Am J Cardiol* 1967;20:457
4. Forrester JS, Diamond GA, Chatterjee K: Medical therapy of acute myocardial infarction by application of hemodynamic subsets. *N Engl J Med* 1976;295:1356
5. Kinch JW, Ryan TJ: Right ventricular infarction. *N Engl J Med* 1994;330:1211
6. Andersen HR, Nielsen D, Falk E: Right ventricular infarction. *Am Heart J* 1989;117:82
7. Dell'Italia LJ, Starling MR, Crawford MH: Right ventricular infarction. *J Am Coll Cardiol* 1984;4:931
8. Goldstein JA, Barzilai, Rosamond TL: Determination of hemodynamic compromise with severe right ventricular infarction. *Circulation* 1990;82:359
9. Tcheng JE, Jackman JD, Nelson CL: Outcome of patients sustaining acute ischemic mitral regurgitation during myocardial infarction. *Ann Intern Med* 1992;117:18
10. Sharma SK, Seckler J, Israel DH: Clinical angiographic and anatomic findings in acute severe ischemic mitral regurgitation. *Am J Cardiol* 1992;70:277
11. Lear J, Feinberg MS, Vered Z: Effect of thrombolytic therapy on the evaluation of significant mitral regurgitation in patients with a first inferior myocardial infarction. *J Am Coll Cardiol* 1993;21:1661
12. Kisdnuke A, Otsuji Y, Kuroiwa R: Two dimensional echocardiographic assessment of papillary muscle contractility in patients with prior myocardial infarction. *J Am Coll Cardiol* 1993;21:932
13. Harrison MR, MacPhail B, Gurley JC: Usefulness of color flow Doppler imaging to distinguish ventricular septal defect from acute mitral regurgitation complicating acute myocardial infarction. *Am J Cardiol* 1989;64:697
14. Gray JM, Sethna D, Matloff JM: The role of cardiac surgery in acute myocardial infarction with mechanical complications. *Am Heart J* 106:723
15. Bates RJ, Beutler S, Resnekov L: Cardiac rupture: challenge in diagnosis and management. *Am J Cardiol* 1977;40:1231
16. Assmann PE, Roelandt JR: Two dimensional and Doppler echocardiography in acute myocardial infarction and its compliations. *Ultrasound Med Biol* 1987;13:507-517
17. Buda AJ: The role of echocardiography in the evaluation of mechanical complications of acute myocardial infarction. *Circulation* 1991;84(Suppl 3):109
18. Pappas PJ, Cerndianu AC, Baldino WA, et al: Ventricular free rupture after myocardial infarction: treatment and outcome. *Chest* 1991;99:892
19. Visser CA, Kan G, David CK, et al: Echocardiographic cineangiographic correlation in detecting left ventricular aneurysm. *Am J Cardiol* 1982;50:337
20. Heras M, Sany G, etriu A, et al: Does left ventricular aneurysm influence survival after acute myocardial infarction. *Eur Heart J* 1990;11:441
21. Arvan S, Varat MA: Persistent ST elevatio and ventricular wall abnormalities: a two-dimensional echocardiographic study. *Am J Cardiol* 1984;53:1142
22. Flaherty JT, Becker LC, Bulkley BH: Randomized prospective trial of intravenous nitroglycerin in patients with AMI. *Circulation* 1983;68:576
23. Jugoutt BI, Warnica JW: Intravenous nitroglycerin therapy to limit myocardial infarct size, expansion and complications. *Circulation* 1988;78:906
24. Gibson RS, Boden WE, Theroux P, et al: Diltiazem and reinfarction in patients with non–Q wave myocardial infarction. *N Engl J Med* 1986;315:423
25. The Multicenter Diltiazem Postinfarction Trial Group: The effect of diltiazem on mortality and reinfarction after myocardial infarction. *N Engl J Med* 1988;319:385
26. The Danish Study Group on Verapamil in Myocardial Infarction: Treatment with verapamil during and after an acute myocardial infarction: a review based on Danish Verapamil Infarction Trials I and II. *J Cardiovasc Pharmacol* 1991;18 (Suppl 6):520
27. Herlity J, Hjalmarson A, Swedberg K, et al: The influence of early intervention in acute myocardial infarction on long term mortality and morbidity assessed in the Goteborg Metoprolol trial. *Int J Cardiol* 1986;10:291
28. Viscoli CM, Horowitz RI Singer BH: Beta blockers after myocardial infarction. *Ann Intern Med* 1993;118:99
29. ISIS-I Collaborative Group: Mechanisms for the early mortality reduction produced by beta blockade started early in myocardial infarction: ISIS-I. *Lancet* 1988;i(8591):921
30. Roberts R, Rogers WJ, Mueller HS, et al: Immediate versus deferred beta blockade following thrombolytic therapy in patients with acute myocardial infarction (TIMI-IIB). *Circulation* 1991;83:422
31. Rackley CE, Russel RO, Rogers WJ: Glucose-insulin-potassium infusion: review of clinical experience. *Postgrad Med* 1979;65:93
32. Henderson A, Campbell RWF, Julian DG: Effect of a highly purified hyaluronidase preparation on electrocardiographic changes in acute myocardial infarction. *Lancet* 1982;i:874
33. The SAVE Investigators: Effect ofcaptopril on mortality and morbidity in patients with left ventricular dysfunction after myocardial infarction. *N Engl J Med* 1992;327:669
34. SwedburgK, Held P, Kjekshus J: Effects of early administration of enalapril on mortality in patients with acute myocardial infarction: results of the Co-operative New Scandinavian Enalapril Survival Study (Consensus-II). *N Engl J Med* 1992; 327:678

35. Grella RD, Becker RC: Cardiogenic shock complicating coronary artery disease: diagnosis, treatment and management. *Curr Probl Cardiol* 1994;12:693

36. Gruppo Italiano Per lo Studio Della Streptochinase Mell Infarcto Miocardio (GISSI): Effectiveness of intravenous streptokinase treatment in acute myocardial infarction. *Lancet* 1986; i:397

37. Cox RH: Mechanical aspects of large coronary arteries. In: Santamore WP, Bove AA (eds). *Coronary Artery Disease*. Baltimore, Urban and Schwartzenberg, 1982:19

38. Strack RS, Califf RM, Hinohara R, et al: Survival and cardiac event rates in the first year after emergent coronary angioplasty for acute myocardial infarction. *J Am Coll Cardiol* 1988;11: 1141

39. Shawl FA, Forman MB, Punja S, et al: Emergent coronary angioplasty in thetreatment of acute ischemic mitral regurgitation. *J Am Coll Cardiol* 1989;14:986

40. Mueller HS, Evans R, Ayres SM: Effects of dopamine on hemodynamics and myocardial metabolism in shock following acute myocardial infarction in man. *Circulation* 1978;57:361

41. Goldberg LO: Cardiovascular and renal actions of dopamine: potential clinical applications. *Pharmacol Rev* 1972;21:1

42. Teba L, Schiebel F, Dedhia HV, et al: Beneficial effect of norepinephrine in the treatment of circulatory shock caused by tricyclic antidepressant overdose. *Am J Emerg Med* 1988;6: 566

43. Horowitz D, Goldberg LI, Sjoerdsm A: Increased blood pressure response to dopamine and norepinephrine produced by MAO inhibitors. *J Lab Clin Med* 1960;56:747

44. Sonnenblick EH, Frishman WH, Lyeintel TH: Dobutamine: a new synthetic cardioactive sympathetic amine. *N Engl J Med* 1979;300:17

45. Mueller H, Ayres S, Giarinelli S, et al: Effect of isoproterenol, L-norepinephrine and intra-aortic balloon counterpulsation on hemodynamics and myocardial metabolism in shock following myocardial infarction. *Circulation* 1972;55:325

46. Kelly RA, Smith TW: Digoxin in heart failure: implications of recent trials. *J Am Coll Cardiol* 1993;22(Suppl 4):107A

47. Sarter BH, Marchinski FE: Redefining the role of digoxin in atrial fibrillation. *Am J Cardiol* 1992;69:71

48. Honerjager P: Pharmacology of bipyridine phosphodiesterase III inhibitors. *Am Heart J* 1991;121:1939

49. Benotti JR, Grossman W, Braunwald E, et al: Hemodynamic assessment of amrinone. *N Engl J Med* 1978;299:1373

50. Klein M, Siskind S, Frishman W: Hemodynamic comparison of intravenous amrinone and dobutamine in patients with chronic congestive heart failure. *Am J Cardiol* 1981;48:160

51. Dage RC, Kariya T, Hsiek CP, et al: Pharmacology of enoximone. *Am J Cardiol* 1987;60:10C

52. Goldstein RE, Skelton CL, Levey GS: Effects of chronic heart failure on the capacity of glucagon to enhance contractility and adenyl cyclase. *Circulation* 1971;44:638

53. Scholtz H: Inotropic drugs and their mechanisms of action. *J Am Coll Cardiol* 1984;4:389

54. De Wood MA, Heit J, Spores J, et al: Anterior transmural myocardial infarction: effects of surgical coronary reperfusion on global and regional left ventricular function. *J Am Coll Cardiol* 1983;1:1223

55. De Wood MA, Notske RN, Berg R, et al: Medical and surgical management of early Q wave myocardial infarction. *J Am Coll Cardiol* 1989;14:65

56. Gray RJ, Sethna D, Matloff JM: The role of cardiac surgery in acute myocardial infarction with mechanical complications. *Am Heart J* 1983;10:723

57. Fox AC, Glassman E, Isom OW: Surgically remediable complications of myocardial infarction. *Prog Cardiovasc Dis* 1979; 21:461

58. Bates RJ, Beutler S, Resnekov L, et al: Cardiac rupture: challenge in diagnosis and management. *Am J Cardiol* 1977; 40:1231

59. Shapiro I, Isakov A, Burke M, et al: Cardiac rupture in patients with acute myocardial infarction. *Chest* 1987;92:219

60. Cohn LH: The role of mechanical devices. *J Cardiac Surg* 1990;5:278

61. Farrar DJ, Hill JD, Gray LA, et al: Heterotopic prosthetic ventricles as a bridge to cardiac transplantation. *N Engl J Med* 1988;318:333

62. Merhige ME, Smalling RW, Cassidy D, et al: Effect of the hemopump left ventricular assist device on regional myocardial perfusion and function. *Circulation* 1989;80(Suppl 3):158

Critical Care, Third Edition, edited by Joseph M. Civetta,
Robert W. Taylor, and Robert R. Kirby.
Lippincott-Raven Publishers, Philadelphia, PA © 1997.

CHAPTER 28

Sepsis and Septic Shock

Janice L. Zimmerman
Robert W. Taylor

IMMEDIATE CONCERNS ■

MAJOR PROBLEMS

Sepsis, the inflammatory response to infection, directly or indirectly contributes to mortality in many critically ill patients. The complex pathophysiologic processes result in a spectrum of findings, ranging from mild systemic toxicity to severe circulatory shock. Toxins from infecting microorganisms activate cellular and humoral immune defenses. Mediators, including cytokines, propagate the response to infection. These processes result in characteristic hemodynamic changes that include an elevated cardiac index, despite evidence of myocardial dysfunction, low systemic vascular resistance, and a normal to low cardiac filling pressure. Clinical manifestations of sepsis are variable, and a high index of suspicion is necessary to recognize early signs and symptoms. Sepsis and septic shock can result in refractory hypotension leading to early death or progressive multiple organ dysfunction leading to a later death.

STRESS POINTS

1. Sepsis often develops in patients compromised by underlying disease, immunosuppressive therapy, or invasive procedures.
2. Sepsis is most commonly caused by bacterial infection. Gram-negative aerobes are the most common pathogens; infection by these microbes has the worst prognosis.
3. Sepsis usually results in a hyperdynamic state with elevated cardiac output, decreased systemic vascular resistance, and normal to low cardiac filling pressure.

Inadequate volume resuscitation or intrinsic myocardial dysfunction may less commonly result in low cardiac output and increased systemic vascular resistance.
4. Reversible myocardial dysfunction in sepsis results in a decreased ejection fraction, biventricular dilatation, and altered ventricular compliance.
5. The systemic response of sepsis may result in significant organ dysfunction including adult respiratory distress syndrome (ARDS), renal failure, encephalopathy, disseminated intravascular coagulation, and gastrointestinal dysfunction.
6. Clinical manifestations of sepsis include systemic findings and clinical signs of local infection. In many patients, no source can be localized by physical examination or routine laboratory tests.

ESSENTIAL DIAGNOSTIC TESTS AND PROCEDURES

1. Appropriate cultures of blood and focal sites should be obtained. Ideally, cultures should be obtained before initiation of antibiotic therapy, but delays should not occur.
2. Laboratory tests such as complete blood cell count, coagulation profile, and serum chemistries should be obtained to assess organ function and acid-base status.
3. Radiographic and other imaging procedures should be obtained as necessary, depending on the clinical suspicion of infected site.
4. A pulmonary artery catheter is helpful to guide therapy in patients with septic shock or evidence of hypoperfusion.

INITIAL THERAPY

1. Infection should be eliminated through early use of appropriate antibiotics and surgical intervention when indicated.
2. Volume resuscitation should be accomplished in all patients with sepsis. The endpoints of resuscitation must be individualized.
3. If hypotension or hypoperfusion persists after volume is optimized, vasoactive drugs should be initiated. Drugs to be considered include vasopressors such as dopamine, norepinephrine, epinephrine, and phenylephrine as well as inotropic agents such as dobutamine.
4. Endpoints of resuscitation in septic shock are controversial. Goals may include an elevated cardiac output, oxygen delivery, or oxygen consumption, or reversal of hypotension and hypoperfusion using clinical and laboratory parameters.
5. In a septic normotensive patient, inotropic support with dobutamine to increase cardiac output may be warranted if there is evidence of hypoperfusion.
6. Mechanical ventilation, dialysis techniques, transfusion of blood products, and early nutritional support should be considered in the septic patient.

EPIDEMIOLOGY AND ETIOLOGY ■

The incidence of sepsis is on the rise. The estimate of 400,000 cases of sepsis per year in the United States is most likely a significant underestimate of the prevalence because of variable reporting.[1] Definitions of sepsis vary, but at an American College of Chest Physicians/Society of Critical Care Medicine Consensus Conference, definitions of sepsis and related conditions were proposed that may allow more uniformity among critical care practitioners[2] (Table 28-1). Sepsis most often claims its victims in the very young or very old and particularly in patients compromised by underlying disease or those receiving immunosuppressive therapy. Common conditions that predispose to sepsis include the following:

Acquired immunodeficiency syndrome
Burns, wounds, and multiple trauma
Diabetes mellitus
Extremes of age
Hepatic failure
Hyposplenism
Immunosuppressive medication
Indwelling urinary catheters
Invasive catheters or devices
Malignancy
Malnutrition
Organ transplantation
Radiation therapy
Renal failure

Shock develops in approximately 40% of patients with sepsis and substantially worsens the prognosis.[3] Sixty percent to 80% of patients with septic shock die.[4]

TABLE 28-1. Definitions

Infection: Microbial phenomenon characterized by an inflammatory response to the presence of microorganisms or the invasion of normally sterile host tissue by those organisms

Bacteremia: The presence of viable bacteria in the blood

Systemic Inflammatory Response Syndrome: The systemic inflammatory response to a variety of severe clinical results. The response is manifested by two or more of the following conditions:
  Temperature >38° or <36°C
  Heart rate >90 bpm
  Respiratory rate >20 breaths/min or $PaCO_2$ <32 mm Hg (<4.3 kPa)
  WBC >12,000 cells/mm^3, <4000 cells/mm^3, or >10% immature (band) forms

Sepsis: The systemic response to infection. This systemic response is manifested by two or more of the following conditions as a result of infection:
  Temperature >38° or <36°C
  Heart rate >90 bpm
  Respiratory rate >20 breaths/min or $PaCO_2$ <32 mm Hg (<4.3 kPa)
  WBC >12,000 cells/mm^3, <4000 cells/mm^3, or >10% immature (band) forms

Severe Sepsis: Sepsis associated with organ dysfunction, hypoperfusion, or hypotension. Hypoperfusion and perfusion abnormalities may include, but are not limited to, lactic acidosis, oliguria, or an acute alteration in mental status.

Septic Shock: Sepsis with hypotension, despite adequate fluid resuscitation, along with the presence of perfusion abnormalities that may include, but are not limited to, lactic acidosis, oliguria, or an acute alteration in mental status. Patients who are on inotropic or vasopressor agents may not be hypotensive at the time that perfusion abnormalities are measured.

Hypotension: A systolic BP of <90 mm Hg or a reduction of >40 mm Hg from baseline in the absence of other causes for hypotension

Multiple Organ Dysfunction Syndrome: Presence of altered organ function in an acutely ill patient such that homeostasis cannot be maintained without intervention

bpm, beats per minute; kPa, kilopascal; BP, blood pressure; WBC, white blood cell count.

Sepsis is most often caused by infection with aerobic or anaerobic bacteria. Both gram-positive and gram-negative organisms are associated with this condition; however, gram-negative aerobes are the most common pathogens, and infection with these organisms has the worst prognosis. *Escherichia coli, Klebsiella* sp., and *Pseudomonas aeruginosa* are the most common gram-negative pathogens in this group. Other microorganisms including mycobacteria, fungi, viruses, rickettsia, and protozoa may produce a syndrome clinically indistinguishable from bacterial sepsis. The most common sites of infection in sepsis are the genitourinary tract, gastrointestinal tract, respiratory tract, wounds, and vascular access sites.

PATHOPHYSIOLOGY ■

The pathophysiologic mechanism of sepsis is complex and only partially understood.[5,6] Intense investigation aimed at unraveling the cascade of events leading to the syndromes of sepsis and septic shock is ongoing. Attention has shifted from the infecting organism to the host response. Fundamentally, the host response to invasion or injury is to preserve "self" and to protect against invasion by "nonself" molecules. This inflammatory process involves several intertwined systems of cellular and humoral immunity (Chap. 20). Sepsis is probably initiated by toxins released from (exotoxin) or associated with (endotoxin) the infecting organism. Exotoxins are released from organisms such as *Staphylococcus aureus*, *Streptococcus pyogenes*, and *Clostridium perfringens*. Endotoxin originates from the cell wall of gram-negative organisms and may activate a variety of cellular and humoral mediators. The macrophage and a group of host-manufactured products termed *cytokines* provide the foundation for the chain of events that produce sepsis.

INITIATING TOXINS

Endotoxin, also referred to as *lipopolysaccharide*, is an important initiator of sepsis.[7] This complex molecule is composed of the O antigen side chain, the R core antigen, and lipid A. The oligosaccharide O antigens vary from one strain to another, but the R core antigen and lipid A are relatively constant across species and strains of gram-negative bacteria. Lipid A, the toxic moiety of endotoxin, interacts with various cells that propagate the response through production of other mediators of sepsis (Table 28-2). Multiple studies

TABLE 28-2. Mediators of Sepsis

MEDIATOR	ACTION
ACTH	May help support blood pressure
Arachidonic acid metabolites	Production of abnormal vasomotor tone
Catecholamines	Alteration in regional blood flow
Complement	Neutrophil aggregation, release of toxic oxygen products
Cytokines	Variety of deleterious actions
Hageman factor	Induction of the intrinsic coagulation pathway and fibrinolysis
Histamine	Vasodilation and increased capillary permeability
Kinins	Vasodilation and increased capillary permeability
Nitric oxide	Vasodilation
Oxygen free radicals	Myocardial and vascular dysfunction, altered capillary permeability
Platelet activating factor	Hypotension and increased capillary permeability

ACTH, corticotropin.

TABLE 28-3. Cytokine Classification

Interleukins 1–10
Tumor necrosis factors
  α (Cachectin)
  β (Lymphotoxin)
Interferons
Colony stimulating factors
  Granulocyte
  Monocyte
Chemotactic factors
  Neutrophil-activating proteins 1 and 2
  Marcophage inflammatory proteins
Variety of growth and differentiating factors

document the deleterious effects of endotoxin; however, clinically similar sepsis is seen in patients invaded by microorganisms that lack endotoxin. Endotoxin is, therefore, an important but not sole initiator of sepsis. Exotoxins, peptidoglycan-teichoic acid complex of gram-positive organisms, and zymosan-like polysaccharides of fungi also are thought to initiate sepsis.

CYTOKINES

Cytokines are soluble regulatory proteins secreted by a variety of cells in response to such insults as infection, trauma, burns, inflammation, and hemorrhage.[7-9] These nonantibody mediators may be secreted from lymphocytes (lymphokines), mononuclear phagocytes (monokines), neutrophils, endothelial cells, or other cell lines. Cytokines may be roughly divided into six classes[7] (Table 28-3). Although interleukin (IL)-1, IL-6, and tumor necrosis factor-alpha (TNF-α) are considered to have primary proinflammatory roles in the pathophysiologic mechanism of sepsis, the contributions and interrelationships of mediators are incompletely elucidated. Animal and human studies document an elevation of cytokines in the systemic circulation during sepsis. The magnitude of the elevation correlates with the severity of sepsis in some studies. When purified cytokines are injected in humans, sepsis results.

ORGAN SYSTEM DYSFUNCTION IN SEPSIS ■

CARDIOVASCULAR

The cardiovascular effects of sepsis and septic shock (Chap. 26) are varied, and the individual's response is dependent on premorbid cardiovascular function, stage of sepsis, adequacy of volume resuscitation, and numerous other factors. Sepsis usually results in a hyperdynamic state with elevated cardiac output, decreased systemic vascular resistance, and normal to low cardiac filling pressures.[6,10] The findings of low cardiac output and increased systemic vascular resistance may be caused by intrinsic myocardial dysfunction or inadequate volume resuscitation, or they may rarely occur as a terminal event in sepsis. Preexisting myocardial dysfunction also may result in a mixed hemodynamic pattern with low cardiac output and low systemic vascular resistance.

Depressed myocardial function in sepsis is common.[6,11,12] Despite a normal or elevated cardiac output, a decreased ejection fraction and biventricular dilatation may be present.[13] The myocardial depression is reversible, resolving if the sepsis clears. Abnormalities in ventricular compliance in response to volume loading also have been observed in sepsis.[14] The reasons for myocardial dysfunction in sepsis are not entirely understood. A circulating substance (or substances) that decreases myocardial contractility has been proposed.[6,15]

Oxygen delivery is usually increased in sepsis because of the hyperdynamic state. However, peripheral oxygen extraction is decreased, as reflected in a narrow arteriovenous oxygen content difference. Tissue hypoxia associated with an elevated lactate level may result, even with an elevated oxygen delivery. Maldistribution of blood flow to tissues has been hypothesized to be responsible for ineffective oxygen utilization, but cellular defects also must be considered. Oxygen consumption in sepsis previously has been thought to be "flow dependent."[16] In other words, as oxygen delivery increases or decreases, oxygen consumption increases or decreases, respectively. This premise has been questioned because of mathematical coupling in calculated values. Direct measurements of oxygen consumption do not always support flow dependency in sepsis (Chap. 24).[17–19]

PULMONARY

Early respiratory changes in sepsis include tachypnea and hyperventilation caused by endotoxin or other mediators. The result of the chest radiograph is often normal at this time; however, gas exchange may be mildly abnormal. Later in the course of sepsis, many patients develop diffuse alveolar damage consistent with the ARDS (Chap. 123).[20–22] From 40% to 60% of patients with gram-negative septic shock develop ARDS. Alveolar–capillary membrane damage allows for leakage of fluid and protein into the pulmonary interstitium. Alveoli are subsequently flooded, causing a marked increase in intrapulmonary shunting, arterial hypoxemia, and reduction in lung compliance. At this stage, the chest radiograph demonstrates diffuse bilateral alveolar infiltrates. Hypoxic pulmonary vasoconstriction, in situ thrombosis, and aggregation of neutrophils and platelets in the pulmonary microvasculature increase pulmonary artery pressures and right ventricular afterload and worsen right ventricular performance.

MULTIPLE ORGAN SYSTEM DYSFUNCTION

In addition to cardiovascular and pulmonary abnormalities in sepsis, the systemic inflammatory process results in other organ dysfunction (Chap. 25).[23,24] Exactly how sepsis leads to individual organ dysfunction or failure is not known. Mediators previously mentioned likely play a central role. Stress ulceration of the gastric mucosa during sepsis may lead to gastrointestinal bleeding. Decreased intestinal peristalsis

occurs. Hepatic dysfunction may manifest as hyperbilirubinemia, elevated aminotransferase levels, cholestasis, or intractable hypoglycemia.[25] Abnormality of the liver's biosynthetic function may be evident as levels of clotting factors, serum albumin, or both, decline. Acalculous cholecystitis has been reported. Oliguria from renal hypoperfusion occurs frequently along with rises in blood urea and creatinine levels. If hypoperfusion is not corrected, acute tubular necrosis and progressive uremia may ensue. Alterations of mental status, ranging from mild disorientation or lethargy to coma and obtundation, may be an early sign of infection, especially in the elderly. The encephalopathy associated with sepsis has been associated with a poor prognosis.[26] Suppression of all bone marrow cell lines occurs during sepsis. A prolonged prothrombin time and partial thromboplastin time, hypofibrinogenemia, elevated level of fibrin split products, and the presence of the D-dimer herald the onset of disseminated intravascular coagulation in sepsis.

CLINICAL MANIFESTATIONS ■

The clinical manifestations of sepsis vary widely and may be subtle or flagrant.[27,28] Common systemic findings are shown in Table 28-4. Fever is the most frequent sign that raises the suspicion of infection. However, normothermia and hypothermia can occur. Hypothermia is more likely in patients at the extremes of age, those with debilitating disease, and those with profound sepsis and is associated with a worse prognosis.[29] Tachycardia is usually present but may be absent in the presence of cardiac conduction disturbances, autonomic dysfunction, or the use of beta-blockers or calcium-channel blockers. Hypotension is initially present or develops in many patients with sepsis. Systemic hypoperfusion may result in oliguria, anuria, or altered mental status.

Systemic signs of sepsis often are associated with or preceded by clinical signs of local infection. Infection of the central nervous system may be associated with headache, seizures, meningism, or focal neurologic findings. Altered mental status often is present but is not specific for central nervous system infections. Respiratory tract infections may result in dyspnea, tachypnea, cough, sputum production, or hemoptysis. Diffuse crackles may herald the presence of ARDS. Focal abnormalities suggest a more localized pneumonic process. Intraabdominal infection may be accompa-

TABLE 28-4. Systemic Signs of Sepsis

Hyperthermia, hypothermia
Tachypnea
Tachycardia
Hypotension
Impaired organ perfusion
Metabolic abnormalities (lactic acidosis)
Multiple organ dysfunction
    Adult respiratory distress syndrome
    Renal insufficiency
    Hepatobiliary dysfunction
    Central nervous system dysfunction

---

nied by pain, distension, nausea with or without vomiting, diarrhea, and anorexia. Findings include diffuse or focal tenderness, rebound tenderness, ileus, or guaiac-positive stool. Upper urinary tract infection is classically associated with flank or abdominal pain, tenderness, and dysuria. Hematuria and oliguria also may be observed. Cutaneous infections may present with erythema, edema, lymphangitis, crepitus, overt abscess, or ecthyma gangrenosum.

Laboratory findings in sepsis reflect the systemic involvement that occurs. No test is specific for the diagnosis of sepsis, but the constellation of results may be suggestive and allow for assessment of organ dysfunction. The common laboratory findings in sepsis are as follows:

Elevated bilirubin and transaminases
Elevated blood urea nitrogen
Elevated prothrombin time and partial thromboplastin time
Elevated white blood cell count, leftward shift, leukopenia
Hyperglycemia
Hypoxemia
Metabolic acidosis (elevated lactate)
Respiratory alkalosis
Thrombocytopenia

DIAGNOSTIC CONSIDERATIONS ■

A presumptive diagnosis of sepsis is usually made based on suggestive clinical findings in a patient with predisposing conditions. Confirmation of the diagnosis involves detection of the source of infection or the causative organism. Identification of the specific offending organism or organisms and their source is vital; however, this task is most often difficult if not frustrating.[30] Bacteremia is not a necessary condition for diagnosis. Physical examination, stains, cultures, and imaging procedures frequently do not convincingly identify the organism, source, or location. Under these circumstances, the diagnostic approach varies widely with little consensus. Repetitive cultures and imaging procedures clearly increase hospital cost. Whether this approach improves outcome is much less clear.[31] Insertion of a pulmonary artery catheter with findings of the characteristic hemodynamic pattern of sepsis may be supportive of the diagnosis. However, noninfectious processes such as pancreatitis, burns, or hyperthyroidism may have similar hemodynamic profiles. Practical guidelines for evaluation of the septic patient requiring thought and decision-making have been published.[32] Laboratory tests such as complete blood cell count, coagulation profile, and serum chemistries should be obtained to assess organ function and acid-base status.

MANAGEMENT OF SEPSIS ■

Treatment of the septic patient often involves most or all of the supportive and many of the therapeutic modalities available to the critical care practitioner.

TREATMENT OF INFECTION

Detailed descriptions of the treatment of all microbiologic causes of sepsis are beyond the scope of this chapter but may be found throughout this text. Therapeutic measures to eliminate infecting organisms should be instituted as soon as possible. Empiric broad-spectrum antimicrobial therapy should be instituted based on clinical suspicion of likely pathogens. Every effort should be made to obtain appropriate cultures before antibiotic administration, but delays in therapy are not acceptable. Antibiotic selection must take into account comorbid organ dysfunction, drug allergies, hospital formulary, and patterns of antibiotic resistance in the individual hospital. Antimicrobial therapy can be more specifically targeted as the patient's clinical condition dictates and as the results of stains, cultures and sensitivities, and imaging procedures become available. Foreign bodies such as catheters may need to be removed, and drainage of closed-space infections may be necessary.

HEMODYNAMIC MANAGEMENT

One half of nonsurvivors of sepsis are estimated to die of refractory hypotension and the other half die of multiple organ failure. Therefore, hemodynamic management of the septic patient to support blood pressure and maintain perfusion to vital organs is a critical aspect of care. However, the methods of achieving these goals and the specific endpoints of therapy remain controversial. Clinical studies documenting improved outcome from different interventions are often lacking. Critical care practitioners must use their best judgment in individualizing treatment for each patient.

Clinical objectives in the hemodynamic management of sepsis include an adequate blood pressure (mean arterial pressure above 60 mm Hg), a decrease in heart rate, adequate renal perfusion as manifested by a urine output over 0.5 mL/kg/hour, an improvement in mental status, or a decrease in lactate level. In most critically ill septic patients, a pulmonary artery catheter is useful to guide therapy. Parameters measured from invasive hemodynamic monitoring also may be used to optimize tissue perfusion. Numerous studies suggest that enhancing hemodynamic variables to "supranormal" levels (oxygen delivery [DO_2] above 600 mL/minute/m^2, oxygen consumption [VO_2] over 170 mL/minute/m^2, and cardiac index more than 4.5 L/minute/m^2) may improve survival in septic patients.[33–35] Although increased DO_2 can be accomplished by various interventions, an improvement in oxygen utilization by tissues (oxygen consumption) may not ensue. The ability to increase oxygen delivery may be a marker of improved survival rather than the increase in DO_2 itself. Other studies have not consistently found improved survival associated with increase in DO_2 or VO_2 or consumption.[36,37] The heterogeneity of septic patients and the variety of methods used to increase DO_2 in different studies make it difficult to arrive at firm conclusions.[35,36] Continuous mixed venous oximetry is generally not useful to guide therapy in sepsis. Despite controversy on the specific endpoints of hemodynamic management, the recommended interventions remain remarkably similar.

The greatest challenge lies in the care of the hypotensive septic patient. The first step in managing these patients is volume resuscitation.[38] Most patients with sepsis have moderate to profound intravascular volume deficits because of vasodilatation and increases in microvascular permeability. Restoration of circulating blood volume enhances preload, cardiac performance, and DO^2. The type and amount of fluid to be given are usually based on individual clinician choice. A clear-cut advantage of colloids (5% albumin, hydroxyethyl starch) or crystalloids (normal saline, lactated Ringer's solution) has not been established. Fluid boluses of 250 to 500 mL can be administered over 10 to 15 minutes and repeated as needed with frequent clinical reassessment. The magnitude of the volume deficit may be extremely large in the first 24 to 48 hours of septic shock.

An optimum pulmonary artery occlusion pressure of 12 to 18 mm Hg has been suggested for fluid resuscitation, but alterations of myocardial compliance must be taken into account. A more specific goal may be the optimization of cardiac performance or oxygen delivery. Volume resuscitation also must take into account pulmonary dysfunction. The presence of ARDS and significant hypoxemia may require a lower pulmonary artery occlusion pressure to minimize pulmonary edema if oxygen concentrations are in a toxic range.

Volume resuscitation should improve oxygen delivery to tissues by increasing cardiac output. However, arterial oxygen content is the other parameter influencing oxygen delivery. Oxyhemoglobin saturation should be optimized (arterial oxyhemoglobin saturation greater than 90%) through use of supplemental oxygen and mechanical ventilation as needed. Transfusion of red blood cells to increase the hematocrit to approximately 30% or greater has been advocated as another means of increasing arterial oxygen content and oxygen delivery. However, clinical studies in septic patients have not supported a parallel increase in oxygen utilization with transfusion.[39,40] Changes in stored blood that decrease red blood cell deformability and oxygen off-loading along with increased blood viscosity may alter microvascular blood flow and impede oxygen delivery.

When volume resuscitation fails to restore hemodynamic stability, vasoactive medications are usually initiated.[41] No universal agreement exists as to how these agents should be used. Dopamine is commonly employed as the initial drug in the hypotensive septic patient. Its beta-adrenergic effects may enhance cardiac performance and its alpha-adrenergic effects may support arterial blood pressure. Norepinephrine, epinephrine, and phenylephrine also have been used effectively as vasopressor or inotropic agents in sepsis.[42-44] Concerns regarding excessive vasoconstriction with norepinephrine seem unwarranted if intravascular volume is optimized. Concurrent administration of low-dose dopamine has been advocated to preserve renal perfusion during use of norepinephrine. Dobutamine as an inotropic agent has been used alone or in combination with other catecholamines to improve cardiac performance.[41] Traditional concepts of therapeutic ranges of vasoactive drugs may require adjustment in the septic patient. The correct dose is best determined by the individual patient response in achieving target endpoints. The response to any one vasoactive drug is often unpredict-

able and the clinician should be willing to use other drugs to optimize management. Vasopressor medications used before restoration of blood volume may worsen tissue perfusion.

A less common, but no less challenging, management problem is the septic patient with adequate blood pressure who continues to have evidence of hypoperfusion. This may be manifested as elevated lactate level, inadequate urine output, or organ dysfunction. A reasonable option in this circumstance may be to increase oxygen delivery by increasing cardiac output with an inotropic agent such as dobutamine. Further objective clinical studies are needed to clarify the hemodynamic management of septic patients. Given the complex pathophysiologic mechanism of sepsis and heterogeneity of patients, it is unlikely that a single regimen will be optimum for all patients.

OTHER IMPORTANT MANAGEMENT ISSUES

Sodium bicarbonate has been administered to patients with septic shock to offset the lactic acidosis. The clinician is cautioned against this practice as a routine.[45,46] Convincing data do not exist documenting an improved outcome with sodium bicarbonate administration. Detrimental effects have been documented and include a leftward shift of the oxyhemoglobin dissociation curve with impaired release of oxygen to tissue, paradoxical intracellular acidosis, and hypertonicity. Attention is more appropriately directed to correcting the causes of impaired perfusion, as outlined above.

Corticosteroids have been recommended in patients with septic shock in the past. Large, prospective, randomized trials document no benefit and suggest detrimental effects in selected patients.[47,48] Nonsteroidal antiinflammatory agents also have been used in patients with septic shock. The available data are promising but preliminary, so these agents cannot be recommended.

Cytoprotection of the gastric mucosa is suggested to prevent stress gastric ulceration. Our preference is use of an H_2 receptor antagonist.

Sepsis results in an increased metabolic requirement. Nutritional support should be instituted early in the septic patient. The route of feeding should be individualized, but the enteral route offers several advantages. Preservation of the intestinal mucosal function may prevent translocation of bacteria or endotoxin, resulting in fewer infections.[49] Parenteral nutrition is associated with more metabolic and infectious complications.

Blood products should be used as necessary in the septic patient. Although disseminated intravascular coagulation is often noted by laboratory parameters, significant bleeding is less common. Platelets and fresh frozen plasma should be used only when significant bleeding occurs or an invasive procedure is necessary.

Intubation and mechanical ventilation often are necessary in septic patients. Indications for initiating mechanical ventilation do not differ significantly from other patients and include the need for airway protection, respiratory muscle fatigue, and hypoxemia. The ventilator mode selected should take into account the hemodynamic status, metabolic demands, acid-base status, and degree of pulmonary dysfunction to optimize oxygenation and ventilation.

Renal dysfunction may pose several problems in the patient with sepsis or septic shock.[50] Choice of antibiotics and dosages must be carefully adjusted to prevent toxicity or renal injury. Volume overload may result from fluid administration in the oliguric patient. Loop diuretics are frequently used in the hemodynamically stable patent to induce a nonoliguric state. Low doses (1 to 3 μg/kg/minute) of dopamine have also been advocated to improve renal perfusion and urine output, but beneficial effects have not been clearly demonstrated. Dialytic therapy may be warranted in the septic patient to manage fluid balance, electrolyte abnormalities, acid-base disturbances, or uremia. Hemodialysis is the most widely used method but may be unsuitable in the hemodynamically unstable patient because of fluctuations in blood pressure. Other techniques such as peritoneal dialysis, continuous arteriovenous hemodiafiltration, or continuous venovenous hemodiafiltration should be considered in the unstable patient.

IMMUNOTHERAPY

Efforts to improve the outcome of sepsis and septic shock have led to the development of agents that target the initiating toxins and mediators.[51] Clinical trials have been conducted with antiendotoxin monoclonal antibodies,[52,53] anti-TNF monoclonal antibodies,[54,55] IL-1 receptor antagonist,[56] bradykinin antagonist, platelet activating factor antagonist,[57] and N-acetylcysteine.[58] Thus far, no agent has convincingly demonstrated a significant improvement in mortality. The need for better therapy supports the continued testing of immunomodulatory agents for sepsis.

CONCLUSION

Although immunotherapy and other modalities promise to favorably impact the outcome from sepsis in the future, a current mortality rate of 30% or higher with the best therapy available is unacceptable. Prevention of sepsis will always be an important ingredient in patients at risk for infection. Vaccination of patients at high risk for gram-negative sepsis is under evaluation. The pneumococcal vaccine may benefit many patients. Aggressive handwashing, aseptic techniques, and appropriate catheter care are crucial.

REFERENCES

1. Increase in national hospital discharge survey rates for septicemia—United States, 1979–1987. *MMWR* 1990;39:31
2. American College of Chest Physicians/Society of Critical Care Medicine Consensus Conference: Definitions for sepsis and organ failure and guidelines for the use of innovative therapies in sepsis. *Crit Care Med* 1992;20:864
3. Kreger BE, Craven DE, McCabe WR: Gram-negative bacteremia. IV. Re-evaluation of clinical features and treatment in 612 patients. *Am J Med* 1980;68:344
4. Young LS, Martin WJ, Meyer RD, et al: Gram-negative rod bacteremia: microbiologic, immunologic, and therapeutic considerations. *Ann Intern Med* 1977;86:456
5. Bone RC: The pathogenesis of sepsis. *Ann Intern Med* 1991;115:457
6. Parrillo JE: Septic shock in humans: advances in the understanding of pathogenesis, cardiovascular dysfunction, and therapy. *Ann Intern Med* 1990;113:227
7. Arai K, Lee F, Miyama A, et al: Cytokines: Coordinators of immune and inflammatory responses. *Annu Rev Biochem* 1990;59:783
8. Filkins JP: Cytokines: mediators of the septic syndrome and septic shock. In: Taylor RW, Shoemaker WC (eds). *Critical Care: State of the Art*, vol 12. Fullerton, CA, Society of Critical Care Medicine, 1991:351
9. Tracey KJ, Lowry SF: The role of cytokine mediators in septic shock. *Adv Surg* 1990;23:21
10. Breslow MJ: Hemodynamic changes in sepsis: pathophysiology and treatment: a critical care medicine review. In: Prough DS, Traystman RJ (eds). *Critical Care: State of the Art*, vol 14. Anaheim, CA, Society of Critical Care Medicine, 1993:299
11. Parker MM, Shelhamer JH, Bacharach SL, et al: Profound but reversible myocardial depression in patients with septic shock. *Ann Intern Med* 1984;100:483
12. Snell RJ, Parrillo JE: Cardiovascular dysfunction in septic shock. *Chest* 1991;99:1000
13. Parker MM, McCarthy KE, Ognibene FP, et al: Right ventricular dysfunction and dilatation, similar to left ventricular changes, characterize the cardiac depression of septic shock in humans. *Chest* 1990;97:126
14. Ognibene FP, Parker MM, Natanson C, et al: Depressed left ventricular performance: response to volume infusion in patients with sepsis and septic shock. *Chest* 1988;93:903
15. Parrillo JE, Burch C, Shelhamer JH, et al: A circulating myocardial depressant substance in humans with septic shock: septic shock patients with a reduced ejection fraction have a circulating factor that depresses in vitro myocardial cell performance. *J Clin Invest* 1985;76:1539
16. Rackow EC, Astiz ME, Weil MH: Cellular oxygen metabolism during sepsis and shock. *JAMA* 1988;259:1989
17. Vermij CG, Feenstra BWA, Adrichem WJ, et al: Independent oxygen uptake and oxygen delivery in septic and postoperative patients. *Chest* 1991;99:1438
18. Ronco JJ, Fenwick JC, Tweeddale MG, et al: Identification of the critical oxygen delivery for anaerobic metabolism in critically ill septic and nonseptic humans. *JAMA* 1993;270:1724
19. Manthous CA, Schumacker PT, Pohlman A, et al: Absence of supply dependence of oxygen consumption in patients with septic shock. *J Crit Care* 1993;8:203
20. Pepe PE, Potkin RT, Rens DH, et al: Clinical predictors of the adult respiratory distress syndrome. *Am J Surg* 1982;144:24
21. Kaplan R, Sahn SA, Petty TL: Incidence and outcome of the respiratory distress syndrome in gram-negative sepsis. *Arch Intern Med* 1979;139
22. Bersten A, Sibbald WJ: Acute lung injury in septic shock. *Crit Care Clin* 1989;5:49
23. Bell RC, Coalson JJ, Smith JD, et al: Multiple organ system failure and infection in adult respiratory distress syndrome. *Ann Intern Med* 1983;99:293
24. Borzotta AP, Polk HC: Multiple system organ failure. *Surg Clin North Am* 1983;63:315
25. Keller GA, West MA, Cerra FB, et al: Macrophage-mediated modulation of hepatic function in multiple-system failure. *J Surg Res* 1985;39:555
26. Young GB, Bolton CF: Septic encephalopathy: what significance in patients with sepsis? *J Crit Illness* 1992;7:668
27. Harris RL, Musher DM, Bloom K, et al: Manifestations of sepsis. *Arch Intern Med* 1987;147:1895

28. Bone RC: Sepsis syndrome. Part I. The diagnostic challenge. *J Crit Illness* 1991;6:525
29. Clemmer TP, Fisher CJ, Bone RC, et al: Hypothermia in the sepsis syndrome and clinical outcome. *Crit Care Med* 1992; 20:1395
30. Meakins JL: Diagnosis and mechanisms of occult sepsis. In: Taylor RW, Shoemaker WC (eds). *Critical Care: State of the Art*, vol 12. Fullerton, CA, Society of Critical Care Medicine, 1991:141
31. Civetta JM, Hudson-Civetta JA: Maintaining quality of care while reducing charges in the ICU. *Ann Surg* 1985;202:524
32. Norwood SH, Civetta JM: Evaluating sepsis in critically ill patients. *Chest* 1987;92:137
33. Tuchschmidt J, Fried J, Astiz M, et al: Elevation of cardiac output and oxygen delivery improves outcome in septic shock. *Chest* 1992;102:216
34. Yu M, Levy MM, Smith P, et al: Effect of maximizing oxygen delivery on morbidity and mortality rates in critically ill patients: a prospective, randomized, controlled study. *Crit Care Med* 1993;21:830
35. Shoemaker WC, Appel PL, Kram HB, et al: Temporal hemodynamic and oxygen transport patterns in medical patients: septic shock. *Chest* 1993;104:1529
36. Hayes MA, Timmins AC, Yau EHS, et al: Elevation of systemic oxygen delivery in the treatment of critically ill patients. *N Engl J Med* 1994;330:1717
37. Bakker J, Coffernils M, Leon M, et al: Blood lactate levels are superior to oxygen-derived variables in predicting outcome in human septic shock. *Chest* 1991;99:956
38. Astiz ME, Galera-Santiago A, Rackow EC: Intravascular volume and fluid therapy for severe sepsis. *New Horizons* 1993; 1:127
39. Marik PE, Sibbald WJ: Effect of stored-blood transfusion on oxygen delivery in patients with sepsis. *JAMA* 1993;269: 3024
40. Lorente JA, Land,n L, DePablo R, et al: Effects of blood transfusion on oxygen transport variables in severe sepsis. *Crit Care Med* 1993;21:1312
41. Vincent JL, Preiser JC: Inotropic agents. *New Horizons* 1993; 1:137
42. Moran JL, O'Fathartaigh MS, Peisach AR, et al: Epinephrine as an inotropic agent in septic shock: a dose-profile analysis. *Crit Care Med* 1993;21:70
43. Desjars P, Pinaud M, Bugnon D, et al: Norepinehrine therapy has no deleterious renal effects in human septic shock. *Crit Care Med* 1989;17:426
44. Gregory JS, Bonfiglio MF, Dasta JF, et al: Experience with phenylephrine as a component of the pharmacologic support of septic shock. *Crit Care Med* 1991;19:1395
45. Mizock BA, Falk JL: Lactic acidosis in critical illness. *Crit Care Med* 1992;20:80
46. Stacpoole PW: Lactic acidosis: the case against bicarbonate therapy. *Ann Intern Med* 1986;105:276
47. The Veteran's Administration Systemic Sepsis Cooperative Study Group: Effect of high-dose glucocorticoid therapy on mortality in patients with clinical signs of systemic sepsis. *N Engl J Med* 1987;317:659
48. Bone RC, Fisher CJ, Clemmer TP, et al: The methylprednisolone severe sepsis study group: a controlled clinical trial of high-dose methylprednisolone in the treatment of severe sepsis and septic shock. *N Engl J Med* 1987;317:353
49. Kudsk KA, Croce MA, Fabian TC, et al: Enteral vs parenteral feeding: effects on septic mortality following blunt and penetrating trauma. *Ann Surg* 1992;215
50. Fischer DB, Badr KF: Managing renal involvement in sepsis: current concepts and future directions. *J Crit Illness* 1992; 7:1446
51. Natanson C: Selected treatment strategies for septic shock based on proposed mechanisms of pathogenesis. *Ann Intern Med* 1994;120:771
52. Zeigler EJ, Fisher CJ, Sprung CL, et al: Treatment of gram negative bacteremia and septic shock with HA-1A human monoclonal antibody against endotoxin. *N Engl J Med* 1991; 324:429
53. Greenman RL, Schein RM, Martin MA, et al: A controlled clinical trial of E5 murine monoclonal IgM antibody to endotoxin in the treatment of gram-negative sepsis. *JAMA* 1991; 266:1097
54. Fisher CJ, Opal SM, Dhainaut JF, et al: Influence of an anti-tumor necrosis factor monoclonal antibody on cytokine levels in patients with sepsis. *Crit Care Med* 1993;21:318
55. Abraham E, Wunderink R, Silverman H, et al: Efficacy and safety of monoclonal antibody to human tumor necrosis factor α in patients with sepsis syndrome. *JAMA* 1995;273:934
56. Fisher CJ, Dhainaut JF, Pribble JP, et al: A study evaluating the safety and efficacy of human recombinant interleukin-1 receptor antagonist in the treatment of patients with sepsis syndrome. Presented at the 13th International Symposium on Intensive Care and Emergency Medicine, Brussels, Belgium, March 23, 1993
57. Dhainaut JF, Tenaillon A, Tulzo YL, et al: Platelet-activating factor receptor antagonist BN 52021 in the treatment of severe sepsis: a randomized, double-blind, placebo-controlled, multicenter clinical trial. *Crit Care Med* 1994;22:1720
58. Spies CD, Reinhart K, Witt I, et al: Influence of N-acetylcysteine on indirect indicators of tissue oxygenation in septic shock patients: results from a prospective, randomized, double-blind study. *Crit Care Med* 1994;22:1738

Critical Care, Third Edition, edited by Joseph M. Civetta,
Robert W. Taylor, and Robert R. Kirby.
Lippincott-Raven Publishers, Philadelphia, PA © 1997.

CHAPTER 29

Fluids and Electrolytes

Gary P. Zaloga
Robert R. Kirby
Walter C. Bernards
A. Joseph Layon

IMMEDIATE CONCERNS

MAJOR PROBLEMS

Fluid and electrolyte disorders are volume related, compositional, or both. Diagnosis and therapy focuses on measurements such as blood pressure, pulse, central venous pressure, serum electrolyte values, arterial blood gas partial pressures, and pH. These are, however, gross indicators of what is really important: normal cellular function and satisfactory, if not optimal, metabolic status.

Normal compensatory responses to fluid and electrolyte abnormalities preserve volume and composition. In the extreme, however, composition (e.g., electrolyte content) is sacrificed to ensure adequate volume. The "volumes" of importance are blood (plasma), interstitial fluid (functional extracellular fluid [FECV]), and intracellular fluid (ICF). Thus, mechanisms that initially act to maintain oxygen delivery at the cellular level ultimately can result in hyperosmolar or hypoosmolar states that may be life-threatening.

STRESS POINTS

1. Total body water (TBW) averages 50% of body weight in normal subjects. ICF comprises 66% of TBW whereas extracellular fluid (ECF) is 34% of TBW. The latter is 75% interstitial and 25% intravascular.
2. In normal subjects, sodium and its accompanying anions, such as chloride and bicarbonate, are responsible for 93% of the total ECF osmolality.
3. The primary intracellular cation is potassium.
4. Normal serum osmolality is 280 to 295 mOsm/kg H_2O. Values below this range represent hypoosmolal, whereas those that are higher are hyperosmolal. Hyperosmolality also can result from excessive glucose, as in diabetes mellitus and nonketotic hyperosmolar syndrome; central or nephrogenic diabetes insipidus; and excessive water loss from any cause.
5. Hyponatremia may occur with normal, elevated, or low serum osmolality.
6. Hypokalemia most commonly results from excessive renal potassium loss. Hyperkalemia is associated with acidosis, increased catabolism, tissue necrosis, and rhabdomyolysis.
7. Hypocalcemia most commonly results from impaired parathyroid secretion or vitamin D synthesis or a circulatory chelator. The fraction of calcium that is ionized (Ca^{2+}) is physiologically most important. Clinical features of hypercalcemia are nonspecific, representing aspects of the underlying disease.
8. Magnesium depletion results primarily by dilution, chelation, redistribution, and renal losses. It is common during cardiopulmonary bypass. Hypermagnesemia occurs in patients with renal disease and after the administration of magnesium-containing antacids, laxatives, enemas, or nutritional products.
9. Hypophosphatemia results from intracellular anabolic shifts, gram-negative bacteremia, alcoholism, alkalosis, and diabetic ketoacidosis or salicylism. Hyperphosphatemia follows decreased renal excretion, hyperthyroidism, ICF to ECF shifts, severe hypo-

thermia, malignant hyperthermia, sepsis, and cancer chemotherapy.

10. In general, acute changes of any electrolyte are more serious than are those of a more chronic nature. Acute and severe hyponatremia can be rapidly lethal. Thus, rapidity of diagnosis and treatment are paramount considerations.

ESSENTIAL DIAGNOSTIC TESTS AND PROCEDURES

Volume

1. Assess skin turgor, mucous membranes, changes in body weight, urine output, blood pressure, and pulse.
2. Invasive measurements (e.g., central venous pressure, pulmonary arterial occlusion pressure) are less frequently necessary than is commonly thought to determine baseline volume status. They can be useful for fine tuning and in situations where a significant abnormality such as renal failure or congestive heart failure complicate diagnosis and treatment.
3. The patient's mental status (alert, oriented, somnolent, confused) may be the most important feature regardless of "the numbers."

Composition

1. Measure serum electrolytes and serum and urine osmolality before diuretics are given. Determine serum glucose.
2. Assessment of osmolality is most important to define the basic problems. Specific electrolyte and glucose abnormalities guide replacement therapy and correction.

INITIAL THERAPY

Volume

1. Restoration of circulatory volume is more important than replenishment of red cell mass. Balanced electrolyte solutions are the key to most resuscitations.
2. In selected patients, hypertonic saline solutions, with or without a colloid such as dextran, may be useful. Hyperosmolality is a possibility. It rarely is a significant side effect of such therapy, unless these solutions are used in excess.
3. Colloid therapy is less favored for early volume restoration. It may play a role in burn therapy after the first

24 hours or in severely hypoalbuminemic states (e.g., albumin level >1.5 to 2.0 g/dL).

Composition

1. Selected ionic abnormalities are addressed by specific fluid regimens. The key to success is serial measurement of the ions in question. Too rapid a correction may produce problems worse than those being treated. Correction of symptomatic hyponatremia at a rate greater than 2 mMol/L/hour is one example.
2. Correction to normal values seldom is necessary. Elevation of pH to 7.2 when severe acidosis is present is sufficient, as is an increase of serum sodium to 125 mMol/L in the treatment of acute hyponatremia.

FLUID COMPARTMENTS ∎

DISTRIBUTION

Total body water makes up 60% of the body weight in an average man and approximately 50% in an average woman. In thin men and women, the values are 65% and 55%, respectively, whereas in obese persons, they are 60% and 50%, respectively. In a 70-kg, lean man, the intracellular compartment contains 66% (28 L) of TBW and the extracellular compartment 34% (14 L). The extracellular compartment is composed of intravascular and interstitial subcompartments. The former contains approximately 3.5 L and the latter approximately 10.5 L (Table 29-1).

EFFECTS OF FLUID ADMINISTRATION

If no solute is present, the added fluid distributes evenly through the TBW until the concentrations of solute in both compartments are equal. Clinically, this sequence only occurs when dextrose solutions are infused.

In the prototypic 70-kg man, 30 minutes after rapid infusion of 1 L of 5% dextrose in water (D_5W), the compartments are enlarged to the following dimensions: TBW, 43 L; intracellular water, 28.8 L; extracellular water, 14.2 L; interstitial water, 10.6 L; and intravascular water, 3.6 L (Table 29-2). After 30 minutes, only 100 mL of additional volume is in the intravascular compartment. In contrast, 30 minutes after rapid infusion of 1 L of Ringer's lactate solution, TBW is 43 L; intracellular water, 28 L; extracellular water, 15 L; interstitial water, 11.2 L; and intravascular water, 3.8 L (see Table 29-2). Here, the intravascular compartment has been

TABLE 29-1.   Normal Distribution of Body Water (70-kg Male Patient)

TOTAL-BODY WATER (TBW)	=	60% Body weight	=	42 L
Intracellular fluid (ICF)	=	66% TBW	=	28 L
Extracellular fluid (ECF)	=	34% TBW	=	14 L
Interstitial fluid	=	75% ECF	=	10.5 L
Intravascular fluid	=	25% ECF	=	3.5 L

TABLE 29-2. Effects of Infusing Various Fluids Into a Normal 70-kg Male Patient

	TOTAL-BODY WATER (L)	INTRACELLULAR COMPARTMENT (L)	EXTRACELLULAR COMPARTMENT	
			Interstitial Fluid (L)	*Intravascular Fluid (L)*
1 L D₅W	43	28.8	10.6	3.6
1 L Ringer's lactate	43	28	11.2	3.8
1 L 3% saline	43	25.5	12.9	4.6
100 mL 25% albumin	42.1	28	10.5 (initial)	3.6
			10.05 (later)	4.05 (later)

D₅W, 5% dextrose in water.

enlarged by 300 mL, or 200 mL more than results from the same volume infusion of D₅W.

This reasoning becomes more complicated when colloid solutions are considered. The half-life of albumin is approximately 20 days in the body but about 16 hours in plasma. Ten percent of infused albumin leaves the vascular space within 2 hours, and 75% within 2 days.[1] The membranes between the fluid compartments are semipermeable; thus albumin, like crystalloid solutions, crosses over, but at a slower rate. If 100 mL of 25% albumin is infused rapidly into a healthy individual, 30 minutes later essentially all of the infused volume is within the intravascular compartment (see Table 29-2). In the 70-kg man, the volume changes are as follows: TBW, 42.1 L; intracellular water, 28 L; extracellular water, 14.1 L; interstitial water, 10.5 L; and intravascular water, 3.6 L. Thus, immediately after infusion, the intravascular compartment is increased by only 100 mL. However, each gram of intravascular albumin is thought to "bind" 18 mL of water because of its oncotic activity.[2] Thus, the 25 g in 100 mL of infused albumin theoretically draws another 450 mL of interstitial fluid into the intravascular space. After equilibration, the extracellular compartment still is composed of 14.1 L; however, the interstitial compartment decreases to 10.05 L, and the intravascular compartment increases to 4.05 L (see Table 29-2).

ELECTROLYTES

Electrolytes are essential for normal cellular function. Alterations in circulating electrolyte concentrations are common in critically ill patients and occur in most patients admitted to the intensive care unit during their hospital stay. Abnormal electrolyte concentrations reflect altered metabolic status. The meaning and treatment of disorders of the primary extracellular and intracellular ions are described in this chapter.

SODIUM

Sodium is the major ion in the ECF, and its normal concentration is 135 to 145 mMol/L. It is primarily responsible for maintaining plasma and ECF osmolality and intravascular

and ECF volume. Serum osmolality can be estimated as follows:

$$2 \times \text{Na (mMol/L)} + \text{glucose (mg/dL)}/18 \quad (1)$$
$$+ \text{BUN (mg/dL)}/2.8$$

where Na is sodium and BUN is blood urea nitrogen. Sodium also plays a physiologic role in the generation of the membrane resting potential, action potential, and glucose and amino acid transport.

Circulating sodium concentration is regulated by the renal and endocrine systems.[3] The kidneys conserve sodium during hypovolemia and states of sodium depletion. Normal kidneys can decrease sodium excretion to less than 10 mMol/day. Sodium conservation effected in the renal tubules is controlled by intrinsic renal mechanisms and influenced by hormones. Aldosterone, the major hormone regulating renal sodium excretion, stimulates distal renal tubule absorption of sodium in exchange for tubule excretion of hydrogen or potassium. Aldosterone does not concentrate urine, because it exchanges one ion for another. The kidneys are also capable of excreting large amounts of sodium during states of sodium overload. Sodium excretion is controlled by intrinsic renal mechanisms, suppression of aldosterone excretion, and stimulation of secretion of atrial natriuretic hormone, a cardiac hormone capable of producing natriuresis.

Antidiuretic hormone (ADH) and thirst do not regulate sodium directly; rather, they control water balance by affecting water absorption in the collecting duct of the nephron or altering water intake.[4] However, absorption and excretion of water do alter the concentration of sodium in the ECF. When positive free water balance lowers the serum sodium concentration to less than 135 mMol/L, cell volume receptors in the hypothalamus inhibit the secretion of ADH. Free water is excreted and circulating sodium is returned to normal levels. ADH secretion and thirst are stimulated by hyperosmolality and volume depletion by parasympathetic input from baroreceptors and volume receptors in the great vessels and heart. Because of differences between the regulation of total-body volume and sodium concentration, it is possible to have hyponatremia or hypernatremia in the face of hypovolemia, euvolemia, or hypervolemia.

Sodium circulates in the plasma as free ions. The normal circulating sodium concentration is between 135 and 145 mMol/L. The serum sodium concentration does not reflect the state of sodium balance; it primarily reflects body water content.[5] The average 70-kg adult has a whole-body sodium content of 5000 to 6000 mMol.

HYPONATREMIA

Causes

Hyponatremia, one of the most common electrolyte disorders, may occur with normal, elevated, or low serum osmolality[6,7] (Fig. 29-1). Hyponatremia occurring with a normal serum osmolality (pseudohyponatremia) usually results from severe hyperlipidemia or markedly elevated serum proteins, as in multiple myeloma. Lipid and protein represent solid components of the blood (normally 7%). Standard laboratory techniques for measuring serum sodium assume a constant solid component of blood. If these components are elevated, these techniques underestimate the true sodium concentration in the liquid portion of the blood. Ion-selective electrode systems measure ion concentrations by activity and are not affected by lipid and protein levels.

Hyponatremia also may result from high concentrations of impermeant solutes (see Fig. 29-1). The impermeant solutes replace sodium as osmotically active particles in the blood and are usually associated with hyperosmolality. The most common causes of hypertonic hyponatremia are glu-cose, mannitol, and toxin ingestion. The osmolar gap is equal to the measured osmolality − calculated osmolality > 10 mOsm/kg H_2O. An osmolar gap indicates additional solute osmoles.[8] Urea and ethanol also may elevate the serum osmolality, but these substances distribute into TBW. They do not cause a shift in water and do not themselves cause hyponatremia. However, disorders associated with excess ethanol or urea concentrations, such as renal failure, may result in hyponatremia because of impaired water excretion.

Hyponatremia is most commonly associated with hypoosmolality and occurs if the intake of free water exceeds free water losses.[5,9] Three categories of hypoosmolar hyponatremia are based on a clinical assessment of total-body volume (see Fig. 29-1).

HYPOVOLEMIC.   Patients with low intravascular volume have hypotension, orthostatic hypotension, tachycardia, or signs of skin dehydration. Fluid loss may result from renal or nonrenal causes and occur with diuretic use, renal tubular dysfunction, and aldosterone deficiency. Nonrenal fluid losses may be caused by gastrointestinal losses (e.g., diarrhea) or skin losses. Volume loss stimulates the secretion of ADH, retention of free water, and dilution of the plasma sodium level. In patients with normal renal function, urine osmolality is high (>500 mOsm/kg) and urine sodium is low (>20 mMol/L). In patients with renal tubular dysfunction

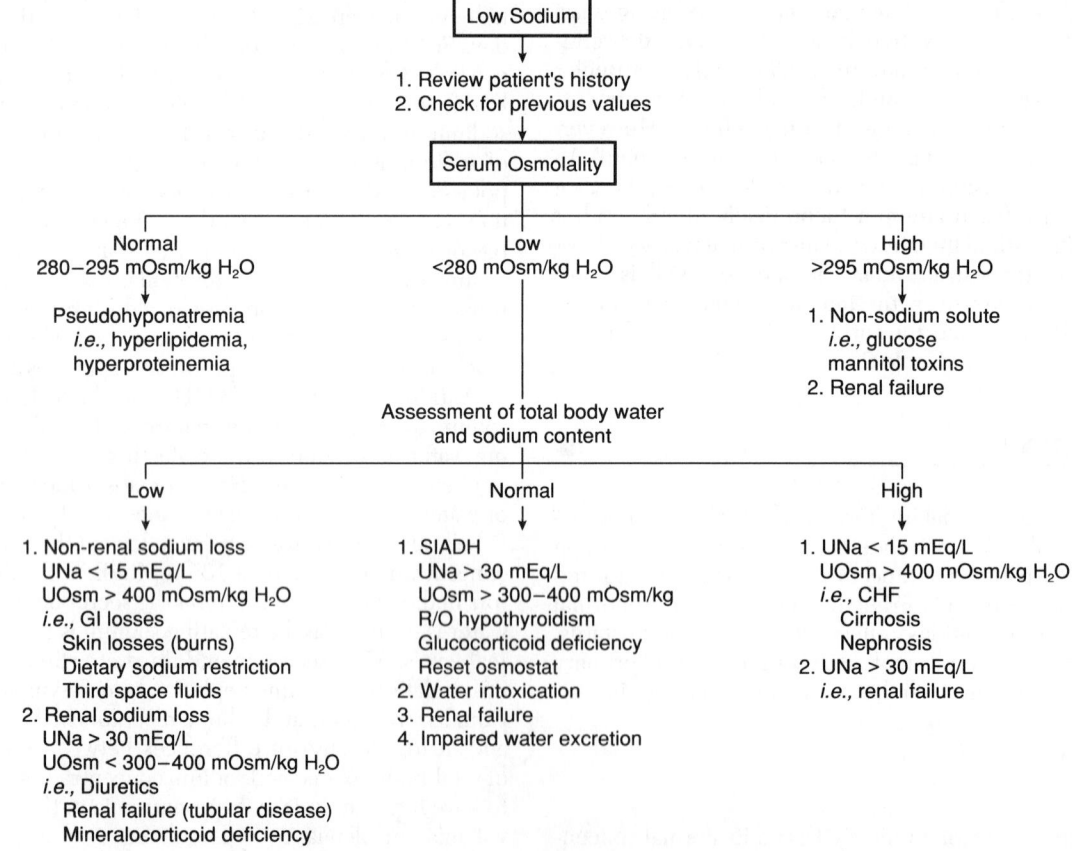

FIGURE 29-1. Evaluation of hyponatremia. R/O, rule out; CHF, congestive heart failure; GI, gastrointestinal; UNa, urinary sodium; UOsm, urinary osmolality; SIADH, syndrome of inappropriate antidiuretic hormone.

and salt wasting, urine sodium is high (>50 mMol/L) and urine osmolality is usually isotonic.

HYPERVOLEMIC. Patients with elevated TBW have edema and include patients with congestive heart failure, cirrhosis, and nephrosis. Although TBW is increased, the effective circulating volume is low, stimulating ADH and aldosterone secretion. The net result is retention of free water and hyponatremia. These patients have low urine sodium levels (less than 20 mMol/L) and high urine osmolality (>500 mOsm/kg).

EUVOLEMIC. *SIADH.* Patients with euvolemia and hyponatremia usually have the syndrome of inappropriate antidiuretic hormone (SIADH).[10,11] ADH secretion is stimulated by nonosmotic, nonvolume factors, and is thus considered inappropriate. SIADH may result from pain, nausea, drugs, central nervous system (CNS) disease, pulmonary disease, or endocrine disease (e.g., glucocorticoid deficiency, hypothyroidism). Patients receiving hypotonic fluids may become acutely hyponatremic resulting from impaired water excretion. Many cases of parenteral water intoxication have been seen after surgery. Anesthesia and surgery are common stimulants to ADH secretion. Women, children, and the elderly are more susceptible to hyponatremia because of a lower body water content. Drugs associated with SIADH include vincristine, oxytocin, carbamazepine, clofibrate, chlorpropamide, morphine, and nonsteroidal antiinflammatory agents.

The kidneys possess a large capacity to excrete free water. In the absence of ADH, urine osmolality usually falls 50 to 100 mOsm/kg H_2O. Given a normal daily diet of 1000 mOsm of solute, a maximally dilute urine allows excretion of 20 L of fluid each day. If water intake exceeds the capacity of the kidneys to excrete it, hyponatremia results. SIADH patients cannot maximally dilute their urine and develop hyponatremia at levels of free water intake that are considered normal. Such patients have high urine sodium levels (>40 mMol/L) and high urine osmolalities (>500 mOsm/kg). Natriuresis results from elevated atrial natriuretic hormone levels and suppressed aldosterone concentrations, and concentrated urine results from high ADH levels.

Water Intoxication. Other causes of hyponatremia associated with euvolemia include water intoxication (e.g., psychotic patients, heavy beer drinkers, absorption of hypoosmolar fluids during prostate resection). These patients have low urine osmolalities (usually <100 mOsm/kg H_2O) and polyuria. Diuretics are an important cause of hyponatremia in euvolemic patients. Thiazides and metolazone block reabsorption of sodium chloride in the distal convoluted tubule, preventing the formation of maximally dilute urine, but they leave intact the ability to excrete maximally concentrated urine.

CNS Effects

Sodium primarily affects osmolality and cellular volumes. The cells most affected by changes in osmolality are those in the CNS. When blood sodium concentration falls, the brain gains fluid and swells. The CNS can compensate for slow or chronic changes in osmolality.[5,12–14] Thus, acute changes in sodium concentration should be treated rapidly and chronic changes more slowly.[5,15,16] Acute hyponatremia may produce lethargy, disorientation, obtundation, coma, impaired mentation, and seizures[5,17–19] (Table 29-3). Other symptoms of hyponatremia relate to the underlying cause and intravascular volume status. Severe acute hyponatremia (<125 mMol/L) is associated with significant morbidity and mortality.[5,20–22] Although less symptomatic, chronic hyponatremia is not synonymous with asymptomatic hyponatremia. Patients with low serum sodium concentrations usually have neurologic symptoms.

Treatment

The treatment of hyponatremia (Table 29-4) is based on correction of the underlying cause and restoration of a normal serum sodium concentration.[7]

HYPOVOLEMIC. Volume depletion is treated by replacing intravascular volume with fluids, which suppresses ADH secretion. Initial therapy involves use of isotonic crystalloids, colloid, or blood. Restoration of volume and treatment of the underlying disease may correct the serum sodium, without the need for additional therapy. After intravascular volume is replenished, further therapy replaces free water with sodium. This goal is best accomplished by restricting free water, preventing free water generation in the kidneys with furosemide, and replacing urine output with isotonic or hypertonic saline. Usually total fluids need not be restricted as long as free water intake is limited. Continued nutritional intake is desirable to blunt catabolism and improve recovery from illness. Hyperglycemia can be corrected with insulin. Other nonsodium solutes, such as toxins, should be treated appropriately. Hyponatremia secondary to mannitol administration usually suggests overdosage with the agent.

TABLE 29-3. Clinical Features of Acute Hyponatremia

NEUROLOGIC FEATURES

Apathy, depressed mentation
Lethargy, obtundation, coma
Confusion, irritability
Disorientation
Seizures
Weakness
Respiratory failure
Headache, nervousness
Cerebral edema
Uncal and tonsillar herniation
Neuronal death

GASTROINTESTINAL FEATURES

Anorexia
Nausea and vomiting

MUSCULAR FEATURES

Cramps
Weakness

TABLE 29-4. Treatment of Hyponatremia

GENERAL MEASURES
> Treat underlying cause
> Remove offending drugs

NORMAL OR HIGH SERUM OSMOLALITY
> Restore volume and free water deficits
> Treat hyperglycemia or elevated mannitol levels
> Treat for nonsodium solutes (e.g., toxin ingestion)
> Treat hyperlipidemic or hyperproteinemic states

LOW SERUM OSMOLALITY
> Elevated total-body sodium
> Restrict sodium and water
>> Increase cardiac output (e.g., β-adrenergic agonists, ACE inhibitors)
>> Diuresis (e.g., furosemide)
> Normal total-body sodium
>> Restrict free water
>> Loop diuretic plus isotonic or hypertonic saline
>> Monitor electrolytes
>> Demeclocycline (300 mg every 6–8 h)
>> Thyroid hormone for hypothyroidism
>> Glucocorticoids for adrenal insufficiency
> Low total-body sodium
>> Restore circulating volume
>> Minimize sodium losses
>> Treat adrenal insufficiency

ACE, angiotensin converting enzyme.

EUVOLEMIC. The cornerstone of therapy for SIADH is correction of the cause (e.g., tumor, pain, nausea, stress), free water restriction, and replacement of water loss with fluids higher in sodium content. The goal is a net negative water balance. Even if the source of ADH secretion cannot be removed or suppressed, water restriction decreases intravascular fluid volume. The result is decreased renal blood flow (RBF) and glomerular filtration rate (GFR), which enhances proximal tubular reabsorption of salt and water, decreases free water generation, and increases aldosterone secretion, enhancing distal tubule sodium reabsorption. However, decreased renal blood flow may predispose the patient to renal failure. Net negative water balance also may be obtained by using furosemide to promote free water loss in the kidney.[11,23,24] Furosemide frequently produces a urine sodium loss of 40 to 70 mMol/L, but the exact amount can be measured every 6 to 12 hours.

Excreted water and salt can be replaced with isotonic or hypertonic saline solution that is more concentrated than the fluid excreted. This technique can rapidly restore serum sodium levels to normal values. Isotonic saline (154 mMol Na/L) alone may not correct hyponatremia, although it is hypertonic compared with the patient's plasma, because the infused sodium can be excreted in a more concentrated form than it is administered. The net effect is further water retention and worsening hyponatremia. Loop diuretics may be useful in these situations by impairing the patient's ability

to concentrate the urine. Loop diuretics also can be combined with hypertonic saline or oral salt. Saline should be used to replace urinary sodium losses and not urine volume, to avoid excess volume expansion.

Care must be taken not to correct chronic hyponatremia too rapidly and to prevent saline overload, which is more common with the use of hypertonic saline.[10,12–15,19–21,25] The adaptations that defend against brain swelling during hyponatremia predispose to complications if a chronic disturbance is corrected too quickly. While serum sodium concentration is corrected, solutes lost in the adaptation to hyponatremia must be recovered. Rapid correction of chronic hyponatremia may result in brain dehydration, cerebral bleeding, demyelination, neurologic injury, or death.

The osmotic demyelination syndrome is a delayed complication of rapid reversal of hyponatremia (i.e., correction by >12 mMol/L/day).[5,21] In this syndrome, hyponatremic symptoms improve during correction of the electrolyte disorder, but improvement is followed within one to several days by neurologic deterioration (e.g., seizures, movement disorders, akinetic mutism, pseudobulbar palsy, quadriparesis, unresponsiveness). Although no consensus has been reached on how rapidly to correct acute hyponatremia (<2-day duration), we recommend that the serum sodium level be corrected no faster than 1 to 2 mMol/L/hour and that the serum sodium be increased to only 130 mMol/L.[26] Hypernatremia should be avoided. In chronic hyponatremia, we recommend a correction rate of less than 12 mMol/L/day. These rates of correction usually can be accomplished by measuring the sodium concentration in urine after 10 to 40 mg of furosemide over 1 to 2 hours and replacing the sodium content with a more concentrated fluid (i.e., 0.9% or 3% saline).

Saline infusion alone often results in only a transient increase in the circulating sodium concentration. In the face of an expanded intravascular volume—which is common in patients with SIADH, aldosterone suppression—and elevated atrial natriuretic hormone levels, the administered saline is quickly excreted in the urine. In addition, the basic fluid problem in SIADH is water overload and not salt depletion.

Demeclocycline (900 to 1200 mg/day) and lithium produce a state of nephrogenic diabetes insipidus and have been used effectively to treat patients with SIADH (usually patients in whom the primary disease cannot be reversed).[27,28] Demeclocycline is better tolerated than lithium, but both drugs have significant toxicities. Occasionally, diphenylhydantoin may inhibit neurohypophyseal release of ADH in a patient with SIADH and may be useful in management.

Psychogenic polydipsia usually autocorrects rapidly by water diuresis after water intake is curtailed. In these patients, it is difficult to prevent rapid correction of the serum sodium level. Hypertonic saline is rarely required.

HYPERVOLEMIC. Patients with hyponatremia and elevated TBW have an excess of salt and water. Sodium should be restricted and free water intake minimized. Therapy is directed at improving effective circulating volume, renal perfusion, cardiac function, and improving distal tubule delivery of sodium (e.g., with diuretics). The combination of furosemide and an angiotensin converting enzyme (ACE) inhibitor is particularly effective. ACE inhibitors blunt the stimulating effect of angiotensin II on thirst and ADH secretion. Thiazides should be avoided in these patients, because the drugs impair the formation of maximally dilute urine. Hypertonic saline may be dangerous because of rapid correction of hyponatremia and volume overload, but it may be indicated in seizures, coma, and water intoxication. Rapid infusion of hypertonic saline should be used only to correct the serum sodium to non–life-threatening levels (i.e., rate <12 mMol/L/day; concentration of 130 mEq/L).

CNS signs of hyponatremia usually improve within 24 to 72 hours after correction of the hyponatremia. A large increase in sodium concentration is not needed to reduce cerebral edema caused by hyponatremia. A small increase in plasma osmolality is sufficient to reduce brain swelling. Because brain water content cannot increase by more than about 10% because of the confines of the skull, a 5% to 10% increase in sodium concentration (i.e., 6 to 12 mMol) can markedly reduce cerebral edema. Continued CNS abnormalities suggest another cause or permanent damage from the hyponatremia. After hyponatremia is corrected, careful monitoring of fluid and electrolyte status is required to prevent recurrence.

HYPERNATREMIA

Causes

Hypernatremia results from the loss of free water or gain of sodium ions in excess of water. The net result is an increase in the concentration of sodium in the blood. Most patients with hypernatremia have impaired thirst or inaccessibility to water. Thirst usually results in increased water intake in awake patients. Hyperosmolality always exists with hypernatremia. Because sodium is an impermeant soluble, hypernatremia

produces cellular dehydration. However, hypernatremia can exist with hypovolemia, euvolemia, or hypervolemia.[29,30] Approximately half the cases of hypernatremia are present on admission to the hospital, and the other half develop after admission. Severe hypernatremia is associated with high mortality (30% to 90%).

Hypernatremic hypovolemia (Fig. 29-2) results from renal water losses (e.g., impaired response to ADH, diabetes insipidus, osmotic diuretics, adrenal failure) or nonrenal water losses (e.g., diarrhea, severe sweating from fever or thyrotoxicosis). Hypernatremia occurring in patients with volume overload (e.g., edematous states) usually results from iatrogenic sodium administration or states of mineralocorticoid excess. Hypernatremia in relative euvolemia usually results from excess skin water losses (e.g., fever), diarrhea, or impaired secretion or response to ADH (e.g., diabetes insipidus).

DIABETES INSIPIDUS. Diabetes insipidus may be central or nephrogenic.[10,31,32] Central diabetes insipidus can be idiopathic or follow head trauma, neurosurgical procedures, brain tumors, CNS granulomatous disease, intracranial aneurysms, or meningitis and encephalitis. Nephrogenic diabetes insipidus frequently develops in patients with sickle cell nephropathy, chronic pyelonephritis, multiple myeloma, hypercalcemia, hypokalemia, or disorders requiring lithium, demeclocycline, amphotericin B, and methoxyflurane.

Most patients with central diabetes insipidus can maintain normal intravascular volume by increasing their intake of water. Intravascular volume depletion only occurs if oral intake is impaired because of obtundation, anesthesia, or other forms of critical illness. Diabetes insipidus is diagnosed by monitoring blood pressure, heart rate, and serum sodium during a period of water deprivation. Patients with diabetes insipidus develop signs of intravascular volume depletion or hypernatremia while continuing to excrete dilute urine.

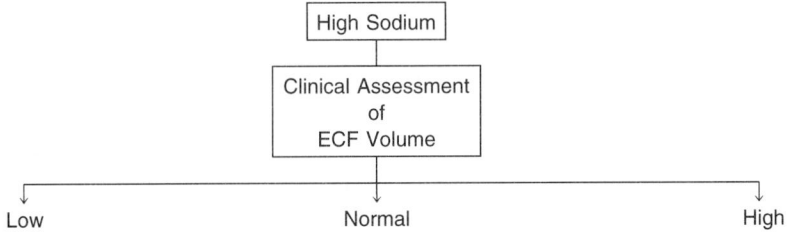

FIGURE 29-2. Evaluation of hypernatremia. ECF, extracellular fluid; UNa, urinary sodium; GI, gastrointestinal; UOsm, urinary osmolality; CAH, congenital adrenal hyperplasia.

Central and nephrogenic diabetes insipidus are differentiated by the effect of ADH on urine osmolality after a period of dehydration.

CNS Dysfunction

Hypernatremia primarily affects CNS function by causing cellular dehydration.[33] Because the CNS can compensate for slow or chronic changes in sodium level, acute changes should be treated acutely and chronic changes should be treated slowly. Clinical features of hypernatremia include impaired mentation, weakness, lethargy, obtundation, coma, and seizures (Table 29-5). Severe brain dehydration puts mechanical traction on cerebral blood vessels and may cause bleeding. Other clinical features reflect the underlying causes of hypernatremia and intravascular volume status. Severe water loss may cause dehydration, oliguria, hypotension, and shock. Salt overload may results in peripheral and pulmonary edema. Patients with diabetes insipidus usually have polydipsia and polyuria. Polyuria may also result from renal water losses (e.g., osmotic diuretics) and salt overload states.

Treatment

Hypernatremia indicates intracellular volume depletion and a relative or absolute need for water. Treatment (Table 29-6) consists of water replacement and addressing underlying medical conditions, associated electrolyte abnormalities, and intravascular volume status. If the patient is hypovolemic, intravascular volume should be replaced with isotonic saline, colloid, or blood. After intravascular volume is restored,

TABLE 29-5. Clinical Features of Hypernatremia

NEUROLOGIC FEATURES

    Thirst
    Weakness
    Lethargy, obtundation, coma
    Irritability
    Seizures
    Respiratory failure
    Focal deficits
    Cerebral hemorrhage
    Cerebral dehydration

CARDIOVASCULAR FEATURES

    Dehydration
    Volume depletion
    Tachycardia
    Hypotension
    Syncope
    Shock
    Edema

RENAL FEATURES

    Polyuria
    Oliguria
    Renal insufficiency

TABLE 29-6. Treatment of Hypernatremia

GENERAL MEASURES

    Treat underlying cause
    Remove offending drugs
    Correct electrolyte abnormalities

SODIUM OVERLOAD STATES

    Remove sodium with loop diuretic or dialysis
    Replace volume with hypotonic fluids

SODIUM-DEPLETED STATES

    Replenish intravascular volume with isotonic saline or colloid
    Give hypotonic fluids if intravascular volume replete

EUVOLEMIC STATES

    Give hypotonic fluids
    Treat diabetes insipidus

water is replaced using hypotonic intravenous fluids (i.e., 5% dextrose in water) or enteral water.

In patients with sodium overload, sodium can be removed from the body with diuretics or dialysis and volume replaced with hypotonic fluids. Hypernatremia resulting from a glucose-induced osmotic diuresis can be treated with insulin after repletion of intravascular volume.[34] The rate of correction depends on how quickly it developed. Acute hypernatremia can be corrected fairly rapidly, but chronic hypernatremia should be corrected slowly to avoid neurologic sequelae such as seizures and cerebral edema. We recommend that chronic hypernatremia be corrected no faster than 1 to 2 mMol/L/hour. The water deficit usually is replaced over 24 to 48 hours.

DIABETES INSIPIDUS.   Management of diabetes insipidus depends on the cause.[10,31,32] Central diabetes insipidus can be treated with hormonal replacement. ADH is available in a variety of forms (Table 29-7). Central diabetes insipidus is usually treated with 1-desamino-8-D-arginine vasopressin (desmopressin acetate or DDAVP), given by nasal, subcutaneous, or intravenous routes. The duration of action of DDAVP is 12 to 24 hours. It is best to wait for the drug effect to diminish (i.e., onset of polyuria) before giving the next dose to avoid fluid overload.

Patients with partial diabetes insipidus may be treated with pharmacologic agents that stimulate ADH secretion (e.g., chlorpropamide, clofibrate). Those with nephrogenic diabetes insipidus are difficult to treat. Occasionally, they respond to DDAVP if resistance is not complete. Frequently, management involves limited salt and water intake and use of diuretics (e.g., thiazides). This therapy causes volume depletion, enhances proximal tubule fluid reabsorption, and diminishes urine output.

POTASSIUM

Potassium is the major cation in the ICF. Normal extracellular potassium concentration is 3.5 to 5.0 mMol, and normal

TABLE 29-7.   Treatment of Diabetes Insipidus

CENTRAL DIABETES INSIPIDUS

    Antidiuretic hormone
        Desmopressin (DDAVP): 10–20 μg every 12–24 h nasally;
            2–4 μg IV or SC every 12–24 h
        Aqueous arginine vasopressin: 5–10 U IV, IM, or SQ every
            2–8 h
        Vasopressin tannate in oil: 2–5 U IM every 24–96 h
        Lysine vasopressin: 1–2 sprays nasally every 3–6 h
    Potentiate antidiuretic hormone action
        Chlorpropamide: 250–750 mg daily, orally (danger of
            hypoglycemia)
        Carbamazepine: 400–800 mg daily, orally
        Clofibrate: 500 mg every 6 h, orally

NEPHROGENIC DIABETES INSIPIDUS

    Restrict salt and water
    Thiazide diuretics: 50–100 mg daily, orally

IV, intravenously; SC, subcutaneously; IM, intramuscularly.

intracellular potassium concentration averages 150 to 160 mMol. Total-body potassium in an average 70-kg adult is approximately 3500 mEq (50 mMol/kg), only 70 mMol of which are in the ECF (and only 10 mMol in the plasma volume). Thus, 98% of body potassium is intracellular. Potassium circulates in plasma as free ions. Blood potassium levels are a poor reflection of total-body potassium in most critically ill patients. However, in patients with chronic hypokalemia, a decrement of 1 mMol/L in serum potassium concentration corresponds to a loss of approximately 200 to 300 mMol in body potassium stores.

Functions

Potassium is important for the generation of transmembrane potentials. Potassium currents maintain the resting membrane potential, prolong the plateau of the action potential, initiate repolarization, and bring about diastolic depolarization. The electrical gradient between the ICF and ECF is maintained by the sodium-potassium (Na-K) ATPase pump, which moves potassium into the cell and sodium out. The potential difference (Em) across the membrane is described by the Nernst equation: $Em = -61.5 \log K_i/K_o$, where K_i represents intracellular potassium and K_o represents extracellular potassium. Changes of 1 to 2 mMol/L in K_o have larger effects on the potential difference than similar alterations in K_i. Thus, the extracellular potassium has the greatest influence on the electrical stability of the heart. When the extracellular potassium falls, the cell membrane becomes hyperpolarized (more negative). The force of muscle contraction and nerve conduction depend on the potential difference. Alterations in K_i/K_o affect muscle and nervous system activity and may result in cardiac arrhythmias.

Potassium plays a role as a cofactor in enzymatic reactions, including those affecting nucleic acid synthesis, protein synthesis, and growth. It contributes most of the intracellular solute and thus is important in maintaining normal cell volume. Intracellular potassium ion concentrations affect intra-

cellular hydrogen ion concentrations and participate in the regulation of intracellular pH.

Regulation

Potassium is regulated by a complex system of interactions involving the kidneys and endocrine glands.[35] These systems maintain the circulating potassium level within a narrow range despite large fluctuations in intake. Short-term control of potassium is mediated by changes in renal excretion by shifting potassium into and out of the ECF compartment. Aldosterone, insulin, and epinephrine (through β2-adrenergic receptors) are important regulators responsible for potassium distribution.[35,36] Long-term control is primarily accomplished by the rate of renal excretion. Renal excretion is influenced by intrinsic renal mechanisms within the kidney and aldosterone action.[36] Renal excretion of potassium can range from a low of 3 to 10 mMol/day to more than 300 mMol/day. The rate of intake of potassium and gastrointestinal absorption is not regulated. Normally, 85% to 90% of ingested potassium is absorbed. A small amount (10% to 15%) is excreted in the feces.

RENAL CONTROL.   Potassium is freely filtered across the glomeruli, and 70% is reabsorbed by the proximal tubules. It enters the renal tubules in the descending limb of the loops of Henle, increasing the amount at the top of the loops compared with the amount filtered. Reabsorption of potassium takes place in the ascending limbs of Henle's loop, reducing the quantity in the tubular fluid to less than 5% to 10% of the amount filtered. For practical purposes, almost all filtered potassium is reabsorbed during passage through the nephron. Thus, renal excretion is independent of the GFR and amount of potassium filtered. Actual regulation takes place in the distal tubules and collecting ducts, where potassium ions are secreted into the tubular lumen (controlled by the Na-K pump). Activity of the Na^+-K^+ pump and renal potassium excretion are stimulated by aldosterone and potassium. Potassium excretion is affected by the rate of tubular flow; the higher the flow rate, the greater the rate of potassium secretion.

Increased flow to the distal tubules decreases intraluminal potassium concentration. The net result is a gradient favoring potassium excretion. This effect has important consequences during changes in sodium balance when changes in ECF volume alter GFR and proximal tubular sodium and water reabsorption. For example, an increase in sodium intake leads to an increase in ECF volume. With volume expansion, GFR increases and proximal tubule reabsorption decreases. The net result is an increase in distal tubular flow and potassium wasting.

The secretion of tubular potassium is affected by the rate of hydrogen ion secretion. During acidosis, intracellular potassium concentrations fall while hydrogen ion concentrations rise. Hydrogen is secreted in place of potassium from renal tubular cells. The reverse occurs during alkalosis; potassium moves into cells and favors urinary potassium wasting. This mechanism explains why potassium deficiency contributes to metabolic alkalosis. A decrease in intracellular potassium concentration favors a shift of hydrogen from the

ECF to the ICF. Increased amounts of nonabsorbable anions (e.g., bicarbonate, sulfate, phosphate) in the lumen of the distal tubule also favor potassium loss in the urine.

Aldosterone alters renal potassium excretion and the distribution of potassium between the ICF and ECF. Secretion of aldosterone is regulated by plasma concentrations of potassium and angiotensin II, with minor effects from ACTH and sodium. Plasma potassium and angiotensin II interact multiplicatively in stimulating aldosterone secretion. If the concentration of either is low, aldosterone secretion is impaired. Aldosterone is involved in two interacting feedback regulatory systems: one controlling sodium balance and one regulating potassium balance. When distal nephron flow rate decreases because of negative sodium balance (e.g., volume depletion), renin–angiotensin–aldosterone secretion is stimulated. Aldosterone augments sodium reabsorption at the expense of potassium. The interaction between potassium and angiotensin II is capable of stimulating the appropriate level of aldosterone to maintain electrolyte balance over wide ranges of sodium and potassium intake. Only in pathologic situations in which sodium balance is severely disturbed is potassium balance affected by alterations in sodium balance.

TISSUES. The tissues primarily involved in ICF–ECF potassium shifts are the skeletal muscle and liver.[35–38] The distribution of potassium between these two compartments is a function of aldosterone concentration. β-Adrenergic agonists also shift potassium into cells and significantly affect potassium distribution during stress states.[35,36,39] The lack of effect of β-adrenergic blockers on circulating potassium during unstressed rest states suggests that β-adrenergic tone is not a major factor controlling potassium distribution under basal conditions. However, use of β-adrenergic agonists and β-blockers in critically ill patients may have significant effects on potassium distribution. This extrarenal β-adrenergic effect is mediated by the β_2-adrenergic receptor (primarily in skeletal muscle). In addition to aldosterone and β-adrenergic agonists, insulin also stimulates potassium movement into cells.

HYDROGEN ION. Extracellular pH affects potassium distribution; an increase in hydrogen ion concentration is associated with an outward movement of potassium.[35] As a general guide, for each acute rise of 0.1 pH units, a fall occurs in serum potassium of 0.8 mMol/L. For each acute fall in pH of 0.1 units, serum potassium rises 0.5 mMol/L. There is an important distinction between mineral acids (e.g., HCl) and organic acids (e.g., lactate, ketones). Organic acids have little effect on circulating potassium levels.[35] Presumably, they enter cells and are metabolized, resulting in little shift of potassium. Acid–base alterations modify renal potassium excretion. Acute respiratory and metabolic acidosis decrease renal potassium excretion whereas acute respiratory and metabolic alkalosis increase renal potassium excretion. Chronic acid–base changes have less effect on renal potassium excretion.

HYPOKALEMIA

Hypokalemia, a common electrolyte disturbance, is defined as a serum or blood potassium level less than 3.5 mMol/ L.[40,41] Because potassium is primarily an intracellular ion, hypokalemia may occur in patients with low, normal, or high total-body potassium. If hypokalemia has been chronic, a decrease in circulating potassium of 1 mMol/L corresponds to approximately a 200- to 300-mMol deficit in total-body potassium.

Causes

Causes of hypokalemia may be divided into those associated with renal potassium conservation and those associated with renal potassium wasting[30,40,41] (Fig. 29-3). A low urinary potassium in the face of hypokalemia suggests extrarenal losses. However, urinary potassium is elevated during diuretic use, and diuretics may have caused hypokalemia and body potassium depletion. After discontinuation of the diuretic, the kidney may appropriately conserve potassium. Sodium depletion may produce a low urinary potassium level, despite the fact that renal potassium loss caused hypokalemia.

LOSS OF POTASSIUM. Obligate loss of potassium from the body is 10 to 20 mMol/day, and hypokalemia may occur if potassium intake is severely limited or losses exceed normal intake. Because of the ubiquitous nature of potassium in the diet, dietary causes of hypokalemia are seen only in patients with extreme starvation. A more common cause of hypokalemia is loss of gastric contents (e.g., prolonged vomiting, gastric suction). Gastric juices contain approximately 10 to 15 mMol/L of potassium. Loss of hydrogen ions also cause metabolic alkalosis, with a resultant shift of potassium into cells and kaliuresis. Potassium deficits of 200 to 300 mMol are commonly encountered in patients receiving continuous gastric suction. Nonrenal potassium losses also occur with rapid gastrointestinal transit, intestinal drains, small intestinal bypass procedures, small bowel fistulae, and malabsorption diseases (e.g., diarrhea). Diarrhea fluid frequently contains 35 to 60 mMol/L of potassium.

The most common causes of hypokalemia are those resulting from renal losses of potassium (see Fig. 29-3). Diuretics are frequently associated with hypokalemia caused by increased renal tubular flow, aldosterone secretion (volume depletion), and alkalosis. Patients receiving diuretics who are at an increased risk for developing life-threatening hypokalemia are those with edema and a brisk diuretic response, high sodium intake, metabolic alkalosis, or simultaneously, receiving two diuretics that have actions in different portions of the nephron.

Mineralocorticoids (e.g., aldosterone) cause significant potassium wasting in the presence of sodium ions. Corticosteroids possess mineralocorticoid activity and frequently cause hypokalemia in patients who are sodium repleted. Renal tubular damage from nephrotoxins (e.g., aminoglycosides, amphotericin B, cyclosporine) may cause renal potassium wasting. Renal magnesium wasting impairs potassium reabsorption and can cause hypokalemia. Large doses of penicillin (poorly reabsorbed anion) produce hypokalemia as a result of renal potassium wasting. Carbonic anhydrase inhibitors promote distal tubular potassium secretion by increasing delivery of sodium and bicarbonate (nonreabsorbable anion). Diabetic ketoacidosis is associated with potassium depletion as a result of an osmotic diuresis and

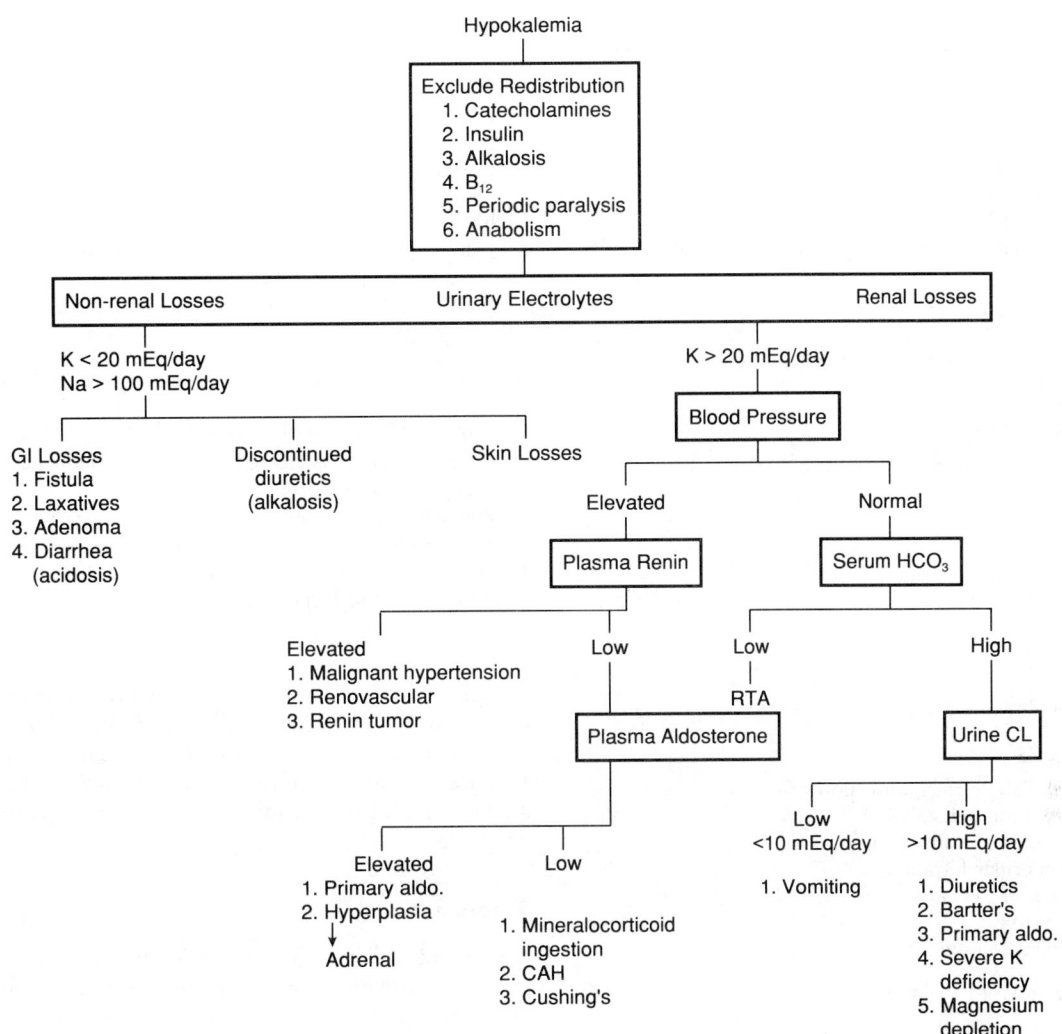

FIGURE 29-3. Evaluation of hypokalemia. K, potassium; Na, sodium; B₁₂, vitamin B₁₂; GI, gastrointestinal; HCO₃, bicarbonate; aldo, aldosteronism; RTA, renal tubular acidosis; CL, clearance; CAH, congenital adrenal hyperplasia.

increased excretion of nonreabsorbable ketoacid anions. Hypokalemia in these patients is frequently masked by a shift of potassium out of cells because of insulin deficiency.

POTASSIUM SHIFTS. Hypokalemia may be precipitated by a shift of potassium from the ECF to the ICF (see Fig. 29-3). Shift stimuli include acute alkalosis, insulin, β-adrenergic agonists, mineralocorticoids, barium poisoning, and vitamin B₁₂. Acute shifts are also seen in patients with hypokalemic periodic paralysis.

Clinical Effects

The clinical features of hypokalemia (Table 29-8) primarily result from increased cellular irritability and muscular weakness. Signs and symptoms are more common with acute alterations in potassium levels than with chronic alterations. If chronic, intracellular and extracellular potassium concentrations fall, diminishing their effects on the membrane potential. Hypokalemia causes skeletal muscle weakness, and it can result in paralysis if severe. Maintenance of potassium levels is important in weaning patients from mechanical ventilation. Severe potassium deficiency may cause rhabdomyolysis.

TABLE 29-8.   Clinical Features of Hypokalemia

CARDIOVASCULAR FEATURES

Arrhythmias
Tachycardias
Delayed conduction
Impaired contraction
Potentiation of digitalis effects
ECG: U wave, flat T wave, ST depression, wide QRS complex, AV block

VASCULAR FEATURES

Impaired pressor responses to catecholamines, angiotensin
Postural hypotension

MUSCULAR FEATURES

Weakness, paralysis, respiratory failure
Myalgias
Cramps
Rhabdomyolysis

NEUROLOGIC FEATURES

Hyporeflexia
Confusion
Depression
Impaired mentation

RENAL FEATURES

Nephrogenic diabetes insipidus (polyuria)
Decreased ureteral peristalsis
Increased ammonia production
Reduced glomerular filtration
Renal damage
Phosphate wasting
Urinary acidification defects

GASTROINTESTINAL FEATURES

Decreased bowel motility, ileus, constipation
Nausea, vomiting, anorexia

METABOLIC FEATURES

Decreased protein synthesis
Negative nitrogen balance
Growth retardation
Glucose intolerance
Metabolic alkalosis
Reduced carbohydrate synthesis

ECG, electrocardiogram; AV, atrioventricular.

TABLE 29-9.   Treatment of Hypokalemia

GENERAL MEASURES

Evaluate and treat underlying disease
Discontinue offending drugs
Correct alkalosis, hypomagnesemia

CORRECT HYPOKALEMIA

If K <2 mMol or ECG abnormalities or muscle weakness/paralysis, give up to 40 mMol/h IV or KCl (in saline)
If K >2 mMol/L and no ECG abnormalities, give up to 10 mMol/h IV KCl

MONITOR SERUM OR BLOOD K, SERUM MAGNESIUM, ECG

REPLACE DEFICITS AND CORRECT EXCESSES

After deficits are corrected, place on maintenance K to cover ongoing losses
For hyperaldosterone states, give spironolactone

IV, intravenously; KCl, potassium chloride; ECG, electrocardiogram; K, potassium.

ectopic arrhythmias, delayed conduction, ventricular tachycardia, and ventricular fibrillation. Other clinical features of hypokalemia include hypodynamic ileus, gastroparesis, impaired pressor responses to catecholamines, digitalis sensitivity, diminished insulin action, and impaired protein synthesis.

Treatment

Treatment of hypokalemia (Table 29-9) involves correction of the underlying abnormality (e.g., offending drugs, diarrhea) and potassium replacement.[40,41] Serum sodium, potassium, magnesium, phosphorus, and calcium should be measured and treated appropriately. Hypokalemia is frequently accompanied by other electrolyte disorders. Blood pH should be measured and acid–base disorders corrected. Patients should be monitored for cardiac arrhythmias.

REPLACEMENT.   Repair of potassium deficits must be undertaken with caution to avoid cardiac arrhythmias and hyperkalemia. Because potassium is primarily an intracellular ion, judging the amount required to replace body stores is difficult. Replacing potassium by the oral or enteral route is safer. The intravenous route is necessary for rapid correction of hypokalemia.

Enteral potassium can be administered in higher amounts than intravenous potassium and rarely causes significant cardiac toxicity (i.e., it has a safer therapeutic–toxicity ratio). For example, many critically ill patients require 160 to 200 mMol of potassium each day to replace ongoing losses; 160 mMol/L can be administered as 40 mMol every 6 hours orally or 6.7 mMol/hour intravenously.

When administered intravenously (see Table 29-7), potassium should not be given faster than 10 to 40 mMol/hour to avoid a dangerous hyperkalemia. To avoid pain, peripheral infusions should be limited to a potassium concentration of less than 60 mMol/L. Intravenous potassium should be administered into a large peripheral or central vein to dimin-

CARDIAC.   Cardiac complications are among the most dangerous side effects of potassium depletion. Hypokalemia hyperpolarizes the resting membrane potential, increases the duration of the action potential, and increases the refractory period.[41,42] Because refractory period prolongation is longer than action potential prolongation, reentrant arrhythmia production is enhanced. Reentry is also encouraged by the delay in conduction velocity and stimulation of automaticity. The increased rate of diastolic depolarization is such that, despite hyperpolarization of the resting membrane potential, the threshold is reached sooner. By this mechanism, ectopic beats may be initiated and arrhythmias induced. Acute hypokalemia may lead to premature ventricular beats,

ish the risk of causing sclerosis. If infusing through a central vein, be sure the catheter is not in the atrium or ventricle to avoid localized hyperkalemia. Potassium is best administered in nonglucose solutions because glucose stimulates insulin secretion and shifts potassium intracellularly.

Potassium is usually replaced using the chloride salt. Patients with concomitant phosphorus deficiency can receive some of their potassium repletion using potassium phosphate. Frequently, potassium needs exceed phosphorus needs, and the physician must be careful not to overload the patient with phosphorus by giving all of the potassium replacement as the phosphate salt. Because magnesium depletion can result in renal potassium wasting, replacement of magnesium deficits is important. Magnesium is also required for cellular potassium entry. A magnesium-deficient patient may normalize the serum potassium but may remain intracellularly potassium deficient until magnesium deficits are replaced. Hyperkalemia is more likely to occur in patients with acidemia, diabetes mellitus, renal tubular acidosis, or those receiving nonsteroidal antiinflammatory agents, angiotensin converting enzyme inhibitors, β-adrenergic blockers, or potassium-sparing diuretics.

The hypokalemia of hyperaldosterone states can be minimized by reducing sodium intake. Spironolactone also may be used to antagonize mineralocorticoid action (i.e., diminished potassium loss) in patients with hyperaldosteronism. Potassium-sparing diuretics may be useful for the management of patients requiring chronic diuretic therapy (e.g., heart failure). Use caution in giving potassium supplements or potassium-sparing diuretics to patients with diabetes mellitus or renal insufficiency, who have a limited ability to compensate for acute potassium elevations. Potassium supplementation should precede correction of acidosis in hypokalemic patients to avoid precipitous decreases in the plasma potassium concentration.

HYPERKALEMIA

Hyperkalemia is defined as a blood potassium level greater than 5.0 mMol/L and may occur with low normal, or elevated total-body potassium stores.[43,44] Pseudohyperkalemia results if potassium is released from cells in the test tube at the time of blood drawing or clotting. This type of hyperkalemia is factitious and requires no treatment. Potassium may be elevated in patients resulting from ex vivo hemolysis or lysis of leukocytes (usually >200,000/mL) or platelets (usually >750,000/mL). These disorders can be diagnosed by comparing a serum potassium (clotted blood) to a plasma or blood potassium (nonclotted blood).

Causes

RENAL DYSFUNCTION. Because the kidneys are the primary organs responsible for potassium excretion (90%), hyperkalemia usually results from renal insufficiency (Fig. 29-4). Hypertrophy of the renal tubule compensates for loss of renal tissue during chronic renal disease. Patients with chronic renal failure can frequently maintain circulating potassium within normal limits until the GFR decreases below 10 mL/minute, provided dietary potassium intake is normal. However, increased potassium intake or tissue release may

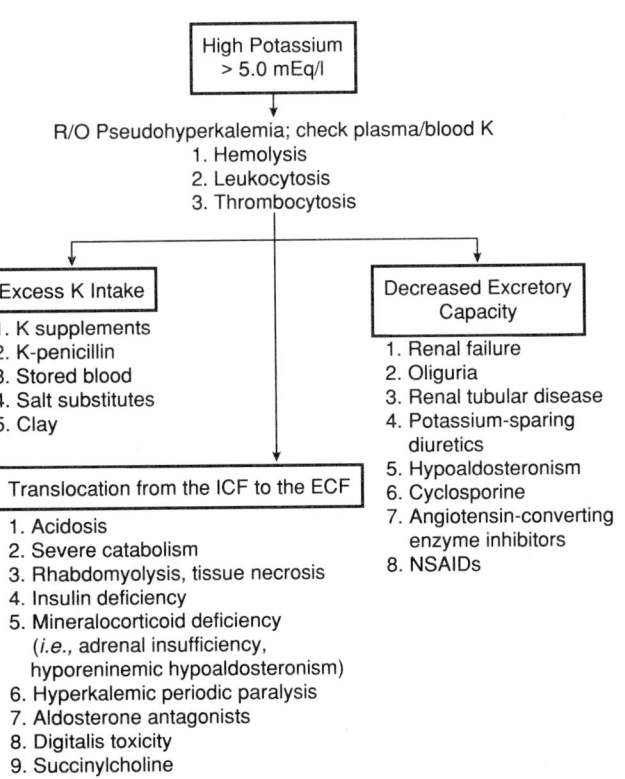

FIGURE 29-4. Evaluation of hyperkalemia. ICF, intracellular fluid; ECF, extracellular fluid; NSAIDs, nonsteroidal antiinflammatory agents.

result in hyperkalemia in patients with higher GFRs. Impaired renal tubular function (e.g., interstitial nephritis) may lead to hyperkalemia despite preserved glomerular filtration. Renal transplant patients are susceptible to hyperkalemia as a result of rejection, hyporeninemic hypoaldosteronism, and use of cyclosporine.

FLUID SHIFTS, HORMONES AND DRUGS. The sudden shift of potassium from the ICF to the ECF may cause hyperkalemia (see Fig. 29-4). Common causes include acidosis, increased catabolism, tissue necrosis, and rhabdomyolysis. Other causes of hyperkalemia include insulin deficiency, discontinuation of catecholamine infusions, cardiac glycoside overdose, succinylcholine, aldosterone deficiency (e.g., adrenal failure, hyporeninemic hypoaldosteronism), and use of aldosterone antagonists (e.g., spironolactone). Hyporeninemic hypoaldosteronism is frequently seen in patients with advanced renal disease. It is also seen in the elderly and in patients with diabetes mellitus, interstitial nephritis, and only mild renal insufficiency. Drug-induced causes of the syndrome include nonsteroidal antiinflammatory drugs, ACE inhibitors, and cyclosporine. Hyperkalemia frequently corrects with fluorocortisone treatment. Adrenal insufficiency may be the result of tumors or infections and can produce hyperkalemia, which is frequently associated with hyponatremia. Succinylcholine inhibits cell membrane repolarization and can precipitate lethal hyperkalemia in patients with trauma, burns, or CNS damage.

SODIUM REABSORPTION.   The potential difference across cells in the distal nephron is important for potassium excretion. Agents like amiloride or triamterene that block sodium reabsorption distally leave the tubule lumen less negative and reduce potassium secretion. Negativity (e.g., bicarbonate or chloride) of the tubule lumen increases potassium secretion. When sodium chloride and bicarbonate are avidly reabsorbed in the proximal nephron (e.g., volume depletion), little reaches the distal nephron, and less potassium can be secreted. Acidosis impairs potassium conductance in the distal nephron and depresses potassium excretion. Acidosis also shifts potassium from the intracellular to the ECF. Hyperosmolality produces cellular contraction, increased cellular potassium levels, and potassium efflux from the cells. This effect may be seen in severely hyperglycemic patients (e.g., diabetes mellitus) and patients receiving mannitol.

During treatment of potassium depletion, intracellular potassium is replaced. Much of the administered potassium is deposited intracellularly. However, if cell stores are repleted, continued replacement may cause hyperkalemia.

Clinical Effects

The electrical excitability of neuromuscular cells depends on the difference between resting membrane potential (E_m) and threshold potential. E_m is determined by the ratio of intracellular to extracellular potassium ($E_m = -61.5 \log K_i/K_o$). High extracellular potassium depolarizes the cell membrane and reduces conduction velocity. Eventually transmission of electrical impulses is inhibited. Unidirectional block in the myocardium can give rise to reentry ventricular tachycardia and fibrillation. Clinically, depolarization block and muscle paralysis may occur. With chronic hyperkalemia, intracellular and extracellular potassium increase, and there is less effect on E_m.

Clinical features of hyperkalemia (Table 29-10) involve primarily the cardiovascular and neuromuscular systems. Symptoms are rare if serum potassium is less than 6 mMol/L. Arrhythmias, conduction abnormalities, cardiac arrest, and

electrocardiographic (ECG) changes, such as peaked T waves, PR prolongation, diminished P wave amplitude, atrial asystole, or widening of the QRS complex, may occur. The effects of hyperkalemia are enhanced by hyponatremia, hypocalcemia, hypermagnesemia, and acidosis. Wide variability exists in the degree of hyperkalemia that results in cardiac toxicity. Because fatal cardiotoxicity is unpredictable, the presence of any ECG changes of hyperkalemia mandates immediate treatment. Neuromuscular manifestations of hyperkalemia include paresthesia, weakness, and paralysis.

Potassium is lost from cells after ischemia. The increase in extracellular potassium concentration may exceed 10 mMol/L within a few minutes of ischemia and accounts for most of the changes in the action potential and electrocardiograph after coronary ischemia. The cellular loss of potassium is believed to result from diminished energy stores. Differences in potassium concentration between ischemic and nonischemic muscle causes different levels of cellular depolarization and sets up currents that may result in arrhythmias.

Treatment

Treatment of hyperkalemia (Table 29-11) is aimed at reversing the membrane effects, removing the cause for the increased potassium load, and removing potassium from the body. The membrane effects can be reversed by depressing the membrane threshold potential with calcium and by translocating potassium from the ECF to the ICF. The effects of calcium are immediate but transient and buy time for more definitive treatments. Potassium can be translocated intracellularly by administering bicarbonate or insulin (and glucose). Inhaled β_2-adrenergic agonists also decrease blood potassium levels (0.5 to 1.0 mMol/L). The onset of action for these methods is 15 to 30 minutes. Potassium can be removed from the body by volume expansion and diuresis (e.g., furosemide), dialysis, or use of gastrointestinal resins that bind potassium, such as sodium polystyrene sulfonate. Mineralocorticoid deficiency can be treated with fluorocortisone (0.025 to 0.1 mg/day).

CALCIUM

Functions

Calcium is the major divalent cation in the ECF. It is an important regulator of cellular function and essential for numerous cellular processes. Calcium is required for excitation–contraction coupling (i.e., muscle contraction), neurotransmission, hormonal secretion, enzyme activation, blood clotting, cell division, cell motility, and wound healing. In general, processes that require movement involve calcium. It contributes to the plateau phase of the cardiac action potential and is responsible for spontaneous depolarization in pacemaker cells. Calcium is an important second and third messenger, linking cellular membrane activation to intracellular events. It is also an important structural component of cellular membranes and bone.

Regulation

The recommended daily oral calcium intake is 1200 mg. Thirty percent to 35% of dietary calcium is normally ab-

---

TABLE 29-10.   Clinical Features of Hyperkalemia

CARDIOVASCULAR FEATURES

   Arrhythmias
   Heart block
   Delayed conduction
   Ventricular standstill
   ECG: peaked T waves, decreased P waves, prolonged PR
      interval, wide QRS complex, sine wave

NEUROMUSCULAR FEATURES

   Paresthesias
   Weakness, respiratory insufficiency
   Flaccid paralysis
   Mental confusion

ECG, electrocardiogram.

TABLE 29-11. Treatment of Hyperkalemia

GENERAL MEASURES

   Treat underlying disease
   Restrict exogenous potassium
   Remove offending drugs

MILD HYPERKALEMIA (K <6 mMol/L)

   Restrict K, liberalize Na and water intake

SEVERE HYPERKALEMIA (K >7 mMol/L; CARDIAC MANIFESTATIONS)

   Reverse membrane effects
      Calcium: 5 mMol IV over 5 min
      Hypertonic saline
   Transfer K into cells
      Glucose and insulin: 250–500 mL/h $D_{10}W$ + 10–20 U regular insulin per 100 g glucose; monitor blood glucose and K
      Sodium bicarbonate: 50–100 mMol over 5–10 min (may cause ionized hypocalcemia)
      Inhaled or infused β_2-agonists
   Remove K from body
      Potassium-binding resins; sodium polystyrene sulfonate (Kayexalate [sodium polystyrene sulfonate]), 20–30 g orally in 50 mL 70% sorbitol every 4 h or 50–100 g in 200 mL water by retention enema every 4 h (danger of sodium overload)
      Loop diuretics (e.g., furosemide)
      Dialysis

MONITOR K, ECG

K, potassium; Na, sodium; IV, intravenously; ECG, electrocardiogram; $D_{10}W$, 10% dextrose in water.

sorbed in the small intestine by vitamin D–dependent and –independent processes. Calcium exits the body in the urine (approximately 150 mg/day) and stool (150 to 200 mg/day). The average healthy adult body contains 1000 to 1400 g of calcium, of which 99% is in the skeleton and 1% is in the soft tissues and extracellular space. Calcium circulates in the blood in three major forms: a protein-bound form, a chelated form, and an ionized form (Ca^{2+}).

The ionized form of calcium is physiologically active and homeostatically regulated.[45–48] Most clinical laboratories measure the total serum concentration of calcium (8.5 to 10.5 mg/dL, or 2.10 to 2.60 mMol/L). Although total serum calcium reliably indicates circulating calcium status in healthy individuals, it is an unreliable indicator of calcium status in sick patients.

Total serum calcium concentrations are a poor predictor of ionized calcium status in critically ill patients.[45–47,49,50] Because calcium binds to albumin and binding is influenced by changes in acid–base status (i.e., decreased by acidosis; increased by alkalosis), many clinicians have attempted to correct total calcium levels for alterations in albumin and pH levels. Unfortunately, these corrections are inaccurate for predicting the true Ca^{2+} level.[49,50] The only valid measure of physiologically active circulating calcium in critically ill patients is a directly measured Ca^{2+} concentration. Many multichannel analyzers are capable of measuring blood gases, Ca^{2+}, potassium, and sodium in whole blood.[51]

CHELATING AGENTS. Changes in circulating levels of chelating agents (e.g., citrate, phosphate, albumin) alter total and ionized calcium levels.[45–48] Total calcium levels remain unchanged or increase with chelators, but ionized calcium values may remain unchanged or decrease. Citrate is used as a blood preservative and anticoagulant. Citrate-induced decreases in Ca^{2+} are usually small and transient in normothermic patients with normal renal and hepatic function.[45–48,52–54] However, ionized hypocalcemia may develop in patients if blood transfusion is rapid, citrate clearance is impaired (e.g., hypothermia, renal or hepatic insufficiency), or there is insufficient parathyroid hormone and vitamin D. Albumin, like citrate, may also chelate calcium and can contribute to ionized hypocalcemia.

PARATHYROID HORMONE. The circulating Ca^{2+} level is regulated primarily by the combined actions of parathyroid hormone and vitamin D on bone.[45–48] Dietary calcium is not essential for the maintenance of a normal ionized calcium level if bone calcium is available. Parathyroid hormone secretion is stimulated by ionized hypocalcemia and mild hypomagnesemia. It is suppressed by ionized hypercalcemia, severe hypomagnesemia, and hypermagnesemia. Parathyroid hormone increases bone resorption, renal tubular calcium reabsorption, and intestinal calcium absorption (by vitamin D).

VITAMIN D. Vitamin D is a fat-soluble vitamin and enters the body by the diet or is synthesized in the skin under the influence of ultraviolet light. Intestinal absorption depends on biliary secretion, pancreatic secretion, and intact fat absorption. Either source of vitamin D can provide adequate vitamin D for metabolic needs. However, if both are inadequate, vitamin D deficiency and hypocalcemia may develop.

Vitamin D undergoes hydroxylation at the 25 position in the liver and at the 1 position in the kidneys to form 1,25-dihydroxyvitamin D (1,25(OH)$_2$D) or calcitriol. Calcitriol is the active form of the vitamin. Renal hydroxylation of 25-hydroxyvitamin D is stimulated by parathyroid hormone and hypophosphatemia. It is suppressed by hyperphosphatemia, acidosis, and elevated calcitriol levels. Calcitriol stimulates bone calcium resorption, renal tubular calcium reabsorption, and intestinal calcium absorption. Renal and hepatic disease may cause hypocalcemia by interfering with the synthesis of calcitriol.

HYPOCALCEMIA

Causes

Hypocalcemia is reflected by ionized calcium levels less than 1.0 mMol/L or total serum Ca less than 8.5 mg/dL (Table 29-12). A common cause, parathyroid insufficiency, is seen most frequently in an acquired form after neck surgery. It may also occur after trauma to the neck and from tumor, sarcoid, and amyloid infiltration. Parathyroid suppression also results from hypomagnesemia and hypermagnesemia, burns, sepsis, and pancreatitis.

Vitamin D–related hypocalcemia is associated with impaired vitamin D activation, as in renal failure, and vitamin D deficiency when this vitamin is not added to intravenous parenteral nutrition solutions. Rhabdomyolysis causes hypocalcemia by inhibiting renal synthesis of 1,25(OH)$_2$D and by causing calcium precipitation in the injured muscle. Finally, many drugs can induce hypocalcemia (Table 29-13).

Clinical Effects

Clinical features of hypocalcemia include weakness, fatigue, and neuromuscular irritability that ranges from muscle spasms to seizures. Chvostek's sign is demonstrated by tapping over the facial nerve where it passes through the parotid gland; ipsilateral contraction of the facial muscles suggests hypocalcemia-induced irritability. Trousseau's sign is evoked when a blood pressure cuff on the upper arm is inflated to a level somewhat above systolic pressure and held there for 3 minutes; myotonic carpal spasm of the wrist muscles is seen. Cardiovascular abnormalities are arrhythmias, digitalis insensitivity, prolongation of the QT and ST segments of the electrocardiogram, and terminal T-wave inversion.

Treatment

Management of severe and symptomatic hypocalcemia includes calcium gluconate, 10 mL of a 10% solution injected intravenously over 10 minutes; or calcium chloride, 10 mL of a 10% solution in 500 mL of D$_5$W, infused over 30 minutes. If symptoms persist, supplemental calcium may be infused at a rate of 1 to 2 mg/kg body weight/hour. When hyperphosphatemia or potassium deficits exist, they also must be corrected (see Table 29-12).

TABLE 29-12. Diagnosis and Treatment of Hypocalcemia

Diagnosis:	Ca^{2+} <1.0 mMol/L (4.0 mg/dL), or serum Ca <2.2 mMol/L (8.5 mg/dL) and albumin levels

Causes:	Parathormone-related
	    Parathyroid insufficiency
	    Parathyroid suppression

	Vitamin D–related
	    Impaired vitamin D activation
	    Increased loss of vitamin D

	Miscellaneous
	    Hyperphosphatemia
	    Drugs
	    Hypoalbuminemia
	    Fat embolism

Management:	Severe, symptomatic
	    Calcium gluconate (10 mL 10% solution over 10 min), or calcium chloride (10 mL 10% solution in 50 mL D$_5$W over 30 min)
	    If symptoms persist: 1–2 mg/kg/h of elemental calcium
	    Correct magnesium and potassium deficits, if present
	    Treat hyperphosphatemia, if present
	    Monitor symptoms and serum total or ionized calcium levels

	Asymptomatic
	    Calcium gluconate or calcium lactate (2–4 g/d, divided doses every 6 h)
	    If needed, add a vitamin D preparation[16]

Complications:	Work-up cause
	Inadequate therapy
	    Seizures
	    Laryngospasm/respiratory arrest
	    Congestive heart failure
	    Arrhythmias

	Excessive therapy
	    Hypercalcemia
	    If hyperphosphatemia present, soft tissue calcification when calcium–phosphate product >40–60

Ca^{2+}, ionized calcium; Ca, calcium; D$_5$W, 5% dextrose in water.

HYPERCALCEMIA

Causes and Clinical Effects

Hypercalcemia is defined by ionized calcium more than 1.3 mMol/L or total serum calcium more than 10.5 mg/dL (Table 29-14). Causes are listed in Table 29-15. Several drugs also significantly increase calcium levels (Table 29-16).

Cardiovascular effects include an increase in peripheral vascular resistance, hypertension, and potentiation of the cardiac effects of digoxin. Electrocardiographic changes include prolongation of the PR interval, widening of the QRS interval, shortening of the ST segment, and a slight flattening

TABLE 29-13. Drugs Associated With Hypocalcemia

AGENT	MECHANISM
Heparin	Pseudohypocalcemia
Phosphate	↑ Phosphate load
Magnesium sulfate	↓ Parathormone secretion/action
Colchicine	
Furosemide	
Calcitonin	
Mithramycin	
Propylthiouracil	
Cimetidine	
Phenytoin	↓ Active vitamin D production/
Phenobarbital	action
Aspirin	
Estrogens	
Glutethimide	
Gentamicin	Hypomagnesemia
Tobramycin	
Capreomycin	
Neomycin	
Carbenicillin	
Cisplatin	
Amphotericin B	
Polymyxin B	
Digitalis	
Diuretics	
Purgatives/laxatives	
Citrate	Chelating agents
EDTA	

EDTA, ethylene diamino tetraacetic acid.
Nanji AA: Drug-induced electrolyte disorders. *Drug Intell Clin Pharmacol* 1983;17:175.

of T waves. Biphasic T waves and QRS voltage increase also are reported.

Treatment

Hypercalcemic crisis involves intravascular volume depletion, renal insufficiency, and coma. Therapy includes intravenous infusion of normal saline, 2 to 3 L over 3 to 6 hours, and furosemide, 40 mg to 100 mg intravenously every 2 to 4 hours (see Table 29-14).

When this therapy is ineffective or contraindicated, administration of mithramycin, 25 μg/kg body weight intravenously every 3 to 4 days, or calcitonin, 4 MRC° units per kg body weight subcutaneously every 12 hours, may be initiated. The calcium-lowering effect with mithramycin is seen within 12 to 24 hours. Significant toxicity—including nephrotoxicity, thrombocytopenia, hepatocellular necrosis, nausea, vomiting, sodium retention, and hypokalemia—can occur with this agent.

° MRC, British Medical Council unit (4 μg pure porcine calcitonin).

TABLE 29-14. Diagnosis and Treatment of Hypercalcemia

Diagnosis:	Ca^{2+} >1.3 mMol/L (5.0 mg/dL)
	Serum Ca >5.4 mMol/L (10.5 mg/dL)
Management:	Emergency treatment
	Normal saline (2–3 L over 3–6 h)
	Furosemide (40–100 mg IV every 2–4 h)
	Mithramycin (25 μg/kg IV every 3–4 d)
	Calcitonin (4 MRC units/kg SC every 12 h)
	Steroids
	Hydrocortisone (3 mg/kg/d in divided doses
	every 6 h)
	Prednisone (40–80 mg/d)
	Hemodialysis or peritoneal dialysis
	Nonemergency treatment
	Adequate fluid intake
	Withdrawal of drugs causing hypercalcemia
	Restriction of oral calcium
	Mobilization, if possible
Complications:	Inadequate therapy
	Severe dehydration
	Renal failure
	Coma and death
	Excessive therapy
	Related to agents used (see text)
	Hypocalcemia

Ca^{2+}, ionized calcium; Ca, calcium; PTH, parathyroid hormone; IV, intravenously; SC, subcutaneously; MRC units, British Medical Council units.

Calcitonin usually results in a decrease in calcium 1 to 2 hours after initiation of therapy. Side effects are less serious with calcitonin than with mithramycin and include nausea, facial flushing, and diarrhea. In patients with renal failure or congestive heart failure, hemodialysis or peritoneal dialysis occasionally is used to decrease serum calcium rapidly.

PHOSPHORUS

Hypophosphatemia

The strict definition of hypophosphatemia includes a serum phosphate less than 3 mg/dL while the patient is in the fasting state (Table 29-17). When the serum phosphate level is less than 2 mg/dL, the urine should contain less than 100 mg of phosphate per day. Amounts in excess of this value suggests hyperparathyroidism or a primary renal dysfunction.

CAUSES

Five major categories of causes are intracellular anabolic shifts (recovery from malnutrition and burns), gram-negative bacteremia, alcoholism, alkalosis (respiratory and metabolic), and diabetic ketoacidosis or salicylate poisoning. Clinical manifestations include acute skeletal myopathy with profound weakness and occasionally respiratory muscle paralysis; cardiomyopathy; neurologic dysfunction; hematologic

TABLE 29-15. Causes of Hypercalcemia

MOST COMMON
    Malignancy
        PTH-like material
            Lung, hypernephroma, lymphoma, multiple myeloma
        Osteoclast activating factor
            Lymphoma, multiple myeloma
            Prostaglandins
            Solid tumors (lung, breast, kidney)
    Endocrine
        Parathyroid hormone
            Primary hyperparathyroidism

LESS COMMON
    Endocrine
        Hyperthyroidism
            Pheochromocytoma
            Adrenal insufficiency
            Acromegaly
    Drug use of intoxication
        Hypervitaminosis (A and D)
        Thiazide diuretics
        Lithium
        Hormonal treatment of cancer
        Milk–alkali syndrome
    Granulomatous diseases
        Berylliosis
        Coccidiodomycosis
        Histoplasmosis
        Sarcoid
        Tuberculosis
    Immobilization
        Especially with underlying bone disease or high bone
            turnover
    Miscellaneous
        Critically ill patients
        Paget's disease
        After renal transplant
        Recovery from acute renal failure
        Phosphate depletion syndrome
        Familial hypocalciuric hypercalcemia

PTH, parathyroid hormone.

TABLE 29-16. Drugs Associated With Hypercalcemia

AGENT	MECHANISM
Intravenous lipid emulsion	Pseudohypercalcemia (when fluorometric technique used to measure calcium)
Self-administered calcium and vitamin D	Factitious
Vitamins D and A	Increased bone reabsorption
Low-dose furosemide (oral)	Decreased urinary calcium excretion
Thiazides	Multifactorial
Chlorthalidone	
Lithium	
Tamoxifen	Unknown
Estrogens	
β-Adrenergic agents	Increased PTH release

PTH, parathyroid hormone.
Nanji AA: Drug-induced electrolyte disorders. *Drug Intell Clin Pharmacol* 1983;17:175.

Hyperphosphatemia

Hyperphosphatemia is defined by a fasting serum phosphate level of more than 4.5 mg/dL (Table 29-18). Common causes are decreased renal phosphate excretion, renal failure, hyperthyroidism, growth hormone excess, use of diphosphonates, and increased intracellular-to-extracellular phosphate shifts, which are seen in rhabdomyolysis, sepsis, severe hypothermia, malignant hyperthermia, sepsis, and tumor chemotherapy. Urinary excretion of phosphate is enhanced by saline infusion and acetazolamide, 500 mg every 6 hours. If hypocalcemia is present, it should be corrected. In renal failure, phosphate may be eliminated through peritoneal dialysis or hemodialysis.

MAGNESIUM

Function

Magnesium is the second most abundant intracellular cation in the body and is required for the maintenance of normal metabolic activity.[45,55,56] It is a cofactor for numerous enzymes that play vital roles in energy metabolism. These enzyme systems include Na-K ATPase and calcium ATPase. It is required for enzymes essential in the maintenance of electrolyte gradients and protein synthesis. Magnesium is essential for enzymes involved in the production of cyclic AMP, regulation of slow calcium channels, secretion of parathyroid hormone, membrane permeability, and action potential generation. It is important for neurochemical transmission, muscle contraction, membrane stability, cell division, and metabolism of protein, fat, and carbohydrate.

Distribution

Magnesium is primarily an intracellular ion and is found mostly in bone and muscle tissue. Less than 1% of magnesium is found in the serum, and circulating levels of magne-

disorders with decreased platelet adhesiveness, phagocytic impairment, and hemolysis of red cells; and, in chronic deficiency states, skeletal dysfunction with increased bone turnover and decreased mineralization.

TREATMENT. Management of profound depletion of phosphorus (serum phosphate <1 mg/dL) includes intravenous potassium phosphate or sodium phosphate in a dose of 2.5 to 5 mg/kg every 6 hours. Serum phosphate, calcium, magnesium, and potassium levels must be measured every 12 hours. Intravenous phosphate must not be given to patients with hypercalcemia; the hypercalcemia must be corrected first to prevent metastatic calcifications.

TABLE 29-17. Diagnosis and Treatment of Hypophosphatemia

Diagnosis:	Serum PO_4 3 mg/dL in fasting state
Causes:	Intracellular shift
	Renal loss
	Gastrointestinal
	Iatrogenic
	Drugs
Management:	Profound depletion <1 mg/dL
	Potassium phosphate or sodium phosphate (2.5–5.0 mg/kg/6 h)
	Follow serum phosphate, calcium, magnesium, potassium levels every 12 h
	When phosphate ≥2 mg/dL, switch to oral agents
	Depletion (≥2 mg/dL)
	Whole cow's milk (1 mg phosphate/mL; 1500–2000 mL/d)
	Neutra-Phos (dibasic & monobasic sodium & potassium phosphates: 250 mg/tablet; 2 tablets every 8–12 h)
	Phsopho-soda (129 mg/mL; give 5 mL every 8–12 h)
Complications:	Metastatic calcifications
	Hyperphosphatemia

PO_4, phosphate.

TABLE 29-18. Diagnosis and Treatment of Hyperphosphatemia

Diagnosis:	Serum PO_4 >4.5 mg/dL in fasting state
Causes:	Decreased renal excretion
	Increased intracellular to extracellular shift
	Increased phosphate ingestion
Management:	Restrict PO_4 intake (<200 mg/d)
	Saline infusion
	Acetazolamide
	Oral phosphate binders
	Correct hypocalcemia
	Peritoneal dialysis or hemodialysis
Complications:	Hypophosphatemia
	Hypocalcemia
	Metastatic calcification

PO_4, phosphate.

sium may not accurately reflect intracellular concentrations. Magnesium circulates in the plasma in three forms: a protein-bound form (30%), a chelated form (15%), and an ionized form (55%). The ionized form is physiologically active and homeostatically regulated. Measuring ionized magnesium is difficult, and most laboratories report magnesium as total magnesium. The normal circulating level for total magnesium is 1.6 to 2.4 mg/dL (0.8 to 1.2 mMol/L).

Human adult magnesium requirements average 5 mg/kg/day or 0.2 mMol/kg/day orally. Requirements are increased in children, pregnancy, critical illness, and states of increased magnesium loss (e.g., diuretics, diarrhea). Magnesium is absorbed in the distal small intestine. Normally, only 33% of ingested magnesium is absorbed. Gastrointestinal absorption is inhibited by phosphates, calcium, and fats. There is little hormonal control over magnesium absorption.

Regulation

Magnesium is regulated primarily by renal excretion, and renal insufficiency is the primary cause of hypermagnesemia. Urinary magnesium excretion is less than 1 mMol/day. The normal kidney is capable of conserving magnesium during states of magnesium deficiency, provided renal magnesium wasting is not the primary cause of the deficiency. Although many agents can influence magnesium metabolism (e.g., parathyroid hormone, vitamin D, thyroid hormone, mineralocorticoids), they are not primary regulators of magnesium excretion.

Magnesium is important for the maintenance of normal potassium metabolism.[55,57–66] It is a cofactor for sodium-potassium transport. Magnesium deficiency results in cellular potassium depletion and renal potassium wasting. Cellular potassium repletion requires magnesium to enable optimal potassium entry into cells. Thus, magnesium deficiency should be corrected in patients with potassium depletion.

Parathyroid gland secretion requires magnesium for optimal function. Although mild hypomagnesemia stimulates parathyroid hormone secretion, severe hypomagnesemia may cause hypocalcemia by impairing hormone secretion.[55,61–63] Hypermagnesemia also impairs parathyroid gland secretion.[64] Moreover, hypomagnesemia causes end-organ resistance to parathyroid hormone and vitamin D.[62,65,66]

HYPOMAGNESEMIA

Magnesium is primarily an intracellular ion, and cellular magnesium deficiency may occur in the presence of normomagnesemia. Hypomagnesemia may occur in the presence of normal cellular magnesium levels, but from a practical standpoint, most hypomagnesemic critically ill patients have some degree of magnesium deficiency, and they usually benefit from magnesium repletion.

Measurement of urine magnesium may be helpful in assessing magnesium status and in delineating the cause of magnesium deficiency[46,55,56] (see Fig. 29-5). Normal kidneys are capable of reducing magnesium excretion to less than 1 mMol/day during states of magnesium deficiency. High urinary excretion of magnesium in the face of hypomagnesemia suggests renal magnesium wasting as the cause for the hypomagnesemia. Low urinary magnesium in the face of hypomagnesemia suggests nonrenal causes for the hypomagnesemia. If cellular magnesium depletion is suspected in normomagnesemia patients, the magnesium retention test may be useful. In a normal magnesium-repleted patient, 75% to 80% of an intravenous magnesium load (30 mMol/12 hour) is excreted in the urine within 24 hours. Magnesium-deficient patients with normal kidneys usually retain more than 25% to 50% of the administered magnesium.

Causes

Magnesium deficiency is one of the most common electrolyte disorders encountered in critically ill patients. The prevalence varies from 10% to 65%, depending on the type of patients studied.[42,55,56,67-70] Magnesium deficiency may result from redistribution of magnesium, excessive gastrointestinal losses of magnesium, or excessive renal losses of magnesium.

MAGNESIUM SHIFTS.   Magnesium may move from the extracellular space into the intracellular space, resulting in hypomagnesemia. Shift of magnesium into cells occurs during recovery from malnutrition, during recovery from hypothermia, and after administration of catecholamines and insulin. Magnesium consumption by bone occurs after parathyroidectomy for hyperparathyroidism (i.e., hungry bone syndrome). Hypomagnesemia may also result from magnesium precipitation or chelation by tissues (e.g., pancreatitis, rhabdomyolysis).

OBLIGATE LOSS.   An obligate loss of magnesium occurs in urine, in stool, and from the skin. Failure to replace magnesium losses can deplete magnesium. Increased loss of magnesium from the gastrointestinal tract or skin can cause hypomagnesemia (see Fig. 29-5). Excess losses may result from malabsorption, diarrhea, fistulas, and gastric suction. Lower gastrointestinal secretions are richer in magnesium (5 to 7 mMol/L) than upper gastrointestinal secretions (0.5 to 1 mMol/L).

RENAL.   Renal loss of magnesium is a common cause of hypomagnesemia. Etiologic agents include diuretics, aminoglycosides, cisplatin, cardiac glycosides, amphotericin B, and cyclosporine.[42,55,56,71] Diseases that interfere with renal tubular reabsorption of magnesium are also common causes of magnesium wasting.

MISCELLANEOUS.   Hypomagnesemia is common in patients undergoing cardiac bypass surgery.[72] Magnesium depletion is caused by dilution and chelation, redistribution, and renal losses. Arrhythmias are decreased in postcardiac surgery patients who are administered magnesium.

Clinical Effects

Magnesium depletion primarily affects the cardiovascular and neuromuscular systems[55,56,73-81] (Table 29-19). Clinical features include cardiac arrhythmias, vasospasm, cardiac ischemia, muscle weakness, spasms, seizures, tetany, obtundation, and coma. Biochemical features include hypocalcemia, hypokalemia, and hypophosphatemia. Magnesium administration has been shown to decrease cardiac arrhythmias during states of myocardial ischemia, such as myocardial infarction and coronary bypass surgery, and improve survival in patients with myocardial infarctions.[74-81] Magnesium has also proved useful in decreasing arrhythmias and improving outcome in patients with nonocclusive coronary artery disease, torsades de pointes, digitalis toxicity, and coronary artery bypass surgery. The antiarrhythmogenic effects of magnesium occur in conditions of normomagnesemia. Concern exists that large doses of magnesium may impair myocardial and smooth muscle function. Overall, magnesium administration at clinically relevant doses has few detrimental hemodynamic actions.[82-85] Cardiac output

TABLE 29-19.   Clinical Features of Hypomagnesemia

CARDIOVASCULAR FEATURES
    Arrhythmias
    Vasospasm
    Angina pectoris

NEUROMUSCULAR FEATURES
    Weakness, respiratory insufficiency
    Spasm, tremor
    Seizures
    Tetany
    Obtundation, coma
    Depression, apathy
    Irritability, psychosis

GASTROINTESTINAL FEATURES
    Anorexia
    Dysphagia
    Nausea

METABOLIC FEATURES
    Hypocalcemia
    Hypokalemia
    Hypophosphatemia

is usually well maintained or slightly increased. Systemic vascular resistance and arterial pressure are maintained or slightly decreased.

Treatment

Treatment of magnesium depletion is based on correcting the cause for magnesium loss and replacing magnesium by the intravenous, intramuscular, or enteral routes[42,55,56] (Table 29-20). Maintenance doses of magnesium for adults are 0.2 mMol/kg/day orally or 0.1 mMol/kg/day parenterally. These requirements assume normal body stores and no unusual losses.

ACUTE SYMPTOMATIC DEPLETION.   Patients with symptomatic magnesium depletion are best treated with parenteral magnesium. In the treatment of acute life-threatening arrhythmias, we recommend giving 1 to 2 g (8 to 16 mMol) intravenous magnesium sulfate over 3 to 5 minutes. The bolus should be followed with an infusion of 1 to 2 g of magnesium sulfate each hour for the next few hours and then reduced to 0.5 to 1.0 g of magnesium sulfate each hour as a maintenance infusion in patients with normal renal function. Potassium should also be monitored and replaced if necessary. Serum magnesium levels must be monitored during therapy to avoid severe hypermagnesemia. In patients with severe but non–life-threatening hypomagnesemia, we recommend beginning with an infusion of 1 to 2 g of magnesium sulfate each hour for 3 to 6 hours and then decreasing the rate to 0.5 to 1.0 g each hour as a maintenance infusion.

CHRONIC DEPLETION.   In less urgent situations and in patients with prolonged magnesium depletion, we recom-

TABLE 29-20.   Treatment of Hypomagnesemia

GENERAL MEASURES

Treat underlying cause
Correct other electrolyte disorders
Remove offending drugs

REPLACE MAGNESIUM

Intravenous/intramuscular magnesium sulfate (maintenance 0.1 mMol/kg/d)°
Enteral (maintenance 0.4 mEq/kg/d)
    Magnesium oxide: 400-mg tab = 10 mMol Mg = 241 mg Mg
    Magnesium gluconate: 500-mg tab = 1.2 mMol Mg = 27 mg Mg; 5 mL = 2.4 mMol Mg = 54 mg Mg
    Magnesium hydroxide: 400-mg tab = 3.5 mMol Mg = 84 mg Mg

tab, tablet.
°Elemental magnesium (Mg): 1 mEq = 0.5 mMol = 12 mg.
Magnesium sulfate: 1 g = 4 mMol = 8 mEq = 98 mg Mg.

mend administering 25 to 50 mMol of magnesium sulfate (600 to 1200 mg of elemental magnesium) each day if renal function is normal. Treatment is usually continued for 3 to 5 days to replace intracellular stores, and then the patient is placed on maintenance doses of magnesium, which depend on magnesium losses from the body. Because bolus intravenous doses of magnesium are quickly excreted by the kidneys, it is better to administer magnesium by continuous intravenous infusion, intramuscularly, or enterally to maintain an elevated blood magnesium concentration. If given enterally, only 30% to 50% of gut magnesium is normally absorbed. Replacing deficits plus ongoing losses is important. Therapy should be guided by the serum magnesium level.

The dose of magnesium is usually decreased in patients with renal insufficiency. Oral magnesium may cause diarrhea. During magnesium repletion, we monitor serum magnesium, calcium, potassium, creatinine, blood pressure, ECG changes, respiratory status, and neurologic status (especially deep-tendon reflexes). Symptoms of hypermagnesemia are unusual unless serum levels exceed 2 to 3 mMol/L.

HYPERMAGNESEMIA

Causes

Hypermagnesemia occurs if the serum magnesium concentration is above 3 mg/dL (0.6 mMol/L).[46,55,86] Hypermagnesemia is rare in patients with normal renal function. Most cases occur in patients with renal disease and result from the administration of magnesium-containing antacids, laxatives, enemas, or nutritional products. Other causes of hypermagnesemia include adrenal insufficiency, hypothyroidism, lithium intoxication, treatment of eclampsia, and premature labor.

Clinical Effects

Hypermagnesemia diminishes neuromuscular transmission and can depress skeletal muscle function and cause neuro-muscular blockade.[46,55,86] Excess magnesium causes vasodilation and hypotension, depressed deep-tendon reflexes, bradycardia, heart block, cardiac arrest, respiratory depression, respiratory failure, paralysis, depressed mentation, and coma. Hypocalcemia may result from parathyroid gland suppression.[55,64] ECG changes include prolongation of PR, QRS, and ST intervals; bradycardia; and heart block.

Treatment

Neuromuscular and cardiac toxicity can be transiently antagonized by intravenous calcium (100 to 200 mg over 5 minutes). Definitive therapy to lower the serum magnesium level consists of stopping all exogenous magnesium and administering saline and loop diuretics to enhance renal excretion. Magnesium may also be removed by dialysis.

INTRAOPERATIVE AND POSTOPERATIVE FLUID THERAPY

In addition to blood, commonly used fluids for intraoperative use are divided into three categories: conventional crystalloids, colloids, and hypertonic solutions. Some less commonly used fluids include blood substitutes. In this section, the choice of initial fluids and the question of glucose utilization are addressed.

CONVENTIONAL CRYSTALLOIDS

Conventional crystalloids are fluids that contain a combination of water and electrolytes. They are divided into "balanced" salt solutions (e.g., Ringer's lactate solution, Plasma-Lyte, and Normosol) and hypotonic solutions (Table 29-21). Either their electrolyte composition approximates that of plasma, or they have a total calculated osmolality that is similar to that of plasma.

Normal saline (0.9%) is actually hypertonic with respect to sodium and especially to chloride, if the osmolality is calculated. However, when normal saline is subjected to a freezing point depression test in an osmometer, its osmolality is approximately 285 mOsm/kg. The *calculated* value is derived by simple addition of its ionic constituents, whereas the measured value is affected by ionic association or dissociation. Sodium chloride has a relative osmolality of 1 compared with that of sodium and chloride, the value of which is 2. Other balanced electrolyte solutions are slightly hypotonic in vitro (265 mOsm/kg) in comparison with their calculated values and normal plasma. Solutions that contain less than the concentration of electrolytes found in Ringer's lactate solution are not used often intraoperatively.

Distribution

The previously described distribution of water after the administration of D_5W, Ringer's lactate solution, hypertonic saline, and albumin is shown in Table 29-2. Notice that when an electrolyte-free solution such as D_5W is administered, less than 10% stays intravascular. Approximately two thirds is

TABLE 29-21. Composition of Selected Intravenous Fluids

	Na (mMol/L)	Cl (mMol/L)	K (mMol/L)	Mg (mMol/L)	Ca (mMol/L)	LACTATE (mMol/L)	OTHER	APPROX pH	mOsm/kg (CALCULATED)
D$_5$W							Dextrose, 5 g/dL	5.0	253
0.9 NaCl	154	154						4.2	308
Ringer's lactate	130	109	4.0		1.5	28		6.5	273
Plasma-lyte	140	98	5.0	1.5			Acetate, 27 mEq/L Gluconate, 23 mEq/L	7.4	294
Hespan	154	154					Hetastarch, 6 g/dL	5.5	310
Dextran 70	154	154						5.5	308
5% Albumin	145	145					Albumin, 5.0 g/dL		308
3% NaCl	513	513						5.0	1027
5% NaCl	855	855						5.6	1710

Na, sodium; Cl, chloride; K, potassium; Mg, magnesium; Ca, calcium; Approx, approximate; D$_5$W, 5% dextrose in water; NaCl, sodium chloride.
From McGough EK, Kirby RR: Fluids and electrolytes. In: Kirby RR, Gravenstein N (eds). *Clinical Anesthesia Practice.* Philadelphia, WB Saunders, 1994:717.

distributed to the intracellular space. Intravascular resuscitation is minimal, and cellular swelling occurs. The administered free water causes a decease in the serum and interstitial electrolyte concentrations (dilutional effect) and may lead to symptomatic hyponatremia.

When solutions such as 0.2% or 0.45% saline are administered, similar, although slightly less pronounced, redistribution occurs. Therefore, a balanced salt solution with a sodium concentration of 130 mMol/L or more is normally chosen when major operative procedures are performed and when excessive blood loss is anticipated. More hypotonic solutions and D$_5$W should be restricted to minor procedures and for some pediatric operations.

COLLOIDS

Colloids commonly used in the United States include albumin, hydroxyethyl starch (HES; also known as hetastarch [Hespan]) and dextran. In Europe, gelatin derivatives are available as well. Colloid molecules are sufficiently large that they normally do not cross capillary membranes in significant numbers. Most of an administered colloid remains intravascular unless an altered permeability condition is present (see Table 29-2). Distribution of fluid throughout the body is dependent on the forces represented in the Starling equation:

$$J_v = K_f[(P_{MV} - P_{is}) - \delta(COP_{MV} - COP_{is})] \quad (2)$$

in which J_v represents the rate of filtration of fluid across the capillaries; K_f is the ultrafiltration coefficient (a measure of permeability); P_{MV} is the hydrostatic pressure within the microvasculature (i.e., the capillaries); P_{is} is the hydrostatic pressure in the interstitial space (the tissues); δ is the reflection coefficient and is a relative value expressing the ability of the semipermeable membrane to prevent movement of

a given solute (in this case, the colloids of interest); COP_{MV} is the colloid oncotic pressure in the microvasculature; and COP_{is} is the colloid oncotic pressure in the tissue.

Distribution

For colloids "to work" as desired (i.e., remain in the intravascular compartment), δ must be large (approaching 1.0). The value of δ varies greatly among tissues; for example, the lungs are moderately permeable ($\delta = 0.6$); muscle is moderately impermeable ($\delta = 0.9$); and the brain and glomeruli are essentially impermeable to protein entry ($\delta = 0.99$ and 1.0, respectively). The δ value for other tissues, such as liver, is low ($\delta \approx 0$).[87]

Changes in Capillary Permeability

During trauma or sepsis, δ values may change significantly. A classic example is the increase in capillary permeability to albumin in the lungs during the acute respiratory distress syndrome. In such a case, administered colloid may freely move across what ordinarily would be moderately permeable membranes in much the same fashion as does a balanced electrolyte solution. Increased capillary permeability (capillary leak) also occurs at the site of surgical trauma, and administered colloid moves out of the capillaries into the involved interstitium. In this setting, colloids are less effective than otherwise would be expected for intravascular expansion. They may increase interstitial edema by exerting a reverse oncotic gradient as they accumulate in the tissues.

Oncotic Pressure Gradients

Once colloid molecules leak into the interstitial space, they must be removed to prevent this reverse oncotic pressure gradient and tissue edema. Rarely does a concentration gradient exist for colloid movement from the interstitial space back into the capillaries. Instead, it must be removed by the lymphatic system. Although many tissues, especially the lungs, have a large capacity for lymphatic drainage, others, including skeletal muscle, do not. Removal of colloid is much slower than that of crystalloid, and persistent edema, even to the point of blood flow interruption, sometimes results. This situation is particularly problematic in major trauma and burns.

THE COLLOID VERSUS CRYSTALLOID DEBATE

Few topics in anesthesia and surgery have generated as much controversy as the relative merits of colloids and crystalloids for intraoperative fluid replacement and resuscitation. Numerous animal and human studies have been undertaken to prove that one or the other is superior.[88-93] In most cases, the choice is based more on personal opinion and dogma rather than on scientific merit.

One noteworthy attempt to sort out this controversy was undertaken by Valanovich.[88] He performed a metaanalysis of mortality for eight previously published human trials in patients receiving either crystalloid or colloid for resuscitation. (A metaanalysis is a statistical technique that involves the combining of data from multiple studies to increase the overall statistical power of the data.) These pooled data showed an overall 5.7% decrease in mortality rate in patients who were resuscitated with crystalloid rather than colloid solutions. When the data were divided into subgroups of trauma/sepsis and elective surgery, a 12.3% decrease in mor-

tality in the former group was demonstrated. Conversely, a 7.8% increase in mortality was found in the crystalloid group undergoing elective surgical procedures (Fig. 29-5).

Valanovich believed that patients with trauma and sepsis have an increase in capillary permeability that allows the administered colloid to leak out of the vasculature, to be less effective as an intravascular volume expander, and to slow resolution of edema from the affected tissues (mentioned earlier). In patients undergoing elective procedures, the amount of capillary leak, in contradistinction to that in major trauma, is more discretely limited to the surgical site; thus, the use of colloids may be more efficacious in increasing intravascular volume. This study does not settle the controversy, but it does provide some insight into specific situations when one or the other may be preferable.

Most colloid advocates do not recommend these substances as the sole resuscitative fluid. The usual protocol involves initial infusion of crystalloids, followed by the administration of colloids when large volumes are necessary to reduce the amount of crystalloids. In general, crystalloids need to be administered in volumes that are approximately two to three times that of isooncotic colloid such as 5% albumin or HES to obtain the same hemodynamic effect. When more concentrated colloid solutions such as 25% albumin are used, this ratio is no longer valid.

Role of Colloid Therapy

The most comprehensive evaluation of colloid therapy was presented in a 1991 workshop on the assessment of plasma volume expander.[94] All of the pertinent clinical trials involving albumin, dextran, and HES were carefully evaluated in

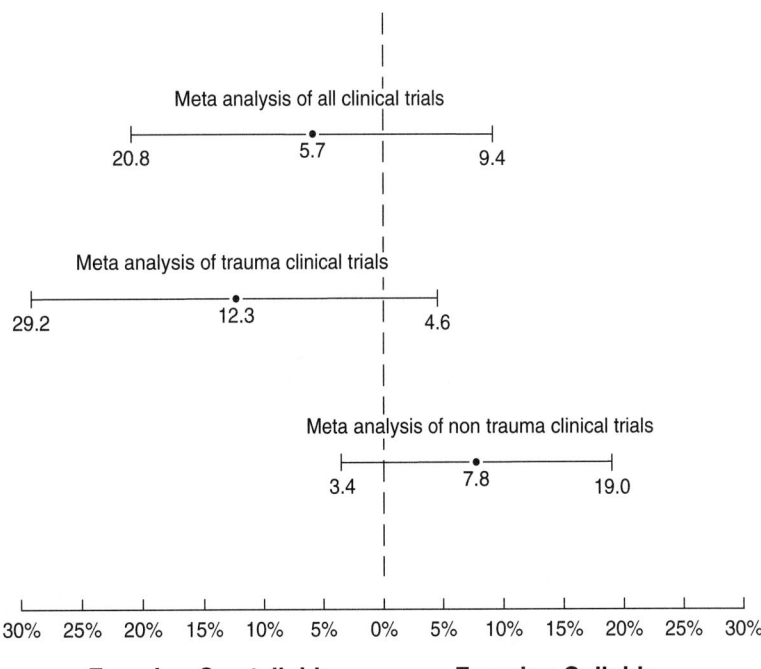

FIGURE 29-5. Metaanalysis of mortality rates for colloid versus crystalloid fluid resuscitation. (From Valanovich V: Crystalloid vs. colloid fluid resuscitation: a meta-analysis of mortality. *Surgery* 1989;105:70.)

terms of efficacy, cost, indications for use, and complications. Little evidence was found for either a short-term or long-term benefit from the use of supplemental colloidal agents in blood loss, burns, cardiopulmonary bypass, pulmonary edema, trauma, and nutrition. No evidence suggested that serum albumin levels as low as 3.0 g/dL were deleterious, and even values as low as 2.0 g/dL have not been clearly shown to be problematic.

PULMONARY EDEMA.   Of particular interest was the discussion relating pulmonary edema and the fact that administration of albumin in hypoalbuminemic patients, by abruptly increasing pulmonary artery perfusion pressure, may produce the very complication it is designed to prevent—interstitial and alveolar flooding.[94]

RENAL FUNCTION.   A rise in the colloid oncotic pressure a little above normal significantly impairs renal salt and water excretion. No congenital hyperalbuminemic states are known, and the body reacts to transient elevations of albumin by immediately stopping production and accelerating catabolism. The adverse renal effects may be associated with the absence of naturally occurring states of excess albumin, whereas those in which albumin level is low are common. However, with one exception,[95] in which albumin supplementation of 900 g occurred over several days, no toxic effect of albumin therapy has been shown. The effects of colloidal products on bleeding and clotting have been mentioned and are discussed in detail later.

COSTS.   Cost is another factor when considering the use of crystalloid and colloid solutions. Table 29-22 gives the approximate 1992 *hospital* cost of the various crystalloid and colloid solutions. Notice that balanced electrolyte solutions are inexpensive (a 1-L bag costs approximately $1.00). The cost of colloid solutions is as much as 200 times that for an equal volume of crystalloid solution or 50 to 100 times that for an equipotent volume of crystalloid solution. The cost to patients is much higher.

Colloids and Hemostasis

Patients who undergo surgery with significant blood loss often have problems with coagulation. However, not all coagulation deficits seen in surgical patients can be related to the use of blood. Colloid solutions have been reported to be responsible in many settings. These deficits are in addition to those expected purely from the dilution associated with large-volume resuscitation.

ALBUMIN.   Johnson and coworkers[96] treated severely injured patients with a standardized resuscitation protocol. Approximately one half of the patients received 150 g/day or additional albumin for 3 to 5 days. The patients given supplemental albumin required greater volumes of whole blood and fresh frozen plasma to obtain normal clotting studies than did those who were resuscitated with crystalloid solutions. Albumin-treated patients had a significant decrease in fibrinogen concentration and prolongation of the prothrombin time that could not be explained by dilution. In

TABLE 29-22.   Approximate Hospital Cost of One Liter of Various Fluids°

Plasma-lyte	$1.66
Ringer's lactate	$0.80
Normal saline	$0.65
5% Albumin	$236.00
Hespan	$83.06
Dextran 70	$17.50
3% NaCl	$1.40

NaCl, sodium chloride.
°January 1992.
From McGough EK, Kirby RR: Fluids and electrolytes. In: Kirby RR, Gravenstein N (eds). *Clinical Anesthesia Practice.* Philadelphia, WB Saunders, 1994:720.

contrast, the prolonged thromboplastin time and decreased platelet counts that also occurred in the albumin-treated group were ascribed to dilution.

The amount of albumin administered in this study was much greater than that usually given in clinical settings. Other investigators, using smaller doses of albumin, reported clotting abnormalities that could be explained solely on the basis of dilution.[97] In addition, in vitro studies found that albumin did not adversely influence clotting nor did it affect the structure of fibrin clots.[98]

Overall, albumin may exert some mild effects on hemostasis; however, these effects seem to be primarily dilutional as a result of volume expansion. When large amounts of albumin are infused, the degree of volume expansion exceeds that obtained with a comparable amount of crystalloid solutions. Therefore, a more pronounced coagulation defect is likely.

DEXTRAN.   Dextran is used not only for volume expansion but as a form of antiaggregant in patients undergoing vascular and microvascular surgical procedures. Clotting deficits associated with dextran probably are related to defects in platelet interaction and to an antithrombotic effect. The platelet–vascular interaction is believed to be primarily associated with an effect on factor VIII.[99-101] Dextran also seems to be incorporated into the polymerizing fibrin clot so that it alters clot structure and enhances fibrinogenolysis.[102-105]

Dextran is commonly supplied in two forms: dextran 70 and dextran 40. The numbers 70 and 40 refer to the average molecular weights (70,000 and 40,000, respectively) of the molecules in solution. Dextran 40 seems to have greater inhibitory effects on coagulation than does Dextran 70. It is used in vascular surgery to prevent thrombosis but is rarely employed as a primary volume expander, alone or in combination with hypertonic saline.

HYDROXYETHYL STARCH.   Hydroxyethyl starch is derived from carbohydrate (usually corn). It is available in the United States as a 6% solution in 0.9% sodium chloride (Hespan). Its effects have been studied in two major groups of patients. The first consists of healthy patients undergoing leukophoresis for donation of white blood cells. These patients usually receive small amounts (approximately 500 mL) of HES. In one study, 10 donors who received HES during leukopheresis had slight but significant prolongation of their prothrombin time and prolonged thromboplastin time (mean increases of 0.6 and 2.5 seconds, respectively).[106] Levels of fibrinogen, factor VIII:C, and factor V were similarly reduced but remained within the normal range. In another report, no defects in platelet function were noticed.[107]

The second includes those who receive larger doses of HES for trauma and surgery. In these patients, a prolonged partial thromboplastin time and up to a 50% decrease in factor VIII:C occurs with an infusion of 1 L of HES.[106,107]

In addition to its effect on levels of factor VIII, HES seems to cause changes in fibrin clot formation and fibrinogenolysis. This characteristic may be related to incorporation of the HES molecules into the clot with subsequent prevention of solid clot formation.

PENTASTARCH. Pentastarch is a new lower molecular weight version of HES that has fewer hydroxyethyl groups per molecule. It is unavailable for volume expansion in the United States but is undergoing clinical trials. It is available in Europe. The anticoagulation effects of pentastarch seem to be similar in type and magnitude to those observed with HES.

HYPERTONIC SOLUTIONS

Hypertonic saline solutions (sodium concentration greater than that found in normal saline) include 1.8%, 3%, 5%, 7.5%, and 10% sodium chloride solutions. Other anions such as lactate and acetate may be incorporated. They are sometimes mixed with colloids such as dextran.[108]

Distribution

Table 29-2 shows the changes that occur when 1 L of 3% sodium chloride solution is administered to a normal 70-kg adult. Because the osmolality of the administered solution exceeds that of intracellular water and because sodium and chloride ions cannot freely cross cell membranes, the ECF becomes slightly hyperosmolar. A gradient for water to pass from the cells into the extravascular compartment is established, and the extracellular volume is expanded by approximately 2.5 L.

Because electrolytes freely cross capillary membranes, the fluid is divided between the intravascular and extravascular compartments according to their relative volumes. Although hypertonic saline solutions increase the intravascular volume more than would the same volume of a balanced salt solution, they do so at the expense of a decreased intracellular volume. If large volumes of previously administered balanced electrolyte solutions have already increased intracellular volume (remember that most are, in effect, slightly hypotonic), hypertonic saline is therapeutic. If not, cellular dehydration can result.

Potential Complications

Hypertonic saline solution use is not widespread. However, there has been a resurgence of interest in these solutions for intraoperative administration and trauma resuscitation.[108–112] A major concern is the potential development of hypernatremia. However, complications associated with hypernatremia have not been reported in the clinical trials. Hypernatremia, when it occurs, is usually transient, especially when these solutions are used with balanced electrolyte or colloid solutions.[108] Comprehensive reviews of many of the aspects of hypertonic saline have been published.[112,113] Hyperchloremic acidosis is of theoretical concern owing to the large chloride load. However, substitution of hypertonic sodium acetate, although transiently improving acid–base parameters, has not been found to improve outcome and, curiously, increases lactemia.[114]

HYPOOSMOLAR STATES ■

DEXTROSE AND WATER IN THE SURGICAL PATIENT

Water intoxication results from the administration of excessive amounts of hypotonic fluids. Excess balanced electrolyte solutions are easily excreted by most surgical patients, whereas excess amounts of D_5W are retained. At least two reasons explain these findings: (1) hyponatremia causes a depression of renal function, and (2) D_5W does not provide the solute that is necessary for urine formation.

Hyponatremia and Renal Function

Schroeder[115] described postsurgical patients with oliguria not responding to large infusions of D_5W, rising BUN, urea clearance of less than 10% of normal, and a progressive decrease of serum sodium concentration. Despite increasing volumes of D_5W, they progressed to anuria and CNS deterioration. The syndrome was reversed by the administration of 6% sodium chloride.

Bristol[116] made dogs hyponatremic, hydrated them with 25 mL of water/kg/hour for 7 hours, and measured the percentage of the fluid load that they excreted during this period. He found that the latter was reduced as the serum sodium level decreased (Table 29-23). In addition to oliguria, animals with the more marked hyponatremia developed nausea and vomiting, apathy, generalized muscle irritability, disorientation, convulsions, and in the absence of salt administration, death.

Ariel and Miller[117] studied normally hydrated surgical and nonsurgical patients made hypochloremic by gastric aspiration, a salt-free diet, and intravenous D_5W. They found that during hypochloremia (serum sodium was not measured), the RBF and GFR fell by about 25%, returning to normal after the administration of saline.

McCance[118,119] and Wilkinson[119] published articles on the effect on man and animals of primary sodium deficiency. McCance's subjects were made sodium-deficient by salt-free diet, sweat-box treatments, and given unlimited tap water. In humans, salt and water were lost together at first, and normal body osmolality was maintained at the expense of a decrease in TBW (about 2 L). With continued sodium loss, osmolality was sacrificed to maintain body water content

TABLE 29-23. Decrease in Excretion of Water Load With Hyponatremia

SERUM SODIUM (mEq/L)	% OF WATER LOAD EXCRETED
140	71
135–139	60
130–134	48
125–129	43
120–124	43
110–119	30

From Bristol WR: Relation of sodium chloride depletion to urine excretion and H_2O intoxication. *Am J Med Sci* 1951; 221:412.

TABLE 29-24. Normal Values for Water and Solute Metabolism and Renal Function

Insensible water loss averages 1000 mL/m²/24 h
Water of oxidation averages 200 mL/m²/24 h
Solute excretion on an average diet varies from 600–800 mOsm/m²/24 h
Solute excretion on IV D_5W averages 200 mOsm/m²/24 h
The maximum range of urinary concentration and dilution in a healthy kidney, in a nonstressed person, is 0.7 to 10 mL of water/mOsm of solute

IV, intravenous; D_5W, 5% dextrose in water.

at its now decreased volume. GFR fell by 30%, and it became difficult to evoke a diuresis after a certain level of sodium deficiency, even when the subjects drank copious amounts of water. In hyponatremic rabbits, a nearly 50% decrease in GFR and marked oliguria occurred.[119]

Hyponatremic dogs maintained chronically at serum sodium concentrations of 15 to 25 mMol/L below normal exhibited a marked reduction in their ability to form urine.[120] On occasion, only 20 mL of a 600-mL water load was voided in 5-hour period.

Stokes and coworkers[121] studied salt depletion without dehydration in dogs and man. They found that hyponatremia caused a reduction in GFR of 30% to 80%. A large infusion of D_5W at the time that the subjects were already hyponatremic resulted in a further depression of the GFR and did not increase the rate of urine flow. In spite of hyponatremia (10 to 30 mMol/L below normal) and overhydration, the urine remained hyperosmotic compared with plasma. Treatment with hypertonic saline resulted in a return to normal of RBF and GFR and led to the excretion of large volumes of hypotonic urine. The authors concluded that the hyponatremia of the postoperative state may significantly affect renal water and solute excretion.

Lack of Solute for Urine Formation

A second cause for oliguria in a patient given only D_5W is the lack of solute available for excretion. A few normal values involving water and solute formation and renal function must be appreciated (Table 29-24).

A healthy patient eating a normal diet is able to maintain body water and solute homeostasis with a water intake varying from 1220 to 8800 mL/m²/24 hour. With a 24-hour restricted water intake of 1220 mL/m² plus 200 mL/m² water of oxidation (a total of 1420 mL/m²), this healthy patient can sustain an insensible loss of 1000 mL/m² and still excrete a dietary solute of 600 mOsm/m² in the remaining 420 mL/m² (0.7 mL/mOsm × 600 mOsm/m² = 420 mL/m²). With an intake of 8800 mL/m²/24 hours, plus 200 mL/m² of water of oxidation, an insensible loss of 1000 mL/m² allows excre-

tion of the excess water at a concentration of 10 mL of water per mOsm of solute (10 mL/mOsm/m² × 800 mOsm = 8000 mL/m²).

If this same person is given intravenous D_5W only, the maximum 24-hour tolerable water load, without change in body osmolality, decreases from 8800 mL/m² to 2800 mL/m². Insensible loss in excess of the water of oxidation takes care of 800 mL/m². However, the 200 mOsm of solute available from metabolism of dextrose in D_5W, if excreted in a maximally dilute urine of 10 mL of water/mOsm, acts as a vehicle for only an additional 2000 mL of water. Thus, if this patient, receiving only D_5W, were given the same 24-hour maximum water load of 8800 mL/m² that he can tolerate when eating a normal diet, he will retain 6000 mL of water/m², developing hyponatremia and water intoxication. This scenario would occur even with completely normal kidneys and renal function.

The postsurgical patient is even more severely limited with respect to the handling of solute-free water. His maximum urinary dilution frequently is in the range of 1.2 to 1.6 mL/mOsm of solute, rather than 10 mL/mOsm in the nonstressed patient. Causative factors include depression of RBF and GFR and hyponatremia. The unreplaced deficit in the FECV plays a part in many patients. Increased ADH secretion undoubtedly is a factor. With a maximum urinary dilution of 1.6 mL/mOsm of solute and 200 mOsm of solute if D_5W is administered, only 320 mL of water/m²/24 hours (a 24-hour urine volume of 550 mL in a 70-kg man) can be excreted. This value is the usual urinary output of a major surgical patient treated only with D_5W intraoperatively and postoperatively. The forcing of additional D_5W to increase urine output is of little avail, because without supplemental insulin, humans normally cannot use more than 50 to 75 g of glucose/m²/24 hours[12,123]; the additional glucose, therefore, does not lead to any appreciable increase in solute production.

Reports of oliguria postoperatively in patients given only D_5W,[124–136] and the occurrence of water intoxication when additional D_5W is "pushed," thus are to be expected. Likewise, the prompt diuresis and symptomatic improvement seen upon the administration of hypertonic saline or other solute is not surprising,[17] although the rapidity with which correction should be achieved is debated.[137]

REFERENCES ■

1. Lewis RT: Albumin-role and discriminative use in surgery. *Can J Surg* 1980;23:322
2. Heyl JT, Gibson JC, Janeway CA: Studies on plasma proteins. *J Clin Invest* 1943;22:763
3. Reineck HJ, Stein JH: Sodium metabolism. In: Maxwell MH, Kleeman CR, Narins RG (eds). *Clinical Disorders of Fluid and Electrolyte Metabolism*, 4th ed. New York, McGraw-Hill, 1987:33
4. Zerbe RL, Robertson GL: Osmotic and nonosmotic regulation of thirst and vasopressin secretion. In: Maxwell MH, Kleeman CR, Narins RG (eds). *Clinical Disorders of Fluid and Electrolyte Metabolism*, 4th ed. New York, McGraw Hill, 1987:61–78
5. Sterns RH: The management of hyponatremic emergencies. *Crit Care Clin* 1991;7:127
6. Anderson RJ, Chung HM, Kluge R, et al: Hyponatremia: a prospective analysis of its epidemiology and the pathogenic role of vasopressin. *Ann Intern Med* 1985;102:164
7. DeFronzo RA, Thier SO: Pathophysiologic approach to hyponatremia. *Arch Intern Med* 1980;140:897
8. Gennari FJ: Serum osmolality: uses and limitations. *N Engl J Med* 1984;310:102
9. Rose BD: New approach to disturbances in the plasma sodium concentration. *Am J Med* 1986;81:1033
10. Moses AM, Notman DD: Diabetes insipidus and syndrome of inappropriate antidiuretic hormone secretion (SIADH). *Adv Intern Med* 1982;27:73
11. Hantman D, Rossier B, Zohlman R, et al: Rapid correction of hyponatremia in the syndrome of inappropriate secretion of anti-diuretic hormone. *Ann Intern Med* 1973;78:870
12. Sterns RH: Neurological deterioration following treatment for hyponatremia. *Am J Kidney Dis* 1989;12:434
13. Sterns RH: The management of symptomatic hyponatremia. *Semin Nephrol* 1990;10:503
14. Sterns RH: Brain dehydration and neurologic deterioration after rapid correction of hyponatremia. *Kidney Int* 1989;35:69
15. Thurston JH, Hauhart RE, Nelson JS: Adaptive decreases in amino acids (taurine in particular), creatinine, and electrolytes prevent cerebral edema in chronically hyponatremic mice: rapid correction (experimental model of central pontine myelinolysis) causes dehydration and shrinkage of brain. *Metab Brain Res* 1987;2:223
16. Berl T: Treating hyponatremia: damned if we do and damned if we don't. *Kidney Int* 1990;37:1006
17. Arieff AI: Hyponatremia, convulsions, respiratory arrest, and permanent brain damage after elective surgery in healthy women. *N Engl J Med* 1986;314:1529
18. Arieff AI, Llach F, Massry SG: Neurologic manifestations and morbidity of hyponatremia: correlation with brain water and electrolytes. *Medicine* 1976;55:121
19. Cluitsman FHM, Meinders AE: Management of severe hyponatremia: rapid or slow correction? *Am J Med* 1990;88:161
20. Sterns RH: Severe symptomatic hyponatremia: treatment and outcome. A study of 64 cases. *Ann Intern Med* 1987;107:656
21. Sterns RH, Riggs JE, Schochet SS: Osmotic demyelination syndrome following correction of hyponatremia. *N Engl J Med* 1986;314:1535
22. Hantman O, Rossier B, Zohlman R, et al: Rapid correction of hyponatremia in the syndrome of inappropriate secretion of antidiuretic hormone: an alternative to hypertonic saline. *Ann Intern Med* 1973;78:870
23. Ayus JC, Olivero JJ, Frommer JP: Rapid correction of severe hyponatremia with intravenous hypertonic saline solution. *Am J Med* 1982;72:43
24. Schrier RW, Lehman D, Zacherle B, et al: Effect of furosemide on free water excretion in edematous patients with hyponatremia. *Kidney Int* 1973;3:30
25. Brunner JE, Redmond JM, Haggar AM, et al: Central pontine myelinolysis and pontine lesions after rapid correction of hyponatremia: a prospective magnetic resonance imaging study. *Ann Neurol* 1990;27:61
26. Arieff AI: Treatment of symptomatic hyponatremia: neither haste nor waste. *Crit Care Med* 1991;19:748
27. Forrest JN, Cox M, Hong C, et al: Superiority of demeclocycline over lithium in the treatment of chronic syndrome of inappropriate secretion of antidiuretic hormone. *N Engl J Med* 1978;298:173
28. White MG, Fetner CD: Treatment of the syndrome of inappropriate secretion of antidiuretic hormone with lithium carbonate. *N Engl J med* 1975;292:390
29. Feig PU, McCurdy DK: The hypertonic state. *N Engl J Med* 1977;297:1444
30. Narins RG, Jones ER, Storn MC, et al: Diagnostic strategies in disorders of fluid, electrolyte, and acid-base homeostasis. *Am J Med* 1982;72:496
31. Ober KP: Diabetes insipidus. *Crit Care Clin* 1991;7:109
32. Hall J, Robertson G: Diabetes insipidus. *Probl Crit Care* 1990;4:342
33. Arieff AI: Central nervous system manifestations of disordered sodium metabolism. *Clin Endocrinol Metab* 1984;13:269
34. Zaloga GP, Chernow B: Insulin and oral hypoglycemics. In: Chernow B (ed). *The Pharmacologic Approach to the Critically Ill Patient*, 2nd ed. Baltimore, Williams & Wilkins, 1988:637
35. Alexander EA, Perrone RD: Regulation of extrarenal potassium balance. In: Maxwell MH, Kleeman CR, Narins RG (eds). *Clinical Disorders of Fluid and Electrolyte Metabolism*, 4th ed. New York, McGraw Hill, 1987:105
36. Field MJ, Berliner RW, Giebisch GH: Regulation of renal potassium metabolism. In: Maxwell MH, Kleeman CR, Narins RG (eds). *Clinical Disorders of Fluid and Electrolyte Metabolism*, 4th ed. New York, McGraw Hill, 1987:119
37. Bia M, DeFronzo RA: Extrarenal potassium homeostasis. *Am J Physiol* 1981;240:F268
38. Young DB: Analysis of long-term potassium regulation. *Endocr Rev* 1985;6:24
39. Brown RS: Potassium homeostasis and clinical implications. *Am J Med* 1984;77(Suppl):3
40. Raymond KH, Kunau RT: Hypokalemic states. In: Maxwell MH, Kleeman CR, Narins RG (eds). *Clinical Disorders of Fluid and Electrolyte Metabolism*, 4th ed. New York, McGraw Hill, 1987:519
41. Freedman BI, Burkart JM: Hypokalemia. *Crit Care Clin* 1991;7:143
42. Helfant R: Hypokalemia and arrhythmias. *Am J Med* 1986;80(Suppl):13
43. DeFronzo RA: Hyperkalemic states. In: Maxwell MH, Kleeman CR, Narins RG (eds). *Clinical Disorders of Fluid and Electrolyte Metabolism*, 4th ed. New York, McGraw Hill, 1987:547
44. Williams ME: Hyperkalemia. *Crit Care Clin* 1991;7:155
45. Zaloga GP: Calcium disorders. *Probl Crit Care* 1990;4:382
46. Zaloga GP, Chernow B: Divalent ions: calcium, magnesium and phosphorus. In: Chernow B (ed). *The Pharmacologic*

Approach to the Critically Ill Patient, 2nd ed. Baltimore, Williams & Wilkins, 1988:603

47. Zaloga GP, Chernow B: Hypocalcemia in critical illness. *JAMA* 1986;256:1924

48. Prielipp R, Zaloga GP: Calcium action and general anesthesia. *Adv Anesth* 1991;8:24

49. Zaloga GP, Chernow B, Cook D, et al: Assessment of calcium homeostasis in the critically ill patient: the diagnostic pitfalls of the McLean Hastings nomogram. *Ann Surg* 1985;202:587

50. Ladenson JH, Lewis JW, Boyd JC: Failure of total calcium corrected for protein, albumin, and pH to correctly assess free calcium status. *J Clin Endocrinol* 1978;46:986

51. Zaloga GP: Evaluation of bedside testing options for the critical care unit. *Chest* 1990;97(Suppl):185

52. Denlinger JK, Nahrwold ML, Gibbs PS et al: Hypocalcemia during rapid blood transfusion in anesthetized man. *Br J Anaesth* 1976;48:995

53. Howland WS, Schweizer O, Jascott D, et al: Factors influencing the ionization of calcium during major surgical procedures. *Surg Gynecol Obstet* 1976;143:895

54. Kahn RC, Jascott D, Carlon GC, et al: Massive blood replacement: correlation of ionized calcium, citrate, and hydrogen ion concentration. *Anesth Analg* 1979;58:274

55. Zaloga GP, Roberts JE: Magnesium disorders. *Probl Crit Care* 1990;4:425

56. Salem M, Munoz R, Chernow B: Hypomagnesemia in critical illness: a common and clinically important problem. *Crit Care Clin* 1991;7:225

57. Whang R, Fink EB, Dycker T, et al: Magnesium depletion as a cause of refractory potassium repletion. *Arch Intern Med* 1985;145:1686

58. Whang R, Morosi HJ, Rodgers D, et al: The influence of continuous magnesium deficiency on muscle K repletion. *J Lab Clin Med* 1967;70:895

59. Ryan MP, Whang R, Yamalis W: Effect of magnesium deficiency on cardiac and skeletal muscle potassium during dietary potassium restriction. *Proc Exp Biol Med* 1973;143:1045

60. Dyckner T, Wester PO: Relationship between potassium, magnesium and cardiac arrhythmias. *Acta Med Scand* 1981;647(Suppl):163

61. Anast CS, Winnacker JL, Forte LR, et al: Impaired release of parathyroid hormone in magnesium deficiency. *J Clin Endocrinol Metab* 1976;42:707

62. Rude RK, Oldham SB, Singer FR: Functional hypoparathyroidism and parathyroid hormone end-organ resistance in human magnesium deficiency. *Clin Endocrinol* 1976;5:209

63. Brown EM, Chen CJ: Calcium, magnesium and the control of PTH secretion. *Bone Miner* 1989;5:249

64. Cholst IN, Steinberg SF, Tropper PJ, et al: The influence of hypermagnesemia on serum calcium and parathyroid hormone levels in human subjects. *N Engl J Med* 1984;310:1221

65. Freitag JF, Martin KJ, Conrades MB, et al: Evidence for skeletal resistance to parathyroid hormone in magnesium deficiency. *J Clin Invest* 1979;64:1238

66. Medalli R, Waterhouse C, Hahn TJ: Vitamin D resistance in magnesium deficiency. *Am J Clin Nutr* 1976;29:854

67. Zaloga GP, Wilkens R, Tourville J, et al: A simple method for determining physiologically active calcium and magnesium concentrations in critically ill patients. *Crit Care Med* 1987;15:813

68. Chernow B, Barmberger S, Stoikso M, et al: Hypomagnesemia in patients in postoperative intensive care. *Chest* 1989;95:391

69. Ryzen E, Wagers PW, Singer FR, et al: Magnesium deficiency in a medial ICU population. *Crit Care Med* 1985;13:19

70. Fiaccadori E, DelCanale S, Coffrini E, et al: Muscle and serum magnesium in pulmonary intensive care unit patients. *Crit Care Med* 1988;16:751

71. Zaloga GP, Chernow B, Pock A, et al: Hypomagnesemia is a common complication of aminoglycoside therapy. *Surg Gynecol Obstet* 1984;158:561

72. Robertie PG, Butterworth JF, Royster RL, et al: Normal parathyroid hormone responses to hypocalcemia during cardiopulmonary bypass. *Anesthesiology* 1991;75:43

73. Zaloga GP: Interpretation of the serum magnesium level. *Chest* 1989;95:257

74. Dyckner T: Serum magnesium levels in acute myocardial infarction: relation to arrhythmias. *Acta Med Scand* 1980;207:59

75. Rasmussen HS, Aurup P, Hojberg S, et al: Magnesium and acute myocardial infarction. *Arch Intern Med* 1986;146:872

76. Bigg RPC, Chia R: Magnesium deficiency: Role in arrhythmias complicating acute myocardial infarction. *Med J Aust* 1981;1:346

77. Morton BC, Nair RC, Smith FM, et al: Magnesium therapy in acute myocardial infarction: a double blind study. *Magnesium* 1984;3:346

78. Rasmussen HS, McNair P, Norregard P, et al: Intravenous magnesium infusion in acute myocardial infarction. *Lancet* 1986;1:234

79. Smith LF, Heagerty AM, Bing RF, et al: Intravenous infusion of magnesium sulfate after acute myocardial infarction: effects of arrhythmias and mortality. *Int J Cardiol* 1986;12:175

80. Abraham AS, Rosenmann D, Kramer M, et al: Magnesium in the prevention of lethal arrhythmias in acute myocardial infarction. *Arch Intern Med* 1987;147:753

81. Rasmussen HS, Suenson M, McNair P, et al: Magnesium infusion reduces incidence of arrhythmias in acute myocardial infarction: a double blind, placebo-controlled study. *Clin Cardiol* 1987;10:351

82. Butterworth JF, Strickland RA, Zaloga GP: Hemodynamic actions and drug interactions of calcium and magnesium. *Probl Crit Care* 1990;4:402

83. Prielipp RC, Zaloga GP, Butterworth JF, et al: Magnesium inhibits the hypertensive but not the cardiotonic actions of low dose epinephrine. *Anesthesiology* 1991;74:973

84. Mroczek WJ, Lee WR, Davidov ME: Effect of magnesium sulfate on cardiovascular hemodynamics. *Angiology* 1977;28:720

85. James MFM, Cork RC, Dennett JE: Cardiovascular effects of magnesium sulfate in the baboon. *Magnesium* 1987;6:314

86. Van Hook JW: Hypermagnesemia. *Crit Care Clin* 1991;7:215

87. Gabel JC, Drake RE: Plasma proteins and protein osmotic pressure. In: Staub NC, Taylor AE (eds). *Edema*. New York, Raven Press, 1984:371

88. Valanovich V: Crystalloid versus colloid fluid resuscitation: a meta-analysis of mortality. *Surgery* 1989;105:65

89. Gammage GW: Crystalloid versus colloid: is colloid worth the cost? *Int Anesthesiol Clin* 1987;25:32

90. Vincent JL: Fluids for resuscitation. *Br J Anesth* 1991;67:185

91. Nearman HS, Herman ML: Toxic effects of colloids in the intensive care unit. *Crit Care Clin* 1991;7:713

92. Falk JL, Rackow EC, Astiz M, et al: Fluid resuscitation in shock. *Cardiothorac Anesth* 1988;2(Suppl):33

93. London MJ: Plasma volume expansion in cardiovascular surgery: practical realities, theoretical concerns. *J Cardiothorac Anesth* 1988;2(Suppl):39

94. Center for Biologics, Food and Drug Administration and National Heart, Lung, Blood Institute, Division of Blood Diseases and Resources. *Workshop on Assessment of Plasma Volume Expanders*. Bethesda, MD, March 25 and 26, 1991

95. Lucas CE, Ledgerwood AM, Higgins RF: Impaired pulmonary function after albumin resuscitation from shock. *J Trauma* 1980;20:446

96. Johnson SD, Lucas CE, Gerrick SJ, et al: Altered coagulation after albumin supplements for treatment of oligemic shock. *Arch Surg* 1979;114:279

97. Strauss RG: Volume replacement and coagulation: a comparative review. *J Cardiothorac Anesth* 1988;2(Suppl):24

98. Carr ME: Turbidimetric evaluation of the impact of albumin on the structure of thrombin-mediated fibrin gelatin. *Haemostasis* 1987;17:189

99. Aberg M, Hedner U, Bergentz S: Effects of dextran on factor VIII (antihemophilic factor) and platelet function. *Ann Surg* 1979;189:243

100. Aberg M, Hedner U, Bergentz S: The antithrombotic effect of dextran. *Scand J Haematol* 1979;34:61

101. Battle J, del Rio F, Lopez-Fernandez F, et al: Effect of dextran on factor VIII/von Willebrand factor structure and function. *Thromb Haemost* 1985;54:697

102. Carr ME, Gabriel DA: The effect of dextran 70 on the structure of plasma derived fibrin gels. *J Lab Clin Med* 1980;96:985

103. Katsuda K, Maeno H: Mechanism for the inhibitory effect of dextran on α_2 plasmin inhibitor activity. *Thromb Res* 1980;19:655

104. Carlin G, Saldeen T: On the interaction between dextran and the primary fibrinolysis inhibitor α_2-antiplasmin. *Thromb Res* 1980;19:103

105. Carlin G, Bang NU: Enhancement of plasminogen activation and hydrolysis of purified fibrinogen and fibrin by dextran 70. *Thromb Res* 1980;19:535

106. Kisker CT, Strauss RG, Kaepke JA, et al: The effects of combined platelet and leukopheresis on the blood coagulation system. *Transfusion* 1978;19:173

107. Maguire LC, Henriksen RA, Strauss RG, et al: Platelet function in donors undergoing intermittent-flow centrifugation plateletpheresis or leukapheresis. *Transfusion* 1980;20:549

108. Holcroft JW, Vassar MJ, Turner JE, et al: 3% NaCl and 7.5% NaCl/dextran 70 in the resuscitation of severely injured patients. *Ann Surg* 1987;206:279

109. Maningas PA, Mattox KL, Pepe PE, et al: Hypertonic saline–dextran solutions for the prehospital management of traumatic hypotension. *Am J Surg* 1989;157:528

110. Jelenko C, Williams JB, Wheeler ML, et al: Studies in shock and resuscitation. I. Use of a hypertonic, albumin-containing, fluid demand regimen (HALFD) in resuscitation. *Crit Care Med* 1979;7:157

111. Cross JS, Gruber DP, Gann DS, et al: Hypertonic saline attenuates the hormonal response to injury. *Ann Surg* 1989;209:684

112. McGough EK: Resuscitation in shock, trauma, and burns. *Probl Crit Care* 1991;5:346

113. McGough EK, Kirby RR: Fluids and electrolytes. In: Kirby RR, Gravenstein N (eds). *Clinical Anesthesia Practice*. Philadelphia, WB Saunders, 1994:714

114. Frey L, Kesel K, Prückner S, et al: Is sodium acetate dextran superior to sodium chloride dextral for small volume resuscitation from traumatic hemorrhagic shock? *Anesth Analg* 1994;79:517

115. Schroeder HA: Renal failure associated with low extracellular sodium chloride: the low salt syndrome. *JAMA* 1949;141:117

116. Bristol WR: Relation of sodium chloride depletion to urine excretion and H_2O intoxication. *Am J Med Sci* 1951;221:412

117. Ariel IM, Miller F: The effects of hypochloremia upon renal function in surgical patients. *Surgery* 1950;28:552

118. McCance RA: Experimental sodium chloride deficiency in man. *Proc R Soc Biol Sci [B]* 1935;119:245

119. Wilkinson BM, McCance RA: The secretion of urine in rabbits during experimental salt deficiency. *Q J Exp Physiol* 1940;30:249

120. Holmes JH: Studies of water exchange in dogs with reduced serum electrolyte concentration. *Am J Physiol* 1940;129:384

121. Stokes JM, Bernard HR, Balfour J: Effects of experimental electrolyte depletion upon renal water and solute excretion. *Arch Surg* 1962;85:540

122. Hayes MA, Williamson RJ, Heidenreich WF: Endocrine mechanisms involved in water and sodium metabolism during operation and convalescence. *Surgery* 1957;41:353

123. Kerrigan GA, Talbot NB, Crawford JD: Role of the neurohypophyseal–antidiuretic hormone–renal system in everyday clinical medicine. *J Clin Endocrinol Metab* 1955;15:265

124. Coller FA, Campbell KN, Vaughan HH, et al: Postoperative salt intolerance. *Ann Surg* 1944;119:533

125. Ariel IM: Effects of a water load administered to patients during the immediate postoperative period. *Arch Surg* 1951;62:303

126. Coller FA, Iob V, Vaughan HH, et al: Translocation of fluid produced by the intravenous administration of isotonic salt solutions in man postoperatively. *Ann Surg* 1945;122:663

127. Cooper DR, Iob VI, Coller FA: Response to parenteral glucose of normal kidneys and of kidneys of postoperative patients. *Ann Surg* 1949;129:1

128. LeQuesne LP: Postoperative water retention—with a report of a case of water intoxication. *Lancet* 1954;i:172

129. LeQuesne LP, Lewis AAG: Postoperative water and sodium retention. *Lancet* 1953;i:153

130. Stewart JD, Rourke GM: The effects of large intravenous infusions on body fluid. *J Clin Invest* 1942;21:197

131. Wynn V, Rob CG: Water intoxication—differential diagnosis of the hypotonic syndromes. *Lancet* 1954;i:587

132. Zimmerman B, Wangensteen OH: Observations on water intoxications in surgical patients. *Surgery* 1952;31:654

133. Hayes MA, Coller FA: The neuroendocrine control of water and electrolyte excretion during surgical anesthesia. *Surg Gynecol Obstet* 1952;95:142

134. Dudley HF, Boling EA, LeQuesne LP, et al: Studies in antidiuresis in surgery: effects of anesthesia, surgery and posteriorpituitary antidiuretic hormone on water metabolism. *Ann Surg* 1954;140:354

135. Ariel IM, Kremen AJ, Wangensteen OH: An expanded interstitial (thiocyanate) space in surgical patients. *Surgery* 1950;27:827

136. Bartholomew LG, Scholz DA: Reversible postoperative neurological symptoms: report of five cases secondary to water intoxication and sodium depletion. *JAMA* 1956;162:22

137. Sterns RH, Riggs JE, Schochet SS: Osmotic demyelination syndrome following correction of hyponatremia. *N Engl J Med* 1986;314:1535

Critical Care, Third Edition, edited by Joseph M. Civetta,
Robert W. Taylor, and Robert R. Kirby.
Lippincott-Raven Publishers, Philadelphia, PA © 1997.

CHAPTER 30

■

Splanchnic Flow and Resuscitation

Orlando C. Kirton
Joseph M. Civetta

Ischemia signifies failure to satisfy the metabolic needs of the cell secondary to either impaired oxygen delivery or the impairment of cellular oxygen extraction and utilization. Incomplete splanchnic cellular resuscitation has been associated with the development of multiple organ system failure and increased mortality in the critically ill patient.[1,2] For many years, the merits of augmenting systemic oxygen delivery and consumption and attainment of supranormal levels have been examined and debated as primary treatment goals.[3-6] There is convincing evidence that systemic hemodynamic and oxygen transport variables fail to accurately portray the complex interaction between energy requirements and the energy supply at the tissue level,[7-9] and that achieving supranormal cardiovascular oxygen transport and utilization indices does not reliably confer improved outcome (i.e., decreased mortality rates and diminished multiple organ system failure) in several clinical conditions (e.g., sepsis, adult respiratory distress syndrome [ARDS]).[10-13] These findings have led to the search for monitoring techniques that directly measure changes in regional tissue bioenergetics.

Gastric or intestinal tonometry has been proposed as a relatively noninvasive index of the adequacy of aerobic metabolism in organs whose superficial mucosal lining is extremely vulnerable to low flow and hypoxemia, and in which blood flow is sacrificed first in both shock and the cytokine milieu of the systemic inflammatory response.[1,14,15] The gastrointestinal tract, therefore, acts like the "canary," displaying early metabolic changes before other indices of adequate oxygen utilization.[16] This chapter reviews the fundamental and clinical underpinnings of gastric tonometry,

the potential applications and limitations of the technology, its use as a prognostic and treatment endpoint, and, finally, a consideration of potential future directions.

THE INTESTINAL MICROCIRCULATION ■

The gastrointestinal tract has three major functions: motility, secretion, and absorption. Blood flow is important for each of these functions, being highest in the small intestines and lowest in the colon. The splanchnic circulation contains approximately 30% of the circulating blood volume at any given moment with the bulk of this volume held in the postcapillary venous capacitance vessels.[17] Resting blood flow in the intestine is ten times higher than in skeletal muscle. Most of the blood flow is delivered to the mucosa and submucosa, reflecting the varying demands for oxygen within the intestinal wall, being highest in the mucosal layer. The arterial supply emanates from an extensive arterial plexus in the submucosa. A *counter-current* blood flow exchange system exists within the superficial mucosal layer between the arterial and venous circulation, rendering this tissue particularly sensitive to neuronal and systemic vasoconstrictors.[18] The arterioles, which run in parallel with the venules in the stalk of the intestinal villus, allow diffusion of oxygen from the arterioles down a concentration gradient to the venules, bypassing the capillary bed at the villus tip; thus, the mucosa at the villus tip is rendered vulnerable to changes in oxygen content. Water also diffuses from arterioles to venules because of an osmotic gradient caused by the absorption of

443

sodium in the capillary bed at the villus tip. Therefore, the sodium concentration is higher in the venules. Plasma water content is then lowered at the villus tip compared with the base of the stalk, predisposing this area to low or absent flow in states of compensated or uncompensated shock when splanchnic circulation is compromised.

Mesenteric vasoconstriction is mediated by alpha-adrenergic postganglionic sympathetic fibers, but, even more dramatically, by the affects of circulating hormones and peptides (Table 30-1). Endogenous vasoconstrictors known to be released in major injury, sepsis, and other physiologically stressful circumstances include catecholamines, angiotensin, vasopressin, myocardial depressant factor, leukotriene D$_4$, thromboxane A$_2$, and serotonin. The high concentration of receptors for these systemically released vasoconstrictors, which affect the splanchnic circulation more than any other tissue beds, has a substantial effect on peripheral (systemic) vascular resistance and hence, on systemic blood pressure by redistributing blood from the splanchnic organs (as well as the peripheral circulation) to the central circulation (i.e., heart and brain). This effect may be compounded by tissue edema and atheroma in the splanchnic arteries. The peptides, angiotensin II and vasopressin, are the most potent splanchnic vasoconstrictors.[14] The splanchnic vasoconstriction induced by these two peptides alone accounted for the most of the increase in total peripheral vascular resistance recorded in animal models of cardiogenic and hemorrhagic shock. The adequacy of gut mucosal oxygenation cannot be reliably inferred from measurements of tissue oxygenation in the skin or of subcutaneous tissue because of their different response to endogenous vasoconstrictors.

Newer techniques, such as laser Doppler flowtometry, have been developed to measure blood flow within the gut. Several of these techniques have confirmed that the gastrointestinal mucosa is the first layer to have its flow reduced in a low flow state. However, absolute measurement of flow rate has not been applied to any formal clinical investigation of splanchnic perfusion in patients who are critically ill. Moreover, direct measurements of blood flow would not provide precise information concerning the adequacy of tissue oxygenation, except by inference in the absence of flow. The level to which perfusion must be lowered to reduce oxygen delivery below the tissue's metabolic requirements depends not only on the rate of blood flow, but also on several other variables, such as the PaO$_2$, the hematocrit, platelet and leukocyte number and function, the integrity of the endothelial lining, the capillary network distribution, the distance between the cell and capillary, the presence or absence of a counter-current exchange system, the metabolic needs of the tissue at the time, and, ultimately, the ability of these tissue cells to utilize the oxygen being delivered to them.[14,19] The tissue PO$_2$ maybe of some value in assessing the adequacy of tissue oxygenation because it usually falls in ischemia. Tissue PO$_2$ cannot, however, be used either to establish or reject a diagnosis of ischemia because vasodilation and increased extraction of oxygen may enable tissues to meet their metabolic demands despite a reduced oxygen delivery.[2]

CELLULAR ENERGY METABOLISM

Cellular energy is stored in the high-energy phosphate bonds of adenosine triphosphate and is readily released at the site of utilization by hydrolysis. Under conditions of oxygen abundance or normoxia, adenosine triphosphate (ATP) synthesis equals ATP hydrolysis, and the intracellular concentrations of adenosine diphosphate (ADP), inorganic phosphate, and hydrogen ions remain minuscule because these metabolites are used to reconstitute ATP in the process of oxidative phosphorylation.[7] Inadequate oxygen supply results in anaerobic glycolysis and systemic lactic acidosis. In the anoxic cell, uncompensated ATP hydrolysis is associated with the intracellular accumulation of ADP, inorganic phosphate, and hydrogen ions with resultant intracellular acidosis.[7,20] These hydrogen ions lead to tissue acidosis as well, with unbound hydrogen ions combining with interstitial bicarbonate to form the weak acid, carbonic acid, that disassociates to produce carbon dioxide (CO$_2$) plus water. These metabolites

TABLE 30-1. Endogenous Vasoconstrictors Known to Be Released in Stressful Circumstances and Their Actions on Different Tissue Beds

VASOCONSTRICTOR	GUT	RENAL	BRAIN	CORONARY	PULMONARY	MUSCLE	SKIN
Cathecholamines	+	+	0	±	±	±	+
Angiotensin II	+	+	0	0	0	0	0
Vasopressin	+	+	?0	+	?	?	+
Myocardial depressant factor	+	0	0	0	0	0	0
Leukotriene D$_4$	+	+	0	+	?	0	0
Thromboxane A$_2$	+	+	+	+	+	+	+
Serotonin	+	+	?	?	+	−	±

+, vasoconstriction; −, vasodilatation; 0, no effect; ±, effect varies.

(From Fiddian-Green RG: Studies in splanchnic ischemia and multiple organ failure. In: Marston A, Bulkley GR, Fiddian-Green RG, et al (eds). *Splanchnic Ischemia and Multiple Organ Failure.* London, Edward Arnold/St Louis, CV Mosby, 1989:349.)

also provide a feedback signal that promotes the anaerobic production of ATP by glycolysis and the creatine and adenylate kinase reactions.[7] Approximately 15,000 mMol of the volatile acid, carbonic acid, dissociates to CO_2 and water, which is excreted by the lungs during ventilation. Ten times as much fixed acid (150,000 mMol of hydrogen ions) is added by the hydrolysis of ATP and associated organic phosphates each day, 1 proton being generated for every inorganic phosphate liberated by hydrolysis. 99.9% (149,850 mMol of hydrogen ions) is balanced by ATP resynthesis during oxidative phosphorylation. The remaining 0.1% of this fixed acid load (150 mMol of hydrogen ions) is excreted by the kidneys.

Investigators have considered serum lactate levels to be a cellular marker of oxygen debt in patients with sepsis. Serum lactate, however, may not be a reliable marker of hypoxia because it represents the net effect of production and elimination. Its level may be elevated in conditions associated with either increased lactate production or decreased clearance, that is, sepsis associated with liver failure. Furthermore, serum lactate level represents a global index and may not be an optimal measure of the adequacy of regional or microvascular perfusion and may transiently rise during therapeutic maneuvers because of a regional washout phenomenon.[21,22] Other metabolic markers include the ATP–ADP ratio and direct plasma measurements of the metabolites resulting from the degradation of adenine nucleotides: for example, inosine, hypoxanthine, xanthine, and uric acid.[20,23] Phosphorus magnetic resonance spectroscopy, reflecting tissue metabolic activity, provides a noninvasive measure of the level of high-energy phosphate in several important tissues, such as the brain and heart.[24] Furthermore, proton magnetic resonance spectroscopy may allow the precise localization and measurement of many biologically active compounds, including tissue lactate levels. Unfortunately, the size and magnetic properties preclude the routine use of theses techniques in the ICU. Direct measurements of tissue pH can be made with pH microprobes placed in the intestinal mucosa. However, this technique is invasive and is limited by local tissue artifact, electrode artifact, and an inability to recalibrates the electrode in vivo, and, therefore, is not applicable clinically.[23,25] Mass spectrometry is another option but is also cumbersome and expensive.

INTESTINAL ISCHEMIA

Intestinal tissue injury can be induced by the initial ischemia (either from inadequate oxygen content or inadequate flow) or by the generation of oxygen derived free radicals during reperfusion.[1,7] Ischemic injury may be progressive, spanning a spectrum from mild injury characterized by increased capillary permeability with no microscopic changes to transmural infarction, depending on the severity and duration of the ischemia.[1,2,26,27]

Intracellular acidosis impairs cellular function by one of several mechanisms: (1) the loss of adenosine nucleotides from mitochondria by the inhibition of the ATP–magnesium/inorganic phosphate carrier; (2) inhibition of sodium–calcium exchange, resulting in the intracellular sequestration of calcium ions; (3) increases in the activity of cyclic adenosine monophosphate (AMP) deaminase and loss of adenine nucleotide precursors from the cell; (4) decreases in the nicotinamide adenine nucleotide pool by the acid-catalyzed destruction of nicotinamide adenine dinucleotide (NAD); and (5) the conversion of intracellular inorganic phosphate to its inhibitory deproteinated form.[7]

Hypoxia renders the superficial gastrointestinal mucosa susceptible to the cytolytic effects of gastric acid, proteolytic enzymes, and bacteria already present in the intestine by impairing cellular mucus and bicarbonate secretion. Disruption of the mucosal barrier is associated with the generation of myocardial depressant factors that cause a low cardiac output syndrome in animals.[14,28,29] Commonly, in low flow and hypoxic states, tissue oxygen consumption ($\dot{V}O_2$) is maintained by adaptive mechanisms that are activated when oxygen delivery ($\dot{D}O_2$) falls below a critical level and oxygen consumption becomes delivery dependent.

Hypoxia also results in intracellular calcium overload by inhibiting ATP-driven membrane transport pumps and sodium–calcium exchange. Increases in intracellular calcium are a pivotal event in cellular dysfunction during hypoxia, because calcium-activated proteases can destroy the sarcolemma and the cellular cytoskeleton.[7] Cellular membrane degradation seems to be related to calcium influx. Calcium stimulates phospholipase A_2 (PLA_2) and phospholipase C, which are known to degrade membrane phospholipids.[30,31] The resultant imbalance between the rate of membrane synthesis and the rate of membrane breakdown results in the accumulation of arachidonic acid, the precursor of thromboxane, prostaglandins and leukotrienes, substances that produce further cellular damage and profound alterations in microvascular control.

REPERFUSION INJURY

During reperfusion, oxygen is the culprit. During normoxia, the enzyme xanthine dehydrogenase catalyzes the resynthesis of ATP through the anabolic process of oxidative phosphorylation. This reaction consumes hydrogen ions by converting hypoxanthine plus NAD^+ to xanthine and NADH, NAD^+ is reduced in the conversion. During ischemia, xanthine dehydrogenase is converted to xanthine oxidase by calcium-activated proteases (the D to O conversion). Hydrogen ions accumulate, and ATP is sequentially degraded to ADP, AMP, adenosine, inosine, and, eventually, hypoxanthine. Hypoxanthine is acted on by xanthine oxidase rather than xanthine dehydrogenase to form xanthine, and xanthine is irreversibly converted to urate. During the process, oxygen is transformed into superoxide ($O_2^{\cdot}$) and hydrogen peroxide (H_2O_2). $O_2^{\cdot}$ plus H_2O_2 interact to form the more reactive oxygen species, hydroxyl radical ($OH^{\cdot}$), in the presence of transition metals such as iron (i.e., the Fenton and Haber-Weiss reactions) (Fig. 30-1). $OH^{\cdot}$ is also formed in a radical–radical reaction in which $O_2^{\cdot}$ combines with nitric oxide (NO) to yield the potent oxidant peroxynitrite anion ($ONOO^{\cdot}$), which spontaneously decomposes to release $OH^{\cdot}$ and nitrous oxide radical ($NO_2^{\cdot}$). These compounds plus ozone are

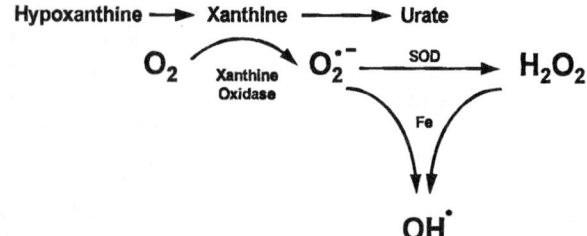

FIGURE 30-1. The sequential conversion of hypoxanthine to urate by the enzyme xanthine oxidase during ischemia–reperfusion, generating superoxide ($O_2^{\cdot-}$). Superoxide is dismutated to hydrogen peroxide (H_2O_2) by superoxide dismutase (SOD). $O_2^{\cdot-}$ and H_2O_2 form hydroxyl radical ($OH^{\cdot}$) in the presence of a transition metal (Fe): (Haber Weiss and Fenton reactions).

loosely grouped together as *oxygen free radicals*. These oxygen free radicals are capable of causing cellular injury through cellular membrane lipid peroxidation and degradation of nucleic acids, eventually leading to increased membrane permeability and cell lysis[31,32,33] Certain species, including $O_2^{\cdot}$ and $OH^{\cdot}$, cause polymorphonuclear cells (PMNs) to attract, adhere, activate, and release proteases which, through their respiratory burst, lead to further tissue injury. Altogether, the free radical pathways, activated during ischemia-reperfusion, prime PMNs, with formation and release of intracellular proteases and lipases capable of autodigestion of cellular components, producing arachidonic acid, leukotrienes, thromboxanes, and prostaglandins through lipid peroxidation[34] (Fig. 30-2). The body's natural antioxidant defenses consist principally of glutathione peroxidase, catalase, and superoxide dismutase.[34–36]

Circulating levels of xanthine oxidase have been demonstrated in critically ill patients with the ARDS.[25,36] Moreover, the ischemic intestine releases large amounts of xanthine oxidase into the portosystemic circulation, potentially becoming a systemic toxic oxygen-metabolite generating system. Elevated plasma malondialdehyde (from membrane lipid peroxidation) and elevated levels of PLA_2 activity also have been identified.[31]

Free radical pathways

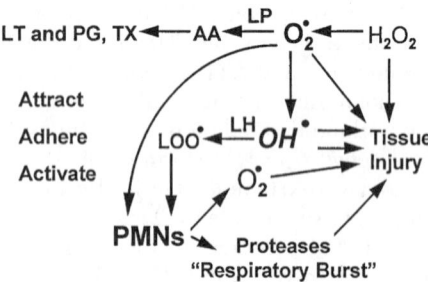

FIGURE 30-2. Free radical pathways leading to tissue injury, both directly and through the formation of the arachidonic acid (AA) metabolites, thromboxane (TX), prostaglandins (PG), and leukotrienes (LT) from lipid perioxidation (LP) and activation of the polymorphonuclear leukocytes (PMNs). H_2O_2, hydrogen peroxide; $OH^{\cdot}$, hydroxyl radical; $O_2^{\cdot}$, superoxide; LH, lipoxygenase; $LOO^{\cdot}$, lipid peroxyl radical.

DYSOXIC VERSUS NORMOXIC STATE ■

Oxygen delivery is the product of cardiac output and the arterial oxygen content. Under normal conditions, oxygen consumption, according to the Fick principle, can be calculated from cardiac output multiplied by the difference in arterial and mixed venous oxygen content, and is independent of oxygen delivery. While oxygen delivery falls, a critical level is reached where consumption becomes dependent on delivery. This *supply-dependent* oxygen consumption is believed to represent a state of oxygen debt and the onset of anaerobic metabolism. There are two types of shock: hemodynamically uncompensated shock, and compensated normotensive shock. Uncompensated shock is characterized by tachycardia, hypotension, oliguria, and peripheral vasoconstriction. The systemic acidosis is secondary to unreversed ATP hydrolysis. In compensated normotensive shock, the patient may have a normal blood pressure, heart rate, and urine output, warm perfused extremities, and no acidemia or metabolic acidosis detected by arterial blood gas analysis, but regional acidosis secondary to unreversed ATP hydrolysis and a progressive oxygen debt may still persist.[37] Failure to reverse compensated normotensive shock is associated with multiple organ system failure and increased mortality.[2]

Tissues with a high perfusion-to-extraction (demand) ratio, such as skeletal muscle, have high capillary densities that act as a microvascular reserve to produce an increase in local blood flow. These organs, in situations of low flow, use a disproportionate share of the cardiac output as increased capillary recruitment lowers local vascular resistance. These tissues are characterized by low oxygen extraction ratios and high mixed venous oxygen saturations. Less "fortunate" tissues, which include the intestinal tract, possess a lower capillary density and are unable to recruit capillaries to augment local blood flow to match increases in metabolic needs. This results in low perfusion-to-oxygen demand ratios and subsequent tissue hypoxia (the "trickle down economy" of systemic oxygenation).[15] The gastrointestinal tract is characterized by a high oxygen extraction ratio, lactate release, and low mixed venous oxygen saturation; it can tolerate severe hypoxemia without a decrease in oxygen consumption but is limited in its ability to respond to decreased blood flow.

GLOBAL PARAMETERS OF DELIVERY AND UTILIZATION: THE CONTROVERSY ■

The determinants of arterial oxygenation include hemoglobin content, inspired oxygen tension, alveolar oxygen tension, pH, temperature, mixed venous oxygen tension, ventilation/perfusion ($\dot{V}/\dot{Q}$) mismatch, physiologic shunting and cellular–interstitial diffusion abnormalities. Indices of adequacy of systemic perfusion include the following: (1) global systemic parameters, such as blood pressure, heart rate, central venous pressure measurements, and urine output; (2) tissue markers, including arterial pH (pHa), base excess, and serum lactate level; and (3) pulmonary artery catheter measurements and derivations, such as cardiac output, oxygen delivery, oxygen consumption, and oxygen extraction. Variables available from a pulmonary artery catheter can be used to differentiate types of systemic uncompensated shock, including the hypovolemic, hemorrhagic, cardiogenic, septic, and neurogenic varieties. The normal ranges are cardiac index, 2.8 to 3.5 L/minute/m^2; oxygen delivery, 400 to 500 mL/minute/m^2; and oxygen consumption, 120 to 140 mL/minute/m^2. The interpretation of oxygen delivery and oxygen consumption measurements is challenging because (1) these parameters do not provide direct information regarding the oxygen requirements of specific tissues; (2) the distribution of oxygen delivery is impacted by local microvascular and neurogenic responses; (3) the unpredictable effect of cytokines and endogenous peptides; and (4) the disease process may affect cellular metabolism directly (i.e., sepsis and ARDS).[38–40] Several prospective studies suggest that failure to achieve supranormal oxygen delivery and utilization parameters in the acute phase of major injury or physiologic stress is associated with increased mortality and shock-related complications, including multiple organ system dysfunction syndrome. The failure to reverse pathologic flow dependency, tissue hypoxia, and oxygen debt has been inferred as the cause of these adverse outcomes.[3–6,41,42] In these prospective studies, both responders and nonresponders achieved normal or hyperdynamic cardiovascular function; however, more cardiovascular interventions were often used in patients who died, so, ultimately, failure of patient response to achieve therapeutic objectives could be considered as the cause of the observed increased mortality and morbidity. Several reports failed to identify either an optimal or a critical value of oxygen delivery or consumption to distinguish survivors from nonsurvivors in critically ill patients.[10–13,29] Adequate or supranormal oxygen delivery may not be tantamount to effective tissue oxygen utilization.

"Critical oxygen delivery" purportedly marks the transition from aerobic to anaerobic metabolism; however, the relationship between oxygen delivery and consumption obtained in critically ill patients with ARDS, sepsis, and heart failure has been linear.[29] The lack of a clearly defined inflection point in a linear $\dot{D}O_2 - \dot{V}O_2$ function makes it impossible to determine a critical level of oxygen delivery that aerobically satisfies cellular energy requirements.

THE GASTROINTESTINAL TRACT AND MULTIPLE ORGAN SYSTEM FAILURE ∎

Multiple organ system failure (defined as failure of two or more vital organs or systems, in sequence or simultaneously, irrespective of the primary disease) and sepsis are distressingly familiar to surgeons who perform major elective cases, as well as to those involved in transplantation and trauma.[43] Uncompensated or compensated shock leading to progressive oxygen debt, ischemia-reperfusion injury, and cellular dysfunction is the underlying unifying pathophysiologic mechanism.[1] Throughout the world, multiple organ system failure has become the most common cause of death in the intensive care unit: the reported mortality rates vary from 30% to 100% with a mean of 50%, depending on the number of organ systems involved; the patients' ICU stay lasts for 6 weeks to many months and, in prior studies, these patients have used nearly 40% of the available ICU days.[43–47] Many hypotheses link the noxious event, whether surgery or trauma, to the development of multiple organ system failure and sepsis. There have also been many attempts to use single agents (e.g., antibiotics, monoclonal antibodies against cytokines and endotoxin) or combinations of these agents to affect the process; unfortunately, no significant progress has been made with these approaches. This may result from the many redundancies in the initiation and promulgation of multiple organ system failure, so that attacking a single pathway is ineffective, or, perhaps, efforts have been started too late in the sequence of events. Bacterial endotoxin in the gut may translocate across the semipermeable mucosa. Besides endotoxins, the products of the damaged mucosa also may contribute to the development of multiple organ system failure and death of the ICU patient. The translocation of enteric bacteria across the ischemic gut seems to be an important cause of nosocomial infection in the critically ill.[14,43] However, reducing the number of nosocomial infections from enteric organisms by selective decontamination does not seem to have a dramatic effect on outcome, that is, "again, the horse is already out of the barn."[48]

While representing an oversimplification, we believe the current hypotheses can be combined. Most current thinking can be categorized as the *gut starter* hypothesis (Fig. 30-3) popularized by Moore and colleagues,[49] and the *gut motor* hypothesis (Fig. 30-4) as described by Deitch, Marshall, and coworkers.[44–46]

In the gut starter hypothesis, the noxious stimulus leads to a neurohumoral response. High levels of catecholamines cause splanchnic vasoconstriction and a decrease in splanchnic flow. This leads to gut ischemia and, depending on the length of the ischemia period, various reactions occur that prime tissue to develop a reperfusion injury once flow is restored. During reperfusion, PLA$_2$ is activated, this in turn activates platelet activating factor (PAF). PAF attracts and primes PMNs in the gut; thereafter, they are released into the systemic circulation, where they undergo activation (the 2 *hit* model) and cause end-organ injury.[49] Therefore, the

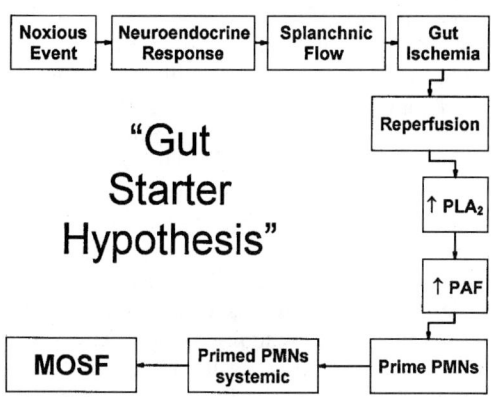

FIGURE 30-3. The gut starter hypothesis of multiple organ system failure (MOSF). PLA$_2$, phospholipase A$_2$; PAF, platelet activating factor; PMNs, polymorphonuclear leukocytes.

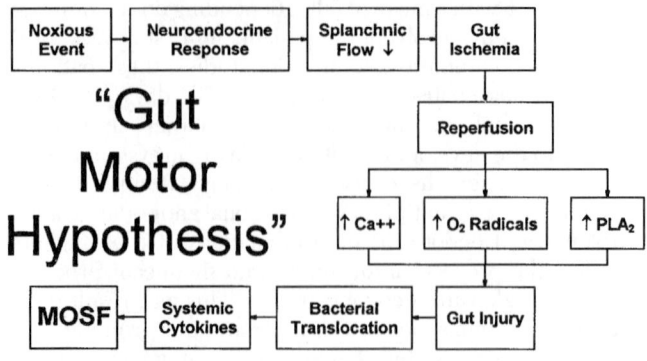

FIGURE 30-4. The gut motor hypothesis of multiple organ system failure (MOSF). PLA$_2$, phospholipase A$_2$; PAF, platelet activating factor; Ca^{++}, calcium; O$_2$, oxygen.

polymorphonuclear leukocyte is implicated as the major effector of cellular damage attributed to ischemia-reperfusion through its respiratory burst and activation of cytokines and arachidonic acid metabolites.

In the gut motor hypothesis, the steps leading to ischemia are the same. During reperfusion, gut mucosal injury results from the accumulation of intracellular calcium, activation of PLA$_2$, and the generation of free oxygen radicals. This leads to bacterial translocation and initial production and amplification of numerous systemic cytokines.[32,50] The end result again is multiple organ system failure. It is likely that these hypotheses are correct, although they are still incomplete explanations.

RELEVANT CLINICAL STUDIES

Acidosis of the gastric mucosa during or after surgery has in recent studies been associated with a high incidence of serious complications after major surgical procedures.[51] The incidence of stress gastritis was monitored in 94 ICU patients needing nasogastric tubes. Bleeding from stress ulceration was seen only in patients whose intramucosal pH (pHi) had fallen below 7.24. In another study of 85 patients, intramucosal acidosis and the duration of hypotension were more sensitive indicators of complications after cardiac surgery than cardiac index, pHa, and urine output during the operation.[52] Guys and colleagues,[53] studying pHi in its relation to sepsis in surgical patients, found significantly higher short-term mortality in patients with a pHi less than 7.32. Moreover, 90% of the septic patients had a pHi less than 7.32. Landow and associates[54] noticed that a low gastric pHi correlated with adverse outcome in patients undergoing cardiopulmonary bypass. Ischemic colitis, a complication after abdominal aortic surgery, often is diagnosed late, and mortality is consequently high. Low sigmoid colon pHi has been documented to predict endoscopically detectable ischemic colitis.[55,56] In another survey of critically ill patients undergoing abdominal aortic surgery, Schiedler and colleagues[57] verified that the severity of the depression and duration of the abnormal sigmoid pHi correlated with the development of isch-

emic colitis and major postoperative morbidity, with a sensitivity rate of 100% and a specificity rate of 92%.

Doglio and associates[58] measured gastric pHi in a heterogenous group of 80 patients at the time of admission ICU and at 12 hours later. A pHi above 7.35 was defined as normal. The group admitted with a low pHi had a greater ICU mortality rate, 65% versus 44% (p <0.04). Furthermore, patients with persistently low pHi at 12 hours after ICU admission had the highest mortality rate (87%). The prevalence of sepsis was also greater in the low pHi group, 59% versus 26% (p <0.01). The study was repeated in patients with acute circulatory failure by Maynard and colleagues[59] who found remarkably similar outcomes (Fig. 30-5). In addition to gastric pHi, Maynard measured hemodynamic oxygen transport and metabolic variables on admission and again at 24 hours. Prediction of outcome was assessed by sensitivity, specificity, and logistic regression. There were significant differences in mean gastric pHi values between survivors and nonsurvivors on admission and at 24 hours, (7.40 versus 7.28, 7.40 versus 7.24 respectively; p <0.001). There was no difference in cardiac index, oxygen delivery, and oxygen uptake between survivors and nonsurvivors. Gastric pHi had a sensitivity of 88% for predicting death and an odds ratio of 2.32, higher than for any other parameter.

In 35 patients undergoing orthotopic liver transplantation, gastric pHi was evaluated as an indicator of graft survival and liver function.[60] The only patient whose pHi remained lower than 7.3 for longer than 3 hours after reperfusion underwent retransplantation the following day. In a level 1 trauma center, Chang and colleagues[61] conducted a prospective study of 20 critically ill patients that compared pHi with base deficit, lactate, oxygen delivery and oxygen consumption, mixed venous oxygen saturation, the oxygen utilization coefficient, and pHa. Patients with pHi less than 7.32 on admission, who did not correct within the initial 24 hours, had a higher mortality than those whose pHi corrected (50% versus 0%; p = 0.03) and a higher incidence of multiple organ system failure (2.6 organs/patient versus 0.62 organs/patient; p = 0.02).

Rouman and associates[62] performed gastric tonometry prospectively in 15 multiple trauma patients. A pHi value less than 7.32 was considered abnormal. Three of 8 patients who developed a low pHi for 6 hours or longer developed major complications, and two subsequently died. The 7 patients who never had an abnormal pHi measurement experienced an uneventful recovery.

There have been only two prospective controlled interventional studies in which therapy was instituted because the pHi was low. Neither of these studies, however, attempted to normalize the pHi, but rather focused on increasing oxygen delivery and utilization. Gutierrez and associates[63] observed that the hospital mortality rate was significantly greater in control patients whose pHi was normal on admission (pHi $\geq$7.35) and then became abnormal during their ICU stay compared with those whose abnormal pHi prompted interventions to increase oxygen delivery. Unfortunately, if admission pHi was low, the mortality rates were the same in both treatment and control groups. The authors chose to increase oxygen delivery rather than restore pHi to normal values.

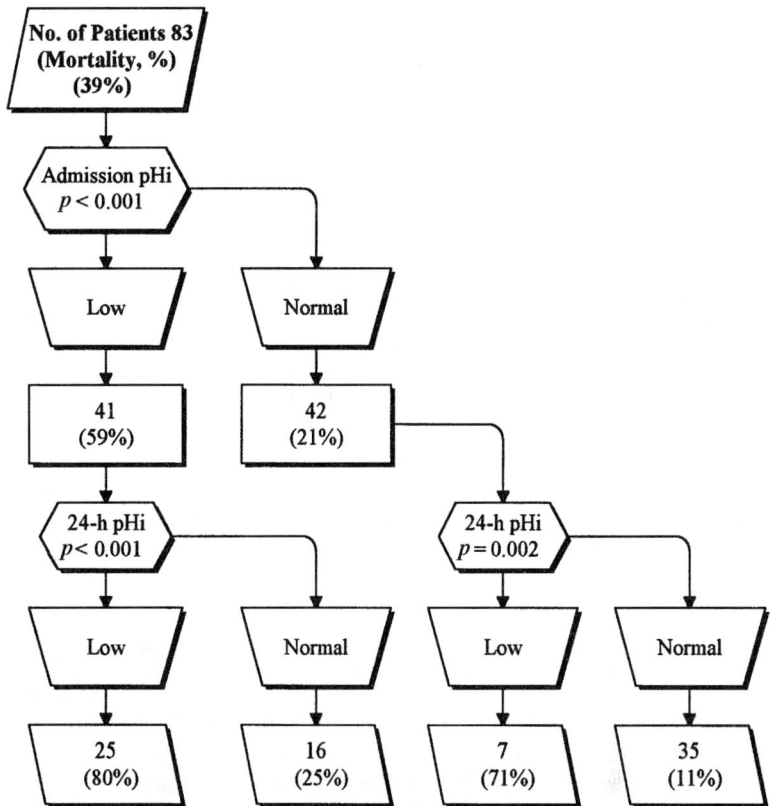

FIGURE 30-5. Mortality according to intramucosal pH on admission and at 24 hours. (From Maynard N, Bihari D, Beale R, et al: Assessment of splanchnic oxygenation by gastric tonometry in patients with acute circulatory failure. *JAMA* 1993;270:1203.)

In addition, they limited the prescribed interventions to three fluid boluses (750 mL total), mean posttreatment hemoglobin levels to 11 g/dL, and dobutamine was limited to a maximum of 10 μg/kg/minute. Neither splanchnic vasodilators nor agents to influence ischemia-reperfusion injury were employed.

Ivatury and others[64] randomized critically ill trauma patients into the following groups: group 1—an endpoint of pHi of 7.3 or more, 11 patients; and group 2—supranormal oxygen delivery parameters (as defined by Shoemaker and others[3]), 16 patients. In the pHi group, goals were met by 24 hours in 10 of 11 patients—9 survived. The incidence rate of multiple organ dysfunction was 18% and the death rate was 9%. In the supranormal oxygen delivery group, goals were met in 14 patients—10 survived. In the 10 surviving patients, pHi values were also 7.3 or more. The incidence rate of multiple organ system failure was 38%; the death rate was 31%. Of interest, if the pHi was less than 7.3, the patient was treated with volume and inotropes. Neither splanchnic vasodilation or ischemia-reperfusion modifications were employed. Seventy-five percent of the patients who developed multiple organ system failure had pHi less than 7.3. In group 2, 4 of the 5 patients who died did achieve supranormal oxygen delivery and consumption goals, but had a pHi less than 7.3 at 24 hours. Moreover, they observed that a late fall in pHi was often associated with a physiologic catastrophe (e.g., intestinal leak, gangrene, bacteremia).

We also confirmed that failure of splanchnic resuscitation correlated with multiple organ system failure and increased length of ICU stay in the hemodynamically unstable trauma patient.[65] The relative risk of death in patients whose pHi was less than 7.32 was 4.5 and the relative risk of developing multiple organ system failure was 5.4 compared with those having a pHi of 7.32 or more. Global parameters of oxygen transport utilization did not distinguish survivors from nonsurvivors nor those patients who developed multiple organ system failure from those who did not.

In a subsequent audit, we evaluated consecutive patients who met state trauma triage criteria, who were admitted to the Ryder Trauma Center at Jackson Memorial Hospital (Miami), and had a nasogastric tube placed during resuscitation. All patients were given 50 mg of ranitidine intravenously on admission. Exclusion criteria included esophageal injury, stomach injury requiring pyloric ablation, major head injury (i.e., Glasgow Coma Scale <8), and death within 24 hours. The trauma patients judged after clinical evaluation to have minimal injury and who were treated in routine care areas were found to have normal pHi on transfer from the resuscitation area. The mean pHi was 7.4 ± 0.11 (>7.2 in 95% of patients; >7.25 in 88%). All patients survived; none developed multiple organ system failure. In this subset of minimally injured patients (Trauma Score: 14.9 ± 1.9, AIS: 8.2 ± 7.2, APACHE II: 3.9 ± 4.8) values below any "cutoff" could represent false-positive results or be artifactually low because of intragastric generation of CO_2 secondary to bicarbonate neutralization in the stomach or duodenum secondary to gastric acid production.

In another audit, we specifically studied ICU patients with persistent uncorrected gastric pHi, who had pulmonary artery catheters to guide resuscitation.[66] The resuscitation protocol, begun on ICU admission, used inotropic and vasodilatory agents to optimize systemic and splanchnic oxygen delivery (e.g., dobutamine, isoproterenol, prostaglandin E, nitroglycerin, and nitroprusside). The xanthine oxidase inhibitor, folate, and the hydroxyl radical scavenger, mannitol, were uniformly administered. Drugs causing splanchnic vasoconstriction (e.g., epinephrine, norepinephrine, Neo-Synephrine [phenylephrine HCl]) were only used to treat severe systemic hypotension (mean arterial pressure <55 mm Hg). We observed a significant reduction in the incidence of multiple organ system failures per patient (1.9 ± 0.4 to 0.9 ± 0.2; p = 0.02), length of ICU stay (35 ± 9 to 18 ± 4 days; p = 0.03), and total hospital stay (51 ± 12 to 29 ± 5 days; p = 0.03) in patients with persistent gastric intramucosal acidosis who were administered agents that increased splanchnic perfusion and that were intended to prevent free radical damage during reperfusion. We conclude that efforts to correct gastrointestinal intramucosal acidosis related to splanchnic hypoperfusion are warranted because multiple organ system failure and mortality were increased in those patients whose pHi never corrected (i.e., pHi <7.25).

THE MONITORING PLAN

A tonometer is comprised of a semipermeable silicone balloon connected to a sampling tube for tonometry, which means the measurement of fluid or vapor pressure. Tonometry was first used by Bergofsky[67] and Dawson and others[68] in 1964 to demonstrate that the gas tension within a hollow viscus approximates that within the mucosa of the viscus. Grum and Fidian-Green[20] extended this concept to the intestinal tract of adults, and Antonnson and others[69] and Hartmann and colleagues[70] performed validation studies demonstrating that both the stomach and small intestine could be used as suitable sites to measure intraluminal P_{CO_2}. They confirmed that intraluminal P_{CO_2} equalled that measured within the intestinal mucosa as well as approximated hepatic vein P_{CO_2}. Moreover, it has been validated that the intramucosal P_{CO_2} rises and falls in parallel with changes in P_{CO_2} in arterial blood.[71] This indirect method of measuring the pH within the intestinal mucosa is based on the fact that CO_2 is a highly permeable gas and on the assumption that this generated CO_2 is the end result of ATP hydrolysis, with neutralization of generated hydrogen ions by intestinal interstitial bicarbonate.[25]

The tonometer balloon permits fluid to be placed into the lumen of gut (stomach, small intestine, or colon) for a sufficient period for the P_{CO_2} in the fluid to equilibrate with the P_{CO_2} in the superficial layers of the mucosa. A dual purpose product—a tonometer in combination with a standard vented gastric sump—is commercially available (TRIP NGS Catheter, Instrumentarium Corp., Helsinki, Finland). The tonometer balloon is primed with normal saline to eliminate air before insertion. Priming involves introduction of normal saline, pointing the tip of the catheter down so that air rises to the top of the balloon in proximity to the connecting tube and aspirating the air first and then saline. It may be necessary to repeat this step until all air is eliminated. Before insertion, the remaining saline is completely aspirated. The catheter is then advanced into the stomach in a manner similar to any nasogastric tube. Next, 2.5 mL of saline is infused into the balloon. Time is allowed for equilibration. The time allowed for equilibration of P_{CO_2} between the superficial layers of the gastric mucosa and the tonometer balloon is called the equilibration period. The tonometer P_{CO_2} is multiplied by an equilibration factor based on the equilibration period to derive the tissue P_{CO_2} value.

The tonometer, however, cannot determine how or where the intraluminal CO_2 is generated. CO_2 can be generated from the buffering of free hydrogen ions by bicarbonate present in either the superficial mucus layer of the stomach lining, or in duodenal–biliopancreatic secretions refluxed into the stomach; both raise the intraluminal CO_2 and increase the P_{CO_2} within the silicone balloon.[71–74] Subsequently, calculation of pHi will be falsely low because the elevated P_{CO_2} is in the denominator of the equation and lowers the quotient. This artifact can be mitigated by administering an H_2 receptor antagonist, a proton pump inhibitor (e.g., omeprazole), or by using a dilute antacid lavage (see later) before obtaining a balloon saline sample for analysis.[75,76] Critically ill patients often still secrete gastric acid. The low pHi calculated from intraluminally generated P_{CO_2} in the hemodynamically stable patient with no signs of compensated shock may represent complete resuscitation with gastric acidity reflecting normal function (i.e., "the low pHi of good health").[74] Hydrogen ion secretion can be detected by measuring the intragastric pH, just as in stress ulcer prophylaxis protocols. If the pH is less than 4.5, acid is being secreted and should be blocked before interpreting the pHi as "low."

The measurement of pHi depends also on the assumption that the bicarbonate concentration in the wall of the organ is the same as that which is delivered to it by arterial blood, and that the dissociation constant (pK) is the same as that in the plasma. Using the Henderson-Hasselbach equation, pHi is calculated as follows:

$$pHi = 6.1 + \log(HCO_3^-/0.03 \times P_{CO_2})$$

pKa is 6.1, and 0.03 is the solubility coefficient for CO_2. The pK in plasma is not the same as that in the cytosol, but the value 6.1 is the best approximation of the pK within the intestinal fluid of the superficial layers of the mucosa.[14,77,78]

Although the premise of equilibrium between luminal and mucosal P_{CO_2} is accepted, the assumption of equality between mucosal and arterial bicarbonate remains disputed.[79,81] Cunningham and others[82] in 1987 simultaneously measured the ileal pHi of the anesthetized pig using the balloon tonometer and a glass pH microelectrode. During a 16-minute period of partial or total mesenteric occlusion and after the injection of *Escherichia coli* endotoxin, tonometrically calculated pHi was greater than the microelectrode measured pHi. Both methods, however, yielded similar pHi values during the 2 hours after release of occlusion. The disparity of pHi measurements was concluded to reflect depletion of interstitial bicarbonate during low or no flow states, such that the arterial bicarbonate overestimated mucosal bicarbonate. Benjamin and associates[80,81] also contend that correction of systemic acidemia by the intravenous administration of sodium bicarbonate or employing hyperventilation can lead to complete normalization of the calculated pHi, even in the presence of advanced gastrointestinal ischemia. The assumption that the interstitial bicarbonate in the stomach mucosa is the same as that in the arterial blood may also be invalid during stimulation of gastric acid secretion when an alkaline tide may be generated. This potential source of error can be avoided by blocking gastric acid secretion. Antacid administration can also induce a local tissue alkalosis, masking an actual tissue acidosis. No data regarding the effect of sucralfate on tonometric reading of mucosal PCO_2 are available. These data have been used by both proponents and detractors of tonometry to validate or to impute the validity of the technique. However, despite these potential sources of error, indirect pHi measurements correlate remarkably well with measurements made by direct puncture.[14,19,77]

The concern that intestinal pHi reflects ischemia-associated metabolic acidosis or simply CO_2 produced by aerobic metabolism was investigated experimentally by Schlichtig and Bowles.[83] They subjected dogs to progressive decreases in intestinal blood flow and measured pHi, oxygen delivery, oxygen consumption, and arterial–mixed venous pH and PCO_2 differences. They found that oxygen delivery less than the minimum capable of sustaining aerobic metabolism coincided with decreased pHi. Furthermore, pHi paralleled the onset of critical $\dot{D}O_2$ implying that decreases in intestinal pHi during progressive flow reduction was also associated with the onset of tissue metabolic acidosis. These findings were corroborated by Antonnson and coworkers[19] in the anesthetized pig. Landow and associates[54] found statistically significant correlations between gastric pHi obtained during cardiopulmonary bypass surgery and hepatic venous lactate, PCO_2, and pHa (r^2 was 0.5, 0.58, and 0.32 respectively).

TROUBLE SHOOTING

Measurement of saline PCO_2 can be an important source of error in the assessment of gastric pHi and depends on both the analyzer and measured intraluminal PCO_2.[84] The pHi calculated by different analyzers may not be the same.[77] These errors are eliminated by using a dedicated analyzer; however, not all manufacturers produce analyzers that produce valid results. A change in gastric pHi of 0.06 pH units can be detected by most analyzers in the clinically relevant PCO_2 range. Calibrated CO_2 containing saline can be used to verify the precision and accuracy of the analyzer. Ten to 20 ampules at three different PCO_2 levels should be used to calibrate the correct and dedicated blood gas analyzer.

The importance of proper handling of the saline sample cannot be overemphasized. The sample should be transported on ice and analyzed immediately, because the capacity of saline to dissolve CO_2 is low. CO_2 lost from the sample during handling and analysis will not be measured, and therefore, the remaining CO_2 measured will lead to overestimation of pHi (the denominator will be falsely low and the quotient falsely high).

If a low pHi value is considered to be inconsistent with the patient's overall clinical picture, the position of the tonometer balloon should be checked and an attempt made to drain the stomach manually. If still in doubt, exclude

factitious PCO_2 generation by administering an H_2 receptor blocker with or without a proton pump inhibitor (e.g., omeprazole) or perform a dilute antacid lavage. The measurement should then be repeated. The antacid lavage we employ consists of a dilute concentration of aluminum or magnesium hydroxide (60 mL suspended in 200 mL of water). The suspension is allowed to dwell in the stomach for 20 minutes and then is aspirated. Hydroxide neutralization of luminal hydrogen ions produces water, not CO_2 as the end result. Verify elimination of intragastric acid by measuring intraluminal pH before accepting a low pHi value to avoid overtreatment based on an artifactually lowered value. However, if the pHi is truly low and the clinical picture is suggestive, the concept of hemodynamically compensated shock must be recognized, which is the fundamental reason for monitoring pHi.

In summary, to minimize errors in pHi monitoring, we recommend the following guidelines:

1. Use the same (dedicated) blood gas analyzer for all pHi determinations, making sure that the type has been validated.
2. Place balloon saline PCO_2 samples on ice, send them to the laboratory, and analyze them immediately after sampling.
3. Adopt a standard written protocol, including potential errors and corrective measures, using a data collection format.
4. Discontinue enteral feeding before PCO_2 sampling.
5. Discontinue suction and clamp the sump port for at least 30 minutes before sampling.
6. Delay sampling for at least 2 hours after intravenous bicarbonate infusion.
7. Do not monitor pHi after pyloric ablation or bypass surgery or in the presence of significant intragastric bleeding.
8. Maintain intragastric pH above 4.5, monitoring with either litmus pH paper or indwelling pH probe, checked simultaneously with each aspirated tonometer saline sample.[85]
9. Administer a H_2 receptor blocker or proton pump inhibitor throughout the monitoring period.

WHO SHOULD BE MONITORED?

Intramucosal pH provides an intermittent measure of the ability of tissues to resynthesize high-energy phosphate compounds utilizing aerobic metabolism. In dysoxic states, protons accumulate and pHi falls, indicative of inadequate oxidative metabolism. If this is recognized and can be reversed, the clinician may be able to prevent or limit the duration of compensated shock. Global measurements of oxygen delivery, oxygen consumption, oxygen extraction ratio, and mixed venous blood hemoglobin oxygen saturation ($S\bar{v}O_2$) are unsatisfactory for this purpose.[75,77] The calculation of pHi can provide clinicians with a metabolic endpoint that may be used to determine whether the milieu is likely to create a reperfusion injury if resuscitation is successful or whether subclinical maldistribution of blood flow persists—a reflection of a still-active neurohumoral response to stress.

Monitoring all patients likely to have had activation of the neurohumeral response and decreased splanchnic blood flow is probably beneficial because they are at risk for a reperfusion injury, multiple organ system failure, and a higher mortality rate.[77] Outcome can be improved by preventing ischemia-reperfusion injury and ensuring that intramucosal acidosis is promptly reversed. Recognize that the window of opportunity for effective therapy is early.[75] Both a preemptive intervention to block and modify the ischemia-reperfusion injury and restoration of splanchnic perfusion must be incorporated into a resuscitation algorithm to reduce the incidence of bacterial translocation and systemic white cell priming before the ensuing systemic inflammatory response.[1] Because early abnormalities in the gastrointestinal intramucosa act as a marker of mortality and morbidity, efforts to correct them may improve outcome and should diminish resource utilization.[86,87] If pHi falls unexpectedly (the canary), look for intraabdominal catastrophes, intraabdominal hypertension, sepsis, tissue necrosis, line sepsis, nosocomial infection, unappreciated excess patient ventilatory work, hypovolemia, and hypoxemia.[64,86,89–91]

APPROACH TO THERAPY

The limited success thus far that has attended attempts to elevate an already depressed pHi and an understanding of the importance of the ischemia-reperfusion injury as a fundamental part of both the gut starter and gut motor hypotheses suggest that a new perspective is needed. Two separate elements must be combined: a preemptive intervention to prevent the ischemia-reperfusion injury in high-risk patients, and restoration of oxidative high-energy phosphate synthesis as judged by a normalizing pHi. As an approach to preventing intramucosal acidosis and ischemic gut mucosal injury, we suggest the following goals: (1) increase global oxygen delivery; (2) increase splanchnic flow; (3) affect ischemia-reperfusion injury by preventing or neutralizing free radicals generation, binding endotoxin, blocking PAF activation, "unpriming" PMNs, and stopping the cytokine cascade before it starts; and (4) judge reversal of ischemia and anaerobic metabolism by restoration of normal pHi—an abnormal pHi is the marker for free radical production.[9,26,32,49,50,92–94]

To increase global oxygen delivery, use isotonic fluids, albumin solutions, and red blood cells. Use high inspired oxygen tensions during resuscitation. Avoid epinephrine or alpha agents, which cause splanchnic vasoconstriction. This also means "tolerating" a lower mean arterial pressure, perhaps 60 mm Hg if there is satisfactory end-organ perfusion. Use vasodilators such as isoproterenol, dobutamine, nicardipine (also a calcium channel blocker), nitroglycerin, nitroprusside, prostaglandin E, or prostacyclin to increase splanchnic flow.[40,95–98] Reperfusion injury can be attenuated by blocking free radical generation with folate or allopurinol and administering free radical scavengers such as albumin, mannitol, vitamin C, vitamin A, and vitamin E.[34,36] Injury

related to PLA_2 activity may be ameliorated by quinacrine, lidocaine, allopurinol, and steroids,[50,99–101] and intracellular calcium content may decreased by calcium channel blockers such as diltiazem and nicardipine, as well as with lidocaine, which binds calcium in cell membranes. Moreover, lidocaine, vitamin C, and vitamin E stabilize cell membranes and prevent increased capillary permeability.

Glutamine has been implicated as sustaining mucosal architecture and function by scavenging free radicals and preventing lipid peroxidation. In addition, glutamine combines with acetyl cystine to form glutathione.[35] In the reaction catalyzed by the selenium containing enzyme, glutathione peroxidase, glutathione is transformed to oxidized glutathione. This then combines with hydrogen peroxide and degrades it to water, preventing hydrogen peroxide from reacting with superoxide to produce a hydroxyl radical. N-acetyl cystine has been reported to favorably affect indirect indicators of tissue oxygenation,[102] perhaps because it is a precursor of glutathione.

Lidocaine has many actions that may be beneficial in preventing reperfusion injury. It has been shown to inhibit the activation of PLA_2, to bind calcium in cell membranes, to decrease capillary permeability, to stop cytokine release from macrophage and PMNs, to block PAF activation, and, finally, to unprime PMNs.[100,101] Hydrocortisone has been implicated in decreasing cytokine release from primed macrophages. Occasionally patients have an inadequate steroid response to stress and an appropriate daily stress dose of glucocorticoid (e.g., 300 mg of hydrocortisone) should be administered. Polymixin B avidly binds endotoxin; in fact, it is used in industry to clear endotoxin during production of various medical devices. Finally, albumin is another free radical scavenger and may have a place in trauma resuscitation if prior therapy can prevent increased capillary permeability. A solution of 5% albumin would then be an effective plasma volume expander while binding free radicals. The iron-dependent reactions can be blocked by deferoxamine, a chelating agent; however, unless it forms a complex with hydroxyethyl starch, its duration of action is too short and its incidence of hypotension has been too great to justify use in patients.[33,50,103]

FUTURE INVESTIGATIONS

Although pHi monitoring has been tested in several clinical applications, fundamental questions remain: Has secreted gastric acid generated CO_2 resulting in a low pHi? What value should be used as the cutoff between low and normal? Should pHi be used to initiate therapy, or represent an end point? At least in the last question, the available data suggest that intervention to prevent the ischemia-reperfusion injury should not wait for an abnormal pHi. Restoration of a normal pHi could be valuable as a marker for the restoration of oxidative metabolism. It is likely that this technique can be used to assess organ preservation and function, as an early prognostic sign for severe acute pancreatitis or to detect complications like pancreatic necrosis. Gastric tonometry may be useful in identifying those critically ill patients who are able to tolerate enteral feedings[14] and conventional weaning from ventilatory support.[86,104]

Because the calculated pHi value markedly depends on the blood gas analyzer used, the proper handling and transport of samples, and eliminating factitious intraluminal CO_2 generation, the use of detailed protocols, which delineate sources of error and their prevention, are important for any multicenter study. Measuring the Po_2 may help assess the accuracy of the saline Pco_2 measurement. Intramucosal Po_2 should be lower than arterial Po_2 because the Po_2 in the lumen reflects the Po_2 in the mucosa, which is less than arterial Po_2. If the saline Po_2 is higher, the Pco_2 is likely to be erroneous. The equilibrium characteristics of Po_2 across the silicone balloon have not been fully characterized and this presents a problem, particularly when equilibration times are less than 90 minutes.

Any ischemia-reperfusion regimen should consist of elements that are relatively inexpensive, essentially nontoxic, can be combined in a multiprong attack, and which will block the pathways of reperfusion injury that sets the stage for the long-term, high-morbidity, high-mortality, and multiple organ system failure. These conditions are necessary because the protocol should be initiated if there is any clinical suspicion that the neurohumoral response has been activated (i.e., is the stress greater than a cholecystectomy?). The neurohumoral response is activated if there has been an Advanced Trauma Life Support Class 2 hemorrhage (1000 mL or more). Initiation of the protocol in the trauma resuscitation area, surgical emergency room, or operating room should be done as soon as this level of insult has occurred. Finally, intraluminal oxygenation may be beneficial in preventing the development of intestinal mucosal injury and may possess some therapeutic promise.[105] Intraluminal balloonless air tonometry remains investigational but may eliminate many of the problems with intermittent saline sampling.[106]

REFERENCES ■

1. Fiddian-Green RG: Association between intramucosal acidosis in the gut and organ failure. *Crit Care Med* 1993;21:S103
2. Fiddian-Green RG: Should measurements of tissue pH and Po_2 be included in the routine monitoring of intensive care unit patients? *Crit Care Med* 1991;19:141
3. Shoemaker W, Appel PL, Kram HB, et al: Prospective trial of supra normal values of survivors as therapeutic goals in high-risk surgical patients. *Chest* 1988;94:1176
4. Tuchschmidt J, Fried J, Astiz M, et al: Elevation of cardiac output and oxygen delivery improves outcome in septic shock. *Chest* 1992;102:210
5. Moore FA, Haenel JB, Moore EE, et al: Incommensurate oxygen consumption in response to maximal oxygen availability predicts post-injury multiple organ failure. *J Trauma* 1992;33:58
6. Boyd O, Grounds M, Bennett ED: A randomized clinical trial of the effect of deliberate perioperative increase of oxygen delivery on mortality in high risk surgical patients. *JAMA* 1993;270:2699
7. Gutierrez G: Cellular energy metabolism during hypoxia. *Crit Care Med* 1991;19:619
8. Gutierrez G, Bismar H, Dantzker DR, et al: Comparison of gastric intramucosal pH with measure of oxygen transport and consumption in critically ill patients. *Crit Care Med* 1992;20:451
9. Fiddian-Green RG, Haglund U, Gutierrez G, et al: Goals for resuscitation of shock. *Crit Care Med* 1993;21:S25
10. Hayes MA, Timmins AC, Yau EHS, et al: Elevation of systemic oxygen delivery in the treatment of critically ill patients. *N Engl J Med* 1994;330:1717
11. Steltzer H, Hiesmayr M, Mayer N, et al: The relationship between oxygen delivery and uptake in the critically ill: is there a critical or optimal therapeutic value? *Anesthesia* 1994;49:229
12. Ronco JJ, Fenwick JC, Tweeddale MG, et al: Identification of the critical oxygen delivery for anaerobic metabolism in critically ill septic and non-septic humans. *JAMA* 1993;270:1724
13. Ronco JJ, Fenwick JC, Wiggs BR, et al: Oxygen consumption is independent of increases in oxygen delivery by dobutamine in septic patients who have normal or increased plasma lactate levels. *Am Rev Respir Dis* 1993;147:25
14. Fiddian-Green RG: Studies in splanchnic ischemia and multiple organ failure. In: Marston A, Bulkley GR, Fiddian-Green RG, et al (eds). *Splanchnic Ischemia and Multiple Organ Failure*. London, Edward Arnold/St Louis, CV Mosby, 1989:349
15. Gutierrez G: Regional blood flow and oxygen transport: implications for the therapy of the septic patient. *Crit Care Med* 1993;21:1263
16. Dantzker D: The gastrointestinal tract: the canary of the body? *JAMA* 1993;270:1247
17. Hjelmquist B, Teder H, Borgstrom A, et al: Indomethacin and pancreatic blood flow. *Acta Chir Scand* 1990;156:543
18. Stephenson RB: The splanchnic circulation. In: Patton HD, Fuchs AF, Hille B, Scher AM, et al (eds). *The Textbook of Physiology*, ed 21, vol 2, no 46. Philadelphia, WB Saunders, 1989:911
19. Antonsson JB, Kuttila K, Niinikoski J, et al: Subcutaneous and gut tissue perfusion and oxygenation changes are related to oxygen transport in experimental peritonitis. *Circ Shock* 1993;41:261
20. Grum CM, Fiddian-Green RG, Pittenger GL, et al: Adequacy of tissue oxygenation in intact dog intestine. *J Appl Physiol* 1984;56:1065
21. Hotchkiss RS, Karl IE: Re-evaluation of the role of cellular hypoxia and bioenergetic failure in sepsis. *JAMA* 1992;267:1503
22. Silverman HJ, Tuma P: Gastric tonometry in patients with sepsis: effects of dobutamine infusions and packed red blood cell transfusions. *Chest* 1992;102:184
23. Grum CM, Simon RH, Dantzker DR, et al: Evidence for adenosine tri-phosphate degradation in critically ill patients. *Chest* 1985;88:763
24. Gutierrez G, Andry JM: Nuclear magnetic resonance measurements: clinical applications. *Crit Care Med* 1989;17:73
25. Grum CM: Tissue oxygenation in low flow states during hypoxemia. *Crit Care Med* 1993;21:S44
26. Fink MD, Kaups KL, Wang H, et al: Maintenance of superior mesenteric arterial perfusion prevents increased intestinal mucosal permeability in endotoxic pits. *Surgery* 1991;110:154
27. Fink MD, Antonsson JB, Wang et al: Increased intestinal permeability in endotoxic pigs: mesenteric hypoperfusion on an etiologic factor. *Arch Surg* 1991;126:211

28. Haglund UH: Myocardial depressant factors. In: Marston A, Bulkley GB, Fiddian-Green RG, et al (eds). *Splanchnic Ischemia and Multiple Organ Failure*. London, Edward Arnold/St Louis, CV Mosby, 1989:229

29. Gutierrez G, Pohil RJ: Oxygen consumption is linearly related to O_2 supply in critically ill patients. *J Crit Care* 1986;1:45

30. Otani H, Prasad MR, Jones RM, et al: Mechanism of membrane phospholipid degradation in ischemic-reperfused rat hearts. *Am J Physiol* 1989;257:H252

31. Otamiri T, Tagesson C: Role of phospholipase A_2 and oxygenated free radicals in mucosal damage after small intestinal ischemia and reperfusion. *Am J Surg* 1989;157:562

32. Flynn WJ, Hoover EL: Allopurinol plus standard resuscitation preserves hepatic blood flow and function following hemorrhage shock. *Trauma* 1994;37:956

33. Hernandez LA, Grisham MB, Granger DN: A role for iron in oxidant-mediated ischemic injury to intestinal microvasculature. *Am J Physiol* 1987;253:G49

34. Grace RA: Ischemia-reperfusion injury. *Br J Surg* 1994;81:637

35. Zimmerman JJ: Therapeutic application of oxygen radical scavengers. *Chest* 1991;100:S190

36. Granger DN, McCord JM, Parks DA, et al: Xanthine oxidase inhibition attenuate ischemia-induced vascular permeability changes in the cat intestine. *Gastroenterology* 1986;90:80

37. Haglund U: Intramucosal pH. *Intensive Care Med* 1994;20:90

38. Steffes CP, Dahn MS, Lange MP: Oxygen transport-dependent splanchnic metabolism in the sepsis syndrome. *Arch Surg* 1994;129:46

39. Mark PE: Gastric intramucosal pH: a better predictor of multiorgan dysfunction syndrome and death than oxygen-derived variables in patients with sepsis. *Chest* 1993;104:225

40. Marik PE, Mohedin M: The contrasting effects of dopamine and norepinephrine on systemic and splanchnic oxygen utilization in hyperdynamic sepsis. *JAMA* 1994;272:1354

41. Bishop MH, Shoemaker WC, Appel PL, et al: Relationship between supranormal circulatory values, time delays, and outcome in severely traumatized patients. *Crit Care Med* 1993;21:56

42. Abramson D, Scalea TM, Hitchcock R, et al: Lactate clearance and survival following injury. *J Trauma* 1993;35:584

43. Carrico CJ, Meakins JL, Marshall JC, et al: Multiple organ failure syndrome. *Arch Surg* 1986;121:196

44. Deitch EA: Overview of multiple organ failure: state of the art. *Crit Care Med* 1993;4:131

45. Marshall JC, Christou NV, Meakins JL: The gastrointestinal tract: the undrained abscess of multiple organ failure. *Am Surg* 1993;218:111

46. Marshall JC, Christou NV, Horn R, et al: The microbiology of multiple organ failure. *Arch Surg* 1988;123:309

47. Meakins JL, Marshall JC: The gut as the monitor of multiple system organ failure. In: Martson A, Bulkley G, Fiddian-Green RG, et al (eds). *Splanchnic Ischemia and Multiple Organ Failure*. London, Edward Arnold/St Louis, CV Mosby, 1989:339

48. Cerra FB, Maddaus MA, Dunn DL, et al: Selective gut decontamination reduces nosocomial infection and length of stay but not mortality or organ failure in surgical intensive care patients. *Arch Surg* 1992;127:163

49. Moore EE, Moore FA, Franciose RJ, et al: The post ischemic gut serves as a priming bed for circulating neutrophils that provoke multiple organ failure. *J Trauma* 1994;37:881

50. Xu D, Lu Q, Deitch EA: Calcium and phospholipase A_2 appear to be involved in the pathogenesis of hemorrhagic shock-induced mucosal injury and bacterial translocation. *Crit Care Med* 1995;23:125

51. Fiddian-Green RG, McGough E, Pittenger G, et al: Predictive value of intramucosal pH and other risk factors for massive bleeding from stress ulceration. *Gastroenterology* 1983;85:613

52. Fiddian-Green RG, Baker S: Predictive value of the stomach wall pH for complications after cardiac operations: comparison with other monitoring. *Crit Care Med* 1987;15:153

53. Guys T, Hubens A, Neels H, et al: Prognostic value of gastric intramural pH in surgical intensive care patients. *Crit Care Med* 1988;16:1222

54. Landow L, Phillips DA, Heard SO, et al: Gastric tonometry and venous oximetry in cardiac surgery patients. *Crit Care Med* 1991;19:1226

55. Fiddian-Green RG, Amelin P, Herman JB, et al: Prediction of the development of sigmoid ischemia on the day of aortic operations: indirect measurements of intramural pH in the colon. *Arch Surg* 1986;121:654

56. Björck M, Hedberg B: Early detection of major complications after abdominal aortic surgery: predictive value of sigmoid colon and gastric intramucosal pH monitoring. *Br J Surg* 1994;81:25

57. Schiedler MG, Cultler BS, Fiddian-Green RG: Sigmoid intramucosal pH for prediction of ischemic colitis during aorta surgery. *Arch Surg* 1987;122:881

58. Doglio GR, Pusajo JF, Egurrola MA, et al: Gastric mucosal pH as a prognostic index of mortality in critically ill patients. *Crit Care Med* 1991;19:1037

59. Maynard N, Bihari D, Beale R, et al: Assessment of splanchnic oxygenation by gastric tonometry in patients with acute circulatory failure. *JAMA* 1993;270:1203

60. Frenette L, Doblar DD, Singer D, et al: The value of gastric intramucosal pH as an indicator of early allograft viability in liver transplant. *Transplantation* 1994;58:292

61. Chang MC, Cheatham ML, Nelson LD, et al: Gastric tonometry supplements information provided by systemic indicators of oxygen transport. *J Trauma* 1994;37:488

62. Rouman RM, Ureugde JPC, Goris JA: Gastric tonometry in multiple trauma patients. *J Trauma* 1994;36:313

63. Gutierrez G, Palizas F, Doglio G, et al: Gastric intramucosal pH as a therapeutic index of tissue oxygenation in critically ill patients. *Lancet* 1992;339:195

64. Ivatury RR, Simon RJ, Havriliak D, et al: Gastric mucosal pH and oxygen delivery and consumption indices in the assessment of adequacy of resuscitation after trauma: a prospective, randomized study. *J Trauma* 1995;39:1

65. Kirton OC, Windsor J, Civetta JM, et. al: Failure of splanchnic resuscitation in the acutely injured trauma patient correlates with multiple organ system failure and death in the intensive care unit. *Chest* 1995;108:104S

66. Kirton OC, Windsor J, Lynn M, et al: Persistent uncorrected intramucosal pH (pHi) in the critically injured: the impact of splanchnic and antioxidant therapy. *J Trauma* 1995;39:1221

67. Bergofsky EH: Determination of tissue O_2 tensions by hollow visceral tonometers: effect of breathing enriched O_2. *J Clin Invest* 1964;43:193

68. Dawson AM, Trenchard D, Guz A: Small bowel tonometry: assessment of small gut mucosal oxygen tension in dog and man. *Nature* 1965;206:943

69. Antonsson JB, Boyle CC, Kruithoff KL, et al: Validation of tonometric measurement of gut intramural pH during endotoxemia and mesenteric occlusion in pigs. *Am J Physiol* 1990;259:G519

70. Hartmann M, Montgomery A, Jonsson K, et al: Tissue oxygenation in hemorrhagic shock measured as transcutaneous oxygen tension, subcutaneous oxygen tension and gastrointestinal pH in pigs. *Crit Care Med* 1991;19:205

71. Stevens MH, Thirlby RC, Feldman M: Mechanism for high pCO_2 in gastric juice: Roles of bicarbonate secretion and CO_2 diffusion. *Am J Physiol* 1987;253:G527

72. Fiddian-Green RG, Pittenger G, Whitehouse WM: Back diffusion of CO_2 and its influence on the intramucosal pH in gastric mucosa. *J Surg Res* 1982;33:39

73. Dalenback J, Olbe L, Sjovall H: Hypovolemia-induced cardiovascular effects on human gastric mucosal acid and HCO_3 release. *Scand J Gastroenterol* 1994;29:595

74. Heard SO: Gastric tonometry in healthy volunteers: effect of ranitidine on calculated intramural pH. *Crit Care Med* 1991;19:27

75. Gutierrez G, Brown SD: Gastric tonometry: a new monitoring modality in the Intensive Care Unit. *J Intensive Care Med* 1995;10:33

76. Kolkman JJ, Groeneveld ABJ, Meuwissen SGM: The effect of ranitidine on basal and bicarbonate enhanced intragastric pCO_2: a tonometric study. *Gut* 1994;35:737

77. Fiddian-Green RG: Tonometry: theory and applications. *Intensive Care World* 1992;9:60

78. Rasmussen LB, Haglund ULF: Early gut ischemia in experimental fecal peritonitis. *Circ Shock* 1992;38:22

79. Shijie, S, Weil WH, Wanchung T, et al: Gastric intramucosal bicarbonate: limitations of the tonometry method. *Crit Care Med* 1992;20:S66

80. Benjamin E, N'Fonoyim JM, Hannon EM, et al: Effects of systemic metabolic alkalosis on gastrointestinal tonometry. *Crit Care Med* 1992;20:S65

81. Benjamin E, Polokoff E, Oropello JM: Sodium bicarbonate administration affects the diagnostic accuracy of gastrointestinal tonometry in acute mesenteric ischemia. *Crit Care Med* 1992;20:1181

82. Cunningham JA, Cousar CD, Joffin E: Extraluminal and intraluminal pCO_2 levels in the ischemic intestines of rats. *Curr Surg* 1987;44:229

83. Schlichtig R, Bowles S: Distinguishing between aerobic and anaerobic appearance of dissolved CO_2 in intestine during low flow. *J Appl Physiol* 1994;76:2443

84. Takala J, Parviainen I, Siloaho M, et al: Saline pCO_2 is an important source of error in the assessment of gastric intramucosal pH. *Crit Care Med* 1994;22:1877

85. Meiners D, Clift S, Kaminski D: Evaluation of various techniques to monitor intragastric pH. *Arch Surg* 1982;117:288

86. Fiddian-Green RG: Tonometry: clinical use and cost implications. *Intensive Care World* 1992;9:130

87. Mythen MG, Webb AR: Intraoperative gut mucosal hypoperfusion is associated with increased post-operative complications and cost. *Intensive Care Med* 1994;20:99

88. Bendahan J, Cotezee CJ, Papagianopoulous C, et al: Abdominal compartment syndrome. *J Trauma* 1995;38:152

89. Diebel L, Saxe J, Dulchavsky S: Effect of intraabdominal pressure on abdominal wall blood flow. *Am Surg* 1992;58:573

90. Diebel LN, Dulchavsky SA, Wilson RF: Effect of increased intraabdominal pressure on mesenteric arterial and intestinal mucosal blood flow. *J Trauma* 1992;33:45

91. Pusajo JE, Bumaschny E, Agurrola A, et al: Postoperative intraabdominal pressure: its relation to splanchnic perfusion, sepsis, multiple organ failure and surgical reintervention. *Intensive Crit Care Dig* 1994;13:2

92. Yee JB, McJames SW: Use of gastric intramucosal pH as a monitor during hemorrhagic shock. *Circ Shock* 1994;43:44

93. Mythen MG, Webb AR: Perioperative plasma volume expansion reduces the incidence of gut mucosal hypoperfusion during cardiac surgery. *Arch Surg* 1995;130:423

94. Gutierrez G, Clark C, Brown S, et al: Effect of dobutamine on oxygen consumption and gastric mucosal pH in septic patients. *Am J Respir Crit Care Med* 1994;150:324

95. Smithies J, Tai-Hwei Y, Jackson L, et al: Protecting the gut and the liver in the critically ill: effects of dopexamine. *Crit Care Med* 1994;22:789

96. Cullen JJ, Ephgrave KS, Broadhurst KA, et al: Captopril decreases stress ulceration without affecting gastric perfusion during canine hemorrhagic shock. *J Trauma* 1994;37:43

97. Hannemann L, Reinhart K, Meier-Hellmann A, et al: Prostacyclin in septic shock. *Chest* 1994;105:1504

98. Boyd O, Grounds M, Bennet ED: The use of dopexamine hydrochloride to increase oxygen delivery perioperatively. *Anesth Analg* 1993;76:372

99. Boros M, Karacsony G, Kaszaki J, et al: Reperfusion mucosal damage after complete intestinal ischemia in the dog: the effects of antioxidant and phospholipase A2 inhibitor therapy. *Surgery* 1993;113:184

100. Mikawa K, Maekawa N, Nishina K, et al: Effect of lidocaine pretreatment on endotoxin-induced lung injury in rabbits. *Anesthesiology* 1994;81:689

101. Sasagawas S: Inhibitory effects of local anesthetics on migration, extracellular release of lysosomal enzyme and superoxide anion production in human polymorphonuclear leukocytes. *Immunopharmacol Immunotoxicol* 1991;13:607

102. Spies CD, Reinhart K, Witt I, et al: Influence of N-acetylcysteine on indirect indicators of tissue oxygenation in septic shock patients: results from a prospective, randomized double-blind study. *Crit Care Med* 1994;22:1738

103. Lelli JL, Pradhan S, Cobb LM: Prevention of post ischemic injury in immature intestine by deferoxamine. *J Surg Res* 1993;54:34

104. Mohsenifar Z, Hay A, Hay J, et al: Gastric intramucosal pH as a predictor of success or failure in weaning patients from mechanical ventilation. *Ann Intern Med* 1993;119:794

105. Haglund U: Therapeutic potential of intraluminal oxygenation. *Crit Care Med* 1993;21:S69

106. Salzman AL, Strong KE, Wang H, et al: Intraluminal balloonless air tonometry: a new method for determination of gastrointestinal mucosal carbon dioxide tension. *Crit Care Med* 1994;22:126

Critical Care, Third Edition, edited by Joseph M. Civetta,
Robert W. Taylor, and Robert R. Kirby.
Lippincott-Raven Publishers, Philadelphia, PA © 1997.

CHAPTER 31

Enteral and Parenteral Nutrition

Patricia M. Byers

K. N. Jeejeebhoy

IMMEDIATE CONCERNS

MAJOR PROBLEMS

Critical illness precipitates a metabolic environment of increased expenditure and protein turnover. Due to the increased metabolic needs of the critically ill, enteral feedings should be initiated within 24 hours of admittance to the ICU whenever possible. Parenteral support should be administered to all patients who will not tolerate an enteral regimen within 5 days of initiating their fast. Patients should be selected based on available predictive models, number of anticipated ventilator days, or fasting prior to ICU entry. Care is simplified when enteral access of the jejunum is obtained intraoperatively. Elemental feedings can be initiated postoperatively at 10–25 cc^3/hour depending on the extent of surgery, resuscitation, edema, or distention.

STRESS POINTS

1. Protein and energy requirements should be met without overfeeding to avoid complications. The initial dosage of protein should be between 1.5 and 2.5 g/kg of ideal body weight/day, with at least half of it as enteral support whenever possible. Energy requirements can be estimated by calculating the basal energy expenditure (BEE) by the Harris-Benedict Equation and multiplying it by 1.1 to 1.4, by giving 25 kcal/kg/day, or by calculating protein requirements and deriving energy needs from a calorie to nitrogen ration of 100 to 1.
2. In patients with energy deficits, Na$^+$ administration

should be limited and supplemental phosphorus, potassium, and magnesium should be given.
3. Gastrointestinal access should be selected based on short-term goals of nutritional therapy, GI function, and whether or not long-term support is anticipated. Enteral formulas should be selected with considerations of cost, absorptive capacity, and potential risk of infections.
4. Patients with renal or hepatic insufficiency require special attention to feeding volumes and composition.
5. Intestinal volvulus and idiopathic gangrene are catastrophic complications of jejunostomy tubes.
6. Bronchopulmonary aspiration is most likely during periods of transfer into and out of ICUs.
7. Diarrhea is a frequent complication of tube-fed patients, but is usually caused by factors other than the tube feeding itself. It is important to assess the patient for *Clostridium difficile* infection.
8. Line sepsis and air embolus are two life-threatening complications that can occur in patients on central total parenteral nutrition (TPN).
9. Intestinal mucosal atrophy and cholestasis may occur in patients on TPN.

ESSENTIAL DIAGNOSTIC TESTS/PROCEDURES

1. Nitrogen balance studies and short-term protein markers may be used to determine the adequacy of protein support. Carbohydrate and lipid administration should be monitored with triglyceride levels, blood sugar lev-

457

els, and PCO_2 levels. Patients should not receive more than 4 mg of carbohydrate/kg/min.

2. It is important to monitor patients for refeeding edema, hypophosphatemia, and hypokalemia.

3. Gastric ileus mandates access into the small bowel, with selection of invasive versus noninvasive access based on the patient's condition and anticipated length of therapy. Patients with edema, severe malnutrition, inflammation, and diarrhea may have decreased absorptive capacity.

4. Renal insufficiency may be diagnosed in patients with evidence of uremic symptoms or oliguria. Hepatic failure is usually diagnosed in patients who are jaundiced with evidence of encephalopathy, high ammonia levels, or abnormal prothrombin times.

5. Abdominal radiographs should be performed on patients with obvious abdominal distention. This finding is more significant if there has been a history of hypoperfusion.

6. Blue food coloring in enteral formulas, acute changes in respiratory status, and the presence of new infiltrates on chest radiographs assist in the diagnosis of aspiration.

7. Diarrhea is defined as more than 200g of stool or 3 large liquid stools in a 24-hour period. Stool titers for *Clostridium difficile* should be obtained and all medications should be reviewed as to whether they contain sorbitol or magnesium.

8. To diagnose line sepsis, the subcutaneous segment of the line is sent for quantitative cultures. Fifteen or more colony-forming units per millimeter are diagnostic for line sepsis. Hemodynamic and respiratory deterioration may be secondary to air embolus after inadvertent line disconnection or removal.

9. Cholestasis may be heralded by elevated alkaline phosphatase and perhaps overt jaundice. Intestinal atrophy may be evident at surgery or by decreased absorption with the initiation of enteral feedings.

INITIAL THERAPY

1. Adjust protein administration to achieve a positive nitrogen balance of 2 to 4 gm. In patients with carbohydrate intolerance, decrease kilocalories to a maximum of 20 to 25 kcal/kg/day and supplement with 30% of the calories as fat. In patients with hypertriglyceridemia, decrease the rate of fat administered by half and follow levels.

2. Nutritional support should always include supplementation of phosphorous, potassium, and magnesium in the absence of renal failure.

3. Nasogastric or nasoenteral access is low risk and satisfactory for short-term support. Elemental feedings should be given if decreased absorptive capacity is suspected.

4. Patients with renal insufficiency should be maintained on required nutritional therapy and continuous hemodialfiltration should be initiated as needed. Fluid restriction should be attempted, but not at the cost of nutrient intake. Patients with hepatic failure should receive special hepatic formulas.

5. Tube feedings should be immediately stopped in patients with abdominal distention. These patients should be carefully observed for improvement, and lack of improvement should prompt further diagnostic tests, including exploratory laparotomy.

6. Early recognition, intubation, removal of particulate matter, and antibiotic therapy can decrease morbidity and mortality from aspiration pneumonia.

7. Enteral metronidazole or vancomycin should be given for *Clostridium difficile* colitis. After completion of therapy, titers should be repeated. Meanwhile the patient should be supplemented with the appropriate intravenous nutrition, fluid, and electrolytes.

8. Upon making the diagnosis of line sepsis, the offending line should be removed and the patient started on appropriate antibiotic coverage. If air embolus is suspected, place the patient in Trendelenburg's position with the right side up and attempt to aspirate air if the line is still in place.

9. To avoid gastrointestinal complications of TPN, it is best to infuse small amounts of enteral feedings concomitantly whenever possible.

INTRODUCTION

Nutritional management is an integral part of intensive care and will continue to gain importance as changes in resource allocation concentrate the highest acuity patients in ICUs. Critically ill and injured patients are severely catabolic and hypermetabolic and thus lose significant body mass daily. The understanding and manipulation of this metabolic response has been an important focus of scientific research in the past decade.[1,2]

With the onset of critical illness, there is a metabolic environment of increased catecholamines and cortisol which are felt to orchestrate an increase in resting energy expenditure and protein turnover.[3] With the resultant insulin resistance, there is decreased peripheral use of glucose and an increase in the rates of lipolysis and proteolysis for the provision of amino acid and fatty acid subunits as fuel. Although the amino acid pool is initially expanded, it rapidly becomes depleted of essential amino acids as the high branched chain amino acids are used as fuel in skeletal muscle while large amounts of glutamine are required for metabolic processes in the intestinal mucosa.[4] This catabolic process is perpetuated by the development of intestinal mucosal derangements and cytokine activation.[5] Traditional therapy with parenteral nutrition has not been shown to effectively reverse this condition. For this reason, the exploration of other modalities such as growth hormone therapy, very early enteral feedings, and specialized immunomodulatory enteral formulas has been undertaken.[6] In this chapter we will discuss some of the new approaches to nutritional support which are currently available. Additionally, more traditional therapy will also be discussed to present a practical overall approach that can be easily applied in the care of the critically ill.

THE IMPORTANCE OF A NUTRITIONAL SUPPORT SERVICE

The expertise and input of a nutritional support team are required to deliver optimal nutritional support to critically ill patients. The team should include: a physician with an understanding of the science of nutrition; a nurse conversant with the management of catheters, infusion sets, and the likely complications of parenteral infusions and enteral feeds; a pharmacist with an understanding of parenteral mixtures and compatibilities of these mixtures; and a nutritionist who is an expert in the metabolic needs of the critically ill patient and the use of enteral formulas.

The team should be responsible for the development of ICU protocols which relate to the initiation of support, routes of administration, catheter selection and care, monitoring protocols, and the selection of products on formulary. These can be incorporated into an ICU handbook created for use by housestaff and students. Ongoing in-service education is required for housestaff, students, and nurses so that nutritional support can be successful and complications minimized. The team can best be used to influence daily nutrient management when the members are able to participate in daily ICU rounds.[7]

In spite of the multiple roles of the nutritional support team in the ICU, its efficacy must be measurable so that its cost can be justified to the hospital administration. The team must also be able to demonstrate that its input promotes cost containment and improves quality of care.[8,9] This may be accomplished by monitoring interventions and using the techniques of continuous quality improvement.

NUTRITIONAL ASSESSMENT AND PATIENT SELECTION

The process of nutritional support in the ICU should be an integrated continuum based on a plan which is developed with the input of the nutritional support team at the moment of each patient's entry. Historic information which includes the patient's premorbid diet, weight, and overall nutritional status should be taken into consideration. The number of days the patient has been without oral intake prior to entering the ICU should be reviewed.

A discussion with the ICU and surgical teams should include whether the length of time of ventilatory support or intestinal ileus can be estimated with some certainty. The overall condition of the patient with attention to the level of hypermetabolism and catabolism must be assessed. According to the American Society of Parenteral and Enteral Nutrition (ASPEN), patients should receive early enteral feedings whenever possible, and parenteral nutrition should be used when enteral feedings are unsuccessful or impossible so that the period of starvation is limited to only 5 to 7 days.[10] Availability and need for intravenous or gastrointestinal access must then be determined.

Due to a multitude of recent controversial literature regarding the efficacy of perioperative parenteral nutrition, there is increased pressure on physicians to provide early enteral support.[11,12] This becomes problematic for the intensivist, when faced with treating a patient who has recently come from surgery and yet has not had gastrointestinal access placed. For this reason, it is logical that the decision to initiate nutritional support in any particular patient should occur preoperatively whenever possible. For elective surgery patients, this can be discussed with the treating surgical team after the preoperative evaluation so that at the time of surgery enteral access will not be overlooked.

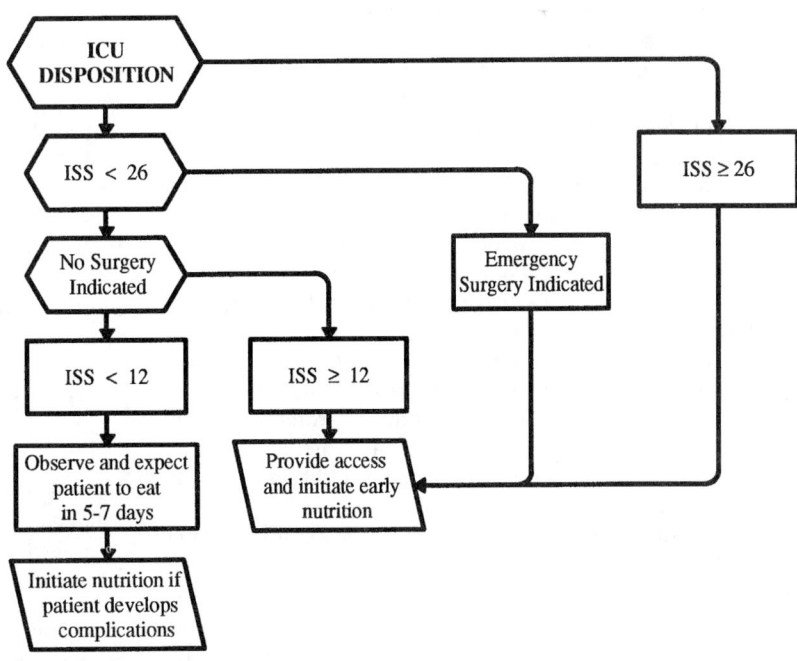

FIGURE 31-1. Nutritional support algorithm for the critically injured patient. ISS, Injury Severity Score based on Automotive Injury Score (AIS) 1990.

However, the ability to plan and discuss enteral access is often not possible in patients scheduled for emergency surgery. In order to circumvent the difficulties in making these decisions, we developed a model for use in patients who have suffered from traumatic injury (Fig. 31-1).[13] We found that 80% of all patients admitted to our trauma intensive care unit require nutritional support based on the ASPEN criteria.[10] All patients who need ICU admission and have an indication for emergency surgery of any type should have enteral access placed at the time of surgery. In addition, any patient without an indication for emergency surgery, but with an Injury Severity Score of 12 or above needs to have an aggressive attempt at early enteral access placement in order to initiate enteral feedings. This simple algorithm has an accuracy rate of 88% in selecting which patients are candidates for early and aggressive nutritional support.

Although short-term parenteral feedings have not been demonstrated to be efficacious, parenteral nutrition remains as a lifesaving therapy in those patients with gastrointestinal failure. Patients with obvious malnutrition or without enteral intake for more than 5 to 7 days are candidates for parenteral nutrition. In addition, immediate parenteral feedings should be initiated in those patients with known compromised bowel function such as massive bowel resection, chronic bowel obstruction, radiation enteritis, necrotizing pancreatitis, extensive intestinal disease, and end-jejunostomy syndrome. In addition, those patients whose ileum and colon have been resected may not be able to concentrate their intestinal contents and will initially need parenteral infusions to maintain hydration, electrolyte, and nutritional balance.

NUTRITIONAL REQUIREMENTS ■

PROTEIN REQUIREMENTS

During critical illness, catabolism erodes body proteins which have structural and functional roles. Studies have shown that dietary protein alone has an anabolic effect independent of energy, and the quantity of nitrogen given is an important determinant of nitrogen balance.[14] Protein support during critical illness maintains an adequate amino acid pool so that immune function, wound healing, and visceral integrity can be maintained.

Although the oral nitrogen requirement for balance in stable adults is only 0.6 g/kg/day, the increase in metabolic rate during critical illness increases nitrogen losses, raising the basal needs for balance. As a first approximation, 1.5 to 2.5 g/kg of ideal body weight/day of protein should be given.[15] If possible, half of the protein administered should be enteral, so that no more than 2g/kg/day of protein is given parenterally. It is somewhat controversial whether optimal support should also include 0.5 g/kg/day of additional protein as enteral glutamine.[4]

The adequacy of this approximation can then be monitored using measurements of plasma proteins and urea nitrogen excretion. Nitrogen balance studies should be done approximately once per week with the level of support stabilized over at least 5 days to allow for equilibration. In order to calculate nitrogen balance, the following formula should be used:

$$\text{Nitrogen (N) balance} = \text{N (in)} - \text{N (out)}$$

$$\text{Nitrogen (N) balance} = \frac{\text{protein}}{6.25}\ (\text{gm/day}) - \text{N (out)}$$

$$\text{N (out)} = \frac{\text{urine urea N}}{0.8}\ (\text{gm/day})$$
$$+ \text{ gastrointestinal losses (2–4 gm/day)}$$
$$+ \text{ cutaneous losses (0–4 gm/day)}$$

In the ICU setting, nitrogen delivery should be attempted with a goal of 2 to 4 grams of positive nitrogen balance daily whenever possible.[16] However, nitrogen balance studies may suffer from cumulative errors due to unmeasured losses which may result in artifactually positive balances during periods of high nitrogen intake.

Serum proteins may also be used to monitor adequacy of protein support. The choice of which marker to use is dependent upon the information desired (Table 31-1). Although albumin is the best prognostic marker, serum levels do not change rapidly in response to changes in dietary intake of protein. Serum proteins such as transferrin, prealbumin, and retinal binding protein have shorter half-lives and are more sensitive to rapid changes in nutritional status.

ENERGY REQUIREMENTS

Energy requirements are dependent on a number of factors, which include height, weight, age, and sex. For normal individuals, needs can be predicted with reasonable accuracy by the Harris-Benedict equation:

Men: kcal/24 hr

$$= 66.5 + (13.8 \times \text{W}) + (5.0 \times \text{H}) - (6.8 \times \text{A})$$

Women: kcal/24 hr

$$= 655 + (9.6 \times \text{W}) + (1.8 \times \text{H}) - (4.7 \times \text{A}),$$

where W is equal to body weight in kilograms, H is equal to height in centimeters, and A is equal to age in years. These caloric requirements approximate the BEE, and to these values must be added the specific dynamic action of food to give resting energy expenditure (REE).

In the past, injury, sepsis, and burns were believed to increase energy requirements by roughly 30%, 60%, and

TABLE 31-1. Visceral Protein Markers

PROTEIN MARKER	NORMAL VALUES	HALF-LIFE (DAYS)
Albumin	>3.5 gm/dL	20
Transferrin	>200 mg/dL	8.5
Prealbumin	20–30 mg/dL	1.3
Retinol-binding protein	4–5 mg/dL	0.4

100%, respectively, but the degree of hypermetabolism in injured and septic patients has come into question recently. Because excess feeding increases the risk of metabolic complications, a more conservative approach is advocated regarding the administration of energy substrate.[17] The mean increase in metabolic rate of injured and septic patients has been shown to exceed the expected value as predicted by the BEE by only 14%.[18] It is recommended that patients not be overfed and that they be supplied with no more calories than the actual REE.[19] Although the use of indirect calorimetry to establish the REE is optimal, measurements in critically ill ventilator-dependent patients is labor intensive, complex, and costly.[20] In the absence of indirect calorimetry, the REE can be estimated by calculating the BEE and multiplying by 1.1 to 1.4, by administering 25 kcal/kg/day of nonprotein calories, or by estimating protein needs and providing nonprotein calories to achieve a kilocalorie to nitrogen ratio of 100 to 1.[10] After the patient is transferred to the ward and anabolism is desired, the energy intake may then be liberalized to achieve weight gain.

ELECTROLYTE REQUIREMENTS

The importance of fluid and electrolyte replacement for promoting tissue perfusion and ionic equilibrium is self-evident. In addition, the processes of malnutrition and refeeding are both associated with major changes in electrolyte balance. With protein-calorie malnutrition there is loss of the intracellular ions potassium, magnesium, and phosphorus, together with a gain in sodium and water. On refeeding patients with an energy deficit, potassium, magnesium, and phosphorous levels may drop precipitously and thus need to be repleted. It should be recognized that potassium and magnesium deficiencies are integral components of malnutrition and must be corrected if nitrogen deficiency is to be treated. Precipitous drops in serum phosphorous may be responsible for the development of tremors, impaired mentation, coma, paresthesias, and muscle weakness with reduced diaphragmatic contractility. Additionally, during refeeding the sodium balance may become markedly positive and cause water retention although diuresis will occur as the nutritional status improves. Information regarding the major compartments of electrolyte distribution, serum concentrations, total body concentration, and deleterious effects of imbalances can be found in Table 31-2.

Sodium

The majority of critically ill patients can be given from 100 to 120 mEq of sodium daily. Patients with abnormal gastrointestinal losses may require further supplementation. However, those patients with severe malnutrition or cardiopulmonary disease should be restricted to 50 or 60 mEq of sodium daily.

Potassium

To determine the patient's potassium requirement during parenteral nutrition, it must be considered that glucose infusions increase the need for potassium and that approximately 3 mEq of K^+ is retained along with each gram of nitrogen. The infusion of as much as 80 to 120 mEq/day may be needed to replenish stores and meet daily needs in patients with large losses.

TABLE 31-2. Major Electrolyte Additives to TPN Solutions

ELECTROLYTE	FLUID COMPARTMENT	EFFECTS OF EXCESSIVE LEVELS	EFFECTS OF DIMINISHED LEVELS
Sodium (Na^+)	Extracellular	Dry mucous membranes Maniacal behavior	Seizures Altered mental status
Potassium (K^+)	Intracellular	Cardiac arrest Peaked T waves on ECG Widened QRS on ECG	Dysrhythmias Muscle weakness
Magnesium (Mg^{2+})	Intracellular	Hypotonia Cardiac dysrhythmias	Hypokalemia Hypocalcemia Seizures
Phosphorus (PO_4^{2-})	Intracellular	Tissue depositon of calcium phosphate (i.e., cardiac, renal) Hypocalcemia	Rhabdomyolysis Altered mental status Muscle weakness Hemolysis Paresthesias
Calcium (Ca^{2+})	Intracellular	Lethargy Constipation	Tetany Hyperreflexia Seizures Cardiac dysrhythmias

Magnesium

Magnesium should always be included in parenteral nutrition regimens. At least 12 to 15 mmol/day should be given with additional quantities added to cover losses in gastrointestinal secretions.

Calcium

It is unnecessary to add large amounts of calcium to daily parenteral nutrition solutions as it can result in precipitation, hypomagnesemia, and phosphate depletion.[21] The addition of 5 mg/day is likely to be sufficient.

Phosphorous

The total needs for phosphorous amount to approximately 14 to 16 mmoles daily when a mixed glucose and lipid source of nonprotein energy is given.[22] These requirements are increased when glucose is given as the sole calorie source. High insulin levels increase cellular uptake of phosphorus while lipid emulsions contain phospholipids, which act as an additional source of phosphorus.

MICRONUTRIENT REQUIREMENTS

The major part of our dietary intake is composed of water, proteins, carbohydrates, fats, and electrolytes. Other substances called micronutrients are ingested in smaller or minute amounts. These may be vitamins which are complex organic compounds, or trace minerals which are inorganic elements. Both are essential because they regulate metabolic processes in many different ways. The majority act as coenzymes or as essential elemental constituents of enzyme complexes regulating the use of carbohydrates, proteins, and fats.

Trace Elements

Iron, zinc, copper, chromium, selenium, iodine, and cobalt are currently known to be necessary for health in man. However, in the seriously ill patient, there are markedly increased requirements for zinc and selenium (Table 31-3).[15,23]

IRON.   Iron is an essential constituent of porphyrin-based compounds incorporated with protein, such as hemoglobin and myoglobin. In addition, smaller amounts of tissue iron associated with enzymes and mitochondria have important metabolic functions. Iron is also an essential component of bacterial cell growth and as such functions as an adjuvant to bacterial infection. Iron deficiency appears to be a normal host defense in response to infection or trauma and should not be replaced.[23]

ZINC.   Zinc is a widely distributed element in the human body and has now been identified as a component of approximately 120 enzymes. Zinc deficiency has a pronounced effect on nucleic acid metabolism, and can alter protein and amino acid metabolism. Growth, cellular immunity, fertility, hair growth, and wound healing are impaired in the absence of zinc.[24,25] Although endogenous stores of zinc are mobilized in the fasting state, these do not meet metabolic needs during stress and anabolism because the net movement of zinc is into tissues and there is little free zinc circulating.

The excretion of zinc occurs mainly in feces, with a smaller amount excreted in urine. Significant losses may also occur in sweat. Zinc losses increase significantly in patients with diarrhea, excessive stoma output, and gastrointestinal fistulas.[26] Urine losses also may increase with catabolism and in patients receiving amino acid infusions. Absorbed zinc is bound to albumin and an alpha$_2$-macroglobulin in the circulation, where it is taken up by the liver and other tissues.[27] With infection, leukocyte endogenous mediator stimulates the uptake of zinc by the liver, reducing plasma concentrations. The presence of abnormal GI losses, hypercatabolism, amino acid infusions, or the clinical syndrome of acrodermatitis enteropathica confirms the need for zinc supplementation.

In patients receiving parenteral nutrition, a minimum of 2.5 mg/day of zinc is required for balance in patients who do not have excessive losses.[26] However, patients who are hypercatabolic will probably require twice that, while those with abnormal gastrointestinal loss will need an additional 15 mg/L of gastrointestinal tract fluid lost. It is important to realize that if supplementation is given orally, only 7% of the intake is absorbed so that dosages must be corrected accordingly.

COPPER.   Copper is widely distributed in human tissues and is part of multiple enzyme systems. Ninety percent of plasma copper is in the form of ceruloplasmin, an iron oxidase. A deficiency in copper may result in a conditioned iron

TABLE 31-3.   Trace Minerals

MINERAL	FUNCTION	REQUIREMENTS
Iron	Constituent of porphyrin-based compounds, enzymes and mitochondria	0–2 mg/day
Zinc	Constituent of multiple enzyme systems	1–15 µg/day
Copper	Constituent of multiple enzyme systems and ceruloplasmin	.1–.5 µg/day
Chromium	Influences insulin sensitivity	10–20 µg/day
Selenium	Integral component of glutathione perioxidase	20–100 µg/day

deficiency, weakened connective tissues, and leukopenia in infants.[28] Plasma copper levels may be unreliable. In critically ill patients, Phillips and Garnys have recommended the administration of 0.5 mg/day, but this should be decreased to 0.1 mg/day in patients with abnormal liver function.[29]

CHROMIUM.   Chromium is important in promoting insulin action in peripheral tissues. Chromium enhances glucose oxidation and lipogenesis in adipose tissue and insulin-stimulated amino acid transport. Chromium deficiency decreases insulin sensitivity and causes a syndrome of glucose intolerance.[30]

Plasma chromium levels are reduced in deficiency and acute infection. However, the only convincing way of assessing chromium deficiency is to demonstrate prolonged glucose clearance that responds to chromium supplementation. The need in patients receiving parenteral nutrition may be as high as 10 to 20 mg daily.[31]

SELENIUM.   Selenium and vitamin E are interrelated in their actions and a deficiency of one can be partially corrected by administering the other. In well-nourished cells, superoxide dismutase (SOD) catalyzes, the conversion of superoxide (O_2) to peroxide (H_2O_2), and the peroxide so formed, is reduced by glutathione peroxidase (GSHPx) to water (H_2O):

$$O_2 + H^+ \xrightarrow{\text{SOD}} H_2O_2 \xrightarrow{\text{GSHPx}} H_2O$$

Glutathione peroxidase is made up of four subunits, each containing selenocysteine as an integral part of the molecule. In association with superoxide dismutase, selenium ultimately affects lipid peroxidation of polyunsaturated fatty acids in cell membranes. Increased losses may occur in wound drainage, pus, and fistula output. Deficiency may result in muscle pains and cardiomyopathy.[32]

Plasma selenium and glutathione peroxidase levels are sensitive to selenium intake and can be used to assess the need for this element.[33] The daily requirement of this element has been estimated to be between 20 to 70 µg/day in humans.[33] However, in those patients with underlying deficiency or increased requirements, replacement doses may be in excess of 100 µg/day.

Vitamins

Vitamins are essential nutrients that are active in minute quantities. Although it is obvious that these substances have to be given in any regimen of TPN to avoid deficiency (with the exception of vitamin D), the optimum dose and frequency of administration during TPN have not been studied in detail (Table 31-4).

VITAMIN E.   As has been previously mentioned, vitamin E is interrelated with selenium and is the second line of defense in controlling the formation of hydroperoxides from the fatty acid residues of phospholipids. This process depends on both the antioxidant role of the vitamin and its structural relation with the membrane phospholipids. Vitamin E is a fat soluble vitamin and its status can be assessed by the level of this vitamin in plasma, as well as by multiple functional means. The RDA of vitamin E is 10 IU of alpha-tocopherol per day; however, TPN patients need as much as 50 IU per day.[34] This requirement has not been studied with varying amounts of selenium in the infusion.

VITAMIN A.   Vitamin A is a fat soluble vitamin which is stored in large quantities in the liver. It is essential for the integrity of epithelial surfaces, synthesis of retinal pigments, and protection against infection. From clinical observations, 2500 IU is the recommended daily dose of this vitamin.

VITAMIN C.   Vitamin C is a water soluble vitamin, a reducing agent in redox reactions, and important in collagen synthesis and normal immune functions. A syndrome of scurvy exists in deficiency states which is characterized by perifollicular hemorrhages in the skin, gingivitis, and increased infections. Although 300 to 500 mg/day is adequate, patients who are seriously ill should receive 1000 mg/daily.[15]

VITAMIN D.   Vitamin D is a fat soluble vitamin and when given intravenously in normal daily dosages causes a syndrome of hypercalciuria, intermittent hypercalcemia, and osteomalacia.[35] For this reason intravenous vitamin D is not recommended; however, the oral intake of 250 IU daily will maintain normal plasma levels of 25-hydroxycholecalciferol, a metabolite of this vitamin.

VITAMIN K.   Vitamin K is a fat soluble vitamin which is required for the synthesis of four factors necessary for coagulation. Although severe deficiency will cause prolongation of prothrombin time and bleeding diathesis, subclinical deficiency may actually predispose to hypercoagulation. Patients who are on TPN for more than two weeks should receive 10 mg per week of a water-soluble analogue of this vitamin.

THIAMINE.   Thiamine is an integral part of the cocarboxylase enzyme system which is necessary for the metabolism of alpha-keto acids such as pyruvate. Cells which depend exclusively on carbohydrate for energy substrate are especially vulnerable to its deficiency. Thiamine deficiency can cause a metabolic acidosis as lactic acid accumulates and it has been observed that thiamine deficiency is associated with an increased mortality in critically ill patients.[36] Although 5 mg/day meets the needs in patients receiving short-term TPN, it is suggested that all patients receive a loading dose of 50 to 250 mg of thiamine on admission to the ICU.[37]

RIBOFLAVIN.   Riboflavin is a component of flavin coenzymes which are necessary for hydrogen transfer in redox systems. Deficiency causes photophobia, glossitis, cheilosis, and pruritus of the skin with inflammation. Five milligrams per day will avoid this deficiency.

NIACIN.   Niacin is a component of nicotinamide-adenine dinucleotide (NAD) and its phosphate (NADP), which are necessary for dehydrogenation reactions occurring in cell respiration. Pellagra develops in deficiency states, with deep red erythema, cracking of the skin, glossitis, stomatitis, diar-

TABLE 31-4. Vitamins

VITAMIN	FUNCTION	DEFICIENCY	REQUIREMENT
Vitamin A	Integrity of epithelial surfaces, synthesis of retinal pigments, and protection against infection	None described in parenterally fed patients	2500 IU/day
Vitamin C	Redox reactions, collagen synthesis, immune function	Scurvy: perifollicular hemorrhages, gingivitis, infections	1000 mg/day
Vitamin D	Bone metabolism	None described in parenterally fed patients	—
Vitamin E	Antioxidant protector of membrane phospholipids	Myonecrosis, cardiomyopathy	50 IU/day
Vitamin K	Synthesis of coagulation factors	Hypercoagulability or bleeding diathesis	10 mg/week
Thiamine	Part of cocarboxylase enzyme system	Lactic acidosis	50–250 mg load, then 5 mg/day
Riboflavin	Component of coenzymes in redox systems	Photophobia, glossitis, cheilosis, anogenital pruritis and inflammation	5 mg/day
Niacin	Component of nicotinamide adenine dinucleotide (NAD) and its phosphate (NADP)	Pellagra: erythema, cracking of skin, glossitis, stomatitis, diarrhea, delerium	50 mg/day
Pantothenate	Component of coenzyme A	Fatigue, mental disturbance, paresthesias and epigastric discomfort	15 mg/day
Pyridoxine	Coenzyme of amino acid metabolism	Dermatitis, intertrigo, seborrhea, irritability, somnolence, neuropathy	5 mg/day
Folic acid	Nucleic acid synthesis	Megaloblastic anemia, glossitis	600 μg/day
Vitamin B_{12}	Nucleic acid synthesis	Megaloblastic anemia, glossitis, neuromyelopathy	12 μg/day
Biotin	Coenzyme of carboxylase	Dermatitis, impetigo-like eruption, hair loss, paresthesias, lethargy	60 μg/day

rhea, and delirium. It is felt that 50 mg/day is a safe intake that will prevent deficiency.

PANTOTHENATE. Pantothenic acid is a component of coenzyme A. The deficiency of this vitamin results in fatigue, mental disturbances, paresthesias, and epigastric discomfort. It is likely that 15 mg/day is a suitable intake.

PYRIDOXINE. Pyridoxine is a coenzyme in many reactions concerned with amino acid metabolism. In the adult human, symptoms of deficiency consist of dermatitis, intertrigo, seborrhea, irritability, somnolence, and neuropathy. An intake of 5 mg/day is sufficient to prevent these symptoms.

FOLIC ACID AND VITAMIN B. Folic acid and vitamin B_{12} are important for the synthesis of nucleic acids. Deficiencies cause megaloblastic anemia and glossitis, while severe vitamin B_{12} deficiency results in neuromyelopathy. The recommended daily parenteral intake is 600 μg of folic acid and 12 μg of vitamin B_{12} daily.

BIOTIN. Biotin deficiency has been described in patients receiving total parenteral nutrition.[38] To prevent this, the American Medical Association has recommended the administration of 60 μg/day to patients on TPN.

ROUTES AND TECHNIQUES OF ADMINISTRATION

ENTERAL VERSUS PARENTERAL NUTRITION

Although for many years it has been intuitively known that enteral feedings were more physiologic than parenteral nutrition, it was not until the last decade that this has been unequivocally demonstrated. Multiple animal and human studies have demonstrated an improved outcome with early enteral feedings, while similar protocols using early parenteral nutrition have shown less than favorable results. Indeed it has been suggested that failure to tolerate enteral feedings heralds a poor prognosis in critically ill patients.[39]

Early work by Dietch that demonstrated bacterial translocation in animals gave insight that gut mucosal atrophy was detrimental.[40] By maintaining mucosal integrity and preventing bacterial translocation, it could be hypothesized that early enteral feedings decrease weight loss, energy expenditure, and hypercatabolism.[40,41] Subsequently it was shown that glutamine is an important intestinal substrate during stress which helps to protect against cellular injury.[42] Numerous clinical trials have demonstrated that patients fed enterally early after operation have decreased infections and improved outcome when compared with patients fed parenterally.[12,43–48] Trials which have not demonstrated an improved outcome with enteral feedings have been flawed in that the enteral feedings were not initiated early (within 12–24 hours) after the insult causing the stress response.[49,50]

ENTERAL NUTRITION

Despite the overwhelming evidence in the literature in support of enteral feedings, they are not always routinely used. It seems that reasons for this are threefold: patient selection, difficulty in attaining access to the gastrointestinal tract, and the added nursing and physician effort that is required for successful administration. To aid in patient selection, prospective clinical models, similar to the one discussed earlier, must be developed to help clinicians in the decision to aggressively pursue therapy with enteral support. Although it is presumed that enteral feedings are more economical than parenteral solutions, the total cost of delivering enteral versus parenteral therapy is no different due to the expense of achieving and maintaining access.[50] Furthermore, protocols must be developed so that adequate feedings are delivered despite diagnostic and therapeutic interventions; for example, it has been demonstrated that enteral feedings did not have to be discontinued for prolonged periods prior to operative interventions in burn patients.[51,52] Although it is easier to initiate parenteral feedings in critically ill patients who have multiple central access catheters in place, and a more reliable quantity of nutrients can be delivered daily, it must be remembered that less nutrient support is needed when nutritional support is delivered enterally.[48,53] Enteral feedings also have the additional therapeutic effect of maintaining an alkaline gastric pH despite being infused distal to the pylorus.[54]

In contrast, parenteral nutrition causes intestinal mucosal atrophy which predisposes to bacterial translocation.[55] For all of the reasons mentioned, all efforts should be made to secure and maintain an upper intestinal access tube to improve delivery of enteral feedings. However, when there is poor tolerance, partial support may be given enterally with the addition of supplemental parenteral nutrition.[53,56]

Gastrointestinal Access

There are multiple operative and nonoperative techniques to achieve access for enteral feedings. In patients without abdominal surgery and adequate gastric emptying, nasogastric feedings with a small bore, flexible, weighted tube are adequate.[57] Nasogastric feeding tubes are usually between 5 to 8 French in diameter, made of silicone rubber or polyurethane, weighted at the end, and have a stylet for insertion. It is wise to lubricate the stylet with mineral oil prior to insertion for ease of withdrawal.

After lubricating the tube and placing anesthetic in the nostril, the tube is advanced through the pharynx and esophagus to about 50 cm. Fifty milliliters of air are then injected and the tube is advanced along the greater curvature of the stomach as close to the pylorus as possible. Note that in patients with severe facial and head trauma the tube may be temporarily placed in the mouth until the time of surgery, when it may be replaced through the nose under direct vision.

When feeding into the stomach, gastric residuals should be measured and not exceed 200 cm^3 when checked every 4 hours. When residuals reach this level, the tube feeding should be reduced to half the rate. Pharmacologic agents such as metoclopramide and erythromycin may be administered to aid in gastric emptying.[58]

Patients with severe head and neck pathology or debilitating brain injury may need long-term gastric access. There is some controversy whether jejunal access is better in head-injured patients because of the risk of aspiration; however, gastric tubes are easier to maintain and replace and allow greater flexibility in the administration of feedings and medications.[59] Ideally gastrojejunal tubes may be used during the acute phase of injury and converted to gastrostomy tubes if needed during the chronic phase. In patients with severe closed head injury, the rapid placement of percutaneous gastrostomy tubes along with tracheostomy has been shown to be safe and effective in decreasing ICU and hospital length of stay.[60] In patients undergoing head and neck surgery, percutaneous endoscopic gastrostomy tubes can be placed preoperatively to allow for nutritional repletion, and then can be available for postoperative use. It is important to note that these procedures have been performed safely in patients who have had previous abdominal surgery, so that surgery solely for the purpose of gastrostomy placement is now rarely indicated.[61]

Patients with gastric atony need to have enteral access established distal to the pylorus. Nasoduodenal tubes may be used to accomplish this and are successfully passed 80% of the time by individuals well-practiced in the technique.[62] The technique is similar to the one described above for nasogastric intubation; however, these tubes should be at least 100 to 110 cm long. Upon passage of the tube to 50 cm, 200 to 300 mL of air is injected to inflate the stomach. The tube is then passed until the point of resistance at the pylorus is met. Upon relaxation of the pylorus, the tube is then advanced to attain positioning in the duodenum. Radiographic confirmation is necessary prior to use and residual measurements should be continued as tube displacement back into the stomach is not uncommon.

Should attempts at blind passage fail, there are specialized tubes that may be passed into the duodenum with the aid of a gastroscope. Although some tubes have a lead string that can be pulled into the duodenum with the biopsy forceps of the gastroscope, a more successful technique is to use a special tube with a weighted tip and central hole which allows it to be passed over a guide wire. The endoscope is passed into the second or third part of the duodenum and a long guide wire is passed through the biopsy channel of the scope. The scope is then withdrawn over the guide wire, which is passed through the nasopharynx to exit from the nose, using a soft flexible tube in the kit. The feeding tube is then lubricated with mineral oil and the central opening at the tip is passed over the guide wire and fed into the duodenum. The position is verified fluroscopically and the guide wire is removed. Because the procedures described above are labor intensive, patients who undergo abdominal surgery should have jejunal access established at the time of operation.[63] The simplest technique is the needle catheter jejunostomy. A 7 French tube should be used which does, however, require frequent flushes and vigilant nursing care to maintain patency. For this reason, some surgeons prefer a more traditional Witzel jejunostomy.

If jejunal access is desired but fixation of the jejunum to the abdominal wall is deemed to be unacceptable, permanent jejunal access can be obtained with a surgical gastrojejunostomy tube. Although these tubes can provide simultaneous gastric decompression, the jejunal tube must be of sufficient length so that the feeding and suction ports are not in close proximity.[64] In patients who need short-term and noninvasive access, nasojejunal tubes can be fed manually by the surgeon during laparotomy.

Selection of Feeding Mixture

After enteral access is attained, the most appropriate enteral feeding mixture should be selected (Fig. 31-2). As blenderized diets are rarely appropriate for the ICU patient, the initial selection is between a lactose-free polymeric diet or an elemental diet. A polymeric diet is composed of whole protein, oils, and corn syrup or sucrose to provide protein, fat, and carbohydrates, respectively, while elemental diets are composed of amino acids or short chain peptides and oligosaccharides or monosaccharides. In polymeric diets, fat calories usually comprise approximately 30% of the total caloric content, while elemental or peptide diets supply the minimum amount of long-chain triglycerides (1–2%) and supply additional fat calories (10–20%) in the form of medium-chain triglycerides. Modules of carbohydrate, protein, or fat are available to add to stock formulas so that specialized

nutritional needs can be met.

In patients with normal gastrointestinal motility and absorption, polymeric diets are acceptable and should be well-tolerated.[65,66] However, any patient with malabsorption or hypomotility of the small or large intestine should be fed with an elemental diet until gastrointestinal function has returned to normal. Situations in the critical care unit which might lead to intestinal dysfunction include major surgery, sepsis, pancreatitis, and resuscitation as well as the presence of underlying intestinal pathology.

There have been recent reports of additives and specialized formulations which may result in improved tolerance of enteral nutrition. The addition of sodium chloride to the formula to attain a final concentration of 100 mmol/L may prevent the development of diarrhea. In addition, many tube feedings now contain dietary fiber, which consists of water-soluble and insoluble compounds that are fermented to varying degrees by colonic bacteria. Fiber may be beneficial to help to assure colon mucosal integrity and aid in carbohydrate absorption of the small intestine, but in the critical care setting it has not been shown to be useful in the therapy of either constipation or diarrhea.[67] If polymeric formulations which contain fiber are available, they can be used as long as the nutritional composition is satisfactory for the patient.

Most recently, a new generation of immunomodulary enteral feeding formulations have been developed. The components which have been added to these formulations include glutamine, arginine, RNA nucleotides, and omega-3 fatty acids.[68] While glutamine is added to many new commercial formulations, it is rarely added in the recommended dosage of 0.5 g/kg/day. Another component, arginine, has a

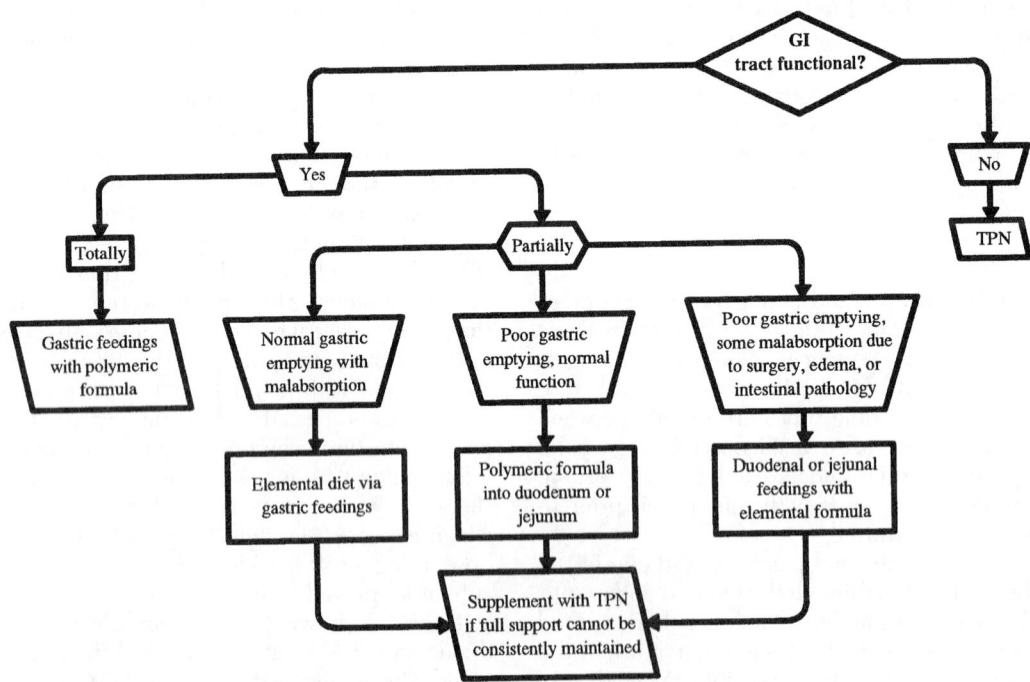

FIGURE 31-2. An algorithm for the selection of enteral feeding route and formula. Selection of enteral feeding technique depends on gastrointestinal motility and absorption.

duel effect; it is known to potentiate the immune system while it is also a substrate for the potent vasodilator nitric oxide. RNA nucleotides and omega-3 fish oils also potentiate the immune system, with the fish oils achieving this by the modification of the inflammatory response. These specialized immunomodulatory products are considerably more expensive than standard enteral formulas and it is questionable as to whether they successfully have been shown to improve outcome by decreasing infectious complications.[69,70]

Delivery of Nutrients

In the ICU setting feedings should only be initiated after the correction of low flow states. They should be initiated as full strength at a rate commensurate with the patient's level of gastrointestinal function. A typical starting rate would be 25 cm³/hr. If this is tolerated well, the rate may be increased by 25 cm³/hr as tolerated every 8 to 12 hours. Observation for tolerance must include residual measurements and evaluation for distention or symptoms of abdominal pain. Enteral pumps should be used to ensure accurate rates of delivery, and bags of enteral feeding should be prepared in a sterile manner and not hang longer than 8 hours to avoid contamination.

PARENTERAL NUTRITION

Parenteral nutrition must be used when the gastrointestinal tract is totally dysfunctional or attempts at enteral feedings fail to provide adequate support. It is optimal to continue small amounts of enteral feeding whenever possible during parenteral therapy. However, a common error is failing to recognize that attempts at enteral nutrition have not been successful and delaying the initiation of parenteral nutritional support.[56]

Intravenous Access

Parenteral nutrition requires hypertonic fluids be infused on a continuous basis into a central venous catheter in the vena cava. Superior vena cava catheters inserted by the infraclavicular subclavian route are least likely to be associated with sepsis and displacement and are thus the preferred route of access for TPN.[71] A second choice is the internal jugular site; the least optimal location is the femoral site due to an increased rate of infectious complications.[71] However, in patients with difficult access, femoral access may be used safely on a short-term basis.[72] Patients with prolonged or repeated ICU admissions may have total or partial occlusions of the internal jugular, subclavian, and femoral veins. In these cases, ultrasound or fluoroscopic guidance can be used to gain access through partially occluded veins. In more extreme circumstances, direct cannulation of the inferior vena cava can be achieved by the translumbar or transhepatic route using fluoroscopic guidance.

Catheter insertion is usually performed using a multilumen catheter. Although these catheters were initially found to have increased infection rates when compared to single lumen catheters, more recent evaluations have proven them

to be acceptable and practical in the critical care setting.[71,73,74] Catheter insertion should be performed by an experienced operator with full aseptic precautions including gown, gloves, mask, and cap. Poor technique, inadequate skin preparation, and contamination during insertion will result in the early development of line sepsis (for details on insertion, see Chapter 35).

Catheter and Tubing Care

The dressing of the catheter exit site should be changed at least once every 72 hours and more frequently if it becomes nonadherent. After handwashing, the nurse puts on a mask and gloves, the old dressing is removed, and the exit site is inspected for infection. The skin and exit site are cleansed and a fresh gauze is placed on the exit site and the plastic occlusive dressing reapplied. The tubing attached to the catheter should be changed at least every 48 hours.

Parenteral Formulations

Parenteral solutions can be mixed with varying concentrations of dextrose and amino acids. Two standard concentrations are 25% dextrose with 4.25% amino acids and 21% dextrose with 7.0% amino acids. However, with the use of an automated compounding system, nutrient base solutions can be tailored to accommodate the protein and caloric needs of each individual patient.

Essential high branch chain amino acids comprise approximately 25% of standard amino acid solutions. Specialized stress formulations with up to 50% of the amino acids being of the high branched chain variety have been developed. Although they have demonstrated metabolic benefits, they have never been shown to influence outcome in critically ill patients and are not advocated.

In selecting the quantity of dextrose and lipid calories, it should be remembered that neither glucose alone or a combined substrate influence whole body protein dynamics.[75] It has been shown that despite glucose administration in injured and septic patients, the respiratory quotient may be low secondary to the use of endogenous fat.[18,76] For this reason, approximately 70% of the energy needs should be supplied as carbohydrate with 30% or less administered as fat with ≥3% of energy requirements composed of essential fatty acids.[15] In patients who are septic, lipid calories should be limited to 15 to 20% of the total calories.

Intravenous lipids are emulsions which come in concentrations of 10% or 20% and contain phospholipid as the emulsifying agent. The polyunsaturated fatty acids in these emulsions are long chained and of the N-6 variety. Because the 10% solutions contain more phospholipid than the 20% solutions (7.2 gm/L and 3.6 gm/L respectively), it is recommended that only 20% emulsions be used.[77] Additionally, previous concerns regarding the effects of lipid emulsions on platelet aggregation have been shown to be unfounded.[78] Thus only two contraindications currently exist regarding lipid emulsions: severe hypertriglyceridemia (>300mg/dL) and pancreatitis secondary to hyperlipidemia.

Delivery of Nutrients

All parenteral solutions should be initiated at a rate of one liter per day (42 cm³/hr) as a continuous infusion. As blood sugar levels and electrolytes are noted to be stable, this rate can be increased by 500 cm³/day until the goal rate is achieved. Parenteral nutrient admixtures are solutions of glucose, amino acids, lipids, and other pharmaceutical agents. Although these solutions offer the advantages of fluid conservation, cost savings, and potential decrease in the risk of infection secondary to reduced catheter manipulation, separate lipid infusions are recommended in critically ill patients. Pharmaceutical agents which are comparable with TPN and may be added to the glucose and amino acid solutions include H-2 blockers, heparin, corticosteroids, and albumin. However, it is important to note that the addition of albumin has never been demonstrated to be of any benefit in this patient population.[79]

NUTRITIONAL THERAPY OF PATIENTS WITH ORGAN SYSTEM DYSFUNCTION ■

VOLUME RESTRICTION

The majority of patients in the ICU with excessive intravascular volume may be treated with either diuretics, ultrafiltration, or hemodialysis. In these patients, as well as in others, it is important to restrict volume intake. Nutritional support can be best accomplished in this setting with high density (2 kcal/cm³) enteral formulas. In patients receiving parenteral support, protein requirements should take priority as most medications can be administered in dextrose solutions and adipose tissue can be mobilized for short-term caloric deficits. The most concentrated TPN formula available should be used providing 30% of the kilocalories with a 20% lipid emulsion.

All compatible maintenance drugs should be added to the parenteral nutrition solutions to decrease the need for additional fluid administration.[80] Additional kilocalories can be administered by infusing prescribed drugs which are compatible in 20% dextrose solutions. In this way concentrated high protein formulas may be administered, as the TPN solution and kilocalorie needs may be supplemented with lipids and the remaining necessary intravenous infusions.

RENAL INSUFFICIENCY

Nutritional management of patients in renal failure has changed with the availability of improved dialytic methods for this patient population. In patients on adequate dialysis therapy, protein restriction is no longer necessary.[81] However, conventional means for the estimation of glomerular filtration rate may not be accurate in this setting because of decreases in creatinine production due to malnutrition and immobilization, or increases in creatine and urea production due to increased catabolism. For this reason more than one method of assessment should be used to evaluate renal function. Despite impairment of renal function, full protein alimentation can be maintained when patients are treated with continuous hemofiltration.[82] When increased catabolism is documented by increased urea production, supplementation with essential branch chain amino acid formulas may be beneficial as these amino acids are often depleted in patients with renal failure.[83] In addition, special attention must be paid to phosphorous, magnesium, potassium, and trace element levels. Protein restriction should only be necessary in those few patients who are not candidates for dialytic therapy.

CARBOHYDRATE INTOLERANCE

The most common manifestation of excessive carbohydrate administration is hyperglycemia with serum blood sugars of 400mg/dL or more.[84] When this occurs, kilocalories should be restricted to 20 to 25 kcal/kg and 30% of caloric requirements should be given as intralipid. If hyperglycemia persists, insulin must be used aggressively in a constant infusion to maintain blood sugars at levels of less than 200mg/dL. Because insulin is compatible with TPN solutions, 2/3 of the daily insulin dosage may be added to the parenteral infusions. In patients on enteral feedings, a high fiber concentrated formula with 40% to 50% of the calories as fat is tolerated best.

Another manifestation of carbohydrate intolerance is increased CO_2 production and resultant hypercapnea. However, multiple studies have shown that if caloric intake is limited to the actual resting energy expenditure and carbohydrate infusion is maintained at a maximum of 4 mg/kg/min, carbon dioxide production will not be increased.[17]

HEPATIC INSUFFICIENCY

Patients with cirrhosis are known to have abnormal substrate oxidation and during periods of hypermetabolism and hypercatabolism are prone to the development of abnormal amino acid profiles.[85] In addition, these patients are often fluid restricted due to excessive total body water and sodium with resultant ascites. Enteral feedings should be used whenever possible and if the patient is awake and alert without evidence of sepsis or hypercatabolism, standard enteral feedings with casein-based protein can be used. However, in patients whose mental status cannot be fully evaluated or who are encephalopathic, a product with supplemental high branch chain amino acids and restricted aromatic amino acids is recommended. In patients with gastrointestinal dysfunction, hepatic failure, and malabsorption or ileus, specialized hepatic parenteral formulas may be necessary.

COMPLICATIONS ■

GENERAL AND METABOLIC

Infectious and metabolic complications frequently occur in critically ill patients on nutritional support. The most common metabolic complication is undernutrition which is associated with respiratory muscle weakness and ventilator dependency.[16] Alternatively, overnutrition may increase carbon dioxide production, increase ventilatory demands, and result in hyperglycemia.[16,17,84] Hyperglycemia usually precipitates glucosuria which, if untreated, will result in an osmotic diuresis and hyperosmolar nonketotic coma. This should be suspected in a hyperglycemic patient with poor tissue turgar, oliguria, confusion, or lethargy. Hyperglycemia may also be detrimental in that it is associated with impaired immune function and increased infections.[86] Although less common than hyperglycemia, hypoglycemia may occur if hypertonic glucose infusions or enteral feedings are abruptly terminated. Symptoms include weakness, trembling, diaphoresis, headaches, chills, tachycardia, and decreased consciousness. Additionally, the excessive administration of protein can produce uremia in the absence of renal dysfunction.[87]

Electrolyte imbalances related to potassium, phosphorous, and magnesium are most common. The levels of these nutrients may fall suddenly due to protein synthesis upon the institution of nutritional support. Excesses may build up rapidly in patients with renal dysfunction.[87] Adjustments should be made through changes in the parenteral nutrition prescription, or by the addition of supplements in patients on enteral feedings. When potassium restrictions are necessary, a low potassium enteral formula should be selected. Trace mineral and vitamin deficiencies may also occur and require supplementation. Thiamine should always be supplemented to avoid metabolic acidosis and folate should also be given to all patients with a history of alcohol abuse.[36]

COMPLICATIONS OF ENTERAL NUTRITION

Complication of Gastrointestinal Access

Dislodgement of enteral access catheters into the peritoneum may be associated with peritonitis.[88] This complication must be anticipated during the first week after access placement or replacement. It is recommended to always obtain radiographic confirmation of tube placement with contrast studies. Occasionally, a leak cannot be adequately treated and fistula formation will occur.

Another catastrophic complication which has been described after jejunostomy placement is small bowel volvulus and infarction. Furthermore, papers have described small bowel infarction secondary to jejunostomy feedings alone, without evidence of concommitant volvulus.[89] This diagnosis must be suspected whenever there is hypoperfusion and abdominal distention. If these symptoms develop, the feedings must be immediately discontinued and abdominal radiographs obtained.

A lesser complication of gastrointestinal access includes catheter occlusion, which is more likely to occur with small bore and needle catheter feeding tubes.[88] Nursing care of these catheters must be meticulous and include frequent flushing with saline. No medications should be administered through them.

Long standing enteral tubes may eventually leak and cause skin breakdown. The placement of a smaller tube will allow the stoma to contract and thus prevent leaking when the original size catheter is replaced.

Gastric Distention and Aspiration

Gastric distention decreases lower esophageal sphincter pressure and predisposes to reflux and pulmonary aspiration. Patients being transferred into or out of the ICU appear to be at highest risk for pulmonary aspiration.[90] By administering continuous feedings and decreasing the rate by half whenever residuals reach 150 to 200 mL, the incidence of aspiration can be reduced. Despite efforts to prevent aspiration, it may occur in 1% to 5% of ICU patients receiving enteral feedings.

The diagnosis of aspiration may be made after a witnessed event, or by the appearance of enteral feedings or gastric secretions in the tracheal aspirate. To aid in the diagnosis, blue food coloring should be added to all feedings. Glucose concentrates in the tracheal aspirate are not predictive of episodes of aspiration.[91] When bronchopulmonary aspiration does occur, early recognition and treatment with expeditious intubation, ventilation, removal of particulate matter, and institution of antibiotics can decrease morbidity and mortality.

Diarrhea and Gastrointestinal Complications

In the ICU, diarrhea is a frequent occurrence in tube-fed patients, although it is usually caused by factors other than the tube feeding itself. Elixer drugs containing sorbitol are most often responsible. When evaluating diarrhea in critically ill patients, it is important to quantitate the stool output. Diarrhea is defined as more than 200 g of stool or 3 large liquid stools in a 24 hour period. It is more likely to occur in patients with a serum albumin of less than 2.5 mg/dL and who have received more than 7 days of antibiotic therapy.[92]

Antibiotic therapy may also predispose patients to *Clostridium difficile* infection. These patients may have an elevated leukocyte count, abdominal pain, or copious liquid stool. Sucralfate administration has been associated with a decreased risk of this infection.[93] Stool cultures and titers should be sent whenever the diagnosis is entertained. One week of enterally administered metronidazole or vancomycin is usually curative; however, repeat studies should be performed at the conclusion of therapy.

Other factors which may be responsible for diarrhea include bacterial overgrowth of the enteral feeding itself, bolus feeding into the stomach resulting in an uncontrolled flow of nutrients into the intestine, malabsorption due to intestinal edema or atrophy, or an intercurrent gastrointestinal problem. Untreated diarrhea will result in volume depletion, hypokalemia, and a hyperchloremic metabolic acidosis. While the diarrhea is undergoing evaluation it is important to supplement the patient with the appropriate intravenous fluids and electrolytes. If malabsorption is a potential factor, the tube feeding formula should be changed to an elemental diet. In the absence of a putative cause or evidence of gastrointestinal disease, antidiarrheal agents should be initiated.

COMPLICATIONS OF PARENTERAL NUTRITION

Complications of Catheter Insertion

During central line placement adjacent anatomic structures may be injured. For example, subclavian and internal jugular line placement may result in pneumothorax or hemothorax. In the intensive care setting, these should always be treated with thoracostomy tube decompression. Occasionally, line placement may occur with the tip in the pleural space. This is easily diagnosed by chest radiograph and treated by catheter removal. However, if the diagnosis was missed and fluids are infused into the pleural space, tube thoracostomy drainage will be necessary. Arterial or venous laceration may occur with subsequent arterial thrombosis and limb ischemia. For this reason distal pulses must be checked frequently and occlusion suspected if there is any change in the caliber of the pulses. Nerve damage may also occur and is treated by catheter removal.

If the thoracic duct is injured during a left subclavian or interal jugular catheter placement, there will be clear lymph drainage from the insertion site or chylothorax formation. Treatment includes catheter removal and, when necessary, evacuation of the pleural space until lymphatic drainage ceases. Injury to the mediastinum may also occur and must be rapidly diagnosed. A compressive hematoma may require evacuation while infiltration will require removal of the line. Cardiac arrhythmias may occur if the guide wire or catheter is placed within the heart itself. However, positioning of the catheter a good distance into the superior vena cava is important to avoid dislodgement and venous thrombosis.

During catheter placement both line embolus and air embolus may occur. Line embolus is avoided by not pulling the line back through an introducing needle. However, with placement kits now using the Seldinger technique, this complication is less common. To avoid air embolus it is optimal to hydrate and position the patient so as to create venous hypertension in the vein being entered. This may be accomplished by placing the patient in the Trendelenburg position for internal jugular and subclavian vein insertions.

Complications of Indwelling Catheters

Line sepsis is the most common complication of indwelling lines and is best diagnosed by using the Maki semiquantitative technique.[94] If 15 or more colony forming units per milliliter grow following culture of the subcutaneous segment, catheter related sepsis is likely, and when bacteremia correlates with these cultures, the diagnosis is definitive.[95] The diagnosis of catheter sepsis necessitates line removal.

Venous thrombosis also may occur with resultant thrombophlebitis and extremity edema and may be treated with extremity elevation, heparin, and thrombolytics as indicated. The usual cause is catheter malposition. Acute pharyngitis has also occurred secondary to thrombophlebitis of the interal jugular vein due to catheter malposition.[96]

Thrombosis of the catheter may also occur and may be treated by instilling 7500 IU of urokinase in 3 mL of normal saline and injecting up to 2.5 mL into the catheter. The catheter is capped for 3 hours and then flushed with saline and heparin. It is important to note that parenteral nutrient admixtures containing intralipids have been implicated in causing catheter occlusion.[97]

Malposition of a central venous catheter in the atrium may cause arrhythmias, infected thrombosis, and atrial perforation. Another serious complication is inadvertent line disconnection. Thus may result in unrecognized hemorrhage or air embolism. The patient should immediately be placed in the Trendelenburg position with the right side up. This may help to prevent the air from occluding the pulmonary artery. If the line remains in place it is warranted to attempt to aspirate air.

Complications of Lipid Emulsions

Patients receiving parenteral nutrition need to receive daily calories in the form of intralipid to prevent essential fatty acid deficiency. The topical application of vegetable oils does not prevent the development of essential fatty acid deficiency.[98] If the patient develops hypertriglyceridemia, the rate of lipid administration is decreased, and the total amount of fat is reduced. Similarly, in cases of hypertriglyceridemia with resultant pancreatitis, lipids are administered in small quantities at a slow rate. Excessive lipid administration in septic patients should be avoided because of studies which have shown that long-chain triglycerides affect host cellular immunity.[99,100] In addition, critically ill patients should never receive parenteral support in the form of three-in-one nutrient admixtures due to the risk of unrecognized precipitation and cracked emulsions.[101]

Gastrointestinal Tract Complications

Gastrointestinal tract complications develop insidiously in patients receiving full parenteral support. Cholestasis, steatosis, jaundice, and alcalculous cholecystitis may occur.[102] Some preliminary studies have shown that this can be partially reversed by the administration of ursodeoxycholic acid.[103] A cheaper and more effective therapy is to maintain slow infusions of enteral feedings.[104] Other complications which may be prevented by the administration of small amounts of enteral feedings is gut mucosal atrophy and impaired pulmonary macrophage function.[105,106]

REFERENCES ∎

1. Wilmore DW: Catabolic illness: strategies for enhancing recovery. *N Engl J Med* 1991;325:695
2. Clevenger FW: Nutritional support in the patient with the systemic inflammatory response syndrome. *Am J Surg* 1993; 165:685
3. Woolf PD, McDonald JV, Feliciano DV, et al: The catacholamine response to multisystem trauma. *Arch Surg* 1992; 127:899
4. Darmaun D, Just B, Messing B, et al: Glutamine metabolism in healthy adult men: response to enteral and intravenous feeding. *Am J Clin Nutr* 1994;59:1395

5. Offenbartl K, Bengmark S: Intraabdominal infections and gut origin sepsis. *World J Surg* 1990;14:191

6. Byrne TA, Morrissey TB, Gatzen C, et al: Anabolic therapy with growth hormone accelerates protein gain in surgical patients requiring nutritional rehabilitation. *Ann Surg* 1993; 218:400

7. Cohen IL: Establishing and justifying specialized teams in intensive care units for nutrition, ventilator management, and palliative care. *Crit Care Clin* 1993;9:511

8. Gales BJ, Gales MJ: Nutritional Support teams: a review of comparative trials. *Ann Pharmacother* 1994;28:227

9. O'Brien DD, Hodges RE, Day AT, et al: Recommendations of nutrition support team promotes cost containment. *JPEN* 1986;10:300

10. ASPEN Board of Directors: Guidelines for use of parenteral and enteral nutrition in adult and pediatric patients. *JPEN* 1993;17:1SA

11. Brennan MF, Disters PW, Posner M, et al: A prospective randomized trial of parenteral nutrition after pancreatic resection for malignancy. *Ann Surg* 1994;220:436

12. Moore EE, Moore FA: Immediate enteral nutrition following multisystem trauma: a decade perspective. *J Am Coll Nutr* 1991;10:633

13. Byers P, Block E, Albornoz J, et al: The need for aggressive nutritional intervention in the injured patient: the development of a predictive model. *J Trauma* 1995;39:1103

14. Greenberg GR, Jeejeebhoy KN: Intravenous protein-sparing therapy in patients with gastrointestinal disease. *JPEN* 1979; 3:427

15. DeBlassee MA, Wilmore DN: What is optimal nutritional support? *New Horiz* 1994;2:122

16. Christman JW, McClain RW: Sensible approach to the nutritional support of mechanically ventilated critically ill patients. *Intensive Care Med* 1993;19:129

17. Guenst JM, Nelson LD: Predictors of total parenteral nutrition-induced lipogenesis. *Chest* 1994;105:553

18. Askanzai J, Carpentier YA, Elwyn DH, et al: Influence of total parenteral nutrition on fuel utilization in injury and sepsis. *Ann Surg* 1980;191:40

19. Frankenfield DC, Wiles CE III, Bagley S, et al: The relationship between resting and total energy expenditure in injured and septic patients. *Crit Care Med* 1994;22:1796

20. Steinhorn DM, Rozenberg AL, Boyle MJ, et al: Modular indirect calorimeter suitable for long-term measurements in multipatient intensive care units. *Crit Care Med* 1991;19: 963

21. Al-Jurf AS, Arapman-Furr F: Magnesium balance and distribution during total parenteral nutrition: effect of calcium additives. *Metabolism* 1985;34:658

22. Aubier M, Murciano D, Lecocguic Y, et al: Effects of hypophosphatemia on diaphragmatic contractility in patients with acute respiratory failure. *N Eng J Med* 1985;313:420

23. Mainous MR, Deitch EA: Nutrition and infection. *Surg Clin North Am*: 1994;74:659

24. Fraker PJ, Gershwin ME, Good RA, et al: Interrelationships between zinc and immune function. *Fed Proc* 1986;45:1474

25. Golden MNH, Golden BE, Jackson AA: Skin breakdown in Kwashiorker responds to zinc. *Lancet* 1980;1:1256

26. Wolman SL, Anderson GH, Marliss EB, et al: Zinc in total parenteral nutrition: requirements and metabolic effects. *Gastroenterology* 1979;76:458

27. Smith KT, Cousins RJ: Quantitative aspects of zinc absorption by isolated, vascularly perfused rat intestine. *J Nutr* 1980; 110:316

28. Mason, KE: A conspectus of research on copper metabolism and requirements in man. *J Nutr* 1979;109:1979

29. Phillips GD, Garnys VP: Parenteral administration of trace elements to critically ill patients. *Anaesth Intensive Care* 1981;9:221

30. Pekarek RS, Hauer EC, Bayfield EJ, et al: Relationship between serum chromium concentrations and glucose utilization in normal and infected subjects. *Diabetes* 1975;24:350

31. Jeejeebhoy KN, Chu RC, Marliss EB, et al: Chromium deficiency, glucose intolerance and neuropathy reversed by chromium supplementation in a patient receiving long-term parenteral nutrition. *Am J Clin Nutr* 1977;30:531

32. Johnson RA, Baker SS, Fallon JT, et al: An accidental case of cardiomyopathy and selenium deficiency. *N Engl J Med* 1981;304:1210

33. Levander OA, Sutherland B, Morris VC, et al: Selenium balance in young men during selenium depletion and repletion. *Am J Clin Nutr* 1981;34:2662

34. Thurlow PM, Grant JP: Vitamin E and total parenteral nutrition. *Ann NY Acad Sci* 1982;393:121

35. Shike M, Sturtridge WC, Tam CS, et al: A possible role of vitamin D in the genesis of parenteral-nutrition-induced metabolic bone disease. *Ann Int Med* 1981;95:560

36. Velez RJ, Myers B, Guber MS: Severe acute metabolic acidosis (acute beriberi): an avoidable complication of total parenteral nutrition. *JPEN* 1985;9:216

37. Cruickshank AM, Telfer AB, Shenkin A: Thiamine deficiency in the critically ill. *Intensive Care Med* 1988;14:384

38. Matsusue S, Kashihara S, Takeda H, et al: Biotin deficiency during total parenteral nutrition: its clinical manifestation and plasma non-esterified fatty acid level. *JPEN* 1985;9:760

39. Chang RW, Jacob S, Lee B: Gastrointestinal dysfunction among intensive care unit patients. *Crit Care Med* 1987; 15:909

40. Dietch EA: Does the gut protect or injure patients in the ICU? *Prospect Crit Care* 1988;1:1

41. Mochizuki H, Trocki O, Dominion L, et al: Mechanism of prevention of postburn hypermetabolism and catabolism by early enteral feeding. *Ann Surg* 1984;200:297

42. Wilmore DW, Smith RJ, O'Dwyer ST, et al: The gut: a central organ after surgical stress. *Surgery* 1988;104:917

43. Moore EE, Jones TN: Benefits of immediate jejunostomy feeding after major abdominal trauma: a prospective, randomized study. *J Trauma* 1986;26:874

44. Grahm TW, Zadrozny DB, Harrington T: The benefits of early jejunal hyperalimentation in the head injured patient. *Neurosurg* 1989;25:729

45. Moore FA, Moore EE, Jones TN, et al: TEN vs TPN following major abdominal trauma: reduced septic morbidity. *J Trauma* 1989;29:916

46. Chiarelli A, Enzi G, Casadei A, et al: Very early nutrition supplementation in burned patients. *Am J Clin Nutr* 1990; 51:1035

47. Moore PA, Feliciano DV, Andrassy J: Early enteral feeding, compared with parenteral, reduces post-operative septic complications: the results of a meta-analysis. *Ann Surg* 1992; 216:172

48. Kudsk KA, Croce MA, Fabian TC, et al: Enteral vs. parenteral feeding: effects on septic morbidity following blunt and penetrating trauma. *Ann Surg* 1992;215:503

49. Eyer SD, Micon LT, Konstantinides FN, et al: Early enteral feeding does not attenuate metabolic response after blunt-trauma. *J Trauma* 1993;39:639

50. Cerra FB, McPherson JP, Konstantinides FN, et al: Enteral nutrition does not prevent multiple organ failure syndrome (MOFS) after sepsis. *Surgery* 1988;104:727

51. Pearson KS, From RP, Symreng T, et al: Continuous enteral feeding and short fasting periods enhance perioperative nutri-

tion in patients with burns. *J Burn Care Rehabilitation* 1992;13:477

52. Jenkins ME, Gottschlich MM, Warden GD: Enteral feeding during operative procedures in therma injuries. *J Burn Care Rehabilitation* 1994;15:199

53. Kemper M, Weissman C, Hyman Al: Caloric requirements and supply in critically ill surgical patients. *Crit Care Med* 1992;20:344

54. Layon AJ, Plorele OG Jr, Day AL, et al: The effect of duodeno-jejunal alimentation or gastric PH and hormones in intensive care unit patients. *Chest* 1991;99:695

55. Alverdy J: The effect of nutrition on gastrointestinal barrier function. *Semin Respir Infect* 1994;9:248

56. Wagner DR, Elmore MF, Tate JT: Combined parenteral and enteral nutrition in severe trauma. *Nutr Clin Pract* 1992;7:113

57. Marian M, Rappaport W, Cunningham D, et al: The failure of conventional methods to promote spontaneous transpyloric feeding tube passage and the safety of intragastric feeding in the critically ill ventilated patient. *Surg Gynecol Obstet* 1993;176:475

58. Stern MA, Wolf DC: Erythromycin as a prokinetic agent: a prospective, randomized controlled study of efficacy in na-soenteric tube placement. *Am J Gastroenterol* 1994;89:2011

59. Kodakia SC, Cassaday M, Shaffer RT: Comparison of foley catheter as a replacement gastrostomy tube with commercial replacement gastrostomy tube: a prospective randomized trial. *Gastrointest Endosc* 1994;40:188

60. D'Amelio LF, Hammond JS, Spain DA, et al: Tracheostomy and percutaneous endoscepic gastrostomy in the management of the head-injured trauma patient. *Am Surg* 1994;60:180

61. Townsend MC, Flancbaum L, Cloutier CT, et al: Early post laparotomy percutaneous endoscopic gastrostomy. *Surg Gynecl Obstet* 1992;174:46

62. Ugo PJ, Mohler PA, Wilson GL: Bedside pyloric placement of weighted feeding tubes. *Nutr Clin Pract* 1992;7:284

63. Montecalvo MA, Steger KA, Farber HW, et al: Nutritional outcome and pneumonia in critical care patients randomized to gastric versus jejunal tube feedings. The Critical Care Research Team. *Crit Care Med* 1992;20:1377

64. Gentilello LM, Cortes V, Castro M, et al: Enteral nutrition with simultaneous gastric decompression in critically ill patients. *Crit Care Med* 1993;21:392

65. Swalts WS, Bell SJ, Baumler J: Clinical comparison of tolerance to elemental or polymeric enteral feedings in the postoperative patient. *JPEN* 1992;16:587

66. Ford EG, Hull SF, Jennings LM, et al: Clinical comparison of tolerance to elemental or polymeric enteral feedings in the postoperative patient. *J Am Coll Nutr* 1992;11:11

67. Frankenfield DC, Beyer PL: Dietary fiber and bowel function in tube-fed patients. *J Am Diet Assoc* 1991;91:590

68. McClave SA, Lowen CC, Snider HL: Immunonutrition and enteral hyperalimentation of critically ill patients. *Dig Dis Sci* 1992;37:1153

69. Bower RH, Cerra FB, Bershadsky B, et al: Early enteral administration of a formula (Impact) supplemented with arginine, nucleotides and fish oil in intensive care unit patients: results of a multicenter, prospective, randomized clinical trial. *Crit Care Med* 1995;23:436

70. Alexander JW: Immunoenhancement via enteral nutrition. *Arch Surg* 1993;128:1242

71. Kemp L, Burge J, Choban P, et al: The effect of catheter type and site on infection rates in total parenteral nutrition patients. *JPEN* 1994;18:71

72. Friedman B, Kanter GM, Titus D: Femoral venous catheters: a safe alternative for delivering parenteral nutrition. *Nutr Clin Pract* 1994;9:69

73. Clark-Christoff N, Watters VA, Sparks W, et al: Use of triple-lumen subclavian catheters for administration of total parenteral nutrition. *JPEN* 1992;16:403

74. Manglano R, Martin M: Safety of triple lumen catheters in the critically ill. *Am Surg* 1991;57:370

75. de Chalain TM, Michell WL, O'Keefe SJ, et al: The effect of fuel source on amino acid metabolism in critically ill patients. *J Surg Res* 1992;52:167

76. Jeejeebhoy KN, Anderson GH, Nakhooda AF, et al: Metabolic studies in total parenteral nutrition with lipid in man: comparison with glucose. *J Clin Invest* 1976;57:125

77. Rotenberg M, Rubin M, Bor A, et al: Physico-chemical characterization of intralipid emulsions. *Biochi Biophys Acta* 1991;1086:265

78. Porta I, Planas M, Padro JB, et al: Effect of two lipid emulsions on platelet function. *Infusionsther Transfusionsmed* 1994;21:316

79. Golub R, Sorrenlo JJ Jr, Cantu R Jr, et al: Efficacy of albumin supplementation in the surgical intensive care unit: a prospective, randomized study. *Crit Care Med* 1994;22:613

80. Broyles JE, Brown RO, Vehe KL, et al: Pharmacist interventions improve fluid balance in fluid-restricted patients requiring parenteral nutrition. *DICP* 1991;25:119

81. Seidner DL, Matarese LE, Steiger E: Nutritional care of the critically ill patient with renal failure. *Semin Nephrol* 1994;14:53

82. Frankenfield DC, Reynolds HN, Wiles CE III: Urea removal during continuous hemodiafiltration. *Crit Care Med* 1994;22:407

83. Riedel E, Hampl H, Nundel M: Essential branched-chain amino acids and alpha-ketoanalogues in hemodialysis patients. *Nephrol Dial Transplant* 1993;7:117

84. Bjerke HS, Shabot MM: Glucose intolerance in critically ill surgical patients: relationship to total parenteral nutrition and severity of illness. *Am Surg* 1992;58:728

85. Griglielmi FW, Mastronuzzi T, De Marco M, et al: Oxidative metabolism in cirrhotic patients with and without hepatocellular carcinoma and effects of malnutrition. *Hepatology* 1992;16:1144

86. Hennessey PJ, Black CT, Andrassy RJ: Nonenzymatic glycosylation of immunoglobulin G impairs complement fixation. *JPEN* 1991;15:60

87. Phelps SJ, Brown RO, Helms RA, et al: Toxicities of parenteral nutrition in the critically ill patient. *Crit Care Clin* 1991;7:725

88. Gerndt SJ, Orringer MB: Tube jejunostomy as an adjunct to esophagectomy. *Surgery* 1994;115:164

89. Gaddy MC, Max MH, Schwab CW, et al: Small bowel ischemia: a consequence of feeding jejunostomy? *South Med J* 1986;79:180

90. Mullan H, Roubenoff RA, Roubenoff R: Risk of pulmonary aspiration among patients receiving enteral nutrition support. *JPEN* 1992;16:160

91. Kinsey GC, Murray MJ, Swensen SJ, et al: Glucose content of tracheal aspirates: implication for the detection of tube feeding aspiration. *Crit Care Med* 1994;22:1557

92. Heimburger DC, Sockwell DG, Geels WJ: Diarrhea with enteral feeding: prospective reappraisal of putative causes. *Nutrition* 1994;10:392

93. Jensen GL, Bross JE, Bourbeau PP, et al: Risk factors for *Clostridium difficile* stool cytotoxin b among critically ill patients: role of sucralfate. *J Infect Dis* 1994;170:227

94. Maki DG, Weise MS, Sarafin HW: A semiquantitative culture method for identifying intravenous-catheter-related infection. *N Engl J Med* 1977;296:1305

95. Gosbell IB, Duggan D, Breust M, et al: Infection associated

with central venous catheters: a prospective survey. *Med J Australia* 1995;162:210

96. Sakaguchi M: Acute pharyngitis, an unusual complication of intravenous hyperalimentation. 1994;108:159

97. Rubin M, Bilik R, Aserin A, et al: Catheter obstruction: analysis of filter content of total nutrient admixture. *JPEN* 1989; 13:641

98. Sacks GS, Brown RO, Colleen P, et al: Failure of typical vegetable oils to prevent essential fatty and deficiency in a critically ill patient recovering long-term parenteral nutrition. *JPEN* 1994;18:274

99. Palmbland J: Intravenous lipid emulsions and host defense: a critical review. *Clin Nutr* 1991;10:303

100. Sedman PC, Somers SS, Ramsden CW, et al: Effects of different lipid emulsions on lymphocyte function during total parenteral nutrition. *Br J Surg* 1991;78:1396

101. Lumpkin MM: Safety alert: hazards of precipitation associated with parenteral nutrition. *Am J Hosp Pharm* 1994;51: 427

102. Murray FE, Stinchcombe SJ, Hawkey CJ: Development of biliary sludge on patients in intensive care unit: results of a prospective ultrasonographic study. *Gut* 1992;33:1123

103. Beau P, Labat-Labourdette J, Ingrand P, et al: Is ursodeoxycholic acid an effective therapy for total parenteral nutrition-related liver disease? *Hepatol* 1994;20:240

104. Zamir O, Nussbaum M, Bhadra S, et al: Effect of enteral feeding on hepatic steatosis induced by total parenteral nutrition. *JPEN* 1994;18:20

105. Mukau L, Talamini MA, Sitzmann JV: Elemental diet may accelerate recovery from total parenteral nutrition-induced gut atrophy. *JPEN* 1994;18:75

106. Shou J, Lappin J, Daly JM: Impairment of pulmonary macrophage function with total parenteral nutrition. *Ann Surg* 1994;219:291

Critical Care, Third Edition, edited by Joseph M. Civetta,
Robert W. Taylor, and Robert R. Kirby.
Lippincott-Raven Publishers, Philadelphia, PA © 1997.

CHAPTER 32

■

Pharmacologic Principles

Subhash K. Todi
Ronald A. Hartmann

Pharmacotherapy plays an essential role in the successful treatment of the critically ill patient. As such, it is incumbent on critical care practitioners to possess a good working knowledge and understanding of certain pharmacokinetic and pharmacodynamic principles as well as the factors that alter them. The ability to apply these principles in the clinical setting is equally important.

Critical care therapeutics often involves the use of multiple pharmacologic agents, each with its own therapeutic purpose, toxicity, and side effects. Many of these agents can be affected by illness-related impairment (acute or chronic) of metabolic organs such as the liver, kidney, and lungs; changes in fluid balance; drug–drug and drug–nutrient interactions; and other factors.

The goal of pharmacotherapy is the attainment of a desired therapeutic response without untoward toxicity. The goal of this chapter is to present principles that will be clinically useful in developing a practical approach to pharmacotherapy in the critically ill patient. Pharmacokinetic principles (with selected examples), drug dosage in renal and hepatic disease, drug–drug interactions, and adverse drug reactions are reviewed.

PHARMACOKINETICS AND PHARMACODYNAMICS ■

Pharmacokinetics can be defined as the quantitative study of the processes of absorption, distribution, biotransformation (metabolism), and elimination of a drug in the body.[1] The use of mathematical models that describe these processes allow predictions to be made about drug concentrations in various parts of the body as a function of dosage, route of administration, clearance, and time.

Pharmacodynamics is the study of the relationship between the concentration of a drug and the biochemical or physiologic response obtained by that drug in a given patient.[2] Some drugs exhibit a linear dose–response relationship (two times the dose equals two times the response) through the entire range of clinically used doses; others may exhibit a linear dose–response relationship to a "maximal" response, above which no additional response is demonstrated. Some agents do not behave in a linear fashion at all. The following are examples of quantifiable pharmacodynamic measurements: decrease in heart rate during betablocker or calcium channel blocker therapy, and decrease in ectopy during antiarrhythmic therapy. Some responses are more difficult to measure, such as the response to corticosteroid or anticonvulsant therapies.

A pharmacokinetic–pharmacodynamic relationship exists in most cases, as demonstrated in Figure 32-1. In general, free (unbound) drug in the plasma is considered to be the pharmacologically active component (both for desired and adverse effects) because it is able to cross into tissues and elicit a pharmacodynamic response. This component is also the only portion available to be metabolized and eliminated.

PHARMACOKINETICS

As stated, pharmacokinetics is the study of the absorption, distribution, metabolism, and elimination of drugs. Much of our knowledge of this subject has resulted from the development of sensitive and specific assays for determining drug concentrations in biological fluids. Conceptual models and mathematical equations have been devised to describe these behaviors[3]; however, the pharmacokinetic parameters described in the literature often are based on data from small numbers of patients or normal volunteers, and these data

475

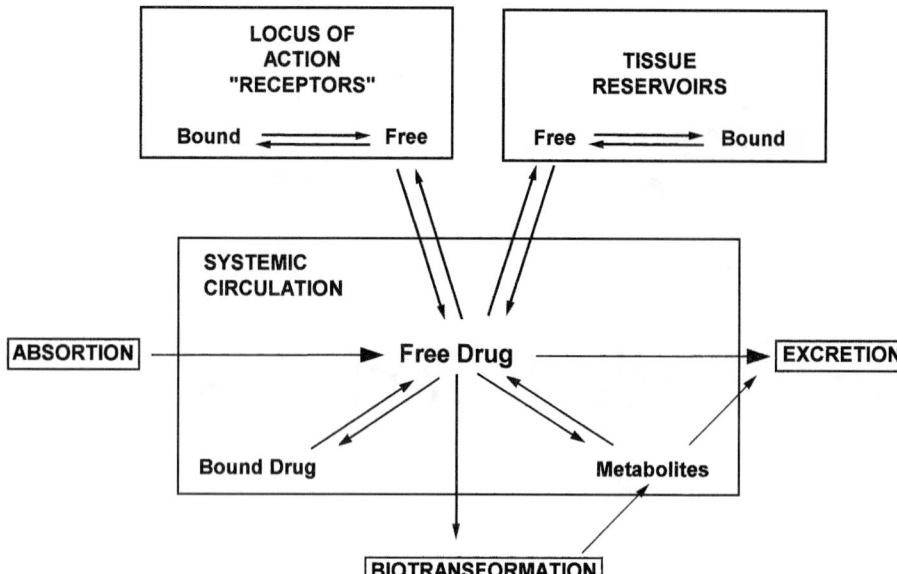

FIGURE 32-1. Schematic representation of the interrelationship of the absorption, distribution, binding, biotransformation, and excretion of a drug and its concentration at its locus of action. Possible distribution and binding of metabolites are not depicted. (Benet LZ, Kroetz DL, Sheiner LB: Pharmacokinetics: The dynamics of drug absorption, distribution and elimination. In: Hardin JG, Limbird LE, Gilman AG, et al (eds). *Goodman and Gilman's The Pharmacologic Basis of Therapeutics*, ed 9. New York, McGraw Hill, 1996:3.)

may not accurately reflect the behavior of that drug in a critically ill patient. Appropriate interpretation of accurately obtained plasma level measurements of a given drug in a specific patient provides significantly more information (with regard to individualizing that patient's drug therapy) than any empiric calculation could provide.

One-Compartment Model

The simplest pharmacokinetic model describes the body as one "compartment." Drugs enter the compartment at rates determined by routes of administration (e.g., intravenous bolus, intravenous infusion, intramuscular, oral, or transdermal) and leave the compartment at rates determined by routes of elimination (e.g., renal, hepatic, or pulmonary).

Two-Compartment Model

A two-compartment model, although an oversimplification in many cases, reasonably describes the behavior of most drugs in humans.[4] In this model, there is a small central compartment consisting of the rapidly perfused organs (heart, lungs, kidney, and endocrine glands) and a larger peripheral compartment consisting of the less rapidly perfused organs (skin, muscle, bone, and fat). After administration, drugs initially distribute into the central compartment and then redistribute into the peripheral compartment, reaching an equilibrium between compartments at a rate that depends on perfusion of peripheral compartment tissues and tissue affinity for the drug.

An assumption of this model is that the drug obeys first-order or linear kinetics, where a constant *proportion* of the drug is removed per unit of time. Rate of elimination of the drug is proportional to serum concentration and diminishes logarithmically over time. The fraction (or percentage) of drug removed per unit of time remains constant, however, and is independent of dose. Also notice that in first-order elimination, both clearance and volume of distribution re-

main constant. Because of this, serum concentration can be adjusted by changing the dose in relation to the desired change in concentration (two times the dose equals two times the concentration).

Some drugs, however, obey zero-order kinetics in which a constant *amount* of drug is eliminated per unit of time, regardless of serum concentration. Others obey saturable (Michaelis-Menten) kinetics. Drugs in the latter category (e.g., ethyl alcohol and phenytoin) exhibit capacity-limited metabolism, and elimination may not be proportional to serum concentration. Phenytoin, for example, exhibits Michaelis-Menten kinetics and demonstrates linear elimination to a point where the patient's hepatic enzyme system is functioning at its maximum rate. After this point, phenytoin serum levels increase out of proportion to dose, so that increasing the dose from 300 to 400 mg/day (a 33% increase) may result in a much greater increase in serum level.

In first-order kinetics, a plot of the logarithm of serum concentration after initial distribution versus time is a straight line. As seen in Figure 32-2, the intravenous injection of a drug results in an initially high serum drug concentration, followed by a rapid decrease because of drug distribution. After the distribution (or alpha) phase, the serum concentration further decreases because of the drug elimination (beta) phase. At any point in time, the serum drug concentration (C_s) can be calculated from the biexponential disappearance function:

$$C_s = Ae^{-\alpha t} + Be^{-\beta t}$$

where α and β are the first-order rate constants for the alpha and beta phases, respectively.[5]

From a practical standpoint, there are four pharmacokinetic parameters of particular value in the application of these principals to clinical practice: volume of distribution, clearance, half-life, and bioavailability.

Volume of distribution (Vd) is that apparent volume of fluid in which a given dose would have to be distributed to achieve the observed serum concentration. This relationship

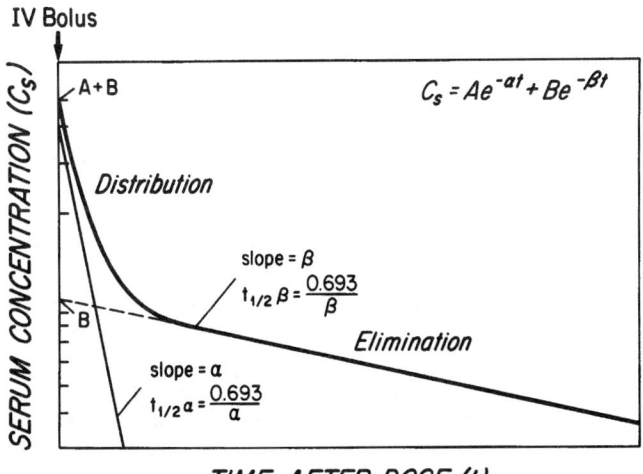

FIGURE 32-2. Schematic graph of serum drug concentrations (C_s) plotted on a logarithmic scale versus time after a single intravenous bolus injection. (Greenblatt DJ, Koch-Weser J: Clinical pharmacokinetics. *N Engl J Med* 1975;293:703.)

is described by the following equations:

$$C_s = \text{dose}/Vd \quad \text{or} \quad Vd = \text{dose}/C_s$$

This volume is not necessarily a physiologic volume because of tissue distribution and binding. Digoxin, for example, has an apparent volume of distribution of 500 to 600 L because of extensive tissue binding. Clinically, volume of distribution is useful for estimating the initial "loading" dose required to achieve a desired serum concentration or for calculating an incremental bolus dose required to raise a patient's serum level by a desired amount. For example, theophylline has a volume of distribution of approximately *0.5 L/kg* in most patients, thus a 60-kg person would have an apparent volume of distribution of 30 L. If the desired serum concentration was 15 mg/L, the loading dose required to achieve this goal would be calculated as follows:

$$\text{Dose} = (Vd)\,(C_s) = (30\ \text{L})\,(15\ \text{mg/L}) = 450\ \text{mg}$$

Drug clearance (Cl) is defined as the volume of blood or serum from which all drug is removed per unit of time. Clearance can be affected by alterations in distribution, biotransformation, or excretion. Specific issues relating to changes in clearance from impairment of renal or hepatic function are discussed later in this chapter.

One of pharmacokinetic's fundamental principles is that at steady state, rate in equals rate out.[6] Based on this principle, drug clearance (rate out) can be useful in determining the amount of drug required to maintain a therapeutic drug level. With an intravenously administered or completely absorbed oral agent, the steady-state serum concentration (C_{ss}) can be determined by the following equations:

$$C_{ss} = \text{dosage rate/clearance, or}$$

$$= \frac{\text{dose}}{(\text{dosage interval})\,(\text{Cl})}$$

Drug half-life ($t_{1/2}$) is a function of both volume of distribution and clearance:

$$t_{1/2} = (0.693)\ Vd/Cl$$

In most cases, this variable refers to elimination half-life, that is, the time required to reduce the initial serum concentration by 50% after the initial distribution phase. The drug half-life can be useful in determining the amount of time required to reach steady-state serum concentration. Four elimination half-lives are required to achieve approximately 94% of steady state. The time required to reach steady-state serum concentration is independent of dose and dosage interval, and whether or not a loading dose was given. As described earlier, it is a function of clearance and volume of distribution. As seen in Figure 32-3, drug accumulation occurs on repeated dosing until an equilibrium or steady state is reached at approximately four to five half-lives. If, in this example, the desired pharmacologic response is observed at a serum concentration of 1 to 2 units, there is a period of time after the initiation of therapy in which the serum concentration is "subtherapeutic." It is generally a

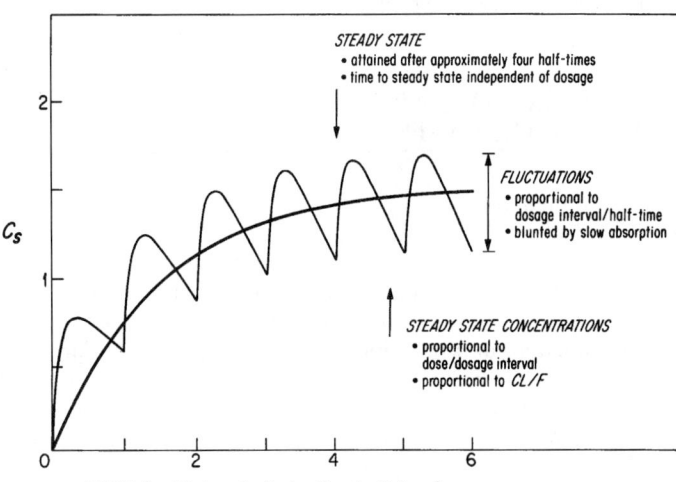

FIGURE 32-3. Fundamental pharmacokinetic relationships for repeated administration of drugs. (Benet LZ, Kroetz DL, Sheiner LB: Pharmacokinetics: The dynamics of drug absorption, distribution and elimination. In: Hardin JG, Limbird LE, Gilman AG, et al (eds). *Goodman and Gilman's The Pharmacologic Basis of Therapeutics*, ed 9. New York, McGraw Hill, 1996:23.)

desirable goal to achieve *therapeutic* levels at the initiation of therapy. To accomplish this, a loading dose may be given as described above, followed by the maintenance doses.

For example, digoxin has an elimination half-life of 36 hours in a patient with normal renal function. A period of 6 days, therefore, would be required to achieve a steady-state drug level with daily dosing. If a loading dose of 1 mg (0.5 mg + 0.25 mg + 0.25 mg) is given, *therapeutic* digoxin concentrations may be achieved more rapidly. It is important to measure a serum digoxin level (allowing at least 6 hours for distribution to take place) to confirm this effect. As stated, steady-state serum concentrations will not be achieved for four to five half-lives.

Bioavailability of a drug is defined as the fraction of a drug dose that reaches the systemic circulation. Bioavailability is a consideration primarily with orally administered agents. Absorption can be affected by many factors relating to the pharmaceutical preparation itself (e.g., tablet, capsule, oral liquid, suspension, or sustained-release product), gastric pH and emptying time, intestinal motility, and drug complex formation with other drugs or nutrients.[7] Many orally absorbed drugs demonstrate a "first-pass" effect with significant metabolism in the liver before the drug enters the systemic circulation. Examples are propranolol, hydralazine, verapamil, and lidocaine. Lidocaine's first-pass effect is so great that it must be administered by the parenteral route. For other drugs like propranolol and verapamil, oral doses need to be substantially higher than parenteral doses to account for this affect. For these drugs, the fraction of drug available to the systemic circulation (F) must be included in the calculation of steady-state serum concentration as follows:

$$C_{ss} = \frac{(F)\,(dose)}{(dosage\ interval)\,(Cl)}$$

Because most pharmacologic agents are administered parenterally in the ICU, the issue of bioavailability does not often need to be considered. It is, however, an important factor to keep in mind when switching a patient from certain parenterally administered dosage forms (with 100% availability) to oral "equivalents" (or vice versa). In addition to verapamil and hydralazine, this is also true for digoxin, levothyroxine, and phenytoin.

PHARMACOTHERAPY IN RENAL DISEASES

Renal dysfunction is often present in critically ill patients. Acute and chronic renal impairment can have profound effects on the pharmacokinetics and pharmacodynamics of many commonly used agents.[8] Drug therapy in patients with renal dysfunction is often more complex than simply reducing the daily dose in proportion to reductions in glomerular filtration rate (GFR).[9] Other factors, such as changes in protein binding or volume of distribution, also can affect the way certain drugs behave in this patient population.[10] Renal disease affects the pharmacokinetic parameters of many drugs used in the ICU. The *absorption* and *bioavailability* of enterally administered drugs can be affected by the higher gastric pH, altered gastric emptying time, vomiting, ileus, or intestinal edema seen in uremic patients. *Distribution* of many drugs also can be significantly altered in renal dysfunction. Because uremic patients generally have a higher percentage of their body mass as water, the apparent volume of distribution for water-soluble drugs is often increased. Also, serum protein binding (mainly of acidic drugs) is often reduced in renal failure, leading to increased free (unbound) levels of agents that are normally highly protein bound with a resulting decrease in the volume of distribution (e.g., phenytoin). As discussed earlier, increased "free" drug levels may cause enhanced activity or toxicity while also making more drug available for metabolism and clearance. If the kidneys or liver are diseased and are unable to handle the increased amount of unbound drug, the drug effect may be further amplified. Free drug concentrations may correlate better with pharmacologic effect than total (free plus bound) concentrations in this setting.

Altered *tissue binding* also may affect the apparent volume of distribution of a drug. For example, digoxin's distribution volume is reduced by 30% to 50% of normal in patients with renal disease.[6] As a result, loading doses should be reduced accordingly (depending on therapeutic intent) to a total of 0.5 mg in most renal failure patients, with maintenance doses reduced as well (often to 0.125 mg three times per week). For most drugs, however, the volume of distribution is *not* significantly altered, and as such, renal failure patients should receive the same loading doses as patients with normal renal function:

$$Loading\ dose\ (mg) = Vd\ (L) \times desired\ C_s\ (mg/L)$$

The major pharmacokinetic effect seen in renal dysfunction is the impaired elimination of drugs and their metabolites by the kidney, resulting in decreased clearance and an increased half-life. Renal clearance of pharmacologic agents is complex, involving one or more of the processes of filtration, tubular secretion, and reabsorption. Few drugs are excreted solely by glomerular filtration. Additionally, tubular secretion and reabsorption for many compounds may vary with the type of renal dysfunction and the administration of other agents (e.g., probenecid). Thus, clearance (expressed as liters per hour per kilogram) may be highly variable in this particular clinical setting.

Extensive references are available to guide practitioners in the appropriate dosing reductions for varying degrees of renal impairment.[11,12] As stated earlier, initial or loading doses are usually not altered in renal impairment. Maintenance dosing schemes should be designed to compensate for the decreased clearance and resulting prolongation of half-life seen in these patients. The optimal regimen may by achieved by prolonging dosing intervals, reducing the standard maintenance dose, or both.

In the ICU, this knowledge is particularly important in the prescribing of antimicrobial agents, cardiovascular drugs, sedatives, analgesics, and H₂ receptor blocking agents. Serum drug concentrations, when available, should be used selectively to monitor therapy (Table 32-1). With regard to

TABLE 32-1. Therapeutic Serum Drug Levels

DRUGS	THERAPEUTIC RANGE
CARDIOVASCULAR DRUGS	
Digitoxin	10–25 ng/mL
Digoxin	0.8–2.0 ng/mL
Disopyramide	207 µg/mL
Lidocaine	1.5–5 µg/mL
Procainamide + NAPA	10–30 µg/mL
Quinidine	2–5 µg/mL
ANTICONVULSANTS	
Carbamazepine	4–12 µg/mL
Ethosuximide	40–100 µg/mL
Phenobarbital	15–40 µg/mL
Phenytoin	10–20 µg/mL
Primadone	5–12 µg/mL
Valproic acid	50–100 µg/mL
ANTIBIOTICS	
5-Flucytosine	50–100 µg/mL
Gentamicin/tobramycin/ netilmicin*	Peak: 5–10 µg/mL Trough: <2 µg/mL
Amikacin	Peak: 20–30 µg/mL Trough: <8 µg/mL
Vancomycin	Peak: 20–40 µg/mL Trough: <15 µg/mL
OTHERS	
Cyclosporine (plasma by RIA)	Trough: 50–300 ng/mL
Lithium	0.5–1.5 mEq/L/mL
Nortriptyline	50–140 µg/mL
Salicylic acid	150–300 µg/mL
Theophylline	5–20 µg/mL

*Aminoglycoside peak ranges based on traditional dosing; NAPA, N-acetyl procainamide; RIA, radioimmunoassay.

serum levels, their use should be judicious and for specific purpose. It may be useful (or necessary) at times to obtain a peak serum level after the initial dose of a drug to assess whether an adequate dose was given. In general, it is best to wait until drug levels accumulate to the point of steady state before obtaining blood samples. As described earlier, steady state is a function of clearance, and it takes approximately four elimination half-lives to reach this point (where rate in equals rate out). In renal impairment, half-lives of renally cleared drugs are prolonged and time to steady state is delayed. For a drug like gentamicin, for example, half-life is increased from 2 to 8 hours when GFR drops from 120 to 25 mL/minute. The amount of time required to reach steady state (regardless of dosing regimen) would, therefore, increase from 8 to 32 hours. For this reason, it would *not* be reasonable to check levels "at the third dose" unless the dosing interval was set at 18 to 24 hours.

For drugs administered by continuous infusion (e.g., lidocaine and theophylline), the time required to reach steady state (four to five half-lives) is the main factor to consider

in deciding when to draw a serum level. Also, if a change is made in the dosing regimen, an additional four to five half-lives must elapse before a new steady state is reached.

CREATININE CLEARANCE

Creatinine is a muscle breakdown product that is produced at a constant rate related primarily to a person's muscle mass, age, and sex. It is cleared from the body (almost completely) by glomerular filtration and has provided clinicians with a useful marker to estimate GFR based on creatinine's clearance.[13] This clearance can be measured directly through timed urine collections, or it can be reasonably accurately estimated using the patient's serum creatinine concentration, along with other parameters. Several estimation methods exist, and clinicians often have differences of opinion as to how to best use them. The method described by Cockcroft and Gault[14] continues to be the most frequently used:

$$\text{CrCl (men)} = \frac{(140 - \text{age})\,(\text{body weight in kg})}{72 \times (\text{serum creatinine in mg/dL})}$$

This value should be reduced by 15% (multiplied by 0.85) for women. Also, it is this author's (R.H.) opinion that for this calculation, body weight equals ideal body weight (IBW) or actual weight if less than ideal:

IBW (m) = 50 kg + 2.3 (height in inches − 60)

IBW (w) = 45.5 kg + 2.3 (height in inches − 60)

Also, when making this calculation, serum creatinine should be rounded up to 1.0 if less than 1.

Notice that serum creatinine values are affected by other factors. An elevated serum creatinine value in a dehydrated patient, for example, may underestimate that patient's ability to eliminate renally cleared drugs. Creatinine values in muscle-wasted patients may also provide misleading overestimations of a patient's clearance abilities. In these situations, accurately obtained serum drug levels, if available, provide a much better estimate of GFR.

Despite the limitations, this indirect estimate of GFR makes it possible to assess the degree of renal impairment in a given patient and to make appropriate decisions on whether to reduce a patient's dose and by how much.

Renal failure requiring dialysis (hemodialysis or peritoneal) presents additional challenges in determining appropriate drug dosing regimens. The following factors lead to enhanced drug clearance by dialysis: high concentration, small volume of distribution, significant water (not lipid) solubility, small molecular size, and low degree of protein or tissue binding.[11] The type of dialyzer and filter also are important.[15] For drugs removed to a significant degree by dialysis, "supplemental" doses are often recommended after dialysis sessions. An alternative approach in many cases is to simply administer the scheduled dose after dialysis.

In summary, renal failure affects many aspects of pharmacotherapy with the most important effect being impaired drug elimination. Designing an appropriate dosage regimen, selectively monitoring drug levels, and being observant for clinical evidence of therapeutic and toxic effects are crucial elements in caring for these patients.

CLINICAL EXAMPLE: GENTAMICIN

Aminoglycoside antibiotics remain valuable tools for the critical care practitioner to use in the treatment of many gram-negative bacillary infections as well as their use as an adjunct in the treatment of certain gram-positive infections. Because the volume of distribution, drug clearance, and half-lives of these agents are similar, the same pharmacokinetic details discussed here can be applied to all of the agents in the group (i.e., gentamicin, tobramycin, netilmicin, and amikacin). Aminoglycosides are excreted almost exclusively by the kidneys through glomerular filtration and have no known metabolites. They have a narrow toxic:therapeutic index with ototoxicity and nephrotoxicity associated with excessive levels, and lack of therapeutic efficacy seen when levels are inadequate to treat the targeted infection. Enhancement of neuromuscular blockade is an additional concern in the ICU. The nephrotoxicity is thought to be caused by the gradual accumulation of drug in renal cortical cells by tubular reabsorption, with resultant acute tubular necrosis. Renal dysfunction, although usually reversible, is enhanced by extracellular volume depletion, hepatic failure, magnesium and potassium depletion, and increased frequency of dosage.[16]

As with all drugs prescribed, specific goals of therapy should guide the choice of dose and interval in an individual patient. In the treatment of most serious gram-negative infections, desirable peak serum gentamicin concentrations are in the range of 6 to 10 μg/mL, and the drug should be dosed accordingly. Lower peak levels are probably adequate for gram-positive synergy and the treatment of some urinary tract infections. Trough levels above 2 μg/mL have been associated with the development of nephrotoxicity and should be avoided. Although somewhat unclear, ototoxicity, once thought to be a result of elevated peak levels (more than 10 μg/mL), may not be related to this factor at all and also may be related to elevated trough concentrations over extended periods of time. Aminoglycosides exhibit concentration-dependent bacterial killing and a postantibiotic effect that allows the depressed bacterial growth to persist after plasma concentrations have fallen below the minimum inhibitory concentration (MIC) of the organism being treated.[17]

Volume of Distribution

Although the reported volume of distribution for aminoglycosides varies widely[18] (0.1 to 0.5 L/kg), a reasonable estimate in most patients is *0.26 L/kg*. Larger distribution volumes are seen in certain critically ill patients, particularly those with significant burn injuries or septic shock. The weight to be used in this calculation is controversial: in patients near or below their ideal body weight, the actual weight should be used; in patients who are more than 25% above their ideal body weight (because of obesity, edema, or third-spaced fluid) a reasonable approach is to add 43% of the "non-lean" weight to the ideal body weight[19]:

$$\text{Dosing weight (kg)} = \text{IBW} + [0.43\,(\text{TBW} - \text{IBW})]$$

From this estimate of volume of distribution (0.26 L/kg), a reasonable loading dose can be calculated based on the desired peak serum level (C_{max}):

$$\text{Loading dose (mg)} = \text{Vd} \times C_{max}$$
$$= 0.26\ \text{L/kg} \times \text{DW (kg)} \times C_{max}$$

where DW is dosing weight (this dose should be rounded to the nearest 10 mg for practical purposes).

CLEARANCE. Aminoglycoside elimination parallels creatinine's clearance in a relationship described by the following equations, where K_{el} is the elimination rate constant that describes the slope of the terminal elimination curve in a log-concentration versus time graph (the term *beta* in Fig. 32-2) and where CrCl is creatinine clearance:

$$K_{el} = [(0.00285 \times \text{CrCl}) + 0.015]$$
$$t_{1/2} = 0.693/K_{el}$$

Because clearance equals K_{el} multiplied by volume of distribution, and volume of distribution remains constant in most cases, aminoglycoside clearance varies nearly proportionally with creatinine clearance. Half-life varies inversely (as creatinine clearance doubles, half-life is cut in half).

CHOICE OF DOSING REGIMEN. The choice of dose and interval should be guided by therapeutic intent. If a peak gentamicin level of 8 mg/L is desired, a dose sufficient to achieve that level should be calculated for the specific patient being treated. Dosing intervals should be practical (8, 12, or 24 hours) and should be selected to allow sufficient time to elapse after a dose for the "trough" level to decline to less than 2 mg/L before re-dosing. In fact, the postantibiotic effect described earlier may allow trough levels to drop to subtherapeutic levels for some part of the dosing interval without compromising efficacy. It is reasonable, therefore, to dose aminoglycosides at 12-hour intervals in most adult patients with estimated creatinine clearance more than 40 mL/minute as long as adequate doses are given. In the absence of patient-specific pharmacokinetic dosing recommendations, a reasonable *empiric* dosing scheme for many patients is to administer *2 mg/kg doses (based on the adjusted dosing weight) every 12 hours*. Patients with estimated creatinine clearance in the 20 to 40 mL/minute range should receive this dose every *24* hours, and if creatinine clearance is less than 20 mL/minute, dosing should be approached cautiously and serum levels monitored closely. In younger patients with creatinine clearance above 120 mL/minute (half-lives less than 2 hours), it may still be reasonable to dose at 8-hour intervals. Serum levels should be obtained at steady state, with trough levels 0 to 30 minutes before the dose and peak levels 30 minutes after a 30-minute infusion. Documentation of accurate sample timing is essential to the interpretation of these levels because doses and intervals may need to be adjusted based on the concentrations measured. General guidelines for dosage adjustment are presented in Table 32-2.

Based on these concepts, some clinicians advocate using large (5 to 7 mg/kg/dose) single doses of gentamicin or

TABLE 32-2. General Guidelines for Adjusting Aminoglycoside Dosing Based on Serum Levels

SCENARIO	PEAK	TROUGH	INTERVENTION
1	OK	OK	No change; recheck trough every 3 d to monitor
2	OK	Low	Probably OK—can shorten interval
3	OK	High	Lengthen interval and probably increase dose
4	Low	OK	Increase dose +/− lengthen interval
5	Low	Low	Increase dose +/− shorten interval
6	Low	High	Increase dose and lengthen interval
7	High	OK	Decrease dose—no change in interval
8	High	Low	Decrease dose—can shorten interval
9	High	High	Lengthen interval +/− decrease dose

tobramycin every 24 to 48 hours to achieve high peaks (often 18 to 25 μg/mL) with low (often undetectable) troughs.[7,20,21] Whereas this approach virtually guarantees reaching "therapeutic" peak levels, there are some concerns with regard to efficacy in patients with excellent renal function (half-life less than 2 hours) who will clear all drug in 8 to 10 hours (does the postantibiotic effect last that long?) as well as safety concerns in treating patients with these high doses for extended (10- to 14-day) courses of therapy. Additionally, this dosing approach has not been shown to be superior to appropriately dosed "conventional" therapy in published reports.[17,22] Data in critically ill patients also are limited. Although unclear, some researchers suggest that optimal aminoglycoside peak levels may be related to ratios of peak to MIC, or area under the curve (AUC) to MIC, which, if correct, will allow for further optimization of aminoglycoside dosing.[22]

PHARMACOTHERAPY IN LIVER DISEASE

The liver plays a pivotal role in the maintenance of body homeostasis through its influence on the metabolism of endogenous and exogenous chemicals. Thus, hepatic disease—both acute and chronic—can affect the bioavailability, distribution, action, and elimination of many drugs.

The bioavailability of some orally administered drugs with extensive first-pass effect, like propranolol and morphine, is greatly increased in liver diseases with large portosystemic shunt. As such, their dosage should be appropriately reduced to prevent adverse side effects.[23] In chronic liver disease with ascites, an increase in the volume of distribution is observed for several drugs; examples include ampicillin, lorazepam, diazepam, and lidocaine. Moreover, hypoalbuminemia is common in cirrhotics, and metabolism of drugs that are highly protein bound (Table 32-3) is adversely affected by this.

The level of drug in the blood is also influenced by the capacity of liver to remove the drug from the circulating blood, expressed by the term *clearance*. Hepatic clearance (ClH) is directly related to hepatic blood flow (Q), and to the amount of drug extracted from the blood as it passes through the liver, referred to as extraction ratio (E), which, in turn, depends on the capacity of hepatic enzymes to metabolize the drug[24]:

$$ClH = Q \times E$$

The metabolic capacity of the liver for drugs with high extraction ratio (more than 0.7) is much greater than the rate at which they are presented to the liver and are often referred to as flow limited[24-26] (Table 32-4). The clearance of these drugs is determined primarily by hepatic blood flow and usually is not affected by mild hepatic impairment, enzyme-inducing or enzyme-inhibiting drugs, or changes in protein binding. Disease states like severe cirrhosis, initial phase of hepatic trauma, and shock state, and the use of vasopressors can all decrease hepatic blood flow, thereby increasing the elimination half-life and bioavailability of drugs with a high extraction ratio, such as verapamil and propranolol. The doses of these drugs should be reduced in such conditions. Low extraction ratio drugs (E less than 0.3) are less dependent on hepatic blood flow but are highly dependent on

TABLE 32-3. Drugs With High Plasma Protein Binding Affinity

Digoxin	Phenytoin	Tolbutamide
Diazoxide	Quinidine	Valproic acid
Hydralazine	Sulfonamides	Warfarin
NSAIDs	Salicylates	

NSAIDs, nonsteroidal antiinflammatory drugs.

TABLE 32-4.   Drug Dosage Adjustment in Hepatic Failure

DRUGS	% PROTEIN BOUND	MECHANISM	METHOD OF ADJUSTMENT
Cefoperazone	90	EL, BS	Decrease dose
Chloramphenicol	60	EL, BS	Decrease dose
Cimetidine	20	FL	Decrease dose if severe
Clindamycin	75	EL, BS	Decrease dose if severe
Diazepam	97	EL, BS	Decrease dose
Erythromycin	80	EL, BS	Decrease dose
Labetalol	50	FL	Decrease dose
Lidocaine	65	FL	Decrease dose
Lorazepam	90	EL, BS	None
Meperidine	65	EL, FL	Decrease dose, avoid if severe
Morphine	35	FL	Decrease dose, avoid if severe
Phenobarbital	50	EL, BI	Decrease dose
Phenytoin	92	EL, BS	Decrease dose
Propranolol	95	FL	Decrease dose
Quinidine	85	EL, FL	Decrease dose
Ranitidine	15	FL	Decrease dose (oral)
Theophylline	52	EL, BI	Decrease dose
Verapamil	92	FL	Decrease dose

EL, enzyme limited; FL, flow limited; BI, binding insensitive; BS, binding sensitive.

Data from Secor JW, Schenker S: Drug metabolism in patients with liver diseases. *Adv Intern Med* 1987;32:379; and Williams RL: Drug administration in hepatic disease. *N Engl J Med* 1983;309:1616.

protein binding and the level of intrinsic clearance (enzymatic capacity) of the liver (see Table 32-4). These drugs are susceptible to changing clearance because of induction or inhibition of liver enzymes and are often referred to as enzyme limited or capacity limited.[27] Hepatic extraction process of some enzyme-limited drugs is termed *binding-sensitive* or *restrictive* when only circulating free drug is removed during passage through the liver. Therefore, a decrease in drug binding causes an almost proportional change in the hepatic extraction of the drug. Drugs that are highly protein bound are subjected to this mechanism[23] (see Table 32-3). In contrast, when extraction is nonrestrictive, that is, when the liver removes not only the free fraction but also the bound drug, the extraction efficiency is less affected by alteration in drug binding. These are *binding-insensitive* drugs.[23] Agents with extraction ratio in the intermediate range (0.3 to 0.7) are effected by both hepatic blood flow and metabolic enzyme activity, the extent depending on the precise extraction ratio.[23]

Table 32-4 contains information on dosage adjustments of some commonly used drugs in liver failure. Unfortunately, there are no markers analogous to creatinine clearance that can guide dosage adjustments in hepatic impairment. Individualized pharmacokinetic determinations, guided by drug levels when possible, and careful pharmacodynamic monitoring are important in this setting.[28,29] An example of this is the dosage adjustment of theophylline in liver disease states. The pharmacokinetics of theophylline are complex. The volume of distribution is approximately 500 mL/kg with 40% to 60% of the drug bound to protein. Theophylline is

metabolized in the liver, with only 10% excreted unchanged in the urine. It is primarily an enzyme-limited and binding-insensitive drug. Therefore, changes in liver function, especially in the mixed-function oxidase enzyme activity, can have a profound effect on the agent's clearance. Factors that reduce hepatic blood flow, including drugs such as cimetidine and congestive heart failure, reduce theophylline clearance.[30–32] In contrast, hepatic enzyme induction by drugs such as barbiturates or smoking increases theophylline clearance. These factors should be considered in regulating theophylline dosage to achieve therapeutic serum levels range from 10 to 20 µg/mL.

ADVERSE DRUG REACTIONS

The term *adverse drug reactions* (ADRs) encompasses a broad range of drug effects, ranging from exaggerated but predictable pharmacologic actions of the drug to toxic effects unrelated to intended pharmacologic effects.[33] As such, the true incidence rate of ADRs is difficult to determine, with estimates ranging from 5% to 30%.[34,35] Only by maintaining a high index of clinical suspicion, keeping the drug therapy to the minimum necessary, and by stopping the suspect drug if possible could one minimize the incidence of ADRs, thereby decreasing patient morbidity, perhaps mortality, and also keeping the cost of therapy low.

A small group of widely used drugs account for a disproportionate number of ADRs: aspirin, anticoagulants, diuretics, digoxin, antimicrobials, steroids, and hypoglycemic agents account for 90% of reactions.[33]

The most frequent ADRs result from the exaggerated but predicted pharmacologic actions of the drug, and, as such, are readily identifiable and often are preventable. Examples of such effects include hemorrhagic complications caused by anticoagulants or hypoglycemia caused by oral hypoglycemic agents or insulin. The most important determinant for such adverse effect is the abnormally high drug concentration at the receptor site. This can occur for a variety of reasons, ranging from errors in drug dosage calculation or administration to alteration in the pharmacokinetics (such as reduction in the volume of distribution, rate of metabolism, or rate of excretion), or because of drug interaction resulting in increased concentration of free drug at receptor site, leading to untoward effects. There are increasing reports of persistent paralysis in some patients after exposure to nondepolarizing neuromuscular blockade in the ICU.[36] Monitoring neuromuscular transmission is strongly recommended during use of paralytic agents to avoid this complication.[37]

Other ADRs result from toxic effects unrelated to the intended pharmacologic actions. These, therefore, often are unpredictable and frequently are severe. There are various mechanisms for such ADRs: genetic, immunologic and nonimmunologic, or idiosyncratic. Genetic susceptibility to certain drugs leading to ADRs sometimes can be encountered in the intensive care setting (Table 32-5). The most relevant of these would be succinylcholine-induced prolonged apnea (suxamethonium sensitivity) and drug-induced malignant hyperthermia (MH). Succinylcholine is a depolarizing muscle relaxant that is rapidly metabolized by plasma pseudocholinesterase with duration of paralysis for 2 to 4 minutes. Approximately 1 in 3200 patients is homozygous for a defective pseudocholinesterase, which has an autosomal recessive transmission, and demonstrates markedly prolonged block with succinylcholine in the range of 3 to 8 hours.[38] MH is a clinical syndrome of muscle rigidity, tachycardia, tachypnea, rapidly increasing temperature, hypoxia, hypercapnia, hyperglycemia, hyperkalemia, hypercalcemia, lactic acidosis,

and eventual cardiovascular collapse that occurs during or after general anesthesia.[39] Several drugs have been implicated in triggering MH, particularly the halogenated inhalational agents (halothane, enflurane, and isoflurane), succinylcholine, and possibly aminoamide local anesthetic (lidocaine or bupivacaine).[40,41]

The cause of MH seems to be an inability of the sarcoplasmic reticulum of skeletal muscle to take up released myoplasmic calcium. When a MH episode is triggered, the myoplasmic levels of calcium rise tremendously, accelerating muscle metabolism and contraction and leading to the clinical manifestations of the syndrome.[39]

Dantrolene is the cornerstone of therapy for MH.[42] It reduces rigidity and restores muscle function by preventing calcium release from the sarcoplasmic reticulum and antagonizes its effects on muscle contraction.[43] Treatment of MH is initiated by discontinuing the anesthetic and other possible triggering agents, ventilating the patient with 100% oxygen, and providing hemodynamic support as needed. Dantrolene sodium, 2.5 mg/kg intravenously, should be given immediately and repeated every 5 minutes until a total of 10 mg/kg is reached or until all manifestations of the syndrome have resolved. Maintenance doses are given every 5 to 8 hours if needed.[44] The mortality rate from the fulminant syndrome was approximately 70% before the use of dantrolene.[45] With early recognition and optimal therapy, it is now reported as 7% to 10%.[45] The use of prophylactic dantrolene prevents MH in most susceptible persons.

Immunologically mediated ADR is epitomized by the classic anaphylactic reaction, which is IgE mediated, and serum sickness-like condition. A similar reaction, but not immunologically mediated, known as *anaphylactoid reaction*, is sometimes seen as an indirect histamine release from the mast cells by morphine, or complement activation leading to mediator release from the mast cell and basophil by aspirin and radiocontrast media. There are a host of drug reactions for which the exact underlying mechanism of toxicity is not well understood, and these are termed *idiosyncratic reactions*. Every organ system can potentially be adversely affected by drug exposures, or ADRs can pres-

TABLE 32-5. Examples of Inherited Disorders Involving an Abnormal Response to Drugs

	DISORDER		
Characteristic	*Suxamethonium Sensitivity*	*Malignant Hyperthermia*	*Warfarin Insensitivity*
Molecular abnormality	Pseudocholinesterase in plasma	Unknown	Altered receptors
Mode of inheritance	Autosomal recessive	Autosomal dominant	Autosomal dominant
Clinical effects	Apnea	Hyperpyrexia, muscle rigidity	Inability to achieve anticoagulation
Drugs producing abnormal response	Succinylcholine	Halothane, succinylcholine, cyclopropane	Warfarin

From Goldstein JL, Brown MS: Genetics and disease. *Harrison's Principles of Internal Medicine,* ed 13. New York, McGraw Hill, 1994:349.

ent with effects on multiple organ systems. Of the multisystem manifestations of ADRs, drug fever, drug withdrawal reactions, and anaphylaxis are worth elaborating.

Drug-induced fever should always be considered in the workup of pyrexia in the intensive care unit, more so when there is no other obvious source. Fever is thought to be relatively rare as a primary or sole manifestation of a drug reaction and is usually associated with other hypersensitivity type reactions like anaphylaxis, serum sickness, rash, or eosinophilia. But sometimes it can be the only manifestation of an ADR. Antibiotics, cardiovascular drugs, and central-acting agents are the largest categories of drugs causing fever.[46] Patients with hypersensitivity-induced drug fever have been observed to have fevers as high as 40°C and yet generally appear well.[47] This finding may be an important clue to the presence of a drug-related fever.

Tolerance and dependence on opiates and benzodiazepines can develop over a short period, and subsequent attempts at withdrawing these medications might be associated with hypermetabolism and "sympathetic overdrive" characterized by fever, hypertension, mental confusion, seizures, and cardiac arrhythmias, a picture that sometimes can be confused with an underlying disease process. This syndrome has recently been reviewed in detail.[48] Management consists of the gradual withdrawal of the drug and substitution longer acting agents; clonidine, a centrally acting drug, has been used recently with some success in these conditions.[49] Anaphylactic drug reactions have been described elsewhere in this text.

Mental confusion is a common problem in the ICU, and the cause is often multifactorial.[50] Drugs that have been reported to alter mood and increase mental confusion, especially in the elderly, include high doses of or withdrawal from corticosteroids, cimetidine, theophylline, barbiturates, benzodiazepines, digoxin, antidepressants, penicillin, lidocaine, antihistamines, quinidine, opiates, and phenothiazines. Drugs like imipenem-cilastatin have been implicated as an inducer or promoter of seizure-like activity.[51]

Some of the antiarrhythmic drugs, particularly quinidine, procainamide, and disopyramide, have a strong proarrythmic effect, and their drug levels should be closely monitored during their use. Torsade de pointes, a form of polymorphic ventricular tachyarrhythmia caused by drugs that can prolong the QTc interval (like phenothiazines and tricyclic antidepressant), could be fatal. Treatment with intravenous magnesium, isoproterenol, and overdrive pacing has been used with some success.

Alteration in acid-base balance with drugs causing metabolic alkalosis (like diuretics and acetate in total parenteral nutrition solutions) can cause depression of respiratory drive, which can become significant in patients with severe lung function impairment, making them difficult to wean off the ventilator. The addition of acetazolamide, a carbonic anhydrase inhibitor that can cause metabolic acidosis, might be useful in these situations.

Drug-induced renal injury remains a major cause of increased morbidity and contributes to overall mortality of the critically ill. The aminoglycoside antibiotics and radiographic contrast agents are the leading cause of acute nephrotoxicity in the ICU. Other risk factors that make patients prone to develop nephrotoxicity include advanced age, prior renal disease, intravascular volume depletion, simultaneous use of other nephrotoxic agents, and certain disease states like congestive heart failure, cirrhosis of liver, and diabetes mellitus.[52]

Drugs can cause abnormalities in any of the formed elements of blood, which can lead to diagnostic confusion in separating these from primary disease processes. Drug-induced pancytopenia, hemolytic anemia, thrombocytopenia, and granulocytopenia all have been well described.[52] Some of these are more pertinent to ICU patients than others. Heparin-induced thrombocytopenia is an example of the latter, with an incidence rate of 5% to 10%.[53] The mechanism is believed to be the induction of platelet-specific IgG antibody by heparin, with subsequent aggregation of platelets causing vascular thrombosis and fall in circulating platelets.[54] It is more common in patients given bovine heparin than in those treated with porcine heparin, and may be related to the heparin lot.[53] It is rarely seen with highly purified low molecular weight heparin, suggesting that high molecular weight components may be responsible. It is also rare in patients given prophylactic minidose heparin, occurring in only 1 of 348 patients.[54] But, once the syndrome is initiated, even trivial amounts of heparin can perpetuate it. Heparin-containing flush solutions, indwelling catheters, and even heparin-bounded pulmonary artery catheters have been reported to sustain the syndrome. The onset of thrombocytopenia is usually on the 3rd to 15th day (mean, day 10) but can occur after several hours in patients previously sensitized. The severity of thrombocytopenia is variable (commonly to 50,000/mm^3) but can be severe (less than 5000/mm^3). Most patients remain asymptomatic but some have major arterial or venous thrombosis or life-threatening hemorrhage. Any time that heparin is given, it is prudent to measure platelet counts on a daily basis. An otherwise unexplained drop in platelet count of 30% has been suggested as the threshold that should prompt discontinuation of therapy.[54] Although platelet counts sometime normalize despite continued heparin administration, the drug should be stopped because potentially catastrophic thrombosis may occur unpredictably. Heparin-dependent platelet antibody should be sought for in patient's serum, but this assay is not routinely available and is not very sensitive, so a negative test result is not helpful. After discontinuation of all heparin, the platelet count usually rises in 2 or 3 days. Platelet transfusions should be avoided even if the patient is bleeding because they may precipitate arterial thrombosis. If continued anticoagulation is necessary, porcine or low molecular weight heparin could be substituted or warfarin treatment begun. Generalized skin reaction of various forms occur as a part of a hypersensitivity reaction to various drugs. The drugs commonly indicted are sulfonamides, penicillins, erythromycin, and phenytoin. Of concern to the intensivists are the three major types of drug-induced skin diseases with the potential for life-threatening complications. These include erythema multiforme (Stevens-Johnson syndrome), toxic epidermal necrolysis, and exfoliative erythroderma.[33] The lesions range from typical target-shaped eruptions to extensive bullous eruptions and large areas of skin sloughing. These are usually associated with hypovolemic shock, hypercatabolic state, and multisystem organ dysfunction; the management is mainly supportive.

DRUG INTERACTIONS

Conventionally, a drug interaction is regarded as the modification of the effect of one drug by prior or concomitant administration of another.[55] Several textbooks[26,56-59] and reviews[60] have compiled extensive listings of potential interactions. Most drug interaction studies report on small numbers of noncritically ill patients or volunteers, and extrapolation of these studies to the ICU setting is undesirable, leading to unnecessary restriction of useful medications. This section reviews clinically significant drug interactions encountered in the ICU.

Drug interactions can result from pharmacokinetic or pharmacodynamic causes. Pharmacokinetic interactions affect the process of drug absorption, distribution, metabolism, and excretion. Pharmacodynamic interactions alter the biochemical or physiologic effect of a drug.

PHARMACOKINETIC INTERACTIONS

Absorption

Many drug interactions affect bioavailability of drugs through effects on absorption. These include adsorption and formation of drug complexes, changes in gastric emptying time and pH, alteration in intestinal motility and mucosal function, and reduction in splanchnic perfusion. Phenytoin absorption has been found to vary with enteral feeding type.[61] Anion exchange resin (cholestyramine) aluminum-containing drugs like sucralfate and antacids, kaolin pectin, activated charcoal, and iron-containing preparations impair absorption of a variety of drugs like digoxin, warfarin, and thyroxine by forming insoluble complexes. It is safest not to give any oral medication within 2 hours of administration of these chelating agents.

Drug incompatibilities in intravenous preparations also can present as drug interaction or absorption problems. Precipitation or chemical alteration may occur before parenteral dosing. Knowledge of in vitro drug incompatibilities is, therefore, essential, and in-depth charts are available.[56] Precipitation of phenytoin in glucose-containing solution is a relevant example.[62]

Distribution

Many drugs circulate in the plasma partly bound to plasma proteins. Because the free or unbound serum concentration of a drug determines its biological activity, changes in protein binding induced by another agent can have an important effect on the drug's pharmacologic response.[63-66] Displacement from a protein of one drug by another depends on the concentration and relative binding affinities of the drugs. A drug with a higher serum concentration and higher protein binding affinity displaces a second drug more readily. For

example, warfarin's displacement by another drug can result in clinical bleeding complications. The acute elevation of free drug concentration in serum often is accompanied by an increased distribution to other tissues or increased elimination by metabolism and excretion until a new steady state is reached. Thus, when a new steady state is reached, the total drug level in the blood will be lower because of less protein bound drug, while the free drug level will be in the therapeutic range. It is critical, therefore, that the drug dose not be titrated into the usual therapeutic range because this leads to excessive response and toxicity. Individualization of drug therapy should rather be based on the clinical response or the plasma concentration of unbound drug, if available. Highly protein-bound drugs are particularly susceptible to these interactions (see Table 32-3).

Metabolism

The metabolism of most drugs occur largely in the liver. Quantitatively, the cytochrome P-450 microsomal enzyme system containing mixed-function oxidases present in smooth endoplasmic reticulum is most important for initial metabolic conversion. The activity of these enzymes can be profoundly influenced by genetic factors and coadministration of many drugs. These enzymes can be induced or inhibited by a variety of agents.[67,68]

Some common enzyme-inducing agents include the anticonvulsants phenytoin, phenobarbital, and carbamazepine; ethanol; phenylbutazone; and rifampin (Table 32-6). Cigarette smoking has been shown to be an excellent inducer of isoenzymes responsible for theophylline metabolism. Enzyme induction increases the rate of elimination of various drugs, leading to lower plasma levels (Table 32-7).

Several compounds (see Table 32-6) inhibit microsomal enzyme function, inhibiting the metabolism of many of the same drugs affected by enzyme induction (see Table 32-7). For example, cimetidine is a potent inhibitor of oxidative metabolism of warfarin, quinidine, nifedipine, lidocaine, theophylline, and phenytoin. Erythromycin inhibits the metabolism of cyclosporine, warfarin, carbamazepine, and theophylline.

Excretion

The most important route of drug excretion is by the kidneys and involves the processes of filtration, secretion, and reabsorption.[69,70] All of these aspects of renal handling of compounds can potentially lead to drug interactions.

Several drugs, such as the aminoglycoside antibiotics, are eliminated almost completely by glomerular filtration. Furosemide, a potent loop diuretic, by causing intravascular volume depletion, can decrease renal perfusion pressure and filtration rate, thereby reducing elimination of gentamicin.

Many drugs are actively secreted in the proximal tubule. The most important of these agents include the organic acids captopril, cephalosporins, sulfonamides, sulfonylureas, penicillins, diuretics, probenecid, and nonsteroidal anti-inflammatory agents. These compounds can block each others' secretions, thus decreasing their urinary excretion. Also,

TABLE 32-6. Drugs Commonly Affecting Metabolizing Enzymes in Liver

INDUCING AGENTS	Acetaminophen	Cyclosporine	Metoprolol
	Barbiturates	Digoxin	Phenytoin
	Carbamazepine	Glucocorticoids	Quinidine
	Cimetidine	Methadone	Rifampin
	Clonazepam		Theophylline
INHIBITING AGENTS	Allopurinol	Ethyl alcohol	Propranolol
	Amiodarone	(acute)	Quinidine
	Chlorpromazine	Erythromycin	Sulfonamide
	Cimetidine	INH	Tolbutamide
	Ciprofloxacin	Ketoconazole	Trimethoprim
	Diltiazem	Oral contraceptives	Verapamil

INH, isoniazid.

From Chernow B (ed): *The Pharmacologic Approach to the Critically Ill Patient.* Baltimore, Williams & Wilkins, 1983.

quinidine decreases the tubular secretion of digoxin. Thus, the coadministration of quinidine and digoxin approximately doubles the serum digoxin concentration. Inhibition of the tubular cation transport system by cimetidine impedes the renal clearance of procainamide and its active metabolite, N-acetyl procainamide.

The reabsorption of filtered or secreted compounds occurs in the distal tubule or collecting duct. It is a function of drug concentration, urinary flow, and pH of the urine. Alteration in distal urine pH can cause ion trapping of certain weak acids or bases and reduce passive reabsorption (passive movement of ionized compounds across membranes is poor). Thus, alkalinization of urine by sodium bicarbonate facilitates excretion of acidic drugs such as phenobarbital, salicylates, and amphetamines.[33]

Lithium is reabsorbed with sodium in the kidney by the same renal mechanism. In case of volume depletion from chronic diuretic use, renal increases in sodium and lithium reabsorption occur, leading to a potentially toxic lithium level.[33]

PHARMACODYNAMIC INTERACTIONS

Pharmacodynamic drug interactions, which are more numerous and complex than pharmacokinetic processes, include additive or synergistic effects, antagonistic effects, or side effects: for example, the benzodiazepine receptor antagonist flumazenil reversing or blocking the receptor agonist diazepam, or the nonsteroidal antiinflammatory drugs, blunting the antihypertensive effects of beta-blockers and natriuretic effects of thiazide diuretics.

TABLE 32-7. Drugs Commonly Affected by Enzyme-Inducing or Enzyme-Inhibiting Agents

Carbamazepine	Lidocaine	Quinidine
Chlorpropamide	Metoprolol	Rifampin
Cyclosporine	Phenytoin	Tolbutamide
Digoxin	Phenobarbital	Theophylline
Glucocorticoids	Propranolol	Warfarin

In summation, drug interactions are common and often unpredictable. One drug may interact with another on a pharmacokinetic or pharmacodynamic basis or both, with potentially disastrous consequences. The practicing intensivist must have a working knowledge of the important drug interactions that might be encountered. An understanding of the drugs at risk, the vulnerable patients, and the mechanism involved provides a convenient framework. However, only careful use of drugs and the avoidance of unnecessary prescribing can protect the patient adequately.

An Approach To Management

Pharmacotherapy is a complex science in the management of the critically ill patient. However, knowledge of pharmacokinetic principles, drug–drug interactions, changes related to systemic diseases, and possible drug toxicities permits the critical care clinician to design an appropriate medication regimen. The considerations listed below are recommended:

1. Review medications daily; check the medication sheets and make sure that the appropriate agents are being administered.
2. Know the therapeutic and toxic effects of each drug.
3. Keep in mind the pharmacokinetics of each drug (first-order versus zero-order kinetics, serum elimination half-life).
4. Remember that systemic disease (renal, hepatic) may create the need alter the dosage regimen: (1) an increase in volume of distribution may increase the required loading dose; and (2) a decrease in clearance may decrease the required maintenance dose.
5. Look for possible drug–drug interactions.
6. Minimize the number of drugs.
7. Substitute equally effective, less expensive medications when possible; use generic drugs if equally effective.
8. Plan an approach to monitoring therapeutic and toxic effects. Check serum levels as appropriate, allowing four to five half-lives for equilibration.

REFERENCES

1. Benet LZ, Kroetz DL, Sheiner LB: Pharmacokinetics: the dynamics of drug absorption, distribution, and elimination. In: Hardin JG, Limbird LE, Gilman AG *Goodman and Gilman's The Pharmacologic Basis of Therapeutics,* ed 9. New York, McGraw Hill, 1996:3

2. Bauer LA: Individualization of drug therapy: clinical pharmacokinetics and pharmacodynamics. In: DiPiro JT, et al (eds). *Pharmacotherapy: A Pathophysiologic Approach,* ed 2. New York: Elsevier, 1992:15

3. Winter ME: Clinical pharmacokinetics. In: *Applied Therapeutics: The Clinical Use of Drugs,* ed 5. Vancouver, WA, Applied Therapeutics, 1992

4. Riegelman S, Loo JCK, Rowland M: Shortcomings in pharmacokinetic analysis by conceiving the body to exhibit properties of a single compartment. *J Pharmacol Sci* 1968;57:117

5. Greenblatt DJ, Koch Weser J: Clinical pharmacokinetics. *N Engl J Med* 1975;293:702

6. Winter ME: *Basic Clinical Pharmacokinetics,* ed 3. Vancouver, WA, Applied Therapeutics, 1994

7. Koch-Weser J: Bioavailability of Drugs. *N Engl J Med* 1974; 291:233

8. Gambertoglio JG: Effects of renal disease: altered pharmacokinetics. In: Benet LZ, Massoud N, Gambertoglio JG (eds). *Pharmacokinetic Basis for Drug Treatment.* New York, Raven Press, 1984:149

9. Matzke GR, Faye RF: Drug dosing in patients with impaired renal function. In: DiPiro JT, et al (eds). *Pharmacotherapy: A Pathophysiologic Approach,* ed 2. New York, Elsevier, 1992: 750

10. Vanholder R, Van Landsehoot N, De Smet R, et al: Drug protein binding in chronic renal failure: evaluation of nine drugs. *Kidney Int* 1988;33:996

11. Benet WM, et al: *Drug Prescribing in Renal Failure: Dosing Guidelines for Adults,* ed 2. Philadelphia, American College of Physicians, 1991

12. Anderson RJ, Schrier RW (eds): *Clinical Use of Drugs in Patients With Kidney and Liver Disease.* Philadelphia, WB Saunders, 1981

13. Rowland M, Tozer TN (eds): *Clinical Pharmacokinetics: Concepts and Applications.* Philadelphia: Lea & Febiger, 1989: 148

14. Cockcroft DW, Gault MH: Prediction of creatinine clearance from serum creatinine. *Nephron* 1976;16:31

15. Matzke GR, Millikin SP: Influence of renal disease and dialysis on pharmacokinetics. In: Evans WE, Schentag JJ, Jusko WJ (eds). *Applied Pharmacokinetics: Principles of Therapeutic Drug Monitoring,* ed 3. Vancouver, WA: Applied Therapeutics, 1992

16. Benet WM: Aminoglycoside nephrotoxicity. *Nephron* 1983; 35:73

17. Bates RD, Nahta MC: Once-daily administration of aminoglycosides. *Ann Pharmacother* 1994;28:757

18. Dager WE: Aminoglycoside pharmacokinetics: volume of distribution in specific adult patient subgroups. *Ann Pharmacother* 1994;28:944

19. Traynor AM, Nafziger AN, Bertino JS: Aminoglycoside dosing weight correction factors for patients of various body sizes. *Antimicrob Agents Chemother* 1995;39:545

20. Rodman DJ, Maxwell AJ, McKnight JT: Extended dosing intervals for aminoglycosides. *Am J Hosp Pharm* 1994;51:2016

21. Marble EL: Large-dose, once-daily administration of aminoglycosides: a decades-old idea whose time is now. *Clin Microbiol Newsletter* 1994;16:50

22. Rotschafer JC, Ryback MJ: Single daily dosing of aminoglycosides: a commentary. *Ann Pharmacother* 1994;28:797

23. Hoyumpa AM, Schenker S: Influence of liver disease on the disposition and elimination of drugs. In: Schiff L, Schiff ER (eds). *Diseases of the Liver,* ed 7. Philadelphia, JB Lippincott, 1993

24. Wilkinson GR, Shand DG: A physiological approach to hepatic drug clearance. *Clin Pharmacol Ther* 1975;18:377

25. Rowland M, Benet LZ, Graham GG: Clearance concepts in pharmacokinetics. *J Pharmacol Biopharm* 1973;1:123

26. Chernow B (ed): *The Pharmacologic Approach to Critically Ill Patient.* Baltimore, Williams & Wilkins, 1983

27. Blashke TF: Protein binding and kinetics of drugs in liver disease. *Clin Pharmacokinet* 1977;2:32

28. Secor JW, Schenker S: Drug metabolism in patients with liver diseases. *Adv Intern Med* 1987;32:379

29. Williams RL: Drug administration in hepatic disease. *N Engl J Med* 1983;309:1616

30. Mangione A, Inhoff TE, Lee RV: Pharmacokinetics of theophylline in hepatic disease. *Chest* 1978;73:616

31. Campbell MA, Plachetka JR, Jackson JE: Cimetidine decreases theophylline clearance. *Ann Intern Med* 1981;95:68

32. Reitberg DP, Bernhard H, Schentag JJ: Alteration of theophylline clearance and half-life by cimetidine in normal volunteers. *Ann Intern Med* 1981;95:582

33. Oates JA, Wood AJ: Adverse reaction to drugs. In: *Harrison's Principles of Internal Medicine,* ed 12, vol 1. New York, McGraw-Hill 1991:373

34. Gray RK, et al: Short-term intense survillance of adverse drug reactions. *J Clin Pharmacol* 1973;13:61

35. Jick H: Adverse drug effects in relation to renal function. *Am J Med* 1977;62:514

36. Segredo V, Caldwell JE, Matthay MA, et al: Persistent paralysis in critically ill patients after long-term administration of vecuronium. *N Engl J Med* 1992;327:524

37. Rupp SM: Monitoring neuromuscular blockade. *Anesthesiol Clin North Am* 1993;11:361

38. Whittaker M: Plasma cholinesterase variants and the anesthetist. *Anesthesia* 1980;35:174

39. Nelson TE, Flewellen EH: The malignant hyperthermia syndrome. *N Engl J Med* 1983;309:416

40. Gronert GA: Malignant hyperthermia. In: Miller RD (ed). *Anesthesia,* ed 2. New York, Churchill Livingstone, 1986:1971

41. Gronert GA: Malignant hyperthermia. *Anesthesiology* 1980; 53:395

42. Kolb ME, Houne ML, Mautz R: Dantrolene in human malignant hyperthermia: a multicenter study. *Anesthesiology* 1982; 56:254

43. Morgan KC, Bryant SH: The mechanism of action of dantrolene sodium. *J Pharmcol Exp Ther* 1977;201:138

44. Britt BA, Kwong FHF, Endreny L: The clinical and laboratory features of malignant hyperthermia management: a review. In: Henschel EO (ed): *Malignant Hyperthermia: Current Concepts.* New York, Appleton-Century-Crofts, 1977:9

45. Gronert GA: Malignant hyperthermia. *Semin Anesth* 1983; 2:197

46. Norwood S: An approach to the febrile patient. In: Civetta JM, Taylor RW, Kirby RR (eds). *Critical Care,* ed 2. Philadelphia, JB Lippincott, 1992:992

47. Mackowiak P, Le Maistre C: Drug fever: a critical appraisal of conventional concepts. *Ann Intern Med* 1987;106:728

48. George C, Robertson D: Clinical consequences of abrupt drug withdrawal. *Med Toxicol* 1987;2:367

49. Bohrer H, Bach A, Layer M, et al: Clonidine as a sedative adjunct in intensive care. *Intensive Care Med* 1990;16:265

50. Easton C, Mackenzie F: Sensory-perceptual alterations: delir-

ium in the intensive care unit. *Heart Lung* 1988;17:229

51. Messing R, Closson R, Simon R: Drug induced seizures: a 10-year experience. *Neurology* 1984;34:1582

52. Albertson TE, Foulke GE, Tharratt S: Pharmacokinetics and iatrogenic drug toxicity in the intensive care unit. In: Hall JB, Schmidt GA, Wood LH (eds). *Principles of Critical Care*, vol 11. New York, McGraw-Hill 1992:2061

53. Green D, Martin GJ, Schoichet SH, et al: Thrombocytopenia in a prospective randomized double blind trial of bovine and porcine heparin. *Am J Med Sci* 1984;288:60

54. Warkentin YE, Keltin JG: Heparin and platelets. *Hematol Oncol Clin North Am* 1990;4:243

55. McInnes GT, Brodie MG: Drug interaction that matters. *Drugs* 1988;36:83

56. Gilman AG, Goodman LS, Rall TW, et al (eds): *The Pharmacologic Basis of Therapeutics*, ed 7. New York, MacMillan, 1985

57. Hansen PD: *Drug Interaction*. Philadelphia, Lea & Febiger, 1979

58. Morselli PL, Garattinni S, Cohen SN: *Drug Interaction*. New York, Raven Press, 1974

59. Stockley I: *Drug Interactions*. Oxford, Blackwell Scientific Publications, 1981

60. Prescott LF: Pharmacokinetic drug interactions. *Lancet* 1969;ii:1239

61. Guidry J, Eastwood T, Curry S: Phenytoin absorption involunteers receiving selected enteral feedings. *West J Med* 1989; 150:659

62. Cloyd JC, Bosch DE, Sawchuk RJ: Concentration-time profile of phenytoin after admixture with small volumes of intravenous fluids. *Am J Hosp Pharm* 1978;35:45

63. Koch-Weser J, Sellers EM: Binding of drugs to serum albumin. *N Engl J Med* 1976;294:311

64. Wood M: Plasma drug binding: implications for anaesthesiologists. *Anesth Analg* 1986;65:786

65. McElnay JL, D'Acry PF: Protein binding displacement interactions and their clinical importance. *Drugs* 1983;25:495

66. MacKichan JJ: Pharmacokinetic consequences of drug displacement from blood and tissue proteins. *Clin Pharmacokinet* 1984;9:32

67. Gelhrter TD: Enzyme induction. *N Engl J Med* 1976;294: 522

68. Burns JJ, Conney AH: Enzyme stimulation and inhibition in the metabolism of drugs. *Proc R Soc Med* 1965;58:955

69. Prescott LF: Mechanism of renal excretion of drugs. *Br J Anesth* 1972;44:246

70. Weiner IM, Mudge GJ: Renal tubular mechanisms for excretion of organic acids and bases. *Am J Med* 1964;36:743

Techniques, Procedures, and Treatment

Critical Care, Third Edition, edited by Joseph M. Civetta,
Robert W. Taylor, and Robert R. Kirby.
Lippincott-Raven Publishers, Philadelphia, PA © 1997.

CHAPTER 33

■

Fundamentals of Cardiopulmonary Resuscitation

Robert R. Kirby
Richard S. Melker

IMMEDIATE CONCERNS ■

MAJOR PROBLEMS

Intact survival is the overriding goal of cardiopulmonary resuscitation (CPR). Biologic survival with a dead brain is a Pyrrhic victory at best and a terrible cost to the patient, surviving family members, friends, and society at large. Despite the array of monitors, drugs, techniques of resuscitation, and general available knowledge, survival and hospital discharge of cardiac arrest victims is little improved over the last 20 to 30 years. The key to improvement in this area is to find out why this observation holds true.

Cerebral survival is the major concern, and why it is often absent or at best partial should prompt insightful questions. Was the problem recognized? Did the persons respond appropriately with fundamentally sound techniques (e.g., airway, breathing, circulation, early defibrillation, and functional equipment)? Was monitoring and assessment adequate and appropriate? Time spent inserting a pulmonary artery catheter during the initial phase of resuscitation is *wasted* time and may hamper airway management, external cardiac compression, and more conventional intravenous access.

A question of significance is the cause of the arrest. Although some similarities are present, clear differences must be recognized in the approach to a person with a myocardial infarction (MI), an individual who has been electrocuted, or one who has near-drowned. Use of available sources for information—family members, bystanders, rescue personnel, physicians, nurses, and respiratory therapists—can be invaluable in the initial diagnosis and treatment. Finally, remember that time is the critical element. Survival probability decreases the longer important and fundamental management is delayed.

STRESS POINTS

1. Remember the ABCs! Clear and maintain the Airway. Ensure that the patient is Breathing (or breathe for the patient). Support the Circulation by whatever means are available.
2. Defibrillate immediately if a defibrillator is available (and the patient is experiencing ventricular fibrillation). This step takes precedence over the airway, breathing, and external compression.
3. In essentially *every* cardiac arrest scenario, epinephrine is *the* drug of choice. Use it early, frequently (every 3 to 5 minutes), and in sufficient dosage (minimum of 1.0 mg bolus for adults).
4. While the resuscitation commences, try to find out what happened. The knowledge may help (i.e., saltwater near-drowning would *not* be a reason to give furosemide although the patient is in pulmonary edema).
5. Be careful with tried-and-true drugs. Current advanced cardiac life support (ACLS) guidelines do *not* support routine use of sodium bicarbonate and seldom

491

recommend calcium chloride. Acid-base disturbances are best managed by proper control of alveolar ventilation.

6. When possible, monitor exhaled gas for carbon dioxide (CO_2). Its presence indicates that an endotracheal tube is correctly placed and also gives a reasonably reliable indication as to the success of your efforts (exhaled CO_2 can only be detected if blood is perfusing the lungs).

7. Measure blood gas partial pressures and pH. Venous values for the partial pressure of carbon dioxide (PCO_2) and pH are as good as (or better) than arterial values. Presumably they reflect the status of the cellular milieu more closely. In addition, if you feel compelled to administer sodium bicarbonate, you at least have some quantifiable basis for therapy.

8. Know your drugs: their indications, potential complications, and side effects. An ounce of prevention (or precaution) really is worth a pound of cure!

ESSENTIAL DIAGNOSTIC TESTS AND PROCEDURES

1. Be alert to potential problems and artifacts. Check electrocardiogram (ECG) leads and connections. Nothing ruins a patient's day more than a well-intentioned physician beating on the patient's chest because a lead is disconnected.

2. Conversely, don't waste an inordinate amount of time ascribing a loss of circulation to lead faults, oximeter probe dysfunction, or deep sleep. Cardiopulmonary arrest generally is pretty easy to detect.

3. Have somebody review the most recent blood gas values, serum electrolyte values, and chest radiograph results. A previously unrecognized abnormality (i.e., tension pneumothorax) may be easily treated and the problem resolved.

4. Find out what you can about the patient's history. In the intensive care unit, such information usually is readily available unless the patient "just came through the door."

5. When the first semblance of control emerges, consider more advanced and invasive monitoring. As stated earlier, however, don't delay basic diagnosis and treatment while attempting to cannulate the internal jugular or subclavian vein.

INITIAL THERAPY

1. ABCs, ABCs, ABCs!! Add defibrillation or cardioversion when indicated, and you'll seldom go wrong.

2. Know the pharmacology of the first-line drugs such as epinephrine, atropine, lidocaine. Be familiar with others such as bretylium, adenosine, procainamide, and verapamil. When used properly, these drugs can be life-saving; when used inappropriately, they can kill the patient.

3. Don't try to memorize all the algorithms. They are too complex and too numerous. Remember that a few drugs (epinephrine, atropine, lidocaine) and a few techniques (defibrillation, chest compression, ventila-tion, and oxygenation) will take care of the overwhelming number of immediately life-threatening emergencies until you can get help.

4. When things aren't working, consider what you may have missed. If help is available, step back and think. Are the monitors providing what I need? Is the oxygen on and connected? Is the equipment working properly? *Don't* substitute algorithms for thought and analysis.

5. ABCs, ABCs, ABCs!!

INITIAL CONSIDERATIONS ■

BASIC LIFE SUPPORT

Basic life support (BLS) creates a patent airway, using mouth-to-mouth ventilation, and uses closed chest cardiac massage in the setting of cardiac arrest. The ABC steps of CPR—A, airway; B, breathing; and C, circulation—constitute the initial management of unconscious patients. Properly executing these skills in the prescribed sequence is essential.

INTERMEDIATE LIFE SUPPORT

Intermediate life support adds some adjuncts of advanced life support. Emergency personnel may be trained to ventilate with a bag-valve-mask but not to perform tracheal intubation, or they may be trained to use an automatic external defibrillator but not to initiate intravenous infusions or give drugs.

ADVANCED LIFE SUPPORT

Advanced life support comprises additional methods of airway management. Prompt diagnosis and, when appropriate, treatment of life-threatening arrhythmias are mainstays of this therapy. Definitive management of these arrhythmias may require defibrillation, cardioversion, pacemaker insertion, and pharmacologic therapy.

AIRWAY PATENCY ■

POSITIONING

Airway patency must be assessed in an unconscious patient. If possible, the patient should be placed in the supine position, preferably on a firm surface, with the neck slightly flexed at the shoulders and extended at the atlantoaxial joint in the sniffing position (Fig. 33-1). This position can be maintained by placing a towel or roll under the victim's occiput. Observe the chest and abdomen for signs of spontaneous respiration or evidence of airway obstruction. The tongue, epiglottis, and soft tissues of the posterior pharynx may completely obstruct the upper airway of an unconscious patient. This simple maneuver must be executed carefully so that the cervical vertebrae and spinal cord are not injured.

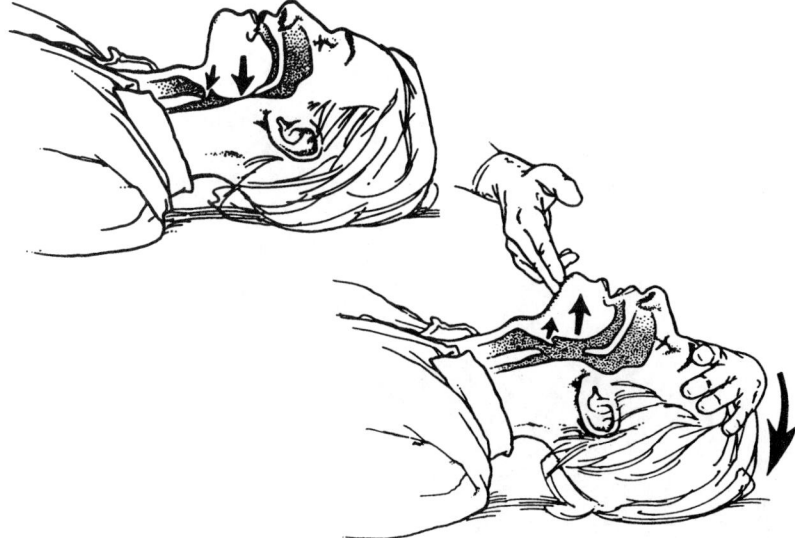

FIGURE 33-1. Opening the airway. (*Top*) Airway obstruction produced by tongue and epiglottis. (*Bottom*) Relief by head tilt and chin lift. (From Adjuncts for airway control, ventilation, and supplemental oxygen. In: Cummins RO [ed]: *Textbook of Advanced Cardiac Life Support,* 2nd ed. Dallas, American Heart Association, 1994, p. 2-1.)

When unconscious patients are spontaneously breathing, rolling them on their side into the *recovery position* is recommended to decrease the likelihood of airway obstruction and aspiration of gastric contents.

If cervical fractures are suspected (i.e., in a trauma victim), the head should *not* be hyperextended because of potential damage to the spinal cord. Lifting or thrusting the jaw forward may move the tongue anteriorly and create a patent airway without hyperextension of the head. When the patient's condition allows both maneuvers to be used, however, the combination of jaw lift and hyperextension usually is more successful.

The upper airway is most patent in infants when the head is maintained in the sniffing position. Hyperextension may collapse the soft trachea, which does not have well-formed rigid cartilaginous rings. Spontaneously breathing unconscious infants and children also can be placed in the recovery position.

NASAL AND OROPHARYNGEAL AIRWAYS

A nasal or oropharyngeal airway often relieves soft tissue obstruction. Insertion of a nasal airway, however, may traumatize the nasal mucosa and cause bleeding, which exacerbates the existing obstruction. Semiconscious patients may tolerate a nasal airway better than an oral airway, which predisposes to gagging and vomiting. An oral airway is probably more effective in unconscious patients. However, when improperly inserted, it can push the tongue back into the pharynx and worsen the airway obstruction.

FOREIGN BODY REMOVAL

Subdiaphragmatic abdominal thrusts (the Heimlich maneuver) have been recommended to dislodge and expel a foreign body that is not readily visible. Slapping blows with the open palm on the midposterior thorax, which may increase airway pressure enough to dislodge the object, are recommended only in infants. Midsternal chest thrusts, in erect or supine patients, may generate enough expulsive air movement from the chest to expel the foreign body and can be used in pregnant or obese patients or in pediatric patients. Abdominal thrusts should not be used in these patients because they increase the risk of injury to the fetus or the abdominal organs.

After these maneuvers are completed, an adult's mouth should be gently probed for any dislodged materials. A child's mouth should not be probed for foreign objects, because they can easily be forced more deeply into the airway. Instead, the pharynx can be examined if the rescuer's thumb is placed over the child's tongue and the jaw is lifted forward. The foreign body, once visualized, should be removed.

TRACHEAL INTUBATION

Tracheal intubation is indicated for patients with an otherwise difficult-to-manage airway and for patients who remain unconscious. An attempt should always be made to ventilate and oxygenate patients before intubation. After intubation, ventilation and chest compression can be performed independently. Intubation techniques are discussed in Chapter 50.

AIRWAY ADJUNCTS

The esophageal obturator airway (EOA) (Fig. 33-2) and other devices are used if tracheal intubation is impossible or the rescuer is not skilled in this technique. These include the esophageal gastric tube airway (EGTA) (Fig. 33-3), the pharyngotracheal lumen airway, the esophageal-tracheal double-lumen airway (the *combitube*), and the laryngeal mask airway[1] (Fig. 33-4). These devices are considered to be acceptable and possibly helpful. However, the full extent of their complications is unknown, and they have not all been well studied in CPR. Tracheal intubation remains the technique of choice for airway control. As much training is needed to properly use alternative adjuncts as to accomplish

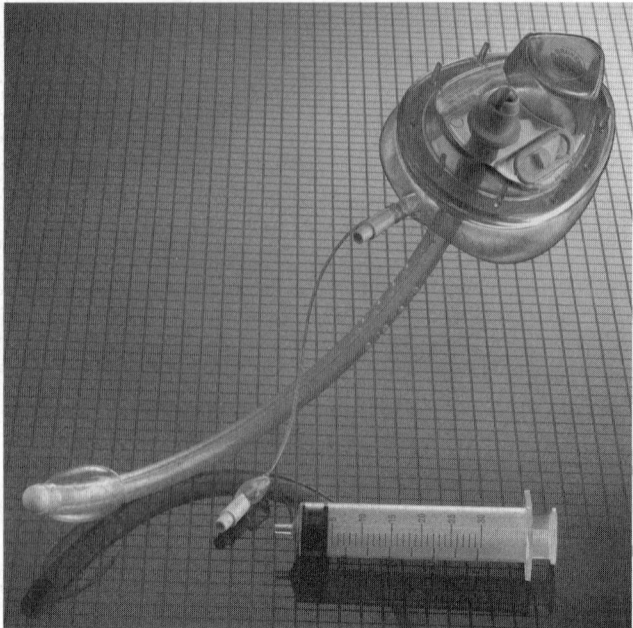

FIGURE 33-2. The esophageal obturator airway facilitates ventilation and prevents regurgitation. (From Melker RJ, Kirby RR, Marshall JR: Cardiopulmonary resuscitation. In: Kirby RR, Gravenstein N [eds]: *Clinical Anesthesia Practice*. Philadelphia, WB Saunders, 1994:837.)

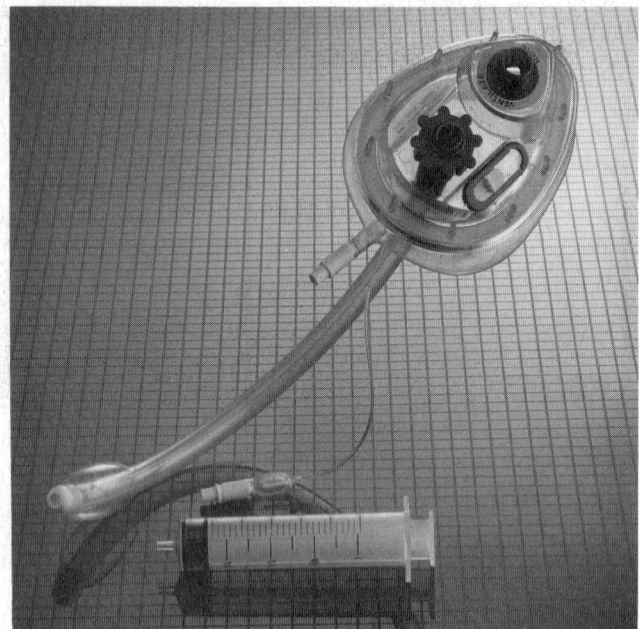

FIGURE 33-3. The esophageal gastric tube airway allows emptying of the stomach through the open end of the tube as opposed to the esophageal obturator airway that has a blind end. (From Melker RJ, Kirby RR, Marshall JR: Cardiopulmonary resuscitation. In: Kirby RR, Gravenstein N (eds). *Clinical Anesthesia Practice*. Philadelphia, WB Saunders, 1994:838.)

tracheal intubation. Although they are seldom used in the ICU, their application should be understood.

The Esophageal Obturator Airway

The EOA is a 15-cm flexible tube that resembles an endotracheal tube; its tip is occluded with an obturator (see Fig. 33-2). It is blindly inserted through the mouth into the esophagus. The adequacy of breath sounds must be confirmed before the cuff is inflated to ensure that the tube is not inadvertently placed within the trachea. The distal cuff is inflated with approximately 35 mL of air, which occludes the esophagus and minimizes the risk of regurgitation.[2]

The proximal tip of the tube extends through a face mask that is securely placed over the person's mouth and nose. Because the tube is occluded at the tip, the inspiratory volume enters the tube at the mask and exits through multiple perforations in the tube wall. If the upper airway is patent, the mask fit is adequate, and the tube was not inadvertently placed in the trachea, the lungs will be inflated. Careless insertion may cause esophageal perforation.[3] Inadvertent placement into the trachea is a potentially lethal complication.[4]

The Esophageal Gastric Tube Airway

The EGTA is a modification of the EOA and has two separate ports in the mask[5] (see Fig. 33-3). One is used for ventilation and the other allows direct access to the esophageal tube. Because a separate port in the mask is used for ventilation, perforations in the tube are unnecessary. When the distal cuff is inflated, breath sounds must be confirmed to verify that the esophagus and not the trachea is obstructed by the tube.

A small nasogastric tube can be inserted through the mask and tube for removing air and liquid from the stomach. Electrodes also can be placed in the tube for transesophageal cardiac monitoring, pacing, and defibrillation.

If a patient requires ventilatory assistance for longer than 2 hours, placement of an endotracheal tube should be attempted. Regurgitation and aspiration can easily occur when the EOA or EGTA is removed. Therefore, the endotracheal tube should be inserted and effective ventilation established before these tubes are removed.

The Laryngeal Mask Airway

The laryngeal mask airway superficially resembles an endotracheal tube (see Fig. 33-4). It is shorter and its tip ends in a miniature inflatable "mask" that conforms in shape to the glottic inlet. It is inserted blindly through the mouth until it seats over the laryngeal aperture (Fig. 33-5). The mask is then inflated through a pilot tube, similar to that which leads to the cuff of an endotracheal tube. With inflation, a relatively firm seal is achieved and an oxygen source is connected to the proximal 15-mm adapter. Current sizes are 1, 2, 2.5, 3, 4, and 5. This device is popular in Great Britain and increasingly so in the United States.

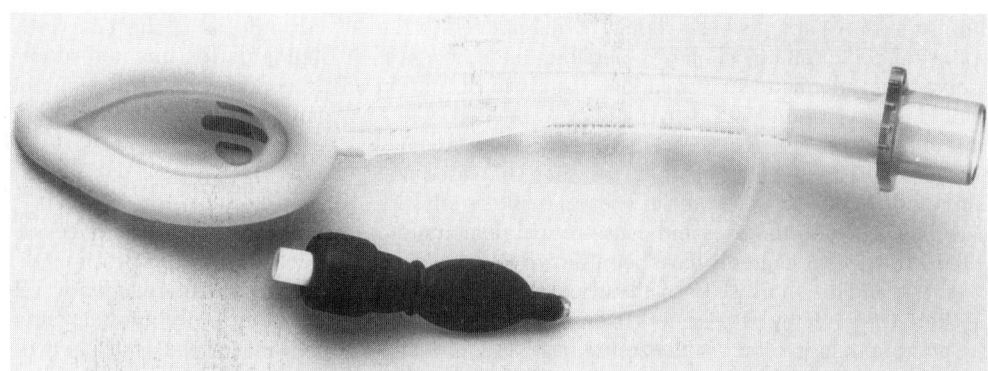

FIGURE 33-4. The laryngeal mask airway. The distal, inflatable mask fits over the glottic opening.

EMERGENCY SURGICAL TECHNIQUES

Cricothyroidotomy and transtracheal catheter ventilation[6-9] may be required in patients who cannot be ventilated with a mask or cannot be intubated, as may occur after face and neck trauma. These procedures can be life-saving, but they are not without hazards. They should be used only when other, less traumatic methods are not feasible and should be performed only by trained individuals. Potential complications include hemorrhage, creation of a false passage, subcutaneous or mediastinal emphysema, perforation of the esophagus, infection, pneumothorax, and subsequent tracheal stenosis. The techniques are discussed in Chapter 50.

BREATHING ■

In some situations, a patient's life may be saved by creating a patent airway that allows the resumption of spontaneous breathing. Frequently, however, a patient's ventilation must be assisted or controlled, often requiring the use of one or more of the previously discussed techniques. If the requisite equipment or skill is unavailable, the following basic concepts apply.

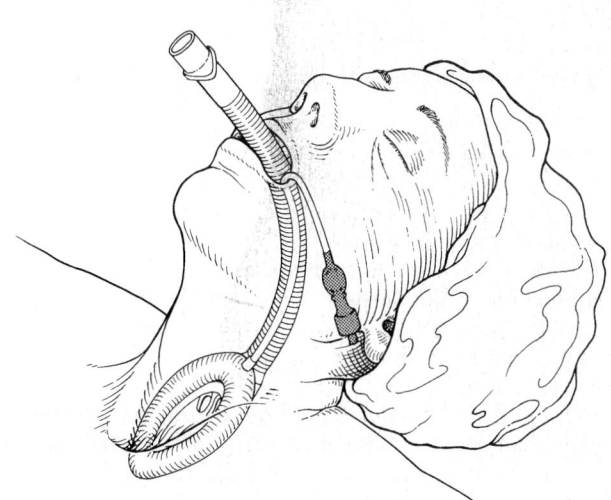

FIGURE 33-5. The laryngeal mask airway as it is positioned for airway maintenance and ventilation.

APNEA

If a victim is not breathing, give two slow, 2-second lung inflations of approximately 800 mL with sufficient time for exhalation between breaths. Positive airway pressure increases the chance of gastric inflation and the incidence of regurgitation and aspiration. Pressure should be kept as low as possible by long inspiratory times (T_Is). Gastric inflation may cause restriction of diaphragmatic excursion, and thus ventilation, particularly in infants.

Ventilation should continue with inflation of the lungs approximately every 5 to 6 seconds (10 to 12/minute) in adults and every 3 seconds (20/minute) in infants. T_I for ventilation in adults should be 1.5 to 2 seconds and in children should be 1 second. The tidal volume (V_T) recommended for nonintubated patients is significantly greater than that used in intubated patients because of the increased dead space produced by dilation of the soft tissues of the mouth and nasopharynx.

TECHNIQUES

Mouth-to-Mouth

Mouth-to-mouth (or mouth-to-nose) ventilation delivers a fraction of inspired oxygen (FIO_2) of about 0.16; this amount usually is sufficient to maintain a life-sustaining arterial oxygen partial pressure but may be associated with significant hypercapnia. Supplemental oxygen must be given as soon as possible. The increased pulmonary shunting and ventilation-perfusion ($\dot{V}/\dot{Q}$) mismatching that are common in victims of cardiac arrest greatly reduce oxygenation.

Mouth-to-Mask

Mouth-to-mask ventilation with one-way valves to prevent rebreathing of exhaled gas by the rescuer delivers higher V_T with longer T_I than does bag-valve-mask ventilation. A port to deliver supplemental oxygen is also recommended.

Bag-Valve-Mask

Bag-valve-mask devices deliver a FIO_2 between 0.21 and 1.0, depending on their construction and whether supplemental oxygen is available. The highest possible FIO_2 should be administered. A patient's head should be maintained in the hyperextended position whenever possible, and the chest observed for adequate lung inflation. If gastric distention is noted, reassessment of airway patency is needed. Close attention must be paid to mask positioning. A loose mask may allow air to escape from beneath it, resulting in inadequate ventilation. Mask pressure on the eyes may interrupt adequate blood flow to the eyes and cause retinal detachment.

These devices repeatedly have been shown to deliver the lowest V_Ts and the shortest T_Is of all devices. When possible, they should be used by two rescuers to ensure adequate mask seal, and two hands should squeeze the bag.[10] Additionally, cricoid pressure should be used during ventilation of nonintubated patients. When patients are intubated by any of the previously described tubes, the mask is detached and the valve adapter connected directly to the 15-mm universal adapter.

CIRCULATION ∎

In many situations, respiratory arrest occurs in conjunction with cardiac arrest or life-threatening arrhythmia. Cardiac function should be assessed by feeling for a carotid pulse. It can be palpated just lateral to the thyroid cartilage. Because of peripheral vasoconstriction associated with a shock state, the radial pulse may be difficult to palpate. The femoral pulse may also be difficult to locate in some patients because of obesity, trauma, or other confounding variables.

In pediatric patients, the precordial, brachial, or temporal artery pulse may be more easily monitored. If the pulse is absent and the patient is unconscious, external cardiac compression should be initiated. In cases with significant hypovolemia, no benefit accrues to the Trendelenburg (head-down) position. Instead, the legs should be elevated to enhance venous return.

CLOSED CHEST CARDIAC COMPRESSION

Adults

External cardiac compression may be totally ineffective or hazardous if performed improperly. The rescuer should place the heel of one hand over the lower half of the sternum approximately 2.5 to 4 cm above the tip of the xiphoid. The heel of the second hand is then placed on top of the first. The arms must be extended with the rescuer's finger tips off the patient's chest. A vertical thrust that displaces an adult's sternum approximately 1.5 to 2 inches should be delivered. Closed cardiac massage must be performed in a regular, deliberate, uninterrupted manner; quick, jabbing thrusts are far less effective.[11]

Infants

Rescuers often place their hands around an infant's chest, positioning both thumbs on the midsternum and exerting a vertical thrust with the thumb tips. Although some studies suggest that compression should take place over the distal sternum, as is the case in adult resuscitation,[12] the 1992 standards for infant resuscitation do not recommend this procedure because of potential damage to abdominal organs.[13] In small children, only the heel of one hand is used.

Effectiveness

Under ideal circumstances of CPR and drug therapy, a cardiac output of approximately 30% of prearrest blood flow can be maintained with effective external compression; therefore, only minimal interruptions are tolerated. Compression of the heart between the sternum and vertebral column (chest pump model) and the increase in intrathoracic pressure during compression (thoracic pump model) cause the forward flow of blood from the chest in some instances; in others, one mechanism or the other predominates. Various adjunctive techniques have been advocated to increase the effectiveness of external compression.

COMPRESSION-RELAXATION CYCLE. The duration of the compression should be 50% of the compression-relaxation cycle. This ratio is most easily achieved at a rate of 80 to 100 per minute. Maintaining this ratio of compression to relaxation with a manual technique is physically exhausting. Commercially available oxygen-powered automatic compression units may be more effective and are not subject to human fatigue. Portable units provide effective compressions interposed with appropriate ventilation.[14]

G-SUITS. Application of a G-suit over the abdominal cavity is thought to improve cardiac output by retarding the retrograde movement of blood from the heart into the large venous plexus in the peritoneal cavity during compression.[15] This suit can be used in combination with the automatic compression unit for an even greater improvement in cardiac output. Clinical studies have not shown improved resuscitation success, however. Intermittent abdominal compression during the relaxation phase of chest compressions improves survival compared with standard CPR for in-hospital patients.[16]

Compression Rate

TWO RESCUERS. If two rescuers are present, one can perform cardiac compressions while the second ventilates the patient. The rate of cardiac compression in this case is 80 to 100 per minute for adults, with a compression-to-ventilation ratio of 5:1. A 1.5- to 2-second pause should be provided for inspiration. Exhalation occurs during chest compression. Simultaneous compression and ventilation previously was evaluated as a means of further increasing cardiac output; it did not improve survival[17] and is not recommended.

Although close attention must be paid to the rate of compression and the ratio of compression to relaxation, the latter probably has a greater influence on cardiac output. The second rescuer must periodically check the carotid pulse to evaluate the effectiveness of the cardiac compressions and to observe the return of spontaneous cardiac activity.

However, a palpable carotid pulse may reflect only external, not internal, carotid artery flow; thus, it does not guarantee effective cerebral circulation.

SINGLE RESCUER. Fifteen chest compressions are performed at a rate of 80 to 100 per minute, followed by two breaths of 1.5 to 2 seconds each. This cycle is repeated four times, followed by reassessment. If CPR is continued, the rescuer should check for pulse and spontaneous breathing every few minutes. In infants, compressions are performed at approximately 100 to 120 per minute, with one breath interposed after every fifth compression. Obviously, single rescuer techniques seldom apply in the ICU.

Support should be continued until the patient has recovered, the rescuers are exhausted, relief rescuers have arrived, or a medical decision to discontinue resuscitative efforts has been made.

Complications

Complications related to closed chest compression include the following: fracture of the xiphoid and sternum; costochondral separation; pneumothorax; hemothorax; lung contusion; laceration of the liver, stomach, heart, and lungs; fat embolization; and cardiac contusion.

Efficacy

No reliable prognostic indicator exists for the efficacy of ongoing CPR efforts. Experimental studies suggest that aortic diastolic and coronary perfusion pressures correlate with successful resuscitation.[18] These findings have been corroborated in a small number of humans. When arterial catheters are present, the diastolic pressure should be optimized, and in instances in which a pulmonary artery catheter is available, arterial minus right atrial diastolic pressure may be an indicator of CPR efficacy and survival.

Capnography is promising to evaluate blood flow during CPR[19,20] and for confirming endotracheal tube placement. Unfortunately, many drugs given during resuscitation and a variable minute ventilation interfere with the interpretation of end-tidal CO_2 measurements during CPR. Despite these caveats, a sudden increase in end-tidal CO_2 is generally the earliest sign of return of spontaneous circulation, unless sodium bicarbonate has just been given.[21] A single 50-mL ampule of the latter can acutely increase mixed venous P_{CO_2} ($P\bar{v}_{CO_2}$) by almost 300 mm Hg.

THE PRECORDIAL THUMP

A precordial thump is most effective when it is performed as soon as possible after the onset of ventricular tachycardia or fibrillation and when the arrhythmia is not secondary to hypoxia.[22] This technique is used only when the rescuer observes the onset of the arrhythmia and a defibrillator is not immediately available in the operating room, postanesthesia care unit, or intensive care unit. It is acceptable for unmonitored patients who have an arrest in the presence of someone who can initiate therapy immediately.

The procedure incorporates a single blow to the midsternum with the fleshy portion of the clenched fist from a distance of 20 to 30 cm. Repeated precordial thumps are not indicated. An effective precordial thump causes ventricular depolarization, followed by a coordinated contraction, frequently of supraventricular origin. The thump in a patient with ventricular tachycardia can, unfortunately, produce ventricular fibrillation, asystole, or pulseless electrical activity.

DEFIBRILLATION AND CARDIOVERSION ■

VENTRICULAR DEFIBRILLATION

Defibrillation is most successful when it is performed immediately after the onset of ventricular fibrillation.[23] However, regardless of the time lapse between the onset of ventricular fibrillation and the initiation of therapy, electrical defibrillation should be performed as soon as possible. A coarse fibrillation pattern, which is usually of more recent onset, may be more easily corrected than a fine pattern. In many cases, a fine fibrillation pattern can be converted to a coarse pattern with an intravenous injection of epinephrine, 1 mg. The treatment algorithm for ventricular fibrillation and pulseless ventricular tachycardia is shown in Figure 33-6.

Precautions

Defibrillation is frequently unsuccessful in the anoxic myocardium and may be more effective after the initiation of CPR. It also is less successful when it is performed in a patient who is severely acidotic. However, immediate defibrillation should be attempted in all situations, if feasible, even before BLS or drug administration. Electrical defibrillation is not indicated in the treatment of asystole unless uncertainty exists as to whether the rhythm is fine ventricular fibrillation or asystole.[24] More than one ECG lead should be viewed to make this determination.

Technique

Before the paddles are placed, conductive electrode paste or saline sponges should be applied to decrease skin impedance and to increase the efficiency of current passage through the thorax. The electrode paste or saline of one paddle must not come into contact with the conductive material of the other paddle, or the amount of current delivered through the myocardium will be reduced and the effectiveness of the defibrillation minimized. Alcohol-soaked sponges should never be used as a conductor because the current may cause them to burst into flames.

Paddle Placement

Two 8- to 12-cm diameter paddles should be placed on the patient's chest, with one paddle to the right of the upper sternum just below the clavicle and the other to the left of the left nipple in the midaxillary line.[25] If the design of the

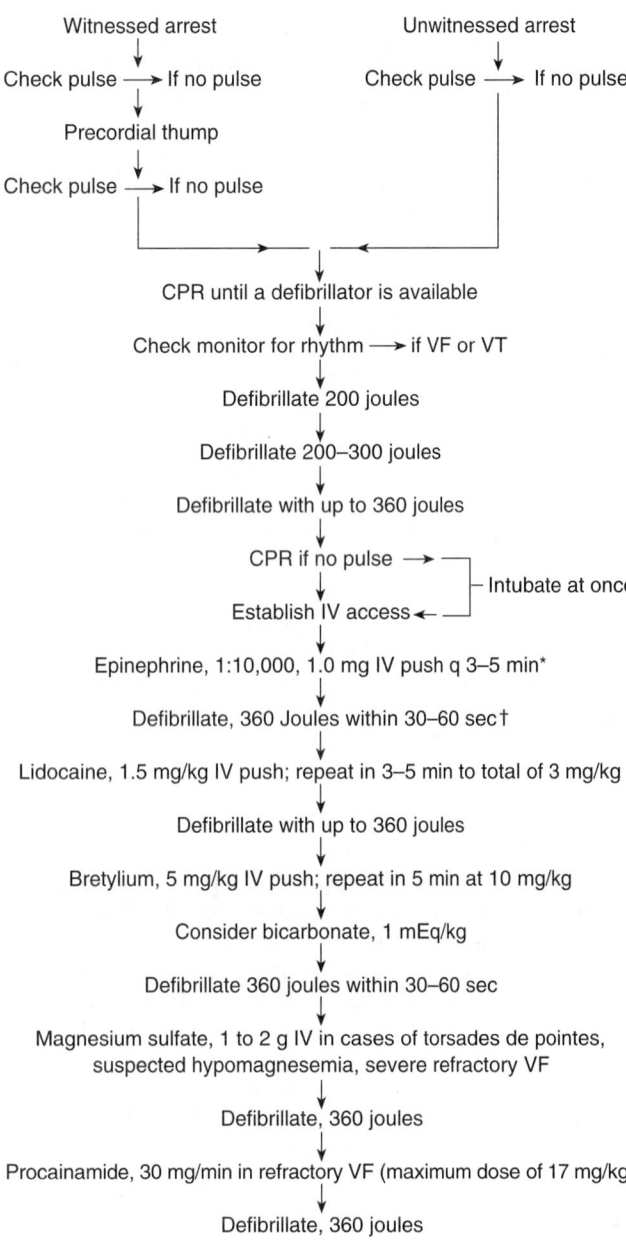

Witnessed arrest		Unwitnessed arrest

Check pulse ⟶ If no pulse Check pulse ⟶ If no pulse

Precordial thump

Check pulse ⟶ If no pulse

CPR until a defibrillator is available

Check monitor for rhythm ⟶ if VF or VT

Defibrillate 200 joules

Defibrillate 200–300 joules

Defibrillate with up to 360 joules

CPR if no pulse ⟶

Establish IV access ⟵ — Intubate at once

Epinephrine, 1:10,000, 1.0 mg IV push q 3–5 min*

Defibrillate, 360 Joules within 30–60 sec†

Lidocaine, 1.5 mg/kg IV push; repeat in 3–5 min to total of 3 mg/kg

Defibrillate with up to 360 joules

Bretylium, 5 mg/kg IV push; repeat in 5 min at 10 mg/kg

Consider bicarbonate, 1 mEq/kg

Defibrillate 360 joules within 30–60 sec

Magnesium sulfate, 1 to 2 g IV in cases of torsades de pointes, suspected hypomagnesemia, severe refractory VF

Defibrillate, 360 joules

Procainamide, 30 mg/min in refractory VF (maximum dose of 17 mg/kg)

Defibrillate, 360 joules

FIGURE 33-6. Suggested treatment of ventricular fibrillation (VF) and pulseless ventricular tachycardia (VT). The algorithm presumes that VF or pulseless VT is continuing and represents suggested management only. °Consider epinephrine, 2 to 5 mg IV push q 3–5 min; or 1 mg to 3 mg to 5 mg IV push sequentially, 3 min apart; or 0.1 mg/kg q 3–5 min if initial approach fails. †Multiple sequential shocks (200 J, 200 to 300 J, 360 J) are acceptable. (From Resuscitation Algorithms (B1–B6). In: Civetta JM, Taylor RW, Kirby RR [eds]. *Handbook of Critical Care.* Philadelphia, JB Lippincott, 1994, as modified from American Heart Association: Guidelines for cardiopulmonary resuscitation and emergency cardiac care. *JAMA* 1992;268:2217.)

paddles permits, one may be placed anteriorly over the heart and the other posteriorly.[25,26] This positioning is preferred by some rescuers, but it is not practical in most emergencies.

The paddles should be firmly placed against the patient's skin, using an estimated 9 to 11 kilograms (20 to 25 pounds) of pressure on each. Smaller paddles should be used in pediatric patients (4.5 cm diameter for infants and 8.0 cm for older children).

Energy Level

The initial defibrillation should employ 200 J of delivered energy.[27] If unsuccessful, a second shock at 200 to 300 J should be attempted immediately. Because the transthoracic resistance is decreased by the first defibrillation attempt, a greater amount of energy is transmitted to the heart during the second attempt, even if the energy level is not increased.[28] If the second attempt, too, is unsuccessful, a third attempt at 360 J is performed (see Fig. 33-6).

Should the third attempt also be unsuccessful, ALS should be initiated. After the administration of epinephrine, a fourth attempt at 360 J is indicated. If it, too, is unsuccessful, intravenous administration of lidocaine, bretylium, or both may terminate the fibrillation or allow subsequent defibrillation attempts to be successful (see Fig. 33-6). For patients who weigh less than 50 kg, the initial attempt should be with 2 J/kg and should be doubled if the first attempt is unsuccessful.[29]

During open chest defibrillation in adults (such as during cardiac surgery), defibrillation should be attempted with 10 J of delivered energy through paddles specifically designed for internal use.[30] The energy may be increased stepwise, if necessary.

ELECTRICAL CARDIOVERSION

Electrical cardioversion rather than pharmacologic therapy may be the treatment of choice for life-threatening arrhythmias causing rapid cardiovascular deterioration. These include ventricular tachycardia (Fig. 33-7) and supraventricular tachycardias, such as paroxysmal atrial tachycardia (PAT, Fig. 33-8), atrial flutter, or atrial fibrillation with a rapid ventricular response.

Technique

Unlike defibrillation, cardioversion must be synchronized with the patient's ECG. The ideal discharge point is during the upstroke of the R wave of the QRS complex. Delivery of the energy during the T wave of the QRS may result in ventricular fibrillation. Most commercially available defibrillators automatically coordinate the discharge to the patient's ECG if the machine is placed in the synchronized mode and if the QRS complex is of adequate size. If the defibrillator does not "sense" the QRS complex, the ECG gain should be increased so that the sensing algorithm functions. Cardioversion should never be attempted with quick-look paddles, because ECG artifact may make synchronization impossible. Unsynchronized cardioversion should only be used when the equipment at hand does not allow synchronization.

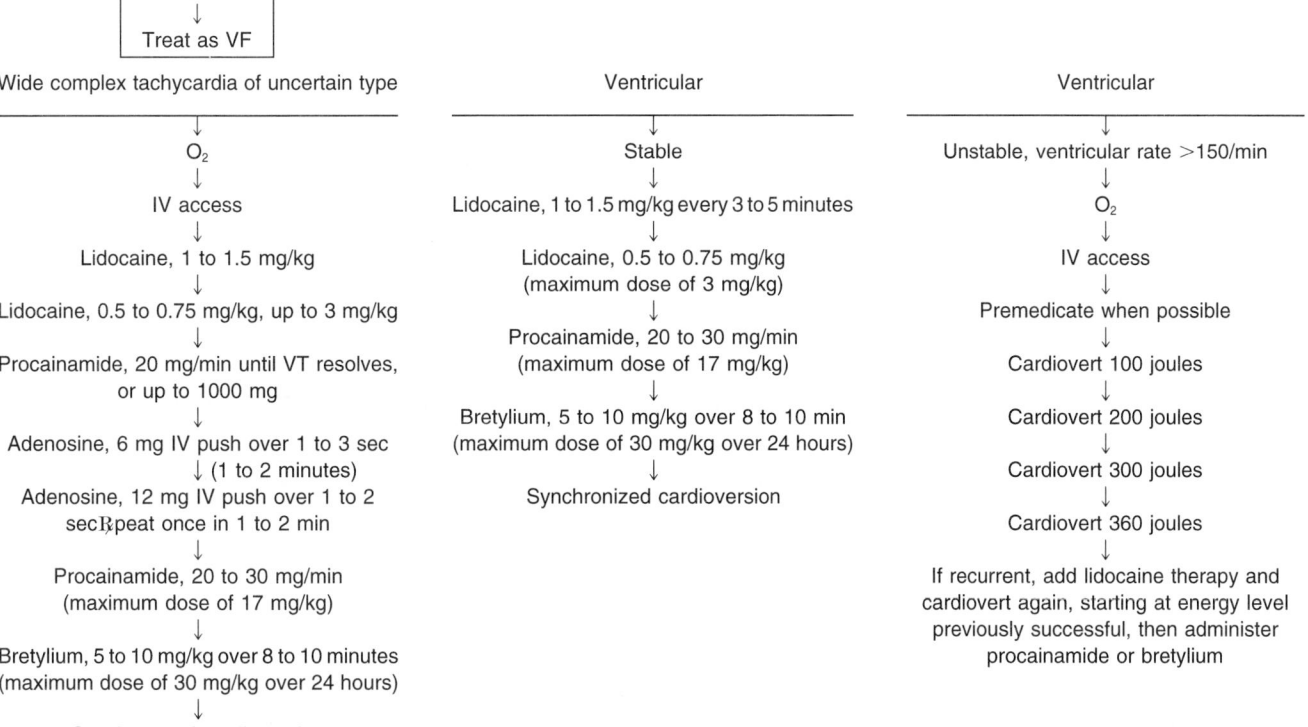

FIGURE 33-7. Suggested treatment of sustained ventricular tachycardia (VT). The algorithm presumes that VT is continuing. Unstable patients include those with chest pain, dyspnea, hypotension (systolic blood pressure <90 mm Hg), congestive heart failure, ischemia, or myocardial infarction. The algorithm represents suggested management only. (From Resuscitation Algorithms (B1–B6). In: Civetta JM, Taylor RW, Kirby RR [eds]. *Handbook of Critical Care.* Philadelphia, JB Lippincott, 1994, as modified from American Heart Association: Guidelines for cardiopulmonary resuscitation and emergency cardiac care. *JAMA* 1992;268:2224.)

Energy Level

The amount of energy recommended for emergency cardioversion varies with the rhythm.[28,31] An initial energy of 100 J is recommended for atrial fibrillation, and 50 J for atrial flutter.[32] Monomorphic ventricular tachycardia responds well to cardioversion, and 100 J should be attempted first (see Fig. 33-7). Pulseless ventricular tachycardia behaves like ventricular fibrillation, and 200 J should be used initially (see Fig. 33-6). For cardioversion in conscious patients, sedation with intravenous diazepam, midazolam, or methohexital is indicated, and the cardioversion accomplished with the lowest energy possible (50–200 J).

PULSELESS ELECTRICAL ACTIVITY, BRADYCARDIA, AND ASYSTOLE ■

The treatment of pulseless electrical activity (including electromechanical dissociation), bradycardia (including heart block), and asystole is summarized in Figures 33-9 through 33-11, respectively.

PHARMACOLOGIC THERAPY ■

EPINEPHRINE

Epinephrine has both α- and β-stimulating properties. The primary cardiovascular effect mediated through stimulation of the α_1-receptors is peripheral vasoconstriction, which increases systemic vascular resistance. Stimulation of β-receptors increases heart rate and myocardial contractile force.

A combination of increased contractile force, increased heart rate, and increased systemic vascular resistance increases blood pressure, cardiac output, and work of the heart. Large doses of epinephrine promote cerebral perfusion more effectively than other drugs and are particularly useful to increase internal carotid artery blood flow.[33] Epinephrine increases myocardial irritability and automaticity

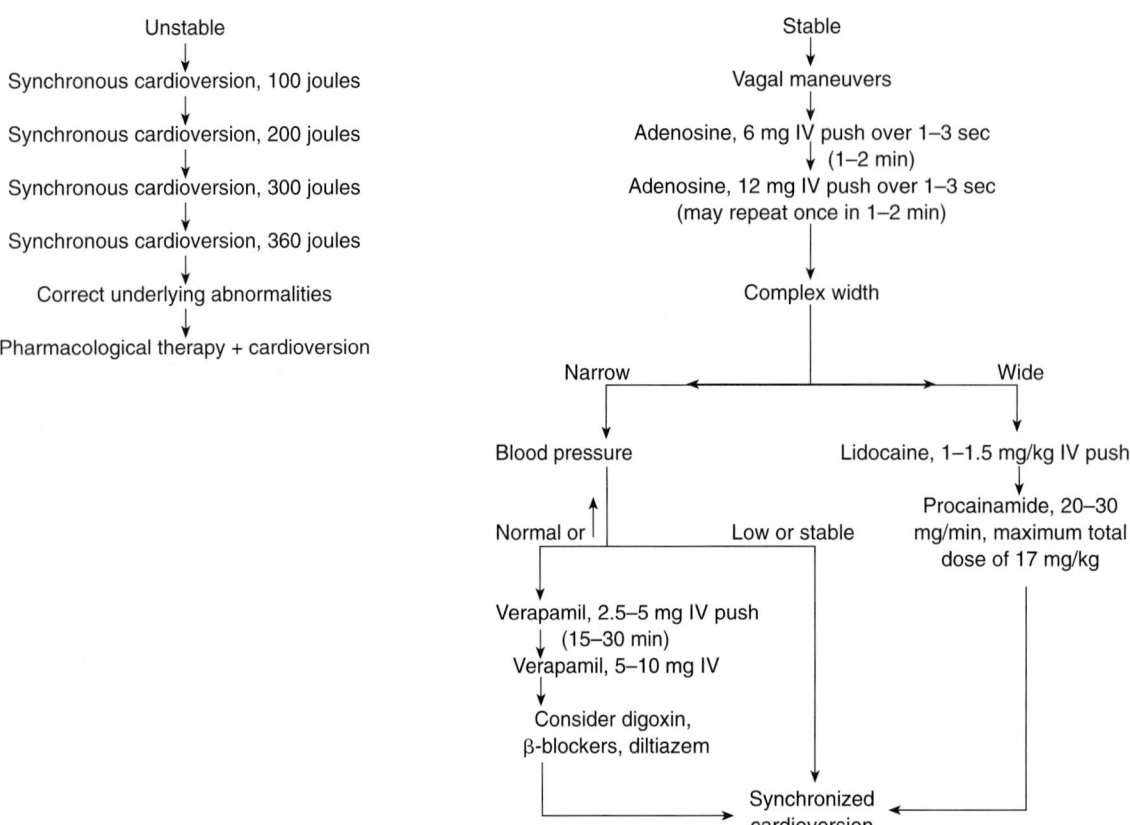

FIGURE 33-8. Suggested treatment of paroxysmal supraventricular tachycardia (PSVT). The flow of the algorithm presumes that PSVT is continuing. The algorithm represents suggested management only. (From Resuscitation Algorithms (B1–B6). In: Civetta JM, Taylor RW, Kirby RR [eds]. *Handbook of Critical Care.* Philadelphia, JB Lippincott, 1994, as modified from American Heart Association: Guidelines for cardiopulmonary resuscitation and emergency cardiac care. *JAMA* 1992;268:2223,2224.)

and may initiate rhythms originating from various ectopic foci, especially the ventricles.

Indications

Epinephrine effectively improves cardiac output in a failing myocardium seen in patients with pulseless electrical activity caused by poor cardiac output. In these patients, although the ECG may appear normal, ventricular contractility is so impaired that a patient is without an effective pulse or blood pressure. Epinephrine increases automaticity when attempts are made to convert cardiac standstill to spontaneous contractions. Also, as observed earlier, it may be useful in converting fine fibrillation to coarse ventricular fibrillation, which generally is thought to be more responsive to electrical defibrillation. The exact mechanism of the change in rhythm is unknown.

Dosage

Before 1992, the recommended dose of epinephrine was 0.5 to 1 mg (5 to 10 mL of a 1:10,000 solution) intravenously or 10 mL (1 mg) intratracheally. Because of the drug's short duration of action, this dose was administered as often as every 5 minutes, and a continuous infusion of 0.04 µg/kg/

minute was recommended to sustain improved contractility in some patients.

The 1992 guidelines recommend an epinephrine dosage of 1.0 mg (10 mL of a 1:10,000 solution) every 3 to 5 minutes.[34] Each peripheral injection should be followed by a 20-mL flush of intravenous fluid to ensure that it is delivered to the central circulation. The dose for tracheal administration is at least 2.5 times greater than the intravenous dose. It should be drawn up from a 1:1000 solution, diluted to 10 mL with sterile water, and administered by a catheter to the tip of the endotracheal tube.

High-dose epinephrine also has been recommended in patients who are refractory to the conventional dosage. Preliminary results from unpublished studies using 0.07 to 0.2 mg/kg on more than 2400 patients in cardiac arrest are disappointing, however. They show no statistically significant difference in survival compared with patients treated with standard doses. Thus, higher doses of epinephrine are acceptable but are neither recommended nor discouraged and should be used at the discretion of the physician.[34]

Route of Administration

Epinephrine is best administered through a central venous catheter. If the tracheal route is used, peripheral bronchial

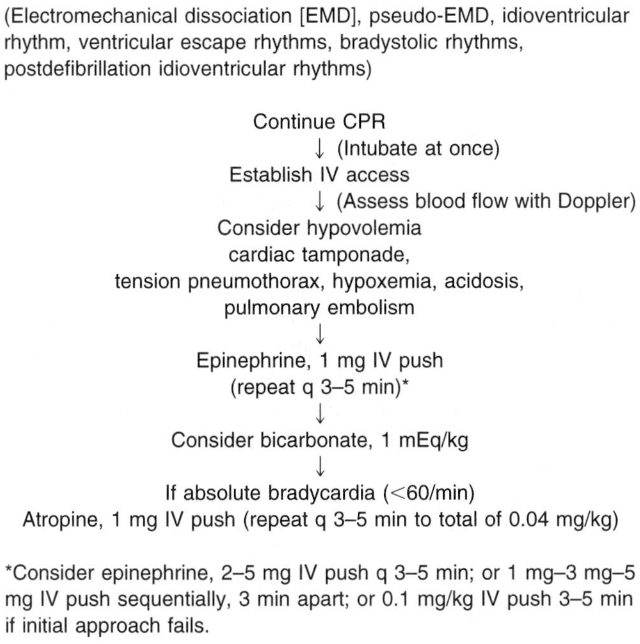

(Electromechanical dissociation [EMD], pseudo-EMD, idioventricular rhythm, ventricular escape rhythms, bradystolic rhythms, postdefibrillation idioventricular rhythms)

Continue CPR
↓ (Intubate at once)
Establish IV access
↓ (Assess blood flow with Doppler)
Consider hypovolemia
cardiac tamponade,
tension pneumothorax, hypoxemia, acidosis,
pulmonary embolism
↓
Epinephrine, 1 mg IV push
(repeat q 3–5 min)*
↓
Consider bicarbonate, 1 mEq/kg
↓
If absolute bradycardia (<60/min)
Atropine, 1 mg IV push (repeat q 3–5 min to total of 0.04 mg/kg)

*Consider epinephrine, 2–5 mg IV push q 3–5 min; or 1 mg–3 mg–5 mg IV push sequentially, 3 min apart; or 0.1 mg/kg IV push 3–5 min if initial approach fails.

FIGURE 33-9. Suggested treatment of electromechanical dissociation (EMD). The flow of the algorithm presumes that EMD is continuing. The algorithm represents suggested management only. (From Resuscitation Algorithms (B1–B6). In: Civetta JM, Taylor RW, Kirby RR [eds]. *Handbook of Critical Care.* Philadelphia, JB Lippincott, 1994, as modified from American Heart Association: Guidelines for cardiopulmonary resuscitation and emergency cardiac care. *JAMA* 1992;268:2219.)

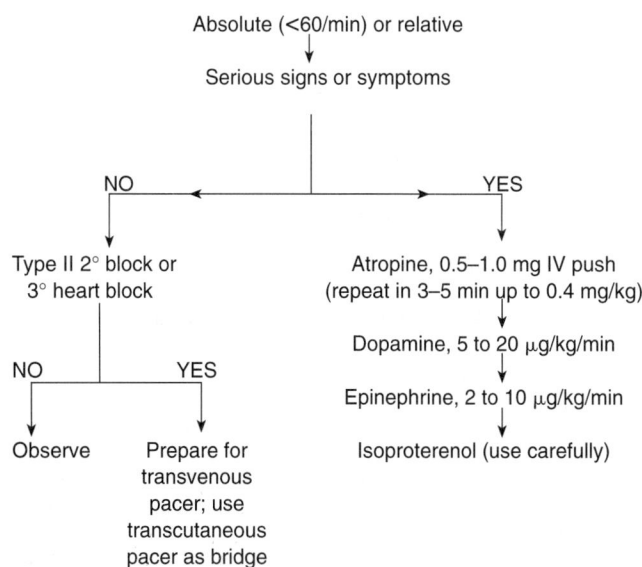

FIGURE 33-10. Suggested treatment of hemodynamically significant bradycardia. Significant signs and symptoms include hypotension (systolic blood pressure <90 mm Hg), premature ventricular contractions, altered mental status, chest pain, dyspnea, ischemia, or myocardial infarction. The use of isoproterenol should be considered as temporizing therapy only. The algorithm represents suggested management only. (From Resuscitation Algorithms (B1–B6). In: Civetta JM, Taylor RW, Kirby RR [eds]. *Handbook of Critical Care.* Philadelphia, JB Lippincott, 1994, as modified from American Heart Association: Guidelines for cardiopulmonary resuscitation and emergency cardiac care. *JAMA* 1992;268:1921.)

administration with a catheter seems to be more efficient than endotracheal.[35] An intracardiac injection of epinephrine may be indicated in a patient in asystole who is unresponsive to intravenous or endotracheal administration. However, the needle piercing the myocardium may be more of a cardiac stimulant than the epinephrine itself. Possible hazards of this route of administration include the following: interruption of cardiac compression and ventilation; pneumothorax; coronary artery laceration; cardiac tamponade; intramyocardial injection; and intractable ventricular fibrillation. It should be the *last* choice of available methods.

SODIUM BICARBONATE

Respiratory and metabolic acidosis usually develop during cardiac arrest. All patients maintained with external cardiac compression have decreased tissue perfusion and tissue hypoxia. Lactic acid is generated through anaerobic metabolism. Inadequate ventilation and the administration of sodium bicarbonate lead to hypercapnia and respiratory acidosis. The latter perturbation is best treated through improved ventilation by reducing CO_2; metabolic acidosis is managed with bicarbonate administration, if the arterial pH is less than 7.10, and hyperventilation.

An elevated CO_2 value probably is more detrimental to myocardial performance than is metabolic acidosis. Because CO_2 is readily diffusible across cell membranes, it rapidly enters the myocardial cells. Intracellular acidosis quickly develops, causing life-threatening derangements of myocar-

dial function. Likewise, cerebrospinal fluid acidosis may occur secondary to the diffusion of CO_2 across the blood-brain barrier, producing postarrest cerebral acidosis. Therefore, administration of sodium bicarbonate without sufficient ventilation and circulation to remove the CO_2 that it produces seems to be more detrimental than helpful.[36]

Indications

Untreated acidosis causes the suppression of spontaneous cardiac activity, decreases the electrical threshold required for the onset of ventricular fibrillation, decreases ventricular contractile force, and may decrease cardiac responsiveness to catecholamines such as epinephrine. Under these circumstances, bicarbonate therapy may be useful but should only be administered after confirmed interventions such as defibrillation, cardiac compression, intubation, ventilation, and more than one trial of epinephrine have been used.[37] Evidence suggests that whatever benefit bicarbonate therapy has may be related more to volume expansion related to its high sodium content rather than to its buffering effects.[38]

Dosage

If arterial blood gas and pH measurements are not available, the recommended initial dose of sodium bicarbonate is 1 mEq/kg intravenously; half of this dose may be repeated at 10-minute intervals. For pediatric patients, this 1 mEq/kg dose should be diluted 1:1 with sterile water to reduce

If rhythm is unclear and if there is possible ventricular fibrillation (VF), defibrillate as for VF. If asystole is present

↓

Continue CPR

↓ (Intubate at once)

Establish IV access

↓

Consider immediate transcutaneous pacing

↓

Epinephrine, 1:10,000, 1.0 mg IV push q 3–5 min*

↓

Atropine, 1.0 mg IV push q 3–5 min up to 0.04 mg/kg

↓

Consider bicarbonate, 1 mEq/kg

↓

Consider termination of efforts†

*Consider epinephrine, 2–5 mg IV push q 3–5 min; or 1 mg–3 mg–5 mg IV push sequentially, 3 min apart; or 0.1 mg/kg q 3–5 min if initial approach fails.

†If patient remains asystolic or has other agonal rhythm after intubation and initial medications and no reversible cause is identified.

FIGURE 33-11. Suggested treatment of asystole. The flow of the algorithm presumes that asystole is continuing. The algorithm represents suggested management only. (From Resuscitation Algorithms (B1–B6). In: Civetta JM, Taylor RW, Kirby RR [eds]. *Handbook of Critical Care.* Philadelphia, JB Lippincott, 1994, as modified from American Heart Association: Guidelines for cardiopulmonary resuscitation and emergency cardiac care. *JAMA* 1992;268:2220.)

the osmolality.

During the initial stage of patient management, when sodium bicarbonate is given empirically, the rescuer must be careful to avoid an excessive dose. As soon as possible, arterial blood gas and pH measurements should be obtained as a guide to further therapy.

Sodium bicarbonate should be given as incremental bolus injections rather than as continuous infusions. This method allows better minute-to-minute control of the quantity administered. It also reduces the possibility of inactivating other drugs such as the catecholamines that cannot be mixed directly with bicarbonate.

Complications

Administration of excessive amounts of sodium bicarbonate can result in metabolic alkalosis, leftward shift of the oxyhemoglobin dissociation curve, interference with tissue oxygenation, hypernatremia, hypokalemia, and worsening of respiratory and myocardial acidosis if adequate ventilation cannot be maintained.

ATROPINE

Atropine is used for its vagolytic actions. A reduced vagal influence on the heart improves both the rate of firing of the sinoatrial node and impulse conduction through the atrioventricular (AV) conduction system, with a resulting increase in heart rate.

Indications

Atropine is most useful in treating sinus bradycardia when it occurs with hypotension or frequent premature ventricular contractions (PVCs) secondary to unsuppressed ectopic electrical activity arising in the area of injured tissue during the prolonged period after repolarization. Sinus bradycardia after a MI may predispose the heart to the onset of ventricular fibrillation.[39]

When profound bradycardia is present, acceleration of the heart rate above 60 beats per minute (bpm) may improve cardiac output and reduce the incidence of ventricular fibrillation. Atropine also may be useful for treating a high-degree AV block with a slow ventricular rate.

Asystole occurring after increased parasympathetic tone that results in suppression of the electrical activity to the heart also frequently responds to atropine.[18] Because heart rate is a major determinant of myocardial oxygen consumption, however, any excessive increase in heart rate in an ischemic myocardium may result in frank infarction. Therefore, care should be taken in selecting the proper dose.

Dosage

The recommended dosage of atropine for bradycardia is 0.5 to 1.0 mg intravenously repeated every 3 to 5 minutes until the desired pulse rate is obtained or a maximum of 0.04 mg/kg has been given. A larger dose has little therapeutic value, and a smaller dose may actually slow the heart rate. Intratracheal atropine also may be given, in which case the dose is 2 to 2.5 mg. In the treatment of asystole, incremental doses of 1 mg are preferred.

Complications

Ventricular tachycardia and fibrillation after intravenous administration of atropine have been reported. In second-degree type II heart block, a paradoxical decrease in ventricular response may result.[36]

LIDOCAINE

By raising the electrical stimulation threshold of the ventricle during diastole, lidocaine renders the myocardial tissue less prone to ectopic electrical activity. In ischemic myocardial tissue after infarction, it may suppress reentrant arrhythmias such as ventricular tachycardia or fibrillation. This effect occurs by an induced delay of conduction through damaged myocardial tissue in the ischemic areas until the surrounding normal tissue is depolarized and refractory to the propagation of an abnormal impulse.

Indications

Lidocaine is the drug of choice for the treatment and prevention of ventricular arrhythmias. Because of its reliability, relatively low incidence of side effects, and ease of administration, it is frequently used for the treatment of monomorphic and polymorphic PVCs, ventricular tachycardia, and ventricular fibrillation.

Dosage

The recommended loading dose of lidocaine is approximately 1 to 1.5 mg/kg given as an intravenous bolus. To control the arrhythmia and to prevent its recurrence, the bolus dose may have to be repeated, up to a total of 3 mg/kg, followed by a continuous infusion of 20 to 40 µg/kg/minute (2 to 4 mg/minute in a 70-kg patient).[39] Only bolus therapy should be used during cardiac arrest. The bolus dose, too, may be administered through the trachea.

Complications

Used in the recommended doses, lidocaine has no significant effect on myocardial contractility, arterial blood pressure, or AV and intraventricular conduction. Excessive doses may induce heart block or depression of sinus node discharge, especially in patients with preexisting conduction disturbances.

Toxicity

Toxicity may occur more easily in oliguric or anuric patients, because the degradation products of lidocaine, which also have pharmacologic effects and toxic potential, cannot be adequately eliminated from the plasma.

Early clinical signs of lidocaine toxicity are related to the drug's central nervous system (CNS) effects and include anxiety, loquacity, tremors, metallic taste in the mouth, and tinnitus. These may be followed by somnolence, respiratory depression, apnea, and, in extreme cases, cardiovascular collapse. If CNS irritability occurs, lidocaine therapy should be withdrawn. A barbiturate or a benzodiazepine may be administered if deemed necessary and if the patient's circulatory status is sufficiently stabilized.

PROCAINAMIDE

The mechanisms of action of procainamide are similar to those of lidocaine. It may decrease the rate of discharge of an ectopic irritable focus. It also blocks reentrant arrhythmias by slowing electrical conduction in the damaged myocardial tissue and by creating a bidirectional block.

Indications

A second-line agent, procainamide is used in the management of PVCs, ventricular tachycardia, and persistent ventricular fibrillation unresponsive to lidocaine or when lidocaine is contraindicated.

Dosage

Incremental bolus injections of procainamide are slowly infused at 20 mg/minute until (1) the arrhythymia is controlled, (2) hypotension occurs, (3) the QRS complex is widened 50%, or (4) a total dose of 17 mg/kg has been given.[40] After initial control of the arrhythmia with the bolus injection, a continuous infusion of 1 to 4 mg/minute may be required

to prevent recurrent arrhythmias. Other effective administration schedules have been tested and approved; all are designed to maintain a therapeutic plasma level of 4 to 8 µg/mL.

Complications

Because of the profound myocardial depressant effects that may occur during administration of procainamide, continuous ECG and arterial blood pressure monitoring are mandatory. Patients may be especially prone to these side effects after a MI, and their treatment requires extreme caution. End points of therapy include hypotension and a greater than 50% widening of the QRS complex.

BRETYLIUM

The pharmacologic effects of bretylium tosylate, a quarternary ammonium compound, are complex. It has both postganglionic adrenergic-blocking properties and a positive inotropic action. After the administration of an initial dose, catecholamine release may increase peripheral resistance and central inotropy. This response is followed by adrenergic blockade and a decrease in peripheral resistance, which frequently produces postural hypotension when the drug is administered to a conscious patient.

A large body of data documents the antifibrillatory effect of bretylium in animals; this effect is less well documented in humans. Clinically, bretylium has been found to be useful in treating ventricular tachycardia and fibrillation. In direct comparisons, it has been found to be no better than lidocaine; thus, it is considered to be a second-line drug.[41]

Indications

Bretylium is recommended in the following cases: if lidocaine and defibrillation fail to convert ventricular fibrillation; if ventricular fibrillation recurs despite lidocaine therapy; or if lidocaine and procainamide fail to control ventricular tachycardia with a pulse. In conjunction with large doses of epinephrine, it may be the drug of choice for malignant bupivacaine-induced ventricular arrhythmias.

Dosage

In refractory ventricular fibrillation, 5 mg/kg are given intravenously as a bolus, followed by attempts at electrical defibrillation. If ventricular fibrillation persists, the dose may be increased to 10 mg/kg and repeated every 5 minutes up to a maximum dose of 35 mg/kg.

In persistently recurring ventricular tachycardia, 5 to 10 mg/kg can be diluted to 50 mL with 5% dextrose in water and given intravenously over 8 to 10 minutes. After the loading dose, bretylium can be administered as a continuous infusion at a rate of 1 to 2 mg/minute.[41]

β-ADRENERGIC BLOCKERS

Three β-blockers (atenolol, metoprolol, and propranolol) have been shown to significantly reduce the incidence of ventricular fibrillation in post-MI patients who did not receive thrombolytic agents. Studies also suggest a potential benefit in patients receiving thrombolytics. β-Blockers act to control rate and to limit infarct size. They also have a role in chronic therapy after MI to reduce mortality rates.

Indications

β-Blockers are used in paroxysmal supraventricular tachycardia (PSVT) after the rate is initially controlled, and in uncomplicated MI.

Dosage

In patients who have had a MI and are not receiving thrombolytic agents, the recommended dosage of atenolol is 5 to 10 mg intravenously over 5 minutes. Alternatively, metoprolol, 5 to 10 mg, can be given as slow intravenous boluses at 5-minute intervals to a total of 15 mg; an oral regimen can then be initiated. Propranolol, in a dosage of 0.1 mg/kg, divided into three equal, slowly administered doses, also can be used, as can esmolol in a dose of 1 to 2 mg/kg, followed by an infusion titrated to maintain the heart rate at the desired level. Oral therapy can then be initiated. Esmolol may be the safest drug to use in patients with chronic obstructive lung disease. It seems to have less potential for inducing bronchospasm than other β-blockers.[42]

Complications

Side effects that should be monitored include bradycardia, AV conduction delays, and hypotension. Cardiovascular decompensation to cardiogenic shock is rarely observed. Contraindications include bradyarrhythmias, greater than first-degree heart block, conduction delays, hypotension, overt congestive heart failure, and lung disease caused by bronchospasm.

CALCIUM CHANNEL BLOCKING AGENTS

Verapamil and diltiazem are the calcium channel blocking agents of choice in emergency cardiac care. Both agents slow conduction and increase refractoriness in the AV node. These actions may terminate reentrant arrhythmias requiring the AV node for their continuation. Verapamil and diltiazem also may be used to control the ventricular response rate in atrial fibrillation and flutter. Because these agents decrease myocardial contractility, they may exacerbate congestive heart failure in patients with severe left ventricular dysfunction, despite their vasodilatory effects.

Indications

Intravenous verapamil is effective in terminating narrow-complex PSVT and can be used to control the ventricular rate in atrial fibrillation. It may not be as effective in controlling atrial flutter. Diltiazem seems to be equally efficacious and may produce less myocardial depression than verapamil.

Dosage

The initial dosage of verapamil is 2.5 to 5 mg intravenously over 2 minutes. In the absence of a response or a drug-induced adverse event, repeated dosages of 5 to 10 mg may be administered every 15 to 30 minutes to a maximum of 20 mg. Diltiazem is given at a dose of 0.25 mg/kg, followed by a second dose of 0.35 mg/kg.

Complications

Verapamil may produce significant hypotension, which can be reversed with calcium chloride, 0.5 to 1 g, given slowly through a central catheter, or 1.5 to 3 g calcium gluconate, given slowly through a peripheral vein.[43]

ADENOSINE

Adenosine, available in the United States only since 1990, is an endogenous purine nucleoside that depresses AV node and sinus node activity. It is effective in terminating common forms of PSVT because they involve a reentry pathway including the AV node (see Fig. 33-8). It does not terminate arrhythmias that are not caused by reentry involving the AV node (e.g., atrial flutter, atrial fibrillation, atrial or ventricular tachycardia) but may produce transient AV or ventriculo-atrial block that clarifies the diagnosis.

Indications

Adenosine is indicated in PSVT and also may be used to differentiate PSVT from other tachyarrhythmias, including ventricular tachycardia.

Dosage

The recommended initial dosage is 6 mg as a bolus over 3 to 5 seconds, followed by a 20-mL saline flush. If no response is observed in 1 to 2 minutes, a 12-mg dose should be given. Larger doses have not been well studied.

Complications

Side effects are common but transient. Flushing, dyspnea, and chest pain are frequently encountered. These side effects rarely last more than 1 to 2 minutes. Sinus bradycardia and ventricular ectopy are common transiently after termination of PSVT. Because the half-life of adenosine is less than 5 seconds, PSVT may recur and require additional adenosine or calcium channel blocker.

Adenosine interacts with methylxanthines, which block the receptor responsible for adenosine's effects. Dipyridamole blocks adenosine uptake and potentiates its effects. Alternative therapy is warranted for patients receiving these drugs.

NITROGLYCERIN

Nitroglycerin relaxes vascular smooth muscle. It is the nitrate of choice for acute angina pectoris. In patients with congestive heart failure, intravenous nitroglycerin produces hemodynamic effects similar to those of sodium nitroprusside. Low dosages (30 to 40 μg/minute) produce predominantly venodilation; high dosages (150 to 500 μg/minute) lead to arteriolar dilation as well.

Indications

Indications for the use of nitroglycerin in emergency cardiac care include congestive heart failure and unstable angina pectoris associated with MI.

Dosage

For suspected angina pectoris, one nitroglycerin tablet is administered sublingually. It may be repeated at 3- to 5-minute intervals if discomfort is unrelieved. Safe administration of intravenous nitroglycerin usually requires hemodynamic monitoring. The initial intravenous dosage is 10 to 20 μg/minute, and the dosage may be increased by 10 μg/minute until the desired response occurs.

Complications

The principal toxic side effect of nitroglycerin is hypotension, which may exacerbate myocardial ischemia. Other potential complications include tachycardia, paradoxical bradycardia, hypoxemia caused by increased V̇/Q̇ mismatch, increased intracranial pressure, and headache.

CALCIUM CHLORIDE

Calcium ions enter the sarcoplasm of muscle from the extracellular space through an intracellular tubular network called the *sarcoplasmic reticulum.* On spread of the excitation impulse in cardiac muscle, the calcium ions travel from the sarcoplasmic reticulum to the points of interaction between the sarcomeric actin and myosin filaments. Calcium interacts there with troponin, a regulatory protein that inhibits the formation of cross-bridges between actin and myosin. When this inhibition is terminated by the action of calcium on troponin, cross-bridges form between the contractile elements of the muscle, and contraction ensues. It is probably through this mechanism that calcium has its positive inotropic effect.

Indications

Calcium chloride is most beneficial in reversing the cardiac effects of hyperkalemia, hypocalcemia, and toxicity resulting from the administration of calcium channel blockers. However, its use is controversial because of the fear that it may produce a tetanic contraction of an irritable myocardium or depression of the sinus node, resulting in asystole. It has been hypothesized that the drug may pass into cells with marginal viability, denaturing intracellular proteins and hastening cell death. This effect is particularly worrisome because the brain is so sensitive to hypoxia.

Dosage

If the drug is to be used, the recommended dose is 2 mL of a 10% solution of calcium chloride (2 to 4 mg/kg). A bolus may be repeated at 10-minute intervals, if necessary. Calcium salts cannot be mixed directly with bicarbonate solution because they precipitate as calcium carbonate.

Several calcium preparations are available for intravenous use; calcium chloride, calcium gluceptate, and calcium gluconate are the most popular. Calcium gluceptate can be given in a dose of 5 to 7 mL, and calcium gluconate in a dose of 6 to 8 mL.

Complications

Rapid administration of a large bolus of calcium chloride, especially through a central venous catheter, may produce severe sinus bradycardia or sinus arrest. Undiluted calcium chloride given through a peripheral vein causes sclerosis and tissue injury; therefore, if a central site is not available, it should either be diluted or administered in a less irritating form (e.g., calcium gluconate). Calcium must also be used cautiously in patients receiving digitalis, because it can produce or accentuate digitalis toxicity. Calcium probably is contraindicated in the management of cardiac arrest, unless documented hypocalcemia or hyperkalemia is present, or calcium channel blocking drug toxicity is thought to be present.[43]

GENERAL REFERENCE ■

Cummins RO (ed): *Textbook of Advanced Cardiac Life Support.* Dallas, American Heart Association, 1994

REFERENCES ■

1. American Society of Anesthesiologists: Practice guidelines for management of the difficult airway: a report of the ASA Task Force on Management of the Difficult Airway. *Anesthesiology* 1993;78:597
2. Smith JP, Bodai BI, Seifkin A, et al: The esophageal obturator airway. *JAMA* 1983;250:1081
3. Kassels SJ, Ropbinson WA, O'Bara KJ: Esophageal perforation associated with the esophageal obturator airway. *Crit Care Med* 1980;8:366
4. Michael TAD: The esophageal obturator airway: a critique. *JAMA* 1981;246:1098
5. Goldenberg IF, Campion BC, Siebold CM, et al: Esophageal gastric tube airway vs endotracheal tube in prehospital cardiac arrest. *Chest* 1986;90:90
6. Walls RM: Cricothyroidotomy. *Emerg Med Clin North Am* 1986;6:725
7. Melker RJ, Banner MJ: Work imposed by breathing through cricothyrotomy tube. 6th World Congress on Emergency and Disaster Medicine, Hong Kong, September 1989
8. Scuderi PE, McLeskey CH, Comer PB: Emergency percutaneous transtracheal ventilation during anesthesia using readily available equipment. *Anesth Analg* 1982;61:867

9. Florete OG Jr: Airway devices and their application. In: Kirby RR, Gravenstein N (eds): *Clinical Anesthesia Practice.* Philadelphia, WB Saunders, 1994:298

10. Jesudian MCS, Harrison RR, Keenen RL, et al: Bag-valve-mask ventilation: two rescuers are better than one. Preliminary report. *Crit Care Med* 1985;13:122

11. Babbs CF, Voorhees WD, Fitzgerald KR, et al: Relationship of blood pressure and flow during CPR to chest compression amplitude: evidence for an effective compression threshold. *Ann Emerg Med* 1983;12:527

12. Orlowski JP: Optimum position for external cardiac compression in infants and young children. *Ann Emerg Med* 1986;15:667

13. Emergency Cardiac Care Committee and Subcommittee, American Heart Association. Guidelines for cardiopulmonary resuscitation and emergency cardiac care. VII: Neonatal resuscitation. *JAMA* 1992;268:2276

14. McDonald JL: Systolic and mean arterial pressures during manual and mechanical CPR in humans. *Ann Emerg Med* 1982;11:292

15. Halperin HR, Tsitlik JE, Guerci AD, et al: Determinants of blood flow to vital organs during cardiopulmonary resuscitation in dogs. *Circulation* 1986;73:539

16. Sack JB, Kesselbrenner MB, Bregman D: Survival from in-hospital cardiac arrest with interposed abdominal counterpulsation during cardiopulmonary resuscitation. *JAMA* 1992;266:379

17. Krischer JP, Fine EG, Weisfeldt ML, et al: Comparison of prehospital conventional and simultaneous compression-ventilation cardiopulmonary resuscitation. *Crit Care Med* 1989;17:1263

18. Paradis NA, Martin GB, Rivers EP, et al: Coronary perfusion pressure and the return of spontaneous ventilation in human cardiopulmonary resuscitation. *JAMA* 1990;263:1106

19. Falk JL, Rackow EC, Weil MH: End-tidal carbon dioxide concentration during cardiopulmonary resuscitation. *N Engl J Med* 1988;318:607

20. Callaham M, Barton C: Prediction of outcome of cardiopulmonary resuscitation from end-tidal carbon dioxide concentration. *Crit Care Med* 1990;18:358

21. Martin GB, Gentile NT, Paradis NA, et al: Effect of epinephrine on end-tidal carbon dioxide monitoring during CPR. *Ann Emerg Med* 1990;19:396

22. Befeler B: Mechanical stimulation of the heart: its therapeutic value in tachyarrhythmias. *Chest* 1978;73:832

23. Kerber RE: Statement on early defibrillation. American Heart Association: Medical scientific statement from the Emergency Cardiac Care Committee. *Circulation* 1991;83:2233

24. Ewy GA, Dahl CF, Zimmerman M, et al: Ventricular fibrillation masquerading as ventricular standstill. *Crit Care Med* 1981;9:841

25. American Heart Association: American Heart Association standards and guidelines for cardiopulmonary resuscitation (CPR) and emergency cardiac care (ECC). *JAMA* 1986;255:2841

26. Kerber KE, Grayzel J, Kennedy J, et al: Elective cardioversion: influence of paddle-electrode location and size on success rates and energy requirements. *N Engl J Med* 1981;305:658

27. Weaver WD, Cobb LA, Copass MK, et al: Ventricular defibrillation: a comparative trial using 176-J and 320-J shocks. *N Engl J Med* 1982;307:1101

28. Sirna SJ, Ferguson DW, Charbonnier F, et al: Electrical cardioversion in humans: factors affecting transthoracic impedance. *Am J Cardiol* 1988;62:1048

29. Gutgesall LHP, Zacker WP, Geddes LA, et al: Energy dose for ventricular defibrillation of children. *Pediatrics* 1976;58:898

30. Kerber RE, Carter J, Klein S, et al: Open-chest defibrillation during cardiac surgery: energy and current requirements. *Am J Cardiol* 1980;46:393

31. Kerber RE, Martins JB, Kienzle MG, et al: Energy, current, and success in defibrillation and cardioversion: clinical studies using an automated impedance-based energy adjustment method. *Circulation* 1988;77:1038

32. Kerber RE, Kienzle MG, Olshansky B, et al: Ventricular tachycardia rate and morphology determine energy and current requirements for transthoracic cardioversion. *Circulation* 1992;85:158

33. Brown CG, Werman HA, Davis EA, et al: Comparative effects of graded doses of epinephrine or regional brain blood flow during CPR in a swine model. *Ann Emerg Med* 1986;15:1138

34. Emergency Cardiac Care Committee and Subcommittee, American Heart Association. Guidelines for cardiopulmonary resuscitation and emergency cardiac care. III. Adult advanced cardiac life support. *JAMA* 1992;268:2208

35. Mazkereth R, Paret G, Ezra D, et al: Epinephrine blood concentrations after peripheral bronchial versus endotracheal administration of epinephrine in dogs. *Crit Care Med* 1992;20:1582

36. Kette F, Weil M, Gazmuri R, et al: Buffer solutions may compromise cardiac resuscitation by reducing coronary perfusion pressure. *JAMA* 1991;266:2121

37. Emergency Cardiac Care Committee and Subcommittee, American Heart Association. Guidelines for cardiopulmonary resuscitation and emergency cardiac care. III. Adult advanced cardiac life support. *JAMA* 1992;268:2210

38. Benjamin E, Oropello JM, Abalos AM, et al: Effects of acid-base correction on hemodynamics, oxygen dynamics, and resuscitability in severe canine hemorrhagic shock. *Crit Care Med* 1994;22:1616

39. Gunnar RM, Passamani ER, Bourdillon PD, et al: American College of Cardiology/American Heart Association Guidelines for the early management of patients with acute myocardial infarction: report of the ACC/AHA Task Force on Assessment of Diagnostic and Therapeutic Cardiovascular Procedures. *Circulation* 1990;82:664

40. Haynes RE, Chinn TL, Copass MK, et al: Comparison of bretylium tosylate and lidocaine in management of out of hospital ventricular fibrillation: a randomized clinical trial. *Am J Cardiol* 1981;48:353

41. Emergency Cardiac Care Committee and Subcommittee, American Heart Association. Guidelines for cardiopulmonary resuscitation and emergency cardiac care. III. Adult advanced cardiac life support. *JAMA* 1992;268:2206

42. Gold MR, Dee GW, Cocca-Spofford D, et al: Esmolol and ventilatory function in cardiac patients with COPD. *Chest* 1991;100:1215

43. Weiss AT, Lewis BS, Halon DA, et al: The use of calcium with verapamil in the management of supraventricular tachyarrhythmias. *Int J Cardiol* 1983;4:275

Critical Care, Third Edition, edited by Joseph M. Civetta,
Robert W. Taylor, and Robert R. Kirby.
Lippincott-Raven Publishers, Philadelphia, PA © 1997.

CHAPTER 34

Clean and Aseptic Technique
at the Bedside

Judith A. Hudson-Civetta
Joseph M. Civetta

Sepsis is recognized as a significant cause of death or a major complicating factor in most intensive care units (ICUs) today. Because of the risk of nosocomial infection, a great deal of attention must be focused on sterile technique and on maintaining a sterile interface at insertion sites of vascular catheters, particularly in the long-term ICU patient. The three relevant factors in the development of a clinical infection are the host, the organism, and the environment. We understand that the patient with multiple system dysfunction who remains in the ICU for protracted periods becomes increasingly susceptible to nosocomial infection because of compromise in immune function, both cellular and humoral elements. Malnutrition and liver dysfunction potentiate the process because of diminished production of acute-phase reactive proteins.

Notwithstanding the importance of the host and organisms, everyone agrees that the *caregiver* plays the major role in transmitting nosocomial infection. In terms of generating innovative countermeasures, however, the effect of this knowledge seems to have been limited. In fact, in 1985, Nahata[1] wrote, "The U.S. Department of Health and Human Services is preparing to launch a nationwide infection control campaign. The campaign, called, 'Handwashing Prevents Infection . . . It Really Does!' uses a teddy bear character to present this important message in an appealing and persuasive manner. The objective of this campaign was to reduce nosocomial infection by 20% by 1990." The campaign consisted of teddy bears, posters, stickers, and buttons proclaiming the message, "T Bear wants *you* to wash your hands . . . he really does!" and "T Bear likes clean hands . . . he

really does!" We have passed 1990, and there are no triumphant reports of decreased nosocomial infection rates.

We address four questions for viewing the problem of implementation of satisfactory handwashing as the primary mechanism to diminish nosocomial infection in intensive care.

QUESTIONS REGARDING HANDWASHING

Is the Problem of Nosocomial Infection Exaggerated and Overemphasized?

In 1985 there were nearly 2,000,000 nosocomial infections in the United States. Nosocomial infections were estimated to cause approximately 30,000 deaths and contribute to another 70,000 deaths each year. The cost of nosocomial infections was then estimated to be approximately $2.5 billion.[2] Further, about one third of these infections were deemed preventable by effective surveillance and control programs.[3,4] A marked increase has occurred in the number of immunocompromised patients treated in intensive care since 1985. The increased number of heart, lung, and bone marrow transplantations, an aging population with ever-diminishing host resistance, and the staggering increase in patients with acquired immunodeficiency syndrome (AIDS) together with the ever-escalating costs of intensive care suggest that the problem is of even greater magnitude and cost today. The problem is not exaggerated and is of such an impact that it cannot be overemphasized *because* it is amenable to change with savings of lives and resources.

Is There Convincing Evidence Linking Handwashing and Nosocomial Infection?

Larson[5] reviewed 423 published articles concerning handwashing and the prevention of infection from 1879 through 1986. Except for specificity, she judged that all of the elements for causality between handwashing and prevention of infection, including temporality, strength of association, consistency of the association, and biologic plausibility, were present. Her principal conclusion was that the emphasis on handwashing as a primary infection control measure had not been misplaced and should continue.

The concepts of hygiene and antisepsis arose from three innovators—Semmelweis, Lister, and Nightingale—at about the same time but apparently independently in the mid-1800s.[6] Puerperal fever was a deadly scourge of lying-in women for centuries. It was viewed by Hippocrates as a fatal inevitable disease, responsible for about two thirds of the deaths of women in childbirth.[7] Semmelweis, a Hungarian obstetrician, joined the staff of the Vienna lying-in hospital and noticed that women attended by medical staff had two to five times the death rate of those attended by midwives (about 2% to 3% mortality). In 1846, one of his associates died of sepsis after being inadvertently stuck with an instrument used for dissection of a woman who had died of puerperal fever. Semmelweis realized that puerperal fever was being transmitted by contact with autopsy material and demonstrated that the discrepancy between the puerperal fever rates was explained by the fact that only physicians performed postmortem examinations. He then required all students and physicians, after autopsies, to soak their hands in chlorinated lime before examining antepartal patients. Within a few months, puerperal fever deaths among women attended by the medical staff had fallen to levels comparable with those of women attended by midwives. His discovery was not widely accepted among his medical peers for 40 years.

The second major innovator, Lister, introduced antisepsis in surgery by applying Pasteur's germ theory to surgical practice. Pus, in those days, was so universal as to be considered essential to healing and was referred to as "laudable."[8] Lister believed that wound contamination emanated from the air; his solution (application of dressings soaked in carbolic acid) had dramatic effects, although the source of contamination was identified erroneously.

Florence Nightingale went to the Scutari Hospital in the Crimea in 1854. Conditions were deplorable: vermin crawling, walls and floors wet with excreta, inadequate food, and little clothing or bedding for patients. Nightingale was a meticulous record keeper and recognized the value of statistics for influencing health policy.[9] When she arrived, the death rate was 42%. Only 4 months later, militant discipline, which she applied to initiate the sanitary administrative changes, resulted in a reduction of the death rate to 2%.[10] She rejected the concept of contagion, however; the idea of person-to-person transmission of disease was repugnant to

her as it did not fit into her concept of the ordered and controlled nature of the universe.[11]

Are There Unrecognized Factors Influencing Behavior?

Whenever logical arguments fail to change behavior conclusively and consistently, perhaps an illogical or, at least, unrecognized factor is at work. Many of us grew up with mothers who required that we wash our hands before meals, demands that intruded on our growing sense of personal autonomy. Perhaps it was not that we did not wish to have clean hands before eating dinner but, rather, we resented the constant reminders. The "child" in the high-tech ICU might conceivably be responding to the constant admonition, "Wash hands between each patient contact," with resentment. It is not difficult to observe the similarities between handwashing as practiced in the ICU and the way that the child, who was stopped on the way to the dinner table, washed with more of an intention to satisfy his mother and get it over with rather than to sit down at the table (or practice at the bedside as an adult) with hygienically clean hands.

Is There Any Hope for the Future?

Let us examine the role of the ICU caregivers to determine why the admonition "Wash hands between each patient contact" is so easy to express, so universally acknowledged, yet so difficult to practice. We must first examine the cast of usual ICU characters. First, attending physicians usually know the dangers of person-to-person contamination and the risks of such infections to the compromised patient; they try to limit unnecessary patient contact. Most ICU personnel should reconsider the frequency of contacts, especially in this day of necessary universal precautions. Nurses know the dangers and are constantly aware, given a two-patient assignment, that they must frequently move between patients—handwashing becomes second nature. In all studies, nurses' compliance has been higher than that of physicians'. On the other hand, because nurses limit their contact to their assigned patients, the risk of cross-contamination is also limited. Physicians outside the unit staff see only their own one or, perhaps, more patients but again have a limited opportunity to spread organisms throughout the ICU. On the other hand, surgeons may need to examine open wounds or do other bedside procedures. Although the use of sterile technique is second nature in the operating room (OR), remembering to stop at the sink *before and after* visiting each bed requires a special conscious effort.

In fact, the group at highest risk to transmit nosocomial infections is the ICU team of physicians. They have the most direct contact with the most ICU patients. Furthermore, given rotations of relatively junior personnel, they may be less knowledgeable with respect to risks of nosocomial infection, aseptic technique, and the technical procedures themselves. It is also truly a Herculean task to remember handwashing between each patient contact because of the sheer number of patient contacts during their tour of duty. Also, it is extremely difficult to place handwashing at the top of

the list when suddenly called to assist in the management
of an emergency. Thus, there are many realistic reasons
why the ICU physicians are the caregivers most likely to
transmit infection.

COMPLIANCE WITH HANDWASHING GUIDELINES. In
1985, the Centers for Disease Control (CDC) published
revised versions of guidelines for handwashing.[12] The difficulty of proposing guidelines is evident in the opening
paragraphs:

> The absolute indications for an ideal frequency of handwash-
> ing are generally not known because of the lack of well-
> controlled studies. Listing all circumstances that may require
> handwashing would be a lengthy and arbitrary task. The
> indications for handwashing probably depend upon the type,
> intensity, duration, and sequence of activity. Generally, su-
> perficial contact with a source not suspected of being con-
> taminated does not require handwashing. In contrast, long
> and intense contact with a patient should probably be fol-
> lowed by handwashing.
>
> The circumstances that require handwashing are fre-
> quently found in high-risk units because patients in these
> units are often infected and colonized with virulent or multi-
> ply resistant microorganisms, and are highly sensitive to in-
> fection because of wounds, invasive procedures, or dimin-
> ished immune function. Handwashing in these units is
> indicated between direct contact with different patients and
> often is indicated more than once in the care of one patient,
> for example, after touching excretions or secretions and be-
> fore going on to another active care activity for the same
> patient.

Recommendations are made in the form of categories:
category I indicates measures that are strongly supported
by well-designed and controlled clinical studies that show
their effectiveness in reducing the risk of nosocomial infection or are viewed as effective by most expert reviewers;
category II refers to measures that are supported by highly
suggestive clinical studies in general hospitals or by definitive
studies in specialty hospitals that might not be representative
of general hospitals. Measures that have not been adequately
studied but have a logical or strong theoretical rationale
indicating probable effectiveness are included in category II.

RECOMMENDATIONS OF THE CDC
I. Handwashing indications
   A. In the absence of a true emergency, personnel
      should *always* wash their hands:
      1. *Before* performing invasive procedures—cate-
         gory I
      2. *Before* taking care of particularly susceptible
         patients, such as those who are severely immu-
         nocompromised and newborns—category I
      3. *Before* and *after* touching wounds, whether sur-
         gical, traumatic, or associated with an invasive
         device—category I
      4. *After* situations during which microbial con-
         tamination of hands is likely to occur, especially
         those involving contact with mucous mem-
         branes, blood or body fluids, secretions, or ex-
         cretions—category I

      5. *After* touching inanimate sources that are likely
         to be contaminated with virulent or epidemio-
         logically important microorganisms; these
         sources include urine-measuring devices or se-
         cretion-collection apparatuses—category I
      6. *After* taking care of an infected patient or one
         who is likely to be colonized with microorgan-
         isms of special clinical or epidemiologic sig-
         nificance (e.g., multiply resistant bacteria)—
         category I
      7. *Between* contacts with different patients in
         high-risk units—category I
   B. Most routine, brief patient care activities involving
      direct patient contact other than that discussed in
      I.A. (e.g., taking a blood pressure reading) do not
      require handwashing—category II
   C. Most routine hospital activities involving indirect
      patient contact (e.g., handling a patient's medica-
      tions, food, other objects) do not require hand-
      washing—category I
II. Handwashing technique

For routine handwashing, a vigorous rubbing together
of all surfaces of lathered hands for at least 10 seconds
followed by thorough rinsing under a stream of water is
recommended—category I

EFFICACY OF HANDWASHING. The effectiveness of removing organisms is related to the duration of washing, the
agent used, and the objectives of the different forms of
cleansing and disinfection. Reybrouck[13] identifies four distinct types of hand disinfection recognized in Europe (although disinfection in the United States is reserved for inanimate objects). *Hygienic disinfection* kills pathogenic
organisms that have been deposited on the hands and are
part of the transient flora. In this context, transient flora[14]
are organisms isolated from the skin but not demonstrated
to be consistently present in most persons. However, in
health care workers, hand carriage of the aerobic gram-
negative rods may not be transient.[15] Therefore, handwashing that merely concentrates on removing organisms acquired during the day may not be sufficient. *Resident flora*[14]
refers to organisms persistently isolated from the skin of most
persons. These organisms are considered to be permanent
residents of the skin and are not readily removed by mechanical friction. These organisms and the *transient flora* may
be affected by the second form of hand disinfection, *hygienic
hand disinfection with residual action.*[13] It kills the pathogenic bacteria present in the transient flora at the time of
washing, reduces the numbers of resident organisms, and
also has some continued activity over time. The aim is to
obtain a continuing residual antibacterial effect on the transient flora, particularly *Staphylococcus aureus.* The third
form of hand disinfection is *surgical hand disinfection,* the
preoperative disinfection of the surgeon's hands.[13] Its aim
is distinctly different because it is effective against the resident and the transient flora. Because most surgical operations are of some duration and because a large percentage
of gloves have been demonstrated to develop perforations,
the aim of *surgical hand disinfection* is to render the sur-

geon's hands as germ free as possible for some hours. To achieve this aim, duration of washing is increased, brushes or sponges are used to mechanically cleanse the hands, and the subungual spaces are carefully cleaned (surgeons also keep their nails closely cropped). It is also important to recognize that cultures taken after *surgical hand disinfection* are expected to show the removal of most organisms. In contrast, the forms of hand disinfection appropriate to the ICU—not having the ultimate goal of many hours of germ-free effect—demonstrate lesser reductions in total bacterial count, in part because of the duration of handwashing and especially the elimination of the routine cleansing of the subungual area. Although a three logarithmic (1000-fold) reduction in organisms may be seen after a typical surgical scrub, perhaps only 50% of organisms can be removed by hygienic hand disinfection because of persistent subungual bacteria.[16]

The last form of hand disinfection is termed *basic disinfection*.[13] This is defined as the effects of repeated applications of a disinfectant, which would cause a greater reduction in the hand flora than can be attained from a single treatment. It is useful for personnel caring for immunocompromised patients in a protective isolation area. The resident flora on the hands of the caregiver should be as low as possible.

Thus, the goals of handwashing in the ICU, in terms of the quantitative aspects, should be to remove as many of the transient flora (transient flora are not necessarily pathogenic) as possible while recognizing a need to decrease the resident flora, because disease-causing organisms can be a part of or become resident flora on the hands of health care workers. Thus, an overall diminution in the number of organisms seems to be desirable.

IMPORTANCE OF NOSOCOMIAL BLOOD STREAM INFECTION

In addition to being one of the most serious complications of intravenous therapy, nosocomial blood stream infection (BSI) is growing at an alarming rate. In 1980, the BSI rate per 100,000 discharges was 186; in 1989, the National Nosocomial Infections Surveillance System reported that the rate had risen to 349.[16]

BSI represent a serious risk to the safety of the ICU patient. Many sources of the bacteria contaminate or infect catheters that may also predispose to BSI. The following factors have been implicated by investigations in the literature:

1. Length of catheterization[17-22]
2. Direct entry of bacteria into the blood stream from contaminated or infected intravascular catheters[17,21,22]
3. Bacteria on the patient's skin near the site of catheter insertion[17,19,21]
4. Contaminated transducer pressure–monitoring systems attached to the catheter[21,23]
5. Another source of infection in the patient coexisting with the catheter[17,20-22]

6. Excessive time intervals between replacement of the catheter's dressing, stopcocks, transducer, or infusion fluid[21,24]
7. Faulty decontamination of transducer components[25]

This list has a common denominator: the caregiver who maintains and uses the catheterization monitoring systems.

SOURCES OF BACTERIA

There are three sources of the bacteria: the patient's own skin; the caregiver; and other sites in the patient. With respect to the patient's own skin, antisepsis is discussed in the section on preparation. Remember, however, that skin cannot be permanently sterilized because bacteria colonize hair follicles and sweat glands. Even if the surface is rendered sterile temporarily, regrowth occurs over time from the depths of the skin appendages, which is an indication for repeating sterilization techniques at specified intervals. The study by Sitzman and associates[26] emphasizes the importance of maintaining surface sterility: there was an 8% incidence of positive results from catheter segment cultures in patients who had negative culture results of the skin site, compared with a 50% rate of positive culture results from catheter segments in patients who had positive cultures from the skin. Thus, the skin surrounding the insertion site is an obvious source of bacteria. If bacterial growth flourishes, organisms can gain entrance through the skin puncture site and grow in the subcutaneous tract; this growth is usually termed *colonization*. Subsequently, this may lead to either signs of local infection or bacteremia if bacteria enter the blood stream through the perforation in the vessel wall caused by catheterization.

The caregiver might also be the source of the bacteria ultimately responsible for nosocomial infection. Common sites of transmission include the skin (especially the hands), hair, nose, and mouth. These are the reasons for the use of gloves, caps, gowns, and masks.

Other sites in the patient, the final source of nosocomial infection, include open wounds and drains, the lungs, urinary tract, the gut, and perineum. Two potential pathways exist for transmission: exogenous and endogenous pathways. Bacteria from an exogenous source arrive at the catheter insertion site through some intermediate steps. For instance, bacteria in tracheostomy secretions may penetrate the dressing overlying a subclavian catheter, or a person wearing sterile gloves during a dressing change may reach up to reconnect the ventilator tubing that "popped off" the endotracheal tube. In doing so, the operator's gloves are accidentally contaminated and, if they are not changed, will contaminate the catheter insertion site.

The second mode of organism spread from one site in a patient to another can be termed *endogenous*. After the development of bacteremia from a distant source (abscesses or pneumonia), organisms may lodge in a fibrin sheath surrounding the intravascular portion of the catheter. This fibrin sheath is more common with the usual central venous and pulmonary artery catheters; the use of less reactive materials such as Silicone elastomers and the incorporation of chlorhexidine and silver sulfadiazine into the catheter surface are attempts to decrease this sheath formation. A cause-and-effect relationship to demonstrate endogenous transmission is difficult for many reasons. Peripheral bacteremia may not be detected, removal of the catheter may strip the fibrin sheath, and culture of the catheter tip (often performed, but on an incorrect specimen) that has only briefly traversed the catheter wound may not reveal the organism.

INSERTION PROTOCOLS ■

A quick glance at an ongoing insertion procedure in the ICU provides a view that seems reasonably similar to sterile technique in the OR. Many factors make this appearance deceiving. First, the patient is usually not asleep so that the field itself does not remain stationary. All of us have experienced unexpected "help" as a patient frees an arm and a hand suddenly enters the sterile field. The actual physical isolation of the sterile area from nonsterile areas is much more difficult than in the OR because they must overlap during continued treatment of the patient. To achieve this separation and isolation in the OR, separate sterile and nonsterile teams are necessary. It is a far cry from the OR team of a surgeon, assistant, scrub nurse, technician, and one or two circulating nurses to the team in the ICU, which is usually limited to the fellow or resident and one nurse. Training in sterile technique is limited in many of the people involved in sterile procedures in the ICU *and* there are fewer "watchdogs," that is, those in the OR assigned to keep an eye on the inexperienced (usually) medical students and junior residents during their first exposures to sterile technique. The time factor must also be considered: in the OR, the need for sterility ends with the end of the procedure, but in the ICU, efforts to maintain sterility must be sustained for all of the days of monitoring—in a difficult environment, with busy personnel, inadequate education and training, less supervision, and hurried techniques.

A PRACTICAL BEDSIDE APPROACH ■

We believe that masks, caps, gowns, and gloves should be used. Separate sterile and nonsterile work areas also should be established. A small table can be used for kits and the necessary additions. For the sterile field, try to create as large a covered area as possible. Remember to talk to the patient ahead of time to provide reassurance and explanations. Remember not to underestimate the duration of the procedure or to minimize the discomfort that the patient might experience. When things do not proceed as quickly as hoped, anxiety may be *created*; do not gloss over or minimize the time and pain to "spare" the patient. Sedation may be necessary, and restraints should be used. Work through as small an opening in the sterile drapes as possible to avoid inadvertent contamination from other pieces of equipment surrounding the patient. Use prepackaged kits whenever

possible. They are easier and faster to assemble and more likely to contain the "right" components; however, the major advantage is that each preassembled connection eliminates another potential source of contamination by the caregiver during assembly.

In invasive catheterization, the focus usually is on the actual insertion procedure. In fact, the physician asks to be called when everything is ready and leaves when the catheter is in place. There is a much broader focus, which we believe is necessary to understand the complete process, many days in duration. From this perspective, the nurse in the ICU is charged with the responsibility of maintaining and caring for the catheter before, during, and after insertion as well as assessing the patient for signs and symptoms of infection.[27] The nurse's responsibilities include the following activities in caring for the critically ill patient:

1. Assembling the transducer pressure–monitoring system with sterile technique
2. Ensuring proper cleaning of the transducer between use (or using sterile, disposable transducers)
3. Assembling the equipment needed for insertion of the catheter using sterile technique
4. Testing the patency and function of the catheter
5. Maintaining sterile technique during insertion
6. Monitoring the patient's physiologic status during insertion
7. Applying the sterile, occlusive dressing and changing the dressing when soiled, saturated, or disturbed or at a specified interval, every 3 days has been chosen in our unit
8. Assessing the catheter–skin interface for signs of inflammation
9. Obtaining pressure measurements from the catheter as the patient's physiologic needs indicate
10. Calibrating the transducer on a periodic basis
11. Obtaining blood samples as indicated
12. Infusing intravenous fluids and medications
13. Obtaining cultures of blood, urine, tracheal aspirate, and wound as indicated for patients with a known or suspected source of infection

PREPARATION OF SITE AND DRESSING ■

Preparing the insertion site with antiseptic solutions seems to be an area of little controversy. Here we present what is commonly accepted, with our own variations and comments.

Shaving before elective surgical operations used to be done the night before. However, nicks and scratches became reddened, and it was observed that if shaving was performed too early, an increased incidence of wound infection resulted.[28] Because sterilization of the site is necessary for days, shaving to add sterilization is not advisable. However, in hirsute patients, shaving may be necessary to enable a dressing to be fastened securely. If necessary, shaving should be done lightly and repeated when necessary. Acetone may be used first, primarily to remove old tape adhesive. Aqueous chlorhexidine (2%) also has been used as a skin antiseptic but is not available commercially.[29] Because it proved superior to povidone-iodine, we use the 4% skin cleanser in all of the steps needing an antiseptic.

TECHNIQUE OF SKIN PREPARATION ■

Each catheter should be inserted by use of a prepackaged kit containing all essential sterile components assembled by a central supply department or by a manufacturer (Fig. 34-1). The individual catheter and the solutions used for preparation of the skin are added after the sterile field is formed.

The kit should be placed on a clean, dry surface. After the outer wrapper is opened, masks, hats, and gloves are distributed to the involved personnel at the bedside before the inner kit is carefully opened. Masks should decrease the transmission of oral and nasal flora onto the sterile field and should be worn by everyone at the bedside (including an extubated patient). In intubated patients, the exhalation port of the ventilator should be directed away from the field.

The physician dons sterile gloves and prepares the kit contents for the procedure. An assistant pours the chlorhexi-

dine solution used for preparation of the skin. The physician begins preparing the skin with acetone if tape adhesive or other substances are in the area intended for catheter insertion with a soaked sterile gauze sponge (4 × 4 in), folded twice and clamped in forceps. The skin is briskly scrubbed in an expanding circular manner, beginning at the proposed insertion point and reaching a diameter of approximately 25 cm. The forceps and gauze are changed, and the cleansing process is repeated in the same manner four times with the chlorhexidine skin cleanser. The final application is allowed to remain in contact with the skin for 2 minutes. The physician removes the "prep" gloves and puts on a sterile gown and a new set of sterile gloves.

The surrounding skin is covered by sterile drapes, and a sterile sheet is placed over the remainder of the patient's body. The sterile drapes provide a large, sterile working area to prevent contamination of the equipment used in insertion (Fig. 34-2). After the preparation has been completed, the catheter is introduced according to defined technique. When the catheter is in correct functional position, it is attached to the appropriate connection. The area is wiped with chlorhexidine skin cleanser to remove blood and other material that may have accumulated during insertion (Fig. 34-3). Povidone-iodine ointment is then applied to the site of insertion on the skin (Fig. 34-4). The method used to secure the placement of the catheter varies according to the type of catheter. A sterile sleeve used with pulmonary artery catheters is attached to the hub of the introducer and is fixed 20 to 30 cm along the catheter body. This leaves a segment enclosed in the sheath so that it can be manipulated later if the tip of the catheter must be readjusted to maintain proper position. The introducer is usually sutured to the skin. Arterial and central venous catheters commonly have flanges for anchoring skin sutures as well. The surrounding skin is dried and then sprayed with tincture of benzoin. The dressing is completed using the following steps: (1) placing a folded 2 × 2 in gauze square over the insertion site and

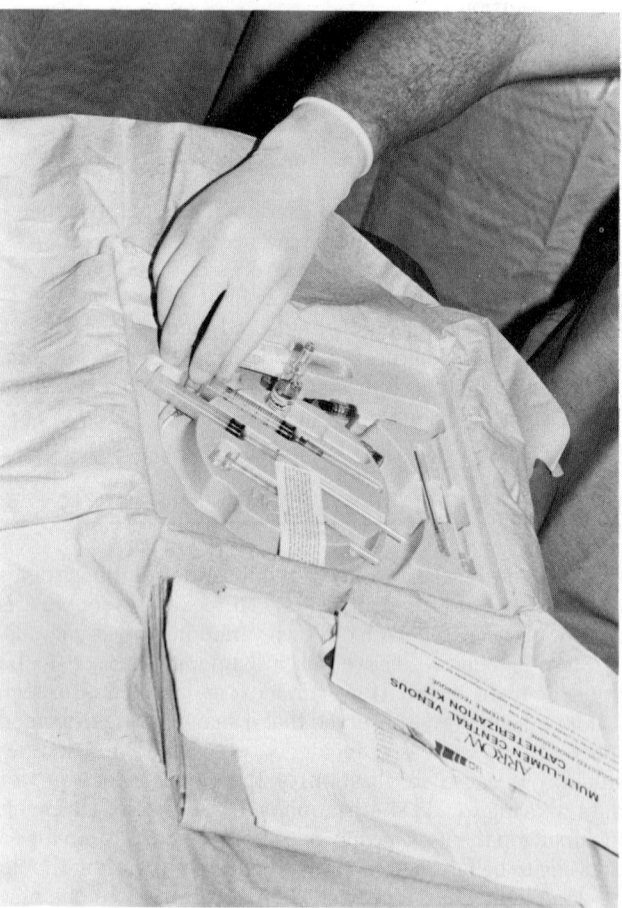

FIGURE 34-1. A prepackaged insertion kit is opened, creating a sterile work area on a bedside table. Not only are these kits faster and easier to use but they contain all of the proper elements needed.

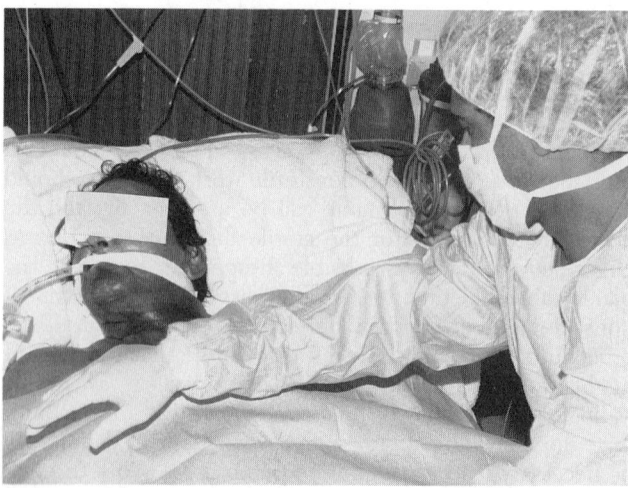

FIGURE 34-2. After preparation of the skin, a sterile sheet is spread over the patient's body, providing a continuous sterile work area from the insertion site to the insertion kit. The proposed insertion site is then covered with a fenestrated drape.

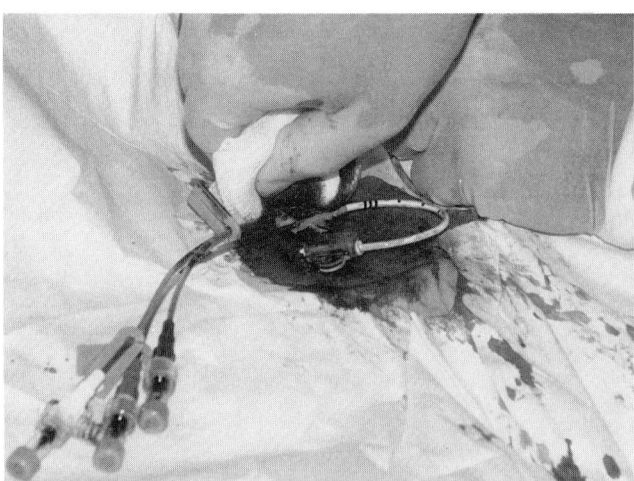

FIGURE 34-3. After insertion, the area is again cleansed with chlorhexidine skin cleanser. This process should remove any inadvertent surface contamination during the insertion process.

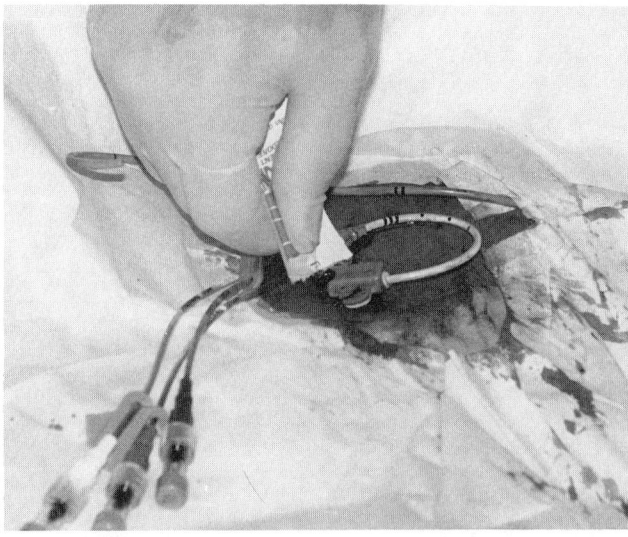

FIGURE 34-4. Povidone-iodine ointment is applied after the catheter has been sutured in place. The skin surface should be dry, and there should be no bleeding from the insertion site or sutures. Sterile gauze is then applied.

antiseptic ointment; (2) applying occlusive tape (Fig. 34-5); and (3) sealing with clear, waterproof tape (Fig. 34-6). The occlusive tape prevents entry of bacteria that are airborne, and the waterproof tape prevents oral or tracheostomy secretions and any other moisture from saturating and contaminating the dressing. The date and time are written on the surface of the dressing. A chest radiograph is obtained to verify the position of the catheter and to rule out complications such as pneumothorax.

Catheters for parenteral nutrition (PN) should never be connected to pressure-monitoring equipment for verification of position to reduce possible contamination; we consider verification by radiograph the only means of establishing the correct position of the catheter tip. Until the correct position is known, 5% dextrose in water should be infused slowly at a keep-open rate. This precaution prevents the

concentrated dextrose solution from being infused into a noncentral vein and should lessen the incidence of thrombotic complications that may result.

Our final connection to the catheter for central venous and arterial catheters is a T-connector. We prefer the T-connector to the stopcock for the patient's safety and to minimize the risk of microbial contamination. A catheter or a dedicated lumen of a multilumen catheter for PN is connected to a "final" filter (0.22 μm) before infusing the nutritional solution. After the PN catheter or lumen is connected to the appropriate filter, tubing, and solution, the system must never be interrupted except to change the dressing, the intravenous tubing, and the final filter. It is

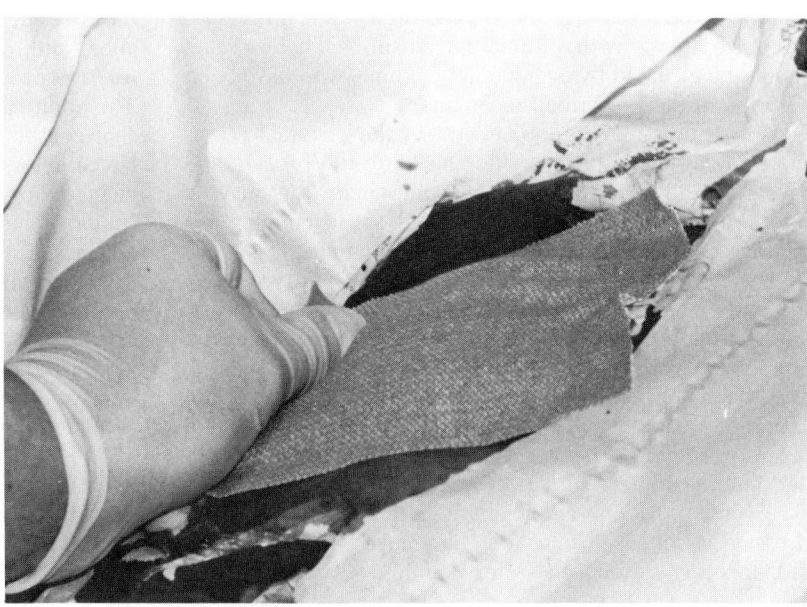

FIGURE 34-5. Elastoplast tape is applied after tincture of benzoin spray.

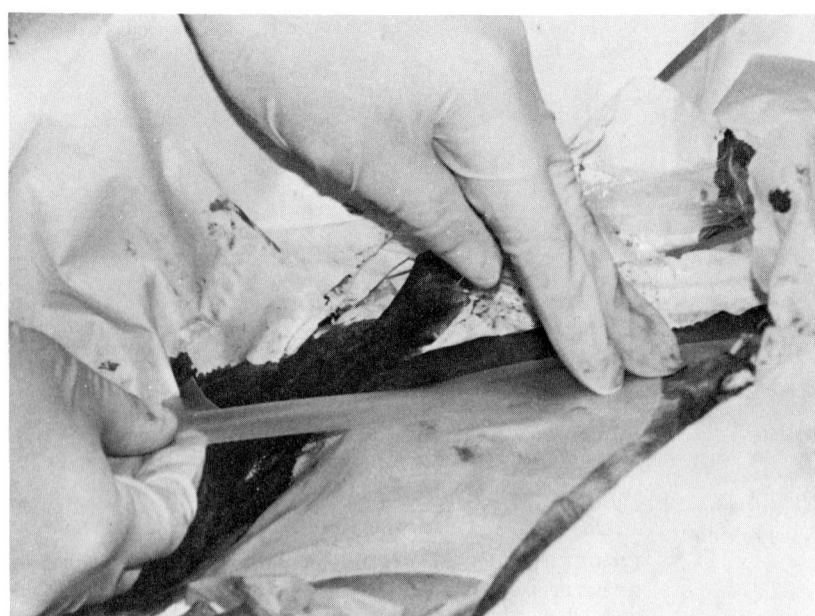

FIGURE 34-6. Waterproof tape is used to finish the dressing. This type of dressing is preferred to transparent dressings (see text).

never used to infuse medication or withdraw blood samples for routine laboratory studies or cultures. Substances are not added to the solution after its preparation in the pharmacy. These precautions have been recommended to prevent bacterial contamination.

MAINTENANCE OF INTRAVASCULAR CATHETERS ■

DRESSING CHANGES

All dressings on invasive intravascular catheters should be handled in a similar manner. We change them every 72 hours or more often if soiled, saturated, or disturbed to minimize the growth of microorganisms.[30] The dressing should be changed by competent personnel who have been certified in the prescribed technique.

We use dressing kits prepackaged by the hospital or commercially available because they facilitate the process and prevent use of scattered available components that may be undesirable. The ready availability of all sterile components decreases the possibility of breaks in technique.

The dressing change kit is placed on a clean, dry surface; the outer package is opened; the packages of gloves, masks, and sterile occlusive tape are removed; and a mask and cap are donned by the practitioner. The inner package is opened, and the practitioner dons sterile gloves and arranges the contents of the kit to position the receptacles for the skin cleansing solutions. The recommended solutions are acetone and chlorhexidine. The gloves are discarded, the solutions are poured, povidone-iodine ointment to be used in the new dressing is squeezed onto a sterile gauze square, and the old dressing is removed. After donning of a new pair of

sterile gloves, the cleansing process is begun. The process is identical to that previously described for inserting a catheter. Care must be taken not to dislodge any catheter that is not sutured.

After the acetone has been applied and the povidone-iodine ointment removed, the site should be visually inspected and palpated for indications of infection. Specifically look for exudate around the site of insertion, redness, or edema, and then palpate for tenderness or warmth. If any abnormal sign is noticed, the catheter should be removed and cultures taken.

After the cleansing process has been completed, the ointment is applied and a new occlusive dressing secured. Quality assurance and surveillance must be maintained routinely by the charge nurse or the infection control nurse to check the dressings (noting date and time of change and appearance) and, on a more formal basis, through the quarterly use of a process audit tool designed by the ICU personnel. The audit can be designed to measure the presence or absence of specific procedures related to the care of intravascular catheters: frequency of dressing change, frequency of change for pressure monitoring and intravenous tubing and solution change, rate and type of positive culture results, and so on.

Intravenous tubing, fluid, filters, and the external system used with pressure-monitoring equipment are replaced every 3 days.[24,31] The same is true for parenteral nutrition, although the bags containing the solution are changed once a day. Any equipment must be replaced if known or suspected contamination has occurred.

We have not adopted the use of transparent polyurethane dressings. A metaanalysis of nine clinical trials concluded that these dressings demonstrate a significantly increased risk of catheter tip colonization, catheter sepsis, and local infection.[32]

SEMIQUANTITATIVE CULTURE SPECIMENS USING GUIDEWIRE EXCHANGE ■

The guidewire exchange technique was devised to obtain the portion of the catheter that resided in the subcutaneous tract. The catheter tip should not be cultured because it does not add meaningful information and may underestimate the number of colonies present.[33]

The dressing is removed, including any remaining antibacterial ointment. The insertion site is scrubbed with chlorhexidine skin cleanser four times and is allowed to remain for 2 minutes. Preparation should include the introducer from the insertion site to the end of the hub, including the tubing of the sidearm (Fig. 34-7). After the skin and introducer have been prepared, the hub is detached from the introducer, and the hub and catheter are removed together (Fig. 34-8). The new catheter is coated with chlorhexidine (Fig. 34-9). The introducer is scored with a scalpel to mark the skin insertion site (Fig. 34-10). The guidewire is then coated with chlorhexidine and inserted into the introducer (Fig. 34-11). The introducer is then removed and a new catheter is threaded over the guidewire. The guidewire is removed and aspiration of all ports of the catheter is used to confirm intravascular location, and the catheter is sutured in place (Fig. 34-12). Using a sterile forceps, grasp the intracutaneous segment (ICS) of the introducer and cut a 2-cm segment proximally and distally with the sterile scissors or a scalpel (Fig. 34-13). The distal cut should be 1 cm below the skin insertion site (Fig. 34-14). Exerting downward pressure, roll the ICS back and forth at least four times across the surface of the agar. Gently press ICS into the agar without breaking its surface (Fig. 34-15). Apply a generous amount of povidone-iodine ointment to the insertion site.

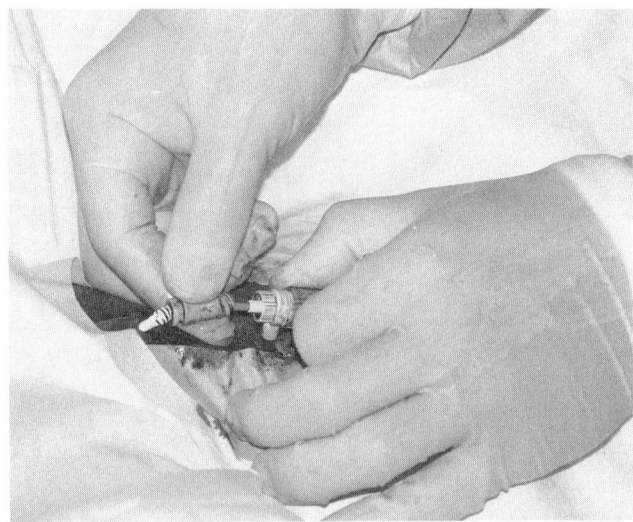

FIGURE 34-8. After the field has been draped with sterile towels, only the scrubbed portions of the catheter should be visible in the field. The hub is detached from the introducer, and the catheter and hub together are withdrawn.

Cover with a dry sterile gauze. Assist the nurse in completing a sterile occlusive dressing, including the date and time of insertion.

The repetitive skin preparations, letting the preparations remain in place for 2 minutes and using antibacterial solutions on the guidewire and new catheter were adopted and modified from the technique described by Norwood and Jenkins.[34] Their results for multiple guidewire exchanges, particularly in long-term septic ICU patients, were better than what has generally been reported and what we had

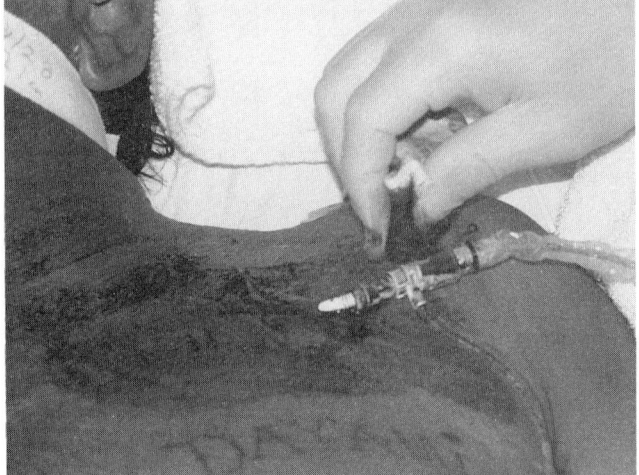

FIGURE 34-7. Wipe away any remaining antibacterial ointment. The skin surrounding the insertion site and the existing introducer, its hub, pulmonary artery catheter sheath, and side arm should be scrubbed vigorously with gauze soaked in chlorhexidine skin cleanser. This should be repeated four times and then allowed to dry completely.

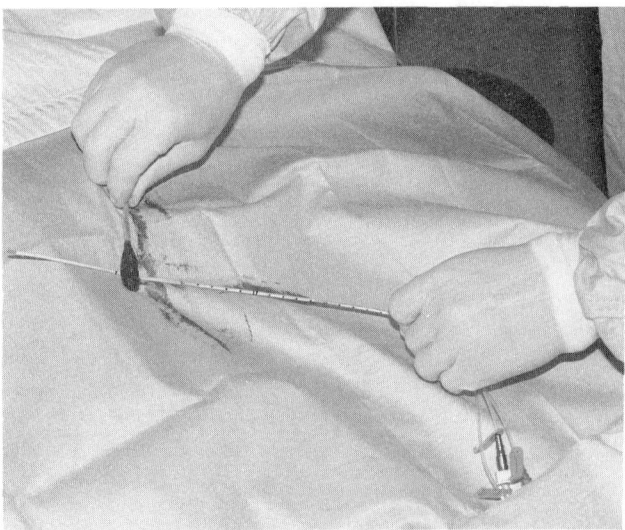

FIGURE 34-9. The new catheter to be inserted is painted with chlorhexidine skin cleanser before its insertion over the guidewire. This can be done in an open area of the wide sterile field with the catheter left in a convenient place for insertion later.

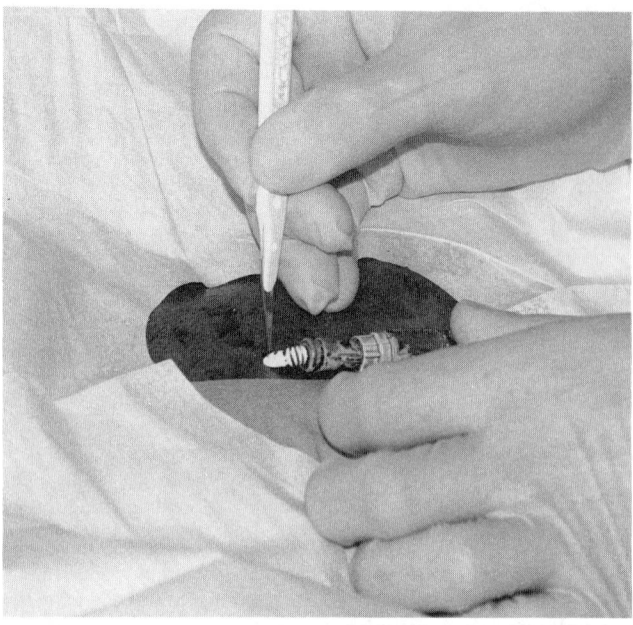

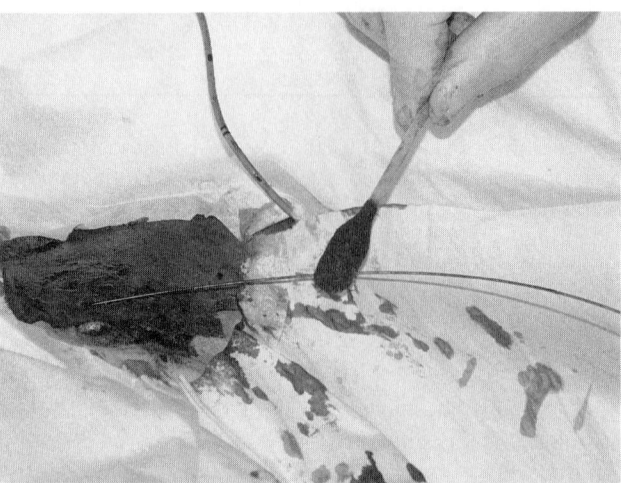

FIGURE 34-11. A swab soaked in chlorhexidine skin cleanser is rubbed over the entire external portion of the guidewire. The new catheter is then threaded over the guidewire.

FIGURE 34-10. A scalpel is used to mark the point at which the introducer perforates the skin surface. This is an important landmark to ensure that the segment used for culture lies completely beneath the surface of the skin. The introducer is removed, leaving the guidewire in place. It can be placed on another portion of the sterile field while the introduction of the new catheter is completed. Alternatively, gauze can be placed over the insertion site with the guidewire in place, and a culture specimen of the segment of the catheter can be taken at this time. The choice is a matter of considering the stability of the patient and the preferences of the insertion team.

observed.[35,36] After adopting their procedures, our rate of positive culture results from catheter segments decreased.[37] We now routinely use multiple guidewire exchanges, stopping when catheters are not needed, clinical signs of infection are evident, or the culture result from the catheter segment is positive. We also have eliminated routine guidewire exchanges for fever. We prefer to use chlorhexidine, silver sulfadiazine impregnated catheters (Arrowgard catheters, Arrow International, Reading, PA) whenever possible. The numbers of catheters used per patient have diminished, and the duration of each catheter's use has increased whereas the percentage of positive catheter segment results has decreased.[38]

It is essential to develop a system in conjunction with the microbiology laboratory by which specimens are logged in,

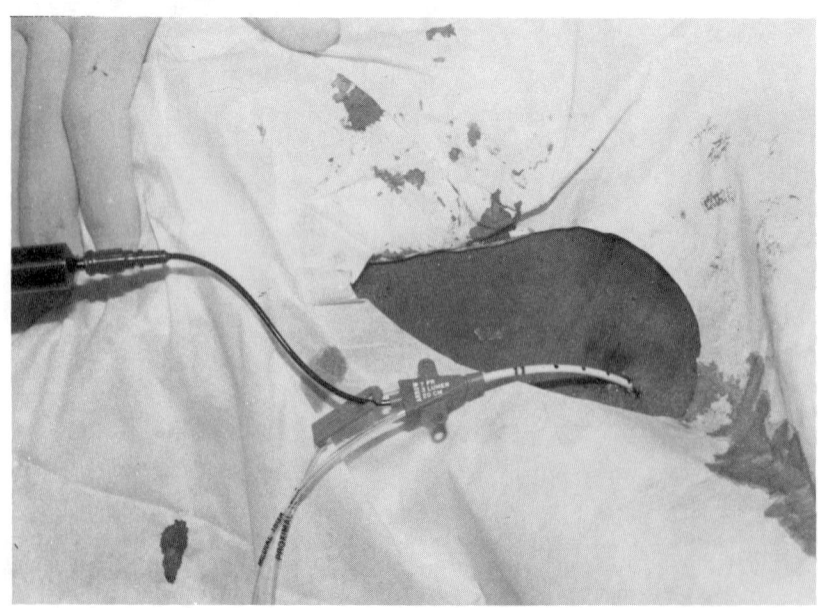

FIGURE 34-12. The guidewire is removed; a syringe is sequentially attached to all ports of the multilumen catheter and aspiration is performed to confirm intravascular location of the new catheter. The catheter is then sutured in place through the holes in the attached flange.

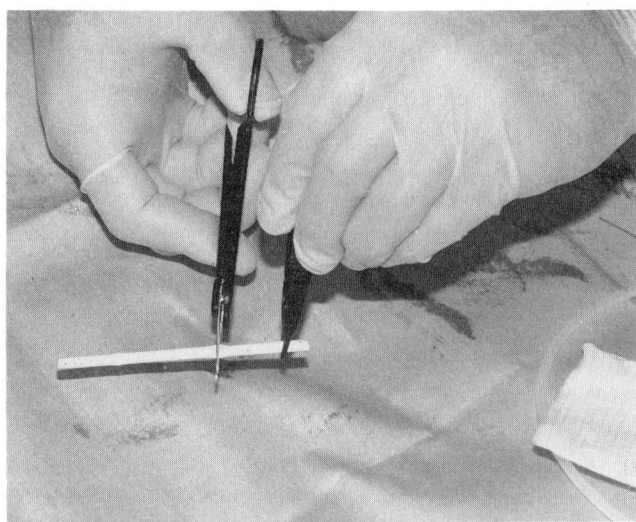

FIGURE 34-13. Using a sterile forceps or hemostat, the intracutaneous segment of the introducer is created by cutting a 2-cm segment proximally and distally from the portion of the introducer that had previously lain beneath the skin surface.

cultured, and results recorded in an easily accessible fashion. These catheter segment cultures must be checked on a daily basis. Normally, growth occurs at 24 hours or not at all. In perhaps only 1 of 50 segments, growth will be reported as negative at 24 hours yet positive some time later. Depending on the time of day that the catheter segment culture is initially performed, however, a negative result the next day may reflect only an insufficient time for growth. We check the cultures for 2 days to be sure.

GUIDELINES FOR THE USE OF GUIDEWIRES

Because the risk of infection of the catheter wound increases with duration of catheterization and a significant risk of bacteremia exists without necessarily any external signs of infection, the "proper" duration of catheterization would

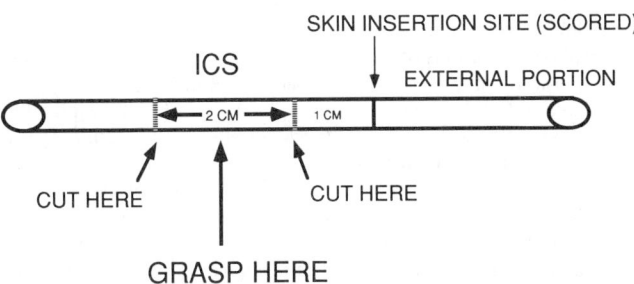

FIGURE 34-14. The landmarks used in identifying the intracutaneous segment are shown diagrammatically. The segment selected should be approximately 2 cm long and be cut from the portion of the introducer that is at least 1 cm below the skin insertion site, which had been previously marked with a scalpel.

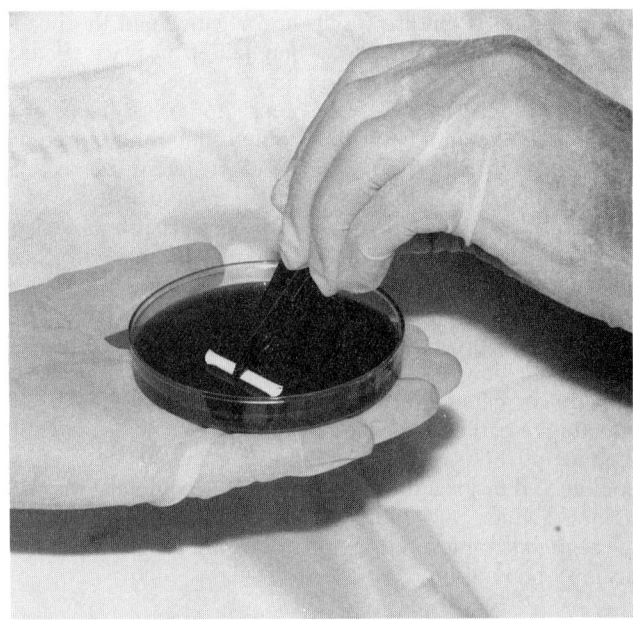

FIGURE 34-15. The intracutaneous segment of the introducer also should be rolled back and forth four times across the surface of the agar and then gently pressed into the agar without breaking its surface.

be difficult to assess based on clinical observation alone. A second insertion procedure contains both risks and added expenses. Exchanging a catheter over a guidewire is a method of separating the catheters with significant bacterial growth from those without, yet maintaining continuity of the tract to avoid the risk of a new insertion procedure. Guidelines for the use of guidewire techniques and careful technique for culturing the removed catheter segments are both mandatory for this approach to be practical. We use the following schema. There are two exclusions: signs of local inflammation and a previous positive catheter segment culture from the same site. Technical problems often develop, particularly with multifunction, multilumen catheters. These catheters may be exchanged within the first day through the same introducer. Repeated exchanges seem to have positive catheter segment rates similar to the cumulative rates attained when new sites are used late in the patient's ICU stay.[37-39] The presence of catheter-related infection may be indicated by a fever but a fever spike is no longer considered a sufficient indication to exchange a catheter. No higher rate of positive catheter segments was found for this indication alone.[37] After eliminating routine changes for fever spikes and using protected catheters (Arrowgard catheters), the incidence of positive segment cultures decreased from 17% to 6% ($p < 0.05$) despite significantly increased duration of catheterization.[38] Even routine guidewire exchanges in nonprotected catheters have not been deemed worthwhile to diminish catheter-related sepsis.[39] If catheter-related sepsis is suspected, a guidewire exchange is performed, primarily to obtain the intracutaneous segment for culture. If culture results are positive (the next day), the replaced catheter should be removed, and a new catheter must be inserted in a new site. If culture results are negative and the fever resolves, the replaced catheter may be left in place. If the culture results are negative and fever persists, however, we would consider catheter-related sepsis to be less likely and would continue an investigation to determine the source of the fever. The patient would have been spared the risk of a second insertion in this case. Certain specific factors, such as coagulopathy or anatomic distortions caused by massive edema or subcutaneous emphysema, may be so severe that delaying the change or removal of a catheter is advisable. In these situations, the risk of insertion to the patient is considered of greater magnitude than the risk of catheter-related infection and bacteremia. The prevalence of positive catheter segment cultures is much higher than either clinical infection or catheter-related bacteremia. Of course, even in the face of these reasons for extension, should bacteremia be detected or local infection appear, the catheter must be removed. Each new catheter may remain in place only if the segments removed from the prior catheter give negative results when cultured.

CONCLUSION ■

Clean and aseptic technique, when applied to invasive catheterizations, is a complex subject in the ICU. The battle against bacteria is not glamorous but must be never ending. Many factors in the environment, in the host, and in the organisms themselves tend to favor infection rather than sterility. We have focused on details beyond the technical aspects of insertion because most physicians seem concerned with the vascular cannulation and consider placing the catheter to be the beginning and end of their role. For long-term catheterization of patients who remain critically ill, this approach is too limited. Ultimately, the success of invasive catheterization depends on a maintained process of clean and aseptic technique. Scrupulous and persistent attention to detail is the only force sufficiently powerful to keep the enemy at bay.

REFERENCES ■

1. Nahata MC: Handwashing prevents infection. *Drug Intell Clin Pharm* 1985;19:738
2. Haley RW, Culver DH, White CW, et al: The nationwide nosocomial infection rate: a new need for vital statistics. *Am J Epidemiol* 1985;121:159
3. Haley RW, Culver DH, White CW, et al: The efficacy of infection surveillance and control programs in preventing nosocomial infections in the U.S. hospitals. *Am J Epidemiol* 1986;121:182
4. Centers for Disease Control: Nosocomial infection surveillance 1980–1982. *CDC Surveill Sum* 1983;32:1
5. Larson E: A causal link between handwashing and risk of infection? Examination of the evidence. *Infect Control Hosp Epidemiol* 1988;9:28
6. Larson E: Innovations in health care: antisepsis as a case study. *Am J Public Health* 1989;79:92
7. Reid R: *Microbes and Men.* New York, Saturday Review Press, 1974
8. Keen WW: Modern antiseptic surgery and the role of experimentation in its discovery and development. *JAMA* 1910;54:1104
9. Cohen IB: Florence Nightingale. *Sci Am* 1984;250:128
10. Nash R: *A Short Life of Nightingale.* New York, Macmillan, 1925
11. Billings JS, Hurd HM: *Hospital Dispensaries and Nursing.* Baltimore, Johns Hopkins University, 1894:449
12. Guidelines for Nosocomial Infections: Handwashing. *Handwashing Hosp Environment Control* 1985;7
13. Reybrouck G: Handwashing and hand disinfection. *J Hosp Infect* 1986;8:5
14. Larson E: APCI guidelines for infection control practice: guideline for use of topical antimicrobial agents. *Am J Infect Control* 1988;16:253
15. Adams BG, Marrie TJ: Hand carriage of aerobic gram-negative rods may not be transient. *J Hyg Camb* 1982;89:33
16. Banerjee S, Emori G, Culver D, et al: Trends in noscomial bloodstream infections (BSI) in the United States, 1980–1989 [abstract 36]. In: *Final Program and Abstracts, 3rd Decennial International Conference on Nosocomial Infections,* Atlanta, 1990:25
17. Maki DG, Weise CE, Sarafin HW: A semiquantitative method for identifying intravenous catheter-related infection. *N Engl J Med* 1977;296:1305
18. Sise MM, Hollingsworth P, Brimon JE, et al: Complications of the flow-directed pulmonary artery catheter: a prospective analysis in 219 patients. *Crit Care Med* 1981;9:315
19. Pinnella JC, Ross DF, Martin T, et al: Study of the incidence of intravascular catheter infection and associated septicemia in critically ill patients. *Crit Care Med* 1983;11:21
20. Caruthers TE, Reno DJ, Civetta JM: Implications of positive blood cultures associated with Swan-Ganz catheters. *Crit Care Med* 1979;7:135
21. Maki DG, Hassemer CA: Endemic rate of fluid contamination and related septicemia in arterial pressure monitoring. *Am J Med* 1981;70:733
22. Applefeld J, Caruthers T, Reno D, et al: Assessment of sterility of long-term cardiac catheterization using the thermodilution Swan-Ganz catheter. *Chest* 1978;74:377
23. Donowitz LG, Marski FJ, Hoyt JW, et al: *Serratia marcescens* bacteremia from contaminated pressure transducers. *JAMA* 1979;242:1749
24. Centers for Disease Control: *National Nosocomial Infections Study Report: Annual Summary 1979.* Atlanta, Centers for Disease Control, March 1982
25. Beck-Sague CM, Jarvis WR: Epidemic bloodstream infections associated with pressure transducers: a persistent problem. *Infect Control Hosp Epidemiol* 1989;10:54
26. Sitzmann JV, Townsend TR, Siler MC, et al: Septic and technical complications of central venous catheterization: a prospective study of 200 consecutive patients. *Ann Surg* 1985;202:766
27. Kenner CV: Multisystem failure. In: Kenner CV, Guzzetta CE, Dossey BM (eds). *Critical Care Nursing: Body–Mind–Spirit.* Boston, Little, Brown, 1981
28. Seropian R, Reynolds BM: Wound infection after preoperative depilatory versus razor preparation. *Am J Surg* 1971;121:251
29. Maki D, Ringer M, Alvarado C: Prospective randomized trial of povidone-Iodine, alcohol and chlorhexidine. *Lancet* 1991;338:339
30. Hudson-Civetta JA, Caruthers TE, Banner TE: Intravascular catheters: current guidelines for care and maintenance. *Heart Lung* 1983;12:466
31. Hudson-Civetta JA, Civetta JM, Martinez OV, et al: Risk and detection of pulmonary artery catheter-related infection in septic surgical patients. *Crit Care Med* 1987;15:29

32. Hoffmann KK, Weber DJ, Samsa GP, et al: A meta-analysis of transparent polyurethane for use as a central venous catheter dressing [abstract 86]. *Final Program and Abstract, 3rd Decennial International Conference on Nosocomial Infections,* Atlanta, 1990;34

33. Shatz D, Civetta J: Efficacy of pulmonary artery catheter tip culture. *Clin Intensive Care* 1993;4(Suppl):9

34. Norwood SH, Jenkins G: An evaluation of triple-lumen catheter infections using a guidewire exchange technique. *J Trauma* 1990; 30:706

35. Civetta JM, Hudson-Civetta JA, Nelson LD, et al: Utility and efficacy of guidewire changes [abstract]. *Crit Care Med* 1987;15:380

36. Civetta JM, Hudson-Civetta JA, Dion L: Duration of illness effects catheter-related infection and bacteremia [abstract 1141]. In: *Program and Abstracts of the 27th Interscience Conference on Antimicrobial Agents and Chemotherapy.* Atlanta, 1987;69

37. Ball S, Hudson-Civetta JA, Civetta J: Re-evaluation of insertion and guidewire exchange protocols effectiveness and validity. *Crit Care Med* 1995;23:S250

38. Ball S, Hudson-Civetta J, Civetta JM: Decreasing catheter-related infection, patient risk and hospital costs by continuous quality improvement. *Crit Care Med* 1996;A24:24

39. Eyer S, Brummitt C, Crossley K, et al: Catheter-related sepsis: a prospective, randomized study of three methods of long-term catheter maintenance. *Crit Care Med* 1990;18:1073

Critical Care, Third Edition, edited by Joseph M. Civetta,
Robert W. Taylor, and Robert R. Kirby.
Lippincott-Raven Publishers, Philadelphia, PA © 1997.

CHAPTER 35

Vascular Cannulation

Bahman Venus
Paul Satish

Vascular cannulation is the cornerstone of monitoring and therapy for most serious illnesses. Although benefits usually exceed risks, benefit-to-risk ratios must be optimized by considering the purpose, complications, urgency, and site of the procedures, together with the availability and experience of the operator and the equipment to be used.

IMMEDIATE CONCERNS

Cannulation involves cognitive, judgmental, and dexterity skills that can only be learned through careful observation and closely supervised practice. Performance improves and complications decrease with experience.[1,2] Hence, formal didactic education, supervision, and certification programs are strongly recommended.[3] Details and related issues beyond the scope of this chapter are available in the cited reviews and in a recently published monograph.[4]

PATIENT PREPARATION
AND INFORMED CONSENT

The operator should discuss the benefits, risks (and measures that will be taken to minimize them), and alternatives with each patient, whenever permitted by the situation and the patient's mental status. If the patient is unable to comprehend, judge, or respond to the discussion, the legal representative or legally responsible next of kin should receive the discussion and make the decision to proceed. In some instances, such as cardiac arrest or profound physiologic instability, the procedure must be accomplished within seconds. Usual preparation and sterility measures must then be abbreviated or omitted.

This discussion should be recorded on the standard form that is signed by the person consenting to the procedure as well as one witness. A progress note by the informing physician, or documentation of phone permission by two witnesses to the discussion, are acceptable alternatives. Informed consent is recommended for all procedures with the exception of peripheral vein cannulation. Discussion of risks should include those short- and long-term complications whose chance of occurring is greater than 1%.[5] Find out if the patient has had adverse reactions to drugs or skin preparation agents that you plan to use and whether there have been difficulties or complications with similar procedures in the past.

After selecting the optimal site and assembling the necessary equipment, request the attendance of a qualified assistant, preferably a registered nurse with intensive care training and experience, for all except peripheral venous cannulation procedures.

ANALGESICS

A local subcutaneous analgesic, such as 1% or 2% lidocaine without epinephrine, is advisable for most cannulation procedures on conscious patients. For peripheral arterial or venous cannulation, use small amounts such as 0.5 mL. Wait 2 to 4 minutes before proceeding. When deeper procedures are planned, draw 4 to 5 mL into a 5-mL syringe through a 20-gauge or larger needle to facilitate rapid filling, change the needle to a 22-gauge or smaller to minimize discomfort, and inject 0.2 to 0.4 mL subcutaneously so that a 1-cm wheal is raised. Slow injection minimizes the initial burning discomfort in sensitive patients.

Inject subsequent 0.2-mL boluses after advancing the needle in 2-mm increments. Always aspirate to detect freely

521

returning blood, which indicates intravascular placement, before injection. Do not exceed 2-mg lidocaine per kg of patient body weight for a procedure. Diphenhydramine (Benadryl) containing 2 mg/mL similarly can be used for patients with previous adverse reactions to other local anesthetics.[6]

Noncooperative, delirious, and anxious patients may require sedation. Appropriate pharmacotherapeutic agents may cause potentially lethal adverse effects and must not be used without close supervision or extensive experience. Reduce dosages in elderly and unstable patients.

The preferred drug for delirium and psychotic agitation is droperidol (Inapsine), 0.1 mg/kg initially, then repeated at 5-minute intervals until the desired degree of sedation is achieved. Low-dose ketamine (2–3 mg/kg) can be considered an alternative for hypotensive patients. Midazolam (Versed), 2 to 4 mg initially, then 2 mg every 2 to 4 minutes, is an alternative for patients with substantial anxiety. Previously preferred agents such as haloperidol (Haldol) and diazepam (Valium) lack rapid onset and therefore do not have the titration capabilities of droperidol and midazolam. Use of any of these drugs mandates careful and continuous observation and monitoring.

SKIN PREPARATION

Two skin regions must be prepared with bacteriocidal soap: the site to be cannulated and the operator's hands. Scrub the cannulation site, including a margin 5 cm peripheral to the anticipated area of the fenestration in the surgical drapes, with a solution of povidone-iodine on sterile gauze or cotton-tipped swabs. Scrub from the intended site of cannulation, outward, in an uninterrupted circular pattern.

The scrub should be completed twice, and the povidone-iodine should be allowed to dry on the skin for optimal bacteriocidal effect. When medical devices abut the sterile field, wash them thoroughly with povidone-iodine solution, then drape the cleaned but nonsterilizable device with povidone-iodine–soaked sterile gauze sponges so that only sterile surfaces are present in and near the cannulation site.

STERILE PREPARATION OF THE OPERATOR AND CANNULATION SITE

In addition to sterile gloves, the operator should don a sterile gown, mask, and cap for all procedures using a guidewire or cannula longer than 5 cm. Otherwise, such devices contact nonsterile wrists or forearms, often without the operator's knowledge. Sterile drapes are not routinely used for peripheral intravenous catheter insertion. A good general rule is to maintain a sterile field with a diameter 10 cm larger than the longest sterile device to be used. This approach is not practical for long catheters and wires. Before catheterization, recently measured electrolytes, coagulation status, arterial blood gas partial pressures, and pH should be evaluated and corrected.

Do not occlude the air supply or field of vision when draping neck areas of conscious patients. An assistant, electronic devices, or both must monitor relevant parameters of the patient's well-being continually through the procedure, because the operator may lose valuable clues while concentrating on the procedure and because much of the patient is obscured by drapes.

ESSENTIAL TECHNIQUES

A plethora of cannulation needles, catheters, and equipment kits is available. The operator must be thoroughly familiar with all available equipment and routine procedures before participating in a cannulation procedure. Each facility or medical center benefits from a critical care organization, committee, or team to coordinate the latest equipment options with the needs of each member of the health-care team.

Standard recommendations for changing vascular cannulas are noted more in their breach than observance. Nonetheless, there is an unacceptable increase in risk of infectious complications after cannulas have been in place for more than 72 hours. We strongly recommend that all central vascular cannulas should be changed routinely, approximately every 3 days. For such changes, the operator must weigh risks versus benefits of the change. In a situation when a cannula may be discontinued in the near future, it can be left in for an additional 1 to 2 days in hope that such a course will obviate the need for a change with its attendant risks and costs.

The modified Seldinger technique is an essential cannulation technique. Its performance is illustrated for femoral vascular cannulation in Figure 35-1 and described in the accompanying legend. Similar principles, equipment, and techniques are used for modified Seldinger techniques for other vascular and tracheal structures.

General guidelines for equipment, care of invasive catheters, and central vascular cannulation are summarized in Tables 35-1 and 35-2.

VENOUS CANNULATION

Venous access can be achieved by cannulating peripheral or central veins. Central veins should be cannulated only when peripheral cannulation does not serve the purpose or is unobtainable.

PERIPHERAL VENOUS ACCESS

Peripheral catheterization is the first choice for intravenous access. It may be initiated by physicians or nurses. Site selection, in the order of most to least preferred, includes the metacarpal, forearm, and pedal veins. Antecubital veins usually are not used because arm flexion often causes discomfort and thrombosis, although this site is excellent for emergency venous access during cardiac resuscitation. Pedal veins cannot be used except in patients at bedrest, because backflow of blood and thrombosis occur frequently in patients who are sitting or standing. Patients who have received previous intravenous therapy are often an excellent source of information concerning preferred locations. If both upper extremities are available, the nondominant side should be used.

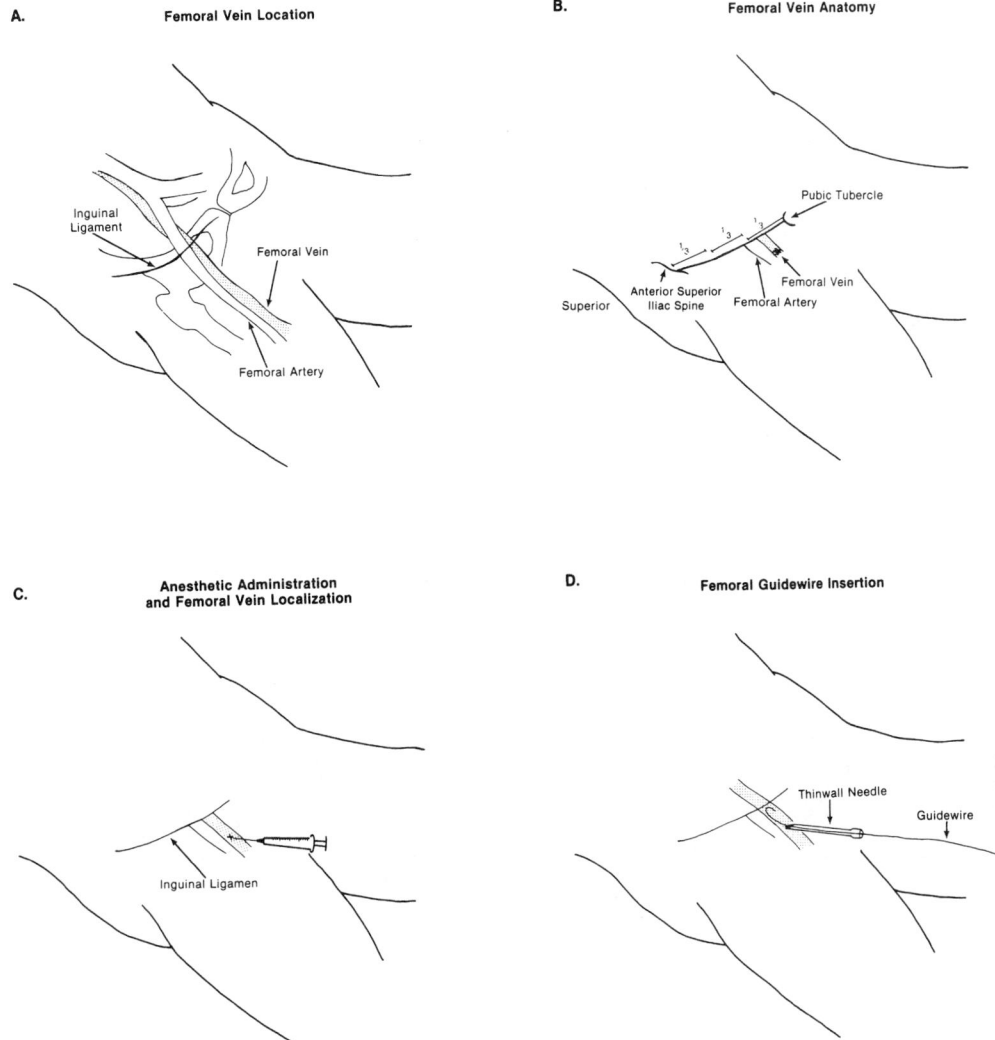

FIGURE 35-1. (**A**) Femoral vein location. At the level of the inguinal ligament, the femoral vein is located medial to femoral artery. (**B**) Femoral vein anatomy. At a level 2 to 3 cm below the inguinal ligament, the femoral artery can be found one third of the way from the pubic tubercle toward the anterior superior iliac spine. The femoral vein is found 1 to 2 cm medial to the artery. (**C**) Anesthetic administration and femoral vein localization. Local lidocaine is administered over the insertion site, and the femoral vein is located. The syringe should be directed at 45-degree angle cranially, staying below the inguinal ligament. Always withdraw on the syringe plunger before injection of lidocaine to avoid inadvertent intravascular injection. (**D**) Femoral guidewire insertion. The femoral vein is cannulated with a needle capable of accommodating a flexible guidewire. The guidewire is gently inserted through the needle. There should be no resistance to the passage of the guidewire. The needle is then removed, leaving the guidewire in place.

(continued)

A cannula or stainless-steel needle is selected, based on an internal diameter that provides adequate flow. Flow through a cannula is related directly to the third power of the diameter and therefore is greatly increased with increasing size. Packed red cells can be administered through needles as small as 23 gauge, although hemolysis may occur from the pressure required to deliver the infusion. Size 18- or 19-gauge needles or catheters permit adequate administration of packed red cells; however, the rates of delivery are insufficient for patients with hemodynamic instability.

Rapid delivery of packed red cells at rates adequate for most resuscitation procedures can be accomplished through 16-gauge or larger cannulas.

The Centers for Disease Control recommend that plastic peripheral intravenous cannulas should be replaced every 48 to 72 hours. The National Intravenous Therapy Association recommends the use of stainless-steel cannulas for short-term or one-dose peripheral intravenous therapy and the use of plastic catheters for more secure routine peripheral therapy.[7,8] Gloves should be worn for all patient contacts.

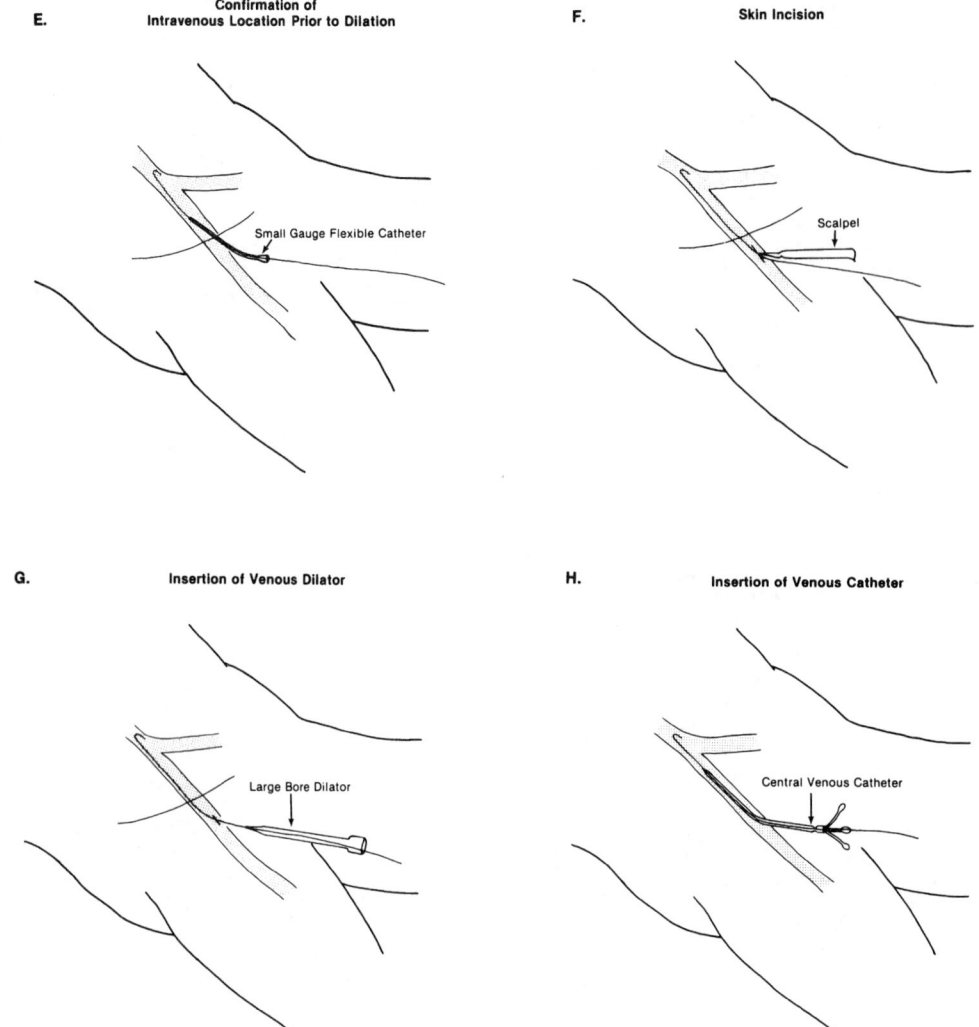

FIGURE 35-1 *(continued).* (**E**) Confirmation of intravenous location before dilation. Intravenous location of the guidewire is confirmed before dilation of the cannulation site by passing a small flexible catheter over the guidewire. The guidewire is then removed, and blood is withdrawn through the catheter. The guidewire is again placed through the catheter, and the catheter is removed (leaving the guidewire in place again in the vein). (**F**) Skin incision. A small (0.25 cm) skin incision is made at the site of entry of the guidewire. (**G**) Insertion of venous dilator. A large-bore dilator is passed over the guidewire. The dilator is then removed, leaving the guidewire in place in the vein. (**H**) Insertion of venous catheter. The central venous catheter is placed over the guidewire. The guidewire is removed and the catheter is sutured securely in place. (From Tribett D, Brenner M; Peripheral and femoral vein cannulation. *Probl Crit Care* 1988;2:266.)

For a venipuncture, the gloves need not be sterile but should fit snugly.

The intravenous site is prepared by trimming nearby hair and cleansing with antimicrobial soap. The vein is distended using gravity or application of a tourniquet. Local analgesia may be applied. The needle is guided into the vein at a 30- to 45-degree angle; once venous blood is observed to flow through the needle, it is lowered so that its axis is parallel to that of the vein. It is then advanced another 2 to 4 mm so that it is securely within the venous lumen before the cannula is advanced (if used) or the steel needle is secured. The site is then dressed and labeled appropriately (see Table 35-1).

CENTRAL VENOUS CANNULATION

Peripherally Inserted Central Venous Catheters

The idea of accessing the major thoracic veins through the peripheral veins is not new. Before introduction of the Seldinger technique, to aid central venous cannulation, physicians mostly used cutdown of antecubital veins to reach major central veins. As the catheter material improved and physicians became more familiar and comfortable with clavicular and jugular approaches, the antecubital approach went out of fashion.

The major disadvantages of centrally placed catheters (Table 35-3) and increased use of ambulatory therapy have

TABLE 35-1. Recommended Equipment and Care of Invasive Catheters

EQUIPMENT

Povidone-iodine or 70% isopropyl alcohol solution
Hat and mask, sterile gloves and gown, and disposable bed protection pad
Sterile drapes, gauze (2 × 2s and 4 × 4s) and a 13-cm (6-in) extension tubing
Lidocaine vial (1–2% without epinephrine), sterile needles (18-, 22-, 25-gauge) and syringes (3, 10, and 20 mL)
Sterile suture (3-0 silk), needle, scalpel, needle holders, scissors; 3-0 silk sutures wedged on a straight cutting needle
Appropriate sterile cannula dilator and guidewire or thin-wall needle-catheter set
Opposite type sterile occlusive dressing, adhesive tape, stopcock
When required, 500 mL normal saline and 200 U pork heparin in a pressure bag connected to an automatic flush system, calibrated transducer, and monitor, through pressure tubings

ROUTINE CHECKS AND CARE

Every 8 h:
   Palpate insertion site for pain, tenderness, heat, drainage, and swelling. Check patient's cannula. The dressing must be changed whenever it appears wet or soiled.
   Check peripheral and distal pulses as well as capillary refill.
   When appropriate, check the waveform, its characteristics, and numeric values.
   Check proper position and alignment of the extremity. Perform range of motion exercises.
Every 48 h:
   Change solutions, tubing, and flush systems.
   Change dressing.
Every 72 h:
   Evaluate for change or discontinuation of the cannula.

DOCUMENTATION

Write a procedure note after every procedure, including the indication, type of sterile preparation, analgesic, and sedatives used, any difficulties encountered.
Write date of insertion and characteristics of the catheter.
Document all routine checks and care in the chart.
Write date of dressing change.

made physicians to look for alternatives. Tunneled silicone catheters, such as Hickman/Broviac and Groshung catheters, were developed to reduce the risk of infection while allowing long-term central venous catheterization for intravenous therapy inside and outside of hospitals.[9] The technique allows the catheter to travel under the skin for 1 to 2 inches before entering the thoracic cavity. This surgical procedure is done by physicians in the operating room and under the guidance of fluoroscopy, which makes it expensive and time consuming.

Since the late 1980s, technological advancement has provided safer, less traumatic catheter insertion methods and catheter materials that are better tolerated in the peripheral venous system. Combined with cost containment issues and expansion of the role of qualified paramedical personnel, there has been an increase in use of peripherally inserted central catheters.[10] The catheters are used when long-term intravenous access is needed.

The catheters are made of silicone, polyurethene, or elastomeric hydrogel. They are available in both single and double lumen with dual port infusion in gauges from 16 to 23. A flexible, blunt-tipped stylet or guidewire is usually provided to help with insertion. The catheters can be inserted by the Seldinger technique, through a peel-away sheath, or using a catheter-over-needle technique. Insertion complications include arterial puncture, catheter embolism, catheter malposition, arrhythmias, thrombophlebitis, and infection.

Compartment syndrome caused by hematoma at insertion site and catheter sheering and knotting are specific complications of peripherally inserted central venous catheters (PICCs). The incidence of catheter-related infection is low despite prolonged length of therapy and is considered the major advantage of PICCs (Table 35-4).

CATHETER INSERTION. Veins below, at, or above the antecubital space, including cephalic, basilic, medial-cephalic, and medial basilic veins, are used for venipuncture and insertion of the PICC. When a midline catheter is placed, a physician's specific order for placement may not be needed because the catheter tip remains in the peripheral circulation and no radiograph is needed. A sterile insertion procedure should be followed. To facilitate catheter advancement, the patient's head must be turned to the side where placement is being made and the chin moved close to the chest. Supine position with arm at 90-degree angle from the body is recommended. Local anesthetics are recommended only when large-gauge introducers are used. Silicone catheters can be placed in a bath of sterile water or saline before insertion to make them easier to slide into the vein.

Devices made of elastomeric hydrogel must not be in contact with fluid before insertion. Catheter advancement should be stopped if any obstruction is encountered. Encouraging the patient to relax, providing a warm comfortable

TABLE 35-2. General Guidelines for Central Vascular Cannulation

1. Avoid sites with previous surgery and trauma or obvious anatomic abnormalities.
2. An agitated patient may predispose to complications. Assure comfort and sedation.
3. Use ample local anesthetics without distorting landmarks or the vessel.
4. Assure optimum position for the patient. Avoid awkward or uncomfortable position for yourself.
5. Assure oxygenation, ventilation, and monitoring under drapes.°
6. Valsalva maneuver, inspiratory hold, volume challenge, and Trendelenburg position are additional techniques to deliver vein-distending forces.°
7. Gauge the depth and angle of insertion by first performing venipuncture with a small-gauge needle. The needle can temporarily be left in place unless it prohibits passage of the cannulating needle or needle/plastic cannula assembly.°
8. Puncture the skin and subcutaneous tissue generously or incise with a no. 11 scalpel blade to avoid skin plugs and to facilitate catheter or introducer passage.
9. If a stab incision is not used initially, inject a small amount of saline to express skin plugs.
10. When attempting to find the vein with a needle or while cannulating the vein, use a small syringe to apply slight negative pressure.°
11. When vascular puncture is accomplished, adjust the needle bevel and guidewire. Lower the needle slightly to move closely parallel to the vascular lumen and advance the needle 2–5 mm further to assure intravascular placement of the lumen.
12. Do not redirect the needle while it is partially inserted to avoid laceration of the vein. When advancement fails, withdraw slowly while observing for blood return. If blood return is not observed after full withdrawal, then vary the technique by slightly altering the needle angulation.
13. If resistance is felt, remove the catheter or guidewire. The location of the catheter or guidewire shape may give clues to the cause of the obstruction. If cannulation is unsuccessful, check the tip of your cannula. A sheared or occluded tip may be the problem.
14. Once in the vessel, never leave the needle or cannula unoccluded. Air embolism can occur through veins, and unacceptable blood loss can occur from arteries.
15. Estimate the safe length of guidewire that can be inserted before attempting the insertion. Always watch the monitor of the length of inserted guidewire to minimize potential arrhythmias.°
16. If resistance is met in advancing or withdrawing of a guidewire, never use force. Gently withdraw the guidewire and the catheter/needle together.
17. Allow yourself three to five attempts for each venous approach. Perhaps 5–10 passes can be reasonably attempted for arterial puncture with a 20-gauge needle. It is better to accept failure than cause a serious complication.
18. For placement of transcardiac or vena cava catheters, always order a stat follow-up radiograph to assure correct catheter tip placement. Right atrial electrocardiography is an acceptable alternative for correct placement of the catheter.

°Applies to venous cannulation only.

environment, and rotating the wrist or moving the arm at different angles from the body may help the catheter to advance. If these maneuvers fail, the catheter should not be forced in, because scarring of the vein or sclerosis may be the cause of obstruction, which dictates abandoning the procedure. A postprocedure radiograph of the chest is a must to confirm optimum positioning of the catheter.

Femoral Vein Cannulation

Femoral vein catheters fell into disfavor in the 1950s because of early references to high catheter infection rates.[11] The report by Shaldon and others[12] brought this site to favor during the 1960s, and currently it is regarded as relatively safe. The femoral vein is an easy site to cannulate, although

TABLE 35-3. Advantages and Disadvantages of Different Types of Central Venous Access

ADVANTAGES/DISADVANTAGES	CIVC	TSC	PICC
Complexity of placement	Moderate	High	Low
Time needed for insertion	Moderate	High	Low
Recommended dwell time	Days	Weeks to months	Weeks to months
Infection rate	High	Low	Low
Complexity of complications	High	High	Low
Complication rate	Moderate	Moderate	Low
Possibility for central pressure monitoring	Yes	No	No
Possibility of bolus injection & fluid resuscitation	Yes	Yes	No
Use in ambulatory/home care setting	No	Yes	Yes
Cost	Moderate	High	Low
Patient tolerance	Moderate	High	High

CIVC, centrally inserted venous catheters; TSC, tunneled silicone catheters; PICC, peripherally inserted central catheters.

TABLE 35-4.   Indications and Contraindications of PICC

INDICATIONS	CONTRAINDICATIONS
Difficult IV access	Skin lesion at or above the insertion site
Long-term (> 7 d) IV antibiotic therapy	Previous ipsilateral venous thrombosis
Hyperalimentation	High fluid volume infusion
Chemotherapy	Rapid bolus IV injection
Continuous narcotic infusion	Hemophoresis/hemodialysis
Hyperosmolar fluid infusion	Crutch walking°
Long-term rehydration	Mastectomy°
Long-term IV access in patients with coagulopathy	Presence of pacemaker wires°

PICC, peripherally inserted central catheters; IV, intravenous.
°Denotes relative contraindication.

it also has the disadvantage of requiring longer catheters to pass the diaphragm. Femoral venous cannulation during resuscitation should be reserved for instances in which attempts for cannulation of other sites have failed.[13]

Humans manifest congenital abnormalities of femoral vascular structures, although most patients possess the anatomic relationships represented in Figure 35-1. In patients with a palpable femoral arterial pulse, the vein can be located by probing just medial to the artery, one third of the way from the pubic tubercle toward the anterior superior iliac spine.

Basic equipment required for central venous cannulation should be assembled (see Table 35-1). The site is prepared by having the patient lie flat while slightly rotating the leg externally. Use a 20-gauge, 5- or 7.5-cm (2- or 3-inch) needle directed toward the vein at an angle 45 degrees above the skin. Withdraw the syringe plunger continuously while advancing the needle. The distal tip should not traverse cephalad to the inguinal ligament to avoid retroperitoneal hematoma.

Once venous blood is obtained, repeat the procedure with a larger needle through which an appropriate J-tipped guidewire can be passed. An alternative method is to use an 18-gauge catheter over a 20-gauge needle, in which case the catheter is slid into the vein. If this option is used, after directing the needle toward a line more nearly parallel to the presumed axis of the vein, the needle should be advanced another 2 to 5 mm to ensure that the cannula tip is securely within the lumen.

The site should be appropriately dressed, and documentation should be completed in the chart. A radiograph is usually not taken because tip placement is reasonably assured to be correct if venous blood can be withdrawn easily. Inadvertent arterial puncture and local hematoma formation can be obviated by placing a 2- to 4.5-kg (5- to 10-lb) sandbag on the hematoma site for approximately 30 minutes.

Be sure to secure the dressing so that urine and fecal contamination does not occur. Transparent dressings are ideal for such purposes. Standard adhesive tape can be used to reinforce adherence of the transparent dressing to the skin, if necessary. The dressing should always be changed whenever the percutaneous entry site appears to be moist or contaminated. Complications are uncommon but can include infection, local or retroperitoneal hemorrhage, thrombosis, and arteriovenous fistula formation.[14]

Internal Jugular Vein Cannulation

Percutaneous cannulation of the internal jugular vein (IJV) has evolved over the last two decades.[15] Currently it is the urgent elective and emergency central venous approach preferred by most anesthesiologists and many intensivists (Table 35-5). The merits and disadvantages of IJV cannulation are always relative and must be weighed against the merits and disadvantages of other central vascular approaches (Table 35-6).

ANATOMY.   A thorough knowledge of regional anatomy is essential before attempting to cannulate the vein. The IJV usually runs beneath the belly of the sternocleidomastoid muscle immediately lateral to the carotid artery. Patients manifest a surprising variety of anatomic variations. The vein may be absent or in an unusual anatomic location, on any one side, in approximately 10% of ICU patients. Nonetheless, most ICU patients have a patent IJV on at least one side.

CANNULATION APPROACHES.   Cannulation can be attempted at relatively high sites (level of the cricoid cartilage) or at lower supraclavicular sites. Higher sites have slightly lower success rates than lower sites where the vein is larger and closer to the skin; however, the high sites have negligible risk of pneumothorax or hemothorax.

In general, high sites should be attempted first, followed by lower sites. We prefer to prepare the skin from the angle of the mandible to below the ipsilateral nipple. This approach gives the operator abundant options for cannulation of the IJV from anterior, central, posterior, and clavicular approaches.

TECHNIQUE.   The IJV usually runs deep to the sternocleidomastoid muscle. It can be approached high or low from three directions: anterior to the sternocleidomastoid muscle, centrally between the bellies of the sternocleidomastoid, or posterior to the sternocleidomastoid (Fig. 35-2). These three approaches are illustrated at the level of the cricoid cartilage. Similar needle orientations are used for lower approaches near the clavicle.

The following steps are recommended:

1. Patient and equipment are prepared.
2. The patient should be flat or slightly hyperextended

TABLE 35-5. Preferred Technique for Specific Clinical Situations

| CLINICAL SITUATIONS | CHOICES (Order of Preference) | | | | |
	1st	*2nd*	*3rd*	*4th*	*5th*
Bleeding diathesis	EJV	IJ	High SC†	Femoral° Large peripheral vein†	—
Obesity or generalized edema	IC	SC	IJ	—	—
Decrease pulmonary reserve; ventilation with PEEP	EJV	IJ	Femoral°	IC	SC
Parenteral nutrition	IC	IJ	SC	EJV	Femoral
Hypovolemia; shock	IC or SC	Femoral	IJ	Large peripheral vein†	—
Cardiopulmonary resuscitation	IJ	EJV	Femoral°	Large peripheral vein†	IC High SC†
Emergency airway management	IC	Femoral°	Large peripheral vein†	—	—
Temporary hemodialysis	IC	IJ	Femoral	SC	—
Multiple catheter insertions	IC	SC	Femoral	IJ	EJV
Pulmonary artery catheter insertion	IC or IJ	SC or IJ	EJV	Femoral	
Temporary pacemaker§	IJ	IC	SC	Femoral	EJV
Tracheostomy or sternal wounds	EJV or IJ	Femoral°	High SC†	IC	—
Short diagnostic techniques	Femoral	IJ	IC	SC	—
Inability to lower the head	EJV	Femoral°	SC	—	—

EJV, external jugular vein; IJ, internal jugular; SC, supraclavicular; IC, infraclavicular; PEEP, positive end-expiratory pressure.
°Femoral approach is suitable for bedridden patients. Short-term use in nonobese patients is possible. During resuscitation, catheter should be long enough to reach the intrathoracic veins.
†High SC refers to skin puncture 1–2 cm above clavicle, thereby allowing easier tamponade for arterial bleeding. The skin puncture site is close to the central IJ technique.
‡Peripheral vein cannulation is useful for volume resuscitation and rarely for hemodynamic monitoring or temporary pacing.
§If IC approach is used, left is preferred over right. If SC or IJ approach is used, the preferred site is the right.

Modified from Novak RA, Venus B: Clavicular approaches for central vein cannulation. *Probl Crit Care* 1988;2:242.

in the maximal modified Trendelenburg position (head down at least 15 degrees) to diminish air embolism risks and to distend the target vein maximally.[16] Contraindications to head-down position include elevated intracranial pressure and pulmonary edema. Such patients may be cannulated while supine or in a semisitting position, as long as central venous pressure is adequate to distend the vein. Rotate the head away from the side of cannulation at approximately 45 degrees. An adhesive tape headband, secured to the bedframe on the operator's side, running across the forehead and secured to the bedframe on the opposite side, is invaluable in securing the head if the patient is unable to cooperate.

3. Wash your hands thoroughly with antimicrobial soap.
4. Complete skin sterilization. We strongly recommend that contiguous internal jugular and clavicular sites be prepared unless one or the other is unavailable. You can then switch to the alternate site without repreparing or redraping if unsuccessful at the first site. Cannulation is likely to be unsuccessful 10% to 40% of the time at any site but is usually successful more than 99% of the time before five different approaches have been used.[17,18] If the vein is not cannu-

lated within the first five needle passes, cannulation at that site is unlikely and another site should be tried.[17]
5. Don the sterile hat, mask, gown, and gloves in that order. While this procedure is accomplished, the povidone-iodine usually is applied as the requisite 3-minute waiting period during which skin sterilization is optimized.
6. Drape the cannulation site, leaving the smallest possible area of skin exposure for palpation, analgesic administration, and cannulation. A sterile drape can be placed over the clavicular approach sites, which then can be removed and replaced over the unsuccessful IJV sites, if necessary.
7. Cannulate the vessel at a relatively low angle, approximately 10 to 20 degrees above the skin plane if possible. The low angle facilitates threading the cannula or wire down the vein and minimizes pneumothorax risks. For anterior and central approaches, the carotid artery should be palpated, if possible, before the cannulating needle is advanced, but not during needle advancement, because doing so diminishes or obliterates the IJV lumen.[16] Gentle negative pressure should be applied to the barrel of the syringe, both during needle advancement and withdrawal.

TABLE 35-6.   Advantages and Disadvantages of Various Venous Approaches

APPROACH	ADVANTAGES	DISADVANTAGES	SUCCESS RATES (%)
External jugular vein	Part of surface anatomy Clotting abnormalities not prohibitive Pneumothorax avoided Head-of-table access Prominent in elderly	High failure rate Not ideal for prolonged central venous access Uncomfortable for patient Dressing and maintenance are difficult Poor landmark in obese or edematous patients Unsuccessful in young patients Difficult for threading central catheters	60–90
Peripheral vein	Part of surface anatomy Clotting abnormalities not prohibitive Pneumothorax avoided Easily accessible	High failure rate during hypotension and shock Not recommended for drug infusion during resuscitation Difficult approach for threading central catheters Not suitable for infusion of irritative drugs	75–99
Internal jugular	Pneumothorax rare High success rate Head-of-table access Control of bleeding is easier Right internal jugular straight path to SVC (easier to pass catheters; less malposition) Continued chest compression during CPR is possible Less failure with inexperienced operator	Not ideal for prolonged central venous access (e.g., TPN) Uncomfortable for patient Dressings and catheter difficult to maintain Left internal jugular increases risk of thoracic duct injury Poor landmarks in obese or edematous patients Difficult access with tracheostomies Contraindicated with intracranial hypertension Vein more prone to collapse with volume depletion or shock Not ideal for temporary hemodialysis Difficult access during emergencies when airway control is being established Carotid artery puncture relatively frequent	58–99
Supraclavicular	Low incidence of pneumothorax High success rate Easier to pass catheter Accessible from head of table Good landmarks No interference with chest compression Anatomic landmarks constant Short path from skin to vein	Control of bleeding difficult Pneumothorax possible Not ideal for prolonged venous access Uncomfortable for patient Dressings and catheter maintenance difficult Thoracic duct puncture possible Not ideal for temporary hemodialysis Not ideal approach when airway control is being established	85–99
Infraclavicular	Easier to maintain dressings and more comfortable for patient Better landmarks in obesity Large vein less collapsible during hypovolemia	Higher risk of pneumothorax Compression of bleeding site difficult Decreased success rate with inexperience Long pass from skin to vein	70–98.8

TPN, total parenteral nutrition; SVC, superior vena cava; CPR, cardiopulmonary resuscitation.

From Novak RA, Venus B: Clavicular approaches for central vein cannulation. *Probl Crit Care* 1988;2:242.

8. Venous blood return is typically dark and low pressured, although even experienced operators can be fooled if the patient is hypoxic or if the cannula or needle is adjacent to an arterial atheromatous plaque. When venous blood is obtained through a search needle, a needle appropriate for cannula insertion can then be inserted parallel to the search needle. The search needle should not be left open to air to prevent risk of air embolism. The modified Seldinger technique is then used to insert the desired catheter into the vein (see Fig. 35-1). Multilumen catheters require two crossing skin incisions adjacent to the wire at 180-degree angles, 5 mm deep and 2 to 3 mm wide, using a no. 11 scalpel blade to facilitate insertion of the dilator through the skin. This step may be omitted if a coagulopathy is present or if the skin is fragile.

9. Needle and cannula hubs must be occluded at all times to reduce the risk of air embolism. All catheter ports should be irrigated with 2 to 3 mL of heparin-

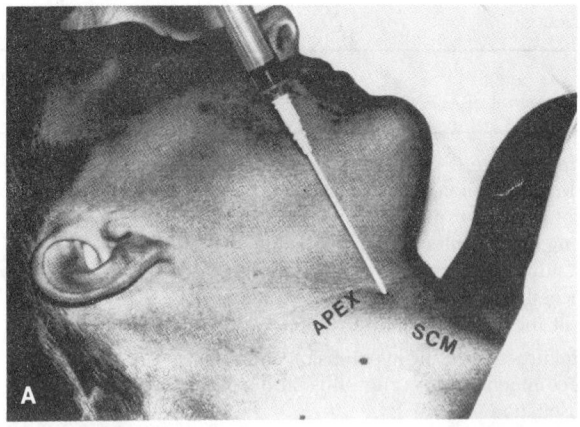

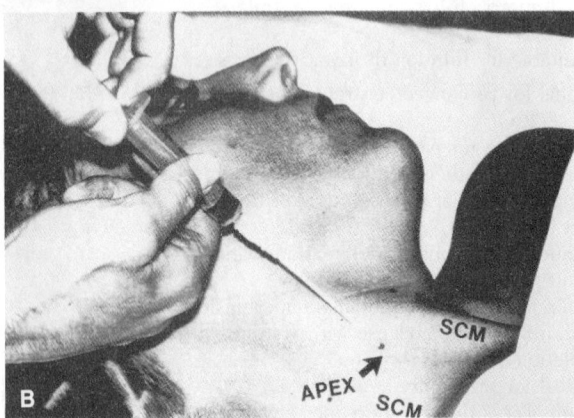

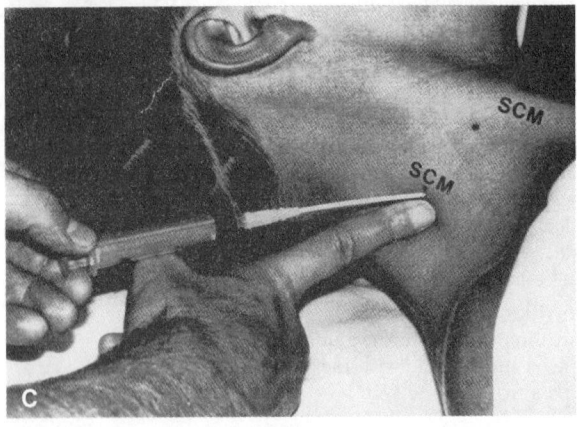

FIGURE 35-2. (A) Demonstration of the anterior approach to internal jugular vein (IJV) cannulation. Direct the needle toward the ipsilateral nipple at an angle approximately 20 degrees above the skin. Deeper insertion angles are occasionally necessary to position the needle below the sternocleidomastoid. Direct the needle just lateral to the carotid artery. **(B)** Demonstration of the central approach to IJV cannulation. The needle is directed toward the ipsilateral nipple 20 to 30 degrees above the skin. In general, the needle should not be directed more medial than a line parallel to the spinal axis to avoid carotid artery puncture. **(C)** Demonstration of the posterior approach to IJV cannulation. Direct the needle across the midline toward the contralateral nipple approximately 15 to 20 degrees above the skin. It is inserted just posterior to the dorsal border of the sternocleidomastoid muscle. Deeper insertion angles are occasionally necessary to position the needle below the sternocleidomastoid (SCM). (From McGee WT, Mallory DL: Cannulation of the internal and external jugular veins. *Probl Crit Care* 1988;2:217.)

flush solution containing 100 to 200 U/mL; alternatively, an intravenous infusion can be initiated immediately after catheter insertion, at a rate not less than 20 mL/hour if a gravimetric pump is used or 3 mL/hour if a mechanical pump is used. Heparin flushes tend to be unsuccessful in keeping introducer sheaths open; hence, the initial heparin flush should be changed to a "keep vein open" order for introducer sheaths. Allow blood to back-fill the cannula to eliminate small air emboli before flushing procedures. If the catheter is not flushed before insertion, speed is important to avoid catheter thrombosis, which usually occurs within 1 to 2 minutes.

10. Do not release the cannula until it is sutured in place. Be careful not to draw the suture tightly against the skin to avoid pressure necrosis with attendant infection, pain, and loss of fixation. We recommend that the cannula be secured to the skin entry site by at least two sutures. This procedure minimizes the four possible types of catheter movement, that is, pitch, yaw, longitudinal axis, and rotational movements. Minimizing such movement is important to reduce the risk of catheter infection.

11. Order and discuss the appropriate dressing with the nurse and properly dispose of all sharp objects used for the procedure.

12. Always write a procedure note that includes the date, time, indication, anesthetic, and any appropriate notations regarding unexpected difficulties, compilations, or follow-up procedures such as radiography.

TIP POSITION.   Triple-lumen or feeding catheters should be inserted so that the tips are approximately 2 cm proximal to the right atrium (for right-sided approaches) and similarly placed or well within the innominate vein but not abutting the inferior vena cava (for left-sided approaches). Right atrial electrocardiography is an excellent means to accomplish ideal placement.[19,20] Such catheter tip placement concomitantly assures that the catheter tip is parallel to the superior vena cava wall, which minimizes the risks of caval perforation.[21]

COMPLICATIONS.   Complications of the IJV procedures are typical for thoracic central catheter placements (Table 35-7). Specifically, the infection rate is 0.5% to 2%; carotid artery puncture rate is approximately 5% (although this is usually inconsequential if the puncture was caused by a 20-gauge or smaller needle); and the pneumothorax rate is less than 0.1%. Rare complications include carotid artery cannulation, endotracheal tube cuff puncture, cannulation of the spinal cord, neck hematomas causing severe compression and obliteration of the trachea, and embolism of fragmented cannula components.[15]

External Jugular Vein Cannulation

The external jugular vein (EJV) is used occasionally for peripheral or central venous access. The EJV is a superficial vein, making it a preferred route in the presence of substantial coagulopathy. Although the EJV is a good site for medica-

TABLE 35-7. Complications of Central Venous and Pulmonary Artery Cannulation

IMMEDIATE

Multiple puncture
Pneumo/hemo/hydro/chylothorax—mediastinum
Arterial puncture—hematoma or bleeding
Air embolism
Cardiac dysrhythmias
Catheter malposition
Catheter knotting
Subcutaneous and mediastinal emphysema
Tracheal puncture-laceration

LATE

Pulmonary artery rupture°
Pulmonary infarction°
Catheter-related sepsis
Balloon rupture°
Endocardial or valvular damage°
Venous thrombosis
Infections (cellulitis, osteomyelitis, endocarditis, thrombophlebitis)
Nerve injury (brachial, phrenic, recurrent, laryngeal, vagus, cranial IX–XII, Horner and Brown-Sequard syndromes)
Cerebrovascular compromise
Cardiac perforation and tamponade
Arteriovenous fistula
Thrombocytopenia

°Applies to pulmonary artery cannulation only.

tion delivery, the superior vena cava can be cannulated only approximately half of the time because of EJV valves and anatomic angles that prevent successful guidewire passage.

The EJV begins just anterior to the ear at the angle of the mandible. It courses obliquely across the anterior surface of the sternocleidomastoid muscle and joins the subclavian vein (SV) behind the medial third of the clavicle (Fig. 35-3).

For cannulation, place the patient in a 15- to 30-degree modified Trendelenburg position with the head turned away from the site of venipuncture. The right side is preferred. The EJV is identified as it crosses the posterior margin of the sternocleidomastoid muscle. If the vein is not visible or palpable, a Valsalva maneuver or inflation hold applied to mechanically ventilated patients may help to distend the vein. If it cannot be visualized or palpated, another approach is preferred.

After introduction of local analgesia, a needle is advanced at an angle approximately 15 to 20 degrees above the skin. While slight negative pressure is maintained in the syringe lumen, the vein is sought. Once it is entered, advance the needle an additional 1 to 2 mm and then either advance the catheter or a guidewire through the needle, according to the selected technique.

If obstruction to guidewire passage is encountered, several maneuvers can be tried, including medial and lateral flexion of the neck as well as sequential or concomitant ipsilateral arm movements (abduction, adduction, internal and external rotation). Another maneuver that is occasionally helpful is withdrawal of the J-wire for approximately 1 cm, followed by rotation and advancement of the wire.

Complications with significant morbidity are rare from this approach. Most complications are associated with catheter placement and catheter maintenance.

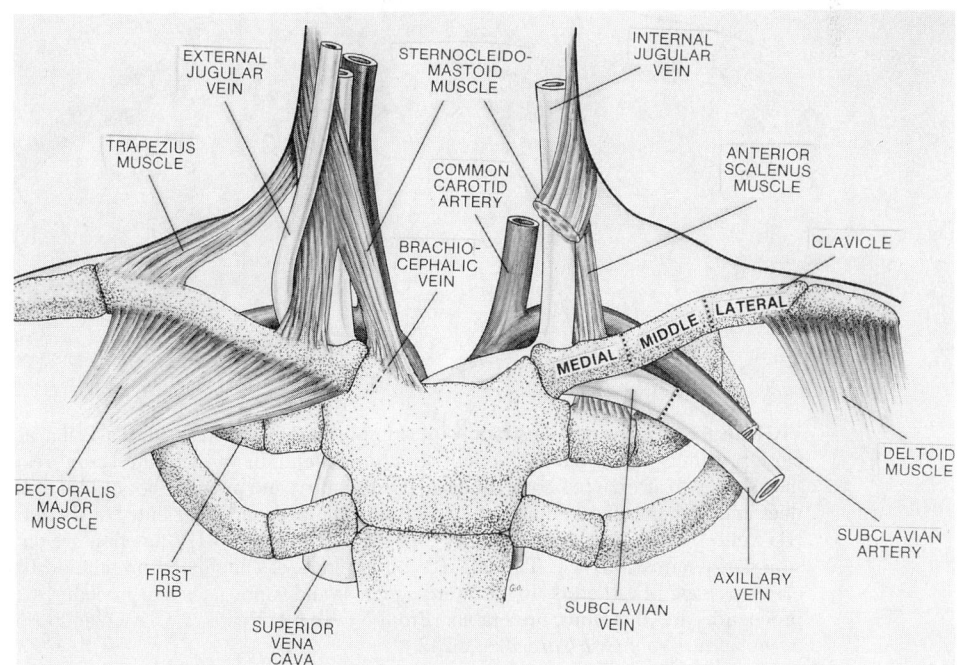

FIGURE 35-3. Relationship of clavicular landmarks and vascular anatomy. Notice the natural "windows" for supraclavicular venipunctures: (1) supraclavicular triangle formed by the clavicle, trapezius, and sternocleidomastoid muscles; (2) clavicular sternocleidomastoid triangle formed by the two bellies of the sternocleidomastoid muscle and the clavicle. See text for discussion of superficial landmarks and vascular anatomy. (From Novak RA, Venus B: Clavicular approaches for central vein cannulation. *Probl Crit Care* 1988;2:242.)

Clavicular Approaches

ANATOMY. Figures 35-3 and 35-4 portray anatomic relationships of the supraclavicular triangle, the clavicle, major vessels, and other pertinent structures. Although the SV is only 3 to 4 cm long, its relationship with the clavicle, first rib, and sternocleidomastoid muscle allows several approaches to venipuncture (see Fig. 35-3). The manubriosternal junction is a surface landmark for the SV–brachiocephalic junction, which is the proper tip position for a SV catheter. The necessary catheter length can be estimated by placing it over the course of the vein with the tip at the junction. The junction of the IJV and the SV is 2 to 3 cm wide (larger than the IJV or SV), making it an ideal structure for venipuncture. In addition, a constant landmark, the clavicular notch, overlies this junction.

The SV begins at the outer aspect of the first rib as a continuation of the axillary vein (see Fig. 35-4). Its direction is medial and slightly superior until it passes anterior to the scalenus anterior muscle at its insertion point on the first rib. This is the highest point of the vein and is just medial to the midpoint of the clavicle. It then passes caudal and slightly anterior to join the IJV, forming the brachiocephalic vein posterior to the sternoclavicular articulation to enter the thorax.

As it passes over the first rib, the SV is anterior to the subclavian artery and brachial plexus and separated from them by the 1- to 1.5-cm thick scalenus anterior muscle (see Figs. 35-3 and 35-4). Medial to the attachment of the anterior scalene muscle to the first rib, the phrenic nerve, internal thoracic artery (not illustrated), and apical pleura are in contact with the posterior jugulosubclavian union and brachiocephalic vein. The thoracic duct and right lymphatic duct cross the anterior scalene to enter the superior margin of the SV near the IJV junction at its lateral aspect (see Fig. 35-4). Anterior to the vein throughout its course is the subclavius muscle, which is covered by the pectoralis muscle and epidermis.

Superiorly, the related structures are the platysma and superficial aponeurosis in the natural windows for venipuncture (see Fig. 35-4); interiorly are the first rib and cupula of the pleura (0.5 cm posterior to the vein) and pulmonary apex (Figs. 35-4 and 35-5). The sagittal plane through the SV describes the costoclavicular–scalene triangle formed by the medial end of the clavicle anteriorly, the broad upper surface of the first rib below, and the anterior scalene muscle posteriorly (see Figs. 35-4 and 35-5). The medial 5 cm (2 inches) of the clavicle cover the vein.

The pleural dome lies caudal to the junction of the IJV and SV and posterior to the subclavian artery. Because the dome of the pleura is lower on the right side and the thoracic duct is smaller, right supraclavicular approaches are preferred (see Fig. 35-4).

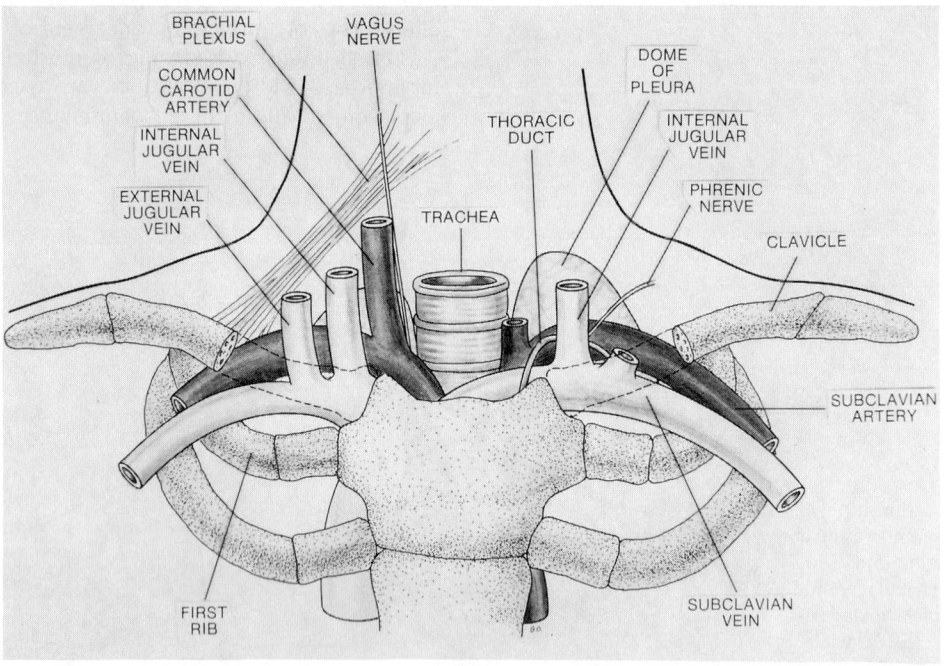

FIGURE 35-4. Anatomic illustrations of side preference rationale for clavicular approaches. Notice the close proximity of arterial and venous structures. Venipunctures in the lateral region of the clavicle are more prone to arterial puncture, brachial plexus injury, and pneumothorax. Notice the prominent thoracic duct and higher pleural cupula on the left and the perpendicular entry of the left internal jugular vein (IJV) into the left subclavian vein (SV). The right IJV and SV–IJV junction are on a straight path to the superior vena cava (SVC). The left SV courses in a less angulated orientation that the right, allowing easier passage of catheters. Right internal jugular and supraclavicular procedures and left infraclavicular procedures are, therefore, preferable. (From Novak RA, Venus B: Clavicular approaches for central vein cannulation. *Probl Crit Care* 1988;2:242.)

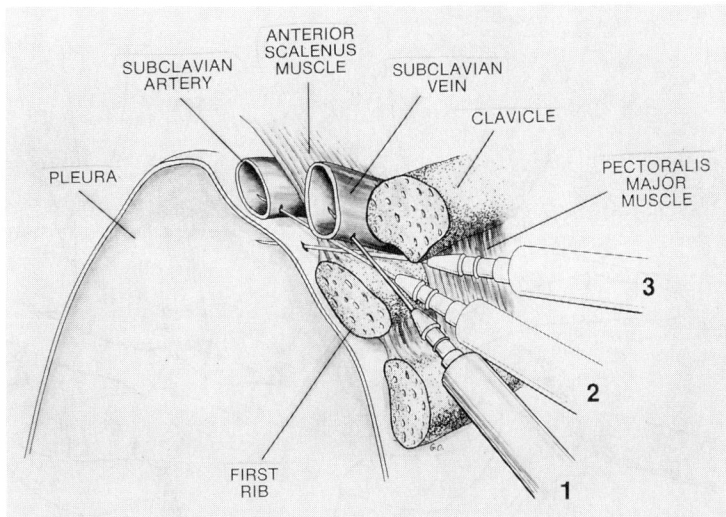

FIGURE 35-5. Sagittal view of subclavian vein and pertinent superficial and deep perivascular anatomy. Safe and unsafe insertions are demonstrated for infraclavicular approach. (1) safe angle and depth of insertion; and (2) unsafe angle and depth of insertion prone to arterial and pleural puncture. (From Novak RA, Venus B: Clavicular approaches for central vein cannulation. *Probl Crit Care* 1988;2:242.)

Puncture of the pleura and artery during supraclavicular and infraclavicular approaches can occur if the angle of the needle incident to the skin is too high or the depth of puncture is too far (Figs. 35-5 and 35-6). In addition, placement of the needle above or behind the vein or penetration through its walls can compromise the lymphatic duct or injure the phrenic nerve (see Fig. 35-4). Placing the needle too far laterally (infraclavicular) or deeply through the anterior scalene muscle may cause penetration of the subclavian artery or injury to the roots of the brachial plexus, respec-

tively (see Figs. 35-5 and 35-6). The vagus nerve courses behind the jugular vein and theoretically can be traumatized by deep insertion of the needle in this region (see Fig. 35-3).

TECHNIQUES

The SV may be entered at six different locations in close proximity from above and below the clavicle.

Supraclavicular Approaches. Supraclavicular approaches are divided into three major techniques by anatomic landmarks and point-of-skin puncture, as illustrated in Figures 35-7 through 35-10. The technique that has been used most extensively is that of Yoffa and Melb[22] (the junctional approach). Slight variations are delineated.

Junctional Technique

1. Position of patient: 10 to 25 degrees with the head down (modified Trendelenburg) unless contraindicated; turn the head slightly to the left or straight up[23]
2. Anatomic landmarks: Lateral border of the clavicular head of the sternocleidomastoid muscle as it inserts on the clavicle
3. Position of operator: Head of the bed on the side of the procedure
4. Depth of puncture required: 0.5 to 5 cm (average, 1 to 2 cm)
5. Puncture point location: At the clavisternomastoid angle (see Fig. 35-7). Variations include the following: (1) 2 to 3 cm superior to the clavicle close to the lateral posterior border of the clavicular head of the sternocleidomastoid muscle[24] (see Fig. 35-8); (2) 1 cm above the superior border of the clavicle and 1 cm lateral to the lateral aspect of the sternocleidomastoid muscle (see Fig. 35-8); and (3) 1 to 1.5 cm above the junction of the clavicle and lateral muscle border[25] (see Fig. 35-9)
6. Angle and direction of puncture: Bisecting the clavi-sternocleidomastoid muscle angle (45 degrees from both the lateral border of muscle and clavicle) and 15 degrees forward to the coronal plane; the needle is

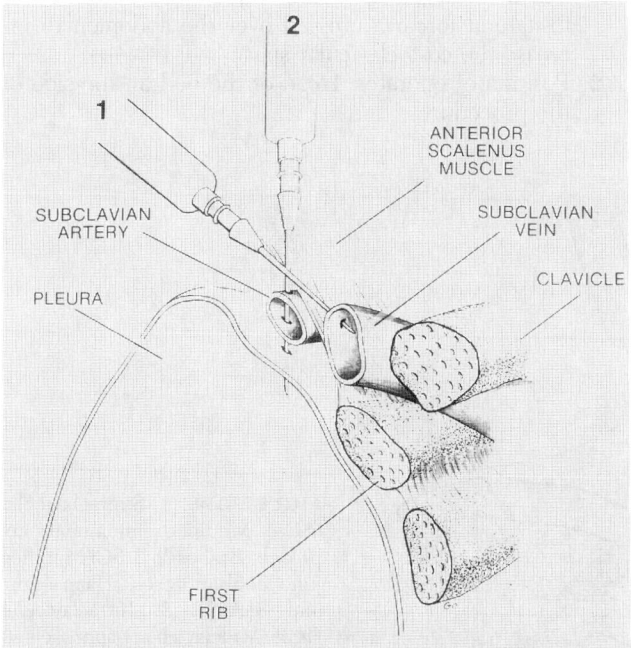

FIGURE 35-6. Same view as Figure 35-5 showing supraclavicular approaches: (1) safe angle and depth of insertion; and (2) unsafe angle and depth of insertion prone to pleural puncture. (From Novak RA, Venus B: Clavicular approaches for central vein cannulation. *Probl Crit Care* 1988;2:242.)

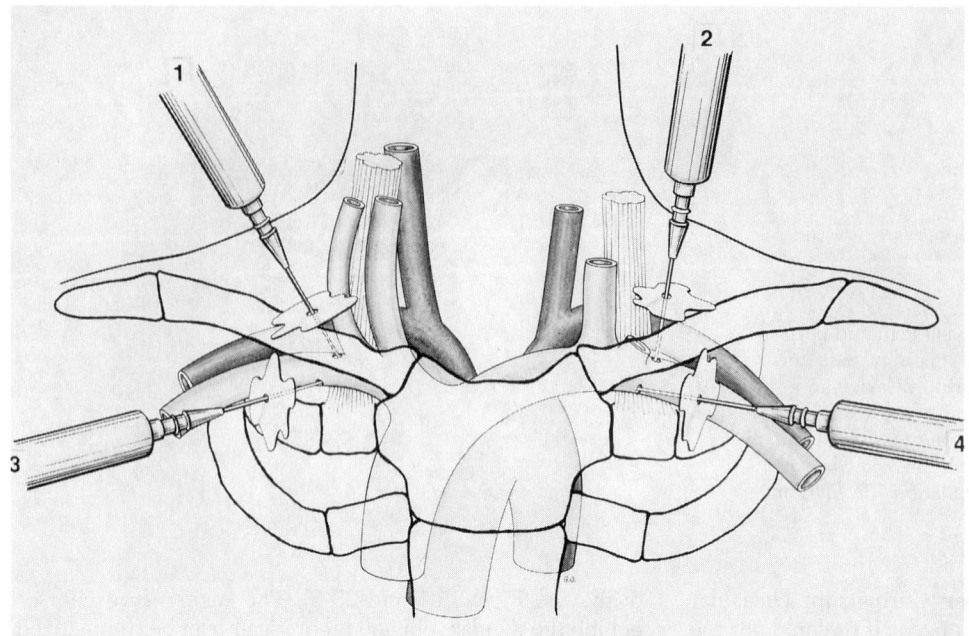

FIGURE 35-7. 1. Supraclavicular (SC): Junctional approach (Yoffa and Melb[22]). 2. SC: Anterior scalene/first rib approach. 3. Midclavicular approach—sternal notch orientation. 4. Infraclavicular: Medial approach—sternal notch orientation. (From Novak RA, Venus B: Clavicular approaches for central vein cannulation. *Probl Crit Care* 1988;2:242.)

pointed toward the retromanubrial area at the level of the sternal angle or sternal notch. In a variation of the technique,[26] the needle and syringe are "swung" laterally 35 degrees from the sagittal plane and depressed slightly below the coronal plane after venipuncture and before passage of a wire or cannula.

If the initial needle pass is unsuccessful, slight redirection is possible. Successful vein entry usually occurs 10 to 20 degrees above the coronal plane.[27] In addition, in elderly patients, the point of entry should be 1 cm back from the angle on the line that bisects it.[22] If the needle is too deep, the subclavian artery may be punctured (see Fig. 35-5). The

anatomy, however, allows application of suitable prolonged pressure in such a case.

Anterior Scalene/First Rib Approach

The anterior scalene/first rib approach is illustrated in Figure 35-7.[28]

1. Position of patient: Head turned to the opposite side and neck flexed approximately 15 degrees with the ipsilateral forearm crossed over the abdomen to increase the costoclavicular space
2. Position of operator: Head of the bed on the side of the procedure

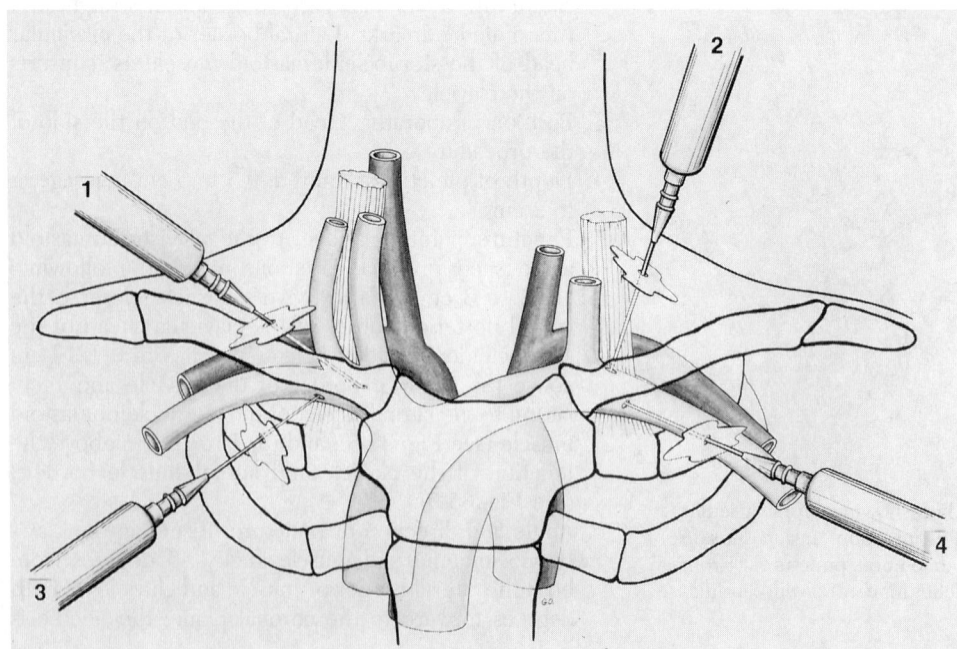

FIGURE 35-8. 1. Supraclavicular (SC): Modified junctional approach (Brahos[24]). 2. SC: Modified junctional approach (Haapaenimi and Slatis[26]). 3. Infraclavicular (IC): Midclavicular approach—clavicular sternocleidomastoid (CSCM) triangle orientation. 4. IC: Medial approach—CSCM triangle orientation. (From Novak RA, Venus B: Clavicular approaches for central vein cannulation. *Probl Crit Care* 1988;2:242.)

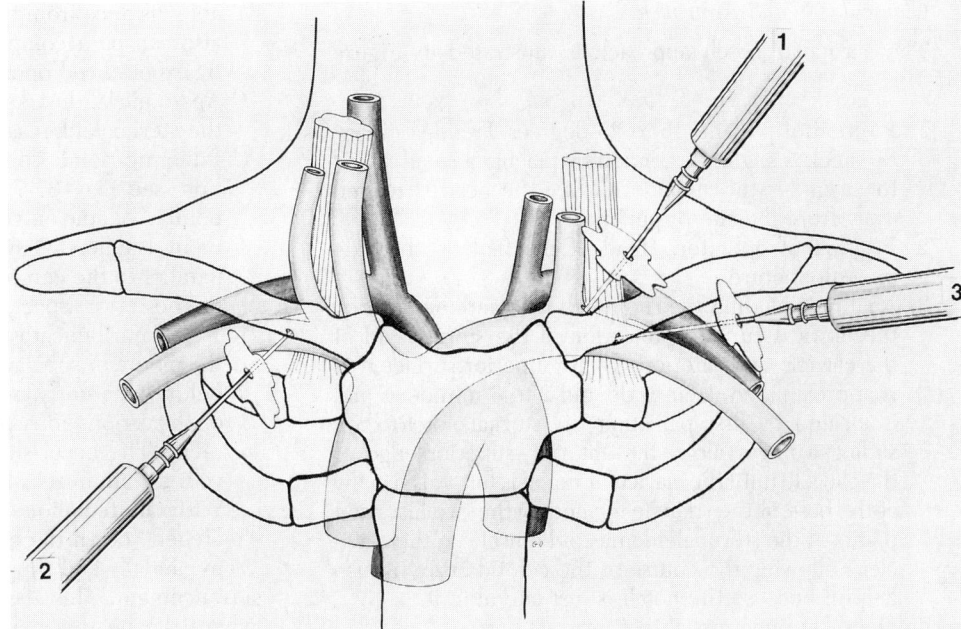

FIGURE 35-9. 1. Supraclavicular (SC): Modified junctional approach (Helmkamp and Sanko[25]). 2. Intraclavicular (IC): midclavicular approach—scalene tubercle orientation. 3. IC: lateral approach. (From Novak RA, Venus B: Clavicular approaches for central vein cannulation. *Probl Crit Care* 1988;2:242.)

3. Anatomic landmarks: Index finger of the left hand is placed at the insertion of anterior scalene muscle on the first rib (scalene tubercle) located behind the insertion point of the clavicular head of the sternocleidomastoid muscle
4. Insertion point, direction, and angle of puncture: The needle is slowly advanced lateral to the scalene tubercle over the first rib until venipuncture is accomplished; it is then lowered toward the shoulder for alignment with the course of the vein, and the catheter is passed.

Parsa and Tabora[28] also describe a modification of their technique that directs the needle perpendicular to the scalene tubercle (see Fig. 35-9), with the site of vein entry intended to be the SV–IJV junction. Again, the needle–syringe assembly is aligned with the course of the vein after the vein is entered.

If the needle is advanced too close to a perpendicular position above the first rib, the bevel can be pressed against the rib, collapsing the wall of the vein and damaging the rib periosteum. A calcified or fibrous mass may result that impairs or prohibits subsequent venipuncture.

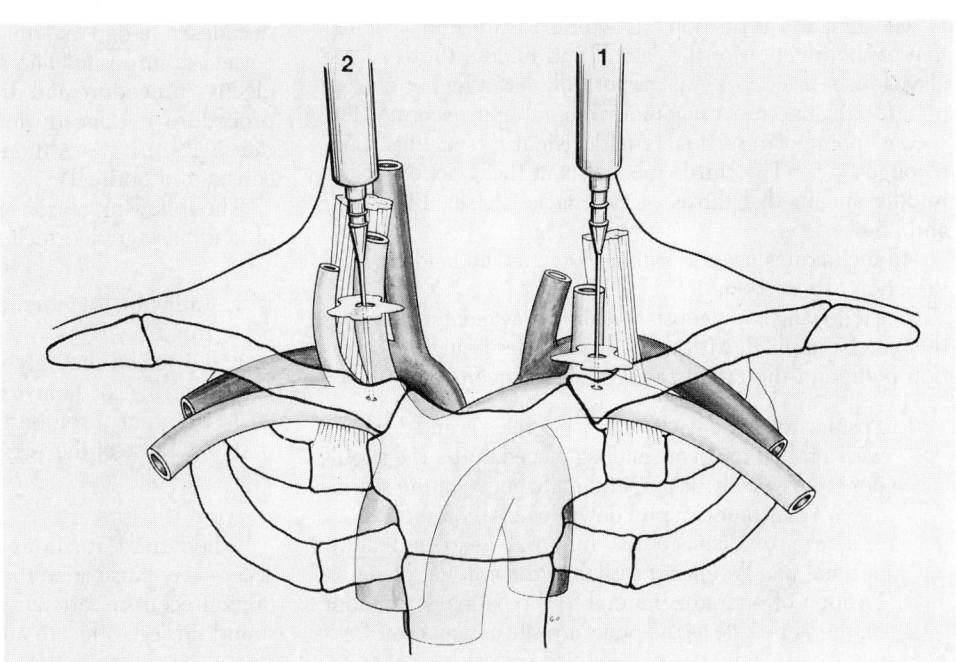

FIGURE 35-10. 1. Supraclavicular (SC): clavicular notch approach. 2. SC: Modified clavicular notch approach. (From Novak RA, Venus B: Clavicular approaches for central vein cannulation. *Probl Crit Care* 1988;2:242.)

Clavicular Notch Approach

The clavicular notch approach is illustrated in Figure 35-10.

1. Position of patient: 15 to 25 degrees Trendelenburg; the neck is slightly extended by placing a small rolled towel under the shoulders while the head is turned away from the site of puncture
2. Position of operator: Head of the bed on the side of venipuncture
3. Anatomic landmarks: The notch is bound medially by the upward curving projection of the sternal end of the clavicle and interiorly by its superior surface.[29] It is approximately 1 cm wide and 2 to 3 mm deep and is located by first palpating the sternal notch, then sliding a finger along the anterior–superior edge of the clavicle until the clavicular notch is felt. It is usually at the base of the triangle formed by the two insertion points of the sternocleidomastoid muscle on the clavicle. Following the course of the carotid artery is also helpful because the notch is just lateral to it.
4. Depth of puncture: 2 to 4 cm
5. Insertion point, direction, and angle of passage: Puncture the skin just above the clavicle, 0.25 to 1 cm lateral to its sternal end. The needle is advanced caudally parallel to the sagittal plane but at a 30- to 40-degree angle to the coronal plane. Puncture of the vein is heralded by a click and confirmed by aspiration of blood. If venipuncture is not accomplished initially, the needle is redirected at the same angle to the coronal plane but slightly lateral to the sagittal plane.

Infraclavicular Approaches. The infraclavicular approaches are illustrated in Figures 35-7 through 35-9. They may be divided into three basic insertion points and three directions or orientations of insertion.[30–32] The angle for all infraclavicular techniques is essentially parallel to the coronal plane.

The first insertion point is lateral to the midclavicular line at the junction of the lateral and middle thirds of the clavicle (see Fig. 35-9) and reportedly has a higher chance of arterial puncture than more medial approaches.[33] The second point of insertion is midclavicular (see Figs. 35-7 through 35-9). The third (medial) is at the junction of the middle and medial thirds of the clavicle[34] (see Figs. 35-7 and 35-8).

All techniques use the sternal notch as the landmark for direction of insertion.

The following is a synopsis of all infraclavicular techniques that can be applied, with the only variables being the insertion point and the target for needle advancement.

1. Position of patient: 10 to 25 degrees Trendelenburg with a rolled towel or sandbag placed under the shoulders transversely or longitudinally between the scapulae. An assistant can pull down (caudal) on the ipsilateral arm to displace the humeral head and allow optimal needle entry parallel to the coronal plane.
2. Position of operator: Lateral to the patient's shoulder on the same side as the puncture site and at a comfortable distance from the point of insertion. Cannulation also can be accomplished from the head of the bed by experienced operators.
3. Anatomic landmarks: Clavicle, suprasternal notch, and the sternocleidomastoid–clavicular triangle
4. Puncture point, depth, direction, and angle of insertion (see Figs. 35-7 through 35-9): Regardless of the point of needle entry and direction of needle advancement, the needle–syringe assembly should be kept as parallel to the coronal plane as possible, just beneath the posterior aspect of the clavicle (the vein is located 1 to 2 cm beneath the clavicle) to avoid puncturing the pleura or subclavian artery. The depth of insertion before vein entry is 2 to 3 cm but varies, depending on the various entry positions and direction of advancement. The bevel should be oriented caudally in the vein to minimize malposition.

With all techniques, the needle should be either "marched" down the clavicle or inserted at a point 1 to 2 cm caudally and slipped just under the clavicle before advancement. This allows the operator to keep track of where the needle is and thereby minimize the risk of subclavian artery puncture and pneumothorax.

Complications

Compared with other methods, clavicular approaches carry a higher incidence of pneumothorax (1% to 8%) and bleeding (1% to 5%).[18] A high index of suspicion should be maintained with alertness to immediate and delayed complications[35–62] (see Table 35-7).

CANNULATION OF THE CENTRAL VEINS WITH THE HELP OF REAL TIME ULTRASOUND

The landmark-guided techniques for central venous catheter access have been used successfully over the last three decades. Guided by the landmarks, the technique has a certain failure rate. The success rate is around 96% for an elective procedure and drops down to about 62% when the procedure is done during emergency.[63] The complication rate is 2% to 8%. Although an acceptable rate, this is not considered optimal.[64]

The following reasons have been reported for the failure of landmark-guided techniques:

1. Individual anatomic variations of the vascular structures
2. Distorted anatomy resulting from contracture, obesity, scarring, or hematoma
3. Inherent thrombosis of the target vessel
4. Collapse of the vessel caused by decreased intravascular volume

When these situations exist, multiple attempts to achieve access may cause operator frustration and result in complications. Recent reports advocate the use of a real time ultrasound device to locate and access the target central vein.

The following are advantages for ultrasound-guided techniques:

1. Anatomic variation can easily be detected and the target vessel exactly located.
2. Inherent thrombosis of the target vein can be ruled out before puncture.
3. Unlike the landmark-guided technique, the seeker needle is not needed.
4. The advancement and proper positioning of the guidewire can be accurately followed.
5. The technique reduces the chance of bleeding, hematoma and barotrauma.

Despite the merits of the real time ultrasound-guided technique, because its use and availability is not practical at all times, a trainee should first learn the conventional landmark-guided approaches in accessing the central veins. Once proficient, then the ultrasound-guided technique should be learned. In patients with distorted anatomy or high risk for complications, the use of ultrasound-guided techniques as the first approach is justified and recommended.

UNUSUAL CIRCUMSTANCES

In emergency circumstances when central catheter placement is planned, a peripheral vein (antecubital is the first choice) should be cannulated if possible and used until central access is accomplished. Surgical placement (cutdowns) should be attempted only if a clinician familiar with the technique is available, while others attempt to gain percutaneous access at other sites. In male patients without peripheral intravenous access, the superficial dorsal vein of the penis may be accessible. It is superficial and cephalad to the corpus cavernosum.

Two-dimensional Doppler ultrasound to guide successful and safe cannulation of the IJV[17] and SV[65] has been reported. In stable patients with a history of difficult cannulation, this technique may be expeditious and safe, provided that the equipment and expertise are available and there is no urgency for gaining central venous access. During emergencies, attempts should be made to cannulate the IJV and SV and, if unsuccessful, the femoral vein. The right femoral vein is preferred because it is shorter. A long catheter should be used to reach the inferior vena cava above the diaphragm.

Endotracheal Routes

If the patient is intubated, the endotracheal route may be used as an alternative to intravenous access for certain medications such as epinephrine, atropine, naloxone, and lidocaine. This route should not be used for administration of fluids, bicarbonate, blood, dopamine, or dobutamine.

Arterial Route

During resuscitation when other attempts have failed, if femoral artery pulsation can be felt during chest compression, the artery can be cannulated and used to infuse colloids, crystalloids, or blood products. Vasoconstrictive drugs should not be infused. If the femoral artery is not accessible, a clinician with expertise in cutdowns may attempt to cannulate an artery of the extremities by direct exposure. If normal blood pressure returns during resuscitation, resuscitative fluids can be infused into the artery using a pressure bag or pump until venous access is obtained.

Right Atrium

A cannula can be inserted directly into the right atrium in a patient with an open chest cavity. The pericardium is incised to expose the right atrium and the catheter inserted and fixed to the atrium by a suture.[3]

Bone Marrow

An alternative route is the bone marrow.[66] The long bones have a rich network of medullary sinusoids that are drained by numerous venous channels that empty into a solitary longitudinal central venous sinus. From there, blood enters the central venous circulation. This method has been successfully used in pediatric and some adult patients. It seems to be safe and effective for infusion of blood, colloids, sodium bicarbonate, 50% dextrose, calcium gluconate, atropine, crystalloids, lidocaine, heparin, corticosteroids, phenytoin, and other resuscitative drugs.[67]

The site of choice in pediatric patients is the proximal tibia 1 to 3 cm below the tibial tubercle, on the flat anteromedial surface. In adults, the medial malleolus of the distal tibia, body of the sternum above the xiphoid, or the lateral aspect of the sixth to the ninth ribs can be used.

A needle sturdy enough to penetrate bony cortex is required. Standard 16- to 19-gauge short spinal and hypodermic needles have the advantage of being readily available and can be used in neonates and young infants up to 2 years of age. In older children and adults, a 13-gauge bone marrow needle (Kormed/Jamshidi disposable bone marrow needle) with stylet is required.

Under sterile conditions, firm rotary pressure is applied to the needle until a loss of resistance indicates entry into the marrow cavity. At this point, the obturator is removed and a syringe is attached to aspirate blood and bone spicules. Standard intravenous tubing can then be connected to the end of the needle for fluid and drug administration.

Potential hazards associated with intraosseous therapy include fat embolization, cellulitis, abscess, subperiosteal infiltration or hematoma, subcutaneous infiltration, and osteomyelitis. The risk of infection is higher with continuous infusion for more than 72 hours or infusion of hypertonic solutions.

Penile Administration

In male patients, the corpus cavernosum of the penis is suggested as a reliable, quickly accessible route for short-term emergency fluid administration.[68] The corpus cavernosum has superficial and deep venous drainage systems that communicate with each other and ultimately drain into the saphenous and hypogastric veins, respectively.

A tourniquet is placed at the base of the penis. An 18- to 21-gauge needle is introduced into the corpus cavernosum in the lateral aspect of the penis. A distinct "click" indicates penetration of the tunica albuginea and correct position of the needle. The tourniquet is then released and the needle is connected to the fluid bag. Subcutaneous hematoma is a possible complication. The safety of administering resuscitative drugs and efficacy of the technique have not been formally evaluated.

All of these methods are temporary and should be replaced by a conventional method as soon as possible.

Converting One Lumen to Multiple Lumina

Resuscitation of critically ill, severely burned, or multiple trauma patients may require emergency placement of two or three central venous cannulas. Once access is established, time can be saved and complications reduced by converting the single cannula to a multiple access one. A large-bore introducer is first inserted using the modified Seldinger technique. A triple-lumen catheter is then inserted through the diaphragm of the introducer, providing four venous ports from a single central-access site.[69]

PULMONARY ARTERY CANNULATION ■

DESCRIPTION

The introduction of a flow-directed, balloon flotation catheter in 1970 allowed right heart catheterization to be performed safely at the bedside.[70] The catheter provides important physiologic information for assessment of cardiac function. Although the basic design of the catheter remains unchanged from its original conception, a variety of modifications provide options to measure intracardiac pressures and cardiac output, continuously monitor pulmonary arterial blood saturation, perform arterial and ventricular pacing, and calculate right ventricular volumes and ejection fraction.

The typical catheter for hemodynamic monitoring is radiopaque, 110 cm long, made of polyvinylchloride, and marked with rings at 10-cm intervals from the tip. A black ring thicker than the rest identifies the 50-cm mark. The distal lumen terminates at the tip, whereas the proximal lumen ends about 30 cm from the tip. In some versions, a third lumen opens at 20 cm (ventricle) or 30 cm (atrium) from the tip and provides an extra site for administration of drugs and fluids, insertion of pacemaker wires, or right ventricular evaluation.

A wire connects a thermistor bead, located 3 to 5 cm from the tip, to an external thermistor connector that, in turn, is linked to a cardiac output computer. Rapid-response thermistors also allow right ventricular volumes and ejection fraction to be calculated.[71] A latex balloon with maximal inflation capacity of 2 mL is positioned near the tip in such a way that, when inflated, it engulfs the tip and prevents endocardial irritation during the passage. The inflated balloon guides the flotation catheter to the pulmonary artery and facilitates measurement of pulmonary arterial occlusion pressure by occlusion of a pulmonary artery branch.

INDICATIONS

Table 35-8 lists the major indications for performing hemodynamic monitoring. A lack of well-controlled, prospective, randomized trials to demonstrate efficacy of hemodynamic monitoring in improving outcome has prompted some critics to suggest limiting its use.[72,73] Currently, invasive hemodynamic monitoring should be employed whenever the patient's stability cannot be accurately determined by clinical means or whenever clinical evidence suggests progressive deterioration. Medical personnel must be able to interpret and apply the needed information correctly to establish a diagnosis and formulate a treatment plan. The hazards, inconvenience, and expense are important considerations that should be evaluated for each patient.

INSERTION TECHNIQUE

Table 35-5 summarizes preferred cannulation approaches for specific clinical situations and recommend proper equipment and care of the pulmonary artery catheter. A variety of different dilator-sheath assemblies are available for introduction. After venipuncture, we use the modified Seldinger technique to place a no. 8 French sheath with a one-way valve at the outer end and a side arm for blood sampling and infusion of fluids or drugs. Introducer and sheath are advanced gently to avoid venous perforation. After proper placement, the introducer is removed.

Before insertion, every catheter should be tested for bends or kinks and integrity of the balloon and thermistor. The catheter is then connected by a three-way stopcock and pressure tubing to an appropriately balanced and calibrated pressure transducer. All lumina are flushed and filled with sterile heparinized saline solution. Finally, the catheter is "shaken and flicked" to assure display of optimum-size pressure tracing. A tightly fitting plastic sleeve is often placed over the catheter before insertion to preserve a sterile length of the catheter outside of the insertion site for subsequent

TABLE 35-8. Indications for Pulmonary Artery Cannulation

CARDIOVASCULAR

    Complicated cardiac surgery
    Dissecting abdominal aneurysm
    Thoracic aneurysmectomy
    Emergency or extensive surgery in patients
    Cardiogenic shock

RESPIRATORY

    Pneumonectomy
    Acute pulmonary edema
    Acute lung injury
    Complicated mechanical ventilation

MISCELLANEOUS

    Severe burns
    Multiple trauma
    Septic shock
    Research
    Preoperative optimization

manipulations. The balloon should remain deflated while inserting the catheter through the sheath until the catheter tip is in an intrathoracic location; the correct location is indicated by increased respiration-related variations.

Once the tip is advanced 20 cm, the balloon is inflated with 1.5 mL of air. The catheter is then slowly and monotonously advanced under continuous electrocardiographic and pressure monitoring across the tricuspid valve, through the right ventricle. As a general guide, the right ventricular tracing should appear about 45 to 55 cm from the antecubital fossa, 40 to 45 cm from the femoral vein, 35 to 40 cm from the IJV, and 30 to 40 cm from the SV (the smaller numbers represent right-sided approaches). Characteristic pressure changes should accompany passage from the right ventricle to the pulmonary artery and into the occlusion position (Fig. 35-11). The occlusion position should be obtained when the balloon is inflated with 1.5 mL air. If occlusion is obtained with less than 1-mL inflation, the catheter is probably too far in the pulmonary artery and needs readjustment.

Once the catheter is in the pulmonary artery, secure it with a suture. Obtain a chest radiograph to document the tip location and to check for pneumothorax. Placement may be difficult in the presence of right atrial or ventricular dilatation, low cardiac output, pulmonary hypertension, or tricuspid regurgitation. Passage during deep, spontaneous inspiration, in the sitting position, or after replacement of air with 1.5 mL of sterile saline may facilitate entrance to the right ventricle.[74] Stiffening the catheter in a cold solution before passage, or using a guidewire (length 120 cm, outer diameter 0.021 inches) under fluoroscopy sometimes helps. Distal migration of the catheter tip, which occurs frequently, can be prevented by removing the catheter slack in the right ventricle.

COMPLICATIONS

Table 35-7 lists early and late complications of pulmonary artery catheterization.[37–42] Sustained ventricular arrhythmias usually result from catheter slack and should be treated by removal. A knotted catheter usually can be removed in a cardiac catheterization laboratory without much difficulty, but occasionally a surgical approach is necessary. The incidence of pulmonary artery rupture is low but should be

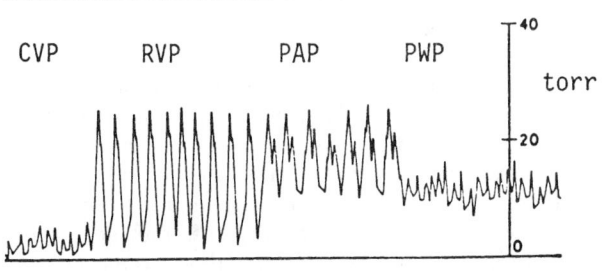

FIGURE 35-11. Pressure waveforms recorded as the pulmonary artery catheter is advanced through the right atrium (central venous pressure [CVP]), right ventricle (right ventricular pressure [RVP]), into the pulmonary artery (pulmonary artery pressure [PAP]), and to the occlusion position (pulmonary artery occlusion pressure [PWP]).

suspected whenever hemoptysis occurs. Mechanical damage to the cardiac valves and endocardium may occur as a result of prolonged catheterization. Valvular ruptures have been reported when the catheter is entrapped in the trabeculae. The balloon should be deflated before withdrawing the catheter at any time.

Pulmonary artery catheters predispose to bacterial colonization and systemic infection. The degree of catheter manipulation and the length of time that it is in place are important factors. In critically ill patients, entrapment of platelets by the catheter may cause clinically significant thrombocytopenia that responds to removal of the catheter.

PERIPHERAL ARTERIAL CANNULATION ■

The management of critically ill patients requires frequent and accurate measurements of blood pressure. Because indirect blood pressure measurements depend on blood flow, whereas intraarterial catheters measure pressures directly; significant differences sometimes occur between arterial pressures measured by indirect and direct, invasive methods.[75,76] The main indications for peripheral arterial cannulation are continuous direct blood pressure measurement, access for repeated blood sampling, and assessment of contractility by visualization of the upstroke of the pressure tracing. Table 35-9 summarizes the advantages and disadvantages of the most common sites of insertion in order of popularity.

Catheterization of an artery may be achieved by surgical cutdown or percutaneous insertion. The latter method is preferred because of a threefold to eightfold lower risk of infection.[77] We suggest that operators familiarize themselves with all of the insertion sites (except for the brachial) and use the most suitable site for each individual patient. Relative contraindications to cannulation include broken or infected skin, presence of an arterial graft, and inadequate collateral flow.

The status of collateral perfusion can be evaluated by performing the modified Allen's test[78,79] before cannulation of radial[80] and dorsalis pedis arteries.[81] However, the reliability of this test as a predictor of hand ischemia after radial artery cannulation is questionable.[82–86] A normal or negative test result does not rule out digital gangrene after insertion of a radial arterial catheter. Arterial catheterization has been performed in patients with a positive test result without ischemic consequences. Furthermore, the Allen test is impossible to evaluate in many situations (shock, jaundice, or intense vasoconstriction). Presence of atrophic changes in the nail bed of the great toe preclude performing the test for evaluating collateral circulation before cannulation of the dorsalis pedis artery. Therefore, we do not advocate routine use of the visual modified Allen test. If an abnormality of the collateral circulation in an extremity is suspected, a Doppler Allen's test or Doppler evaluation of the palmar arch, ulnar artery, or posterior dorsalis pedis can be performed before cannulation. The operator should document the impression of collateral circulation in the procedure note.

TABLE 35-9. Peripheral Arterial Cannulation Sites: Advantages and Disadvantages

SITE	ADVANTAGES	DISADVANTAGES
Radial	Highly accessible Easily visible	Relatively high complication rate High degree of disability if complication occurs
Femoral	Relatively low complication rate Longer catheter function More accurate readings High cannulation success rate	Decreased mobilization of patient Possibly higher contamination rate Occult bleeding
Axillary	Low complication rate Longer catheter function More accurate readings	Low accessibility and visibility High degree of disability if complication occurs. Possibly higher contamination rate. Occult bleeding
Dorsalis pedis	Easily visible Highly accessible	Congenital absence in more than 12% of population High rate of cannulation failure. Decreased mobilization of patient
Temporal	Low complication rate	Difficult cannulation Short catheter function
Brachial	Highly accessible	Inadequate collateral circulation High degree of disability if complication occurs. Not recommended by most authors

INSERTION TECHNIQUES

Cannulation should be attempted using a 20-gauge catheter if possible. The artery is palpated at two points 2.5 cm (1 inch) apart, and a small incision is made midway between them using a pointed scalpel or 18-gauge needle. This technique prevents shearing and damage of the tip of the catheter during penetration of the skin and subcutaneous tissue. The cannula is then advanced through the puncture site along the course of the artery at 30- to 45-degree angles to the skin. Cannulation can be achieved by transfixing, direct threading, pressure-curve–directed, liquid stylet, or modified Seldinger techniques. All are acceptable, and no difference in sequelae has been found.[87]

In the transfixation technique, the anterior and posterior walls of the artery are penetrated before the inner needle is withdrawn. The outer plastic cannula is then withdrawn slowly until blood flows freely from the end. The cannula then can be advanced further up the arterial lumen.

With direct insertion, only the anterior wall of the artery is penetrated. To assure position of the cannula within the arterial lumen, bring the needle and catheter to the skin level and place it 2 or 3 mm further in the artery before advancing the catheter. We suggest a 30- to 45-degree angle between the needle and the skin for arterial puncture. Advancement of the cannula into the vessel should be done at a lower angle (15 to 30 degrees) to facilitate smooth passage.

The third technique for cannulation is pressure-curve directed. The catheter with inner needle is connected to a transducer and a pressure monitor display. After flushing the catheter, it is advanced while pressure is monitored. Appearance of a blood pressure tracing signals that the anterior wall of the artery has been penetrated. Cannulation is then achieved using the direct insertion technique.[88]

The liquid stylet technique was initially described for "catheters that won't thread."[89] A 3-mL syringe is filled with saline and is attached to the cannula after the anterior wall of the artery is penetrated. After confirming the intraarterial position by aspiration of blood, saline is injected slowly and steadily while the catheter is advanced slowly by the other hand.

The modified Seldinger technique employs threading of a guidewire into the artery after penetration. If the wire meets resistance at the end of the needle, try advancing the needle 1 to 2 mm and rethread the wire while making a series of 90-degree rotations to alleviate the possibility that the bevel is just proximal to an intimal flap. Never try to thread it against even slight resistance. When placement is achieved, remove the needle and thread the catheter over the guidewire. Assure adequate opening of the skin and subcutaneous tissue to prevent fraying and shearing the tip.

After cannulation, withdraw the wire and cover the cannula hub with a sterile finger until the transducer-flush system can be connected. After each unsuccessful attempt, local fingertip pressure should be applied long enough to prevent hematoma formation. If vasospasm occurs, another site should be tried. Alternatively, a delay of 15 minutes may allow return of a good pulse.

Arterial catheters should be changed every 5 to 7 days or earlier if distal ischemia, local infection, or difficulty with the pressure tracing or blood withdrawal is encountered. Before an arterial catheter is removed, pressure should be applied proximally and distally to the insertion site. A syringe should be attached to the catheter and suction applied while it is removed. This procedure decreases the incidence of arterial thrombotic occlusion after catheter removal by removing developed clots. After catheter removal, fingertip pressure must be applied to the site for as long as it is necessary to achieve complete hemostasis.

The following specific points should be kept in mind regarding different insertion sites.

Radial Artery

Cannulation of the nondominant hand of the patient should be attempted first. Hyperextension of the wrist to about 20 degrees diminishes arterial tortuosity. Cannulate the artery 1 to 2 cm proximal to the proximal flexion skin fold, where it is less tortuous and has a lower risk of digital ischemia because of better collateral circulation.

Femoral Artery

The femoral artery runs directly across the midpoint of a line drawn between the superior iliac spine and the symphysis pubis. It should be punctured below the inguinal ligament. Punctures above this level carry a higher incidence of retroperitoneal hemorrhage. The artery is usually reached 3 to 5 cm from the skin. The modified Seldinger technique is usually required for femoral cannulation.

Axillary

The artery should be cannulated as high as possible in the axilla, close to the thoracic apex. Risk of distal ischemia is less with this method than with the brachial approach because of a rich anastomotic network surrounding the artery.[90] However, pneumothorax and thromboembolism from the catheter tip to the radial or ulnar artery are possible complications. Hematoma from a puncture leak of the artery can fill the axillary sheath around the neurovascular bundle and compress the brachial plexus, resulting in nerve damage and peripheral neuropathy. The left axillary artery should be chosen first because the risk of cerebral air embolism from inadvertently injected air is higher with right-sided catheterization.

Dorsalis Pedis Artery

This small artery is congenitally absent in 12% of the population and is often difficult or impossible to cannulate. It should be avoided in the absence of a posterior tibial artery pulse.[91] Blood pressure measured in the dorsalis pedis artery differs significantly from that measured in more central arteries.

Brachial Artery

Because of inadequate collateral circulation, obstruction of the brachial artery results in poor or absent flow to the radial and ulnar arteries. Therefore, few authors recommend its utilization.[92]

Temporal Artery

Rich collateral circulation and easy accessibility makes the temporal artery an attractive site for cannulation. Tortuosity and its location, however, make cannulation and maintenance extremely difficult.

TABLE 35-10. Complications of Peripheral Arterial Cannulation

Local ischemia, inflammation, or infection
Arterial spasm
Hematoma formation and infection
Bleeding from cannula disconnection
Thrombosis
Distal embolism
Limb ischemia and necrosis
Sepsis
Pseudoaneurysm
Arteriovenous fistula
Cerebral air embolism
Peripheral neuropathy

COMPLICATIONS

Unlike central venous cannulation, arterial catheterization is a technically straightforward procedure, and its complications seem to be operator independent.[93] Among the complications (Table 35-10), ischemic necrosis[94,95] and infection[96,97] are of most concern. Several factors are known to increase the chance of complications (Table 35-11). Reversible subclinical arterial occlusion or decrease of flow is common after catheter removal, and up to 25% of arteries show signs of occlusion 1 week later.[94,95] Ischemic necrosis occurs less than 1% of the time.[98] It is noteworthy that the reported incidence of thrombosis has steadily decreased. The most recent study incidence rate is only 2.5%.[99] Improvement may result from use of continuous heparin-flush systems, better catheter material and design, and shorter duration of cannulation.[100]

Several types of infection are caused by arterial catheters. Local infection at the catheter site and catheter colonization have a reported incidence rate of 10% to 15%.[77] The incidence rate of catheter-related sepsis varies from 0.2% to 5%.[77,96] The duration of catheterization and contamination of the infusate are the dominant causes of bacteremia.

Median nerve neuropathy associated with radial artery catheterization may be caused by stretching of the nerve

TABLE 35-11. Factors Increasing the Chance of Complications After Peripheral Arterial Cannulation

Low perfusion state
Use of vasopressors
Intrinsic vascular disease
Cannula/vessel diameter ratio
Tapered catheters
Catheter material (non-Teflon)
Long duration of cannulation
Repeated cannulation attempts
Reusable transducer systems
Insertion by cutdown
Presence of bacteremia
Bleeding diathesis or hypercoagulable states
Use of dextrose solutions for flush systems
Flush system close to insertion site

during wrist hyperextension or nerve compression by blood in the carpal tunnel.[101] Pseudoaneurysm of the radial artery usually is a delayed complication, occurring up to 2 weeks after catheter removal.[102]

REFERENCES ■

1. Eisenhauer ED, Derveloy RJ, Hastings PR: Prospective evaluation of central venous pressure (CVP) catheters in a large city–county hospital. *Ann Surg* 1982;196:560
2. Sznajder JI, Zveibil FR, Bitterman H, et al: Central vein catheterization. *Arch Intern Med* 1986;146:259
3. Parsa KMH, Tabora F: Central venous access in critically ill patients in the emergency department. *Emerg Clin North Am* 1986;4:709
4. Venus B, Mallory DL: Vascular cannulation. *Probl Crit Care* 1988;2:1
5. Howe EG: Forensic issues in critical care medicine. *Probl Crit Care* 1988;2:171
6. Wilson GL: Preparation of the patient for vascular cannulation. *Probl Crit Care* 1988;2:211
7. National Intravenous Therapy Association: *Intravenous Nursing Standards of Practice.* Cambridge, NITA, 1981:9
8. Centers for Disease Control guidelines for the prevention of intravascular infections. In: Farber B (ed). *Infection Control in Intensive Care.* New York, Churchill Livingstone, 1987:50
9. Press OW, Ramsey RG, Larson EB, et al: Hickman catheter infections in patients with malignancies. *Medicine* 1984; 63:189
10. Ryder MA: Peripherally inserted central venous catheters. *Nurs Clin North Am* 1993;28:937
11. Bansmer MD, Keith BA, Tesluk MD: Complications following use of indwelling catheters of inferior vena cava. *JAMA* 1958;167:1606
12. Shaldon S, Chjiandussi L, Higgs B: Hemodialysis by percutaneous catheterization. *Lancet* 1961;ii:857
13. Emerman CL, Bellon EM, Lukens TW, et al: A prospective study of femoral versus subclavian vein catheterization during cardiac arrest. *Ann Emerg Med* 1990;19:27
14. Tribett D, Brenner M: Peripheral and femoral vein cannulation. *Probl Crit Care* 1988;2:266
15. McGee WT, Mallory DL: Cannulation of the internal and external jugular veins. *Probl Crit Care* 1988;2:217
16. Mallory DL, Shawker TH, Evans RG, et al: Effects of clinical maneuvers on sonographically determined internal jugular vein size during venous cannulation. *Crit Care Med* 1990; 18:1269
17. Mallory DL, McGree WT, Shawker TH, et al: Ultrasound guidance improves the success rate of internal jugular vein cannulation. *Chest* 1990;98:157
18. Patel C, Laboy V, Venus B, et al: Acute complications of pulmonary artery catheter insertion in critically ill patients. *Crit Care Med* 1986;14:195
19. McGee WT, Mallory DL, Johans TG, et al: Safe placement of central venous catheters is facilitated using right atrial electrocardiography. *Crit Care Med* 1988;16:434
20. Wilson RG, Gaer JAR: Right atrial electrocardiography in placement of central venous catheters. *Lancet* 1988;i:462
21. Mallory DL, McGee WT, et al: A multi-center study evaluated the safety and technical aspects of central vascular cannulation. *Chest* 1989;96:295S
22. Yoffa D, Melb MB: Supraclavicular subclavian venipuncture and catheterization. *Lancet* 1965∞:614
23. Patterson DLH: The supraclavicular approach to the subclavian vein and temporary cardiac pacemaker electrode. In: Peters JL (ed). *A Manual of Central Venous Catheterization and Parenteral Nutrition.* Boston, LPSG, 1983;70
24. Brahos GJ: Central venous catheterization via the supraclavicular approach. *J Trauma* 1977;17:872
25. Helmkamp BF, Sanko SR: Supraclavicular central venous catheterization. *Am J Obstet Gynecol* 1985;153:751
26. Haapaniemi L, Slatis P: Supraclavicular catheterization of the superior vena cava. *Acta Anaesthesiol Scand* 1974;18:12
27. James PM, Myers RT: Central venous pressure monitoring: complication and a new technique. *Am J Surg* 1983;39:75
28. Parsa MH, Tabora F: Establishment of intravenous lines for long term intravenous therapy and monitoring. *Surg Clin North Am* 1985;65:835
29. Rao TLK, Wong AY, Salem MR: A new approach to percutaneous catheterization of the internal jugular vein. *Anesthesiology* 1977;46:362
30. Mogil RA, DeLaurentis DA, Rosemond GP: The infraclavicular venipuncture: value in various clinical situations including central venous pressure monitoring. *Arch Surg* 1967;95:320
31. Jacob AS, Schweiger MJ: A method for inserting two catheters, pulmonary arterial and temporary pacing, through a single puncture into a subclavian vein catheter. *Cardiovasc Diagn* 1983;9:6111
32. Kinyon GE, Jones RA, Spraul GL, et al: Subclavian techniques of central venous pressure monitoring. *Acta Anaesthesiol Scand Suppl* 1966;24:191
33. Borja AR, Honshaw JR: A safe way to perform infraclavicular subclavian vein catheterization. *Surg Gynecol Obstet* 1970; 130:673
34. Mooseman DL: The anatomy of infraclavicular subclavian vein catheterization and its complications. *Surg Gynecol Obstet* 1973;136:71
35. Novak RA, Venus B: Clavicular approaches for central vein cannulation. *Probl Crit Care* 1988;2:242
36. Kasten GW, Owens E, Kennedy D: Ventricular tachycardia resulting from central venous catheter tip migration due to arm position changes: report of two cases. *Anesthesiology* 1985;62:185
37. Childs D, Wilkes RG: Puncture of the ascending aorta: a complication of subclavian venous cannulation. *Anesthesia* 1986;41:331
38. Herbst CA: Indications, management, and complications of percutaneous subclavian catheters. *Arch Surg* 1978;113:1421
39. Brown CQ: Inadvertent prolonged cannulation of the carotid artery. *Anesth Analg* 1982;61:150
40. Bernard RW, Stahl WM: Subclavian vein catheterization: a perspective study. I. Non-infectious complications. *Ann Surg* 1971;173:184
41. Jay AWL, Aldridge HE: Perforation of the heart or vena cava by central venous catheters inserted for monitoring or infusion therapy. *Can Med Assoc J* 1986;135:1143
42. Aldridge HE, Jay AWL: Central venous catheters and heart perforation. *Can Med Assoc J* 1986;135D:1145
43. Karnauchow PN: Cardiac tamponade from central venous catheterization. *Can Med Assoc J* 1986;135:1082
44. Hermosura B, Vanags L, Dicket NW: Measurement of pressure during intravenous therapy. *JAMA* 1966;195:321
45. Paschall RM, Mandel S: Brachial plexus injury from percutaneous cannulation of the internal jugular vein. *Ann Emerg Med* 1983;12:112
46. Sato O, Tada Y, Sudo K, et al: Arteriovenous fistula following central venous catheterization. *Arch Surg* 1986;121:729
47. Robinson PN, Jewkes DA, Kendall B: Vertebrovertebral arte-

riovenous fistula: a complication of internal jugular catheterization. *Anaesthesia* 1984;39:46

48. Horrow JC, Laucks SO: Coronary air embolism during venous cannulation. *Anesthesiology* 1982;56:212

49. Morgan RNW, Morrell DF: Internal jugular catheterization. *Anaesthesia* 1981;36:512

50. Hansbrough JF, Narrod JA, Rutherford R: Arteriovenous fistulas following central venous catheterization. *Intensive Care Med* 1983;9:287

51. Conahan TJ: Air embolization during percutaneous Swan-Ganz catheter placement. *Anesthesiology* 1979;50:360

52. Feliciano DV, Mattox KL, Graham JM, et al: Major complication of percutaneous subclavian vein catheters. *Am J Surg* 1979;173:184

53. Maki DG: Pathogenesis, prevention, and management of infections due to intravascular devices used for infusion therapy. In: Bisno A, Waldrogel F (eds). *Infections Associated With Indwelling Medical Devices.* Washington, DC, American Society of Microbiology, 1989:161

54. Dimesnil JG, Proulx G: A new nonsurgical technique for untying tight knots in flow-directed balloon catheters. *Am J Cardiol* 1984;53:395

55. O'Toole JD, Wurtxbacher JJ, Wearner NE, et al: Pulmonary-valve injury and insufficiency during pulmonary artery catheterization. *N Engl J Med* 1979;301:1167

56. Greene JF, Cummings KC: Aseptic thrombotic endocardial vegetations. *JAMA* 1973;225:1525

57. Lange HW, Galliani CA, Edwards JE: Local complications associated with indwelling Swan-Ganz catheters: autopsy study of 36 cases. *Am J Cardiol* 1983;52:1108

58. Kellky TF, Morris GC, Crawford ES, et al: Perforation of the pulmonary artery with Swan-Ganz catheters. *Ann Surg* 1981;193:686

59. Gore JM, Matsumoto AH, Layden JJ, et al: Superior vena cava syndrome: its association with indwelling balloon-tipped pulmonary artery catheters. *Arch Intern Med* 1984;144:506

60. Miller JJ, Venus B, Mathru M: Comparison of the sterility of long-term central venous catheterization using single lumen, triple lumen, and pulmonary artery catheters. *Crit Care Med* 1984;12:634

61. Mangano DT: Heparin bonding and long-term protection against thrombogenesis. *N Engl J Med* 1982;307:894

62. Koehler PJ, Wizngarrd PRA: Brown-Sequard syndrome due to spinal cord infections after subclavian vein catheterization. *Lancet* 1986;ii:914

63. Denys BG, Uretsky BF, Reddy PS: Ultrasound-assisted cannulation of the internal jugular vein: a prospective comparison to the external landmark-guided technique. *Circulation* 1993;87:1557

64. Leon Skolnick M. The role of sonography in the placement and management of jugular and subclavian central venous catheters: review article. *AJR* 1994;37:291

65. Sukgar M, Yamazaki T, Hatanaka M, et al: Ultrasonic real time guidance for subclavian venipuncture. *Surg Gynecol Obstet* 1988;167:239

66. Parrish GA, Turkewitz D, Skiendzielewski JJ: Intraosseous infusion in the emergency department. *Am J Emerg Med* 1986;4:59

67. Heinild S, Sondergard TD, Tudrad F: Bone marrow infusion in childhood: experience from a thousand infusions. *J Pediatr* 1947;30:400

68. Godec CJ: The penis: a possible alternative emergency venous access for males? *Am J Emerg Med* 1982;11:266

69. Landers DF, Boskovski N: Volume replacement in patients with limited venous access. *Anesth Analg* 1989;68:412

70. Swan HJC, Ganz W, Forrester JS, et al: Catheterization of the heart in man with the use of flow-directed balloon-tipped catheters. *N Engl J Med* 1970;283:447

71. Vincent JL, Thirion M, Brimiwell S, et al: Thermodilution measurement of right ventricular ejection fraction with a modified pulmonary artery catheter. *Intensive Care Med* 1986;12:33

72. Robin ED: The cult of the Swan-Ganz catheter: overuse and abuse of pulmonary flow catheters. *Ann Intern Med* 1985;103:445

73. Podick DM: Physiologic and prognostic indications of invasive monitoring: Undetermined risk benefit ratio in patients with heart disease. *Am J Cardiol* 1980;46:173

74. Venus B, Mathru M: A maneuver for bedside pulmonary artery catheterization in patients with right heart failure. *Chest* 1982;82:803

75. Venus B, Mathru M, Smith RA, et al: Direct versus indirect blood pressure measurements in critically ill patients. *Heart Lung* 1985;14:228

76. Brunner JMR, Krenis LJ, Kunsman JM: Comparison of direct and indirect methods of measuring arterial blood pressure. *Med Instrum* 1981;15:11

77. Band JD, Maki DG: Infections caused by arterial catheters used for pressure monitoring. *Am J Med* 1970;67:735

78. Allen EV: Thromboangiitis obliterans: methods of diagnosis of chronic occlusive arterial lesions distal to the wrist with illustrative cases. *Am J Med Sci* 1929;178:237

79. Clarke W, Freund PR, Wasse L: Assessment of adequacy of ulnar arterial flow prior to radial artery atheterization [abstract]. *Anesthesiology* 1982;55:A38

80. Ejrup B, Fischer B, Wright IS: Clinical evaluation of blood flow to the hand: the false positive Allen test. *Circulation* 1966;33:778

81. Husum B, Eriksen T: Percutaneous cannulation of the dorsalis pedis artery. *Br J Anaesth* 1979;51:1055

82. Mandel MA, Dauchot PJ: Radial artery cannulation in 1000 patients: precautions and compilations. *J Hand Surg [Am]* 1977;2:482

83. Slogoff S, Keats AS, Arlund C: On safety of radial artery cannulation. *Anesthesiology* 1983;59:42

84. Wilkins RG: Radial artery cannulation and ischaemic damage: a review. *Anaesthesia* 1985;40:896

85. Baker RJ, Chunprapah B, Nyhus LM: Severe ischemia of the hand following radial artery catheterization. *Surgery* 1976;80:449

86. Kamienski RW, Barnes RW: Critique of the Allen test for continuity of the palmar arch assessed by Doppler ultrasound. *Surg Gynecol Obstet* 1976;142:861

87. Jones RM, Hill AB, Nahrwold ML, et al: The effect of method of radial artery cannulation on postcannulation blood flow and thrombus formation. *Anesthesiology* 1981;55:76

88. Kondo K: Percutaneous radial artery cannulation using a pressure-curve-directed technique. *Anesthesiology* 1984;61:639

89. Stirt TA: "Liquid stylet" for percutaneous radial artery cannulation. *Can Anaesth Soc J* 1982;29:492

90. Bryan-Brown CW, Kwun KB, Lumb PD, et al: The axillary artery catheter. *Heart Lung* 1983;12:492

91. Youngberg J, Miller E: Evaluation of percutaneous cannulations of the dorsalis pedis artery. *Anesthesiology* 1976;44:80

92. Barnes RW, Foster EJ, Janssen GA, et al: Safety of brachial arterial catheters as monitors in the intensive care unit: prospective evaluation with the Doppler ultrasonic velocity detector. *Anesthesiology* 1976;44:260

93. Puri VK, Carlson RW, Bander JJ, et al: Complications of vascular catheterization in the critically ill. *Crit Care Med* 1980;8:495

94. Gardner RM, Schwartz R, Wong HC, et al: Percutaneous

indwelling radial-artery catheters for monitoring cardiovascular function. *N Engl J Med* 1974;290:1227

95. Bedford RF: Radial artery function following percutaneous cannulation with 18 and 20 gauge catheters. *Anesthesiology* 1977;47:37
96. Weinstein RA, Stamm WE, Kramer L: Pressure monitoring devices: Overlooked sources of nosocomial infection. *JAMA* 1976;236:936
97. Shinozaki T, Deane R, Mazuzan JE, et al: Bacterial combination of arterial lines: a prospective study. *JAMA* 1983;249:223
98. Shapiro BA: Monitoring gas exchange in acute respiratory failure. *Respir Care* 1983;28:605
99. Weiss BM, Gattiker RI: Complications during and following radial artery cannulation: a prospective study. *Intensive Care Med* 1986;12:424
100. Sladen A: Complications of invasive hemodynamic monitoring in the intensive care unit. *Curr Probl Surg* 1988;17:69
101. Marshall G, Edelstein G, Hirshman CA: Median nerve compression following radial arterial puncture. *Anesth Analg* 1980;59:953
102. Russell RC, Steichen JB, Sook EG: Radial artery pseudoaneurysms: their diagnosis, treatment and prevention. *Orthop Rev* 1979;8:49

Critical Care, Third Edition, edited by Joseph M. Civetta,
Robert W. Taylor, and Robert R. Kirby.
Lippincott-Raven Publishers, Philadelphia, PA © 1997.

CHAPTER 36

■

Temporary Cardiac Pacemakers

W. Ross Davis

IMMEDIATE CONCERNS ■

MAJOR PROBLEMS

Temporary pacemakers are useful in the critical care environment when one of several problems occurs.[1] The most commonly seen problem is bradycardia with symptoms of hypoperfusion. Less commonly, bradycardia may cause unstable angina or congestive heart failure. Potential for abrupt progression of moderate bradycardia to threatening levels or asystole may occasionally compel a decision for prophylactic pacing. Although usually the province of the cardiologist, certain types of tachyarrhythmias also may respond to temporary pacing.

STRESS POINTS

1. The evaluation of the rhythm involves determining the type of arrhythmia and detecting and correcting reversible causes.
2. In rapid succession or simultaneously, the arrhythmia's effect on the patient is evaluated, and a decision of appropriate initial therapy can be made.
3. After evaluating the rhythm, determining the effects on the patient, and assessing the risk of progression to more dangerous rhythms, the intensivist must decide on the advisability of temporary pacing.

INITIAL THERAPY

1. If the patient is not significantly compromised and the cause of the bradycardia can be determined and

effectively treated in a short time, drug treatment alone may be appropriate (Chap. 119).
2. However, if there is any doubt about the effect of the arrhythmia, its reversibility, or the potential for progression to more severe bradycardia, temporary pacing is appropriate.
3. If the patient is likely to remain bradycardic for some time or if the patient is seriously compromised by the bradycardia, temporary pacing is established.
4. Several methods of pacing are available, including external pacing, transvenous pacing, and transthoracic pacing. Each is useful when thoughtfully employed.

INDICATIONS FOR TEMPORARY PACING ■

Table 36-1 outlines the usual ICU indications for temporary pacing. These can be classified as significant bradycardias, prophylactic pacing, and control of tachycardia.

SIGNIFICANT BRADYCARDIA

The most common indication for temporary pacing is bradycardia. The decision to institute pacing is based on assessment of the patient, not just the rhythm strip or electrocardiogram (ECG). The most common underlying causes of bradycardias are discussed in Chapter 119.

545

TABLE 36-1.   Indications for Temporary Cardiac Pacing

SYMPTOMATIC BRADYCARDIA

    Profound sinus bradycardia
    Sinus arrest with junctional bradycardia or ventricular escape
      rhythm
    Complete heart block
    Mobitz II heart block

PROPHYLAXIS

    Asymptomatic Mobitz II heart block
    After cardiac surgery
    During right heart catheterization in patients with left bundle
      branch block
    MI with bifascicular or trifascicular block

TACHYCARDIAS

    Atrial flutter
    Paroxysmal atrial tachycardia
    Ventricular tachycardia
    Ectopic atrial tachycardia

MI, myocardial infarct.

PROPHYLACTIC PACING

When symptomatic bradycardia is likely, temporary pacing is indicated (Fig. 36-1). Settings where prophylactic pacing is appropriate include Mobitz II atrioventricular (AV) block,[2] after cardiac surgery, during right heart catheterization in patients with left bundle branch block, and bifascicular block or trifascicular block in acute myocardial infarction (MI).[3] Bifascicular block is defined as right bundle branch block with either left anterior or left posterior fascicular block. Trifascicular block is defined as either of the above with first-degree AV block, left bundle branch block with first-degree AV block, or alternating right and left bundle branch block. Prophylactic pacing with new left bundle branch block in acute anterior MI is controversial.[4,5]

TACHYCARDIAS

Temporary pacing can be used to terminate, prevent, or control tachycardia.[6] Many reentrant arrhythmias such as atrial flutter, paroxysmal atrial tachycardia, or ventricular tachycardia sometimes can be terminated by pacing the chamber primarily involved at a rate higher than the arrhythmia (Figure 36-2). Once an arrhythmia is abolished, it can frequently be avoided by pacing the chamber at rates higher than the intrinsic rate, thus preventing premature systoles from triggering the reentrant arrhythmia. The ventricular response to automatic atrial arrhythmias can be controlled by pacing the atrium faster than the intrinsic rhythm at rates, resulting in functional AV block. For example, if a patient has an ectopic atrial tachycardia with a rate of 170 that conducts 1:1, one may be able to pace the atrium at 200 pulses per minute (ppm) and induce 2:1 AV conduction, reducing the ventricular rate to 100.

ELECTRODE CATHETERS AND EXTERNAL PACEMAKER UNITS

Electrode catheters and external pulse generators are the equipment required for temporary transvenous cardiac pacing. Transvenous electrode catheters are available in various sizes (most commonly, 4 to 6 French) and vary in flexibility (Fig. 36-3). Electrode catheters constructed of woven Dacron are relatively firm, whereas extruded plastic electrodes are soft and pliable. The placement of a balloon between the proximal and distal electrodes of an extruded plastic catheter allows blood flow–assisted catheter placement. Softer catheters are less maneuverable and less stable once positioned, so woven Dacron firm catheters are preferable, although even with fluoroscopic guidance one must be careful not to perforate vessels or endocardium during insertion. When fluoroscopic equipment is not available and urgent

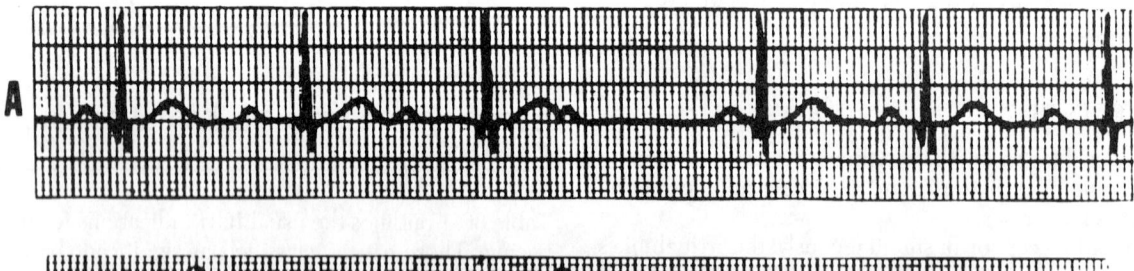

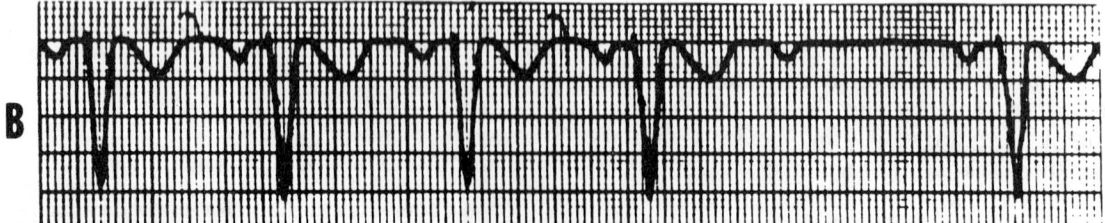

FIGURE 36-1. Prophylactic temporary cardiac pacing. (**A**) Mobitz type I second-degree atrioventricular (AV) block. This form of second-degree AV block rarely progresses to high-degree AV block, and thus temporary pacing is rarely indicated. (**B**) Mobitz II second-degree AV block. This form of AV block is usually associated with a QRS morphology of greater than 120 msec and indicates a need for prophylactic temporary pacing, especially in the setting of an acute myocardial infarction.

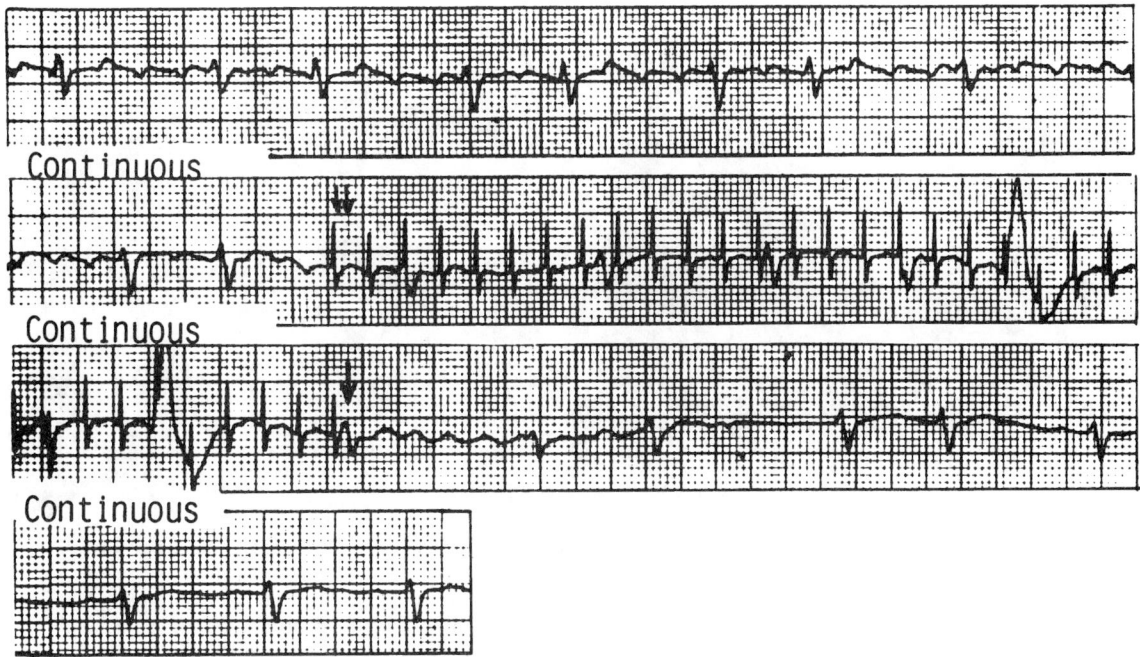

FIGURE 36-2. Temporary pacing is used to terminate a tachyarrhythmia. Atrial flutter is terminated by atrial pacing. At the double arrow, atrial pacing is begun at a rate about 25% faster than the flutter rate. Pacing is terminated at the single arrow. The atrial flutter has been converted to atrial fibrillation, which then spontaneously converts to sinus rhythm.

transvenous pacing is needed, a balloon-tipped electrode catheter may be used,[7] although transcutaneous pacing may be more quickly established.

Most temporary electrode catheters are bipolar, that is, both the distal (cathode) and proximal (anode) electrodes are within the heart chamber being paced. Unipolar catheters have only one distal electrode used for cathode stimulation (i.e., the electron source) with a patch on the skin serving as the anode. Bipolar electrodes are preferred because they are less susceptible to external electrical interference. If needed, a bipolar catheter can be converted to a unipolar

catheter by connecting the proximal lead from the external pacing unit to a skin electrode (Fig. 36-4).

Most ICU pacing needs can be met with ventricular, and, less commonly, atrial single-chamber pacing. However, for specialized needs, modified pacing catheters are available. Multielectrode catheters with electrodes positioned so that both atrial and ventricular endocardial contact occur allow temporary AV pacing with a single catheter (Fig. 36-5). Preformed electrode catheters have been designed to facilitate placement into the right atrial appendage or coronary sinus, thus allowing atrial pacing (Fig. 36-6). Electrode cath-

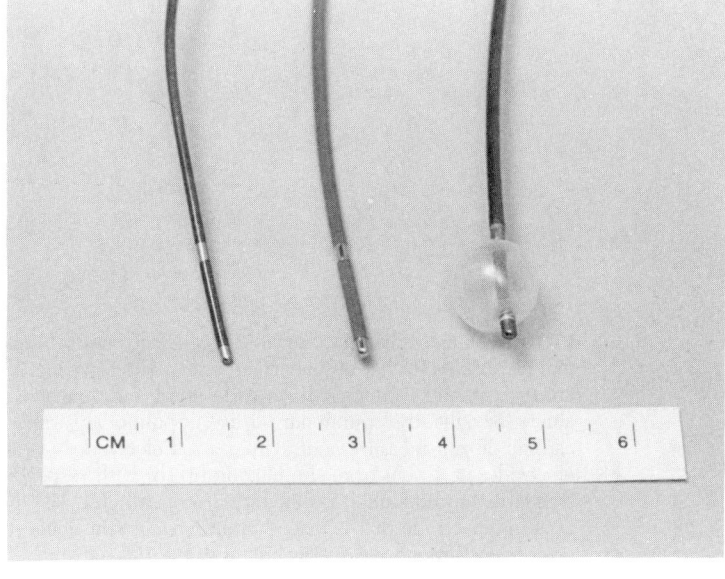

FIGURE 36-3. Electrode catheters. Transvenous electrode catheters are available in various sizes (commonly 4–6 French). The left electrode catheter is constructed of woven Dacron and is a firm, relatively nonpliable catheter. The middle catheter is formed from extruded plastic and is soft and pliable. The electrode catheter on the right is formed from extruded plastic and has a balloon located between the distal and proximal electrodes to allow blood flow–assisted catheter placement.

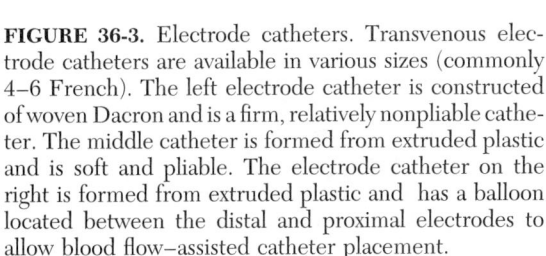

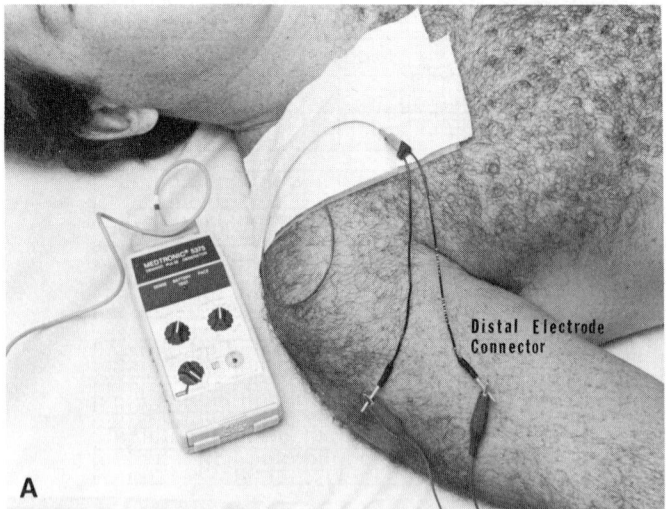
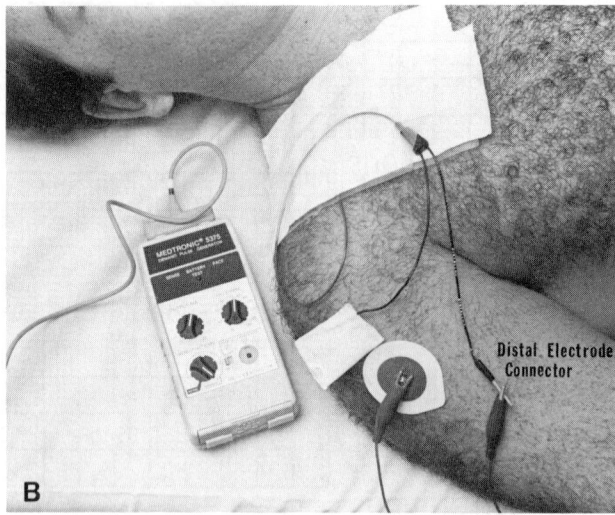

FIGURE 36-4. Converting a bipolar to a unipolar pacemaker. Conversion of a bipolar electrode to a unipolar electrode is sometimes useful if undersensing of the bipolar electrogram occurs or if one electrode becomes electrically disrupted, thus preventing the electrical circuit from being completed. (**A**) Typical bipolar connection. Attachment of the negative and positive poles of the generator to the respective distal and proximal catheter electrodes is shown using connecting cable and alligator clamps. (**B**) Conversion to a unipolar pacemaker. The alligator connector to the distal electrode remains unchanged, whereas the proximal electrode pin is covered with adhesive tape (or other insulator). Connecting the other alligator connector to a skin electrode allows completion of the circuit back to the generator.

eters incorporating a lumen also are available and allow fluid or drug administration and pressure determinations.

The external temporary pacemaker unit controls the stimulus output, stimulus frequency, and the threshold for sensing intrinsic activity (Fig. 36-7). The range of output varies from 0 to 20 mA. The frequency can be adjusted from 30 to 180 ppm. Sensing threshold can be varied from no sensing (asynchronous) to less than 1.5 mV.

PROCEDURES FOR ESTABLISHING TEMPORARY PACING

TRANSVENOUS PACING

Temporary transvenous pacing electrode catheters can be inserted from several venous access sites including brachial, femoral, subclavian, internal jugular, or external jugular

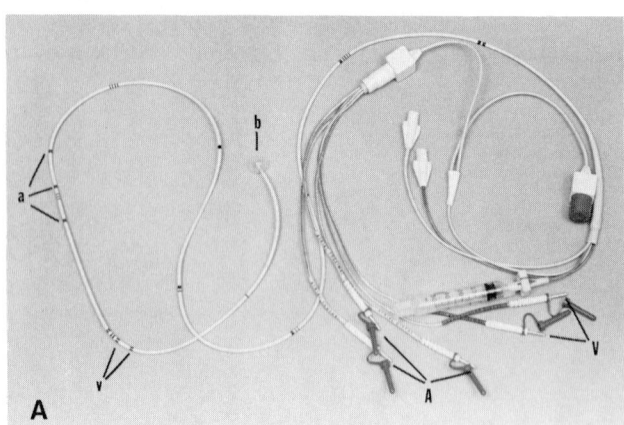
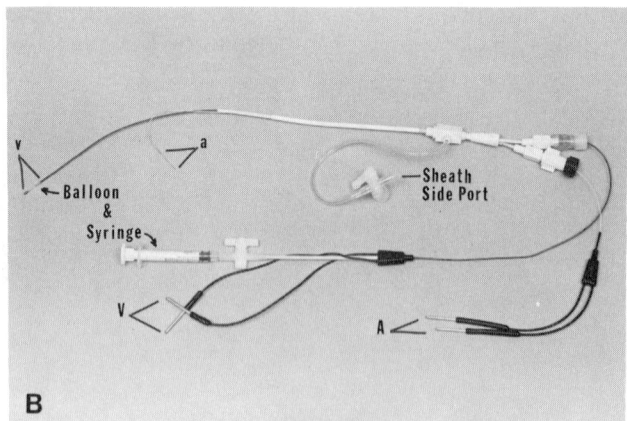

FIGURE 36-5. Multielectrode catheters. Electrode catheters have been designed with distal and proximal electrodes so that atrioventricular sequential pacing can be performed. (**A**) A "pacing pulmonary artery" catheter, designed to provide atrial and ventricular sequential pacing while maintaining the ability for right atrial, pulmonary artery, or pulmonary artery occlusion pressure as well as thermodilution cardiac output measurement. Three atrial electrodes (a) at approximately 30 cm and two ventricular electrodes at 20 cm from the balloon tip (b) with respective pin connectors (A, V) are additions to a standard thermodilution pulmonary artery catheter. (**B**) The system shown has a ventricular balloon flotation electrode that is placed into the right ventricular apex. A small atrial J electrode then can be positioned through a catheter lumen in the right atrium.

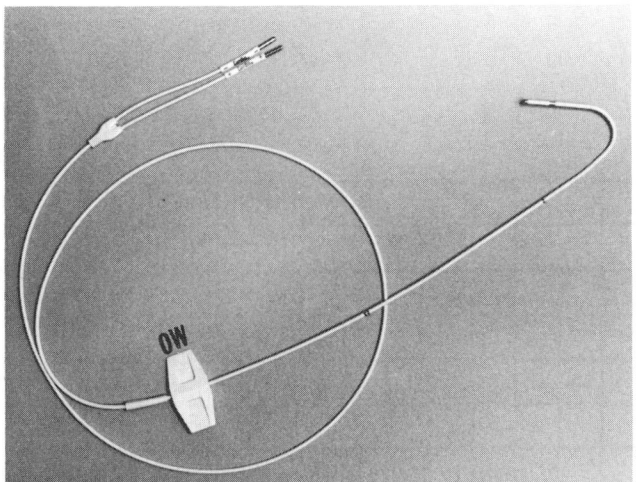

FIGURE 36-6. Atrial pacing electrodes. Preformed electrode catheters have been designed with a permanent "J" to facilitate placement into the right atrial appendage. The "orientation wing" (OW) provided with this electrode catheter allows relatively easy placement into the right atrial appendage, in experienced hands, even without fluoroscopic guidance. Because of stability, these preformed atrial J wires are a preferred form of atrial pacing.

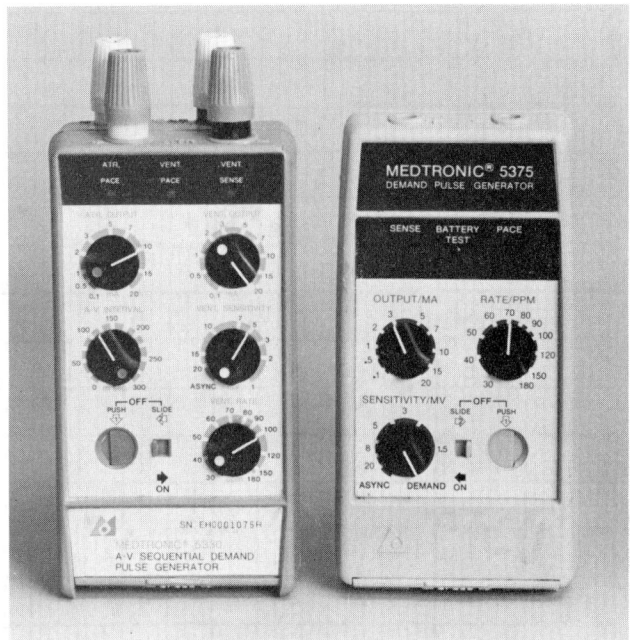

FIGURE 36-7. External temporary pacemaker generators. External pulse generators provide reliable output and pacing rates. Powered by a 9-V battery; they can provide 20-mA output and pacing rates of up to 800 pulses per minute (specially designed units not shown here). Dual channel units (*left*) are provided that allow atrioventricular (AV) synchronous pacing while controlling the AV interval (in milliseconds), ventricular sensitivity, and AV outputs.

veins using the techniques described in Chapter 35. Virtually all temporary ventricular pacing electrodes are positioned in the right ventricular apex, and atrial temporary pacing electrodes are positioned in the right atrial appendage.[8-13]

Preparation

The pacing system should be checked before proceeding. The lead should be examined for any breaks or manufacturing defects. A new battery should be installed in the pulse generator. It should be turned on, and all switches and controls should be tested. A long connector cable should be available. Continuous electrocardiographic monitor and a defibrillator at the bedside are required. Ideally, fluoroscopic placement should be used, but if this is not available, a balloon-tipped electrode catheter can be used.

Insertion

The standard central venous cannulation approach can be modified by the Seldinger technique to facilitate the placement of an introducer sheath. In this approach, a needle is inserted into the vein and a flexible guidewire is inserted through the needle and passed gently into the venous lumen, then the needle is removed. A small puncture wound in the skin is made with a scalpel blade at the guidewire insertion, and blunt dissection used to create a pathway for the dilator and sheath. A tapered vessel dilator with a surrounding sheath is then introduced over the guidewire and inserted into the vessel. The dilator and wire are removed and the sheath remains. The temporary electrode catheter then can be placed into the vascular system through the sheath.

Catheter Position

Whichever venous approach is used, the ideal catheter position for ventricular pacing is at the right ventricular apex where the electrode catheter tip becomes wedged in the trabeculae and endocardial contact is better maintained. Electrodes placed in the outflow tract or along the free wall are less stable. These sites also are more prone to ventricular perforation, especially if any excessive pressure is placed on the electrode tip. The natural sweep of the electrode catheter from the superior vena cava helps to stabilize the lead at the right ventricular apex without undue pressure.

It is best to position catheters into the right ventricular apex under fluoroscopic control; however, the use of a balloon-flotation catheter with electrocardiographic monitoring during catheter insertion is sometimes necessary. In this technique, standard limb electrocardiographic leads are attached to the patient. Using alligator clips, the distal electrode of the catheter is connected to one of the precordial chest electrocardiographic leads (usually V_1). Using an electrocardiographic machine, intracardiac electrograms can be displayed for reference while the lead is advanced (Fig. 36-8). When the electrode catheter is in the superior vena cava, the atrial deflection is negative, and in the inferior vena cava it is positive. The deflections in the right atrium are more rapid, discrete, and larger than in either vena cava. While the electrode catheter is advanced into the right ventricle, there is a much larger ventricular electrogram and the atrial electrogram becomes small. When the electrode

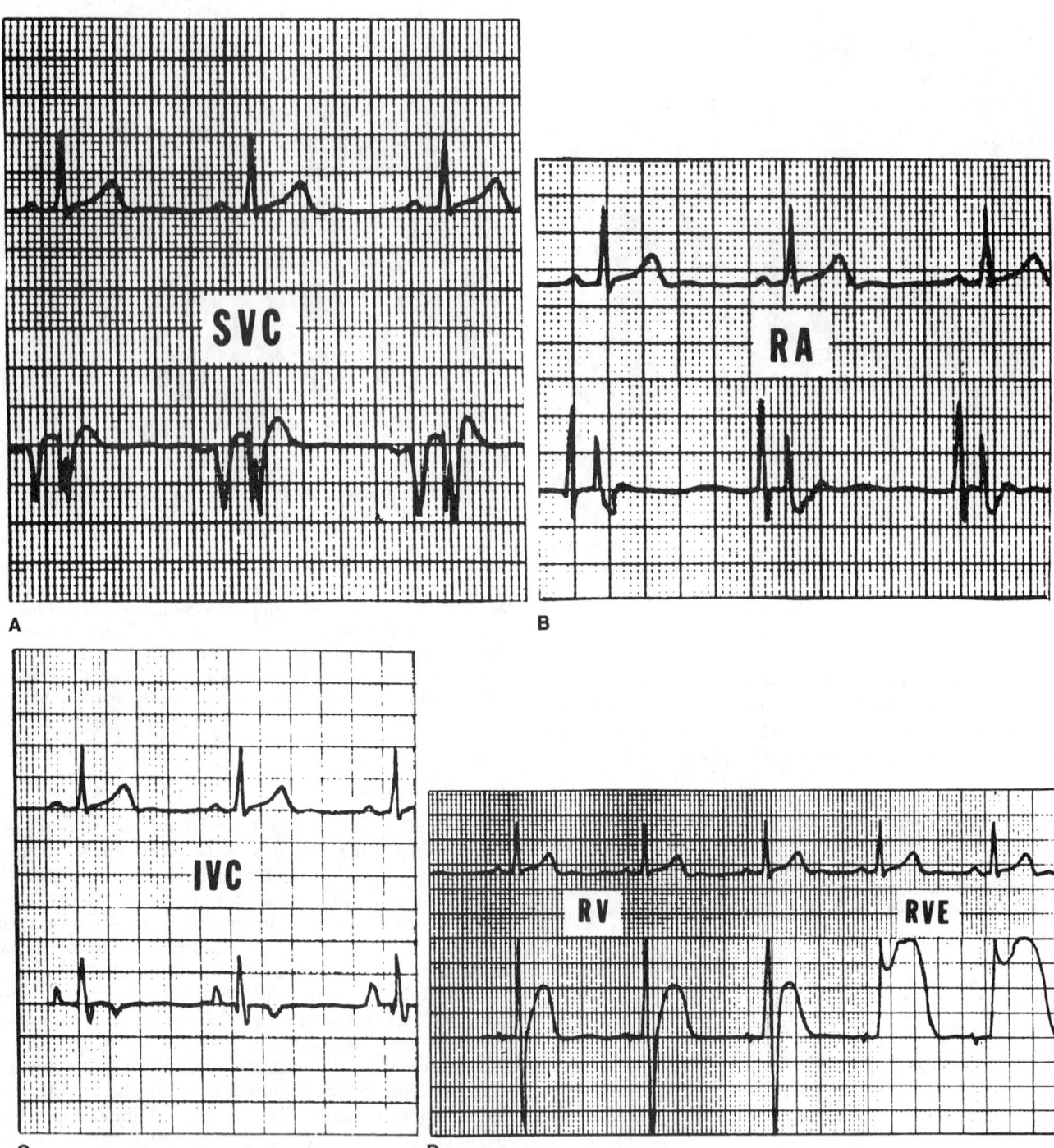

FIGURE 36-8. Electrocardiographic monitoring during electrode catheter positioning. A unipolar electrogram, obtained by attaching lead V_1 of the electrocardiographic machine to the distal pole of the electrode catheter, can be of use in positioning the catheter into the appropriate position. Using an electrocardiographic machine that can give simultaneous limb lead recordings is helpful to those unfamiliar with atrial and ventricular electrograms. (**A**) An electrogram obtained in the superior vena cava (SVC) shows a negative atrial deflection, whereas (**C**) in the inferior vena cava (IVC), the atrial electrogram is positive. (**B**) The deflections in the right atrium (RA) are more rapid, discrete, and larger than in either vena cava. (**D**) As the catheter is advanced into the right ventricle (RV), the ventricular electrogram is much larger and the atrial electrogram barely detectable. When the electrode catheter is against the right ventricular endocardium (RVE), ST segment elevation is seen (**D**, last two complexes).

catheter touches the right ventricular wall, ST segment elevation is seen. A simultaneously recorded limb lead provides an easy reference for recognition of the atrial and ventricular electrograms.

A variety of new electrode catheters are available for atrial pacing. Catheters with several electrodes positioned 10 to 20 cm proximal to the distal-tip electrodes have been designed (see Fig. 36-5A). These electrodes are positioned to lie along the lateral right atrial wall, allowing atrial sensing and pacing. An innovative modification of this technique allows for a small atrial J wire to be placed through an opening in the right atrium in a catheter with distal electrodes already positioned in the right ventricular apex (see Fig. 36-5B). Both of these types of catheter adaptations have been developed to allow a "one venous stick" approach to AV pacing. However, the atrial electrodes provided by these catheters often do not reliably pace the atrium. Therefore, in patients with significant right ventricular or large anterior MIs who require pacing and need AV synchronous pacing, a second electrode catheter should be placed in the atrium. A preformed J-shaped electrode catheter has been developed for transvenous temporary right atrial pacing (see Fig. 36-6).

Pacing and Sensing Threshold Determinations

After obtaining good anatomic positioning of the pacemaker catheter electrode, a stimulation threshold should be determined. With continuous electrocardiographic monitoring, pacing should begin at a rate at least 10 beats per minute faster than the patient's intrinsic heart rate with the output set at 5 mA. The output of the pacemaker is gradually decreased until the stimuli fail to produce ventricular (or atrial) capture. The milliampere current setting at which capture fails to occur is called the pacing threshold and should be less than 1 mA. The pacemaker output should be set at three to five times the pacing threshold.

If the pacemaker is to be used in a demand mode, it is also important that there is adequate sensing of the endocardial electrogram. To ensure good sensing, the pacing rate is set slower than the patient's intrinsic rate, and the sensitivity of the pulse generator is set at its most sensitive level and then is decreased (higher numbers) gradually. The setting at which the pacemaker fails to sense and begins pacing competitively with the patient's intrinsic rhythm is the sensing threshold. For demand pacing, the sensitivity should be set at a more sensitive level (lower number) than the sensing threshold.

Postinsertion Care

The electrode catheter and its introducer should be secured to the skin. Standard bandaging techniques may be followed. Coiling the proximal electrode catheter around the insertion site and firmly taping to the skin prevents inadvertent dislodgement of the distal electrode catheter. An extension cable should be used to connect the catheter electrode pins to the pulse generator. The pulse generator should be secured to the bed and not to the patient. The plastic shield provided with the pulse generator should be slipped over its controls to prevent accidental control movement. Covering of the entire pacemaker unit (including shield) with a plastic see-through glove prevents exposure of the generator to liquids.

A portable chest radiograph should be obtained to ensure proper positioning of the electrode catheter and to exclude complications, particularly pneumothorax. A baseline 12-lead ECG should be obtained to document the QRS morphologic features with the electrode catheter in proper position. A change in the morphology of the paced QRS may be the first sign of electrode displacement. Continuous telemetry monitoring of the patient is imperative.

Daily evaluation should include inspection of the entry site, cardiac auscultation, threshold determinations, and evaluation of intrinsic rhythm. Complications of the pacemaker often can be determined by auscultation. For example, a pericardial friction rub may indicate ventricular penetration, and a clicking sound may imply intercostal muscle stimulation. Marked changes in thresholds may occur with catheter movement or perforation, requiring catheter repositioning. Any significant changes should be evaluated with an ECG and chest roentgenogram. The intrinsic rhythm can be evaluated by reducing the rate of the pacemaker until the underlying rhythm emerges.

TRANSTHORACIC PACING

Although the transthoracic approach (Fig. 36-9) has been used successfully on many occasions, it is uncommon that temporary pacing is of such an acute need that the risk of this procedure is warranted.[14] This seems especially true since the introduction of effective noninvasive temporary cardiac pacing. When required, the approach can be made from the precordium or from the subxiphoid region. When using the precordial approach, a needle and stylet are inserted in the fourth intercostal space along the upper rib margin, near the left margin of the sternum. The needle is held perpendicular to the chest wall. With the subxiphoid approach, the needle and stylet are inserted below the xiphoid at a 45-degree angle to the chest wall and are directed toward the left shoulder. Connecting the stylet and needle

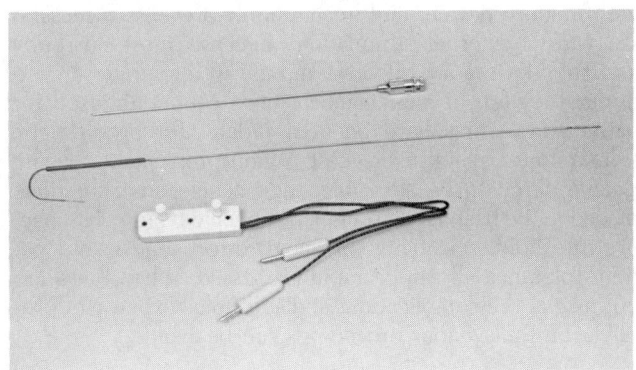

FIGURE 36-9. Transthoracic temporary pacing. Transthoracic pacing "kits" are provided, supplying a needle with stylette (*top*), pacing electrode (*middle*), and electrode connector (*bottom*). The transthoracic approach is rarely indicated, especially since the introduction of the external noninvasive pacing (see Fig. 36-10).

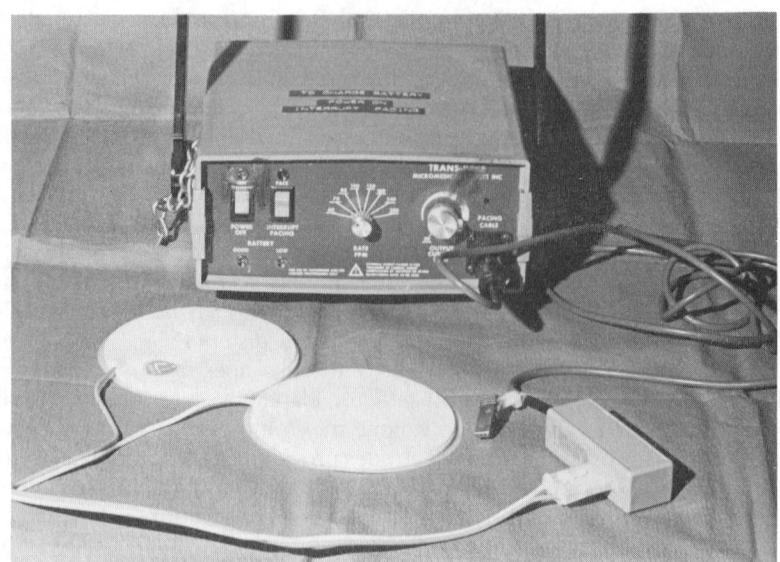

FIGURE 36-10. External noninvasive pacing. Large electrode patches are attached to the anterior and posterior chest walls, and the output is adjusted upward to obtain ventricular capture. Technically effective pacing can be obtained in nearly 80% of patients; however, patient discomfort can limit long-term use.

to the V_1 lead of a standard electrocardiograph provides a current of injury pattern on penetration of the right ventricular wall, providing that there is not complete ventricular asystole. Removal of the stylet and aspiration of blood verifies intracardiac positioning. The pacing catheter is then passed through the needle, the needle is removed, and the electrodes are connected to a standard pacing box. There are several severe potential complications, including pneumothorax, coronary artery perforation, mediastinal bleeding, and cardiac tamponade. This approach should be used only when other pacing options are not available.

EXTERNAL NONINVASIVE APPROACH

External transcutaneous pacing was first attempted in the 1950s, before other pacing techniques were developed. Modifications have been made regularly in the available devices with resultant good stimulation thresholds, patient comfort, and stimulation effectiveness (Fig. 36-10).[15] Pectoral muscle stimulation is common but is usually tolerable with modern devices and uncommonly prevents successful short-term external stimulation. Because most currently available devices are effective and are well tolerated by patients, they are becoming much more commonly used for patients who may have been candidates for prophylactic transvenous pacing in the past. When prophylactic pacing is considered to be advisable, the pacing pads should be placed and a trial of transcutaneous pacing begun. The pacing threshold, sensitivity threshold, effectiveness, and patient tolerance all can be rapidly assessed. When these are optimized, the complications and additional expense of prophylactic transvenous procedures can be avoided.

REFERENCES ∎

1. Zipes DP, Duffin EG: Cardiac pacemakers. In: Braunwald E (ed). *Heart Disease*. Philadelphia, WB Saunders, 1984:744

2. Langendorf R, Pick A: Atrioventricular block type II (Mobitz): its nature and clinical significance. *Circulation* 1968;38:819
3. Atkins J, Leshin S, Blomqvist G, et al: Ventricular conduction blocks and sudden death in acute myocardial infarction. *N Engl J Med* 1973;288:281
4. Nimitz A, Shubrooks S, Hutter A, et al: The significance of bundle branch block during acute myocardial infarction. *Am Heart J* 1975;90:439
5. Hindman MD, Wagner GS, JaRo M, et al: The clinical significance of bundle branch block complicating acute myocardial infarction. II. Indications for temporary and permanent pacemaker therapy. *Circulation* 1978;58:689
6. Batchelder J, Zipes DP: Treatment of tachyarrhythmias by pacing. *Arch Intern Med* 1975;135:1115
7. Schnitzler RN, Caracta AR, Damato AN: "Floating" catheter for temporary transvenous ventricular pacing. *Am J Cardiol* 1973;31:351
8. Bilitch M, Berens SC: Insertion techniques and electrode placement. In: *Temporary Transvenous Cardiac Pacing: A Clinical Update*. Pro Clinica, 1981:14
9. Rosenberg AS, Grossman JI, Escher DJW, et al: Bedside transvenous cardiac pacing. *Am Heart J* 1969;77:697
10. Rao G, Zikria EA: Technique of insertion of pacing electrode through the internal jugular vein. *J Cardiovasc Surg* 1973; 14:294
11. Killip T, Kimball JT: Percutaneous techniques for introducing flexible electrodes for intracardiac pacing. *Ann NY Acad Sci* 1969;167:597
12. Weinstein J, Gnoj J, Mazzarra JT, et al: Temporary transvenous pacing via the percutaneous femoral vein approach: a prospective study of 100 cases. *Am Heart J* 1973;85:695
13. Littleford PO, Pepine CJ: A new temporary atrial pacing catheter inserted percutaneously into the subclavian vein without fluoroscopy: a preliminary report. *Pace* 1981;4:458
14. Roberts R: Emergency transthoracic pacemaker: review. *Ann Emerg Med* 1981;10:600
15. Zoll PM, Zoll RH, Falk RH, et al: External non-invasive temporary cardiac pacing: clinical trials. *Circulation* 1985;71: 937

Critical Care, Third Edition, edited by Joseph M. Civetta,
Robert W. Taylor, and Robert R. Kirby.
Lippincott-Raven Publishers, Philadelphia, PA © 1997.

CHAPTER 37

Important Intensive Care Unit Procedures

Neil S. Yeston
Richard L. Grotz
Laurie A. Loiacono

This chapter describes and discusses diagnostic and therapeutic procedures commonly performed in the intensive care unit (ICU). In general, attention to anatomic detail and sterile technique yields favorable results with minimal complications. The following methods for thoracentesis, tube thoracostomy, Heimlich catheter placement, peritoneal lavage, paracentesis, intraabdominal pressure measurement, cardioversion and defibrillation, venous cutdown, pericardiocentesis, and transtracheal aspiration are safe and effective.

THORACENTESIS

The pleural cavity normally is a potential space between the visceral and parietal pleura of the lung. The pleura respond to various disease processes with an outpouring of fluid, resulting in a pleural effusion.

The diagnosis of pleural fluid can be made during physical examination. Percussion dullness, reduced or absent breath sounds, and reduced transmission of whispered voice are usual findings. Grocco's triangle, or the presence of a triangle of dullness on the contralateral hemithorax, is caused by the bulging of fluid into the posterior mediastinal pleura and is considered pathognomonic of pleural effusion.[1] Characteristic radiographic findings include a partial or complete opacification of the hemithorax, which usually layers out on lateral decubitus projections. Computed tomography and ultrasonography are often helpful in diagnosing and localizing free or loculated pleural effusions.

Thoracentesis can be diagnostic (i.e., differentiate an exudate from a transudate) or therapeutic (i.e., when drainage of a restrictive effusion relieves respiratory compromise).

PROCEDURE

The diaphragm inserts along the thorax at approximately the level of the eighth ribs anteriorly, tenth ribs laterally, and the 12th ribs posteriorly.

> *Posterior Approach:* The patient is placed in the sitting position with the arms supported on a bedside table (Fig. 37-1).
>
> *Posterolateral Approach:* If sitting is impossible, a supine position with the head of the bed elevated as close to a 90-degree angle as possible may be used. Thoracentesis is approached along the posterior axillary line.

The level of thoracentesis should be one or two interspaces below the percussed fluid level but not lower than the eighth intercostal space. Count the ribs downward from the second rib anteriorly and upward from the 12th rib posteriorly. Prepare the skin with povidone-iodine (Betadine) and create a sterile field with drapes. Administer local anesthesia with a 25-gauge needle and 1% lidocaine, creating a skin wheal and then penetrating into the subcutaneous tissues. The total volume of lidocaine should not exceed 4.5

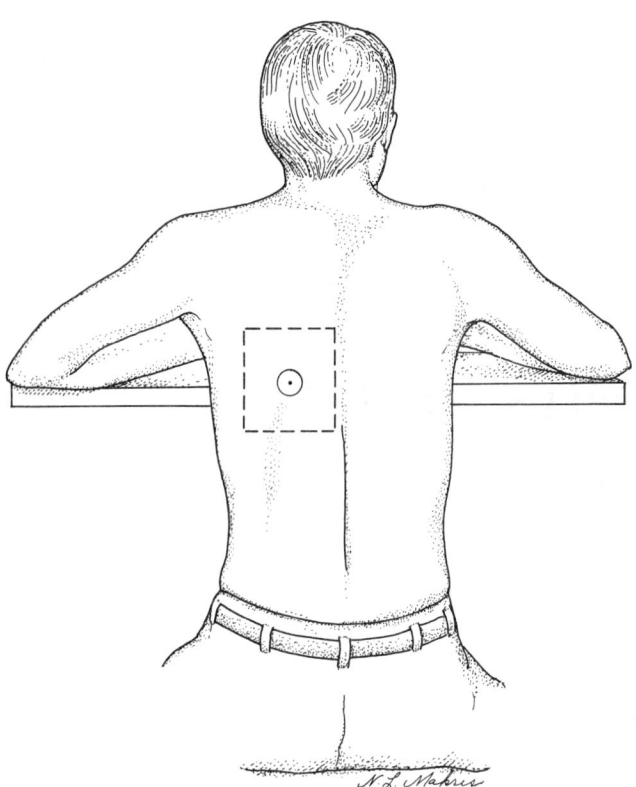

FIGURE 37-1. The patient is placed in the sitting position with the arms supported on a bedside table.

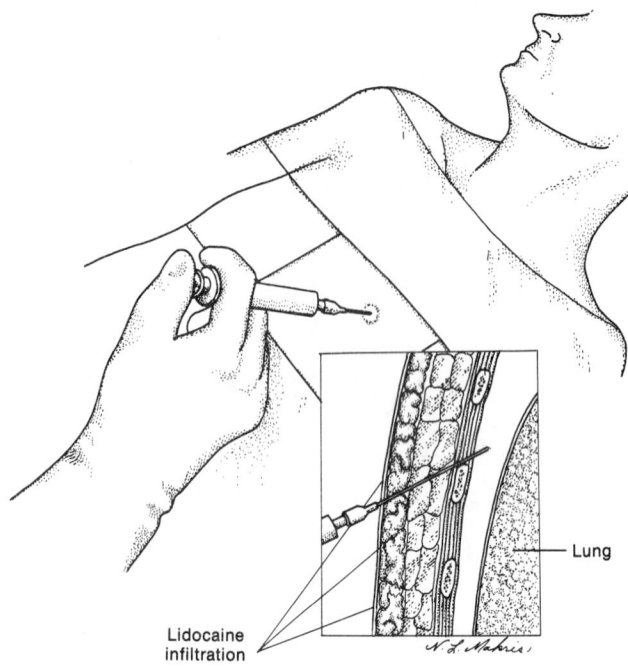

FIGURE 37-2. Inject the local anesthetic and aspirate to confirm the presence of fluid. Mark the needle depth with a Kelly clamp.

mg/kg (without epinephrine) or 7 mg/kg (with epinephrine). Use a 20-gauge needle to anesthetize the deeper tissues. Inject the local anesthetic over and along the periosteum of the middle of the rib. "Walk" the needle up and over the superior margin of the rib to avoid the more inferior neurovascular bundle. Aspirate frequently to avoid intravascular infusion of lidocaine. Infiltrate generously through the pleura (a "pop" may be felt when the pleura has been entered). At this point, the patient may complain of some discomfort. Aspirate to confirm the presence of fluid, mark the needle depth with a clamp, and withdraw the needle (Fig. 37-2).

A pleural effusion can be drained by thoracentesis using several different methods. One method uses a catheter within a needle (i.e., Deseret Intracath, 14-gauge needle, 16-gauge/8-inch catheter)[2] (Fig. 37-3). Place a 10-mL non–Luer-lock syringe on an Intracath needle. Mark the needle depth with a second clamp to prevent excess penetration, and insert it with the bevel downward. Remove the syringe, occlude the needle with a finger to avoid creating a pneumothorax, and insert the catheter into the needle. During expiration, advance the catheter into the pleural space, then slide the needle back over it. Never pull the catheter back through the needle because it may be sheared. A three-way stopcock may be attached so that the pleural fluid can be withdrawn into the syringe and injected into intravenous (IV) tubing connected to a sterile container[3] (Fig. 37-4). Alternatively, a vacuum bottle can be used for a rapid, effi-

cient method of collection (Fig. 37-5). The catheter is connected to clamped IV tubing attached to a vacuum bottle, after which the tubing clamp is released.

An 18- or 20-gauge needle within the catheter also can be used to perform thoracentesis. Attach the syringe to the hub of the needle and insert as previously discussed. When fluid returns, advance the catheter over the needle. Withdraw the needle and place a finger over the hub of the catheter. Evacuate the pleural effusion using the three-way stopcock or vacuum system as described earlier. Obtain a chest radiograph after completion of the procedure.

Fluid should be sent for blood cell count, Gram's stain, tuberculosis and fungal smears, culture (aerobic, anaerobic, fungal, and *Mycobacterium*), cytologic study and cell block, pH, and to determine levels of protein, glucose, lactate dehydrogenase (LDH), and amylase. Obtain samples for pH anaerobically and place them on ice.

Guidelines for examination of pleural fluid for infection, although variable, have been extensively evaluated. Most empyemas develop in patients with bacterial pneumonia. Up to 40% of patients with pneumonia have been noted to have a pleural effusion during the course of their illness.[4] A parapneumonic process should be considered in all patients with bacterial pneumonia in whom the posterior costophrenic angle is obliterated on a chest radiograph.[5] If an effusion is documented on the lateral decubitus radiograph, perform a diagnostic thoracentesis.

The effusion is considered an exudate if the pleural LDH/serum LDH is more than 0.6[6] and the pleural protein/serum protein ratio is more than 0.5. Diagnostic criteria of an empyema generally include the presence of frank pus; organisms present on Gram stain[5]; and pleural fluid glucose less

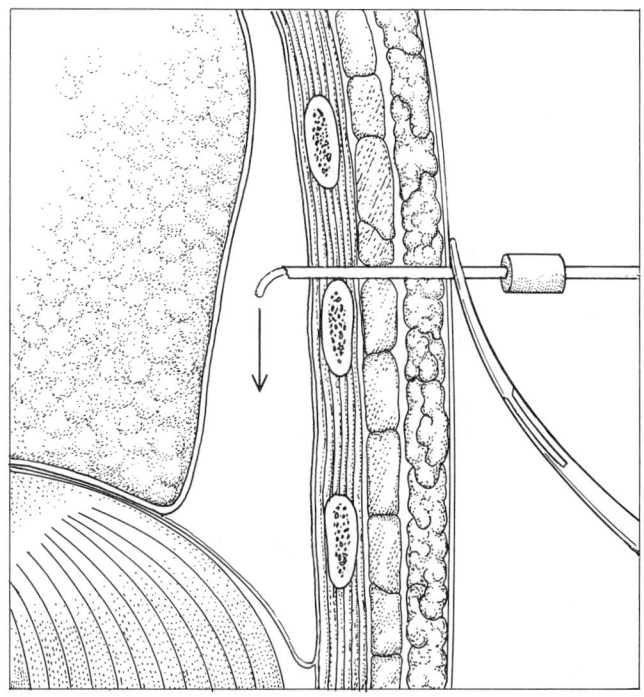

A

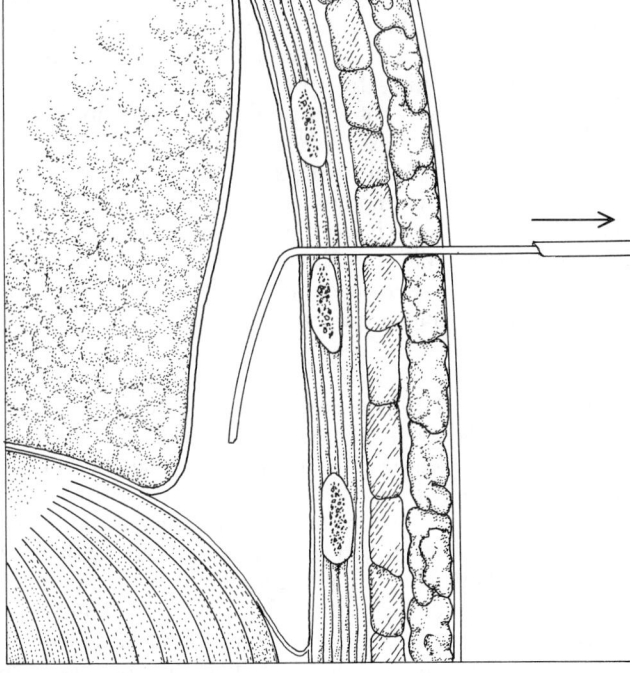

B

FIGURE 37-3. (**A**) Insert the thoracentesis needle. Advance the cannula into the pleural space during expiration. (**B**) Slide the needle back over the catheter.

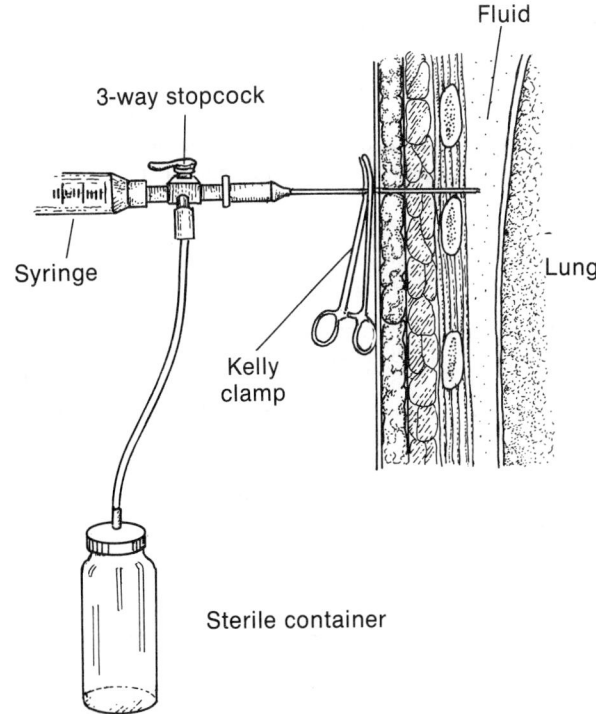

FIGURE 37-4. A three-way stopcock may be attached so the pleural fluid can be withdrawn into the syringe. The fluid is then injected into intravenous tubing connected to a sterile container.

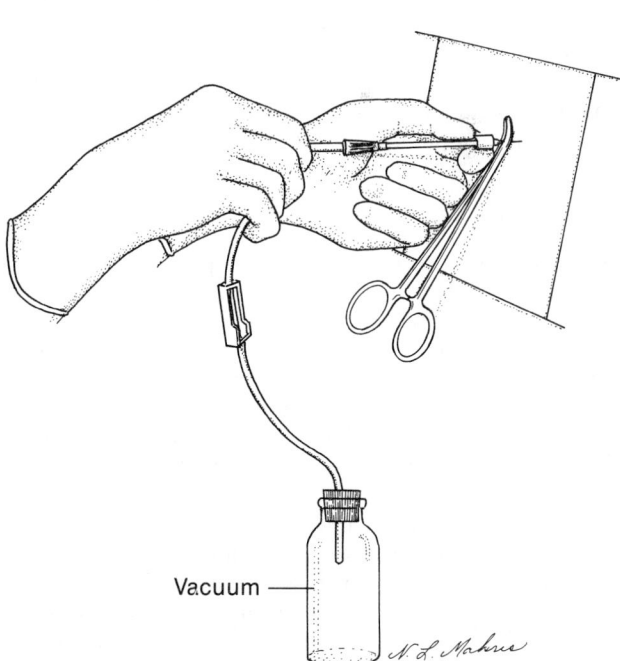

FIGURE 37-5. A vacuum bottle can be used for rapid, efficient collection.

than 40 mg/dL, pleural fluid pH less than 7.20, or both.[7] The pleural fluid pH generally falls before the pleural glucose.[8,9] Patients with tuberculosis and rheumatoid or malignant effusions may have a low pleural fluid pH.[8] Thus, pH alone is unreliable in determining the presence of empyema. Early initiation of tube thoracostomy is recommended for therapy of an empyema, because it becomes more loculated with time.[5,10]

COMPLICATIONS

Complications of thoracentesis include pneumothorax, hemothorax, and hepatic or splenic punctures. The incidence of pneumothorax is 3% to 20%[11,12] and is less likely if the effusion is not completely drained.[13] No more than 1000 to 1500 mL are initially removed to prevent reexpansion pulmonary edema and hypotension.[14] Contraindications to thoracentesis include bleeding diathesis and lack of patient cooperation.[15]

TUBE THORACOSTOMY ■

Closed-tube thoracostomy, or chest tube drainage, was first described by Hewett in 1876[16] but did not become commonplace until World War II.[17] Although variations have developed in technique and indications, the basic principles remain the same.

INDICATIONS

Indications for tube thoracostomy include the need to remove air or liquid (blood, effusion, chyle, and pus) from the pleural space or to instill chemotherapeutic agents after removal of malignant effusions. Prophylactic chest tubes are inserted in patients with penetrating thoracic injuries or multiple rib fractures before nonthoracic surgery, even without evidence of pneumothorax.

Pneumothorax

SPONTANEOUS OR TRAUMATIC. A pneumothorax is the most common indication for chest tube placement.[18] Spontaneous pneumothoraces are most commonly seen in men with tall, slender builds[19] and are thought to result from rupture of fragile, small subpleural blebs.[20] Traumatic pneumothoraces, both penetrating and nonpenetrating, are usually associated with some degree of hemothorax.[21,22] Pneumothoraces caused by blunt trauma are almost always associated with rib fractures.[21]

Minimal respiratory embarrassment may be present in patients with spontaneous or traumatic pneumothorax, but the diagnosis is rarely made incidentally. The history of spontaneous pneumothorax may include sudden onset of pleuritic chest pain. Usual clinical signs include diminished breath sounds, hyperresonance to percussion (most diagnostic), tracheal deviation, and tachypnea.[21] A chest radiograph is required to rule out a minor pneumothorax, usually best seen on an upright view taken during expiration[21,23]; however, the chest radiograph does not take priority over deteriorating clinical signs, and tube thoracostomy should be performed without radiographic confirmation if a pneumothorax is suspected in a patient with worsening respiratory distress.

A minimal pneumothorax, defined as less than 25% total collapse (less than 4-cm apical collapse, or less than 1-cm lateral collapse), may be observed without treatment, providing the patient will not require positive-pressure ventilation. Reabsorption of air occurs at the rate of about 1.25% of the lung volume per day.[24] Resorption rate may be increased through the use of supplemental oxygen therapy.[25] Unfortunately, estimates of the size of the pneumothorax are neither accurate nor reproducible.[26,27] Consideration of tube thoracostomy is then dependent on increase in the size of the pneumothorax and respiratory embarrassment.

TENSION. A tension pneumothorax results when the communication between the lung parenchyma and the pleural cavity acts as a one-way valve, allowing air to enter the cavity during inspiration but not to exit during expiration. Air builds up in the pleural space under pressure, the diaphragm flattens, and the mediastinum shifts to the opposite side.[28] The trachea is shifted to the side opposite the tension, and little or no air movement is auscultated on the affected side. Jugular venous distension and arterial hypotension develop. While the contralateral lung and great vessels become compressed, ventilation and venous return are compromised, leading to hypoxia and circulatory collapse.[21,29] Conscious patients may become extremely dyspneic and cyanotic. Mechanically ventilated patients present initially with sudden increases in airway pressures[30] and later with hemodynamic compromise. The diagnosis is usually apparent in advanced cases of tension pneumothorax and represents a life-threatening emergency for which immediate treatment is required. A large-bore needle–catheter assembly may be placed in the second intercostal space anteriorly to decompress the pleural space while preparing to perform a tube thoracostomy.[21]

IATROGENIC. Iatrogenic causes of pneumothorax have increased with the advent of mechanical ventilation and central venous catheterization. The incidence of pneumothorax in patients who are mechanically ventilated is 3% to 4% and approaches 23% in those treated with mechanical ventilation and end-expiratory pressure.[31,32] Tension pneumothorax is present in 50% of ventilator-associated pneumothoraces. Subclavian vein catheterization has a 3% to 6% incidence of pneumothorax.[33,34] Many other procedures have been noticed to cause pneumothoraces, including thoracentesis, pleural biopsy, pulmonary artery catheterization,[35] invasive cardiac electrophysiologic procedures,[36] cardiopulmonary resuscitation (CPR), unusual gastroduodenal feeding tube placement,[37] esophageal obturator airways,[38] nerve conduction studies,[34] colonoscopy,[39] esophagoscopy,[40] acupuncture,[41] and aspiration of breast cysts.[42]

Pneumothorax also has been observed in patients who are IV drug abusers[43] and generally results from attempted central vein injection. Pneumothorax secondary to "free-base" cocaine use[44,45] that required deep inspiration and Valsalva maneuver has also been reported.

Hemothorax

Most cases of traumatic hemothorax can be managed with tube thoracostomy alone. A large-caliber chest tube is needed (32 to 40 French) along with −20 cm H_2O of suction. Intrathoracic bleeding usually stops spontaneously with simple reexpansion of the lung because of the low-pressure pulmonary vascular system.[46,47] The hemothorax must be completely drained; failure to do so can result in fibrothorax and significant impairment of respiratory function. Recommendations for a clotted hemothorax include a limited thoracotomy for evacuation.[48]

Persistent bleeding is an indication for open thoracotomy, although guidelines vary regarding specific volumes of blood loss. The amount of the initial blood loss with insertion of tube thoracostomy and evidence of continued bleeding are included in most formulas. Siemens and associates[49] recommend open thoracotomy for an initial blood loss of more than 800 mL or for hypotension on presentation (systolic blood pressure less than 90 mm Hg). Others use an initial blood loss of 1000 to 1500 mL and continued loss of at least 150 to 200 mL/hour for longer than 4 hours as an indication for thoracotomy.[50-54] Autotransfusion is available for massive hemothorax after traumatic injury[55,56] or after open heart surgery using sterile collection devices.[57]

Chylothorax

Chylothorax is the accumulation of lymphatic fluid in the pleural space. The problem is uncommon and usually related to trauma or malignant disease.[29,58] Filariasis, tuberculosis, and subclavian vein obstruction also are associated with chylothorax.[59] Lymphosarcoma is the most common malignancy associated with chylothorax, followed by metastatic disease and bronchogenic carcinoma.[59] Chylothorax usually does not resolve spontaneously, and its presence rarely requires emergency action. Treatment includes repeated thoracentesis or tube thoracostomy and dietary restriction with enteral replacement of medium-chain triglycerides.[60] Thoracotomy and ligation of the thoracic duct are indicated if more conservative measures fail. Pleuroperitoneal shunts also have been successfully used for chylothorax.[61]

PROCEDURE

Place the patient in the supine position with the arm abducted to 90 degrees. The preferred site for placement of the chest tube is the fourth or fifth intercostal space in the anterior axillary line. An alternate site is the second or third intercostal space in the midclavicular line, but this approach is useful only when pneumothorax is present (Fig. 37-6). Prepare the skin with povidine-iodine solution and create a sterile field with drapes. Measure the chest tube from the lateral chest wall to the apex and mark it with a suture tied at the estimated intrathoracic distance. Local anesthesia with

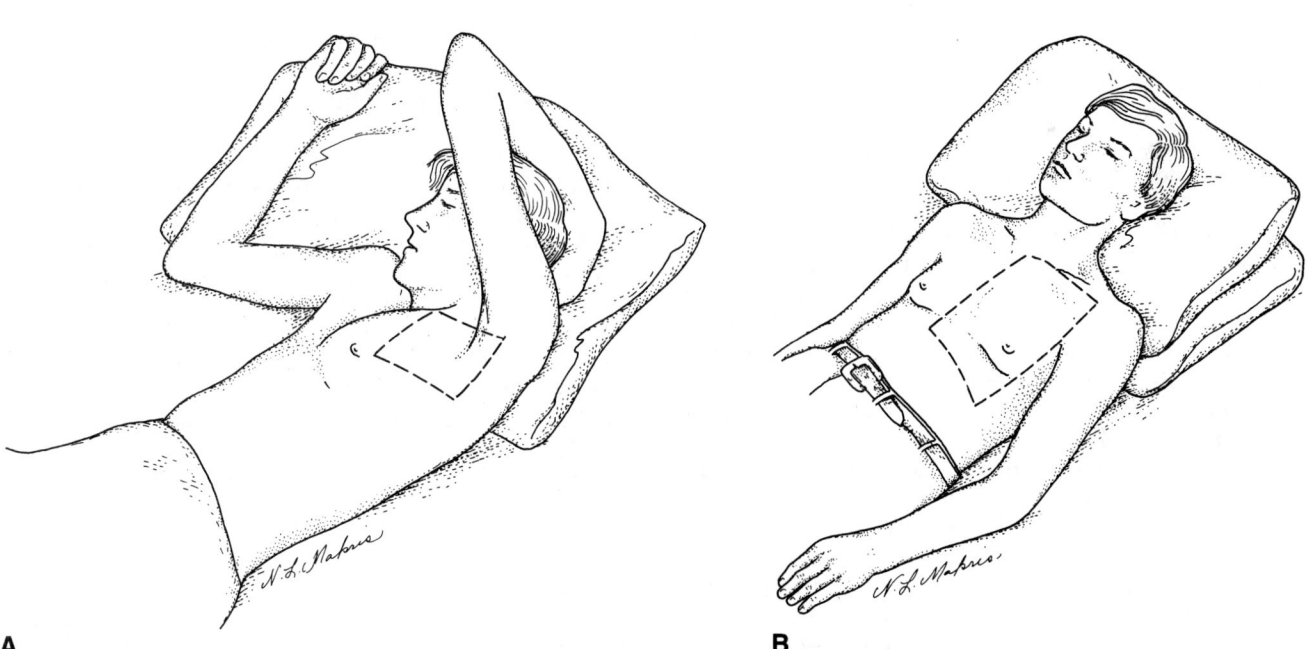

A   **B**

FIGURE 37-6. (**A**) The preferred site for placement of the chest tube is the fourth or fifth intercostal space in the midclavicular line. (**B**) The second or third intercostal space is an alternate site for thoracostomy when pneumothorax alone is present.

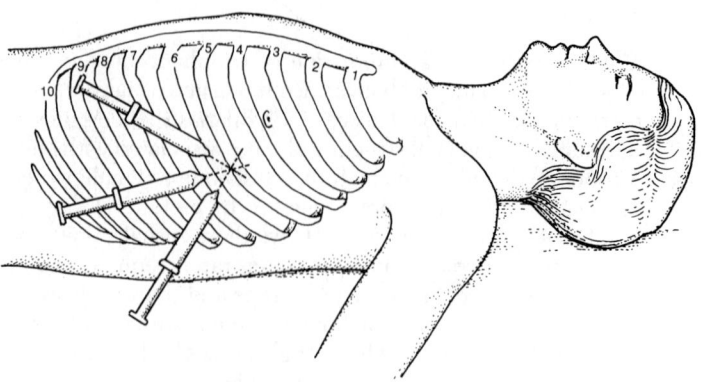

FIGURE 37-7. Local anesthesia should include the skin, subcutaneous tissue, intercostal muscles, periosteum, and pleura.

1% lidocaine using a 25-gauge needle should include the skin, subcutaneous tissue, intercostal muscles, periosteum, and pleura (Fig. 37-7).

Make a 2-cm incision in the anterior axillary line in the midportion of the rib just inferior to the interspace that the tube will traverse. Do not enter the space from the midaxillary to posterior axillary line because the patient will lie on the tube, causing discomfort and kinking.

Fashion a subcutaneous tunnel with blunt dissection using a Kelly clamp; the trocar method is not recommended. Entry into the pleural space is just over the superior margin of the lower rib to avoid injury to the neurovascular bundle (Fig. 37-8). Slipping over the superior margin of that rib, bluntly perforate the pleura with a Kelly clamp (Fig. 37-9). Once the instrument has entered the pleural cavity, open the pleura about 1 cm by spreading the handles of the Kelly clamp. As the pleura is entered, a "gush" of air may be heard if a tension pneumothorax was present.

Place a gloved finger into the pleural space to confirm thoracic penetration. Palpate the lung medially (Fig. 37-10). If unable to confirm thoracic penetration, consider intraabdominal penetration. Using the gloved finger, sweep away any intrapleural adhesions, which opens the intrapleural space and allows safe entrance of the chest tube. Grasp the tip of the thoracostomy tube with a Kelly clamp and direct it into the pleural space posteriorly and superiorly (Fig. 37-11) to aspirate a pneumothorax or posteriorly and inferiorly to drain fluid. Care should be taken not to introduce the catheter along the subcutaneous tissue outside the chest wall. Place the tube deeply enough so that the last hole in the catheter is well inside the pleural space and not in the subcutaneous tissue, thereby avoiding the development of subcutaneous emphysema.

The catheter is connected to a standard collection apparatus that has a high-volume flow, adjustable level of suction, and an underwater seal with a compartment for accurately measuring liquid that drains from the chest tube. A heavy nonabsorbable suture, such as O silk, is used to secure the chest tube to the skin. The wound is dressed with petrolatum gauze, 4 × 4 sterile gauze, and elastic bandage or heavy tape. All connection sites are taped together and secured to the patient's abdomen. Obtain a chest radiograph to evaluate tube placement and function. Never clamp the chest tube during transportation because a tension pneumothorax may develop. Two chest tubes may be needed if a massive air leak or residual intrathoracic fluid is present after single chest tube insertion.

CHEST TUBE CARE

A chest tube should not be advanced further into the pleural cavity after the procedure has been completed, but the tube can be withdrawn, with care taken not to expose the drainage holes. A new site is necessary if a new tube must be inserted. The tube should not be clamped during transportation but left on water seal. Moreover, the drainage system should not be placed higher than the thorax. Movement of the fluid column with respiration is evidence for chest tube function. If respiratory variation is not present, the tube should be removed or replaced.

SUGGESTIONS

In the absence of a formal pleural fluid collection system, an emergency one-way valve can be constructed by tying a rubber glove over the external end of the chest tube and cutting a small hole in the end of a glove finger. This apparatus functions as a one-way exit valve, providing temporary control of a simple or tension pneumothorax. A Penrose drain can be used in similar fashion.

The Heimlich valve, a one-way flutter valve placed at the distal end of the chest tube, was first developed in 1968 and used successfully in Vietnam and Israel.[20] Although designed for emergency treatment, the valve is used in selected patients for the outpatient management of spontaneous pneumothorax.[25,62] The major drawback of this approach is the inability of the valve to keep the lung expanded in the face of a persistent air leak. Even in carefully selected patients, outpatient management fails in 25% of cases.[63]

COMPLICATIONS

Bleeding

Technical complications associated with insertion of chest tubes approach 1% when performed by experienced physicians.[64] Bleeding is generally caused by the inadvertent laceration of an intercostal or internal mammary vessel.[64] This complication can be prevented if care is taken to guide the instruments along the superior edge of the rib, avoiding the

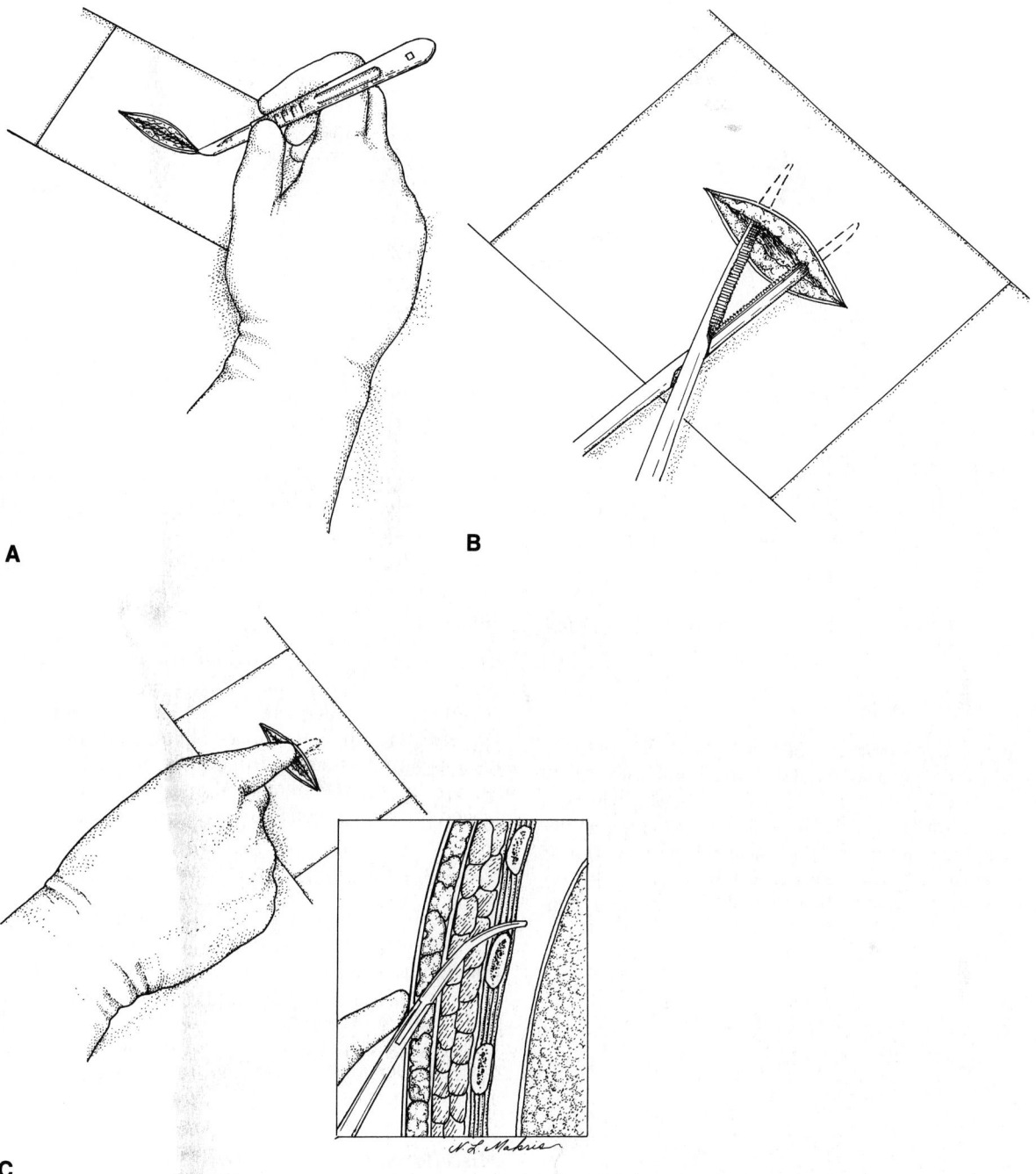

FIGURE 37-8. (**A**) A 2-cm incision is made in the anterior axillary line, just inferior to the rib that the tube will traverse. (**B**) A subcutaneous tunnel is fashioned with a Kelly clamp. (**C**) The entrance point into the pleural space should be just over the superior margin of the upper rib.

intercostal vessels, and by placing the anterior chest tube no closer to the sternum than the midclavicular line. Intercostal and long thoracic nerve injury is prevented by careful blunt dissection.[14] Laceration of the lung can be avoided by grasping the clamp used to puncture the pleura so that the distance from hand to tip is just greater than the chest wall thickness.[65] Finding the proper tract with finger exploration will prevent improper placement of the tube. Ectopic placement of the chest tube into the lung parenchyma, heart, or abdominal viscera is rare but more commonly seen with the use of a trocar for insertion.[63] Chest tube occlusion can be prevented by stripping the tube hourly and ensuring that

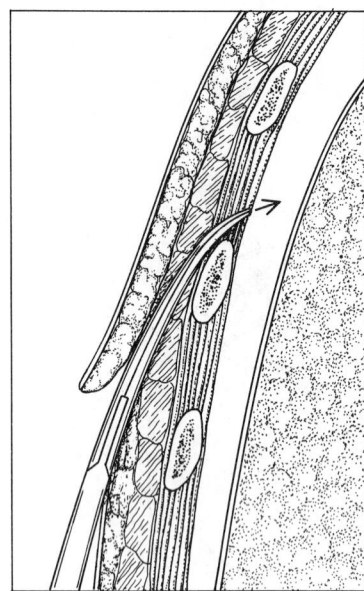

FIGURE 37-9. The pleural space is then entered using a Kelly clamp.

a large tube is used for either a hemothorax or viscous pleural effusion.[65]

Bronchopleural Fistula

Persistent pneumothorax can be caused by a large bronchopleural fistula and may require thoracotomy for surgical closure. In general, a continued massive air leak (diagnosed as inadequate lung reexpansion on a chest radiograph) despite two adequately functioning chest tubes on suction is an indication for early thoracotomy. Continued air leak after 1 week of treatment with a chest tube also may be an indication for thoracotomy.

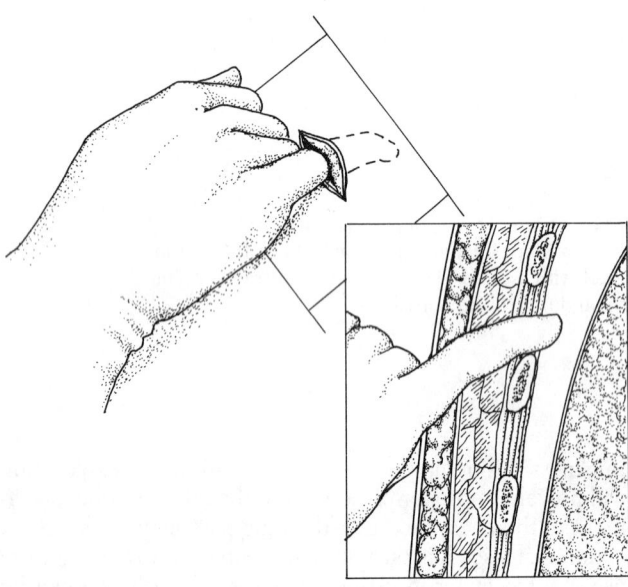

FIGURE 37-10. A gloved finger is placed into the pleural space, confirming thoracic penetration.

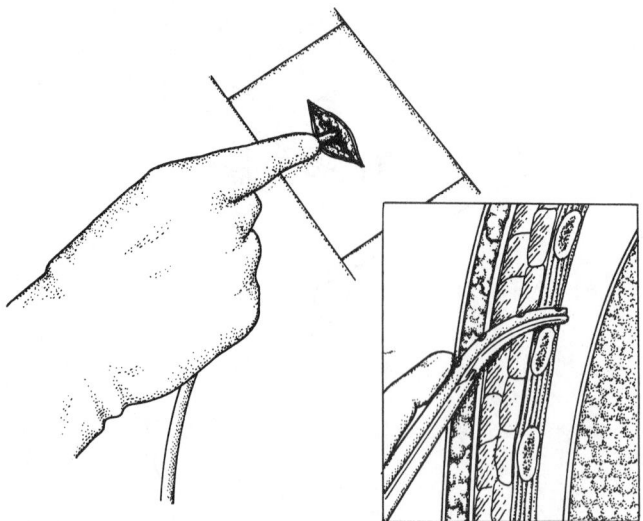

FIGURE 37-11. The tip of the thoracostomy tube is grasped with a Kelly clamp and directed into the pleural space posteriorly and superiorly.

Infection

The incidence of intrapleural infection is reported to be 1% to 16%[66–68]; however, most series report an incidence of less than 3%.[66] Adequate pleural drainage and pulmonary reexpansion with pleural space obliteration are important in preventing infection.[67,69] In general, prophylactic antibiotic therapy is not recommended for thoracostomy, whether placed for spontaneous pneumothorax or trauma.[70–72]

Recurrent Pneumothorax

Chest tube removal may result in recurrent pneumothorax, but the incidence is uncommon (2.4%).[73] Higher recurrent pneumothorax rates occur after traumatic chest injury.[69] The most common abnormality seen after removal of a chest tube is the presence of pleural thickening or pleural fluid. Occasional atelectasis may be seen on follow-up chest radiograph. Fibrothorax results from the inadequate drainage of a hemothorax.

Miscellaneous

Atelectasis from splinting secondary to pain at the chest tube insertion site is common and can be easily avoided when appropriate analgesia is provided.

Reexpansion pulmonary edema after tube thoracostomy usually presents 2 to 3 hours after insertion and may be avoided by gradual evacuation of pleural fluid.[14]

HEIMLICH CATHETER INSERTION   ■

Heimlich catheters are useful in elective circumstances associated with intrapleural fluid or air.[18] Advantages include ease of insertion with less patient discomfort,[74] low cost,[75] and greater freedom of movement.[76–78] Drawbacks include incomplete fluid and air evacuation, catheter malposition, kinking, and occlusion. Heimlich one-way valves can be substituted for the suction apparatus when a pneumothorax is treated, but they are more appropriate for outpatient management rather than the ICU.

PROCEDURE

The patient is positioned and a sterile site is prepared similar to that for tube thoracostomy. The skin, subcutaneous tissue, intercostal muscles, periosteum, and pleura are anesthetized with 1% lidocaine. A small skin incision is made, and a 16-gauge Teflon catheter with side holes is inserted using the inner trocar through the soft tissues above the superior margin of the rib. A pop is felt as the trocar and catheter pass through the pleura into the pleural space. The trocar is advanced no further. The catheter is advanced over the trocar into the pleural space, the trocar is removed, and the lumen of the catheter is occluded with a finger. Sterile IV connecting tubing with a three-way stopcock is attached to the hub of the catheter (the valve must be off to prevent air entry into the pleural space). The IV tubing is connected to the pleural drainage system, the valve is turned on, and wall suction is applied to the system. The catheter is sutured to the chest wall with a 2-0 silk and a sterile dressing is applied. Connections are secured with tape. A chest radiograph is outlined to verify catheter position and function.

An alternative approach is insertion without a trocar. A 14-gauge needle attached to a 10-mL syringe is inserted through the chest wall incision into the pleural cavity similar to the trocar method (Fig. 37-12A). Entry into the pleural space is verified by aspiration of fluid or air. The syringe is removed and the catheter lumen is occluded until a J-wire is inserted through the needle into the pleural space. The needle is removed, leaving the guidewire in place (see Fig. 37-12B). After the catheter is advanced over it (see Fig. 37-12C), the guidewire is removed and the catheter lumen is occluded until the connecting tubing is attached. The pleural drainage system is then connected, the catheter is secured to the chest wall, and a chest radiograph should be obtained.

CHEST TUBE BOTTLES ■

Although the three-bottle drainage system generally has been replaced by plastic portable units, the physical principles remain the same. The functioning chest drainage setup requires that the drainage tube from the chest be inserted beneath the level of water in a container. While the tubing is progressively submerged within the bottle, greater intrapleural pressure is needed to allow evacuation of the pleural contents. The usual distance is 1 to 2 cm under the surface[77] (Fig. 37-13). If the pressure in the chest rises above 1 to 2 cm H_2O, fluid or air will be evacuated. If the pressure within the chest falls below atmospheric pressure, fluid will be drawn up into the tube by an equivalent amount. The usual configuration of chest tube drainage systems is illustrated in Figure 37-14.

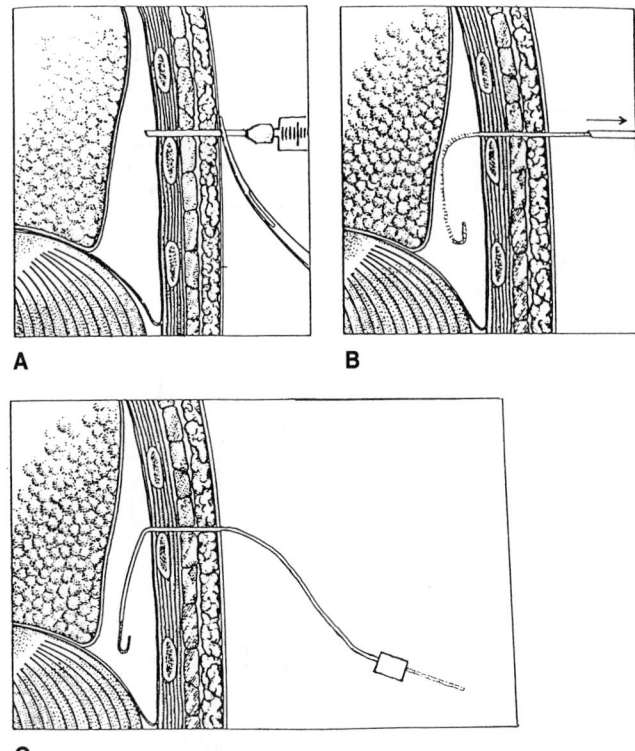

FIGURE 37-12. (**A**) Insert the needle into the pleural cavity. (**B**) The needle is removed after insertion of the J-wire. (**C**) The catheter is advanced over the wire.

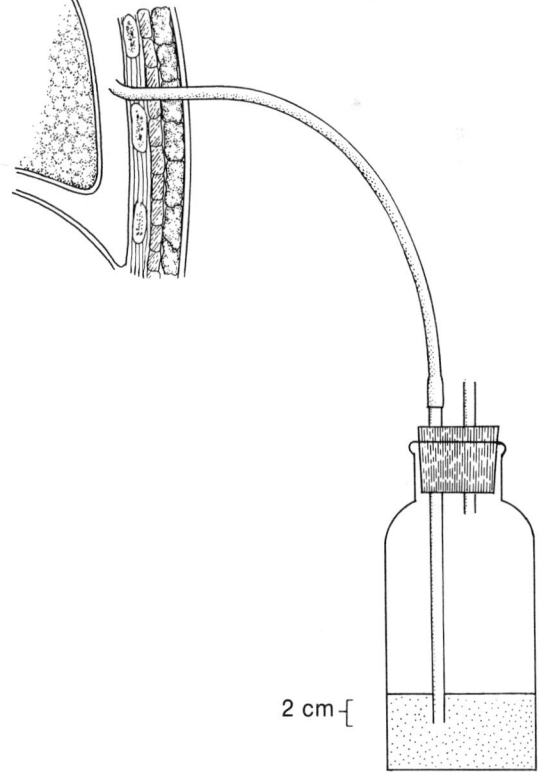

2 cm

FIGURE 37-13. Underwater seal drainage.

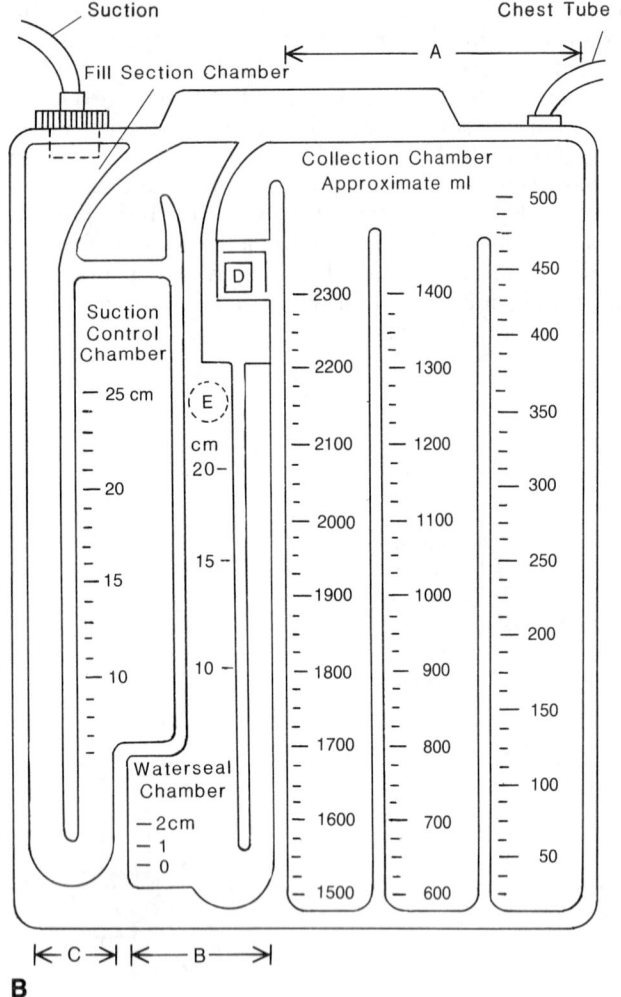

FIGURE 37-14. (**A**) Three bottle drainage system. (**B**) Portable unit embodying same principles of operation. Removal of the second and third bottles (**A**) leaves a simple water seal drainage system. The effective suction pressure is equal to the difference in levels of bottles 1 and 2. The third bottle serves as a trap.

PARACENTESIS

Diagnostic paracentesis often is used in patients with ascites. Particular attention is directed toward the patient with unexplained fever or leukocytosis who is thought to have spontaneous bacterial peritonitis.[79] Paracentesis is also recommended in patients with a rapid increase in ascitic fluid that was previously well controlled with medical therapy (diuretics and sodium restriction). Therapeutic paracentesis may be performed on patients with respiratory compromise caused by massive ascites.

Usual precautions in the performance of paracentesis include choosing an avascular site on the abdominal wall (preferably in the lower abdomen just lateral to the rectus abdominis muscle), correcting any underlying coagulopathy, and ensuring that the urinary bladder is well drained before the procedure.

PROCEDURE

Place the patient in the supine position. Confirm the presence of ascitic fluid at the site intended for paracentesis by physical examination (i.e., percussion). Ultrasound guidance also may be used. Prepare the skin with povidine-iodine and create a sterile field with drapes (Fig. 37-15). Using a 25-gauge needle, inject 1% lidocaine with epinephrine, first creating a skin wheal. Stretch the skin about 1 cm inferior to the point of the wheal (the z-track technique), which makes the needle track discontinuous and lessens the chance of an ascitic leak. Inject the lidocaine with a 21-gauge needle, first through the wheal, then through the fascia and peritoneum (a pop may be felt). Aspirate as the needle is advanced, stopping when ascitic fluid is returned. Remove the needle.

Next, advance a 20-gauge needle with the catheter attached to a 10-mL syringe through the anesthetized area. Aspirate continuously. When ascitic fluid is returned, advance the catheter over the needle. Remove the needle and connect a 50-mL syringe to the catheter. The catheter should not be pulled back over the needle because this action may

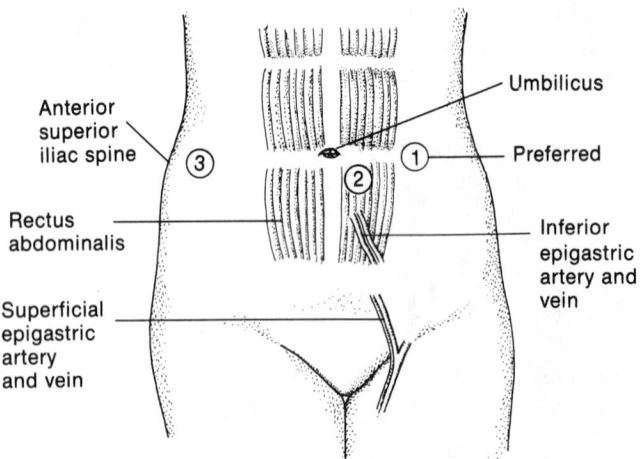

FIGURE 37-15. The preferred site for paracentesis is in the lower abdomen just lateral to the rectus abdominis muscle.

TABLE 37-1.   Ascitic Fluid Characteristics in Various Disease States

| | | | | CELL COUNT | | |
CONDITION	GROSS APPEARANCE	SPECIFIC GRAVITY	PROTEIN (g/dL)	Red Blood Cells (>10,000/mm³)	White Blood Cells (per mm³)	OTHER TESTS
Cirrhosis	Straw-colored or bile-stained	<1.016 (95%)°	<2.5 (95%)	1%	<250 (90%)°: predominantly endothelial	
Neoplasm	Straw-colored, hemorrhagic, mucinous, or chylous	Variable, >1.016 (45%)	>2.5 (75%)	20%	>1000 (50%): variable cell types	Cytology, cell block, peritoneal biopsy
Tuberculous peritonitis	Clear, turbid, hemorrhagic, chylous	Variable, >1.016 (50%)	>2.5 (50%)	7%	>1000 (70g): usually >70% lymphocytes	Peritoneal biopsy, stain and culture for acid-fast bacilli
Pyogenic peritonitis	Turbid or purulent	If purulent, >1.016	If purulent, >2.5	Unusual	Predominantly polymorphonuclear leukocytes	+ Gram's stain, culture
Congestive heart failure	Straw-colored	Variable, <1.016 (60%)	Variable, 1.5–5.3	10%	<1000 (90%): usually mesothelial, mononuclear	
Nephrosis	Straw-colored or chylous	<1.016	<2.5 (100%)	Unusual	<250: mesothelial, mononuclear	If chylous, ether extraction, Sudan staining
Pancreatic ascites (pancreatitis, pseudocyst)	Turbid, hemorrhagic, or chylous	Variable, often >1.016	Variable, often >2.5	Variable, may be blood stained	Variable	Increased amylase in ascitic fluid and serum

°Because the conditions of examining fluid and selecting patients were not identical in each series, the percentage figures (in parentheses) should be taken as an indication of the order of magnitude rather than as the precise incidence of any abnormal finding.

shear the tip of the catheter within the peritoneal cavity. Withdraw 50 mL of fluid (diagnostic tap) or the desired amount (therapeutic tap). Withdraw the catheter and cover with a sterile dressing.

The ascitic fluid should be sent to have the following tests performed: specific gravity, protein level, cell count, cytologic study, cell block, Gram stain and culture, stain and culture for acid-fast bacilli, and amylase level (Table 37-1). Unless the patient has glycosuria or proteinuria, ascites will test positive and urine will test negative for protein and glucose, confirming that the bladder has not been tapped inadvertently.

COMPLICATIONS

Complications include bleeding, infection, bowel or bladder perforation, persistent ascitic leak, and increased fluid requirements secondary to reaccumulation of ascites after aspiration of larger volumes. With the use of smaller catheters, morbidity is less common.[80] Rare complications include exacerbation of encephalopathy, hyponatremia, renal failure, and hypotension in cirrhotic patients.[81]

DIAGNOSTIC PERITONEAL LAVAGE   ■

The need for accurate detection of intraabdominal injury in the trauma patient was first emphasized by Williams and Zollinger[82] in 1959. In 200 patients with blunt abdominal trauma, 80% of deaths were noticed to be secondary to intraabdominal hemorrhage, and one half of those were associated with a delay in diagnosis and treatment. Four-quadrant taps (paracentesis) were known to have a high false-negative rate, failing to produce a representative sample of peritoneal fluid. Giacobine and Siler[83] showed a linear relationship in dogs between the amount of blood in the peritoneal space and a positive tap rate. An equivalent of 50 mL of defibrinated intraperitoneal blood yielded no true positive results with paracentesis, and a 500-mL equivalent yielded a positive tap rate of only 78%. Root and colleagues[84] demonstrated a 100% accuracy in detecting intraperitoneal blood with 1 L of lavage fluid, thus establishing peritoneal lavage as an efficacious method of evaluating intraabdominal hemorrhage in the trauma patient.

Peritoneal lavage is routinely used to evaluate patients with blunt abdominal trauma and altered sensorium as a result of an associated head injury, drug or alcohol ingestion, or shock. In addition, peritoneal lavage is used to diagnose intraabdominal trauma in patients with multiple injuries who require anesthesia for extraabdominal procedures. Diagnostic lavage also has been used in situations involving penetrating abdominal trauma, lower thoracic and flank trauma, unexplained hypotension, and equivocal findings on physical examination, and in the intensive care setting to evaluate nontraumatic intraabdominal processes.

The only true contraindication to diagnostic peritoneal lavage is predetermined laparotomy. Relative contraindications include a gravid uterus, lower midline abdominal scar (find another entry site), and abdominal wall hematomas (false positive).

OPEN TECHNIQUE

Place the patient in the supine position. Insert a Foley catheter to prevent inadvertent puncture of the bladder. A nasogastric tube is inserted to prevent gastric perforation. Prepare the skin with povidine-iodine solution and apply sterile drapes. For local anesthesia, administer 1% lidocaine with epinephrine (to minimize skin bleeding at the incision site, which may contribute to a false-positive result) using a 25-gauge needle.

A 3- to 4-cm midline infraumbilical skin incision is created, which can be incorporated into a standard midline incision if laparotomy is necessary (Fig. 37-16). Select a different site if a surgical scar is present in the lower midline or if the abdomen is enlarged because of pregnancy. A midline incision above the umbilicus is an acceptable alternative, but do not extend it too far cephalad (to avoid encountering the falciform ligament). Continue the incision through

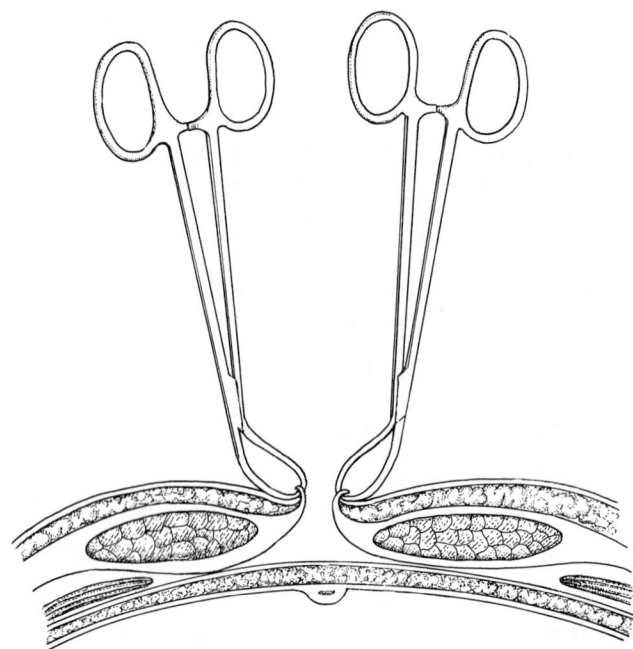

FIGURE 37-17. The fascial edge is grasped with towel clips and elevated to lift the abdominal wall away from the intraabdominal structures.

the subcutaneous tissue and through the linea alba. A periumbilical approach can be used by retracting the rectus muscle laterally and visualizing the posterior fascia.

Grasp the fascial edge on each side firmly with towel clips and elevate it to lift the abdominal wall away from the intraabdominal structures (Fig. 37-17). Isolate the underlying peritoneum, and open it under direct vision (Fig. 37-18). Introduce a gloved finger into the peritoneal cavity to assure that adhesion is not present and to ensure a safe pathway for the lavage catheter. Insert the catheter without the trocar through the small peritoneal rent, and carefully advance it into the pelvis (Fig. 37-19). Place a purse-string suture through the peritoneum around the catheter with a 3-0 chromic suture (Fig. 37-20). Attach a 10-mL syringe to the dialysis catheter for aspiration. If 10 mL gross blood is aspirated, no further procedure is necessary and laparotomy is indicated. If not, connect an IV infusion set to the catheter and infuse 1 L of normal saline. Leave a small amount of the lavage fluid to establish a siphon effect when the container is placed on the floor. Lower the nearly empty saline bottle to the floor for return of the lavage fluid by gravity siphonage (Fig. 37-21). At least 300 mL lavage effluent should be withdrawn. Using large-bore irrigation tubing, fluid may be more rapidly infused and withdrawn compared with standard IV tubing.[85] Lavage return is submitted to the laboratory for analysis of red blood cell (RBC) and white blood cell (WBC) counts, amylase level, and presence of bile, bacteria, or particulate matter. After removing the catheter, tie the purse-string suture, approximate the linea alba with 2-0 suture material, and close the skin.

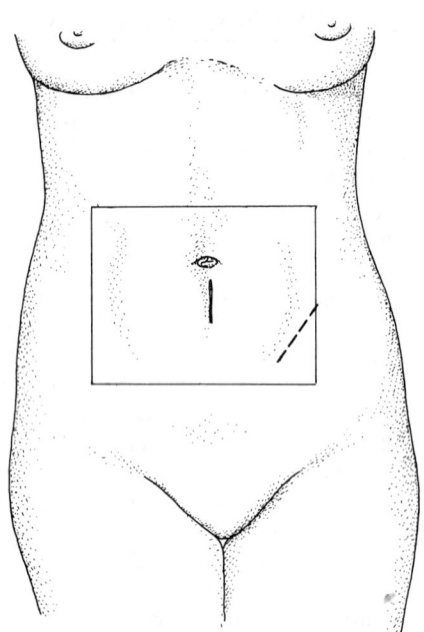

FIGURE 37-16. A 3- to 4-cm midline infraumbilical skin incision is created, which can be incorporated into a standard midline incision if laparotomy is necessary. A different site is selected if a surgical scar is present in the lower midline.

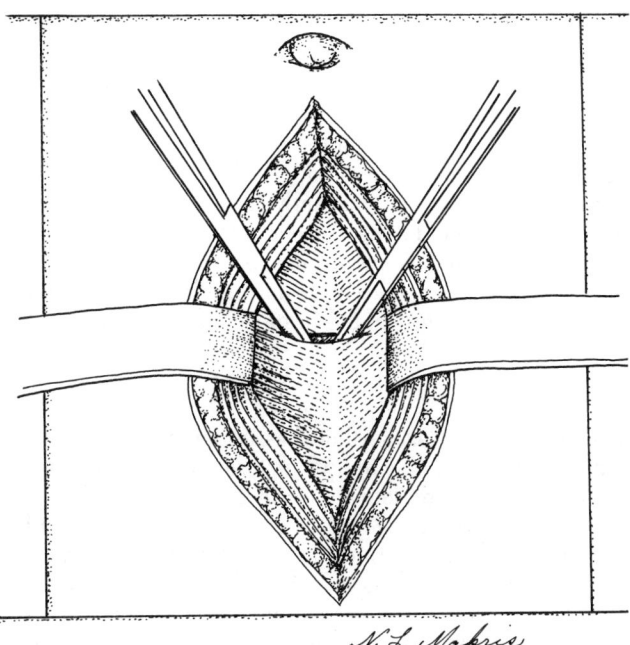

FIGURE 37-18. The underlying peritoneum is isolated and opened under direct vision.

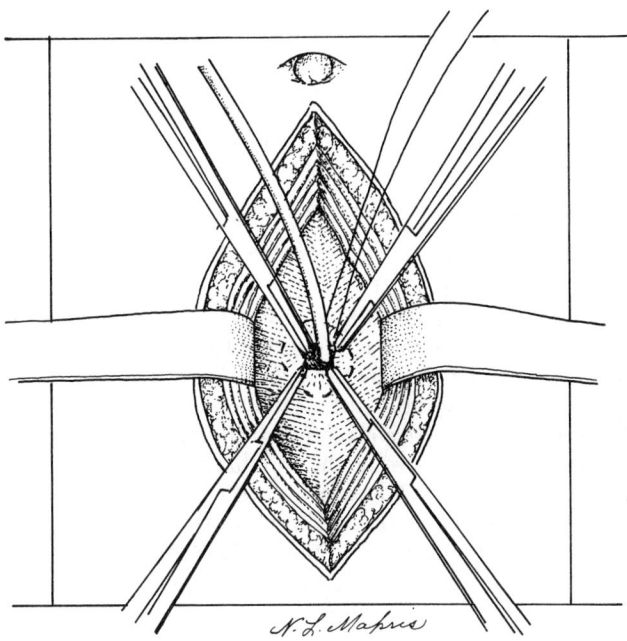

FIGURE 37-20. A purse-string suture is placed through the peritoneum, around the catheter with a 3-0 chromic suture.

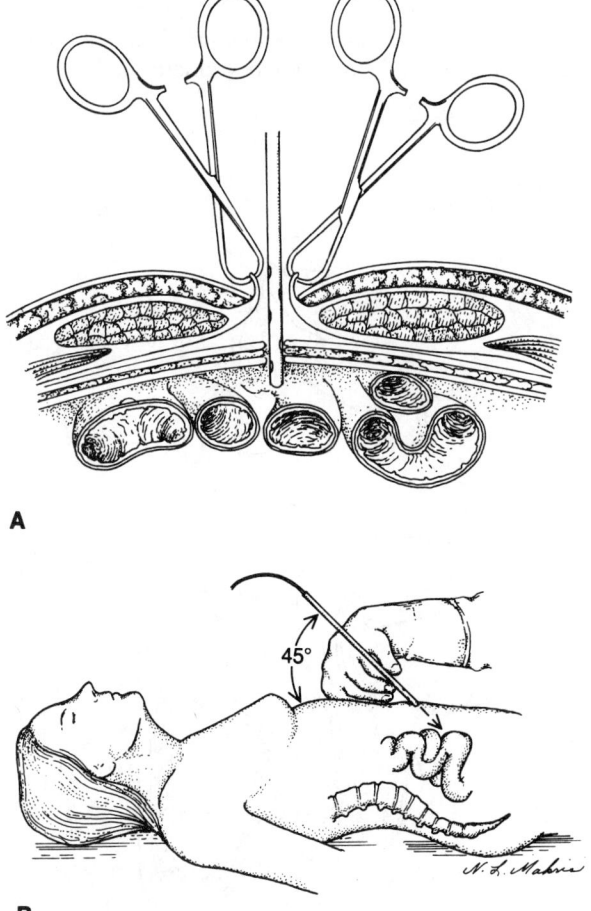

A

B

FIGURE 37-19. The catheter without the trocar is inserted through the small peritoneal rent and directed into the pelvis.

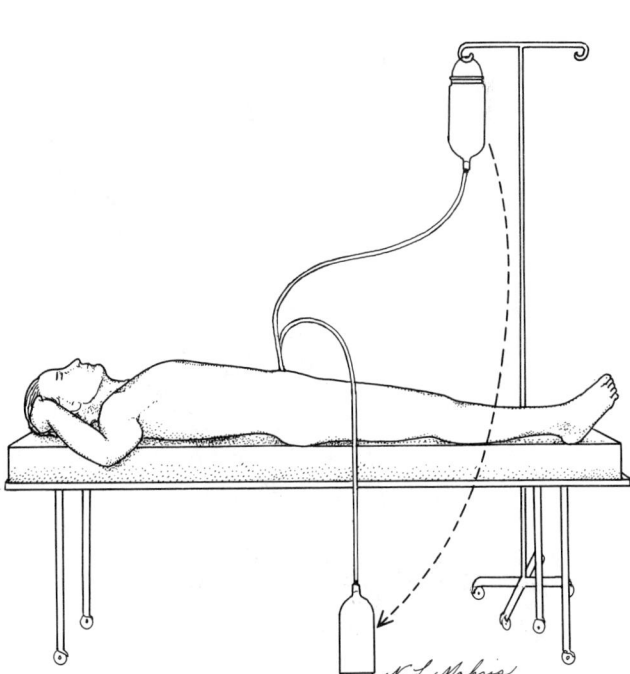

FIGURE 37-21. The saline bottle is lowered to the floor for return of the lavage fluid by gravity siphonage.

CLOSED TECHNIQUE

Two methods are available: a prepackaged kit (Arrow International, Reading, PA) and a dialysis catheter kit with a trocar (Trocath-McGaw). The skin preparation, draping, and local anesthesia are the same as for the open technique, as is the decompression of the bladder and stomach.

Dialysis Catheter and Trocar Method

Use a no. 11 scalpel to incise the skin 2 to 3 cm inferior to the umbilicus in the midline. A supraumbilical location is used if a pelvic fracture is suspected. Continue the incision to the linea alba. Administer more local anesthesia below the linea alba. Insert the trocar/catheter at a 45-degree angle toward the pelvis. Give a controlled thrust with both hands and stop all pressure when the pop through the peritoneum is felt (Fig. 37-22). Advance the catheter over the trocar into the peritoneal cavity, and remove the trocar (Fig. 37-23). Connect the catheter to the infusion set, and carry out the procedure identically to that of the open method.

Prepackaged Kit

Make a 3-mm skin incision with a no. 11 blade. Introduce the 18-gauge needle into the peritoneal cavity and angle it toward the center of the pelvis (Fig. 37-24). Then introduce a 15-cm J-tipped guidewire through the needle (Fig. 37-25). If the wire does not advance easily, remove it and advance the needle. Remove the needle when half of the wire has been introduced. Place the catheter over the guidewire, and thread it with a twisting motion to go past the fascia. Remove the guidewire when the catheter is within the abdomen. Proceed with the remainder of the procedure as with the open method.

COMPLICATIONS

Technical complications occur at a rate of 1% to 3%[86] and include wound bleeding, misplacement of the catheter into the preperitoneal space, and perforation of the bowel, bladder, and vessels.[87] Although the open technique is generally safer than the closed technique,[88,89] the closed approach using the guidewire is significantly faster.[90] When complications such as wound dehiscence and failure to return lavage fluid are considered, some studies report a complication rate of 9%.[88,91] A false-positive lavage may result in an unnecessary surgical exploration, leading to morbidity.[92]

RESULTS

Interpretation of lavage fluid has undergone considerable refinement since the technique first was introduced. Initially, positive results were determined by the presence of intraabdominal hemorrhage alone in blunt trauma. Many studies showed that 20 mL of freely aspirated gross intraperitoneal blood had a 100% correlation with intraperitoneal injury.[93–95] Peritoneal lavage for blunt trauma has an accuracy rate of 96%.[89] The organ systems most commonly involved in false-negative studies include ruptured diaphragm, ruptured spleen, lacerated liver, and intraperitoneal bladder rupture.[88,96] Retroperitoneal injuries also may be missed by peritoneal lavage. When history and physical examination alone are used, the error rate is 25% to 45%.[97–100]

The RBC count should be measured rather than estimated, and counted on a hemocytometer rather than by

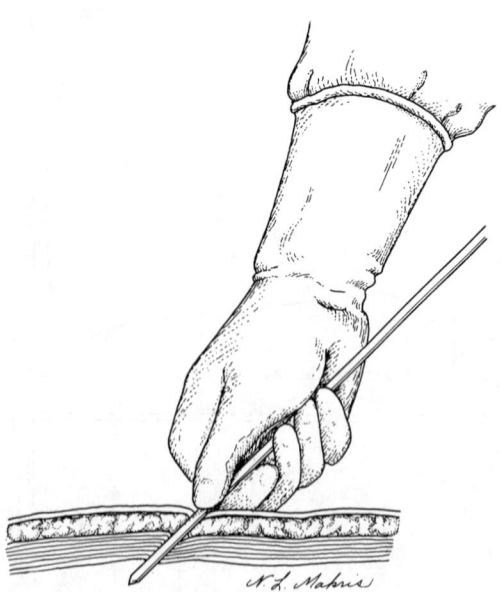

FIGURE 37-22. The catheter is inserted with a controlled thrust at a 45-degree angle toward the pelvis.

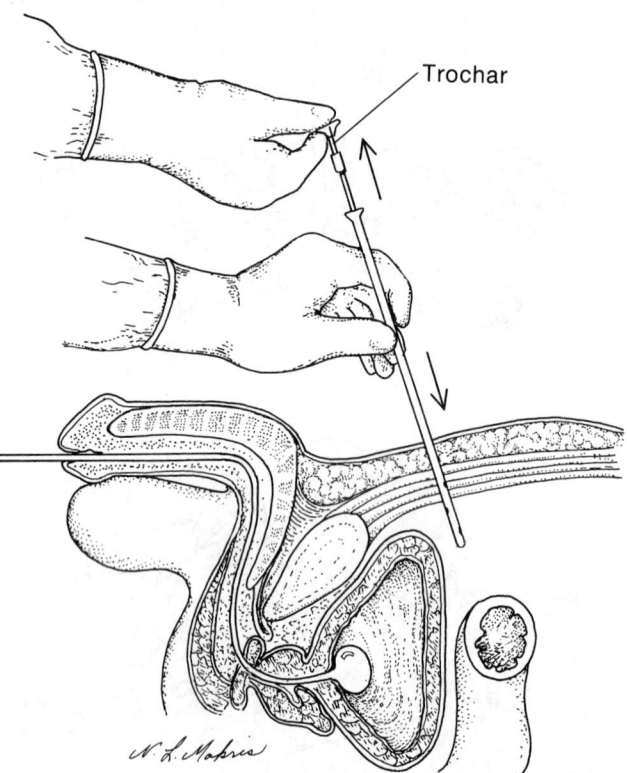

FIGURE 37-23. The catheter is advanced over the trocar into the peritoneal cavity, and the trocar is removed.

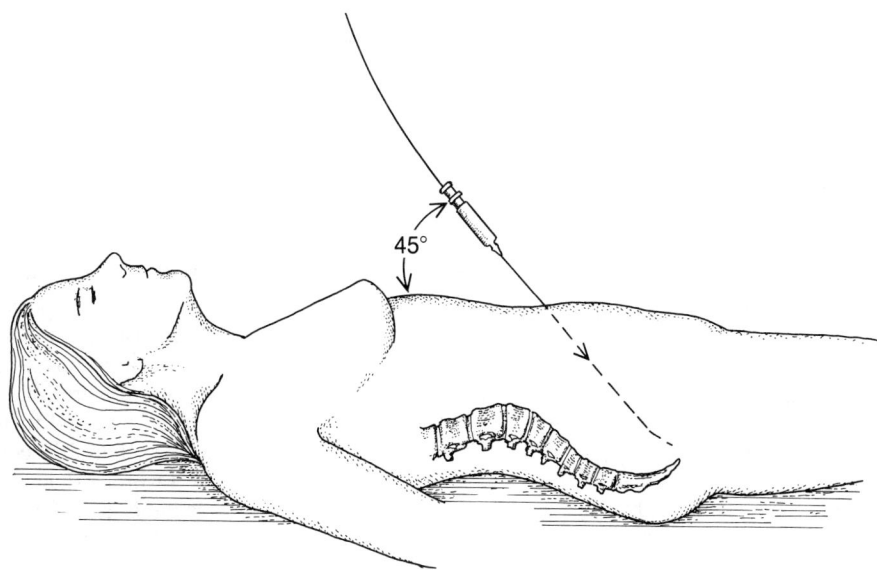

FIGURE 37-24. The 18-gauge needle is introduced into the peritoneal cavity and angled toward the center of the pelvis.

Coulter counter, because the latter may falsely increase the count by including macrophages and debris.[101] Other recommendations include attempting to read newsprint through IV tubing and spinning a hematocrit of the lavage fluid. Cell counts remain the most accurate method of determining a positive lavage[93] (Table 37-2).

Studies in animals have shown that after injury resulting from a perforated viscus, it may take 3 hours for the WBC count to become elevated enough to produce a positive result.[102] Most diagnostic peritoneal lavage procedures are performed within several hours of injury, raising concern as to the potential for false-negative studies. However, Engrav

and colleagues[103] demonstrated an 83% correlation of significant intraperitoneal injury with an elevated lavage WBC count (more than 500 cells/mm^3) in early peritoneal lavage (although an unspecified number also had significant hemoperitoneum).

All patients with a positive lavage are prepared for exploratory laparotomy. The management of indeterminate lavage results remains controversial, and some have suggested repeated lavage in several hours.[104,105]

Several studies have evaluated the efficacy of diagnostic peritoneal lavage in penetrating trauma. Most institutions consider gunshot wounds to the anterior abdomen as an

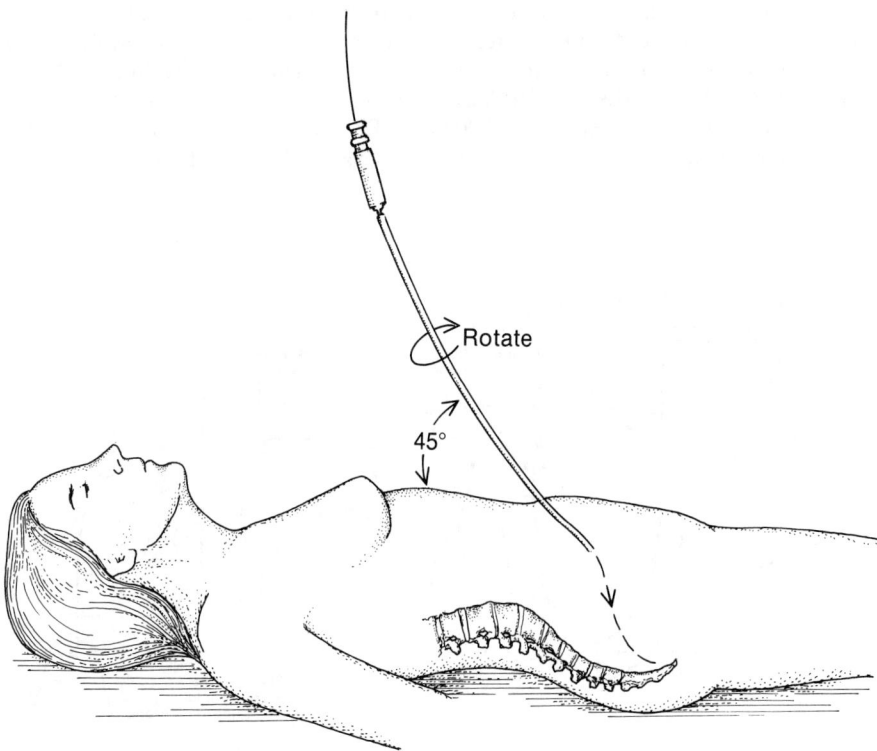

FIGURE 37-25. A 15-cm guidewire is introduced through the needle. The needle is removed when half of the wire has been introduced. The catheter is placed over the guidewire and threaded with a twisting motion to go past the fascia.

TABLE 37-2.   Interpretation of Peritoneal Lavage

POSITIVE

Aspiration of >10 mL of blood
Lavage fluid exits by means of Foley catheter or chest tube
Grossly bloody lavage return
RBC >100,000/mm^3
WBC >500/mm^3
Amylase >175 U/dL
Presence of bile, bacteria, or particulate matter

NEGATIVE (NONPENETRATING TRAUMA)

RBC <50,000/mm^3
WBC <100/mm^3
Amylase <75 U/dL

INDETERMINANT

Dialysis catheter fills with blood
RBC >50,000–<100,000/mm^3
WBC >100–<500/mm^3
Amylase >75–<175 U/dL

RBC, red blood cell (count); WBC, white blood cell (count).

absolute indication for exploratory laparotomy. Thal and associates[106] performed diagnostic peritoneal lavage in patients with gunshot wounds to the lower chest and anterior abdomen before exploratory laparotomy and found a false-negative rate of 25% using a lavage fluid RBC count greater than 100,000 RBC/mm^3 as criteria for a positive result.

Merlotti and coworkers[107] performed diagnostic peritoneal lavage on patients with penetrating trauma between the nipples and subcostal margins, with flank and back trauma, and with tangential gunshot wounds to the anterior abdominal wall. In this study, an RBC count greater than 10,000 RBC/mm^3 was considered a positive result. There was a 13.6% false-positive and 1% false-negative rate, with an overall accuracy of 96.6%. If 1,000,000 RBC/mm^3 had been interpreted as diagnostic of a positive lavage, there

would have been no false positive results but a prohibitively high false-negative rate of 11.1%.

Similarly, Thal[108] evaluated patients with stab wounds below the fifth intercostal space between anterior axillary lines, or if local exploration of an anterior abdominal stab wound showed penetration of the posterior fascia. With greater than 100,000 RBC/mm^3 considered as a positive lavage, the false-positive rate was 2.4%. However, the false-negative rate of 4.9% included patients with serious injuries that could have caused significant morbidity if missed.

Diagnostic peritoneal lavage recently has been observed to be useful for evaluating suspected nontraumatic peritonitis in elderly patients or in those with altered sensorium and an uninterpretable abdominal examination.[109,110] In general, surgery was performed if there was an elevated WBC count (more than 500 cells/mm^3) in the lavage fluid.

Overall, diagnostic peritoneal lavage is believed to be reliable, safe, and efficacious in rapidly detecting intraabdominal injury and leads to an organized plan of care in the trauma patient.

INTRAABDOMINAL PRESSURE MEASUREMENT ■

Massive elevation of intraabdominal pressure has been associated with renal, respiratory, and cardiac dysfunction.[111] Causes of high intraabdominal pressure include intraabdominal hemorrhage, massive ascites and pneumoperitoneum, edematous bowel loops, intraabdominal tumors, retroperitoneal hematomas, and external compression (military antishock trousers [MAST]).

Myocardial dysfunction is related to decreased stroke volume, left ventricular contractility, and depressed cardiac output.[111] Causes of cardiac compromise include inferior vena caval compression, decreasing filling pressures,[112,113] and diaphragmatic elevation compressing the heart and great vessels.[111] Respiratory impairment is manifested by high peak inspiratory pressure, low compliance, high minute ventilation, and ventilation-perfusion abnormalities.[111] Acute renal

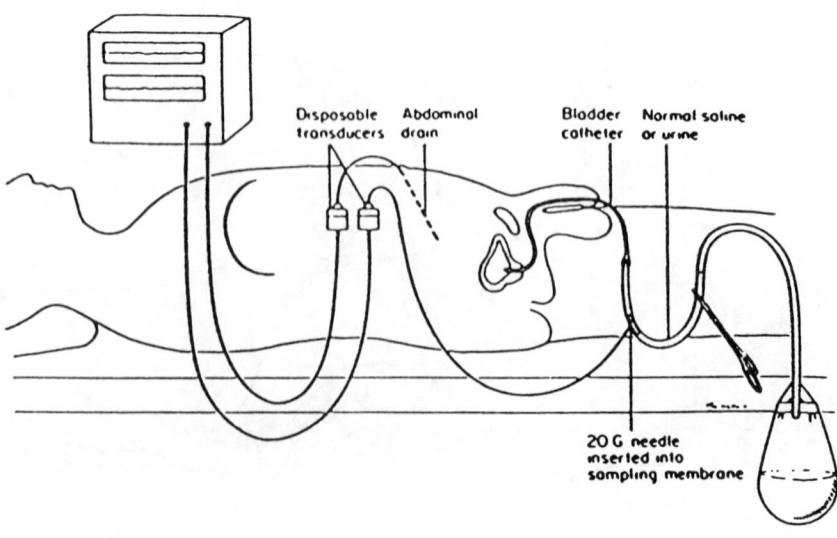

FIGURE 37-26. Schematic illustration of a patient in the supine position showing the closed-system drain and transurethral bladder pressure monitoring technique.

insufficiency may be related to impaired renal blood flow and decreased glomerular filtration rate.[114] Blood flow is redistributed to the upper torso, with resulting hypoperfusion of the abdominal viscera and lower extremities.[115]

Measurement of intraabdominal pressure can identify patients who may benefit from laparotomy and decompression. Pressure initially was measured with closed-system abdominal drains or dialysis catheters. Recently, transurethral bladder catheters have been shown to be accurate and less invasive.[115–117]

Normal intraabdominal pressure is zero to subatmospheric.[114] After laparotomy, intraabdominal pressure measures 3 to 15 mm Hg.[115] Hemodynamic, pulmonary, and renal dysfunction appear with intraabdominal pressures above 25 mm Hg.

PROCEDURE

The bladder is drained with an indwelling transurethral catheter. The catheter is clamped distal to the sampling membrane. A 20-gauge needle is inserted through the membrane and attached to a three-way stopcock connected to sterile IV tubing leading to a pressure transducer. The symphysis pubis is used as the zero point in the supine patient (Fig. 37-26). With the stopcock turned on to the transducer, the pressure is recorded.

VENOUS CUTDOWN ■

The need to perform venous cutdowns has diminished as a result of the improved techniques and technology for cannulating the central vasculature. On occasion, a cutdown may be helpful in caring for the markedly hypovolemic patient who requires urgent IV therapy when the veins are collapsed and a large-caliber conduit is needed for fluid and blood administration, or in the rare instance when percutaneous central or peripheral venous cannulation is unsuccessful (Table 37-3). Advantages include ease of cannulation and avoidance of pneumothorax, hemothorax, or brachial plexus injury. Peripheral access may be difficult in obese patients, IV drug abusers, patients receiving chemotherapy, or those with large body-surface burns.[118] Contraindications include overlying cellulitis and adjacent unstable fracture. Multiple access sites are available, and anatomic knowledge and attention to technique are essential for successful cannulation.

PROCEDURE

Prepare the skin with povidine-iodine and apply sterile drapes. Administer 1% lidocaine without epinephrine as local anesthesia using a 25-gauge needle (Fig. 37-27). Make a 2- to 3-cm transverse incision over the vein (Fig. 37-28). Mobilize a 2-cm segment of the vein with blunt dissection (Fig. 37-29). Pass two silk ligatures beneath the vein and place the distal suture on tension by attaching it to the drapes with a Kelly clamp (Fig. 37-30). Insert the catheter percutaneously through the skin distal to the cut-down incision. Place tension on the distal ligature and insert the cannula into the vein with the bevel facing the back wall (Fig. 37-31). Relax the proximal ligature and advance the plastic catheter. Remove the inner needle. Assure good backflow of blood to confirm the position of the catheter in the lumen of the vein. Connect the IV tubing and suture the skin with 3-0 nylon. Secure the cannula to the skin at the exit point.

Alternatively, use a catheter within the needle. Pass a 14-gauge needle through the skin, from inside out (Fig. 37-32), then pass the catheter through the needle, from the outside in. Remove the needle (Fig. 37-33). Incise the vein with a no. 11 blade, first by hemisecting the vein in the horizontal plane and then by turning the blade 90 degrees upward. This technique creates a flap that extends through the radius of the vein and allows easy access for the venous cannula (Fig. 37-34). Insert the cannula into the vein. A mosquito clamp may be needed to dilate the vein and guide the catheter (Fig. 37-35). Close the skin and secure as described above.

Preferred veins include the median basilic, basilic, and cephalic. The proximal saphenous vein can be used when other sites are not available or when IV tubing is inserted in the vein directly to achieve high infusion rates ("Vietnam" lines).

Ankle

The saphenous vein begins at the junction of the medial end of the dorsal venous arch of the great toe. It ascends anterior to the medial malleolus, where it lies on tough periosteum (Fig. 37-36). The only associated structure at this point is the terminal segment of the saphenous nerve supplying sensation along the medial aspect of the foot.[119]

The advantage of using this vein is that it can be cannulated during a cardiac arrest situation when most of the clinical activity is centered around the upper torso. The

TABLE 37-3. Saline Flow Rates Through Various Catheters

CATHETER TYPE	DIAMETER	LENGTH (cm)	FLOW RATE (GRAVITY) (mL/s)	FLOW RATE (PRESSURE) (mL/s)
Deseret Intracath	16 gauge	20	1.6	2.5
Vicra Quik-Cath	14 gauge	5	2.9	4.8
McGaw Extension Set	3 mm	30	3.6	6.5

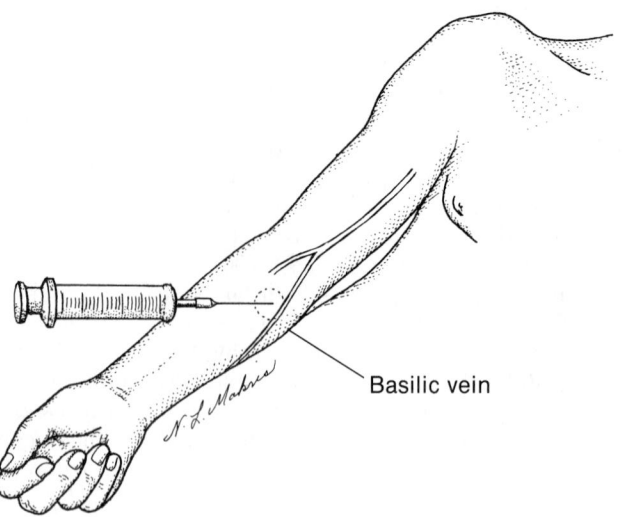

FIGURE 37-27. Lidocaine 1% is used as local anesthesia.

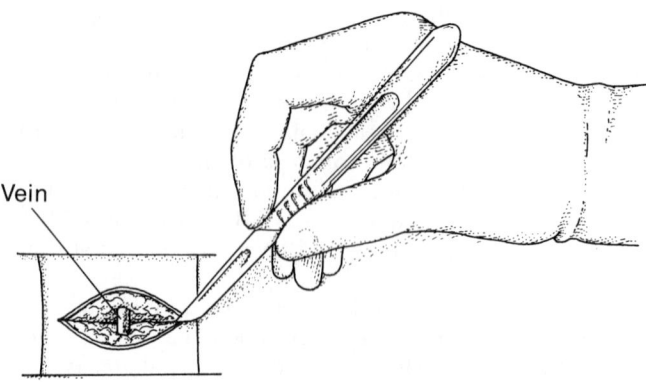

FIGURE 37-28. Make a 2- to 3-cm transverse incision over the vein.

MAST has not been shown to impede fluid infusion in the lower extremity.[120] Access using this vein should be converted to another site when clinically feasible. Potential disadvantages include thrombophlebitis and loss of a vein valuable for arterial bypass. This site should not be used if there is a suspicion that the inferior vena cava, iliac, or femoral veins are disrupted.[121]

Groin

The proximal saphenous vein is 4 to 5 mm in diameter and joins the femoral vein 7 to 8 cm inferior to the inguinal ligament, along the anteromedial aspect of the thigh. The proximal saphenous vein may be confused with the anterior lateral femoral vein, which is smaller (2 to 3 mm) and more anterior.[119] Rotate the thigh externally and make a transverse

incision in the anterior medial thigh 5 cm distal to the femoral pulse. The saphenous vein is medial to the femoral artery (Fig. 37-37). If no pulse is palpable, make the incision 5 cm below the junction of the medial and middle thirds of the inguinal ligament. The incision should be 5 to 7 cm long. Alternatively, a transverse incision beginning where the scrotal or labial fold meets the medial thigh is extended lateral to the femoral pulse.[122] Bluntly dissect the subcutaneous tissue (Fig. 37-38).

The Vietnam catheter uses a beveled IV extension tubing inserted 8 to 12 cm into the vein. This device is used when maximal fluid and blood infusion rates are needed.[123] The disadvantages of this method include anatomic variability and loss of a potential vein for arterial bypass surgery and dialysis.[121]

Antecubital Fossa

The basilic vein is a continuation of the ulnar end of the dorsal venous arch of the hand. The vein ascends along the ulnar border of the forearm into the antecubital fossa ante-

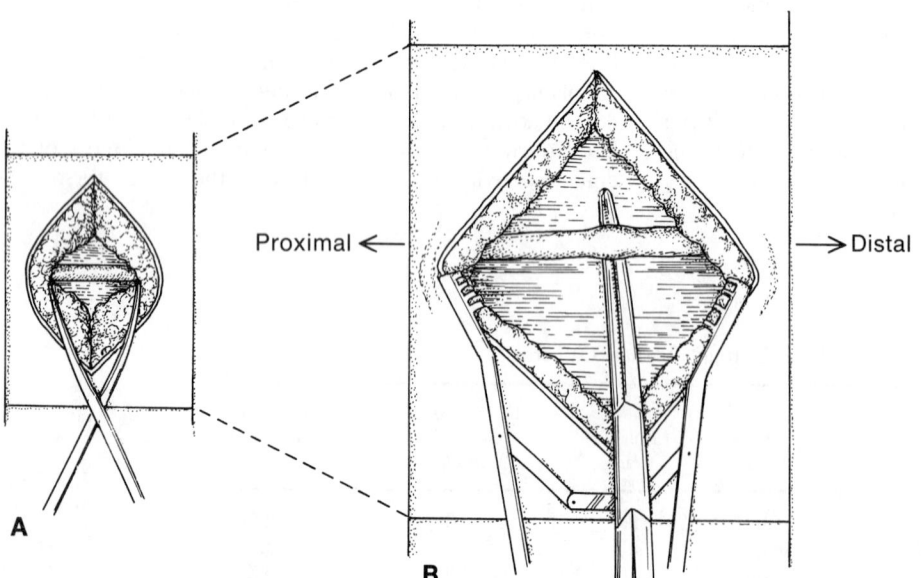

FIGURE 37-29. The vein is immobilized with blunt dissection.

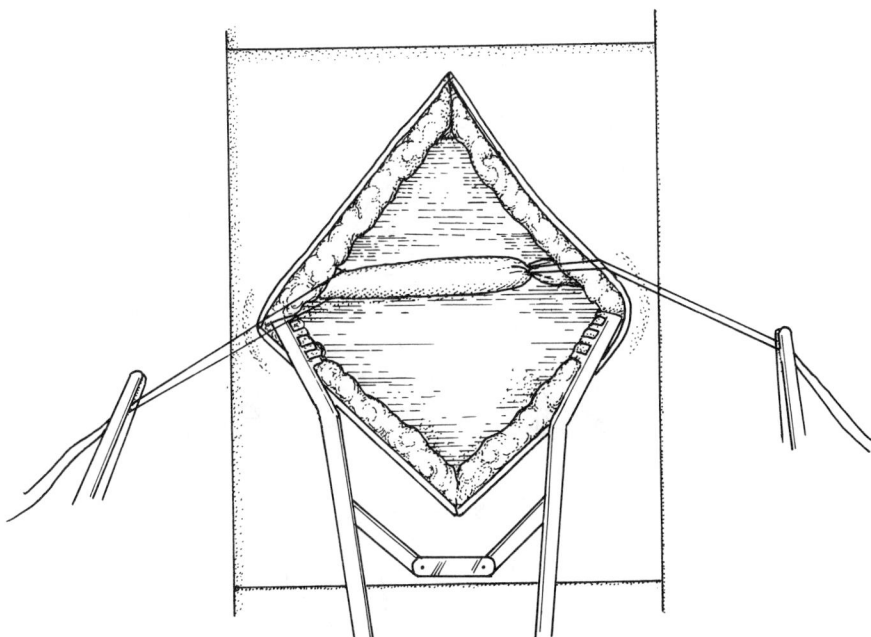

FIGURE 37-30. Pass two silk ligatures beneath the vein and place the distal suture on tension by attaching to the drape with a Kelly clamp.

rior to the medial epicondyle. After the vein is joined by the median antecubital vein, it ascends in the bicipital groove, accompanied by the medial cutaneous nerve[119] (Fig. 37-39). Make the incision 1 to 2 cm lateral and superior to the medial epicondyle of the humerus. Alternatively, extend the skin incision from the brachial artery pulse at the proximal flexor crease of the antecubital fossa toward the medial epicondyle.

The advantages of this approach are the consistently large diameter of the vein, the superficial location, and the capabil-

ity to place a long catheter for central venous pressure measurement.[121] A disadvantage includes a longer time to isolate the basilic vein compared with the saphenous vein.[122] Damage to the medial cutaneous nerve results in loss of sensation over the medial aspect of the forearm. Deeper dissection presents a risk to the brachial artery and median nerve.

The cephalic vein is a radial continuation of the dorsal venous arch of the hand and ascends parallel to the brachio-radialis muscle into the antecubital fossa. Where it connects with the basilic vein by the obliquely ascending median

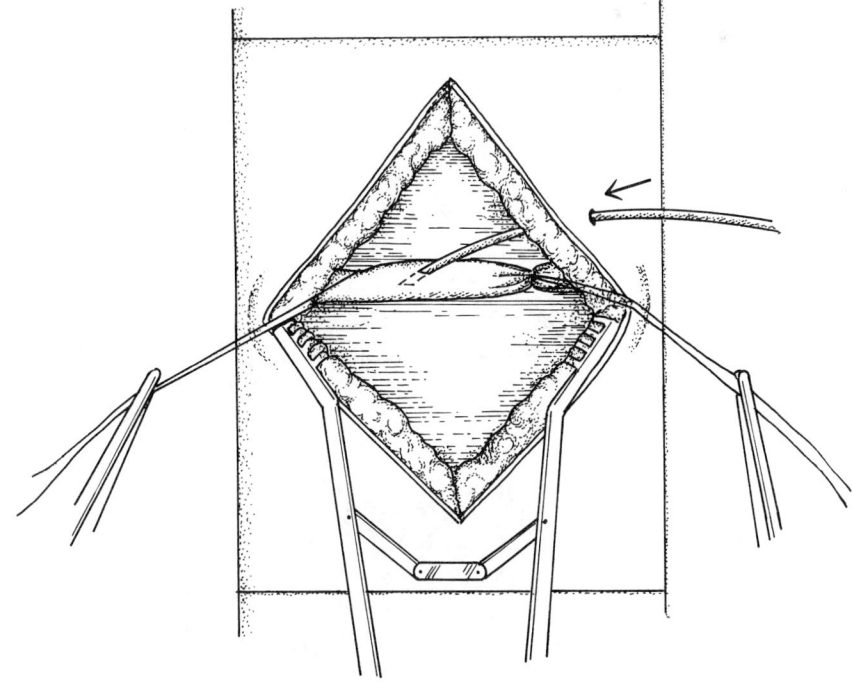

FIGURE 37-31. Insert the catheter percutaneously through the skin distal to the cutdown incision. Place tension on the distal ligature, and insert the cannula into the vein with the bevel facing the back wall.

Intracath
needle

Intracath
cannula

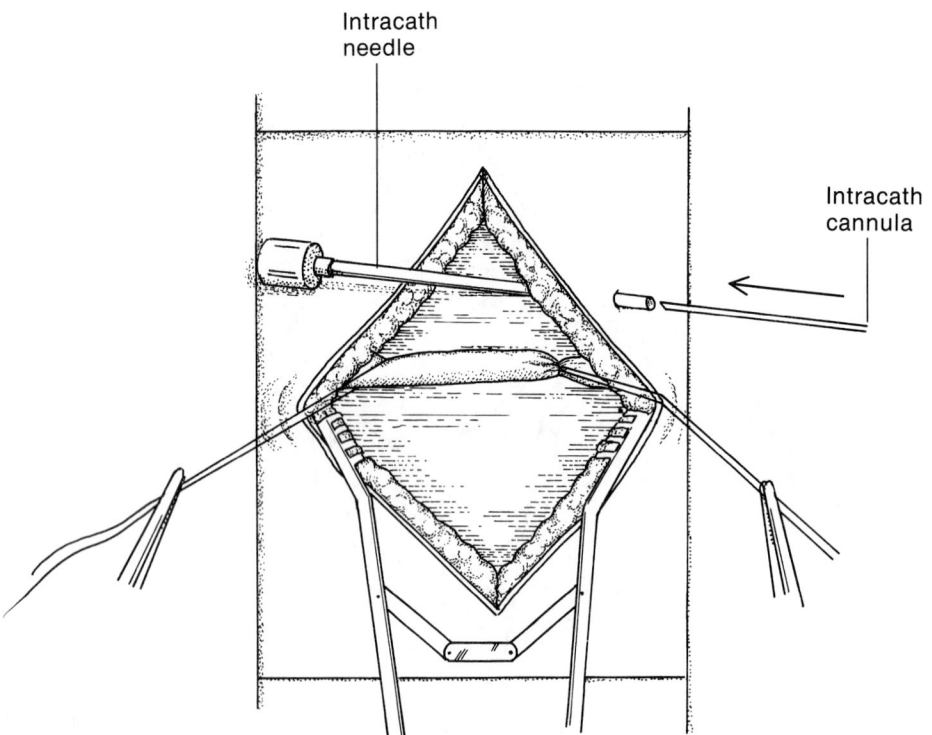

FIGURE 37-32. The 14-gauge needle is passed through the skin, from inside out.

cubital vein, the diameter may be greatly reduced in size. The vein ascends in the lateral bicipital groove to a superficial location in the deltopectoral groove and empties into the axillary vein[121] (see Fig. 37-39). Make the incision at the distal flexor crease of the antecubital fossa lateral to the midline. Alternatively, the cephalic vein can be identified with a transverse incision over the deltopectoral groove.[124]

The disadvantage of this approach is the variability in size of the vein. In addition, this method cannot be used easily for central venous access because the vein traverses the clavipectoral fascia at right angles, making passage into the central venous system difficult.[119]

COMPLICATIONS

Complications of venous cutdown include thrombophlebitis, local hematoma, and cellulitis. Because most cutdowns are placed during initial fluid resuscitation of hemorrhagic

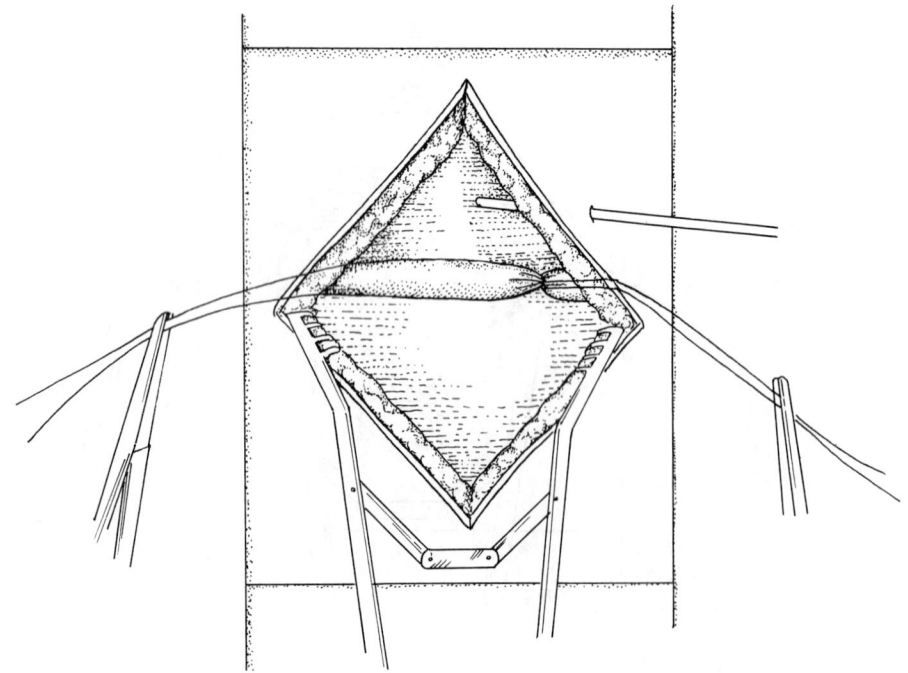

FIGURE 37-33. The cannula is passed through the needle, from outside in, and the needle is removed.

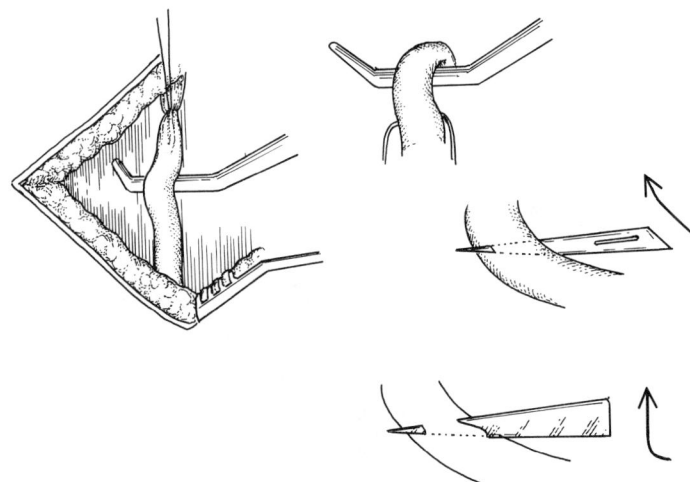

FIGURE 37-34. Incise the vein by hemisecting the vein in the horizontal plane and turning the blade 90 degrees upward.

shock, sterile technique is often compromised, leading to an increased incidence of phlebitis. Therefore, emergency cutdown catheters should be removed within 24 hours.[121]

Generalized sepsis is a more serious complication. In addition to early removal of contaminated or infected catheters, precautionary measures to prevent contamination include secure fixation of the cannula to avoid to-and-fro movement, keeping the puncture site dry and sterile, and avoiding antibiotic ointment, which encourages fungal growth.[125]

DEFIBRILLATION

Ventricular fibrillation is the most disorganized of all arrhythmias and is thought to be maintained by a "critical mass" of fibrillating myocardium.[126] The only practical treatment for ventricular fibrillation is electrical fibrillation, which is dependent on depolarizing a sufficient portion of the fibrillating ventricle to allow the dominant pacemaker to control the rhythm.[127]

Defibrillation was first described in 1899 by Prevost and Batelli.[128] The first successful human defibrillation was in 1947 with an open-chest technique.[129] Initially, alternating-current defibrillators were used but have been replaced by direct-current monophasic defibrillators, which are more effective, portable, and less dangerous.[130,131] The strength of energy delivery is expressed in joules (J) or watt-seconds (product of power and duration) and produces several thou-

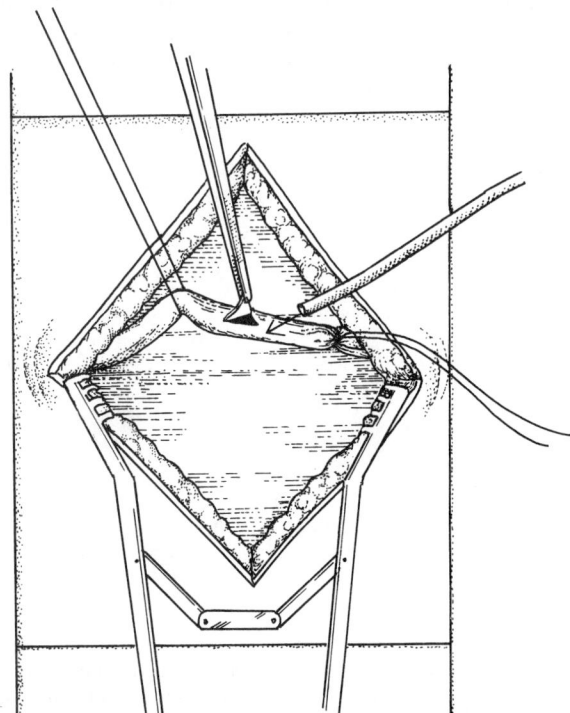

FIGURE 37-35. Insert the cannula into the vein.

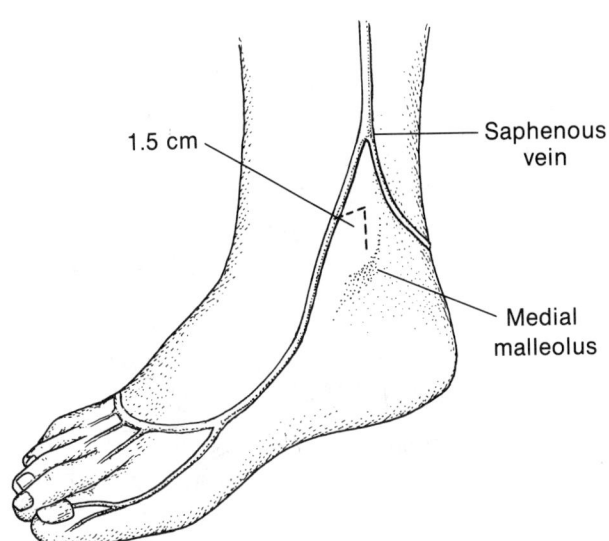

FIGURE 37-36. The saphenous vein.

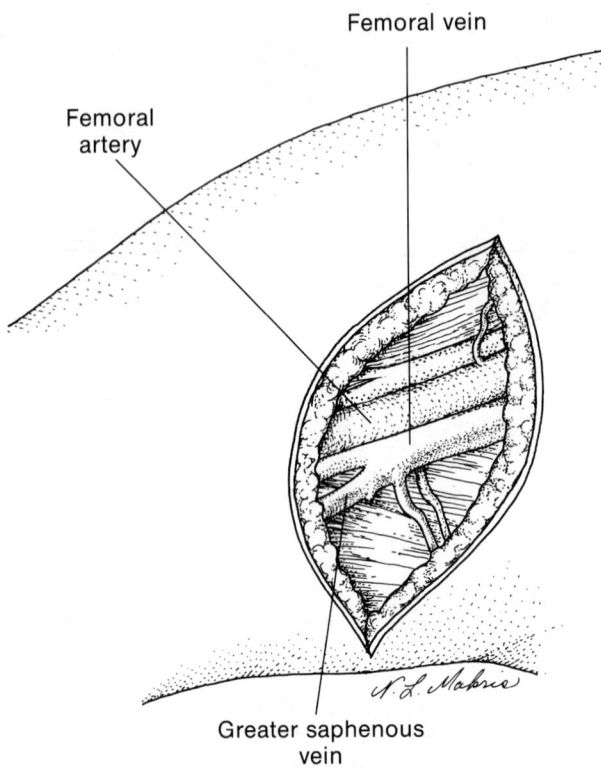

FIGURE 37-37. The proximal saphenous vein.

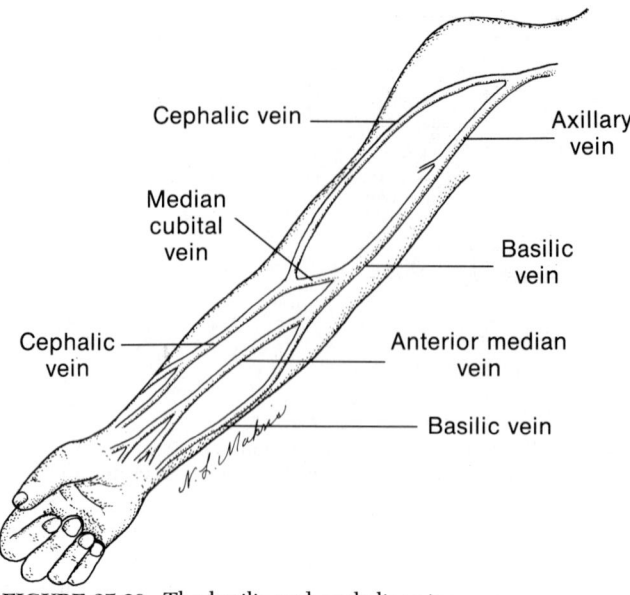

FIGURE 37-39. The basilic and cephalic veins.

sand volts during a 4- to 12-millisecond monophasic energy delivery.[132]

The indication for defibrillation is ventricular fibrillation that does not revert with a precordial thump.[133] The patient is defibrillated initially with 200 J; if ventricular fibrillation continues, the patient is defibrillated again immediately with 200 to 300 J while the transthoracic resistance is low.[134] CPR is continued if ventricular fibrillation persists and subsequent defibrillations are attempted with 360 J.

PROCEDURE

Turn the cardioverter on and the synchronizer switch off. Select the appropriate energy level. Apply electrode jelly to the paddles. Do not use alcohol pads. Apply one paddle below the right clavicle and the second just lateral to the left nipple in the anterior axillary line (Fig. 37-40). Be sure that the operator and assistants have no patient or bed contact. Administer the shock. Check the pulse, electrocardiogram (ECG), and airway. If unsuccessful, continue CPR and repeat defibrillation using the Advanced Cardiac Life Support protocol (see Chap. 33).

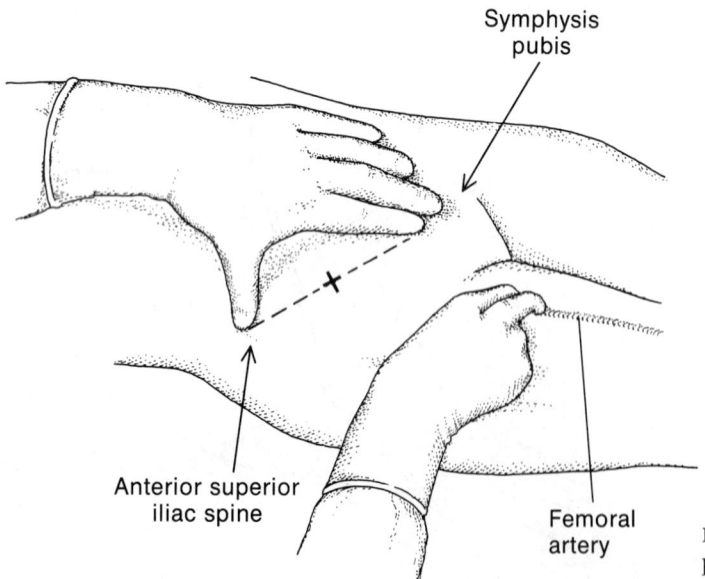

FIGURE 37-38. Femoral artery runs directly across the midpoint of the line drawn between anterior superior iliac spine and symphysis pubis.

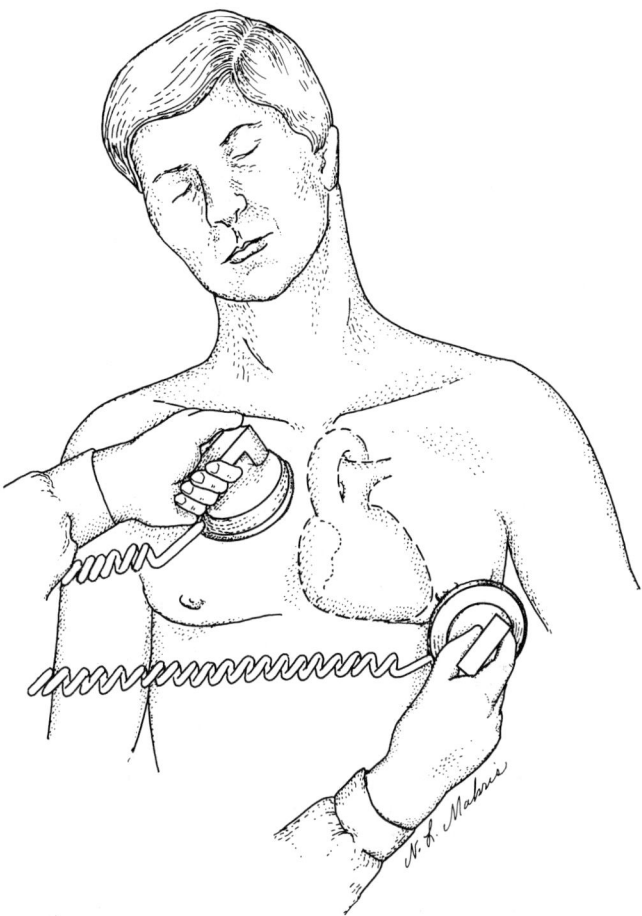

FIGURE 37-40. Apply the paddles: one below the right clavicle just lateral to the upper sternum and one just lateral to the left nipple in the anterior axillary line.

COMPLICATIONS

Complications include asystole, unsuccessful defibrillation, and skin burns from inadequate electrode contact to skin (caused either by arcing or inadequate electrode contact with electrode jelly).[135]

Pacemaker failure and elevated pacing threshold have been noticed infrequently after defibrillation.[136] Diodes were incorporated into the pacer circuitry in the early 1960s, giving them a degree of safety from shocks of less than 400 J.[137] Recommendations for defibrillation in pacemaker patients include use of low energy, placement of the paddles in the anterior–posterior position at least 10 cm from the electrodes and pulse generator, reconfirmation of pacemaker function after shock, and availability of a standby temporary pacemaker.[137–143]

The success of defibrillation depends on many factors. Longer duration of ventricular fibrillation makes successful defibrillation less likely.[133] The environment and the condition of the myocardium are extremely important, and poor outcome is associated with hypoxemia, acidosis, hypothermia, electrolyte imbalance, and drug toxicity.[144] Fine fibrillation (low amplitude) is less likely to respond to defibrillation than is coarse fibrillation (high amplitude).[145,146] A larger heart size is associated with a larger critical fibrillating mass and is thought to require more energy delivery for defibrillation.[147] Increased energy delivery leads to a higher rate of successful defibrillation. A relation between body weight and energy requirements has been shown in animal studies, although this association has not been proved in humans.[148,149]

Previous countershocks tend to diminish transthoracic resistance, thereby decreasing energy requirements.[150] Transthoracic resistance is also lowered if defibrillation is delivered during expiration.[151] The ideal paddle size for defibrillators in adults has yet to be established, but current recommendations suggest a 10- to 13-cm diameter.[152,153] The paddle–skin interface is best with a low-impedance medium.[154,155] Alcohol may ignite and should not be used. Firm pressure with the paddles can improve energy delivery, and paddle contact pressure of about 10 kg (25 lb) can decrease the transthoracic resistance by 25%.[153] Preapplied self-adhesive, dual ECGs, and defibrillator pads developed in 1984 by Kerber and coworkers[156] may lower intrathoracic impedance, improve defibrillation success rates, and increase operator safety.[157]

CARDIOVERSION

Cardioversion is used to treat ventricular and supraventricular tachyarrhythmias in clinical settings that mandate rapid arrhythmia termination to prevent further clinical deterioration (i.e., severe hypotension or chest pain).

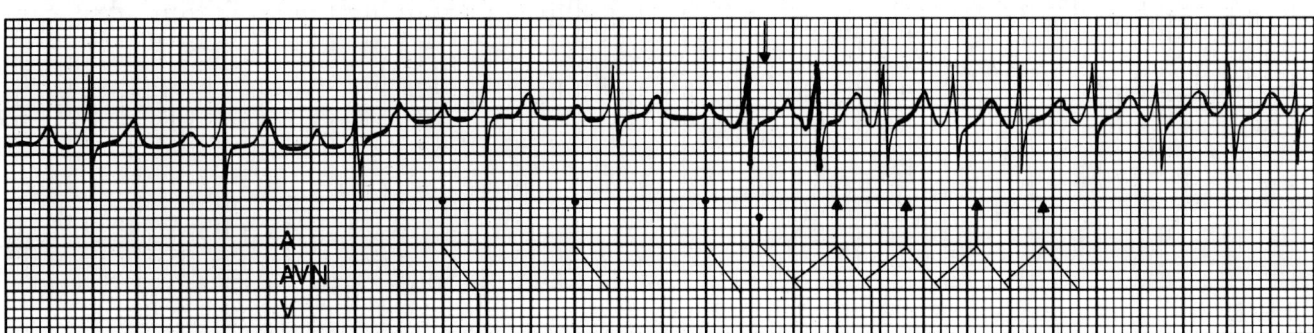

FIGURE 37-41. Atrial tachycardia. Initially, normal sinus rhythm is present. This is interrupted by a premature atrial contraction (*arrow*), which initiates episode of atrial tachycardia with rate of 185/minute. The proposed reentry mechanism at atrioventricular node level is illustrated in ladder diagram.

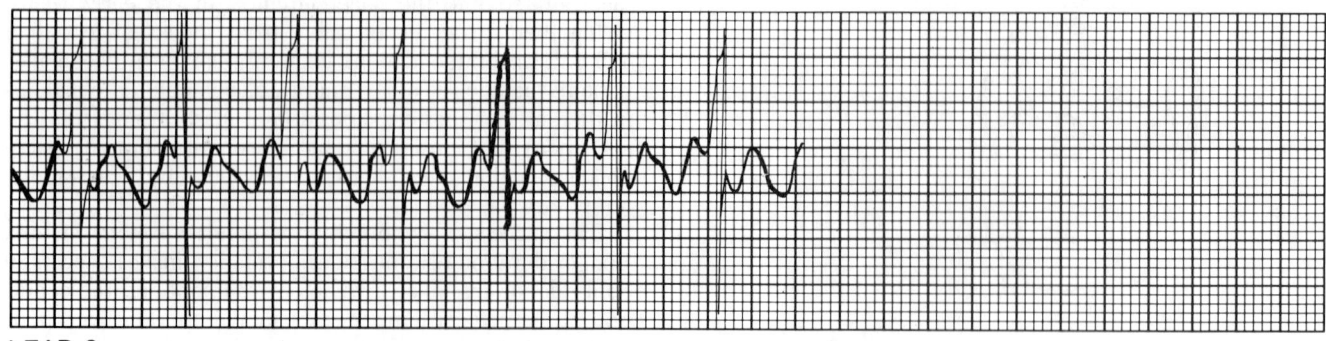

LEAD 2

FIGURE 37-42. Atrial flutter. Atrial rate is 250/minute and rhythm is regular. Every other F wave is conducted to ventricles (2:1 block), resulting in regular ventricular rhythm at rate of 125/minute.

Paroxysmal atrial tachycardia is characterized by the sudden onset of repeated episodes of atrial tachycardia[158,159] (Fig. 37-41). The episodes last several minutes to hours and usually end abruptly. The arrhythmia is thought to be caused by a reentrant phenomenon, and the ECG findings include 1:1 atrioventricular conduction or 2:1 conduction when the atrial rate exceeds 200/minute.

Atrial flutter is caused by reentry at the atrial level and seldom occurs without organic heart disease[133] (Fig. 37-42). Atrial flutter is usually the intermediate rhythm between normal sinus rhythm and atrial fibrillation. Characteristic ECG findings include flutter waves at a regular rate of about 300/minute. The ventricular rate is regular with constant conduction, usually at a ratio of 2:1.

Atrial fibrillation results from multiple ectopic foci, each depolarizing only a small islet of atrial myocardium[133] (Fig. 37-43). Impulses are randomly transmitted through the atrioventricular node, causing an irregular rhythm with no visible P waves.

Ventricular tachycardia is defined as three or more consecutive beats of ventricular origin[160] (Fig. 37-44). The arrhythmia may be well tolerated or may be life threatening, depending on the presence or absence of underlying myocardial dysfunction. Cardioversion is not indicated for arrhythmias possibly related to digitalis toxicity.

A synchronizing circuit allows delivery of a countershock to be "programmed" during a specific part of the QRS complex. This has been shown to reduce energy requirements and secondary complicating arrhythmias.

PROCEDURE

Attach the patient's electrodes to the cardioverter for sensing. Turn the cardioverter and the synchronizer switch on. Use the lead with an upright QRS complex and maximum R wave height, because the inverted QRS complex may not trigger the synchronizing circuit or may cause discharge on the T wave.

Select the appropriate energy level: ventricular tachycardia, 200 J; atrial arrhythmias, begin at 10 J if the patient has been treated with digitalis, and increase sequentially to 50, 100, 200, 300, or 400 J if needed. Ninety-five percent of patients with atrial flutter have their rhythm corrected with less than 50 J, whereas 95% of patients with atrial fibrillation revert with less than 200 J.[135]

If the patient is awake, give an amnesic drug, such as diazepam or midazolam, until sedation and amnesia are obtained, or methohexital, while monitoring blood pressure and respiratory rate. Apply electrode jelly to the paddles. Assure that the operator has no patient or bed contact.

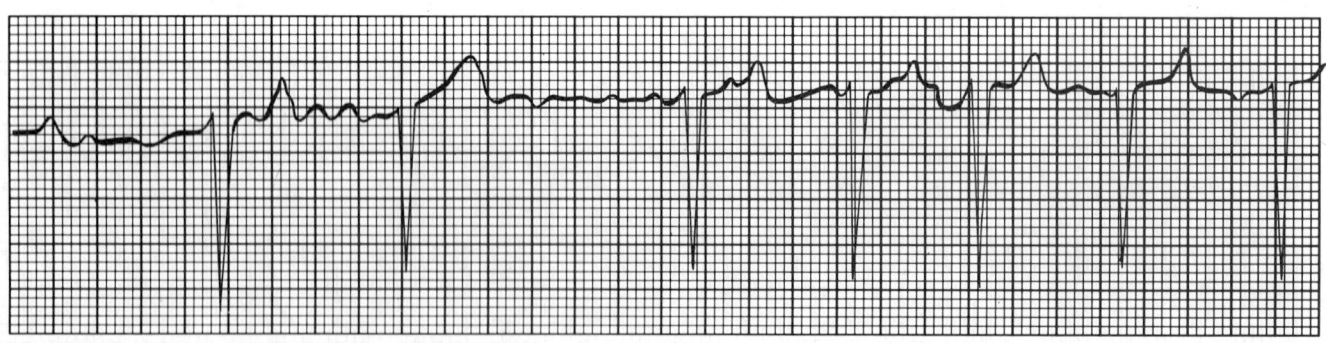

LEAD V₁

FIGURE 37-43. Atrial fibrillation with controlled ventricular response. Notice irregular undulations of baseline representing atrial electrical activity (F waves). The F waves vary in size and shape and are irregular in rhythm. Conduction through the atrioventricular node occurs at random, hence ventricular rhythm is irregular.

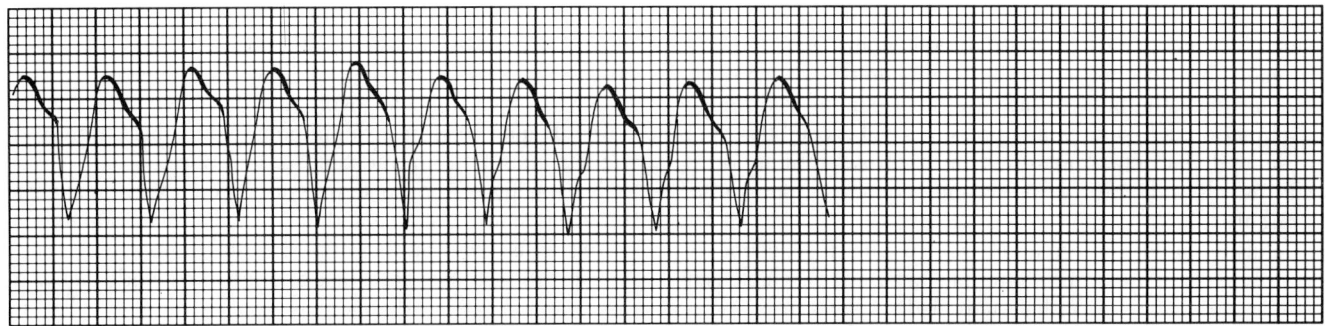

FIGURE 37-44. Ventricular tachycardia. The rhythm is regular at rate of 158/minute. The QRS complex is wide. No evidence of atrial depolarization is seen.

Administer the shock, holding the firing buttons down until the patient receives the current. Check the pulse, ECG, and airway. If the rhythm does not revert, increase the energy level and repeat the cardioversion. Should ventricular fibrillation develop, turn off the synchronizer circuit and defibrillate as previously described. Pulseless ventricular tachycardia should be treated similar to ventricular fibrillation.

COMPLICATIONS

Complications include additional arrhythmias, most being transient and innocuous.[161] Delivery of more than one countershock does not predispose to additional postshock arrhythmias.[162] Serious arrhythmias are related to high electrical discharge, overdigitalization, severity of heart disease, and electrolyte abnormalities. Postshock bradycardia exacerbated by antiarrhythmic drugs rarely requires support with pacing.[162] Animal studies have demonstrated a 2000-fold increase in sensitivity to electrical discharge with ouabain toxicity, manifested by ventricular tachycardia.[163] Ventricular fibrillation after cardioversion is usually related to improper synchronization and begins immediately after the shock.[161] Late onset of ventricular fibrillation suggests digitalization or quinidine toxicity.[164–167]

Transient elevations of creatine kinase and LDH enzymes have been observed with repeated high-energy shocks,[168,169] but cardioversion rarely obscures the diagnosis of myocardial infarction, and rarely are both enzymes elevated from cardioversion alone. Pulmonary edema may occur immediately or up to several hours after cardioversion.[170] The cause is not known but is postulated to be related to delayed return of left atrial function. Systemic embolization after cardioversion in patients with atrial fibrillation occurs in 1.2% to 1.5% of those reverted to sinus rhythm.[171,172] Anticoagulation is recommended for 3 weeks before and 4 weeks after cardioversion if the atrial fibrillation has been present for more than a week.[161]

PERICARDIOCENTESIS ■

Pericardiocentesis is indicated for the relief of cardiac tamponade or when a fluid sample is needed for diagnosis of a pericardial effusion. The pericardial sac normally contains up to 50 mL of fluid, which has the same composition as serum.[173] Pericardial tamponade results from the accumulation of fluid within the pericardial sac, which restricts ventricular diastolic filling and reduces stroke volume, cardiac output, and arterial blood pressure.[174–177] The fluid emanates from trauma, infection, renal failure, or neoplastic diseases.[178] While intrapericardial pressure rises, systemic arterial pressure declines and cardiac output is maintained with increasing tachycardia. Beck's triad of hypotension, increased venous pressure, and muffled heart sounds is fulfilled in less than 50% of the patients with tamponade.[179] Volume infusion to increase ventricular filling pressure is likely to help maintain adequate systemic pressure while the clinician prepares for pericardiocentesis.[180]

The earliest response to increased intrapericardial pressure is a compensatory increase in venous pressure; thus, an elevated central venous pressure is seen in most cases of cardiac tamponade.[174–178,181] Low-pressure tamponade may occur in volume-depleted patients with a central venous pressure less than 10 mm Hg.[178] The Y descent in the venous pulse and early filling dip in the ventricles are diminished with inhibition of early ventricular filling and atrial emptying

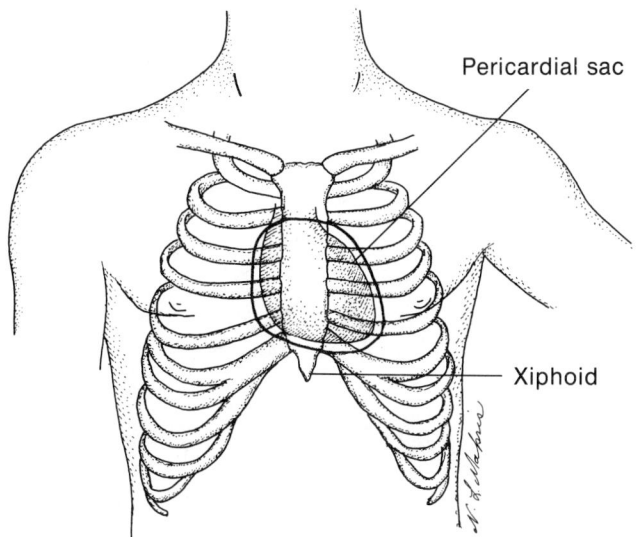

FIGURE 37-45. The paraxiphoid approach is most common and avoids both the pleura and coronary vessels.

during diastole. Diastolic equalization of intracardiac pressures (central venous, right atrial, right ventricular, and pulmonary artery occlusion) can be documented when a pulmonary artery catheter is in place. In the face of left ventricular dysfunction, left-sided filling pressures will exceed the right atrial and ventricular pressures, but right-sided filling pressures will still be elevated and equal to pericardial pressures.[174–178,181]

Pulsus paradoxus (greater than 10 mm Hg decline in systolic arterial pressure with normal inspiration), which usually is present in pericardial tamponade, results from a leftward shift of the septum while the ventricles compete for space within the distended pericardial sac. This change leads to selective impairment of ventricular filling.[174–178,181] Reduced ventricular filling also results from increased pulmonary capacitance because of the discrepancy in intrapericardial pressure and pulmonary venous pressure.[174–178,181] Pulsus paradoxus may be difficult to detect in the presence of severe hypotension, cardiac arrhythmias, or erratic respiratory patterns. Direct arterial pressure tracings may be more sensitive

in detecting respiratory variation than is cuff measurement. Pulsus paradoxus occurs in other disease states, such as obstructive airway disease, restrictive cardiomyopathy, constrictive pericarditis, hypovolemia, or mechanical ventilation.[181] It may be seen with pulmonary embolism, right ventricular infarction, mitral stenosis, and obesity.[178]

Narrowing of the pulse pressure occurs with rising systemic vascular resistance and decreased stroke volume. Hypotension is a late finding in pericardial tamponade.[174–178,181] Nonspecific findings of cardiac tamponade include tachycardia, cyanosis, pallor, diaphoresis, cool extremities, oliguria, and impaired sensation.

The chest radiograph may show evidence of a pericardial effusion with an enlarged cardiac silhouette, but it is rarely helpful in acute pericardial tamponade. Although bulging sac-like and globular heart shapes are characteristic for pericardial effusion, no size or shape is obligatory.[182] Lung fields are clear. Patients with acute tamponade can die with as little as 200 mL of pericardial fluid, yet 300 mL or more may be present without a detectable increase in cardiac

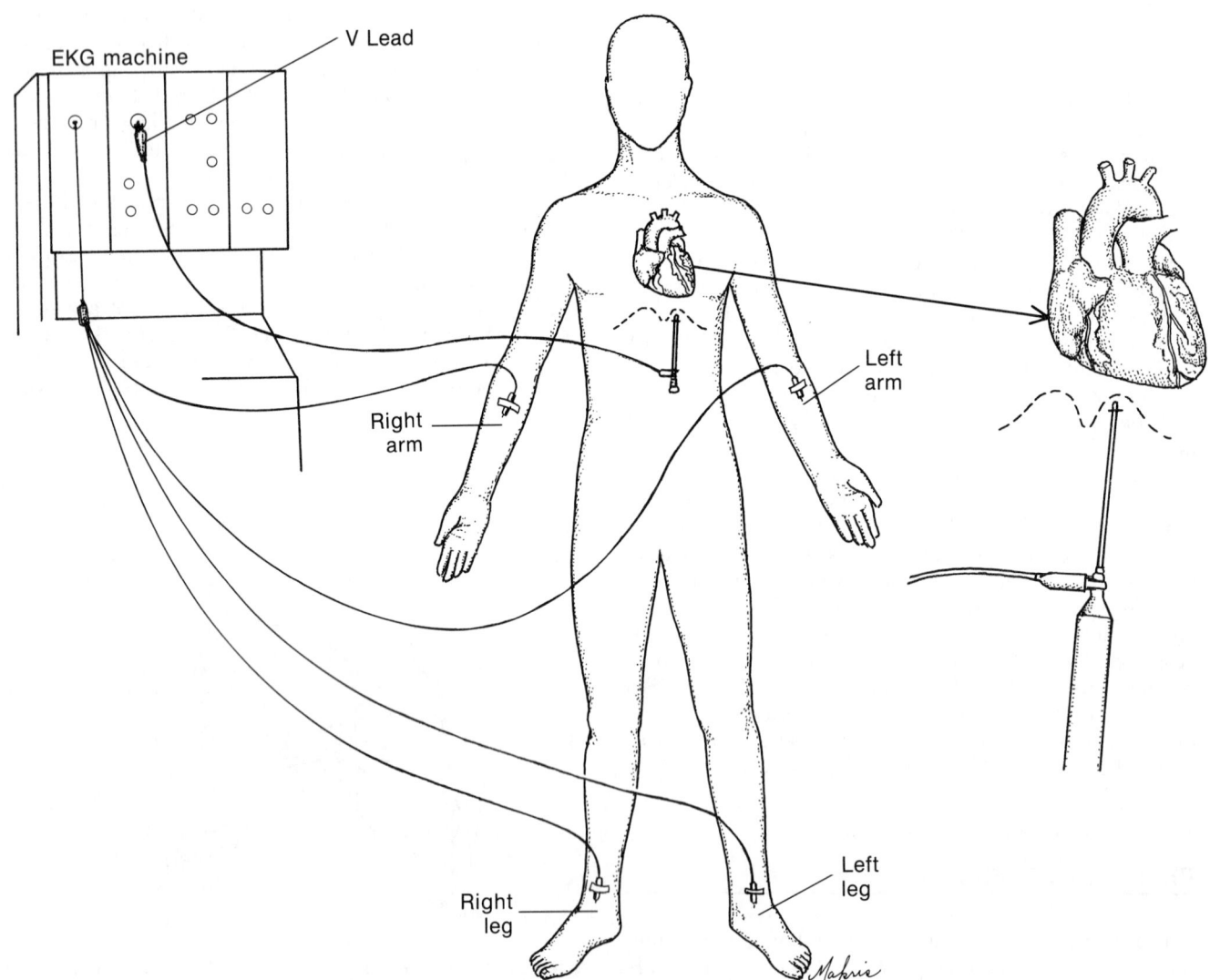

FIGURE 37-46. Connect the metal needle to the V lead of the electrocardiogram with a sterile alligator clip and place a 10-mL syringe on the needle.

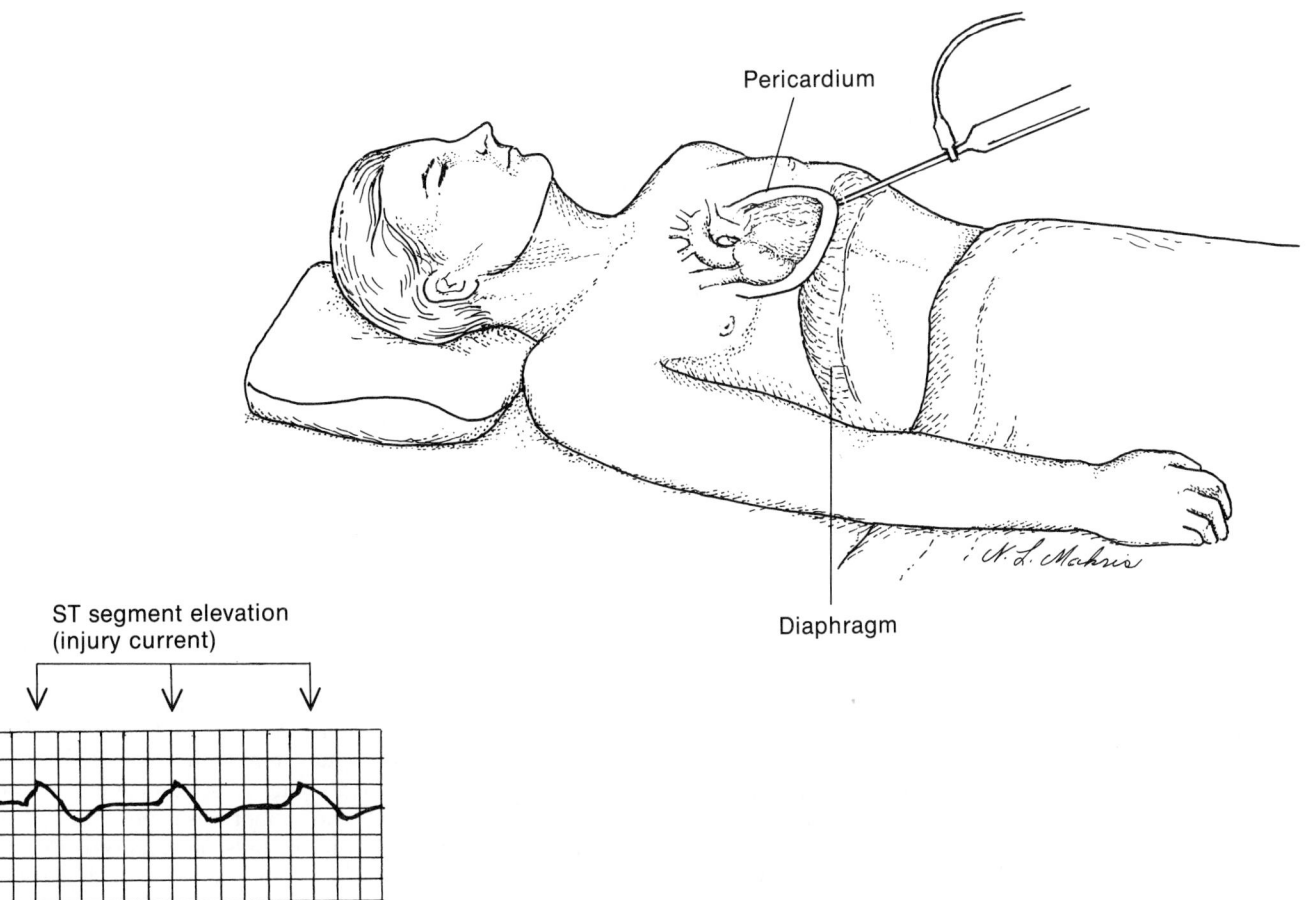

FIGURE 37-47. ST segment elevation is present with ventricular epicardial elevation.

silhouette. Subtle clues may be observed acutely, such as a central venous catheter lodged against a right atrial wall but more than 5 mm from the cardiac silhouette, indicating an effusion.[182]

Echocardiography is sensitive in diagnosing tamponade and also may be useful in guiding needle drainage of the pericardial sac.[183] Pericardial effusion with right ventricular implosion during end-diastole and expiration are diagnostic of cardiac tamponade.[184] Nonspecific findings of tamponade include decreased left ventricular end-diastolic dimension, "swinging heart," electrical alternans, and reciprocal respiratory variations in right and left ventricular end-diastolic dimensions.[184] The right ventricular compression resolves after pericardiocentesis.

The ECG may show low voltage and nonspecific ST-T wave changes. Electrical alternans may be present, showing beat-to-beat changes in the axis as the heart swings within the pericardial effusion.[185] Electromechanical dissociation may be a manifestation of pericardial tamponade.[174–178,181]

Needle pericardiocentesis is indicated for cardiac tamponade when it is life threatening or when it is progressive and produces increasingly severe hemodynamic impairment. Pericardiocentesis should be performed for any patient with acute tamponade in whom systolic blood pressure has fallen more than 30 mm Hg from the baseline level.[173,186]

PROCEDURE

Place the patient in the supine position or with the upper torso elevated 20 to 30 degrees. Atropine may be used as a premedication to prevent vagal reactions associated with pericardial puncture. Lidocaine without epinephrine should be used as the local anesthetic. The paraxiphoid subcostal approach is most common and avoids both the pleura and the coronary vessels (Fig. 37-45). The left parasternal approach through the fourth intercostal space also can be used.

Attach a long (12- to 18-cm), large-bore (16- to 18-gauge) cardiac needle with a short bevel (to minimize the risk of cardiac laceration) to a 50-mL syringe. Connect the metal needle to the V lead of the ECG with a sterile alligator clip and place a 10-mL syringe on the needle (Fig. 37-46). For the paraxiphoid approach, enter the skin just below the costal margin adjacent to the xiphoid and advance the needle slowly at a 45-degree horizontal angle under the ribs toward the midpoint of the left clavicle. Apply gentle suction to the syringe.

For the left parasternal approach, advance the needle slowly through the fourth intercostal space at the sternal border and perpendicular to the chest wall. Insert the needle in the anesthetized tract. When the needle tip is deep to the costal arch, depress the hub and advance the needle toward the left shoulder, aspirating during advancement. Monitor for injury current. ST elevation is present with ventricular epicardial contact (Fig. 37-47), and PR segment elevation is present with atrial epicardial contact. After epicardial contact, withdraw the needle slightly or reposition. If fluid is not obtained, redirect the needle toward the head or right shoulder. A characteristic resistance of the pericardium may often be felt at the needle tip. A popping sensation may be noted as the pericardium is penetrated.

When fluid is returned, the needle is stabilized by attaching a hemostat at the skin surface, preventing inadvertent overpenetration and also providing depth reference for future aspiration attempts. Removal of as little as 25 to 50 mL of blood may result in immediate improvement in the patient's condition, with a decrease in venous pressure and rise in systolic pressure.

The beating heart usually defibrinates blood in the pericardial space. Clotting suggests that a cardiac chamber has been entered inadvertently. Massive intrapericardial bleeding may not defibrinate and thereby clots, preventing needle aspiration. In such a case, drainage using a subxiphoid approach or thoracotomy is necessary. If no improvement in the patient's condition occurs after aspiration for suspected acute tamponade, immediate thoracotomy is mandatory. Pericardiocentesis to remove bloody fluid after trauma should be considered a temporary measure to be followed in most cases by thoracotomy. If V-lead monitoring from the pericardiocentesis needle is not feasible, an alternate approach utilizes a 20-gauge spinal exploring needle over which a 14-gauge needle has been placed. Once the pericardial space has been entered with the spinal needle, the large-bore needle is advanced over the spinal needle into the epicardial space and the spinal needle is removed.

COMPLICATIONS

A complication of pericardiocentesis includes ventricular puncture, which usually has no sequelae. The patient should be observed for tamponade.[187] Cardiac arrhythmias and laceration of the cardiac chambers or coronary vessels are potential complications, as are hemothorax and pneumothorax.[186,187]

TRANSTRACHEAL ASPIRATION ■

Transtracheal aspiration was first described by Pecora and Brook[188] in 1959 after the discovery that sputum specimens did not accurately reflect the bacteriologic makeup of the lower respiratory tract because of contamination with mouth organisms. Bartlett and coworkers[189] subsequently showed that transtracheal aspiration is efficacious in documenting anaerobic pulmonary infections.

Transtracheal aspiration may diagnose pulmonary infection, thereby avoiding bronchoalveolar lavage and lung biopsy, which are associated with a higher morbidity.[190] Transtracheal aspiration is used to obtain a sputum specimen in the nonintubated patient who cannot raise sputum or who is likely to be infected with an unusual organism. False-negative cultures approach 14% in patients treated with antibiotics but are present in only 1% of untreated patients.[191]

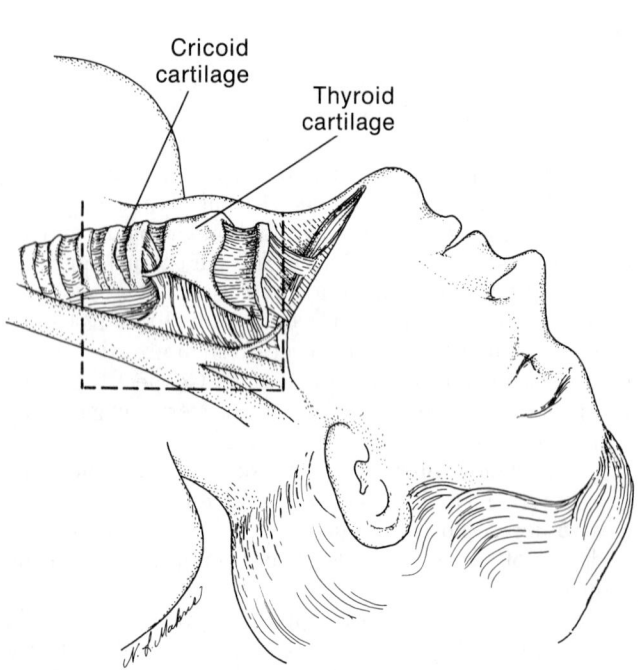

FIGURE 37-48. Locate the cricothyroid space.

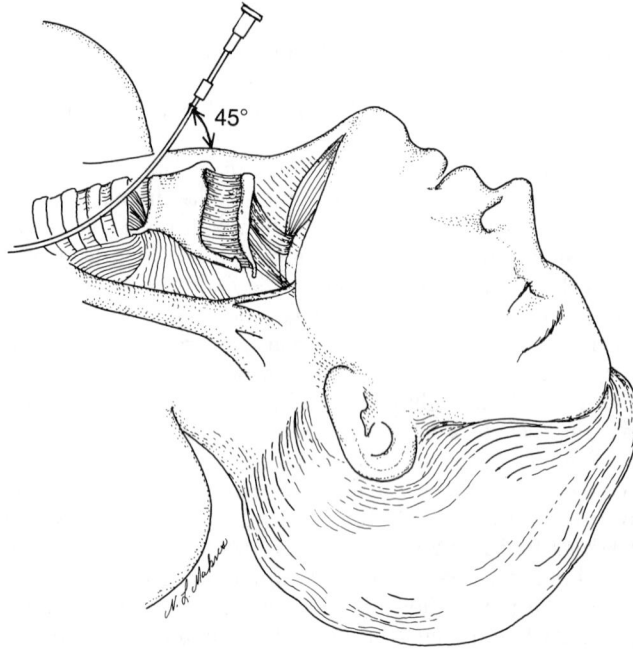

FIGURE 37-49. Thread the catheter down into the trachea. Remove the stylet, and slide the needle out of the trachea over the cannula.

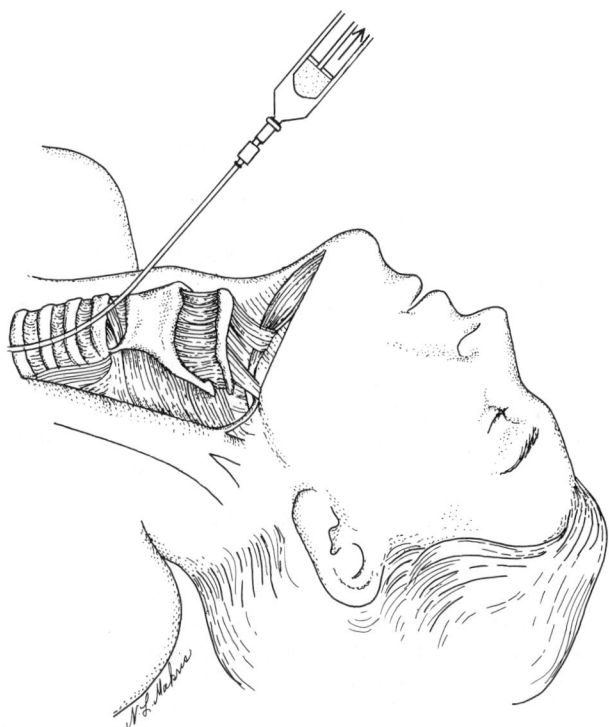

FIGURE 37-50. Aspirate the specimen during cough only.

PROCEDURE

Place the patient in the supine position with a pillow or roll under the shoulders to extend the neck. Locate the cricothyroid space (Fig. 37-48). Inject the local anesthetic, first raising a skin wheal, then infiltrating down to the cricothyroid membrane. Avoid injecting lidocaine into the trachea—it is bacteriostatic and dilutes the specimen. Puncture the membrane with a 14-gauge Intracath needle attached to a syringe with the bevel up. Aim caudally and 45 degrees to the skin. Thrust the needle through the membrane. Aspirate to confirm intratracheal position. Remove the syringe. Quickly thread the catheter down into the trachea. Remove the stylet, and slide the needle from the trachea over the cannula (Fig. 37-49). Aspirate the specimen during coughing only. If the specimen is inadequate (two to three drops of secretions are necessary for processing), inject 2 to 3 mL of sterile, nonbacteriostatic saline and aspirate again (Fig. 37-50). Remove the syringe, and inoculate the culture media immediately. Withdraw the catheter and needle as a single unit, and apply a dressing.

COMPLICATIONS

Complications are related to the needle puncture site, catheter placement in the lower airways, and vasovagal reactions precipitating cardiac arrest.[192] Paroxysmal coughing and hypoxemia may result from catheter irrigation. Minor hemoptysis is self-limiting. Local abscess and cellulitis are rare.

Subcutaneous emphysema, the most frequent complication, has been reported to be more prominent in patients with persistent coughing after the procedure; the incidence was less if the patient was placed at bedrest for 8 to 12 hours.[193,194] Fatal hemorrhage has occurred.[195]

Contraindications include bleeding diathesis, marked hypoxemia, severe hemoptysis, and inability to cooperate.[192] Caution is necessary in pediatric patients because of the smaller airway caliber and difficulty with cooperation.[192]

REFERENCES ■

1. Langston HT: The thorax, pleura and lungs. In: Davis L (ed). *Christopher's Textbook of Surgery.* Philadelphia, WB Saunders, 1968
2. Gott PH: A simplified method for thoracentesis and pleural fluid drainage. *Am Rev Respir Dis* 1965;92:295
3. Hoffman L: A modified thoracentesis technique. *Am Rev Respir Dis* 1964;89:106
4. Light RW, Girard WM, Jenkinson SG, et al: Parapneumonic effusions. *Am J Med* 1980;69:507
5. Light RW: Parapneumonic effusions and empyema. *Clin Chest Med* 1985;6:55
6. Light RW, MacGregor MI, Luchsinger PC, et al: Pleural effusions: the diagnostic separation of transudates and exudates. *Ann Intern Med* 1972;77:507
7. Light RW, Ball WC Jr: Glucose and amylase in pleural effusions. *JAMA* 1973;225:257
8. Light RW, MacGregor MI, Ball WC Jr, et al: Diagnostic significance of pleural fluid pH and pCO$_2$. *Chest* 1973;64:591
9. Potts DE, Levin DC, Sahn SA: Pleural pH in parapneumonic effusions. *Chest* 1976;70:328
10. Light RW: Management of parapneumonic effusions. *Chest* 1976;70:325
11. Seneff MG, Corwin RW, Gold LW, et al: Complications associated with thoracentesis. *Chest* 1986;90:97
12. Collins TR, Sahn SA: Thoracentesis: Clinical value, complications, technical problems, and patient experience. *Chest* 1987;91:837
13. Health and Public Policy Committee, American College of Physicians: Diagnostic thoracentesis and pleural biopsy in pleural effusions. *Ann Intern Med* 1985;103:799
14. Dalbec DL, Krome RL: Thoracostomy. *Emerg Med Clin North Am* 1986;4:441
15. The American Thoracic Society: Guidelines for thoracentesis and needle biopsy of the pleura. *Am Rev Respir Dis* 1989;140:257
16. Hewett FC: Thoracentesis: the plan of continuous aspiration. *Br Med J* 1876;1:317
17. Betts RH, Less WM: Military thoracic surgery in forward area. *J Thorac Surg* 1946;15:44
18. Kovarik JL, Brown RK: Tube and trocar thoracostomy. *Surg Clin North Am* 1969;49:1455
19. Melton LJ III, Hepper WG, Offord KP: Influence on height on risk of spontaneous pneumothorax. *Mayo Clin Proc* 1981;56:678
20. Hinsaw HC, Murray JF: *Diseases of the Chest.* Philadelphia, WB Saunders, 1980
21. Rutherford RB, Campbell DN: Thoracic injuries. In: Zuidema GD, Rutherford RB, Ballinger WF (eds). *The Management of Trauma,* 4th ed. Philadelphia, WB Saunders, 1973:391

22. Cordice JWV, Cabezon J: Chest trauma with pneumothorax and hemothorax: review of experience with 502 cases. *J Thorac Cardiovasc Surg* 1965;50:316

23. Kattan KR: Trauma of the bony thorax. *Semin Roentgenol* 1978;13:69

24. Kircher LT Jr, Swartzel RL: Spontaneous pneumothorax and its treatment. *JAMA* 1954;155:24

25. Light RW: Management of spontaneous pneumothorax. *American Review of Respiratory Disease.* 1993;148(1):245-8

26. Greene R, McCloud TC, Stark P: Pneumothorax. *Semin Roentgenol* 1977;12:313

27. Rhea JT, DeLuca SA, Greene RE: Determining the size of pneumothorax in the upright patient. *Radiology* 1982;144:733

28. Sabiston DC, Spencer FC: *Gibbon's Surgery of the Chest*, 3rd ed. Philadelphia, WB Saunders, 1976

29. Vukich DJ: Pneumothorax, hemothorax, and other abnormalities of the pleural space. *Emerg Med Clin North Am* 1983;1:431

30. Vukich DJ: Diseases of the pleural space. *Emerg Med Clin North Am* 1989;7:309

31. Zimmerman JE, Dunbar RS, Klingermaier CH: Management of subcutaneous emphysema, pneumomediastinum and pneumothorax during respiratory therapy. *Crit Care Med* 1975; 3:69

32. Zwilich DW, Pierson DJ, Creagh CE, et al: Complications of assisted ventilation: a prospective study of 354 consecutive cases. *Am J Med* 1974;57:161

33. Bernard RW, Stahl WM: Subclavian vein catheterizations: a prospective study. I. Noninfecting complications. *Ann Surg* 1971;173:184

34. Christenson KH: Complications of percutaneous catheterization of the subclavian vein in 129 cases. *Acta Chir Scand* 1967;113:615

35. Farber DL, Rose DM, Bassell GM, et al: Hemoptysis and pneumothorax after removal of a persistently wedged pulmonary catheter. *Crit Care Med* 1981;9:494

36. Dimarco JP, Hasan G, Ruskin JN, et al: Complications of patients undergoing cardiac electrophysiologic procedures. *Ann Intern Med* 1982;97:490

37. Culpepper JA, Veremakis C, Guntapalli KK, et al: Malpositioned nasogastric tube causing pneumothorax and bronchopleural fistula [letter]. *Chest* 1982;81:389

38. Sarr MG: Bilateral pneumothoraces after resuscitation with esophageal airway [letter]. *JAMA* 1980;243:2154

39. Thomas JH, Perce GE, MacArthur RI: Bilateral pneumothoraces secondary to colonic endoscopy. *J Natl Med Assoc* 1979;71:701

40. McDonald HF: Right pneumothorax following fiberoptic oesophageal dilation. *Endoscopy* 1978;10:130

41. Ritter HG, Tarala R: Pneumothorax after acupuncture. *Br Med J* 1978;2:602

42. Orr KB, Magarey CJ: Pneumothorax after aspiration of breast cysts [letter]. *Med J Aust* 1978;1:101

43. Lewis JW, Elliott JF Jr, Obeid FN: Complications of attempted central venous injections by drug abusers. *Chest* 1980;78:613

44. Cohen S: Coca past and freebase: new fashion in cocaine use. *Drug Abuse Alcoholism Newsletter* April 9, 1980

45. Shesser R, David C, Edelstein S: Pneumomediastinum and pneumothorax after inhaling alkaloid cocaine. *Ann Emerg Med* 1981;10:213

46. Graham JM, Mattox KL, Beall AC: Penetrating trauma to the lung. *J Trauma* 1979;19:665

47. Griffith GL, Todd EF, McMillin RD, et al: Acute traumatic hemothorax. *Ann Thorac Surg* 1978;26:204

48. Coselli JS, Mattox KL, Beall AC Jr: Reevaluation of early evacuation of clotted hemothorax. *Am J Surg* 1984;148:786

49. Siemens R, Polk HC, Gray LA, et al: Indications for thoracotomy following penetrating thoracic injury. *J Trauma* 1977;17: 493

50. McNamara JJ, Messersmith JK, Dunn RA, et al: Thoracic injuries in combat casualties in Vietnam. *Ann Thorac Surg* 1970;10:389

51. Sandrasagra FA: Management of penetrating stab wounds of the chest: An assessment of the indication for early operation. *Thorax* 1978;33:474

52. Webb WR: Thoracic trauma. *Surg Clin North Am* 1974;54: 1179

53. Oparah SS, Mandal AK: Penetrating stab wound of the chest in civilian practice: experience with 200 consecutive cases. *J Trauma* 1976;16:868

54. Oparah SS, Mandal AK: Penetrating gunshot wounds of the chest in civilian practice: experience with 250 consecutive cases. *Br J Surg* 1978;65:45

55. Symbas PN: Autotransfusion from hemothorax: experimental and clinical studies. *J Trauma* 1972;12:689

56. Jacobs LM, Hsieh JW: A clinical review of autotransfusion and its role in trauma. *JAMA* 1984;251:3283

57. Schaff HV, Hauer JM, Bell WR, et al: Autotransfusion of shed mediastinal blood after cardiac surgery: a prospective study. *J Thorac Cardiovasc Surg* 1978;75:632

58. Schulman P, Cheng E, Cvitkovic E, et al: Spontaneous pneumothorax as a result of cytotoxic chemotherapy. *Chest* 1979;75:194

59. McFarlane JR, Cranston WH: Chylothorax. *Am Rev Respir Dis* 1972;105:207

60. Bessone LN, Ferguson TB, Burford TH: Chylothorax. *Ann Thorac Surg* 1971;12:527

61. Murphy MC, Newman BM, Rodgers BM: Pleuroperitoneal shunts in the management of persistent chylothorax. *Ann Thorac Surg* 1989;48:195

62. Mercier C, Page A, Verdant A, et al: Outpatient management of intercostal tube drainage in spontaneous pneumothorax. *Ann Thorac Surg* 1976; 22:163

63. Symbas PN: Chest drainage tubes. *Surg Clin North Am* 1989;69:41

64. Millikan JS, Moore EE, Steiner E, et al: Complications of tube thoracostomy for acute trauma. *Am J Surg* 1980;140:739

65. VanderSalm TJ: Chest tube insertion (closed thoracostomy). In: VanderSalm TJ, Cutler BS, Wheeler HB (eds). *Atlas of Bedside Procedures*. Boston, Little, Brown, 1979:193

66. Beall AC Jr, Crawford HW, DeBakey M: Considerations in the management of acute traumatic hemothorax. *J Thorac Cardiovasc Surg* 1966;52:351

67. Beall AC Jr, Bricker DL, Crawford WH, et al: Considerations in the management of penetrating thoracic trauma. *J Trauma* 1968;8:408

68. Grover FL, Richardson JD, Fewel JG, et al: Prophylactic antibiotics in the treatment of penetrating chest wounds. *J Thorac Cardiovasc Surg* 1977;74:528

69. Levitsky S, Annable CA, Thomas PA: The management of empyema after thoracic wounding: observation on 25 Vietnam casualties. *J Thorac Cardiovasc Surg* 1970;59:630

70. Helling TS, Gyles NR, Eisenstein CL, et al: Complications following blunt and penetrating injuries in 216 victims of chest trauma requiring tube thoracostomy. *J Trauma* 1989;29:1367

71. LoCurto JJ, Tischler CD, Swan KG, et al: Tube thoracostomy and trauma: antibiotics or not? *J Trauma* 1986;26:1067

72. LeBlanc KA, Tucker WY: Prophylactic antibiotics and closed tube thoracostomy. *Surg Gynecol Obstet* 1985;160:259

73. Daly RC, Mucha P, Pairolero PC, et al: The risk of percutaneous chest tube thoracostomy for blunt thoracic trauma. *Ann Emerg Med* 1985;14:865

74. Bernstein A, Waqaruddin M, Shah M: Management of spontaneous pneumothorax using a Heimlich flutter valve. *Thorax* 1973;28:386

75. Vallee P, Sullivan M, Richardson H, et al: Sequential treatment of a simple pneumothorax. *Ann Emerg Med* 1988;17:936

76. Heimlich HJ: Valve drainage of the pleural cavity. *Dis Chest* 1968;53:282

77. Nealon TF Jr: Diagnostic procedures. In: Nealon TF Jr (ed). *Fundamental Skills in Surgery*, 3rd ed. Philadelphia, WB Saunders, 1979

78. Guyton SW, Paull DL, Anderson RP: Introducer insertion of minithoracostomy tubes. *Am J Surg* 1988;155:693

79. Glickman RM, Isselbacker KJ: Abdominal swelling and ascites. In: Petersdorg RG, Adams RD, Braunwald E, et al (eds). *Harrison's Principles of Internal Medicine*, 10th ed. New York, McGraw-Hill, 1983

80. Runyon BA: Paracentesis of ascitic fluid: a safe procedure. *Arch Intern Med* 1986;146:2259

81. Gines P, Arroyo V, Quintero E, et al: Comparison between paracentesis and diuretics in the treatment of cirrhotics with tense ascites. *Gastroenterology* 1987;93:234

82. Williams RD, Zollinger RM: Diagnostic and prognostic factors in abdominal trauma. *Am J Surg* 1959;97:575

83. Giacobine JW, Siler VE: Evaluation of diagnostic abdominal paracentesis with experimental and clinical studies. *Surg Gynecol Obstet* 1960;110:676

84. Root HD, Keizer PJ, Perry JF: The clinical and experimental aspects of peritoneal response to injury. *Arch Surg* 1967;95:531

85. Cotter CP, Hawkins ML, Kent RB, et al: Ultrarapid diagnostic peritoneal lavage. *J Trauma* 1989;29:615

86. Drew T, Perry JF Jr, Fischer RP: The expediency of peritoneal lavage for blunt trauma in children. *Surg Gynecol Obstet* 1977;145:885

87. Ryan JJ, Kyes FN, Horner WR, et al: Critical analysis of open peritoneal lavage in blunt abdominal trauma. *Am J Surg* 1986;151:221

88. Fischer RP, Beverlin BC, Engrav LH, et al: Diagnostic peritoneal lavage: 14 years and 2586 patients later. *Am J Surg* 1978;136:701

89. Perry JF, DeMeules JE, Root HD: Diagnostic peritoneal lavage in blunt abdominal trauma. *Surg Gynecol Obstet* 1970;131:742

90. Howdieshell TR, Osler TM, Demarest GB: Open versus closed peritoneal lavage with particular attention to time, accuracy, and cost. *Am J Emerg Med* 1989;7:367

91. Cochran W, Sobat WS: Open versus closed diagnostic peritoneal lavage. *Ann Surg* 1984;200:24

92. Lowe RJ, Boyd DR, Folk FA, et al: The negative laparotomy for abdominal trauma. *J Trauma* 1972;12:853

93. Engrav LH, Benjamin CI, Strate RG, et al: Diagnostic peritoneal lavage in blunt abdominal trauma. *J Trauma* 1975;15:854

94. Olsen WR, Redman HC, Hildreth DH: Quantitative peritoneal lavage in blunt abdominal trauma. *Arch Surg* 1972;104:536

95. Thal ER, Shires GT: Peritoneal lavage in blunt abdominal trauma. *Am J Surg* 1973;125:64

96. Fischer RP, Freeman T: The inadequacy of peritoneal lavage in diagnosing acute diaphragmatic rupture. *J Trauma* 1976;16:538

97. Parvin S, Smith D, et al: Effectiveness of peritoneal lavage in blunt abdominal trauma. *Ann Surg* 1975;181:255

98. Bivins BA, Jona JZ, Belin RP: Diagnostic peritoneal lavage in pediatric lavage. *J Trauma* 1976;16:739

99. Olsen WR, Hildreth DM: Abdominal paracentesis and peritoneal lavage in blunt abdominal trauma. *J Trauma* 1971;11:824

100. Pacey J, Forward AD, Preto AD: Peritoneal tap and lavage in patients with abdominal trauma. *Can Med Assoc J* 1971;105:365

101. Jergens ME: Peritoneal lavage. *Am J Surg* 1977;133:365

102. Marx JA, Moore EE, Bar-Or D: Peritoneal lavage in penetrating injuries of the small bowel and colon: value of enzyme determinations. *Ann Emerg Med* 1983;12:13

103. Engrav LH, Benjamin CI, Strate RG, et al: Diagnostic peritoneal lavage in blunt abdominal trauma. *J Trauma* 1975;15:854

104. Hornyak SW, Shaftan GW: Value of "inconclusive lavage" in abdominal trauma management. *J Trauma* 1979;19:329

105. Alyono DA, Perry JF: Significance of repeating diagnostic peritoneal lavage. *Surgery* 1982;91:656

106. Thal ER, May RA, Beesinger D: Peritoneal lavage: its unreliability in gunshot wounds of the lower chest and abdomen. *Arch Surg* 1980;115:430

107. Merlotti GJ, Marcet E, Sheaff CM, et al: Use of peritoneal lavage to evaluate abdominal penetration. *J Trauma* 1985;25:228

108. Thal ER: Evaluation of peritoneal lavage and local exploration in lower chest and abdominal stab wounds. *J Trauma* 1977;17:642

109. Lobbato V, Cioroiu M, LaRaja RD, et al: Peritoneal lavage as an aid to diagnosis of peritonitis in debilitated and elderly patients. *Am Surg* 1985;51:508

110. Richardson JD, Flint IM, Polk HC: Peritoneal lavage: a useful diagnostic adjunct for peritonitis. *Surgery* 1983;94:826

111. Cullen DJ, Coyle JP, Teplick R, et al: Cardiovascular, pulmonary and renal effects of massively increased intra-abdominal pressure in critically ill patients. *Crit Care Med* 1989;17:118

112. Doppmann J, Robinson RM, Rockoff SD, et al: Mechanism of obstruction of the infradiaphragmatic portion of the inferior vena cava in the presence of increased intra-abdominal pressure. *Radiology* 1966;1:37

113. Suazzi M, Polese A, Magrini F, et al: Negative influence of ascites on the cardiac function of cirrhotic patients. *Am J Med* 1975;59:165

114. Harman PK, Kron IL, McLachlan HD, et al: Elevated intra-abdominal pressure and renal function. *Ann Surg* 1982;196:594

115. Kron IL, Harman PK, Nolan SP: The measurement of intra-abdominal pressure as a criterion for abdominal re-exploration. *Ann Surg* 1984;199:28

116. Celoria G, Steingrub J, Dawson JA, et al: Oliguria from high intra-abdominal pressure secondary to ovarian mass. *Crit Care Med* 1987;15:78

117. Iberti TJ, Lieber CE, Benjamin E: Determination of intraabdominal pressure using a transurethral bladder catheter: clinical validation of the technique. *Anesthesiology* 1989;70:47

118. Arrighi DA, Farnell MB, Mucha P, et al: Prospective, randomized trial of rapid venous access for patients in hypovolemic shock. *Ann Emerg Med* 1989;18:927

119. Woodburn RT: *Essentials of Human Anatomy*, 5th ed. New York, Oxford University Press, 1973

120. Tucker JF, Danzl DF, Teague E, et al: Infusion of intravenous fluids distal to pneumatic anti-shock trousers. *Emerg Med* 1984;2:79

121. Moore FA: Venous access. In: Moore EE, Eisman B, Van Way CW III (eds). *Critical Decisions in Trauma*. St. Louis, CV Mosby, 1984

122. Simon RR, Hoffman JR, Smith M: Modified new approaches for rapid intravenous access. *Ann Emerg Med* 1987;16:44

123. Dronen SC, Yee AS, Tamlovich MC: Proximal saphenous vein cutdown. *Ann Emerg Med* 1981;10:238
124. Au FC: The anatomy of the cephalic vein. *Ann Surg* 1989;55:638
125. Ellis BW, Dudley HAF: Intravenous therapy and blood transfusion. In: Dudley HAF (ed). *Hamilton Bailey's Emergency Surgery*, 10th ed. Chicago, Year Book Medical Publishers, 1977:25
126. Zipes DP, Fischer J, King RM, et al: Termination of ventricular fibrillation in dogs by depolarizing a critical amount of myocardium. *Am J Cardiol* 1975;36:37
127. Seger JJ, Griffin JC: Electrical therapy of arrhythmias. *Cardiol Clin* 1985;3:617
128. Prevost JL, Batelli F: Sur quelques effets des decharges electriques sur le coeur des mammiferers. *CR Acad Sci (Paris)* 1899;129:1267
129. Beck CS, Pritchard WH, Feil H: Ventricular fibrillation of long duration abolished by electrical shock. *JAMA* 1947;135:985
130. Lown B, Neuman J, Amarasingham R, et al: Comparison of alternating current with direct current electroshock across the closed chest. *Am J Cardiol* 1962;10:223
131. Nachias MM, Box HH, Mower MM, et al: Observations on defibrillators, defibrillation and synchronized countershock. *Prog Cardiovasc Dis* 1966;9:64
132. *American National Standard for Cardiac Defibrillator Devices*. Arlington, VA, American Association for the Advancement of Medical Instrumentation, 1981
133. American Heart Association: *Textbook of Advanced Cardiac Life Support*, 3rd ed. Dallas, American Heart Association, 1994
134. Dahl CF, Ewy GA, Ewy MD, et al: Transthoracic impedance to direct current discharge: effect of repeated countershocks. *Med Instrum* 1976;10:151
135. DeSilva RA, Graboys TB, Podrid PJ, et al: Cardioversion and defibrillation. *Am Heart J* 1980;100:881
136. Ewy GA: Electrical therapy for cardiovascular emergencies. *Circulation* 1986;74(Suppl 4):111
137. Lau FY: Protection of implanted pacemakers from excessive electrical energy of DC shock. *Am J Cardiol* 1969;23:244
138. Cordis Corporation: *Cordis Gemini Pulse Generator Technical Manual*. Miami, Cordis Corporation, 1983
139. Cordis Corporation: *Cordis Sequicor Pulse Generator Technical Manual*. Miami, Cordis Corporation, 1982
140. Gould L, Patel S, Gomes GI: Pacemaker failure following external defibrillation. *PACE* 1981;4:575
141. Medtronic, Inc: *Medtronic Mirel VL 5988/5989 Pulse Generator Technical Manual*. Minneapolis, Medtronic, 1978
142. Medtronic, Inc: *Medtronic Spectrax SXT Pulse Generator Technical Manual*. Minneapolis, Medtronic, 1978
143. Springrose S: *CPI Technical Issues, Technical Memorandum and Recommendations for Defibrillator Procedures for Pacemaker Patients*. St. Paul, Cardiac Pacemakers, 1979
144. Lown B, Amarasingham R, Neuman J: New methods for terminating cardiac arrhythmias: use of synchronized capacitor discharge. *JAMA* 1962;182:548
145. Weaver WD, Zia M, Green D, et al: Coarse and fine ventricular fibrillation during cardiac arrest. *Circulation* 1982;66(Suppl 2):348
146. Weaver WD, Cobb LA, Dennis D, et al: Amplitude of ventricular fibrillation waveform and outcome after cardiac arrest. *Ann Intern Med* 1985;102:53
147. Zipes DP: Electrophysiological mechanisms involved in ventricular defibrillation. *Circulation* 1975;52(Suppl 13):120
148. Geddes LA, Tacker WA, Rosborough JP, et al: Electrical dose for ventricular defibrillation of large and small animals using precordial electrodes. *J Clin Invest* 1974;53:310
149. Lown B, Crampton RS, DeSilva RA, et al: The energy for ventricular defibrillation: too little or too much? *N Engl J Med* 1978;298:1252
150. Geddes LA, Tacker WA, Cablar P, et al: The decrease in transthoracic impedance during successive ventricular defibrillation trails. *Med Instrum* 1975;9:179
151. Kerber RE, Hoyt R, Grayzel J, et al: Effects of repeated paddle shocks and paddle contact pressure. *Circulation* 1979;59(Suppl 2):127
152. Thomas ED, Ewy GA, Dahl CF, et al: Effectiveness of direct current defibrillation: role of paddle electrode size. *Am Heart J* 1977;93:463
153. Kerber RE, Grayzel J, Hoyt R, et al: Transthoracic resistance in human defibrillation: effects of body weight, chest size, same-energy shocks, paddle size, and paddle contact pressure [abstract]. *Med Instrum* 1980;14:56
154. Patton JN, Pantridge JF: Current required from ventricular defibrillation. *Br Med J* 1979;1:513
155. Ewy GA, Taren D: Impedance to transthoracic direct current discharge: a model for testing interface material. *Med Instrum* 1978;12:47
156. Kerber RE, Martini JB, Kelly KJ, et al: Self-adhesive preapplied electrode pads for defibrillation and cardioversion. *J Am Coll Cardiol* 1984;3:815
157. Dalzell GWN, Cunningham SR, Anderson J, et al: Electrode pad size, transthoracic impedance and success of external defibrillation. *Am J Cardiol* 1989;64:741
158. Marriott HJ, Myerburg RJ: Recognition and treatment of cardiac arrhythmias and conduction disturbances. In: Hurst JW, Logue RB, Schlant TC (eds). *The Heart, Arteries and Veins*, 4th ed. New York, McGraw-Hill, 1978
159. Goldreyer BN, Bigger JT Jr: Site of reentry in paroxysmal supraventricular tachycardia in man. *Circulation* 1971;43:15
160. Wellens HF, Bar FW, Lie KI: The value of the electrocardiogram in the differential diagnosis of a tachycardia with a widened QRS complex. *Am J Med* 1978;64:27
161. Lown B, DeSilva RA: The technique of cardioversion. In: Hurst JW (ed). *The Heart*. New York, McGraw-Hill, 1986
162. Waldecker B, Brugada P, Zehender M, et al: Dysrhythmias after direct-current cardioversion. *Am J Cardiol* 1986;57:120
163. Lown B, Cannon RL III, Rossi MA: Electrical stimulation and digitalis drugs: repetitive response in diastole. *Proc Soc Exp Biol Med* 1967;126:698
164. Regan TJ, Markov A, Oldewurtel HA, et al: Myocardial K loss after countershock and the relation to ventricular arrhythmias after nontoxic doses of acetyl strophanthidin. *Am Heart J* 1969;77:367
165. Rabbino MD, Likoff W, Dreifus LS: Complications and limitations of direct current countershock. *JAMA* 1964;190:147
166. Ross EM: Cardioversion causing ventricular fibrillation. *Arch Intern Med* 1964;114:811
167. Castellanos A, Lamberg L, Gilmore H, et al: Countershock exposed quinidine syncope. *Am J Med Sci* 1965;260:254
168. Ehsani A, Ewy GA, Sobe BE: Effects of electrical countershock on serum creatinine phosphokinase (CPK) isoenzyme activity. *Am J Cardiol* 1976;37:12
169. Reiffel JA, McCarthy DM, Leakey EB: Does cardioversion affect isoenzyme recognition of myocardial infarction? *Am Heart J* 1974;97:810
170. Resnekov L, McDonald L: Complications in 220 patients with cardiac dysrhythmias treated by phased direct current shock and indications for electroversion. *Br Heart J* 1967;29:926
171. Lown B: Electrical reversion of cardiac arrhythmias. *Br Heart J* 1967;29:469
172. Goldman MJ: The management of chronic atrial fibrillation: indications for and method of conversion to sinus rhythm. *Prog Cardiovasc Dis* 1960;2:465

173. Roberts WC, Spray TL: Pericardial heart disease: a study of its causes, consequences, and morphologic features. *Cardiovasc Clin* 1976;7:11

174. Fowler NO: Physiology of cardiac tamponade and pulsus paradoxus. II. Physiological, circulatory, and pharmacological responses in cardiac tamponade. *Mod Concepts Cardiovasc Dis* 1978;47:115

175. Shabetai R: The pathophysiology of cardiac tamponade and constriction. *Cardiovasc Clin* 1976;7:67

176. Shabetai R, Fowler NO, Guntheroth WG: The hemodynamics of cardiac tamponade and constrictive pericarditis. *Am J Cardiol* 1970;26:480

177. Fowler NO: Physiology of cardiac tamponade and pulsus paradoxus in cardiac tamponade. *Mod Concepts Cardiovasc Dis* 1978;47:109

178. Spodick DH: Pericarditis, pericardial effusion, cardiac tamponade, and constriction. *Crit Care Clin* 1989;5:455

179. Peper WA, Obeid FN, Horst HM, et al: Penetrating injuries of the mediastinum. *Am Surg* 1986;52:359

180. Cooper FW, Stead EA, Warren JV: Beneficial effect of intravenous infusions in acute pericardial tamponade. *Ann Surg* 1944;120:822

181. Hancock EW: Management of pericardial disease. *Mod Concepts Cardiovasc Dis* 1979;48:1

182. Spodick DH: Acute cardiac tamponade: pathologic physiology, diagnosis and management. *Prog Cardiovasc Dis* 1967;10:64

183. Zobel G, Stein J, Beitze A, et al: Echocardiography controlled pericardiocentesis. *Int Care Med* 1987;13:297

184. Schiller NB, Botvinick EH: Right ventricular compression as a sign of tamponade: an analysis of echocardiographic ventricular dimensions and their clinical implications. *Circulation* 1977;56:774

185. Usher BW, Popp RL: Electrical alternans: mechanism in pericardial effusion. *Am Heart J* 1972;83:459

186. Kilpatrick ZM, Chapman CB: On pericardiocentesis. *Am J Cardiol* 1965;16:722

187. Pories WJ, Guadiani VA: Cardiac tamponade. *Surg Clin North Am* 1975;55:573

188. Pecora DV, Brook R: A method of securing uncontaminated tracheal secretions for bacterial examination. *J Thorac Surg* 1959;37:653

189. Bartlett JG, Rosenblatt JE, Finegold SM: Percutaneous transtracheal aspiration in the diagnosis of anaerobic pulmonary infection. *Ann Intern Med* 1973;79:535

190. De Vivo F, Pond GD, Rhenman B, et al: Transtracheal aspiration and fine needle aspiration biopsy for the diagnosis of pulmonary infection in heart transplant patients. *J Thorac Cardiovasc Surg* 1988;96:696

191. Bartlett JG: Diagnostic accuracy of transtracheal aspiration bacteriologic studies. *Am Rev Respir Dis* 1977;115:777

192. Bartlett JG: Diagnosis of bacterial infections of the lung. *Clin Chest Med* 1987;8:119

193. Kalinske RW, Parker RH, Brandt D, et al: Diagnostic usefulness and safety of transtracheal aspiration. *N Engl J Med* 1967;276:604

194. Spencer CD, Beaty HN: Complications of transtracheal aspiration. *N Engl J Med* 1972;286:304

195. Schillner RF, Iacovoni VE, Conte RS: Transtracheal aspiration complicated by fatal endotracheal hemorrhage. *N Engl J Med* 1976;295:488

Critical Care, Third Edition, edited by Joseph M. Civetta,
Robert W. Taylor, and Robert R. Kirby.
Lippincott-Raven Publishers, Philadelphia, PA © 1997.

CHAPTER 38

Interventional Radiology

Diego Nunez
Kimberly A. Lentz
Alejandro Zuluaga

This chapter offers the critical care physician a working repertory of available imaging and image-guided procedures that can provide extended diagnostic information or therapy in various medical problems that commonly affect the critically ill patient. To facilitate the discussion on the applications of interventional radiology in critical care medicine, the disease entities and related procedures are considered under vascular and nonvascular categories.

VASCULAR PROCEDURES

The vascular emergencies amenable to radiologic endovascular management include the following: pulmonary embolism, acute ischemia, gastrointestinal (GI) bleeding, intravascular catheters and foreign body manipulations, and traumatic vascular injuries.

PULMONARY EMBOLISM

Thromboembolic disease is a common complicating problem in the setting of the intensive care unit (ICU) and in critically ill patients with a variety of serious medical illnesses. Although there has been considerable progress in its clinical management and a decreasing incidence of the disease, advanced medical care also has enhanced the survival of patients with predisposing, severe conditions such as advanced malignancy, multisystem trauma, and extensive surgery. The diagnosis must be precise because the patient can be left at risk of a fatal outcome if misdiagnosed, or at risk of the morbid effects of therapy if over diagnosed. Yet, controversy remains as to the most effective way to provide the diagnosis with certainty.

Diagnosis

The chest radiograph combined with the ventilation/perfusion ($\dot{V}/\dot{Q}$) radionuclide scan are the imaging examinations initially requested for the evaluation of pulmonary embolism. The interpretation of these tests is difficult, particularly in a patient in whom a preexisting disease may mimic the clinical presentation of pulmonary embolism. Multiple diagnostic criteria have been recently proposed, which led to a prospective multicenter study that was undertaken to establish the diagnostic utility of the $\dot{V}/\dot{Q}$ scan.[1] The results supported the importance of combining the clinical evaluation with the $\dot{V}/\dot{Q}$ findings to obtain a more accurate diagnosis of pulmonary embolism.

Conclusions derived from the study include the following: (1) a high-probability $\dot{V}/\dot{Q}$ scan usually indicates the presence of pulmonary embolism; (2) a normal- or low-probability $\dot{V}/\dot{Q}$ scan in the setting of low clinical suspicion makes the diagnosis of pulmonary embolism unlikely; and (3) an indeterminate or intermediate probability, or a low probability with high clinical suspicion, usually does not establish or exclude the diagnosis of pulmonary embolism.

Because more than 60% of the patients entered into the study were in the nondiagnostic categories, the fact remains that most patients undergoing $\dot{V}/\dot{Q}$ scans need additional studies for a precise diagnosis of pulmonary embolism.

Pulmonary Arteriography

The following situations should be considered to be indications for pulmonary arteriography: (1) the presence of contraindications for anticoagulation; (2) the need to confirm the diagnosis before other performing therapeutic procedures such as caval filter placement, ligation, or thrombectomy; and (3) an indeterminate- or intermediate-probability lung scan, or when disparity exists between the radionuclide scan findings and the degree of clinical suspicion.

When performing pulmonary arteriography, access is usually gained through a femoral approach, providing that there is no proven evidence of caval or iliofemoral thrombosis. An upper extremity or jugular vein also can be used if necessary. A pigtail or a Grollman-type catheter is advanced to the right atrium and through the tricuspid valve into the right ventricle and pulmonary outflow tract. Selective injections during rapid filming sequences are required for proper evaluation. Typical volumes of iodinated contrast material are 40 to 50 mL injected at a rate of 20 to 25 mL/second. Physiologic monitoring during pulmonary angiography should include arterial pressure, continuous electrocardiography, and pulse oximetry. Pulmonary artery pressures are obtained before injections. Patients with elevated pressures are considered at higher risk of mortality during the procedure. Values at or above 50 mm Hg require special considerations such as limited selective injections using nonionic contrast or balloon occlusion arteriography.

The angiographic diagnosis is established by demonstrating an intraluminal filling defect or an abrupt interruption of a pulmonary artery branch. A normal arteriogram finding remains a reliable indicator to rule out pulmonary embolism.

Other Interventions

The interventional radiologist can also participate in more aggressive endovascular therapy of pulmonary embolism, such as vena caval filtration, thrombolysis, and thombectomy. Chemical fibrinolysis[2,3] and mechanical removal of clot[4] have been advocated in the acute stage of thromboembolic disease for rapid restoration of perfusion. Both procedures have limitations and shortcomings. Mechanical catheter devices fail to achieve complete removal of distal or peripheral thrombi, and thrombolytic therapy may not achieve recanalization despite prolonged therapy, which also produces an increased risk for bleeding. Recently, a rheolytic thrombectomy catheter based on the effects of high-velocity jets of saline solution has been used in both in vitro and in vivo experiments.[5] It offers potential advantages in comparison with other devices, such as reduction of vessel wall trauma, ability to lyse clots that are at least 1 week old, and collection of thrombotic debris through a central lumen.

In some patients, anticoagulant therapy is contraindicated; others have significant hemodynamic instability despite adequate anticoagulant therapy. In the latter subset of patients, vena caval filters have been used. Trapping of thrombi can be accomplished by inserting a filter percutaneously into the vena cava. The indications for caval interruption include the following:

1. Contraindication for anticoagulant therapy
2. Failure of anticoagulation manifested by recurrent pulmonary emboli
3. The development of complicating events such as GI bleeding
4. Evidence of massive pulmonary emboli

5. Prophylaxis in high-risk patients (i.e., elderly, oncology, history of deep vein thrombosis) before extensive surgery
6. Protection of high-risk trauma patients

Factors that place trauma patients in particularly high risk include pelvic, spine, and long bone fractures, and head and spinal cord injuries, all of which lead to prolonged immobilization. The risk of bleeding from the listed injuries precludes anticoagulation. Venous compressive devices may not be effective or suitable if multiple extremity fractures are present. Prophylaxis, which is considered to be vital, may be limited to the placement of intracaval filters.[6]

Different types of filters with variations in design for specific situations are commercially available. The most commonly used include the titanium Greenfield filter, the bird's nest (stainless steel wires), the LGM, and the nitinol filters. The LGM filters are more commonly used at our institution. They are easily deployed and can be inserted using a 12-French delivery system. Because of its wider diameter, the bird's nest type is usually reserved for patients with larger venae cavae.

Ideally, the filter should be placed using a right femoral approach, immediately below the renal veins. In other unusual situations (i.e., upper extremity thrombi), the filter can be positioned in the superior vena cava. For all filter placements, cavography should be performed routinely to define the venous anatomy and to assess proper positioning of the filter.

ACUTE ISCHEMIA

Low flow conditions and occlusion of major arterial flow may be amenable to transcatheter therapy. Thrombolysis can be indicated in acute peripheral arterial occlusions, specifically for thrombosed grafts and for thrombus in distal runoff vessels. Significant advances have been made in local transcatheter fibrinolytic therapy, which has become a useful preliminary step before revascularization for graft and native vessel occlusions. Urokinase is accepted as the agent of choice, although the protocols and delivery systems vary considerably between different institutions. The use of high-dose urokinase thrombolysis has gained acceptance, as well as the use of multiple side hole catheters and infusion wires. Newer agents such as tissue plasminogen activator with more fibrin-specific characteristics are being developed. Protocols of treatment are discussed elsewhere in this book (Chaps. 41 and 77).

Acute mesenteric ischemia is another surgical emergency that may benefit from transcatheter intervention. Mesenteric ischemia may result from embolic or thrombotic occlusion of the superior mesenteric artery but is more commonly related to a low flow state. The latter, nonocclusive ischemia, can be effectively treated by transcatheter infusion of a vasodilator such as papaverine. Nonocclusive ischemia is characterized by significant vasoconstriction in association with narrowing of the proximal branches of the superior mesenteric artery. When this diagnosis is established angiographically, a bolus of 50 mg of papaverine can be followed by an infusion of 1 mg/minute for a total of 30 minutes. A repeat arteriogram should be performed with comparable settings to the preinfusion arteriogram to obtain an optimal comparison of the effects of the treatment. The infusion of papaverine can be continued under close monitoring in the ICU for up to 48 hours. The angiographic changes of nonocclusive ischemia may reverse after the intraarterial infusion of papaverine. However, a failure to respond may imply that intestinal infarction has already occurred. Bowel ischemia has been seen more frequently in low flow states related to drugs such as cocaine and heroin. Prompt angiographic diagnosis and drug infusion into the mesenteric artery to promote bowel perfusion is mandatory to avoid the evolution of ischemia to infarction.

GASTROINTESTINAL BLEEDING

Interventional radiology has had a place in the management of GI bleeding for many years. At first, angiography was used for identification of the bleeding site, but eventually it developed into a therapeutic modality in upper and lower GI hemorrhage.

In acute GI bleeding, keep in mind that most patients (75% to 80%) stop bleeding with conservative management. Angiography becomes a useful option in patients who continue to bleed despite conservative management. Because of the different therapeutic implications, acute GI bleeding can be classified into three categories: (1) upper GI bleeding of arterial or capillary origin, (2) upper GI bleeding caused by gastroesophageal varices, and (3) lower GI bleeding. For specific demonstration of the bleeding site, three diagnostic modalities are usually available: endoscopy, radionuclide scanning, and angiography. The angiographic diagnosis of the GI bleeding is based on the demonstration of contrast extravasation, which increases throughout the arterial phase and into the venous phase. Realize, however, that the patient must be actively bleeding for an angiogram result to be positive. A rate of 0.5 mL/minute during the angiographic examination has been considered the minimum for a bleeding point to be shown angiographically.[7]

Upper Gastrointestinal Bleeding

When dealing with upper GI bleeding, emergency endoscopy should be the initial diagnostic examination. In the ideal situation, endoscopy localizes the point of bleeding, and then angiography can be used for subsequent transcatheter therapy. Once the bleeding site has been determined, angiographic therapy can be used to avoid an emergency operative procedure. The modalities for the angiographic control of bleeding include the infusion of vasopressin and occlusion of the bleeding vessel by embolization. The tip of the catheter used for infusion of vasopressin should be as close as possible to the bleeding point for the most effective results. This implies selective catheterization of the left gastric artery or the gastroduodenal artery, depending on the type and location of the bleeding lesion. Vasopressin is usually infused selectively into the bleeding vessel at a rate of 0.2 units/minute for a total of 20 minutes. After this time, the arteriogram is repeated and, if bleeding continues, the dose can be repeated at the same rate or increased to 0.4 units/minute

for an additional 20 minutes. Once the bleeding is controlled, the patient should be managed in an ICU with the catheter left in place. The infusion should be continued over the next 12 to 36 hours. If bleeding continues after the initial or double-dose infusion, embolization, endoscopic control, or surgery should be considered.

Typically, patients with gastric mucosal hemorrhage have a better chance for control of bleeding when treated by vasopressin infusion than those with actively bleeding duodenal ulcers.

If intraarterial infusion of vasopressin fails to control upper GI hemorrhage, arterial embolization may be considered. Absorbable gelatin, preferably formed into small plugs, can be used after the catheter has been positioned selectively with the tip in the vessel, demonstrating extravasation. Embolization has distinct advantages over vasopressin infusion because it provides a more effective reduction of blood flow to the bleeding lesion and avoids the complications related to prolonged catheterization required for the infusion. The patient who responds to embolization therapy may not require ICU admission, as is usual for continued infusion of vasopressin. Many authors[8–10] consider embolization to be the angiographic therapeutic modality of choice in upper GI bleeding from peptic ulcers because the results with vasopressin infusion are not as effective as in the bleeding secondary to hemorrhagic gastritis or more superficial ulcerations.

If the patient is shown to have gastroesophageal varices and no extravasation is identified in the angiographic examination, the bleeding may be assumed to be from the varices. Vasopressin can be infused intravenously at a rate of 0.3 units/minute for 24 hours, with progressive reduction over 72 hours. A recent alternative to control bleeding varices is the transjugular intrahepatic portosystemic shunt (TIPS), which has been shown to reduce portal venous pressure promptly and to decrease the frequency of recurrent hemorrhage from gastroesophageal varices.[11] In addition, it has a beneficial effect on ascites. A combined multicenter survey in 1750 patients was recently analyzed to evaluate the current status of TIPS.[12] Main indications included acute or recurrent bleeding and, to a lesser extent, ascites and Budd-Chiari syndrome. In all of the institutions, a wallstent was preferred to establish the shunt because of its more flexible and self-expanding nature. In the same series, patients presenting with acute variceal bleeding had hemorrhage controlled 91% of the time. However, later rebleeding has been a problem, occurring at a rate of 16% during the first year. The impact of this procedure in the management of bleeding esophageal varices is yet to be determined. Currently, the intervention is performed in all symptomatic patients with recurrence of bleeding and ascites. Contraindications include right-sided heart failure, severe liver failure, thrombosed portal vein, and severe encephalopathy.

Lower Gastrointestinal Bleeding

In patients with bleeding distal to the ligament of Treitz, angiography is usually the procedure of choice to determine the bleeding site because endoscopy has a limited value. Most of these patients bleed from diverticular lesions or from colonic angiodysplasia. Other less frequent causes of bleeding are anastomotic sites, aortoduodenal fistula after vascular surgery, GI tumors, and miscellaneous inflammatory diseases. Bleeding from hemorrhoids, anal fissures, or other local rectal problems can be excluded by proctosigmoidoscopy before other more involved diagnostic procedures are considered. Radionuclide scanning, either by the administration of technetium ^{99m}Tc sulfur colloid or by ^{99m}Tc–labeled red blood cells, plays an important role in the initial investigation of the patient with lower GI bleeding. The test is considered more sensitive and specific than angiography, and it can detect bleeding rates lower than those required for angiographic demonstration.[13] We believe it should be used as the preliminary screening procedure for patients with lower GI bleeding. In patients with positive radionuclide scan results, arteriography is indicated for the precise localization, to further define the nature of the bleeding lesion, and finally, for definitive therapy in some cases. Selective superior and inferior mesenteric artery injections are necessary for complete angiographic evaluation. A bleeding diverticulum can be diagnosed by the presence of a relatively localized extravasation that at times may even pool within the diverticulum. Colonic angiodysplasia is usually diagnosed by the finding of early opacification of draining veins, usually from the cecum or the ascending colon, with persistent opacification into the late venous phase. The association of clusters of small arteries and capillaries in the ileocecal area supports the diagnosis.

Bleeding colonic and small bowel lesions are amenable to treatment with vasopressin infusion. The dose is the same as that used in upper GI bleeding. Unlike bleeding duodenal ulcers, diverticular hemorrhage and bleeding angiodysplasias have a satisfactory response to vasopressin infusion. Approximately 80% of patients respond to the initial selective mesenteric infusion of vasopressin. Patients with recurrent hemorrhage may require surgical treatment and exclusion of a neoplasm or other associated lesion.

INTRAVASCULAR CATHETERS AND FOREIGN BODY MANIPULATION

Advances in fluoroscopic imaging and catheter instrumentation have allowed safe and effective percutaneous removal of intravascular foreign bodies. Embolized catheter fragments frequently become lodged in the pulmonary circulation or cardiac chambers that would entail a major open surgical procedure for removal. The angiographic removal has become a relatively simple procedure with lowered morbidity and costs. A wide variety of complications are known to occur with catheter fragment embolization, intravascular bullet fragments, or other intravascular foreign bodies. Cardiac arrhythmia and arrest, pulmonary emboli, caval thrombosis, sepsis, endocarditis, and vascular perforation are among the common complications. Immediate consultation with the vascular-interventional radiologist is warranted once the diagnosis is made. Homemade loop snares were used initially, but a variety of materials for retrieval are commercially available. The most popular devices are the retrieval baskets, loop snares, and hook-shaped catheters with deflecting systems.

Grasping forceps and Fogarty balloon catheters may occasionally be used.

VASCULAR TRAUMA

Angiography remains the method of choice for evaluating vascular injuries. The development of dedicated level I trauma centers with on-site availability of state-of-the-art digital angiography has expanded the indications for diagnostic and therapeutic vascular procedures for the acutely traumatized patients.

Angiography is usually performed to rule out a posttraumatic vascular lesion or to establish the extent of injury to select the appropriate treatment. Depending on the type and extent of vascular insult, the angiographic features of trauma-induced injury may include intimal flap, pseudoaneurysm, contrast extravasation, arteriovenous fistula, and occlusion.

When a lesion is identified and a catheter can be advanced to the injured or bleeding vessel, an endovascular intervention can often be considered as an alternative to surgical treatment. Because uncontrolled hemorrhage accounts for a significant number of deaths among traumatized patients, such an intervention should be performed immediately, without unnecessary delays. The control of arterial bleeding can be safely and effectively accomplished by transcatheter embolization. Not all agents currently used in the more elective embolization procedure are appropriate in the acute trauma setting. Absorbable gelatin can serve as a long-term nonpermanent agent, but steel coils provide more permanent occlusion and, in larger vessels, are usually more effective for angiographic hemostasis. Rarely, balloon-tipped catheters may be required.

Indications for embolization after vascular trauma include the following:

1. Management of bleeding or occluded vertebral carotid arteries; before the embolization of these vessels, the integrity of the contralateral and potential collateral circulation must be evaluated
2. Active extravasation from upper and lower extremity branches, providing that they do not represent the main arterial supply to the limb
3. Recurrent postoperative bleeding or hemobilia after hepatic trauma
4. Posttraumatic hematuria when a pseudoaneurysm or a renal arteriovenous fistula is suspected
5. Uncontrolled hemorrhage associated with pelvic fractures (Fig. 38-1)

NONVASCULAR PROCEDURES ■

There are two general types of percutaneous nonvascular procedures: catheter drainage of fluid collections including postoperative abscesses, enteric abscesses, pancreatic collections, and various noninfected collections; and access to various organ systems including biliary procedures, gastrostomy, and nephrostomy.

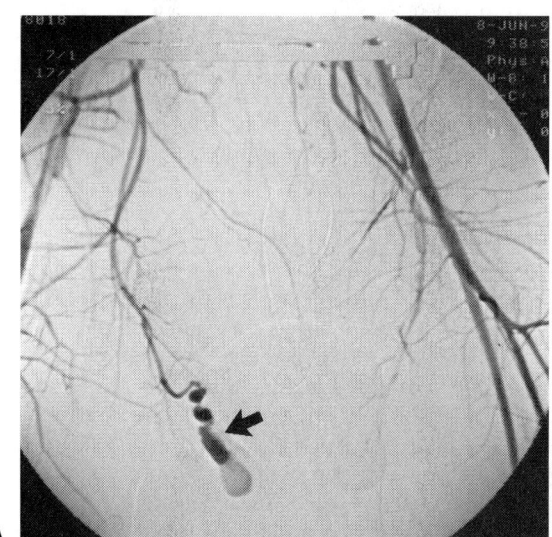
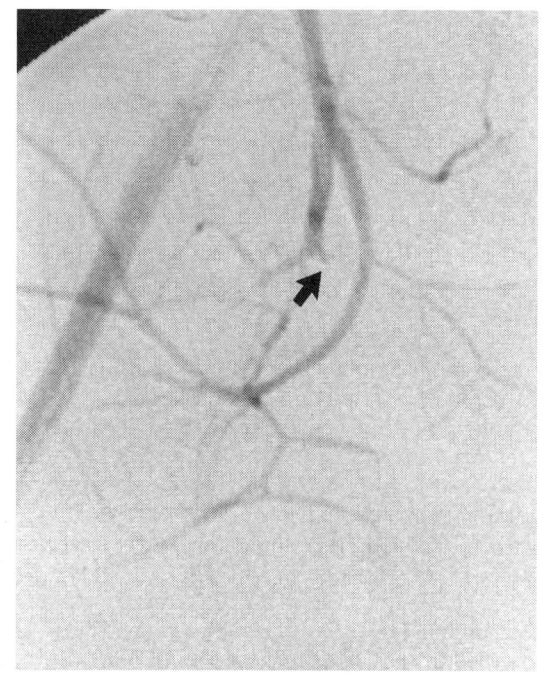

FIGURE 38-1. (**A**) Pelvic arteriogram in a patient with multiple fractures. Contrast extravasation from the right internal pudendal artery indicates active bleeding (*arrow*). Selective catheterization of the right internal iliac artery was performed, and the catheter tip was positioned distal to the origin of the superior gluteal artery. Small pieces of Gelfoam were advanced through the catheter, and occlusion of the bleeding vessel (*arrow*) is demonstrated in the follow-up angiogram (**B**).

PERCUTANEOUS CATHETER DRAINAGE

Percutaneous catheter drainage (PCD) of abscesses and fluid collections has become an indispensable procedure in the management of the critically ill patient.[14,15] For percutaneous drainage, infected and noninfected collections can be categorized as simple or complex, based on their imaging features. Simple collections are defined as unilocular, well-demarcated, superficial, and having an easy or direct access route. Complex collections are multilocular or multiple, poorly demarcated, and have either difficult access because of the depth or associated fistulas.

Historically, complex collections were not considered amenable to percutaneous drainage.[16–24] Extensive clinical research along with recent technical advances have resulted in an expanding list of potentially drainable collections. Abdominal abscesses complicating surgery are the most common indication for PCD, currently the treatment of choice. The percutaneous drainage of noninfected fluid collections including pancreatic pseudocysts, hematomas, bilomas, urinomas, and lymphoceles also has been accepted. Prior concern of infecting a sterile collection has not been validated.[25]

Separating collections into simple and complex is important for predicting successful drainage. Cure rates range from 82% to 100% for simple collections.[14,16,26,27] Lower success rates (45% to 85%) should be expected for complex collections. The complexity, rather than the source, determines the success of drainage.[14]

A frequently reported advantage of PCD is its temporizing effect in patients with complex abscesses.[14,15,28] In particular, the critically ill patient has been shown to benefit from a combined radiologic–surgical approach. PCD can improve the clinical status by "debulking" an infected peritoneum and by directing antibiotic selection. In selected patients, laparotomy is performed after clinical improvement; it is then safer and less time consuming.[15,29]

Imaging

Ultrasound (US) and computed tomography (CT) are the modalities used for diagnosis and localization of suspected collections. CT offers fine anatomic detail and accurate localization in axial planes. Simple collections are easily drained using CT, but it is especially advantageous for PCD of complex collections, in which factors such as deep location, difficult access, and multiple pockets are present. The use of CT is not limited by the presence of stomas, surgical dressings, or open wounds. However, CT requires in-hospital transport of the critically ill patients with its inherent risks.

US is also used for PCD. It offers the advantages of a fast, portable examination and intervention that can be performed at the bedside. This is especially beneficial in the critically ill patient. US provides cross-sectional anatomic detail and easily distinguishes fluid from solid material. The catheter insertion may be performed under direct real time imaging. US is most effective when used for the drainage of simple, unilocular collections, especially for those that are superficial in location.

Technique

After selecting the appropriate imaging technique for guidance, the procedure is performed either at the bedside or in the radiology department. Under local anesthesia and after any indicated premedication has been given, drainage is performed using either the modified Seldinger technique or the trocar catheter technique.

In the modified Seldinger technique, confirmatory aspiration with a sheathed 18-gauge needle is performed and a floppy guidewire is inserted through the sheath into the cavity. The tract is then enlarged by passing progressively larger dilators over the wire, and then an appropriately sized, multihole pigtail catheter is inserted into the cavity. With the trocar technique, aspiration also can be performed through an 18- or 20-gauge needle. The collection can then be entered in a tandem approach or directly with a trocar catheter combination using the path predetermined from the CT or US images. The trocar is removed, leaving a self-retaining catheter coiled in the cavity.

After catheter placement using either technique, the collection is aspirated completely and lavage is performed several times using normal saline solution. As with open surgical drainage, the major benefit is achieved at the time of initial drainage if complete aspiration of the contents can be performed.[30] Further clinical improvement may be seen over the next hours if additional drainage occurs or if the systemic inflammatory response abates. These techniques allow for placement of catheters ranging in size from 6 to 14 French, although catheters as large as 24 French have been used for more complex collections with thicker contents. Catheter choice depends on the size, depth, location, and contents of the collection to be drained. Samples of the aspirate should be sent for immediate gram stain and culture, as well as other desired laboratory analyses.

Catheter Maintenance

Normal saline flushes of 5- to 10-mL are used to maintain catheter patency. Initial reports stressed the importance of routine repeat imaging (CT/US) and injection under fluoroscopic control (abscessograms) to evaluate cavity size, catheter position, and potential fistulous tracts. Alternatively, careful clinical assessment of the catheter output has been shown to be sufficient. Any abrupt change, especially cessation of drainage, warrants contrast injection under fluoroscopy or CT/US evaluation. Catheters are removed when drainage ceases, there is clinical improvement, or repeat radiographic imaging indicates complete resolution of the cavity.

Complications

The complication rate associated with PCD ranges from 5% to 15%,[31–34] and the types vary depending on the nature and location of the drainage. In general, minor complications include bacteremia (at the time of placement), skin infection,

and minor bleeding. Major complications occur in less than 5% of cases[26] and include massive hemorrhage or inadvertent visceral injury related to the initial puncture. These complications usually can be managed nonoperatively. The reported mortality rate is less than 1%.

Locations and Types of Collections

Some specific locations and types of collections deserve special consideration because of their prevalence in the traumatized and acutely ill patient.

POSTOPERATIVE ABDOMINAL ABSCESSES. Abdominal abscesses complicating surgery are the most common indication for PCD. The diagnosis is usually established with CT during a workup for sepsis. In evaluating patients with fever of unknown origin, its accuracy rate is 93% with sensitivity and specificity rates of 97% and 91%, respectively.[16,25] US, by comparison, has an accuracy rate of 68% and sensitivity and specificity rates of 44% and 79%, respectively. PCD has become the treatment of choice for postoperative abscesses (Fig. 38-2) because of its low associated morbidity and mortality, along with the added advantage of avoiding surgery and general anesthesia.[14,16,18]

PANCREATIC AND PERIPANCREATIC COLLECTIONS. Percutaneous drainage of a pancreatic pseudocyst has become a widely used procedure. The cure rate for PCD of noninfected pseudocysts is approximately 90% and compares favorably with the success of open surgical drainage.[35] The indications for PCD of pseudocysts depend on size, duration, and the presence of symptoms. Pseudocysts less than 4 cm may be observed with follow-up CT or US (1- to 2-week intervals). A pseudocyst that is larger than 4 to 5 cm or one that causes symptoms may be selected for PCD. Large, persistent pseudocysts are unlikely to resolve spontaneously and are prone to serious complications such as infection, hemorrhage, and rupture.[35–37] Whereas surgical drainage usually is performed after a 6-week delay to allow a mature capsule to form, PCD may be performed earlier, once criteria for drainage are met.

The pathogenesis of a pseudocyst involves disruption of the pancreatic duct with leakage of pancreatic fluid. The fluid is sequestered and a collection forms. Drainage of pancreatic pseudocysts should, therefore, follow guidelines for the management of fistulous collections, specifically, closure of the fistula before catheter removal. Duration of catheter drainage for a simple pseudocyst is approximately 2 to 3 weeks. To ensure complete drainage and closure of the fistula, the patient can undergo imaging after the catheter has been clamped for 1 to 3 days and no reaccumulation is shown. Prolonged drainage may be expected for large and communicating pseudocysts.

Infected pancreatic collections represent a spectrum of disease, ranging from an infected pseudocyst to complex pancreatic abscess. Treatment and success depends largely on the complexity. Infected pancreatic pseudocysts and pancreatic abscesses encompass the most challenging of drainage procedures because they frequently lack easy access and have a propensity for marked tissue destruction, loculations,

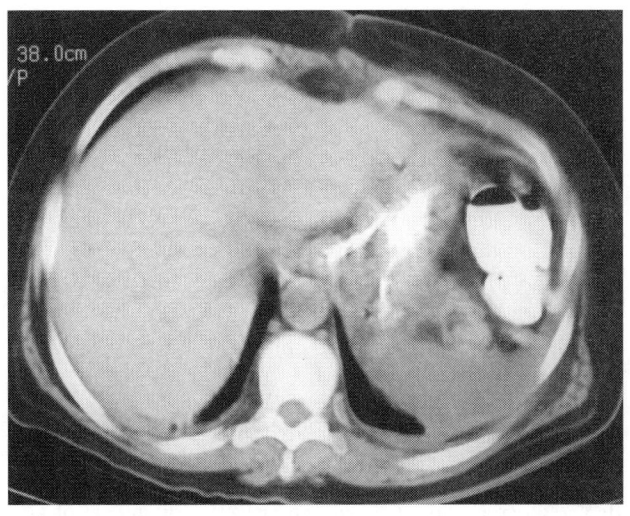
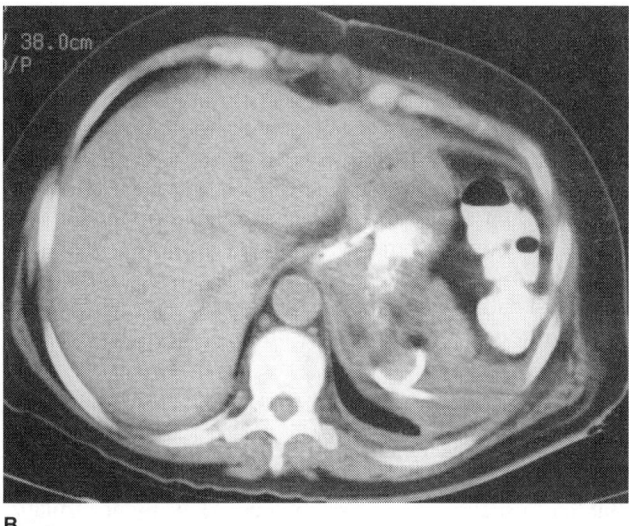

A
B

FIGURE 38-2. (**A**) Computed tomography scan in a patient with signs of sepsis, 7 days after splenectomy. A left subphrenic fluid collection is demonstrated. (**B**) Computed tomography–guided insertion of a percutaneous catheter was performed for drainage of a subphrenic abscess.

and septations. Although lower cure rates are reported (32% to 94%), PCD can be used as the initial means of therapy for infected pseudocysts and simple pancreatic abscesses. It also may provide microbiologic data or may simply be a temporizing method before definitive surgery for more complex pancreatic collections.[15,35,38] CT provides the accurate localization and characterization required for successful drainage. Multiple and often large-bore catheters are used to drain complex collections. Because of underlying pancreatitis, prolonged catheter drainage should be expected. Complex abscesses may benefit from an aggressive radiologic–surgical approach. Drainage of fluid collections followed by open debridement of necrotic debris has been shown to be an effective form of management.[29,39] Phlegmon and pancreatic necrosis are predominantly solid tissues and are not amenable to PCD.

Complications of pancreatic drainage include superinfection of noninfected collections, managed by catheter exchange and continued drainage. Bleeding is rarely encountered but may occur because of vascular perforation by the catheter or to the effect of proteolytic enzymes.[39] Necrotic debris or persistent fistulous communication with the pancreatic duct or the GI tract may result in failure of PCD.

ENTERIC ABSCESSES. Enteric abscesses are the result of bowel perforation. Types of enteric abscesses include periappendiceal, diverticular, and those related to Crohn's disease. Less common etiologies are perforated colon carcinomas and gastric ulcers. These abscesses have in common the presence of a fistulous communication with the diseased bowel. By definition, these collections with associated fistulae are complex and radiologic intervention should be planned accordingly. CT is usually chosen when drainage is planned. Often these collections are deeply situated and in close proximity to bowel loops. The rare superficial collection may be accessed using US guidance. Successful PCD is

accomplished in 70% to 93%[40–43] of patients, but this is only possible if the fistulous communication closes, as demonstrated by fluoroscopic catheter injections. Traditionally, the treatment of these abscesses required a two-stage operative procedure: open surgical drainage and alimentary diversion followed by bowel resection and reanastomosis. The goal of PCD is to avoid the first step of this two-stage procedure. The definitive treatment may be performed on an elective basis.[15,28,40] Nonoperative resolution of sepsis is particularly advantageous in the critically ill patient.

NONINFECTED COLLECTIONS. The postoperative or posttrauma patient may develop various noninfected fluid collections. Those often considered for PCD include the following: pleural effusions, hematomas, bilomas, urinomas, and lymphoceles. In these cases, PCD is performed for diagnosis, symptomatic relief, or to remove a potential source of infection.

Thoracic Collections. Radiographically guided PCD of thoracic collections is an alternative to thoracentesis, closed-tube thoracostomy, or open thoracotomy/thoracoscopy. Either CT or US may be used for guidance. Catheter drainage is useful for both pleural effusions and empyemas. Effusions are generally drained for diagnosis of possible infection or relief of dyspnea. Free layering pleural fluid is easily drained using US and often can be performed at the bedside. Successful PCD of empyemas has been reported ranging from 80% to 92% of treated patients.[44–46] Success may follow failed thoracostomy tube drainage. As with pleural effusions, free layering empyemas may be drained using US. Loculated collections are best drained under CT guidance.

Hematomas. Indications for drainage of a postoperative or posttraumatic hematoma include suspected superinfection in a septic patient or relief from bothersome symptoms. The ability of a hematoma to be drained depends on the degree of liquefaction that has taken place. Liquefied hematomas are easily drained; however, fresh or clotted hematomas are particularly difficult to drain, even if large-bore catheters are used. Both US and CT can be unreliable for determining liquefaction. Fresh, clotted hematomas may appear echofree by US mimicking a liquefied collection. CT may be similarly imprecise, and liquefaction may only be determined on initial aspiration. Prolonged catheter drainage, ranging from 10 to 39 days,[47] is usually required for hematomas. Instillation of thrombolytic agents such as urokinase has been effective at reducing drainage time in refractory cases.[29,47]

Bilomas. Bilomas are localized collections of bile within the peritoneal cavity and are usually the result of bile duct disruption, usually secondary to hepatic trauma or surgery.[48] Bilomas usually present as unilocular, well-encapsulated fluid collections. Although usually located in the right upper quadrant, bilomas may be seen in the left subphrenic space, paracolic gutters, or the lesser sac. Drainage is indicated when infection is suspected or symptoms develop. CT is generally advocated for guidance, but US can be used for the larger, more superficial collections.[49,50] Prolonged drainage is necessary when an active bile leak is present. A continuous leak can be determined by the character and the amount of drainage. Confirmation with a biliary scan is seldom required. To treat an active leak, the disrupted bile duct may have to be drained selectively by a percutaneous or endoscopic approach.[48,51]

Urinoma. Urine extravasation into the retroperitoneum either from the upper or lower urinary tract can result in urinoma formation. PCD may be used if significant secondary symptoms develop or in the event of continuous accumulation and expansion of the collection. Also, PCD may help determine if the urinoma is infected. Once an urinoma is drained, the integrity of the urinary tract must be documented to exclude the possibility of a continuous urine leak. If disruption and extravasation are demonstrated, a percutaneous nephrostomy should be inserted and ureteral stenting may be used to avoid urine flow through the injured segment and to promote healing around the stent. In many cases, simple aspiration or short-term drainage is sufficient.

Lymphoceles. Pelvic surgery, retroperitoneal lymphadenectomy, or renal transplant surgery may be complicated by the formation of a lymphocele. The diagnosis is usually made several weeks after surgery. Therefore, they present later than urinomas and hematomas.[52,53] US easily detects lymphoceles because they are usually pelvic or retroperitoneal in location. Drainage is indicated if infection is suspected, for persistence or increase in size on sequential studies (1- to 2-week intervals), and if signs of ureteral or venous obstruction develop. Drainage may be performed under CT or US guidance. Successful drainage requires long-term catheter placement. Simple aspiration and short-term catheter drainage result in recurrences. Catheter drainage has been reported for 120 days.[54] Sclerosing agents such

as tetracycline, alcohol, sodium salts, and povidone-iodine solution have been shown to be safe and beneficial.[53–55] PCD results in nonoperative cure in 85% to 95% of patients.[53,54]

PERCUTANEOUS ACCESS TO VARIOUS ORGAN SYSTEMS

Imaging-guided interventions can provide access to different organs for diagnostic purposes or for palliative or definitive therapy.

Percutaneous Cholecystostomies

Critically ill patients are particularly susceptible to acute acalculous cholecystitis. Prolonged fasting leads to bile stasis and sludge accumulation within the gallbladder. Bile inspissation results in cystic duct obstruction and acute cholecystitis.[56,57] Despite this well-known risk, the diagnosis of acute cholecystitis continues to be elusive in the ICU patient. Clinical evaluation, sonography, and nuclear scintigraphy are used for diagnosis. Clinical evaluation often reveals persistent signs of sepsis and other nonspecific findings such as vague abdominal pain and tenderness. Sonography may show gallbladder distension, sludge, gallbladder wall thickening, pericholecystic fluid, and a sonographic Murphy's sign. These signs are also nonspecific. Gallbladder wall thickening and pericholecystic fluid may be seen in other processes such as hypoalbuminemia, ascites, and hepatitis.

The accuracy rate of US has been reported to be as low as 58% in this population of patients.[56,58] Although usually accurate in the diagnosis of acute cholecystitis, gallbladder scintigraphy is associated with a false-positive rate as high as 92% in critically ill patients.[59–62] Severe intercurrent illness, prolonged fasting, and the use of total parenteral nutrition result in "nonvisualization" of the gallbladder.

Because of the difficulties in diagnosis and the importance of early treatment, some studies advocate a trial of percutaneous cholecystostomy (PCC) for this subset of patients.[56] Selection criteria include persistent sepsis of unknown origin and gallbladder distension. A sonographic Murphy's sign or clinical evidence of abdominal tenderness are strongly suggestive of acute cholecystitis. However, these symptoms are usually difficult to elicit from the ICU patient. Clinical improvement in the patient with suspected acute cholecystitis should occur in 24 hours, as indicated by defervescence of fever and disappearance of abdominal pain.

The trocar technique with small 6- to 7-French catheters is unique to PCC, and the use of US provides a safe and expedient bedside method. Although bile leak is a potential complication, PCC is considered a low-risk procedure.[57,63,64] The risk of this complication can be minimized by using a transhepatic approach and by entering the bare area of the gallbladder. The catheter should be left in place for 2 to 4 weeks to allow a mature tract to form.[56]

Although more liberal criteria for PCC results in more "normal" gallbladders drained, approximately 60% of patients benefit from drainage. In the remaining patients, the gallbladder has been excluded as the source of sepsis by a low-risk procedure.[56,63,64]

Percutaneous Gastrostomy and Transgastric Jejunostomy

Gastrostomy is an effective method for enteral feeding[65] and GI decompression.[66,67] Three different methods can be used to establish a gastrostomy:

1. *Surgical*: Technically simple and well-established for many years, the surgical method is associated with significant morbidity and mortality because of the patient's poor physical condition (debilitated and malnourished),[68,69] especially if general anesthesia is chosen.
2. *Endoscopic*: Percutaneous endoscopic gastrostomy, introduced in 1980,[70] is a safe procedure, but it cannot be carried out in patients with obstructive lesions of the upper alimentary tract.
3. *Radiologic*: First described in 1983,[71–73] the radiologic method has been shown to be a safe and effective way to gain access into the stomach.

Percutaneous gastrostomy is mainly indicated for nutritional support[73–78] in patients with a variety of conditions that limit oral intake:

1. Impaired swallowing secondary to cerebrovascular accidents, anoxic brain damage, or trauma
2. Head and neck tumors and malignant esophageal obstruction[79,80]
3. Impaired appetite from anorexia nervosa, severe depression, or advanced malignancy;
4. Gastric or small bowel motility disorder and small bowel disease that does not tolerate normal oral intake but accepts slowly infused enteral feedings delivered to the small bowel[81]
5. Patients with scleroderma, short gut syndrome, radiation enteritis, and Crohn's disease
6. Decompression of the stomach or small bowel in chronic small bowel obstruction[74] and gastric carcinoma[75]

Percutaneous gastrostomy is contraindicated if the colon or liver is interposed between the anterior gastric wall and the abdominal wall.[74,76,77,82] The presence of previous gastric surgery may be a relative contraindication[76,77,83,84] as is neoplastic involvement of the gastric wall, which can preclude the air distention necessary for the puncture. CT can be a valuable tool to define the regional anatomy when fluoroscopy and endoscopy are considered unsafe or difficult to perform in placing a percutaneous gastrostomy.[85] A bleeding diathesis and severe gastric varices also are considered contraindications for percutaneous gastrostomy.

TECHNIQUE. Preparation includes coagulation tests, overnight fasting, and the placement of a nasogastric tube. Whenever possible, the tube is inserted on the day before the gastrostomy to aspirate gastric contents and to minimize peritoneal spillage during the procedure. In patients with obstructive lesions of the upper alimentary tract, there are two options: a catheter–guidewire combination to transverse the obstructive segment under fluoroscopic observation, or direct puncture of the stomach performed under CT guidance. When selecting the entry site, interposition of bowel or liver must be excluded by fluoroscopic or sonographic assessment. The procedure is performed under mild sedation and local anesthesia. The stomach is accessed using the Seldinger technique, and a suitable guidewire is introduced to allow for subsequent dilatation of the percutaneous tract. When percutaneous gastrostomy is performed for decompression, large-bore catheters (24 to 28 French) should be used.[74] For enteral feeding, a smaller catheter (10 to 14 French) with a Cope loop device is used.[86,87]

A percutaneous gastrojejunostomy tube instead of a percutaneous gastrostomy tube has been proposed to provide protection against reflux of gastric contents into the esophagus. Positioning of the tip of the feeding tube distal to the ligament of Treitz prevents gastric reflux.[88] Some authors routinely advance the feeding tube into the jejunum[77–89] whereas others choose jejunal placement only when the patient has a significant risk for aspiration.[87–90] Jejunal placement may be more time-consuming and technically more involved, but it reduces aspiration, and feeding can be begun immediately after the procedure.

Unlike surgical or endoscopic gastrostomy, the percutaneous technique described does not appose the anterior gastric wall to the abdominal wall. Brown and colleagues[91] describe a percutaneous method to simulate surgical apposition by a nylon t fastener (a specially designed 18-gauge needle with a 5-mm longitudinal side slot cut from the heel of the bevel to load the fastener). Saini and colleagues[76] advocate the routine use of gastropexy fixation; other authors report successful percutaneous gastrostomy without the use of fixation.[74,77,83,92,93]

Most authors report high success rates (98% to 100%) and a low rate of complications.[94] Major complications have been reported in 0% to 6% of cases, including peritonitis requiring laparotomy, GI bleeding, and deep stomal infection. Minor complications occur in 4% to 12% of patients and include fever, catheter malfunction, pain, and superficial infection of the stoma. The procedure-related mortality rate is 0% to 2%.[74,76,77,95] Gastrostomy function was maintained as long as clinically required in 89.5% of the patients (34 of 38), with an average duration of 10.75 weeks.[96]

Ho and others[83] encountered significantly fewer complications with the percutaneous method compared with surgical gastrostomy. The endoscopic technique does not reduce aspiration and infectious complications but can be performed at bedside for critically ill patients.

Percutaneous Nephrostomy

Percutaneous nephrostomy is a useful and safe procedure that has been primarily used in patients with urinary obstruction associated with azotemia or sepsis.[97–101] It has been used in benign disease as a temporary measure before definitive treatment, but the indications in the preterminal oncology patient remain less defined.[102–106] The procedure is indicated for the emergency management of urinary tract obstruction. In particular, patients with pyonephrosis show prompt clinical improvement after percutaneous drainage, and patients with azotemia secondary to obstruction benefit from external drainage of urine through nephrostomy catheters.

Catheters are inserted using a posterolateral approach under fluoroscopic or ultrasonographic control. Access to the renal pelvis is gained through a posterior calyx. The angiographic Seldinger technique is preferred, with self-retaining catheters advanced over a guidewire, after progressive dilatation of the percutaneous tract. In difficult cases or in patients with altered anatomy, CT may be useful for guidance.

A success rate of more that 98% has reported in several series,[107-110] and complications requiring specific treatment occurred in 4% of patients.[111] Hemorrhage is the most common complication and, when severe, must be treated aggressively with blood transfusions and direct surgical intervention or transcatheter embolization. Other significant complications include septicemia, pneumothorax, and urinoma formation. Mechanical problems with the catheters such as obstruction and dislodgement are reported to occur between 12% and 18% of patients.[110]

REFERENCES ■

1. The Pioped Investigators: Value of the ventilation/perfusion scan in acute pulmonary embolism. *JAMA* 1990;263:2753
2. Urokinase Pulmonary Embolism Trial: a national cooperative study. *Circulation* 1973;47(Suppl 2):1
3. Urokinase-Streptokinase Pulmonary Embolism Trial: phase II results. *JAMA* 1974;229:1606
4. Bildsoe MC, Moradian GP, Hunter DW, et al: Mechanical clot dissolution: a new concept. *Radiology* 1989;171:231
5. Drasler WJ, Jenson ML, Wilson GJ, et al: Rheolytic catheter for percutaneous removal of thrombus. *Radiology* 1992;182:263
6. Winchell RJ, Hoyt DB, Walsh JC, et al: Risk factors associated with pulmonary embolism despite routine prophylaxis. *J Trauma* 1994;37:600
7. Baum S, Nussbaum M: The control of gastrointestinal hemorrhage by selective mesenteric infusion of vasopressin. *Radiology* 1971;98:497
8. Baum S: Angiography and gastrointestinal bleeding. *Radiology* 1982;143:569
9. Gomes AS, Lois JF, Meloy RD: Angiographic treatment of gastrointestinal hemorrhage: comparison of vasopressin infusion and embolization. *AJR* 1986;146:1031
10. Okazaki M, Furui S, Higashihara H: Emergert embolotherapy of small intestinal hemorrhage. *Gastrointest Radiol* 1992;17:223
11. Ritcher GM, Palmaz JC, Noeldge G, et al: The transjugular intrahepatic portosystemic shunt. *Radiology* 1989;29:406
12. Rosch J: Current status of TIPS. Presented at the *Seventh Interventional Symposium on Vascular Diagnosis and Intervention*. Miami Beach, Florida, January 1995
13. Winzelberg GG, Fruelich JW, McKusick KA: Radionuclide localization of lower gastrointestinal hemorrhage. *Radiology* 1981;139:465
14. Gerzof SG, Johnson WC, Robbins AM, et al: Expanding the criteria for percutaneous abscess drainage. *Arch Surg* 1985;120:227
15. van Sonnenberg E, Wing VW, Casola G, et al: Temporizing effect of percutaneous drainage of complicated abscesses in critically ill patients. *AJR* 1984;142:821
16. Johnson WC, Gerzof SG, Robbins AM, et al: Treatment of abdominal abscesses: comparative evaluation of operative drainage versus percutaneous catheter drainage guided by computed tomography and ultrasound. *Ann Surg* 1981;194:510
17. Aeder MI, Wellman JL, Haager JR, et al: Role of surgical and percutaneous drainage in the treatment of abdominal abscesses. *Arch Surg* 1983;118:273
18. Gerzof SG, Robbins AH, Birkett DH, et al: Percutaneous catheter drainage of abdominal abscesses guided by ultrasound and computed tomography. *AJR* 1979;133:1
19. Glass CA, Cohn I: Drainage of intra-abdominal abscesses: a comparison of surgical drainage and computerized tomography guided catheter drainage. *Am J Surg* 1984;147:315
20. Saini S, Kellum JM, O'Leary MP, et al: Improved localization and survival in patients with intraabdominal abscesses. *Am J Surg* 1983;145:136
21. Glick PL, Pellegrini CA, Stein S, et al: Abdominal abscesses: a surgical strategy. *Arch Surg* 1983;118:646
22. Hinsdale JG, Jaffe BM: Reoperation for intra-abdominal sepsis. *Ann Surg* 1984;199:31
23. Welch CE: Catheter drainage of abdominal abscesses. *N Engl J Med* 1981;305:694
24. Halasz NA, van Sonnenberg E: Drainage of intra-abdominal abscesses: tactics and choices. *Am J Surg* 1983;146:112
25. Pruett TL, Simmons RL: Status of percutaneous catheter drainage of abscesses. *Surg Clin North Am* 1988;68:89
26. van Sonnenberg E, Mueller PR, Ferrucci JT: Percutaneous drainage of 250 abdominal abesses and fluid collections. Part I. Results, failures and complications. *Radiology* 1984;151:337
27. Gerzof SG, Robbins AH, Johnson WC, et al: Percutaneous catheter drainage of abdominal abscesses: a 5 year experience. *N Engl J Med* 1981;305:637
28. Flancbaum L, Nosher JL, Brolin RE: Percutaneous catheter drainage of abdominal abscesses associated with perforated viscus. *Am Surg* 1990;56:52
29. van Sonnenberg E: Advances in percutaneous abscess drainage. In: *Syllabus: A Categorical Course in Interventional Radiology*. Ed. RSNA, 1991
30. Mueller PR, van Sonnenberg E, Ferrucci JT: Percutaneous drainage of 250 abdominal abscesses and fluid collections. Part II. Current proceedural concepts. *Radiology* 1984;131:343
31. Brolin RE, Nosher JL, Leiman S, et al: Percutaneous catheter versus open surgical drainage in the treatment of abdominal abscesses. *Am Surg* 1984;50:102
32. Gerzof SG, Johnson WC, Robins AH, et al: Intrahepatic pyogenic abscesses: treatment by percutaneous drainage. *Am J Surg* 1985;149:48
33. Gerzof SG, Robbins AM, Johnson WC, et al: Percutaneous catheter drainage of abdominal abscesses. *N Engl J Med* 1981;305:653
34. Pruett TL, Rotstein OD, Crass J, et al: Percutaneous aspiration and drainage for suspected abdominal infection. *Surgery* 1984;96:731
35. van Sonnenberg E, Wittich GR, Casola G, et al: Percutaneous drainage of infected and noninfected pancreatic pseudocysts: experience in 101 cases. *Radiology* 1989;170:757
36. Sankaran S, Walt AJ: The natural and unnatural history of pancreatic pseudocysts. *Br J Surg* 1975;62:37
37. Bradley EL, Gonzalez AC, Clements JL: Acute pancreatic pseudocysts: incidence and implications. *Ann Surg* 1976;184:734
38. Freeny PC, Lewis GP, Traverso LW, et al: Infected pancreatic fluid collections: percutaneous catheter drainage. *Radiology* 1988;167:435

39. Steiner E, Mueller PR, Hahn PF et al: Complicated pancreatic abscesses: problems in interventional management. *Radiology* 1988;167:443
40. Neff CC, van Sonnenberg E, Casola G, et al: Diverticular abscesses: percutaneous drainage. *Radiology* 1987;163:15
41. Casola G, van Sonnenberg E, Neff CC, et al: Abscesses in Crohn disease: percutaneous drainage. *Radiology* 1987; 163:19
42. Jeffrey RB, Federle MP, Tolentino CS: Periappendiceal inflammatory masses: CT directed management and clinical outcome in 70 patients. *Radiology* 1988;167:13
43. van Sonnenberg E, Wittich GR, Casola G, et al: Periappendiceal abscesses: percutaneous drainage. *Radiology* 1987;163:23
44. Merriam MA, Cronan JJ, Dorfman GS, et al: Radiographically guided percutaneous catheter drainage of pleural fluid collections. *AJR* 1988;151:1113
45. van Sonnenberg E, Nakamoto SK, Mueller PR, et al: CT and ultrasound guided catheter drainage of empyemas after chest-tube failure. *Radiology* 1984;151:349
46. Westcott JL: Percutaneous catheter drainage of pleural effusion and empyema. *AJR* 1985;144:1189
47. Garcia-Vila J, Saiz-Paches V, Domenech-Iglesias MA, et al: Infected intraabdominal hematomas: percutaneous drainage. *Abd Imag* 1993;18:313
48. Mueller PR, Ferrucci JT, Cronan JJ, et al: Detection and drainage of bilomas: special considerations. *AJR* 1983;140:715
49. Gold L, Patel A: Ultrasound detection of extrahepatic encapsulated bile: "biloma." *AJR* 1979;139:1014
50. Zager HB, Kurtz AB, Perlmutter GS, et al: Ultrasonic characteristics of bilomas. *JCU* 1981;9:21
51. van Sonnenberg E, Casola G, Wittich GR, et al: The role of interventional radiology for complications of cholecystoctomy. *Surg* 1990;107:632
52. Meyers AM, Levine E, Myburgh JA, et al: Diagnosis and management of lymphoceles after renal transplantation. *Urology* 1977;10:497
53. van Sonnenberg E, Wittich GR, Casola G, et al: Lymphoceles: imaging characteristics and percutaneous management. *Radiology* 1986;161:593
54. White M, Mueller PR, Ferrucci JT, et al: Percutaneous drainage of postoperative abdominal and pelvic lymphoceles. *AJR* 1985;145:1065
55. McDowell GC, Babaian RJ, Johnson DE: Management of symptomatic lymphocele via percutaneous drainage and sclerotherapy with tetracycline. *Urology* 1991;37:237
56. Lee MJ, Saini S, Brink JA, et al: Treatment of critically ill patients with sepsis of unknown cause: value of percutaneous cholecystostomy. *AJR* 1991;156:1163
57. Long TN, Heimbach DM, Carrico CJ: Acalculous cholecystitis in criticaly ill patients. *Am J Surg* 1987;136:31
58. Mirvis SE, Vainright JR, Nelson AW, et al: The diagnosis of acute acalculous cholecystitis: a comparison of sonography, scintigraphy, and CT. *AJR* 1986;147:1171
59. Weissman HS, Frank MS, Berstein LH, et al: Rapid and accurate diagnosis of acute cholecystitis with 99m-Tc HDA cholescintigraphy. *AJR* 1979;32:523
60. Larsen MJ, Klingensmith WC, Kuni CC: Radionuclide hepatobiliary imaging: nonvisualization of the gallbladder secondary to prolonged fasting. *J Nucl Med* 1982;23:1003
61. Kalff V, Froelich JW, Lloyd R, et al: Predictive value of an abnormal hepatobiliary scan in patients with severe intercurrent illness. *Radiology* 1983;146:191
62. Shuman WP, Gibbs R, Rudd TG, et al: PIPIDA scintigraphy for cholecystitis: false positives in alcoholism and total parenteral nutrition. *AJR* 1982;138:1
63. Boland GW, Lee MJ, Leung J, et al: Percutaneous cholecys-

tostomy in critically ill patients: early response and final outcome in 82 patients. *AJR* 1994;163:339
64. Browning PD, McGahan JP, Gerscovich ED: Percutaneous cholecystostomy for suspected acute cholecystitis in the hospitalized patient. *JVIR* 1993;4:531
65. Torosian MH, Rombeau JL: Feeding by tube enterostomy. *Surg Gynecol Obstet* 1980;150:918
66. Kumar SS: Tube gastrostomy: a routine adjunct in major abdominal operations. *Am Surg* 1985;51:201
67. Tunca JC, Buchler DA, Mack EA, et al: The management of ovarian-cancer caused bowel obstruction. *Gynecol Oncol* 1981;12:186
68. Wasilgew BK, Ujiki GT, Beal JM: Feeding gastrostomy: complications and mortality. *Am J Surg* 1982;143:194
69. Shellto PC, Malt RA: Tube gastrostomy: technique and complications. *Ann Surg* 1985;201:180
70. Gauderer WL, Ponsky JL, Izant RJ: Gastrostomy without laparotomy: a percutaneous endoscopic technique. *J Pediatr Surg* 1980;15:872
71. Ho CS: Percutaneous gastrostomy for jejunal feeding. *Radiology* 1983;149:595
72. Tao HH, Gulie RR: Percutaneous feeding gastrostomy. *AJR* 1983;141:793
73. Willis JS, Oglesby JT: Percutaneous gastrostomy. *Radiology* 1983;149:449
74. O'Keffe F, Carrasco CH, Charngangavet C, et al: Percutaneous drainage and feeding gastrostomies in 100 patients. *Radiology* 1989;172:341
75. Wills JS: Percutaneous gastrostomy: application in gastric carcinoma and gastroplasty stoma dilatation. *AJR* 1986;147:826
76. Saini S, Mueller PR, Gaa J, et al: Percutaneous gastrostomy with gastropexy: experience in 125 patients. *AJR* 1990;154:1003
77. Halkier BK, Ho Cs, Nee ACN: Percutaneous feeding gastrostomy with the Seldinger technique: review of 252 patients. *Radiology* 1989;171:359
78. Ho Cs, Gray RR, Goldtmger M, et al: Percutaneous gastrostomy for enteral feeding. *Radiology* 1985;156:349
79. O'Dwyer F, Gullane P, Ho CS: Percutaneous feeding gastrostomy in patients with head neck tumors: a 5 year review. *Laryngoscope* 1990;100:29
80. Luctzow AM, Chaffo RA, Young H: Percutaneous gastrostomy: the Stanford experience. *Laryngoscope* 1988;98:1035
81. Purdum PP III, Kirby DF: Short bowel syndrome: a review of the role of nutritional support. *J Parenter Enter Nutr* 1990;15:93
82. Wills JS, Oglesby JT: Percutaneous gastrostomy. *Radiology* 1988;167:41
83. Ho CS, Yee AC, McPherson R: Complications and surgical and percutaneous nonendoscopic gastrostomy: review of 233 patients. *Gastroenterology* 1988;95:1206
84. Foutch PG, Talbert GA, Wanng JP, et al: Percutaneous endoscopic gastrostomy in patients with prior abdominal surgery: virtues of the safe tract. *Am J Gastroenterol* 1988;83:147
85. Sanchez RB, Van Sonnenberg E, D'Agostino HB, et al: CT guidance for percutaneous gastrostomy and gastroenterostomy. *Radiology* 1992;184:201
86. Yeung EY, Ho CS: Percutaneous gastrostomy: an underutilized technique? *J Intervent Radiol* 1991;6:43
87. Gray RR, St Louis EL, Grosman H: Modified catheter for percutaneous gastroenterostomy. *Radiology* 1989;173:276
88. Gustke RF, Varma RR, Soergel KH: Reflux during perfusion of the proximal bowel. *Gastroenterology* 1970;59:890
89. Alzate GD, Coons HG, Elliot J, et al: Percutaneous gastrostomy for jejunal feeding: a new technique. *AJR* 1986;147:822
90. Olson DL, Krubsack AS, Stewart ET: Percutaneous enteral

alimentation: gastrostomy vs gastrojejunostomy. *Radiology* 1993;187:105

91. Brown AS, Muellar PR, Ferrucci JT: Controlled percutaneous gastrostomy: nylon T-fastener for the fixation of the anterior gastric wall. *Radiology* 1986;158:543

92. Moote DJ, Ho CS, Felice V: Fluoroscopically guided percutaneous gastrostomy: is gastric fixation necessary? *Can Assoc Radiol* 1990;41:363

93. Deutsch LS, Kannegreter L, Vanson DT, et al: Simplified percutaneous gastrostomy. *Radiology* 1992;184:181

94. Ho CS, Yeung EY: Percutaneous gastrostomy and transgastric jejunostomy. *AJR* 1992;158:251

95. Hicks ME, Surratt RS, Picus D, et al: Fluoroscopically guided percutaneous gastrostomy and gastroenterostomy: analysis of 158 consecutive cases. *AJR* 1990;154:725

96. McLoughlin RF, Gibney RG: Fluoroscopically guided percutaneous gastrostomy: tube function and malfunction. *Abd Imag* 1994;19:195

97. Almgard LE, Fernstroin I: Percutaneous nephrostomy. *Acta Radiol* 1974;126:639

98. Barbaric ZL, Wood BP: Emergency percutaneous nephrostomy: experience with 34 patients and review of the literature. *AJR* 1977;128:453

99. Irving HC, Arthur RJ, Thomas DFM: Percutaneous nephrostomy on pediatrics. *Clin Radiol* 1987;38:245

100. Stables DP: Percutaneous nephrostomy: techniques, indications and results. *Urol Clin North Am* 1982;9:15

101. Teenan RP, Ramsey A, Deane RF: Percutaneous nephrostomy in the management of malignant ureteric obstruction. *Br J Urol* 1989;64:238

102. Chapman ME, Reid JM: Use of percutaneous nephrostomy in malignant ureteric obstruction. *Br J Radiol* 1991;64:318

103. Cullain JD, Wheeler JS, Marsons RE, et al: Percutaneous nephrostomy for palliation of metastatic ureteric obstruction. *Urology* 1987;30:229

104. Fallon B, Olney L, Culp DA: Nephrostomy in cancer patients: to do or not to do. *Br J Urol* 1980;52:237

105. Keidan DR, Greenberg RE, Hoffman JP, et al: Is percutaneous nephrostomy for hydronephrosis appropriate in patients with advanced cancer? *Am J Surg* 1988;156:206

106. Soper JT, Blaszyk TM, Oke E, et al: Percutaneous nephrostomy in gynecologic oncology patients. *Am J Obstet Gynecol* 1988;158:1127

107. Stables DP, Ginsberg NJ, Johnson ML: Percutaneous nephrostomy: a series and review of the literature. *AJR* 1978;130:75

108. Ekelund L, Karp W, Klefsgard U, et al: Percutaneous nephrostomy indicational and technical considerations. *Urol Radiol* 1980;1:227

109. Hildell J, Aspelin R, Sigfussor B: Percutaneous nephrostomy. *Acta Radiol* 1980;21:485

110. Kehinde EO, Newland CJ, Tery TR, et al: Percutaneous nephrostomies. *Br J Urol* 1993;71:664

111. Stables DF: Percutaneous nephrostomy. In: *Syllabus: A Categorical Course in Genitourinary Radiology*. Ed. RSNA, 1978

Critical Care, Third Edition, edited by Joseph M. Civetta,
Robert W. Taylor, and Robert R. Kirby.
Lippincott-Raven Publishers, Philadelphia, PA © 1997.

CHAPTER 39

■

Feeding Tube Placement

Scott A. Shikora

IMMEDIATE CONCERNS ■

MAJOR PROBLEMS

For critically ill patients, enteral nutrition is preferable to
parenteral in terms of cost, complications, gut mucosal maintenance, and metabolic and immune function. However, it
has not been widely employed in this patient population.
This is partly because of the success of current parenteral
nutrition and the difficulties encountered with enteral feedings. Feeding the patient using the gastrointestinal tract is
more difficult than through a central vein. Enteral feeding
is commonly frustrated by gastric dysmotility, aspiration,
diarrhea, and occasionally by intestinal ileus. Feeding intolerance, fluid restrictions, metabolic derangements, and hyperglycemia further frustrate attempts to establish total enteral support. Appropriate gastrointestinal access also can be
challenging to obtain and maintain and may require surgical
placement. Often, after successful tube placement, feeding
tubes occlude, dislodge, or are inadvertently removed.

The choice of tube type, access site, and placement techniques is not always simple and will depend upon a number
of considerations. These include each patient's unique requirements, the status of the gastrointestinal tract, clinician
preference, and even available resources. Currently, there
are a multitude of commercially available tube designs and
a variety of placement techniques to meet most needs. No
single system has been shown to be uniformly superior to
another. A different approach may be indicated for each
patient. The large variety of options available should insure

that all critically ill patients will be able to have enteral
access established.

STRESS POINTS

1. The initial consideration for determining the choice
   of an enteral access system is the anticipated duration
   of enteral feeding.
2. Patients predicted to need enteral feeding for 2 weeks
   or less are said to have short-term requirements.
   These patients are best served with bedside placement of a nasoenteric tube.
3. Patients thought to need enteral feeding for greater
   than 6 to 8 weeks are described as having long-term
   requirements. Percutaneous or surgically placed tubes
   are most appropriate for this subgroup of patients.
4. Patients with the anticipated need for enteral feeding
   for greater than 2 weeks but less than 6 to 8 weeks
   are said to have an intermediate requirement. These
   patients are well served by nasally, percutaneously,
   or surgically placed feeding tubes.
5. Thirty percent to 70% of critically ill patients have
   gastric emptying dysfunction. For these patients, enteral tubes must be placed beyond the pylorus.
6. Several bedside techniques have been described to
   aid in achieving postpyloric placement of tubes inserted through the nose. These techniques are highly
   successful in experienced hands.
7. Fluoroscopic or endoscopic support may be necessary for passing the tip of the nasoenteric tube beyond
   the pylorus. Even with the assistance of these modalities, success is not guaranteed.
8. Percutaneous gastrostomy has been shown to be less
   costly and less time-consuming and has fewer complications than surgical gastrostomy.

The opinions expressed herein are those of the author and do
not necessarily reflect the opinions of the United States Air Force
or the Department of Defense.

599

9. Currently, the percutaneous jejunostomy tube has not been shown to be a reliable long-term access option.
10. Surgically placed jejunostomy tubes are excellent for long-term feeding but expose the critically ill patient to the risks and complications of an operative procedure.

ESSENTIAL DIAGNOSTIC TESTS AND PROCEDURES

1. Auscultation of air instilled into the nasogastric or nasoenteric tube is useful for determining proper tube placement. It is important to confirm that the tube was not inadvertently placed into the bronchial tree.
2. After placement of a nasogastric or nasoenteric feeding tube, a chest radiograph should be obtained to confirm proper tube location before infusing enteral formula.
3. If there is concern that a nasoenteric tube has migrated back into the stomach, its position must be clarified with a radiograph.
4. Food coloring can be added to enteral formulas to discern whether patients are aspirating feeds or oropharyngeal secretions.

INITIAL THERAPY

1. Determine whether the patient can tolerate enteral nutrition.
2. Based on the patient's overall condition, associated medical conditions, the functional status of the gastrointestinal tract, and available hospital resources, the most appropriate type of feeding tube and placement technique can be chosen.
3. If the attempted placement technique is unsuccessful, reconsider the above and choose another enteral access option.

OVERVIEW

Critically ill patients will invariably require nutritional intervention. Traditionally, enteral nutrition has not been widely employed in this patient population. This is due in part to the success of present-day parenteral nutrition, and to difficulties encountered with enteral feedings. While parenteral nutrition can effectively administer protein and calories, it does not prevent intestinal mucosal atrophy.[1,2] It is now well-recognized that the healthy gut mucosal layer provides a barrier to pathogen invasion.[3,4] Microbial invasion through the gut into the systemic circulation is thought to represent a major cause of the nosocomial sepsis, and possibly the multiple organ dysfunction, seen with critical illness.[5-8]

Recent evidence has demonstrated that enteral nutrition is preferable to parenteral in terms of cost, complications, gut mucosal maintenance, and metabolic and immune function.[9-12] However, feeding the patient via the gastrointestinal tract is more difficult than through a central vein. Enteral

feeding is commonly frustrated by gastric dysmotility, aspiration, diarrhea, and occasionally, by intestinal ileus.[13] Feeding intolerance, fluid restrictions, metabolic derangements and hyperglycemia further frustrate attempts to establish total enteral support. Appropriate gastrointestinal access can also be challenging to obtain and maintain, and may require surgical placement. Often, after successful access placement, feeding tubes occlude, dislodge or are inadvertently removed. Despite these obstacles, it is clear that the benefits of enteral nutrition outweigh the concerns.

Fortunately, there are a multitude of commercially available tube designs and a variety of placement techniques to meet most needs. The choice of tube type, access site, and placement technique will depend upon a number of considerations including each patient's unique requirements, clinician preference, and even available resources. This chapter will review the assortment of tube types, the differences between gastrointestinal placement sites, and the variety of access options available to choose from. In addition, it will describe the decision-making process required to choose the best combination of tube, site, and method of placement.

DETERMINING THE MOST APPROPRIATE TUBE TYPE, SITE, AND PLACEMENT TECHNIQUE

When considering the initiation of enteral feeding, the clinician must first decide on the most appropriate type of tube to employ, the region in the gastrointestinal tract to place the tube, and the technique to access the lumen. Several factors influence the ultimate decision[14]:

Duration of enteral feeding
Current status of the patient
Coexisting medical conditions
Functional status of the gastrointestinal tract
Previous abdominal surgeries
Tube brands in stock
Availability of radiologic, gastroenterologic, and surgical support

The initial consideration is the anticipated duration of enteral feeding. Based on the patient's current status and comorbidity, it must be estimated whether the access requirement is to be short term, intermediate, or long term. The distinction between the three classifications is somewhat artificial and there are no absolute time separations. Short term usually implies the need for enteral feeding for up to 2 weeks in duration. Short-term enteral feeding is commonly used for patients who tend to be free of significant underlying medical conditions, such as trauma victims and younger patients who undergo uncomplicated major surgery. In most of these patients, access requirements can be satisfied by placing the tube into the gastrointestinal tract using the nasal approach. These tubes are considered to be temporary in that they can be easily removed when they are no longer required. Placement techniques tend to be inexpensive, minimally invasive, and carry a low complication rate. Although these tubes easily dislodge, replacement is often easy.

Long-term enteral access can be defined as the need to administer enteral nutritional support for an extended period of time or even permanently. Some authors describe long-term support as that requiring access for more than 4 to 6 weeks.[15,16] Whether one defines this category as access use greater than 4 weeks, 6 weeks, or 2 months, the important consideration for these patients is that the tube needs to be more permanently secured. In most cases, nasally placed tubes are not adequate. For this subgroup of patients, tube placement tends to be more invasive and more expensive and has greater potential for complications. It also usually requires surgical or percutaneous procedures. Patients requiring long-term enteral nutrition are those whose illness is such that recovery will be delayed or permanently incomplete. These patients typically are older, have significant comorbid conditions or end-stage organ dysfunction, and have had a serious acute event.

Intermediate duration is also a relative term but encompasses all patients with requirements for enteral feeding access for greater than 2 weeks but less than 6 to 8 weeks. These patients can be served by any of the available access routes. Whereas nasally placed tubes are less secure, the ease of replacement can often extend their use for the duration of their necessity. Tubes placed percutaneously or surgically tend to be considered permanent but can be removed without much difficulty should feeding access no longer be necessary. In most cases, the decision can be based on factors such as previous abdominal surgery and the availability of resources.

Although the patient's current medical status and comorbid conditions indirectly influence the choice of tube by their effects on the duration of tube utilization, these factors also directly impact the choice of placement site and technique. The more critically ill patients are less likely to tolerate a surgical or endoscopic procedure. In these patients, if enteral feeding is desired (but usually should not be initiated in patients who are hemodynamically unstable), less invasive techniques such as nasal access can be used temporarily until conditions are more conducive to long-term access placement. Patients with complications such as intestinal fistula, laparotomy wound infections, open abdomens, or sepsis from other sources also may be inappropriate for surgically or percutaneously placed tubes. Other groups at increased risk for complications with surgically or percutaneously placed tubes include the obese and patients with diabetes, cancer, malnutrition, immunocompromised conditions, end-stage liver disease, cirrhosis, ascites, renal failure, uremia, thrombocytopenia, coagulopathy states, and significant heart disease.

Another important consideration when determining the best choice of feeding tube, access site, and placement technique is the functional status of the gastrointestinal tract. Although gastric feeding is generally preferable to jejunal feeding because it is more physiologically suitable for normal digestion and nutrient absorption, many conditions mandate postpyloric or jejunal feeding. Many critically ill patients have gastric emptying dysfunction as a consequence of their illness. Interleukin-1, a cytokine released during stressed states, has been shown to delay gastric emptying when administered to rats fed a liquid diet.[17] Many underlying conditions such as diabetes mellitus, medication use, gastritis, sepsis, and electrolyte abnormalities also affect gastric emptying.[18] Feeding into the stomach in these circumstances may increase the risk of regurgitation and aspiration. Patients with normal gastric emptying but diminished ability to protect their airways, such as those with neurologic disorders, also may require postpyloric tube placement.

Inadequate gastric emptying has been reported to occur in as many as 30% to 70% of patients.[18] With the high incidence of gastric emptying abnormalities, many clinicians favor jejunal feeding.[5,19] In a randomized, prospective study, Montecalvo and colleagues[20] demonstrated that critically ill patients fed through jejunostomy tubes received more total calories, had a greater increase in serum prealbumin concentrations, and had a lower rate of pneumonia than those fed through a gastrostomy tube. Jejunal feeding also may provide more reliable nutrition support because, unlike gastric feeding, it does not have to be interrupted for procedures, surgeries, or high gastric residuals.

The functional status of the gastrointestinal tract also may influence the technique of tube placement. Gastroesophageal disease or obstruction may preclude the ability to pass tubes nasally and may also make percutaneous tube placement using the endoscopic approach difficult or impossible. Adhesions from previous upper abdominal surgeries or the anatomic alterations seen after procedures like gastrectomy or pancreaticoduodenectomy diminish the likelihood of endoscopic and radiologic placement and may make a surgical placement more complicated.

Hospital resources—both supplies and personnel—also influence the decision-making process. Hospitals may have a limited selection of tube products. Product cost is becoming an ever more significant determinant of hospital purchasing. Because many tube designs are similar, substitutions can be successful, and the inability to obtain a specific tube should not preclude the use of enteral nutrition. Human resources also vary from facility to facility. Not all hospitals offer equal expertise in each of the support services required. The choice between radiologic, gastroenterologic, or surgical support may be based to some degree on the strength and weaknesses of these departments within the hospital.

The selection of the most appropriate tube type, access site, and placement technique for the critically ill is based on the consideration of these interrelated factors. Therefore, the final decision varies from patient to patient. Success is never ensured but occurs most often when all of the dependent variables are considered and the approach is flexible to allow for change when the situation warrants creativity. To aid in the decision-making process, a useful algorithm is provided (Fig. 39-1).

TUBE OPTIONS

Currently, a large variety of tube designs are commercially available. For nasal placement, tubes tend to be thin, soft, and flexible. Most are polyvinyl chloride, silicone, or polyurethane. Many are weighted at the tip with mercury whereas others are unweighted. Most contain a thin metal stylet to

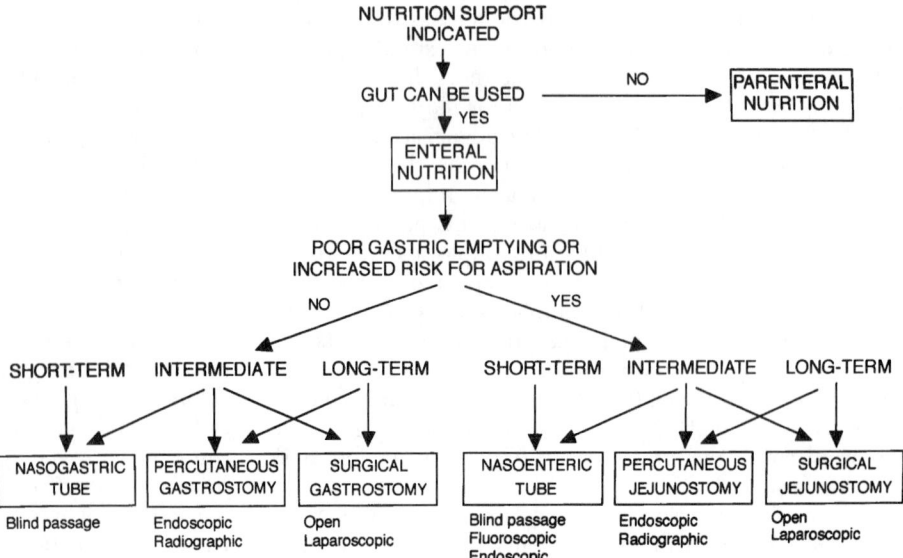

FIGURE 39-1. Algorithm for determining appropriate enteral access for the critically ill.

assist in placement. All are radiopaque to enable confirmation of position by radiographic study. Their soft, flexible construction and narrow diameter enables these tubes to be well tolerated by the patient, and they rarely contribute to sinus infections or obstruct breathing. However, these tubes are prone to occlusion. This occurs particularly if feeding is interrupted without irrigating the tube free of formula and when the tube is used for the delivery of crushed or dissolved medications.

Percutaneously placed tubes also come in a variety of commercially prepared designs. These tubes tend to be wider in diameter than those used for nasal placement, which decreases but does not prevent the likelihood of occlusion. Placement requires fluoroscopic or endoscopic assistance to direct the tube into the appropriate lumen after skin puncture. These tubes are more socially acceptable and less likely to dislodge but can leak, cause pain at the insertion site, and induce a local soft tissue infection. With long-term use they also may begin to deteriorate. Some models have separate ports for simultaneous jejunal feeding and gastric decompression. Most are secured from within the lumen of the viscus by a small flange or balloon contained within the tip. Removal may require endoscopy.

The choices for surgical access are also extensive. Balloon and mushroom-tipped soft rubber tubes are commonly used for gastrostomy tubes. These have a wide bore and are flexible. Like their percutaneously placed cousins, they may leak, cause pain at the insertion site, and induce a local soft tissue infection. The rubber tubes also have been known to deteriorate with time. Some models on the market have multiple lumen and ports to allow for gastric decompression and jejunal nutrient infusion.

Feeding tubes used for jejunal access tend to be smaller in diameter than surgically placed gastrostomy tubes but wider than the nasally inserted models. In the early 1970s, the needle catheter jejunostomy was introduced.[21] It consisted of a tube similar in design to those used for nasal insertion in that it was extremely narrow in diameter. Al-

though easy to insert, the needle catheter jejunostomy has fallen from favor because it is a poor conduit for most enteral formulas. The small tube size employed was prone to kink and frequently was too narrow to allow rapid flow of the more viscous feeding solutions.[14,22] Many surgeons, including myself, have abandoned its use. Other acceptable options for jejunostomy placement include soft rubber tubes and biliary T tubes. Their wider internal diameter improves infusion and decreases the likelihood of occlusion. Tube deterioration, site infection, or leakage also are possible. Red rubber or Robinson catheters are excellent choices. Unfortunately, these tubes are prone to dislodgement. Balloon and mushroom-tipped tubes are less susceptible to inadvertent removal because their tips are wider than their shafts and anchor them in place. Although popular with some, these tubes are disdained by many. The widened tip can potentially obstruct the narrow lumen or erode the wall of the jejunum. The biliary T tube provides some of the security of the balloon and mushroom-tipped tubes with less risk of intestinal obstruction or erosion.

PLACEMENT TECHNIQUE OPTIONS

The myriad techniques available for feeding tube placement ensure the potential for obtaining enteral access in nearly all critically ill patients. As stated earlier, the many factors involved in choosing the most appropriate tube type and access site also determine the technique for placement.

NASOGASTRIC

The least complicated and quickest feeding access is the nasogastric tube. Although the stiffer, wider tubes used for gastric decompression also can be used for feeding, it is preferable to replace these tubes with the thin, softer, more flexible tubes. The former has several potential complications, including increased risk of sinusitis, gastroesophageal

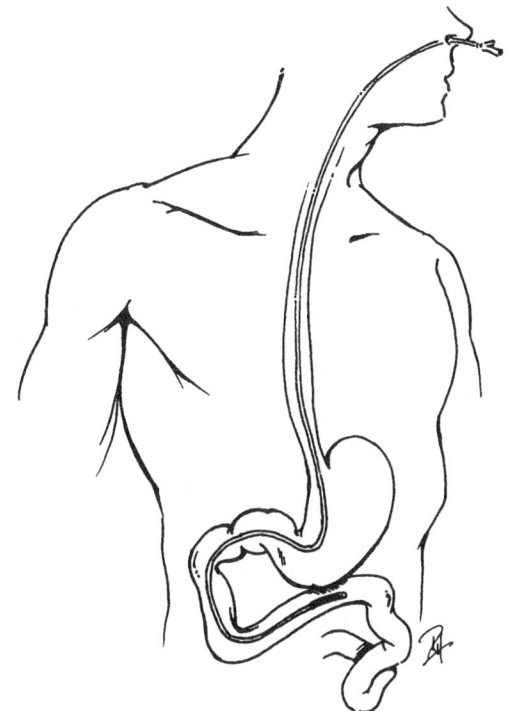

FIGURE 39-2. Nasoenteric feeding tube.

reflux and aspiration, nasal skin erosion, and obstruction to breathing. Placement is similar to that of the drainage sump tubes. The tube is lubricated and then passed blindly through a nostril. It travels down the posterior pharynx into the esophagus and then into the stomach. Placement is aided by wire stylets or weighted tips. Complications are similar to those of the sump tube such as epistaxis, rhinitis, esophageal perforation or hemorrhage, pneumothorax, and inadvertent placement into the trachea or bronchus.

NASODUODENAL AND NASOJEJUNAL

Zaloga[23] found that only 5% of weighted small-bore feeding tubes pass spontaneously through the pylorus. Manually passing the soft, thin, flexible tube across the length of the stomach and beyond the pylorus is not always easy. Often, the tube coils back into the fundus or cannot easily be negotiated through the antrum and pylorus. In most cases, the difficulty in tube advancement into the duodenum is related to the blind nature of the passage and to the inability to steer or guide the tube (Fig. 39-2). Success varies from 49% to 60%.[24] Some authors claim to have improved success with simple maneuvers such as placing the patient in the right lateral decubitus position, by giving the tube a gentle clockwise twist as it is being passed or bending the tip of the stylet.[23,25] One author claims to be able to "feel" the tube pass through the pylorus.[23]

When simple methods fail, more detailed maneuvers may be necessary. Several techniques have been described to aid in passage. One approach involves administering a promotility agent in conjunction with tube advancement. Lord and others[26] describe an 88% success rate when 10 mg of met-

oclopramide was administered 10 minutes before inserting a unweighted tube. However, Kittinger and associates[27] found that when metoclopramide was given after tube insertion into the stomach, it improved tube passage only in diabetic patients. Continuous pH monitoring using a specially designed tube that has a built-in pH sensor in the tip has been described to facilitate passage by enabling recognition of the tube tip location.[28,29] Generally, lower pH values are found in the stomach compared with the duodenum. This device may obviate the need for radiographic confirmation of tube location. Whereas the need for fewer radiographs may save money, the requirement for specialized tubes and a pH monitor may offset any savings. These tubes are generally two to three times more expensive than traditional tubes, and most pH monitors cost a few hundred dollars.

Serial or continuous pH monitoring also can be used to indicate if the tube has migrated back into the stomach. Strong and coworkers[29] report a 100% correlation between the radiographic documentation of tube location with the measured pH in 8 patients. In that study, all changes in tube tip location as interpreted by pH were confirmed by radiography. However, the ability to use pH values to determine location may be less accurate in the setting of H_2 blocker administration or with achlorhydria, where the stomach has less acid production, hence higher than normal pH readings. Despite the advantages of knowing tube tip location, Heiselman and coworkers[28] were still only 79% successful in getting the tip of the tube beyond the pylorus. Other indicators of duodenal placement were compared by Welch and coworkers.[24] They reviewed the accuracy of auscultation, the vacuum effect, and fluid aspiration for color and pH. They were 80% successful in achieving postpyloric tube placement. In addition, they found that whereas all four methods had positive predictive values greater than 80%, they also had negative predictive values no less than 28%. In a similar study, Thurlow[25] reports an 87% success rate in achieving duodenal placement with a technique that utilizes bending the stylet tip, placing the patient in the right lateral decubitus position, corkscrewing the tube on placement, and auscultation for location. Zaloga,[23] also using a combination of these techniques, achieved a 92% success rate in 231 patients. Whereas in experienced hands these techniques may be more accurate than more standard methods, they still have their limitations. Therefore, confirmatory radiographs cannot be omitted.

The literature has no consensus as to whether weighted or unweighted tubes pass into the duodenum more often. Levenson and coworkers[30] demonstrated that there was no apparent difference in the likelihood of tube passage between weighted and unweighted tubes. Lord and coworkers[26] found that with the addition of preinsertion metoclopramide, unweighted tubes were significantly more likely to pass than weighted (84% versus 36%, respectively). In contrast, Whatley and associates[31] found that 80% of weighted tubes passed when metoclopramide was given before insertion.

Fluoroscopic guidance is an excellent method for placing the tip of the feeding tube beyond the pylorus.[32] Because the tubes are radiopaque, they are easily seen under fluoroscopy. Tube passage can then be guided by "direct vision." Whereas this technique increases the likelihood of success, it has several drawbacks: the critically ill patient must be transported to the radiology department, or the the radiography equipment must be brought to the patient. It also exposes the patient to radiation. Endoscopy provides an alternate means of delivering the tube past the pylorus, but it is also the most invasive. After positioning the tube into the stomach, an esophagogastroscopy is performed. The tip of the tube, or a suture secured to the tip, can then be grasped with a biopsy forceps that was passed through the endoscope and dragged into the duodenum. Although this technique is effective, the tube may get pulled back into the stomach by the withdrawal of the endoscope, and the procedure places the patient at risk for all of the complications associated with endoscopy, including injury to the esophagus, stomach, or duodenum; perforation; bleeding; and aspiration. Nasoenteric tubes also can be placed at time of laparotomy for patients requiring temporary jejunal access.

Even after the successful nasoenteric placement, tubes easily can be inadvertently removed or pulled back into the stomach. No method for tube immobilization (i.e, sutures, bridles, or taping) is completely secure. Fortunately, the tube can be replaced with little effort.

PERCUTANEOUS GASTROSTOMY

Although surgically placed gastrostomy tubes have long been heralded as the "gold standard" for obtaining stable long-term gastric luminal access, numerous published reports demonstrate that percutaneous placement offers all of the same advantages but with a significantly lower complication rate. This technique involves the placement of an access tube into the gastric lumen using a direct puncture of the skin, abdominal, and gastric walls. Endoscopic or radiographic assistance is essential. Percutaneous endoscopic gastrostomy (PEG) tube placement generally requires one of two techniques. These are termed "push" and "pull." There are numerous commercially available insertion kits that contain the tube and the equipment necessary for placement. A formal esophagogastroduodenoscopy is performed first to rule out upper gastrointestinal disease that precludes tube placement. The endoscope is then steered against the anterior gastric wall to transilluminate the stomach's position through the abdominal wall and skin. If successful, a small needle is then passed through a skin puncture into the gastric lumen. With the pull technique, a long nylon guidewire is the inserted through the needle and grabbed with a snare that was fed through the endoscope. The guidewire is then dragged out of the patient's mouth. It is then used to guide the tube down the esophagus, into the stomach, and out the skin. With the push method, the catheter is passed directly over the guide wire with a peel-away sheath.

The incidence of major complications with this technique is generally described as 1% to 3%, and the reported mortality rate is about 0.5%.[33,34] Complications include colonic injury, gastric perforation, hemorrhage, leakage with peritonitis, necrotizing fasciitis, and skin infection.[33–36] In addition to having a lower complication rate than the open technique, the PEG procedure has been shown to require less time (10 to 30 minutes) to perform and has a lower cost overall.[34,37,38] It

also can usually be performed under local or intravenous sedation. Conditions that preclude the ability to perform upper endoscopy such as obstruction, varices, and severe *Candida* esophagitis also are contraindications to this procedure. Upper abdominal surgery is a relative contraindication because the adhesions that form after surgery may prevent the stomach from being manipulated up to the abdominal wall. If transillumination cannot be achieved, the procedure should be aborted.

An alternative method for percutaneous gastrostomy is the radiographic approach. The stomach is distended with air using a nasogastric tube. Radiopaque contrast is then instilled in the stomach to enable it to be seen with fluoroscopy. The abdominal wall then can be pressed down onto the stomach. A needle is passed into the lumen and a guidewire inserted through the needle. The tract is dilated to the appropriate diameter and the tube is pushed into the lumen. This technique eliminates the need for endoscopy; however, many of the same contraindications and complications apply. In addition, this method does not allow inspection of the mucosa before tube placement or direct visualization of tube position after it is in place.

PERCUTANEOUS JEJUNOSTOMY

With the success of the percutaneous gastrostomy, an interest arose in applying the same technology to jejunal access for patients with a significant risk of aspiration or abnormal gastric motility. In most cases, the procedure begins by placing a percutaneous gastrostomy tube. After this is completed, a thin, flexible tube is passed either through or alongside the gastrostomy tube and steered beyond the pylorus. In addition to the more common endoscopic technique, the percutaneous jejunostomy tube also can be inserted with radiographic assistance.[39]

Despite the similarity of the percutaneous endoscopic jejunostomy (PEJ) technique with percutaneous gastrostomy placement, the procedure has been found to have a much higher complication rate. The published rate of tube dysfunction ranges from 30% to 85%.[40–42] Ironically, there seemed to be no decrease in aspiration rate with these jejunal tubes for patients with an increased aspiration risk. This may not be indicative of a failure of the tube in preventing the reflux of feeding formula. In fact, formula is rarely recovered from the tracheal aspirate. In all likelihood, the lack of improvement in aspiration suggests that the aspiration is mainly oral and pharyngeal secretions. In addition, like nasojejunal access, passage of these tubes through the pylorus is not always successful, and they have been known to migrate back into the stomach.

In one study of PEJ tubes, DiSario and coworkers[41] describe a 95% serious complication rate, a 50% mortality rate, and a 70% incidence rate of tube failure. The alarmingly high mortality rate resulted predominantly from aspiration. However, the investigators did not make the distinction as to whether patients aspirated feeds or oropharyngeal secretions. In addition, they did not radiographically check tube position after aspiration to see if the tip had migrated back into the stomach. Tube failure was also a significant problem in this study. Occlusion represented greater than half of the tube complications. This was attributed to using the tube to deliver crushed tablets and to inspissated feeding solutions. Proper use of the catheters should minimize these problems. Wolfsen and coworkers[40] also report a higher incidence of complications with PEJ catheters compared with PEG tubes. However, in contrast to the DiSario study, they reported a 36% incidence of tube dysfunction and a 17% incidence of aspiration. Although complications were more likely to occur in patients with PEJ versus PEG tubes, the study was not randomized and the differences may be related more to the underlying diseases of the patients than to the tubes themselves. The significant complication and tube failure rates reported in the literature suggest that currently the percutaneous endoscopically placed jejunostomy tube may not be the best option for long-term feeding.[42]

SURGICAL GASTROSTOMY

Before the development of safe and effective methods for percutaneous tube placement, surgical techniques were the most commonly employed. After entering the abdominal cavity, a large-bore tube is placed directly into the gastric lumen and then pulled through the abdominal wall and out through the skin. The tubes used are usually balloon or mushroom-tipped to prevent dislodgement. To minimize the risk of leakage and peritonitis, the tube is secured with two or three concentric pursestring sutures, and the anterior wall of the stomach is tacked to the undersurface of the abdominal wall to obliterate any potential space around the tube. This technique is generally referred to as the Stamm gastrostomy.

The overall complication rate varies from 2.5% to 24% in the literature, with a major complication rate of about 10%.[33,34] However, the wide range may be more indicative of the severity of illness of the patient populations than from the procedure itself. In addition to the complications associated with any gastric tube, surgical placement adds the increased risks associated with surgery and anesthesia. For patients requiring laparotomy for other reasons, the gastrostomy tube can be inserted at that time with minimal additional time or morbidity. However, for patients not requiring abdominal surgery, this technique requires a laparotomy and an anesthetic. In patients without previous abdominal surgery, the procedure can be brief and limited. The incision can be either a limited vertical midline or a small left upper quadrant transverse one. Many surgeons can perform this procedure with local anesthesia, which avoids the risk associated with general anesthetics. Patients who have had previous abdominal surgery may pose a greater risk for complications because the procedure may be more involved. Adhesions—scar tissue that forms in the abdominal cavity as a result of surgery—may extend the incision size and the length of time necessary for tube placement. In addition, it increases the likelihood of injury to the stomach or intestines.

Recently, new minimally invasive techniques have been described using laparoscopy.[43] These procedures have a decreased morbidity compared with the traditional open techniques because they do not require the laparotomy incision. However, they require a surgeon with experience in laparoscopic surgery and may be impossible in patients with previ-

ous abdominal surgery. In addition, the decreased morbidity must be balanced with the significantly increased cost because laparoscopic surgery is dependent on costly equipment.

SURGICAL JEJUNOSTOMY

Like the surgically placed gastrostomy, the technique for open jejunostomy tube placement is generally safe; however, it can be more risky in patients who have had abdominal surgery and may require general anesthesia. The most commonly employed techniques minimize the risks of leak from the bowel around the tube by either placing a pursestring suture around the tube (Stamm), or by creating a serosal tunnel from the bowel wall overlying a portion of the tube (Witzel). After tube insertion into the jejunal lumen, the bowel is plicated to the undersurface of the anterior abdominal wall with three to four silk sutures placed circumferentially around the tube to further minimize the risk of leak and peritonitis (Fig. 39-3). The bowel is also carefully positioned for plication to prevent kinking or tube erosion.

To facilitate tube placement and minimize the risk of leak, the needle catheter jejunostomy technique was developed. It was first described by Delaney and coworkers[21] in 1973 as a safe and simple alternative to standard jejunostomy tube placement. This method employs a narrow tube that is inserted by needle puncture through the antimesenteric border of the jejunal wall obliquely to create a subserosal tunnel. The tube is secured with a pursestring suture and then passed through the abdominal wall and skin. Few major complications were reported with this technique. Page and others[44] had a 1% major and 1.5% minor complication rate in 199 patients. As stated earlier, these tubes tend to be unreliable and therefore are unpopular with many surgeons.

I prefer the use of a large-bore soft flexible catheter placed into the jejunal lumen with a single pursestring su-

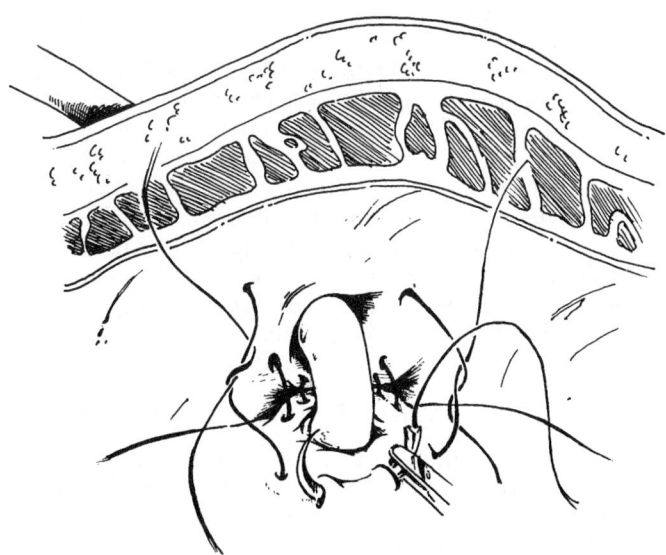

FIGURE 39-3. Plication of the jejunum to the anterior abdominal wall. By suturing the jejunum to the abdominal wall circumferentially around the tube, the risk of leakage is decreased.

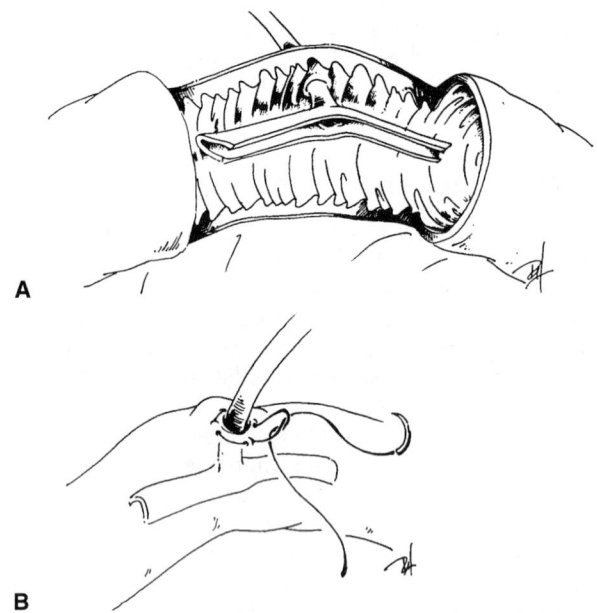

FIGURE 39-4. A surgically placed jejunostomy tube using a biliary T tube.

ture. A biliary T tube is a good choice of tube for jejunal feeding in that it is less likely to dislodge than the straight tube but unlikely to obstruct the lumen (Fig. 39-4). The limbs are cut to approximately 3 cm in length each, and the back of the T limb is slit lengthwise to facilitate removal. After tube insertion into the jejunal lumen, the bowel is plicated as described earlier.

As with gastrostomy tube placement, laparoscopic insertion techniques also have been developed. One such procedure attaches the jejunum to the anterior abdominal wall with four specially designed T fasteners. After this is completed, a large-bore needle is inserted into the jejunal lumen. A guidewire is then threaded through the needle and the catheter passed over a guidewire with the use of a peel-away introducer.[45]

Jejunostomy tubes often become occluded, leak, or are removed either deliberately or inadvertently. Replacement is most easily performed with fluoroscopic assistance.[39] This technique can even be successful for reinserting tubes that have been removed in the distant past. Because the jejunal limb used for the jejunostomy is routinely fixed to the under-surface of the abdominal wall, luminal access can be achieved by passing a needle catheter through the skin site or scar. Once the tip of the needle is in the lumen, a long guidewire is then directed into the lumen and used to direct the tube.

NOVEL APPROACHES TO ENTERAL ACCESS

Although not endorsed by myself, a few novel approaches to enteral access are included for completeness. These techniques were performed in patients unable to have access established with more conventional methods. In two case reports, the duodenal lumen was safely cannulated by fluoroscopy- or computed tomography–guided puncture using a lumbar approach.[46,47]

CONCLUSION

Enteral nutrition is increasingly recognized as an important addition to the comprehensive care of the critically ill and the preferred means of nutritional support. However, the successful establishment of secure and dependable enteral feeding access may be challenging. Several factors, including the patient's current condition, past medical and surgical history, status of the gastrointestinal tract, and the hospital resources available to the clinician determine the best tube type, access choice, and placement method. Fortunately, several options are currently available so that there should be few reasons (short of gastrointestinal tract dysfunction) that preclude the use of enteral nutrition.

No single enteral access combination is superior to the others. None guarantees success in all instances. Using a flexible strategy based on the unique characteristics of the patient and the patient care environment will maximize the likelihood of success. Persistence also pays dividends. Failure of one attempt should not be a cause to abandon enteral feeding. A fresh new approach, possibly using another access option, may ultimately succeed. Only with patience, determination, and an understanding of the available access options will the greatest number of critically ill patients reap the benefits of enteral nutrition.

ACKNOWLEDGMENT

The author would like to thank Ryan Hagino, MD, for his excellent illustrations, which greatly add to the quality of this chapter.

REFERENCES

1. Moore FA, Moore EE, Jones TN, et al: TEN versus TPN following major abdominal trauma-reduced septic morbidity. *J Trauma* 1989;29:916
2. Kudsk KA, Croce MA, Fabian TC, et al: Enteral versus parenteral feeding: effects on septic morbidity after blunt and penetrating abdominal trauma. *Ann Surg* 1992;215:503
3. Gianotti L, Alexander JW, Nelson JL, et al: Role of early enteral feeding and acute starvation on postburn bacterial translocation and host defense: prospective, randomized trials. *Crit Care Med* 1994;22:265
4. Heyland DK, Cook DJ, Guyatt GH: Enteral nutrition in the critically ill patient: a critical review of the literature. *Intensive Care Med* 1993;19:435
5. Babineau TJ, Blackburn GL: Time to consider early gut feeding. *Crit Care Med* 1994;22:191
6. Grant JP, Snyder BA: Use of L-glutamine in total parenteral nutrition. *J Surg Res* 1988;44:506
7. Johnson LR, Copeland EM, Dudrick JT, et al: Structural and hormonal alterations in the gastrointestinal tract of parenterally fed rats. *Gastroenterology* 1975;68:1170
8. Wilmore DW, Smith RJ, O'Dwyer ST, et al: The gut: a central organ after surgical stress. *Surgery* 1988;104:917
9. Page CP: The surgeon and gut maintenance. *Am J Surg* 1989;158:485
10. Deitch EA: Multiple organ failure: pathophysiology and potential future therapy. *Ann Surg* 1992;216:117

11. Carrico J, Meakin JL: Multiple organ failure syndrome. *Arch Surg* 1986;121:196
12. Border JR, Hassett J, LaDuca j, et al: The gut origin septic states in blunt multiple trauma (ISS = 40) in the ICU. *Ann Surg* 1987;206:427
13. Marshall JC, Christou NV, Meakins JL: The gastrointestinal tract: the "undrained abscess" of multiple organ failure. *Ann Surg* 1993;218:111
14. Thibault A: Care of feeding tubes. In: Borlase BC, Bell SJ, Blackburn GL, et al (eds). *Enteral Nutrition.* New York, Chapman & Hall, 1994:197
15. Koruda MJ, Guenter P, Rombeau JL: Enteral nutrition in the critically ill. *Crit Care Clin* 1987;3:133
16. Minard G: Enteral access. *NCP* 1994;9:172
17. Nompleggi D, Teo TC, Blackburn GL, et al: Human recombinant interleukin-1 decreases gastric emptying in the rat. *Gastroenterology* 1988;94:A326
18. McClave SA, Snider HL, Lowen CC, et al: Use of residual volume as a marker for enteral feeding intolerance: prospective blinded comparison with physical examination and radiographic findings. *J Parenter Enter Nutr* 1992;16:99
19. Borlase BC, Bell SJ, Lewis EJ, et al: Tolerance to enteral tube feeding diets in hypoalbuminemic critcally ill, geriatric patients. *Surg Gynecol Obstet* 1992;174:181
20. Montecalvo MA, Steger KA, Farber HW, et al: Nutritional outcome and pneumonia in critical care patients randomized to gastric versus jejunal tube feedings. *Crit Care Med* 1992;20:1377
21. Delaney HM, Carnevale NH, Garvey JW: Jejunostomy by a needle catheter technique. *Surgery* 1973;73:786
22. Jones TN, Moore EE, Moore FA: Early postoperative feeding. In: Borlase BC, Bell SJ, Blackburn GL, et al (eds): *Enteral Nutrition.* New York, Chapman & Hall, 1994:78
23. Zaloga GP: Bedside method for placing small bowel feeding tubes in critically ill patients: a prospective study. *Chest* 1991;100:1643
24. Welch SK, Hanlon MD, Waits M, et al: Comparison of four bedside indicators used to predict duodenal feeding tube placement with radiography. *J Parenter Enter Nutr* 1994;18:525
25. Thurlow PM: Bedside enteral feeding tube placement into duodenum and jejunum. *J Parenter Enter Nutr* 1986;10:104
26. Lord LM, Weser-Maimone A, Pulhamus M, et al: Comparison of weighted vs unweighted enteral feeding tubes for efficacy of transpyloric intubation. *J Parenter Enter Nutr* 1993;17:271
27. Kittinger JW, Sandler RS, Heizer WD: Efficacy of metoclopramide as an adjunct to duodenal placement of small-bore feeding tubes: a randomized, placebo-controlled, double-blind study. *J Parenter Enter Nutr* 1987;11:33
28. Heiselman DE, Vidovich RR, Milkovich G, et al: Nasointestinal tube placement with a pH sensor feeding tube. *J Parenter Enter Nutr* 1993;17:562
29. Strong RM, Gribbon R, Durling s, et al: Enteral tube feedings utilizing a pH sensor enteral feeding tube. *Nutr Suppl Serv* 1988;8:11
30. Levenson R, Turner WW, Dyson A, et al: Do weighted nasogastric feeding tubes facilitate duodenal intubations? *J Parenter Enter Nutr* 1988;12:135
31. Whatley K, Turner WW, Dey M, et al: When does metoclopramide facilitate transpyloric intubation? *J Parenter Enter Nutr* 1984;8:679
32. Grant JP, Curtas MS, Kelvin FM: Fluoroscopic placement of nasojejunal feeding tubes with immediate feeding using a nonelemental diet. *J Parenter Enter Nutr* 1983;7:299
33. Larson DE, Burton DD, Schroeder KW, et al: Percutaneous endoscopic gastrostomy: indications, success, complications, and mortality in 314 consecutive patients. *Gastroenterology* 1987;93:48
34. Grant JP: Comparison of percutaneous endoscopic gastrostomy with Stamm gastrostomy. *Ann Surg* 1988;270:598
35. Peasarini AC, Dittler HJ: Feeding tube perforation as a complication of percutaneous endoscopic gastrostomy. *Endoscopy* 1992;24:235
36. Saltzberg DM, Anand K, Juvan P, et al: Colocutaneous fistula: an unusual complication of percutaneous endoscopic gastrostomy. *J Parenter Enter Nutr* 1987;11:86
37. Cass OW, Steinberg SE, Onstad GR: A long-term follow-up of patients with percutaneous endoscopic gastrostomy (PEG) or surgical (Stamm) gastrostomy (SG) [abstract]. *Gastrointest Endosc* 1986;32:147
38. Kirby DF, Craig RM, Tsang T-K, et al: Percutaneous endoscopic gastrostomies: a prospective evaluation and review of the literature. *J Parenter Enter Nutr* 1986;10:155
39. Lambiase RE, Dorfman GS, Cronan JJ, et al: Percutaneous alternatives in nutritional support: a radiologic perspective. *J Parenter Enter Nutr* 1988;12:513
40. Wolfsen HC, Kozarek RA, Ball TJ, et al: Tube dysfunction following percutaneous gastrostomy and jejunostomy. *Gastrointest Endosc* 1990;36:261
41. DiSario JA, Foutch PG, Sanowski RA: Poor results with percutaneous endoscopic jejunostomy. *Gastrointest Endosc* 1990;36:257
42. Henderson JM, Strodel WE, Gilinsky NH: Limitations of percutaneous endoscopic jejunostomy. *J Parenter Enter Nutr* 1993;17:546
43. Reiner DS, Leitman IM, Ward RJ: Laparoscopic Stamm gastrostomy with gastropexy. *Surg Laparosc Endosc* 1991;1:189
44. Page CP, Carlton PK, Andrassy RJ, et al: Safe, cost-effective postoperative nutrition: defined formula diet via needle catheter jejunostomy. *Am J Surg* 1979;138:939
45. Duh Q-Y, Way LW: Laparoscopic jejunostomy using T-fasteners as retractors and anchors. *Arch Surg* 1993;128:105
46. Cwikiel W: Percutaneous duodenstomy-alternative route for enteral nutrition. *Acta Radiol* 1991;32:153
47. Koolpe HA, Dorfman D, Kramer M: Translumbar duodenostomy for enteral feeding. *AJR* 1989;153:299

Critical Care, Third Edition, edited by Joseph M. Civetta,
Robert W. Taylor, and Robert R. Kirby.
Lippincott-Raven Publishers, Philadelphia, PA © 1997.

CHAPTER 40

∎

Mechanical Cardiac
Assist Devices

Thomas L. McKiernan
William H. Wehrmacher

Complacency with the old therapeutic agents, which failed to reduce the greater than 90% mortality rate when cardiogenic shock complicates myocardial infarction (MI), is no longer justifiable when several new techniques providing mechanical assistance to the heart are available. Intractable unstable angina, hemodynamic decompensation after angioplasty, prophylaxis before bypass surgery, high-risk percutaneous transluminal coronary angioplasty (PTCA) and noncardiac surgery, and acute mitral insufficiency may likewise require mechanical assistance. The problem is significant because shock may occur in as many as 10% to 15% of the 1.5 million patients sustaining heart attacks in the United States each year.

Between 1 in 70 and 1 in 100 patients who cannot be weaned from cardiopulmonary bypass despite adequate volume loading, metabolic stabilization, electronic pacing, and inotropes may need the intraaortic balloon pump (IABP).

When the IABP falls short of providing adequate assistance for the ventricle, temporary additional assistance can be provided by surgically introduced temporary ventricular assist devices (VADs), which can help the heart recover from injuries that would be irreversible with conventional therapy.

PURPOSE ∎

Although low blood pressure may be well tolerated in some situations, true shock is characterized by severe circulatory impairment, tissue hypoperfusion, and cell necrosis. Blood pressure measurements by the peripheral cuff blood pressure sphygmomanometer often are unreliable, correlating poorly with intraarterial pressure measurements in shock. True cardiogenic shock after acute MI is characterized by the following: systolic pressure less than 90 mm Hg, pulmonary artery occlusion pressure greater than 12 mm Hg, and peripheral perfusion impairment (cold, clammy, pale skin; cloudiness of thought; oliguria; and diminished cardiac index to less than 2 L/m²/minute). Ten percent to 15% of patients with acute MI are candidates for circulatory support by an IABP.

Consider that other causes of hypotension—including vasovagal reactions, pericardial tamponade, tension pneumothorax, pulmonary embolism, dissecting aortic aneurysm, and several types of shock (hemorrhagic, hypovolemic, septic, or anaphylactic)—need exclusion not only for diagnostic accuracy, but also for selection of specific therapy that is effective when appropriately applied but does not work for cardiogenic shock. The converse is true: IABP is a poor treatment for noncardiogenic shock.

Large and progressive myocardial injuries produced by ischemia lead to severe pumping inadequacy. Collateral circulation is usually inadequate, and distant ischemia further impairs left ventricular function, producing a vicious cycle. The compensatory mechanisms for one difficulty create new problems: the impaired contractility of the heart, with reduced cardiac output, leads to hypotension. Immediately, hypotension has the favorable effect of reducing the load on the impaired muscle, but it also quickly and unfavorably further impairs myocardial perfusion and increases the amount of heart in jeopardy. At the border zones, there is

609

inadequate collateral flow; and further infarction in this border area may occur, further reducing effective contraction, leading to further hypotension, shock, and, ordinarily, to death. This vicious cycle must be interrupted at every opportunity if the currently unacceptable mortality rate is to be reduced. Mechanical assist devices—the IABP and VAD—can interrupt this vicious cycle.

Myocardial assistance devices have been employed since 1962 when S.D. Moulopoulas and others from W. Kolff's laboratory in Cleveland[1] suggested intraaortic balloon pumping as a means of dealing with intractable cardiogenic shock. Among the many devices perfected in that laboratory (including hemodialysis), the IABP has been used throughout the world, and particularly since A. Kantrowitz and coworkers[2] demonstrated in 1968 that poor left ventricular indices could be positively influenced. The IABP augments diastolic blood flow, particularly to the coronary vessels, and reduces impedance to systolic ejection from the left ventricle.

Originally, the intraaortic balloons were introduced surgically through the femoral arteries by open arteriotomy; but, in 1979, introduction percutaneously around a central wire was established. This percutaneous method was rapidly improved in subsequent years. It is appropriate for use by the invasive cardiologist, the surgeon, or the critical care specialist using modified Seldinger technique and reliably prepackaged, sterilized devices (which became available after 1981, featuring dual-lumen catheters with a flexible lumen incorporated inside the catheter to be advanced over a 0.0836-cm [0.038-inch] J-tip guidewire).

The prepackaged device for percutaneous use contains detailed instruction for introduction through the femoral artery and use. The cephalic end of the balloon should be placed just below the left subclavian artery, a position that can be approximated by measuring the distance between the point of introduction to the sternal angle of Louis. Higher position risks cerebral embolization or introduction into the left subclavian artery with laceration; a lower position risks reduction in effective diastolic counterpulsation or blockage of major tributary vessels. A radiograph or other imaging method can determine whether optimal position has been achieved. Fluoroscopy with image intensification is helpful during insertion to ensure appropriate placement of the balloon—ideally between a cephalad level just distal to the exit of the left subclavian artery and a caudad level at a maximum distance above the bifurcation of the aorta (Fig. 40-1).

In special circumstances, the balloon may be introduced surgically through femoral or iliac arteries, through the left subclavian artery, or transthoracically through previous exposure of the aortic arch into the lateral wall of the ascending aorta and secured by purse-string suture.

The balloon is connected to a pneumatic pump that produces phasic changes in its helium volume, synchronized appropriately with heart beat by the patient's electrocardiogram. Rapid inflation during ventricular diastole increases aortic diastolic pressure and augments coronary perfusion pressure. The sudden deflation in systole reduces resistance to left ventricular emptying, enhancing cardiac output and reducing myocardial oxygen needs. Ordinarily, the cardiac output increases by 10% to 20%; the mean aortic pressure is unchanged, but with decreased systolic pressure and in-

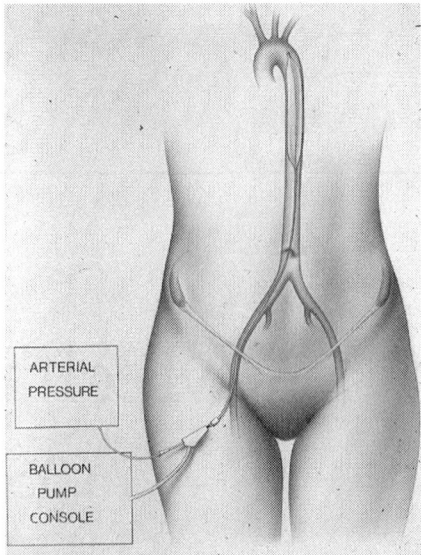

FIGURE 40-1. Balloon catheter in position in the descending thoracic aorta, distal to the left subclavian artery. (Courtesy of Datascope, Cardiac Assist Division, Fairfield, NJ.)

creased diastolic pressure; and the ventricular end-diastolic pressure decreases by 5 to 15 mm Hg.

The function of the IABP can be monitored remotely, even in the cardiologist's bedroom, with special telecommunications software such as Datascope's PC-IABP software, which was reported on and made available during the 44th Annual Scientific Session of the American College of Cardiology (ACC) held in New Orleans in March 1995.[3] The system permits faster physician response, provides nursing staff with reassurance, reduces hospital costs, affords better patient care, and minimizes potential legal liability.

INDICATIONS FOR IABP

Indications for IABP include cardiogenic shock, intractable unstable angina, impending MI, hemodynamic decompensation after angioplasty, prophylaxis before bypass surgery or before hazardous cardiac catheterization, high-risk PTCA and noncardiac surgery, weaning from cardiopulmonary bypass, refractory ventricular failure, and acute mitral insufficiency. It may be useful for treating complications of MI such as (1) left-to-right shunt from infarction of septum, and (2) papillary muscle rupture with acute mitral regurgitation while preparing for surgical correction. It is useful for intraoperative pulsatile flow generation. Although it has been recommended for ischemia resulting from intractable arrhythmia, the problems of creating adequate synchronization often are insurmountable.

CONTRAINDICATIONS FOR IABP

Contraindications for IABP include aortic regurgitation, aortic aneurysm, severe calcific disease of the aorta, and obstructed peripheral vessels. Tachyarrhythmias and irregular heart rhythms are relative contraindications. Introduction of the IABP without the use of an introducer sheath is not recommended for patients with severe obesity, scarring in the groin, or other contraindications to percutaneous insertion.

COMPLICATIONS WITH IABP

Complications that may occur with use of the IABP include damage or perforation of aortic wall, ischemia distal to insertion of the catheter, peripheral embolization, thrombosis, thrombocytopenia, and hemolysis. Ischemia distal to insertion of the catheter and thromboses are more likely to occur in small patients and in those with disease of the aortoiliac arterial system. Perforation of the balloon can be extremely hazardous: continued pumping can produce a large blood clot and require surgical removal. Membrane damage can result from sharp objects, membrane fatigue, or unusual (biaxial) folding of the balloon during use; contact with calcific plaque may abrade the surface or perforate the balloon membrane. There may be femoral thrombi requiring embolectomy; arterial occlusion; false aneurysms; aortic dissection; paraplegia; infection; or improper placement of the balloon with occlusion of mesenteric, renal, or internal mammary arteries. Complications are infrequently encountered, however.

SYNCHRONIZED CORONARY VENOUS RETROPERFUSION

Synchronized coronary venous retroperfusion has received little attention, despite the extensive and expanding experience of the research group of Elliot Corday and Samuel Meerbaum during the last 20 years.[4] Diastolic-augmented coronary venous retroperfusion with arterial blood provided significant but not complete restoration of function in ischemic segments in animal studies of 75 minutes of left anterior descending coronary artery occlusion. In 1991, Kar and others[5] reported both the efficacy and the safety of synchronized coronary venous reperfusion among 30 patients undergoing angioplasty. In 1994, Freedman and coworkers[6] from St. Frances Cabrini Hospital in Alexandria, Louisiana, reported combined retroperfusion with intraaortic balloon counterpulsation for three patients with severe cardiogenic shock. All three were temporarily improved and stabilized, and long-term survival was seen in two of the patients. Coronary venous retroperfusion deserves more consideration than it has received among the cardiologic community.

VENTRICULAR ASSIST DEVICES

Temporary ventricular support by an electrically or pneumatically driven pump allows the heart to recover from injuries that would otherwise be irreversible by conventional therapy. Consideration and employment of less invasive procedures, including the IABP, should first be employed if reasonably adequate. Suitable candidates for VADs include (1) patients in cardiogenic shock after MI, (2) patients with potentially reversible metabolic cause (e.g., digitalis intoxication, hyperkalemia) for cardiac failure, (3) patients who cannot be weaned from cardiopulmonary bypass after otherwise successful cardiac surgery, and (4) patients with many types

of low cardiac output syndrome, particularly that which develops within 48 hours after cardiac surgery.

As reported to the ACC in 1995,[3] there are 15,000 to 20,000 potential candidates for heart transplantation yearly in the United States. Only *2000* donor hearts become available each year. Almost half of the candidates die while awaiting transplantation. For them, VADs can provide a better chance of surviving long enough to get one of the precious transplants. Furthermore, many other patients could benefit from VADs, although the devices do not meet current requirements of the Food and Drug Administration (FDA) to receive financial support, except in an investigational environment.

VADs should reduce ventricular preload and afterload, reduce ventricular wall stress, augment myocardial oxygen delivery, and maintain physiologic systemic cardiac output more effectively than the IABP and inotropic drugs. By supporting the failing ventricle for hours or days, one seeks to overcome problems with an ischemic (not yet infarcted) ventricle, limit the magnitude of the infarct, and arrest the vicious cycle of low cardiac output, ischemia, lower output cycling, and eventual death.

The VAD is being developed further while extension of its indications are being sought. This development has been slow since the first left ventricular bypass device was introduced at Baylor College of Medicine (Waco, Texas) in 1963; that device was donated to the Smithsonian Institute in 1964.[7] Reporting to the ACC in New Orleans in 1995,[3] Dr. Glenn Pennington of St. Louis considered it more appropriate to make the decision as to whether to provide biventricular support or univentricular support at the outset. He said that chances of survival were better if the decision was better made in the operating room rather than 14 to 24 hours later. He pointed out that the right ventricle ordinarily recovers more quickly than the left, and this recovery may require removal of the right ventricular device to prevent clotting within the patient's own right ventricle. Ordinarily, late right ventricular dysfunction could be treated effectively with drugs. Dr. Pennington left the group with the unanswered question as to whether one should put the biventricular device into place for all patients; however, his consideration of the differences in complications and costs provided a conundrum that could not be answered.[3]

Also, in a report to the ACC in 1995, Jack C. Copeland[3] of the Arizona Health Science Center in Tucson followed Dr. Pennington to report current and future trends in support devices, including interactions with the FDA. He emphasized that we have finally reached a situation where patients with VADs can leave the hospital. This possibility helps to control the otherwise almost overwhelming costs. It is not, as he says, the cost of the device, but rather the costs of hospitalization, around $3000 per day, that stand in the way of wider use of VADs. He calls them a "great weapon" to treat end-stage congestive heart failure. He called on the profession to exert pressure on the FDA to "make them realize how *important* and *urgent* it is that we get on with permanent implantation of these devices." He indicated that the FDA so far only allows their use as a "bridge to transplantation," but that the total artificial heart (TAH) should be made available for treatment of end-stage heart failure soon. He said that the Novocor totally implantable system, currently not approved by the FDA, has the greater applicability for permanent implantation as a *TAH* for end-stage heart failure. Funds, he lamented, are unfortunately being cut back at this time when success seems to have become so close at hand. Furthermore, he pointed out that any change of even a single component in the system brings restrictive legal requirements to duplicate all of the preliminary work before adding the new component to a device under development—a restriction that has not similarly retarded applications in Europe.

Other uses also were reported to the assembly: (1) for dilated cardiomyopathy by Johannes Muller and coworkers from the German Heart Institute in Berlin; (2) for acute fulminate myocarditis by Takahito Sone from Ogaki, Japan; (3) for cardiogenic shock by Paul A. Overlie and coworkers from Methodist/St. Mary Hospitals, Lubbock, Texas; (4) as assisted circulatory support for complicated multivessel angioplasty in cardiogenic shock by Fayaz A. Shawl and coworkers from Takoma Park, Maryland; (5) for elective coronary intervention by Erminia M. Guarneri and coworkers from the Scripps Clinic in LaJolla, California; and (6) for heart failure by Stuart D. Katz, Howard Levin and Milton Packer from Columbia University in New York City. Valluvan Jeevanandam and coworkers from Temple University in Philadelphia suggested the use of the biocompatible mechanical left ventricular support device as a potential alternative to transplantation, stating that it "improves hemodynamics and can bridge patients in preimplant cardiogenic shock to transplantation . . . [and] as the donor shortage continues . . . [it] may provide an alternative to cardiac transplantation."

Implanted into the upper abdomen, chest, or elsewhere, a VAD ordinarily is used to assist the left ventricle, connected by large cannulas, and to deliver blood into the aorta. The VAD is coordinated with ventricular contraction to optimize both the function of the heart and the device. Inside its rigid casing, an electrically powered mechanism squeezes a plastic blood sac between two plates. The direction of blood movement is controlled by two valves of the same type as used for implantation into the heart. Electric power is transmitted through the skin (in a transformer-like arrangement in Novocor's design) to charge an internal rechargeable battery that continues to operate for 20 to 30 minutes for emergency use or during bathing. External rechargeable batteries are carried on a belt and can provide power for 6 to 8 hours. A volume compensator or compliance chamber is implanted to accommodate air displacement of each filling stroke of the pump.

Loyola University Stritch School of Medicine (Maywood, Illinois) began using the Jarvik-7 TAH and the Symbion VAD as bridges to transplantation because of the substantial numbers of potential recipients dying while awaiting a donor organ (25 patients between 1984 and 1987) and because of published results: 15 TAHs and three VADs were used as bridges to transplantation in October 1990. The average support was 10 days (range, 1 to 34 days). The investigators concluded that "the TAH and VAD are excellent mechanical bridges to transplantation."[8]

On January 11, 1980, the FDA withdrew its approval for its clinical use; but in January 1991, National Heart Lung and Blood Institute (NHLBI) funding for work on the TAH was restored. The "HeartMate," developed by Thermo Cardiosystems in Woburn, Massachusetts, was designed for temporary use in patients awaiting transplantation. It is completely portable, and has unique textured blood contacting surfaces to prevent thrombosis and a special access device intended to reduce the likelihood of infection around the electrical leads from the battery power for the device. The FDA approved the first heart-assist device as a bridge to heart transplantation, the HeartMate Implantable, in February 1995. It is approved for use in patients with irreversible heart failure whose death is likely to occur within 24 to 48 hours. Patients must be on their hospital's transplant list to qualify for this device.

SUMMARY ■

No longer can one remain complacent with conventional therapy under the desperate circumstances produced by cardiogenic shock. Mechanical cardiac assist devices provide substantial additional benefits when cardiogenic shock or postinfarction angina complicates MI or for intractable unstable angina, hemodynamic decompensation after angioplasty, or in high-risk PTCA. The IABP has become accepted for critical care almost everywhere, and VADs are becoming more widely employed. Ultimate selection of appropriate candidates will become more obvious as the devices are more widely employed, but many of their benefits can be seen today.

ACKNOWLEDGMENT ■

Preparation of this chapter was supported by the James DePauw Research Fund and the Bane Charitable Research Fund of Chicago.

REFERENCES ■

1. Moulopoulas SD, Ropaz SD, Kolff WJ: Diastolic balloon pumping with carbon dioxide in the aorta: a mechanical assistance to the failing circulation. *Am Heart J* 1962;63:669
2. Kantrowitz A, Tjonneland S, Freed PS, et al: Initial clinical experience with intra-aortic balloon pumping in cardiogenic shock. *JAMA* 1968;203:113
3. Wehrmacher WH: Ventricular assist devices (VADs) provide new hope for heart disease patients. *Intern Med World Rep* 1995;10:1
4. Meerbaum S, Lang TX, Osher JV, et al: Diastolic retroperfusion of acutely ischemic myocardium. *Am J Cardiol* 1976;37:588
5. Kar S, Drury JK, Hajduczki I, et al: Synchronized coronary venous retroperfusion for support and salvage of ischemic myocardium during elective and failed angioplasty. *J Am Coll Cardiol* 1991;18:271
6. Freedman RJ Jr, Laorda DM, O'Neill WW: Combined intraaortic balloon counterpulsation with synchronized retroperfusion: the United States experience. *Cathet Cardiovasc Diagn* 1994; 33:362
7. Hall CW: When did artificial heart implants begin? *JAMA* 1988;259:1650
8. Pifarre R, Sullivan HJ, Montoya A, et al: The use of the Jarvik-7 total artificial heart and the Symbion ventricular assist device as a bridge to transplantation. *Surgery* 1990;108:681

Critical Care, Third Edition, edited by Joseph M. Civetta,
Robert W. Taylor, and Robert R. Kirby.
Lippincott-Raven Publishers, Philadelphia, PA © 1997.

CHAPTER 41

Antithrombotic and Thrombolytic Therapy

Steven J. Trottier

IMMEDIATE CONCERNS

MAJOR PROBLEMS

Antithrombotic and thrombolytic agents are commonly administered in the intensive care unit, and over the last decade, major advances involving these agents have transpired. The Antiplatelet Trialists' Collaboration documented a statistically significant decrease in vascular events and mortality in selected groups of patients receiving aspirin.

STRESS POINTS

1. The administration of heparin to patients with venous thromboembolic disease should be guided by the recently developed heparin nomogram.
2. The international normalized ratio (INR) has standardized the monitoring of oral anticoagulation.
3. The development of low molecular weight heparin (LMWH) may revolutionize the treatment of thrombotic and embolic disorders.
4. Several prospective randomized trials document a decreased incidence of stroke in patients with nonvalvular atrial fibrillation receiving oral anticoagulation.
5. Thrombolytic trials involving acute myocardial infarction document improved survival of patients receiving thrombolytic agents.
6. This chapter highlights these advances and provides practical guidelines for the administration of antithrombotic and thrombolytic therapy.

ANTIPLATELET THERAPY

ASPIRIN

Aspirin has been in clinical use for over 200 years. The mechanism of action and pharmacodynamics of aspirin have been recently reviewed.[1] This section focuses on the antiplatelet rather than the antiinflammatory or antipyretic properties of aspirin, although these actions may be interrelated. The antiplatelet action of aspirin is mediated by the irreversible inhibition of platelet cyclooxygenase (prostaglandin G/H synthetase). Platelet cyclooxygenase converts arachidonate to prostaglandin G_2, and ultimately, thromboxane A_2 and prostaglandin H_2 are produced. Thromboxane A_2 is a potent inducer of irreversible platelet aggregation.[2] Furthermore, aspirin reduces eicosinoid production (prostaglandin E_2, prostacyclin, and thromboxane A_2) in different tissues, accounting for a variety of pharmacologic effects.

The therapeutic and toxic effects of aspirin are mediated by these actions. A single dose of 162 to 325 mg of aspirin completely inhibits platelet cyclooxygenase. Subsequent doses of 70 to 325 mg/day (medium dose) provide complete and continued suppression of platelet cyclooxygenase. Higher doses of aspirin do not confer enhanced antiplatelet activity but may translate into increased toxicity. When aspirin is administered as an antiplatelet agent, the gastrointestinal tract, kidneys, and coagulation system are the main targets of toxicity. Gastrointestinal distress seems to be related to dose, duration, and preparation. In non–critically ill patients, aspirin doses of 75 mg/day do not increase the frequency of gastrointestinal distress compared with placebo, but doses of greater than 325 mg/day may increase the frequency of gastrointestinal bleeding.[3,4] Unlike most nonsteroidal antiinflammatory agents, aspirin only weakly affects renal prostaglandin production. Unfortunately, the gastrointestinal or renal effects of medium-dose aspirin in critically ill patients has not been fully evaluated. Gastrointestinal prophylaxis for stress ulceration should be considered in high-risk patients receiving aspirin. Aspirin renders the hemostatic action of platelets ineffective. Aspirin should be discontinued and a bleeding time should be ordered in patients sustaining a clinically significant hemorrhage. Normalization of a prolonged bleeding time secondary to aspirin may take 5 to 10 days after the discontinuation of aspirin.[5] If the situation warrants immediate normalization of platelet function, then platelet transfusions is required. Although aspirin is usually administered by using the upper gastrointestinal tract, critically ill patients frequently experience gastroparesis or ileus and thus may require a suppository form of aspirin.

Clinical recommendations regarding aspirin therapy for patients at high risk for occlusive vascular disease and vascular events (nonfatal myocardial infarction, nonfatal stroke, or vascular death) have been made by the Antiplatelet Trialists' Collaboration.[6,7] This metaanalysis found a statistically significant reduction of vascular events in all categories evaluated. The data revealed a reduction of nonfatal myocardial infarction by one third, nonfatal stroke by one third, and vascular death by one sixth (Table 41-1). If tolerated, patients at high risk for occlusive vascular disease and vascular events should receive medium-dose aspirin therapy indefinitely.

Currently, aspirin is not recommended for venous thromboembolism prophylaxis.[8] A recently completed metaanalysis evaluating aspirin as a prophylactic agent against deep vein thrombosis found a statistically significant reduction of deep vein thrombosis in patients receiving aspirin versus placebo.[9] Overall, aspirin is less effective than standard venous thromboembolism prophylaxis (subcutaneous heparin,

pneumatic compression stockings, or warfarin), yet further evaluation of this agent is warranted.

Critical care physicians must assure that patients presenting with an acute myocardial infarction or unstable angina receive immediate (162 mg or more) and continued (75 mg/day or more) aspirin therapy. The administration of aspirin reduces mortality by 25% in patients sustaining acute myocardial infarctions (Fig. 41-1). In addition, long-term aspirin therapy should be administered to the patient groups listed in Table 41-1.

TICLOPIDINE

Clinical trials have documented the beneficial antiplatelet effects of ticlopidine. Ticlopidine, a thienopryidine, irreversibly interferes with adenosine diphosphate–mediated platelet activation and thus prevents platelet aggregation and clot retraction.[10] Unlike aspirin, the thienopryidines do not affect arachidonic acid metabolism in platelets or prostacyclin metabolism in the vasculature. Maximal platelet inhibition occurs at 3 to 5 days after initiating ticlopidine and dissipates within a week after discontinuing the drug. The side effects are reversible and include rash, diarrhea, and neutropenia (1%). Neutropenia typically occurs during the first 3 months of therapy; therefore, close monitoring of the white blood cell count is strongly recommended during this time. Two large clinical trials have documented the effectiveness of ticlopidine as a secondary stroke prevention agent in patients with recent stroke or transient ischemic event.[11,12] Furthermore, data demonstrate that ticlopidine is an effective agent for patients with unstable angina, coronary artery bypass grafting, and peripheral vascular disease.[13–15] Currently, ticlopidine should not be administered as a first-line antiplatelet agent but should be reserved for patients intolerant of aspirin. The enteral dose of ticlopidine is 250 mg twice a day. Clopidogrel, a successor drug to ticlopidine, is currently under investigation.

TABLE 41-1. Antiplatelet Therapy

CATEGORY	PATIENTS	VASCULAR EVENT°	
		Aspirin[†] *(%)*	*Control (%)*
AMI	20,000	10	14
History of AMI	20,000	13	17
Stroke–TIA	10,000	18	22
Unstable angina	4000	9	14
Relevant medical history[‡]	16,000	6	8

AMI, acute myocardial infarction; TIA, transient ischemic attack.
°Vascular death, myocardial infarction, stroke.
[†]All values $2p < 0.00001$.
[‡]Stable angina, vascular surgery, angioplasty, atrial fibrillation, valvular disease, peripheral vascular disease.

From Antiplatelet Trialists' Collaboration: Collaborative overview of randomized trials of antiplatelet therapy. I. Prevention of death, myocardial infarction, and stroke by prolonged antiplatelet therapy in various categories of patients. *Br Med J* 1994;308:81.

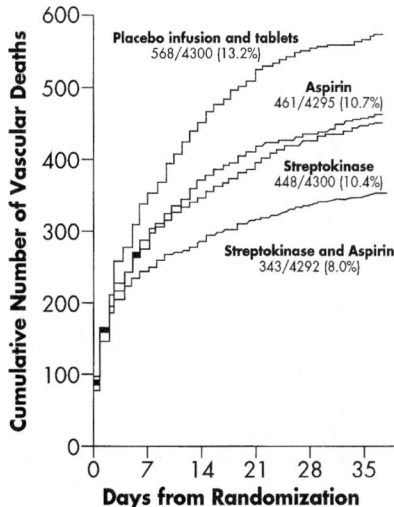

FIGURE 41-1. The administration of aspirin or streptokinase to patients with an acute myocardial infarction reduces the mortality rate by 25%, and the combination of aspirin and streptokinase reduces the mortality rate by 42%. (From ISIS-2 [Second International Study of Infarct Survival] Collaborative Group: Randomised trial of intravenous streptokinase, oral aspirin, both, or neither among 17,187 cases of suspected acute myocardial infarction: ISIS-2. *Lancet* 1988;ii:349.)

OTHER AGENTS

Monoclonal antibody to platelet glycoprotein IIb/IIIa receptor has been recently reviewed.[16] The glycoprotein IIb/IIIa receptor appears to be the final common pathway of platelet aggregation, irrespective of the platelet stimulus. Preliminary data from coronary trials suggest that the monoclonal antibody to glycoprotein IIb/IIIa is an effective antiplatelet agent in patients with unstable angina or myocardial infarction or who are undergoing angioplasty.[17–19] A chimeric monoclonal antibody to glycoprotein IIb/IIIa receptor, abciximab or c7E3, was recently approved by the Food and Drug Administration. On review of the reported clinical trials, data do not support the use of dipyridamole as an antiplatelet agent.[20] Dextran, a synthetic glucose polymer, decreases platelet aggregation and the release of platelet granules. Clinically, dextran is an effective agent for deep vein thrombosis prophylaxis.[21]

ANTITHROMBOTIC THERAPY ■

HEPARIN

Heparin has been in clinical use for over 50 years and is a ubiquitous agent in the intensive care unit. Heparin has been administered therapeutically to patients with embolic or thrombotic disorders and more recently for venous thromboembolism prophylaxis. Derived from bovine or porcine sources, this glycosaminoglycan may be administered intravenously or subcutaneously. Once in the circulation, a unique pentasaccharide sequence of heparin binds to anti-

thrombin III, forming a complex that inactivates clotting factors (II, IX, X, XI, and XII).[22] The metabolism of heparin is variable and incompletely understood. Heparin binds to macrophages, endothelial cells, and a variety of proteins including von Willebrand factor, vitronectin, fibronectin, and histidine-rich glycoprotein. Heparin is inactivated by platelet factor 4, partially excreted renally, and partially metabolized by the reticuloendothelial system. The half-life of heparin is approximately 60 to 90 minutes.[23]

The activated partial thromboplastin time (APTT) is used to measure the anticoagulant effect of heparin. The commonly recommended therapeutic range is an APTT ratio of 1.5 to 2.5 times the control value, which should correspond to a heparin blood level of 0.2 to 0.4 U/mL.[24] Routine determination of heparin levels by protamine titration is impractical, and thus the APTT is used clinically. However, individual thromboplastin reagents used to perform the APTT vary widely in their response to heparin. That is, a therapeutic APTT (1.5 to 2.0 times control) may not correlate with a heparin blood level of 0.2 to 0.4 U/mL for a given reagent unless the reagent is properly standardized. To properly standardize a given thromboplastin reagent, individual laboratories must establish that a therapeutic APTT correlates to a heparin blood value of 0.2 to 0.4 U/mL by the protamine titration assay.[25] The APTT provides a meaningful guide to anticoagulation only when properly standardized.

Complications of heparin therapy are well defined and include hemorrhage, thrombocytopenia, osteoporosis, hypoaldosteronism, elevated transaminases, and allergic reactions.[26–29] Advancing age, risk factors for bleeding, and co-morbid conditions such as hepatic or renal failure predispose patients to hemorrhagic events while receiving heparin. The average risk for major bleeding has been estimated to be 0.8% per day of therapeutic anticoagulation. Diagnostic evaluation of gastrointestinal bleeding or gross hematuria should be considered because one third of cases are caused by a previously unknown lesion.[26] In the case of life-threatening hemorrhage, heparin anticoagulation may be reversed with protamine sulfate. Approximately 1 mg of protamine sulfate neutralizes 100 U of heparin in the plasma. Protamine sulfate should be infused slowly (not more than 50 mg over 10 minutes); more rapid infusions may precipitate hypotension, bradycardia, dyspnea, and flushing. Rarely, anaphylaxis occurs secondary to protamine sulfate. Critically ill patients requiring heparin anticoagulation should receive gastrointestinal prophylaxis for stress ulceration.[30]

Approximately 5% of patients receiving heparin develop thrombocytopenia. Intravenous, subcutaneous, flush, or catheter-bound heparin may precipitate thrombocytopenia. Heparin-induced thrombocytopenia exists in two forms, idiosyncratic and nonidiosyncratic. Nonidiosyncratic heparin-induced thrombocytopenia is theoretically caused by heparin-induced platelet aggregation. Platelet counts gradually fall by 10% to 20% and subsequently return to normal despite continued heparin exposure. No therapy is required. Idiosyncratic heparin-induced thrombocytopenia, on the other hand, occurs on day 6 to 12 of heparin exposure, is immune related, and requires immediate cessation of heparin. Thrombocytopenia may develop sooner in patients previously exposed to heparin. Platelet counts should be monitored routinely during the administration of heparin. A platelet count less than 100,000/mL^3 should be treated as idiosyncratic heparin-induced thrombocytopenia. Recent data provide new insight into the pathogenesis of heparin-induced thrombocytopenia.[31] After the intravenous administration of heparin, levels of platelet factor 4 rise. Platelet factor 4 is found in the alpha granules of platelets and the surface of endothelial cells. Platelet factor 4, a heparin-binding protein, combines with heparin, and in most circumstances, this complex is of no clinical significance. Unfortunately, certain patients develop specific IgG antibodies targeting the heparin–platelet factor 4 complex. The formation of these immune complexes activates platelets, releases platelet factor 4, and results in thrombocytopenia. Excess platelet factor 4 combines with endothelial cell proteoglycans, which may ultimately result in antibody-mediated endothelial injury predisposing to thrombosis. Up to 20% of patients with idiosyncratic heparin-induced thrombocytopenia may develop paradoxical arterial or venous thrombosis. The diagnosis of heparin-induced thrombocytopenia is fraught with difficulties. Platelet-associated IgG antibody is usually elevated in patients with heparin-induced thrombocytopenia, a sensitive but nonspecific finding. The heparin-dependent release of platelet ^{14}C serotonin is a more sensitive test but not widely available. A recently developed solid-phase assay that uses complexes of heparin and platelet factor 4 as targets for the detection of heparin-induced antibodies seems promising.[31] Thus, the diagnosis of heparin-induced thrombocytopenia relies on sound clinical judgment in addition to laboratory data.

Venous Thromboembolism Prophylaxis

Essentially all patients in an intensive care unit should receive venous thromboembolism prophylaxis. Critically ill patients are inherently at moderate to high risk of developing deep vein thrombosis (Table 41-2). Compared with placebo, subcutaneous heparin (5000 U every 8 to 12 hours) effectively reduces deep vein thrombosis by 67% and pulmonary embolism by 50% in moderate- to high-risk patients.[32] Furthermore, combination prophylaxis (pharmacologic or nonpharmacologic) has been recommended for high-risk patients[33,34] (Table 41-3). Despite the vast literature supporting

venous thromboembolism prophylaxis, recent data documented that only 32% of patients in medical intensive care units receive adequate prophylaxis.[35] Venous thromboembolism prophylaxis decreases but does not eliminate deep vein thrombosis and pulmonary embolism; thus, a high clinical suspicion for venous thromboembolism must be maintained in critically ill patients.

Venous Thromboembolism

The method of heparin administration to patients with venous thromboembolic disease has evolved significantly. Provided that there are no contraindications to anticoagulation, patients clinically suspected of a pulmonary embolism or deep vein thrombosis should receive an intravenous heparin bolus followed by a heparin infusion. The diagnostic evaluation of patients suspected of venous thromboembolism should proceed after the institution of heparin. The "standard" approach to anticoagulation (5000-U bolus followed by 1000 U/hour) should be abandoned and replaced by a heparin-dosing nomogram. The standard approach achieved therapeutic anticoagulation in 40% of patients within the first 24 hours of therapy compared with 66% of patients treated by following a heparin-dosing nomogram.[36] Inadequately anticoagulated patients are 10 to 15 times more likely to sustain recurrent venous thromboembolism compared with patients receiving adequate anticoagulation.[24,37] Hull and coworkers[38] modified the original heparin-dosing nomogram and achieved therapeutic anticoagulation in 98% of patients during the initial 24 hours of therapy (Table 41-4). Instead of the original 1300 U/hour, 1680 U/hour were administered unless risk factors for bleeding were present. If risk factors for bleeding were present, then 1240 U/hour were initially infused. Subsequent changes in the infusion rate were directed by the original heparin nomogram (Table 41-5). Interestingly, patients receiving supratherapeutic anticoagulation (APTT ratio of 2.5 or more) had equivalent bleeding complications compared with therapeutically anticoagulated patients. Evaluation of a recently developed weight-based heparin-dosing nomogram found similar results.[39] Therapeutic heparin anticoagulation should be administered for a minimum of 5 days.[40] Provided that no invasive procedures are anticipated, oral anticoagulation can be instituted within 48 hours of heparin anticoagulation and

TABLE 41-2.   Venous Thromboembolism Risk

EVENT	LOW RISK°	MODERATE RISK†	HIGH RISK‡
Calf-vein thrombosis (%)	2.0	10–40	40–80
Proximal DVT (%)	0.4	2–8	10–20
Clinical PE (%)	0.2	1–8	5–10
Fatal PE (%)	0.002	0.1–0.4	1–5

DVT, deep vein thrombosis; PE, pulmonary embolism.
°Younger than 40 years of age, less than 30 minutes of surgery. No other risk factors.
†Older than 40 years of age, greater than 30 minutes of surgery, other risk factors.
‡Same as †: spinal cord injury, pelvic or lower extremity long bone fractures, stroke, prior DVT or PE, major orthopedic surgery, extensive malignant disease.

TABLE 41-3. Venous Thromboembolism Prophylaxis

LOW RISK	MODERATE RISK	HIGH RISK
Ambulation	Low-dose heparin°	LMWH
Elastic stockings	Intermittent pneumatic compression	Adjusted-dose heparin[‡]
	Dextran	Warfarin[‡]
		Combination therapy
		Inferior vena caval filter[§]

LMWH, low molecular weight heparin; APTT, activated partial thromboplastin time; INR, international normalized ratio.
°5000 U subcutaneously every 8 to 12 h, starting 1–2 h before surgery.
[‡]Subcutaneous heparin administered every 8 h to maintain APTT at high-normal values.
[‡]Minidose warfarin 1 mg 10–14 d before surgery, then increased to an INR = 2.0–3.0 postoperatively: moderate-dose warfarin start 5 to 10 mg the day of or after surgery aiming for INR = 2.0–3.0.
[§]Placement of an inferior vena caval filter may be considered in selected high-risk orthopedic–trauma patients in whom other forms of prophylaxis would be contraindicated or ineffective.

continued for 3 to 6 months, depending on the clinical circumstances.[41]

Cardiovascular Disorders

Patients with certain cardiovascular conditions should be treated with heparin anticoagulation, including those with acute myocardial infarction, unstable angina, non–endocarditis-related cardiac embolism, mechanical heart valves, and those who have had an angioplasty. The American College of Cardiology and the American Heart Association Task Force recommend the administration of heparin (APTT 1.5 to 2.5 times control) to patients with an acute myocardial infarction not receiving thrombolytic agents, provided that there are no contraindications to anticoagulation.[42] Patients not receiving therapeutic heparin anticoagulation should receive subcutaneous heparin (not less than 7500 U every 12 hours) for 7 days or until fully ambulatory.[43] Patients sustaining large acute anterior myocardial infarctions, severe left ventricular dysfunction, or echocardiographic evidence of mural thrombus should receive therapeutic heparin anticoagulation followed by oral anticoagulation for 3 months

TABLE 41-4. Heparin Protocol for Patients With Venous Thromboembolism

1. Initial intravenous heparin bolus: 5000 U
2. Continuous intravenous heparin infusion: Commence at 42 mL/h of 20,000 U (1680 U/h) in 500 mL of normal saline (a 24-h heparin dose of 40,320 U), except in the following patients, in whom the heparin infusion is commenced at a rate of 31 mL/h (1240 U/h; i.e., a 24-hour dose of 29,760 U):
   a. Patients who have undergone surgery within the previous 2 wk
   b. Patients with a previous history of peptic ulcer disease, gastrointestinal bleeding, or genitourinary bleeding
   c. Patients with recent stroke (i.e., thrombotic stroke within 2 wk previously)
   d. Patients with a plate count <150,000/mm³
   e. Patients with miscellaneous reasons for a high risk of bleeding (e.g., invasive line, hepatic failure)
3. APTT is performed in all patients as outlined below:
   a. 4 h after commencing heparin; the heparin dose is then adjusted according to the nomogram shown in Table 41-5
   b. 4–6 h after implementing the first dosage adjustment
   c. APTT is then performed as indicated by the nomogram (Table 41-5) for the first 24 h of therapy
   d. Thereafter, APTT is performed once daily, unless the patient is subtherapeutic, in which case APTT should be repeated 4 h after increasing the heparin dose

APTT, activated partial thromboplastin time.
Modified from Hull R, Raskob G, Rosenbloom D, et al: Optimal therapeutic level of heparin therapy in patients with venous thrombosis. *Arch Intern Med* 1992;152:1589.

TABLE 41-5. Heparin Nomogram for Patients With Venous Thromboembolism°

APTT (s)	IV INFUSION		ADDITIONAL ACTION
	Rate Change (mL/h)	*Dose Change (U/24 h)*	
≤45	+6	+5760	Rebolus with 5,000 U, Repeat APTT in 4–6 h
46–54	+3	+2880	Repeat APTT in 4–6 h
55–85	0	0	None
86–110	−3	−2880	Stop heparin for 1 h; repeat APTT 4–6 h after restarting heparin
>110	−6	−5760	Stop heparin for 1 h; repeat APTT 4–6 h after restarting heparin

IV, intravenous; APTT, activated partial thromboplastin time.
°Using Actin-FS APTT reagent (Dade, Mississauga, Ontario). Heparin concentration 20,000 U in 500 mL (40 units/mL). During the first 24 h, repeat APTT in 4–6 hours; thereafter, the APTT is done once daily, unless subtherapeutic.

From Hull R, Raskob G, Rosenbloom D, et al: Optimal therapeutic level of heparin therapy in patients with venous thrombosis. *Arch Intern Med* 1992;152:1589.

and then be reevaluated for the need of continued anticoagulation.[44]

The current practice in the United States is to administer intravenous heparin and oral aspirin as adjuvants to thrombolytic therapy to patients with acute myocardial infarction.[45] Early and maintained patency of the infarct-related artery may confer improved survival for patients with acute myocardial infarctions.[46,47] Intravenous heparin seems to improve the patency rate of the infarct related artery when tissue plasminogen activator is administered compared with streptokinase.[48] In addition, data show that the simultaneous administration of aspirin, heparin, and a thrombolytic agent may result in increased bleeding complications.[49] The clinician faces difficult decisions based on these complex data. The current recommendations include the administration of therapeutic heparin anticoagulation (APTT 1.5 to 2.5 times control value) concomitantly with tissue plasminogen activator. In uncomplicated cases, heparin anticoagulation is continued for 24 to 48 hours after thrombolysis. The concomitant administration of intravenous heparin to patients receiving streptokinase for an acute myocardial infarction is not supported in the literature and cannot be recommended.[50] Standard venous thromboembolism prophylaxis should be administered after a streptokinase infusion. Questions regarding the optimal agent, route, dose, risks, and benefits of concomitant antithrombin therapy for acute myocardial infarction patients receiving aspirin and a thrombolytic agent warrant further evaluation.

If tolerated, patients diagnosed with unstable angina should receive therapeutic heparin anticoagulation and aspirin therapy. Data evaluating the administration of each agent to patients with unstable angina reveal a reduction in recurrent ischemic events.[51,52]

Patients undergoing angioplasty of a coronary, renal, or peripheral artery should receive aspirin and therapeutic heparin anticoagulation.[53-55] Heparin is usually discontinued 12 to 24 hours after angioplasty and, if indicated, aspirin is continued indefinitely. Complicated angioplasty cases may require a longer course of heparin.

Patients sustaining non–endocarditis-related cardiac embolism should receive heparin followed by oral anticoagulation.[56] Before initiating anticoagulation, imaging the central nervous system is mandatory to exclude an intracerebral hemorrhage in patients suspected of cardiac emboli. Heparin anticoagulation has been administered for the prophylaxis of cardiac emboli in patients with mechanical heart valves undergoing surgery.[57] Oral anticoagulation is discontinued 1 to 5 days before surgery, and when the INR becomes subtherapeutic, heparin is started to maintain anticoagulation. Two hours before surgery, heparin is discontinued. Depending on the clinical circumstances, heparin is resumed 12 to 48 hours postoperatively followed by oral anticoagulation.

Central Nervous System Disorders

The data evaluating heparin administration to patients diagnosed with transient ischemic attacks, acute completed strokes, or evolving strokes are controversial and conflicting. The American Heart Association recently approved guidelines for the management of patients diagnosed with transient ischemic attacks and acute strokes.[55,58] Heparin anticoagulation was not routinely recommended for patients with a single transient ischemic attack or an ischemic stroke, acutely or as long-term therapy. Because of insufficient data regarding the use of heparin in patients with a single transient ischemic attack or an acute ischemic stroke, no recommendations were offered. The committee stated that the use of heparin in these patients remains a matter of physician preference with the understanding that neurologic outcome may not be altered. In 1989, a survey of randomly selected neurologists in the United States documented that 22% of responders administered heparin to patients with an acute ischemic stroke.[59] The ongoing International Stroke Trial may provide data on which to base decisions regarding heparin therapy in acute ischemic stroke.

Patients diagnosed with a transient ischemic attack who display continued symptoms despite antiplatelet therapy should be considered as candidates for heparin anticoagulation. In addition, heparin anticoagulation should be considered in patients with central nervous system ischemia secondary to occlusive disease of the vertebral basilar system.

Patients sustaining acute cardioembolic ischemic strokes should receive anticoagulation, provided that the embolism is not secondary to infective endocarditis. Regardless of therapy, single or multiple transient ischemic attacks in the presence of high-grade ipsilateral carotid artery stenosis (70% or more) is an indication for carotid endarterectomy.[60]

Before administering anticoagulation to patients with signs of focal cerebral ischemia, an imaging procedure to exclude intracranial hemorrhage is mandatory. Data describing the hemorrhagic transformation of ischemic strokes from anticoagulation are difficult to secure. Large ischemic strokes, uncontrolled hypertension, and excessive anticoagulation seem to increase the risk of hemorrhagic transformation.[61] Seizure activity or acute neurologic change in a patient receiving anticoagulation should prompt an evaluation to exclude intracranial hemorrhage.

Miscellaneous Disorders

Coagulation disorders are commonly encountered in the intensive care unit. The management of disseminated intravascular coagulation is complex, and the use of subcutaneous or intravenous heparin remains controversial.[62] Intensive care unit patients frequently require central venous catheterization. Unfortunately, catheter-related deep vein thrombosis is not prevented by heparin flush, subcutaneous heparin, low-dose or full-dose heparin infusions, or heparin-bound catheters.[63–66] Recent data demonstrated a decreased incidence of catheter-related deep vein thrombosis with the use of low-dose warfarin (1 mg/day) in cancer patients with chronic indwelling catheters.[67] Whether these data apply to intensive care unit patients with short- or long-term intravenous catheters is unknown.

LOW MOLECULAR WEIGHT HEPARIN

Low molecular weight heparin (LMWH) is derived from standard unfractionated heparin by an enzymatic process. The average molecular weight of standard unfractionated heparin is 15,000 daltons (d) compared with 4500 d for LMWH. Similar to standard unfractionated heparin, LMWH complexes with antithrombin III to inactivate clotting factors. Standard unfractionated heparin–antithrombin III complex inactivates activated factor X (factor Xa) and thrombin (factor IIa) in an equimolar basis. Inactivation of factor IIa requires the formation of a tertiary complex between the heparin–antithrombin III complex and factor IIa (Fig. 41-2). Heparin molecules larger than 18 saccharide units are necessary to form the tertiary complex. Only a few

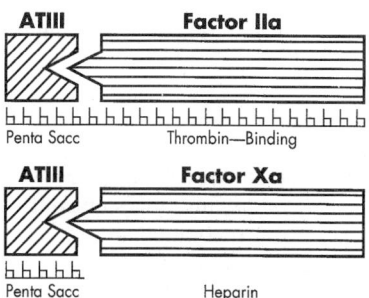

FIGURE 41-2. Heparin–antithrombin III complex. Penta Sacc, pentasaccharide sequence. (From Hirsh J: From bench to bedside: history of development of LMWH. *Pharmacol Ther* 1994;19:40S.)

LMWH molecules are larger than 18 saccharide units, and thus, the inactivation of factor IIa by LMWH is minimal compared with standard unfractionated heparin. The antifactor Xa activity correlates with the antithrombotic property of the heparin preparation, whereas the antifactor IIa activity is related to bleeding complications. Therefore, an equivalent antithrombotic dose of LMWH compared with unfractionated heparin should theoretically be associated with less bleeding complications.[68–69] Unfortunately, clinical trials have demonstrated equal bleeding complications between LMWH and standard heparin. An antifactor Xa activity level of 0.35 to 0.7 U/mL provides therapeutic anticoagulation. Measuring an antifactor Xa activity level is unnecessary because of the excellent bioavailability and predictable levels of LMWH. The anticoagulant effect of LMWH results mainly from the inactivation of factor Xa and, therefore, the APTT is seldom prolonged and does not require monitoring. LMWH has a prolonged half-life and can be subcutaneously dosed once or twice daily. Compared with standard heparin, LMWH causes less platelet aggregation, less vascular permeability changes, and equivalent hemorrhagic complications.[70] The anticoagulant effect of LMWH cannot be reversed by protamine sulfate because the smaller heparin molecules are not bound and inactivated by protamine. The safety of LMWH during pregnancy and the risk of osteoporosis during chronic administration requires further evaluation. Although heparin-induced thrombocytopenia may occur with the administration of LMWH, recent data found a lower incidence of thrombocytopenia secondary to LMWH compared with standard unfractionated heparin.[71]

Several studies have documented that LMWH is equally efficacious compared with standard heparin for venous thromboembolism prophylaxis.[72] Two recent metaanalyses reviewed the randomized control trials comparing LMWH versus standard unfractionated heparin for the treatment of deep vein thrombosis.[73,74] Mortality, recurrent venous thromboembolism, and major bleeding were found to be equal between LMWH and standard unfractionated heparin. Studies evaluating LMWH in patients with ischemic strokes, myocardial infarctions, and angioplasty have found favorable results. Currently, the only LMWH approved by the Food and Drug Administration for venous thromboembolism prophylaxis in patients undergoing total hip arthroplasties is exoxaparin. The recommended dose is 30 mg subcutaneously twice a day.[75]

HIRUDIN

Originally extracted from the salivary glands of the medicinal leech *Hirudo medicinalis*, hirudin is currently produced by bacteria or yeast as a recombinant protein. Hirudin is a direct tight-binding inhibitor of thrombin. Unlike heparin, hirudin does not require a cofactor (antithrombin III), is not neutralized by platelet factor 4, and produces a more predictable dose response than heparin. Hirudin may be administered subcutaneously or intravenously, has a half-life of 30 to 45 minutes, and is cleared by the kidneys.[76] Initial clinical studies have found hemorrhage to be the major complication of hirudin therapy.[77,78]

Data defining the indications, optimal route of administration, dosing, and monitoring of this antithrombin agent are forthcoming. Hirulog and the hirugens are the derivatives of hirudin currently under investigation.

WARFARIN

The oral anticoagulant most often used in the United States is warfarin. The indications, mechanism of action, and complications associated with warfarin have been recently reviewed.[79] Administered enterally, warfarin has excellent bioavailability and a predictable onset of action. The peak concentration of warfarin occurs in 90 minutes after ingestion, and the half-life is 36 to 42 hours. The anticoagulant effect of warfarin is mediated by the inhibition of vitamin K epoxide reductase and possibly vitamin K reductase. The inhibition of these enzymes limits the gamma-carboxylation of the vitamin K–dependent coagulation factors (II, VII, IX, and X). Subsequently, hepatic production and secretion of partially carboxylated coagulation factors with limited coagulant activity occur. The anticoagulant effect of warfarin may be detected within 6 hours of ingestion and results primarily from decreased factor VII levels. Factor VII is the coagulant factor with the shortest half-life (approximately 6 hours). The peak anticoagulant effect of warfarin is delayed for 72 to 96 hours. Anticoagulant proteins C and S are also vitamin K–dependent factors with half-lives similar to factor VII. Large initial doses of warfarin (more than 10 mg) may potentially result in a procoagulant milieux because of decreased levels of protein C and protein S early on, relative to the coagulation factors. Concomitant heparin administration or smaller initial doses of warfarin may avoid this theoretic procoagulant state.[80]

The effective administration of warfarin to complex intensive care unit patients is influenced by multiple factors. Gastrointestinal function and integrity are frequently altered in critical illness, which may cause erratic absorption of warfarin. The tube feeding, administered concomitantly with warfarin, may bind the warfarin and usually contains vitamin K, resulting in a decreased anticoagulant effect.[81] Critically ill patients frequently receive multiple drugs, including antibiotics, antifungals, or anticonvulsants, which may alter the anticoagulant effect of warfarin (Table 41-6). When multiple factors influence the anticoagulant effect of warfarin, the

temporary administration of intravenous heparin may be more prudent.

Monitoring the anticoagulant effect of warfarin has been standardized by the INR:

$$INR = \left(\frac{Patient\ prothrombin\ time}{Control\ prothrombin\ time} \right)^{ISI}$$

where ISI represents the international sensitivity index for the thromboplastin reagent used to perform the prothrombin time. The ISI is a measure of responsiveness of a given thromboplastin reagent to the reduction of vitamin K–dependent factors compared with an international reference preparation (IRP). The IRP (human brain thromboplastin) has an ISI value of 1.0. To provide greater precision in prothrombin time testing, thromboplastin reagents with low ISI values (1.0 to 1.2) are preferred. The therapeutic INR of warfarin is 2.0 to 3.0 except for mechanical prosthetic heart valves, which is 2.5 to 3.5. The INR is the best available method to monitor warfarin anticoagulation.[82]

The major complications of warfarin therapy are hemorrhage and warfarin-induced skin necrosis. The average risk for major bleeding during warfarin therapy is approximately 3% per year. During the first month of warfarin therapy, the risk for bleeding is tenfold higher than it is after the first year of therapy. Age, comorbid conditions, and intensity of anticoagulation are patient-specific risk factors for bleeding. Patients sustaining gross hematuria or gastrointestinal bleeding while receiving warfarin anticoagulation should undergo a diagnostic evaluation because one third of these patients will have an underlying lesion responsible for the hemorrhage.[26] Critically ill patients receiving warfarin anticoagulation should receive stress ulcer prophylaxis.[30] Warfarin-induced skin necrosis is fortunately an uncommon occurrence. In 3 to 8 days after the initiation of warfarin anticoagulation, patients typically complain of pain in the areas of skin overlying the breast, thigh, or buttock. Subsequently, these areas devitalize and the skin sloughs. The pathogenesis is unknown but involves extensive thrombosis of small veins, venules, and capillaries. Acutely ill women, patients with protein C deficiency, and patients receiving large initial doses of warfarin (more than 10 mg) are at risk for this complication. Treatment involves the discontinuation of warfarin, administration of parenteral vitamin K, and continuation or initiation of heparin, if indicated.[83]

Venous Thromboembolism Prophylaxis

Warfarin administered to selected patients following specific recommendations is an effective mode of venous thromboembolism prophylaxis. Data support the use of warfarin in patients after hip surgery or major gynecologic surgery.[84,85] A two-step regimen has been described for patients undergoing elective hip surgery. Patients initially receive low-dose warfarin (approximately 3 mg/day) to prolong the prothrombin time 1 to 3 seconds preoperatively, and postoperatively the anticoagulation is increased to an INR of 2.0 to 3.0. Patients scheduled to undergo nonelective hip surgery should receive warfarin prophylaxis (INR 2.0 to 3.0) after surgery. Warfarin given in a fixed minidose (1 mg/day) or

TABLE 41-6. Factors Altering the Pharmacokinetics and Pharmacodynamics of Warfarin

GUT	PLASMA	LIVER		HEMOSTATIC PLUG

Anticoagulant effect potentiated
  Low vitamin K intake
  Reduced vitamin K absorption in fat malabsorption
Anticoagulant effect counteracted
  Increased vitamin K intake
  Reduced absorption of warfarin by cholestyramine
	Anticoagulant effect unchanged
	  Displacement of warfarin from albumin binding does not influence anticoagulant effect of coumarins
		Anticoagulant effect potentiated
		Drugs
		  Phenylbutazone
		  Metronidazole
		  Sulfinpyrazone
		  Trimethoprim–sulfamethoxazole
		  Disulfiram
		  Amiodarone
		  Erythromycin
		  Anabolic steroids
		  Clofibrate
		  Cimetidine
		  Omeprazole
		  Thyroxine
		  Ketoconazole
		  Fluconazole
		  Isoniazid
		  Piroxicam
		  Tamoxifen
		  Quinidine
		  Vitamin E (mega doses)
		  Phenytoin
		Liver disease
		Hypermetabolic states
		Pyrexia
		Thyrotoxicosis
			Anticoagulant effect counteracted
			Drugs
			  Barbiturates
			  Rifampin
			  Griseofulvin
			  Carbamazepine
			  Penicillin
			  Alcohol
				Impaired hemostatic plug formation
				Impaired coagulation
				  Reduced vitamin K dependent
				  Coagulation factors
				  Reduction in concentration of other coagulation factors
				  Other anticoagulants: heparin, ancrod
				Impaired platelet function
				  Thrombocytopenia
				  Aspirin
				  Other nonsteroidal antiinflammatory drugs
				  Ticlopidine
				  Moxalactam
				  Carbenicillin and high doses of other penicillins

From Hirsh J, Dalen JE, Deykin D, et al: Oral anticoagulants mechanism of action, clinical effectiveness, and optimal therapeutic range. *Chest* 1992;102:312S.

to maintain an INR of 1.5 to 2.5 has been shown to be effective in patients after major gynecologic surgery.

Venous Thromboembolism

Standard clinical practice for the treatment of venous thromboembolic disease includes immediate heparin anticoagulation followed by the institution of oral anticoagulation within 24 to 48 hours. Heparin is discontinued after a minimum of 5 days, provided that oral anticoagulation is therapeutic (INR of 2.0 to 3.0). Oral anticoagulation is continued for 3 to 6 months, depending on the clinical circumstances. Recurrent life-threatening venous thromboembolic disease or documented venous thromboembolism secondary to a hypercoagulable state mandates lifelong anticoagulation.[86]

Atrial Fibrillation

Several prospective studies investigating the safety and efficacy of oral anticoagulation for stroke prevention in patients with nonvalvular atrial fibrillation have been recently completed.[87-92] Low-intensity warfarin therapy (INR of 2.0 to 3.0) consistently reduced the incidence of stroke risk by approximately 70% (Fig. 41-3). Pooled analysis of these data found that diabetes mellitus, hypertension, transient ischemic attacks, stroke, and increasing age are independent risk factors for the development of stroke. In addition, patients with angina, myocardial infarction, or congestive heart failure had stroke rates three times higher than did patients without these factors. The risk of stroke in elderly patients (older than 75 years of age) is paralleled by the risk of intracranial hemorrhage and, therefore, careful attention to the INR in this patient group should be emphasized. Patients at risk for stroke who cannot tolerate oral anticoagulation should be placed on aspirin (325 mg/day) if possible. Patients younger than 60 years of age without the aforementioned risk factors (lone atrial fibrillation) have a low risk of stroke (less than 0.5% per year) and do not require anticoagulation.[93]

Patients undergoing elective cardioversion for atrial fibrillation of 2 days' duration or longer should receive oral anticoagulation (INR of 2.0 to 3.0) 3 weeks before and 4 weeks after cardioversion.[94] Because of the low risk of embolism, patients with atrial flutter do not require anticoagulation for elective cardioversion. Recent data suggest that cardioversion of atrial fibrillation without anticoagulation may be safe in the absence of intracardiac clot demonstrated by trans-

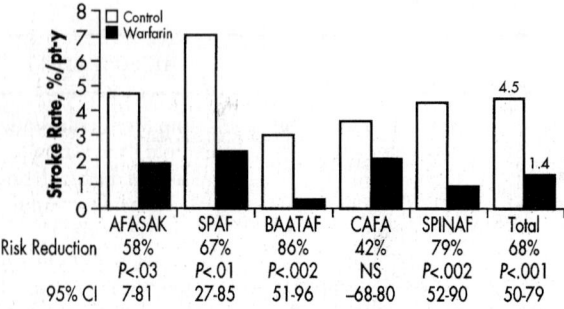

FIGURE 41-3. Risk reduction of stroke in patients with atrial fibrillation treated with warfarin versus placebo. (From Albers GW: Atrial fibrillation and stroke: three new studies, three new questions. *Arch Intern Med* 1994;154:1443.)

| TABLE 41-7. | Secondary Hypercoagulable States |

Cancer
Pregnancy
Oral contraceptives
Nephrotic syndrome
Myeloproliferative disorders
Hyperlipidemias
Diabetes mellitus
Paroxysmal nocturnal hemoglobinuria
Postoperative states
Vasculitis
Antiphospholipid syndrome
Increased levels of factor VII and fibrinogen
Anti-cancer drugs
Heparin thrombocytopenia
Obesity

From Nachman RL, Silverstein R: Hypercoaguable states. *Ann Intern Med* 1993;119:819.

esophageal echocardiography.[95] Data corroborating these findings are warranted.

Prosthetic Heart Valve

Patients receiving bioprosthetic mitral valve replacement should receive warfarin (INR 2.0 to 3.0) postoperatively for 3 months and then subsequently be placed on an enteric-coated aspirin (325 mg/day) indefinitely. Anticoagulant therapy for patients with bioprosthetic aortic valve replacement is optional. Lifetime oral anticoagulation (INR 2.5 to 3.5) is required for patients receiving mechanical heart valves.[96,97] The addition of low-dose aspirin (100 mg/day) to oral anticoagulation recently has been shown to decrease mortality in major systemic embolism in patients with mechanical heart valves and in high-risk patients with bioprosthetic heart valves. The addition of low-dose aspirin increased the risk of bleeding but was offset by the considerable benefit of decreased stroke.[98] Before formal recommendations can be made, the ultimate role of aspirin in these patients requires further study.

Myocardial Infarction

The administration of long-term oral anticoagulation after myocardial infarction remains controversial. However, patients with anterior Q wave myocardial infarction, left ventricular ejection fraction less than 40%, acute left ventricular aneurysm, or echocardiographic documentation of a mural thrombosis should receive intravenous heparin followed by oral anticoagulation.[99] The duration of oral anticoagulation depends on the clinical circumstances and should be reevaluated periodically. If oral anticoagulation is discontinued, aspirin should be instituted and continued indefinitely. The association between dilated cardiomyopathy, left ventricular thrombus, and systemic embolization is well established. Unfortunately, the lack of randomized trials prevents firm recommendations regarding anticoagulant therapy. The use of anticoagulants in this patient population should be individualized.[44]

Hypercoagulable States

The hypercoagulable state defines a group of prethrombotic clinical disorders associated with an increased risk for thrombosis. The major inherited disorders include protein C deficiency, protein S deficiency, antithrombin III deficiency, and recently described factor V resistance to the anticoagulant action of activated protein C.[100] Factor V resistance to the anticoagulant action of activated protein C seems to be the most common inherited factor predisposing patients to thrombotic events.[101] Secondary hypercoagulable states are listed in Table 41-7. Patients with an inherited or persistent secondary hypercoagulable state who sustained two or more documented spontaneous thrombotic events or a single life-threatening thrombotic event should receive oral anticoagulation indefinitely. The management of asymptomatic patients with documented hypercoagulable states remains controversial.

THROMBOLYTIC THERAPY ■

Over the last 20 years, tremendous advances relating to the clinical use of thrombolytic agents have transpired, most notably involving patients with acute myocardial infarction. The administration of thrombolytic agents is routinely performed in the intensive care unit. Individual thrombolytic agents, including their indications and complications, are discussed in the following sections.

THROMBOLYTIC AGENTS

Hemostasis may be divided into primary (vasculature and platelets) and secondary (coagulation pathways) phases that ultimately result in the formation of fibrin, providing the framework for a permanent hemostatic plug. The hemostatic process is balanced by the endogenous anticoagulants and the fibrinolytic system. When the proenzyme plasminogen is converted to the active enzyme plasmin, fibrin is lysed. Thrombolytic agents refer to a heterogeneous group of substances that convert plasminogen into plasmin. Clinically available thrombolytic agents include streptokinase, urokinase, tissue plasminogen activator, and anisoylated plasminogen streptokinase activator complex. Single-chain urokinase plasminogen activator is not yet clinically available (Table 41-8).

Streptokinase is synthesized by the beta-hemolytic streptococci of the Lancefield group C. After intravenous administration, streptokinase complexes with plasminogen in an equimolar basis, and this complex activates fibrin-bound and free plasminogen to plasmin. Although fibrin is the primary target of plasmin, degradation of fibrinogen, factor V, factor VIII, and other factors occurs. Streptokinase–plasminogen complex is the most efficient activator of free plasminogen to plasmin. Theoretically, this should cause higher rates of hemorrhagic complications compared with the more fibrin-specific activators such as tissue plasminogen activator. Clinical data have not supported this theory; in fact, the hemorrhagic complications between thrombolytic agents seems equal. Streptokinase is hepatically metabolized and has an 18- to 23-minute half-life. Streptokinase is antigenic, and postinfusion antibody production should be anticipated. Antibody titers may remain significantly elevated for 6 months. Streptokinase infusion during this period may result in a decreased clinical effect in addition to allergic reactions. Approximately 4% to 5% of patients receiving streptokinase sustained allergic reactions. Streptokinase is the least expensive thrombolytic agent available.[102]

Isolated from human melanoma cells by Collen in 1981, tissue plasminogen activator is commercially produced by recombinant technology and endogenously produce by vascular endothelial cells. Tissue plasminogen activator is nonantigenic and relatively fibrin specific regarding the activation of plasminogen to plasmin. Fibrin enhances the affinity of tissue plasminogen activator for plasminogen at the clot surface, which strikingly increases the rate of conversion of plasminogen to plasmin. Theoretically, the relative fibrin specificity of tissue plasminogen activator should translate into lower hemorrhagic complications compared with nonspecific plasminogen activators. However, clinical data have found roughly equal bleeding complications between tissue plasminogen activator and less fibrin-specific thrombolytic agents. Tissue plasminogen activator has a half-life of 3 to 4 minutes and is hepatically metabolized. Tissue plasminogen activator is the most expensive thrombolytic agent available.[103]

Anisoylated plasminogen streptokinase activator complex, a second-generation thrombolytic agent, consists of streptokinase bound to plasminogen to form an activator complex. The anisoylated form is inactive and protected from plasmin inhibitors. Once in the circulation, the inactive form becomes active by deacylation. Compared with streptokinase, anisoylated plasminogen streptokinase activator complex can be administered more swiftly and has a prolonged half-life (70 to 120 minutes). The antigenic properties of anisoylated plasminogen streptokinase activator complex are similar to streptokinase, and the cost of this agent is comparable with tissue plasminogen activator.[104]

In 1947, urokinase was isolated from human urine. Currently, urokinase is synthesized from human fetal renal tissue culture. Fibrinolysis occurs by direct nonspecific activation of plasminogen to plasmin, producing a fibrinolytic state that is less than what occurs with streptokinase. Metabolized by the liver, urokinase is nonantigenic, expensive to produce, and has a half-life of 14 to 20 minutes.

Newer thrombolytic agents such as recombinant plasminogen activator, mutant tissue plasminogen activator, and recombinant vampire bat salivary plasminogen activator are currently under investigation.[105]

TABLE 41-8. Characteristics of Thrombolytic Agents

	STREPTOKINASE	UROKINASE	TISSUE PLASMINOGEN ACTIVATOR	APSAC
Source	Group C streptocci	Recombinant human fetal kidney	Recombinant human	Group C streptocci Plasminogen, anisoylated
Molecular weight (kd)	47	35–55	63–70	131
Half-life (min)	18–23	14–20	3–4	70–120
Metabolism	Hepatic	Hepatic	Hepatic	Hepatic
Plasminogen binding	Indirect	Direct	Direct	Indirect
Fibrin specificity	Minimal	Moderate	Moderate	Minimal
Antigenicity	Yes	No	No	Yes

APSAC, anisoylated plasminogen streptokinase activator complex.

Modified from Granger CB, Califf RM, Topol EJ: Thrombolytic therapy for acute myocardial infarction. *Drugs* 1992;44:293.

Acute Myocardial Infarction

The administration of thrombolytic agents to patients with an acute myocardial infarction was recently reviewed.[106–108] The pathogenesis of acute myocardial infarction involves atherosclerotic plaque disruption, platelet deposition, and thrombus formation, resulting in an occluded artery. Intravenous thrombolysis reestablishes coronary artery patency in 50% to 80% of patients with acute myocardial infarction and decreases the infarct-related mortality by approximately 30% compared with patients treated without thrombolytic agents.[109–111] The current indications and contraindications for the administration of thrombolytic agents to patients with acute myocardial infarction are listed in Table 41-9.

The early and efficient delivery of thrombolytic agents to patients with acute myocardial infarction is the cornerstone of therapy, not necessarily the particular agent administered. Recent data demonstrated a reduction in mortality and infarct size in patients with acute myocardial infarction receiving thrombolysis within 70 minutes of symptom onset compared with patients receiving thrombolysis after this time.[112] Although early administration of thrombolytic therapy has been emphasized, patients benefit from thrombolysis

TABLE 41-9. Suggested Guidelines for Thrombolytic Therapy in Myocardial Infarction

CRITERIA	INDICATED	POSSIBLY INDICATED	CONTRAINDICATED
Duration of chest pain or discomfort	Within 12 h of onset	12–24 h with ongoing pain and ST elevation (>0.1 mV), or stuttering pattern	After 24 h
Age	No upper limit		
ECG criteria	ST elevation (>0.1 mV) in 2 or more contiguous leads LBBB or RBBB (new or old) with clinical picture of MI	Reversion of ST segments to baseline after nitroglycerin	Repeatedly normal or nonspecific tracing over at least 30 min
Congestive heart failure	No CHF Mild to moderate CHF	Pulmonary edema (direct PTCA an alternative)	Cardiogenic shock if PTCA available within 2–3 h
Recent surgery	None	Surgery more than 2 wk likely to rebleed	Surgery, organ bx within 2 wk Any intracranial operation
CPR	Defibrillation Limited CPR (<10 min)		Traumatic or prolonged CPR
Hypertension	Transiently elevated systolic (150–180); diastolic (90–110)	Transiently elevated systolic (180–210); diastolic (110–120)	Persistently elevated systolic (>180); diastolic (>110) Any systolic >210, diastolic >120
Stroke and intracranial disease	None	Nonhemorrhagic CVA >6 mo	Recent head trauma (2 mo) Intracranial neoplasm, AV malformation, aneurysm Nonhemorrhagic CVA within 6 mo
Gastrointestinal disorders	Heme-positive stool without symptoms or active bleeding; normal Hb	History of ulcers >6 mo ago	Active peptic ulcer disease Ulcerative colitis Esophageal varices, severe liver disease
Other	"Clean" jugular, femoral, or radial punctures Active menstruation	"Clean" subclavian vein punctures Chronic warfarin therapy Minor trauma within 2 wk	Pregnancy Retinal detachment or hemorrhagic retinopathy Known or suspected aortic dissection Pericarditis, endocarditis Active bleeding Major trauma within 2 wk Known coagulopathy

ECG, electrocardiogram; LBBB, left bundle branch block; RBBB, right bundle branch block; CHF, congestive heart failure; PTCA, percutaneous transluminal coronary angioplasty; CPR, cardiopulmonary resuscitation; CVA, cerebrovascular accident; MI, myocardial infarction; Hb, hemoglobin; AV, arteriovenous; bx, biopsy.

From Jafri SM, Walters BL, Borzak S: Medical therapy of acute myocardial infarction. Part I. Role of thrombolytic and antithrombotic therapy. *J Intensive Care Med* 1995;10:54.

up to 12 hours from the symptom onset of an acute myocardial infarction.[113,114]

In general, 30% to 40% of patients with acute myocardial infarction are eligible for thrombolysis, yet, approximately 10% of these hospitalized patients receive a thrombolytic agent in the United States.[115,116] The Food and Drug Administration–approved dosing of thrombolytic agents can be found in Table 41-10. The recently reported Global Utilization of Streptokinase and Tissue Plasminogen Activator for Occluded Coronary Arteries Trial demonstrated an improved survival of patients receiving recombinant tissue plasminogen activator in an accelerated dosing schedule with simultaneous aspirin and intravenous heparin administration.[48] According to the National Registry of Myocardial Infarction, recombinant tissue plasminogen activator is the most widely used thrombolytic agent for acute myocardial infarction in the United States.[45] Ten percent to 15% of patients experience reocclusion of the infarct-related coronary artery after thrombolysis. Repeat thrombolysis with tissue plasminogen activator, coronary angiography followed by percutaneous transluminal coronary angioplasty, or coronary artery bypass grafting should be considered in these patients.

The administration of adjuvant antiplatelet or antithrombotic therapy to patients receiving thrombolytic agents for acute myocardial infarction is of paramount importance. Whether or not thrombolysis is administered, all patients with acute myocardial infarction should receive immediate (162 to 325 mg) and continued aspirin (70 to 325 mg/day) therapy. Concomitant heparin anticoagulation is recommended for all acute myocardial infarction patients receiving tissue plasminogen activator. Typically, intravenous heparin is discontinued after 24 to 48 hours in patients with uncomplicated acute myocardial infarcts. According to current data, intravenous heparin anticoagulation is not recommended for acute myocardial infarction patients receiving streptokinase.[49,50] Venous thromboembolism prophylaxis should be initiated after the infusion of streptokinase. Currently, studies have failed to demonstrate benefit of thrombolysis for patients with unstable angina or non–Q wave myocardial

TABLE 41-10. Thrombolytic Agents for Myocardial Infarction

AGENT	DOSAGE
Tissue plasminogen activator	IV bolus of 15 mg followed by 0.75 mg/kg over 30 min (not to exceed 50 mg), and then 0.5 mg/kg (up to 35 mg) over the next 60 min
Streptokinase	IV infusion of 1.5 million U over 1 h
APSAC	IV infusion of 30 U over 5 min
Urokinase	IV bolus of 1 million U followed by 1 million U over 1 h

APSAC, anisoylated plasminogen streptokinase activator complex; IV, intravenous.

infarction; therefore, thrombolysis cannot be recommended for these patients.[117]

Venous Thromboembolic Disease

The Urokinase Pulmonary Embolism Trial documented increased hemorrhagic complications and equivalent mortality in patients receiving thrombolytic agents versus anticoagulation for documented pulmonary emboli.[118] Recent data challenge these results, providing renewed interest in the administration of thrombolytic agents to patients with venous thromboembolic disease.

The administration of thrombolytic agents to patients with documented deep vein thrombosis was recently reviewed.[119] Proponents of thrombolytic therapy for the treatment of deep vein thrombosis cite data demonstrating improved venous patency and preservation of valve function in patients receiving thrombolysis versus heparin. Opponents cite data demonstrating no difference in the postphlebitic syndrome in patients receiving either agent and emphasize the increased risk of hemorrhage in patients receiving thrombolysis. The characteristics of patients with deep vein thrombosis most likely to benefit from thrombolysis include an initial deep vein thrombosis with a short duration of symptoms (less than 5 days), proximal versus distal thrombus, and a nonocclusive versus occlusive thrombus. Contraindications to thrombolysis are listed in Table 41-9. The optimal dose, duration of therapy, and agent used remain to be defined. The dose and duration of streptokinase, the most widely evaluated agent, includes a loading dose of 250,000 U infused over 30 minutes followed by 100,000 U/hour for 72 hours. After the streptokinase infusion, standard anticoagulation for deep vein thrombosis is administered.

Unfortunately, there are no formal guidelines governing the administration of thrombolytic agents to patients with documented pulmonary emboli. In 1980, the National Institutes of Health Consensus Conference recommended thrombolytic therapy in patients for whom the benefits of thrombolysis outweighed the risks, specifically, in patients with at least 40% of obliteration of the pulmonary vasculature.[120] Recently, investigators have recommended that thrombolytic therapy should be given to patients with refractory hypoxemia, hemodynamic compromise, or echocardiographic evidence of right ventricular failure secondary to pulmonary embolism.[121] Administration of streptokinase, tissue plasminogen activator, or urokinase for pulmonary embolism is approved by the Food and Drug Administration; dosing recommendations are listed in Table 41-11. Infusion of the thrombolytic agent directly into the pulmonary artery has not shown to be more efficacious or safer than a peripheral infusion. In fact, this technique is associated with more bleeding complications and, therefore, cannot be recommended.[122] The reported advantages of thrombolytic therapy compared with standard anticoagulation include improved pulmonary perfusion, enhanced clot lysis, and improved right ventricular function.[123,124] Future studies will determine whether patients without hemodynamic compromise or refractory hypoxemia may benefit from thrombolysis. Standard anticoagulation for venous thrombolic disease should follow the administration of thrombolytic therapy.

TABLE 41-11. Thrombolytic Agents for Pulmonary Embolism

AGENT	DOSAGE
Tissue plasminogen activator	IV infusion of 100 mg over 2 h
Streptokinase	IV bolus of 250,000 U over 30 min followed by a maintenance dose of 100,000 U/h for 12 to 24 h
Urokinase	IV bolus of 4000 U/kg over 20 min followed by a maintenance infusion of 4000 U/kg/h for 12–24 h

IV, intravenous.

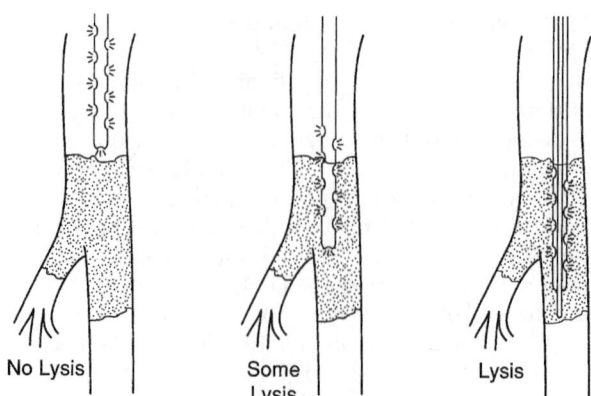

FIGURE 41-4. The catheter is placed within the substance of the thrombus, including all of the infusion holes. Lysis is rare when the infusion holes are not within the substance of the clot. A tip-occluding guidewire can be positioned to force the agent through the side holes. (From Ouriel K: Thrombolytic therapy in the management of peripheral arterial occlusion. In: Yao JS, Pearce WH (eds). *The Ischemic Extremity.* Norwalk, CT, Appleton & Lange, 1995:527.)

Peripheral Vascular Disease

Controversy surrounds the medical versus surgical management of patients with acute lower limb ischemia. Coordination of care between the vascular surgeon and interventional radiologist is essential. In selected patients, medical therapy with a thrombolytic agent effectively decreases the mortality and amputation rate of patients with acute lower limb ischemia.[55] Typically, a multiple side-hole catheter, placed in the contralateral femoral artery, is advanced to the occluded artery and embedded into the substance of the thrombus (Fig. 41-4). The thrombolytic agent most commonly infused for percutaneous intraarterial thrombolysis is urokinase. Peripheral heparin anticoagulation is administered simultaneously. The effectiveness of thrombolysis is assessed by serial angiography and clinical examinations. The critical care physician should frequently assess these patients for hemorrhagic complications, a development of postthrombolysis compartment syndrome, and the adequacy of hydration because of the need for serial angiography. Hemorrhagic complications occur in 3% of patients receiving percutaneous intraarterial thrombolysis and frequently involve the catheterization site.

Miscellaneous

Catheter and venous thrombosis are well recognized complications of indwelling central venous catheters required for chemotherapy, total parenteral nutrition, prolonged antibiotic therapy, or dialysis. The use of thrombolytic agents to restore patency of thrombosed catheters is well established. Typically, occluded catheters are filled with a predetermined volume of urokinase (5000 U/mL). The volume of urokinase required (the catheter volume) can usually be found inscribed on the catheter. After a dwell time, the thrombolytic agent is aspirated and catheter patency assessed. Care must be taken to avoid the systemic administration of the thrombolytic agent. This protocol may be repeated several times. Restoration of catheter patency is reported to be 57% to 100%.[125]

The administration of thrombolytic agents to patients with axillary subclavian vein thrombosis, superior vena caval syndrome, and mesenteric, renal, and hepatic vein thrombo-

sis has been reported, although no controlled data exist. The use of thrombolysis for patients with acute ischemic stroke remains experimental. Several prospective studies are underway evaluating the safety and efficacy of thrombolysis in patients with acute ischemic stroke.

Complications of Thrombolytic Agents

The two most common complications of thrombolysis are hemorrhage and allergic reactions. Four percent to 6% of patients receiving streptokinase or anisoylated plasminogen streptokinase activator complex experience allergic reactions. These reactions consist of fever, arthralgia, leukocytoclastic vasculitis, and occasionally renal failure. Fortunately, anaphylaxis occurs rarely (0.1% to 0.7%). Preformed streptococcal antibodies from a prior streptococcal exposure are thought to be responsible for these allergic phenomena. Pretreatment of patients with corticosteroids to prevent allergic reactions is ineffective.

Hemorrhagic complications may be divided into systemic and intracranial hemorrhage. Systemic hemorrhage is usually related to invasive procedures or preexisting disease. If patients eligible for thrombolysis are carefully screened, the incidence rate of major hemorrhage is approximately 1%. Intracranial hemorrhage occurs in 0.3% to 0.7% of patients receiving thrombolytic agents and carries a significant mortality (63%).[126] Age older than 75 years, recent stroke, uncontrolled hypertension, concomitant heparin therapy, and intracranial disease are risk factors for intracranial hemorrhage. Sudden neurologic change in a patient receiving thrombolytic therapy should be treated as intracranial bleeding. Thrombolytic therapy and anticoagulation should be discontinued, and imaging of the brain should be performed immediately. Clinical management of hemorrhage secondary to thrombolysis is described in Table 41-12.[127]

TABLE 41-12.   Management of Bleeding During Thrombolysis

MINOR BLEEDING: RELATED TO VASCULAR PUNCTURE

1. Manual compression for 15–30 min
2. Establish intravenous access
3. Draw blood for APTT, platelet count, type, and crossmatch
4. Treat as major bleeding if persistent

MAJOR BLEEDING: PERSISTENT BLEEDING OR HEMODYNAMIC COMPROMISE

1. Manual compression if possible
2. Stop thrombolytic agent, heparin, and aspirin
3. Administer protamine (standard dose: 1 mg for every 100 U of heparin received in last 4 h intravenously—not more than 50 mg over 10 min) if patient has received heparin in the past 4 h
4. Establish large-bore intravenous access and administer crystalloid
5. Transfuse packed RBCs to maintain hematocrit level of 25 mL/dL or more
6. If bleeding persists, transfuse 10 U cryoprecipitate, especially if APTT is elevated
7. If bleeding persists, transfuse 2 U fresh frozen plasma
8. If bleeding persists and bleeding time is more than 9 min, transfuse platelets
9. If bleeding persists despite the previously noted steps, consider aminocaproic acid (standard dose: 0.1 g/kg body weight given intravenously over 30–60 min, followed by a continuous infusion of 0.5–1.0 g/h)

MAJOR BLEEDING: INTRACRANIAL HEMORRHAGE

1. Follow steps 1 through 5 as just mentioned
2. Administer cryoprecipitate, fresh frozen plasma, platelets, and aminocaproic acid (standard dose as mentioned in step 9 noted previously)
3. Arrange for CT scan of head to document intracranial hemorrhage

APTT, activated partial thromboplastin time; RBCs, red blood cells; CT, computed tomography.

Modified from Sane DC, Califf RM, Topol EJ, et al: Bleeding during thrombolytic therapy for acute myocardial infarction: mechanisms and management. *Ann Intern Med* 1989;111:1010.

REFERENCES

1. Patrono C: Aspirin as an antiplaelet drug. *N Engl J Med* 1994;330:1287
2. FitzGerald GA: Mechanisms of platelet activation: thromboxane A_2 as an amplifying signal for other agonists. *Am J Cardiol* 1991;68:11B
3. Juul-Moller S, Edvardsson N, Jahnmatz B, et al: Double-blind trial of aspirin in primary prevention of myocardial infarction in patients with stable chronic angina pectoris. *Lancet* 1992;340:1421
4. The United Kingdom transient ischaemic attack (UK-TIA) aspirin trial: final results. *J Neurol Neurosurg Psychiatry* 1991;54:1044
5. Hirsh J, Salzman EW, Harker L, et al: Aspirin and other platelet active drugs: relationship among dose, effectiveness, and side effects. *Chest* 1989;95:12S
6. Antiplatelet Trialists' Collaboration: Collaborative overview of randomized trials of antiplatelet therapy. I. Prevention of death, myocardial infarction, and stroke by prolonged antiplatelet therapy in various categories of patients. *Br Med J* 1994;308:81
7. Antiplatelet Trialists' Collaboration: Collaborative overview of randomised trials of antiplatelet therapy. II. Maintenance of vascular graft or arterial patency by antiplatelet therapy. *Br Med J* 1994;308:159
8. Clagett GP, Anderson FA, Levine MN, et al: Prevention of venous thromboembolism. *Chest* 1992;102:391S
9. Antiplatelet Trialists' Collaboration: Collaborative overview of randomised trials of antiplatelet therapy. III. Reduction in venous thrombosis and pulmonary embolism by antiplatelet prophylaxis among surgical and medical patients. *Br Med J* 1994;308:235
10. McTavish D, Faulds D, Goa K: Ticlopidine: an updated review of its pharmacology and therapeutic use in platelet-dependent disorders. *Drugs* 1990;40:238
11. Hass WK, Easton JD, Adams HP, et al: A randomized trial comparing ticlopidine hydrochloride with aspirin for the prevention of stroke in high-risk patients. *N Engl J Med* 1989;321:501
12. Gent M, Blackley JA, Easton JD, et al: The Canadian American Ticlopidine Study (CATS) in thromboembolic stroke. *Lancet* 1989;i:1215
13. Balsano F, Rizzon P, Violi F, et al: Antiplatelet treatment with ticlopidine in unstable angina. *Circulation* 1990;82:17
14. Limet R, Jean-Louis D, Magotteaux P, et al: Prevention of aorta-coronary bypass graft occlusion: beneficial effect of ticlopidine on early and late patency rates of venous coronary bypass grafts. A double-blind study. *J Thorac Cardiovasc Surg* 1987;94:773
15. Arcan JC, Blanchard J, Boissel JP, et al: Multicenter double-blind study of ticlopidine in the treatment of intermittent claudication and the prevention of its complications. *Angiology* 1988;39:802
16. Lefkovits J, Plow EF, Topol EJ: Platelet glycoprotein IIb/IIIa receptors in cardiovascular medicine. *N Engl J Med* 1995;332:1553

17. Kleiman NS, Ohman EM, Califf RM, et al: Profound inhibition of platelet aggregation with monoclonal antibody 7E3 fab after thrombolytic therapy. *J Am Coll Cardiol* 1993;22:381

18. Simoons ML, Jan de Boer M, Van den Brand M, et al: Randomized trial of a GPIIb/IIIa platelet receptor blocker in refractory unstable angina. *Circulation* 1994;89:596

19. The EPIC Investigators: Use of a monoclonal antibody directed against the platelet glycoprotein IIb/IIIa receptor in high-risk coronary angioplasty. *N Engl J Med* 1994;330:956

20. Fitzgerlad GA: Dipyridamole. *N Engl J Med* 1987;316:1247

21. Myrvold HE, Persson JE, Svensson B, et al: Prevention of thrombo-embolism with dextran 70 and heparin in patients with femoral neck fractures. *Acta Chir Scand* 1973;139:609

22. Rosenberg RD: The heparin-antithrombin system: a natural anticoagulant mechanism. In: Colman RW, Hirsh J, Marder VJ, et al (eds). *Hemostasis and Thrombosis: Basic Principles and Clinical Practice*, ed 2. Philadelphia, JB Lippincott, 1987:1372

23. Hirsh J: Heparin. *N Engl J Med* 1991;324:1565

24. Hull RD, Raskob GE, Hirsh J, et al: Continuous intravenous heparin compared with intermittent subcutaneous heparin in the initial treatment of proximal-vein thrombosis. *N Engl J Med* 1986;315:1109

25. Brill-Edwards P, Ginsberg JS, Johnston M, et al: Establishing a therapeutic range for heparin therapy. *Ann Intern Med* 1993;119:104

26. Landefeld CS, Beyth RJ: Anticoagulant-related bleeding: clinical epidemiology, prediction, and prevention. *Am J Med* 1993;95:315

27. Oster JR, Singer I, Fishman LM: Heparin-induced aldosterone suppression and hyperkalemia. *Am J Med* 1995;98:575

28. Swiet MD, Ward PD, Fidler J, et al: Prolonged heparin therapy in pregnancy causes bone demineralization. *Br J Obstet Gynaecol* 1983;90:1129

29. Dukes GE, Sanders SW, Russo J, et al: Transaminase elevations in patients receiving bovine or porcine heparin. *Ann Intern Med* 1984;100:646

30. Cook DJ, Fuller HD, Guyatt GH, et al: Risk factors for gastrointestinal bleeding in critically ill patients. *N Engl J Med* 1994;330:377

31. Visentin GP, Ford SE, Scott JP, et al: Antibodies from patients with heparin-induced thrombocytopenia/thrombosis are specific for platelet factor 4 complexed with heparin or bound to endothelial cells. *J Clin Invest* 1994;93:81

32. Collins R, Scrimgeour A, Yusuf S, et al: Reduction in fatal pulmonary embolism and venous thrombosis by perioperative administration of subcutaneous heparin. *N Engl J Med* 1988;318:1162

33. Clagett GP, Anderson FA, Heit J, et al: Prevention of venous thromboembolism. *Chest* 1995;108:312S

34. Goldhaber SZ, Morpurgo M: Diagnosis, treatment, and prevention of pulmonary embolism. *JAMA* 1992;268:1727

35. Keane MG, Ingenito EP, Goldhaber SZ: Utilization of venous thromboembolism prophylaxis in the medical intensive care unit. *Chest* 1994;106:13

36. Cruickshank MK, Levine MN, Hirsh J, et al: A standard heparin nomogram for the management of heparin therapy. *Arch Intern Med* 1991;151:333

37. Basu D, Gallus A, Hirsh J, et al: A prospective study of the value of monitoring heparin treatment with the activated partial thromboplastin time. *N Engl J Med* 1972;287:324

38. Hull RD, Raskob GE, Rosenbloom D, et al: Optimal therapeutic level of heparin therapy in patients with venous thrombosis. *Arch Intern Med* 1992;152:1589

39. Raschke RA, Reilly BM, Guidry JR, et al: The weight-based heparin dosing nomogram compared with a "standard care" nomogram. *Ann Intern Med* 1993;119:874

40. Hull RD, Raskob GE, Rosenbloom D, et al: Heparin for 5 days as compared with 10 days in the initial treatment of proximal venous thrombosis. *N Engl J Med* 1990;322:1260

41. Schulman S, Rhedin A, Lindmarker P, et al: A comparison of 6 weeks with 6 months of oral anticoagulant therapy after a first episode of venous thromboembolism. *N Engl J Med* 1995;332:1661

42. Gunnar RM, Bourdillon PD, Dixon DW, et al: Guidelines for the early management of patients with acute myocardial infarction: a report of the American College of Cardiology/American Heart Association Task Force on assessment of diagnostic and therapeutic cardiovascular procedures (subcommittee to develop guidelines for the early management of patients with acute myocardial infarction). *J Am Coll Cardiol* 1990;16:249

43. Cairns JA, Hirsh J, Lewis HD, et al: Antithrombotic agents in coronary artery disease. *Chest* 1992;102:456S

44. Raskob GE, Comp PC: Preventing systemic embolism in patients with abnormal ventricular function. *Cardiol Clin* 1994;12:477

45. Rogers WJ, Chandra NC, Gore JM: National registry of myocardial infarction (NRMI): what have we learned from the first 100,000 patients. *J Am Coll Cardiol* 1993;21:349A

46. The Gusto Angiographic Investigators: The effects of tissue plasminogen activator, streptokinase, or both on coronary-artery patency, ventricular function, and survival after acute myocardial infarction. *N Engl J Med* 1993;329:1615

47. White HD, Cross DB, Elliott JM, et al: Long-term prognostic importance of patency of the infarct-related coronary artery after thrombolytic therapy for acute myocardial infarction. *Circulation* 1994;89:61

48. The Gusto Investigators: An international randomized trial comparing four thrombolytic strategies for acute myocardial infarction. *N Engl J Med* 1993;329:673

49. Ridker PM, Hebert PR, Fuster V, et al: Are both aspirin and heparin justified as adjuncts to thrombolytic therapy for acute myocardial infarction? *Lancet* 1993;341:1574

50. Ward SR, Topol EJ: How best to use heparin in MI patients given thrombolysis. *J Crit Illness* 1995;10:385

51. Theroux P, Quimet H, McCans J, et al: Aspirin, heparin, or both to treat acute unstable angina. *N Engl J Med* 1988;319:1105

52. The Risk Group: Risk of myocardial infarction and death during treatment with low dose aspirin and intravenous heparin in men with unstable coronary artery disease. *Lancet* 1990;336:827

53. Tegtmeyer CJ, Sos TA: Techniques of renal angioplasty. *Radiology* 1986;161:577

54. Barry WL, Sarembock IJ: Antiplatelet and anticoagulant therapy in patients undergoing percutaneous transluminal coronary angioplasty. *Cardiol Clin* 1994;12:517

55. McNamara TO, Bomberger RA, Merchant RF: Intra-arterial urokinase as the initial therapy for acutely ischemic lower limbs. *Circulation* 1991;83:106I

56. Feinberg WM, Albers GW, Barnett JM, et al: Guidelines for the management of transient ischemic attacks. *Stroke* 1994;25:1320

57. Eckman MH, Beshansky JR, Durand-Zaleski I, et al: Anticoagulation for noncardiac procedures in patients with prosthetic heart valves. *JAMA* 1990;263:1513

58. Adams HP, Brott TG, Crowell RM, et al: Guidelines for the management of patients with acute ischemic stroke. *Stroke* 1994;25:1901

59. Marsh EE, Adams HP, Biller J, et al: Use of antithrombotic

drugs in the treatment of acute ischemic stroke: a survey of neurologists in practice in the United States. *Neurology* 1989;39:1631

60. Moore WS, Barnett HJM, Beebe HG, et al: Guidelines for carotid endarterectomy. *Stroke* 1995;26:188

61. Korczyn AD: Heparin in the treatment of acute stroke. *Neurol Clin* 1992;10:209

62. Bick RL: Disseminated intravascular coagulation. *Hematol Oncol Clin North Am* 1992;6:1259

63. Karnik R, Valentin A, Winkler WB, et al: Duplex sonographic detection of internal jugular venous thrombosis after removal of central venous catheters. *Clin Cardiol* 1993;16:26

64. Mollenholt P, Eriksson I, Andersson T: Thrombogenicity of pulmonary-artery catheters. *Intensive Care Med* 1987;13:57

65. Chastre J, Cornud F, Bouchama A, et al: Thrombosis as a complication of pulmonary-artery catheterization via the internal jugular vein. *N Engl J Med* 1982;306:278

66. Ruggiero RP, Aisenstein TJ: Central catheter fibrin sleeve-heparin effect. *J Parenter Enter Nutr* 1983;7:270

67. Bern MM, Lokich JJ, Wallach SR, et al: Very low doses of warfarin can prevent thrombosis in central venous catheters. *Ann Intern Med* 1990;112:423

68. Hirsh J: Rationale for development of low-molecular-weight heparins and their clinical potential in the prevention of post-operative venous thrombosis. *Am J Surg* 1991;161:512

69. Mammen EF: Why low molecular weight heparin? *Semin Thromb Hemost* 1990;16:1

70. Hirsh J: From bench to bedside: history of development of LMWHs. *Pharmacol Ther* 1994;19:40S

71. Warkentin TE, Levine MN, Hirsh J, et al: Heparin-induced thrombocytopenia in patients treated with low-molecular-weight heparin or unfractionated heparin. *N Engl J Med* 1995;332:1330

72. Jorgensen LN, Jorgensen PW, Hauch O: Prophylaxis of post-operative thromboembolism with low molecular weight heparins. *Br J Surg* 1993;80:689

73. Leizorovicz A, Simonneau G, Decousus H, et al: Comparison of efficacy and safety of low molecular weight heparins and unfractionated heparin in initial treatment of deep venous thrombosis: a meta-analysis. *Br Med J* 1994;309:299

74. Lensing AW, Prins MH, Davidson BL, et al: Treatment of deep venous thrombosis with low-molecular-weight heparins. *Arch Intern Med* 1995;155:601

75. Noble S, Peters DH, Goa KL: Enoxaparin: a reappraisal of its pharmacology and clinical applications in the prevention and treatment of thromboembolic disease. *Drugs* 1995;49:388

76. Fareed J, Walenga JM, Hoppensteadt D, et al: Neutralization of recombinant hirudin: some practical considerations. *Semin Thromb Hemost* 1991;17:137

77. Antman EM: Hirudin in acute myocardial infarction safety report from the thrombolysis and thrombin inhibition in myocardial infarction (TIMI) 9A trial. *Circulation* 1994;90:1624

78. The Global Use of Strategies to Open Occluded Coronary Arteries (GUSTO) IIa Investigators: Randomized trial of intravenous heparin versus recombinant hirudin for acute coronary syndromes. *Circulation* 1994;90:1631

79. Hirsh J: Oral anticoagulant drugs. *N Engl J Med* 1991;324:1865

80. Hull RD, Pineo G: Current concepts of anticoagulation therapy. *Clin Chest Med* 1995;16:269

81. Kuhn TA, Garnett WR, Wells BK, et al: Recovery of warfarin from an enteral nutrient formula. *Am J Hosp Pharm* 1989;46:1395

82. Hirsh J, Poller L: The international normalized ratio. *Arch Intern Med* 1994;154:282

83. Eby C: Warfarin-induced skin necrosis. *Hematol Oncol Clin North Am* 1993;7:1291

84. Francis CW, Marder VJ, McCollister C, et al: Two-step warfarin therapy. *JAMA* 1983;249:374

85. Poller L, McKernan A, Thomson JM, et al: Fixed minidose warfarin: a new approach to prophylaxis against venous thrombosis after major surgery. *Br Med J* 1987;295:1309

86. Hirsh J: The optimal duration of anticoagulant therapy for venous thrombosis. *N Engl J Med* 1995;332:1710

87. Stroke Prevention in Atrial Fibrillation Investigators: Warfarin versus aspirin for prevention of thromboembolism in atrial fibrillation: stroke prevention in atrial fibrillation II study. *Lancet* 1994;343:687

88. The Boston Area Anticoagulation Trial for Atrial Fibrillation Investigators: The effect of low-dose warfarin on the risk of stroke in patients with nonrheumatic atrial fibrillation. *N Engl J Med* 1990;323:1505

89. Connolly SJ, Laupacis A, Gent M, et al: Canadian atrial fibrillation anticoagulation (CAFA) study. *J Am Coll Cardiol* 1991;18:349

90. Ezekowitz MD, Bridgers SL, James KE, et al: Warfarin in the prevention of stroke associated with nonrheumatic atrial fibrillation. *N Engl J Med* 1992;327:1406

91. Petersen P, Boysen G, Godtfredsen J, et al: Placebo-controlled, randomised trial of warfarin and aspirin for prevention of thromboembolic complications in chronic atrial fibrillation. *Lancet* 1989;i:175

92. Stroke Prevention in Atrial Fibrillation Investigators: Stroke prevention in atrial fibrillation study. *Circulation* 1991;84:527

93. Albers GW: Atrial fibrillation and stroke. *Arch Intern Med* 1994;154:1443

94. Arnold AZ, Mick MJ, Mazurek RP, et al: Role of prophylactic anticoagulation for direct current cardioversion in patients with atrial fibrillation or atrial flutter. *J Am Coll Cardiol* 1992;19:851

95. Manning WJ, Silverman DI, Gordon PF, et al: Cardioversion from atrial fibrillation without prolonged anticoagulation with use of transesophageal echocardiography to exclude the presence of atrial thrombi. *N Engl J Med* 1993;328:750

96. Turpie AG, Gunstensen J, Hirsh J, et al: Randomised comparison of two intensities of oral anticoagulant therapy after tissue heart valve replacement. *Lancet* 1988;i:1242

97. Saour JN, Sieck JO, Mamo LAR, et al: Trial of different intensities of anticoagulation in patients with prosthetic heart valves. *N Engl J Med* 1990;322:428

98. Turpie AGG, Gent M, Laupacis A, et al: A comparison of aspirin with placebo in patients treated with warfarin after heart-valve replacement. *N Engl J Med* 1993;329:524

99. Cairns JA, Hirsh J, Lewis HD, et al: Antithrombotic agents in coronary artery disease. *Chest* 1993;102:456S

100. Nachman RL, Siverstein R: Hypercoagulable states. *Ann Intern Med* 1993;119:819

101. Dahlback B: Inherited thrombophilia: resistance to activated protein C as a pathogenic factor of venous thromboembolism. *Blood* 1995;85:607

102. Granger CB, Califf RM, Topol EJ: Thrombolytic therapy for acute myocardial infarction. *Drugs* 1992;44:293

103. Gillis JC, Wagstaff AJ, Goa KL: Alteplase a reappraisal of its pharmacologic properties and therapeutic use in acute myocardial infarction. *Drugs* 1995;50:102

104. Ferres H: Preclinical pharmacological evaluation of anisoylated plasminogen streptokinase activator complex. *Drugs* 1987;33(Suppl 3):33

105. Verstraete M, Lijnen HR, Collen D: Thrombolytic agents in development. *Drugs* 1995;50:29

106. Habib GB: Current status of thrombolysis in acute myocardial

infarction. I. Optimal selection and delivery of a thrombolytic drug. *Chest* 1995;107:225

107. Habib GB: Current status of thrombolysis in acute myocardial infarction. II. Optimal utilization of thrombolysis in clinical subsets. *Chest* 1995;107:528

108. Habib GB: Current status of thrombolysis in acute myocardial infarction. III. Optimalization of adjunctive therapy after thrombolytic therapy. *Chest* 1995;107:809

109. Wilcox RG, Lippe G, Olsson CG, et al: Trial of tissue plasminogen activator for mortality reduction in acute myocardial infarction. *Lancet* 1988;ii:525

110. ISIS-2 (Second International Study of Infarct Survival) Collaborative Group: Randomised trail of intravenous streptokinase, oral aspirin, both, or neither among 17 187 cases of suspected acute myocardial infarction: ISIS-2. *Lancet* 1988; ii:349

111. Gruppo Italiano Per Lo Studio Della Streptochinasi Nell Infarto Miocardico (GISSI): Effectiveness of intravenous thrombolytic treatment in acute myocardial infarction. *Lancet* 1986;i:397

112. Weaver WD, Cerqueira M, Hallstrom AP, et al: Prehospital-initiated vs hospital-initiated thrombolytic therapy. *JAMA* 1993;270:1211

113. EMERAS (Estudio Multicentrico Estreptoquinasa Republicas de America del Sur) Collabortive Group: Randomised trial of late thrombolysis in patients with suspected acute myocardial infarction. *Lancet* 1993;342:767

114. LATE (Late assessment of thrombolytic efficacy) Study Group: Late assessment of thrombolytic efficacy (LATE) study with alteplase 6-24 hours after onset of acute myocardial infarction. *Lancet* 1993;342:759

115. Grines CL, DeMaria AN: Optimal utilization of thrombolytic therapy for acute myocardial infarction: concepts and controversies. *J Am Coll Cardiol* 1990;16:223

116. Muller DW, Topol EJ: Selection of patients with acute myocardial infarction for thrombolytic therapy. *Ann Intern Med* 1990;113:949

117. Effects of tissue plasminogen activator and a comparison of early invasive and conservative strategies in unstable angina and non-q-wave myocardial infarction. *Circulation* 1994;89:1545

118. National Heart, Lung, and Blood Institute: Urokinase pulmonary embolism trial: Phase one results. *JAMA* 1970;214:2163

119. Rogers LQ, Lutcher CL: Streptokinase therapy for deep vein thrombosis: a comprehensive review of the english literature. *Am J Med* 1990;88:389

120. National Institutes of Health Consensus Development Conference: Thrombolytic therapy in thrombosis. *Ann Intern Med* 1980;93:141

121. Kelley MA, Abbuhl S: Massive pulmonary embolism. *Clin Chest Med* 1994;15:547

122. Leeper KV, Popovich J, Lesser BA, et al: Treatment of massive acute pulmonary embolism. *Chest* 1988;93:234

123. Goldhaber SZ, Haire WD, Feldstein ML, et al: Alteplase versus heparin in acute pulmonary embolism: randomised trial assessing right-ventricular function and pulmonary perfusion. *Lancet* 1993;341:507

124. Sharma GV, Burleson VA, Sasahara AA: Effect of thrombolytic therapy on pulmonary-capillary blood volume in patients with pulmonary embolism. *N Engl J Med* 1980;303:842

125. Monturo CA, Dickerson RN, Muller JL: Efficacy of thrombolytic therapy for occlusion of long-term catheters. *J Parenter Enter Nutr* 1990;14:312

126. Sobel BE: Intracranial bleeding, fibrinolysis, and anticoagulation: causal connections and clinical implications. *Circulation* 1994;90:2147

127. Sane DC, Califf RM, Topol EJ, et al: Bleeding during thrombolytic therapy for acute myocardial infarction: mechanisms and management. *Ann Intern Med* 1989;111:1010

Critical Care, Third Edition, edited by Joseph M. Civetta,
Robert W. Taylor, and Robert R. Kirby.
Lippincott-Raven Publishers, Philadelphia, PA © 1997.

CHAPTER 42

∎

Renal Replacement Therapies

Sudarshan Hebbar
Richard S. Muther

IMMEDIATE CONCERNS ∎

MAJOR PROBLEMS

Five renal replacement therapies are available for use in
the intensive care unit (ICU): intermittent hemodialysis,
continuous hemodialysis, continuous hemofiltration, continuous hemodiafiltration and peritoneal dialysis. They share a
similar design: a selectively permeable membrane separates
the patient's blood from a second compartment. The therapies alter the composition of the patient's blood by establishing concentration or pressure gradients that direct solute
movement across the membrane by diffusion or convection.
They are integral to the treatment of patients with acute
renal failure whenever severe azotemia or uremia occurs
and when hyperkalemia, metabolic acidosis, and hypervolemia are refractory to medical therapy. The renal replacement therapies also provide an alternative to the traditional
management of hypothermia.[1] In addition, intermittent hemodialysis is an effective therapy for patients intoxicated
with methanol, ethylene glycol, salicylates, lithium, and
theophylline.

STRESS POINTS

1. Intermittent hemodialysis and continuous hemodiafiltration control volume and azotemia in ICU patients
   with acute renal failure. Continuous hemofiltration
   and peritoneal dialysis may not adequately control azotemia in a severely catabolic patient, but they effectively treat hypervolemia.
2. Studies have not defined what constitutes adequate
   control of azotemia in patients with acute renal failure.
   One study suggests that an intensive prescription does

not improve survival in patients with acute renal failure, but the findings may not apply to the ICU.
3. Cellulose membranes activate the complement system
   when they come into contact with blood. Complement
   activation worsens the prognosis for survival in patients
   with acute renal failure. Because synthetic membranes
   do not activate the complement system, they are the
   standard of care.
4. An episode of hypotension during a renal replacement
   therapy may retard the recovery of renal function in
   patients with acute renal failure because kidneys cannot autoregulate blood flow.
5. No studies compare the outcome of patients with acute
   renal failure treated with intermittent hemodialysis or
   one of the continuous therapies. Therefore, there is
   no proof that one type of therapy is superior to another.
   An ICU should have the ability to tailor the type of
   therapy to the patient's condition. The choice of therapy should take advantage of the merits of each type of
   therapy. To avoid complications, continuous therapies
   must be performed regularly in ICUs.

ESSENTIAL PROCEDURES

1. Define the goals of treatment for the renal replacement therapies. Select the renal replacement therapy
   that best suits the goals of treatment. In critically ill
   patients, negotiate a trial of therapy and clearly define
   a successful endpoint for the trial.
2. The extracorporeal therapies require a vascular access
   that accommodates the blood flow necessary for adequate solute control. A double-lumen catheter cannulated into a central vein provides the necessary blood
   flow for intermittent hemodialysis and the continuous

venovenous (VV) therapies. The continuous arteriovenous (AV) therapies require an arterial access such as a catheter in a central artery or a Scribner shunt. Peritoneal dialysis requires a peritoneal catheter placed into the peritoneum.

3. Although anticoagulation is not mandatory for the extracorporeal therapies, heparin is routinely administered. Alternate strategies exist for patients who are at risk to bleed from an underlying condition but need anticoagulation because the extracorporeal circuit continually clots.

INITIAL THERAPY

1. To avoid the dialysis disequilibrium syndrome, gradually increase urea clearance. Limit the blood flow rate used during the initial session and the length of the session.

2. To avoid hypotension during intermittent hemodialysis, prevent excessive interdialytic fluid gain, remove fluid slowly, and use isolated ultrafiltration, a dialysate with a higher sodium concentration, or a colder dialysate.

3. To treat hypotension during intermittent hemodialysis, lower the ultrafiltration rate and infuse isotonic or hypertonic fluids back into the patient. If the hypotension does not resolve, use clinical signs and symptoms to broaden the differential diagnosis for the cause of hypotension.

PHYSIOLOGY

The various renal replacement therapies share a similar design: a selectively permeable membrane separates the patient's blood from a second compartment. The membrane may be part of a dialyzer incorporated into an extracorporeal circuit, or it may exist within the patient, as does the peritoneal membrane. The second compartment may contain dialysate or form a simple reservoir that collects ultrafiltrate from plasma. The therapies alter the composition of the patient's blood by establishing concentration or pressure gradients that direct solute movement into the second compartment using either diffusion or convection.

Diffusion is the primary mechanism of solute removal during dialysis. How well a solute diffuses depends on the size of the solute, the slope of the concentration gradient from blood to dialysate, and the membrane's resistance to transport. Because the rate of diffusion is inversely proportional to the molecular weight of a solute, smaller molecules such as urea diffuse more rapidly than larger molecules. Diffusion reduces the total mass of a solute in the patient's body and the concentration of a solute in the patient's blood.

Convection is the primary mode of solute transport during ultrafiltration. Ultrafiltration refers to the movement of water from the patient's blood that results from either a hydrostatic or osmotic pressure gradient directed toward the second compartment. The resulting flux of water molecules drags solutes through the membrane at a concentration equal to that in blood. The degree of the pressure gradient

and the sieving characteristics of the membrane determine the extent of convective transport. Convection removes larger molecules from the patient's blood than does diffusion, but it is not as efficient in removing smaller molecules such as urea. Convection reduces the total mass of a solute in the patient's body, but the concentration in the blood does not change.

The clearance represents a hypothetical volume of blood that a therapy clears of a solute each minute, or for peritoneal dialysis, each day. It is a measure of how efficiently a therapy removes a solute and is a marker of comparison between therapies. For the extracorporeal therapies, the clearance of a solute is the product of the blood flow rate and the difference in solute concentration of the blood entering and leaving the dialyzer. The relationship between the clearance and blood flow rate is not completely linear because the efficiency of the dialyzer and the dialysate flow rate limit increases in solute clearance at higher blood flows. For peritoneal dialysis, the clearance is the product of the volume of dialysate removed from the peritoneal cavity and the ratio of the solute concentrations in the dialysate and the venous blood.

EXTRACORPOREAL THERAPIES

Intermittent hemodialysis is the renal replacement therapy most frequently used in the ICU. In patients with acute renal failure, the goals of intermittent hemodialysis are to provide adequate solute and fluid removal while avoiding complications that may impair the recovery of renal function. Before initiating therapy, the nephrologist must place a suitable vascular access, choose an appropriate dialyzer, select the composition of the dialysate, and prescribe the blood flow rate and the length of the hemodialysis session.

Intermittent hemodialysis requires a vascular access that can accommodate a blood flow of 200 to 350 mL/minute. A recent study emphasizes the importance of an adequate vascular access by documenting that vascular access dysfunction is the most frequent cause for ICU patients to receive inadequate renal replacement therapy.[2] The most popular method of obtaining vascular access is to cannulate a large-bore, double-lumen catheter into a large vein such as the femoral, subclavian, or internal jugular vein. An alternate technique for obtaining vascular access is to surgically implant polyethylene tubes into an extremity artery and a nearby vein. When connected, the tubes form an external shunt, commonly referred to as a Scribner shunt. The Scribner shunt decreases blood flow to the distal portion of the extremity and may precipitate ischemia in the presence of underlying arterial insufficiency. Because it is easier to insert a double-lumen catheter, the Scribner shunt has become largely obsolete for use with acute intermittent hemodialysis. Patients who do not recover adequate renal function after an episode of acute renal failure should receive a long-term vascular access such as a "permanently" placed central venous catheter or an AV fistula or graft.

Dialyzers contain selectively permeable membranes that vary in permeability to solutes and water because they differ in surface area and pore size. For each dialyzer, the mass transfer area coefficient describes how efficiently urea crosses its membrane and the ultrafiltration coefficient expresses how permeable the membrane is to water. High-efficiency dialyzers employ membranes that have a larger surface area so that small solutes may diffuse more rapidly. They are useful in patients who need a high urea clearance while on intermittent hemodialysis. High-flux dialyzers incorporate membranes that have larger pores, and their use yields higher clearances of water and larger solutes.

Dialysis membranes also vary in their ability to activate the complement system on contact with blood. Of the four types of materials that form membranes (cellulose, substituted cellulose, cellulosynthetic, and synthetic), cellulose activates complement to the greatest degree. The use of cellulose membranes adversely affects the outcome of acute renal failure. In a rat model of ischemic renal failure, complement-activating membranes caused sequestration of neutrophils in the glomerulus and delayed recovery of renal function.[3] When patients with acute renal failure received intermittent hemodialysis with a cellulose membrane, they had a longer duration of renal failure and a lower survival rate when compared with patients who received hemodialysis with a synthetic membrane.[4] Although it is not clear whether there are clinically significant differences between synthetic membranes and substituted cellulose or cellulosynthetic membranes, we recommend using synthetic membranes in patients with acute renal failure.

During intermittent hemodialysis, the composition of the dialysate creates the concentration gradients necessary to remove solutes from blood. Dialysate consists of highly purified water, dextrose, and selected concentrations of electrolytes, which typically include sodium, potassium, chloride, bicarbonate, calcium, and magnesium. Dialysate may contain acetate as an alternate base, but the use of acetate is falling out of favor because it aggravates hypotension during intermittent hemodialysis and causes hypoventilation, thereby inducing hypoxemia. Dialysate must be sterile; if bacteria contaminate the solution, the back-leak of endotoxin and other bacterial products[5] may cause the patient to develop a fever or become hypotensive while receiving therapy.

The dialysate flows continuously at a rate of 500 to 800 mL/minute in a direction countercurrent to the flow of blood. The continuous flow of dialysate maintains the concentration gradients that would otherwise diminish as solutes diffuse from blood, and the countercurrent direction of flow prevents concentration equilibrium—with the consequent back-leak of solutes to blood—from being reached in the distal portion of the dialyzer. The dialysate may make a single pass through the dialyzer before being discarded, or it may pass through a sorbent cartridge that regenerates fresh dialysate by adsorbing waste products before returning to the dialyzer. The sorbent cartridge system is useful in hospitals that lack a dialysis facility or in the ICU, which may lack the capacity to purify the large amounts of water—up to 120 L—needed for a single-pass system.

The prescription for intermittent hemodialysis centers on achieving adequate urea clearance and fluid removal while avoiding complications. What constitutes adequate urea clearance for patients with acute renal failure is controversial. A controlled study suggests that an intensive intermittent hemodialysis prescription that keeps the blood urea

nitrogen level below 60 mg/dL does not improve survival in patients with acute renal failure when compared with a prescription that maintains the blood urea nitrogen level at 100 mg/dL.[6] Therefore, most nephrologists aim to maintain the blood urea nitrogen level below 100 mg/dL. However, there are two shortcomings of the study[7] that caution against generalizing the conclusions to practice in the ICU: (1) the severity of illness of patients in each treatment arm of the study is unclear, and (2) the patients received intermittent hemodialysis with cellulose membranes. Additional research is needed to clarify the issue by studying ICU patients and using synthetic membranes and newer renal replacement therapies.

In patients with severe azotemia, a goal of intermittent hemodialysis is to lower the blood urea nitrogen level without causing the dialysis disequilibrium syndrome. This syndrome occurs during the hemodialysis session or shortly thereafter and produces symptoms ranging from headaches, nausea and vomiting, and muscle cramps to seizures and coma. The syndrome seems to result from cerebral edema, but how intermittent hemodialysis produces cerebral edema remains uncertain.[8] Because the patient has an increased risk of developing the syndrome when the predialysis blood urea nitrogen level is high and the level falls by more than 35% with therapy, a nephrologist should limit the length of the initial hemodialysis session to 2 or 3 hours and the blood flow rate to 200 mL/minute. The subsequent sessions can be longer and employ a higher blood flow.

In patients with acute renal failure who are hypervolemic, the goal of intermittent hemodialysis is to remove fluid without causing hypotension. When a normal individual has a rapid decrease in plasma volume, sympathetic reflexes maintain blood pressure by increasing the cardiac output and the total peripheral resistance. As the plasma volume decreases in the uremic patient, however, sympathetic reflexes fail to increase the total peripheral resistance[9] and the blood pressure falls. In addition, the rapid decrease in plasma osmolarity during hemodialysis stimulates intracellular movement of water, further aggravating hypotension. An episode of hypotension may have serious consequences for patients with acute renal failure because it may retard the recovery of renal function. Animal studies of acute renal failure suggest that episodes of hypotension delay the recovery of renal function because kidneys have lost the ability to autoregulate blood flow[10] and experience further ischemic damage from the decrease in blood pressure.[11] A nephrologist can diminish the likelihood of hypotension by preventing excessive interdialytic fluid gain, limiting the volume of ultrafiltration during a session, and removing fluid at a constant rate. Other techniques to minimize the risk of hypotension include isolated ultrafiltration without simultaneous dialysis (so-called "dry ultrafiltration"), raising the sodium concentration in the dialysate, and lowering the temperature of the dialysate.

Despite these efforts, hypotension remains the most frequent complication of an intermittent hemodialysis session. The most common cause for dialysis-associated hypotension is rapid or excessive ultrafiltration. Therefore, when treating a hypotensive patient on intermittent hemodialysis, the first step is to reduce the ultrafiltration rate, place the patient in the Trendelenburg position, and infuse isotonic or hypertonic fluids into the patient. If the patient remains hypotensive despite volume resuscitation, the next step is to institute vasopressor therapy while considering other causes that either impair cardiac output or decrease the systemic vascular resistance (Table 42-1).

Another important complication of intermittent hemodialysis is hypoxemia. During a session of intermittent hemodialysis, the arterial Po_2 falls by 5 to 20 mm Hg. The drop in arterial oxygen tension reaches a nadir during the first hour of a hemodialysis session and resolves 1 to 2 hours after a patient completes the session. The etiology of the fall in the Po_2 is uncertain, but two possible causes are complement activation and hypoventilation.[12] The complement system activates within a few minutes of starting the hemodialysis session with a cellulose membrane, causing leukocytes to sequester in the lung and the pulmonary capillaries to become more permeable to fluid. The resulting intrapulmonary abnormalities widen the alveolar-to-arterial oxygen gradient. However, complement activation is not the sole explanation for the hypoxemia because the alveolar-to-arterial gradient returns to normal before the nadir in Po_2 occurs, and intermittent hemodialysis with a synthetic membrane also results in hypoxemia. A decrease in the minute ventilation is an additional explanation for the hypoxemia. Patients hypoventilate during hemodialysis with acetate because carbon dioxide diffuses from blood to dialysate, whereas patients hypoventilate during hemodialysis with bicarbonate because alkalinization of the blood depresses the respiratory center. The fall in the Po_2 with a bicarbonate bath is not as great as with an acetate bath. To minimize the clinical impact of the fall in Po_2, patients with a compromised cardiopulmonary system should receive supplemental oxygen during intermittent hemodialysis.

TABLE 42-1. Differential Diagnosis of Hypotension During Intermittent Hemodialysis

---

DECREASED INTRAVASCULAR VOLUME

Excessive or rapid ultrafiltration
GI hemorrhage
Hemolysis

DECREASED CARDIAC OUTPUT

Myocardial ischemia
Decreased myocardial contractility
Diastolic dysfunction
Arrhythmias
Pericardial tamponade
Air embolism
Beta-blockers

DECREASED VASCULAR RESISTANCE

Septicemia
Acetate dialysate
Autonomic neuropathy
Dialyzer reaction
Antihypertensive medications given before hemodialysis
Increased nitric oxide production

GI, gastrointestinal.

The *continuous renal replacement therapies* (Fig. 42-1) have gained increasing favor as a treatment for renal dysfunction in the ICU because they provide greater hemodynamic stability than intermittent hemodialysis[13] and they allow aggressive fluid and nutritional support without the worry of pulmonary edema. As with intermittent hemodialysis, the nephrologist must define the goals of therapy, place a vascular access, and select equipment before starting the continuous therapy.

Three continuous therapies are widespread in use: continuous hemofiltration, continuous hemodialysis, and continuous hemodiafiltration. Each type of continuous renal replacement therapy has an AV and a VV form (see Figs. 42-1A and 42-1B). A continuous AV therapy uses the mean arterial pressure to drive blood flow through the extracorporeal circuit. To perform continuous AV therapy, a nephrologist accesses the patient's arterial system with either an arterial catheter or a Scribner shunt. In hypotensive patients, a femoral artery catheter produces a greater driving force for blood flow than a Scribner shunt. A continuous VV therapy uses a pump rather than the patient's blood pressure to drive blood flow from a double-lumen catheter cannulated into a central vein. A pump adds complexity to the continuous therapy and may not improve urea clearance, but its use avoids the complications of an arterial access: laceration of the artery, thrombosis of the artery with embolization, peripheral ischemia from arterial insufficiency, and exsanguination if blood lines accidentally disconnect and clamps are not immediately available.[14]

Continuous hemofiltration (see Figs. 42-1A and 42-1B) uses convection to drive solute and fluid removal. The therapy directs a pressure gradient across a highly permeable membrane to create an ultrafiltrate of plasma. Because the ultrafiltrate has a solute composition similar to plasma, the volume of ultrafiltrate determines solute clearances. To adequately control azotemia in patients with acute renal failure, continuous hemofiltration must produce 15 to 20 L of ultrafiltrate per day. As the volume of ultrafiltrate increases, infusion of replacement solution becomes necessary to reconstitute the patient's intravascular volume. The difference between the volume of ultrafiltrate and the volume of replacement solution equals the net amount of fluid lost by the patient. The infusion of replacement solution also replenishes essential electrolytes such as bicarbonate and calcium. Replacement solutions such as lactated Ringer's and peritoneal dialysis solution replace the bicarbonate lost in the ultrafiltrate with lactate, which metabolizes to bicarbonate. If a patient has poor liver function, lactate may not convert to bicarbonate and a metabolic acidosis may develop. In patients at risk for developing metabolic acidosis, we replace essential electrolytes by alternating every hour (1) the infusion of a 5% dextrose solution mixed with two to three ampules of sodium bicarbonate, and (2) the infusion of a normal saline solution with added calcium and other depleted electrolytes, such as magnesium and potassium. Infusion of the replacement solution into the tubing proximal to the dialyzer (predilution hemofiltration) instead of distal to the dialyzer (postdilution hemofiltration) has a theoretic advantage of decreasing clotting in the dialyzer. However, predilution hemofiltration is less efficient at clearing solutes

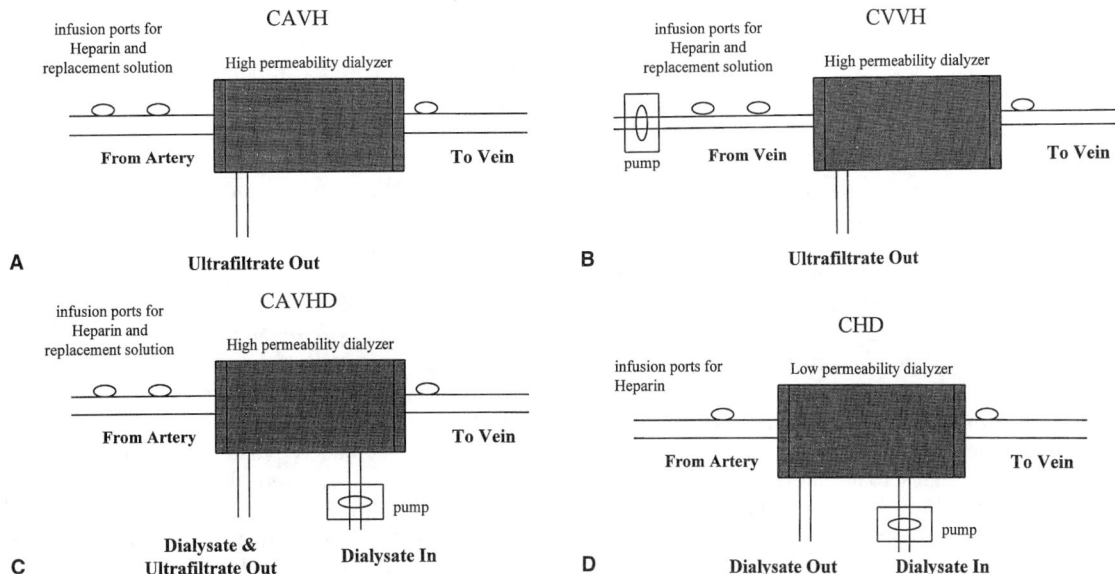

FIGURE 42-1. Continuous renal replacement therapies. CAVH, continuous arteriovenous hemodiafiltration; CVVH, continuous venovenous hemodiafiltration.

than postdilution hemofiltration and obligates a greater volume of ultrafiltrate to achieve similar solute clearances.

In a severely catabolic patient, continuous hemofiltration may not adequately control azotemia.[15] To control azotemia with continuous hemofiltration, a nephrologist may resort to intermittent hemodialysis for additional urea clearance or pump dialysate (usually peritoneal dialysis solution) through the dialyzer countercurrent to blood flow. With the addition of dialysate, continuous hemofiltration transforms into *continuous hemodiafiltration* (see Fig. 42-1*C*) where both convection and diffusion occur. Because dialysate flows through the dialyzer at a rate of 1 to 2 L/hour, which is significantly slower than blood traveling through the extracorporeal circuit, the dialysate flow rate is the most important determinant of urea clearance.[16] Increasing the dialysate flow rate augments urea clearance. Like continuous hemofiltration, continuous hemodiafiltration produces a large volume of ultrafiltrate and requires the infusion of replacement solution to restore the patient's intravascular volume. The flow of dialysate obviates the need to replenish bicarbonate and other electrolytes. When the continuous hemodialysis circuit incorporates a membrane with a low permeability to water, ultrafiltration rates are limited (so that replacement fluid is unnecessary) and only diffusive transport of solutes occurs. This is *continuous hemodialysis* (see Fig. 42-1*D*). Both continuous hemodialysis and continuous hemodiafiltration effectively control azotemia in the severely catabolic patient.[17]

Anticoagulation is a routine component of the extracorporeal therapies. The extracorporeal circuit is thrombogenic because it primes platelets to release procoagulants and initiates the intrinsic clotting cascade. The configuration of the circuit may heighten the risk of clotting: longer tubing exposes blood to a larger surface area of thrombogenic material, and infusion ports create turbulent blood flow and increase the resistance in the circuit by decreasing the diameter of the tubing. Additional risk factors for clotting are a

slow blood flow through the circuit, a high hematocrit, a high ultrafiltration rate, and the transfusion of blood into the extracorporeal circuit. When an extracorporeal circuit clots, the patient receives suboptimal care because the therapy fails to deliver the intended prescription. Measures to keep the circuit functioning include inserting a vascular access that provides rapid blood flow, using predilution hemofiltration, keeping blood lines short, and administering anticoagulants.

The standard anticoagulant is heparin. During intermittent hemodialysis, a common anticoagulation regimen maintains the activated clotting time at 1.5 times the baseline value by giving a bolus of 3000 IU of heparin at the start of the procedure and supplementing the level of anticoagulation with either a continuous infusion of heparin or repeat boluses. Because such a regimen results in systemic anticoagulation, it increases the risk that a patient will bleed from a predisposing condition. A "tight" heparin regimen decreases the risk by using smaller doses of heparin so the activated clotting time remains at 1.2 times the baseline value. During a continuous therapy, an accepted protocol infuses heparin into the tubing proximal to the dialyzer at an initial rate of 250 to 500 IU per hour and raises the dose if a circuit continues to clot. As with intermittent hemodialysis, avoiding systemic anticoagulation is preferable in patients who are predisposed to bleed.

In patients who have a high risk of bleeding, the nephrologist may opt not to use anticoagulants, or may apply alternate strategies of anticoagulation such as regional heparinization[18] or citrate regional anticoagulation.[19] Whereas there is considerable experience in performing intermittent hemodialysis without anticoagulants,[20] only recently have reports suggested that anticoagulants are not absolutely necessary for the optimal function of a continuous therapy.[21,22] The technique of regional heparinization infuses heparin into the tubing proximal to the dialyzer and protamine sulfate distal to the dialyzer. Protamine sulfate is a protein that prevents systemic anticoagulation by binding to heparin and forming an inactive complex. The side effects of protamine include hypotension, flushing, bradycardia, dyspnea, and, if the heparin protamine complex dissociates, rebound anticoagulation. Citrate regional anticoagulation prevents clotting in the dialyzer by lowering the ionized calcium, a cofactor in the coagulation cascade. The procedure interrupts the coagulation cascade only in the dialyzer because it infuses trisodium citrate into the tubing proximal to the dialyzer and calcium chloride distal to the dialyzer. When performing citrate anticoagulation, the dialysate should be free of calcium and the serum calcium concentration should be frequently monitored. Trisodium citrate may produce hypernatremia and metabolic alkalosis unless the dialysate has a low sodium and bicarbonate concentration.

Anticoagulation strategies that may be available in the future include prostacyclin,[23] low molecular weight heparin,[24] and heparin-coated circuits. Prostacyclin and low molecular weight heparin are anticoagulants not yet commercially available in the United States. Prostacyclin anticoagulates blood by inhibiting platelet aggregation. It is an ideal anticoagulant because it has a half-life of 3 to 5 minutes, but side effects such as hypotension, chest pain, headaches, flushing, and nausea may limit its use. Low molecular weight heparin accrues from the degradation of heparin. Because the drug selectively inhibits the coagulation cascade without affecting thrombin formation, it reduces the risk of bleeding. Heparin-coated extracorporeal circuits currently are being tested in clinical trials for their efficacy in preventing clotting.

PERITONEAL DIALYSIS ■

Peritoneal dialysis uses the peritoneal membrane as a dialyzer to remove solutes and fluid. The therapy requires the insertion of a catheter into the peritoneal cavity. There are two types of catheters: an "acute" catheter that is rigid and easy to place percutaneously, and a "chronic" catheter that is more flexible and is tunneled through the subcutaneous fat. Many nephrologists prefer to use a chronic catheter in patients with acute renal failure because an acute catheter has a high risk of peritonitis, especially when it remains in the peritoneum for longer than 3 days. Although a nephrologist may insert a catheter at the bedside, surgical placement is safer, particularly in patients who have had previous abdominal surgeries.

The peritoneal dialysis procedure infuses dialysate into the peritoneal cavity and periodically exchanges the dialysate with fresh solution. As dialysate dwells in the peritoneal cavity, solutes diffuse from blood down concentration gradients until the gradients dissipate. By exchanging dialysate, peritoneal dialysis maintains the concentration gradients that drive solute removal. The glucose in the dialysate drives ultrafiltration by creating an osmotic gradient. The osmotic gradient decreases with a longer dwell time because the peritoneum absorbs glucose. If the dialysate dwells long enough, there is a net influx of fluid into the peritoneum. Unlike the extracorporeal therapies, anticoagulation is not a routine component of peritoneal dialysis.

A standard prescription of peritoneal dialysis in patients with acute renal failure exchanges dialysate every 2 to 3 hours. In a severely catabolic patient, the nephrologist enhances the urea clearance that peritoneal dialysis provides by increasing the frequency of exchanges. As the frequency increases, the concentration of urea in each exchange decreases, but the urea clearance improves because the procedure exchanges a greater volume of dialysate. An alternate approach to augment urea clearance is to enlarge the volume of dialysate infused into the peritoneal cavity, but the approach causes atelectasis and abdominal hernias. By increasing the frequency of exchanges, peritoneal dialysis effectively controls a patient's volume status, but it still may fail to provide adequate urea clearance in a catabolic adult patient. For this reason, the continuous extracorporeal therapies have largely replaced peritoneal dialysis as the alternate treatment to intermittent hemodialysis for patients with acute renal failure.

Peritoneal catheter infections and peritonitis are common complications of peritoneal dialysis. Peritoneal catheter infections manifest as erythema and tenderness at the exit site or in the subcutaneous tunnel. Peritonitis presents as abdominal pain or fever with an elevated polymorphonuclear cell count in the dialysate. If peritonitis supervenes, ICU patients should receive aggressive nutritional support because protein losses during peritoneal dialysis approach 10 to 20 grams per day. The antibiotic therapy for peritoneal catheter infections and peritonitis presumptively covers skin organisms and gram-negative bacteria until cultures identify the organism. Fungal peritonitis usually requires removal of the peritoneal catheter and discontinuation of peritoneal dialysis.

CHOICE OF THERAPY ■

Because intermittent hemodialysis uses rapid blood flows to clear solutes quickly, it is the therapy of choice for treating isolated hyperkalemia, hypothermia, and drug intoxications. Controversy exists over the choice of therapy for ICU patients with acute renal failure. There is concern that intermittent hemodialysis delays the recovery of renal function[25] and limits the ability to provide adequate nutritional support. Therefore, some have advocated that the choice of therapy for most critically ill patients should be one of the continuous therapies.[26] This is supported by retrospective data demonstrating similar survival in patients treated with continuous arteriovenous hemodiafiltration (CAVHD) versus intermittent hemodialysis, despite a greater severity of illness and a higher probability of death in the CAVHD group.[27] However, no prospective, randomized control trials examine the outcome of patients with acute renal failure treated with intermittent hemodialysis compared with the outcome of patients treated with one of the continuous therapies. Therefore, until a study clarifies the issue, the choice of therapy should depend on the technical expertise of the ICU. Remember that the number of complications during a continuous therapy increases if the continuous therapy is not performed frequently in the ICU.[28] We recommend that an ICU have the capability of offering both types of extracorporeal therapies, and that the best approach is to tailor the type of therapy to the condition of the patient. For example, in a hypotensive patient with acute renal failure as a part of multisystem organ failure, a continuous therapy may be the initial choice of therapy because it provides greater hemodynamic stability than intermittent hemodialysis. The type of continuous therapy depends on whether the primary goal of treatment mandates ultrafiltration or solute removal: we use continuous hemofiltration for ultrafiltration, continuous hemodialysis for solute removal, and continuous hemodiafiltration for both ultrafiltration and solute removal. As the patient improves, intermittent hemodialysis may become the preferred therapy because it permits greater mobility.

The nephrologist must determine if the therapy will favorably improve the prognosis for survival. When ICU patients require renal replacement therapy for acute renal failure, mortality rates approach 50%.[29] Several studies have attempted to clarify the prognostic variables that predict survival, but the results have been inconsistent because the studies have defined survival differently and only a few studies have used a severity of illness scoring system to compare patients. The need for mechanical ventilation seems to be the most powerful predictor of whether the patient dies.[30] However, the studies do not provide complete certainty about predicting survival in an individual patient. Therefore, we believe that it is prudent to negotiate a trial of therapy with the patient or family on the understanding that if the patient does not improve, the nephrologist will withdraw therapy. By setting a time limit on the trial and clearly defining a successful endpoint, the nephrologist eases the burden on the family if the time arrives to withdraw therapy from the patient.

REFERENCES ■

1. Hernandez E, Praga M, Alcazar JM, et al: Hemodialysis for treatment of accidental hypothermia. *Nephron* 1993;63:214
2. Paganini EP, Pudelski B, Bednarz D: Dialysis delivery in the ICU: are patients receiving the prescribed dialysis dose? *J Am Soc Nephrol* 1992;3:384
3. Schulman G, Gung A, Fogo A, et al: Cuprophane membrane delays the resolution of ischemic acute renal failure in the rat. *Kidney Int* 1990;37:494
4. Hakim RM, Wingard RL, Parker RA: Effect of the dialysis membrane in the treatment of patients with acute renal failure. *N Engl J Med* 1994;331:1338
5. Pereira B, Snodgrass BR, Hogan PJ, et al: Diffusive and convective transfer of cytokine-inducing bacterial products across hemodialysis membranes. *Kidney Int* 1995;47:603
6. Gillum DM, Dixon BS, Yanover MJ, et al: The role of intensive dialysis in acute renal failure. *Clin Nephrol* 1986;25:249
7. Metha R: Therapeutic alternatives to renal replacement for critically ill patients in acute renal failure. *Semin Nephrol* 1994;14:64
8. Arieff AI: Dialysis disequilibrium syndrome: current concepts on pathogenesis and prevention. *Kidney Int* 1994;45:629
9. Daugirdas JT: Dialysis hypotension: a hemodynamic analysis. *Kidney Int* 1991;39:233
10. Adams PL, Adams FF, Bell PD, et al: Impaired renal blood flow autoregulation in ischemic acute renal failure. *Kidney Int* 1980;18:68
11. Kelleher SP, Robinette JB, Miller F, et al: Effect of hemorrhagic reduction in blood pressure on recovery from acute renal failure. *Kidney Int* 1987;31:725
12. Cardoso M, Vinay P, Vinet B, et al: Hypoxemia during hemodialysis: a critical review of the facts. *Am J Kidney Dis* 1988;11:281
13. Davenport A, Will EJ, Davison AM: Effect of renal replacement therapy on patients with combined acute renal and fulminant hepatic failure. *Kidney Int* 1993;43(Suppl 41):S245
14. Bellomo R, Parkin G, Love J, et al: A prospective comparative study of continuous arteriovenous hemodiafiltration and continuous venovenous hemodiafiltration in critically ill patients. *Am J Kidney Dis* 1993;21:400
15. Golper TA: Continuous arteriovenous hemofiltration in acute renal failure. *Am J Kidney Dis* 1985;6:373
16. Sigler MH, Teehan BP: Solute transport in continuous hemodialysis: a new treatment for acute renal failure. *Kidney Int* 1987;32:562
17. Ronco C: Continuous renal replacement therapies in the treatment of acute renal failure in intensive care patients. II. Clinical indications and prescription. *Nephrol Dial Transplant* 1994;9 (Suppl 4):S201
18. Kaplan AA, Petrillo R: Regional heparinization for continuous arteriovenous hemofiltration. *Trans Am Soc Artif Intern Organs* 1987;33:312
19. Ward DM, Mehta RL: Extracorporeal management of acute renal failure patients at high risk of bleeding. *Kidney Int* 1993;43(Suppl 41):S237
20. Sanders PW, Taylor H, Curtis JJ: Hemodialysis without anticoagulation. *Am J Kidney Dis* 1985;5:32
21. Paganini EP: Continuous renal replacement therapy: ultrafiltration, hemofiltration and hemodialysis. In: Parillo JE, Bone RC (eds). *Critical Care Medicine*. St Louis, CV Mosby, 1995
22. Martin PY, Chevrolet JC, Suter P, et al: Anticoagulation in patients treated by continuous venovenous hemofiltration: a retrospective study. *Am J Kidney Dis* 1994;24:806
23. Davenport A, Will EJ, Davison AM: Comparison of the use of standard heparin and prostacyclin anticoagulation in spontaneous and pump-driven extracorporeal circuits in patients with combined acute renal and hepatic failure. *Nephron* 1994;66:431
24. Nurmohamed Mt, ten Cate J, Steven P, et al: Long term efficacy and safety of a low molecular weight heparin in chronic hemodialysis patients: a comparison with standard heparin. *ASAIO Trans* 1991;37:M459
25. Conger JD: Does hemodialysis delay recovery from acute renal failure? *Semin Dial* 1990;3:146
26. Harris DCH: Acute renal replacement: which treatment is best? *Aust N Z J Med* 1990;20:197
27. VonBommel EFH, Bouvy ND, So KL, et al: Acute dialytic support for the critically ill: intermittent hemodialysis versus continuous arteriovenous hemofiltration. *Am J Nephrol* 1995;15:192
28. Health and Public Committee, American College of Physicians: Clinical competence in continuous arterio-venous hemofiltration. *Ann Intern Med* 1988;108:900
29. Barton IK, Hilton PJ, Taub NA, et al: Acute renal failure treated by hemofiltration:factors affecting outcome. *Q J Med* 1993;86:81
30. Spiegal DM, Ullian ME, Zerbe GO, et al: Determinants of survival and recovery in acute renal failure patients dialyzed in intensive care units. *Am J Nephrol* 1991;11:44

Critical Care, Third Edition, edited by Joseph M. Civetta,
Robert W. Taylor, and Robert R. Kirby.
Lippincott-Raven Publishers, Philadelphia, PA © 1997.

CHAPTER 43

■

Transfusion Therapy

Richard C. Dennis
David Clas
Joan M. Niehoff
Neil S. Yeston

IMMEDIATE CONCERNS ■

MAJOR PROBLEMS

Current transfusion practices are deeply rooted in tradition; many lack scientific support, and recommendations are often conflicting. For decades, transfusion equated to the infusion of whole blood. Eventually, the concept that packed red blood cells diluted with saline satisfied the need to increase oxygen-carrying capacity led to the concept of component therapy. Thus, a unit of donor blood could be fractionated so that more than one patient received the benefit of specific therapy. Blood banking entered a new age, and techniques for salvage and preservation increased dramatically.

Subsequently, concerns about the safety of transfused blood and blood products became a major issue, not so much with respect to typing and crossmatching errors, but more so from a concern about disease transmission. Acquired immunodeficiency syndrome (AIDS) and blood-borne hepatitis (B and non-A, non-B) are household concerns resulting in new testing methodology and, ultimately, vastly improved safety for the recipient.

New transfusion guidelines significantly reduced the transfusion trigger. For years, a hemoglobin of 10 g/dL was considered the point at which red cell transfusion should be initiated. Currently, however, experimental and clinical evidence suggests that most patients can have blood administration withheld until the hemoglobin falls to 7 g/dL or, rarely, even less. The result should be a reduction in the amount of blood administered and even less risk.

One major problem afflicting both the operating room and ICU has been the tendency of clinicians to administer fresh frozen plasma (FFP) and platelets prophylactically to forestall bleeding and clotting problems. This practice generally is discouraged by experts in the field but still is widely employed. Similarly to be discouraged is the administration of FFP for intravascular volume expansion.

STRESS POINTS

1. Be selective when transfusing. Use red blood cells to increase oxygen-carrying capacity, *not* for volume expansion.
2. For patients without suspected or documented significant cardiopulmonary disease, reduce your transfusion trigger. A hemoglobin of 7 g/dL usually is sufficient so long as plasma volume is adequate and cardiac output can increase.
3. Except in patients who undergo massive transfusion associated with shock, hypothermia, or prolonged hypotension, don't give FFP prophylactically. Follow bleeding and clotting studies serially whenever possible. The resulting therapy will be much more cost-effective physiologically and in terms of money spent.
4. Beware of hypothermia in a bleeding patient. Platelet function is affected adversely. Rewarming of a cold patient usually reverses this functional platelet defect.
5. Type O uncrossmatched blood and type-specific blood can be administered safely when time does not allow

a full crossmatch. If more than 4 units of type O blood have been given, recrossmatch before giving type-specific blood or blood that was crossmatched with an earlier sample.

6. After massive transfusion, observe closely for excessive bleeding. Severity is related to the duration and magnitude of shock, if it is present.

7. Hemolytic reactions generally are related to clerical errors. Clinical manifestations (i.e., fever, back pain, chills, and dyspnea) often can be masked in anesthetized or heavily sedated patients. Treatment includes increased fluid administration, mannitol, furosemide, or ethacrynic acid, and pressor agents as necessary.

8. Metabolic complications of blood transfusion usually are fleeting. Exceptions include intravascular volume overload (usually related to ancillary fluid administration) and citrate intoxication (reduction of serum ionized calcium). Be reasonably sure of the diagnosis and severity in the latter case. The cure (calcium administration) may be more problematic than the problem.

9. Patients with a platelet count less than $50,000/mm^3$ who are scheduled for surgery or for large-bore central vascular catheter monitoring probably should receive prophylactic platelet transfusion to a level of $100,000/mm^3$ or greater.

ACUTE MASSIVE HEMORRHAGE ■

Case 1: A 60-year-old man has been transferred directly from the emergency department to the ICU with an upper gastrointestinal (GI) bleed. He is somewhat stuporous, cold, and clammy, and has a heart rate of 140 beats per minute; his systolic blood pressure is 80 mm Hg by palpation, and his respiratory rate is 38 breaths per minute. Fresh blood and blood clots are in the emesis basin that accompanied him to the ICU. He takes aspirin three times daily for arthritis, had a heart attack last year, and began vomiting blood 1 hour earlier.

Clearly, this is not the time to obtain an extensive history and physical examination. His upper GI bleed may be complicated by a platelet defect as a result of aspirin ingestion; he is markedly hypovolemic (>40% blood loss), he has an open airway (he breathes), and he has circulation (he talks). The rest of the history and physical examination should be performed *while* therapy is initiated.

MECHANICS OF TREATMENT

First, ascertain that the airway is adequate, then insert a large 14- or 16-gauge catheter (preferably 14-gauge) in the upper extremity (Table 43-1). Using a 20-mL syringe to start the intravenous (IV) infusion allows blood samples to be drawn immediately. Fill the syringe, then attach the IV tubing with a macrodrip chamber to the cannula. Initially, give normal saline or lactated Ringer's solution "wide open."

Use a pressure bag or a stopcock and 50-mL syringe to achieve high flow rates (>100 mL/minute).

The blood specimen must be sent for type and crossmatch (red top tube), complete blood cell count (CBC; purple top), prothrombin time (PT) and partial thromboplastin time (PTT; blue top), and levels of blood urea nitrogen, creatinine, sodium, potassium, chloride, and bicarbonate (usually red top). Other studies also may be useful, so save any extra blood in a red top tube. Your responsibility includes being certain that the tube for type and crossmatch is properly labeled. The second most common cause of major transfusion reactions is failure to label this tube properly. Also, the blood bank will not release blood for your patient unless labeling is complete.

Considerations of speed and safety strongly favor the use of arm veins. If no suitable arm vein can be found, the femoral vein is a second choice. Internal jugular or subclavian vein approaches have greater risks, take longer, require the Trendelenburg position, and in general use smaller catheters incapable of the rapid flow rates that can be obtained through 4 cm–long 14- or 16-gauge catheters. A single 16-gauge catheter has a larger cross-sectional area and allows higher flow rates than two 18-gauge catheters.[1]

During the 15 minutes it takes to infuse the first 2 L of fluid, insert a second large-bore IV catheter and ascertain pertinent information regarding allergies, medication, and past medical history. Aspirin, warfarin, nonsteroidal antiinflammatory agents such as ibuprofen, and other drugs may profoundly affect bleeding and therapy. The initial hematocrit in an active bleeding patient may be an indicator of preexisting blood loss; it does not measure the magnitude of the current blood loss.

Vital signs are usually obtained at this point. Tachycardia and hypotension may not reflect the severity of blood loss. Young patients in particular maintain perfusion pressure by vasoconstriction. Cool extremities and a base deficit may be better indicators of significant hemorrhage than a change in vital signs. The pulse rate is misleading in patients taking beta-adrenergic blocking drugs, and cardiac output may not increase in response to anemia. The patient's premorbid state of health and nutrition should be assessed to determine any preexisting volume or red cell deficits. Patients with signs and symptoms of malnutrition may be hypovolemic and anemic on the basis of a catabolic state. These losses must be replaced in addition to the measured and estimated losses caused by the acute hemorrhagic event.

The best resuscitation strategy for acute bleeding is to stop the bleeding while replacing the volume loss. Soon after the initial presentation, you must decide if the patient needs to go for surgery or interventional radiologic workup. If a procedure is necessary to stop the bleeding, the outcome generally will be better if it is performed early, thereby avoiding a large-volume resuscitation. Apply direct pressure on external sites of hemorrhage when possible. Bleeding from pelvic fractures and perhaps other intraperitoneal sites may benefit from application of the pneumatic antishock garment. In all cases of acute hemorrhage, obtain a surgical consultation and decide on the most appropriate method to stop the bleeding.

TABLE 43-1. Management of Massive Hemorrhage

1. Establish an adequate airway and ensure adequate ventilation.
2. Obtain initial vital signs.
3. Insert a large (14- or 16-gauge) intravenous catheter, preferably in an arm vein. Simultaneously obtain a blood sample and request type and crossmatch, CBC, PT, PTT, BUN, creatinine, sodium, potassium, chloride, and bicarbonate.
4. Give 1–2 L of crystalloid rapidly (>100 mL/min) unless blood pressure rises and is stable.
5. Evaluate the need for surgery now! Put direct pressure on the site of hemorrhage when possible. Evaluate use of interventional radiologic or endoscopic procedures now.
6. Estimate the present volume deficit and the deficit in 40–60 min at present rate of hemorrhage. Order the appropriate no. of RBC units.
7. Insert a second large intravenous cannula.
8. If hemorrhage continues, give crossmatched packed RBCs as soon as they are available.
9. If hemorrhage is massive, order universal donor packed cells (O positive for male patients, O negative for female patients; ready in 10 min). Type-specific RBCs (20 min) also can be ordered.
10. Heat the room, warm all solutions (crystalloid and blood products), and use a warming blanket. Maintain body temperature at 37°C!
11. After 6 to 8 units of packed RBCs are transfused, give fresh frozen plasma at a ratio of 1 to 2 units for each additional 2 units of packed cells. Fresh frozen plasma must be ordered 35 to 45 min before it is needed. Anticipate!
12. After replacing 8 to 10 units of packed red cells, give platelets at a ratio of 1:1 (i.e., 6 units of platelets with the 14th, 20th, and 26th units of RBCs). Fresh platelets or liquid stored platelets <48 h old are recommended.
13. If the patient had a deficiency in plasma volume, red cell mass, platelets, or clotting factors before the hemorrhagic event, replace them at the initiation of resuscitation.
14. Measure hematocrit, PT, PTT, Ca^{2+}, and platelet count periodically and modify therapy as necessary.
15. Give 1 ampule of calcium *slowly* after every 4 to 6 units of packed RBCs *only* if the rate of infusion approaches 1 unit every 5 min. Follow Ca^{2+} levels when possible; otherwise, monitor QT intervals.
16. Reconsider surgical or interventional radiologic methods to stop the hemorrhage.
17. Consider using blood salvage and rapid infusion systems.
18. Maintain patient temperature.

CBC, complete blood cell count; PT, prothrombin time; PTT, partial thromboplastin time; BUN, blood urea nitrogen; Ca^{2+}, calcium; RBCs, red blood cells.

ESTIMATING THE ACUTE DEFICIT

Shock is manifested by inadequate organ perfusion. Progressive peripheral vasoconstriction occurs to preserve blood flow to the kidneys, heart, and brain. Cool extremities from the vasoconstriction and tachycardia to maintain cardiac output are the earliest measurable manifestation of hypovolemic shock. Inadequate perfusion at the cellular level causes metabolic acidosis. Although these responses may not be maximal at the time the patient presents, or the volume loss may be ongoing, an initial estimate of the volume deficit is possible based on the physiologic parameters listed in Table 43-2.[2] Significant hemorrhage may not be accompanied by clinically apparent changes in vital signs.[3,4] You must consider the possibility that even "stable" patients are hemorrhaging actively. The physiologic response to hemorrhage takes time to become manifest. Therefore, once treatment begins, the response to the initial fluid resuscitation is the key to determining subsequent therapy (Table 43-3).

Initial Therapy

A 15% to 30% blood loss (1.5 to 3 units of blood) results in tachycardia, tachypnea, and a decrease in pulse pressure. Most of such patients require transfusion. However, they can be easily stabilized with crystalloid during the initial resuscitation. An acute blood loss of 30% to 40% of blood volume (3 to 4 units) results in a reduction in systolic blood pressure, significant tachycardia, and tachypnea. Transfusion is usually required. A loss of more than 40% (over 4 units of blood) is life threatening, with symptoms including marked tachycardia, significant depression of systolic blood pressure, narrow pulse pressure, and, frequently, unobtainable auscultatory diastolic pressure. The skin is cold and pale.

Initial therapy is based on an evaluation of the severity of shock according to the criteria found in Table 43-2. Subsequent therapy must be titrated to the response to initial fluid resuscitation (see Table 43-3). If the initial blood loss was less than 20%, a rapid response to the initial fluid resuscita-

TABLE 43-2. Estimated Fluid and Blood Requirements in a 70-kg Man°

	CLASS I	CLASS II	CLASS III	CLASS IV
Blood loss (mL)	<750	750–1500	1500–2000	≥2000
Blood loss (% BV)	<15%	15–30%	30–40%	≥40%
Pulse rate	<100	>100	>120	≥140
Blood pressure	Normal	Normal	Decreased	Decreased
Pulse pressure (mm Hg)	Normal or increased	Decreased	Decreased	Decreased
Capillary blanch test	Normal	Positive	Positive	Positive
Respiratory rate	14–20	20–30	30–40	>35
Urine output (mL/h)	30 or more	20–30	5–15	Negligible
CNS–mental status	Slight anxious	Mildly anxious	Anxious and confused	Confused and lethargic
Fluid replacement (3.1 rule)	Crystalloid	Crystalloid	Crystalloid + blood	Crystalloid + blood

BV, blood volume.

From *Advanced Trauma Life Support Program for Physicians: Instructor Manual.* American College of Surgeons Committee on Trauma, 1993:8.

°Applied blindly, these guidelines can result in excessive or inadequate fluid administration. For example, a patient with a crush injury to the extremity will have hypotension out of proportion to blood loss and will require fluids *in excess* of the 3:1 guidelines, but a paient whose ongoing blood loss is being replaced will require *less* than 3:1. The use of bolus therapy with careful monitoring of the patient's response can moderate these extremes.

tion should occur. In the absence of ongoing bleeding, blood transfusion should not be required. The need for surgery varies with the etiology of the bleeding. A transient response to the initial fluid bolus indicates either inadequate resuscitation or ongoing blood loss. In both cases, the severity of the hemorrhage was underestimated. These patients have lost 20% to 40% of their blood volume and may die without blood transfusion and surgical treatment. Patients who do not respond to the initial fluid bolus need immediate blood transfusion (uncrossmatched type-specific or type O blood if no crossmatched blood is available) and most likely require emergency surgery.

Our hypothetical patient has a blood loss greater than 40%, with no evidence that the bleeding has stopped. Eight units of packed red blood cells should be ordered immediately and transfusion begun as soon as the blood is available.

TABLE 43-3. Responses to Initial Fluid Resuscitation°

	RAPID RESPONSE	TRANSIENT RESPONSE	NO RESPONSE
Vital signs	Return to normal	Transient improvement: recurrence of ↓BP and ↑HR	Remain abnormal
Estimated blood loss	Minimal (10–20%)	Moderate and ongoing (20–40%)	Severe (>40%)
Need for more crystalloid	Low	High	High
Need for blood	Low	Moderate–high	Immediate
Blood preparation	Type and crossmatch	Type–specific	Emergency blood release
Need for operative intervention	Possibly	Likely	Highly likely
Surgical consultation	Yes	Yes	Yes

BP, blood pressure; HR, heart rate.

From *Advanced Trauma Life Support Program for Physicians: Instructor Manual.* American College of Surgeons Committee on Trauma, 1993:8.

°2000 mL Ringer's lactate in adults or 20 mL/kg Ringer's lactate in children, over 10 to 15 min.

Crystalloids should be infused rapidly in the interim period. Colloid therapy is controversial and has not proven to be more efficacious than crystalloid infusion. It is also significantly more expensive.[5,6] Give 1 to 2 L of crystalloid and, if the blood pressure rises, continue this infusion until red cells are available. If the blood pressure falls again or fails to rise with rapid infusion of 2 L of crystalloid, order type-specific or universal donor blood.[1] The use of such blood is associated with a less than 1% incidence rate of complications.[7] Nevertheless, most patients in the ICU can be stabilized long enough to wait for fully crossmatched blood.

Bleeding and Clotting

If stabilization is not easily achieved and more than 10 to 12 units of blood probably will be required because of continued bleeding, order FFP and platelets. Thirty to 45 minutes are necessary to thaw, prepare, and deliver FFP, and 1 to 3 hours may be needed to obtain platelets. Accordingly, early anticipation of the patient's needs prevents significant delays in treating a coagulopathy that results from platelet and other clotting factor deficits. Platelets should be ordered earlier if any antiplatelet drugs have been ingested (e.g., aspirin, ibuprofen). At least 2 units of FFP and 10 mg of subcutaneous or IV vitamin K should be administered if warfarin has been taken recently.

Hypothermia may have a significant negative impact on the success of resuscitation. With a volume deficit of 40%, the skin is cool (near room temperature) because of vasoconstriction. With rehydration, warmer core blood flows through the periphery and is rapidly cooled, effectively reducing the core temperature. Platelets have a marked, but reversible, functional impairment as a result of hypothermia. In addition, the complex chemical reactions of the clotting mechanism are temperature dependent. Thus, hypothermia may inhibit hemostasis.

All fluids should be warmed to 37°C and efforts made to maintain body temperature from the outset. The most practical means of raising body temperature are increasing the room temperature, using blood warmers for all IV solutions, warming and humidifying inspired gas, and applying a hyperthermia blanket or a warm air blower over exposed body surface. However, these measures are inefficient in warming a cold patient, serving only to help maintain the current temperature.

SUBACUTE BLOOD VOLUME DEFICIENCY

Case 2: A preoperative evaluation is performed on a 45-year-old man scheduled for drainage of a pelvic abscess. Two weeks earlier he underwent emergency sigmoid colon resection and colostomy for perforated diverticulitis and initially did well. On day 5 he began eating, but he developed nausea and vomiting 2 days later. On day 9, parenteral nutrition was initiated. A computed tomography scan reveals a small pelvic abscess. The patient has no history of cardiac, renal, or pulmonary disease. He feels well, has had several loose bowel movements, has taken some oral fluids, and has a temperature of 37.5°C.

Examination suggests that he is well hydrated and has clear lungs, a nontender abdomen, and slight peripheral edema. His hematocrit is 34%, white blood cell count is 10,000/mm[3], and serum albumin is 3.6 g/dL; the rest of his laboratory study results are normal. You determine that this man is a good operative risk, needs no preoperative ICU evaluation, and wonder why you were asked to see him, because antibiotics have already been started.

At 3 AM, the patient is transferred on an emergency basis to the ICU with a temperature of 39.5°C and a systolic blood pressure of 70 mm Hg by palpation. You rule out bleeding and cardiogenic shock, and take all the appropriate steps to treat sepsis. The patient responds, and by 7 AM he is alert and hemodynamically stable, with a normal urine output, cardiac output, and pulmonary artery occlusion pressure. To your astonishment his hematocrit is now 23%, and his albumin is 2.8 g/dL. Where did all that blood go?

CAUSES

Blood volume deficiency (Table 43-4) in the hospitalized and chronically ill patient results from poor nutrition, GI losses, fever or inadequate volume replacement, and chronic vasoconstriction.[8,9] Routine, frequent phlebotomy to obtain blood for diagnostic tests reduces blood volume significantly.

TABLE 43-4. Algorithm for Subacute Blood Volume Deficiency

1. Chronic blood volume deficiency is common in hospitalized, chronically ill patients.

2. The deficit is difficult to diagnose; it can be 20–30% or more of the normal blood volume.

3. Heart rate, systolic and diastolic blood pressure, respiratory rate, hematocrit, albumin, urine output, central venous pressure, pulmonary artery occlusion pressure, and cardiac output can be near normal.

4. The diagnosis can be made by measuring blood volume using ^{51}Cr-labeled red cells, a test often not readily available. High index of suspicion must prevail.

5. Subacute deficiencies are almost routine in patients with mild chronic sepsis, prolonged bowel preparations, intestinal fistulae, long-term total parenteral nutrition, advanced cancer, prolonged ICU stays, and poor nutrition.

6. Patients with marked subacute deficiencies tolerate anesthesia, hemorrhage, and stress poorly.

7. The most effective treatment is replacement with packed red cells; such therapy is controversial.

8. Treatment with crystalloid or colloid increases urine output without increasing blood volume.

9. Assume a subacute deficiency is present if a relatively small stress or hemorrhage causes a greater than expected physiologic derangement.

10. Be prepared to transfuse packed cells early in patients undergoing second operations or those who are in the ICU for prolonged periods.

The deficit can be as much as 20% to 40% of normal blood volume.[8] Routine clinical assessment, including heart rate, systolic and diastolic pressure, respiratory rate, hematocrit, and urine output are generally near normal. The diagnosis of blood volume deficit can be assessed more accurately using ^{51}Cr-labeled red cells, but this test is not readily available.

DIAGNOSIS

The deficit should be suspected in any chronically ill hospitalized patient. Accordingly, you must have a high index of suspicion and assume a preexisting deficit, especially when relatively small hemorrhagic events or stress cause greater than expected changes in physiologic parameters. Crystalloid infusions increase urine output but do not expand blood volume significantly. Indirect confirmation of this syndrome occurs when infusion of 1 to 2 units of packed red blood cells fails to increase the hematocrit. Presumably, the red cells expand the peripheral circulation and recruit plasma proportionally, resulting in an unchanged hematocrit.

TRANSFUSION

Clinicians often are reluctant to transfuse patients with hematocrits over 30%. This decision is rational, provided that the plasma volume is normal. However, if a *total* volume deficit of 30% is present, restoration of the *plasma* volume yields a hematocrit of only 21%. (Total blood volume equals 60 mL/kg times 70 kg, or 4250 mL. A 30% deficit, or 4250 mL times 70% of normal, yields a blood volume of 2975 mL. If the measured hematocrit is 30%, the red cell mass is 900 mL. When blood volume is expanded to normal, the new hematocrit is 900/4250 times 100, equaling 21%). Few would argue against transfusion when the "true" hematocrit is 21%.

Anticipate the need to transfuse packed cells early in patients undergoing secondary operations or those requiring prolonged stays in the ICU. For the syndrome described, therapy continues to be controversial. No prospective studies demonstrate the efficacy of restoring red cell mass and plasma volume to normal in critically ill patients. Disease transmission through blood products has reduced the enthusiasm for transfusion. Prospective studies are in progress to determine whether these large, subacute deficiencies require treatment. Until the risk of transfusion is proven to be justified in these relatively asymptomatic patients, realize that 20% to 40% blood volume deficits may exist and be prepared to transfuse immediately when patients become symptomatic.

CHRONIC ANEMIA ∎

The problem of chronic anemia is not of major concern in the ICU. An algorithm for its evaluation and treatment is summarized in Table 43-5.[10]

TABLE 43-5. Algorithm for Chronic Anemia

1. In an asymptomatic patient with no major stress, no treatment is indicated until the cause is determined. Determine iron, iron binding capacity, vitamin B_{12}, folate, red cell indices, Coombs' test, and reticulocyte count. A thorough history and physical examination, including stool guaiac, often reveal the cause.

2. Young, previously healthy patients can tolerate a stable hematocrit of 20% after an acute hemorrhage event.

3. If further stress is anticipated in an asymptomatic anemic patient (e.g., rebleed, second operation, sepsis), give oral iron.

4. If further stress is anticipated, transfuse to a hematocrit of 30% before surgery.

5. Patients with chronic renal failure tolerate hematocrits of 18–22% well and do not require transfusion prior to surgery. Patients who have received 2 to 3 units of packed red cells depleted of 2,3-DPG for an acute hemorrhage event may no longer have an elevated P_{50}. They may require higher hematocrit during and immediately after the acute hemorrhagic event for adequate oxygen transport.

6. Patients with severe coronary artery disease may need a hematocrit of 35% to control angina.

7. Patients with severe chronic lung disease often have hematocrits above 50% and often need hematocrits above 40% to wean from ventilator support.

HISTORY OF BLOOD TRANSFUSION ∎

Descriptions of the mystical qualities of blood appeared as early as 200 A.D., when bloodletting was performed to rid the body of evil humors.[11] The properties of blood also were thought to impose positive effects and to embody the physical and mental attributes of the donor[12]; for example, Romans drank the blood from slain gladiators to acquire their physical prowess. Exchanging "old blood" for new was reported in the 1400s when blood from three young boys was given to Pope Innocent VIII as a rejuvenator.[13] The boys died from exsanguination and the pope, whose "rejuvenation" failed, died shortly thereafter.

After Harvey demonstrated that blood circulated in the body, the first successful blood transfusion was performed in humans. Before the Royal Society in London, Richard Lower transfused blood from a lamb into Arthur Loga, "a mildly melancholy insane man," to improve his unbalanced character. The patient did well and returned to the Society 6 days later to report his progress.[14]

In contrast to this positive experience, John Baptiste-Denis, in the same year, transfused blood from a calf into Antoin Mauroy, who was then suffering from "rage."[15] Baptiste-Denis reasoned that the docile quality of the calf's blood might provide a calming effect on the maniacal Mauroy. After suffering a well-documented transfusion reaction, Mauroy was given a repeat blood transfusion that resulted in his death. Discouraged and dishonored, Baptiste-Denis was accused of murder by Mauroy's wife (perhaps the first reported malpractice case) and was subsequently arrested.

As a result, species-nonspecific blood transfusions lost favor for approximately 200 years.

In 1818, James Blundell initiated the first species-specific (human-to-human) transfusion for acute hemorrhage.[16] Blundell, an obstetrician-gynecologist, successfully used homologous blood transfusions to resuscitate women from exsanguinating postpartum hemorrhage. Despite these successes, transfusions of homologous blood frequently resulted in severe and often fatal reactions.

Not until 1900 did Landsteiner[17] recognize the importance of ABO blood grouping. In 1911, Ottenberg[18] developed the concept and practice of preliminary crossmatching of blood before its administration. In 1937, Fantis[19] established the first blood bank at the Cook County Hospital in Chicago, and modern storage and distribution of blood for the general population became available.

RED BLOOD CELL TRANSFUSION

RATIONALE

The primary indication for transfusing red cells is to maintain or restore the blood's oxygen-carrying capacity. Oxygen delivery to the tissues is directly dependent on cardiac output and the arterial oxygen content of the blood. Most oxygen is hemoglobin bound, whereas a small portion is dissolved in the plasma. The most important functional feature of hemoglobin is its ability to bind reversibly with oxygen. The hemoglobin molecule releases oxygen to the tissues more easily when it is fully saturated; a marked increase in oxygen affinity occurs when it is only partially saturated.

The partial pressure of oxygen at which the hemoglobin is 50% saturated (P_{50}) is a measure of oxygen affinity. The normal adult value is 26 mm Hg. Fever, acidosis, and increased levels of 2,3-diphosphoglycerate (2,3-DPG) diminish oxygen-hemoglobin affinity, facilitating oxygen release when tissue oxygen requirements are increased. Tissue oxygen consumption is calculated from the product of cardiac output and the difference between the arterial and the mixed venous oxygen contents, $C(a - \bar{v})O_2$.

The normal oxygen transport system has a large reserve capacity that responds to physiologic stress and provides a margin of safety if any portion of the system becomes impaired. This feature is best demonstrated by the relationship between normal oxygen consumption (250 mL/minute) and oxygen delivery (1000 mL/minute). The amount of available oxygen is four times that which is normally consumed.

However, if one looks more closely at the supply side of the equation, that is, oxygen delivery, we notice that it is defined as arterial oxygen content (CaO_2) times cardiac output. Content is further defined as the amount of oxygen that is carried by hemoglobin (Hgb):

$$CaO_2 = (Hgb \times 1.39 \times SaO_2) + (0.0031 \times PaO_2)$$

where 1.39 equals milliliters of oxygen per gram of Hgb; SaO_2 equals Hgb saturation with oxygen; and 0.0031 equals milliliters per deciliter solubility of oxygen in plasma at 37°C.

The solubility coefficient of oxygen in plasma is so low that the contribution of oxygen partial pressure relative to total oxygen delivery is almost insignificant. For example, if a patient has a hemoglobin concentration of 14 g/dL, an arterial oxyhemoglobin saturation of 100%, a PaO_2 of 100 mm Hg, and a cardiac output of 5 L/minute, the amount of delivered oxygen is 988 mL/minute. If the PaO_2 increases by 20%, that is, from 100 to 120 mm Hg, while the hemoglobin concentration and cardiac output remain the same, oxygen delivery increases only 1.6%, to 1004 mL/minute. Thus, an increase in PaO_2 gained by increasing the fraction of inspired oxygen does not dramatically augment oxygen delivery.

Conversely, alterations in the hemoglobin concentration may impact significantly on oxygen delivery. For example, a 20% increase in hemoglobin concentration from 14 to 16.8 g/dL, assuming the negligible effect of PaO_2 and given a constant cardiac output of 5 L/minute, yields a 20% increase in oxygen delivery (973 to 1167 mL/minute). A similar relationship can be found for cardiac output.

HEMOGLOBIN CONCENTRATION AND BLOOD VOLUME

The relationship between hemoglobin concentration and blood volume is also of critical importance. A normal hemoglobin concentration and a reduced blood volume are more deleterious than a reduced hemoglobin concentration and normal blood volume. Reference to the oxygen delivery formula shows that if a hemoglobin concentration of 15 g/dL is reduced to 10 g/dL (assuming a PaO_2 of 60 mm Hg and a SaO_2 of 90%), oxygen delivery falls from 990 to 612 mL/minute.

Minimally Acceptable Hemoglobin

Examples such as this were used in the past to justify the concept that a hemoglobin concentration of 10 g/dL, with a SaO_2 of 90% or greater, was optimal for oxygen delivery. However, if the hemoglobin concentration of 10 g/dL was associated with a cardiac output of 3 L/minute as a result of a reduction in blood volume (SaO_2 of 90% and PaO_2 of 60 mm Hg), oxygen delivery would fall from 610 to 366 mL/minute, clearly an inadequate value despite a minimally acceptable hemoglobin concentration. Conversely, even if the hemoglobin concentration was reduced to 8 g/dL, as long as the body compensated with an increase in cardiac output (i.e., 6 L/minute), oxygen delivery could be sustained at 600 mL/minute.

Thus, a normal or minimally acceptable hemoglobin concentration associated with a reduced blood volume may not be adequate to meet cellular demands, whereas a reduced hemoglobin concentration associated with a normal blood volume (and an appropriately compensated cardiac output) often meets the challenge of oxygen delivery.

The importance of the association between hemoglobin concentration and blood volume was recently illustrated by Spence and colleagues[20] who, while caring for a group of Jehovah's Witnesses, failed to identify a difference in outcome in patients undergoing major surgical procedures whose preoperative hemoglobin concentration exceeded 10 g/dL, compared with those whose values were less than 10 g/dL but greater than 6 g/dL of hemoglobin. However, if blood volume was reduced intraoperatively (defined as greater than 500 mL of blood loss), mortality rate rose from 0% to 7.4%.

Optimal Hemoglobin Concentration

EXPERIMENTAL STUDIES.   The concept of optimal hemoglobin concentration has been challenged. Until recently (as observed earlier), most clinicians supported a "transfusion trigger" of 10 g/dL despite experimental and clinical data that supported efficacy at lower hemoglobin levels. To identify the limits of cardiac compensation in acute anemia, Wilkerson and colleagues,[21] using a paralyzed, anesthetized, normovolemic, anemic primate model, identified a net positive increase in myocardial lactate production when hematocrit fell below 10%. They further noted that compensatory mechanisms for low hemoglobin concentration (increase in cardiac output, decrease in systemic vascular resistance, increase in left ventricular blood flow, and decrease in left ventricular resistance) did not occur until the hemoglobin concentration fell below 7 g/dL (hematocrit 21%).

The animals used were healthy primates that were anesthetized, paralyzed, and euthanized within 6 hours; thus, correlation with the clinical setting was unclear. Accordingly, the same investigators again selected a normovolemic, anemic, primate model, but attempted to recreate surgical stress and anemia by performing laparotomy on 19 adult baboons, followed by an exchange transfusion of 6% hetastarch, yielding a final hematocrit of 15%. The animals were then observed for 2 months. The results indicated no morbidity or mortality, with all hematocrits approaching baseline at the conclusion of the study.[22]

CORONARY ARTERY DISEASE.   Animals might survive extremely low hemoglobin concentrations as a result of having presumably normal coronary arteries with the ability to increase myocardial oxygen delivery in compensation for maximal oxygen extraction. What are the compensatory mechanisms, if any, in persons who sustain acute anemia and who, in addition, have coronary artery disease? This scenario has been best described by Case and associates,[23] who in a canine model identified that the association between coronary artery stenosis and anemia produced a far greater depression in myocardial performance than either anemia alone or the combination of coronary artery stenosis and normal hemoglobin concentration. They conclude that there is no universal (optimal) hemoglobin concentration. Rather, a transfusion trigger must be individualized in response to the variability in comorbidity associated with most critically ill patients.

The young, healthy trauma victim, who in most instances can be assumed to have normal coronary artery anatomy, may safely sustain hemoglobin concentrations far below 10 g/dL, provided that a normal blood volume exists. However, persons with coronary artery disease, who usually cannot augment coronary artery blood flow in compensation for acute anemia, may require higher hemoglobin concentra-

tions and should undergo transfusion. A hematocrit less than 28% was significantly associated with myocardial ischemia and cardiac death in high-risk vascular patients in an ICU.[24]

Recommendations

This conclusion has been supported by the National Institutes of Health Consensus Development Conference.[25] The group concluded the following:

> . . . the decision to transfuse a specific patient should take into consideration the duration of anemia, the intravascular volume, the extent of the operation, the probability for massive blood loss, and the presence of coexisting conditions such as pulmonary function, inadequate cardiac output, myocardial ischemia, and cerebral vascular or peripheral circulatory output, myocardial ischemia, and cerebral vascular or peripheral circulatory disease. These factors are representative of the universe of considerations that compromise clinical judgment. No single measure can replace good clinical judgment for decisions regarding perioperative transfusion. However, current experience would suggest that otherwise healthy patients with hemoglobin values of 10 g/dL or greater rarely require perioperative transfusion. Whereas those with acute anemia with resulting hemoglobin values of less than 7 mg/dL frequently required red blood cell transfusions, it appears that some patients with chronic anemia, such as those with chronic renal failure, tolerate hemoglobin values of less than 7 g/dL. The decision to transfuse red blood cells depends on clinical assessment that is aided by laboratory data such as arterial oxygenation, mixed venous oxygen tension, cardiac output, the oxygen extraction ratio, and blood volume when indicated.

2,3-DIPHOSPHOGLYCERATE

Reduced red cell 2,3-DPG causes increased hemoglobin-oxygen affinity and diminished tissue oxygen release. Levels of 2,3-DPG rapidly decrease in red cells stored in the liquid state to less than 10% after 2 weeks.[26] Transfusion of 2,3-DPG–depleted red cells is reported to have potentially adverse clinical implications.[27] Restoration of 2,3-DPG in circulating transfused red cells may take 24 to 48 hours in healthy persons and considerably longer in metabolically deranged patients.[28]

Proponents of infusion of 2,3-DPG–enriched red blood cells suggest that near-normal oxygen release is critical during the acute phase of resuscitation, when oxygen delivery is impaired because of decreased red cell mass and diminished cardiac output.[29] Fresh blood, citrate-phosphate-dextrose-adenine (CPDA) blood less than 14 days old, and cryopreserved red cells provide enough 2,3-DPG for nearly normal oxygen release when it is most needed.

STORAGE AND CONVENTIONAL PRESERVATION

Fresh, warm whole blood most effectively restores red cell mass, plasma volume, platelets, and clotting factors. However, the blood bank cannot be expected to have donors of each blood type available at a moment's notice. In addition, the requirement for testing blood for hepatitis and AIDS requires storage, during which time platelets and clotting factors rapidly deteriorate. Therefore, fresh whole blood is not currently available, and component therapy is the mainstay of blood banking practice (Table 43-6).

Whole blood is collected from a donor into a closed system of plastic bags containing an anticoagulant. Packed red blood cells (hematocrit of 70% to 80%) are prepared by removing approximately 200 mL of plasma by either centrifugation or gravity sedimentation. The cells usually are stored in a liquid state at 4°C. Anticoagulation is achieved with either citrate-phosphate-dextrose (CPD) or CPD plus adenine, glucose, mannitol, and sodium chloride (Adsol). Red cells preserved in CPD for 1, 2, or 3 weeks yield 90%, 80%, and 70% 24-hour posttransfusion cell survivals, respectively.[30] Those stored in Adsol for 42 days have only a 65% 24-hour red cell survival. Thus, 10 units of 42-day-old, Adsol-preserved red blood cells effectively donate 6.5 units of blood to the recipient 24 hours following transfusion.

Clinicians have difficulty assessing the therapeutic effectiveness of blood product transfusions because of biologic variability, the diverse disease processes treated, and the lack of standardization of blood product "units." A unit of whole blood is defined as 450 mL (±10%) plus 63 mL of anticoagulant. If one donor has a borderline low but acceptable hemoglobin of 12.5 g/dL and a "short draw" of 405 mL, whereas another has a hemoglobin of 17 g/dL and a "large draw" of 495 mL, the hemoglobin in the acceptable unit varies from 50.6 to 84.1 g. In other words, 8 small-volume, low-hemoglobin units are equivalent to 5 large-volume, high-hemoglobin units.

To confuse matters even more, not all transfused red cells survive. Taking these variables into account, one can devise a clinical scenario in which 6.7 small, 50.6-g hemoglobin units transfused near the end of their storage period are required to provide the same number of red cells as 3 large

units transfused after a brief storage period. Small wonder that the incremental rise in hemoglobin after transfusion often differs from the predicted norm. Clinicians have little control over donors, collection, processing, storage, and distribution of the blood products ordered. The development of strict standards of blood banking is essential to quality and quantity assurance.

Cryopreservation

Cryopreservation has the potential to provide the optimally stored red cell product. Red cells stored at −80°C in 40% glycerol for as long as 21 years demonstrate acceptable in vitro storage criteria and clinical efficacy. The 24-hour posttransfusion survival of cryopreserved red cells ranges from 80% to 90%.[30] Oxygen release is similar to that of fresh whole blood because the 2,3-DPG level is normal. Antigenic immune reactions are minimized by the near elimination of platelets and leukocytes. Large quantities of red blood cells, including rare blood types, can be stockpiled. Recognizing these distinct advantages, the Department of Defense approved cryopreserved red cells for routine preservation.

Leukocyte-Depleted and Washed Packed Red Blood Cells

Leukocyte-depleted red cells can be prepared by passing packed red blood cells through cellulose acetate, polyester, or cotton wool filters during packed cell preparation or during administration of the unit, although the latter process slows the transfusion. Leukocyte-depleted red cells decrease the risk of immune suppression and do not cause nonhemolytic transfusion reactions. A decreased risk of transmission of certain viral diseases associated with white blood cells

TABLE 43-6. Characteristics of Component Therapies

BLOOD COMPONENT	CONTENT	VOLUME (mL)	HEMATOCRIT (%)	PLASMA		
				Platelets	*mL*	*Shelf-life*
Whole blood	450 mL blood: RBCs, plasma, WBCs	500	40–45	Nonviable	108–305	42 d in Adsol
CPDA	Platelets; 63 mL CPD, 60 g hemoglobin	—	—	—	—	21 days in CPD at 4°C
RBCs	RBCs, WBCs, platelets; 60 g hemoglobin	250–350	70	Nonviable	40–115	42 d in Adsol; 35 d in CPDA; 21 d in CPD
Frozen RBCs	RBCs, minimal WBCs and platelets, no plasma; 54 g hemoglobin	170–190	90	None	0	24 y at −80°C 72 h at 4°C
Platelets, single donor	Platelets; some WBCs, plasma, and RBCs	300	0	$3–8 \times 10^{11}$	250	24 h at 22°C, open

RBCs, red blood cells; WBCs, white blood cells; CPD, citrate–phosphate–dextrose; CPDA, CPD + adenine.

such as cytomegalovirus (CMV), Epstein-Barr virus (EBV), and possibly human immunodeficiency virus (HIV) should occur.[31]

Leukocyte-depleted packed red blood cells may be useful in patients with repeated allergic and febrile transfusion reactions, or in patients who have an increased risk for transfusion-associated viral transmission. Such cases include CMV, seronegative pregnant women, premature infants born to CMV-seronegative mothers, and patients who are immunosuppressed because of transplantation or AIDS.

Washing of red cells removes most of the plasma. Fewer plasma proteins, particularly antibodies, remain. This fact may be of importance in ABO-mismatched bone marrow recipients or in patients with blood admixture after transfusion of uncrossmatched type O blood.

Designated Donation

The major infectious risk of transfused blood, in terms of incidence and mortality, is hepatitis, not AIDS. The risk of becoming infected with hepatitis has greatly declined in the last decade, whereas the risks of transmission of AIDS after transfusion is low. Nonetheless, the general public has become fascinated with the risks of acquiring AIDS through blood transfusion. Hence, a demand for intraoperative blood salvage, preoperative autologous blood donation, and directed donation from relatives has increased.

Blood donations from relatives or friends designated for use by a specified recipient present several ethical and practical dilemmas.[32,33] Asking family members or friends to donate blood to replenish the blood bank after a loved one has received blood is to be encouraged. However, the notion that the friends or relatives of a patient requiring transfusion are somehow immune from high-risk behavior unknown to the recipient is dubious. These designated units may not meet Food and Drug Administration or local blood bank criteria for acceptable blood donation and if unused should be discarded.

Blood bank questions about high-risk behavior may discriminate against certain groups and represents an infringement of civil rights. This process ultimately may change the risk–benefit ratio of designated donations. That designated units are safer has not been shown; in fact, they may carry more risk than routine units. They are more expensive, because if they are not used for the specified patient, they are discarded.

Preoperative Autologous Donation

Preoperative autologous blood donation is the planned collection of blood from a patient scheduled for elective surgery who is likely to require blood transfusion. Patients undergoing elective procedures in which a preoperative crossmatch is usually required are candidates for autologous donation. They should be healthy enough to undergo elective surgery and have a hemoglobin higher than 11 g/dL.[34] Bacteremia is an absolute contraindication for autologous blood donation because bacteria can proliferate during storage. Homologous blood may still be required, and patients should be counseled about this possibility.

Autologous blood is generally collected starting at 6 weeks and continuing up to 3 days before surgery. Blood can be collected as often as every 3 days, but weekly donation is more common. Patients need to be monitored closely because anemia may preclude the donation of an adequate number of units. Vasovagal reactions associated with blood donation increase the morbidity of patients with cardiac or cerebrovascular disease. Recombinant human erythropoietin may increase the ability to donate blood preoperatively.[35]

Testing of autologous blood is the same as for homologous blood donations. Units that test positive will be released for autologous use with a written prescription from the patient's physician.[34] The addition of unused autologous units to the blood pool does not significantly increase the availability of blood. Furthermore, autologous blood units have a lower red cell mass and represent a lower quality product than the usual units collected by blood banks. Unused autologous units are destroyed, thus adding cost over that of "routine" blood.

FRESH FROZEN PLASMA ■

Fresh frozen plasma is removed from a unit of whole blood within 6 hours of collection and frozen at −18°C. Freezing protects factors V and VIII (the remainder of the coagulation factors are stable during liquid storage). All of the components of the coagulation, fibrinolytic, and complement systems, as well as the proteins that maintain oncotic pressure and modulate immunity, are present in FFP. Fats, carbohydrates, and minerals are present in concentrations similar to those in the donor.

INDICATIONS

Treatment with FFP is indicated for deficiencies of factors II, V, VIII, IX, and XI to reverse the effects of warfarin for antithrombin III deficiency; to treat thrombotic thrombocytopenic purpura; and to correct humoral immunodeficiencies. Administration of FFP after massive transfusion (more than one blood volume within several hours) is suggested, but supportive data for this recommendation are limited. In such patients, thrombocytopenia probably is more important than the depletion of plasma coagulation factors. FFP is not indicated as a volume expander or as a nutritional source.

Abnormal Clotting

Although numerous formulas are designed to guide FFP administration, few stand up to scientific scrutiny. Some investigators have suggested that FFP be administered in response to abnormal clotting parameters, that is, PT more than 16 seconds or PTT more than 60 seconds in patients about to undergo major surgical procedures.[36] Yet, the sensitivity and specificity of these laboratory determinations (PT and PTT) are 40% to 63% and 47% to 67%, respectively, when used preoperatively in predicting perioperative bleeding.[37] However, a strong correlation between postoperative bleeding and preoperative abnormal clotting tests has been observed if the PT and PTT were more than one and one half times normal[38] (these values are associated with factor V and VIII levels less than 20% of normal, as well as fibrinogen levels in the range of 75 mg/dL). Patients with preoperative PT and PTT not in excess of one and one half times normal failed to show evidence of significant postoperative bleeding.

The lack of correlation between abnormal clotting parameters and significant clinical bleeding can be explained as a result of adequate levels of clotting factors (30% to 50% of baseline) being available despite the prolongation of PT and PTT (as long as these values are less than one and one half times normal). Unfortunately, few studies support conclusive scientific recommendations. Accordingly, the patient who exhibits significantly abnormal clotting parameters in the perioperative period (approaching one and one half times control) should have those values corrected with FFP, although such therapy may result in some unnecessary transfusions.

Replacement of Coagulation Factors

Conflicting data exist with respect to the replacement of coagulation factors after massive transfusion. Here the outcome (control of hemorrhage or postoperative coagulopathy) has been evaluated clinically when shed blood has been replaced with whole blood, modified whole blood, or packed red blood cells. Some studies fail to reveal the type of blood replaced. Accordingly, comparisons among studies are difficult.

Counts and colleagues[39] failed to confirm levels of coagulation factors below adequate values in massively transfused patients receiving modified whole blood as replacement. They suggest that nonsurgical bleeding was a consequence of thrombocytopenia or disseminated intravascular coagulation (DIC) rather than dilutional coagulopathy.

Others have failed to reveal any significant differences of coagulation parameters in patients receiving FFP replaced by formula (1 unit FFP for every 3 units of fresh whole blood or packed red blood cells transfused) compared with those receiving whole blood or packed red blood cells alone.[40] This observation may be explained by the fact that 37% of initial plasma constituents remain in the circulation despite a full blood volume exchange transfusion.[41]

Prophylactic Administration

Most reports fail to support the prophylactic administration of FFP for the prevention of dilutional coagulopathy in the massively transfused patient if less than 2 blood volume equivalents have been replaced. However, if shock, hypotension, hypothermia, or previous liver disease is associated with massive transfusion (as is frequently the case), prophylactic administration of FFP may be warranted. In evaluating 36 trauma patients with at least 1 blood volume replacement, Harke and Rihman[42] failed to correlate abnormalities in the coagulation profile with perioperative bleeding. However, a strong association between the duration of hypotension and the development of a perioperative coagulopathy was noted.

We agree with Phillips and colleagues,[43] who suggest that one cannot predict which patients will develop a significant perioperative coagulopathy as a consequence of massive transfusion, especially those with prolonged hypotension, hypothermia, or shock. Because the risk of death from coagulopathy, once established, far exceeds the risk of disease transmission as a consequence of unnecessary FFP administration, the balance is clearly in favor of erring on the side of the prophylactic administration of FFP in this patient population. An example of such a schema can be found in Table 43-1. If the goal of prophylaxis is to replace clotting factors to adequate levels, volumes in the range of 10 to 15 mL/kg of FFP should be administered.

The major hazard of FFP administration is disease transmission. The risk of AIDS and hepatitis from FFP is thought to be the same as with the transfusion of red blood cells. Posttransfusion hepatitis, mainly non-A, non-B varieties, ranges up to 0.5% per unit. Allergic reactions vary from urticaria to fatal noncardiac pulmonary edema. Alloimmunization and volume overload also are possible complications.

CRYOPRECIPITATE

Cryoprecipitate is a plasma concentrate consisting primarily of factor VIII and fibrinogen in approximately 10 mL of plasma. A single unit of cryoprecipitate contains approximately 100 clotting units of factor VIII and 250 mg of fibrinogen. A clotting unit of factor VIII is the amount of factor VIII in 1 mL of fresh normal plasma. Cryoprecipitate is stored frozen and can be prepared for infusion at 37°C (complete thawing) in 10 minutes. Temperatures greater than 37°C cause a loss of factor VIII activity.

Cryoprecipitate is recommended for the replenishment of factor VIII, or fibrinogen. An average adult dose is 8 to 10 units, which results in an increase of 2% per unit in the factor VIII level. The most satisfactory way to judge the amount required is to measure the patient's circulating factor VIII level. Cryoprecipitate carries a greater risk of disease transmission because it is pooled from multiple donors.

PLATELETS

Platelets initiate vasoconstriction and platelet aggregation at sites of damaged vascular endothelium. The platelet is a small, disk-like structure with a life span of 10 days. One third of the platelets released from the marrow into the vascular space are stored in the spleen. When additional platelets are required to maintain hemostasis, splenic platelets are released. Marrow production increases if platelet mobilization is inadequate.

COLLECTION

Platelets are removed from a unit of fresh whole blood, first by differential centrifugation into platelet-rich plasma, then by repeat centrifugation, at which time most of the plasma is removed. The platelet pellet is resuspended in 50 mL of residual plasma and stored at 22°C. Platelets also can be collected by single-donor platelet pheresis. Heparinized, citrated donor blood flows into a continuous centrifuge that separates the blood into its components. The platelets are harvested, and the plasma and remaining cells are reinfused into the donor. Platelets so collected must be used within 24 hours of collection or they must be frozen. An advantage of this system is that 6 to 8 units of platelets can be collected from a single donor, presumably reducing the danger of disease transmission, compared with the collection of platelet transfusions from six or eight different donors.

CONCENTRATION

The number of platelets present in a unit to be transfused is variable. Guidelines state that a unit of platelets should contain 5.5×10^{10} platelets. A normal platelet count ranges between 15 and 44×10^{10}/L. A small unit from a donor with a low normal platelet count may contain only 6×10^{10} platelets, whereas a large unit from a donor with a high normal count may contain 22×10^{10} platelets. Platelet units contain only 70% of the platelets present in the original unit of whole blood; thus, a fresh unit of platelets can be as small as 4×10^{10} or as large as 15×10^{10}. Because donor platelet counts are not routinely measured, the variability can be even greater. Because platelet units are stored for up to 5 days in the blood bank, their therapeutic effectiveness deteriorates. A fresh, large unit can have many times the number of functional platelets available as a stored smaller unit.

FUNCTION

As a result of the release of thromboxane A_2 (a prostenoid instrumental in the initiation of the vasoconstriction phase of the clotting mechanism),[44] as well as aggregation resulting in a platelet plug, platelets effectively initiate clotting. They are released from the bone marrow and have a 10-day survival time. When available in adequate numbers (greater than 100,000 thrombocytes/mm³) and free from thrombocytopathy, platelets reduce the bleeding time to normal (5 to 8 minutes).

Platelet counts below 50,000/mm³ correlate with increased bleeding time.[45] Levels below 20,000/mm³ render the person to be at risk for microvascular bleeding and, in general, signal the need for prophylactic platelet transfusion.[46] Patients scheduled for surgery or those who are about to receive large-bore central hemodynamic monitoring catheters and who have platelet counts less than 50,000 platelets/mm³ are deserving of prophylactic platelet transfusions. In general, transfusion of platelets to achieve a posttransfusion platelet count of 100,000/mm³ or greater is the accepted norm.[47] By and large, 1 unit of administered platelets results in a net gain of 10,000 or more platelets/mm³ after transfusion.

Platelet Mass

The concept of platelet mass is critically important to the understanding of platelet function. Large platelets contain a greater number of platelet granules than smaller platelets. Because platelet granules are partly responsible for platelet function, large platelets are more hemostatically effective than smaller ones. Consequently, a low platelet count of predominantly large platelets can be as hemostatically effective as a higher platelet count comprising primarily small platelets. Thus, the platelet mass, as well as the number, should be considered before transfusion therapy is undertaken.

Storage

The collection and storage of platelets have an important effect on platelet function. For example, liquid-stored platelets (stored at room temperature for 24 to 48 hours) when transfused to aspirin-treated persons (aspirin inhibits thromboxane synthesis and prevents vasoconstriction such that bleeding time increases) fail to effect a reduction in bleeding time for 2 to 4 hours after transfusion. However, in the ensuing 18 to 20 hours of circulation, platelets regain their functional ability and effectively reduce bleeding time to normal.[47] Accordingly, the hemostatic effect of platelet transfusion in the acutely bleeding patient with an abnormal bleeding time may not be apparent immediately, and the administration of yet additional platelets within the first 4 hours of transfusion is not warranted. Extending the shelf-life to 5 days at room temperature, although associated with adequate viability, yields platelets with a reduced ability to synthesize thromboxane A_2.[44] Consequently, if transfusion of 5-day-old, liquid-stored, room temperature platelets fails to correct bleeding, fresh platelets may be required.

Hypothermia

Valeri and colleagues[48] showed that hypothermia produces a platelet defect characterized by the platelets' inability to synthesize thromboxane. The defect is totally reversible with rewarming. Reed and associates[49] failed to demonstrate the benefit of platelet transfusion in persons receiving more than 12 units of blood in a 12-hour period. Because the acute administration of 12 units of blood generally reduces the platelet count to levels below 100,000/mm³ and correspondingly increases bleeding time, the transfusion of functionally adequate platelets should have corrected the bleeding diathesis. However, because most massively transfused patients are rendered hypothermic as a result of inadequate warming techniques, the lack of efficacy of platelet transfusions may have resulted from the hypothermic effect rather than the platelets' inability to function normally. Similarly, if the platelets transfused in these studies had shelf-lives approaching 5 days, the storage defect itself may have been responsible for the lack of efficacy.

Because most recent studies fail to demonstrate a benefit of platelet administration in the massively transfused patient, any formula for platelet therapy based on units of blood transfused is unsubstantiated (assuming the bone marrow is functioning normally). In patients whose bone marrow production of platelets may be depressed, prophylactic platelet transfusions are indicated.

We suggest that platelets should not be transfused to the hypothermic patient who has adequate platelet numbers and a prolonged bleeding time and who continues to bleed. The return to normothermia should reverse the platelet defect as well as the abnormality in bleeding time. Similarly, in patients who are thrombocytopenic and hypothermic, we suggest active, aggressive rewarming in addition to platelet transfusion. However, if bleeding persists in a normothermic patient with adequate platelets and a prolonged bleeding time after transfusion with routinely collected and stored platelets, freshly collected platelets (up to 48 hours' shelf-life) should be administered.

Future Trends

Experimental cryopreservation of platelets has yielded a product with a normal linear life span and adequate hemostatic properties. Current research efforts are centered about the reduction in toxicity of dimethyl sulfoxide used as the preservative. Platelets that have been stored in the frozen state for 2 years effectively reduce the bleeding time in aspirin-treated patients.[50] Frozen, single-donor, pheresed platelets ultimately may prove to be the most versatile and reliable functional product.

DDAVP

1-Desamino-8-D-arginine-vasopressin (DDAVP, Desmopressin) has been shown to reduce significantly the bleeding time in patients with von Willebrand's disease,[51] uremia,[52] primary or acquired platelet disorders, and aspirin ingestion.[53] In addition, it has been shown to decrease intraoperative and postoperative blood loss in patients undergoing Harrington rod insertion[54] or cardiac bypass surgical procedures.[55] The mechanism of efficacy is probably related to an overall increase in the von Willebrand factor released from endogenous storage pools as a result of DDAVP stimulation.[56]

Few studies are available for wholesale recommendations. However, Rocha and colleagues[57] report that infusions of 0.3 or 0.4 μg/kg of DDAVP reduced the bleeding time to normal within 1 hour in 75% of patients with chronic renal failure and prolonged bleeding time. Most patients subsequently returned to baseline bleeding time levels within 8 hours. In most cases, tachyphylaxis occurs with prolonged therapy. In addition, DDAVP has been shown to be associated with mild to moderate hypertension[58] as well as hyponatremia because of its antidiuretic properties.[53]

TECHNICAL ASPECTS OF BLOOD PRODUCT ADMINISTRATION

A written order should be entered before the transfusion. In situations where this is not possible, the administration of blood products must be clearly documented. In the operating room, transfusions are recorded on the permanent anesthesia record. Indications for the use of blood products should be tested along with the transfusion order. Transfusion orders must take into consideration not only the current hematocrit but also ongoing blood loss, preexisting blood loss, and the patient's clinical condition, particularly with respect to cardiac and pulmonary comorbid states. With proper documentation, transfusion committees generally do not question a transfusion, even if the hematocrit is above 30%.

DILUTION OF PACKED RED BLOOD CELLS

Packed red blood cells can be administered as supplied by the blood bank. However, the fibrinogen and other plasma proteins increase viscosity. Diluting packed cells allows more rapid administration. Red blood cell concentrates should be diluted with 0.9% normal saline. Ringer's lactate does not contain sufficient calcium to cause clotting of citrated packed cells with hematocrits of less than 90%.[35] Blood can safely be administered through an IV administration set containing Ringer's lactate. Plasmalyte can be used to dilute packed cells because it contains magnesium and not calcium.

Dextrose in water might cause red blood cells to become agglomerated and thus slow the rate of blood transfusion, but it does not hemolyze red cells.[59] However, red blood cells transfused in 5% dextrose have decreased survival. In an emergency situation, one can safely infuse blood through a set that previously contained Ringer's lactate or dextrose in water. This approach is preferable to a delay in administering the transfusion or the loss of IV access caused by changing and flushing IV tubing sets.

RATE OF ADMINISTRATION

Blood products should be administered as rapidly as needed. There is no maximal safe rate of blood transfusion. If rapid blood administration is required in severe hemorrhagic shock, not only should consideration be given to diluting the packed red cells,[60] but the standard 170-μm screen filter should be removed from the infusion system. This filter is used to trap large microaggregates whose role in pulmonary complications of transfusion is unclear.[61] Rapid infusion systems and larger bore cannulae may be necessary (i.e., a 7-French introducer).

EMERGENCY TRANSFUSION IN HEMORRHAGIC SHOCK

In most cases of acute blood loss, a full crossmatch can be performed during the initial resuscitation with crystalloid. However, some patients who need immediate blood transfusion may die while waiting for a crossmatch to be completed. Type O uncrossmatched blood is immediately available and has been in routine use by the military for over 50 years.[62] Ideally, type O blood should be available in the resuscitation area before the arrival of the patient.[63] Type-specific blood can be available in less than half the time needed for full crossmatch. Of the over 60,000 transfusions of type O blood in 1952 during the Korean conflict, only four transfusion reactions occurred.[64]

During the Vietnam conflict, not only was a similar record of safety maintained, but almost all the transfusion reactions occurred after the use of group-specific blood and not type O blood.[64] Furthermore, type O reactions resulted from the accidental use of high-titer type O blood. Whereas civilian uncrossmatched blood use has been more restrained than military usage, a similar pattern of safety has been documented after administration of type O Rh-negative blood in women and type O Rh-positive in men.[63,65] If type O Rh-positive blood must be administered to reproductive-age women, they should receive human immune globulin containing IgC anti-D antibodies (RhoGAM) to prevent Rh immunization.

Type O blood contains antibodies to both type A and type B red cells antigen. The use of low antibody titer type O packed red blood cells minimizes the amount of antibody administered to the patient. Nonetheless, a hemolytic transfusion reaction can occur in patients who have had massive quantities of uncrossmatched blood. The presence of the antibodies can also create difficulties in the subsequent determination of the native blood type.

How much uncrossmatched blood can be transfused before problems develop with admixture of antibodies, and how much time must elapse before the problem resolves are unclear. A patient who has received more than 4 units of type O blood should be recrossmatched before receiving type-specific blood or blood crossmatched with a sample sent before the administration of type O blood. A safer practice may be to continue giving type O blood in massively transfused patients or in patients with residual antibody to the native blood type.[66]

INCOMPLETE CROSSMATCHED BLOOD

Incompletely crossmatched type-specific blood has an excellent safety record[65] and is preferred for emergency blood resuscitation by the American Association of Blood Banks.[67] Only 5 to 10 minutes are required to ensure major blood group compatibility. Additional time is necessary to draw and transport a clot to the blood bank and return with several units of packed cells. In a well-organized emergency department, this 20-minute or less delay does not jeopardize patient outcome. Fewer problems result with subsequent transfusion because the amount of uncrossmatched type O blood administered is minimized.[62]

TRANSFUSION COMPLICATIONS ◼

AGE OF TRANSFUSED BLOOD

To maintain blood stores and to avoid waste, the blood bank transfuses units that are the closest to their outdating period. A 24-hour posttransfusion red cell survival of greater than 70% is the only standard required. Whereas the real risks of transfusion have decreased, we are more aware of the potential risks. Transfused blood should be of the highest quality. Valeri[35] recommends that the 24-hour posttransfusion red cell survival be greater than 80% with normal oxygen transport function. To achieve this goal, blood must not be liquid-preserved at 4°C for more than 2 weeks.

Recent investigations purport to show an increased morbidity[68] or mortality[69] from the use of old stored blood units.[70] In one study, the median age of blood received by ICU patients who died had been stored significantly longer than the blood received by survivors.[71] The median age of blood units transfused was 16 days in survivors of septic shock compared with 25 days in patients who died. The number of units received by both groups was the same. Prolonged ICU stay is significantly associated with increased median age of transfused blood.[68] Survivors received fewer units that were more than 14 days old. These studies point to a potential benefit from using freshly processed blood.

MASSIVE TRANSFUSION

Massive transfusion is defined as the administration of more than 10 units of packed cells in less than 24 hours.[62] This value represents the entire blood volume of a 70-kg man. Complications include coagulopathy, thrombocytopenia, disease transmission, and abnormalities of oxygen transport, electrolytes, acid base status, and body temperature.[48] The effect of massive transfusion on the need for specific blood products has been discussed primarily in the sections on FFP and platelets.

Excessive bleeding is the most common complication observed after massive transfusion. This coagulopathy is related to the duration and the severity of the hemorrhagic shock and may not be corrected by red cell transfusion, platelets, and clotting factors.[42,49] Acidemias from hypoperfusion and hypothermia from cold volume resuscitation impair platelet function and coagulation.[48,70,71] Because the PT and PTT are determined at 37°C, they may not reflect a hypothermic coagulopathy.[72] Resuscitation and rewarming may be necessary before the coagulopathy is reversed.

IMMUNOLOGIC TRANSFUSION REACTIONS

Acute Hemolytic

Most hemolytic reactions result from clerical errors. A small percentage of reactions results from laboratory "failures." Clinical manifestations of hemolysis are immediate symptoms that start after 50 mL or less of blood have been given and include fever and chills, followed sometimes by clinical or subclinical icterus. More severe manifestations are headache, severe back pain, substernal tightness, dyspnea, and shock. Few symptoms may be present in anesthetized or obtunded patients. Objective findings include facial flushing, cyanosis, distended neck veins, tachycardia, and profound shock, usually occurring within 1 hour of transfusion. DIC may follow. Hemoglobinuria, hemoglobinemia, jaundice, oliguria, anuria, and acute renal failure may supervene. The severity of the reaction depends on the antibody titer, the affinity (strength of binding) of the antibody, and the "dose" of offending red cells that has been administered. Hemolytic reactions caused by interdonor incompatibility involve mostly the ABO and Kell blood groups.

RENAL FAILURE. Renal failure associated with hemolysis is thought to be caused by the stroma–antibody complexes released into the circulation, rather than hemoglobin precipitation in the tubular lumina. Damage probably results from a combination of hypotension and vasoconstriction, leading to a reduction in renal blood flow and the deposition of fibrin thrombi. The severity of renal dysfunction ranges from mild (quickly resolving diminution of urine output with little alteration in the clearance of metabolites) to acute tubular necrosis and bilateral renal cortical necrosis.

MANAGEMENT. Management depends on the prompt recognition of symptoms and immediate discontinuation of the transfusion. The blood should be quickly checked against the patient's identification, then returned to the blood bank along with another sample of the patient's blood for repeat typing and crossmatch. Blood bank personnel then test for a hemolytic antibody, and blood and urine are checked for free hemoglobin. Often the urine test is positive for free hemoglobin because of the presence of red blood cells related to a Foley catheter or surgical trauma. The simple technique of centrifuging a tube of urine and identifying pink discoloration of the supernatant aids in the diagnosis.

Some authorities recommend infusion of 25 g of mannitol over 5 minutes as soon as a hemolytic reaction is suspected. Others suggest the use of furosemide or ethacrynic acid because these drugs may be more effective in maintaining renal blood flow. IV fluids should be increased to maintain urine output of more than 100 mL/hour. Hypotension should be corrected with crystalloids or plasma expanders. Vasoactive drugs may be necessary. Additional blood transfusions should be avoided until the blood bank evaluation is complete. If renal failure develops, dialysis or hemofiltration may be required.

Delayed

Delayed transfusion reactions occur 3 to 21 days after blood is infused and result in a hemolytic anemia. Symptoms include malaise and fever; shock and renal complications are rare. Laboratory studies reveal an elevation of the indirect bilirubin fraction, failure of the hematocrit to reach expected levels, and the conversion of Coombs' test results from negative to positive.[73] Serologically detectable incompatibility is not present. Some patients have no detectable alloantibodies but do manifest shortened red cell survival. An anamnestic immune response seems to explain all delayed reactions and is not based on a primary immunologic response. Therapy is conservative, and additional transfusion should be avoided unless absolutely necessary.

Nonhemolytic/Noninfectious

Febrile reactions caused by antileukocyte antibodies represent most of the untoward reactions and are seen in nearly 7% of all blood product recipients. Prior transfusions contribute to the development of the responsible antibodies. The incidence of developing antileukocyte antibodies is high and increases with repeated exposure.

Signs and symptoms include chills, fever, and tachycardia. Patients may also develop hypotension, cyanosis, tachypnea, transient leukopenia, and a syndrome of self-limited fibrinolysis. A high level of leukoagglutinins in donor plasma may contribute to the reaction. Severity depends on the magnitude of the antibody titers, increased numbers of leukocytes, and rapidity of the transfusion. The differential diagnosis includes red cell incompatibility, bacterial contamination, and an unrelated disease process. Treatment is supportive but includes stopping the transfusion and retesting the donor blood. Aspirin and diphenhydramine can prevent future reactions, as can leukocyte-poor blood.

Allergic

A blood transfusion recipient may demonstrate an allergic reaction to either medication or food ingested by the donor. The reaction may vary in severity from urticaria to frank anaphylaxis. Alternatively, allergic transfusion reactions develop as a result of the passive transfer of sensitizing antibodies. The recipient subsequently encounters the allergen to which the antibody has developed, and an allergic reaction ensues. Ramirez[74] reported the first case of such a phenomenon in 1919 when a patient who had been recently transfused from a donor known to be allergic to animal dander developed wheezing during a carriage ride. Several months later, no sensitivity was present.

Graft-Versus-Host Disease

CAUSES. Graft-versus-host disease (GVHD) follows infusion of immunocompetent cells into an immunoincompetent recipient who is incapable of rejecting the foreign cells. Consequently, the infused immunocompetent cells initiate rejection of the host's normal tissues. Blood product transfusions into patients with cell mediated immune deficiency may cause GVHD. Acute GVHD also occurs in recipients of allogeneic bone marrow transplants, and in persons with primary immunodeficiencies who receive viable allogeneic lymphocytes.

Blood products placing the patient at risk are whole blood, packed red blood cells, buffy coats, granulocytes, fresh plasma, and platelets. In animal studies, the number of lymphocytes transfused seems critical. GVHD is not seen after transfusion of frozen blood, FFP, cryoprecipitate, or washed red cells. Irradiated blood products also may be given safely.[75]

CLINICAL PRESENTATION. Clinical presentation of GVHD involves many organ systems, including the skin, liver, GI tract, and bone marrow. Fever occurs first, with a skin rash developing 24 to 48 hours after that. The rash is a generalized erythroderma starting on the face (frequently behind the ears), then spreading to the trunk and extremities. Bullous formation can occur. Skin biopsies show extensive lymphocytic infiltration. Anorexia, nausea, vomiting, diarrhea, hepatocellular dysfunction manifested by elevated liver enzymes, and pancytopenia also occur.

MORBIDITY AND MORTALITY. Posttransfusion GVHD occurs approximately 2 to 30 days after transfusion.[75] Fifty percent of the patients with reported GVHD received cytotoxic drugs before the transfusion. When they develop GVHD, the bone marrow does not regain its function. The high mortality rate results from bone marrow aplasia, severe hypoplasia, and failure of bone marrow regeneration. Secondary infections occur as a result of agranulocytosis. GVHD is not seen in healthy, immunologically normal persons or in those lacking only humoral immunity.[76] Apparently, the person must lack the ability to reject histoincompatible cells.

Immune Suppression

The association between red blood cell transfusion and immune suppression has received increasing attention during the last decade. Nonviable red blood cells, as well as particulate matter found in red cell transfusions, have been suggested to impede the reticuloendothelial system's ability to clear bacteria, thereby predisposing the organism to the risk of sepsis.[77,78]

ORGAN TRANSPLANTATION. Immunocompetent lymphocytes present in recipients of repeated red blood cell donor red blood cell transfusions depress natural killer cell activity.[79,80] As a result, potentially altered immune function may result from red blood cell transfusion. Opels and colleagues[81,82] demonstrated that renal homograft survival increased dramatically at 36 months if patients received homologous red blood cell transfusions in the preoperative period.

TUMOR RECURRENCE.   This exciting benefit of the apparent immunoregulatory activity of blood has been countered, however, by a negative view that the same immunosuppression may have an adverse effect on tumor recurrence and mortality in the cancer patient. A similar hypothesis has been brought to the fore regarding bacterial killing in the potentially septic person.[83–85] Numerous reports suggest an increase in tumor recurrence and a decrease in survival in patients burdened with cancer of the colon, rectum, breast, cervix, lung, prostate, and head and neck who have received red blood cell transfusions.[86–92] Similar data have been shown in patients with sarcoma.[93] Perhaps stored plasma or cellular debris is associated with the negative outcome. Blumberg and Heal[94] showed that transfusion with whole blood confers a worsened prognosis when compared with packed red blood cells (less than 3 units) in patients operated for carcinoma of the colon, prostate, and cervix.

SEPTIC COMPLICATIONS.   Red cell transfusions are associated with an increase in septic complications in patients undergoing surgical procedures for carcinoma of the colon[95] as well as in multiply traumatized[96–98] patients or those with orthopedic injury.[99] All current studies, however, have been noncontrolled and retrospective. Prospective studies are warranted before wholesale recommendations can be made. In our opinion, the data are nevertheless sufficient to warrant a concern for the potential association between blood transfusions and an altered immune response. Hence, additional caution should be raised in the clinician's mind before the administration of any homologous blood products.

POSTTRANSFUSION PURPURA

Posttransfusion purpura results from acute hemorrhagic thrombocytopenia, usually occurring 1 week after blood transfusion. The patient is generally an older woman (fourth to eighth decade) with a prior history of pregnancy but no prior history of transfusions. This reaction occurs after an uneventful transfusion and may recur with subsequent transfusions. The clinical presentation includes severe thrombocytopenia ($<$10,000 platelets/mm^3) with skin and mucous membrane bleeding. Megakaryocytes are normal or increased. Most patients lack the PL^{A1} antigen that is present in 98% of the normal population. The precise mechanism is unknown, and the thrombocytopenia lasts from 10 days to 2 months. Exchange transfusion and plasmapheresis seem to abbreviate the period of thrombocytopenia. Platelet transfusions are contraindicated and can be associated with life-threatening febrile reactions and an autoimmune thrombocytopenia.

PULMONARY REACTIONS

Pulmonary insufficiency is often attributed to microaggregates in stored, transfused blood. Canine models show increased shunt and diminished pulmonary diffusing capacity after transfusion that can be prevented with a micropore filter.[100,101] However, primates resuscitated with stored blood administered without a micropore filter do not develop pulmonary insufficiency.[102] A retrospective analysis of combat injuries concludes that the volume of blood transfused was less closely related to the development of pulmonary dysfunction than to the magnitude and location of injuries incurred.[103]

A prospective, randomized, double-blind study comparing transfusion of washed or unwashed packed red blood cells in patients undergoing abdominal aortic aneurysmectomy showed no difference in postoperative pulmonary function between both groups.[104] Thus, microaggregates or other particles in stored blood do not directly impair pulmonary function. The exact role of blood transfusions in the development of pulmonary dysfunction remains unsolved.

METABOLIC

Metabolic complications of blood transfusion are citrate "intoxication" (hypocalcemia), hyperkalemia, hypothermia, circulatory overload, transfusion iron overload, and acid base abnormalities.

Hypocalcemia

Rapid infusion of citrated blood products ($>$100 mL/minute) can produce citrate intoxication manifested by acute hypocalcemia.[2] The patient may develop involuntary muscle tremors, ST segment prolongation, T wave delay, decreased cardiac output, electromechanical dissociation, and ventricular fibrillation. Supplemental calcium therapy corrects the problem and should be monitored by measurement of serum ionized calcium or of the QT interval. The total dose of calcium administered should not exceed 1 g unless signs of hypocalcemia are evident. Some authorities suggest that calcium should rarely be given to improve cardiac function, except in patients undergoing open heart surgery.[2] Be cautious when administering calcium to avoid hypercalcemic cardiac toxicity.

Hyperkalemia/Hypokalemia

The concentration of potassium in a unit of packed red blood cells approaches 70 mMol/L after storage for 35 days in CPDA-1 as a consequence of cell membrane adenosine triphosphatase (ATPase) pump inactivation.[10] However, because only 100 mL of plasma is present in a unit of packed red blood cells, 10 units of blood must be infused to administer the 70 mMol of potassium. After infusion, the pump is restored and red cells regain their normal electrolyte concentration. Subsequently, hypokalemia may be seen after massive transfusion with older blood.

Hypothermia

In surgical patients, large volumes of cold blood precipitate ventricular arrhythmias more often than does warmed blood. Hypothermia impairs citrate metabolism and aggravates the leftward shift in the hemoglobin–oxygen dissociation curve, thereby diminishing oxygen release. During massive transfusion, blood should be warmed.

Iron Deposition

A unit of packed red blood cells contains approximately 250 mg of iron. Normal iron excretion is 1 to 2 mg/day. Patients with a long history of transfusion for chronic anemia may develop iron overload. Deposition of iron in parenchymal cells results in damage to the myocardium, endocrine organs, and liver. Serum ferritin levels are markedly elevated and the total iron binding capacity is fully saturated. The iron chelating agent, disferroxamine, is ineffective when given intramuscularly but decreases iron levels when given by subcutaneous injection. Orally ingested chelating agents are ineffective. Transfusing "neocytes" (young red blood cells with a longer in vivo half-life) reduces the frequency of transfusion and therefore decreases the rate of iron accumulation.[105]

INFECTIONS

An infectious complication should be considered in patients with fever, chills, leukocytosis, or hypotension. However, all of these can be manifestations of transfusion reactions or allergic reactions. Specific early treatment may be required, as discussed earlier in this chapter. Blood transfusion alone can be associated with a leukocytosis that is noninfectious.[106] Careful clinical evaluation of patient is needed before initiating treatment.

Bacterial Contamination

Bacterial contamination is a rare complication of blood transfusions. Cold-growing, gram-negative, endotoxin-producing bacteria are generally the cause. Bacteremia in the donor is a potential hazard for the recipient, and donors are screened for a history of recurring fever, recent dental work, and other signs. Contamination also may stem from organisms on the skin of the donor at the site of the venipuncture, or from airborne organisms. Double-prepping the donor puncture site and the use of closed-system plastic bags with integral tubing and needles virtually eliminate this problem.

Bacterial contamination of FFP is exceptionally rare. Packed red blood cells and platelets stored at room temperature are at increased risk for bacterial contamination. Platelet pools are 12 times more likely to be associated with sepsis in the recipient than apheresis platelet units, not only because of an increased donor exposure but also because of longer storage time.[107]

Clinical manifestations include shock, hemoglobinuria, DIC, and renal failure. The diagnosis is suspected when the patient develops shaking chills, fever, hypotension, and shock shortly after the transfusion begins. Observation of organisms in gram-stained plasma from the residual donor blood confirms the diagnosis. The transfusion must be stopped immediately, and supportive treatment begun. Mortality rate is 50% to 80%, despite aggressive measures.

Acquired Immunodeficiency Syndrome

Several components contribute to the risk of AIDS from blood transfusion: potentially infected donors may not be identified during screening; a unit of donated blood may carry the virus; the unit may not be identified during testing; the infected unit may be received and seroconversion may follow; the patient may die from other causes before converting; and the seropositive state may not be diagnosed. Hence, we cannot evaluate the true risk of transfusion at this time. A review of 700,000 donor units that screened antibody negative at U.S. Army blood donor centers identified two cases of transfusion-associated HIV-1 infection in which HIV-1 RNA was detected in the donor units when they were retested.[108]

All blood banks in the United States currently eliminate donors with known risk factors and screen blood products for HIV. Both the enzyme-linked immunosorbent assay (ELISA) and the Western blot tests are available. The ELISA is 99% sensitive and has a specificity rate of 93% to 97%. Recent data suggest the risk of acquiring HIV through blood transfusion in the United States to be between 1 in 60,000 and 1/600,000 per unit of blood transfused.[109] The risk may be 1/100 in West Africa[110] and varies with the seropositivity rate of the donor pool.

Because current testing requires antibody detection to determine the potential for disease transmission, the fact that viremia can occur for a significant interval without antibody production in certain persons helps to explain why screening is not 100% effective. The risk of disease transmission must be balanced by sound indications and clinical judgment when transfusion is being contemplated.

Hepatitis

The incidence rate of posttransfusion hepatitis had been 5% to 10% nationwide,[77,111] with great regional variation. Now that an anti–hepatitis C monoclonal antibody screening test exists, the incidence rate of posttransfusion hepatitis is much lower, probably less than 0.5% per unit.[112] Fifteen percent to 20% of patients developing posttransfusion hepatitis progress to chronic active hepatitis, with 6% to 20% of those patients developing cirrhosis. Of the latter group, as many as 15% die.[113] Transmission of hepatitis A virus by blood transfusion is extremely low.

Other Viral Infections

Cytomegalovirus, human herpesvirus 6 (HHV-6), EBV (HHV-4), and human parvovirus B19 are associated with posttransfusion infection and are transmitted by lymphocytes. Antibodies to these viruses are present in 50% to 90% of adults. Transmission and clinical symptoms occur primarily in compromised recipients such as premature infants, seronegative pregnant women, immunosuppressed transplant patients, and after splenectomy in seronegative patients.[114]

CMV infection in immunocompromised patients ranges from a mild, self-limited febrile illness to extensive disseminated disease resulting in death. Fifty-one percent to 72% of donors have anti-CMV antibodies, but only 5% are capable of transmitting the infection. However, which seropositive donors are infectious cannot be predicted. High-risk seronegative patients should receive blood from CMV seronegative patients. Some investigators believe that seronegative blood should be administered to all transplant recipients regardless of the status of their antibodies, because prior CMV disease does not protect against new infection. Apparently, only the cellular elements of blood from CMV-seropositive donors are potentially infectious. Filtering units of packed cells to remove the white blood cells may decrease the transmission of CMV.[114]

Rickettsiae

Blood collected during the asymptomatic incubation period from persons with a chronic carrier state potentially can transmit a rickettsial agent. This problem, at worst, is minimal.

Syphilis

Posttransfusion syphilis is possible only from blood products stored at room temperature (platelets) because the infective agent cannot survive cooler temperatures. In the last 40 years, only one possible case of transfusion-associated syphilis has been reported.[42] Because most of the serologic test results for syphilis are negative during the phase of the disease when spirochetemia occurs, routine screening is ineffective. The American Association of Blood Banks has eliminated this requirement in its standards.

Parasites

Posttransfusion malaria is not a significant cause of morbidity in blood recipients. Blood banks screen and exclude donors with a history of travel in areas in which malaria is endemic.

REFUSAL OF TRANSFUSION

Two common clinical scenarios occur in which patients refuse transfusion. The first involves patients with cardiac or pulmonary comorbidity who need a transfusion for a low or decreasing hematocrit and who refuse transfusion out of fear of disease transmission. Appropriate education and counseling about the medical risks of transfusion usually convinces such patients that transfusion is necessary to avoid cardiac complications. The second involves Jehovah's Witnesses.

JEHOVAH'S WITNESSES

Jehovah's Witnesses are proscribed by their religion from accepting whole blood and packed red blood cell transfusion. They cite several Biblical references for justification of this proscription, believing that acceptance of blood or blood products makes them ineligible for resurrection and eternal salvation. They will not accept their own blood if it has left the continuity of their body, and will not accept preoperative autologous blood donation. Most Witnesses will accept intraoperative autotransfusion if the collection and return circuits remain in continuity. Transplantation, immunization, and vaccination remain less well defined by church rules. Crystalloid solutions, dextran and synthetic colloids, desmopressin, erythropoietin, and iron are acceptable to the Jehovah's Witness. Some Witnesses will accept albumin, although many do not.

Mentally competent adults have the right to refuse a treatment even if that refusal results in their death. The difficulties arise when dealing with minors and noncompetent adults. Case law rulings have not always been consistent and have not always agreed with freedom of religion as guaranteed by the Bill of Rights.[115] Therefore, each case needs to be evaluated individually, thus raising moral, ethical, and legal issues. The operating strategy may need to be altered to avoid excessive blood loss. Hypotensive anesthesia and hemodilution are encouraged. Hyperbaric chambers and synthetic blood substitutes have been employed, but their use is still investigational. Decreasing oxygen demand through paralysis, hypothermia, or barbiturate coma also has been tried in severely anemic patients.[116]

REFERENCES

1. Schwab CW, Shayne JP, Turner J: Immediate trauma resuscitation with type O uncrossmatched blood: a two year prospective experience. *J Trauma* 1986;26:897
2. *Advanced Trauma Life Support Program for Physicians*, In-

structor Manual. American College of Surgeons Committee on Trauma, 1993:8

3. Shenkin HA, Cheney RH, Govons SR, et al: On the diagnosis of hemorrhage in man: a study of volunteers bled large amounts. *Am J Medical Sci* 1944;208:421

4. Wo CCJ, Shoemaker WC, Appel PL, et al: Unreliability of blood pressure and heart rate to evaluate cardiac output in emergency resuscitation and critical illness. *Crit Care Med* 1993;21:218

5. Fald JL, Rackow EC, Weil MH: Colloid and crystalloid fluid resuscitation. *Acute Care* 1983/84;10:59

6. Ross AD, Angaran DM: Crystalloids versus colloids: a continuing controversy. *Drug Intell Clin Pharmacol* 1984;18:202

7. Isbister JP: Haemotherapy for acute haemorrhage. *Anaesth Intensive Care* 1984;12:217

8. Valeri CR, Altshule MD: *Hypovolemic Anemia of Trauma: The Missing Blood Syndrome*. Boca Raton, CRC Press, 1981

9. Cordts PR, LaMorte WW, Fisher JB, et al: Poor predictive value of hematocrit and hemodynamic parameters for erythrocyte deficits after extensive elective vascular operations. *Surg Gynecol Obstet* 1992;175:243

10. Steinbronn K, Heustis D: Rationale in blood component therapy. *Contemp Anesth Pract* 1983;6:151

11. Wintrobe MM: *Blood: Pure and Eloquent*. New York, McGraw-Hill, 1980:659

12. Dreyfus C: *Some Milestones in the History of Hematology*. New York, Grune & Stratton, 1957

13. Hutchin P: History of blood transfusion: a tercentennial look. *Surgery* 1968;64:685

14. Hoff EC, Hoff PM: The life and times of Richard Lower, physiologist and physician (1631–1691). *Bull Med Hist* 1936;4:517

15. Siewers AB: A case of madness cured by blood transfusion. *Bull Med Hist* 1928;6:1010

16. Jones AW, Mackmull G: The influence of James Blundell on the development of blood transfusion. *Ann Med Hist* 1928;10:242

17. Landsteiner K: Individual differences in human blood. *Science* 1931;73:403

18. Ottenberg R: Studies in isoagglutination. I. Transfusion and the question of intravascular agglutination. *J Exp Med* 1911;13:425

19. Fantis B: The therapy of Cook County Hospital. Blood preservation. *JAMA* 1937;109:128

20. Spence RK, Carson JA, Poses R, et al: Elective surgery without transfusion: influence of preoperative hemoglobin level and blood loss on mortality. *Am J Surg* 1990;159:320

21. Wilkerson DK, Rosen AL, Sehgal LR, et al: Limits of cardiac compensation in anemic baboons. *Surgery* 1988;103:665

22. Levine E, Rosen A, Seagal L, et al: Physiologic effects of acute anemia: implications for a reduced transfusion trigger. *Transfusion* 1990;30:11

23. Case RB, Berglund E, Sarnoff SJ: Ventricular function: changes in coronary resistance and ventricular function resulting from acutely induced anemia and the effect thereon of coronary stenosis. *Am J Med* 1955;55:397

24. Nelson AH, Fleisher LA, Rosenbaum SH: Relationship between postoperative anemia and cardiac morbidity in high-risk vascular patients in the intensive care unit. *Crit Care Med* 1993;21;860

25. National Institutes of Health Concensus Development Conference Statement: *Perioperative Red Cell Transfusion*. Bethesda, MD, U.S. Department of Health and Human Services, Public Health Service, 1988;7:1

26. Beutler E, Meul A, Wood LA: Depletion and regeneration of 2,3-diphosphoglyceric acid in stored red blood cells. *Transfusion* 1969;9:109

27. Weisel RD, Dennis RC, Manny J, et al: Adverse effects of transfusion therapy during abdominal aortic aneurysectomy. *Surgery* 1978;83:682

28. Valeri CR, Hirsch NM: Restoration of in vivo erythrocyte adenosine triphosphate, 2,3-diphosphoglycerate, potassium ion, and sodium ion concentration following transfusion of acid-citrate-dextrose stored human red blood cells. *J Lab Clin Med* 1969;73:722

29. Dennis RC, Hechtman HB, Berger RL, et al: Transfusion of 2,3 DPG–enriched red blood cells to improve cardiac function. *Ann Thorac Surg* 1978;26:17

30. Valeri CR: *Blood Banking and the Use of Frozen Blood Products*. Boca Raton, CRC Press, 1976

31. Sayers MH: Transfusion-transmitted viral infections other than hepatitis and human immunodeficiency virus infection. *Arch Pathol Lab Med* 1994;118:346

32. Page PL: Directed blood donations: *Con Transfusions* 1989;29:65

33. Goldfinger D: Directed blood donations: *Pro Transfusion* 1989;26:70

34. The National Blood Resource Education Program Expert Panel: The use of autologous blood. *JAMA* 1990;263:414

35. Valeri CR: Physiology of blood transfusion. In: Barie PS, Shires GT (eds). *Surgical Intensive Care*. Boston, Little, Brown, 1993:681

36. Coffin CM: Current issues in transfusion therapy. *Postgrad Med* 1987;8:343

37. Braunstein AH, Oberman HA: Transfusion of plasma components. *Transfusion* 1984;249:281

38. Murray DJ, Olson J, Strauss R, et al: Coagulation changes during packed red cell replacement of major blood loss. *Anesthesiology* 1988;69:839

39. Counts RB, Haisch C, Simoa TL, et al: Hemostasis in massively transfused trauma patients. *Ann Surg* 1979;190:91

40. Mannucci PM, Federici AB, Sirchia G: Hemostasis testing during massive blood replacement: a study of 172 cases. *Vox Sang* 1982;42:113

41. Marsaglia G, Thomas ED: Mathematical consideration of cross circulation and exchange transfusion. *Transfusion* 1971;11:216

42. Harke H, Rihman S: Hemostatic disorders in mass transfusions. *Bibl Haematol* 1980;46:179

43. Phillips TF, Soulier G, Wilson RF: Outcome of massive transfusion exceeding two blood volumes in trauma and emergency surgery. *J Trauma* 1987;27:903

44. Giorgio A, Finegold H, Ragno G, et al: *Effect of autologous fresh- and liquid-preserved platelets on an aspirin-induced thrombocytopathy in the baboon*. American Association of Blood Banks Joint Congress. Los Angeles, November 10–15, 1990:S-164

45. Harker LA, Schlicter SJ: The bleeding time as a screening test for evaluation of platelet function. *N Engl J Med* 1972;287:155

46. Daly PA: Platelet transfusion: clinical applications in the oncology setting. *Am J Med Sci* 1980;280:130

47. Handin RI, Valeri CR: Hemostatic effectiveness of platelets stored at 22°C. *N Engl J Med* 1971;285:538

48. Valeri CR, MacGregor H, Cassidy G, et al: Effects of temperature on bleeding time and clotting time in normal male and female volunteers. *Crit Care Med* 1995;23:698

49. Reed RL, Ciavarella D, Heinbach D, et al: Prophylactic platelet administration during massive transfusion: the prospective randomized double-blind clinical study. *Ann Surg* 1986;203:40

50. Melarangno AJ, Carciero R, Feingold H, et al: Cryopreservation of human platelets using 6% dimethyl sulfoxide and storage at −80°C: effects of two years of frozen storage at −80°C and transportation in dry ice. *Vox Sang* 1985;49:245

51. Mannucci PM, Ruggeri ZM, Pareti FI, et al: 1-Desamino-8-D-arginine vasopressin: a new pharmacological approach to the management of haemophilia and von Willebrand's disease. *Lancet* 1977;i:869

52. Mannucci PM, Remuzzi G, Pusinieri F, et al: Desamino-8-D-arginine vasopressin shortens the bleeding time in uremia. *N Engl J Med* 1983;308:8

53. Kobrinsky NL, Israels ED, Gerrard JM, et al: Shortening of bleeding time by 1-desamino-8-D-arginine vasopressin in various bleeding disorders. *Lancet* 1984;i:1185

54. Kobrinsky NL, Letts RM, Patel LR, et al: 1-Desamino-8-D-arginine vasopressin (desmopressin) decreases operative blood loss in patients having Harrington rod spinal fusion surgery. *Ann Intern Med* 1987;107:446

55. Saltzman EW, Weinstein MJ, Weintraub RM, et al: Treatment with desmopressin acetate to reduce blood loss after cardiac surgery: a double-blind randomized trial. *N Engl J Med* 1986;314:1402

56. Mannucci PM: Desmopressin (DDAVP) for treatment of disorders of hemostasis. *Prog Hemost Thromb* 1986;8:19

57. Rocha E, Llorens R, Paramo JA, et al: Does desmopressin acetate reduce blood loss after surgery on patients on cardiopulmonary bypass? *Circulation* 1988;77:1319

58. D'Alauro FS, Johns RA: Hypotension related to desmopressin administration following cardiopulmonary bypass. *Anesthesiology* 1988;69:962

59. Jones JH, Kilpatrick GS, Franks EH: Red cell aggregation in dextrose solutions. *J Clin Pathol* 1962;15:161

60. Calkins JM, et al: Critical importance of diluting packed RBC for transfusion. *Anesthesiology* 1980;53:S169

61. Grindlinger GA, Vegas AM, Churchill WH Jr, et al: Is respiratory failure a consequence of blood transfusion? *J Trauma* 1980;20:627

62. Barnes A: Transfusion of universal donor and uncrossmatched blood. *Bibl Haematol* 1980;46:132

63. Lefebre J, McLellan BA, Coovadia AS: Seven years' experience with group O unmatched packed red blood cells in a regional trauma unit. *Ann Emerg Med* 1987;16:1344

64. Barnes A Jr: Status of the use of universal blood donor transfusion. *Crit Rev Clin Lab Sci* 1973;4:147

65. Gervin AS, Fischer RP: Resuscitation of trauma patients with type-specific uncrossmatched blood. *J Trauma* 1984;24:327

66. Barnes A Jr, Allen TE: Transfusion subsequent to administration of universal donor blood in Vietnam. *JAMA* 1968;204:147

67. American Association of Blood Banks: *Technical Manual*, 11th ed. 1993:416

68. Martin CM, Sibbald WJ, Lu X, et al: Age of transfused red blood transfused in septic ICU patients. *Clin Invest Med* 1994;17:B20

69. Purdy Fr, Tweeddale Mg, Merrick PM: Association of mortality with age of blood cells is associated with ICU length of stay. *Clin Invest Med* 1994;17:B21

70. Ferrara A, MacArthur JD, Wright HK, et al: Hypothermia and acidosis worsen coagulopathy in the patient requiring massive transfusion. *Am J Surg* 1990;160:515

71. Valeri CR, MacGregorH, Cassidy G, et al: Effects of temperature on bleeding time and clotting time in normal male and female volunteers. *Crit Care Med* 1995;23:698:704

72. Rohrer MJ, Natale AM: Effect of hypothermia on the coagulation cascade. *Crit Care Med* 1992;20:1402

73. Giblett ER: Blood groups and blood transfusion. In: Braunwald E, Isselbacker KJ, Petersdorf RG (eds): *Harrison's Principles of Internal Medicine*, 11th ed. New York, McGraw-Hill, 1987:1483

74. Ramirez MA: Horse asthma following blood transfusion: report of a case. *JAMA* 1919;73:984

75. Brubaker DB: Human posttransfusion graft-versus-host disease. *Vox Sang* 1983;45:401

76. Hong M, Gatti RA, Good RA: Hazards and potential benefits of blood transfusion in immunologic deficiency. *Lancet* 1968;ii:388

77. Rutledge R, Sheldon GF, Collins ML: Massive transfusion. *Crit Care Clin* 1986;4:791

78. Collins, JA: Recent developments in the area of massive transfusion. *World J Surg* 1987;11:75

79. Waymack JP, Rapien J, Garnett D, et al: The effect of transfusion on immune function in a traumatized animal model. *Arch Surg* 1986;121:50

80. Kaplan J, Sarniak S, Gitlin J, et al: Diminished helper/suppressor lymphocyte ratios and natural killer activity in recipients of repeated blood transfusions. *Blood* 1984;64:308

81. Opelz G, Sengar DPS, Mickey MR, et al: Effect of blood transfusion on subsequent kidney transplants. *Transplant Proc* 1973;5:253

82. Opelz G, Terasaki PI: Improvement of kidney grafts survival with increased number of blood transfusions. *N Engl J Med* 1978;299:799

83. Waymack JP, Yurt RW: The effect of blood transfusions on immune function. V. The effect on the inflammatory response to bacterial infections. *J Surg Res* 1990;48:147

84. Waymack JP, Warden GD, Miskell P, et al: Effect of varying number and volume of transfusions on mortality rate following septic challenge in an animal model. *World J Surg* 1987;11:387

85. Waymack JP, Robb E, Alexander JW: Effect of transfusion on immune function in a traumatized animal model. II. Effect of mortality rate following septic challenge. *Arch Surg* 1987;122:935

86. Sallo M: Immunosuppressive effects of blood transfusion in anesthesia and surgery. *Acta Anesthesiol Scand* 1988;32 (Suppl 89):26

87. Schriemer PA, Longnecker DE, Mintz PD: The possible immunosuppressive effects of perioperative blood transfusion in cancer patients. *Anesthesiology* 1988;68:422

88. Harford FJ, Williams LF, Woodward SC, et al: Recurrence of colon carcinoma after curative resection and blood transfusion: proposal for a prospective study. *Transplant Proc* 1988;20:2210

89. Wu HS, Little AG: Perioperative blood transfusions and cancer recurrence. *J Clin Oncol* 1988;6:1348

90. van Aken WG: Does perioperative blood transfusion promote tumor growth? *Transfusion Med Rev* 1989;3:243

91. Tartter PI: The association of perioperative blood transfusion with colorectal cancer recurrence. *Ann Surg* 1992;216:633

92. Weiden PL: Do perioperative blood transfusions increase the risk of cancer recurrence? *Eur J Cancer* 1993;26:987

93. Rosenberg SA, Seipp CA, White DE, et al: Perioperative blood transfusions are associated with increased rates of recurrence and decreased survival with high-grade soft-tissue sarcomas of the extremities. *J Clin Oncol* 1985;3:698

94. Blumberg N, Heal JM: Transfusion and host defenses against cancer recurrence and infection. *Transfusion* 1989;29:236

95. Tartter PI: Blood transfusion and infectious complications following colorectal cancer surgery. *Br J Surg* 1988;75:789

96. Dawes LG, Aprahamian C, Condon RE, et al: The risk of infection after colon injury. *Surgery* 1986;100:796

97. Nichols RL, Smith JW, Klein DB, et al: Risk of infection after penetrating abdominal trauma. *N Engl J Med* 1984;311:1065

98. Dellinger EP, Oreskovich MR, Wertz MJ, et al: Risk of infection following laparotomy for penetrating abdominal injury. *Arch Surg* 1984;119:20

99. Dellinger EP, Miller SD, Wertz MJ, et al: Risk of infection after open fracture of the arm or leg. *Arch Surg* 1988;123:1320

100. Snyder EL, Underwood PA, Spivack M, et al: An in vivo evaluation of microaggregrate blood filtration during total hip replacement. *Ann Surg* 1979;190:75

101. Rosario MD, Rumsey EW, Arakaki G, et al: Blood microaggregates and ultrafilters. *J Trauma* 1978;18:498

102. Ketai LH, Grum CM: C3a and adult respiratory distress syndrome after massive transfusion. *Crit Care Med* 1986;14:1101

103. Collings JA, James PM, Bredenberg CE: The relationship between transfusion and hypoxemia in combat casualties. *Ann Surg* 1978;188:513

104. Krausz MM, Dennis RC, Utsunomiya T, et al: Cardiopulmonary function following transfusion of three red blood cell products in elective abdominal aortic aneurysmectomy. *Ann Surg* 1981;194:616

105. National Institute of Health: Use of neocytes decreases frequency of transfusion to reduce iron overload. *JAMA* 1979; 242:2669

106. Fenwick JC, Cameron M, Naiman SC, et al: Blood transfusion as a cause of leukocytosis in critically ill patients. *Lancet* 1994;344:855

107. Wagner SJ, Friedman LI, Dodd RY: Transfusion-associated bacterial sepsis. *Clin Microbiol Rev* 1994;7:290

108. Roberts CR, Longfield JN, Platte RC, et al: Transfusion-associated human immunodeficiency virus type 1 from screened antibody negative donors. *Arch Pathol Lab Med* 1994;118:1188

109. Nelson KE, Donahue JG, Munoz A, et al: Transmission of retroviruses from seronegative donors by transfusion during cardiac surgery: a multicenter study of HIV-1 and HTLV-I/II infections. *Ann Intern Med* 1992;116:554

110. Savarit D, De Cock KM, Schutz R, et al: Risk of HIV infection from transfusion with blood negative for HIV antibody in a West African city. *Br Med J* 1992;305:498

111. Stevens CE, Aach RD, Hollinger FB, et al: Hepatitis B virus antibody in blood donors and the occurrence of non-A non-B hepatitis in transfusion recipients. *Ann Intern Med* 1984; 101:733

112. Morris JA Jr, Wilcox TR, Reed GW, et al: Safety of the blood supply: surrogate testing and transmission of hepatitis C in patients after massive transfusion. *Ann Surg* 1994;219:517

113. Alter HJ, Purcell RH, Shih JW, et al: Detection of antibody to hepatitis C virus and prospectively followed transfusion recipients with acute and chronic non-A non-B hepatitis. *N Engl J Med* 1989;321:1494

114. Sayers MH: Transfusion-transmitted viral infections other than hepatitis and human immunodeficiency virus infection. *Arch Pathol Lab Med* 1994;118:346

115. Rothenberg DM: The approach to the Jehovah's Witness patient. *Anesth Clin North Am* 1990;8:589

116. Bragg LE, Thompson JS: Management strategies in the Jehovah's Witness patient. *Contemp Surg* 1990;36:45

Critical Care, Third Edition, edited by Joseph M. Civetta,
Robert W. Taylor, and Robert R. Kirby.
Lippincott-Raven Publishers, Philadelphia, PA © 1997.

CHAPTER 44

∎

Decreasing the Need for Homologous Blood Transfusion

Stephen F. Flaherty
Richard C. Dennis

IMMEDIATE CONCERNS ∎

MAJOR PROBLEMS

Transfusion of blood products is common in critically ill patients. Transfusion therapy is closely monitored; hospitals have transfusion committees to identify, among other things, "unnecessary transfusions." Blood products are a source of infectious risks (hepatitis, human immunodeficiency virus, *Yersinia*, cytomegalovirus, and bacteria) to patients and staff. Immunologic considerations include anaphylaxis and immunosuppression. Finally, costs in collecting, preparing, and administering blood products are substantial.

In the public's view, the acquired immunodeficiency syndrome (AIDS) is the biggest risk from transfusion. Concern over this fear has led to changes in transfusion practice over the last 10 years. The blood banking industry believes that the blood supply has never been safer and that the risk of transmission of infectious disease, although real, continues to decrease. The diseases most often contracted through transfusion are hepatitis B and C. Routine testing of blood products and the availability of tests for non-A and non-B hepatitis and the human immunodeficiency virus have decreased the incidence of such transmission (Table 44-1)[1,2] (personal communication, American Red Cross, Boston Chapter). Nevertheless, the risk of blood transfusion can be eliminated totally only if *no* transfusion is given.

STRESS POINTS

1. The most obvious and effective method to avoid the need to transfuse blood products is to limit blood loss. This approach requires strict attention to detail.
2. Preparation for surgery should include an assessment of previous treatments that may increase the risk of blood loss (radiation, known or suspected significant adhesions, a re-do operation).
3. Considerations include whether an approach can be planned to avoid operating through the affected areas, and whether the patient has recently ingested aspirin, warfarin (Coumadin), or other drugs known to affect coagulation.
4. Surgical technique must be fastidious. Tissues must be handled properly to minimize bleeding. When bleeding does occur, expeditious control is essential. Application of direct pressure is a simple, effective technique that should not be forgotten.
5. Other methods such as electrocautery, suture ligature, oxidized cellulose, and microfibrillar collagen powder (Avitene) should be applied as needed.
6. When a central catheter is inserted, don't aspirate a syringe full of blood to confirm that the needle is within the vein; 2 mL is adequate.
7. Don't watch a surface wound bleed for several hours, hoping that it will stop.

TABLE 44-1. Estimated Incidence of Transmission of Disease per Unit of Blood Product Transfused

Hepatitis C	1 : 3300
Hepatitis B	<1 : 250,000
Hepatitis A	<1 : 1,000,000
HIV	1 : 420,000–600,000
Yersinia	<1 : 1,000,000
Plasmodia	<1 : 1,000,000

HIV, human immunodeficiency virus.

8. The intensivist must be familiar with operative procedures in general and with the specific operative procedure in particular, including any unusual intraoperative hemorrhage.
9. If postoperative bleeding is suspected, the intensivist must assess and, if necessary, correct a possible coagulopathy. If bleeding continues, alert the surgeon to consider early operative reintervention.
10. The intensivist must not replace continuing blood loss without keeping the surgeon informed. Early reexploration often limits blood loss.

ESSENTIAL DIAGNOSTIC TESTS AND PROCEDURES

1. Factors that contribute to coagulopathy include excessive intraoperative blood loss replaced with red cells without clotting factors (massive transfusion, use of a high-volume blood reclamation device, and hypothermia).
2. At a minimum, measure hematocrit, platelet count, prothrombin time, partial thromboplastin time, and body temperature.
3. In general, an elevated prothrombin time can be corrected with intravenous or intramuscular vitamin K and fresh frozen plasma (FFP). An increased partial thromboplastin time can be treated with FFP and, if caused by heparin therapy, with protamine sulfate.
4. A platelet count of 50,000/mm³ without thrombocytopathy is adequate for hemostasis. Thrombocytopathies are most commonly caused by aspirin, other nonsteroidal antiinflammatory drugs, and hypothermia.[3]
5. In hypothermia-induced thrombocytopathy, rewarming (warm room, warm fluids, and warm air blown over the patient) reverses the coagulopathy. Aspirin-poisoned platelets may require platelet transfusion.

INITIAL THERAPY

1. Epsilon aminocaproic acid (EACA) inhibits the activity of plasmin and the conversion of plasminogen to plasmin, thus prolonging the life of formed clot. Patients undergoing cardiopulmonary bypass are thought to have increased bleeding partly because of increased plasminogen activator, which leads to hyperfibrinolysis.
2. Some reports show that EACA decreases postoperative bleeding after coronary artery bypass surgery.[4] Recommended dosage is a 4- to 5-g loading dose followed by 1 g hourly.
3. The mechanism of action of tranexamic acid is similar to that of EACA, but this drug is more potent with a longer duration of action. It has the added benefit of preserving platelet ADP, thus helping to preserve platelet function.[5] The usual intravenous dosage is 25 mg/kg every 6 to 8 hours. Dosage is reduced for patients in renal failure.
4. Desmopressin (DDAVP) is a synthetic analogue of vasopressin that does not demonstrate vasoconstrictor activity. It causes the release of preformed factor VIII and von Willebrand factor from endothelial cells.
5. DDAVP should be given in a dose of 0.3 µg/kg and can be given either intravenously or as a nasal spray. When given intravenously, it should be infused over 15 minutes, because hypotension may result if infused more rapidly.
6. Because DDAVP only causes release of preformed factor, tachyphylaxis develops if it is administered more than twice in a 48-hour period.
7. Whereas some studies have shown decreased need for red cell transfusion when DDAVP is used,[6,7] others have shown neither decreased operative blood loss nor decreased transfusion requirement.[8,9]
8. Aprotinin (Traysylol) is a serine protease inhibitor derived from bovine pancreas that acts by inhibiting plasmin and kallikrein. It also is thought to preserve platelet adhesion receptors, an effect that may make it a useful adjunct in patients who take aspirin.[10] A 1-mL test dose (10,000 KI units) is followed by a 200-mL loading dose administered over 20 minutes, and an infusion of 50 mL/hour. Lesser doses are being assessed.
9. Complications of aprotinin include a need to use large doses, which raises cost; hypotension during infusion; and renal damage from accumulation in the kidneys.[11]
10. Several materials are available to obtain hemostasis. Aggressive bleeding must first be controlled using techniques such as direct pressure, electrocautery, suture ligation, or argon beam coagulation. These agents are then used to reinforce the hemostatic plug.[11]
11. Fibrin glue is a gel-like compound formed by combining fibrinogen with thrombin. Fibrinogen can be obtained from FFP or cryoprecipitate; thrombin is available commercially. The reaction occurs quickly, so the mixture needs to be made at the site of application. Once formed, it adheres firmly and is effective in controlling bleeding, especially from solid organs such as liver.
12. Bone wax is available as a solid plug material in use for many years and is inexpensive. Bone wax is usually used on cut or broken bone ends, such as from median sternotomy. It has no native hemostatic property

but is simply pressed onto the bone end and acts to tamponade bleeding.

13. Absorbable gelatin (Gelfoam) is a gelatin sponge matrix. It also has no hemostatic property. Blood is absorbed into the matrix where the expanded surface area facilitates clot formation.

14. Gelfoam is available as pads of various sizes. They may be left in vivo where the gelatin liquefies and is reabsorbed with little tissue reaction or scarring. Caution should be exercised, however, regarding the amount of pad left in place because any foreign material can lead to increased infection rates.

15. SurgiCel is an oxidized cellulose product. It is available in woven strips and is simply laid on the area and held in place. The material has an acidic property that is thought to cause small vessel contraction and local deposition of fibrin.[12] However, the woven fiber also expands surface area for clot formation.

OPTIMIZATION OF RED CELL PRODUCTION ■

Normal marrow production of red cells is the safest and least expensive method to correct anemia. Nutritional support, including not only adequate calories and protein, but also iron and vitamins, is required. Manipulation of the hormonal milieu is also possible.

NUTRITION

Vitamins

Adequate protein and calorie nutrition is essential. To maximize production of red blood cells in the otherwise healthy patient, appropriate iron stores, vitamins, and trace elements must be available.

FOLATE.   Folate refers to a group of compounds with nutritional activities similar to folic acid. It is important in the synthesis of DNA and is required for two different steps in purine formation. Enteral or parenteral administration can be used with a recommended dose of 1 mg/day. Leafy green vegetables, liver, and kidney are good dietary sources.

VITAMIN B_6.   Vitamin B_6 (pyridoxine, pyridoxamine, and pyridoxal) is required for heme synthesis. It can be administered either parenterally or enterally. This vitamin complex is found in meats and grains. It is usually given as a multivitamin preparation.

VITAMIN B_{12}.   Vitamin B_{12} in a complex with intrinsic factor binds to a receptor in the brush border of the distal ilium for absorption. In diseases such as pernicious anemia (lack of intrinsic factor), vitamin B_{12} absorption does not occur. It is required as an essential cofactor for DNA synthesis. Normally, vitamin B_{12} is stored in the liver, but in cases of chronic disease or malabsorption syndrome, it must be administered as a monthly injection of 1 mg. Dietary sources include red meat, liver, egg, and cheese. Although some bacteria can produce vitamin B_{12}, this vitamin is not available from higher plants.

Iron

Iron can be administered as a supplement of ferrous gluconate or ferrous sulfate to stimulate erythropoiesis. These compounds are given orally over time; after 10 to 14 days, they stimulate red cell production above the normal level. The usual dose is 325 mg orally one to three times per day. Although intravenous compounds have been used, they are not generally recommended and are not commonly given in the ICU. Critically ill patients with chronic illnesses often need supplemental iron, usually in the form of red cell transfusions.

HORMONAL THERAPY

Erythropoietin, a naturally occurring hormone synthesized in the kidneys, is a potent stimulus for red blood cell production. A genetically engineered version of this hormone is available as epoetin alfa (r-HuEPO; PROCRIT®, Ortho Biotech Inc.; Epogen®, Amgen Inc.) and can be used to help restore and maintain red cell volume. Epoetin alfa has various uses and indications globally. In the United States, epoetin alfa is indicated for the treatment of anemia, and reduction of transfusion, due to chronic renal failure at a recommended starting dose of 50–100 U/kg three times a week (T.I.W.), administered either subcutaneously (SC) or intravenously (IV). For the treatment of anemia, and reduction of transfusion, in zidovudine-treated, HIV-infected patients epoetin alfa can be administered at a dose of 100–300 U/kg SC or IV T.I.W. For the treatment of chemotherapy-induced anemia, and reduction of transfusion, in cancer patients, epoetin alfa can be administered at a dose of 150–300 U/kg SC T.I.W. And, for the treatment of anemic (hemoglobin >10 to ≤ 13 g/dL) patients scheduled to undergo elective, noncardiac, nonvascular surgery to reduce the need for allogeneic blood transfusions epoetin alfa has two dosing regimens for the perisurgical indication. First, 600 U/kg SC weekly, starting day -21, -14, -7, and the day of surgery (total of four doses). An alternative dosing regimen is also indicated, 300 U/kg SC daily starting 10 days prior to surgery, the day of surgery, and four days after surgery (total of 15 doses).[13] A dose-dependent effect on red cell production results in reticulocytosis at 3 to 4 days and a change in hematocrit after 7 days.[14] When using epoetin alfa, ensure adequate iron stores for maximal effect. One special situation in which epoetin alfa may also be useful is severely anemic Jehovah's Witnesses. Although the preparation of epoetin alfa does involve a small amount of human albumin, it generally has been accepted by people with this religious belief.[15,16]° Beyond these indications epoetin alfa is being explored in other clinical settings, including critical care.

° Further information on Jehovah's Witnesses and blood transfusion or Epogen can be obtained from the Watch Tower Bible and Tract Society at (718) 625–3600, extension 25136, during normal business hours, or (718) 624–8100 after business hours.

AUTOTRANSFUSION ■

Autotransfusion is the process of collecting and reinfusing the patient's own blood for intravascular volume replacement. Descriptions date back to the early 1800s. Advantages in the event of acute hemorrhage include immediate availability of blood without the need to type and crossmatch, as well as elimination of the risks of alloimmunization and transmission of infectious diseases. Finally, the patient receives blood containing higher levels of 2,3-DPG than those present in banked units. The term *autotransfusion* includes preoperative collection of blood for administration during a procedure using both fresh and frozen storage techniques, as well as salvage and processing of shed blood both intraoperatively and in the ICU.

PREDONATION

Predonation, or predeposit autologous transfusion, requires blood donation before surgery. The blood may be stored in the liquid phase for up to 42 days in Adsol (adenine-glucose-mannitol-sodium chloride), or cryopreserved, stored up to 20 years, and then made available at the time blood loss is anticipated. This process is suitable only for elective surgery. Recently increased public awareness of disease transmission by blood products (AIDS; hepatitis B; non-A, non-B hepatitis; and cytomegalovirus) has renewed interest in the concept of autologous blood banking.

Recommendations

Whereas recommendations for predonation candidates are similar to those of routine homologous donation at most centers, they are not requirements. Patients may, in some cases, predonate even if they have low hematocrits, take medications, or have diseases that would exclude them from routine donation. In general, patients are candidates for predonation if their hemoglobin concentration is 11 g/dL or greater (hematocrit 33%). Numerous schemata are available for predonation schedules. They can allow blood donation every fourth day[17] (provided the previous hemoglobin and hematocrit criteria are met) or, more commonly, 1 unit per week.[18] In general, the final phlebotomy is performed 3 days before the surgical event.

In one study, human recombinant erythropoietin administered in the preoperative period to patients scheduled for elective orthopedic surgery resulted in increased mean numbers of autologous units collected per patient.[19] The mean red cell volume was clinically and statistically greater in the erythropoietin group when compared with those in the control group. However, the role of erythropoietin in the predonation schema needs further clarification.

Complications

Few complications have arisen as a result of predonated blood, and most donors are acceptable. Although some centers have reported predonations in patients with coronary artery disease, pregnancy, and the extremes of age as being free from complications,[20] others find predonation in these groups to be relatively contraindicated.[21]

Errors in identification of blood can occur during phlebotomy, processing, or transfusion. The true cost of autologous transfusion probably exceeds that of homologous transfusions, because donor recruitment is only a small percentage of the cost of transfusion therapy. In addition, red cells stored by cryopreservation are estimated to be three to four times more costly than liquid-preserved red cells. Routine type and crossmatch, as well as disease testing, should be done, even with autotransfusion units as a precaution in case improper identification has occurred.

Advantages

Because predonation of autologous blood generally is safe and effective, many believe the practice is grossly underutilized throughout the country. Despite the growth of autologous blood donation from 30,000 units in 1982 to 397,000 units in 1987,[22] Toy and associates[23] found that only 5% of patients who were scheduled for major elective surgery and who were potential candidates for predonation actually received autologous blood. If those same patients had donated autologous blood preoperatively and received their blood when indicated, the incidence of homologous blood transfusions would have been reduced by 68%.

Risk and Cost:Benefit Ratios

The risk:benefit ratio of predonated autologous blood is positive when compared with the many known associated complications of homologous red cell transfusion. Unfortunately, the cost is high, because if the predonated unit is not transfused into the donor, it must be discarded (the patient/donor is not considered "voluntary" and may not have met the strict criteria of a usual voluntary donor). A cost analysis of predonation has shown it to be considerably more expensive than use of blood bank blood.[24]

NORMOVOLEMIC HEMODILUTION

Hemodilution is a technique that results in a net loss of fewer red blood cells per given volume of blood loss than would otherwise be lost. Whole blood is collected from the patient, generally in the operating room just before operation. This blood is replaced with crystalloid to maintain normovolemia. As the operation proceeds, if the patient requires transfusion (to treat hypotension or improve oxygen delivery), the patient's own blood is returned. For example, an 80-kg man with a hematocrit of 45% has a red cell volume of 2520 mL (80 kg × 70 mL/kg × 0.45). One liter of blood removed before an operative procedure contains 450 mL of red blood cells (1000 mL × 0.45). The patient would be given crystalloid solution at a ratio of 3:1 to maintain a normal blood volume of 5600 mL (80 kg × 70 mL/kg) with a new hematocrit of 37%.

This calculation assumes that two thirds of the crystalloid given leaves the vascular space rapidly. Blood lost during the procedure has fewer red cells per volume of loss. In our hypothetical patient, a 1-L intraoperative blood loss with a hematocrit of 37% would represent 370 mL of red cells, which postoperatively can easily be replaced by the 450 mL of red cells already saved. Ness and coworkers[25] and Hur and associates[26] have shown this technique to reduce the need for transfusion of homologous blood.

SALVAGE OF SHED BLOOD

Indications

Candidates for emergency autotransfusion of shed blood include the following: patients injured by blunt or penetrating chest trauma with an acute chest tube blood loss of 1000 mL or more; those experiencing an acute blood loss with no available homologous blood; and those who have massive blood loss when homologous blood is available but is insufficient for resuscitation.

Methodology

A sterile basin and syringe were used as the first autotransfusion system. Clots were removed by straining through gauze.[27] Although several automated devices are available, the general principles remain the same. Blood is collected, anticoagulated, stored with or without processing, and reinfused. Some systems collect and reinfuse whole blood whereas others return washed red cells.

The Bentley autotransfusion system was the first commercially available device.[28] Blood was collected and stored in a reservoir. It was then infused into the patient at a rate of 700 to 800 mL/minute. An alarm sounded when the blood in the reservoir was less than 200 mL. Despite safety measures, cases of air embolism were reported. Although most of these resulted from operator error, clots were observed to obscure the photoelectric cell on the alarm, rendering the system unreliable. It was subsequently removed from the market.

The currently available Sorenson system consists of a soft inner collection bag contained in a rigid outer canister.[29] Anticoagulant is either added by drip to the suction tubing or contained in the collection bag. The system must be monitored closely because insufficient or excessive amounts can be administered inadvertently. The Sorenson system is relatively inexpensive, can be employed in a variety of clinical situations, and is easy to use.

The IBM blood cell processor centrifuges and washes blood collected by the Sorenson or other salvage systems. Up to 500 mL of blood can be washed in each cycle; depending on the amount of debris, more than one cycle may be required. A cycle takes approximately 15 minutes. The final product is washed red blood cells suspended in saline. This system is expensive, but it does not require constant operator attention, and the processor can be used for other blood banking purposes.

The Haemonetics Cell Saver is a dedicated cell washing unit that provides a product similar to the IBM system. Shed blood is anticoagulated and aspirated directly into the apparatus. It is then washed, concentrated, and stored in a transfer pack. Up to 3 units of blood can be processed for retransfusion in 9 minutes. The device is expensive, as is the disposable

software. Both the IBM and Haemonetics units yield red cells with virtually no plasma, clotting factors, or oncotic properties.

Complications

THROMBOCYTOPENIA. The most reproducible hematologic complication of autotransfusion is thrombocytopenia.[30] Platelet counts approach 50,000/mm^3 when patients receive more than 4000 mL of autologous processed blood.[31,32] Platelets collected from the Sorenson autotransfusion system function abnormally in vitro yet aggregate normally in vivo after transfusion. Hypofibrinogenemia is the most reproducible coagulation factor abnormality.[28] Platelet counts and fibrinogen levels, however, return to normal by 48 to 72 hours.[29] In an evaluation of autotransfusion patients with traumatic hemothorax, Symbas[32] found that no patient demonstrated evidence of a coagulopathy as long as the autotransfused volume was less than 50% of the patient's total blood volume (5 units).

DISSEMINATED INTRAVASCULAR COAGULATION. Although good data are lacking, it is reasonable to speculate that devices returning partially activated, filtered whole blood (Sorenson) are more likely to produce disseminated intravascular coagulation and less likely to produce dilutional coagulopathy than systems returning washed red cells (IBM, Haemonetics). In addition, dilutional thrombocytopenia may occur earlier in systems that wash red cells in saline. Some authors recommend administering FFP after 4 to 6 units of autologous washed red cells are transfused.[33] Platelets also may be given after a 6- to 8-unit replacement.

INCREASED PLASMA-FREE HEMOGLOBIN. Red cells hemolyze from prolonged exposure to serosal surfaces and from mechanical trauma in the autotransfusion systems.[34] Elevated plasma-free hemoglobin, generally falling in the range of 25 to 30 mg/dL but occasionally much higher, is a consistent finding. Increased plasma-free hemoglobin is associated with an increased risk of acute tubular necrosis, particularly when accompanied by shock or acidosis. In normal subjects, free hemoglobin is excreted by the kidneys when plasma levels exceed 100 mg/dL. For this reason, some authorities suggest that renal insufficiency is a relative contraindication to autotransfusion. During autotransfusion, the hematocrit falls in direct proportion to the quantity of blood transfused,[34,35] decreasing by as much as 50% when patients receive an average of 6 units.

NONHEMATOLOGIC. Nonhematologic complications of autotransfusion include sepsis, air embolization, tumor embolization, particulate microemboli, and disseminated intravascular coagulation.[29,36] The risk of sepsis from autotransfusion seems to be minimal after an isolated thoracic injury. Blood has been transfused without incident after contamination, but this practice is not advisable.[37]

Platelet or fat microemboli can be eliminated by the use of a micropore filter.[38] Air embolism has been reported in systems using automated roller pumps when the aspirate reservoir was allowed to run dry. Air emboli are rare with standard gravity-assisted reinfusion techniques but have been lethal when the primary collection bag was pressurized by a pneumatic cuff for rapid infusion. If pressure infusion is necessary, the blood should be drained into a standard transfer pack.

PASSIVE BLOOD LOSS IN THE ICU ■

Ongoing "passive" blood loss in the ICU can result in blood loss requiring transfusion. Attention to detail eliminates much of this loss. Avoiding unnecessary or frequent laboratory blood tests save a considerable amount of blood. The clearing of an arterial pressure tubing of flush solution before drawing blood can waste 4 to 6 mL per sample.[39] Several devices are commercially available that allow aspirated blood/flush solution to be reinfused safely into the patient, thus eliminating this source of blood.[40]

Another source of blood loss is the use of older laboratory equipment that requires serum or plasma and larger samples. This methodology not only adds to the health care bill but also, over a period of days, may create the need for blood transfusion in the patient.[41] Newer generations of blood gas analyzers allow smaller samples (as small as 210 μL) and provide multiple analyses including Po_2, pH, Pco_2, hematocrit, sodium, potassium, chloride, calcium, glucose, blood urea nitrogen, and lactate in less than 2 minutes. These tests are run on heparinized whole blood. "Point of care" testing refers to analyzers in close proximity to the patient. Devices not in contact with the patient do not conserve blood. Implanted electrodes, however, can provide near real-time results and consume no blood.

BLOOD SUBSTITUTES ■

A discussion of blood "substitutes" cannot begin without first asking the question, "For what action are we substituting?" Most commonly, the term *blood substitute* refers either to the ability of blood to carry oxygen or to act as a colloid.

COLLOID

Increased colloid oncotic pressure in the intravascular space can be replaced by synthetic colloids or by blood products. Hydroxyl ethyl starch (Hespan) is the most common synthetic colloid material and is routinely given during operative procedures to replace blood loss. Limitations include a dose-dependent coagulopathy. Generally, no more than 1000 mL is given per 24-hour period. It is not recommended for the chronically ill patient but has been useful during operative procedures with a limited blood loss of less than 30% of the blood volume. Hespan has been shown to interfere with subsequent crossmatching.

Whereas FFP contains albumin, globulin, and other proteins, has a normal colloid oncotic pressure, and is an excellent plasma expander, the risk of disease transmission and its high expense make it unsuitable for volume expansion. Albumin, although acquired from human blood, is heat treated, thereby eliminating the risk of infectious disease transmission. Although albumin is safe, it remains an expensive plasma substitute and has a short intravascular half-life. The therapeutic use of albumin as a colloid substitute is further diminished by the observation that the "sicker" the ICU patient, the more rapidly albumin is lost from the vascular space.

OXYGEN CARRIERS

An ideal solution would supplement the oxygen-carrying capacity of blood, have a long half-life in vitro and in vivo, be nonimmunogenic, and be disease-free. Current research focuses on two main approaches. The first creates a solution that is able to hold a larger amount of dissolved oxygen than human plasma; the second creates a purified hemoglobin solution.

Perfluorocarbons

Perfluorocarbon solutions consist of a carbon skeleton saturated with fluorine, which makes them relatively inert; yet they have a solubility for oxygen that is up to 20 times that of water.[42] Unfortunately, perfluorocarbons are not soluble in plasma. To overcome this problem, an emulsified solution is required. The emulsification process, however, yields a solution that is only 10% to 20% perfluorocarbon, thus decreasing the enhanced oxygen solubility to approximately six times that of plasma.

Perfluorocarbon solutions are cleared rapidly by the reticuloendothelial system, with a circulating half-life of less than 24 hours. However, they remain within the reticuloendothelial system for months to years, thus limiting our ability to give large quantities of perfluorocarbon.

Hemoglobin Solutions

Separating the red cell membrane and other intracellular material from hemoglobin yields a solution of "stroma free" hemoglobin, advantageous because residual red cell stroma is thought to cause nephrotoxicity associated with these solutions. Because the ABO, Rh, and other antigens are contained on the red cell membrane, hemoglobin solutions do not require crossmatching.[43] One disadvantage of separating hemoglobin from the stroma, however, is that it loses its 2,3-DPG, resulting in impaired release of oxygen from the hemoglobin molecule. This problem can be partially corrected by adding pyridoxal-5-phosphate to the solution, which raises the P_{50}.

A second disadvantage of free monomer hemoglobin solution is that the individual molecules raise the colloid oncotic pressure of the solution to a range that is too high for clinical application. The individual hemoglobin molecules are small enough to be filtered by the kidneys, thus causing osmotic diuresis and nephrotoxicity. This problem can be overcome by polymerizing the hemoglobin molecules into longer chains. The final result is a solution of polymerized pyridoxilated stroma-free hemoglobin. Several products are in clinical trials and look promising. Other experimental approaches include the encapsulation of hemoglobin with a liposome.

REFERENCES ■

1. Management of surgical blood loss. *American Red Cross Scientific Forum.* Washington DC, American Red Cross, 1994

2. Gillon J, Greenburg AG: Transfusions: infectious complications. *Blood* 1992;19:28

3. Valeri CR, MacGregor H, Cassidy G, et al: Effects of temperature on bleeding time and clotting time in normal male and female volunteers. *Crit Care Med* 1995;23:698

4. Del Rossi AJ, Cernaianu AC, Botros S, et al: Prophylactic treatment of postperfusion bleeding using EACA. *Chest* 1989;96:27

5. Ereth MH, Oliver WC, Santrach PJ: Perioperative interventions to decrease transfusion of allogenic blood products. *Mayo Clin Proc* 1994;69:575

6. Salzman EW, Weinstein MJ, Weintraub RM, et al: Treatment with desmopressin acetate to reduce blood loss after cardiac surgery: a double blind randomized trial. *N Engl J Med* 1986;314:1402

7. Czer LSC, Bateman TM, Gray RJ, et al: Treatment of severe platelet dysfunction and hemorrhage after cardiopulmonary bypass: reduction in blood product usage with desmopressin. *J Am Coll Cardiol* 1987;9:1139

8. Hackman T, Gascoyne RD, Naiman SC, et al: A trial of desmopressin (1-desamino-8-D-arginine vasopressin) to reduce blood loss in uncomplicated cardiac surgery. *N Engl J Med* 1989;321:1437

9. Rocha E, Llorens R, Paramo JA, et al: Does desmopressin acetate reduce blood loss after surgery in patients on cardiopulmonary bypass? *Circulation* 1988;77:1319

10. Wildevuur RH, Eijsman L, Gu YJ, et al: Aprotinin reduces bleeding during cardiopulmonary bypass in aspirin treated patients. *J Cardiovasc Surg* 1990;31:34

11. Spence RK, Cernaianu AC: Pharmacological agents as adjuncts to bloodless vascular surgery. *Semin Vasc Surg* 1994;7:114

12. Helmkamp BF, Krebs HB, Loughner JE: Effectiveness of topical hemostatic agents. *Contemp Obstet Gynecol* 1985;4:171

13. Procrit® package insert. Raritan, NJ: Ortho Biotech, Inc.; 1998 Dec.

14. Goodnough LT: Erythropoietin as a pharmacologic alternative to blood transfusion in the surgical patient. *Transfusion Med Rev* 1990;4:288.

15. Jim RTS: Use of erythropoietin in Jehovah's Witness patients. *Hawaii Med J* 1990;49:209

16. Akingbola OA, Custer JR, Bunchman TE, et al: Management of severe anemia without transfusion in a pediatric Jehovah's Witness patient. *Crit Care Med* 1994;22:524

17. Autologous blood transfusions council on scientific affairs. *JAMA* 1986;256:2378

18. Lonser RE, Taber B: Autologous transfusion in a community hospital. In: *Proceedings of Haemonetics Research Advanced Component Seminar,* Boston, 1980

19. Goodnough LT, Rudnick S, Price TH, et al: Increased preoperative collection of autologous blood with recombinant human erythropoietin therapy. *N Engl J Med* 1989;321:1163

20. Pendyck J, Avorn J, Kuriyan N, et al: Blood donation in the elderly. *JAMA* 1987;257:1186

21. Mann M, Sacks HJ, Goldfinger D: Safety of autologous blood donation prior to elective surgery for a variety of potentially high risk patients. *Transfusion* 1983;23:229

22. Surgenor DM, Wallace EL, Hao SHS, et al: Collection and transfusion of blood in the United States 1982–1988. *N Engl J Med* 1990;322:1646

23. Toy PTCY, Strauss RG, Stehling LC, et al: Predeposited autologous blood for elective surgery: a national multicenter study. *N Engl J Med* 1987;316:517

24. Etchason J, Petz L, Keeler E, et al: The cost effectiveness of preoperative autologous blood donations. *N Engl J Med* 1995;332:719

25. Ness PM, Bourke DL, Walsh PC: A randomized trial of perioperative hemodilution versus transfusion of perioperatively depository of autologous blood in elective surgery. *Transfusion* 1991;31:226

26. Hur SR, Huizenga BA, Major M: Acute normovolemic hemodilution combined with hypotensive anesthesia and other techniques to avoid homologous transfusion in spinal fusion surgery. *Spine* 1992;17:867

27. Duncan J: On reinfusion of blood in primary and other amputations. *Br Med J* 1886;1:192

28. Klebanoff G, Watkins D: A disposable autotransfusion unit. *Am J Surg* 1968;116:475

29. Noon GP, Solis RT, Natelson EA: A simple method of intraoperative autotransfusion. *Surg Gynecol Obstet* 1976;143:65

30. Bell W: The hematology of autotransfusion. *Surgery* 1978;84:695

31. Davidson SJ: Emergency unit autotransfusion. *Surgery* 1978;84:703

32. Symbas PN: Extraoperative autotransfusion from hemothorax. *Surgery* 1978;84:722

33. Young GP, Purcell TB: Emergency autotransfusion. *Ann Emerg Med* 1983;12:180

34. Stillman RN, Wrezlewicz WW, Stanzcewski: The haematological hazard of autotransfusion. *Br J Surg* 1976;63:651

35. Smith RN, Yaw PB, Glover JL: Autotransfusion of contaminated intraperitoneal blood: an experimental study. *J Trauma* 1978;18:341

36. Dowling J: Autotransfusion: its use in the severely injured patient. In: *Proceedings of the First Annual Bentley Autotransfusion Seminar.* San Francisco, 1972:11

37. Glover JL, Smith R, Yaw PB, et al: Autotransfusion of blood contaminated by intestinal contents. *JACEP* 1978;7:142

38. Raines S, Buth J, Brewster DC, et al: Intraoperative autotransfusion: equipment protocol and guidelines. *J Trauma* 1976;16:616

39. Dennis RC, Yeston NM, Statland B: Effect of sample dilutions on arterial blood gas determinations. *Crit Care Med* 1985;13:1067

40. Peruzzi WT, Parker MA, Lichtenthal PR, et al: A clinical evaluation of a blood conservation device in medical intensive care unit patients. *Crit Care Med* 1993;21:501

41. Smoller BR, Kruskall MS: Phlebotomy for diagnostic laboratory tests in adults. *N Engl J Med* 1986;314:1233

42. Gould SA, Rosen AL, Sehgal LR, et al: Fluosol-DA as a red cell substitute in acute anemia. *N Engl J Med* 1986;315:1653

43. Rabinovici R, Neville LF, Rudolph AS, et al: Hemoglobin-based oxygen-carrying resuscitation fluids. *Crit Care Med* 1995;23:801

Critical Care, Third Edition, edited by Joseph M. Civetta,
Robert W. Taylor, and Robert R. Kirby.
Lippincott-Raven Publishers, Philadelphia, PA © 1997.

CHAPTER 45

Extracorporeal Circulation for Respiratory or Cardiac Failure

Joseph B. Zwischenberger
Aravind B. Sankar
Robert H. Bartlett

IMMEDIATE CONCERNS

MAJOR PROBLEMS

Should extracorporeal membrane oxygenation (ECMO) be considered for the patient with severe respiratory failure unresponsive to optimal management? Definitely yes, if the patient is a newborn infant over 34 weeks' gestational age. Possibly, if the patient is a child or adult with treatable and reversible pulmonary disease of less than 5 days' duration. Definitely not, if the patient has extensive pulmonary fibrosis or other incurable disease, necrotizing pneumonitis, or if the patient has been treated with a ventilator with high pressure and high oxygen concentration for 1 week or more.

If the patient is a candidate for ECMO, how do you do it? *If you have to ask, do not do it!* Transfer the patient to a center where ECMO is routinely practiced. Although the necessary equipment is simple, this is not a procedure that can be done on the spur of the moment. Currently, many centers throughout the world are capable of treating neonates and children. Only a few centers successfully treat adult patients.

STRESS POINTS

1. What is ECMO? *Extracorporeal membrane oxygenation* is the term used to describe prolonged extracorporeal cardiopulmonary bypass achieved by extrathoracic vascular cannulation.[1]

2. A modified heart-lung machine is used, consisting of a distensible venous blood drainage reservoir, a servo-regulated roller pump, a membrane lung to exchange oxygen and carbon dioxide, and a countercurrent heat exchanger to maintain temperature. The patient must be maintained with continuous heparin anticoagulation to prevent thrombosis within the circuit.

3. Is extracorporeal circulation helpful for cardiac failure? Yes, in all age groups and disease categories, but only if there is reason to believe that the patient will recover from cardiac disease within a few days.

4. Severe left ventricular failure may be better managed by left atrial–aortic extracorporeal circulation or a total artificial heart, as a bridge to transplantation.

5. Total venoarterial (VA) ECMO is reserved for patients with right ventricular or biventricular failure, unresponsive to other modes of therapy, in which heart recovery or replacement is anticipated within 5 to 7 days.

6. Although most ECMO centers are experienced in the treatment of neonatal respiratory failure, local expertise and need dictate the availability of pediatric ECMO for respiratory or cardiac support, or adult ECMO for respiratory failure.

7. Alternate treatment modalities for severe respiratory failure, including nitric oxide, high-frequency ventilation, surfactant, new ventilation techniques, and management protocols have impacted the potential ECMO patient population.

This chapter briefly reviews the pertinent history of extra-corporeal circulation for cardiac and respiratory support and describes the current techniques of ECMO. Most of the description refers to ECMO for newborn respiratory failure, because ECMO has been established as a standard treatment for this group of patients. The principles described in the discussion of infant ECMO also apply to the use of ECMO for children and adults. Also, commentary is added for adult patients and the potential for expanded application of ECMO in trauma. The use of ECMO for cardiac failure after repair of congenital heart defects and for perioperative support in pediatric heart transplantation is described.

BACKGROUND ■

Gibbon[2] and others developed the heart-lung machine in 1937 and opened the era of cardiac surgery in 1954. The use of an artificial pump and lung, however, was limited to 1 to 2 hours—not because of the pump but because of the oxygenator, which severely altered blood cells and proteins. The first membrane oxygenator built and used clinically was reported in 1956 by Clowes and his coworkers.[3] With the introduction of silicone rubber as a membrane for gas transfer, the membrane oxygenator became practical for long-term cardiopulmonary bypass.[4]

NEONATAL APPLICATION

Bartlett and associates[5] began clinical trials of ECMO in 1972 and reported the first successful use of ECMO in newborn respiratory failure in 1976; subsequently, several groups were successful using their method. As of January 1995, the technique had been used in the management of over 9900 neonates in 89 centers in the United States (and 20 outside the United States) with an overall survival rate of 81%.[6] This observation alone is sufficient to establish ECMO as therapeutically effective, because infants in these centers are treated after they meet criteria thought to predict an 80% mortality.

Bartlett and coworkers[7] conducted the first prospective randomized study of ECMO in newborn infants. The statistical method used in this study (randomized play-the-winner),[8] which for ethical considerations progressively weights the more successful treatment, directed 11 patients to the ECMO group (all survived) and one patient to the control group (died). O'Rourke and coworkers[9] completed a prospective randomized study comparing ECMO with conventional mechanical therapy with 6 of 10 survivors in the conventional treatment group and 28 of 29 survivors in the ECMO group. In 1986, Bartlett and others[10] published their first 100 cases of ECMO for neonatal respiratory failure, 72% of whom survived.

ADULT APPLICATION

A multicenter prospective randomized study of ECMO in adults with acute respiratory failure (ARF) was reported in 1979.[11] Ninety adults with severe ARF were admitted into the study, which specified management of the control group (continuing conventional mechanical ventilation) and the study group (ECMO). The survival rate with ECMO was 9.5% compared with 8.3% with conventional treatment. Overall national experience at that time was only marginally better, with a reported pooled survival rate of 15%.[12] ECMO did not change the outcome in a group of patients with ARF for whom therapy was begun after several days of high-pressure mechanical ventilation and high oxygen concentration.

The cause of death in patients in the ECMO and control groups was pulmonary fibrosis or necrotizing pneumonitis. ECMO provided safe and stable life support, and it seemed that ECMO would be effective for high-risk patients if begun early, before pulmonary fibrosis or necrosis occurred. Because of several key factors—new equipment, a more clinically homogeneous study group, earlier intervention, a lower fraction of inspired oxygen (FIO_2), and less traumatic ventilator settings—many investigators believe survival rates with ECMO can be improved.[13]

Gattinoni and coworkers,[14] using a modified ECMO technique (low-frequency positive-pressure ventilation with extracorporeal carbon dioxide removal [LFPPV–ECCO$_2$R]) achieved 49% survival in adult ARF. Based on these results, Bartlett and colleagues developed a protocol for ECMO in adult respiratory failure that yielded a 55% recovery rate with an overall survival of 45%. Surviving patients typically were younger and placed on ECMO early in their disease.[15] The worldwide experience with adult ECMO (VA and venovenous), which totals over 171 patients, reports an overall survival rate that is comparable (42%).[6]

With this information at hand, a controlled trial of a three-step therapy for adult respiratory distress syndrome was initiated by Morris and associates.[16] In this trial, patients were randomly assigned to a control arm of protocol-controlled continuous positive-pressure ventilation or a new treatment arm of pressure-controlled inverse-ratio ventilation; if the patient failed to improve, LFPPV–ECCO$_2$R was used.[16] The overall survival rate was 39% in ECCO$_2$R and conventional therapy groups. Detailed and specific protocols for respiratory management to ensure consistent and uniform respiratory care may yield superior results to historical or nonprotocol-controlled critical care and may decrease the need for extracorporeal support.[17]

PEDIATRIC APPLICATION

Concurrent with the adult collaborative study, ECMO was evaluated in children. Bartlett and coworkers[18] and Kolobow and others[19] reported an ECMO survival rate of 30% in children and infants beyond the neonatal period with ARF whose predicted survival rate with conventional therapy was thought to be less than 10%. Pediatric clinical trials are subject to many of the same problems experienced in adult populations, notably diverse underlying disease processes and initiation of therapy after the onset of irreversible pulmonary changes. Investigators are using ECMO for selected children with overall reported survival rate of 54% for respiratory failure and 42% for children with congenital heart disease treated for cardiac failure after open-heart surgery.[6]

TRAUMA

Respiratory failure adds significant morbidity, mortality, and cost to the care of patients with multiple trauma. High peak airway pressures, FIO_2 values, and respiratory rates are often needed to maintain oxygenation and carbon dioxide removal, all of which are associated with barotrauma and oxygen toxicity.[19] ECMO can provide cardiorespiratory support for the trauma patient, allowing reduction of ventilatory support to less-damaging levels.[20,21] The primary risk with advanced cardiac life support (ACLS) in trauma patients is severe bleeding because of the need for systemic heparinization. Anderson and associates[20] published their experience with 24 moribund pediatric and adult patients with respiratory failure from trauma. Fifteen patients (63%) survived to discharge. As would be expected, early intervention was the key factor in successful outcome.

PATHOPHYSIOLOGY ■

The beneficial effects of ECMO in respiratory failure are clearly related to decreasing the lung injury associated with mechanical ventilation. Oxygen and carbon dioxide transfer are accomplished, and systemic perfusion is well supported, but the actual amounts of gas transfer are similar to those in the immediate pre-ECMO period. However, gas exchange during ECMO takes place at ventilator settings that "rest" the lungs in both the newborn and adult populations.

NEONATES

Persistent fetal circulation (PFC), also known as persistent pulmonary hypertension of the newborn, is a major pathophysiologic mechanism of hypoxemia in full-term infants, regardless of whether the primary condition is diaphragmatic hernia, meconium aspiration, respiratory distress syndrome, sepsis, or primary PFC.[22] In this condition, pulmonary arteriolar spasm results in high pulmonary vascular resistance and right-to-left shunting through the patent ductus arteriosus and foramen ovale. During ECMO, the lungs are exposed to a low FIO_2, low ventilator rate, and low airway pressures, allowing reversal of PFC and promoting recovery by minimizing the harmful effects of high-pressure mechanical ventilation.

ADULTS

In adults and children, the challenge is to identify the causes of ARF that may be reversible within the safe time limits of extracorporeal support. Conditions treated successfully by ECMO techniques include bacterial and viral pneumonia, fat and thrombotic pulmonary embolism, thoracic or extrathoracic trauma, shock, sepsis, and near-drowning. As in neonates, lung rest from the harmful effects of excessive positive-pressure ventilation (high FIO_2, positive end-expiratory pressure [PEEP], peak inspiratory pressure [PIP], and minute ventilation) may be the universal benefit of ECMO in neonates and adults.[23]

PATIENT SELECTION ■

Patients selected for ECMO must have a potentially reversible underlying pathologic process. Indications for ECMO support include acute reversible respiratory or cardiac failure unresponsive to optimal ventilator and pharmacologic management, but from which recovery can be expected within a reasonable period (10 to 20 days) of extracorporeal support. The requirement for systemic heparinization limits the population for whom ECMO is appropriate to patients without bleeding complications, thereby relatively excluding premature infants (younger than 35 weeks' gestation)[24] and patients with active bleeding. Other contraindications include those which are incompatible with normal life after lung recovery (such as major brain injury), congenital or acquired immunodeficiency state, and mechanical ventilation for more than 5 to 10 days (as an indication of irreversible ventilator-induced lung injury).[25]

NEONATES

Extracorporeal membrane oxygenation has been applied to infants with a mortality risk of 80% or greater by retrospective analysis of local patient populations. Included were neonates who, despite optimum medical management, demonstrated acute deterioration ($Po_2 < 40$ mm Hg or pH < 7.15 for 2 hours), failure to improve ($Po_2 < 55$ mm Hg and hypotension requiring inotropic support), uncontrolled air leak, pneumomediastinum, or deterioration after diaphragmatic hernia repair.

Excessive alveolar-to-arterial oxygen gradients $P(A - a)O_2$ have been proposed as a qualification for ECMO. In a retrospective review by Krummel and associates,[26] a $P(A - a)O_2$ greater than 620 mm Hg for 12 consecutive hours correlated with over 90% mortality rate. We currently use the oxygenation index: mean airway pressure $\times$ FIO_2 $\times$ 100 divided by postductal PaO_2. Based on data generated before ECMO availability, after optimal conventional therapy, an oxygenation index consistently over 25 implies a 50% mortality rate, and over 40 defines an 80% mortality rate.

Contraindications to ECMO include any evidence of intracerebral hemorrhage, other brain damage, multiple congenital anomalies, and irreversible lung damage. In congenital diaphragmatic hernia, PFC cannot be distinguished from pulmonary hypoplasia; therefore, in most centers all patients with diaphragmatic hernias are treated who otherwise meet local ECMO criteria.[27] In some centers, a PaO_2 value higher than 70 mmHg or a $PaCO_2$ less than 80 mm Hg is required at some time in the neonate's life as evidence of sufficient functional pulmonary parenchyma to avoid infants with fatal pulmonary hypoplasia. Potential ECMO candidates are evaluated with cranial ultrasound to rule out intraventricular hemorrhage and cardiac ultrasound to rule out congenital cardiac anomalies. Entry criteria should be evaluated at each hospital before ECMO therapy is begun because of regional differences in patient populations and treatment protocols.

ADULTS

The indication for ECMO in adults is severe ARF of a few days' duration with a predicted mortality rate of 80% or greater. Reversible ARF in adults is difficult to define; therefore, adult criteria for ECMO are controversial.[18,23,28] Most investigators use the entry criteria from the National Institutes of Health ECMO Study (shunt > 0.30 despite optimum treatment).[11] Many use a PaO_2:FIO_2 ratio less than 100. Care must be taken to avoid therapy in patients with established pulmonary fibrosis. Lung biopsy may be necessary to determine the diagnosis and to measure the extent of fibrosis. Patients with the potential for bleeding or those with major destruction of lung tissue are not candidates for ECMO.

TECHNIQUES AND MANAGEMENT ■

NEONATES

Circuit Preparation

After the medical decision to begin ECMO is made, the necessary parental consent is obtained while the circuit is prepared and primed with approximately 350 mL of heparin-ized blood. Because the blood volume in the circuit is as much as twice the blood volume of the neonate, the appropriate hematocrit, pH, and electrolyte concentration must be adjusted before cardiopulmonary bypass is instituted. VA ECMO is the most common technique in use (Fig. 45-1); however, single-cannula venovenous ECMO is preferred by many as a primary technique of extracorporeal support.

Surgical Preparation

A surgical and operating room support team performs the dissection and cannulation under local anesthesia in the intensive care unit. An oblique incision in the right side of the neck anterior to the sternocleidomastoid muscle exposes the internal jugular vein and common carotid artery. The infant is given a 100-U/kg bolus of heparin as a loading dose. The vessels are ligated distally, and cannulas are inserted in a proximal direction from the ligation site. The venous cannula is threaded through the right internal jugular vein into the right atrium, and the arterial cannula is threaded into the common carotid artery so that its tip rests at the entrance to the aortic arch (Fig. 45-2). The largest catheters that fit "comfortably" inside the artery and vein are used. Catheter positions are confirmed by chest radiograph or ultrasonography. Positioning and flow resistance of the venous drainage catheter determine the maximum blood flow; the catheter should be capable of delivering total cardiac support of 120 mL/kg/minute. The right common carotid artery in a neonate can be successfully ligated with a relatively low complication rate, presumably because of abundant collateral flow.[29]

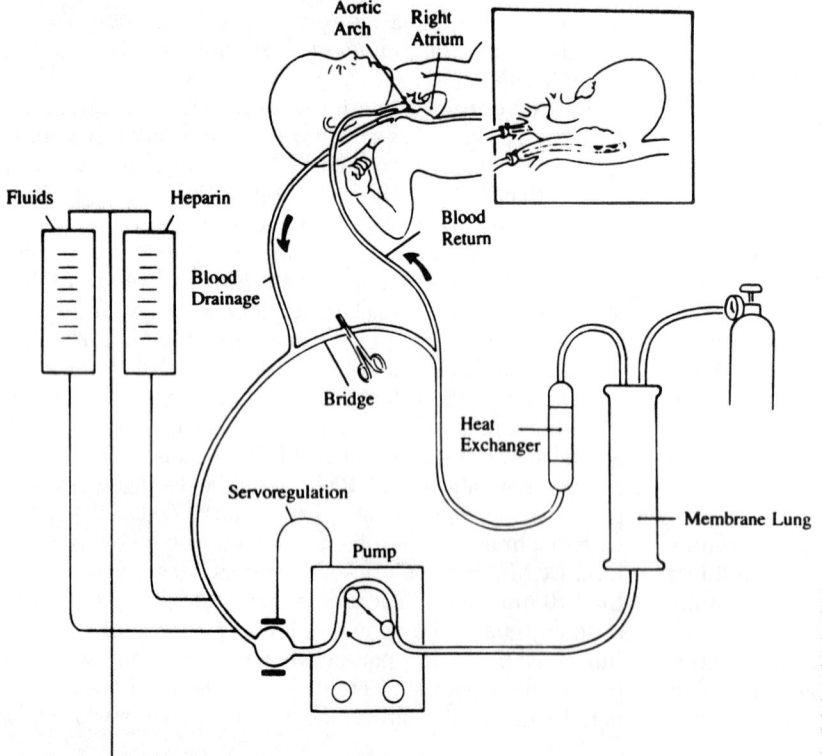

FIGURE 45-1. Venoarterial extracorporeal membrane oxygenation (ECMO) circuit. A modified heart-lung machine is used, consisting of a venous blood drainage reservoir, a servoregulated roller pump, a membrane lung to exchange oxygen and carbon dioxide, and a heat exchanger to maintain temperature.

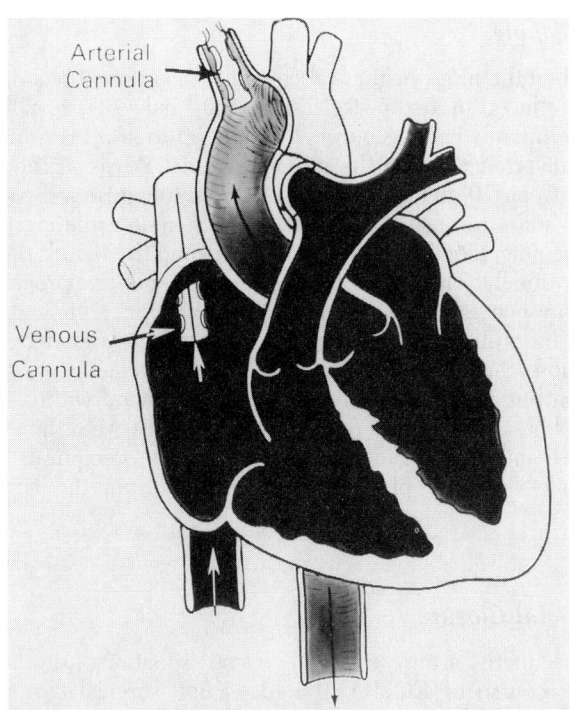

FIGURE 45-2. Venoarterial ECMO. Blood is drained from the right atrium through a catheter placed in the right internal jugular vein, with the tip of the catheter in the right atrium. The blood is oxygenated and returned to the patient through the right common carotid artery into the aortic arch.

Circulation

After cannulation is accomplished and bypass initiated, blood drains by gravity through the venous catheter to a servoregulated roller pump. The pump then perfuses the blood through a 0.6-, 0.8-, 1.5-, 2.5-, 3.5-, or 4.5-m² membrane lung (Avecor Cardiovascular, Minneapolis, MN) matched to the size of the patient. Gas exchange occurs in the membrane lung where oxygen is added to the blood and water vapor and carbon dioxide are removed. Because carbon dioxide removal is much more efficient than oxygen transfer, exogenous carbon dioxide often must be added to the oxygen inflow to avoid hypocapnic alkalosis.

The blood then passes through a heat exchanger and returns to the patient. Blood flow is gradually increased during the initial 15 to 20 minutes of bypass until approximately 80% of the infant's cardiac output flows through the circuit (Fig. 45-3). Oxygenated blood from the circuit then mixes in the aortic arch with poorly oxygenated blood from the left ventricle and ductus arteriosus to yield a mixed oxygen content adequate for the infant's metabolic requirements.[30]

Mechanical Ventilation

After extracorporeal support is established and appropriate pH, PaO_2, and $PaCO_2$ values are obtained, ventilator settings are reduced to minimize barotrauma and oxygen toxicity (PIP, 20 cm H_2O; rate 10/minute; FIO_2 0.3). The optimum PEEP level is uncertain, but many programs use high PEEP (12 to 15 cm H_2O) with mean airway pressures of 13 to 16 cm H_2O, based on experimental studies in a neonatal lamb model of meconium aspiration[31] that showed decreased time on ECMO and no increased barotrauma. A prospective, randomized study in neonates concluded that higher PEEP safely prevents deterioration of pulmonary function during ECMO and results in a more rapid lung recovery.[32]

FIGURE 45-3. Hemodynamic changes during venoarterial bypass. Total flow and arterial pulse pressure are shown during various levels of bypass. As blood is diverted from the right atrium to the extracorporeal circuit, pulmonary blood flow (and consequently left ventricular flow) decreases to the point where there is no flow during total bypass. Pulse amplitude decreases, reaching a nearly nonpulsatile state during total bypass. (Bartlett RH, Gazzaniga AB: In: Ionescu M, Wooler C [eds]. *Current Techniques in Extracorporeal Circulation.* London, Butterworths, 1976.)

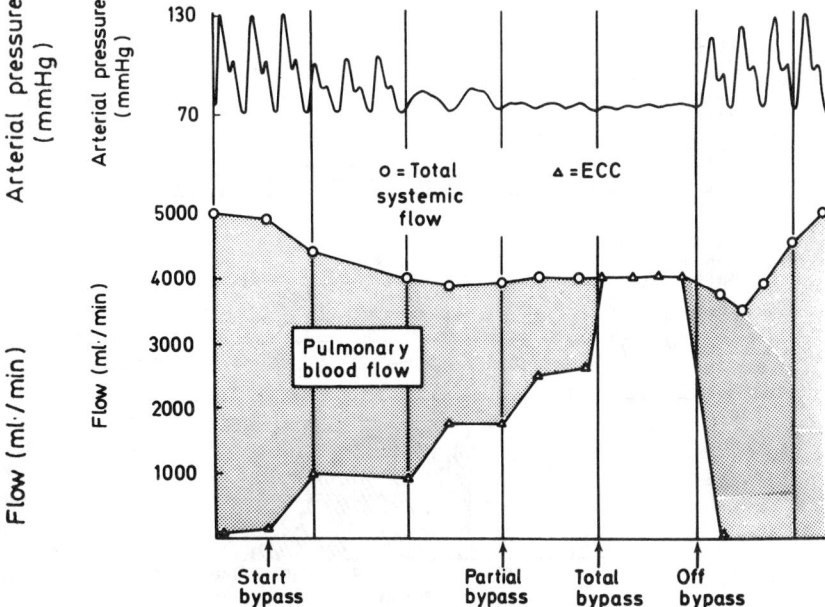

Therapeutic Endpoints

The ECMO flow is maintained at a level that achieves full respiratory support until lung improvement occurs (Fig. 45-4). The usual flow for full support is 80 to 120 mL/kg/minute (average 300 to 400 mL/minute) and is set to maintain PaO_2 between 70 and 90 mm Hg. Adequate support is defined as that level of extracorporeal flow that results in normal arterial and mixed venous oxygenation, mean arterial pressure, and organ function. During ECMO, chest physiotherapy continues, and suctioning is accomplished through the endotracheal tube. Paralyzing agents and vasoactive drugs are discontinued, and patients are maintained alert and awake.

Anticoagulation, Transfusion, and Fluid Therapy

Anticoagulation must be maintained during the entire course of treatment. Heparin is administered into the circuit with a loading dose (100 U/kg) followed by a constant infusion of approximately 30 U/kg/hour. Whole blood activated clotting time (ACT) is measured each hour and maintained at two to three times normal values. Platelets, which may be destroyed by the membrane lung, are administered when thrombocytopenia of 100,000 (or 150,000—the exact number is controversial) or less is observed. Hematocrit is maintained between 35% and 45% with packed red blood cell transfusions. Maintenance intravenous fluids are delivered directly into the bypass circuit, as is total parenteral nutrition, which is begun on the second or third day of life. Antibiotics (ampicillin and gentamicin) are administered until ECMO is completed. A chest radiograph and cranial ultrasound study are obtained daily.

Weaning

When the lungs begin to recover, extracorporeal blood flow is reduced in a stepwise fashion until only 10% to 20% of the infant's cardiac output (usually 50 to 100 mL/minute) is diverted through the circuit. Arterial PO_2 is maintained between 70 and 90 mm Hg. After an idling period of 8 to 12 hours to ensure continued lung function, the circuit is disconnected, the cannulas removed, and the vessels ligated proximally. The vessels can be repaired, but this procedure is not necessary, based on available follow-up data, and may be harmful if thrombi form and embolize. After decannulation, the infant is maintained with mechanical ventilation but is usually weaned to an oxygen hood within 48 to 72 hours. During the first 3 to 4 days off ECMO, the platelet count must be monitored closely for a precipitous drop while damaged platelets are removed from the circulation.

Ductal Closure

The ductus arteriosus usually closes spontaneously during the course of ECMO. If it does not, surgical closure is indicated while the patient is still on bypass. Termination of ECMO is indicated when the lungs have recovered or when signs of irreversible brain damage, uncontrollable bleeding, or irreversible lung damage (when the patient is dependent on ECMO for more than 20 days) are present. ECMO may be continued longer than 20 days if progressive improvement is seen or if open-lung biopsy demonstrates a reversible condition.

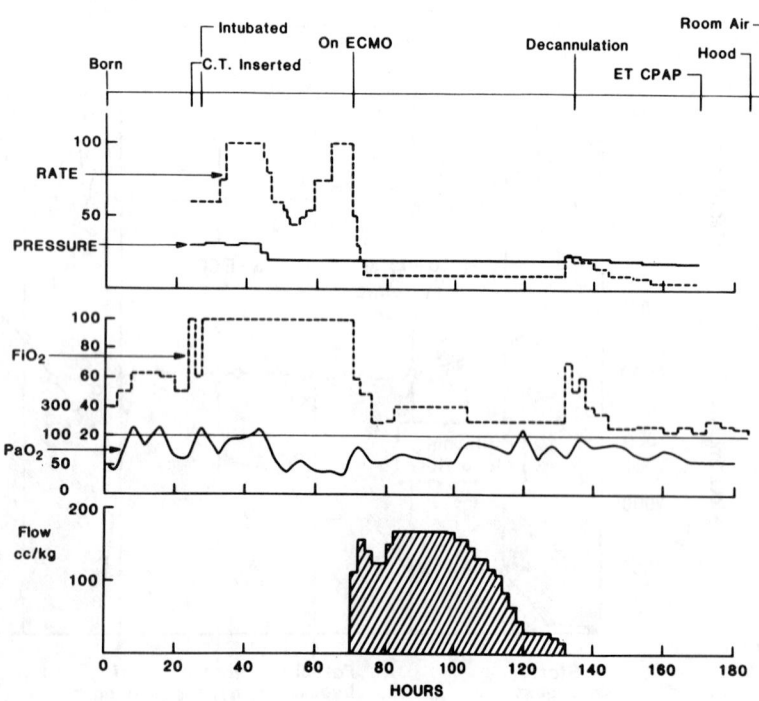

FIGURE 45-4. ECMO course of a typical neonate with persistent fetal circulation. ECMO permits "lung rest" with low pressure and low fraction of inspired oxygen (FIO_2). Between hours 100 and 130, extracorporeal flow is decreased as pulmonary blood flow im-

ADULTS

The general principles described for infants also apply to adult patients. Vascular access is achieved under local anesthesia, and recently available percutaneous introducer kits have increased the ease of bedside cannulation. For VA bypass, the same vessels used for neonatal ECMO are cannulated to deliver the oxygenated blood into the aortic arch. The femoral artery is not the best access site unless a long cannula is used. For venovenous access, we prefer the right internal jugular vein for drainage and the right femoral vein for reinfusion. In adults, 80 to 100 mL/kg/minute is often an adequate blood flow rate. As in the neonate, the extracorporeal flow is increased until satisfactory gas exchange is achieved with low ventilator settings. Management and weaning of adults is similar to neonates, but survivors require a longer time on ECMO. Complications are related to bleeding and circuit component failure.

VENOVENOUS ECMO ■

RATIONALE

The technique of venovenous ECMO, as performed by Kolobow and coworkers[13] and Gattinoni and associates,[14] is different from that of VA ECMO.[33] The rationale of this technique is to prevent damage to diseased lungs by reducing their motion (pulmonary rest), although three to five "sighs" with LFPPV are provided each minute to preserve the functional residual capacity. With this method, oxygen uptake and carbon dioxide removal are dissociated: oxygenation is accomplished primarily through the lungs, whereas carbon dioxide is cleared through extracorporeal removal ($ECCO_2R$). This combination ($LFPPV–ECCO_2R$) is performed at an extracorporeal blood flow of 20% to 30% of cardiac output. Vascular access may be jugulofemoral, femoral–femoral, or saphenosaphenous. Venovenous access emphasizing carbon dioxide removal is promising in adults, although most infants and children go through a phase of diminished lung function that may require systemic oxygenation as well. Bartlett currently uses venovenous ECMO for all applications of respiratory support (from newborns to adults). VA ECMO is used only when cardiac support is required.

ADVANTAGES

If the lungs are not functioning, all gas exchange requirements can be achieved during venovenous bypass by increasing the flow to 120% of cardiac output. Systemic oxygen saturation is decreased because of the recirculation fraction, but this decrement is offset by the increased extracorporeal flow. Venovenous ECMO has the advantage of maintaining normal pulmonary blood flow and avoiding arterial cannulation with its risk of systemic microemboli. Total support of gas exchange with venovenous perfusion, returning the perfusate blood into the venous circulation through the femoral vein or a modified jugular venous drainage catheter, also has the advantage of avoiding carotid artery ligation.[34]

Bartlett's group has developed a polyurethane double-lumen catheter for single-site cannulation of the internal jugular vein[35,36] (Fig. 45-5). A tidal flow venovenous system with a single-lumen catheter[34] has been developed to aid venous gas exchange. Efficient wire-wound cannulas, which are capable of sufficient flow for total gas exchange, can be inserted in large children (>15 kg) and adults by percutaneous insertion (Seldinger technique). Although jugulofemoral venovenous bypass is feasible in neonates, the advantages did not outweigh the disadvantages.[33] The occasional need for better cardiopulmonary support, and the extra complexity of two-vein venovenous bypass led us to favor VA bypass for hemodynamically unstable neonates as well.

OUTCOME

Since the 14-French venovenous double-lumen catheter (VVDL) became commercially available in 1989, over 1100 neonates have been treated with a 90% overall survival. A multicenter retrospective comparison of VA access to VVDL for newborns with respiratory failure undergoing ECMO was undertaken.[37] Overall survival in patients undergoing VA bypass was 87%, whereas survival in patients undergoing VVDL was 95%. Eleven patients required conversion from VVDL to VA because of insufficient support with ten survivors. Average bypass time for newborns on VA bypass was 132 ± 7.4 hours versus 100 ± 5.1 hours on VVDL bypass. Neurologic complications were more common in VA bypass. Hemorrhagic, cardiopulmonary, and mechanical complications, other than kinking of the VVDL catheter, occurred with equal frequency in each group.

When the entire Extracorporeal Life Support Organization (ELSO) registry experience of VA versus VVDL were compared, the survival for VA (1990 to 1992, n = 3146) was 81%, whereas that for VVDL (1990 to 1992, n = 576) was 91%.[38] The average duration of VA ECMO was 141 ± 89 hours and of VVDL was 120 ± 64 hours. Comparison of specific mechanical complications demonstrated that VVDL had a significantly higher prevalence of restrictive sutures (2% VVDL versus 0% VA) and kinking in the cannulas (9% VVDL versus 1% VA). When comparing the specific patient complication rates between techniques, VVDL had a much lower rate of major neurologic complications. The prevalence and survival rates with seizures (6% and 89% VVDL versus 13% and 61% VA, respectively) or cerebral infarction (9% and 69% VVDL versus 14% and 46% VA, respectively) were significantly lower with VVDL and seemed to have a substantial impact on overall survival. Therefore, during the initial experience, VVDL ECMO had a higher survival rate and a lower rate of major neurologic complications.[38]

Although cases in which this technique was used may have been more carefully selected and "more stable" than VA ECMO cases, the early success of the technique is encouraging. The less-invasive VVDL technique may lead to an important conceptual change in the use of ECMO technology. The current practice of waiting until the natural lungs become severely dysfunctional and then having to support cardiopulmonary function almost completely, as with VA ECMO, may give way to the concept of early lung

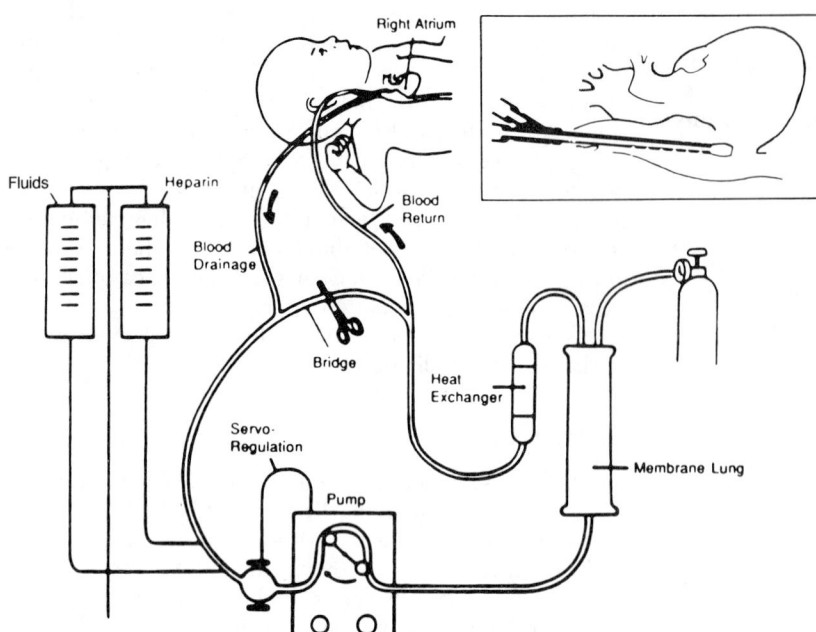

FIGURE 45-5. Venovenous extracorporeal life support (ECLS) circuit using the double-lumen catheter. *Inset:* Cannulation of the right atrium by way of the right internal jugular vein with this catheter. Side holes on the return lumen of the catheter direct oxygenated blood toward the tricuspid valve and foramen ovalis. (Anderson HL, Dtsu T, Chapman RA, et al: Venovenous extracorporeal life support in neonates using a double lumen catheter. *ASAIO Trans* 1989;35:650.)

assistance. Single-site cannulation may soon become the method of choice for most newborn patients. Likewise, continued catheter development will soon allow percutaneous access for VVDL ECMO.

THE ECMO TEAM

The complex and challenging care of patients treated with ECMO requires a highly trained and skilled team including physicians, perfusionists, ICU nurses, and ECMO specialists (Fig. 45-6). Maintaining the procedure without mistakes requires constant, diligent concentration. Providing this mode of care is not feasible for many hospitals because of the expense and commitment involved in training personnel. The technique cannot be undertaken on the spur of the moment by an unprepared team. In our institution, the training of the ECMO specialist alone requires a minimum of 80 hours of class and laboratory work.

A nurse and ECMO specialist are assigned to care for the ECMO patient. The nurse is responsible for ongoing assessment, hemodynamic monitoring, data collection, and pulmonary care. The ECMO specialist is responsible for monitoring the circuit, adjusting gas and pump flow, maintaining heparinization, drawing blood specimens, administering fluids and medications into the ECMO circuit, and documentation. Future technical development in the ECMO circuit includes simplification with more servoregulation and

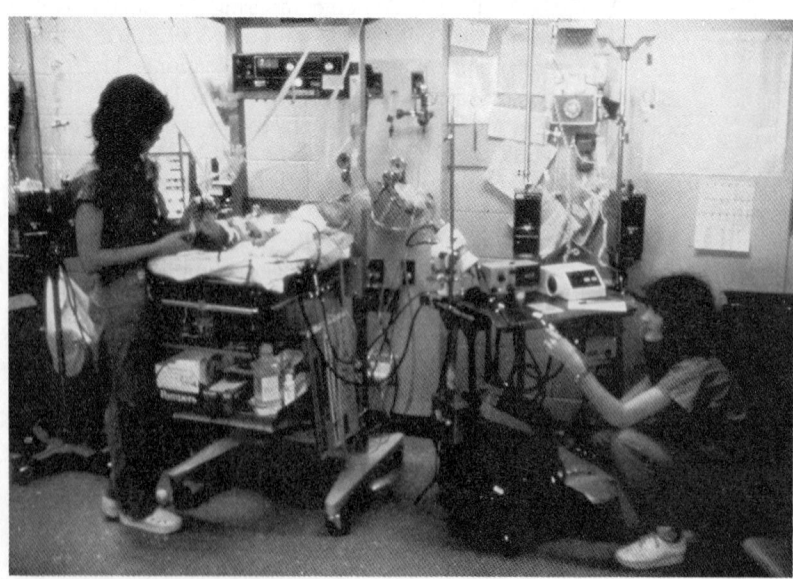

FIGURE 45-6. The ECMO system in use for neonatal respiratory failure.

automatic monitoring, so that a nurse with appropriate technical training can care for the infant and monitor the circuit.

COMPLICATIONS ■

NEONATES

Technical

The average duration of ECMO is 126 hours. Mechanical complications, in descending order of frequency of occurrence as reported in the National Registry, are listed in Table 45-1. Notice that mechanical complications not specifically attributable to a single-circuit component are the leading cause of problems, emphasizing the need for diligent and skilled bedside care of the circuit.[38] Air in the circuit (air embolism), power failure, malposition of the venous or arterial cannulas requiring repositioning, and unintentional decannulation are included in this group.

The overall incidence rate of mechanical complications is approximately 24%.[6] Although this figure seems high, it includes all problems encountered from any component of a complex circuit that is run for an average of over 5 days. Technical complications are rarely a direct cause of mortality; however, interrupting ECMO to change an oxygenator or ruptured tubing often causes physiologic instability. Patient complications in descending order of frequency are shown in Table 45-2. The medical management of the ECMO patient spans the entire field of critical care.[39]

Bleeding

Because of systemic heparinization, bleeding complications are common. Intracranial bleeding occurs primarily in premature infants less than 2 kg birth weight or less than 35 weeks' gestation.[30] Oozing at the cannulation site is present in many patients. Bleeding from other sites, however, occurs in approximately 14% of cases. Significant bleeding is managed by lowering the heparin dose to allow the ACT to be approximately 160 to 180 seconds and by increasing the platelet count to greater than 150,000.[40] We also consider discontinuing heparin for 1 to 2 hours. These measures may lead to clotting in the circuit, particularly the membrane lung, or even systemic embolization! Heparin-bonded circuits, including oxygenators using the Carmeda process, have become available commercially for short-term use. The risk–

benefit ratio of using a heparin-bonded circuit for ECMO (although intellectually appealing) remains to be defined.

Cardiovascular

When pulmonary vasospasm relaxes, recovery of lung function begins; flow through the ductus reverses (becoming left to right), and the ductus usually closes within 24 hours. The ductus may remain patent with major left-to-right shunting occurring in approximately 20% of patients. When persistent for more than 48 hours, we perform ductus ligation during ECMO.

Other complications include hypoxic cardiac arrest requiring cardiopulmonary resuscitation during cannulation, systemic hypertension requiring vasoactive drugs, hemopericardium with tamponade, and global myocardial dysfunction. We have not observed any major complications related to decannulation or vessel ligation, but brief paralysis is induced to minimize the chance of air embolism. Renal failure may be treated with dialysis or continuous hemofil-

TABLE 45-1. Mechanical Complication Rates in Neonates

Oxygenator failure	14%
Pump malfunction	1%
Heat exchange malfunction	1%
Clots in circuit	65%
Cracks in connectors	5%
Cannula problems	17%
Hemofilter malfunction	3%
Kinking in cannula	1%
Other mechanical	19%

TABLE 45-2. Patient Complication Rates During ECMO in Neonates

GI hemorrhage	2%
Cannula site bleed	11%
Surgical site bleed	10%
Hemolysis	30%
Other hemorrhagic	4%
Seizures	8%
Infarct or bleed by HUS	13%
Infarct or bleed by CT/MRI	10%
Other neurologic	1%
Creatinine >1.5 mg/dL	7%
Dialysis/hemofiltration	20%
Pulmonary hemorrhage	4%
CPR required	2%
Myocardial stun	4%
Cardiac arrhythmia	1%
Symptomatic PDA	6%
Hypertension	16%
Other cardiopulmonary	4%
Pneumothorax	3%
Other pulmonary	7%
Infection	12%
WBC suspect	5%
Other infectious	2%
K^+ <2.5 mMol/L	5%
K^+ >6.0 mMol/L	2%
Na^+ >150 mMol/L	3%
Ca^{2+} <6	1%
Blood glucose >240 mg/dL	2%
pH <7.2	4%
pH >7.6	5%
Hyperbilirubinemia	9%
Other metabolic	1%

GI, gastrointestinal; HUS, hemolytic–uremic syndrome; CT, computed tomography; MRI, magnetic resonance imaging; CPR, cardiopulmonary resuscitation; PDA, patent ductus arteriosus; WBC, white blood cell count; K^+, potassium; Na^+, sodium; Ca^{2+}, calcium.

tration through the ECMO circuit. This procedure is successful in removing extracellular fluid, and we use hemofiltration freely for symptomatic fluid overload unresponsive to diuretics.

After 20 days of ECMO support, the complication rate may exceed the potential benefit, although the absolute limits of ECMO have not been determined. Because of our experience with intracranial hemorrhage and major bleeding, we believe that intracranial hemorrhage (more than grade I), active gastrointestinal bleeding, and a gestational age younger than 35 weeks are relative contraindications to ECMO.

ADULTS

Bleeding and mechanical circuit problems occur even more commonly in adults. Intracranial bleeding is unlikely except in patients with recent cranial trauma. Gastrointestinal and nasopharyngeal bleeding likewise are more common. Platelet transfusion is less frequent in adults than in neonates.

RESULTS ■

NEONATAL SURVIVAL

From January 1973 to January 1995, more than 9900 newborn infants were treated with ECMO at over 109 centers. The survival rate for the entire series, including all of the early cases, is 81%.[6] Bartlett's experience up to January 1995 includes over 500 newborn cases, ranging from patients with cardiac arrest to those for a prospective controlled randomized study managed under a variety of protocols. Meconium aspiration is the most common form of respiratory failure treated with ECMO (35%) and the most successful of reported cases.[6]

Results in infants weighing less than 2 kg at birth and who are less than 35 weeks' gestation are poor. In the early experience of Bartlett and coworkers,[10] only 3 of 16 patients in this group survived. Almost all the deaths resulted from intracranial hemorrhage or cerebral edema. Intracranial bleeding is often a terminal event in critically ill premature infants and may be aggravated by thrombocytopenia and anticoagulation during ECMO. Our current entry criteria for ECMO may favor a high incidence of intracranial hemorrhage because of the moribund state of many patients.

Cost

The quality of life for survivors seems to be the same or better than that reported for conventional respiratory care, and the cost may be less. Short and Pearson[41] evaluated the effect of ECMO therapy on hospital charges. By decreasing average length of stay and essentially eliminating bronchopulmonary dysplasia and other chronic lung damage secondary to maximum ventilator support, ECMO therapy reduced total hospital and physician charges considerably. The length of hospitalization for survivors of routine therapy and ECMO therapy were 75.8 and 25.0 days, respectively. Total charges

were 43% lower for ECMO patients. Cumulative experience has reinforced these conclusions.

Follow-Up

Follow-up on the 72 survivors from Bartlett and associates' initial 100 neonatal cases ranges from 3 months to 11 years.[10] Of these 72 infants, 45 (63%) are normal or near normal. Seven late deaths have occurred. Twelve patients (17%) had major neurologic dysfunction and developmental delay. Eight had pulmonary dysfunction (needed supplemental oxygen at the time of hospital discharge).

Glass and coworkers[42] reported the outcome in 42 patients at 1 year of age. Using the Bayley Scales with a score greater than 90 considered normal, they found that 25 of 42 patients (60%) were normal and that 8 infants were suspect for delay (19%). The suspect patients generally had a mild motor delay with normal scores on the mental scale. They also identified three factors that were associated with a poor outcome at 1 year of age: pre-ECMO diagnosis of sepsis, chronic lung disease, and abnormal cranial ultrasound or computed tomographic scan.

The results of Adolph and colleagues[43] are consistent with the previous reports of outcome in neonatal ECMO patients. Using the Bayley, the McCarthy, and the Gessell scales, they found that 74% of 57 patients were normal. Only one patient (2%) was profoundly delayed.

A prospective, controlled study of outcome was performed to quantify the degree and frequency of developmental disabilities in ECMO survivors compared with a matched group. Mean scores of ECMO infants were well within the average range, and 77% of the ECMO infants were developmentally normal. These data suggest that early developmental morbidity in ECMO survivors is low, considering the severity of their neonatal illness.[44]

Differentiation between preexisting deficits and those secondary to ECMO remains difficult. However, some infants at high risk for brain damage (low Apgar scores, perinatal cardiac arrest, prolonged or profound hypoxia, prolonged fetal distress) have normal mental function; therefore, definitive predictors of outcome remain to be determined. The normal function of most survivors is encouraging and suggests that ECMO support can be accomplished safely and that subsequent normal development is frequent. An ECMO registry has been established with the ELSO to continue tabulation of multicenter early and late results.

PEDIATRIC SURVIVAL

The Pediatric Respiratory ECMO Registry lists 883 children treated with ECMO, with a survival rate for the series of 52%. Outcome by primary respiratory diagnosis reveals the best outcome for aspiration (56/87, 64%) and the worst for *Pneumocystis* infection (5/13, 38%).[6]

ADULT SURVIVAL

The results from a multicenter ECMO trial in adults are not nearly as favorable. Approximately 10% of adults treated with ECMO recovered and survived.[11,12] Successful applications usually involved situations in which ECMO was used early in conditions characterized primarily by interstitial pulmonary edema rather than major interstitial disease or lung destruction. However, as observed earlier, Gattinoni and associates[14] report a 49% survival rate in an uncontrolled series of adults with ARF who were treated with LFPPV–ECCO$_2$R. Anderson's group[15] has recently reported a 45% survival rate. In adult ECMO survivors, pulmonary and cerebral function usually return to normal within a few months after hospital discharge.

LABORATORY INVESTIGATION

Current laboratory efforts include investigation of measures other than systemic heparinization to prevent thrombosis of the extracorporeal circuit and the membrane lung.[45-47] Heparin and other anticoagulant surface coatings have been tested experimentally, and the results demonstrate that this principle is sound.

Development and refinement of ECMO technology are not limited to newborns with respiratory failure. Vascular access techniques, methods of clotting time measurement, and low-resistance membrane oxygenators are used in cardiopulmonary bypass for cardiac surgery. The servocontrol mechanism, heparin-coated circuits, and perfusion technology gained from the ECMO experience also have potential application in cardiac surgery. Similarly, measurements of whole blood ACT and techniques of prolonged continuous perfusion are useful in hemodialysis, hyperthermic perfusion, and hemofiltration.

CARDIAC SUPPORT

Mechanical circulatory support systems, intraaortic balloon counterpulsation, and ventricular assist devices for acute postcardiotomy ventricular failure effectively reduce postoperative mortality in adult populations. Technologic barriers, particularly size constraints, currently limit the clinical application of these devices to adult patients. ECMO provides univentricular or biventricular cardiac, as well as respiratory support, and has extended application of ECMO to infants and children who develop refractory postoperative cardiogenic shock after repair of congenital heart defects.[48] Several anecdotal reports noting survival using ECMO for postoperative cardiogenic shock appeared in the 1970s; however, Pennington and others[49] first reported four patients of pediatric age in 1984 with three survivors. Several groups soon reported results averaging 50% survival.[50,51] Klein and co-workers[52] treated 36 children, with 22 (61%) surviving to extubation. All had adequate surgical repair and were believed to have little chance for survival without mechanical support.

ECMO has also been used for perioperative support in pediatric heart transplantation. In a report of the known cases of ECMO used as an adjunct to pediatric cardiac transplantation, Galantowitz and Stolar[53] reported on 16 children with cardiac failure refractory to conventional therapy who underwent ECMO support for a mean of 63 hours in the perioperative period. In four cases, ECMO was used as a bridge to transplant with no late survivors. In 11 cases, ECMO was used for postoperative allograft support; there were eight deaths and three long-term survivors, all with normal cardiac function.

OUTCOME

The Cardiac ECMO Registry lists 1401 patients treated with ECMO with a survival rate for the entire series of 37%.[6] Outcome by primary cardiac diagnosis includes postcardiac surgery 451 of 1084 (42%), postcardiac transplant 34/79 (43%), myocardiopathy 35/60 (58%), myocarditis 23/43 (53%), and other 63/135 (47%). The Registry does not distinguish the cardiac abnormality or the surgical repair for patients after cardiac surgery. There are no specific preoperative predictors of a need for ECMO, or predictors of mortality in children after repair of congenital heart defects.

Improved survival is observed when ECMO for cardiac support can be initiated 6 to 24 hours after weaning from cardiopulmonary bypass. This process selects a group with better cardiac function than those who cannot wean off bypass and allows normalization of coagulation parameters. The general consensus among physicians involved in the care of these patients is that, without mechanical circulatory support, mortality rate would exceed 90%. All patients displayed signs and symptoms of inadequate cardiac output: systemic arterial hypotension, oliguria, poor peripheral perfusion, lactic acidemia, and diminished venous oxygen saturation.

TECHNIQUES

Venoarterial perfusion is used exclusively for cardiopulmonary support with gravity drainage from the right atrium and return of oxygenated blood to the aortic arch. The ECMO circuit described by Bartlett[54] is used in most institutions for neonatal pulmonary support and is generally used for postoperative patients, as previously described. Several cannulation sites can be used for VA bypass in the postoperative cardiac patient. A transthoracic approach with the heart still exposed after cardiac repair is convenient because cannulas can be placed or retained in the aorta and right atrium directly. Cannulas are brought through the sternotomy and the skin loosely approximated. However, this approach seems to have a higher incidence of postoperative hemorrhagic complications. Femoral artery and femoral vein cannulation can be performed through a groin incision. Also, the right common carotid artery and internal jugular vein, similar to neonatal cannulation through a lateral neck dissection, can be used. Venous drainage by internal jugular vein cannulation and arterial cannulation through the right axillary artery also can be used. Currently, most experienced investigators recommend neck cannulation when technically feasible. Some groups are reporting repair of the carotid artery and jugulovenous cannulation sites after ECMO support.[55-59]

After ECMO is initiated, inotropic support and ventilatory support are weaned. Cardiac recovery is determined by echocardiographic variables for an overall assessment of contractility and cardiac function. These variables are clinically correlated with the hemodynamic consequences of diminished ECMO flow rates with or without inotropic support to determine weaning.

COMPLICATIONS

Hemorrhage remains the most serious complication with ECMO after cardiac surgical procedures. Most hemorrhagic complications occur in patients who have transthoracic cannulation, which may reflect the need for ECMO intraoperatively or the constant cardiac motion at the venous and arterial cannulation sites. Most programs prefer right carotid artery and jugular venous cannulation. Besides bleeding complications, all other complications previously observed during ECMO have been reported. Patients who require circulatory support at the time of weaning from cardiopulmonary bypass in the operating room or shortly thereafter seem to be at the greatest risk of not recovering with ECMO support (only a few of these patients have survived).

Long-term follow-up is preliminary but seems to parallel the neonatal population, with most patients experiencing normal growth and development. Contraindications to ECMO for postcardiotomy support are unknown; however, conditions such as hypoplastic left heart syndrome seem to rule out patients who are otherwise good candidates for ECMO, unless neonatal heart transplantation becomes well established. Relative contraindications to ECMO include severe coagulopathies or known neurologic dysfunction.

CONCLUSION ■

With further experience, the indications, techniques, and outcome will be more reliably identified. Bleeding—the most serious complication of ECMO—may be significantly reduced by new extracorporeal devices that will permit ECMO with reduced systemic anticoagulation. These advances in technique and technology may facilitate the use of ECMO in other environments, such as the trauma room and cardiac catheterization laboratory.

REFERENCES ■

1. Zwischenberger JB, Bartlett RH: Extracorporeal circulation and oxygenation. In: Civetta JM, Taylor RW, Kirby RR (eds). *Critical Care*, 2nd ed. Philadelphia, JB Lippincott, 1992:1629
2. Gibbon JH Jr: Artificial maintenance of circulation during experimental occlusion of pulmonary artery. *Arch Surg* 1937;34:1105
3. Clowes GHA Jr, Hopkins AL, Neville WE: An artificial lung dependent upon diffusion of oxygen and carbon dioxide through plastic membranes. *J Thorac Surg* 1956;32:630
4. Kolobow T, Bowman RL: Construction and evaluation of an alveolar membrane artificial heart-lung. *Trans Am Soc Artif Intern Organs* 1963;9:238
5. Bartlett RH, Gazzaniga AB, Jefferies MR, et al: Extracorporeal membrane oxygenation (ECMO) cardiopulmonary support in infancy. *ASAIO Trans* 1976;22:80
6. ECMO Registry Report of the Extracorporeal Life Support Organization. Ann Arbor, MI, January 1995
7. Bartlett RH, Roloff DW, Cornell RG, et al: Extracorporeal circulation in neonatal respiratory failure: a prospective randomized study. *Pediatrics* 1985;76:479
8. Cornell RG, Landenberger BD, Bartlett RH: Randomized play-the-winner clinical trials. *Comm Stat Theory Methods* 1986;1:159
9. O'Rourke PT, Crone RK, Vacanti JP, et al: A prospective randomized study of extracorporeal membrane oxygenation (ECMO) and conventional medical therapy in neonates with persistent pulmonary hypertension of the newborn: a prospective randomized study. *Pediatrics* 1989;84:957
10. Bartlett RH, Gazzaniga AB, Toomasian JM, et al: Extracorporeal membrane oxygenation (ECMO) in neonatal respiratory failure: 100 cases. *Ann Surg* 1986;204:236
11. Zapol WM, Snider MT, Hill JD: Extracorporeal membrane oxygenation in severe acute respiratory failure: a randomized prospective study. *JAMA* 1979;242:2193
12. Peirce EC: Is extracorporeal membrane oxygenation a viable technique? *Ann Thorac Surg* 1981;31:102
13. Kolobow T: An update on adult extracorporeal membrane oxygenation-extracorporeal CO_2 removal. *ASAIO Trans* 1988;34:1004
14. Gattinoni L, Pesenti A, Mascheroni D, et al: Low-frequency positive-pressure ventilation with extracorporeal CO_2 removal in severe acute respiratory failure. *JAMA* 1986;256:881
15. Anderson H, Steimle C, Shapiro M, et al: Extracorporeal life support for adult cardiorespiratory failure. *Surgery* 1993:114;161
16. Morris AH, Menlove RL, Rollins RJ, et al: A controlled clinical trial of a new 3-step therapy that includes extracorporeal CO_2 removal for ARDS. *ASAIO Trans* 1988;34:48
17. Morris AH, Wallace CJ: Randomized clinical trial of pressure-controlled inverse ratio ventilation and extracorporeal CO_2 removal for adult respiratory distress syndrome. *Am J Respir Crit Care Med* 1994;149:295
18. Bartlett RH, Gazzaniga AB, Wetmore NE, et al: Extracorporeal membrane oxygenation (ECMO) in the treatment of cardiac and respiratory failure in children. *ASAIO Trans* 1980;26:578
19. Kolobow T, Stool EW, Sacks KL, et al: Acute respiratory failure, survival following ten days' support with a membrane lung. *J Thorac Cardiovasc Surg* 1975;69:947
20. Anderson HL, Shapiro MB, Delius RE, et al: Extracorporeal life support for respiratory failure after multiple trauma. *J Trauma* 1994;37:266
21. Anderson HL, Coran AG, Schmeling DJ, et al: Extracorporeal life support (ECLS) for pediatric trauma: experience with five cases. *Pediatr Surg* 1990;5:302
22. Bartlett RH: Respiratory support extracorporeal membrane oxygenation in newborn respiratory failure. In: Welch K, Randolph J, Ravitch M, et al (eds). *Pediatric Surgery*, 4th ed. Chicago, Year Book Medical Publishers, 1986:74
23. Kolobow T: Acute respiratory failure: on how to insure healthy lungs (and prevent sick lungs from recovering). *ASAIO Trans* 1988;34:31
24. Cilley RE, Zwischenberger JB, Andrews AF, et al: Intracranial hemorrhage during extracorporeal membrane oxygenation in neonates. *Pediatrics* 1986;78:699
25. Bartlett RH, Anderson HL: Extracorporeal life support in pediatric trauma. In: Coran AG, Harris BH (eds). *Pediatric Trauma*. Proceedings of the Third Nutritional Conference, 1990:142
26. Krummel TM, Greenfield LJ, Kirkpatrick BV, et al: Alveolar-arterial oxygen gradients versus the neonatal pulmonary insufficiency index for prediction of mortality in ECMO candidates. *J Pediatr Surg* 1984;19:380

27. Lally KP, Paranka MS, Roden J, et al: Congenital diaphragmatic hernia: stabilizations and repair on ECMO. *Ann Surg* 1992;216:569

28. Bone RC: Extracorporeal membrane oxygenation for acute respiratory failure [editorial]. *JAMA* 1986;256:910

29. Campbell LR, Bunyapen C, Holmes GL, et al: Right common carotid artery ligation in extracorporeal membrane oxygenation. *J Pediatr* 1988;113:110

30. Cilley RE, Wesley JR, Zwischenberger JB, et al: Metabolic rates of newborn infants with severe respiratory failure treated with extracorporeal membrane oxygenation. *Curr Surg* 1987; Jan/Feb:48

31. Kolobow T, Moretti MP, Mascheroni D, et al: Experimental meconium aspiration syndrome in the preterm fetal lamb: successful treatment using the extracorporeal artificial lung. *ASAIO Trans* 1983;29:221

32. Keszler M, Ryckman FC, McDonald JV, et al: A prospective multicenter randomized study of high vs. low positive end-expiratory pressure during extracorporeal membrane oxygenation. *J Pediatr* 1992;120:107

33. Klein MD, Andrews AF, Wesley JR, et al: Venous perfusion in ECMO for newborn respiratory insufficiency: a clinical comparison with venoarterial perfusion. *Ann Surg* 1985;201:520

34. Zwischenberger JB, Toomasian JM, Drake K, et al: Total respiratory support with single cannula venovenous ECMO: double lumen continuous flow vs. single lumen tidal flow. *ASAIO Trans* 1985;31:610

35. Otsu T, Merz SI, Hultquist KA, et al: Laboratory evaluation of a double lumen catheter for venovenous neonatal ECMO. *ASAIO Trans* 1989;35:647

36. Anderson HL III, Otsu T, Chapman RA, et al: Venovenous extracorporeal life support in neonates using a double lumen catheter. *ASAIO Trans* 1989;35:650

37. Anderson HL, Snedecor SM, Otsu T, et al: Multicenter comparison of conventional venoarterial access versus venovenous double-lumen catheter access in newborn infants undergoing extracorporeal membrane oxygenation. *J Pediatr Surg* 1993;28:530

38. Zwischenberger JB, Nguyen T, Upp JR, et al: Complications of neonatal extracorporeal membrane oxygenation. *J Thorac Cardiovasc Surg* 1994;107:838

39. Upp JR, Bush PE, Zwischenberger JB: Complications of neonatal extracorporeal membrane oxygenation. *Perfusion* 1994;9:241

40. Sell LL, Cullen ML, Whittlesey GC: Hemorrhagic complications during extracorporeal membrane oxygenation: prevention and treatment. *J Pediatr Surg* 1986;21:1087

41. Short BL, Pearson GD: Neonatal extracorporeal membrane oxygenation: a review. *J Int Core Med* 1986;1:47

42. Glass P, Miller MK, Short BL: Morbidity for survivors of extracorporeal membrane oxygenation: neurodevelopmental outcome at one year of age. *Pediatrics* 1989;83:72

43. Adolph V, Edelund C, Smith C: Developmental outcome of neonates treated with extracorporeal membrane oxygenation. *J Pediatr Surg* 1990;25:43

44. Wildin SR, Landry SH, Zwischenberger JV: Prospective, controlled study of developmental outcome in survivors of extracorporeal membrane oxygenation: the first 24 months. *Pediatrics* 1994;93:404

45. Shanley CJ, Hultquist KA, Rosenberg DM, et al: Prolonged extracorporeal circulation without heparin: evaluation of the medtronic minimax oxygenator. *ASAIO Trans* 1992;38:M311

46. Mottaghy K, Oedekoven B, Poppel K, et al: Heparin free long-term extracorporeal circulation using bioactive surfaces. *ASAIO Trans* 1989;35:635

47. Montoya JP, Shanley CJ, Merz SI, et al: Plasma leakage through microporous membranes: role of phospholipids. *ASAIO J* 1992; 38:M399

48. Toomasian JM, Haiduc NJ, Zwischenberger JB, et al: Techniques of extracorporeal membrane oxygenation for cardiac failure. *Proc Am Acad Cardiovasc Perf* 1986;7:105

49. Pennington DG, Merjauy JP, Codd JE, et al: Extracorporeal membrane oxygenation for patients with cardiogenic shock. *Circulation* 1984;70(Suppl 1):130

50. Rogers AJ, Trento A, Siewers RD, et al: Extracorporeal membrane oxygenation for postcardiotomy cardiogenic shock in children. *Ann Thorac Surg* 1989;47:903

51. Weinhaus L, Canter C, Noetzel M, et al: Extracorporeal membrane oxygenation for circulatory support after repair of congenital heart defects. *Ann Thorac Surg* 1989;48:206

52. Klein MD, Shaheen KW, Whittlesey GC, et al: Extracorporeal membrane oxygenation (ECMO) for the circulatory support of children after repair of congenital heart disease. *J Thorac Cardiovasc Surg* 1990;100:498

53. Galantowitz ME, Stolar CJ: Extracorporeal membrane oxygenation for perioperative support in pediatric heart transplantation. *J Thorac Cardiovas Surg* 1991;102:148

54. Bartlett RH: Extracorporeal life support for cardiopulmonary failure. *Curr Probl Surg* 1990;27:10

55. Crombleholme TM, Adzick NS, deLorimier AA, et al: Carotid artery reconstruction following extracorporeal membrane oxygenation. *Am J Dis Child* 1990;144:872

56. Spector ML, Wiznitzer M, Walsh-Sukys MC, et al: Carotid reconstruction in the neonate following ECMO. *J Pediatr Surg* 1991;26:357

57. Moulton SL, Lynch FP, Cornish JD, et al: Carotid artery reconstruction following neonatal extracorporeal membrane oxygenation. *J Pediatr Surg* 1991;26:794

58. Schaupp W, Brands W, Wirth H, et al: Reconstruction of the arteria carotis communis in newborn following extracorporeal membrane oxygenation (ECMO). *Eur J Pediatr Surg* 1992;2:78

59. DeAngelis GA, Mitchell DG, Merton DA, et al: Right common carotid artery reconstruction in neonates after extracorporeal membrane oxygenation: color Doppler imaging. *Radiology* 1992;182:521

Critical Care, Third Edition, edited by Joseph M. Civetta,
Robert W. Taylor, and Robert R. Kirby.
Lippincott-Raven Publishers, Philadelphia, PA © 1997.

CHAPTER 46

∎

Fiberoptic Bronchoscopy

J. Steven Hata
David A. Schenk
R. Phillip Dellinger

IMMEDIATE CONCERNS ∎

The fiberoptic bronchoscope is an essential diagnostic and therapeutic tool in the intensive care unit (ICU). Airway management indications are of particular importance, including intubation, changing of endotracheal tubes, and extubation over the fiberoptic bronchoscope. From a diagnostic standpoint, it can identify the etiology of hemoptysis and the cause of pulmonary infection. Therapeutic benefits, in addition to intubation, include treatment of atelectasis, hemoptysis (in the patient who is not a candidate for surgery), and initiation of independent lung ventilation. Although larger diameter fiberoptic bronchoscopes have logistic disadvantages, they afford greater suction/instrument passage channel diameter. Advances in technology have facilitated a larger channel size to bronchoscope outer diameter ratio as well as greater inflection and extension range of the instrument. Compared with rigid bronchoscopy, fiberoptic bronchoscopy offers enhanced visualization of the distal bronchi and can be performed at the bedside, averting the need for general anesthesia and operating room resources. Fiberoptic bronchoscopy in the intensive care setting can be invaluable in managing patients with atelectasis unresponsive to conventional forms of chest physiotherapy, in removing a foreign body from the peripheral airways, and in initial or replacement tracheal intubation. Fiberoptic bronchoscopy may be necessary for confirming mycobacterial disease, localizing the source of hemoptysis, identifying a specific cause of pneumonia in compromised and noncompromised hosts, or assessing tracheobronchial trauma, upper airway obstruction, and acute inhalation injury.

The availability of video bronchoscopy has allowed better resolution of image because of the greater number of pixels on the charge-coupled device for image acquisition. In contrast, the resolution of the traditional fiberoptic bronchoscope is determined by the diameter of the optical fiber and seems to have reached its limit. With the video bronchoscope, observation by multiple parties is possible, decreasing the possibility of missed findings. It also facilitates teaching and education. This is particularly advantageous in the ICU at teaching institutions where time may be of the essence with a limited time window for accomplishing the procedure. Images can be frozen, and most clinicians report that manipulation is easier with the video bronchoscope. Those who wear corrective lenses find this system an advantage, and there is a lower risk of contamination from the working channel, which is an important factor in this day of potential viral illness transmission. The manipulative advantage of the video system and the ease of operation is primarily associated with the direct type of video bronchoscopes that have the charge-coupled device chip on their tips. Many of these advantages are lost with indirect video bronchoscopes, which require a camera mount on the proximal end of the bronchoscope. The optical system is in particular better with the charge-coupled device chip. The two primary shortcomings of video bronchoscopes are increased expense and occasional problems with color reconstruction, especially the resolution of red, the color of blood. When cost is factored in, however, it has not been convincingly shown that the difference in resolution between video bronchoscopy and traditional fiberoptic bronchoscopy offers significant clinically advantages.[1,2]

To minimize airway resistance and high inflation pressures during bronchoscopy in patients requiring mechanical ventilation, an endotracheal tube or tracheostomy tube with an inner diameter of at least 8 mm is recommended. Bronchoscopy performed through a tube with a smaller inner diameter increases airway resistance, predisposing the patient to hypoventilation, barotrauma, and hypotension. Hypoventilation may occur when tidal volumes decrease. The decrease in tidal volume invariably occurs when the breath being delivered is a pressure-limited, time-cycled breath and occurs when flow-limited, volume-cycled breaths become pressure-limited. To reliably assure tidal volume delivery, volume-cycled breaths should be used during bronchoscopy. Because the increase in peak pressure is dissipated along the endotracheal tube and does not represent an increased risk for barotrauma, the peak pressure limit can be significantly elevated to ensure delivery of tidal volume. The high peak pressures seen during bronchoscopy are not reflective of pressures distal to the endotracheal tube. The problem with high peak pressures is pressure limiting, resulting in decrease in effective tidal volume. Decreasing inspiratory flow rate decreases pressure limiting but increases predisposition to automatic positive end-expiratory pressure (auto PEEP). Barotrauma and hypotension may occur if the bronchoscope-added expiratory resistance leads to auto PEEP. The presence of auto PEEP produces hyperinflation as a risk for barotrauma and increases intrathoracic pressure as a potential for hypotension. The larger the internal diameter of the endotracheal tube or tracheostomy tube and the smaller the outer diameter of the fiberoptic bronchoscope, the lower the risk of air trapping (auto PEEP) and the potential for hypotension and barotrauma, and the less likely is pressure-limiting during volume-cycled ventilator breaths. A special in-line adapter provides sealed access to the airway, maintaining a relatively closed system. In mechanically ventilated patients, adequate sedation and airway anesthesia minimize cough and patient discomfort. Airway suctioning should be minimized (predisposition to hypoxemia) and the fraction of inspired oxygen (FIO_2) increased to 1.0 during the procedure to ensure adequate alveolar oxygenation.

COMPLICATIONS

With appropriate care, fiberoptic bronchoscopy is an extremely safe procedure. The incidence rate of major complications ranges from 0.08% to 0.15%, and the mortality rate from 0.01% to 0.04%. Minor complications (e.g., vasovagal reaction, fever, bleeding, nausea, vomiting) occur in as many as 6.5% of these patients.[3–5] Fiberoptic bronchoscopy in patients with respiratory failure on mechanical ventilation has the potential for life-threatening complications (Table 46-1), including hypoxemia, hypercapnia, barotrauma, cardiac arrhythmias, myocardial ischemia, intracranial hypertension, local anesthetic toxicity, and pulmonary hemorrhage.

Careful patient selection, meticulous preparation before the procedure, and vigilant physiologic monitoring during the procedure limits complications and mortality. Characteristics of high-risk patients are summarized in Table 46-2. A

TABLE 46-1.   Complications of Fiberoptic Bronchoscopy in the ICU

Hypoxemia	Hypercapia
Barotrauma	Hypotension
Hypertension	Hemorrhage
Aspiration	Intracranial hypertension
Infection	Laryngospasm
Loss of FOB equipment	Cardiac arrhythmias

ICU, intensive care unit; FOB, fiberoptic bronchoscopy.

recent, prospective clinical trial[6] in critically ill, mechanically ventilated patients with adult respiratory distress syndrome (ARDS) provides important background with regard to the safety of bronchoalveolar lavage (BAL) and protected specimen brush (PSB) biopsy specimens in defining pneumonia with bronchoscopy. Careful attention was directed toward maintenance of minute ventilation and the limitation of auto PEEP during the procedure. Severe hypoxemia or hypotension were seen in 4.5% and 3.6% of patients, respectively. No significant reduction occurred in postprocedure pulmonary function, such as static compliance or PaO_2/FIO_2 ratio. No deaths resulted attributed to the procedure. The incidence of pneumothorax was 0.9% (1 of 110 patients). No serious bleeding was encountered with the restriction of PSB biopsy if platelet count less than 50,000/mm³.

These results contrast other investigators who have shown the potential for significant decline in oxygenation, which can persist for up to 2 hours after the procedure.[7] In healthy patients, the arterial partial pressure of oxygen (PaO_2) may decline by 20 to 30 mm Hg during fiberoptic bronchoscopy.[7] In critically ill patients, the decrement in PaO_2 can exceed 30 to 60 mm Hg.[8,9]

Meticulous preoperative preparation and intraoperative assessment during the bronchoscopic procedure are essen-

TABLE 46-2.   Characteristics of Increased-Risk Patients for Bronchoscopy on Mechanical Ventilation

Pulmonary
   PaO_2 <70 mm Hg with FIO_2 >0.70
   PEEP >10 cm H_2O
   Auto PEEP >15 cm H_2O
   Active bronchospasm
Cardiac
   Recent myocardial infarction (<48 h)
   Unstable arrhythmia
   Mean arterial pressure <65 mm Hg on vasopressor therapy
Coagulopathy
   Platelet count <20,000/mm³
   Increase of prothrombin time or partial thromboplastin time >1.5 times control
Central nervous system
   Increased intracranial pressure

FIO_2, fraction of inspired oxygen; PEEP, positive end-expiratory pressure.

Adapted from Meduri GU, Chastre J: The standardization of bronchoscopic techniques for ventilator-associated pneumonia. *Chest* 1992; 102:557S.

tial to avoid morbidity. In all patients, avoidance of intraoperative hypoxemia is fundamental, facilitated by initiating F_{IO_2} of 1.0 several minutes before and during the procedure. This is combined with an effective exhaled minute ventilation and an endotracheal tube adapter to limit bronchoscopy-associated volume loss. If hypoxemia is caused by excessive airway secretions, bronchoscopy can improve oxygenation through secretion clearance. Hypoxemia from prolonged suctioning reduces the effective tidal volume and functional residual capacity. Endotracheal instillation of saline or lidocaine also reduces arterial oxygen levels. Hypoxemia- and hypercapnia-induced increased sympathetic tone can result in arrhythmias, myocardial ischemia, hypotension, and cardiac arrest. Bronchoscopy-associated hypoxemia may be minimized by providing 100% oxygen during the procedure, shortening bronchoscopy time, and frequently withdrawing the bronchoscope from the airway to allow adequate ventilation. Adequate tidal volume delivery should be monitored by observing chest excursions and exhaled tidal volumes in patients undergoing mechanical ventilation. Tidal volume and flow rates must be adjusted to provide adequate ventilation.[7,10,11] Unacceptably high intrathoracic pressures are avoided by limitation of tidal volume, reduction of peak inspiratory gas flow, and adjustment of ventilator "pop-off valves." To minimize barotrauma and hypoventilation in patients undergoing mechanical ventilation, fiberoptic bronchoscopy has been performed through endotracheal tubes with inner diameters less than 8 mm by using a 70% helium and 30% oxygen ventilating gas mixture. The use of a helium–oxygen mixture during bronchoscopy may obviate the need to reintubate patients before the procedure.[12]

In contrast to outpatient bronchoscopy, effective sedation and judicious use of neuromuscular blocking drugs facilitate the procedure on mechanical ventilation. In this group of patients, it is difficult to predict effectiveness of cough suppression with sedation alone, with its potential adverse effect on oxygenation and hemodynamic parameters. Administration of a rapidly acting intravenous anesthetic or benzodiazepine combined with an intermediate acting neuromuscular blocker at the start of the procedure minimizes the cough reflex and associated sequelae. This method avoids the use of lidocaine, minimizing toxicity and the potential limitations on microbiologic cultures.

All patients require intensive monitoring, emphasizing pulse oximetry, continuous electrocardiographic (ECG) monitoring, serial measurement of blood pressure, exhaled tidal volume, and peak inspiratory pressures. ECG ST segment analysis is enhanced with the V_5 and II positions with the five-lead system in patients at high risk for myocardial ischemia. If a three-lead ECG system is employed, the central subclavicular lead (CS_5) can be used for anterior and inferior ischemia.[13] If the procedure is prolonged, capnometry can identify a trend of worsening hypercapnia secondary to reduced alveolar ventilation.

In critically ill patients with respiratory failure, it is prudent to be well prepared for complications of bronchoscopy and bronchoscopic intubation. The mnemonic "MSMAID" reminds the clinician of the essential tools for the carefully planned bronchoscopic procedure (Table 46-3).

Complications associated with the administration of premedication and local anesthesia include hypotension, allergic

TABLE 46-3. Materials for Bronchoscopic Intubation

M:	"Machine" including mechanical ventilator, bag-mask resuscitator with supplemental oxygen
S:	"Suction" including a Yankour and endotracheal catheters
M:	"Monitors" with pulse oximetry, ECG monitor, blood pressure
A:	"Airway" equipment including several sizes of endotracheal tubes, a William's airway, and a laryngoscope; and a bronchoscopic adaptor for endotracheal tube
I:	"Intravenous line" with a macrodrip infusion setup
D:	"Drugs" including necessary sedatives, bronchodilators, and necessary resuscitation medications in case of emergency (e.g., epinephrine, atropine, nitroglycerine, adenosine)

ECG, electrocardiographic.

reactions, hypoventilation, and hypoxemia from oversedation and respiratory depression. The overzealous use of local anesthetic agents within the airways has potential for toxicity with the rapid uptake of these agents into the systemic circulation from the bronchial mucosa.[14] Lidocaine is the most commonly used airway anesthetic, with decreased risks of toxicity with total doses of less than 4 mg/kg of body weight.[15] The duration of airway anesthesia induced by lidocaine is approximately 20 to 40 minutes. It avoids the allergic risks associated with the ester group of local anesthetics (e.g., compared with procaine, tetracaine, and cocaine). In patients not receiving intravenous lidocaine to suppress ventricular arrhythmias, toxicity from airway anesthesia is rare. Serum levels of anesthetic agents applied to bronchial mucosa approach those obtained with intravenous use, with peak levels occurring at 10 to 15 minutes after application. Lidocaine can cause sinus arrest and atrial ventricular block, especially in patients with underlying heart disease. Other potential adverse reactions include respiratory arrest, seizures, laryngospasm, and, rarely, hypersensitivity reactions.

Although rarely associated with bronchoscopy, arrhythmias are more likely to occur in critically ill patients.[15,16] Major cardiac arrhythmias occur in 3% to 11% of all patients undergoing bronchoscopy. Hypoxemia is the major risk factor for the development of arrhythmias.[17,18]

Laryngospasm (in the nonintubated patient) or bronchospasm can occur in any patient undergoing fiberoptic bronchoscopy, but are more common in patients with preexisting reactive airway disease. Preoperative bronchodilator therapy significantly reduces the risk of bronchoscopy-induced bronchospasm in most patients with reactive airway disease.[19]

Although transbronchial biopsy is a relatively safe procedure in patients with normal hemostasis and pulmonary vascular pressures, it is associated with 2.7% and 0.12% risks of morbidity and mortality, respectively.[20] Hemorrhage (more than 50 mL) is more likely to occur in patients who undergo transbronchial biopsy. Risk factors for hemorrhage include thrombocytopenia, azotemia, pulmonary hypertension, and the superior vena cava syndrome. Transbronchial biopsy should be restricted to nonazotemic patients with platelet counts greater than 50,000/mm^3 who have normal prothrombin times and activated partial thromboplastin times.[3,20–22] The incidence rate of bronchoscopy-related hemorrhage in normal hosts approaches 1.4%. In compromised hosts, it ranges from 25% to 29%, and hemorrhage occurs in as many as 45% of uremic patients.[3,23,24] Pneumothorax occurs in fewer than 5% of patients undergoing transbronchial biopsy. Tube thoracostomy is required in approximately half of these patients.[3,6] A major risk factor for pneumothorax is positive-pressure ventilation, especially if PEEP is used. Fluoroscopic guidance may diminish the risk of pneumothorax.[25] No patient should undergo bilateral transbronchial biopsy procedures at the same setting because of the small risk of bilateral pneumothorax.

Desmopressin can temporarily reverse the uremic effect on platelet function and normalize bleeding time to permit minor surgical procedures in patients with hemophilia A, von Willebrand's disease, or renal failure.[26,27] Maximal correction of bleeding time is achieved after 15 to 30 minutes of intravenously administered desmopressin (0.3 μg/kg). The response is diminished if the dose is repeated more frequently than every 48 hours. Desmopressin given intravenously seems to be safe and effective for temporary correction of coagulation defects. However, no controlled studies have confirmed the safety of performing transbronchial biopsy in uremic patients pretreated with desmopressin.

If severe hemorrhage occurs, the patient should be placed with the bleeding side dependent. The bronchoscope should be wedged into the involved distal bronchus with suction applied.[3] A dose of 2 to 3 mL of 1:10,000 epinephrine can be administered locally into the bleeding segmental orifice.[28] If necessary, a Fogarty catheter can be directly positioned into the bleeding orifice by the bronchoscope.

Postbronchoscopy fever occurs in as many as 16% of patients. Bronchoscopy-related pneumonia is rare, occurring in fewer than 5%. Risk factors for fever include advanced age, endobronchial abnormalities, and bronchial brushing.[6] Bacteremia is exceedingly rare.[29,30] In general, endocarditis prophylaxis is not required with fiberoptic bronchoscopy.[31]

Neurosurgical patients are at risk for intracranial hypertension, a result of bronchoscopy-induced elevation of intrathoracic pressure, arterial hypertension, and hypercapnia. Bronchoscopy-associated cough or retching therefore must be avoided. If bronchoscopy is deemed necessary under these circumstances, sedation and neuromuscular blockade can be required, as discussed in the following sections.

FIBEROPTIC BRONCHOSCOPY IN AIRWAY MANAGEMENT ■

Fiberoptic bronchoscopy can provide an efficient and effective means to secure a difficult airway, change an endotracheal tube, and inspect an airway during extubation. Endotracheal intubation, typically performed orally or nasally with a laryngoscope, can be technically difficult in select patient groups (Table 46-4). Importantly, fiberoptic endotracheal intubation can be the initial choice of intubation for those skilled in the technique, using either a nasal or oral approach. Previous studies have shown that nasal intubation can be performed relatively quickly by those experienced in fi-

beroptic bronchoscopy with a mean time of 3.0 minutes[32] (Figs. 46-1 and 46-2). After preparation of the nasal mucosal with a local anesthetic and a mucosal vasoconstrictor, the bronchoscope (which has been passed through the nares) is situated directly above the glottic opening. It is then passed into the trachea and the endotracheal tube is passed over the bronchoscope into the trachea. The major limitation of this approach in many ICU patients with concomitant abnormalities of coagulation is epistaxis and the potential for sinusitis with prolonged nasal intubation. When epistaxis occurs, its impairment of the fiberoptic examination can seriously hamper subsequent nasal attempts at intubation as well as a laryngoscopic intubations. Other difficulties associated with nasal intubation include adenoid dislocation and difficulty passing the endotracheal tube in patients with limited nares' diameter. Oral fiberoptic intubation effectively avoids these difficulties associated with nasal intubation. It is facilitated by topical and regional anesthesia as well as the use of an oral airway intubator.[33] The oral airway intubator directs the fiberoptic bronchoscopy past the tongue and directly over the larynx, facilitating endotracheal intubation. Previously, it has been used successfully and efficiently with topical anesthesia and general anesthesia.[34] A special facial mask with a diaphragm for the bronchoscope has been developed for the critically ill and for use in the operating room.[35] It is useful for bronchoscopic intubation in sedated or comatose patients and with limited respiratory reserve, providing a tight seal for assisted ventilation during the procedure. Another adaptation taken from the operating room is the laryngeal mask, an innovative apparatus that can secure an airway and has been used for fiberoptic intubation.[35]

The fiberoptic bronchoscope allows endotracheal tube changes in patients with endotracheal tube cuff leaks, inadequate internal diameters, and nasotracheal tube–associated sinusitis. Before bronchoscopy, the oropharynx should be suctioned thoroughly. For oral tracheal intubation, the endotracheal tube should be shortened 2 to 3 cm at its proximal end and advanced over the bronchoscope before its placement in the pharynx. The bronchoscope tip is advanced to the level of the cuff of the existing endotracheal tube, and secretions are aspirated through the suction channel. If necessary, the cuff is deflated and the bronchoscope advanced into the tracheal lumen. The endotracheal tube is then withdrawn with the cuff fully deflated, the bronchoscope tip advanced to the carina, and the new endotracheal tube advanced over the fiberoptic bronchoscope into the trachea. Adequate positioning of the tube 3 to 4 cm proximal to the carina is confirmed by the bronchoscope and the cuff inflated. After intubation, a chest radiograph is not required to confirm adequate placement of the endotracheal tube.[36,37] Tube changes by the oral or nasal routes are possible. Contralateral nasal reintubation, however, may be difficult because of the lateral displacement of the septum by the existing nasotracheal tube.

Fiberoptic bronchoscopy can be extremely useful in the placement of a double-lumen endotracheal tube (Fig. 46-3). If a right-sided tube is used, adequate positioning of the tube with the tracheal port proximal to the carina and bronchial port proximal to the right upper lobe orifice can be confirmed by using a small-diameter (3.5-mm outer diam-

TABLE 46-4. Factors Associated With Difficult Endotracheal Intubations

ANATOMIC

  Short muscular neck
  Receding mandible
  Prominent upper incisors
  Microglossia
  Limited mandible movement
  Large breasts
  Cervical rigidity

CONGENITAL ABNORMALITIES

  Absence of nose
  Choanal atresia
  Macroglossia

INFECTIOUS

  Bacterial retropharyngeal abscess
  Epiglottis
  Diphtheria
  Infectious mononucleosis
  Croup
  Leprosy

NONINFECTIVE INFLAMMATION

  Rheumatoid arthritis
  Instability of cervical spine
  Cervical fixation
  Temporomandibular disease
  Cricoarytenoid disorders
  Hypoplastic mandible
  Ankylosing spondylitis

NEOPLASIA

  Laryngeal papillomatosis
  Stylohyoid ligament calcification
  Laryngeal carcinoma
  Mediastinal carcinoma

TRAUMA

  Mandibular fracture
  Maxillary fracture
  Laryngeal and tracheal trauma
  Mediastinal carcinoma

ENDOCRINE

  Obesity
  Acromegaly
  Thyromegaly

Adapted from Latto IP, Rosen M: Difficulties in Tracheal Intubation. London, Baillere Tindall, 1985.

eter) fiberoptic bronchoscope to inspect the airway through each lumen.[38,39]

Fiberoptic bronchoscopy provides an excellent opportunity to inspect airways at the time of extubation in patients at risk for airway compromise, including those intubated for inhalation injury, trauma, subglottic stenosis, and laryngeal edema. The bronchoscope is advanced through the endotracheal tube to its most distal aspect, and the tube and bronchoscope are withdrawn slowly together to allow inspection of the airway. If bronchoscopy confirms persistent mucosal edema or extrinsic airway compression, the endotracheal tube can be readvanced over the bronchoscope into the tracheal lumen and secured, with extubation postponed until a later time.[40,41]

ANESTHESIA FOR BRONCHOSCOPY

Effective anesthesia can facilitate the ease and safety of the bronchoscopic examination in the ICU patient. The basic goals of the anesthetic include (1) inhibiting coughing, (2) amnesia, (3) limiting excessive sympathetic nervous system activity, and (4) blunting the "protective reflexes" of the upper airway and tracheobronchial tree (e.g., coughing and laryngospasm). Effective anesthesia allows for a controlled examination of the bronchopulmonary tree in an unhurried

fashion and provides for greater patient comfort. Furthermore, it can prevent hemodynamic compromise, such as tachycardia and hypertension, that may stress patients with underlying ischemic heart disease. Bronchospasm and severe coughing in the mechanically ventilated patient with respiratory failure can result in life-threatening hypoxemia and barotrauma. Although many outpatient bronchoscopic examinations can be performed using a nasal approach, the critically ill patient with borderline respiratory function can benefit from bronchoscopic oral intubation as an integral part of the procedure. The presence of an endotracheal tube has multiple benefits, including the following: (1) the enhancement of oxygenation and ventilation in the high-risk patient; (2) an increased margin of safety in patients who require higher doses of intravenous sedation; (3) the rapid insertion and removal of the bronchoscopy, required by excessive secretions or hemoptysis; (4) a decreased risk pulmonary aspiration of gastric contents; and, finally (5) a controlled airway in the event that the patient requires mechanical ventilation at the conclusion of the procedure.

Understanding nerve innervation of the upper airway can contribute to effective analgesia during the bronchoscopic examination. The maxillary division and ophthalmic division of the trigeminal nerve innervate the nose. Branches of the trigeminal division, facial, glossopharyngeal, vagus, and

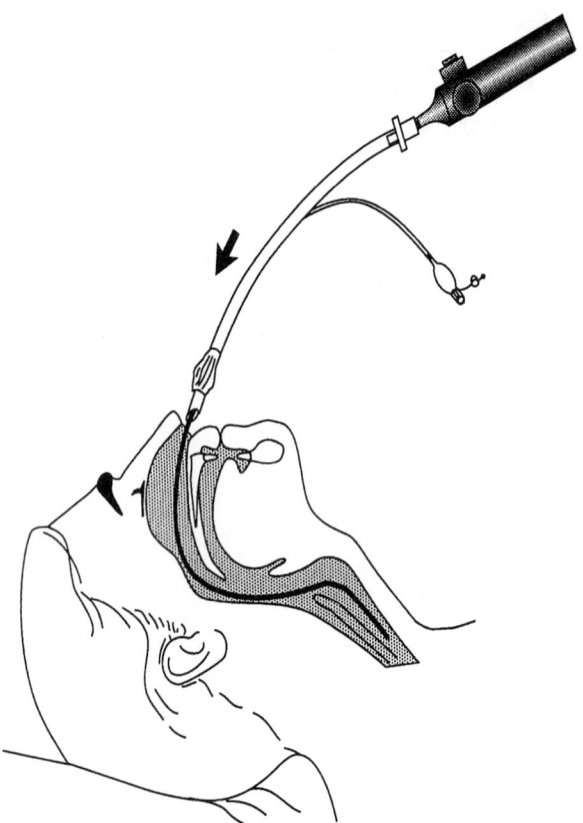

FIGURE 46-1. Bronchoscopic nasotracheal intubation. The bronchoscope tip is positioned in the midtrachea, and the endotracheal tube is carefully advanced into the trachea using the bronchoscope as a guide. Before bronchoscopy, the endotracheal tube can be prepositioned within the nasopharynx.

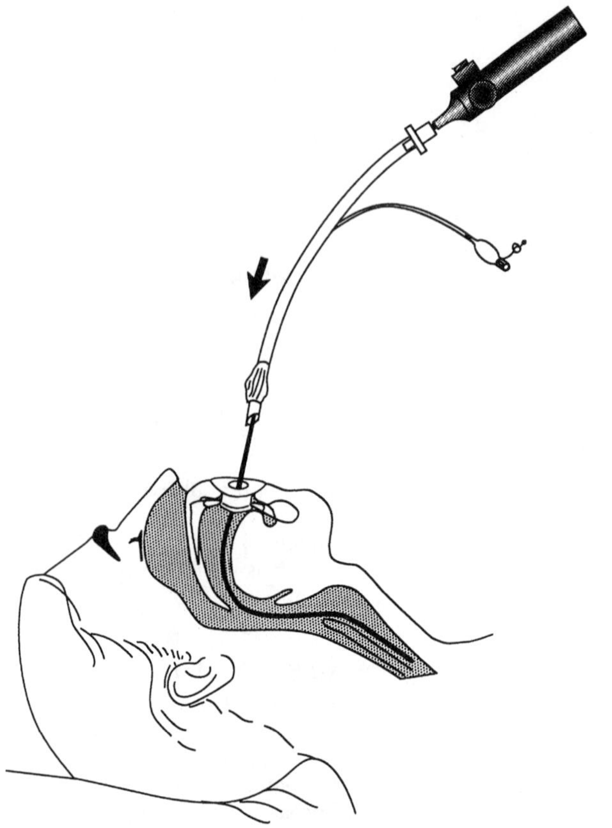

FIGURE 46-2. Bronchoscope-directed orotracheal intubation. The bronchoscope is passed into the trachea through a bite-block and the endotracheal tube advanced over the bronchoscope. Correct placement of the endotracheal tube tip 3 to 4 cm proximal to the carina is visually confirmed before removing the bronchoscope.

hypoglossal nerves supply innervation to the mouth and tongue. The superior laryngeal nerve, a branch of the vagus nerve, supplies sensation of the larynx and vocal cords. The recurrent laryngeal nerves supply innervation below the vocal cords into the trachea.[15] For example, regional anesthesia using local anesthetic blockade of the superior laryngeal nerve may limit sedation requirements of intubation.

A variety of pharmacologic options are available to provide appropriate conditions for fiberoptic bronchoscopic intubation, as summarized in Table 46-5. Lidocaine is an effective topical anesthetic with a favorable risk-to-benefit ratio. When given by nebulizer, it can provide anesthesia for the mouth, larynx, and trachea. Supplementation with internal or external superior laryngeal nerve blockade can provide further anesthesia above the larynx. Because of lidocaine's apparent bacteriostatic effects, it is common practice to limit the use of this drug below the vocal cords before obtaining the microbiologic specimens. Lidocaine (e.g., 2 mL of 4% concentration) can be injected transtracheally. This, however, can be associated with significant coughing and cardiovascular response.

The benzodiazepines (e.g., midazolam, diazepam, and lorazepam) offer sedation and amnestic effects. Midazolam

offers rapid onset with effective amnesia with a half-life much shorter than lorazepam and diazepam. With its mild vasodilator properties, it has the potential for hypotension, which can be pronounced in the elderly. It should be titrated to the desired level of sedation during the course of the bronchoscopic study. If necessary, its effects can be antagonized with flumazenil, a competitive inhibitor of the γ-aminobutyric acid–benzodiazepine receptor in the central nervous system within minutes of administration. Notice that the effective half-life of flumazenil is much shorter than the duration of effect of diazepam and lorazepam. Vigilance therefore is necessary for potential of recurrent sedation when these latter drugs are used; repetitive doses of the antagonist flumazenil may be required.[42]

Atropine and glycopyrrolate, both with anticholinergic properties, are used as premedication for bronchoscopy to minimize oropharyngeal and bronchial secretions. Atropine is efficacious when given intravenously or by intramuscular injection. Its vagolytic properties can result in tachycardia with resultant myocardial ischemia in patients with ischemic heart disease. Glycopyrrolate, given intramuscularly or intravenously, similarly is an effective antisialagogue. It seems to have less chronotropic effects than atropine. Additionally, it

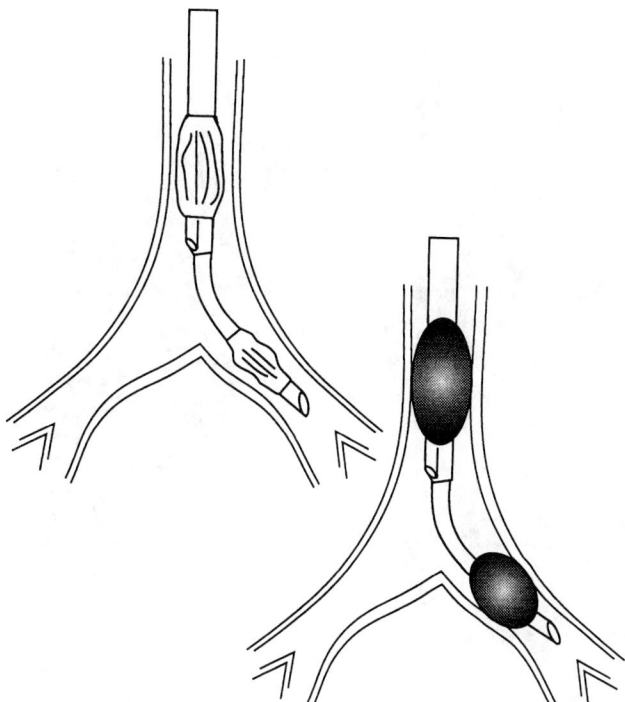

FIGURE 46-3. A left-sided, double-lumen endobronchial tube. The proximal port is correctly positioned within the distal trachea, and the distal port is within the left mainstem bronchus. Correct positioning of the tube can be confirmed by passing a pediatric bronchoscope through each lumen.

does not cross the blood–brain barrier and, unlike atropine, is not associated with delirium.

Intravenous lidocaine has been shown to be effective in minimizing the hypertension and tachycardia associated with laryngoscopy when given at 1.5 mg/kg.[43] Combined with topical lidocaine, the potential for toxicity with systemic absorption still exists. Because of this, it is not recommended as a routine practice.

ATELECTASIS

Segmental or lobar atelectasis presents radiographically as a parenchymal density associated with some combination of shift of an interlobar fissure, crowding of vessels or bronchi, or elevation of the diaphragm or the mediastinum (Figs. 46-4 and 46-5). Predisposing conditions include inadequate inspiratory effort (pain, sedation, muscle weakness), obesity, excessive airway secretions, preexisting airway disease, and intrabronchial obstructing lesions. Atelectasis of a segment or lobe produces hypoxemia by right-to-left vascular shunting and ventilation/perfusion mismatching. The clinical significance of atelectasis is directly related to its extent and to the preexisting pulmonary reserve of the patient. Patients with underlying pulmonary disease may develop clinically significant atelectasis after upper abdominal or thoracic surgical procedures. Postoperative failure to inspire deeply secondary to "splinting" and poor coughing associated with abdominal or chest wall pain can result in the accumulation of secretions in the affected atelectatic segment or lobe. Atelectasis can also develop in patients who are sedated or who are unable to perform intermittent deep breathing or sighs.

The exact mechanism for postoperative pulmonary compromise remains uncertain, but diaphragmatic dysfunction may play a role. Cephalad shift of the diaphragm has been demonstrated after induction of anesthesia.[44] Diaphragmatic dysfunction can alter pleural pressures, especially at the bases, producing distending pressure for alveoli that is less than that for alveoli in more superior regions of the lung. The smaller, dependent alveoli therefore receive a proportionately smaller fraction of the tidal volume, resulting in microatelectasis. The development of microatelectasis may be enhanced by the administration of gas mixtures containing a low-nitrogen–high-oxygen concentration that increases the likelihood of alveolar collapse by adsorption atelectasis.

Much of the evidence supporting the role of fiberoptic bronchoscopy in the treatment of atelectasis is anecdotal. It may be most effective in secretion removal by inducing

TABLE 46-5. Pharmacology for Bronchoscopy in the ICU

RATIONALE	DRUG OF CHOICE	COMMENTS
Topical analgesia	4% lidocaine 1% lidocaine	Toxicity can occur with doses >4 mg/kg
Bronchodilator	Albuterol	
Analgesia	Morphine Fentanyl	Potential for histamine release No histamine release
Sedation/amnesia	Midazolam	Shorter half-life than diazepam and lorazepam
Antisialogogue	Glycopyrrolate	Less vagolytic effects than atropine
General anesthesia	Sodium thiopental Etomidate	Can be combined with an intermediate-acting neuromuscular blocker

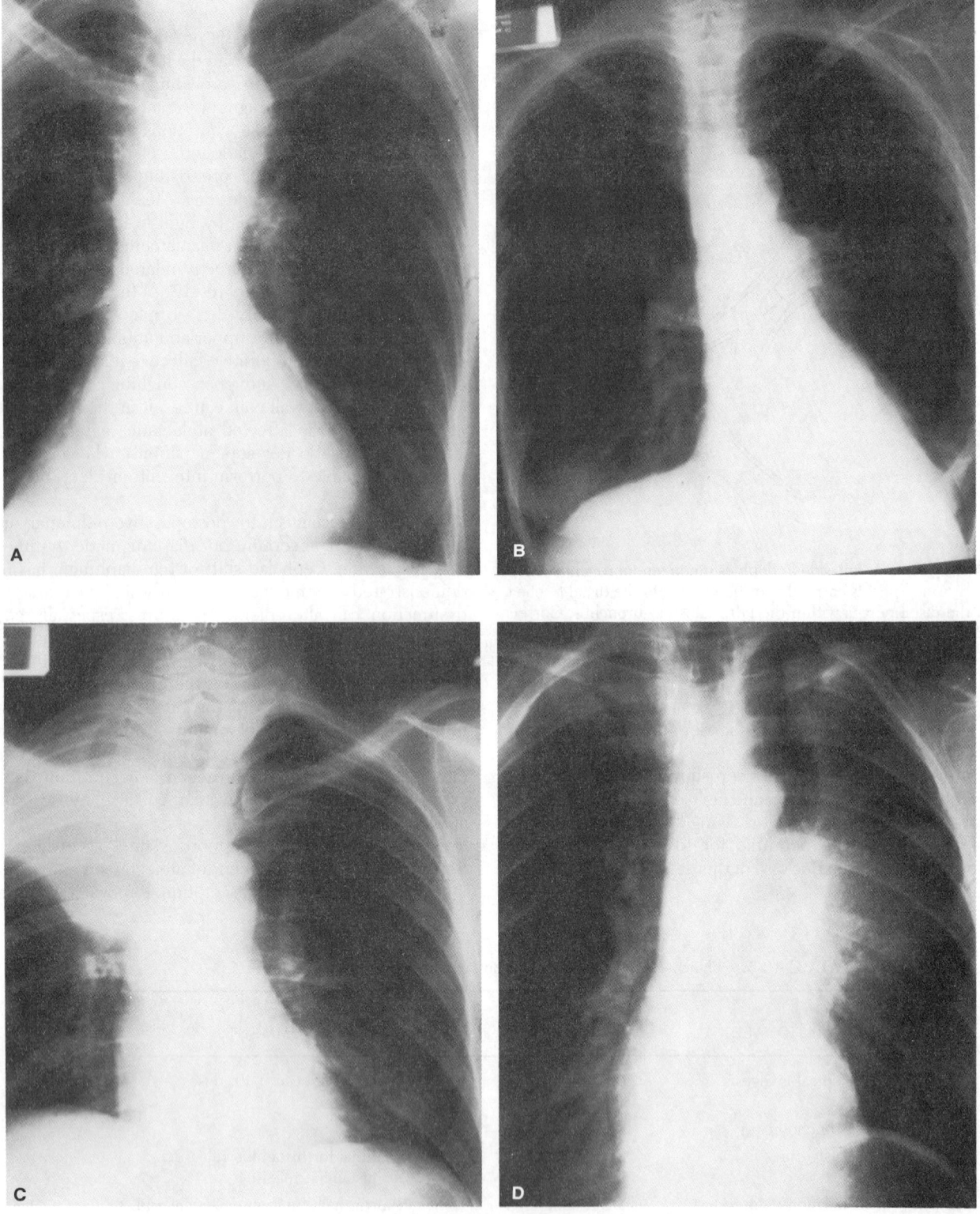

FIGURE 46-4. (**A**) Right lower lobe atelectasis with obscuration of the right hemidiaphragm and heart border, (**B**) Left lower lobe atelectasis manifested by a retrocardiac density and partial obscuration of the left hemidiaphragm. (**C**) Partial right upper lobe collapse with superior-medial positioning of the minor fissure. (**D**) Left upper lobe collapse. The left hilum is indistinct because of the superimposed atelectatic left upper lobe. The left diaphragm is elevated.

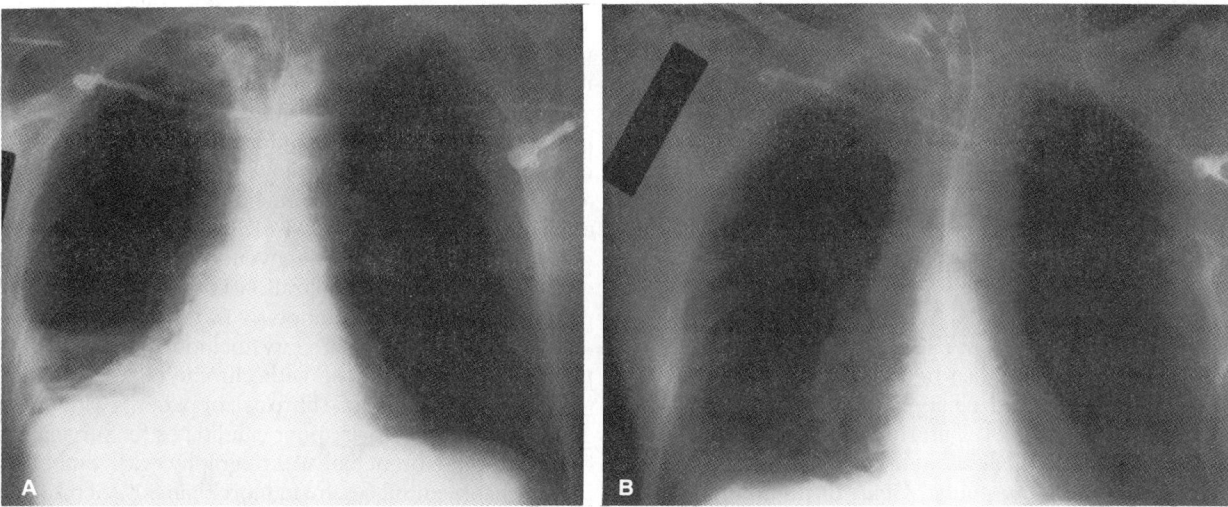

FIGURE 46-5. (**A**) Right middle lobe atelectasis. (**B**) After fiberoptic bronchoscopy and removal of a thick mucous plug, the right middle lobe has reexpanded.

cough and deep breathing. If the larger central airways are not obstructed by mucous plugs, bronchoscopy may be fruitless. In general, bronchoscopy is no more efficacious than more conservative measures in resolving atelectasis.[45] Instillation of saline or a dilute solution of acetylcysteine (2% to 10%) through the suction channel may clear thick, tenacious secretions. Acetylcysteine is a bronchial irritant, however, and may exacerbate bronchospasm in patients with reactive airways disease.[46,47] We use 10- to 20-mL aliquots of saline as the irrigant to facilitate clearing of mucous plugs. If this fails, the options include acetylcysteine or gentle teasing of the plug with a biopsy forceps, being careful not to advance the biopsy forceps against significant resistance. Occasionally, holding suction while withdrawing the bronchoscope through the endotracheal tube allows removal of large mucous plugs that cannot be withdrawn directly through the suction channel. This is practical only if the patient is endotracheally intubated; however, we recommend that intubation usually should accompany bronchoscopy in critically ill patients, especially for treatment of atelectasis. Patients with segmental or lobar atelectasis who are unresponsive to more conservative measures (such as deep breathing to total lung capacity, tracheal suctioning, and chest physiotherapy with chest percussion and postural drainage if indicated) may be candidates for fiberoptic bronchoscopy.

In patients with preexisting conditions such as cervical spine injuries, chest trauma with multiple rib fractures, and thoracic burns that compromise the ability to perform adequate pulmonary toilet, fiberoptic bronchoscopy may be the initial treatment of choice. Air bronchograms in the atelectatic segment or lobe makes fiberoptic bronchoscopy a less attractive procedure because central airway occlusion by mucous plugging is unlikely in these circumstances.[45] Turner and colleagues[48] use a combination of fiberoptic bronchoscope and chest physiotherapy. They use 10 to 40 mL of

normal saline instilled directly into lobar segmental bronchi, followed by bronchial hygiene by a physiotherapist. Bronchial hygiene consists of vibration and chest hyperinflation techniques. They reported full reexpansion in 71% of patients and improvement in a further 18%.[48]

Selective intrabronchial insufflation by the fiberoptic bronchoscope (preceded by suctioning of mucous from large airways) has been used in patients with refractory atelectasis. A recent surgical ICU study using air insufflation for lobar collapse reports an overall effectiveness of 82% with 92% effectiveness when collapse was less than 72 hours' duration.[49] Although only minor clinically insignificant complications have been described, selective positive-pressure insufflation does carry the potential risk of barotrauma.[50–52]

HEMOPTYSIS

Massive hemoptysis may be defined as bronchial bleeding exceeding 200 to 600 mL over a 24-hour period. In practice, the rapidity of bleeding and ability to maintain a patent airway are critical factors, and life-threatening hemoptysis can be defined as the amount of bleeding that compromises ventilation. Most patients who die from massive hemoptysis do so from asphyxiation secondary to airway occlusion by clot and blood, not exsanguination. The causes of massive hemoptysis are listed in Table 46-6. Infections associated with bronchiectasis, lung abscess, and necrotizing pneumonitis are commonly responsible for the massive bleeding. Other causes include bronchogenic carcinoma, mycetoma, invasive fungal diseases, chest trauma, cystic fibrosis, and broncholithiasis. Airway patency must be assured in patients with massive hemoptysis. Appropriate maneuvers include placing the patient in Trendelenburg position with the bleeding side down and isolating the nonbleeding side by selective contralateral mainstem intubation.

TABLE 46-6. Causes of Massive Hemoptysis

COMMON CAUSES	UNCOMMON CAUSES
Tuberculosis	Iatrogenic
Bronchiectasis	Alveolar hemorrhage syndrome
Pulmonary abscess	Cardiovascular disease
Mycetoma	Bronchial adenoma
Bronchogenic	Metastatic carcinoma
carcinoma	Foreign-body aspiration
Cystic fibrosis	Pulmonary contusion
Broncholithiasis	Tracheobronchial tree trauma

In patients with persistent massive hemoptysis, management by rigid endoscopy had been preferred traditionally because of the enhanced ability to suction and ventilate through the large channel. Unfortunately, rigid bronchoscopy affords limited visualization of the more distal airways and requires general anesthesia. Goals of fiberoptic bronchoscopy should be to identify a definitive cause for the bleeding, to localize the bleeding site, and to provide therapeutic intervention. In most instances of massive hemoptysis, a large-bore endotracheal tube should be positioned in the trachea or, if necessary, the mainstem bronchus contralateral to the bleeding side to assure airway patency. Rarely, fiberoptic bronchoscopy directed placement of a double-lumen endotracheal tube may be considered to isolate the bleeding lung. A small-diameter bronchoscope is passed through each lumen to confirm appropriate placement of the tube. The relatively small diameter of each lumen may compromise the ability of the patient to clear blood and clots. In addition, fiberoptic bronchoscopic placement may be handicapped by poor visibility with ongoing hemorrhage. An endotracheal tube incorporating a bronchial blocker is easier to insert than many double-lumen endotracheal tubes, providing selective one-lung ventilation.

Endobronchial tamponade with fiberoptic bronchoscopy offers a life-saving technique in patients who cannot be transferred because of logistical problems or who have rapidly deteriorated in the ICU. Endobronchial tamponade can be achieved with a 4-French Fogarty balloon-tipped catheter. This is passed directly through the suction channel of the bronchoscope or passed adjacent to the bronchoscope held in place by biopsy forceps extending just beyond the distal suction port. Care must be taken not to perforate the catheter or balloon by the forceps. The catheter tip is inserted into the bleeding segmental orifice, and the balloon is filled with 0.75 mL of sterile saline solution. If passed through the suction channel, the proximal end of the catheter is clamped with a hemostat, the hub cut off, and a straight pin inserted into the catheter channel proximal to the hemostat to maintain saline inflation of the balloon catheter. The clamp is removed, and the bronchoscope is carefully withdrawn from the bronchus with the Fogarty catheter remaining in position, providing endobronchial hemostasis.[53,54] The catheter can safely remain in position until hemostasis is assured by surgical resection of the bleeding segment or bronchial artery embolization. Refinements in catheter development continue to occur.[55]

A relatively new technique designed to provide hemostasis is intrabronchial selective coagulative therapy. The bronchoscope is wedged into the bleeding segmental bronchus, and thrombin or a fibrinogen–thrombin mix is injected directly through the suction channel into the bleeding segment. It was successful in a high percentage of patients in one study and is apparently quick, safe, and simple.[56] Fibrin precursors sprayed directly into the bleeding bronchus also have been successfully employed to achieve hemostasis in a few patients. These fibrin sealant plugs undergo fibrinolysis after about 8 to 10 days.[57] Further controlled studies are necessary to confirm the effectiveness of coagulative therapy.

Bronchial artery embolization is the primary treatment modality for massive hemoptysis in the nonsurgical candidate. Patients in this category include those with limited pulmonary reserve, those with chronic bilateral inflammatory processes (e.g., cystic fibrosis), or patients with bronchogenic carcinoma who are poor candidates for surgical resection. Selective bronchial arteriography with embolization therapy has been successful in more than 80% of these cases. It is associated with a low recurrence rate of bleeding and reduced mortality among severely ill patients. Occasionally, pulmonary and bronchial arteries must be visualized to localize the bleeding source. A rare but significant risk associated with bronchial artery embolization is inadvertent occlusion of the anterior spinal artery.[58–61]

In patients with moderate hemoptysis, controversy exists about the appropriate timing of diagnostic bronchoscopy. Although bronchoscopy is difficult with massive hemoptysis, it can, despite the presence of moderate bleeding, diagnose the segmental location of hemorrhage in a high percentage of cases. The bleeding site can be directly visualized or localized to a specific segment in more than 90% of patients who undergo bronchoscopy during active hemoptysis.[62] Potential bias exists in the study of this condition because patients with massive hemoptysis are less likely to undergo fiberoptic bronchoscopy. The addition of high-resolution computed tomography scan may be helpful in identifying a specific cause of bleeding.[63]

THE DIAGNOSIS OF PNEUMONIA

Fiberoptic bronchoscopy provides an essential tool for the diagnosis of pneumonia in the ICU. Although commonly attributed to pneumonia, the chest radiographic finding of alveolar infiltrates in the ICU patient can represent a broad differential diagnosis, requiring a wide range of therapies. Standard clinical criteria for the diagnosis of pneumonia, such as new pulmonary infiltrates, hypoxemia, leukocytosis or leukopenia, fever, and pathogenic bacteria in respiratory secretions, previously have been associated with a significant rate of misdiagnosis when compared with postmortem histologic study.[64] Bacterial colonization of the upper airways and endotracheal tube can confound the reliability of the Gram stain on specimens obtained from the intubated patient. Classifying the results of Gram stains on nonbronchoscopically obtained sputum from the intubated patient in terms of number of bacteria, neutrophils, intracellular organisms, and quantitative bacterial cultures is a promising modality, but has the potential for overlap between colonized versus the infected patients. An incorrect diagnosis of pneumonia in the critically ill patient—based on the standard clinical criteria of fever, lung infiltrate on chest radiograph, and purulent secretions—can result in unnecessary antibiotic treatment of noninfected patients.[65] A recent consensus statement suggests that the routine use of bronchoscopy for diagnosis of community-acquired pneumonia is generally not indicated.[66] In the severely ill patient, however, who is not responding to antibiotic therapy or is immunocompromised, bronchoscopy can diagnose *Legionella pneumophila* and *Mycobacterium tuberculosis*, as well as resistant or unusual pathogens. In patients who have failed empiric antibiotic therapy early or late in their treatment course, bronchoscopy has been reported to be diagnostically beneficial in 41% in a recent clinical study.[67]

The diagnostic utility of fiberoptic bronchoscopy in patients with infectious pulmonary infiltrates has been advanced through the development of semiquantitative culture techniques of specimens obtained by the PSB catheter and BAL. The diagnosis of bacterial pneumonia in critically ill patients by bronchoscopy is difficult because of bacterial contamination of the bronchoscope during its passage through the oropharynx or nasopharynx, endotracheal tube, and upper tracheobronchial tree. Culture and Gram stain of standard bronchial washings typically fail to identify the etiologic agent causing pneumonia and are frequently misleading and unreliable. The use of a PSB allows sampling of selected bronchopulmonary segments, while avoiding the potential bacterial colonization of the upper tracheobronchial tree.[68] The PSB catheter combines a brush recessed within an inner catheter, itself within an outer catheter protected by a biodegradable plug. The PSB can be directed into the involved bronchopulmonary segment, which can be identified by pulmonary infiltrate on chest radiograph or with fluoroscopic guidance, or by purulent drainage from the involved bronchopulmonary segment. Selectively placed, the inner catheter is extended, expelling the plug. The PSB samples the distal tracheobronchial tree in the area of the infiltrate. On removal of the PSB from the tracheobronchial tree, a Gram stain can be performed with a sterile slide. The PSB is then placed into 1 mL of solution for obtaining immediate quantitative cultures.[68] Collective reviews of PSB combined with quantitative bacterial cultures have shown sensitivity rates between 65% and 100% with specificity rates of 80% to 100%.[69] Importantly, the reference standards with which PSB was compared varied from evaluation of clinical response to actual lung histologic features. Clinical trials to date are supportive that a quantitative threshold of greater than or equal to 10^3 colony forming units (CFUs) per milliliter correlate with pathologically proven pneumonia.[70] To maximize the diagnostic yield of this technique, it is useful to limit intratracheal lidocaine secondary to its bacteriocidal effect.[71] Furthermore, the sensitivity of the PSB technique seems to be limited by previous use of antibiotic therapy. The diagnostic sensitivity therefore is increased by performance of the procedure before use of antibiotics as well as withholding antibiotics for longer than 48 hours after antibiotic administration. Limiting bronchoscopic suctioning can avoid upper airway contamination and potential false-positive culture results.

TABLE 46-7. Diagnostic Stain Preparation of Bronchoalveolar Lavage

STAIN	APPLICATION
Gram stain	Bacteria
Acid-fast bacilli	Mycobacteria and *Nocardia* organisms
Papanicolaou	CMV and herpes viruses *Pneumocystis* organisms Fungi Malignant cells
Romanovsky (modified Diff-Quick)	Cell differential Cytologic study
Oil-red-O technique	Lipoid pneumonia or fat embolism
Mucicarmine	*Cryptococcus* organisms Mucin-producing neoplasm
May-Grünwald Giemsa	Alveolar cell population
KOH	Elastin fibers

CMV, cytomegalovirus; KOH, potassium hydroxide.

Adapted from Henry-Stanley MJ: Laboratory processing of BAL fluids. In: Stanley MW, Henry-Stanley MJ, Iber C (eds). *Bronchoalveolar Lavage: Cytology and Clinical Applications*. New York, Igaku-Shoin, 1991:213.

BAL is an invaluable diagnostic tool in the immunocompromised host (Tables 46-7 and 46-8), especially in patients infected with the human immunodeficiency virus (HIV) who have opportunistic infections such as *Pneumocystis carinii* and *Mycobacterium avium-intracellulare*. Up to 250 mL of nonbacteriostatic normal saline is instilled in 20- to 50-mL aliquots through the suction channel of a bronchoscope wedged into a segmental orifice. The fluid is retrieved after each instillation by a large hand-held syringe. A small aliquot of the lavage specimen is quantitatively cultured, and Gram staining is performed after cytocentrifuge. Visualization of more than one bacterium per high-powered field on Gram

TABLE 46-8. Bronchoalveolar Lavage as a Diagnostic Tool

INFECTIOUS ORGANISMS DIAGNOSED BY BAL ISOLATION

Mycobacterium tuberculosis	*Mycoplasma*
Legionella	Influenza virus
Pneumocystis carinii	Respiratory syncytial virus
Toxoplasma gondii	*Strongyloides*

INFECTIOUS ORGANISMS ISOLATED BY BAL REQUIRING SUPPORTING CLINICAL CRITERIA FOR DIAGNOSIS

Bacteria	Atypical mycobacteria
Aspergillus	Herpes simplex
Cryptococcus	Cytomegalovirus

BAL, bronchoalveolar lavage.

Adapted from American Thoracic Society: Clinical role of bronchoalveolar lavage in adults with pulmonary disease. *Am Rev Respir Dis* 1990;142:481.

stain of the cytocentrifuge preparation predicts significant culture growth.[72-75] BAL, in combination with quantitative bacterial cultures, provides sensitivity and specificity similar to the PSB. A quantitative culture threshold of greater or equal to 10^4 CFUs/mL support the diagnosis of ventilator-associated pneumonia.[68] The initial lavage fluid (e.g., the first 20 mL) is discarded by some investigators because of its potential for airway contamination and lack of correlation with alveolar pathologic findings.[68] Although frequently analyzed with BAL specimens, the cell count and associated differential of leukocytes (for example, the percentage of neutrophils) on BAL do not seem distinguishing features in the diagnosis of pneumonia. The differential cell count, however, can be useful in the support of other noninfectious diagnoses mimicking nosocomial pneumonia. For example, a BAL finding showing a high percentage of eosinophils (40% or more) is supportive of the diagnosis of eosinophilic pneumonia,[69] particularly if other stains and cultures do not support a microbiologic process.

The percentage of BAL-derived cells containing intracellular organisms can provide a helpful clue in the identification of pneumonia.[68] Available before the growth of cultures, it is proposed that bacteria present in greater than 7% of total BAL cells supports the diagnosis of pneumonia.[76] The Gram stain results of the BAL fluid seem to correlate with quantitative culture results, supporting its routine use in the diagnosis of ventilator-associated pneumonia.[68] The presence of elastin fibers was originally proposed as a sensitive tool for the diagnosis of pneumonia, but these also are identified in uninfected patients with ARDS.[68]

To avoid bronchial contamination, a protected bronchoalveolar lavage (PBAL) catheter has been studied, with initial promising results.[77] Similar to BAL, PBAL uses a protected balloon-tipped catheter to sample distal airway secretions with minimal proximal airway contamination. Quantitative cultures of the PBAL specimens had a diagnostic sensitivity rate of 97% and specificity rate of 92%, with a positive predictive value of 92% in a prospective series of 49 patients. Gram stain results of the PBAL specimens were positive in all but 1 patient with pneumonia and negative in all but 1 patient without infection, allowing diagnosis of pneumonia before culture results were available. Concurrent antibiotic therapy did not affect the results of PBAL cultures, unlike that observed for the protected brush specimens.[78]

Another study involving 55 patients compared PBAL with the PSB during 78 suspected episodes of nosocomial pneumonia. Using 10^3 CFUs/mL or more as the criterion for pneumonia, the sensitivity and specificity rates of the plugged telescoping catheter were 100% and 82.2%, and those of the PSB were 64.7% and 93.5%, respectively.[79]

Proper use of PSB and BAL with careful processing of the specimen are important to a successful yield. The methods of processing bronchoscopic specimens are key components for diagnostic success, requiring input from the intensive care clinician, the pathologist, and the microbiologist. The organization of the specimens' processing should be well detailed in advance to avoid delayed processing, "forgotten" microbiologic stains, or "lost" specimens. In a recent report, Baselski and colleagues[80] carefully review the details of laboratory handling of bronchoscopically obtained samples. No-

tice that direct microscopic study of the bronchoscopic samples can result in an expeditious diagnosis. Available microbiologic and cytologic stains are summarized in Table 46-7.[81] Normal saline or Ringer's solution are typically used, but these may not be ideal for fastidious organisms.[82] Delayed transport of specimens for quantitative culture has been associated with a tenfold reduction in bacteriologic yield.[83]

In addition to the information provided by microbiologic and cytologic analysis, BAL also shows potential uses in fundamental investigation of lung inflammation. A recent study has shown the BAL cytokine measurements of tumor necrosis factor-alpha, interleukin (IL)-1β, IL-6, and IL-8 correlate with severity and prognosis of ARDS.[84]

The transbronchial forceps biopsy can provide a histopathologic diagnosis in the mechanically ventilated patient,[85,86] although its use is controversial in this group of patients with only small clinical trials available. In a previous study of 13 patients, all of whom required mechanical ventilation with an PaO_2/FIO_2 ratio of less than 150 with PEEP levels of 7 to 12 cm H_2O, the biopsy result was helpful in 10 of 13 patients (73%). In another published series, a diagnosis was established in 33% of patients. Morbidity in both of these trials included infrequent pneumothorax (3.6%) and self-limited pulmonary hemorrhage with no associated deaths. No large series compare transbronchial biopsy with the previously described techniques of PSB and BAL in mechanically ventilated patients.

THE DIAGNOSIS OF PNEUMONIA IN THE IMMUNOCOMPROMISED HOST

The possible causes for pulmonary infiltrates in the immunosuppressed patient are myriad (Table 46-9). As a diagnostic first step, fiberoptic bronchoscopy is a reasonable choice, employing BAL and PSB with quantitative cultures in patients without contraindications. Transbronchial lung biopsy adds additional risk to the procedure with a potential increase in diagnostic yield. A specific diagnosis allows for the withdrawal of unnecessary antibiotics as well as institution of appropriate therapy for newly discovered pathologic processes. In all instances, the risks and benefits of invasive diagnostic procedures, including bronchoscopy and open-lung biopsy, must be carefully weighed.

Pulmonary infection is common in the immunocompromised host. It has been associated with a high mortality, especially when lung involvement is diffuse. As many as one third of these infected patients have more than one type of pathogen present.[46] The overall diagnostic accuracy of bronchoscopy in this heterogeneous group of patients varies widely. This is a consideration when therapy is dictated by a single, specific opportunistic infection as diagnosed by bronchoscopy.

In patients with acquired immunodeficiency syndrome (AIDS), open-lung biopsy is rarely required because of the extremely high diagnostic yield of fiberoptic bronchoscopy. In AIDS patients, BAL has a sensitivity rate in diagnosing *P carinii* pneumonia of approximately 85% to 90%, and for transbronchial biopsy, the diagnostic yield approaches 87% to 95%. When BAL and transbronchial biopsy are performed

TABLE 46-9. Pulmonary Infiltrates in the Immunocompromised Host

INFECTIONS	RADIATION INJURY
Bacterial	Pneumonitis
Fungal	Fibrosis
Parasitic	
Viral	MALIGNANCY
	Metastatic (hematogenous)
DRUG-INDUCED	Direct extension
Chemotherapeutic agents	Lymphangitic spread
Bleomycin	
Busulfan	IDIOPATHIC
Cyclophosphamide	Usual interstitial
Mitomycin	pneumonitis
Methotrexate	Desquamative interstitial
Procarbazine	pneumonitis
Chlorambucil	
Melphalan	PULMONARY HEMORRHAGE
Antibiotics	
Nitrofurantoin	PULMONARY EDEMA
Sulfonamides (rarely)	Cardiogenic
Amiodorone	Noncardiogenic (ARDS)
Tocainide	
Lidocaine	ASPIRATION
Aspirin	
Diphenylhydantoin	PULMONARY EMBOLI OR
Carbamazepine	INFARCTION
Hydrochlorothiazide	
Opiates	VASCULITIS
Heroin	
Methadone	LEUKOSTASIS
Propoxyphene	
Penicillamine	UNDERLYING DISEASE
Gold salts	PROGRESSION
Colchicine	

ARDS, adult respiratory distress syndrome.

in AIDS patients with *P carinii* pneumonia, the diagnostic yield is 95% to 98%. The diagnostic yield of bronchoscopy for all other pathogens in this patient population approaches 65%.[87-90] Patients considered to be at increased risk when performing transbronchial biopsy (e.g., those with bleeding diathesis or on mechanical ventilation with positive-pressure ventilation) can safely undergo BAL. BAL is the most sensitive procedure (70%) for establishing the diagnosis of pulmonary cryptococcosis.[72,91]

Bronchoscopy can significantly increase the diagnostic yield in patients with sputum smear–negative tuberculosis, invasive aspergillosis, coccidioidomycosis, cryptococcosis, and viral pneumonia. In immunosuppressed patients with prolonged granulocytopenia and focal infiltrates, recovery of *Aspergillus* in BAL specimens is sufficient to warrant the diagnosis of invasive infection and the institution of antifungal therapy.[92,93]

Bronchoscopy with transbronchial biopsy, BAL, and bronchial brushings can effectively confirm the diagnosis of infection, cytotoxic lung injury, malignant infiltrates, vasculitis, and bronchiolitis obliterans with organizing pneumonia. BAL can be useful in diagnosing some pulmonary malignan-

cies, including acute myelomonocytic leukemia and bronchoalveolar cell carcinoma.[94,95] The overall diagnostic yield with lavage alone for malignancies approaches 40%.[96]

Open-lung biopsy provides a higher diagnostic yield than fiberoptic bronchoscopy in immunocompromised patients who present with pulmonary infiltrates. Although open-lung biopsy can provide a specific diagnosis in as many as 45% of the patients who have undergone nondiagnostic bronchoscopy, only a few patients benefit as a direct result of the procedure.[97] Fiberoptic bronchoscopy has its highest diagnostic yield (50%) in patients with diffuse pulmonary infiltrates.[98-100] Bronchoscopy has a reasonably good diagnostic yield in non-AIDS patients, especially if transbronchial biopsies and BAL are used.[75,91,96,101-103] Rapid detection of pathogenic viruses (e.g., cytomegalovirus) by BAL can be enhanced by a monoclonal antibody method, and the need for open-lung biopsy may be negated in many patients. If the results of the BAL and transbronchial biopsy are nondiagnostic, open-lung biopsy can subsequently be performed.[103]

TRACHEOBRONCHIAL TRAUMA

The classic signs of tracheobronchial disruption include shortness of breath, massive subcutaneous emphysema, persistent pneumothorax despite chest tube insertion, and a large air leak after tube thoracoscopy. On occasion, however, only subtle signs exist, even in the presence of significant injury. Fiberoptic bronchoscopy should be performed early in any patient with chest trauma in whom airway injury may have occurred.[104] Signs and symptoms of tracheobronchial injury are listed in Table 46-10. Tracheobronchial disruption rarely occurs as an isolated injury.[105] There is usually a history of a rapid deceleration injury, such as a motor vehicle accident with the patient's chest striking the steering wheel or dashboard. In patients with tracheal or bronchial disruption, early bronchoscopy can reliably detect the site of airway injury.[106-111] Fiberoptic bronchoscopy should be performed by an experienced bronchoscopist who is familiar with normal oropharyngeal, tracheal, and bronchial anatomy and who is skilled in the technique of endotracheal intubation using the fiberoptic bronchoscope as a guide. Prompt diagnosis

TABLE 46-10. Signs and Symptoms of Tracheobronchial Injury

Fracture of upper ribs
Fracture of clavicle or sternum
Chest wall contusions
Chest radiograph
    Subcutaneous emphysema
    Pneumothorax
    "Sagging" lung
    Pneumomediastinum
    Atelectasis
    Pulmonary contusion
Hemoptysis
Bronchopleural fistula
Dyspnea
Cough

and surgical correction or tracheobronchial disruption produce a better outcome, and delay in diagnosis is usually detrimental to the patient.[105] Patients with partial tracheal or bronchial disruption may be relatively asymptomatic and present with a paucity of physical findings. Delays in diagnosis unfortunately are common and have been associated with decreased frequency of successful repair. Failure to diagnose disruption may result in a delayed stricture formation at the site of injury, resulting in distal atelectasis, chronic recurrent infections, and bronchiectasis.

The pathogenesis of tracheobronchial rupture in blunt chest trauma is caused by shearing, wrenching, or compressive forces, acting alone or in concert. Rapid deceleration results in shearing forces, acting predominantly at the distal trachea near the carina where the relatively fixed trachea joins the more mobile distal airways.[112,113] The lungs may be suddenly pulled apart by rapid compression of the chest, with subsequent narrowing of the anteroposterior diameter and widening of the transverse diameter. If the trachea and mainstem bronchi are crushed between the chest wall and vertebral column and the glottis closed, airway pressure suddenly increases, with resultant rupture of the airway.[105]

If an airway injury is suspected, fiberoptic bronchoscopy should be performed through an endotracheal tube prepositioned on the bronchoscope to assess tracheal or bronchial disruption. If a persistent bronchopleural fistula exists because of proximal airway trauma, the cuff of the endotracheal tube sometimes can be positioned just distal to the rupture site and inflated, and adequate ventilation can be established before surgical repair.[106,114–116] Cervical tracheal rupture is less common than rupture of the intrathoracic trachea. Cervical tracheal rupture, however, may be more difficult to diagnose once the patient is intubated because of proximal location of the tear, and may itself be an impediment to intubation.[117] Emergency room intubation attempts have been reported to be unsuccessful in as many as 75% of patients with cervical tracheal disruption when using standard intubation techniques.[118]

Lin and colleagues[119] retrospectively reviewed bronchoscopy performed on 30 consecutive patients with acute chest trauma. Physical and radiographic findings that indicated a high probability of positive bronchoscopic findings included open wound over the chest, subcutaneous emphysema, decreased breath sounds, bilateral pneumothorax, pneumomediastinum, and signs of tracheobronchial separations. Thirty-three percent of trauma patients were judged to benefit from early bronchoscopy as it related to management decisions. Unfortunately, the physical and radiographic findings were not specific enough to highly predict which patients would benefit from bronchoscopy. In an editorial accompanying that report, Prakash[120] commented that the primary indication for diagnostic bronchoscopy in patients with acute or recent chest trauma is to exclude significant damage to the tracheobronchial tree. Difficulty or inability to intubate the trachea or to adequately ventilate and oxygenate despite proper intubation should increase suspicion of disruption of the tracheobronchial tree. The role of rigid bronchoscopy also was identified as to its value in aligning proximal and distal transected segments to allow ventilation through the rigid bronchoscope in preparation for surgical repair.

BRONCHOPLEURAL FISTULA

Most bronchopleural fistulas present subacutely as a chronic air leak manifested by chest tube thoracostomy. If conservative measures, such as prolonged negative intrapleural pressure administered by chest tube thoracostomy and chemical pleurodesis, fail to close the fistula by 1 to 3 weeks, surgery is usually undertaken. Several techniques can be employed by bronchoscopy to localize the proximal endobronchial site of the fistulous tract. Occasionally, air bubbles can be seen emanating from the segmental bronchus. Washing the suspected segment with normal saline and coughing may accentuate the bubbling. A balloon-tipped catheter (e.g., a 4-French Fogarty) can be selectively positioned in suspected segmental orifices. The catheter can be passed through the suction channel of the fiberoptic bronchoscope or adjacent to the bronchoscope held in place by a biopsy forceps extending through the distal tip of the suction channel. It can then be advanced under direct visualization into the suspect segment and the balloon carefully inflated to occlude the orifice, with cessation of bubbling observed in the water seal chamber.[121]

After the offending segmental orifice has been localized, a variety of techniques can be used to temporarily obstruct the segment minimizing the air leak. These include fibrin glue, gel foam, lead shot plugs, an autologous blood patch, or balloon-tipped catheter.[122–132] Biologic "glue" prepared from pooled plasma is not currently available in the United States because of the potential risk of transmitting hepatitis B, HIV, or other diseases. Single-donor cryoprecipitate can provide a high concentration of fibrinogen and factor VIII. Two milliliters of fibrinogen is injected through the distal port of a pulmonary artery catheter wedged into the proximal orifice of the segment subtending the bronchopleural fistula. Subsequently, 0.5 mL (500 U) of topical thrombin is injected, followed by 2 mL of air. One milliliter of epsilon aminocaproic acid may then be administered in a similar fashion to diminish fibrinolysis of the tissue "clot" and enhance the endobronchial tamponade. This technique has proven effective in selected patients with persistent bronchopleural fistula.[127]

Instillation of tetracycline or doxycycline, followed by fresh nonheparinized autologous blood through a wedged balloon-tipped catheter introduced by bronchoscopy, also has effectively closed persistent bronchopleural fistulas. This technique is easily performed at the bedside with little risk to the patient, averting the need for surgical intervention in selected cases.[133,134]

FOREIGN-BODY ASPIRATION

Risk factors for foreign-body aspiration include age younger than 3 years, altered consciousness, trauma, and disordered swallowing mechanisms. Although occurring less frequently in adults than in children, tracheobronchial foreign bodies are problematic in adults.[135] Patients may present with dyspnea, coughing, wheezing, or stridor. Foreign-body aspiration may be relatively occult, with no obvious history for aspiration. Radiographically, there may be evidence of atelectasis, bronchiectasis, or recurrent pneumonitis.

Bronchoscopy performed to remove an aspirated foreign body should be performed by an experienced bronchoscopist. Traditionally, rigid bronchoscopy under general anesthesia has been the method of choice for removing foreign bodies in adults and has enjoyed almost exclusive utility in infants with foreign bodies. Castro and others[136] have recently reported a small series demonstrating the potential success of fiberoptic bronchoscopic removal of foreign bodies from pediatric airways. Two of the 6 patients were younger than 1 year of age. The 3.6-mm external diameter fiberoptic bronchoscope was used. In these small children, the foreign body was grasped with a ureteral basket, and after withdrawal to the distal tip of the endotracheal tube, the endotracheal tube was removed. The ability to pass the ureteral basket alongside the fiberoptic bronchoscope also exists. It is appropriate to use a fiberoptic bronchoscope for foreign-body removal in children when attempts with the rigid instrument have failed. Fiberoptic bronchoscopy offers potential advantage with a peripherally placed foreign body or its localization in the upper lobe segment that cannot be visualized with the rigid bronchoscope. For most situations, however, the rigid bronchoscope remains the instrument of choice.[136] In adults fiberoptic bronchoscopy has clearly been shown to be an effective diagnostic and therapeutic tool in cases of suspected foreign-body aspiration. Several extraction devices are available for use through the fiberoptic bronchoscope. Compared with rigid bronchoscopy, fiberoptic bronchoscopy offers an enhanced visualization of the more peripheral airways, can be performed at the bedside, averts the need for general anesthesia and operating room facilities, and is associated with less morbidity.[137,138] Occasionally, flexible fiberoptic bronchoscopy and rigid endoscopy are required jointly to enhance retrieval of the foreign body.[139]

INHALATION INJURY

Exposure to fire or smoke in an enclosed environment puts the patient at risk for thermal airway injury. Patients with singed nasal hairs, facial burns around the nose or mouth, oral/nasopharyngeal burns, carbonaceous sputum, or hoarseness should be suspect for subclinical upper airway injury. Stridor, wheezing, or other manifestations of upper airway symptomatology may imply impending ventilatory failure. In patients with suspected inhalation injury, fiberoptic bronchoscopy should be performed early by an experienced bronchoscopist to identify evidence of thermal airway injury. Fiberoptic bronchoscopy allows direct examination of the supraglottic and infraglottic areas. The need for intubation should be anticipated and an endotracheal tube placed over the bronchoscope before examining the airways. If intubation is deemed necessary, the bronchoscope can function as a guide for endotracheal tube placement. Serial examinations may be necessary in patients with apparent minimal thermal airway injury on initial evaluation.[140] Signs indicating impending airway obstruction include inflammation, edema, ulceration, or hemorrhage of the upper airway mucosa.[141-144]

By using fiberoptic bronchoscopy, inhalation injury can be classified into acute, subacute, and chronic phases.[145] In the acute stage, upper airway obstruction from mucosal edema and respiratory failure from pulmonary edema and hemorrhage are the main characteristics. Soot deposition in the airways and carbon monoxide poisoning also may be found. The subacute stage, which last from hours to several days, is manifested by necrosis of the tracheobronchial mucosa, hemorrhagic tracheal bronchitis, persistent pulmonary edema with or without hemorrhage, and secondary infection. Scaring and stenosis of the tracheobronchial tree with formation of granulation tissue and bronchiectasis in bronchiolitis obliterans are the hallmarks of the chronic stage.[145,146] Fiberoptic bronchoscopy may offer significant utility in identifying these three stages of significant injury.[147] Mesanes and colleagues[148] performed fiberoptic bronchoscopy on 130 consecutive patients with inhalation injury. They showed that inhalation injury can be diagnosed within a few hours of the accident and that microscopic and histologic aspects of the bronchial mucosa are independent of hemodynamic status. They demonstrated that macroscopic soot deposits in the airways are always associated with histologic signs of ventilation injury, even when the appearance of the mucosa is normal. They also compared the association of absence of cough reflex in smoke inhalation injury with the absence of pain in full-thickness burns of the skin.

In the intubated patient, repeat airway examination by bronchoscopy may be necessary before extubation to assure airway patency and resolution of the supraglottic or laryngeal edema. The endotracheal tube can be withdrawn over the bronchoscope while inspecting the airway mucosa and replaced if the airway is compromised.[149]

In patients with inhalation injury, fiberoptic bronchoscopy is not useful for predicting either the degree of respiratory insufficiency or the required length of mechanical ventilation. Its value lies predominantly in identifying the need for establishing a stable airway.[150]

ACUTE UPPER AIRWAY OBSTRUCTION

Causes of upper airway obstruction include epiglottitis, bilateral vocal cord paralysis, laryngeal edema, and a foreign body. Fiberoptic bronchoscopy may be diagnostic and therapeutic in these circumstances. The exception is that upper airway obstruction related to foreign body is best treated with rigid bronchoscopy. In the pediatric patient, subglottic stenosis secondary to croup also must be considered. Fiberoptic bronchoscopy may be particularly helpful for diagnosis and therapeutic intubation in upper airway obstruction after burn and smoke inhalation injury, as well as trauma to the face and neck. The fiberoptic bronchoscope affords immediate direct visualization of the upper airway, and if performed through a previously positioned endotracheal tube, it affords visualization and guidance for endotracheal intubation. If epiglottitis is suspected, it may be prudent to perform bronchoscopy in the surgical suite with the surgical team available for emergency tracheostomy in case of failure. When performing bronchoscopic intubation in suspected upper airway obstruction, the nasotracheal approach may be preferable because the turbinates offer stabilization and a more controlled approach to the area of acute airway obstruction.[151] Guidice and associates[151] used a 5.2-mm fiberoptic bronchoscope and the transnasal approach in 22 adult patients with suspected acute upper airway obstruction. They used an 8-mm nasotracheal tube for broncho-scopic intubation. All 8 patients with life-threatening upper airway obstruction were successfully intubated. There was no mortality and no significant morbidity. Three patients had slight bleeding in the nares. Preparing the nares with vasoconstrictor and inserting the nasotracheal tube into the posterior nasopharynx before inserting the bronchoscope may minimize bleeding complications. In the Guidice study, the average time of the procedure was 15 minutes. The nasotracheal approach is optimum for patient tolerance, angle of approach to the glottic area, and decreased irritation and trauma of the upper airway.[151] Fiberoptic bronchoscopic intubation in upper airway obstruction also may be performed in the sitting position with decreased posterior displacement of the epiglottis over the compromised upper airway when compared with laryngoscopic examination in the supine position. If foreign-body obstruction is known or suspected as the cause of the upper airway obstruction, rigid bronchoscopy should be the bronchoscopy method of choice.

STATUS ASTHMATICUS

The usefulness of bronchoscopy in patients with status asthmaticus is the subject of controversy.[152,153] Success has been reported with bronchial lavage in patients with obstructive airway disease who could not be weaned from ventilatory support.[154,155] Bronchial lavage may benefit selected patients with thick, tenacious secretions who are unresponsive to aggressive bronchodilator therapy, requiring mechanical ventilatory support.[156,157] Mucus plugs impacted in airways may be expelled using the fiberoptic bronchoscope for lavage, thus improving ventilation and oxygenation.[158,159] Critically ill mechanically ventilated asthmatic patients are, however, poor candidates for bronchial lavage. The procedure is likely to produce a significant increase in auto PEEP and worsening of hypoxemia. The extolled benefits of lung lavage are limited to case reports.[47,160,161] Normal saline lavage solution has been traditionally used, but diluted N-acetylcysteine may enhance mucus clearance from the airways by a mucolytic effect.[47,156] N-acetylcysteine should be used with caution because it may provoke bronchospasm in patients with reactive airways disease.

Asthmatics should receive aggressive bronchodilator therapy including beta-agonists, corticosteroids, and anticholinergic agents before bronchoscopy.

TUBERCULOSIS

Fiberoptic bronchoscopy should be performed in patients suspected of having active tuberculosis who manifest negative sputum results on smears or cultures or from whom adequate sputum specimens are impossible to obtain. The primary value of fiberoptic bronchoscopy in the diagnosis of tuberculosis is in its ability to enhance the early recognition of disease by obtaining material for staining from more distal airways. The diagnosis of infection can be accomplished by demonstration of mycobacteria in bronchoscopy specimens or in postbronchoscopy sputum samples. Bronchial washings of sputum smear–negative patients with tu-

TABLE 46-11. Diagnostic and Therapeutic Uses of Fiberoptic Bronchoscopy in the Intensive Care Unit

DIAGNOSTIC EVALUATION	METHOD
Etiology of hemoptysis	Direct observation
Degree of inhalation injury	Direct observation
Evaluation of placement of endotracheal tube	Direct observation
Airway obstruction	Direct observation
Tracheobronchial trauma	Direct observation
Atelectasis	Direct observation
Diagnosis of pneumonia Ventilator-associated pneumonia Nonimmunocompromised host Immunocompromised host	BAL and protected specimen brush with quantitative cultures; special stains; transbronchial biopsy
Evaluation of suspected neoplastic mass in endobronchial, mediastinal, and parenchymal locations	Cytologic brush biopsy, BAL, transbronchial forceps biopsy, and transtracheal needle biopsy

THERAPEUTIC USE	ASSOCIATED TECHNIQUES
Emergency airway management	Oral or nasal route; use of oropharyngeal airway; high-frequency jet ventilation
Foreign body retrieval	Biopsy forceps, wire basket, Fogarty balloon catheter
Hemoptysis	Endobronchial blocker; laser therapy; vasoconstrictor drug application; tissue glue
Localization and treatment of bronchopleural fistula	Fogarty balloon localization; tissue glue, blood patch, lead shot
Initiation of independent lung ventilation	Placement of double lumen ETT; placement of bronchial blocker

BAL, bronchoalveolar lavage; ETT, endotracheal tube.

berculosis are smear positive in 12% to 42% of patients and culture positive in 66% to 95%.[162] In one third to one half of initially sputum smear–negative patients, bronchoscopy specimens yield the only positive source of mycobacterial tuberculosis.[163–165] Overall, the sensitivity rate of fiberoptic bronchoscopic washings and BAL fluid culture ranges from 83% to 95%. Immediate identification of *M tuberculosis* by bronchoscopy may approach 90%.[163–166] The use of the polymerase chain reaction has potential for rapid diagnosis of smear-negative tuberculosis.[166] Further studies are required to examine the utility of this technique.

CONCLUSION

Fiberoptic bronchoscopy is an extremely important diagnostic and therapeutic tool in the management of seriously ill and injured patients (Table 46-11). It provides an opportunity to establish a stable, secure airway and allows sampling of pulmonary specimens for diagnostic studies. Fiberoptic bronchoscopy facilitates the timely management of patients having a variety of traumatic and inhalation injuries. It can be safely performed at the bedside and has supplanted rigid bronchoscopy as the diagnostic and therapeutic procedure of choice for a variety of pulmonary problems. Video bronchoscopy offers additional advantages for ICU bronchoscopy. Bronchoscopic experience and skill are necessary to provide optimal care and management. The future holds promise of further therapeutic and diagnostic bronchoscopic advancements that may favorably influence patient survival in the ICU.

REFERENCES

1. Kato H, Kobayashi T, Konaka C: Video (CCD) flexible bronchoscopy versus standard flexible bronchoscopy: pro video-bronchoscope. *J Bronchol* 1995;2:328
2. Edell ES: Video (CCD) flexible bronchoscope versus standard flexible bronchoscope: pro standard bronchoscope. *J Bronchol* 1995;2:331
3. Credle WF, Smiddy JF, Elliott RC: Complications of fiberoptic bronchoscopy. *Am Rev Respir Dis* 1974;109:67
4. Udaya BS, Prakash MD, Stubbs SE: Bronchoscopy: indications and technique. *Semin Respir Med* 1981;3:17
5. Pereira W, Kovnat DM, Snider GL: A prospective cooperative study of complications following flexible fiberoptic bronchoscopy. *Chest* 1978;73:813
6. Steinberg KP, Mitchell DR, Maunder RJ, et al: Safety of bronchoalveolar lavage in patients with adult respiratory distress syndrome. *Am Rev Respir Dis* 1993;148:556
7. Albertini RE, Harrell JH, Kurihara N: Arterial hypoxemia induced by fiberoptic bronchoscopy. *JAMA* 1974;230:1666
8. Albertini R, Harrell JH, Moser KM: Hypoxemia during fiberoptic bronchoscopy. *Chest* 1974;65:117
9. Ghows MB, Rosen MJ, Chuang MT, et al: Transcutaneous oxygen monitoring during fiberoptic bronchoscopy. *Chest* 1986;89:543
10. Lindholm CE, Ollman B, Snyder JV, et al: Cardiorespiratory effects of flexible fiberoptic bronchoscopy in critically ill patients. *Chest* 1978;74:363
11. Dubrawsky C, Awe RJ, Jenkins DE: The effect of bronchofiberscopic examination on oxygenation status. *Chest* 1976;67:137
12. Pingleton SK, Bone RC, Ruth WC: Helium-oxygen mixtures during bronchoscopy. *Crit Care Med* 1980;8:50
13. Kaplan JA, Thys DM: Electrocardiography. In: Miller RD (ed). *Anesthesia*, 3rd ed. New York, Churchill Livingstone, 1990:1101
14. Wu FL, Razzaghi A, Souney PF: Seizure after lidocaine for bronchoscopy: case report and review of the use of lidocaine in airway anesthesia. *Pharmacotherapy* 1993;13:72
15. Latto IP, Rosen M: *Difficulties in Tracheal Intubation*. London: Bailliere Tindall, 1985
16. Barrett CR: Flexible fiberoptic bronchoscopy in the critically ill patient. *Chest* 1978;73:746
17. Shrader DL: The effect of fiberoptic bronchoscopy on cardiac rhythm. *Chest* 1978;73:821
18. Katz AS, Michelson EL, Stawick J, et al: Cardiac arrhythmias: frequency during fiberoptic bronchoscopy and correlation with hypoxemia. *Arch Intern Med* 1981;141:603
19. Belen J, Neuhaus A, Markowitz D, et al: Modification of the effect of fiberoptic bronchoscopy on pulmonary mechanics. *Chest* 1981;79:516
20. Zavala DC: Pulmonary hemorrhage in fiberoptic transbronchial biopsy. *Chest* 1976;70:584
21. Fulkerson WJ: Current concepts: fiberoptic bronchoscopy. *N Engl J Med* 1984;311:511
22. Koontz CH, Joyner LR, Nelson RA: Transbronchial lung biopsy via the fiberoptic bronchoscope in sarcoidosis. *Ann Intern Med* 1978;85:64
23. Landa JF: Indications for bronchoscopy. *Chest* 1978;73:687
24. Johnston H, Reisz G: Changing spectrum of hemoptysis: underlying causes in 148 patients undergoing diagnostic flexible fiberoptic bronchoscopy. *Arch Intern Med* 1989;149:1666
25. Sanderson DR, Fontana RS, Woolner LB, et al: Bronchoscopic localization of radiographically occult lung cancer. *Chest* 1974;65:608
26. Mannucci PM, Remuzzi G, Pusineri F, et al: Deamino-8-D-arginine vasopressin shortens the bleeding time in uremia. *N Engl J Med* 1983;308:8
27. Kobrinsky NL, Gerrard JM, Watson CM, et al: Shortening of bleeding time by 1-deamino-8-D-arginine vasopressin in various bleeding disorders. *Lancet* 1984₂:1145
28. Zavala DC: Bronchoscopy and cytology. In: Clark TSH (ed). *Clinical Investigation of Respiratory Disease*. London, Chapman & Hall, 1981:337
29. Pereira W, Kovnat DM, Khan MA, et al: Fever and pneumonia after flexible fiberoptic bronchoscopy. *Am Rev Respir Dis* 1975;112:59
30. Kane RC, Cohen MH, Fossieck BE, et al: Absence of bacteremia after fiberoptic bronchoscopy. *Am Rev Respir Dis* 1975;111:102
31. Dajani AS, Bisno AL, Chung KJ, et al: Antimicrobial prophylaxis for the prevention of bacterial endocarditis in patients with underlying cardiac conditions. *JAMA* 1990;264:2919
32. Ovassapian A, Yelick SJ, Dykes MHM, et al: Fiberoptic nasotracheal intubation: incidence and causes of failure. *Anesth Analg* 1983;62:692
33. Williams RT, Maltabey JR: Airway intubator. *Anesth Analg* 1983;61:309
34. Rogers SN, Benumof JL: New and easy techniques for fiberoptic endoscopy–aided tracheal intubation. *Anesthesiology* 1983;59:569
35. Ovassapian A, Randel GI: The role of the fiberscope in the critically ill patient. *Crit Care Clin* 1995;11:29
36. Shinnick JP, Johnson RF, Oslick T: Bronchoscopy during

mechanical ventilation using the fiberscope. *Chest* 1974;65: 613

37. O'Brien D, Registrar S, Curran J, et al: Fiberoptic assessment of tracheal tube position: a comparison of tracheal tube position as estimated by fiberoptic bronchoscopy and by chest x-ray. *Anaesthesia* 1985;40:73

38. Shinnick JP, Freedman AP: Bronchofiberscopic placement of a double-lumen endotracheal tube. *Crit Care Med* 1981;10:544

39. Ovassapian A: Fiberoptic bronchoscope and double-lumen tracheal tubes. *Anesthesia* 1983;38:1104

40. Stauffer JI, Olson DE, Petty TL: Complications and consequences of endotracheal intubation and tracheotomy. *Am J Med* 1981;70:65

41. Amikam B, Landa J, West J, et al: Bronchofiberscopic observations of the tracheobronchial tree during intubation. *Am Rev Respir Dis* 1972;105:747

42. Krenzelok EP: Principles of toxicology and therapeutics. In: Chernow B. *The Pharmacologic Approach to the Critically Ill Patient*. 3rd ed. Baltimore, Williams & Wilkins, 1994:223

43. Hamill JF, Bedford RF, Weaver DC, et al: Lidocaine before endotracheal intubation: intravenous or laryngotracheal? *Anesthesiology* 1981;55:578

44. Froese AB, Bryan AC: Effects of anesthesia and paralysis on diaphragmatic mechanics in man. *Anesthesiology* 1974;41: 242

45. Marini JJ, Pierson DJ, Hudson LD: Acute lobar atelectasis: a prospective comparison of fiberoptic bronchoscopy and respiratory therapy. *Am Rev Respir Dis* 1979;119:971

46. Marini JJ, Wheeler AP: Fiberoptic bronchoscopy in critical care. In: Clark TSH (ed). *Clinical Investigation of Respiratory Disease*. London, Chapman & Hall, 1981

47. Niederman MS, Gambino A, Lichter J, et al: Tension ball valve mucus plug in asthma. *Am J Med* 1985;79:131

48. Turner JS, Willcox PA, Hayhurst MD, et al: Fiberoptic bronchoscopy in the intensive care unit: a prospective study of 147 procedures in 107 patients. *Crit Care Med* 1994;22:259

49. Haenel JB, Moore FA, Moore EE, et al: Efficacy of selective intrabronchial air insufflation in acute lobar collapse. *Am J Surg* 1992;164:501

50. Harada K, Mutsuda T, Saoyama N, et al: Re-expansion of refractory atelectasis using a bronchofiberscope with a balloon cuff. *Chest* 1983;84:725

51. Millen JE, Vandree J, Glauser FL: Fiberoptic bronchoscopic balloon occlusion and re-expansion of refractory unilateral atelectasis. *Crit Care Med* 1978;6:50

52. Chang-Yao Tsao T, Tsai Ying-Huang, Lan RS, et al: Treatment for collapsed lung in critically ill patients. *Chest* 1990;97:435

53. Gottlieb LS, Hillberg R: Endobronchial tamponade therapy for intractable hemoptysis. *Chest* 1975;67:482

54. Saw EC, Gottlieb LS, Yokoyama T, et al: Flexible fiberoptic bronchoscopy and endobronchial tamponade in the management of massive hemoptysis. *Chest* 1976;70:589

55. Freitag L: Development of a new balloon catheter for management of hemoptysis with bronchofiberscopes. *Chest* 1993;103:593

56. Tsukamoto T, Sasaki H, Nakamura H: Treatment of hemoptysis patients by thrombin and fibrinogen-thrombin infusion therapy using a fiberoptic bronchoscope. *Chest* 1989;96:473

57. Bense L: Intrabronchial selective coagulative treatment of hemoptysis. *Chest* 1990;97:990

58. Uflacker L, Kaemmerer A, Neves C, et al: Management of massive hemoptysis by bronchial artery embolization. *Radiology* 1983;146:627

59. Ferris EJ: Pulmonary hemorrhage. *Chest* 1981;80:710

60. Muthuswamy PP, Akbik F, Franklin C, et al: Management of major or massive hemoptysis in active pulmonary tuberculosis by bronchial arterial embolization. *Chest* 1987;92:77

61. Sweezey NB, Fellows KE: Bronchial artery embolization for severe hemoptysis in cystic fibrosis. *Chest* 1990;97:1322

62. Selecky PA: Evaluation of hemoptysis through the bronchoscope. *Chest* 1978;73:741

63. Flower CDR, Smith IE, Chan AP, et al: Hemoptysis: comparative study of the role of CT and fiberoptic bronchoscopy. *Radiology* 1993;198:677

64. Andrews CP, Coalson JJ, Smith JD, et al: Diagnosis of nosocomial bacterial pneumonia in acute, diffuse lung injury. *Chest* 1981;80:254

65. Fagon JY, Chastre J, Hance AJ, et al: Detection of nosocomial lung infection in ventilated patients: use of a protected specimen brush and quantitative culture techniques in 147 patients. *Am Rev Respir Dis* 1988;138:110

66. American Thoracic Society: Guidelines for the initial management of adults with community-acquired pneumonia: diagnosis, assessment of severity, and initial antimicrobial therapy. *Am Rev Respir Dis* 1993;148:1418

67. Ortqvist A, Kalin M, Lejdeborn L, et al: Diagnostic fiberoptic bronchoscopy and protected brush culture in patients with community-acquired pneumonia. *Chest* 1990;97:576

68. Meduri GU, Chastre J: The standardization of bronchoscopic techniques for ventilator-associated pneumonia. *Chest* 1992;102:557S

69. American Thoracic Society: Clinical role of bronchoalveolar lavage in adults with pulmonary disease. *Am Rev Respir Dis* 1990;142:481

70. Fagon JY, Chastre J, Hance AJ, et al: Detection of nosocomial lung infection in ventilated patients: use of a protected specimen brush and quantitative culture techniques in 147 patients. *Am Rev Respir Dis* 1988;138:110

71. Teague RB, Wallace RJ, Awe RJ: The use of quantitative sterile brush culture and Gram stain in the diagnosis of lower respiratory tract infection. *Chest* 1981;79:157

72. Rankin JA: Role of bronchoalveolar lavage in the diagnosis of pneumonia. *Chest* 1989;95:187S

73. Thorpe JE, Baughman RP, Frame PT, et al: Bronchoalveolar lavage for diagnosing acute bacterial pneumonia. *J Infect Dis* 1987;155:855

74. Kahn FW, Jones JM: Diagnosing bacterial respiratory infection by bronchoalveolar lavage. *J Infect Dis* 1987;155:862

75. Thorpe JE, Baughman RP, Frame PT, et al: Bronchoalveolar lavage for diagnosing acute bacterial pneumonia. *J Infect Dis* 1987;155:855

76. Chastre J, Fagon JY, Soler P, et al: Quantification of BAL cells containing intracellular bacteria rapidly identifies ventilated patients with nosocomial pneumonia. *Chest* 1989;95:190S

77. Meduri GU, Wunderink RG, Leeper KV, et al: Management of bacterial pneumonia in ventilated patients: protected bronchoalveolar lavage as a diagnostic tool. *Chest* 1992;101:500

78. Meduri GU, Beals DH, Maijub AG, et al: A new bronchoscopic technique to retrieve uncontaminated distal airway secretions. *Am Rev Respir Dis* 1991;143:855

79. Pham LH, Brun-Buisson C, Legrand P, et al: Diagnosis of nosocomial pneumonia in mechanically ventilated patients. *Am Rev Respir Dis* 1991;143:1055

80. Baselski VS, El-Torky M, Coalson JJ, et al: The standardization of criteria for processing and interpreting laboratory specimens in patients with suspected ventilator associated pneumonia. *Chest* 1992;102:571S

81. Henry-Stanley MJ: Laboratory processing of BAL fluids. In: Stanley MW, Henry-Stanley MJ, Iber C, (eds). *Bronchoalveolar Lavage: Cytology and Clinical Applications*. New York, Igaku-Shoin, 1991:213

82. Rein MF, Mandell GL: Bacteria killing by bacteriostatic saline solutions: potential for diagnostic errors. *N Engl J Med* 1973; 298:794

83. Baughman RP, Thorpe JE, Staneck J, et al: Use of the protected specimen brush in patients with endotracheal or tracheostomy tubes. *Chest* 1987;135:233

84. Meduri GU, Kohler G, Headley S, et al: Inflammatory cytokines in the BAL of patients with ARDS. *Chest* 1995;108:1303

85. Papin TA, Grum CM, Weg JC: Transbronchial biopsy during mechanical ventilation. *Chest* 1986;89:168

86. Pincus PS, Kallenbach JM, Hurwitz MD, et al: Transbronchial biopsy during mechanical ventilation. *Crit Care Med* 1987; 15:1136

87. Ognibene FP, Shelhamer J, Gill V, et al: The diagnosis of *Pneumocystis carinii* pneumonia in patients with the acquired immunodeficiency syndrome using subsegmental bronchoalveolar lavage. *Am Rev Respir Dis* 1984;129:929

88. Stover DE, White DA, Romano PA, et al: Diagnosis of pulmonary disease in acquire immune deficiency syndrome (AIDS). *Am Rev Respir Dis* 1984;130:659

89. Wollschlager C, Khan F: Diagnostic value of fiberoptic bronchoscopy in acquired immunodeficiency syndrome. *Cleve Clin Q* 1985;52:489

90. Broaddus C, Dake MD, Stulbarg MS, et al: Bronchoalveolar lavage and transbronchial biopsy for the diagnosis of pulmonary infections in the acquired immunodeficiency syndrome. *Ann Intern Med* 1985;102:747

91. Chechani V, Kamholz SL: Pulmonary manifestations of disseminated cryptococcosis in patients with AIDS. *Chest* 1990; 98:1058

92. Kahn FW, Jones JM, England DM: The role of bronchoalveolar lavage in the diagnosis of invasive pulmonary aspergillosis. *Am J Clin Pathol* 1986;86:518

93. Andrews CP, Weiner MH: *Aspergillus* antigen detection in bronchoalveolar fluid from patients with invasive aspergillosis and aspergillomas. *Am J Med* 1982;73:372

94. Rossi GA, Balbi B, Risso M, et al: Acute myelomonocytic leukemia: demonstration of pulmonary involvement by lavage. *Chest* 1985;87:259

95. Springmeyer SC, Hackman R, Carlson JJ, et al: Bronchoalveolar cell carcinoma diagnosed by bronchoalveolar lavage. *Chest* 1983;83:278

96. Stover DE, Zaman MB, Hajdi SI, et al: Bronchoalveolar lavage in the diagnosis of diffuse pulmonary infiltrates in the immunocompromised host. *Ann Intern Med* 1984;101:1

97. Nishio JN, Lynch JP: Fiberoptic bronchoscopy in the immunocompromised host: the significance of a "nonspecific" transbronchial biopsy. *Am Rev Respir Dis* 1980;121:307

98. Lauver GL, Hasan FM, Morgan RB, et al: The usefulness of fiberoptic bronchoscopy in evaluating new pulmonary lesions in the compromised host. *Am J Med* 1979;86:580

99. Wilson WR, Cockerill FR, Rosenow EC: Pulmonary disease in the immunocompromised host [second of two parts]. *Mayo Clin Proc* 1985;60:610

100. Feldman NT, Pennington JE, Ehrie MG: Transbronchial lung biopsy in the compromised host. *JAMA* 1977;238:1377

101. Stover DE, Zaman MB, Hajdu SL, et al: Bronchoalveolar lavage in the diagnosis of diffuse pulmonary infiltrates in the immunosuppressed host. *Ann Intern Med* 1984;101:1

102. Wallace JM, Catanzaro A, Moser KM, et al: Flexible fiberoptic bronchoscopy for diagnosing pulmonary coccidioidomycosis. *Am Rev Respir Dis* 1981;123:286

103. Martin WJ, Smith TF, Brutinel M, et al: Role of bronchoalveolar lavage in the assessment of opportunistic pulmonary infections: utility and complications. *Mayo Clin Proc* 1987; 62:549

104. Barmada H, Gibbons JR: Tracheobronchial injury in blunt and penetrating chest trauma. *Chest* 106:74

105. Baumgartner F, Sheppard B, de Virgilio C, et al: Tracheal and main bronchial disruptions after blunt chest trauma: presentation and management. *Ann Thorac Surg* 1990;50: 569

106. Hara KS, Prakash UBS: Fiberoptic bronchoscopy in the evaluation of acute chest and upper airway trauma. *Chest* 1989; 96:627

107. Ecker RR, Libertini RV, Rea WJ, et al: Injuries of the trachea and bronchi. *Ann Thorac Surg* 1971;11:280

108. Grover FL, Ellestad C, Arom KV, et al: Diagnosis and management of major tracheobronchial injuries. *Ann Thorac Surg* 1979;28:384

109. Kelly JP, Webb WR, Moulder PV, et al: Management of airway trauma: combined injuries of the trachea and esophagus. *Ann Thorac Surg* 1987;43:160

110. Jones WS, Mavroudis C, Richardson JD, et al: Management of tracheobronchial disruption resulting from blunt trauma. *Surgery* 1984;95:319

111. Roxburgh JC: Rupture of the tracheobronchial tree. *Thorax* 1987;42:681

112. Caster R, Wareham EE, Brewer LA: Rupture of the bronchus following closed chest trauma. *Am J Surg* 1962;104:212

113. Kirsh MM, Orringer MB, Douglas MB, et al: Management of tracheobronchial disruption secondary to nonpenetrating trauma. Current review: tracheobronchial disruption from blunt trauma. *Ann Thorac Surg* 1976;22:93

114. Heffner JE: When to consider fiberoptic bronchoscopy in the ICU: today's indications for infection, trauma, hemoptysis, atelectasis. *J Crit Illness* 1988;3:69

115. Lumpe DH, Sang OK, Wayman SA: A characteristic pulmonary finding in unilateral complete bronchial transection. *Am J Roentgenol* 1970;110:704

116. Luce JM: Chest trauma. *Pulmonary Crit Care Update* 1990;5:2

117. Major CP, Floresguerra CA, Messerschmidt WH, et al: Traumatic disruption of the cervical trachea. *J Tenn Med Assoc* 1992;85:517

118. Reece GP, Shatney CH: Blunt injuries of the cervical trachea: review of 51 patients. *South Med J* 1987;18:1542

119. Lin MC, Lin HC, Lan RS, et al: Emergent flexible bronchoscopy for the evaluation of acute chest trauma. *J Bronchol* 1995;1:188

120. Prakash UBS: The role of bronchoscopy in patients with chest trauma [editorial]. *J Bronchol* 1995;2:179

121. McManigle JE, Fletcher GL, Tenholder MF: Bronchoscopy in the management of bronchopleural fistula. *Chest* 1990;97: 1235

122. Jessen C, Sharma P: Use of fibrin glue in thoracic surgery. *Ann Thorac Surg* 1985;39:521

123. Glover W, Chavis TV, Daniel TM, et al: Fibrin glue application through the flexible fiberoptic bronchoscope: closure of bronchopleural fistulas. *J Thorac Cardiovasc Surg* 1987;93: 470

124. Onotera RT, Unruh HW: Closure of a post-pneumonectomy bronchopleural fistula with fibrin sealant (Tisseel). *Thorax* 1988;43:1015

125. Regel G, Sturm JA, Neumann C, et al: Occlusion of bronchopleural fistula after lung injury: a new treatment by bronchoscopy. *J Trauma* 1989;29:223

126. McCarthy PM, Trastek VF, Bell DG, et al: The effectiveness of fibrin glue sealant for reducing experimental pulmonary air leak. *Ann Thorac Surg* 1988;45:203

127. Matar AF, Hill JH, Duncan W, et al: Use of biological glue to control pulmonary air leaks. *Thorax* 1990;46:670

128. Jones DP, David I: Gelfoam occlusion of peripheral bronchopleural fistulas. *Ann Thorac Surg* 1986;42:334
129. Ratliff JL, Hill J, Tucker H, et al: Endobronchial control of bronchopleural fistula. *Chest* 1977;71:98
130. Lan R, Lee C, Tsai Y, et al: Fiberoptic bronchial blockade in a small bronchopleural fistula. *Chest* 1987;92:944
131. Pace R, Rankin RN, Finley RJ: Detachable balloon occlusion of bronchopleural fistulae in dogs. *Invest Radiol* 1983;18:504
132. Ellis JH, Sequeira FW, Weber TR, et al: Balloon catheter occlusion of bronchopleural fistulae. *Am J Radiol* 1982;138:157
133. Lan RS, Lee CH, Tsai YH, et al: Fiberoptic bronchial blockade in a small bronchopleural fistula. *Chest* 1987;92:944
134. Martin WR, Siefkin AD, Allen R: Closure of a bronchopleural fistula with bronchoscopic instillation of tetracycline. *Chest* 1991;99:1040
135. Limper AH, Prakash UBS: Tracheobronchial foreign bodies in adults. *Ann Intern Med* 1990;112:604
136. Castro M, Midthun DE, Edell ES, et al: Flexible bronchoscopic removal of foreign bodies from pediatric airways. *J Bronchol* 1994;1:92
137. Cunanan OS: The flexible fiberoptic bronchoscope in foreign body removal. *Chest* 1978;73:725
138. Lan RS, Lee CH, Chiang YC, et al: Use of fiberoptic bronchoscopy to retrieve bronchial foreign bodies in adults. *Am Rev Respir Dis* 1989;140:1734
139. Wood RE: Flexible bronchoscopy to remove foreign bodies in children: yes, maybe—but...[editorial]. *J Bronchol* 1994;1:87
140. Hunt JL, Agee RN, Pruitt BA Jr: Fiberoptic bronchoscopy in acute inhalation injury. *J Trauma* 1975;15:641
141. Wald PH, Balmes JR: Respiratory effects of short-term, high-intensity toxic inhalations: smoke, gases, and fumes. *J Intensive Care Med* 1987;2:260
142. Crapo RO: Smoke-inhalation injuries. *JAMA* 1981;246:1694
143. Hunt JL, Agec RN, Pruitt BA Jr: Fiberoptic bronchoscopy in acute inhalation injury. *J Trauma* 1975;15:641
144. Williams DO, Vanecko RM, Glassroth J: Endobronchial polyposis following smoke inhalation. *Chest* 1983;84:774
145. Prakash UBS: Chemical warfare and bronchoscopy. *Chest* 1991;100:1486
146. Freitag L, Firusian N, Stamatis G, et al: The role of bronchoscopy in pulmonary complications due to mustard gas inhalation. *Chest* 1991;100:1436
147. Sueoka N, Kato O, Aoki Y, et al: Fiberoptic bronchoscopy in inhalation injury. *J Jpn Soc Bronchol* 1994;16:454
148. Mesanes MJ, Legendre C, Lioret N, et al: Using bronchoscopy and biopsy to diagnose early inhalation injury: macroscopic and histologic findings. *Chest* 1991;107:1365
149. Dellinger RP: Fiberoptic bronchoscopy in adult airway management. *Crit Care Med* 1990;18:882
150. Bingham HG, Gallagher TJ, Powell MD: Early bronchoscopy as a predictor of ventilatory support for burned patients. *J Trauma* 1987;27:1286
151. Giudice JC, Komansky H, Gordon R, et al: Acute upper airway obstruction: fiberoptic bronchoscopy in diagnosis and therapy. *Crit Care Med* 1981;9:878
152. Sahn SA, Scoggin C: Fiberoptic bronchoscopy in bronchial asthma: A word of caution. *Chest* 1976;69:39
153. Dubrawsky C, Awe RJ, Jenkins DE: The effect of bronchofiberscopic examination on oxygenation status. *Chest* 1975;67:137
154. Lang, DM, Simon RA, Mathison DA, et al: Safety and possible efficacy of fiberoptic bronchoscopy with lavage in the management of refractory asthma with mucous impaction. *Ann Allergy* 1991;67:324
155. Henke CA, Hertz M, Gustafson P: Combined bronchoscopy and mucolytic therapy for patients with severe refractory status asthmaticus on mechanical ventilation: a case report and review of the literature. *Crit Care Med* 1994;22:1880
156. Millman M, Goodman AH, Goldstein IM, et al: Status asthmaticus: use of acetylcysteine during bronchoscopy and lavage to remove mucous plugs. *Ann Allergy* 1983;50:85
157. Shridharani M, Maxson TR: Pulmonary lavage in a patient in status asthmaticus receiving mechanical ventilation: a case report. *Ann Allergy* 1982;49:157
158. Millman M, Goodman AH, Goldstein IM, et al: Status asthmaticus: use of acetylcysteine during bronchoscopy and lavage to remove mucous plugs. *Ann Allergy* 1983;50:85
159. Weinstein HJ, Bone RC, Ruth WE: Pulmonary lavage in patients treated with mechanical ventilation. *Chest* 1977;72:583
160. Millman M, Goodman AH, Goldstein IM, et al: Bronchoscopy and lavage for chronic bronchial asthma. *Immunol Allerg Pract* 1981;3:10
161. Brashear RE, Meyer SC, Manion MW: Unilateral atelectasis in asthma. *Chest* 1973;63:847
162. Danek JJ, Bower JS: Diagnosis of pulmonary tuberculosis by fiberoptic bronchoscopy. *Am Rev Respir Dis* 1979;119:677
163. Jett JR, Cortese DA, Dines DE: The value of bronchoscopy in the diagnosis of mycobacterial disease. *Chest* 1981;80:575
164. Pant K, Chawla R, Mann PS, et al: Fiberbronchoscopy in smear-negative miliary tuberculosis. *Chest* 1989;95:1151
165. de Gracia J, Curull V, Vidal R, et al: Diagnostic value of bronchoalveolar lavage in suspected pulmonary tuberculosis. *Chest* 1988;93:329
166. Uddenfeldt M, Lundgren R: Flexible fiberoptic bronchoscopy in the diagnosis of pulmonary tuberculosis. *Tubercle* 1981;62:197

Critical Care, Third Edition, edited by Joseph M. Civetta,
Robert W. Taylor, and Robert R. Kirby.
Lippincott-Raven Publishers, Philadelphia PA © 1997.

CHAPTER 47

■

Oxygen Therapy

Robert A. Smith

IMMEDIATE CONCERNS ■

Oxygen is given to increase arterial blood oxygen partial pressure (PaO_2). Except for patients undergoing extracorporeal membrane oxygenation or intravascular oxygenation, the only means to increase PaO_2 is with oxygen-enriched inspired gas delivered across the alveolar–capillary barrier. The usual indication for oxygen therapy is potential or established hypoxemia. Hypoxemia arbitrarily is considered to be present when the arterial oxyhemoglobin saturation (SaO_2) is less than 90%, corresponding to a PaO_2 less than 60 mm Hg when blood pH and hemoglobin kinetics are normal. Hypoxemia resulting from alveolar hypoventilation, ventilation-perfusion ($\dot{V}/\dot{Q}$) mismatch, or oxygen diffusion limitation is potentially responsive to increased inspired oxygen therapy. Oxygen therapy is also indicated in treating carbon monoxide poisoning, because hyperoxia accelerates dissociation of carboxyhemoglobin. Hypoxemia from intrapulmonary or intracardiac shunting of mixed venous blood is not significantly affected by oxygen therapy.

STRESS POINTS

1. Atmospheric air contains an oxygen fraction of 0.209 that exerts a partial pressure (PO_2) determined by the ambient barometric (PB) and water vapor (PH_2O) pressures.
2. Inspired oxygen partial pressure (PIO_2) is equal to the product of the fraction of inspired oxygen (FIO_2) and $P(B - H_2O)$ and diminishes while inspired gas traverses the airways. Alveolar oxygen partial pressure (PAO_2) depends on the PIO_2, rates at which oxygen ($\dot{V}O_2$) and carbon dioxide ($\dot{V}CO_2$) are exchanged between pulmonary capillary blood and alveolar gas, and the alveolar ventilation ($\dot{V}A$).

3. Normally the respiratory gas exchange ratio ($R = \dot{V}CO_2/\dot{V}O_2$) is 0.8, but R may be altered by the composition of catabolized nutrients, gas exchanging efficiency of the lungs, and during low cardiac output states when the mixed venous-to-arterial carbon dioxide partial pressure gradient is significantly increased.[1]
4. Normal barometric pressure at sea level is 760 mm Hg and the PIO_2 of dry gas is 160 mm Hg. Water vapor (47 mm Hg at 37°C) and carbon dioxide (40 ± 5 mm Hg) partial pressures in alveolar gas reduce PAO_2 to approximately 100 to 105 mm Hg.
5. Oxygen transfer across the alveolar–capillary barrier is determined by the PAO_2 and pulmonary capillary blood oxygen partial pressure and solubility (principally dependent on oxyhemoglobin reaction kinetics). Pulmonary capillary PO_2 varies from approximately 35 to 40 mm Hg (mixed venous blood in the pulmonary artery [$P\bar{v}O_2$]) to a level similar to PAO_2 if the blood equilibrates with alveolar gas (oxygenated blood in distal pulmonary capillaries [$Pc'O_2$]).
6. An equilibration deficit between PAO_2 and $Pc'O_2$ may be caused by a diffusion limitation, for example, hydrostatic pulmonary edema.[2] Clinically, however, $Pc'O_2$ is assumed to equal PAO_2. Elevating the FIO_2 by 0.01 increases the PIO_2 by approximately 8 mm Hg and the PAO_2 by approximately 7 mm Hg at sea level.

ESSENTIAL DIAGNOSTIC TESTS AND PROCEDURES

1. Ideal PAO_2 is calculated with the equation:

$$PAO_2 = PIO_2 - (PACO_2/R) + PACO_2 \times FIO_2(1 - R)/R$$

where $PACO_2 = 0.863\dot{V}CO_2/\dot{V}A$ (the factor 0.863 accounts for $\dot{V}CO_2$ and $\dot{V}A$ being calculated at ATPD and BTPS, respectively).

2. Clinically, arterial blood carbon dioxide partial pressure ($PaCO_2$) is considered to be an adequate estimate of $PACO_2$, and R is assumed to be normal; PAO_2 is often estimated as follows:

$$PAO_2 = PIO_2 - (PaCO_2 \times 1/R) = PIO_2 - (PaCO_2 \times 1.25).$$

3. Thebesian and bronchial venous drainage into the pulmonary veins produces a normal partial pressure gradient between alveolar gas and arterial blood [$P(A - a)O_2$] and results in a PaO_2 of about 90 to 95 mm Hg. The alveolar–arterial oxygen partial pressure gradient is often used as an index of pulmonary function.

4. When $P\bar{v}O_2$ is normal, and assuming $PAO_2 = Pc'O_2$, a $P(A - a)O_2$ gradient of 20 mm Hg represents a venous admixture of approximately 1% if the patient breathes 100% oxygen (although breathing hyperoxic gas may induce $\dot{V}/\dot{Q}$ mismatch and increase venous admixture (*infra vide*).

INITIAL THERAPY

1. Oxygen therapy with jet mixing is commonly employed, but the FIO_2 is variable at any pressure other than atmospheric.
2. The FIO_2 is stable when an air-oxygen, high-pressure blender is used.
3. Nasal cannulae and catheters increase the FIO_2 about 0.03 to 0.04/L of oxygen flow. The maximum tracheal FIO_2 achievable is about 0.45-0.5.
4. Mask oxygen delivery provides a FIO_2 varying from 0.35 to 0.5 for simple masks, and up to 0.8 to 0.95 with nonrebreathing masks. Air entrainment masks provide a FIO_2 of 0.24 to 0.70, depending on the oxygen flow and the amount of air entrained.
5. Nebulization and humidification are employed commonly with oxygen delivery devices but, in the absence of an endotracheal tube or tracheotomy tube, are relatively ineffective. Most of the water "rains out" in the oral, nasal, and pharyngeal passages.
6. Complications of oxygen therapy include hypercapnia, absorption atelectasis, and pulmonary oxygen toxicity.

THERAPEUTIC CONSIDERATIONS ■

TECHNIQUES OF AIR-OXYGEN BLENDING

Jet Entrainment

Blending of oxygen and air to deliver a desired FIO_2 can be accomplished with jet entrainment or proportional mixing of compressed air and oxygen. Jet mixing is accomplished with either an injector (Venturi mechanism) or a jet mixing device. The most frequently used air entrainment mechanism employs jet mixing. The jet exit is in or near the plane of the entrainment port; at this point and within the mixing chamber, pressure is ambient. Thus, air entrainment does not result from high-velocity jet flow (Venturi effect) but from viscous shearing between dynamic and static air layers. The dynamic gas (oxygen) imparts kinetic energy to the

static air mass, thus *dragging* ambient air into the moving stream. Accuracy of air entrainment devices requires operation at atmospheric pressure. Elevation in delivery circuit pressure above ambient pressure causes less air to be entrained whereas oxygen flow remains unaltered. Thus, FIO_2 will fluctuate. Oxygen delivery devices vulnerable to this problem are discussed later.

Mechanical Blending

A method of FIO_2 control unaffected by circuit pressure fluctuations uses mechanical blending of compressed air and oxygen. Blenders are commonly powered by 50-psi gauge air and oxygen sources (Fig. 47-1). Source gases are balanced to the lowest pressure by reducing valves, and air and oxygen at equal pressure are proportioned to a selected FIO_2. Blended gas is then directed to the outlet port for delivery by a flow meter.

OXYGEN DELIVERY SYSTEMS

Supplemental oxygen administration is provided with either fixed or variable performance devices. Fixed performance systems deliver a predictable and consistent FIO_2 independent of fluctuations in the patient's breathing pattern. These are large-capacitance systems providing gas flow that exceeds peak inspiratory flow demand. Variable systems (i.e., small

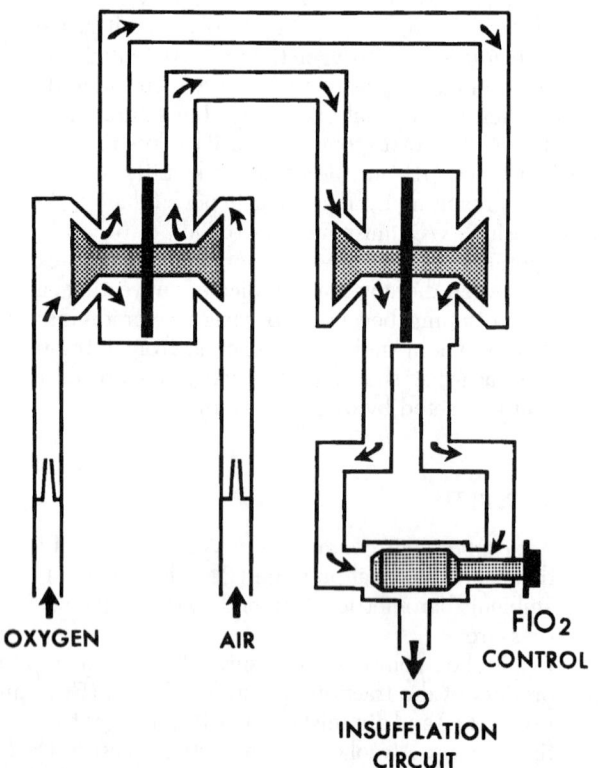

FIGURE 47-1. Schematic representation of an air-oxygen blender. High-pressure air and oxygen are equilibrated by pressure regulators; each is then interfaced with the fraction of inspired oxygen (FIO_2) control valve for delivery to the circuit.

or noncapacitance) are patient dependent. A noncapacitance device, such as a nasal catheter or cannula that provides a low flow rate (e.g., ≤ 4 L/minute) yields insufficient storage of oxygen during exhalation to affect the next inspiration substantially. Therefore, oxygen enrichment is a function of the patient's gas flow rate and the oxygen flow rate. A nasal or pharyngeal oxygen delivery device may provide some capacitance at flow rates greater than 4 L/minute. An oxygen mask or face tent increases capacitance to a variable extent that is dependent on the presence of a reservoir.

Nasal Cannula and Catheter

Supplemental oxygen may be administered with a cannula or catheter. An oxygen cannula consists of two prongs placed approximately 1 cm into the nares and held stationary by an elastic head strap. The catheter should be lubricated with water-soluble jelly and then inserted into a naris until its tip is just visible below the soft palate. It is secured to the upper lip or nose with tape. Cannulas and catheters should be changed at least every day and more frequently if crusting of the outlet ports occurs.

The FIO_2 administered with either device depends on oxygen flow rate, the patient's inspiratory flow, respiratory rate, exhalation time, and the anatomic reservoir (i.e., nasopharyngeal volume). Higher FIO_2 may be realized with a nasal cannula when patients breathe with their mouth closed.[3] A rule of thumb for cannula or catheter systems is that the FIO_2 is increased by 0.03 to 0.04 for each liter per minute of oxygen flow rate. However, maximum tracheal FIO_2 is unlikely to exceed 0.50; therefore, flow rates greater than 8 L/minute are unlikely to increase delivered oxygen further, may prove uncomfortable, and often lead to mucous membrane desiccation.

Transtracheal Catheter

Oxygen may be delivered through a transtracheal catheter. Transtracheal oxygen delivery involves administration of oxygen percutaneously through a catheter inserted in the suprasternal trachea.[4-7] Transtracheal delivery of oxygen permits adequate oxygenation of patients at lower flow rates than are required for delivery by nasal cannulas. Transtracheal oxygen therapy seems to be a relatively safe approach for oxygen administration.

Face Masks

Four types of face masks are used to supplement oxygen delivery: simple, partial rebreather, nonrebreather, and air entrainment (high-flow oxygen-enrichment masks).

SIMPLE MASKS. Simple oxygen masks do not contain valves or a reservoir. They provide FIO_2 of 0.35 to 0.50 when the oxygen flow rate is 6 to 10 L/minute. Oxygen flow must exceed the patient's minute ventilation to minimize expired gas rebreathing.[8] The mask augments the anatomic reservoir volume by providing supplemental oxygen about the nose and mouth; however, variation in the patient's inspiratory flow and respiratory rate can alter FIO_2.

PARTIAL REBREATHING MASKS. Partial rebreathing masks provide delivery of a relatively high FIO_2. These masks incorporate an oxygen reservoir bag from which the patient breathes (Fig. 47-2). An advantage of the partial rebreather is that it provides a high FIO_2 while conserving the oxygen supply. Oxygen flow rate is regulated to permit the initial one third of the exhaled tidal volume (i.e., anatomic dead space) to distend the reservoir maximally. Thus, entry of gas-containing carbon dioxide is prevented and, instead, exits through side ports in the mask. Theoretically, this mask reduces the oxygen requirement by approximately 30%, making it suitable for applications such as patient transport where the availability of oxygen is limited. A mean FIO_2 between 0.70 and 0.85 may be obtained with proper application of this device.

NONREBREATHING MASKS. Nonrebreathing masks have unidirectional valves on each side of the mask that permit venting of exhaled tidal volume and prevent inspiration of room air. Another one-way valve separates the reservoir bag from the mask to prevent retrograde flow of expired gas. Oxygen flow rate should be adequate to sustain the reservoir bag volume. When a disposable, bubble-through humidifier is employed, oxygen is vented to ambient environment through the pressure valve in the delivery unit at flow rates greater than 15 L/minute. Therefore, if a patient's minute ventilation exceeds that level, the humidifier must be bypassed or another one interfaced to provide sufficient gas flow. For short periods, the former solution is quick and generally innocuous for an hour or so. A mean FIO_2 of 0.80 to 0.95 is attainable with correct application of this system.

AIR ENTRAINMENT MASKS. Oxygen-powered air entrainment masks are designed to provide a high flow of gas at a

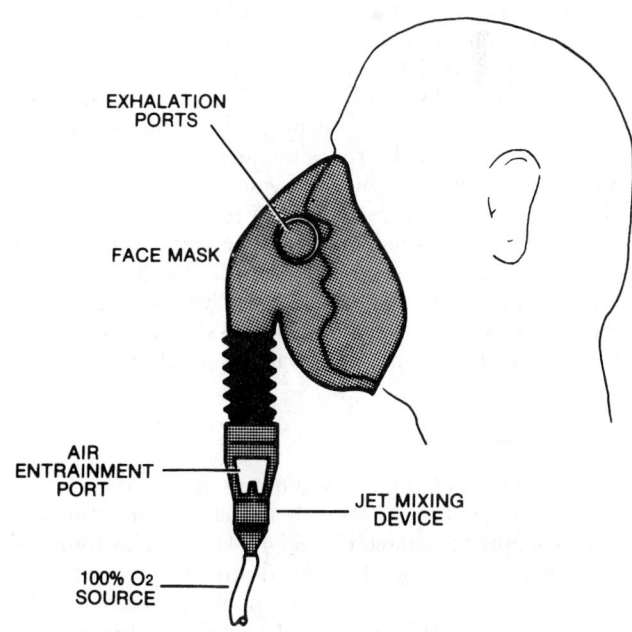

FIGURE 47-2. Partial rebreathing reservoir and mask systems provide delivery of almost 100% oxygen.

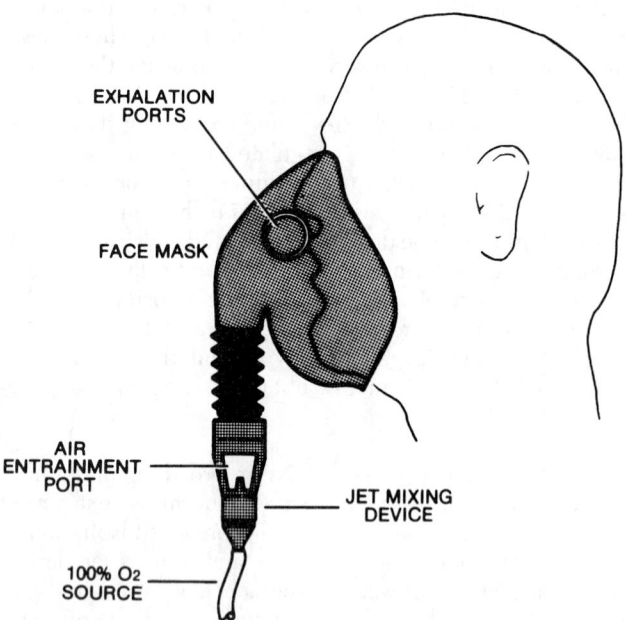

FIGURE 47-3. Air-entrainment masks are powered by 100% oxygen, which is diluted by air entrained through a jet-mixing device.

known FIO_2 (Fig. 47-3). Oxygen is delivered to a small tube or jet mixing device (previously discussed) that increases gas velocity. While the high-velocity stream exits from the jet nozzle, ambient air is entrained and dilutes the stream of pure oxygen. This high flow of mixed gas into the mask substantially exceeds the patient's minute ventilation. Thus, no valve or reservoir is necessary to prevent rebreathing. The high flow also promotes a consistent FIO_2 despite fluctuations in a patient's ventilatory pattern (i.e., it provides high capacitance of oxygen-enriched gas).

Often, these masks are called ventimasks, implying that a Venturi mechanism is used, but the air-dilution mechanism actually occurs by jet mixing. Commercial air entrainment masks provide delivery of oxygen with a FIO_2 from 0.24 to 0.70. The level is controlled by graded adjustment of an entrainment port or by specific injector attachments. The latter masks are accompanied by several color-coded and labeled jets that produce a known FIO_2 at a given flow rate of oxygen. The desired injector is connected to the inlet hose of the mask and powered by the designated oxygen flow. Most air entrainment masks also have an adapter that permits aerosol therapy at a lower FIO_2 than is possible with conventional oxygen-powered wall-mounted nebulizers.

NEBULIZATION

Wall-mounted nebulizers are often used to administer humidified oxygen to patients with artificial airways through a Briggs's adapter (T-adapter) (Fig. 47-4) or tracheotomy collar. Compressed oxygen is directed through a restricted orifice, creating a jet stream. It then passes across one end of a small-diameter tube immersed in water and produces a subatmospheric pressure immediately adjacent to the tube. Because water surface pressure is atmospheric, liquid is

drawn up the tube; droplets are continuously fractured (aerosolized) by the jet stream and delivered to the inspiratory circuit.

Oxygen-powered nebulizers have an adjustable air entrainment port. At maximum air entrainment, the FIO_2 is generally 0.35. Higher FIO_2 may be delivered by manually reducing the size of the entrainment port. Two considerations are important. Because of inherent resistance, only 14 to 16 L/minute of oxygen at 50-psi gauge can flow through the jet. Normally, the patient's peak inspiratory flow is approximately three to four times resting minute ventilation (i.e., 10 to 30 L/minute).

When total gas flow is less than the patient's inspiratory flow, ambient air is inhaled, thus decreasing the FIO_2. This problem frequently occurs when a tachypneic patient is treated with a high FIO_2 (total gas flow is decreased). If a low-capacitance device (mask or tracheostomy collar) is used, two nebulizers may be linked to provide double gas flow. In T-adapter circuits, the problem is solved by adding sufficient reservoir tubing to the distal end of the T-adapter.

HUMIDIFICATION

Humidity refers to moisture or water vapor in a gas. Saturated gas at 37°C contains 43.8 mg of water per liter of gas and produces a vapor pressure of 47 mm Hg. Alveolar gas has a relative humidity of 100% at 37°C. When the water content of inspired gas is less than 43.8 mg/L at 37°C, vapor pressure is less than 47 mm Hg. Thus, a pressure gradient (e.g., humidity deficit) is created between the inspired gas and respiratory mucosa. The amount of mucosal evaporation depends on this deficit. Mucosal dehydration increases mucus viscosity and reduces mucociliary clearance.

Oxygen that is delivered with a nasal cannula or catheter, partial rebreathing or nonrebreathing mask, or air entrainment mask is often humidified by passing gas through room temperature water. Use of a humidifier with an air entrainment mask is optional because the gas mixture is partially humidified by entrained air. Usually, oxygen is directed into

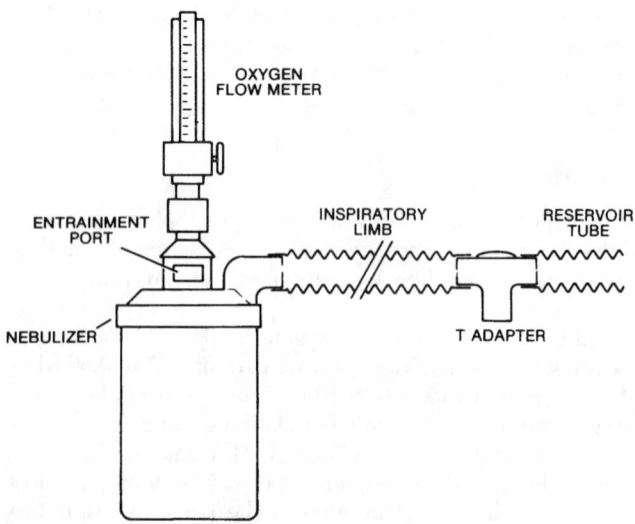

FIGURE 47-4. Jet nebulizer circuit with large water reservoir.

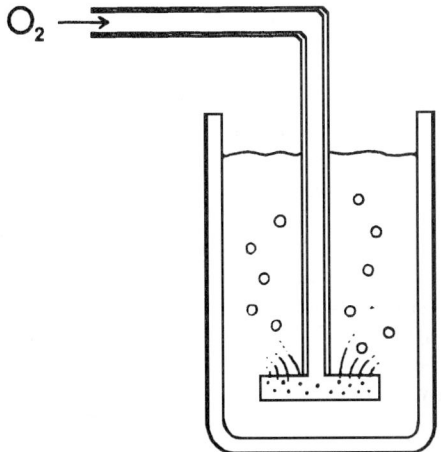

FIGURE 47-5. Schematic illustrating the mechanism of a bubble-diffusion humidifer. Dry gas is fractionated by a submerged diffusion grid into small bubbles, which are dispersed through water.

a submerged grid (diffuser) that fractionates the gas into many bubbles and increases the gas–liquid interface area (Fig. 47-5). Bubble-diffusion humidifiers increase the relative humidity of compressed oxygen from zero to approximately 80% to 90% at room temperature.

Warming, filtration, and humidification of inspired air occur in the upper respiratory tract. When this conditioning system is partially bypassed by an artificial airway, adequate humidification must be ensured to minimize the humidity deficit. Under these conditions, a heated humidifier or an aerosol generator should be used. An effective heated humidifier incorporates a bubble-diffusion mechanism (*supra vide*) and a 0.5- to 1.0-L reservoir of sufficiently warm water to provide an inspired temperature of approximately 37°C. Ideally, reservoir water temperature is controlled by a servo system incorporating a thermistor located near the patient's airway.

POTENTIAL COMPLICATIONS

HYPERCAPNIA

Patients with severe chronic obstructive lung disease (COLD) develop progressive hypoxemia and hypercapnia. Despite these alterations, arterial and cerebrospinal fluid pH are normal because of increased bicarbonate levels. Patients with COLD may become *desensitized* to the respiratory stimulant effects of carbon dioxide and presumably maintain ventilation by a reflex ventilatory response to a decrease in PaO_2 originating in the carotid and aortic bodies (hypoxemic drive). If the hypoxemic drive is suppressed by oxygen administration so that the PaO_2 exceeds 55 to 60 mm Hg, ventilation is reduced significantly, carbon dioxide retention is exacerbated, and narcosis can result.

Another cause of hypercapnia in chronically hypoxemic patients who receive supplemental oxygen (hyperoxic hypercapnia) is thought to involve impedance of the vascular adjustment of the $\dot{V}/\dot{Q}$ ratio (blocking of hypoxic pulmonary

vasoconstriction).[9] This vascular autoregulatory mechanism becomes inactive as a result of increased alveolar Po_2, and the resulting failure to direct blood flow away from hypoventilated lung areas increases carbon dioxide retention. Nevertheless, potential ventilatory depression should never contraindicate oxygen therapy in severe hypoxemia. If hypercapnia is a major problem, other support measures, including mechanical ventilation, can be employed.

ABSORPTION ATELECTASIS

Underventilated alveoli ($\dot{V}/\dot{Q} < 0.1$) tend to remain patent because of the presence of nitrogen, which exhibits little tendency to volume change (nitrogen splinting). However, these lung units become unstable and collapse when high concentrations of oxygen rapidly denitrogenate alveoli. If oxygen flow into pulmonary capillary blood exceeds oxygen flow into the alveoli, atelectasis occurs.[10] This phenomenon has been reported in healthy persons at a FIo_2 greater than 0.60[10] and probably occurs at lower levels in patients with acute respiratory insufficiency.[11,12]

PULMONARY OXYGEN TOXICITY

In 1775, Joseph Priestley recognized that

> "Though pure dephlogisticated air might be useful as a medicine, it might not be so proper for use in the usually healthy state of the body; for, as a candle burns out much faster in dephlogisticated than in common air, so we might live out too fast, and the animal powers be too soon exhausted in the pure kind of air. A moralist may say that the air which nature has provided for us is as good as we deserve."[13]

Oxygen-Free Radicals

The dependence of living organisms on oxygen is paradoxical. Although it is essential for aerobic metabolism, hyperoxia, or inappropriate oxygen metabolism, can be toxic. Thus, survival in an oxygen environment involves a complex interaction between the biologic generation of reactive chemical species called *free radicals* (atoms or molecules with one unpaired electron occupying an outer orbit) and the ability to harness these substances. Mammals derive most of their cellular adenosine triphosphate by controlled, four-electron reduction of oxygen and the formation of hydrogen peroxide (H_2O_2) by the mitochondrial electron transport system. During the course of normal metabolism, oxygen can accept less than four electrons to form reactive species that may be cytotoxic to cells. Toxic products of oxygen reduction include: $O_2^{\cdot-}$, $OH^{\cdot}$, $^1O_2$, H_2O_2, and $HO_2^{\cdot}$.

The lone electron present in the outer orbit of a free radical produces unusual chemical reactivity and physical characteristics.[14] Free radical reactivity is accounted for by the strong tendency of this electron to pair with another, forming a chemical bond. These metabolites may be responsible for the inactivation of sulfhydryl enzymes, the peroxidation of unsaturated membrane lipids and accompanying loss of membrane integrity, and the disruption of DNA synthesis.[15]

Antioxidant Enzymes

Cells, however, contain protective antioxidants such as the enzymes superoxide dismutase (SOD), catalase, and glutathione reductase.[16] Lung antioxidant enzyme levels are correlated with tolerance to hyperoxia, as shown by investigations with agents that induce production of these enzymes.[17,18] Pretreatment of rats with *Salmonella* endotoxin produces decreased SOD and oxygen tolerance.[19] Laboratory animals exposed to 80% oxygen for several days increase SOD production and have increased survival rates when subsequently exposed to a near–lethal dose treatment schedule of hyperoxia.[20]

Other Antioxidants

Alpha tocopherol (the most active form of vitamin E), ascorbic acid (vitamin C), and beta carotene (vitamin A) also are important in the scavenging and conversion of free radicals to less harmful forms.[15] During hyperoxia, increased free radical production presumably overwhelms intracellular scavenging and detoxification, precipitating cell damage and death.

Granular Pneumocytes

Granular pneumocytes (type II cells) may be inherently resistant to hyperoxia.[15] Because ultrastructural changes appear relatively late, their response may be adaptive rather than toxic.[21,22] They are thought by some to produce most antioxidants available in the lungs. Thus, lungs with a high ratio of type II to type I pneumocytes (infants and patients recently exposed to hyperoxia or acute lung injury) seem to exhibit significant resistance to oxygen toxicity. Increases of lung enzyme activity in oxygen-tolerant and oxygen-adapted animals apparently reflect alterations in the antioxidant capacity of individual cells or an increase in the number of cells exhibiting high antioxidant enzyme activity (e.g., type II cells and alveolar macrophages).

Pulmonary Effects

Substantial evidence suggests that hyperoxia for prolonged periods can produce deleterious effects on the lungs. The degree of pulmonary cytotoxicity is related to Pa_{O_2} rather than FI_{O_2}. Tolerance to a low-pressure, pure oxygen environment (e.g., manned space flights) has produced evidence that 100% oxygen at 0.3 atmosphere absolute (ATA) is not hazardous to lung function.[23] Histologic damage occurs at PI_{O_2} greater than 428 mm Hg ($FI_{O_2} = 0.60$ at 1 ATA), although individual susceptibility varies substantially, and more subtle alterations may occur at lower PI_{O_2}.[14]

Early Manifestations

The earliest manifestation of pulmonary hyperoxic toxicity is tracheobronchitis. Associated physiologic alterations include decreased mucociliary clearance, chest pain (usually subeternal), cough, and reduced vital capacity. These changes develop within 24 hours at a FI_{O_2} of 1.0. Continued hyperoxic

exposure between 48 and 72 hours produces progressive cellular changes, and areas of capillary endothelium and alveolar epithelium may become denuded. These histologic alterations are accompanied by interstitial fluid accumulation, decreased lung compliance and gas transfer, and polymorphonuclear leukocyte infiltration.[24]

Pulmonary cytotoxicity is unlikely to develop in humans at a FI_{O_2} less than 0.5 at atmospheric pressure, even with prolonged exposure. Singer and colleagues[25] observed no alterations in venous admixture or lung compliance in postoperative patients who received mechanical ventilation with 100% oxygen for 15 to 48 hours. Certainly, under most clinical conditions, hypoxemia is a greater threat than oxygen toxicity.

Death

Death that occurs after approximately 72 hours of breathing a high FI_{O_2} is attributed to pulmonary edema and respiratory failure. However, Harabin and associates[26] described a similar occurrence in which dogs exposed to a FI_{O_2} approximately 1.0 manifested significant lactic acidemia despite a Pa_{O_2} greater than 400 mm Hg, normal cardiac output, and normal blood pressure. They observed an abrupt reduction in terminal Pa_{O_2}, but the metabolic acidemia clearly preceded the reduction in oxygenation. Factors other than pulmonary may have played an etiologic role.

REFERENCES ■

1. Wiklund L, Jorfeldt L, Sternstrom H, et al: Gas exchange as monitored in mixed venous and arterial blood during experimental cardiopulmonary resuscitation. *Acta Anaesthesiol Scand* 1992;36:427
2. Turnage S, Thrush D, Smith RA: Gas exchange during experimental cardiogenic edema. *Anesthesiology* 1994;81:A296
3. Dunlevy CL, Tyl SE: The effect of oral versus nasal breathing on oxygen concentrations received from nasal cannulas. *Respir Care* 1992;37:357
4. Heimlich JH, Carr GC: Transtracheal catheter technique for pulmonary rehabilitation. *Ann Otol Rhinol Laryngol* 1985;94:502
5. Christopher KL, Spofford BT, Brannin PK, et al: Transtracheal oxygen therapy for refractory hypoxemia. *JAMA* 1986;256:494
6. Couser JI Jr, Make BJ: Transtracheal oxygen decreases inspired minute ventilation. *Am Rev Respir Dis* 1989;139:627
7. Hoffman LA, Johnson JT, Wesmiller SW, et al: Transtracheal delivery of oxygen: efficacy and safety for long-term continuous therapy. *Ann Otol Rhinol Laryngol* 1991;100:108
8. Jensen AG, Johnson A, Sandstedt S: Rebreathing during oxygen treatment with face mask: the effect of oxygen flow rates on ventilation. *Acta Anaesthesiol Scand* 1991;35:289
9. Aubier M, Murciano D, Melic-Emili J, et al: Effects of administration of O_2 on ventilation and blood gases in patients with chronic obstructive pulmonary disease during acute respiratory failure. *Am Rev Respir* Dis 1980;122:747
10. Douglas ME, Downs JB, Dannemiller FJ, et al: Change in pulmonary venous admixture with varying inspired oxygen. *Anesth Analg* 1976;55:688
11. Register SD, Downs JB, Stock MC, et al: Is 50% oxygen harmful? *Crit Care Med* 1987;15:598

12. Baker AB, McGinn A, Joyce C: Effect on lung volumes of oxygen concentration when breathing is restricted. *Br J Anaesth* 1993;70:259

13. Priestly J: Experiments and observations on different kinds of air. Reprinted in: *The Discovery of Oxygen: Part 1*. London, Gurney and Jackson, 1923:5

14. Brigham KL: Role of free radicals in lung injury. *Chest* 1986; 89:6

15. Nickerson PA, Matalon S, Farhi LE: An ultrastructural study of alveolar permeability to cytochrome C in rabbit lung: effect of exposure to 100% oxygen at one atmosphere. *Am J Pathol* 1981;102:1

16. Beckman JS, Freeman BA: Antioxidant enzymes as mechanistic probes of oxygen-dependent toxicity. In: Taylor AE, Matalon S, Ward PA (eds). *Physiology of Oxygen Radicals*. Bethesda, MD, American Physiological Society, 1986:39

17. Massaro D, Massaro GD: Biochemical and anatomical adaptation of the lung to oxygen-induced injury. *Fed Proc* 1978;37:26

18. Fisher AB, Forman HJ: Oxygen utilization and toxicity in the lungs. In: Fishman AP, Fisher AB (eds). *The Respiratory System*, vol 1. Bethesda, MD, American Physiological Society, 1985:231

19. Frank L, Summervile J, Massaro D: Protection from oxygen toxicity with endotoxin: the role of the endogenous antioxidant enzymes of the lung. *J Clin Invest* 1980;65:1104

20. Crapo JD, Barry BE, Foscue HA, et al: Structural and biochemical changes in rat lungs occurring during exposures to lethal and adaptive doses of oxygen. *Am Rev Respir Dis* 1980; 112:123

21. Kaplan HP, Robinson FR, Kapanci Y, et al: Pathogenesis and reversibility of the pulmonary lesions of oxygen toxicity in monkeys. I. Clinical and light microscopic studies. *Lab Invest* 1969;20:94

22. Kapanci Y, Weibel ER, Kaplan HP, et al: Pathogenesis and reversibility of the pulmonary lesion of oxygen toxicity in monkeys. II. Ultrastructual and morphometric studies. *Lab Invest* 1969;20:101

23. DuBois AB, Hyde RW, Hendler E: Pulmonary mechanics and diffusing capacity following simulated space flight of two weeks' duration. *J Appl Physiol* 1963;18:696

24. Pratt PC, Vollmer RT, Shelburne JD, et al: Pulmonary morphology in a multihospital collaborative extracorporeal membrane oxygenation project. I. Light microscopy. *Am J Pathol* 1979;95:191

25. Singer MM, Wright F, Stanley LK, et al: Oxygen toxicity in man: a prospective study in patients after open-heart surgery. *N Engl J Med* 1970;283D:1473

26. Harabin AL, Homer LD, Bradley ME: Pulmonary oxygen toxicity in awake dogs: metabolic and physiologic effects. *J Appl Physiol* 1984;57:1480

Critical Care, Third Edition, edited by Joseph M. Civetta,
Robert W. Taylor, and Robert R. Kirby.
Lippincott-Raven Publishers, Philadelphia, PA © 1997.

CHAPTER 48

◼

Mechanical Ventilation

Michael J. Banner
Samsum Lampotang
Paul B. Blanch
Robert R. Kirby

IMMEDIATE CONCERNS ◼

MAJOR PROBLEMS

When a normal adult lies supine, the functional residual capacity (FRC) decreases by as much as 500 mL. If this person subsequently is paralyzed and manually or mechanically ventilated, significant alveolar ventilation/perfusion ($\dot{V}_A/\dot{Q}$) alterations occur. Blood flow is directed predominantly to the posterior dependent areas, whereas ventilation is distributed primarily to anterior or nondependent regions. The resulting changes produce increased dead space (areas of ventilation without perfusion), shunt (areas of perfusion without ventilation), or both. This problem can be further exacerbated by pregnancy, tumor, or ascites, all of which reduce venous return, or by overzealous lung inflation, which further reduces cardiac output and hyperinflates the lungs.

A similar, but sometimes worse, situation prevails when the patient is placed in the lateral "kidney rest" position and is mechanically ventilated during surgical procedures. Here, the dependent (down) lung receives most of the pulmonary blood flow while the nondependent (up) lung is maximally ventilated. Venous return often is compromised, and significant hypoxemia may result. Increased hydrostatic pressure to the dependent lung sometimes results in the so-called "down lung" syndrome (unilateral pulmonary edema), which persists into the postoperative period.

Many abnormalities of ventilation are not associated with pulmonary parenchymal changes. When the etiologic factor is removed, lung function and breathing quickly revert to normal. Several disorders produce damage to lung structure, however, and the respiratory insufficiency that results may be profound, life threatening, and not easily reversed. Critical care personnel often are called on to deal with such patients, either in primary or consulting status, and should have a working knowledge of the pathophysiology and treatment of acute respiratory failure.

Reductions of the partial pressures of arterial oxygen (Pa_{O_2}) and carbon dioxide (Pa_{CO_2}) are characteristic of the early stage of acute respiratory distress syndrome (ARDS). Later, Pa_{CO_2} increases, and in the terminal throes of the disease it cannot be returned to normal by the most vigorous attempts at mechanical ventilation. Hypoxemia results from continued perfusion of lung regions with decreased to absent ventilation.

STRESS POINTS

1. Peak inflation pressure (PIP) generated during mechanical inflation varies directly with respiratory system *elastance* (E_{RS}—reciprocal of compliance) and *resistance*. Acute respiratory failure is primarily associated with increases in elastance (or decreases in lung compliance, chest wall compliance, or both); chronic respiratory failure is associated with increases in airway resistance (Raw).

2. *Time*-cycled ventilators cycle "OFF" when a preselected inhalation time elapses. *Pressure*-cycled ventilators cycle OFF when a preselected pressure is generated. *Volume*-cycled ventilators cycle OFF when a

711

preselected volume is delivered. *Flow*-cycled ventilators cycle OFF when the inspiratory flow rate ($\dot{V}I$) decreases to a critical preselected level.

3. Microprocessor-controlled ventilators employ microprocessor chips to control the overall operation and supervision of the system, similar to personal computers. Modes of ventilation and cycling mechanisms are software dependent, and hardware components are relatively simple in design.

4. Conventional mechanical ventilation includes *controlled mechanical ventilation* (CMV), with or without positive end-expiratory pressure (PEEP), and *patient-triggered (assisted) mechanical ventilation*, with or without controlled backup ventilation.

5. *Pressure-controlled* mechanical ventilation may be applied with a normal or inverse inhalation-to-exhalation (I:E) time ratio. The latter condition is referred to as pressure-controlled inverse ratio ventilation (PC-IRV).

6. *Intermittent* and *synchronized intermittent mandatory ventilation* (IMV/SIMV) allow the patient to breathe spontaneously as desired with mechanical inflations supplied at regular preset intervals.

7. *Pressure support ventilation* (PSV) *ventilates* the lungs and *unloads* the respiratory muscles. Thus, it decreases the work of breathing to a tolerable level, which, for many adults, corresponds to a normal value. For a given level of PSV, the faster the rates of flow and pressure rise, the less the work of breathing and vice versa.

8. *Pressure augmentation*, used during PSV, provides a guaranteed tidal volume (VT) per breath (a *safety net*).

9. *Proportional assist ventilation* (PAV), an experimental support mode used during PSV, allows the patient to control $\dot{V}I$ demand, breathing frequency, VT, minute ventilation, and the *level of pressure applied* to the airway.

10. *Mandatory minute volume* (MMV) guarantees the patient a preselected minute volume through spontaneous ventilation, positive pressure breaths from the ventilator, or a combination of the two.

11. *Airway pressure release ventilation* (APRV) provides alveolar ventilation by intermittently *decreasing* airway pressure from a preselected level of continuous positive airway pressure (CPAP). PIP never exceeds the level of CPAP. Spontaneous breathing occurs with CPAP with or without supplemental ventilation.

PEAK INFLATION PRESSURE ■

Positive pressure is any pressure greater than atmospheric. Mechanical ventilators facilitate the movement of gas in and out of the lungs by generating positive pressure. Evolving from simple oxygen-powered breathing devices, modern mechanical ventilators are complex microprocessor-controlled systems capable of providing a variety of ventilatory techniques. An understanding of these devices and the

modes of mechanical and spontaneous positive-pressure ventilation is essential for critical care practitioners.

During mechanical inhalation, a positive-pressure difference is generated between the airway opening and the alveoli. The PIP results from lung–thorax compliance (CLT) and Raw (impedance) interacting with the VT, $\dot{V}I$, and baseline airway pressure. These factors may be represented mathematically as follows:

$$PIP = \frac{VT}{CLT} + (Raw \times \dot{V}I) + Baseline\ Pressure \quad (1)$$

Example A, Normal compliance and Raw (adult values):

$$PIP = \frac{1\ L}{0.1\ L/cm\ H_2O}$$
$$+ [2\ cm\ H_2O/L/second \times 1\ L/second]$$
$$+ 0\ cm\ H_2O = 12\ cm\ H_2O$$

Example B, *Decreased* compliance (e.g., acute lung injury):

$$PIP = \frac{1\ L}{0.02\ L/cm\ H_2O}$$
$$+ (2\ cm\ H_2O/L/second \times 1\ L/second)$$
$$+ 10\ cm\ H_2O$$
$$= 62\ cm\ H_2O$$

Example C, *Increased* Raw (e.g., chronic obstructive lung disease [COLD]):

$$PIP = \frac{1\ L}{0.1\ L/cm\ H_2O}$$
$$+ (20\ cm\ H_2O/L/second \times 1\ L/second)$$
$$+ 5\ cm\ H_2O$$
$$= 35\ cm\ H_2O$$

VENTILATOR CLASSIFICATION ■

CYCLING MECHANISMS

Time, volume, pressure, and flow rate are interrelated variables used to describe positive-pressure ventilation (Table 48-1). The changeover from the mechanical inhalation to the exhalation phase, i.e., the process used to cycle the ventilator OFF, is a means by which mechanical ventilators are classified. Time, volume, pressure, or flow cycling mechanisms have been employed on a variety of ventilators. Time- and volume-cycled ventilators are the more common types.

Time

Time-cycled inhalation is terminated after a preselected inspiratory time (T_I) elapses. The timing mechanism may be pneumatic or electronic. Duration of the inspiratory phase is selected by the operator and is not influenced by the PIP, CLT, and Raw. VT is the product of T_I (seconds) and $\dot{V}I$ (mL/second).

TABLE 48-1. Parameters Used to Describe Ventilation

PRESSURE

A measure of the impedance to flow rate encountered in the patient's airways and lungs

A measure of force applied per unit area by a gas

Expressed in cm H_2O, mm Hg, or kPa (1 cm H_2O = 1.36 mm Hg, 7.6 mm Hg = 1 kPa)

VOLUME

Measure of the tidal volume delivered by the ventilator to the patient

Expressed in milliliters for tidal volume and in liters for minute volume

FLOW RATE

Rate at which gas volume is delivered to the patient

Refers to the volume change per unit time

Expressed in L/s or L/min

TIME

Divided into inspiratory (T_I) and expiratory time (T_E) periods

Expressed in seconds or by the relationship of T_I to T_E defined as an I:E ratio

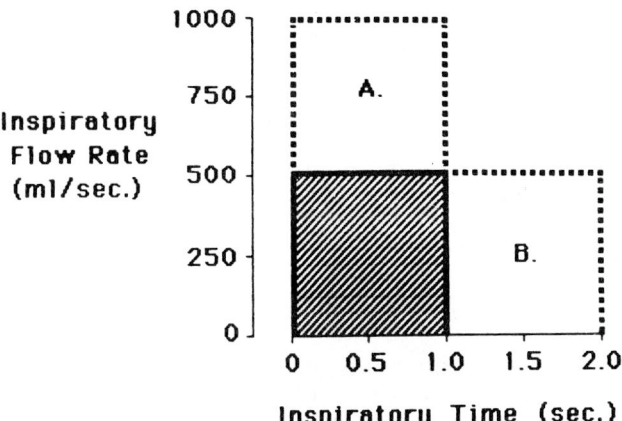

FIGURE 48-1. With a time-cycled ventilator, mechanical inhalation terminates after a preset inspiratory time has elapsed. Tidal volume is the product of inspiratory flow rate and inspiratory time and is represented as the area under the curve. The shaded rectangle represents a tidal volume of 500 mL. Tidal volume may be increased to 1000 mL either by increasing flow rate as shown in *A,* or by increasing inspiratory time as shown in *B.* (Banner MJ, Desautels DA: Special ventilatory techniques and considerations. In: Kirby RR, Banner MJ, Downs JB [eds]. *Clinical Applications of Ventilatory Support.* Philadelphia, JB Lippincott, 1990:247.)

$$V_T = T_I \times \dot{V}_I \qquad (2)$$

An example of this formula is the following:

$$V_T = 2 \text{ seconds} \times 500 \text{ mL/second}$$

$$= 1000 \text{ mL}$$

When C_{LT} decreases, T_I is unaffected, but PIP increases (equation 1). Under these conditions $\dot{V}_I$ may decrease as a result of increased back pressure in the system, with a resultant decreased V_T. V_T can be restored to the initial value by increasing either T_I, $\dot{V}_I$, or both (Fig. 48-1).

Volume

Volume-cycled inhalation is terminated after a preselected V_T has been delivered by the ventilator, irrespective of the PIP, T_I, and $\dot{V}_I$ (e.g., Puritan-Bennett MA-1). The patient's V_T does *not* remain constant with increases in PIP. During inhalation, the delivered V_T is distributed to the ventilator breathing circuit tubing and the patient's lungs. Increases of the PIP cause a greater fraction of V_T to be compressed or "left behind" in the breathing circuit, with less volume delivery to the patient (Fig. 48-2). Compliant breathing tubing results in more volume compressed in the tubing and less volume received by the patient. When high PIP is required, noncompliant (nondistensible) tubing should be used, and the humidifier should be full to minimize gas compression.

Pressure

Pressure-cycled inhalation is terminated when a preselected PIP is achieved within the ventilator breathing circuit, irrespective of the V_T, T_I, or $\dot{V}_I$. The delivered V_T and T_I are

related directly to C_{LT} and inversely to R_{aw}. V_T may be expressed as the product of the change (Δ) in airway pressure and C_{LT}:

$$V_T = \Delta\text{Pressure} \times C_{LT} \qquad (3)$$

An example is the following:

$$V_T = 10 \text{ cm } H_2O \times 50 \text{ mL/cm } H_2O$$

$$= 500 \text{ mL}$$

Either a decrease in C_{LT}, an increase in R_{aw}, or both predispose to a decrease in T_I and V_T.

Flow

Flow-cycled inhalation is terminated when the $\dot{V}_I$ delivered by the ventilator decreases to a preselected critical value, irrespective of T_I and V_T. Flow cycling is employed by microprocessor-controlled mechanical ventilators operating in the PSV mode. When the ventilator is patient-triggered "ON," an abrupt increase in airway pressure occurs, and a high peak $\dot{V}_I$ is delivered. The inhalation phase continues until the $\dot{V}_I$ decelerates to a predetermined percentage of the initial peak $\dot{V}_I$ (e.g., 25%); at this critical level, $\dot{V}_I$ ceases, and the ventilator flow cycles OFF.

INSPIRATORY FLOW WAVEFORMS

Sinusoidal, constant, decelerating, and accelerating flow waveforms, influenced to some degree by the flow delivery mechanism, may be delivered during mechanical inhalation (Table 48-2 and Fig. 48-3). Microprocessor-controlled proportional flow valves in newer ventilators allow a variety of inspiratory flow waveforms.

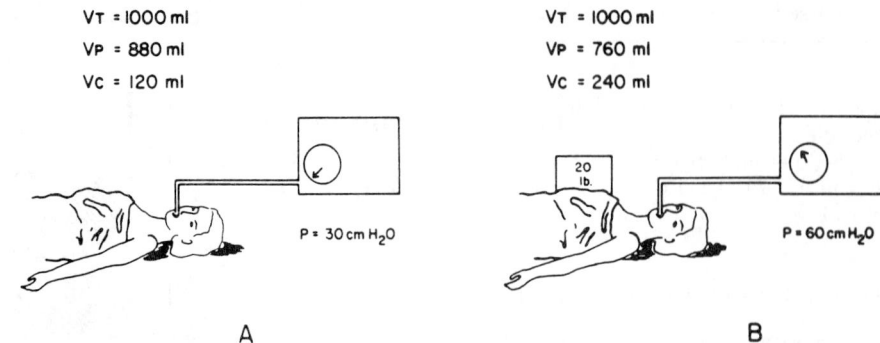

FIGURE 48-2. Effect of changing compliance (simulated by a weight on the chest) on patient ventilation. (**A**) Volume-cycled ventilator is set to deliver a tidal volume of 1000 mL, of which 880 mL reaches the patient and 120 mL is compressed within the ventilator circuit. Notice that the peak inflation pressure (P) is 30 cm H_2O. (**B**) A 9-kg weight is placed on the patient's chest to simulate a decrease in C_{LT}. The ventilatory again delivers the 1000-mL tidal volume but, because of the patient's decreased compliance, a pressure of 60 cm H_2O is required and only 760 mL reaches the patient, whereas 240 mL is compressed or left behind in the breathing-circuit tubing. In this example, the compression factor is 4 mL/cm H_2O; i.e., 4 mL/cm H_2O × 60 cm H_2O = 240 mL. V_T, set tidal volume; V_P, patient tidal volume; V_C, compression volume. (Kirby RR, Smith RA, Desautels DA: mechanical ventilation. In: Burton GG, Hodgkin JE [eds]. *Respiratory Care*, 2nd ed. Philadelphia, JB Lippincott, 1984:564.)

TABLE 48-2.   Mechanisms in Mechanical Ventilators for Providing Gas Flow

---

INJECTOR

Based on the Bernoulli principle, i.e., as gas accelerates through a Venturi, subambient pressure is generated; as a result, additional gas is entrained and the total flow rate output is delivered directly to the patient (referred to as a direct drive or single-circuit system), e.g., Bird Mark series ventilators, IMV Bird, high-frequency jet ventilators.

INJECTOR—BELLOWS

Outflow from an injector is directed to a chamber where a gas-filled bellows is compressed delivering its contents to the patient (referred to as an indirect drive or double-circuit system), e.g., Puritan-Bennett MA-1 and MA-2 (Fig. 48-4). Outflow from an injector may also be used to compress a bladder, e.g., Engström Erica.

STEPPER MOTOR FLOW VALVE

Signals from a microprocessor control a motor that rotates a shaft using a series of discrete rotational steps. Each rotational step is converted into a linear motion, thus modulating the valve orifice size and hence the flow rate. Flow rate through the valve is in L/min per rotational step (Fig. 48-5). The valve regulates inspiratory time, flow rate, and waveform during mechanical inhalation and gas flow rate on demand during spontaneous inhalation, e.g., Bird 6400 ST, Bear 5. These valves are not necessarily controlled by a microprocessor. For example, the Siemens 900 C uses a stepper motor that actuates a lever arm of a hinged clamp device that pinches a silicone rubber tube to regulate gas flow rate.

PISTON

By regulating the excursion of a piston, a specific volume of gas with each stroke is displaced into the breathing circuit to the patient (direct drive), e.g., IMV Emerson (see Fig. 48-6).

SOLENOID (ON/OFF OR OPEN AND CLOSED FLOW VALVE)

During mechanical inhalation, the valve opens, directing gas flow from a regulated pressure source through a peak flow rate control device and into the breathing circuit, e.g., Bear-1. (These valves are also used in high-frequency jet ventilators.)

MICROPROCESSOR-CONTROLLED FLOW VALVE

By altering the voltage or current supplied to these valves, it is possible to regulate precisely the internal orifice size and hence flow rate. The microprocessor, after referencing (consulting) each of the preselected ventilatory parameters, modulates the valve to produce the desired inspiratory time, flow rate, and waveform during mechanical inhalation and gas flow rate on demand during spontaneous inhalation, e.g., BEAR 1000, Puritan-Bennett 7200a, Hamilton Veolar, and Amadeus (see Fig. 48-6).

IMV, intermittent mandatory ventilation.

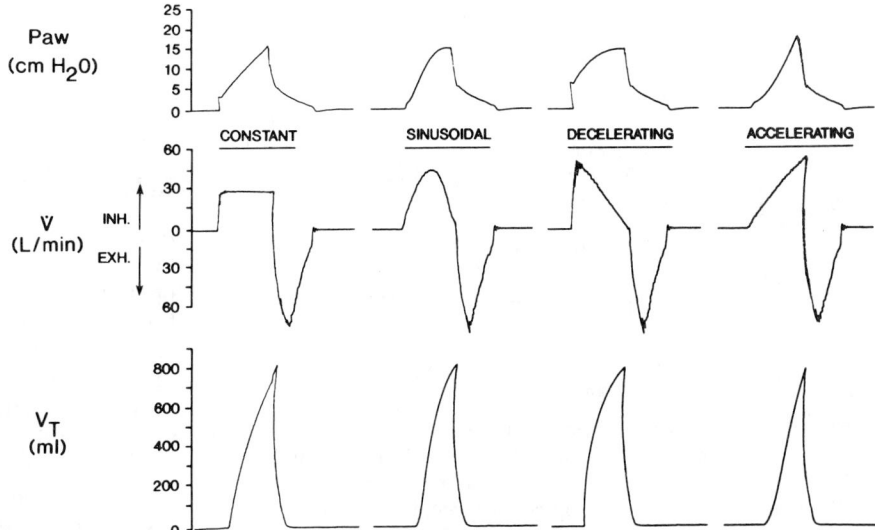

FIGURE 48-3. Airway pressure (Paw), flow rate ($\dot{V}$), and tidal volume (VT) are shown for constant, sinusoidal, decelerating, and accelerating inspiratory flow waveforms. Inspiratory time and VT were held constant. Peak inspiratory pressure was highest with the accelerating waveform and lowest with the decelerating one; however, mean airway pressure was highest with the latter inspiratory flow waveform. INH, inhalation; EXH, exhalation.

Whether a particular flow waveform can improve the distribution of ventilation, $\dot{V}_A/\dot{Q}$ matching, and gas exchange is controversial. Discrepancies in many reports are related to a host of confounding variables. In some studies, altering the inspiratory flow waveform may have affected T_I, I:E ratio, peak $\dot{V}_I$, VT, and minute ventilation. Some investigators compared various inspiratory flow waveforms and found little difference in the distribution of ventilation.[1] However, T_I is increased by an end-inspiratory pause, suggesting that T_I is as important, if not more so, than the inspiratory flow waveform.[2]

Studies of multiple lung compartment models with different airway resistances show improved distribution of ventilation with a decelerating T_I waveform compared with other waveforms.[3,4] These data may be relevant in treating patients with COLD. Clinical reports suggest similar findings.[5–7] In one investigation in which VT, T_I, I:E ratio, and ventilator rate were held constant, PIP, Pa_{CO_2}, dead space–to–VT ratio (VD/VT), and alveolar-to-arterial oxygen pressure gradient, $P(A - a)O_2$, were significantly lower with a decelerating inspiratory flow waveform than with a constant inspiratory flow waveform.[6] However, mean airway pressure was greater, predisposing to potentially adverse hemodynamic effects.

MICROPROCESSOR-CONTROLLED VENTILATORS ■

BASIC OPERATION

Pneumatic and microprocessor technologies have resulted in the previously mentioned new generation of microprocessor-controlled mechanical ventilators.[8,9] The basic differences between a microprocessor-controlled ventilator and a conventional ventilator are illustrated comparing Figures 48-4 and 48-5. Some microprocessor-controlled ventilators incorporate several microprocessors. Besides providing multiple modes of ventilation and computerized monitoring, these ventilators can acquire, process, store, and retrieve data. The choice of several ventilatory modes, coupled with real-

time monitoring of pertinent variables (e.g., CLT, Raw, ventilatory work, end-tidal CO_2 partial pressure [$P_{ET}CO_2$], airway pressure, flow rate, and VT waveforms), suggests that ventilatory therapy for critically ill patients should be facilitated with these ventilators. However, clear documentation of this hypothesis is yet to be achieved. Potential advantages are summarized in Table 48-3.

Central Processing Unit

The microprocessor or central processing unit (CPU) is the "brain" of a microprocessor-controlled ventilator. Computations and overall supervision of the system are performed here. Considering its tremendous computing power, the physical size of a microprocessor is surprisingly small. Dimensions are measured in centimeters, and it weighs only a few grams. Microprocessor costs range from about $5 for an Intel 8088 (Intel Corp., Santa Clara, CA) to $300 for more powerful units. A microprocessor is a general-purpose device, mass-produced at low cost, and programmed for

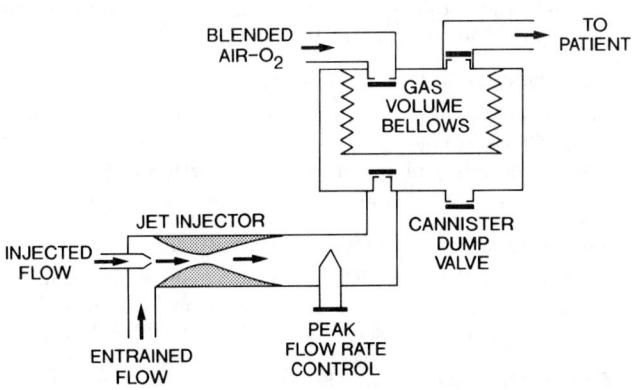

FIGURE 48-4. Example of a conventional nonmicroprocessor-controlled ventilator (Puritan-Bennett MA-1) is illustrated. During mechanical inhalation, flow rate from a jet injector is directed into a rigid canister to compress a bellows, the contents of which are directed to the breathing circuit and the patient.

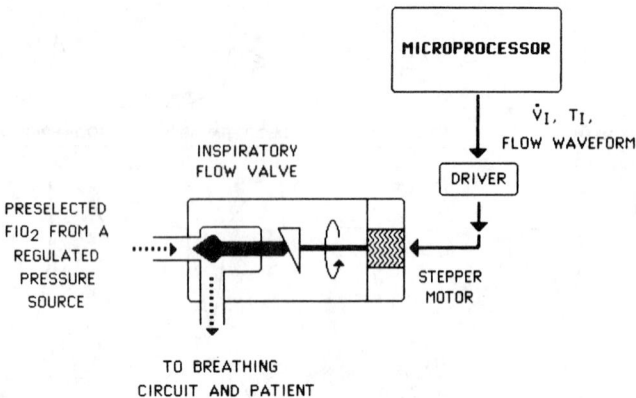

FIGURE 48-5. Microprocessor-controlled stepper motor inspiratory flow valve as used in the Bird 6400 ST and 8400 STi and Bear 5 ventilators. Preselected ventilatory parameters from the control panel are directed to a microprocessor that, in turn, controls the operation of the stepper motor via a driver mechanism to regulate inspiratory flow rate ($\dot{V}I$), time (T_1), and the flow waveform during mechanical inhalation. Gas flow also is provided on demand from the stepper motor flow valve during spontaneous inhalation.

specific tasks using software modifications. The same microprocessor used in an automobile engine system may also control a ventilator. Microprocessor systems in mechanical ventilators are sometimes called *microcontroller* or *embedded controller systems*.

DATA MANIPULATION AND LOGIC

Relational Operations

A microprocessor can perform arithmetic (addition, subtraction, multiplication, and division) and relational and logical operations. It controls the operation, and the flow of information within the system. A relational operation assesses the "truth" of a relational expression like x < y?, x = y? or x > y?. A relational expression can be either "TRUE" or "FALSE." For example, x might be the measured airway pressure and y the high airway pressure alarm limit. If the answer to x > y? is TRUE, a predetermined set of instructions (e.g., sounding an alarm and perhaps aborting the inspiratory phase) is carried out. If it is FALSE, the next set of commands in the ventilator control algorithm (e.g., measure exhaled V_T) is performed.

Logical Operations

Logical operations include "NOT," "AND," "OR," and operate on the result of relational expressions. They have the

---

TABLE 48-3. Potential Advantages of Microprocessor-Controlled Ventilators

GENERAL VERSATILITY

    Capable of providing various modalities of mechanical and spontaneous positive-pressure ventilation
    Ability to ventilate with a variety of inspiratory flow waveforms
    Choice of cycling mechanisms
    Capability of being reprogrammed and upgraded, depending on current trends
    Ability to ventilate adult and pediatric patients

MONITORING CAPABILITY

    Real-time monitoring of a variety of ventilatory parameters
    Ability to calculate and monitor lung–thorax compliance (CLT), airways resistance (Raw), minute exhaled ventilation, work of breathing
    Permits self-checking and cross-checking to ensure proper function of computer and pneumatic operations
    Computer memory permits the storage and retrieval of ventilation data for trend analysis

COMPUTER CORRECTION CAPABILITY

    Allegedly able to perform automatic corrections to maintain the inspiratory flow rate, waveform as PIP increases because of changes in CLT and Raw
    Measured tidal and minute volumes corrected to BTPS
    Allegedly, volume losses in the ventilator breathing circuit secondary to compression may be calculated and/or compensated

DISPLAY AND COMMUNICATIONS CAPABILITY

    Computer-controlled LED indicating all current ventilatory parameters, alarms, and limits
    Communication with separate microcomputers available for the monitoring and storage of data
    Ability to easily interface with a CRT terminal for data display

REPAIRS AND MAINTENANCE

    System down-time reduced to the relative case of diagnosing and troubleshooting ventilation programs and the minimal number of moving components in a microprocessor-controlled ventilator
    Modular components facilitate repair

PIP, peak inflation pressure.

same meaning as their counterparts in the English language and follow the rules of *Boolean algebra* or logic. For example, NOT TRUE is FALSE and NOT FALSE is TRUE. The "AND" function operates on two relational expressions and requires that both expressions must be TRUE for the result to be TRUE; TRUE AND TRUE is TRUE; TRUE AND FALSE is FALSE. The "OR" function requires that at least one of the two relational expressions is TRUE for the result to be TRUE; TRUE OR FALSE is TRUE and FALSE OR FALSE is FALSE.

As an example, if "measured exhaled VT has decreased" is TRUE, and "VT has not changed" is TRUE, then "possible leak in breathing circuit" is TRUE. With these simple building blocks, which form the fundamental elements of computer language, powerful algorithms (instructions to perform a specific function) are written as computer programs (software) in languages like Assembly, Basic, Pascal, and C (Fig. 48-6).

Some microprocessor ventilators use 8-bit microprocessors, whereas others use more powerful 16-bit microprocessors. One might assume that a ventilator incorporating a more powerful microprocessor is necessarily better. However, a ventilator using an older, less powerful microprocessor benefits from its "maturity," that is, there is less likelihood that flaws are present in the system because previous users will have identified them. Costs are also lower. Although 32-bit microprocessors like the Intel 80386c are available, they are not yet incorporated into commercially manufactured ventilators.

Microprocessor Control

Ventilators such as the Hamilton Amadeus and the PPG Biomedical Systems IRISA have more than one microprocessor. The Puritan-Bennett 7200a is the only ventilator to have only one microprocessor. In a multimicroprocessor ventilator, the main microprocessor controls overall ventilator operation, whereas the subsystem microprocessors perform tasks such as front panel control and display, actuator control, and so forth. The subsystem microprocessors offload some of the processing tasks from the main microprocessor. Multimicroprocessor ventilators may offer an increased measure of safety, because the microprocessors can cross-check each other's proper operation.

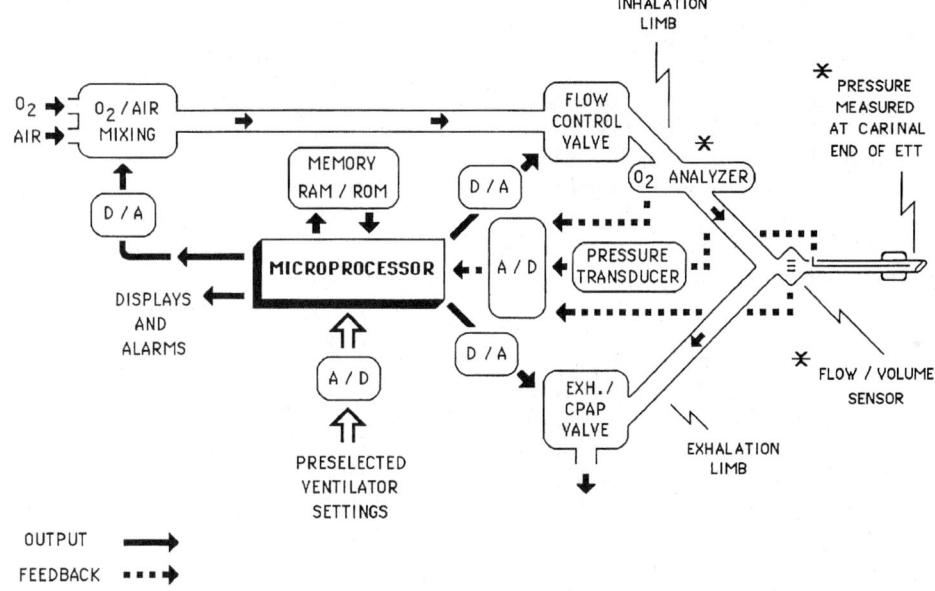

FIGURE 48-6. Diagrammatic representation showing the operation of a microprocessor-controlled ventilator. Preselected ventilator settings, entered as analog signals via knobs on the front panel, are converted to digital data via an analog-to-digital converter (A/D) and then directed to the *microprocessor,* which controls the overall operation of the ventilator. The data are, in turn, directed to random access memory (RAM). The general ventilator control program can be stored on read only memory (ROM). *Output* control data (solid lines), via digital-to-analog conversion (D/A), are then directed from the microprocessor to the oxygen/air mixing system, inspiratory flow control valve, and exhalation/continous positive airway pressure (CPAP) valves. *Feedback* data (dashed lines), via A/D conversion, are directed back to the microprocessor from the oxygen analyzer, airway pressure transducer, and flow/volume sensor. Ideally, the ventilator should function as a closed-loop feedback control system. On most ventilators, the sites of pressure and flow/volume measurement are either inside the ventilator on the exhalation limb of the breathing circuit or at the Y piece. For greater accuracy, it is recommended to measure airway pressure at the *carinal* end of the endotracheal tube (ETT) and a flow/volume at the Y piece of the breathing circuit (see Figs. 48-26 and 48-27).

MICROPROCESSOR SYSTEMS

The microprocessor system includes the microprocessor and its supporting hardware.

Memory

Memory is essential for the operation of microprocessor-controlled ventilators. A trend for PIP over a given period can be displayed only if the ventilator can "remember" previous PIP values. Memory provides data storage for later retrieval. Memory locations or cells each have a unique *address*.

RANDOM ACCESS AND READ ONLY. Random-access memory (RAM) and read-only memory (ROM) are found in microprocessor-controlled ventilators and computers (Fig. 48-7). The flow of data between RAM and the microprocessor is bidirectional. The microprocessor can write data into RAM for storage and can also retrieve data by reading from the memory locations of interest. When new data are placed into a memory cell, old data stored in that cell are written over and lost. RAM is volatile; when electrical power is switched off, all stored data are lost. Because it is possible to write into RAM, parts of the ventilator control program could accidentally be written over and deleted, resulting in ventilator malfunction. Thus, RAM is unsuitable for storage of a ventilator control program.

The ventilator control program can be stored in ROM. Because the software is self-contained in the ROM *module*, an upgrade consists simply of replacing the old ROM-type device with a new chip containing the improved software. The relative ease of software alteration, without expensive hardware changes, allows ventilator manufacturers to be more responsive to design suggestions and requests for new features.

DATA TRANSFER, ACCESS, AND CONTROL. In a microprocessor system, data are transferred by the *data bus*. A data bus consists of a set of parallel wires that carry data in the form of bit patterns. The *address bus* is used to indicate which component of the microprocessor system needs to be accessed. For that purpose, each of the input and output ports and each memory location is assigned a unique address. The *control bus* carries timing signals and coded instructions that coordinate the operation of the system and specify what operation is to be performed. For example, if data need to be read from memory, the desired memory location is addressed by the address bus. The control bus then relays instructions that data are to be read from that memory location. Finally, stored data are transferred by the data bus to the microprocessor.

DIGITAL AND ANALOG SIGNALS

The concepts of *digital* and *analog* signals are essential in understanding the operation of microprocessor-controlled ventilators. A digital signal is discrete in both time and magnitude. A microprocessor processes *only* digital signals encoded in the form of bits (Table 48-4). With digital data, the number of bits taken at a time determines the number

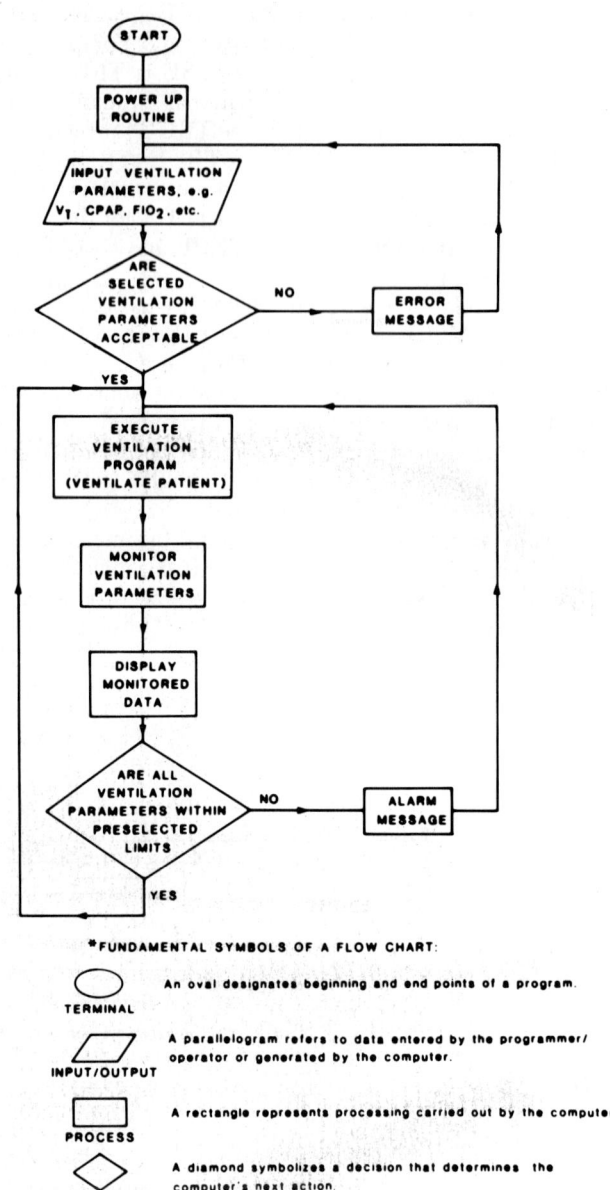

FIGURE 48-7. Flow chart of a generic ventilation control program (software) for microprocessor-controlled ventilation. (Lampotang S: Microprocessor-controlled ventilation systems and concepts. In: Kirby RR, Banner MJ, Downs JB [eds]. *Clinical Applications of Ventilatory Support.* New York, Churchill Livingstone, 1990:107.)

of combinations possible. If 8 bits taken at a time are used to represent digital information, then only $2^8 = 256$ combinations are possible. Because each combination can be assigned to represent a unique value, only 256 specific values can be encoded. Therefore, an 8-bit digital signal having a range of 0 to 1 V can only have 256 values represented within that range. If the values are equally spaced, the voltages represented will be 0, 1/256, 2/256, . . . 254/256, 255/256 V, and the resolution is 1/256 V.

The real world is an analog world. By definition, an analog signal is continuous in both time and magnitude. Commonly encountered physical variables like flow rate, pressure, and

TABLE 48-4. Data Terminology

ANALOG

Analog signal: An analog signal is *continuous* both in time and magnitude, e.g., physical variables like changes in flow rate, pressure, and voltage are analog in nature.

DIGITAL°

Digital signal: A digital signal is *discrete* both in time and magnitude. Digital data are encoded in the form of binary digit (bit) patterns.
Bit pattern: A combination of "0" and "1" that is used to encode digital information (base 2). The number (n) of bits determines the number of combinations possible (2^n), e.g., for 12 bits, 2^{12} or 4096 combinations are possible.
Byte: Defined as eight bits and permits representation of 2^8 or 256 possible digital combinations.
ASCII code: By assigning a specific meaning to each unique combination or bit pattern in a byte, a code is created for communicating data. For example:

Character	ASCII Code
"A"	01000001
"3"	00110011

ASCII, American Standard Code for Information Interchange.

°Microprocessors process *only* digital data in form of bits. Thus, analog signals must first be converted to digital data using an analog-to-digital converter to enable the microprocessor to "understand" the data.

voltage are analog in nature. In an analog signal, an infinite number of values exists between any two values, because any interval between two numbers can always be divided into even smaller intervals ad infinitum. Hence, no restriction is imposed on the magnitude an analog signal may assume, that is, the signal is unquantized.

Analog-to-Digital Converters

Because a microprocessor works only with digital signals, analog signals must be transformed into equivalent digital signals by an analog to digital (A/D) converter. The A/D converter samples an analog signal at a given frequency or rate and converts the resulting signal to a digital signal that the microprocessor can process (see Fig. 48-6).

Digital-to-Analog Converters

The digital data from a microprocessor are meaningless to the outside world. Therefore, a digital to analog (D/A) converter is required to transform digital data into an analog voltage. A D/A converter functions opposite to an A/D converter. The power output of a D/A converter is usually too low to drive an *actuator*, for example, the ventilator's inspiratory flow valve. An amplifier interposed between the D/A converter and the actuator is used to amplify the output from the D/A converter to the required level (see Fig. 48-6).

CONVENTIONAL MECHANICAL VENTILATORY TECHNIQUES ■

CONTROLLED VENTILATION

Operational Principles

Mechanical ventilation is indicated if spontaneous ventilation is inadequate (or absent) and $PaCO_2$ and arterial pH (pHa) cannot be maintained at acceptable levels. CMV deliv-

ers a preselected ventilatory rate independent of the patient's spontaneous effort, if any (Fig. 48-8). It does not permit normal spontaneous breathing and requires that the patient be hyperventilated, sedated, or paralyzed to blunt spontaneous attempts to breathe.

Indications for CMV include apnea secondary to central nervous system depression (brain, spinal cord, or both), drug overdose, or neuromuscular dysfunction (drug induced or pathology induced). Accidental circuit disconnection or a mechanical malfunction represents a potentially life-threatening situation when the patient is apneic. Therefore, a *disconnect* or a *failure-to-cycle* alarm is crucial.

Clinical Applications

Continuous positive-pressure ventilation (CPPV) like CMV, delivers a positive-pressure breath at a preselected rate followed, when the ventilator cycles off, by a fall in airway pressure to a preset end-expiratory pressure above zero (see Fig. 48-8). Like CMV, CPPV does not permit normal spontaneous breathing and requires that the patient's spontaneous attempts to breathe be eliminated. This technique was popularized by Ashbaugh and coworkers[10] for the treatment of ARDS to prevent alveolar collapse during the ventilator's exhalation phase, thereby improving and maintaining $\dot{V}_A/\dot{Q}$ relationships.

PATIENT-TRIGGERED VENTILATION

Operational Principles

Patient-triggered or assisted ventilation provides a mechanical V_T when the patient initiates inspiration (see Fig. 48-8). It does not allow spontaneous breathing. If the patient does not initiate a breathing effort, however, the ventilator *will not* deliver a mechanical breath; thus, apnea can be fatal with this mode of ventilation.

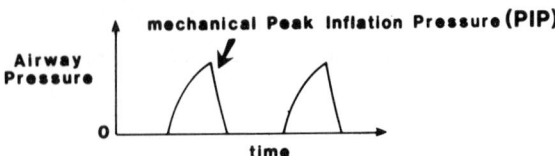

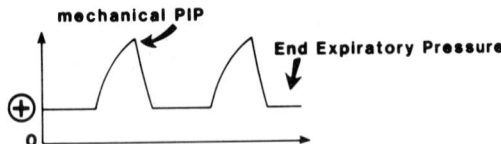

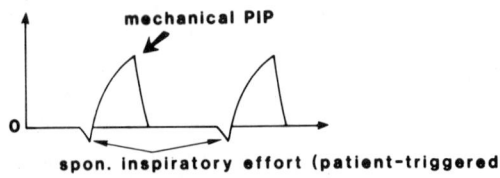

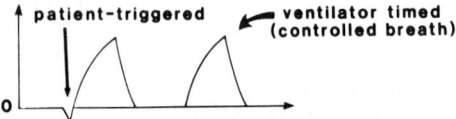

FIGURE 48-8. Mechanical ventilatory airway pressure patterns. (**A**) Controlled mechanical ventilation (CMV). Mechanical ventilator rate, tidal volume (VT), and inspiratory flow rate are preset and cannot be affected by the patient's respiratory efforts. (**B**) CMV with end-expiratory pressure or continous positive pressure ventilation. When mechanical inhalation ends, pressure drops to a set positive-pressure plateau, i.e., the end-expiratory pressure level. (**C**) Assisted (patient-triggered) mechanical ventilation. VT is preset and cannot be affected by the patient. If the patient does not initiate inhalation, the ventilator does not switch ON. (**D**) Patient-triggered with controlled back-up ventilation. The ventilator may be triggered to mechanical inhalation by the patient's inspiratory efforts or by a timing device, whichever comes first. The patient may trigger the ventilator as often as desired, and the timing device determines the minimum ventilator cycling rate.

Clinical Applications

This technique has been employed as intermittent positive-pressure breathing for short-term delivery of gases and therapeutic aerosols to patients with pulmonary parenchymal or airway disease. It is infrequently used for support of patients with acute or chronic respiratory failure.

Patients treated with patient-triggered mechanical ventilation tend to develop respiratory alkalemia, the deleterious effects of which are increased Raw and oxygen consumption; decreased cardiac output, coronary blood flow, cerebral blood flow, serum potassium, and ionized calcium; and left-

ward shift of the oxygen-hemoglobin dissociation curve (increased oxyhemoglobin affinity).

CMV Backup

Patient-triggered ventilation with controlled backup ventilation may be provided; the ventilator is triggered ON by the patient's spontaneous inspiratory efforts or by a timing device, whichever comes first (see Fig. 48-8). The patient can initiate cycling at any time, but the timer determines a minimal preselected rate. Thus, CMV acts as a backup should the patient become apneic or attempt to breathe at a lower rate than that set by the timer.

Potential Problems

Patient-triggered ventilation and CMV predispose to ventilator-induced $\dot{V}A/\dot{Q}$ abnormalities. This untoward effect is related to the maldistribution of ventilation. A disproportionate amount of the VT is delivered anteriorly to nondependent lung regions with decreased perfusion when the patient is supine.[11]

Conversely, spontaneous ventilation tends to promote more normal $\dot{V}A/\dot{Q}$ distribution. Some studies have demonstrated that dead space increases during mechanical ventilation with or without positive expiratory pressure.[12,13] Downs and Mitchell[12] showed that increases of dead space ventilation were related to the rate of mechanical cycling, regardless of the ventilatory pattern and whether positive expiratory pressure was employed.

END-INSPIRATORY PAUSE

Operational Principles

Postinflation hold, end-inspiratory plateau, or *end-inspiratory pause* refer to a period of time after mechanical inhalation when no flow is delivered from the ventilator, positive pressure is maintained in the lungs, and the opening of the exhalation valve is delayed (Fig. 48-9). End-inspiratory pause is an extension of the mechanical inhalation phase because exhalation does not occur until the end-inspiratory pause is terminated. The duration of the end-inspiratory pause is designated in seconds or as a percentage of the total time of the respiratory cycle.

With end-inspiratory pause, the PIP is generated when VT delivery is completed. During the pause time, airway pressure decreases to the static elastic recoil pressure or plateau pressure of the respiratory system. PIP and elastic recoil pressure are useful in determining CLT and Raw (Table 48-5).

Clinical Applications

End-expiratory pause has been advocated as a method to improve VT distribution and to decrease PaCO$_2$ and VD/VT.[14] If inhalation is sufficiently prolonged to exceed the time constant of slow-filling spaces in the lung, gas distribution is improved.[2] Collateral ventilation and Pendelüft flow, also thought to enhance the distribution of ventilation, occur

END INSPIRATORY PAUSE (EIP)

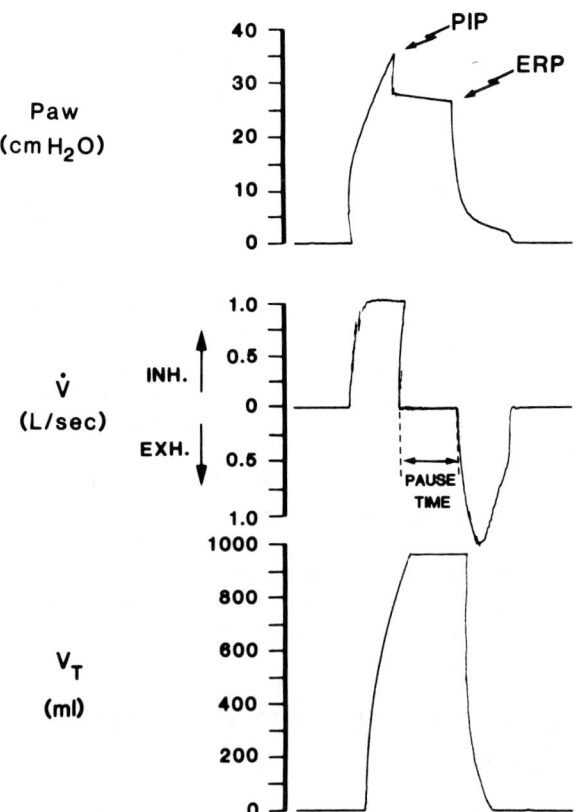

FIGURE 48-9. Airway pressure (Paw), flow rate (V̇), and tidal volume (VT) during end-inspiratory pause. Peak inflation pressure (PIP) is generated (35 cm H_2O), whereas gas flows from the ventilator. During the pause, no flow is delivered to the patient and airway pressure decreases to the level of the static elastic recoil pressure (ERP) or plateau pressure of the respiratory system (27 cm H_2O). The greater the decrease from PIP to ERP, the greater the airways resistance. After the previously determined pause time, the exhalation valve opens, permitting passive exhalation. INH, inhalation; EXH, exhalation. (Banner MJ, Blanch P, Desautels DA: Mechanical ventilators. In: Kirby RR, Banner MJ, Downs JB [eds]. *Clinical Applications of Ventilatory Support.* Philadelphia, JB Lippincott, 1990:414.

more readily when time is allowed for pressure to equalize throughout the lungs during the end-inspiratory pause interval.

Collateral ventilation occurs when gas enters alveoli through collateral channels; these may be channels in the alveolar walls (Kohn's pores) or communications between the bronchioles and alveoli (Lambert's canals). Pendelüft flow occurs when, during the end-inspiratory pause, surplus volume from fast-filling spaces redistributes and flows to slow-filling spaces. Gas flow between different regions of the lung is caused by instantaneous pressure gradients resulting from inequalities of time constants among these regions.

TABLE 48-5. Measurements of Compliance and Airways Resistance

Definition: End-inspiratory pause may be used to differentiate dynamic (Cdyn) (L/cm H_2O) from static lung–thorax compliance (Cst) (L/cm H_2O) and to determine airways resistance (Raw) (cm H_2O/L/s).

1. Cdyn = VT (PIP − baseline airway pressure)
   Where: VT = exhaled tidal volume (L)
   PIP = peak inflation pressure (cm H_2O)
   Baseline airway pressure = atmospheric pressure, or the continuous positive airway pressure (CPAP) (cm H_2O) level
   *e.g., Cdyn = 1 L/35 cm H_2O − 0 cm H_2O
   = 0.028 L/cm H_2O

2. Cst = VT (ERP − baseline airway pressure)
   Where: ERP = static elastic recoil pressure of the respiratory system (cm H_2O)
   *e.g., Cst = 1 L/27 cm H_2O − 0 cm H_2O
   = 0.037 L/cm H_2O

3. Raw = (PIP − ERP) V̇I
   Where: V̇I = inspiratory flow rate (L/s)
   *e.g., Raw = (35 cm H_2O − 27 cm H_2O)L/s
   = 8 cm H_2O/L/s

*See Fig. 48-9.

PRESSURE-CONTROLLED INVERSE RATIO VENTILATION

Operational Principles

Pressure-controlled mechanical ventilation may be applied with a normal or inverse I:E ratio. The latter is referred to as PC-IRV. With PC-IRV the mechanical inhalation phase is pressure limited and time cycled, and a decelerating inspiratory flow waveform is generated (Fig. 48-10). As with CMV, the patient cannot breathe spontaneously because most ventilators do not provide gas flow on demand in the PC-IRV mode. Furthermore, the long inhalation phase makes this technique incompatible with spontaneous breathing. Sedation, neuromuscular paralysis, or both must be induced to assure patient acceptance.

Clinical Applications

This mode frequently is used in the management of infants with hyaline membrane disease.[15] Several studies report improvements in oxygenation with lower PIP using I:E ratios as high as 4:1.[16,17] It also has been applied in adults, although experience in this group is limited.[18,19] Beneficial effects are thought to result from an elevation in mean airway and transpulmonary pressures. FRC is improved with PC-IRV as with CPAP, but this effect probably results from the decreased expiratory time, which prevents full exhalation.[20] Notice that in Figure 48-10, the expiratory flow waveform is not at zero at end-exhalation before the ventilator's initiation of the next mechanical breath. Full exhalation has not occurred, resulting in intrinsic or auto PEEP and potential air trapping.

PRESSURE CONTROLLED - INVERSE RATIO VENTILATION (PC - IRV)

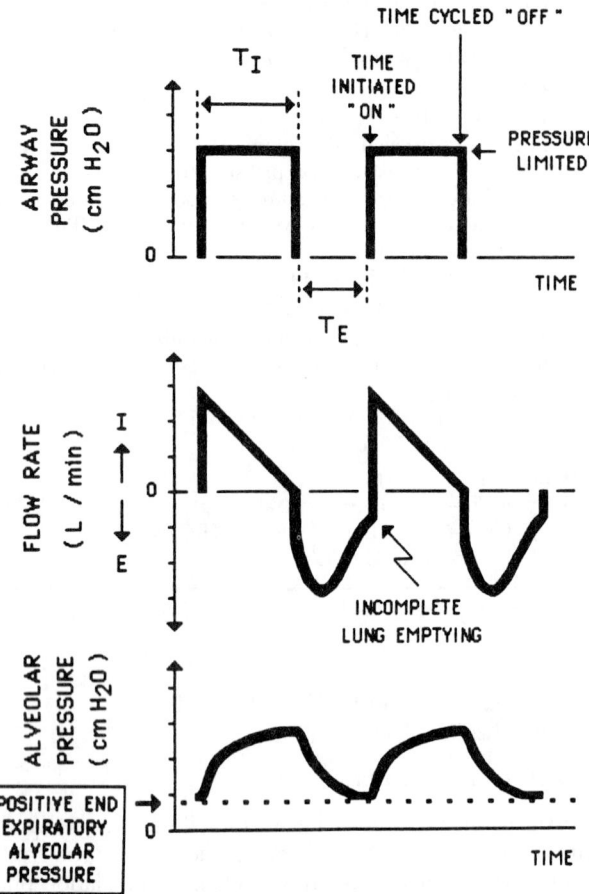

FIGURE 48-10. Illustrated are idealized representations of airway pressure, inspiratory (I) and expiratory (E) flow, and alveolar pressure waveforms for pressure-controlled inverse ratio ventilation (PC-IRV). In this example, the inhalation time (T_I) is approximately twice as long as the exhalation time (T_E); hence, the inhalation-to-exhalation time raito (I:E) is 2:1. the mechanical inhalation phase is time-initiated ON, pressure-limited, time-cycled OFF, and a decelerating inspiratory flow waveform is generated. With PC-IRV, the patient is *not* allowed to breathe spontaneously and the ventilator rate is controlled. Because of decreased exhalation time that prevents full exhalation, the lungs empty incompletely (notice the expiratory flow waveform is *not* at zero at end-exhalation before ventilator's initiation of the next mechanical breath), resulting in air trapping and positive end-expiratory alveolar pressure or intrinsic or auto PEEP.

Advantages and Disadvantages

The major proposed advantage of PC-IRV is that adequate arterial oxygenation and ventilation can be achieved at lower PIP and baseline pressures (CPAP).[18–22] Alveolar recruitment, improved distribution of ventilation, and a decreased V_D/V_T allegedly result. Alveolar recruitment should result in a better matching of $\dot{V}_A/\dot{Q}$, leading to a reduction in venous admixture and correction of hypoxemia. Improved ventilation probably results from increased duration of the inhalation phase, allowing areas of longer T_I constants to achieve greater flow than would otherwise occur with conventional ventilation techniques using normal (decreased) I:E ratios.[19]

The inspiratory pressure and flow waveform characteristics with this mode of ventilation may also be instrumental in improving gas exchange. A constant (square) inspiratory pressure waveform combined with a decelerating flow wave are thought to promote better distribution of ventilation relative to using a constant inspiratory flow waveform at a similar I:E ratio.[5,6]

A major disadvantage is that spontaneous breathing is precluded by the need for deep sedation and muscle paralysis. Reduced exhalation time predisposes to inadequate emptying of lung regions with long expiratory time constants, air trapping, and intrinsic PEEP. Regions so affected often become overdistended and are likely to rupture, resulting in pulmonary barotrauma. Tharatt and associates[18] report a 26% incidence of barotrauma with PC-IRV, which is similar to the levels of barotrauma commonly noted with CMV.[23,24] Although lower PIPs are used, mean airway pressure usually is increased or remains unchanged. Therefore, circulatory function is similar to that during CMV.[25,26]

Surprisingly, no controlled clinical trials have been conducted to support the use of PC-IRV. Until such studies have been performed, this mode of ventilation must be considered investigational in adults.[27]

INTERMITTENT MANDATORY VENTILATION

Operational Principles

Originally proposed as a method to ventilate infants with hyaline membrane disease[28,29] and adults who were difficult to wean from ventilators.[30] IMV allows the patient to breathe spontaneously, with mechanical inflations supplied at regular, preset intervals. The preselected mechanical rate (IMV breaths) cannot be influenced by the patient; thus, they are analogous to CMV. Between sequential mechanical breaths, an unrestricted flow rate of gas equal to or greater than the patient's peak $\dot{V}_I$ demand must be provided to allow spontaneous breathing and to minimize the associated work.

Clinical Applications

The IMV rate should be titrated to deliver only that support that, in conjunction with spontaneous breathing, maintains acceptable alveolar ventilation, $PaCO_2$, and pHa. When used in patients with antecedent pulmonary disease (emphysema, chronic bronchitis), IMV is useful in regulating $PaCO_2$ and pHa compared with patient-triggered ventilation.[31,32]

Other proposed physiologic advantages include improved right ventricular filling and cardiovascular function because of lower inspiratory intrapleural pressure and decreased rate of mechanical ventilator cycling. When IMV is combined with CPAP (Fig. 48-11), the cardiopulmonary effects are improved compared with CPPV, and higher expiratory positive pressure with fewer deleterious effects on venous return and cardiac output results.[33,34] Finally, spontaneous breathing with IMV also promotes more normal $\dot{V}_A/\dot{Q}$ matching than does CMV.[11,25]

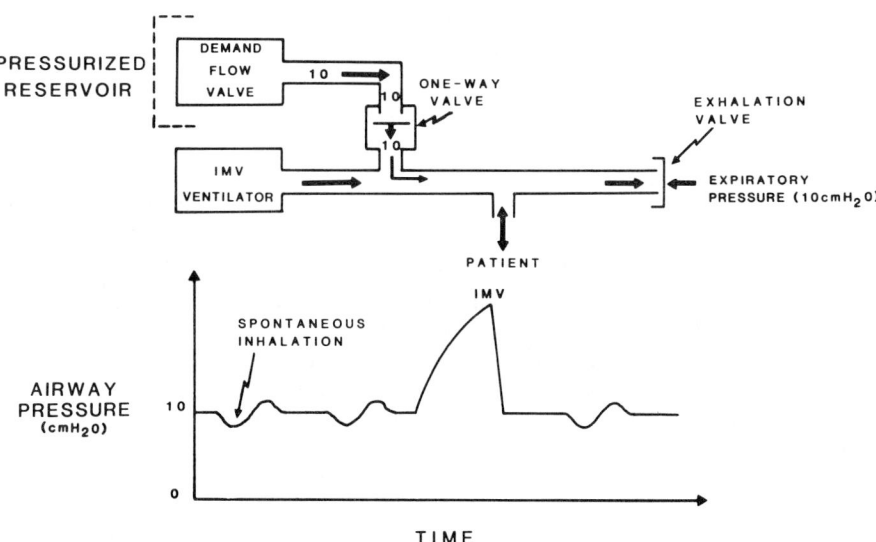

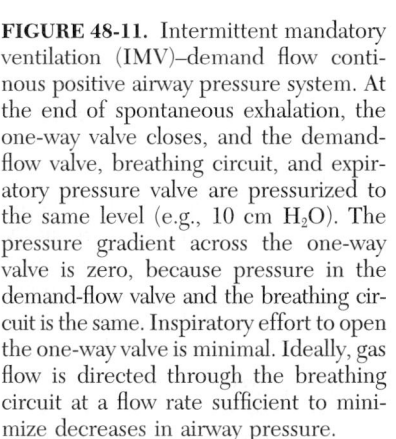

FIGURE 48-11. Intermittent mandatory ventilation (IMV)–demand flow continuous positive airway pressure system. At the end of spontaneous exhalation, the one-way valve closes, and the demand-flow valve, breathing circuit, and expiratory pressure valve are pressurized to the same level (e.g., 10 cm H_2O). The pressure gradient across the one-way valve is zero, because pressure in the demand-flow valve and the breathing circuit is the same. Inspiratory effort to open the one-way valve is minimal. Ideally, gas flow is directed through the breathing circuit at a flow rate sufficient to minimize decreases in airway pressure.

Equipment

GAS FLOW. Sufficient gas flow rate must be provided through the IMV circuit to satisfy the patient's peak spontaneous V̇ı demand, just as with CPAP circuits. Gas flow rates of two to three times the patient's minute ventilation usually are sufficient. Also, as with CPAP circuitry, the resistance to gas flow through the IMV system must be minimal during spontaneous breathing (i.e., highly resistant humidifiers, one-way valves, narrow-bore breathing circuit tubing, and right-angled connectors should *not* be used). Systems that cannot provide adequate gas flow rate increase the patient's work of breathing to intolerably high levels and can result in failure of the technique.

HUMIDIFICATION. Full humidification of inspired gas during spontaneous and mechanical inspiration must be provided. Two problems arise with humidifiers in IMV systems: the capability to humidify gas sufficiently during high-flow rate conditions (≥ 60 L/minute), which on occasion is necessary to satisfy spontaneous inspiratory demand; and flow resistance characteristics of the humidifier itself. Poulton and Downs[35] studied several commercially available humidifiers. The Bird heated-wick humidifier delivered acceptable humidity with negligible flow resistance during high-flow rate conditions. Other humidifiers failed to provide sufficient humidity or imposed excessive resistance to gas flow, either of which precludes their use in an IMV system. High-flow resistance is not a problem during CMV because the ventilator provides essentially all the work of breathing. However, during spontaneous inhalation with IMV, the patient must provide this work.[36]

OUTFLOW VALVES. The IMV system should be capable of pressurizing the inspiratory reservoir to the CPAP level. A continuous-flow or demand-flow system (see Fig. 48-11) can be used. Most commercially available IMV-CPAP systems are of the latter design. Low-resistance, threshold resistor exhalation valves are advisable for two reasons. First, high-resistance valves significantly increase expiratory airway pressure (especially during coughing). Second, large de-

creases in airway pressure occur during spontaneous inhalation with continuous gas flow directed through high-resistance valves. During spontaneous inhalation, some of the continuous flow passing through the valve is diverted to the patient. Because pressure in the circuit is proportional to both resistance and flow rate, the reduction of flow rate through the valve results in a substantial reduction of inspiratory pressure and a corresponding increase in the patient's work of breathing.[37]

SYNCHRONIZED INTERMITTENT MANDATORY VENTILATION

Operational Principles

SIMV also allows spontaneous breathing between mechanically delivered ventilator breaths. At regular intervals, the mandatory breath is synchronized to begin with the patient's next spontaneous inspiratory effort in the same fashion as the patient-triggered method described earlier. This technique was introduced because of concern that a mechanical breath might be superimposed on a spontaneous breath (stacking), causing increases in PIP and mean airway and intrapleural pressures. Similar concerns existed if the mechanically delivered volume was added at the peak of spontaneous exhalation.

Subsequently, investigations were conducted to examine the clinical efficacy of SIMV. Shapiro and colleagues[38] noted that mean intrapleural pressure, assessed with an esophageal balloon, was substantially lower with SIMV than with IMV in normal volunteers. However, Hasten and coworkers[39] compared SIMV with IMV in 25 critically ill patients and found that although PIP was greater with IMV than with SIMV, cardiovascular variables (blood pressure, cardiac output, stroke index, central venous pressure, and pulmonary artery pressure) did not differ significantly.

In another study, Heenan and colleagues[40] studied anesthetized, near-drowned dogs ventilated with IMV or SIMV. Again, no differences between the two modes were noted with respect to cardiac output, stroke volume, intrapleural pressure, and intrapulmonary shunt. PIP and mean airway pressure were significantly increased with IMV and some breath stacking occurred, but without demonstrable adverse effects. Based on these data, SIMV does *not* seem to offer any physiologic advantages compared with IMV.

PRESSURE SUPPORT VENTILATION

Operational Principles

PSV is used to unload the ventilatory muscles and to decrease the work of breathing of patients with decreased C_{LT} and increased Raw.[41] It also augments spontaneous breathing by offsetting the work imposed by the resistance of breathing circuits and smaller than optimal size artificial airways.[42,43] When the ventilator is patient-triggered ON, an abrupt rise in airway pressure to a preselected positive-pressure limit results from a variable flow rate of gas from the ventilator.

As long as the patient maintains an inspiratory effort, airway pressure is held constant at the preselected level. Gas flow from the ventilator ceases when the patient's $\dot{V}_I$ demand decreases to a predetermined percentage of the initial peak mechanical $\dot{V}_I$ (e.g., 25%). The ventilator is thus flow-cycled OFF in the PSV mode. Once the preselected inspiratory pressure limit is set, the patient *interacts* with

the pressure-assisted breath and retains control over T_I and flow rate, expiratory time, frequency, V_T, and minute volume (Figs. 48-12 and 48-13; Table 48-6).

Clinical Application

Two approaches are described: (1) low-level PSV (5 to 30 cm H_2O), to assist spontaneous breathing between IMV/SIMV breaths and to decrease patient work of breathing by *partially* unloading the ventilatory muscles; and (2) high-level PSV (20 to 50 cm H_2O), as an independent or stand-alone mechanical ventilatory mode to unload the ventilatory muscles *totally*[44,45] (Fig. 48-14). Some overlap occurs.

LOW-LEVEL PSV.   The rationale for low-level PSV include offsetting the increased work imposed by endotracheal tubes and poorly designed demand-flow systems (low flow rate on demand, long response time, and a highly resistant breathing circuit). Increased flow resistance associated with these devices produces undesirable high pressure–volume workloads, further compromising ventilatory muscle function.

Partial unloading of the ventilatory muscles results when, after the initial decrease in intrapleural pressure at the onset of inhalation, the ventilator is patient-triggered ON and airway pressure rises abruptly to the preselected positive-pressure level. (Integration of airway pressure with respect to V_T represents work performed by the ventilator.) A further decrease in intrapleural pressure is indicative of work performed by the patient, who thus interacts with the positive-pressure assisted breath to regulate V_T. (Integration of intrapleural pressure with respect to V_T represents work performed by the patient.) Thus, total work is performed partly by the ventilator and partly by the patient.

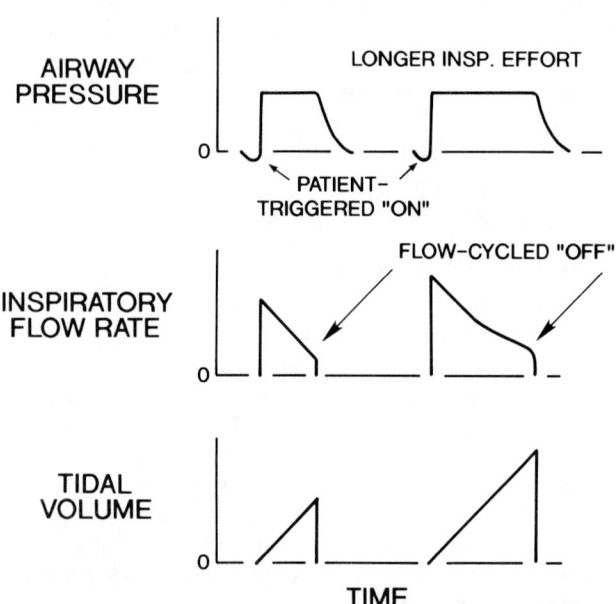

FIGURE 48-12. Pressure support ventilation (PSV). The ventilator is patient-triggered ON and, as long as inspiratory effort is maintained, airway pressure stays constant with a variable flow rate of gas from the ventilator. The ventilator cycles OFF when the patient's inspiratory flow rate demand decreases to a predetermined percentage of the peak inspiratory flow rate, i.e., the ventilator is flow-cycled OFF. In the PSV mode, the airway pressure level is preselected, while the patient retains control over inspiratory time and flow rate, tidal and minute volume, and ventilator rate. On the right, the patient increases inspiratory effort and generates a longer inspiratory time compared with the PSV breath on the left. Because tidal volume equals inspiratory time times inspiratory flow rate, a greater tidal volume is delivered than with the previous breath. Although peak inflation pressure is constant from breath to breath, tidal volume is thus variable with patient effort.

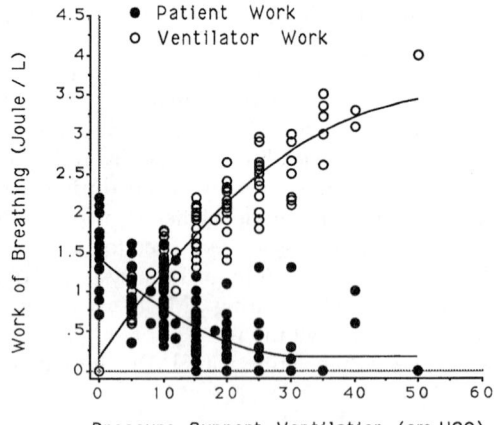

FIGURE 48-13. Relationships between patient and ventilator work of breathing at incremental levels of pressure support ventilation (PSV) for 30 adults are illustrated. Patient work decreases while ventilator work increases as the level of PSV increases. Patient work of breathing is in a near-normal range (0.3 to 0.6 J/L) at approximately 15 cm H_2O for this group of patients with moderate respiratory failure.

TABLE 48-6. Ventilators Incorporating Pressure Support Ventilation

VENTILATOR	PSV RANGE (cm H₂O)
Puritan-Bennett 7200a	1–70
Bird 6400 ST	1–50
Bourns BEAR-5	1–72
Hamilton Veolar	1–50
Hamilton Amadeus	1–100
Ohmeda CPU-1	1–30
PPG IRISA	1–80
Engström Erica	1–30
Siemens 900C	1–100

PSV, pressure support ventilation.

HIGH-LEVEL PSV. Alternatively, the level of PSV may be set high enough to unload the ventilatory muscles completely, provide essentially all the work of breathing, and allow the patient to rest. High levels of PSV have been defined as that pressure sufficient to provide a VT of 10 to 12 mL/kg (maximum PSV [PSV_{max}]).[45] A negligible amount of work is performed by the patient to trigger the ventilator ON. Pressure levels greater than 40 cm H₂O have been used in patients with large minute ventilation demands and severely impaired pulmonary mechanics.[46] Used in this manner, PSV is similar to conventional patient-triggered positive-pressure ventilation, but with a pressure limit.

APNEA. When used as an independent mode of ventilation on most ventilators (except the Puritan Bennett 7200a, Hamilton Veolar, and Ohmeda CPU-1), no safety or backup mechanism to ventilate the patient exists in the event of apnea. Thus, PSV is contraindicated for patients with an unstable respiratory drive (central neurologic disorders or respiratory depression associated with sedative or narcotic drugs). Because *all breaths* are initiated by the patient, apnea is life threatening.

Assessment of Work of Breathing

The level of PSV may be adjusted to provide an optimal muscle load. However, in clinical practice this setting often is difficult to determine. The proper level of muscle unloading is that which encourages muscle reconditioning and prevention of atrophy while avoiding the development of fatigue.[47] Respiratory rate has been advocated as a method to assess ventilatory muscle load[45,48]: a slow rate suggests that the patient is experiencing a subfatiguing load (15 to 25 breaths/minute), whereas a higher rate (>30 breaths/minute) is an inference of an intolerable load on the ventilatory muscles. Abdominal paradox and the use of accessory muscles are also indicative of increased ventilatory muscle loading and the onset of fatigue.

In one carefully performed clinical study, an optimal muscle load for patients with ventilatory failure was imposed by adjusting the levels of PSV from 10 to 20 cm H₂O.[41] PSV was applied to spontaneously breathing patients to unload the ventilatory muscles and to prevent diaphragmatic fatigue by diminishing work of breathing and oxygen consumption. Optimal PSV was defined as the level that maintained maximal diaphragmatic electrical activity without fatigue. Ventilatory muscle fatigue is associated with a frequency shift in the electromyographic power spectrum of the diaphragm from higher to lower frequency.[48] Thus, the lowest PSV level at which no reduction in the high/low power spectrum ratio occurred was chosen.

Another approach to provide appropriate ventilatory muscle loads is to titrate PSV while monitoring intrapleural pressure.[47] A greater decrease of inspiratory intrapleural pressure is associated with increased patient work of breathing. While PSV is increased (ventilator work), less decrease of intrapleural pressure should be seen. At PSV_{max}, intrapleural pressure may decrease imperceptibly or may increase during inhalation.

Flow Rate and Pressure Rise

Rates of flow and pressure rise during PSV affect breathing pattern, patient–ventilator synchrony, and work of breath-

FIGURE 48-14. Two setting options for pressure support ventilation (PSV) are to (1) *partially* unload the respiratory muscles, and (2) *totally* unload the muscles; both options are achievable based on real time measurements of the work of breathing. Work of breathing performed by the patient (N = 30 adults) decreased (*) and work performed by the ventilator (X) increased significantly (*p* <0.05) when the respiratory muscles were partially unloaded while the level of PSV was raised from 0 to 18 ± 7 cm H₂O; work was performed in part by the patient and in part by the ventilator (work sharing approach). Partial unloading may be defined as patient work of breathing in a normal range (0.3 to 0.6 J/L). A nonfatiguing workload was performed by the patients under these conditions. Patient work of breathing decreased further to 0 J/L (+) (*p* <0.05) and ventilator work increased when the muscles were totally unloaded at a PSV level of 31 ± 8 cm H₂O. Data are mean ± SD.

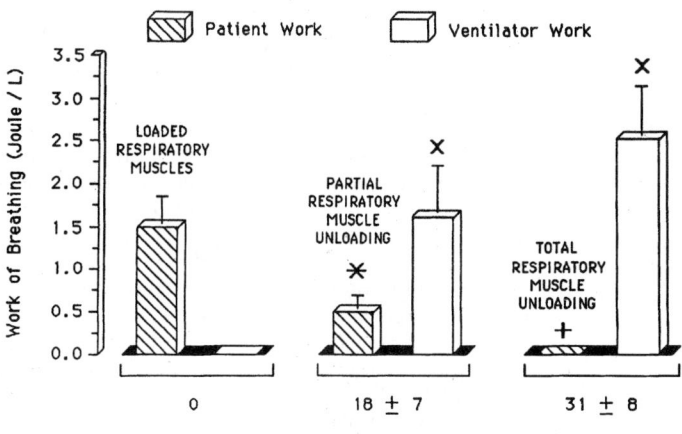

ing. The rate of flow rise is the manipulated or independent variable, whereas the corresponding rate of pressure rise is the response or dependent variable during PSV. An optimal flow rate, and thus rate of pressure rise for a given level of PSV, is defined as that which results in the patient obtaining the maximal pressure and volume from the ventilator, that is, the work of breathing performed by the ventilator to inflate the respiratory system.[49] Flow rates above or below the optimal flow rate are associated with faster breathing frequencies, shorter T_Is, smaller V_Ts, and a tendency for airway pressure to not reach the preselected level of PSV.

The optimal rate of flow rise during PSV is highest in patients with the lowest compliance and highest $\dot{V}_I$ demand. These findings were affirmed by Cohen and researchers[50] and Branson and associates,[51] who concluded that titration of ventilator flow rate *supply* to patient $\dot{V}_I$ *demand* improves patient–ventilator synchrony during PSV. A means to adjust flow rate output and thus the rate of pressure rise should be incorporated into ventilators.

Czervinske and colleagues[52] applied PSV at a fast rate of pressure rise to infants and noted that the breaths terminated prematurely. This finding was attributed to excessive ventilator flow rates (>90 L/minute) directed into narrow internal diameter endotracheal tubes (3 to 4 mm). Ventilator $\dot{V}_I$ supply was greatly in excess of patient $\dot{V}_I$ demand. When a lower flow rate was applied, ventilator supply and patient demand were in better balance, and T_I and V_T increased while breathing frequency decreased.

In patients with a low peak $\dot{V}_I$ demand, an inappropriately high ventilator flow rate supply results in too rapid a rate of pressure rise causing "ringing" in the pressure waveform (transient overshooting, rapidly oscillating, or spiking phenomenon). Disruption of the inspiratory muscle contraction pattern results in premature termination of inspiratory muscle effort and patient discomfort. A lower, more gradual rate of flow rise during PSV seems to be appropriate.

Patient and Ventilator Interaction

The rate of airway pressure rise is affected by the interaction of ventilator flow rate supply and patient $\dot{V}_I$ demand. When ventilator flow rate supply is appropriately high to satisfy a patient's peak $\dot{V}_I$ demand, a fast rise in pressure and a square shaped pressure waveform during PSV decreases patient work of breathing. Conversely, when the ventilator flow rate supply is inappropriately less than the patient's peak $\dot{V}_I$ demand, a slower rise in pressure and a concave or "scooped-out" pressure waveform results, predisposing to increased patient work of breathing (Figs. 48-15 and 48-16).

In one report, as ventilator $\dot{V}_I$ supply (rate of flow rise) came into better balance with patient $\dot{V}_I$ demand, the corresponding rates of pressure rise increased from slow to fast and patient work of breathing decreased.[53] A fast rate of pressure rise or square-shaped pressure waveform, in the absence of excessive ringing, was associated with the lowest patient work of breathing.

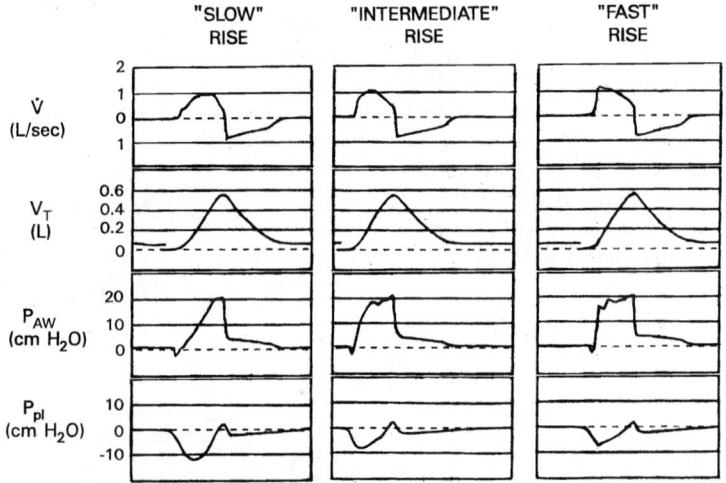

FIGURE 48-15. Slow, intermediate, and fast rates of airway pressure (Paw) rise during pressure support ventilation (PSV) at 20 cm H_2O are shown. Tidal volume (V_T), inspiratory time, and peak inspiratory flow rate ($\dot{V}$) are essentially the same during all conditions. Notice that with a slow rate of pressure rise the airway pressure waveform is linear and somewhat concave in shape. With a fast rate of pressure rise the airway pressure waveform is square shaped. Notice that during the slow rate of pressure rise, the flow wave form is sinusoidal and the peak flow point is shifted to the right of center; during the intermediate condition, the peak flow point is to the left of center; and during the fast rate of pressure rise, a decelerating flow wave form results and the peak flow rate is provided at the *onset* of the breath. The change in intrapleural pressure (Ppl), and thus *patient* work of breathing, is greatest during the slow condition, less during the intermediate condition, and least during the fast condition. The area under the Paw time curve, proportional to *ventilator* work of breathing, is least during the slow condition, greater during the fast condition. For a given level of PSV, meeting a patient's peak inspiratory flow rate demand *early* in a pressure supported breath lessens patient work of breathing. Also, the faster the rate of pressure rise, the lower the patient work and the greater the ventilator work of breathing.

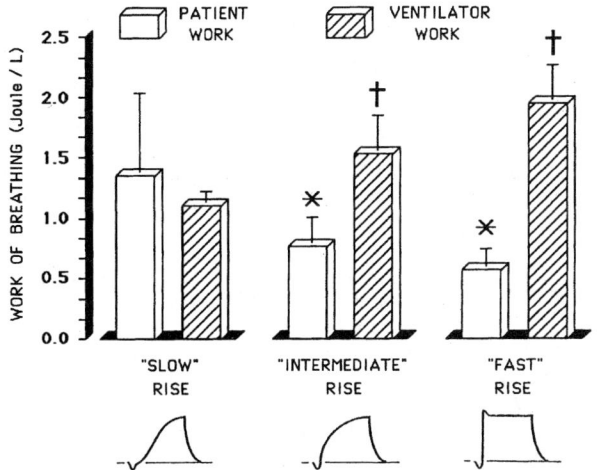

FIGURE 48-16. Influence of the rates of pressure and flow rise during pressure support ventilation (PSV) on patient ventilator work of breathing for ten adults diagnosed with acute respiratory failure, PSV level = 16 ± 4 cm H_2O. Patient work was measured along the method described by Campbell, whereas ventilator work was measured by integrating the change in airway pressure and tidal volume. For each patient, the level of PSV was held *constant* whereas slow, intermediate, and then fast rates of pressure and flow rise were applied in random order. Patient work decreased whereas ventilatory work increased significantly, comparing the slow to the intermediate and fast conditions. $p < 0.05$ compared with patient work during the slow condition (*) and compared with ventilator work during the slow condition (†).

Messida and associates,[54] when comparing patient work of breathing using slower and faster rates of ventilator flow and pressure rise, noticed that patient work of breathing was approximately 78% greater with the slower compared with the faster rate of flow and pressure rise. Cane and others[55] report that as the rates of flow and pressure rise were increased, significant decrease in patient work of breathing, change in esophageal pressure (inference of intrapleural pressure), and the pressure time product resulted. Stenz and coworkers[56] also report significant decreases in patient work of breathing and the pressure time product, as well as significant increases in ventilator work of breathing while the rates of flow and pressure rise were increased.

During PSV, work is *shared* between the ventilator and patient; while ventilator work increases, patient work decreases and vice versa (see Fig. 48-16). When an appropriately fast rate of flow rise greater than a patient's peak $\dot{V}I$ demand is applied, a fast airway pressure rise and a square-shaped pressure waveform results. Under these conditions, more work is provided by the ventilator to inflate the respiratory system, resulting in proportionately smaller changes of intrapleural pressure and decreased workload for the patient. This finding is in accordance with MacIntyre and Ho's[49] definition of an optimal flow rate and rate of pressure rise during PSV, that is, maximal work of breathing performed by the ventilator for a given level of PSV.

Independent control of the rate of flow and pressure rise during PSV are available with three commercially available ventilators:[57] BEAR 1000 (pressure slope control), Siemens 300 (inspiratory rise time control), and EVITA (Draeger) (percent increase time control). We believe that all future ventilator designs should incorporate such control mechanisms to optimize patient—ventilator synchrony and the work of breathing.

NEW OR EXPERIMENTAL TECHNIQUES ■

PRESSURE AUGMENTATION

Pressure augmentation provides a *guaranteed* VT per breath during PSV.[57] This mode is available only with the BEAR 1000 ventilator. When PSV is used as a stand-alone mode or combined with CPAP, decreases in VT and minute volume may occur as a result of decreases in the level of consciousness, inspiratory effort, and pulmonary mechanics. Hypoxemia, hypercapnia, acidemia, and their associated sequelae may result secondary to inappropriately low minute volume.

Operational Principles

Pressure augmentation may be available in the "background" or actively operating during PSV to protect the patient from hypoventilation. For this mode, a level of PSV that is deemed appropriate for the patient is preselected. Next, a minimum VT and a backup $\dot{V}I$ are chosen. If the VT during the PSV breath is greater than the minimum VT setting, no augmentation of pressure above the PSV level occurs; the breath is terminated or cycled OFF in the usual manner by flow. If VT is less than the minimum volume setting after the initial phase of the pressure supported breath, a constant flow rate of gas (backup inspiratory flow setting) is directed to the patient until the minimum VT is delivered. As a result, airway pressure is augmented above the level of PSV and the breath is cycled OFF by volume. With pressure augmentation the breath looks like a conventional PSV breath with the volume feature activated only when necessary (Fig. 48-17).

Pressure augmentation guarantees VT delivery during PSV and represents a sensible safety precaution. Future ventilator designs will likely incorporate pressure augmentation or a similar mode to protect against hypoventilation. In addition to setting a minimum VT and backup $\dot{V}I$, a backup respiratory rate setting is recommended to protect the patient in the event of apnea.

PROPORTIONAL ASSIST VENTILATION

When properly adjusted, PAV optimizes the relationship between respiratory muscle workloads and ventilatory response. This optimal relationship applies for only one specific set of physiologic conditions. If patient work of breathing changes as a result of changes in Raw, E_{RS}, $\dot{V}I$ demand, or VT, the clinician must readjust the level of PSV (up or down) to maintain an optimal and nonfatiguing respiratory muscle workload. Because one or more of the above respiratory parameters may change on a frequent basis, maintaining the precise level of PSV required to optimize respiratory muscle workloads is difficult at times.

PRESSURE AUGMENTATION*

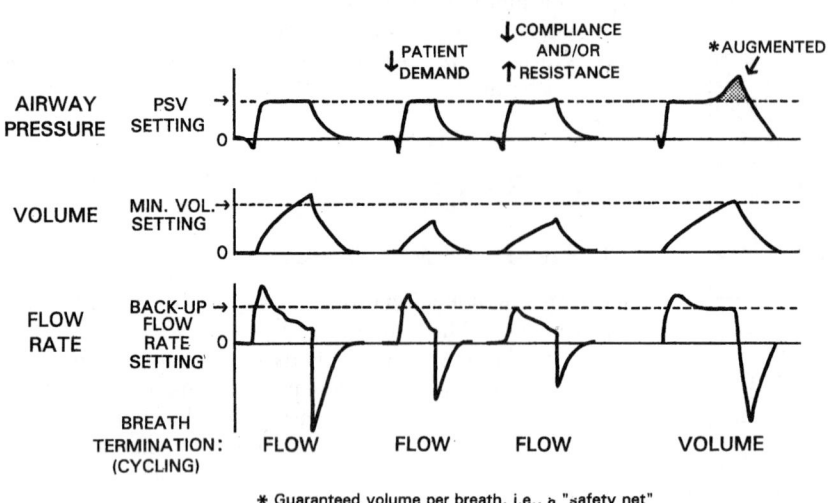

* Guaranteed volume per breath, i.e., a "safety net"

FIGURE 48-17. Pressure augmentation (BEAR 1000 ventilator) is a ventilatory mode that provides a *guaranteed* tidal volume per breath during pressure support ventilation (PSV). For this mode, a level of PSV, minimum volume, and back-up inspiratory flow rate are set. In the first breath, tidal volume is greater than the minimum volume setting, and no augmentation of pressure above the PSV level occurs; the breath is terminated or cycled OFF by flow. In the second and third breaths, tidal volume is less than the minimum volume setting as a result of decreased patient effort/demand and decreased compliance or increased airway resistance, respectively. In the fourth breath, a continous flow rate is directed to the patient after the initial phase of the breath until the minimum tidal volume is delivered; as a result, pressure is augmented above the level of PSV (shaded area); the breath is terminated or cycled OFF by volume.

Operational Principles

A favorable relationship between respiratory muscle workloads and alveolar ventilation at all times is an important and desirable therapeutic objective. An experimental technique known as PAV may eventually prove superior to PSV in accomplishing this objective.[58,59] By design, a ventilator capable of PAV continuously manipulates the level of PSV applied to the airway (Paw) throughout the course of each spontaneous inhalation. In contrast, conventional PSV applies a single pressure level throughout the entire inspiratory phase. During PAV, Paw is varied in response to the patient's respiratory muscle pressure or effort (Pmus) which is affected by Raw (change in pressure/flow rate), E_{RS} (change in pressure/change in volume), $\dot{V}I$, and VT. Mathematically, the relationship between these variables and the ventilator's response is described by the following equation of motion for the respiratory system:

$$Paw + Pmus = (\dot{V}I \times Raw) + (VT \times E_{RS}) \qquad (4)$$

To use PAV (and solve the equation of motion), the clinician must first accurately measure the patient's Raw and E_{RS}. Two controls on the PAV ventilator are then adjusted: one, referred to as the *resistive gain control*, based on the measured Raw; and the second, the *elastic gain control*, based on the measured E_{RS}. With this information and real-time feedback from airway pressure, flow rate, and volume sensors that are correctly positioned in the breathing circuit (see Fig. 48-6), the ventilator automatically adjusts the applied pressure (PSV) either up or down to maintain the specific relationship defined by the equation of motion.

Consider an adult whose E_{RS} increases to 50 cm H_2O/L (normal, approximately 10 cm H_2O/L) and Raw increases to 10 cm H_2O/L/second (normal, approximately 2 cm H_2O/L/second). To "normalize" this particular patient, the elastic gain control would be set to 40 cm H_2O/L (measured E_{RS} minus normal E_{RS}), thereby causing the ventilator to assume the extra elastic work resulting from the increase in E_{RS}. The resistive gain control would be set to approximately 8

cm H_2O/L/second (measured Raw minus normal Raw). The total resistive work, or pressure drop, that the patient must generate across the airways and breathing apparatus to achieve a desired $\dot{V}I$ would thereby be reduced.

During PAV, like PSV, the patient interacts with the pressure-supported breath and retains control over $\dot{V}I$, T_I, breathing frequency, VT, and minute ventilation. Unlike PSV, the patient regulates the applied airway pressure level as well, thus retaining control over *all* ventilatory parameters during PAV.

Clinical Applications

With PAV, the elastic and resistive gain controls can be set in several different ways, based on the patient's individual needs. Chronically fatigued respiratory muscles can be totally unloaded to allow a period of rest simply by adjusting the gain controls to assume the total work of breathing. The respiratory muscles may be partially unloaded by adjusting the gain settings to allow only work that the patient can tolerate. Finally, the gain settings can be adjusted to "exercise" the patient's respiratory muscles by periodically forcing a greater than normal work of breathing.

Potential Problems

As with other ventilatory approaches, PAV is not without shortcomings. It requires real-time airway pressure, flow rate, and volume signals from the "Y" piece of the breathing circuit. Loss of, or alteration in any or all of these signals, could jeopardize the patient. Accurate measurements of Raw and E_{RS} also are necessary. Accuracy in obtaining these measurements dictates a totally relaxed patient, which in general, may involve temporary pharmacologic intervention. Furthermore, PAV is similar to setting a level of PSV in that the gain controls must be readjusted to accommodate changes in either Raw, E_{RS}, or both.

Other potential problems include the following: a dependency on patient spontaneous effort (without spontaneous effort PAV cannot function); or a tendency to "run-away" (e.g., a leak in the breathing circuit or around the endotracheal tube could "fool" the ventilator into providing inappropriately high flow rates in response to the leak rather than patient effort). Finally, PAV does not control either V_T or breathing rate and therefore has no direct control over a patient's breathing pattern.

MANDATORY MINUTE VOLUME

Operational Principles

Hewlett and colleagues[60] described MMV, a technique by which the patient is guaranteed a preselected minute volume with spontaneous ventilation, positive-pressure breaths from the ventilator, or a combination of the two. If the desired minute volume is breathed spontaneously, no mandatory ventilation is provided by the ventilator. If not, that portion of the preselected minute volume that is not breathed spontaneously is provided by the ventilator and delivered automatically. Theoretically, weaning with MMV is simplified because the clinician is not required to make periodic adjustments of the ventilator rate as spontaneous ventilation changes.[61] Microprocessor-controlled ventilators that incorporate MMV are the Hamilton Veolar, Bourns Bear-5, Ohmeda CPU-1 and Advent, Engström Erica, and the PPG Biomedical Systems IRISA.

Various algorithms are used to regulate ventilator frequency and thus modify the amount of support in the MMV mode.[62] The Hamilton Veolar ventilator, for example, incorporates PSV in the MMV mode. After every eight breaths, a microprocessor compares the spontaneous minute volume with the preselected MMV and corrects any differences between the two by automatically adjusting the level of PSV in increments of approximately 2 cm H_2O.

Selecting an appropriate target minute volume is essential when using MMV. Unfortunately, few data exist as a guide for determining this value. A reasonable approach is to ensure that adequate ventilation is provided to patients with fluctuations in their ventilatory drive; the target minute volume should, therefore, be that which results in an acceptable $Paco_2$.[62]

Clinical Application

Potentially, MMV is a useful ventilatory technique. Because it ensures a minimal level of support, it has been advocated for weaning patients from mechanical ventilation. However, it is not without possible problems. Patients may become tachypneic and breathe with a small V_T; under these conditions, the spontaneous minute volume can equal or exceed the preselected MMV.

Consider an adult at a preselected MMV of 8 L/minute; if the spontaneous breathing frequency and V_T are 40/minute and 225 mL, respectively, the spontaneous minute volume would equal 9 L/minute and thus exceed the level of MMV. Although indicated, *no* mechanical ventilation would be provided.

SPONTANEOUS BREATHING

CPAP AND PEEP

CPAP and spontaneous PEEP (sPEEP) are positive-pressure modes used with spontaneous breathing. They can be employed individually or in conjunction with IMV/SIMV. With CPAP, both inspiratory and expiratory pressure are positive, although the inspiratory level is less than is the expiratory level. With sPEEP, airway pressure is zero or negative (subambient) during inspiration but increases at the end of expiration to the predetermined positive pressure (Fig. 48-18). The level of CPAP or sPEEP used is designated by the value measured at end-exhalation. Both are designed to increase expiratory transpulmonary pressure and lung volume (FRC). Inspiratory and mean airway pressures do not reflect the total alveolar distending pressure at end-exhalation (Fig. 48-19).

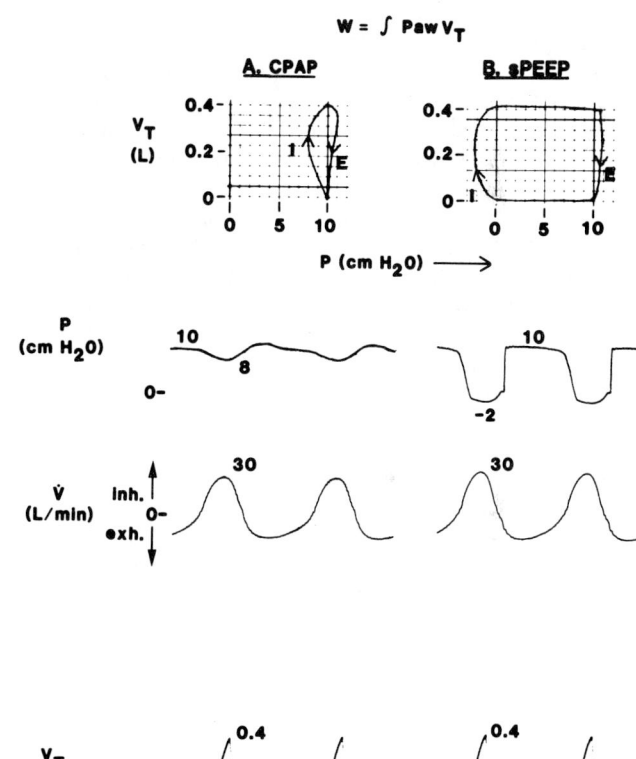

FIGURE 48-18. Work (W) imposed by the system during spontaneous breathing with continuous positive airway pressure (CPAP) and spontaneous positive end-expiratory pressure (sPEEP). End-expiratory airway pressure is 10 cm H_2O, and tidal volume (V_T) and inhaled and exhaled flow rates ($\dot{V}$) are the same for both modes. During spontaneous inhalation (I) with CPAP, pressure (P) decreases to 8 cm H_2O. With sPEEP, P decreases to -2 cm H_2O. During exhalation (E), P returns to 10 cm H_2O in both modes. For the same changes in V_T, a greater change in airway pressure occurs during sPEEP, resulting in a larger pressure–volume loop. The areas within these loops represent W. For CPAP, W is 0.25 kg/m/minute; for sPEEP, W is 1.56 kg/m/minute, a 524% increase.

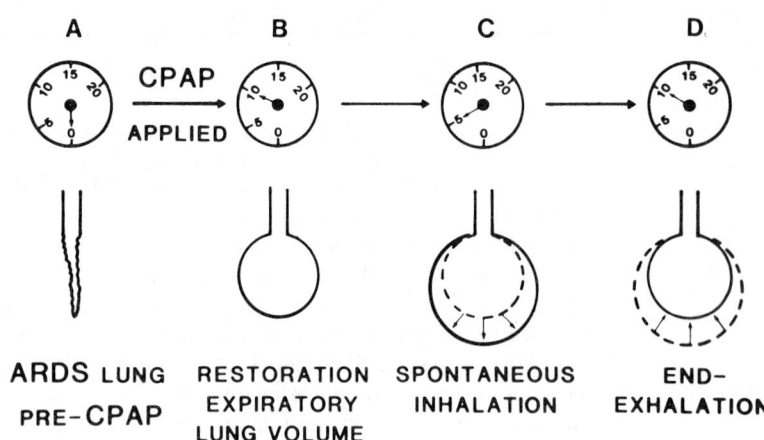

A CPAP APPLIED **B** → **C** → **D**

ARDS LUNG PRE-CPAP   **RESTORATION EXPIRATORY LUNG VOLUME (FRC)**   **SPONTANEOUS INHALATION**   **END-EXHALATION**

FIGURE 48-19. Pressure and volume changes in the lung during spontaneous ventilation with continuous positive airway pressure (CPAP). (**A**) With acute respiratory distress syndrome (ARDS), the lung characteristically has reduced functional residual capacity (FRC); airway pressure is zero. (**B**) CPAP increases the airway pressure to 10 cm H_2O, for example, and restores FRC to normal. (**C**) During spontaneous inhalation, airway pressure decreases to 5 cm H_2O whereas inspiratory transpulmonary pressure and lung volume increase. (**D**) At end-exhalation, airway pressure returns to 10 cm H_2O and the lung volume to FRC.

Equipment

Several mechanical devices are used to deliver CPAP. A common and convenient method, with or without a ventilator, uses continuous gas flow (usually 10 to 20 L/minute at a specified fractional inspired oxygen concentration [FIO_2]), and a reservoir bag, one-way valve, humidifier, and expiratory pressure valve (Fig. 48-20). FIO_2 and gas flow rate are precisely regulated by an air-oxygen blender with a back pressure–compensated flow meter. The gas is directed into a 3-L bag that acts as a reservoir for the patient's breathing. It then passes through the one-way valve, which opens during spontaneous inhalation and closes during exhalation. Expiratory closure of the one-way valve precludes retrograde flow to the reservoir bag and maintains a fairly nondistensible breathing circuit, with only the expiratory pressure valve influencing airway pressure.

Expiratory Pressure Valves

Expiratory pressure valves regulate the level of airway pressure during CPAP and sPEEP, as well as during mechanical ventilation with PEEP. They are characterized as threshold resistors and flow resistors.[63,64] In theory, threshold resistors

generate pressure (P) without associated additional flow resistance.[65] Pressure from a threshold resistor results from a force (F), expressed in newtons (N), applied over a discrete surface area (SA), expressed in square meters (m^2) (100 N/m^2 = 1 cm H_2O):

$$P = F/SA \qquad (5)$$

Exhaled gas passes freely through the completely open threshold resistor orifice until the balance of forces on opposite sides of the valve mechanism changes at end-exhalation.[64] At this point, the valve closes abruptly, preventing further gas loss from the airways and lungs (Fig. 48-21).

In contrast, flow resistors generate P by imposing resistance (R) to exhaled flow rate ($\dot{V}$) by an adjustable orifice (Fig. 48-22):

$$P = R\dot{V} \qquad (6)$$

Assuming $\dot{V}$ is constant, P varies directly with R. This relationship holds true only under laminar flow conditions and within a given range of flow rates. For example, if R is 10 cm H_2O/L/second and exhaled $\dot{V}$ is 1 L/second, so long as these conditions prevail, P = 10 cm H_2O. A threshold resistor should maintain a set pressure regardless of variations in exhaled flow rate,[65] as opposed to a flow resistor in

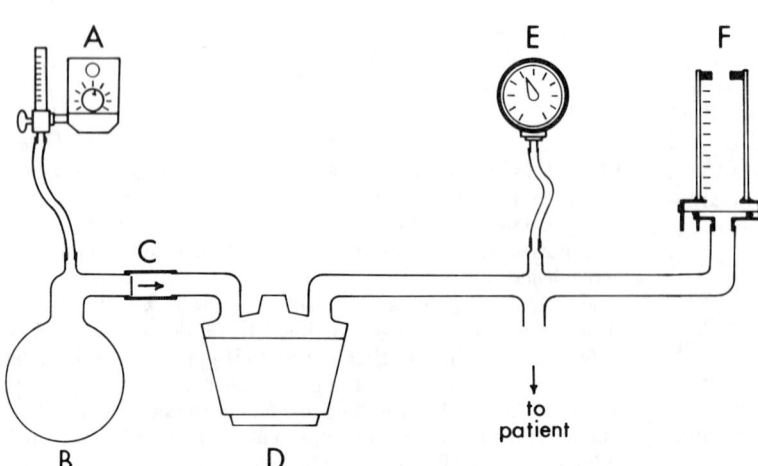

A **C** **E** **F** **B** **D** to patient

FIGURE 48-20. Reservoir bag continuous positive airway pressure system. (**A**) air–oxygen blender and flow meter; (**B**) 3-L reservoir bag; (**C**) one-way valve; (**D**) humidifier; (**E**) aneroid pressure manometer; (**F**) threshold resistor expiratory pressure valve (Emerson).

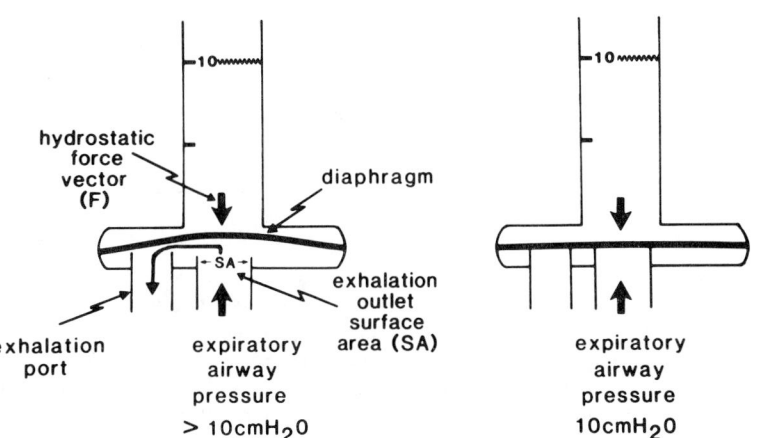

A BEGINNING EXHALATION   **B** END-EXHALATION

FIGURE 48-21. Emerson water column threshold resistor (P = F/SA). Positive pressure (P) results from a force (F) applied to a surface area (SA). Opening and closing the valve diaphragm is dependent on the balance of forces across it. (**A**) At the beginning of exhalation, force resulting from the patient's airway pressure against the bottom side of the diaphragm is greater than the hydrostatic F vector, resulting from pressure of the water column against the upper surface. Consequently, the diaphragm rises, allowing exhalation. (**B**) At end-exhalation, the balance of forces acting across the valve is changed, and the diaphragm descends, occluding the exhalation outlet.

which deviations in airway pressure occur when gas flow rate through the system is changed.

A third type of expiratory pressure valve is the pneumatic balloon valve. Balloon valves combine the properties of threshold and flow resistors.[63,66,67]

Resistance to exhaled flow rate varies widely with all three types of valves. This observation led us to further reclassify threshold resistors as high- or low-flow resistant valves. The equation describing the operation of the threshold resistors was revised to the following:

$$P = F/SA + R\dot{V} \qquad (7)$$

The $R\dot{V}$ component of this expression determines whether valves are high- or low-flow resistant types.

When exhaled $\dot{V}$ is increased, as with coughing, high airway pressures may result,[68] possibly predisposing the patient to an increased risk of barotrauma. Gal[69] reports that intubated patients can generate peak exhaled flow rates up to 240 L/minute (4 L/second) during coughing.

Consider two threshold resistor valves with resistances of 10 and 1 cm H_2O/L/second, respectively, at a preselected level of CPAP of 10 cm H_2O. If valve no. 1 is used, and the patient suddenly coughs, generating a peak exhaled flow rate of 4 L/second, the expiratory pressure increases instantane-

ously to 50 cm H_2O (50 cm H_2O = 10 cm H_2O + [10 cm H_2O/L/second × 4 L/second]). Under the same conditions with valve no. 2, pressure increases to only 14 cm H_2O (14 cm H_2O = 10 cm H_2O + [1 cm H_2O/L/second × 4 L/second]). Obviously, resistance, even with threshold resistors, is variable. Only low-resistance threshold resistors should be used in CPAP systems (e.g., Vital Signs, Hamilton, and Emerson)[67,68] to maintain airway pressure essentially constant in the face of variations in expiratory flow rate.

Work of Breathing

The relationship between the rate of gas inflow provided to the breathing circuit and the rate of the patient's $\dot{V}I$ is a factor that determines whether CPAP or sPEEP results. If the rate of gas inflow to a low-resistance breathing circuit is greater than the patient's peak spontaneous $\dot{V}I$, CPAP results (i.e., pressure is always positive during spontaneous inhalation). Conversely, when the rate of inflow to the breathing circuit is less than the patient's peak $\dot{V}I$, sPEEP results (i.e., pressure at the peak of inhalation is zero or subambient) (Fig. 48-23). In the latter situation, increased inspiratory work of breathing results[70] (see Fig. 48-18).

An increase in imposed work (e.g., work necessary to initiate gas flow, overcome circuit resistance) superimposed on the patient's intrinsic flow resistance and elastic work of breathing is associated with a greater decrement of airway pressure (increased total work of breathing). Because the fundamental goal in treating patients with acute respiratory failure is to reduce respiratory work, careful attention must be paid when delivering CPAP to maintain positive pressure at end-inhalation. A low-resistance breathing system providing high flow on demand (usually greater than two to three times the patient's minute ventilation) during spontaneous inhalation usually meets the requirements.[36]

Demand-Flow Valves

Demand-flow valves can provide CPAP. These systems were introduced during World War II as a means of increasing altitude tolerance by delivering oxygen under pressure to

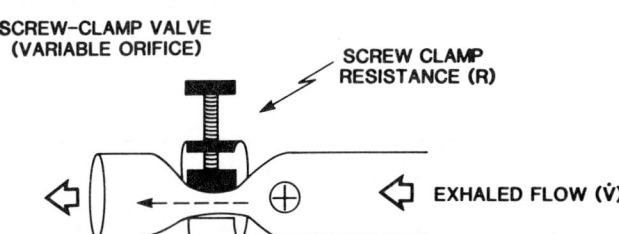

SCREW-CLAMP VALVE (VARIABLE ORIFICE)

SCREW CLAMP RESISTANCE (R)

EXHALED FLOW ($\dot{V}$)

FIGURE 48-22. A flow resistor (P = R$\dot{V}$) screw-clamp variable orifice generates expiratory positive pressure (+) dependent on the product of resistance (R) and flow rate ($\dot{V}$) directed through the valve. Resistance varies inversely with orifice size. A smaller exhalation orifice increases R and P (assuming constant flow rate) and vice versa. (Banner MJ, Lampotang S, Boysen PG, et al: Flow resistance of expiratory positive pressure valve systems. *Chest* 1986;90:212.)

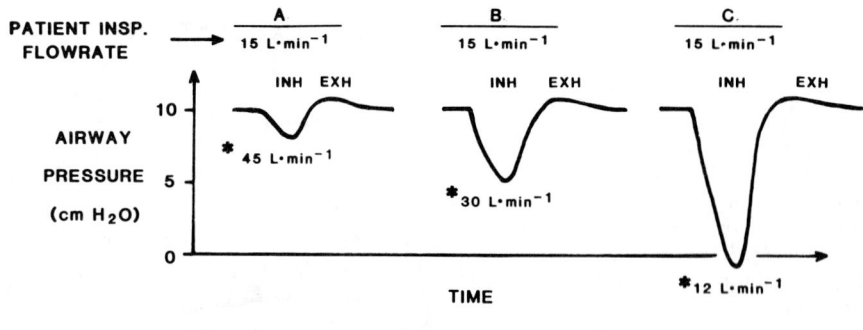

FIGURE 48-23. Spontaneous breathing with continuous positive airway pressure (CPAP) and spontaneous positive end-expiratory pressure (sPEEP). In all three examples, the patient's peak inspiratory flow rate is presumed constant at 15 L/min, and end-expiratory pressure is 10 cm H_2O. (**A**) The system flow rate is three times the patient's demand; during spontaneous inhalation, airway pressure decreases to approximately 8 cm H_2O; during exhalation, pressure returns to 10 cm H_2O. (**B**) System flow rate is twice the patient's demand; during inhalation, airway pressure decreases to 5 cm H_2O. (**C**) System flow rate is less than the patient's demand; during inhalation, airway pressure is less than zero. **A** and **B** represent CPAP, whereas **C** is sPEEP.

face masks worn by pilots. Some 30 years later, Dr. Forrest M. Bird and Mr. Jack Emerson introduced similar devices as alternatives to the continuous-flow reservoir bag apparatus. Demand-flow valves function as pressurized, high-capacity reservoirs to provide intermittent $\dot{V}I$ at a level sufficient to reduce spontaneous inspiratory work and to maintain high inspiratory positive airway pressure. The rate of gas flow should accelerate and decelerate automatically in response to the patient's $\dot{V}I$ requirements.

A demand-flow CPAP system offers two theoretical advantages. First, because the valve and the breathing circuit are pressurized at the same level, inspiratory effort is negligible. Thus, a decrease of 1 cm H_2O or less below the baseline pressure provides instantaneous gas flow at any level of CPAP (see Fig. 48-11). Second, significant gas loss—inherent in continuous high-flow reservoir bag CPAP systems—does not occur because flow is intermittent and only on demand.

Overall, however, some poorly designed demand-flow valve CPAP systems actually predispose to increased inspiratory work.[71-75] If the flow output is inadequate, greater inspiratory effort results as patients struggle to meet their peak $\dot{V}I$ requirements. Such demand-flow valves, in combination with high-resistance humidifiers and low-flow air-oxygen blenders, lead to intolerably high resistance to flow and failure of CPAP or to overstressed and fatigued patients.

Reports involving healthy volunteers,[71,72] lung models,[73,74] and patients[75] demonstrate significant variability in the operational characteristics of commercially available demand-flow CPAP systems. In some of these reports, a continuous flow (60 L/minute) reservoir bag system with a low-resistance threshold resistor expiratory pressure valve (Emerson) required less inspiratory effort, maintained higher inspiratory airway pressure, and was associated with less work of breathing than several demand-flow systems.[71-73,75] The desirable characteristics of a demand-flow system are listed in Table 48-7.

AIRWAY PRESSURE RELEASE VENTILATION

Operational Principles

Conventional modes of mechanical ventilation use positive pressure to inflate the lungs; however, high PIP and mean airway pressures predispose to increased risk of barotrauma and adverse hemodynamic changes.[76-78] Downs and oth-

TABLE 48-7. Desirable Characteristics of a Demand-Flow Valve CPAP System

Response time	Delay time from the onset of spontaneous inhalation to DFV opening and gas flow to patient (<0.2 s)
Triggering pressure	1–2 cm H_2O below end-expiratory pressure
Flow rate output	≥120 L/min during spontaneous inhalation; must be able to accelerate and decelerate flow on patient demand
CPAP range	0 ≥ 30 cm H_2O (upper limit has not been established)
Expiratory pressure valve	Low-resistance threshold resistor (e.g., Vital Signs, Hamilton, and Emerson)
Air-oxygen blender	High-flow ouptut (≥120 L/min), directly related to flow rate output of DFV
Resistance characteristics of breathing circuit	Low-flow resistive components in the breathing circuit (e.g., humidifier, one-way valves, propery sized diameter tubing, avoidance of right-angle and narrow-bore endotracheal tube connectors)

CPAP, continuous positive airway pressure; DFV, demand-flow valve.

ers[79-82] conceived APRV as a unique mode of ventilatory support that provides alveolar ventilation by intermittently *decreasing* airway pressure from a preselected level of CPAP. Peak inspiratory pressure during APRV never exceeds the level of CPAP, and the maximum lung volume corresponds to the FRC. Therefore, the incidence of pulmonary barotrauma should be minimal. APRV allows spontaneous breathing during CPAP with or without supplemental ventilation.

Equipment

A system to provide APRV is shown in Figure 48-24. Oxygen from a 50-psig gas source powers a Venturi (Downs flow generator; Vital Signs), entraining sufficient ambient air to produce a continuous flow rate of 90 to 100 L/minute. Regulation of the oxygen–air entrainment ratio controls the F_{IO_2}. Gas, heated to body temperature and at 100% relative humidity, is directed to the patient's airway, then through a low-flow resistant threshold resistor expiratory pressure valve (Vital Signs).[68]

At regular, preset intervals, an electronically controlled release (solenoid) valve on the exhalation limb of the breathing circuit opens, and airway pressure (CPAP) is released (see Fig. 48-24). The release valve must have low-flow resistance to allow adequate emptying of the lungs during pressure release. It is fully opened or closed in less than 10 milliseconds. When the valve opens, a sudden drop in CPAP to ambient pressure (or to a lower preselected level of CPAP) allows gas to leave the lungs and carbon dioxide to be excreted. When the release valve closes, a rapid increase in airway pressure to the original level of CPAP causes the lungs to reexpand (see Fig. 48-24).

Tidal Volume Control

Release VT is the product of the change in airway pressure and CLT (equation 8). Consider a patient breathing with CPAP of 10 cm H_2O and a CLT of 50 mL/cm H_2O. When the release valve in the breathing circuit opens and the circuit pressure decreases to zero, the change in airway pressure is 10 cm H_2O, resulting in an exhaled volume of 500 mL (Fig. 48-25):

$$\text{Volume} = \text{Change in airway pressure} \times C_{LT}$$

$$= 10 \text{ cm } H_2O \times 50 \text{ mL/cm } H_2O \qquad (8)$$

$$= 500 \text{ mL}$$

Release volume with APRV varies with the change in airway pressure (the difference between CPAP and release pressure level), total compliance, total resistance, and release time. A greater change in Paw produces a greater exhaled volume (assuming constant total compliance and resistance). In our experience, a release volume of about 8 to 10 mL/kg seems to be sufficient for most adults.[83,84]

Release volume varies directly with release time. The pressure release time is set in seconds and must equal the time required for adequate lung emptying (approximately 3 or 4 expiratory time constants) to ensure that a sufficient volume of gas is exhaled. A release time of about 1.5 to 2.0

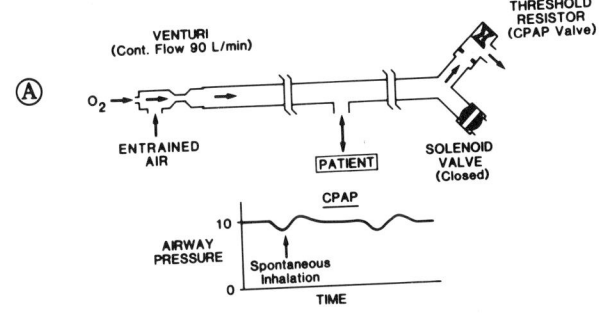

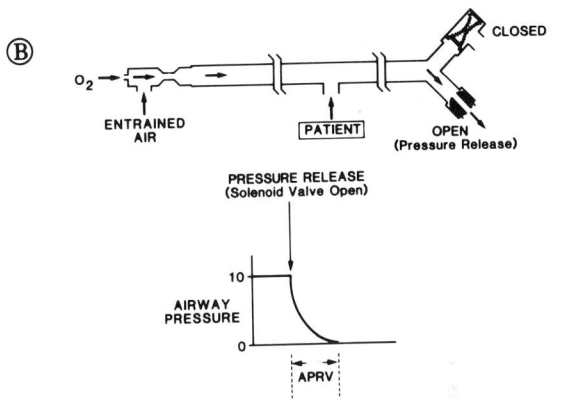

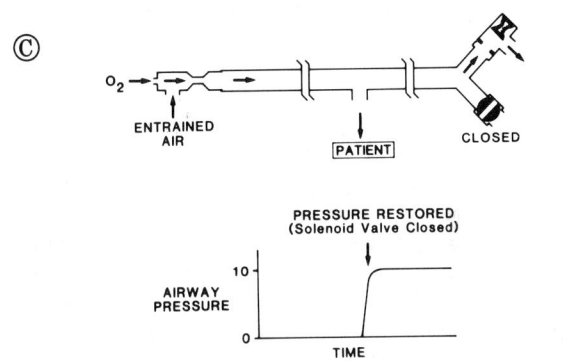

FIGURE 48-24. Principles of airway pressure release ventilation (APRV). Venturi device (Downs Flow Generator, Vital Signs) provides gas at high continuous (Cont) flow rate and controls the fraction of inspired oxygen (F_{IO_2}). Gas flows through the humidifier (not shown) and then to the patient. On the expiratory limb of breathing circuit, a threshold resistor valve with low resistance to flow controls the level of continuous positive airway pressure (CPAP). (**A**) A release (solenoid) valve also attached to expiratory limb is closed, and patient is allowed to breathe spontaneously as desired with CPAP. (**B**) Release valve opens; thus, airway pressure and volume from lungs are released. (**C**) Release valve closes, airway pressure is restored, and patient is allowed to breathe with CPAP. (Florete OG, Banner MJ, Banner TE, et al: Airway pressure release ventilation in a patient with acute pulmonary injury. *Chest* 1989; 96:679.)

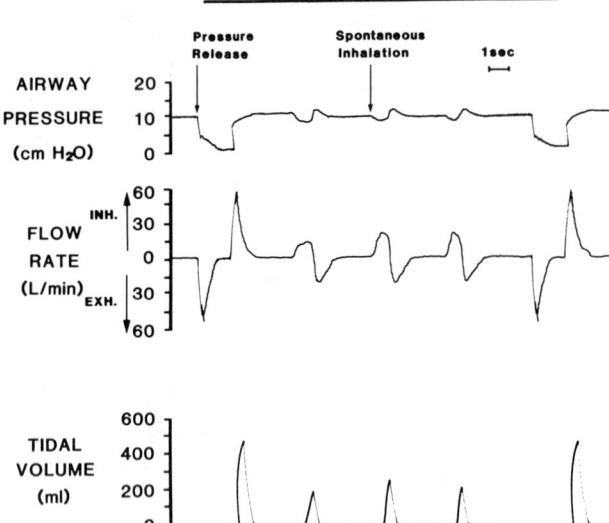

APRV with SPONTANEOUS BREATHING

AIRWAY PRESSURE (cm H₂O)
FLOW RATE (L/min)
TIDAL VOLUME (ml)

FIGURE 48-25. Airway pressure, flow rate, and tidal volume waveforms of a spontaneously breathing patient receiving airway pressure release ventilation (APRV). With APRV, the patient is allowed to breathe spontaneously as desired on continuous positive airway pressure (CPAP). At regular preselected intervals, a release valve opens; thus, pressure, flow, and volume from the lungs are released. After a preselected release time has elapsed, the release valve closes and the level of CPAP is restored, gas flow fills the lungs, and a tidal volume is applied.

seconds seems to be appropriate for adult patients with acute respiratory failure.[82–84]

Selection of CPAP

The level of CPAP is adjusted with two goals in mind: oxygenation and ventilation. "Optimum" CPAP is defined as that level required to optimize arterial oxygenation, the work of breathing, and pulmonary mechanics without depressing cardiac function. It is also adjusted so that the difference between the CPAP level and the release pressure level is appropriate to produce the desired change in volume.

In one study involving 51 patients, APRV was administered so that the difference between CPAP and the release pressure remained constant and equal to the value of the optimum CPAP.[85] Thus, if the patient was receiving 10 cm H₂O CPAP, the difference between that and the release pressure would remain 10 cm H₂O. If arterial oxygenation deteriorated, CPAP and release pressures were increased simultaneously to keep the difference constant and equal to the optimum CPAP value. Used in this manner, an acceptable change in volume was provided and gas exchange was increasingly normal. In our experience with APRV, CPAP levels seem to be one and one half to two times greater than are required for IMV with CPAP in adults with acute respiratory failure.[83,84]

Selection of Patients

Adjusting the APRV rate is similar to adjusting IMV, that is, the rate is decreased to augment spontaneous breathing

or is increased to maximize mechanical support. However, in contrast to IMV, increasing the APRV rate decreases mean airway pressure, because the system is depressurized more frequently. Although APRV allows spontaneous breathing, the patient's minute volume can be controlled by increasing the release-valve opening rate. Thus, APRV can be used in paralyzed patients.

As with IMV, the APRV rate is decreased commensurate with the patient's ability to resume spontaneous ventilation. When mechanical ventilation is no longer required, the release valve is deactivated (i.e., continuously closed), and the system provides constant-flow CPAP.

Comparison With PC-IRV

As previously described, the release valve usually stays open for 1.5 to 2.0 seconds. Thus, the CPAP:release pressure time ratio is usually about 3:1 to 5:1. When the patient is apneic and makes no spontaneous ventilatory effort, the airway pressure waveforms for APRV and PC-IRV are indistinguishable. However, once the patient begins to breathe spontaneously, the difference becomes apparent. APRV allows unrestricted spontaneous breathing during all parts of the ventilatory cycle, whereas PC-IRV requires muscle paralysis, heavy sedation, or both, because no fresh gas flow is available for spontaneous breathing.

Cardiorespiratory Effects

Respiratory and hemodynamic effects of APRV and conventional mechanical ventilation have been compared. After acute lung injury in dogs, APRV was associated with less physiologic dead space, lower airway pressures, and better arterial oxygenation than was conventional ventilation with PEEP.[80] Hemodynamic function was similar during both modes.

After coronary artery bypass grafting, patients were ventilated with APRV and with positive-pressure ventilation and 5 cm H₂O CPAP. APRV was delivered using 10 to 12 cm H₂O CPAP from which airway pressure was released to 2 cm H₂O for 1.5 seconds. Positive-pressure ventilation with CPAP was delivered with a VT of 12 mL/kg. Gas exchange, acid-base status, and hemodynamic function were indistinguishable between the two modes. However, lower airway pressures resulted with APRV.[70]

In another study, 28 adult patients in acute respiratory failure were ventilated with APRV, followed by IMV with CPAP at a similar minute ventilation. Lower PIP and mean airway pressures were noted with APRV. No significant differences in gas exchange and hemodynamic function occurred.[83] An evaluation in adults with more severe acute respiratory failure revealed similar findings.[85]

THE WORK OF BREATHING

The breathing apparatus, which may be defined as the *endotracheal tube*, breathing circuit tubing and valves, and ventilator, represents a series of resistors over which a pressure decrease must be generated by the patient to spontaneously inhale. The endotracheal tube is the primary resistor.[86-89]

MEASUREMENT OF PRESSURE

To accurately assess airway pressure changes during spontaneous breathing with CPAP, pressure should be measured at the tracheal or carinal end of the endotracheal tube (Fig. 48-26). Measuring pressure inside the ventilator or at the Y piece of the breathing circuit (commonly used pressure measuring sites) results in significant *underestimations* of pressure compared with measuring at the carinal end of the endotracheal tube.[90] This observation is especially true when narrow internal diameter endotracheal tubes are used and peak $\dot{V}_I$ demands are high. The narrower the tube and the greater the flow rate demand, the greater the discrepancy in measured pressure inside the ventilator or at the Y piece compared with the carinal end of the endotracheal tube[91,92] (Fig. 48-27).

Rationale

The further from the trachea that pressure is measured, the smaller the deviations in pressure that occur during spontaneous breathing with CPAP, and thus, the more spurious the value in imposed work of breathing, that is, resistive work performed by the patient to breathe spontaneously through the breathing apparatus (calculated by integrating the change in pressure measured at the carinal end of the endotracheal tube and V_T).[91] For example, smaller deviations in pressure and, thus, imposed work are measured at the Y

piece of the breathing circuit compared with the carinal end of the endotracheal tube. Such small deviations during spontaneous inhalation may lead the clinician to conclude, erroneously, that the flow rate provided on demand by the ventilator is sufficient and that the imposed work of breathing is minimal when, in fact, large deviations in a pressure and a high workload are present. The clinician is "blinded" to this situation because of the inappropriate site used for pressure measurement.

The site of pressure measurement also influences the PIP measured during *mechanical* ventilation.[92] During volume-cycled ventilation, PIP varies directly with total resistance (breathing apparatus plus airway) and inversely with C_{LT}. Pressure measured inside the ventilator is generated by the series resistance of the breathing circuit, endotracheal tube, the patient's airways, and the patient's total compliance.

Pressure measured at the carinal end of the endotracheal tube results from the patient's airway resistance and compliance only. Consequently, the PIP measured inside the ventilator will always be greater than at the carinal end of the endotracheal tube (see Fig. 48-27). The narrower the internal diameter of the endotracheal tube, and the greater the mechanical $\dot{V}_I$, the greater the discrepancy in PIP measured inside the ventilator compared with the carinal end of the endotracheal tube.

CARINAL PRESSURE. Two approaches for measuring airway pressure at the carinal end of the endotracheal tube have been described. Endotracheal tubes with a pressure measuring lumen embedded in the sidewall and opening at the carinal end of the tube are commercially available (e.g.,

A. PRESSURE MEASURING SITE: EXHALATION LIMB OF VENTILATOR

SMALLER CHANGE IN AIRWAY PRESSURE

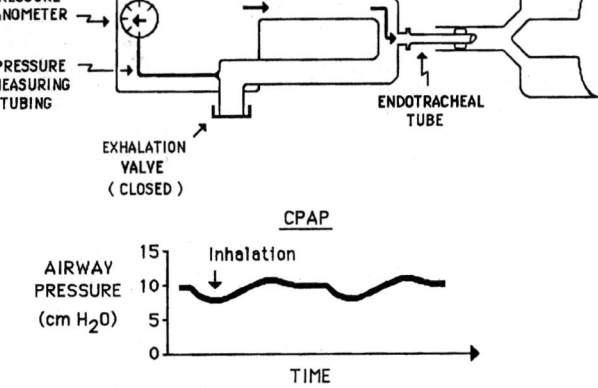

B. PRESSURE MEASURING SITE: TRACHEAL END OF ENDOTRACHEAL TUBE

LARGER CHANGE IN AIRWAY PRESSURE

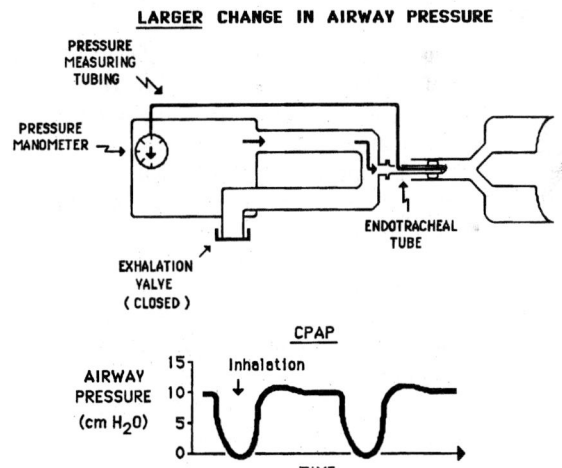

FIGURE 48-26. Effect of the *site* of pressure measurement on changes in airway pressure are illustrated. (**A**) Pressure changes during spontaneous inhalation with continuous positive airway pressure (CPAP) are measured inside the ventilator on the exhalation limb of the breathing circuit (an approach used on many ventilators) and (**B**) in the endotracheal tube at the carinal or tracheal end of the tube. Under similar peak inspiratory flow rate demands, larger changes in pressure are measured at the carinal site because of the resistance of the endotracheal tube. The *true* change in pressure on the airways is at the carinal site, not inside the ventilator. Spuriously smaller changes in pressure are measured inside the ventilator and, thus, should *not* be used.

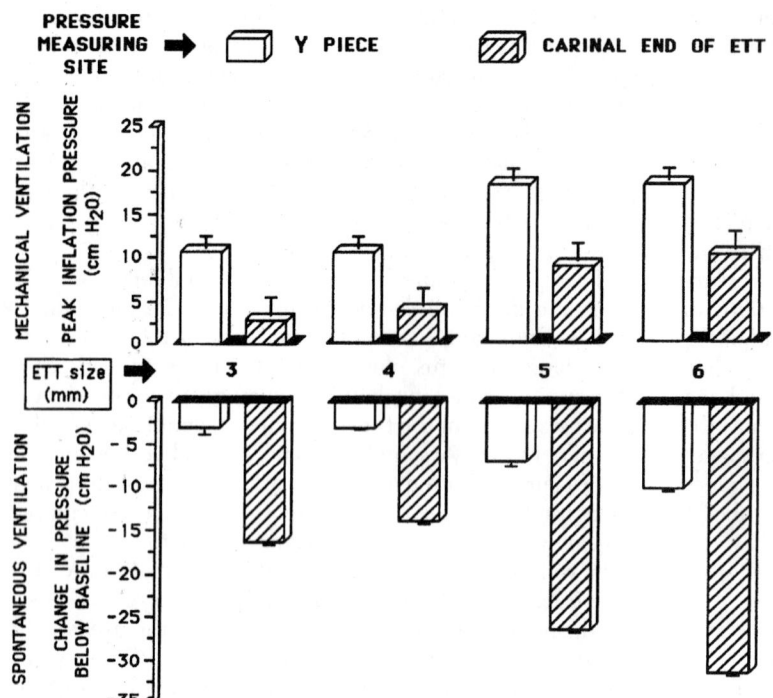

FIGURE 48-27. Comparison of pressure changes measured simultaneously at the Y piece of the ventilator breathing circuit and at the carinal end of the endotracheal tube (ETT) during mechanical and spontaneous inhalation with pediatric-size ETTs. For all ETT sizes, during mechanical inhalation peak inflation pressure is *smaller* at the carinal end of the ETT than at the Y piece; during spontaneous inhalation, *larger* changes in pressure below the baseline are measured at carinal end of the ETT than at the Y piece. The resistance of the ETT is the cause for the discrepancies in pressure. The *true* change in pressure on the airways is at the carinal end of the ETT, *not* at the Y piece.

NCC Malinkrodt, Argyle, NY). This approach has been successfully employed with the Bunnell infant ventilator (Bunnell, Inc, Salt Lake City, Utah) for several years. The other approach is to insert a 1-mm outside diameter catheter into the endotracheal tube (e.g., Bicore Monitoring Inc, Irvine, CA). We have successfully used this approach on adults.[93]

TRIGGERING INSPIRATORY FLOW

Pressure

Initiation of flow during spontaneous inhalation with most demand-flow CPAP systems is accomplished by decreasing the baseline airway pressure to a preselected sensitivity level, that is, the ventilator is pressure-triggered ON. Normally, the pressure measuring/triggering site is *inside* the ventilator on the inspiratory or expiratory limb of the breathing circuit. To initiate flow from the demand-flow system, the patient must overcome the series resistance of the breathing apparatus by generating a pressure differential across the endotracheal tube, breathing circuit tubing, connectors, and valves. This additional workload is the imposed resistive work of the breathing apparatus.

Flow

In addition to providing pressure-triggered spontaneous ventilation, some ventilators provide an option of flow-triggering the ventilator ON. This method of triggering is referred to as *flow-by* triggering with the Puritan-Bennett 7200a ventilator. Flow sensitivity is used to trigger the breaths instead of pressure sensitivity. As an example, a continuous flow rate of 6 L/minute is directed through the breathing circuit, and a triggering sensitivity of 3 L/minute

is preselected. The demand-flow system is triggered ON when, at the onset of inhalation, the patient diverts at least 3 L/minute of gas flow rate from the breathing circuit into the endotracheal tube. The system is flow cycled OFF when the total exhaled flow rate exceeds the preselected continuous flow rate by 2 L/minute.[94]

Modifications

Pressure triggering the ventilator may also be accomplished by moving the triggering site to the carinal or tracheal end the endotracheal tube (see Fig. 48-26*B*). Pressure triggering ON at the carinal end of the endotracheal tube decreases the work of breathing by decreasing the imposed resistance of the endotracheal tube and the remainder of the breathing apparatus.[95–97] Although a different pressure measuring site is used, this approach is similar to the conventional pressure-triggering method described above. The response characteristics of the ventilator's demand-flow system are improved by moving the pressure measuring/triggering site physically closer to the respiratory muscles, that is, at the carinal end of the endotracheal tube.[95,98,99]

Clinical Applications

A clinical study of adults diagnosed with respiratory failure evaluated the effects on total (physiologic plus imposed work), physiologic, and imposed work of breathing comparing conventional pressure, flow, and tracheal pressure triggering methods.[3] Tracheal pressure triggering decreased imposed work to approximately zero and total work decreased significantly by 35% compared with conventional and flow triggering. With tracheal pressure triggering only, a PSV-like effect of approximately 6 cm H_2O occurred, which explained the decrease in work of breathing (Fig. 48-28). Endotracheal tube resistance is effectively eliminated by triggering the ventilator ON at the carinal end of the endotracheal tube.

SPECIAL TECHNIQUES ■

HIGH-FREQUENCY VENTILATION

The term *high-frequency ventilation* is a generic one encompassing three primary techniques: high-frequency positive-pressure ventilation (HFPPV), high-frequency jet ventilation (HFJV), and high-frequency oscillation.[100] Most adult clinical experience in the United States is with HFJV. Gas is accelerated through an injector cannula, and lateral pressure decreases below the ambient level at the nozzle or orifice of

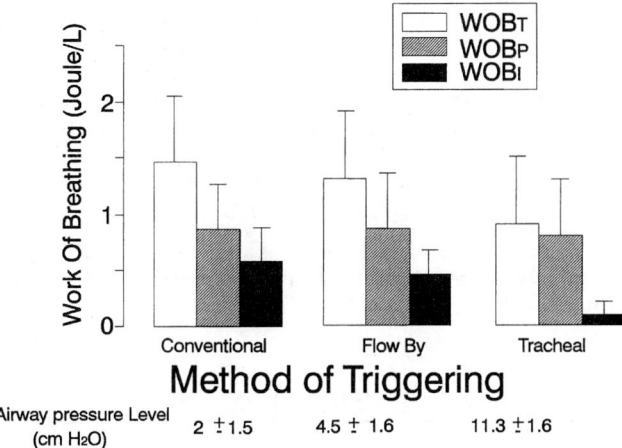

FIGURE 48-28. Comparison of the total work of breathing (WOBT), physiologic WOB (WOBP), and imposed WOB (WOBI) of 14 patients when evaluating three methods of triggering ON a demand-flow continuous positive airway pressure (CPAP) system (Puritan-Bennett 7200ae ventilator) are illustrated. (WOBT equals WOBP plus WOBI.) The level of CPAP was set at 5 cm H_2O for all methods of triggering. *Conventional* triggering relies on measuring a decrease in pressure (triggering pressure) at the onset of the breath *inside* the ventilator (exhalation limb of breathing circuit). *Flow by* triggering relies on measuring a decrease in continuous flow rate (triggering flow rate) at the onset of the breath *inside* the ventilator. *Tracheal* triggering relies on measuring a decrease in pressure (triggering pressure) at the onset of the breath at the *carinal end of the endotracheal tube* (actual airway pressure). The triggering pressure or sensitivity was set at −2 cm H_2O for the conventional and tracheal pressure triggering methods. The continuous and triggering flow rates for flow by triggering were set at 6 and 3 L/minute, respectively. With conventional and flow by triggering, no clinically significant differences in WOBT, WOBP, and WOBI resulted. With tracheal pressure triggering, WOBI decreased significantly. Airway pressure was highest during tracheal pressure triggering, lower during flow by, and least during conventional pressure triggering during spontaneous inhalation. A pressure support ventilation-like effect of approximately 6 cm H_2O resulted during tracheal pressure triggering causing the decrease in WOB. All data are mean ± SD.

the injector. The result is additional gas entrainment, which contributes significantly to the $\dot{V}_I$ and V_T[101] (Fig. 48-29).

Jet Ventilators

A fairly constant inspiratory flow waveform is delivered with HFJV; however, if CLT decreases, Raw increases, or both occur, peak flow delivery and V_T are decreased, and Paw is increased (at the same jet drive pressure and T_I).[101] V_T also decreases as the level of PEEP/CPAP is increased, with constant drive pressure, probably because jet entrainment is inhibited by increased airway–alveolar back pressure.[102,103]

CONTROLS. Three controls are common to most high-frequency jet ventilators: drive pressure, frequency, and percent inspiratory time (%T_I). The drive pressure directly affects V_T and PIP (i.e., increased drive pressure increases V_T and PIP). The %T_I control regulates the duration of inspiration. At a frequency of 100 breaths/minute, the entire ventilatory cycle is 0.6 seconds; if a 20% T_I is selected, T_I is 0.12 seconds and expiratory time is 0.48 seconds. Thus, the I:E ratio is approximately 1:4 or 0.25. Such values commonly are employed in adult patients. Overall characteristics of HFJV are summarized in Table 48-8.

POTENTIAL PROBLEMS. Indications and complications of HFJV are listed in Table 48-9. Inadequate humidification is one of the more common problems reported. Anhydrous gas delivered at high flow rates causes secretions to "cake," particularly in the endotracheal tube. In some instances, total occlusion has occurred, requiring immediate extubation and reintubation. Deleterious effects on the respiratory mucosa and the airways result from breathing dry gas. To minimize this problem, water is infused into the jet stream and nebulized directly into the airway (see Fig. 48-29). Humidity is easily controlled by regulating the drip rate of the water infusion pump; however, care must be taken to avoid fluid overload. An infusion rate of approximately 20 to 30 mL/hour seems satisfactory for most patients.

Another potential complication arises when a specially designed injector lumen endotracheal tube is used. If the

TABLE 48-8. Characteristics of High-Frequency Jet Ventilation

Frequency	100–150 breaths/min
Injector type	(1) 14-gauge steel cannula (internal diameter = 1.7 mm; length = 10 cm)
	(2) Lumen embedded in side wall of a special endotracheal tube
Cycling mechanism	Time
% Inspiratory time	20–30% respiratory cycle
Drive pressure	5–50 psig (directly affects airway pressure, tidal volume, and minute volume)
Tidal volume	Injector flow plus entrained flow (100–300 mL)
Inspiratory flow waveform	Square
Exhalation	Passive

HFJV System

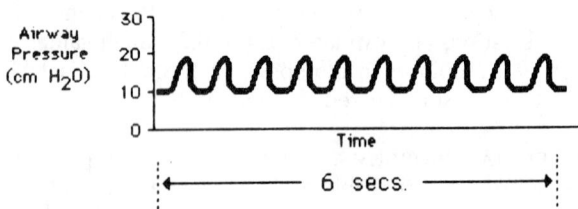

D P: Drive pressure control

FIGURE 48-29. High-frequency jet ventilation (HFJV) system. Gas under pressure (50 pounds per square inch gauge [psig]) at a known fraction of inspired oxygen (FIO_2) is directed to the HFJV ventilator and a flow meter. Drive pressure, adjustable from 5 to 50 psig, is directed into the ventilator's solenoid valve. The opened/closed rate (ventilator rate) and the duration the solenoid valve is open (inspiratory time) are electronically controlled. Tidal volume (VT) is directly proportional to the drive pressure and inspiratory time settings. A continuous flow rate from the flow meter (15 to 20 L/minute) is sent through the circuit. During inhalation, gas is accelerated through a 14-gauge injector that creates subatmospheric pressure at its outlet and causes additional gas to be entrained. VT equals injector volume plus entrained volume. Airway pressure is measured in the endotracheal tube about 15 cm distal to the injector outlet (not shown). Humidification is provided by infusing water (20 to 30 mL/hour) directly into the jet stream and entraining nebulized water. A threshold resistor valve is used to control the level of CPAP. An HFJV rate of 100 breaths/minute with a CPAP of 10 cm H_2O is shown above. (Banner MJ, Desautels DA: Special ventilatory techniques and considerations. In: Kirby RR, Banner MJ, Downs JB [eds]. *Clinical Applications of Ventilatory Support*. Philadelphia, JB Lippincott, 1990:242.)

tip of the endotracheal tube is at or near the carina, and the orifice of the injector lumen is "aimed" toward a main stem bronchus, the bulk of the insufflated flow is directed to one lung, predisposing to maldistribution of ventilation. This problem can be minimized by positioning the endotra-

cheal tube an appropriate distance (approximately 10 cm) from the carina.

TRANSPORT VENTILATION

Ventilation during transport is often administered with a manual self-inflating bag (e.g., Ambu), a flow-inflating (Mapleson) system, or an oxygen-powered breathing apparatus (Elder demand valve or similar device). However, because the VT, respiratory rate, minute ventilation, PIP, and FIO_2 delivered by these devices may vary from breath to breath, a portable time-cycled ventilator is a better alternative.

Mechanical ventilators typically used in the intensive care unit are large and cumbersome and therefore impractical for the transportation of ventilator-dependent patients. Certain characteristics are desirable for a transport ventilator (Table 48-10). It must be light enough for one person to carry easily, compact enough to be stored in a locker or on a bed, and suitable for both adults and for children.[104,105] In addition, the ventilator controls must be easily identified and used.

A variety of portable ventilators have been designed specifically for transporting ventilator-dependent patients. These ventilators range in cost, size, complexity of operation, and modalities of ventilation that can be provided. The Hamilton adult/pediatric transport ventilator (Max) typifies this group of miniature ventilators (Fig. 48-30). It is small (2.5 × 7.5 × 5.5 in); lightweight (1.8 kg [4 lb]); pneumatically (E-size oxygen cylinder) and battery powered; time cycled; and can provide IMV, CMV, sPEEP, and CPPV at a FIO_2

TABLE 48-9. Indications for and Complications of High-Frequency Jet Ventilation

ESTABLISHED INDICATIONS

Bronchopleural fistula
Bronchoscopy
Laryngoscopy

POSSIBLE INDICATIONS

Excessive PIP—may predispose to pulmonary barotrauma, decreased cardiac output, and increased intracranial pressure; lower airway pressures with HFJV might minimize these problems
Hyaline membrane disease—low PIP with HFJV may decrease the incidence of bronchopulmonary dysplasia
Emergency percutaneous transtracheal jet ventilation—for upper airway obstruction, crushed larynx, and similar conditions

COMPLICATIONS

Inadequate humidification
Damage to tracheal mucosa—shear forces from the high-velocity jet pulses may damage these tissues

PIP, peak inflation pressure; HFJV, high-frequency jet ventilation.

TABLE 48-10. Characteristics of a Transport Ventilator

PSV 1–30 cm H_2O
CPAP 15–20 cm H_2O (an upper limit has not been established)
Demand flow rate capabilities ≥120 L/min during spontaneous
 ventilation
Time cycled
Range of IMV of 2–45 breaths/min
PIP ≥150 cm H_2O
Peak mechanical inspiratory flow rate ≥120 L/min
A range of F_{IO_2} of 0.21–1.0
Humidification capabilities
Pneumatically powered
Lightweight (approximately 4.5–9 kg [10–20 lb])
Gas consumption should be minimal
High PIP and disconnect alarms

IMV, intermittent mandatory ventilation; CPAP, continuous
positive airway pressure; PIP, peak inflation pressure; F_{IO_2}, fraction
of inspired oxygen.

of 1.0. (Variable F_{IO_2} may be provided by using an air-oxygen blender.)

SIDE EFFECTS AND COMPLICATIONS ■

SPONTANEOUS BREATHING

An understanding of the effects of any form of airway pressure support must be preceded by a thorough knowledge of events transpiring during spontaneous breathing. With inspiration at ambient pressure, a pressure gradient is established from the mouth to the pleural space, and air flows into the lungs. During expiration, the gradient is reversed.

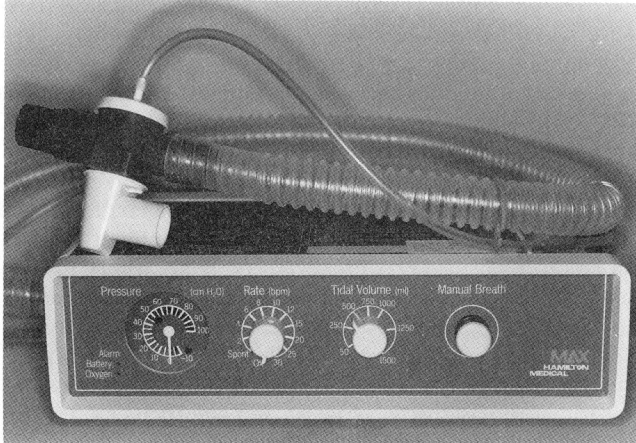

FIGURE 48-30. An example of a portable, easy-to-operate transport ventilator for adult and pediatric (not newborn) patients (Max, Hamilton Medical, Reno, NV). One control sets the ventilator rate, and the other the tidal volume. A demand-flow valve automatically provides gas flow for spontaneous breathing with or without continuous positive airway pressure.

Hemodynamic

Return of venous blood to the heart generally is dependent on the gradient of pressure between the peripheral vasculature and the right atrium. If mean systemic pressure (MSP) rises or right atrial pressure (RAP) falls, venous return increases. Conversely, a fall in MSP or an increase in RAP results in a decrease of venous return. Because blood flow from the right ventricle is dependent on venous return to it, any factors that alter MSP and RAP also affect cardiac output.[106]

INTRAPLEURAL PRESSURE CHANGES. A decrease in intrapleural pressure during inhalation is associated with a similar decrease in RAP, and venous return is thereby augmented. During exhalation, as intrapleural and atrial pressures increase, venous return decreases. These respiratory fluctuations are familiar to anyone who has viewed the direct recording of central venous pressure in a spontaneously breathing patient.

VENTRICULAR INTERDEPENDENCE. Because the right and left ventricles are surrounded by the pericardium, volume changes in one chamber affect the other. An increase of right ventricular volume during inspiration "pushes" the interventricular septum to the left (posteriorly), increasing left ventricular pressure (which decreases left ventricular filling), and changing the spatial configuration and compliance of the left ventricle.

LEFT VENTRICULAR AFTERLOAD. The decrease in intrapleural pressure is also transmitted to the left ventricle. At the peak of spontaneous inspiration (lowest intrapleural pressure), the left ventricular end-diastolic pressure is reduced correspondingly. In contrast, the pressure that must be developed by the ventricle to perfuse the systemic vessels outside the thoracic cavity remains the same. Because the ventricle is initiating contraction from a lower baseline pressure, however, the gradient of pressure that must be generated is increased.

The increment in necessary wall tension represents an increase of left ventricular afterload and may be tolerated poorly by patients with coronary ischemia and compromised ventricular function. Spontaneous breathing with sPEEP, which requires greater decrements in airway and pleural pressures for gas to flow, predisposes to this chain of events. Conversely, a properly functioning CPAP system, with lesser decrements in airway and intrapleural pressures, minimizes such changes.

PULMONARY VASCULAR CHANGES. Expansion of the lungs also affects hemodynamic function. Alveolar vessels are compressed and elongated while pressure and alveolar volume increase. Extraalveolar vessels, however, are pulled open by lung inflation with a consequent decrease in their resistance. When the alveolar vessels are engorged, inspiration decreases net pulmonary blood volume, and pulmonary venous return to the left ventricle may be increased. Conversely, when the alveolar vessels contain less blood, spontaneous inspiration changes alveolar blood volume very little, but a net increase in total pulmonary blood volume and a concomitant decrease in pulmonary venous flow to the left ventricle occurs.

CLINICAL IMPLICATIONS.   Such changes in normal persons during quiet breathing are associated with slightly decreased arterial pressure during inspiration and slightly increased pressure with exhalation. Pathologic conditions that cause exaggerated intrapleural pressure fluctuations (i.e., asthma, COLD, and occluded airway) alter the normal variations described, as do changes in transmitted airway pressure associated with positive-pressure ventilatory support.

Notwithstanding deficiencies in our understanding, a reasoned hypothesis of the cardiovascular effects of sPEEP and CPAP may be advanced, keeping in mind the effects of normal, spontaneous ventilation. Hemodynamic abnormalities involve five major areas[106,107]:

1. *Decreased venous return*: Most studies support the notion that the increase in intrapleural pressure resulting from applied airway pressure reduces the MSP–RAP gradient, impeding venous return. A fall in cardiac output reflects the fact that less blood is returning to the heart.
2. *Decreased right ventricular function*: Acute respiratory failure, positive-pressure ventilation, and PEEP/CPAP may increase pulmonary vascular resistance, singly or in combination. Conceivably, the right ventricle might fail under these conditions. Right ventricular failure, however, is probably not a major direct cause of positive-pressure–induced cardiovascular insufficiency.
3. *Decreased left ventricular function*: Left ventricular dysfunction may result from increased airway pressure, but the changes usually are a result of right ventricular dilatation and interventricular septal shift. The mechanism presumably is similar to that which was earlier described for normal spontaneous breathing. Some investigators question this hypothesis, however. Prewitt and Wood[108] suggest that in selected instances (high PEEP), 50% of the reduction in cardiac output results from left ventricular dysfunction. Clearly, the mechanisms are complex and incompletely understood.
4. *Neural and humoral depression*: In canine cross-circulation studies, PEEP applied to one dog's lungs produced a reduction of cardiac output in both animals.[109] The nature of the depressant substances is unknown.
5. *Reduction of endocardial blood flow*: In some patients, this mechanism may be operative, presumably because of a compromised coronary artery blood supply.[110] Such a decrease has been demonstrated experimentally during PEEP therapy.

Prior cardiac status also has a significant effect on the response of a patient to airway pressure changes. Patients were studied who underwent double aortocoronary bypass grafting and postoperatively were treated with CMV, IMV, and IMV with 5 cm H_2O PEEP.[111] Patients with normal ventricular function before surgery had a large increase in cardiac and stroke volume indices when changed from CMV to IMV, presumably because of increased venous return. Conversely, patients with preoperative left ventricular dysfunction had a significant fall in the same parameters and blood pressure, and a marked rise in RAP and pulmonary artery occlusion pressure (PAOP). Apparently, acute right ventricular overload resulting from resumption of spontaneous breathing produced adverse effects on left ventricular function (ventricular interdependence), possibly by an excessive increase in volume return to the right ventricle. Changeover to IMV returned cardiovascular performance to the CMV levels.

sPEEP AND CPAP.   Most studies show that sPEEP does not affect circulatory function adversely, as long as patients are not hypovolemic. These observations, which seemingly conflict with much of what already has been discussed, may reflect the differences that occur when sPEEP or CPAP is applied to patients with normal or abnormal lungs. In the former case, FRC is increased significantly above normal, and increases in pulmonary vascular resistance result. Also, a maximal transmission of airway pressure to the pleural space occurs with concomitant depression of venous return. Patients with stiff lungs, however, begin with a lower than normal lung volume. As sPEEP or CPAP is applied and lung volume returns toward normal, pulmonary vascular resistance may decrease and unloading of the right ventricle may occur.

Sturgeon and colleagues[112] evaluated the effects of 15 cm H_2O sPEEP or CPAP compared with zero pressure in spontaneously breathing patients after coronary artery bypass grafting. They found that patients had a cardiac output that averaged almost 1 L/minute more with sPEEP compared with either zero pressure or CPAP. Transmural PAOP (PAOP minus intrapleural pressure) decreased by 6 mm Hg with CPAP, indicating that effective preload had been reduced. Presumably, the large inspiratory decrease in pleural pressure during sPEEP compared with either zero pressure or CPAP resulted in enhanced venous return. Also, as pleural pressure increased during expiration, ventricular compression might result and, to some extent, aid ejection.

As was already mentioned, however, the large decrease in intrapleural pressure can be deleterious because of an increase of left ventricular afterload. The net effect on cardiac function of any spontaneous breathing pattern thus depends on many factors. One can postulate that the worst situation for a patient with severe coronary artery disease and left ventricular dysfunction is spontaneous breathing using a high-pressure sPEEP circuit. Under these circumstances, the sharply decreased inspiratory intrapleural pressure floods the right ventricle because of increased venous return, whereas the increase in left ventricular afterload (increased myocardial wall tension) impairs left ventricular output. Substitution of a properly functioning CPAP circuit, all other things remaining equal, would effectively unload the left ventricle and decrease preload in the right ventricle, thereby decreasing the possibility of pulmonary edema formation.

MECHANICAL VENTILATION

Hemodynamic

FALLING PRESSURES. When a ventilator delivers a positive-pressure inflation, airway pressure is raised above ambient pressure or PEEP, intrapleural pressure increases, and right ventricular volume decreases. With maximal transmission of pressure (normal lungs), excessive PEEP or mechanical ventilation increases FRC above normal, decreases overall heart size, and causes the heart to appear small on chest radiographs. Interpretation of ventricular filling pressures is difficult because of the increase in intrapleural pressure and the direct effect of the overexpanded lungs pressing on the pericardium. Thus, CVP and PAOP may be elevated when actual ventricular diastolic volumes (and hence stroke volumes) are decreased.

VENTRICULAR FUNCTION. Transmission of high airway pressure from a mechanical breath increases right ventricular afterload and decreases venous inflow to the right heart. At the same time, transmural aortic pressure and left ventricular afterload are reduced and end-systolic left ventricular volume decreases. The reduced volume of both ventricles can be restored by intravascular volume expansion. However, if the ventilator is removed from a patient with a severely compromised left ventricle, the sudden reduction of airway pressure and transmural pulmonary vascular pressure may predispose to acute pulmonary edema.[113]

Robotham and coworkers[114] summarized the known and postulated effects of the inspiratory phase of IPPV on cardiopulmonary function (Table 48-11). They conclude that the concept of the ventilator acting as a (relatively) noninvasive left ventricular assist device deserves further evaluation.

IMV/SIMV/CPAP. The distinction between the hemodynamic effects of spontaneous breathing, with or without CPAP, and those occurring during positive-pressure ventilation, with or without CPAP, are complicated by IMV/SIMV. Presumably, the additive effects depend on the relative contributions of spontaneous breathing and the mechanical components in a given case, as well as the absolute values of inspiratory and expiratory pressure, VT, baseline cardiovascular status, intravascular volume, and so forth. Also,

ventilator circuit design plays a major role in determining the characteristics of airway (and hence intrapleural) pressure changes during spontaneous breathing, just as is the case with sPEEP and CPAP without positive-pressure mechanical ventilation.[115]

A continuous-flow, low-resistance circuit employing a threshold-resistor expiratory pressure valve generally should enhance cardiovascular function to a greater extent in patients with any degree of left ventricular dysfunction. A poorly functioning demand-flow valve that requires a major inspiratory effort by the patient is relatively contraindicated, both because of the potentially adverse hemodynamic effects and the increased work of breathing associated with its use.

Pulmonary Barotrauma

Pulmonary barotrauma includes pneumothorax, pneumomediastinum, pneumopericardium, pneumoperitoneum and pneumoretroperitoneum, subcutaneous emphysema, and air embolization (venous or arterial). Increased pressure, per se, is not the only cause of barotrauma. Alveolar distension resulting from large VT delivery probably is equally important. No increase in the incidence of barotrauma occurs when positive-pressure ventilation and CPAP are used compared with positive-pressure ventilation alone.[116,117] Pneumothorax frequently occurs during the recuperative phase of ARDS when ventilator pressures and CPAP are decreased but lung volume is increased. The published incidence rate of barotrauma in the mid-1970s was 10% to 20%, but most clinicians believe that it has decreased substantially since that time.

Several iatrogenic complications may predispose a patient to barotrauma. Bronchial intubation that results in the entire VT delivery to one lung is perhaps most obvious. A similar result is possible in the case of unilateral lung disease wherein the decreased compliance and increased Raw of the diseased lung is associated with excess VT delivery to the contralateral healthy lung. If only one lobe of a lung is involved, the adjacent lobes become increasingly distended until alveolar rupture finally takes place. Flow-resistor expiratory pressure valves produce a large rise in airway pressure during coughing and straining, particularly when a high, continuous gas flow rate is present.[68]

A purported advantage to high-frequency ventilation is that lower airway pressure and VT should result in a decreased incidence of barotrauma. Thus far, however, this advantage has not been confirmed, perhaps because an unknown amount of inadvertent PEEP or intrinsic PEEP is generated by air trapping within the lung that is not detectable at the proximal airway. A similar phenomenon is described in adult patients with COLD who develop air trapping because of decreased expiratory time during mechanical ventilation at too rapid a breathing rate.

TABLE 48-11. Beneficial Cardiopulmonary Effects of IPPV

Decreases left ventricular afterload
Improves left ventricular compliance
Compresses heart, aids ejection of blood
"Squeezes" pulmonary vessels, augments left atrial filling
Decreases venous return, pulmonary congestion
Improves oxygenation
Decreases work of breathing

IPPV, intermittent positive pressure ventilation.

(Patten MT, Liebman PR, Hectman HB: Humorally mediated decrease in cardiac output associated with positive end-expiratory pressure. *J Microvase Res* 1977;13:137).

REFERENCES ■

1. Dammann JF, McAslan TC: Optimal flow pattern for mechanical ventilation of the lungs. *Crit Care Med* 1977;5:128

2. Banner MJ, Lampotang S: Clinical use of inspiratory and expiratory flow waveforms. In: Kacmarek RM, Stoller JK (eds). *Current Respiratory Care*. Philadelphia, BC Decker, 1988:139

3. Hedenstierna G, Johansson H: Different flow patterns and their effect on gas distribution in a lung model study. *Acta Anaesthesiol Scand* 1973;17:190

4. Jansson L, Jonson B: A theoretical study of flow patterns of ventilators. *Scand J Respir Dis* 1972;55:237

5. Al-Saady N, Bennett ED: Decelerating inspiratory flow waveform improves lung mechanics and gas exchange in patients on intermittent positive-pressure ventilation. *Intensive Care Med* 1985;11:68

6. Baker AB, Colliss JE, Cowie RW: Effects of varying inspiratory flow waveform and time in intermittent positive-pressure ventilation. II. Various physiologic variables. *Br J Anaesth* 1977;49:1221

7. Johansson H, Lofstrom JB: Effects on breathing mechanics and gas exchange of different inspiratory gas flow patterns during anesthesia. *Acta Anaesthesiol Scand* 1975;19:8

8. Lampotang S: Microprocessor-controlled ventilation systems and concepts. In: Kirby RR, Banner MJ, Downs JB (eds). *Clinical Applications of Ventilatory Support*. New York, Churchill Livingstone, 1990:105

9. Kacmarek RM, Meklaus G: Microprocessor-controlled mechanical ventilators. *Probl Crit Care* 1990;4:161

10. Ashbaugh D, Bigelow D, Petty T, et al: Acute respiratory distress in adults. *Lancet* 1967;2:319

11. Froese AB, Bryan AC: Effects of anesthesia and paralysis on diaphragmatic mechanics in man. *Anesthesiology* 1974;41:242

12. Downs JB, Mitchell LA: Pulmonary effects of ventilatory pattern following cardiopulmonary bypass. *Crit Care Med* 1976;4:295

13. Murphy EJ, Downs JB: Ventilator induced ventilation-perfusion mismatching. *Anesthesiology* 1976;45:A345

14. Fuleihan SF, Wilson RS, Pontoppidan H: Effect of mechanical ventilation with end-inspiratory pause on blood gas exchange. *Anesth Analg* 1976;55:122

15. Boros SJ: Variations in inspiratory:expiratory ratio and airway pressure waveform during mechanical ventilation: the significance of mean airway pressure. *J Pediatr* 1979;94:114

16. Reynolds EOR: Effect of alterations in mechanical ventilator settings on pulmonary gas exchange in hyaline membrane disease. *Arch Dis Child* 1971;46:159

17. Spahr RC, Klein AM, Brown DR, et al: Hyaline membrane disease: a controlled study of inspiratory to expiratory ratio and its management by ventilator. *Am J Dis Child* 1980;134:373

18. Tharatt RS, Allen RP, Albertson TE: Pressure controlled inverse ratio ventilation in severe adult respiratory failure. *Chest* 1988;94:755

19. Gurevitch MJ, Van Dyke J, Young ES, et al: Improved oxygenation and lower peak airway pressure in severe adult respiratory distress syndrome: treatment with inverse ratio ventilation. *Chest* 1986;89:211

20. Cole AGH, Welle SF, Sykes MK: Inverse ratio ventilation compared with PEEP in adult respiratory failure. *Intensive Care Med* 1984;10:227

21. Ravizza AG, Carugo D, Cerchiari EL, et al: Inverse ratio and conventional ventilation: comparison of the respiratory effects [abstract]. *Anesthesiology* 1983;59:A523

22. Greaves TH, Gramolina GM, Walker DH, et al: Inverse ratio ventilation in a 6 year old with severe post-traumatic adult respiratory distress syndrome. *Crit Care Med* 1989;17:588

23. Mathru M, Venus B: Ventilator-induced barotrauma in con-trolled mechanical ventilation versus intermittent mandatory ventilation. *Crit Care Med* 1983;11:359

24. Pepe PE, Hudson LD, Carrico CJ: Early application of positive end-expiratory pressure in patients at risk for the adult respiratory distress syndrome. *N Engl J Med* 1984;311:281

25. Rasanen J, Downs JB: Modes of mechanical ventilatory support. In: Kirby RR, Banner MJ, Downs JB (eds). *Clinical Applications of Ventilatory Support*. New York, Churchill Livingstone, 1990:173

26. Abraham E, Yoshihara G: Cardiorespiratory effects of pressure controlled inverse ratio ventilation in severe respiratory failure. *Chest* 1989;96:1356

27. Kacmarek RM, Hess D: Pressure-controlled inverse ratio ventilation: panacea or auto-PEEP? *Respir Care* 1990;35:945

28. Kirby RR, Robison E, Schulz J: Continuous flow ventilation as an alternative to assisted or controlled ventilation in infants. *Anesth Analg* 1972;51:871

29. Kirby RR, Robison E, Schulz J: A new pediatric volume ventilator. *Anesth Analg* 1971;50:533

30. Downs JB, Klein EF, Desautels D: Intermittent mandatory ventilation: a new approach to weaning patients from mechanical ventilators. *Chest* 1973;64:331

31. Groeger JS, Levinson MR, Carlon GC: Assist control versus synchronized intermittent mandatory ventilation during acute respiratory failure. *Crit Care Med* 1989;17:607

32. Kirby RR: Synchronized intermittent mandatory ventilation versus assist control: just the facts, ma'am. *Crit Care Med* 1989;17:706

33. Kirby RR, Perry JC, Calderwood HW: Cardiorespiratory effects of high positive end-expiratory pressure. *Anesthesiology* 1975;43:533

34. Kirby RR, Downs JB, Civetta JM: High level positive end-expiratory pressure (PEEP) in acute respiratory insufficiency. *Chest* 1975;67:156

35. Poulton TJ, Downs JB: Humidification of rapidly flowing gas. *Crit Care Med* 1981;9:59

36. Downs JB: Ventilatory patterns and modes of ventilation in acute respiratory failure. *Respir Care* 1983;28:586

37. Banner MJ, Downs JB, Kirby RR: Effects of expiratory flow resistance on inspiratory work of breathing. *Chest* 1988;93:795

38. Shapiro BA, Harrison RA, Walton JR: Intermittent demand ventilation (IDV): a new technique for supporting ventilation in critically ill patients. *Respir Care* 1976;21:521

39. Hasten RW, Downs JB, Heenan TJ: A comparison of synchronized and nonsynchronized intermittent mandatory ventilation. *Respir Care* 1980;25:554

40. Heenan TJ, Downs JB, Douglas ME: Intermittent mandatory ventilation: is synchronization important? *Chest* 1980;77:598

41. Brochard L, Harf A, Lorino H, et al: Inspiratory pressure support prevents diaphragmatic fatigue during weaning from mechanical ventilation. *Am Rev Resp Dis* 1989;139:513

42. Kacmarek RM: The role of pressure support ventilation in reducing work of breathing. *Respir Care* 1988;33:99

43. Fiastro JF, Habib MP, Quan SF: Pressure support compensation for inspiratory work due to endotracheal tubes and demand continuous positive airway pressure. *Chest* 1988;93:499

44. MacIntyre NR: Respiratory function during pressure support ventilation. *Chest* 1986;89:677

45. MacIntyre NR: Weaning from mechanical ventilatory support: volume-assisting intermittent breaths versus pressure-assisting every breath. *Respir Care* 1988;33:121

46. MacIntyre NR: Pressure support ventilation. *Probl Crit Care* 1990;4:225

47. MacIntyre NR, Nishimura M, Usada Y, et al: The Nagoya conference on system design and patient-ventilator interac-

tions during pressure support ventilation. *Chest* 1990;97:1463

48. Cohen CA, Zaglebaum G, Gross D, et al: Clinical manifestations of inspiratory muscle fatigue. *Am J Med* 1982;73:308

49. MacIntyre NR, Ho L: Effects of initial flow rate and breath termination criteria on pressure support ventilation. *Chest* 1991;99:134

50. Cohen IL, Bilen Z, Krishnamurthy S: The effects of ventilator working pressure during pressure support ventilation. *Chest* 1993;103:588

51. Branson RD, Campbell RS, Davis K, et al: Altering flow rate during maximum pressure support ventilation: effects on cardiorespiratory function. *Respir Care* 1990;35:1056

52. Czervinske MP, Shreve J, Lester KB, et al: Effects of working pressure on respiratory pattern and airway pressure during pressure support ventilation in infants with chronic lung disease [abstract]. *Respir Care* 1988;33:930

53. Banner MJ, Blanch PB, Kirby R: Work of breathing during pressure support ventilation affected by rises in pressure and flow rate [abstract]. *Anesthesiology* 1994;81:A270

54. Messida A, Ben-Ayed M, Brochard L, et al: Comparison of the efficacy of two waveforms of inspiratory pressure support: slow vs fast pressure wave [abstract]. *Am Rev Respir Dis* 1990;141:A519

55. Cane R, Campbell R, Goldsberry D, et al: Effect of inspiratory rise time (IRT) setting during pressure support ventilation (PSV) on patient work of breathing [abstract]. *Crit Care Med* 1995;23:A120

56. Stenz R, Calzia E, Lindner KH: Effect of pressure increase time and trigger threshold on work of breathing and pressure time product during pressure support ventilation [abstract]. *Crit Care Med* 1995;23:A124

57. MacIntyre NR, Gropper C, Westfall T: Combining pressure-limiting and volume-cycling features in a patient-interactive mechanical breath. *Crit Care Med* 1994;22:353

58. Younes M: Proportional assist ventilation: a new approach to ventilatory support. *Am Rev Respir Dis* 1992;145:114

59. Younes M, Puddy A, Roberts D, et al: Proportional assist ventilation. *Am Rev Respir Dis* 1992;145:121

60. Hewlett AM, Platt AS, Terry VG: Mandatory minute volume: a new concept in weaning from mechanical ventilators. *Anesth Analg* 1977;32:163

61. Forette TL, Cairo JM: Mandatory minute volume: a conceptual approach. *Curr Rev Respir Crit Care* 1988;10:163

62. Quan SF, Parides GC, Knoper SR: Mandatory minute volume (MMV) ventilation: an overview. *Respir Care* 1990;35:898

63. Kacmarek RM, Dimas S, Reynolds J, et al: Technical aspects of positive end expiratory pressure (PEEP). I. Physics of PEEP devices. *Respir Care* 1982;27:1478

64. Kirby RR: Positive airway pressure: system design and clinical application. In: Shoemaker WC (ed). *Critical Care: State of the Art*, vol 5. Fullerton, CA, Society of Critical Care Medicine, 1985:61

65. Mushin WW, Rendell-Baker L, Thompson PW: *Automatic Ventilation of the Lungs*, 3rd ed. Oxford, Blackwell Scientific Publications, 1980:105

66. Marini JJ, Culver BH, Kirk W: Flow resistance of exhalation valves and positive end expiratory pressure devices used in mechanical ventilation. *Am Rev Respir Dis* 1985;131:850

67. Banner MJ, Lampotang S, Boysen PG, et al: Resistance characteristics of expiratory pressure valves [abstract]. *Anesthesiology* 1986;65:A80

68. Banner MJ: Expiratory positive-pressure valves: flow resistance and work of breathing. *Respir Care* 1987;32:431

69. Gal TJ: Effects of endotracheal tube intubation on normal cough performance. *Anesthesiology* 1980;52:324

70. Douglas M, Downs JB: Special correspondence. *Anesth Analg* 1978;57:347

71. Gibney RTN, Wilkson RS, Pontoppidan H: Comparison of work of breathing on high gas flow and demand valve continuous positive airway pressure systems. *Chest* 1982;82:692

72. Cox D, Niblett DJ: Studies on continuous positive airway pressure breathing systems. *Br J Anaesth* 1984;56:905

73. Op't Holt TB, Hall MW, Bass JB, et al: Comparison of changes in airway pressure (CPAP) between demand valve and continuous flow devices. *Respir Care* 1982;27:1200

74. Gjerde GE, Katz JA, Kramer RW: Inspiratory work and airway pressure with continuous positive airway pressure delivery systems [abstract]. *Crit Care Med* 1984;12:272

75. Henry WC, West GA, Wilson RS: A comparison of the oxygen cost of breathing between a continuous flow CPAP system and a demand-flow CPAP system. *Respir Care* 1983;28:1273

76. Zwillich CW, Pierson DJ, Creagh CE, et al: Complications of assisted ventilation: a prospective study of 354 consecutive episodes. *Am J Med* 1974;57:161

77. Fleming WH, Bowen JC: Early complications of long-term respiratory support. *J Thorac Cardiovasc Surg* 1972;64:729

78. Cournand A, Motley HL, Werko L, et al: Physiological studies of the effect of intermittent positive-pressure breathing on cardiac output in man. *Am J Physiol* 1948;152:162

79. Downs JB, Stock MC: Airway pressure release ventilation: a new concept in ventilatory support [editorial]. *Crit Care Med* 1987;15:459

80. Stock MC, Downs JB, Frolicher DA: Airway pressure release ventilation. *Crit Care Med* 1987;15:462

81. Garner W, Downs JB, Stock MC, et al: Airway pressure release ventilation: a human trial. *Chest* 1988;94:779

82. Stock MC, Downs JB: Airway pressure release ventilation. *Probl Crit Care* 1990;4:217

83. Banner MJ, Kirby RR, Banner TE: Airway pressure release ventilation in patients with acute respiratory failure. *Crit Care Med* 1989;17:S32

84. Florete O, Banner MJ, Banner TE, et al: Airway pressure release ventilation in a patient with acute pulmonary injury. *Chest* 1989;96:679

85. Räsänen J, Cane R, Downs JB, et al: Airway pressure release ventilation in severe acute respiratory failure. *Crit Care Med* 1989;17:S32

86. Bolder PM, Healy EJ, Bolder AR, et al: The extra work of breathing through adult endotracheal tubes. *Anesth Analg* 1986;65:853

87. Fiastro JF, Habib MP, Quan SF: Pressure support compensation for inspiratory work due to endotracheal tubes and demand continuous positive airway pressure. *Chest* 1988;93:499

88. Bersten AD, Rutten AJ, Vedig AE, et al: Additional work of breathing imposed by endotracheal tubes, breathing circuits, and intensive care ventilators. *Crit Care Med* 1989;17:671

89. Shapiro M, Wilson RK, Casar G, et al: Work of breathing through different sized endotracheal tubes. *Crit Care Med* 1986;14:1028

90. Banner MJ, Kirby RR, Blanch PB: Site of pressure measurement during spontaneous breathing with continuous positive airway pressure: effect on calculating imposed work of breathing. *Crit Care Med* 1992;20:528

91. Banner MJ, Blanch PB, Kirby RR: Imposed work of breathing and methods of triggering demand-flow, continuous positive airway pressure system. *Crit Care Med* 1993;21:183

92. Saqer JG, Banner MJ, Blanch PB, et al: Effect of pressure measuring *SITE* on change in airway pressure during spontaneous and mechanical ventilation. *Crit Care Med* 1995;23 (Suppl 1):A187

93. Banner MJ, Kirby RR, Blanch PB, et al: Decreasing imposed work of the breathing apparatus to zero using pressure-support ventilation. *Crit Care Med* 1993;21:1333

94. *Puritan-Bennett Corporation Technical Manual*, no. 20535 B. Carlsbad, CA, Puritan-Bennett Corporation, 1989:5

95. Banner MJ, Blanch PB, Kirby RR: Imposed work of breathing and methods of triggering a demand-flow, continuous positive airway pressure system. *Crit Care Med* 1993;21:183

96. Messinger G, Banner MJ, Gabrielli A, et al: Tracheal pressure triggering a demand-flow CPAP system decreases work of breathing. *Anesthesiology* 1994;81:A272

97. Messinger G, Banner MJ, Blanch PB, et al: Using tracheal pressure to trigger the ventilator and control airway pressure during continuous positive airway pressure decreases work of breathing. *Chest* 1995;108:509

98. Kacmarek RM, Shimada Y, Ohmura A, et al: The second Nagoya conference: triggering and optimizing mechanical ventilatory asst. *Respir Care* 1991;36:45

99. MacIntyre N, Nishimura M, Usada Y, et al: The Nogoya conference on system design and patient-ventilator interactions during pressure support ventilation. *Chest* 1990;97:1463

100. Froese AB: High frequency ventilation: a critical assessment. In: Shoemaker WC (ed). *Critical Care: State of the Art*, vol 5. Fullerton, CA, Society of Critical Care Medicine, 1984:1

101. Carlon GC, Miodownik S, Ray C: High frequency jet ventilation. In: Carlon GC, Howland WS (eds). *High Frequency Ventilation in Intensive Care and During Surgery*. New York, Marcel Dekker, 1985:77

102. Schlacter MD, Perry ME: Effect of continuous positive airway pressure on lung mechanics during high frequency jet ventilation. *Crit Care Med* 1984;12:755

103. Hamilton LH, Londino JM, Linehan JH: Pediatric endotracheal tube designed for high frequency ventilation. *Crit Care Med* 1984;12:988

104. Murphy EJ, Desautels DA, Modell JH: A compact ventilator and headboard ventilator transport system. *Crit Care Med* 1978;6:387

105. Downs JB, Marston AW: A new transport ventilator: an evaluation. *Crit Care Med* 1977;5:112

106. Pinsky MR: Cardiovascular effects of ventilatory support and withdrawal. *Anesth Analg* 1994;79:567

107. Pick RA, Handler JB, Friedman AS: The cardiovascular effects of positive end-expiratory pressure. *Chest* 1982;82:345

108. Prewitt RM, Wood LH: Effects of positive end-expiratory pressure on ventricular function in dogs. *Am J Physiol* 1972;236:H534

109. Patten MT, Liebman PR, Hechtman HB: Humorally mediated decrease in cardiac output associated with positive end-expiratory pressure. *J Microvasc Res* 1977;13:137

110. Laver MB: The pulmonary response to trauma and mechanical ventilation: its consequences on hemodynamic function. *World J Surg* 1983;7:31

111. Mathru M, Rao TLK, El-Etr AA, et al: Hemodynamic response to changes in ventilatory patterns in patients with normal and poor left ventricular reserve. *Crit Care Med* 1982;10:423

112. Sturgeon CL, Douglas ME, Downs JB, et al: PEEP and CPAP: cardiopulmonary effects during spontaneous ventilation. *Anesth Analg* 1977;56:633

113. Beach T, Millen E, Grenvik A: Hemodynamic response to discontinuation of mechanical ventilation. *Crit Care Med* 1973;1:85

114. Robotham JL, Cherry D, Mitzner W, et al: A reevaluation of the hemodynamic consequences of intermittent positive-pressure ventilation. *Crit Care Med* 1983;11:783

115. Katz JA, Marks JD: Inspiratory work with and without continuous positive airway pressure in patients with acute respiratory failure. *Anesthesiology* 1985;63:598

116. Kumar A, Pontoppidan H, Falke KJ, et al: Pulmonary barotrauma during mechanical ventilation. *Crit Care Med* 1973;1:181

117. Kirby RR: Best PEEP: issues and choices in the selection and monitoring of PEEP levels. *Respir Care* 1988;33:569

Critical Care, Third Edition, edited by Joseph M. Civetta,
Robert W. Taylor, and Robert R. Kirby.
Lippincott-Raven Publishers, Philadelphia, PA © 1997.

CHAPTER 49

◾

Ventilatory Support Modes

Orlando C. Kirton

The decision to initiate ventilatory support, until recently, usually meant intubation, based on the need to manage hypoxemic or hypercapnic respiratory insufficiency, to decrease the patient's work of breathing, or to assure airway patency and facilitate pulmonary toilet. In most applications of ventilatory support, the objectives are to normalize alveolar ventilation and to achieve and maintain a level of adequate arterial oxygenation by augmenting inspiratory and expiratory lung volumes respectively. This chapter does not address every one of the varied and complex modes available, but provides a basis for understanding the setup parameters, advantages, and limitations of the most common modes; this includes the noninvasive techniques, which do not require intubation, as well as the truly assisted and near-total ventilatory support modalities.

NONINVASIVE TECHNIQUES ◾

FACE MASK CONTINUOUS POSITIVE AIRWAY PRESSURE

Continuous positive airway pressure (CPAP) elevates airway pressure above atmospheric pressure throughout spontaneous inspiration and exhalation. It increases lung volume and improves oxygenation by elevating functional residual volume above the closing volume, thereby preventing airway closure and alveolar collapse.[1] CPAP is also used to reduce the pressure gradient between the mouth and the alveoli in patients with air trapping. Because it only assists spontaneous breathing, it requires an intact respiratory drive and adequate alveolar ventilation.

Setup Parameters

Setup parameters include pressure level, flow rate, sensitivity, and amount of inspiratory pressure descent (demand

valves or flow triggered system) or flow rate (continuous-flow system).

Suggested Initial Settings

The demand-flow system requires a minimal triggering effort, approximately 1 cm H_2O (or slightly more to avoid auto cycling); the flow rate is adjusted to avoid deflection of more than 2 to 4 cm H_2O below baseline during peak inspiration; set the continuous-flow system to 2.5 to 3 times minute volume and titrate to produce a 2 to 4 cm H_2O pressure drop during inspiration; the larger the deflection during inspiration, the greater the work for the patient.

Advantages

CPAP offers the benefit of positive end-expiratory pressure (PEEP) to spontaneously breathing patients. It improves oxygenation if hypoxemia is caused by decreased lung volume. It may help reduce the work of breathing in patients with dynamic hyperinflation and auto PEEP.

Disadvantages

Hyperinflation, barotrauma, and carbon dioxide (CO_2) retention may occur secondary to fatigue in patients with marginal ventilatory reserve.

Work of Breathing

Excessive expiratory work may result if excessive CPAP levels are used. High flow resistance or inadequate inspiratory flow rates may increase inspiratory work of breathing.[2]

Data suggest that the work of breathing is reduced with systems incorporating a continuous-flow system in comparison with demand-flow systems.[3] Active contraction of expir-

745

atory muscles (and associated expiratory work) will occur if CPAP levels increase the functional residual capacity above normal.

NASAL CPAP

When CPAP is required in extubated patients in the ICU, it is commonly applied by full face mask. Whereas the efficiency of full face mask CPAP is widely accepted, the mask is often poorly tolerated by patients.[4] Nasal continuous positive airway pressure (N-CPAP) is extensively used in treating the sleep apnea syndrome and has been successfully applied to managing patients with pulmonary atelectasis secondary to neurologic disease and exacerbated chronic obstructive lung disease (COLD), patients who have had cardiac surgery, and patients with *Pneumocystis* infection and viral pneumonia.[4-8]

Setup Parameters

A 5 cm H_2O end-expiratory pressure (EEP) pop-off valve is positioned in close proximity to the nasal mask (Fig. 49-1). Connection is best made using an Adams pillow. This nasal bridge cushion provides improved patient comfort and a more reliable seal around the nares. The pillows are held in position with a standard headgear assembly. Circumferential cushioned plastic masks are also available. Humidified gas is necessary to avoid drying of the nasal mucosa. Nasogastric tubes are not used for airway pressures of less than 15 cm H_2O to preserve an airtight seal.

Suggested Initial Settings

For the patient with hypoxemic respiratory failure, the initial settings of CPAP can be 5 cm H_2O. Oxygen flows at 5 to 15 L/minute are used. Nasal settings then are adjusted for optimal comfort and oxygenation using the following guidelines: for the patient with hypoxemic respiratory failure, CPAP is raised in 2–cm H_2O steps until satisfactory oxygenation is achieved (pulse oximetry oxygen saturation [SpO_2] >0.92; fraction of inspired oxygen [FIO_2] <0.4).

Advantages

The nasopharyngeal pressure generated with N-CPAP does not differ significantly from that produced during full face mask CPAP. The continued use of N-CPAP by patients with the sleep apnea syndrome suggests that it is well tolerated.[9] Therefore, it may find a role in situations where the advantage of CPAP is outweighed by the discomfort of a full face mask. Examples of this include the prevention of episodic obstructive apnea after opiate administration and as an adjunct to physiotherapy in the treatment of pulmonary atelectasis after abdominal surgery.

Disadvantages

The role of N-CPAP in the severely hypoxemic, nonintubated, critically ill patient needs to be clarified. The N-CPAP system does not generate high levels of PEEP as reliably as a full face mask CPAP system without high inspiratory flow rates, which are expensive and may lead to patient discomfort. In addition, major disadvantages of N-CPAP are the loss of airway pressure during mouth breathing and the requirement for patient cooperation. By tensing the soft palate, patients can completely obstruct the flow of gas from the N-CPAP system. This may limit its usefulness in patients with severely impaired pulmonary oxygen transfer. A full face mask, if tolerated, produces a more continuous level of positive airway pressure. CO_2 retention may occur with N-CPAP as with face mask CPAP. In addition, hyperinflation and barotrauma can occur.

Work of Breathing

Similar to face mask CPAP, N-CPAP reduces the inspiratory work of breathing and, in patients with obstructive airway disease, the expiratory work of breathing.

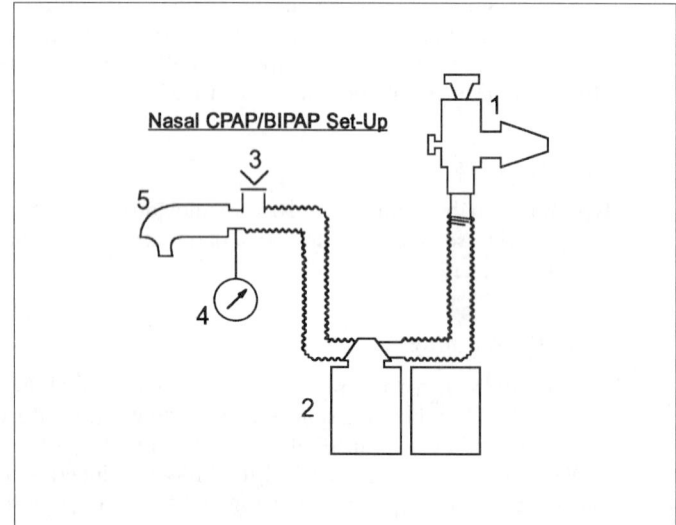

FIGURE 49-1. Nasal continuous positive airway pressure (CPAP)–bilevel positive airway pressure (BIPAP) circuit: (1) Downs adjustable flow generator; (2) Concha thermal humidifer; (3) CPAP [expiratory positive airway pressure (EPAP)] valve; (4) pressure monitor; (5) nasal mask attachment.

BILEVEL POSITIVE AIRWAY PRESSURE

The goals of bilevel positive airway pressure (BIPAP) are to improve patient comfort while providing inspiratory and end-expiratory lung volume augmentation, without the physical and psychological trauma associated with tracheal intubation.[10] The improvement in gas exchange with BIPAP is comparable with that of conventional mechanical ventilation in the hemodynamically stable patient with respiratory failure. BIPAP has been successfully used in treating patients with sleep apnea, acute respiratory failure, nocturnal muscle fatigue, and COLD.[11]

Setup Parameters

The BIPAP ventilatory support system is based on a standard nasal CPAP flow generator (see Fig. 1). A valve sets two pressure levels, the expiratory positive airway pressure (EPAP) level (equivalent to PEEP in conventional mechanical ventilation), and the inspiratory positive airway pressure (IPAP) level (equivalent to pressure support ventilation), even in the presence of rapidly changing flows. In this spontaneous mode setting, the unit cycles from EPAP to IPAP when the patient's inspiratory flow exceeds 40 mL/second for more than 30 milliseconds. The IPAP level is maintained for more than 180 milliseconds and will return to EPAP when (1) the inspiratory flow decreases below a threshold level, (2) an active expiratory effort is detected, or (3) BIPAP has lasted 3 seconds. The mask usually consists of a triangular, solid plastic shell with a light-weight, flexible silicon rubber attachment such that the rubber can conform to the facial contour. A head band secures the nasal mask firmly in place so that no or little gas leaks at the mask/face junction. The gas must be delivered through a tightly fitting mask.

Suggested Initial Settings

For the patient with hypoxemic respiratory failure, the initial settings of the BIPAP system can be 5 cm H_2O EPAP and 10 cm H_2O IPAP. For the patient with hypercapnic respiratory failure, set EPAP at 2 cm H_2O and IPAP at 10 cm H_2O with oxygen flows at 5 to 15 L/minute. To improve oxygenation by augmenting functional residual capacity (FRC), EPAP can be raised in 2 to 5 cm H_2O increments while IPAP is kept at a fixed increment above EPAP (approximately 5 to 10 cm H_2O difference). For the patient with hypercapnic respiratory failure, IPAP is increased by 2 cm H_2O intervals with EPAP held constant. Nasal fittings are then adjusted for optimal comfort. If the patient's inspiratory effort fails to trigger the IPAP phase, the mode of ventilation is changed to timed, and the rate set to two breaths per minute less than the estimated spontaneous respiratory rate, the percentage of IPAP is set to 30%.

Advantages

Bilevel positive airway pressure has been used successfully in patients with mild to moderate hypoxemic or hypercapnic respiratory failure, associated with a low incidence of complications (e.g., gastric distention, aspiration or mask disloca-

tion).[10,11] This noninvasive ventilatory technique allows speech and feeding without mask removal, as well as continuous support for patients unable to tolerate periodic discontinuation.

Disadvantages

The most persistent complication of BIPAP has been abrasion of the bridge of the nose, which limits the application to intermittent use; however, by applying a patch of wound care dressing, the problem can be eliminated and a continuous support mode can be used. A major disadvantage of nasal BIPAP is the loss of airway pressure during mouth breathing. This may limit its usefulness in patients with severely impaired pulmonary oxygen transfer, where a full face mask will, if tolerated, produce more continuous level of CPAP.[10]

Work of Breathing

Relative to CPAP, BIPAP does provide a theoretic advantage in that the work of inspiration is assisted by positive-pressure support ventilation. BIPAP provides inspiratory pressure support, allows afterload reduction of the ventilatory muscles, and decreases the patient's work of breathing.

TRULY ASSISTED VENTILATION ■

INTERMITTENT MANDATORY VENTILATION

Intermittent mandatory ventilation (IMV) is a mode of ventilation that combines a preset number of ventilator-delivered mandatory breaths of predetermined tidal volume (VT) and patient-generated spontaneous breaths.[12] Minute ventilation is the summation of patient-initiated (high pressure–low volume, if compliance is low) breaths and preset ventilator (high volume–high pressure) breaths.[13] Several ventilators offer pressure-targeted breaths instead of volume-targeted breaths during mandatory cycles. If the mandatory breaths are patient triggered, the technique is termed synchronized (SIMV).

Setup Parameters

Parameters of IMV include VT, flow rate or inspiratory time (T_I), frequency of controlled breaths, and demand-valve sensitivity (Fig. 49-2). When pressure-targeted breaths are used, pressure level and T_I must be set.

Suggested Initial Settings

The following are the suggested settings for IMV: set VT, 10 to 12 mL/kg; T_I, 1.5 to 2 seconds (or flow rate adjusted to provide this T_I with the set VT); initial IMV rate (postoperative), four breaths per minute if the patient is awake to eight breaths per minute if still anesthetized or paralyzed; trigger effort, 1 cm H_2O or more to prevent auto cycling (SIMV); FIO_2, 0.4 (unless hypoxic in operating room); PEEP, 5 cm H_2O; and high-pressure limit approximately 25% above peak inspiratory pressure.

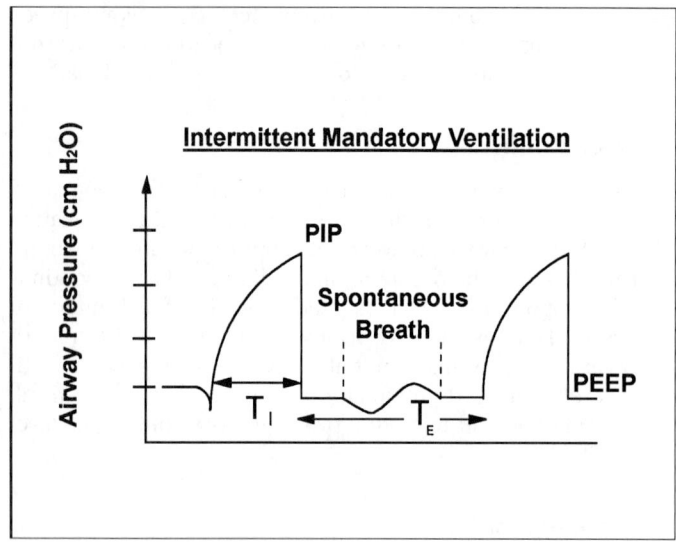

FIGURE 49-2. Intermittent mandatory ventilation. PEEP, positive end-expiratory pressure; PIP, peak inflation pressure; T_I, inspiratory time; T_E, expiratory time.

Advantages

Advantages of IMV are that the patient performs a variable amount of respiratory work yet there is the security of the preset mandatory volume cycled ventilator breaths. IMV or SIMV allows varying support from continuous mechanical ventilation (IMV rates >10/minute) to spontaneous breathing (IMV rate = 0) and thus can be used as a weaning tool.

Disadvantages

With IMV, the machine-delivered volume may be provided at the peak of a spontaneous breath and are high volume, high pressure.[14] This combination has been associated with barotrauma and progressive lung injury.[15,16] Worsening dynamic hyperinflation has been described in patients with COLD.[17] The spontaneous V_T in a patient with poor compliance may not exceed dead space and may add nothing to alveolar ventilation.

Work of Breathing

During IMV, minute ventilation is fractionated in a horizontal axis and represents the summation of preset, ventilator-delivered, volume-limited breaths (high volume–high pressure) and the patient's spontaneous (high pressure–low volume) breaths. Spontaneous breaths have a high associated work. Extra work may be imposed on the patient during spontaneous breathing because of the presence of a poorly responsive demand-valve system, suboptimal ventilator circuit, or inappropriate flow delivery. This can be minimized or abolished with the addition of pressure support. The total work performed by the patient is dependent on the number of mandatory breaths. The work of breathing may be less with the use of pressure-targeted mandatory breaths.[12]

PRESSURE SUPPORT VENTILATION

Pressure support ventilation (PSV) is a pressure-triggered, pressure-targeted, flow-cycled mode of ventilation.[13] It is used as a mode of ventilation during stable ventilatory support periods and in weaning. PSV can be used to unload the ventilatory muscles and decrease the inspiratory work of breathing and total oxygen consumption.[18] This ventilatory technique augments spontaneous breaths and offsets the work imposed by the endotracheal tube and breathing apparatus. Because the PSV is designed to assist spontaneous breathing, the patient must have an intact respiratory drive. At initiation of inspiration, the pressure rises rapidly to the preselected positive airway pressure that is maintained for the remainder of inspiration. Gas flow from the ventilator cycles off, when the patient's inspiratory flow rate decreases to a predetermined percentage of the initial inspiratory flow rate, usually 25%. The patient and the ventilator work in synchrony to achieve the total work required for each breath.

Setup Parameters

Parameters of PSV include pressure level and sensitivity; no mandatory PSV rate is set (Fig. 49-3). In some ventilators, it is possible to adjust the rate of rise in the pressure at the beginning of inspiration or to adjust the flow threshold for cycling from inspiration to expiration. Many ventilators incorporate volume-targeted backup modes in the event of apnea.

Suggested Initial Settings

The following are the suggested initial settings in PSV: set trigger level at 1 cm H_2O or more to prevent auto cycling; flow triggering, set (as instructed by device manufacturer's recommendation) so that minimal inspiratory effort (1 to 2 cm H_2O) will initiate the breath; the initial level of PSV can be estimated by this author's formula, selecting a value corresponding to one half of the peak inflation pressure (PIP) minus PEEP during a mechanical breath, adjusting as necessary to provide initial augmented V_Ts of 7 to 8 mL/kg; add one SIMV breath at a V_T of 10 to 12 mL/kg (sigh breath to prevent atelectasis); and set T_I and flow rate to

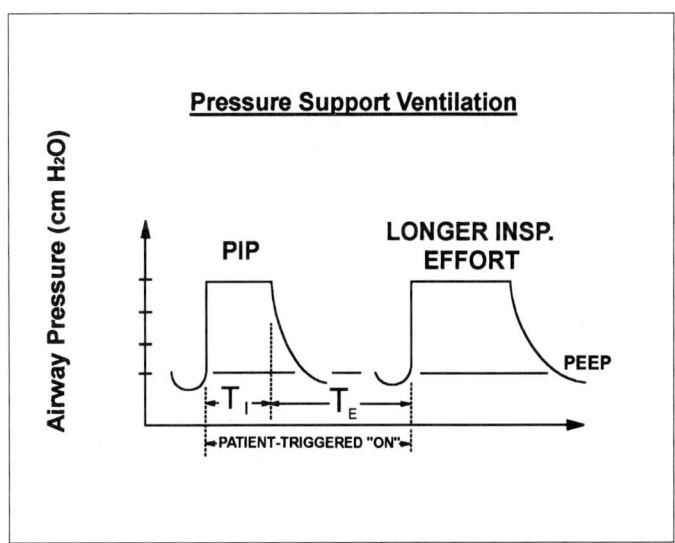

FIGURE 49-3. Pressure support ventilation. PEEP, positive end-expiratory pressure; PIP, peak inflation pressure; T_I, inspiratory time; T_E, expiratory time.

allow Vᴛ to be delivered in 1.5 to 2.0 seconds. Titrate pressure support to unload the respiratory muscles to negate the imposed work of breathing while maintaining physiologic work of breathing (0.5 to 1 J/L).

Advantages

With PSV, improved patient ventilator synchrony and comfort have been identified in published literature and clinical practice. The patient interacts with the pressure-assisted breath but retains control over T_I and flow rate, expiratory time (T_E), frequency, Vᴛ, and minute ventilation. Pressure-limited ventilation using a rapidly decelerating flow delivery pattern is associated with lower peak airway pressure and more rapid improvement in static thoracic compliance compared with IMV or CMV.[14] PSV should also be used to compensate for the imposed work produced by the endotracheal tube, the demand-valve system, and breathing circuit. It permits variation from nearly total ventilatory support to essentially spontaneous breathing. PSV may be useful in patients who are difficult to wean.

Disadvantages

In PSV, Vᴛ is not controlled and varies with compliance, cycling frequency, and synchrony between the patient and ventilator. Backup mandatory ventilation is recommended for unstable patients. One or two volume-cycled breaths (10 to 12 mL/kg) per minute may prevent atelectasis. PSV may be poorly tolerated in patients with high-airway resistance because of the preset high initial flow and terminal respiratory flow algorithms. Adjustment of initial flow rates, which is possible in newer systems, may ameliorate this problem.

Work of Breathing

Increasing PSV level decreases inspiratory respiratory efforts. PSV can be used alone or in combination with SIMV to neutralize the additional work of breathing caused by the endotracheal tube and the demand valve, that is, the imposed work of breathing. PSV can be used during weaning to reload the respiratory muscle pump while preserving a normal physiologic work of breathing. With PSV, the total minute ventilation is fractionated in a vertical plane in which each spontaneous breath is supplemented by positive pressure. Total work of breathing also is decreased secondary to improved ventilator patient synchrony. Work of breathing is less with flow triggering compared with pressure triggering.[3]

AIRWAY PRESSURE RELEASE VENTILATION

Airway pressure release ventilation (APRV) is another technique that minimizes lung expansion.[19] APRV is a pressure-controlled, time-triggered, pressure-limited, time-cycled ventilation that allows spontaneous breathing throughout the ventilator cycle. In this mode, CPAP (usually 10 to 20 cm H_2O) is maintained until the time release valve opens, allowing the pressure in the system to fall to a lower preset level, usually the functional residual capacity or a lower preset EEP. When the release valve closes again, insufflation rapidly restores the original airway inflation pressure.[20] This form of mechanical ventilation is the opposite of the intermittent positive-pressure ventilation methods in terms of the direction of lung volume change. In conventional and spontaneous ventilation, inspiration increases lung volume to eliminate CO_2; APRV achieves this goal by decreasing lung volume and eliminates large volume changes above the optimal resting lung volume. The goal of APRV is to limit peak airway pressures, thereby minimizing barotrauma and cardiac compromise. There are two types of pressure release ventilation: APRV during which pressure release time is preset and intermittent mandatory pressure release ventilation (IMPRV),[21] which is integrated into the ventilator circuit, providing EEP change according to the patient's spontaneous breathing activity. Oxygenation is improved by increasing CPAP, lengthening T_I, or increasing FIO_2 while CO_2 elimination is effected by increasing the APRV rate and the airway pressure change (i.e., release pressure). When compared with conventional intermittent positive-pressure ventilation plus PEEP, APRV was shown to produce comparable oxygenation and hemodynamic effects at lower peak and EEPs but similar mean airway pressures in patients with acute respiratory failure.[22]

Setup Parameters

Respiratory monitoring and alarms are available with APRV (Fig. 49-4). During APRV, the following respiratory parameters are preset: upper and lower airway pressure levels (i.e., CPAP and EEP, respectively), T_I, frequency of pressure release, and pressure release time (T_E). During IMPRV, the following respiratory parameters are preset: upper and lower PEEP levels, frequency of PEEP changes, and sensitivity of the trigger. Ventilatory assistance is progressively decremented by decreasing the spacing of PEEP-CPAP changes (e.g., positive airway pressure released every two, three, four, five, six ventilatory cycles, and so forth, to spontaneous expiration).

Suggested Initial Settings

The following are suggested initial settings in APRV: set F_{IO_2} to maintain Pa_{O_2} at 65 mm Hg or higher; set CPAP initially at 20 cm H_2O; EEP (FRC), 0 to 10 cm H_2O; release pressure; T_E fixed at 1.5 seconds to three or more times the T_E constant of the patient (airway resistance [Raw] × lung compliance [C_L]) to avoid auto PEEP; set APRV rate of four to eight breaths per minute, depending on level of sedation. The following formula can be used: T_I (in seconds) = 60 (seconds)/frequency (breaths per minute) − T_E (in seconds).

Advantages

An advantage of APRV is that it allows spontaneous breathing. The potential for alveolar hyperinflation and iatrogenic lung injury is minimized. Also, there is improved matching of ventilation and perfusion at lower peak and EEPs, and theoretically, less hemodynamic compromise.

Disadvantages

Airway pressure release ventilation has not been evaluated in patients with poor compliance. It is not applicable in patients with severe airflow obstruction. Minute ventilation must be carefully monitored. Excessive auto PEEP may develop if the respiratory frequency increases above 30 breaths/minute. Spontaneous inspiration coinciding with airway pressure release may cause sustained hyperinflation or may be compensated by an increased ventilatory drive during APRV. Synchronization of spontaneous inspiration increases ventilatory efforts and decreases respiratory drive.[17]

Work of Breathing

Spontaneous breathing ensures sustained patient effort and prevents atrophy. Imposed work of breathing is minimal. Fatigue can occur if the APRV frequency is set too low.

NEAR-TOTAL VENTILATORY SUPPORT ■

ASSIST CONTROL VENTILATION

In assist control (A/C) ventilation, every patient breath is supported by the ventilator. The ventilator delivers a breath, either when triggered by the patient's inspiratory effort (assist) or independently, if such an effort does not occur within a preselected period (control). Volume-cycled and pressure-limited or pressure-targeted modes are available.

Setup Parameters

Using volume-targeted A/C ventilation, the V_T, inspiratory flow rate, flow wave form, sensitivity, and mandatory ventila-

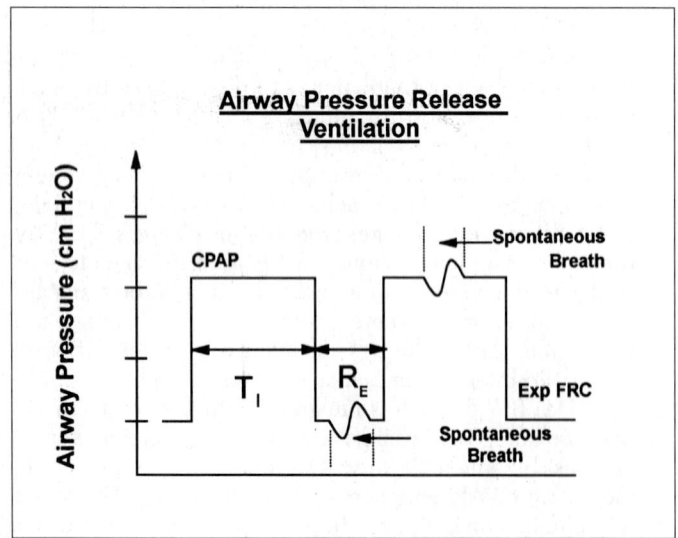

FIGURE 49-4. Airway pressure release ventilation. Spontaneous breaths are shown. PIP, peak inflation pressure; PEEP, positive end-expiratory pressure; CPAP, continuous positive airway pressure; T_I, inspiratory time; T_E, expiratory time; R_E, release (expiratory) time; Exp FRC, expiratory functional residual capacity.

tory rate are set (Fig. 49-5). With pressure-limited or pressure-targeted A/C modes, pressure level, T_I, mandatory ventilatory rate, and sensitivity are set.

Suggested Initial Settings

The suggested initial settings are as follows: set backup rate, six to eight breaths per minute; flow rate (60 to 80 L/minute) commensurate with patient's spontaneous inspiratory flow demand or to achieve inspiratory–expiratory (I:E) ratio of at least 1:2 to avoid auto PEEP; V_T, 8 to 10 mL/kg; high-pressure limit 20% greater than peak inspiratory pressure; and trigger, 1 cm H_2O or more to avoid auto cycling.

Advantages

Assist control ventilation combines the security of controlled ventilation with the possibility of synchronizing the breathing rhythm of the patient and ventilator, and it ensures ventilatory support during each breath.

Disadvantages

Excessive patient work occurs in cases of inadequate peak flow or inspiratory sensitivity setting, especially if the patient's respiratory drive is excessive. Volume-targeted A/C ventilation may be poorly tolerated in awake, nonsedated patients and may require sedation to ensure synchrony of patient and machine cycle lengths. This mode of ventilatory support can be associated with respiratory alkalosis and may potentially lead to stacking of breaths, air trapping, and barotrauma. Pressure-targeted A/C ventilation may result in inadequate minute ventilation during changes in lung impedance, patient-ventilatory drive, or patient-ventilatory dyssynchrony.[13]

Work of Breathing

Patient work of breathing or effort during volume-targeted A/C ventilation is dependent on the ability of the ventilator to rapidly recognize patient effort (demand-valve sensitivity) and provide sufficient flow to meet inspiratory demand (flow rate <40 L/minute should probably be avoided) and the respiratory drive of the patient. Improper ventilator setup or malfunction (i.e., inadequate flow rate or demand-valve sensitivity) may cause a significant imposed work load, resulting in either dyspnea, tachypnea, and hyperventilation or ventilator intolerance and fatigue with eventual hypercapnic respiratory failure. Concern with excessive patient work is potentially minimized by using pressure-targeted A/C ventilation. Pressure-targeted A/C ventilation, once triggered, is more likely to provide sufficient flow to allow the set pressure plateau level to be achieved rapidly. When properly functioning, however, a major disadvantage is that the patient essentially performs no work. If A/C ventilation is continued for more than 1 or 2 weeks, muscle atrophy may develop. Weaning will then be more difficult and prolonged.

INVERSE RATIO VENTILATION

Inverse ratio ventilation (IRV) uses T_Is greater than exhalation, thus reversing the normal ratio of inhalation to exhalation of 1:2 (see Fig. 49-5). It may be created by pressure-controlled or volume-cycled modes. Pressure-controlled IRV with a rapidly decelerating inspiratory flow pattern is more widely used than volume-cycled IRV in patients with adult respiratory distress syndrome (ARDS).[23] There is a lack of convincing data to support any outcome superiority of IRV over conventional ventilation, although it is popular because it limits peak inspiratory pressures.[24] Because high volume, rather than high pressure, has been identified as causing pulmonary damage, limiting peak inspiratory pressure has no proven advantage.[16] In addition, inversion of conventional I:E ratios produces no significant improvement in the overall cardiorespiratory profile. Its proposed clinical

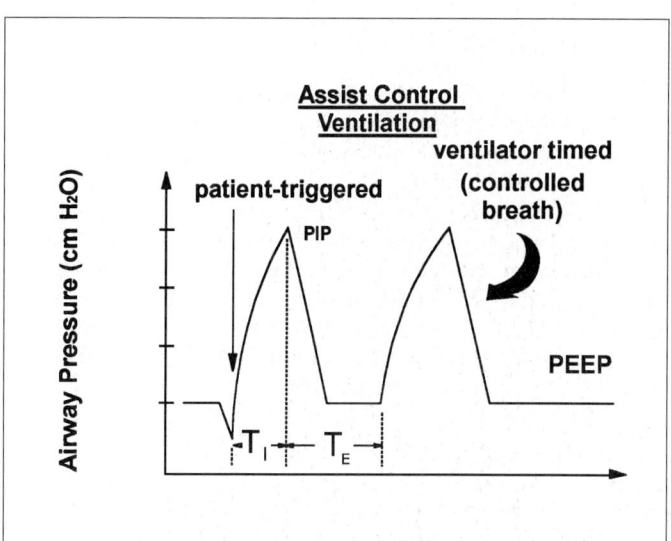

FIGURE 49-5. Assist-control ventilation. PEEP, positive end-expiratory pressure; PIP, peak inflation pressure; T_I, inspiratory time; T_E, expiratory time.

use is in advanced ARDS with refractory hypoxemia or hypercapnia.[25]

Setup Parameters

The following are the setup parameters for IRV. Choose the pressure limit desired. Increase time of inspiration or inspiratory hold incrementally until oxygen and CO_2 elimination are in desired range (Fig. 49-6). Deep sedation or paralysis is nearly always required in most patients to avoid dyssynchrony with the ventilator. Careful monitoring of peak airway pressure and end-inspiratory plateau pressure are required during volume-control IRV. The high-pressure alarm should be set at 10 cm H_2O above intended peak airway pressure. Careful monitoring of minute ventilation is required during pressure-control IRV; V_T is markedly dependent on the patient's respiratory mechanics. Auto PEEP may develop as the I:E ratio increases and should be regularly measured. Because auto PEEP and increased mean airway pressure associated with IRV may compromise cardiac function, hemodynamic status should be assessed using a pulmonary artery catheter when IRV is implemented.

Suggested Initial Settings

The following are the suggested initial settings for IRV: set pressure limit arbitrarily at half the prior peak inspiratory pressure; the I:E ratio should be 1.5:1 to 2:1 with either T_I control or flow rate control; trigger effort is usually not synchronized to patient's inspiratory effort; set high-pressure alarm at 10% above pressure limit; adjust PEEP and FIO_2 (<50%) to maintain a PaO_2 of 65 mm Hg or more.

Advantages

The advantages of IRV are that peak airway (alveolar) pressures are minimized while maintaining relatively high mean airway pressure, and prolongation of inspiration allows recruitment of lung units with long-time constants.

Disadvantages

Disadvantages of IRV include excessive gas trapping, which can cause auto PEEP and barotrauma. Cardiac output and tissue oxygen delivery may fall while mean airway pressure and auto PEEP increase, although several studies report no significant alteration in oxygen transport.[26,27] V_T varies with changing respiratory mechanics, therefore minute ventilation must be monitored carefully. With pressure-controlled IRV, progressive atelectasis can occur in the presence of poor lung compliance. Deep sedation or paralysis are frequently required, which produces the potential for atrophy and detraining of the respiratory musculature.

Work of Breathing

Patient effort is minimal with IRV because this form of ventilatory support usually requires moderate sedation or paralysis.

HIGH-FREQUENCY VENTILATION

High-frequency ventilation (HFV) uses small V_Ts (1 to 3 mL/kg) at high frequencies (100 to 300 breaths/minute). The mechanism of gas transfer changes from conventional bulk flow to other types when V_T is less than the volume of dead space (V_D). Proposed mechanisms include coaxial flow, Taylor dispersion, pendelluft, and augmented molecular diffusion. The V_T and frequency product is usually much higher than during conventional mechanical ventilation. Alveolar ventilation seems to be influenced more by V_T than frequency. Several types of high-frequency ventilation exist. The three most common are high-frequency oscillation; high-frequency positive-pressure ventilation, which is used in anesthesia; and high-frequency jet ventilation, which is used in anesthesia and in the critically ill patient with acute respiratory failure.[28]

Setup Parameters

In HFV, the clinician sets the driving pressure, T_I, respiratory rate, FIO_2, and PEEP. Adequate humidification of delivered gases is mandatory if high-frequency jet ventilation is to be administered for periods longer than 8 hours. Mean airway pressure, which approximates alveolar pressure, should be continuously monitored using an endotracheal catheter located at least 5 cm from the injection site. PaO_2 is affected by altering the FIO_2 and PEEP. Increase in the I:E ratio and the driving pressure increase the V_T and decrease the partial pressure of carbon dioxide ($PaCO_2$). Increasing respiratory frequency, decreasing the driving pressure, and decreasing T_I, decrease V_T and increases $PaCO_2$. FRC also can be increased by increasing the I:E ratio, driving pressure, and respiratory frequency.

Suggested Initial Settings

Follow the manufacturer's device-specific algorithms or recommendations because settings vary with type of high-frequency ventilator and type of circuit used. The following settings may be used initially: HFV, T_I of 0.3 seconds; ventilatory frequency 80 to 100/minute; drive pressure, 30 to 40 psi; titrate to achieve acceptable low mean airway pressure and adequate alveolar ventilation; adjust PEEP and FIO_2 (<50%) to maintain PaO_2 of 65 mm Hg or more.

Advantages

High-frequency ventilation is useful during laryngoscopy, bronchoscopy, tracheal surgery, bronchopleural fistula, and tracheoesophageal fistula.[28] A prospective randomized study comparing high-frequency jet ventilation with conventional ventilation performed in a nonhomogeneous population of cancer patients with ARDS did not demonstrate any significant advantage over conventional methods.[29] Ultrahigh-frequency ventilation (up to rates of 900 breaths/minute) has improved oxygenation and the elimination of CO_2 at lower airway pressures, but no clinical trials have shown superior outcome. A subset of patients with hypovolemia may be more likely to tolerate high-frequency jet ventilation compared with CMV.

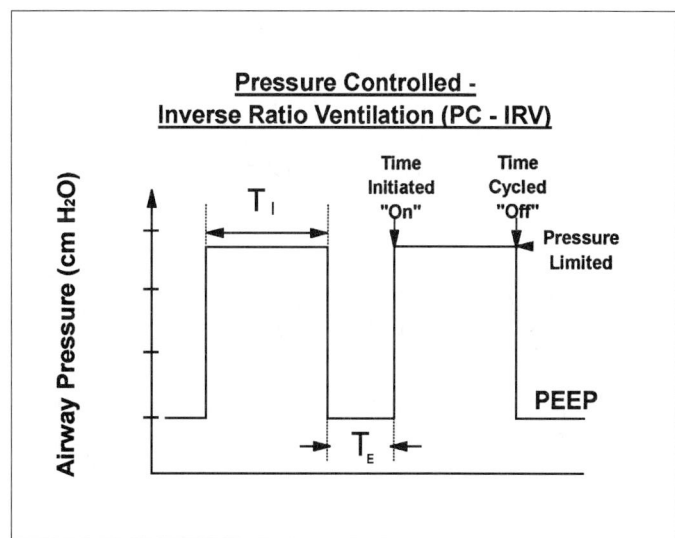

FIGURE 49-6. Pressure controlled–inverse ratio ventilation. PEEP, positive end-expiratory pressure; T_I, inspiratory time; T_E, expiratory time.

Disadvantages

Outflow obstruction can rapidly lead to increases in lung volume, which can cause hemodynamic compromise and barotrauma. Air trapping is especially of concern in patients with compliant lungs and airway obstruction. It can be assessed by measuring airway opening pressure under static conditions after airway occlusion by monitoring esophageal pressure, or by measurements of lung volume obtained at the chest wall (e.g., inductive plethysmography). Inadequate humidification can induce severe necrotizing tracheobronchitis. Long-term jet ventilation can result in squamous metaplasia with submucosal inflammatory cell infiltration.

Work of Breathing

Patients do no work of breathing whether paralyzed or not. Some work is done while driving pressure is decreased. Work is increased when the patient is switched to conventional weaning.

MINIMAL EXCURSIONARY VENTILATION

If alveolar hyperinflation is the primary etiologic factor causing the structural lung injury associated with positive-pressure ventilation, a reduction in cyclical volume expansion during mechanical ventilation should be expected to be beneficial.[16] This approach has been called minimal excursionary ventilation (MEV); several approaches are available (Chap. 45).

PERMISSIVE HYPERCAPNIA

The term *permissive hypercapnia* is inaccurate and it is suggested that it be termed *iatrogenic hypercapnia*. The choice of increasing continuous mechanical ventilation with paralysis (whether this is called pressure control or volume preset ventilation) or intentionally diminishing or providing

inadequate Vts as a means to limit peak inspiratory pressure, may both result in increased V_D/V_T and retention of CO_2. The retention of CO_2 is not permitted, but rather is caused by the physician who selects that mode of ventilatory support. The simplest method of minimal excursionary ventilation is controlled hypoventilation. In this approach, total minute ventilation is reduced and the consequent rise in $PaCO_2$ is accepted, provided the pH is greater than 7.2. $PaCO_2$ as high as 90 mm Hg has been reported[15]; if bicarbonate is conserved, pH will increase, just as in the metabolic compensation for the respiratory acidosis associated with COLD.

EXTRACORPOREAL CO_2 REMOVAL WITH VENOVENOUS BYPASS USING A MEMBRANE OXYGENATOR

Carbon dioxide is removed by a membrane oxygenator while arterial oxygenation by the native lung is enhanced by CPAP. Mechanical Vts are limited by 45 cm H_2O peak inflation pressure. The reduction in lung volume excursions during ventilatory support result in less injury visualized at pathologic examination. This technique, first described by Gattinoni and others,[30] has not been found superior to conventional mechanical ventilation in prospective controlled trials. Also, extracorporeal CO_2 removal is expensive, effort intensive, and entails complications, especially related to the systemic heparinization.[31]

IVOX (INTRAVASCULAR OXYGENATOR)

This technique of extrapulmonary gas exchange does not require an extracorporeal circuit. The intravascular oxygenator is a device made of several hundred gas-permeable hollow fibers that are inserted into the vena cava by femoral cut-down. Flow of gas through each fiber adds oxygen and removes carbon dioxide from the bloodstream. Insertion of the IVOX was found to decrease cardiac index and systemic oxygen delivery despite maximum fluid and inotropic support in a study by Gentilello and coworkers.[32] Mortality was

80%. Although some gas exchange occurred, the device did not allow significant reduction in the level of mechanical ventilatory support and adversely affected systemic oxygen transport. It is unclear what role IVOX may eventually play in the treatment of severe respiratory failure, although the concept is exciting because it does not require extracorporeal circulation.

SPONTANEOUS AUGMENTED LOW-VOLUME VENTILATION

I prefer spontaneous augmented low-volume ventilation, using PSV as the primary ventilatory support mode. Spontaneous ventilation directs flow of gas to regions of low ventilation–perfusion, increasing efficiency in gas exchange.[33] Positive-pressure ventilation, on the other hand (i.e., IMV, A/C, CMV), directs ventilation to areas of high $\dot{V}/\dot{Q}$ ratios, increasing dead space ventilation and potentially worsening hypoxemia. In addition, high-volume ventilation should be avoided because it has been associated with increased lung damage. PSV can augment V_T to provide adequate alveolar ventilation. I monitor patient work of breathing using a microprocessor-based monitor (CP_{100}, Bicore Inc., Irvine, CA) and titrate the level of PSV to ensure that the patient always performs an acceptable physiologic work of breathing (thus avoiding disuse atrophy). PSV is also adjusted to avoid a fatiguing work load (use dystrophy) resulting from the imposed work of breathing (endotracheal tube, breathing circuit, demand valve system) and the increased work of underlying parenchymal and chest wall disease. PEEP is used to recruit FRC, decrease intrapulmonary shunt, and improve ventilation to areas of low $\dot{V}/\dot{Q}$ ratios. This allows F_{IO_2} to be decreased to less than 0.4, which avoids exacerbating injury caused by free radicals and late absorption atelectasis. PSV monitored by patient work of breathing combined with PEEP should create less injury from lower V_T, usually 5 to 6 mL/kg, to achieve a breathing frequency less than 38 breaths/minute and near-normal Pa_{CO_2}. Reversing or preventing atelectasis is important in correcting hypoxemia and in modifying (limiting) the progression of the underlying pathophysiologic process; accordingly, one 10 mL/kg IMV breath per minute is included. It is clear that underinflation is equally deleterious to the injured lung as alveolar overinflation. Spontaneous augmented low-volume ventilation does allow for iatrogenic hypercapnia in situations where mean alveolar pressure or peak inspiratory pressure needs to be limited (i.e., hemodynamic compromise).

I believe that this philosophy avoids the heavy-handed approach of over-ventilation and prevents atrophy and ventilator dependency; I hope it will be cheaper and more effective, and it should result in more survivors who have less residual pulmonary damage. Ventilatory support is withdrawn by decreasing PSV, allowing reloading of the ventilatory muscles while the patient maintains work of breathing within an acceptable range. The patient is not subjected to the clinician's perception that support can be discontinued and weaning begun. Rather, mechanical supplementation is only added if the patient cannot accomplish the full work of breathing needed to overcome the disease and is withdrawn as the disease resolves. Extubation follows without a separate weaning process.

REFERENCES ■

1. Devita MA, Friedman Y, Petrella V: Mask continuous positive airway pressure in AIDS. *Crit Care Clin* 1993;9:137
2. Moran JL, Homan S, O'Fathartaigh M, et al: Inspiratory work imposed by continuous positive airway pressure (CPAP) machines: the effect of CPAP level and endotracheal tube size. *Intensive Care Med* 1992;18:148
3. Banner MJ, Blanch PB, Kirby RR: Imposed work of breathing and methods of triggering a demand-flow, continuous positive airway pressure system. *Crit Care Med* 1993;21:183
4. Thomas AN, Ryan JP, Doran BRH, et al: A nasal CPAP system: description and comparison with facemask CPAP. *Anesthesia* 1992;47:311
5. Lucas P, Tarancón C, Puente L, et al: Nasal continuous positive airway pressure in patients with COPD in acute respiratory failure: a study of the immediate effects. *Chest* 1993;104:1694
6. Baratz RM, Westbrook PR, Shah PK, et al: Effect of nasal continuous positive airway pressure on cardiac output and oxygen delivery in patients with congestive heart failure. *Chest* 1992;102:1397
7. Thomas AN, Ryan JP, Doran BRH, et al: Nasal CPAP after coronary artery surgery. *Anesthesia* 1992;47:316
8. Petrof BJ, Kimoff RJ, Levy RD, et al: Nasal continuous positive airway pressure facilitates respiratory muscle function during sleep in severe chronic obstructive pulmonary disease. *Am Rev Respir Dis* 1991;143:928
9. Kribbs NB, Pack AI, Kline LR, et al: Effects of one night without nasal CPAP treatment on sleep and sleepiness in patients with obstructive sleep apnea. *Am Rev Respir Dis* 1993;147:1162
10. Pennock BE, Kaplan PP, Carlin BW, et al: Pressure support ventilation with a simplified ventilatory support system administered with a nasal mask in patients with respiratory failure. *Chest* 1991;100:1371
11. Lien TC, Wang JH, Chang MT, et al: Comparison of BIPAP nasal ventilation and ventilation via iron lung in severe stable COPD. *Chest* 1993;104:460
12. Sassoon CSH, Del Rosario N, Fei R, et al: Influence of pressure-and on flow-triggered synchronous intermittent mandatory ventilation on inspiratory muscle work. *Crit Care Med* 1994;22:1933
13. Slutsky AS: ACCP consensus conference mechanical ventilation. *Respir Care* 1993;38:1389
14. Rappaport SH, Shipner R, Yoshihara G, et al: Randomized, prospective trial of pressure-limited versus volume-controlled ventilation in severe respiratory failure. *Crit Care Med* 1994;22:22
15. Bray JG, Cane RD: Mechanical ventilatory support and pulmonary parenchymal injury: positive airway pressure or alveolar hyperinflation. *Intensive Crit Care Dig* 1993;12:33
16. Dreyfuss D, Soler P, Bassett G, et al: High inflation pressure pulmonary edema/respective effects of high airway pressure, high tidal volume and positive end-expiratory pressure. *Am Rev Respir Dis* 1988;137:1159
17. Putensen C, Leon MA, Putensen-Himmer: Timing of pressure release affects power of breathing and minute ventilation dur-

ing airway pressure release ventilation. *Crit Care Med* 1994; 22:872

18. Tokioka H, Saito S, Kosaka F: Comparison of pressure support ventilation and assist control ventilation in patients with acute respiratory failure. *Intensive Care Med* 1989;15:364

19. Davis K, Johnson DJ, Branson RD, et al: Airway pressure release ventilation. *Arch Surg* 1993;128:1348

20. Cane RD, Peruzzi WT, Shapiro BA: Airway pressure release ventilation in severe acute respiratory failure. *Chest* 1991; 100:460

21. Rouby JJ, Ameur MB, Jawish D, et al: Continuous positive airway pressure (CPAP) vs intermittent mandatory pressure release ventilation (IMPRV) in patients with acute respiratory failure. *Intensive Care Med* 1992;18:69

22. Räsänen J, Cane RD, Downs JB, et al: Airway pressure release ventilation during acute lung injury: a prospective multi-center trial. *Crit Care Med* 1991;19:1234

23. Papadakos PJ, Halloran W, Hessney JI, et al: The use of pressure-controlled inverse ratio ventilation in the surgical intensive care unit. *J Trauma* 1991;31:1211

24. Marcy TW, Marini JJ: Inverse ratio ventilation in ARDS: rationale and implementation. *Chest* 1991;100:494

25. Chan K, Abraham E: Effects of inverse ratio ventilation on cardiorespiratory parameters in severe respiratory failure. *Chest* 1992;102:1556

26. Abraham E, Yoshihara G: Cardiorespiratory effects of pressure controlled inverse ratio ventilation in severe respiratory failure. *Chest* 1989;96:1356

27. Mercat A, Graini L, Teboul JL, et al: Cardiorespiratory effects of pressure controlled ventilation with and without inverse ratio in the adult respiratory distress syndrome. *Chest* 1993; 104:871

28. Standiford TJ, Morganroth ML: High-frequency ventilation. *Chest* 1989;96:1380

29. Carlon GC, Howland W, Ray C Jr, et al: High frequency jet ventilation: a prospective randomized evaluation. *Chest* 1983; 84:551

30. Gattinoni L, Kolobow T, Tomlinson T, et al: Low frequency positive pressure ventilation with extra corporeal CO_2 removal in severe acute respiratory failure. *JAMA* 1986;256:881

31. Pesenti A, Gattinoni L, Bombino M: Long term extracorporeal respiratory support: 20 years of progress. *Intensive Crit Care Dig* 1993;12:15

32. Gentilello LM, Jurkovich GJ, Gubler KD, et al: The intravascular oxygenator (IVOX): preliminary results of a new means of performing extra pulmonary gas exchange. *J Trauma* 1993;35: 399

33. Hubmayr RD, Abel MD, Rheder K: Physiologic approach to mechanical ventilation. *Crit Care Med* 1990;18:103

Critical Care, Third Edition, edited by Joseph M. Civetta,
Robert W. Taylor, and Robert R. Kirby.
Lippincott-Raven Publishers, Philadelphia, PA © 1997.

CHAPTER 50

Airway Management

Orlando G. Florete
Robert R. Kirby

IMMEDIATE CONCERNS

MAJOR PROBLEMS

Maintenance of the airway and circulatory homeostasis are
two of the most essential goals of critical care. Failure to
achieve either renders other efforts academic at best. Airway
functions are numerous, and yet many are overlooked. The
airway is often thought of as a passive conduit that primarily
effects the exchange of oxygen and carbon dioxide. Yet it
also regulates temperature, warms and humidifies inspired
gas, traps and expels foreign particles, permits phonation,
protects against foreign body entry into the lungs through
a complex array of reflex responses, and fosters the senses
of smell and taste.

Many of these functions are altered or lost in critically
ill patients. Airway obstruction can result from infection,
trauma, laryngospasm, soft tissue edema, and aspiration of
gastric or other noxious materials. Protective reflexes may
be lost as a result of disease and depression with narcotics,
sedatives, or paralytic agents. Humidification can be lost as
various appliances that bypass the nose, pharynx, and upper
airway are inserted to maintain patency. Clinicians must then
employ methods to maintain airway hydration, including
humidifiers, nebulizers, and heat-moisture exchangers.
These devices introduce additional problems such as nosocomial infections and increased work of breathing.

Finally, efforts to improve lung function by artificial airways, positive-pressure ventilation, positive end-expiratory
pressure, and continuous positive airway pressure predispose to possible airway trauma and bleeding, pulmonary
barotrauma, circulatory compromise, and death.

STRESS POINTS

1. Assurance of airway patency is the overriding and
   primary concern. Failure to do so has tragic, often
   lethal, consequences.
2. Familiarity with the equipment and techniques to
   sustain the airway is mandatory. Not all critical care
   practitioners have to be adept at all aspects of cardiopulmonary support (consultants are available), but
   they must be able to deal with a lost airway. The
   latter condition offers little time, as is attested to by
   a high incidence of permanent neurologic damage
   and death.
3. Remember that in cardiopulmonary resuscitation,
   the first two considerations are airway and breathing.
   The same analysis applies to critical care in general.
4. Know how to provide oxygenation and ventilation
   with common equipment: face masks; oral, nasal,
   and pharyngeal airways; and endotracheal tubes. Be
   familiar and comfortable with laryngoscopes and
   curved and straight laryngoscope blades (at least
   one each).
5. Have a working knowledge of fiberoptic laryngoscopes
   and bronchoscopes, lightwands, tube changers, and
   techniques of percutaneous cricothyroidotomy. Leave
   surgical cricothyroidotomy and tracheotomy to experts with surgical training.
6. If you *think* an endotracheal tube is obstructed or
   malpositioned (i.e., in the esophagus), it is! Remove
   it and replace it.
7. Be able to use proper techniques of tracheal suction,
   occlusive cuff inflation, and detection of esophageal

or mainstem bronchial intubation. Failure to do so will lead to potentially disastrous consequences, some immediate and some long term.

8. Ask for assistance when faced with a difficult airway problem. This is one situation in which too many cooks seldom spoil the broth. Each involved individual brings a different perspective and additional skills that may be life-saving.

9. Communicate with your patient whenever possible. The patient is the one individual who can tell you if things are okay. Don't treat restlessness or combativeness that may result from a compromised airway by giving more narcotics and sedatives.

10. Always have all equipment and drugs necessary to secure and maintain the airway immediately available. If you have to send someone to the operating room to obtain succinylcholine or a different sized endotracheal tube, the delay may be fatal.

ESSENTIAL DIAGNOSTIC TESTS AND PROCEDURES

1. Observe your patient. Look for sternal and intercostal retractions, sternocleidomastoid contraction, nasal flaring, and paradoxical breathing. Listen for wheezing, asymmetrical breath sounds, or absent breath sounds.

2. Use your monitors appropriately. Remember that cardiovascular changes (bradycardia, hypotension) are *late* signs of airway compromise and hypoxemia. In this regard, pulse oximetry and, when available, capnography are invaluable.

3. Arterial blood gas analysis is still the gold standard for the assessment of oxygenation, ventilation, and airway function. However, it cannot be obtained instantaneously. Don't make a major change (i.e., intubation) and wait an hour before ordering a blood gas analysis. The effects of the change should be demonstrable within 5 minutes.

4. Use chest radiographs judiciously. The too frequent every-morning chest radiograph is a costly waste of time. However, a stat radiograph to check tube placement, tracheal dilatation from an overinflated cuff, atelectasis from an occluded bronchus, and air trapping can be useful and lifesaving.

5. Monitor occlusive cuff pressures frequently. Beware of an ever-increasing requirement for additional air in the cuff. Tracheal erosion into the esophagus or brachiocephalic artery still occurs, and tracheal stenosis from ischemic cuff damage is seen even with high-volume, low-pressure cuffs.

INITIAL THERAPY

1. Administer oxygen with a bag-valve-mask before attempting to intubate. This important step can be taken while somebody else prepares the laryngoscope and endotracheal tube. Oral and nasal pharyngeal airways can make this task easier.

2. Procedures involving the airway are at best uncomfortable and at worse excruciatingly painful. Be humane with liberal but judicious administration of narcotics, sedatives, and anxiolytics. Consider lidocaine nebulization. Superior laryngeal and glossopharyngeal nerve blocks are simple and useful. A comfortable patient is a more cooperative patient.

3. Get all the help you can. If the possibility of an emergency cricothyroidotomy or tracheotomy seems real, have an ear, nose, and throat surgeon available whenever possible.

4. Be gentle. Traumatic damage to the nose or pharynx with subsequent bleeding adds an incredible amount of difficulty. Fiberoptic techniques frequently are rendered useless, and what began as an urgent but reasonably controlled situation may become an emergent, uncontrolled one.

5. Remember the alternatives to intubation such as the laryngeal mask airway (LMA). The technique for insertion generally requires less skill than does tracheal intubation, and the devices may help to convert an emergent situation back to urgent.

6. Also, use your monitors while performing your tasks. They are your best indicators when things are going right or wrong.

7. Don't panic. Do the best you can. To try and to fail is better than not to intervene. Some patients cannot be intubated or ventilated. They are rare, but they do exist.

GENERAL PRINCIPLES ■

Primum non nocere (first do no harm) applies most fittingly to the airways of critically ill patients. The intensivist must not only be knowledgeable in respiratory pathophysiology but also should possess technical skill and sound judgment in airway management. Various options are available, including bag-valve-mask ventilation, translaryngeal intubation (oral or nasal), tracheotomy, and cricothyroidotomy. Adjunctive drugs such as local anesthetics, narcotics, benzodiazepines, barbiturates, muscle relaxants, ketamine, and propofol play an important role. Their use facilitates airway control and improves respiratory support.

In most instances, bag-valve-mask ventilation precedes tracheal intubation. Immediate correction of hypoxemia can be achieved by application of a mask and initiation of bag ventilation while equipment for intubation is prepared. An appropriate mask provides a tight seal around the nose and mouth, and the colorless plastic with soft and pliable edges allows visualization of the mouth and secretions. The mask is attached to a standard self-inflating bag with an oxygen reservoir. During manual inflation, this system supplies almost a 1.0 fraction of inspired oxygen (FIO_2).[1] Proper inflation requires two hands: one to hold the mask firmly in place against the patient's face, and the other to compress the bag[2] (Fig. 50-1). The mandible must be lifted to create a seal without airway occlusion. An oropharyngeal or nasal

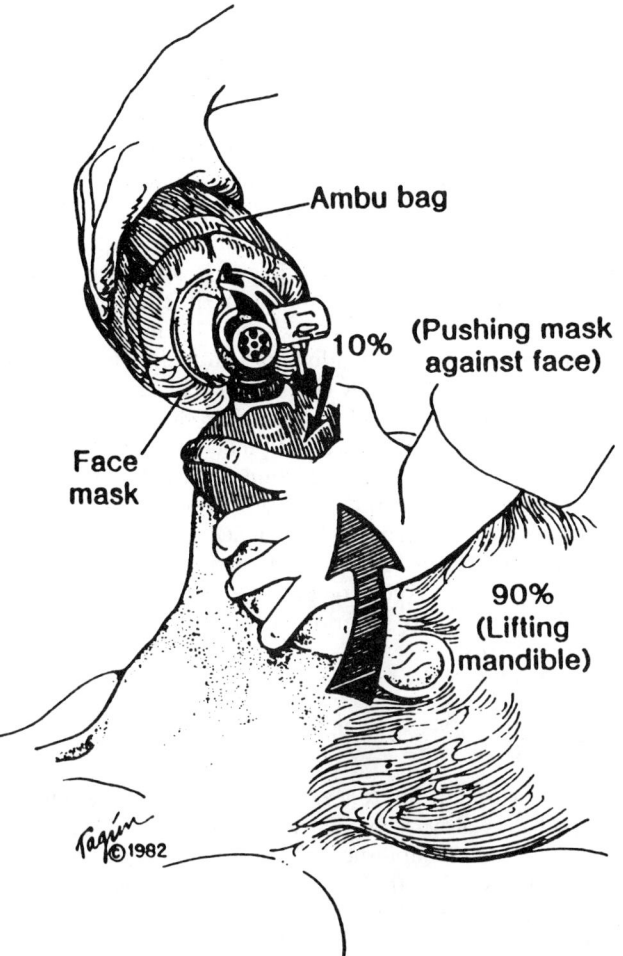

FIGURE 50-1. Proper technique of bag-valve-mask ventilation. (Hayes HR: Cardiopulmonary resuscitation. In: Wilkens GW [ed]. *Emergency Medicine.* Baltimore, Williams & Wilkins, 1989:10.)

TABLE 50-1. Indications for Tracheal Intubation

Open an obstructed airway
Provide airway pressure support to treat hypoxemia
   PaO_2 <60 with FIO_2 >0.5
   Alveolar to arterial oxygen gradient 300 mm Hg
   Intrapulmonary shunt >15–20%
Provide mechanical ventilation
   Respiratory acidosis
   Inadequate respiratory mechanics
      Respiratory rate >30/min
      FVC <10 mL/kg
      PNP >−20 cm H_2O
   V_D/V_T >0.6
Facilitate suctioning
Prevent aspiration
   Gag and swallow reflexes absent

FIO_2, fraction of inspired oxygen; FVC, forced vital capacity; PNP, peak negative pressure; V_D/V_T, dead space/tidal volume ratio.

Epinephrine, atropine, lidocaine, and naloxone exert their pharmacologic effects after tracheal administration.[6–9]
Contraindications to conventional tracheal intubation exist in patients with traumatic or severe degenerative disorders of the cervical spine; in those with acute infectious processes such as acute supraglottitis or intrapharyngeal abscess; and in patients with extensive facial injury and basal skull fracture.[10,11] Blind nasal intubation may be contraindicated in upper airway foreign body obstruction because the tube may push the foreign body distally and exacerbate airway compromise.[12,13] Malignant tumors of the upper airway may be seeded into the pulmonary tree and can spread into surrounding structures or metastasize to distant sites through vascular breach during intubation.

ANATOMIC CONSIDERATIONS ■

ADULT

Specific anatomic characteristics may determine the ease or difficulty of intubation. The intensivist sometimes does not have the flexibility to examine and assess the airway at leisure but must act quickly with skill and confidence. A good working knowledge of the anatomy of the mouth, neck, cervical spine, and pulmonary tree is mandatory for a successful and safe intubation.
Evaluation of the mouth should include examination of the surrounding bony structures (teeth, maxilla, and mandible) and the tongue. Teeth and dental plates are susceptible to injury and dislodgement, perhaps accounting for the most common complication of intubation.[14] Facial, pharyngeal, and glossal congenital anomalies may result in difficult intubation. Temporomandibular joint mobility should be rapidly evaluated by opening the patient's mouth as wide as possible. Adequate jaw opening generally is present when the distance

airway facilitates oxygen delivery by bypassing or retracting the tongue.[3] Forceful bag compression should be avoided to prevent gastric distention and possible pulmonary aspiration. Gentle insufflation allows clinical assessment of lung compliance and minimizes complications.
Contraindications to bag-valve-mask ventilation include airway obstruction, pooling of blood or secretions in the pharynx, and severe facial trauma.[4] Preferably, immediate intubation should be carried out in any of these situations.
Critically ill patients require tracheal intubation for several reasons[5] (Table 50-1). When inadequate ventilation is observed, tracheal intubation becomes necessary. It provides airway patency, facilitates tracheobronchial suctioning, and minimizes aspiration of blood, gastric contents, or secretions into the pulmonary tree. Oxygen administration and mechanical ventilation correct hypoxemia and hypercapnia, improve the alveolar-to-arterial oxygen partial pressure gradient, and reduce intrapulmonary shunting. In emergency situations in which intravascular access is absent, drug administration into the endotracheal tube can be lifesaving.

between the upper and lower incisors is equal to or greater than 40 mm (two finger-breadths).[15]

Examination of cervical spine mobility includes flexion and extension. Neck flexion aligns the pharyngeal and tracheal axes, whereas head extension on the neck and opening

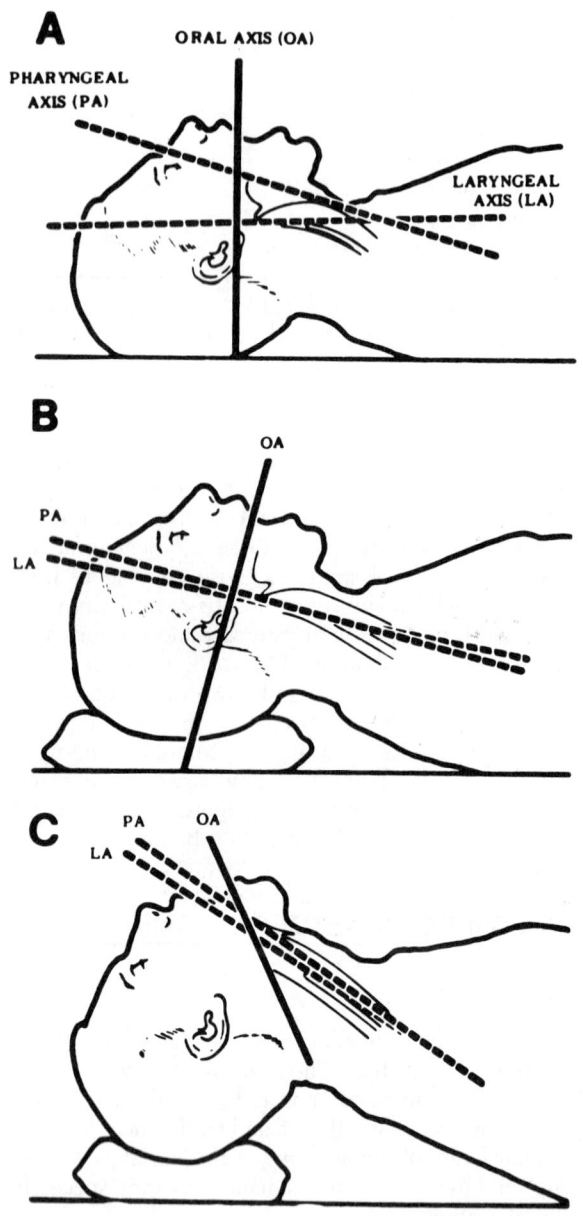

FIGURE 50-2. Proper head position is important for successful orotracheal intubation. (**A**) The oral (OA), pharyngeal (PA), and laryngeal (LA) axes must be aligned for direct laryngoscopy. (**B**) Elevate the head 10 cm above the shoulders with a folded towel to align the pharyngeal and laryngeal axes. (**C**) Extend the atlanto-occipital joint to achieve the straightest possible line from the incisors to the glottis.

of the mouth align the oral passage with the pharyngeal and tracheal axes.[16] This maneuver places the patient in a "sniffing position"[17,18] (Fig. 50-2). Incorrect positioning of the head and neck accounts for one of the common errors in orotracheal intubation.[19] Flexion and extension of the head decreases 20% by 75 years of age. Degenerative arthritis limits cervical spine motion, more so with extension than flexion.[20–22] Movement of the spine is contraindicated in the presence of potential cervical spine injury, precluding visualization other than with fiberoptic endoscopy as a means of intubation. Rheumatoid arthritis may reduce motion and can cause atlantoaxial instability and reduced mouth opening.

Important anatomic landmarks may help the physician during direct laryngoscopy (Fig. 50-3). The cricoid, a circle of cartilage above the first tracheal ring, can be compressed to occlude the esophagus (Sellick maneuver), thereby preventing passive gastric regurgitation into the trachea during intubation.[24] The epiglottis, a large cartilaginous structure, lies in the anterior pharynx. The vallecula, a furrow between the epiglottis and base of the tongue, is the placement site for the tip of a curved laryngoscope blade.[25] The larynx is located anterior and superior to the trachea and contains the vocal cords.

PEDIATRIC

Several anatomic differences exist between the adult and the pediatric airways. Pediatric patients have a relatively large head and flexible neck.[26] The air passages are small, the tongue is large, the epiglottis is floppy, and the glottis is slanted, making intubation more difficult. Mucous membranes are softer, looser, more fragile, and readily become edematous when an oversized endotracheal tube is used.

Adenoids and tonsils in a child are relatively larger than those in the adult. The epiglottis and larynx of infants lie more cephalad and anterior, and the cricoid cartilage ring is the narrowest portion of the upper airway. In contrast, the adult glottic opening is narrowest. Additionally, the pediatric vocal cords have a shorter distance from the carina, angulating symmetrically at the mainstem at 55 degrees. In adults, the right mainstem angulates at 25 degrees and the left at 45 degrees. The cupulae of the lungs are higher in the infants neck, increasing the risk of lung trauma.

ASSESSMENT

A relatively simple way to grade the ease of laryngoscopy and intubation has been proposed by Mallampati and co-workers.[27,28] The Mallampati signs and classifications (Fig. 50-4) are based on the ability to visualize the faucial pillars, soft palate, and base of the uvula to predict the degree of difficulty in laryngeal exposure. The extent of glottic exposure during laryngoscopy is also graded. Although originally applied to preoperative airway evaluation, it can be useful in the intensive care unit (ICU) as well.

Radiographically, the posterior depth of the mandible (distance between the alveolus immediately behind the third

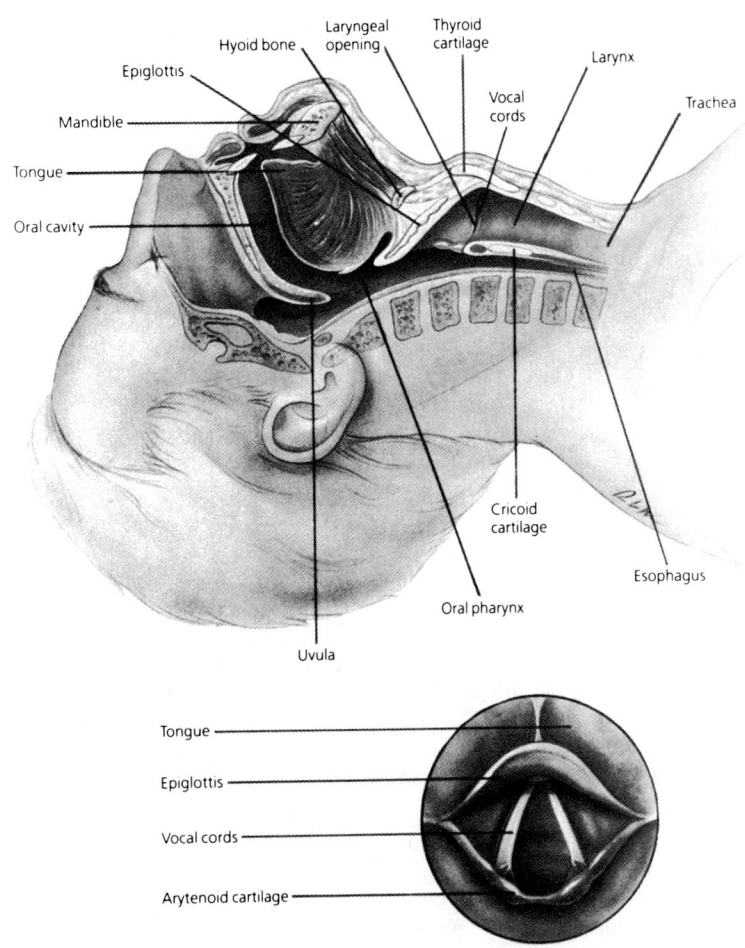

FIGURE 50-3. Anatomic landmarks of the head and neck. (Hines D, Bone RC: The technique of endotracheal intubation. *J Crit Illness* 1986;1:60.)

Mallampati		Structures visible
Class I	Class I	soft palate, fauces, uvula, pillars
Class II	Class II	soft palate, fauces, uvula
	Class III	soft palate, base of uvula
Class III	Class IV	hard palate, soft palate not visible

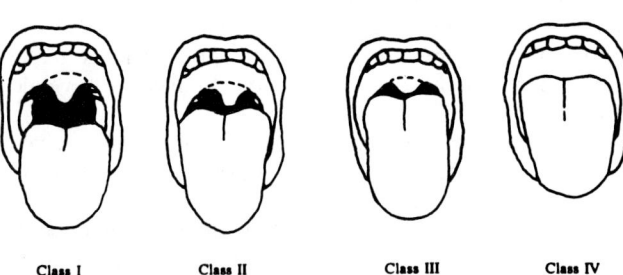

Class I Class II Class III Class IV

FIGURE 50-4. Mallampati signs and classifications. (Modified from Mallampati SR, Batt SP, Gugino LD, et al: A clinical exam to predict difficult tracheal intubation: a prospective study. *Can Anaesth Soc J* 1985;32:429.)

molar and the lower mandibular border) is the most important factor in determining the ease of laryngoscopy.[29] An increased depth hinders soft tissue displacement by the laryngoscope blade.

The Difficult Airway

In most instances, a difficult airway can be predicted by history and physical examination. A short muscular or obese neck, full set of teeth, and receding lower jaw with obtuse mandibular angles often preclude an easy intubation.[30] Overgrowth of the premaxilla with upper incisor protrusion and poor mobility of the mandible caused by arthritis, trismus, infection, or inflammation make laryngoscopy difficult. Additionally, a long arched palate associated with a narrow mouth, increased anterior and posterior depth of the mandible, and limited mobility of the head and cervical spine may result in problematic intubation. Other adverse prognostic signs are decreased interspinous gap of the atlanto-occipital joint, decreased distance from the mandibular symphysis to the thyroid notch, tumor, infection, upper airway trauma, and pathologic signs of airway obstruction. Practice guidelines for difficult airway management have been published.[30,31]

DRUGS ■

To avoid delay and minimize complications, all anticipated equipment and drugs must be available for the planned intubation technique (Table 50-2). Additionally, a bronchoscope or fiberoptic laryngoscope should be readily available. An assistant must assess vital signs and provide cricoid pressure.

The pharynx, larynx, and trachea contain a rich network of sensory innervation, necessitating the use of anesthesia, analgesia, sedation, and sometimes muscular paralysis during intubation of a spontaneously breathing, awake, or semiconscious patient.[22] Drugs commonly used are local anesthetics, sodium thiopental, opioid narcotics, benzodiazepines (diazepam and midazolam), muscle relaxants (depolarizing and nondepolarizing agents), and miscellaneous agents such as ketamine and propofol.

LOCAL ANESTHETICS

Aerosolized 1% to 4% lidocaine can readily achieve nasopharyngeal and oropharyngeal anesthesia. Transtracheal (cricothyroid membrane) instillation of 2 to 4 mL of 4% lidocaine with a 22-gauge needle causes sufficient coughing-induced reflux to anesthetize the larynx and posterior pharynx in 90% of patients.[32] Cocaine solution, 4%, provides topical anesthesia for nasal intubation and promotes mucosal and vascular shrinkage, thus facilitating tube passage through the nasopharynx.[33] Phenylephrine combined with lidocaine also causes vasoconstriction and anesthesia of the nasal mucosa and may be used in lieu of cocaine.[34] Lidocaine ointment applied to the base of the tongue with a tongue blade allows performance of direct laryngoscopy.

BARBITURATES

Sodium thiopental, an ultra–short-acting barbiturate, decreases the level of consciousness and provides amnesia without analgesia after an intubation dose of 4 to 7 mg/kg body weight. The onset of action is rapid, occurring 20 to 50 seconds after administration. Its short duration of action (5 to 10 minutes) makes it ideal for short procedures such

TABLE 50-2. Equipment and Drugs for Translaryngeal Intubation

A means to ventilate the patient manually (bag-valve-mask)
Oxygen source with circuitry
Suction apparatus
Selection of oral and nasal airways
Assortment of laryngoscope blades and endotracheal tubes
Tape, stylet, lubricant, syringes, tongue depressors
Monitors (ECG, blood pressure monitor, pulse oximeter, and if available, capnograph) and defibrillator
An adjustable bed
A drug tray or cart with vasoconstrictors, topical anesthetics, sedatives, muscle relaxants, emergency, and other adjuvant drugs
14-Gauge intravenous catheter over needle, scalpel handle, and blade

as intubation. Thiopental, however, can cause hypotension in critically ill patients; antianalgesia during recovery; and respiratory depression, especially when combined with a narcotic.[35]

NARCOTICS

Narcotics such as morphine, fentanyl, alfentanil, and sufentanil reduce pain perception and allay anxiety, making intubation less stressful. In addition, they have some sedative effect, suppress cough, and relieve dyspnea.[31,36–38] Fentanyl, sufentanil, and alfentanil have a more rapid onset and shorter duration of action than morphine. Unlike morphine, they do not cause histamine release and thus do not produce significant hypotension. Narcotics cause respiratory depression, occasional muscular rigidity that may hamper ventilation, and, rarely, bradycardia.

BENZODIAZEPINES

Benzodiazepines such as diazepam and midazolam have excellent amnestic and sedative properties.[39,40] They do not provide analgesia and should be combined with an analgesic agent during intubation. Midazolam largely has replaced diazepam for intubation because of its more rapid onset and shorter duration of action. Hypotension may occur in hypovolemic patients and potential narcotic-induced respiratory depression.

MUSCLE RELAXANTS

Occasionally, muscle relaxation may be necessary to achieve intubation. Indications include agitation or lack of cooperation, increased muscle tone (seizures, tetanus, and neurologic diseases), and avoidance of intracranial hypertension. Neuromuscular blockers may cause depolarization of the motor end-plate (succinylcholine) or prevent depolarization (pancuronium, tubocurarine, vecuronium, atracurium). Succinylcholine has a rapid onset and short duration of effect, making it useful in the critical care setting; however, it may raise serum potassium levels by 0.5 to 1.0 mEq/L. It is contraindicated in bedridden patients and in those with preexisting hyperkalemia, burns, or recent neurologic deficits.[41,42] Other side effects are elevation of intragastric and intraocular pressures, muscle fasciculation, myalgia, malignant hyperthermia, cardiac bradyarrhythmias, and myoglobinuria.

Nondepolarizing muscle relaxants like pancuronium, vecuronium, atracurium, and D-tubocurarine have longer onset and duration of action. Because they can cause loss of spontaneous ventilation and airway integrity, their use during intubation may be hazardous if the clinician does not have extensive knowledge, training, and familiarity with the drugs. Muscle relaxants must be used cautiously in patients with partially obstructed airways because they produce apnea and occasional total airway obstruction. Newer agents such as mevicurium and rocuronium have been little used in the ICU but are rapid–acting and of short duration.

KETAMINE

Ketamine, a phencyclidine derivative, provides profound analgesia, amnesia, and dissociative anesthesia.[43] The patient may appear awake but is uncommunicative. Airway reflexes are often, but not always, preserved. Ketamine has a rapid onset and relatively short duration of action. Its use is limited by cardiovascular stimulation, resulting from increased sympathetic outflow, and a high incidence of dreams, hallucinations, and emergence delirium. The latter problems, however, are rare with a single induction dose.

PROPOFOL

Propofol also is useful during intubation.[44,45] After intravenous administration of 1.5 to 3 mg/kg body weight, unconsciousness occurs in less than 60 seconds. Awakening is observed in 4 to 6 minutes with minimal lingering sedation. Side effects include pain on injection, involuntary muscle movement, coughing, hiccups, and, rarely, hypotension and bradycardia.

ESOPHAGEAL, PHARYNGEAL, AND LARYNGEAL TUBES

Several devices for maintenance of a patent airway are available, but their role in the ICU is undefined. They are confined mainly to emergency situations and out-of-hospital resuscitation and include the esophageal obturator airway (EOA), the pharyngeal tracheal lumen airway (PTLA), and the esophageal tracheal combitube (ETC). The binasal pharyngeal airway (BNPA) and LMA have been used with success in the operating room but have not been applied widely in the ICU. However, the LMA seems to be promising.

ESOPHAGEAL OBTURATOR AIRWAY

The EOA is a 34-cm plastic tube with a balloon at its distal end designed to be inflated in the esophagus[46] (Fig. 50-5). Sixteen 3-mm diameter holes are present in the upper third of the tube and allow passage of air during ventilation. The EOA is attached to a self-sealing face mask and is inserted blindly into the esophagus at a level just distal to the carina. Insertion is facilitated by grasping the mandible between the thumb and the index finger and lifting it forward while the tube is directed into the esophagus with the other hand. The balloon is inflated with 30 mL of air once the tube is in place, and the mask is fitted to the face. Air is blown through the small holes in the upper part of the tube into the airways. Inflation of the balloon prevents gas passage into the stomach.

Complications, some of which are fatal, include esophageal rupture, inadvertent tracheal intubation and occlusion, massive gastric distension, vomiting, and aspiration.[47-49]

PHARYNGEAL TRACHEAL LUMEN AIRWAY

The PTLA is a modification of the EOA. This device consists of two tubes: an endotracheal tube and a shorter tube that is designed to terminate in the hypopharynx.[50] A large, 150-

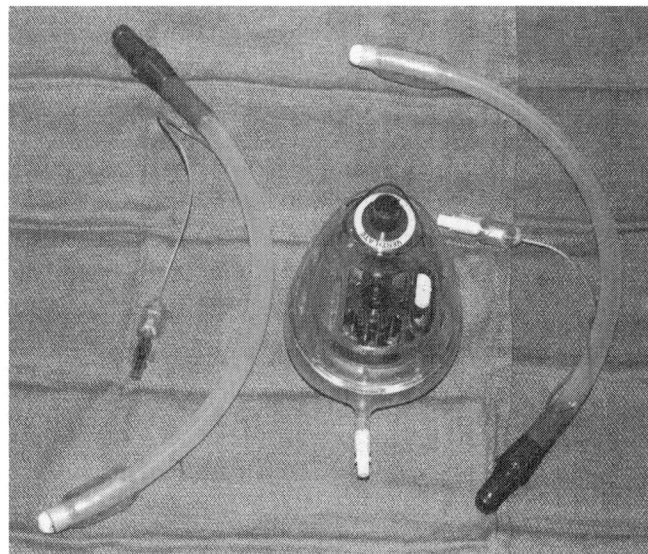

FIGURE 50-5. The esophageal obturator airway. (From Florete OG Jr: Airway devices and their application. In: Kirby RR, Gravenstein N [eds]. *Clinical Anesthesia Practice.* Philadelphia, WB Saunders, 1994:300.)

to 200-mL cuff is attached proximal to the port of the pharyngeal tube; inflation prevents oral and nasal secretions from entering the airway and prevents oral escape of air delivered by the pharyngeal tube.[51] A smaller, 30-mL distal cuff is attached to the endotracheal tube.

The PTLA also is inserted blindly, allowing placement of the endotracheal tube component into the trachea or esophagus. Once the airway is in position, the oropharyngeal and endotracheal tube cuffs are inflated. Air is then blown into the pharyngeal tube. If lung inflation occurs, a resuscitator bag is attached to the tube, and ventilation is continued. If lung inflation does not occur when the pharyngeal tube is ventilated, the endotracheal tube is in the trachea. The resuscitator bag is then attached to it and ventilation initiated, after which the pharyngeal balloon is deflated. The face mask is not required to maintain an effective seal.

ESOPHAGEAL TRACHEAL COMBITUBE

The ETC is a variant of the PTLA. Its proximal cuff is smaller than that of the PTLA and is placed between the base of the tongue and the hard palate.[52] It is inserted in the same manner as the PTLA. Ventilation is similar to that of the EOA except for the absence of a face mask.

BINASAL PHARYNGEAL AIRWAY

The BNPA is made up of two soft nasopharyngeal tubes connected to a suitable 15-mm male adapter.[53] It is inserted in both nares in a similar manner to that for a single nasal airway. This airway has been successfully used to ventilate patients in the operating room.[54] Gastric dilatation is unlikely because excess air escapes through the mouth. The BNPA is recommended only during difficult intubation when skilled personnel or more sophisticated equipment is not available.

LARYNGEAL MASK AIRWAY

The LMA consists of a shortened endotracheal tube attached to a shallow mask[54] (Fig. 50-6). It conforms to the shape of the laryngeal inlet and is passed through the mouth downward to the larynx. Inflation of the cuff holds the device in place over the glottis, and the position of the mask is adjusted if a good seal is not obtained. The sequence is shown in Figure 50-7. It is expensive but can be sterilized in the autoclave and is reusable. It is widely used in the United Kingdom for airway management during general anesthesia[55] and is gaining popularity in the United States. The LMA is available in sizes 1, 2, 2^1/$_2$, 3, 4, and 5 for neonates, infants, children, and adults.

The LMA seems to be associated with fewer episodes of desaturation, less difficulty in maintenance of a patent airway, and decreased arm and hand fatigue when compared with a conventional face mask.[56] It can serve as an emergency airway during difficult intubation or when ventilation is not possible with a standard face mask and bag.[57–59] It also can serve as an airway conduit for an intubating tracheal stylet or fiberoptic bronchoscope, through which an endotracheal tube may be passed when airway management or intubation is difficult.[60–62] Fiberoptic diagnostic visualization of the airway and fiberoptic laser ablation of tracheobronchial tree tumors are facilitated, as is management of patients with facial burns and those who need multiple anesthetics in a short period of time.[62–65] It may be useful in patients with unstable cervical spines, because its insertion does not require neck manipulation. Recent work suggests that it is better tolerated and produces few cardiovascular side effects than does tracheal intubation.[66]

The most common problem during insertion is failure to achieve correct placement as a result of inadequate anesthesia or inadequate relaxation, with failure to negotiate the 90-degree turn from the posterior pharynx to the hypopharynx (see Fig. 50-7C), and with the selection of the wrong LMA size.[60] The device is difficult to insert in patients with small mouths, large tongues or tonsils, or a posteriorly displaced pharynx. The esophagus may be exposed to positive pressure, resulting in gastric dilatation and regurgitation. Failed insertion occurs in up to 5% of attempts.

The LMA is contraindicated in patients with pharyngeal or laryngeal pathology; in patients who are at risk of regurgitation or aspiration or who have blood in the upper airway; or when more than 25 cm H_2O peak inflation pressure is required to ventilate the lungs. It is relatively contraindicated for situations in which tracheal intubation cannot be performed immediately.[67]

TRACHEAL INTUBATION ◼

During emergencies, orotracheal intubation is the preferred procedure to establish an airway because it usually can be performed rapidly, allows direct visualization of the glottis, and requires no surgery. It has fewer complications when compared with the nasal approach.

Before attempting to intubate, all anticipated equipment and drugs must be prepared. The patient may be intubated when fully anesthetized and relaxed, after sedation and analgesia, or when awake. Critically ill patients often require less medication for intubation. Careful intravenous titration prevents hemodynamic depression, loss of consciousness, apnea, and aspiration.

EQUIPMENT

Laryngoscopes

A laryngoscope is used to expose the glottis. The instrument is made of metal and consists of a handle, a blade, and a light source. The handle contains batteries to provide current for a light bulb that is fitted into the tip of the blade, the latter with a hook-on attachment to the handle. The C-

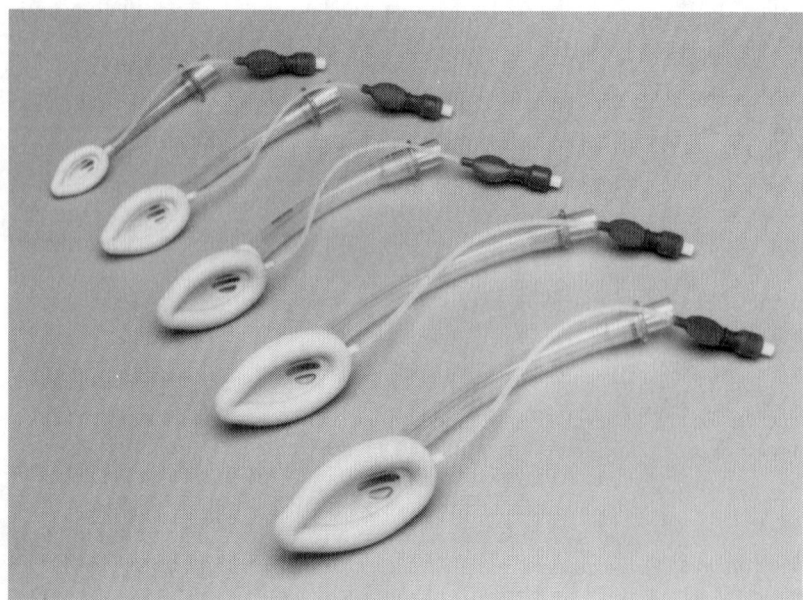

FIGURE 50-6. The laryngeal mask airway. Shown are sizes 1, 2, 2.5, 3, and 4.

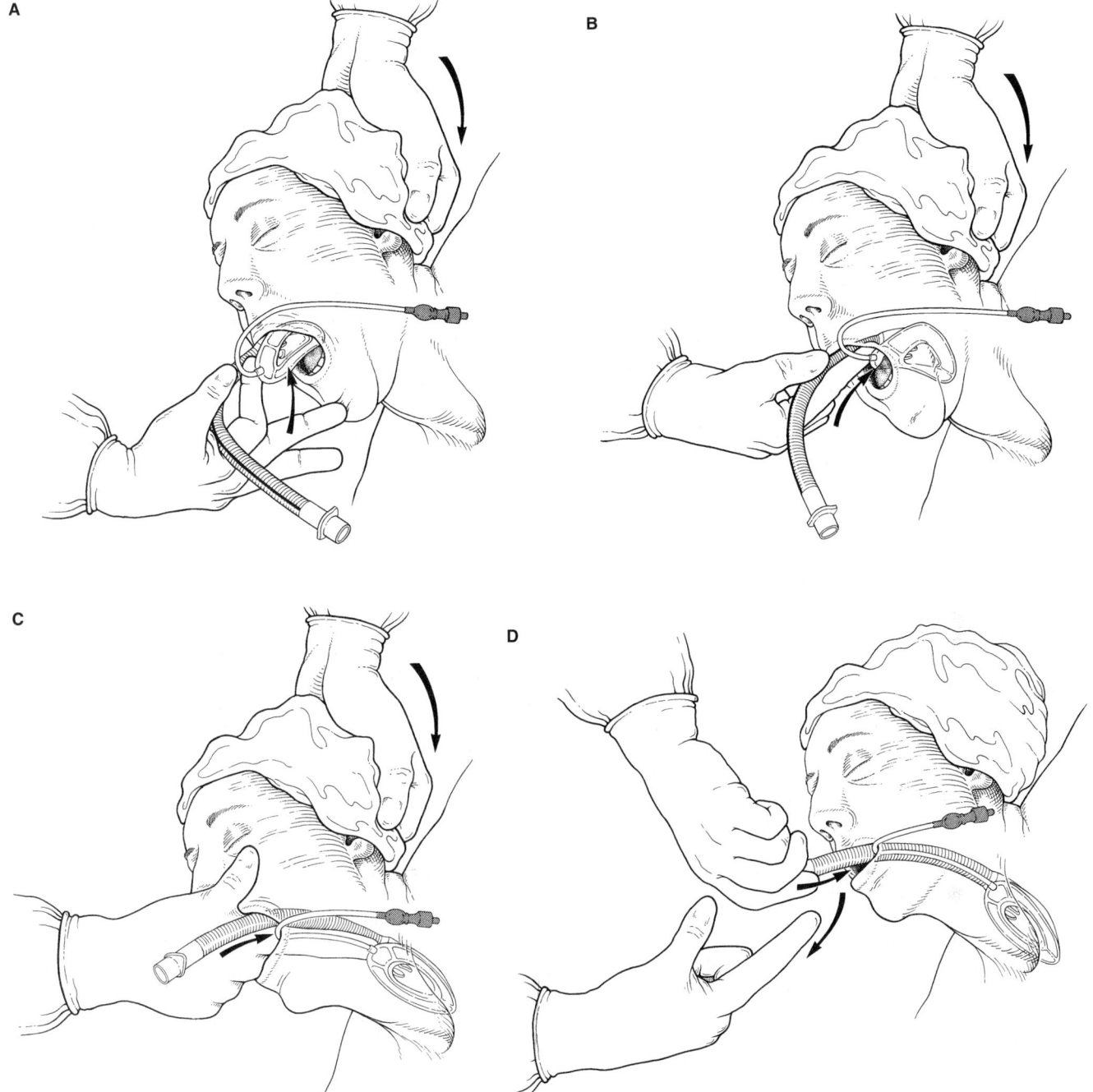

FIGURE 50-7. Sequential steps for insertion and positioning of the laryngeal mask airway.

shaped cross-section displaces the tongue to the left away from the path of vision, which is kept open to the right for passage of a tracheal tube.

BLADES. Laryngoscope blades are of two principal kinds, curved and straight, varying in size for use in infants, children, or adults (see Fig. 50-7). Many varieties of both the curved and straight blades have been designed to facilitate passage of a tracheal tube. However, an accomplished practitioner can manage with two or three blades at most. Dispos-

able blades are available to avoid transmission of infectious disease.

Tracheal Tubes

Most tracheal tubes are disposable and are made of clear, pliable polyvinylchloride, with little tendency to kink. They are sterilized by the manufacturer with ethylene oxide and thoroughly vented before use. At body temperature, the tubes mold to the contour of the upper airway and present a smooth interior to easy passage of suction catheters or a flexible bronchoscope.

Tracheal tubes are of measured length, marked in 0.5-mm increments according to diameter, with inflatable cuffs optional above 5 mm, and with a Magill's or Murphy's tip. The latter has an opening opposite the bevel. They are usually longer than necessary when received from the manufacturer and benefit from shortening to lessen the possibility of bronchial intubation or to prevent kinking at the nose or mouth. If the proximal end of the tube is cut, the connector should be reinserted firmly.

Built-in cuffs are used in adults and older children; when inflated, the cuff ensures a closed system, permitting easy control of ventilation and minimizing the possibility of aspiration of vomitus or blood. Cuffs may be of the high- or low-pressure variety, depending on the volume of air required for their inflation. When inflated, a high-pressure cuff has a short length; thus, a small surface is in contact with the tracheal wall and a high internal cuff pressure is required to seal the trachea. Low-pressure cuffs offer a larger volume and diameter plus a broad contact with the tracheal wall.

TECHNIQUES

The method of intubation is predicated not only on the site of operation but also on the projected need for postoperative ventilation.

Orotracheal

Before induction of anesthesia, all necessary equipment should be tested and readied for use. A tube of appropriate diameter and length should be selected: in women, a 7.5-mm inside diameter; and in a man, 8 to 9 mm. The tube should be examined for patency and the cuff inflated to detect air leak. The adapter placed in the proximal end should fit snugly. The tube is kept in its sterile wrapper and not handled until ready for insertion.

CURVED BLADE. The moistened or lubricated laryngoscope blade is introduced at the right side of the mouth and advanced in the midline, displacing the tongue to the left. The epiglottis is seen at the base of the tongue and the tip of the blade inserted into the vallecula. The wrist is held rigid to avoid using the upper teeth as a fulcrum for the laryngoscope blade. A forward and upward lift of the laryngoscope and blade stretches the hyoepiglottic ligament, thus folding the epiglottis upward and further exposing the glottis. As a result, the larynx is suspended on the tip of the blade by the hyoid bone.

The tracheal tube, with cuff deflated and concavity directed anterolaterally, is passed to the right of the laryngoscope through the glottis into the trachea until the cuff passes 2 to 3 cm beyond the vocal cords. The glottis occasionally is not fully visible, but intubation is possible when only the arytenoid cartilages and posteriori commissure are seen. A curved stylet helps to direct the tube anteriorly.

STRAIGHT BLADE. Intubation with a straight blade involves the same maneuvers but with one major difference.

The blade is slipped *beneath* the epiglottis, and exposure of the larynx is accomplished by an upward and forward lift at a 45-degree angle. Again, leverage must not be applied against the upper teeth.

With either technique, the common causes of failure to intubate include inadequate position of the head; misplacement of the laryngoscope blade; inadequate muscle relaxation; insufficient depth of general anesthesia; an obscuring of the glottis by the tongue; and lack of familiarity with the anatomy, especially where pathologic changes are present. Inserting a laryngoscope blade too deeply results in lifting of the entire larynx and esophagus if the tip of the blade is not placed in the vallecula. Familiar landmarks are lost and a sense of panic may ensue. Under these circumstances, withdraw the blade and start over.

Nasotracheal

Nasotracheal intubation is commonly used in oral and maxillofacial operations and in emergency situations outside the operating room. Although nasotracheal intubation is indicated in a patient with trismus or a fractured jaw, it is avoided in patients with a basilar skull fracture, a fractured nose, or nasal obstruction. It is also contraindicated in the presence of acute sinusitis or mastoiditis, because the infection may be spread to the rest of the airway.

The technique may be applied either with a patient awake and well sedated or after induction of general anesthesia and use of a neuromuscular blocker. Nasal intubation may be performed blindly or under direct vision using a laryngoscope or flexible fiberoptic bronchoscope. In either case, the tube should be smaller in diameter than that required for oral intubation, soft and pliable to avoid injuring the nasal mucosa or turbinates, but of a consistency to resist compression and to maintain a reasonable curvature. These conditions can be met by warming the tube in hot water just before intubation.

BLIND. For blind intubation, the tube is introduced with its concavity forward and the bevel directed laterally; advancement is slow and gentle, with rotation when resistance is encountered. Rough maneuvers, large-bore rigid tubes, poor lubrication, and use of force against obstruction easily induce epistaxis. Rotation of the tube and manual depression or elevation of the larynx may be required to succeed. Voluntary or hypercapnic-induced hyperpnea helps if the patient is awake because maximal abduction of the cords is present during inspiration. Entry into the trachea is signified by consistent breath sounds transmitted by the tube and inability to speak if the patient is breathing, as well as by lack of resistance, often accompanied by cough. One can then feel the inflation of the tracheal cuff below the larynx and above the manubrium sterni, followed by connecting the tube to the rebreathing system and expanding the lungs.

DIRECT VISION. Nasotracheal intubation under direct vision is accomplished during laryngoscopy frequently with Magill's forceps. The tube is inserted through one nostril into the oropharynx, with the bevel pointing laterally. The vocal cords are then exposed, and the tube is advanced under direct vision into the trachea. If it does not progress, Magill's forceps are used to direct the tip toward the glottis, with an assistant then advancing the tube. They may also be useful during conscious nasotracheal intubation under direct vision.

COMPLICATIONS

Tracheal intubation is an important source of morbidity and occasionally of mortality.[68–77] Complications occur in four time periods: during intubation, after placement, during extubation, and after extubation (Table 50-3). Several predisposing factors have been identified. Patients with smaller airways, especially infants and children, have a higher incidence of complications. They are also more susceptible to upper airway obstruction secondary to glottic edema and subglottic stenosis.

Certain adverse anatomic features such as facial or cervical abnormalities, short neck, receding chin, obesity, and face and neck congenital anomalies increase the risk of complications. Patients with upper airway or lung infection, coagulation abnormalities, poor tissue perfusion, or chronic debilitating illness are more prone to complications.

Cuffed tube usage for prolonged intubation and artificial ventilation substantially increases the rate of tracheal and laryngeal injury. The extent of injury is dependent on duration of exposure, the presence of infected secretions, and severity of respiratory failure. Cuff pressures above 25 to 35 mm Hg further add to risk by compressing tracheal capillaries, which predisposes to ischemic mucosal damage.[78–89] High-volume, low-pressure cuffs allow tracheal tube usage for prolonged periods. They have changed the pattern of complications associated with tracheal intubation.

Selection of the correct size tube is mandatory (Table 50-4). Too large a tube can cause a higher incidence of postoperative sore throat, laryngeal damage, and tracheal stenosis. These problems are especially true in female patients because of their smaller airway compared with male

TABLE 50-4. Recommended Sizes for Endotracheal Tubes

PATIENT AGE	INTERNAL DIAMETER OF TUBE (mm)*
Newborn	3.0
6 mo	3.5
18 mo	4.0
3 y	4.5
5 y	5.0
6 y	5.5
8 y	6.0
12 y	6.5
16 y	7.0
Adult female	8.0–8.5
Adult male	8.5–9.0

*One size larger or one size smaller should be allowed for individual intraage variations.

patients of comparable size. Women should be intubated with an endotracheal tube one full size smaller than that used for a comparable-sized man. Red rubber and double-lumen endotracheal tubes, stylets, and tube changers predispose to injury.[90–92]

Other factors of importance include the duration of intubation, reintubation, route of intubation (nasal intubation produces more complications), excessive tube movement, trauma during procedures, and poor tube care. Clinicians unskilled in intubation techniques increase the complication rate.

During Intubation

TRAUMA. Tracheal intubation dangers begin at the time of initial tube insertion. Direct airway trauma depends on skill and the degree of difficulty encountered during intubation.[93,94] Injuries include bruised or lacerated lips and tongue,

TABLE 50-3. Risks of Tracheal Intubation

TIME	TISSUE INJURY	MECHANICAL PROBLEMS	OTHER
Tube placement	Corneal abrasion; nasal polyp dislodgement; bruise/laceration of lips/tongue; tooth extraction; retropharyngeal perforation; vocal cord tear; cervical spine subluxation or fracture; hemorrhage; turbinate bone avulsion	Esophageal/endobronchial intubation; delay in cardiopulmonary resuscitation	Arrhythmia; pulmonary aspiration; hypertension; hypotension
Tube in place	Tear/abrasion of larynx, trachea, bronchi	Airway obstruction; migration of tube; ignition of tube during laser surgery	Bacterial infection (secondary) Gastric aspiration Paranasal sinusitis Problems related to mechanical ventilation (e.g., pulmonary barotrauma)
Extubation	—	Difficult extubation; airway obstruction from blood, foreign bodies, dentures, or throat packs	Pulmonary aspiration; laryngeal edema; laryngospasm; tracheomalacia

inadvertent tooth extraction, upper airway hemorrhage, vocal cord tears, and nasal polyp dislodgement. Inadvertent contact of the cornea by the operator's hand may cause abrasion. Nasopharyngeal mucosa perforation can create a false passage, whereas a tear in the pyriform fossa mucosal lining may lead to mediastinal emphysema and tension pneumothorax.[95] Fracture or subluxation of the cervical spine can result from careless movement of the head or forceful hyperextension during attempts to improve laryngeal exposure.

DELAY. Excessive delay in cardiopulmonary resuscitation may occur while an inexperienced practitioner tries to visualize the vocal cords. If intubation cannot be accomplished within 15 seconds, a more experienced person should make the attempt whenever possible. Multiple intubation attempts by an unskilled person make subsequent attempts more problematic.

ASPIRATION OF GASTRIC CONTENTS. Aspiration of gastric contents may occur in high-risk patients.[96,97] Factors that predispose the patient to aspiration include poorly functioning cardioesophageal sphincter, full stomach, acute intestinal obstruction, difficult intubation, and loss of consciousness and gag reflex.

MISPLACEMENT. A major complication is accidental tube misplacement. Because it is less angulated from the trachea, the right mainstem bronchus is the more common site of mainstem intubation.[98-100] Tube misplacement may cause hypoxemia secondary to contralateral lung collapse and hyperinflation of the intubated lung with possible pulmonary barotrauma. Another problem is accidental esophageal intubation followed by gastric distention.[101]

ARRHYTHMIAS. Premature ventricular contractions have been observed in 5% to 15% of intubations. Patients with myocardial ischemia seem particularly susceptible to significant arrhythmias. Adequate preoxygenation and lidocaine prophylaxis (100 mg intravenous bolus just before intubation) may preclude complications. Bradyarrhythmias are relatively common because of stimulation of the laryngeal branches of the vagus nerve, especially in younger patients. Although both hypotension and hypertension occur, prophylactic use of vasoactive drugs does not seem warranted and may cause more hemodynamic problems.

After Intubation

OBSTRUCTION. The most common and most serious complication after intubation is tube obstruction.[102,103] It may be caused by biting or abutment against the tracheal wall. A bite block in the patient's mouth or slight rotation of the tube may correct the obstruction. Kinking of the tube or herniation of the cuff can occlude the airway and compromise ventilation, as can blood clots, tissue, dried secretions, tube lubricants, and foreign bodies. Suctioning removes most obstructing material. Signs of tube obstruction are high inflation pressure, absent or impaired chest excursion,

marked respiratory effort with paradoxic movement, cyanosis, and venous congestion.

DISPLACEMENT/EXTUBATION. Tube displacement out of the trachea or migration of the tube tip into a bronchus may compromise the airway.[104,105] Appropriate securing and notation of tube markings in relation to the lip minimizes this complication,[105,106] and follow-up chest radiograph confirms tip location. Ideally, the tube tip should lie midway between the glottis and the carina. Hyperextension of the head may cause migration of the endotracheal tube tip away from the carina toward the pharynx; head flexion and extension is associated with an average 1.9-cm movement of the tube.[107] Lateral rotation of the head causes the tube to move 0.7 cm away from the carina. Chest radiographs should be taken with the patient's head in its usual position to assess tube placement.

Accidental extubation, another potentially lethal complication after intubation, occurs in 8% to 13% of intubated, critically ill patients. To prevent unplanned extubation, secure the tube by taping circumferentially around the upper neck. Benzoin improves adhesiveness of the tape to the skin and the tube. Restraining the patient's hands, care in turning and moving the patient, and good nursing practices minimize this complication.

LARYNGEAL/TRACHEAL DAMAGE. Prolonged intubation may cause laryngeal or tracheal injury.[106,108-112] Excessive cuff pressure and prolonged intubation can initiate mucosal erosion, cartilage necrosis, and eventually tracheal stenosis. Movement of the tube during assisted ventilation may erode the trachea, usually in the posterior membranous portion. Tracheal or bronchial rupture occurs more frequently in infants, the elderly, or in patients with chronic obstructive lung disease. Because signs and symptoms may be delayed, chest radiographs and prompt endoscopy can confirm the diagnosis.

NOSOCOMIAL INFECTION. A complication dreaded during long-term tracheal intubation is the development of nosocomial pulmonary infection.[113-115] Infection results from oropharyngeal colonization and bacterial aspiration. Certain microorganisms such as *Pseudomonas*, *Acinetobacter*, and *Staphylococci* produce glycocalyx, a molecular cement that allows organisms to stick to each other, the wall of the endotracheal tube, and the respiratory tract. Adhesive colonization of the tube may be a significant factor in the pathogenesis of nosocomial pulmonary infection. Diagnosis is often difficult: sputum cultures, transthoracic needle aspiration, and protected specimen brushes have been used, but none has been entirely satisfactory. Antibiotic prophylaxis only facilitates the selection and acquisition of bacterial resistance that makes treatment more difficult and infection more likely.

MISCELLANEOUS. Other problems encountered during intubation are aspiration of gastric contents secondary to silent regurgitation and leakage past the cuff. Paranasal sinusitis develops in 2% to 5% of nasally intubated patients[116-118] and commonly involves the maxillary sinus. Most patients have gram-negative polymicrobial infection. Signs and symptoms include fever and purulent nasal discharge, which appear 2 days after nasal and oral intubation. An infrequently reported complication is middle ear infection.[119,120] The incidence reaches as high as 30%, with *Pseudomonas*, *Klebsiella*, and *Enterobacter* accounting for most infecting organisms. Infection results from bacterial reflux into the Eustachian tube, followed by contiguous spread into the middle ear.

Nasotracheal intubation can cause avulsion of the turbinate bone[121] when the tube engages the anterior end of the middle turbinate's lateral attachment in the nose and forces the avulsed turbinate into the nasopharynx. Additionally, prolonged nasotracheal intubation often causes naris ulceration related to the duration of intubation or because of poor tube fixation and support.[122]

During Extubation

Problems during extubation arise secondary to mechanical damage, which develops while the tube is in place or in response to tissue injury. Failure to deflate the cuff, adhesion of the tube to the tracheal wall, or transfixation of the tube by a suture to a nearby structure may result in difficult or impossible extubation.[123] Laryngospasm represents the most serious complication during this period. It may cause airway obstruction, especially if laryngeal edema is still present. Other causes of airway obstruction after extubation are blood clots, foreign bodies, dentures, and throat packs lodged in the airway. Passive regurgitation or active vomiting at extubation may result in gastric content aspiration.

After Extubation

Complications after extubation are divided into early (up to 72 hours) and late (more than 72 hours).

EARLY.   Early complications are listed in Table 50-5. Mechanical irritation to the pharyngeal mucosa causes sore throat.[124] This common, benign intubation sequela develops in 40% to 100% of cases. It affects female patients more than male patients and typically resolves in 48 to 72 hours. Pressure on the hypoglossal or lingual nerve may result in numbness of the tongue, which can persist for up to 2 weeks after extubation. In 45% of cases, laryngitis develops because of local mucosal damage.

Laryngeal edema, although not always clinically important in adults, may compromise the already small laryngeal opening in children. Edema can involve the supraglottic, retroarytenoidal, and subglottic areas. Severe respiratory obstruction may occur after extubation and frequently requires urgent reintubation or tracheotomy. Steroid use in the prevention and treatment of laryngeal edema is controversial.[71] Intravenous dexamethasone reportedly has prevented traumatic laryngeal edema and hastened resolution of existing traumatic edema.[125]

Vocal cord paralysis can also occur after extubation.[125,126] Paralysis may be unilateral or bilateral, with the left cord twice as frequently affected as the right. Male patients are

TABLE 50-5. Tracheal Intubation Complications After Extubation

TIME OF OCCURRENCE	COMPLICATIONS
Early (0–72 h)	Numbness of tongue
	Sore throat
	Laryngitis
	Glottic edema
	Vocal cord paralysis
Late (>72 h)	Nostril stricture
	Laryngeal ulcer, granuloma, or polyp
	Laryngotracheal webs
	Laryngeal or tracheal stenosis
	Vocal cord synechiae

seven times more likely to experience this problem than female patients. Recurrent laryngeal nerve injury can have several effects. Damage to the external laryngeal nerve may cause lasting voice change, and unilateral nerve injury usually causes hoarseness. Paralysis can result and, if the injury is bilateral, may lead to airway obstruction. The patient usually recovers in 4 to 5 weeks.

LATE.   Late postextubation complications include laryngeal ulcer, granuloma, polyp, synechiae (fusion) of the vocal cords, laryngotracheal membrane webs, laryngeal or tracheal fibrosis, and nostril stricture from damage of the alae.[127–129] Laryngeal ulcerations or granulomas are more commonly located at the posterior region of the vocal cords where the endotracheal tube tends to have more continual contact. The patient may complain of foreign body sensation, fullness or discomfort at the back of the throat, and persistent hoarseness.

Granuloma formation may lead to chronic hoarseness; it seems to be related to the type of tube material rather than duration of intubation. If the posterior third of the vocal cords fuse, aphonia and respiratory obstruction can occur. The gravest extubation sequela, tracheal stenosis, occurs with or without laryngeal stenosis.[68–72,129] Symptoms of progressive respiratory obstruction appear as late as 45 to 60 days after extubation. Occasionally, the problem escapes attention for years. In the subglottic area and particularly the trachea, the lesion is circumferential at the previous level of the cuff. After the lumen narrows to less than 5 mm, stridor is common. Although dilatation can provide relief, surgical intervention often is required.

TRACHEOTOMY   ■

Although tracheotomy is one of the oldest surgical procedures, its role in airway management of critically ill patients remains controversial. It carries a mortality rate of 2% to 5% with potentially lethal complications.[130–132] Reported indications for elective tracheotomy are relief of upper airway obstruction, improved suctioning, decreased work of breathing, provision of airway access for prolonged mechanical ventilation, decreased dead space, improved patient comfort, and assistance in weaning mechanically ventilated patients with marginal pulmonary function.

Indications for emergency tracheotomy include rare instances of direct laryngeal trauma and emergent airway control in infants.[133] The procedure remains within the surgical domain and requires skill and thorough knowledge of regional anatomy to avoid serious iatrogenic complications. Contraindications include patients with fresh sternotomies, because of the danger of infection spread from the stoma to the sternotomy site and mediastinum. It should be avoided in most cases of emergency airway access because of a high morbidity and complication rate.[134,135]

The timing for tracheotomy in translaryngeally intubated patients is controversial. Proponents of early tracheotomy argue that prolonged transtracheal intubation causes greater risk from laryngeal injury; this problem is more difficult to treat after recovery from respiratory failure. They suggest that tracheotomy offers better patient comfort, simplifies patient care, and carries a decreased risk of laryngeal damage.[136,137] When the procedure is performed under optimal conditions by properly trained surgeons, complications are markedly reduced; tracheotomy is thus urged after 5 days of intubation.[138]

Proponents of delayed tracheotomy, beyond 2 or more weeks of translaryngeal intubation, argue that the procedure is risky. It exposes the patient to surgical and medical complications, promotes long-term tracheal injury, causes bacterial colonization of the airway, and prolongs intubation unnecessarily because of the reluctance to expeditiously discontinue a surgically placed airway.[139-141] Berlauk[142] emphasizes the safety of translaryngeal intubation for up to 3 weeks; others report uncomplicated intubation lasting 2 to 6 months.[143,144]

CRICOTHYROIDOTOMY

Percutaneous or surgical cricothyroidotomy is a standard approach during emergencies when translaryngeal intubation is difficult, impossible, or contraindicated.[145-148] The procedure requires access to the airway at the level of the cricothyroid membrane. Although faster, easier, and safer than emergency tracheotomy, cricothyroidotomy generates some degree of trepidation because the procedure and indications are rare. Because of a reportedly high incidence of subglottic stenosis, chronic tracheal cannulation with cricothyroidotomy has not gained widespread acceptance.[149-151]

Cricothyroidotomy is indicated when nasal or oral intubation fails or is contraindicated for relief of upper airway obstruction; during traumatic facial injuries where other techniques of emergency airway access are difficult to perform; and in those with recent sternotomy who require airway access. Patients in whom cricothyroidotomy is contraindicated are relatively few and include those who have been translaryngeally intubated for more than 3 days because of the propensity to develop subglottic stenosis; those with laryngeal injury; and infants and small children in whom anatomic landmarks are difficult to palpate.[146,152]

CUFF INFLATION

Common to most airway tubes are inflatable cuffs at the distal end. The cuff serves two purposes. Once inflated, it creates a seal against the underlying tracheal mucosa, making aspiration of pharyngeal or gastric contents into the trachea less likely. It also helps to prevent air leak, thereby facilitating positive-pressure ventilation. Problems of cuff inflation damage to the trachea have been mentioned earlier but are discussed in detail in the following section.

HIGH-PRESSURE, LOW-VOLUME CUFFS

Cuffs are classified as high-pressure or low-pressure. High-pressure cuffs have low volume and compliance and can exert as much as 180 to 250 mm Hg of pressure on the tracheal mucosa before creating an effective seal. When inflated, these cuffs are spherical and narrow and have a small area of tracheal contact. They expand the trachea until the normal C-shaped tracheal contour is lost, at which point the trachea is forced to assume the cuff's shape.[78]

High cuff pressure transmission exceeds the capillary perfusion pressure (normally 25 to 35 mm Hg), and ischemia results. Persistent ischemia leads to tracheal necrosis, stricture, or tracheoesophageal fistula formation. The mechanism of high pressure–induced tracheal injury is illustrated in Figure 50-8.[153] Low compliance cuffs may also expand asymmetrically, deforming the trachea and producing tracheal dilatation. When tracheal injury occurs, the rigid, nonyielding tracheal wall becomes more extensively damaged than does the posterior membranous portion.[153-155]

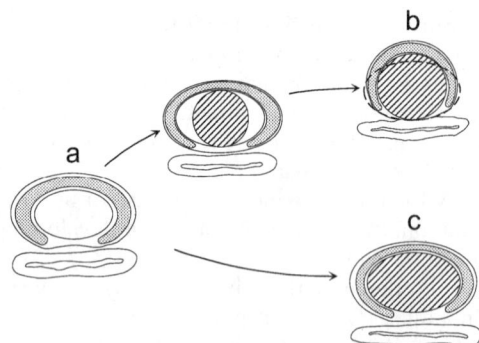

FIGURE 50-8. Mechanism of tracheal injury by high-pressure cuff inflation. A high-pressure cuff produces a narrow, spherically shaped structure with a small area of tracheal contact. It expands the trachea until the normal C shape of the tracheal form is lost and the trachea assumes the cuff's shape. Pressure on the tracheal wall exceeds capillary perfusion pressure, resulting in mucosal ischemia, inflammation, hemorrhage, and ulceration. This ultimately leads to tracheal dilatation, granuloma formation, tracheomalacia, tracheal stenosis, and, in some instances, erosion into the innominate artery. (From Cooper JD, Grillo HC: The evolution of tracheal injury due to ventilatory assistance through cuffed tubes: a pathologic study. *Ann Surg* 1969;169:334.)

LOW-PRESSURE, HIGH-VOLUME CUFFS

Low-pressure, high-volume cuffs adapt to the tracheal contour without deforming its shape. When used correctly, they inflate symmetrically and provide a seal with the trachea at relatively low intraluminal cuff pressures. Their sausage-like shape allows the pressure to be transferred to the trachea over a wide area, causing a lower tracheal wall pressure at any given point. The lower pressure causes less obstruction to mucosal blood flow than occurs with high-pressure cuffs.[156-158] Pressures above 25 to 35 mm Hg cause at least partial obstruction to tracheal mucosal perfusion.[159-162]

Even at low cuff pressures, normal tracheal mucosal architecture may be disrupted. Superficial histologic damage and ciliary denudation have been observed at the cuff site when pressure was less than 25 mm Hg.[159,163] Figure 50-9 shows the comparison of the pressure volume curves of high-pressure and low-pressure cuffs before and after placement in the trachea, clearly illustrating the significant difference in intracuff pressure necessary to create a seal.[81]

Cuff Size

Although available modern endotracheal tubes are classified as low-pressure and high-volume, not all behave the same way under different clinical settings.[88] Cuffs of nearly identical diameter (internal diameters one and one half times that of the trachea) but of different lengths provide an equal and adequate tracheal seal at peak inflation pressures less than 25 mm Hg. When lung compliance is reduced and peak inflation pressure is increased to 80 cm H_2O, shorter cuffs need an inflation pressure of nearly 50 mm Hg compared with only 30 mm Hg in longer cuffs. The difference in performance is attributed to the length of their tracheal contact. The distal ends of both cuffs collapse when the peak airway pressure is increased, whereas the proximal end bulges outward, changing the cuff shape from cylindric to conical[88] (Fig. 50-10).

Inflation Volume and Pressure

Ideally, the cuff should be inflated to a point that allows a seal without jeopardizing tracheal mucosal blood flow. Careful monitoring and control of cuff pressure is necessary to prevent significant changes. Patients with poor lung compliance, high airway resistance, or both may require higher pressure to seal, thus limiting the protection afforded by low-pressure, high-volume cuffs.[88] During general anesthesia with nitrous oxide, intracuff pressure increases because of nitrous oxide diffusion into the cuff.[164-166] This problem can be prevented by inflating the cuff with gas from the breathing circuit rather than with air[167,168] or by periodic cuff deflation and reinflation.

After prolonged intubation, cuff pressures have been observed to decrease with time, although the magnitude of decrease and time were not correlated.[169] This reduction is believed to result from diffusion of gas and from slow movement (creeping) of plastic in the cuff. Intermittent increases occur during positive-pressure ventilation if the airway pressure exceeds that in the cuff. Transient large increases are seen during coughing, chest physiotherapy, and when a patient struggles with the ventilator.[170]

Measurement of Pressure and Volume

Measurement and monitoring of intracuff volume and pressure are necessary during prolonged periods of tracheal intubation. The equipment is simple and composed of an aneroid manometer and a syringe attached to the female port of a three-way stopcock.[171] The male element of the stopcock is attached to the pilot balloon in the closed position to prevent air escape from the pilot line. After suctioning the pharynx free of secretions, the stopcock is opened, and the entire air volume is aspirated and measured. The air is then reinjected back into the cuff, and the stopcock is again turned to the off position. The stopcock is then rotated to the sec-

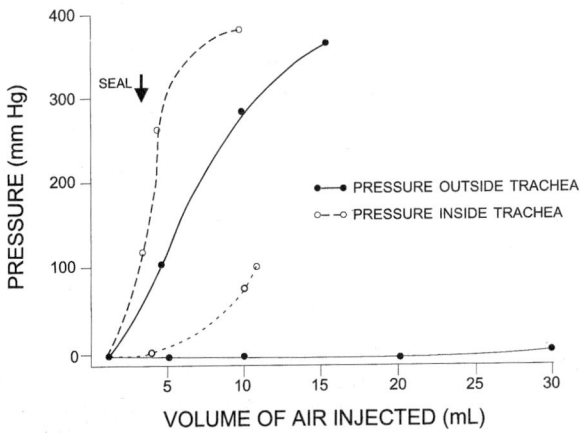

FIGURE 50-9. Difference in volume and pressure curves of low-pressure and high-pressure endotracheal tube cuffs. Solid and dotted lines show the volume and pressure curves of low-pressure and high-pressure cuffs, respectively. (From Dunn CR, Dunn DL, Moser KH: Determinants of tracheal injury by cuffed tracheostomy tubes. *Chest* 1974;65:128.)

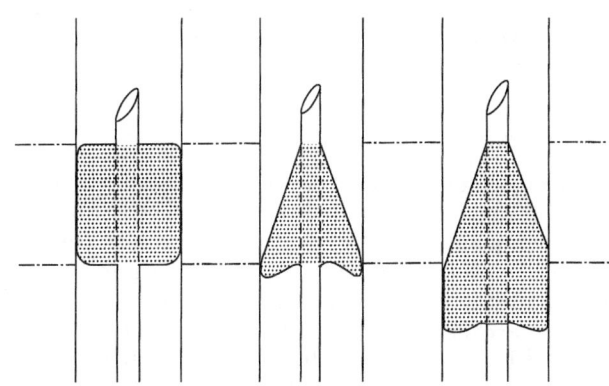

FIGURE 50-10. Effect of increased peak airway pressure on an endotracheal tube cuff's shape. (From Guyton DC: Endotracheal and tracheotomy tube cuff design: influence on tracheal damage. *Crit Care Updates* 1990;1:1.)

ond orifice to allow cuff pressure to be measured by the manometer. It is then rotated again to allow air from the cuff to be aspirated into the syringe.

The volume obtained at this point is lower than the original volume because some of the air filling the pressure-measuring system previously was in the cuff. Additional air is reinjected into the cuff to compensate for that lost to the manometer tube, and the stopcock is again rotated to the position that allows pressure to be read from the manometer. This pressure is higher than the initial reading and is the true intracuff pressure, compensating for the volume of air in the manometer.

Minimal Leak Cuff Inflation

To minimize the possibility of an excessively high intracuff pressure, the minimal leak inflation technique is increasingly preferred. The cuff is inflated during positive-pressure ventilation until total occlusion occurs between the cuff and the tracheal wall. Air is then gradually aspirated until minimal air leak is heard at peak inspiratory pressure. The tidal volume is then adjusted to compensate for the minimal loss through the leak in this system. This approach minimizes tracheal damage at low to moderate peak inflation pressure but not when high ventilatory pressure is necessary.

No Leak Cuff Inflation

In some clinical situations, the minimal leak technique may not be helpful, and total occlusion is desirable, particularly for patients who aspirate repeatedly, have poor lung compliance, or require high levels of positive end-expiratory pressure to maintain adequate ventilation and oxygenation. In these instances, a "no leak" technique with minimal occluding volume is used to inflate the cuff. This approach requires frequent, round-the-clock monitoring of intracuff pressure and volume.

To assure that minimum pressure and volume are used, the cuff is inflated and deflated in a similar manner as for the minimal leak technique. Once a minimal leak is observed, an additional volume of air is slowly injected until no leak is appreciated. This process is periodically repeated. This technique of cuff pressure inflation is prevalent in the operating room to avoid contamination of the room with anesthetic gases.

Intermittent Cuff Inflation

This approach involves injection of a small, static volume of gas into the cuff at a pressure below that which is associated with tracheal mucosal ischemia. A specially constructed cuff inflator that cycles on synchronously with each mechanical inflation injects whatever additional gas volume is necessary to reach peak airway pressure without an air leak.[89] When the ventilator cycles to exhalation, the added gas is aspirated from the cuff, leaving only the baseline "safe" volume with acceptable intracuff pressure. Thus, tracheal perfusion is maintained throughout exhalation. Massive tracheal dilatation from a chronically hyperinflated cuff has been managed successfully by this approach.[171]

REFERENCES ■

1. Campbell TP, Stewart RD: Oxygen enrichment of bag valve mask units during positive pressure ventilation: a comparison of various techniques. *Ann Emerg Med* 1988;17:232
2. Hayes H: Cardiopulmonary resuscitation. In: Wilkens EW (ed). *Emergency Medicine.* Baltimore, Williams & Wilkins, 1989:10
3. Hocbaum SR: Emergency airway management. *Emerg Clin North Am* 1986;4:411
4. Jorden RC: Airway management. *Emerg Clin North Am* 1988;6:671
5. Florete OG: Airway management. In: Civetta JM, Taylor RW, Kirby RR (eds). *Critical Care,* 2nd ed. Philadelphia, JB Lippincott, 1992:1419
6. Hasegawa EA: The endotracheal use of emergency drugs. *Heart Lung* 1986;15:66
7. Greenberg MI: Endotracheal drugs: state of the art. *Ann Emerg Med* 1984;13:789
8. Greenberg MI, Mayeda DV, Chrzanowski R, et al: Endotracheal administration of atropine sulfate. *Ann Emerg Med* 1982;10:546
9. Powers RD, Donowitz LG: Endotracheal administration of emergency medications. *South Med J* 1983;77:340
10. Dauphine K: Nasotracheal intubation. *Emerg Clin North Am* 1988;6:715
11. Moore EE, Eiseman B, Vanuy CW: *Critical Decisions in Trauma.* St Louis, CV Mosby, 1984:30
12. Donlon JV: Anesthetic management of patients with compromised airways. *Anesth Rev* 1980;VII:22
13. Linscott MS, Horton WC: Management of upper airway obstruction. *Otolaryngol Clin North Am* 1979;12:351
14. Lockhart PB, Feidbau EV, Sabel RA, et al: Dental complications during and after tracheal intubation. *J Am Dental Assoc* 1986;23:480
15. Block C, Brechner VL: Unusual problems in airway management. II. The influence of the temporomandibular joint, the mandible and associated structures on endotracheal intubation. *Anesth Analg* 1971;50:14
16. Bannister FB, Macbeth RG: Direct laryngoscopy and intubation. *Lancet* 1944ₓ:651
17. Stone DJ, Gal TJ: Airway management. In: Miller RD (ed). *Anesthesia,* 4th ed, vol 2. New York, Churchill Livingstone, 1994:1408
18. Magill IW: Technique in endotracheal anesthesia. *Br Med J* 1930;2:817
19. Salem MR, Mathrubhutham M, Bennet EJ: Difficult intubation. *N Engl J Med* 1975;295:879
20. Brechner VL: Unusual problems in the management of airways. I. Flexion-extension mobility of the cervical vertebrae. *Anesth Analg* 1968;47:363
21. Bogetz MS, Kalz JA: Airway management of the trauma patient. *Semin Anesth* 1985;4:114
22. Kastendieck JG: *Emergency Medicine,* ed 2. St Louis, CV Mosby, 1987:41
23. Natanson C, Shelhamer JH, Parillo JE: Intubation of the trachea in the critical care setting. *JAMA* 1985;253:1160
24. Sellick BA: Cricoid pressure to control regurgitation of stomach contents during induction of anesthesia. *Lancet* 1961ₓ:404
25. MacIntosh RR: New laryngoscope. Lancet 1943;i:205
26. Barkin RM: Pediatric airway management. *Emerg Med Clin North Am* 1988;6:687
27. Mallampati SR, Gatt SP, Gugino LD, et al: A clinical sign to predict difficult tracheal intubation: a prospective study. *Can Anaesth Soc J* 1985;32:429

28. Mallampati SR: Clinical sign to predict difficult tracheal intubation (hypothesis). *Can Anaesth Soc J* 1983;30:316

29. White A, Kander PL: Anatomical factors in difficult direct laryngoscopy. *Br J Anaesth* 1975;47:468

30. Benumof JL: Management of the difficult adult airway. *Anesthesiology* 1991;75:1087

31. Practice guidelines for management of the difficult airway: a report by the American Society of Anesthesiologists Task Force on management of the difficult airway. *Anesthesiology* 1993;78:597

32. Gold MI, Buechel DR: Translaryngeal anesthesia: a review. *Anesthesiology* 1959;20:181

33. Stoelting RK: Local anesthetics. In: *Pharmacology and Physiology in Anesthetic Practice*, 2nd ed. Philadelphia, JB Lippincott, 1991:148

34. Gross JB, Hartigan ML: A suitable substitute for 4% cocaine before blind nasotracheal intubation: 3% lidocaine-0.25% phenylephrine nasal spray. *Anesth Analg* 1984;63:915

35. Marshall BE, Wollman H: General anesthetics. In: Gilman AG, Goodman RS, Rall RW (eds). *The Pharmacologic Basis of Therapeutics*. New York, Macmillan, 1985:276

36. Flacke JW, Bloor BC, Kripke E-A, et al: Comparison of morphine, meperidine, fentanyl and sufentanil in balanced anesthesia: a double blind study. *Anesth Analg* 1985;64:897

37. Stanski DR, Hug CC: Alfentanil: a kinetically predictable narcotic analgesic. *Anesthesiology* 1982;87:435

38. Foldes FF, Tarda TAG: Comparative studies with narcotics and narcotic antagonists in man. *Acta Anaesthesiol Scand* 1965;9:121

39. Greenblatt DJ: Benzodiazepines. *N Engl J Med* 1974;291:1011

40. Reves JG, Fragen RJ, Vinik HR, et al: Midazolam: pharmacology and uses. *Anesthesiology* 1981;54:66

41. Cooperman LH, Strobel GE, Kennel EM: Massive hyperkalemia after administration of succinylcholine. *Anesthesiology* 1970;32:161

42. Gronert GA, Theye RA: Pathophysiology of hyperkalemia induced by succinylcholine. *Anesthesiology* 1975;65:89

43. Collier BB: Ketamine and the conscious mind. *Anaesthesia* 1972;27:120

44. Sebel PS, Lowdon JD: Propofol: a new intravenous anesthetic. *Anesthesiology* 1989;71:260

45. Taylor MB, Grounds RM, Dulrooney PD, et al: Ventilatory effects of propofol during induction of anaesthesia: comparison with thiopentone. *Anaesthesia* 1986;41:816

46. Smith JP, Bodai BI, Seifkin A, et al: The esophageal obturator airway: a review. *JAMA* 1983;250:1081

47. Harrison EE, Ward HJ, Bleman RW: Esophageal perforation following use of the esophageal obturator airway. *Ann Emerg Med* 1980;9:21

48. Jancey W, Wear SR, Kamajian G: Unrecognized tracheal intubation: a complication of the esophageal obturator airway. *Ann Emerg Med* 1980;9:18

49. Key GK: Use of the esophageal obturator airway with a report of an unusual complication. *Postgrad Med* 1980;67:189

50. Niemann JT, Rosborough JP, Myers R, et al: The pharyngeotracheal lumen airway: preliminary investigation of a new adjunct. *Ann Emerg Med* 1984;13:591

51. Bartlett RL, Martin SD: The pharyngeo-tracheal lumen airway: an assessment of airway control in the setting of upper airway hemorrhage. *Ann Emerg Med* 1987;16:343

52. Frass M, Frenzer R, Zdrahl F, et al: The esophageal tracheal combitude: preliminary results with a new airway for CPR. *Ann Emerg Med* 1987;16:768

53. Elam JO, Titel JH, Feingold A, et al: Simplified airway management during anaesthesia or resuscitation: a binasal pharyngeal system. *Anesth Analg* 1969;48:407

54. Brain AIJ: The laryngeal mask: a new concept in airway management. *Br J Anaesth* 1983;55:801

55. Leach AB, Alexander CA: The laryngeal mask: an overview. *Eur J Anaesthesiol Suppl* 1991;4:19

56. Smith I, White PF: Use of the laryngeal mask airway as an alternative to a face mask during outpatient arthroscopy. *Anesthesiology* 1992;77:850

57. Brain AIJ: The laryngeal mask: a new concept in airway management. *Br J Anaesth* 1983;55:801

58. Calder I, Ordman AJ, Jackowski A, et al: The brain laryngeal mask airway: an alternative to emergency tracheal intubation (case report). *Anaesthesia* 1990;45:137

59. Riley RH, Swan HD: Value of the laryngeal mask during thoracotomy (Letter). *Anesthesiology* 1992;77:1051

60. Benumof JL: Laryngeal mask airway: indications and contraindications. *Anesthesiology* 1992;77:843

61. Benumof JL: Management of the difficult airway: with special emphasis on the awake tracheal intubation. *Anesthesiology* 1991;75:1087

62. Brimacombe J: The laryngeal mask airway and flexible bronchoscopy [letter]. *Thorax* 1991;46:591

63. Walker RWM, Murrel D: Yet another use for the laryngeal mask airway. *Anaesthesia* 1991;46:591

64. Tanigawa K, Inoue Y, Iwata S: Protection of recurrent laryngeal nerve during neck surgery: a new combination of neutracer, laryngeal mask airway, and fiberoptic bronchoscope [letter]. *Anesthesiology* 1991;74:918

65. Grebenik CR, Ferguson C, White A: The laryngeal mask airway in pediatric radiotherapy. *Anesthesiology* 1990;72:474

66. Cork RC, Depa RM, Standen JR: Prospective comparison of use of laryngeal mask and endotracheal tube for ambulatory surgery. *Anesth Analg* 1994;79:719

67. Fisher JS, Ananthanarayan C, Edelist G: Role of the laryngeal mask in airway management. *Can J Anaesth* 1992;39:1

68. Blanc FB, Tremblay NAG: The complications of tracheal intubation: a new classification with a review of the literature. *Anesth Analg* 1974;53:202

69. Gaylor EB, Greenberg SB: Untoward sequelae of prolonged intubation. *Laryngoscope* 1985;95:1461

70. Donnelly WH: Histopathology of endotracheal intubation. *Arch Pathol* 1969;88:511

71. McGovern FH, Fitz-Hugh GS, Edgemon LJ: The hazards of endotracheal intubation. *Ann Otolaryngol* 1971;80:556

72. Rashkin MC, Davis T: Acute complications of endotracheal intubation: relation to reintubation, route, urgency, and duration. *Chest* 1986;89:165

73. Zwillich CW, Pierson DJ, Creagh CE et al: Complications of assisted ventilation: a prospective study of 354 consecutive episodes. *Am J Med* 1974;57:161

74. Stewart RD, Paris PM, Winter PM, et al: Field endotracheal intubation by paramedical personnel: success rates and complications. *Chest* 1984;85:341

75. Taryle DA, Chandler JE, Good JT, et al: Emergency room intubations: complications and survival. *Chest* 1979;75:541

76. Lewis FR, Schlobohm RM, Thomas AN: Prevention of complications from prolonged tracheal intubation. *Am J Surg* 1978;135:452

77. Ching NPH, Ayers SM, Spina CR, et al: Endotracheal damage during continuous ventilatory support. *Ann Surg* 1974;179:123

78. Cooper JD, Grillo HC: Analysis of problems related to cuffs on intratracheal tubes. *Chest* 1972;62(Suppl):21S

79. Shelly WM, Dawson RB, Macy IA: Cuff tubes as a cause of tracheal stenosis. *J Thorac Cardiovasc Surg* 1969;57:623

80. Seegobin RD, van Hasselt GL: Endotracheal cuff pressures and tracheal mucosal blood flow: endoscopic study of effects of four large volume cuffs. *Br Med J* 1984;288:965
81. Dunn CR, Dunn CL, Moser KM: Determinants of tracheal injury by cuffed tracheostomy tubes. *Chest* 1974;65:84
82. Cox PM Jr, Schatz ME: Pressure measurements in endotracheal cuffs: a common error. *Chest* 1974;65:84
83. Bernhard WN, Yost L, Turndorf H, et al: Cuffed tracheal tubes: physical and behavioral characteristics. *Anesth Analg* 1982;61:36
84. Deane RS, Schinozoki T, Morgan JG: An evaluation of cuff characteristics and incidence of laryngeal complications using a new nasotracheal tube in prolonged intubation. *J Trauma* 1977;17:311
85. Lederman DS, Klein EF Jr, Drury WD, et al: A comparison of foam and air-filled endotracheal tube cuffs. *Anesth Analg* 1974;53:521
86. Tonnessen AS, Vereen L, Arens JF: Endotracheal tube cuff residual volume and lateral wall pressure in a model trachea. *Anesthesiology* 1981;55:680
87. Crawley BE, Cross DE: Tracheal cuffs: a review and dynamic pressure study. *Anaesthesia* 1975;30:4
88. Guyton DC: Endotracheal and tracheotomy tube cuff design: influence on tracheal damage. *Crit Care Update* 1990;1:1
89. Kirby RR, Robison EJ, Schulz J: Intermittent cuff inflation during prolonged positive-pressure ventilation. *Anesthesiology* 1970;32:364
90. Wagner DL, Gammage GW, Wong ML: Tracheal rupture, following the insertion of a disposable double endotracheal tube. *Anesthesiology* 1985;63:698
91. Clapham MCC, Vaughan RS: Bronchial intubation: a comparison between polyvinyl chloride and red rubber double-lumen tubes. *Anaesthesia* 1985;40:1111
92. Heiser M, Steinberg JJ, MacVaugh H, et al: Bronchial rupture, a complication of use of the Robertshaw double-lumen tube. *Anesthesiology* 1979;51:88
93. Samsoon GLT, Young JRB: Difficult tracheal intubation: a retrospective study. *Anaesthesia* 1987;42:487
94. Cormack RS, Lehane J: Difficult tracheal intubation in obstetrics. *Anaesthesia* 1984;39:1105
95. Stauffer JL, Petty TL: Accidental intubation of the pyriform sinus: a complication of "roadside" resuscitation. *JAMA* 1977;237:2324
96. Gotein KJ, Rein AJ-JT, Gornstein A: Incidence of aspiration in endotracheally intubated infants and children. *Crit Care Med* 1984;12:19
97. Wynne JW, Modell JH: Respiratory aspiration of stomach contents. *Ann Intern Med* 1977;87:466
98. Seto K, Goto H, Hacker DC, et al: Right upper lobe atelectasis after inadvertent right main bronchial intubation. *Anesth Analg* 1983;62:851
99. Gandhi SK, Munshi CA, Kampine JP: Early warning sign of an accidental endobronchial intubation: a sudden drop or sudden rise in PaCO$_2$? *Anesthesiology* 1986;65:114
100. Owen RL, Cheney FW: Endobronchial intubation: a preventable complication. *Anesthesiology* 1987;67:255
101. Pollard BJ, Junius F: Accidental intubation of the oesophagus. *Anaesth Intens Care* 1980;8:183
102. Glinsman D, Pavlin EG: Airway obstruction after nasal-tracheal intubation. *Anesthesiology* 1982;56:229
103. Kemmots O: Six cases of endotracheal tube obstruction. *Jpn J Anesthesiol* 1971;21:259
104. Greene ER Jr, Gutierez FA: Tip of polyvinyl chloride double-lumen endotracheal tube inadvertently wedged in left lower lobe bronchus. *Anesthesiology* 1986;64:406
105. Brodsky JB, Shulman MS, Mark JBD: Malposition of left-sided double-lumen endotracheal tubes. *Anesthesiology* 1985;62:667
106. Hedden M, Erosoz CEJ, Donnelly WH, et al: Laryngotracheal damage after prolonged use of orotracheal tubes in adults. *JAMA* 1969;207:703
107. Conrardy PA, Goodman LR, Lainge F, et al: Alteration of endotracheal tube position: flexion and extension of the neck. *Crit Care Med* 1976;4:8
108. Dubick MN, Wright BD: Comparison of laryngeal pathology following long term oral and nasal endotracheal intubation. *Anesth Analg* 1978;57:663
109. Kastanos N, Miro RE, Perez AM, et al: Laryngotracheal injury due to endotracheal intubation incidence, evolution and predisposing factors: a prospective long term study. *Crit Care Med* 1983;11:362
110. Thompson DS, Read RC: Rupture of the trachea following intratracheal intubation. *JAMA* 1968;204:137
111. Kumar SM, Pandit SK, Cohen PJ: Tracheal laceration associated with endotracheal anesthesia. *Anesthesiology* 1977;47:298
112. Freiberger JJ: An unusual presentation of an airway tear. *Anesthesiology* 1984;61:204
113. Matthew EB, Holstrom FMG, Kaspar RL: A simple method for diagnosing pneumonia in intubated or tracheotomized patients. *Crit Care Med* 1977;5:76
114. Brook I: Bacterial colonization, tracheobronchitis and pneumonia following tracheostomy and long-term intubation in pediatric patients. *Chest* 1979;76:420
115. Sottile FD, Marie TJ, Prough DS, et al: Nosocomial pulmonary infection: possible etiologic significance of bacterial adhesion to endotracheal tubes. *Crit Care Med* 1986;14:265
116. Caplan ES, Hoyt NJ: Nosocomial sinusitis. *JAMA* 1982;247:839
117. Gallagher TJ, Civetta JM: Acute maxillary sinusitis complicating nasotracheal intubation: a case report. *Anesth Analg* 1976;55:885
118. Grindlinger GA, Niehoff J, Hughes SL, et al: Acute paranasal sinusitis related to nasotracheal intubation of head-injured patients. *Crit Care Med* 1987;15:214
119. Balkany TJ, Berman SA, Simmons MA, et al: Middle ear effusion in neonates. *Laryngoscope* 1978;88:398
120. Lucks D, Consiglio A, Stankiewecz J: Incidence and microbiological etiology of middle ear effusion complicating endotracheal intubation and mechanical ventilation. *J Infect Dis* 1988;157:368
121. Scamman FL, Babin RW: An unusual complication of nasotracheal intubation. *Anesthesiology* 1983;59:352
122. Sherry KM: Ulceration of the inferior turbinate: a complication of prolonged nasotracheal intubation. *Anesthesiology* 1983;59:148
123. Lee C, Schwartz J, Mok MS: Difficult extubation due to transfixation of a nasotracheal tube by a Kirschner wire. *Anesthesiology* 1977;46:427
124. Loeser EA, Orn DL, Bennett GM, et al: Endotracheal tube cuff design and postoperative sore throat. *Anesthesiology* 1976;45:684
125. Hahn FW, Martin JT, Lillie JC: Vocal cord paralysis with endotracheal intubation. *Arch Otolaryngol* 1970;92:226
126. Salem MR, Wong AY, Barangan VC, et al: Postoperative vocal cord paralysis in paediatric patients. *Br J Anaesth* 1971;43:696
127. Jackson C: Contact ulcer granuloma and other laryngeal complications of endotracheal anesthesia. *Anesthesiology* 1953;14:425
128. Klainer AS, Turndorf H, Wu W-H, et al: Surface alterations due to endotracheal intubation. *Am J Med* 1975;58:674

129. Rainer WG, Sanchez M, Lopez L: Tracheal stricture secondary to cuffed tracheotomy tubes. *Chest* 1971;59:115

130. Frost EAM: Tracing the tracheostomy. *Ann Otol Rhinol* 1976;85:618

131. Heffner JE, Miller KS, Sahn SA: Tracheostomy in the ICU. II. Complications. *Chest* 1986;90:430

132. Selecky PA: Tracheostomy: a review of present-day indications, complications, and care. *Heart Lung* 1974;3:272

133. Piotrowski JJ, Moore EE: Emergency department tracheostomy. *Emerg Med Clin North Am* 1988;6:737

134. Heffner JE, Miller KS, Sahn SA: Tracheostomy in the intensive care unit. I. Indications, technique, management. *Chest* 1986;90:269

135. Heffner JE, Sahn SA: The technique of tracheostomy and cricothyroidotomy. *J Crit Care Illness* 1987;2:79

136. Burns HP, Dayal VS, Scott A, et al: Laryngotracheal trauma: observation on its pathogenesis and its prevention following prolonged endotracheal intubation in the adult. *Laryngoscope* 1979;89:1316

137. White RE: A prospective study of laryngotracheal sequelae in long term intubation. *Laryngoscope* 1984;94:367

138. El-Naggar M, Sadagopa S, Levin H, et al: Factors in influencing choice between tracheostomy and prolonged translaryngeal intubation in acute respiratory failure: a prospective study. *Anesth Analg* 1976;55:195

139. Stauffer JL, Olsen DE, Petty TL: Complications and consequences of endotracheal intubation and tracheostomy: a prospective study of 150 critically ill adult patients. *Am J Med* 1981;70:65

140. Brooks R, Bartlett RH, Gazzaniga AB: Management of acute and chronic disorders of the trachea and subglottis. *Am J Surg* 1988;150:24

141. Dayal VS, Masri W: Tracheostomy in intensive care setting. *Laryngoscope* 1986;96:58

142. Berlauk JF: Prolonged endotracheal intubation vs. tracheostomy. *Crit Care Med* 1986;14:742

143. Via-Reque E, Pattenborg CC: Prolonged oro- or nasotracheal intubation. *Crit Care Med* 1981;9:637

144. Skaggs JA: Tracheostomy: management, mortality, complications. *Am Surg* 1969;35:393

145. Walls RM: Cricothyroidotomy. *Emerg Clin North Am* 1988;6:725

146. Mace SE: Cricothyrotomy. *J Emerg Med* 1988;6:309

147. Collicot PA, Aprahamian C, Carrico CJ, et al: Upper airway management. In: *Advanced Trauma Life Support Course.* Chicago, American College of Surgeons, 1984:155

148. Roven AN, Clapham MC: Cricothyroidotomy. *Ear Nose Throat J* 1983;62:68

149. Boyd AD, Romita MC, Conlan AA, et al: A clinical evaluation of cricothyrotomy. *Surg Gynecol Obstet* 1979;149:365

150. Essess BA, Jafek BW: Cricothyroidotomy: a decade of experience in Denver. *Ann Otol Rhinol Laryngol* 1987;96:519

151. O'Connor JV, Redy K, Ergin MA, et al: Cricothyroidotomy for prolonged ventilatory support after cardiac operations. *Ann Thorac Surg* 1988;39:353

152. Sise MJ, Shaelford SR, Cruickshank JC, et al: Cricothyroidotomy for long term tracheal access. *Ann Surg* 1984;200:13

153. Cooper JD, Grillo HC: The evolution of tracheal injury due to ventilatory assistance through cuffed tubes: a pathologic study. *Ann Surg* 1969;169:334

154. Cooper JD, Grillo HC: Experimental production and prevention of injury due to cuffed tracheal tubes. *Surg Gynecol Obstet* 1969;129:1235

155. Grillo HC, Cooper JD, Geffin B, et al: A low pressure cuff for tracheostomy tubes to minimize tracheal injury. *J Thorac Cardiovasc Surg* 1971;62:898

156. Ching NP, Nealon TB Jr: Clinical experience with new low-pressure, high-volume tracheostomy cuffs: importance of limiting intracuff pressure. *NY State J Med* 1974;74:2379

157. Dobrin P, Canfield T: Cuffed endotracheal tubes: mucosal pressure and tracheal wall blood flow. *Am J Surg* 1977;133:562

158. Leigh JM, Maynard JP: Pressure on the tracheal mucosa from cuffed tubes. *Br Med J* 1979;1:1173

159. Nordin U: The trachea and cuff-induced tracheal injury. *Acta Otolaryngol Suppl (Stockh)* 1977;345:1

160. Bjorkund S, Ekedahl C, Hansson PG, et al: Experimental tracheal wall injury. *Acta Otolaryngol* 1973;75:387

161. Dobrin P, Canfield T: Cuff endotracheal tubes: mucosal pressures and tracheal wall blood flow. *Am J Surg* 1972;133:562

162. Nordin U, Lindholm CE, Wolfgast M: Blood flow in the rabbit tracheal mucosa under normal conditions and under the influence of tracheal intubation. *Acta Anaesth Scand* 1977;21:8

163. Klainer AS, Turndorf H, Wen-Hsien WV, et al: Surface alterations due to endotracheal intubation. *Am J Med* 1975;58:674

164. Stanley TH, Kawamura R, Graves C: Effects of nitrous oxide on volume and pressure of endotracheal tube cuffs. *Anesthesiology* 1974;41:256

165. Stanley TH: Effects of anesthetic gases on endotracheal tube cuff gas volumes. *Anesth Analg* 1974;53:480

166. Stanley TH: Nitrous oxide and pressures and volumes of high and low pressure endotracheal tube cuffs in intubated patients. *Anesthesiology* 1975;42:637

167. Stanley TH, Liu WS: Tracheostomy and endotracheal tube cuff volume and pressure changes during thoracic operations. *Ann Thorac Surg* 1975;20:144

168. Ravenas B, Lindholm CE: Pressure and volume changes in tracheal tube cuffs during anesthesia. *Acta Anaesthesiol Scand* 1976;20:321

169. Jacobsen L, Greenbaum R: A study of intracuff pressure measurements, trends and behaviour in patients during prolonged periods of tracheal intubation. *Br J Anaesth* 1981;53:97

170. MacKenzie CF, Klose S, Browne DRG: A study of inflatable cuffs on endotracheal tubes. *Br J Anaesth* 1976;48:105

171. Jaeger JM, Wells NC, Kirby RR, et al: Mechanical ventilation of a patient with decreased lung compliance and tracheal dilatation. *J Clin Anesth* 1992;4:147

Critical Care, Third Edition, edited by Joseph M. Civetta,
Robert W. Taylor, and Robert R. Kirby.
Lippincott-Raven Publishers, Philadelphia, PA © 1997.

CHAPTER 51

Hyperbaric Medicine

Luis A. Matos

IMMEDIATE CONCERNS

MAJOR PROBLEMS

Hyperbaric medicine (HM) evolved into a clinical specialty developed from undersea medicine. Initially, HM was limited to the treatment of air embolism and decompression sickness (DCS) in divers and flyers. However, in the 1980s and 1990s, its scope has broadened dramatically, and managing problem wounds has become an integral part of clinical medicine. This evolution occurred because we understand the pivotal role that oxygen plays in wound repair and resistance to infection. Since the 1960s, systematic, in vitro, randomized, controlled animal studies have elucidated mechanisms that subsequently have been confirmed by clinical experience.

Currently, clinical HM services provide hyperbaric oxygen (HBO) therapy for diseases enumerated in the Guidelines of the Undersea and Hyperbaric Medical Society[1] (Table 51-1). Diagnostic transcutaneous oximetry (TCO) and a comprehensive wound management program are tools that facilitate proper patient selection and improve the effectiveness of HBO treatment for problem wounds in which hypoxia or infection play a significant etiologic role.

STRESS POINTS

1. Basic components of HBO therapy include the mechanical effect of pressure, used to compress bubbles, and the increased partial pressure of gases, particularly oxygen, that increases tissue oxygen partial pressure (PO_2).
2. The compression of gas-filled bubbles present in patients with DCS or air embolism is a reflection of Boyle's law: As pressure increases inside the hyperbaric chamber, the volume and diameter of a gas bubble in the body decreases (Table 51-2).
3. Typically, the maximum chamber pressure used to treat DCS is 2.8 atmospheres absolute (ATA), which is equivalent to 60 feet of sea water (fsw). For air embolism, the pressure is 6 ATA (165 fsw). At a pressure of 6 ATA, a gas bubble is reduced to approximately one sixth (16%) of its original volume and to about 50% of its original diameter. This reduction in bubble size improves blood flow and aids in bubble resolution.
4. Bubble resolution is faster if 100% oxygen is breathed. Because oxygen is toxic at high pressures, breathing pure oxygen is usually limited to chamber treatment pressures of 3 ATA (66 fsw) or less.
5. Increased PO_2 increases the amount of oxygen physically dissolved in plasma, thereby improving tissue oxygenation and correcting tissue hypoxia, as well as increasing the PO_2 gradient from blood to tissues.
6. At normal sea level pressure, arterial PO_2 (PaO_2) is about 100 mm Hg, hemoglobin is about 97% saturated with oxygen, and blood oxygen content is about 19.5 mL/dL. When hemoglobin is 100% saturated, 1 dL of blood transports 20.1 mL of oxygen in association with hemoglobin (20.1 mL/dL).
7. Because hemoglobin can be fully saturated by breathing oxygen at 1 ATA, HBO therapy does not increase oxyhemoglobin. However, dissolved oxygen in the plasma, which is normally only 0.31 mL/dL at 100 mm Hg PO_2, can be significantly increased during HBO therapy. The amount of oxygen dissolved in plasma is determined by its solubility coefficient and the partial pressure of respired oxygen, as defined by Henry's law.
8. Hyperbaric oxygen exposure in typical clinical treatment is 2 to 3 ATA, which is equivalent to 33 to

TABLE 51-1. Hyperbaric Oxygen Indications

1. Clostridial myonecrosis (gas gangrene)
2. Necrotizing soft tissue infections (subcutaneous tissue, muscle, fascia)
3. Crush injury, compartment syndrome, and other acute traumatic ischemias
4. Enhancement of healing in selected problem wounds
5. Compromised skin grafts and flaps
6. Radiation tissue damage
7. Air or gas embolism
8. Decompression sickness
9. Carbon monoxide poisoning and smoke inhalation
10. Refractory osteomyelitis
11. Thermal burns
12. Exceptional blood loss (anemia)

66 fsw (Table 51-3). This exposure increases alveolar oxygen partial pressure (PAO_2) to 1400 to 2200 mm Hg, enabling large amounts of oxygen, ranging from 4.4 to 6.8 mL/dL, to dissolve in plasma. This example illustrates the effects of Henry's law: In a hyperbaric chamber, as pressure increases, more oxygen dissolves in the plasma during 100% oxygen breathing.

9. This significant increase in dissolved oxygen increases the pericapillary diffusion gradient and drives oxygen into avascular areas. Such a gradient can be achieved only by HBO therapy, thus forming the basis for its use in hypoxic or infected problem wounds.

ESSENTIAL DIAGNOSTIC TESTS, PROCEDURES, AND THERAPY

1. Hyperbaric oxygen therapy requires informed consent. The patient or family members need to understand the risks of the hyperbaric environment such as ear, sinus, and pulmonary barotrauma and oxygen toxicity.
2. The chest radiograph should be assessed to identify pneumothorax, severe chronic obstructive lung disease (COLD), blebs, or active pulmonary infection.

Patients with pneumothorax must have a chest tube inserted to prevent tension pneumothorax during therapy.

3. Myringotomies and placement of pressure equalization tubes must be performed in intubated patients to prevent middle and inner ear barotrauma. Patients who are unable to autoinflate their middle ears (Eustachian tube dysfunction) also require this procedure.
4. To prevent loss of airway control from compression of air in the cuffs, endotracheal and tracheotomy tube cuffs should be filled with saline.
5. If an extubated patient is not alert and has questionable airway control, the trachea should be intubated and the patient placed on ventilatory support. The ventilator should be small and lightweight, simple to operate, pneumatically powered, and unaffected by pressure. The Penlon-Oxford ventilator is safe and reliable in the hyperbaric environment. It is a pressure-driven, time-cycled, volume-set ventilator to which alarms are easily added.
6. If a patient is not hemodynamically stable, invasive arterial and central pressure monitoring should be established. The Marquette (Tram) monitor can be used inside the chamber for cardiac and hemodynamic monitoring. Chest tubes should be properly secured and connected to water seal. They should not be removed before treatment.
7. The number of intravenous catheters should be minimized to prevent introduction of air into the vascular system if any become accidentally disconnected. I use infusion pumps for delivery of vasoactive substances and other intravenous therapy.
8. Adequate sedation and pain control are important when the patient is combative or significant pain is present. Morphine with midazolam or diazepam works well. A combative patient can be paralyzed with vecuronium.
9. Frequent suctioning for significant pulmonary secretions is necessary in the chamber to prevent air trapping and pulmonary barotrauma during the ascent phase.
10. If a seizure occurs during HBO therapy, 100% oxygen should be stopped; it may have precipitated the seizure. Anticonvulsive therapy usually is not required.

TABLE 51-2. Bubble Volume and Diameter Relative to Total Pressure Applied

DEPTH PRESSURE		RELATIVE VOLUME (%)	RELATIVE DIAMETER (%)
(feet)	ATA		
Sea Level	1	100	100
33	2	50	79.3
45	2.36	42.4	75.7
66	3	33.3	69.3
165	6	16.6	55

ATA, atmospheres absolute.

TABLE 51-3. Ideal Dissolved Oxygen Content in Blood and the Alveolar Oxygen Pressure

TOTAL PRESSURE		AIR (mL/dL)	100% O_2 (mL/dL)	PAO_2 (mm Hg)
ATA	*fsw*			
1	0	0.31	2.09	673
2	33	0.81	4.44	1433
2.36	45	0.99	5.29	1707
3	66	1.31	6.80	2193

ATA, atmospheres absolute; fsw, feet of sea water.

Chamber pressure should not be altered during a seizure or bronchospasm; pulmonary barotrauma can occur.

11. Claustrophobia can be problematic in some patients. It usually can be resolved by reassurance, sedation, or both.

CLINICAL APPLICATION ■

MECHANISM OF ACTION

Local tissue hypoxia (tissue Po_2 below 30 to 40 mm Hg) and infection in wound healing impair polymorphonuclear white blood cell and fibroblast function.[2] HBO therapy increases the Po_2 of hypoperfused or infected wounds and promotes the wound repair process[3] (Table 51-4). When tissue Po_2 is raised above 40 mm Hg with HBO therapy, wound healing is stimulated by directly enhancing fibroblastic replication, collagen synthesis, and epithelialization. Hyperbaric oxygen also stimulates angiogenesis in the ischemic wound. This effect seems to be mediated by an increase in the Po_2 gradient between the functional capillaries and the wound space.[4,5]

Disruption in wound oxygen delivery increases susceptibility to infection.[6] A reduction of tissue Po_2 below 30 to 40 mm Hg impairs the oxygen-dependent leukocyte bacterial killing mechanisms for common aerobic organisms found in wound infections and abscesses.[7,8] Hypoxia also allows anaerobic organisms to flourish. By increasing tissue Po_2, HBO therapy increases leukocyte bacterial activity and oxygen radicals that have direct bactericidal or bacteriostatic effects on anaerobic organisms.

TRANSCUTANEOUS OXIMETRY

HBO therapy does not accelerate tissue repair in wounds with normal Po_2 and will be effective only in hypoxic wounds in which the tissue Po_2 can be elevated to therapeutic levels. Thus, measuring Po_2 in the periwound soft tissue envelope helps to decide if HBO treatment has a role.

TCO is a simple, reliable, noninvasive diagnostic technique that provides an objective assessment of local tissue oxygenation and perfusion. It can be used repetitively to assess problem wounds (e.g., ischemic compromised flaps and grafts, marginal wound dehiscence, amputation sites, traumatic degloving injuries, compromised diabetic foot, and ischemic lower extremities).

Transcutaneous Po_2 is measured by placing the electrode of a transcutaneous oxygen pressure ($TcPo_2$) monitor over the skin area to be evaluated. Usually, one electrode is placed on the anterior chest wall as a control, and several electrodes are placed near the wound site over intact skin. Measurements also may be obtained while the patient is breathing 100% oxygen at normobaric pressures (1 ATA) and during HBO therapy.

In general, wounds in the lower extremities with $TcPo_2$ values below 30 mm Hg (air breathing) have a low probability of healing, whereas values higher than 40 mm Hg usually

TABLE 51-4. Hyperbaric Oxygen Therapy: Mechanisms of Action

Decrease bubble size

Elevate tissue oxygen partial pressure
    Promote fibroblastic activity and collagen synthesis
    Neovascularization
    Enhance leukocyte bacterial killing
    Vasoconstriction
    Inhibit growth of anaerobic bacteria

predict a successful wound outcome. TCO is used to determine the degree of hypoxia, the wound healing potential, the selection of amputation level, and the prediction of response to HBO therapy.[9]

Hauser[10] prospectively assessed 159 wounds in 113 high-risk patients with diabetes mellitus and peripheral vascular disease. In this study, the regional perfusion index (RPI, or wound $TcPo_2$ divided by chest $TcPo_2$) was compared with the leg to brachial blood pressure index (BPI). Surgical wound management consisted of 93 local debridements (48 healed) and 66 amputations (45 healed). When the RPI was greater than 0.8, all wounds healed. When the ratio was between 0.6 and 0.8, 94% healed. With values between 0.4 and 0.6, 58% healed. When the RPI value was below 0.4, primary wound healing was achieved in only 3% of the procedures. The RPI was a more accurate predictor of healing than was the BPI. The author believed that the use of RPI values would have dramatically reduced the rate of wound failure.

A study of extremity major vascular trauma by Mathieu and colleagues[11] suggests that transcutaneous oxygen measurements obtained in the HBO environment are a valuable adjunctive method for prediction of the final outcome. Patients whose wounds healed had $TcPo_2$ increase from 31 ± 19 mm Hg (breathing air) to 425 ± 292 mm Hg with HBO therapy, whereas those whose wounds did not heal had 34 ± 46 mm Hg (breathing air) to 113 ± 148 mm Hg ($p < 0.05$).

Robla and associates[12] used TCO to assess soft tissue injury in open tibial fractures. $TcPo_2$ less than 85 mm Hg (breathing oxygen) and a wound-to-chest ratio less than 25% was found to correlate with the development of complications in the study group. Wattel and coworkers[13] studied 59 diabetic patients with soft tissue infection or gangrenous changes of the foot. Values greater than 450 mm Hg obtained during HBO therapy predicted successful outcome. Increases in TCO during HBO therapy also predict healing.

TCO reliably determines tissue viability and allows maximum tissue preservation, particularly in limb salvage situations. $TcPo_2$ enhances the ability of the physician specializing in hyperbaric medicine to properly select patients for therapy by identifying tissue hypoxia at ambient pressures and its correction by HBO therapy. It can also assist orthopedic surgeons in their decision to débride or amputate the severely compromised lower extremity, or to consider revascularization as an alternative, if a functional extremity can be achieved.

INDICATIONS ■

GAS GANGRENE AND NECROTIC SOFT TISSUE INFECTIONS

Clostridial myonecrosis and rapidly spreading necrotizing soft tissue infections are surgical emergencies that carry high morbidity and mortality. A successful outcome is based on prompt recognition of the disease process, early surgical debridement, appropriate intravenous antibiotics, HBO therapy, and aggressive wound management.

Gas gangrene is produced most frequently by *Clostridium perfringens*, a facultative anaerobic organism that can grow freely in tissue with a Po_2 up to 30 mm Hg, and in a restricted manner in tissue Po_2 up to 70 mm Hg. Its devastating tissue effect is caused by the continuous production of alpha exotoxin, which is hemolytic and tissue necrotizing. Gas gangrene begins in areas of low tissue Po_2, including wounds with severe extensive soft tissue damage, necrotic muscle, or significant vascular compromise.

Hyperbaric oxygen therapy that produces tissue hyperoxia ($Po_2 > 250$ mm Hg), inhibits clostridial alpha toxin production. Tissue Po_2 above 300 mm Hg can be achieved during HBO therapy at 3 ATA (66 fsw). The significant increase in Po_2 and subsequent oxygen-free radical formation is lethal to most anaerobic organisms that lack the enzymes superoxide dismutase, catalases, and peroxidases.

In a landmark study, De Mello and colleagues[14] established the efficacy of HBO therapy in a large controlled, randomized study using a dog model of lethal *C. perfringens* infection. A combination of surgery, antibiotics, and HBO therapy achieved 95% survival rate, the highest of any treatment modality studied.

Hart and associates[15] showed that the lowest morbidity and mortality in a large clinical series were obtained with early HBO therapy plus conservative surgical debridement and intravenous antibiotic therapy. An 80% salvage rate of extremities with posttraumatic clostridial myonecrosis was demonstrated, together with a 5% mortality rate and a 70% survival rate for gas gangrene involving the head and trunk.

Treatment should be started as soon as the presumptive diagnosis (clinical findings and gram-positive rods) of clostridial myonecrosis is made. The initial operative intervention should be limited to debridement of grossly necrotic tissue and fasciotomies of the involved extremity to prevent vascular compromise. Therapy should include penicillin G as part of a double or triple antibiotic regimen directed against a presumed polymicrobial flora.

Hyperbaric oxygen therapy should follow the initial surgical debridement. The chamber is pressurized to 3 ATA and the patient breathes 100% oxygen for 90 minutes. The treatment schedule consists of three treatments during the first 24 hours, followed by two treatments daily until the infection is completely controlled. Seven treatments are usually given during a 3-day period. Early HBO therapy disrupts the anaerobic tissue environment and halts advancing margins of the infection. This protocol produces early tissue demarcation that minimizes tissue loss and prevents major extremity amputation or excessive debridement. Mortality is decreased because alpha toxin production is interrupted and less radical surgery is required in critically ill patients.

If a hyperbaric chamber is not available, transfer to a hospital with a clinical hyperbaric facility should be considered.

NECROTIZING FASCIITIS

Necrotizing fasciitis is a polymicrobial soft tissue infection with high morbidity and mortality.[16] This progressive, rapidly spreading infection causes significant undermining and tracks along fascial planes. Necrosis is secondary to an occlusive endarteritis that creates local hypoxia and severely impairs leukocyte function.

The accepted management of necrotizing fasciitis is wide excision of all necrotic fascia and the nonviable soft tissue envelope. In addition, appropriate intensive antibiotic therapy is required. Hyperbaric oxygen therapy should be considered in patients who do not respond to standard treatment or when high morbidity is expected. I advocate HBO therapy for patients with diabetes mellitus, vascular compromise, or immunosuppression.

Riseman and associates[17] report that HBO therapy reduced the mortality and number of debridements in necrotizing fascitis. Although patients in the HBO group were more severely ill, their mortality was significantly lower (23%) compared with those in the control group (66%) ($p < 0.02$). Only 1.2 debridements were required to achieve infection control in the HBO group compared with 3.3 debridements in the control group.

In life- or limb-threatening situations, I treat the patient at 2.36 ATA (45 fsw) with 100% oxygen for 90 minutes twice a day to stop the progression of infection and to minimize tissue loss. Thereafter, I continue daily treatments until a clean, granulating soft tissue envelope is suitable for grafting.

The rationale for adjunctive HBO therapy in necrotizing fasciitis also applies to other polymicrobial necrotizing soft tissue infections such as Fournier's gangrene, non-clostridial myonecrosis, and progressive bacterial gangrene.

SELECTED TRAUMATIC INJURIES

The importance of a comprehensive, multidisciplinary approach to managing crush injuries, acute traumatic ischemia, and complex open fractures of the extremities cannot be overemphasized. Vascular compromise reinforces a hostile environment through hypoxia, thereby reducing host resistance to infection, halting wound healing, and increasing posttraumatic edema. Hyperbaric oxygen therapy enhances the viability of compromised tissues. In HBO therapy (2.36 ATA), a Po_2 of 1500 mm Hg can be achieved. This 15-fold increase in Po_2 increases the oxygen diffusion gradient to areas with severely compromised blood flow.

HBO therapy–associated vasoconstriction reduces blood flow by 20% but provides enough oxygen dissolved in plasma to maintain the compromised tissue. The reduction in flow minimizes edema and enhances microcirculatory blood entry. Hyperbaric therapy maximizes the viability of marginal tissue, prevents or controls wound infection, decreases the soft tissue losses, and provides a well-vascularized recipient bed for successful reconstruction and bone grafting. Such therapy must be used early to be useful. Adjunctive HBO therapy is based on physiologic data,[18] supported by animal studies,[19–21] and limited clinical experience.[22,23]

For limb-threatening injuries, I use adjunctive HBO therapy at 2.36 ATA (45 fsw) with 100% oxygen for 90 minutes twice a day. Once the threat of limb loss has passed, HBO therapy is used daily to improve the soft tissue envelope quality.

If soft tissue reconstruction is performed and the graft or muscle flap becomes compromised, therapy should be used to enhance flap or graft viability and to minimize tissue loss. I have treated several patients with low TcPo₂ values and large traumatic subcutaneous skin flaps (i.e., the medial border of the tibia). Tissue viability has been preserved until soft tissue perfusion is improved. This approach facilitates extremity reconstruction. Adjunctive HBO therapy is also beneficial in eliminating soft tissue infection after aggressive debridement of necrotic and infected bone in osteomyelitis.

PROBLEM WOUNDS

Problem wounds result from varying degrees of tissue ischemia and infection. The most important management principles are to determine the underlying cause and to identify and treat any correctable risk factors disrupting the wound healing process. Baroni and associates[24] showed that HBO therapy was efficacious in the management of diabetic feet (Wagner classification types III and IV). Hyperbaric oxygen resulted in a significantly higher healing rate and lower amputation rate. In addition, Hammarland and Sundberg[25] report that HBO therapy was a valuable adjunct to conventional treatment in refractory nondiabetic wounds.

COMPROMISED FLAPS AND GRAFTS

Hyperbaric oxygen therapy is effective in increasing survival of compromised grafts and flaps. If signs of necrosis, infection, ischemia, or dehiscence occur, HBO therapy can significantly increase tissue Po₂. As discussed earlier, this effect stimulates angiogenesis and seems to close arteriovenous shunts in nonischemic areas, thereby increasing perfusion to ischemic tissue distally.

In a controlled randomized animal study, Nemiroff and Lungu[26] found that the absolute number and size of blood vessels in skin flap microvasculature was significantly greater in the HBO-treated group. Bowersox and associates[27] reviewed 105 patients with threatened flaps or grafts who received HBO therapy. Eighty-nine percent of the flaps and 91% of the skin grafts were salvaged; patients with a poor outcome had three or more wound healing risk factors. When flap or graft viability is in question, HBO therapy should be started as soon as possible to be effective. Once significant tissue necrosis or progressive infection is observed, such therapy generally has a marginal effect.

As with life-threatening necrotizing fasciitis, I use HBO treatments at 2.36 ATA with 100% oxygen for 90 minutes twice a day. Once the tissue appears more viable, and risk factors are corrected, treatment is continued on a daily basis. It is stopped when tissues are clearly demarcated and the recipient bed is stable.

RADIATION INJURY

Irradiated tissue becomes hypocellular, hypovascular, and hypoxic. With time, spontaneous wound breakdown may occur. Therapeutic radiation abolishes the oxygen gradient between adjacent normal soft tissue envelope and the wound space that is required for revascularization of the wounded tissue. Irradiated tissue (>5000 cGy) does not have the capacity for normal wound healing.

Therapy with HBO creates a steep oxygen gradient into the wound space, as documented by Marx and colleagues.[5] In irradiated tissue, the capillary density is approximately 20% to 40% that of nonirradiated tissue. Twenty HBO treatments induce vascular proliferation and increase the density to 75% to 85% of normal.

The outcome for patients undergoing surgery in a previously irradiated field has been improved significantly by HBO therapy. Marx[28] assessed three types of wound complications in patients undergoing major surgery or flap placement into irradiated tissue (>6900 cGy). Wound infection occurred in 16% of the patients in the control group and in 2.5% of the patients in the HBO group. Wound dehiscence was seen in 33% of the patients in the control group and 3.5% of the patients in the HBO group. Finally, delayed wound healing was documented in 55% of the patients in the control group compared with 11% of the patients in the HBO group.

At the University of Miami, the Marx protocol provides 20 HBO treatments before surgery to induce the maximum possible angiogenesis and 10 treatments after surgery to meet the increase in metabolic demands of the wounded tissues.

CARE BEFORE HBO THERAPY ■

Successful management of the critically ill patient requires a team approach and meticulous attention to detail. Transportation from the ICU to the hyperbaric chamber can be a dangerous event. The risk versus benefit of HBO therapy and the risk of patient transport must be carefully evaluated. Transport should be performed by an ICU team with the necessary monitoring equipment (Chap. 52).

TECHNIQUES

The multiplace chamber is a metal vessel designed to accommodate several patients and medical personnel simultaneously. It usually has at least two compartments (locks) to allow passage of other medical personnel, equipment, and medications to the treatment compartment while it remains pressurized. Hyperbaric therapy is provided by administering 100% oxygen intermittently through a plastic hood, double-seal face mask, or endotracheal tube to the patients inside the chamber, which is pressurized with compressed air.

A monoplace chamber occasionally is used. This is a small, cylindrical, single-compartment vessel in which a patient can be treated by pressurization with 100% oxygen. No means of direct patient access are available while the chamber is pressurized.

WOUND MANAGEMENT

A wound care program based on wound healing physiology is critical to promote tissue viability and minimize complications such as infection, dehiscence, and amputation. Wound management doesn't mean just dressing changes! Assessment of the problem wound should start with the identification and correction of risk factors that inhibit tissue repair.

Nutritional Deficits

Nutritional deficits impair tissue repair and increase susceptibility to infection. Dickhaut and colleagues[29] found that if the serum albumin was 3.5 g/dL and the total lymphocyte count was at least 1500/μL, the amputation healing rate was 86%. When these criteria were not met, the healing rate was 18%. If clinical evidence of malnutrition is present, deficiency of other critical nutrients such as vitamins C and A, zinc, iron, and folate may be present. Specific essential nutrients should be replaced.

Soft Tissue Infection

The presence of invasive wound infection (bacterial concentration greater than 10^5 organisms per gram of tissue) impairs tissue repair and leukocyte function.[30] Proper wound management and specific antimicrobial therapy reduces the bacterial load and promotes wound healing. Patients with systemic diseases such as diabetes mellitus[31] have an increased susceptibility to infection and slower wound healing. Supplemental oxygen should be considered to improve host antibacterial defenses. Strict glycemic control is required in the diabetic patient to optimize wound healing.

Radiation Damage

Previous exposure to radiation causes progressive tissue ischemia (see earlier discussion). Surgery performed in previously irradiated tissue is associated with significantly increased postoperative complications. If an operation is necessary, it should be done between 6 weeks and 4 months after radiation therapy, when complications are less likely.

Immunosuppression

Adrenocortical steroids inhibit all phases of wound healing. Chemotherapeutic agents also produce significant impairment of tissue repair. Whenever possible, chemotherapy should be withheld until the early phases of wound repair have been completed. Hunt and colleagues[32] found that topical application of vitamin A counteracts the effects of steroids on open wounds.

Foreign Bodies

Retained foreign bodies increase the risk of wound infection. In general, the foreign body must be removed to control the infection and allow healing. A foreign body must be considered if a wound fails to heal in the absence of any other known risk factor.

Ischemia and Hypoxia

In the presence of clinically significant ischemia and TCO values of less than 30 to 40 mm Hg, or an ischemic index less than 0.45, revascularization may be indicated. If hypoxia persists after revascularization, normobaric supplemental oxygen or HBO therapy may be indicated.

Wound Care

Aggressive and meticulous wound care is essential to preserve marginal tissue and to control infection in the problem wound. Aseptic technique should include cap, mask, and sterile gloves; a wound care room with adequate lighting and table; and all sterile instruments and supplies readily available.

Guidelines should be followed by ICU personnel or the surgical team primarily involved with the patient's care. Because wound care is so critical, to obtain maximum benefit from HBO therapy I have cataloged my own practices:

1. Wound cleansing with noncytotoxic solutions (e.g., Saf-Clens).
2. Wound inspection and gentle exploration to assess tissue viability; determine the presence or absence of necrotic tissue; search for purulent material within the wound space or a foreign body; and to evaluate soft tissue envelope for signs of cellulitis, ischemic changes, or rubor.
3. Sharp debridement to remove all necrotic and devitalized tissue.
4. Opening and drainage of all abscesses.
5. High-pressure wound irrigation. A simple, inexpensive, and effective manual high-pressure wound irrigation system consists of a sterile 50-mL syringe and 18-gauge catheter over needle. The wound irrigation is performed with sterile normal saline. Pressure exerted by fluid delivered through this system is approximately 400 mm Hg. This system is more useful to remove particulate matter (small bits of necrotic debris) and bacteria than is low-pressure irrigation. It does not create tissue damage or embed material into deeper tissues.
6. Usually, normal saline wet-to-dry dressings are adequate. When the wound is colonized with *Pseudomonas*, one eighth percent to one fourth percent acetic acid can be used without affecting the wound healing process. Cytotoxic agents detrimental to tissue repair should not be used. They include hydrogen peroxide, povidone-iodine solution (Betadine), or Dakin's solution.
7. Supplemental oxygen therapy that may increase tissue PO_2 should be used in patients at high risk for wound

failure or infection. For supplemental oxygen to be effective, blood flow must be optimized. I believe that supplemental oxygen has played a significant role in healing refractory hypoxic, infected wounds.

8. Antibacterial therapy may be required to control infection, but it is not a substitute for aggressive wound care.

9. The frequency of wound care is dictated by the severity and extent of the soft tissue injury and degree of infection.

AIR EMBOLISM

Presentation

Air embolism involves the entry of air bubbles into the vascular system as a consequence of pulmonary overpressure accidents in divers[33] and as an iatrogenic surgical event in patients.[34] The presentation ranges from subtle to sudden death. Diagnosis requires a high index of suspicion to recognize the temporal relationship between the introduction of air and the appearance of a sudden neurologic deficit. Most cases of air embolism develop symptoms within 5 to 10 minutes of the event. In divers, the typical scenario involves a sudden loss of consciousness with seizures or altered mental status and a motor or sensory deficit on surfacing or immediately thereafter.

In surgery and anesthesia, air embolism should be suspected when patients do not regain consciousness or a neurologic deficit appears. It should also be considered when sudden dramatic changes in neurologic or cardiovascular status are seen after invasive procedures such as arterial or venous central catheter placement, coronary angiography and angioplasty, upright neurosurgical or head and neck procedures, cardiopulmonary bypass, and mechanical ventilation (Table 51-5). Air embolism also occurs after penetrating chest trauma.

Clinical Manifestations

Clinical manifestations of air embolism are caused by the mechanical effects of bubbles in the vascular system. The dramatic cardiac and neurologic effects result from obstruction of coronary or cerebral blood vessels. In addition to obstruction by gas bubbles, direct endothelial damage occurs, followed by extravasation of fluids into extravascular spaces. This damage is amplified by the complex biochemical sequence of events that occur at the blood–bubble interphase.[33] Ultimately, a loss of blood supply with resultant ischemia follows.

Hyperbaric oxygen therapy is effective because it reduces bubble size. One hundred percent oxygen breathing creates a favorable nitrogen diffusion gradient from the bubble to the surrounding milieu, thus decreasing its size and enhancing resolution. In time, this process reestablishes blood flow and provides tissue hyperoxia.

Treatment

The definitive treatment of air embolism is HBO.[35,36] All other modalities are adjunctive. Once the diagnosis is made,

TABLE 51-5. Causes of Air Embolism

Sudden decrease in ambient pressures
  Breathing compressed air
    Scuba divers
    Workers in compressed air
  Sudden loss of aircraft cabin pressure
  Hyperbaric/altitude chamber exposure
Iatrogenic
  Neurosurgical invasive procedures
  Central catheter insertions
  Cardiopulmonary bypass
  Mechanical ventilation
  Arterial catheter insertions
  Angiography or angioplasty

the patient should be placed in the supine position and 100% oxygen should be administered immediately with a double-sealed mask. A balanced electrolyte solution should be infused, especially in divers, because volume depletion may be significant.

If the patient requires air transportation to a hyperbaric facility, the aircraft cabin pressure should be maintained at normal atmospheric pressure or no "higher" than one thousand feet above sea level. Even a slight increase in altitude (decrease of barometric pressure) increases bubble size, causes further deterioration, and adversely affects outcome.

Most favorable outcomes are obtained when HBO treatment is initiated within 4 to 6 hours of the incident. However, we have had several successful cases although treatment could not be initiated for up to 24 hours. If air embolism is suspected, a physician specializing in hyperbaric/diving medicine should be consulted immediately to assess the clinical situation and coordinate patient management. The patient is taken to a depth of 6 ATA (165 fsw). Hyperbaric therapy is provided according to a United States Navy Treatment Table 6A or initiated at 2.8 ATA (60 fsw) with the manual's Table 6, which uses 100% oxygen instead of air or a nitrox gas mix.[35] Treatment as outlined in the manual's Table 6 provides maximum tissue oxygenation without increasing the nitrogen load in the tissues. A typical case lasts 5 to 6 hours.

Treatments should be continued if neurologic deficits persist. Continue daily therapy until full neurologic recovery occurs or no further improvement is achieved while the patient is inside the chamber undergoing treatment. Severe cases may require 7 to 10 days of therapy. The patient should be followed by a neurologist to document the neurologic status.

DECOMPRESSION SICKNESS

DCS is a disease of scuba divers and, to a lesser extent, aviators. It is produced by a reduction in ambient pressure sufficient to cause formation of bubbles from gas dissolved in the blood and body tissues. Typically, it results from inadequate elimination of dissolved gas after a dive.

Presentation

The clinical patterns have been classically divided into type I DCS (bends) and type II (serious DCS).[37] Type I DCS, the most common type, involves localized pain in the musculoskeletal system, typically described as a deep, dull, extremity joint pain. The most common involved sites are the shoulder, elbow, wrist, hip, knee, and ankle. Type II DCS includes central nervous, respiratory, or cardiovascular manifestations.

Typical neurologic manifestations include paresthesia, muscle weakness, paralysis, alterations in mental status, and inner ear and visual disturbances. In divers, the spinal cord is more frequently affected, whereas lesions in the brain are more commonly seen in aviators.

Pulmonary manifestations of DCS are called chokes; they are life threatening, but fortunately are rare. The triad of substernal chest pain, dry nonproductive cough, and dyspnea is classically described. Vestibular DCS causes dizziness, nausea, and vomiting; tinnitus and loss of hearing also may be present.

Diagnosis and Treatment

The diagnosis of DCS is suggested by an exposure to a depth greater than 2 ATA (33 fsw) and a temporal relationship between the exposure and onset of symptoms. DCS occurs within 3 hours of exposure in 60% of cases; 98% occur within 24 hours.[35] Once the diagnosis is established, HBO therapy should be started as soon as possible. Administration of 100% oxygen with a double-sealed mask and intravenous fluids should be initiated during transportation to a hyperbaric facility. The patient is treated according to United States Navy Tables 5 or 6, depending on the severity of illness.[35,36]

CARBON MONOXIDE POISONING

Carbon monoxide (CO) poisoning is the most common type of poisoning in the United States and has a significant morbidity and mortality.[38] The diagnosis is difficult because CO is colorless, odorless, and tasteless, and the clinical picture is nonspecific. Generally, it is made because of a history of exposure in an environment associated with CO, such as an enclosed room with a natural gas-fueled space heater. It is documented by elevated carboxyhemoglobin (COHb) levels.

Severity

The severity of intoxication depends on the CO concentration in the environment, duration of exposure, and the rate and depth of breathing. No direct correlation exists between COHb levels and the severity of CO intoxication. However, patients with COHb levels less than 10% are usually asymptomatic. With COHb levels up to 20%, the patient often exhibits nausea and vomiting, mild headache, and general malaise. When levels are above 25%, altered mental status, dyspnea, chest pain, and loss of consciousness may be present. Patients in this category are more likely to develop neurologic sequelae.

Treatment

Treatment includes the administration of 100% oxygen to hasten the dissociation of CO from hemoglobin and to correct tissue hypoxia. Hyperbaric oxygen therapy significantly increases carboxyhemoglobin dissociation at a rate that cannot be achieved with 100% oxygen at normal atmospheric pressure. In addition, it improves underlying cellular dysfunction and immediately provides enough oxygen dissolved in plasma to meet tissue metabolic demands. To decrease delayed neurologic sequelae and mortality, HBO therapy is recommended specifically for patients with altered mental status or neurologic signs, cardiac ischemia, or a history of unconsciousness.[38,39]

REFERENCES ■

1. *Hyperbaric Oxygen Therapy: A Committee Report*. Bethesda, MD, Undersea and Hyperbaric Medicine Society, 1992
2. Hunt TK: The physiology of wound healing. *Ann Emerg Med* 1988;17:1265
3. Sheffield PJ: Tissue oxygen measurements. In: Davis JC, Hunt TK (eds). *Problem Wounds: The Role of Oxygen*. New York, Elsevier, 1988:17
4. Knighton D, Silver I, Hunt TK: Regulation of wound healing angiogenesis: effect of oxygen gradients and inspired oxygen concentration. *Surgery* 1981;90:262
5. Marx RE, Ehler WJ, Tayapongsak P, et al: Relationship of oxygen dose to angiogenesis induction in irradiated tissue. *Am J Surg* 1990;160:519
6. La Van FB, Hunt TK: Oxygen and wound healing. *Clin Plast Surg* 1990;17:463
7. Jonsson K, Hunt TK, Mathes SJ: Oxygen as an isolated variable influences resistance to infection. *Ann Surg* 1988;208:783
8. Knighton DR, Halliday B, Hunt TK: Oxygen as an antibiotic: the effect of inspired oxygen on infection. *Arch Surg* 1984;119:199
9. Matos LA, Nunez AA: Enhancement of healing in selected problem wounds. In: Kindwall EP (ed). *Hyperbaric Medicine Practice*. Flagstaff, AZ, Best Publishing, 1994:590
10. Hauser CJ: Tissue salvage by mapping of skin surface, transcutaneous oxygen tension index. *Arch Surg* 1987;122:1128
11. Mathieu D, Wattel F, Bouachour G, et al: Post traumatic limb ischemia: prediction of final outcome by transcutaneous oxygen measurements in hyperbaric oxygen. *J Trauma* 1990;30:307
12. Robla J, Zych GA, Matos A: Assessment of soft tissue injury in open tibial shaft fractures by transcutaneous oximetry. *Clin Orthop* 1994;304:222
13. Wattel FE, Mathieu DM, Neviere RR: Transcutaneous oxygen pressure measurements. *J Hyperbaric Med* 1991;6:269
14. De Mello FJ, Haglin JJ, Hitchcock CR: Comparative study of experimental *Clostridium perfringens* infection in dogs treated with antibiotics, surgery and hyperbaric oxygen. *Surgery* 1973;73:936
15. Hart GB, Lamb RC, Strauss MB: Gas gangrene. I. A collective review. II. A 15-year experience with hyperbaric oxygen. *J Trauma* 1983;23:991
16. Sutherland ME, Meyer AA: Necrotizing soft tissue infections. *Surg Clin North Am* 1994;74:591
17. Riseman JA, Zamboni WA, Surtis A, et al: Hyperbaric oxygen therapy for necrotizing fasciitis reduces mortality and need for débridement. *Surgery* 1990;108:847
18. Boerema I, Meijne G, Brummelkamp K, et al: Life without

blood: study of the influence of high atmospheric pressure and hypothermia on dilution of the blood. *J Cardiovasc Surg* 1960;1:133

19. Nylander G, Lewis D, Nordstrom H, et al: Reduction of post-ischemic edema with hyperbaric oxygen. *Plast Reconstr Surg* 1985;76:595
20. Strauss MB, Hargens AR, Gershuni DH, et al: Reduction of skeletal muscle necrosis using intermittent hyperbaric oxygen in a model compartment syndrome. *J Bone Joint Surg* 1983; 65A:656
21. Skyhar MJ, Hargens AR, Strauss MB, et al: Hyperbaric oxygen reduces edema and necrosis of skeletal muscle in compartment syndromes associated with hemorrhagic hypotension. *J Bone Joint Surg* 1986;68A:1218
22. Shupak A, Gozal D, Ariel A, et al: Hyperbaric oxygenation in acute peripheral posttraumatic ischemia. *J Hyperbaric Med* 1987;2:7
23. Strauss MB: Role of hyperbaric oxygen therapy in acute ischemias and crush injuries: an orthopedic perspective. *HBO Rev* 1981;2:87
24. Baroni G, Porro T, Faglia E, et al: Hyperbaric oxygen in diabetic gangrene treatment. *Diabetes Care* 1987;10:81
25. Hammarlund C, Sundberg T: Hyperbaric oxygen reduced size of chronic leg ulcers: a randomized double blind study. *Plast Reconstr Surg* 1994;93:829
26. Nemiroff PM, Lungu AL: The influence of hyperbaric oxygen and irradiation on vascularity in skin flaps: a controlled study. *Surg Forum* 1987;38:565
27. Bowersox JC, Strauss MB, Hart GB: Clinical experience with hyperbaric oxygen therapy in the salvage of ischemic skin flaps and grafts. *J Hyperbaric Med* 1986;1:141
28. Marx RE: Radiation injury to tissue. In: Kindwall EP (ed). *Hyperbaric Medicine Practice*. Arizona: Best Publishing, 1994:448
29. Dickhaut S, DeLee JC, Page CP: Nutritional status: importance in predicting wound-healing after amputation. *J Bone Joint Surg* 1984;66A:71
30. Robson MC, Stenberg BD, Heggers JP: Wound healing alterations caused by infection. *Clin Plast Surg* 1990;17:485
31. Morain WD, Coley Lawrence B: Wound healing in diabetes mellitus. *Clin Plast Surg* 1990;17:493
32. Hunt TK, Erlich P, Garic JA, et al: Effect of vitamin A on reversing the inhibitory effect of cortisone on healing of open wounds in animals and man. *Ann Surg* 1969;170:633
33. Bradley ME: Pulmonary barotrauma. In: Bove AA, Davis JC (eds). *Diving Medicine*. Philadelphia: WB Saunders, 1990: 188
34. Murphy BP, Harford FJ, Cramer FS: Cerebral air embolism resulting from invasive medical procedures: treatment with hyperbaric oxygen. *Ann Surg* 1985;201:242
35. U.S. Navy Diving Manual. Arizona: Best Publishing, 1993;1:18
36. Davis JC: Treatment of decompression sickness and arterial gas embolism. In: Bove AA, Davis JC (eds). *Diving Medicine*. Philadelphia: WB Saunders, 1990:249
37. Francis TJ, Dutka AJ, Hallenbeck JM: Pathophysiology of decompression sickness. In: Bove AA, Davis JC (eds). *Diving Medicine*. Philadelphia: WB Saunders, 1990:170
38. Myers R, Thom SR: Carbon monoxide and cyanide poisoning. In: Kindwall EP (ed). *Hyperbaric Medicine Practice*. Arizona: Best Publishing, 1994:343
39. Hardy KR, Thom SR: Pathophysiology and treatment of carbon monoxide poisoning. *Clin Toxicol* 1994;32:613

Critical Care, Third Edition, edited by Joseph M. Civetta,
Robert W. Taylor, and Robert R. Kirby.
Lippincott-Raven Publishers, Philadelphia, PA © 1997.

CHAPTER 52

Intrahospital Transport

Gregory M. Gullahorn

IMMEDIATE CONCERNS

MAJOR PROBLEMS

The modern intensive care unit (ICU) concentrates specialized health care professionals who use an array of monitors to assess not only the physiologic status of patients, but also the functional performance of ventilators and other life-support equipment as well. We feel relatively comfortable caring for even the most critically ill patients in the ICU and the operating room (OR), largely because of the monitors and other resources immediately available to diagnose and respond to emergencies or functional changes. This focused care may also be applied to an extent in the postanesthesia care unit (PACU) and emergency room (ER), areas where the intensivist may routinely be involved. Unfortunately, many of our critical care resources are fixed, and the prospect of transporting patients between critical care areas or to other diagnostic and therapeutic locations within the hospital is sure to evoke anxiety.

Technological development has dramatically improved the information available from diagnostic testing such as computed tomography (CT), magnetic resonance imaging (MRI), angiography, cardiac catheterization, and nuclear imaging, as well as a variety of interventions that can be made using these tools. As a result, critically ill patients are, with increasing frequency, moving not only between the ICU and OR, but often on longer journeys to remote locations throughout the hospital. By understanding the problems that can arise during the transport process, we can avoid and lessen the severity of many of these complications.

Such patients are at risk for rapid changes in their physiologic status, and moving them may only magnify such risks. Rather than letting down our guard for the quick trip from the OR to the ICU, we must, if anything, increase our vigilance. Hypoxemia is common in patients after anesthesia, even during the brief transfer from the OR to the PACU. Other sedated or obtunded patients are similarly vulnerable. Patients who are intubated and ventilated frequently experience hemodynamic changes, hypocapnia, and alkalemia during transport.

Patients brought to the ICU after major surgical procedures often develop hypotension, hypertension, and heart rate and ventilatory changes during transfer from the OR. Physiologic changes may increase morbidity, mortality, and expenditure of health care resources. Patients with head injuries are particularly susceptible to secondary insults during transport, and many preventable deaths are attributed to mishaps after arrival in the hospital

STRESS POINTS

1. The transport process should be broken down into three phases: planning and preparation, transport, and stabilization. Adequate attention to the first phase minimizes problems in the other two.
2. Concerns during transport should be individualized depending on the physiologic status of the patient and the nature of the procedure.
3. Planning should involve the physician, nurses, and other health professionals. Communication between parties is vital.
4. Patients should be stabilized as much as possible before transport, and particular attention should be paid to assessment of the airway and the adequacy of intravenous access.
5. Resuscitative and scheduled medications, fluids, monitors, life-support equipment, and adequate personnel need to be assembled. Airway supplies, including

equipment for intubation and ventilation and an oxygen supply, are essential.

6. Ventilator-dependent patients may require a transport ventilator, or even an ICU ventilator, to maintain adequate oxygenation during transport and in the OR.

7. A physician should accompany any unstable patient.

8. Patients remain at risk after return to the ICU, and particular care should be taken during this restabilization period.

ESSENTIAL DIAGNOSTIC TESTS AND PROCEDURES

1. The value of clinical observation should not be overlooked. Monitoring should duplicate that which is present in the ICU as much as possible. Pulse oximetry, electrocardiography, and blood pressure measurement are mandatory in the critically ill. Determination of intracranial pressure (ICP), central venous pressure, and pulmonary artery pressure may be necessary in some patients.

2. Airway pressure monitoring is important in ventilated patients, and spirometry and capnography may be helpful to maintain minute ventilation and avoid swings in arterial blood pressure and Pco_2.

3. Organization, planning, and communication are the most essential procedures and cannot be overemphasized.

OVERVIEW ■

BASIC ISSUES

Patients who are sedated or anesthetized, or who have serious illness or injury may have altered organ system function and abnormal responses to physiologic stress.[1,2] As a general philosophy, we use monitors as an extension of our senses to evaluate an individual patient's physiologic status and homeostatic mechanisms. In doing so, we identify trends or problems that require intervention, and then assess the effects of our therapy. The most efficacious monitors follow trends and functions for which our treatment may have a significant impact, such as pulse oximeters in patients with compromised respiratory status or electrocardiographic (ECG) tracings in patients with arrhythmias.

Anticipation of a patient's response may dictate the use of specific monitors; we would be apprehensive if faced with performing laryngoscopy and intubating a patient with an unclipped intracranial aneurysm or inducing anesthesia in a shock/trauma patient without being able to frequently measure blood pressure. At the completion of surgery, or once a patient is "stabilized" during a resuscitation, less attention may be paid to monitoring for the "quick trip" from the OR to the ICU or PACU. If extensive transport monitoring is not immediately available, a tendency to rush to the destination is often present because of the presumed brief time frame of the transport. I doubt, however, that the potential for physiologic changes with alterations in cardiac rhythm, rate, blood pressure, oxygenation, or ICP are re-

duced during the transport process, nor are their consequences likely to be less severe. The risks of transient untreated hypertension during emergence of a neurosurgical patient after resection of an arteriovenous malformation are potentially severe. Yet, changes are likely related to varying levels of stimulation and to anesthetic elimination (especially volatile agents).[3] A recently extubated, morbidly obese patient emerging from anesthesia may have tenuous oxygenation during a prolonged transfer and transport process. These admittedly extreme examples illustrate the point.

In any situation, simple inspection of the patient is noninvasive and forms the basis of all other monitoring. A precordial or esophageal stethoscope, pulse oximeter, electrocardiograph, blood pressure measurement (invasive or noninvasive), and capnograph are standard monitors in the OR.[4] Neuromuscular response, temperature monitoring, and fluid balance may be followed as dictated by anesthetic technique, the patient's status, and the surgery. Critical care areas provide a setting where we can investigate physiologic changes and where an array of pharmaceutical and other agents are available to address these changes.

COMMON PROBLEMS

Oxygenation

We are taught that airway and breathing are of highest priority, yet hypoxemia is common in sedated patients after anesthesia. Hensley and others[5] found that 60% of patients prepared for coronary bypass surgery became hypoxemic with a Spo_2 less than 90% during placement of invasive monitors after a standard premedication with morphine and scopolamine. All patients were judged to be alert or easily arousable, and 40% actually required additional sedation for comfort during insertion of monitors.[4] Notwithstanding an average transport time of less than 1 minute, 84% of adult patients experienced "modest" desaturation while being moved from the anesthesia induction room to the OR. Two of 25 patients (all of whom were apneic or breathing room air) experienced a decrease to less than 90%.[6] Tyler and coworkers[7] report that in a series of adult patients recovering from anesthesia, 12% desaturated to a Spo_2 of less than 85%, and fully 35% of patients to a Spo_2 of less than 90% during transport from the OR to the PACU.

Healthy pediatric patients are no less at risk. Despite administering 100% oxygen for 3 minutes after surgery, Kataria and colleagues[8] found a significant age-related fall in Spo_2 during a 120- to 180-second transfer to the PACU, with the mean Spo_2 being 88% in children younger than 6 months of age. Studying healthy children with American Society of Anesthesiologists physical status I or II, Tomkins and associates[9] found that 24% became hypoxemic ($Spo_2 <$ 90%) during the first 10 minutes after anesthesia. Significantly, clinical signs of respiratory compromise such as cyanosis or upper airway obstruction correlated poorly with measured hypoxemia.

Administering supplemental oxygen empirically to sedated patients or during the brief transfer from the OR to the PACU minimizes the risk of hypoxemia, and thus I have made this a routine practice. When a longer transit time is anticipated, such as transfer from the OR or ER to the ICU, the potential for adverse events increases. In these circumstances, administering oxygen without monitoring its effects may not be adequate and may provide a false sense of security.

Cardiovascular

Cardiovascular changes seem to be common. Insel and co-workers[3] studied patients being transferred from the OR to the ICU after either major general or vascular surgery, carotid endarterectomy, or coronary artery bypass, comparing them to ICU patients undergoing transport for diagnostic or other nonoperative procedures. In the major postoperative groups, significant alterations occurred in blood pressure and pulse and were associated with noted initial lability. Despite continuous arterial blood pressure monitoring, 20% of patients in the major vascular and general surgery group required vigorous fluid resuscitation for hypotension on arrival in the ICU, whereas 36% required either nitroglycerin or nitroprusside for control of hypertension. Patients in all groups, except nonoperative transport, were also found to be mildly hypothermic.

Central Nervous System

Certain groups of patients are at particularly high risk from mishaps. Secondary insults such as hypoxia, hypotension, or decreased cerebral perfusion pressure are devastating in head-injured patients (Table 52-1). Gentleman and Jennet[10] found that "suboptimum care" was responsible for most avoidable deaths after head trauma, and that more than one third of deaths in neurotrauma patients had avoidable factors. In a large audit of head-injured patients, these investigators report compromised airways in over 25% of victims arriving in the neurosurgical unit, with 15% to 22% demonstrating hypoxemia. Andrews and associates[11] report secondary insults occurring in 47% of neurotrauma patients during transport from the ER, and that fully 80% of patients had insults within the first 4 hours after transfer.[11] Clearly, if factors leading to secondary insults can be identified and controlled, improved monitoring and optimal preparation

for transport might have a dramatic impact on outcome in neurotrauma.

TRANSPORT SCENARIOS

Experienced physicians may feel that the likelihood of clinically significant problems occurring during an expeditious transfer from the OR is remote, except in specific subsets of patients. In most cases, clinical observation is sufficient; the challenge is to identify the patients and the types of transports that carry an increased risk. In developing a rational approach, consider different common scenarios for intrahospital transport, such as those defined by Venkataraman and Orr[12] (Table 52-2).

TRANSFER FROM CRITICAL CARE AREAS

Vigilance and anticipation are basic attributes of critical care medicine and are vital in the safe conduct of each transport. Differences exist, however, in the physiologic status of patients likely to be encountered, as well as the expected stressors imposed by the move. Individuals transferring from a critical care area no longer need the extensive monitoring they had in the ICU or OR. They should not be experiencing cardiovascular or respiratory instability, and may be expected to continue a process of improvement. Major concerns are alterations in level of consciousness and development of airway problems.

TRANSFER TO CRITICAL CARE AREAS

Patients moving to critical care areas present a different set of challenges. Physiologic status may change rapidly, as in the patient with sepsis who has deteriorated on the ward, or the trauma victim who is being resuscitated in the ER. In this setting, the potential for adverse events or secondary insults likely will increase through the transport process, and the breadth of monitoring and preparation required is increased. Clearly, the data in head-injured patients point out the importance of vigilance in this scenario.

TABLE 52-1. Secondary Insults and Poor Outcomes in Head Injury

| PATIENT SUBGROUP | % PATIENTS DEAD/VEGETATIVE/ SEVERELY DISABLED | |
	No Insult	Insult
All	44% (158)	76% (33)
GCS 3–5	66% (68)	100% (15)
GCS 6–8	28% (90)	56% (18)
Operated hematoma	61% (57)	86% (7)
Diffuse injury	35% (101)	73% (26)

GCS, Glasgow Coma Scale.

TABLE 52-2. Intrahospital Transport Scenarios

One-way transfer to critical care areas	ER to ICU or OR Ward to ICU
Transfer between critical care areas	OR to ICU ICU to OR
Round-trip transfer from critical care to noncritical care areas and return	ICU to CT scan and back ICU to cardiac catheterization laboratory and back OR to angiography to ICU
Transfer from critical care areas	OR to PACU or ward

ER, emergency room; OR, operating room; CT, computed tomographic; PACU, postanesthesia care unit.

TRANSPORT FROM CRITICAL CARE AREAS

The critical care unit has evolved to provide multiple life-support modalities, including ventilation, pharmacotherapy, and cardiopulmonary support. These have developed along with progressively sophisticated monitoring systems and personnel who are experienced in treating the severely ill or injured. As we become better at resuscitation and support, we increase the patient pool and, perhaps, the severity of illness of patients who must journey outside of the ICU for various diagnostic and therapeutic interventions. Those of us involved in critical care are justifiably uncomfortable with the transport of patients from the ICU to other parts of the hospital and back. Any intensivist may be called on to assist in this process. Sedation or full general anesthesia may be required for combative or unstable patients who must undergo MRI or CT, angiography, or a variety of invasive radiologic procedures and radiation therapy.

Transport of anesthetized patients to and from ancillary areas poses special clinical and logistical challenges; measures must be taken to ensure the continued adequacy of anesthesia and to assess the impact of anesthetic agents in an already compromised individual. Before such a move is undertaken, the critical care team must carefully weigh the potential for misadventure against the potential of the procedure to improve outcome. Adverse events or mishaps during transport may be related to physiologic changes or to technical or equipment problems.[12] Minor changes in heart rate or blood pressure may have little impact; however, unplanned extubation or loss of intravenous access for pressor support can have lethal consequences. Problems may occur and must be anticipated for any organ system (Table 52-3). Early detection of such changes and rapid intervention are critically important to outcome.

Wadell[13] studied critically ill ICU patients and postoperative patients in the 1970s who had undergone at least one intrahospital transport. Over a 5-month period, at least one critically ill patient a month died or experienced a cardiac arrest from causes directly attributed to the transport process.

Manual Versus Mechanical Techniques

In a prospective study of ventilator-dependent patients who underwent procedures outside the ICU, Braman and colleagues[14] examined changes in arterial blood gas partial pressures and hemodynamic parameters in two treatment groups. Group 1 was ventilated manually during transport, and group 2 by a portable volume-limited ventilator (with settings matched to the bedside ventilator). Significant changes in arterial Pco_2 (> 10 mm Hg) and pH were common in both groups, as was hypotension. However, the incidence rate was clearly greater in the manually ventilated group (75% versus 44%), and two of the group 1 patients developed new cardiac arrhythmias. Blood gas deterioration correlated strongly with the development of hypotension and new arrhythmias. Gervais and coworkers[15] compared manual ventilation with and without spirometry for tidal volume monitoring, and mechanical ventilation with a portable device that allowed tidal volume to be set but had no capacity for measurement. Both groups without spirometry developed significant decreases in $Paco_2$ and increases in pH. When manual ventilation with tidal volume monitoring was used to approximate the minute ventilation patients received in the ICU, no significant changes were observed.[14]

Physiologic Impact

Positive airway pressure impacts venous return, ventricular interdependence, blood pressure, and intracranial elastance. Unintentional changes in arterial Po_2, Pco_2, pH, and blood pressure can be deleterious for patients with cerebrovascular or coronary artery disease, and especially for victims of head injury. These patients are likely to undergo multiple trips for MRI, CT, or angiography, or to the OR.

Contributing Factors

Gentleman and Jennet's[10] case audit revealed that over a third of deaths in patients referred to a neurosurgical unit had avoidable contributing factors. Examining secondary insults in head injury, Andrews and colleagues[11] showed that the occurrence of pretransfer insults (i.e., episodes of hypotension, hypoxia, or intracranial hypertension) in the ER or ICU was predictive of increased ICP during transport and strongly associated with further insults during the first 4 hours after return to the ICU. The authors echo the admonition that adequate resuscitation and stabilization are vital before transport.

Studying factors related to mishaps, Smith and associates[16] prospectively followed a series of 125 intrahospital transports from the ICU. Mishaps were defined as events having a detrimental effect on patient stability (e.g., ventilator disconnection, extubation, intravenous catheter infiltration or disconnection, vasoactive infusion disconnection, invasive monitor or catheter-related mishap, or monitor failure). Twenty-four percent of patients were believed to be less stable on return to the ICU. Eleven percent of transports had multiple misadventures, and over one third involved at least one mishap.

"RED FLAGS." This series revealed several interesting trends. Transports to the CT scanner were more likely to involve mishaps than any other destination, particularly if any delays occurred at the site. Contributing factors were believed to include the physical isolation of the patient during the procedure and the transfer of the patient from the bed to the scanner and back. Overall, 75% of mishaps occurred at the remote study site. Surprisingly, emergent transports were not more likely to have mishaps, nor was a correlation observed between the number of catheters and monitors and the incidence of mishaps. This observation may be indicative of increased awareness and vigilance in such scenarios.[16]

CRITICAL CARE TRANSPORTS

Transfers of patients between critical care areas (from the OR to ICU or from the ICU to OR) are unlikely to isolate patients in remote areas of the hospital with limited resources. Issues involving the transport process itself are still

TABLE 52-3. Potential Complications During Transport

CARDIOVASCULAR

Physiologic
  Hypertension
  Hypotension
  Hypervolemia
  Hypovolemia/bleeding
  Arrhythmias
  Congestive heart failure/pulmonary edema
  Decreased cardiac output/inadequate tissue perfusion
  Ischemia/Infarction
  Compromise of vascular anastomoses/grafts/bypasses

Technical
  ECK lead disconnect or artifact
  Monitor failure
  Arterial catheter/central venous catheter disconnect
  Vasoactive drug infusion error or disconnect
  Pacer malfunction
  IABP malfunction
  Inability to fit IABP into elevator or ancillary location
  Loss of invasive monitoring catheters

RESPIRATORY

Physiologic
  Hypoxemia/desaturation
  Hypercapnia/respiratory acidosis
  Hypocapnia/respiratory alkalosis
  Tachypnea
  Bronchospasm
  Loss of functional residual capacity
  Increased airway pressures/hemodynamic compromise
  Pneumothorax
  Aspiration

Technical
  Loss of unprotected airway
  Extubation/endotracheal tube obstruction
  Loss of oxygen gas supply
  Inability to match bedside ventilator mode
  Ventilator malfunction
  Lack of house gas lines at remote or diagnostic locations
  Chest tube occlusion or loss

NEUROLOGIC

Physiologic
  Increased intracranial pressure
  Decreased cerebral perfusion pressure
  Inadequate cerebral blood flow
  Excessive cerebral blood flow
  Seizures
  Cerebral edema
  Hemorrhage
  Stroke
  Herniation

Technical
  ICP monitor loss or malfunction
  Inability to maintain adequate head-up positioning
  Errors with pentobarbital infusion during induced coma
  Loss of electrophysiologic monitoring capabilities
  Difficulty in temperature control

OTHER

Physiologic
  Metabolic acidosis/alkalosis
  Hyperglycemia/hypoglycemia
  Hypothermia/hyperthermia
  Oliguria/diabetes

Technical
  Pulled nasogastric or feeding tube
  Pulled Foley catheter
  Pulled surgical drain/catheter
  Tangled infusion and monitoring catheters
  Loss of hyperalimentation source
  Compression stocking malfunction
  Bed malfunction
  Transport elevator malfunction

ECG, electrocardiogram; IABP, intraaortic balloon pump; ICP, intracranial pressure.

relevant, however, and the nature of events leading to such transports makes these patients imminently at risk. Much as Insel and colleagues[3] demonstrated hemodynamically significant changes in adults during transfer from the OR to ICU, Venkataraman and Orr[12] described major cardiorespiratory changes in children going from the OR to the ICU. Many of these required significant interventions such as ventilator changes or vasoactive infusions for stabilization.[12–19] Petre and coworkers[17] noted that patients undergoing complex cardiothoracic procedures could leave the OR with multiple inotropic or vasoactive infusions, invasive monitors, pacemakers, and even intraaortic balloon pumps or ventricular assist devices, all requiring monitoring and adjustment during the transport process. They observed that patients were frequently unstable when they arrived in the ICU.

After complex neurovascular procedures, tight control of blood pressure—with moderate induced hypotension (or in some cases, hypertension)—often is required throughout emergence from anesthesia, transport to the ICU, and transfer to the critical care team. After resection of high-flow arteriovenous malformations, this approach may be vital to prevent hemorrhage or edema, and requires meticulous attention.

The same potential for physiologic deterioration is present when patients are transferred from the ICU to the OR, frequently compounded by the urgency or emergency of the transfer. The transport and transfer process may be thought of as an extension of our care, and clearly places patients at risk for physiologic changes that are at least as great as in the areas between which they are being transported.

COST AND BENEFIT

Cost–benefit relationships exist with both monitors and monitoring.[1,2] The costs may be physical (iatrogenic injury to the patient), economic (related to the equipment itself), or a combination of the two (increased time or personnel requirements, delay of procedures). Benefits may be measured in similar terms and are related to shorter ICU and hospital stays, reduced complications, improved patient care, and ideally, better outcome. We may be asked continually to revisit these issues from a societal perspective as well as that of individual patients.

Although the risks and costs of monitors increase as we move from simple clinical observation, through noninvasive equipment–assisted monitoring, to invasive monitors, the potential benefits may not. Merely increasing the level of monitoring for all patients does not necessarily improve outcome. Decisions about appropriate monitors to use during transport must be individualized based on each patient's physiologic status and the stresses imposed by disease process, injury, surgery, and medications. The anticipated length of the transport, as well as the type and purpose of transport, may also mitigate these needs.

In any situation, every effort should be made to stabilize patients before transport.[10–14,16,18,19] In the healthy patient after elective surgery who is moving from the OR to PACU or ward, all that may be required is a regular heart rate and rhythm, adequate airway with regular respirations, and acceptable blood pressure before transfer.

PLANNING: PREPARATORY PHASE ▪

GENERAL CONSIDERATIONS

Transport of the critically ill may be broken down into three phases: the preparatory phase, the transfer phase, and post-transport stabilization.[12] Preparation begins with careful evaluation of the risks and benefits of the transport by the primary members of the critical care, trauma, or surgical team (including the anesthesiologist). A thorough review of systems should then be performed to determine if any further interventions can optimize the patient's stability.

Vasoactive infusions should be addressed to obtain a steady state before any elective transport. Intravascular volume resuscitation should be well under way in patients with shock caused by trauma, and large-bore vascular access catheters should be in place before movement. When blood

pressure cannot be stabilized, surgical exploration and control of bleeding must take precedence over any further diagnostic procedures.[10,11]

The hypotensive trauma patient with obvious, severe head injury may be further evaluated by placement of a ventriculostomy catheter during surgical exploration in the OR. This process allows measurement and potential treatment of increased ICP, and can be used to diagnose a lateralizing mass lesion by performing an air ventriculogram. Alternatively, diagnostic burr holes may be placed.

Careful assessment of the patient's airway is critical, and adequate oxygenation and ventilation should be assured. In patients who are combative or who show decreased levels of consciousness for whatever reason, careful consideration should be given to electively securing the airway before transport. Similarly, elective intubation should be entertained in patients with significant burn injuries (especially inhalation burns), chest trauma, or respiratory distress.

As a rule, all anticipated procedures should be performed in the critical care area before transport. An apparently insignificant pneumothorax can progress rapidly, particularly if the patient is receiving positive-pressure ventilation; tube thoracostomy should be considered. Once in place, chest tubes may be transported under water seal, and then, ideally, reattached to suction during any therapeutic or diagnostic procedure. They should never be clamped for transport.

PERSONNEL

Adequate and appropriate personnel should be gathered to accompany the patient, including a minimum of two people, one of whom is the patient's critical care nurse.[20] Nursing care plays a vital role in the ICU and must be continued throughout the transport process to ensure proper administration of scheduled medications, titration of vasoactive infusions, and accurate record keeping. A trained physician must accompany any unstable patient who requires extensive acute interventions. If the patient is at risk for airway problems, a physician skilled in tracheal intubation should be present.[18,19,21] Specific problems may dictate the need for a respiratory therapist or perfusionist as well.

COMMUNICATION

Communication and coordination are essential to the safe conduct of transport. When a patient is transferred to or from a critical care area, or between critical care areas, information should be passed from physician to physician and nurse to nurse regarding the patient's condition, treatment, and management.[20] Timing of arrival and procedures should be confirmed with personnel at the patient's destination, especially when CT, angiography, or nuclear medicine (mishaps are more likely when delays occur) are involved. Ideally, patient escort or security may arrange to clear the transport route and to have elevators standing by. If the responsible physician does not accompany the patient, the physician must at least be aware when the transport is taking place. The reasons for the transport should be documented in the patient's chart.

EQUIPMENT AND SUPPLIES

A standard set of equipment should be available for most critical care transports. Basic resuscitation drugs such as epinephrine, atropine, and lidocaine, along with a cardiac monitor and defibrillator, are appropriate for most transfers to or between critical care areas. Airway support supplies, including a self-inflating resuscitation bag, masks, airways, and a functioning laryngoscope with appropriate blades and endotracheal tubes, are mandatory. An adequate oxygen supply should allow full support during the anticipated duration outside the ICU, with a 30-minute reserve time. No excuse exists for exhausting the patient's oxygen supply during transport; the potential consequences are too severe.[18,20] A self-inflating bag is an important safety feature to allow ventilation in the event that a temporary interruption of the compressed gas source occurs.

Intravenous fluids should include maintenance requirements, as well as isotonic crystalloids, colloids, and blood products as indicated for resuscitation. Medications given by infusion should be continued by battery-operated volumetric pumps. All scheduled and anticipated medications (e.g., insulin, antibiotics, sedatives, and muscle relaxants) also should accompany the patient, and guidelines should be established for administration if the physician is not present.

MONITORS

Transport Beds

Parameters to be followed during transport must be transferred to portable monitors. Specialized transport beds incorporating built-in monitors seem attractive; however, their use requires an additional transfer of the patient from the ICU bed, with the inherent risk of dislodging catheters and the endotracheal tube, or of inducing changes in ICP. As a result, patients should be transported in their ICU bed if possible. Neonatal transport units that allow full monitoring and ventilatory support, as well as tight control of thermal regulation, are a notable exception. Self-contained critical care transport carts that can quickly be attached or detached from the ICU bed are a modification of this approach. They consolidate monitors, compressed gas cylinders, transport or ICU ventilators, infusion pumps, and a battery power source into a single unit.[22–25] These systems do not avoid brief periods of blackout for the parameters being monitored as they are transferred and transducers rezeroed.

TRAM System

The transport remote acquisition monitor (TRAM) system was developed to ease the problem of monitor transfer and reduce the number of equipment systems with which the transport team must be familiar. The TRAM is centered around a self-contained data acquisition and processing module to which ECG leads, pulse oximeter probes, invasive or noninvasive pressure transducers, temperature probes, and other monitoring modalities may be attached. The module can be "slaved" to a portable TRAM LED display while still plugged into the fixed bedside or OR monitor. When the patient is moved, the processing module is simply removed from the permanent monitor, following the patient without the need to detach any of the monitoring catheters or transducers, thus avoiding monitoring gaps.[26]

Temporary duplication of monitoring between the bedside and transport systems also can be used to avoid blackouts. If cardiac rhythm is a concern, a separate set of ECG pads may be placed and attached to the transport monitor leads, and blood pressure may be followed noninvasively while transducers are transferred. The TRAM system shows its full utility when multiple invasive monitors are to be followed in the unstable patient, or when the patient is to be transported to an intermediate location (e.g., CT or angiography suite) en route between the OR and ICU.

ENTROPY

In addition to the various monitoring catheters and cables, care must be taken to ensure that the intravenous infusion catheters are organized and readily identifiable. Most of us are acutely aware of the medical corollary to the Second Law of Thermodynamics, and the tendency for infusions to become disordered. Patient safety dictates that we not allow intravenous access catheters to become confused; an inadvertent bolus of a vasoactive infusion can have disastrous consequences.

Our approach is to simplify. Ideally, one intravenous access route, free from infusions, should be maintained in all patients. If possible, all necessary infusions should be administered through a separate, single port. Any further access ports may be flushed and capped if not required during the transport. Bundling of catheters and cables may be helpful, and proper labeling is essential. I have found that tubing from an anesthesia breathing circuit (or ventilator circuit) can be useful in organizing monitoring cables and is reusable as long as it is not contaminated.

INTEGRATED APPROACHES

To increase efficiency and safety during the transfer of cardiac surgery patients, The Cleveland Clinic (Cleveland) developed an elegant system centered around the ICU bed as the primary transport tool (Fig. 52-1). A bracket system is incorporated into the bed so that all patient monitoring transducers and a TRAM display screen may be mounted at the head of the bed in clear view and with easy access. The TRAM system forms the basis of monitoring in the OR, ICU, and during transport as the processing module is inserted in a receptacle under the bed.

All intravenous fluids and infusions are supported by an infusion rack that contains volumetric pumps and hooks for fluids. The rack attaches to the side of the bed for transport, but is suspended from ceiling mounts in the OR and ICU. The monitoring system and infusion/medication systems are thus integrated into the ICU bed and follow the patient as a unit. Despite a cost in 1988 of over $1000 per bed in hardware alone, the system was believed to be cost-effective in the Cleveland Clinic because of an estimated 50% time savings in the transport process and increased ability of transport personnel to focus on the patient rather than on movement of equipment.[17,27]

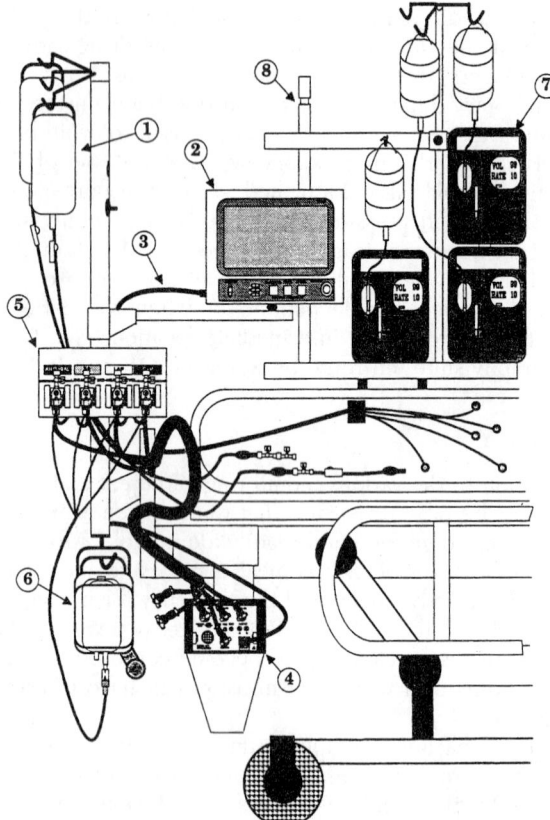

FIGURE 52-1. Integrated transport system. Support pole at head (1) holds pressure transducer mount (5), pressurized flush solution, (6) and hooks for intravenous solutions. The TRAM display screen (2) is mounted on the pole by a moveable sidearm and connected to the transport remote acquisition monitor (TRAM) module (4) by a telephone cord (3). the infusion bracket (8) is mounted on the side of the bed and can support multiple intravenous solutions and up to six infusion pumps (7). (From Hendren W, Higgins T: Immediate postoperative care of the cardiac surgical patient. *Semin Thorac Cardiovasc Surg* 1991;3:63.)

Although the design of this system may be too complex for many institutions to find worthwhile, the concept of maintaining continuous and uninterrupted monitoring and infusions through the transport process is laudable. Recent development of small, battery-operated monitors and multichannel infusion pumps allow us to approximate this concept using more standard ICU beds (Fig. 52-1).

Care should be taken to assure that the ICU bed provides easy access to the head for airway management and to the chest should cardiopulmonary resuscitation be necessary. These factors should be kept in mind throughout transport, as when "squeezing" onto an elevator. Many ICU beds have attached poles and may include support trays for placing monitors. Beds should have manual or dual controls to allow Trendelenburg positioning or leg elevation, even if no power source is available. Radiolucency and the ability to perform fluoroscopy through the bed are also desirable features, which decrease transferring the patient simply to perform radiographs or fluoroscopy.

HOT TOPIC

A final note in the preparation phase is the importance of taking steps to maintain body temperature. Heat may be lost through radiation, convection, or conduction throughout transport, and administering warm intravenous fluids or heated ventilator gases may be difficult. Covering the patient during movement and at remote sites, and increasing ambient temperature at any location where the patient will be stationary may help. The transport team must watch for hypothermia and treat it aggressively should it occur.

ON THE ROAD AGAIN: TRANSPORT PHASE ■

The goal during the transport phase is to maintain the same level of care as the patient had in the critical care area. As much as possible, we should strive to achieve the following: (1) maintain patient stability through monitoring, (2) continue the present, ongoing management, and (3) avoid iatrogenic mishaps.[12] In transports from the ICU to and from ancillary locations, every attempt should be made to return monitoring and care to the ICU level during the procedure. Modalities such as pulmonary artery pressure, which may be difficult to follow in a moving patient, can again be monitored in a stationary location. By adhering to the principles of thorough preparation and minimizing time spent during the transport phase, we should decrease the potential for complications.

HOME AT LAST: POSTTRANSPORT STABILIZATION ■

When a patient returns to the ICU no less attention should be paid to the posttransport stabilization phase than to other components of the process, or to the new arrival of a potentially unstable patient. Patients are frequently judged to be unstable on arrival in the ICU and may require urgent hemodynamic or ventilatory interventions.[3,10,12,16] Furthermore, they may continue to be at increased risk of secondary insults through the first 4 hours after return.[10] At the same time these events are taking place, monitored parameters are transferred to bedside monitors, intravenous catheters and infusions are examined and resecured, and the patient is connected to a bedside ICU ventilator. To reestablish order, we must not neglect the principles followed during preparation for transport. Ideally, no monitoring blackout should occur during this transition period, or at least only a *minimal* blackout period should occur with no more than one modality unmonitored at a time.

Additional issues may arise, and communication is essential. The primary team may be unaware of all of the problems that began in the OR or during a transport, or important new findings may follow from a diagnostic procedure. The transport team members must review these issues with the full critical care team, including the nurses who will be working with the patient. This communication is especially important for the trauma patients, who may have physicians from several disciplines involved in their care.[21]

INDIVIDUALIZING APPROACHES ■

Monitoring and transport procedures may appropriately be tailored to individual patients. Much information can be gained from observation alone, including skin color, evidence of tissue perfusion, and normal regular respirations, without rocking or signs of upper airway obstruction. Through patient interaction we may assess level of consciousness and the ability to follow commands. Touch, palpation, and auscultation all yield valuable information as to heart rate and rhythm, some idea of blood pressure, and adequacy of ventilation.

Patients in all age groups are unquestionably at risk for hypoxemia during emergence from anesthesia; thus, it is rational to routinely administer supplemental oxygen during transport from the OR to the PACU. Extension of this argument to patients who are sedated or who have altered levels of consciousness may be prudent. I tend to use oxygen empirically in this group if monitoring is not readily available. If underlying pulmonary disease is present, or the nature of the surgery raises concern that a patient may not be able to maintain adequate oxygenation with simple face mask or "blow-by" oxygen, observation in the OR combined with pulse oximetry and the proposed transport mode of supplemental oxygen are advisable.

During transport, one can gauge the rate and depth of respirations by feeling exhalations on the palm of the hand while supporting the airway (Fig. 52-2). Addition of a precordial stethoscope allows simultaneous monitoring of heart rate, rhythm, and breath sounds. Lateral positioning with the occiput cushioned tends to pull soft tissues forward and away from the airway, decreasing obstruction and allowing secretions (or emesis, should it occur) to drain out of the corner of the mouth.[1] This approach may be useful in the obtunded but nonintubated patient and for those emerging from anesthesia (see Fig. 52-2).

Even during brief transfer to the PACU, additional monitors may be desirable in individual patients; generally, however, observation and a stethoscope suffice. A pulse oximeter is advisable if a longer transfer is required when a patient is anesthetized at an outlying location. Automated noninvasive blood pressure (NIBP) monitoring and electrocardiography

can be performed easily with lightweight transport monitors, and are desirable to follow rhythm or when intravascular volume shifts or bleeding may occur during transport. This may be the case after invasive radiologic or angiographic procedures.

Patients being transferred from critical care areas or the PACU to the ward should require only careful observation, unless they are moving to a telemetry or step-down unit. In general, monitoring should be maintained similarly to that which will be employed at the destination; thus, pulse oximetry, ECG, or NIBP monitoring may be appropriate. Patients receiving supplemental oxygen should continue to do so, unless they have clearly demonstrated a sustained ability to maintain oxygenation while they breathe room air before discharge.

CRITICAL MONITORS

Perhaps more than any other patients, the critically ill demand that we individualize monitoring schemes, support systems, and the transport process. Guidelines have been accepted that set the minimum acceptable standards[20] (Table 52-4). Specific circumstances (patients with an evolving myocardial infarction, recent cardiac surgery, or high thoracic/cervical spinal cord injury) may indicate the need for an external cardiac pacemaker to be available.

Some portable monitors are sophisticated. I have had favorable experience using such devices under austere conditions in third world environments. These lightweight, battery-operated devices can be used as a stand alone monitor in the OR or ICU, and are easily moved with the patient without disconnection. In their present advanced configuration (Fig. 52-3), they provide ECG, pulse oximetry, NIBP monitoring, temperature, two invasive pressures, and capnography, with an optional printer.

VENTILATOR-DEPENDENT PATIENTS

Ventilator-dependent patients are at high risk for mishaps and clinical deterioration during transport. How ventilation should be accomplished during transport and what additional monitors should be used are critically important questions. Alterations in arterial blood gas partial pressures and hemodynamic function, which can accompany unmonitored manual ventilation or use of a transport ventilator, have been discussed. Gervais and associates[15] found that spirometry

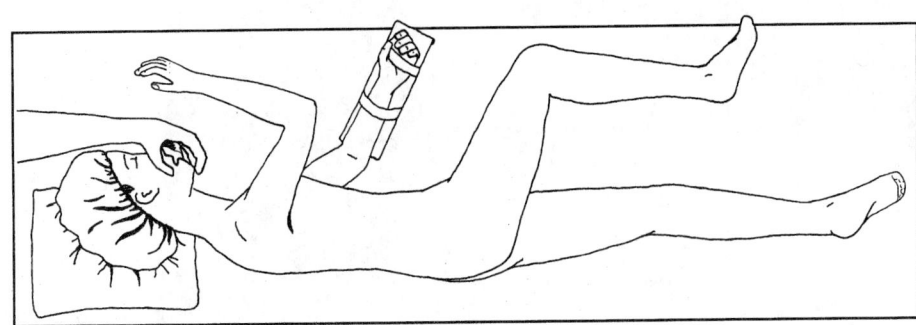

FIGURE 52-2. Positioning for transport of the unconscious patient. A precordial stethoscope follows heart tones and breath sounds while the supporting hand senses exhalation. (From Gravenstein JS, Paulus DA: *Monitoring Practice in Clinical Anesthesia,* 2nd ed. Philadelphia, JB Lippincott, 1987:20.)

TABLE 52-4.   Monitoring During Transport

Patients should receive the same physiologic monitoring during transport as in the ICU, to the extent technically possible

Minimum levels of monitoring shall include:
  Continuous monitoring and periodic documentation of ECG and pulse oximetry
  Intermittent measurement and documentation of BP, respiratory rate, pulse rate

Selected monitoring based on clinical status:
  Capnography
  Continuous measurement of BP, pulmonary artery pressure, ICP, $S\bar{v}o_2$
  Intermittent measurement of central venous pressure, pulmonary artery occlusion pressure, and cardiac output

Intubated patients should have airway pressure monitored
  Transport ventilators should have disconnect and high airway pressure alarms

---

$S\bar{v}o_2$, saturation with oxygen (mixed venous); ECG, electrocardiogram; BP, blood pressure; ICP, intracranial pressure.

measurement alerted practitioners to these changes during manual ventilation. Weg and Haas[28] note that an experienced respiratory therapist could maintain stable respiratory status and blood pressure for most patients with manual ventilation by matching minute ventilation and inspired oxygen fraction (Fio_2) to the bedside ventilator. Others have found significant trends toward hyperventilation with manual ventilation compared with the use of a transport ventilator[29] (Table 52-5).

In my experience, most ventilator-dependent patients can be managed adequately using a Mapleson D or modified Jackson-Reese circuit in conjunction with an airway pressure gauge. This combination allows the physician or respiratory therapist to apply modest controlled positive end-expiratory pressure (PEEP) or continuous positive airway pressure (CPAP) while minimizing the risk of barotrauma. With few exceptions, 100% oxygen may be used throughout the transport process, simplifying equipment needs and providing an added margin of safety. Neonatal transport, however, may require air-oxygen mixtures to lower Fio_2 and decrease the risk of retinopathy of prematurity.

VENTILATORS

Critically ill patients with respiratory failure frequently require high levels of CPAP or complex ventilatory modes such as pressure-control ventilation with inverse inhalation-to-exhalation (I:E) ratios to maintain oxygenation. Manual ventilation is not likely to be effective in these patients, and a transport ventilator should be used. Branson and McGough[29] conducted an extensive review of available transport ventilators (Table 52-6). A recent addition to this armamentarium is the Bird Avian, a time- or volume-cycled, pressure-limited, 4.5-kg (10-lb) ventilator with controlled mechanical ventilation, synchronized intermittent mandatory ventilation, assist/control, and CPAP modes. This device offers potential for interhospital and intrahospital transport (Fig. 52-4).

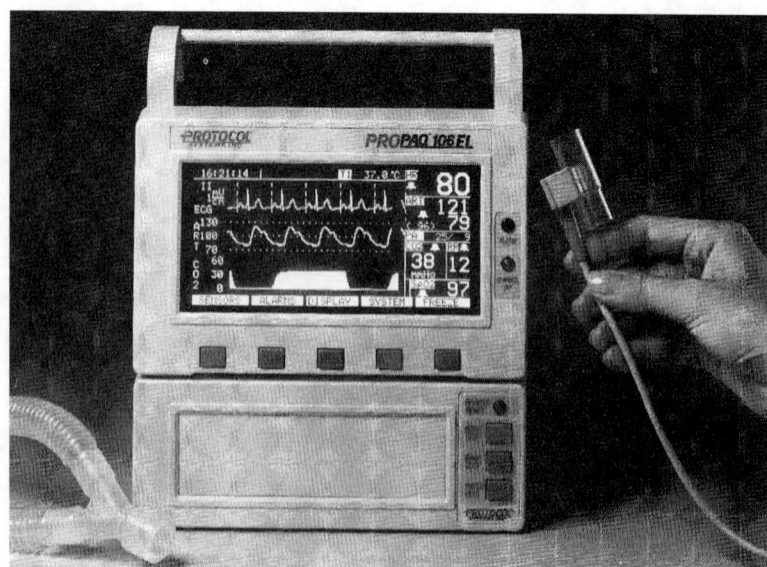

FIGURE 52-3. PROPAQ 106 portable monitor. Battery-operated transport monitor capable of electrocardiogram, noninvasive blood pressure, pulse oximetry, two invasive pressures, temperature, and continuous capnography. Weight less than 4.5 kg (10 lbs). (Courtesy of Protocol Systems, Beaverton, Ore.)

TABLE 52-5. Comparison of Self-Inflating Bag and Transport Ventilators

	CONVENTIONAL VENTILATION BEFORE TRANSPORT	SELF-INFLATING BAG USED DURING TRANSPORT	TRANSPORT VENTILATOR USED DURING TRANSPORT
pHa	7.39 ± 0.3	$7.51 \pm 0.2°$	7.40 ± 0.3
Paco$_2$ (mm Hg)	39 ± 4	$30 \pm 3°$	39 ± 3
Pao$_2$ (mm Hg)	116 ± 17	109 ± 24	117 ± 20
Heart rate (bpm)	106 ± 23	115 ± 19	109 ± 25
Systolic BP (mm Hg)	130 ± 36	112 ± 24	136 ± 31
Diastolic BP (mm Hg)	86 ± 12	73 ± 10	81 ± 20

pHa, arterial pH; BP, blood pressure.

° $p < 0.05$ compared with conventional ventilation.

(From Branson RD, McGough EK: Transport ventilators. *Probl Crit Care* 1990;4:261).

Unfortunately, matching the characteristics or "advanced" modes of an ICU ventilator (pressure support ventilation, pressure control ventilation, airway pressure release ventilation) or the control over CPAP/PEEP, flow rates, and I:E ratio may be difficult to impossible. Use of the ICU ventilator for transport, and in the OR for any surgical or other procedure, is the safest course in such cases. The ventilator can move as part of a transport cart, bound to any necessary compressed gas tanks and power supply,[24] or independently with personnel to ensure that disconnects do not occur.

Airway pressure and SpO$_2$ should be continuously monitored in ventilated transport patients. A pneumotachograph or simple spirometer should be used at least intermittently to verify tidal volume and minute ventilation. Capnometry, with a calorimetric carbon dioxide detector, should be readily available as a minimum standard. Patients with impaired intracranial elastance or those who are critically ill may benefit from continuous end-tidal carbon dioxide monitoring.[24,30]

SPECIAL CIRCUMSTANCES

Hemodynamically Unstable Patients

The importance of stabilization before transport cannot be overemphasized. Adequate large bore venous access, resuscitation fluids, and blood products must be available throughout the transport. One person may need to be assigned the sole task of managing blood and fluid administration, especially if any significant amount of time is to be spent at an ancillary location.

Patients with cardiovascular collapse may require multiple vasopressor and inotropic infusions that must be available for adjustment during transport, and may at times be moved to the OR with cardiopulmonary resuscitation in progress. Recently, we have seen increased transport use of the intraaortic balloon pump or cardiopulmonary support system, which at times may be placed in remote locations such as the cardiac catheterization laboratory. A perfusionist should accompany such patients during transport, and advance planning is necessary to ensure that probable transfer routes to the OR or ICU are feasible (i.e., that all associated equipment will fit through passageways and on elevators).

Neurotrauma

HEAD. Head injury is common in all age groups and remains a leading cause of morbidity and mortality in young adults; these patients are at particular risk for secondary injury.[10,11] The most reliable monitor of neurologic status is the clinical examination. However, sedation and even neuromuscular blockers may be needed to perform a complete evaluation in an uncooperative patient. Clinical examination capabilities will be lost if surgery is required for other associated injuries. Unless the patient remains hemodynamically unstable, a stop for CT is often planned en route to the OR if neurologic injury is suspected. In the combative or obtunded patient, sedation and intubation should be handled in a controlled setting before transport to the CT scanner or another ancillary location. In my experience, short-acting sedatives such as propofol are especially useful, allowing rapid titration and emergence so that the clinical examination is not obscured.

Patients with severe head injuries or other causes of increased ICP should be intubated to protect the airway and control ventilation. An ICP monitor usually is placed, and management may include hyperventilation, positioning with the head up 20 to 30 degrees, or both. Additional modalities include jugular bulb oximetry, somatosensory evoked potentials, and brain stem auditory evoked potentials. Although jugular bulb and evoked potential monitoring are unnecessary during the movement phase of transport, other monitoring and treatment modalities should be held as constant as possible. The physiologic goal is to maintain optimum cerebral perfusion pressure and substrate delivery.

Maintenance of adequate oxygenation and blood pressure is vital, and capnography should be used to avoid fluctuations in PCO$_2$. If head-up positioning is used, it should be continued. ICP changes are common during transport[11]; these

(text continues on p. 800)

TABLE 52-6. Ventilatory and Monitoring Characteristics of Transport Ventilators

VENTILATOR	CYCLING VARIABLES	MODES	RATE (BREATHS PER MINUTE)	TIDAL VOLUME (mL)	MINUTE VOLUME (L/min)*	I:E RATIO (MINIMUM)
Hamilton MAX	Time	IMV, CMV	2–30	50–1500	45.0	1:1
Biomed IC2A	Time	CMV, IMV, CPAP	1–66	130–2500	37.5	4:1
Healthdyne 105	Time	IMV, CPAP, CMV	1–150	10–1000	20.0	4:1
Impact Universal	Time	CMV	14, 20, 30 child; 12, 18 adult	10–1250	22.5	1:2
Life Support Products Auto Vent 2000	Time	IMV, CMV	8–20	400–1200	24.0	1:1
Life Support Products Auto Vent 3000	Time	IMV, CMV	9–27 child; 8–20 adult	200–600 child; 400–1200 adult	24.0 adult; 16.0 child	1:1
Newport E100i	Time or pressure	IMV, CMV, A/C, CPAP	1–90	100–3600	36.0	1:1
Ohmeda Logic 07	Time	CMV	10–40	100–2000	20.0	1:2
Penlon 350	Time	CMV	10–85	10–300 neonate/ child; 50–2000 adult	0.1–9.0 neonate/ child; 1.0–3.0 adult	2:1
Pneupac Model 2-R	Time	CMV	11, 12, 13, 14, 16, 19, and 21	340–1450	16.0	1:1.5
Stein-Gates	Time	CMV	1–150	30–3000	20.0	2:1
Bird Space Technologies Mini-TXP	Time	CMV	4–15	50–2500	30.0	1:2

I:E, inspiration-to-expiration; F_{IO_2}, fraction of inspired oxygen; PEEP, positive end-expiratory pressure; IMV, intermittent mandatory ventilation; CMV, controlled mechanical ventilation; CPAP, continuous positive airway pressure; A/C, assist/control.

*Maximum available minute volume with an I:E of 1:1.

[†]PEEP can be provided in all ventilators with an external PEEP valve.

[‡]During spontaneous inhalation, the ventilator cycles "on," but the exhalation valve remains depressurized to allow venting of gas to the atmosphere. Depending on the inspiratory flow rate and time settings, gas flow rate for a specific duration of time is available for spontaneous breathing. The system does not function as a demand-flow valve.

(From Branson RD, McGough EK: Transport ventilators. In: Banner M (ed). *Problems in Critical Care*. Philadelphia, JB Lippincott, 1990:264).

PEAK FLOW RATE (L/min)	FIO₂	PEEP (cm H₂O)†	ALARMS	MONITORING	DEMAND-FLOW VALVE	MANUAL BREATH
90	1.0	No	Low inlet pressure and low battery (audible and visual) High airway pressure (audible)	Airway pressure	Yes	Yes
7.5	1.0	0–25	None	Airway pressure	No‡	Yes
60	0.21–1.0	0–20	Audible/visual; low/high pressure; low inlet pressure, system interrupt, insufficient expiratory time, reverse I:E, power loss, disconnect	Airway pressure	No, continuous flow only	Yes
90	1.0	No	Visual low battery; audible high pressure	None	No	Yes
48	1.0	No	High pressure audible	None	Yes	No
48	1.0	No	High pressure audible	None	Yes	No
72	0.21–1.0	0–25	Visual/audible; high/low pressure, inspiration time too long	Airway pressure	No, continuous flow only	Yes
6.5	0.5 or 1.0	No	Audible high pressure	Airway pressure	No	No
60	1.0	No	Audible high pressure	Airway pressure	No	No
40	0.45 or 1.0	No	Audible high pressure	None	No	No
45	1.0	No	None	None	No	No
120	0.45–0.8	No	None	None	No	Yes

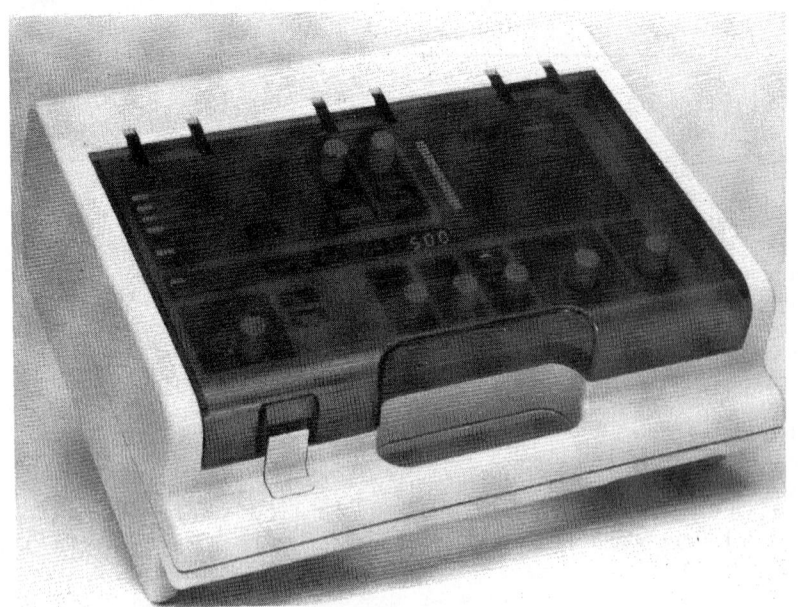

FIGURE 52-4. Bird AVIAN transport ventilator. Modes include control, assist/control, synchronized intermittent mandatory ventilation, and continuous positive airway pressure in time cycled or volume cycled configuration. Battery powered with alarms for low/high airway pressure, disconnect, apnea, PEEP not set, low power. Weight, 5 kg. Circuit and power source not shown. (Courtesy of Bird Products Corporation, Palm Springs, CA)

patients frequently require transport for diagnostic procedures not available in the ICU or to the OR; thus, ICP monitoring should not be interrupted. Newer fiberoptic devices facilitate this process, but careful attention to transducer height and monitor function allow a ventriculostomy catheter or Richmond bolt to be used.

SPINAL CORD.   Spinal cord–injured patients are also at risk for progression of their injuries or deficits and require the same meticulous attention to physiologic variables as those who are head injured. In addition, they present special logistical concerns related to the traction and stabilization devices that may be employed. Movement or transport is ideally performed in concert with a member of the neurosurgical team. Concern about airway protection in spinal cord injury must also take into consideration the potential for progressive ventilatory muscle insufficiency. Although this problem is unlikely to progress rapidly, the issue needs to be addressed before any prolonged transport. Bradycardia, heart block, and distributive shock are additional special concerns that must be anticipated, especially in patients with high thoracic or cervical cord injuries.

Magnetic Resonance Imaging

MRI can provide invaluable diagnostic information but poses multiple management problems for the critically ill because of the effects of the magnetic field on monitoring and life-support equipment, physical isolation of the patient, and the frequently remote location of the scanner. If MRI is deemed essential, careful planning is essential.

With minor modification, most monitoring techniques are adaptable to the MRI suite. Cathode ray displays may be disrupted by the powerful magnetic fields currently in use; thus, monitoring screens should be placed outside the MRI room. Placing nonferrous ECG leads close together and using twisted (not coiled) graphite and copper leads

may minimize artifact and decrease the potential for burns or electric shock from the antenna effect. Pulse oximeters have been widely used in the MRI environment, and most may be placed within 2 m of the magnet. Oscillometric NIBP monitoring functions well in the MRI suite when extended tubing is used and the monitor is placed far from the magnet. A plastic precordial or esophageal stethoscope can be useful; however, ambient noise may be troublesome.[31]

Tobin and colleagues[32] report the safe, continuous use of invasive arterial blood pressure monitoring and vasopressor administration in critically ill patients undergoing MRI by the addition of appropriate-length extension tubing. Several of their patients also had combined fiberoptic ventriculostomy ICP monitors in place, and manometric measurement of ICP was maintained during the scan.

Because of patient isolation during the scan, particular attention should be paid to airway assessment. Ventilation is most often supported by manual use of a Mapleson D circuit; if compressed gas tanks are used, they must be placed outside of the MRI room. Nonferrous anesthesia ventilators have been developed, and the Siemens 900 ventilator has been used successfully when placed at least 1.2 meters from the magnet.[31] It may be helpful to consult an anesthesiologist who is familiar with the MRI environment when such procedures are contemplated on critically ill patients.

REFERENCES   ■

1. Gravenstein J, Paulus D: *Monitoring Practice in Clinical Anesthesia.* Philadelphia, JB Lippincott, 1982
2. Blitt C: A philosophy of monitoring. In: Blitt C (ed). *Monitoring in Anesthesia and Critical Care Medicine.* New York, Churchill Livingstone, 1985:1
3. Insel J, Weissman C, Kemper M, et al: Cardiovascular changes during transport of critically ill and postoperative patients. *Crit Care Med* 1986;14:539

4. American Society of Anesthesiologists: *Standards for Basic Anesthesia Monitoring.* Approved by House of Delegates Oct 21, 1986 and last amended Oct 13, 1993. Park Ridge, IL, American Society of Anesthesiologists:384

5. Hensley FA, Dodson DL, Martin DE, et al: Oxygen saturation during placement of invasive monitoring in the premedicated, unanesthetized cardiac patient. *Anesthesiology* 1986;65:A22

6. Riley R, Davis N, Finucane K, et al: Arterial oxygen saturation in anaesthetised patients during transfer from induction room to operating room. *Anaesth Intensive Care* 1988;16:182

7. Tyler I, Tatisara B, Winter P, et al: Continuous monitoring of arterial oxygen saturation with pulse oximetry during transfer to the recovery room. *Anesth Analg* 1985;64:1108

8. Kataria B, Harnik E, Mitchard R, et al: Postoperative arterial oxygen saturation in the pediatric population during transportation. *Anesth Analg* 1988;67:280

9. Tomkins D, Gaukroger P, Bentley M: Hypoxia in children following general anesthesia. *Anaesth Intensive Care* 1988;16:177

10. Gentleman D, Jennet B: Audit of transfer of unconscious head-injured patients to a neurosurgical unit. *Lancet* 1990;335:330

11. Andrews P, Piper I, Dearded N, et al: Secondary insults during intrahospital transport of head-injured patients. *Lancet* 1990;335:327

12. Venkataraman S, Orr R: Intrahospital transport of critically ill patients. *Crit Care Clin* 1992;8:525

13. Waddel G: Movement of critically ill patients within hospital. *Br Med J* 1975;2:417

14. Braman S, Dunn S, Amico C, et al: Complications of intrahospital transport in critically ill patients. *Ann Intern Med* 1987;107:469

15. Gervais H, Eberle B, Konietzke D, et al: Comparison of blood gases of ventilated patients during transport. *Crit Care Med* 1987;15:761

16. Smith I, Fleming S, Cernaianu A: Mishaps during transport from the intensive care unit. *Crit Care Med* 1990;18:278

17. Petre J, Bazaral M, Estafanous F: Patient transport: an organized method with direct clinical benefits. *Biomedical Instrum Technol* 1989;23:100

18. Melker R, Gallagher TJ: Transport of the critically ill/injured patient. In: Civetta J, Taylor R, Kirby R (eds). *Critical Care,* 2nd ed. Philadelphia, JB Lippincott, 1992:1797

19. Fromm R, Dellinger R: Transport of critically ill patients. *J Intensive Care Med* 1992;7:223

20. Guidelines Committee for the American College of Critical Care Medicine–Society of Critical Care Medicine and American Association of Critical-Care Nurses Transfer Guidelines Task Force: Guidelines for the transfer of critically ill patients. *Crit Care Med* 1993;21:931

21. Watson C, Norfleet E: Anesthesia for trauma. *Crit Care Clin* 1986;2:717

22. Kondo K, Herman S, O'Reilly P, et al: Transport system for critically ill patients. *Crit Care Med* 1985;13:1081

23. Vandermeersch E, Muller E, Mulier J, et al: A new mobile artificial respiration and monitoring system for transporting critically ill (emergency) patients. *Anasthesiol Intensivmed Notfallmed Schmerzther* 1988;23:276

24. Link J, Krause H, Wagner W, et al: Intrahospital transport of critically ill patients. *Crit Care Med* 1990;18:1427

25. Schirmer U, Heinrich H, Siebeneich H, et al: Safe intraclinical transfer of intensive care patients: a concept to avoid monitoring and treatment gaps. *Anasthesiol Intensivmed Notfallmed Schmerzther* 1991;26:112

26. Weinfurt P: TRAM: a new concept in transport monitoring. *Int J Clin Monit Comput* 1987;4:149

27. Hendren W, Higgins T: Immediate postoperative care of the cardiac surgical patient. *Semin Thorac Cardiovasc Surg* 1991;3:3

28. Weg J, Haas C: Safe intrahospital transport of critically ill ventilator-dependent patients. *Chest* 1989;96:631

29. Branson RD, McGough EK: Transport ventilators. *Probl Crit Care* 1990;4:254

30. End-tidal carbon dioxide measurement in emergency medicine and patient transport. *Health Devices* 1991;20:35

31. Patteson SK, Chesney JT: Anesthetic management for magnetic resonance imaging: problems and solutions. *Anesth Analg* 1992;74:121

32. Tobin JR, Spurrier EA, Wetzel RC: Anaesthesia for critically ill children during magnetic resonance imaging. *Br J Anaesth* 1992;69:482

Critical Care, Third Edition, edited by Joseph M. Civetta,
Robert W. Taylor, and Robert R. Kirby.
Lippincott-Raven Publishers, Philadelphia, PA © 1997.

CHAPTER 53

Interhospital Transport of the Critically Ill

Robert E. Fromm

IMMEDIATE CONCERNS

MAJOR PROBLEMS

Critically ill patients present to facilities with varying clinical capabilities. Thus, some critically ill patients must be transported to receive needed care. The transport environment poses additional stresses on the patient and medical equipment. Knowledge of the personnel, vehicles, and equipment is necessary for safe, efficient transports.

STRESS POINTS

1. Typically, two transport modes are available: ground and air. Ground ambulances are usually less expensive but staffed by prehospital personnel who must be augmented by hospital staff in many instances.
2. Helicopter transport systems usually are based at referral centers and are well equipped for critical care transports. They are generally expensive and add the concerns of pressure, acceleration, and additional vibration.
3. Air transports for distances exceeding 200 miles are usually more efficiently accomplished by airplane.
4. The following must be reviewed before the transport: the needs of the patient (oxygen, fluids, skeletal traction, gastrointestinal, and closed airspace drainage); and the needs of the required equipment (gases, power source), together with the specific environment and vehicle contemplated for the transport.

ESSENTIAL PROCEDURES

1. Contact the appropriate physicians before transferring the patient.
2. Confirm supplies and power needs with the transport team.
3. Decompress all closed airspaces and the gastrointestinal tract, as appropriate.
4. Protect the airways of those at risk *before* transport.
5. Find alternatives for medical appliances that may pose a danger to vehicle occupants (i.e., skeletal traction).
6. Ensure that all possible stabilizing therapy has been initiated before transport.

OVERVIEW

The transport of critically ill patients is a regular occurrence in current medical practice. Subjecting the critically ill the expense and potential problems of an interhospital transport requires that the responsible physician have a clear understanding of the potential risks and benefits. Interhospital transports may occur by ground or by air and are commonly accomplished by practitioners with whom the intensivist has little familiarity, using equipment foreign to the hospital environment. Safe and efficient transports require the intensive care physician and nurse to be involved in the patient's care before, during, and after the patient's arrival at the receiving hospital.

The relevance of transport of the critically ill has increased over the last decade. The diagnostic and therapeutic armamentarium of the physician in the hospital has improved substantially. New technologies in cardiology and diagnostic and interventional radiology, to name a few, have made important contributions to patient care. However, because of the substantial expenditures necessary for equipment, facilities, and recruitment of qualified personnel to perform these services, they may be available only in larger community hospitals and regional referral centers. Prospective payment and other changes in health care finance have led to an increasing number of hospital closures. In fact, it was estimated in 1986 that 10% of the nation's 5000 hospitals would face bankruptcy or closure before 1991.[1,2] Thus, advances in medical technology and facility closures have combined to increase the need to transport critically ill.[1] Data from helicopter transport programs provide ample evidence of the large population of transported critically ill patients. During the time period from 1980 to 1989, the number of hospital-based helicopter transport programs increased from 31 to 170 with a total fleet of 210 helicopters, and the number of patient transports exceeded 125,000 in 1989.[3,4] The number of critically ill patients transported by ground also likely increased during this same period, although the exact number of critical care transports accomplished by ground is an illusive figure. Data from the National Association of State Emergency Medical Services Directors and the Council of State Governments indicate that an excess of 12,000 ground transport ambulance services exist in the United States with nearly 35,000 ambulance vehicles.[5]

The transport of the critically ill is commonly accomplished by paramedics and other health care providers who most frequently practice in the prehospital setting. A basic understanding of the history, constraints, and practitioners involved in ground and air interhospital transport is necessary if we are to comprehend the issues involved.

PREHOSPITAL PRACTITIONERS   ■

The era of advanced prehospital emergency medical services (EMS) and, thus, the involvement of prehospital providers in the transport of the critically ill, is scarcely two decades old in the United States. Yet, it is commonly taken for granted by the medical community and the populous at large.[6] Advanced prehospital care had its genesis in 1967 with the use of mobile coronary care units in Belfast by Pantridge and Geddes.[7] This development marked a transition from simple first aid (provided by ambulance attendants in vehicles that were, in many cases, directly descended from the funeral home hearse and often in the United States were run by funeral homes),[8] to sophisticated medical care previously unavailable outside of the hospital environment. These early experiments in extending the hospital into the field demonstrated that advanced cardiac care could be provided outside of the hospital. The Vietnam conflict[9] demonstrated the success of rapid, efficient extrication and transportation of trauma victims. Subsequently, public debates

sparked by the report of the American Academy of Sciences National Research Council on *Accidental Death and Disability: The Neglected Disease of Modern Society*[9,10] led to several federal funding programs for the development of pilot EMS. Nearly every metropolitan area possesses some element of advanced prehospital care, and these practitioners are commonly involved in interhospital transport.[9,11]

It is extremely rare in the United States for physicians to directly provide care in ground ambulances. Most of the injury cases evaluated by EMS personnel do not require advanced skills, and the use of physician resources in this setting would be inefficient. Several allied health personnel with varying degrees of training attend patients in the prehospital setting.[12] Because these practitioners are frequently the care givers during transport, an understanding of their skills and training is important. The regulation of prehospital care occurs at the state level; thus, there is considerable variation in qualifications and training requirements for EMS personnel in different states. Most states grant certification in two major categories for EMS personnel: basic emergency medical technician (EMT-A) and paramedic (EMT-P).

BASIC EMERGENCY MEDICAL TECHNICIANS

Although standards and training requirements are set by the state, the U.S. Department of Transportation has developed minimum standards and objectives for basic EMT training. In addition, a national registry exists (National Registry of Emergency Medical Technicians) that grants a nationally recognized certification for reciprocity purposes. Basic emergency medical technician training generally totals 120 hours, 80 hours of which involves didactic education and skills laboratories. Clinical exposure in the patient care environment (emergency room, ICU, labor and delivery) is typically limited to approximately 40 hours. Certification usually requires completion of a written test and skills examination. The level of care provided by the EMT is commonly denoted as basic life support and includes basic extrication and immobilization of trauma victims, advanced first aid maneuvers, emergency childbirth, and the use of oxygen and bag-valve-mask devices. These practitioners have limited experience and training in patient monitoring and titrated care and are not trained in intravenous therapy, advanced airway maneuvers, or pharmacology; thus, they are generally inappropriate as primary care givers during interhospital transport of the critically ill.

PARAMEDICS

Training programs for EMT-P may be as little as 500 hours or as long as 3000 hours of training. A typical curriculum provides 300 hours of job-specific didactic training including pharmacology, physiology, and pathophysiology of body systems; and approximately 200 hours of clinical participation in prehospital and intrahospital care. The typical paramedic has training in endotracheal intubation, peripheral intravenous catheter placement, electrocardiographic rhythm assessment, drug administration (including drugs commonly associated with the management of cardiac arrest), use of the external DC defibrillator, and the skills previously ascribed to basic life-support personnel. The level of care provided by EMT-P is commonly denoted as advanced life support. These practitioners are generally not trained in the use of invasive monitoring devices, mechanical ventilation, or the broad pharmacopeia generally used in the ICU. For most critically ill patients requiring interhospital transport, the capabilities of these practitioners must be augmented by other health care providers if a similar level of care is to be maintained during transport as in the hospital.

GROUND AMBULANCES

Removal of battlefield victims by horseback and wheeled carts is likely as old as human conflict. However, the first motorized ambulances were constructed in the early 1900s.[6] The types of vehicles used have varied considerably over the years, ranging from a Harley-Davidson motorcycle side-car unit constructed in the mid-1920s to the current truck-type configurations.[12] No matter what configuration of ground ambulance vehicle is used, space limitations are of concern.

Equipment in ambulances varies. Basic and advance life-support units alike are equipped with some method of delivering oxygen to the patient. This is usually accomplished with oxygen from compressed gas cylinders. Many ground ambulances for both basic and advanced life support have inverter systems for the provision of 110-V AC electric power in the patient care area. Advanced life-support equipment also includes a cardiac monitor–defibrillator device, endotracheal tubes, drugs used for resuscitation, intravenous fluid and tubing, as well as syringes, needles, catheters, bandages, and splinting materials. Noninvasive blood pressure monitors and pulse oximeters also may be carried.

Critical care in the typical ground ambulance is constrained by the following factors:

1. *Sophistication of the prehospital care provider*: Although generally highly motivated and skilled in the areas in which they practice, prehospital providers are trained to use and interpret a limited number of monitoring modalities and critical care therapeutic strategies. This limitation may be overcome by adding higher level practitioners to the transport team.
2. *Space constraints*: The ground ambulance must transport all of the equipment necessary for the care of the patient throughout the transport. Although, ambulances built under current specifications are roomy compared with their forbearers, cartage of an unlimited quantity of supplies and devices clearly is not possible.
3. *Power*: Although electrical systems are frequently found in ambulance vehicles, they are not universal or of unlimited capacity.
4. *Vibration/acceleration*: The moving ambulance is subjected to varying magnitudes of vibration and acceleration, which can result in damage to sensitive instruments and erroneous monitoring measurements.

AIR MEDICAL TRANSPORT ■

The first heavier-than-air aircraft flight occurred December 17, 1903 by the Wright brothers, but the concept of air medical evacuation preceded this historic event.[9] In March 1784, the Montgolfier brothers demonstrated balloon flight to the medical faculty of Montpelier,[13] and it is commonly believed that balloons were used to evacuate the wounded during Bismarck's siege of Paris in 1870 (although careful investigation of the facts reveals that balloon evacuation of patients from Paris never occurred[14]). Early use of both airplane and helicopter to transport patients occurred in the military.[15-19] Subsequently, helicopter air medical evacuation has become an integral part of the EMS system in many communities.

Modern air medical transport uses both fixed wing (airplane) and rotor wing (helicopter) transport modes. For distances greater than 200 miles, fixed wing transport is generally more efficient.[4] Unfortunately, fixed wing transports must originate and end at airports. Thus, they all involve at least some brief ground transport of the patient. Many different types of airplanes are used. None were specifically designed for air medical transport.[20] Most of these aircraft are not configured for easy care of the patient. In many instances, power for medical equipment is not available in the main cabin. Storage and restraint of equipment is commonly makeshift.

Short transports of less than 200 miles are ideal for helicopter use. The helicopter has three clear advantages in transporting patients[4]:

1. *Speed*: Rotor wing aircraft commonly used in air medical transport are capable of sustained speeds in excess of 150 miles per hour. This raw speed advantage, combined with the unique ability to travel point to point, offers the potential for decreased total transport time over surface transport alternatives.
2. *Accessibility*: "Vertical takeoff and landing" capabilities of helicopters permit these vehicles to extract patients who are inaccessible to surface vehicles. This quality is of great value in rescue operations in remote regions, but is also significant in large metropolitan areas made inaccessible by the urban gridlock of rush-hour traffic.
3. *Specialized personnel and equipment*: Helicopter transport services routinely operate out of regional referral centers. They are commonly staffed by highly skilled, trained personnel and carry sophisticated monitoring and therapeutic equipment. The helicopter allows a single crew and payload to provide service to a much larger geographic area and patient population than is possible when using surface conveyances.

With the advantage of flight comes some disadvantages. Environmental factors and forces acting on the aircraft in flight also affect the contents of the aircraft including the patient, the care giver, and instrumentation. These forces must be considered in discussing transport of the critically ill.

AIR MEDICAL ENVIRONMENT

The Atmosphere

The earth's gravity holds a mixture of gases about the earth that we term the atmospheric envelope. The atmosphere extends from the surface of the earth to approximately 700 kilometers (430 miles), above which it is no longer considered to be a continuous medium.[21–23] The dry composition of the earth's atmosphere is constant from sea level to about 15,000 m (50,000 feet), containing approximately 21% oxygen. What does change importantly with altitude is ambient pressure. Gravitational forces pull the atmosphere toward the surface of the planet while solar radiation heats the atmosphere and acts to expand it into the surrounding vacuum of space. The gases closest to the surface of the planet are compressed through gravitational forces, leading to the highest pressures at or below sea level and decreasing pressures with increasing altitude. The altitude–pressure relationship is depicted in Figure 53-1.

Changes in pressure with increasing altitude have numerous effects on patients and on the other contents of the aircraft. Hypoxia is the greatest threat to anyone who flies and occurs eventually with rising altitude, even in healthy individuals.[24] Representative pressures at various altitudes, as contained in the U.S. Standard Atmosphere, are shown in Table 53-1. As can be seen in the table, significant hypoxemia may develop in healthy individuals at altitudes well within the reach of the simplest of aircraft. A nomogram for depicting in-flight arterial PO_2 levels from preflight PAO_2 measures has been published.[25] However, continuous pulse oximetry seems prudent during air medical evacuation.

Ambient pressure changes also affect gases in closed spaces. Boyle's law states that the volume of gas varies inversely with pressure at a constant temperature. These gas volume changes may produce several medical problems: cuffed medical appliances expand during ascent and contract during descent, medications stored in gas filled containers may leak, and mechanical ventilators may not deliver prescribed tidal volumes.[26] Cabin pressurization is helpful but does not eliminate these concerns because cabins are routinely pressurized to "cabin altitudes" of 1800 to 2400 m (6000 to 8000 feet) and not to sea level.[27–29] As noted in Table 53-1, this exposes the occupants and instruments of the aircraft to substantially reduced pressures.

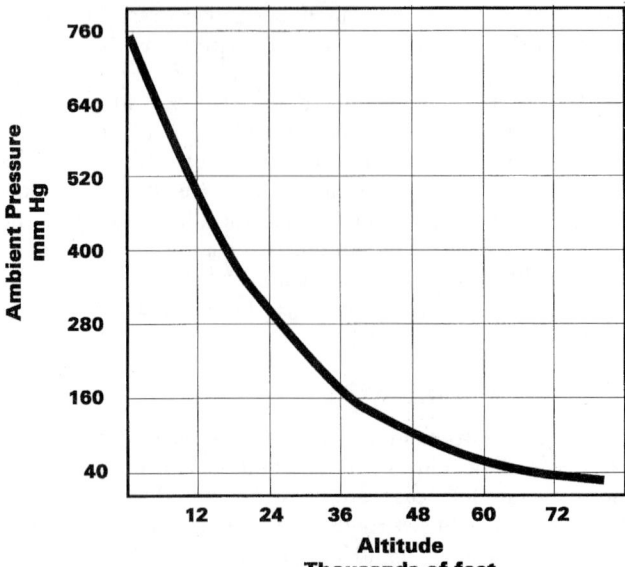

FIGURE 53-1. Relationship between altitude and ambient pressure in the Standard Atmosphere.

Temperature

Temperature falls with increasing altitude at a rate of approximately 2°C per 300 m (1000 feet).[30] Fortunately, modern aircraft are equipped with efficient heaters to make cabin temperatures comfortable.

Acceleration

A passenger seated in an airplane as it accelerates down the runway, or executes a coordinated maneuver in flight, experiences a change of velocity and thus an acceleration. The effect of sustained acceleration is related to the magnitude and the direction of the force. Commonly, acceleration is measured in units of "G." One G is equal to the acceleration of a free-falling object near the surface of the earth. Aerospace physiologists and others dealing with the forces of acceleration have adopted a system for describing these forces based on lettered axes.[31] High levels of acceleration, particularly in the head-to-foot direction ($+G_z$) may have

TABLE 53-1.   Representative Pressures at Various Altitudes in the U.S. Standard Atmosphere

	BREATHING ROOM AIR				BREATHING 100% OXYGEN		
Altitude	Barometric Pressure	Tracheal PO_2	PAO_2	Altitude	Barometric Pressure	Tracheal PO_2	PAO_2
Sea level	760	149	103	33,000	196	149	109
5000	632	122	79	36,000	170	123	85
10,000	523	100	61	39,000	148	100	64
15,000	429	80	46	42,000	128	811	48
20,000	349	63	33	45,000	111	64	34
22,000	321	57	30	46,000	106	59	30

important cardiovascular effects.[32] Fortunately, routinely experienced accelerations are of little concern.

Vibration

Vibration is a repeating, alternating form of motion that has direction, intensity, and frequency. Vibration levels commonly encountered in the air medical environment contribute to flight crew fatigue, motion sickness, and malfunction of monitoring equipment.[33–35]

NOISE

Noise is also of concern in the air medical environment. Noise is measured with sound level meters, which determine sound pressure using a decibel (dB) scale. Ambient noise levels in helicopter cabins are so high as to require the routine use of protective headphones and intercom systems for communications. Helicopter noise also may compromise communication immediately outside of the cabin. Airplane cabins and ground ambulances are also noisy environments. Noise is an important issue in the transport of the critically ill because it may preclude using auditory feedback for physiologic signals (e.g., auscultated blood pressure) and may mask alarms.[36,37]

ISOLATION AND CABIN CONSTRAINTS

Aircraft cabins, like ground ambulances, are physically constrained. In addition, acceleration forces experienced in aircraft may result in unrestrained medical devices becoming dangerous missiles during flight. The need to restrain monitoring equipment, therefore, also must be considered in air medical transport. Business aircraft may not have electrical power available in the cabin, and what is available may not be sufficient to supply the needs of specialized medical equipment.

APPROACH TO THE TRANSPORT OF THE CRITICALLY ILL ■

When considering transportation of the critically ill, the following questions must be answered:

1. *Is transport indicated?* Transport of the critically ill is a risk–benefit decision. The clinician considering transport must weigh the added benefit of moving the patient against the risks inherent in the transport. This is often a difficult decision and requires considerable judgment.
2. *What is the appropriate mode of transport?* For critically ill patients, this question usually is one of ground-versus-air transport. The capabilities of these modes generally differ with higher level practitioners, and more sophisticated equipment typically available in the air transport arena. The specific clinical needs of the patient may dictate one mode over the other.
3. *How do we prepare the patient for and manage the patient during transport to maximize the potential for*

success? Preparation of the patient for transport begins with contacting the receiving physician's institution. The transporting organization also should be contacted. If the patient is to be transported by air, careful consideration of the effects of pressure and the other forces of the air medical environment should be considered, and closed gas spaces should be decompressed. Oxygen supply and calculated usage must be considered as well as the power needs of any specialized equipment that is required. The makeup of the transport team should be determined based on the anticipated needs of the patient.

The transport of the critically ill patient encompasses all of the difficulties of the ICU with the additional problems of the transport environment. Like most situations, planning is the key to minimizing the risk of transport. Knowledge of the transport resources available in the community and a careful consideration of the clinical situation are vital to successful critical care transports.[38]

REFERENCES ■

1. American Hospital Association Hospital Data Center: *Hospital Closures: A Statistical Profile*. Chicago, American Hospital Association, 1989
2. Sabatino F: Bankruptcy, boards, physicians, and CEO's. *Hospital* 1986;60:103
3. Collett M: The conference cometh. *Hospital Aviation* 1989;8:5
4. Fromm RE, Varon J: Air medical transport. *J Fam Pract* 1993; 36:313
5. The National EMS Clearing House: *Emergency Medical Services Transportation Systems and Available Facilities*. Lexington, KY, National Association of State EMS Directors and the Council of State Governments, 1988
6. Pepe PE: Pre-hospital and inter-hospital transport of the trauma patient. *Probl Critical Care* 1990;4:556
7. Pantridge JF, Geddes JS: A mobile intensive care unit in the management of myocardial infarction. *Lancet* 1967;ii:271
8. Stewart RD: Facilities and regionalization: emergency medical services systems. *Emerg Med Clinic North Am* 1990;8:33
9. Lam DM: Wings of life and hope: a history of aeromedical evaluation. *Probl Critical Care* 1990;4:556
10. National Academy of Sciences/National Research Council: *Accidental Death and Disability: The Neglected Disease of Modern Society*. Washington, DC, National Academy of Sciences, 1966
11. Pepe PE, Almaguer DR: Emergency medical services: personnel and ground transport ethics. *Probl Crit Care* 1990;4:470
12. Federal Specifications for Star of Life Ambulances, KKK-1822-C. Washington, DC, General Accounting Office, 1990
13. Durieux J: Essai sur l'usage des aerostats et ses applications en medicine. *Paris Medical* 1913;12:833
14. Lam DM: To pop a balloon: air evacuation during the siege of Paris, 1870. *Aviat Space Eviron Med* 1988;59:988
15. Blanchard R: Transport des blesses en aeroplane. *Paris Medical* 1916;21:54
16. Clark DM: Helicopter in air evacuation. *Air Surgeon Bull* 1944;6:694
17. Neel S: Helicopter evacuation in Korea and its effect on the future. *Mil Surg* 1952;110:323

18. Neel S: Army aeromedical procedures in Vietnam: implications for rural America. *JAMA* 1968;204:309
19. Meyers RN, et al: A civilian aeromedical lifesaving plan, HELP. *Penn Med J* 1965;68:51
20. Walker VB, Fromm RE: Aircraft, airmen and aviation aspects of aeromedical transport. *Probl Crit Care* 1990;4:508
21. Strughold H: The earth's environment and aviation. In: Randel HW (ed). *Aerospace Medicine*, ed 2. Baltimore, Williams & Wilkins, 1971:22
22. Fromm RE, Duvall JO: Medical aspects of flight for civilian aeromedical transport. *Probl Crit Care* 1990;7:495
23. Armstrong HG: The atmosphere. In: Armstrong HG (ed). *Aerospace Medicine*. Baltimore, Williams & Wilkins, 1961:109
24. Harding RM, Mills JF: Problems of altitude. I. Hypoxia and hyperventilation. *Br Med J* 1983;286:1408
25. Henry JN, Krenis LJ, Cutting RT: Hypoxemia during aeromedical evacuation. *Surg Gynecol Obstet* 1973;136:49
26. Bradshaw M, Dyer LL, Gortter W, et al: Effect of altitude on pneumatically powered fluidic controlled versus electronically powered microprocessor-controlled volume ventilators. *Aeromed J* 1988;Sept/Oct:43
27. AMA Commission on Emergency Medical Services:Medical aspects or transportation aboard commercial aircraft. *JAMA* 1982;247:1007
28. Cottrell JJ: Altitude exposures during aircraft flight: flying higher. *Chest* 1988;93:81
29. MacMilian AJF: The pressure cabin. In: Ernsting J, King P (eds). *Aviation Medicine*. London, Butterworth, 1988:112
30. Welch BE: The biosphere. In: DeHart RL (ed). *Fundamentals of Aerospace Medicine*. Philadelphia, Lea & Febinger, 1985:63
31. Gell C: Table of equivalents for acceleration terminology, recommended for general international use by the aerospace medicine panel AGARD. *Aerospace Med* 1961;32:1109
32. Leverett SD, Whinery JE: Biodynamics: sustained acceleration. In: DeHart RL, King P (eds). *Fundamentals of Aerospace Medicine*. Philadelphia, Lea & Febiger, 1985:202
33. Stott JRR: Vibration. In: Ernsting J, King P (eds). *Aviation Medicine*. London, Butterworth, 1988:185
34. Von gierke HE, Clarke NP: Effects of vibration and buffeting on man. In: Randel HW (ed). *Aerospace Medicine*, ed 2. Baltimore, Williams & Wilkins, 1971:198
35. Wayle S, Guntupalli K: Physiologic monitoring during prehospital and inter-hospital transport of critically ill patients. *Probl Critical Care* 1990;4:459
36. Rood GM: Noise and communication. In: Ernsting J, King P (eds). *Aviation Medicine*. Philadelphia, Lea & Febiger, 1985;353
37. Laufer MD, Croes CE: A device to improve scene call communications. *J Air Med Transport* 1989;8:58
38. Fromm RE, Dellinger RP: Transport of critically ill patients. *J Intensive Care Med* 1992;7:223

Critical Care, Third Edition, edited by Joseph M. Civetta,
Robert W. Taylor, and Robert R. Kirby.
Lippincott-Raven Publishers, Philadelphia, PA © 1997.

CHAPTER 54

Pain Control

David L. Brown
James F. Flynn

IMMEDIATE CONCERNS

MAJOR PROBLEMS

Providing effective pain relief in the critical care unit is one of the most direct methods of decreasing postoperative complications and health care costs in high-risk surgical patients.[1-3] Nevertheless, the production of effective analgesia is elusive. Traditionally, analgesia care is viewed as an extra expense rather than as a means of saving health care funds.

For years, a common routine for critically ill patients undergoing high-risk operations was to prescribe sedatives and analgesics as necessary while a tracheal tube was maintained and mechanical ventilation used during the first days postoperatively. This routine was theorized as preferable to extubating high-risk patients, who required sophisticated monitoring. Often, however, a considerable portion of the monitoring, prolonged airway maintenance, and ventilatory interventions were mandated by the choice of unconsciousness and mechanical ventilation as the means of treating the patient's "incision defect."

Similarly, analgesia has not been a principal concern in traumatized patients, except in those with flail chest. Such an approach is understandable because, after significant trauma, cardiovascular, neurologic, and coagulation function are often ill-defined; this approach also limits the interest in neuraxial blocks, which are the mainstay of effective intensive care unit (ICU) analgesia. The essential feature of providing analgesia is to tailor the method to the patient, procedure, personnel, and institution.

STRESS POINTS

1. Historically, pain control has been poorly managed. Although intramuscular narcotics have been the standard analgesic regimen for decades, approximately 75% of hospitalized patients receiving intramuscular narcotics remain in moderate to severe pain.[4,5]

2. Ineffective analgesia results from a reluctance by physicians and nurses to give sufficient doses of narcotics. This reluctance seems to result from an exaggerated fear of narcotic addiction; surveys demonstrate that most physicians overestimate the risk of narcotic addiction in postoperative patients by 10 to 100 times.[4,6]

3. A survey of both surgical residents and nurses on a postoperative surgical ward showed only 20% of each group aimed for complete pain relief postoperatively.[7]

4. Although attaining the goal of complete pain relief after operation or injury may be in the future, pain has detrimental physiologic impact that must be understood before prescribing an analgesic technique for a critically ill patient.

5. Patients undergoing thoracic or upper abdominal procedures or those sustaining blunt chest trauma are the ones who have the most marked ventilatory compromise after operation or injury. In these patients, pain results in acute restrictive pulmonary disease. This incision or trauma defect produces patients with increased respiratory rate and decreased tidal volume, vital capacity, forced expiratory volume, and functional residual capacity (FRC).

6. After upper abdominal or thoracic operations, vital capacity is the first parameter to change and is proportionally the most severely reduced of the pulmonary measurements. Decreases to 40% to 60% of preoperative values are common after operation and do not return to normal for at least 2 weeks. In

addition to the vital capacity changes, the residual volume, FRC, and forced expiratory volume are reduced, reaching their nadir between 24 and 48 hours postoperatively. In patients with an uncomplicated course, these parameters return to near-normal levels by the seventh to tenth day.

7. Loss of FRC seems to unify most pulmonary complications in the postoperative period. Intraoperatively, some decrease in FRC is predictable[8]; however, in the absence of complications, the anesthetic-induced change should return toward normal shortly after emergence, even after an upper abdominal operation[9] (Table 54-1).

8. While FRC diminishes, the resting lung volume approaches that lung volume necessary to prevent small airway closure, that is, the closing volume. If FRC decreases below closing volume, atelectasis and ventilation-perfusion ($\dot{V}/\dot{Q}$) abnormalities result; the end result is hypoxemia.

9. Mechanisms responsible for the predictable decrease in FRC after surgery are controversial and poorly understood, but the decrease seems to result from at least two factors: an ill-defined, pain-related neural reflex producing increased tone in the abdominal muscles during expiration[10]; and a decrease in diaphragmatic function.[11] Effective postoperative analgesia should focus on the first of these two factors to minimize the detrimental impact.

10. Ventilation alterations are not the only detrimental effects of pain. The perioperative stress response is closely tied to pain experienced after operation. Biochemical components of the stress response include elevated levels of catecholamines; hypercoaguability; systemic and often coronary vasoconstriction; metabolic shifts to a catabolic, protein-wasting state; and immunosuppression.[12]

11. Although this stress response may be beneficial and self-protective in some situations, it often is counterproductive postoperatively. Early in the twentieth century, Crile and Lower[13] were proponents of reducing this adverse response to pain when they promoted their concept of anociassociation. Their early ideas have been substantiated by others, including those

at Johns Hopkins[14] (Fig. 54-1) and in Europe.[15] Experimental and clinical evidence is accumulating that further outlines the adverse effects of postsurgical pain.[16–18]

ESSENTIAL DIAGNOSTIC TESTS AND PROCEDURES

1. Few diagnostic tests and procedures are necessary unless specific abnormalities are possible. Vertebral column abnormalities are important when considering central neuraxial techniques. An assessment of coagulation parameters may also be indicated, although the precise implication of somewhat abnormal findings is debated.

2. Time spent talking to the patient and explaining the options is well worthwhile. Many individuals reject some techniques because they fear "a needle in the back."

INITIAL THERAPY

1. Plan your approach carefully. Recognize the positive benefits of effective pain relief, but don't consider it to be a cure-all.

2. Be prepared to treat adverse side effects (e.g., respiratory depression) or frank complications (e.g., pneumothorax, total spinal). Make sure nurses, respiratory therapists, and others know what to anticipate when "bad things" happen.

3. Titrate drugs (and antidotes such as naloxone) to their appropriate effects. Small, incremental doses are always better than a "slam-dunk."

TABLE 54-1.   Timing of FRC Decrease After Cholecystectomy in 11 Patients

TIME AFTER OPERATION	MEAN FRC (L)
Preoperative value	2.18
4 h	2.20
10 h	2.25
16 h	1.70
24 h	1.63
3 d	1.65
5 d	2.00

FRC, functional residual capacity.

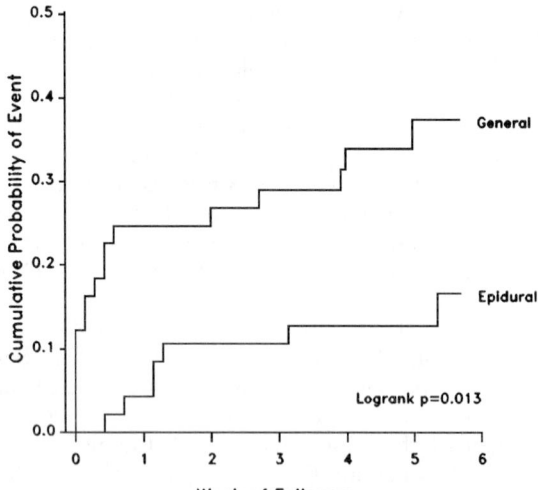

FIGURE 54-1. Frequency of reoperation (regrafting, thrombectomy, or amputation) after major vascular surgery when comparing routine general anesthesia and narcotic analgesia with epidural anesthesia and analgesia. Reoperation was significantly more frequent after general than after epidural anesthesia. (From Christopherson R, Beattie C, Frank SM, et al: Perioperative morbidity in patients randomized to epidural or general anesthesia for lower extremity vascular surgery. *Anesthesiology* 1993;79:422.)

4. Don't withhold therapy for fear of narcotic addiction. To do so is inhumane and is not based on established fact. Practice the golden rule.
5. When in doubt, ask for help. Pain management is a major anesthesiology subspecialty and is of increasing interest to other physicians. Somebody usually is available to provide consultation.

PATIENT SELECTION

In some ways, analgesia can be prescribed for critically ill patients more easily than for their healthier counterparts. The typical intensive monitoring and observation of these patients by highly skilled nurses allows the risk–benefit decisions to move toward more potent analgesic techniques, such as neuraxial narcotic–local anesthetic mixtures. In contrast, for a ward patient, the risk and benefit analysis of these techniques is necessarily more problematic. Conversely, admission to an ICU postoperatively should not automatically encourage the use of a potent technique; the physiologic impairment of the patient must be weighed against expected benefits of the analgesic technique. Typically, more potent techniques are appropriate for thoracotomy, major upper abdominal surgery, major vascular surgery, or abdominal surgery in patients with pulmonary compromise from intrinsic lung disease, obesity, or old age (Table 54-2). Our previous concept that pain control alone was important in reducing perioperative or critical care morbidity and mortality seems clinically unsophisticated. Rather, it is clear that perioperative (critical care) rehabilitation, which may include earlier enteral nutrition, physical therapy, and stress attenuation, demands more than simple pain control. Even the most effective pain control is likely to have limited benefit if the surgical rehabilitation aspect is neglected.

Postoperative patients are not the only critically ill patients for whom analgesia decisions are appropriate. Multiple-system trauma patients are also admitted to ICUs. Although the multiple injuries and possible coagulation alterations after a significant injury and resuscitation limit neuraxial analgesia techniques, an assortment of peripheral blocks may be appropriate for painful body wall or extremity injuries.

TABLE 54-2. ICU Patients at High Risk if Analgesia Is Ineffective

Thoracic surgery
Major upper abdominal surgery
Major vascular surgery
Abdominal surgery in
　Pulmonary disease, chronic
　Morbid obesity
　Extreme aging
Blunt thoracic trauma

ANALGESIC TECHNIQUE

The techniques of postoperative analgesia appropriate to critical care patients can be classified into two principal areas: (1) narcotic analgesia, and (2) local anesthetic analgesia. Additionally, these two types are increasingly being combined, that is, mixtures of local anesthetics and narcotics in neuraxial infusions, to minimize side effects and optimize analgesia.

NARCOTIC THERAPY

Intramuscular

On-demand (PRN) intramuscular narcotic therapy is the traditional method of analgesia. The major advantage of this technique is its simplicity. Nevertheless, computed tomographic analysis has demonstrated that most ($\geq$85%) of the injections are not intramuscular but subcutaneous.[19] This finding helps to explain the wide variation in dose–response curves repeatedly found in intramuscular injection studies. As an example, when similar narcotic doses are injected, peak drug concentrations vary as much as fivefold, and the time to reach peak blood levels varies threefold to sevenfold.[20] These studies also demonstrate that blood meperidine concentrations were in excess of the minimum analgesic concentration for only about 35% of each 4-hour dosing interval when meperidine, 100 mg, was administered in the traditional intramuscular fashion.[21] Thus, despite their ease of use, the extreme variability in absorption and general tendency to underdose make it difficult to achieve adequate pain control.

Intravenous

The one-to-one or one-to-two registered nurse–to–patient ratio found in most ICUs facilitates frequent intravenous dosing of narcotics. Thus, a more stable and effective blood level of narcotic is possible. In effect, the nurse-administered narcotic mimics the popular patient-controlled analgesia (PCA) techniques used widely by many postoperative ward patients. By anticipating and administering additional drug proactively before painful experiences (such as moving about and coughing), thus improving overall pain relief, critical care nurses are able to provide a similar service with intravenous narcotics to critically ill patients.

Epidural or Intrathecal

Opioid receptors in the substantia gelatinosa of the spinal cord[22] (Fig. 54-2) allow selective, segmental spinal (neuraxial) analgesia to be produced. The narcotic drugs have a specific spinal action characterized by intense analgesia, an attractive property because of the absence of motor and sympathetic blockade and the central nervous system and cardiovascular toxicity sometimes associated with neuraxial local anesthetic use. Presynaptic and postsynaptic receptors in the substantia gelatinosa of the dorsal horn are the site of neuraxial narcotic action. The lipid-soluble agents, fentanyl and sufentanil, diffuse to the opioid receptors more

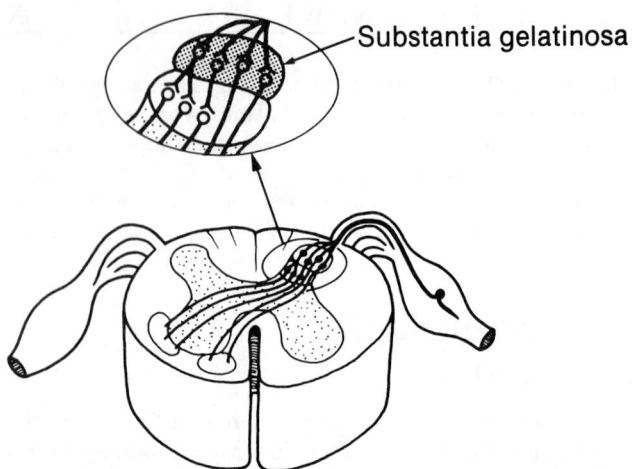

Substantia gelatinosa

FIGURE 54-2. Cross-section view of spinal cord with expanded view of area of dorsal horn that contains the substantia gelatinosa. This area contains a high concentration of opioid receptors and is the region where intraspinal opioids are most effective in producing analgesia.

rapidly than morphine and need to be applied nearer the intended level of analgesia. Thus, thoracic epidural catheters may be needed for upper abdominal or thoracic pain managed with fentanyl or sufentanil. Morphine, because of the water solubility conferred on it by hydroxyl groups, remains in the cerebrospinal fluid longer and thus allows rostral spread, with the potential for respiratory depression. Although this insolubility gives morphine a slower onset, it confers a longer duration of analgesia.

The overall cost–benefit value to society associated with this therapy remains to be clarified; in the short run, neuraxial narcotic therapy seems more expensive than traditional PRN narcotic therapy. Nevertheless, Yeager and colleagues' data[1] suggest that the aggregate costs of care may be reduced by decreasing the incidence of postoperative complications in high-risk patients (Table 54-3). Data from Johns Hopkins Hospital showed fewer reoperations when effective analgesia was used in vascular surgery patients, supporting the concept that health care costs can be lowered if pain control is considered in high-risk patients.[2] Nevertheless, additional information is needed in larger numbers of patients relating how analgesia choices affect health care costs.

LOCAL ANESTHETIC BLOCKS

Local anesthetics also have a place in providing analgesia to critically ill patients. Principally, these techniques are useful when combined narcotics and local anesthetics are administered for neuraxial techniques, during intercostal nerve blocks, or when a peripheral block catheter technique can be used for extremity pain.

Epidural

Epidural local anesthetics, used without added narcotics and administered as a continuous infusion, are of limited usefulness postoperatively. Analgesia provided in this manner results in patients who have a significant sympathectomy with potential cardiovascular side effects and an inability to ambulate caused by motor blockade. These effects may be appropriate for some time interval postoperatively in certain patients; however, the increasing trend is to provide neuraxial analgesia care with narcotics alone or in combination with dilute concentrations of local anesthetics not associated with extensive cardiovascular and motor side effects.

Peripheral

Peripheral regional blocks also can be used, often with continuous infusions using catheters inserted percutaneously.[23] These techniques have been shown to be useful for upper extremity pain and, in some instances, lower extremity pain. Again, however, the popularity and efficacy of neuraxial narcotic techniques limits interest in developing lower extremity plexus techniques using only local anesthetics.

TECHNIQUES AND PROCEDURES

Intravenous Narcotics

Intravenous narcotic therapy for critically ill patients must rely heavily on nursing personnel to titrate the drug. A flexible dosing regimen should be prescribed so that the variabil-

TABLE 54-3. Results From Analgesia Comparison Among Yeager and Colleagues' Patients

VARIABLE	GENERAL AND OPIOID	EPIDURAL AND EPIDURAL ANALGESIA
Intubation	81.8 ± 186 h	7.1 ± 1.7 h°
ICU stay	5.7 + 9.3 d	2.5 + 1.8 d
Hospital stay	15.8 + 12.3 d	11.4 + 4.6 d
Hospital costs	$20,380 + 20,343	$11,218 + 5738°
Physician costs	$5134 + 2939	$3,801 + 1342°
Mortality	4 per 25 patients	0 per 28 patients°
Morbidity	19 per 25 patients	9 per 28 patients°

°$p < 0.05$.

(From Yeager MP, Glass DD, Neff RK, et al: Epidural anesthesia and analgesia in high risk surgical patients. *Anesthesiology* 1987;66:729).

ity in patient narcotic requirements can be addressed effectively. Nurses should provide a basal dosing interval, with additional PRN narcotic administered for painful treatments or manipulations, as is done with PCA pumps. A clear advantage for a particular narcotic in critical care patients is not apparent; thus, familiarity with your institution's narcotic preference is probably more important than having a long list of agents on the hospital formulary.

Peripheral Local Anesthetic Block

Peripheral block with local anesthetics has the advantage of producing analgesia without respiratory depression. Intercostal nerve block or continuous thoracic epidural analgesia can be used to provide analgesia for blunt chest injuries (flail chest injuries), whereas extremity injuries can be blocked with either a continuous brachial (upper extremity) or epidural (lower extremity) technique. In either instance, lower concentrations of long-acting local anesthetics (bupivacaine 0.125% to 0.25%) can be used, because motor block is unnecessary; sensory blocking concentrations will suffice. Continuous intrapleural analgesia also has received considerable attention as a means of providing chest wall analgesia; however, its place in the ICU needs further delineation before the simplicity of the technique promotes an overzealous use in critical care patients.

INTERCOSTAL.   Intercostal nerve block should be learned from an experienced anesthesiologist; however, it is not difficult to perform. Although intercostal nerves can be blocked anywhere along their anatomic course, the technique is usually performed with a blunt 22-gauge needle at the angle of the rib, that is, approximately 8 to 10 cm lateral to the posterior midline where the paraspinous muscles attach to the ribs. Here the nerve is most easily accessible, and the risk of pneumothorax is minimized. It is typically performed with 3 to 5 mL of local anesthetic injected for each intercostal nerve. One should plan ahead so that a suitable concentration of local anesthetic is chosen, thus minimizing problems with local anesthetic systemic toxicity. Postoperatively, patients are usually placed in a lateral decubitus position, with the side to be blocked uppermost. If the block is being placed preoperatively in a high-risk patient, it is usually performed with the patient in a prone position.

AXILLARY CATHETER.   When a catheter technique for upper extremity analgesia is chosen, it is inserted 6 to 10 cm into the axillary sheath once a paresthesia is obtained. Although such single injection site techniques sometimes do not produce effective surgical anesthesia, their usefulness in producing upper extremity analgesia seems well established, and more anesthesiologists are using the infraclavicular approach to continuous postoperative brachial plexus analgesia.[23]

Neuraxial Technique

ANATOMY.   The 12 thoracic and 5 lumbar vertebrae make up the bony reference for neuraxial techniques. All vertebrae have similar basic structure, although they vary in shape and size according to position and function. A vertebra is made up of a vertebral body and bony arch, which consists of two pedicles anteriorly and two laminae posteriorly, the junctions of which form the transverse processes (Fig. 54-3). The laminae join to form the spinous process, which varies from almost a horizontal position in the lumbar and lower thoracic region to one of steep caudal angulation in the midthoracic region (Fig. 54-4). Ligamentous structures join the vertebrae and are used clinically, particularly in epidural placement (Fig. 54-5), to facilitate needle placement.

The lateral decubitus position is used most frequently in performing lumbar puncture and epidural catheterization. In a critically ill patient, this is often the only way in which the patient can be positioned. The patient is placed in the fetal position by flexing the knees to the chest and flexing the neck. Every effort should be made to reduce lumbar lordosis maximally, while keeping the patient's back perpendicular to the floor (Fig. 54-6A).

Less frequently, especially in the ICU, the sitting position is used. It is usually chosen in patients who are obese or with significant scoliosis to more precisely identify midline vertebral anatomy (see Fig. 54-6B). The patient should sit on the bed with the feet supported and the neck and back maximally flexed. Blood pressure changes may occur during this positioning, and a strong, facile assistant is mandatory, as is the need for appropriate monitoring and life-support equipment. Again, of practical importance is the concept that each of these positions is an attempt to increase the vertebral interlaminar gap by reducing the lumbar lordosis.

EQUIPMENT.   A hospital-prepared or commercial tray should be used with utmost care to ensure asepsis. The choice of tray depends on local preference, utilization, and the economics of the situation. Whichever tray is available, the items listed in Table 54-4 should be included.

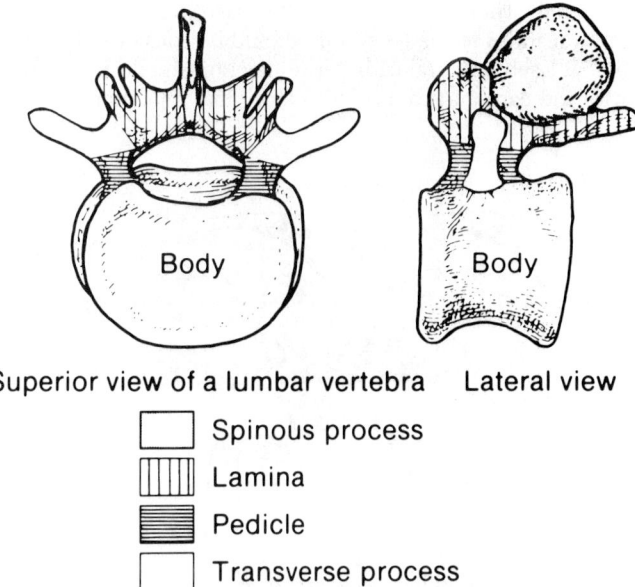

Superior view of a lumbar vertebra   Lateral view

☐ Spinous process

▥ Lamina

▤ Pedicle

☐ Transverse process

FIGURE 54-3. Superior and lateral view of a lumbar vertebra.

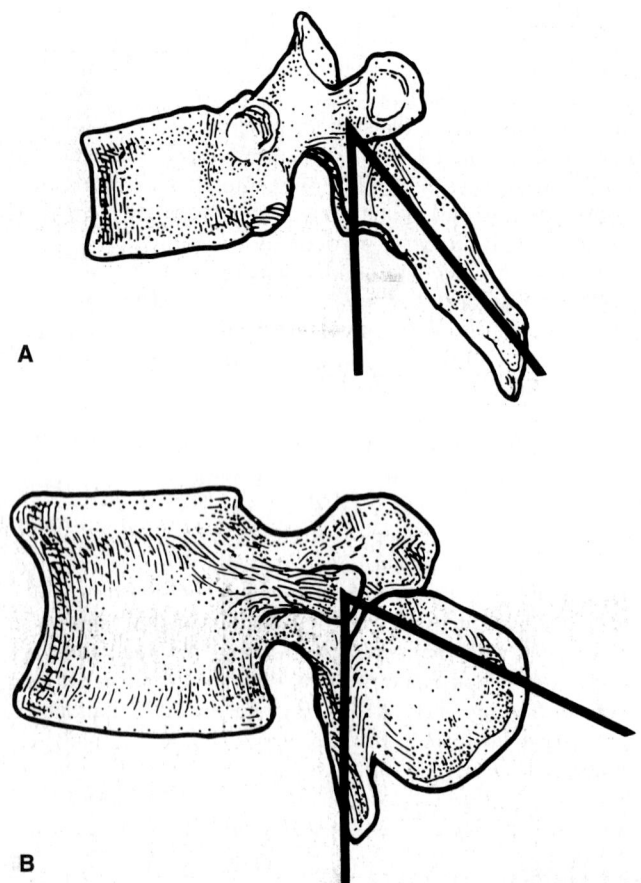

FIGURE 54-4. Comparison of spinous process angulation: (**A**) midthoracic and (**B**) lumbar vertebrae.

EPIDURAL PUNCTURE.   Epidural nerve blockade carried out in the ICU should have complete monitoring and resuscitative equipment available for treatment of complications, especially when a local anesthetic is used. Additionally, contraindications to the technique should be considered (Table 54-5). Each epidural catheter reinjection should be treated with the care and caution of the original injection.

The loss of resistance technique (Fig. 54-7A) is the most common method for identification of the epidural space. Because the epidural space is entered "blindly," the trained hand of the operator must be used to guide the needle. A ground-glass syringe containing saline (preferred) or air is attached to an epidural needle placed within the interspinous ligament. Injection of the solution will be difficult if the needle tip is within the midline ligaments. With the noninjecting hand firmly against the patient's back and thumb and index or middle finger holding the needle hub, the needle is advanced slowly with the noninjecting hand, while constant pressure is applied to the syringe plunger with the other thumb. While the needle enters the ligamentum flavum, an increased resistance to injection can be appreciated. While the needle traverses the ligament and enters the epidural space, injection of solution occurs with ease (Fig. 54-7B).

The negative (subambient) pressure found in the epidural space, which is lowest in the thoracic region, is the basis of the hanging-drop epidural technique. A drop of fluid is placed in the hub of the epidural needle once the needle is seated within the interspinous ligament. Increased resistance to advancement is observed when the ligamentum flavum is encountered; when the needle enters the epidural space, the fluid is drawn into the space by the negative pressure. Many anesthesiologists believe this technique is less reliable than is the loss of resistance for epidural space identification.

Midline Approach.   The patient is appropriately positioned with assistance. The most easily palpable interspace from L-2 to L-5 is identified and an intradermal wheal is raised in its midpoint. After skin puncture is made with a sharp, large-bore needle, an epidural needle is advanced with care through this skin entry site in the midline of the back. Once the needle is placed in the interspinous ligament with a 5- to 10-degree cephalad angulation, it is advanced to the ligamentum flavum; the epidural space is entered using the chosen technique. The usual cause of failure of needle advancement is striking the lamina when the needle is off the midline. Midline needle placement and modification of

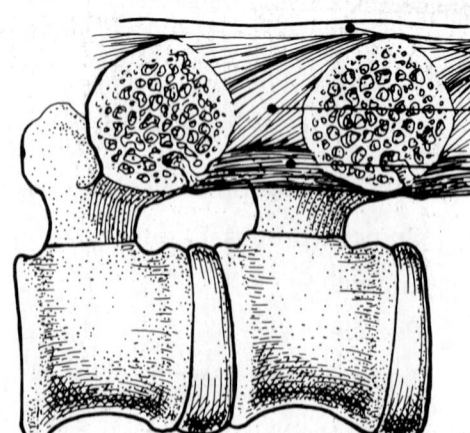

Supraspinous ligament

Interspinous ligament

Ligamentum flavum

FIGURE 54-5. Vertebral ligaments.

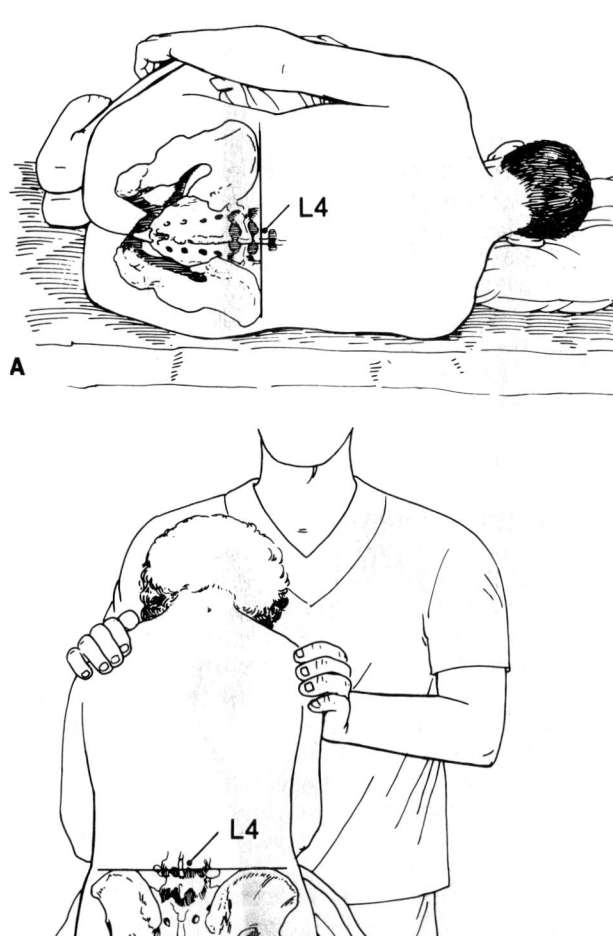

whose lumbar flexion is limited by life-support equipment. The paramedian approach frees the operator from dependency on maximal patient cooperation needed to produce spinal flexion and is especially valuable if a thoracic epidural technique is being performed. In the lumbar region, skin infiltration is carried out 1 cm lateral and 1 cm caudad to the caudad tip of the cephalad spinous process of the chosen interspace. Advancing the needle parallel to the midline until the bony lamina is reached provides an indication of the depth of the ligamentum flavum. The epidural needle is then withdrawn, reinserted with a medial angulation of 10 degrees, and "walked" off the lamina into the ligamentum flavum (see Fig. 54-8*B*), and then into the epidural space using your chosen technique.

Thoracic Approach. A thoracic epidural approach is indicated when a selective block of the thoracic and upper abdominal areas is desired. This technique has the advantage of minimizing the dose of local anesthetic, narcotic, or both, and decreasing the spread of denervation to sacral and lumbar segments, causing less impairment of sympathetic tone. Because of the rare but potential hazard of spinal cord injury, only clinicians with considerable epidural experience should use this technique. The spinous processes in the midthoracic region have an extreme downward angulation, making the paramedian approach preferred. The patient is placed in a lateral decubitus position with head on a pillow and thorax bowed toward the operator. The inferior angle of the scapula is approximately at the level of T-7. A skin wheal is produced at a point 1 cm lateral and 1 cm caudad to the chosen spinous process. Infiltration of local anesthetic to the level of the lamina identifies its depth. The epidural needle is inserted with an angulation of 10 to 15 degrees medially and 45 to 60 degrees in the sagittal plane, again walking off the lamina into the ligamentum flavum and subsequently into the epidural space.

EPIDURAL CATHETER TECHNIQUE. Most ICU applications of epidural analgesia require catheter placement. Catheters are biologically inert, radiopaque Teflon or nylon and pass through a standard thin-wall 18- or 19-gauge epidural needle. They have distance markers to guide the depth of insertion and may have a metal stylet to provide rigidity. If

FIGURE 54-6. Patient positioning for peridural techniques. (**A**) Lateral position. (**B**) Sitting position.

cephalocaudal angulation should permit entry through the intralaminar space (Fig. 54-8*A*).

Paramedian Approach. Patients are encountered in whom a midline approach remains difficult even with ideal positioning. This problem is especially common in the elderly with marked calcification of the supraspinous and intraspinous ligaments, those with rigid spines, and in critically ill patients

TABLE 54-4. Equipment Needed for Peridural Techniques

Skin preparation material
Sterile towels for draping
Local anesthetic and 25- to 26-gauge needle and syringe for skin infiltration
Epidural needle, 18- or 19-gauge (Touhy, Weiss, or Crawford)
Epidural catheter
Syringe for loss of resistance (preferably ground-glass barrel and plunger with Luer-lok connector)

TABLE 54-5. Contraindications to Peridural Techniques

ABSOLUTE	RELATIVE
Patient refusal	Hypovolemia (LA)
Infection of skin or underlying tissue at insertion site	Hypotension (LA)
Full anticoagulation or severe coagulopathy	Preexisting central nervous system disease (e.g., multiple sclerosis)
Raised intracranial pressure	Allergy to drug
	Systemic infection (catheter technique)
	Spinal deformities (technical difficulties)

LA, when using local anesthetics.

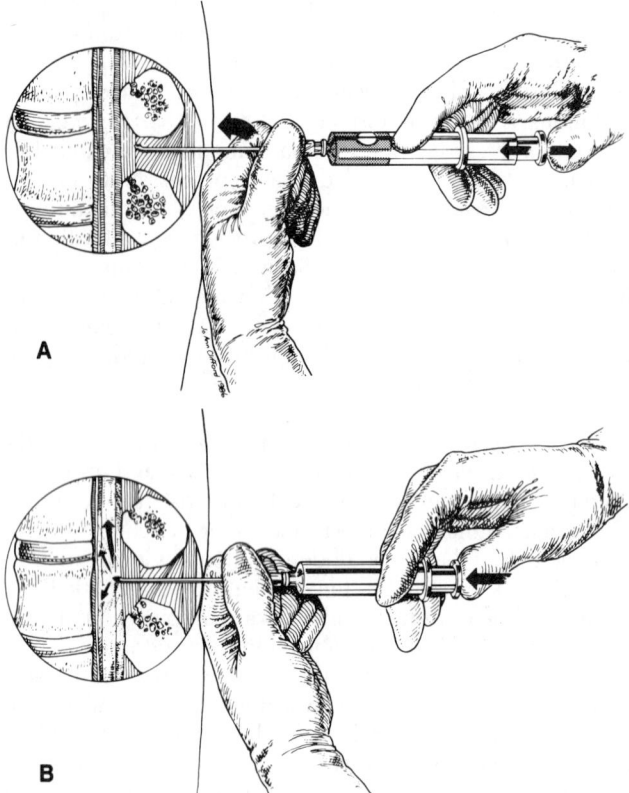

FIGURE 54-7. Loss of resistance technique for epidural space localization. (**A**) Needle seated in interspinous ligament and ligamentum flavum. (**B**) Entry of needle into epidural space.

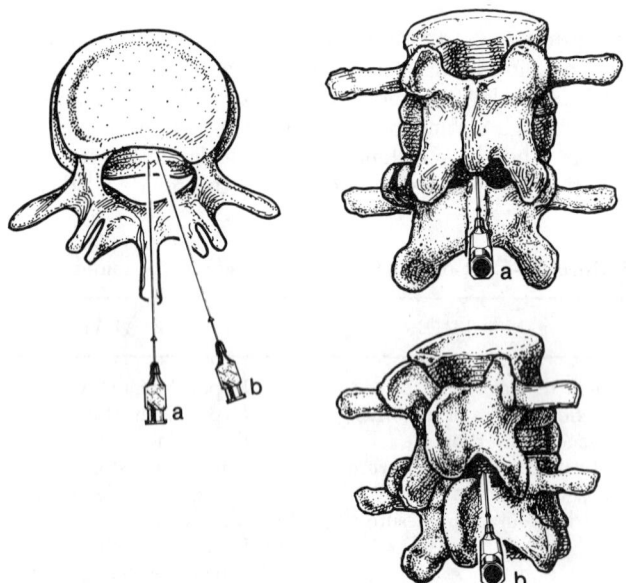

FIGURE 54-8. Peridural technique. (**A**) Midline approach. (**B**) Paramedian approach.

a stylet is used, it should be withdrawn from the catheter tip before insertion, thereby minimizing the chance of unintentional dural puncture. After the needle is placed in the epidural space, the catheter is advanced to the cephalad-directed needle tip; while it passes beyond the tip, a slight resistance to further advancement may be felt. Three to four centimeters of catheter are then inserted, the needle is withdrawn over the catheter, and the catheter is taped securely to the patient's back.

Once an epidural catheter has been inserted beyond the tip of an epidural needle, it should never be withdrawn through the needle because catheter shearing may occur. If resistance is encountered in removing a catheter, increased flexion of the spine may help. Should a catheter break in the epidural space, because of the catheter's inert nature, there is no reason to remove it surgically. Postoperative analgesia management is simplified by noting at what depth the catheter was secured.

SPINAL PUNCTURE. On occasion, spinal puncture and subsequent subarachnoid catheter insertion may be indicated to provide intrathecal narcotic analgesia. The appropriate place of this analgesia management technique is probably years away, because the equipment continues to be refined. No convincing evidence demonstrates significant advantages to spinal catheters and intrathecal drug administration in preference to the epidural route.

Nevertheless, if subarachnoid puncture is required, the cannulation is carried out in a manner similar to that used for an epidural technique. When the needle passes through the ligamentum flavum, it is advanced until the "pop" of passing through the dura is appreciated by the fingers inserting the spinal needle. To assure subarachnoid location of the needle tip, it is helpful if cerebrospinal fluid is able to be aspirated throughout a 360-degree rotation of the needle.

CLINICAL MANAGEMENT ■

INADEQUATE ANALGESIA

The most difficult aspect of assessing patient requirements for analgesia is attempting to predict the variation in requirements between patients for what is estimated to be an equivalent pain-producing event. A fourfold to sixfold variation in acute postoperative narcotic requirements has been demonstrated between patients.[24] This difference seems to extend to most forms of analgesia care. Additionally, postoperative analgesia requirements are influenced by other patient variables. For example, Melzack and coworkers[25] outlined a subgroup of older, medically compromised patients who exhibited persistent postoperative pain (i.e., significant pain lasting more than 4 days) in contrast with younger and healthier patients who responded in a more traditional manner.

When focusing on patients as individuals, an area of analgesia research that needs further definition is the patient's preference for analgesia techniques. A report by Eisenach and associates[26] emphasizes this point. These investigators compared intramuscular, epidural, and narcotic PCA in patients recovering from cesarean section. Analgesia was most complete with epidural opioid analgesia; however, this group had more pruritus, whereas the PCA group was more sedated. Despite the sedation, the patients seemed to prefer the PCA technique. Postoperative analgesia prescription thus is more complicated than simply providing the technique with the lowest postoperative pain scores.

NEURAXIAL TECHNIQUES

One of the keys to using neuraxial narcotics (with or without added local anesthetic) is to have the block in place at the completion of operation. Additionally, it seems most effective clinically if a significant local anesthetic–induced epidural block is not present at the conclusion of operation in patients scheduled for neuraxial postoperative analgesia. This observation is important, because an early assessment of analgesia related to the neuraxial opioid or dilute local anesthetic is not possible if a local anesthetic block is well established and providing analgesia. We recommend establishing the neuraxial regimen before operation and then planning the anesthetic and analgesic regimen to minimize intense local anesthetic block at the time of emergence. This concept allows an earlier assessment of the adequacy of pain relief and minimizes pain control problems in the early evening hours, when pain service personnel are least likely to be available.

Neuraxial Side Effects

The incidence of nausea and vomiting after neuraxial narcotic analgesia is reported in as many as 50% of patients. This incidence rate, however, is comparable with that reported with parenteral opioid analgesia. With repeat dosing, the incidence rate decreases (and is extremely low in cancer patients). Nausea is usually treatable with naloxone. Urinary retention, similar to respiratory depression, is more common in the postoperative period or acute care setting, as compared with neuraxial narcotic analgesia in patients with chronic pain. The reported incidence rate ranges from 25% to 50% and also is reversible with naloxone. Pruritus is one of the most bothersome neuraxial narcotic side effects, with as many as 50% of patients admitting to it on direct ques-

TABLE 54-6. Factors Conferring an Increased Risk of Respiratory Depression With Peridural Narcotics

---

Intrathecal administration
Advanced age (>70 y)
High doses (>10 mg morphine)
Residual effects of parenteral narcotics
Residual effects of central nervous system depressant drugs
Lack of tolerance to opioids
Preexisting respiratory disease

(From Cousins MJ, Mather LE: Intrathecal and epidural administration of opioids. *Anesthesiology* 1984;61:276).

tioning. Again, it is less of a problem in chronic pain patients. The itching responds poorly to antihistamine therapy, although somewhat better to naloxone. Reversal of side effects can be obtained by titrating naloxone to effect and then beginning an infusion of from 5 to 10 µg/kg/hour.[27]

PROBLEMS AND RELATED COMPLICATIONS ■

RESPIRATORY DEPRESSION

Although respiratory depression was reported shortly after the clinical introduction of neuraxial narcotic analgesia and remains the most feared complication, its incidence may be no different than when compared with intramuscular or intravenous narcotic therapy.[28] Conversely, evidence suggests that regional block with local anesthetic is associated with less of a decrease in oxygen saturation during the first postoperative day than when intravenous narcotic analgesia was used in patients undergoing upper abdominal and hip surgery.[29] Because these patients did not receive supplemental oxygen during the intervals that oxygen saturation was measured, perhaps the correct interpretation of this work is that patients receiving postoperative narcotic analgesia should receive supplemental oxygen.

Respiratory depression with neuraxial morphine is a biphasic phenomenon. The initial phase is caused by systemic absorption from the epidural space during the first hour, whereas the later event occurs more frequently 6 to 10 hours after administration. Migration of the narcotic from the epidural space rostrally through the cerebrospinal fluid produces direct depression of the respiratory centers. This respiratory depression can be reversed with naloxone. A 5 µg/kg/hour intravenous infusion of naloxone prevents neuraxial narcotic respiratory depression and does not interfere with neuraxial narcotic analgesia in patients undergoing cholecystectomy.[27] Factors associated with an increased likelihood of respiratory depression are listed in Table 54-6.[30] The overall incidence of respiratory depression was less than 0.5% in one series of more than 6000 patients.

HEADACHE

Unintentional dural puncture may occur in 1% to 2% of epidural attempts and often results in a postdural puncture headache. The headache is believed to be the result of a persistent cerebrospinal fluid leak through the dural hole and is characteristically occipital or circumferential, may have a delayed onset, and worsens when the patient rises from the supine position. It usually resolves with conservative therapy, bedrest, fluids, and analgesics, but in selected cases an epidural blood patch should be performed. Using strict aseptic technique, 5 to 15 mL of autologous blood, drawn aseptically from the patient's arm, should be injected into the epidural space at the site of prior dural puncture. This treatment is effective in 90% of patients after one injection. Repeat injection brings the success rate to over 95%.

NEUROLOGIC DEFECTS

Epidural block or lumbar puncture is rarely followed by neurologic deficit. The most common cause of postoperative neurologic damage is neuropathy unrelated to the epidural block. Nevertheless, needle trauma can occur and usually involves a single spinal nerve. Danger of direct trauma to the cord is remote if the puncture is performed below the level of the conus medullaris (L1-2). Any patient complaint of pain during needle insertion or with injection of any solution must be taken as an urgent signal to stop and to evaluate the nature of the pain. This warning may be obscured in patients who are obtunded or sedated.

EPIDURAL HEMATOMA

Epidural hematomas occur spontaneously in apparently normal patients but are more likely to occur during anticoagulant therapy. The principal clinical features are severe backache associated with progressive paraplegia. This problem constitutes a surgical emergency, and diagnosis followed by surgical decompression is urgent. Total systemic anticoagulation or a coagulopathy is a contraindication to neuraxial techniques. The frequent use of *minidose* heparin raises frequent concern about the safety of combining neuraxial techniques.

Some authorities consider any form of systemic heparin therapy a contraindication to neuraxial techniques. Conversely, nearly 6000 vascular surgery patients received intravenous heparin and perioperative centroneuraxis catheters without development of an epidural hematoma.[31–33] Avoiding epidural catheterization for fear of causing an epidural hematoma in patients receiving minidose heparin therapy does not seem justified to us. Continued communication with surgical and anesthesiology colleagues is important, because not all share this view of the data.[34,35]

EPIDURAL ABSCESS

Epidural abscess has been reported after uneventful lumbar puncture and epidural block but more frequently results from hematogenous spread from distant infectious foci.[36] The usual presentation is a patient with fever, leukocytosis, and a progressive backache resulting in paraplegia. This complication also constitutes a surgical emergency. One unanswered question involves the role of epidural catheterization in the face of systemic infection and whether the catheter can be a focus for epidural infection. Most anesthesiologists believe systemic infection is a contraindication to epidural catheterization. Rarely, subarachnoid infection may occur after a lumbar puncture or epidural technique. It usually is caused by an unusual bacteria and requires meticulous evaluation.

INTERRUPTION OF BLOOD SUPPLY

The blood supply of the spinal cord is occasionally tenuous and easily compromised. The anterior spinal artery derives its main lumbar supply from the artery of Adamkiewicz, and interruption of this blood supply, although rare, can occur. The combination of arteriosclerosis and low blood flow states may cause disruption of this blood supply and an immediate painless paraplegia. In critically ill patients, interruption of spinal cord blood flow during an abdominal surgical procedure is more common than interruption from the use of a neuraxial technique.

ADHESIVE ARACHNOIDITIS

Adhesive arachnoiditis is a serious, albeit rare, condition that may progress to disability, with pain, paralysis, and impairment of bowel and bladder function. It usually follows injection of an irritant solution into the cerebrospinal fluid. Several compounds, including pyrogen-contaminated dextrose and detergents for cleaning needles, have been implicated. The disorder is a proliferative reaction of the arachnoid mater, followed by fibrosis and distortion of the arachnoid space. Clinical signs and symptoms may not become apparent for weeks after the precipitating event.

LOCAL ANESTHETIC—RELATED PROBLEMS

Toxicity

The epidural space is highly vascular, and the needle or catheter occasionally may be placed unknowingly within a vessel lumen. Intravascular injection of local anesthetic is the most common cause of serious toxicity. Central nervous system effects are the most commonly recognized manifestation of a toxic reaction, with a spectrum of symptoms ranging from lightheadedness and circumoral numbness to seizures and coma. The cardiovascular system may show direct myocardial depression and peripheral vasodilation. Rapid development of severe hypoxemia and acidosis is a result of seizure activity and has been shown to be a major factor in myocardial depression. Early and aggressive control of the airway with supplemental oxygen improves outcome.

As a precaution, every injection through a needle or catheter should include gentle aspiration and an appropriate test dose of 15 µg of epinephrine. A positive test dose result is defined as a heart rate increase of 30% within 30 seconds of injection or an increase in blood pressure in β-blocked patients. Incremental injection and constant verbal contact with the patient, in conjunction with a negative test dose, significantly reduces the risk of unrecognized intravascular injection.

Total Spinal Block

Total or high spinal block is most commonly caused by the unintentional subarachnoid injection of local anesthetic. Reports citing several uneventful injections through an epidural catheter, followed by a subsequent injection causing a total spinal, presumably reflect migration of the catheter through the dura. A negative aspiration, followed by a 3- to 5-mL injection of local anesthetic and a 5-minute period of observation, helps in avoiding subarachnoid injection. If an unintentional subarachnoid injection does occur, a profound degree of sensory and motor blockade develops within 5 minutes of injection of the local anesthetic. When the block reaches the upper cervical segments, diaphragmatic paralysis may be produced. Appropriate cardiopulmonary resuscitation, including positive-pressure ventilation, stabilizes the patient until the block recedes.

Hypotension

The most common side effect of epidural local anesthetic analgesia is a decrease in blood pressure. The decrease is attributed to dilation of both resistance and capacitance vessels from the sympathetic blockade. A block extending above the level of T-5 limits compensatory vasoconstriction and affects the cardiac accelerator fibers arising in the T-1 to T-5 segments. Judicious use of intravascular volume preload, limitation of the extent of the neural blockade, and estimation of preblock volume status should reduce such problems.

Pupillary Effects

Local anesthetics can sometimes produce effects that mimic neurologic events. In critically ill patients, unless the possibility of local anesthetic change is considered, a needless evaluation of unequal pupils may ensue. Pupillary changes may result from spread of local anesthetic to the sympathetic chain through thoracic epidural, some brachial, and, occasionally, intercostal blocks. Likewise, unintentional total spinal anesthesia often produce pupillary dilation, mimicking "fixed and dilated" pupils for hours after the event.

Subdural Catheter Placement

The subdural space is a potential space, because the arachnoid is in close contact with the dural sheath and is separated from it only by a thin film of serous fluid. Cases of massive epidural (total spinal) blocks have followed the injection of small volumes of epidural local anesthetics subdurally. A subdural injection differs from the rapid onset of high spinal block accompanying unintentional subarachnoid injection. With subdural injection, total block does not occur for 20 to 30 minutes after injection. Management should be the same as for high or total spinal block.

PNEUMOTHORAX

Pneumothorax after intercostal nerve block does occur, although it is rarely life threatening and most often can be managed by observation or, occasionally, small-catheter evacuation of the air. Chivers'[37] report suggests that the frequency of pneumothorax was almost 19%, which has done more to limit the block's appropriate use than any other data. Conversely, in a study of more than 4000 patients undergoing intercostal nerve block, the incidence of symptomatic pneumothorax was less than 1 in 1000 patients.[38] This incidence is approximately the same as that of severe respiratory depression from narcotic analgesia. Thus, using pneumothorax as a reason not to provide analgesia with intercostal nerve block seems inappropriate.

SPECIAL CONSIDERATIONS ■

ANALGESIA SERVICE FUNCTION

Providing analgesia care through a distinct postoperative pain management service has many similarities with provision of critical care in an ICU. Collaboration of nurses and physicians must be facilitated, and a *sharing of patients* is essential for effective analgesia and overall medical care. The people leading the acute pain service effort must anticipate spending considerable time during its inception, providing education to nurses and physicians, if it is to be effective.[39] Essential features of an acute pain service are 24-hour availability of personnel and standardization of analgesia care.

ADVANCES IN NEURAXIAL PHARMACOLOGY

Spinal cord pharmacology remains in a developmental stage, with our understanding growing yearly. Neuraxial analgesia is more complicated than matching a narcotic and epidural catheter to patient and procedure. The adrenergic nervous system, through its α-adrenergic component, is being studied as a possible means of augmenting or supplanting segmental neuraxial narcotic analgesia. α_2-Adrenergic agonists seem to produce nociception through a nonopiate action at the α_2-receptors in the dorsal horn of the spinal cord. These receptors may be synergistic with the opiate system.[40]

REFERENCES ■

1. Yeager MP, Glass DD, Neff RK, et al: Epidural anesthesia and analgesia in high risk surgical patients. *Anesthesiology* 1987;66:729
2. Christopherson R, Beattie C, Frank SM, et al: Perioperative morbidity in patients randomized to epidural or general anesthesia for lower extremity vascular surgery. *Anesthesiology* 1993;79:424
3. Tuman KJ, McCarthy RJ, March RJ, et al: Effects of epidural anesthesia and analgesia on coagulation and outcome after major vascular surgery. *Anesth Analg* 1991;73:696
4. Cohen FL: Postsurgical pain relief: patients' status and nurses' medication choices. *Pain* 1980;9:265
5. Marks RM, Sachar EJ: Undertreatment of medical inpatients with narcotic analgesics. *Ann Intern Med* 1973;78:173
6. Porter J, Jick H: Addiction rare in patients treated with narcotics. *N Engl J Med* 1980;302:123
7. Weis OF, Sriwatanakul K, Alloza JL, et al: Attitudes of patients, housestaff, and nurses toward postoperative analgesia care. *Anesth Analg* 1983;62:70
8. Rehder K, Sessler AD, Marsh HM: Lung disease. In: Muray JF (ed). *State of Art: General Anesthesia and the Lung.* New York, American Lung Association, 1975–1976
9. Ali J, Weisel RD, Layug AB, et al: Consequences of postoperative alterations in respiratory mechanics. *Am J Surg* 1974;128:376
10. Duggan J, Drummond GB: Activity of lower intercostal and abdominal muscles after upper abdominal surgery. *Anesth Analg* 1987;66:852

11. Dureuil B, Desmonts JM, Mankikian B, et al: Effects of aminophylline on diaphragmatic dysfunction after upper abdominal surgery. *Anesthesiology* 1985;62:242

12. Woloski BM, Smith EM, Meyer WJ, et al: Corticotropin-releasing activity of monokines. *Science* 1985;230:1035

13. Crile GW, Lower WE: *Anoci-Association.* Philadelphia, WB Saunders, 1914

14. Rosenfeld BA, Beattie C, Christopherson R, et al: The Perioperative Ischemia Randomized Anesthesia Trial Study Group: The effects of different anesthetic regimens on fibrinolysis and the development of postoperative arterial thrombosis. *Anesthesiology* 1993;79:435

15. Bush DJ: Pre-emptive analgesia: local anaesthesia given before general anaesthesia may reduce severity of postoperative pain. *Br Med J* 1993;306:285

16. Wall PD: The prevention of postoperative pain [editorial]. *Pain* 1988;33:289

17. McQuay HJ, Carroll D, Moore RA: Postoperative orthopaedic pain: the effect of opiate premedication and local anaesthetic blocks. *Pain* 1988;33:291

18. Anand KJS, Hickey PR: Halothane-morphine compared with high-dose sufentanil for anesthesia and postoperative analgesia in neonatal cardiac surgery. *N Engl J Med* 1992;326:1

19. Cockshott WP, Thompson GT, Howlett LJ, et al: Intramuscular or intralipomatous injections? *N Engl J Med* 1982;307:356

20. Austin KL, Stapelton JV, Mather LE: Relationship between blood meperidine concentrations and analgesic response: a preliminary report. *Anesthesiology* 1980;53:460

21. Austin KL, Stapleton JV, Mather LE: Multiple intramuscular injections: a major source of variability in analgesic response to meperidine. *Pain* 1980;8:47

22. Yaksh TL, Rudy TA: Analgesia mediated by a direct spinal action of narcotics. *Science* 1976;192:1357

23. Raj PP, Montgomery SJ, Nettles D, et al: Infraclavicular brachial plexus block: a new approach. *Anesth Analg* 1973;52:897

24. White PF: Patient-controlled analgesia: a new approach to the management of postoperative pain. *Semin Anesth* 1985;4:255

25. Melzack R, Abbott FV, Zackon W, et al: Pain on a surgical ward: a survey of the duration and intensity of pain and the effectiveness of medication. *Pain* 1987;29:67

26. Eisenach JC, Grice SC, Dewan DM: Patient-controlled analgesia following cesarean section: a comparison with epidural and intramuscular narcotics. *Anesthesiology* 1988;68:444

27. Rawal N, Schott U, Dahlstrom B, et al: Influence of naloxone infusion on analgesia and respiratory depression following epidural morphine. *Anesthesiology* 1986;64:194

28. Ready LB: Acute peridural narcotic therapy. *Probl Anesth* 1988;2:327

29. Catley DM, Thorton C, Jordan C, et al: Pronounced, episodic oxygen desaturation in the postoperative period: its association with ventilatory pattern and analgesic regimen. *Anesthesiology* 1985;63:20

30. Cousins MJ, Mather LE: Intrathecal and epidural administration of opioids. *Anesthesiology* 1984;61:276

31. Odoom JA, Sih IL: Epidural analgesia and anticoagulant therapy: experience with one thousand cases of continuous epidurals. *Anesthesia* 1983;38:254

32. Rao TLK, El-Etr AA: Anticoagulation following placement of epidural and subarachnoid catheters: an evaluation of neurologic sequela. *Anesthesiology* 1981;55:618

33. Baron HC, LaRaja RD, Rossi G, et al: Continuous epidural analgesia in the heparinized vascular surgery patient: a retrospective review of 912 patients. *J Vasc Surg* 1987;6:144

34. Bunt TJ, Manczuk M, Varley K: Continuous epidural anesthesia for aortic surgery: thoughts on peer review and safety. *Surgery* 1987;101:706

35. Owens EL, Kasten GW, Hessel EA: Spinal subarachnoid hematoma after lumbar puncture and heparinization: a case report, review of the literature, and discussion of anesthetic implications. *Anesth Analg* 1986;65:1201

36. Baker AS, Ojemann RG, Swartz MN, et al: Spinal epidural abscess. *N Engl J Med* 1975;293:463

37. Chivers EM: Pulmonary complications following regional anesthesia for abdominal operations. *Br J Anaesth* 1946;20:55

38. Moore DC, Bridenbaugh LD: Intercostal nerve block in 4,333 patients: Indications, technique, and complications. *Anesth Analg* 1962;41:1

39. Ready LB, Oden R, Chadwick HS, et al: Development of an anesthesiology-based postoperative pain management service. *Anesthesiology* 1988;68:100

40. Ossipov MH, Suarez LJ, Spaulding TC: Antinociceptive interactions between alpha-2-adrenergic and opiate agonists at the spinal level in rodents. *Anesth Analg* 1989;68:194

Critical Care, Third Edition, edited by Joseph M. Civetta,
Robert W. Taylor, and Robert R. Kirby.
Lippincott-Raven Publishers, Philadelphia, PA © 1997.

CHAPTER 55

Sedation and Paralysis

Antoni M. Nejman

IMMEDIATE CONCERNS

MAJOR PROBLEMS

Choices for ICU sedation require diagnosis of the underlying disorder. Life-threatening physiologic abnormalities must be eliminated before attempting pharmacologic intervention. Make sure the patient is adequately ventilated and oxygenated and that no other potentially correctable processes are ongoing. Most patients have pain, anxiety, or both; thus analgesia and anxiolysis must be addressed adequately. Assess the patient's mental status, then choose your sedation technique.

Paralytic drugs, when chosen, must be used in concert with sedation and analgesia, because alone they provide only neuromuscular blockade. Their use must be tailored carefully to the condition at hand, and the level of blockade must be monitored closely, especially in the patient with renal failure. Many other medications act to increase the effect of paralytics and should be taken into account when chemical immobilization is employed.

STRESS POINTS

1. Analgesics provide some sedation as a side effect, but if the patient is awake, addition of a benzodiazepine generally is indicated.
2. Intravenous diazepam works faster than midazolam, which works faster than lorazepam. However, the half-life ($T^1/2$) of the drugs is as follows: diazepam $>>$ lorazepam $>$ midazolam. Infusions of midazolam seem to last longer than lorazepam; diazepam is not recommended for infusion.
3. Haloperidol (Haldol) is a good choice for the frankly psychotic patient and can be administered intrave-

nously in bolus form, 5 to 10 mg every 30 minutes, or as an infusion. Advantages also may be seen during ventilator weaning when sedation without major depression of respiratory drive is important. Problems include some degree of vasodilation, extrapyramidal reactions (infrequently), neuroleptic malignant syndrome (seldom), and cardiac arrhythmias such as torsades de pointes (rarely).

4. Propofol is a useful drug in the ICU. Remember, however, once the dose is much greater than 50 μg/kg/minute, you are providing general anesthesia.
5. Paralytic drugs must be tailored to the indication at hand and, above all else, monitored from the inception of therapy to avoid the problem of long-term paralysis.
6. Choose these agents appropriately, and most complications can be avoided. Whereas atracurium is the only drug with little renal excretion, chances are that if drug administration is titrated to a one– or two–nerve stimulator twitch response, long-term problems will not develop with any agent.

ESSENTIAL DIAGNOSTIC TESTS, PROCEDURES, AND THERAPY

1. Presedation workup requires the analysis of the patient's baseline status, including reevaluation of medications that may exacerbate confusion or compound the sedative profile. Physical examination is needed to rule out any potential intracranial disease or obvious surgically correctable conditions. Electrolytes and blood gas partial pressures should be analyzed to eliminate obvious causes of confusion that may have more sinister overtones.
2. Neuromuscular blockade is optimal when a nerve stimulator is applied before and during drug adminis-

tration. Without analysis of baseline stimulator function, it is impossible to determine whether medication, stimulator malfunction, or the patient is the cause of decreased muscle twitching.

3. Aim for one to two nerve stimulator–induced twitches during infusion for adequate paralysis. Once all twitches are lost, the dose administered is 100% to 300% more than necessary for adequate relaxation.

4. Different muscle groups have different sensitivities to paralysis and stimulation, so total peripheral paralysis may not mean total diaphragmatic paralysis.

5. Treat any underlying derangements, orient your patient as best as is possible and then, if needed, choose your medications and deliver them with a specific target in mind (e.g., comfort, sedation, analgesia, amnesia, obtundation). Always keep the patient's airway patency and hemodynamic status as top-of-the-line priorities.

6. Never paralyze a patient without airway control, analgesia, and amnesia.

SEDATION ■

The ICU is an uncomfortable and frightening environment. Patients are confined to a bed, often for prolonged periods, commonly are intubated, usually are attached to a multitude of tubes and wires, and frequently are subjected to painful and unfamiliar invasive procedures. Added to this scenario are the constant auditory onslaught and fragmentation of sleep-wake cycles, which make the goal of patient tranquility unlikely at best.

THERAPEUTIC GOALS

The goals of sedation in this setting should be patient comfort from and amnesia of traumatic events. Adequate analgesia must be considered as a given before evaluating the patient for further sedation requirements. Narcotics are useful for analgesia and secondary sedative effects. Nociception is only a part of the stress that contributes to the release of catecholamines and stress hormones. Pain and anxiety affect the immune system and wound healing.[1,2] Analgesics and sedatives may decrease morbidity, and perhaps mortality, by decreasing endorphin release, which has been implicated in alteration of the immune response.[3] Anxiety, fear, distress, hallucinations, disorientation, confusion, agitation, and loss of personal control are deleterious parts of the critical care experience that should be eliminated.

Patients report distorted perceptions of time, surroundings, and procedures. One individual recounted to us his perceived experience of being on a barbecue spit, basted, and stabbed with sharp forks. Another tried to extubate himself because he thought that his endotracheal tube was connected to the patient in the bed next to him. Many instances of agitation and what physicians see as inappropriate behavior may be rational to patients who have lost their ability to think clearly.

INDICATIONS AND EVALUATION

Verbal reassurance and communication are important to keep the patient oriented and in touch with reality. Sedation in concert with this verbal reassurance often requires pharmacologic agents (Table 55-1). Common points of reference are useful in monitoring sedated patients. The most frequently used method is a graded assessment such as the Ramsay Scale[4]:

Level 1, Anxious and agitated
Level 2, Cooperative, oriented, tranquil
Level 3, Responds only to verbal commands
Level 4, Asleep with brisk response to light stimulation
Level 5, Asleep with sluggish response to stimulation
Level 6, Asleep with no response to stimulation.

Apparent calm and tranquility should not be construed as such; they may represent paralysis. In a study by Loper and coworkers,[5] 5% of the physician house staff and 10% of the ICU nurses believed that pancuronium relieved anxiety, leading to a relaxed and passive patient. We should strive to reduce anxiety and pain while rendering a patient calm but able to cooperate.

Behavioral Disturbances

Diagnosis of the behavioral disturbance makes the choice of pharmacologic agent somewhat easier[6] (Table 55-2).

ANXIETY.   Anxiety is apprehension, tension, or uneasiness from anticipation of danger, the source of which is largely unknown or unrecognized. Most patients in the critical care setting experience anxiety or agitation from a variety of conditions and drugs (Tables 55-3 and 55-4).

TABLE 55-1.   Indications for Sedation

Mechanical ventilation
    With modes that require paralysis
    With modes that control the patient's respiratory mechanics
Invasive procedures
    Wound debridement
    Dressing changes
    Tracheostomy
    Tube thoracostomy
    Diagnostic laparoscopy/endoscopy
Acute events
    Resuscitation
    Intubation
    Cardioversion
Decreasing O_2 requirements
Prevention of self-harm in the agitated, confused patient
During therapeutic paralysis
Supplementation of analgesia
Terminal care
Control of physiologic parameters

TABLE 55-2. Indications for Specific Drugs

BEHAVIORAL DISTURBANCE	MEDICATION
Pain	Analgesics
Anxiety	Benzodiazepines
Agitation	Sedative hypnotics
Delusions, hallucinations, delirium	Neuroleptics
Withdrawal	Benzodiazepines

DELIRIUM. The clouding of consciousness with reduced capacity to focus and sustain attention to environmental stimuli constitutes delirium. It tends to develop over a short period of time (hours to days) and to fluctuate over the course of the day. At least two of the following conditions must be present to make the diagnosis: perceptual disturbances, including misinterpretations, illusions or hallucinations; speech that is at times incoherent; disturbances of sleep-wakefulness cycles; and increased or decreased psychomotor activity. Disorientation and memory impairment also are included in the diagnostic criteria.

PSYCHOSIS. Multiple categories of neurobehavioral abnormalities are encompassed. They manifest with delusions, hallucinations, incoherence, marked loosening of associations, poverty of thought content, and bizarre behavior.

TABLE 55-3. Conditions That Induce or Mimic Anxiety

CARDIOVASCULAR	PULMONARY
Angina pectoris	Asthma
Hypertension	COLD
Mitral valve prolapse	Hyperventilation
Myocardial infarction	Hyperoxia
Supraventricular tachycardia	Pulmonary insufficiency
ENDOCRINE & METABOLIC	**OTHER ORGANIC DISORDERS**
Adrenal dysfunction	Anemia
Hyper/hypocalcemia	Carcinoid syndrome
Hyperkalemia	Chronic infection
Hyperthyroidism	Drug intoxication/withdrawal
Hypoglycemia	Fever
Hyponatremia	Fear
Parathyroid dysfunction	Pheochromocytoma
Pituitary dysfunction	Pain
Porphyria	Rheumatoid arthritis
	SLE
NEUROLOGIC	
Cerebral neoplasms & trauma	
Huntington's disease	
Multiple sclerosis	
Seizure disorder	
Vascular disorders	
Wilson's disease	

COLD, chronic obstructive lung disease; SLE, systemic lupus erythematosus.

AGITATION. Excessive motor activity, usually nonpurposeful and associated with internal tension, reflects agitation. The term *agitation* refers only to the motor manifestations and not the psychological state. The term is often used incorrectly in the ICU to categorize more serious disturbances such as delirium or psychosis.

BENZODIAZEPINES

General Considerations

Treatment of anxiety includes reassurance, elimination of compounding contributory factors, and, if needed, administration of an appropriate anxiolytic agent. Benzodiazepines are the agents of choice for anxiety, but they are also useful for insomnia, irritability, seizures, ethanol withdrawal, and adjustment disorders. They prevent memory consolidation, thus providing amnesia.

SITE OF ACTION. Benzodiazepines act in the cerebral cortex, substantia nigra, hippocampus, cerebellum, and the spinal cord. The benzodiazepine receptor is a complex described as a benzodiazepine–gamma aminobutyric acid (GABA)–chloride ionophore. When benzodiazepines are present, the receptor has an increased affinity for GABA, which increases the cellular inflow of chloride.[7] The resultant hyperpolarization decreases overall neuronal excitation in

TABLE 55-4. Drugs That May Induce Anxiety

ACE inhibitors	Ethanol (and withdrawal)
Amphetamines	GABA antagonists
Analgesics	H_2-receptor antagonists
Anorexants	Hallucinogens
Antibiotics (especially fluoroquinolones)	Heterocyclic antidepressants
Anticholinergics	Interferon-α
Anticonvulsants	Mefloquine
Anti-Parkinson agents (especially deprenyl/ selegiline)	Metrizamide
	MAOIs
	Neuroleptics
Baclofen	Opiate abstinence syndrome
Benzodiazepines (withdrawal)	Pergolide
β-Agonists	Procaine derivatives
Bromocriptine	Quinacrine
Caffeine (and caffeine withdrawal)	Sulfonamides
	Sympathomimetic amines
Chemotherapeutic agents	Theophylline/aminophylline
Cocaine	Thyroid supplements
Corticosteroids	Tobacco/nicotine (withdrawal)
Cycloserine	Vasopressors
Digitalis	
Dronabinol (and cannabis)	

ACE, angiotensin-converting enzyme; GABA, gamma aminobutyric acid; MAOIs, monoamine oxidate inhibitors.

the areas of the brain that modulate anxiety, arousal, and behavioral inhibitions.

SAFETY. Benzodiazepines are safe agents that can be titrated predictably for a range of effects from anxiolysis, amnesia, anticonvulsance, decreased reaction time, and controlled psychomotor activity. The major side effects of these drugs are cardiovascular and respiratory depression. When benzodiazepines are used with opioids, blood pressure decreases are greater than with benzodiazepines alone. Respiratory depressant effects are synergistic when opioids and benzodiazepines are used together.

EFFICACY. Approximately 30 benzodiazepines are available worldwide, but only three (diazepam, midazolam, and lorazepam) are available for parenteral use in the United States (Table 55-5). These three drugs are highly protein bound (96% to 98%) and have volumes of distribution from 0.8 to 1.5 L/kg. Alterations in protein binding during sepsis may change the apparent volume of distribution, require a different drug dose, and explain the variability of the drug response and efficacy in the critically ill patient. Many benzodiazepines are available for oral administration (Table 55-6).

Midazolam is better for short-term infusions, whereas lorazepam may be more appropriate for long-term administration. Patients in one study with infusions of 3 to 4.5 days returned to their baseline condition after discontinuation of lorazepam in 4.5 hours, whereas a midazolam comparison group took up to 30 hours,[8] probably because of midazolam's increased fat solubility. Remember that benzodiazepine requirements fluctuate through the course of the ICU stay; a standard infusion for all patients is inappropriate.

Onset of action after bolus injection of these drugs depends on the rate at which uptake occurs in the brain. Electroencephalographic analysis under identical clinical conditions suggests that maximal effects of diazepam occur by the time the injection is ending. Midazolam effect peaks about 5 minutes after the injection, whereas that of lorazepam requires 30 minutes.[9,10] This comparison is important to remember when the need arises for immediate effect from a benzodiazepine or when titrating the drug to effect (see Table 55-5).

Parenteral Agents

DIAZEPAM. This agent is insoluble in water but dissolves in propylene glycol, ethyl alcohol, benzyl alcohol, and sodium benzoate. In solution, it has a pH of 6.6 to 6.9. Injection may be painful, and intramuscular absorption is variable and unpredictable.

Diazepam is metabolized by hepatic microsomal enzymes by oxidative N-desmethylation to desmethyldiazepam and oxazepam. Desmethyldiazepam (with an elimination half-life of 48 to 96 hours), is only slightly less potent than diazepam and is probably responsible for the frequently observed secondary drowsiness. Oxazepam activity is significant only after repeat doses of diazepam. As a rough guide, the $T^{1/2}$ of diazepam in hours is equivalent to the patient's age in years; the physician should exercise prudence when administering this drug to older patients. The prolonged elimination $T^{1/2}$, in combination with an active metabolite, which also has a long $T^{1/2}$ (36 to 90 hours) may make diazepam an inappropriate choice for continuous infusions.

Respiratory depression with increases in the partial pressure of arterial carbon dioxide ($PaCO_2$) are seen with varying doses, depending on the patient's physiologic status. Intravenous doses of 0.5 to 1.0 mg/kg produce minimal reductions in blood pressure but may interfere with compensatory responses in hypovolemic patients. Administration of diazepam followed by intravenous opioid is associated with decreases in systemic vascular resistance and blood pressure greater than that seen with the opioid alone. Skeletal muscle relaxation occurs and is mediated by a diminution of the spinal gamma neuron output, thereby decreasing skeletal muscle tone. Finally, the anticonvulsant properties of diazepam may result from increased release of GABA, which acts as an inhibitory neurotransmitter.

MIDAZOLAM. Midazolam is a water-soluble benzodiazepine mixed in sodium chloride solution, disodium ethylene

TABLE 55-5. Characteristics of Benzodiazepines

AGENT	METABOLISM	HALF-LIFE ELIMINATION (h)	DOSING EQUIVALENT (mg/kg IV)	AVERAGE BOLUS DOSE IN ADULTS	INFUSION DOSE	COMMENTS
Diazepam	Hepatic oxidation	21–37	0.3–0.5	2–20 mg IV/IM; intramuscular absorption unreliable	1 mg/kg/24 h	Increased effect in elderly, delayed clearance with H_2 blockade
Midazolam	Hepatic oxidation	1–4	0.15—0.3	1–5 mg IV, 30% less with narcotics	0.05–0.15 mg/kg/h	H_2 receptor antagonists do not interfere with metabolism
Lorazepam	Conjugation	10–20	0.05	1–4 mg IV	0.01–0.1 mg/kg/hr	Less affected by hepatic function

IM, intramuscularly; IV, intravenously.

TABLE 55-6. Oral Benzodiazepines

DRUG	ROUTE	INITIAL DOSE (mg)	DOSING INTERVAL (hours)
Alprazolam	PO	0.25–0.5	8
Chlordiazepoxide	PO	5–25	6–8
Clonazepam	PO	0.5	8
Diazepam	PO	2–10	6–8
Flurazepam	PO	15–30	3–4
Lorazepam	PO	1–3	24
Oxazepam	PO	10–15	4–6
Prazepam	PO	10–15	6–8
Quazepam°	PO	7.5–15	24
Temazepam°	PO	15–30	24
Triazolam°	PO	0.125–0.25	24

PO, orally.
°Used primarily for insomnia.

diamine tetraacetic acid, and benzyl alcohol and adjusted to a pH of 3. Its effects are similar to diazepam with a slightly slower onset. It is two to four times as potent as diazepam but has an elimination half-life of 1 to 4 hours. Midazolam is metabolized by hepatic microsomal oxidation to 1-hydroxymidazolam and 4-hydroxymidazolam. Both metabolites are active, but their contribution to clinical effects is being evaluated.[11] Renal failure does not alter the clearance, elimination half-life, or volume of distribution.[12]

Ventilatory depression is similar to diazepam; apnea can result from rapid intravenous injection of approximately 0.15 mg/kg. Midazolam seems to produce greater decreases in blood pressure than does diazepam, especially when hypovolemia is present. It will not prevent the heart rate and blood pressure increases associated with tracheal intubation.

LORAZEPAM.   Lorazepam is a more potent amnestic than diazepam. Its elimination half-life is 10 to 12 hours. The effects on ventilation and cardiovascular function are similar. It is conjugated with glucuronic acid to form inactive metabolites. Metabolism is not entirely dependent on hepatic microsomal enzymes; thus, it is less likely to be affected by hepatic function, age, or interfering drugs such as cimetidine.

Reversal With Flumazenil

Flumazenil is a specific competitive antagonist of all benzodiazepine effects. When administered intravenously, the onset of reversal is usually evident within 1 to 2 minutes, whereas peak effects occur at 6 to 10 minutes. The duration of effect is related to the plasma level of flumazenil and the dose of benzodiazepine initially administered. Dosing should be started at 0.2 mg and titrated to a maximum total of 1 mg.

Keep in mind that flumazenil administration may expose benzodiazepine dependence and possibly result in seizure activity. The duration of antagonism is short, and resedation remains a concern, especially when a longer acting benzodiazepine has been given in a large, single dose or over a prolonged period. A second course of 1 mg in 0.2-mg increments is appropriate 30 minutes after the initial dosing.

Flumazenil is hepatically metabolized by glucuronide conjugation. Its activity is not significantly affected by gender, age, renal failure, or hemodialysis that has been started 1 hour after the drug is given.

SEDATIVES, HYPNOTICS, AND ANESTHETICS

Many of these drugs are used primarily in the operating room as general anesthetics but also have been used for specific tasks in the ICU (Table 55-7).

Barbiturates

Barbiturates are used to control intracranial hypertension and seizures. Hypotension in a hypovolemic patient results from direct myocardial depression. These drugs are potent hepatic enzyme inducers, produce tachyphylaxis, have poor amnestic effects, and are associated with frequent infectious complications. The ultra short-acting barbiturates, although useful for the rapid induction of unconsciousness and the termination of seizure, are redistributed to fat stores if continued for long periods. This property prolongs their effect and can result in coma that lasts for weeks after several days of thiopental infusion.

Etomidate

Etomidate is a nonbarbiturate, carboxylated, imidazole-containing compound. It is associated with relative cardiovascu-

TABLE 55-7. Intravenous Sedatives, Hypnotics, and Anesthetics

DRUG	GA INDUCTION DOSE (mg/kg)	BOLUS SEDATION DOSE (mg/kg)	INFUSION DOSE (mg/kg/min)
Thiopental	2–5	0.5–2	Not recommended
Methohexital	1–2	0.25–1	Not recommended
Etomidate	0.2–0.4	0.05–1	Not recommended
Ketamine	2–4	0.2–1	0.01–0.1°
Propofol	2–2.5	0.05–0.4	0.01–0.2

GA, general anesthesia.
°Infrequently used for prolonged infusion.

lar stability as an agent for the induction of unconsciousness but is inappropriate as an infusion sedative because of its suppression of adrenocortical function.[13,14]

Ketamine

Ketamine is a phenylcyclidine derivative used to create dissociation between the thalamocortical and limbic systems. Patients may appear awake but are noncommunicative and amnestic. Analgesia is intense. Administration of ketamine stimulates the hepatic enzymes responsible for the breakdown of the drug. This effect explains the development of tolerance to its analgesic effects. Its effects on the cardiovascular system resemble those of the sympathetic nervous system, with increases in systemic and pulmonary blood pressure, heart rate, and cardiac output. In the patient who is catecholamine-depleted, direct myocardial depressant effects may be unmasked with an unexpected drop in blood pressure and cardiac output.

Ketamine does not significantly depress respiration or upper airway skeletal muscle tone, but aspiration can occur. Salivary secretions and tracheobronchial mucus are increased. Thus, an antisialagogue may be needed when ketamine is used.

Emergence delirium is a common problem (5% to 30%)[15] for up to 24 hours after the administration of ketamine. Patients often complain of vivid, morbid hallucinations and dreams. Benzodiazepines given before ketamine seem to be the most effective drug for prevention of delirium. Ketamine doses of 0.5 mg/kg/hour or less are seldom associated with such problems.

Propofol

Propofol is a substituted isopropylphenol administered as a 1% solution in an aqueous solution of 10% soybean oil, 2.25% glycerol, and 1.2% purified egg phosphatide. It was initially introduced as an anesthetic induction agent. It produces unconsciousness in 30 seconds when administered in intravenous doses of 2 to 2.5 mg/kg. The elimination half-life is short at 0.5 to 1.5 hours and is not affected by cirrhosis, nor is its clearance influenced by renal failure. It has a modest cumulative effect, especially in the elderly. Propofol has become popular because of its rapid onset and prompt recovery.

Propofol sedation in the ICU is useful in patients who remain severely agitated despite no underlying or uncorrected cause (e.g., pain, hypoxia) and who are not responding to apparently adequate doses of other sedative or antipsychotic drugs. The patient's airway should be secured because propofol is a profound respiratory depressant, especially in concert with narcotics and other sedatives.

Administration should be started slowly to minimize hypotension and overdose. Whereas a range of 5 to 50 μg/kg/minute is usually adequate, higher doses may be required. Start at 5 μg/kg/minute and increase the infusion in increments of 5 to 10 μg/kg, waiting 5 to 10 minutes between increases to achieve peak drug effect. Several precautions should be observed and considerations followed when using propofol:

1. Airway control and monitoring are essential to detect and offset early cardiovascular depression.
2. Adequate narcotic supplementation is required because propofol is not an analgesic.
3. Elevation of serum triglycerides may occur with prolonged administration (1.0 mL of propofol emulsion contains 1.1 kcal as 0.1 g of fat).
4. Strict asepsis is required when handling the vials, syringes, and administration tubing because the emulsion is an ideal culture medium.
5. Avoid in patients with soybean or egg allergies.
6. Use central venous catheter access when possible to avoid the transient pain often associated with administration through a peripheral intravenous catheter.
7. Red-brown or green discoloration of the urine may result from the quinol metabolites.
8. Waking the patient and assessing central nervous system (CNS) function should be carried out daily to determine the minimum necessary dose for sedation.

Diphenhydramine

Diphenhydramine, a common ethanolamine antihistamine, is used for H_1-receptor blocking properties and for its sedative side effect. The intravenous or deep intramuscular dose is 10 to 50 mg with a daily maximum of 400 mg.

Haloperidol

Haloperidol is a butyrophenone neuroleptic antipsychotic that blocks dopaminergic transmission at postsynaptic CNS receptor sites. It may inhibit central catecholamine reuptake and has α-blocking properties that can produce hypotension. Its $T^{1/2}$ is 12 to 38 hours.

Apparent indifference or slowing of responses to external stimuli and diminution of initiative and anxiety without a change in the awake state, consciousness, or intellectual faculties constitute the psychological profile attributable to neuroleptic drugs. Patients generally appear more calm, are more capable of appropriate response, and are without major respiratory depression.

Haloperidol has been used intravenously for over 30 years to manage delirium.[16] Large doses have been administered to critically ill patients without harmful side effects.[17-19] Riker and others[20] have described its use in agitated patients to facilitate weaning from the ventilator. However, the United States Food and Drug Administration has not approved the drug for intravenous use.

DOSE.   An appropriate intravenous dosing regimen for haloperidol can be given according to the level of agitation: mild, starting dose of 0.5 to 2.0 mg IV; moderate, 2 to 5 mg IV; and severe, 5 to 10 mg IV. Guidelines for its administration are as follows:

1. Eliminate potential underlying causes of agitation.
2. Use lower starting doses in the elderly.
3. Allow 20 to 30 minutes between doses.
4. After three doses, add 0.5 to 1 mg of lorazepam intravenously concurrently or every other dose.

TABLE 55-8. Causes of Torsades de Pointes

MEDICATIONS	MEDICAL CONDITIONS
Quinidine	Hypokalemia
Procainamide	Hypomagnesemia
Disopyramide	Hypocalcemia
Phenothiazines	Hypokalemia
Tricyclic antidepressants	Ingestion of liquid protein
	Acute ischemia
	Bradycardia
	Amyloidosis
	Acute myocarditis
	Mitral valve prolapse
	CNS disease

CNS, central nervous system.

5. Once the patient is controlled, add the total dose of haloperidol and administer that amount over the next 24 hours.
6. If the patient remains calm, reduce the dose by 50% each 24 hours.
7. The oral dose is twice the intravenous dose.

If, after control is achieved, the patient cannot be maintained on a 4-hour dosing schedule, a continuous infusion should be considered. The infusion should be started at 10 mg/hour and increased by 1 mg/hour every 20 minutes to effect control. If agitation continues, repeat intravenous boluses of 5 to 10 mg are appropriate. Remember that weaning needs to be addressed early so that the patient's degree of agitation, delirium, and recovery can be ascertained. In difficult patients, a continuous infusion can decrease the dosing from 23 doses per 24 hours, using intermittent boluses, to 7 dosing adjustments per 24 hours.[20]

SIDE EFFECTS. Side effects of haloperidol include cardiac arrhythmias, hypotension as a result of its α-blocking properties, hypoglycemia, and extrapyramidal syndrome with in-

creased muscle tone in 16%,[21] (more frequently in cocaine abusers).[22] Side effects are decreased with intravenous administration.[23] Less common side effects include cholestatic jaundice, photosensitivity, rash, weight gain, convulsions, and neurotoxicity in hyperthyroid patients.

COMPLICATIONS
Torsades de Pointes. Of the cardiac arrhythmias, the most worrisome is torsades de pointes (polymorphic ventricular tachycardia). It is often self-terminating but may degenerate into ventricular fibrillation. The rhythm is frequently heralded by QT prolongation. Whereas the prolongation is usually congenital, several drugs and abnormalities also cause it (Table 55-8).

Treatment of the arrhythmia must be directed at the cause. Discontinue the drug, correct electrolyte abnormalities, and administer magnesium sulfate as a 2-g bolus.[24] Bretylium may be effective. Although cardioversion does not always prevent repeat bouts of the arrhythmia, definitive treatment is atrial overdrive pacing with initial rates of 110 to 150 beats per minute.[25]

Neuroleptic Malignant Syndrome. Neuroleptic malignant syndrome rarely develops over 24 to 72 hours after administration of haldoperidol or other potent neuroleptics. The syndrome is characterized by hyperthermia, generalized skeletal muscle hypertonicity, tachycardia and arrhythmias, fluctuating levels of consciousness, increased levels of creatine kinase and liver enzymes, autonomic dysfunction, tachycardia, labile blood pressure, profuse sweating, dyspnea, and incontinence. Mortality is 20% to 30%.

Treatment is symptomatic, including discontinuation of the drug, airway control, intravenous fluids for hypotension, cooling techniques, and intravenous sodium dantrolene, 2 mg/kg, repeated every 5 to 10 minutes to a maximum dose of 10 mg/kg. Acute dyskinesia and dystonia are treated with intravenous diphenhydramine, 25 to 50 mg every 6 hours. Chronic dysfunction may respond to anticholinergic drugs

TABLE 55-9. Cost Comparison of Common Sedative and Analgesic Agents

DRUG	$/BOTTLE	mg/BOTTLE	%/mg	AVG DOSE mg/h (70-kg MALE)	DAILY INFUSION COST ($)
Propofol	15.28	500	0.03056	420	308.04
Ketamine°	7.98	500	0.01596	—	—
Haloperidol	0.33	5	0.066	5	7.92
Meperidine°	0.549	100	0.00549	50	6.59
Morphine	12.5	500	0.025	10	6.00
Alfentanil°	5.79	1	5.79	1	138.96
Sufentanil°	21.66	0.25	86.64	0.015	31.19
Fentanyl	0.4	0.1	4	0.1	9.60
Midazolam	44.98	50	0.8996	2	43.18
Lorazepam	5.52	4	1.38	1	33.12
Diazepam°	1.57	10	0.157	2	7.54

These are wholesale costs for a large teaching institution.
° Not often used as infusions in ICU.

such as benztropine, 1 to 2 mg orally or intravenously, trihex-yphenidyl, 2 to 5 mg orally, or procyclidine, 2.5 mg orally three times a day. Akathisia (intense restlessness) is a common extrapyramidal effect that may respond to propranolol if the other anticholinergics are not effective.

Cost

In times of cost constraints, physicians should be aware of overall and individual item costs (Table 55-9). Expenses can mount quickly if costs are not monitored. Significant cost containment can result when these agents are used in combination, depending on the patient's underlying abnormalities. Narcotic analgesics, benzodiazepines, and other sedatives in appropriate doses usually result in a tranquil, pain-free patient.

PARALYSIS ■

GENERAL CONSIDERATIONS

Neuromuscular blockade interrupts the transmission of impulses from motor nerves to muscle, thus achieving a decrease or elimination of muscle activity. These agents have absolutely no analgesic, anxiolytic, amnestic, sedative, or analgesic properties.

A study of 265 facilities that had pulmonary medicine training programs[26] showed that neuromuscular blocking agents (NMBAs) were used frequently in approximately 30% of ICUs and at least occasionally in 70% of hospitals. Use has increased dramatically with the advent of newer, safer, shorter acting drugs that have an excellent track record in the operating room. In the critical care setting, if used properly, these drugs facilitate patient care and recovery.

Prolonged paralysis is avoidable with diligent monitoring and the tailoring of the agent to the patient. Yet only 34% of critical care–trained anesthesiologists used peripheral nerve stimulators to monitor their patient's degree of paralysis in a study published in 1992.[27] The overall rate of the peripheral nerve stimulator monitoring is lower in units without anesthesiologists. A 1991 study showed that in pulmonary care units, only 21% of the patients were monitored with peripheral nerve stimulators.[26]

The evolution of ventilatory management from controlled mechanical ventilation in the 1960s; intermittent mandatory ventilation and positive end-expiratory pressure in the 1970s; and computerized ventilators capable of administering pressure support, pressure control, and inverse-ratio ventilation in the 1980s and 1990s also heralded modifications in NMBA use. In an era of less ventilation and more patient-driven respiratory function, paralysis is not always appropriate. However, certain situations are improved by the appropriate administration of sedation, analgesia, and paralysis.

INDICATIONS

Indications for pharmacologically induced neuromuscular paralysis in the ICU follow:

Decrease oxygen consumption and metabolism
Improve chest compliance in adult respiratory distress syndrome
Control intracranial pressure
Supplement some forms of mechanical ventilation (pressure-controlled ventilation, pressure-controlled inverse-ratio ventilation, and high-frequency jet ventilation)
Control severe agitation not controlled by sedatives
Facilitate procedures
Maintain delicate surgical grafts until stable

No question about the patient's level of consciousness should exist when paralysis is instituted. As observed previously, one study showed that 5% of the physician house staff and 10% of ICU nurses believed that pancuronium relieved anxiety.[5] The patient must have pain relief and be sedated, preferably with anxiolytic or amnestic agents, before the induction of paralysis. Monitoring of blood pressure and heart rate may not be reliable as a means of determining the level of fear or anxiety in the paralyzed patient.[28] Auditory-evoked potentials[29] or an enhanced electroencephalogram may be better choices to delineate the level of consciousness. However, they are somewhat prohibitive in cost and ease of implementation.

PHYSIOLOGY AND PHARMACOLOGY OF NEUROMUSCULAR TRANSMISSION

Acetylcholine (Ach) is synthesized in nerve fibers and stored within nerve fiber endings. Baseline Ach release is increased by the arrival of a nerve impulse. Ach diffuses across the neuromuscular junctional cleft and binds to the nicotinic Ach receptors on the postsynaptic membrane (motor end plate). This receptor binding causes a change in the membrane receptor's ionic permeability, which, in turn, causes an increase in the resting membrane potential from -90 mV to -45 mV. Once this threshold potential is reached, the propagated action potential spreads over the surface of the muscle fiber causing contraction.

Two types of postjunctional nicotinic Ach receptors respond to NMBAs: (1) those found on the postjunctional membrane, and (2) those found extrajunctionally. The extrajunctional receptors appear throughout skeletal muscle after denervation. These receptors are responsible for many of the complications seen when succinylcholine is administered to such patients.

Prejunctional nicotinic receptors found on motor nerves influence the release of neurotransmitters and may facilitate mobilization of Ach from the site of synthesis to the site of release. NMBAs may interfere with Ach function presynaptically and postsynaptically.

Depolarizing Blockade

SUCCINYLCHOLINE. The primary depolarizing NMBA is succinylcholine. Succinylcholine attaches to the postjunctional nicotinic receptor and mimics the action of Ach, depolarizing the membrane, which then can no longer respond to endogenous Ach. Sustained configurational changes in the receptor allow the leakage of K^+ from the muscle cell, causing an increase in serum K^+ of approximately 0.5 mEq/L.

In the face of an increased number of extrajunctional receptors (after denervation, burns, and sepsis), this K^+ increase can be significant and may cause life-threatening cardiac arrhythmias. Second and third repeat doses of succinylcholine are sometimes associated with sinus bradycardia, junctional rhythms, and sinus arrest.

Succinylcholine is hydrolyzed by plasma cholinesterase (pseudocholinesterase), which is responsible for the drug's brief duration of action (3 to 5 minutes). Reductions in hepatic production of plasma cholinesterase or genetically programmed atypical plasma cholinesterase may result in slowed hydrolysis and prolonged succinylcholine effect. Treatment of the prolonged effect is intubation and ventilation until the paralysis resolves.

Nondepolarizing Blockade

Nondepolarizing reversible blockade is thought to occur when the NMBA binds reversibly to the postsynaptic nicotinic receptor without inducing agonist activity. These drugs compete for the binding sites with endogenous Ach. At high doses, the drug molecules may block the receptor channels as opposed to just binding to the receptor. Up to 70% of the receptors may be blocked without producing neuromuscular blockade, as evidenced by twitch monitoring.

Nondepolarizing NMBAs are subdivided into two main groups: (1) benzylisoquinolines (mivacurium, atracurium, D-tubocurarine, metocurine, and doxacurium); and (2) those with a steroid nucleus (rocuronium, vecuronium, pancuronium, and pipecuronium). These groups are then further subdivided into short, intermediate, and long-acting agents.

BENZYLISOQUINOLINES

Mivacurium. Mivacurium, a short- to intermediate-acting NMBA, has an effective dose in 95% of patients studied (ED_{95}) of 0.08 mg/kg. It is metabolized by plasma cholinesterase. Administration of three times the ED_{95} over 10 to 15 seconds causes enough histamine release to lower blood pressure transiently.

Atracurium. Atracurium is an intermediate-acting NMBA with an ED_{95} of 0.2 mg/kg. It undergoes ester hydrolysis and Hoffmann elimination (spontaneous degradation in vivo to laudanosine and electrophilic acrylates). This degradation is dependent on pH and temperature; it is slowed by acidosis and cold and is enhanced by alkalosis and increased temperature. Laudanosine also is a product of ester hydrolysis, but this hydrolysis probably plays only a minor role.

Atracurium also is a histamine releaser when given rapidly as a bolus injection. Lack of renal metabolism may make this the drug of choice in the face of renal failure. Laudanosine in high plasma concentrations may cause epileptic spike activity at 10 µg/kg and seizure activity at 17 µg/kg.[30] The laudanosine level seen with a paralyzing dose of atracurium is approximately 0.3 µg/kg, which is 30 times less than the plasma

concentration causing epileptiform activity. Thus laudanosine is unlikely to present a real problem.

D-Tubocurarine. D-Tubocurarine is the prototype nondepolarizing NMBA. It is seldom used in critical care. One of its major drawbacks is histamine release, which is significant when a drug bolus is administered.[31] It is predominantly excreted by the kidneys with a minor biliary component to elimination. The ED_{95} is 0.51 mg/kg.

Metocurine. Metocurine is a trimethylated derivative of D-tubocurarine. Although it is twice as potent as D-tubocurarine (the ED_{95} is 0.28 mg/kg), it releases far less histamine. It is excreted by the kidneys with no hepatic metabolism. Its use in the ICU has been limited.

Doxacurium. Doxacurium is a long-acting, extremely potent NMBA without histamine-releasing properties. It has an ED_{95} of 25 to 30 µg/kg and is dependent on renal clearance. It has a duration similar to pancuronium.

STEROID NUCLEUS

Rocuronium. Rocuronium is the most recent addition to this family of drugs and has an ED_{95} of 0.25 to 0.3 mg/kg. The onset of action almost rivals succinylcholine but is shorter than vecuronium. It is becoming popular for rapid-sequence intubations when succinylcholine is contraindicated. Duration of action is comparable with vecuronium. Because its metabolism is primarily hepatic, it is not affected by renal failure.

Vecuronium. An aminosteroid NMBA with very little cardiovascular effect, vecuronium has become popular in the ICU. It has an ED_{95} of 50 µg/kg and can be used intermittently or by infusion. It is metabolized by the liver to 3-desacetyl, 17-desacetyl, and 3,17-desacetyl vecuronium. The 3-desacetyl form is 50% as active as the parent compound. The metabolites are excreted renally. As such, they tend to accumulate in patients with renal failure.

Pancuronium. The oldest of the aminosteroid nucleus group, pancuronium is a long-acting NMBA. It is associated with tachycardia and increases in blood pressure. Pancuronium has a metabolite, 3-OH-pancuronium, which is 50% as active as the parent drug. Both the original and the metabolic by-product are primarily excreted by the kidney and also tend to accumulate when the kidneys fail.

Pipecuronium. Pipecuronium is an aminosteroid NMBA with a duration of action somewhat longer than pancuronium. ED_{95} is 50 µg/kg. It is not associated with cardiovascular side effects or histamine release. The drug and its metabolites are renally excreted. Few published reports describe its use in the ICU.

The NMBA properties are shown in Table 55-10. Table 55-11 lists their relative costs. Drugs and conditions affecting NMBA effects are shown in Table 55-12.[32–35]

TABLE 55-10. NMBA Properties

DRUG	DURATION OF ACTION	LOADING DOSE (mg/kg ED$_{95}$)	STARTING INFUSION (µg/kg/min)	METABOLISM	RENAL EXCRETION (% UNCHANGED)	SIDE EFFECTS
Succinylcholine	Ultrashort	0.6–1.5 mg/kg for intubation	0.5 mg/min, short times only	Plasma cholinesterase	10	Beware phase II blockade
BENZYLISOQUINOLINES (BF)						
Mivacurium	Short–Intermed	0.08	2	Plasma cholinesterase	Insignificant	Histamine release
Atracurium	Intermed	0.23	5	Hoffmann elimination & ester hydrolysis	Insignificant	Histamine release
D-Tubocurare	Intermed–long	0.51	2	Hepatic degradation	45	Histamine release
Metocurine	Intermed–long	0.28	Insuff data	Renal 80%–10%	43	Histamine release
Doxacurium	Long	0.025	Insuff data	Renal 60%–90%	70	Extremely potent, slower onset
STEROID NUCLEUS						
Rocuronium	Intermed	0.3	3	Primarily hepatic excretion		Rapid onset
Vecuronium	Intermed	0.05	1	Renal 10%–20% Hepatic 70% active metabolite	15–25	Minimal cardiovascular
Pancuronium	Long	0.07	0	60%–80% renal 15%–40% hepatic 50% active metabolite		Tachycardia, hypertension
Pipecuronium	Long	0.05	Insuff data	Renal 60%–90%	70	Potent

ED$_{95}$, effective dose in 95% of patients studied; Intermed, intermediate; Insuff, insufficient; NMBAs, neuromuscular blocking agents.

MONITORING

Monitoring of neuromuscular blockade is common in anesthesiology.[36] Quantifying the effects of NMBAs includes the following: determining grip strength,[37] assessing voluntary efforts of the rectus abdominis, use of spirometric study, fluorescent screen imaging of diaphragmatic movement, determining negative inspiratory force (peak negative pressure),[38] and assessing the patient's ability to maintain a sustained head lift.[39,40] These methods require cooperation and response, both of which are difficult to obtain in sedated, critically ill patients (Table 55-13).

The most useful and commonly practiced technique for monitoring the level of paralysis involves stimulation of a peripheral motor nerve and evaluation of the innervated muscle response. Connection of a force transducer to the

TABLE 55-11. Relative Costs of NMBAs

	VAH BOTTLE ($)	mg/BOTTLE	$/mg	AVG DOSE (mg/h) (70-kg MAN)	24-h COST ($)
Atracurium	28.12	100	0.2812	40	269.95
Doxacurium	14.8	5	2.96	1	71.04
Pancuronium	0.81	10	0.081	2	3.88
Pipecuronium	10.6	10	1.06	2	50.88
Rocuronium	11.19	50	0.2238	50	268.56
Succinylcholine	0.31	100	0.0031	—	—
Vecuronium	12.8	10	1.28	4	122.28

NMBAs, neuromuscular blocking agents; VAH, Veterans Affairs Hospital.

TABLE 55-12. Drugs Enhancing NMBA Effects

Antihypertensives
  Ganglionic blockers
  Calcium channel blockers
  β-blockers
  Furosemide[59]
Antiarrhythmics
  Quinidine[60]
  Bretylium
  Procainamide
  Local anesthetics in large doses
Antibiotics
  Aminoglycoside antibiotics[61]
  Polymyxin B
  Clindamycin
  Tetracycline
  Azathioprine
Miscellaneous drugs
  Cyclosporin[62]
  Steroids
  Volatile anesthetics
  Dantrolene
  Magnesium
  Lithium

PHYSIOLOGIC ALTERATIONS OR DISEASE PROCESSES

Enhancing NMBAs
  Hypokalemia[59]
  Hypocalcemia
  Hypothermia[63]
  Respiratory acidosis
  Myasthenia gravis
  Eaton Lambert syndrome
  Muscular dystrophy
  Myotonic syndromes
  Multiple sclerosis
  Neurofibromatosis
  Acute intermittent porphyria
  Amyotrophic lateral sclerosis
  Poliomyelitis
  Adrenocortical dysfunction
  Renal failure (variable prolongation)
  Hepatic failure
Drugs that antagonize NMBAs
  Phenytoin
  Carbamazepine
  Sympathomimetics
  Chronic exposure to NMBAs[64]

NMBA, neuromuscular blocking agent.

muscle allows the graphic representation and quantification of the response; this technique is used clinically and in research.

Electromyography (EMG) also can be used to evaluate the muscle response to stimulation. Advances in computer technology and miniaturization may prove this technique to be a practical method for evaluating the degree of neuromuscular blockade. It does not require a force transducer and tension device that are awkward in the ICU with the multiplicity of devices and lines. EMG also is useful for the monitoring of a dense blockade.

Understanding the Twitch Response

I have chosen a more practical approach for the evaluation of muscle response that is "low tech," easy to accomplish, and low in cost, but requires human intervention. The evaluation involves primarily visual and tactile sensing of muscle twitches elicited by a standard intraoperative nerve stimulator.

Stimulation of the motor nerve at the appropriate location causes release of Ach at the neuromuscular junction and contraction of innervated muscle. Multiple stimuli cause multiple contractions, and tetanic stimulation (50 to 100 Hz) produces sustained release of Ach and tetanic muscle contraction without fade. Five patterns of electrical stimulus—single twitch, tetany, train-of-four (TOF), posttetanic count (PTC), and double-burst stimulus (DBS)—are available. Only the last three are commonly used.

Train-of-Four

Train-of-four monitoring entails a supramaximal square wave stimulus (15 to 40 mA) of four twitches, 0.5 seconds apart, with a duration less than that of the neuromuscular junction refractory period. The stimuli provide a series of four muscular contractions, which can be seen or felt (Fig. 55-1).

When the patient has a partial depolarizing neuromuscular blockade, a fade in the second, third, and fourth twitch amplitudes occurs. The ratio of the fourth twitch height or strength to the first twitch defines the TOF ratio. A sustained response to tetanic stimulation is closely related to a TOF ratio of 0.7 and suggests normal neuromuscular function in most patients. Some patients are unable to sustain a 5-second head lift until a ratio of 0.8 is reached.

Double-Burst Suppression

Double-burst stimulation (DBS) allows easier tactile detection of minor degrees of paralysis. The fade is easier to feel with DBS. In the unparalyzed patient, two 50-Hz, 60-millisecond trains separated by 750 milliseconds cause two contractions of equal strength. Absence of tactile fade to DBS usually excludes clinically significant blockade.

Posttetanic Count

Intensive neuromuscular blockade without any twitch can sometimes be evaluated by amplification of the Ach at the neuromuscular junction using a tetanic stimulus of 50 Hz for 5 seconds. If the tetanic stimulus is followed by a single stimulus at 1 Hz, a twitch response may be seen. Counting the total number of twitches after tetany allows an estimate of the level of paralysis. Blockade intense enough to paralyze the diaphragm will have no posttetanic response. While the block recedes and before the return of the first TOF twitch, this amplified PTC will be palpable. A correlation exists between the number of posttetanic twitches and the degree of blockade. In general, the first TOF will reappear when the PTC is 8 to 12.

TABLE 55-13.   Methods to Assess Neuromuscular Blockade

TEST	ESTIMATED % RECEPTORS OCCUPIED BEFORE TEST IS ABNORMAL	DISADVANTAGES
V_T	75–80	Insensitive
Tetanic stimulation (50 Hz)	75	Painful
TOF	75–80	Moderate sensitivity; requires <50% T_u/T_1 for visibility
Peak negative pressure	50	Unreliable
Head lift–5 seconds	33	Needs cooperation
Vital capacity	75–80	Needs cooperation

TOF, train-of-four; V_T, tidal volume.

Electrode Placement

The electrode placed over the nerve is designated the *active electrode*. The other electrode is the *inactive electrode* and can be placed away from the nerve. If the active electrode is negative, for a given current the force of the muscle contraction will be greater than if the active electrode is positive.[41] If both the electrodes are placed close together over the nerve, there is no difference.

Clinical Applications

The most commonly used nerve muscle combinations for twitch monitoring are the *ulnar nerve–adductor pollicis* (Fig. 55-2) and the *facial nerve–orbicularis oculi* (Fig. 55-3). Muscle groups vary in their response to blockade so that NMBA dosing for complete blockade of one muscle group may not be adequate for all muscle groups. This difference may be related to the type of muscle fiber (fast twitch versus slow twitch), blood flow to the muscle, and the receptor–muscle fiber ratio. In a study by Donati and associates[42]

evaluating TOF reductions with two doses of vecuronium, differing muscle group sensitivities were demonstrated (Table 55-14). The time for recovery was similar between the diaphragm and the orbicularis oculi but prolonged at the adductor pollicis.

The differences in twitch responses becomes less significant while the dosing of NMBA increases, with all skeletal muscles becoming blocked at higher dosages. If the goal of paralysis is to completely suppress any diaphragmatic movement, the orbicularis oculi-facial nerve combination may be more appropriate to monitor. During paralysis, ulnar nerve stimulation often results in no twitch, whereas diaphragmatic movement is still detected by ventilatory monitors. The laryngeal musculature is similar to the orbicularis oculi, and facial nerve monitoring is optimal to determine the onset of laryngeal blockade when intubating.[43]

Application of adhesive stimulating electrode pads is effective in most patients as long as the pads are placed on clean, nonedematous areas over the nerve to be stimulated. Cleaning the skin before application facilitates the electrical contact. In the edematous patient, needle electrodes are

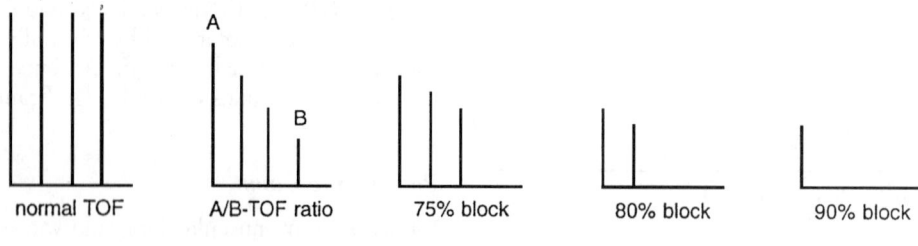

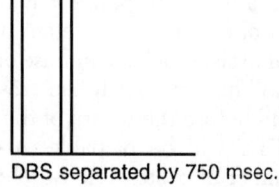

DBS separated by 750 msec.

FIGURE 55-1. Relative twitch heights seen with nondepolarizing neuromuscular blocking agents. DBS, double-burst stimulus; TOF, train-of-four.

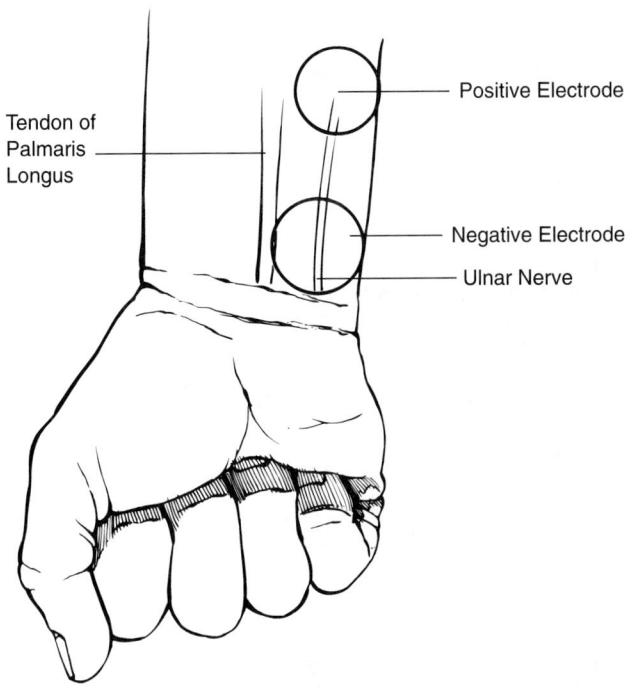

FIGURE 55-2. Electrode placement for the ulnar nerve–adductor pollicis muscle.

sometimes necessary, but these should be placed subcutaneously and not in the nerve itself. Infection is a potential problem, but more importantly, direct damage to the nerve can occur if the needle punctures it.

Titration of Paralysis

The degree of paralysis should be tailored to the indication. Titration to obliteration of ventilatory response is often more than is necessary. By contrast, minimizing oxygen consumption may necessitate a much greater depth of paralysis than control of a patient's dangerous thrashings. A one-to-two twitch response at the ulnar nerve adductor pollicis is usually adequate for all but the most complex problems. If a greater degree of neuromuscular blockade is needed, the PTC should be used, and at least twice a day the patient should recover one to two twitches without tetanic potentiation to assure the maintenance of normal neuromuscular function.

CAUSES OF PROLONGED PARALYSIS

Reports of prolonged paralysis in critical care have become more frequent.[32,33,35,44–49] Causes include critical illness polyneuropathy, generalized myopathy associated with the use of steroids or steroid nucleus NMBAs, and many other medical conditions (Table 55-15).

Overdose

Avoidance of excessive administration and accumulation of active metabolites is best accomplished with the continuous infusion of the chosen agent in concert with neuromuscular

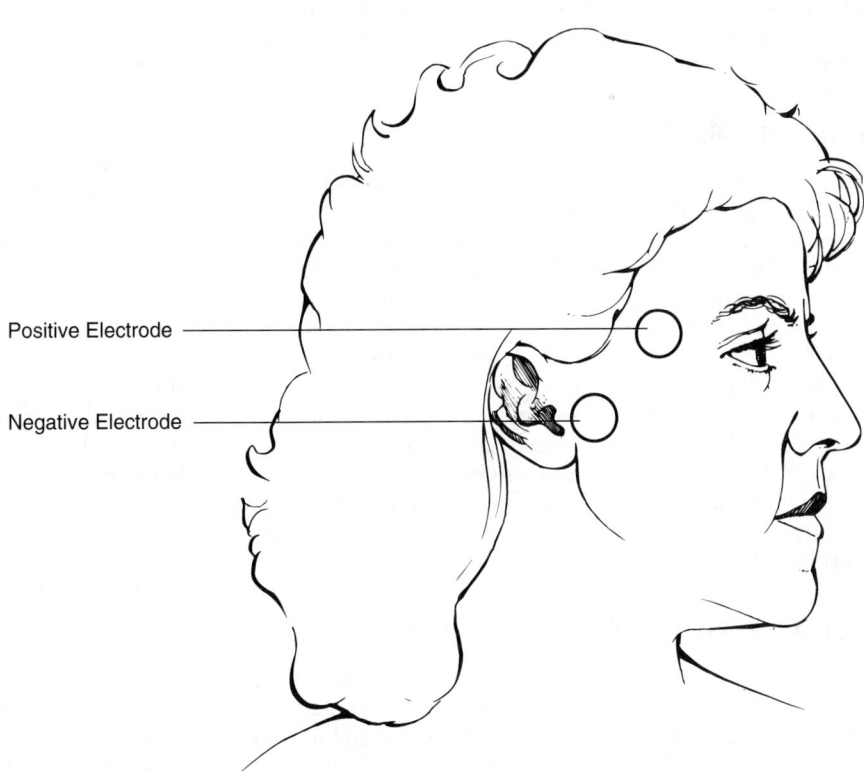

FIGURE 55-3. Electrode placement for facial nerve–orbicularis oculi muscle.

TABLE 55-14. Percent Reduction in TOF Response With Two Different Doses of Vecuronium

MUSCLE	0.04 mg/kg	0.07 mg/kg
Adductor pollicis	84%	95%
Diaphragm	78%	95%
Orbicularis oculi	62%	82%

TOF, train-of-four.

blockade monitoring. Segredo and coworkers[33] describe 7 of 16 ICU patients with prolonged paralysis after the discontinuation of vecuronium infusions. These patients all had significant renal failure and metabolic acidosis with the probable accumulation of the active metabolite of vecuronium (3-desacetylvecuronium).

Myopathy

Prolonged paralysis in asthmatics treated with steroids and muscle relaxants, along with other descriptions of acute myopathy after high doses of corticosteroids alone,[48-52] may support the theory of an adverse interaction between muscle relaxants and corticosteroids. As stated by Hansen-Flaschen and others,[45] corticosteroids may cause a myopathy in critically ill patients that is amplified by NMBAs. Yet no reports describe prolonged paralysis with ICU use of atracurium in concert with steroids. The structural differences between atracurium quaternary ammonium molecule and the vecuronium–pancuronium aminosteroid nucleus are well known. The structural similarity of vecuronium to the steroids may play a role in the myopathy seen with vecuronium and pancuronium.

Critical Illness

Suffice it to say that critically ill, paralyzed patients are at risk for prolonged neuromuscular malfunction. At particularly high risk are those with sepsis and multiorgan system dysfunction (critical illness polyneuropathy), those with renal failure (accumulation of renally excreted active metabolites), those with hepatic failure (hepatically metabolized agents), and those concomitantly receiving corticosteroids.

Evaluation of patients with prolonged blockade should include a review of their history, an assessment of their neuromuscular function (physical examination, nerve stimulation, EMG), and, on occasion, muscle and nerve biopsy. Although no specific treatment for the condition exists, it usually clears in a matter of weeks to months. In some cases, permanent disability results.

ANTAGONISM OF RESIDUAL BLOCKADE

Based on studies in the 1970s, a TOF ratio of 0.7 has become accepted as a useful measure of muscle strength and adequate mechanical respiratory reserve.[53,54] Although this value may represent a starting point, safety dictates that a TOF

TABLE 55-15. Causes of Prolonged Paralysis

Encephalopathy
  Septic
  Anoxic-ischemic, etc.
Myelopathy
  Anoxic-ischemic
  Trauma
  Sepsis
Neuropathy
  Critical illness polyneuropathy
  Thiamine deficiency
  Vitamin E deficiency
  Nonspecific nutritional deficiency
  Pyridoxine abuse
  Hypophosphatemia
  Aminoglycoside toxicity
  Penicillin toxicity
  Guillain-Barré syndrome
  Motor neuron disease
  Porphyria
  Carcinomatous polyneuropathy
  Compressive neuropathy
  Diphtheria
Neuromuscular Transmission Defects
  Neuromuscular blocking agent
  Anesthetic drugs
  Aminoglycoside toxicity
  Myasthenia gravis
  Eaton-Lambert syndrome
  Hypocalcemia
  Hypomagnesemia
  Organophosphate poisoning
  Wound botulism
  Tick bite paralysis
Water and Electrolyte Disturbances
  Potassium
  Phosphate, calcium
  Magnesium
Other
  Steroid myopathy
  Muscular dystrophy
  Polymyositis
  Acid maltase deficiency

ratio not less than 0.8 to 0.9 should be used to indicate return to more normal function.

Pharmacologic antagonism of neuromuscular blockade can be effective as long as the physician takes into account the duration of action of the NMBA and interindividual variation. Long-acting drugs are less completely antagonized than intermediate ones given the same starting level of blockade (i.e., TOF ratio) and equivalent doses of neostigmine. Bartkowski[55] showed that anticholinesterases do not have an unlimited capacity to antagonize curare-like drugs. Some NMBAs are better antagonized by specific anticholinesterases; atracurium and mivacurium are well antagonized by edrophonium.[56,57]

These agents act by decreasing acetylcholinesterase activity, thereby allowing an increase in the available Ach for the postjunctional receptor stimulation. When a nondepolarizing NMBA is administered, increased Ach availability allows

TABLE 55-16. Dosing of NMBA Reversing Drugs

DRUGS	IV DOSE	TIME TO PEAK	DURATION
Edrophonium	0.5–1 mg/kg	1 min	45 min
Neostigmine	0.05 mg/kg to max of 5 mg	7 min	60 min
Pyridostigmine	0.25 mg/kg	12 min	100 min
Atropine	15 µg/kg	70 s	1–2 h
Glycopyrrolate	10–20 µg/kg	4 min	2–4 h

IV, intravenous; max, maximum; NMBA, neuromuscular blocking agent.

competition with the NMBA, therefore providing an increase in the level of muscular activity and return of more normal function. The anticholinesterase should have a longer duration of action than the NMBA that is being reversed or reparalysis will occur.

Anticholinesterases also create Ach responses at the muscarinic receptors that may present unwanted side effects (i.e., increased secretions, bronchoconstriction, miosis, increased gastrointestinal and genitourinary tone, and bradycardia). These problems are avoided by administering a muscarinic blocking agent with the reversal agent. The two most commonly used are atropine and glycopyrrolate. Atropine onset is much faster than glycopyrrolate. If the physician chooses to use glycopyrrolate with edrophonium, the glycopyrrolate must be given three or four minutes before the edrophonium.

Atropine and edrophonium go well together, whereas glycopyrrolate and neostigmine or pyridostigmine seem well suited with respect to onset profiles. Dosing regimens for reversal agents are summarized in Table 55-16. Several physiologic abnormalities common to ICU patients also may antagonize NMBA activity: alkalosis, extensive burns, diabetes, hepatic failure with ascites, hemiplegia, denervation syndromes, hyperkalemia, and hypercalcemia.[58-61]

REFERENCES

1. Riley V: Psychoneuroendocrine influences on immunocompetence and neoplasia. *Science* 1981;212:1100
2. Watkins J, Glynn LE: Symposium on trauma, stress, and immunity at Bath. *Anesthesiology* 1981;36:647
3. Demling RH: What are the functions of endorphins following thermal injury (discussion). *J Trauma* 1984;24S:172
4. Ramsay MA, Savege TM, Simpson BR, et al: Controlled sedation with alphaxalone/alphadolone. *Br Med J* 1974;2:256
5. Loper KA, Butler S, Nessly M: Paralyzed with pain: the need for education. *Pain* 1989;37:315
6. Barkin RL: Pharmacologic management considerations for the critical care patient with symptoms of anxiety. In: Yardley PA. *Recognition, Assessment, and Treatment of Anxiety in the Critical Care Patient.* New York, The Medicine Group USA, 1993
7. Mohler H, Richards JG: The benzodiazepine receptor: a pharmacological control element of brain function. *Eur J Anaesthesiol* 1988;15:356
8. Pohlman AS, Simpson KP, Hall JB: Continuous intravenous infusion of lorazepam versus midazolam for sedation during mechanical ventilatory support: a prospective randomized study. *Crit Care Med* 1994;22:1241
9. Greenblatt DJ, Ehrenberg BL, Gunderman J, et al: Kinetic and dynamic study of intravenous lorazepam: Comparison with intravenous diazepam. *J Pharmacol Exp Ther* 1989;250:134
10. Greenblatt DJ, Ehrenberg BL, Gunderman J, et al: Pharmacokinetic and electroencephalographic study of intravenous diazepam, midazolam, and placebo. *Clin Pharmacol Ther* 1989;45:356
11. Reves JG, Fragen RJ, Vinik HR, et al: Midazolam: pharmacology and uses. *Anesthesiology* 1985;62:310
12. Vinik HR, Reves JG, Greenblatt DJ, et al: The pharmacokinetics of midazolam in chronic renal failure patients. *Anesthesiology* 1983;59:390
13. Wagner RL, White PF, Kan PB, et al: Inhibition of adrenal steroidogenesis by the anesthetic etomidate. *N Engl J Med* 1984;310:1415
14. Fragen RJ, Shanks CA, Molteni AMJA: Effects of etomidate on hormonal responses to surgical stress. *Anesthesiology* 1984;61:652
15. White PF, Way WL, Trevor AJ: Ketamine: its pharmacology and therapeutic uses. *Anesthesiology* 1982;56:119
16. Settle EC, Ayd FJ: Haloperidol: a quarter century of experience. *J Clin Psychiatry* 1983;44:440
17. Tesar GE, Murray GB, Cassem NH: Use of high dose Haldol in the treatment of agitated cardiac patients. *J Clin Psychopharmacol* 1985;5:344
18. Sos J, Cassem NH: Managing postoperative agitation. *Drug Therapy* 1980;10:103
19. Menza MA, Murray GB, Holmes VF: Decreased extrapyramidal symptoms with intravenous haloperidol. *J Clin Psychiatry* 1987;48:278
20. Riker RR, Fraser GL, Cox PM: Continuous infusion of haloperidol controls agitation in critically ill patients. *Crit Care Med* 1994;22:433
21. Swett MP: Drug induced dystonia. *Am J Psychiatry* 1975;132:532
22. Kumor K, Sherer M, Jaffe J: Haloperidol-induced dystonia in cocaine addicts. *Lancet* 1986;2:1;341
23. Dubin WR, Feld JA: Rapid tranquilization of the violent patient. *Am J Emerg Med* 1989;7:313
24. Tzivoni D, Keren A: Suppression of ventricular arrhythmias by magnesium. *Am J Cardiol* 1990;65:1397
25. Smith WM, Gallagher JJ: "Les Torsades de Pointes": an unusual ventricular arrhythmia. *Ann Intern Med* 1980;93:578
26. Hansen-Flaschen JH, Brazinsky S, Lanken PN: Use of sedating drugs and neuromuscular blocking agents in patients requiring mechanical ventilation for respiratory failure: a national survey. *JAMA* 1991;266:2868
27. Klessig HT, Geiger HJ, Murray MJ, et al: A national survey on the practice patterns of anesthesiologist intensivists in the use of muscle relaxants. *Crit Care Med* 1992;20:1341

28. Kulli J, Koch C: Does anesthesia cause loss of consciousness? *Trends Neurosci* 1991;14:6

29. Sneyd JR, Wang DY, Edward D: Effect of physiotherapy on auditory evoked response in the intensive care unit. *Br J Anaesth* 1992;68:349

30. Chapple DJ, Miller AA, Ward JB, et al: Cardiovascular and neurological effects of laudanosine: studies in mice and rats, and in conscious and anaesthetized dogs. *Br J Anaesth* 1987;59:218

31. Basta SJ, Savarese JJ, Ali HH: Histamine-releasing potencies of atracurium and dimethyl-tubocurarine. *Br J Anaesth* 1983;55:105

32. Kupfer Y, Namba T, Kaldawi E, et al: Prolonged paralysis after long term infusion of vecuronium. *Ann Intern Med* 1992;117:484

33. Segredo V, Caldwell JE, Miller R: Persistent paralysis in critically ill patients after long term administration of vecuronium. *N Engl J Med* 1992;327:524

34. Vandenbrom RHG, Wierda MKH: Pancuronium bromide in the intensive care unit: a case of overdose. *Anesthesiology* 1988;69:996

35. Watling SM, Dasta JF: Prolonged paralysis in intensive care unit patients after the use of neuromuscular blocking agents: a review of the literature. *Crit Care Med* 1994;22:884

36. Churchill-Davidson HC, Christie TH: The diagnosis of neuromuscular block in man. *Br J Anaesth* 1959;31:290

37. Mushin WW, Wein R: Curare-like actions of tri(diethylaminoethoxy)-benzene triethyliodide. *Lancet* 1949;1:726

38. Bendixen HH, Surtees AD, Oyama T, et al: Postoperative disturbances in ventilation following the use of muscle relaxants in anesthesia. *Anesthesiology* 1959;20:121

39. Dam WH, Guldman N: Inadequate post-anesthetic ventilation. *Anesthesiology* 1961;22:699

40. Johansen SH, Jorgensen M, Molbech S: Effect of tubocurarine on respiratory and nonrespiratory muscle power in man. *J Appl Physiol* 1964;19:990

41. Berger JJ, Gravenstein JS, Munson ES: Electrode polarity and peripheral nerve stimulation. *Anesthesiology* 1982;56:402

42. Donati F, Meistemiman C, Plaud B: Vecuronium neuromuscular blockade at the diaphragm, the orbicularis oculi, and adductor pollicis muscles. *Anesthesiology* 1990;73:870

43. Donati F, Meistemiman C, Plaud B: Vecuronium muscular blockade at the adductor muscles of the larynx and adductor pollicis. *Anesthesiology* 1991;74:833

44. Benzing G, Iannaccone ST, Bove KE, et al: Prolonged myasthenic syndrome after one week of muscle relaxants. *Pediatr Neurol* 1990;6:190

45. Hanson-Flaschen J, Cowen J, Raps EC: Neuromuscular blockade in the intensive care unit. *Am Rev Respir Dis* 1993;147:234

46. Partridge BL, Abrams JH, Bazemore C, et al: Prolonged neuromuscular blockade after long-term infusion of vecuronium bromide in the intensive care unit. *Crit Care Med* 1990;18:1177

47. Witt NJ, Zochodyne DW, Bolton CF, et al: Peripheral nerve function in sepsis and multiple organ failure. *Chest* 1991;99:176

48. Hirano M, Ott B, Raps E, et al: Acute quadriplegic myopathy: a complication of treatment with steroids, nondepolarizing blocking agents, or both. *Neurology* 1992;42:2082

49. Knox AJ, Mascie-Taylor BH, Muers MF: Acute hydrocortisone myopathy in acute severe asthma. *Thorax* 1986;41:411

50. MacFarlane IA, Rosenthal FD: Severe myopathy after status asthmaticus. *Lancet* 1977;2:615

51. Kupfer Y, Okren DG, Twersky RA, et al: Disuse atrophy in a ventilated patient with status asthmaticus receiving neuromuscular blockade. *Crit Care Med* 1987;15:795

52. Williams TJ, O'Hehir RE, Czarny D, et al: Acute myopathy in severe acute asthma treated with intravenously administered corticosteroids. *Am Rev Respir Dis* 1988;137:460

53. Brand JB, Cullen DJ, Wilson NE, et al: Spontaneous recovery from nondepolarizing neuromuscular blockade: correlation between clinical and evoked responses. *Anesth Analg* 1977;56:55

54. Ali HH, Wilson RS, Savarese JJ, et al: The effect of tubocurarine on indirectly elicited train-of-four muscle response and respiratory measurements in humans. *Br J Anaesth* 1975;56:570

55. Bartkowski RR: Incomplete reversal of pancuronium neuromuscular blockade by neostigmine, pyridostigmine, and edrophonium. *Anesth Analg* 1987;66:594

56. Kopman AF: Tactile evaluation of train-of-four count as an indicator of reliability of antagonism from vecuronium or atracurium-induced neuromuscular blockade. *Anesthesiology* 1991;75:588

57. Cook DR, Chakravorti A, Brandom BW, et al: Effects of neostigmine, edrophonium, and succinylcholine on the in vitro metabolism of mivacurium: clinical correlates. *Anesthesiology* 1992;77:A948

58. Miller RD, Roderick L: Diuretic-induced hypokalaemic pancuronium neuromuscular blockade and its antagonism by neostigmine. *Br J Anaesth* 1978;50:541

59. Berg DK, Hall ZW: Increased extrajunctional acetylcholine sensitivity produced by chronic post-synaptic neuromuscular blockade. *J Physiol (Lond)* 1975;244:659

60. Atallah MM, Daif AA, Saied MMA: Neuromuscular blocking activity of tubocurarine in patients with diabetes mellitus. *Br J Anaesth* 1992;68:567

61. Hogue CWJ, Itani MS, Martyn JA: Resistances to D-tubocurare in lower motor neuron injury is related to increased acetylcholine receptors at the neuromuscular junction. *Anesthesiology* 1990;73:703

Monitoring: Practical Applications

Critical Care, Third Edition, edited by Joseph M. Civetta,
Robert W. Taylor, and Robert R. Kirby.
Lippincott-Raven Publishers, Philadelphia, PA © 1997.

CHAPTER 56

∎

Invasive Pressure Monitoring

Reed M. Gardner

Invasive pressure monitoring, now routinely performed at the patient's bedside, incorporates more advanced technology than was formerly used in heart cardiac catheterization laboratories. The monitoring enables the clinician to have a better understanding of the relationship between the pressure and blood flow in the patient's cardiovascular system. However, every measuring system can produce false information. Constant vigilance and understanding of such systems is the best prescription for ensuring acquisition of high-quality pressure monitoring information.

Arterial blood pressure can be measured by both invasive and noninvasive means. However, central venous pressure, pulmonary artery (PA), and pulmonary artery occlusion pressure (PAOP) currently can be measured only by invasive means.

Continuous and accurate assessment of blood pressures can only be made invasively. Having continuous pressure data available permits timely detection of dangerous hemodynamic events and provides the information necessary to initiate and titrate patient therapy. Nevertheless, invasive pressure monitoring provides valuable information *only* when correct techniques are used to obtain accurate data.

This chapter covers the technical aspects of invasive monitoring. Details about catheter insertion techniques are presented in Chapter 57. Complications associated with pressure physiologic measurements, clinical understanding, and managing patient-related problems also are discussed in other chapters of this book.

EQUIPMENT ∎

The components used for invasive pressure monitoring are shown in Figure 56-1.[1,2] This diagram illustrates an arterial site, but a similar setup is appropriate for PA pressure measurement. The components known as the "plumbing system" (see Fig. 56-1, points 1 through 6) must be kept sterile because they come in direct contact with the patient's blood. Usually, these components are disposable. The other components (see Fig. 56-1, points 7 through 10) in the system are used for processing and displaying pressure waveforms and for obtaining derived hemodynamic parameters.

CATHETER

Arterial and PA catheters provide access to the patient's blood vessels for pressure monitoring and provide a site for withdrawing blood samples for blood gas analysis and other tests.

STOPCOCK NO. 1

Stopcock no. 1 is used as a site for withdrawing blood for analysis. When filling the plumbing system with fluid, precautions must be taken to be sure that all central switching cavities of the stopcock are fluid filled. All entrapped air bubbles must be removed. Stopcocks are particularly vulnerable sources of patient contamination. Therefore, stopcocks should be handled with extreme care; ports not in active use should be covered with sterile caps, and the open ports should never be touched.

PRESSURE TUBING

The catheter and stopcock are normally attached to the continuous flush device and pressure transducer by nonelastic pressure tubing. To optimize the dynamic response of the plumbing system, avoid long lengths of tubing.

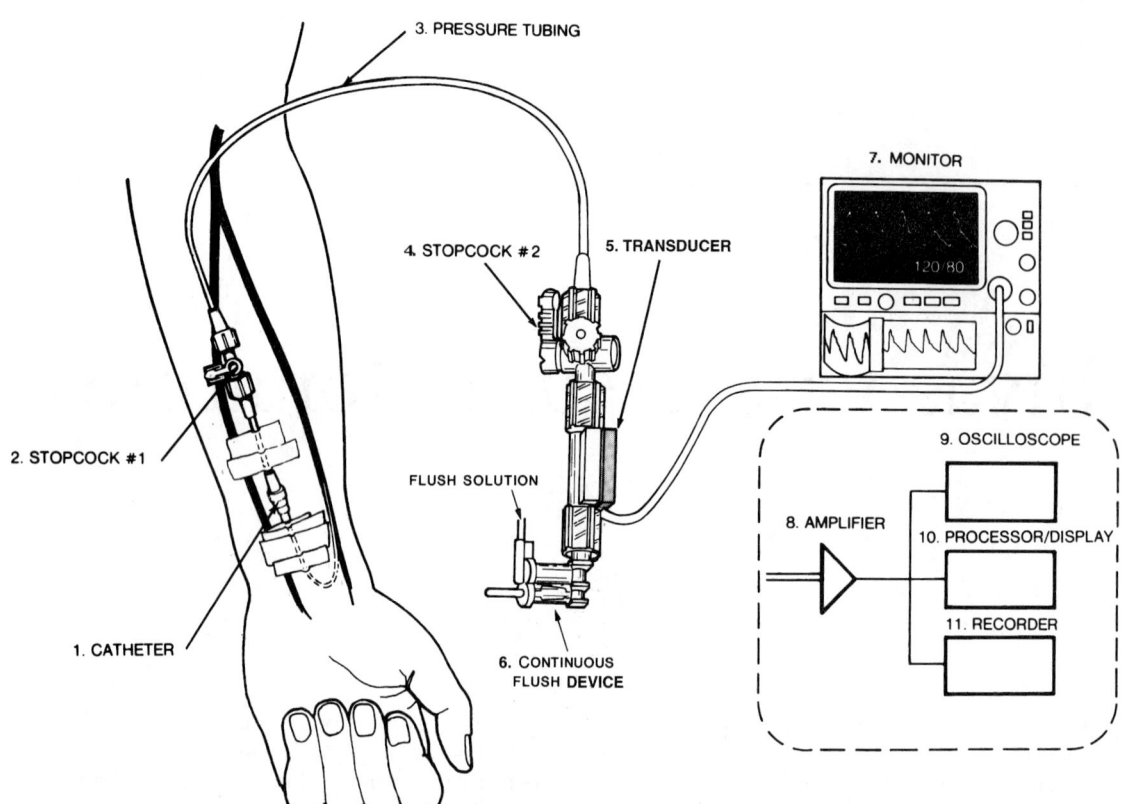

FIGURE 56-1. Components used to monitor blood pressure directly are nearly the same, independent of whether the catheter is in an artery (radial, brachial, or femoral) or in the pulmonary artery. The size of the transducer and plumbing components were enlarged for the illustration. (Adapted from Gardner RM, Hollingsworth KW: Optimizing ECG and pressure monitoring. *Crit Care Med* 1986;14:651.)

STOPCOCK NO. 2

If the transducer is patient mounted when measuring arterial pressures, stopcock no. 2 may not be necessary.

CONTINUOUS FLUSH DEVICE

The continuous flush device is used to fill the pressure monitoring system with fluid and helps prevent blood from clotting in the catheter by continuously flushing fluid through the system at a rate of from 1 to 3 mL/hour.

PRESSURE TRANSDUCER

Most pressure transducers currently used for monitoring are miniature, rugged, disposable devices.[3-7] Because of their miniature size, they can be patient mounted. All currently available disposable pressure transducers are resistive devices that convert the movement of their sensing diaphragm into an electrical signal.[8] Standards for blood pressure transducers have been developed by the Association for the Advancement of Medical Instrumentation (AAMI) and adopted by the American National Standards Institute (ANSI).[3-5] Because of such standardization, transducers from different vendors can be used interchangeably with any modern moni-

tor.[9] In fact, errors of less than ±3% typically result from the use of such transducers *without* calibration.[9,10]

AMPLIFIER SYSTEM

Output voltage from the transducer required to drive an oscilloscope or strip recorder is furnished by an amplifier system inserted between the transducer and display. Transducer excitation is provided either from a direct current or alternating current source, with voltages ranging from of from 4 to 8 V. Most amplifier systems include low-pass filters that filter out unwanted high-frequency signals. Pressure amplifier frequency response should be "flat"—from 0 to 50 Hz—to avoid pressure waveform distortion.[1,2]

OSCILLOSCOPE DISPLAY

Pressure waveforms are best visualized on a calibrated oscilloscope.

PROCESSOR/DIGITAL DISPLAY

Digital displays provide a simple method for presenting quantitative data from the pressure waveform. They are found on most modern pressure monitoring equipment. Systolic, diastolic, and mean pressure are derived from the pressure waveforms.

RECORDER

Strip chart recorders often are used to document dynamic response characteristics, respiratory variations in PA pressures, and aberrant rhythms and pressure waveforms.

EQUIPMENT SETUP ■

ZEROING THE TRANSDUCER

The accuracy of blood pressure requires the establishment of an accurate reference point from which all measurements are made. The patient's midaxillary line (right heart level) is the reference point most commonly used. The "zeroing" process is used to compensate for offset caused by hydrostatic pressure differences or offset in the pressure transducer, amplifier, oscilloscope, recorder, or digital displays. Zeroing is accomplished by opening an appropriate stopcock to atmosphere and aligning the resulting air–fluid interface with the midaxillary reference point.[1,2,11] Figure 56-2 shows two methods that can be used to zero the transducer.[1,2]

Once the system is zeroed, the appropriate stopcock can be switched to allow the patient's waveform to be displayed. Because PA and PAOP are especially susceptible to improper zeroing, the zero should be verified with each measurement. Although disposable transducers have stable zero characteristics,[7,12] it is wise to zero transducers before each right heart measurement and reestablish the zero at least once per day for arterial pressures.

CALIBRATION

The sensitivity of the AAMI/ANSI disposable blood pressure transducer is fixed at 5.0 μV/V/mm Hg and calibrated by the manufacturers to within ±3%.[5] When using transducers that meet the AAMI/ANSI standard and modern monitors

that interconnect with standardized transducers, there is no need to "calibrate" the transducer or monitoring system.[9] Based on current data, fixed calibration pressure monitoring systems should be purchased and maintained and fixed calibration disposable pressure transducers should be used.

If pressure transducer or monitor calibration errors are suspected in the clinical situation, the following steps are recommended: the pressure transducer should be replaced and "tested" in the laboratory situation; if the monitor module is suspect, it should be tested with a high-accuracy pressure transducer "simulator" and, if faulty, replaced and repaired.

CHECKING AND OPTIMIZING DYNAMIC RESPONSE CHARACTERISTICS

Catheter–tubing–transducer plumbing setups used in the ICU are underdamped second-order dynamic systems.[1,2,13–15] Characteristics of second-order systems are described mathematically by a second-order differential equation with characteristics determined by three mechanical parameters: elasticity, mass, and friction. These same parameters apply to a catheter–tubing–transducer system where the natural frequency (Fn in Hz) and damping coefficient zeta (ζ) determine the dynamic characteristics of the plumbing system.

Dynamic response characteristics of catheter–tubing–transducer systems are expressed by two interrelated techniques. One specifies a bandwidth (frequency) and requires that the system's frequency response be flat up to a given frequency so that a specified number of harmonics—usually 10—of the original pulse wave can be reproduced without distortion (Fig. 56-3). The second specifies the Fn and ζ.[13] The resulting plot of Fn and ζ is shown in Figure 56-4.[13] If the characteristics of the plumbing system fall in the adequate or optimal area of the graph, the pressure waveforms will be adequately reproduced. If this point falls in any of the remaining three areas, there will be pressure waveform distortion.

Catheter–tubing–transducer plumbing systems assembled under optimal conditions are usually underdamped, although a few fall into the unacceptable area. Methods

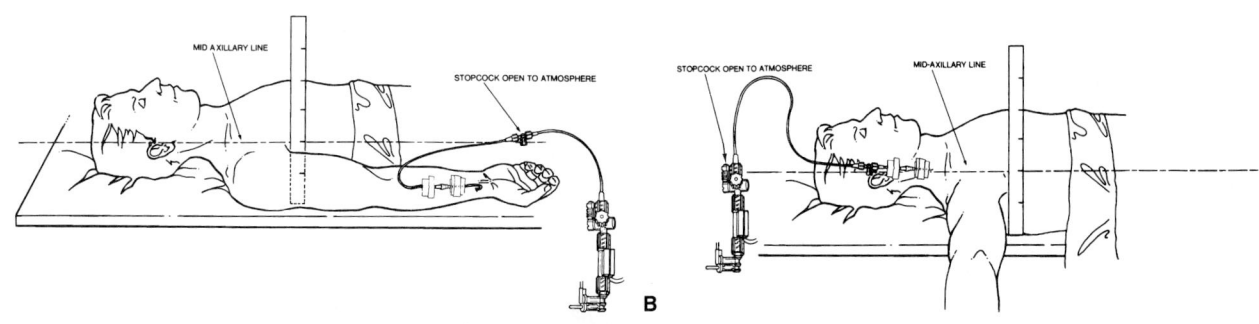

A   **B**

FIGURE 56-2. Two methods of zeroing a pressure transducer. Notice the place at which the water–air interface occurs should always be at the mid-axillary line when zeroing. (**A**) The stopcock near the catheter is placed at the mid-axillary line. (**B**) The stopcock is placed near the transducer at the mid-axillary line. (Adapted from Gardner RM, Hollingsworth KW: Optimizing ECG and pressure monitoring. *Crit Care Med* 1986;14:651.)

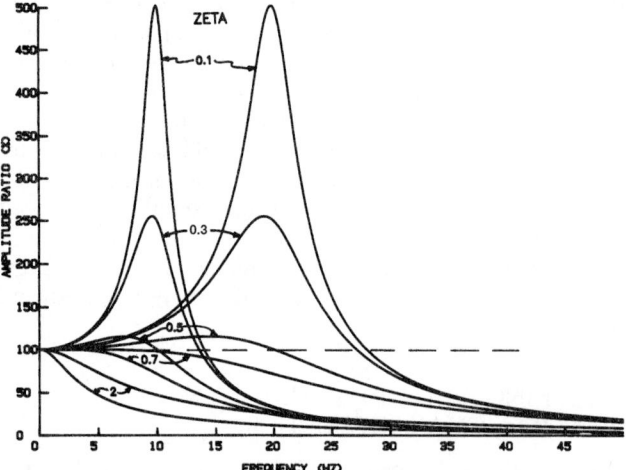

FIGURE 56-3. Family of frequency versus amplitude ratio plots for five different damping coefficients (zeta, ζ) and two different natural frequencies of 10 and 20 Hz. A damping coefficient of 0.1 occurs if the system is very underdamped, whereas a damping coefficient of 2.0 occurs when a system is overdamped. The ideal or "flat" frequency versus amplitude response is shown (*dashed line*). Notice that the response of the system with a 10-Hz natural frequency can be brought closer to the ideal "flat" response if the damping coefficient is between 0.5 and 0.7. However, by increasing the natural frequency to 20 Hz, the range of damping coefficients can be widened still further and gives nearly the same "flat" frequency response.

for optimizing the plumbing system components have been outlined.[1,13–15] In the clinical setting, there are dramatic differences between each monitoring system setup; therefore, it is mandatory to test the adequacy of each pressure monitoring system. This can be done easily using the fast-flush technique. A fast-flush is produced by opening the valve of the continuous flush device (e.g., by quickly releasing the fast-flush valve on the continuous flush system). The rapid

closure generates a square wave from which the Fn and ζ of the plumbing system can be measured.

Once the fast-flush test has been executed two or three times, the dynamic response characteristics (Fn and Z) can be quickly and easily determined.[1,13] Fn can be estimated by measuring the period of each full oscillation on a strip chart recorder (Fig. 56-5A) after a fast-flush, and calculating the frequency from the period. To determine the ζ, any two successive peak amplitudes are measured and an amplitude ratio obtained by dividing the measured height of the lower peak by that of the amplitude of the larger peak (see Fig. 56-5B). This ratio is then converted to the ζ.

Once the Fn and the ζ have been determined, the data can be plotted on the graph in Figure 56-4 to ascertain the adequacy of dynamic response. Some bedside monitors and recorders may compromise the fast-flush technique with their built-in low-pass filters. These filters should be expanded to at least 50 Hz.

Several factors lead to poor dynamic responses: air bubbles in the system, usually caused by a poor initial fluid filling of the plumbing system; pressure tubing that is too long, too elastic, or has a diameter that is too small; and pressure transducers that are too elastic. The best way to enhance the system's dynamics is to maximize its Fn.

CLINICAL VERSUS LABORATORY MEASUREMENT OF DYNAMIC RESPONSE

Several investigators have studied the dynamic response characteristics of catheter–transducer systems.[1,2,13–17] Some investigators have evaluated the dynamics of pressure monitoring systems by evaluating only one element in the system. However, recent studies have examined the *complete* pressure monitoring plumbing system.[15,17]

The results of these studies show that the simpler the mechanical plumbing setup of a pressure monitoring system, the higher its fidelity.[17] The more complex the plumbing

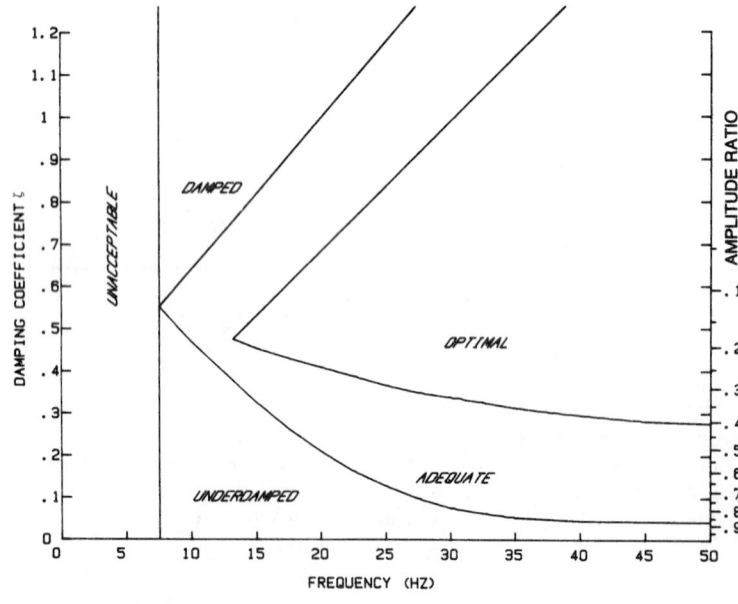

FIGURE 56-4. Plot shows the range of damping coefficient (ζ) and natural frequencies outlining the regions that indicate the type distortion of the pressure wave (see Fig. 56-5 for examples).

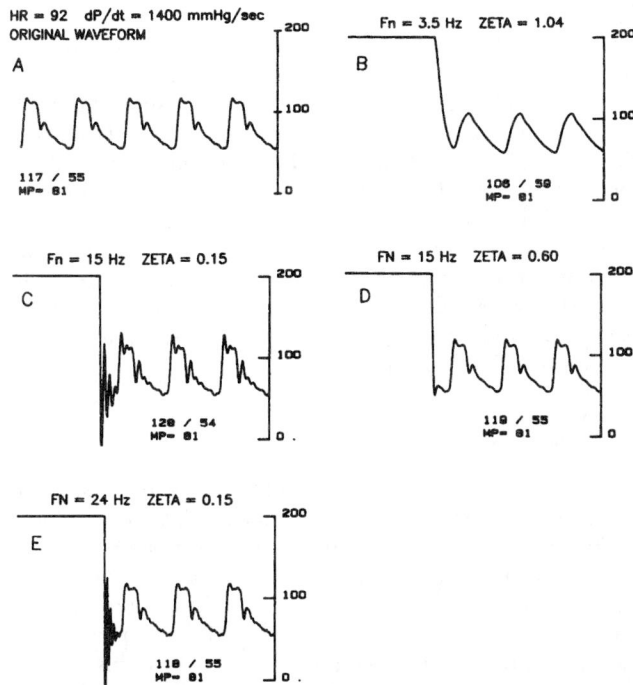

HR = 92 dP/dt = 1400 mmHg/sec
ORIGINAL WAVEFORM

A

117 / 55
MP= 81

Fn = 3.5 Hz   ZETA = 1.04

B

106 / 59
MP= 81

Fn = 15 Hz   ZETA = 0.15

C

128 / 54
MP= 81

FN = 15 Hz   ZETA = 0.60

D

119 / 55
MP= 81

FN = 24 Hz   ZETA = 0.15

E

119 / 55
MP= 81

FIGURE 56-5. Arterial pressure waveforms recorded with different pressure monitoring systems. Patient heart rate is 92 with a maximum rate of change of pressure with time (dP/dt) of 1400 mm Hg/second. (**A**) The original patient waveform is shown as it might be recorded with a catheter-tipped pressure transducer. The systolic pressure is 118 mm Hg; diastolic, 55 mm Hg; and mean pressure, 81 mm Hg. (**B**) The same patient's arterial pressure waveform recorded with an "overdamped" plumbing system. ζ is 1.04 and natural frequency (Fn) is 3.5 Hz. Notice the "fast-flush" signal (*upper left*) returns slowly to the patient waveform. Systolic pressure is underestimated at 106 mm Hg, diastolic pressure is overestimated at 59 mm Hg, but mean pressure is unchanged at 81 mm Hg. (**C**) An "underdamped" condition is shown with a low damping coefficient of 0.15 and a natural frequency of 15 Hz. After the fast-flush, the pressure waveform oscillates rapidly and returns to the original waveform shape quickly. Systolic pressure is overestimated at 128 mm Hg, diastolic is nearly the same as the original at 54 mm Hg, and the mean pressure is unchanged at 81 mm Hg. (**D**) Same as in *C*, but a damping device has been inserted and adjusted.[1] The waveform is optimally damped with a damping coefficient of 0.60 and a natural frequency of 15 Hz. (**E**) An "underdamped" condition is shown but with high natural frequency of 24 Hz. Notice the pressure waveform is only slightly distorted and that the pressures are close to the true pressures.

system, that is, the greater the number of components within the system, the greater the susceptibility of that system to have degraded dynamic performance. Lack of tubing or shorter lengths of tubing minimize the chances of air bubble entrapment. Chances for setup error also were minimized with simpler plumbing systems.

The dynamic response characteristics of a system that uses catheters or elastic tubing or systems with air bubbles in them are known to have large volume displacement (Vd). Systems that use long, narrow catheters (such as the PA catheter) or have long lengths of small-diameter pressure

tubing are not desirable because Fn decreases and ζ increases. Conversely, if the catheters and tubing are nonelastic and short, with large diameters and no air bubbles, then the Fn increases and ζ decreases.

Figure 56-6 illustrates the effects of tubing length and air bubbles entrapped in the system. As the Vd increases, Fn decreases and ζ increases. The magnitude of the change is multiplied for systems with long catheters or tubing (PA catheter and radial catheter with 183-cm [72-inch] tubing). For the short radial arterial catheter, the effect of tubing length is also apparent. Increasing the tubing from 30 to

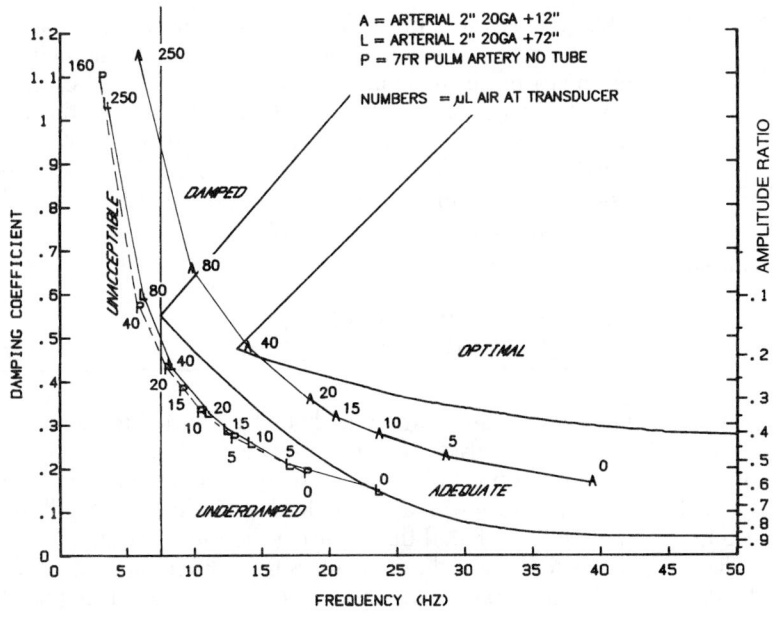

FIGURE 56-6. Plot of natural frequency versus damping coefficient for one pulmonary artery and two arterial monitoring systems showing the effect of inserting small bubbles into the transducer dome. The volumes (Vd) of air inserted in microliters are shown near the marks on the curves. The curves were generated using the modeling techniques of Taylor and coworkers. Results are presented for short radial catheters (Deseret 5cm [2 in]) with 30 cm (12 in) (index A) and 183 cm (72 in) (index L) of pressure tubing. The results from a pulmonary artery catheter system without extension tubing are shown as index P. For all situations, the operating point moves upward and to the left with the addition of air into the system. The best condition is always when *no* air is in the system.

183 cm (12 to 72 inches) with no air bubbles in the system reduces the Fn from 39 to 23 Hz. For a PA catheter system without pressure tubing, the effect of increasing air bubble size (Vd) on the system is shown. In every case, the operating point moves upward and to the left. Despite what is taught in some centers, adding air to the transducer to "damp" the pressure waveform is *not* a good idea.

The use of extension tubing for PA lines was found to be especially detrimental to the system's response. The adverse effects of long tubing are compounded because of the long length of the PA catheter. The use of extension tubing, which affords greater freedom of mobility from the transducer to the catheter, seems to be contraindicated.

This same study found that each clinical catheter–tubing–transducer system must have its dynamic response verified at frequent intervals.[17] There can be vast differences in fidelity of systems between the ideal laboratory setting and the clinical setting where the system is subject to changes over time, human assembly error, repeated blood sample withdrawal, and air entrapment. The fast-flush method of determining the dynamic response characteristics is a simple, rapid, and safe testing modality that can be easily incorporated clinically.[1,2,13,15] By performing the fast-flush testing on each clinical system, one can verify the adequacy of dynamic response and optimize it if necessary. If the fast-flush testing produces dynamic response characteristics that are inadequate, the user can take the opportunity to troubleshoot the system (i.e., remove excessive tubing length or purge air bubbles until acceptable dynamic characteristics are obtained).

SELECTING BLOOD PRESSURE TRANSDUCERS

The objective of the recently published AAMI/ANSI blood pressure transducer standards was to provide labeling and performance requirements, testing methods, and terminology to ensure that health care professionals are supplied with safe, accurate, disposable blood pressure transducers that can be used interchangeably with any monitor.[5,7,9] Fortunately, all of the current disposable transducers meet these new standards.

COMPLICATIONS OF INVASIVE PRESSURE MONITORING ■

The three most important risks associated with vascular cannulation and direct blood pressure monitoring are air embolism, thrombosis, and infection.

AIR EMBOLISM

Air embolism is the introduction of air into the circulatory system. Air insufflation can occur in a variety of ways into either the venous or arterial portion of the circulation. Venous air embolism may reduce or stop the flow of blood through the heart or may cause neurologic complications. The exact amount of venous air that is fatal to adults is unknown but is estimated to be between 300 and 1600 mL.[18]

The rate of air injection into the venous circulation is of primary importance. Death appears to be caused by the right ventricle compressing air rather than pumping blood.

The complication from arterial air embolism is different. Air entering the left side of the heart passes quickly into the aorta. Then, depending on the position of the patient, the air may flow into the coronary arteries, cerebral arteries, or both.[18] Air entering these vessels then obstructs the blood flow to areas supplied by these vessels. In dogs, small amounts of air—between 0.05 and 1.0 mL—injected into the coronary circulation have been fatal.[18] Air embolism is best prevented by using continuous flush systems and keeping the plumbing systems closed.[18-20]

THROMBOSIS

Thrombosis can be caused by an invasive catheters, yet is an infrequent complication of arterial or PA catheterization. Embolization of clots formed on a catheter can be flushed retrograde into the central circulation from radial arterial cannulation sites. To minimize thrombus formation, continuous flush systems have been developed to keep catheters patent and prevent the need to use syringes to flush catheters.[19,21] PA catheters have had heparin bonding added to their surface to minimize thrombus formation.[22] There has been considerable discussion about the use of heparin in the flush solution and its effects on minimizing clot formation in the catheter tip.[23,24] Reports conflict regarding the need to heparinize the flush solution.[23,24] In my experience, over the last 4 years, heparin was not used in the flush solution for arterial catheters. Since heparin was eliminated, there has not been an increased rate of thrombus formation or loss of catheter function. If heparin is used in the flush solution, clinicians must be aware that a discard volume of 5 times the dead space of the catheter and tubing must be withdrawn to minimize effects on coagulation studies.[25]

INFECTION

Although invasive pressure monitoring provides valuable monitoring information, such systems also can result in bacteremia from contamination of catheters, stopcocks, pressure transducers, and flush solutions.[26-35] Most of the reported cases of pressure transducer–related infections were traced to "reusable" devices. Thus, use of totally disposable assemblies is recommended and monitoring systems should be manipulated as little as possible.[35]

SIGNAL AMPLIFICATION, PROCESSING, AND DISPLAY ■

Once the pressure signal has been transmitted to the transducer, the bedside monitor operates on that signal. Most monitors display the heart rate and systolic, diastolic, and mean pressure with a digital display. Evaluation of bedside monitors has found that applying the same pressure waveforms to each of three monitors gave different results.[36] In addition, it was found that none of the monitors recognized and rejected the following artifact conditions: (1) zeroing the transducer, (2) fast-flushing the system, and (3) drawing blood from the patient. These conditions occur several times daily during normal patient care and result in false alarms and erroneous trend data logging.[37]

To eliminate these problems, new algorithms are being developed for bedside pressure monitors. Preliminary testing has shown that these enhanced algorithms produce dramatic improvements in the bedside monitor's ability to evaluate pressure waveforms in the clinical setting.[38]

REFERENCES ■

1. Gardner RM, Hollingsworth KW: Optimizing ECG and pressure monitoring. *Crit Care Med* 1986;14:651
2. Gardner RM: Hemodynamic monitoring: from catheter to display. *Acute Care* 1986;12:3
3. Gardner RM, Kutik M: *American National Standard for Blood Pressure Transducers: General.* Arlington, VA, Association for the Advancement of Medical Instrumentation (AAMI), and American National Standards Institute (ANSI), 1986
4. Gardner RM, Kutik M: *American National Standard for Interchageability and Performance of Resistive Bridge Type Blood Pressure Transducers.* Arlington, VA, Association for the Advancement of Medical Instrumentation (AAMI), and American National Standards Institute (ANSI), 1986
5. Cooper T, Paulsen AW: *American National Standard for Blood Pressure Transducers.* Arlington, VA, Association for the Advancement of Medical Instrumentation (AAMI), and American National Standards Institute (ANSI), 1994
6. Disposable pressure transducers. *Health Devices* 1984;13:268
7. Disposable pressure transducers: evaluation. *Health Devices* 1988;17:75
8. Gardner RM, Hujcs M: Fundamentals of physiologic monitoring. In: Susan G. Osguthorpe (ed). *Concepts of Physiological Monitoring/Hemodynamic Pressure Monitoring Systems: Physiological Monitoring. AACN Clinical Issues in Critical Care Nursing.* Philadelphia, JB Lippincott, 1993:11
9. Gardner RM: Accuracy and reliability of disposable pressure transducers coupled with modern pressure monitors. *Crit Care Med* 1996 (May, in press)
10. Bailey RH, Bauer JH, Yanos J: Accuracy of disposable pressure transducers used in the critical care setting. *Crit Care Med* 1995;23:187
11. Geddes LA: The significance of a reference in the direct measurement of blood pressure. *Med Instrum* 1986;20:331
12. Ahrens T: How often is it necessary to zero-balance a disposable transducer used for intravascular and intracardiac pressure readings? *Crit Care Nurse* 1994;14:98
13. Gardner RM: Direct blood pressure measurement: dynamic response requirements. *Anesthesiology* 1981;54:227
14. Kleinman B: Understanding natural frequency and damping and how they relate to the measurement of blood pressure. *J Clin Monit* 1989;5:137
15. Kleinman B, Powell S, Kumar P, et al: The fast flush does measure the dynamic response of the entire blood pressure monitoring system. *Anesthesiology* 1992;77:1215
16. Taylor BC, Ellis DM, Drew JM: Quantification and simulation of fluid-filled catheter/transducers systems. *Med Instrum* 1986;20:123
17. Gibbs NC, Gardner RM: Dynamics of invasive pressure monitoring systems: clinical and laboratory evaluation. *Heart Lung* 1988;17:43
18. Toll MO: Direct blood-pressure measurements: risks, technology evolution and some current problems. *Med Biol Eng Comput* 1984;22:2
19. Gardner RM, Bond EL, Clark JS: Safety and efficacy of continuous flush systems for arterial and pulmonary artery catheters. *Ann Thorac Surg* 1977;23:534
20. Disposable blood pressure transducers: calibration methods. *Health Devices* 1993;22:97
21. Gardner RM, Warner HR, Toronto AF, et al: Catheter flush system for continuous monitoring of central arterial pulse waveform. *J Appl Physiol* 1970;29:911
22. Hoar PF, Wilson RM, Mangano DT, et al: Heparin bonding reduces thrombogenicity of pulmonary-artery catheters. *N Engl J Med* 1981;305:993
23. Hook ML, Reuling J, Luettgen ML, et al: Comparison of patency of arterial lines maintained with heparinized and non-heparinized infusions. *Heart Lung* 1987;16:693
24. Clifton GD, Branson P, Kelly HJ, et al: Comparison of normal saline and heparin solution for maintenance of arterial catheter patency. *Heart Lung* 1991;20:115
25. Reihnardt ACR, Tonneson AS, Goodnough SKC: Minimum discard volume from arterial catheters to obtain coagulation studies free of heparin effect. *Heart Lung* 1987;16:699
26. Weinstein RA, Stam WE, Kramer L, et al: Pressure monitoring devices: overlooked source of nosocomial infection. *JAMA* 1976;236:936
27. Hekker TA, van Overhagen W, Schneider AJ: Pressure transducers: an overlooked source of sepsis in the intensive care unit. *Intensive Care Med* 1990;16:511
28. Thomas F, Burke JP, Parker J, et al: The risk of infection related to radial vs. femoral sites for arterial catheterization. *Crit Care Med* 1983;11:807
29. Sommers MS, Baas LS: Nosocomial infections related to four methods of hemodynamic monitoring. *Heart Lung* 1987;16:13
30. Simmons BP: Centers for Disease Control: guidelines for prevention of infections related to intravascular pressure-monitoring systems. *Infect Control* 1982;3:68
31. Luskin RL, Weinstein RA, Nathan C, et al: Extended use of disposable pressure transducers: a bacteriologic evaluation. *JAMA* 1986;255:916
32. Maki DG, Botticelli JT, LeRoy ML, et al: Prospective study of replacing administration sets for intravenous therapy at 48 vs 72 hour intervals: 72 hours is safe and cost effective. *JAMA* 1987;258:1777
33. O'Malley MK, Rhame FS, Cerra FB, et al: Value of routine pressure monitoring system changes after 72 hours of continuous use. *Crit Care Med* 1994;22:1424
34. Mermel LA, Maki DG: Epidemic bloodstream infections from hemodynamic pressure monitoring: signs of the times. *Infect Control Hosp Epidemiol* 1989;10:47
35. Mermel LA, Maki DG: Infectious complications of Swan-Ganz pulmonary-artery catheters: pathogenesis, epidemiology, prevention, and management. State of the art. *Am J Resp Crit Care Med* 1994;149:1020
36. Maloy L, Gardner RM: Monitoring systemic arterial blood pressure: strip recording versus digital display. *Heart Lung* 1986;15:627
37. Gardner RM, Monis SM, Oehler P: Monitoring direct blood pressure: algorithm enhancements. *IEEE Comput Cardiol* 1986;13:607
38. Ellis DM: Interpretation of beat-to-beat blood pressure values in the presence of ventilatory changes. *J Clin Monit* 1985;1:65

Critical Care, Third Edition, edited by Joseph M. Civetta,
Robert W. Taylor, and Robert R. Kirby.
Lippincott-Raven Publishers, Philadelphia, PA © 1997.

CHAPTER 57

■

Arterial, Central Venous, and Pulmonary Artery Catheters

Albert J. Varon

IMMEDIATE CONCERNS ■

MAJOR PROBLEMS

Invasive bedside hemodynamic monitoring permits the acquisition of information concerning cardiorespiratory performance and the effects of therapy in critically ill patients. An arterial catheter is indicated whenever a need exists for continuous monitoring of blood pressure, frequent sampling of arterial blood, or both. In addition, observation of the arterial pressure waveform permits a qualitative assessment of the patient's cardiovascular status. When myocardial contractility is diminished, the upslope of the arterial pressure tracing decreases. When a patient is hypovolemic and has a small stroke volume, the pressure waveform becomes smaller. Analysis of the systolic blood pressure (SBP) variation during mechanical ventilation may also offer important information as to the nature of low-flow states. The normal decrease in SBP after a mechanical breath is more pronounced during hypovolemia and is practically nonexistent during congestive heart failure.

Although central venous catheters are placed primarily for venous access, useful information can be obtained by measuring the central venous pressure (CVP). CVP is usually decreased in patients with hypovolemia. It is increased in patients with hypervolemia, right ventricular failure or infarction, tricuspid regurgitation, and pericardial tamponade. CVP cannot be used to assess left ventricular function reliably in critically ill patients, because ventricular disparity and independence of right atrial pressure and left atrial pressure (LAP) have been confirmed repeatedly in such individuals. Furthermore, the CVP reading is a single parameter, in contradistinction to the more complete information available with pulmonary artery catheters.

STRESS POINTS

1. A pulmonary artery catheter is indicated whenever the data obtained will improve therapeutic decision-making without unnecessary risk. Table 57-1 represents the indications most often noted in the medical literature.
2. The information obtained with a pulmonary artery catheter includes CVP, pulmonary artery diastolic pressure, pulmonary artery systolic pressure, mean pulmonary artery pressure, pulmonary artery occlusion pressure (PAOP), cardiac output (CO) by thermodilution, mixed venous blood gas partial pressure and pH by intermittent sampling, and continuous mixed venous oximetry.
3. To determine if the catheter is in the "wedge" position, the waveform should be inspected. The mean PAOP should be lower than the mean pulmonary artery pressure and lower than or equal to the pulmonary artery diastolic pressure (unless large v waves are present). When in doubt, aspiration of pulmonary capillary blood from the wedge position confirms the position, because at this level the oxygen partial pressure and pH are higher and the carbon dioxide partial pressure (PCO_2) lower than pulmonary arterial (mixed venous) blood.
4. When the pulmonary artery catheter balloon is inflated (1.5 mL), the blood flow in a distal segment of the pulmonary artery is occluded, creating a conduit

847

TABLE 57-1.   Conditions for Which Pulmonary Artery Catheterization Has Been Recommended

GENERAL

Shock unresponsive to perceived adequate fluid therapy
Oliguria unresponsive to perceived adequate fluid therapy
Assessment of the effect of intravascular volume on cardiac function
Delineation of cardiovascular contribution to multiple organ system dysfunction

SURGICAL

Preoperative cardiovascular assessment and perioperative management of high-risk patients undergoing extensive surgical procedures
Cardiac or major vascular surgery
Postoperative cardiovascular complications
Multisystem trauma
Severe burns

PULMONARY

To differentiate ARDS from cardiogenic pulmonary edema
To assess effects of high levels of ventilatory support on cardiovascular status

CARDIAC

Complicated myocardial infarction
Unstable angina requiring intravenous nitroglycerin therapy
Congestive heart failure unresponsive to conventional therapy, to guide preload and afterload therapy
Pulmonary hypertension, for diagnosis and monitoring during acute drug therapy

ARDS, acute respiratory distress syndrome.

through which LAP can be measured. In the absence of mitral valve disease or premature mitral valve closure from aortic regurgitation, the LAP reflects the left ventricular end-diastolic pressure (LVEDP).

5. If no alterations in left ventricular compliance occur, LVEDP reflects left ventricular end-diastolic volume (LVEDV). In the intact ventricle, LVEDV reflects the end-diastolic stretch of the muscle fiber, which represents the true preload. Thus, changes in PAOP are frequently used as an estimate of changes in left ventricular preload.

6. Because changes in ventricular compliance may affect the relationship between LVEDP and LVEDV, caution should be exercised in the interpretation of the PAOP as the sole measure of left ventricular preload.

7. In clinical practice, judgments concerning preload adequacy are best made empirically by observing the responses of PAOP and indices of cardiac performance to a rapid alteration of intravascular volume.

8. In patients with acute respiratory insufficiency, compliance is often diminished and the "stiff" lungs do not transmit alveolar pressure as readily to the heart and pulmonary circulation.

9. Because intrathoracic vascular pressure measurements are affected by pressure swings during respira-

tion, they should be performed at end-expiration and obtained from a calibrated strip-chart recorder or oscilloscope rather than a digital display.

10. When mixed venous blood is sampled, it should be withdrawn from the most proximal pulmonary artery location possible and at a slow rate to avoid contamination with arterialized pulmonary capillary blood.

ESSENTIAL DIAGNOSTIC TESTS, PROCEDURES, AND THERAPY

1. Critical analysis of the pressure waveform components obtained with arterial, central venous, and pulmonary artery catheters provides valuable insight into cardiovascular pathophysiology.

2. In addition to the information directly provided by catheterization, numerous additional values can be calculated (e.g., systemic and pulmonary vascular resistances, left and right ventricular stroke work).

3. Measured and derived hemodynamic and gas analysis parameters are termed the cardiopulmonary profile. Normal values are listed in Tables 57-2 and 57-3.

4. These data can be used to formulate a plan of intervention designed to improve oxygen delivery relative to myocardial and systemic oxygen needs. This analysis is a dynamic process that evolves as new data are obtained and appropriate therapy instituted.

5. Invasive hemodynamic monitoring cannot be expected in and of itself to improve outcome. A meticulous clinical protocol is necessary. Most importantly, a thoughtful analysis of the data is essential. Don't simply "massage" the numbers.

6. Only certain patients need to be monitored. Catheters must be inserted correctly; the monitoring system must produce accurate numbers; abnormal values need to be recognized; pathophysiologic causes have to be identified; the need for therapy must be appreciated; and a specific form of therapy must be selected and administered appropriately.

INTRODUCTION ■

Critically ill patients represent a major clinical challenge. Traditional clinical evaluation, usually the initial assessment tool, may be unreliable, because major changes in cardiovascular function are not always accompanied by obvious clinical findings.

Invasive bedside hemodynamic monitoring permits the acquisition of information concerning cardiorespiratory performance and the effects of therapy. The decision to monitor involves a careful clinical process and should not be taken lightly because of patient risk and expense. In addition, the gathered data must be accurate, and the clinician must use this information in an appropriate manner.

This chapter reviews the indications and clinical utility of arterial, central venous, and pulmonary artery catheters. Special attention is given to interpretation and problems that can be encountered during monitoring. The relevance

TABLE 57-2. Measured and Derived Cardiopulmonary Parameters

PARAMETER (ABBREVIATION)	UNIT	NORMAL RANGE
Systolic blood pressure (SBP)	mm Hg	100–140
Diastolic blood pressure (DBP)	mm Hg	60–90
Mean arterial blood pressure (MAP)	mm Hg	70–105
Pulmonary artery systolic pressure (PASP)	mm Hg	15–30
Pulmonary artery diastolic pressure (PADP)	mm Hg	4–12
Mean pulmonary artery pressure (MPAP)	mm Hg	9–16
Right ventricular systolic pressure (RVSP)	mm Hg	15–30
Right ventricular end-diastolic pressure (RVEDP)	mm Hg	0–8
Central venous pressure (CVP)	mm Hg	0–8
Pulmonary artery occlusion pressure (PAOP)		
Diastolic mean	mm Hg	2–12
a wave	mm Hg	3–15
Cardiac output (CO)	L/min	°
Stroke volume (SV)	mL/beat	°
Cardiac index (CI)	L/min/m^2	2.8–4.2
Stroke index (SI)	mL/beat/m^2	30–65
Left ventricular stroke work index (LVSWI)	g·m/m^2	43–61
Right ventricular stroke work index (RVSWI)	g·m/m^2	7–12
Systemic vascular resistance (SVR)	dyne·sec·cm^{-5}	900–1400
Pulmonary vascular resistance (PVR)	dyne·sec·cm^{-5}	150–250
Arterial blood oxygen tension (Pao$_2$)	mm Hg	70–100
Arterial hemoglobin oxygen saturation (Sao$_2$)	(fraction)	>0.92
Arterial blood oxygen content (Cao$_2$)	mL O$_2$/dL blood	16–22
Mixed venous blood oxygen partial pressure (P$\bar{v}$o$_2$)	mm Hg	35–45
Mixed venous hemoglobin O$_2$ saturation (S$\bar{v}$o$_2$)	(fraction)	0.65–0.80
Mixed venous blood oxygen content (C$\bar{v}$o$_2$)	mL O$_2$/dL blood	12–17
Arterial–venous oxygen content difference		
C(a − $\bar{v}$)O$_2$	mL O$_2$/dL blood	3.5–5.5
Oxygen delivery ($\dot{D}$o$_2$)	mL/min	700–1400
Oxygen consumption ($\dot{V}$o$_2$)	mL/min	180–280
Oxygen utilization (O$_2$ Util)	(fraction)	0.23–0.32
Physiologic shunt (venous admixture)		
($\dot{Q}$sp/$\dot{Q}$t)	(fraction)	0.03–0.05

°Varies with size.

TABLE 57-3. Formulas Derived from Blood Gas Analysis

Alveolar O$_2$ tension	$PAo_2 = FIo_2 (PB - PH_2O) - \dfrac{Paco_2}{RQ}$
Pulmonary capillary O$_2$ content	$Cc'o_2 = (Hgb \times 1.39)° + (0.0031 \times PAo_2)$
Arterial O$_2$ content	$Cao_2 = (Hgb \times Sao_2 \times 1.39) + (0.0031 \times Pao_2)$
Mixed venous O$_2$ content	$C\bar{v}o_2 = (Hgb \times S\bar{v}o_2 \times 1.39) + (0.0031 \times P\bar{v}o_2)$
Arterial–venous content difference	$C(a - \bar{v})O_2 = Cao_2 - C\bar{v}o_2$
O$_2$ delivery	$\dot{D}o_2 = Cao_2 \times CO \times 10$
O$_2$ consumption	$\dot{V}o_2 = C(a - \bar{v})O_2 \times CO \times 10$
O$_2$ utilization	$O_2\,Util = \dfrac{\dot{V}o_2}{\dot{D}o_2} = \dfrac{C(a-\bar{v})O_2 \times CO}{Cao_2 \times CO} = \dfrac{C(a-\bar{v})O_2}{Cao_2}$
Physiologic shunt (venous admixture)	$\dot{Q}sp/\dot{Q}t = \dfrac{Cc'o_2 - Cao_2}{Cc'o_2 - C\bar{v}o_2}$

FIo$_2$, inspired O$_2$ fraction; PB, barometric pressure; PH$_2$O, partial pressure of water vapor (47 mm Hg at 37°C); Paco$_2$, arterial blood CO$_2$; RQ, respiratory quotient (CO$_2$ production/O$_2$ consumption); Hgb, hemoglobin concentration; Sao$_2$, arterial hemoglobin O$_2$ saturation; Pao$_2$, arterial blood O$_2$ partial pressure; S$\bar{v}$o$_2$, mixed venous hemoglobin O$_2$ saturation: P$\bar{v}$o$_2$, mixed venous blood O$_2$ partial pressure; CO, cardiac output,

°Assumes 100% Hgb saturation.

of the cardiopulmonary profile and the calculation of the derived hemodynamic parameters are also discussed.

Techniques of vascular cannulation and complications of arterial, central venous, and pulmonary artery catheters are discussed in Chapter 35, and the technical aspects of invasive pressure monitoring systems in Chapter 56.

ARTERIAL CATHETERS

INDICATIONS

Conditions in which precise and continuous blood pressure data are necessary include acute hypertensive crises, shock of any etiology, use of potent vasoactive or inotropic drugs, hypotensive anesthesia, aggressive respiratory support (high intrathoracic pressure), and any situation in which factors affecting cardiac function are rapidly changing.[1]

Sequential analysis of blood gas partial pressures and pH is necessary in acute illness involving cardiovascular or respiratory dysfunction or when hyperventilation is instituted in patients with central nervous system injuries.

Insertion of an arterial catheter is a relatively safe and inexpensive procedure. No absolute contraindications exist, although bleeding diatheses and anticoagulant therapy may increase the risk of hemorrhagic complications. Severe occlusive arterial disease with distal ischemia, the presence of a vascular prostheses, and local infection are contraindications to specific sites of catheterization.

CLINICAL UTILITY

Pressure Measurements

The peak SBP is determined by volume and velocity of left ventricular ejection, peripheral arteriolar resistance, arterial wall distensibility, blood viscosity, and the arterial system end-diastolic volume. Subsequent diminution in pressure during diastole is, in turn, influenced by blood viscosity, arterial distensibility, systemic vascular resistance (SVR), and the cardiac cycle length.[2]

Direct measurements of arterial pressure correlate poorly with indirect measurements. The disparities partly result from physiologic considerations but are largely conditioned by the frequency response of the monitoring systems.[3] Because blood pressure trends are probably more important than absolute values, the most important aspect of direct arterial pressure monitoring is that it constantly reminds the clinician to pay attention to the patient, to think about what is happening, and to reason why changes are occurring.[4]

To obtain accurate data when measuring any pressure within the vascular system, one must have an understanding of the monitoring system and methods of calibration. Seemingly minor details, such as the use of long tubing and the presence of air bubbles or blood clots in the system, can make the measurements unreliable (Chap. 56).

Waveform Analysis

Observation of the arterial pressure waveform obtained with an arterial catheter and monitoring system may permit a qualitative assessment of the patient's cardiovascular status.

The arterial pulse wave begins with aortic valve opening and the onset of left ventricular ejection. Aortic pressure increases rapidly in early systole because the left ventricular stroke volume enters the aorta faster than it flows to the distal sites. The rapid-rising portion of the arterial pressure curve is referred to as the *anacrotic limb*. After its peak, aortic pressure declines as ventricular ejection slows and peripheral blood flow continues. During isovolumetric relaxation, a transient reversal of flow from the central arteries toward the ventricle just before aortic valve closure is associated with an *incisura* on the descending limb of the aortic pressure pulse. The subsequent smaller, secondary positive wave has been attributed to the elastic recoil of the aorta and aortic valve, but is partially caused by reflected waves from more distal arteries. Subsequently, aortic pressure decreases again as further runoff in the peripheral circulation occurs in diastole.[5]

CONTOUR CHANGES. As the normal aortic pulse wave is transmitted peripherally, significant changes in its contour occur (Fig. 57-1). The pulse pressure and systolic amplitude increase, and the ascending limb of the pulse wave becomes steeper. The incisura of the central aortic pulse is gradually replaced by a smoother, somewhat later, *dicrotic notch* that occurs at lower pressure levels. The dicrotic notch and the subsequent positive secondary or dicrotic wave probably result from the summation of the forward pulse wave and reflected waves from the peripheral vessels.[5] Thus, the term *incisura* should be used for the dip in aortic pressure corres-

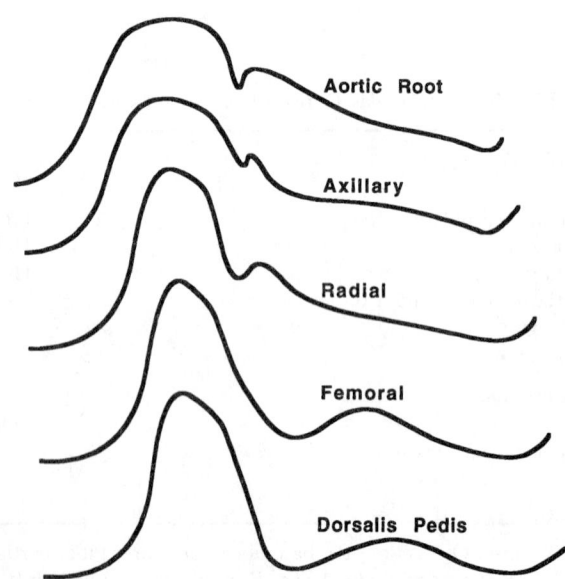

FIGURE 57-1. Configuration of the pressure-pulse wave at various sites in arterial tree. See text for a description of the changes as the aortic pulse wave is transmitted peripherally.

ponding to aortic valve closure, and the term dicrotic notch should be used for the dip in the peripheral pressure waveform that is caused by resonant behavior of peripheral arterial walls.

Major factors responsible for changes in the arterial pulse contour are (1) distortion of the components of the pulse waves as they travel peripherally; (2) different rates of transmission of various components of the pulse wave; (3) amplification or distortion of different components of the pulse by standing or reflected waves; (4) differences in elastic behavior and in the caliber of arteries; and (5) conversion of some kinetic energy to hydrostatic energy.[6] In general, the farther into the periphery blood pressure is measured, the narrower the waveform appears, the greater the increase in the systolic and pulse pressures, and the lower the diastolic and mean values. Although the *mean* pressure measured in the periphery is close to the value in the aortic arch, the peripheral SBP does not accurately reflect aortic arch SBP.

ANALYSIS OF STROKE VOLUME. The shape of the arterial pressure tracing represents a particular stroke volume ejected at a particular state of myocardial contractility. Qualitative interpretation may be made in a hypovolemic patient with a small stroke volume, which thus creates a smaller pressure wave. As intravascular volume is replenished, stroke volume increases, as does the arterial pressure tracing until it attains normal shape. If myocardial contractility is diminished, the rate of increase in aortic pressure will diminish, and the upslope of the arterial pressure tracing will decrease.

Quantitation of stroke volume has been attempted using computers to relate the shape of the arterial pressure tracing to actual stroke volume ejected. However, in addition to the factors that modify the aortic pulse contour as it travels peripherally, critical illness introduces too many variables for this measurement to be reliable. Although the location of the dicrotic notch on the arterial waveform has been advocated as an indicator of the SVR, Gerber and associates[7] were unable to demonstrate any statistically significant correlation.

Effects of Positive-Pressure Ventilation

A single positive-pressure breath normally affects the arterial waveform in a biphasic manner. Blood pressure increases during early inspiration, then decreases in late inspiration and early expiration. Clinically, it is well recognized that the decrease in SBP after a mechanical breath is more pronounced in hypovolemic states. Perel and colleagues[8] define the *systolic pressure variation* as the difference between the maximum and minimum values of SBP after a single positive-pressure breath (Fig. 57-2A). The systolic pressure variation can be further divided into two components: the delta (Δ) up and the Δ down, by using the SBP after a short apneic period or during the preinspiratory period as a reference value. The Δ down is the difference between SBP during apnea and the lowest value of the SBP after a mechanical breath (see Fig. 57-2B). The Δ up is the difference between maximal SBP and the SBP value during apnea (see Fig. 57-2C). In normotensive, normovolemic patients who are

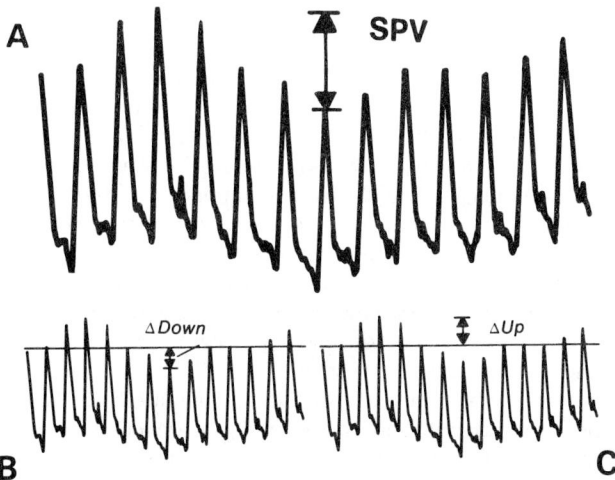

FIGURE 57-2. (**A**) The systolic pressure variation (SPV) is the difference between the maximal and minimal systolic blood pressure during one ventilatory cycle. The sum of (**B**) Δ down and (**C**) Δ up constitute the SPV. The horizontal reference line indicates systolic blood pressure during end-expiration. (Reproduced with permission from Perel A, Segal E, Pizov R: Assessment of cardiovascular function by pressure waveform analysis. In: Vincent JL [ed]. *Update in Intensive Care and Emergency Medicine.* New York, Springer-Verlag, 1989:542.)

mechanically ventilated with conventional tidal volumes, the Δ down and the Δ up are about 5 mm Hg each and the systolic pressure variation is about 10 mm Hg (approximately 10% of the SBP during apnea).

PHYSIOLOGIC SIGNIFICANCE. The Δ up and the Δ down components have different physiologic significance because they reflect events that occur in the heart after a mechanical breath. The initial response to a mechanical breath involves squeezing of the pulmonary blood into the left heart. This transient increase in left ventricular preload leads to an increase in the stroke output for two or three beats and a brief increase in the arterial blood pressure (Δ up). Other explanations for the observed increase in left ventricular stroke output during early inspiration include decreased left ventricular afterload, increased left ventricular compliance, and physical compression of the heart by the expanding lungs.

While the preload to the left side increases during early inspiration, the elevated intrathoracic pressure diminishes venous return so that the preload to the right heart is reduced. This transient reduction in the right ventricular stroke output leads, a few beats later, to a smaller left ventricular stroke output and a brief reduction in arterial blood pressure (Δ down).

Increases in the systolic pressure variation and its Δ down component have been reported to be accurate indicators of hypovolemia in ventilated dogs subjected to hemorrhage[9] and in supine surgery patients during deliberate hypotension.[10] This observation suggests that changes in the arterial pressure waveform during mechanical ventilation may constitute an additional parameter in the evaluation of hypovolemic patients. However, the increase in the systolic pressure variation from a greater Δ down component may be caused by conditions other than hypovolemia. These include the deliberate or inadvertent use of large tidal volumes, air trapping, decreased chest wall compliance, and nodal rhythm.

In another study, Pizov and associates[11] observed that the disappearance of the Δ down component of the systolic pressure variation was characteristic of congestive heart failure. They suggested that analysis of the systolic pressure variation may offer important information as to the nature of low-flow states; specifically, that the Δ down component would be prominent during hypovolemia and practically nonexistent during congestive heart failure.

Recently, Coriat and associates[12] compared the systolic pressure variation and transesophageal echocardiographic estimates of end-diastolic left ventricular size in patients after aortic surgery. They found that the magnitude of both the systolic pressure variation and its Δ down component correlated well with the left ventricular preload assessed by transesophageal echocardiography.

Arterial Blood Sampling

An indwelling arterial catheter provides ready means for arterial blood gas measurement. The preanalytic error—that which occurs before the arrival of the sample in the laboratory—has been observed to be higher in "single-stick" samples than in samples obtained from arterial catheters, especially in patients with unstable cardiac or respiratory status.[13]

Prothrombin time and partial thromboplastin time (PTT) assays in specimens obtained through these catheters are accurate in patients not receiving therapeutic doses of heparin.[14] However, conflicting data exist about the necessary volume (4 to 10 mL) of flush-blood solution to be discarded before sampling for the tests can be regarded as reliable. Blood-conserving arterial catheter systems provide clinically reliable blood samples for the measurements of PTT and hematocrit with no evidence of hemodilution or heparin contamination. By eliminating the need for an initial volume of blood to be discarded, these systems reduce blood loss in the intensive care unit (ICU).[15]

Newer technologies that eliminate preanalytic errors and the need for arterial sampling include continuous intraarterial[16] and extracorporeal[17] in-line blood gas monitoring. Although the results of early studies are encouraging, further revaluation is needed to determine the utility of these systems in the day-to-day management of the critically ill patient.

CENTRAL VENOUS CATHETERS ■

INDICATIONS

The most common indications for central venous catheterization in the critically ill are to secure access for fluid therapy, drug infusions, or parenteral nutrition, and for CVP monitoring. Central venous catheters also have been used for insertion of cardiac pacemakers or inferior vena cava

filters for hemodialysis access and for aspiration of air in case of embolism during sitting neurosurgical procedures.

No absolute contraindications exist for central venous catheter placement although coagulopathy, thrombocytopenia, and anticoagulant or thrombolytic therapy are factors that increase the risk of hemorrhagic complications. Vessel thrombosis, local infection of inflammation, and distortion by trauma or previous surgery are considered contraindications to specific sites of catheterization.

CLINICAL UTILITY

Pressure Measurements

The CVP usually is decreased in patients with hypovolemia and is increased in patients with hypervolemia, right ventricular failure or infarction, tricuspid regurgitation, and pericardial tamponade.

A properly placed CVP catheter can be used to measure right atrial pressure, which, in the absence of tricuspid valve disease, reflects the right ventricular end-diastolic pressure. CVP, therefore, can give information regarding the relationship between intravascular volume and *right* ventricular function. It cannot be used to assess left ventricular function in critically ill patients, because, as was observed previously, ventricular disparity and independence of right and LAPs have been confirmed repeatedly in these patients.[18-20]

For CVP monitoring, the catheter should be attached to a pressure transducer for electronic measurement rather than to a water manometer. Water manometry does not permit visualization of the pressure tracing and cannot provide reliable measurements because of the frequency response limitations of a fluid-filled column that cannot respond to the full range of pressure variations.[21]

Waveform Analysis

A critical analysis of the components of the CVP waveform can provide valuable insight into cardiovascular pathophysiology.[5,22-24] A normal CVP waveform consists of five phasic events: three peaks (*a*, *c*, *v*) and two descents (*x*, *y*) (Fig. 57-3). The *a* wave results from atrial systole and follows the P wave of the electrocardiogram (ECG). The *c* wave occurs concomitant with tricuspid valve closure at the onset of ventricular systole and follows the onset of the QRS complex. The *x* descent results from a combination of atrial relaxation and downward displacement of the atrioventricular junction during the early part of ventricular systole. The *v* wave is caused by venous filling of the right atrium while the tricuspid valve is closed and occurs during the late part of ventricular systole. The peak of the *v* wave occurs near the end of the electrocardiographic T wave. Finally, the *y* descent results from rapid atrial emptying after opening of the tricuspid valve. During spontaneous inspiration, the mean atrial pressure declines because of the decrease of intrathoracic pressure, whereas the *a* and *v* waves, as well as the *x* and the *v* descents, frequently become more prominent.

CARDIAC ARRHYTHMIAS. Cardiac arrhythmias often cause recognizable changes in the atrial pressure tracings

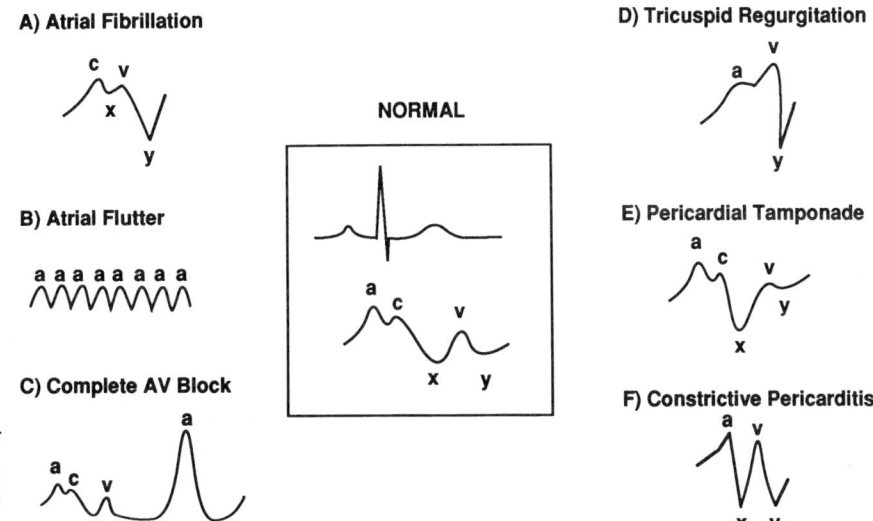

FIGURE 57-3. Schematic representation of normal and abnormal right atrial pressure waveforms. See text for definition of *a*, *c*, and *v* waves and the *x* and *y* descents.

that can be used to diagnose the arrhythmia and to understand its hemodynamic consequences. The *a* wave is absent in patients with atrial fibrillation (see Fig. 57-3*A*). Flutter *a* waves at a regular rate of 250 to 300 per minute frequently are observed in patients with atrial flutter and varying degrees of atrioventricular block (see Fig. 57-3*B*). Large *a* waves occur when the atria contract while the atrioventricular valves are closed during ventricular systole. Such *cannon a* waves may occur regularly in junctional rhythm or irregularly when atrioventricular dissociation accompanies premature ventricular beats, ventricular tachycardia, or complete heart block (see Fig. 57-3*C*).

TRICUSPID INSUFFICIENCY. With tricuspid insufficiency, the right atrial *v* wave becomes prominent, the *x* descent is obliterated, and the *y* descent is steep (see Fig. 57-3*D*). When tricuspid regurgitation is severe, these changes may appear as a single, large positive wave on the right atrial pressure tracing. Significant regurgitation may cause difficulty in passing a pulmonary artery catheter through the tricuspid valve and makes CO measurements by thermodilution unreliable.

PERICARDIAL TAMPONADE. Pericardial tamponade causes elevation and equalization of diastolic filling pressures. The *x* descent on the right atrial pressure tracing is preserved; however, the *y* descent is damped or absent because of restricted early ventricular filling (see Fig. 57-3*E*). During inspiration, the mean right atrial pressure usually declines.

CONSTRICTIVE PERICARDITIS. Constrictive pericarditis also causes elevation and equalization of diastolic pressures. The *a* and *v* waves are followed by prominent *x* and *y* descents, resulting in a typical "M" waveform (see Fig. 57-3*F*). Unlike tamponade, the *y* descent is prominent because no restriction of early ventricular filling is present. In addition, the right atrial pressure may increase with inspiration (Kussmaul's sign).

Right ventricular failure is the most common cause of the Kussmaul's sign and produces a CVP waveform similar to that of pericardial constriction: prominent *a* and *v* waves and *x* and *y* descents. The diagnosis of right ventricular failure is suggested by a disproportionate elevation of CVP compared with PAOP.

PULMONARY ARTERY CATHETERS ■

INDICATIONS

Several studies in critically ill patients have shown that clinical assessment accurately predicts CO, PAOP, and SVR less than 50% of the time. Not surprisingly, as a result of the information obtained by pulmonary artery catheterization, the planned therapy is changed in 45% to 58% of the cases.[25–27]

Although the pulmonary artery catheter permits accurate hemodynamic assessment and modification of therapy as a result, these facts do not prove that overall patient outcome is improved. Currently available evidence from published research provides incomplete information about the effectiveness of pulmonary artery catheterization.[28] Table 57-4 summarizes the results of the controlled studies of pulmonary artery catheterization with clinical outcomes. Although no carefully designed study has established the benefit of hemodynamic monitoring to the individual patient, it is reasonable to assume that more precise bedside knowledge of fundamental cardiovascular parameters permits earlier diagnosis, guides therapy, decreases morbidity, and improves survival. However, improved cardiovascular function, the end result of early diagnosis and intervention, does not always achieve ultimate success when measured by survival.

Risks of pulmonary artery catheterization result from complications of catheter insertion and use, and from misinterpretation of hemodynamic data after catheterization.[29] In addition, concern exists about the financial cost of invasive monitoring in an era of finite resources (Chap. 11). There-

TABLE 57-4. Controlled Studies of Pulmonary Artery Catheterization and Clinical Outcome

STUDY	SETTING	DESIGN	OUTCOME	PROBLEMS
Moore et al. (1978)	Surgery for left main coronary artery stenosis (N = 28)	Observational–historical controls; study cohort vs previous year	Lower rates of perioperative MI, ventricular fibrillation, and deaths in patients with PAC	Historical controls, nonrandom selection
Rao et al. (1983)	Noncardiac surgery in patients with prior MI (N = 733)	Observational–historical controls; 1977–1982 cohort vs 1973–76 cohort	Lower perioperative reinfarction and mortality in patients with PAC	Historical controls, random selection
Gore et al. (1987)	Patients with complicated MI (N = 3263)	Observational; PAC vs no PAC	Higher mortality and longer hospital stay in patients with PAC	Retrospective, nonrandom selection
Hesdorffer et al. (1987)	Abdominal aortic reconstruction (N = 61)	Observational–historical controls; 1983–1984 cohort vs 1980–82 cohort	Lower perioperative hypotensive episodes, renal failure and mortality in patients with PAC	Historical controls, nonrandom selection
Shoemaker et al. (1988)	High-risk surgical patients (N = 146)	RCT. CVP–control vs PAC–control vs PAC–protocol	Lower postoperative mortality, complications, ICU and hospital stay, ventilator use, and costs in PAC–protocol group	Uncertain methodology and case mix
Tuman et al. (1989)	Elective CABG surgery (N = 1094)	Controlled prospective cohort; PAC vs CVP	No difference	Nonrandom selection, uncertain case mix
Pearson et al. (1989)	Elective cardiac surgery (N = 226)	RCT; CVP vs PAC vs oximetric PAC	No difference	Small number of patients, significant group crossover
Isaacson et al. (1990)	Abdominal aortic reconstruction (N = 102)	RCT; CVP vs PAC	No difference	Small number of patients
Joyce et al. (1990)	Abdominal aortic reconstruction (N = 40)	RCT; CVP vs PAC	No difference	Small number of patients
Scalea et al. (1990)	Geriatric blunt multiple trauma (N = 30)	Observational–historical controls; 1987–88 cohort vs 1986 cohort (early vs delayed insertion of PAC)	Lower mortality rate in patients that received early insertion of PAC	Historical controls, nonrandom selection
Berlauk et al. (1991)	Peripheral vascular surgery (N = 89)	RCT; PAC 12 h and <3 h before surgery vs no preoperative PAC	Fewer intraoperative hemodynamic disorders, less postoperative cardiac morbidity and graft thrombosis in preoperative PAC patients	Inconsistencies in data reporting of cardiac morbidity

MI, myocardial infarction; CABG, Coronary artery bypass graft; PAC, pulmonary artery catheter; CVP, central venous pressure catheter; RCT, randomized clinical trial.

fore, the decision to use bedside pulmonary artery catheterization must involve a careful assessment of the risks and benefits for the individual patient.

In general, a pulmonary artery catheter is indicated whenever the data obtained will improve therapeutic decision-making, without unnecessary risk. Table 57-2 represents the indications most often noted in the medical literature. Pulmonary artery catheterization may also be of value in obstetric patients with severe preeclampsia complicated by refractory hypertension, pulmonary edema, or persistent oliguria.[30] Absolute contraindications to pulmonary artery cath-

eterization are rare, but the same cautions as those attached to central venous access apply.

CLINICAL UTILITY

The pulmonary artery catheter provided a quantum leap in the physiologic information available for the management of critically ill patients.[21] The information that can be obtained, in addition to the standard values described earlier, include right ventricular pressures and hemoglobin oxygen saturation that can be measured during catheter insertion and removal. On the basis of this information, a multitude of derived parameters also can be obtained.

Catheters are most commonly placed percutaneously into a central vein. This procedure has been facilitated by the use of introducer assemblies. Once the catheter tip reaches a central venous location and the balloon is inflated, it usually passes through the right ventricle and into the appropriate pulmonary artery position rapidly. Maneuvers often employed to facilitate passage through the pulmonary valve include elevation of the head of the bed, performance of the Valsalva maneuver, and the administration of inotropic drugs.

The techniques of vascular cannulation and complications of pulmonary artery catheterization are discussed in Chapter 35. Clean and aseptic technique and maintenance of intravascular catheters are discussed in Chapter 34.

Pressure Measurement

With a pulmonary artery catheter and monitoring system, the central venous and pulmonary artery pressures can be displayed continuously, and the PAOP can be obtained by inflating the balloon intermittently. To determine if the catheter is in the wedge position, the waveform needs to be inspected. The mean PAOP should be lower than the mean pulmonary artery pressure and lower than or equal to the pulmonary artery diastolic pressure (unless large v waves are present). When in doubt, aspirate pulmonary capillary blood from the distal port of the balloon-inflated catheter to confirm the wedge position.[31] The specimen should have a higher oxygen partial pressure and pH and a lower carbon dioxide partial pressure than pulmonary arterial (mixed venous) blood slowly withdrawn from the balloon-deflated catheter. Aspiration of pulmonary capillary blood, however, is not an absolute criterion for a wedge position, because incomplete "arterialization" of the sample may occur if the tip of the pulmonary artery catheter is wedged in a low ventilation-perfusion ($\dot{V}/\dot{Q}$) region.

CLINICAL APPLICATIONS. When the pulmonary artery catheter balloon is inflated (1.5 mL), the blood flow in a distal segment of the pulmonary artery is occluded, creating a conduit throughout which LAP can be measured (Fig. 57-4A). In a tubular system, flow can be created only when a pressure differential is present at the entrance and exit. If no pressure differential is present, flow is absent. Using this principle in reverse, a *stagnant* system in which no forward flow is present permits an accurate measurement of a distal pressure from a proximal location[32] (see Fig. 57-4B). Simultaneous PAOP and LAP measurements in patients validate this principle.[33]

In the absence of mitral valve disease or premature mitral valve closure caused by aortic regurgitation, LAP reflects LVEDP. In the absence of alterations in left ventricular compliance, LVEDP reflects LVEDV. In the intact ventricle, LVEDV reflects the end-diastolic stretch of the muscle fiber, which represents the true preload.

WEST'S ZONES. The PAOP reflects LAP as long as the column of blood distal to the pulmonary artery catheter tip

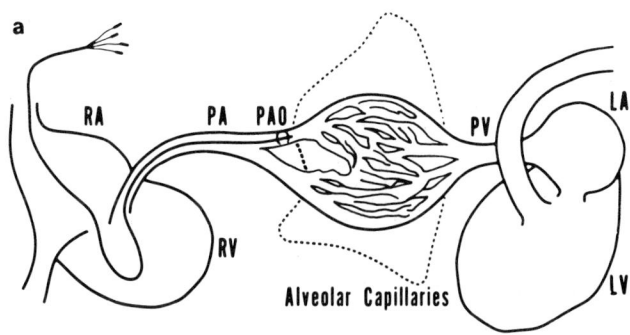

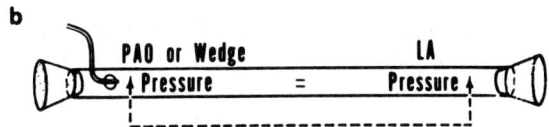

FIGURE 57-4. (**A**) Diagrammatic representation of a pulmonary artery catheter in the correct position. Notice that although the tip of the catheter lies in a pulmonary artery, with the balloon inflated, no flow exists in the system, and that (**B**) in a "closed pipe" analogy, pressure readings throughout the system would be equal. (Reprinted with permission from Sprung CL, Rackow EC, Civetta JM: Direct measurements and derived calculations using the pulmonary artery catheter. In: Sprung CL [ed]. *The Pulmonary Artery Catheter: Methodology and Clinical Application.* Rockville, Aspen Publishers, 1983:105.)

is patent to the left atrium. This relationship may not hold if the catheter is positioned in an area of the lung where the alveolar pressure exceeds pulmonary venous pressure (West's zone 2[34]) (Fig. 57-5) or both pulmonary artery and venous pressures (West's zone 1), causing intermittent or continuous collapse of the pulmonary capillaries. Under such conditions, PAOP may reflect alveolar pressure and not LAP. This fact is particularly important in patients who have low pulmonary vascular pressures (i.e., hypovolemia), are receiving high PEEP, or both.

Because the pulmonary artery catheter is "flow-directed," it is most likely to pass into dependent areas of the lung where blood flow is high and both pulmonary artery and venous pressures exceed alveolar pressure (West's zone 3). In this location, the continuous column of blood between the distal lumen of the catheter and the left atrium remains patent and the PAOP reflects LAP.

A second factor favoring appropriate catheter position results from supine positioning in which the volume of lung located above the heart and the hydrostatic gradient favoring the formation of zones 1 and 2 is decreased.[35] If doubt remains, a lateral chest radiograph can be used to determine the location of the balloon-inflated catheter tip in relation to the left atrium. If the tip of the catheter is below this chamber, zone 3 conditions exist even if high levels of PEEP are used.[36]

Another method to help confirm the location of the catheter tip in zone 3 is to calculate the ratio between the change in PAOP and that in pulmonary artery systolic pressure during positive-pressure ventilation.[37] If the pulmonary artery catheter is located in zone 3, the ratio will be close to

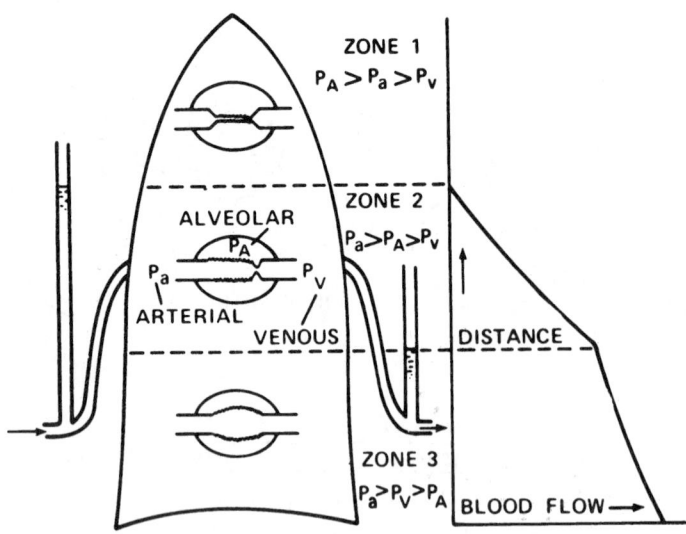

FIGURE 57-5. Model to explain the uneven distribution of blood flow in the lung based on the pressures affecting the capillaries. In zone 1, alveolar pressure (PA) exceeds pulmonary arterial (Pa) and venous (Pv) pressures so that the collapsible vessels are held closed and no flow occurs. In zone 2, pulmonary arterial pressure exceeds alveolar, but alveolar exceeds venous. Under these conditions, a constriction occurs at the downstream end of each collapsible vessel. In zone 3, pulmonary arterial and venous pressures exceed alveolar pressure, and the collapsible vessels are held open. (Reproduced with permission from West JB, Dollery CT, Naimark A: Distribution of blood flow in isolated lung: relation to vascular and alveolar pressures. *J Appl Physiol* 1964;19:713.)

1, because the change in pleural pressure with mechanical ventilation will be transmitted to both the PAOP and the pulmonary artery pressure. However, if the pulmonary artery catheter is not in zone 3, the alveolar pressure will be directly transmitted to the PAOP, making the ratio much greater than 1. O'Quinn and Marini[35] have suggested that non–zone 3 conditions should be suspected if the measured PAOP increases by more than one half of an applied increment in PEEP.

PAOP, LAP, AND LVEDP.   The PAOP is a reliable index of LAP, even in the presence of elevated pulmonary vascular resistance (PVR).[38] Although the pulmonary artery diastolic pressure also has been used as an index of LAP, it is not as reliable as the PAOP.[33] The inconsistency between pulmonary artery diastolic pressure and LAP can be explained by a lack of time for pressure equalization across the pulmonary vascular bed during tachycardia (heart rates greater than 115 beats per minute) or by an abnormally increased PVR. A right bundle branch block can also cause discrepancies between pulmonary artery end-diastolic pressure and the LAP.[39]

LAP may overestimate LVEDP when mitral valve obstruction prevents equilibration of atrial and ventricular pressures at end-diastole or when the mitral valve becomes acutely incompetent, causing retrograde ejection of blood into the left atrium. Conversely, LAP may underestimate LVEDP when severe aortic regurgitation causes the mitral valve to close prematurely while the ventricle continues to fill retrograde from the aorta.

Disparity between LAP and LVEDP can also occur in the presence of impaired left ventricular compliance. In this situation, the end-diastolic atrial contraction is exaggerated and may substantially increase the LVEDP while having a significantly lesser effect on the mean LAP.[40] Careful analysis of the PAOP waveform may help determine the best approximation of the LVEDP in some of these situations.

Raising the intrathoracic pressure introduces an artifact that affects all intrathoracic vascular pressures to an extent that depends on the state of pulmonary compliance. In pa-

tients with acute respiratory insufficiency, compliance is often diminished and the stiff lungs do not transmit alveolar pressure as readily to the pulmonary circulation.[41] In these patients, the PEEP artifact on the PAOP measurement usually should not exceed 1 mm Hg for every 5 cm H_2O PEEP applied.[21] A greater discrepancy can be seen if the patient is hypovolemic or if the catheter is malpositioned, as described earlier.

Transmural PAOP

When high intrathoracic pressure is present, more accurate "transmural" PAOP readings may be obtained. The transmural pressure is the difference between pressures inside and outside of the heart and intrathoracic vessels. Pressure surrounding the heart and intrathoracic vessels is approximated by measuring the pleural pressure, which can be assessed directly by a catheter in the pleural space or indirectly by a balloon in the distal esophagus. The transmural PAOP may then be calculated by subtracting the intrapleural pressure from the measured PAOP. Methods of measuring pleural pressure, however, have many technical limitations and are not widely applied in clinical practice.

PEEP Artifact

Another method to evaluate the effects of PEEP involves observation of the decrement in PAOP when PEEP is briefly removed. Presumably, this decrement remains relatively constant and can be subtracted from subsequent pressure measurements. Although removal of PEEP may decrease arterial oxygen partial pressure and increase physiologic shunt, these changes are rapidly reversible.[42] The immediate nadir or "pop-off" PAOP after the abrupt disconnection from PEEP closely approximates the actual transmural pressure during the application of PEEP.[43]

How much influence this knowledge might have on patient management is unclear, because an isolated PAOP reading, like CVP, has little clinical value, unless it is very high or low. Instead, clinical decision-making should be based on how changes in the PAOP correlate with other hemodynamic and oxygen transport parameters.[44] If a physician believes that the PAOP should be measured off-PEEP, this maneuver probably should be performed when PEEP is discontinued for other reasons (suctioning or changing breathing circuits), and increased concentrations of oxygen should be given before and after PEEP is stopped. Patients receiving high levels of PEEP or whose condition deteriorates when PEEP is discontinued should not have PEEP removed exclusively to measure PAOP.

Timing of Measurement

Because intravascular pressure measurements are affected by the intrathoracic pressure swings during respiration, they should be performed at end-expiration. At this point, intrathoracic pressure is closest to atmospheric pressure, regardless of whether positive pressure or spontaneous ventilation is occurring. In most patients, end-expiration can be easily identified by examining the pressure tracing or by watching the patient and the ventilator while the data are collected. Measurements should be obtained from a calibrated strip-chart recorder or oscilloscope rather than a digital display.[45] Most digital displays are inaccurate, because of the selective nature of time-based electrical sampling and averaging. Designed primarily for use with systemic blood pressure signals, the electronic circuits of bedside monitors identify the highest, lowest, and mean values over a predetermined interval (typically 1 to 4 seconds), regardless of the relationship of the predetermined interval to the respiratory cycle. Although sophisticated electronic algorithms have been incorporated into monitors to eliminate the respiratory artifact, they are inaccurate or fail completely under some conditions, such as high respiratory rates.

PAOP and Pulmonary Capillary Pressure

Usually, the vascular pressure gradient across the pulmonary circulation is so small that PAOP is close to the pulmonary capillary hydrostatic pressure (Pc). The Pc is the major force determining the rate of fluid filtration from the pulmonary capillaries into the interstitium and air spaces of the lung. Therefore, PAOP can be used to estimate the tendency for hydrostatic pulmonary edema. The PAOP, however, may

underestimate Pc whenever an increase in PVR occurs. This problem should be suspected when an increased difference between the pulmonary artery diastolic pressure and the PAOP is present; a difference of less than 2 to 3 mm Hg means the PAOP more closely approximates the Pc.[46]

Cope and coworkers[47] describe a bedside method for estimating Pc by observing the pressure transient after inflation of the balloon on a pulmonary artery catheter. When the balloon is inflated, a rapid initial drop in pressure results, followed by a more gradual decline in pressure until the *classic* PAOP is attained. The inflection point or transition from fast to slow decline is thought to reflect the Pc. Many influences, however, most notably respiratory artifact, make it difficult to determine Pc with certainty in most patients.[46] No data prove that Pc estimates are clinically more useful than PAOP measurements in the management of critically ill patients.[48]

Waveform Analysis

A careful analysis of the components of the pressure waveform obtained with the pulmonary artery catheter also provides significant information regarding cardiovascular pathophysiology.[22–24] The waveform reveals an initial systolic pressure caused by flow of blood into the pulmonary artery from the right ventricle. When right ventricular pressure drops below the pulmonary pressure, the pulmonary valve closes, resulting in the incisura. Pressure in the pulmonary artery then falls gradually as blood flows through the pulmonary arteries and veins into the left atrium and ventricle. The nadir of this pressure in late diastole is termed the *end-diastolic pulmonary artery pressure* (Fig. 57-6).

A wedged pulmonary artery catheter records cyclic LAP events, just as CVP records cyclic right atrial pressure events. However, LAP waves arrive at the wedged catheter both damped and delayed because of the interposed pulmonary vascular bed (see Fig. 57-6). As a result, the *c* waves may not be apparent and the peak of the *v* wave will occur *after* the T wave of the ECG has been inscribed. Otherwise, one can substitute PAOP for CVP, left for right, and mitral for tricuspid to analyze PAOP tracings.

ACUTE MITRAL INSUFFICIENCY. In acute mitral insufficiency, a large *v* wave may be present in the PAOP that

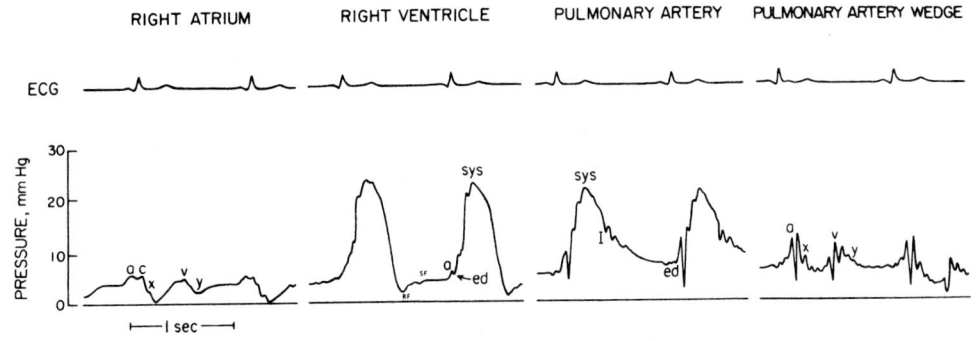

FIGURE 57-6. Normal pressure waveforms from the right heart and pulmonary artery. sys, systolic; ed, end-diastolic. (Reproduced with permission from Grossman W, Barry WH: Cardiac catheterization. In: Braunwald E [ed]. *Heart Disease: A Textbook of Cardiovascular Medicine.* Philadelphia, WB Saunders, 1988:250.)

is attributed to the regurgitant blood flowing across the incompetent mitral valve into a relatively noncompliant left atrium. The *v* wave may mimic the pulmonary artery waveform and, if not recognized, may be misinterpreted as the catheter being in the pulmonary artery position. This error can result in permanent wedging of the catheter, with the associated risk of pulmonary infarction, or it may cause the operator to make further attempts to wedge the catheter, with the attendant risk of pulmonary artery rupture. Careful examination of the pressure waveform and observation of its relationship to the ECG are necessary to avoid this pitfall.

The peak of the pulmonary artery systolic wave occurs within the T wave of the ECG, whereas the peak of the *v* wave occurs after the T wave has been inscribed. At the bedside, the *v* wave is observed to "move away" from the QRS complex when the pulmonary artery catheter balloon is inflated (Fig. 57-7). When large *v* waves are present, the *a* wave on the PAOP trace may be used to estimate the LVEDP.[49] Remember that large *v* waves in the occlusion pressure tracing are not always indicative of mitral insufficiency. Mitral obstruction, congestive heart failure, and ventricular septal defect may all be associated with large *v* waves in the absence of significant mitral regurgitation. Detection of a significant increase (10% or more) in the hemoglobin oxygen saturation between the right atrium and the pulmonary artery may help differentiate acute ventricular septal defect from acute mitral insufficiency.

DECREASED LEFT VENTRICULAR COMPLIANCE. When left ventricular compliance decreases, the *a* wave of the PAOP trace may increase. The exaggerated atrial contraction is capable of increasing LVEDP without a proportionate increase in the mean LAP. In this situation, the *a* wave of the PAOP trace provides a more reliable assessment of the LVEDP than will the mean PAOP.[50]

RIGHT VENTRICULAR FAILURE. With right ventricular failure, right ventricular end-diastolic pressure may be so high that during catheter insertion, the right ventricular pressure waveform may resemble the pulmonary artery tracing[51] (Fig. 57-8). Careful observation of the distance that the catheter is introduced and absence of the incisura on the waveform should help identify this situation.

HYPOVOLEMIC SHOCK. In hypovolemic shock, extremely low right ventricular and pulmonary artery pressures may be observed. It may be difficult to ascertain the location of the catheter during insertion (Fig. 57-9). In this condition, an extremely small difference between right ventricular end-diastolic and pulmonary artery diastolic pressures is present. Rapid fluid administration sometimes makes the recognition of this situation easier and provides primary therapy for the underlying disorder. A bubble in the system may cause damping sufficient to produce an identical tracing. Therefore, the entire monitoring system should be inspected to be sure that this tracing is real and not caused by artifact.

PULMONARY HYPERTENSION. In pulmonary hypertension, the catheter tip may be difficult to position correctly and can even reverse its direction and again traverse the pulmonary valve, leaving a loop in the pulmonary artery. If the catheter is advanced, the tip may impinge on the right ventricular musculature. Damping of the tracing may be assumed to represent wedge position. A chest radiograph should reveal the catheter malposition in this instance.

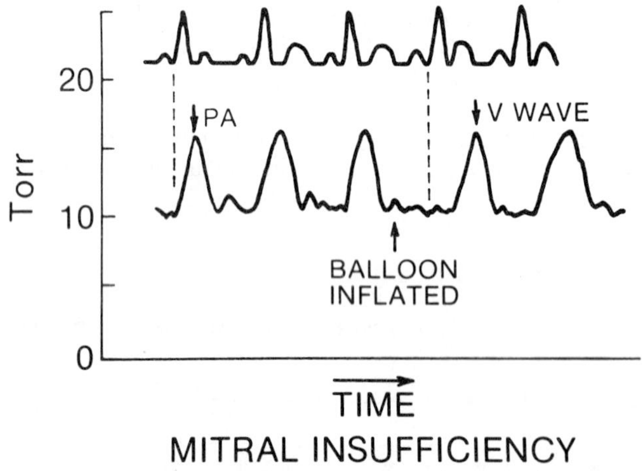

FIGURE 57-7. Representation of a pressure tracing in a patient with mitral insufficiency. After the balloon has been inflated and the pulmonary artery occlusion pressure tracing obtained, the *v* wave moves away from the QRS complex. (Reprinted with permission from Civetta JM: Pulmonary artery catheter insertion. In: Sprung CL [ed]. *The Pulmonary Artery Catheter: Methodology and Clinical Applications.* Rockville, Aspen Publishers, 1983:21.)

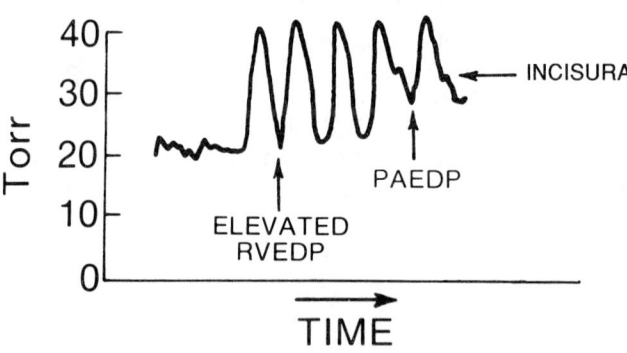

RIGHT VENTRICULAR FAILURE

FIGURE 57-8. Representation of a pressure tracing in a patient with right ventricular failure. Notice that the right ventricular end-diastolic pressure (RVEDP) exceeds 20 mmHg. In this circumstance the right pressure waveform may be misinterpreted to be the pulmonary artery tracing. The absence of an incisura on the waveform and the distance that the catheter is introduced should make this distinction clear. PAEDP, pulmonary artery end-diastolic pressure. (Reprinted with permission from Civetta JM: Pulmonary artery catheter insertion. In: Sprung CL [ed]. *The Pulmonary Artery Catheter: Methodology and Clinical Applications.* Rockville, Aspen Publishers, 1983:21.)

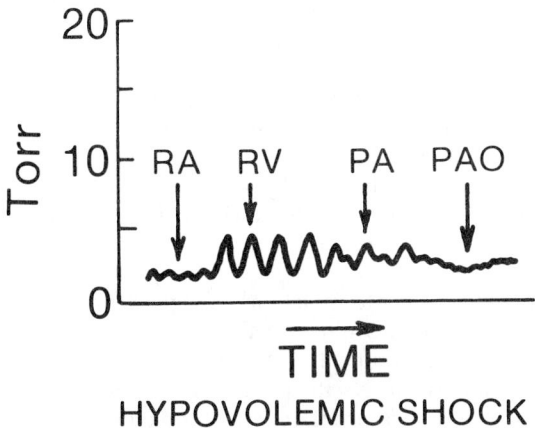

HYPOVOLEMIC SHOCK

FIGURE 57-9. Representation of a pressure tracing obtained in a patient with hypovolemic shock. Notice that the right atrial (RA), right ventricular (RV), and pulmonary artery (PA) pressures are all low, making interpretation of the tracing more difficult. PAO, pulmonary artery occlusion. (Reprinted with permission from Civetta JM: Pulmonary artery catheter insertion. In: Sprung CL [ed]. *The Pulmonary Artery Catheter: Methodology and Clinical Applications.* Rockville, Aspen Publishers, 1983:21.)

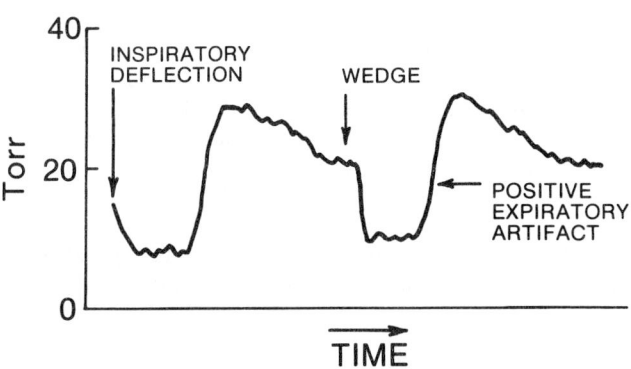

FIGURE 57-11. Representation of the pulmonary artery occlusion pressure tracing after treatment of bronchospasm. The magnitude of the positive expiratory artifact has diminished, permitting a better assessment of the pulmonary artery occlusion pressure tracing. (Reprinted with permission from Civetta JM: Pulmonary artery catheter insertion. In: Sprung CL [ed]. *The Pulmonary Artery Catheter: Methodology and Clinical Applications.* Rockville, Aspen Publishers, 1983:21.)

CHRONIC OBSTRUCTIVE LUNG DISEASE. In chronic obstructive lung disease with bronchospasm or in asthmatic states, intrathoracic pressure during exhalation can increase significantly. This pressure will be transmitted to the catheter, making interpretation of the pulmonary artery occlusion tracing extremely difficult (Fig. 57-10). Careful inspection of the pressure tracing after treatment of this condition can be helpful in resolving the conflict (Fig. 57-11).

TACHYCARDIA. In patients with severe tachycardia, the pressure tracing may be extremely "busy," especially if catheter whip artifact is present. In this circumstance, an accu-

rate position determination for measuring PAOP is often difficult (Fig. 57-12). In addition, the *a* and *v* waves, as well as the *x* and *y* descents, may be difficult to separate.

Mixed Venous Blood Sampling

The pulmonary artery catheter can be used to obtain true mixed venous blood samples for gas analysis. The oxygen partial pressure of mixed venous blood ($P\bar{v}O_2$) and the oxygen saturation of mixed venous hemoglobin ($S\bar{v}O_2$) provide valuable diagnostic information and are necessary for the calculation of various oxygen transport parameters.

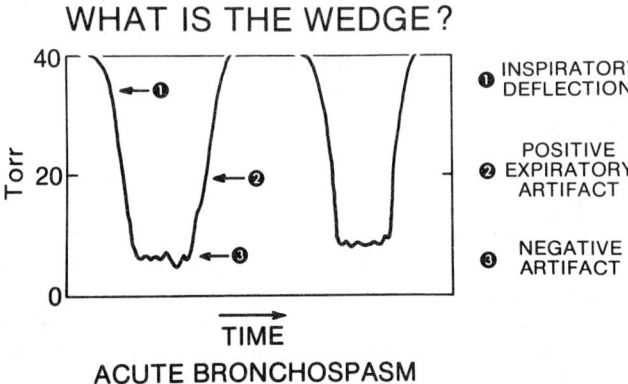

ACUTE BRONCHOSPASM

FIGURE 57-10. Representation of a pulmonary artery occlusion pressure tracing in a patient with severe bronchospasm and marked elevation of intrathoracic pressure during exhalation. The positive-pressure artifact makes interpretation of the pulmonary artery occlusion pressure tracing difficult. (Reprinted with permission from Civetta JM: Pulmonary artery catheter insertion. In: Sprung CL [ed]. *The Pulmonary Artery Catheter: Methodology and Clinical Applications.* Rockville, Aspen Publishers, 1983:21.)

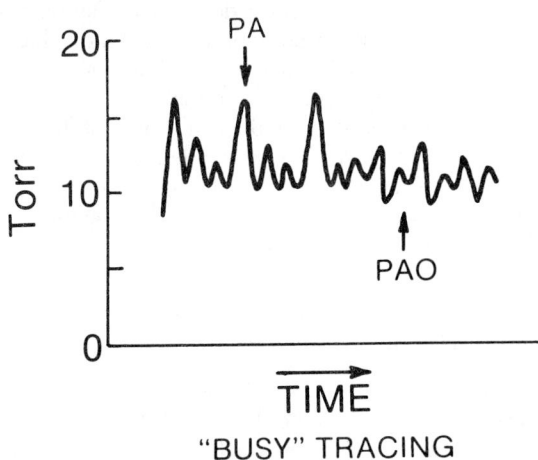

"BUSY" TRACING

FIGURE 57-12. Representation of a "busy" pulmonary artery pressure tracing. The numerous waveforms make interpretation of the tracing particularly difficult. (Reprinted with permission from Civetta JM: Pulmonary artery catheter insertion. In: Sprung CL [ed]. *The Pulmonary Artery Catheter: Methodology and Clinical Applications.* Rockville, Aspen Publishers, 1983:21.)

Sampling technique is important. Blood should be withdrawn from the most proximal pulmonary artery location possible and at a slow rate. A fast rate of blood withdrawal or a malpositioned catheter (distal migration or wedging) may cause a falsely elevated $P\bar{v}O_2$. This error is caused by *contamination* of the mixed venous blood with arterialized pulmonary capillary blood. Shapiro and associates[52] have identified contaminated samples by comparing the carbon dioxide partial pressures in blood obtained from systemic ($PaCO_2$) and pulmonary ($P\bar{v}CO_2$) arteries. A $P\bar{v}CO_2$ value equal to or lower than a simultaneous $PaCO_2$ value suggests contamination of pulmonary arterial blood by pulmonary capillary blood.

Cardiac Output Measurements

The CO is measured by the thermodilution technique, which correlates well with both the Fick and the dye dilution methods. Thermodilution represents application of the indicator dilution principle in which a change in the heat content of the blood is induced at one point of the circulation and the resulting change in temperature is detected at a point downstream. This change is produced by a rapid injection of known volume of fluid at a known temperature (colder than the body) into the right atrium by the proximal port of the pulmonary artery catheter. The change in temperature is registered by a thermistor embedded in the catheter wall approximately 4 cm proximal to the catheter tip. This lowered temperature decreases the electrical resistance of the thermistor and generates a thermodilution curve. A computer integrates the area under this curve, and the resulting calculation is displayed as the CO. If for any reason the fluid bolus cannot be injected through the atrial port of the pulmonary artery catheter (i.e., obstructed lumen), it can be administered through the venous infusion port,[53] the right ventricular port,[54] or the introducer side port.[55]

Newer approaches that permit continuous measurement of CO with a pulmonary artery catheter include continuous thermodilution,[56] thermodeprivation,[57] and Doppler technology.[58] The continuous thermodilution technique has been reported to be accurate and safe in animal models and in critically ill patients.[59] Although animal data on the use of the continuous arterial thermodeprivation system (KATS) are also encouraging, studies are needed to assess the accuracy of this system in the ICU. The Doppler technique failed for economic reasons and is not presently available.

CO measurement technology is discussed in more detail in Chapter 58.

Right Ventricular Ejection Fraction

Pulmonary artery catheters equipped with rapid-response thermistors and ECG electrodes permit the measurement of right ventricular ejection fraction.[60] This technique is based on a model using the response of a single pulsatile chamber (the right ventricle) to a pulsed input (cold water) bolus. The mathematical result gives a single, first-order, exponential washout curve that indicates the residual fraction of the indicator in the chamber.

After a first-order, exponential curve fit is established on the downslope of the thermodilution curve, the residual fraction occurring within each R-R ECG interval is computed. The ejection fraction is then obtained by subtracting the average residual fraction from unity. CO is computed from the same thermodilution curve, and the stroke volume is calculated by dividing CO by heart rate. Finally, the right ventricular end-diastolic volume (RVEDV) is *calculated* by dividing the stroke volume by the ejection fraction.

APPLICATION. Determinations of right ventricular ejection fraction may prove to be valuable in patients in whom right ventricular dysfunction limits overall cardiac performance, such as those with pulmonary hypertension, right ventricular ischemia or infarction, chronic obstructive lung disease, and pulmonary embolism. Although right ventricular dysfunction has been reported in patients with septic shock, these data may only demonstrate that overall myocardial function is impaired in sepsis.[61]

Some investigators advocate right ventricular ejection fraction catheters in patients who receive high levels of PEEP because of the potential for right ventricular dysfunction. However, a recent study[62] in patients with posttraumatic hypoxemia could not demonstrate right ventricular dysfunction caused by PEEP from 15 cm H_2O up to 35 cm H_2O.

Investigators have reported a stronger correlation of RVEDV index (RVEDVI) with stroke volume index (SVI) and cardiac index (CI) than CVP and PAOP. However, the high correlation could be easily explained by the mathematical coupling that occurs when one or more parameters are included in both x and y variables (i.e., CO included in the calculation of both RVEDVI and CI). Civetta and associates[63] report that after accounting for common elements, the correlations of RVEDV with SVI and CI were no longer statistically significant.

Other Uses

DUAL OXIMETRY. Pulmonary artery catheters that incorporate optical fibers allow $S\bar{v}O_2$ to be continuously measured (Chap. 60). An oximetric pulmonary artery catheter used in conjunction with a pulse oximeter (dual oximetry) allows real-time evaluation of the patient's cardiorespiratory system and response to various therapeutic maneuvers.

EMBOLIC SYNDROMES. Some investigators have used a wedged pulmonary artery catheter to recover fetal squamous cells in patients with amniotic fluid embolism, fat globules in patients with fat embolism, and malignant cells in patients with lymphangitic carcinomatosis.[64] However, the presence of squamous cells or small amounts of fat in the pulmonary circulation of these patients is not pathognomonic, and cancer cells may be difficult to distinguish from megakaryocytic nuclei.[64-66]

Pulmonary artery pressure monitoring has been found helpful in the detection of venous air embolism during neurosurgical procedures in the seated position. Increases in pulmonary artery pressure can provide a semiquantitative estimate of the volume of venous air embolism, and the pulmonary artery pressure return toward baseline can be used as a guide of physiologic recovery from the embolic episode.[67]

Bedside pulmonary angiography using a standard flow-directed pulmonary artery catheter has been successful in diagnosing pulmonary emboli.[68] However, a false-negative diagnosis may be made if the catheter lodges in a segmental pulmonary vessel that does not contain an embolus.

CARDIAC PACING.   A multipurpose pulmonary artery catheter that incorporates pacing electrodes is available. This catheter can provide atrial, ventricular, or atrioventricular sequential pacing and may also be used to obtain an intracavitary ECG. Another system (Paceport, Baxter Healthcare Corp., Edwards Critical Care Division, Irvine, CA) provides right atrial and ventricular ports that allow the introduction of wires for emergency pacing.

DERIVED CARDIOPULMONARY PARAMETERS

Although heart rate, blood pressure, and respiratory rate may provide an overview of ICU patient stability, traditional vital signs do little to suggest therapy. For the most prompt and effective therapy to be implemented, one needs not only the physiologic variables obtained by direct monitoring but also those calculated from the original variables. The derived hemodynamic parameters aid in quantitating the relationships among heart rate, filling pressures, resistance, contractility, and CO. Parameters derived from gas analysis help the physician to estimate the adequacy of oxygen delivery and pulmonary function. This collection of measured and derived cardiopulmonary parameters, the cardiopulmonary profile, has been mentioned; normal values are presented in Table 57-3.

HEMODYNAMIC PARAMETERS

The first parameter usually derived from the measured hemodynamic parameters is the mean pressure (MP). MPs may be measured electronically by the bedside monitor or calculated from the SBP and diastolic blood pressure (DBP) by the formula:

$$MP = DBP + \frac{SBP - DBP}{3} \qquad (1)$$

Often, MP, rather than SBP and DBP, is recorded because it is less influenced by the dynamic response of the monitoring system.

An index is a method used to eliminate the effect of body size and provide "normal" ranges. Dividing a parameter by the body surface area (BSA) is one accepted method. The BSA may be obtained using a height (Ht)-weight (Wt) nomogram or by using the classic Du Bois formula[69]:

$$BSA(m^2) = 0.007184 \times Ht(cm)^{0.725} \times Wt(kg) \qquad (2)$$

A simpler calculation can estimate BSA in adults with reasonable accuracy when compared with the standard Du Bois formula[70]:

$$BSA(m^2) = \frac{Ht(cm) + Wt(kg) - 60}{100} \qquad (3)$$

Cardiac index is then equal to the CO divided by the BSA. Similar indices have been used for SVR and PVR, right and left ventricular stroke work, and stroke volume.

CO is the sum of all stroke volumes ejected in a given time. It is usually represented as the product of average stroke volume and heart rate (beats per minute), where stroke volume is the amount of blood ejected by the heart with each contraction. When CO and heart rate (HR) are known, mean stroke volume (SV) can be calculated:

$$SV(mL/beat) = \frac{CO}{HR} \qquad (4)$$

The primary determinants of stroke volume are ventricular preload, afterload, and contractility.

Preload

Preload is the passive load that establishes the initial muscle length of the cardiac fibers before contraction.[6] It is not measured directly in critically ill patients. On the basis of the work by Otto Frank and others, Starling describes the relationship between the resting fiber length of the myocardium and ventricular work.[71] As resting fiber length increases, an increase in work performed on the subsequent contraction occurs. Beyond a certain point, however, further increases in fiber length will not increase external mechanical work, and work may decrease—a description of cardiac failure. The end-diastolic fiber length is proportional to the end-diastolic volume. If no change in ventricular compliance is present (the relationship between pressure and volume), LVEDV is proportional to LVEDP.

Because in most clinical circumstances PAOP provides a reliable measure of LVEDP, changes in PAOP are frequently used as an estimate of changes in left ventricular preload. In critically ill patients, however, changes in ventricular compliance may affect the relationship between LVEDP and LVEDV.[46,49,72] Therefore, caution should be exercised in the interpretation of PAOP as the sole measure of left ventricular preload. In clinical practice, judgments concerning preload adequacy are often best made empirically by observing the responses of PAOP and indices of cardiac performance to a rapid alteration of intravascular volume.

Afterload

The second determinant of stroke volume is afterload. Afterload is the sum of all the loads against which the myocardial fibers must shorten during systole, including aortic impedance, arterial wall resistance, SVR, end-diastolic pressure, the mass of blood in the aorta and great arteries, and the blood viscosity.[6] The most commonly used clinical measure of ventricular afterload is the SVR. Changes in SVR usually reflect either altered blood viscosity or a change in the radius of the vascular circuit. SVR, however, does not necessarily reflect left ventricular loading conditions because the true measure of ventricular afterload must consider the interaction of factors internal and external to the myocardium.[73] Although it is not physiologically correct to speak of afterload in terms of SVR, it is clinically useful to relate changes in SVR to changes in ventricular afterload. Resistance may be calculated by using an analogy derived from Ohm's law, which relates voltage, current flow, and resistance in electrical circuits. The pressure differential across the system is substituted for voltage and CO for current flow, then resistance is calculated according to the following formulas. For the left ventricle (SVR):

$$SVR(dyne \cdot second \cdot cm^{-5}) =$$

$$\frac{MBP - CVP}{CO} \times 80 \qquad (5)$$

For the right ventricle (PVR):

$$PVR(dyne \cdot second \cdot cm^{-5}) =$$

$$\frac{MPAP - PAOP}{CO} \times 80 \qquad (6)$$

Because the sympathetic control of the circulation mediated by peripheral baroreceptors is designed to maintain blood pressure within relatively narrow limits, CO is inversely proportional to SVR when this control is functioning. However, in the human circulatory system, additional factors are present so often that this relationship should not be assumed to be a substitute for direct measurements and repeated calculations.

Contractility

Contractility, the final determinant of stroke volume, may be estimated in the laboratory by the maximum velocity of contraction of the cardiac muscle fibers. At the bedside, we only have inferences based on the stroke work performed by the ventricle as filling pressure changes. Plotting the work of the ventricle for each beat of LVSWI or RVSWI against an estimate of preload, and comparing that point with a normal range, may be useful in assessing overall ventricular function. An upward shift to the left has been interpreted as an improvement in ventricular performance. A shift downward and to the right has been considered as declining ventricular performance. Work is equal to the force times distance; when fluids are involved, the units are pressure change and volume:

$$LVSWI(g \cdot m/m^2) =$$

$$\frac{SV \times (MAP - PAOP)}{BSA} \times 0.0136 \qquad (7)$$

$$RVSWI(g \cdot m/m^2) =$$

$$\frac{SV \times (MPAP - CVP)}{BSA} \times 0.0136 \qquad (8)$$

Ventricular function curves are influenced by changes in ventricular afterload and compliance and therefore do not reflect true contractility. The method for assessing myocardial contractility that is most widely considered load dependent is the end-systolic pressure-volume relationship.[74] However, the logistical difficulty in obtaining frequent ventricular volume measurements in the ICU limits the clinical usefulness of this method. Thus, plotting PAOP and stroke work against normal curves is an appropriate use of data currently available in the ICU. The underlying physiology is better understood if it is considered in terms of the ventricular pressure-volume relationship.

CLINICAL APPLICATION

An appreciation of the determinants of stroke volume permits a rational approach in the management of patients with low-perfusion states. The first and most common intervention used to increase stroke volume is to increase preload by augmentation of intravascular volume. The level of PAP that corresponds to optimal left ventricular preload can be determined only by sequentially assessing the effects of acute hemodynamic interventions on cardiac function and may vary over time in any particular patient. Fluid can be administered rapidly in predetermined increments while changes in PAOP and in the indices of cardiac performance are monitored.

A major increase in PAOP during infusion suggests a high risk of pulmonary edema with further volume infusion. However, if the PAOP rises modestly, if indices of cardiac performance improve, and if PAOP returns to within several mm Hg of the original value within 10 minutes of stopping the infusion, additional fluid can be given without significant risk of exacerbating pulmonary venous congestion. After a brief observation period, this sequence can be repeated until the hemodynamic parameters are adequate or the PAOP shows an unacceptable rise.[35] If tissue perfusion remains inadequate after volume optimization, augmentation of stroke volume may be accomplished by increasing myocardial contractility with inotropic drugs, decreasing ventricular afterload with vasodilators, or both.

Other derived hemodynamic parameters are the rate-pressure product (RPP) and the coronary perfusion pressure. The goal of most cardiopulmonary interventions is to increase peripheral oxygen delivery at minimal cost in terms of myocardial oxygen consumption ($M\dot{V}o_2$). However, the effect of interventions on the balance between myocardial oxygen delivery and $M\dot{V}o_2$, must be considered. Although no currently available measurement is suitable for routine bedside assessment of $M\dot{V}o_2$, the RPP is proportional in experimental situations and can be used to estimate changes caused by our interventions:

$$RPP = HR \times SBP \qquad (9)$$

Myocardial oxygen delivery is not measured at the bedside, but because coronary blood flow is pressure-dependent in patients with fixed coronary vascular resistance from occlusive disease, the change in coronary perfusion pressure may be inferred to represent the most likely direction of change in coronary blood flow resulting from an intervention. The coronary perfusion pressure (CPP) is usually defined as the aortic diastolic blood pressure (DBP) minus the LVEDP. Using PAOP as an estimate of LVEDP:

$$CPP = DBP - PAOP \qquad (10)$$

Elevation of the LVEDP decreases the gradient of blood flow to the vulnerable subendocardium during diastole as much as an equal decrease in the diastolic blood pressure.

PARAMETERS BASED ON ANALYSIS OF BLOOD GAS PARTIAL PRESSURE

Just as the derived hemodynamic parameters can be used to evaluate the choice and effects of hemodynamic interventions, parameters derived from blood gas analysis yield information regarding the adequacy of cardiopulmonary function in meeting tissue demands for oxygen. Blood gas values are usually reported in terms of directly measured partial pressures (Po_2 or Pco_2) and calculated saturations (So_2). Saturations may also be measured directly in a cooximeter or continuously by using transmission or reflectance spectrophotometry. The formulas for the calculation of these parameters are reviewed in Table 57-3. A detailed discussion of the assessment of oxygen transport balance can be found in Chapter 60.

The measured and derived data can be used to formulate a plan of intervention designed to improve oxygen delivery relative to myocardial and systemic oxygen needs. This analysis is a dynamic process that evolves as new data are obtained and appropriate therapy instituted.

CONCLUSION

Hemodynamic monitoring is an integral part of the diagnosis and management of critically ill patients. The monitoring devices, however, are not amulets that by themselves protect the patient or improve outcome. Clearly, a clinical process is necessary: physicians should select only certain patients to be monitored; the catheters must be inserted correctly; the monitoring system must produce accurate numbers; abnormal values need to be recognized; pathophysiologic causes have to be identified; the need for therapy must be appreciated; and a specific form of therapy must be selected and administered appropriately. The sequence still is based on the clinician's knowledge, but unless hemodynamic monitoring is initiated, the potential for improvement in outcome can never be realized.

REFERENCES ■

1. Cohn JN: Blood pressure measurement in shock. *JAMA* 1967; 199:972
2. Nutter DO: Measurement of the systemic blood pressure. In: Hurst JW (ed). *The Heart*, 5th ed. New York, McGraw-Hill, 1982:182
3. Bruner JMR, Krenis LJ, Kunsman JM, et al: Comparison of direct and indirect methods of measuring arterial blood pressure. III. *Med Instrum* 1981;15:182
4. Bruner JMR: *Handbook of Blood Pressure Monitoring*. Boston, PSG Publishing, 1978
5. O'Rourke RA, Silverman ME, Schlant RC: General examination of the patient. In: Schlant RC, Alexander RW, Hurst JW (eds). *Hurst's the Heart*, 8th ed. New York, McGraw-Hill, 1994:217
6. Schlant RC, Sonnenblick EH: Normal physiology of the cardiovascular system. In: Schlant RC, Alexander RW, Hurst JW (eds). *Hurst's the Heart*, 8th ed. New York, McGraw-Hill, 1994:113
7. Gerber MJ, Hines RL, Barash PG: Arterial waveforms and systemic vascular resistance: is there a correlation? *Anesthesiology* 1987;66:823
8. Perel A, Segal E, Pizov R: Assessment of cardiovascular function by pressure waveform analysis. In: Vincent JL (ed). *Update in Intensive Care and Emergency Medicine.* New York, Springer-Verlag, 1989:542
9. Perel A, Pizov R, Cotev S: Systolic blood pressure variation is a sensitive indicator of hypovolemia in ventilated dogs subjected to graded hemorrhage. *Anesthesiology* 1987;67:498
10. Pizov R, Segal E, Kaplan L, et al: The use of systolic pressure variation in hemodynamic monitoring during deliberate hypotension in spine surgery. *J Clin Anesth* 1990;2:96
11. Pizov R, Ya'ari Y, Perel A: The arterial pressure waveform during acute ventricular failure and synchronized external chest compression. *Anesth Analg* 1989;68:150
12. Coriat P, Vrillon M, Perel A, et al: A comparison of systolic blood pressure variations and echocardiographic estimates of end-diastolic left ventricular size in patients after aortic surgery. *Anesth Analg* 1994;78:46
13. Shapiro BA: Monitoring gas exchange in acute respiratory failure. *Respir Care* 1983;28:605
14. Lew JKL, Hutchinson E, Lin ES: Intra-arterial blood sampling for clotting studies: effects of heparin contamination. *Anaesthesia* 1991;46:719
15. Silver MJ, Jubran H, Stein S, et al: Evaluation of a new blood-conserving arterial line system for patients in intensive care units. *Crit Care Med* 1993;21:507
16. Larson CP, Vender J, Seiver A: Multisite evaluation of a continuous intraarterial blood gas monitoring system. *Crit Care Med* 1994;81:543
17. Shapiro BA, Mahutte CK, Cane RD, et al: Clinical performance of a blood gas monitor: a prospective, multicenter trial. *Crit Care Med* 1993;21:487
18. Berglund E: Balance of left and right ventricular output: relation between left and right atrial pressures. *Am J Physiol* 1954;178:381
19. Civetta JM, Gabel JC, Laver MB: Disparate ventricular function in surgical patients. *Surg Forum* 1971;22:136
20. Forrester JS, Diamond G, McHugh TJ, et al: Filling pressures in the right and left sides of the heart in acute myocardial infarction. *N Engl J Med* 1971;285:190
21. Civetta JM: Invasive catheterization. In: Shoemaker WC, Thompson WL (eds). *Critical Care: State of the Art*, vol 1. Fullerton, CA, Society of Critical Care Medicine, 1980:1
22. Sharkey SW: Beyond the wedge: clinical physiology and the Swan-Ganz catheter. *Am J Med* 1987;83:111
23. Grossman W, Barry WH: Cardiac catheterization. In: Braunwald E (ed). *Heart Disease: A Textbook of Cardiovascular Medicine*, 4th ed. Philadelphia, WB Saunders, 1992:180
24. Mark JB: Central venous pressure monitoring: clinical insights beyond the numbers. *J Cardiothorac Vasc Anesth* 1991;5:163
25. Eisenberg PR, Jaffe AS, Schuster DP: Clinical evaluation compared to pulmonary artery catheterization in the hemodynamic assessment of critically ill patients. *Crit Care Med* 1984;12:549
26. Steingrub JS, Celoria G, Vickers-Lahti M, et al: Therapeutic

impact of pulmonary artery catheterization in a medical/surgical ICU. *Chest* 1991;99:1451

27. Mimoz O, Rauss A, Rekik N, et al: Pulmonary artery catheterization: a prospective analysis of outcome changes associated with catheter-prompted changes in therapy. *Crit Care Med* 1994;22:573

28. Task Force on Guidelines for Pulmonary Artery Catheterization: Practice guidelines for pulmonary artery catheterization: a report by the American Society of Anesthesiologists Task Force on Pulmonary Artery Catheterization. *Anesthesiology* 1993;78:380

29. Iberti TJ, Fischer EP, Leibowitz AB, et al: A multicenter study of physicians' knowledge of the pulmonary artery catheter. *JAMA* 1990;264:2928

30. Clark SL, Cotton DB: Clinical indications for pulmonary artery catheterization in the patient with severe preeclampsia. *Am J Obstet Gynecol* 1988;158:453

31. Morris AH, Chapman RH: Wedge pressure confirmation by aspiration of pulmonary capillary blood. *Crit Care Med* 1985;13:756

32. Eidelman LA, Sprung CL: Direct measurements and derived calculations using the pulmonary artery catheter. In: Sprung CL (ed). *The Pulmonary Artery Catheter: Methodology and Clinical Applications*, 2nd ed. Closter, NJ, Critical Care Research Associates, 1993:101

33. Lappas D, Lell WA, Gabel JC, et al: Indirect measurement of left-atrial pressure in surgical patients: pulmonary-capillary wedge pressure and pulmonary-artery diastolic pressures compared with left-atrial pressure. *Anesthesiology* 1973;38:394

34. West JB, Dollery CT, Naimark A: Distribution of blood flow in isolated lung: relation to vascular and alveolar pressures. *J Appl Physiol* 1964;19:713

35. O'Quinn R, Marini J: Pulmonary artery occlusion pressure: clinical physiology, measurement, and interpretation. *Am Rev Respir Dis* 1983;128:319

36. Tooker J, Huseby J, Butler J: The effect of Swan-Ganz catheter height on the wedge pressure–left atrial pressure relationship in edema during positive pressure ventilation. *Am Rev Respir Dis* 1978;117:721

37. Teboul JL, Besbes M, Andrivet P, et al: A bedside index assessing the reliability of pulmonary artery occlusion pressure measurements during mechanical ventilation with positive end-expiratory pressure. *J Crit Care* 1992;7:22

38. Levin RI, Glassman E: Left atrial—pulmonary wedge pressure relation: effect of elevated pulmonary vascular resistance. *Am J Cardiol* 1985;55:856

39. Herbert WH: Pulmonary artery and left heart end-diastolic pressure relations. *Br Heart J* 1970;32:774

40. Rahmitoola SH: Left ventricular end-diastolic and filling pressure in assessment of ventricular function. *Chest* 1973;63:858

41. Teboul JL, Zapol WM, Brun-Buisson C, et al: A comparison of pulmonary artery occlusion pressure and left ventricular end-diastolic pressure during mechanical ventilation with PEEP in patients with severe ARDS. *Anesthesiology* 1989;70:261

42. De Campo T, Civetta JM: The effect of short-term discontinuation of high level PEEP in patients with acute respiratory failure. *Crit Care Med* 1979;7:47

43. Pinsky M, Vincent JL, De Smet JM: Estimating left ventricular filling pressure during positive end-expiratory pressure in humans. *Am Rev Respir Dis* 1991;143:25

44. Leatherman JW, Marini J: Pulmonary artery catheter: pressure monitoring. In: Sprung CL (ed). *The Pulmonary Artery Catheter: Methodology and Clinical Applications*, 2nd ed. Closter, NJ, Critical Care Research Associates, 1993:119

45. Schmitt EA, Brantigan CO: Common artifacts of pulmonary artery and pulmonary artery wedge pressures: recognition and interpretation. *J Clin Monit* 1986;2:44

46. Tuman KJ, Carroll GC, Ivankovich AD. Pitfalls in interpretation of pulmonary artery catheter data. *J Cardiothorac Vasc Anesth* 1989;3:625

47. Cope DK, Allison RC, Parmentier JL, et al: Measurement of effective pulmonary capillary pressure using the pressure profile after pulmonary artery occlusion. *Crit Care Med* 1986;14:16

48. Glauser FL: Derived pulmonary capillary hydrostatic pressure: time for clinical application? *Crit Care Med* 1991;19:1335

49. Raper R, Sibbald WJ: Misled by the wedge? The Swan-Ganz catheter and left ventricular preload. *Chest* 1986;89:427

50. Fisher ML, DeFelice CE, Parisi AF: Assessing left ventricular filling pressure with flow-directed (Swan-Ganz) catheters. *Chest* 1975;68:542

51. Civetta JM: Pulmonary artery catheter insertion. In: Sprung CL (ed). *The Pulmonary Artery Catheter: Methodology and Clinical Applications*. Rockville, MD, Aspen Publishers, 1983:21

52. Shapiro HM, Smith G, Pribble AH, et al: Errors in sampling pulmonary arterial blood with a Swan-Ganz catheter. *Anesthesiology* 1974;40:291

53. Pesola GR, Ayala B, Plante L: Room-temperature thermodilution cardiac output: proximal injectate lumen vs proximal infusion lumen. *Am J Crit Care* 1993;2:132

54. Pesola GR, Carlon GC: Thermodilution cardiac output: proximal lumen versus right ventricular port. *Crit Care Med* 1991;19:563

55. Hunn D, Gobel FL, Pedersen W, et al: Thermodilution cardiac output values obtained by using a centrally placed introducer sheath and right atrial port of a pulmonary artery catheter. *Crit Care Med* 1990;18:438

56. Yelderman ML, Ramsay MA, Quinn MD, et al: Continuous thermodilution cardiac output measurement in intensive care unit patients. *J Cardiothorac Vasc Anesth* 1992;6:270

57. Miyasaka K, Takata M, Miyasaka K: Flow velocity profile of the pulmonary artery measured by continuous cardiac output monitoring catheter. *Can J Anaesth* 1993;40:183

58. Segal J, Nassi M, Ford AJ, et al: Instantaneous and continuous cardiac output in humans obtained with a Doppler pulmonary artery catheter. *J Am Coll Cardiol* 1990;16:1398

59. Boldt J, Menges T, Wollbruck M, et al: Is continuous cardiac output measurement using thermodilution reliable in the critically ill patient? *Crit Care Med* 1994;22:1913

60. Dhainaut JF, Brunet F, Monsallier JF, et al: Bedside evaluation of right ventricular performance using a rapid computerized thermodilution method. *Crit Care Med* 1987;15:148

61. Pinsky MR: The role of the right ventricle in determining cardiac output in the critically ill. *Intensive Care Med* 1993;19:1

62. Kirton O, Hudson-Civetta J, DeHaven B, et al: Post traumatic hypoxemia treated with positive end expiratory pressure (PEEP): effect on right ventricular function [abstract]. *Crit Care Med* 1995;23:A134

63. Civetta JM, Kirton O, Hudson-Civetta J, et al: Mathematical coupling: why correlations of right ventricular function are so good [abstract]? *Crit Care Med* 1995;23:A126

64. Masson RG, Ruggieri J: Pulmonary microvascular cytology: a new diagnostic application of the pulmonary artery catheter. *Chest* 1985;88:908

65. Clark SL, Pavlova Z, Greenspoon J, et al: Squamous cells in the maternal pulmonary circulation. *Am J Obstet Gynecol* 1986;154:104

66. Gitin TA, Seidel T, Cera PJ, et al: Pulmonary microvascular fat: the significance? *Crit Care Med* 1993;21:673

67. Marshall WK, Bedford RF: Use of a pulmonary-artery catheter for detection and treatment of venous air embolism. *Anesthesiology* 1980;52:131

68. Dougherty JE, La Sala AF, Fieldman A: Bedside pulmonary angiography utilizing an existing Swan-Ganz catheter. *Chest* 1980;77:43

69. Du Bois D, Du Bois EF: A formula to estimate the approximate surface area if height and weight be known. *Arch Intern Med* 1916;17:863

70. Mattar JA: A simple calculation to estimate body surface area in adults and its correlation with the Du Bois formula. *Crit Care Med* 1989;17:846

71. Starling EH. The Linacre Lecture on the Law of the Heart. Presented at Cambridge, 1915. London, Longmans, Green, 1918

72. Calvin JE, Driedger AA, Sibbald WJ. Does the pulmonary capillary wedge pressure predict left ventricular preload in critically ill patients? *Crit Care Med* 1981;9:437

73. Lang RM, Borow KM, Neumann A, et al: Systemic vascular resistance: an unreliable index of left ventricular afterload. *Circulation* 1986;74:1114

74. Sagawa K. End-systolic pressure-volume relationship in retrospect and prospect. *Fed Proc* 1984;43:2399

Critical Care, Third Edition, edited by Joseph M. Civetta,
Robert W. Taylor, and Robert R. Kirby.
Lippincott-Raven Publishers, Philadelphia, PA © 1997.

CHAPTER 58

Assessment of Cardiopulmonary Function

Nikolaus Gravenstein
Michael L. Good
Tina E. Banner

The prevalence of invasive monitors in the intensive care unit (ICU) is striking. Easily overlooked and often not considered is the fact that much of the same information also can be obtained by noninvasive means. The basis of acute, noninvasive assessment of cardiopulmonary function is physical examination for a palpable pulse and unobstructed airway, supplemented by pulse oximetry, blood pressure determination, electrocardiography, and capnometry. If these parameters are normal, a serious adverse event probably is not imminent.

Why, then, is the use of invasive devices so common? Several differences can be seen between clinical assessment, noninvasive monitoring, and invasive monitoring (Table 58-1). In general, the disadvantages of noninvasive assessment are that it is labor intensive, intermittent, includes subjective assessments, and may not incorporate alarm capabilities. Advantages of noninvasive assessment and devices include immediate availability, relatively low cost, and low risk.

Patients of greatest concern are those who have just arrived in the ICU, have been there for some time and remain unstable, or are at risk for becoming unstable from a cardiopulmonary standpoint. Often, invasive monitors are already in place, which may prompt the physician to forgo a detailed physical examination and noninvasive assessment of cardiopulmonary function. This temptation should be resisted because much information can be gleaned from such assessment.

RELATIVE ATTRIBUTES

The immediate application and data return from clinical assessment and noninvasive monitors are obvious attributes. With invasive monitors, site preparation, catheter or probe placement, and calibration of the monitor cause delays. The invasively monitored patient may also have a partial or complete data hiatus during transport. Clinical assessment and noninvasive monitors are particularly helpful during these periods. The stethoscope can be used to identify a displaced endotracheal tube and previously undiagnosed bronchospasm, mucus plug, or pneumothorax. A manual or automated noninvasive blood pressure measurement can quickly assess systolic blood pressure, which can change because of alterations in patient position, ventilation pattern, and fluid or drug administration rate. The pulse oximeter immediately ascertains the adequacy of oxygenation, and the peak exhaled carbon dioxide (CO_2) displayed by a capnometer helps to verify that transport ventilation is adequate.

USER INVOLVEMENT

User involvement can be viewed as a downside of clinical assessment because it is a labor-intensive method. Invasive monitoring also requires labor and time to initiate, but after it is in place, it generally functions without additional work

TABLE 58-1.   Features of Different Monitoring Modalities

CHARACTERISTIC	CLINICAL MONITORING	NONINVASIVE MONITORING	INVASIVE MONITORING
Availability	Immediate	Immediate	Delayed
User involvement	Active	Passive	Passive/active
Frequency	Highly intermittent	Intermittent/ continuous	Continuous/ intermittent
Objectivity	Objective/ subjective	Objective	Objective
Alarms	No	Yes	Yes
Risk	No	No	Yes
Cost	Low	Intermediate	High

on the part of the user. There are some exceptions, for example, thermodilution cardiac output (CO) determinations.

DATA ACQUISITION

With respect to data acquisition, clinical assessment is the least frequent, whereas noninvasive monitors provide a range of frequency: the electrocardiogram (ECG) is continuous, but the noninvasive blood pressure method is intermittent. Invasive monitors also provide a spectrum of data frequency from continuous intraarterial blood pressure measurement to highly intermittent CO determinations. In terms of objectivity, the clinical examination provides the entire spectrum, from objective (pulse rate) to subjective (quality of sounds); noninvasive and invasive monitors report objective, although not necessarily accurate, data.

ALARM CAPABILITIES

Clinical monitoring does not provide alarm functions and thus is not a reliable passive indicator of acute changes in patient status, unless they fortuitously occur during a period of observation or assessment. Noninvasive and invasive monitors do provide alarm capability; however, this feature should not be overvalued, because alarms are only useful if they are activated and if the alarm limits are tailored to the particular patient rather than used in the generic default mode. For discontinuous monitoring, the alarm usefulness is largely a function of the frequency at which data are collected.

RISK

Clinical assessment is without risk; nevertheless, if it is improperly performed, an error in diagnosis can occur. Noninvasive monitoring is also virtually without risk, but invasive monitoring always involves some risk and may cause considerable excess mortality.[1]

COST

If clinical assessment is performed by those caring for the patient, it does not increase cost, unless more manpower is required because of it. Noninvasive monitoring is also virtu-

ally "free," because after the instrument is purchased, the sensors are typically reusable (blood pressure cuff) or relatively inexpensive and disposable (ECG electrodes). With capnometry and pulse oximetry readily available, clinicians should question whether the expensive routine use of an intraarterial catheter is necessary for every case of mechanical ventilation of an otherwise stable patient.

CLINICAL ASSESSMENT OF CARDIOPULMONARY FUNCTION ■

The approach to evaluation with clinical assessment and noninvasive monitors assumes that the patient's history has been reviewed.

PULMONARY

Inspection

During pulmonary assessment, inspection immediately identifies several common clinical signs of respiratory distress:

Tachypnea
Stridor
Suprasternal or intercostal retraction
Discoordination between chest and abdominal movements
Flared nostrils
Airway sputum or edema
Prolonged expiration
Pursed lip breathing
Breathlessness during speech

TACHYPNEA.   Tachypnea usually is defined arbitrarily as a respiratory rate greater than 30 breaths per minute. Care should be taken that the respiratory rate is accurately counted. If respirations are counted for only 5 seconds and multiplied by 12 to arrive at the breaths per minute, an error of one counted respiration becomes an error of 12 in the calculated respiratory rate. If an abnormality is suspected, counting for at least 15 or 30 seconds limits this mathematical error to four or two breaths per minute, respectively, for each one breath error in counting. The best way to determine respiratory rate is by auscultation, not inspection. This practice eliminates counting chest or abdominal movements that seem to be associated with airway gas movement but are not.

STRIDOR.   Stridor, a high-pitched airway sound that suggests partial obstruction, can result from a mass effect, causing external tracheal compression, or from accumulated secretions in the natural airway or endotracheal tube. Stridor combined with tachypnea is particularly ominous because it implies inadequate gas exchange. Flared nostrils and suprasternal or intercostal retractions are also manifestations of respiratory distress. Secretions in the airway partially obstruct gas flow and should not be ignored. Resistance to airflow in a tube increases as a function of decreasing radius (R). In turbulent flow occurring with partial obstructions, the resistance for any given flow rate is proportional to $1/R^5$. A reduction in airway diameter from secretions in an endotracheal tube can easily cause a dramatic increase in airway resistance.

EDEMA AND AIRWAY OBSTRUCTION.   Edema fluid, classically described as pink and frothy when observed in an endotracheal tube, identifies an alveolar capillary leak. Respiratory patterns that include a prolonged expiratory phase or pursed lip breathing suggest bronchospasm or premature airway closure. Inspect the uncooperative, intubated patient to verify that an oral airway or bite block is present to prevent obstruction of the endotracheal tube through biting and that the patient is restrained to forestall unplanned extubations.

DISCOORDINATE BREATHING.   Discoordinate breathing is present if the abdomen and chest do not rise synchronously during inspiration; this pattern commonly occurs with residual neuromuscular blockade and also after phrenic nerve or spinal cord injury. Another form of asymmetric breathing may be seen with pneumothorax or rib fracture, in which one hemithorax moves less than the other. A useful rule of thumb for nonintubated patients is that respiratory distress is not severe if the patient can carry on a *normal* conversation without appearing breathless (i.e., neither tachypneic nor stridorous).

Palpation

Palpation of the neck may detect deviation of the trachea (e.g., pneumothorax, hematoma) or subcutaneous air that manifests as crepitation. If the examiner's hands are placed on the anterior aspect of each hemithorax, discrepancies and asymmetry in excursion are readily detected. If discoordination of the abdominal and thoracic excursions is suspected, placement of one hand on the abdomen and the other on the chest may more accurately identify discoordinated breathing than inspection alone.

PERCUSSION.   We classify percussion under palpation and use it to elicit hyperresonance (e.g., air trapping, pneumothorax) or dullness (e.g., hemothorax, hydrothorax, pleural effusion, consolidation). Palpation or percussion of the upper abdomen also may detect gastric distension, which can contribute to respiratory compromise.

TUBE PLACEMENT.   A quick method can be used to verify that a cuffed tracheal tube is not inserted too far.[2] While palpating the anterior trachea between the larynx and suprasternal notch with one finger and holding the endotracheal tube pilot balloon halfway compressed in the fingers of the other hand, the endotracheal tube cuff position is identified when tracheal ballotement causes maximal fluctuation in the pilot balloon. If this position is in the suprasternal notch, the endotracheal tube tip is *not* in a mainstem bronchus. The technique, however, does not differentiate tracheal from esophageal intubation. If it is impossible to identify fluctuations in the pilot balloon, the tube tip may be in a mainstem bronchus or in the larynx.

CUFF INFLATION.   It is also appropriate at this time to palpate the pilot balloon of the endotracheal tube to verify qualitatively that it is not grossly overinflated. A better practice is to deflate the cuff and then reinflate with the minimal volume needed to prevent air leak around the cuff at peak manual or mechanical inspiration. If this maneuver is performed, a more precise manometric determination of endotracheal tube cuff pressure is unnecessary in our view, although some believe that intracuff pressure measurement is mandatory to prevent complications of overinflated or underinflated cuffs.[3]

Auscultation

Stethoscopic examination is the sine qua non of pulmonary assessment. The initial goal is to verify air movement in each hemithorax and to ascertain that the intensity and quality of the sound is approximately symmetric. These findings are particularly important in the intubated patient, in whom esophageal or endobronchial placement may occur. Regardless of whether capnometry is in use, both sides of the chest should be auscultated after intubation or tube repositioning. Although bronchial intubation may not be catastrophic, it can worsen the respiratory status and exacerbate intrapulmonary shunting.

Attention should be directed to identifying breath sounds in all lung fields. Wheezing, rales, or rhonchi suggest various diagnoses and treatments. If bronchial intubation, pneumothorax, or hemothorax is suspected, breath sounds should be auscultated from the axillae. Over the anterior chest, they may seem bilateral and symmetric as a consequence of their transmission across the precordium. Clinical examination, although not sufficiently sensitive to obviate the many indications for a chest radiograph, is immediately available, and in some cases, significant changes, such as rales with pulmonary edema, may become manifest or disappear from the clinical examination hours before radiographic changes catch up.

CARDIAC

Inspection

The inspection component of cardiac assessment begins with identifying whether the patient is conscious (i.e., circulation is adequate for cerebration) and then focuses on dependent edema, jugular venous distension, color of the extremities, and evidence of hypovolemia (e.g., sunken eyes, dry mucous membranes).

Jugular venous pressure assessment is helpful in estimating central venous pressure; if elevated, hypervolemia, right heart failure, cardiac tamponade, and superior vena cava obstruction should be considered. The head of the patient's bed should be elevated to a point at which the fluid meniscus is visible in the external jugular vein. If the vertical height of this meniscus above the sternal manubrium plus 5 cm (i.e., the average distance from the sternomanubrial junction to the right atrium) is more than 15 cm at end-expiration, one of the above diagnoses should be considered. Conversely, if the external jugular veins are flat in a supine patient at the end of expiration, these diagnoses are less likely and the patient may be hypovolemic.

Palpation

Absent or weak and rapid peripheral pulses and cool extremities are indicators of a hypovolemic state. Bounding pulses and warm extremities make this situation unlikely. Palpation of peripheral pulses also allows determination of the heart rate and regularity of cardiac rhythm. Heart rate determination by peripheral palpation is subject to limitations analogous to respiratory rate assessment by inspection or palpation. Ideally, a central pulse (carotid or femoral) is palpated or a stethoscope is used on the precordium, especially in patients with irregular rhythms, because "smaller" pulses (e.g., premature ventricular contractions) may not transmit with sufficient force peripherally to be palpated and counted. If significant fluctuations in pulse intensity are related to the respiratory cycle, they suggest hypovolemia or cardiac tamponade and should be followed by a quantitative determination of the pulse paradox.

Auscultation

The heart examination is incomplete without auscultation, which can identify valvular incompetence or stenosis, pathologic heart sounds, and pericardial friction rubs. Cardiac auscultation is also the best clinical way to determine the heart rate and rhythm. Palpation of the carotid pulse during cardiac auscultation is an important aid, particularly in the tachycardic patient in whom it is often difficult to separate systolic and diastolic. The marked difference in treatment for a patient with valvular insufficiency instead of stenosis highlights the importance of correctly characterizing a murmur during the clinical examination.

SUMMARY

The two most significant shortcomings of the clinical examination are that its components are intermittent and subjective in most cases. A need for more continuous and objective methods to assess cardiopulmonary function leads to the use of noninvasive monitors in the ICU that supplement the clinical evaluation alone or in concert with invasive monitors. These devices are listed in Table 58-2.

TABLE 58-2. Noninvasive Cardiopulmonary Monitors

Blood pressure	Capnometer
Manual	Cardiac output
Automated—	Transthoracic Doppler
intermittent	Transtracheal Doppler
Automated—continuous	Bioimpedance
Electrocardiograph	Cardiac imaging
Pulse Oximeter	Echocardiograph

NONINVASIVE BLOOD PRESSURE MEASUREMENT ■

CONVENTIONAL MANUAL TECHNIQUE

Sphygmomanometric blood pressure determination remains a standard assessment in all patients, including those with an invasive arterial pressure monitoring system in use. This measurement can be made in a variety of ways with an aneroid or mercury manometer. Several factors influence the accuracy of manual blood pressure determination, including blood pressure cuff size in relation to the measurement site, manometer calibration, blood pressure cuff deflation rate, and Korotkoff sound interpretation.

Cuff Size

In performing manual blood pressure determinations, the importance of correct blood pressure cuff size should not be overlooked. In general, a blood pressure cuff should be at least 20% wider than the diameter or 40% longer than the circumference of the limb around which it is applied. The length of the cuff should be twice the cuff width, and the bladder within the cuff must be over the artery and cover at least 40% of the arm circumference.[4] Characteristically, a too-small blood pressure cuff yields artifactually high values, and one which is too large tends to yield low readings. The error associated with a too-small cuff is greater than that associated with a too-large cuff.[5] Contrary to popular belief, a loosely applied cuff does not adversely affect blood pressure measurement.[6]

If the correct size cuff is not available, we place the available cuff on an extremity whose size is appropriate for the cuff. Most commonly, this adjustment involves placing a normal adult cuff (13 × 24 cm bladder) on the midforearm of an obese patient.[4] For acute monitoring during transport or resuscitation, the forearm cuff location does not interfere with an antecubital intravenous site.

If the cuff is located on the forearm or calf just above the malleoli, the radial, dorsalis pedis, or posterior tibial arteries also can be auscultated or palpated in analogous fashion to the brachial artery during conventional upper arm blood pressure determination.

In supine patients, blood pressure values from various sites, particularly the mean arterial pressure (MAP), correlate well if the appropriate size of cuff is used in each location. If an appropriate match of cuff and patient is not possible, even an improper cuff size allows trend monitoring, because the offset from the true pressure is relatively constant.

Manometer Calibration

The aneroid manometer is a mechanical device and should be calibrated to verify its accuracy. In one series, 13% of aneroid instruments provided erroneous measurements of 7 mm Hg or more; most readings were low.[7] Mercury manometers also can be inaccurate; they read low if the air vent for the mercury column is obstructed or the mercury reservoir is low. This problem may occur after the device falls over. Because aneroid and mercury manometers are often used to calibrate invasive monitors, their accuracy should be periodically verified.

Cuff Deflation

The variability in blood pressures that results from a pathophysiologic influence must be differentiated from that which is a consequence of user measurement technique. Technique artifact can be limited by keeping the manometer deflation rate at 2 to 3 mm Hg/second or, ideally, 2 to 3 mm Hg per heart beat.[8] The latter approach reduces the measurement error in patients with slower heart rates.

Consider the patient with a systolic blood pressure of 100 mm Hg. If the cuff is deflated from 101 to 90 mm Hg or more between consecutive heartbeats, the systolic pressure is recorded as 90 mm Hg, giving a 10% error. The heart rate, therefore, is an important consideration in choosing a cuff deflation rate.

Accurate blood pressure determinations are time-consuming if the cuff is inflated to 200 mm Hg and slowly deflated (2 mm Hg per heart beat) to 60 mm Hg. For a patient with a heart rate of 60 beats per minute, measurement would take over 2 minutes. We recommend an initial quick deflation to determine the approximate systolic pressure, followed by a more precise measurement as circumstances permit.

Interreader variability is another source of technique artifact that occurs if repeated blood pressure measurements are made from different sites, particularly in patients with atherosclerosis. In one series, 25% of patients with a history of peripheral vascular disease had an interarm blood pressure discrepancy of more than 15 mm Hg, and 41% had at least a 10–mm Hg interarm difference.[9] Some patients without peripheral vascular disease also may have discrepancies, but these are usually less than 10 mm Hg. This observation has important implications for invasive monitoring and for comparing invasive and noninvasive determinations. If time permits, a quick reading on each arm, leaving the blood pressure cuff on the arm or placing the arterial catheter on the side where the higher reading is obtained, prevents confusing data.

Cuff reinflation after an incomplete deflation also causes technique artifact. A bias toward progressively higher values results from venous congestion, which increases limb diameter. Ideally, a minute or two should pass between determinations to let venous congestion and postocclusion reactive hyperemia resolve.

Korotkoff Sounds

Incorrect interpretation of Korotkoff sounds is another common source of error (Fig. 58-1). The American Heart Association recommends that systolic pressure be recorded as the cuff pressure when "tapping" sounds are first heard (phase 1) and that diastolic pressure be recorded when the sounds disappear completely (phase 5). If they do not disappear, the pressure at which they become abruptly muffled is substituted (phase 4).[4] Because the Korotkoff sounds are low frequency, they are best identified using the bell head of the stethoscope.[10]

An auscultatory gap is a cuff pressure range of up to 50 mm Hg in which the initial phase 1 sounds are absent or disappear.[11] This phenomenon is most likely to occur in hypertensive patients and can cause dramatic underestimation of systolic pressure if cuff inflation never exceeds the auscultatory gap or diastolic overestimation if the beginning of the auscultatory gap is interpreted as the diastolic pressure. The auscultatory gap also can confuse the diagnosis of pulsus paradoxus, an important finding in hypovolemia and cardiac tamponade.

The physiologic basis for the auscultatory gap is unknown. Its impact on clinical monitoring in patients with apparent elevated diastolic pressures can be minimized by palpating the radial artery during an initial quick check to elicit the cuff pressure at which the palpable pulse disappears, followed by cuff deflation to less than 80 mm Hg during auscultation.

The normal pulse paradox (i.e., the systolic pressure variation associated with respiration) is 10 mm Hg or less during spontaneous breathing. It is determined by inflating the cuff 30 mm Hg above systolic pressure and deflating it slowly. The difference between the cuff pressure at which the phase 1 sounds are first heard intermittently and the highest cuff pressure at which they are heard continuously throughout the respiratory cycle is the pulse paradox.

Unlike the auscultatory gap, in which the pulse is palpable but not audible, the palpable pulse is intermittently lost during pulse paradox changes in systolic blood pressure. We are unaware of any reports describing the upper limit for the normal pulse paradox value during mechanical ventilation. It is reasonable to expect that it is somewhat higher than during spontaneous breathing.

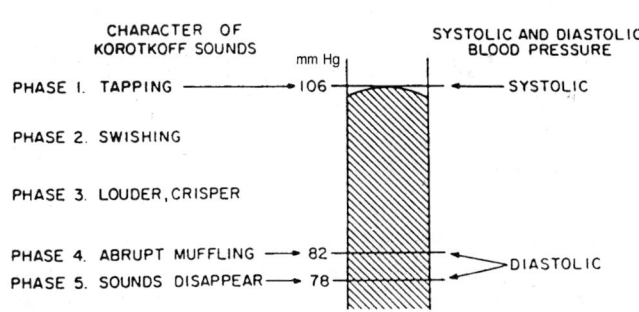

FIGURE 58-1. Graphic representation of the relationship of the Korotkoff sounds to blood pressure measurement. (From Whelton PK, Russell RP: In: Harvey AM, Johns RJ, Mckusik VA, et al [eds]: *The Principles and Practice of Medicine,* 21st ed. Norwalk, CT, Appleton-Century-Crofts, 1984:279.)

Auscultatory blood pressure determinations may be impossible to obtain or may significantly underestimate true intraarterial pressure in patients with shock and high total peripheral resistance or in whom a vasopressor infusion is being used.[12] In these circumstances, invasive monitoring should be considered.

Mean Arterial Pressure

A derived value of physiologic importance is the MAP. This value is the pressure that encompasses one half of the area under the arterial pressure curve during a cardiac cycle. If manual blood pressure determinations are used, MAP is estimated as follows:

$$MAP = DBP + \frac{1}{3}(SBP - DBP) \qquad (1)$$

or

$$MAP = \frac{SBP + 2(DBP)}{3} \qquad (2)$$

where DBP is the diastolic blood pressure and SBP is the systolic blood pressure.

OTHER MANUAL TECHNIQUES

Palpation

Palpation of an artery distal to the blood pressure cuff is the fastest way to assess systolic pressure. The artery is palpated as the cuff is inflated, and the cuff pressure at which the pulse disappears is noted. The cuff is inflated an additional 30 to 40 mm Hg and then deflated at 2 to 3 mm Hg per heart beat or second, and the pressure at which the pulse returns is recorded. Some clinicians average the pulse occlusion and pulse reappearance pressures to arrive at systolic pressure. Both pressures reasonably estimate systolic pressure, with a slight bias toward underestimation because the palpable pulse is lost a little before flow actually ceases and returns a little after flow actually returns.

Doppler Detection of Blood Flow

Doppler-enhanced detection of loss or return of flow is accomplished in analogous fashion to palpation; because it is more sensitive to flow, it is more accurate. This technique, however, requires a Doppler instrument, probe, and a liquid or gel interface.

Photoplethysmography

Another technique is to use the photoplethysmographic pulse detector within a pulse oximeter. The pulse oximeter is observed for loss of signal as the cuff is slowly inflated. The cuff pressure at loss of signal during cuff inflation (not deflation) correlates best with Doppler determination of systolic pressure.[13] Using the pulse oximeter to determine systolic pressure during cuff deflation can result in underestimation of true systolic pressure. This error is caused by

the delay in signal reacquisition by the signal-processing algorithm.

Palpation and pulse oximeter methods cannot be used to determine diastolic pressures or MAPs. Doppler-determined diastolic pressure can be made if the piezoelectric transmitter-detector is placed under the distal portion of the occlusive cuff, thereby detecting both arterial wall motion and blood flow.

AUTOMATED TECHNIQUES

Automated noninvasive blood pressure devices generally use an auscultatory or oscillometric technique or a combination of both; a photooscillometric technique also is available.

Oscillometry

The oscillometric technique is most commonly used. These automated devices are particularly useful because they cycle automatically at a programmed frequency and emit an audible alarm if a limit is exceeded. Auscultatory devices provide automated cycling and determination of the Korotkoff sounds and calculate MAP. They are sensitive to sensor placement over the artery but are not as reliable in calf or forearm placements because the Korotkoff sounds are often less audible.

Oscillometric devices do not require extremely careful positioning and work equally well on all extremities and on the digits if the appropriate cuff size is used (Fig. 58-2). They assess the pressure of the cuff and minute pressure oscillations within the cuff[14] (Fig. 58-3). Initial cuff inflation just exceeds systolic pressure. During slow, graded cuff deflation, systolic pressure is recorded as the cuff pressure at which the minute oscillations first increase in amplitude; mean pressure is indicated when the oscillations are maximal

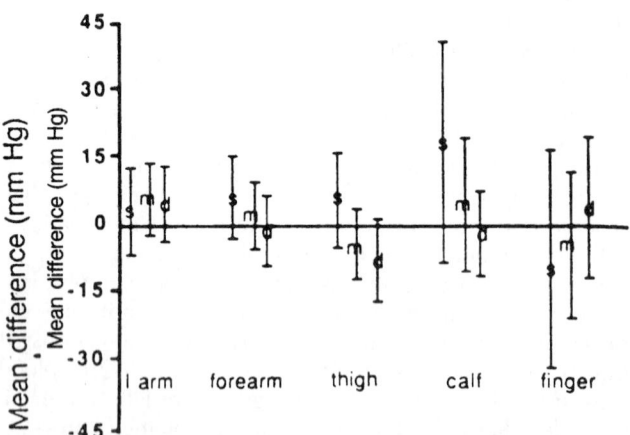

FIGURE 58-2. Mean difference ± SD in mm Hg for systolic (s), mean (m), and diastolic (d) pressures at nonstandard cuff sites, with cuff sizes appropriate for the sites. (From Zornow MH, Schubert A, Todd MM: Intraoperative oscillometric arterial blood pressure monitoring using nonstandard cuff locations. *Anesthesiology* 1986;65:A135.)

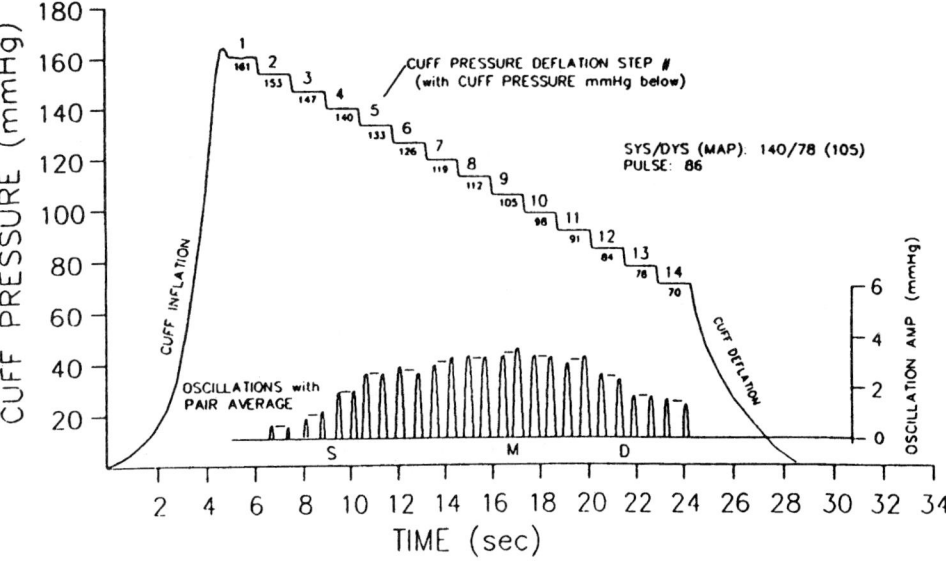

FIGURE 58-3. Blood pressure measurement diagram, illustrating the ideal measurement condition with no artifact. The cuff pressure and oscillation amplitude (AMP) are plotted on the same time axis, with the cuff pressure amplitude axis on the left and the oscillation amplitude axis on the right. Mean arterial pressure (MAP, M) is calculated from systolic (SYS, S) and diastolic (DYS, D) pressures. (From Ramsey M: Blood pressure monitoring: automated oscillometric devices. *J Clin Monit* 1991; 7:56.)

and diastolic pressure when the oscillations rapidly diminish or disappear.

With oscillometric devices, the MAP is a direct measurement and is generally the most accurate; diastolic pressure is the least accurate by this method.[15] In patients who are hypovolemic, hypotensive, or who have a narrow pulse pressure, these devices may only report MAP because this parameter has the greatest signal-to-noise ratio. It should be considered accurate, even if it is not accompanied by companion systolic and diastolic values.

Automated-Continuous Method

The arterial volume clamp method allows virtually continuous, noninvasive determination of arterial blood pressure. The device uses a finger cuff with a light source and detector on opposite sides of the digit. The thumb is most commonly used because of its greater vascular supply and tissue mass.[16] Cuff inflation is maintained at the point where the blood volume of the digit, as determined by the photoplethysmograph, is held constant. The required cuff pressure is the instantaneous pressure in the underlying digital arteries. A rapid-acting servosystem tracks the entire arterial pressure waveform beat to beat, with systolic, diastolic, and mean arterial pressures recorded.

As appealing as continuous noninvasive blood pressure determinations by this method may appear, it is unreliable, inaccurate, or even impossible in patients with peripheral vasoconstriction. In others, it may become inaccurate with peripheral circulatory changes, even after displaying accurate values initially. Despite these shortcomings, the continuous availability of blood pressure data may offer some advantage to patients in whom an adequate signal is obtained over more intermittent but comparably accurate oscillometric devices.[17] Other noninvasive continuous blood pressure measurement technologies are also available but less well tested.

ELECTROCARDIOGRAPHY

PRINCIPLES OF OPERATION

Few ICU patients are without continuous ECG monitoring because they are considered to be at increased risk for significant disturbances in heart rate, rhythm, or perfusion. Despite continuous monitoring, clinicians are unaware of over 75% of arrhythmias and ischemic episodes detected.[18-20] This problem is compounded by the fact that patients are usually asymptomatic during these episodes, and neither their prehospital angina history nor routine diagnostic testing reliably characterize their arrhythmias or ischemic pattern.[18-20]

A standard ECG recording is only a 20-second snapshot of an 86,400-second day. The ECG monitor, in contrast, with appropriate alarm limits set, warns when rate limits are exceeded *if* the alarms are activated. Another critical observation is that ischemic episodes most commonly occur without significant changes in other hemodynamic variables. There is rarely an inciting factor like tachycardia or hypertension.[18]

Ischemia, as detected by the ECG, is usually defined as ST segment depression of 1 mm (0.1 mV) 60 to 80 milliseconds past the J point, lasting at least 60 seconds. Most ischemia manifests as ST segment depression, with the exception of acute myocardial infarction and after cardiopulmonary bypass. The presence of left bundle branch block or left ventricular hypertrophy obscures the diagnosis of ischemia because of repolarization changes in the baseline ST segment. T wave changes are remarkably common perioperatively (20% incidence rate) and are not in and of themselves diagnostic of ischemia or infarction.[21]

Electronic filtering of the signal, such as occurs when the ECG is used in the monitoring rather than the diagnostic mode or when only the oscilloscope display is viewed, may suggest ischemia that, in fact, is not present. Conversely, the ECG may appear normal on the oscilloscope tracing, although clear evidence of ST segment depression is evident on a strip chart recording. If the screen display of an ECG monitor is filtered, there is no substitute for a properly calibrated strip chart recording. The admission 12-lead ECG may be used for comparison with subsequent ICU tracings if the lead placement is identical, the calibration is standardized, and the patient's position is similar to that at the time of the baseline recording.

Automated arrhythmia detection and ST segment trending systems faithfully alert ICU personnel to ECG abnormalities, even if they have resolved at the time of inspection. These systems, if used in conjunction with a calibrated strip chart recording, provide hard-copy documentation on which to base treatment. Arrhythmia detection is possible with most ECG leads. Lead II (right arm negative, left leg positive) typically gives the best P wave, which is useful in characterizing supraventricular arrhythmias. However, an esophageal or pacing wire lead, if available, is even better.

DETECTION OF ISCHEMIA

Lead V₅

If it is common practice in your ICU to monitor lead II for its clear P wave, identification of ST segment changes will be compromised significantly. If a patient is at greater risk for ischemia than arrhythmia, lead V_5 is preferred. This unipolar lead is correctly positioned in the fifth intercostal space on the anterior axillary line. Proper positioning of V_5 is not a trivial issue, because the sensitivity of all other leads to detect ischemia is significantly less; in fact, several leads are virtually worthless in this regard[22,23] (Fig. 58-4).

The most compelling study supports the preferred use of V_5.[23] In this study, 61 patients with known coronary artery disease underwent treadmill testing with 87 surface ECG electrodes placed over the torso. Each patient experienced

significant ST segment changes in at least one lead; 87% of these changes were observed in unipolar lead V_5, which was the most sensitive. Interestingly, even in patients in whom specific anatomic knowledge of coronary artery vessel involvement was available, the lead in which ST segment changes occurred did not predictably correlate with the site of the anatomic lesion. Therefore, even angiography cannot be used to predict reliably in which lead ST segment changes may manifest.

Our approach is to monitor V_5 in all patients at risk for myocardial ischemia unless we have specific information, such as an exercise stress test, that a particular patient's ischemia manifests in some other lead. If we have the luxury of a two-lead system, we monitor leads V_5 and V_4, because this approach increases sensitivity by 90% or more and is the single best two-lead combination.[22] No two combined leads have 100% sensitivity for ischemia detection.

Modified V₅ Lead

In some ICUs and in most transport situations, the ECG monitor often has only three leads. In this case, if the left arm lead is placed in the V_5 position and the lead selector switch is set to lead I, a modified V_5 lead (bipolar) is displayed (Fig. 58-5). If a rhythm disturbance occurs and lead II is preferred, it can still be obtained without moving electrodes or wires by changing the lead selector switch to lead II. Be sure to document which lead is monitored and indicate to those taking care of the patient the implications and potential benefits of monitoring the specific lead selected.

Trouble-Shooting

Commonly, an ECG signal is of poor quality or includes 60-cycle or muscle artifact noise. This problem usually can be prevented or corrected by the following: (1) skin preparation

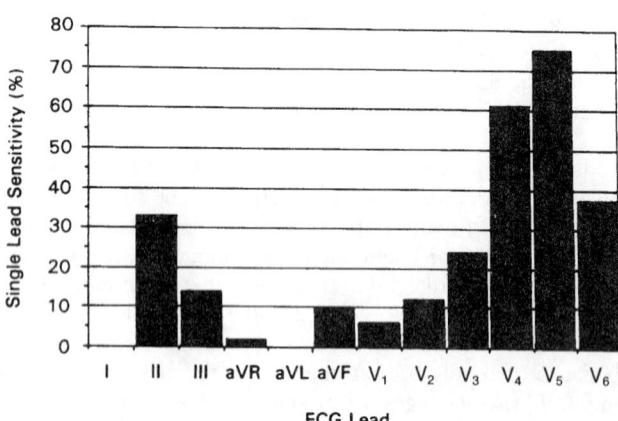

FIGURE 58-4. The distribution of ischemic ST segment changes in each of the 12 leads. The estimated sensitivity was calculated from the number of changes in a single lead as a percentage of the total number of episodes. (From London MJ, Hollenberg M, Wong MG, et al: Intraoperative myocardial ischemia: localization by continuous 12-lead electrocardiography. *Anesthesiology* 1988; 69:232.)

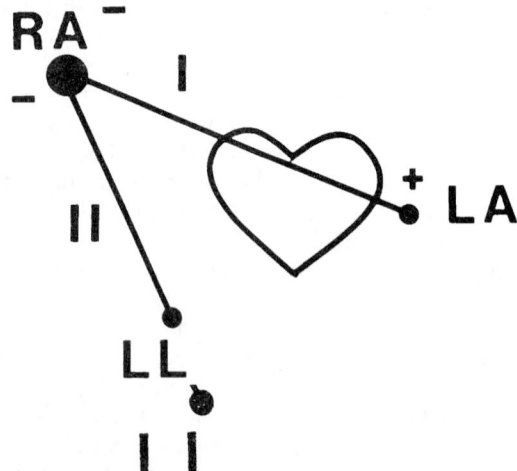

FIGURE 58-5. A three-lead system can be modified to create a bipolar (modified) V_5 lead by placing the left arm electrode (+) in the V_5 position and setting the lead selector switch to lead I, thereby monitoring right arm (RA) (−) → V_5(+). LA, left arm; LL, left leg.

that includes degreasing; (2) use of a single electrode type, which prevents a "battery" effect, because patients from the operating or emergency room often have some electrodes in place that may be of a different brand; (3) keeping other electrical cables away from the ECG cable, because they may otherwise act as an antenna for electrical noise; and, (4) use of a bipolar lead.

PULSE OXIMETRY ■

Cyanosis is an unreliable and late end point to use in diagnosing hypoxemia.[24] For this reason, pulse oximetry, introduced clinically in the mid-1980s, enjoys immense popularity. Severinghaus and coworkers[25] describe it as the most important technologic advancement ever made in monitoring the well-being of patients during anesthesia, recovery, and critical care. This opinion, articulated in 1987, still holds true today. The pulse oximeter is a standard of basic intraoperative and postanesthesia care unit monitoring, and an emerging standard in ICU monitoring.[26]

PRINCIPLES OF OPERATION

Reduced hemoglobin (Hgb) absorbs light differently from oxyhemoglobin ($HgbO_2$). Most pulse oximeters determine oxygen saturation by measuring and comparing the amount of light transmitted at 650 and 940 nm from two light-emitting diodes through a tissue bed to a photodetector. To differentiate light absorption not caused by arterial blood, the instrument algorithm considers only the pulsatile component of the measurement cycle. This beat-to-beat change in local blood volume from the inflow of arterial blood affects the intensity of transmitted light (Fig. 58-6). The ratio of the absorption of this pulsatile component of the signal at these two wavelengths of light corresponds to the ratio of $HgbO_2$ to Hgb, which is converted to percent saturation. This method of arterial oxygen saturation determination is designated as SpO_2 to differentiate it from that determined by gas analysis of arterial blood using the co-oximeter (SaO_2).

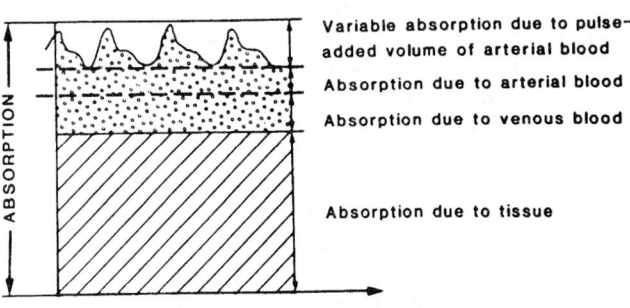

FIGURE 58-6. Tissue composite, showing dynamic and static components affecting light absorption during pulse oximetry. (Adapted from *Ohmeda 3700, Pulse Oximeter Users Manual.* Madison, WI, Ohmeda, 1989:22.)

ARTIFACTUAL READINGS

A pulse oximeter can be applied to any site that allows proper orientation of the light-emitting diodes and photodetector directly opposite one another across an "arterialized" tissue. If the tissue is too thick and attenuates the light before it reaches the detector, the oximeter cannot function. Success has been reported using fingers, toes, ears, lips, cheeks, and the bridge of the nose.

Motion

Motion artifact tends to make light absorption at both wavelengths similar; because an absorption ratio of 1 corresponds to a saturation of 85%, it is common for patients to experience apparent (artifactual) desaturation when motion occurs at the probe site. The response to decreased saturation in a patient who is moving should include assessment that the photoplethysmograph is free of artifacts and that the ECG-derived heart rate matches that of the pulse oximeter. If it does, it is unlikely that desaturation results from motion artifact. Chest compression in cardiopulmonary resuscitation (CPR) induces arterial and venous pulsations. The latter makes the pulse oximeter an unreliable monitor of saturation in this setting.

Position and Ambient Light

Several other factors may interfere with SpO_2 monitoring. Dependent positioning of the monitoring site may cause venous pooling and cause a lower reading from enhanced venous pulsations. Excessive ambient light is corrected by applying the probe so that the photodetector is over the palmar surface of the fingertip and in complete contact with the finger pad rather than on the nail surface. It can also be shielded with a towel or the opaque wrapper from an alcohol wipe.

Nail Polish

Nail polishes, especially those with blue color, may cause low SpO_2 measurements by absorbing light of the wavelengths used by the pulse oximeter. Therefore, nail polish should be removed before monitoring, although what appears to be a normal signal may be obtained despite its presence.

Carboxyhemoglobin

Carboxyhemoglobin may interfere because the pulse oximeter does not differentiate carboxyhemoglobin from $HgbO_2$ and, therefore, overestimates the true $HgbO_2$ fraction. If a patient is at risk for increased carboxyhemoglobin, blood gas analysis using a co-oximeter is needed to determine the actual SaO_2. Interestingly, although the level of bilirubin in jaundice affects the co-oximeter, it does not affect the pulse oximeter.

Penumbra Effect

Kelleher and Ruff[27] describe another common cause of misleading saturations—the penumbra effect. This is an artifactually low saturation that results from improper probe application. If the photodetector is not positioned over a well-arterialized tissue bed, (e.g., the patient with long fingernails in whom the sensing site is across the fingertip instead of the finger), optical shunting or sufficient contamination by venous pulsations can cause low saturation readings. Warm patients with bounding pulses seem to be most susceptible.

Peripherally vasoconstricted patients are least susceptible to this phenomenon, perhaps because no data are obtained unless the probe is ideally positioned over pulsating arterioles.[26] Repositioning the probe readily corrects the problem. In the vasoconstricted patient in whom a pulse oximeter reading cannot be obtained, a digital nerve block using 1% lidocaine without epinephrine into the web space on each side of the digit often restores sufficient pulsatile flow within several minutes to enable SpO_2 monitoring.[28]

ACCURACY

Pulse oximetry differentiates saturation from desaturation. It offers no resolution for PaO_2 above 100 mm Hg because Hgb is already essentially 100% saturated at this level (Fig. 58-7). Thus, an increase in shunting causing a patient's PaO_2 to drop from 160 to 110 mm Hg is not identified by pulse oximetry. More importantly, a drop in PaO_2 from 100 to 60 mm Hg results in significant changes in SaO_2 and SpO_2, yielding a saturation of 90% by both methods. This observation is reassuring because a 90% saturation corresponds to a PaO_2 of 60 mm Hg, a common threshold for clinical intervention. The lack of SpO_2 resolution for changes in PaO_2 above 100 mm Hg is more than compensated for by the sensitivity of SpO_2 to changes in PaO_2 lower than 100 mm Hg. For SpO_2 between 90% and 60%, PaO_2 is approximately equal to SpO_2 minus 30.

The accuracy of pulse oximeters is typically within 2% for values in the 90% to 100% range and progressively less for lower saturations. The sensitivity of the $HgbO_2$ dissociation curve to changes for PaO_2 less than 100 mm Hg suggests that, in patients breathing room air or those whose PaO_2 is less than 100 mm Hg, a pulse oximeter can be used to monitor oxygenation and ventilation. This suggestion arises from the linked effect a change in $PaCO_2$ has on PaO_2, as predicted by the alveolar gas equation during room air breathing:

$$PaO_2 < PAO_2 = FIO_2 \times (PB - 47) \frac{PaCO_2}{R}$$

$$= 0.21 \times (760 - 47) = \frac{40}{0.8}$$

$$= 100 \qquad (3)$$

in which PAO_2 is the alveolar PO_2, FIO_2 is the inspired oxygen fraction, PB is the barometric pressure, and R is the respiratory quotient. If $PaCO_2$ increases by 10 and R = 0.8, the PaO_2 must decrease by 12. Such a change is readily observed by SpO_2 changes at PaO_2 less than 100 mm Hg, and hypoventilation should be included in the differential diagnosis of a saturation change. Conversely, hyperventilation causes an increase in PaO_2 by the opposite effect on this equation.

ASSESSMENT OF PERFUSION

The pulse oximeter also has application as a blood pressure and perfusion monitor. The pressure at which the pulsatile signal is lost during blood pressure cuff inflation correlates well with systolic pressure determined by the Doppler method.[13] A pulse oximeter placed on the thumb also enables a passive Allen's test to be performed; if the signal persists after ipsilateral radial artery occlusion, the hand has collateral blood flow by the ulnar artery. This technique only identifies that collateral flow is present; it does not quantify it. In the patient who has had a vascular procedure, a pulse oximeter placed distal to the anastomosis can aid in identifying a perfusion disturbance.

Pulse oximeters display heart rate and SpO_2, and they give some indication of the pulse photoplethysmogram in digital or analog form. Devices with an analog waveform display, especially if the scale factor can be set, may serve as pulse volume monitors and thereby allow pulse waveform (analogous to systolic pressure waveform) cycling to be observed noninvasively[29] (Fig. 58-8). It can then be quantified by a formal pulse paradox determination.

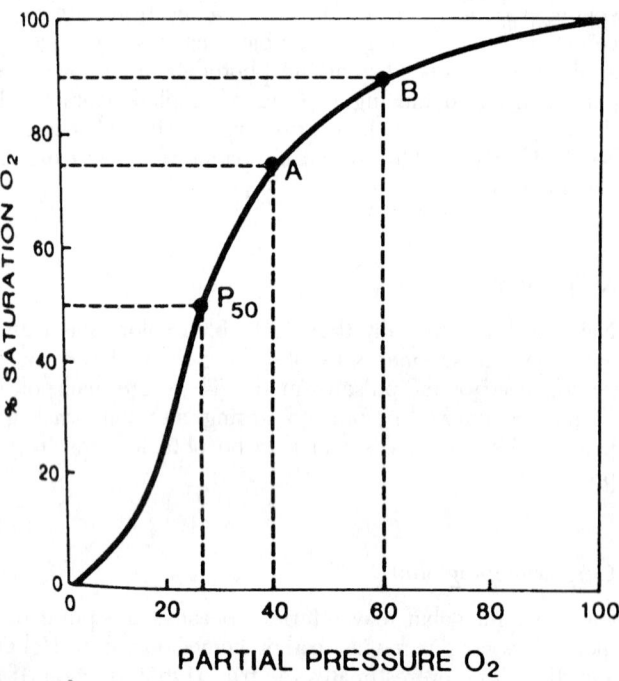

FIGURE 58-7. Oxyhemoglobin dissociation curve for normal adult hemoglobin. Point A: $PO_2 = 40$ (75% saturation). Point B: $PO_2 = 60$ (90% saturation). Point C: $PO_2 = 28$ (50% saturation, i.e., the P_{50} value). (From Bowe EA, Klein EF Jr: Acid-base, blood gas, electrolytes. In: Barash PG, Cullen BF, Stoelting RK (eds): *Clinical Anesthesia.* Philadelphia, JB Lippincott, 1989:679.)

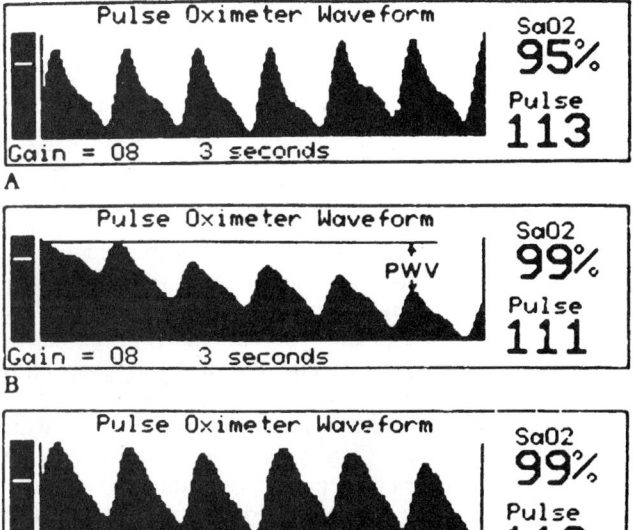

FIGURE 58-8. Pulse oximeter waveform representation. (**A**) When the patient arrived in the operating room, central venous pressure (CVP) was 8 mm Hg. Little variation was seen in the waveform with positive-pressure ventilation. (**B**) After third space transloca-tion and blood loss, CVP was 4 to 5 mm Hg. The pulse waveform varied with respiration. The method for measuring pulse waveform variation is shown. (**C**) After fluid resuscitation, CVP was 8 mm Hg. The pulse waveform no longer shows significant variation with respiration. SaO2, arterial blood saturation with oxygen. (From Partridge BL: Use of pulse oximetry as a noninvasive indicator of intravascular volume status. *J Clin Monit* 1987;3:263.)

CLINICAL APPLICATIONS

Because saturation monitoring is continuous and noninva-sive, requires no calibration, is available within seconds of application, and is a sensitive indicator of hypoxemia, it is indispensable to those caring for patients at risk for hypo-xemia (SpO2 ≤90%, i.e., PaO2 ≤60). The onset or worsening of respiratory failure, acute pulmonary embolism, or failure to wean from ventilatory support resulting in hypoxemia are all immediately identified. Even in patients who are otherwise stable, SpO2 monitoring indicates when a change in the patient's position or care (e.g., suctioning) causes desaturation.

In cases of desaturation, we prefer to use the pulse oxi-meter in the fast response mode. The data displayed repre-sent a 2-second running average rather than the longer 6- to 10-second default averaging interval. We find this change helpful in warning sooner that the saturation is decreasing and in demonstrating improvement of saturation more rap-idly after the inciting factor is corrected. Most devices allow the user to select a response time other than the typical factory default setting of 6 to 10 seconds. Placing the sensor on the ear or nose also enhances the response time of the pulse oximeter, because desaturated blood arrives at these sites as much as 1 minute sooner than peripheral sites, especially in vasoconstricted patients.[30]

SpO2 monitoring has been used successfully in conjunc-tion with capnometry to decrease the need for frequent blood gas analysis and to accelerate weaning from mechani-cal ventilation.[31,32] As equipment becomes available, we think that every patient treated with supplemental oxygen should have pulse oximetry monitoring.[33] Supplemental oxygen does not always correct hypoxemia, and the pulse oximeter readily identifies this deficiency. Intubated patients may develop hypoxemia as a result of mucus plugging, bronchospasm, aspiration, and loss of airway pressure. The effective deliv-ered FIO2 often varies from the FIO2 setting, and masks or cannulas are frequently displaced. The physiologic conse-quences of such abnormalities can be rapidly and reliably detected by SpO2 monitoring.

CAPNOMETRY ■

In the operating room, almost half the critical incidents that can lead to morbidity are related to the airway.[34–37] Routine capnometry, the measurement of CO2 in the respired gas, has been touted as decreasing airway-related critical inci-dents. Since 1991, it has been an intraoperative standard of care to "identify carbon dioxide in the expired gas" every time an endotracheal tube is inserted, and since 1996, con-tinual end-tidal carbon dioxide analysis has been required from the time of intubation until extubation or transfer to a postoperative care location.[26] If in the operative setting the patient lies quietly, is attended one-on-one, and cap-nometry is an accepted standard, it is hard to argue that the intubated ICU patient should be monitored any differently. Capnometry is useful in assessing endotracheal tube place-ment, ventilation, weaning from mechanical ventilation, and the adequacy of CPR.[38]

PRINCIPLES OF OPERATION

Capnometers used in the ICU are usually electronic or occa-sionally chemical. Most electronic capnometers measure CO2 by sending a beam of infrared light through an airway adapter on the endotracheal tube (mainstream or in-line devices) or through a flow of gas sampled from the airway (sidestream devices). CO2 strongly absorbs infrared light at a wavelength of 4300 nm. By continuously comparing the baseline intensity of the infrared light to that transmitted through the respired gas, a CO2 concentration or partial pressure value (capnometer) or graph (capnogram) results (Fig. 58-9). Chemical devices detect CO2 by the chemical reaction,

$$CO_2 + CO_3^- + H_2O \rightarrow 2HCO_3^- \qquad (4)$$

This acid-base reaction drives a pH indicator color change to one of six color zones that correspond to a CO2 of 0.03% or less (purple) to 4% or more (yellow). Table 58-3 compares features of mainstream, sidestream, and chemical CO2 monitors.

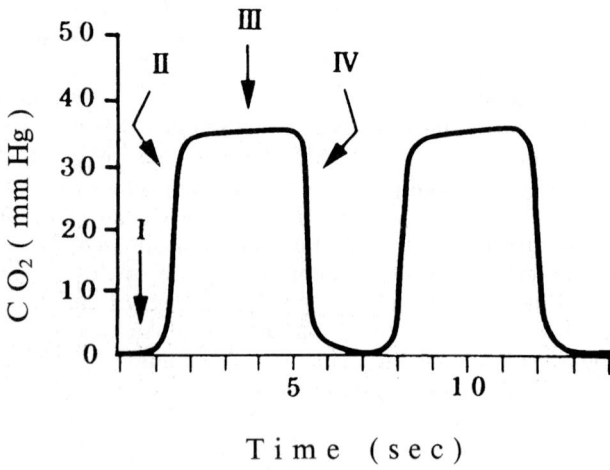

FIGURE 58-9. Phases of the capnogram. Inspiratory baseline (I), expiratory upstroke (II), expiratory plateau (III), and inspiratory downstroke (IV). (From Good ML: Capnography: uses, interpretation, and pitfalls. In: Barash PG, Deutsch S, Tinker J [eds]. *Refresher Courses in Anesthesiology*, vol. 18. Park Ridge, IL, American Society of Anesthesiologists, 1990:179.)

Chemical Monitors

Chemical indicators are disposable, require no calibration, and give instantaneous breath-by-breath results.[39] The adult-size devices have a shelf life of 15 months and add approximately 38 mL of dead space to the airway. These CO_2 indicators are useful during emergent intubations, but they provide only semiquantitative information. The color chart used for interpretation varies depending on fluorescent or other ambient lightning, and its useful life is limited to 10 minutes (manufacturer's specifications) because water vapor degrades the chemicals in the indicator. The device will function for 5 hours if the humidity to which the detector is exposed is limited, as by the interposition of an artificial nose in the circuit between patient and detector.[40]

Chemical CO_2 detectors offer no resolution for CO_2 of 4% or more; therefore, they cannot be used to quantitate hypercapnia. Color changes may be subtle or equivocal with low expired CO_2 concentrations, such as those accompanying CPR or low CO states. Although obvious, repetitive color

changes synchronized with ventilation confirm tracheal intubation, absent or ambiguous color changes do not rule it out; decisions should be supported by clinical evaluation (e.g., auscultation over thorax and left upper quadrant of the abdomen) before replacing the endotracheal tube.[41]

Electronic Monitoring

Electronic CO_2 monitors, in addition to providing high-resolution (1 mm Hg) quantitative data, also provide a waveform and have alarm, respiratory rate, and trending capabilities. Getting your money's worth out of capnometry means having a waveform display (i.e., capnograph) and then inspecting the capnogram like an ECG tracing.

After intubation, tracheal placement is confirmed by the recurring presence of CO_2 after each ventilatory cycle (see Fig. 58-9). Esophageal placement gives either no waveform or rapidly diminishing amounts of exhaled CO_2 and irregular waveforms caused by washout of gastric CO_2. In the emergency room, "esophageal capnograms" may be obtained after esophageal intubation in the patient who has recently ingested a carbonated beverage. The exhaled CO_2, however, is not sustained.[41] If CO_2 is not observed after intubation, failure to ventilate the lungs (e.g., esophageal intubation, obstructed tube, apnea, a disconnection) or circulatory failure must be assumed. Capnograph failure can be ruled out by exhaling your own breath through the airway adapter or into the sampling line.

CAPNOGRAPHIC PHASES. The four phases of the capnogram are identified in Figure 58-9: inspiratory baseline (I); expiratory upstroke (II); expiratory plateau (III); and inspiratory downstroke (IV). The typical shape of a normal capnogram depends on the breathing system being used.

Inspiratory Baseline. A functioning ICU ventilator is a nonrebreathing system, and the inspiratory baseline is expected to be zero. It may not be zero if the patient is ventilated with a Mapleson D system (Fig. 58-10A) unless a fresh gas flow in excess of twice the minute ventilation with a slow respiratory rate is used (see Fig. 58-10B).

The inspiratory baseline is also elevated if water or mucus accumulates in the infrared light path. With sidestream cap-

TABLE 58-3. Chemical and Electronic Carbon Dioxide Monitors

CHARACTERISTIC	CHEMICAL DEVICES	SIDESTREAM ELECTRONIC DEVICES	MAINSTREAM ELECTRONIC DEVICES
Breath-by-breath	+	+	+
Increased dead space	+ +	−	±
Quantitative	−	+	+
Long-term use	−	+	+
Requires calibration gas	−	+	−
Respiratory rate	−	+	+
Alarm	−	+	+
Diagnose hypercapnia	−	+	+
Power requirement	−	+	+

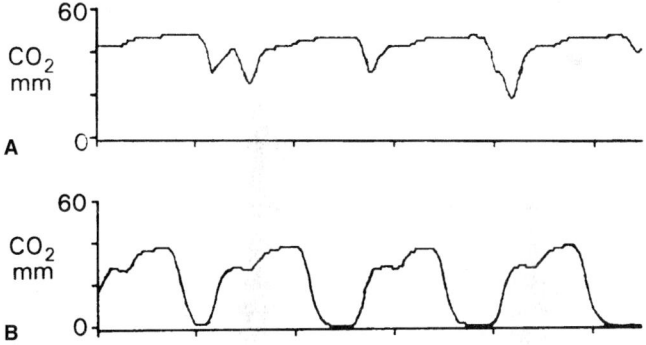

FIGURE 58-10. Capnogram from a patient ventilated with a Mapleson D system using (**A**) 1 L/min fresh gas flow and (**B**) 10 L/min fresh gas flow.

nography, this artifact is best avoided by using a filter in the sampling line and a heat and moisture exchanger between the patient and sampling site. If a humidifier is included in the breathing circuit, the sampling site should be in a nondependent position. With mainstream sensors, moisture accumulation in the light path is inhibited by keeping the windows of the airway adapter oriented perpendicular to the floor and by heating the adapter.

Expiratory Upstroke. The second phase of the capnogram (see Fig. 58-9) signals exhalation of alveolar gas; if normal, it rises rapidly. A slanted upstroke suggests obstruction in the breathing system (e.g., kinked or plugged endotracheal tube) or in the patient's airways (e.g., chronic obstructive lung disease [COLD] or bronchospasm).

Expiratory Plateau. The third phase should be relatively flat. The end of the plateau (end tidal) normally has the highest CO_2 concentration and correlates best with $Paco_2$. If the plateau phase does not level off, it suggests incomplete emptying of the lungs and makes the peak exhaled CO_2 value a much less reliable predictor of $Paco_2$. If the plateau phase is slanted, the patient and breathing circuit should be examined for bronchospasm or partial obstruction. If the patient's breathing pattern is irregular, a discrepancy is often observed between the reported (often averaged or last breath only) peak exhaled CO_2 and the highest value observed on inspection of the capnogram. If this difference occurs, the highest value is always the most representative of $Paco_2$.[42]

With slow respiratory rates and long expiratory pauses, irregularities in the capnogram plateau and plateau decay are commonly seen. These irregularities have no diagnostic significance and are caused by small air movements in the airway from changes in thoracic volume associated with the cardiac cycle and a net gas flow into the lungs; they are called cardiogenic oscillations. Decay of plateau phase in this setting also occurs if sidestream capnography is used because the constant sampling flow continuously draws fresh gas from the breathing circuit forward to the sampling line.

Inspiratory Downstroke. Like the expiratory upstroke, the inspiratory downstroke should be brisk (see Fig. 58-9). A slanted downstroke suggests slow airflow from partial obstruction or partial rebreathing, as with a Mapleson D breathing system (see Fig. 58-10).

Capnometry and the Mapleson D Breathing System

Mapleson D breathing systems provide effective ventilation but usually produce some rebreathing of CO_2. If the rebreathing is excessive or the desired end-tidal CO_2 cannot be obtained, increasing the fresh gas flow, not the respiratory rate, is often the best treatment (see Fig. 58-10). Figure 58-11 demonstrates the relationship between fresh gas flow and minute ventilation with a Mapleson D–type breathing apparatus. At low minute ventilation, $Paco_2$ depends on minute ventilation, but at higher minute ventilations, the $Paco_2$ is independent of minute ventilation, depending instead on fresh gas flow. Capnography allows an appropriate fresh gas flow and minute ventilation combination to be chosen. Increased fresh gas flow is immediately accompanied by a decrease in the inspiratory baseline, signaling a decrease in rebreathing (see Fig. 58-10).

Nonintubated Patients

Sidestream, but not mainstream or chemical CO_2 monitoring systems, can be used to monitor patients who are not intubated. Under ideal circumstances, peak exhaled CO_2 obtained from a nasal sampling catheter corresponds well with that from an endotracheal tube or arterial blood sample.[43] Important features of this technique are that nasal sampling is done from patients who are not mouth breathers, from the most patent side (administer a vasoconstrictor first), and from sufficiently far within the nose so the expired gas sample

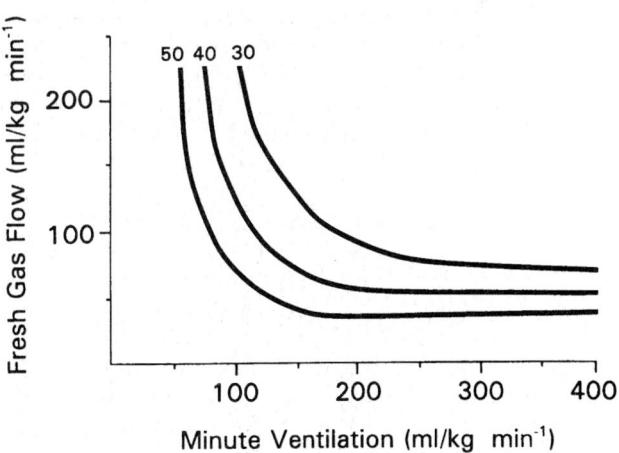

FIGURE 58-11. Nomogram predicting $Paco_2$ at any combination of fresh gas flow rate and minute ventilation with a Mapleson D–type circuit and controlled ventilation. The three curves are $Paco_2$ isopleths at $Paco_2$ = 30, 40, and 50 mm Hg. (Modified from Seeley HF, Barnes PK, Conway CM: Controlled ventilation with the Mapleson D systems: a theoretical and experimental study. *Br J Anaesth* 1977;49:107.)

is not contaminated by ambient air or supplemental oxygen administration.

CLINICAL APPLICATION

Assessing Adequacy of Ventilation

Assessing the adequacy of ventilation is predicated on determining the discrepancy between the desired $PaCO_2$ and the actual $PaCO_2$. The capnometer is a useful tool to aid in this assessment, but it must be used with an understanding of factors that are responsible for the difference between $PaCO_2$ and peak exhaled or end-tidal PCO_2 ($PETCO_2$). In patients with healthy lungs, the $PaCO_2 - PETCO_2$ difference is usually 6 mm Hg or less. The ICU patient often does not fall into this category and frequently manifests differences of 10 mm Hg or more.[44] Therefore, if it is clinically important to know the precise $PaCO_2$, capnometry cannot replace arterial blood gas analysis. However, this fact should not be perceived as negating the usefulness of capnometry in the ICU; after the difference is quantified, it provides insight into the offset between $PaCO_2$ and $PETCO_2$ under current clinical and physiologic conditions. If these conditions change significantly, the $PaCO_2 - PETCO_2$ difference is easily reassessed by subsequent blood gas analysis.

Causes of the $PaCO_2 - PETCO_2$ Difference

The $PaCO_2 - PETCO_2$ difference occurs from three component sources[45] (Fig. 58-12). The first and most important is the difference brought about by ventilation/perfusion ($\dot{V}/\dot{Q}$) mismatching. An increase in $\dot{V}/\dot{Q}$ (dead space) has a much greater effect on the difference than does a decrease (shunt). In the case of increased dead space (e.g., pulmonary embolism, decreased CO), alveolar CO_2 is diluted with alveolar gas containing no CO_2, thereby decreasing $PETCO_2$ and increasing the $PaCO_2 - PETCO_2$ difference. The amount of alveolar CO_2 dilution is a function of the degree of $\dot{V}/\dot{Q}$ change that, if large, increases the difference substantially. An increase in shunting, on the other hand, only causes an increased admixture of venous and arterial blood (i.e., arterial blood cannot have its CO_2 raised beyond that of mixed venous blood, which is usually only 5 mm Hg higher than arterial). Thus, exhaled CO_2 is virtually unaffected.

The second factor that can affect the $PaCO_2 - PETCO_2$ difference is a discrepancy between the alveolar PCO_2 and the CO_2 of the gas delivered to the upper airway. In this case, mixed alveolar gas is not delivered to the gas sampling system (e.g., high respiratory rate or shallow breathing).

The third source of the $PaCO_2 - PETCO_2$ difference is the instrument itself and includes improper calibration, inadequate frequency response, or leaks in the sampling system. Sampling system leaks entrain ambient air, diluting the gas sampled from the patient.

DIFFERENTIATION. The $\dot{V}/\dot{Q}$ mismatch contribution to the $PaCO_2 - PETCO_2$ difference can be identified only by blood gas analysis. Differences from abnormal lung emptying and shallow breathing or high breathing rates should be expected if the capnogram does not reach a horizontal pla-

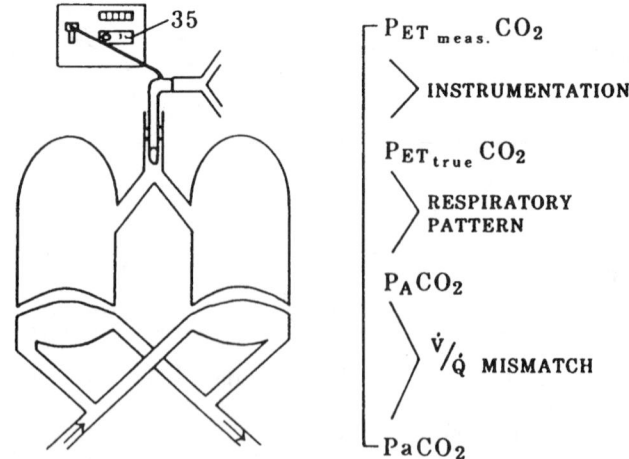

FIGURE 58-12. The difference between arterial and end-tidal CO_2 ($PaCO_2 - PETCO_2$) can be divided into three component sources. The first is the difference between arterial and alveolar CO_2. Ventilation to perfusion mismatching causes this component of the $PaCO_2 - PETCO_2$ difference to increase. The second component is the difference between alveolar and true end-tidal CO_2. Respiratory patterns that do not deliver mixed alveolar gas to the upper airway increase this component of the $PaCO_2 - PETCO_2$ difference. The third component is the difference between true end-tidal and measured end-tidal CO_2. This component of the $PaCO_2 - PETCO_2$ difference increases with problems related to instrumentation. (From Good ML: Capnography: uses, interpretation, and pitfalls. In: Barash PG, Deutsch S, Tinker J [eds]. *Refresher Courses in Anesthesiology,* vol 18. Park Ridge, IL, American Society of Anesthesiologists, 1990:185.)

teau. During mixed breathing patterns, the highest $PETCO_2$ value observed over several minutes is the best indicator of $PaCO_2$[42] (Fig. 58-13). If high-frequency jet ventilation is in use, the periodic interposition of a normal breath produces a $PETCO_2$ that is a reasonable indicator of $PaCO_2$. In patients with COLD, measurement of CO_2 partial pressure at maximal expiration markedly improves the correlation between $PETCO_2$ and $PaCO_2$.[46] This effect can be achieved through a voluntary maneuver by a cooperative patient or by interposing an expiratory pause after a mechanical breath if the patient is unable to cooperate. Interruption of ventilation to achieve a maximal exhaled CO_2 also has been proposed by Chopin and others[44] as a technique to rule out the diagnosis of pulmonary embolism. These investigators suggest that an R value less than 5% eliminates pulmonary embolus as a consideration when

$$R = ([1 - PemCO_2/PaCO_2) \times 100 \qquad (5)$$

where $PemCO_2$ is the maximal expired CO_2 determined by an interruption of mechanical ventilatory support in sedated, paralyzed COLD patients with acute respiratory failure[44] (Fig. 58-14).

To rule out an instrument source of $PaCO_2 - PETCO_2$ difference, the instrument can be calibrated with a known gas or by analyzing the operator's own peak exhaled CO_2. If this value is 30 to 35 mm Hg, a significant calibration error is unlikely. If a respiratory rate of 16 or higher is present, some devices have an inadequate frequency re-

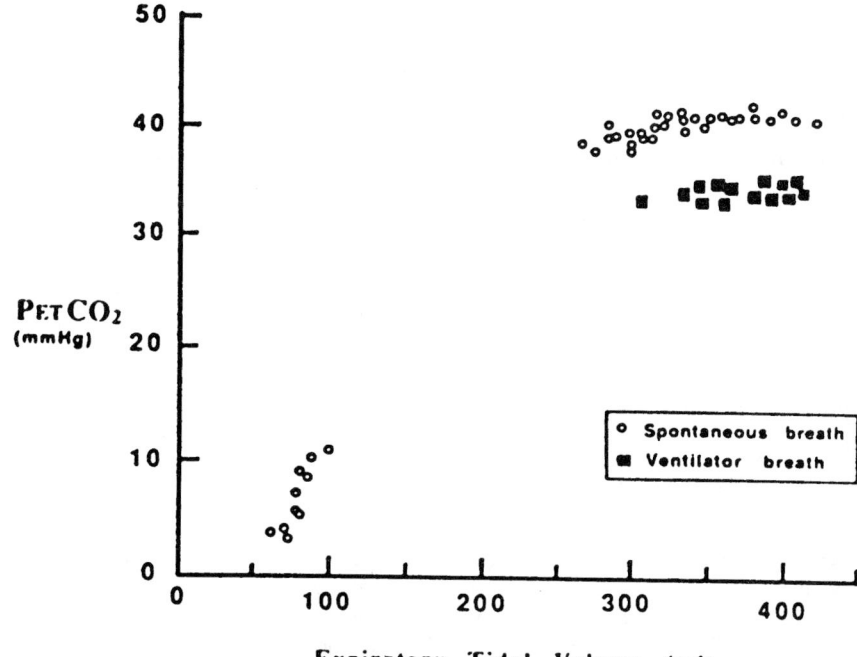

FIGURE 58-13. The end-tidal pressure of carbon dioxide (PETCO2) versus expiratory tidal volume plot is presented for a representative subject. The graph demonstrates the two classes of spontaneous breaths. The PETCO2 for spontaneous breaths with moderate tidal volumes is generally greater than that for ventilator breaths. (From Weinger MB, Brimm JE: End-tidal carbon dioxide as a measure of arterial carbon dioxide during intermittent mandatory ventilation. *J Clin Monit* 1987;3:77.)

sponse, manifested by a rounded waveform and the artifactual appearance of inspired CO_2.[47] Hence, the monitor does not return to zero during inspiration. When this problem occurs, we make a partial correction by summing inspired and peak expired CO_2 to get a better estimate of $PaCO_2$.

Capnography During Transport

Capnography assists the clinician in many ways during the transport of intubated ICU patients. Because of the battery-operated capability of most devices, it can indicate changes in ventilation. Blood gas values (pH and $PaCO_2$) commonly

change during transport.[48] If manual ventilation is used, $PaCO_2$ and pH changes are more likely to be associated with a hemodynamic effect than is a change in PaO_2[48] because of the almost universal use of 100% oxygen during transport. The resulting increase in PaO_2 is harmless, and decreases in PaO_2, if they occur, are evident by pulse oximetry. $PaCO_2$, on the other hand, may change from alterations in either total or effective minute ventilation; the latter situation occurs when a Mapleson D breathing system is used with an insufficient fresh gas flow to prevent rebreathing of CO_2.

Transport also exposes the intubated patient to the risk of extubation and esophageal reintubation. Hyperventilated neurosurgical patients are at particular risk for increased

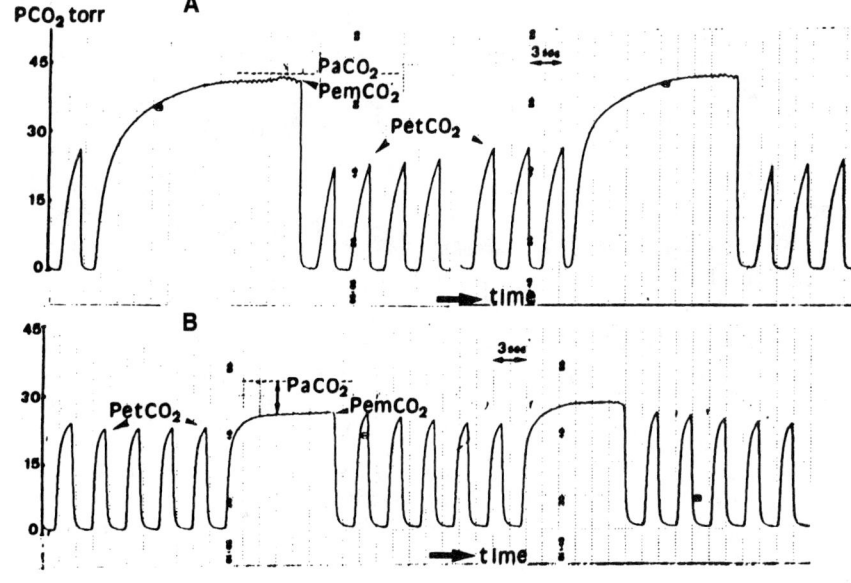

FIGURE 58-14. Two examples of the maximal expired carbon dioxide pressure (PemCO2) measurement, showing typical capnographic recordings. (**A**) Chronic obstructive lung disease (COLD) patient without PE; PaCO2 is 43 mm Hg, PemCO2 is 42 mm Hg, P(a − em)CO2 is 1 mm Hg (i.e., R = 2%). (**B**) COLD patient with PE; PaCO2 is 32 mm Hg, PemCO2 is 25 mm Hg, P(a − em)CO2 is 7 mm Hg (i.e., R = 22%). (From Chopin C, Fesard P, Mangalaboyi J, et al: Use of capnography in diagnosis of pulmonary embolism during acute respiratory failure of chronic obstructive pulmonary disease. *Crit Care Med* 1990;18:353.)

intracranial pressure because they may no longer be in a head-elevated position and may receive inadequate ventilation. During radiographic studies, ICU patients frequently are isolated from ICU personnel. The capnograph in this situation provides an additional benefit by displaying data visible from a safe position behind protective shielding.

Capnography During Cardiopulmonary Resuscitation

Carbon dioxide monitoring during CPR provides interesting and clinically useful data. Cardiac arrest stops pulmonary and systemic blood flow. If the patient is ventilated at this time, exhaled CO_2, over the course of the next few breaths, decreases in a stepwise fashion until it becomes zero or circulation is restored[49] (Fig. 58-15). Cardiac arrest creates an infinite $\dot{V}/\dot{Q}$ ratio (i.e., $\dot{Q} = 0$).

CARDIAC OUTPUT.   In the presence of *constant* minute ventilation and CO_2 production, changes in P_{ETCO_2} reflect changes in CO, and P_{ETCO_2} reflects the circulatory status during and after CPR.[50] Although some form of mechanical ventilation would be ideal, monitoring P_{ETCO_2} during CPR with relatively constant valved-bag ventilation has proven clinically useful.[49] In the intubated patient during CPR, capnography also can verify tracheal intubation.

OUTCOME PREDICTION.   End-tidal CO_2 during CPR before the return of spontaneous circulation ranges from 0.5% to 2.5%. If P_{ETCO_2} is 15 mm Hg or more at the beginning of CPR, it may predict the eventual return of a pulse.[50] Other investigators are less convinced that P_{ETCO_2} levels achieved during CPR predict survival.[51] The P_{ETCO_2} during CPR is variable between patients and is subject to the ventilation pattern. Some survivors had a P_{ETCO_2} maximum of less than 10 mm Hg. Thus, P_{ETCO_2} alone should not be used to decide when to terminate CPR.[50] After spontaneous

circulation resumes, P_{ETCO_2} at least doubles almost instantaneously because of increased flow of hypercarbic venous blood to the lungs.[49,51]

Failure to achieve recovery of P_{ETCO_2} during CPR should prompt a consideration of the differential diagnoses of an end-tidal CO_2 value less than 1% during CPR:

> Esophageal intubation
> Hypovolemia
> Cardiac tamponade
> Tension pneumothorax
> Massive pulmonary embolus
> Ineffective CPR
> Hyperventilation

Hypovolemia, cardiac tamponade, pneumothorax, and massive pulmonary embolus may contribute to ineffective CPR by preventing adequate cardiac filling.[52] A low P_{ETCO_2} is seen with ineffective CPR, which may result from poor technique (e.g., improper compression location, compression depth, compression relaxation ratio) or from resuscitator fatigue, suggesting that another available person take over.[53] Another cause of low P_{ETCO_2} in this setting is alveolar hyperventilation, which easily occurs during CPR because of the low pulmonary blood flow. If a mechanical ventilator is not available, clinical judgment regarding appropriate ventilation should prevail.

RETURN OF INTRINSIC CIRCULATION.   Another advantage of capnography during CPR is that it almost instantaneously heralds the return of intrinsic circulation in an unambiguous fashion, unlike palpation of a pulse, and does so without requiring that CPR be periodically interrupted. Unlike the ECG, capnography is relatively immune to mechanical artifact. The only false-positive elevations of P_{ETCO_2} in this setting follow a significant decrease in ventilation or occur immediately after bicarbonate administration. A 50-mL ampule liberates more than 1 L of CO_2 as acid neutralization occurs:

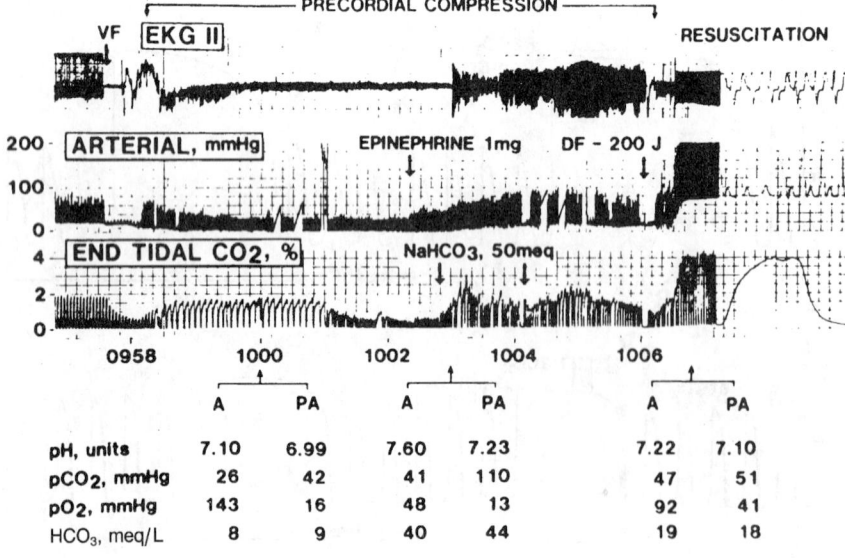

	A	PA		A	PA		A	PA
pH, units	7.10	6.99		7.60	7.23		7.22	7.10
pCO₂, mmHg	26	42		41	110		47	51
pO₂, mmHg	143	16		48	13		92	41
HCO₃, meq/L	8	9		40	44		19	18

FIGURE 58-15. Serial changes in the end-tidal carbon dioxide concentration ($ETCO_2$) and arterial (A) and mixed venous (PA) blood gases in a representative patient before and immediately after cardiac arrest, during precordial compression, and after defibrillation (DF) and resuscitation. The transient increase in the $ETCO_2$ after the administration of sodium bicarbonate ($NaHCO_3$) is also demonstrated. The original tracing has been modified because of space limitations. (From Falk JL, Rackow EC, Weil MH: End-tidal carbon dioxide concentration during cardiopulmonary resuscitation. *N Engl J Med* 1988;318:608.)

$$HCO_3^- + H^+ \rightleftharpoons H_2O + CO_2 \qquad (6)$$

SUMMARY

We think that every intubated patient should be monitored with capnometry and capnography. This approach is especially true for those who are chemically paralyzed and in whom a minor change in $PaCO_2$ may be hazardous (e.g., a neurosurgical patient being hyperventilated to decrease intracranial pressure). Why capnography, a standard for intubated patients in every operating room where patients are observed continuously, is not a standard in ICUs, where patients are less frequently observed, is unclear. The ICU patients are usually more active than the patients in the operating room and at even greater risk for endotracheal tube displacement; moreover, they are often just as dependent, or even more so, on airway support as their counterparts in the operating room.

NONINVASIVE ASSESSMENT OF CARDIAC OUTPUT

The simplest form of noninvasive CO assessment includes relatively simple observations, such as normal mentation, urine output, and circulation time. Circulation time is assessed by administering a substance by a central or peripheral route and timing the administration-effect onset time. A normal arm–heart or brain circulation time is 20 seconds or less.

In one prospective comparison of clinical and pulmonary artery (PA) catheter assessment of hemodynamic values, 53% of clinical CO assessments were incorrect.[54] In half of the patients studied, planned therapy based on clinical observation was altered using objective data from a PA catheter. CO is one of the variables derived from the PA catheter that is also available from several noninvasive devices that use Doppler or bioimpedance technology.

DOPPLER-DETERMINED CARDIAC OUTPUT

A properly positioned Doppler probe can be used to measure the velocity of blood flow in a vessel. If that vessel is the ascending aorta and if the cross-sectional area of that vessel is known (measured) or estimated (nomogram), CO can be continuously and noninvasively determined using this equation:

$$CO = SVI \times \text{aortic cross-sectional area} \times \text{heart rate} \qquad (7)$$

where SVI represents the systolic blood velocity integral that, when multiplied by the cross-sectional area of the aorta, equals the stroke volume.

Methodology

The Doppler technique has been used with the probe placed in the suprasternal notch, the esophagus, or the trachea. If the transesophageal echocardiography (TEE) approach is used, the SVI data reflect descending aortic blood flow; thus, a correction must be made to account for the brachiocephalic blood flow that exits the aorta proximal to the measurement site. This approach requires a reference thermodilution or suprasternal Doppler determination and assumes that the relationship between ascending and descending aortic blood flow and the aortic diameter remain constant. Considerable doubt exists concerning whether either of these assumptions predictably holds true.[55,56] Transtracheal Doppler measurement is accomplished by a special endotracheal tube with a Doppler probe at its distal end.

Accuracy

Substantial literature compares the various Doppler CO technologies with thermodilution.[56-61] Review of these data suggests that, although each of these technologies shows promise as noninvasive CO monitors, none yields data consistently within 10% of that derived from simultaneous thermodilution measurements in adult patients. Therefore, these Doppler technologies are not yet a routine alternative to invasive CO determination. Factors that decrease the correlation between Doppler CO and thermodilution CO are listed here[62:]

Mechanical ventilation
Arrhythmia
Heart rate over 120 beats per minute
Open heart surgery
Aortic surgery
Aortic valve disease
Estimated aortic area
Operator inexperience
Labile blood pressure

BIOIMPEDANCE-DETERMINED CARDIAC OUTPUT

Determination of stroke volume by impedance cardiography was first reported in the 1960s.[63] This technique is based on the observation that blood flow in the thoracic aorta can be quantified by continuously assessing the impedance to an alternating electrical current applied to the thorax. In its current versions, it usually requires that only four electrode pairs be applied to each side of the neck and thorax (Fig. 58-16). One electrode in each pair applies current while the other measures the voltage, allowing calculation of impedance.[62]

Bioimpedance monitoring requires that the patient's height and weight be known to model the thoracic volume as a truncated cone. Some investigators report a systematic tendency for this technique to underestimate thermodilution CO,[64,65] whereas others have reported an unpredictable bias.[66] Bioimpedance-determined CO, however, has good correlation if it is calibrated against a thermodilution device. Bioimpedance technology continues to improve, and in its current form, it seems to function well as a continuous CO trend monitor, even if it is not calibrated to thermodilution values; its continuous function is believed by some to more

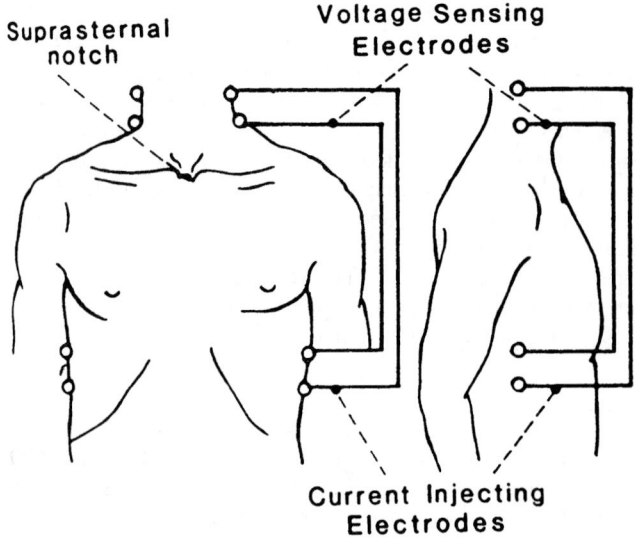

FIGURE 58-16. Thoracic bioimpedance electrode placement. Adjacent electrodes are 5 cm apart. (From Wong DH, Tremper KK, Stemmer EA: Noninvasive cardiac output: simultaneous comparison of two different methods with thermodilution. *Anesthesiology* 1990;72:789.)

than make up for its shortcomings.[67] Several factors have been associated with diminishing the correlation between bioimpedance and thermodilution CO, when it is important to know the "precise" CO, rather than just the trend[62]:

Improper electrode placement
Extreme of body habitus
Pacemaker
Heart rate over 120 beats per minute
Arrhythmia
Open heart surgery
Aortic surgery
Abnormal anatomy
Change in hematocrit
Pleural Effusion

SUMMARY

Because currently available noninvasive CO measurement techniques are sufficiently inconsistent without periodic thermodilution correlation, we cannot recommend them for routine intensive care use in place of thermodilution CO.

ECHOCARDIOGRAPHY ■

Echocardiography offers another method to assess cardiac preload and function. It is used to image the cardiac structures and pericardium from a transthoracic (TTE) or transesophageal (TEE) approach. Echocardiography is the only monitoring instrument available to the ICU clinician that allows anatomic, functional, and hemodynamic diagnoses to be made simultaneously.

PRINCIPLES OF OPERATION

The echocardiograph bombards the heart with high-frequency ultrasound waves, and an echocardiographic image is computer constructed from the reflected ultrasound waves. The transducer consists of an array of piezoelectric crystals that transmit and receive ultrasound waves. The transmitted wave propagates well through tissues but poorly through air or bone. Waves reflect to the transducer crystals from tissue interfaces. By timing the return of reflected waves with their emission, a two-dimensional image can be constructed. Because this process is repeated continuously, a moving picture is produced. In systems that include color flow capability, transvalvular, transseptal, and blood flow directions and patterns can be imaged. This capability enhances the diagnosis and grading of valvular function and septal defects.

CHOICE

The choice of TTE or TEE is a function of probe availability, but it also has implications for the clinician and patient. TTE has a significantly inadequate study (visualization) rate in patients who are obese, have COLD, are elderly, have chest wall deformity, are undergoing treatment with positive end-expiratory pressure, or must maintain a supine position. Examination of prosthetic valves often is inadequate because of artifact and poorer resolution than with TEE. In patients evaluated for atrial thrombus, the left atrial appendage is not visualized well by TTE.

TEE, in general, provides a much better image and higher successful study rate, but it exposes the patient to the passage of a gastroscope. This procedure is uncomfortable and has been associated with a 17% incidence rate of bacteremia.[68] However, in only one of four cases was the same organism identified in dual cultures. Subsequent prospective investigations have shown positive blood culture rates during TEE to be no higher than the background contamination rate observed in the same patient population before the procedure.[69] The TEE approach is relatively contraindicated in patients with esophageal disease or varices because of the potential for esophageal trauma. Studies of TEE in animals and humans indicate that pressures of 10 to 17 mm Hg are exerted by the transducer on the esophagus.[70]

CLINICAL APPLICATIONS

The resolution of TTE and TEE images is good enough that a relatively long list of potential assessment applications should be considered:

Preload
Emboli
Endocarditis (vegetation)
Valvular heart disease
Prosthetic valve dysfunction
Pericardial effusion
Internal jugular vein localization/cannulation
Ventricular function assessment
Dissection of the aorta

Dissecting Thoracic Aneurysms

Diagnosis and classification of dissecting thoracic aortic aneurysms can be made using combined TEE and TTE. The TTE approach alone is not sufficient because the entire thoracic aorta cannot be visualized in approximately one third of patients. Both methods allow diagnosis of aortic dissection, comparing favorably with diagnoses by computed tomography and angiography (Table 58-4). Images generated by newer biplanar TEE transducers are particularly effective in evaluating aneurysm extension into the aortic arch vessels.[71]

Infective Endocarditis

The diagnosis of infective endocarditis is a common but often frustrating challenge for the intensivist. TEE overcomes the reduced image quality problems that hamper TTE examination of the heart valves. It confirms endocarditis more frequently than TTE (Table 58-5) and is particularly effective if the TTE examination is inconclusive[72] (Fig. 58-17).

Valvular Heart Disease

In the ICU, as in the operating room, TEE allows excellent visualization of the heart valves, even in patients with emphy-sema or in those whose lungs are mechanically ventilated. Combining TEE with color flow Doppler imaging allows assessment of the severity of regurgitant valvular lesions. Because of better image resolution, TEE tends to provide better assessment of prosthetic values than does TTE.

Pericardial Effusion and Cardiac Tamponade

Both TTE and TEE can be used to diagnose pericardial effusion or cardiac tamponade, and the imaging technique can guide needle placement during pericardiocentesis. One group of investigators mounted a needle guide on the TTE transducer to help maintain the needle path in the center of the sector scan.[73] Continued assessment after pericardiocentesis enables the clinician to detect reaccumulation of the pericardial effusion. A TTE transducer can be used to great advantage to visualize the internal jugular vein and to guide cannulation.[74,75]

Ventricular Function

Ventricular function can be assessed in the ICU using TEE or TTE, although TTE examination is often unsatisfactory in critically ill patients. Global function, or contractility, is assessed by calculating the left ventricular fractional area change, typically at the midpapillary muscle level. Regional

TABLE 58-4. Diagnosis Employing Transesophageal Echocardiography, Computed Tomography, and Aortography in Patients With Aortic Dissection

RESULTS FOR PATIENT GROUPS	TRANSESOPHAGEAL ECHOCARDIOGRAPH (%)	COMPUTED TOMOGRAPHY (%)	ANGIOGRAPHY (%)
SURGERY/AUTOPSY			
Sensitivity	98	77	89
Specificity	88	100	87
Positive predictive accuracy	97	100	96
Negative predictive accuracy	93	33	68
WITHOUT SURGERY/AUTOPSY			
Sensitivity	100	93	85
Specificity	100	100	97
Positive predictive accuracy	100	100	94
Negative predictive accuracy	100	98	92
TOTAL STUDY GROUP			
Sensitivity	99	83	88
Specificity	98	100	94
Positive predictive accuracy	98	100	96
Negative predictive accuracy	99	86	84

(From Rennollet R, Engberding R, Visser CA, et al: Transesophageal imaging of the thoracic aorta in aortic dissection. In: Erbel R, Khandheria BK, Brennecke R, et al (eds). *A New Window to the Heart.* Berlin, Springer-Verlag, 1989:140.)

TABLE 58-5.   Positive Findings in Infective Endocarditis by Transthoracic and Transesophageal Methods

INVESTIGATION	NO. OF PATIENTS	DISEASED VALVES	TTE POSITIVE (%)	TEE POSITIVE (%)
Daniel et al	88[*]	A, M, T	60 (16.9)[§]	94 (2)[§]
Erbel et al	20[*]	A, M, T	55	100
Maisch et al	19[*,†]	A, M, T	68	84
	87[‡]	A, M, T	15 (85)[§]	60

TTE, transthoracic; TEE, transesophageal; A, aortic; M, mitral; T, tricuspid.
[*]Confirmed at surgery or necropsy.
[†]Positive blood culture: clinical evidence highly indicative of infective endocarditis.
[‡]Inconclusive TTE clinical symptoms suggesting infective endocarditis.
[§]Questionable findings.
(From: Maisch B, Ertle G, Kleinert C, et al: Sensitivity and specificity of transesophageal echocardiography in the diagnosis of vegetations and abscesses in infective endocarditis. In: Erbel R, Khandheria BK, Brennecke R, et al (eds). *Transesophageal Echocardiography: A New Window to the Heart.* Berlin, Springer-Verlag, 1989:102.)

myocardial function is assessed by apportioning the ventricular muscle into segments and examining these for hypokinetic, akinetic, or dyskinetic wall motion abnormalities. The midpapillary muscle short axis image also is used to detect wall motion changes, because myocardium perfused by each of the three major coronary arteries is visualized in this view. This image level does not provide insight into apical and basal myocardial function, which must be assessed by separately examining the ventricle in these planes.

Ventricular preload is assessed by measuring the left ventricular end-diastolic area, which relates to end-diastolic volume independently of ventricular compliance. The capability to determine ventricular preload noninvasively in critically ill patients has been demonstrated.[76] These investigators used TEE to obtain a long-axis, four-chamber view and then used transmitral pulsed Doppler echocardiography

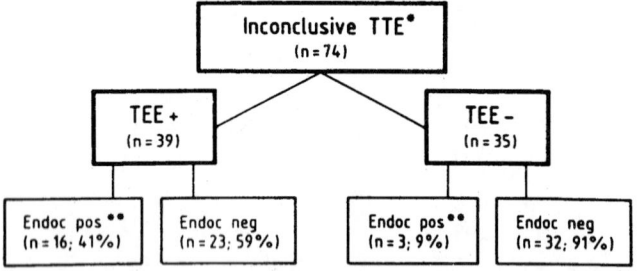

FIGURE 58-17. Findings in patients with inconclusive transthoracic (TTE) results but with indications of infective endocarditis. The transesophageal (TEE) approach is helpful in sorting out patients with old (sterile) or new (infected) vegetations. *, in patients with target symptoms; **, confirmed at surgery or necropsy or positive blood cultures. Endoc pos, positive for infective endocarditis; Endoc neg, negative for infective endocarditis. (From Maisch B, Erth G, Kleinert C, et al: Sensitivity and specificity of transesophageal echocardiography in the diagnosis of vegetations and abscesses in infective endocarditis. In: Erbel R, Khandheria BK, Brennecke R, et al [eds]: *Transesophageal Echocardiography: A New Window to the Heart.* Berlin, Springer-Verlag, 1989:103.)

to measure indices of diastolic inflow to the left ventricle. The A/E ratio of late diastolic active (A wave) to early diastolic passive (E wave) transmitral flow correlated in a highly significant and linear fashion with pulmonary artery occlusion pressure as determined by right heart catheterization[76] (Fig. 58-18). The investigators conclude that data obtained noninvasively from TEE can be used as a reliable measurement of pulmonary artery occlusion pressure.

SUMMARY

Current technologic constraints make TTE and TEE more useful as diagnostic techniques and less so as continuous monitors. The TTE probe must be held in position, and the TEE probe is sufficiently large and uncomfortable that patients need anesthesia or heavy sedation. Both systems are expensive. However, with continued research and development, one hopes for smaller, less expensive echocardiographic instruments in the future.

INVASIVE CARDIAC OUTPUT DETERMINATIONS ■

THERMODILUTION

Cardiac output can be easily measured at the bedside by the thermodilution technique by using a multiple-lumen PA catheter. To use this method with accuracy and reproducibility, one must be aware of and consider the underlying technology and associated opportunities for technical errors.

Principle of Operation

The thermodilution method for measuring blood flow was first described by George Fegler in 1954.[77] Introduced into clinical medicine in 1971 by Ganz and coworkers,[78] this method for measuring CO has been evaluated by investiga-

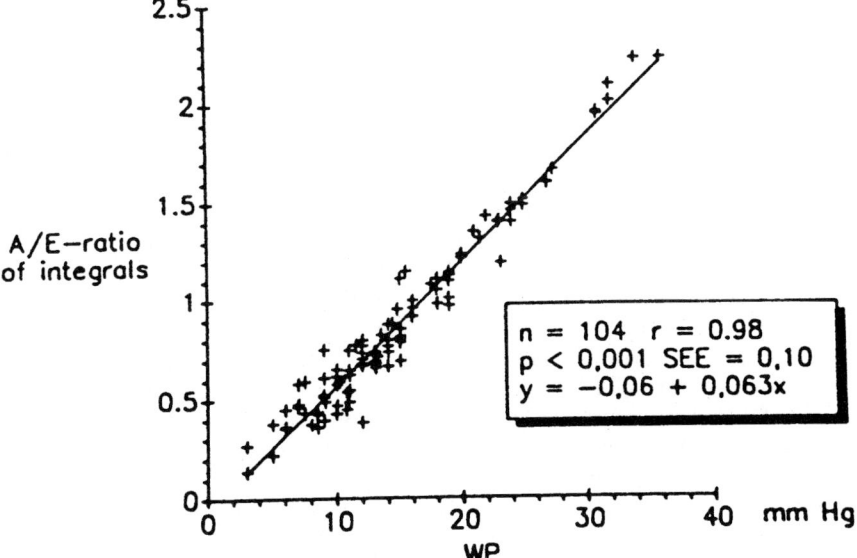

FIGURE 58-18. Regression of pulsed Doppler echocardiograph determined the A/E ratio of transmitral flow integrals to invasively determined pulmonary artery occlusion pressure. (From Störk TV, Müller RM, Piske GJ, et al: Noninvasive determination of pulmonary artery wedge pressure: comparative analysis of pulsed Doppler echocardiography and right heart catheterization. *Crit Care Med* 1990;18:1161.)

tors[78-83] for almost 30 years and is the most widely used technique for measuring CO in the clinical setting.

The principle of thermodilution is an extension of indicator dilution, in which a known amount of indicator (e.g., "cold") is injected at a specified site "upstream" (e.g., right atrium), and the resultant dilutional effect of the indicator as it mixes with blood at a "downstream" location (e.g., PA thermistor) is measured (Fig. 58-19). Using a thermal indicator (cold), CO can be calculated according to the Stewart-Hamilton indicator dilution formula[84]:

$$CO = \frac{V_I(T_B - T_I)K_1K_2}{\int \Delta T_B dt} \qquad (8)$$

where V_I is injectate volume; T_B is the blood (PA) temperature; T_I is injectate temperature; $\Delta T_B dt$ is the change in

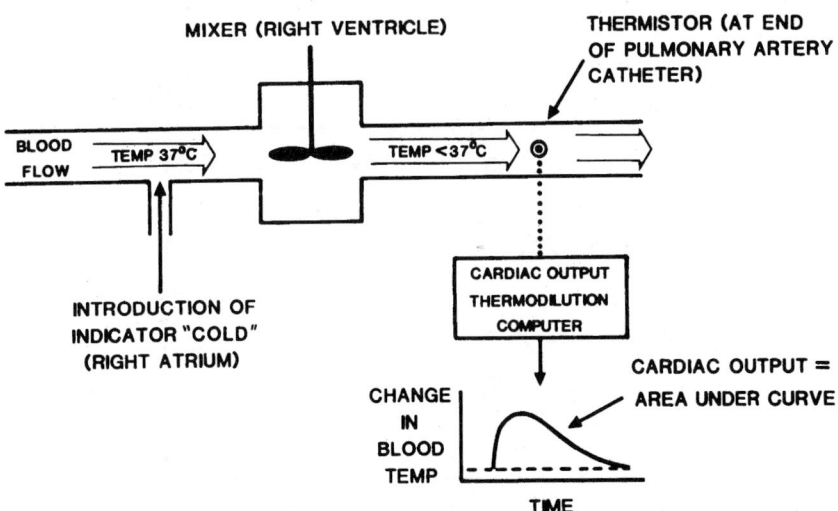

FIGURE 58-19. Thermodilution principle for measuring cardiac output. In this model, a change in the temperature of the blood is created at one point in the circulation (right atrium) by injecting a bolus of "cold" (lower than blood temperature) indicator. The resultant change in blood temperature is detected by the thermistor at a point "downstream" in the pulmonary artery (PA). As the "thermodiluted" (temperature-reduced) blood flows by the thermistor, a transient change in blood temperature with respect to time is detected by the thermistor altering its resistance and generating an appropriate curve. The area under this curve is integrated, and cardiac output is calculated using the Stewart-Hamilton indicator dilution formula. (Modified from Banner MJ, Gallagher TJ: Respiratory failure in the adult: ventilatory support. In: Kirby RR, Smith RA, Desautels [eds]: *Mechanical Ventilation.* New York, Churchill Livingstone, 1985:232.)

blood temperature as a function of time; K_1 is the density factor (injectate/blood); and K_2 is the computation constant.

Familiarity with the components of this formula provides an understanding of the fundamental principles and technical aspects of thermodilution CO measurement and potential sources of errors.

The thermistor of the catheter represents one of four resistors in a Wheatstone bridge electrical circuit (Fig. 58-20). The catheter connected to the CO computer then functions as a complete Wheatstone bridge circuit. Before injection, baseline blood temperature must be determined. In currently available CO computers and catheters, T_B is measured at the PA thermistor once this lumen is connected to the CO computer.

The temperature reference probe continuously measures and enters T_I. At baseline, before the injection, the Wheatstone bridge is said to be balanced, that is, no voltage difference exists across the bridge. Decreased blood temperature resulting from the injection of the cold indicator ($T_B - T_I$) lowers the resistance of the thermistor, resulting in a voltage differential that describes a curve over time. The computer integrates the area under this curve ($\int \Delta T_B dt$), and the resulting calculation is displayed on the monitor as CO in liters per minute.

With this technique, CO varies inversely with the temperature–time integral change (and thus resistance change) created by the cold injection. Thus, the greater the blood flow over time, the smaller the temperature–time integral, the smaller the area under the curve and the greater the CO, and vice versa. In actuality, right ventricular output is being measured: in the absence of intracardiac shunting, right and left ventricular outputs are equivalent, so that CO is assessed based on right ventricular performance. The accuracy and reproducibility of the measurement are highly dependent on correct technique.

Preparation

INJECTATE. Either 5% dextrose in water (D_5W) or normal saline may be used for injection. CO computers accept room temperature or iced (0°C) injectate as a thermal indicator. An injectate reference probe from the CO computer is placed in the same temperature conditions as the injectate solution.

If a room temperature injectate is used, the probe may be placed in a nonsterile infusion bag (not to be used for patient injection because the probe is not sterile) at room temperature in proximity (preferably side by side) to the sterile solution to be used as injectate. Neither solution should be placed on or near electrical equipment, which could warm it. In commercially available systems, the injectate sensor is attached to the connecting tubing; the temperature is sensed as the solution enters the PA catheter.

If iced injectate is used, the reference temperature probe should be placed in a nonsterile solution bag in an iced bath. The reference probe and injectate temperatures must be identical. Commercially available systems for iced injectate are available. Prefilled syringes also may be used as an alternate method for injectate preparation. Injectate temperature, measured by the reference probe, is displayed on the computer.

COMPUTATION CONSTANT. Once the catheter model number and injectate temperature and volume are known, refer to the manufacturer's reference table to determine the appropriate computation constant. This information can be obtained from the computer manual or the pamphlet accom-

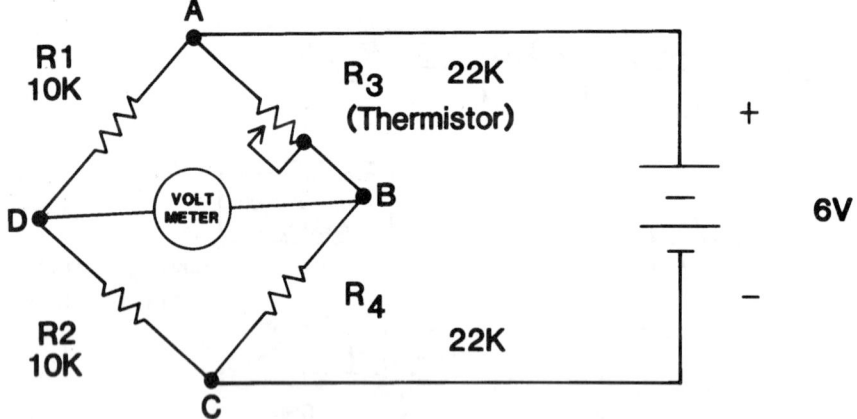

FIGURE 58-20. Wheatstone bridge electrical circuit in which R_1 and R_2 are resistors of 10 kiloohms (k) each, and R_4 is a resistor of 22 k. Resistor R_3 is variable, that is, resistance is proportional to changes in temperature (lower the temperature, lower the resistance). The R_3 leg of the bridge represents the thermistor of the pulmonary artery catheter. At baseline, the resistance of R_3 is assumed to be 22 k. When a driving voltage of, for example, 6 V is placed across the bridge at points marked A and C, currents develop in the circuit with one current flowing through R_3 and R_4 and a second current flowing through R_1 and R_2. As long as the ratio of R_4/R_3 and R_2/R_1 is equal, (22/22 = 10/10), the voltage difference developed (measured by a voltmeter) between points B and D will be null. The bridge is then considered balanced. Any variation in the resistance of the thermistor causes the bridge to become unbalanced, resulting in a voltage difference across points B and D.

panying each PA catheter in the packaging. A copy of this table should be permanently attached to the CO computer to provide quick reference. After determining the computation constant, the appropriate value is entered into the CO computer.

CATHETER POSITION.   Catheter position should be verified by observing a characteristic PA waveform. For accurate CO values, the catheter tip should lie in a main branch of the PA (using radiographic verification).

PATIENT POSITION.   The thermodilution technique should accurately reflect CO regardless of the patient's position. However, CO should be measured in the same position in which the other hemodynamic parameters are measured.

COMPUTER CHECK.   The thermistor lumen of the PA catheter is connected to the CO computer cable. Most computers have a self-test mechanism that indicates whether the integrity of the system is acceptable. If the integrity of the system is inadequate, a fault message will appear on the display screen, after which all connections should be rechecked. If these are intact, the problem may be a defective thermistor.

Procedure

The procedure for measuring CO by thermodilution is straightforward, but the accuracy of the method is highly dependent on adherence to proper technique. Once the described preparations are completed, the following CO procedure may be initiated:

1. Check that the computer is in the measurement mode and is "ready."
2. If room temperature injectate is used, the bolus may be withdrawn at any time, providing the filled syringe remains at room temperature. (Never place filled syringes on electronic equipment.) In commercial systems, the syringe remains attached to the closed system, which includes the infusion bag, one-way valve, connecting tubing, and injectate probe. If iced injectate is used, the bolus for injection should be withdrawn from the solution rapidly and injected immediately to prevent warming. The iced injectate bolus should be withdrawn and injected completely within 15 seconds.

    The exact amount of solution should be injected and air bubbles or excess fluid should be removed. Avoid holding the filled syringe, because heat transfer from the hand can warm the fluid (particularly iced solutions) and induce an error in the technique.
3. The computer is activated and the solution injected rapidly into the proximal central venous pressure catheter lumen. Injection should be smooth and continuous without stopping or changing the rate. It should be completed within 2 to 4 seconds. These aspects of actual injection technique are crucial to the accuracy and reproducibility of the method.
4. CO is displayed on the computer in liters per minute.

INJECTATE TEMPERATURE.   Several investigators have demonstrated the accuracy and reproducibility of room air and iced injectate temperatures,[82,85–89] even during hypothermia, hypotension, and low CO conditions once thought to be exceptions to the use of room temperature injectate. These studies showed that despite the maximized signal-to-noise ratio (Fig. 58-21) associated with an iced injectate, in most cases it provides no particular advantage over room temperature injectate when 10-mL bolus volumes are used. However, when 5-, 3-, or 1-mL injectate volumes are used, iced temperature injectates may result in greater reproduc-

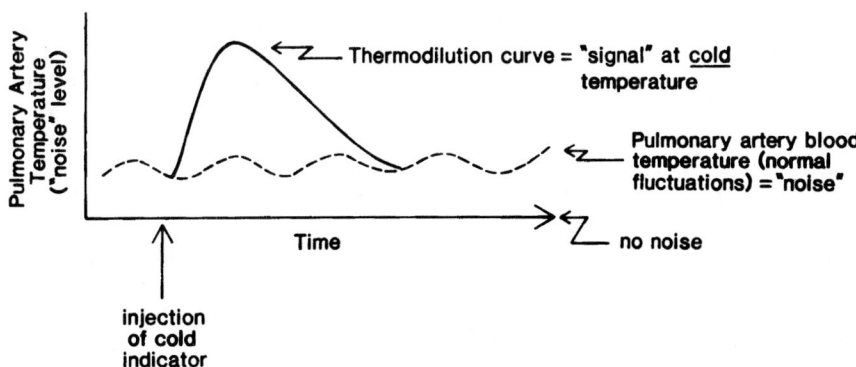

FIGURE 58-21. Diagrammatic representation of signal-to-noise ratio as related to the thermodilution cardiac output technique. Signal-to-noise ratio is the ratio of the amplitude of a signal after detection to the amplitude of the noise accompanying the signal. Relating this definition to thermodilution, signal-to-noise ratio could be described as the ratio of the thermistor resistance change created by the injection of cold indicator ("signal") and the temperature variations occurring in the PA ("noise"). The greater the difference between the temperature change resulting from the injection of cold indicator and the baseline PA temperature, the greater the signal-to-noise ratio and vice versa. Iced injectates result in a greater signal-to-noise ratio than room temperature injectates; larger injectate volumes produce a greater signal-to-noise ratio than smaller volumes.

ibility than room temperature injectate because of the greater signal-to-noise ratio.[88]

Room temperature injectate solutions offer several advantages:

1. There is less chance of obtaining spurious CO values, which can result when the injectate bolus is warmed as it is withdrawn through warm tubing or from handling the syringe or injection delay.[84]
2. Cost is minimized because no special equipment is required to maintain iced temperature, and efficiency is improved because there is no need to wait for temperature equilibration. (It takes about 45 to 60 minutes for syringes or infusion bags in an iced bath to reach equilibration at 0° to 4°C.)
3. Arrhythmias that have been reported to occur with iced temperature injectate are eliminated.[90,91]

INJECTATE SOLUTION AND VOLUME. Either D_5W or normal saline may be used as injectate. The density factor (K_1: the ratio of the product of the specific heat and specific gravity of the injectate to that of blood) for each solution is similar,[79] allowing either to be used. The V_1 used is determined by patient size and fluid status. In adult patients without fluid restrictions, 10-mL boluses are generally used. For pediatric or fluid-restricted patients requiring frequent CO determinations, smaller volumes (5, 3, or 1 mL) may be used. Iced injectate volumes as small as 1 and 3 mL in pediatric patients yield accurate and reproducible results.[92,93] However, smaller volumes (5 mL or less) with room temperature injectate may reduce the signal-to-noise ratio sufficiently to result in less accurate CO measurements.[88,94] Therefore, consider iced injectate when smaller volumes are used.

The volume of injectate must be measured accurately to avoid spurious results. Moreover, it must be injected in its entirely (i.e., no leakage during injection). The injection of less indicator than specified produces falsely high CO values because less cooling of the blood is interpreted electronically as a higher than actual flow. Errors in delivered injectate volume are minimized with larger volumes (e.g., a 0.1-mL error is 1% of 10 mL; the same 0.1-mL error in volume is 3.3% of 3 mL).

In clinical practice, indicator commonly is injected through a stopcock rather than directly into the proximal lumen port. Although direct catheter port injection would appear ideal, it "opens" the system to potential contamination and, because no stopcock closes the system, blood tends to back up through the catheter lumen. For these reasons, this method is less desirable.

If injection is through a stopcock port and iced injectate is used, the injectate syringe should be connected to the stopcock port nearest the proximal lumen port to minimize stopcock dead space, in which the solution is at room temperature. For example, 0.13 mL (with a Pharmaseal stopcock [American Pharmaseal Co, Valencia, CA]) to 0.2 mL (Luer-type stopcock) of injectate remains in the stopcock after injection. This volume is 1.3% to 2%, respectively, of a 10-mL injectate. With smaller injectate volumes, the stopcock content percentage of the bolus volume is increased. How-

ever, with 5-mL injectate volumes, injection directly into the catheter port may be advisable when iced injectates are used. Minimization of errors in injectate temperature and volume is achieved through attention to accurate and reproducible technique.

COMPUTATION CONSTANT. The K_2 is different for each manufacturer, computer, catheter model, T_I, and V_I. It must be determined and adjusted before measurement. The constant is obtained by referring to the manufacturer's table, usually included in each catheter packaging, and in the CO computer operations manual. This constant takes into consideration a correction to the units of measurement (liters per minute), injection or proximal lumen dead space, heat transfer, injection rate, and volume and temperature of injectate.

The proximal lumen should be fluid filled at all times. That portion of lumen within the body contains fluid at body temperature, whereas the portion of lumen lying outside the body contains fluid near room temperature. During injection, these two segments of fluid are injected as part of the indicator, and an equivalent amount of indicator remains in this dead space at the completion of injection. An exchange of temperature also occurs during and after injection between the catheter wall and the surrounding blood. This "indicator loss" at both room or iced injectate temperature and various bolus volumes is considered in deriving the constant.

THERMODILUTION CURVE. Reference to the Stewart-Hamilton formula (equation 8) for calculating CO makes it clear that the numerator variables (V_I, T_I, and K_I) are largely predetermined before the actual injection has been selected; K_2 is entered into the computer; and, once connected to the computer, the catheter thermistor measures T_B. The remaining determination is predominantly the denominator of the equation, or the integration of the thermodilution curve produced by the injection of the cold indicator that determines the CO. Notice that faults in the actual injection technique can alter numerator variables, thus yielding possible erroneous CO values.

Most CO computers actually terminate the processing of the descending portion of the thermodilution curve when it reaches a point equivalent to 30% of the upstroke. The decay of the curve from this point is assumed to be exponential, and the total area, using this assumption, is then integrated. This feature was designed to eliminate potential artifact (e.g., "noise") that may occur during this portion of the curve as a result of PA temperature changes related to other factors such as respiration.

The shape of the curve is of vital importance because the area under the curve is integrated. A normal curve is smooth and typically consists of a rapid upstroke or peak, followed by a slower decay and return to baseline (Fig. 58-22A). Grossly irregular curves are not reliable and are frequently associated with inadequate mixing of the indicator with total blood flow (see Fig. 58-22B). However, small irregularities are common and are the result of normal variations in PA blood temperature. Evaluating the individual thermodilution curves for accuracy and consistency is recommended.

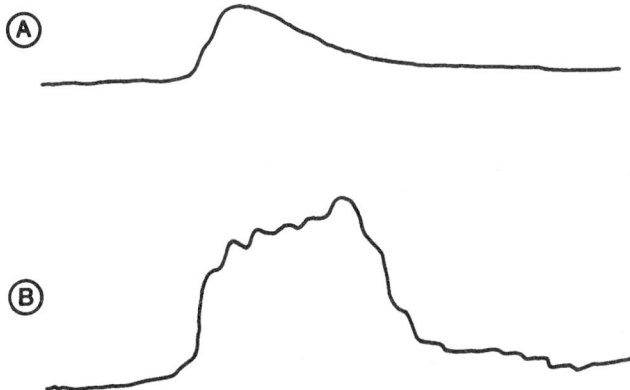

FIGURE 58-22. Examples of thermodilution curves. The curve results from the thermistor resistance change created by the injection of "cold" indicator in the right atrium. Characteristically, the curve should be smooth and consist of a steep upstroke, followed by a slower decline toward baseline. (**A**) Normal curve. (**B**) Irregular curve. (From Levett JM, Replogle RL: Thermodilution cardiac output: a critical analysis and review of the literature. *J Surg Res* 1979;27:392.)

Injection Technique

Ganz and Swan[79] demonstrated that when the injectate is delivered smoothly and continuously within a 2- to 4-second period, CO measurements are accurate and reproducible. Injection rates that are too slow can influence K_2 in the indicator-dilution formula. Smooth and continuous curves are more readily obtained when pressure to the syringe plunger during injection is applied with the thenar eminence, as opposed to the thumb itself. Room temperature injectate does not warm to any significant extent from the time of filling the syringe to injection. However, the temperature of iced injectate does increase during this period but is minimal if injection is completed in less than 30 seconds (from initial withdrawal to completion of injection).[84]

Automatic injector devices show improved injection time, rate, and consistency in comparison with manual injection.[95] These devices may control variations between and within individuals performing manual injections. However, CO values are not statistically different when automatic injection is compared with manual injection performed by experienced personnel.

Injectate Systems

Three types of injectate systems are generally used for the maintenance and delivery of injectate: prefilled syringe, open two-bag, and closed injectate systems.

PREFILLED SYRINGES. Measurements obtained with 10-mL prefilled iced syringes and 10-mL prefilled room temperature syringes are comparable.[96] Syringes can be prefilled and stored in an iced temperature environment or at room temperature.

The major disadvantage of this system is the potential for contamination of the syringe contents. When syringes are chilled directly in ice baths, syringe hubs can become contaminated once the needle and cover or Luer-tip cap is removed; contamination of the catheter or stopcock port may then result.[97] In addition, bacterial growth has been reported to occur in an iced water bath after 3 hours.[97] No differences in contamination rates occur between capped-syringe and closed-loop techniques,[98] but meticulous attention to the capped-syringe technique by the nursing staff is essential. Syringes wrapped in plastic bags before immersion in the iced bath may be less subject to contamination.

When prefilled syringes are maintained at room temperature, 16% become contaminated within the first 24 hours and 45% become contaminated when stored more than 72 hours.[99] The higher "incubation" temperature (room temperature) may predispose this system to increased bacterial growth.

OPEN SYSTEMS. For iced temperature injectate, two intravenous infusion bags (D_5W or normal saline) are generally stored in an iced bath. One is maintained as a sterile source from which injectate is aspirated immediately before a CO measurement; the temperature reference probe is placed in the second bag. Maintained in the same iced environment, the temperature of each bag, despite removal of fluid from the injectate bag, should not vary more than 0.5°C.[100]

The injectate may be aspirated either by a needle introduced into the bag or through some type of intravenous extension tubing. Two sources of injectate temperature error can occur with this setup. First, if extension tubing is used, it must also be immersed in the iced bath; otherwise, warmer (room temperature) fluid will comprise part of the injectate bolus. For example, one commonly used type of tubing with a three-way stopcock has a capacity of 3.6 mL. If all of the tubing is in contact with room temperature rather than iced temperature, 36% of a 10-mL bolus will be at room temperature, creating a significant injectate temperature error.

Second, the syringe itself should be precooled by aspirating cold solution back and forth several times. Aspirating the cold solution directly into a room temperature syringe allows for some amount of cold transfer to the syringe material and, thus, another source of "warming" of the injectate.

Microbial growth occurs in 35% of injectate bags within 48 hours using an open system for iced injectate.[101] Moreover, greater numbers of CO measurements increase the likelihood of contamination because each measurement represents a "break" in the system. The incidence of microbial growth in open room temperature systems has not been demonstrated. However, given the incidence reported with open iced systems and the incidence with room temperature prefilled syringes, it is probably substantial.

CLOSED SYSTEMS. Commercially available closed systems for the maintenance and delivery of injectate are available (Fig. 58-23). These systems provide a sterile conduit from the injectate source to the catheter and are ideal for iced temperature injectate solutions. In addition, an in-line thermistor located near the injection lumen port measures the injectate temperature as it is delivered into the catheter. Many of the temperature errors commonly associated with iced injectate are thereby minimized. For room temperature

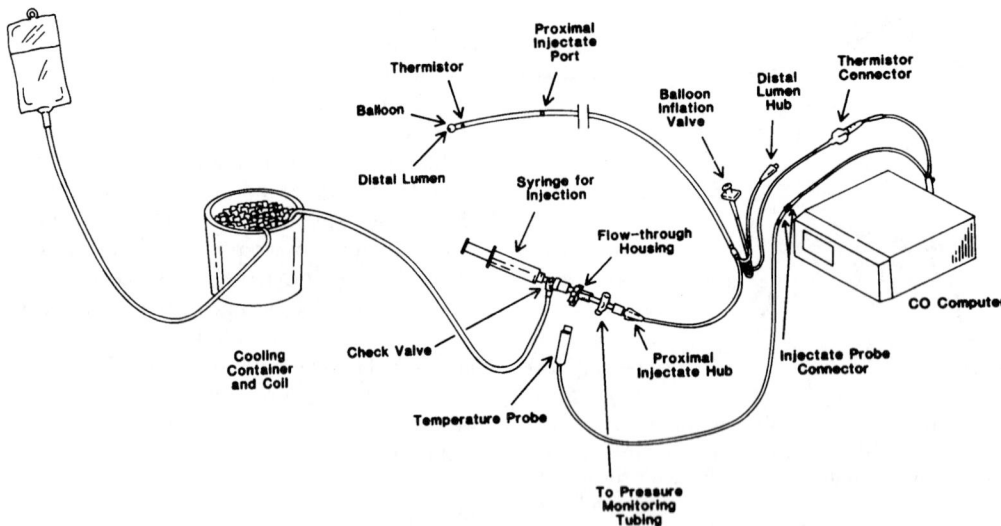

FIGURE 58-23. Example of a commercially available closed–iced injectate delivery system.* The coil of tubing filled with injectate is immersed in an ice bath. Injectate is withdrawn from the iced coiled tubing by the "check valve" and, when ready, is injected through the "flow-through housing" into the proximal lumen. Injectate temperature is monitored by an in-line temperature probe positioned proximal to the catheter port. (*Modified from Co-Set, American Edwards Laboratories, Santa Ana, CA.)

injectates, closed systems can be easily assembled (Fig. 58-24) at minimal cost.

Microbiologic testing of a commercially available closed system for iced injectate (CO-set, American Edwards Laboratories, Santa Ana, CA) showed that only 1 patient in 20 yielded a positive culture result within a 48-hour period (this patient had 61 CO determinations).[101] Another study demonstrated microbial growth in only 1 of 81 samples (1.2%) within a 48-hour period when a closed system was used for room temperature injectate.[99] These data indicate

that closed systems can be maintained and changed every 48 hours without a significant incidence of bacterial growth.

Technique-Related Errors

INJECTATE TEMPERATURE.   Whenever the delivered injectate is warmer or cooler than the temperature selected and used in determining the computation constant, or is warmer or cooler than the temperature reference probe, errors in CO measurement occur. The most frequent tem-

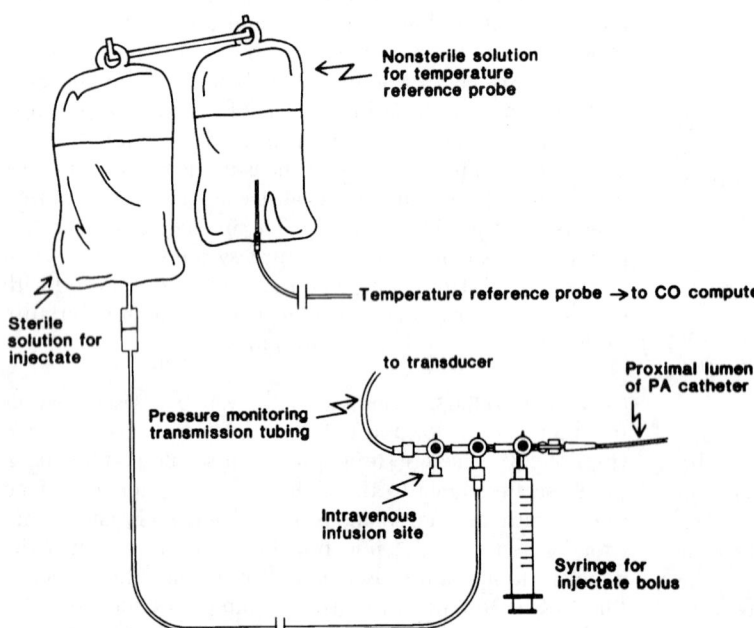

FIGURE 58-24. Example of a closed system for room temperature injectate delivery. The sterile solution bag for injectate is hung side by side with the nonsterile solution bag used for the injectate temperature reference probe (both bags are at the same temperature). Without "opening" the system, injectate can be withdrawn from the sterile source through stopcocks and injected into the proximal lumen. A third stopcock can be added for intravenous infusions. The syringe injection port must be that closest to the proximal lumen port to minimize catheter–stopcock dead space.

perature errors probably occur when iced temperature inject-ate is used, because the latter is predisposed to inadvertent warming of the injectate bolus before injection. Ten-milli-meter iced injectate samples warm from 0.6° to 1.0°C within 30 seconds after removal from an iced bath and warm 1°C every 13 seconds when clasped in a warm hand.[84,85] If all other factors are unchanged, a 10-mL bolus of iced injectate that has warmed before delivery into the circulation can yield a 2% to 3% error per degree warmed (e.g., injectate delivered at 7°C: the error is almost 20%). Thus, meticulous attention to syringe handling and time lapse after withdrawal is essential when using iced injectate solutions.

Use of room temperature injectate solutions minimizes some of the potential temperature errors with iced tempera-ture. Warming of room temperature injectate is not affected by time lapse from solution withdrawal to injection. Holding a room temperature syringe in a warm hand results in a temperature increase of 1C per minute, an unlikely period of delay in clinical practice. Injected boluses that are warmer than the reference temperature yield spuriously high CO values. The converse happens if the injectate is colder than the reference temperature.

INJECTATE VOLUME ERRORS. The selected injectate vol-umes should be accurately measured. If the delivered bolus volume (irrespective of temperature) is less than that chosen, falsely high CO values result (the thermistor detects less cold and interprets it as higher flow).

A common source of injectate volume error occurs when the injected bolus leaks from the site of connection to the catheter or stopcock during forceful injection. Obtained val-ues should be disregarded and the measurement repeated. Another potential error may occur when intravenous infu-sion flow rates are altered immediately before or after injec-tion, that is, a non–steady-state condition.

A change in fluid administration rate just before or during CO determination has a similar effect to that of changing injectate volume in the same direction. Concurrent steady-state infusions do not pose a problem.[102] In patients receiving a vasoactive drug infusion through the injectate lumen, the proximal lumen should be aspirated before injecting the indicator so that a vasoactive bolus is not injected during CO measurement.

Computation Constant Errors

Another source of operator error is entering an incorrect computation constant. A constant that is set too high yields falsely high COs. Measurements already performed with an incorrect constant can be adjusted once the correct constant is determined, as follows[103]:

$$\text{CO}_{\text{correct}} = \frac{\text{computation constant}_{\text{correct}}}{\text{computation constant}_{\text{incorrect}}} \times \text{CO}_{\text{incorrect}} \quad (9)$$

CATHETER INTRODUCER INFLUENCE ON INJECTATE VOLUME. A source of error associated with the use of side-port introducers occurs if the in vivo portion of the introducer sheath covers the proximal (right atrial) exit port or orifice. If this event occurs, the indicator may not be

delivered rapidly or entirely into the circulation.[104] The re-sulting error produces a falsely high CO value because less indicator is detected. This problem is more likely to occur when PA catheters are inserted in the subclavian or internal jugular veins, in which case a shorter in vivo catheter distance is present. Introducer sheaths are usually between 10 and 15 cm in length.

By examining the PA catheter marking at the skin level and knowing the proximal lumen exit port location (usually 30 cm), one can determine the in vivo length and anticipate this problem. For example, if the PA catheter skin level is less than 45 cm in a catheter with the proximal exit port at 30 cm from the tip, the in vivo catheter distance to the proximal exit port is less than 15 cm, and the sheath will cover the proximal exit port.

Hunn and associates[105] compared thermodilution CO measurements in 15 adult patients using a 10-cm introducer sheath and the proximal (right atrial) port located 30 cm from the tip for indicator injection. Statistical correlation ($r^2 = 0.88, p < 0.0001$) and no statistical difference was obtained between measurements obtained less than 3 minutes apart (mean absolute difference 0.3 ± 0.3 L/minute). These data suggest that when the right atrial port of a PA catheter is nonfunctional, thermodilution CO measurement obtained using a centrally placed introducer sheath offers a reliable alternative.

Patient-Related Factors

EFFECTS OF VENTILATION

PA Blood Temperature. Fegler[106] describes a large error that could be introduced into the thermodilution calculations when respiratory movement is significant. Ganz and Swan[79] showed cyclic changes with respiration in PA blood tempera-ture that were negligible during quiet spontaneous breathing but could be greatly amplified in the presence of abnormal respiratory patterns. Snyder and Powner[107] have identified unstable PA blood temperatures in patients receiving me-chanical ventilation and undergoing coronary artery bypass surgery. Alterations in intrathoracic pressures and venous return also have been demonstrated to change baseline PA blood temperature.[108]

These fluctuations in PA blood temperature, probably related to variations in thoracic venous inflow, represent a physiologic "noise" that lowers the signal-to-noise ratio and results in baseline T_B drifts that may affect the reproducibil-ity of CO measurements.[79,109] Most currently available CO computers moderate the potential baseline temperature drift problems by electronically averaging these values over a short period before indicator injection.[103]

Timing of Injection. Minimization of errors and variations resulting from respiratory-induced fluctuations in PA blood temperature may be accomplished by injecting the indicator at a consistent point in the ventilatory cycle, preferably at end-exhalation.[107,108] Unlike intracardiac pressure readings, which are more easily synchronized with end-exhalation, the thermodilution technique requires approximately 8 to 12 seconds of transit time for the injectate bolus to flow past the thermistor.[103] During this time, several cycles of ventilation may occur, making it impossible to obtain an instantaneous end-exhalation value.

Jansen and coworkers[110] could not determine any satisfactory moment during the ventilatory cycle for injection during mechanical ventilation. Reproducibility is best accomplished by averaging CO values obtained at regularly spaced intervals during the ventilatory cycle, especially when mechanical ventilation is employed.[107,108]

When distortion by respiratory movement is large, especially when it affects the steepest part of the thermodilution curve, a large error is introduced into the calculation.[106] Hence, the actual injections should coincide with a period without mechanical ventilation, if possible. The injection should ideally begin at the onset of exhalation during mechanical ventilation, particularly with higher mechanical ventilatory rates. In this manner, the greatest amount of temperature change (i.e., the steepest part of the curve) would be integrated during the end-exhalation phase of the ventilatory cycle.

Rapid-Volume Infusions. An additional source of error is the effect on baseline temperature fluctuations when rapid-volume infusions are administered concurrently with CO determinations.[111] In such situations, as previously mentioned, infusions should either be maintained at a constant rate or temporarily reduced before and during CO determinations.

ARRHYTHMIAS. Arrhythmias may result in CO measurement variability because values reflect the cardiac rhythm and resulting right ventricular output during the computation time only. Although extremely rare, bradycardia[90] and atrial fibrillation[91] have been reported to develop after the right atrial injection of iced injectate solutions. The exact mechanisms are unclear; however, the alternative choice of a room temperature injectate might be considered in such situations.

HYPOTHERMIA. Accuracy in thermodilution CO measurements during hypothermia has been confirmed.[112] In hypothermic adult patients, both 10- and 5-mL injectate volumes at either iced or room temperature correlate well, even at core temperatures between 30.3° and 34.8°C.[85,86] However, when fluid restriction is not a concern, 10-mL injectate volumes are recommended to maximize the signal-to-noise ratio.

HIGH AND LOW FLOW STATES. Few reports have evaluated the accuracy of thermodilution using iced or room temperature injectate when CO was less than 3 L/minute. Above 3 L/minute, no difference in reproducibility and accuracy is observed when 10-mL iced or 10-mL room temperature injectate is used.[94] Variability in measurements increases when smaller volumes (5 mL and, especially, 3 mL) of injectate are used, and even more so if smaller volumes of room temperature injectate are used.[94]

A strong correlation exists between iced and room temperature injectate volumes when CO is measured in hyperdynamic cirrhotic patients, with CO ranging from 6.4 to 11.2 L/minute.[113]

PATIENT POSITION. Measurements obtained in supine and semierect positions show no significant differences in mean values.[114] However, this study did show significant intrapatient changes in some individuals. The thermodilution technique reflects CO in any position.

INTRACARDIAC SHUNTS. Caution should be observed in performing thermodilution CO procedures in patients with intracardiac shunting. If this situation occurs and thermodilution CO measurements are performed, errors may result. With right-to-left shunting, indicator injected into the right atrium may be "lost" to the left side of the heart and never pass the thermistor, resulting in falsely high CO values. With left-to-right shunting, recirculation of cold may occur, as "cooled" blood flowing through the right heart and PA reaches the left side of the heart, passes back to the right side, and is then recirculated through the PA past the thermistor. This situation can produce a second peak in the thermodilution curve, which becomes uninterpretable by the computer. In the case of undiagnosed septal defect, the previously described findings after thermodilution injections might suggest this possibility.

RIGHT HEART VALVULAR DYSFUNCTION. Tricuspid or pulmonic valvular regurgitation may prevent accurate CO measurements because of indicator loss resulting from retrograde flow. In situations associated with significant right heart valvular regurgitation flow, the thermodilution technique may not be accurate.

Pediatric Considerations

Freed and Keane[92] and Wyse and colleagues[93] compared thermodilution to Fick CO measurements in critically ill children and infants and demonstrated that thermodilution is an accurate and reproducible technique for measuring CO ($r^2 = 0.76$ and 0.69, respectively). For intensive care management, 4- and 5-French thermodilution catheters with lumina for hemodynamic monitoring and indicator injection are available. These catheters also may be procured with proximal or right atrial orifice (exit port) locations at 10 or 15 cm from the catheter tip, enabling appropriate catheter selection for different body sizes (7-French catheters are also available with proximal orifice locations of 15 and 20 cm for large children or small adults).

As was mentioned previously, proximal lumen orifice position in the right atrium is an important factor in the accuracy of thermodilution. Location of the proximal orifice in the right ventricle may result in incomplete mixing of the indicator with total blood flow, yielding erroneous CO values. Proximal orifice location in the introducer sheath results in the loss of indicator.

The volume of injectate should be determined by fluid requirements and the weight of the child or infant. The potential for fluid overload in small infants can be minimized by using 1-mL injectate volumes. Excessive injectate volumes in hyperdynamic small children and infants may result in CO errors caused by recirculation.

Because of the small volumes used, most studies in children have employed iced injectate temperatures. Room temperature injectate, however, has yielded accurate thermodilution values when compared with Fick CO determinations.[93] In selecting the appropriate injectate temperature, consider the previously described signal-to-noise ratio factors to ensure or enhance the accuracy of the technique.

OTHER INVASIVE TECHNIQUES

Right Ventricular Ejection Fraction

A PA catheter with a fast-response thermistor and two intracardiac electrocardiogram electrodes to sense the R wave allows measurement of right ventricular ejection fraction (RVEF) and CO. An additional proximal lumen, terminating in a port located 21 or 24 cm from the distal tip of the catheter, is used for injecting indicator and facilitates mixing of the cold bolus above the tricuspid valve. When connected to a single-purpose ejection fraction/CO computer, values can be obtained for right ventricular end-diastolic volume, right ventricular end-systolic volume, right ventricular stroke volume, and RVEF, in addition to CO.

Vincent and colleagues[115] demonstrated significant relatively poor correlation between RVEF measured by thermodilution compared with radionuclear techniques ($r^2 = 0.45$, $p < 0.01$); values obtained by thermodilution were usually lower, especially when RVEF was high. They concluded (questionably) that although some discrepancy was found, thermodilution techniques allow simple, accurate, and repetitive bedside measurements of right ventricular volumes in critically ill patients.

Fick Technique

In 1870, Adolph Fick promulgated a theory for quantitating blood flow that he never used in the laboratory: "The total uptake or release of a substance by an organ is the product of the blood flow to the organ and the arteriovenous concentration of the substance."[116] The Fick technique is a form of indicator dilution. In this method, oxygen entering the pulmonary circulation is the indicator that is measured in the pulmonary blood flow. According to the Fick principle, CO (liters per minute) is equal to the oxygen consumption ($\dot{V}O_2$) divided by the arteriovenous oxygen content $C(a - \bar{v})O_2$ difference multiplied by 100:

$$CO = \frac{\dot{V}O_2}{C(a - \bar{v})O_2} \times 100 \quad (10)$$

If $\dot{V}O_2$ is 250 mL/minute, arterial blood oxygen content is 20 mL/dL, and mixed venous blood oxygen content is 15 mL/dL, then

$$CO = \frac{250 \text{ mL/minute}}{5 \text{ mL}} \times 100 \quad (11)$$

$$= 5000 \text{ mL/minute (or 5 L/minute)}$$

The normal basal $\dot{V}O_2$ (mL/minute) divided by body surface area ranges from 110 to 150 mL O_2/minute/m^2. An error analysis reveals the average error in $\dot{V}O_2$ measurement is approximately 6%, and the error for $C(a - \bar{v})O_2$ is approximately 5%, making the total error in measurement of CO by this technique about 10%, which is somewhat better than the thermodilution technique. The Fick technique is

generally used in the cardiac catheterization laboratory and is most accurate in low CO states in which the $C(a - \bar{v})O_2$ is large.[117]

Dye Dilution

In the indicator dye dilution technique, indocyanine green dye (the indicator) is injected rapidly as a bolus into the right atrium or PA. Its appearance and concentration in a peripheral artery is detected by a cuvette densitometer. The result is a time-concentration curve resulting from the appearance and the gradual disappearance of the dye. Because of recirculation, the curve characteristically includes a second rise. The true "first pass" (of the dye) curve is considered for CO calculations as follows:

$$CO = \frac{\text{quantity of indicator}}{(\bar{c})(t)} \quad (12)$$

where $\bar{c}$ is the average concentration of the indicator during its first pass and t is the total duration of the curve $[(\bar{c})(t)]$ equals the area under the first pass curve). As with other indicator-dilution techniques, CO values are falsely high if the indicator is lost. Recirculation, which has not been considered, results in the indicator concentration being detected twice, yielding falsely low CO values.[41]

Errors with this technique are more common in patients with extremely low CO, severe mitral or aortic regurgitation, or intracardiac shunting.[117] Use of this technique is generally limited to cardiac catheterization laboratories. This method is associated with the risk of allergic reactions to the dye. Repetitive injections also may result in dye accumulation in the blood that can affect later measurements.

Continuous Thermodilution (Heated Filament)

In continuous thermodilution,[118] a PA catheter is modified to include a filamentous heating element in the right ventricle. The filament is intermittently heated, and the heat transfer to the blood results in a temperature change that is detected downstream in the PA as in the conventional thermodilution technique. To filter out background "thermal noise," which is primarily respiratory-induced temperature fluctuations in the PA, this filament heating is done in an intermittent, pseudorandom manner. The heating of the blood by the filament causes approximately a 0.02°C temperature change of the thermistor. The heating coil temperature is limited to 44°C. The uniqueness of this technique is that it uses a "warm" thermal indicator and provides continuous CO data—a distinct advantage over other technologies. This technique/device has undergone considerable testing and, when correctly placed with the heating filament positioned in the right atrium and right ventricle, seems to be sufficiently accurate and reliable to represent a real clinical advance.[119-121] The 75% response time to an in vivo change in CO is 10.5 minutes and may, therefore, initially obscure an acute change. This characteristic is much better than a random check and is a trivial criticism, because the device also has traditional thermodilution capability for the user interested in an instantaneous rather than an averaged value.[122]

REFERENCES ■

1. Robin ED: Death by pulmonary artery flow-directed catheter: time for a moratorium (editorial)? *Chest* 1987;94:727

2. Pollard RJ, Lobato EB: Endotracheal tube location verified reliably by cuff palpation. *Anesth Analg* 1995;81:135

3. Fernandez R, Blanch L, Mancebo J, et al: Endotracheal tube cuff pressure assessment: pitfalls of finger estimation and need for objective measurement. *Crit Care Med* 1990;18:1423

4. Kirkendall WM, Feinleib M, Freis ED, et al: Recommendations for human blood pressure determination by sphygmomanometers. *Circulation* 1980;54:1245A

5. Geddes LA, Whistler SJ: The error in indirect blood pressure measurement with the incorrect size of cuff. *Am Heart J* 1978;96:4

6. Banner TE, Gravenstein JS: How tightly to wrap a blood pressure cuff. *Anesthesiology* 1989;71:A352

7. Perlman LV, Chiang BJ, Keller J: Accuracy of sphygmomanometers in hospital practice. *Arch Intern Med* 1970;125:1000

8. Young PG, Geddes LA: The effect of cuff pressure deflation rate on accuracy in indirect measurement of blood pressure with the auscultatory method. *J Clin Monit* 1987;3:155

9. Frank SM, Norris EJ, Christopherson R, et al: Right and left arm blood pressure discrepancies in vascular surgery patients. *Anesthesiology* 1991;75:457

10. Prineas RJ, Jacobs D: Quality of Korotkoff sounds: bell vs. diaphragm, cubital fossa vs. brachial artery. *Prev Med* 1983;12:715

11. Askey JM: The auscultatory gap in sphygmomanometry. *Ann Intern Med* 1974;80:94

12. Cohn JN: Blood pressure measurement in shock: mechanism of inaccuracy in auscultatory and palpatory methods. *JAMA* 1967;199:118

13. Talke P, Nichols RJ Jr, Traber DL: Does measurement of systolic blood pressure with a pulse oximeter correlate with conventional methods? *J Clin Monit* 1992;8:147

14. Ramsey M: Blood pressure monitoring: automated oscillometric devices. *J Clin Monit* 1991;7:56

15. Venus B, Mathru M, Smith RA, et al: Direct versus indirect blood pressure measurements in critically ill patients. *Heart Lung* 1985;14:228

16. Kurki T, Smith NT: Noninvasive continuous blood pressure measurement from the finger: optional measurement conditions and factors affecting reliability. *J Clin Monit* 1987;3:6

17. Gorback MS, Quill TJ, Lavine ML: The relative accuracies of two automated noninvasive arterial pressure measurement devices. *J Clin Monit* 1991;7:13

18. Shea MJ, Deanfield JE, Wilson R, et al: Transient ischemia in angina pectoris: frequent silent events with everyday activities. *Am J Cardiol* 1985;56:34E

19. Berger JJ, Donchin M, Morgan LS, et al: Perioperative changes in blood pressure and heart rate. *Anesth Analg* 1984;63:647

20. Knight AA, Hollenberg M, London MJ, et al: Perioperative myocardial ischemia: importance of the preoperative ischemic pattern. *Anesthesiology* 1988;68:681

21. Breslow MJ, Miller CF, Parker SD, et al: Changes in T-wave morphology following anesthesia and surgery: a common recovery-room phenomena. *Anesthesiology* 1986;64:398

22. London MJ, Hollenberg M, Wong MG, et al: Intraoperative myocardial ischemia: localization by continuous 12-lead electrocardiography. *Anesthesiology* 1988;69:232

23. Kubota I, Ikeda K, Ohyama T, et al: Body surface distributions of ST segment changes after exercise in effort angina pectoris without myocardial infarction. *Am Heart J* 1985;110:949

24. Comroe JH, Botelho S: The unreliability of cyanosis in the recognition of arterial anoxemia. *Am J Med Sci* 1947;214:1

25. Severinghaus JC, Honda Y: Pulse oximetry. *Int Anesthesiol Clin* 1987;24:212

26. *Standards for Basic Intraoperative Monitoring: Directory of Members.* Park Ridge, IL, American Society of Anesthesiologists, 1996:394

27. Kelleher JF, Ruff RH: The Penumbra effect: vasomotion-dependent pulse oximeter artifact due to probe malposition. *Anesthesiology* 1989;71:787

28. Freund PR, Bowdle TA, Neuenfeld T, et al: Reversal of intraoperative pulse oximetry failure by digital nerve block. *Anesth Analg* 1991;72:581

29. Partridge BL: Use of pulse oximetry as a noninvasive indicator of intravascular volume status. *J Clin Monit* 1987;3:263

30. Wilkins CJ, Moores M, Hanning CD: Comparison of pulse oximeters: effects of vasoconstriction and venous engorgement. *Br J Anaesth* 1989;62:439

31. Niehoff J, Del Guercio C, La Morte W, et al: Efficacy of pulse oximetry and capnometry in postoperative ventilatory weaning. *Crit Care Med* 1988;16:701

32. Rotello LC, Warren J, Jastremski MS: Pulse oximetry weaning of ventilated patients from high FIO₂. *Crit Care Med* 1991;19:562

33. Moore FA, Haenel JB, Moore EE, et al: Hypoxic events in the surgical intensive care unit. *Am J Surg* 1990;160:647

34. Cooper JB, Newbower RS, Kitz RJ: An analysis of major errors and equipment failures in anesthesia management: considerations for prevention and detection. *Anesthesiology* 1984;60:34

35. Birmingham PK, Cheney FW, Ward RJ: Esophageal intubation: a review of detection techniques. *Anesth Analg* 1986;65:886

36. Holland R, Webb RK, Runciman WB: Oesophageal intubation: an analysis of 2000 incident reports. *Anaesth Intensive Care* 1993;21:608

37. Tinker JH, Dull DL, Caplan RA, et al: Role of monitoring devices in prevention of anesthetic mishaps: a closed claims analysis. *Anesthesiology* 1989;71:541

38. Sanders AB: Capnometry in emergency medicine. *Ann Emerg Med* 1989;18:1287

39. Strunin L, Williams T: The FEF end-tidal carbon dioxide detector. *Anesthesiology* 1989;71:621

40. Ponitz A, Gravenstein N, Banner MJ: Humidity affecting a chemically based monitor of exhaled carbon dioxide. *Anesthesiology* 1990;73:A515

41. Sum Ping ST, Mehta MP, Symreng T: Reliability of capnography in identifying esophageal intubation with carbonated beverage or antacid in the stomach. *Anesth Analg* 1991;73:333

42. Weinger MB, Brimm JE: End-tidal carbon dioxide as a measure of arterial carbon dioxide during intermittent mandatory ventilation. *J Clin Monit* 1987;3:73

43. Bowe FA, Boysen PG, Broome JA: Accurate determination of end-tidal carbon dioxide during administration of oxygen by nasal cannulae. *J Clin Monit* 1989;105:110

44. Chopin C, Fesard P, Mangalaboyi J, et al: Use of capnography in diagnosis of pulmonary embolism during acute respiratory failure of chronic obstructive pulmonary disease. *Crit Care Med* 1990;18:353

45. Good ML: Capnography: uses, interpretation, and pitfalls. In: Barash PG, Deutsch S, Tinker J (eds). *Refresher Courses in Anesthesiology*, vol 18. Park Ridge, IL, American Society of Anesthesiologists, 1990:175

46. Tulou PP, Walsh PM: Measurement of alveolar carbon dioxide tension at maximal expiration as an estimate of arterial carbon dioxide tension in patients with airway obstruction. *Am Rev Respir Dis* 1970;102:921

47. From RP, Scammon FL: Ventilatory frequency influences accuracy of end-tidal CO_2 measurements. *Anesth Analg* 1988;67:884

48. Braman SD, Dunn SM, Amico CA, et al: Complications of intrahospital transport in critically ill patients. *Ann Intern Med* 1987;104:469

49. Falk JL, Rackow EC, Weil MH: End-tidal carbon dioxide concentration during cardiopulmonary resuscitation. *N Engl J Med* 1988;318:607

50. Callaham M, Barton C: Prediction of outcome of cardiopulmonary resuscitation from end-tidal carbon dioxide concentration. *Crit Care Med* 1990;18:358

51. Garnett AR, Ornato JP, Gonzalez ER, et al: End-tidal carbon dioxide monitoring during cardiopulmonary resuscitation. *JAMA* 1987;257:512

52. Leiplin MG, Vasilyev AV, Vildinov A, et al: End-tidal carbon dioxide as a non-invasive monitor of circulatory status during cardiopulmonary resuscitation: a preliminary clinical study. *Crit Care Med* 1987;15:958

53. Kalenda Z: The capnogram as a guide to the efficiency of cardiac massage. *Resuscitation* 1978;6:259

54. Celoria G, Steingrub JS, Vickers-Lahti M, et al: Clinical assessment of hemodynamic values in two surgical intensive care units: effects on therapy. *Arch Surg* 1990;125:1036

55. Greenfield JC, Patel DJ: Relation between pressure and diameter in the ascending aorta of man. *Circ Res* 1962;10:778

56. Thys DM, Hillel Z: Can the K-factor be a source of inaccuracy in the determination of esophageal Doppler cardiac output? *Anesthesiology* 1988;69:A2392

57. Siegel LC, Fitzgerald DC, Engström RH: Simultaneous intraoperative cardiac output by thermodilution and transtracheal Doppler. *Anesthesiology* 1991;74:664

58. Abrams JH, Weber RE, Holmes KD: Continuous cardiac output determination using transtracheal Doppler: initial results in humans. *Anesthesiology* 1989;71:11

59. Kamal GD, Symreng T, Starr J: Inconsistent esophageal Doppler cardiac output during acute blood loss. *Anesthesiology* 1990;72:95

60. Huntsman LL, Stewart DK, Banes DR, et al: Noninvasive Doppler determinations of cardiac output in man. *Circulation* 1983;67:593

61. Perrino AC, Fleming J, La Mantia KR: Transesophageal Doppler ultrasonography: evidence of improved cardiac output monitoring. *Anesth Analg* 1990;71:651

62. Wong DH, Tremper KK, Stemmer EA: Noninvasive cardiac output: simultaneous comparison of two different methods with thermodilution. *Anesthesiology* 1990;72:784

63. Kubicek WG, Karnegis JN, Patterson RP, et al: Development and evaluation of an impedance cardiac output system. *Aerospace Med* 1966;1:208

64. Spahn DR, Schmid ER, Tornic M, et al: Noninvasive versus invasive assessment of cardiac output after cardiac surgery: clinical validation. *J Cardiothorac Anesth* 1990;4:46

65. Preiser JC, Daper A, Parquier J-N, et al: Transthoracic electrical bioimpedance versus thermodilution technique for cardiac output measurement during mechanical ventilation. *Intensive Care Med* 1989;15:221

66. Atallah MM, Demain AD: Cardiac output measurement: lack of agreement between thermodilution and thoracic electric bioimpedance in two clinical settings. *J Clin Anesth* 1995;7:182

67. Shoemaker WC, Wo CCJ, Bishop MH, et al: Multicenter trial of a new thoracic electrical bioimpedance device for cardiac output estimation. *Crit Care Med* 1994;23:1

68. Görge G, Erbel R, Henrichs KJ, et al: Positive blood cultures during transesophageal echocardiography. *Am J Cardiol* 1990;64:1404

69. Steckelberg JM, et al: Prospective evaluation of the risk of bacteremia associated with transesophageal echocardiography. *Circulation* 1991;84:177

70. Urbanowicz JH, Kernoff RS, Oppenheim G, et al: Transesophageal echocardiography and its potential for esophageal damage. *Anesthesiology* 1990;72:40

71. Seward JB, Khanderia BK, Edwards WD, et al: Biplanar transesophageal echocardiography: anatomic correlations, image orientation, and clinical applications. *Mayo Clin Proc* 1990;65:1193

72. Maisch B, Ertl G, Kleinert C, et al: Sensitivity and specificity of transesophageal echocardiography in the diagnosis of vegetations and abscesses in infective endocarditis. In: Erbel R, Khandheria BK, Brennecke R, et al (eds). *Transesophageal Echocardiography: A New Window to the Heart.* Berlin, Springer-Verlag, 1989

73. Hanaki Y, Kamiya H, Todoroki H, et al: New two-dimensional, echocardiographically directed pericardiocentesis in cardiac tamponade. *Crit Care Med* 1990;18:750

74. Troianos CA, Savino JS: Internal jugular vein cannulation guided by echocardiography. *Anesthesiology* 1991;74:787

75. Sulek CA, Gravenstein N, Blackshear RH, et al: Head rotation during internal jugular vein cannulation and the risk of carotid artery puncture. *Anesth Analg* 1996;82:119

76. Störk TV, Müller RM, Piske GJ, et al: Noninvasive determination of pulmonary artery wedge pressure: comparative analysis of pulsed Doppler echocardiography and right heart catheterization. *Crit Care Med* 1990;18:1158

77. Fegler G: Measurement of cardiac output in anaesthetized animals by a thermo-dilution method. *Q J Exp Physiol* 1954;39:153

78. Ganz W, Donoso R, Marcus HS, et al: A new technique for measurement of cardiac output by thermodilution in man. *Am J Cardiol* 1971;27:392

79. Ganz W, Swan HJC: Measurement of blood flow by thermodilution. *Am J Cardiol* 1972;29:241

80. Kohanna FH, Cunningham JN: Monitoring of cardiac output by thermodilution after open-heart surgery. *J Thorac Cardiovasc Surg* 1977;73:451

81. Sorensen MB, Bille-Brahe NE, Engell HC: Cardiac output measurement by thermal dilution. *Ann Surg* 1976;183:67

82. Stetz CW, Miller RG, Kelly GE, et al: Reliability of the thermodilution method in the determination of cardiac output in clinical practice. *Am Rev Respir Dis* 1982;126:1001

83. Vandermoten P, Bernard R, De Hemptinne J, et al: Cardiac output monitoring during the acute phase of myocardial infarction: accuracy and precision of the thermodilution method. *Cardiology* 1971;62:291

84. Levett JM, Replogle RL: Thermodilution cardiac output: a critical analysis and review of the literature. *J Surg Res* 1979;27:392

85. Nelson LD, Anderson HB: Patient selection for iced versus room temperature injectate for thermodilution cardiac output determinations. *Crit Care Med* 1985;13:182

86. Shellock FG, Riedinger MS: Reproducibility and accuracy of using room-temperature vs. ice-temperature injectate for thermodilution cardiac output determinations. *Heart Lung* 1983;12:175

87. Vennix CV, Nelson DH, Pierpont GL: Thermodilution cardiac output in critically ill patients: comparison of room-temperature and iced injectate. *Heart Lung* 1984;13:574

88. Elkayam U, Berkley R, Azen S, et al: Cardiac output by thermodilution technique: effect of injectate's volume and temperature on accuracy and reproducibility in the critically ill patient. *Chest* 1983;84:418

89. Shellock FG, Riedinger MS, Bateman TM, et al: Thermodilution cardiac output determination in hypothermic postcardiac surgery patients: room vs. ice temperature injectate. *Crit Care Med* 1983;11:668

90. Nishikawa T, Dohi S: Slowing of heart rate during cardiac output measurement by thermodilution. *Anesthesiology* 1982; 57:538

91. Todd MM: Atrial fibrillation induced by the right atrial injection of cold fluids during thermodilution cardiac output determination: a case report. *Anesthesiology* 1983;59:253

92. Freed MD, Keane JF: Cardiac output measured by thermodilution in infants and children. *J Pediatr* 1978;92:39

93. Wyse SD, Pfitzner J, Rees A, et al: Measurement of cardiac output by thermal dilution in infants and children. *Thorax* 1975;30:262

94. Pearl RG, Rosenthal MH, Nielson L, et al: Effect of injectate volume and temperature on thermodilution cardiac output determination. *Anesthesiology* 1986;64:798

95. Nelson LD, Houtchens BA: Automatic vs. manual injections for thermodilution cardiac output determinations. *Crit Care Med* 1982;10:190

96. Barcelona M, Patague L, Bunoy M, et al: Cardiac output determination by the thermodilution method: comparison of ice-temperature injectate versus room-temperature injectate contained in prefilled syringes or a close injectate delivery system. *Heart Lung* 1985;14:232

97. Mattea EJ, Paruta AN, Worthen LR: Sterility of prefilled syringes for thermal dilution cardiac output measurements. *Am J Hosp Pharm* 1979;36:1156

98. Yonkman CA, Hamory BH: Sterility and efficiency of two methods of cardiac output determination: closed loop and capped syringe methods. *Heart Lung* 1988;17:121

99. Burke KG, Larson E, Maciorowski L, et al: Evaluation of the sterility of thermodilution room-temperature injectate preparations. *Crit Care Med* 1986;14:503

100. Ray C, Carlon GC, Campfield PB, et al: Multiple determinations of cardiac output using a two-bottle technique. *Crit Care Med* 1979;7:33

101. Nelson LD, Martinez OV, Anderson HB: Incidence of microbial colonization in open versus closed delivery systems for thermodilution injectate. *Crit Care Med* 1986;14:291

102. Pearl RG, Rosenthal MH, Nielson L, et al: Effect of injectate volume and temperature on thermodilution cardiac output determination. *Anesthesiology* 1986;64:798

103. *American Edwards Laboratories—Models 9520 and 9520A: Cardiac Output Computer Operations and Troubleshooting Manual.* Santa Ana, CA, American Edwards, 1983

104. Bearss MG, Yonutas DN, Allen WT: A complication with thermodilution cardiac outputs in centrally-placed pulmonary artery catheters (letter). *Chest* 1982;81:527

105. Hunn D, Gobel FL, Pedersen W, et al: Thermodilution cardiac output values obtained by using a centrally placed intro-ducer sheath and right atrial port of a pulmonary artery catheter. *Crit Care Med* 1990;18:4

106. Fegler G: The reliability of the thermodilution method for determination of the cardiac output and the blood flow in central veins. *Q J Exp Physiol* 1957;42:254

107. Snyder JV, Powner DJ: Effects of mechanical ventilation on the measurement of cardiac output by thermodilution. *Crit Care Med* 1982;10:677

108. Armengol J, Man GCW, Balsys AJ, et al: Effects of the respiratory cycle on cardiac output measurements: reproducibility of data enhanced by timing the thermodilution injections in dogs. *Crit Care Med* 1981;9:852

109. Wessel HU, Paul MH, James GW, et al: Limitations of thermal dilution curves for cardiac output determinations. *J Appl Physiol* 1971;30:643

110. Jansen JRC, Schreuder JJ, Bogaard JM, et al: Thermodilution technique for measurement of cardiac output during artificial ventilation. *J Appl Physiol* 1981;51:584

111. Wetzel RC, Latson TW: Major errors in thermodilution cardiac output measurement during rapid volume infusion. *Anesthesiology* 1985;62:684

112. Merrick SH, Hessel EA, Dillard DH: Determination of cardiac output by thermodilution during hypothermia. *Am J Cardiol* 1980;46:419

113. Keen JH: The effect of injectate temperature on thermodilution cardiac output measurements in hyperdynamic cirrhotics (abstract). *Heart Lung* 1986;15:312

114. Grose BL, Woods SL, Laurent DJ: Effect of backrest position on cardiac output measured by the thermodilution method in acutely ill patients. *Heart Lung* 1981;10:661

115. Vincent JL, Thirion M, Brimioulle S, et al: Thermodilution measurement of right ventricular ejection fraction with a modified pulmonary artery catheter. *Intensive Care Med* 1986;12:33

116. Franch RH, King SB, Douglas JS: Techniques of cardiac catheterization including coronary arteriography. In: Hurst JW (ed). *The Heart, Arteries, and Veins,* 5th ed. New York, McGraw-Hill, 1982;1851

117. Barry WH, Grossman W: Cardiac catheterization. In: Braunwald E (ed). *Heart Disease: A Textbook of Cardiovascular Medicine.* Philadelphia, WB Saunders, 1984;289

118. Yelderman M: Continuous measurement of cardiac output with the use of stochastic system identification techniques. *J Clin Monit* 1990;6:322

119. Jakobsen CJ, Melsen NC, Andresen EB: Continuous cardiac output measurements in the perioperative period. *Acta Anaesthiol Scand* 1995;39:485

120. Milhaljevic T, vanSegesser LK, Tonz M, et al: Continuous versus thermodilution cardiac output measurements: a comparative study. *Crit Care Med* 1995;23:944

121. Thrush D, Downs JB, Smith RA: Continuous thermodilution cardiac output: agreement with Fick and bolus thermodilution methods. *J Cardiothorac Vasc Anesth* 1995;9:399

122. Holler M, Zollner C, Briegel J, et al: Evaluation of a new continuous thermodilution cardiac output monitor in critically ill patients: a prospective criterion study. *Crit Care Med* 1995;23:860

Critical Care, Third Edition, edited by Joseph M. Civetta,
Robert W. Taylor, and Robert R. Kirby.
Lippincott-Raven Publishers, Philadelphia, PA © 1997.

CHAPTER 59

Continuous ST Segment Monitoring

David V. Shatz
Valerie R. Wells

Despite decades of research and advanced technology, coronary artery disease (CAD) continues to be a significant source of morbidity and mortality. Nearly two million hospital procedures are performed every year to diagnose or treat CAD; events related to myocardial ischemia account for more than two million hospital admissions annually in the United States. These ischemic events account for more than 13 million hospital days used in this country.[1] Approximately 50,000 patients undergoing noncardiac surgery annually in the United States sustain a perioperative myocardial infarction (MI), and nearly half of the 40,000 perioperative deaths are a direct result of an acute MI.[2] As the baby-boomer generation of the 1950s and 1960s grows older, increasing the average age of our population and the overall number of people at risk for cardiac disease, these statistics will attain an even greater significance. And, as available health care dollars shrink, serious concerns are raised regarding cost of medical care, with a major shift in focus to preventive care. Although it is unlikely that CAD will ever be eradicated, detection of disease and prevention of serious complications, such as debilitating MI, will contribute to the reduction in health care spending. However, to contain health care dollars, diagnostic methods must not be cost-prohibitive. An acceptably predictive, cost-effective preoperative cardiac evaluation should accompany all at-risk patients scheduled for operative procedures. Perioperative noninvasive ST segment monitoring has proven to be a reliable, safe means by which myocardial ischemia, silent or otherwise, can be detected. This should allow appropriate early interventions to curtail the ischemic event and prevent long-term morbidity or mortality.

PREVALENCE OF SILENT ISCHEMIA

The symptoms of CAD are certainly familiar to all physicians, and even most patients recognize the association of radiating substernal chest pain and diaphoresis with cardiac disease. A major concern however, is the frequency with which there are no symptoms, that is, the ischemia is silent. The true incidence is unknown, but studies suggest that as many as 25% of acute MIs occur in the absence of symptoms, detected only by the presence of electrocardiographic (ECG) changes.[3] These are often patients with diabetes or hypertension and without prior angina. The incidence of silent ischemic episodes in patients with typical angina and positive stress tests is well documented and is disturbingly high. As seen in Table 59-1, preoperative ischemic episodes are frequently without symptoms, with some studies reporting the incidence rate of silent ischemia in patients scheduled for coronary artery bypass grafting as high as 93%.[2] Hospitalized patients with unstable angina receiving medical therapy exhibit ST segment depression without accompanying chest pain almost 90% of the time.[3,4]

Of further concern is that episodes of silent ischemia occur at times when they are least expected, in other words, not only during exercise or periods of stress, but even at low heart rates. The Multicenter Investigation of Limitation of Infarct Size showed a marked circadian pattern of MI episodes, with diurnal peaks in the morning (between 8:00 AM and noon) and early evening (6:00 PM to 8:00 PM). The peak occurrence period at 6:00 AM had a 300% higher incidence than at trough periods (11:00 PM). Although the mechanism for this variation is poorly understood, several

TABLE 59-1.   ST Segment Alterations During
Ambulatory ECG Monitoring

REFERENCE	NO. OF ISCHEMIC EPISODES	NO. OF SILENT EPISODES
ST DEPRESSION		
Allen et al[4]	109	67 (61%)
Carboni et al[5]	85	60 (71%)
Cecchi et al[6]	170	116 (68%)
Chierchia et al[7]	278	226 (81%)
Cocco et al[8]	256	138 (54%)
Deanfield et al[9]	1934	1464 (76%)
Ribeiro et al[10]	92	72 (78%)
Schang and Pepine[11]	411	310 (75%)
Selwyn et al[12]	703	590 (84%)
Von Arnim et al[13]	165	107 (65%)
ST ELEVATION		
Carboni et al[5]	14	11 (79%)
Cocco et al[8]	142	87 (61%)
Von Arnum et al[13]	56	37 (66%)
TOTAL	4415	3285 (74%)

theories have been postulated.[14-16] An increase in platelet aggregation in conjunction with a decrease in fibrinolytic activity in the morning hours suggests a tendency toward increased thrombosis.[17,18] Also, peaking in a similar diurnal pattern are circulating serum catecholamines,[19] providing another possible explanation for the increased frequency of ischemic events during these times of what would otherwise be considered low-stress periods.[20]

Several studies also have documented myocardial ischemia occurring at lower heart rates in day-to-day life than during treadmill stress tests. The average heart rate at which ST segment changes appeared was 20 beats per minute less in the ambulatory versus the stress-tested patients[9-12]; nearly 75% of the episodes of ST segment depression in the ambulatory patients were silent. Even mental stimulation has increased the frequency of ischemic events during periods of what would otherwise be considered low stress times; studies have demonstrated coronary vasoconstriction during the performance of mental mathematical exercises in patients with coronary vascular disease.[21,22] In one study, all patients demonstrated perfusion deficits on exercise and 75% demonstrated the same deficits on mathematical computations alone.[22]

One plausible explanation of how ischemia occurs during times of normal myocardial oxygen demand may lie in nitric oxide (previously known as endothelial relaxant factor), a vasodilator present in healthy endothelium.[23-25] This molecule is absent in the endothelium overlying atherosclerotic plaque, resulting in an altered response to endothelial-dependent coronary vasodilators. This would not preclude response to endothelial-independent vasodilators such as nitroglycerin and calcium channel blockers. At the same time that atherosclerotic vessels are incapable of responding to endogenous vasodilators, the abundant supply of alpha-ad-

renergic receptors present on stenotic coronary arteries results in an enhanced vasoconstriction sensitivity to neurohumoral influences. The circadian fluxes of catecholamines and increased levels during mental stress may, therefore, result in ischemic episodes during these periods not by increasing myocardial oxygen demand, but instead by further limiting its supply. Ultimately, the clinical importance lies in the fact that ischemic episodes in patients with CAD may occur even during periods in which no ischemia would be expected.

SIGNIFICANCE OF PERIOPERATIVE ISCHEMIA   ■

Angina in patients with CAD leads to a heightened level of concern and more in-depth perioperative workup and monitoring in the surgical patient. However, patients with disease manifested only by silent ischemia may not be recognized as high risk, and, therefore, may not undergo extensive monitoring, often resulting in an unfortunate, unexpected, postoperative myocardial event.

Raby and associates[26] studied consecutive patients scheduled for surgical repair of peripheral vascular disease and found that patients without preoperative ischemia rarely (1%) had a postoperative cardiac injury. However, 38% of those with preoperative ischemia (97% of the events were asymptomatic) had major postoperative events, all within 48 hours. Preoperative ischemia was most likely to occur in elderly patients (older than 70 years of age) or those with a history of hypertension, previous carotid surgery, angina, congestive heart failure, MI, coronary bypass surgery, or any degree of CAD. However, logistic regression analysis indicated that only preoperative ischemia correlated with postoperative events, and that hypertension, hypercholesterolemia, and noncarotid surgery were of borderline significance. Fleisher and coworkers[27] also found a 38% rate of postoperative adverse myocardial events in patients with preoperative silent ischemia. Preoperative evaluation of high-risk patients can, therefore, be valuable in predicting postoperative adverse cardiac events and in directing therapeutic and monitoring plans.

Patients experiencing postoperative ischemia have significantly worse outcomes than those who do not. In fact, a nearly threefold increase in the odds of experiencing an adverse outcome accompanies myocardial ischemia in the first 48 postoperative hours. Additionally, the risk of a major ischemic event is increased ninefold. The Study of Perioperative Ischemia research group[28] conducted a large-scale analysis of perioperative ambulatory electrocardiographic monitoring and demonstrated that postoperative ischemic changes most accurately correlated as an independent variable with in-hospital death, nonfatal MI, and unstable angina. In the same study, postoperative ischemia was silent in nearly all cases, detected only by ST segment changes. Landesberg and others[29] suggest that the duration of the ischemic event, and not simply the presence of one, was the most significant factor. The number and duration of ischemic events were similar among patients who did not experience cardiac events. In patients who did experience cardiac complications, the number of ischemic episodes was greater and the cumulative duration longer, with the latter being the variable most associated with adverse cardiac outcome in multivariate logistic regression analysis. Eight of 13 patients had ischemic episodes of greater than 5 hours. ST segment depression, rather than elevation, was also the only electrocardiographic manifestation of ischemia, and coupled with the long duration of the event, led these researchers to believe that the inciting cause was not acute coronary artery occlusion, but rather subendocardial ischemia.

Whereas most experts agree that postoperative myocardial events occur within the first 48 to 72 hours, many have demonstrated a bimodal distribution, with the second peak at 6 to 7 days.[30–32] After coronary artery bypass grafting for CAD, ischemic episodes occur most often during the first 48 hours, peaking during the first 2 hours after revascularization.[32] The cause of the immediate ischemia is unclear, but may be a result of reperfusion injury, or of significantly elevated levels of circulating catecholamines and stress steroids. Volume shifts and physiologic stresses peak around the third postoperative day, adding additional work to an already strained myocardium. Of the possible factors, tachycardia seems to be most often associated with ischemia in this early period. Indeed, in noncardiac surgical patients, Mangano and colleagues[33] found nearly all ischemic episodes to be unaccompanied by symptoms but associated with tachycardia. Although a second peak of ischemic episodes has been demonstrated at 1 week, the significance of these episodes may be different. Similar to early ischemia, late ischemia is most commonly clinically silent. In the cardiac surgical group, episodes seem to be less frequent, and in general, not associated with adverse cardiac outcomes.[32] On the contrary, for those occurring in noncardiac surgical patients, although the ischemic burden was highest early in the postoperative course, marked ischemia persisted as long as 1 week postoperatively in the Mangano study.[33] Whether cardiac monitoring is beneficial or cost-effective for this extended period of time is certainly debatable.

PATHOPHYSIOLOGIC BASIS OF ELECTROCARDIOGRAPHIC CHANGES ■

Electrocardiographically, myocardial ischemia may manifest as the appearance of Q waves, deviation of the ST segment, or T wave changes. Deep and wide Q waves, in leads positioned toward the necrotic area, reflect myocardial necrosis. Simply represented, normal ventricular depolarization may be thought of as a small initial force moving from left to right through the septum, followed by a much larger force moving from right to left through the free wall of the left ventricle. A qR complex results when an electrode, oriented toward the left ventricle, detects a small force moving away through the septum, followed by a larger upward deflection (a tall R wave), which is triggered by the spread of the force through the free wall of the left ventricle toward the electrode. Necrotic tissue cannot be depolarized and is electrically inert. A raised and hollowed ST segment in leads oriented toward the injured area suggests myocardial injury.

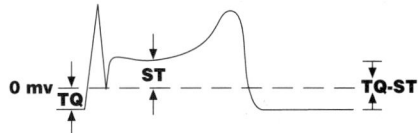

FIGURE 59-1. Electrocardiographic tracing of ischemic tissue. Whether "ST elevation" is actually the TQ depression of diastole or the combined TQ-ST changes of diastole plus systole is unclear.

An inverted, sharply pointed and symmetrical T wave suggests myocardial ischemia. An infarcted region (necrotic tissue, surrounded by injured tissue, and in turn surrounded by ischemic tissue) reflects the three patterns associated with its component tissues: the pathological Q waves of myocardial necrosis, the raised and hollowed ST segment of myocardial injury, and the sharply inverted and symmetrical T wave of myocardial ischemia.

Whether the generation of electrocardiographic changes during periods of coronary artery occlusion are a systolic or diastolic event is not completely understood, but probably results from a combination of progressive decreases in resting membrane potentials and altered action potentials in ischemic cells. The electrical charge of the intracellular milieu of normal cells is positive in comparison with that of ischemic cells, thereby establishing an intercellular current flow toward ischemic cells. This alteration in electrical charge follows the release of intracellular potassium in ischemic cells to the extracellular space. Because of coronary occlusion, potassium is not cleared and, therefore, concentrations rise rapidly, decreasing the resting membrane potential. This decrease in resting membrane potential is seen as a depression of the TQ segment (diastole) on the electrocardiogram.[30,34] Action potential configuration remains unchanged initially, but with approximately 4 minutes of coronary occlusion (this time frame varies depending on the degree of collateralization present), action potential upstroke is progressively reduced to a small amplitude and is evidenced by ST segment (systole) elevation. In situ, these changes occur much more rapidly, with subendocardial TQ depression beginning in 20 seconds and ST elevation between 1 and 2 minutes. Subepicardial TQ depression appears in about 1 minute, with ST elevation appearing at 2 to 3 minutes.[35] Because no distinction can be made between the two on AC amplifiers or monitors, the classic "ST elevation" of myocardial ischemia may actually be TQ depression alone, or a combination of TQ depression and ST elevation (Fig. 59-1).

ADVANTAGES OF ST SEGMENT MONITORING ■

Continuous monitoring of ST segments in intensive care unit (ICU) patients has several benefits. What is believed to be routine daily care for most patients may, in fact, be a significant strain on some. For example, routine suctioning of the endotracheal tube may not be tolerated well in some patients whose myocardia may be prone to ischemia, but which may not otherwise be noted without continuous monitoring of the ST segments. Hence, this monitoring modality provides a means for gauging a patient's ability to tolerate activity and procedures. Once ischemia is detected, the inciting activity can be terminated or modified.

Although seen by nursing personnel, ischemic episodes are often resolved by the time a 12-lead electrocardiogram can be obtained or a physician summoned to the bedside. Monitors capable of recording ST segment changes should also be capable of producing hard copies, and most times should automatically produce a printed copy when the limits of deviation are violated. These printed copies can then be used to verify the ischemic episodes and analyze repeat episodes occurring throughout the patient's ICU stay.

Even when monitored by an experienced physician, ST segment changes on standard monitors often go undetected. In a European study,[36] cardiologists were presented rhythm strips in groups of four along with two other tracings not related to the study. Only 48% of the episodes were detected. Ninety-two percent of the episodes were recognized if only one ECG wave was presented on the screen, and 71% were detected if accompanied by chest pain, thereby calling attention to the event. The low rate of detection is attributed to the presentation of several ECGs at once and to fatigue. For anesthesiologists, the rate of nondetection is presumably considerably higher, because their attention is not solely focused on the monitor screen. Therefore, with violations of preset ST segment limitations and audible alarms to announce these violations, the detection of ischemic events should be markedly higher.

With immediate detection of myocardial ischemia comes the ability to provide immediate therapy. This may be in the form of medication (i.e., coronary vasodilators, afterload reduction, beta-blockade) or simply the cessation of the offending activity. This may be provided at a nursing or physician level, with the ability to analyze both the event and the response to therapy at a later, convenient time. Printed copies attached to the medical records also provide medicolegal documentation, should it be a necessary part of the record.

LIMITATIONS OF ST SEGMENT MONITORING ■

Whereas continuous monitoring of ST segments provides a decided benefit in selected patients, this monitoring modality also has its limitations. Although some of these limitations may be nothing more than annoyances, some acute changes may indicate physiologic changes other than ischemia that are, nonetheless, clinically disastrous in their later stages. For example, ST monitor alarms will activate in the face of T wave changes in hyperkalemia, although no ST segment changes, nor ischemia, have occurred. These early, subtle T wave changes may otherwise be overlooked without ST monitoring.

Several other nonischemic conditions exist that affect the ST segment. The earliest recognizable change of pericarditis is the elevation of ST segments in leads reflecting the in-

volved epicardial surface. Although the configuration of the ST segment differs in pericarditis versus MI (concave versus convex), electrocardiographic changes often precede clinical signs and can alert medical personnel to the developing problem. Hyperthyroidism also can result in elevated ST segments and may be caused by the hyperdynamic state associated with thyroid overactivity. Pulmonary embolism with resulting right ventricular strain (acute cor pulmonale) may be manifested as elevated ST segments with T wave inversion in the precordial leads.[37] This can often be confused with inferior wall MI and must be differentiated by suspicion, clinical examination, and 12-lead ECG.

Several nonischemic conditions can lead to ST segment depression. Digitalis effects are characterized by rounded, scooped ST segments, and are expected in therapeutically digitalized patients. For unclear reasons, hypothermia also results in ST segment depression. As in 12-lead ECGs, bundle branch blocks make it nearly impossible to interpret ST segment morphologic changes. However, with continuous ST segment recordings, trend analysis may become valuable in detecting new ischemic events.

INDICATIONS FOR MONITORING ■

Whereas ST segment monitoring has not been accepted as a preoperative screening tool, it can be used to monitor high-risk surgical patients (hypertension, diabetes mellitus, previous MI, and carotid artery surgery) whose ischemia may not be symptomatic (i.e., silent ischemia). Postoperative continuous ST segment monitoring can then identify within that group those patients likely to experience major adverse cardiac events and for whom early directed therapy can be provided.

In light of the significant incidence of postoperative adverse cardiac events in patients with cardiac disease, we believe that all such patients should undergo both intraoperative and postoperative ST segment monitoring. Similarly, any other high-risk patients should be monitored. Additionally, continuous evaluation of efficacy can be obtained in patients undergoing thrombolytic therapy or percutaneous transluminal coronary angioplasty using ST segment monitoring. Patients with difficult-to-control potassium levels may also benefit because of the earlier detection of ECG changes associated with hyperkalemia.

LEAD PLACEMENT ■

Current technology limits the ability to do continuous monitoring of all 12 leads. Therefore, proper selection of leads influences the accuracy of ST segment values and is crucial if one is to have the greatest chance of identifying all valid ischemic events. Upper limb leads are positioned inferior to the clavicle and laterally, avoiding placement over bony structures and the heart. Minor changes in the position of limb lead electrodes have, in actual practice, produced little or no significant alterations in the ST segment. Care should be exercised, however, not to reposition the V lead (precordial) electrodes, because changes in placement may reflect electrical activity in areas of the heart other than those desired. Some ICUs have opted to mark electrode location in indelible ink on the patient's chest; it is usually unnecessary to do this, but may be assessed on an individual basis.

Appropriate lead selection is vital to obtaining information related to vulnerable areas of the heart. Leads to be monitored for ischemic changes should be chosen in accordance with the patient's coronary vascular (angiographic) history, when available, or knowledge of previous myocardial events. Table 59-2 details leads representative of specific coronary vessels and associated areas of the heart; this information is used in lead selection when cardiac history is known. Occlusion of the right coronary artery leads to inferior wall infarction, whereas occlusion of the left coronary system results in either massive left ventricular infarction (left main coronary artery), apical, anterior, or septal infarction (left anterior descending artery), or lateral, inferolateral, or true posterior wall infarction (left circumflex artery). It follows, therefore, that optimal lead placement reflects the areas of highest probability for disease. In patients undergoing percutaneous transluminal angioplasty, Krucoff[38] has documented the incidence of ST segment changes corresponding to specific vascular occlusions. With occlusion of the left anterior descending artery, approximately 95% of patients had ST deviation in V_2, 65% had changes in V_5, and 70% showed change in the aVF lead. Occlusion in the right coronary artery was associated with a 78% incidence rate of ST segment changes in V_2, 68% in V_5, and 86% in the aVF lead. In the circumflex artery, 90% had changes anteriorly, 70% had ST deviation in the V_5 lead, and 72% had changes in aVF.

Frequently, patients have risk factors associated with myocardial ischemia but unidentified coronary vascular lesions or ischemic episodes. In this case, the leads to be monitored are not as easy to identify. Krucoff's results[38] discourage the use of single-lead monitoring. In his studies, if only the V_2 lead was monitored over the entire population, ST elevation would be missed in about one third of the events and ST depression would be missed in approximately 40% of coronary occlusions. Using the V_5 lead alone would miss 81% of the occlusions. Using aVF alone, ST elevation is missed in about 50% of the cases and ST depression in

about 30% of the cases, with the total (about 80%) roughly the same as with the V_5 lead. Two-channel monitoring improves the detection and definition of ischemic episodes. Simultaneous recording of V_2 and V_5 leads captures 59% of ST changes, missing some elevation in 17% and depressions in 23%. Combining V_2 and aVF leads gives the best yield for complete definition (87%), missing a small percentage each of elevation and depression. Monitoring of V_5 and aVF leads defined ST episodes in 45% of cases, missing approximately one quarter each of ST elevations and depressions. London and coworkers[39] found dual-lead monitoring of V_4 and V_5 leads to be 90% sensitive to ST changes, with I and V_5 at 80%. Lead V_5 was the most sensitive single lead, reflecting 75% of changes. Others[40] recommend including V_1 in the leads selected. Although the V_1 lead is not as sensitive in ischemia detection, it is recommended to facilitate arrhythmia recognition. It is suggested that V_1 in combination with an anterior lead such as I, and an inferior lead such as II, III, or aVF, would meet monitoring needs for both arrhythmias and ischemia. In addition, choosing the anterior–posterior lead combination of I and aVF allows for axis determination, thereby affording the ability to distinguish between ventricular tachycardia and wide-complex supraventricular tachycardia.

In selecting the optimal leads for patients with undocumented cardiac histories, the clinician must consider all important electrocardiographic needs as well as the limitations of available bedside monitoring systems. Examples of these limitations include (1) the number of leads that may be simultaneously monitored, (2) the number of precordial leads that may be simultaneously monitored, and (3) the presence of a mandatory precordial channel that the user is unable to change to a limb lead. Optimally, comprehensive quantitation of total ischemic burden requires monitoring of a minimum of three lead locations. In our experience, with equipment capable of monitoring only two locations, leads II and V_5, provide reasonable sensitivity for ischemia and arrhythmia detection. If one is able to monitor three leads, leads II, aVF, and V_5 are used.

MONITOR SETUP

MEASURING POINTS

After having selected the leads to be monitored, the next step in monitor setup is the designation of measuring points and related reference points. Methods of measurements and setup vary from one type of equipment to another, but all compare a point on the isoelectric line with a point on the ST segment. The amplitude difference between the isoelectric point and ST point reflects the degree of ST elevation or depression in each lead; this variation is displayed by the monitor as a positive or negative value (Figs. 59-2 and 59-3).

When the monitor is turned on, it defaults to factory or user-programmed measuring points. These points should be examined to ensure that the isoelectric point falls on a flat baseline (usually on the PR segment, but the user may choose to use the TP segment), which is a "zero" point, and

TABLE 59-2. Optimal Leads for Specific Coronary Vascular Monitoring

LOCATION	CORONARY ARTERY	LEADS
Anterior	LAD	V_1, V_2, V_3, V_4
Lateral	LCA, circumflex	I, aVL, V_5, V_6
Inferior	RCA, left circumflex	II, III, aVF
Septal	LAD	V_1, V_2, V_3
Posterior	RCA	V_1, V_2, V_3 (reciprocal changes)
Right ventricle	RCA	V_{4R}, V_{6R}

LAD, left anterior descending; LCA, left coronary artery; RCA, right coronary artery.

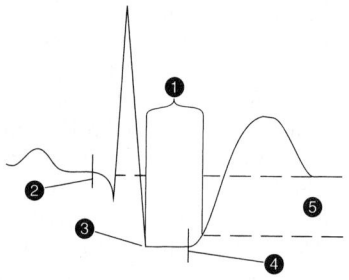

FIGURE 59-2. Key points on the QRS tracing for continuous ST segment monitoring. 1, ST segment; 2, PR point (isoelectric); 3, J-point (end of QRS complex); 4, ST point; 5, ST deviation from PR point.

that the ST point actually lies on the ST segment. These points should be manually altered if necessary. A monitor may not allow movement of the ST point independent of the J-point, that is, it allows only the manipulation of the ST point from J-point plus 60 milliseconds to J-point plus 80 milliseconds (Figs. 59-4 and 59-5). The user should then adjust the J-point location as needed until the ST point accurately reflects ST segment location (Figs. 59-6 and 59-7), because the J-point is merely a reference point.

The monitoring system analyzes the isoelectric and ST points continuously and updates the digital display every 15 to 30 seconds. This time frame may be prolonged if a specific number of "good" beats are not obtained within the window.

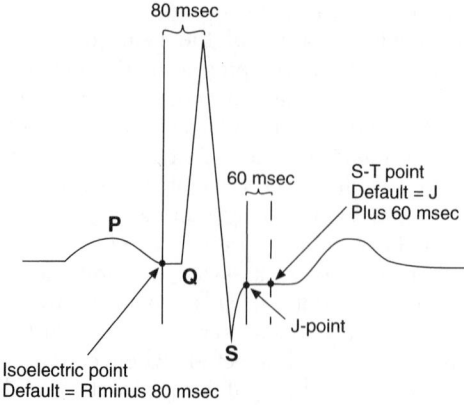

FIGURE 59-4. Monitoring systems have factory or user-programmed default settings. These settings are based on electrocardiographic landmarks such as the R wave or the J-point. The locations of these preset points should be examined on initiating ST monitoring and may be manually adjusted to ensure accuracy.

ALARM LIMITS

The final step in setup is selection of alarm limits. Because the normal ST segment ranges between 0 and −0.5 mm, and a depression of −1 mm is considered a clinically significant deviation, the negative alarm limit should be set at −1.5 mm. Similarly, a 2-mm elevation is significant; therefore, limits of −1.5 and +2.0 mm have been selected and used clinically with decreased incidence of false alarms, allowing clinicians to recognize and treat significant ST variations. Some conditions, however, require deviation from these standard limits. Examples of these limits include atrial fibrillation, use of digoxin, or bundle branch block (see "Limitations of ST Segment Monitoring"). After careful examination of a baseline ECG, alarm limits may be set 1 mm positive

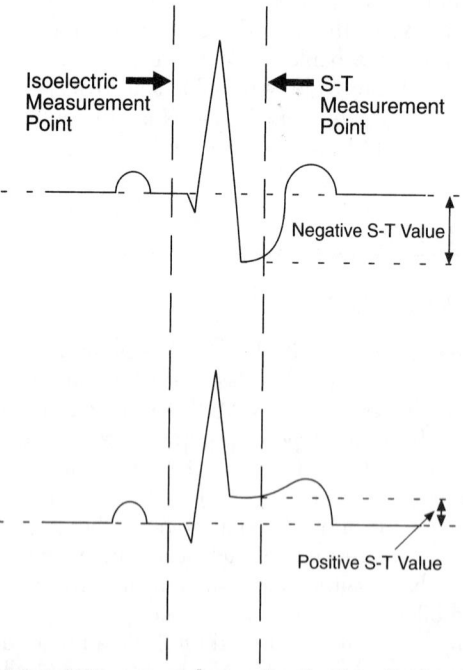

FIGURE 59-3. ST segment depression (*top*) is displayed by the monitor as a negative value; ST segment elevation (*bottom*) is displayed as a positive value. Each is derived by analyzing the difference in millimeters between the isoelectric and ST points.

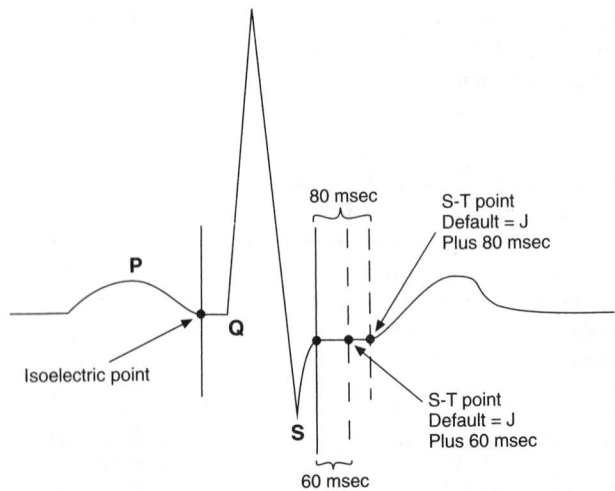

FIGURE 59-5. Whereas some monitors allow adjustment of the ST point independent of the J-point, others limit choices of ST points to preset distances from the J-point.

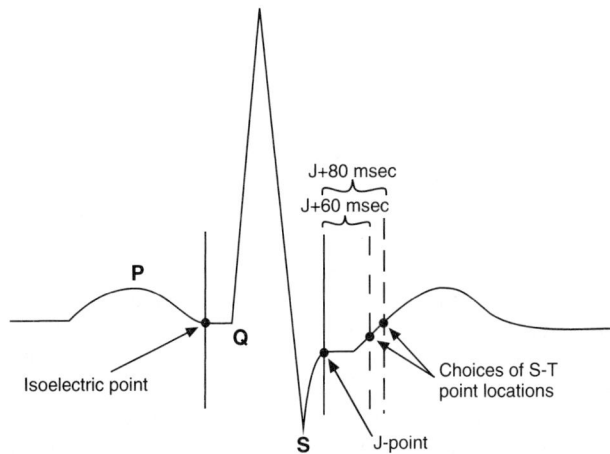

FIGURE 59-6. In this figure, the ST segment has shortened such that the ST point falls on the upslope of the T wave instead of on the ST segment. This situation may occur with monitors that do not allow for movement of the ST point independently of the J-point.

and negative of the patient's baseline[40] (Fig. 59-8). Thus, a 1-mm ST deviation will sound the alarms.

TROUBLESHOOTING ALARM CONDITIONS ■

When preset alarm parameters are violated and the monitor alarm sounds, troubleshooting techniques should be employed before assuming the occurrence to be an ischemic episode. Electrodes should be examined for proper placement. Patients who have turned so as to be positioned directly on top of an electrode (particularly V lead electrodes) may occasionally falsely trigger an alarm; resolution of the

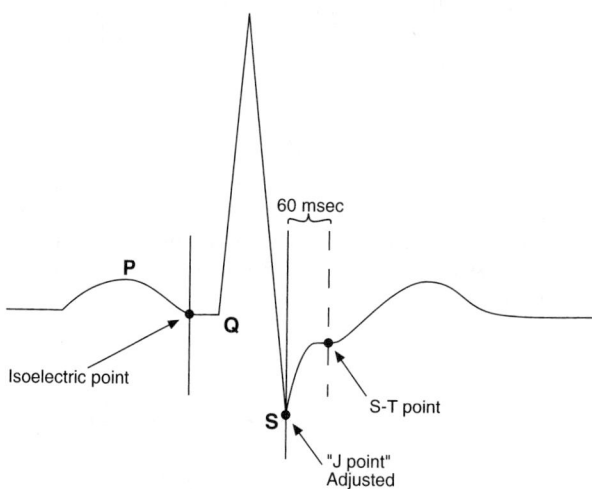

FIGURE 59-7. The falsely elevated ST segment value produced by the erroneous ST point settings in Figure 59-6 are easily corrected. The user should simply move the J-point to the left until the ST point is lying on the ST segment.

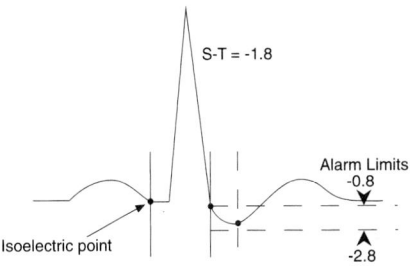

FIGURE 59-8. The electrocardiograph of a patient receiving digoxin therapy. The "scooped-out" appearance of the ST segment may trigger alarms in the absence of ischemia. Alarm limits are adjusted 1 mm above and 1 mm below the patient's ST segment value.

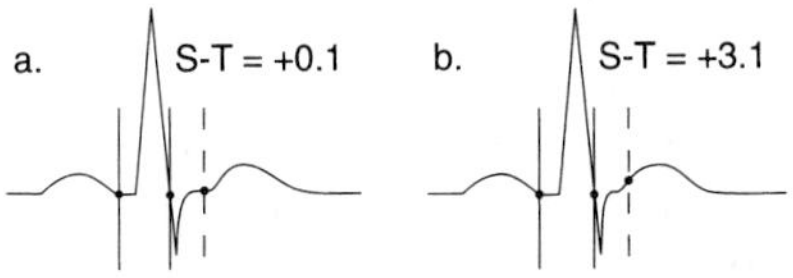

false alarm condition should occur when the patient resumes the previous position. Another troubleshooting measure is to visually assess the ECG configuration that the monitor has analyzed during alarm conditions. Current systems are successful in rejecting most artifacts. More importantly, the measuring points on the ECG waveform should be reexamined. Conditions such as tachycardia may shorten PR and QT intervals, and hypocalcemia may prolong the ST segment such that the monitor identifies an erroneous isoelectric or ST point (Fig. 59-9). Lastly, other conditions that alter the ST segment should be considered and ruled out.

Monitoring systems produce a hard copy of the configuration triggering the alarm. Many allow for a comparison with baseline configurations, as well as the retrieval of past waveforms and associated measuring points for visual examination. When these waveforms are printed, the clinician should ensure that they are of standard voltage (0.1 mV = 1 mm). Waveforms are frequently enlarged for screen-viewing convenience and will alter the clinician's visual interpretation of the data.

Physicians who are not yet comfortable with relying on ST monitoring tend to order a standard 12-lead ECG when bedside monitoring indicates an ST deviation. This increases cost, is rarely necessary, and is sometimes detrimental. With correct electrode placement, printouts from the bedside monitoring system are extremely accurate. Moreover, standard 12-lead ECG machines are rarely immediately available at the bedside, and will miss the ischemic event by the time the ECG is done. If this false-negative ECG is believed, true episodic ischemia will go untreated.

a. S-T = +0.1   b. S-T = +3.1

FIGURE 59-9. (**A**) Electrocardiograph of a patient in normal sinus rhythm. (**B**) The same patient has become tachycardic, inducing a shortened ST segment. Visualization of the measuring points (isoelectric and ST points) indicates that ST segment elevation and the digital display are incorrect.

DEFINITION OF ISCHEMIC EVENTS ▪

As discussed previously, the mere presence of an ischemic event does not necessarily portend an adverse cardiac event. Therefore, a definition of which ST segment changes represent a more likely predictor of poor outcome, and therefore, which events require intervention, needs to be established. Based on data by Landesberg and associates,[29] we have chosen the following definitions of "significant" ST segment changes, that is, those requiring attention, with good success:

1. A single episode with a duration greater than 4 minutes
2. In any given hour, five or more episodes of 1-minute duration and 1-mm deviation, or greater
3. Any single deviation of greater than 2.5 mm

THERAPEUTIC OPTIONS ▪

Interpretation of any test must be done with the possibility of false-positive and false-negative results in mind and is no different for ST segment monitoring. In patients with typical angina and symptomatic coronary disease, depression of the ST segment has a high likelihood of accuracy, with a low false-positive rate. This has been verified by a study by Deanfield and others,[41] in which patients with typical angina and ST segment depression had a demonstrable perfusion deficit on positron emission scans. However, the likelihood that ST segment changes represent actual cardiac ischemic events decreases in patients with asymptomatic disease or nonanginal chest pain. Mathematically, the probability of an event representing a specific condition with a low prevalence results in a high false-positive rate. Bayes' theorem states that the predictive value of a test, that is, the probability that a patient with a positive test result actually has the disease, is dependent on (1) the probability that an event will happen and (2) the probability that the disease is present.[42] Therefore, whereas the development of ST segment changes is highly correlated with perfusion defects in patients with typical angina and positive exercise test results, this high association may not necessarily hold true for patients without such clinical findings. Therefore, the evaluation of, and decision to treat, ST segment changes should be made with this in mind. In the ICU setting, more emphasis is placed on ST segment *trends* rather than on isolated events. Under some circumstances, a cause-and-effect relationship can be seen leading to the ST segment change. In these cases, treatment is probably immediately justified. In others, a high degree of suspicion coupled with the potential for a catastrophic event may justify therapy. In yet others, an analysis of trends or evaluation of past such events may be warranted before aggressive therapy is instituted.

As with data obtained with continuous mixed venous oxygen saturation monitoring, we have learned with continuous ST segment monitoring that procedures performed on an everyday basis may not be entirely benign, and, in fact, many patients develop silent ischemia during routine nursing procedures. A change in approach, or termination of the procedure, may be indicated based on evidence from the ST segment monitor and evaluated based on the clinical importance of the task.

Magnesium sulfate has been shown to be an effective agent in decreasing the risk of serious ventricular arrhythmias and cardiac death after MI.[43,44] Magnesium is an important ion in several basic energy-demanding physiologic processes, and its influence on cardiac arrhythmias may occur through a direct action, through interaction with potassium, or as a naturally occurring calcium channel blocker.[45] Infusion of magnesium retards impulse formation from the sinus node and slows intraatrial and intraventricular conduction, thereby increasing the duration of the absolute refractory period and decreasing the relative refractory period. Thus, the duration of the vulnerable period in the heart cycle is reduced. Magnesium is also known to decrease the tendency toward abnormal impulse formation and increase the threshold for ventricular fibrillation. Accordingly, all patients at risk for ischemia, arrhythmias, or both should receive magnesium sulfate. Patients without known risk but who develop significant ST segment changes during their hospitalization should similarly be treated with 1 g daily of magnesium sulfate, intravenously, for each of 3 days.

Tachycardia-induced ischemia detected by ST segment changes should be treated immediately and aggressively. Relief of anxiety or pain may the only therapeutic intervention necessary, but intravenous beta-blockade with a short-acting agent, such as esmolol, may be indicated. Heart rate and ischemia may be controlled with appropriate titration of beta-blockers, with reversal of ischemia documented by return to baseline of the ST segment.

Increasing afterload, seen clinically as hypertension, can put undo strain on the left ventricle, increasing the myocardial oxygen consumption and inducing ischemia. Control of the hypertension (reduction of the afterload) may be necessary to mitigate ongoing cardiac ischemia and further functional compromise. Systemic beta-blockade with such agents as labetalol, or calcium channel blockers such as nifedipine or diltiazem, may effectively lower systemic vascular resistance, with resulting reduction in ischemic insult monitored by ST segment return to baseline. More aggressive and rapid control can be obtained with sodium nitroprusside.

If ST segment changes do not seem to be the result of extracoronary disease, coronary artery vasodilation with nitroglycerin may reverse or improve the ischemic condition. Once again, recognition of the pathologic condition, and effectiveness of therapy, can result directly from judicious and aggressive ST segment monitoring.

CONCLUSION ▪

Silent ischemia is so prevalent that one must never rely on the onset of symptoms in high-risk ICU patients to guide therapy. This is even more applicable in postoperative surgical patients whose pain perception or mental status may be altered with narcotics given to minimize incisional pain. Noninvasive, continuous ST segment monitoring of leads II, V₅, and aVF will provide an accurate, low-cost means of detecting ischemic events and lead to early directed therapy and possible prevention of catastrophic cardiac dysfunction.

REFERENCES ■

1. National Hospital Discharge Survey: Annual Summary 1992. U.S. Department of Health and Human Services. Vital and Health Statistics, series 13, no. 119, 1994
2. National Center for Health Statistics: Health, United States, 1988. In: Advance Data From Vital and Health Statistics. Washington DC: U.S. Government Printing Office, 1989:10-17 (DHSS publication no. [PHS] 89-1232)
3. Kannel AWB, Abbott RD: Incidence and prognosis of unrecognized myocardial infarction: an update on the Framingham study. *N Engl J Med* 1984;311:1144
4. Allen RD, Gettes LS, Phalan C, et al: Painless ST segment depression in patients with angina pectoris: correlation with daily activities and cigarette smoking. *Chest* 1976;69:467
5. Carboni GP, Celli P, D'Ermo M, et al: Combined cardiac cineflouroscopy, exercise testing and ambulatory ST-segment monitoring in the diagnosis of coronary artery disease: a report of 104 symptomatic patients. *Int J Cardiol* 1985;9:91
6. Cecchi AC, Dovellini EV, Marchi F, et al: Silent myocardial ischemia during ambulatory electrocardiographic monitoring in patients with effort angina. *J Am Coll Cardiol* 1983;1:934
7. Chierchia S, Smith G, Morgan M, et al: Role of heart rate in pathophysiology of chronic stable angina. *Lancet* 1984;2:1353
8. Cocco GX, Braun S, Strozzi C, et al: Aymptomatic myocardial ischemia in patients with stable and typical angina pectoris. *Clin Cardiol* 1982;5:403
9. Deanfield JE, Selwyn AP, Chierchia S, et al: Myocardial ischemia during daily life in patients with stable angina: its relation to symptoms and heart rate changes. *Lancet* 1983;2:753
10. Ribeiro P, Shea M, Deanfield JE, et al: Different mechanisms for the relief of angina after coronary bypass surgery: physiological versus anatomical assessment. *Br Heart J* 1984;52:502
11. Schang SJ Jr, Pepine CJ: Transient asymptomatic ST segment depression during activity. *Am J Cardiol* 1977;39:396
12. Selwyn AP, Fox K, Eves M, et al: Myocardial ischemia in patients with frequent angina pectoris. *Br Med J* 1978;2:1594
13. Von Arnim T, Hofling B, Shreiber M: Characteristics of episodes of ST elevation or ST depression during ambulatory monitoring in patients subsequently undergoing angiography. *Br Heart J* 1985;54:484
14. Muller JE, Stone PH, Turi ZG, et al: Circadian variation in the frequency of onset of acute myocardial infarction. *N Engl J Med* 1985;313:1315
15. Chierchia S, Lazzari M, Freedman B, et al: Impairment of myocardial perfusion and function during painless myocardial ischemia. *J Am Coll Cardiol* 1983;1:924
16. Gottlieb SO, Weisfeldt ML, Duyang P, et al: Silent ischemia as a marker for early unfavorable outcomes in patients with unstable angina. *N Engl J Med* 1986;314:1214
17. Petralito A, Mangiafico RA, Giblino S, et al: Daily modifications of plasma fibrinogen, platelet aggregation, Howell's time, PPT, PT, and antithrombin III in normal subjects and in patients with vascular disease. *Chronobiologia* 1982;9:195
18. Rosing DR, Brakma P, Redwood DR, et al: Blood fibrinolytic

19. activity in man: diurnal variation and the response to varying intensities of exercise. *Circ Res* 1970;27:171
19. Turton MB, Deegan T: Circadian variations of plasma catecholamine, cortisol, and immunoreactive insulin concentrations in supine subjects. *Clin Chim Acta* 1974;55:389
20. Quyyumi AA, Mockus L, Wright C, et al: Morphology of ambulatory ST segment changes in patients with varying severity of coronary artery disease: investigation of the frequency of nocturnal ischemia and coronary spasm. *Br Heart J* 1985;53:186
21. Rebecca GS, Wayne R, Zebede J, et al: Pathogenic mechanisms causing transient myocardial ischemia with mental arousal in patients with coronary artery disease [abstract]. *Clinica e Investigacion en Arteriosclerosis* 1986;34:338A
22. Deanfield JE, Kensett M, Wilson RA, et al: Silent myocardial ischemia due to mental stress. *Lancet* 1984ₓ:1001
23. Cherry PD, Furchgott RF, Zawadzi JV, et al: Role of endothelial cells in relaxation of isolated arteries by bradykinin. *Proc Natl Acad Sci USA* 1982;79:2106
24. Furchgott RF: Role of endothelium in responses of vascular smooth muscle. *Circ Res* 1983;53:557
25. Kilbourn RG, Fonseca GA, Griffith OW, et al: N^G-methyl-L-arginine, an inhibitor of nitric oxide synthase, reverses interleukin-2-induced hypotension. *Crit Care Med* 1995;23:1018
26. Raby KE, Goldman L, Creager MA, et al: Correlation between preoperative ischemia and major cardiac events after peripheral vascular surgery. *N Engl J Med* 1989;321:1296
27. Fleisher L, Rosenbaum SH, Nelson AH, et al: The predictive valve of preoperative silent ischemia for postoperative ischemic cardiac events in vascular and non-vascular surgical patients. *Am Heart J* 1991;122:980
28. Mangano DT, Browner WS, Hollenberg M, et al: Association of perioperative myocardial ischemia with cardiac morbidity and mortality in men undergoing noncardiac surgery. *N Engl J Med* 1990;323:1781
29. Landesberg G, Luria MH, Cotev S, et al: Importance of long-duration postoperative ST-segment depression in cardiac morbidity after vascular surgery. *Lancet* 1993;341:715
30. Holland RP, Brooks H: TQ-ST segment mapping: critical review and analysis of current concepts. *Am J Cardiol* 1977;40:110
31. Knight AA, Hollenberg M, London MJ, et al: Perioperative myocardial ischemia: importance of the preoperative ischemic pattern. *Anesthesiology* 1988;68:681
32. Smith RC, Leung JM, Mangano DT, et al: Postoperative myocardial ischemia in patients undergoing coronary artery bypass graft surgery. *Anesthesiology* 1991;74:464
33. Mangano DT, Wong MG, London MJ, et al: Perioperative myocardial ischemia in patients undergoing noncardiac surgery. II. Incidence and severity during the first week after surgery. *J Am Coll Cardiol* 1991;17:851
34. Janse MJ: Electrical activity immediately following myocardial infarction. In: Rosen MR, Janse MJ, Wit AL. *Cardiac Electrophysiology: A Textbook*. Mount Kisco, NY: Futura, 1990
35. Cinca J, Figueras J, Senador G, et al: Transmural DC electrograms after coronary artery occlusion and latex embolization in pigs. *Am J Physiol* 1984;246:H475
36. Biagini A, L'Abbate A, Testa R, et al: Unreliability of conventional visual electrocardiographic monitoring for detection of transient ST segment changes in coronary care units. *Eur Heart J* 1984;5:784
37. Marriott HJ: *Practical Electrocardiography*, 8th ed. Baltimore, Williams & Wilkins, 1988
38. Krucoff M: Identification of high-risk patients with silent myocardial ischemia after percutaneous transluminal coronary

angioplasty by multilead monitoring. *Am J Cardiol* 1988;61:29F

39. London MJ, Hollenber M, Wong MG, et al: Intraoperative myocardial ischemia: localization by continuous 12-lead electrocardiography. *Anesthesiology* 1988;69:232

40. Tisdale L, Drew B: ST segment monitoring for myocardial ischemia. *AACN Clin Issues* 1993;4:34

41. Deanfield JE, Shea M, Ribiero P, et al: Transient ST-segment depression as a marker of myocardial ischemia during daily life. *Am J Cardiol* 1984;54:1195

42. Dawson-Saunders B, Trapp RG: *Basic and Clinical Biostatistics*. Norwalk, CT: Appleton & Lange, 1990

43. Smith LF, Heagerty AM, Bing RF, et al: Intravenous infusion of magnesium sulphate after myocardial infarction: effects on arrhythmias and mortality. *Int J Cardiol* 1986;12:175

44. Abraham AS, Rosenmann D, Kramer M, et al: Magnesium in the prevention of lethal arrhythmias in acute myocardial infarction. *Arch Intern Med* 1987;147:753

45. Wester PO: Magnesium: effect on arrhythmias. *Int J Cardiol* 1986;12:181

Critical Care, Third Edition, edited by Joseph M. Civetta,
Robert W. Taylor, and Robert R. Kirby.
Lippincott-Raven Publishers, Philadelphia, PA © 1997.

CHAPTER 60

Venous Saturation Monitoring and Usage

Joseph M. Civetta
Loren D. Nelson

IMMEDIATE CONCERNS ■

MAJOR PROBLEMS

Patient Selection for Continuous Venous Oximetry

Continuous venous oximetry is likely to be most useful in patients at greatest risk of oxygen transport imbalance, namely: (1) patients at increased risk for cardiopulmonary dysfunction, including patients with cardiac disease, severe respiratory disease, patients with underlying risk factors who are undergoing major surgical procedures, and patients who are undergoing therapy that may interfere with their ability to increase oxygen delivery during times of stress; and (2) patients who have demonstrated deficits in oxygen transport, including patients receiving resuscitation from shock, those with acute respiratory failure receiving high levels of ventilatory support, and patients requiring hemodynamic support using inotropes, vasodilators, or vasopressors.

Goals of Venous Oximetry Monitoring

The goals of the continuous venous oximetry vary with the initial condition of the patient. In patients monitored because of risk factors but who have been clinically and physiologically stable, continuous venous oximetry may be used as an on-line assurance that oxygen transport balance is being maintained. Repeated determinations of cardiac output (CO) and arterial and mixed venous blood gases to confirm their stability are not necessary. In the next group of patients

who do become unstable, continuous venous oximetry may be used as an early warning signal regarding the onset of oxygen transport imbalance. As with the first group of patients, a stable and normal value for the mixed venous oxygen saturation ($S\bar{v}O_2$) indicates that further measurements are unnecessary. However, an abrupt decrease in $S\bar{v}O_2$ becomes a warning that more data (CO, arterial oxygen saturation [SaO_2], and hemoglobin [Hgb] concentration) are needed to interpret the change in $S\bar{v}O_2$ and to assess the cause of the oxygen transport imbalance. Finally, in patients undergoing therapy for hemodynamic or respiratory instability, continuously measured $S\bar{v}O_2$ may be used as an on-line indicator of the adequacy of therapy. In these patients, it is necessary to assess initially CO, SaO_2, Hgb, and oxygen consumption ($\dot{V}O_2$) to determine which of these factors is most responsible for the imbalance between oxygen supply and demand (abnormal $S\bar{v}O_2$) so that specific therapy may be directed toward the underlying disorder. Steadily improving $S\bar{v}O_2$ indicates that therapy is effective. Decreasing or unchanging $S\bar{v}O_2$, while seemingly appropriate therapy is being applied, indicates that more information is needed and that all of the individual determinants of oxygen transport balance need to be reassessed.

STRESS POINTS

1. Reflectance spectrophotometry, the principle used today for *continuous in vivo* $S\bar{v}O_2$ measurement, requires that multiple wave lengths of light transmitted at known intensity by the fiberoptic bundles, be re-

909

flected from red blood cells flowing past the tip of the catheter.

2. There are four determinants of $S\bar{v}O_2$: CO, Hgb concentration, arterial oxygen content, and oxygen consumption.

3. In the critically ill patient, an abrupt change in $S\bar{v}O_2$ indicates that a change in oxygen transport–demand balance has occurred but does not identify which determinant has changed.

4. Values in the normal range (0.68 to 0.77) suggest that the balance between oxygen delivery and consumption is normal.

5. A decrease in $S\bar{v}O_2$ may be caused by a decrease in CO, Hgb concentration, and arterial oxygen content or an increase in oxygen demand.

6. An increase in $S\bar{v}O_2$ is more difficult to interpret. Patients may have a high CO, low oxygen consumption, or high arterial oxygen content, especially a large amount of dissolved oxygen during anesthesia of mechanical ventilation.

7. In patients with cirrhosis and sepsis, abnormal distribution of peripheral blood flow may impair oxygen uptake so that $S\bar{v}O_2$ remains high. In these patients, concomitant lactic acidosis indicates that the oxygen delivery transport balance is not functioning normally.

8. Pulse oximetry and continuous mixed venous oximetry can be combined into a tool of great use to provide inferences concerning cardiac and respiratory function.

9. The difference between arterial and venous saturation ($Sa - S\bar{v}$) is an estimation of arterial venous oxygen content difference and is inversely proportional to CO and directly proportional to oxygen consumption.

10. The ventilation perfusion index ($\dot{V}/\dot{Q}$ I) gives an estimate of interpulmonary shunt.

11. Using saturation as an inference of oxygen content, respiratory dysfunction ($\dot{V}/\dot{Q}$ I) can be estimated from the equation $(1 - Sa)/(1 - S\bar{v})$.

ESSENTIAL DIAGNOSTIC TESTS AND PROCEDURES

1. Continuous mixed venous oximetry measurements may drift. Daily calibration using laboratory co-oximetry should be performed.

2. Calibration should also be verified anytime the optical module is disconnected, or whenever the measurement is thought to be erroneous.

3. Distal migration of the pulmonary artery (PA) catheter tip may cause error.

4. Decreased light intensity signal or damping of the PA tracing may indicate migration distally.

5. If irrigation of catheter does not correct the artifact, the catheter should be withdrawn and repositioned.

6. If the light source reflects off the vessel wall instead of the blood, low-intensity light alarm will result and must be corrected by repositioning of the catheter.

7. A change in $S\bar{v}O_2$ of greater than 0.10 in either direction requires investigation.

8. Sudden decrease may be associated with position change, shivering, or suctioning—all transient events that can be identified at the bedside.

9. Physiologically important changes include decreased CO, decreased Hgb concentration, decreased arterial saturation and content, and increased oxygen consumption.

10. Increase in $S\bar{v}O_2$ may indicate artifact caused by positioning, increased CO, or decreased oxygen consumption.

11. Decreased oxygen consumption in association with sepsis, high CO, and low peripheral resistance, especially if associated with lactic acidosis, is an ominous sign.

INITIAL THERAPY

1. If $S\bar{v}O_2$ is low in association with a low CO, response to fluids or inotropic agents should occur within a few minutes.

2. Of greater importance, when titrating inotropic infusions, *a lack of response* ($S\bar{v}O_2$ does not increase) suggests that the chosen infusion rate has not had a desired effect. Remeasure CO and increase inotropic support rapidly.

3. In cases of respiratory dysfunction, arterial saturation should respond to therapy such as increased positive end-expiratory pressure (PEEP) within 8 to 10 minutes.

4. If SaO_2 does not increase or if $S\bar{v}O_2$ decreases, respiratory therapy has been ineffective or CO may be compromised.

5. After improvement in respiratory function, if the patient is receiving a high inspired oxygen tension, this may be decreased every 10 to 20 minutes if arterial and venous saturation remains stable. Increased Sa minus $S\bar{v}$ usually correlates with a sudden decrease in CO.

6. A decrease in Sa minus $S\bar{v}$ in response to measures trying to increase CO usually indicate a successful intervention.

PHYSIOLOGY OF OXYGEN TRANSPORT   ■

The process of oxygen transport includes loading oxygen into the red blood cells and delivering it to the tissue, as well as utilization of the oxygen in the periphery and the return of desaturated blood to the right side of the heart.[1] Several terms must be defined to understand the components of oxygen transport:

Oxygen demand: cellular oxygen requirement to avoid anaerobic metabolism

Oxygen consumption ($\dot{V}O_2$): the calculated (Fick) volume of oxygen consumed each minute [$C(a - \bar{v})O_2 \times CO \times 10$]

Oxygen uptake: measured volume of oxygen removed from inspired gas each minute

Oxygen delivery ($\dot{D}o_2$): volume of oxygen delivered from the left ventricle each minute [$CO \times Cao_2 \times 10$]

Oxygen utilization coefficient (extraction ratio): fraction of delivered oxygen that is consumed [$\dot{V}o_2/\dot{D}o_2$]

Oxygen transport: processes contributing to oxygen delivery and oxygen consumption.

Oxygen demand is the amount of oxygen *required* by the body tissues to function under conditions of aerobic metabolism. Because oxygen demand is determined at the tissue level, it is difficult to quantify clinically. $\dot{V}o_2$, on the other hand, is the amount of oxygen *consumed* by the tissue as calculated by the Fick equation (CO times arterial–venous oxygen content difference). $\dot{V}o_2$ is a mechanism by which the body "protects" the oxygen demand created at the tissue level.[2] Factors associated with increases in $\dot{V}o_2$ are associated with increased survival,[3] whereas low $\dot{V}o_2$ is associated with a mortality as high as 80%. $\dot{V}o_2$ may increase by increasing CO, widening the arterial–venous oxygen content difference, or both. In the normal state, both CO and arterial–venous oxygen difference may increase by about threefold, providing a total increase of $\dot{V}o_2$ during times of stress to about ninefold above the resting state. Normally, $\dot{V}o_2$ and oxygen demand are equal; however, in times of great oxygen demand or times in which either CO or arterial–venous oxygen content difference cannot increase to meet the oxygen demand of the cells, oxygen demand may exceed $\dot{V}o_2$. When this occurs, anaerobic metabolism and lactic acidosis ensue.[2]

Oxygen uptake differs slightly from $\dot{V}o_2$ in that the latter is a *calculated* value (from the Fick equation) and the former is the *measured* volume of oxygen taken up by the patient each minute. Oxygen uptake is measured by analyzing inspired and expired gas concentrations and inspired and expired volumes. Measurement of oxygen uptake may be useful for metabolic studies because it can be performed continuously for long periods to account for variation in $\dot{V}o_2$ owing to activity and the like.

Oxygen delivery ($\dot{D}o_2$) is the volume of oxygen delivered from the heart each minute and is calculated as the product of CO and arterial oxygen content. Oxygen utilization or extraction ratio is the *fraction* of delivered oxygen that is consumed ($\dot{V}o_2$ divided by $\dot{D}o_2$). Therefore, the oxygen utili-zation coefficient defines the balance between oxygen supply (delivery) and demand (consumption).

ASSESSMENT OF OXYGEN TRANSPORT BALANCE ■

Oxygen transport balance may be assessed on several levels. First, examination of the patient may reveal signs of hypoperfusion, including altered mentation, cutaneous hypoperfusion, oliguria, tachycardia, and, when all compensatory systems have failed, hypotension. Unfortunately, these clinical signs are often late, nonspecific, and at times uninterpretable in critically ill patients. A more physiologic approach is to assess the determinants of oxygen transport balance individually by using the Fick equation. The arterial–venous oxygen content difference may be used to assess the relative balance between CO and $\dot{V}o_2$. An increase in the arterial–venous oxygen content difference indicates that either flow is decreased or consumption is increased.

Although oxygen demand cannot be measured, the relative balance between consumption and demand is best indicated by the presence of excess lactate in the blood. Lactic acidosis means that demand exceeds consumption and anaerobic metabolism is present.[2] The relative balance between oxygen supply and demand can be assessed by the oxygen utilization coefficient.[1] Calculation of this coefficient, however, requires the measurement of CO, Hgb, Sao_2, Pao_2, $S\bar{v}o_2$, and mixed venous oxygen tension.

When the Fick equation is solved for $S\bar{v}o_2$ (Table 60-1), it becomes apparent that an inverse linear relation exists between $S\bar{v}o_2$ and oxygen utilization coefficient[4] if Sao_2 is maintained at a high level. $S\bar{v}o_2$ measured continuously is, therefore, an on-line indicator of the adequacy of the oxygen supply and of the demand in perfused tissues. The determinants of $S\bar{v}o_2$ are $\dot{V}o_2$, Hgb, CO, Sao_2, and, to a small degree, Pao_2.

$S\bar{v}o_2$ represents the flow-weighted average of the venous oxygen saturations from all perfused tissues.[1] Therefore, tissues that have high blood flow but relatively low oxygen extraction (kidney) will have a greater effect on $S\bar{v}o_2$ than will tissues with low blood flow, although the oxygen extraction of these tissues may be high (myocardium). The interpretation of $S\bar{v}o_2$ requires consistent and intact vasoregula-

TABLE 60-1. Derivation of $S\bar{v}o_2$ from Fick Equation

1. $\dot{V}o_2 = C(a - \bar{v})o_2 \times CO \times 10$	{Fick equation
2. $\dot{V}o_2/(CO \times 10) = C(a - \bar{v})o_2$	{Divide by CO $\times$ 10
3. $\dot{V}o_2/(CO \times 10) = Cao_2 - C\bar{v}o_2$	{Definition of C(a $- \bar{v}$)o$_2$
4. $\dot{V}o_2/(CO \times 10) - Cao_2 = -C\bar{v}o_2$	{Subtract Cao$_2$
5. $C\bar{v}o_2 = Cao_2 - [\dot{V}o_2/(CO \times 10)]$	{Multiply by -1
6. $C\bar{v}o_2 = 1 - \dot{V}o_2/(CO \times 10 \times Cao_2)\}$	{Divide by Cao$_2$
7. $C\bar{v}o_2/Cao_2 = 1 - \dot{V}o_2/\dot{D}o_2$	{Definition of $\dot{D}o_2$
8. $S\bar{v}o_2 = 1 - \dot{V}o_2/\dot{D}o_2$	{Definition of $S\bar{v}o_2$ if $Sao_2 = 1.0$

CO, cardiac output.

tion.[5] When vasoregulation is altered (such as in sepsis), oxygen uptake may be severely altered, causing a marked increase in $S\bar{v}O_2$. This increase, however, should not be interpreted to mean that all tissues are being well oxygenated; coexisting lactic acidosis demonstrates that this is not the case.

MONITORING OXYGEN TRANSPORT ■

Patients admitted to intensive care units (ICUs) may be grouped into three large categories.[6] Category 1 consists of patients requiring intensive observation or monitoring. These patients may have major risk factors or may be admitted because of the nature of their illness or the nature of the therapy they are receiving. Category 2 patients require intensive nursing care and often specialized technology and care facilities to direct therapy for major systemic illness. Category 3 patients need continuous physician intervention for hemodynamic and other instabilities. Continuous venous oximetry may have clinical applications in each of these broad classes of patients.

The three major objectives of monitoring critically ill patients are (1) to assure that the patient is stable; (2) to provide an early warning system regarding untoward events; and (3) to evaluate the efficiency and efficacy of interventions performed. The role of the three monitoring objectives differs in the three categories of patients being monitored.

Patients undergoing hemodynamic and oxygen transport monitoring only because of underlying risk factors who have a normal and stable $S\bar{v}O_2$ have an intact balance between oxygen supply and demand. Further assessment of CO and arterial and mixed venous blood gas analysis to reach that conclusion can be eliminated, and there is "safety in no (other) numbers."[7] If the patient becomes "unstable" as manifested by a decreasing $S\bar{v}O_2$, the monitoring system will meet the second objective by providing an early warning[8] of the imbalance in oxygen supply and demand. In this situation, although an alert has been given, the cause of the oxygen transport imbalance is not necessarily clear. The change in $S\bar{v}O_2$ is sensitive but not specific. In this clinical situation, it may be necessary to measure CO, SaO_2, and Hgb. When the cause of the imbalance is identified, specific therapy may be instituted to restore the oxygen supply–demand balance. When therapy is instituted to correct an oxygen supply–demand imbalance, continuous venous oximetry demonstrates its greatest efficacy.[9] While interventions are applied, the on-line assessment of supply–demand balance may be used to evaluate the efficacy of the intervention. Because the measurement is continuous, the evaluation of responses to therapy is instantaneous rather than delayed by blood gas analysis. New, continuous CO methodology should supplement but not supplant mixed venous oximetry. In association with pulse oximetry, more information is available and fewer inferences and intermittent tests are needed. This is particularly important in critical illness, defined as a nonsteady state,[10] when changes in all elements of oxygen transport and utilization can be expected.

CLINICAL USEFULNESS OF CONTINUOUS $S\bar{v}O_2$ MONITORING ■

Reflectance spectrophotometry is the technology currently used for continuous venous oximetry (Fig. 60-1). Transmitting and receiving fiberoptic bundles are located in the wall of the PA catheter. Light from the transmission bundle is emitted in two or three specific wavelengths that correspond to the maximum reflectance of oxyhemoglobin and deoxyhemoglobin. While red blood cells flow past the tip of the catheter, light is reflected from the cells to the receiving fiberoptic bundle.[11] The microprocessor uses the relative reflectances to calculate the oxyhemoglobin and total Hgb, the fraction of which represents $S\bar{v}O_2$.

As is the case with most monitoring devices, the continuous oximetry system must be calibrated before use. This may be done in vitro by positioning the catheter tip next to a target that reflects the transmitted light in such a manner that the microprocessor can be calibrated.[12] When this is done (before insertion of the catheter), the oxygen saturation of the central venous system, right atrium, right ventricle, and PA can be measured while the catheter is being floated into the proper position. These measurements during the insertion of the catheter may be useful to rule out intracardiac left-to-right shunts.

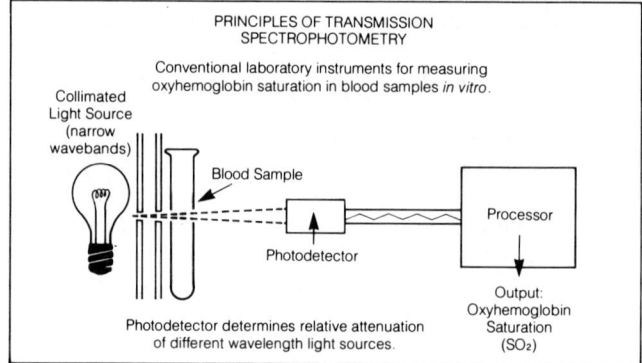

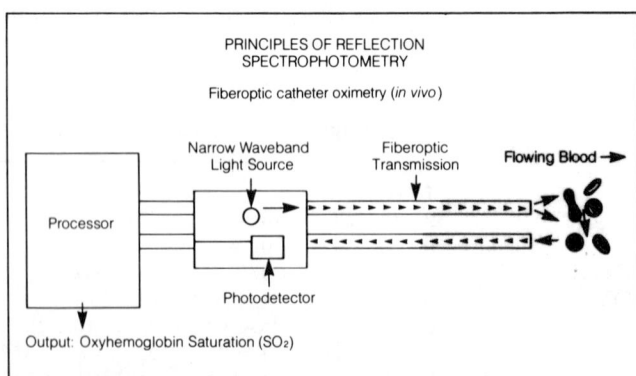

FIGURE 60-1. Principle of reflectance spectrophotometry. (Courtesy of Abbott Critical Care, Mountain View, CA.)

Once the PA catheter is in proper position, blood may be sampled through the distal port to calibrate or to verify the calibration of the system. A mixed venous sample is withdrawn and analyzed by laboratory co-oximetry. The value obtained by the microprocessor at the time the blood sample is drawn is retained by the system. This may be compared against the value obtained from the laboratory sample, and, if a significant (greater than 4%) difference exists, the instrument may be recalibrated to the laboratory co-oximeter value. The calibration should be verified at any time the optical module is disconnected from the catheter, whenever the measurement is suspected of being erroneous, and every 24 hours to ensure stability of the system.[11]

Because it is crucial that red blood cells be flowing past the tip of the catheter, proper positioning of the catheter in the PA is necessary. Distal migration of the PA catheter tip is a common source of error. When the catheter tip advances into the distal segments of the PA, a high or increased $S\bar{v}O_2$, a decreased light intensity signal, or damping of the PA tracing may become evident.[9] If these signs are encountered, the distal lumen of the catheter should be vigorously irrigated with flush solution because fibrin formation on the catheter tip also may cause these artifacts. If the pressure waveform is not restored to a proper PA tracing by irrigation, the catheter should be slowly withdrawn until the PA pressure tracing is restored. At this point, the PA catheter balloon may be slowly inflated until the pulmonary artery occlusion (PAO) tracing is observed. If this tracing is not produced by inflation of the balloon to maximum volume (1.5 mL), the catheter should be slowly advanced until an occlusion pressure tracing is observed. At that point, the balloon can be deflated again and then slowly reinflated until a PAO tracing occurs. The volume required to restore this tracing should be at least 75% of the total capacity of the balloon. Using the maximum balloon volume to attain a PAO tracing ensures that the catheter is in the proximal section of the PA and is, in fact, a "physiologic confirmation" of the catheter tip position.[13]

Distal migration of the PA catheter may cause an artifactually high oxygen saturation because highly saturated pulmonary capillary blood is analyzed. The catheter tip may be lodged against a vessel wall or bifurcation, causing an alteration in the light intensity received by the fiberoptic bundles. A low light intensity alarm must be corrected before the venous saturation measurement is considered to be reliable or before the system is recalibrated. Large fluctuations in the light intensity signal may indicate that the catheter tip is malpositioned but also may indicate a condition of intravascular volume deficit that allows compression or collapse of the pulmonary vasculature (especially during positive-pressure ventilation).

INTERPRETATION OF VENOUS OXYGEN SATURATION

Mixed venous oxygen saturation values within the normal range (0.68 to 0.77) indicate a normal balance between oxygen supply and demand, provided that vasoregulation is intact and a normal distribution of peripheral blood flow is present. Values of $S\bar{v}O_2$ greater than 0.77 indicate an excess of $\dot{D}O_2$ over $\dot{V}O_2$ and are most commonly associated with syndromes of vasoderegulation such as cirrhosis and sepsis. High values also are seen in states of low $\dot{V}O_2$ (hypothermia, muscular paralysis, sedation, coma, or a combination of these factors), hyperoxygenation, high CO, and, rarely, cyanide toxicity.

Uncompensated changes in any of the four determinants of $S\bar{v}O_2$ may result in a decrease in the measured value, but in complex, critically ill patients, the correlation between changes in $S\bar{v}O_2$ and changes in any of the individual determining factors is low. In a study of the patients in a surgical ICU,[14] no statistical correlation existed between changes in either PaO_2 or SaO_2 and $S\bar{v}O_2$. Although there was a statistically significant correlation between changes in $S\bar{v}O_2$ and CO and $\dot{D}O_2$, the coefficients of determination (r^2) were too low to allow prediction of CO, oxygen consumption, or oxygen delivery from $S\bar{v}O_2$. Also, no statistical correlation existed between $S\bar{v}O_2$ and either arterial–venous oxygen content difference or calculated $\dot{V}O_2$. There was a significant inverse correlation between $S\bar{v}O_2$ and oxygen utilization coefficient, confirming the accuracy of the measurement and the reliability of $S\bar{v}O_2$ as an estimation of the oxygen utilization ratio—as long as arterial oxygen saturation is near 100% (Fig. 60-2). The determinants of $S\bar{v}O_2$ are multifactorial and, in critically ill patients, the degree of compensation for changes in one variable cannot be predicted.

It is useful, however, to appreciate the magnitude of change in $S\bar{v}O_2$ that would occur with an isolated change in any of the individual determinants. If no compensatory changes occur in $\dot{V}O_2$ or CO, Hgb must decrease by almost 50% (13 to 7.5 g) before $S\bar{v}O_2$ decreases before the lower limit of the normal range (Table 60-2). In actuality, the changes would be even smaller because CO should increase in response to the acute anemia. However, if CO is fixed because of underlying cardiovascular disease, a decrease in Hgb will be reflected by a decrease in $S\bar{v}O_2$.

The effect of arterial oxygen tension on $S\bar{v}O_2$ in the absence of other compensatory changes is demonstrated in Table 60-3. As long as SaO_2 is maintained in a relatively normal range, the direct effect on $S\bar{v}O_2$ is minimal. However, when there is sufficient arterial hypoxemia to produce arterial desaturation, the $S\bar{v}O_2$ falls in direct proportion to the change in SaO_2. Similarly, changes in CO (Table 60-4) and $\dot{V}O_2$ (Table 60-5) may be shown to affect directly $S\bar{v}O_2$, although the magnitude of changes in any of these individual parameters does not predict the magnitude of change in $S\bar{v}O_2$ because compensatory factors are usually involved.

A decrease in $S\bar{v}O_2$ greater than 0.10 is likely to be clinically significant regardless of the initial value. A change from 0.70 to 0.60 may be associated with a large fractional change in CO (assuming, for argument, that other factors did not change). On the other hand, although a change from 0.60 to 0.50 is associated with a much smaller fractional change in CO, it occurs at a time of greatly limited oxygen transport reserve. Although $S\bar{v}O_2$ is a sensitive indicator in oxygen transport balance, it cannot specifically determine the actual change of any of the individual components of $\dot{D}O_2$ or $\dot{V}O_2$. Therefore, because a sustained decrease in $S\bar{v}O_2$ of greater

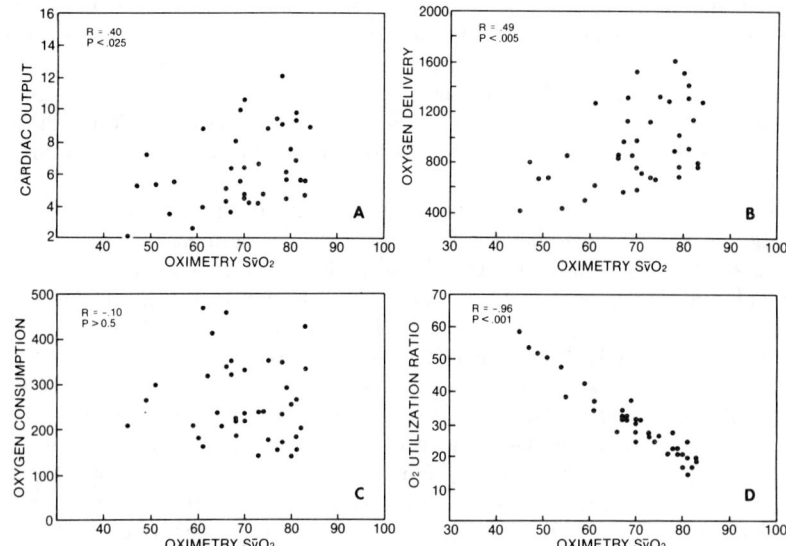

FIGURE 60-2. Correlation between oxygen transport variables and $S\bar{v}O_2$. (**B**) No statistically significant correlation exists between oxygen consumption and $S\bar{v}O_2$ (**B**), and a low correlation exists between either cardiac output (**A**) or oxygen delivery (**C**) and $S\bar{v}O_2$. A highly significant inverse correlation exists between oxygen utilization ratio (**D**) and $S\bar{v}O_2$. (Reproduced with permission from Nelson LD: Continuous venous oximetry in critically ill surgical patients. *Ann Surg* 1986;203: 329.)

than 0.10 does not explain the cause for the imbalance in oxygen supply and demand, this change should alert the clinician to the need for further evaluation of the individual factors likely to affect oxygen transport balance. The first step in this evaluation should be to rule out artifact in the measurement caused by the catheter positioning, low light intensity, or miscalibration of the microprocessor. When a change in $S\bar{v}O_2$ is determined to be clinically significant and valid, measurement of SaO_2, Hgb, and CO, used in conjunction with the $S\bar{v}O_2$ measurement, will provide the database necessary to evaluate the cause for the change in $S\bar{v}O_2$. Continuous CO technology usually provides an average CO value over either a manufacturer-determined or user-selected time interval. Thus, a sudden decrease in $S\bar{v}O_2$ still is an early warning to prompt an instantaneous CO determination. When the derived cardiopulmonary parameters of arterial–venous oxygen content difference, $\dot{V}O_2$, intrapulmonary shunt fraction (venous admixture), and oxygen extraction or utilization coefficient are calculated, the clinician should be able to interpret the oxygen transport imbalance identified by continuous venous oximetry and institute immediate therapy.

Continuous $S\bar{v}O_2$ monitoring helps to assess the *adequacy* of oxygen delivery. Just as the adequacy of fuel in an airliner is defined by the amount of fuel left on landing, the adequacy of oxygen delivery is defined by the amount of oxygen in the venous circulation after extraction by peripheral tissues.

Mixed venous oximetry helps to answer three fundamental questions regarding oxygen transport. First, is oxygen delivery adequate to maintain $\dot{V}O_2$? The oxygen utilization coefficient (extraction ratio) defines the fraction of delivered oxygen that is consumed, and because $S\bar{v}O_2$ correlates inversely with this coefficient, it can be used to define the balance between consumption and delivery of oxygen[14] (Fig. 60-3).

When oxygen delivery is inadequate for consumption (i.e., $S\bar{v}O_2$ is low), the cause for the inadequacy (Hgb, SaO_2, CO) must be determined. The arterial–venous oxygen content difference defines the balance between $\dot{V}O_2$ and CO. When $S\bar{v}O_2$ is low and arterial–venous oxygen content difference is high, it may be inferred that the problem is one of inadequate CO (likely) or markedly increased $\dot{V}O_2$.

The third important balance is between $\dot{V}O_2$ and oxygen demand at the cellular level. If increases in $\dot{V}O_2$ are considered to be protective in keeping the amount of oxygen *used* by the tissues equal to the amount *needed* by the tissues, matching of $\dot{V}O_2$ and oxygen demand is an essential part of treatment. When demand exceeds consumption, anaerobic

TABLE 60-2. Effect of Changes in Hemoglobin Concentration on $S\bar{v}O_2$°

HEMOGLOBIN	13	10	7.5	5
CaO_2	18	14	10.5	7
$C\bar{v}O_2$	14	10	6.5	3
$S\bar{v}O_2$	0.77	0.71	0.61	0.42

°Calculated change in $S\bar{v}O_2$ caused by a change in hemoglobin (g/dL), assuming no compensatory changes in other determinants of $S\bar{v}O_2$; PaO_2 = 100 mm Hg, SaO_2 = 0.98, $C(a - \bar{v})O_2$ = 4.0 mL/dL, and $\dot{V}O_2$ and cardiac output are not changed.

TABLE 60-3. Effect of Variation in PaO_2 on $S\bar{v}O_2$°

PaO_2	600	200	100	80	60	40
SaO_2	1.0	1.0	0.98	0.95	0.90	0.75
CaO_2	19.8	18.6	17.9	17.3	16.3	13.6
$C\bar{v}O_2$	15.9	14.6	13.9	13.3	12.3	9.6
$S\bar{v}O_2$	0.87	0.81	0.77	0.73	0.68	0.53

°Calculated change in $S\bar{v}O_2$ caused by an uncompensated change in PaO_2 (mm Hg), assuming hemoglobin = 13 g/dL, $C(a - \bar{v})O_2$ = 4.0 mL/dL, and $\dot{V}O_2$ and cardiac output are unchanged.

TABLE 60-4.   Effect of Cardiac Output on $S\bar{v}O_2$°

CO	10	7.5	5.0	4.0	3.0	2.0
$C(a-\bar{v})O_2$	2.5	3.3	5.0	6.3	8.3	12.5
CaO_2	18.3	18.3	18.3	18.3	18.3	18.3
$C\bar{v}O_2$	15.8	15.0	13.3	12.0	10.0	5.8
$S\bar{v}O_2$	0.87	0.83	0.73	0.66	0.55	0.31

°Calculated effect of uncompensated changes in cardiac output (L/min) on $S\bar{v}O_2$, assuming hemoglobin = 13 g/dL, PaO_2 = 100 mm Hg, SaO_2 = 0.98, and $\dot{V}O_2$ is fixed at 250 mL/min.

TABLE 60-5.   Effect of Oxygen Consumption on $S\bar{v}O_2$°

$\dot{V}O_2$	150	200	250	300	400	500
$C(a-\bar{v})O_2$	3.0	4.0	5.0	6.0	8.0	10.0
CaO_2	18.3	18.3	18.3	18.3	18.3	18.3
$C\bar{v}O_2$	15.3	14.3	13.3	12.3	10.3	8.3
$S\bar{v}O_2$	0.85	0.79	0.74	0.68	0.57	0.46

°Effect of uncompensated changes in $\dot{V}O_2$ (mL/min) on $S\bar{v}O_2$, assuming hemoglobin = 13 g/dL, PaO_2 = 100 mm Hg, SaO_2 = 0.98, and cardiac output is fixed at 5 L/min.

metabolism must occur and the eventual result is lactic acidosis. The lactate level, therefore, defines the balance between $\dot{V}O_2$ and oxygen demand. An elevated lactate implies either ongoing anaerobic metabolism (shock) or prior anaerobic metabolism and oxygen debt. A normal $S\bar{v}O_2$ implies the latter and a low $S\bar{v}O_2$, the former, in states of lactic acidosis, except in situations in which unloading cellular uptake or mitochondrial utilization are impaired.

PITFALLS IN CONTINUOUS VENOUS OXIMETRY

The most common sources of error in the continuous measurement of $S\bar{v}O_2$ are calibration and catheter malposition. Before instituting major therapeutic changes, it is prudent to confirm that the $S\bar{v}O_2$ value displayed is actually correct by performing co-oximetry on a mixed venous blood sample and comparing the value with that from the on-line instrument. Calibration should be done only after correcting any light intensity alerts.[12] The finding of a normal or high $S\bar{v}O_2$ when the light intensity alert is present should be viewed with skepticism.[9]

Although there are no differences in insertion techniques between fiberoptic and other PA catheters,[14] the fiberoptic catheters may require more frequent repositioning (unreported data). This may result from differences in the handling characteristics of the catheters or may be related to the fact that alarms caused by distal migration of the catheter tip alert the clinical team as to the need for repositioning. Finally, there are no differences in complications reported between traditional and fiberoptic catheters.[15]

Another reported pitfall of continuous $S\bar{v}O_2$ measurements is a poor correlation with CO in some clinical situations. As discussed previously, a high correlation between $S\bar{v}O_2$ and CO should not be expected in patients with changing $\dot{V}O_2$, SaO_2, and Hgb concentration.

COST EFFECTIVENESS

The increased cost of the fiberoptic catheter over other types of flow-directed PA catheters must be justified in the current cost-minded medical care. It is difficult to prove cost effectiveness of any new technology in terms of time to recovery or improved mortality. However, if savings can be shown in other areas because of the use of the new technology, it may be cost effective. With continuous venous oximetry, the potential for cost savings lies in decreased use of other modes for assessing oxygen transport balance (i.e., CO measurements and blood gas analyses).

For venous blood gas analyses to be saved, it must be possible to estimate, rather than measure, $P\bar{v}O_2$. Because dissolved oxygen contributes so little to the oxygen content of mixed venous blood (about 1%), wide differences in estimated $P\bar{v}O_2$ produce only minimal changes in the derived oxygen transport variables (Table 60-6). If $P\bar{v}O_2$ is assumed to be 35 mm Hg, the theoretical errors are halved.[16] Using this assumption, we found that the number of venous blood gas analyses in our surgical ICU was reduced by 4.9 during a 72-hour study period, resulting in a charge reduction of $245 per patient. In this same population, we were able to decrease the number of CO measurements by 2.5 in the same 72-hour period, resulting in an estimated cost reduction to the hospital (for venous blood gas analysis alone) of $104 per catheter and an estimated charge savings to the patient of $278 per catheter. Other studies have confirmed similar savings,[17] and one study has also demonstrated savings of arterial blood gas analyses.[18] Recently, continuous $S\bar{v}O_2$ monitoring has been reported to decrease CO determinants by 69%, resulting in annualized savings of $87,500 for the institution.[19]

Several studies have suggested that the increased cost of the fiberoptic catheter (about $100) is not justifiable in terms of cost savings. Although no evidence supports that rapid

ASSESSMENT OF OXYGEN TRANSPORT

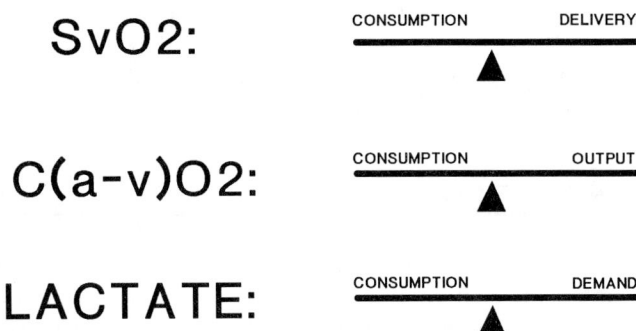

FIGURE 60-3. The three fundamental balances of oxygen transport.

TABLE 60-6. Percentage of Error Resulting
From Estimation of $P\bar{v}O_2$°

	MEASURED VALUES		
FACTOR	$S\bar{v}O_2 = 0.50$	$S\bar{v}O_2 = 0.75$	$S\bar{v}O_2 = 0.85$
$C\bar{v}O_2$	1.2	0.8	0.7
$C(a - \bar{v})O_2$	1.2	2.6	4.8
$\dot{V}O_2$	1.2	2.6	4.8
$\dot{Q}_{sp}/\dot{Q}_t$	0.9	1.0	3.0

°Theoretical maximum errors (%) in derived parameters if $P\bar{v}O_2$ is estimated at 20 and 50 mm Hg for each saturation value measured. Maximum error is only 4.8% at the extreme of estimating $P\bar{v}O_2$ to be 20 mm Hg when $S\bar{v}O_2$ is 0.85. The maximum error would be one half of this amount if $P\bar{v}O_2$ is estimated to be 35 mm Hg in all cases. These maximum predicted errors are not clinically significant.

titration of goal-directed therapy using $S\bar{v}O_2$ (or any monitoring technique) improves patient outcome or reduces morbidity, little doubt exists that physiologic end points may be reached more quickly using continuous monitors. If these end points relate to oxygen transport, $S\bar{v}O_2$ must be measured by some technique. Traditionally, this has been done by blood gas analysis, each therapeutic change being followed by an arterial and possibly a venous measurement. Although charges for each analysis are high ($60 to $125), the cost is also relatively high (estimated at $12 to $20). It does not take many pairs of blood gas analyses to result in cost savings in a critically ill patient. Costs will not be reduced when the system is inappropriately applied to patients who would not be assessed by traditional laboratory monitoring. Thus, in predictably stable populations, the additional venous oximetry would be neither of value nor cost effective. In fact, PA catheterization itself, not merely the capability for venous oximetry, should be carefully evaluated and, in many instances, omitted entirely without jeopardizing patient safety. Cost and charge calculations are always amenable to different interpretations. Whether charges are recoverable under managed care is no longer the issue. Intermittent blood gas measurements and CO determinations require personnel time and use of supplies. A continuous technique frees up the nurse, technician, respiratory therapist, physician, or medical student to perform other tasks. The early warning is an added benefit of recognition of response (or nonresponse) to presumed therapeutic interventions and renders care simpler and more efficient. These efforts are especially important in the developing health care environment, independent of cost calculations.

COMBINED VENOUS AND PULSE OXIMETRY

Pulse oximetry and continuous mixed venous oximetry can be combined into a useful tool if we understand the underlying physiology that allows certain inferences to be made and

specific limitations resulting from the same physiology. The two devices together provide the capacity to evaluate simultaneous changes in the patient's cardiovascular and respiratory systems. Arterial oxygen tension and arterial oxygen saturation are related through the familiar oxyhemoglobin dissociation curve. SaO_2 values in the range of 70 to 95 reflect changes in PaO_2, and are useful in monitoring cardiorespiratory disease and directing therapy. Large changes in PaO_2 (80 to 600 mm Hg) can occur with no change in SaO_2. We must adjust inspired oxygen tension so that the saturation values range between 80% and 95% to correspond to changes in PaO_2. However, to maintain arterial oxygen delivery, we commonly try to restrict SaO_2 values to the narrow range of 90% to 95%. Below 90%, desaturation diminishes arterial oxygen content and oxygen delivery; above 95%, SaO_2 values no longer track PaO_2 values. At a Hgb value of 13 g/dL, fully saturated Hgb would carry 18.07 mL of oxygen. If arterial PO_2 was 100 mm Hg, an additional 0.31 mL would be dissolved in plasma for a total content of 18.38 mL. If PaO_2 fell to 75 and SaO_2 concomitantly dropped to 95%, Hgb carried oxygen would be 18.07 × 0.95, or 17.17 mL. The dissolved oxygen would be 75 × 0.003, or 0.23, and total oxygen content would be 17.4 mL. In the first example, total oxygen content was 18.38 mL. If the second oxygen content, 17.4 mL, is divided by 18.38 mL, the quotient is 0.95; thus, total oxygen content changed the same amount as did the arterial saturation. We can obtain the *same information* by comparing changes in SaO_2 alone without following either PaO_2 or calculating total oxygen content. The same is true for $S\bar{v}O_2$ and mixed venous oxygen content.

ARTERIAL VENOUS OXYGEN CONTENT DIFFERENCE ■

From the Fick principle, we learned that CO was equal to oxygen consumption divided by arterial venous oxygen content difference $(Ca - \bar{v})O_2$. Even in the critically ill patient, it is unlikely that Hgb or total body oxygen consumption can change sufficiently minute-to-minute to affect the calculations. Therefore, $(Ca - \bar{v})O_2$ should reflect changes in CO. In addition, immediate response to therapy—or lack thereof—can help us tailor therapy more precisely and more rapidly.

The contribution of dissolved oxygen can be ignored in the clinically relevant ranges, and the factor, Hgb × 1.39, occurs in both formulas and can be dropped from the calculation. Thus, $(Ca - \bar{v})O_2$ can be estimated by subtracting the output values of pulse oximetry and continuous mixed venous oximetry, $Sa - S\bar{v}$.

INTRAPULMONARY SHUNT ■

Although PaO_2 is affected by changes in respiratory function (intrapulmonary shunt), PaO_2 is also affected by changes in CO. If oxygen consumption remains constant, arterial venous oxygen content difference varies inversely to CO. Because arterial blood is usually nearly completely saturated, arterial venous content difference is changed, principally increased by greater extraction, leaving a decreased mixed venous oxygen content. This venous blood, now desaturated to a greater degree passing through the same areas of intrapulmonary shunting in the lung, has a greater "dilutional" effect on pulmonary capillary oxygen content when mixing occurs in the left side of the heart. Thus, although no change in pulmonary function has occurred, a decrease in CO (or even any factor that decreases venous oxygen content) lowers PaO_2 and increases the alveolar to arterial oxygen tension gradient. Thus, PaO_2 may decrease without deterioration in lung function or increase in intrapulmonary shunt.[20]

The formula for intrapulmonary shunt seems to be a simple equation:

$$\dot{Q}sp/\dot{Q}t = \frac{Cc - Ca}{Cc - C\bar{v}}$$

where $\dot{Q}sp/\dot{Q}t$ is physiologic shunt, Cc is capillary oxygen content, Ca is arterial oxygen content, and $C\bar{v}$ is venous oxygen content. We can form an approximation of the shunt equation, again ignoring the calculation of Hgb-carried oxygen by dropping (Hgb × 1.39) and substituting saturations of 100% for the pulmonary capillary saturation, pulse oximetry for arterial saturation, and mixed venous oximetry for $S\bar{v}O_2$. The entire equation for pulmonary capillary content can be replaced by the term 1 (or 100% Hgb saturation). Because we have already substituted Sa for arterial content and $S\bar{v}$ for venous content, this estimation of physiologic shunt (the $\dot{V}/\dot{Q}$ I)[21] can be represented by the equation:

$$\dot{V}/\dot{Q}\ I = \frac{1 - Sa}{1 - S\bar{v}}.$$

For instance, if arterial saturation was 90% (or .9) and venous saturation was 60% (or .6) the calculation would be

$$\frac{1 - .9}{1 - .6} = \frac{.1}{.4} = 25\%$$

This estimation fails to reflect the severity of respiratory failure as judged by the need to use a high fraction of inspired oxygen (FIO_2) to compensate for and to correct arterial hypoxemia. The severity of respiratory failure is to append the FIO_2 to the $\dot{V}/\dot{Q}$ I. Thus, the statement, "$\dot{V}/\dot{Q}$ I of 0.25 at $FIO_2 = 1.0$," indicates a more serious disturbance of gas exchange than "$\dot{V}/\dot{Q}$ I of 0.25 at $FIO_2 = .3$."

APPLICABILITY ■

There are many valuable bedside uses for simultaneous oximetry. For instance, if a patient's respiratory function has improved, high FIO_2 may be weaned quickly. We have found that changes can be made every 5 minutes. This contrasts to the usual clinical scenario using blood gases: change in FIO_2, 15-minute "equilibration" period, drawing and labeling of arterial specimen, transport of specimen to blood gas laboratory, and awaiting of results—commonly a 30- to 40-minute process for each change. If patients have severely depressed oxygenation, PEEP therapy also can be augmented much more rapidly. In the case of cardiovascular collapse associated with low $S\bar{v}O_2$, the response to blood and other fluid infusions as well as vasoactive drugs can be judged rapidly. If the intervention does not increase $S\bar{v}O_2$ quickly (within a few minutes), it probably has not been effective. Increased CO may result in increased oxygen consumption without a change in (Sa − $S\bar{v}$) but whenever this is suspected, we can measure CO directly. This ability to judge the effectiveness of interventions quickly is certainly attractive and often gratifying to the clinician.

APPENDIX 1 ■

NORMAL RANGE, UNITS, AND DERIVATION FOR COMMON OXYGEN TRANSPORT TERMS

PARAMETER	NORMAL RANGE	UNITS	DERIVATION
PaO_2	(varies with FIO_2)	mm Hg	Measured
SaO_2	>0.92	(fraction)	Measured
CaO_2	16–22	mL/dL	$(SaO_2 \times Hgb \times 1.38) + PaO_2 \times 0.0031)$
$P\bar{v}O_2$	35–45	mm Hg	Measured
$S\bar{v}O_2$	0.68–0.77	(fraction)	Measured
$C\bar{v}O_2$	12–17	mL/dL	$(S\bar{v}O_2 \times Hgb \times 1.38) + (P\bar{v}O_2 \times 0.0031)$
$C(a - \bar{v})O_2$	3.5–5.5	mL/dL	$CaO_2 - C\bar{v}O_2$
$\dot{V}O_2$	180–280	mL/min	$C(a - \bar{v})O_2 \times CO \times 10$
$\dot{D}O_2$	700–1400	mL/min	$CaO_2 \times CO \times 10$
OUC	0.23–0.32	(fraction)	$\dot{V}O_2/\dot{D}O_2$

PaO_2, arterial oxygen tension; SaO_2, arterial oxygen saturation; CaO_2, arterial oxygen content; $P\bar{v}O_2$, mixed venous oxygen tension; $S\bar{v}O_2$ = mixed venous oxygen saturation; $C\bar{v}O_2$ = mixed venous oxygen content; $C(a - \bar{v})O_2$, arterial–venous oxygen content difference; $\dot{V}O_2$, oxygen consumption; $\dot{D}O_2$, oxygen delivery; OUC, oxygen utilization coefficient (extraction ratio); FIO_2, fraction of inspired oxygen; Hgb, hemoglobin; CO, cardiac output.

°Normal ranges are approximate and may vary between laboratories.

APPENDIX 2   ■

CLINICAL EXAMPLES

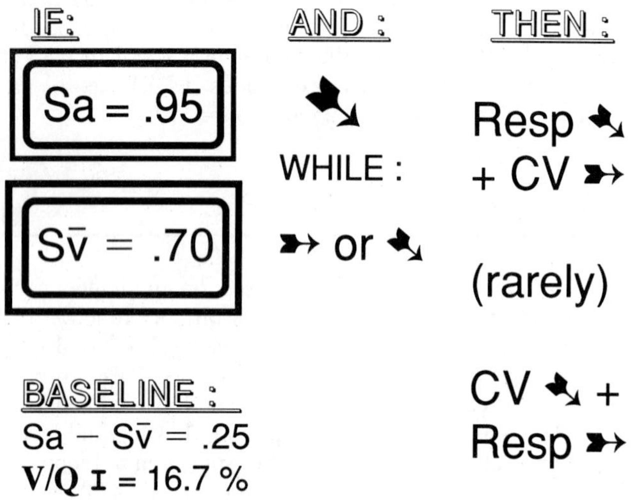

IF:

$Sa = .95$

$S\bar{v} = .70$

AND :

WHILE :

➳ or ➘

THEN :

Resp ➘
+ CV ➳

(rarely)

CV ➘ +
Resp ➳

BASELINE :
$Sa - S\bar{v} = .25$
$V/Q\ I = 16.7\ \%$

FIGURE 60-4.
WHAT'S THE BASELINE?
Conditions are satisfactory: arterial oxygenation (if a nontoxic in-spired oxygen concentration is used) and satisfactory cardiac out-put (CO), as estimated indirectly by an $Sa - S\bar{v}$ value of 0.25. $\dot{V}/\dot{Q}$ index is 0.05/0.30 or 16.7%.
WHAT'S HAPPENING?
Arterial saturation is decreasing while venous saturation is decreas-ing similarly or perhaps somewhat less.
WHAT'S THE INTERPRETATION?
The most likely cause would be a worsening of respiratory function leading to an increased intrapulmonary shunt and decrease in arte-rial oxygen tension and thus arterial oxygen saturation. If no other changes occur in the factors affecting venous saturation, a concomi-tant and equal decrease in venous saturation would be expected. However, if cardiac output increased and oxygen consumption remained the same, $Sa - S\bar{v}$ might diminish and given the lower Sa, $S\bar{v}$ might remain the same.

If, however, intrapulmonary shunt is moderately elevated, per-haps 20% to 30% (higher than in this example) and then cardiac output decreased, we might anticipate that venous saturation would fall and arterial saturation would decrease. In fact, the higher the shunt, the more significant the effect will be. Thus, two possibilities exist: (1) arterial saturation fell first, followed by a fall in venous saturation indicating worsening respiratory function or (2) the op-posite, that is, a fall in venous saturation followed by a fall in arterial saturation reflecting worsening cardiovascular function. It is often difficult to distinguish between the two; therefore, measurements of cardiac output or arterial blood gases may be necessary to help sort out the possibilities. It is clearly important to do so because inappropriate PEEP therapy directed at a perceived worsening in respiratory function may further compromise a decreased cardiac output if that, indeed, was the primary cause. Of even greater significance is that therapy directed against the wrong cause leaves the primary etiology, in this postulation, a depressed cardiac output, undetected and, therefore, untreated.

Worsening respiratory function will be manifested by a decrease in SaO_2 followed by a decrease in $S\bar{v}O_2$ (followed, one hopes, by PEEP therapy). If cardiac function decreases, $S\bar{v}O_2$ falls first and SaO_2 may follow. Augmentation of CO is necessary.

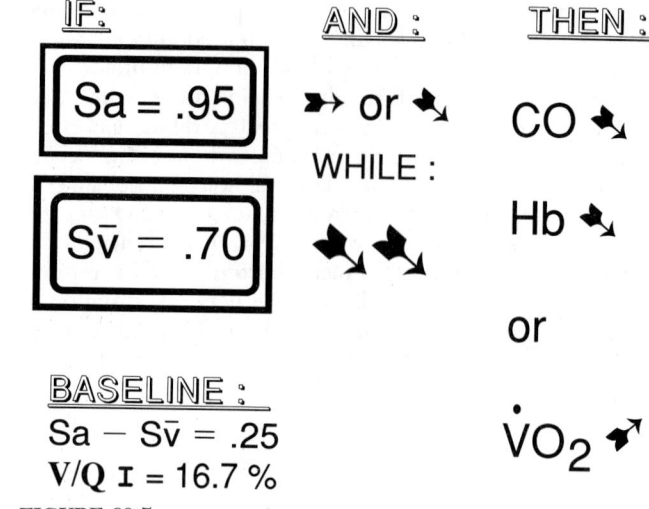

FIGURE 60-5.
WHAT'S THE BASELINE?
Satisfactory arterial oxygenation and a normal value for $Sa - S\bar{v}$ of 0.25. $\dot{V}/\dot{Q}$ index = 0.05/0.30 or 16.7%.
WHAT'S HAPPENING?
In this situation, arterial saturation stays the same or decreases while venous saturation markedly decreases.
WHAT'S THE INTERPRETATION?
The same three factors as in Figure 60-4 must be investigated. A decrease in cardiac output or increase in oxygen consumption may be compensated by an increase in arteriovenous oxygen content difference as estimated by the increasing $Sa - S\bar{v}$. In the presence of moderate to severe respiratory dysfunction, a fall in venous saturation may be accompanied by a fall in arterial saturation. Without respiratory insufficiency, however, arterial saturation is usually well maintained and the compensatory mechanism is seen solely as a fall in venous saturation. Another alternative is that arteriovenous oxygen content difference remains the same but, because of a decreasing hemoglobin concentration, an increased percentage of arterial oxygen must be extracted and the $Sa - S\bar{v}$ value increases but does not reflect a change in arteriovenous oxygen content difference. For instance, arterial content of 15 mL would be associated with an arterial saturation of approximately 0.95 and a hemoglobin of 11 g. If arterial venous oxygen content difference was 5 mL, venous saturation would be approximately 0.65, giving an $Sa - S\bar{v}$ value of 0.30. If the hemoglobin fell to 7 g, arterial oxygen content would be 10 mL, again, at a saturation of approximately 0.95. To maintain the 5-mL arteriovenous oxygen content difference, venous saturation would have to decrease to 0.50, resulting in an $Sa - S\bar{v}$ value of 0.45, which is still associated with an AVO_2 difference of 5 mL. Although a fall in venous satura-tion may not be the typical method of detecting postoperative bleeding (reflected by a decreasing hemoglobin level), it is not uncommon when resuscitative efforts maintain a normal intravascu-lar volume with repeated fluid boluses. This results in an acute normovolemic anemia, which may be manifested by a falling venous saturation. Again, confirmation of a decreased cardiac output or a decreased hemoglobin can be attained by appropriate testing, and changes in oxygen consumption can be inferred from changes in temperature or correction of a metabolic acidosis reflecting an increased oxygen consumption to pay off the oxygen debt.

Fever, chills, rewarming, and agitation can produce marked de-creases in venous saturation. Look for these and treat if necessary, especially in the elderly patient with compromised cardiac function.

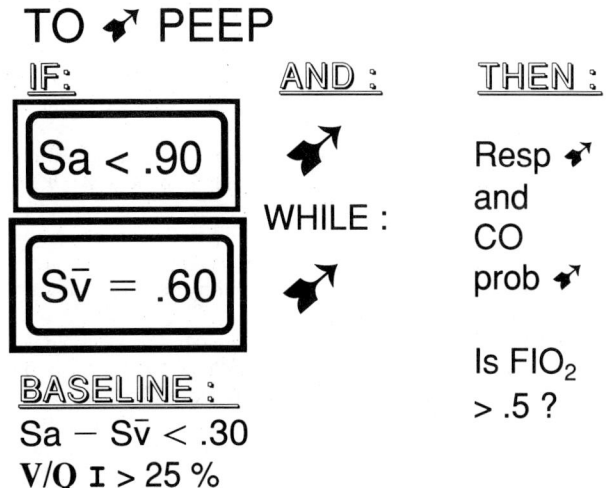

FIGURE 60-6.

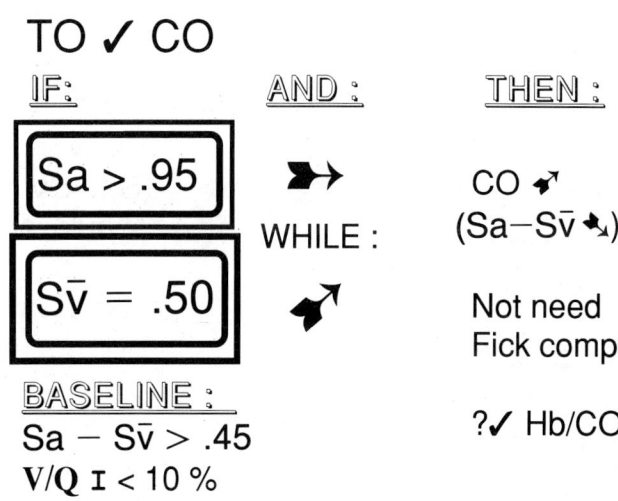

FIGURE 60-7.

WHAT'S THE BASELINE?

So far we have described acute respiratory insufficiency manifested by arterial desaturation without response to therapy. $\dot{V}/\dot{Q}$ index is >25% with Sa − $\bar{v}$ <0.30.

WHAT'S HAPPENING?

Arterial saturation increases with a further increment in PEEP. Additionally, venous saturation may increase a similar amount or to even a greater degree, thus narrowing Sa − S$\bar{v}$.

WHAT'S THE INTERPRETATION?

Finally, we have seen a favorable response to augmentation of PEEP resulting in a decreased intrapulmonary shunt and improvement in respiratory function. If this results in an increase in oxygen delivery, cardiac output might increase, which would be reflected by a diminished Sa − S$\bar{v}$. In this situation, because Sa is increasing, we would not expect that S$\bar{v}$ increased to a greater degree than Sa. Why would cardiac output increase in response to PEEP therapy? First, the improvement in oxygen delivery might improve cardiac function but more likely, especially if PEEP therapy had previously been augmented significantly without affecting respiratory function, some measures at improving cardiac output may have been instituted. Thus, the improvement in cardiac output reflects concomitant therapy directed at both cardiac and respiratory components of the illness. As a rule, when possible, make one intervention at a time. The sequence is to make an intervention, watch for effect; if no effect, increase level; if no effect at maximal dose or level, change interventions. Make the changes quickly and consecutively.

Finally, the goal of therapy is adequate arterial saturation at nontoxic inspired oxygen concentrations. Often, when dealing with acute desaturation, we elevate FIO_2 to compensate for this desaturation. Remember that once saturations improve, the next step is to lower FIO_2 keeping SaO_2 in the range of 0.90 to 0.95 until inspired oxygen concentration is less than 0.50.

WHAT'S THE BASELINE?

We postulate isolated cardiac dysfunction as manifested by normal arterial saturation and a high value for Sa − S$\bar{v}$, >0.45. We have chosen an intervention that we hope will increase cardiac output and we hope to detect it by a diminished Sa − S$\bar{v}$ value. $\dot{V}/\dot{Q}$ index remains <10% (<0.05/0.50).

WHAT'S HAPPENING?

Arterial saturation remains the same, that is, near its maximum of 1.0. Sv, however, increases. We interpret this as diminished need to extract oxygen because of an increase in cardiac output.

WHAT'S THE INTERPRETATION?

The decrease in Sa − S$\bar{v}$ reflects decreased oxygen extraction from the arterial blood, which we believe is caused by the increased delivery caused by the increased cardiac output. Thus, the body no longer needs to use the compensatory mechanism expressed in the Fick principle to maintain oxygen uptake. Reciprocal changes in Sa − S$\bar{v}$ and cardiac output occur only if oxygen consumption remains constant. However, in cases of cardiovascular collapse when we are most likely to want to use Sa − S$\bar{v}$ measurements to estimate cardiac output changes, we can easily think of a number of other factors that complicate this simplistic interpretation. For instance, if oxygen delivery had been low and the body had switched from aerobic to anaerobic metabolism, lactic acidosis and an oxygen debt would also be present. It would be physiologically appropriate to maintain a high oxygen extraction even when cardiac output increased so that this oxygen debt could be paid off more rapidly. Hyperthermia and hypothermia, again, are common and alter oxygen consumption. Hypothermia can diminish oxygen consumption or oxygen consumption can be markedly increased as a hypothermic patient rewarms. Therefore, although we confine observations to the minute-to-minute changes that make it more likely that Sa − S$\bar{v}$ correlates inversely with changes in cardiac output, the best approach is to fill in the blanks between cardiac output measurements rather than to base our overall interpretations of changes in the complicated oxygen transport/oxygen utilization balance on this single measurement.

DOUBLE EFFECT :

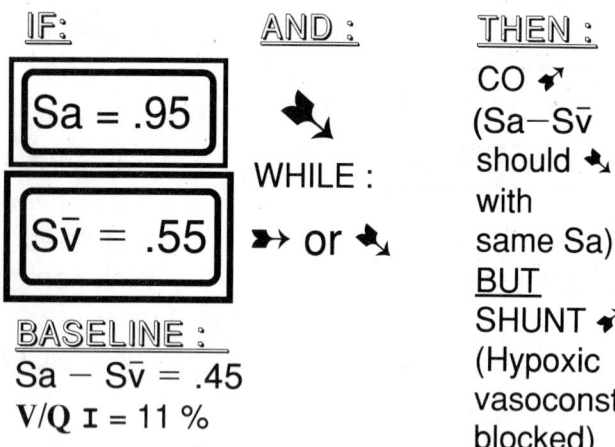

IF:

$Sa = .95$

$S\bar{v} = .55$

BASELINE :

$Sa - S\bar{v} = .45$

$\dot{V}/\dot{Q}$ ɪ = 11 %

AND :

WHILE :

THEN :

CO ↗

(Sa–S̄v should ↘ with same Sa)

BUT

SHUNT ↗

(Hypoxic vasoconst blocked)

FIGURE 60-8.

WHAT'S THE BASELINE?
Arterial oxygen saturation is satisfactory at 0.95 if the F_{IO_2} is <0.5. However, with an $S\bar{v}$ value of 0.55, $Sa - S\bar{v}$ is elevated at 0.40, perhaps indicating a low cardiac output. Indeed, on subsequent measurement, cardiac output is 3.0 L/min in association with an elevated systemic vascular resistance. Sodium nitroprusside is chosen as a vasodilating agent to decrease resistance with the expectation that cardiac output would increase. $\dot{V}/\dot{Q}$ index = 0.05/0.45 or 11%.

WHAT'S HAPPENING?
An immediate and marked decrease in arterial saturation occurs. Concomitantly, a lesser decrease in mixed venous saturation occurs.

WHAT'S THE INTERPRETATION?
This is a problem of combined respiratory and cardiovascular dysfunction and an example of divergent effects resulting from a single intervention. A decrease in vascular resistance, particularly in a patient with compromised myocardial function, would be expected to increase cardiac output through diminished impedance to aortic flow (afterload). In this case, measured cardiac output increased to 4.2 L, associated with a drop in Sa to 0.90, an increase in $S\bar{v}$ to 0.60, and a fall in $Sa - S\bar{v}$ to 0.30. However, the vasodilating agents are not specific to the systemic circulation. Occasionally, patients have a degree of hypoxic pulmonary vascular constriction; sodium nitroprusside, administered for its systemic effect, unfortunately also negates this constriction, which usually occurs in areas of low $\dot{V}/\dot{Q}$ ratios. When this reflex is abolished by the administration of a vasodilator, perfusion increases thus creating an increase in intrapulmonary shunt or at least increasing $\dot{V}/\dot{Q}$ mismatch. Indeed, the $\dot{V}/\dot{Q}$ index in this example increased from 11% (0.05/0.45) to 25% (0.10/0.40). Notice that the fall in arterial saturation is greater than the fall in venous saturation. If no improvement had occurred in cardiac output, $Sa - S\bar{v}$ would not have been narrowed, and the fall in arterial saturation would have been mirrored by a similar decrease in venous saturation.

REFERENCES ■

1. Nelson LD: Venous oximetry. In: Snyder JV (ed). *Oxygen Transport in the Critically Ill Patient.* Chicago, Year Book Medical Publishers, 1986
2. Kandel G, Aberman A: Mixed venous oxygen saturation: its role in the assessment of the critically ill patient. *Arch Intern Med* 1983;143:1400
3. Wilson RF, Christensen C, LeBlanc LP: Oxygen consumption in critically ill surgical patients. *Ann Surg* 1972;276:801
4. Nelson LD: Continuous venous oximetry in critically ill surgical patients. *Ann Surg* 1986;203:329
5. Snyder JV, Carroll GC: Tissue oxygenation: a physiologic approach to a clinical problem. *Curr Probl Surg* 1982;19:650
6. Civetta JM: The inverse relationship between cost and survival. *J Surg Res* 1973;14:265
7. Civetta JM: Continuous mixed venous saturation: neither too little nor too much [panel]. Chicago, Society of Critical Care Medicine, May 1985
8. Watson CB: The PA catheter as an early warning system. *Anesthesiol Rev* 1983;10:34
9. Nelson LD: Continuous venous oximetry. I. Physiology and technical considerations. *Curr Rev Respir Ther* 1986;8:99
10. Civetta JM: Critical illness: the nonsteady state. *Surg Forum* 1972;23:153
11. Baele PL, McMichan JC, Marsh HM, et al: Continuous monitoring of mixed venous oxygen saturation in critically ill patients. *Anesth Analg* 1982;61:513
12. Oximetrix, Inc: *Shaw Catheter Oximetry System Instruction Manual.* Mountain View, CA, Oximetrix, 1981
13. Nelson LD, Snyder JV: Technical problems with data acquisition. In: Snyder JV (ed). *Oxygen Transport in the Critically Ill Patient.* Chicago, Year Book Medical Publishers, 1986
14. Nelson LD: Clinical use of mixed venous oximetry. In: Vincent JL (ed). *Update in Intensive Care and Emergency Medicine.* Berlin, Springer-Verlag, 1990
15. McMichan JC, Baele PL, Wignes MW: Insertion of pulmonary artery catheters: a comparison of fiberoptic and nonfiberoptic catheters. *Crit Care Med* 1984;12:517
16. Nelson LD: Continuous venous oximetry. II. Clinical applications. *Curr Rev Respir Ther* 1986;8:106
17. Orlando R: Continuous mixed venous oximetry in critically ill surgical patients: "high-tech" cost-effectiveness. *Arch Surg* 1986;121:470
18. Fahey PJ, Harris K, Vanderwarf C: Clinical experience with continuous monitoring of mixed venous oxygen saturation in respiratory failure. *Chest* 1984;86:748
19. Arnoldi D, Dechert R, Wise C, et al: Use of continuous SvO_2 monitoring can decrease requirements for cardiac output determination in surgical ICU patients. *Crit Care Med* 1995;23:1(Suppl), A22.
20. Norwood SH, Civetta JM: Ventilatory support in patients with ARDS. *Surg Clin North Am* 1985;65:895
21. Rasaner J, Downs JB, Malec DJ, et al: Real time continuous estimation of gas exchange by dual oximetry. *Intensive Care Med* 1988;14:11

Critical Care, Third Edition, edited by Joseph M. Civetta,
Robert W. Taylor, and Robert R. Kirby.
Lippincott-Raven Publishers, Philadelphia, PA © 1997.

CHAPTER 61

■

Blood Gas Analysis

Barry A. Shapiro
William T. Peruzzi

Respiration is the diffusion of oxygen (O_2) and carbon dioxide (CO_2) across permeable membranes. Respiratory homeostasis is an essential metabolic balance in which the quantities of CO_2 and O_2 exchanged in the lungs are a "mirror image" of cellular respiration. Critically ill patients often require therapeutic interventions to maintain respiratory homeostasis, a clinical demand that depends mostly on proper monitoring and interpretation of the arterial "blood gas values" (arterial pH [pHa], $PaCO_2$, and PaO_2).

INTERPRETIVE GUIDELINES ■

EVALUATION OF ARTERIAL pH AND $PaCO_2$

Normal adult metabolism produces more than 12,000 mMol of H^+ per day. Nearly 99% of that acid load is attributable to CO_2 production. Most of the blood's CO_2 exists in sundry chemical combinations primarily within the erythrocytes; less than 5% of the CO_2 exists in physical solution, the form that directly exerts a partial pressure. The complex interrelationships between the dissolved and the chemically combined CO_2 are such that the $PaCO_2$ is a reliable means of evaluating the extent to which the blood has increased or decreased CO_2 content. The pHa is a measure of free H^+ concentration that must exist within a narrow range for cellular life processes to be maintained.

Normal adult values for $PaCO_2$ and pHa are listed in Table 61-1. Because the $PaCO_2$ varies directly and predictably with the plasma H_2CO_3 concentration, measurement of pHa and $PaCO_2$ allows calculation of plasma bicarbonate (HCO_3^-). Minor variations from these "normal" values rarely influence therapeutic judgments in critically ill patients.

Thus, the concept of "clinically acceptable" ranges (see Table 61-1) is widely accepted. Also listed are the terms used to indicate when these clinically acceptable ranges have been exceeded. Table 61-2 lists the traditional nomenclature for acid–base imbalances.

Acidosis and alkalosis are pathophysiologic processes in which the normal quantities of acid and base are skewed, but the pH may be normal. When abnormal pH values are present (acidemia or alkalemia), an anomalous free hydrogen ion concentration exists, denoting an uncompensated acidosis or alkalosis. Significantly abnormal pH values (<7.30 or >7.50) are potentially life-threatening because (1) enzyme systems may malfunction; (2) electrophysiologic mechanisms may be disrupted; (3) electrolyte balance may be altered; (4) acute pulmonary hypertension may be manifest; and (5) autonomic receptors may not react predictably to exogenous drugs.

Table 61-3 outlines our recommended procedure for initial evaluation of arterial blood gas values: first, classify the ventilatory status ($PaCO_2$); then, subclassify that ventilatory state in conjunction with the acid–base status (pHa).

EVALUATION OF ARTERIAL PaO_2

Precise use of the term *hypoxemia* denotes an insufficient amount of O_2 in the blood. Assuming an adequate hemoglobin content, arterial hypoxemia denotes a PaO_2 below a clinically acceptable level while the individual breathes at least 20.9% O_2 at sea level. Table 61-4 lists these acceptable values at various ages. Table 61-5 lists the minimal PaO_2 that would result from various inspired O_2 concentrations in a normal adult. In ideal circumstances, raising the fraction of inspired O_2 (FIO_2) by 0.1 increases the ideal alveolar PO_2 (PAO_2) by

TABLE 61-1. Interpretative Guidelines for Critically Ill Patients

	pHa	PaCo$_2$ (mm Hg)	HCO$_3^-$ (mMol/L)	BE (mMol/L)
Mean	7.40	40	25	0
Normal range	7.35–7.45	35–45	23–27	+/−3
Clinically acceptable	7.30–7.50	30–50	20–30	+/−10
Alkalemia	>7.50			
Acidemia	<7.30			
Ventilatory failure (respiratory acidosis)		>50		
Alveolar hyperventilation (respiratory alkalosis)		<30		
Acute ventilatory failure	<7.30	>50		

BE, base excess.

TABLE 61-2. Traditional Acid–Base Nomenclature

NOMENCLATURE	pH	Pco$_2$ (mm Hg)	BICARB (mMol/L)	BE (mMol/L)
METABOLIC ACIDOSIS				
Uncompensated (acute)	↓	N	↓	↓
Partly compensated (subacute)	↓	↓	↓	↓
Completely compensated (chronic)	N	↓	↓	↓
METABOLIC ALKALOSIS				
Uncompensated (acute)	↑	N	↑	↑
Partly compensated (subacute)	↑	↑	↑	↑
Completely compensated (chronic)	N	↑	↑	↑
RESPIRATORY ACIDOSIS				
Uncompensated (acute)	↓	↑	N	N
Partly compensated (subacute)	↓	↑	↑	↑
Completely compensated (chronic)	N	↑	↑	↑
RESPIRATORY ALKALOSIS				
Uncompensated (acute)	↑	↓	N	N
Partly compensated (subacute)	↑	↓	↓	↓
Completely compensated (chronic)	N	↓	↓	↓

BICARB, bicarbonate; BE, base excess; N, normal; ↑, increase; ↓, decrease.

TABLE 61-3. Evaluation of Ventilatory Status and Metabolic Acid–Base Status

CLASSIFICATION OF Paco$_2$

Paco$_2$ <30 mm Hg	Alveolar hyperventilation (respiratory alkalosis)
Paco$_2$ 30–50 mm Hg	Acceptable alveolar ventilation
Paco$_2$ >50 mm Hg	Ventilatory failure (respiratory acidosis)

CLASSIFICATION OF VENTILATORY STATE IN CONJUNCTION WITH pH

1. Alveolar hyperventilation (Paco$_2$ <30 mm Hg)

pH >7.50	Acute alveolar hyperventilation
pH 7.40–7.50	Chronic alveolar hyperventilation
pH 7.30–7.40	Compensated metabolic acidosis
pH <7.30	Partly compensated metabolic acidosis

2. Acceptable alveolar ventilation (Paco$_2$ 30–50 mm Hg)

pH >7.50	Metabolic alkalosis
pH 7.30–7.50	Acceptable ventilatory and metabolic acid–base status
pH <7.30	Metabolic acidosis

3. Ventilatory failure (Paco$_2$ >50 mm Hg)

pH >7.50	Partly compensated metabolic alkalosis
pH 7.30–7.50	Chronic ventilatory failure
pH <7.30	Acute ventilatory failure

approximately 50 mm Hg. When oxygen therapy is applied, the PaO$_2$ may be greater than 80 mm Hg, although hypoxemia would be present if room air was breathed. Multiplying the FIO$_2$ by 500 estimates the minimal PaO$_2$ expected in a normal person; a measured PaO$_2$ of less than the predicted minimal value indicates that the patient would be hypoxemic when breathing room air.

Table 61-6 lists the suggested acceptable limits and nomenclature for evaluating the PaO$_2$ during room air breathing and when oxygen therapy is being administered. Decreasing the FIO$_2$ administered to a significantly hypoxemic patient is potentially dangerous and unnecessary for evaluation of hypoxemia.

TABLE 61-4. Acceptable Arterial Oxygen Tensions at Sea Level Breathing Room Air (21% Oxygen)

ADULT AND CHILD	
Normal	97 mm Hg
Acceptable range	>80 mm Hg
Hypoxemia	<80 mm Hg
NEWBORN	
Acceptable range	40–70 mm Hg
ELDERLY	Acceptable range
60 years old	>80 mm Hg
70 years old	>70 mm Hg
80 years old	>60 mm Hg
90 years old	>50 mm Hg

TABLE 61-5. Generalized Inspired Oxygen–Arterial Tension Relationship°

F_{IO_2} (%)	PREDICTED MINIMAL Pa_{O_2} (mm Hg)
0.3 (30)	150
0.4 (40)	200
0.5 (50)	250
0.8 (80)	400
1.0 (100)	500

F_{IO_2}, fraction of inspired oxygen.

°If Pa_{O_2} is less than $F_{IO_2} \times 500$, the patient can be assumed to be hypoxemic while breathing room air.

TABLE 61-6. Evaluation of Hypoxemia

ROOM AIR: PATIENT YOUNGER THAN 60 YEARS OLD°

Mild hypoxemia	Pa_{O_2} <80 mm Hg
Moderate hypoxemia	Pa_{O_2} <60 mm Hg
Severe hypoxemia	Pa_{O_2} <40 mm Hg

OXYGEN THERAPY

Uncorrected hypoxemia	Pa_{O_2} <Room air acceptable limit
Corrected hypoxemia	Pa_{O_2} >Room air minimal limit; <100 mm Hg
Excessively corrected hypoxemia	Pa_{O_2} <Room air minimal limit; <minimal predicted

°For each year over 60 years, subtract 1 mm Hg for limits of mild and moderate hypoxemia. At any age, a Pa_{O_2} <40 mm Hg indicates severe hypoxemia.

ARTERIAL OXYGENATION

Most of the O_2 in the blood exists in chemical combination with hemoglobin, whereas less than 5% is dissolved in the plasma. The quantity of O_2 that moves into (or out of) the blood depends on three factors: (1) the amount of dissolved O_2 (P_{O_2}), (2) the amount of O_2 combined to the hemoglobin (%$HgbO_2$), and (3) the degree to which the hemoglobin attracts O_2 (Hgb–O_2 affinity).

OXYGEN CONTENT CALCULATION

The number of milliliters of O_2 contained in 100 mL of blood is defined as O_2 content (mL/dL). Calculation of O_2 content is illustrated in Table 61-7 and requires measurement of P_{O_2} (mm Hg), %$HgbO_2$, and the hemoglobin (g/dL).

OXYHEMOGLOBIN MEASUREMENT

The sixth valence bond between the ferrous ion within the heme molecule and the imidazole nitrogen on the amino acid chain is capable of reversibly combining with an O_2 molecule. When O_2 is attached, it is called oxyhemoglobin ($HgbO_2$) and when a H^+ is attached, it is called "reduced" (nonoxygenated) hemoglobin. Two other conditions commonly alter the hemoglobin's ability to transport O_2: (1) car-

TABLE 61-7. Calculating Oxygen Content

STEPS

1. Hemoglobin content (g/dL) $\times$ 1.34 $\times$ $HgbO_2$ = oxygen attached to hemoglobin (mL/dL)
2. P_{O_2} $\times$ 0.003 = oxygen dissolved in plasma (mL/dL)
3. Steps 1 + 2 = oxygen content (mL/dL)

EXAMPLE 1: Hgb 15 g/dL, P_{O_2} 100 mm Hg, Hgb_{O_2} 100%

1.	$15 \times 1.34 \times 1.00 =$	20.10 mL/dL
2.	$100 \times 0.003 =$	0.30 mL/dL
3.		20.40 mL/dL

EXAMPLE 2: Hgb 15 g/dL, P_{O_2} 50 mm Hg, Hgb_{O_2} 85%

1.	$15 \times 1.34 \times 0.85 =$	17.09 mL/dL
2.	$50 \times 0.003 =$	0.15 mL/dL
3.		17.24 mL/dL

Grams percent (g%) = grams of hemoglobin per deciliter (dL).
Volumes percent (vol%) = milliliters of oxygen per deciliter (dL).

boxyhemoglobin (HgbCO), where carbon monoxide (CO) is attached at the sixth valence site; and (2) methemoglobin, where iron is oxidized to the ferric state and thereby loses the sixth valence.

The %$HgbO_2$ is the portion, expressed as a percentage, of the total hemoglobin that is oxygenated. The gold standard for measuring %$HgbO_2$ is multiwavelength oximetry, which measures $HgbO_2$, reduced hemoglobin, HgbCO, and methemoglobin. When $HgbO_2$ is calculated, the assumption usually is made that only $HgbO_2$ and reduced hemoglobin exist. This assumption may be incorrect in the critically ill patient.

HEMOGLOBIN–OXYGEN AFFINITY

Hemoglobin has a strong affinity for O_2 that can be altered by numerous factors. A decreased Hgb–O_2 affinity (shift to the right, or increased O_2 partial pressure at which hemoglobin is 50% saturated [P_{50}]) results in a diminished O_2 content that may further limit O_2 delivery; an increased Hgb–O_2 affinity increases the O_2 content but potentially inhibits O_2 unloading to the tissues. Because numerous factors in critically ill patients modify Hgb–O_2 affinity, the presence of hypoxemia demands that both P_{O_2} and %$HgbO_2$ be assessed. Assuming an adequate hemoglobin content (8 to 10 g/dL), a Pa_{O_2} of more than 60 mm Hg reliably reflects the arterial oxygenation status because %$HgbO_2$ is approaching maximum (Fig. 61-1); a hypoxemic Pa_{O_2} reliably reflects O_2 content *only* if the Hgb–O_2 relationship is normal. A "shift to the left" should never diminish clinical concern when significant hypoxemia is present.

ASSESSMENT OF HYPOXEMIA

Because cellular oxygenation is dependent on cardiac output and capillary perfusion in addition to the arterial O_2 content, Pa_{O_2} values greater than 60 mm Hg do not significantly

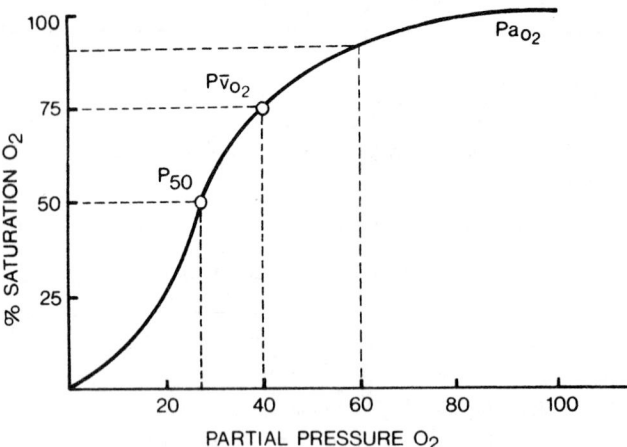

FIGURE 61-1. The hemoglobin dissociation curve. This curve shows the relationship of plasma oxygen partial pressure to the degree to which potential oxygen-carrying hemoglobin sites have oxygen attached (% saturation oxygen). This nonlinear relationship accounts for most of the oxygen reserves in blood. Normally, hemoglobin is 50% saturated at a plasma, Po of approximately 27 mm Hg; this is designated P_{50}. Normal mixed venous blood has an oxygen partial pressure ($P\bar{v}_{O_2}$) of 40 mm Hg and an oxyhemoglobin saturation of 75%. A Po_2 of 60 mm Hg normally results in approximately 90% saturation. Normal arterial blood has an oxygen partial pressure (Pao_2) of 97 mm Hg and an oxyhemoglobin saturation of 97%.

increase the capability for O_2 delivery and are generally considered acceptable in the critically ill. Deficiencies in arterial oxygenation that demand increased cardiac work to ensure tissue oxygenation are deemed clinically significant. Assuming adequate hemoglobin concentrations, significant hypoxemia is defined by Pao_2 less than 60 mm Hg or %$HgbO_2$ less than 90%. Pao_2 of less than 40 mm Hg (most often associated with %$HgbO_2$ below 75%) reflects a significantly decreased O_2 content and hemoglobin molecules that are less able to release O_2. Such severe hypoxemia is a direct threat to tissue oxygenation. A Pao_2 from 40 to 60 mm Hg may threaten tissue oxygenation if other functions such as cardiac output cannot sufficiently compensate for the diminished O_2 content.

VENTILATION ∎

The essential role of CO_2 excretion to the maintenance of acid–base balance was fully appreciated by the turn of the century and led to the traditional concepts of respiratory acidosis and alkalosis. However, advances in cardiopulmonary supportive care have demanded clinical acceptance of the reality that *respiratory acid–base imbalance is primarily a ventilatory malfunction.*

ESSENTIAL PHYSIOLOGY

Ventilation is gas movement in and out of the pulmonary system. In critically ill patients, it is most readily measured as the gas volume exhaled in 1 minute ($\dot{V}E$). The portion of

the $\dot{V}E$ that respires (removes CO_2 from the blood and transfers O_2 to the blood) is referred to as alveolar ventilation ($\dot{V}A$). The portion of the $\dot{V}E$ that does not respire is designated dead space ventilation ($\dot{V}D$).

Alveolar Ventilation and PaCO₂

Because metabolism determines the rate of CO_2 diffusion into the blood and $\dot{V}A$ determines the rate of CO_2 removal from the blood, $Paco_2$ reflects the adequacy with which $\dot{V}A$ balances CO_2 production.

Significantly abnormal CO_2 production must be identified when interpreting the $Paco_2$ in critically ill patients. Consider, for example, that: (1) temperature deviation directly alters CO_2 production approximately 10% per degree Celsius change; (2) excessive muscular activity (shivering, rigor, or seizure) can increase CO_2 production threefold to fivefold; (3) generalized "stress" responses can increase CO_2 production; and (4) sepsis is known to alter CO_2 production. Furthermore, changes in CO_2 stores can allow homeostasis to exist while intracellular, extracellular, blood, and alveolar Pco_2 ($Paco_2$) values are abnormal. Such changes in CO_2 stores are discussed later in this chapter. This initial presentation assumes a relatively normal CO_2 production and normal CO_2 stores.

Dead Space Ventilation

Ventilation is always the sum of alveolar and dead space components:

$$\dot{V}E = \dot{V}A + \dot{V}D \qquad (1)$$

$\dot{V}E$ can be measured, with $Paco_2$ used as a reflection of $\dot{V}A$, but a clinically meaningful assessment of the ventilatory status must include consideration of increases in $\dot{V}D$, which requires an increase in $\dot{V}E$ to maintain a consistent $\dot{V}A$. The common circumstances that increase $\dot{V}D$ are (1) acutely diminished cardiac output, which creates a greater portion of lung that is poorly perfused (high ventilation/perfusion [$\dot{V}/\dot{Q}$] matching); (2) acute pulmonary emboli, which create unperfused or ventilated alveoli; (3) acute pulmonary hypertension, which creates less perfusion of nongravity-dependent lung (high $\dot{V}/\dot{Q}$); (4) severe acute lung injury (acute respiratory distress syndrome [ARDS]), which creates zero $\dot{V}/\dot{Q}$, low $\dot{V}/\dot{Q}$, and high $\dot{V}/\dot{Q}$, causing significant intrapulmonary shunting and $\dot{V}D$; and (5) positive-pressure ventilation, which favors ventilation to nongravity-dependent lung to an extent that significantly increases $\dot{V}D$.

Two practical methods for clinical assessment of increases in $\dot{V}D$ are available. Although both methods are qualitative and subject to significant error, experience has shown their value when properly applied and interpreted.

$\dot{V}E$–$Paco_2$ DISPARITY. Clinical observation that $\dot{V}E$ is increased *without* an appropriate decrease in $Paco_2$ raises the possibility of increased $\dot{V}D$. Table 61-8 shows the expected $\dot{V}E$–$Paco_2$ relationships when CO_2 production remains normal and consistent. In our clinical experience (1) when the measured $\dot{V}E$ is associated with a $Paco_2$ significantly greater than predicted in Table 61-8, and increased CO_2 production

TABLE 61-8. Exhaled Minute Volume to Arterial Carbon Dioxide Tension Relationships in the Normal Nonexercising Human

$\dot{V}_E$	Pa_{CO_2} (mm Hg)	RANGE (mm Hg)
Normal	40	35–45
Twice normal	30	25–35
Quadruple normal	20	15–25

can be reasonably ruled out, increased $\dot{V}_D$ is the most likely explanation; (2) when the $\dot{V}_E$ is associated with a Pa_{CO_2} significantly less than predicted in Table 61-8, diminished CO_2 production or depleted CO_2 stores should be suspected.

$P(a - ET)CO_2$ DISPARITY. Figure 61-2 shows a normal CO_2 exhalation curve in a healthy young person. In the absence of significant pulmonary disease, the "end-tidal" P_{CO_2} (PET_{CO_2}) is several millimeters of mercury less than the Pa_{CO_2}. Acute increases in this $P(a - ET)CO_2$ gradient reflect increases in $\dot{V}_D$. This analysis is useful in the ICU and operating room, provided that baseline values are available for comparison.

WORK OF BREATHING

Breathing is the process by which cyclic respiratory muscle contractions that require energy expenditure produce ventilation. This to-and-fro valveless pump is so inefficient that in the normal resting state, only about 10% of the energy expended actually achieves physiologic ventilation, whereas the other 90% is lost as heat. Furthermore, as $\dot{V}_E$ is increased, the work of breathing (WOB) increases exponentially, so that fatigue limits are readily attainable even in normal persons.

In essence, we breathe to ventilate and ventilate to respire. WOB provided within the limits of cardiopulmonary reserves improves $\dot{V}/\dot{Q}$ matching and augments venous return to the heart, factors that can be considered beneficial to the maintenance of respiratory homeostasis. However, if WOB places demands on the cardiopulmonary system that

exceed functional reserves, the result is often detrimental to the maintenance of respiratory homeostasis.[1] Detrimental WOB can result from any circumstance in which increased $\dot{V}_E$ is required (e.g., increased metabolic rate or compensation for metabolic acidemia) or in which ventilatory reserves are reduced (e.g., lung disease, neuromuscular disease, postthoracoabdominal surgery).

Extreme degrees of detrimental WOB are clinically recognized as acute respiratory distress (progressive tachypnea, tachycardia, dyspnea, hypertension, intercostal retraction, use of accessory muscles of ventilation, diaphoresis, and mental status changes). The patient is often described as appearing "fatigued" or "tiring out." Lesser degrees of detrimental WOB are manifested by progressive increases in respiratory rate, heart rate, and systolic blood pressure, onset of diaphoresis and mental confusion, delirium, or even obtundation. Patients able to communicate invariably complain of dyspnea. The progression of clinical signs is an important element in the diagnosis of detrimental WOB.

ACUTE VENTILATORY FAILURE

The Pa_{CO_2} values of more than 50 mm Hg reflect a clinically significant failure of the cardiopulmonary system to adequately satisfy the metabolic requirements for CO_2 excretion. Traditional physiology terms this process *respiratory acidosis;* however, because the life-threatening process that must be treated is inadequate $\dot{V}_A$, a more clinically relevant term is *ventilatory failure.*

Respiratory failure is a clinical diagnosis implying that the pulmonary system is failing to provide adequate exchange of O_2, CO_2, or both to meet metabolic requirements. Ventilatory failure (respiratory acidosis) is a blood gas diagnosis that refers only to failure of the pulmonary system to provide adequate CO_2 excretion. As defined in Table 61-1, when the pH_a of less than 7.30 is in concert with an Pa_{CO_2} of more than 50 mm Hg, acute ventilatory failure exists and represents a potentially life-threatening circumstance.

In such life-threatening cases, the following factors must be immediately considered: (1) the need for ventilatory assistance if the patient is spontaneously breathing; (2) the adequacy of ventilatory assistance if the patient is mechanically ventilated, especially the presence of significant $\dot{V}_D$; (3) the

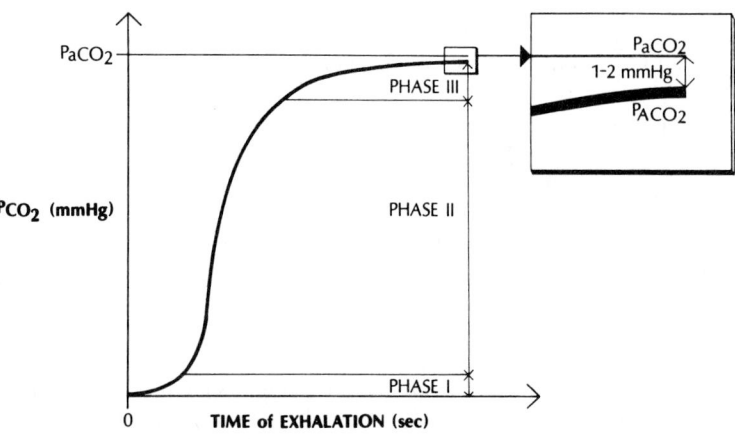

FIGURE 61-2. A normal exhaled CO_2 curve. *Phase I* represents deadspace. *Phase II* represents the increasing CO_2 tension as the exhaled gas becomes composed of increasingly more alveolar gas. *Phase III* represents the CO_2 plateau where the exhaled gas is composed primarily of gas from the alveoli. Inset shows the normal relationship between Pa_{CO_2} (arterial carbon dioxide tension) and the carbon dioxide tension of end-exhalation (end-tidal) gas. The normal disparity is less than 3 mm Hg. Increases in this disparity probably reflect increases in alveolar deadspace ventilation.

presence of tissue hypoxia if hypoxemia is documented; and (4) the probability of concomitant metabolic acidosis secondary to inadequate perfusion or detrimental WOB.

IMPENDING VENTILATORY FAILURE

The clinical suspicion of detrimental WOB in a patient with a still-acceptable $PaCO_2$ suggests that if no therapeutic interventions to reduce WOB are instituted, acute ventilatory failure will ensue. This circumstance represents impending ventilatory failure.[2] Metabolic acidemia, hypoxemia, or both are common in patients with impending ventilatory failure and are rapidly reversed when appropriate ventilatory assistance is instituted.

ACUTE RESPIRATORY ALKALOSIS ■

Clinically significant acute respiratory alkalosis ($PaCO_2$ <30 mm Hg; pH >7.50) represents acute alveolar hyperventilation and usually indicates an increased WOB. Three common causes of acute alveolar hyperventilation are recognized in the critically ill patient: (1) response to arterial hypoxemia, (2) response to metabolic acidosis; and (3) central nervous system (CNS) malfunction. The latter two are seldom concomitant with hypoxemia.

ACUTE RESPIRATORY ALKALOSIS WITHOUT HYPOXEMIA

These blood gas values are most commonly secondary to intracranial disease, anxiety, or pain. However, severe anemia, CO poisoning, and methemoglobinemia should be ruled out.

ACUTE RESPIRATORY ALKALOSIS WITH HYPOXEMIA

Blood gas findings indicating acute respiratory alkalosis are mostly attributable to cardiopulmonary disease.

Acute Pulmonary Disease

When hypoxemia results from a pulmonary process that is responsive to oxygen therapy (asthma, bronchitis, noncardiogenic edema, retained secretions, early pneumonia), administering O_2 should decrease WOB, increase $PaCO_2$, and decrease heart rate and blood pressure toward normal. The PaO_2 approaches 60 mm Hg but seldom exceeds that value until cardiopulmonary work has been significantly reduced.

When hypoxemia is caused by a pulmonary process that is refractory to oxygen therapy (consolidated pneumonia, lobar atelectasis, ARDS), the blood gases and WOB do not significantly change with O_2 administration.

Acute Myocardial Disease

Acute decreases in cardiac output result in diminished mixed venous oxygenation because the tissues must extract the required O_2 from less blood. Any degree of preexisting intrapulmonary shunting has greater hypoxemic effects on the arterial blood because the shunted blood is less oxygenated. If the heart is unable to increase cardiac output in response to hypoxemia, the pulmonary system increases $\dot{V}E$ and produces acute alveolar hyperventilation with hypoxemia. Hypoxemia attributable to acute myocardial infarction, acute heart failure, and interstitial pulmonary edema should respond to oxygen therapy and significantly decrease cardiopulmonary work. Pulmonary edema producing fluid-filled alveoli may be refractory to oxygen therapy.

METABOLIC ACID–BASE IMBALANCES ■

Carbonic acid can be readily formed from (or transformed to) CO_2, allowing excretion of this *volatile* acid load to be dependent on lung function (respiratory acid–base balance; Chap. 17). Approximately 1% to 2% of the normal acid load and all pathologic acid metabolites are *nonvolatile* acids that depend primarily on renal excretion (metabolic acid–base balance).

ESSENTIAL ACID–BASE PHYSIOLOGY

Renal Buffers

The renal system regulates acid–base changes by HCO_3^- reclamation and H^+ secretion. The bulk of filtered HCO_3^- is reabsorbed in the proximal tubule. Renal epithelial cells contain carbonic anhydrase, an enzyme that accelerates the hydration and dehydration of CO_2, thereby ensuring a high rate of intracellular carbonic acid and HCO_3^- formation:

$$H_2O + CO_2 \rightleftarrows H_2CO_3 \rightleftarrows HCO_3^- + H^+ \qquad (2)$$

The secretion of H^+ in the proximal tubule is largely related to sodium (Na^+) reabsorption. Simply stated, HCO_3^- and Na^+ are reabsorbed into the blood, whereas H^+ is excreted into the tubular lumen.

Because the kidneys cannot produce urine with a pH below 4.4, less than 1% of urinary acid excretion occurs as free H^+. In essence, excretion of nonvolatile acids depends on phosphate and ammonium (NH_4^+) urinary buffers. In plasma, the ratio of HPO_4^{-2} to $H_2PO_4^-$ is 4:1; as tubular fluid is acidified to a pH of 6.8, the ratio becomes 1:1 by the end of the proximal tubule. At a pH of 4.8, the ratio is 1:100. Renal tubular cells generate NH_3, a highly diffusible gas and a strong base, by deamination and deamidization of glutamine. Ammonia readily diffuses into the tubular fluid, where it reacts with H^+ to form NH_4^+. Ammonium ion is relatively nondiffusible and largely remains in the tubular fluid.

Base Excess/Deficit

The blood normally contains a large buffering capacity that allows significant changes in acid content, with little change in free H^+ concentration (pH). As deviation from the normal buffering capacity ensues, a greater pH change results from any given change in H^+ content. This buffering capacity depends not only on the HCO_3^- concentration, but also on the red blood cell mass and other factors. The concept of base excess/deficit is founded on the premise that the degree of deviation from the normal total buffer base availability can be calculated independently of compensatory PCO_2 changes. A negative base excess is referred to as a base deficit.

An abnormal pH with a base excess within ±5 mMol/L denotes a relatively balanced *metabolic* acid–base status. An abnormal pH with a base excess outside ±10 mMol/L denotes a clinically significant metabolic acid–base imbalance that must be investigated and corrected.

ESTIMATING BASE EXCESS. The PCO_2–pH relationship is predictable and can be approximated as shown in Table 61-9 if a baseline PCO_2 of 40 mm Hg with a pH of 7.40 are assumed. An acute 10 mm Hg increase in the PCO_2 results in a pH decrease of approximately 0.05 U; an acute decrease in PCO_2 of 10 mm Hg results in a pH increase of 0.10 U. Under normal circumstances, a 10 mMol/L variance from the normal buffer baseline represents a metabolic pH change of approximately 0.15 U. Moving the pH decimal point two places to the right results in a 2:3 relationship (10:15). The steps for estimating the base excess are illustrated in Table 61-10.

Estimating Bicarbonate Deficiency

When sodium bicarbonate ($NaHCO_3$) or hydrochloric acid is administered to correct severe metabolic acid–base imbalance, quantifying the abnormality is essential as a guide to therapy. Table 61-11 demonstrates our recommended procedure for quantifying extracellular HCO_3^- deficit. It is generally prudent to administer one half to two thirds of the calculated deficit, and then obtain another blood gas sample in 5 minutes and reevaluate.

Anion Gap

The anion gap represents a calculated disparity between cations and anions, resulting from the fact that only Na^+, potassium (K^+), chloride (Cl^-), and HCO_3^- are routinely measured. Because there are normally more unmeasured anions than cations, an "anion gap" of about 15 mMol/L normally exists. An increased anion gap usually results from an increase in uncalculated anions secondary to metabolic

TABLE 61-10. Estimating the Base Excess

1. DETERMINE PCO_2 VARIANCE

   Difference between measured PCO_2 and 40; move decimal point two places to the left

2. DETERMINE PREDICTED pH

   If PCO_2 over 40, subtract half PCO_2 variance from 7.40. If PCO_2 under 40, add PCO_2 variance to 7.40.

   Examples

pH 7.04, PCO_2 76	pH 7.47, PCO_2 18
$76 - 40 = 36 \times \frac{1}{2} = 0.18$	$40 - 18 = 22 = 0.22$
$7.40 - 0.18 = 7.22$	$7.40 + 0.22 = 7.62$

3. ESTIMATE BASE EXCESS/DEFICIT

   Determine difference between measured and predicted pH; move decimal point two places to the right. Multiply by $\frac{2}{3}$

   Examples

   $7.22 - 7.04 = 0.18 \times \frac{2}{3} = 12$ mMol/L base deficit

   $7.62 - 7.47 = 0.15 \times \frac{2}{3} = 10$ mMol/L base deficit

acidosis (increased lactate, ketones), renal failure (increased sulfates, phosphates), excessive organic salt therapy (Ringer's lactate solution, sodium acetate, carbenicillin, high-dose penicillin), and dehydration. Occasionally, an increased anion gap may be caused by decreased uncalculated cations such as calcium and magnesium.

A decreased anion gap is commonly caused by decreased uncalculated anions seen with hypoalbuminemia and severe dilution. Increased uncalculated cations are less common but are seen with lithium toxicity, increased calcium and magnesium, polymyxin B administration, bromide toxicity, severe hypernatremia, and hyperviscosity.

METABOLIC ACIDEMIA

Typical room air–breathing arterial blood gas values and pH are

pHa <7.30
$PaCO_2$ <40 mm Hg
PaO_2 >60 mm Hg
Base excess > −10 mMol/L

TABLE 61-9. Approximate $PaCO_2$–pH Relationship

$PaCO_2$ (mm Hg)	pH	$[HCO_3^-]p$ (mMol/L)
80	7.20	28
60	7.30	26
40	7.40	24
30	7.50	22
20	7.60	20

TABLE 61-11. Quantifying Extracellular Bicarbonate Deficit

1. Base deficit (negative base excess) represents the mMol/L of bicarbonate ion required to restore the extracellular water to the normal buffer base status
2. Approximately 20% of the adult's total body weight expressed in kilograms is equivalent to the extracellular water expressed in liters

$$\frac{\text{Base deficit} \times \text{weight (kg)}}{5} = \text{Calculated extracellular bicarbonate (or hydrogen ion) deficiency}$$

Metabolic acidemia is the result of base loss or nonvolatile acid accumulation. Renal failure is the most common cause in hospitalized patients. These patients usually have compensated acidosis because of adequate ventilatory reserves. Therefore, acidemia (uncompensated acidosis) with renal failure usually denotes a sudden deterioration in ventilatory function.

Metabolic acidemia is a potentially life-threatening condition and must be aggressively treated. Immediate evaluation of cardiopulmonary function is warranted because metabolic factors alone rarely create pH below 7.20 when adequate cardiopulmonary reserves are present. O_2 content will be less than predicted because of decreased Hgb-O_2 affinity (shift to the right), requiring an increased cardiac output to ensure O_2 delivery. As stated previously, if hypoxemia is present, tissue hypoxia must be assumed! With the exception of lactic acidosis, metabolic acidosis is rarely caused by pulmonary disease and usually is not associated with severe hypoxemia.

Except during cardiopulmonary resuscitation (CPR) and low cardiac output states, the major therapeutic intervention for metabolic acidemia is administration of $NaHCO_3$, which should be guided by blood gas measurements as follows: (1) a base excess above -10 mMol/L does not require $NaHCO_3$ therapy; (2) a pHa greater than 7.20 does not require $NaHCO_3$ unless concomitant cardiovascular instability exists; (3) when indicated, half the calculated extracellular deficiency (see Table 27-11) should be administered and blood gas measurements repeated in 5 minutes; and (4) $NaHCO_3$ administration is contraindicated during CPR.

METABOLIC ALKALEMIA

Typical room air–breathing arterial blood gas values are

pHa >7.50
$PaCO_2$ 40 to 50 mm Hg
PaO_2 >60 mm Hg
Base excess > -10 mEq/L

Metabolic alkalemia is the most common acid–base abnormality in critically ill patients. A pH of less than 7.60 rarely causes electrophysiologic or enzymatic dysfunction in an otherwise normal patient, but may be significant to an already diseased myocardium or CNS. Acute changes in pH can be disastrous, even when the change is toward normal. Therefore, metabolic alkalemia should be slowly reversed unless the patient is already unstable. In the unconscious, semicomatose, or severely debilitated patient, metabolic alkalemia may precipitate marked alveolar hypoventilation.

ELECTROLYTE ABNORMALITIES

Potassium Loss

Inadequate K^+ replacement, tubular diuretics, carbonic anhydrase inhibitors, and persistent gastric suctioning commonly deplete K^+ in the critically ill patient. As much as 20% of total body K^+ may be lost before serum K^+ falls below the normal range. Intracellular K^+ loss causes H^+ diffusion into the cell and results in (1) metabolic alkalemia,

(2) intracellular acidosis, (3) ventricular arrhythmia, and (4) muscular weakness. Recommended therapy is intravenous K^+ replacement: 40 to 80 mEq every 6 to 8 hours; more rapid administration requires careful ECG monitoring.

Chloride Loss

Hypochloremia increases renal excretion of H^+, producing metabolic alkalemia without concomitant intracellular acidosis. However, inadequate Cl^- availability hinders renal tubular exchange and promotes K^+ loss. Therapy consists of adequate water, Cl^-, and K^+ replacement.

Bicarbonate Excess

HCO_3^- excess was a common problem when $NaHCO_3$ was recommended during CPR. "Waiting" is the treatment of choice because normal renal function can readily excrete excess HCO_3^-. K^+ depletion must be avoided.

Specific Therapy

Although seldom required, recommended therapy for averting cardiovascular collapse from severe alkalemia (pH >7.70) is central venous administration of 0.1 M hydrochloric acid (100 mMol H^+/L). Dilute 8.35 mL of hydrochloric acid (USP) with 20 mL of unpreserved sterile water (USP); inject through a millipore filter into 1 L of isoosmotic solution. Administer 20% of the calculated deficit (see Table 61-11) over 30 to 60 minutes and repeat blood gas measurements.

Ammonium chloride may rapidly improve metabolic alkalemia but concurrently increases renal K^+ excretion. Therefore, ammonium chloride is contraindicated in a K^+-depleted patient and requires adequate K^+ replacement whenever administered.

CLINICAL ASSESSMENT OF OXYGENATION

The *tissue oxygenation status* is a global concept that cannot be directly measured. No single value or combination of measurements can reliably reflect the oxygenation status of vital tissues in critically ill patients. Therefore, all clinical assessments of oxygenation must begin with an evaluation of the arterial blood (see Tables 61-4 through 61-7).

LUNGS AS OXYGENATORS

Blood that goes from the right to left heart without contacting alveolar gas (zero $\dot{V}/\dot{Q}$ matching, "true shunt") creates hypoxemia by mixing in the left heart with blood that has been oxygenated in the lungs. The degree of hypoxemia is determined by the amount of blood that is shunted and the $HgbO_2$ saturation of the shunted blood. Alveoli that are underventilated in relation to perfusion (low $\dot{V}/\dot{Q}$ matching) will have less than ideal PaO_2. Blood that respires with these alveoli is oxygenated to a lesser degree than if exposed to perfect alveoli and causes hypoxemia ($\dot{V}/\dot{Q}$ inequity, shunt effect).

Arterial oxygenation is the result of three primary factors: O_2 transfer in the lungs, cardiac output, and O_2 consumption. The latter two are considered in the discussions concerning O_2 extraction and mixed venous O_2 saturation. Critical care medicine demands the ability to assess the degree to which abnormal lung function is contributing to hypoxemia. Calculation of the physiologic shunt ($\dot{Q}sp/\dot{Q}t$) represents the best available means of delineating the extent to which the pulmonary system contributes to hypoxemia.

SHUNT CALCULATION

The topic of shunt calculation and nomenclature is controversial, confused, and arbitrary. The following is a reasonable overview: True shunt ($\dot{Q}s/\dot{Q}t$) represents calculation of the intrapulmonary shunt at a FIO_2 of 1.0; the physiologic shunt ($\dot{Q}sp/\dot{Q}t$) represents calculation of the intrapulmonary shunt at a FIO_2 less than 1.0 and, therefore, includes both the true shunt and $\dot{V}/\dot{Q}$ mismatch (shunt effect). Venous admixture ($\dot{Q}va/\dot{Q}t$) is exactly the same as the $\dot{Q}sp/\dot{Q}t$ shunt but is preferred by some to avoid the use of the term "physiologic" when addressing abnormal states.

The shunt equation is

$$\frac{\dot{Q}sp}{\dot{Q}t} = \frac{Cc'o_2 - Cao_2}{Cc'o_2 - C\bar{v}o_2} \quad (3)$$

$Cc'o_2$ is the ideal pulmonary end-capillary O_2 content that is calculated using the ideal alveolar gas equation to determine the ideal Po_2. This equation calculates that portion of the cardiac output that traverses from the right heart to the left heart without increasing O_2 content. The mathematics assume that the nonshunting blood perfectly oxygenates by exchanging with perfect alveolar gas. Although the intrapulmonary shunt calculation does not reflect regional relationships as does the $\dot{V}/\dot{Q}$ concept, it does reflect the degree to which the lungs deviate from ideal as oxygenators of pulmonary blood. This quantitative ability to look at the lung as an oxygenator makes the shunt calculation unique and valuable in the clinical setting.

INTERPRETIVE GUIDELINES

1. A calculated shunt less than 0.1 (10%) is clinically compatible with normal lungs.
2. A calculated shunt of 0.1 to 0.19 (10% to 19%) denotes a degree of disease that seldom requires significant support.
3. A calculated shunt of 0.2 to 0.29 (20% to 29%) may be life-threatening in a patient with limited cardiovascular or nervous system function.
4. A calculated shunt greater than 0.3 (30%) is potentially life-threatening and usually requires significant cardiopulmonary supportive therapy.
5. When significant shunt effect mechanisms are present, the calculated shunt significantly increases as the FIO_2 is decreased from 0.5.

TABLE 61-12. Comparison of Gas Exchange Indices

PARAMETER	MEAN (+/−SD)	RANGE MIN–MAX	r
$\dot{Q}sp/\dot{Q}t$ (%)	22.3 (11.2)	3.0–53.0	
Est shunt (%)	27.6 (11.3)	2.7–62.3	+0.94
RI	3.1 (2.6)	0.3–14.0	+0.74
Pao_2/Pao_2	0.3 (0.2)	0.06–0.77	−0.72
Pao_2/FIO_2	1.8 (0.9)	0.1–4.3	−0.71
$P(A - a)o_2$ (mmHg)	222.8 (141.7)	32–611	+0.62

MIN, minimum; MAX, maximum; RI, respiratory index.
$\dot{Q}sp/\dot{Q}t$ physiologic shunt (venous admixture).

ALTERNATIVES TO THE SHUNT CALCULATION

The most significant factor limiting the widespread clinical use of shunt calculations is that O_2 analysis of pulmonary artery blood is required. O_2 partial pressure–based indices (e.g., $P[A - a]o_2$, Pao_2/Pao_2, and Pao_2/FIO_2) do not require mixed venous O_2 analysis, but they have significant limitations to reliably reflect shunt fractions in critically ill patients.[3] The popularity of these indices is not based on their accuracy or reliability, but on the fact that mixed venous O_2 measurements are not required.

The estimated shunt

$$\text{EST } \dot{Q}sp/\dot{Q}t = \frac{Cc'o_2 - Cao_2}{[Cc'o_2 - Cao_2] + C(a - \bar{v})o_2} \quad (4)$$

is an O_2 content–based index derived by mathematical manipulation of the shunt equation that places the arterial–mixed venous O_2 content difference $[C(a - \bar{v})o_2]$ in the denominator. A value of 3.5 mL/dL reflects the mean $C(a - \bar{v})o_2$ in large populations of critically ill patients with clinically adequate perfusion states.[4] As shown in Table 61-12, the estimated shunt is far superior to O_2 partial pressure–based indices in reflecting changes in the $\dot{Q}sp/\dot{Q}t$.[3] However, the estimated shunt is not an adequate substitute for $\dot{Q}sp/\dot{Q}t$ calculation.

HYPOXEMIA AND OXYGEN THERAPY ■

The Pao_2 results from the dynamic equilibrium between O_2 molecules delivered to the alveoli (ventilation) and those diffusing into the pulmonary capillary blood. All other factors remaining constant, increasing the FIO_2 increases Pao_2.

Hypoxemia caused by true $\dot{Q}sp/\dot{Q}t$ (zero $\dot{V}/\dot{Q}$ matching) is refractory to increased FIO_2 because the nonshunting blood theoretically is ideally oxygenated (%$HgbO_2$ >95). Increasing the Pao_2 adds insignificant quantities of O_2 to the pulmonary capillary blood and none to that blood which is shunted. Hypoxemia secondary to shunt effect mechanisms (low $\dot{V}/\dot{Q}$ matching) is caused by diminished Pao_2; therefore, the resulting arterial hypoxemia is responsive to increasing FIO_2.

The therapeutic range of O_2 administration is essentially limited to less than 50%. The Pao_2 of low $\dot{V}/\dot{Q}$ alveoli is usually greater than 80 mm Hg with FIO_2 values up to 0.5, and denitrogenation atelectasis becomes significant at FIO_2 values of 0.5 or greater.

HYPOXIC PULMONARY VASCONSTRICTION

Vasoconstriction of blood vessels in diseased lung areas is a known phenomenon that accomplishes minimal perfusion of poorly or nonventilated alveoli. Although the exact mechanisms remain unknown, it is most probable that oxygen-sensitive receptors on or near the epithelium modulate pulmonary arteriolar and capillary smooth muscle contraction. Hypoxic pulmonary vasoconstriction (HPV) begins when PaO_2 drops below 80 mm Hg; as the PaO_2 diminishes, pulmonary vascular resistance increases until the phenomenon is maximal when the lung is ventilated with pure nitrogen.

In nonventilated alveoli, HPV is modulated by the pulmonary arterial (mixed venous) PO_2 ($P\bar{v}O_2$).[5] Perfusion to a true shunt (zero $\dot{V}/\dot{Q}$ matching) area of lung varies directly with $P\bar{v}O_2$ changes. Because $P\bar{v}O_2$ tends to increase as cardiac output increases, a relatively greater portion of the improved cardiac output will perfuse the zero $\dot{V}/\dot{Q}$ areas. Such an increase in $\dot{Q}sp/\dot{Q}t$ with increasing cardiac output is well documented but seldom of clinical significance. However, significant increases in $\dot{Q}sp/\dot{Q}t$ (and concomitant hypoxemia) are often seen when vasodilating drugs are administered to patients with large intrapulmonary shunts.

DENITROGENATION ABSORPTION ATELECTASIS

Nitrogen is inert and freely diffusible so that nitrogen partial pressures are nearly equal in the alveoli, blood, and cellular water. When increased FIO_2 values are administered, nitrogen is rapidly eliminated from the body. This denitrogenation process can result in the collapse of alveoli with low $\dot{V}/\dot{Q}$ matching.[6] It is the best explanation for the observation that most patients with shunt effect mechanisms (low $\dot{V}/\dot{Q}$ matching) causing hypoxemia demonstrate only transient increases in PaO_2 when the FIO_2 is increased above 0.5. Increases in oxygenation that otherwise would occur are offset by the resulting alveolar collapse.

TISSUE OXYGENATION ■

Our limited abilities to assess the tissue oxygenation status requires traditional blood gas analysis of both arterial and pulmonary arterial blood plus cardiac output measurement. Obtaining these values allows a variety of useful calculations.

OXYGEN DELIVERY

Oxygen delivery ($\dot{D}O_2$) is the volume of O_2 presented to the tissues in 1 minute (CaO_2 multiplied by the cardiac output). Oxygen consumption ($\dot{V}O_2$) is the volume of O_2 consumed in 1 minute. Data support the assumption that when $\dot{D}O_2$ is three to four times greater than $\dot{V}O_2$, tissue O_2 needs are reasonably satisfied in nonseptic patients.[7]

OXYGEN EXTRACTION

O_2 extraction represents the O_2 transferred to the tissues from a deciliter of blood. On a global scale, this relationship can be quantified as the $C(a - \bar{v})O_2$ and varies inversely with the cardiac output. Critically ill patients with adequate cardiac reserves have values for $C(a - \bar{v})O_2$ in the range of 3 to 4 mL/dL (Table 61-13).[8] In the absence of anemia and sepsis in a patient with clinically adequate peripheral perfusion, a $C(a - \bar{v})O_2$ of 3 to 4 mL/dL suggests adequate cardiac reserve to meet additional stress if required. A $C(a - \bar{v})O_2$ value greater than 5 mL/dL suggests inadequate cardiac response to the stress.

MIXED VENOUS OXYGEN SATURATION

The relationship between the $\dot{D}O_2$ and $\dot{V}O_2$ is reflected in the mixed venous oxygen saturation ($S\bar{v}O_2$) when the hemoglobin content is greater than 10 g/dL.[9] The basic physiologic response to an increasing O_2 demand is an increase in O_2 supply by increasing cardiac output. Because $\dot{D}O_2$ and $\dot{V}O_2$ are increasing in this circumstance, $S\bar{v}O_2$ remains relatively unchanged and can be conceptualized as providing a measure of "oxygen reserve" to meet further increases in O_2 demand. A general guideline is that a $S\bar{v}O_2$ value greater than 65% represents adequate reserve; 50% to 65% represents limited reserve; 35% to 50% represents inadequate reserve; and less than 35% probably reflects inadequate tissue oxygenation.[10]

When O_2 delivery is stable, any increase in $\dot{V}O_2$ results in a fall in $S\bar{v}O_2$. In patients with optimal O_2 content and limited cardiac output, increased ventilatory muscle activity, shivering, convulsions, rewarming after hypothermia, and even movement during routine nursing procedures may result in considerable decreases in $S\bar{v}O_2$. When arterial oxygenation and $\dot{V}O_2$ are normal, decreases in cardiac output will be closely paralleled by decreases in $S\bar{v}O_2$, a phenomenon especially obvious in low flow states.

Documentation of these $S\bar{v}O_2$ changes and their relationships to the tissue oxygenation status has been interpreted by some as suggesting that the $S\bar{v}O_2$ is an essential value to continuously measure in the critically ill. Although little data support such a stance, continuous $S\bar{v}O_2$ monitoring in conjunction with pulse oximetry is considered to be clinically useful by many clinicians.

TABLE 61-13. Pulmonary Arterial Oxygenation Values

CARDIOVASCULAR STATUS	$P\bar{v}O_2$ (mmHg)	$C(a - \bar{v})O_2$ (mL/dL)
Healthy resting human volunteer	40 (37–43)	5.0 (4.5–6.0)
Critically ill, adequate C–V	37 (35–40)	3.5 (2.5–4.5)
Critically ill, borderline C–V	32 (30–35)	5.0 (4.5–6.0)
Critically ill, inadequate C–V	<30	>6.0

C–V, cardiovascular; $P\bar{v}O_2$, partial pressure of oxygen (mixed venous blood); $C(a - \bar{v})O_2$, arterial–mixed venous oxygen content difference.

OXYGEN DEMAND: A NEW CONCEPT

The "traditional" measurements involved with ensuring O_2 delivery and extraction do not take into account that metabolic demand for O_2 may be significantly altered from the norms assumed for traditional guidelines. Some data suggest that $\dot{D}o_2$ can be increased with measurable increases in $\dot{V}o_2$ until the O_2 demands are met, beyond which point an increase in $\dot{D}o_2$ will not result in an increased $\dot{V}o_2$.[11] A clinical endpoint of increasing $\dot{D}o_2$ until the $\dot{V}o_2$ no longer increases may be more useful in critically ill patients whose intracellular O_2 utilization is significantly different from normal.

NONINVASIVE MONITORING ■

Availability of practical and reliable electrodes to measure blood pH, Pco_2, and Po_2 occurred in the 1950s and revolutionized the clinical application of cardiopulmonary supportive techniques. Critical care medicine cannot be practiced in the 1990s without the ability to measure (or reflect) arterial blood gas partial pressures. However, despite the reality of self-calibrating equipment and adequate quality assurance, arterial blood gas and pH measurements require blood removal, are subject to significant preanalytic error,[8] and require at least a 5- or 10-minute interim before the results are available. The values thus represent a previous isolated point in a dynamic physiologic continuum that may hold little current relevance.

These limitations have resulted in the development of methods that continuously and noninvasively "reflect" $Paco_2$ and Pao_2. Although these techniques have significantly improved respiratory monitoring, they have supplemented, not replaced, arterial blood gas and pH measurement. Furthermore, the use of any such monitors demands interpretation by persons with in-depth knowledge of respiratory pathophysiology who appreciate the limitations of the devices.

PULSE OXIMETRY

The pulse oximeter combines a dual wavelength spectrophotometer with plethysmographic capabilities that functions by placing a pulsating arterial vascular bed between the diode and a light detector. For practical purposes, it is designed to detect the oxygenated portion of the hemoglobin "available" for carrying O_2 in the arterial blood (Sao_2), in contradistinction to the laboratory multiwavelength oximeter that measures the percent of "total" hemoglobin that is oxygenated ($\%Hgbo_2$). This is an important distinction because a patient with 20% HgbCO and a Pao_2 of 200 mm Hg might have an "80% saturation" reported by the laboratory ($\%Hgbo_2$) whereas the pulse oximeter reports "99% saturation" (Sao_2). Both values are correct; the clinician must understand the difference.

The generally reliable performance of pulse oximeters as trend monitors for Sao_2 has been improperly interpreted by many clinicians to mean that the device is accurate and reliable under all circumstances in which the equipment is properly functioning. Pulse oximetry has added a significant dimension to bedside monitoring of arterial oxygenation and deserves wide application and use. However, available data indicate that the pulse oximeter should be limited to monitoring changes in arterial oxygenation and should not be used as a quantitative substitute for arterial blood analysis when hypoxemia is present or suspected.

CAPNOGRAPHY

Alveoli empty in parallel at differing rates and degrees, making it impossible to sample "true" alveolar gas. The $Paco_2$ is accepted as the physiologic representation of the true $Paco_2$. Figure 61-2 depicts the ideal exhalation capnogram in which phase I represents primarily apparatus and anatomic dead space gas, phase II represents increasing CO_2 concentrations resulting from progressive emptying of alveoli, and phase III represents alveolar gas. A normal capnogram shows a $Petco_2$ within several mm Hg of the $Paco_2$. The capnogram is significantly influenced by the change in rate and sequence of alveolar emptying that accompany lung disease. Notice that an abnormal capnogram finding is more clinically reliable as an indicator of $\dot{V}/\dot{Q}$ inequalities than as a reflection of the $Paco_2$.

Capnography offers two major clinical advantages: it is noninvasive and it provides continuous real-time information about CO_2 elimination. Emphasis must be placed on the limitations of this monitor in commonly applied clinical circumstances: (1) to reflect the $Paco_2$, and (2) to trend changes in $\dot{V}d$.

End-Tidal and Arterial Pco₂

In patients without lung disease and with stable cardiovascular function, capnography provides a simple noninvasive method to monitor the adequacy of $\dot{V}a$ rapidly and continuously. These circumstances are most commonly found in patients receiving general anesthesia, in patients requiring elective hyperventilation for intracranial diseases, in neurologically diseased patients requiring ventilatory assistance, and in patients with apnea monitoring.

Use of capnography in patients with pulmonary disease or unstable cardiovascular function is limited because when the emptying pattern of the lung or $\dot{V}d$ is abnormal, the $Petco_2$ does not reliably reflect $Paco_2$. However, while the shape of the capnogram remains unchanged, the $Petco_2$ can be used as a "trending" monitor, provided that cardiovascular function is consistent. No clinical data currently justify use of $Petco_2$ as a replacement for $Paco_2$ measurement in patients with cardiopulmonary disease.

Trending Dead Space Ventilation

Changes in the arterial-to-alveolar Pco_2 gradient, as reflected by the $P(a - et)co_2$, must be attributed to changes in $\dot{V}d$. The most common causes of such alterations are lung disease, pulmonary embolic phenomena, and changes in cardiac output. When the $P(a - et)co_2$ changes in conjunction with capnogram configuration alterations, it is reasonable to assume that dead space changes are attributable to lung disease (Fig. 61-3). When the shape of the curve is

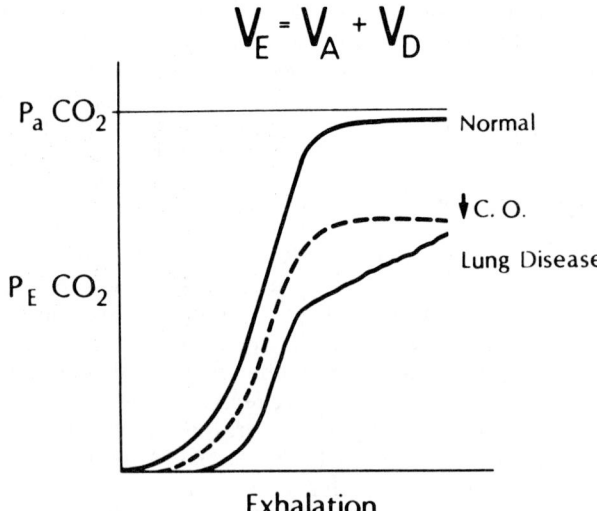

$$V_E = V_A + V_D$$

Exhalation

FIGURE 61-3. Total ventilation ($\dot{V}E$) is composed of both alveolar ventilation ($\dot{V}A$) and deadspace ventilation ($\dot{V}D$). The $PaCO_2$ ($PETCO_2$) is the expired PCO_2 ($PECO_2$) at the end of the plateau. An increase in V_D will be manifest as an increase in $PaCO_2 - PETCO_2$ gradient.

The two most common causes of increased deadspace ventilation are decreased cardiac output and lung disease. A decreased pulmonary perfusion results in more alveoli having lower PCO_2; the net result is a decreased expired PCO_2 but no change in lung emptying pattern. This is depicted as the *dashed curve* with a shape similar to the normal curve. Lung disease involves changing emptying patterns and thus a change in the curve.

unchanged, an increased $P(a - ET)CO_2$ most likely results from diminished cardiac output or pulmonary embolus.

THE TRANSCUTANEOUS O_2 ELECTRODE

In adults, the transcutaneous PO_2 ($PtcO_2$) parallels PaO_2 changes, with the actual value being 80% to 95% of the PaO_2 in hemodynamically stable patients. However, decreases in cardiac output result in diminished $PtcO_2$ values independent of the actual PaO_2, making the technology an unreliable trend monitor of the PaO_2 in critically ill adult patients. In addition, a change of skin site every 4 to 6 hours, a 20- to 30-minute equilibration time whenever the site is changed, and periodic electrode maintenance by skilled personnel make the device clinically unpopular.

THE TRANSCUTANEOUS CO_2 ELECTRODE

Although the practical problems are the same as with the O_2 electrode, the $PtcCO_2$ electrode is accurate and provides a reliable trend of $PaCO_2$ when the device is properly used and maintained.

CARBON DIOXIDE STORES ■

Both intracellular and extracellular water have partial pressures of nitrogen, O_2, and CO_2, which means that some amount of each gas is "stored" in the tissues. Nitrogen stores

change when the inspired fraction of nitrogen is altered (as with oxygen therapy), and O_2 stores change at such rapid rates that steady-state conditions are usually present within the confines of biologic variability. However, CO_2 stores change at a relatively slow pace and are influenced by several clinically relevant physiologic mechanisms, making their consideration clinically significant in the interpretation of blood gas values.[12]

CENTRAL CO_2 STORES

The central CO_2 stores are comprised of the blood CO_2 content, which includes carbamino compounds, the carbonic acid–bicarbonate system, and dissolved CO_2. When $PaCO_2$ is abruptly changed, the central CO_2 stores abruptly change; however, changes in $\dot{V}A$ for less than several hours have little effect on the peripheral CO_2 stores. This fact explains why the $PaCO_2$ and mixed venous PCO_2 can rapidly return to baseline after relatively transient changes in $\dot{V}A$.

PERIPHERAL CO_2 STORES

Peripheral CO_2 stores are estimated to be approximately 110 L in a 70-kg person. Most (up to 100 L) is stored in bone and fat, which have relatively poor perfusion. Therefore, significant changes in these stores would be expected to take days. Skeletal muscle represents the next largest component (approximately 5 L), and changes can occur in hours. Visceral tissue stores account for the remainder, in which changes occur within minutes.

Assuming a normal CO_2 production, Table 61-14 demonstrates the relationships between CO_2 stores, minute ventilation, and $PaCO_2$. Notice that depleted CO_2 stores allow a normal $\dot{V}E$ to result in an unexpectedly low $PaCO_2$; conversely, increased CO_2 stores allow a normal $\dot{V}E$ to result in a greater $PaCO_2$ than expected.

Depletion

Depletion of peripheral stores occurs when CO_2 excretion exceeds CO_2 production for significant periods of time; skeletal muscle depletion is seen in a few hours and bone depletion within several days. These changes occur slowly enough that blood gas values at any point in time reflect CO_2 balance as if a stable equilibrium were present.

TABLE 61-14. Theoretical Relationship of PCO_2 Changes When Peripheral CO_2 Stores Are Altered[*]

CO_2 STORES	TISSUE PCO_2	$P\bar{v}CO_2$	$PaCO_2$	$PaCO_2$
Normal	50	46	40	40
Decreased	40	36	30	30
Increased	60	56	50	50

$P\bar{v}CO_2$, partial pressure of oxygen (mixed venous blood).

[*]CO_2 production and minute ventilation are assumed to be normal.

When a significant depletion of peripheral CO_2 stores occurs, the alveolar, arterial, and venous PCO_2 values all are decreased. However, the diminished $PaCO_2$ is secondary to diminished tissue CO_2 rather than to increased $\dot{V}A$. Therefore, normal $\dot{V}E$ and normal $\dot{V}D$ are present in conjunction with a diminished PaO_2. Patients with these findings usually have a decreased $PaCO_2$ (respiratory alkalosis) in conjunction with a normal or decreased $\dot{V}E$. This combination is common in patients with CNS disease who spontaneously hyperventilate to $PaCO_2$ values of 28 to 30 mm Hg for 48 hours or more. During this time, more CO_2 is excreted than produced, depleting skeletal muscle CO_2 stores. Although the $PaCO_2$ remains constant, the $\dot{V}E$ decreases by almost 50%. This situation emphasizes the necessity for measuring $\dot{V}E$ and arterial blood gas values in critically ill patients.

Peripheral CO_2 stores tend to be repleted within several days after reversal of the underlying disease. The reversal process is important because as the stores are replenished, either the $PaCO_2$ must increase back to normal, or the $\dot{V}E$ must increase to maintain the lower $PaCO_2$. If the patient is unable to increase ventilatory work readily, significant cardiopulmonary and CNS deterioration may result. Appropriate interpretation of the blood gas values can alert the clinician to these potential dangers.

Increase: The "CO_2 Retainer"

Chronic hypercapnia ($PaCO_2$ >50 mm Hg; pHa >7.35) is mostly seen in patients with chronic obstructive lung disease; however, it is also seen in those with chronic restrictive pulmonary disease, morbid obesity (Pickwickian syndrome), and rare CNS disorders. The increased peripheral CO_2 stores allow the patient to maintain CO_2 homeostasis (lung excretion equal to cellular production) while maintaining an increased $PaCO_2$. Minute ventilation is less than would be required with normal CO_2 stores.

Chronic hypercapnia involves intracellular adaptation to increased PCO_2. Such adaptation seems to involve maintenance of mitochondrial function despite significantly diminished $\dot{D}O_2$, because affected patients are usually hypoxemic. Extracellular acid–base balance is maintained by accumulating an increased HCO_3^- concentration and Cl^- deficiency. Available data suggest that water and Cl^- shifts between intracellular and extracellular spaces result in a slightly greater extracellular pH than the normal population.[13] Stable chronic hypercapnia is most commonly seen in conjunction with pHa above 7.40.

ACUTE-ON-CHRONIC VENTILATORY FAILURE

Typical room air breathing arterial blood gas values are

> pHa <7.35
> $PaCO_2$ >60 mm Hg
> PaO_2 <40 mm Hg

Patients with acute-on-chronic ventilatory failure have chronic lung disease with increased $\dot{V}D$ and shunting as well as increased CO_2 stores. Above all, they have a limited capability to increase cardiopulmonary work. Although a significant proportion of these persons do not acutely hypoventilate when given O_2, the drug must be carefully administered.

The severity of acute-on-chronic ventilatory failure must be judged by the degree of acidemia. Regardless of the PCO_2 level, a pH above 7.30 denotes a tolerable change from baseline. If the pH falls below 7.20, evaluation for ventilatory assistance is mandatory. Although lactic acidosis is common in these patients, $NaHCO_3$ administration is contraindicated before supporting ventilation because of the added CO_2 load.

ACUTE ALVEOLAR HYPERVENTILATION-ON-CHRONIC VENTILATORY FAILURE

Typical room air breathing arterial blood gas values are

> pHa >7.50
> $PaCO_2$ >40 mm Hg
> PaO_2 <50 mm Hg

These values would initially be interpreted as a "partly compensated metabolic alkalosis with significant hypoxemia." However, diseases causing metabolic alkalemia rarely cause significant hypoxemia. Consideration should be given to the probability that a patient with chronic ventilatory failure, responding to an acute cardiopulmonary insult by relatively hyperventilating, will "unmask" the underlying base excess.

CARBON MONOXIDE POISONING ■

The hemoglobin molecule's affinity for CO is 200 to 250 times greater than that for O_2. An alveolar PCO of 1 mm Hg may result in $HgbCO$ levels of 40% or greater if exposure extends for several hours. Because the rate of dissociation of CO from hemoglobin is extremely slow, $HgbCO$ results in a decreased arterial O_2 content that cannot be rapidly reversed. In addition, high levels of $HgbCO$ cause the $HgbO_2$ dissociation to shift markedly to the left, further impairing O_2 delivery to tissues.

The definitive diagnosis of CO poisoning is accomplished by measurement of $HgbCO$. These levels are readily determined by a multiple band spectrophotometer, which should be available in any appropriately equipped laboratory providing blood gas measurements. The use of a pH–PCO_2 nomogram to calculate an assumed $HgbO_2$ saturation (SaO_2) is totally misleading in the presence of significant $HgbCO$, because the nomogram assumes all hemoglobin is available to combine with O_2.

A $HgbCO$ level greater than 15% usually produces symptoms, and a level above 20% is considered CO poisoning. At levels greater than 40% $HgbCO$, more severe neurologic sequelae of ataxia, cortical blindness, and behavioral disturbances manifest themselves. Levels in excess of 50% $HgbCO$ may produce irreversible CNS damage. Recent evidence suggests that CO may have a disrupting effect on cellular oxidative metabolism by interfering with the function of intracellular cytochrome oxidase systems.[14] This problem may account for occasional discrepancies between the severity of the patient's clinical status and the measured level of blood HgbCO.

The definitive treatment of CO poisoning is to facilitate elimination of the gas through the lungs. Because there is less than a 2 mm Hg gradient from blood to alveolar gas, and the hemoglobin has an enormous CO affinity, the HgbCO half-life is approximately 5 hours when room air is breathed. For example, a 30% HgbCO is reduced to approximately 15% in 5 hours and to approximately 7% in another 5 hours when the patient breathes room air at one atmosphere. High arterial O_2 partial pressure increases competition for the hemoglobin sites occupied by CO. Breathing 100% O_2 at one atmosphere decreases the HgbCO half-life to less than 1 hour. Thus, administration of near 100% O_2 is the most important factor in CO elimination. Hyperbaric oxygen therapy is also useful in severe cases of CO poisoning.

ABERRANT INTRACELLULAR METABOLISM ■

Increases and decreases in metabolic rate are seen with temperature variation, thyroid dysfunction, and physical activity. These represent quantitative rather than qualitative metabolic changes, because intracellular pathways remain essentially normal. General rules applied to the interpretation of pHa, Pco_2, and Po_2 remain valid when the metabolic rate is altered because the hemostatic relationship of CO_2 production to O_2 consumption remains constant. However, arterial blood gas interpretation requires additional considerations when intracellular metabolism involves aberrant pathways, particularly with sepsis, lactic acidosis, and parenteral hyperalimentation.

SEPSIS

Hyperdynamic sepsis, or "warm shock," involves a decreased $C(a - \bar{v})O_2$, which is most likely secondary to decreased oxidative metabolism. The result is an increased $S\bar{v}O_2$ and thereby an improved arterial oxygenation status. Acute alveolar hyperventilation (acute respiratory alkalosis) is most commonly seen with the hyperdynamic phase of septic shock. Blood lactate levels are seldom increased significantly, and a major component of metabolic acidosis is rare. Most of the guidelines for assessing oxygenation are not applicable because O_2 extraction is decreased independent of the adequacy of cellular oxygenation. The relationship between PaO_2 and tissue oxygenation is thus unpredictable and unreliable.

"Cold septic shock" involves cellular hypoperfusion and manifests blood gas values similar to those seen in all hypoperfusion states.

LACTIC ACIDOSIS

Krebs cycle metabolism requires O_2 utilization and produces CO_2 as the major metabolite. Anaerobic metabolic pathways are less efficient in calorie production, but are most important for producing H^+ and lactate ions as metabolites.

Thus, inadequate availability of O_2 at the mitochondrial level results in anaerobic metabolism and lactic acid production.

The most common cause of anaerobic metabolism is cellular hypoperfusion, clinically referred to as "shock" (hypovolemic, cardiac, or septic). Hypoxemia and anemia may produce anaerobic metabolism by themselves, but usually are combined with a degree of hypoperfusion.

Cellular production of lactic acid is difficult to quantify by laboratory analysis of arterial or central venous blood because organ system perfusion and hepatic function are variable. An adequately oxygenated and perfused liver metabolizes lactic acid to carbonic acid. Thus, if some organ systems (e.g., muscle, gastrointestinal tract, skin) produce lactic acid, normal hepatic function may prevent significant accumulation in the core circulation.

The presence of increased blood lactate indicates anaerobic metabolism; however, the absence of increased blood lactate does not imply the absence of anaerobic metabolism. Metabolic acidosis in a patient with severe hypoxemia, poor perfusion status, or both must be assumed to be lactic acidosis until proven otherwise.

Lactic acidosis in a patient with shock, seizures, or shivering is a dire circumstance. The absence of metabolic acidemia implies that vital organs may still be reasonably oxygenated, but by no means is that a certainty.

PARENTERAL HYPERALIMENTATION

Carbohydrates and proteins are associated with a respiratory quotient (RQ) of 1.0, whereas lipids have a RQ of 0.7. The Krebs cycle in humans averages a RQ of 0.8 because carbohydrates, proteins, and fats all are normally utilized. Hypertonic glucose solution is usually the principal source of nonprotein calories with total parenteral nutrition (TPN) and leads to an increased level of CO_2 production because the excess glucose must be stored as lipid. Because the metabolic pathway changing carbohydrates to fat has a high RQ (approaching 8.0), the overall RQ significantly increases independent of the relatively stable RQ producing energy. Patients receiving TPN in which the nonprotein source is primarily glucose have an increased CO_2 production. This problem can be remedied by providing sufficient nonprotein calories as lipid.[15]

Patients with increased CO_2 production are required to increase $\dot{V}E$ to maintain a normal $PaCO_2$. In patients receiving TPN, this potentially produces an $\dot{V}E-PaCO_2$ disparity similar to that seen with increased $\dot{V}D$.

CARDIOPULMONARY RESUSCITATION AND LOW FLOW STATES ■

Lung function is usually the limiting factor in CO_2 excretion, and normally the venous to $PaCO_2$ gradient [$P(\bar{v} - a)CO_2)$ is 8 mm Hg or less. However, no matter how well the lung functions, a minimal perfusion is required to excrete the CO_2 being produced. A low cardiac output can limit lung perfusion to the point that blood flow becomes the limiting factor to CO_2 excretion. This circumstance generally is limited to profound cardiogenic shock and CPR.

Closed-chest cardiac compression, in conjunction with positive-pressure ventilation, has been the standard CPR technique for more than a quarter of a century. The acid–base abnormalities coincident with CPR are unique and demand separate consideration when interpreting arterial blood gas values.

ACID–BASE BALANCE DURING CPR

Venous Respiratory Acidosis

During CPR with normal lungs and increased $\dot{V}E$, venous "respiratory acidosis" occurs in conjunction with an arterial "respiratory alkalosis."[16] In spontaneously breathing patients with poor cardiac output, the $P(\bar{v} - a)CO_2$ has been observed to increase 50% to 100%; a threefold to tenfold increase has been observed in patients receiving CPR.[16] An acute increase in venous PCO_2 results in a decreased venous pH with little change in plasma HCO_3^- concentration. Because systemic capillary blood is similar to venous blood, it is implied that tissue PCO_2 and pH values will be similar to venous values.

Metabolic Acidosis

Inadequate tissue perfusion inevitably leads to anaerobic metabolism and the production of lactic acid, and traditionally has been considered the primary cause of acidosis during CPR. However, a significant plasma HCO_3^- depletion caused by lactic acid accumulation is seldom present in the first 10 to 15 minutes of CPR.[17] The best explanation for this observation is that hepatic function metabolizes lactate to CO_2 as long as liver oxygenation is adequate; as liver oxygenation diminishes, lactic acid gradually accumulates. Early lactate production probably increases CO_2 production by the liver and thereby contributes to the venous respiratory alkalosis.

The plasma HCO_3^- deficit attributable to metabolic acidosis is essentially equal in both the venous and arterial blood. This means that the "paradoxic" venous pH and pHa values seen in early CPR are caused by the differences of PCO_2.

ARTERIAL BLOOD GASES DURING CPR

Arterial blood gas measurements during CPR are of limited value.

Arterial pH

Mixed venous pH (pH$\bar{v}$) is always less than the pHa. During CPR, a pHa less than 7.20 reflects severe tissue acidosis and is a poor prognostic sign.[16] An alkalemic pHa during CPR usually results from low $PaCO_2$ and does not reflect the tissue acid–base state. HCO_3^- deficiency (metabolic acidosis) will not have a significant disparity between the arterial and

venous blood; therefore, the degree of metabolic acidosis in arterial blood is reflective of total body metabolic acidosis.

Arterial Pco₂

The poor cardiac output coincident with CPR greatly increases physiologic dead space. Therefore, a significant increase in total ventilation (minute ventilation) is required to maintain a normal $PaCO_2$ of 40 mm Hg. In CPR dog models with normal lungs, arterial acidemia can be avoided for up to 18 minutes by providing the required increase in minute ventilation.[17]

Because the $P(\bar{v} - a)CO_2$ greatly increases during CPR, blood going from the right heart to the left heart without exchanging with alveolar gas (true shunt, zero $\dot{V}/\dot{Q}$ matching) enters the left heart with a PCO_2 significantly greater than the blood that has exchanged with alveolar gas. If $\dot{Q}sp/\dot{Q}t$ is more than 20%, the $PaCO_2$ may be greatly increased despite adequate minute ventilation.

The $PaCO_2$ during CPR cannot be considered to be a reflection of total body CO_2 homeostasis. No particular comfort can be validly derived from a $PaCO_2$ less than 40 mm Hg, whereas a $PaCO_2$ greater than 40 mm Hg reflects either inadequate $\dot{V}E$ or intrapulmonary shunting.

Arterial PO₂

The PaO_2 should be as high as possible to deliver maximal O_2 to the heart and brain during CPR. Therefore, PaO_2 remains an important measurement during CPR. A PaO_2 less than 100 mm Hg with a FIO_2 greater than 0.60 suggests either inadequate lung ventilation or significant intrapulmonary shunting. True shunting in excess of 25% is associated with hypoxemia despite high FIO_2 values.

VENOUS BLOOD GASES DURING CPR

Arterial blood gas values are sensitive to rapid changes occurring in the pulmonary capillary bed, whereas mixed venous blood gas values are sensitive to changes occurring in the systemic capillary bed. With the exception of cardiovascular collapse, arterial blood gas partial pressures reasonably reflect respiratory homeostasis because lung function determines CO_2 excretion.

Bicarbonate Administration

When $NaHCO_3$ is administered intravenously, it immediately adds H_2CO_3 to the blood. Bicarbonate ions are added to the blood *only* after the "CO_2 load" inherent in the $NaHCO_3$ solution is eliminated by the lungs. To illustrate this point, if $NaHCO_3$ is administered to a spontaneously breathing patient with acute respiratory acidosis (acute ventilatory failure), the $PaCO_2$ increases and pHa decreases because the CO_2 load cannot be eliminated. A similar circumstance seems to occur during CPR because the low cardiac output limits CO_2 excretion. $NaHCO_3$ causes the $P\bar{v}CO_2$ to increase and pH$\bar{v}$ to decrease.[18,19] Furthermore, serum osmolarity, serum Na^+, and excess HCO_3^- remain after perfusion has been restored.

TEMPERATURE CORRECTION ■

Transport of CO_2 and O_2 involves both gas solution and complex chemical reactions that are affected by temperature variation. Simply stated, a blood sample of given O_2 and CO_2 contents manifests different gas partial pressures when analyzed at various temperatures. Table 61-15 lists the temperature correction values for normal blood.

DEFINING TEMPERATURE CORRECTION

An *open system* allows gas exchange with the adjacent environment, for example, capillary blood or a blood sample exposed to the air. A *closed system* does not allow such exchange of gas content, for example, arterial blood or a gas-tight syringe. In vitro blood samples are in a closed system in which temperature-induced gas changes occur without changes in the gas content. In vivo blood gas changes from temperature variation occur in an open system in which gas contents can change.

To obtain true in vivo blood gas values, the measuring electrode's temperature would have to be adjusted to that of the patient, a process that would add at least 30 minutes to each measurement and would complicate quality assurance. To avoid these undesirable factors, the pH, P_{CO_2}, and P_{O_2} electrodes are encased in a constant 37°C environment to which the blood sample chamber is also exposed. Thus, independent of the patient's temperature, the pH, P_{CO_2}, and P_{O_2} are analyzed in a closed system at 37°C.

The term *temperature correction* refers to mathematical adjustments to the measured 37°C values for obtaining a more accurate reflection of the in vivo gas partial pressures. Although the derivation of temperature correction formulas is empiric in reference to in vitro changes in a closed system, the formulas are generally thought to be reasonably accurate within the clinically relevant ranges.

TABLE 61-15. Temperature Correction Values for Normal Blood

°C	°F	pH	P_{CO_2}	P_{O_2}
20	68	7.65	19	27
25	77	7.58	24	37
30	86	7.50	30	51
35	95	7.43	37	70
36	97	7.41	38	75
37	99	7.40	40	80
38	100	7.39	42	85
39	102	7.47	44	91
40	104	7.36	45	97

PHYSIOLOGIC CONSIDERATIONS

Interpretation of a biologic measurement depends on identification of a normal range. Therefore, before judging the clinical relevance of temperature correction, the degree to which we understand and can identify physiologic variations induced by temperature change must be examined.

Oxygenation

Because O_2 homeostasis at 37°C has been extensively studied, we are capable of defining minimal levels of Pa_{O_2} that should adequately oxygenate tissues at that temperature. A normothermic adult maintains O_2 delivery to tissues with an Pa_{O_2} of 60 mm Hg or greater, as long as hemoglobin content and cardiovascular function are adequate. In contrast, identification of such minimal levels of P_{O_2} at various body temperatures are poorly documented and confounded by concomitant pathophysiology and therapeutic intervention.

Hyperthermia

The effect of temperature change on adult O_2 consumption is approximately 10% per degree Celsius or 7% per degree Fahrenheit. Thus, hyperthermia requires an increased $\dot{V}o_2$, which is generally associated with an increased cardiac output and $\dot{V}E$.

When the initial P_{O_2} is normoxic, increasing temperature increases P_{O_2}; %$HgbO_2$ changes little or not at all because of near total saturation to begin with; and Hgb-O_2 affinity decreases (shift to right). Theoretically, the blood should be better capable of unloading O_2 to the tissues. When the initial P_{O_2} is in the hypoxemic range, the shift to the right decreases arterial O_2 content for any P_{O_2} and, theoretically, threatens tissue oxygenation. The net physiologic advantage or disadvantage of these changes is completely unknown.

Hypothermia

During hypothermia, the Pa_{O_2} can be expected to decrease whereas O_2 unloading is potentially impeded by an increased Hgb-O_2 affinity. However, data from accidental hypothermia in humans illustrate that several cardiopulmonary factors may contribute to the observed arterial hypoxemia in addition to those directly attributable to temperature change.[20] On the one hand, physiologic principles dictate that as $\dot{V}o_2$ falls with temperature, the changes in gas solubility result in an increasing amount of dissolved O_2. On the other hand, pathophysiologic factors like hypoventilation, vasoconstriction, and uneven tissue temperatures predispose toward inadequate O_2 delivery. There are no data to determine the minimal Pa_{O_2} required to prevent tissue hypoxia under hypothermic conditions.

Acid–Base Balance

The pHa rises and Pa_{CO_2} falls during hypothermia when the analysis is made at actual body temperature. However, this "alkalotic" change with hypothermia does not occur when the measurements are made at 37°C. In warm-blooded animals, the pH of intracellular and extracellular water, as well as the neutral pH of water, undergo parallel changes with temperature variation.[21] This finding indicates that these observed pH changes with temperature do not represent deviation from normal acid–base balance. Likewise, the coincident changes in PCO_2 with temperature variation are assumed to be an integral part of the process of maintaining electrochemical neutrality, and therefore do not represent deviation from normal CO_2 homeostasis. Furthermore, blood subjected to in vitro temperature variation demonstrates no evidence of change in acid–base and electrolyte equilibrium, despite significant pH and PCO_2 changes.[22]

Reasonable interpretation of these complex data suggests that the normal pH is not constant with temperature variation but varies in a predictable fashion. This concept further suggests that if the acid–base status is normal at any in vivo temperature, the in vitro pH and PCO_2 at 37°C should approach 7.40 and 40 mm Hg, respectively. Conversely, in vivo acid–base abnormalities should be appropriately reflected in the 37°C measurements. Available human and animal data pertaining to biochemical and physiologic changes coincident with temperature variation demonstrate that pH and PCO_2 values measured at 37°C probably best reflect the in vivo acid–base status, regardless of body temperature.

CLINICAL RELEVANCE

Justification for temperature correction of pH and blood gas values is based on the belief that "knowing" the in vivo status is an advantage to patient care. Such a belief implies that either the normal ranges for pH, PCO_2, and PO_2 remain constant regardless of temperature, or that the normal ranges are well established for all temperatures. Neither of these alternatives is valid.

Acid–Base Interpretation

The pH and PCO_2 changes attributable to temperature variation do not affect the calculated HCO_3^- value. Therefore, the 37°C values for pH and PCO_2 reliably reflect the in vivo metabolic acid–base status at the patient's actual temperature. Because temperature-corrected pH and PCO_2 values have no established physiologic reference points, the clinical application of such values is without foundation and is confusing.

PCO₂ and Ventilation

When the $PaCO_2$ is used to reflect the adequacy of $\dot{V}A$, our established guidelines are predicated on a normal CO_2 production at 37°C. Because both CO_2 production and $PaCO_2$ undergo parallel changes with temperature variation, clinical assessment of $\dot{V}A$ is most reliably reflected by applying the well established homeostatic reference points at 37°C. Even in the circumstances where hypocapnia is desired to minimize the intracranial blood volume by cerebral vasoconstriction, the $PaCO_2$ measurement and reference points at 37°C are as clinically reliable as the temperature-corrected values.

Interpretation of End-Tidal PCO₂

Exhaled gas measurements reflect the in vivo (temperature-corrected) PCO_2. With normal $\dot{V}A$ and a body temperature of 30°C, the $PETCO_2$ is 28 mm Hg, whereas the uncorrected $PaCO_2$ is 40 mm Hg. The clinician must be aware of this circumstance so that the $PETCO_2$ is not inappropriately interpreted. We recommend temperature-correcting the $PETCO_2$ and comparing that value with the 37°C blood gas values.

Oxygenation

In the absence of data quantifying changes in the balance between O_2 delivery and demand at temperature other than 37°C, the clinician should assume that temperature-induced changes do not significantly alter this balance. Clinical decisions concerning hypoxemia based on 37°C requirements (e.g., PaO_2 maintained at 60 to 80 mm Hg) are the best guidelines available, even in conditions of significant hyperthermia or hypothermia. Temperature-correcting PO_2 values does *not* improve our ability to make clinically relevant interpretations!

OXYGEN CONTENT. Because blood O_2 content in a closed system must remain the same despite temperature changes, variations in $\%HgbO_2$ and PO_2 can only occur by transfer of O_2 molecules between the dissolved state and the combined state. In a closed system, the $\%HgbO_2$ changes by less than 2% over a temperature range of 0° to 42°C.[23] Because O_2 content can be accurately calculated from 37°C values regardless of patient temperature, temperature correction of the blood gas values is unnecessary to obtain O_2 content based indices such as the $C(a - \bar{v})O_2$ and $\dot{Q}sp/\dot{Q}t$.

OXYGEN PARTIAL PRESSURE INDICES. When oxygen partial pressure indices are used, the PaO_2 should be temperature-corrected to reflect the true difference with the calculated alveolar PAO_2.

RECOMMENDATION

The popularity of temperature-correcting pH, PCO_2, and PO_2 values is based on the observation that large differences in the blood gas values are present when the patient's temperature is profoundly hypothermic or hyperthermic. This observation leads many clinicians to conclude that the 37°C values are "wrong." The danger in this superficial thought process is the unfounded conclusion that temperature-corrected values are "right." Although temperature correction of blood gases cannot be considered wrong, the process involves several practical disadvantages. First, the assumption that the laboratory has received the patient's true temperature at the time of sampling is not borne out in our experience. Second, temperature-corrected values can be confused with uncorrected values, and vice versa.

The scientific truth is that with significant changes in patient temperature, we do not fully understand the complexity of effects on metabolism, vascular function, and respiration. Therefore, both corrected and uncorrected blood gas values are of uncertain usefulness in patients with significant deviations in body temperature. No logical or scientific basis justifies assuming that temperature-corrected values are better than the 37°C values. In fact, the available technical and biologic data lead to the conclusion that no clinical advantage is derived from using values other than those at 37°C.

POINT OF CARE ANALYZERS AND BLOOD GAS MONITORS ■

Although there is no serious debate concerning the clinical usefulness of pH and blood gas measurements in caring for the critically ill, the *frequency* required for optimal patient care remains a controversy. Blood gas analyzers impose three impediments to frequent serial measurements: (1) each analysis requires permanent blood loss; (2) each analysis is associated with implicit costs; and (3) availability of results involves a significant delay in time. Solid-state transportable analyzers are available that allow nonlaboratory personnel to reliably and consistently perform blood gas measurements at or near the site of patient care.[24] These "point of care" analyzers significantly decrease the delay in obtaining results at the bedside and are preferred over laboratory-based devices. There remain two major reasons that point of care analyzers should limit the frequency of serial blood gas measurements: blood loss and cost.

Laboratory medicine defines an *analyzer* as an in vitro device that performs measurements on fluids, excrement, or tissue permanently removed from the body. A *blood gas monitor* has been defined as an in vivo device that measures pHa, $PaCO_2$, and PaO_2 without permanently removing blood and without additional cost for multiple measurements.[25] Optode microsensing allows measurement of changes in analyte concentration by photochemical reactions altering light absorption, reflection, or reemission (fluorescence). Fluorescent optodes have significant advantages because their stability minimizes drift and pledges reliable calibration, they have a fast response time to changes in analyte concentrations (60 to 90 seconds), and they do not require reagent replacement because they are not consumed by the measurement process.

Fluorescent-based intraarterial blood gas monitors were shown to be clinically feasible in 1989,[26] but the extent to which the intraarterial milieu prevents reliable function in all patients, all of the time, remains an open question. An extraarterial device that locates the optodes in series with the arterial catheter tubing allows intermittent measurements without permanently removing blood from the patient. A prospective, multicenter study[27] of this extraarterial device concludes that the device performed as well as conventional blood gas analyzers in all patients, all of the time.

In vivo blood gas monitors provide serial measurements without blood loss or additional cost. For patients with arterial catheters in place, the correctness of blood gas monitors is obvious as long as there is no requirement to alter the size, location, or placement of the arterial catheter, and the routine use of the arterial catheter system is unaffected. Further, personnel exposure to the patient's blood, and the risk of nosocomial infection from contaminated arterial cath-

eters, should be reduced because the integrity of the arterial line system is not interrupted to obtain blood gas values.

Availability of both blood gas monitors and point of care analyzers should significantly reduce therapeutic decision time (the interval from ordering the test to initiating a therapeutic action based on the test results), thereby, enabling rapid titration of common therapeutic modalities such as O_2 administration, positive-pressure ventilation, positive end-expiratory pressure, and anti-acidemia therapy. In our opinion, the transfer of blood gas measurements from laboratory-based analyzers to the combination of point of care analyzers and monitors should have as profound an impact on acute respiratory care as did the introduction of laboratory-based blood gas analyzers over 30 years ago. However, we must be sure these devices are reliable, consistent, and cost beneficial to avoid widespread adoption of new technology that provides more data, more cost, and questionable patient benefit.

REFERENCES ■

1. Shapiro BA, Kacmarek RM, Cane RD, et al: *Clinical Application of Respiratory Care*, 4th ed, pp 255–260. Chicago, Mosby-Year Book, 1991
2. Shapiro BA, Peruzzi WT, Templin R: *Clinical Application of Blood Gases*, 5th ed. Chicago, Year Book Medical Publishers, 1994
3. Cane RD, Shapiro BA, Templin R, et al: Unreliability of oxygen tension–based indices in reflecting intrapulmonary shunting in critically ill patients. *Crit Care Med* 1988;16:1243
4. Harrison RA, Davison R, Shapiro BA, et al: Reassessment of the assumed A-V oxygen content difference in the shunt calculation. *Anesth Analg* 1975;54:198
5. Domino KB, Wetstein L, Glasser SA: Influence of mixed venous oxygen tension ($P\bar{v}_2$) on blood flow to atelectatic lung. *Anesthesiology* 1983;59:428
6. Markello P, Winter P, Olszowka A: Assessment of ventilation-perfusion inequalities by arterial-venous nitrogen differences in intensive care patients. *Anesthesiology* 1972;37:4
7. Shoemaker WC, Appel PL, Waxman K, et al: Clinical trial of survivors, cardiorespiratory patterns as therapeutic goals in critically ill postoperative patients. *Crit Care Med* 1982;10:398
8. Walton JR, Shapiro BA, Wine C: Pre-analytic error in arterial blood gas measurement. *Respir Care* 1981;26:1136
9. Stock MC, Shapiro BA, Cane RD: Reliability of $S\bar{v}O_2$ in predicting A − VDO_2 and the effect of anemia. *Crit Care Med* 1986;14:402
10. Schmidt CR, Frank LP, Forsythe SB, et al: Continuous $S\bar{v}O_2$ measurement and oxygen transport patterns in cardiac surgical patients. *Crit Care Med* 1984;12:523
11. Schumacker PT, Cain SM: The concept of a critical oxygen delivery. *Intensive Care Med* 1987;13:223
12. Farhi LE: Gas stores in the body. In: *Handbook of Physiology: Respiration*, vol 1. Baltimore, Williams & Wilkins, 1965;873
13. Robin ED: Abnormalities of acid-base regulation in chronic pulmonary disease, with special reference to hypercapnia and extracellular alkalosis. *N Engl J Med* 1963;268:917
14. Goldbaum KR, Ramirez RG, Absalom KB: What is the mechanism of carbon dioxide toxicity? *Aviat Space Environ Med* 1975;46:1289
15. Askanazi J, Nordstrom J, Rosenbaum SH, et al: Nutrition for the patient with respiratory failure: glucose vs. fat. *Anesthesiology* 1981;54:373

16. Weil MH, Rackow EC, Trevino R, et al: Difference in acid-base state between venous and arterial blood during cardiopulmonary resuscitation. *N Engl J Med* 1986;315:153

17. Sanders AB, Ewy GA, Taft TV: Resuscitation and arterial blood gas abnormalities during prolonged cardiopulmonary resuscitation. *Ann Emerg Med* 1984;13:676

18. Emergency Cardiac Care Committee and Subcomittees, American Heart Association: Guidelines for cardiopulmonary resuscitation and emergency cardiac care. III. Adult advanced cardiac life support. *JAMA* 1992;268:2210

19. Cummins RO (ed): *Section 7. Cardiovascular Pharmacology. I. American Heart Association: Textbook of Advanced Cardiac Life Support.* Dallas, American Heart Association, 1994:14

20. McNicol MW, Smith R: Accidental hypothermia. *Br Med J* 1964;1:19

21. Rahn H, Reeves RB, Howell BJ: Hydrogen ion regulation, temperature, and evaluation. *Am Rev Respir Dis* 1975;112:165

22. Reeves RB: Temperature-induced changes in blood acid-base status = pH and PCO$_2$ in a binary buffer. *J Appl Physiol* 1976;40:752

23. Roiughton FJW, Severinghaus JW: Accurate determination of O$_2$ solubility in unmodified human blood from 0 to 37°C. *J Appl Physiol* 1973;35:861

24. Zaloga GP, Dudas L, Roberts P, et al: Near-patient blood gas and electrolyte analyses are accurate when performed by non-laboratory-trained individuals. *J Clin Monit* 1993;9:341

25. Shapiro BA: In-vivo monitoring of arterial blood gases and pH. *Respir Care* 1992;37:165

26. Shapiro BA, Cane RD, Chomka CM, et al: Preliminary evaluation of an intra-arterial blood gas system in dogs and humans. *Crit Care Med* 1989;17:455

27. Shapiro BA, Mahutte CK, Cane RD, et al: Clinical performance of a blood gas monitor: a prospective, multicenter trial. *Crit Care Med* 1993;21:487

Critical Care, Third Edition, edited by Joseph M. Civetta,
Robert W. Taylor, and Robert R. Kirby.
Lippincott-Raven Publishers, Philadelphia, PA © 1997.

CHAPTER 62

Neurologic Monitoring

Thomas Grissom
Joyce Grissom
J. Christopher Farmer

Advances in monitoring technology allow us to follow detailed neurophysiologic responses in the critically ill patient. The ability to monitor change in cerebral function, perfusion, and metabolism, however, does not always lead to an improved outcome. The need to establish clear links between technologic advancements and change in outcome remains a high priority in a cost-sensitive environment. This chapter focuses not only on the ability of different monitoring modalities to differentiate between the diseased and normal state, but on the links, if any, between the use of these technologies and subsequent outcome.

CEREBRAL FUNCTION ■

The assessment of cerebral function begins with a thorough neurologic examination. The introduction and improvement of sophisticated neurophysiologic monitoring techniques such as electroencephalography (EEG) and evoked potential (EP) monitoring have not diminished the importance of obtaining a complete examination.[1-5] Use of a simple standardized scoring system based on the physical examination, like the Glasgow Coma Scale (GCS),[6] provides a means of following repeated neurologic assessments where any deterioration in score prompts a more thorough examination and review of ancillary information. The institution of sedation or neuromuscular paralysis, however, negates the usefulness of this clinical approach. Electrophysiologic monitoring attempts to address this situation where the clinician cannot assess cerebral function readily because of the nature of the injury or concurrent therapy. In addition, the use of electrophysiologic monitoring in some situations may

guide treatment, aid in diagnosis, or provide prognostic information.

NEUROLOGIC EXAMINATION

The GCS, described by Teasdale and Jennett in 1974,[6] has become the most widely used bedside screening examination. The GCS assigns number scores for eye opening, motor response, and verbal response (Table 62-1), which are summed to provide the total score. References to the total score should reflect factors such as endotracheal intubation, facial trauma, focal deficits, and the use of neuromuscular relaxants that impact on the final score. Although originally designed to quantify the severity of head injury, the GCS allows for categorization of patients with neurologic dysfunction from other forms of brain injury[7,8] and nonneurologic conditions.[9-11]

Impairment of consciousness can be prognostically divided into three groups: mild (GCS 13 to 15), moderate (GCS 9 to 12), or severe (GCS 3 to 8). The GCS has good interobserver reliability, although the inexperienced examiner may make consistent errors averaging as much as 1 point on the 4- and 5-point scales.[12] The objective criteria of the GCS provide a more consistent set of criteria than many other scales,[7] particularly when care is taken while performing the different sections of the examination. Eye opening, limited by swelling or trauma, may result in an inappropriate score. When motor responses are asymmetric, the examiner notes the best response but should also record the differential responses in the record. If required to assess the motor response, the painful stimulus must be applied in a consistent manner. Motor responses to deep pressure

TABLE 62-1.   The Glasgow Coma Scale

EYE OPENING (E)

Spontaneous	4
To voice	3
To pain	2
None	1

MOTOR RESPONSES (R)

Obeys commands	6
Localizes pain	5
Normal flexion (withdrawal to pain)	4
Abnormal flexion (decorticate)	3
Extension (decerebrate)	2
None (flaccid)	1

VERBAL RESPONSE (V)

Oriented	5
Confused conversation	4
Inappropriate words	3
Incomprehensible sounds	2
None	1

Glasgow Coma Scale (GCS) score = E + M + V; best score = 15; worst possible = 3

applied to the nail bed, sternum, or nipples fall into one of the following patterns: localized, withdrawal, abnormal flexor, abnormal extension, or no movement. The abnormal flexor and extensor responses are sometimes respectively referred to as decorticate and decerebrate postures. In this setting, the clinician should avoid these terms because they imply a specific anatomic lesion.

In the setting of head injury, the GCS does have prognostic value. A recent analysis of the Major Trauma Outcome Study,[13] which includes data on 59,713 patients with mild to severe head injury, confirms an exponential increase in mortality with lower GCS scores (Fig. 62-1). A score of greater than 7 on the GCS denotes a 90% probability of obtaining a good final outcome or being only moderately

disabled.[14] A score of 7 or less suggests a marked increase in mortality or a resulting persistent vegetative state approaching 60% to 90% for a GCS score of 3.[13,15,16]

When used to assess prognosis for nontraumatic brain injury, the GCS seems to have some utility. In the Brain Resuscitation Clinical Trials I Study Group, the investigators recorded GCS scores in comatose patients up to 7 days after successful resuscitation.[17] A GCS score of 5 or less on admission had a 69% positive predictive value for either severe cerebral disability, persistent vegetative state, or death. The predictive value increased to 100% by day 3, which agrees with other studies[18] showing increased predictive value of the GCS over time after cardiac arrest. The GCS is also predictive of neurologic dysfunction and increased mortality in human immunodeficiency virus–infected patients[19] and in pediatric patients with Reye's syndrome[20] admitted to the ICU with neurologic failure.

ELECTROPHYSIOLOGIC MONITORING

Electroencephalography

The EEG is a sensitive indicator of brain function. It is simple, inexpensive, and free of significant risk or discomfort to the patient. It may complement information obtained from imaging studies better suited to demonstrate structural lesions. In the intensive care unit (ICU), the EEG is useful in the management of refractory status epilepticus and the diagnosis and treatment of nonconvulsive status epilepticus. In addition, certain EEG patterns may provide clues to the cause of certain toxic or metabolic encephalopathies. The EEG may be of some prognostic value in coma and may be an adjunctive tool in confirming the diagnosis of brain death.

Summation of synaptic potentials generated by pyramidal cells in the granular layer of cerebral cortex generates the measured EEG signal. These synaptic potentials are the responses of cortical cells to rhythmic discharges of thalamic nuclei. The particular arrangements of excitatory and inhibitory interconnections between thalamic cells determine the frequencies and amplitudes of the thalamic discharges, and

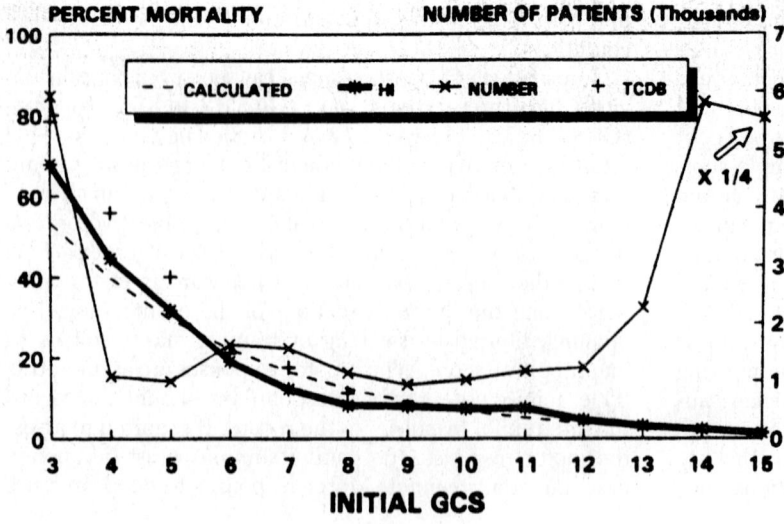

FIGURE 62-1. Number (×), percentage mortality (°), and calculated mortality (dashed line) for head-injured patients compared with initial Glasgow Coma Scale score from the Major Trauma Outcome Study. Data from the Traumatic Coma Data Bank (TCDB) are represented by the pluses (+) for comparison. (From Gennarelli TA, Champion HR, Copes WS, et al: Comparison of mortality, morbidity, and severity of 59,713 head injured patients with 1114,447 patients with extracranial injuries. *J Trauma* 1994;37:962; and Marshall LF, Gautille T, Klauber MR, et al: The outcome of severe closed head injury. *J Neurosurg* 1991;75:S28.)

by extension, the cortical potentials. EEG recording electrodes are large and record at some distance from cortical generator cells. Thus, they only detect the summated activities of numerous pyramidal cells oriented perpendicular to the coritcal surface. Traditional clinical EEG uses a strip chart plot of voltage versus time. Sixteen to 20 channels are recorded simultaneously from electrodes positioned over the scalp in standardized placement according to the 10-20 system of the International Federation of Societies for EEG and Clinical Neurophysiology. Frequency, amplitude, distribution, rhythmicity, and symmetry describe the recorded waveforms. Specific normal and pathologic patterns have been described in adults and children when awake, asleep, or in a coma.

The EEG has some utility in the diagnosis and, possibly, the prognosis of coma. Electrocerebral silence (ECS)—described as a flat, apotential EEG—has considerable, generally ominous significance.[21,22] ECS is not, however, an absolute indication of brain death, and recovery is possible after ECS in cases of hypothermia or barbiturate coma.[23] Burst suppression is an EEG pattern where high-voltage slow-activity bursts and sharp waves regularly alternate with low-amplitude slow-background activity (Fig. 62-2). It is characteristi-

cally seen during deep anesthesia but also may be present in Wernicke's encephalopathy and after cardiac arrest, head injury, or anoxia.[24] An EEG burst suppression pattern frequently accompanies myoclonic status epilepticus after cardiac arrest. Myoclonic status in such patients indicates the presence of severe anoxic cortical damage and is an agonal phenomenon.[25]

Alpha coma is a rhythmic, diffuse, or frontally predominant alpha-frequency pattern unresponsive to auditory, photic, or noxious stimuli in the comatose patient (Fig. 62-3). It may be replaced by a more favorable slow delta-theta wave patterns or may alternate with burst suppression. In general, the prognosis of patients in alpha coma seems to be similar to other patients with similar depths of coma.[26,27] By contrast, a normal or near-normal reactive, occipitally dominant alpha-frequency pattern in a patient appearing comatose may be seen in a brain stem lesion sparing the upper midbrain (locked-in syndrome). Additionally, this pattern can be seen with functional conditions such as catatonic stupor or conversion reaction. Spindle coma, a pattern resembling slow wave sleep, may be present after head injury, where it has a more favorable prognosis. When requested for prognosis after a hypoxic cerebral injury, the EEG should not be performed earlier than 6 hours after the insult.

The EEG pattern in the encephalopathic patient is usually nonspecific but may sometimes provide clues narrowing the differential diagnosis. Periodic patterns can be seen in subacute sclerosing panencephalitis, Jacob-Creuzfeldt disease, and herpes simplex encephalitis. Periodic phenomena also may be present with myoclonic epilepsy, hepatic coma, subdural hematoma, and cerebral lipidosis or after grand mal seizures.[24] Acute lesions of the cerebral hemisphere such as stroke may manifest with unilateral periodic discharges on the corresponding side. Repetitive "blunt spike-wave" activity can transiently be seen in hepatic encephalopathy.[28] In general, excessive frontal beta activity appears in the presence of barbiturates, benzodiazepines, or other sedative-hypnotics.

Cerebral ischemia, as seen in cardiac arrest, is sufficiently prevalent in the ICU patient to warrant further discussion. Normally, the adult brain receives an average global cerebral blood flow (CBF) of 50 mL/100 g/minute and consumes on average 3.5 mL/100 g/minute of oxygen. When perfusion falls below 40% of normal, cerebral neuronal activity decreases significantly. Below 25% to 30% of normal CBF, neuronal activity ceases, although the cells may be metabolically viable for some time. In the setting of a normal body temperature, without the use of cerebroprotective agents, cellular damage occurs within 4 to 5 minutes as CBF falls below 20% of normal. During cardiac arrest, EEG activity begins to change within 15 to 30 seconds.[29] Typically, there is an initial loss of high-frequency activity that progresses to an increase in relatively synchronized delta activity and a subsequent decrease in the amplitude of all activity. Prompt restoration of blood flow and oxygen delivery usually restores EEG activity to normal. Restoration of perfusion after neuronal damage produces a spectrum of abnormal EEG patterns, ranging from diffuse slowing of normal background activity to more ominous patterns, such as epileptiform activity, alpha coma, burst suppression, or ECS.

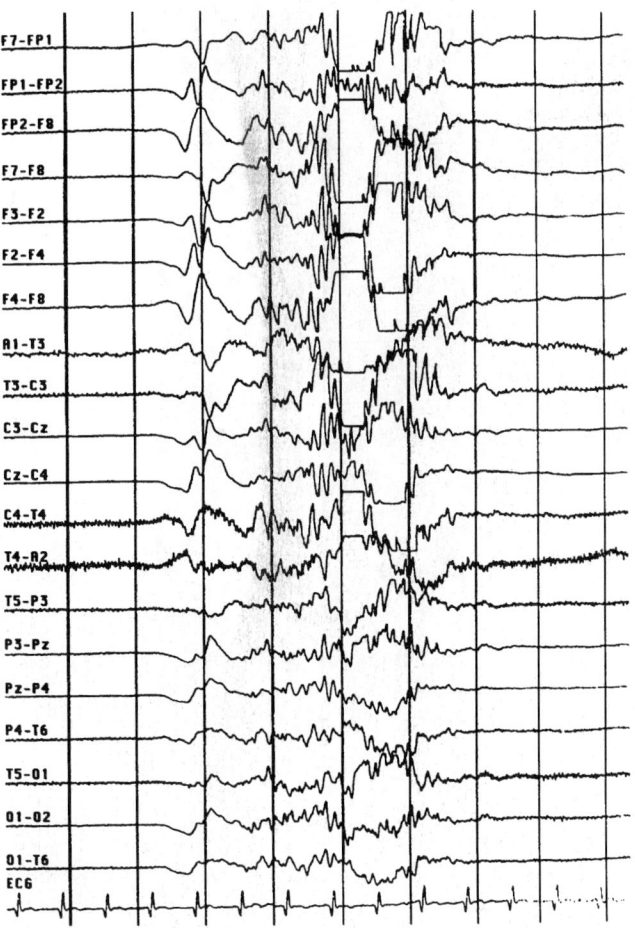

FIGURE 62-2. Burst suppression seen in a 22-year-old man after cardiopulmonary arrest and resuscitation.

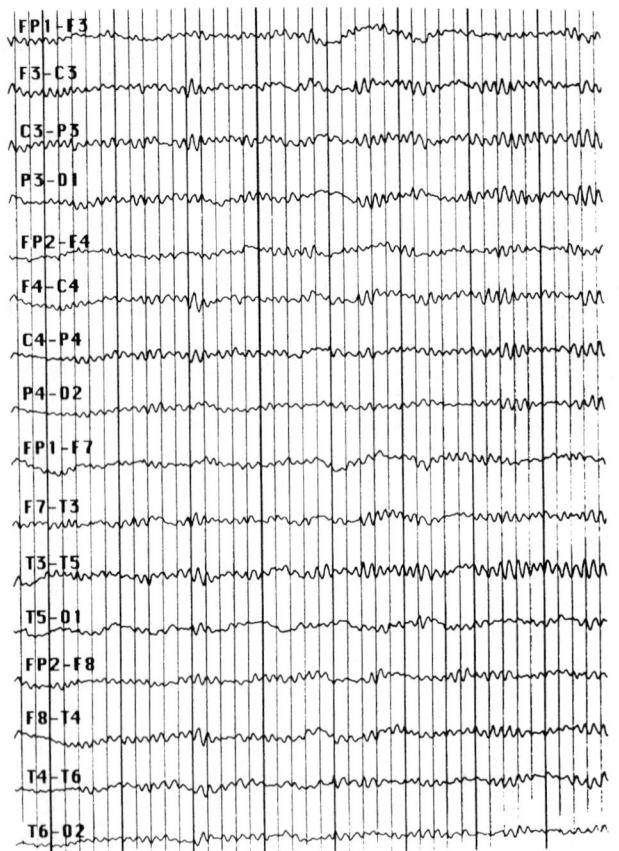

FIGURE 62-3. Alpha-frequency pattern present in an unresponsive 41-year-old woman after respiratory arrest secondary to an acute asthma exacerbation. This is representative of alpha coma and carries a poor prognosis.

Hypoxia is physiologically different from ischemia. The EEG activity does not change significantly until arterial hemoglobin saturation falls below 60%.[30] Systemic hypoxemia progressively, but reversibly, slows EEG activity. Prolonged hypoxemia leads to ECS followed by neuronal necrosis. With gradual onset of hypoxemia, the EEG activity may transiently accelerate before slowing.[31]

EEG is useful in determining a therapeutic endpoint during barbiturate coma for refractory status epilepticus or cerebral protection after severe head injury. By using EEG monitoring, the lowest effective pentobarbital dose can be used to maintain burst suppression. This minimizes the risk of dose-related pentobarbital toxicity.[31]

Frequency Domain Analysis

Raw EEG monitoring produces enormous quantities of information, which makes it difficult to use as a continuous monitor in the ICU. Frequency domain analysis translates these complex waveforms into spectra that display power versus frequency for a given time period. Cooley and Tukey[32] created fast Fourier transform algorithms that produce a set of frequency bins, each containing the power of the signal at that particular frequency. The compressed spectral array (CSA) displays the data as a "hill and valley" or three-dimen-

sional plot of frequency versus power versus time (Fig. 62-4). The final result is a compact, graphical representation of the EEG activity that is more readily evaluated by physicians not trained in standard EEG interpretation. Density spectral array uses gray or color scales to depict the EEG in each frequency at each epoch. Both techniques display essentially the same data, and both have the advantage of significantly compressing EEG information. Spectral EEG analysis does not require a full 20-electrode headset. Information can be obtained using two to four EEG channels. Frequency domain analysis requires less paper and simplifies analysis, an obvious advantage where continuous monitoring is desired over hours or days.

These frequency domain analyses obscure the nuances of the raw EEG signal but may enhance the detection of trends, particularly by physicians without training in clinical neurophysiology required for interpretation of standard EEG. Frequency domain EEG analysis has been used to predict prognosis in patients with traumatic and nontraumatic coma. Prediction of outcome by GCS or by EEG is not reliable during the first few days of unconsciousness.

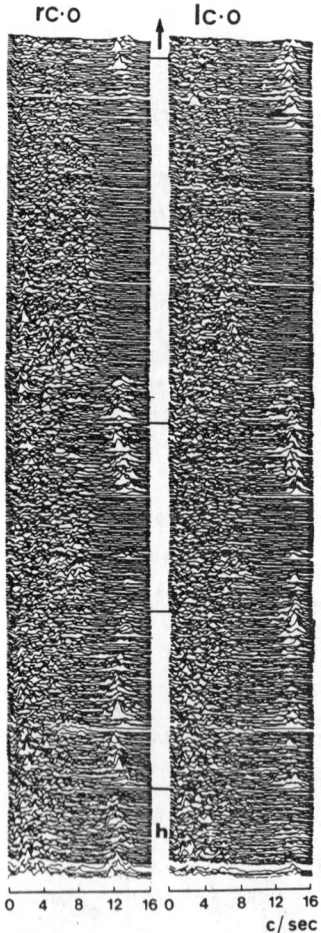

FIGURE 62-4. Changeable spectrogram with sleep-like pattern in a comatose patient after head injury. (Printed with permission from Bricolo A: Clinical application of compressed spectral array in long-term EEG monitoring of comatose patients. *EEG Clin Neurophysiol* 1978;45:211.)

Monotonous, slow, unreactive activity on the CSA correlates significantly with poor outcome.[33,34] The predictive value of CSA may be more sensitive than the GCS in mild cases of head injury whereas the GCS seems to prognosticate poor recovery more accurately.[35] Continuous CSA monitoring can be used to monitor for burst suppression as an endpoint during barbiturate coma. Frequency domain analysis has been used in cardiac arrest and resuscitation, but its use in this setting has not been standardized.[36] Outside of the research setting, few institutions employ this technology routinely.

Evoked Potentials

Evoked potentials are electrical responses of the nervous system to sensory stimulation. Baseline EEG activity obscures the very low amplitude of a single response to a single stimulus. EPs are extracted from unrelated EEG activity by computer-averaging repeated stimuli. Because the EP is time-locked to the the stimulus, averaging has the effect of decreasing the amplitude of unrelated, spontaneous EEG activity and increasing the amplitude of the time-locked response. Clinical EPs are usually elicited using visual or auditory stimuli, or by electrical stimulation of sensory nerves. The averaged responses consist of a series of waveforms or deflections that are characterized by latency and, to a lesser extent, amplitude.

EPs may detect dysfunction in visual, auditory, and somatosensory pathways not detected by clinical examination or other laboratory techniques. They may localize lesions to particular segments of central sensory pathways. The clinician can perform these tests at the bedside, although the electrically "hostile" nature of the ICU environment can produce artifacts making interpretation of the resultant data difficult.

VISUAL EVOKED RESPONSES. Flashing lights or alternating checkerboard patterns produce stimulation of the visual pathways. Leads placed on the scalp over the occiput detect a positive cortical potential at approximately 100 milliseconds. Visual evoked responses can be used differentiate optic neuritis from papilledema[37] and to follow visual function.[38] The presence of normal visual evoked responses in a comatose patient demonstrates intact visual pathways. These are not common in the ICU setting.

BRAIN STEM AUDITORY EVOKED RESPONSES. Repetitive clicks delivered to either ear provide the stimuli for brain stem auditory evoked responses (BAERs) while simultaneously recording over the auditory cortex. Short latency BAERs present in the first 10 seconds after the click are thought to be generated in structures from the cochlear nerve through the thalamus. Central transmission is divided into a caudal component (waves I and II) representing conduction from the cochlear nerve to the pons and a rostral component (waves III through V) representing conduction from the pontine to midbrain structures (Fig. 62-5). Waves VI and VII reflect activity in the thalamus and thalamocortical radiations to primary auditory cortex.[39] Although the exact generators of the BAER waveforms are not known, abnormalities of the the BAERs have localizing value. Short-latency BAERs are resistant to sedatives, anticonvulsants,

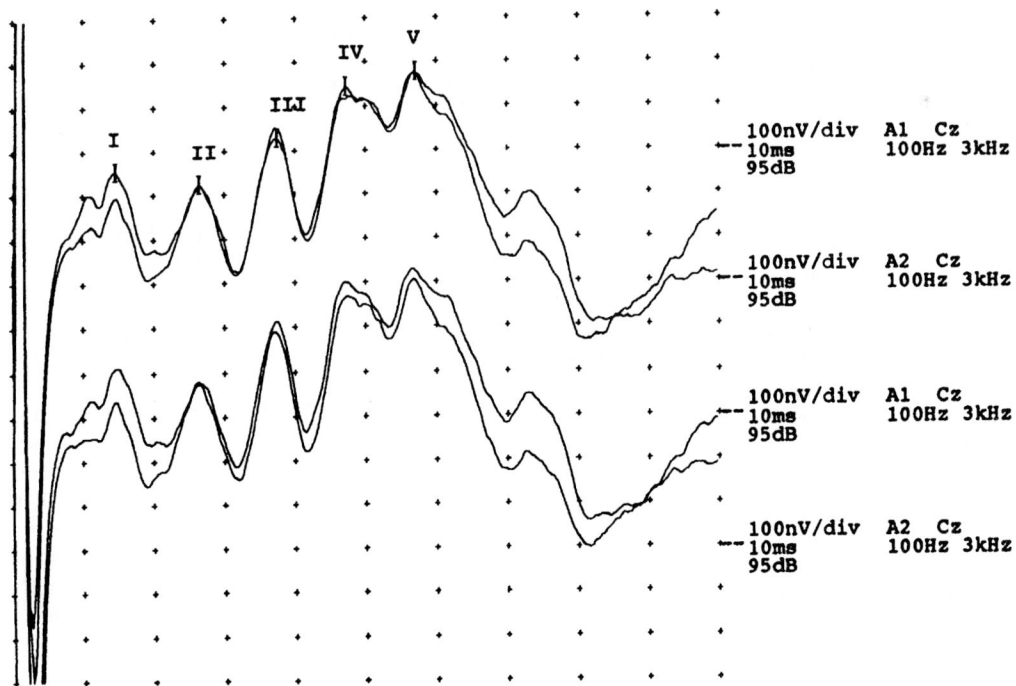

FIGURE 62-5. Normal brain stem auditory evoked response. Caudal components of the overall waveform are represented by I and II whereas conduction from the pons to the auditory cortex is represented by waves III to V.

and barbiturates.[39] BAERs are frequently used to monitor posterior fossa surgery. Abnormal BAERs may indicate brain stem ischemia, transtentorial herniation, or brain death.[40,41]

SOMATOSENSORY EVOKED POTENTIALS. Somatosensory evoked potentials (SSEPs) in the comatose patient most frequently involve median nerve stimulation. Recording from the clavicular area (Erb's point) allows assessment of the peripheral stimulus as it arrives at the brachial plexus approximately 9 milliseconds after stimulation. Recording from the neck demonstrates lower brain stem activity at approximately 13 to 16 milliseconds and somatosensory cortex activity at approximately 20 milliseconds.

Amplitude does not provide an indicator for normality. Large amplitude differences between sides, however, may suggest a lesion along the pathway on the side with the lower amplitude. The precise anatomic generators of the components of the SSEP are debated; however, absence of clavicular, cervical, and scalp components of the SSEP indicates a lesion of the peripheral nerve if technical problems are excluded. Similarly, a delayed clavicular potential with normal conduction time to the cervical and scalp potentials indicates a peripheral process. Increased clavicular to cervical and clavicular to scalp conduction times with normal peripheral conduction time is a reliable indicator of a lesion of the spinal roots or the cervical cord. Increased cervical to scalp conduction time with normal peripheral conduction localizes the lesion to the central nervous system above the lower medulla and below the somatosensory cortex.

Stimulation of the tibial nerve can similarly localize dysfunction in the lower spinal cord and is sometimes used in the monitoring of spinal cord function during orthopedic, neurosurgical, or vascular surgery procedures. Notice that SSEPs can detect only dysfunction in the posterior (sensory) part of the cord and do not exclude anterior (motor) cord dysfunction.

SSEPs, alone[42,43] or with other EPs,[44,45] have been used to evaluate the severity and prognosis of traumatic brain injury. Serial recordings that demonstrate reductions in central conduction time or increase in the number of peaks generally indicate imminent return of function.[46] Central conduction times increase in patients with subarachnoid hemorrhage (SAH) when the condition and prognosis of the patient are poor. Abolishment or reduction of scalp SSEPs may have some prognostic value in Reye's syndrome.[47] Early recovery of short latency peaks indicates survival whereas recovery of peaks with latencies over 100 milliseconds predicts satisfactory recovery in most patients with this disease.[48] SSEPs are abnormal in most asphyxiated newborns, the degree of abnormality corresponding to the degree of asphyxiation. SSEPs also have been used to monitor the brain during carotid endarterectomy and aneurysm surgery.

Abnormal SSEPs and auditory brain stem EPs in comatose patients with normal visual EPs suggest that cortical function is better than brain stem function. Conversely, abnormal somatosensory and visual EPs in the presence of normal auditory EPs suggest that cortical dysfunction is the cause of the comatose state. Multimodality EPs have been used as a prognostic adjunct to the neurologic examination, imaging, and other physiologic parameters in traumatic

coma.[45] This prognostic use of EPs is not routine in most ICUs.

Finally, it is possible to stimulate the motor cortex with electrical or magnetic stimuli. Electrical stimulation may be either transcranial or direct with craniotomy. Magnetic stimulation is transcranial. Resultant motor EPs can be recorded from the spinal cord, peripheral, nerve and muscle. Direct or transcranial cerebellar stimulation can produce descending nonpyramidal cerebellar EPs. Levy[49] described the use of these modalities to monitor pyramidal and nonpyramidal motor function during supratentorial, posterior fossa, and spine surgery. Use of these EPs to evaluate motor pathways is not routine at this time. Further study will define the clinical utility of these newer modalities in the operating room and ICU settings.

CEREBRAL PERFUSION

When assessing cerebral perfusion in the patient with neurologic dysfunction, several monitoring techniques provide valuable information. Currently, there is no single, practical, bedside monitoring modality that provides an easily interpretable and consistently accurate assessment of regional perfusion adequacy. Techniques exist that measure CBF, blood velocity, oxygenation, and perfusion pressure, but individually these provide only a part of the overall picture. Measurement of a normal or even elevated cerebral perfusion pressure (CPP) does not necessarily imply adequate cerebral perfusion relative to oxygen consumption. This is particularly true in the setting of vasospasm.[50] Conversely, global measurements of cerebral oxygenation, which have been studied in acute brain trauma, do not guide therapy toward improving oxygenation without some knowledge of CBF or CPP.[51] Multimodality monitoring, therefore, provides the best summary of the adequacy of cerebral perfusion.[52]

CEREBRAL BLOOD FLOW

The presence of an acceptable level of CBF is usually inferred, rather than measured directly, because of the complexity and expense of available CBF measurement techniques. Estimation of CBF is possible using several techniques including ^{133}Xenon clearance, the nitrous oxide (N_2O) saturation technique, or single-photon emission computer tomography (SPECT).[53-55] Knowledge of the CBF may be helpful in predicting the outcome of patients after traumatic head injury. Patients with moderately reduced CBF in the first 24 hours after injury demonstrate a higher mortality rate.[54,56] Extremely low values usually appear only within the first 8 to 12 hours.[57] Elevations of CBF also have been linked with a worsened neurologic outcome, although the time course and significance of these elevations are not clear.[58]

Nitrous Oxide Saturation

Originally described in the 1940s by Kety and Schmidt,[59] the N_2O saturation technique for determination of CBF relies on an interpretation of the Fick principle where "the amount of inert gas taken up by the tissue per unit of time is equal to the quantity brought to the tissue by the arterial blood minus the quantity carried away in the venous blood."[60] With this technique, N_2O is administered in a low, constant concentration over several minutes until the brain and its effluent blood are in equilibrium. This process takes approximately 10 minutes in most situations, and multiple samples of arterial and mixed cerebral venous (jugular bulb) blood are drawn to determine the arteriovenous difference over time. This technique provides an assessment of global CBF with an error of 5%, but it has been largely supplanted by other methods of CBF determination.[61]

Xenon 133 Clearance

The most common technique for assessing CBF in the ICU is based on the clearance of the freely diffusible, poorly soluble, inert radioisotope ^{133}Xe from brain tissue. The original technique involved injection of the ^{133}Xe into the internal carotid artery; however, inhalation or intravenous injection is the norm.[62] External detection using an array of scintillation counters provides regional CBF measurements. Significant technical demands, relatively high cost, concerns over use of radionuclides, and inability to perform rapid measurements have kept this technique from gaining wider use despite the ability to produce accurate results at the bedside.

Stable Xenon-Enhanced Computed Tomography

Stable xenon-enhanced computed tomography (Xe-CT) avoids some of the disadvantages of the ^{133}Xe clearance technique. Xe-CT offers the advantage of improved spatial resolution and better information on blood flow in deeper regions of the brain. Because Xe-CT can be obtained as an additional study during conventional computed tomography (CT) scanning, this technique provides an opportunity for early assessment of CBF in the acute injury stage.[53] Concerns over transportation to a scanner and the safety of xenon inhalation in the critically ill patient limit the usefulness of this technique even when available.

Single-Photon Emission Computer Tomography

With SPECT, radiopharmaceuticals incorporating isotopes that emit single-photon radiation mostly are administered intravenously or by inhalation. Modern tomographs then rapidly survey the entire cranial vault contents, providing regional CBF information. In addition, this technology goes beyond the determination of CBF because receptor distribution and cerebral volume also can be determined through use of different agents. SPECT evidence of decreased CBF correlates with angiographic evidence of vasospasm after SAH.[63] It is still possible to have evidence of vasospasm or ischemia even without evidence of hypoperfusion by SPECT.[64]

INTRACRANIAL PRESSURE

The intracranial compartment has a fixed volume for a given individual that consists of the brain substance, cerebrospinal fluid (CSF), and blood. As the intracranial mass increases,

there is an accompanying displacement in CSF and intracranial blood, which provides a "buffering" effect on the intracranial pressure (ICP). Once the maximum volume shift is attained, further increases in intracranial volume elicit a marked rise in ICP during a phase of decompensation (Fig. 62-6).

Although the focus is often on the ICP, the CPP is equally, if not more, important. CPP is the mean arterial blood pressure minus the ICP. The work of some investigators suggests that maintaining CPP at or above 70 mm Hg by either reducing ICP or increasing the mean arterial blood pressure does not adversely affect outcome and may improve survival.[65–67] More recent work by Cruz and others,[68] however, failed to demonstrate any statistical relationship between CPP and CBF or cerebral metabolic rate of oxygen consumption ($CMRo_2$).

Besides allowing the determination of CPP, measurement of ICP may be useful in determining the patient's position on the ICP–intracranial volume curve where the patient may be close to decompensation yet display no change in clinical signs. Because there is a measurable risk associated with ICP monitoring, suitable criteria for instituting this invasive procedure have been proposed for traumatic head injury. In 1982, Narayan and colleagues[69] reviewed their experience in 207 severely head-injured patients. They reported a 53% to 63% incidence rate of ICP elevation (above 20 mm Hg) in patients with abnormal CT scans who were unable to obey commands or utter recognizable words after initial resuscitation and stabilization. This study included patients with low-density (i.e., diffuse or focal edema and swelling) and high-density (i.e., subdural, epidural, or intracerebral hematomas) lesions. Most notably, they reported a low risk (13%) for ICP elevations in patients with normal results from CT scans on admission. In this population, they identified several factors associated with an increased

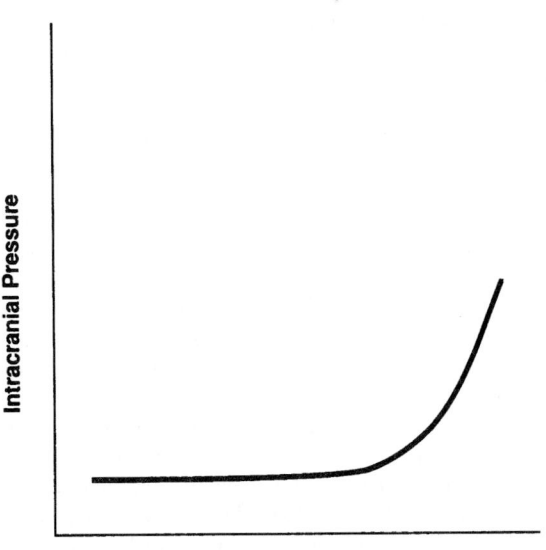

FIGURE 62-6. Diagrammatic representation of the intracranial pressure–volume relationship. A period of decompensation occurs with an expanding intracranial lesion, leading to a marked rise in intracranial pressure.

incidence of intracranial hypertension including age older than 40 years, systolic blood pressure of 90 mm Hg or less, and motor posturing. With two or more of these features, the risk of intracranial hypertension rose to 60%, leading the authors to recommend ICP monitoring in this subpopulation. Other researchers have generally supported these findings[70,71] with the caveat that repeat CT scanning be performed within 12 to 24 hours after the initial scan.[69]

Techniques allowing for the measurement of ICP have been available for several years.[72] They have been extensively used in the management of severe head injury, SAH, Reye's syndrome, hepatic encephalopathy, and other disorders producing elevations in ICP.[73–75] By far, the most extensive use of ICP monitoring is seen in the patient with severe closed head injury where elevations in ICP over 20 mm Hg have been found to correlate with increased morbidity and mortality.[76] In a recent survey of critical care management of head-injured patients, however, only 40% of surveyed institutions reported using ICP monitoring in more than 75% of comatose patients with severe head injury.[77] Even following the guidelines proposed by Narayan and colleagues listed above, this would represent underutilization of this monitoring modality. The authors proposed several issues behind the low utilization rate of ICP monitoring in this clinical setting. The labor-intensive nature of ICP monitoring, as well as the known risks of infection and hemorrhage, may discourage its use in some institutions, whereas the question of proven efficacy still exists in some individual's minds.

Despite the lack of prospective, controlled clinical trials assessing the benefit of invasive ICP monitoring, it is difficult to ignore the accumulating evidence that controlling ICP (less than 20 mm Hg) results in an improved outcome. In 1982, Saul and Ducker[78] published a report comparing two consecutive time periods at the same institution. The only significant variable between the two periods was the level of ICP required to institute more aggressive therapy. The investigators treated all patients with the same protocol with the exception of the target ICP used during each period. Between 1977 and 1978 (127 patients) there was no strict ICP management protocol, whereas between 1979 and 1980 (106 patients) there was a strict protocol instituted for ICP greater than 16 mm Hg for 10 minutes. The mortality rate in the earlier series was 45% compared with 28% (*p* <0.0005) in the series with a strict ICP management protocol. In contrast, a prospective study from Australia treated 100 consecutive patients presenting with a GCS of 8 or less within 48 hours after injury with various strategies but without ICP monitoring.[79] Their reported mortality rate of 34% compares favorably to that reported by other institutions[80] using invasive ICP monitoring to guide therapy during that period. The long transport distances involved in this study, however, provide a serious criticism because the patients most likely to survive transport were being transferred and entered into the study. Given all of the available information, it then becomes hard to design a clinical trial examining the value of ICP monitoring without meeting serious ethical questions.

Once the decision has been made to initiate ICP monitoring, the clinician must select an appropriate device. Several monitoring systems are available including the following:

1. Catheters (intraventricular or subdural)
2. Hollow screw or bolt (Richmond screw, Philly bolt, Leeds screw, Landy screw)
3. Fiberoptic transducer tip (Camino)

These devices can be placed into several sites (Fig. 62-7). The following sites are associated with the different devices:

1. Lateral ventricle: ventricular catheter, fiberoptic device
2. Intraparenchymal: fiberoptic device
3. Subdural or subarachnoid: Richmond bolt, catheter, fiberoptic device
4. Epidural: Gaeltech, Ladd, Philips
5. Anterior fontanelle (in infants): Gaeltech, Ladd, Philips

Numerous comparisons between different ICP monitoring systems are available. The intraventricular catheter remains the gold standard for accuracy in monitoring with the added benefit of allowing CSF drainage as needed to control ICP. We employ ventricular catheters in most cases, although the Camino fiberoptic device is sometimes employed in combination with a ventricular catheter to allow for continuous ICP monitoring. This allows for drainage of CSF in selected patients. Use of fiberoptic transmission from a miniature pressure transducer in a flexible catheter allows the Camino system to move with the patient without requiring a rezero after every move. The Camino system has several other advantages over other ICP monitors (Table 62-2). It has proven to be an acceptable alternative to ventriculostomy placement while maintaining a lower rate of infection and, an otherwise, similar complication profile.[81] A recent survey shows that intraparenchymal monitoring is almost as popular as ventriculostomy for monitoring the patient with severe head injury.[77]

The most frequent significant complications of ICP monitoring are infection and hemorrhage. The overall infection rate for ventricular catheter placement is 5% to 6% with the incidence increasing with time.[82–84] Hematoma formation or intraventricular hemorrhages occur in less than 2% of insertions and are often asymptomatic.[69,82] Other complications including misplacement and neurologic deficits bring

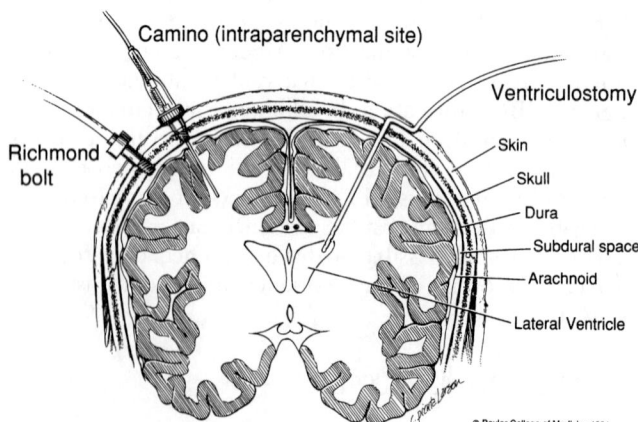

FIGURE 62-7. Intracranial pressure monitors.

TABLE 62-2. Intracranial Pressure Monitors

ICP MONITOR	ADVANTAGES	DISADVANTAGES
Ventricular catheter	Gold standard for accuracy Allows drainage of CSF for ICP control, CSF sampling, monitoring infection	Sometimes difficult to cannulate ventricle Requires fluid-filled column, which can get blocked by air, bubbles, debris Needs transducer repositioning with change in head position
Subarachnoid bolt	Does not enter brain tissue Lower infection rate No need to cannulate ventricle	Blocking of port by swollen brain may artificially lower readings Artifact from tube movement Needs transducer repositioning with change in head position
Fiberoptic device	Can be placed subdurally, intraparechymally, or intraventricularly Minimal artifact and drift High resolution of waveform No need to reposition transducer with change in head position	Inability to check calibration after inserted unless a ventriculostomy is used simultaneously Fiber breakage

CSF, cerebrospinal fluid; ICP, intracranial pressure.

the total complication rate up to 10%, of which most are minor.[69]

TRANSCRANIAL DOPPLER

A recent addition to the tools available for neurologic monitoring is transcranial Doppler (TCD) assessment of CBF velocity in certain intracranial arteries. Using the same principles as Doppler ultrasound, TCD employs sound waves that are transmitted through the skull. When these waves encounter moving objects such as red blood cells, they reflect back at varying frequencies dependent on the velocity of the moving object. Higher frequencies (4 to 10 MHz) facilitate the determination of structure, but this results in a lower depth of penetration. In 1982, Aslid and colleagues[85] introduced TCD using lower frequencies of around 2 MHz that permitted the evaluation of flow velocities at sites where the cranium is usually thin and devoid of cancellous bone. Depth control is accomplished by varying the time interval and allows sampling from 15 to 155 mm from the transducer.

The TCD probe is capable of both transmitting the sound waves and receiving the reflected echoes in pulses. Measurements can be made intermittently or by use of a stationary probe holder, may be continuous. Because the recorded velocity is equal to the actual velocity only when the probe is in line with the flow (i.e., the angle of insonation is 0 or 180 degrees relative to the examined vessel, the recorded value usually is less than the actual value. Thus, the highest velocity obtained most likely approaches the true velocity. The actual vessels that can be examined are limited to those in proximity to a "window." The temporal window, located just superior to the zygomatic arch, allows evaluation of the ipsilateral middle cerebral artery (MCA), terminal internal carotid artery, anterior cerebral artery, and the posterior cerebral artery (Fig. 62-8). The transorbital window, which

is accessed through the closed eyelid, provides information on the ophthalmic artery and the carotid siphon. Finally, the vertebral and basilar arteries can be insonated, with some difficulty, through the suboccipital window at the skull base. Successful examinations through the temporal window are somewhere between 5% and 10%.[86,87]

Data obtained from a TCD study typically include the systolic velocity (V_S), the mean velocity (V_{mean}), the diastolic velocity (V_D), and the pulsatility index (PI) where

$$PI = \frac{V_S - V_D}{V_{mean}}$$

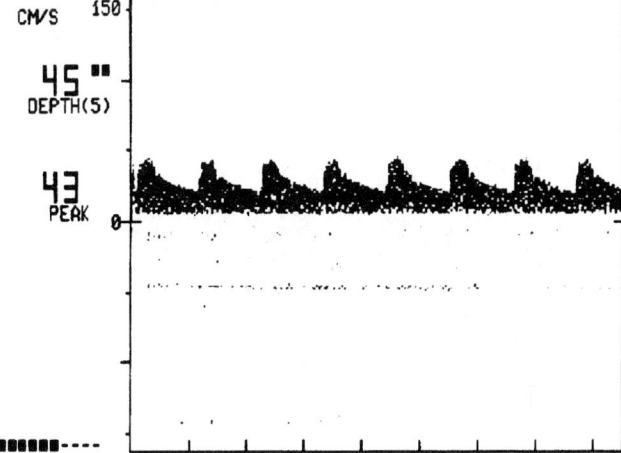

NL:15 DR:20 2.00 MHZ PW POWER: 75% VOL: 32% FLOW
CM/S 150
45
DEPTH(5)
43
PEAK 0

FIGURE 62-8. Transcranial Doppler pattern obtained during examination of the middle cerebral artery in a 46-year-old woman under general anesthesia before thoracotomy.

Pulsatility describes the degree of variability in the maximal velocity that occurs during a cardiac cycle and depends on the blood inflow and the peripheral or "downstream" resistance. The PI is one method of quantifying specific aspects of the overall waveform and has been used to follow trends of cerebrovascular resistance.

TCD monitoring is extensively used for the detection and monitoring of vasospasm after SAH. Numerous investigators report correlation between increased blood velocities in the basilar cerebral arteries, most notably the MCA, and angiographic evidence of vasospasm.[87–89] Reported normal flow velocities vary widely between 50 and 80 cm/second with an extreme of 120 cm/second.[85,86] Flow velocities between 80 and 120 cm/second are believed to be subcritical whereas velocities greater than 140 cm/second predict evidence of significant narrowing on the angiogram. Severe vasospasm occurs most commonly with velocities more than 200 cm/second. Lennihan and coworkers[87] report a sensitivity rate of 86% and specificity rate of 98% for the presence of vasospasm in the MCA distribution using these TCD criteria compared with angiography. However, the utility of TCD was markedly diminished in the anterior cerebral artery circulation, particularly after rupture of an anterior communicating aneurysm, with a sensitivity rate of only 13%.

Unfortunately, the presence of vasospasm, as documented by elevated blood velocities, does not necessarily correlate with the presence of a neurologic deficit.[90] The presence of flow velocities more than 200 cm/second was not associated with delayed ischemic deficits in 8 of 66 patients studied by Laumer and others,[86] whereas 16 of 24 patients developed deficits with normal TCD values. To provide more accurate predictive value, several investigators examined the rate of increase in TCD velocity. Velocity increases equal to or greater than 50 cm/second in a 24-hour period seemed to improve the prognostic value of the studies.[90] Nevertheless, the predictive value was still poor. Despite the unclear association between TCD monitoring and outcome in the patient with a recent SAH, it is being used clinically to noninvasively diagnose vasospasm[91] and to guide therapy.[92] It may also be used to document the presence of cerebral emboli (Fig. 62-9).

TCD also has been used to monitor patients with severe head injury. As ICP increases and the CPP decreases, characteristic changes occur in the TCD profile (Fig. 62-10). During moderate increases in ICP, the blood velocity waveform typically shows an increase in the PI and V_S with a decrease in the V_D. Severe increases in ICP lead toward a decrease in all velocities. The PI correlates best with CPP and, when arterial pressure is relatively stable, may provide some information concerning the ICP.[93,94] Despite this correlation, there is still insufficient evidence at this time to recommend the replacement of more invasive measures of ICP with TCD monitoring in the setting of severe head injury. Multimodality monitoring using jugular venous bulb saturation monitoring combined with TCD may aid in distinguishing patients with global hyperemia from those with decreased global CBF.[94] The use of TCD may be useful as a noninvasive method for documenting deterioration of CPP and could be included in protocols for brain death.[95]

LASER DOPPLER FLOWMETRY

One final method of monitoring regional CBF deserves mention because of its potential for providing continuous bedside measurement of this important variable. Laser Doppler flowmetry (LDF) provides a continuous measure of relative microcirculatory flow. This is accomplished by transmission of coherent laser light through a transmitting fiberoptic bundle that is scattered by biological tissue. Moving red blood cells produce a Doppler shift in the transmitted light while surrounding static tissue does not alter the reflected component. An afferent fiberoptic bundle collects these reflected signals and delivers them to a photodetector. Final analysis of these signals requires various algorithms described in detail elsewhere.[96]

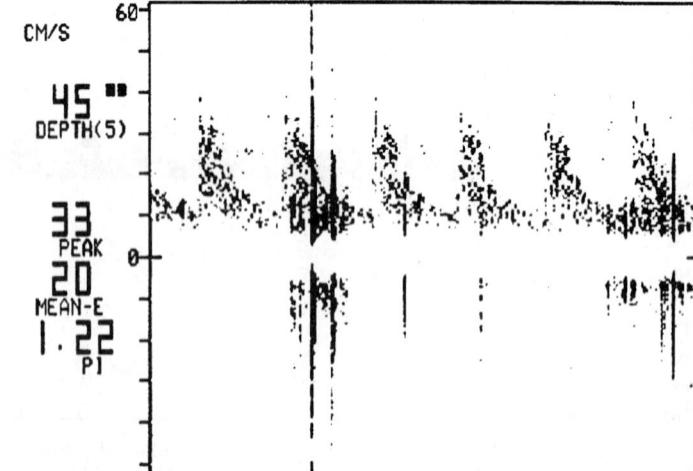

FIGURE 62-9. Characteristic pattern of cerebral emboli noticed during aortic valve replacement in a 68-year-old man. The high-intensity spiking activity is indicative of air emboli.

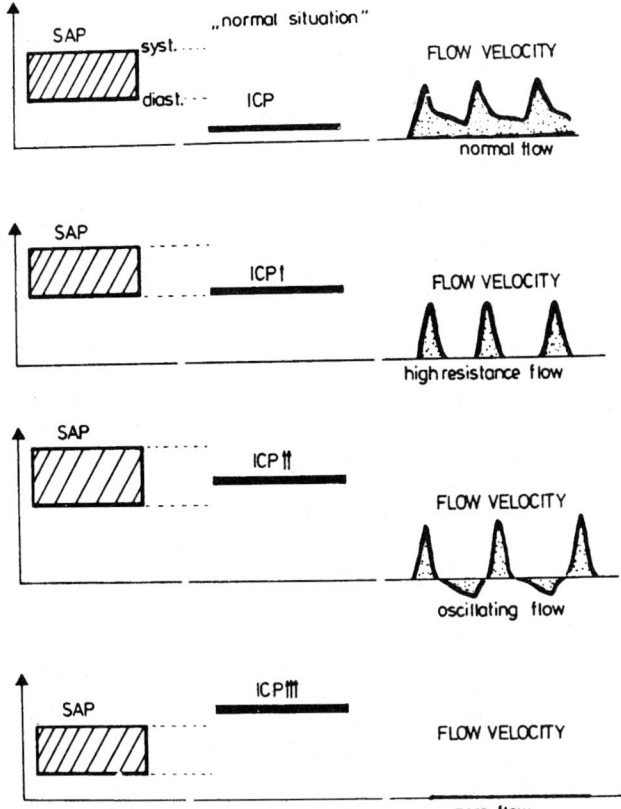

FIGURE 62-10. Relationship between systemic arterial blood pressure (SAP), intracranial pressure (ICP), and flow velocity as measured in the middle cerebral artery by transcranial Doppler ultrasound. Upward deflections in the spectra indicate blood flow toward the Doppler probe, and downward deflections appear with flow directions away from the probe. (From Hassler W: Transcranial Doppler ultrasonography in raised intracranial pressure and intracranial circulatory arrest. *J Neurosurg* 1990;68:745.)

The values obtained from this technique are not qualitative and provide information only on relative changes in CBF. In addition, the area being sampled is extremely limited and may encompass as little as 1 mm^3 of tissue.[97] The output signal most frequently used to quantitate the flow reflects the relative nature of these measurements, flux. Flux describes the number of red cells times their average velocity.

Preliminary reports appearing in the literature describe initial observations and problems with this monitoring modality.[97–99] Meyerson and others[99] report the use of LDF in monitoring regional cortical CBF in four comatose patients. They observed an inverse relationship between ICP and flux in the early stages, which they believed reflected a disruption in autoregulation. This response resolved during the recovery phase and flux changes in the conscious patient were synchronous with the arterial pulse. In contrast to these findings, Steinmeier and colleagues[97] reported several patterns of relationship between flux and other measured parameters affecting CPP. They noted both spatial and temporal heterogeneity of the functional microvascular response. These observations, along with difficulty obtaining consis-

tent LDF signals, were believed to complicate a simple and straightforward interpretation of the measured values. Further observations and refinement of probes and insertion techniques will better define the utility of this monitoring technique.

CEREBRAL METABOLISM ■

As stated earlier in this chapter, knowledge of CBF or CPP does not always allow the clinician to conclude that CMRo$_2$ is adequate. Monitoring modalities that provide an assessment of either regional or global cerebral oxygen metabolism can be triggers to reassess changes in CBF or perfusion. CBF and the cerebral arteriovenous oxygen content difference are related according to the following equation:

$$CMRo_2 = CBF \times (Cao_2 - Cjo_2)$$

where Cao$_2$ is the arterial oxygen content and Cjo$_2$ is the jugular venous content. Rearranged, the equation becomes

$$Cjo_2 = \frac{Cao_2 - CMRo_2}{CBF}$$

Making the assumption that hemoglobin levels are stable, jugular venous saturation (Sjo$_2$) then represents a potential monitor of the cerebral circulation because Cjo$_2$ is a function of CBF, Cao$_2$, and CBF. The ability to cannulate the jugular bulb in a retrograde fashion in combination with the capability to continuously monitor Sjo$_2$ with an oximetry catheter provides a method of assessing global cerebral oxygen metabolism. Near-infrared spectroscopy also has been applied using an external approach to examine focal cerebral oxygenation.[100]

Many of the conditions encountered in the neurologic or neurosurgical ICUs involve focal lesions where global metabolic measurements have significant limitations. Newer techniques, such positron emission tomography, may be able to provide more regional estimates of not only oxygen but glucose metabolism.[101] Currently, these studies are not only expensive but require transport to a usually remote location, making it difficult to obtain repeated measurements.

JUGULAR VENOUS SATURATION

Cannulation of the jugular bulb for intermittent (standard intravascular catheters) or continuous (fiberoptic oximetry catheters) monitoring of jugular venous is a safe and technically simple procedure.[102] Strict positioning of the catheter requires frequent repositioning of the head, neck, and shoulders to minimize artifactual changes. Because the measured saturation reflects a global average from a variety of brain regions, marked regional hypoperfusion may not be represented by a change in this parameter.

Several authors have reported extensively on their experience with the use of continuous cerebral oxygenation monitoring. To date, there have been no controlled trials comparing the utility of these measurements with those from more conventional monitoring systems in guiding therapy or altering outcome. Gopinath and colleagues[56] examined the association of jugular venous desaturation with worsened neurologic outcome. Although unable to establish a cause and effect relationship, the incidence of desaturation (SjO_2 less than 50%) was significantly associated with a poor outcome. Profound neurologic deterioration occurs with desaturation to a value of 30% or less.[103]

Combined arterial and jugular venous saturation monitoring has been evaluated during the use of mannitol[104] and hyperventilation[105] in acute brain injury. Cruz and associates[104] noted improvements in cerebral oxygenation and ICP after the administration of mannitol for acute elevations in ICP over 20 mm Hg associated with a decrease in SjO_2. This occurred in some cases even when CPP was in a normal range. In a follow-up study, Cruz[105] was able to demonstrate an increase in $CMRo_2$ in patients with a decreased cerebral oxygen extraction ("luxury perfusion") who were hyperventilated in response to ICP elevations. Thus, jugular venous saturation may be useful as a guide for therapeutic interventions that alter cerebral oxygenation, although the ability of these manipulations to alter outcome is not as clear.

NEAR-INFRARED SPECTROSCOPY

Near-infrared spectroscopy is a relatively new and potentially valuable technique for noninvasive monitoring of cerebral tissue oxygenation. First described in 1977 by Jobsis,[106] this technology has been used in the assessment of neonates for several years,[107,108] and encouraging reports have appeared concerning its use in adult patients.[109,110] Similar to pulse oximetry, near-infrared spectroscopy uses differential light absorbance of oxyhemoglobin and deoxyhemoglobin to detect changes in cerebral oxygenation. Reflectance spectroscopy, such as that used in mixed venous saturation pulmonary artery catheters, is more complex than that based on absorption. The intensity of reflected light depends both on the concentration of the solute and on the depth the light penetrates (optical path length) into the solution or tissues. Near-infrared wavelengths are best suited for this application because they are transmitted easily through bone and muscle and demonstrate characteristic absorption bands for the above forms of hemoglobin as well as cytochrome oxidase in cerebral tissue. Possible information to be gained from this technology includes not only cerebral oxygen saturation, but estimates of total cerebral blood volume. These estimates are based on changes in total oxyhemoglobin over time after gradual change of inspired oxygen and cerebral utilization of delivered oxygen based on the cytochrome redox state.[111]

Technical limitations continue to provide significant roadblocks to full implementaion of this technology. Because scattering and absorption of the light occurs, calculation of the precise optical path length is problematic. In addition, the contribution of extracranial changes in blood flow and oxygenation may be sufficient to affect its reliability in clinical practice.[112] Ongoing improvements, however, seek to address these issues and may one day provide continuous bedside measurements.

NEUROLOGIC IMAGING

Although not considered a "monitoring" modality, emergency imaging studies are routinely obtained as part of the initial evaluation process in patients with acute head injury to determine whether a surgically correctable lesion exists. CT is currently the procedure of choice because it is faster and more readily available. It also more easily accommodates emergency equipment than magnetic resonance imaging (MRI). Both CT and MRI also play a role in the evaluation of nontraumatic CNS disturbances such as severe headaches, seizures, CNS tumors, focal neurologic deficits, and alteration in mental status. Use of these imaging studies not only guides therapeutic interventions, but may aid in establishing prognosis.

The CT scan is a necessity in evaluating trauma. Not only does it identify the presence of intracranial hemorrhage, but it allows for the evaluation of fractures and shifts of intracranial contents, and it may guide prognosis. After stabilization, it is vital to obtain a CT scan of the head in all comatose patients and in patients with pupillary inequality, persistent neurologic deficit, depressed skull fracture, open cranial wound, or a deteriorating level of consciousness.[113] In the setting of acute hemorrhage, CT scanning has more sensitivity than MRI for detecting blood during the acute phase, whereas MRI has been shown to be more sensitive in detecting nonhemorrhagic contusions.[114] MRI can be useful in detecting hemorrhage in many cases, however, as demonstrated by Goromi and colleagues.[115] After minor head injury, CT scanning can help determine whether ICU admission and observation would be useful. In one study examining 2766 patients with isolated minor head injury, not a single patient with a normal result on CT scan and a normal neurologic examination (933 patients) or a normal CT scan result (1170 patients) required an operative procedure.[116] Of the 2112 patients with a normal neurologic examination, 59 required craniotomy for lesions found on CT.

Effacement of the basal cisterns, ventricular asymmetry, or the degree of midline shift are a good indication of the likelihood of sustained elevations of ICP after severe head injury.[117,118] Abnormal cisterns are associated with a threefold risk of abnormal ICP compared with patients with normal cisterns. Extracerebral masses are more ominous predictors of a poor outcome than intracerebral masses. The demonstration of subarachnoid blood increases the risk of dying by twofold compared with patients without subarachnoid blood.[119]

CONCLUSION

Frequent clinical and physiologic assessment of the critically ill patient with intracranial disease remains the mainstay of neurologic monitoring in the ICU. The role of electrophysiologic monitoring is still being refined and assessed. ICP monitoring seems to have established a more fixed role despite the lack of definitive evidence linking monitoring to outcome. Recently, the use of TCD monitoring is undergoing the same scrutiny for the evaluation of vasospasm after SAH. The full cost–benefit ratio of such monitoring modalities is yet to be proven and will continue to be questioned by some experts.

REFERENCES ■

1. Rocca B, Martin C, Viviand X, et al: Comparison of four severity scores in patients with head trauma. *J Trauma* 1989;29:299
2. Hakkinen VK, Kaukinen S, Heikkila H: The correlation of EEG compressed spectral array to Glasgow Coma Scale in traumatic coma patients. *Int J Clin Monit Comput* 1988;5:97
3. Newlon PG, Greenberg RP: Evoked potentials in severe head injury. *J Trauma* 1984;24:61
4. Jordan KG: Continuous EEG and evoked potential monitoring in the neuroscience intensive care unit. *J Clin Neurophysiol* 1993;10:445
5. Narayan RK, Greenberg RP, Miller JD: Improved confidence of outcome predition in severe head injury: a comparative analysis of the clinical examination, multimodality evoked potentials, CT scanning and intracranial pressure. *J Neurosurg* 1981;54:751
6. Teasdale G, Jennett B: Assessment of coma and impaired consciousness. *Lancet* 1974;ii:81
7. Lindsay KW, Teasdale GM, Knill-Jones RP: Observer variability in assessing the clinical features of subarachnoid hemorrhage. *J Neurosurg* 1983;58:57
8. Krieger D, Adams HP, Schwarz S, et al: Prognostic and clinical relevance of pupillary responses, intracranial pressure monitoring, and brainstem auditory evoked potentials in comatose patients with acute supratentorial mass lesions. *Crit Care Med* 1993;21:1944
9. Barnett GH, Ropper AH, Romeo J: Intracranial pressure and outcome in adult encephalitis. *J Neurosurg* 1988;68:585
10. Duncan CC, Ment LR, Shaywitz BA: Evaluation of level of consciousness by the Glasgow coma scale in children with Reye's syndrome. *Neurosurgery* 1983;13:650
11. Lee H, Hawker FH, Selby W, et al: Intensive care treatment of patients with bleeding esophageal varices: results, predictors of mortality, and predictors of the adult respiratory distress syndrome. *Crit Care Med* 1992;20:1555
12. Rowley G, Fielding K: Reliability and accuracy of the Glasgow Coma Scale with experienced and inexperienced users. *Lancet* 1991;337:535
13. Gennarelli TA, Champion HR, Copes WS, et al: Comparison of mortality, morbidity, and severity of 59,713 head injured patients with 114,447 patients with extracranial injuries. *J Trauma* 1994;37:962
14. Salcman M, Schepp RS, Ducker TB: Calculated recovery rates in severe head trauma. *Neurosurgery* 1981;8:301
15. Jane JA, Rimel RW: Prognosis in head injury. *Clin Neurosurg* 1982;29:346
16. Marshall LF, Becker DP, Bowers SA, et al: The National Traumatic Coma Data Bank. I. Design, purpose, goals, and results. *J Neurosurg* 1983;59:276
17. Edgren E, Hedstrand U, Kelsey S, et al: Assessment of neurological prognosis in comatose survivors of cardiac arrest: BRCT I Study Group. *Lancet* 1994;343:1055
18. Niskanen M, Kari A, Nikki P, et al: Acute Physiology and Chronic Health Evaluation (APACHE II) and Glasgow Coma Scores as predictors of outcome from intensive care after cardiac arrest. *Crit Care Med* 1991;19:1465
19. Bedos JP, Chastang C, Lucet JC, et al: Early predictors of outcome for HIV patients with neurological failure. *JAMA* 1995;273:35
20. Mayer T, Walker ML: Emergency intracranial pressure monitoring in pediatrics: management of the acute coma of brain insult. *Clin Pediatr* 1982;21:391
21. Andriola MR: The role of the electroencephalogram in neurologic practice. *Semin Neurol* 1990;10:156
22. Hockaday JM, Potts F, Epstein E, et al: Electroencephalographic changes in acute cerebral anoxia from cardiac or respiratory arrest. *Electroencephalogr Clin Neurophysiol* 1965;18:575
23. Bird TD, Plum F: Recovery from barbiturate overdose coma with a prolonged isoelectric electroencephalogram. *Neurology* 1968;18:456
24. Kiloh LG, McComas AJ, Osselton JW, Upton ARM: Infective and non-infective encephalopathies. In: Kiloh LG (Ed). *Clinical Electroencephalography*. Boston, Butterworth, 1981:165
25. Wijdicks EF, Parisi JE, Sharbrough FW: Prognostic value of myoclonus status in comatose survivors of cardiac arrest. *Ann Neurol* 1994;35:239
26. Westmoreland BF, Klass DW, Sharbrough FW, et al: Alphacoma: electroencephalographic, clinical, pathologic, and etiologic correlations. *Arch Neurol* 1975;32:713
27. Obeso JA, Iragui MI, Marti-Masso JF, et al: Neurophysiological assessment of alpha pattern coma. *J Neurol Neurosurg Psychiatry* 1980;43:63
28. Bickford RG, Butt HR: Hepatic coma: the electroencephalographic pattern. *J Clin Invest* 1955;34:790
29. Rampil IJ: What every neuroanesthesiologist should know about electroencephalograms and computerized monitors. *Anesth Clin North Am* 1992;10:683
30. Cohen PJ, Alexander SC, Smith TC, et al: Effects of hypoxia and normocarbia on cerebral blood flow and metabolism in conscious man. *J Appl Physiol* 1967;23:183
31. Winer JW, Rosenwasser RH, Jimenez F: Electroencephalographic activity and serum and cerebrospinal fluid pentobarbital levels in determining the therapeutic end point during barbiturate coma. *Neurosurgery* 1991;29:739
32. Cooley JW, Tukey JW: An algorithm for the machine calculation of complex Fourier series. *Math Comput* 1965;19:297
33. Karnaze DS, Marshall LF, Bickford RG: EEG monitoring of clinical coma: the compressed spectral array. *Neurology* 1982;32:289
34. Cant BR, Shaw NA: Monitoring by compressed spectral array in prolonged coma. *Neurology* 1984;34:35
35. Hakkinen VK, Kaukinen S, Heikkila H: The correlation of EEG compressed spectral array to Glasgow Coma Scale in traumatic coma patients. *Int J Clin Monit Comput* 1988;5:97
36. Young WL, Ornstein E: Compressed spectral array EEG monitoring during cardiac arrest and resuscitation. *Anesthesiology* 1985;62:535
37. Chiappa KH: Pattern shift visual, brainstem auditory, and short-latency somatosensory evoked potentials in multiple sclerosis. *Neurology* 1980;30:110
38. Feinsod M, Auerbach E: Electrophysiological examinations of the visual system in the acute phase after head injury. *Eur Neurol* 1973;9:56
39. Spehlmann R: The normal BAEP. In: Spehlmann R (ed). *Evoked Potential Primer: Visual, Auditory, and Somatosensory Evoked Potentials in Clinical Diagnosis*. Boston, Butterworth, 1985:204

40. Starr A: Auditory brain-stem responses in brain death. *Brain* 1976;99:543

41. Goldie WD, Chiappa KH, Young RR, et al: Brainstem auditory and short-latency somatosensory evoked responses in brain death. *Neurology* 1981;31:248

42. Rumpl E, Prugger M, Gerstenbrand F, et al: Central somatosensory conduction time and short latency somatosensory evoked potentials in post-traumatic coma. *Electroencephalogr Clin Neurophysiol* 1983;56:583

43. Moulton RJ, Shedden PM, Tucker WS, et al: Somatosensory evoked potential monitoring following severe closed head injury. *Clin Invest Med* 1994;17:187

44. Cusumano S, Paolin A, Di Paola F, et al: Assessing brain function in post-traumatic coma by means of bit-mapped SEPs, BAEPs, CT, SPET and clinical scores: prognostic implications. *Electroencephalogr Clin Neurophysiol* 1992;84:499

45. Narayan RK, Greenberg RP, Miller JD, et al: Improved confidence of outcome prediction in severe head injury: a comparative analysis of the clinical examination, multimodality evoked potentials, CT scanning, and intracranial pressure. *J Neurosurg* 1981;54:751

46. Spehlmann R: Abnormal SEP's to arm stimulation. In: *Evoked Potential Primer: Visual, Auditory, and Somatosensory Evoked Potentials in Clinical Diagnosis.* Boston, Butterworth, 1985:300

47. Goff WR, Shaywitz BA, Goff GD, et al: Somatic evoked potential evaluation of cerebral status in Reye syndrome. *Electroencephalogr Clin Neurophysiol* 1983;55:388

48. Hrbek A, Karlberg P, Kjellmer I, et al: Clinical application of evoked EEG responses in newborn infants. II. Idiopathic respiratory distress syndrome. *Dev Med Child Neurol* 1978;20:619

49. Levy WJ Jr: Clinical experience with motor and cerebellar evoked potential monitoring. *Neurosurgery* 1987;20:169

50. Martin NA, Doberstein C, Zane C, et al: Posttraumatic cerebral arterial spasm: transcranial Doppler ultrasound, cerebral blood flow, and angiographic findings. *J Neurosurg* 1992;77:575

51. Cruz J, Raps EC, Hoffstad OJ, et al: Cerebral oxygenation monitoring. *Crit Care Med* 1993;21:1242

52. Miller JD, Piper IR, Jones PA: Integrated multimodality monitoring in the neurosurgical intensive care unit. *Neurosurg Clin North Am* 1994;5:661

53. Bouma GJ, Muizelaar JP, Stringer WA, et al: Ultra-early evaluation of regional cerebral blood flow in severely head-injured patients using xenon-enhanced computerized tomography. *J Neurosurg* 1992;77:360

54. Robertson CS, Contant CF, Gokaslan ZL, et al: Cerebral blood flow, arteriovenous oxygen difference, and outcome in head injured patients. *J Neurol Neurosurg Psychiatry* 1992;55:594

55. Oder W, Goldenberg G, Podreka I, et al: HM-PAO-SPECT in persistent vegetative state after head injury: prognostic indicator of the likelihood of recovery? *Inten Care Med* 1991;17:149

56. Gopinath SP, Robertson CS, Contant CF, et al: Jugular venous desaturation and outcome after head injury. *J Neurol Neurosurg Psychiatry* 1994;57:717

57. Bouma GJ, Muizelaar JP, Choi SC, et al: Cerebral circulation and metabolism after severe traumatic brain injury: the elusive role of ischemia. *J Neurosurg* 1991;75:685

58. Overgaard J, Tweed WA: Cerebral circulation after head injury. IV. Functional anatomy and boundary-zone flow deprivation in the first week of traumatic coma. *J Neurosurg* 1983;59:439

59. Kety SS, Schmidt CF: The determination of cerebral blood flow in man by the use of nitrous oxide in low concentrations. *Am J Physiol* 1945;143:53

60. Kety SS: The theory and application of the exchange of inert gas at the lungs and tissues. *Pharmacol Rev* 1951;3:1

61. Bell BA: Early study of cerebral circulation and measurement of cerebral blood flow. In: Wood JH (ed). *Cerebral Blood Flow: Physiologic and Clinical Aspects.* New York, McGraw-Hill, 1987:3

62. Austin G, Laffin D, Rouhe S: Intravenous isotope injection method of cerebrospinal fluid measurement: accuracy and reproducibility. In: Langfitt TW, McHenry LCJ, Reivich M (eds). *Cerebral Circulation and Metabolism.* New York, Springer-Verlag, 1975:391

63. Soucy JP, McNamara D, Mohr G: Evaluation of vasospasm secondary to subarachnoid hemorrhage with technetium ^{99m}-hexamethyl-propyleneamine oxime (HMPAO) tomoscintigraphy. *J Nucl Med* 1990;31:972

64. Tranquart F, Ades PE, Groussin P, et al: Postoperative assessment of cerebral blood flow in subarachnoid haemorrhage by means of ^{99m}Tc-HMPAO tomography. *Eur J Nuc Med* 1993;20:53

65. Rosner MJ, Daughton S: Cerebral perfusion pressure management in head injury. *J Trauma* 1990;30:933

66. Rosner MJ, Coley I: Cerebral perfusion pressure: a hemodynamic mechanism of mannitol and the postmannitol hemogram. *Neurosurgery* 1987;21:147

67. Changaris DG, McGraw CP, Richardson JD, et al: Correlation of cerebral perfusion pressure and Glasgow Coma Scale to outcome. *J Trauma* 1987;27:1007

68. Cruz J, Jaggi JL, Hoffstad OJ: Cerebral blood flow, vascular resistance, and oxygen metabolism in acute brain trauma: redefining the role of cerebral perfusion pressure? *Crit Care Med* 1995;23:1412

69. Narayan RK, Kishore PR, Becker DP, et al: Intracranial pressure: to monitor or not to monitor? A review of our experience with severe head injury. *J Neurosurg* 1982;56:650

70. Lobato RD, Sarabia R, Rivas JJ, et al: Normal computerized tomography scans in severe head injury: prognostic and clinical management implications. *J Neurosurg* 1986;65:784

71. Klauber MR, Toutant SM, Marshall LF: A model for predicting delayed intracranial hypertension following severe head injury. *J Neurosurg* 1984;61:695

72. Lundberg N: Continuous recording and control of ventricular fluid pressure in neurosurgical practice. *Acta Psychiatr Neurol Scand* 1960;36(Suppl 149):1

73. Kanter MJ, Narayan RK: Management of head injury. Intracranial pressure monitoring. *Neurosurg Clin North Am* 1991;2:257

74. Chi CS, Law KL, Wong TT, et al: Continuous monitoring of intracranial pressure in Reye's syndrome: 5 years' experience. *Acta Paediatr Jpn* 1990;32:426

75. Lidofsky SD, Bass NM, Prager MC, et al: Intracranial pressure monitoring and liver transplantation for fulminant hepatic failure. *Hepatology* 1992;16:1

76. Marmarou A, Anderson RL, Ward JD, et al: Impact of ICP instablilty and hypotension on outcome in patients with severe head trauma. *J Neurosurg* 1991;75(Suppl):S59.

77. Ghajar J, Hariri RJ, Narayan RK, et al: Survey of critical care management of comatose, head-injured patients in the United States. *Crit Care Med* 1995;23:560

78. Saul TG, Ducker TB: Effect of intracranial pressure monitoring and aggressive treatment on mortality in severe head injury. *J Neurosurg* 1982;56:498

79. Stuart GG, Merry GS, Smith JA, et al: Severe head injury managed without intracranial pressure monitoring. *J Neurosurg* 1983;59:601

80. Miller JD, Butterworth JF, Gudeman SK, et al: Further experience in the management of severe head injury. *J Neurosurg* 1981;54:289

81. Yablon JS, Lantner HJ, McCormack TM, et al P: Clinical experience with a fiberoptic intracranial pressure monitor. *J Clin Monit* 1993;9:171

82. Paramore CG, Turner DA: Relative risks of ventriculostomy infection and morbidity. *Acta Neurochir (Wein)* 1994;127:79

83. Schultz M, Moore K, Foote AW: Bacterial ventriculitis and duration of ventriculostomy catheter insertion. *J Neurosci Nurs* 1993;25:158

84. Kanter RK, Weiner LB, Patti AM, et al: Infectious complications and duration of intracranial pressure monitoring. *Crit Care Med* 1985;13:837

85. Aaslid R, Markwalder TM, Nornes H: Noninvasive transcranial Doppler ultrasound recording of flow velocity in basal cerebral arteries. *J Neurosurg* 1982;57:769

86. Laumer R, Steinmeier R, Gonner F, et al: Cerebral hemodynamics in subarachnoid hemorrhage evaluated by transcranial Doppler sonography. I. Reliability of flow velocities in clinical management. *Neurosurgery* 1993;33:1

87. Lennihan L, Petty GW, Fink ME, et al: Transcranial Doppler detection of anterior cerebral artery vasospasm. *J Neurol Neurosurg Psychiatry* 1993;56:906

88. Hutchison K, Weir B: Transcranial Doppler studies in aneurysm patients. *Can J Neurol Sci* 1989;16:411

89. Aaslid R, Huber P, Nornes H: Evaluation of cerebrovascular spasm with transcranial Doppler ultrasound. *J Neurosurg* 1984;60:37

90. Grosset DG, Straiton J, McDonald I, et al: Use of transcranial Doppler sonography to predict development of a delayed ischemic deficit after subarachnoid hemorrhage. *J Neurosurg* 1993;78:183

91. Seiler R, Grolimund P, Huber P: Transcranial Doppler sonography: an alternative to angiography in the evaluation of vasospasm after subarachnoid hemorrhage. *Acta Radiol Suppl (Stockh)* 1986;369:99

92. Nowak G, Schwachenwald R, Arnold H: Early management in poor grade aneurysm patients. *Acta Neurochir (Wein)* 1994;126:33

93. Homburg AM, Jakobsen M, Enevoldsen E: Transcranial Doppler recordings in raised intracranial pressure. *Acta Neurol Scand* 1993;87:488

94. Chan KH, Miller JD, Dearden NM, et al: The effect of changes in cerebral perfusion pressure upon middle cerebral artery blood flow velocity and jugular bulb venous oxygen saturation after severe brain injury. *J Neurosurg* 1992;77:55

95. Feri M, Ralli L, Felici M, et al: Transcranial Doppler and brain death diagnosis. *Crit Care Med* 1994;22:1120

96. Nilsson GE: Signal processors for laser Doppler tissue flowmeters. *Med Biol Eng Comput* 1987;22:343

97. Steinmeier R, Bondar I, Bauhuf C: Assessment of cerebral haemodynamics in comatose patients by laser Doppler flowmetry: preliminary observations. *Acta Neurochir Suppl (Wein)* 1993;59:69

98. Kirkpatrick PJ, Smielewski P, Czosnyka M, et al: Continuous monitoring of cortical perfusion by laser Doppler flowmetry in ventilated patients with head injury *J Neurol Neurosurg Psychiatry* 1994;57:1382

99. Meyerson BA, Gunasekera L, Linderoth B, et al: Bedside monitoring of regional cortical blood flow in comatose patients using laser Doppler flowmetry. *Neurosurgery* 1991;29:750

100. McCormick P, Stewart M, Goetting M, et al: Noninvasive cerebral optical spectroscopy for monitoring cerebral oxygen delivery and hemodynamics. *Crit Care Med* 1991;19:89

101. Fulham MJ: Clinical applications of PET in neurology. In: Hubner KF, Collman J, Buonocore E, et al (eds). *Clinical Positron Emission Tomography.* St Louis, Mosby–Year Book, 1992:42

102. Sheinberg M, Kanter JM, Robertson CS, et al: Continuous monitoring of jugular venous oxygen saturation in head-injured patients. *J Neurosurg* 1992;76:212

103. Cruz J: Continuous versus serial global cerebral hemometabolic monitoring: applications in acute brain trauma. *Acta Neurochir Suppl (Wein)* 1988;42:35

104. Cruz J, Miner ME, Allen SJ, et al: Continuous monitoring of cerebral oxygenation in acute brain injury: injection of mannitol during hyperventilation. *J Neurosurg* 1990;73:725

105. Cruz J: Combined continuous monitoring of systemic and cerebral oxygenation in acute brain injury: preliminary observations. *Crit Care Med* 1993;21:1225

106. Jobsis FF: Non-invasive, infrared monitoring of cerebral and myocardial oxygen sufficiency and circulatory parameters. *Science* 1977;198:1264

107. Rolfe P, Wickramasinghe YA, Thorniley M: The potential of near infra-red spectroscopy for detection of fetal cerebral hypoxia. *Eur J Obstet Gynecol Reprod Biol* 1991;42(Suppl):S24

108. Brazy JE: Cerebral oxygen monitoring with near infrared spectroscopy: clinical application to neonates. *J Clin Monit* 1991;7:325

109. Elwell CE, Owen-Reece H, Cope M, et al: Measurement of adult cerebral haemodynamics using near infrared spectroscopy. *Acta Neurochir Suppl (Wein)* 1993;59:74

110. Ausman JI, McCormick PW, Stewart M, et al: Cerebral oxygenation metabolism during hypothermic arrest in humans. *J Neurosurg* 1993;79:810

111. Wahr JA, Tremper KK: Noninvasive oxygen monitoring techniques. *Crit Care Clin North Am* 1995;11:199

112. Germon TJ, Kane NM, Manara AR, et al: Near-infrared spectroscopy in adults: effects of extracranial ischaemia and intracranial hypoxia on estimation of cerebral oxygenation. *Br J Anaesth* 1994;73:503

113. McMicken DB: Emergency CT head scans in traumatic and atraumatic conditions. *Ann Emerg Med* 1986;15:274

114. Snow RB, Zimmerman RD, Gandy SE, et al: Comparison of magnetic resonance imaging and computed tomography in the evaluation of head injury. *Neurosurgery* 1986;18:45

115. Gomori J, Grossman RI, Goldberg HI: Intracranial hematomas: imaging by high field MR. *Radiology* 1985;57:87

116. Shackford SR, Wald SL, Ross SE, et al: The clinical utility of computed tomographic scanning and neurologic examination in the management of patients with minor head injuries. *J Trauma* 1992;33:385

117. Chesnut RM, Marshall LF, Klauber MR, et al: The role of secondary brain injury in determining outcome from severe head injury. *J Trauma* 1993;34:216

118. Bullock R, Golek J, Blake G: Traumatic intracerebral hematoma: which patients should undergo surgical evacuation? CT scan features and ICP monitoring as a basis for decision making. *Surg Neurol* 1989;32:181

119. Eisenberg HM: Initial CT findings in 753 patients with severe head injury. *J Neurosurg* 1990;73:688

Critical Care, Third Edition, edited by Joseph M. Civetta,
Robert W. Taylor, and Robert R. Kirby.
Lippincott-Raven Publishers, Philadelphia, PA © 1997.

CHAPTER 63

Radiographic Imaging

Carl E. Ravin

Diagnostic imaging is firmly established as a keystone in evaluating and monitoring the critically ill patient.[1] Because of limitations in the physical evaluation of severely traumatized or critically ill patients, the use of diagnostic imaging techniques has grown dramatically during the last decade. Plain film radiography remains the foundation of such imaging, but newer technologies have emerged, which, when used appropriately, can be of great assistance in the evaluation and assessment of these patients.

Because of limitations in positioning the critically ill patient, the inability to obtain multiple views of many anatomic areas, and the difficulties inherent in bringing imaging equipment to the bedside, judicious use must be made of the available imaging technologies.[2] Such use begins with clear recognition of the advantages and limitations of each imaging technique, and most important, with a clear formulation of the question to be answered by the imaging study requested. Failure to formulate the question clearly, and then to ascertain whether the imaging study requested is actually capable of answering the question being asked, are probably the most commonly made errors in using diagnostic imaging in the critically ill patient.

PLAIN CHEST RADIOGRAPH

The conventional radiograph of the chest remains the most valuable study for evaluating and monitoring critically ill patients.[3] The radiographic equipment required to perform the examination is available in all ICUs and is relatively inexpensive. Mobile radiography equipment is widely available and reliable and, in competent hands, can produce chest radiographs of reasonably high quality. Radiation exposure to the patient and support personnel is well within acceptable limits if simple precautions are observed. From the patient's

standpoint, the area exposed to the radiographic beam should be confined to that anatomic area being evaluated, and relatively high-speed film/screen combinations and higher kilovoltage techniques should be used whenever possible. The safety of the support personnel (nurses, physicians, and technologists) can be ensured by the simple precaution of remaining out of the direct beam and away from the patient being radiographed.

The intensity of scattered radiation, generated while the beam passes through the patient, falls off with the square of the radius from the source (the patient). Therefore, by moving away from the patient, a significant reduction in radiation exposure can be achieved. Moving 60 cm (2 feet) away from the patient reduces the radiation exposure by a factor of four, and further distance results in proportionally greater dose reductions. In addition, the use of protective gowns, whenever possible, is highly advisable.

As a rule, the conventional chest radiograph is used to answer certain general questions, as discussed later.

DIMINISHED OR IMPAIRED RESPIRATORY FUNCTION

With diminished or impaired respiratory function, the radiograph is used to exclude easily treated causes of respiratory compromise, such as pneumothorax or large pleural effusion, or to confirm disease processes suspected clinically such as acute respiratory distress syndrome (ARDS), pneumonia, or atelectasis.

Simple Pneumothorax

The hallmark of pneumothorax is displacement of visceral pleura away from the parietal pleura by air within the pleural space.[4] The visceral pleura is imaged as a thin white line on chest radiographs, outlined between air within the pleural space on one side and air within the lung parenchyma on the other (Fig. 63-1*A*). Exposing the film in expiration frequently enhances visualization of the pneumothorax because the collection of air occupies a larger percentage of the hemithorax (see Fig. 63-1*B*). In patients radiographed in an upright position, air collects over the apex of the lung in a characteristic pattern.

The radiographic appearance of pneumothorax may be mimicked by skin folds created when redundant skin is compressed against the film cassette (Fig. 63-2). However, skin folds can be differentiated from pneumothorax in that the thin white line, representing the visceral pleura, is not imaged in this situation. Rather, the skin fold produces a gradual increase in opacity medially because air is seen only on the lateral side. In addition, pulmonary vessels are often seen projecting across the skin fold, confirming that the opaque edge is produced by soft tissues outside the thorax rather than by the edge of the lung. If there is any question as to the correct diagnosis, a repeat chest radiograph with the patient in a lateral decubitus position (affected side uppermost) can help to confirm the artifactual nature of the skin fold.

Notice that most radiographs are performed in ICUs with the patient in a supine position. In this case, the highest portion of the thorax is no longer over the apex of the lung but is in the anterior costophrenic sulcus. This sulcus runs laterally in an oblique and inferior direction from approximately the level of the 7th costal cartilage anteriorly to the midaxillary line at the level of the 11th rib laterally. This orientation is shown in the skeletal representation in Figure 63-3. Air collecting in the pleural space tends to rise toward the highest portion of the thorax and, thus, collect in the

anterior costophrenic sulcus. This distribution of air is more difficult to recognize radiographically because the visceral pleural line is generally not seen. Rather, the collection of air in the anterior costophrenic sulcus produces an increased lucency over the upper abdominal quadrant (Fig. 63-4) and sharply outlines the inferior margins of the anterior costophrenic sulcus. The lateral costophrenic sulcus appears deeper and more lucent than normal, an appearance that has been described as the "deep sulcus sign" (Fig. 63-5*A*).

The apex of the heart and associated pericardial fat pads often are more sharply outlined by such a collection of air. It is important to look for this sort of air collection in patients radiographed in the supine position and, again, if there is any doubt as to the correct diagnosis, a lateral decubitus radiograph with the suspicious side up is most helpful, because air in the pleural space outlines the visceral pleura in this position. If there is associated fluid, an air–fluid level can be demonstrated (see Fig. 65-5*B*).

Pleural Effusion

The characteristic appearance of fluid in the pleural space on radiographs obtained in the upright position is well known to most physicians and consists of blunting of the costophrenic angle in a characteristic miniscoid configuration. However, in the critically ill patient, it is often necessary to obtain radiographs in the supine position. In such cases, pleural fluid layers posteriorly in the pleural space, creating a uniform increase in opacity over one lung (Fig. 63-6*A*). Recognition of this generalized increased opacity can aid in identifying large pleural effusions. If there is doubt as to the diagnosis, confirmation may be obtained using a lateral

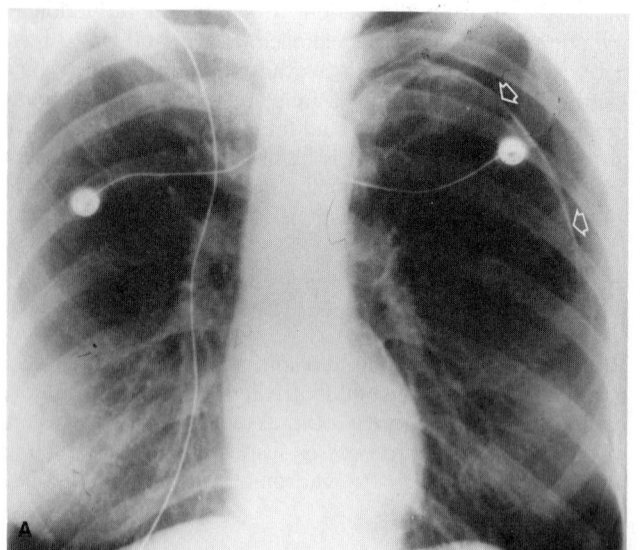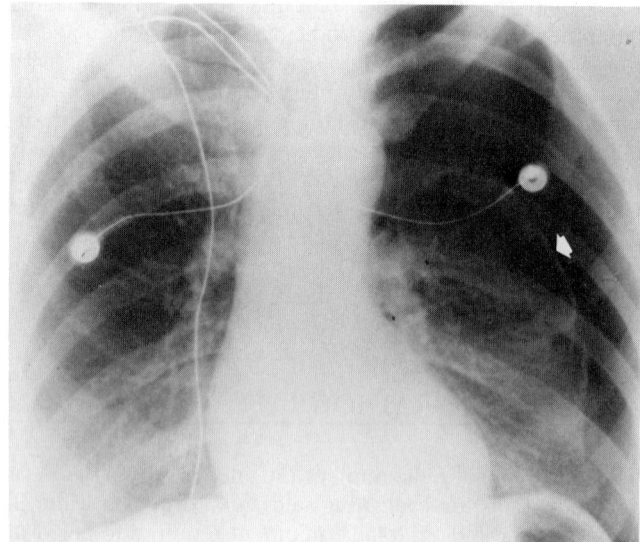

FIGURE 63-1. (**A**) Simple pneumothorax on the left. The characteristic thin white line representing the visceral pleura is readily identified (*open arrows*). (**B**) Same patient with film exposed in expiration. The visceral pleural line (*arrow*) can again be easily identified. The pneumothorax occupies proportionally a larger percentage of the hemithorax, which is reduced in size by exposing the film at expiration. If there is a question about the presence or absence of pneumothorax, exposing a film in expiration often enhances visualization of the pneumothorax.

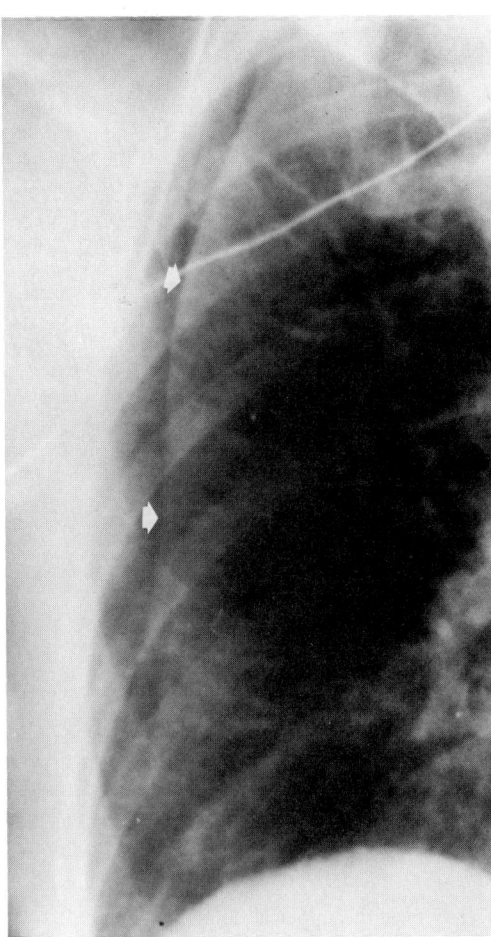

FIGURE 63-2. Skin fold mimicking pneumothorax. The appearance of a skin fold (*arrows*) can be distinguished from a true pneumothorax in that the thin white line of the visceral pleura is not seen, but rather, the opacity fades medially. Compare with that of the classic simple pneumothorax shown in Figure 63-1A.

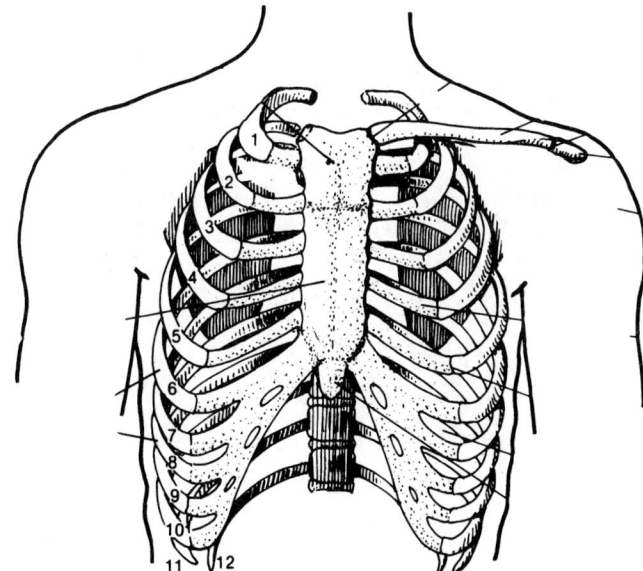

FIGURE 63-3. Anterior view of the skeletal thorax showing relationship of ribs and costal cartilages. Anterior costophrenic sulcus runs approximately from the seventh costal cartilage laterally and obliquely to the midaxillary line at the 11th rib.

Tension Pneumothorax

Tension pneumothorax is generally a clinical diagnosis.[5] However, the diagnosis may be suggested radiographically by a shift of structures such as the heart and mediastinum to the contralateral side, by a flattening of the cardiomediastinal contour, and by a depression or inversion of the ipsilateral hemidiaphragm (Fig. 63-8).

decubitus radiograph with the suspected side of abnormality placed in the dependent position (see Fig. 63-6B).

Hydropneumothorax

The presence of fluid and air in the pleural space produces a characteristic air–fluid level when radiographs are obtained in the upright position. However, when radiographs are obtained in the supine position the radiographic appearance depends on the relative quantities of air and fluid present. If sufficient air is present within the pleural space to outline the visceral pleura laterally, a sharp pleural line can be seen, suggesting pneumothorax (Fig. 63-7). The additional presence of fluid is suggested by a relative increase in opacity on the involved side. If the quantity of air is small, the lateral edge of the lung is less likely to be seen, and the line of the visceral pleura may not be identified. In this case, only the features of hydrothorax can be appreciated on the radiograph.

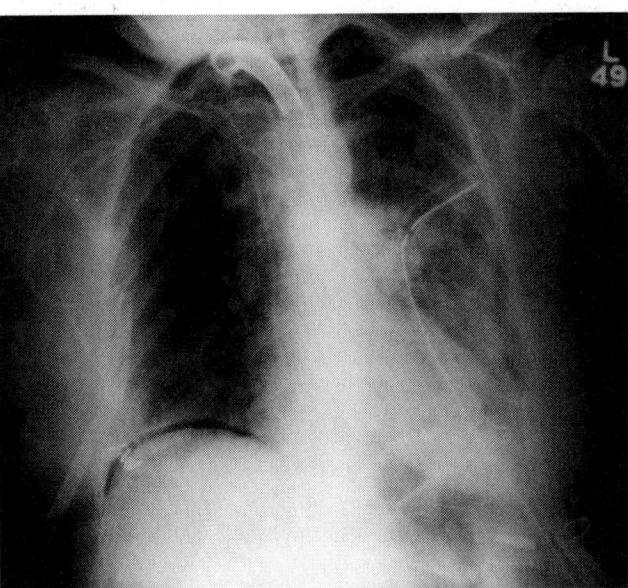

FIGURE 63-4. Persistent pneumothorax despite tube thoracostomy in a patient with severe ARDS and a bronchopleural cutaneous fistula. Notice the obvious lucency above the right hemidiaphragm.

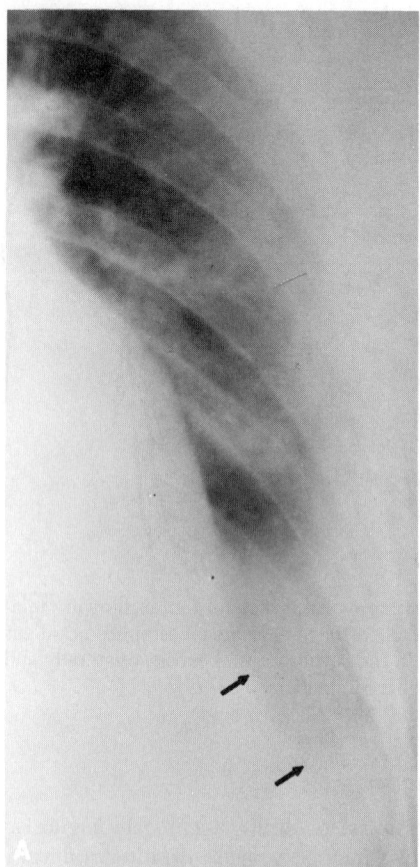
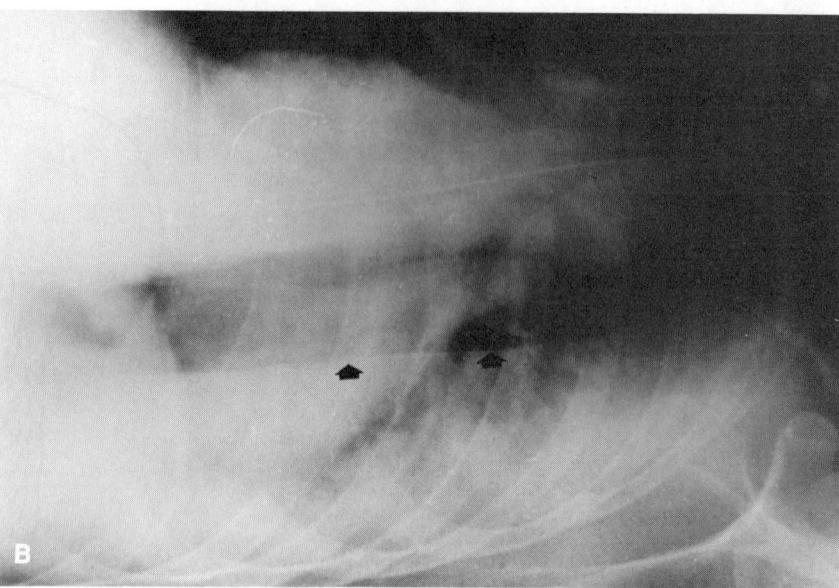

FIGURE 63-5. (**A**) Left hemithorax demonstrates increased lucency over the upper abdomen with the lateral costophrenic sulcus (*arrows*) appearing deeper and more lucent than normal. This radiographic appearance has been referred to as the "deep sulcus sign" of pneumothorax in the supine position. (**B**) Lateral decubitus film with the affected side down in this same patient clearly demonstrates an air–fluid level, confirming the presence of air and fluid in the left hemithorax.

CONGESTIVE HEART FAILURE

The diagnosis of congestive heart failure (CHF) can often be suggested by or suspected from the plain chest radiograph, although clearly appropriate clinical correlation is required to establish the diagnosis. The diagnosis is particularly difficult on radiographs obtained in the supine projection, and, therefore, whenever this diagnosis is suspected, attempts should be made to obtain a radiograph with the patient in the upright position. Such positioning ensures easier and more accurate analysis of pulmonary vascular distribution and allows for a longer, more conventional focal–film distance, which, in turn, makes analysis of cardiac size more accurate. In most instances of CHF the heart is enlarged, although again this is more easily appreciated on upright films exposed at the conventional 180-cm (6-foot) focal–film distance. In this situation, the difference between an anterior–posterior radiograph and the conventional posterior–anterior radiograph results in only minimal (5% or less) magnification; thus, the heart should not exceed 50% of the thoracic diameter. On the other hand, with anterior–

posterior supine radiographs done at short focal–film distance (generally 102 to 122 cm [40 to 48 in]), there is considerable magnification, and accurate evaluation of cardiac size often is difficult.

Pulmonary Vasculature

Evaluation of the pulmonary vasculature is the most critical element in establishing the radiographic diagnosis of CHF. Increase in pulmonary venous pressure results in redistribution of flow to the upper lung zones, as evidenced by the increase in size and number of vessels in these areas (Fig. 63-9). The normal ratio of upper lung zone vessels to lower lung zone vessels is about 1:3 to 1:4. This is a reflection of gravitational diversion of blood flow toward the lung bases caused by hydrostatic pressure differences between upper and lower lung zones, superimposed on the normally low-resistance, low-pressure pulmonary circulation. However, when the patient is in the supine position, the hydrostatic gradient from lung apex to base does not exist (the gradient

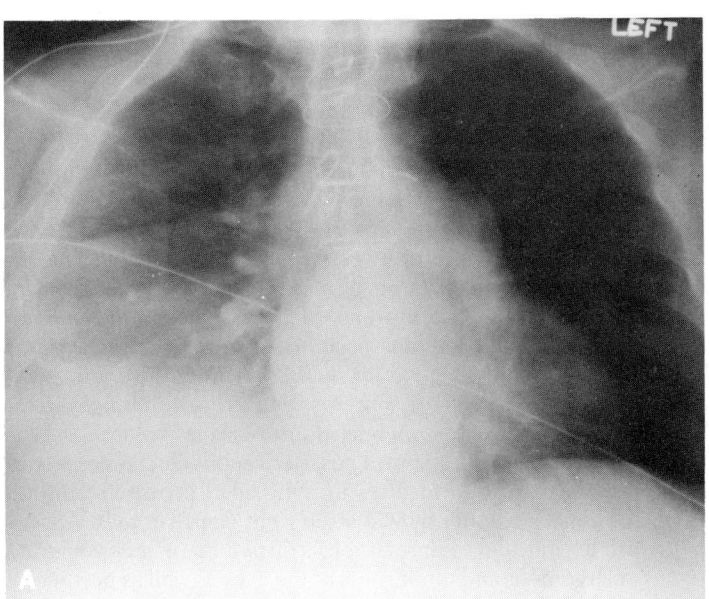

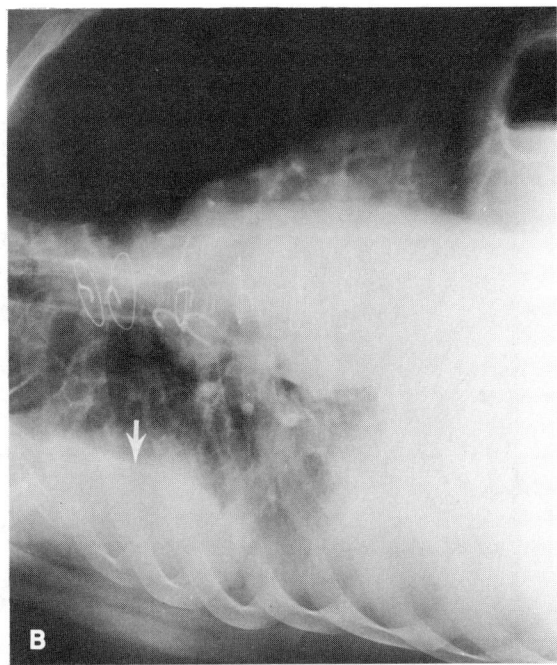

FIGURE 63-6. (**A**) Chest radiograph obtained with patient in supine position. Notice the increased opacity over the entire right hemithorax characteristic of a free pleural effusion layering uniformly in the pleural space posteriorly. (**B**) In the lateral decubitus projection, with the affected side in the dependent position, the fluid (*arrow*) layers along the lateral chest wall, confirming the presence of a large free pleural effusion.

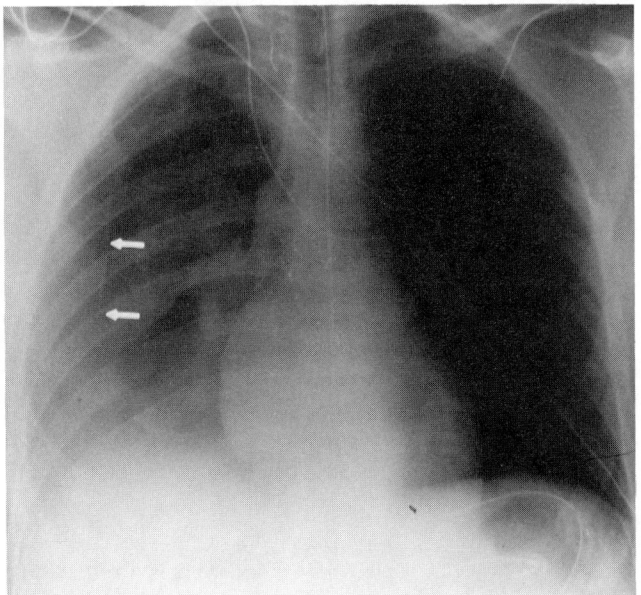

FIGURE 63-7. Chest radiograph with patient in supine position demonstrates opacity over the right hemithorax as well as a thin white line (*arrows*) representing the visceral pleura. This combination of findings is diagnostic of a large free pleural effusion and an associated large pneumothorax.

is from anterior to posterior in this position), and, thus, pulmonary blood flow tends to equalize between upper and lower lung zones. This is evident radiographically as an increase in size and number of vessels in the upper lung zones. Therefore, identification of flow redistribution on a supine radiograph is not indicative of pulmonary venous hypertension or left ventricular failure but can be attributed to positioning alone.

Pulmonary Edema

To establish the diagnosis of CHF on a supine radiograph, signs of pulmonary edema must be identified. Such edema begins by fluid collecting in the interstitial spaces of the lung. This is evidenced radiographically as thickening of normal interstitial structures. Fluid accumulating in the perivascular space results in indistinct margins of the vessels and may be identified at a relatively early stage. In addition, fluid collecting in the interstitium results in thickening of bronchial walls seen on end, an appearance commonly noticed in the perihilar region. Beyond this, fluid may thicken the septa between secondary pulmonary lobules, resulting in visualization of septal lines. These lines, depending on location, may abut the pleura, particularly in the lower lung zones (so-called Kerley B lines; Fig. 63-10), or radiate outward from the hila in the upper lung zones (Kerley A lines). In addition, fluid in the subpleural lymphatics often renders the interlobar fissures more visible, again suggesting the possibility of interstitial pulmonary edema. As fluid accumulates further, alveolar spaces begin to fill, resulting in a more homogeneous opacity of the lungs. As fluid enters the air

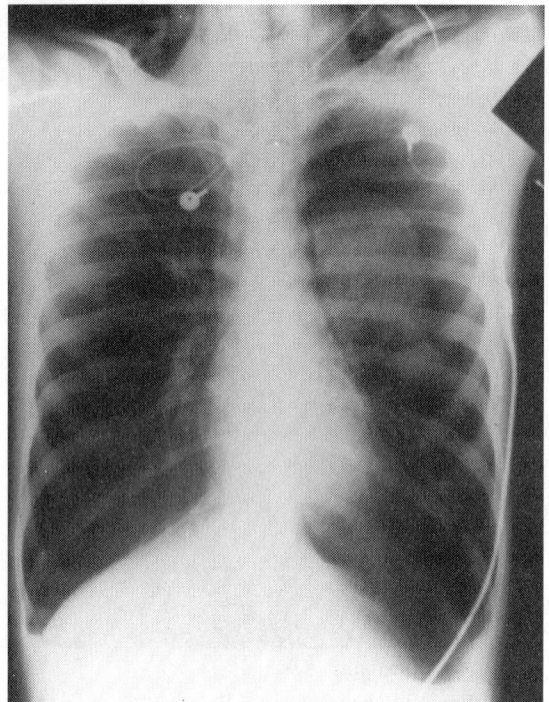

FIGURE 63-8. Tension pneumothorax with complete collapse of left lung, diaphragmatic inversion, and cardiomediastinal flattening.

spaces and airways, clinical correlates become evident such as rales, rhonchi, and, eventually, frothy sputum if the edema is severe enough.

Azygous Vein

An additional radiographic clue to the diagnosis of CHF is enlargement of the azygous vein seen on end as it arches forward over the right main stem bronchus to empty into the back wall of the superior vena cava (Fig. 63-11). On upright radiographs, the transverse diameter of the azygous vein rarely exceeds 7 mm, although 10 mm is generally given at the upper limit of normal. This increases somewhat with the patient in the supine position but, again, a large azygous vein is reasonably good evidence of increased venous pressures. In addition, the superior vena cava often bulges laterally, again reflecting increased intravascular volume and increased venous pressure. The latter venous changes are more reflective of abnormalities in right-sided pressures and are seen more frequently when the right ventricle fails. Appropriate clinical correlates, such as distention of neck veins and enlargement and tenderness of the liver as well as peripheral edema, are generally available in this setting.

ACUTE RESPIRATORY DISTRESS SYNDROME

Acute respiratory distress syndrome has as its radiographic correlate diffuse confluent opacities distributed symmetri-

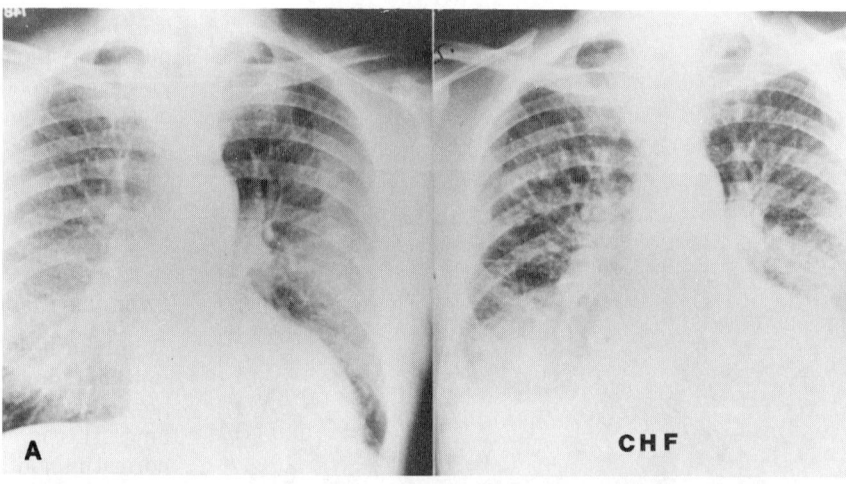

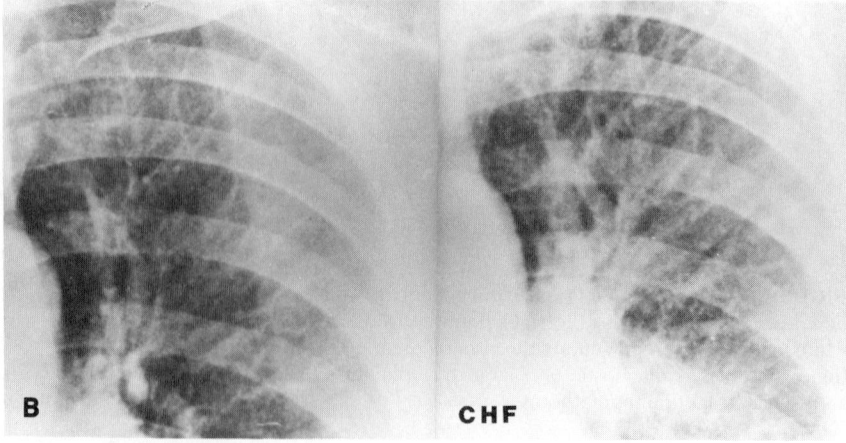

FIGURE 63-9. (**A**) Composite figure showing frontal chest radiographs before and during frank congestive heart failure. Notice that with the onset of congestive heart failure, fluid accumulates in the air spaces at both lung bases, and decreased lung compliance is evidenced by elevation of the hemidiaphragms. In addition, there is striking redistribution of pulmonary blood flow to the upper lung zones. (**B**) Composite view of the left upper lobe demonstrates the striking redistribution that occurs in association with congestive heart failure.

cally throughout both lungs (see Fig. 63-4).[6] In general, there is a latent period of 12 to 24 hours between the time that clinical symptoms first begin and the time that radiograph becomes abnormal. During this period, respiratory compromise increases and lung compliance decreases, both of which are evident clinically. The importance of the radiograph in the early phase of ARDS is to exclude other more treatable problems such as CHF and pulmonary edema. When diffuse radiographic opacity develops after a latent period, a diagnosis of ARDS may be reasonably suspected.

Once this diagnosis is suspected, it is important to continue careful monitoring of the patient for potential complications of the therapy instituted, particularly pneumothorax or pneumomediastinum, which may occur in association with mechanical ventilatory support superimposed on lungs with markedly decreased compliance. The radiographic findings of pneumothorax have been described previously. However, notice that in this setting of so-called stiff lungs, a relatively small pneumothorax may have significant physiologic consequence.[7] Therefore, evaluation of the pneumothorax in terms of "percentage" or size is inappropriate. Rather, it is critical to recognize the presence of a pneumothorax in this setting so that appropriate therapy to relieve it may be instituted rapidly.

PNEUMOMEDIASTINUM

Pneumomediastinum is recognized radiographically as vertically oriented lucencies paralleling and extending along mediastinal fascial planes (Fig. 63-12). Often, air may dissect along the pericardium, suggesting the possibility of pneumopericardium; however, in general, this is a far less common complication. Pneumomediastinum can be differentiated from pneumopericardium by identifying extension of air above the normal insertions of the pericardium at the root of the aorta as well as by identifying air dissecting upward into the soft tissues of the neck. Pneumomediastinum is usually more easily recognized on the lateral projection, although this view is frequently not available in the ICU. However, if the diagnosis is of concern, a cross-table lateral view can be obtained, even in a critically ill patient.

PNEUMONIA

Pneumonia in the critically ill patient is similar in appearance to that seen in other patient groups and is generally recognized as increased radiopacity in the lung. When extensive, it may involve several lobes and, if extremely widespread, may be difficult to differentiate from pulmonary edema on a radiographic basis. Obviously, clinical correlation is critical in these situations. The intensivist should recognize, however, that it is impossible to distinguish pneumonia superimposed on preexisting pulmonary edema. Both appear as diffuse radiographic opacities, and, unless there is a focal nature to the process, it is almost impossible to recognize an inflammatory process superimposed on generalized edema.

On occasion, pneumonia occurs in a location that raises the question of aspiration. In supine patients, the most common location for an aspiration pneumonia is the superior segment of the lower lobe because the bronchus supplying this segment runs straight posteriorly in the supine position.

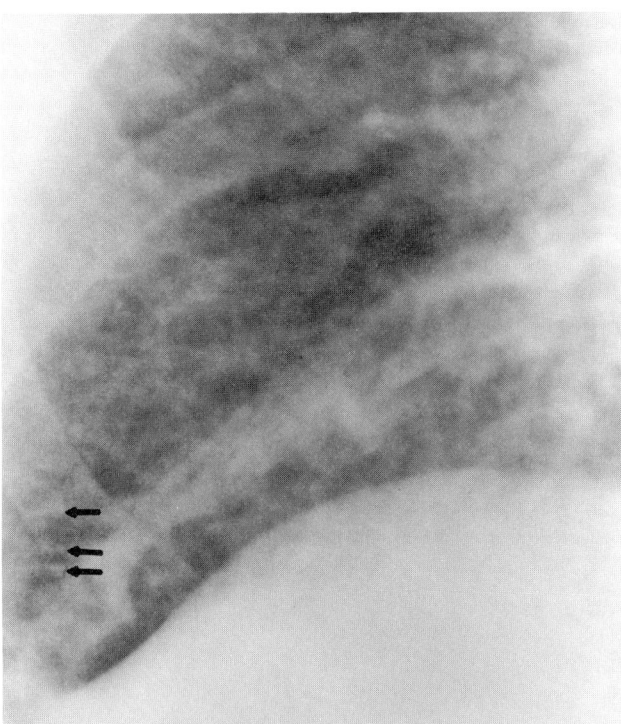

FIGURE 63-10. Close-up view of the left lower zone demonstrates Kerley B lines. These are identified as horizontally oriented thin white lines that abut the pleura and are approximately 1 to 2 cm in overall length.

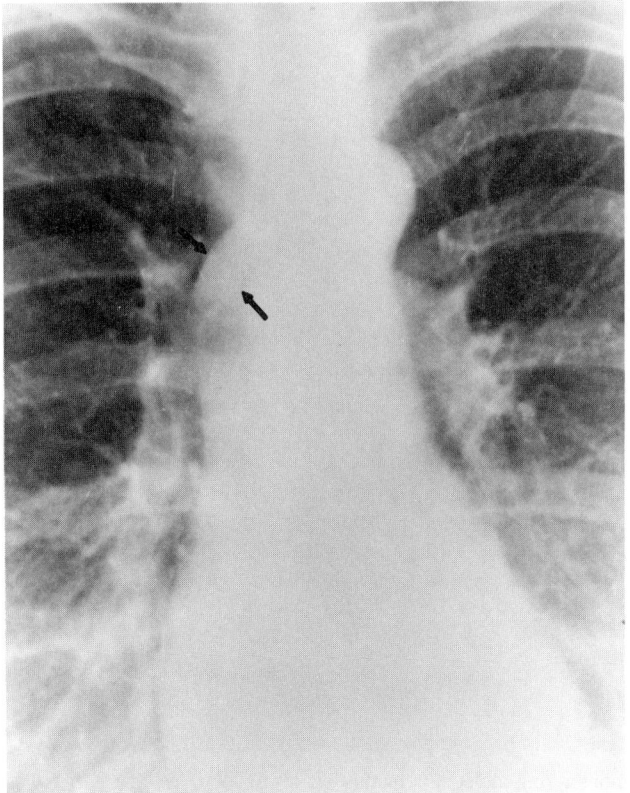

FIGURE 63-11. Enlarged azygous vein measuring 12 mm in transverse diameter (*arrows*). The vein is seen on end as it arches forward to empty into the back wall of the upper vena cava.

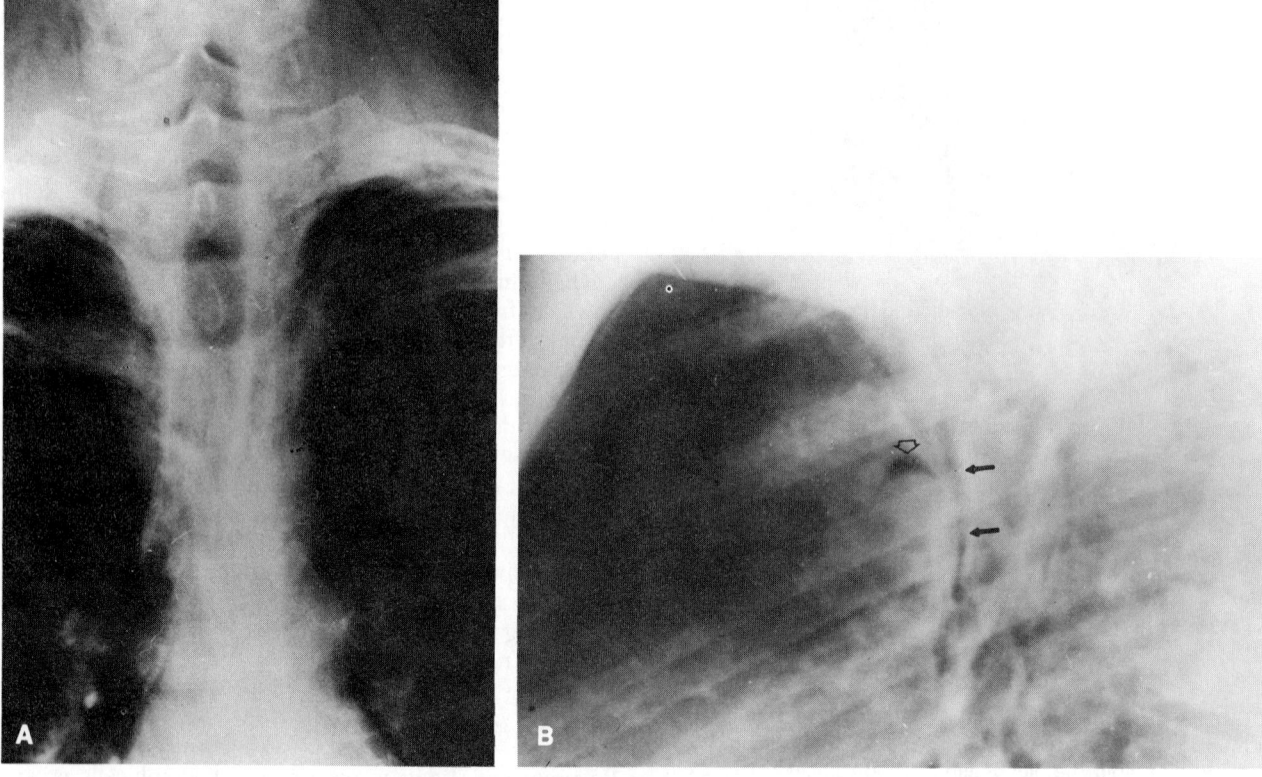

FIGURE 63-12. (**A**) Frontal view of the upper mediastinum shows numerous vertically oriented lucencies (*black lines*) representing air dissecting along fascial planes to extend into the neck. (**B**) Lateral view demonstrates air dissecting in mediastinal fascial planes (*solid arrows*) and accumulating over the right pulmonary artery (*open arrow*).

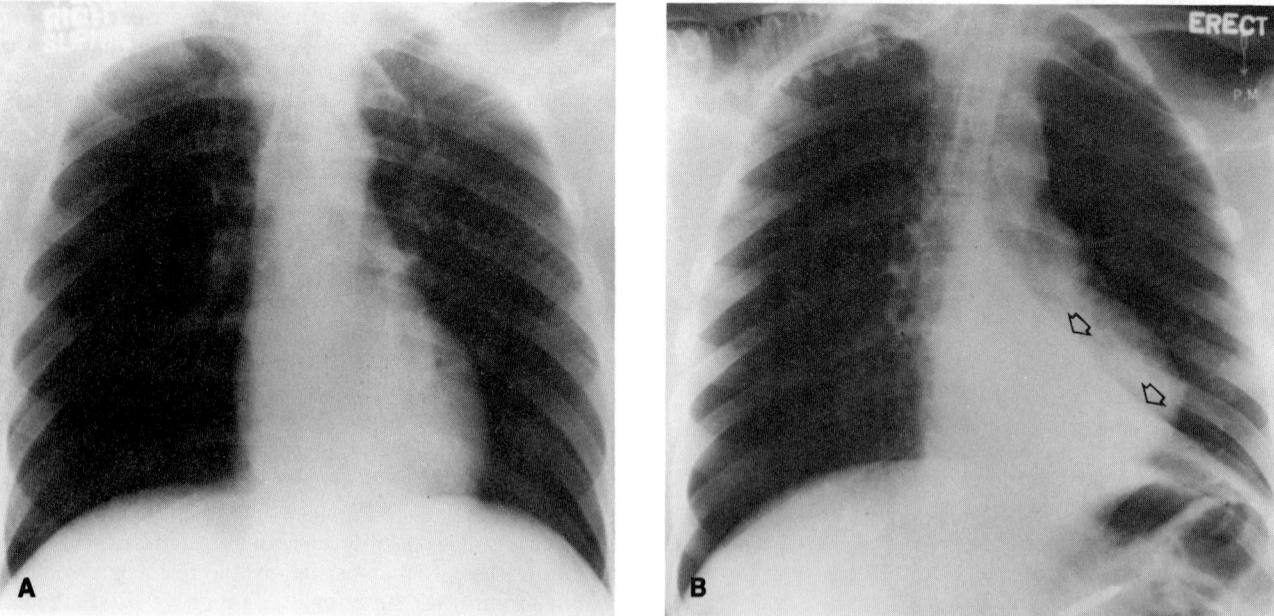

FIGURE 63-13. (**A**) Postoperative chest radiograph demonstrating atelectasis in the left lower lobe, as evidenced by increased opacity in the retrocardiac region. (**B**) Subsequent radiograph demonstrates complete collapse of the left lower lobe, producing a characteristic triangular opacity (*arrows*) behind the heart. Collapse was secondary to a central mucous plug and resolved when the plug was removed.

Additional common locations for aspiration pneumonia are the lower lobes, although the area of the lung that is dependent at the time of aspiration is at risk.

LOBAR COLLAPSE

Patients either seriously traumatized or critically ill are at risk for mucus plugs, which may obstruct segmental or lobar bronchi. Obstruction of these bronchi results in atelectasis, which, in general, has a characteristic appearance, depending on the lobe obstructed. The left lower lobe seems particularly vulnerable, presumably because of compression resulting from the overlying heart, and is recognized characteristically as a triangular-shaped opacity in the retrocardiac area (Fig. 63-13). The right middle lobe, when collapsed or involved by pneumonia, creates an increased opacity over the right lower lung zone which obliterates the normal border of the right heart while preserving the right hemidiaphragm (Fig. 63-14). Right upper lobe collapse is recognized by upward displacement of the minor fissure in a characteristic pattern (Fig. 63-15). Left upper lobe collapse may be among the most difficult to recognize on a single supine view but is seen as a perihilar opacity (Fig. 63-16).

Because the left upper lobe bronchus supplies both the upper lobe and the lingula, both tend to become atelectatic, resulting in obliteration of the left heart border by the increased opacity in the adjacent lingula. Thus, left upper lobe collapse may be recognized by obliteration of the left heart border with associated preservation of the aortic arch, which lies more posteriorly in the chest. Right lower lobe collapse seems to be the most difficult to recognize and is usually identified by noting displacement of the normal major fissure medially and inferiorly.

EVALUATION OF LIFE-SUPPORT AND MONITORING DEVICES ■

A second major role for the conventional chest radiograph in the ICU is to evaluate the various life-support and monitoring devices used in these patients. A reasonable argument can be made for daily confirmation of position of the various tubes and catheters, and indeed, a radiograph to confirm location of these devices is mandatory after their initial placement. In addition, potential complications are associated with all the various support and monitoring devices. Because

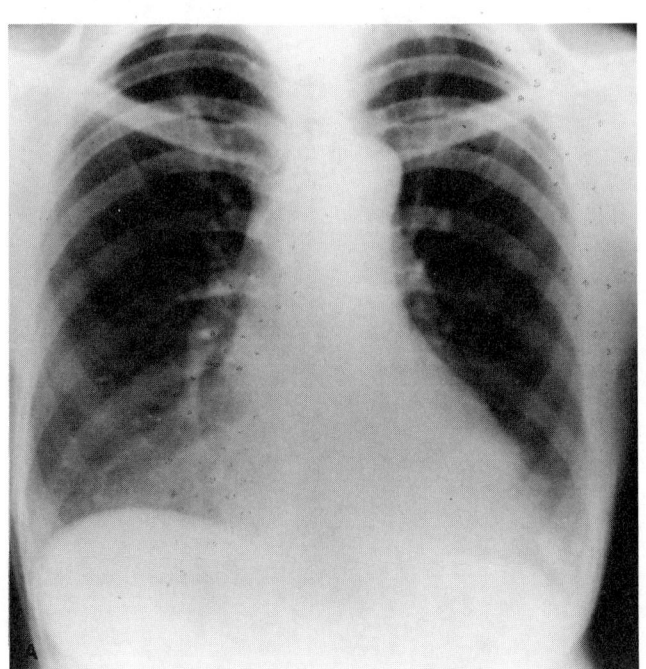 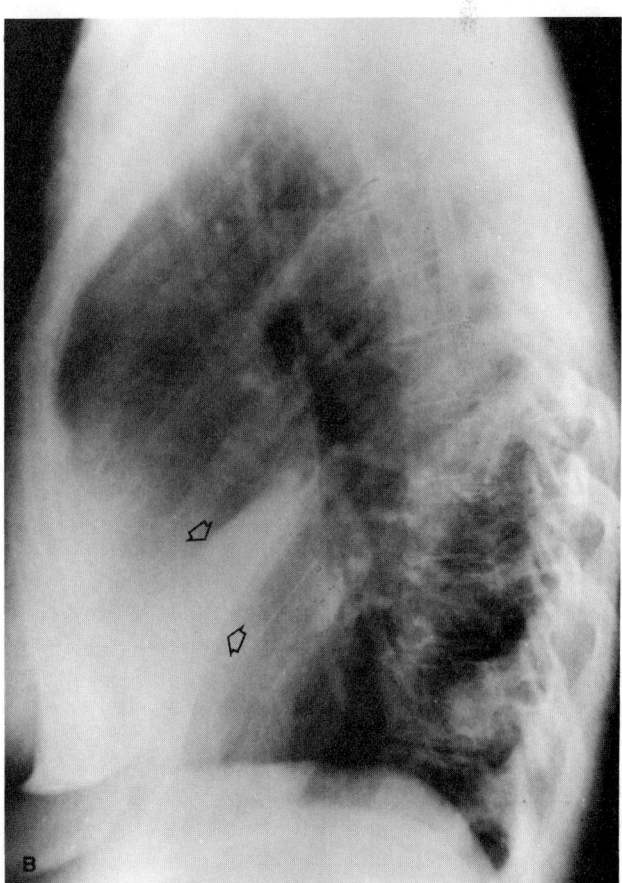

FIGURE 63-14. (**A**) Right middle lobe collapse on the frontal view. Notice that the normally well-defined right heart border is obliterated, whereas the right hemidiaphragm is preserved. (**B**) On the lateral view, a characteristic triangular-shaped opacity (*arrows*) is seen, representing the collapsed right middle lobe.

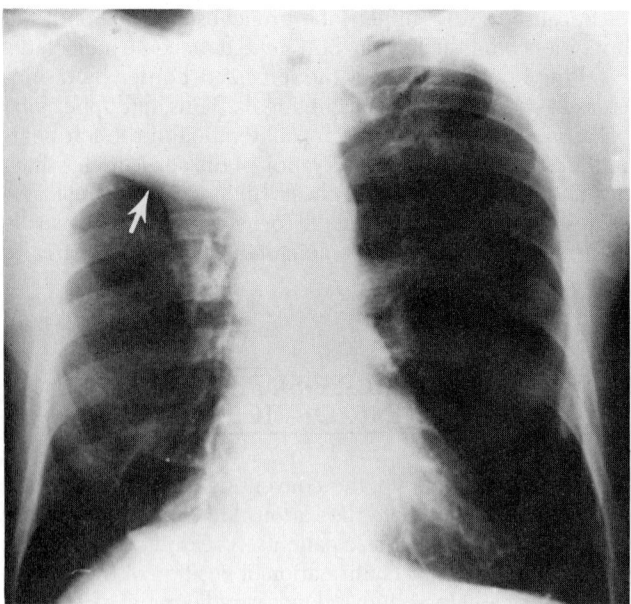

FIGURE 63-15. Characteristic right upper lobe collapse, demonstrating upward displacement of the minor fissure (*arrow*) and displacement of the trachea toward the right.

clinical examination is frequently difficult and unrewarding in this patient group, potential complications often can be recognized only radiographically. The intensivist must make a compulsive and rigorous check of every catheter and tube in each patient on every radiograph.

VENTILATORY SUPPORT TUBES

Inadvertent Bronchial Intubation

Among the most commonly used of the various life-support tubes are the ventilatory support tubes (endotracheal and tracheostomy tubes). The major complications encountered with these tubes generally result from inappropriate positioning. Because of its greater length, incorrect placement is more commonly encountered radiographically with the endotracheal tube. The major problem is that the tube is often inadvertently advanced into the main stem bronchus (right more frequently than left). Such placement can result in various degrees of obstruction of the contralateral bronchus, either by the tube itself or by the balloon cuff, with consequent decreased or absent ventilation. Such obstruction can, in turn, result in rapid and often complete atelectasis of the left lung (Fig. 63-17). The rapidity of collapse

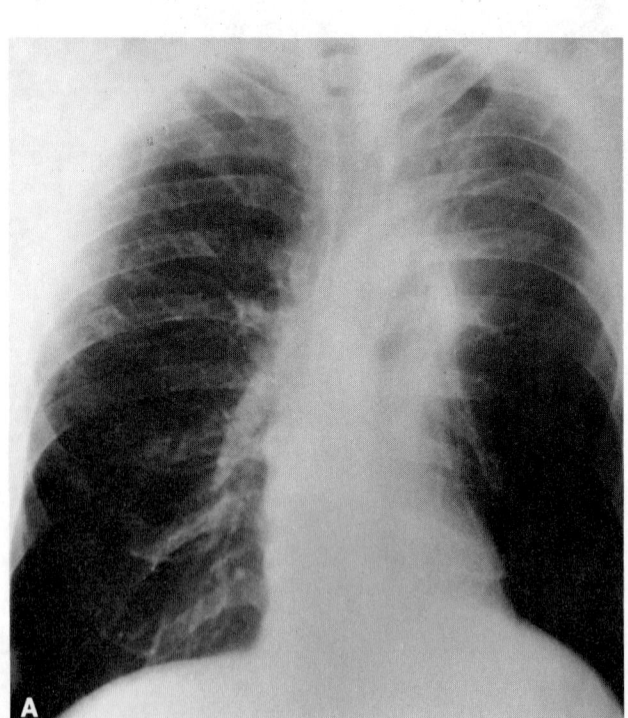

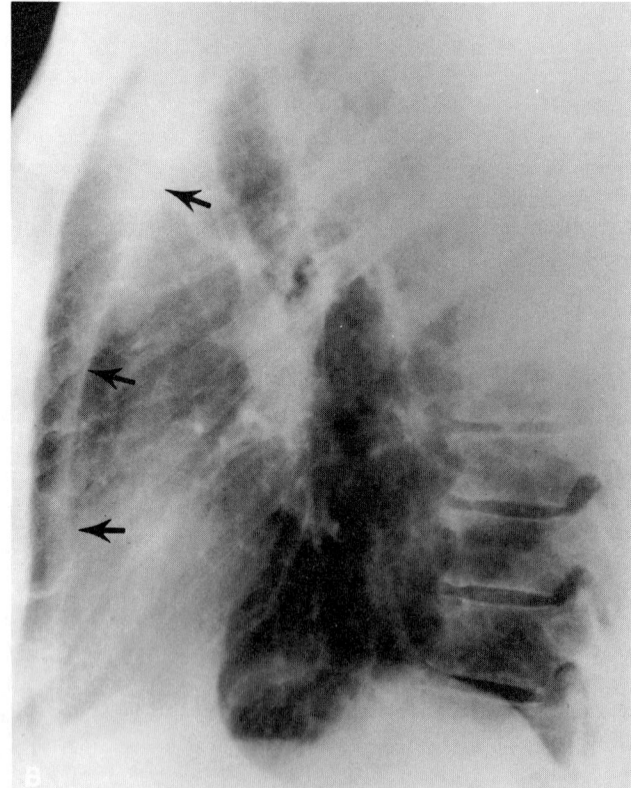

FIGURE 63-16. Left upper lobe collapse. (**A**) Frontal view demonstrating perihilar opacity. Notice preservation of the aortic arch but indistinctness of the left heart border in its uppermost portions where it is in contact with the upper lobe and lingula. (**B**) Lateral projection shows forward displacement of the major fissure (*arrows*) secondary to collapse.

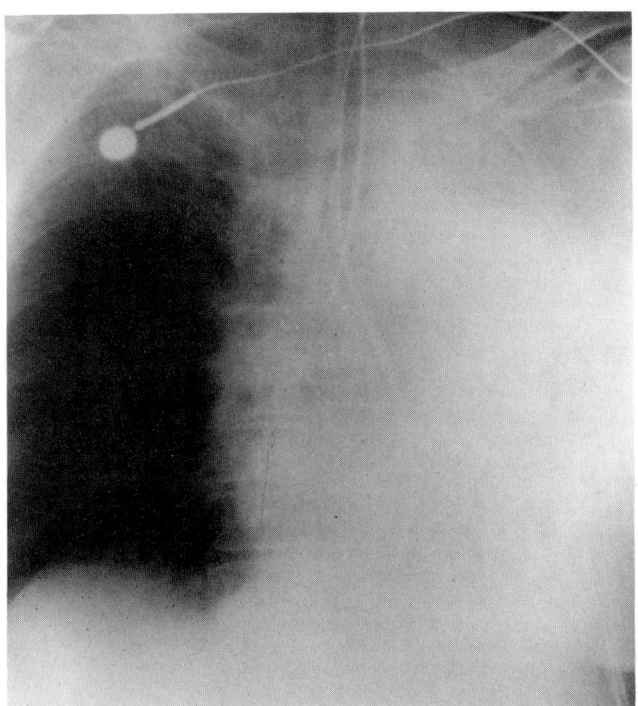

FIGURE 63-17. Endotracheal tube was inadvertently advanced into the right mainstem bronchus, resulting in obstruction of the left mainstem bronchus and subsequent atelectasis of the left lung.

is enhanced by the fact that intubated patients are often ventilated with gas mixtures containing increased amounts of oxygen and proportionately decreased amounts of nitrogen. The rapid resorption of this oxygen from the air spaces of the lung results in more rapid collapse as the normal "splinting" effect of nitrogen is lost.

Incorrect placement of the endotracheal tube can occur either at the time of initial insertion or later, secondary to patient motion or inadvertent movement of the tube. Therefore, a postintubation radiograph is required to ensure appropriate initial placement, and careful evaluation of all subsequent radiographs is required to ensure that there has been no later displacement of the tube. Satisfactory placement in the adult patient is generally accepted as having the distal tip of the tube lying at least 3 cm distal to the vocal cords and 2.5 cm proximal to the carina. However, notice that the position of the patient's head at the time this evaluation is made is important in defining these limits. With flexion of the head, the endotracheal tube moves downward toward the carina. The tube is displaced upward while the head is moved from flexion to a neutral position and is displaced further cephalad while the head is extended. Total movement of the tip of the endotracheal tube may be as much as 4 cm from full flexion to full extension.[8,9] Therefore, evaluation of the adequacy of endotracheal tube placement also must include assessment of the head position.

Esophageal Intubation

Although inadvertent placement of the endotracheal tube into one of the mainstem bronchi is the most common mal-

position noticed radiographically, it is also possible to inadvertently intubate the esophagus (Fig. 63-18). Although most of such episodes are detected clinically, occasionally cases go undetected and are first noticed radiographically. The typical radiographic evidence is that the tube projects outside the tracheal wall and that significant gastric distention is present.

PULMONARY ARTERY CATHETERS

The flow-directed pulmonary artery catheter has greatly facilitated the hemodynamic management of critically ill patients. The major problem detected radiographically with use of these catheters involves either coiling of the catheter in the heart or distal positioning of the catheter tip.[10] Coiling of the catheter within the right atrium or ventricle (Fig. 63-19) can occur when the catheter is advanced too far without appropriate change in recorded pressure to indicate passage across a valve into the next chamber or the pulmonary artery. If the catheter coils in the right ventricle, the potential for cardiac arrhythmia secondary to irritation of the conducting bundle is significant. Therefore, prompt recognition and repositioning of the catheter is necessary if such coiling is identified.

A more common problem is caused by inadvertent distal positioning of the catheter tip. Ideally, the catheter should be maintained in a large central pulmonary artery that is

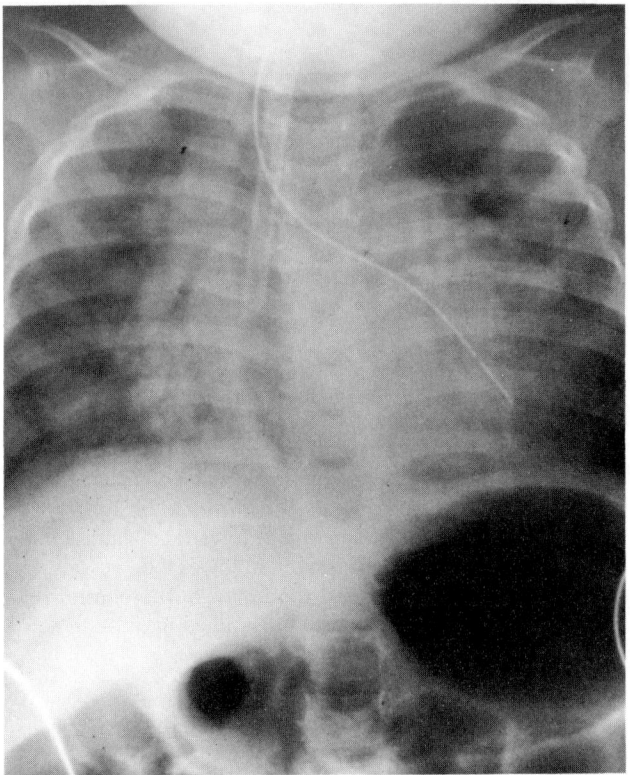

FIGURE 63-18. Inadvertent intubation of the esophagus. The esophagus is filled with air, and there is considerable air in the stomach and gastrointestinal tract. In addition, in this patient, a nasogastric tube has been inadvertently positioned in the left lower lobe.

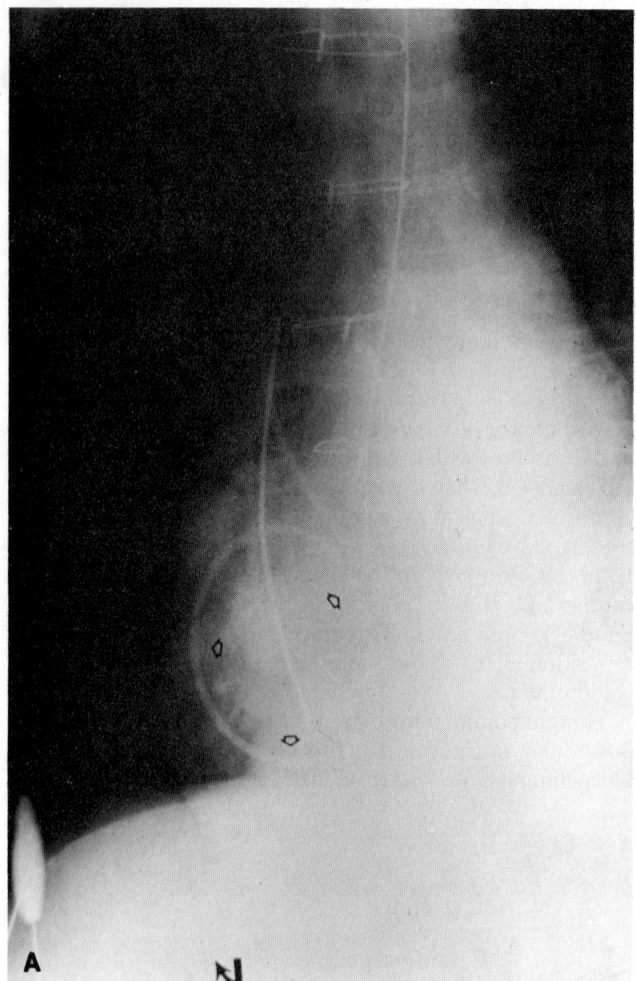

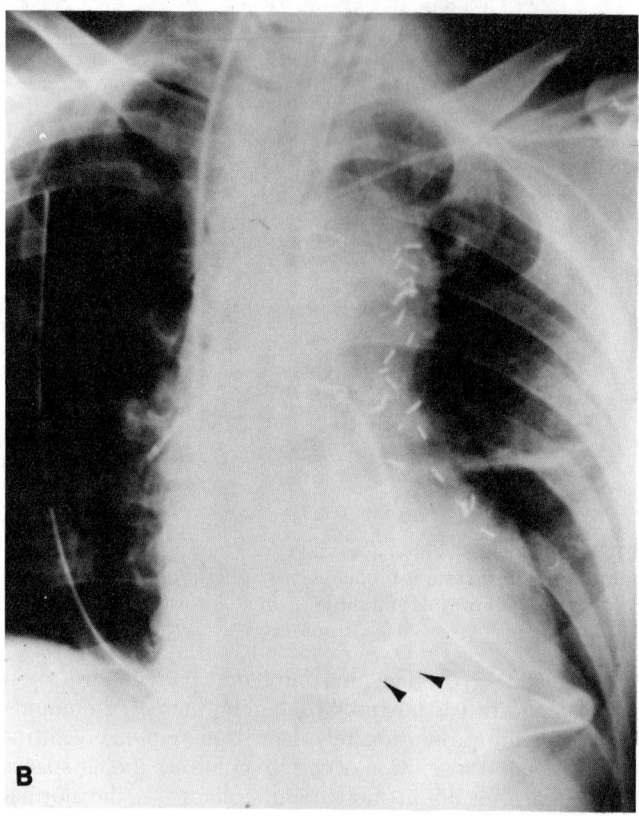

FIGURE 63-19. (**A**) Pulmonary artery catheter was coiled in the right atrium (*open arrows*). The distal tip of the catheter ended in the hepatic veins (*curved arrow*). (**B**) Pulmonary artery catheter was coiled in the right ventricle, resulting in a persistent arrhythmia, which was relieved when the catheter was withdrawn.

occluded when the balloon tip is inflated. The catheter should remain in one of the larger pulmonary arteries on deflation of the balloon tip. Inadvertent distal positioning increases the risk of pulmonary infarction distal to the catheter tip and should be avoided. Notice that the distal tip of the catheter must be evaluated in terms of distance from the hilum rather than advancement toward the lateral chest wall. Catheters that are positioned in lower lobe vessels may lie fairly medially but extend too far from the central hilar area and thus be positioned too distally (Fig. 63-20).

CENTRAL VENOUS PRESSURE CATHETERS

In modern ICUs, central venous pressure catheters are less commonly used for pressure measurement but often are placed to deliver various medications and fluids. Prospective studies have demonstrated that at least one third of these catheters are incorrectly positioned at the time of initial insertion. Not only does this result in inaccurate pressure

measurements if they are made, but more importantly, this may result in infusion of potentially toxic substances into vessels with insufficient flow to quickly dilute the solution. The most common aberrant locations include the internal jugular veins, the hepatic veins, and the subclavian veins distal to the venous valves.[11] Regarding the latter position, notice that valves are found in both the subclavian and internal jugular veins approximately 2.5 cm from their junction to form the brachiocephalic vein. The location of the valve in the subclavian vein corresponds closely to the anterior portion of the first rib and thus can be approximated with reasonable accuracy on the conventional chest radiograph. Also notice that the medial edge of the first rib defines the anterior thoracic inlet for the subclavian vein. Thus, a catheter that does not cross the medial edge of the anterior first rib (Fig. 63-21) has not entered the thorax and, therefore, cannot accurately measure intrathoracic central venous pressure. Moreover, the catheter lies distal to a venous valve, which may interfere with fluid infusion and with withdrawal of blood for venous sampling through the catheter.

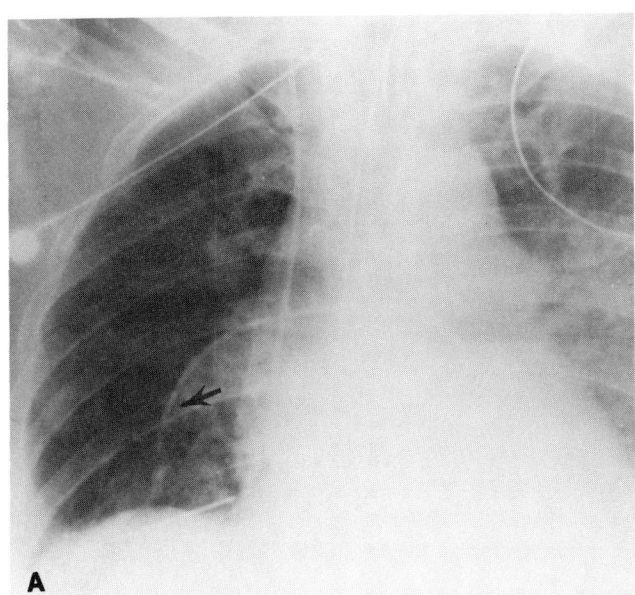
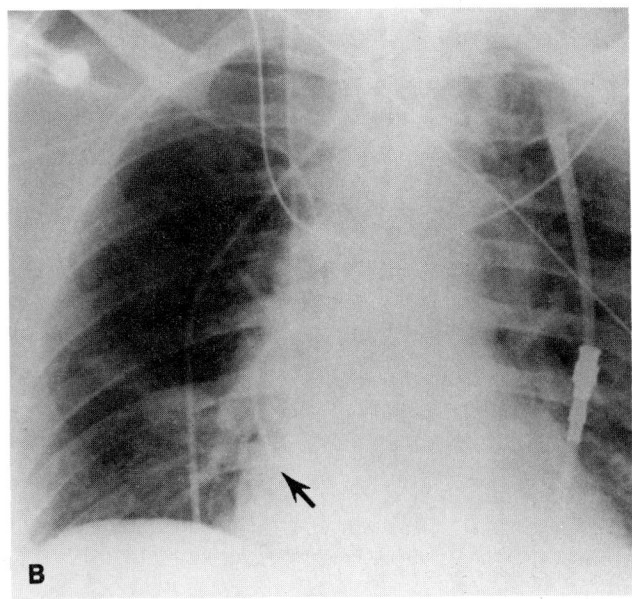

FIGURE 63-20. Pulmonary artery catheter positioned distally. (**A**) Distal positioning of the type generally recognized in that the catheter tip (*arrow*) extends too far toward the lateral chest wall. (**B**) A distal positioning that may be overlooked because the catheter tip is medial (*arrow*) but still extends too far from the hilum, which is the critical measurement.

Subclavian Catheters

The subclavian vein, a large vessel with good blood flow and a consistent anatomic position, potentially provides rapid access to the central venous system. However, because of anatomic features of the region in which the vein lies, percutaneous venipuncture risks several major complications. Anatomically, the vein arches over the medial portion of the first rib to join the internal jugular vein behind the sternoclavicular joint to form the brachiocephalic vein. The subclavian vein is separated from its companion artery as it crosses the first rib by the anterior scalenus muscle. The pleura overlying the apex of the lung lies only 5 mm deep to the vein. The technique for catheter placement involves directing a needle from the midpoint of the clavicle toward the suprasternal notch. Slight posterior angulation of the needle thus may inadvertently lacerate the pleura and result in pneumothorax. Certainly, pneumothorax is the most common complication recognized radiographically and, interestingly, is one that may be overlooked clinically. Therefore, it is mandatory to obtain a chest radiograph after either successful or unsuccessful placement of a subclavian catheter; certainly, a radiograph should be obtained before placement on the opposite side is attempted.

It is also possible to inadvertently place a catheter into either the pleural space or the mediastinum with resultant infusion of fluid into either area. In general, these adverse placements are not clearly delineated radiographically and are more likely to be detected clinically. The major clinical clue seems to be difficulty withdrawing blood through the catheter, although infusion of fluid may be easy. If there is any question as to the position of the catheter, installation of a small amount of intravenous contrast material through the catheter clearly delineates its position. This may be done using conventional radiography with a film exposed immediately after infusion of 5 to 10 mL of material.

INTRAAORTIC COUNTERPULSATION BALLOON

The intraaortic counterpulsation balloon has become increasingly popular for a variety of conditions characterized by low-output cardiac failure. By augmenting diastolic coronary artery perfusion and reducing impedance to ventricular ejection, the device can markedly improve cardiac output. Although various complications are possible with this device, most are not detectable radiographically. The major problem to search for radiographically is inappropriate positioning.[12] Ideally, the catheter tip should be positioned just distal to the origin of the left subclavian artery in the arch of the aorta. In this position, maximum counterpulsation is achieved without risk of embolization of clot from the catheter into the great vessels of the head. Positioning more proximally risks cerebral embolization, or the catheter may inadvertently enter the proximal left subclavian artery (Fig. 63-22) and lacerate the vessel. Distal positions result in decreased effectiveness of diastolic counterpulsation.

ABDOMINAL RADIOGRAPHY ■

Abdominal radiography can be performed at the bedside in ICUs, although because of equipment limitations, it is generally less satisfactory than thoracic imaging. The major problem is that the relatively limited power of mobile radiography units requires longer exposure times, and the thickness of the abdomen enhances the problem even further, often

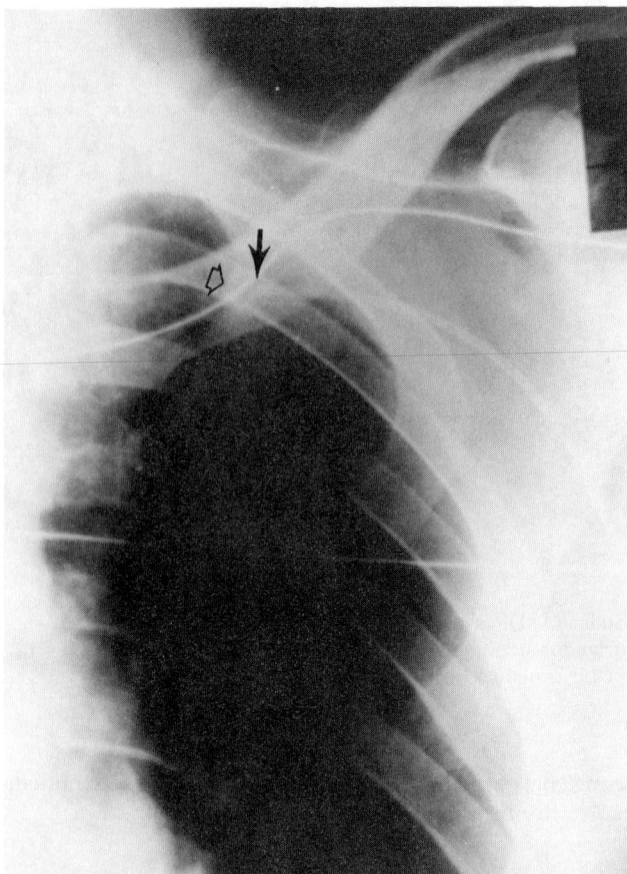

FIGURE 63-21. Central venous pressure catheter that terminates (*solid arrow*) before crossing the medial end of the first rib (*open arrow*) and thus has not entered the thoracic cavity. In addition, there is a valve in the subclavian vein at this same location that may interfere with pressure measurements and fluid infusion or withdrawal.

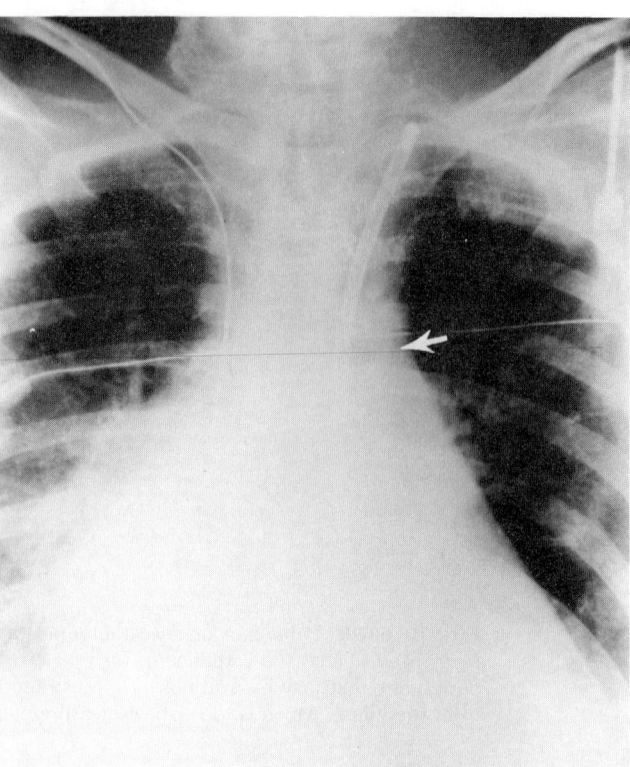

FIGURE 63-22. Intraaortic catheter pulsation balloon shown to extend far above the level of the aortic arch (*arrow*). The catheter extends into the left subclavian artery and may lacerate it when the balloon is inflated.

resulting in considerable motion artifact on the final radiograph. Nonetheless, for certain questions, a plain film abdominal radiograph may provide an accurate answer.[13,14]

FREE INTRAPERITONEAL AIR

Because of the supine position in which most patients are radiographed, detection of free air becomes more difficult, and larger amounts are required before detection is possible. Air generally accumulates in the highest portions of the abdomen, which in the supine position are generally more central. Radiographic signs such as visualization of both sides of a bowel wall (seen between intraluminal air and air in the peritoneal cavity[15]; Fig. 63-23), visualization of the falciform ligament, or generalized increased lucency over the abdomen (Fig. 63-24) are ways in which the diagnosis of free intraperitoneal air may be suspected from a conventional radiograph of the abdomen exposed in the supine position.

Smaller amounts of air are detected by obtaining a lateral decubitus radiograph. It is generally best to place the right side upward so that air may accumulate over the liver, making detection of smaller amounts of air easier. The upright chest radiograph, if it can be obtained, is probably the best

method for detecting small amounts of air, which are readily identified between the diaphragm above and the liver below (Fig. 63-25).

ABDOMINAL DISTENTION

Often, abdominal distention occurs in critically ill patients, and the question is raised as to whether this represents a generalized adynamic ileus of the bowel or bowel obstruction. Distinction is made radiographically by analysis of which portions of the bowel are affected. A generalized ileus occurring from any cause usually affects both large and small bowel. Therefore, distended loops of both colon and small bowel are visualized (Fig. 63-26). The air in the bowel generally extends all the way to the rectum. Occasionally, air may accumulate in the cecum, resulting in disproportionate distention (Fig. 63-27). When the transverse diameter of the cecum exceeds 9 cm, there is an increased risk of rupture. Conversely, with small bowel obstruction, only the small bowel is affected, and the colon is generally collapsed and relatively free of air (Fig. 63-28). Small amounts of air may be seen within the colon, but distention of the small bowel is disproportionate to that seen in the colon.

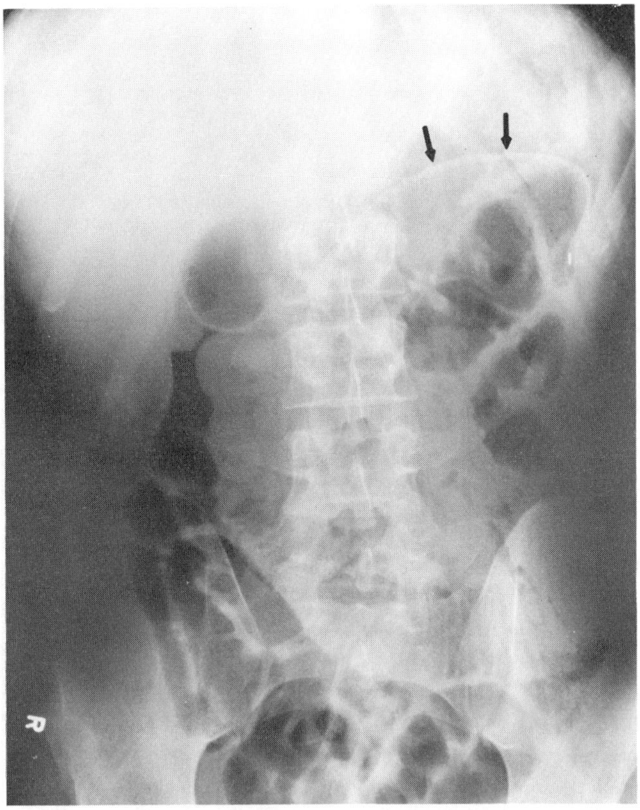

Finally, remember that the obstruction may lie within the colon, and, thus, a portion of the colon also may be distended. However, the portion of the colon distal to the obstruction is relatively gasless and certainly not distended. Rectal examinations, which are generally performed in these patients before radiographic evaluation, may introduce a small amount of gas into the distal rectum, but this should not confuse the overall radiographic pattern.

ISCHEMIC DISEASE

The critically ill patient is also at risk for catastrophic vascular accident, and the bowel gas pattern should be examined for evidence of edema in the bowel wall. This is variously referred to as thumbprinting or thickening of bowel wall loops and occasionally can be recognized with a high degree of certainty. However, because edema takes time to develop, it is a late sign of ischemia or infarction.

NEWER IMAGING TECHNOLOGY

The last 20 years have seen the introduction and refinement of several important new imaging technologies. Although conventional radiography remains the foundation of diagnostic imaging in critically ill patients, judicious use of newer technologies has assumed an important role in their evaluation. Both computed tomography (CT) and ultrasonography have become widely used in the management of severely traumatized or critically ill patients. Magnetic resonance imaging (MRI) has emerged as a powerful imaging technol-

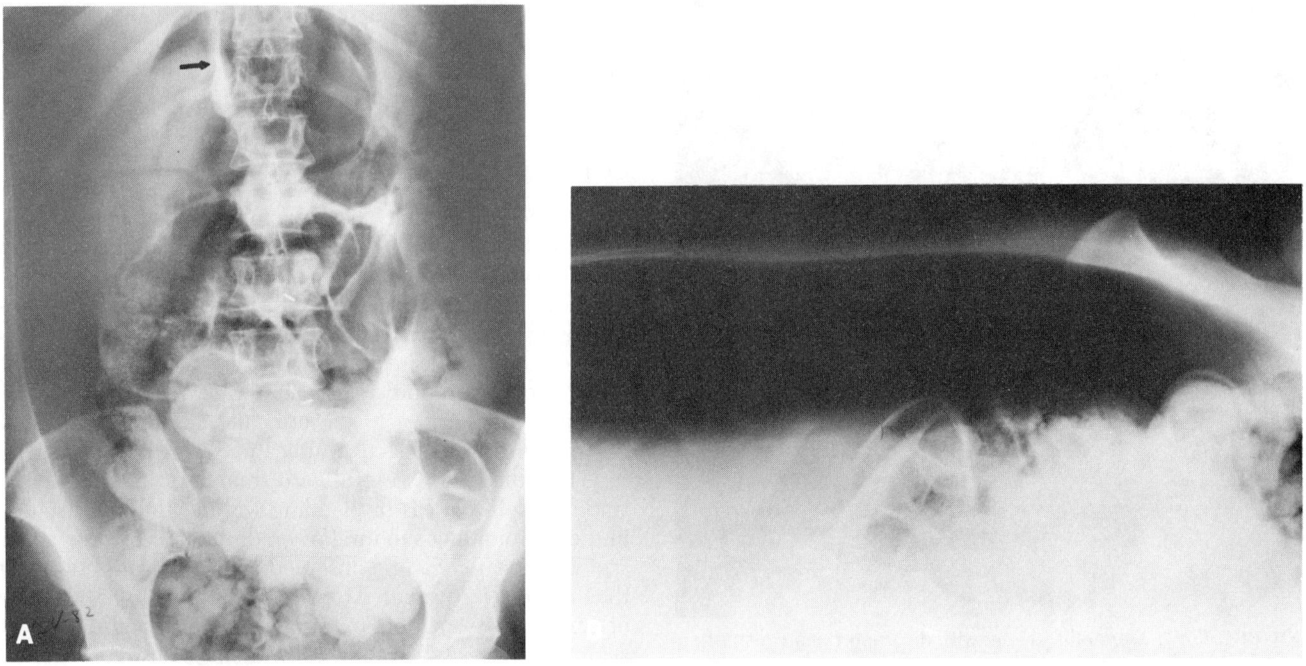

FIGURE 63-23. Free intraperitoneal air demonstrated on a supine radiograph of the abdomen. Notice characteristic visualization of both sides of bowel wall (*arrows*) seen because of air in the bowel lumen on the inside and air free in the peritoneal space on the outside.

FIGURE 63-24. (**A**) Massive amount of free intraperitoneal air as evidenced by increased lucency over the entire abdomen, visualization of both sides of bowel walls in multiple locations, and visualization of the falciform ligament (*arrow*). (**B**) Lateral decubitus view in same patient again demonstrates a massive amount of free intraperitoneal air.

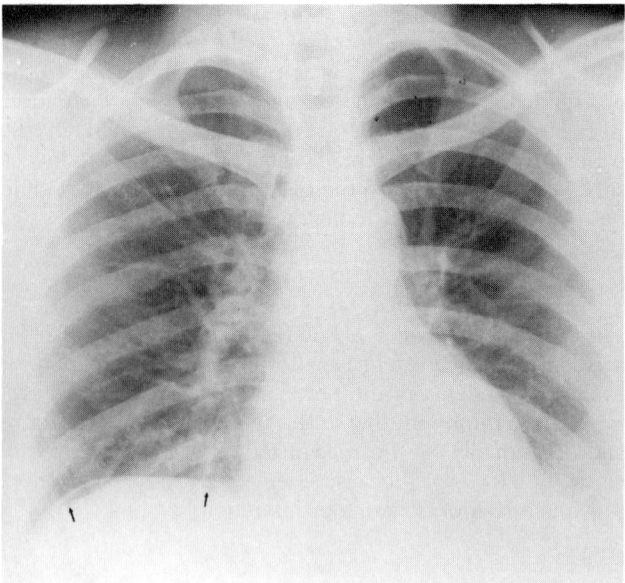

FIGURE 63-25. Small amounts of free intraperitoneal air are best demonstrated on the erect chest radiograph. Air (*arrows*) is contrasted between the liver below and the diaphragm above. If possible, the upright position should be maintained for 5 to 10 minutes to allow the air to move into the subdiaphragmatic area.

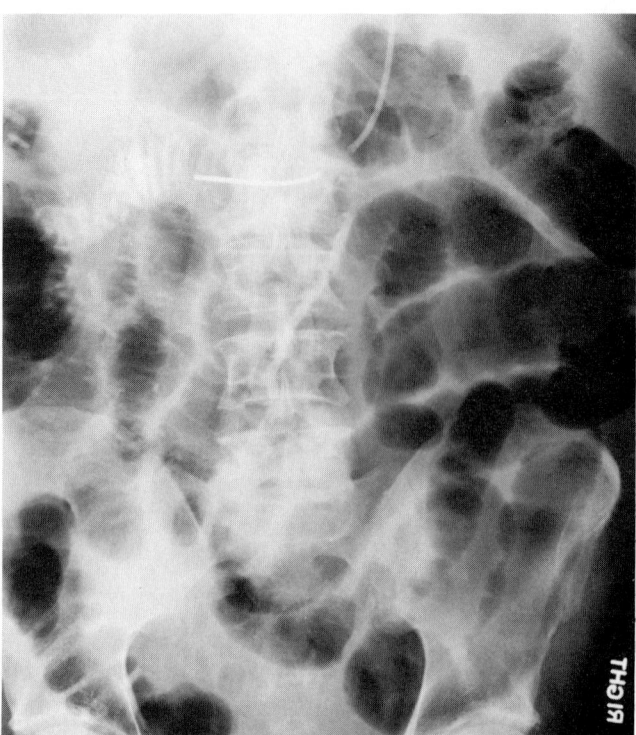

FIGURE 63-26. Adynamic ileus. Supine radiograph of the abdomen demonstrating distention of large and small bowel loops. The small bowel is recognized by the numerous closely spaced lines crossing the lumen. The colon is recognized by haustral markings and its characteristic location along the outer sides of the abdomen. Distention of large and small bowel suggests an ileus.

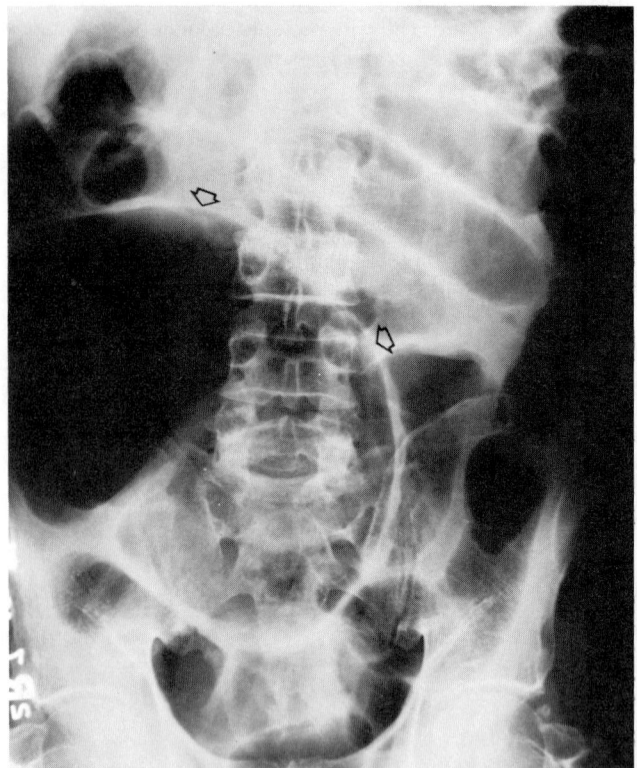

FIGURE 63-27. Generalized ileus with disproportionate distention of the cecum (*open arrows*). When the cecal diameter exceeds 9 cm, there is increased risk of rupture. Changing the patients' position so that the cecum is not uppermost, because it is often in the supine position, may relieve the condition, although more frequently colonoscopy is required to decompress the cecum.

ogy with limited but definite indications in critically ill patients.[16,17] The development of self-shielded magnets and of support and monitoring devices compatible with strong magnetic fields has allowed application of the technology to this patient population.

COMPUTED TOMOGRAPHY

Computed tomography has revolutionized diagnostic imaging since its introduction in the early 1970s. Rapid refinement in the technology has resulted in scan times routinely in the range of 2 to 10 seconds. The axial images produced provide an exquisite look at the underlying body parts. Although the technology has been used throughout the medical community to answer a wide range of diagnostic questions, application to the critically ill patient has been reserved for more selective indications.

CT of the head is useful with trauma or altered mental status to detect areas of bleeding within the brain itself or in the surrounding subdural or epidural spaces. Ventricular size and position can be observed, and the overall status of the brain can be evaluated for remote infarctions or evidence of atrophy. Evaluation of paranasal sinuses also can be achieved; this may be useful in identifying sinusitis associated with infection or nasotracheal intubation.

Scanning of the abdomen may detect abscesses that are recognized as localized collections of fluid and, occasionally, of gas. Opacification of the gastrointestinal tract with contrast

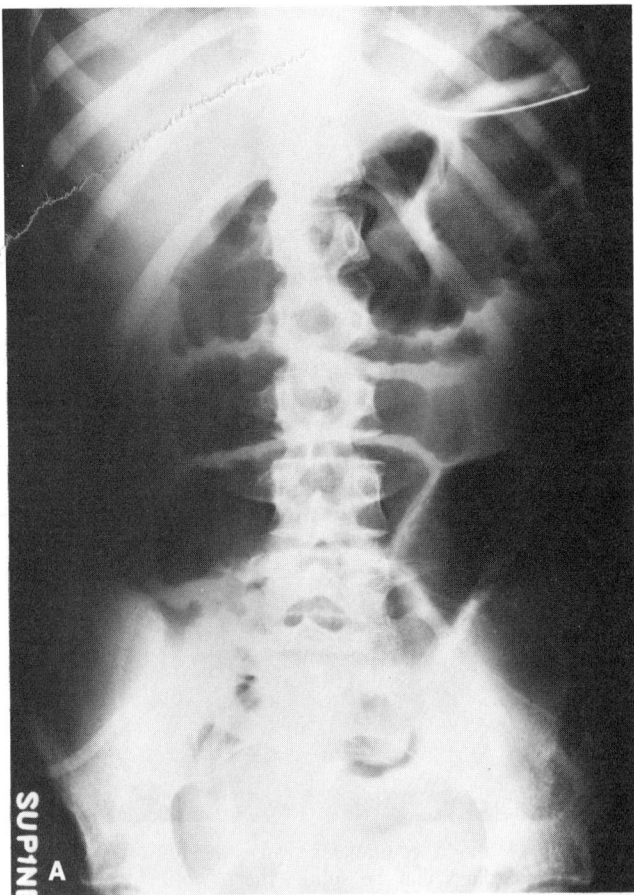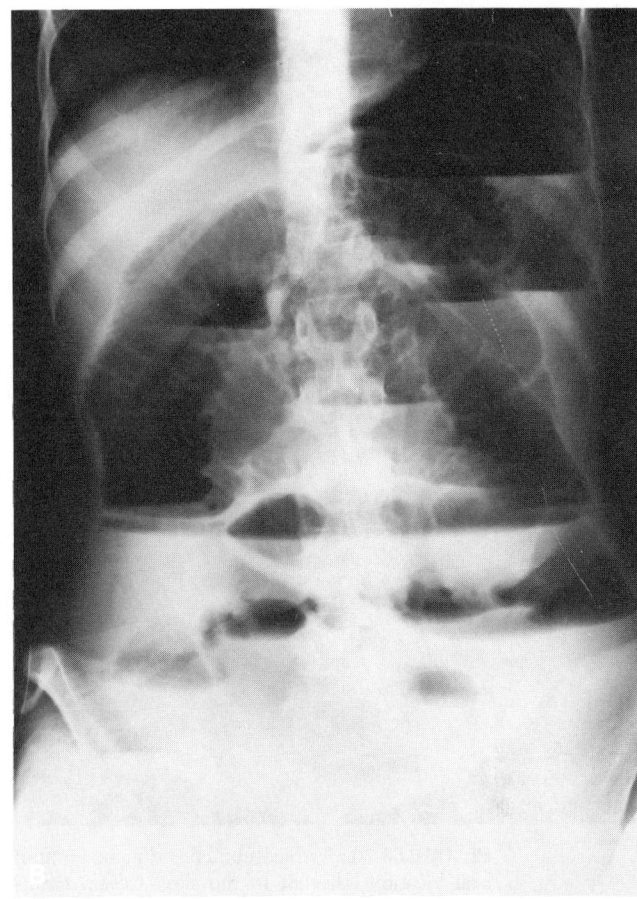

FIGURE 63-28. (**A**) Classic small bowel obstruction. Multiple loops of small bowel are distended. There is no gas in the colon. (**B**) On the erect view, multiple air–fluid levels are seen throughout the small bowel.

material is necessary to distinguish this pattern from the bowel. In addition to diagnosis, percutaneous catheter aspiration guided by the CT may be definitive therapy for intraabdominal abscesses. Abdominal CT also is used in patients with abdominal trauma.

Head

Computed tomography of the head is useful in trauma or altered mental status to detect areas of bleeding within the brain itself or in the surrounding subdural or epidural spaces. Ventricular size and position can be noted, and the overall status of the brain can be evaluated for remote infarctions or evidence of atrophy. Evaluation of paranasal sinuses can also be achieved; this may be useful in identifying sinusitis associated with infection or nasotracheal intubation.

Before the advent of CT, conventional skull radiography offered only a crude method of assessing the underlying brain. Although a fracture likely indicated significant trauma to the head, its presence did not indicate with certainty the status of the brain, and its absence in no way precluded significant underlying injury. With CT, a direct view of the brain became possible. In most ICUs, head CT has been applied to evaluate the the brain for areas of bleeding, either within the brain substance itself (Fig. 63-29) or in the sur-

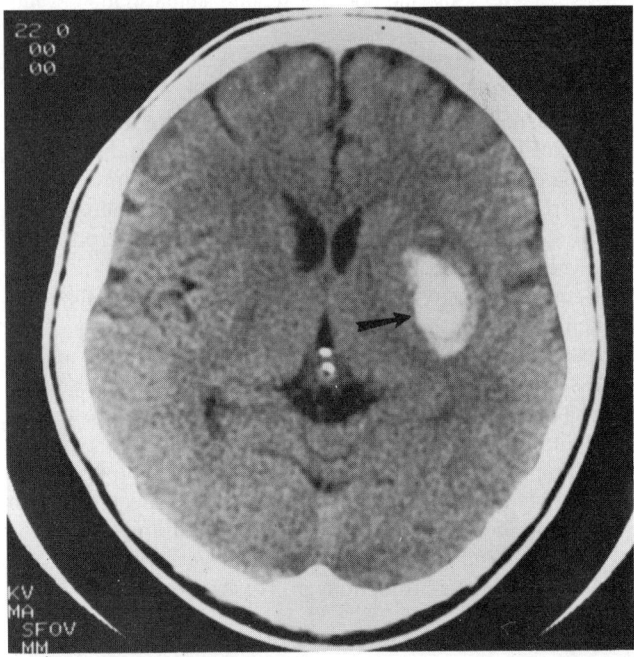

FIGURE 63-29. Classic hypertensive bleed demonstrated by computed tomography scanning. A large area of intracerebral blood is identified (*arrow*). Characteristically, in this setting blood accumulates in the basal ganglia.

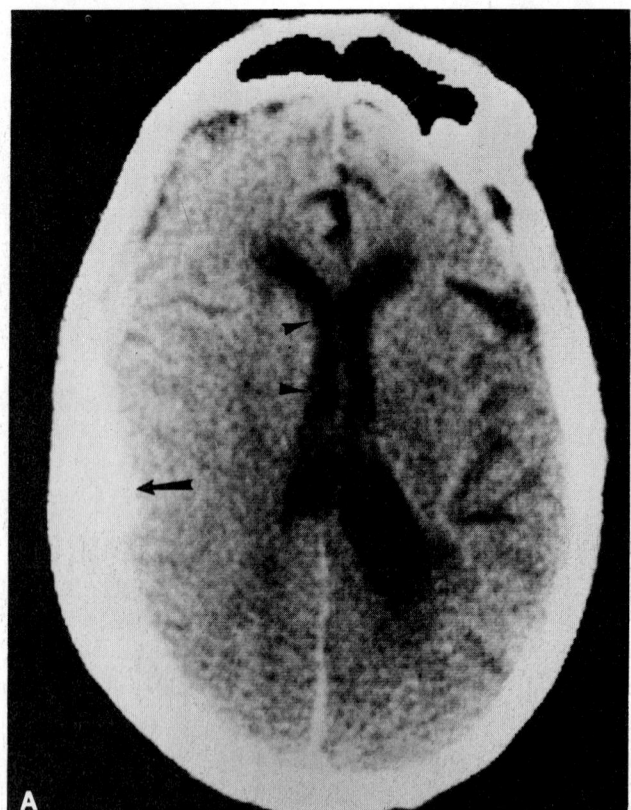 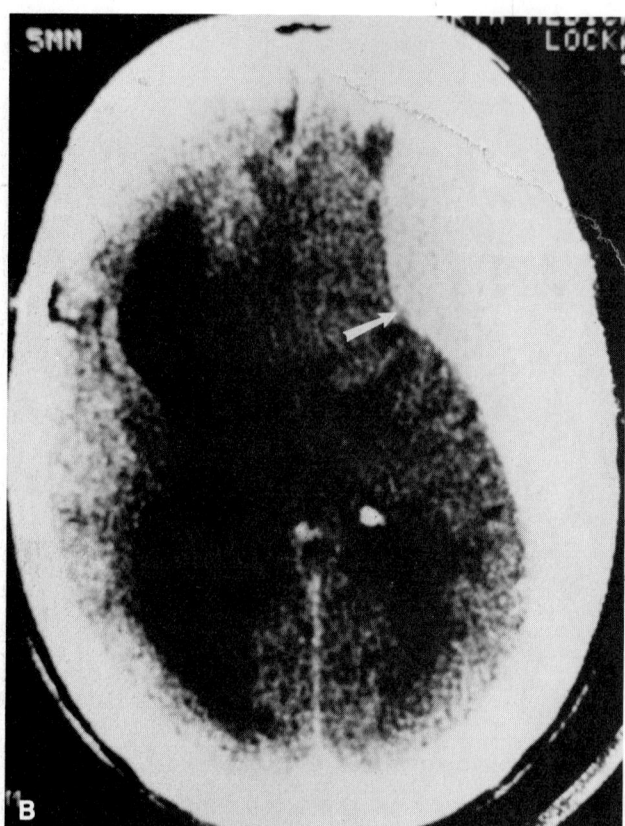

FIGURE 63-30. Extracerebral bleeding on computed tomography. (**A**) Blood accumulates in an extracerebral location adjacent to the skull (*black arrow*). Although the findings may be subtle, the obvious asymmetry is immediately evident. In addition, there is compression of underlying sulci as well as mass effect on the ipsilateral ventricular system (*arrowheads*). These findings allow the diagnosis of subdural hematoma to be made. (**B**) Large extracerebral collection of blood (*white arrow*) compressing underlying brain parenchyma and resulting in midline shift. Acute bleeding is readily imaged on computed tomography scans and does not require administration of intravenous contrast material.

rounding subdural or epidural spaces (Fig. 63-30). Blood is readily visualized on the CT scan in all but the most anemic patients. Thus, intracerebral hemorrhage can be readily identified,[17] as can recent bleeding into the subdural or epidural spaces. The ventricular size also can be evaluated, as can the overall status of the brain for remote infarctions or for evidence of atrophy (Fig. 63-31).

Because changes in mental status are often extremely difficult to evaluate in critically ill patients, the ability of CT to exclude diseases requiring prompt intervention and to assess chronic changes such as remote cerebrovascular accidents (Fig. 63-32) or generalized brain atrophy is most helpful in ultimately directing management of such patients. Scanning of the head also can reveal various other causes of change in mental status, such as unsuspected tumor masses or metastases (Fig. 63-33). In addition, evaluation of the paranasal sinuses is readily achieved, which may be important in certain infectious processes involving the brain.

Abdomen

In most situations in the critically ill but nontraumatized patient, CT has been used to evaluate the abdominal and

pelvic cavities for the presence of abscess. The problem of unexplained fever in the critically ill patient is relatively common, and the ability to exclude an abscess that might require surgery is most valuable. Abscesses are recognized as localized collections of fluid and occasionally gas (Fig. 63-34). Because the bowel can give a similar radiographic appearance, it is necessary to opacify the gastrointestinal tract with radiographic contrast material. If the stomach and large and small bowel are completely opacified, then recognition of an abscess within the peritoneal or pelvic spaces is relatively easy. It is also possible to detect abscesses outside of these areas, either in solid organs (Fig. 63-35) or in surrounding muscle groups or soft tissue.

The ability of CT to detect an abscess and to define its extent is extremely helpful in managing patients with abdominal abscesses. Although in the past an abscess generally required surgery, the recent introduction of percutaneous drainage techniques often allows a focal abscess to be drained (see Fig. 63-34) without having to take the patient to the operating room. Insertion of catheters into abscess cavities under CT guidance has become an accepted technique and is used successfully in appropriate cases. Percutaneous catheter aspiration guided by CT may be definitive therapy for intraabdominal abscesses.

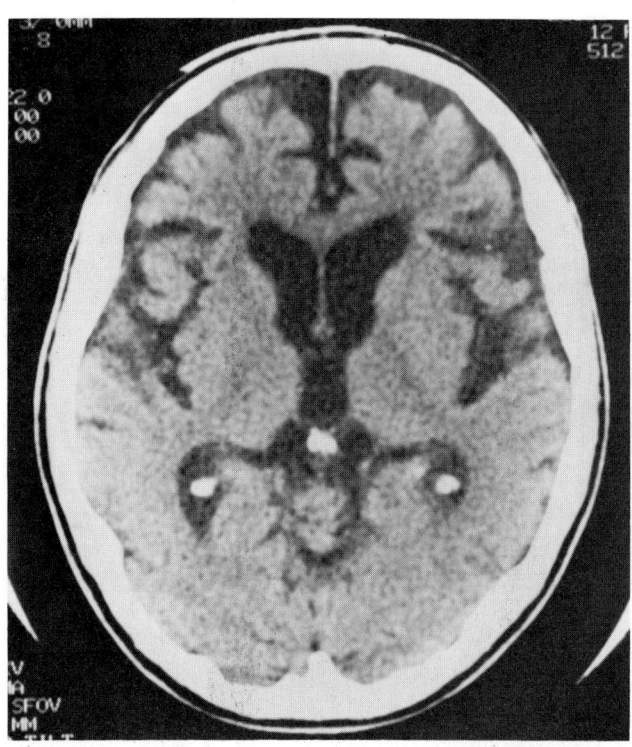

FIGURE 63-31. Moderate atrophy of the brain. Notice increased size of the sulci and the ventricular system. There is no evidence of mass effect. This generalized atrophy is commonly seen in older patients.

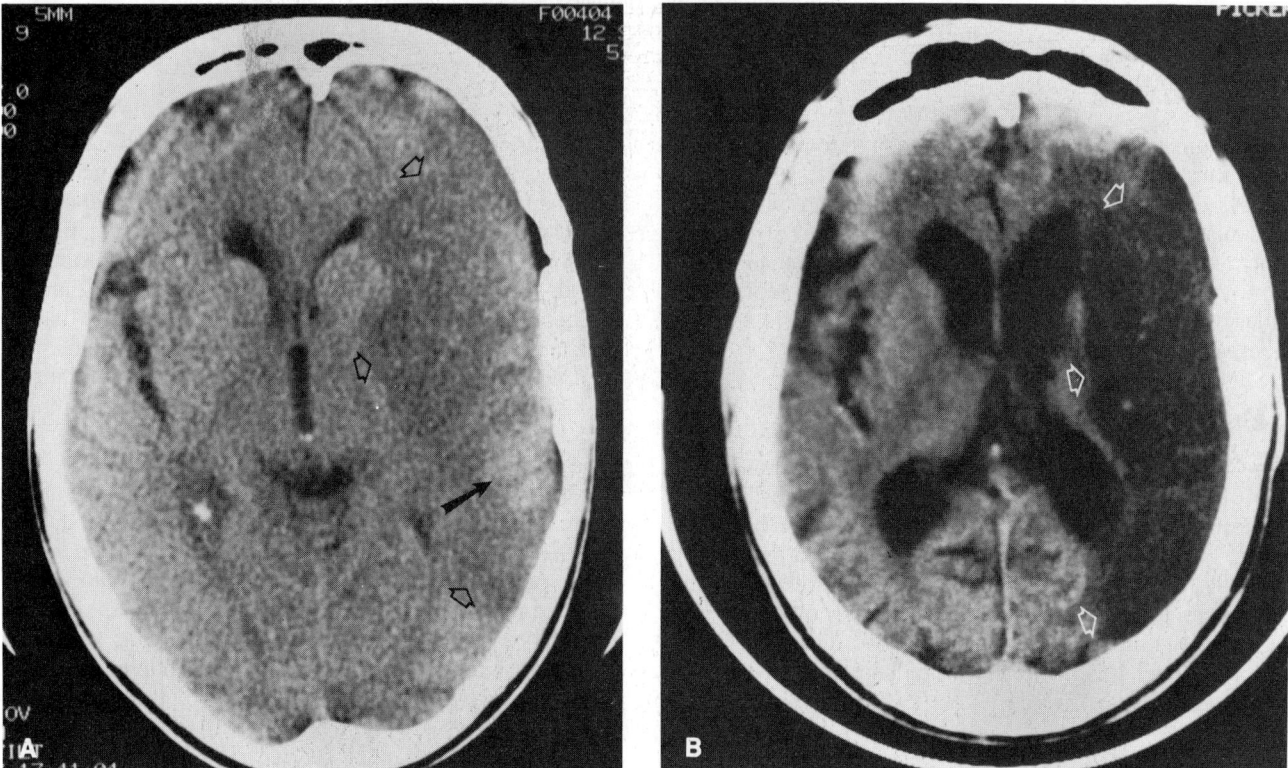

FIGURE 63-32. (**A**) Acute cerebral infarction as evidenced by decreased opacity and edema involving the distribution of the left middle cerebral artery (*open arrows*). An area of increased signal secondary to bleeding within the infarct is also demonstrated (*black arrow*). This represents a hemorrhagic infarction. Also notice evidence of mass effect on the ipsilateral ventricle. (**B**) Remote infarct demonstrating lucency throughout the distribution of the middle cerebral artery (*open white arrows*), with associated enlargement of the ventricular system.

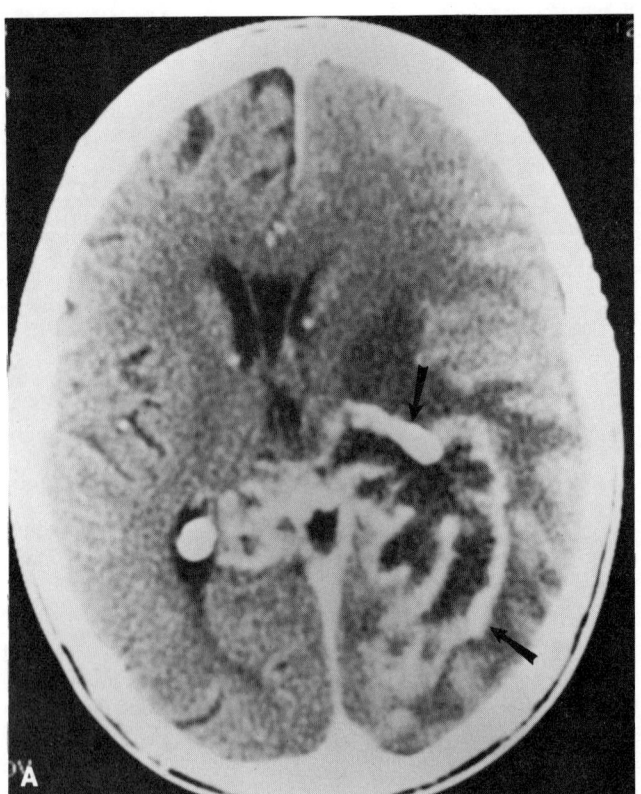
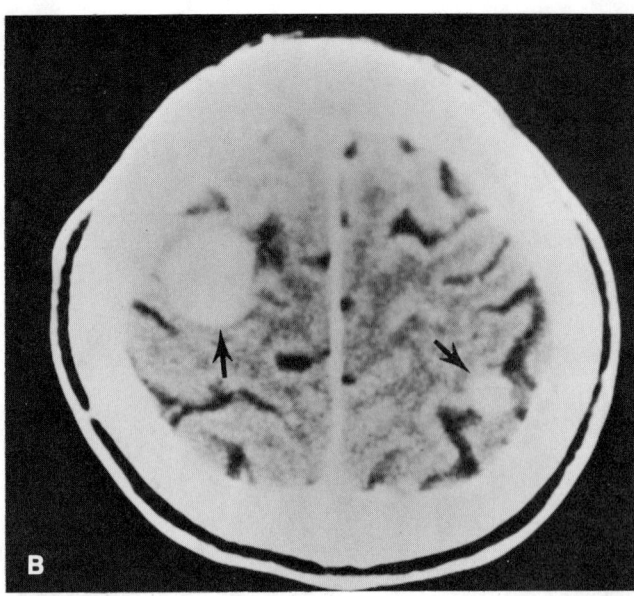

FIGURE 63-33. (**A**) Primary brain tumor (*arrows*). Histologically, this proved to be an astrocytoma of the left parietooccipital lobe that crossed the midline through the corpus callosum. Notice also the effect on the ventricles and midline shift. (**B**) Two metastatic foci (*arrows*) secondary to a primary carcinoma of the lung.

In traumatized patients, CT may be used to rapidly assess the status of many organs such as the liver, spleen, and kidneys and to preclude the need for angiography.[18] It is particularly useful to evaluate retroperitoneal structures, which are difficult to evaluate by physical examination and even peritoneal lavage.[19] A retroperitoneal hematoma secondary to a fractured transverse process can be seen in Figure 63-36.

Limitations of Computed Tomography

The CT scanner itself is extremely expensive (average cost over $1 million), thus limiting to some extent the availability of the technology. In addition, the patient must be transported from the protected ICU environment to receive CT scanning. This is often difficult, given the instability of the patient and the monitoring and life-support equipment and requiring significant forethought and coordination of support personnel. Also, metal foreign bodies may interfere with imaging.

ULTRASONOGRAPHY

Ultrasonography is an outgrowth of sonar technology developed during World War II. Since being introduced to medical practice in the mid-1970s, it has quickly assumed a place in the assessment of various medical conditions. Although conventional or computer-assisted radiographic techniques and ultrasound produce images that demonstrate similar anatomy, they rely on significantly different principles to produce their final image. Unlike methods that depend on attenuation of the radiographic beam by intervening tissues, ultrasonic techniques depend on the acoustical properties of body tissues to provide the basis for the resulting image.

The advantage of ultrasonography lies in the fact that no ionizing radiation is involved, making the technique feasible for pregnant women and young patients. It also eliminates the risk to support personnel. In addition, the equipment is mobile and may easily be brought to the bedside of a critically ill patient. Finally, it is relatively inexpensive and thus can be widely available. The major disadvantage of the technique is that it is extremely operator-dependent, that is, the quality of the examination is almost totally dependent on the person doing the study. In addition, the ultrasound beam cannot be effectively passed through either air or bone. Therefore, the technique can be limited in certain anatomic areas or if considerable intraabdominal gas is present.

ASSESSMENT OF THE KIDNEYS

Impaired renal function and a rising creatinine level in critically ill patients often raise the question of acute obstruction of the ureter. This diagnostic possibility can rapidly be assessed using ultrasound because both kidneys are generally easily visualized (Fig. 63-37A). Numerous echoes generally

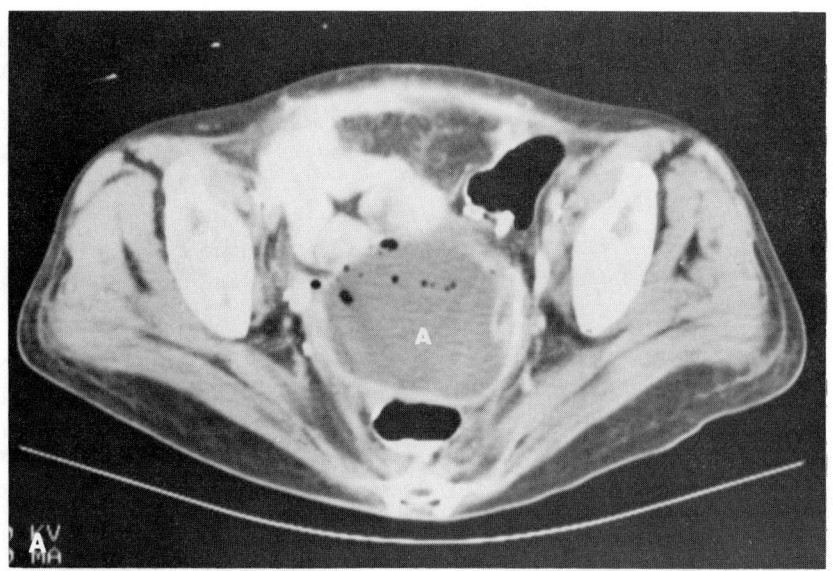

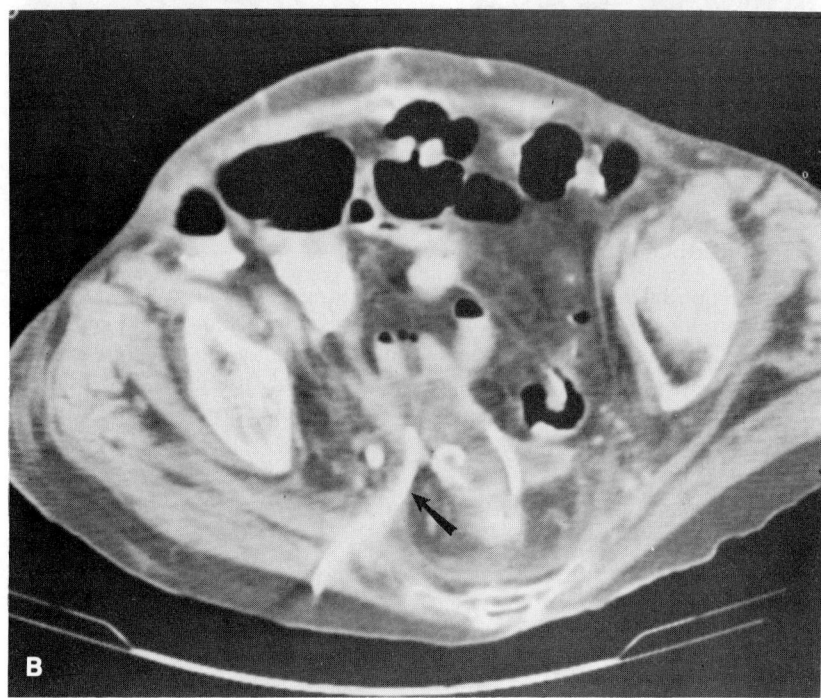

FIGURE 63-34. (**A**) Large localized collection of fluid with gas within it representing an abscess (*A*). (**B**) Drainage catheter (*arrow*) has been placed into the abscess cavity percutaneously to drain it. Notice the marked reduction in size of the abscess seen in *A*.

emanate from the fat surrounding the central collecting system within the kidneys, and dilatation of these collecting systems is easily appreciated on ultrasonic examination (see Fig. 63-37*B*). Conversely, kidneys affected by various disease processes damaging the renal parenchyma show an increased echogenicity in the parenchyma surrounding the more central fat but no evidence of dilatation of the collecting systems.[20]

DETECTION OF GALLSTONES

Ultrasonography has become the method of choice for evaluating suspected cholelithiasis (Fig. 63-38).[21–24] Identification of echogenic foci within the gallbladder, accompanied by

acoustic shadowing distal to the echogenic focus and movement of the foci, is virtually 100% diagnostic of gallstones. The test is easily performed and provides a rapid method of establishing this diagnosis.

BILIARY DUCT OBSTRUCTION

The liver is also readily amenable to ultrasonic evaluation[25] (Fig. 63-39*A*). Dilated bile ducts are easily visualized within the liver parenchyma, and the technique can quickly demonstrate obstructed biliary ducts in a convincing fashion (see Fig. 63-39*B*). In addition, it is often possible to follow the dilated ducts to the level of obstruction making subsequent

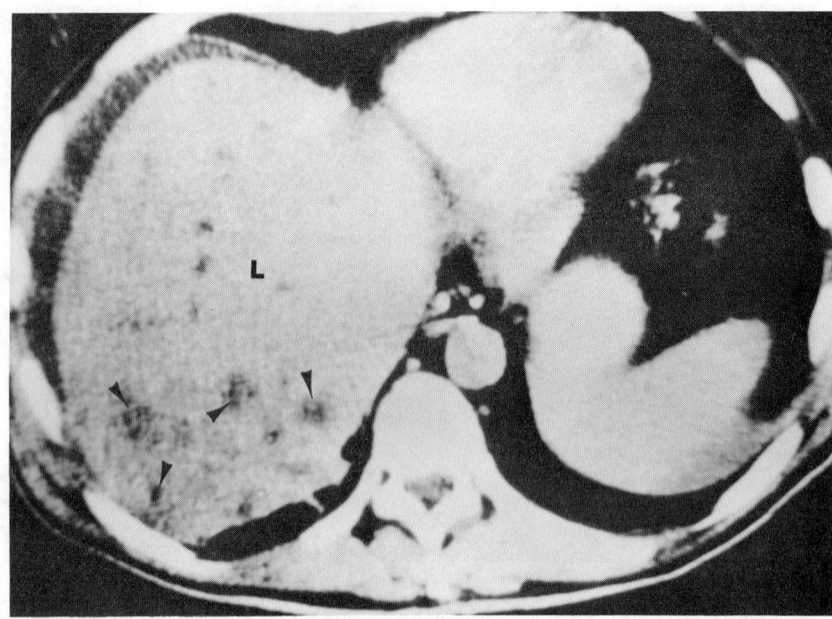

FIGURE 63-35. Multiple abscesses (*arrowheads*) within the liver (L).

surgery much easier. A variety of intrahepatic masses may also be demonstrated by ultrasound.

USE IN PREGNANCY

Because no ionizing radiation is involved, ultrasonic techniques are ideal for evaluation of pelvic organs in pregnant women. The uterus, ovaries, and adjacent adnexal areas are readily assessed. The technique has been reasonably useful in distinguishing intrauterine pregnancies from ectopic preg-

nancies (Fig. 63-40). It can rapidly establish the diagnosis of ectopic pregnancy.

MAGNETIC RESONANCE IMAGING ■

Magnetic resonance imaging has been another dramatic step forward in the realm of diagnostic imaging. Initially, application to evaluation of the critically ill patient was precluded by the fact that devices to support and monitor patients

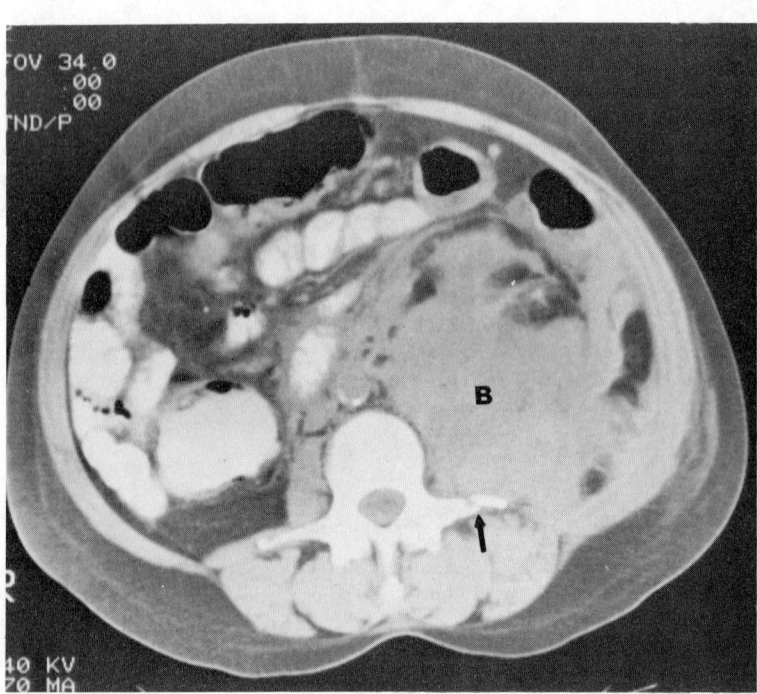

FIGURE 63-36. Retroperitoneal bleed (B) into the left psoas muscle enlarges and distorts it. The bleed was secondary to trauma evidence by the associated fractured left transverse process (*arrow*).

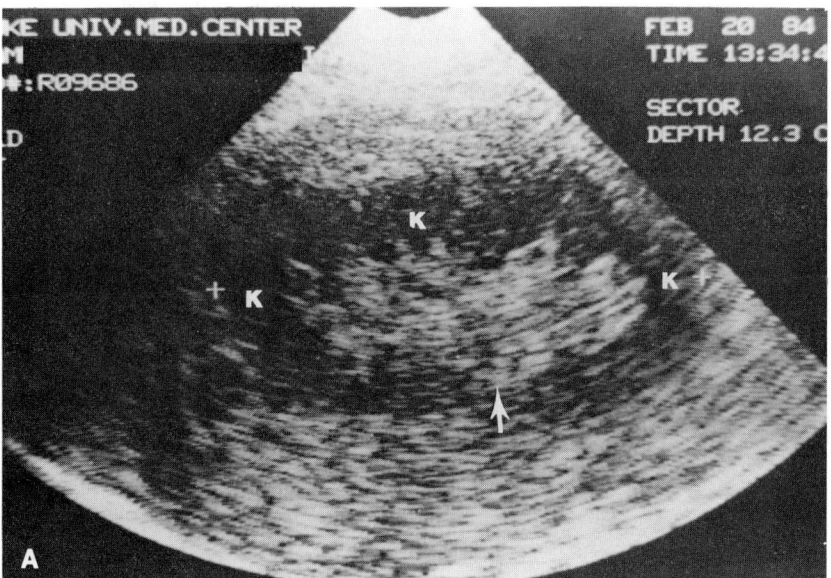

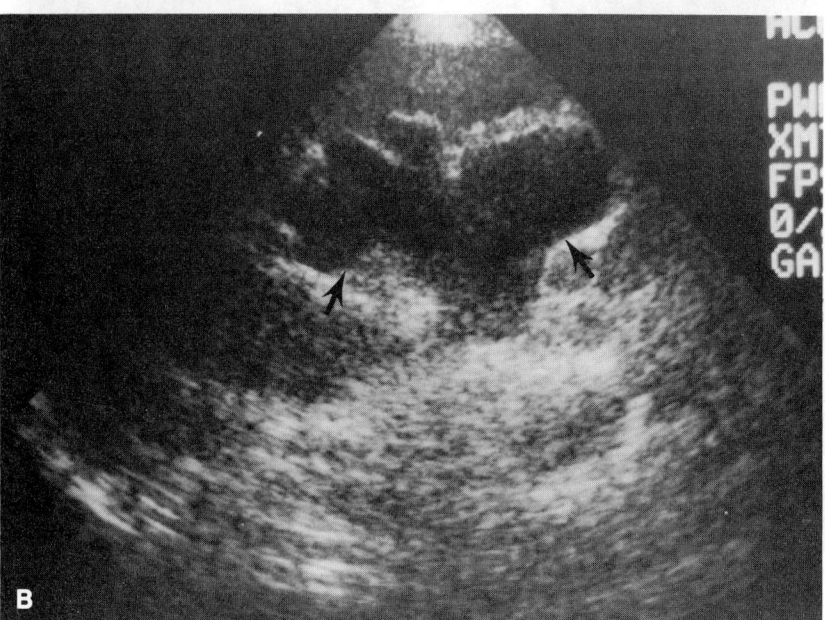

FIGURE 63-37. (**A**) Normal result of ultrasound of the kidney demonstrates increased echogenicity in the central renal sinus (*white arrow*) when sound is reflected off fat in the renal hilum. The cortex of the kidney (**K**) is seen normally as a less echogenic area surrounding the central ring of sinus fat. (**B**) Grossly dilated collecting system. In this case, the hydronephrotic collecting system (*arrows*) distorts and obliterates the central fat.

while in strong magnetic fields were nonexistent. However, because of the great value of MRI, devices have been created that allow ventilatory support and cardiovascular monitoring, even while the patient is in a magnetic field. In addition, some magnets are self-shielded, allowing conventional support and monitoring equipment to be moved into the imaging area.

MRI takes advantage of predictable alterations in protons when placed within strong magnetic fields and perturbed by radiofrequency pulses. The technique has several distinct advantages, including the ability to image large areas of the body quickly and to acquire data in three dimensions, allowing for display in which every projection provides the greatest information. This capability is to be contrasted with CT in which images are routinely obtained in axial projection

and generally displayed in a similar format. In addition, there is no ionizing radiation with MRI, making it particularly applicable to young children and pregnant women.

The major applications of MRI to assessment of the critically ill patient thus far have focused on evaluation of the central nervous system, particularly the spinal cord. In addition, the ability of the technique to visualize cartilage and ligaments has made it an excellent method for evaluation of joint injuries, particularly in the knee. Its ability to visualize the vascular system has made it useful in detection of deep venous thrombosis and a variety of abnormalities of large arteries and veins.

Potential disadvantages of the technique include the considerable expense of the equipment and the fact that it is not mobile, thereby requiring moving the patient to the

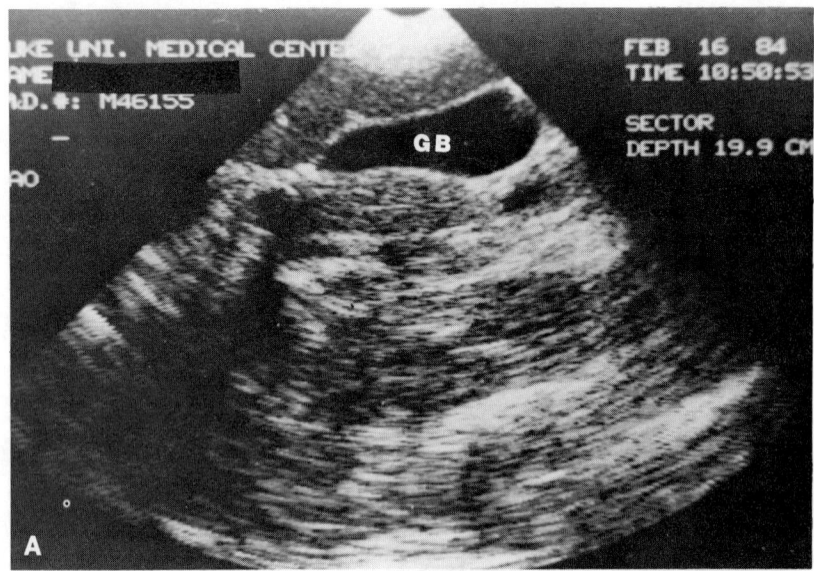

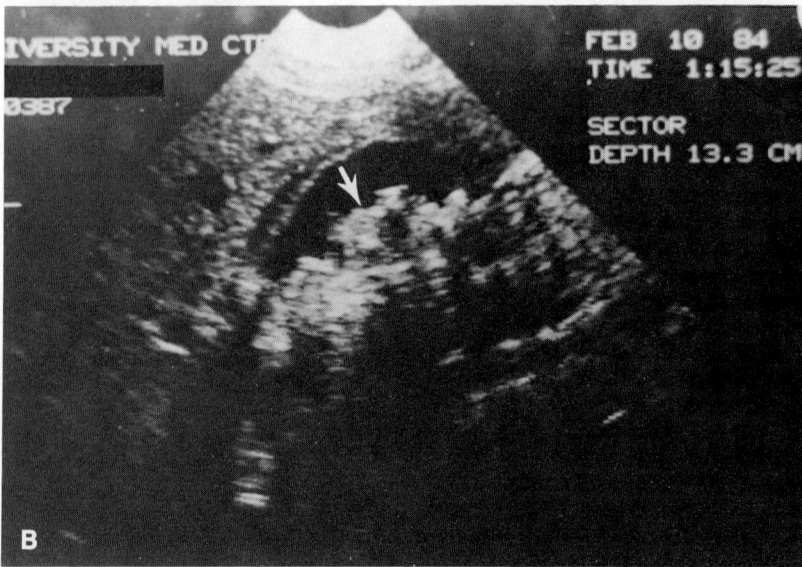

FIGURE 63-38. (**A**) Normal examination of the gallbladder (GB). (**B**) Multiple gallstones within the gallbladder. The gallstones (*arrow*) are visualized as areas of increased echogenicity with distal acoustic shadowings that move with changes in patient position.

equipment rather than vice versa. In addition, specialized equipment must be used to support and monitor the patient.

SPINAL CORD IMAGING

The major application of MRI in the critically ill patient has been for analysis of the central nervous system, particularly the spinal cord. As observed earlier, most abnormalities of the brain in the critically ill patient can be readily and effectively analyzed using CT. However, particularly in cases of spinal trauma or neoplastic disease involving the spinal canal, MRI offers significant advantages. It allows visualization of the entire spinal cord and, in addition, provides display of the information in an easily understood format. In the setting of trauma, lesions within the spinal cord can be readily discerned (Fig. 63-41), and extradural blocks that previously

required myelography for elucidation can be readily demonstrated (Fig. 63-42).

MUSCULOSKELETAL INJURY

Magnetic resonance imaging has become the technique of choice for evaluating soft tissue and cartilage injuries including ligament tears and meniscal injuries in the knee, although these are rarely of clinical importance in the critically ill patient.

VASCULAR ABNORMALITIES

Magnetic resonance imaging has replaced contrast venography as the imaging technique of choice for the evaluation of deep venous thrombosis in the lower extremities and

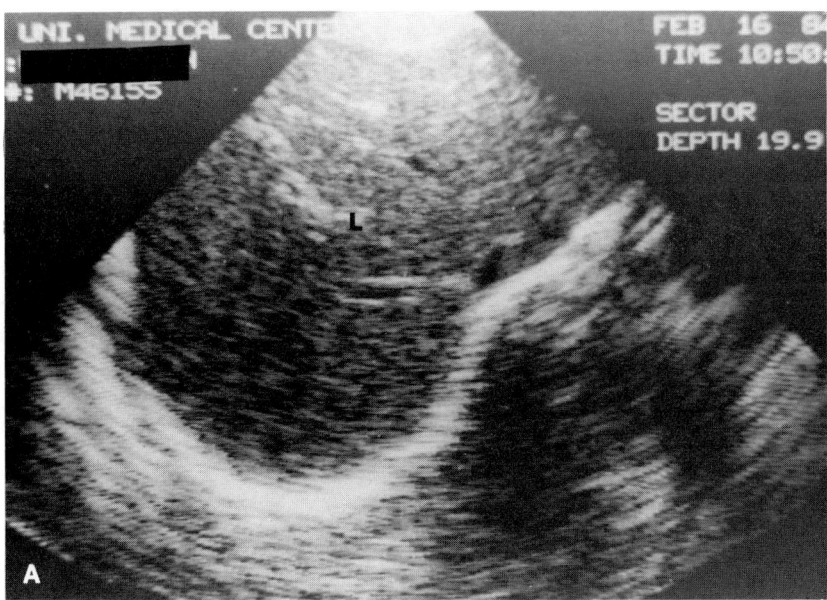

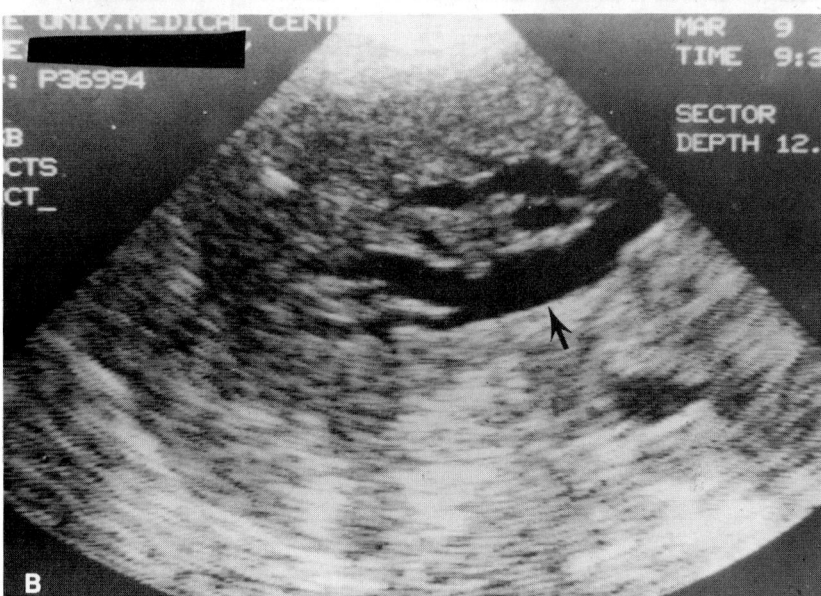

FIGURE 63-39. (**A**) Ultrasound of the liver (L) shows homogeneous echogenicity. (**B**) Markedly dilated biliary ducts (*arrow*) within the liver.

provides reasonable assessment of great vessels in both the abdomen and the thorax. Preliminary investigations suggest that this technique will also be useful in the assessment of pulmonary emboli; preliminary clinical studies to confirm this possibility are underway.

CONCLUSION ■

The conventional chest radiograph provides much valuable information in the evaluation and management of the critically ill patient. In certain selected situations, conventional abdominal radiography also may be valuable. Bedside exami-

nations of other areas, such as the skull, are generally less rewarding because of equipment limitations, resulting in prolonged exposure times and considerable motion indistinctness on the final image. Evaluation of extremities, particularly for fractures, can be done at bedside, although it is important to obtain right-angle views whenever possible because fractures may be missed on a single projection.

The newer imaging modalities have clearly established themselves in diagnostic imaging of the critically ill. They are used to answer specific questions, and each has significant advantages and disadvantages.[26-29]

The exquisite images provided by CT must be weighed against the difficulties in moving the patient to the scanner and maintaining the patient during the examination. Ex-

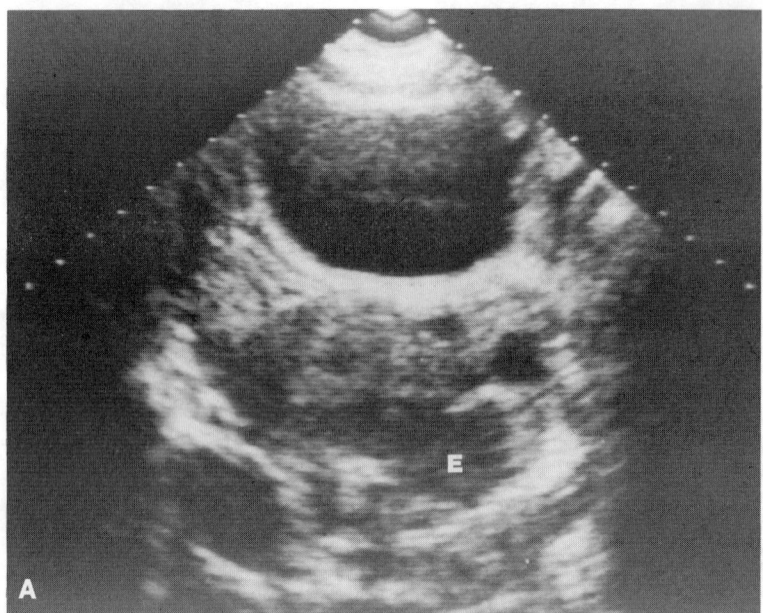

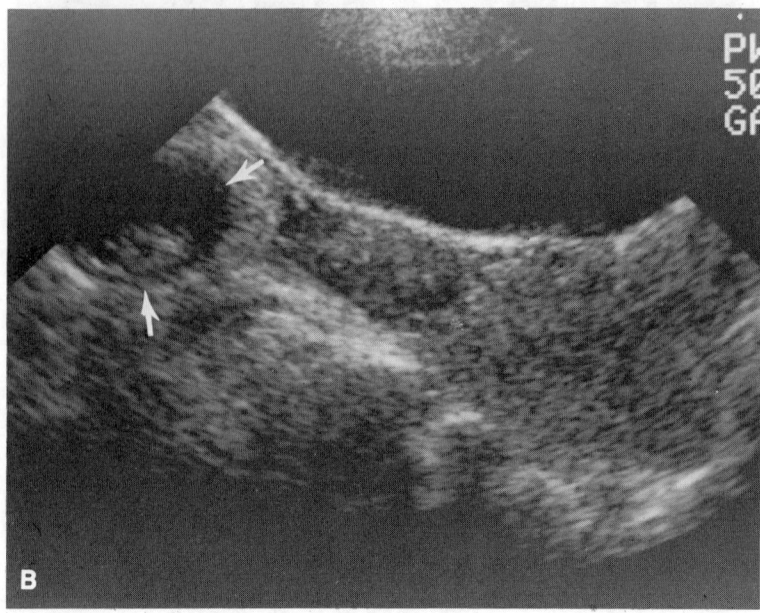

FIGURE 63-40. (**A**) Ectopic pregnancy visualized ultra-sonographically as a mass (E) in the adnexal area. (**B**) Living ectopic pregnancy (*arrows*) lying outside the normal uterus.

penses associated with the equipment itself have, to some extent, limited the availability of this powerful imaging technology.

The advantages of ultrasound lie in its mobile nature, which allows it to be brought to the bedside of the critically ill patient, and the lack of ionizing radiation that makes it exceedingly safe for the patient and medical personnel. In addition, the equipment is of relatively low cost. The disadvantages of the technology lie in its inability to examine all areas of the body because of poor transmission of the ultrasound beam through either air or bone and the tremendous dependence of the technology on the individual opera-

tor. The requirements for highly skilled personnel to obtain meaningful studies, as well the higher degree of difficulty in interpretation of the results, have limited to some extent the widespread application of this technology.

MRI is being applied to the analysis of critically ill patients. The development of monitoring and support devices compatible with magnetic fields has allowed application of the technique, particularly in the analysis of suspected spinal cord abnormalities. The ability to image large areas of the body and to display these images in easily understood formats has enhanced the application of this technology to assessment of the critically ill patient.

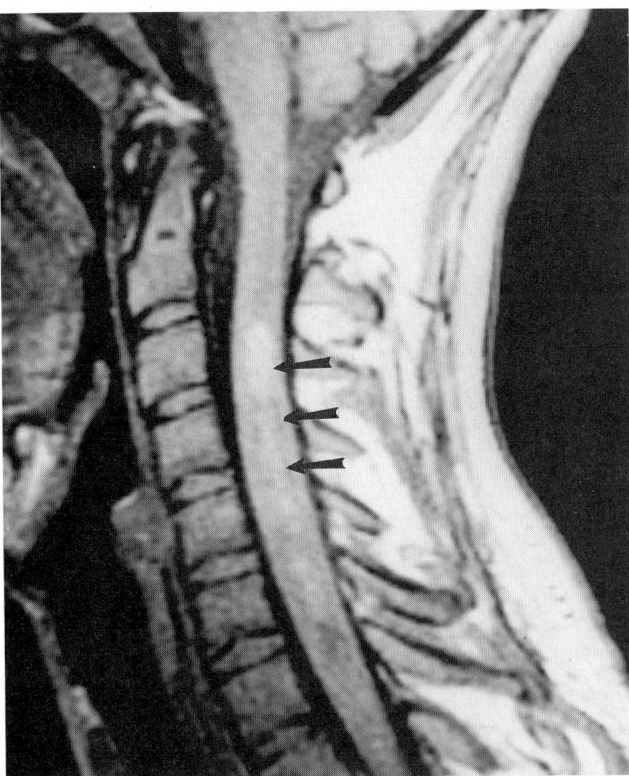

FIGURE 63-41. Magnetic resonance imaging sagittal section through the neck of a patient after trauma. No fractures are present, but the high signal intensity within the spinal cord (*arrows*) reflects subacute hemorrhage (hematomyelia).

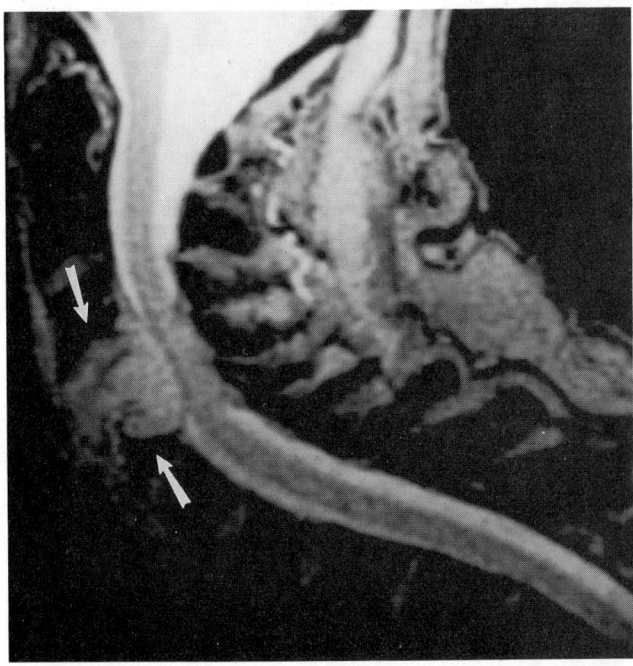

FIGURE 63-42. Magnetic resonance imaging sagittal image of the cervical spine in a patient with quadriparesis. A plasmacytoma of the C-3 vertebral body (*arrows*) is demonstrated impinging on the adjacent spinal cord.

REFERENCES

1. Goodman LR, Putman CE: *Intensive Care Radiology: Imaging of the Critically Ill*, 2nd ed. Philadelphia, WB Saunders, 1983
2. Ravin CE, Putman CE, McLoud TC: Hazards of the intensive care unit. *AJR* 1976;126:423
3. Milne ENC: Chest radiology in the surgical patient. *Surg Clin North Am* 1980;60:1503
4. Chiles C, Ravin CE: Radiographic recognition of pneumothorax in the intensive care unit. *Crit Care Med* 1986;14:677
5. Rohlfing BM, Webb WR, Schlobohm RM: Ventilator-related extra-alveolar air in adults. *Radiology* 1976;121:25
6. Putman CE, Ravin CE: Adult respiratory distress syndrome. In: Goodman LR, Putnam CE (eds). *Intensive Care Radiology: Imaging of the Critically Ill*, 2nd ed. Philadelphia, WB Saunders, 1983:114
7. McLoud TC, Barash PG, Ravin CE: PEEP: Radiographic features and associated complications. *AJR* 1977;129:209
8. Conrardy PA, Goodman LR, Laing FC, et al: Alteration of endotracheal tube position. *Crit Care Med* 1976;4:8
9. Goodman LR, Conrardy PA, Laing FC, et al: Radiographic evaluation of endotracheal tube position. *Am J Roentgenol* 1976;127:433
10. McLoud TC, Putman CE: Radiology of the Swan-Ganz catheter and associated pulmonary complications. *Radiology* 1975;116:19
11. Langston CS: The aberrant central venous catheter and its complications. *Radiology* 1971;100:55
12. Hyson EA, Ravin CE, Kelley MJ, et al: The intra-aortic counter-pulsation balloon: radiographic considerations. *AJR* 1977;128:915
13. Johnson CD, Rice RP: Acute abdomen: plain radiographic evaluation. *Radiographics* 1985;5:259
14. Kelvin FM, Rice RP: Radiologic evaluation of acute abdominal pain arising from the alimentary tract. *Radiol Clin North Am* 1978;16:25
15. Rice RP, Thompson WM, Gedgaudas RK: Diagnosis and significance of extraluminal gas in the abdomen. *Radiographics* 1982;2:819
16. Alfidi RJ, Huaga JR: Symposium on magnetic resonance imaging. *Radiol Clin North Am* 1984;22:765
17. Davis JM: Vascular lesions: intracerebral hemorrhage. In: Taveras JM, Ferrucci JT (eds). *Radiology*, vol 45. Philadelphia, JB Lippincott, 1986
18. Federle MP: Computed tomography of blunt abdominal trauma. *Radiol Clin North Am* 1983;21:461
19. Federle MP: CT of upper abdominal trauma. *Semin Roentgenol* 1984;19:269
20. Jeffrey RB, Federle MP: CT and ultrasonography of acute renal abnormalities. *Radiol Clin North Am* 1983;21:515
21. Berk RN, Ferrucci JT, Fordtran JS, et al: Radiological diagnosis of gallbladder disease: an Imaging symposium. *Radiology* 1981;141:49
22. Cooperberg P, Golding RH: Advances in ultrasonography of the gallbladder and biliary tract. *Radiol Clin North Am* 1982;20:611
23. Laing FC: Diagnostic evaluation of patients with suspected acute cholecystitis. *Radiol Clin North Am* 1983;21:477
24. Laing FC, Federle MP, Jeffrey RB, et al: Ultrasonic evaluation of patients with acute right upper quadrant pain. *Radiology* 1981;140:449
25. Leopold GR: Ultrasonography of jaundice. *Radiol Clin North Am* 1979;17:127

26. Mueller PR, Simeone JF: Intraabdominal abscess: diagnosis by sonography and computed tomography. *Radiol Clin North Am* 1983;21:425

27. Posteraro RH, Ravin CE: Magnetic resonance imaging in critically ill patients. In: Gallagher TJ, Shoemaker WC (eds). *Critical Care: State of the Art*, vol 9. Fullerton, CA, Society of Critical Care Medicine, 1988:273.

28. von Sonnenberg E, Mueller PR, Ferrucci JT: Percutaneous drainage of 250 abdominal abscesses and fluid collections. Parts I, II. *Radiology* 1984;151:337

29. Whitley WO, Shatney CH: Diagnosis of abdominal abscesses in patients with major trauma: the use of computed tomography. *Radiology* 1983;147:179

The Surgical Patient

Critical Care, Third Edition, edited by Joseph M. Civetta,
Robert W. Taylor, and Robert R. Kirby.
Lippincott-Raven Publishers, Philadelphia, PA © 1997.

CHAPTER 64

Perioperative Pulmonary Function Testing and Consultation

Philip G. Boysen
Robert R. Kirby

IMMEDIATE CONCERNS

MAJOR PROBLEMS

Whereas the mechanisms by which reductions of vital capacity, functional residual capacity (FRC), and arterial Po_2 (PaO_2) occur postoperatively are not fully understood, a factor of major importance is the site of the surgical incision. Patients undergoing upper abdominal and thoracic procedures (particularly partial or complete lung resection) are at increased risk of these changes and associated pulmonary complications. Such problems are even more likely in the presence of advanced age, obesity, cigarette smoking, and preexisting pulmonary disease. Individuals with any of the aforementioned risk factors may benefit from preoperative pulmonary function testing and occasionally from a pulmonary medicine consultation.

The decision for such testing or consultation should be based on rational assessment. A 70-year-old thin nonsmoker with no history of chronic or recurrent respiratory dysfunction does not require such an evaluation. At most, brief application of a pulse oximeter probe while the patient breathes room air to assess the percentage of oxyhemoglobin saturation, and a quick review of the chest radiograph that someone else probably ordered, are all that are necessary. (If the chest radiograph *wasn't* obtained, *don't* order one).

If you think pulmonary function tests are indicated, be selective. In most cases, screening spirometric studies (with bronchodilator if indicated) and an arterial blood gas analysis suffice. The criteria that concern risk based on the reported values are well defined for abdominal and thoracic surgery. If removal of lung tissue is a real possibility, regional pulmonary function studies (i.e., bronchospirometry, ventilation-perfusion scintigraphy) may be useful. This approach may help to resolve some problems preoperatively (e.g., promote bronchodilatation with selective β_2 agonists); help with intraoperative management (insertion of a double-lumen endotracheal tube, technique of ventilation); and provide some objective input as to whether the patient needs postoperative mechanical ventilatory support.

STRESS POINTS

1. Don't substitute pulmonary function testing for careful clinical assessment. Focus on the patient's relevant history and physical findings.
2. Be aware that some tests can be misleading or in error. A patient with a chest wall injury or abdominal incision may be unable to perform a satisfactory vital capacity maneuver because of pain. Such information is useful but doesn't tell you about intrinsic lung function.
3. The type of surgery and the patient's position during the operation are important factors to consider. All other things being equal, a lithotomy, Trendelenburg, or lateral decubitus position may predispose to prob-

lems that usually don't occur when the patient is supine.

4. If the patient regularly takes β_2 agonists or theophylline preparations, order them right up to the time of surgery. Also, have them immediately available for postoperative care.

5. If time permits, encourage smokers to stop smoking. However, this effort must be made 4 to 6 weeks before surgery for maximum beneficial effects to occur.

6. Teach incentive spirometry (sustained maximal inflation) or whatever techniques you employ. The therapy may not be useful postoperatively, but it certainly is easier to learn while the patient is awake, alert, and pain-free.

7. Recognize the importance of pain management and encourage discussion with the anesthesiologist, surgeon, or any other involved physician. If a pain management group is available, consult its staff early.

8. The drugs used by anesthesiologists (sedatives, hypnotics, narcotics, muscle relaxants, and inhalation agents) depress ventilation by a variety of mechanisms. Look for their residual effects in a postoperative patient who is not breathing well.

ESSENTIAL DIAGNOSTIC TESTS AND PROCEDURES

1. Find out if there is preexisting pulmonary dysfunction. A patient breathing 14 times a minute with a "room air sat" of 98% does not have a major problem.

2. Put things into perspective before embarking on costly and unnecessary testing. Childhood asthma that disappeared 25 years ago is unlikely to be a risk factor. Persistent episodes of wheezing and sputum production probably do represent a risk.

3. Decide what testing is needed. Spirometry and blood gas analysis should suffice in most cases. Knowledge that the patient is obstructed, restricted, or both, and to what degree should be enough. *Rarely*, diffusion studies and other more esoteric tests may be indicated.

4. Use bronchodilators for diagnostic (and therapeutic) purposes. A reversible component of airway obstruction is much easier to deal with than one that is not.

5. Make sure all involved practitioners (physicians, nurses, and respiratory therapists) collaborate in their care preoperatively and postoperatively. The anesthesiologist is at the crossroad of this activity: make sure he or she is in the loop.

INITIAL THERAPY

1. If respiratory depression is present and you don't plan to keep the patient intubated and ventilated, reverse whatever drug effects you can. Agents such as naloxone (for narcotics), flumazenil (for benzodiazepines), and anticholinesterases (for muscle relaxants) can be helpful.

2. Conversely, don't let the patient remain in agonizing pain to stimulate respiratory activity. This approach is counterproductive and inhumane.

3. Try to restore lung volumes by whatever technique you prefer. No single method works for everybody. However, positive-pressure breathing using an endotracheal tube, nasal mask, or face mask is effective in most patients.

4. If the patient is intubated, make sure the tube tip is above the carina and below the larynx. A misplaced tube creates havoc. When in doubt, obtain a chest radiograph.

5. Control the amount of oxygen you give, not because of oxygen toxicity, which probably takes days to develop, but to avoid resorption (absorption) atelectasis.

6. Consider removing the tube when the patient indicates that the tube should come out. However, some procedures (e.g., cervical corpectomy) are associated with major pharyngeal and glottic edema that does not manifest while the tube is in place. A swollen, protruding tongue can be a tipoff. When in doubt, look.

GENERAL CONSIDERATIONS ■

The decision to measure some aspect of pulmonary function preoperatively has several implications. Data should indicate surgical risk in terms of postoperative morbidity, mortality, or both. Pulmonary function abnormalities may require therapy preoperatively to improve these variables or postoperatively to forestall pulmonary complications. Prophylactic measures are designed to counter the anticipated postoperative pathophysiologic changes that would otherwise devastate a patient with compromised pulmonary function. Alterations in pulmonary function and outcome after thoracotomy differ from those encountered after abdominal surgery.

The incidence rate of postoperative pulmonary complications ranges from 2% to 70%, depending on the criteria used to identify them.[1] Preoperative evaluation of pulmonary function and consultation with a pulmonary specialist can be helpful for several reasons. Assessment of chronic pulmonary disease is useful to design the preoperative regimen, alter intraoperative management, and plan postoperative respiratory care. In addition, documentation of changes in pulmonary function can be useful to assess risk and, in combination with the pulmonary consultation, to better advise patients of the benefits, risk, and outcome of the surgical procedure. A pulmonary consultant can help to assess the benefits of therapy before surgery.

PREOPERATIVE PULMONARY CONSULTATION

Because pulmonary function testing has become more available, the patients who are candidates for assessment of preoperative pulmonary function and possible evaluation by a pulmonary consultant have increased in number.

Patients for Thoracic and Upper Abdominal Surgery

Routine performance of pulmonary function testing for all patients who are scheduled for thoracic surgery generally is considered reasonable, especially if its intention is to resect functional lung tissue.[2] Patients about to undergo upper abdominal surgical procedures also may benefit from preoperative evaluation of pulmonary function. The cost of such testing must be balanced against the likelihood of gaining useful information.

In thoracic or upper abdominal surgery, a major element of postoperative pulmonary function abnormalities involves alterations of normal diaphragmatic muscle activity. This phenomenon may be transient but relatively severe in the early postoperative period, particularly in patients whose pulmonary function is already compromised.

Smokers and Obese Patients

Patients with a history of heavy smoking and cough may also benefit from preoperative pulmonary function testing as a means of documenting dysfunction. A pulmonary consultation may be necessary to design a preoperative regimen of bronchopulmonary toilet. Obese patients can have severe restrictive lung disease as well as chronic obstructive lung disease (COLD) if they smoke. Such individuals are particularly affected shortly after the operation.

Older Patients and Those With Preexisting Pulmonary Disease

Patients with other types of restrictive or obstructive pulmonary disease also are candidates for pulmonary function testing and preoperative consultation. Advanced age, per se, might require pulmonary function testing. Such patients can be at increased risk because they have lost elastic recoil as a result of aging of lung tissue and are, therefore, more prone to postoperative pulmonary complications.

The Downside

If the intent of preoperative pulmonary function testing and pulmonary consultation is to maximize function before the surgical procedure, such testing and consultation are superfluous if the recommendations are not followed and the goals are not met. In the event that chronic organ dysfunction has been previously identified and documented by pulmonary function testing and lung function has been maximized by therapy, additional consultation has little to offer.

ASSESSMENT FOR LUNG RESECTION ■

The early studies of evaluation before thoracotomy included many patients with pulmonary tuberculosis. Currently, the diagnosis is most often lung cancer with coexistent COLD, both of which have resulted from cigarette smoking. Despite improved chemotherapeutic techniques, surgical resection still offers the best hope for long-term survival, except for patients with the histopathologic diagnosis of oat cell carcinoma of the lung, which commonly has widespread metastases.

Patients are classified according to standards of resectability and operability. Resectability implies an absence of distant metastases and local extension, and clinical evidence should indicate the possibility of resecting the patient's tumor. Operability indicates the patient's ability to undergo surgery. Besides the transient alteration in pulmonary function caused by the surgical incision, a permanent loss of functional lung tissue results from resection. If the patient has severe COLD, a resection for surgical cure must leave the patient with adequate lung function. Otherwise, permanent disability characterized by hypoxemia, increased pulmonary vascular resistance, and heart failure (cor pulmonale) is the expected outcome.

The degree of lung resection required cannot be completely evaluated until the surgeon assesses the patient's anatomy directly; therefore, all patients scheduled for thoracotomy should be evaluated as if a pneumonectomy is required. Because spirometry quantifies airflow obstruction, spirometric measurements for dysfunction correlate strongly with morbidity and mortality. Specific guidelines based on pulmonary function testing can be used to assign a level of risk.

FORCED VITAL CAPACITY

The forced vital capacity (FVC) is easily measured during spirometric testing and is highly reproducible. Data derived from a specific patient can be compared with those from subjects of the same height, weight, and age. A decreased FVC suggests a restrictive ventilatory defect or a severe obstructive defect with hyperinflation. A FVC less than 50% or an absolute value less than 1.75 to 2.0 L indicates a higher risk of postoperative pulmonary complications (Table 64-1). Mittman[3] showed that patients with a FVC of 70% or less than predicted had a 28% mortality rate; van Nostrand and colleagues[4] report a mortality rate of 12% for FVC readings less than 2 L. Gaensler and associates[5] retrospectively identified 30% to 40% of patients who died after resection for pulmonary tuberculosis.

TABLE 64-1. Increased Risk of Pulmonary Complications After Pneumonectomy

Forced vital capacity	<50% predicted or <1.75–2 L
Forced expired volume in 1 s	>2 L, mortality = 10%
	<2 L, mortality = 20–45%
	<0.8 L, nonoperable
Maximum voluntary ventilation	<50–60% predicted, mortality = 5–32%

FORCED EXPIRATORY VOLUME IN 1 SECOND

Although the FVC is an index of a restrictive ventilatory defect, the forced expiratory volume in 1 second (FEV_1) is a more direct measurement of airflow obstruction. The ratio of FEV_1/FVC is used as the diagnostic hallmark of obstructive lung disease. Patients with a FEV_1 of less than 800 mL have been excluded from any type of thoracic resection.[6,7] Patients with a FEV of 2 L can be considered to have a moderate obstructive ventilatory defect. A FEV_1 that exceeds 2 L is associated with a mortality rate of approximately 10%. Values less than this level predict a mortality rate of 20% to 45%.[8,9] Although measurement of the FEV_1 is useful in predicting postoperative pulmonary function, this test should not be used as the sole criterion to establish risk.

MAXIMAL VOLUNTARY VENTILATION

The effectiveness of the maximal voluntary ventilation (MVV) test, which evaluates obstructive and restrictive physiology, depends on the ability of the patient to cooperate and to perform the maneuver. The nonspecificity may actually make this a useful test.[3] In one series, no patients who had a MVV more than 50% died, and in another, the mortality rate was only 5%.[3,5] Didolkar and associates[9] report that a MVV less than 60% of predicted was associated with a 32% mortality rate; the mortality rate was 10% for MVV values that exceeded this level. It was 25% when the absolute value of the MVV was less than 70 L/minute, and 8% when it was greater.[8]

These retrospective studies indicate that the MVV can predict 66% of all deaths. Other data confirm that this test is sensitive and specific and that it predicts morbidity and mortality. It is a common practice to estimate the MVV, which usually involves some multiple of the FEV_1. A great disparity between this estimated level and the actual MVV may be related to restriction, pain, general debilitation, or the altered mental status that is typical of carcinomatous patients.

MIDFLOW MEASUREMENTS

Midflow measurements can also be derived from a spirogram. These include the maximal midexpiratory flow rate and the forced expiratory flow between 25% and 75% of the exhaled volume ($FEF_{25\%-75\%}$). These tests are sensitive indicators of small airway dysfunction.[10,11] Midflow measurements are always abnormal in COLD. A value less than predicted indicates a higher risk of postoperative complications after thoracic or abdominal surgical procedures.[11] The $FEF_{25\%-75\%}$ is a highly specific indicator of postoperative complications.[8]

BRONCHODILATORS

The immediate response to nebulized bronchodilators by COLD patients is assessed as part of routine testing. This response has both diagnostic and prognostic importance, because improvement in airflow obstruction may indicate a better postoperative prognosis. Some patients who show little or no response to nebulized bronchodilators eventually improve after an intensive regimen of bronchodilators, hydration, antibiotic therapy, and cessation of smoking. Using the best values for FEV_1 and FVC that can be obtained is advisable, and testing can be done immediately or after bronchodilator therapy has been optimized. Patients whose $FEF_{25\%-75\%}$ or MVV do not improve after such a therapeutic regimen have a higher incidence of postoperative pulmonary complications.[11]

Midflow measurements refine the clinical impression of obstructive airway disease, although restrictive diseases also can decrease midflow measurements. The combination of all available spirometric data enhances the clinical assessment.[12,13]

LUNG VOLUMES AND CAPACITIES

Patients with abnormalities in spirometric measurements often have coexisting changes in lung volumes or capacities and in their normal ratios. Increases in the ratio of residual volume to total lung capacity (RV/TLC) and of functional residual capacity to total lung capacity (FRC/TLC) indicate hyperinflation and gas trapping. A RV/TLC ratio more than 40% retrospectively identified 8% of postoperative deaths.[3] A RV/TLC ratio greater than 50% was associated with a 36% mortality rate. Other inquiries have not shown this ratio to be as sensitive or as useful. By the time hyperinflation and gas trapping are evident, the FEV_1, and possibly the FVC, are severely abnormal. However, lung volumes that improve dramatically after intensive bronchodilator therapy should be considered a good prognostic sign.

DIFFUSING CAPACITY

Diffusing capacity can be low in restrictive or obstructive conditions. With restricted physiology, a lower diffusing capacity suggests an impediment to gas transfer, specifically to the transfer of oxygen at the alveolar-capillary membrane. With obstructive physiology, a low diffusing capacity reflects less effective area for gas transfer. A diffusing capacity less than 15 mL/minute/mm Hg is associated with an 18% mortality rate; for larger values, the mortality rate was 7%. However, the test is not always a good index of obstructive airway disease or postoperative morbidity and mortality.[14]

EXERCISE

Exercise testing may yield valuable prognostic data.[15,16] In one protocol, patients negotiated seven stages of treadmill testing by walking for 2 minutes at each stage, for a total of 14 minutes.[17] Total power output was estimated at 185 W for a 70-kg man. Patients who completed the protocol had no morbidity or mortality after the operation. Among 7 patients who did not complete 4 minutes of testing, 3 died, 3 survived after many complications, and 1 had no postoperative pulmonary complications. The results suggest that exercise testing can indicate increased risk and morbidity.

In a study that quantified stair climbing and related it to power output during treadmill testing, the critical level of exercise correlated with a postbronchodilator FEV_1 of 1700 mL.[18] This finding is consistent with published spirometric and clinical data and indicates that some patients who cannot complete the exercise study can undergo successful operation.

The close correlation between FEV_1 and exercise level has not been shown in other studies of preoperative testing in which perioperative mortality seems to be closely linked to maximal oxygen consumption ($\dot{V}O_2$ max) during exercise testing. Preoperative $\dot{V}O_2$ max under 1000 mL/minute seems to indicate a high risk of morbidity and mortality.[19,20] The $\dot{V}O_2$ max expressed in mL/kg/minute seems to offer better discrimination. Below 15 mL/kg/minute, complications are frequent, but if $\dot{V}O_2$ max exceeds 20 mL/kg/minute, most patients can tolerate surgery without incident.[21]

In borderline cases, preoperative maximal exercise testing added to routine pulmonary function testing should provide a good overall assessment of the patient's status. This approach seems reasonable because exercise testing depends on the patient's cardiovascular system, pulmonary system, peripheral vascular system, and ability to cooperate to do the testing. Exercise provides an integrated measure of physiologic capabilities.

Exercise testing can be considered a stress factor designed to precipitate signs of cardiopulmonary dysfunction. It follows that other physiologic measurements during exercise also may be important. For example, an elevated pulmonary artery pressure at rest or during exercise should indicate a poor prognosis. In fact, a pulmonary artery pressure greater than 30 mm Hg is often associated with elevated right ventricular pressure and cor pulmonale.[22] Because postoperative cor pulmonale is the complication that is most feared, these measurements may be useful before surgery.

Uggla[23] measured pulmonary artery pressure in 109 patients at rest and during 15 W of exercise on a bicycle ergometer. He then attempted to duplicate the hemodynamic changes expected to occur with pulmonary resection by inflating a balloon in the main pulmonary artery of the affected side. Proximal to this occlusion, he measured pulmonary artery pressure at rest and during exercise. A significant elevation in pressure (>53 mm Hg) at rest or during exercise indicated an inability to survive resection. If pulmonary artery pressure was less than 35 mm Hg, survival was likely. Because of the direct approach to abnormal physiology from COLD, this test is the benchmark and the final avenue of investigation before operation and resection.

TESTS OF REGIONAL LUNG FUNCTION

The value of right and left lung differential studies is clear. Split-function studies are used in a predictive fashion. In many cancer patients, most of the gas exchange occurs in the uninvolved lung. Therefore, patients often are not greatly debilitated by the complete removal of the cancerous lung, which contributes little to overall pulmonary function. In addition to balloon occlusion studies, three techniques have been used to compare right and left pulmonary function: bronchospirometry, lateral position testing, and ventilation-perfusion scintigraphy.

Bronchospirometry

Bronchospirometry involves the use of a double-lumen tracheal tube positioned so that one lumen with an occlusive cuff lies in a main bronchus whereas the other lumen supplies the contralateral bronchus. Each lumen can be connected to a separate spirometer.[22,23] Pulmonary perfusion can be assessed, because oxygen uptake is proportional to blood flow to the given lung. Bronchospirometry also has been used to predict MVV and FEV_1 postoperatively.[24,25]

Lateral Position Test

The lateral position test relies on gravity-dependent variations in lung volume to assess the relative contributions of each lung to total pulmonary function. FRC is altered in either lateral decubitus position because of the gradations in pleural pressure throughout both lungs resulting from gravity. If both lungs contribute the same amount to overall pulmonary function, the function change in the right and left lateral decubitus positions should be the same.

The test is performed by determining the FRC with the patient supine; the patient is turned to the left lateral decubitus position and the FRC is calculated again; after another calculation with the patient supine to reestablish the baseline, the right lateral decubitus position is calculated in the same fashion. Changes in FRC in these decubitus positions are added, and the proportional contribution of each side of the lung to overall ventilation is determined.

The lateral position test is easy, noninvasive, and requires minimal patient cooperation. Initial studies showed good correlation between this test and bronchospirometry or radionuclide determination of split function.[27,28] A fixed mediastinum or pleura involvement can produce inaccurate results but may indicate local invasion of the mediastinum that would not be resectable.[29,30] However, in patients with advanced disease, the lateral position test does not correlate well with bronchospirometric determination of oxygen uptake.[31] Nevertheless, it can be useful if additional testing is not possible.

Ventilation-Perfusion Scintigraphy

Nuclear medicine techniques also can provide valuable information about overall pulmonary function and split-function techniques. Initially, radioactive ^{133}Xe, an insoluble gas, was used. With a scintillation camera centered over the mediastinum, a bolus of ^{133}Xe in solution is injected while the breath is held. A split crystal in line with the scintillation camera enables a functional estimate of right and left perfusion, because the gas is rapidly transported and diffuses into alveoli. The patient then breathes, and washout from each lung is recorded. This test can assess ventilation and perfusion.

Even with COLD and severe ventilation-perfusion abnormalities, a good match between ventilation and perfusion for a given lung is usually found. Because perfusion testing is simpler, cheaper, and more widely available (using ^{99}Tc or ^{131}I), it alone has been used as a means of assessing right and left lung functions. A prediction of overall postoperative function after a pneumonectomy can be established by multiplying the FEV_1 or the FVC by the percent of ventilation or perfusion to the remaining lung. The test with the lowest estimate probably determines the limiting factor, although results of the various tests usually are not widely disparate.

CLINICAL APPLICATION

One study evaluated the relative efficacy of all the described techniques, from routine pulmonary function to split function, using radiospirometry with [131]Xe and unilateral pulmonary artery occlusion at rest and with exercise.[7] The investigation assumed that a pneumonectomy would be required in 53 patients. Thirteen patients eventually required pneumonectomy, and 40 patients had lobectomies or lesser surgery. Postoperatively, 2 of the 13 patients died in the first 30 days, but neither died of respiratory failure. The best indicators of high risk from the pulmonary function data were the FEV_1 and the MVV. In predicting postoperative FEV_1, the perfusion scan seemed to be as good as the ventilation scan.[32] This observation prompted a test of the hypothesis that routine pulmonary function studies, combined with perfusion lung scanning, might obviate the need for more invasive testing, such as bronchospirometry and balloon occlusion of the pulmonary artery.[33]

Perfusion scanning alone was used prospectively to compare right and left function in 33 patients who required pneumonectomy.[34] The predicted postoperative FEV_1 was calculated as follows:

$$\text{Preoperative } FEV_1 \times \text{\%perfusion of uninvolved side} = \text{Predicted postoperative } FEV_1$$

As in the previous studies, a predicted postoperative FEV_1 greater than 800 mL was required, although others had used 1000 mL. Overall, 5 (15%) of 33 patients died perioperatively, but none died of respiratory failure. No patients with a predicted FEV_1 of 800 to 1000 mL died during the first 30 postoperative days. Of the 5 patients who died, 3 had MVV values lower than would have been estimated by using a multiple of the FEV_1.

Of the remaining patients, no deaths from primary respiratory failure occurred during the first postoperative year.[34] At the end of the first year, a significant number of patients had evidence of metastatic disease despite an intense investigation to prove resectability. The 5-year survival rate was 15%, which compares favorably with data from patients not judged to be at high risk. These simple principles seem to offer an effective, noninvasive means of evaluation and an adequate estimation of pulmonary function with a greater certainty of outcome. Patients who do not pass these criteria may also be surgical candidates, but additional testing, such as temporary unilateral pulmonary artery occlusion, must be performed. Perhaps exercise testing is most beneficial if the predicted postoperative FEV_1 is 800 to 1200 mL.

The patient who does not require a pneumonectomy may be fortunate, but evaluation is not as straightforward. Determining the contribution of bronchopulmonary segments has proven difficult. With sophisticated radiospirometric techniques, measured values exceeded predicted values

at 6 months.[35] In the early postoperative period, patients were hampered by transient but severe atelectasis and edema in remaining lung tissue on the operative side. These patients can be compromised just as if pneumonectomy had been performed.[36] Aggressive respiratory care showed first rapid, then gradual improvement over a 3-month period. The eventual level of pulmonary function can be estimated at the 3-month interval by dividing the right lung into ten bronchopulmonary segments and the left lung into eight segments and using the following formula:

$$\text{Functional loss} = [(\text{preoperative } FEV_1 \times \text{\%perfusion cancerous lung}) \times (\text{segments resected/total segments of cancerous side of lung})]$$

ASSESSMENT FOR ABDOMINAL SURGERY ∎

Surgical invasion of the chest wall causes disorders in pulmonary function to some degree in all patients and has significant implications for the patient with marginal pulmonary reserve. Why abdominal surgery causes significant changes in postoperative pulmonary function is less clear. Attempts to assign risk levels according to a given test have not been fruitful. A combination of risk factors, however, can help to assess risk, if not predict outcome, and the measurement of pulmonary function is an integral part of evaluation.

Postoperative pulmonary complications occur even in patients with normal lungs. Repeatedly, studies have shown an overall incidence rate of pulmonary complications of 6% to 8% in postoperative patients.[37] This incidence is greatly influenced by two factors: incision site and a history of smoking. The site of incision is related directly to the incidence of complications.[38] For nonabdominal surgery, the risk of subsequent pulmonary complications is less than 1%. As the incision site approaches the diaphragm, the incidence rate of complications rises to approximately 20% for an upper abdominal incision. The second important factor is cigarette smoking. The incidence of complications doubles for the smoker and quadruples if the smoker has COLD.

Postoperative assessments are confounded by the definitions of postoperative pulmonary complications. Bronchospasm, pulmonary edema, pulmonary embolism, and complications of tracheal intubation have been used in these definitions. All are difficult respiratory care problems, but the emphasis is more appropriately oriented toward anticipating atelectasis and infection (e.g., bronchitis, pneumonia).

CLINICAL APPLICATION

Given that preoperative therapy may alter outcome and indicate postoperative risk, two questions are pertinent: (1) Which patients should be subjected to testing? and (2) Which test should be performed? In the latter case, the best information can be obtained with simple spirometric testing before and after bronchodilators and with arterial blood gas analysis. From the spirogram, an assessment of obstructive and restrictive physiologic features can be obtained and the FVC, FEV_1, FEV/FVC ratio, and $FEF_{25\%-75\%}$ can be calcu-

TABLE 64-2. Abdominal Surgery: Moderately Increased Risk

$FEV_1 > 1 < 2$ L
FVC <50% predicted
$FEV_1/FVC > 35\% < 50\%$ predicted
$FEF_{25\%-75\%}$ <50% predicted

FEV_1, forced expired volume in 1 s; FVC, forced vital capacity; $FEF_{25\%-75\%}$, forced expired volume between 25% and 75% of the exhaled volume.

TABLE 64-3. Abdominal Surgery: High Risk

FEV_1 <1 L
FVC <1.5 L or 20 mL/kg
FEV_1/FVC <35% predicted
MVV <50% predicted or <50 L/min
CO_2 retention

FEV_1, forced expired volume in 1 s; FVC, forced vital capacity; MVV, maximum voluntary ventilation; $FEV_{25\%-75\%}$ = forced expired volume between 25% and 75% of the exhaled volume.

lated. Then data are combined with information from the patient's history and physical examination, other laboratory data, and chest radiographs. A preoperative regimen of bronchopulmonary toilet can be instituted if deemed appropriate and retesting performed after a therapeutic interval in borderline cases.

Before an abdominal procedure (particularly an upper abdominal procedure), guidelines other than those used before a thoracotomy may be useful. Increased risk is suggested by FEV_1 less than 2.0 L or less than 50% of the predicted value; increased risk is also indicated by FVC, FEV_1/FVC, or $FEF_{25\%-75\%}$ less than 50% of their predicted values (Table 64-2). These patients usually can be treated successfully with careful attention to detail.

Guidelines that suggest indicators of high risk include FEV_1 below 1.0 L, FVC less than 1.5 L or 20 mL/kg, $FEV_1/$FVC ratio below 35% of the predicted value, MVV below 50% of predicted or less than 50 L/minute, $FEF_{25\%-75\%}$ less than 1 L/second, and carbon dioxide retention (Table 64-3). Even a cholecystectomy in these patients can be life-threatening, and any upper abdominal incision almost always produces respiratory failure and requires postoperative mechanical ventilation. Given the data that demonstrate the duration of diaphragmatic dysfunction and lung volume changes, mechanical ventilatory support is probably necessary for 48 to 72 hours after the operation.

Another useful approach has been outlined by Shapiro and coworkers[39] (Table 64-4). Reasoning that the evaluation

TABLE 64-4. Classification System for Risk of Pulmonary Complications After Thoracic and Abdominal Procedures

	ASSESSMENT	POINTS*
Expiratory spirogram	Normal: FVC% + $FEV_1/FVC\%$ >150	0
	FVC% + $FEV_1/FVC\%$ = 100–150	1
	FVC% + $FEV_1/FVC\%$ <100	2
	Preoperative FVC <20 mL/kg	3
	Postbronchodilator FEV_1/FVC <50%	3
Cardiovascular system	Normal	0
	Controlled hypertension, myocardial infarction without sequelae for more than 2 y	0
	Dyspnea on exertion, orthopnea, paroxysmal nocturnal dyspnea, dependent edema, congestive heart failure, angina	1
Nervous system	Normal	0
	Confusion, obtundation, agitation, spasticity, discoordination, bulbar malfunction	1
	Significant muscle weakness	1
Arterial blood gas values	Acceptable	0
	$PaCO_2$ >50 mm Hg or PaO_2 <60 mm Hg with room air	1
	pH >7.5 or <7.3	1
Recovery	Ambulation (at minimum, sitting at bedside) expected within 36 h	0
	Complete bed confinement expected for at least 36 h	1

FVC, forced vital capacity; FEV, forced expiratory volume; FEV_1, forced expiratory volume in 1 s; $PaCO_2$, arterial partial pressure of carbon dioxide; PaO_2, arterial partial pressure of oxygen.

*0 points, low risk; 1–2 points, moderate risk; >3 points, high risk.

Modified from Clinical Application of Respiratory Care, 4th ed. Shapiro BA, Kacmarek RM, Cane RD, et al (eds). Chicago, Mosby-Year Book Medical Publishers, 1989.

of the thoracotomy patient required attention to pulmonary and cardiovascular clinical variables, they devised a scale accounting for these changes and other clinical modifiers that might affect abdominal surgery. Although no data have been generated to assess outcome of patients graded by this scale, it is a useful and reasonable approach. Attention is focused on the variety of factors that must be considered in any preoperative evaluation, and the scale alerts the physician to possible postoperative complications. This approach is likely to prompt precautionary arrangements for an intensive care bed and a reasonable postoperative plan.

Which patients should have pulmonary function testing preoperatively is open to question. Spirometric testing is easily performed, inexpensive compared with other so-called routine testing, and is usually more informative than either the electrocardiogram or a chest radiograph at approximately half the price. Spirometry has been recommended for any patient scheduled for thoracotomy or upper abdominal surgery, with documented history of upper abdominal surgery, or previous lung disease, smoking, or chronic cough.[40] This recommendation is too generalized; not all individuals in these classes require such testing. However, they should receive careful attention to ascertain those who do.

SPECIFIC THERAPEUTIC MEASURES ■

BRONCHODILATORS

Several issues must be addressed preoperatively for patients with chronic pulmonary disease. First is documentation of the degree of pulmonary dysfunction. Second is an attempt to maximize pulmonary function before the operative procedure is begun. Along these lines, control of bronchospasm and infections is of utmost importance.

A patient's response to bronchodilator therapy may range from minimal to impressive. Evaluation of pulmonary function and the objective response to bronchodilation are important in this regard. Currently, intermittent use of nebulized β_2-agonists by metered-dose inhaler is the most popular means of achieving maximum bronchodilation (Table 64-5). These drugs and this form of delivery are usually effective, well tolerated, and easy to use if patients are properly instructed.[41] Relative to other drugs and considering their minimal side effects, the cost of metered-dose inhalers is reasonable.

In preparation for surgery, maximal bronchodilation usually can be accomplished by coaching and by adequate instruction and administration of the metered dose during deep inspiration. Use of a chambered collection device, which maintains the vapor in the proximity of the patient's airway and facilitates introduction of the volatilized agent to the alveoli, may be most beneficial. Administration of these drugs through intermittent positive-pressure ventilation is no longer routinely recommended. However, some patients who are unable to breathe deeply are best able to receive the nebulized bronchodilator by this technique.

Improvement in airflow after nebulized bronchodilator therapy may indicate a more favorable postoperative prognosis. Some patients with minimal improvement in midflow measurements respond to intensive use of bronchodilators, hydration, antibiotics, and cessation of smoking. For those whose $FEF_{25\%-75\%}$ or MVV does not improve, a higher incidence of postoperative pulmonary complications is to be anticipated.

TABLE 64-5.   Metered-Dose Bronchodilators

DRUG	TRADE NAME	CONCENTRATION/PUFF
Terbutaline	Brethaire	200 μg
Albuterol	Proventil	90 μg
	Ventolin	
Metaproterenol	Alupent	650 μg
	Metaprel	
Isoetharine	Bronkometer	340 μg
Bitolterol	Tornalate	370 μg
Isoproterenol	Isuprel	130 μg
	Mistometer	
	Medihaler-Iso	75 μg
Isoproterenol and phenylephrine	Duo-Medihaler	160 μg
		240 μg Phenyl
Epinephrine°	Asthmahler	160 μg
	Bronitin Mist	
	Bronkaid Mist	
	Medihaler-Epi	
	Primatene Mist	
Ipratropium	Atrovent	18 μg

°Other concentrations available: 200 μg, 270 μg

From Gold ML, Marcial E: An anesthetic adaptor for all metered dose inhalers [letter]. *Anesthesiology* 1988;68:965.

INFECTION CONTROL

Infection control is important because of the tendency for patients who have bacterial colonization to develop postoperative bronchitis and pneumonia. Antibacterial agents and clearance of secretions are important in alleviating such complications. Bronchodilatation is usually effective in allowing an effective cough after a deep breath and facilitates clearance of secretions. Adequate attention to hydration is also beneficial, whereas the use of other agents administered into the airway is not generally efficacious.

Many organisms colonize the upper airways. If a patient has been hospitalized, these organisms are often gram negative. The cost and efficacy of culturing have been debated. Antibiotic therapy administered preoperatively seems prudent, assuming that the surgical procedure is elective, without incurring the cost and delay of first culturing airway secretions.

Ampicillin, tetracycline, trimethoprim/sulfamethoxazole, and other broad-spectrum antibiotics are recommended as reasonable therapeutic agents. Purulent sputum is enough of an indication to begin such therapy. The sputum should clear and decrease if appropriate antibiotic therapy has been instituted. This change should, in turn, improve the postoperative outcome.

CESSATION OF SMOKING AND LOSS OF WEIGHT

If adequate time exists before surgery, smoking cessation is often recommended. However, the ability to affect outcome by discontinuation of smoking is controversial.[42-44] Recovery from the effects of cigarettes is a long and slow process, but mucociliary escalation begins to improve almost immediately. This change should ensure more effective and complete removal of airway secretions. However, cessation of smoking is of more benefit and is an issue better addressed as a long-term goal to maintain pulmonary function than to alter postoperative management and immediate postoperative outcome.[42] Similarly, weight reduction may be appropriate. Outcome is improved if a patient undergoes a surgical procedure after considerable weight loss, particularly the morbidly obese. In either case, however, prolonged waiting periods are necessary to achieve the desired improvement before the operation.

POSTOPERATIVE CARE ■

MAINTENANCE OF LUNG VOLUME

The main feature of postoperative care emphasizes continuation of preoperative and intraoperative therapeutic regimens with particular attention to lung inflation. This goal may be achieved by encouraging deep-breathing exercises, by passive lung inflation with intermittent positive-pressure breathing, continuous positive airway pressure (CPAP), or sustained maximum inspiration (incentive spirometry).[45] The key element is postoperative pulmonary function maintenance, recovery of the FRC, and clearance of secretions.

Because coughing is often painful, and when not associated with a deep inspiration, may be counterproductive (i.e., decreases lung volume and collapses small airways), patients should be coached to take a maximum inspiration and to hold it as long as possible. This maneuver creates the longest duration of subambient intrapleural pressure and best restores the FRC.

If a patient is instructed to perform these maneuvers several times an hour and is able to comply, incentive spirometry devices become almost superfluous. Mobilization of secretions and early ambulation are necessary to maximize bronchopulmonary toilet. Bronchodilatation by previously described techniques is aggressively maintained in the early postoperative period.

PAIN RELIEF

Adequate analgesia in the early postoperative period is an essential part of care. Whether for emotional or physiologic reasons, patients who are undergoing a painful postoperative course are more prone to bronchospasm. Adequate analgesia can be provided in several ways (Chap. 54). An extensive review of pain control after thoracic surgery has been published recently and is highly recommended for additional reading.[46]

Intramuscular and Intravenous Narcotics

The classic approach uses intramuscular or intravenous drug therapy. Such therapy is problematic. High plasma levels of narcotics, resulting in suppression of ventilatory drive, give way to a later period of subtherapeutic blood levels and return to the painful state.[47] Low-dose infusion of narcotics is helpful in this regard.

Patient-Controlled Analgesia

Some patients benefit from a patient-controlled analgesia (PCA) technique,[48] with or without a baseline infusion of narcotic. Intermittent on-demand boluses of low doses of narcotic have a psychotherapeutic benefit because of the control exerted by the patient. A lower overall dose of narcotic is required to achieve adequate pain relief. Some patients, however, cannot or will not cooperate with such devices. Other mechanisms of pain relief may be useful. These include local anesthetic infiltration, regional block therapy, or cryoanalgesia.

Epidural Narcotics

Of major benefit to many compromised, elderly, postoperative patients is the administration of epidural narcotics.[49,50] Nociception is altered at spinal narcotic receptor sites that are occupied by the introduction of these agents into the epidural space. Some absorption occurs, but to a much lesser degree than with intravenous or intramuscular administration.

Although morphine migrates rostrally, producing biphasic suppression of ventilation, this complication is extremely uncommon unless parenteral narcotics have been used intraoperatively. Epidural analgesia leaves patients wide awake and alert but with minimal perception of pain. Morphine, meperidine, fentanyl, and sufentanil have been used to achieve this effect.

Effects on Pulmonary Function

Adequate pain management has an additional benefit that has been underemphasized. PCA and epidural narcotics seem to have a salutary effect on pulmonary function. With epidural narcotics, the breathing pattern is slowed, the tidal volume is increased, and patients are more cooperative in trying to achieve deep lung inflation. PCA is associated with increased FRC and vital capacity and improved outcome.

These changes may result from alleviation of pain and subsequent deep inspiration without splinting. Some neurogenic inhibitory reflex mediated at the spinal cord seems to alter diaphragmatic function postoperatively. Epidural narcotics occupying receptor sites along the spinal cord may interrupt this inhibitory reflex so that improved diaphragmatic function is achieved. Whatever the reason, adequate pain management, combined with physical examination and assessment of a patient's breathing rate, tidal volume, and capacity for deep inspiration, is a useful means to achieve and assess therapeutic goals in the early postoperative time frame.

MECHANICAL VENTILATION AND THE WORK OF BREATHING ■

The most severe alteration in postoperative pulmonary function occurs during the first 3 postoperative days. During this 72-hour interval, reduction in lung volumes, particularly FRC and, in some cases, total lung capacity occurs, in conjunction with other changes[51] (Table 64-6). Loss of lung volume leads to stasis of pulmonary secretions and results in a right-to-left intrapulmonary shunt and subsequent hypoxemia.

Therapy is specifically focused on achieving deep lung inflation and reclaiming lung volumes. This approach should minimize the intrapulmonary shunt. The nadir of these changes usually occurs within the first 24 hours. Intensive respiratory care and mechanical ventilation may be necessary.

Reduction in lung volume and alteration in breathing patterns are associated with a significant increase in the mechanical work of breathing. Compromised patients may be unable to assume this extra ventilatory workload, and respiratory failure can ensue. By assuming muscle work and maintaining lung inflation with mechanical ventilation and some form of PEEP or CPAP, patients can often overcome (or be supported through) the most severe period of respiratory compromise.

Careful assessment of breathing systems is essential in the event that patients are allowed to trigger the ventilator or are supported by intermittent or synchronized intermittent mandatory ventilation.[52] Pressure support ventilation may be advantageous, because it allows patients to control respiratory rate, respiratory flow rate, and tidal volume during spontaneous breathing with mechanical ventilation. This support can be varied from maximum, in which almost total support is provided (i.e., a tidal volume of 10 to 12 mL/kg), through lesser amounts designed to overcome only the imposed work from the ventilator circuit and endotracheal tube.[53-55]

A major therapeutic goal is to reduce the oxygen cost of breathing and to minimize energy expenditure, achieving deep lung inflation and delivering a fraction of inspired oxygen at a frequency sufficient to result in the desired arterial blood gas partial pressures. Adequate attention to control of pain is essential with the hope that subsequent withdrawal of ventilatory therapy can be accomplished within 48 to 72 hours. The frequency with which patients who have been extubated successfully are readmitted to the ICU on the second or third postoperative day because of inadequate pain management is impressive. Elderly and obese patients are particularly problematic.

Thus, documentation of organ function by pulmonary function testing is essential to assess the degree of compromise and the response to therapy. In such cases, extubation criteria such as those listed in Table 64-7 may be used. The values listed are guidelines that must be modified by clinical assessment.

TABLE 64-6. Postoperative Pathophysiologic Pulmonary Changes After Abdominal Surgery

Decreased	Forced vital capacity
	Lung volumes, especially functional residual capacity and total lung capacity
	Tidal volume
	Lung compliance
	↓ PaO_2
	↓ $PaCO_2$

TABLE 64-7. Criteria for Weaning and Tracheal Extubation

Respiratory muscle strength	PNP >20–30 cm H_2O
Ventilatory mechanics	VC >10–15 mL/kg
	V_T >5 mL/kg
	Cst >30 mL · cm H_2O
Ventilatory reserve	MVV >2 × $\dot{V}_E$ and normal (for patient) $PaCO_2$ and pHa
Minute ventilation	$\dot{V}_E$ with normal $PaCO_2$ and pHa
	<10 L/min
	<180 mL/kg/min
Dead space	V_D/V_T <0.6

PNP, peak negative pressure; VC, vital capacity; V_T = tidal volume; Cst, static compliance; $\dot{V}_E$, minute ventilation; V_D/V_T = dead space to tidal volume ratio; $PaCO_2$, arterial partial pressure of carbon dioxide; pHa, arterial pH; MVV, maximum voluntary ventilation.

CONCLUSIONS

The results of these simple tests should guide preoperative and intraoperative therapy and provide some indication of risk. Postoperative therapy should include maintenance of the measures begun before surgery (e.g., bronchodilation and antibiotics) but should further emphasize the importance of ambulation and deep breathing. A deep-breathing regimen can reverse postoperative pathophysiology and lessen the incidence of postoperative pulmonary complications. Spontaneous breathing with sustained maximal inflation is preferable because of the resulting transpulmonary pressure changes and distribution of inspired gas.

If this regimen cannot be achieved, lung inflation can be accomplished by positive-pressure breathing or CPAP. The results should be monitored by clinical examination, chest radiograph, and arterial blood gas analysis, if necessary.

REFERENCES

1. Latimer RG, Dickman M, Day WC, et al: Ventilatory patterns and pulmonary complications after upper abdominal surgery determined by preoperative and postoperative computerized spirometry and blood gas analysis. *Am J Surg* 1971;122:622
2. Tisi GM: Preoperative evaluation of pulmonary function: validity, indications, and benefits. *Am Rev Respir Dis* 1979;119:293
3. Mittman C: Assessment of operative risk in thoracic surgery. *Am Rev Respir Dis* 1961;84:197
4. van Nostrand D, Kjelsberg MO, Humphrey EW: Preresectional evaluation of risk from pneumonectomy. *Surg Gynecol Obstet* 1968;127:306
5. Gaensler EA, Cugell DW, Lindgren I, et al: The role of pulmonary insufficiency in mortality and invalidism following surgery for pulmonary tuberculosis. *J Thorac Surg* 1955;29:163
6. Kristersson S, Lindell SE, Svanberg L: Prediction of pulmonary function loss due to pneumonectomy using ^{133}Xe-radiospirometry. *Chest* 1972;62:694
7. Olsen GN, Block AJ, Swenson EW, et al: Pulmonary function evaluation of the lung resection candidate: a prospective study. *Am Rev Respir Dis* 1975;111:379
8. Boushy SF, Billig DM, North LB, et al: Clinical course related to preoperative and postoperative pulmonary function in patients with bronchogenic carcinoma. *Chest* 1971;59:383
9. Didolkar MS, Moore RH, Takita H: Evaluation of the risk of pulmonary resection for bronchogenic carcinoma. *Am J Surg* 1974;127:700
10. McFadden ER Jr, Kiker R, Holmes B, et al: Small airway disease: an assessment of the tests of peripheral airway function. *Am J Med* 1974;57:171
11. Gracey DR, Divertie MB, Didier EP: Preoperative pulmonary preparation of patients with chronic obstructive pulmonary disease: a prospective study. *Chest* 1979;76:123
12. Miller WF, Wu N, Johnson RL: Convenient method of evaluating pulmonary ventilatory function with a single breath test. *Anesthesiology* 1956;17:480
13. Redding JS, Yakaitis RW: Predicting the need for ventilatory assistance. *Md State Med J* 1970;19:53
14. Karliner JS, Coomaraswamy R, Williams MH Jr: Relationship between preoperative pulmonary function studies and prognosis of patients undergoing pneumonectomy for carcinoma of the lung. *Dis Chest* 1968;54:112
15. Olsen GN: The evolving role of exercise testing prior to lung resection. *Chest* 1989;95:218
16. Boysen PG, Clark CA, Block AJ: Graded exercise testing and postthoracotomy complications. *J Cardiothorac Vasc Anesth* 1990;4:68
17. Reichel J: Assessment of operative risk of pneumonectomy. *Chest* 1972;62:570
18. Johnson AN, Cooper DF, Edwards RHT: Exertion of stair climbing in normal subjects and in patients with chronic obstructive bronchitis. *Thorax* 1977;32:711
19. Eugene J, Brown SE, Light RW, et al: Maximum oxygen consumption: a physiologic guide to pulmonary resection. *Surg Forum* 1982;33:260
20. Brown SE, Prager RS, Eugene J, et al: Exercise capacity before and after thoracotomy for lung cancer [Abstract]. *Chest* 1983;84:353
21. Smith TP, Kinasewitz GT, Tucker WY, et al: Exercise capacity as a predictor of post-thoracotomy morbidity. *Am Rev Respir Dis* 1983;129:730
22. Semb C, Erikson H, Bergan F, et al: Cardiorespiratory function in pulmonary surgery. *Acta Chir Scand* 1955;109:235
23. Uggla LG: Indications for and results of thoracic surgery with

regard to respiratory and circulatory function tests. *Acta Chir Scand* 1956;111:197

24. Svanberg L: Bronchospirometry in the study of regional lung function. *Scand J Respir Dis* 1966;62(Suppl):91

25. Svanberg L: Regional functional decrease in bronchial carcinoma. *Ann Thorac Surg* 1972;13:170

26. Neuhaus H, Cherniack NS: A bronchospirometric method of estimating the effect of pneumonectomy on the maximum breathing capacity. *J Thorac Cardiovasc Surg* 1968;55:144

27. Hazlett DR, Watson RL: Lateral position test: a simple, inexpensive, yet accurate method of studying the separate functions of the lungs. *Chest* 1971;59:276

28. Walkup RH, Vossel LF, Griffin JP, et al: Prediction of postoperative pulmonary function with the lateral position test: a prospective study. *Chest* 1980;77:24

29. Marion JM, Alderson PO, Lefrak SS, et al: Unilateral lung function: comparison of the lateral position test with radionuclide ventilation-perfusion studies. *Chest* 1976;69:5

30. Solomon DA, Goldman AL: Use of lateral position test and perfusion lung scan in predicting mediastinal metastases. *Chest* 1981;79:406

31. DeMeester TR, Van Heertum RL, Karas JR, et al: Preoperative evaluation with differential pulmonary function. *Ann Thorac Surg* 1974;18:61

32. Olsen GN, Block AJ, Tobias JA: Prediction of postpneumonectomy pulmonary function using quantitative macroaggregate lung scanning. *Chest* 1974;66:13

33. Boysen PG, Block AJ, Olsen GN, et al: Prospective evaluation for pneumonectomy using the 99m technetium quantitative perfusion lung scan. *Chest* 1977;72:422

34. Boysen PG, Harris JO, Block AJ, et al: Prospective evaluation for pneumonectomy using perfusion scanning: follow-up beyond one year. *Chest* 1981;80:163

35. Ali MK, Mountain CF, Ewer MS, et al: Predicting loss of pulmonary function after pulmonary resection for bronchogenic carcinoma. *Chest* 1980;77:337

36. Boysen PG: Pulmonary resection and postoperative pulmonary function [editorial]. *Chest* 1980;77:718

37. Wightman JAK: a prospective survey of the incidence of postoperative pulmonary complications. *Br J Surg* 1968;55:85

38. Ali J, Weisel RD, Layug AB, et al: Consequences of postoperative alterations in respiratory mechanics. *Am J Surg* 1974;128:376

39. Shapiro BA, Kacmarek RM, Cane RD, et al (eds): *Clinical Application of Respiratory Care*, 4th ed. Chicago, Mosby–Year Book, 1989

40. Latimer RG, Dickman M, Day WC, et al: Ventilatory patterns and pulmonary complications after upper abdominal surgery determined by preoperative and postoperative computerized spirometry and blood gas analysis. *Am J Surg* 1971;122:622

41. Myers DL: Pharmacologic therapy of respiratory failure. In: Kirby RR, Taylor RW (eds). *Respiratory Failure*. Chicago, Year Book Medical Publishers, 1986:482

42. Ashley K, Kannel WB, Sorlie PD, et al: Pulmonary function: relation to aging, cigarette habit, and mortality. *Ann Intern Med* 1975;82:739

43. Chodoff P, Margand PMS, Knowles CL: Short term abstinence from smoking: its place in preoperative preparation. *Crit Care Med* 1976;3:131

44. Wheatley IC, Hardy KJ, Barter CE: An evaluation of preoperative methods of preventing postoperative pulmonary complications. *Anaesth Intensive Care* 1977;5:56

45. Stock MC, Downs JB, Gauer PK, et al: Prevention of postoperative pulmonary complications with CPAP, incentive spirometry, and conservative therapy. *Chest* 1985;87:151

46. Kavanagh BP, Katz J, Sandler AN: Pain control after thoracic surgery: a review of current techniques. *Anesthesiology* 1994;81:737

47. Austin KL, Stapleton JV, Mather LE: Relationship between blood meperidine concentrations and analgesic response: a preliminary report. *Anesthesiology* 1980;53:460

48. Stanton-Hicks M: Is PCA an effective method of treating postoperative pain? *Curr Rev Clin Anesth* 1994;15:41

49. Ready LB: Acute peridural narcotic therapy. In: Brown DL (ed). *Perioperative Analgesia: Problems in Anesthesia 1988*. Philadelphia, JB Lippincott, 1988:327

50. Cousins MJ, Mather LE: Intrathecal and epidural administration of opioids. *Anesthesiology* 1984;61:276

51. Boysen PG: Pulmonary resection and postoperative pulmonary function [editorial]. *Chest* 1980;77:718

52. MacIntyre NR, Stock MC: Weaning mechanical ventilatory support. In: Kirby RR, Banner MJ, Downs JB (eds). *Clinical Application of Ventilatory Support*. New York, Churchill Livingstone, 1990:263

53. Banner MJ, Kirby RR, MacIntyre NR: Patient and ventilator work of breathing and ventilatory muscle loads at different levels of pressure support ventilation. *Chest* 1991;100:531

54. Banner MJ, Blanch PB, Kirby RR, et al: Decreasing imposed work of the breathing apparatus to zero using pressure support ventilation. *Crit Care Med* 1993;21:1333

55. Banner MJA, Jaeger MJ, Kirby RR: Components of the work of breathing and implications for monitoring ventilator dependent patients. *Crit Care Med* 1994;22:513

Critical Care, Third Edition, edited by Joseph M. Civetta,
Robert W. Taylor, and Robert R. Kirby.
Lippincott-Raven Publishers, Philadelphia, PA © 1997.

CHAPTER 65

■

Preoperative Evaluation of High-Risk Surgical Patients

David L. Brown
Stephen O. Heard
Donald S. Stevens
Robert R. Kirby

IMMEDIATE CONCERNS ■

MAJOR PROBLEMS

The overall perioperative mortality rate is 0.5% to 1.9% for elective surgical procedures. It increases significantly for urgent and emergent operations, particularly when complicating factors such as congestive heart failure, recent myocardial infarction, or severe pulmonary disease are present. Added to these considerations is the ever increasing percentage of elderly patients undergoing surgery. Whereas age, per se, is difficult to quantitate as a risk factor, diseases associated with the aging process present problems to surgeons, anesthesiologists, and critical care physicians.

Although mortality is frequently discussed, perhaps because the endpoint is definite and quantifiable, morbidity may be just as important, or even more so, from a societal standpoint. Few patients die from complications related to their surgical experience, but many incur long and expensive hospitalizations and sometimes permanent disability. If preoperative assessment can detect and lead to correction of premorbid conditions, it represents time and money that is well spent. If such assessment instead leads merely to an almost random testing and screening process, it is unlikely to be anything but costly. The trick is to find the middle ground and stick to it, escalating the investigative process only when one is reasonably certain to obtain useful information that leads to improvement of care.

STRESS POINTS

1. Talk to the patient, family member, guardian, or anybody who knows the individual. More can be obtained from a well-taken history than from most physical examinations.
2. Review the medical records. Read the nurses' notes. They often contain much more useful information than the perfunctory scribbling of a busy (or careless) physician.
3. If alleged medication "allergies" are present, check them out carefully. Most of them represent side effects, not true anaphylactic or anaphylactoid reactions. It's important to know, whenever possible, what medications really can or can't be given.
4. Investigate possible arrhythmia problems. Drugs administered by the anesthesiologist, coupled with the stress of surgery, can lead to intraoperative difficulties that persist into the postoperative period. If the patient has a pacemaker, find out why, how long, the type, and location. When in doubt, call a cardiologist in consultation.
5. Explore the limits of exercise tolerance. We have seen patients with reported ejection fractions of 20% or less who walk 2 miles a day, mow their lawn, or play golf on a regular basis. Is this incongruity possible? Maybe. Is it likely? No.
6. Inquire as to a history of myocardial infarction. All

999

other things being equal, a recent myocardial infarction (6 months or less) mitigates against *elective* surgery. To "push" forward with such a procedure is medically and ethically unconscionable.

7. Make sure that the anesthesiologist finds out about any anesthetic-related problems, familial or personal. Anesthetic mortality is low: 1 in 10,000 to 1 in 100,000 or less. For the person to whom it occurs, however, it's 100%.

8. Know the patient's medications. Medications begun years previously may have no current indication. If the drugs in question are taken for valid reasons, few need to be stopped before surgery.

9. Remember that too little knowledge can be harmful. Know as much as you can.

ESSENTIAL DIAGNOSTIC TESTS AND PROCEDURES

1. Few tests are truly essential. Routine testing is not cost-effective. If a test value is "abnormal," place it into the overall patient perspective. A serum potassium of 3 mMol/L (unchanged for 3 years) in a patient taking thiazide diuretics is not grounds for cancellation or for starting a potassium infusion.

2. An electrocardiogram (ECG) is reasonable for patients ages 45 years or older. It is not a good screening test for younger individuals.

3. Routine chest radiographs are low-yield tests that cannot be justified. Like the ECG, their value may increase with patient age, particularly in smokers or those with a history of lung problems.

4. Tests performed within a year of the planned surgery probably are sufficient as long as the patient has been medically stable. The key word is "stable," which may have different meanings to patients and physicians.

5. Be selective with pulmonary function tests and arterial blood gas analysis. Use the pulse oximeter.

INITIAL THERAPY

1. Remember that although the operation may be the most therapeutic part of the care provided, it can lead to postoperative complications such as atelectasis or other pulmonary problems.

2. Protect the airway. Clean it out. You'll seldom have as good an opportunity as in the anesthetized, intubated, and paralyzed patient.

3. Assess the patient's fluid status and administer fluids liberally but judiciously. "Third space" losses, coupled with preoperative fluid restriction and purges, can lead to a many-liter deficit.

4. Have your patient's respiratory status in as good a shape as possible before surgery. Pulmonary complications are still the leading cause of postoperative morbidity. The leading cause of low urine output is too little fluid, the wrong fluid, or both.

5. Remember antibiotic prophylaxis when it is appropriate. Timing and types of drugs are equally important.

OVERVIEW ∎

Preoperative evaluation of a critically ill patient may vary from rapid diagnosis and resuscitation for a life-threatening emergency to a detailed analysis of the suitability of a physiologically compromised patient to undergo major operation. In the first case, preoperative evaluation involves therapy, is brief, and is narrowly focused.

Physicians caring for patients in the perioperative period know that morbidity and mortality occur, although they often underestimate risk by tenfold to 100-fold.[1] Ten percent of surgical patients experience a complication.[2,3] This morbidity is difficult to quantify, and a consensus view on its clinical importance is not available. Mortality, on the other hand, is a more easily defined endpoint, more information is available for analysis, and most occurs in the postoperative period.[4]

Perioperative mortality rate for elective surgical procedures ranges from 0.001% to 1.9%.[4-6] It is dependent on numerous modifying factors, including patient age and concurrent diseases, surgical procedure, institution, and postoperative care. In a series of more than 100,000 patients, the perioperative mortality rate was 0.5% if no concurrent preoperative medical condition was present; it increased to 2.1% with obesity, 7% with ischemic heart disease, and 15.8% with cardiac failure.[6] Mortality rate was further increased two to five times for each of these conditions if the operation was emergent rather than elective. The reported mortality rate for patients older than 70 years of age is 1.25% to 2.5%.[7] If mortality rate is compared with the data of Farrow and others,[6] age seems to identify patients at increased risk for perioperative death, although most of the increased risk results from concurrent diseases in these older patients[7,8] (Table 65-1).

The American Society of Anesthesiologists (ASA) physical status classification system (class I [normal] through class V [moribund]) was not intended to be a measure of risk, yet increasing numerical values correlate with increasing perioperative mortality[9] (Tables 65-2 and 65-3). Similarly, increasing ASA class identifies an increasingly ill patient population.

The impact of the proposed surgical procedure on a high-risk patient should also be understood if appropriate perioperative management is to be attained. Goldman and colleagues[10] outline a cardiac risk stratification system for patients undergoing a variety of noncardiac surgical procedures, which is widely used as an estimate of cardiac risk.

TABLE 65-1. Risk of Dying Within 7 Days of Operation in a Series of 112,000 Patients Analyzed by Multivariate Analysis

VARIABLE	RISK INDEX
<60 y	1.0
60–69 y	2.3
>80 y	3.3
ASA III or IV	11.0

ASA III or IV, American Society of Anesthesiologists class III or IV.

(Modified from Cohen MM, Duncan PG, Tate RB: Does anesthesia contribute to operative mortality? *JAMA* 1988;260:2859).

TABLE 65-2. Definitions of American Society of Anesthesiologists' (ASA) Physical Status Classification

PHYSICAL STATUS	DEFINITION
I	Healthy patient
II	Mild systemic disease; no functional limitation
III	Severe systemic disease; definite functional limitation
IV	Severe systemic disease that is constant threat to life
V	Moribund patient; unlikely to survive 24 h, with or without operation

CONCURRENT DISEASE ■

When considering patients at higher risk, do general guidelines exist to direct the preoperative evaluation? Two important variables—age and urgency of the operation—cannot be altered. Therefore, direct your evaluation to variables in which improvement is possible: concurrent disease, anesthesia, operative procedure, and postoperative care, including the postoperative analgesia plan. The increased risk associated with aging may indicate that a more detailed evaluation is desirable. Infections in high-risk patients are not covered in detail in this chapter. Nevertheless, they are involved in many delayed perioperative deaths. Every effort should be made to prevent them if they have not occurred, and to treat them if they have.

Concurrent diseases associated with the most significant perioperative complications or the highest mortality are those involving the cardiovascular, pulmonary, and neurologic systems. When organ-system dysfunction is examined in each of these areas, some common signs and symptoms seem to be useful as indicators of increased risk or the need for a more detailed preoperative evaluation (Table 65-4). Additionally, some high-risk operations demand a more detailed evaluation either preoperatively or intraoperatively, even in healthy asymptomatic patients.

CARDIOVASCULAR

Cardiovascular complications contribute to a significant percentage of perioperative mortality because of their prevalence within the surgical population and their immediate life-threatening nature. If we are to limit the impact of cardiovascular complications on perioperative morbidity and mortality, we must recognize when cardiovascular disease is present.

History and Physical Examination

The key to successful patient management encompasses a good history and thorough physical examination. In high-risk patients, this dictum also holds true. Certain facts within the history point to increased risk. The data of Goldman

However, Jeffrey and associates[11] evaluated Goldman's index in a select group of patients undergoing aortic surgery, and documented that the cardiac risk was underestimated from threefold to sevenfold, depending on the Goldman class. This work indicates that the physiologic impact of different procedures needs to be considered when determining the appropriateness of preoperative evaluation in high-risk patients.

Qualification of the physicians caring for the patient also should be ascertained. Slogoff and Keats[12] report that perioperative myocardial infarction varied sevenfold among anesthesiologists practicing in the same institution. Thus, although seldom considered in risk stratification, physicians caring for a patient (anesthesiologists, internists, and surgeons alike) are important determinants of the type and extent of preoperative evaluation that is appropriate for an individual high-risk patient.

Similarly, data suggest that the type of institution may affect mortality.[13] Adjusted mortality rates were significantly higher in for-profit hospitals and public hospitals than for private, nonprofit hospitals. These analyses attempted to adjust patient characteristics and case-mix differences between hospitals; however, whether the data can be directly applied to high-risk patients must be questioned, at least at this time.

TABLE 65-3. Perioperative Mortality in Patients Stratified According to ASA Classification

PHYSICAL STATUS	ANESTHETICS	DEATHS	MORTALITY RATE	MORTALITY FACTOR°
I	50,703	43	0.08%	NA
II	12,601	34	0.27%	3.4
III	3626	66	1.8%	22.5
IV	850	66	7.8%	97.5
V	608	57	9.4%	117.5

°The factor mortality was increased over that in ASA I patients.

(Modified from Vacanti CJ, Van Houten RJ, Hill RC: A statistical analysis of the relationship of physical status to postoperative mortality in 68,388 cases. *Anesth Analg* 1970;49:564).

TABLE 65-4. Indicators of Increased Perioperative Risk and Need for More Detailed Preoperative Evaluation in High-Risk Patients

CARDIOVASCULAR	PULMONARY	NEUROLOGIC
S_3 gallop	Chronic lung disease	CNS injury
Jugular venous distention	$FEV_1 < 2.0$ L	Carotid bruit†
MI within 6 mo	Obesity	
Arrhythmias°	Hypercarbia at rest	
Age > 70 y	Age >70 y	
Emergency operation	Site of operation	
Important aortic stenosis	Smoking history	
Poor general health		

MI, myocardial infarction; CNS, central nervous system; FEV_1, volume of gas exhaled in 1 s during the execution of a forced vital capacity.
°Other than sinus or premature atrial contractions, or premature ventricular contractions >5/min.
†As a marker for ischemic heart disease.
(Modified from Goldman et al,[10] Tisi,[19] and Wolf el al.[30])

and others[10] indicate that the two most significant risk factors for cardiac complications are congestive heart failure and recent myocardial infarction, both of which may be identifiable by history.

Physical examination *may* be helpful if signs point toward a diagnosis of congestive heart failure, but often is of limited value if one attempts to rely on it to predict other cardiovascular functions. Some data suggest that correct predictions of cardiac index and pulmonary artery occlusion pressure are possible, based on physical findings alone, in patients with acute myocardial infarctions.[14] Yet, in critically ill patients, the predictive value of the physical examination seems limited. Conners and coworkers[15] evaluated such persons without myocardial damage. Physical examination was associated with a correct prediction of cardiac index and pulmonary artery occlusion pressure only in 44% and 42% of patients, respectively. The number of correct predictions did not correlate with observer experience; residents and attending staff were equally ineffective. Thus, the concept that physician experience allows more accurate prediction of cardiovascular function is open to question.

Laboratory Examination

Laboratory tests of the cardiovascular system should be directed toward assessment of the functional state of the patient's myocardium and the adequacy of blood pressure control. Blood pressure can be quantified more easily and less expensively than can myocardial function. If control of blood pressure is poor, more sophisticated laboratory investigation may be necessary, including blood and urine tests, rapid sequence urography, renal arteriography, and abdominal computed tomographic scanning or magnetic resonance imaging. Goldman and Caldera suggest that in patients receiving general anesthesia and undergoing elective operation, hypertension does not result in an increased risk, provided

that (1) diastolic blood pressure is stable and not more than 110 mm Hg, and (2) intraoperative and immediate postoperative blood pressures are closely monitored and treated to prevent blood pressure changes of more than 50% above or 33% below the preoperative value for more than 10 minutes.[16]

Assessment of myocardial function often is more extensive and in many ways more limited than assessment of other biologic functions. Most of the significant preoperative cardiovascular diseases involve myocardial ischemia. Most available tests are limited by the point in time at which they are obtained. Ischemic heart disease is a dynamic process, with myocardial dysfunction occurring intermittently. Tests such as preoperative electrocardiography, two-dimensional echocardiography, and cardiac catheterization can provide only a picture of the myocardium at a fixed point in time. Preoperative stress testing may improve the dynamic nature of the examinations; this is possible with electrocardiography, echocardiography, and nuclear myocardial scans. Complicating perioperative assessment is recognition that possibly most of myocardial ischemia is "silent" and unaccompanied by typical angina.[17]

The nature of the patient's symptoms and physical findings should dictate the extent of the preoperative laboratory assessment. Because congestive heart failure, recent myocardial infarction, and aortic stenosis carry a significantly increased risk at operation, they should be ruled out or their severity defined by available laboratory testing. Some data suggest that physiologic testing (heart rate changes with 2 minutes of bicycle ergometry) may be a more reliable predictor of cardiovascular complications in elderly, noncardiac surgical patients than more sophisticated testing.[18]

PULMONARY

The nearly universal impairment of pulmonary function in the perioperative period makes pulmonary risk assessment central to a complete preoperative evaluation. The perioperative pulmonary complication rate varies range from 2% to 70%, depending on the criteria used for identification.[19] Despite this wide variation, high-risk patients can be identified and management altered to lessen the risk of pulmonary problems.

History and Physical Examination

A careful medical history-taking often directs the preoperative evaluation of the high-risk surgical patient. Limited exercise tolerance, increased sputum production, and a history of wheezing demand a more thorough examination before surgery. Obesity, age, smoking history, and the site of operation are additional risk factors that can be identified before laboratory testing. The physical examination reinforces the history; however, as is the case with certain cardiovascular measurements, it may not allow prediction of cardiopulmonary function in patients with chronic obstructive lung disease.[20]

Intensive care unit patients with documented respiratory problems often require urgent or emergent surgical procedures. Evaluation of their respiratory status before induction of anesthesia is important so that early respiratory muscle fatigue can be detected. In these patients, a characteristic increased respiratory rate is followed by paradoxic (inward) movement of the abdomen during inspiration.[21] An alternation between primarily chest and primarily abdominal expansion often is observed, after which $PaCO_2$ increases and respiratory rate and minute ventilation decrease as respiratory muscle fatigue supervenes.

Chest expansion normally is symmetrical. Conditions associated with asymmetric expansion include atelectasis, pneumothorax, pulmonary consolidation, airway obstruction, and a paralyzed hemidiaphragm. The acquisition of additional laboratory data is indicated in this setting.

Laboratory Examination

BLOOD GASES AND PH. Through the years, one pulmonary function test has been sought that allows assessment of the suitability for operation in the compromised pulmonary patient. Currently, however, the most practical approach is to combine several examinations. Arterial blood gas and pH measurements assess oxygenation and ventilatory adequacy. Hypoxemia is not as predictive of high perioperative risk as is hypercapnia. Hypercapnic patients have significantly more perioperative pulmonary complications than those who can maintain normal alveolar ventilation.[19]

SPIROMETRY. Pulmonary spirometry often is performed on patients undergoing routine operation. Rarely do spirometry values alter perioperative management unless a reversible bronchospastic component is present. Even when a patient is identified as high risk for pulmonary complications, pulmonary function testing may not be predictive of clinical outcome. However, a forced expiratory volume at 1 second (FEV_1) of less than 2 L suggests the strong possibility of postoperative pulmonary dysfunction.[22] Because thoracic and upper abdominal surgery impose approximately the same decrement on postoperative pulmonary function, at least during the immediate postoperative period, use of this decrement as a general guide seems appropriate. Additional information may be obtained if maximal voluntary ventilation is measured.[23]

In general, a reduction in forced vital capacity (FVC) is associated with a restrictive physiologic defect, whereas a reduction in FEV_1 suggests airway obstruction. A better definition of pulmonary reserve involves calculation of the FEV_1/FVC ratio, which normally is 0.85 or greater. If this value improves after the administration of a bronchodilator, aggressive preoperative therapy (when time allows) may lessen perioperative risk. The importance of such evaluation and treatment is obvious when the immediate postoperative changes in pulmonary function are considered. Recall that in upper abdominal surgery, a significant reduction of FVC and FRC occurs. The reduction of lung volumes is related not only to pain, but also to apparent diaphragmatic dysfunction.[24,25]

SPLIT-LUNG FUNCTION STUDIES. When a high-risk patient is scheduled to undergo pulmonary resection, more specialized pulmonary function testing may be indicated. In addition to the older split-lung function technique of bronchospirometry, radioisotope lung scanning techniques (ventilation and perfusion scans) can be used.[26] Right heart catheterization, which allows measurement of pulmonary artery pressures and cardiac function, also helps to stratify patients with serious pulmonary impairment. Such tests should be performed when routine pulmonary function testing shows FVC to be less than 50% predicted (or less than 15 mL/kg), FEV_1 less than 50% predicted (or less than 2 L), and maximal voluntary ventilation less than 50% predicted (or less than 50 L/minute).

NEUROLOGIC

Exacerbation of major neurologic disease in the perioperative period is not as common, and often not as immediately life-threatening as are major cardiovascular or pulmonary complications. Nonetheless, significant time is spent screening patients preoperatively for cerebrovascular disease. This effort may be related to the deeply ingrained concept that perioperative strokes are caused by intraoperative hypotension in combination with carotid arterial disease.[27] However, cerebral infarctions related to carotid arterial disease more commonly are caused by artery-to-artery thromboembolism.

History and Physical Examination

The history and physical examination must be used to screen patients for neurologic disease because routine laboratory testing of central nervous system function is not available. Up to 1 in 6 patients older than 55 years of age has a carotid bruit or neurologic symptoms suggestive of carotid arterial disease.[28] Because cerebral angiography is not indicated or logistically possible in all of these patients, how should screening progress? When the patient is asymptomatic but has a carotid bruit, no further investigation seems necessary if the data of Ropper and others[28] can be extrapolated to high-risk surgical patients (Table 65-5). If symptoms of extra-

TABLE 65-5. Incidence of Carotid Bruit and Stroke in Elective Surgical Patients

AUSCULTATION OF NECK	STROKE	
	n	*%*
Carotid bruit (n = 104)	1	0.96
No carotid bruit (n = 631)	4	0.63
Total (n = 735)	5°	0.68

°Strokes occurred only in patients undergoing coronary artery bypass grafting.

(Modified from Ropper AH, Wechsler LR, Wilson LS: Carotid bruit and risk of stroke in elective surgery. *N Engl J Med* 1982;307:1388).

cranial carotid vascular disease are present, further diagnostic workup may be required.

Laboratory Examination

Methods of assessing the extracranial carotid circulation involve estimates of flow (ophthalmodynamometry and ultrasonic carotid artery Doppler) and anatomy (ultrasonic B-mode imaging and carotid arteriography). Noninvasive measures generally are considered adequate except in the presence of more than 70% luminal narrowing of one carotid, more than 50% narrowing of both carotids, or significant ulceration (>0.5 cm in diameter). If these features are present, arteriography is indicated.[29] Perhaps more important is the recognition that carotid bruits are often a marker of potentially life-threatening ischemic heart disease. Myocardial infarction occurs two and a half times more frequently in patients with asymptomatic bruits than in age-matched controls without bruits.[30]

MANAGEMENT ■

WHEN TO EVALUATE

For preoperative management to effect a measurable change in a patient's preoperative medical condition, the initial evaluation must occur at some minimum time before the scheduled operation. The correct diagnostic algorithms in perioperative care of the high-risk patient are useless if time to alter organ system function is not available. Conversely, on occasion, only a brief period of preoperative hemodynamic and respiratory evaluation in the intensive care unit before an operation may provide useful information. One example of the latter situation involves placement of a thermodilution pulmonary artery catheter and application of military anti-shock trousers (MAST). Maximal inflation of MAST produces an acute increase of left ventricular afterload (and perhaps an increase of arterial blood volume). The effects on myocardial performance, in terms of changes in pulmonary artery pressures and cardiac output, can be instantaneously documented and translated into an assessment of myocardial reserve under conditions of stress. If deterioration occurs, a return to baseline is achieved immediately by deflation of the MAST.

Del Guercio and Cohn[31] preoperatively assessed oxygen transport and hemodynamic variables by using arterial and pulmonary artery catheterization. One hundred forty-eight patients older than 65 years who were scheduled for major surgery were studied to determine their suitability for operation. All 148 patients had been previously "cleared for operation" by a physician. The patients were stratified into four groups according to the measured and calculated cardiopulmonary parameters (Table 65-6). As expected, compromised patients had increasingly high perioperative mortality rates (Table 65-7). They suggest that pulmonary artery catheters were justified in 86% of the patients because such monitoring provided information not attainable by any other means. However, they could not demonstrate that this added information improved patient management or outcome. About

TABLE 65-6. Summary of Elderly Patients Scheduled for Major Operations Evaluated by Del Guercio and Cohn: Definition of Classes

STAGE	DEFINITION
I	No functional deficits, no limits to suggested surgery
II	Mild functional deficits; surgery need not be delayed but monitoring with pulmonary artery and arterial catheter indicated
III	Mild to moderate functional deficits; surgery delayed to "fine tune" the patients
IV	Moderate to advanced functional deficits that were not correctable and major surgery should not be performed

(From Del Guercio LRM, Cohn D: Monitoring operative risk in the elderly. *JAMA* 1980;243:1350).

10% of the previously "cleared" patients had unrecognized "chronic lung disease of severe degree," that was identifiable only by invasive monitoring. Complicating the analysis of these data is the inclusion of patients younger than 65 years of age who were studied because the investigators deemed them "physiologically" older than 65 years.

HOW TO EVALUATE

Many physicians perceive, as exemplified by Del Guercio and Cohn's investigation,[31] that increasingly invasive monitoring is somehow protective during the perioperative period. Nevertheless, little definitive information supports this view. Rao and colleagues[32] suggest that such an approach is beneficial; however, their use of pulmonary artery and arterial catheters in patients at high risk for perioperative myocardial infarction was accompanied by many other therapeutic interventions. Furthermore, they dealt with one type of patient with a specific cardiac lesion in a highly controlled environment.

Other prospective, randomized investigation fails to document that improvements in outcome necessarily follow more invasive monitoring. Additionally, with recognition that most perioperative morbidity occurs postoperatively rather than intraoperatively, other explanations for the improved out-

TABLE 65-7. Summary of Elderly Patients Scheduled for Major Operations Evaluated by Del Guercio and Cohn

STAGE	PATIENTS	MORTALITY RATE
I	20 (13.5%)	0%
II and III	94 (63.5%)	8.5%
IV	34 (23%)	100%°

°In the 8 patients in whom major operation was performed, even against evidence.

(From Del Guercio LRM, Cohn D: Monitoring operative risk in the elderly. *JAMA* 1980;243:1350).

TABLE 65-8. Measurements and Derived Calculations Available From Arterial and Pulmonary Artery Catheters

MEASUREMENTS	DERIVED CALCULATIONS	
Arterial pressure (Pa)	Stroke volume (SV):	Cardiac output/heart rate
Arterial hemoglobin saturation and PaO_2	Left ventricular stroke work:	$SV \times (MAP - PAOP) \times 0.0136$
Pulmonary artery pressures (PAP)	Right ventricular stroke work:	$SV \times (MPAP - CVP) \times 0.0136$
Pulmonary artery occlusion pressure (PAOP)	Systemic vascular resistance:	$(MAP - CVP) \times 80/\text{cardiac output}$
Central venous pressure (CVP)	Pulmonary vascular resistance:	$(MPAP - PAOP) \times 80/\text{cardiac output}$
Cardiac output	Arterial O_2 content (CaO_2)	$Hgb \times \%Sat \times 1.34 + 0.003 \times PaO_2$
Midex venous oxygen saturation ($S\bar{v}O_2$)	Mixed venous O_2 content ($C\bar{v}O_2$):	$Hgb \times \%Sat \times 1.34 \times P\bar{v}O_2$
(photospectrometric and laboratory)	Pulmonary end-capillary O_2 content ($Cc'O_2$):	$Hgb \times \%Sat \times 1.34 + 0.003 \times PaO_2$
	Shunt ($\dot{Q}s/\dot{Q}t$):	$Cc'O_2 - CaO_2/Cc'O_2 - C\bar{v}O_2$

MAP, mean arterial pressure; MPAP, mean pulmonary artery pressure; %Sat, percent saturation; Hgb, hemoglobin; PaO_2, partial pressure of oxygen in the alveoli.

come in Rao and coworkers' patients are possible. For example, invasive monitoring perhaps mandated a stay in the ICU for these patients, thereby permitting more timely analgesia care than was possible on the wards during the time interval studied.

Nevertheless, the discrimination that invasive monitoring provides allows a more rational (scientific) basis for decision-making in sick patients. A controlled study demonstrating statistical and clinical improvement associated with perioperative assessment and monitoring in such patients may be impossible. However, carefully selected invasive hemodynamic monitoring in specific conditions probably does allow improvements in patient care. Never forget that such techniques are not without risk and should not be undertaken in a cavalier fashion.[33,34]

The number of devices available for perioperative use continues to expand. Arterial and pulmonary artery catheterization allow measurement and calculation of the variables listed in Table 65-8. Esophageal positioning of an ultrasonic crystal on the distal end of a 9.5-mm modified gastroscope (transesophageal echocardiography) allows real time 2-D and M-mode echocardiography, as well as Doppler flow measurements. With such capabilities, continuous assess-

ment of cardiac wall-motion abnormalities and blood flow is possible in patients receiving general anesthesia. Such monitoring requires special training and a high level of skill.

Intraoperative, noninvasive cardiopulmonary monitors primarily measure airway pressure, inspiratory and expiratory gas volumes and partial pressures, and continuous "pulsed" arterial oxygen saturation (SpO_2). Arterial and pulmonary artery catheters allow oxygen transport assessments and continuous mixed venous oxygen saturation measurements ($S\bar{v}O_2$).

The emphasis on technologically advanced monitoring techniques tends to deemphasize the importance of clinical observation. Despite the limitations of physical assessment, much useful potentially lifesaving information can be obtained by the classic methods. Thus, in a severely traumatized patient who has sustained an undetermined loss of blood, initial and frequent sequential documentation of the pulse, urine flow, overall appearance, and behavior provides a simple, elegant, and inexpensive appraisal of the need for and effects of blood replacement (Table 65-9).

Monitoring of CNS function intraoperatively long has included electroencephalography. Despite many new methods of electroencephalogram information display, the tech-

TABLE 65-9. Evaluation of Hemorrhage (70-kg Man)

	CLASS I	CLASS II	CLASS III	CLASS IV
% Blood loss	≤15	15–30	30–40	>40
Amount (mL)	<800	800–1500	2000–2800	>3000
Signs/symptoms	Normal or slightly increased pulse; with other fluid shifts, symptoms can occur.	Pulse >100; respiratory rate 20–30; ↓ pulse pressure; capillary blanching; urine flow 20–30 mL/h	Pulse 120; respiratory rate 30–40; ↓ systolic and pulse pressures; urine flow 5–15 mL/h; anxiety/confusion	Pulse >140; respiratory rate 35; mean blood pressure <60mm Hg; skin pale, cool; urine flow 0; confusion/lethargy (more than 50% loss leads to loss of consciousness, blood pressure, and pulse)

(Modified from *Advanced Trauma Life Support Program Instructor Manual.* Chicago, Committee on Trauma, American College of Surgeons, 1989:57).

nique is not used by most anesthesiologists. Recently, somatosensory-evoked potentials have increased the scope of CNS monitoring to include the spinal cord and brain stem. A limiting factor in many of these useful applications is the lack of sufficient numbers of physicians and technicians skilled in interpreting the data provided by these monitors.

PREVENTION OF COMPLICATIONS ■

To prevent perioperative complications in high-risk patients, one must know what produces them. Nothing is gained by the monitoring of cardiovascular function in patients undergoing pulmonary resection if they die of pneumonia secondary to the inadequate clearing of bronchial secretions postoperatively. Likewise, the most elegant intraoperative anesthetic and surgical care will be for naught if postoperative pain is permitted to induce tachycardia leading to perioperative myocardial ischemia. To identify the factors most responsible for perioperative complications, an organ-system approach again should be used.

CARDIOVASCULAR

Congestive Heart Failure

Major cardiovascular complications principally involve the heart. Congestive heart failure and perioperative myocardial infarction are associated with high perioperative mortality rates, and every reasonable effort should be made to prevent them. Congestive heart failure frequently accompanies significant valvular heart disease. Goldman and coworkers[35] documented a 20% incidence rate of new or worsening congestive heart failure in the perioperative period in patients with significant valvular heart disease. Additional information revealed that significant mitral valve stenosis in those older than 40 years of age was associated with a 7% perioperative mortality rate for persons with noncardiac surgery. In patients with aortic stenosis, the associated mortality rate was 13%.[10]

Perioperative Myocardial Reinfarction

The incidence of perioperative myocardial reinfarction is related to the passage of time from a patient's previous infarction (Fig. 65-1). Patients with a previous myocardial infarction have a reinfarction risk 30 to 300 times higher than age-matched controls. This risk is quadrupled if the operation is emergent.[36] Specific risk depends on the proximity of the previous infarction to the current surgical procedure. Data from the 1960s and 1970s suggest that surgery taking place less than 3 months after a myocardial infarction was associated with a reinfarction rate of about 35%; when surgery was performed 3 to 6 months after infarction, the rate decreased to 18%; when it was delayed for more than 6 months, the reinfarction rate reached a minimum of 5%.[37,38] These widely quoted figures have been reevaluated in light of more recent data.

Rao and coworkers[32] demonstrated that the incidence rate of reinfarction within 1 to 3 months of a previous myocardial

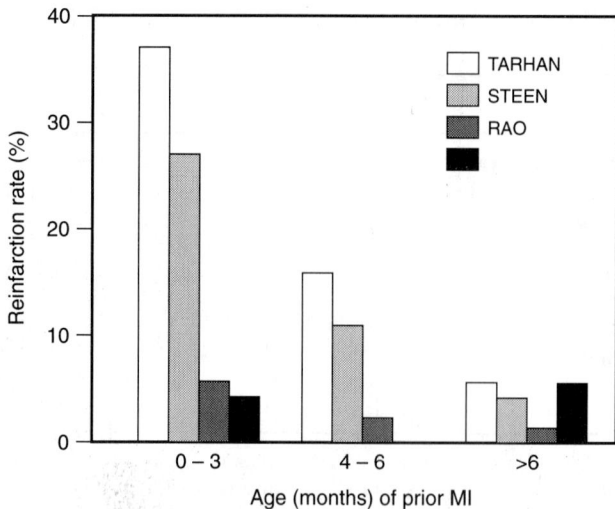

FIGURE 65-1. Reinfarction rates from several studies (Tarhan and others [1972],[37] Steen and others [1978],[38] Rao and others [1983],[32] Shah and others [1990][33]) in patients who have had prior myocardial infarction. (Adapted from McCullough HA, Sprague DH: Myths in vascular anesthesia. *Probl Anesth* 1991;5:453.)

infarction decreased to 5.8% if invasive hemodynamic monitoring was used perioperatively and vasoactive drugs were administered to maintain or restore hemodynamic function to normal (heart rate, blood pressure, and pulmonary artery pressures) during the first 3 or 4 days postoperatively (Table 65-10). Shah and others[33] report similar findings but without a reduction of the incidence of reinfarction 6 or more months after an infarction. Their patient group contained a disproportionate number of high-risk vascular surgery patients.

Slogoff and Keats[12] also presented data suggesting that hemodynamic perturbations, both blood pressure and heart rate, are linked to the risk of perioperative myocardial infarction in patients undergoing myocardial revascularization. Invasive monitors may provide information that helps to decrease perioperative complications if they are used "wisely." Shoemaker and colleagues[39] suggest that wisely means manipulating hemodynamic function perioperatively in high-risk patients to produce supranormal values and

TABLE 65-10. Perioperative Myocardial Reinfarction Studies: Incidence of Time-Related Reinfarction°

PRIOR MI	MAYO SERIES[36]	LOYOLA SERIES[32]
0–3 mo earlier	35%	5.8%
3–6 mo earlier	18%	2.3%
>6 mo earlier	5%	1.9%

MI, myocardial infarction.
°The differences in the Loyola series were (1) pulmonary artery catheters were used routinely; (2) patients were monitored in the ICU for 72–96 h postoperatively; and (3) vasoactive and chronotropic drugs used immediately to treat hemodynamic perturbations.

thereby improve outcome (Table 65-11). Perhaps the stress of the perioperative period demands an alteration of what are normal values perioperatively.

Pain and Analgesia

As previously highlighted by Rao and coworkers,[32] data may be interpreted to suggest that intensive care unit personnel provide more effective analgesia than do ward personnel. This interpretation is given additional credence by information suggesting that traditional postoperative parenteral opioid administration is associated with frequent arterial oxygen desaturation,[40] which may be associated with clinically significant heart rate increases.[41] Yeager and colleagues[42] have also confirmed that analgesia therapy can reduce the incidence of cardiovascular complications in high-risk patients.

PULMONARY

Mechanical Ventilation

Routine postoperative mechanical ventilation does not appear to maintain FRC or to reduce complications. No data indicate that some arbitrary length of postoperative mechanical ventilation is protective. To the contrary, evidence has been published suggesting that such therapy is not productive.[43] The data of Yeager and coworkers can also be interpreted to support the lack of efficacy of routine postoperative mechanical ventilation.[42] They randomly assigned their patients to two groups: one received a moderate- to high-dose fentanyl anesthetic that was associated with longer episodes of mechanical ventilation; the other received a combined epidural and general anesthetic that allowed earlier extubation (Table 65-12). The increased cost, duration of intubation, and complications in the mechanically ventilated group were impressive.

TABLE 65-11. Comparison of Hemodynamic and Selected Outcome Variables in High-Risk Surgical Patients Monitored With Pulmonary Artery Catheters in a Study by Shoemaker and Others

VALUE	NORMAL (n = 30)	SUPRANORMAL (n = 28)
Cardiac index, L/m²/min	2.8–3.5	>4.5
$\dot{D}o_2$ (mL/m²/min)	400–550	>600
$\dot{V}o_2$ (mL/m²/min)	120–140	>170
ICU (d)	15.8	10.2
Ventilator (d)	9.4	2.3
Intraoperative deaths	1	0
Postoperative deaths	10	1
Average costs/survivor	$58,950	$28,690

$\dot{D}o_2$, oxygen delivery; $\dot{V}o_2$, oxygen consumption.

(Modified from Shoemaker WC, Appel PL, Kram HB, et al: Prospective trial of supranormal values of survivors as therapeutic goals in high-risk surgical patients. *Chest* 1988;94:1176).

TABLE 65-12. Comparison of Pulmonary Variables and Costs in Randomized Patients in Two Groups

GROUP	TIME TO EXTUBATION (h)	FREQUENCY OF PULMONARY COMPLICATIONS	HOSPITAL COSTS ($)
I°	7.1	4	11,218
II†	81.8	17	20,380

°Combined epidural and general anesthesia plus epidural analgesia postoperatively.
†General anesthesia and parenteral opioid analgesia postoperatively.
(Modified from Yeager MP, Glass DD, Neff RK, et al: Epidural anesthesia and analgesia in high-risk surgical patients. *Anesthesiology* 1980;52:135).

Pain and Analgesia

Perioperative pulmonary complications are widespread as a result of decreased FRC, atelectasis, and pneumonia. Such changes most often do not take place intraoperatively; rather, they result in part from postoperative pain that produces abdominal and thoracic muscle splinting. Thus, to minimize the postoperative decrement in pulmonary function in the patient at risk for complications, adequate analgesia should be the principal concern.

Several methods provide improved perioperative analgesia, including peridural opioids, intercostal nerve blocks, patient-controlled analgesia, and more liberal use of "on-demand" opioids. Pulmonary "stir-up" regimens should be incorporated into the analgesia management. Increasingly, we are convinced that intermediate care units, allowing improved analgesic management of patients who are not yet critically ill but who are at risk, are needed. Some centers have introduced analgesia wards. We believe that over time they will be shown to be cost-effective by decreasing expensive complications related to inadequate analgesia.

SPECIAL CONSIDERATIONS ■

ASPIRATION OF GASTRIC CONTENTS

One of the most feared anesthetic complications is pulmonary aspiration of gastric contents. The anesthesiologist must determine whether the patient is at risk for the development of aspiration pneumonitis should regurgitation and aspiration occur during anesthesia and surgery. Pain, recent injury, insufficient duration of fasting, diabetes mellitus, obesity, pregnancy, narcotics, β-adrenergic agents, and anticholinergic drugs can delay gastric emptying and alter lower esophageal sphincter tone, and thus potentially increase the risk of aspiration.[44,45] A hiatal hernia is believed to increase the risk for aspiration, but reflux symptoms (i.e., heartburn), rather than the hiatal hernia itself, probably identify the patient at risk.[46]

ADRENAL SUPPRESSION

In patients with diseases in which corticosteroid use is common (e.g., asthma, ulcerative colitis, or rheumatoid arthritis), the anesthesiologist should inquire as to the dose and the time of last use of corticosteroids. The incidence of adrenal suppression is not predictable. It depends on the potency and frequency of steroid dose and the length of therapy. Suppression can occur with cumulative doses of prednisone less than 0.4 g and can last up to a year after cessation of steroids.[47]

BLEEDING AND CLOTTING PROBLEMS

Questions about previous bleeding problems and about the need for blood transfusions almost always identify the patient at risk for perioperative hemorrhage.[48] In addition, if the preoperative assessment is performed sufficiently early, the anesthesiologist and surgeon can identify a patient who is suitable for preoperative autologous blood donation. This procedure should be used more frequently.[49,50] Use of recombinant erythropoietin increases the efficiency of preoperative autologous blood donation.[51]

MEDICATIONS

Antihypertensives

In general, antihypertensive agents other than diuretics should be continued up to the time of surgery. Many studies have documented the adverse hemodynamic effects of discontinuing β-adrenergic blockers or clonidine in the perioperative period.[52,53]

Diuretics

Diuretics usually are stopped before surgery. Patients taking thiazide diuretics have frequent hypokalemia regardless of potassium supplementation or potassium-sparing agents.[54] Serum potassium concentrations less than 3.5 mMol/L occur in 15% of patients, and concentrations less than 3.0 mMol/L occur in 10%.

The perioperative consequences of hypokalemia are not as severe as once was believed.[55,56] Delay of surgery probably is not justified for patients at low risk for perioperative cardiac complications whose preoperative serum potassium concentration is in the range of 3 to 3.5 mMol/L.[57] However, for patients thought to be at higher risk, the potassium concentration should be more than 3.5 mMol/L. The incidence of ventricular arrhythmias increases when serum potassium is less than 3.0 mMol/L compared with more than 3.0 mMol/L.[54] Acute changes are more problematic than chronic ones.

Bronchodilators

The role of aminophylline in the management of the patient with bronchospastic disease is controversial.[58] Although it is an effective bronchodilator, it does not add significantly to the bronchodilating effects of inhaled β-adrenergic or anticholinergic agents.[59]

Because halothane sensitizes the myocardium to circulating catecholamines, the combined use of aminophylline and halothane may result in ventricular arrhythmias.[60] Toxic serum concentrations of aminophylline may occur in the perioperative period, resulting from alterations in the liver's drug metabolism, which were induced by changes in parenteral nutritional content or a persistent low-flow state.[61]

We give aminophylline only if a patient is receiving a stable dose preoperatively. Otherwise, we avoid aminophylline and instead use aerosolized bronchodilators and corticosteroids for bronchospasm secondary to reactive airway disease. If a patient uses aerosolized medications routinely, we administer them 30 to 60 minutes preoperatively and have them available in the operating room.

Insulin

The optimal management of blood glucose levels in the diabetic patient remains controversial; "tight" and "loose" control regimens have been proposed.[62] Those who favor tight control argue that better management of perioperative blood glucose level results in decreased postoperative morbidity, including fewer wound infections and enhanced wound healing.[63]

Those who favor loose control believe that sound data supporting the notion that tight control reduces perioperative morbidity are lacking, the resources needed for tight control are too expensive, and that without these resources, the danger of hypoglycemia is significant.[64] If the patient has adult-onset insulin-dependent diabetes mellitus, one half the usual dose of insulin is administered on the morning of surgery after an intravenous infusion of a dextrose-containing crystalloid solution has been begun.

Oral Hypoglycemics

Oral hypoglycemic agents should not be administered on the day of surgery, particularly those agents with a long duration of action, such as chlorpropamide, glipizide, and glyburide. They bind ionically to serum albumin and may be displaced from their binding sites by drugs used in the perioperative period.[65] Asymptomatic hypoglycemia can occur in the somnolent postoperative patient who has been taking long-acting oral hypoglycemic drugs.

Corticosteroids

Patients receiving corticosteroids or corticotropin should receive appropriate perioperative corticosteroid replacement.[66] If the corticosteroid potency equivalent is more than 300 mg of hydrocortisone per day, hydrocortisone is not substituted for perioperative steroid treatment. Instead, the routine steroid dose can be administered. For example, if a patient takes 3 mg of dexamethasone every 6 hours, this daily dose meets the stress dose requirements of surgery and protects from adrenal insufficiency as long as it is continued perioperatively.

Antiinflammatory Drugs

Antiinflammatory agents affect coagulation through their effect on platelets. Acetylsalicylic acid (aspirin) irreversibly acetylates the platelet enzyme cyclooxygenase, resulting in decreased platelet aggregation for 7 to 10 days.[67]

Other nonsteroidal antiinflammatory drugs (NSAIDs) seem to inhibit the same enzyme but do so reversibly, with effects lasting at most 2 days after a single NSAID dose.[68] Whether aspirin or other NSAIDs increase bleeding during and after surgery is controversial,[69] but "minor hemorrhagic complications" of epidural anesthesia seem to be increased.[70] This effect is also important when small amounts of bleeding may be detrimental in intracranial or ocular procedures.

Aspirin should be stopped at least 7 days before elective surgery, and other NSAIDs at least 48 hours before surgery. A test of bleeding time should be measured before performance of a major regional nerve block if such medications have been continued.

Anticoagulants

In general, anticoagulants should be discontinued before a surgical procedure. In some cases, their effects may require reversal before surgery can proceed. If the patient is receiving warfarin and surgery is urgent, fresh frozen plasma should be given for quick reversal of the anticoagulant effect. If surgery is elective, an oral dose of 5 mg of phytonadione (vitamin K_1) should return the prothrombin time to normal within 24 hours.[71] Vitamin K_1 administration, however, makes anticoagulation after surgery more difficult.

A heparin infusion should be stopped 3 to 4 hours before surgery to allow sufficient time for the return of normal coagulation parameters. If reversal is urgently needed, protamine sulfate can be used. We do not stop heparin therapy in patients with unstable angina or recent myocardial infarction who are undergoing coronary artery bypass grafting. The risk of intracoronary thrombosis before the institution of cardiopulmonary bypass precludes this option.

Antibiotics

If the patient is at risk for the development of infective endocarditis, appropriate antibiotic prophylaxis should be instituted. Table 65-13 provides the most recent American Heart Association guidelines for perioperative endocarditis prophylaxis.[72] Many patients receive preoperative prophylactic antibiotics to reduce the incidence of wound- or prosthetic device–related infections. Such antibiotics must be given 2 hours or less before incision; otherwise, their effectiveness is reduced.[73]

Aspiration Prophylaxis

Patients at risk for vomiting and aspiration of gastric contents should receive prophylaxis with nonparticulate antacids or histamine$_2$ blockers with or without metoclopramide.[74] Proton pump inhibitors such as omeprazole are also effective in keeping gastric pH above 2.5.[75]

Prophylaxis for Venous Thrombosis

Some patients are at high risk for thrombophlebitis in the perioperative period. Prophylactic measures should be used. Various methods include the use of low-dose heparin, intermittent calf compression, warfarin (particularly in total hip replacements), or dextran.[76,77] Recent studies indicate that methods to prevent venous thromboembolism are underused.[78]

THE DO-NOT-RESUSCITATE PATIENT

Approximately 15% of patients with do-not-resuscitate orders undergo a surgical procedure.[79] These patients present a special problem to anesthesiologists and surgeons: Should the do-not-resuscitate orders be suspended during anesthesia and surgery?

Because anesthesia involves potent cardiovascular depressants and often requires some degree of resuscitation (whether it be with fluids, inotropes, or vasopressors), some anesthesiologists recommend that do-not-resuscitate orders be suspended in the perioperative period.[79–82] However, in the preoperative evaluation, the patient's do-not-resuscitate status should be clarified. If the goals of surgery and anesthesia are consistent with that clarification, and if the patient and health care team agree, the operation can proceed. Appropriate resuscitative and supportive measures can then be undertaken should hemodynamic instability or arrest oc-

TABLE 65-13. Bacterial Endocarditis Prophylaxis

A. CONDITIONS FOR WHICH PROPHYLAXIS IS RECOMMENDED

1. Prosthetic heart valves, including bioprosthetic and homograft valves
2. Previous bacterial endocarditis
3. Most congenital cardiac malformations
4. Rheumatic and other acquired valvular dysfunction
5. Hypertrophic cardiomyopathy
6. Mitral valve prolapse with valvular regurgitation

B. SURGICAL PROCEDURES FOR WHICH PROPHYLAXIS IS RECOMMENDED

1. Dental procedures known to induce gingival or mucosal bleeding
2. Tonsillectomy and/or adenoidectomy
3. Surgical procedures that involve intestinal or respiratory mucosa
4. Bronchoscopy with a rigid bronchoscope
5. Sclerotherapy for esophageal varices
6. Esophageal dilatation
7. Gallbladder surgery
8. Cystoscopy
9. Urethral dilatation
10. Urethral catheterization if urinary tract infection is present
11. Prostatic surgery
12. Incision and drainage of infected tissue
13. Vaginal hysterectomy
14. Vaginal delivery in the presence of infection

(continued)

TABLE 65-13. *(continued)*

C. STANDARD PROPHYLACTIC REGIMEN FOR PATIENTS AT RISK

DRUG	DOSING REGIMEN
Amoxicillin	3.0 g orally 1 h before procedure, then 1.5 g at 6 h after initial dose

AMOXICILLIN/PENICILLIN–ALLERGIC PATIENTS

| Erythromycin *or* | Erythromycin ethylsuccinate, 800 mg, or erythromycin stearate, 1.0 g, orally 2 h before procedure, then one half this dose 6 h later |
| Clindamycin | 300 mg orally 1 h before procedure, then 150 mg at 6 h after initial dose |

PATIENTS UNABLE TO TAKE ORAL MEDICATIONS

| Ampicillin | IV or IM administration of ampicillin, 2.0 g, 30 min before procedure, then IV or IM administration of ampicillin, 1.0 g at 6 h after initial dose |

AMPICILLIN/AMOXICILLIN/PENICILLIN–ALLERGIC PATIENTS UNABLE TO TAKE ORAL MEDICATIONS

| Clindamycin | IV administration of clindamycin, 300 mg, 30 min before procedure and an IV or oral administration of 150 mg at 6 h after initial dose |

PATIENTS CONSIDERED HIGH RISK AND NOT CANDIDATES FOR STANDARD REGIMEN

| Ampicillin | IV or IM administration of ampicillin, 2.0 g, and gentamicin, 1.5 mg/kg^{-1} (not to exceed 80 mg), 30 min before procedure, followed by amoxicillin, 1.5 g, orally at 6 h after initial dose; alternatively, the parenteral regimen may be repeated 8 h after initial dose |

AMPICILLIN/AMOXICILLIN/PENICILLIN–ALLERGIC PATIENTS CONSIDERED HIGH RISK

| Vancomycin | IV administration of 1.0 g over 1 h, starting 1 h before procedure; no repeat dose necessary |

ALTERNATIVE LOW-RISK PATIENT REGIMEN

| Amoxicillin | 3.0 g orally 1 h before procedure, then 1.5 g at 6 h after initial dose |

IV, intravenous; IM, intramuscular.

(Modified from Dajani AS, Bisno AL, Chung KJ, et al: Prevention of bacterial endocarditis: recommendations by the American Heart Association. *JAMA* 1990;264:2919).

cur in the perioperative period as a result of the anesthesia or surgery.

If the cause of the arrest is the patient's underlying condition or is believed to be irreversible, resuscitative efforts do not have to be instituted.[80] The most important point that needs to be emphasized is good preoperative communication and agreement among physicians, the patient, and family members.[79,80]

REFERENCES

1. Kronlund SF, Phillips WR: Physician knowledge of risks of surgical and invasive diagnostic procedures. *West J Med* 1985;142:565
2. Cohen MM, Duncan PG, Pope WDB, et al: A survey of 112,000 anaesthetics at one teaching hospital (1975–1983). *Can Anaesth Soc J* 1986;33:22
3. Pederson T, Eliasen K, Henriksen E: A prospective study of risk factors and cardiopulmonary complications associated with anaesthesia and surgery: risk indicators of cardiopulmonary morbidity. *Acta Anaesthesiol Scand* 1990;34:144
4. Spence AA: The lessons of CEPOD [editorial]. *Br J Anaesth* 1988;60:753
5. Farrow SC, Fowkes FGR, Lunn JN, et al: Epidemiology in anaesthesia. II. Factors affecting mortality in the hospital. *Br J Anaesth* 1982;54:811
6. Farrow SC, Fowkers FGR, Lunn JN, et al: Epidemiology in anaesthesia. III. Mortality risk in patients with co-existing disease. *Br J Anaesth* 1982;54:819
7. Cohen MM, Duncan PG, Tate RB: Does anesthesia contribute to operative mortality? *JAMA* 1988;260:2859
8. Tiret L, Desmonts JM, Hatton F, et al: Complications associated with anaesthesia: a prospective survey in France. *Can Anaesth Soc J* 1986;33:336
9. Vacanti CJ, VanHouten RJ, Hill RC: A statistical analysis of the relationship of physical status to postoperative mortality in 68,388 cases. *Anesth Analg* 1970;49:564
10. Goldman L, Caldera DL, Nussbaum SR, et al: Multifactorial index of cardiac risk in non-cardiac surgical procedures. *N Engl J Med* 1977;297:845
11. Jeffrey CC, Kunsman J, Cullen DJ, et al: A prospective evaluation of cardiac risk index. *Anesthesiology* 1983;68:462
12. Slogoff S, Keats AS: Does perioperative myocardial ischemia lead to postoperative myocardial infarction? *Anesthesiology* 1985;62:107
13. Hartz AJ, Krakauer H, Kuhn EM, et al: Hospital characteristics and mortality rates. *N Engl J Med* 1989;321:1720
14. Forrester JS, Diamond GA, Swan HJC: Correlative classification of clinical and hemodynamic function after acute myocardial infarction. *Am J Cardiol* 1977;39:137
15. Conners AF, McCaffree DR, Grey BA: Evaluation of right-heart catheterization in the critically ill patient without myocardial infarction. *N Engl J Med* 1983;308:263
16. Goldman L, Caldera DL: Risks of general anesthesia and elective operation in the hypertensive patient. *Anesthesiology* 1979;50:285
17. Mangano DT: Perioperative cardiac morbidity. *Anesthesiology* 1990;72:153
18. Gerson MC, Hurst JM, Hertzberg VS, et al: Cardiac prognosis in noncardiac geriatric surgery. *Ann Intern Med* 1985;103:832
19. Tisi GM: Preoperative evaluation of pulmonary function: validity, indications, and benefits. *Am Rev Respir Dis* 1979;119:293
20. Unger K, Shaw D, Karlinger JS, et al: Evaluation of left ventricular function in patients with chronic obstructive lung disease. *Chest* 1975;68:135
21. Cohen CA, Zagelbaum G, Gross D, et al: Clinical manifestations of inspiratory muscle fatigue. *Am J Med* 1982;73:308
22. Boushy SF, Billeq DM, North LB, et al: Clinical course related to preoperative and postoperative pulmonary function in patients with bronchogenic carcinoma. *Chest* 1971;59:383
23. Didolkar MS, Moore RH, Takita H: Evaluation of the risk in pulmonary resection for bronchogenic carcinoma. *Am J Surg* 1974;127:700

24. Simmoneau G, Vivien A, Sartene R, et al: Diaphragm dysfunction induced by upper abdominal surgery: role of postoperative pain. *Am Rev Respir Dis* 1983;128:899

25. Dureuil B, Desmonts JM, Mankikian B, et al: Effects of aminophylline on diaphragmatic dysfunction after upper abdominal surgery. *Anesthesiology* 1985;62:242

26. Tisi GM: *Pulmonary Physiology in Clinical Medicine.* Baltimore, Williams & Wilkins, 1980:109

27. Toole JF: Surgery for patients with carotid-artery murmurs [editorial]. *N Engl J Med* 1982;307:1401

28. Ropper AH, Wechsler LR, Wilson LS: Carotid bruit and risk of stroke in elective surgery. *N Engl J Med* 1982;307:1388

29. Toole JF: Management of cervical atherosclerosis [editorial]. *Mayo Clin Proc* 1982;57:267

30. Wolf PA, Kannel WB, Sorlie P, et al: Asymptomatic carotid bruit and risk of stroke: the Framingham study. *JAMA* 1981; 245:1442

31. Del Guercio LRM, Cohn D: Monitoring operative risk in the elderly. *JAMA* 1980;243:1350

32. Rao TLK, Jacobs KH, El-Etr AA: Reinfarction following anesthesia in patients with myocardial infarction. *Anesthesiology* 1983;59:499

33. Shah KB, Kleinman BS, Sami H, et al: Reevaluation of perioperative myocardial infarction in patients with prior myocardial infarction undergoing noncardiac operations. *Anesth Analg* 1990;71:231

34. Robin ED: The cult of the Swan-Ganz catheter: overuse and abuse of pulmonary flow catheters. *Ann Intern Med* 1985; 103:445

35. Goldman L, Caldera DL, Southwick FS, et al: Cardiac risk factors and complications in non-cardiac surgery. *Medicine* 1977;57:357

36. Lowenstein E, Yusuf S, Teplick RS: Perioperative myocardial infarction: a glimmer of hope, a note of caution [editorial]. *Anesthesiology* 1983;59:493

37. Tarhan S, Moffitt EA, Taylor WF, et al: Myocardial infarction after general anesthesia. *JAMA* 1972;220:1451

38. Steen JA, Tinker JH, Tarhan S: Myocardial reinfarction after anesthesia and surgery. *JAMA* 1978;239:2566

39. Shoemaker WC, Appel PL, Kram HB, et al: Prospective trial of supranormal values of survivors as therapeutic goals in high-risk surgical patients. *Chest* 1988;94:1176

40. Catley DM, Thornton C, Jordan C, et al: Pronounced, episodic oxygen desaturation in the postoperative period: its association with ventilatory pattern and analgesic regimen. *Anesthesiology* 1985;63:20

41. Rosenberg J, Dirkes WE, Kehlet H: Episodic arterial oxygen desaturation and heart rate variations following major abdominal surgery. *Br J Anaesth* 1989;63:651

42. Yeager MP, Glass DD, Neff RK, et al: Epidural anesthesia and analgesia in high-risk surgical patients. *Anesthesiology* 1987;66:729

43. Quasha AL, Loeber N, Feeley TW, et al: Postoperative respiratory care: a controlled trial of early and late extubation following coronary-artery bypass grafting. *Anesthesiology* 1980;52:135

44. Olsson GL, Hallen B, Hambraeus-Jonzon K: Aspiration during anaesthesia: a computer-aided study of 185,358 anesthetics. *Acta Anaesthesiol Scand* 1986;30:84

45. Knieriem K, Stehling L: Aspiration pneumonitis. *Semin Anesth* 1990;9:54

46. Cohen S, Harris LD: Does hiatus hernia affect competence of the gastroesophageal sphincter? *N Engl J Med* 1971;284:1053

47. Schlaghecke R, Kornely E, Santen RT, et al: The effect of long-term glucocorticoid therapy on pituitary-adrenal responses to exogenous corticotropin-releasing hormone. *N Engl J Med* 1992;326:226

48. Rapaport SI: Preoperative hemostatic evaluation: which tests, if any? *Blood* 1983;61:229

49. The National Blood Resource Education Program Expert Panel: The use of autologous blood. *JAMA* 1990;263:414

50. Owings DV, Kruskall MS, Thurer RL, et al: Autologous blood donations prior to elective cardiac surgery: safety and efficacy of subsequent blood use. *JAMA* 1989;262:1963

51. Goodnough LT, Rudnick S, Price TH, et al: Increased preoperative collection of autologous blood with recombinant human erythropoietin therapy. *N Engl J Med* 1989;321:1163

52. Kaplan JA, Dunbar RW, Bland JW Jr, et al: Propranolol and cardiac surgery: a problem for the anesthesiologist? *Anesth Analg* 1975;54:571

53. Goldman L: Noncardiac surgery in patients receiving propranolol: case reports and a recommended approach. *Arch Intern Med* 1981;141:193

54. Siegel D, Hulley SB, Black DM, et al: Diuretics, serum and intracellular electrolyte levels, and ventricular arrhythmias in men. *JAMA* 1992;267:1083

55. Vitez TS, Soper LE, Wong KC, et al: Chronic hypokalemia and intraoperative dysrhythmias. *Anesthesiology* 1985;63:127

56. Hirsch IA, Tomlinson DL, Slogoff S, et al: The overstated risk of preoperative hypokalemia. *Anesthesiology* 1988;67:131

57. McGovern B: Hypokalemia and cardiac arrhythmias. *Anesthesiology* 1985;63:127

58. Rossing TH: Methylxanthines in 1989. *Ann Intern Med* 1989; 110:502

59. Lam A, Newhouse MT: Management of asthma and chronic airflow limitation: are methylxanthines obsolete? *Chest* 1990; 98:44

60. Roizen MF, Stevens WC: Multiform ventricular tachycardia due to interaction of aminophylline and halothane. *Anesth Analg* 1978;57:738

61. Pantuck EJ, Pantuck CB, Weissman C, et al: Effects of parenteral nutritional regimens on oxidative drug metabolism. *Anesthesiology* 1984;60:534

62. Roizen MF: Anesthetic implications of concurrent disease. In: Miller RD (ed). *Anesthesia*, 4th ed. New York, Churchill Livingstone, 1994:903

63. Palumbo PJ: Blood glucose control during surgery. *Anesthesiology* 1981;55:94

64. Roizen MF: Is tight perioperative control of diabetes warranted? *Anesthesiology* 1982;56:242

65. Stoelting RK: *Pharmacology and Physiology in Anesthetic Practice*, 2nd ed. Philadelphia, JB Lippincott, 1991:436

66. Chin R: Corticosteroids. In: Chernow B (ed). *The Pharmacologic Approach to the Critically Ill Patient*, 2nd ed. Baltimore, Williams and Wilkins, 1988:559

67. Macdonald R: Aspirin and extradural blocks. *Br J Anaesth* 1991;66:1

68. Cronberg S, Wallmark E, Soderberg I: Effect on platelet aggregation of oral administration of 10 non-steroidal analgesics to humans. *Scand J Haematol* 1984;33:155

69. Dahl JB, Kehlet H: Non-steroidal anti-inflammatory drugs: rationale for use in severe postoperative pain. *Br J Anaesth* 1991;66:703

70. Horlocker TT, Wedel DJ, Offord KP: Does preoperative antiplatelet therapy increase the risk of hemorrhagic complications associated with regional anesthesia? *Anesth Analg* 1990;70:631

71. O'Reilly RA: Anticoagulant, antithrombotic, and thrombolytic drugs. In: Gilman AG, Goodman LS, Rall TW, et al (eds). *Goodman and Gilman's The Pharmacologic Basis of Therapeutics*, 7th ed. New York, MacMillan, 1985:1338

72. Dajani AS, Bisno AL, Chung KJ, et al: Prevention of bacterial endocarditis: recommendations by the American Heart Association. *JAMA* 1990;264:2919

73. Classen DC, Evans S, Pestotnik SL, et al: The timing of prophylactic administration of antibiotics and the risk of surgical-wound infection. *N Engl J Med* 1992;326:281

74. Davies JM, Davison JS, Nimmo WS, et al: The stomach: factors of importance to the anaesthetic. *Can J Anaesth* 1990;37:896

75. Moore J, Flynn RJ, Sampaio M, et al: Effect of single-dose omeprazole on intragastric acidity and volume during obstetric anaesthesia. *Anaesthesia* 1989;44:559

76. National Institutes of Health Consensus Conference: Prevention of venous thrombosis and pulmonary embolism. *JAMA* 1986;256:744

77. Hyers TM, Hull RD, Weg JC: Antithrombotic therapy for venous thromboembolic disease. *Chest* 1986;89(Suppl):26S

78. Anderson FA, Wheeler HB, Goldberg RJ, et al: Physician practices in the prevention of venous thromboembolism. *Ann Intern Med* 1991;115:591

79. Truog RD: "Do-Not-Resuscitate" orders during anesthesia and surgery. *Anesthesiology* 1991;74:606

80. Cohen CB, Cohen PJ: Do-not-resuscitate orders in the operating room. *N Engl J Med* 1991;325:1879

81. Couper C: DNR in the OR. *JAMA* 1992;267:1465

82. Franklin C, Rothenberg DM: DNR in the OR. *JAMA* 1992;267:1465

Critical Care, Third Edition, edited by Joseph M. Civetta,
Robert W. Taylor, and Robert R. Kirby.
Lippincott-Raven Publishers, Philadelphia, PA © 1997.

CHAPTER 66

■

Anesthesia: Physiology and Postanesthesia Problems

Eran Segal
A. Joseph Layon

IMMEDIATE CONCERNS

MAJOR PROBLEMS

Modern anesthesia is a complex art and science that involves exposing patients to various drugs and procedures in a controlled and safe environment. Even under the best of circumstances, some complications occur. The overall risk of death from anesthesia is between 1 in 112,000 and 1 in 450,000.[1] Anesthetic-related morbidity is even more common, with respiratory depression being seen in between 1 in 500 to 1 in 1100 patients receiving epidural narcotics, and 1 in 100 patients given parenteral opioids.[1] Patients who sustain an anesthetic complication may require treatment in the ICU.

Airway problems are the most common causes for critical perioperative anesthetic mishaps. Maintaining an adequate airway is the first priority in all anesthetic management. An algorithm for airway management during anesthesia has been formulated by the American Society of Anesthesiologists[2] (Fig. 66-1).

In the immediate postoperative period, residual anesthetic and muscle relaxant effects may result in airway obstruction that should be quickly diagnosed and treated. Hypoventilation is also a common problem. Patients should be aggressively monitored, preferably with a pulse oximeter, and oxygen should be given to postoperative patients until they are shown to have adequate ventilatory drive and lung function.

STRESS POINTS

1. Postoperative acute respiratory failure is an uncommon but dramatic complication. Several clinical diagnoses should be explored in these situations.
2. Pulmonary edema can occur in the early postoperative period. It is more common in patients with hypertension who develop an acute elevation in blood secondary to the stress response, lack of significant analgesia, or cardiac ischemia.
3. Pulmonary edema has other causes, including "negative pressure" in a patient with partial or complete airway obstruction, aspiration of gastric contents during induction or emergence, and, in special situations, a neurogenic origin in head trauma, or after evacuation of a large pleural effusion.
4. Treatment in any case of hypoxemia entails delivering a high fraction of inspired oxygen (FIO_2) to ensure a saturation of at least 90% (i.e., a PaO_2 of about 60 mm Hg), and in more extreme cases, continuous positive airway pressure applied by mask or tracheal intubation, with or without mechanical ventilation. Although some of these complications may resolve rapidly, patients who develop significant hypoxemia after anesthesia and surgery should be closely monitored in an ICU for at least a day after the event.
5. Cardiac complications also are a frequent cause of perioperative morbidity and mortality. Arrhythmias may occur anytime. Ischemia, arrhythmia, heart fail-

1013

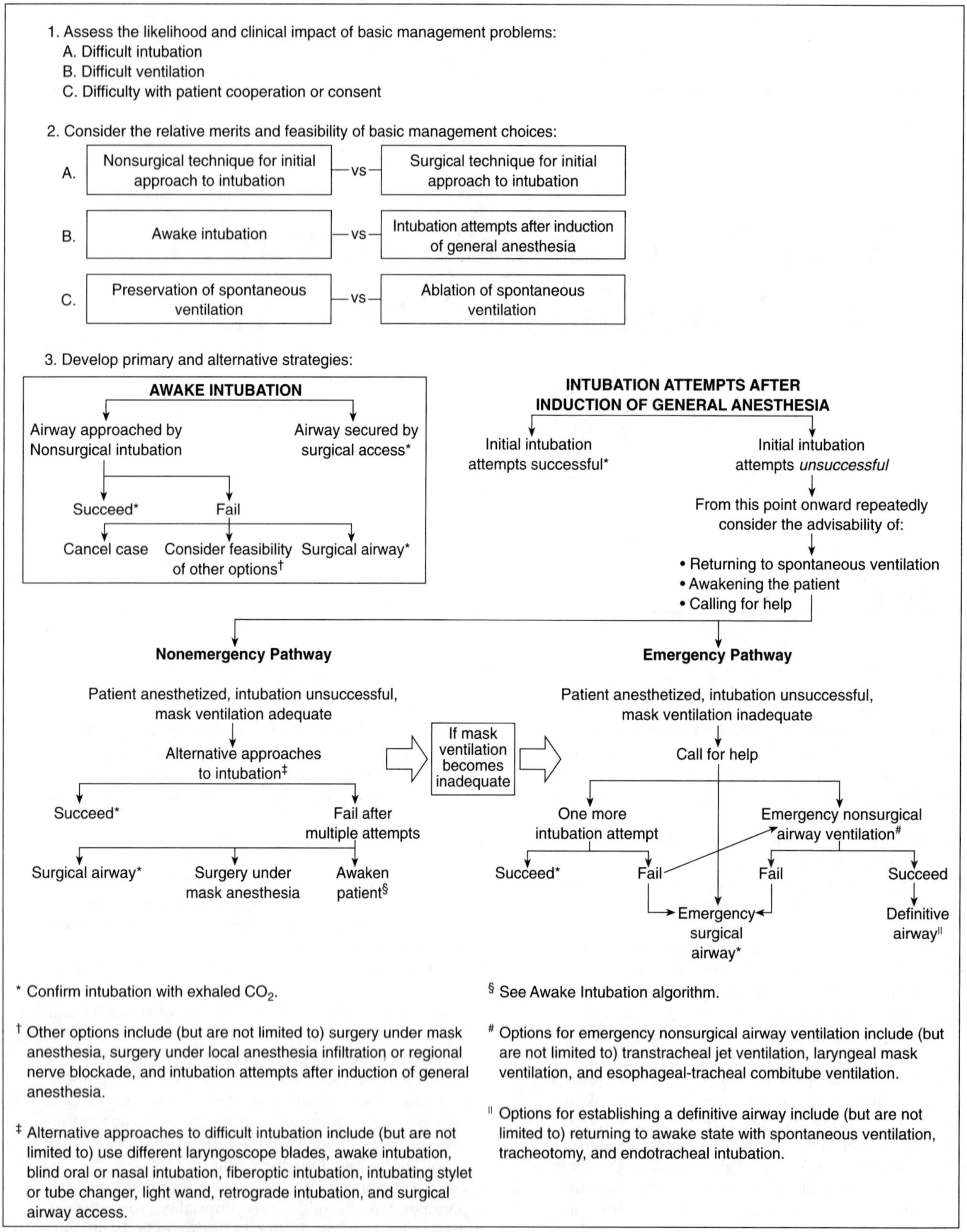

1. Assess the likelihood and clinical impact of basic management problems:
   A. Difficult intubation
   B. Difficult ventilation
   C. Difficulty with patient cooperation or consent

2. Consider the relative merits and feasibility of basic management choices:

A. | Nonsurgical technique for initial approach to intubation | —vs— | Surgical technique for initial approach to intubation |

B. | Awake intubation | —vs— | Intubation attempts after induction of general anesthesia |

C. | Preservation of spontaneous ventilation | —vs— | Ablation of spontaneous ventilation |

3. Develop primary and alternative strategies:

AWAKE INTUBATION

Airway approached by Nonsurgical intubation | Airway secured by surgical access*

Succeed* | Fail

Cancel case | Consider feasibility of other options† | Surgical airway*

INTUBATION ATTEMPTS AFTER INDUCTION OF GENERAL ANESTHESIA

Initial intubation attempts successful* | Initial intubation attempts *unsuccessful*

From this point onward repeatedly consider the advisability of:
• Returning to spontaneous ventilation
• Awakening the patient
• Calling for help

Nonemergency Pathway

Patient anesthetized, intubation unsuccessful, mask ventilation adequate

Alternative approaches to intubation‡

Succeed* | Fail after multiple attempts

Surgical airway* | Surgery under mask anesthesia | Awaken patient§

→ If mask ventilation becomes inadequate →

Emergency Pathway

Patient anesthetized, intubation unsuccessful, mask ventilation inadequate

Call for help

One more intubation attempt | Emergency nonsurgical airway ventilation#

Succeed* | Fail | Fail | Succeed

Emergency surgical airway* | Definitive airway‖

* Confirm intubation with exhaled CO_2.

† Other options include (but are not limited to) surgery under mask anesthesia, surgery under local anesthesia infiltration or regional nerve blockade, and intubation attempts after induction of general anesthesia.

‡ Alternative approaches to difficult intubation include (but are not limited to) use different laryngoscope blades, awake intubation, blind oral or nasal intubation, fiberoptic intubation, intubating stylet or tube changer, light wand, retrograde intubation, and surgical airway access.

§ See Awake Intubation algorithm.

Options for emergency nonsurgical airway ventilation include (but are not limited to) transtracheal jet ventilation, laryngeal mask ventilation, and esophageal-tracheal combitube ventilation.

‖ Options for establishing a definitive airway include (but are not limited to) returning to awake state with spontaneous ventilation, tracheotomy, and endotracheal intubation.

FIGURE 66-1. American Society of Anesthesiologists difficult airway algorithm.

ure, and myocardial infarction occur most commonly 3 to 5 days after surgery.

6. In the patient at risk for a cardiac complication, monitoring directed toward the diagnosis of silent ischemia or infarction may be useful. When a complication occurs, aggressive diagnostic and therapeutic cardiac interventions may be life-saving.

7. Hypertension in the immediate postoperative period commonly results from lack of adequate analgesia. This problem should be treated without delay, because heart failure and cardiac ischemia may result from an acute hypertensive crisis.

8. Patients with malignant hyperthermia (MH) may develop the syndrome at any time after exposure to a triggering agent (i.e., potent inhalational agents, succinylcholine). When MH is suspected, all triggering agents must be stopped. If possible, surgery should be cancelled, and dantrolene should be administered.[3] A MH hot line is available in many countries and can be contacted for assistance in caring for these patients.

UPTAKE AND DISTRIBUTION OF INHALATIONAL AGENTS ■

The goal of inhalational anesthesia is to develop a critical partial pressure of the agent within the brain. Brain levels are determined by several discrete steps[4] (Table 66-1). The anesthesia system is designed to present a suitable mixture of the anesthetic agent with air, oxygen, nitrous oxide, or a combination of these agents.[5,6] It must deliver a predictable concentration of agents, eliminate carbon dioxide, closely control and maintain a predictable F_{IO_2}, and allow monitoring and control of ventilation.

DELIVERY

Alveolar Partial Pressure

The brain partial pressure is responsible for the depth and some of the side effects of anesthesia, and correlates closely with the end-tidal partial pressure.

TABLE 66-1. Factors Governing Uptake and Distribution of Inhaled Agents

---

DELIVERY
  Inspired concentration
  Concentration effect
  Second gas effect
  Ventilation

UPTAKE FROM LUNGS
  Solubility
  Cardiac output
  Alveolar–mixed venous partial pressure gradient

DISTRIBUTION TO TISSUES
  Solubility of agent in tissue
  Blood flow to tissue

CONCENTRATION EFFECT. The inspired concentration is important to the rate of rise of anesthetic agent concentration in the lungs. This relationship is termed the concentration effect and has two important elements. Consider an ideal alveolus filled with 1 mL of nitrous oxide and 9 mL of oxygen. Assume that 50% of the nitrous oxide is rapidly taken up by the circulation and oxygen is not taken up at all. On completion, 0.5 mL of nitrous oxide and 9 mL of oxygen remain. Thus, the nitrous oxide concentration is decreased to 5%, whereas the oxygen concentration is increased to 95%.

Clearly, this situation is ideal and is used only for explanatory purposes. If, however, 8 mL of gas is nitrous oxide, 2 mL is oxygen, and 50% of the nitrous oxide is taken up rapidly, 4 mL of nitrous oxide and 2 mL of oxygen remain. Under these circumstances, the remaining gas is 66% nitrous oxide and 33% oxygen. As a rule, a higher initial inspired concentration of the agent results in a higher alveolar level in spite of uptake from the lung.

SECOND GAS EFFECT. When large amounts of an anesthetic agent such as nitrous oxide are rapidly taken up, the lungs do not collapse. Instead, a subatmospheric alveolar pressure is generated as a result of the rapid removal of this gas by the pulmonary blood flow, and a passive inflow of additional gas from the anesthesia circuit replaces that which is taken up. This second gas effect may have important consequences and can be used to clinical advantage. When another anesthetic agent is administered, its partial pressure increase is also more rapid than when it is administered alone because it is drawn into the lungs with the first agent.

ALVEOLAR VENTILATION. Another primary factor influencing the delivery of the anesthetic agent is alveolar ventilation ($\dot{V}_A$). In other words, a greater $\dot{V}_A$ increases the rate at which the alveolar partial pressure approaches the inspired partial pressure. This factor is limited only by lung volume; that is, a larger functional residual capacity decreases the "wash-in" rate of the agent.

UPTAKE FROM THE LUNGS

Solubility

Solubility describes the extent to which the anesthetic agent dissolves in blood and tissues (Table 66-2; see Table 66-1); the more soluble the agent is in blood, the more is dissolved in the pulmonary blood, and the longer it takes to reach a necessary partial pressure of agent in the lungs and brain. This fact represents the key difference between inhaled agents and other commonly used drugs. For example, 2 g of ampicillin given intravenously is dissolved in blood, carried to the site of infection, and produces the desired pharmacologic effect. The partial pressure of the anesthetic agent reaching the brain is the determinant of its desired effect, but is controlled by the partial pressure achieved in the alveoli. Thus, the greater the amount of anesthetic dissolved

TABLE 66-2. Partition Coefficients of Selected Inhalational Agents (at 37° ± 0.5°C)

AGENT	BLOOD/GAS	TISSUE/BLOOD
Nitrous oxide	0.47	Brain: 1.06
Isoflurane	1.41	Brain: 2.6
		Fat: 45.0
Enflurane	1.78	Brain: 1.45
		Fat: 36.2
Halothane	2.36	Brain: 2.6
		Fat: 60
Sevoflurane	0.69	Brain: 1.7
		Fat: 48
Desflurane	0.42	Brain: 1.3
		Fat: 27

in the blood (taken away from the alveoli), the longer it takes to develop adequate alveolar (and brain) partial pressures to produce anesthesia.

An agent such as nitrous oxide, with a blood/gas partition coefficient of 0.47, is relatively insoluble, and its alveolar partial pressure increases rapidly compared with that of halothane, which has a blood/gas partition coefficient of 2.36. The speed of induction of a more soluble agent can be increased by increasing the inspired fraction to a level well in excess of that required for maintenance of anesthesia.

Cardiac Output

A high cardiac output increases uptake, thereby decreasing the alveolar partial pressure of the agent. This effect is greater with more soluble inhalational anesthetics. Thus, a longer induction time is required for a patient with high cardiac output (as in thyrotoxicosis). Conversely, a patient with a low cardiac output (as with compensated congestive cardiomyopathy) has a rapid increase of alveolar partial pressure, resulting in a rapid induction and possible overdose if care is not taken.

Alveolar–Mixed Venous Anesthetic Partial Pressure Gradient

The last major factor of importance is the influence of the alveolar to central mixed venous anesthetic partial pressure gradient. This factor relates the size of the anesthetic "sink" to the increase or decrease in uptake from the lungs. At the beginning of induction when the tissue anesthetic level is zero, most of the anesthetic in the arterial blood is removed. Thus, the venous anesthetic partial pressure is much lower than that in the arterial blood, and a large uptake of anesthetic occurs as the venous blood passes through the lungs. The alveolar partial pressure of the anesthetic agent, accordingly, is reduced. However, as the tissue sinks become filled, the alveolar to venous anesthetic partial pressure difference decreases, and this effect is minimized.

DISTRIBUTION

Tissue Solubility and Blood Flow

The tissue distribution (delivery) of the anesthetic is dependent on two major factors (see Table 66-1). The greater the solubility of an anesthetic in a tissue, the larger the capacity of that tissue for the agent. If the tissue has a large capacity but low blood flow, equilibration takes a long time; if the tissue has a small capacity and large blood flow, equilibration is rapid. Tissues can be categorized according to the blood flow they receive. The vessel-rich group comprises the brain, liver, heart, and kidneys. An intermediate group includes muscle and skin. The vessel-poor group incorporates skeletal elements, ligaments, and cartilage, all of which have minimal blood supply. Finally, fat has a poor blood supply but a great capacity.

Based on this division, one can easily determine when the different groups equilibrate with the inspired fraction of anesthetic agent, that is, when they cease removing appreciable amounts of the anesthetic. Nitrous oxide equilibration with the vessel-rich group occurs within 5 to 15 minutes from the beginning of induction. The muscle group equilibrates within approximately 1 hour, and the vessel-poor group and fat group equilibrate within 2 to 3 hours. When a highly fat-soluble agent such as halothane is used for a long case in an obese patient, significant amounts of agent are stored in fat and are released slowly after the agent is discontinued; emergence from anesthesia is thereby prolonged. At the end of surgery, the factors that affect elimination of the agent from the body are the same as those that govern the uptake and distribution at the beginning. Hypoventilation lengthens the period of emergence, as do increased cardiac output, use of a highly soluble anesthetic agent, and an increased alveolar to venous anesthetic concentration gradient.

Diffusion Hypoxia

Diffusion hypoxia may be apparent at the conclusion of an anesthetic if the patient is allowed to breathe room air while large quantities of nitrous oxide diffuse into the alveoli and dilute the oxygen that is present. This problem is significant only for approximately 10 minutes and can be alleviated by having the patient breathe 100% oxygen after discontinuation of the nitrous oxide.

EFFECTS OF ILLNESS

Changes in Ventilation

Organ system dysfunction can affect the uptake and distribution of inhaled anesthetic agents. For example, to control intracranial pressure (ICP) in brain-injured patients, tracheal intubation and mechanical hyperventilation frequently are used. For each 1 mm Hg decrease in the $PaCO_2$ caused by an increase in $\dot{V}A$, an approximate 3% to 4% decrease in cerebral blood flow (CBF) occurs. If the patient is taken to the operating room, and if hyperventilation is continued, a change in the length of time of anesthetic induction results from three factors: increased $\dot{V}A$, decreased CBF, and solubility of the inhaled agents used for induction. The induction time for a moderately soluble agent like halothane is decreased because the increased $\dot{V}A$ produces a more rapid rise in end-tidal halothane partial pressure that offsets the decrease in CBF. For a relatively nonsoluble agent such as nitrous oxide, induction time is increased because the modest increase in end-tidal nitrous oxide partial pressure obtained by hyperventilation is more than offset by the decrease in CBF.

Changes in Cardiac Output

This particular example can become complicated by a decrease in cardiac output, secondary to hyperventilation-induced alkalemia, and a decrease in venous return, resulting from fluid restriction and the effects of mechanical ventilation. The decrease in cardiac output yields an increase in the agent's end-tidal partial pressure, whereas a decrease in CBF decreases transfer of the agent from the lungs to the brain. With halothane, the increase in the end-tidal partial pressure is sufficient to balance the decrease in CBF; thus, the initial rise in brain partial pressure may be normal. Eventually, no matter what agent is used, the increased end-tidal partial pressure resulting from the decrease in cardiac output and increase in $\dot{V}A$ is enough to overcome the decrease in CBF.

Alterations in Ventilation/Perfusion Ratios

Consider a person with a 50% intrapulmonary shunt ($\dot{Q}s/\dot{Q}t$) and two idealized alveoli, one of which is completely obstructed, the second of which is ventilated, and both of which are perfused. With a relatively soluble agent such as halothane and a ventilation/perfusion ($\dot{V}/\dot{Q}$) ratio of 1:1 in the second alveolus, a normal amount of anesthetic agent will be taken up. When blood from this alveolus is mixed with blood from the first alveolus, with a $\dot{V}/\dot{Q}$ ratio of zero (no ventilation), the resultant "pooled" blood partial pressure will be a value well below that which would be obtained if both alveoli had been ventilated. Conversely, with nitrous oxide, equilibration occurs so rapidly and its solubility is so poor that further uptake is limited, and compensation cannot occur.[5]

INHALATION AGENTS AND ORGAN SYSTEM FUNCTION ■

The differential effects of various inhalation agents on organ system function must be compared at equipotent doses. The minimum alveolar concentration (MAC) is the amount of an inhalational agent that prevents movement in 50% of patients in response to surgical incision (Table 66-3). In neonates, the MAC is less than in children, adolescents, and

TABLE 66-3. Minimum Alveolar Concentration in Patients Aged 31 to 55 Years

Halothane	0.75%
Isoflurane	1.15%
Enflurane	1.68%
Nitrous oxide	110%°
Desflurane	6%
Sevoflurane	2.05%

°Obtainable only under hyperbaric conditions.

young adults. After approximately 31 years of age, the MAC value begins to decrease; theoretically, the value for a patient 100 years of age is only 25% to 50% that of a young adult.

CIRCULATORY EFFECTS

Myocardial Contractility

All inhalational anesthetic agents decrease myocardial contractility. Mean maximal velocity (Vmax) and mean maximal developed force (F_M) are decreased at 1 MAC halothane in vitro by 45% and 40%, respectively. Isoflurane at 1 MAC decreased Vmax and F_M by approximately 35% and 40%, respectively; enflurane decreases them by 10% and 35%, respectively. When isolated myocardium from cats with congestive heart failure has been exposed to isoflurane, Vmax and F_M decrease approximately 55%.

Hemodynamic Function

In vivo studies are somewhat more complicated (Table 66-4). Isoflurane seems to have the least effect on myocardial function. Nitrous oxide (under hyperbaric conditions) and isoflurane minimally affect cardiac output, whereas halothane and enflurane decrease cardiac output by 20% to 40% of the awake value. Nitrous oxide, isoflurane, and enflurane all increase heart rate, whereas halothane does not. Stroke volume is unaffected by nitrous oxide, is decreased most (40% to 60%) by enflurane, and is intermediately affected (20% to 40%) by isoflurane and halothane.

If these parameters are studied in the spontaneously breathing patient, a greater increase in heart rate and cardiac output as a percentage of awake values occurs compared with values seen with controlled mechanical ventilation. Desflurane, a new potent inhaled anesthetic agent, seems to have cardiac properties similar to those of isoflurane.

Although the effect of inhalational agents on coronary artery blood flow is another area of controversy, published studies suggest that at 1 MAC, isoflurane, enflurane, and halothane all blunt autoregulation of coronary artery blood flow but that isoflurane does so to a greater extent.

Cardiac Rhythm

Of the several methods for evaluation of the effects of inhalational agents on cardiac rhythm, a common procedure is to

TABLE 66-4. Respiratory and Circulatory Effects of the Inhalation Agents

	N₂O	HALOTHANE	ENFLURANE	ISOFLURANE
Respiratory				
V̇E	↓	↓	↓ ↓ ↓	↓ ↓
% awake response to CO₂	↓ ↓	↓ ↓	↓ ↓	↓ ↓
% awake response to hypoxia	—	↓	↓ ↓	↓ ↓
Circulatory				
% awake ballistocardiogram	—	↓	↓ ↓	θ
% awake cardiac output	θ	↓	↓	θ
% awake stroke volume	θ	↓	↓ ↓	↓
μg/kg epinephrine for ≥3 PVCs	—	2.1–3.7	10.9	6.7

—, no data; θ, no change, ↓ , decrease of ≤33%; ↓ ↓ , decrease of ≤66; ↓ ↓ ↓ , decrease of ≥66%; PVCs, premature ventricular contractions; N₂O, nitrous oxide; V̇E, expired volume per min; CO₂, carbon dioxide.

determine the dose of epinephrine required to produce three or more premature ventricular contractions in 50% of normal patients breathing oxygen and anesthetized at 1.25 MAC (see Table 66-4). With halothane, 2.1 μg/kg body weight of epinephrine is required to produce rhythm abnormalities; if the epinephrine is given with 0.5% lidocaine, the required dose increases to 3.7 μg/kg. With isoflurane, 6.7 μg/kg of epinephrine is needed; and with enflurane, approximately 10.9 μg/kg is required. The new agents, desflurane and sevoflurane, have properties similar to those of enflurane. Thus, halothane is the most and enflurane, desflurane, and sevoflurane are the least arrhythmogenic of the potent inhalation anesthetic agents.

Hypoxic Pulmonary Vasoconstriction

Hypoxic pulmonary vasoconstriction (HPV) may be impaired when potent agents are used. If inhaled concentrations of halothane or enflurane are increased in vitro from 1 to 2 MAC, and $PaCO_2$ is held constant, the local response to hypoxia is unchanged. With isoflurane, HPV seems to be significantly impaired; with desflurane, HPV is inhibited in a concentration-dependent fashion.[7] However, the conclusion that isoflurane is worse for patients with atelectasis and pneumonia has not been documented clinically.

RESPIRATORY EFFECTS

All inhalational agents are respiratory depressants. Decreases in minute ventilation at 1 MAC are 20% with nitrous oxide, 28% with halothane, 34% with isoflurane, and 71% with enflurane. The ventilatory response to an elevation in $PaCO_2$ at 1 MAC is decreased by 50% with nitrous oxide, 60% with halothane, 35% with isoflurane, and 45% with enflurane (see Table 66-4). The response to hypoxia is depressed by 30% with halothane, 40% with isoflurane, and 45% with enflurane. Finally, and of some interest, is that oxygen consumption at 1 MAC also decreases with all three potent agents.

HEPATIC EFFECTS

On the first postanesthetic day, volunteers undergoing 11.7 MAC hours (e.g., 11.7 MAC hours equals 1 MAC for 11.7 hours, or 2 MAC for 5.85 hours) of halothane showed a significant increase in the bromsulphthalein retention, but not after 9.6 MAC hours of enflurane or 8 MAC hours of isoflurane. No clinically significant hepatic dysfunction was noted. Enzyme values (alanine aminotransferase [ALT] and aspartate aminotransferase [AST]) also significantly increased on the first postanesthetic day with enflurane, but not with halothane and isoflurane.

Patients who underwent surgery and anesthesia with isoflurane and halothane manifested a slight increase in ALT, AST, and lactate dehydrogenase. The changes seen with halothane may be greater than those observed with isoflurane. A statistically significant increase in bromsulphthalein retention on the second postoperative day also was seen with halothane and isoflurane. The increase was greater with halothane. Neither desflurane nor sevoflurane seem to have hepatotoxic properties, although this observation needs further confirmation.

So-called halothane hepatitis is a complicated issue and cannot be adequately reviewed in this chapter.[8,9] Nonetheless, halothane is a time-tested, safe anesthetic agent, a conclusion that was supported by the National Halothane Study that reported a fatal halothane-related hepatic necrosis incidence of only 1 per 35,000 patients.

RENAL EFFECTS

All potent inhalation agents result in a dose-dependent decrease in renal blood flow (25% to 50%), glomerular filtration rate (23% to 40%), and urine flow (35% to 67%). No change in creatinine clearance or ability to concentrate urine in response to subcutaneous injection of vasopressin occurs after the use of isoflurane, halothane, or enflurane.

Fluorinated inhalation agents place the patient at some risk of nephrotoxicity, depending on the degree to which they are metabolized.[10] The classic example is methoxyflurane, no longer commonly used. Nephrotoxicity correlates with the serum inorganic fluoride (Fl⁻) concentration. With methoxyflurane, no nephrotoxicity occurs with a serum Fl⁻ value below 40 μMol/L; fluoride levels of 50 to 80 μMol/L result in subclinical toxicity; and levels of 90 to 120 μMol/ L produce serum hyperosmolality, hypernatremia, polyuria, and low urine osmolality—the so-called vasopressin-resistant, polyuric renal failure.

Patients anesthetized with enflurane for approximately 10 MAC hours have peak Fl⁻ levels up to 34 μMol/L in the postanesthetic period. Thus, a relatively nonmetabolized inhalational agent such as isoflurane, or intravenous agents, probably should be used in patients with preexisting renal disease. Although still under study, the two new potent inhaled anesthetic agents, desflurane and sevoflurane, do not seem to be nephrotoxic even though Fl⁻ levels peak at more than 50 μMol/L with sevoflurane.

IMMUNE FUNCTION

Anesthesia and surgery impair immune system functioning (Table 66-5). However, serious questions as to cause and effect and the relevance to clinical outcome have been raised. There are many effects on nonspecific immune system components.[11] For example, mucocilliary escalator function is impaired by inhalational anesthesia, atropine, and high concentrations of inspired oxygen. Malnutrition in the perioperative period also affects immune function and is associated with increased morbidity and mortality.[12] Patients who are nutritionally repleted before their surgical procedure may have a lower incidence of postoperative complications. An element of immune dysfunction may be caused by stress, with elevations in norepinephrine, epinephrine, steroids, and other mediators of the stress response.[11,12] If this supposition is true, perhaps different anesthetic techniques,[13] or even the use of sympathetic blockade, might ameliorate these responses perioperatively and thus decrease some of the reported abnormalities.

Phagocytosis

Phagocytosis reportedly is depressed perioperatively, perhaps because of surgical stress and the direct effects of inhalation anesthetic agents.[11] Everson and colleagues[14] showed increased monocytic function in the first 24 hours postoperatively in patients who had undergone an operative procedure for nonmalignant disease. Patients who underwent surgery for carcinoma had no change in monocytic function. Shenniv and others[15] believe that some members of the mononuclear phagocytic system are affected by the stress of nutritional depletion and may take up to 3 weeks to recover. How standard measures of immunocompetence correlate with the functioning of the alveolar macrophage, abnormalities of which may put the patient at risk for pulmonary infection, is unclear.

Killer Cells

NATURAL KILLER CELLS. Natural killer (NK) cells are cytotoxic to target cells and do not require the presence of complement or specific antibody to perform their killing function. A paucity of information exists concerning the effects of surgery and anesthesia on the NK cell function of peripheral blood mononuclear cells (see Table 66-5). Tonnessen and associates[16] showed that NK activity increased in the perioperative period, returning toward normal by the second postoperative day after intravenous anesthesia. The reasons for and significance of these changes are unclear. On the other hand, Katzav and colleagues[17] showed that mice exposed to ketamine or halothane, but not to nitrous oxide or sodium thiopental, had significantly decreased NK cell function 5 days after exposure. This decrement in NK cell function was significantly improved by treatment of exposed mice with polyinosinic-polycytidylic acid (100 μg intraperitoneally). Polyinosinic-polycytidylic acid is a NK cell modulator that augments activity through interferon induction. Page and colleagues[18] also found that surgical stimulation depleted NK cell number and decreased NK activity; the use of morphine for pain control mitigated the measured immunologic effects of surgical stress. Other work suggests that the decrement in NK activity seen with the cortisol component of the stress response is reversible with epinephrine.[19]

ADCC K CELLS. Another killer cell of importance is the antibody-dependent cellular cytotoxicity (ADCC) K cell.

TABLE 66-5. Effects of Inhalation Agents on Immune Function

	N₂O	HALOTHANE	ENFLURANE	ISOFLURANE
Monocyte function	?	↓	?	?
Natural killer cell activity	↑°	↓, ?	?	?
ADCC K-cell activity	?	?	?	?
Neutrophil function	?	↓	↓	↓
Lymphocyte function	θ°	↓, ?	↓, ?	?

θ, no change; ↑, activity/function increased; ↓, activity/function decreased; ?, needs study; ADCC, antibody–dependent cellular cytotoxicity; N₂O, nitrous oxide.
°Used with intravenous anesthesia.

These cells attack their targets in the presence of specific IgG anti-target cell antibody. Data on the effects of surgery and anesthesia on this function also are sketchy. McCredie[20] reports that the ADCC K cell activity is decreased in critically ill surgical patients, and patients who died had lower initial and final values. Septic patients who lived or died had the same initial values on admission to the ICU, but those who died had lower final values. Operative procedures have no effect on ADCC K cell selectivity in patients with normal activity preoperatively. In patients with decreased ADCC in the preoperative period, a decrease in selectivity was observed as late as 5 days postoperatively, with recovery in approximately 15 days. How inhalation anesthetic agents affect ADCC K cell activity is entirely unclear.

Neutrophils

Data on neutrophil function during and after surgery and anesthesia are more abundant but also conflicting (see Table 66-5). Nakagawara and associates[21] report that halothane, enflurane, and isoflurane depress superoxide production, in part because of a decrease in the mobilization of intracellular calcium (superoxide is the reactive oxygen species produced by neutrophils during phagocytosis). In an accompanying editorial, Welch[22] suggests that calcium-blocking properties of potent inhalational agents may cause neutrophil dysfunction. He noted that the volatile anesthetics, whose potency is correlated with lipid solubility, may prevent the release of membrane-bound intracellular calcium, as well as calcium influx, by occupying hydrophobic sites in the cellular membranes.

A second possibility is that the proteins involved in calcium transport are directly inactivated by the potent agents. Using intravenous anesthetic agents, van Dijk and coworkers[23] found no changes in neutrophil phagocytosis, chemotaxis, or chemoluminescence. Perttilä and colleagues,[24] using "balanced" anesthesia, consisting of both intravenous and relatively small doses of inhalation anesthetic agents, found minimally depressed neutrophil function that returned to preinduction values by the third postoperative day. Our work,[25] using Ficoll gradient–separated neutrophils exposed to isoflurane (0.5%), O$_2$:N$_2$O (50%:50%), or air, suggested no difference in phagocytoses of *Escherichia coli* between control and anesthetic-exposed cells.

Lymphocytes

Lymphocyte function is believed to be impaired in the critically ill. Lymphocyte abnormalities in surgical patients reported by McIrvine and Mannick[26] included anergy, impaired resistance to infection by poorly encapsulated gram-negative organisms (i.e., *Pseudomonas*), and impaired ability to eliminate facultative intracellular pathogens (i.e., *Listeria monocytogenes*). Surgical procedures, including corneal transplantation, dilation and curettage, transurethral resection of the prostate, arthroplasty, open heart procedures, cholecystectomy, nephrectomy, herniorrhaphy, and others, show a decrease in lymphocyte response to mitogens, such as phytohemagglutinin and concanavalin A, which stimulate most T cells, and pokeweed mitogen, which stimulates proliferation of T cells and B cells.

MIXED LYMPHOCYTE REACTION. The mixed lymphocyte reaction exploits the fact that T lymphocytes are stimulated to grow and divide in the presence of another cell (such as a B lymphocyte), which carries foreign class II histocompatibility antigens. A decreased response occurs and suggests impaired lymphocyte function. Delayed hypersensitivity also is decreased. The mechanisms by which suppression of lymphocyte function occur are unclear currently but may include the following: hormonal effects (serum cortisol or a natural endogenous suppressor substance); drugs (antibiotics such as aminocycline, oxytetracycline, cimetidine, and aspirin); anesthesia; and nutritional factors.[26]

HEMORRHAGIC STRESS-INDUCED SERUM FACTOR. Abraham and Chang[27] report a hemorrhagic stress-induced serum factor that depresses lymphocyte proliferation, is heat-stable and dialyzable, and has a molecular weight between 13,000 and 23,000 daltons. This factor, or group of factors, seems to suppress lymphocyte proliferation in a rapid and irreversible manner, and may have some significance in the suppression of cell-mediated immunity in response to the stress of anesthesia and surgery. Recently, extension of this work showed that after an approximate 30% loss of calculated blood volume, mice exposed to bacterial antigen produce significantly less antigen-specific antibody than did exposed but nonhemorrhaged animals.[28] Potent inhalation agents also may cause lymphocyte dysfunction. However, this area is poorly studied and controversial.

POLYCLONAL ACTIVATORS. In a further attempt to clarify these effects, we have investigated lymphocyte responses to polyclonal activators after in vivo exposure to 1.5 MAC of isoflurane or halothane. Healthy BALB/c mice were exposed to one of the two agents in 100% oxygen or, with the same handling, breathed air. After 1.5 hours, the animals were returned to their cages and killed immediately, or at 1, 12, or 24 hours after the exposure was terminated. Spleen cells were cultured in the presence of polyclonal activators, paradigms of antigen, and then pulsed with ^{3}H-thymidine. A second group of animals was exposed to the same anesthetic agents and then injected intraperitoneally with a sublethal dose of *E. coli*.

Our preliminary data suggest that although selective immune defects may be described from the cultures, no increase in mortality occurred in animals exposed to either isoflurane or halothane when compared with that of control (air exposed) animals. Our interpretation of this information is that exposure to clinically useful concentrations of isoflurane or halothane does not significantly impair immune function. Whether this finding holds true in immune-compromised animals is still unclear. Thus, as stated in the first and second editions of this book, no credible data suggest that one anesthetic technique is "safer" than another with regard to its effects on immune system function. Further studies, both phenomenological and mechanistic, are required.

INTRAVENOUS AGENTS

NARCOTICS

General Properties

Although opiates have been used for thousands of years, morphine sulfate was first isolated from opium in 1803. Near the end of the 19th century, morphine and scopolamine, in doses of 1 to 3 mg/kg, were used intramuscularly or intravenously to provide "complete" anesthesia. Because of the increasing operative morbidity and mortality seen with this technique, it rapidly fell into disfavor. However, the use of high-dose narcotics for anesthesia again was popularized in the 1970s.

Problems with morphine include recall, histamine release, prolonged postoperative respiratory depression, hypertension, and increased blood and fluid requirements because of vasodilation. Newer phenylpiperidine narcotics such as fentanyl and sufentanil do not induce histamine release, nor do they increase blood and fluid requirements. Anesthetic induction with opioids is based on the premise that these agents provide hemodynamic stability in patients with heart disease.[29] Incomplete amnesia with either low- or high-dose phenylpiperidine opioids does occur, but pain is rare.

Generally speaking, healthier patients require larger doses of drugs than sicker, older patients. If 30 μg/kg of fentanyl are given to patients ages 18 to 31 years, 57% lose consciousness; if, however, the same dose is given to patients over 60 years, 100% lose consciousness. Loss of consciousness, however, cannot be equated with anesthesia. The latter is obtained when analgesia, amnesia, muscle relaxation, and hemodynamic stability are achieved. Because narcotics do not provide either amnesia or muscle relaxation, other agents such as benzodiazepines and neuromuscular blockers are required.

A further complicating factor in anesthetic induction is that acute tolerance may occur. As a result, awakening or absence of analgesia occurs at plasma opioid levels higher than those associated with the initial loss of consciousness or onset of analgesia. Profound analgesia and apnea can be produced without satisfactory anesthesia. Although supplemental drugs such as nitrous oxide, benzodiazepines, butyrophenones, or a combination thereof, make amnesia more likely, they do not guarantee it. Our impression, based on the literature and personal experience, is that awareness is less common when potent inhalational agents are used.

Pharmacokinetics/Pharmacodynamics

Selected pharmacokinetic data for three commonly used opioids are summarized in Table 66-6. Similarities between the redistribution and elimination half-lives and the clearance and steady-state volume of distribution are noteworthy. The major difference is in lipid solubility, which correlates with potency. Interestingly, the peak respiratory depressant effect of morphine is 15 to 30 minutes after injection, but with fentanyl, it occurs at 5 to 10 minutes.[30] The depressant effect from morphine usually lasts longer, although that of

TABLE 66-6. Selected Pharmacokinetic Data for Three Opioids

	MORPHINE	FENTANYL	SUFENTANIL
Lipid solubility°	1.4	814	1778
$t_{1/2}$ π (min)[†]	0.9–2.4	1–3	0.5–2
$t_{1/2}$ α (min)[‡]	10–20	5–20	5–15
$t_{1/2}$ β (hr)[§]	2–4	2–4	2–3
Clearance (mL/kg/min)	10–20	10–20	10–12
Vd_{ss} (L/kg)[‖]	3–5	3–5	2.5

°Proportional to ease with which agent crosses blood–brain barrier and, hence, potency.

[†]$t_{1/2}$ π, rapid redistribution half-life.

[‡]$t_{1/2}$ α, slow redistribution half-life.

[§]$t_{1/2}$ β, elimination half-life.

[‖]Vd_{ss}, steady-state volume of distribution.

fentanyl can be seen even after the analgesic effect of that drug has dissipated.

A narcotic-induced respiratory depression may occur in natural sleep. Potentiation of the natural "right shift" in the carbon dioxide ventilatory response curve occurs with sleep in patients older than 60 years of age and in those with hypocapnic hyperventilation. In the latter group, the prolonged respiratory depression seems to result from decreased hepatic blood flow, resulting in increased effective duration of the drug.

Hemodynamic Effects

Hypotension is a significant problem with morphine in a dose of 1 to 4 mg/kg. During induction of anesthesia, systolic blood pressures are less than 70 mm Hg in 10% of patients. Possible mechanisms include vagal-induced bradycardia, vasodilation, and splanchnic blood sequestration. The rate of infusion seems to be important, because hypotension seldom occurs at rates of 5 mg/minute or less, but is seen frequently at rates of 10 mg/minute.

Some of these effects seem to result from histamine release. After a 1 mg/kg intravenous dose of morphine, histamine increases four to nine times above the control values. Treatment with H_1 (diphenhydramine) and H_2 (cimetidine) blockers attenuates the cardiovascular response to histamine. Fentanyl, 30 to 100 μg/kg, rarely causes hypotension, even in patients with poor left ventricular function, perhaps because it does not cause histamine release. No significant changes in contractility, heart rate, cardiac output, or systemic or pulmonary artery occlusion pressure occur. When blood pressure decreases with fentanyl, it is often secondary to a decrease in heart rate and is attenuated with a vagolytic agent.

Respiratory Effects

Significant dose-dependent respiratory depression can occur with opioids. Both the end-tidal partial pressure of carbon dioxide and the apneic threshold, defined as the $PaCO_2$ below which spontaneous ventilation is not initiated unless hypoxia is present, are increased. Hypoxic ventilatory drive is decreased and the increase in ventilatory drive seen with increased airways resistance is blunted. The pontine and medullary centers for respiratory rhythmicity also are impaired. Increased respiratory pauses and delayed exhalation produce irregular and periodic breathing.

With regard to respiratory depression, fentanyl is probably worse than enflurane. Opioids also have effects on the distal respiratory tract that may be of some significance. Morphine, and probably other opioids, decrease mucocilliary escalator function. Fentanyl, because of its antihistaminergic, antiseritoninergic, and antimuscarinic effects, may be more useful than morphine in patients with bronchospastic diseases.

Neurologic Effects

Alterations in neurophysiology are common with opioids. Morphine (1 to 3 mg/kg) with 70% nitrous oxide has no effect on CBF, cerebral metabolic rate for oxygen ($CMRO_2$), or cerebral metabolic rate for glucose (CMR_G). Fentanyl, with or without droperidol, causes a small decrease in CBF and cerebral metabolic rate in a canine model.

Muscle rigidity is commonly seen with fentanyl but can occur with other opioids. The mechanism is not well understood, but apparently does not result from a direct effect of the opioid on muscle fibers or on the neural components of muscle. Rather, it may result from stimulation of gamma-aminobutyrate (GABA) receptors located on interneurons. Neuroexcitatory phenomena have been described with the opioids, but the clinical significance of this observation is questionable.

Gastrointestinal Effects

The effects of analgesic doses of opioids on the gastrointestinal system are well known and include the following: emesis secondary to stimulation of the chemoreceptor trigger zone in the area postrema of the medulla; increased gastrointestinal secretions; decreased motility that also may affect emetic action; and increased smooth muscle tone of the gastrointestinal tract and the sphincter of Oddi. Reports suggesting that the agonist–antagonist narcotics (nalbuphine or butorphanol) cause less increase in gastrointestinal tract tone are controversial.

Stress

The effect to which a given drug ameliorates the surgical stress response may be important to immune system function and nutritional balance; however, the associated clinical relevance, as with the potent inhalational agents, remains controversial. The effects of morphine and fentanyl on metabolic responses are shown in Table 66-7. These data are drawn from several series, including those with patients undergoing cardiac surgery.

Immune Function

As is the case with inhalational agents, controversy exists concerning the narcotic effects on cellular immune system

TABLE 66-7. Opioid Effect on Stress Response

	MORPHINE (1–4 mg/kg)	FENTANYL (50–100 μg/kg)
Catecholamines	↑ ↓	θ to ↑
Cortisol	θ to ↑	↓
HGH	θ	↓
ADH	↑	θ

θ, no change; ↑, activity/function increased; ↓, activity/function decreased; HGH, human growth hormone; ADH, antidiuretic hormone.

function. McDonough and coworkers[31] and Brown and colleagues[32] suggest that a transient impairment of in vitro cellular immunity is demonstrable in opiate addicts. After treatment of lymphocytes with naloxone, or after cessation of intravenous opiate administration, the response to mitogen stimulation returns toward normal.

Whether this apparent impairment of cellular immune function is caused by contaminants in the intravenous opioid obtained by drug abusers or whether it is a more specific effect of opioids in general is unclear. Balanced anesthesia, including fentanyl, has no depressive effects on the mitogen responses of lymphocytes. When atropine and meperidine are used as premedication, a small number of patients show a decrease in lymphocyte response to mitogens. Thus, narcotics (at least fentanyl and meperidine) affect cellular immune function minimally, if at all.

Renal Effects

Whereas changes in renal function occur with opioids in animal models, changes in humans probably are secondary to alterations in systemic and renal hemodynamics rather than to direct effects of these agents on the kidneys.

BARBITURATES

Thiobarbiturates (sodium thiopental and methohexital) are frequently used. In contradistinction to other barbiturates, the thiopental ring structure has a sulfur atom in place of the oxygen atom at carbon-2. Methohexital, while retaining its carbon-2 oxygen atom, has a methyl group that replaces the hydrogen at the nitrogen-1 position of the ring. These chemical changes confer ultrashort onset and offset action compared with other barbiturates. Sodium thiopental usually comes in a 2.5% solution with a pH greater than 10, causing the drug to be irritating if accidentally extravasated. Methohexital is two to three times more potent than thiopental.

Pharmacokinetics/Pharmacodynamics

The pharmacokinetics of thiopental, as well as other commonly used nonnarcotic, intravenous anesthetic agents, are summarized in Table 66-8. Thiopental is a highly lipophilic agent with a pKa of 7.6 and is 60% nonionized at pH 7.4. With a standard clinical dose of 3 to 5 mg/kg, loss of consciousness occurs within one arm–brain circulation time (10

TABLE 66-8.   Selected Pharmacokinetic Data for Nonopioid Intravenous Anesthetics

	THIOPENTAL	PROPOFOL	DIAZEPAM	LORAZEPAM	MIDAZOLAM	KETAMINE
$t^{1/2}$ α (min)*	2–4	2–4	10–15	3–10	7–15	7–17
$t^{1/2}$ β (h)[†]	10	1–3	20–40	10–20	2–4	2–3
Clearance (mL/kg/min)[‡]	2.6–2.8	20–40	0.2–0.5	0.7–1	4–8	18–20
Vd_{ss} (L/kg)[‡§]	1.4–2.8	2.8–7.1	0.85–1.4	0.7–1.3	1–1.8	2.8–3.6

*$t^{1/2}$ α, slow redistribution half-life.

[†]$t^{1/2}$ β, elimination half-life.

[‡]Vd_{ss}, steady-state volume of distribution.

[§]Assume a 70-kg person.

Modified from White PF: Propofol: pharmacokinetics and pharmacodynamics. *Semin Anesth* 1988;7(Suppl):4.

to 15 seconds). The short duration of action of this drug (5 to 10 minutes) is secondary to its redistribution from the brain to muscle, skin, and, to a lesser extent, fat. Less than 1% of the administered drug appears unchanged in the urine; hepatic metabolism is important for its inactivation. Seventy percent to 85% of thiopental is albumin-bound in the blood. Thus, factors that decrease albumin binding also decrease the amount of drug needed for the appropriate anesthetic effect. Renal and hepatic impairment also decrease the amount of drug necessary as a result of decreased albumin.

Methohexital is only slightly less lipid soluble than sodium thiopental and is somewhat less ionized at pH 7.4. The onset and duration of loss of consciousness are approximately the same as with thiopental because of its rapid redistribution (elimination half-life is 3 to 5 minutes). Because it is more dependent on hepatic blood flow for clearance, any changes in flow are more significant for its final elimination.

Neurologic Effects

The mechanisms of action of the barbiturates are multiple and dose-related. At clinically relevant doses, two effects are seen: facilitation of action of inhibitory neural transmitters (i.e., GABA) and inhibition of excitatory neural transmitter action. Barbiturate-induced increase in GABA neuronal hyperpolarization is believed to be related to an increase in the time that chloride (Cl^-) ion channels remain open. Specifically, barbiturates seem to decrease the frequency of channel opening, while increasing the duration of opening. Within the central nervous system (CNS), sodium thiopental effects a decrease in $CMRO_2$, CBF, and ICP. Thiopental also has an antianalgesic or hyperalgesic action at low doses (25 to 150 mg), such that the threshold to pain produced by gradual tibial pressure is decreased.

Cardiorespiratory Effects

Cardiovascular effects of thiopental are of some significance. Increases in coronary blood flow, heart rate, and myocardial oxygen consumption occur, together with a decrease in the inotropic state of the myocardium. The result is a 10% to 25% decrease in cardiac output, blood pressure, and stroke volume at clinically relevant doses. Venous tone may also

decrease, resulting in decreased preload. At doses of 3 to 5 mg/kg, the responses to carbon dioxide elevation and hypoxia are impaired. After injection of thiopental, patients usually take two to three deep breaths (and often yawn), then become apneic.

Other Effects

Renal and hepatic effects of these drugs are insignificant. No clinically significant interactions between thiopental and any neuromuscular blocking drugs occur, making this drug safe for use in cesarean sections.

PROPOFOL

Propofol is an intriguing intravenous anesthetic agent. It is a sedative–hypnotic agent, similar to the thiobarbiturates and benzodiazepines that may be used for induction and maintenance of anesthesia. The agent is not antianalgesic (as are the thiobarbiturates) but is reported to have minimal amnestic effects.[33] The reader is referred to a recent comprehensive review of this drug.[34]

An alkylphenol, propofol is virtually insoluble in aqueous media and thus is provided in a 1% weight/volume (Intralipid) emulsion. The emulsion is composed of 1% diisopropylphenol (propofol), 10% soybean oil, 2.25% glycerol, and 1.2% purified egg phosphatide. Histamine release is not a problem with this formulation. Propofol is 95% to 99% plasma protein–bound; whereas the pH of the emulsion is 7 to 8.5, the drug itself is slightly acidic.

Pharmacokinetics/Pharmacodynamics

The basic pharmacokinetic data of propofol are shown in Table 66-8. Like the thiobarbiturates, propofol is extensively distributed into vessel-rich tissues, and ultimately redistributed to lean muscle and fat. The pharmacokinetic data suggest that accumulation occurs with repeated bolus injections or continuous infusion. Propofol is metabolized to water soluble, highly polar glucuronide and sulfate conjugates; the metabolites are not thought to be active and are excreted in the urine. Almost none of the parent drug is found in urine (<0.3%) or stool (<2%). Extrahepatic metabolism or extrarenal elimination might occur.

Comparing propofol with the other agents in Table 66-8, one observes the high clearance and the short elimination half-life. This profile, one of the reasons that the agent is so appealing, may be increased by age (decreased clearance and dose requirement), obesity (increased clearance and volume of distribution), type of procedure (with major intraabdominal surgery, volume of distribution increases and the elimination half-life is prolonged), and use of narcotics and potent inhaled anesthetic agents (decreased hepatic blood flow with a prolonged elimination half-life).

With intravenous injection in a nonpremedicated patient, a propofol dose of 2 to 2.5 mg/kg results in loss of consciousness in less than 60 seconds; rapid intravenous injection of 1 to 1.5 mg/kg in the elderly or a patient who has been given narcotic or benzodiazepine premedication is often sufficient for induction.

Anesthetic depth is assessed by changes in the respiratory rate in spontaneously breathing patients, or by increases in heart rate, blood pressure, and autonomic activity in those receiving a balanced anesthetic technique. A need to increase the anesthetic depth may be met by increasing the infusion rate or augmenting with 20- to 40-mg boluses intravenously. A relatively linear relationship exists between maintenance infusion rate of propofol and the resultant blood levels of the agent. Nonetheless, as with other intravenous agents, interpatient variability is such that a given dosage rate can result in levels that vary by threefold to sixfold.

A fairly predictable relationship also exists between the adequacy of anesthetic depth and the blood levels of propofol. For example, to achieve an adequate level of anesthesia, blood levels of the drug must be higher (3 to 6 μg/mL) for major as opposed to superficial (2 to 4 μg/mL) surgical procedures. The former blood level is frequently obtained, notwithstanding interpatient variability, with infusion rates between 100 and 150 μg/kg/minute.

Finally, the probability of awakening is reasonably predicted by observing blood levels. More than 50% of persons are awake with a level of 1 μg/mL, over 95% are awake and oriented with a level of 0.5 μg/mL, and most will have recovered baseline psychomotor function when the propofol level is 0.2 μg/mL. For propofol, the effective dose in 50% of patients studied (ED_{50}), which is analogous to MAC for potent inhalation agents, is 53.5 μg/kg/minute (95% confidence limits; 39.9 to 63 μg/kg/minute).[35]

Neurologic Effects

The mechanisms of action of propofol is unclear. Propofol can cause desynchronization of the awake electroencephalographic (EEG) pattern when a loading dose of 2.5 mg/kg, followed by an infusion of 100 to 200 μg/kg/minute are used; this effect is seen within 60 seconds of intravenous administration. Propofol in a dosage of more than 150 μg/kg/minute results in EEG burst suppression lasting 15 seconds or longer; the EEG returns to the awake state within about 11 minutes after the drug infusion is discontinued.

Some evoked potentials are altered by the drug. The latency of the primary complex may be increased and its amplitude decreased in median nerve and posterior tibial nerve somatosensory evoked potentials. Although the latencies of the brain stem auditory-evoked potential are not affected by propofol, the cortical middle latency potential of the auditory response is attenuated in amplitude and increased in latency.[36]

Although some controversy remains as to whether the decreased CBF (26% to 51% decrement) is paralleled by an adequate decrement in the $CMRO_2$ (18% to 36% decrease) and CMR_G,[34,35,37] this agent is used in patients with intracranial disease and is frequently employed in the ICU for long-term sedation.

Cardiovascular Effects

Like thiopental, propofol produces a dose-dependent decrease in systolic, diastolic, and mean arterial blood pressure; this effect is enhanced by narcotic premedication. Profound cardiovascular depression may be seen when propofol is used in elderly or hypovolemic patients and those with impaired ventricular function. Despite the decrease in blood pressure, heart rate remains relatively stable; this response is thought to be caused by a central sympatholytic or vagotonic effect rather than by impaired baroreceptor sensitivity.

The agent is a negative inotrope and, when used in patients with ischemic heart disease, has been associated with an increase in myocardial lactate production. Yet, a recent study describes the hemodynamic effects of propofol infusion on critically ill adults and reports no significant reductions in cardiac output, oxygen delivery, oxygen consumption, or arterial blood lactate concentrations.[38]

Respiratory Effects

Apnea is seen on induction with propofol in 30% to 60% of unpremedicated patients, and in virtually 100% of those premedicated with narcotics. Whereas the incidence of apnea is about the same as that seen with the thiobarbiturates, the duration tends to be somewhat longer. When breathing resumes, the tidal volume is decreased and the slope of the carbon dioxide response curve is decreased by 40% to 60%. The response to hypoxia is also significantly blunted by propofol.[39] Adjuvant use of narcotics further depresses respiratory drive.

Other Effects

Propofol does not seem to have any clinically relevant adverse effect on the production of cortisol. It does not affect the coagulation profile as measured by the thrombin time, prothrombin time, partial thromboplastin time, fibrinogen level, titer of fibrin degradation products, and platelet number and function.

Up to 58% of patients with an intravenous catheter in the dorsum of the hand reported pain on injection of propofol; this number decreased to about 10% if the drug was injected through a vein in the antecubital fossa. Administration of lidocaine through the cannula just before injection of propofol may decrease the pain.

Propofol did not seem to be immunosuppressive at clinical doses when in vitro cellular immune response was studied.[40]

BENZODIAZEPINES

The benzodiazepines of most significance in anesthesia and critical care are diazepam, lorazepam, and midazolam (see Table 66-8). Diazepam and lorazepam are insoluble in water. Midazolam, because of its imidazole ring, is water soluble at a pH of less than 4. The onset of CNS effects is slow and irregular for reasons that are unclear. Lorazepam is less lipid soluble than diazepam, and its slow entry into the CNS may be significant to its delayed onset of action.

Pharmacokinetics/Pharmacodynamics

DIAZEPAM. The sedative properties of diazepam make it useful as a premedicant; peak plasma levels are seen 30 to 60 minutes after an oral dose. Intramuscular injection is painful, and absorption is erratic. Clearance involves oxidation to active metabolites. Cimetidine inhibits the oxidative metabolism of diazepam. The free fraction of diazepam is only 1% to 2%; the rest is bound to albumin. Therefore, changes in albumin binding affect the clearance and half-life of this drug.

With hepatic disease, the volume of distribution increases and metabolism decreases, resulting in an increase in the half-life from 40 to 80 hours. With significant renal disease, an increase in the unbound fraction of diazepam results in a twofold to threefold increase in hepatic clearance and a resultant decrease in the half-life. The significance of these changes is hard to document, however, because no simple relationship can be demonstrated between the plasma levels of diazepam, its metabolites, and the clinical effect.

LORAZEPAM. Lorazepam is useful in oral, intramuscular, and intravenous forms. This agent is directly metabolized in the liver to inactive, glucuronide-conjugated metabolites. The kinetics of this drug are unaltered by age or renal disease, but hepatic disease increases the half-life.

MIDAZOLAM. Midazolam also can be administered by intramuscular, intravenous, or oral routes. The drug undergoes extensive metabolism to active and inactive metabolites. We have extensive experience using this drug as an induction agent in thermally injured patients. Loss of consciousness is rapid after an intravenous loading dose of 300 μg/kg, followed by either ketamine or, more often, a narcotic such as fentanyl in a dose of 2 to 5 μg/kg/hour after a loading dose of 5 to 10 μg/kg.

Neurologic Effects

Like barbiturates, the benzodiazepines have multiple, dose-dependent effects on the CNS and potentiate inhibitory GABA neurotransmission. They increase the frequency but not the duration of chloride channel opening. In addition, at least two specific benzodiazepine receptors have been identified: type 1, which is a postsynaptic receptor found in the cerebellum; and type 2, which is a presynaptic receptor found in the hippocampus and descending GABA pathways from the caudate nucleus to the substantia nigra. The clinical significance of these receptors is under investigation.

CNS effects of the benzodiazepines compared with those of the barbiturates are minimal. As mentioned previously, loss of consciousness occurs 2 to 3 minutes after an intravenous induction dose of diazepam, lorazepam, or midazolam (notwithstanding the more rapid onset of unconsciousness in burned patients given a large dose, as mentioned earlier). Antegrade amnesia is seen with all of the benzodiazepines, but more so with lorazepam.

Cardiorespiratory Effects

When the benzodiazepines are used alone, cardiovascular effects are reported to be insignificant; however, cardiovascular depression has been observed when they are used in conjunction with other anesthetic agents. Respiratory effects are also minimal. Some decrease in the ventilatory response to carbon dioxide may occur after the use of these agents, but data are conflicting in this regard. No difference in recovery time or duration of action of either depolarizing or nondepolarizing muscle relaxants occur when the benzodiazepines are used.

KETAMINE

Pharmacokinetics/Pharmacodynamics

Ketamine is the only arylcyclohexylamine used in anesthesia. It is structurally related to phencyclidine, known in street vernacular as angel dust. The pKa of ketamine is 7.5, and it is about ten times more water soluble than thiopental. Its pharmacokinetics are summarized in Table 66-8. Ketamine is approximately ten times more lipid soluble than thiopental; however, its onset of action is somewhat slower. After an intravenous dose of 2 mg/kg, consciousness is lost in little more than one arm–brain circulation time and returns 10 to 15 minutes later. Ketamine is 45% to 50% protein-bound.

Recovery of consciousness probably results from rapid drug redistribution into muscle and other tissues. However, 95% of the injected drug ultimately is metabolized by the liver, and less than 5% is recovered unchanged in the urine. At least eight different metabolites of the parent compound have been identified, the most important of which is norketamine, which has approximately one third the potency of ketamine.

Neurologic Effects

The exact mechanism of action of ketamine is not well understood. Apparently it does not facilitate GABA inhibitory neurotransmitters, as do the benzodiazepines and barbiturates. Like barbiturates, however, ketamine blocks ion channels in the open position. Specific arylcyclohexylamine receptors in the brain may be related to the σ subclass of opioid receptors. Ketamine increases CBF and so must be used with caution in individuals with elevated ICP.

Cardiovascular Effects

Ketamine causes an increase in systemic blood pressure and cerebrovasodilation, resulting in increased ICP. It also causes central stimulation of the sympathetic arm of the autonomic nervous system. The cardiovascular effects are primarily related to CNS stimulation. Ketamine inhibits the uptake of catecholamines by the postganglionic adrenergic neurons and the uptake of extraneuronal norepinephrine.

Because of the dose-related increase in arterial blood pressure, heart rate, and coronary vasodilation and overall unchanged peripheral vascular resistance associated with ketamine administration, the drug often is thought not to be a myocardial depressant. Nonetheless, with sympathetic blockade or in patients in prolonged shock with a significantly stressed autonomic nervous system, cardiac depression can be seen with ketamine. Pulmonary vascular resistance and right ventricular stroke work also are frequently increased.

Respiratory Effects

Although ketamine is not commonly thought of as a respiratory depressant when used in anesthetic doses of 1 to 2 mg/kg, a moderate decrease in the PaO_2 may occur. The ventilatory response to carbon dioxide is maintained, and ketamine potentiates the bronchodilatory effects of catecholamines. It also increases oral secretions so that an anticholinergic agent may be necessary.

Other Effects

Ketamine enhances the effect of depolarizing and nondepolarizing neuromuscular blocking drugs. The drug has been used safely in patients with MH. Postanesthetic emergence reactions (nightmares and hallucinations) may occur in 5% to 30% of patients. A benzodiazepine and 2 mg/kg (or less) doses of ketamine seem to decrease the incidence of this problem.

IMMUNE SYSTEM FUNCTION

As with the potent inhalation and opioid anesthetics, controversy exists regarding the effects of barbiturates, benzodiazepines, and ketamine on immune function. Sodium thiopental at clinically relevant doses in vitro decreases the mitogenic response of lymphocytes to phytohemagglutinin and inhibited cytotoxicity. Neither ketamine nor diazepam has any adverse effects. In experimental animals, both thiopental (tumor-bearing mice) and pentobarbital (dogs) decrease lymphocyte function. The in vivo response of lymphocytes in patients exposed to thiopental, nitrous oxide, oxygen, droperidol, fentanyl, and muscle relaxants shows no adverse effect. However, balanced anesthesia, including sodium thiopental, halothane or enflurane, nitrous oxide, oxygen, and a muscle relaxant in healthy volunteers and adult patients, results in decreased lymphocyte response to nonspecific mitogens. Although we have not discussed regional anesthetic techniques, brachial plexus block in adult patients undergoing minor orthopedic procedures has no effect on lymphocyte response to either phytohemagglutinin or concanavalin A.

PREFERRED ANESTHETIC TECHNIQUES FOR CRITICALLY ILL PATIENTS ■

Should any agent or technique be used or, conversely, avoided in critically ill patients? Almost no data conclusively support one technique over another. Yet, although we prefer not to muddy the waters (any more than they already are), we believe it makes sense in a hemodynamically unstable patient to shy away from the potent inhalation agents and to use in their place an intravenous technique of either ketamine or one of the phenylpiperidine narcotics. Furthermore, in brain-injured patients, we use intravenous barbiturates and narcotics with isoflurane, and employ hyperventilation; ketamine, enflurane, or halothane are avoided for the reasons discussed previously.[41]

The less-than-adequate data suggest avoidance of potent inhalation anesthetic agents in patients with questionable perioperative immune function. In such cases, intravenous narcotics or ketamine may be useful. However, no outcome studies show that potent inhalation agents increase morbidity or mortality more than agents with no demonstrated adverse effects on in vitro immune function. Finally, because surgical stress has been shown to affect immune function, we do not hesitate to place epidural catheters to facilitate sympathetic blockade.[42]

POSTANESTHETIC PROBLEMS ■

Difficulties in the early postoperative period are common. Postanesthetic complications have been found to occur in 5% to 30% of patients; the wide range results from lack of uniform criteria defining complications, different practices in individual institutions, differences in the strictness of observational practice, and possible significant differences in populations studied.[43]

HYPOXEMIA

Postoperative hypoxemia may result from myriad etiologies. Hypoventilation caused by residual anesthetic or muscle relaxant effects and atelectasis, which may have resulted from a one-lung intubation during surgery, are diagnoses to be considered and treated aggressively in the immediate postoperative period. Consideration should be given to pulmonary edema resulting from heart failure in susceptible patients, noncardiogenic pulmonary edema from aspiration, acute respiratory distress syndrome, infection, trauma, blood reaction, or head injury (neurogenic pulmonary edema).

Negative-Pressure Pulmonary Edema

Pulmonary edema may develop after a strenuous inspiratory effort against an obstructed airway. This type of pulmonary edema may appear immediately or up to 10 hours after the episode of airway obstruction. It most commonly is associated with laryngospasm during anesthetic induction of or emergence from anesthesia; therefore, it frequently is diagnosed in the postanesthesia care unit or ICU.[44]

The pathophysiologic mechanism of negative pressure pulmonary edema is not completely understood, although a common explanation is that the negative intrapleural pressure generated during airway obstruction shifts the balance in the Starling forces toward a large fluid transudation from the intravascular to the interstitial space. The increase in extravascular lung water causes a reduction in lung compliance and an increase in shunt.

The diagnosis of negative pressure pulmonary edema is based on the history and clinical picture of pulmonary edema in patients without heart failure or predisposition for acute respiratory distress syndrome from other causes. Typically, the patient is a young, vigorous adult who sustains an episode of laryngospasm either before intubation or after extubation.[45] The radiologic picture in negative-pressure pulmonary edema has been described as alveolar and interstitial edema, which rarely occur unilaterally. The heart size is normal, but the vascular pedicle is enlarged.[46]

Treatment of negative-pressure pulmonary edema is mainly supportive. Patients should be given oxygen to maintain an arterial oxyhemoglobin saturation of at least 90%. Some patients require reintubation and mechanical ventilation with positive pressure to assure oxygenation and to reduce work of breathing. Diuretics are not recommended in these cases. In most cases, the edema resolves within 24 hours.

PAIN AND PERIOPERATIVE STRESS

Early postoperative pain remains a serious concern. Up to 75% of patients receiving parenteral narcotics for moderate to severe pain have significant residual pain after the drug is administered.[47,48] Whereas some might say that uncontrolled pain is no more than an inconvenience (especially those who have never experienced significant pain or watched loved ones experience it), potentially serious physiologic consequences may result from it.[38] For example, sympathetic nervous system stimulation that accompanies uncontrolled pain leads to elevated plasma catecholamine levels, tachycardia, hypertension, increased systemic vascular resistance, and an increase in myocardial oxygen requirements. In the patient with underlying coronary artery disease, this increased oxygen demand may not be met, resulting in ischemia or infarction.

Surgical procedures on the upper abdomen and thorax may have profound effects on the respiratory system. Because of the pain and surgical muscular alterations, vital capacity and functional residual capacity may be decreased by as much as 60% and 20%, respectively. Although these changes may not be evident with resting tidal respiration, the ability to deep breathe (sigh) and cough is impaired, resulting in atelectasis and retained secretions. Decreased oxygenation and the potential for pulmonary parenchymal infection may follow.

Stress Response

An area less clearly understood and described, but likely no less important with regard to postoperative pain, is the stress response to surgery. Weissman[49] reviews the intriguing and manifold physiologic changes observed with an operative intervention. Surgery, as any trauma, was classically described as being composed of two stages[50]: an initial "ebb phase" is characterized by a shock state with low metabolic activity and cardiac output; and a second period termed the "flow phase" characterized by a hyperdynamic state from the endocrine, metabolic, and cardiovascular standpoints.

The endocrine parameters of the latter stage are an increase in catecholamine levels, an increased secretion of corticotropin and steroids, and resultant hyperglycemia. An increase in antidiuretic hormone (ADH) secretion enables conservation of water by the kidneys.[51] Other aspects of the response to surgery and anesthesia are an increase in growth hormone and a slight increase in thyroxine, with a decrease in triiodothyronine levels. Beta-endorphin levels are increased as is the plasma level of prolactin.[52]

The systemic response to trauma also includes an important component of immune depression, which can appear early after the stressful event[53] and is mediated through several different pathways.[54,55] Traditionally, the stress response was thought to be beneficial for homeostatic stability. Perhaps an evolutionary advantage accrued to the organism that could mount this response to major trauma, blood loss, and organ dysfunction. Currently, however, data show that the metabolic response to trauma may often be exaggerated and thus disadvantageous.

In the otherwise well-controlled diabetic patient, for example, one may see hyperglycemia that is extremely difficult to regulate. An increase in catecholamine secretion that increases myocardial work and oxygen consumption may result in ischemia in patients with coronary artery disease. Increased ADH secretion may result in a picture similar to the syndrome of inappropriate ADH secretion with significant hyponatremia, particularly in patients treated with hypotonic solutions after surgery.[56] The hyponatremic syndrome has been described in a group of children after spinal surgery[57] and also in thermally injured patients.[58]

These data suggest (although we note that significant controversy exists) that the stress response to surgery should at least be attenuated if the detrimental effects are to be avoided. Different anesthetic techniques may affect this response in various ways; thus, the choice of an anesthetic may affect the patient's course in the postoperative period and in the surgical intensive care unit (SICU).

GENERAL ANESTHESIA.   Patients studied under a variety of general anesthetics show an increase in corticotropin, corticosteroids, beta-endorphins, and catecholamines in response to intubation, skin incision, intraabdominal manipulation, and on emergence.[42] Nevertheless, some researchers believe that a well-maintained general anesthetic can blunt the stress response or at least some components of it. Roizen and coworkers[59] have used the acronym MAC-BAR, indicating the minimal alveolar concentration at which the adrenergic response is blocked; it is usually observed at approximately 2 MAC for most inhalational agents. Furthermore, others have shown that graded surgical stress causes minimal endocrine response.[60] Therefore, patients who undergo relatively less stressful surgery under adequate anesthesia do not mount a deleterious stress response.

High-dose narcotic techniques, commonly used in cardiac anesthesia or for patients with ischemic heart disease, have been shown to blunt the endocrine response to stress inasmuch as plasma levels of various stress hormones are not increased.[61] With any general anesthetic technique, the metabolic response is triggered on emergence, even if attenuated during the surgical procedure itself. In the SICU, patients may begin to mount the metabolic-endocrine response in the postoperative period.

REGIONAL ANESTHESIA.   The stress response to surgery is triggered by several mechanisms. Among these, an important one is that of direct neural activation by transmission of noxious stimuli from the traumatized area. This event occurs even when patients receive a general anesthetic and, therefore, are not consciously aware of the noxious stimulus. Blunting the response can be achieved by blocking this neural pathway.

Analgesia and anesthesia achieved with a regional technique does attenuate the stress response when compared with general techniques. Kehlet and colleagues[62,63] have studied this relationship extensively and found major differences in levels of corticosteroids, catecholamines, aldosterone, rennin, growth hormone, prolactin, and ADH in patients undergoing surgery with epidural anesthesia compared with those given general anesthesia. Some aspects of the immune depression after surgery also have been shown not to occur with regional as opposed to general anesthesia.[64]

COMBINED ANESTHESIA.   The advantages of regional anesthesia may be put to use in surgery on the extremities and lower abdomen. A purely regional technique is seldom used for upper abdominal surgery; some anesthesiologists do not use regional techniques in a prolonged surgical procedure if it involves uncomfortable positioning or if immobility is important. In the latter procedures, a common approach is to use regional anesthesia, with control of the airway by intubation, inhalational agents, and positive-pressure ventilation; this approach is called combined anesthesia. The term was coined by Crile in 1921 and involves the block of surgical stimulus by a regional technique, combined with loss of consciousness achieved by light general anesthesia.[65]

Applications

Whereas combined anesthesia usually refers to a general anesthetic combined with a spinal or epidural anesthetic technique, the regional anesthetic might also be a brachial plexus or any other nerve block. Proving that combined anesthesia is successful in obtunding the stress response to trauma is more difficult than in studies comparing regional anesthesia with general anesthetic techniques. This observation probably results from several factors: (1) obtaining control of the airway (the intubation) may itself elicit a strong stress response; (2) the surgical field may include areas that are not well anesthetized; and (3) part of the stress response may be mediated by the release of humoral factors from the locally injured area.

Potential Advantages

The possible advantages of combined anesthesia over a purely general technique are controversial. An important study in this field is that of Yeager and colleagues,[66] who compared major abdominal and vascular procedures done under a general anesthetic technique with those done under combined general and epidural techniques. They found significant differences in the ICU course and in outcome between the two patient groups. The combined group required less time to extubation and a shorter ICU stay; they had less infectious complications and a lower mortality. Expense per patient was considerably lower. Thus, the anesthetic choice becomes an important ICU issue. Some studies did not find an advantage to this approach,[67] whereas one found specific benefits of epidural anesthesia, such as a reduced propensity for thrombosis of vascular grafts.[68]

Cardiac Output and Oxygen Delivery

An important body of data regarding the significance of the stress response in terms of outcome has been generated by Shoemaker.[69] He demonstrated that patients surviving high-risk surgery, sepsis, and shock states are those in whom measured parameters of cardiac function and oxygen delivery are highest. Moreover, patients with low oxygen delivery developed an oxygen deficit during surgery that was more pronounced in those who developed complications and died. Thus, hemodynamic values may be of use in predicting outcome.

GOAL-ORIENTED THERAPY.   Other investigators have shown that the early use of invasive monitoring may be helpful in the management of elderly[70] and young[71] trauma patients using goal-directed therapy. In a prospective study,[72] three groups of general surgical patients were followed. The first group was managed with central venous pressure monitoring; the second group had a pulmonary artery catheter inserted, but therapy was directed by the surgical service according to conventional clinical criteria; and the third group was managed with a pulmonary artery catheter using a rigid protocol to maintain oxygen delivery at supranormal values. The results reported are of interest. The mortality rate decreased from about 30% in both control groups to 4% in the protocol group. Other indicators such as length of hospital stay, utilization of resources, and hospital charges per patient were also significantly lower in the protocol group compared with either the central venous pressure–monitored or conventional criteria groups.

Conclusions

Although these data at first glance seem to contradict the concept of the beneficial effects of stress reduction, a unified view is that in the postoperative period, monitoring and therapy should be aggressive and appropriate to ensure adequate systemic oxygen delivery on the one hand, with strict control of the patient's stress on the other. Modifying risk by blunting the stress response should not lead to a compromise in terms of hemodynamic function and oxygen delivery. Thus, although some reduction of the stress response should reduce postoperative adverse events, prospective randomized studies are necessary to confirm this view.

Specific Techniques of Pain Management

The use of pharmacologically active agents to relieve pain is as ancient as medicine itself. This chapter is not the place for a historical review of pain control; rather, we comment on the newer methods of treating and, more importantly, preventing pain in the perioperative period (Chap. 54).

PREOPERATIVE. Preoperatively, pain is usually emotional and amenable to two modes of therapy. The anesthesiologist and surgeon are obliged to provide the patient with as much detail about the procedure as the patient desires. Allowing the patient time to ask questions and voice concerns, with the physician providing honest and straightforward responses to these subjects, is of utmost importance. Data exist, if any were needed, that spending time with a person before anesthetic induction results in a less nervous patient.[73] Based on our experience with critically ill surgical and thermally injured patients, time spent with conscious adults and older children before a procedure is time well invested.

For some patients, time and talk are not enough, and a pharmacologic agent is desirable before surgery. Our bias (and it is just that) is toward the benzodiazepines. Although many of these drugs exist, we prefer lorazepam in a dose of 0.025 to 0.05 mg/kg (maximum of 4 mg except in thermally injured patients), given either intravenously or by mouth. Subgroups of patients exists for whom preoperative sedation seems unwise. These include children younger than 1 year of age, most outpatients, patients with decreased levels of consciousness or intracranial disease, patients with severe chronic lung disease, and those with hypovolemia. Other classes of agents such as narcotics, barbiturates, butyrophenones, or antihistamines may be used.

We have four general rules for sedation:

1. When *sedation* is required (rather than analgesia) a sedative is used, not an analgesic.
2. Intramuscular injections in adults usually are not necessary and are often ineffective.
3. In children, intramuscular and rectal administration of sedatives usually are not indicated (except in mentally retarded or combative individuals).
4. Intramuscular injections in children are, in general, inhumane.

POSTOPERATIVE. For pain control to be successful postoperatively, one must attempt to prevent, rather than treat the pain. Traditionally, the surgeon writes orders for postoperative analgesics. Intramuscular or intravenous doses of morphine or meperidine on an as-needed basis result in

unnecessary discomfort.[74] Although intravenous narcotics administered by the nursing staff on an as-needed basis may provide adequate control of postoperative pain, if they are adequately dosed and if the nurse is able to respond in a timely manner to the request, our preference is to use one of two more effective modalities: epidural placement of narcotics or patient-controlled analgesia (PCA). Other techniques such as intercostal nerve blocks and the newer intrapleural analgesia are discussed elsewhere.[60]

Epidural Analgesia. Epidural analgesia was first described in the 1940s but was largely unappreciated until the 1960s, when it was used to provide relief from the pain of labor and delivery. The technique involves placement of a catheter into the lumbar or thoracic epidural space through a hollow needle. The epidural space is rich with blood vessels, lymphatics, and spinal roots as they pass from the spinal cord into the foramina; a thin and adherent dura is all that separates the cerebral spinal fluid (CSF) from epidurally injected drugs.

Epidural placement of preservative-free narcotics results in their diffusion into the CSF and from there onto the presynaptic and postsynaptic narcotic receptors of the substantia gelatinosa in the dorsal horn of the spinal cord. The more lipid soluble the narcotic (fentanyl more so than morphine), the more rapidly it is taken up by narcotic receptors in the spinal cord, thus making ascent of the agent in the CSF to the brain stem respiratory control center less likely. Local anesthetics injected into the epidural space are primarily taken up by spinal nerve roots, where they act to prevent transmission of nociceptive impulses from the peripheral to the CNS. Sympathetic blockade occurs with these agents.

Epidural analgesia is most useful with abdominal, thoracic, or lower extremity operative procedures. Because of the different sites of action of epidural narcotics and local anesthetics, we prefer to use them in a combined approach to postoperative pain. The phenylpiperidine narcotic fentanyl is mixed in a saline solution containing 1/32% to 1/8% bupivacaine; the final concentration of the narcotic is 5 to 7.5 μg/mL. This solution is then administered as an initial bolus of fentanyl, 1 to 2 μg/kg, followed by continuous infusion based on the site of the operative procedure: 8 mL/hour for hip and lower abdominal procedure; 10 mL/hour for upper abdominal procedure; 15 mL/hour for knee or thoracic procedure.

We use fentanyl rather than morphine because of its rapid onset (about 15 minutes) and, in case of side effects, its rapid offset (about 60 minutes). Fentanyl delivered through the epidural space may be absorbed to the blood and effect analgesia systemically rather than through a specific effect on the spinal cord.[75,76] We prefer not to use a total dosage of fentanyl above 2 μg/kg/hour. With a properly placed catheter, over 90% of patients have adequate pain control.

Side effects of epidural drug placement are respiratory depression (0.2% to 1%), urinary retention (30% to 50%), nausea (10%), vomiting, and pruritus (common).[60] Fentanyl rather than morphine generally is preferable because its greater lipid solubility limits cephalad ascension and possible resultant respiratory depression.

Pulse oximetry and frequent neurologic checks by the nursing staff are used to monitor potential CNS depression associated with epidural narcotics. When supplemental oxygen is required, the lowest F_{IO_2} that keeps the continuous pulsed arterial oxygen saturation (SpO_2) at 93% to 95% is used. Urinary retention may require decreasing the dose of narcotic, performing "in and out" bladder catheterization every 4 hours, or placing an indwelling urinary bladder catheter. In our clinical areas (SICU and burn intensive care unit), most patients have indwelling urinary catheters. Pruritus may be treated with diphenhydramine (12.5 to 25 mg intravenously) or naloxone 5 to 10 µg/kg/hour without reversing analgesia.

Patient-Controlled Analgesia. PCA allows the patient to self-administer small doses of narcotics. The device used for this technique consists of an electronically controlled pump with a timer. The patient usually is given a loading dose of narcotic, followed by a preset amount of drug every time a trigger is depressed. A predetermined "lockout" time period must elapse between doses so that the patient does not redose until the first dose has had time to exert its maximal effect. In practice, we usually administer a loading dose of morphine at 0.1 to 0.15 mg/kg intravenously; the PCA pump is then programmed at 0.05 to 0.075 mg/kg/hour with a 10-minute lockout period. Thus, a 70-kg patient receives 7 to 12 mg of morphine and may redose with approximately 1 to 1.5 mg every 10 minutes.

This type of pain control eliminates the waiting period bounded by the patient feeling pain and calling the nurse, who then determines that pain is present, goes in search of keys to the narcotic cabinet, and finally administers the drug. The risks of respiratory depression are low (unless a family member sits by the patient's bedside and depresses the PCA pump trigger). This technique can be helpful in other than postoperative pain control, such as management of terminal cancer patients.

AGITATION AND SEDATION

Evaluation

Delayed emergence from anesthesia and agitation are different loci on the same continuum. The former problem may result from significant residual anesthetic agent; the same factors governing anesthetic uptake and distribution also govern anesthetic offset. For the potent inhaled anesthetic agents, a decrease to 60% or less of the MAC value of the agent is required before healthy volunteers respond to commands and protect their airway. If supplemental drugs such as benzodiazepines or narcotics have been used, the percentage of MAC compatible with awakening is lower still. Residual, partial neuromuscular blockade can result in significant agitation. After the possibility of residual drug effect has been eliminated (sometimes it cannot be totally ruled out), one must consider other possible causes (Table 66-9).

The key to evaluating the patient who has not awakened from anesthesia or who is agitated is to rule out treatable and life-threatening causes immediately. Thereafter, the patient

TABLE 66-9. Etiology of Postoperative Mental Status Alteration

Drugs	In the patient emergently anesthetized from the ER, street drugs such as alcohol, narcotics, cocaine may have been present on induction; residual neuromuscular blockade must also be considered.
Postseizure	A seizure under anesthesia may be easily missed. One must consider the delayed emergence as a possible postictal event.
Glucose	Hyperglycemia or hypoglycemia can result in altered mental status.
Metabolic causes	Hypoxia, hypercarbia, hypernatremia or hyponatremia, hypercalcemia, hypothermia (usually at or below 31°C) are several examples.
Trauma	Again in the patient emergently anesthetized from the ER, head trauma must be considered.
Infection	Agitation in an infected patient is sometimes seen; this is no less so in the postoperative period.
Psychogenic causes	Rarely, a patient will feign unconsciousness for some secondary gain. This may only be diagnosed after other life-threatening and treatable causes have been ruled out.
Hemodynamic instability	Hypotension, and sometimes severe hypertension, may cause mental status changes. The former may result from hypovolemia, anaphylaxis, sepsis, or ischemia.
Pain	Pain at the operative site, a full bladder, or gastric distention can result in agitation.

ER, emergency room.

may be placed under expectant observation. Agitation caused by pain or residual instrumentation/cannulation (endotracheal tube, indwelling urinary bladder catheter) must be differentiated from that caused by hypoxemia/hypercapnia.

Treatment

If treatment is considered, several previously discussed therapeutic modalities are available. Although propofol is an attractive drug for continuous sedation, it is expensive. This fact makes some intensivists hesitant to use it frequently.

A recent report compared propofol with midazolam for continuous sedation of postoperative, mechanically ventilated patients. Results were similar for both drugs, although some advantages were claimed for propofol in terms of tolerance of the ICU environment and duration to complete wakefulness after discontinuation of sedation.[77]

For continuous propofol sedation, a loading dose of 1 to 2 mg/kg is administered over 1 to 2 minutes, followed by an infusion of 50 to 100 µg/kg/minute; the dose is titrated up or down so that, with stimulation, the patient awakens. Midazolam is dosed at 0.25 to 3 mg/hour in a 70-kg adult. The use of neuromuscular blocking agents without sedation to abort nonpurposeful movement is wrong and inhumane.

RESIDUAL NEUROMUSCULAR BLOCKADE

Residual neuromuscular blockade usually presents in one of three ways: (1) delayed return to consciousness, which should have been noted in the operating room by both the surgeon and anesthesiologist; (2) respiratory difficulty with hypercapnia (Table 66-10); and (3) muscle weakness (Table 66-11). The major point in the diagnosis of this entity is to consider it; the major point in treatment is to protect the airway (if necessary, by replacing the endotracheal tube) while the differential diagnosis is worked through.

Diagnosis

Most anesthesiologists monitor the depth of neuromuscular blockade with a twitch-stimulating device or a group of clinical signs. Nevertheless, some persons arrive in the SICU with residual neuromuscular blockade. This condition may take the form of an apparent alteration in mental status (see Table 66-9), hypoventilation with hypercapnia, or a seemingly awake and alert status with adequate breathing but a weak or "floppy" appearance. Both depolarizing (succinylcholine) and nondepolarizing (e.g., pancuronium, curare, vecuronium, and atracurium) neuromuscular blockers act at the neuromuscular junction (end plate).[78]

Junction occupancy by these agents can be monitored by applying a supramaximal electrical stimulus to a motor nerve; in the operating room, the ulnar nerve is stimulated to con-

TABLE 66-10. Etiology of Postoperative Hypercapnia

I. Central respiratory depression
   Intravenous (narcotic) anesthetics
   Inhaled anesthetic agents

II. Respiratory muscle dysfunction
   Site of incision (upper abdominal, thoracic)
   Residual neuromuscular blockade
   Use of drugs that enhance neuromuscular blockade
      (gentamicin, clindamycin, neomycin, furosemide)
   Physiologic factors that prevent reversal of neuromuscular
      blockade (hypokalemia, respiratory acidosis) or enhance
      the blockade (hypothermia, hypermagnesemia)

III. Physical factors
   Obesity
   Gastric dilatation
   Tight dressings
   Body cast

IV. Increased production of carbon dioxide
   Sepsis
   Shivering
   Malignant hyperthermia

V. Underlying hyperthermia
   Chronic obstructive pulmonary disease with CO_2 retention
   Neuromuscular—chest cage dysfunction (kyphoscoliosis)
   Acute or chronic respiratory failure of any etiology

Modified from Feeley TW: The recovery room. In: Miller RD (ed). *Anesthesia*, 2nd ed. New York, Churchill Livingstone, 1986:1921; and Wyngaarden JB, Smith LH Jr. (eds): *Cecil Textbook of Medicine*, 18th ed. Philadelphia, WB Saunders, 1988:417, 472, 474.

TABLE 66-11. Etiology of Prolonged Neuromuscular Blockade

I. Nondepolarizing neuromuscular blocking agents
   Intensity of neuromuscular blockade
   Renal failure (decreased metocurine and pancuronium
      excretion)
   Hepatic failure (decreased pancuronium and vecuronium
      excretion)
   Residual potent inhaled anesthetic agent
   Inadequate dose of reversal agents
   Hypothermia
   Acid–base state
   Hypokalemia, hypermagnesemia
   Drugs
      Antibiotics (gentamicin, clindamycin, and multiple other
         drugs with several mechanisms)
      Local anesthetics
      antiarrhythmics (quinidine)
      Furosemide
      Dantrolene
      Trimethaphan (possibly)
   Underlying diseases (myasthenia gravis, myasthenic
      syndrome, familial periodic paralysis)

II. Depolarizing neuromuscular blocking agents (succinylcholine)
   Decreased effective pseudocholinesterase
   Phase II block
   Hypermagnesemia
   Local anesthetics

Modified from Miller RD, Savarese JJ: Pharmacology of muscle relaxants and their antagonists. In: Miller RD (ed). *Anesthesia,* 2nd ed. New York: Churchill Livingstone, 1986:889.

tract the adductor pollicis brevis. If the equipment is properly set up, a single supramaximal stimulus at 50 Hz for 5 seconds that produces contraction without fade seems to correlate with signs of clinical recovery from neuromuscular blockade.

Other more quantitative estimations of neuromuscular blockade use the train-of-four stimulus (four supramaximal stimuli in 2 seconds with each stimulus lasting 0.2 seconds), or double-burst stimulation. With the train-of-four stimulus, when the ratio of the fourth contraction to the first is more than 60%, patients are able to sustain a head lift for over 3 seconds; when the ratio is more than 75%, adequate clinical recovery is present (Table 66-12).

Treatment

If residual neuromuscular blockade is present, an attempt to reverse it may be in order. If blockade results from succinylcholine, reversal agents are unlikely to be of any benefit. The patient is mechanically ventilated and gently sedated until neuromuscular function returns. If a nondepolarizing blocking agent was used, reversal may be attempted with anticholinesterases and anticholinergics (Table 66-13).

An important issue with regard to neuromuscular blocking agents is that of prolonged paralysis in patients who have received neuromuscular blockers for a long period in the ICU. Although controlled studies addressing this prob-

TABLE 66-12. Clinical Signs of Recovery From Neuromuscular Blockade

I. Awake patient
  Opens eyes widely
  Coughs effectively
  Sustains tongue protrusion
  Sustains hand grip
  Sustains head lift for >5 s
  Vital capacity of ≥15 mL/kg
  (PNP) of ≥20 cm H₂O
  Sustained 50 Hz tetanic stimulation for 5 s
II. Patient who is asleep or unable to follow commands
  Tidal volume of 5–10 mL/kg
  PNP of ≥25 cm H₂O
  Sustained 50 Hz tetanic stimulation for 5 s

PNP, peak negative pressure.
Modified from Ali HH, Miller RD: Monitoring of neuromuscular function. In: Miller RD (ed). *Anesthesia,* 2nd ed. New York, Churchill Livingstone, 1986:871.

lem have not been published, several risk factors for the development of prolonged paralysis have been delineated. Among these are renal failure, concomitant drug use, length of administration, monitoring technique used, and the use of steroids in patients receiving steroid-based drugs such as pancuronium or vecuronium. The best way to prevent this distressing complication is to avoid neuromuscular blockers as much as possible and to monitor all patients receiving these drugs with a peripheral nerve stimulator. Some investigators believe that intermittent discontinuation of the drugs, as well as the use of short-acting drugs, may prevent complications (see Chap. 55).[79]

MALIGNANT HYPERTHERMIA

Malignant hyperthermia may be divided into early, late, and postcrisis manifestations (Table 66-14). The differential diagnosis of MH includes sepsis, light anesthesia, thyrotoxicosis, myotonias, neuroleptic malignant syndrome, and pheochromocytoma.

TABLE 66-13. Reversal Agents Used With Neuromuscular Blocking Agents

ANTICHOLINESTERASE	ANTICHOLINERGIC
Neostigmine 35–70 μg/kg (maximum, 5 mg)	Atropine 20 μg/kg or
Edrophonium 500–1000 μg/kg	Glycopyrrolate 10 μg/kg
Pyridostigmine 175–350 μg/kg (maximum, 20 mg)	

Modified from Miller RD, Savarese JJ: Pharmacology of muscle relaxants and their antagonists. In: Miller RD (ed). *Anesthesia,* 2nd ed. New York, Churchill Livingstone, 1986:889.

Background

Malignant hyperthermia is a pharmacogenetic clinical syndrome that usually occurs during general anesthesia. Its onset may be delayed for several hours; thus, the initial presentation may be in the SICU. The hallmark of the syndrome is rapidly increasing temperature caused by uncontrolled skeletal muscle metabolism that can result in rhabdomyolysis and death. After exposure to a triggering agent, a dramatic increase in aerobic metabolism occurs in the skeletal muscle of susceptible persons. Oxygen consumption can increase threefold, whereas blood lactate may increase 15- to 20-fold. The mechanism for this entity involves myoplasmic calcium accumulation and a failure of calcium uptake by the sarcoplasmic reticulum.

The incidence of MH varies; fulminant cases are seen in from 1 in 250,000 to 1 in 62,000 anesthetics (the latter incidence when triggering agents are used); suspected MH occurs in 1 in 6000 anesthetics overall and 1 in 4200 anesthetics with triggering agents. A 24-hour per day emergency phone number for consultations has been set up by the Malignant Hyperthermia Association of the United States: 209-634-4917.

Evaluation of susceptibility includes the family history and measurement of baseline creatine kinase level (elevated in 70% of those affected). The definitive test is a muscle biopsy for contracture studies after exposure to halothane,

TABLE 66-14. Signs of Malignant Hyperthermia

EARLY SIGNS	LATE SIGNS	POSTCRISIS SIGNS
Skeletal muscle rigidity	Hyperpyrexia—may exceed 43°C (109.4°F)	Muscle pain, edema
Tachycardia and hypertension	Cyanosis	Central nervous system damage
Elevated PETCO₂	Serum electrolyte abnormalities	Renal failure
Acidosis	Elevated serum creatinine phosphokinase	Continued electrolyte imbalance
Arrhythmias	Myoglobinuria	
	Coagulopathy	
	Cardiac failure and pulmonary edema	

PETCO₂, end tidal pressure of carbon dioxide.

caffeine, halothane plus caffeine, or potassium. Although laboratory standardization of contracture testing is not complete, patients who have negative in vitro contracture tests for MH appear to have no adverse anesthetic outcome when subsequently exposed to triggering anesthetic agents.[80]

Diagnosis

Treating MH is easier than making the clinical diagnosis because the presenting signs may be mistaken for benign conditions, and MH is relatively uncommon. When triggering anesthetic drugs (potent inhaled anesthetic agents, succinylcholine) are used, MH must be considered in the presence of unexplained tachycardia, tachypnea, arrhythmias, mottling, cyanosis, hyperthermia, muscle rigidity, diaphoresis, or hemodynamic instability. The presence of more than one sign must initiate arterial and central venous blood gas analysis for metabolic and respiratory acidosis and for hyperkalemia. Central venous oxygen and carbon dioxide partial pressures change more dramatically than do those of arterial blood.

TABLE 66-15. Acute Therapy for Malignant Hyperthermia

I. Discontinue all anesthetic agents
  Hyperventilate with an F_{IO_2} of 1
  CO_2 is increased so hyperventilate to achieve a normal Pa_{CO_2}

II. Dantrolene
  Intravenously 2 mg/kg every 5 min to a total of 10 mg/kg
  Effective dosage should be repeated every 10–15 h for at least 48 h

III. Sodium bicarbonate
  Initial dose (mEq) = [base excess × (body weight in kg)]/4
  Give half the calculated dose; repeat as determined by arterial blood gas studies.

IV. Control fever
  Iced fluids
  Surface cooling
  Cooling of body cavities with sterile iced saline
  Heat exchanger with a pump oxygenator
  Dantrolene

V. Monitor urinary output
  At least 0.5 mL/kg/h
  If myoglobinuria is present, at least 1 mL/kg/h

VI. Further therapy
  Guided by blood studies, temperature, urine output
  (Blood studies include blood gases, electrolytes, liver profile, coagulaton studies [including DIC studies], serum hemoglobin and myoglobin, and urine hemoglobin and myoglobin)

DIC, disseminated intravascular coagulation; F_{IO_2}, fraction of inspired oxygen.
Modified from Askanazi J: Principles of nutritional support. In: Barash PG, Deutsch S, Tinker J (eds). *Refresher Courses in Anesthesiology*, vol. 14. Philadephia, JB Lippincott, 1986:1.

Treatment

Mortality rate has decreased from 80% to approximately 10% because of improved therapy (Table 66-15). After brief administration of a triggering agent, discontinuation may abort the attack. With fulminant MH (Pa_{CO_2} above 60 mm Hg and increasing; base excess more than −5 mEq/L; and a body temperature that is increasing by approximately 1 C° every 15 minutes), specific therapy with dantrolene is required. Dantrolene is a hydantoin analogue that inhibits sarcoplasmic reticulum calcium release without affecting re-uptake[81]; it is the key to successful MH treatment. Notice that the preparation of dantrolene for intravenous use requires the full attention of at least one person. Thus, help must be requested as soon as the diagnosis is tentatively made.

REFERENCES ■

1. Brown DL: Risk and outcome analysis: myths and truths. In: Kirby RR, Gravenstein N (eds). *Clinical Anesthesia Practice*. Philadelphia, JB Lippincott, 1994:62
2. Benumof JL: Management of the difficult airway: with special emphasis on awake tracheal intubation. *Anesthesiology* 1991; 75:1087
3. Higuchi H, Sumikura H, Sumita S, et al: Renal function in patients with high serum fluoride concentrations after prolonged sevoflurane anesthesia. *Anesthesiology* 1995;83:449
4. Coleman AJ: Uptake and distribution of inhalational anesthetic agents. In: Churchill-Davidson HC (ed). *A Practice of Anaesthesia*, 5th ed. Chicago, Year Book Medical Publishers, 1984: 223
5. Dripps RD, Eckenhoff JE, Vandam LD: Techniques of inhalational anesthesia. In: *Introduction to Anesthesia*, 6th ed. Philadelphia, WB Saunders, 1982:136
6. Linton RAF: Pulmonary ventilation. In: Churchill-Davidson HC (ed). *A Practice of Anaesthesia*, 5th ed. Chicago, Year Book Medical Publishers, 1984:32
7. Loer SA, Scheeren TWL, Tarnow J: Desflurane inhibits hypoxic pulmonary vasoconstriction in isolated rabbit lungs. *Anesthesiology* 1995;83:552
8. Brown BR: Halothane hepatitis revisited [editorial]. *N Engl J Med* 1985;313:1347
9. Gelman S: Halothane hepatotoxicity—again [editorial]? *Anesth Analg* 1986;65:831
10. Halperin BD, Feeley TW: The effect of anesthesia and surgery on renal function. *Int Anesthesiol Clin* 1984;22:157
11. Walton B: Effects of anesthesia and surgery on immune status. *Br J Anaesth* 1979;51:37
12. Askanazi J: Principles of nutritional support. In: Barash PG, Deutsch S, Tinker J (eds). *Refresher Courses in Anesthesiology*, vol 14. Philadelphia, JB Lippincott, 1986:1
13. Hamberger B, Järnberg P-O: Plasma catecholamines during surgical stress: differences between neurolept and enflurane anaesthesia. *Acta Anaesthesiol Scand* 1983;27:307
14. Everson NW, Neoptolemos JP, Scott DJA, et al: The effect of surgical operation upon monocytes. *Br J Surg* 1981;68:257
15. Shenniv H, Mulder DS, Chiu RC-J: Replenishing the starved patient: when do lung immune cells recover [editorial]? *Chest* 1985;87:138
16. Tonnesen E, Mickley H, Grunnet N: Natural killer cell activity during premedication, anaesthesia, and surgery. *Acta Anaesthesiol Scand* 1983;27:238

17. Katzav S, Shapiro J, Segal S, et al: General anesthesia during excision of a mouse tumor accelerates postsurgical growth of metastases by suppression of natural killer cell activity. *Isr J Med Sci* 1986;22:339

18. Page GC, Ben-Eliyahy S, Liebeslund JC: The role of LGL/NK cells in surgery-induced promotion of metastases and its attenuation by morphine. *Brain Behav Immun* 1994;8:241

19. Nomoto Y, Krasawa S, Uehara K: Effects of hydrocortisone and adrenaline on natural killer cell activity. *Br J Anaesth* 1994;73:318

20. McCredie JA: Antibody-dependent cellular cytotoxicity in critically ill surgical patients. *Surgery* 1980;88:544

21. Nakagawara M, Takeshige K, Takamatsu J, et al: Inhibition of superoxide production and Ca^{++} mobilization in human neutrophils by halothane, enflurane, and isoflurane. *Anesthesiology* 1986;64:4

22. Welch WD: Inhibition of neutrophil cidal activity by volatile anesthetics [editorial]. *Anesthesiology* 1986;64:1

23. van Dijk WC, Verbrugh HA, van Rijswijk REN, et al: Neutrophil function, serum opsonic activity, and delayed hypersensitivity in surgical patients. *Surgery* 1982;92:21

24. Perttilä J, Lilius E-M, Salo M: Effects of anaesthesia and surgery on serum opsonic capacity. *Acta Anaesthesiol Scand* 1986;30:173

25. Clark P, Layon AJ, Duff P: Effect of isoflurane on neutrophil phagocytic function during pregnancy. *Infec Dis Obstet Gynecol* 1993;1:98

26. McIrvine AJ, Mannick JA: Lymphocyte function in the critically ill surgical patient. *Surg Clin North Am* 1983;63:245

27. Abraham E, Chang Y-H: Cellular and humoral basis of hemorrhage-induced depression of lymphocyte function. *Crit Care Med* 1986;14:81

28. Abraham E, Chang Y-H: Effects of intravenous immunoglobulin on hemorrhage-induced alterations in plasma cell repertoires. *Crit Care Med* 1990;18:1252

29. Bailey PL, Stanley TH: Pharmacology of intravenous narcotic anesthetics. In: Miller RD (ed). *Anesthesia*, 2nd ed. New York, Churchill Livingstone, 1986:745

30. McClain DA, Hug CC: Pharmacodynamics of opiates. *Int Anesthesiol Clin* 1984;22:75

31. McDonough RJ, Madden JJ, Falek A, et al: Alteration of T and null lymphocyte frequencies in the peripheral blood of human opiate addicts. *J Immunol* 1980;125:2539

32. Brown SM, Stimmel B, Taub RN, et al: Immunologic dysfunction in heroin addicts. *Arch Intern Med* 1974;134:1001

33. White PF: Propofol: pharmacokinetics and pharmacodynamics. *Semin Anesth* 1988;7(Suppl 1):4

34. Smith I, White PF, Nathanson M, et al: Propofol: an update on its clinical use. *Anesthesiology* 1994;81:1005

35. Coates DP: Diprivan (propofol) infusion anesthesia. *Semin Anesth* 1988;7(Suppl 1):73

36. Sebel PS, Lowdon JD: Propofol: a new intravenous anesthetic. *Anesthesiology* 1989;71:260

37. Van Hemelrijck J, Fitch W, Mattheussen M, et al: Effect of propofol on cerebral circulation and autoregulation in the baboon. *Anesth Analg* 1990;71:49

38. Nimmo GR, Mackenzie SJ, Grant IS: Haemodynamic and oxygen transport effects of propofol infusion in critically ill adults. *Anaesthesia* 1994;49:485

39. Blouin RT, Seifert HA, Babenco HD, et al: Propofol depresses the hypoxic ventilatory response during conscious sedation and isohypercapnia. *Anesthesiology* 1993;79:1177

40. Pirttikangas CO, Salo M, Riutta A, et al: Effects of propofol and intralipid on immune response and prostaglandin E$_2$ production. *Anaesthesia* 1995;50:317

41. Piatt JH, Schiff SJ: High dose barbiturate therapy in neurosurgery and intensive care. *Neurosurgery* 1984;15:427

42. Engquist A, Fog-Møller F, Christiansen C, et al: Influence of epidural analgesia on the catecholamine and cyclic AMP responses to surgery. *Acta Anaesthesiol Scand* 1980;24:17

43. Chaplan S, Feeley TW: Complications in the postanesthesia care unit. *Semin Anesth* 1990;9:98

44. Halow KD, Ford EG: Pulmonary edema following postoperative laryngospasm: a case report and review of the literature. *Am Surg* 1993;59:443

45. Holmes JR, Hensinger RN, Wojtys EW: Postoperative pulmonary edema in young athletic adults. *Am J Sports Med* 1991;19:365

46. Cascade PN, Alexander GD, Mackie DS: Negative pressure pulmonary edema after endotracheal intubation. *Radiology* 1993;186:671

47. Marks RM, Sachar EJ: Undertreatment of medical inpatients with narcotic analgesics. *Ann Intern Med* 1973;78:173

48. Bryan-Brown CW: Development of pain management in critical care. In: Cousins MJ, Phillips GD (ed). *Acute Pain Management*. New York, Churchill Livingstone, 1986:1

49. Weissman C: The metabolic response to stress: an overview and update. *Anesthesiology* 1990;73:308

50. Weissman C, Hollinger I: Modifying systemic response with anesthetic techniques. *Anesth Clin North Am* 1988;6:222

51. Haas M, Glick SM: Radioimmunoassayable plasma vasopressin associated with surgery. *Arch Surg* 1978;113:597

52. Omaya T, Wakayama S: The endocrine response to general anesthesia. *Int Anesth Clin* 1981;26:176

53. Abraham E, Freutas AA: Hemorrhage in mice induces alterations in immunoglobulin-secreting B-cells. *Crit Care Med* 1989;17:1015

54. Schmand JF, Ayala A, Chaudry IH: Effects of trauma, duration of hypotension, and resuscitation regimen on cellular immunity after hemorrhagic shock. *Crit Care Med* 1994;22:1076

55. Wan W, Vriend CY, Wetmore L, et al: The effects of stress on splenic immune function are mediated by the splenic nerve. *Brain Res Bull* 1993;30:101

56. Chung HM, Kluge R, Schrier RW, et al: Postoperative hyponatremia: a prospective study. *Arch Intern Med* 1986;146:333

57. Burrows FA, Shutack JG, Crone RK: Inappropriate secretion of antidiuretic hormone in a postsurgical pediatric population. *Crit Care Med* 1983;11:527

58. Shirani KZ, Vaughan GM, Robertson GL, et al: Inappropriate vasopressin secretion (SIADH) in burned patients. *J Trauma* 1983;23:217

59. Roizen MF, Horrigan RW, Frazer BM: Anesthetic doses blocking adrenergic (stress) and cardiovascular responses to incision: MAC-BAR. *Anesthesiology* 1981;54:390

60. Chernow B, Alexander R, Smallridge RC, et al: Hormonal responses to graded surgical stress. *Arch Intern Med* 1987;147:1273

61. Stanley TA, Berman L, Green O, et al: Plasma catecholamine and cortisol responses to fentanyl-oxygen anesthesia for coronary artery operations. *Anesthesiology* 1980;53:250

62. Kehlet H, Brandt MR, Prange-Hansen A, et al: Effect of epidural analgesia on metabolic profiles during and after surgery. *Br J Surg* 1979;66:543

63. Kehlet H: Epidural analgesia and the endocrine metabolic response to surgery: update and perspectives. *Acta Anaesthesiol Scand* 1984;28:25

64. Hole A, Unsgaard G: The effect of epidural and general anesthesia on lymphocyte functions during and after major orthopedic surgery. *Acta Anaesthesiol Scand* 1983;27:135

65. Brown DL, Thompson GE: Anesthetic choice. In: Brown DL (ed). *Risk and Outcome in Anesthesia*. Philadelphia, JB Lippincott, 1988:152

66. Yeager MP, Glass DD, Neff RK, et al: Epidural anesthesia and analgesia in high risk surgical patients. *Anesthesiology* 1987;66:729

67. Baron JL, Bertrand M, Barre E, et al: Combined epidural and general anesthesia versus general anesthesia for abdominal aortic surgery. *Anesthesiology* 1991;75:611

68. Tuman KJ, McCarthy RJ, March RJ, et al: Effects of epidural anesthesia and analgesia on coagulation and outcome after major vascular surgery. *Anesth Analg* 1991;73:696

69. Shoemaker WC: Pathophysiology, monitoring, outcome prediction, and therapy of shock states. *Crit Care Clin* 1987;3:307

70. Scalea TM, Simon HM, Duncan AO, et al: Geriatric blunt trauma: improved survival with early invasive monitoring. *J Trauma* 1990;30:129

71. Abou-Khalil B, Scalea TM, Trooskin SZ, et al: Hemodynamic responses to shock in young trauma patients: need for invasive monitoring. *Crit Care Med* 1994;22:633

72. Shoemaker WC, Appel PL, Kram HB, et al: Prospective trial of supranormal values of survivors as therapeutic goals in high risk surgical patients. *Chest* 1988;94:1176

73. Egbert LD, Battit GE, Turndorf H, et al: The value of the preoperative visit by an anesthetist. *JAMA* 1963;185:553

74. Lutz LJ, Lamer TJ: Management of postoperative pain: review of current techniques and methods. *Mayo Clin Proc* 1990;65:584

75. van Lersberghe C, Camu F, de Keersmaecker E, et al: Continuous administration of fentanyl for postoperative pain: a comparison of the epidural, intravenous, and transdermal routes. *J Clin Anesth* 1994;6:308

76. Guinard JP, Carpenter RL, Chassot PG: Epidural and intravenous fentanyl produce equivalent effects during major surgery. *Anesthesiology* 1995;82:377

77. Ronan KP, Gallagher TJ, George B, et al: Comparison of propofol and midazolam for sedation in intensive care unit patients. *Crit Care Med* 1995;23:286

78. Hanson CW III: Pharmacology of neuromuscular blocking agents in the intensive care unit. *Crit Care Clin* 1994;10:779

79. Watling SM, Dasta JF: Prolonged paralysis in intensive care unit patients after the use of neuromuscular blocking agents: a review of the literature. *Crit Care Med* 1994;22:884

80. Allen GC, Rosenberg H, Fletcher JE: Safety of general anesthesia in patients previously tested negative for malignant hyperthermia susceptibility. *Anesthesiology* 1990;72:619

81. Britt BA: Dantrolene. *Can Anaesth Soc J* 1984;31:61

Critical Care, Third Edition, edited by Joseph M. Civetta,
Robert W. Taylor, and Robert R. Kirby.
Lippincott-Raven Publishers, Philadelphia, PA © 1997.

CHAPTER 67

Initial Triage
of the Trauma Patient

Larry C. Martin

IMMEDIATE CONCERNS ■

MAJOR PROBLEMS

The care of trauma patients is optimal in an environment in which the prehospital evaluation and transport are systematic and efficient. It is also essential for designated hospitals in a trauma network to be capable of providing emergency coverage on a 24-hour basis, so that victims can be transported to appropriate facilities for the degree of injury sustained.

Evaluation and triage of trauma victims should occur in an organized fashion. Attention should be focused on life-threatening injuries during the primary survey so that airway, breathing, and circulation problems are addressed expeditiously and treated promptly. The resuscitation of the patient with isotonic fluids and blood as required should be started as soon as possible during this phase of the assessment. After this, attention can be turned to elimination of any type of secondary injury that may have occurred as a result of central nervous system or orthopedic trauma.

STRESS POINTS

1. The assessment and control of the airway is the main priority of the primary survey and must be accomplished before attention is turned to any other potential injuries. Care must be taken to avoid manipulation of the cervical vertebrae, because an unstable fracture may be present.
2. Breathing should be carefully assessed to ascertain the presence of a tension pneumothorax, flail chest, or

open pneumothorax. These life-threatening injuries require intervention before radiography in most cases.
3. The circulatory status of the trauma victim can be assessed by blood pressure and pulse measurements. Often, however, it is not feasible to obtain a blood pressure reading, and assessment of the character of the peripheral pulses can give an indication of perfusion. The heart rate is also a good indication of hypovolemia, especially in the young trauma patient, in whom 30% or more of the blood volume may be lost before a decrease in the systolic blood pressure is noted.
4. Most trauma patients require two large-bore, 14- to 16- gauge percutaneous intravenous (IV) catheters placed in a peripheral location to provide adequate resuscitation.
5. Resuscitation of the patient should begin with isotonic salt solution, preferably Ringer's lactate. If the patient has been hypotensive, blood transfusions should be considered early in the resuscitation phase.
6. The use of hypertonic saline, albumin, or other volume expansion solutions such as hetastarch (Hespan) or dextran is usually not indicated. Combinations of hypertonic saline with dextran have been investigated and found useful in small volumes, but the role of this solution in the routine resuscitation of the trauma patient is unclear.
7. After the assessment of circulation and beginning of the resuscitation phase, a rapid neurologic assessment is appropriate. It is important first to evaluate pupillary size and activity, motor and sensory responsiveness, and the patient's level of consciousness.
8. The complete assessment of the trauma patient in-

volves a thorough examination for occult injury. Each patient should have clothes fully removed so that no injuries escape attention. Missed injuries can be devastating.

9. After the patient has been examined appropriately, protection from the environment must be provided to prevent hypothermia.

ESSENTIAL DIAGNOSTIC TESTS AND PROCEDURES

1. A patient who is awake and answers questions has an adequate airway, but any patient who is unconscious as a result of head injury or alcohol or drug use may be at risk for aspiration, hypoxia, and airway obstruction and should have the airway protected early.

2. If oral or nasal intubation fails and the patient cannot maintain adequate ventilation and oxygenation, or if there is a large amount of soft tissue damage to the face, a cricothyroidotomy should be performed.

3. The assessment of breathing involves physical examination of the chest, including inspection for symmetric chest motion, palpation for crepitus or chest wall deformity, and auscultation to determine whether breath sounds are present in each hemothorax and whether they are equal.

4. The diagnosis of tension pneumothorax should be made based on the clinical findings, because there often is no time to obtain a radiograph of the chest to confirm the clinical suspicions. The typical presentation of tachypnea, tracheal deviation to the contralateral side, and distended neck veins with signs of hypotension may not be present initially because of hypovolemia caused by ongoing hemorrhage. However, if the patient is given resuscitative fluids, distended neck veins should be identified as the volume status of the patient is restored. If the patient remains hypotensive, a tension pneumothorax should be suspected.

5. The quickest way to relieve a tension pneumothorax is to insert a 14- or 16-gauge, 6.25-cm IV catheter into the second intercostal space at the midclavicular line, withdraw the needle, and leave the Teflon catheter in place.

6. Flail chest is caused by multiple fractures at three or more adjacent ribs that result in paradoxical chest wall movement in the areas of the fractures.

7. An open pneumothorax, often referred to as a "sucking chest wound," results when a chest wall defect is present, allowing air to enter and exit the chest during respiration. Often, during the prehospital phase, the chest wall defect is covered by a Vaseline gauze or other occlusive dressing on three sides, so that air may exit the chest but not enter.

INITIAL THERAPY

1. If an injury to the cervical spine has been excluded or is not suspected, the oral route is preferred for securing the airway. If a cervical spine injury is likely, then nasotracheal intubation may be preferred. If these maneuvers fail, cricothyroidotomy may be necessary.

2. Tension pneumothorax and open pneumothorax can be alleviated by a tube thoracostomy.

3. Treatment of flail chest requires pain control for the rib fractures and supportive therapy for any underlying pulmonary injury secondary to contusion.

4. After IV access has been established, administration of fluids is begun at a rapid rate to restore tissue perfusion as required. Usually, in the young trauma patient who presents with hypotension, crystalloid volume expansion is necessary and blood is often required in the early phases of resuscitation. The adult patient should rapidly be given 2 to 3 L of isotonic salt solution, with monitoring of the response during infusion.

5. Inotropes and vasopressors are rarely indicated in the initial resuscitation of the trauma patient. The mainstay of resuscitation is adequate volume expansion; these agents only further compromise tissue perfusion and worsen the metabolic acidosis associated with hypovolemia.

Injury is the leading cause of death in the first four decades of life.[1] Numerous studies have documented a preventable death rate of 20% to 30% in patients with injuries that would have been survivable if the proper treatment had been rendered. Only recently have systematic efforts been made to address this issue.[2,3] The publication of *Accidental Death and Disability: The Neglected Disease of Modern Society* in 1966 pointed out the need for a concerted effort to organize trauma care.[4] Further, the Committee on Trauma of the American College of Surgeons has established standards for trauma center designation, so that only those institutions willing to participate in the care of the injured patient are included.[5] In an effort to further organize trauma care and alleviate the problem of preventable deaths, the American College of Surgeons has established the Advanced Trauma Life Support (ATLS) course to standardize the early care of the injured patient.[6]

Approximately 90% of patients who present to the emergency department after sustaining some degree of trauma do not have life-threatening injuries. These patients can be managed in the usual triage scheme of the emergency department. However, the remainder of patients do have life-threatening injuries, some of which may be occult, and they require the mobilization of an organized team, working in an orderly, systematic fashion to identify any life-threatening injuries that may be present.

The most useful, systematic approach to the trauma patient is that taught in the ATLS course,[6] in which the assessment of the trauma victim is broken down into the primary survey, resuscitation, the secondary survey, and definitive management. This chapter deals with the primary survey and the identification of life-threatening injuries that need immediate attention after a patient is transported to the emergency department. The initial assessment and primary survey of the trauma victim often involve what is commonly referred to as the ABCs: **A**irway, with cervical spine control; **B**reathing and ventilation; **C**irculation and control of hemorrhage; **D**isability, which refers to a brief neurologic examination and immobilization of the patient; and **E**xposure, referring to the complete undressing of the patient and quick examination to assess for other unsuspected injuries. The resuscitation phase is usually begun during assessment of circulation and continued throughout the remainder of the primary survey of the patient.

The secondary survey involves a more complete and thorough physical examination, in which all the injuries are categorized and documented so that they can be appropriately evaluated after the patient attains a stable condition. This assessment may include plain radiographs, computed tomography, diagnostic peritoneal lavage, abdominal ultrasound, or angiography. Finally, the definitive care phase involves triage of the patient to an appropriate area for further management. This may involve transport to the operating room, to the intensive care unit, to the surgical ward, or to another facility at which the appropriate care can be provided.

PREHOSPITAL PHASE

Paramedical personnel often can provide the basic skills necessary for identification and treatment of life-threatening injuries at the scene of an accident. These individuals are trained in the use of advanced methods of cardiac resuscitation, such as administration of drugs, establishment of IV routes, and administration of IV fluids. Furthermore, they are trained in endotracheal intubation to provide airway control in the emergency situation. Many of the techniques were initially instituted for the care of cardiac patients, in which stabilization of the patient before transport was thought to be important. However, for the trauma patient, prompt transport to facilitate treatment may be optimal. Many surgeons believe that a "scoop-and-run" protocol is more appropriate for the care of trauma victims. Many of the studies regarding on-scene stabilization versus scoop-and-run tactics have concerned the administration of IV fluid therapy as the most important technique used in the field.[7-14] However, airway obstruction and breathing abnormalities may be appropriately treated in this setting, even during short transports. The most important point is the delivery of the patient to the trauma center rapidly to prevent excessive blood loss, hypothermia, and coagulopathy. These conditions result in multiple organ failure if the patient survives the initial insult, and the prevention of these factors may, ultimately, be lifesaving. The decision to transport to a trauma center or to a community hospital can be of critical importance. In both an urban and rural environment, rotorcraft aeromedical transport in addition to ground transport can be critical in delivery of the traumatized patient to an appropriately equipped facility.[15-20]

Various criteria have been applied regarding mechanism of injury and physiologic status of the patient to identify those patients who require transport to a trauma center. These criteria are reflected in the American College of Surgeons guidelines for trauma patient transport (Table 67-1). As useful as these criteria are, they have been modified by many centers to streamline patient management in particular situations. The criteria currently in use at the University of Miami/Jackson Memorial Medical Center are listed in Table

TABLE 67-1. American College of Surgeons Guidelines for Triage of the Trauma Patient

ASSESSMENT OF VITAL SIGNS

Glasgow Coma Scale score <13
Systolic blood pressure <90
Respiratory rate <10 or >29

ANATOMY AND MECHANISM OF INJURY

Penetrating injury to chest, abdomen, head, neck or groin
Two or more proximal long-bone fractures
Burns of face/airway or > 15% total body surface area
Evidence of flail chest
Evidence of high impact
  Falls ≥20 feet
  Crash speed ≥20 mph: 20 in. deformity of automobile
  Passenger compartment intrusion 20 in. on patient side of car
  Ejection of patient
  Rollover
  Death of same car occupant
  Pedestrian hit at ≥20 mph

CONSIDER TRANSPORT TO TRAUMA CENTER

Age <5 or >55
Known cardiac or respiratory risk factors

67-2. The inclusion of paramedic judgment usually takes into account those severely injured patients who do not meet specific trauma criteria based on physiologic status or mechanism of injury. It is probably of utmost importance for paramedic prehospital personnel to be in radio contact with the receiving hospital to help in these decisions in which patients may not meet any specific trauma criteria but may have life-threatening injuries nevertheless.

IN-HOSPITAL PHASE

Preparation for the care of the trauma patient should be made before arrival. Equipment should be organized, tested, and set up where it is immediately available. The capability for warming IV fluids and blood and for rapid infusion should be set up in advance. The proper laboratory and radiology resources should be ready to care for severely injured patients. Also, transfusion services should be able to provide uncrossmatched blood immediately and to provide crossmatched blood quickly and in large quantities.

Universal precautions should be exercised to protect all those who come in contact with the patient from the trans-

TABLE 67-2. Dade County, Florida Trauma Triage Criteria

Systolic blood pressure <90
Glasgow Coma Score <13
Respiratory rate <10 or >29
Burns >15% total body surface area
Evidence of paralysis
Ejection from a motor vehicle
Amputations proximal to the wrist or ankle

mission of communicable diseases, especially hepatitis and the human immunodeficiency virus. This equipment must be available before the patient's arrival, so that the personnel are dressed and ready for patient care when the patient actually arrives.

PATIENT HISTORY

Immediately after patient arrival, it is often difficult to obtain a pertinent history of the traumatic event. However, this may be the only opportunity to question emergency medical services personnel or others who may have been present at the scene of the trauma. Often fire rescue personnel can provide information regarding the type of trauma sustained and events that occurred at the scene, as well as medical therapy rendered by them. Further, they can place the events in a proper time frame (e.g., the elapsed time from initial trauma until transport).

A reasonable guide to obtaining a rapid history is represented by the mnemonic AMPLE:

Allergies
Medications currently being taken by the patient
Past illnesses
Last meal
Events preceding the accident

It is important to determine whether the patient has any allergies before the administration of any medications, including antibiotics. Medications taken by the patient may reflect prior medical conditions that need appropriate initial treatment, or they may alter the response to stress or hypovolemia. Further, patients who are taking cardiac medications may have had a cardiac event before the accident. It is obviously important to inquire about past illnesses and operations in order to plan an adequate management scheme for each patient.

PRIMARY SURVEY

During the primary survey, those conditions that present an immediate threat to the patient's life are identified and dealt with in an expeditious manner. The primary survey and the initial resuscitation are accomplished simultaneously out of necessity in the patient with multiple injuries. Trauma management is a team effort, and many tasks can be accomplished simultaneously. However, a leadership role should be taken by a general surgeon with trauma management experience, especially during this initial phase of patient care. Many of the decisions reached at this time are instrumental in the treatment of life-threatening injuries and subsequent outcome.

Airway With Cervical Spine Control

The evaluation of the airway is distinctly different from the evaluation of breathing. Assessment of the airway is the highest priority item in the assessment of the trauma patient, and establishment of a patent airway, the most important aspect of the primary survey, must be accomplished before proceeding on to the other areas. A patient who is awake and answers questions has an adequate airway, but any patient who is unconscious as a result of head injury or alcohol or drug use may be at risk for aspiration, hypoxia, and airway obstruction and should have the airway protected early. Severe facial injuries and neck trauma may compromise the airway. In patients with these injuries, potential obstruction should be considered and intubation performed early; otherwise, severe swelling may make intubation impossible at a later time, and cricothyroidotomy may then be required.

The most common cause of obstruction of the upper airway in the unconscious trauma patient is the tongue. Also, blood, loose teeth, vomitus, foreign bodies, or an expanding hematoma may cause airway obstruction. The maneuver employed initially may involve a chin lift or jaw thrust. The chin lift is performed by placing the fingers of one hand under the mandible, which is then gently lifted upward, bringing the chin up anteriorly. The thumb of the same hand slightly depresses the lower lip to open the mouth. If the chin lift is unsuccessful, the forward jaw thrust maneuver may be accomplished by grabbing the angles of the jaw and displacing the mandible forward. These maneuvers are in no way definitive, and any patient who does not respond initially to them will require establishment of an airway for ventilation. The neck must be maintained in the neutral position during all these maneuvers to open the airway. This protects the cervical spine and avoids creation of a spinal cord injury if a bony injury is present. The cervical spine can be maintained in the neutral position with sand bags or by binding the head to a backboard with tape. Also, a hard cervical collar may be used, but this does not prevent some movement of the cervical spine in the combative patient.[21]

In an unconscious patient who is wearing a bicycle or motorcycle helmet, the helmet should be left in place until the cervical spine has been appropriately evaluated radiologically. If the patient requires an airway immediately and there is no time for radiographs to be obtained, the helmet must be removed using the two-person technique, which requires one person below to immobilize the neck and one person above to remove the helmet. In the unconscious patient with a suspected cervical spine injury, endotracheal intubation often must be performed in an emergency fashion. If the neck has not been properly evaluated with radiographs and there is a possibility of a cervical spine fracture, the neck must be held immobile during the intubation process by in-line traction. Although up to 20% of patients who are unconscious and have injuries above the clavicles have a cervical spine fracture, approximately 80% who sustain a cervical cord injury do so at the time of the impact.[22]

If the patient's airway appears stable and does not require emergency intubation, then major injury to the cervical spine can virtually be excluded by performing a cross-table lateral radiograph. All seven cervical vertebrae to the C7-T1 interface must be visualized. Often this requires relaxation of the patient's shoulders and pulling down on the shoulders while the radiograph is being taken. If this view is not adequate, additional radiographs should be taken, including a "swimmer's view." This is taken by placing the patient's arm above the head and placing the x-ray tube in the angle toward the C7-T1 junction. If this radiograph is inadequate, then computed tomography can be used to identify fractures in this area. The patient's cervical spine should remain immobilized until adequate studies can be performed.

Conscious patients can usually maintain their airways but often require a change to a sitting or a leaning-forward position. These patients should not be required to lie supine, because this position may obstruct the airway. Airway control in these patients can be difficult, especially if there is a large amount of soft tissue damage. The skilled physician may be able to pass a tube with a patient in the upright position, but often fiberoptic intubation is necessary in this situation. If an injury to the cervical spine has been excluded or is not suspected, the oral route is the preferred technique for securing the airway. If a cervical spine injury is highly suspected, then nasotracheal intubation may be preferred. The patient must be actively breathing so that the nasotracheal tube can be passed blindly into the trachea. However, it is extremely uncommon to cause any neurologic damage during endotracheal intubation, even if an unstable cervical spine fracture is present.[23,24] Intubation may be greatly facilitated by the use of chemical paralysis, because results are significantly better if the patient is anesthetically relaxed.[25]

If oral or nasal intubation fails and the patient cannot maintain adequate ventilation and oxygenation, or if there is a large amount of soft tissue damage to the face, a cricothyroidotomy should be performed. This is a reasonably fast and safe technique that can be used if other maneuvers fail to provide an adequate airway.[26,27] After the airway has been secured, attention can then be turned to other details of the primary survey.

Breathing

After the airway has been secured, breathing should be assessed. This involves physical examination of the chest, including inspection for symmetric chest excursion, palpation for crepitus or chest wall deformity, and auscultation to determine whether breath sounds are present in each hemothorax and whether they are equal. The patient's respiratory effort should be assessed, and the presence of tachypnea, distended neck veins, or tracheal deviation should be noted.

Tension pneumothorax is the most common life-threatening injury that is identified during the assessment of breathing. It typically occurs results from a parenchymal lung injury, in which air from the lung accumulates in the pleural space but cannot escape this area. Increasing pressure within the pleural space causes collapse and inadequate ventilation of the affected lung. Because of increased pressure in the mediastinum, the mediastinal structures shift to the contralateral side, causing a tension pneumothorax, which in turn results in diminished venous return to the right side of the heart due to distortion of the vena cava. The result is a lower cardiac output and hypotension. Tension pneumothorax is commonly seen in blunt thoracic trauma, and rib fractures may be present. However, the absence of rib fractures does not exclude a tension pneumothorax. Tension pneumothorax may also be seen after penetrating injuries if there is a parenchymal lung injury or a bronchial injury and the chest wall wound has become sealed so that air cannot escape from the pleural space.

The diagnosis of tension pneumothorax should be made based on the clinical findings, because there is often no time to obtain a radiograph of the chest to confirm the clinical suspicions. The typical presentation of tachypnea, tracheal deviation to the contralateral side, and distended neck veins with signs of hypotension may not be present initially owing to hypovolemia from ongoing hemorrhage. However, as the patient is resuscitated, distended neck veins should be identified as the volume status of the patient is restored. If the patient remains hypotensive, tension pneumothorax or pericardial tamponade should be suspected. Certainly, in the advanced stages, in which hypotension is present and the patient is hemodynamically unstable, the affected chest should be decompressed before any radiographs are obtained.

The quickest way to relieve a tension pneumothorax is to insert a 14- or 16- gauge, 6.25-cm IV catheter into the second intercostal space at the midclavicular line, withdraw the needle, and leave the Teflon catheter in place. A sudden rush of air confirms the diagnosis of tension pneumothorax, and the patient's hemodynamic status should improve immediately. After insertion of the needle and relief of the pneumothorax, the patient requires a tube thoracostomy. The tube is usually placed at the level of the fourth or fifth intercostal space, which is directly lateral to the nipple in the anterior to midaxillary line. This procedure is often easier than placing an anterior tube in the second intercostal space in the midclavicular line. A tube in this lateral position effectively clears blood and air from the pleural space. After the tube has been inserted, it should be checked initially for amount of blood present in the pleural space and for the presence of any air leak. A chest radiograph should be obtained to confirm the location of the tube and to identify whether there is residual air or blood remaining in the chest cavity, which may require a second tube for evacuation.

Flail chest may also present with signs of respiratory difficulty requiring immediate therapy during the initial assessment. Flail chest is caused by multiple fractures in three or more adjacent ribs and produces paradoxical chest wall movement in the areas of the fractures. A flail chest can result in multiple problems, all of which require therapy. The most immediate of these are the rib fractures, which may cause a pneumothorax and should be treated by a tube thoracostomy. Also, pain from the fractured ribs may impair ventilation. Finally, the underlying lung beneath the rib fractures may become contused and impair oxygenation and ventilation. Patients who present with hypoxemia caused by a pulmonary contusion usually can be assumed to have a massive injury and should be intubated for oxygenation and ventilation as soon as possible. Those patients who remain stable initially and do not have hypoxemia should be monitored closely for any deterioration in their respiratory status, because intubation may become necessary during the next 24 to 48 hours. Continuous pulse oximetry can be used to rapidly determine and follow the oxygen saturation in this situation and may provide an early indication of deterioration and the need for intubation.[28,29]

An open pneumothorax, often referred to as a sucking chest wound, results when a chest wall defect is present, allowing air to enter and exit the chest during respiration. Often, during the prehospital phase, the chest wall defect is covered by a Vaseline gauze or other occlusive dressing on three sides, so that air may exit the chest but not enter. This effectively relieves most of the problems resulting from open pneumothorax. After the patient is evaluated in the emergency department and the diagnosis is made, a tube thoracostomy should be performed, usually in the lateral position in the fourth or fifth intercostal space, as previously described. Very large defects in the chest wall may require intubation of the patient for initial stabilization, and the defects may require closure in the operating room.

Circulation

Assessment of the circulatory status of the patient includes obtaining the vital signs as well as control of external hemorrhage, if possible, and restoration of adequate tissue perfusion by volume infusion through large-bore IV catheters. The physical findings include the condition of the skin, the character of the pulse, and the mental status of the patient; it is often not possible to obtain a blood pressure reading in the initial phase of the assessment of the circulation.

Skin perfusion is often a reliable indicator of shock, but it may be difficult to assess in the hypothermic trauma patient. Vasoconstriction of the vessels of the skin and muscles is one of the earliest physiologic findings after volume loss and can be identified by pale and cool skin, often with diaphoresis. Pressure on the thenar or hypothenar eminences of the hand until the skin blanches and then quick release of the pressure can be used to identify poor skin perfusion. The color should return to normal within 2 seconds in normovolemia.

Adequate perfusion can also be assessed by determining the quality, rate, and regularity of the pulse. The pulse is a sensitive indicator of hypovolemia; the blood pressure, however, can remain in the normal range even with the loss of up to 30% of the blood volume. In a young patient, heart rates of 160 to 180 beats per minute (bpm) may be present with a normal blood pressure, indicating severe hypovolemia and vasoconstriction. It is often appropriate to assume that hypovolemia is present if there is a pulse rate faster than 120 bpm in an adult. Elderly patients may not be able to raise the pulse rate above 130 to 140 bpm, and the presence of a pacemaker or cardiac medications may limit the tachycardic response to hemorrhage in these patients. Often, a blood pressure reading cannot be obtained in the initial assessment of the circulation, and it is useful to examine the pulses present at the radial, femoral, and carotid areas. A palpable radial pulse corresponds to a blood pressure in the range of 80 to 90 mm Hg, a palpable femoral pulse to at least 70 mm Hg, and a palpable carotid pulse to at least 60 mm Hg.

Altered mental status can be used as an indicator to identify the hypovolemic patient. However, this sign is often unreliable, because the patient may have a central nervous system injury, be intoxicated with alcohol or drugs, or have some degree of hypoxemia that may contribute to the change in mental status. Urinary output can also be a good indication of tissue perfusion, but it is not feasible to monitor the urinary output over time. However, after insertion of a urinary catheter, the color and concentration can quickly be assessed to identify the state of hydration of the patient in the initial phase of resuscitation.

During the initial assessment of circulation, any external bleeding should be controlled, if possible. Control of hemorrhage is achieved by direct pressure over the bleeding site; tourniquets or external devices are rarely indicated. Attempts during the initial evaluation to clamp bleeding vessels in the depths of wounds, without adequate exposure or lighting, are fraught with danger from increased bleeding, adjacent nerve injury, and soft tissue destruction. Large bleeding wounds can be controlled with the use of a sterile compressive dressing, held in place with an elastic wrap, until the patient can be taken to the operating room and an adequate exposure obtained. Scalp lacerations are a common site for major blood loss. One of the most effective ways to control hemorrhage from scalp wounds is to close the skin edges quickly with a skin stapling device. If a cosmetic closure is required at a later time, the staples can be removed and the wound closed in a more appropriate fashion.

Resuscitation

The resuscitation of the patient occurs during the primary survey and simultaneously with control of the airway, breathing, and circulation. Often, oxygen delivery is impaired because of blood loss, decreased cardiac output, or thoracic injuries. During the initial evaluation, all patients should be placed on supplemental oxygen by face mask therapy unless the patient requires immediate intubation.

The basis of resuscitation of the trauma patient is establishment of adequate IV access and IV fluid therapy. Most trauma patients require two large-bore, 14- to 16-gauge percutaneous IV catheters placed in a peripheral location to provide adequate resuscitation. Certain patients present in a hemodynamically stable condition with no apparent injuries, and one IV catheter may be sufficient. However, if there is any suspicion that the patient may have significant ongoing hemorrhage, two catheters should be placed. It is important to obtain blood specimens for a type and crossmatch, hematocrit, and other necessary blood tests at the time the IV lines are started, so that crossmatched blood may be available as soon as possible. The placement of the catheters should be dictated by the location of the injuries. Patients presenting with upper extremity neck or chest trauma should have IV catheters placed on the contralateral side. In patients with upper torso injuries, catheters may be placed in the lower extremities, in the saphenous vein if possible. In the patient with abdominal trauma, however, it may not be appropriate to place any IV catheters in the lower extremities, because adequate therapy may not be achieved if the fluid is infused distal to the area of the injury (e.g., an intraabdominal vena caval injury).

Placement of percutaneous IV catheters is often difficult in the vasoconstricted patient who is hypovolemic. In this situation, a cutdown may be performed at the saphenous vein at the ankle or at the saphenofemoral junction in the groin. A large IV catheter can be inserted in the vein in either of these locations, or an IV extension tube, with the male end cut off, can be inserted directly into the saphenous vein for rapid fluid infusion. The use of percutaneous central catheters has become increasingly popular in the trauma patient. Large 9-French catheters can be inserted by the Seldinger technique in the subclavian or femoral location to provide rapid fluid infusion during resuscitation.[30] These catheters are often useful during rapid infusion, because the fluids are often administered under great pressure, which may not be tolerated by the peripheral veins. Further, these central catheters can be accessed by an anesthesiologist if the patient requires transportation to the operating room. They may also facilitate passage of a pulmonary artery catheter subsequently, if needed for hemodynamic monitoring. Great care must be taken during insertion of these lines in the hypovolemic patient, and only skilled personnel should attempt this technique.

Fluid Resuscitation

The fundamental therapy for fluid resuscitation in the trauma patient is the infusion of Ringer's lactate solution. This fluid replaces loss of isotonic fluid from both the vessels and the interstitial space and restores the intravascular volume so that adequate tissue perfusion may be maintained. Hypertonic saline, albumin, or other volume expansion solutions such as hetastarch or dextran are usually not indicated.[31] Combinations of hypertonic saline with dextran have been investigated and found useful in small volumes, but the role of this solution in the routine resuscitation of the trauma patient is unclear.[32]

After IV access has been established, fluid administration is begun at a rapid rate to restore tissue perfusion. Usually, in the young trauma patient who presents with hypotension, crystalloid volume expansion is necessary and blood is often required in the early phases of resuscitation. The adult patient should rapidly be given 2 to 3 L of isotonic salt solution, with monitoring of the response during infusion. One of the most reliable indicators of improving volume status is a decrease in the heart rate, which should be continuously monitored with a electrocardiographic monitor during resuscitation. If there is minimal or no response in the patient's hemodynamic status during infusion of 2 L of isotonic fluid, then the patient should be given uncrossmatched type O, Rh-negative packed red blood cells as soon as they are available. Although this is not the optimal blood replacement, it is reasonably safe and well tolerated.[33,34] After type-specific blood is available, it should be used until the patient's crossmatched blood can be obtained. Usage of blood must be monitored very closely in order to have blood available at all times for the hemorrhaging trauma patient.

Inotropes and vasopressors are rarely indicated in the initial resuscitation of the trauma patient. The mainstay of resuscitation is adequate volume expansion; these agents only further compromise tissue perfusion and worsen the metabolic acidosis associated with hypovolemia.

Another useful indicator of adequate resuscitation after the blood pressure and pulse have normalized is the base deficit as determined by arterial blood gas analysis. This measure is a reflection of the severity of initial trauma and correlates with mortality[35] as well as with unsuspected blood loss and the need for further resuscitation in the hemodynamically stable patient.[36,37]

Disability

After the assessment of circulation and the beginning of the resuscitation phase, a rapid neurologic assessment is appropriate. It is important first to evaluate pupillary size and activity, motor and sensory responsiveness, and the patient's level of consciousness. During this phase, there is no time to do a complete neurologic examination or to assess the patient's Glasgow Coma Score; however, a quick assessment provides evidence of significant cerebral injury and a baseline with which to compare any changes that may occur during the resuscitation and treatment of the patient. The ATLS course uses the mnemonic AVPU: **A**lert, Responds to **V**ocal Stimuli, Responds to **P**ainful Stimuli, and **U**nresponsive. This scale provides a quick assessment of the patient's mental status until the patient has been stabilized and a complete evaluation, including calculation of the Glasgow Coma Score, can be carried out.

Exposure

The complete assessment of the trauma patient involves a thorough examination for occult injury. Each patient should have clothes fully removed so that no injuries escape attention. Missed injuries can be devastating, and it is not unusual for patients to have suffered multiple types of trauma; for example, a gunshot wound to the back or head may have been the inciting event leading to a single-car accident. Patients should be rolled with care to protect the spine so that the back can also be examined. After the patient has been examined appropriately, protection from the environment must be provided to prevent hypothermia. After the core temperature drops below 32F, it is very difficult to rewarm the patient, which has a direct correlation with increased mortality.[38]

SUMMARY ■

The initial assessment of the trauma patient should proceed in an organized and efficient manner. This is best outlined by the American College of Surgeons Committee on Trauma and the ATLS course, in which priority is directed to the identification and treatment of life-threatening injuries. The ABCs of assessment and resuscitation regarding airway, breathing, and circulation determine which injuries require immediate lifesaving intervention and form the backbone of excellent trauma care.

REFERENCES ■

1. Committee on Trauma Research: *Injury in America*. Washington, DC, National Academy Press, 1985
2. Cales RH: Trauma mortality in Orange County: the effect of implementation of a regional trauma system. *Ann Emerg Med* 1981;13:1
3. Shackford SR, Hollingsworth-Fridlund P, Cooper GF, et al: The effect of regionalization upon the quality of trauma care as assessed by concurrent audit before and after institution of

a trauma system: a preliminary report. *J Trauma* 1986;26:812

4. Committee on Trauma and Committee on Shock, Division of Medical Sciences: *Accidental Death and Disability: The Neglected Disease of Modern Society*. Washington, DC, National Academy of Sciences, 1966

5. Hospital and prehospital resources for optimal care of the injured patient. *Bull Am Coll Surg* 1983;68:11

6. American College of Surgeons Committee on Trauma: *Advanced Trauma Life Support Course*. Chicago, American College of Surgeons, 1993

7. Gervin AS, Fischer RP: The importance of prompt transport in salvage of patients with penetrating heart wounds. *J Trauma* 1982;22:443

8. Aprahamian C, Thompson BM, Towne JB: The effect of a paramedic system in mortality of major open intra-abdominal vascular trauma. *J Trauma* 1983;23:687

9. Jacobs LM, Sinclair A, Beiser A: Prehospital advanced life support: benefits in trauma. *J Trauma* 1984;24:8

10. Pons PT, Honigman B, Moore EE, et al: Prehospital advanced trauma life support for critical penetrating wounds to the thorax and abdomen. *J Trauma* 1985;25:828

11. Lewis FR: Prehospital intravenous fluid therapy: physiological computer modeling. *J Trauma* 1986;26:804

12. Pons PT, Moore EE, Cusick JM, et al: Prehospital venous access in an urban paramedic system: a prospective on-scene analysis. *J Trauma* 1988;28:1460

13. Smith JP, Bodai BI, Hill AS, et al: Prehospital stabilization of critically injured patients: a failed concept. *J Trauma* 1985; 25:65

14. Martin RR, Bickell WH, Pepe PE, et al: Prospective evaluation of preoperative fluid resuscitation in hypotensive patients with penetrating truncal injury: a preliminary report. *J Trauma* 1992;33:354

15. Uhlhorn RW, Jacobs LM: Helicopters: extending the prehospital transportation system. *Med Instrum* 1982;16:202

16. Cleveland HC, Bigelow DB, Dracon D: A civilian air emergency service: a report of its development, technical aspects, and experience. *J Trauma* 1976;16:452

17. Trunkey DD: Trauma. *Sci Am* 1983;249:28

18. Baxt WG, Moody P: The impact of rotorcraft aeromedical emergency care service on trauma mortality. *JAMA* 1983; 249:3047

19. Baxt WG, Moody P, Cleveland HC, et al: Hospital-based rotorcraft aeromedical emergency care services and trauma mortality: a multicenter study. *Ann Emerg Med* 1985;14:859

20. Urdaneta LF, Sandberg MK, Cram AE, et al: Evaluation of an emergency air transport service. *Am Surg* 1984;50:183

21. Cline JR, Scheidel E, Bigsby EF: A comparison of methods of cervical immobilization used in patient extrication and transport. *J Trauma* 1985;25:649

22. Shaftan GW: The initial evaluation of the multiple trauma patient. *World J Surg* 1983;7:19

23. Holley J, Jorden R: Airway management in patients with unstable cervical spine fractures. *Ann Emerg Med* 1989;18:1237

24. Wright SW, Robinson GG 2d, Wright MB: Cervical spine injuries in blunt trauma patients requiring emergent endotracheal intubation. *Am J Emerg Med* 1992;10:104

25. Ligier B, Buchman TG, Breslow MJ, et al: The role of anesthetic induction agents and neuromuscular blockade in the endotracheal intubation of trauma victims. *Surg Gynecol Obstet* 1991;173:477

26. De Laurier GA, Hawkins ML, Treat RC, et al: Acute airway management: role of cricothyroidotomy. *Am Surg* 1990;56:12

27. Burkey B, Esclamado R, Morganroth M: The role of cricothyroidotomy in airway management. *Clin Chest Med* 1991;12:561

28. Jay GD, Hughes L, Renzi FP: Pulse oximetry is accurate in acute anemia from hemorrhage. *Ann Emerg Med* 1994;24:32

29. Mateer JR, Olson DW, Stueven HA, et al: Continuous pulse oximetry during emergency endotracheal intubation. *Ann Emerg Med* 1993;22:675

30. Pappas P, Brathwaite CE, Ross SE: Emergency central venous catheterization during resuscitation of trauma patients. *Am Surg* 1992;58:108

31. Velanovich V: Crystalloid versus colloid fluid resuscitation: a meta-analysis of mortality. *Surgery* 1989;105:65

32. Vassar MJ, Perry CA, Holcroft JW: Prehospital resuscitation of hypotensive trauma patients with 7.5% NaCl versus 7.5% NaCl with added dextran: a controlled trial. *J Trauma* 1993; 34:622

33. Schwab CW, Shayne JP, Turner J: Immediate trauma resuscitation with type O uncrossmatched blood: a two-year prospective experience. *J Trauma* 1986;26:897

34. Lefebre J, McLellan BA, Coovadia AS: Seven years experience with group O unmatched packed red blood cells in a regional trauma unit. *Ann Emerg Med* 1987;16:1344

35. Rutherford EJ, Morris JA Jr, Reed GW, et al: Base deficit stratifies mortality and determines therapy. *J Trauma* 1992; 33:417

36. Davis JW, Shackford SR, Holbrook TL: Base deficit as a sensitive indicator of compensated shock and tissue oxygen utilization. *Surg Gynecol Obstet* 1991;173:473

37. Davis JW, Shackford SR, Mackersie RC, et al: Base deficit as a guide to volume resuscitation. *J Trauma* 1988;28:1464

38. Jurkovich GJ, Greiser WB, Luterman A, et al: Hypothermia in trauma victims: an ominous predictor of survival. *J Trauma* 1987;27:1019

Critical Care, Third Edition, edited by Joseph M. Civetta,
Robert W. Taylor, and Robert R. Kirby.
Lippincott-Raven Publishers, Philadelphia, PA © 1997.

CHAPTER 68

∎

Secondary Triage
of the Trauma Patient

Marc D. Palter
Vicente Cortes

IMMEDIATE CONCERNS ∎

MAJOR PROBLEMS

Trauma patients often arrive in the intensive care unit (ICU) incompletely evaluated because of operative or radiologic interventions for life-threatening injuries. Good communication between the intensivist, the trauma team leader, and the anesthesiologist is essential if the process of diagnosis and treatment is to continue at an adequate pace and in the right direction.

Most trauma patients require further resuscitation on their arrival in the ICU. Therapeutic maneuvers often must be carried out based on clinical grounds without radiologic or laboratory confirmation. Persistent shock despite resuscitation is a poor prognostic sign, and a cause must be sought aggressively.

Delayed diagnosis of compartment syndrome leads to significant disability and, in severe cases, to limb amputation. Intraabdominal compartment syndrome, if left untreated, can lead to multisystem organ failure. Missed injuries are not uncommon, and the intensivist should maintain a high index of suspicion at all times. The physician should actively search for those injuries that are commonly missed instead of waiting for complications to occur.

STRESS POINTS

1. Therapy and diagnosis should be carried out simultaneously. A treatment plan should be initiated that pri-

oritizes therapy and further diagnostic evaluation according to the greatest threat to life or limb and the stability of the patient.
2. Airway maintenance is crucial, because reintubation may be difficult owing to injuries and airway edema.
3. Hypovolemia secondary to hemorrhage is the most common cause of hemodynamic instability in the trauma patient. Despite what appears to be massive resuscitation with crystalloid and blood, invasive hemodynamic monitoring reveals persistent hypovolemia and inadequate oxygen transport.
4. Blood and crystalloid solutions are both necessary to resuscitate severely injured trauma patients adequately. Although some physicians add colloid solutions to the resuscitation regimen, they cannot replace either blood or crystalloid.
5. Severe acidosis can result in hemodynamic instability despite adequate resuscitation. Serial blood gas analyses are invaluable to evaluate the resuscitative process. If the pH is less than 7.20, myocardial performance may be compromised because of acidemia.
6. Myocardial contusion is significant only if it results in arrhythmias or hemodynamic instability.
7. Massive transfusion of more than 10 units of packed red blood cells is associated with a multifactorial coagulopathy. Citrate toxicity may develop in patients who are massively transfused, hypothermic, and in shock.
8. Bleeding from pelvic fractures may not be readily apparent, but it can be the source of exsanguinating

hemorrhage. The pelvis is normally shaped like a closed ring, but fractures allow it to expand so that the possibility of tamponade is lost.

ESSENTIAL DIAGNOSTIC TESTS AND PROCEDURES

1. The airway and breathing should be assessed immediately on arrival of the patient in the ICU. Pulse oximetry, capnography, and auscultation of air entry to both lungs can be used for initial evaluation until a chest radiograph and arterial blood gas analysis can be obtained.
2. Heart rate, blood pressure, and urine output can be used initially to gauge the response to resuscitative efforts administered before ICU admission. If there has not been steady improvement, a pulmonary artery catheter should be inserted. Improved pH, lactate level, or base deficit can be used as an indicator of the response to resuscitation.
3. Persistent shock is most often secondary to insufficient volume replacement. Physical examination should be used to rule out other causes, such as tension pneumothorax or cardiac tamponade. If the cause is not apparent, then invasive hemodynamic monitoring is necessary to obtain further information.
4. Any injured extremity should be considered at risk for development of a compartment syndrome. Compartment pressures should be measured to confirm the presence or absence of elevated pressures.
5. Massive transfusion and hypothermia often result in severe coagulopathy, which is often apparent because of bleeding from wound and intravenous (IV) catheter sites. Laboratory evaluation, consisting of prothrombin time, partial thromboplastin time, platelet count, and fibrinogen determinations, is useful in guiding therapy.

INITIAL THERAPY

1. Direct laryngoscopy and reintubation may be necessary if the endotracheal tube is malpositioned or occluded. Transtracheal jet ventilation by needle cricothyroidotomy may provide enough time to allow intubation of the difficult airway. However, should this fail, the ICU physician should be prepared to gain access by cricothyroidotomy.
2. Hemodynamic instability or persistent shock should be treated with liter boluses of Ringer's lactate solution while a search is made for the cause. A needle or tube thoracostomy to relieve a suspected tension pneumothorax should be performed based on clinical evaluation, without waiting for a chest radiograph. The decision whether to continue resuscitation with fluid and blood or to add inotropic support is made based on information supplied by the pulmonary artery catheter.
3. The treatment for compartment syndrome is fasciotomy extending the entire length of the extremity segment and including all compartments. Intraabdominal compartment syndrome is treated by reopening the abdominal incision and placing a bioprosthetic material.
4. Rewarming should be the initial treatment for most coagulopathic trauma patients because of hypothermia-induced platelet dysfunction. Transfusion of fresh frozen plasma and cryoprecipitate should be used to correct the prothrombin time to less than 16 seconds and the fibrinogen to more than 100 mg/dL. Platelet transfusions should be used to maintain the platelet count higher than 100,000 per cubic millimeter if there are signs of bleeding.
5. The first step in limiting blood loss in patients with pelvic fractures is application of an external fixator. If this is not possible or if bleeding continues, the patient should undergo angiography and embolization of any bleeding sites that are identified. Finally, the military antishock trousers (MAST) can be applied in an attempt to externally tamponade ongoing hemorrhage if other therapies have failed.

Trauma is the leading cause of death in the United States population during the first four decades of life. Because it commonly affects people in their peak years of productivity, its cost must be measured in terms not only of treatment and rehabilitation expenses, but also of lost potential productivity, wages, and taxes. Mortality from trauma has a trimodal distribution. The first peak, occurring seconds to minutes after the traumatic event, is produced by injuries that are essentially lethal despite emergency medical treatment; mortality can be significantly affected only by preventive measures. The second peak occurs minutes to hours after the traumatic event and is produced by injuries of potentially lethal nature (e.g., neurologic injury, hemorrhage) that can be averted by rapid recognition and treatment during the so-called "golden hour." The third peak, days or weeks after the traumatic event, is caused by sepsis and multiple system organ failure; medical knowledge, resources, persistence, and attention to detail play a crucial role in reducing its impact.

Increased awareness of these facts has led to the development of trauma systems with four basic components: access to care, prehospital care, hospital care, and rehabilitation.[1] A systematic and organized approach to the trauma patient, in the form of a basic and advanced Prehospital Trauma Life Support course for paramedics and emergency medical technicians and an Advanced Trauma Life Support (ATLS) course for physicians, has been developed by the National Association of Emergency Medical Technicians and the Committee on Trauma of the American College of Surgeons.[2,3] The ATLS course offers an acceptable, structured, and consistent approach to the initial hospital evaluation of the trauma victim. It establishes assessment and management priorities by dividing the care into three steps: (1) simultaneous rapid primary survey (ABCs) and restoration of vital functions, (2) detailed secondary survey and diagnostic evaluation, and (3) definitive care.[3]

The emergency department staff and trauma team are usually involved directly in the care of the trauma patient during the golden hour and often complete the three steps of the evaluation and early care. However, multiple trauma patients often leave the emergency department before receiving a complete evaluation because of the need for surgical control of hemorrhage in the operating room or for diagnosis of potentially devastating injuries (e.g., intracranial hematoma) by computed tomography (CT). Persistent instability secondary to cardiogenic or neurogenic shock may require interruption of the evaluation and immediate transfer to the ICU so that invasive monitoring procedures and advanced methods of cardiovascular and respiratory support can be provided. The decision to stabilize the patient in the ICU before further radiologic evaluation or operative treatment is based on value judgments about which injury or pathophysiologic process has the most life-threatening potential. As a result, the patient may arrive in the ICU with undiagnosed injuries. The intensivist is, at this point, involved in the care of a trauma victim who has not had a detailed secondary survey.

Two examples are given here to indicate the types of situations that may be encountered in the ICU. In the first scenario, a patient involved in a motor vehicle accident arrives in the emergency department profoundly hypotensive. The patient's hemodynamic instability does not improve despite appropriate airway management, restoration of respiratory function, and initial volume resuscitation. Physical examination and chest and pelvic radiographs do not reveal any explanation for the patient's instability. A diagnostic peritoneal lavage (DPL) is positive for blood, and the patient undergoes immediate laparotomy for hemorrhage control. At exploration, a massive liver injury is encountered. At the completion of the surgical procedure, the patient is hemodynamically unstable, hypothermic, profoundly acidotic, and has a severe coagulopathy. This patient is best cared for in the ICU, where further evaluation for other possible injuries can occur simultaneously with ongoing resuscitation.

In the second scenario, a patient arrives in a similarly unstable situation after having sustained obvious blunt torso trauma and multiple extremity injuries, some of which are open fractures. Bilateral chest tubes are inserted for markedly decreased breath sounds, evacuating bilateral pneumothoraces and minimal hemothoraces. A DPL is grossly negative. A supine chest radiograph shows multiple bilateral rib fractures and a widened mediastinum. The electrocardiogram (ECG) shows ST- and T-wave changes, frequent premature ventricular contractions, and a right bundle branch block. The patient remains hemodynamically unstable despite fluid resuscitation. This patient needs an aortogram to rule out an aortic injury and multiple radiographs to evaluate the orthopedic injuries as well as irrigation and debridement of open fractures. Instead of proceeding with this sequence, the patient must be rapidly transferred to the ICU for invasive monitoring and treatment of the blunt cardiac injury with pump failure. Ideally, this can occur during the time needed by the radiologist to prepare for the angiographic study.

OBTAINING THE PATIENT'S HISTORY AND HISTORY OF INJURY ■

Patient and event histories represent 90% of the diagnostic evaluation. Allergies, medications, past illness, mechanism of the injury, events and environment related to the accident, details of the prehospital course, and positive and negative findings of the workup constitute crucial information. Although intensivists usually cannot get complete firsthand information from the intubated or obtunded patient or from the prehospital personnel, they may create a collage of facts obtained from the members of the emergency department staff, trauma team, anesthesia team, and operating room staff, usually well in advance of the arrival of the patient at the ICU. This information must be shared with other key ICU team members, such as the charge nurse, primary care nurse, house staff, and respiratory therapist. The more information they gather, the better prepared they will be to care for the patient.

Intensivists cannot expect to obtain the needed information by reviewing the chart at the time of admission of the patient to the ICU, because they will be directly assessing and resuscitating the patient. Furthermore, documentation usually lags behind the course of events in unstable patients. Evaluation of the patient in the operating room or emergency room helps the ICU physician to prioritize therapeutic and diagnostic procedures that will be needed when the patient arrives in the ICU. To better anticipate the challenges they are about to face, intensivists should obtain a report of the most recent events from the trauma team leader or anesthesiologist in charge.

REASSESSING THE ABCs WHILE MAINTAINING VITAL FUNCTIONS ■

Trauma patients transferred directly from the emergency department or from the operating room are best approached initially by repeating the primary survey—that is, with a quick reassessment of their airway (with cervical spine control), breathing and ventilation, circulation (with hemorrhage control), disability (neurologic status), and exposure (complete undressing)—while simultaneously intervening to maintain vital functions and normothermia. This must be followed by a head-to-toe evaluation (the secondary survey) while there is ongoing reevaluation of the adequacy of resuscitation.

AIRWAY

Prompt recognition and correction of airway obstruction is imperative. Despite a variety of methods used to secure endotracheal tubes, they can easily become displaced during transport of the patient. Auscultation of both lung fields and the epigastrium during manual ventilation of the patient with a bag-valve device or the ventilator is the simplest way to confirm correct placement and patency of the endotracheal tube. If capnography is immediately available, it also may be used to confirm proper tube placement. If any doubt exists about correct tube placement, direct laryngoscopy must be performed by a clinician experienced in airway management. A completely obstructed airway (endotracheal tube or tracheostomy cannula) must be changed without delay, with the use of a tube changer or by direct laryngoscopy. Any question of partial obstruction of an airway must be resolved before proceeding any further in the evaluation by passage of a large-bore suction cannula and, if doubt remains, by fiberoptic bronchoscopy.

When dealing with an airway crisis, the worst-case scenario (inability to intubate) and its resolution with a surgical airway (cricothyroidotomy) must be anticipated and a contingency plan made for that eventuality. Transtracheal jet ventilation by needle cricothyroidotomy with a 14-gauge catheter or percutaneous cricothyroidotomy tube and a 50-psi oxygen source can be used as a temporizing measure. A pressure of 50 psi is necessary to permit adequate oxygen flow. The most common complication is bleeding. This can be avoided by puncturing the cricothyroid membrane inferiorly and avoiding the blood vessels that are located superiorly. Other complications include subcutaneous emphysema caused by incorrect catheter placement and perforation of adjacent structures such as the esophagus.

In the patient with multisystem trauma, particularly with blunt injuries above the clavicle, a bony or ligamentous cervical spine injury should be assumed until proven otherwise by report of the trauma team leader, personal review of radiologic studies by a competent specialist, or official radiologic report. Meanwhile, appropriate immobilization measures must be instituted or maintained.

BREATHING

The "look, listen, and feel" techniques are used for initial assessment. An arterial blood gas specimen should be sent for analysis as early as possible to assess respiratory function, oxygenation, and ventilation. Pulse oximetry can be used to assess rapidly the adequacy of oxygenation. However, poor peripheral perfusion is often present and may limit the ability of the oximeter to function properly until the patient has been adequately resuscitated. In the nonintubated patient, an unacceptable breathing pattern (i.e., respiratory distress) is an indication for intubation and mechanical ventilatory support regardless of the arterial blood gas analysis.

It is safer to use a high fraction of inspired oxygen (FIO_2) in the patient with marginal respiratory status until the actual partial pressure of oxygen (PO_2) or hemoglobin saturation is verified by arterial blood gas analysis or pulse oximetry. However, high FIO_2 may have a detrimental effect on ventilation-perfusion mismatch (absorption atelectasis) and may potentiate acute lung injury as a result of hyperoxia. It should not be continued beyond initial resuscitation unless necessary to maintain oxygenation. The paradoxical motion of a flail chest segment may have been missed in the trauma room or may not become apparent until the progressive hypoxemia caused by the underlying pulmonary contusion increases minute ventilation and makes it more obvious. The proper therapy here is not just intubation and positive-pressure ventilation, but rapid titration of positive end-expiratory pressure (PEEP) to correct the hypoxemia.

Patients with multisystem trauma are often placed on a ventilator while still in the emergency department or are ventilated by an anesthetic machine while in the operating room. During transport to the ICU, these patients are manually ventilated with a bag-valve device. Lung compliance may have changed dramatically, especially if blunt chest

trauma is present, and even if mechanical ventilation was sufficient, hand bagging may be inadequate to maintain adequate oxygenation and ventilation. The typical result is a patient who decompensates just as he or she arrives in the ICU secondary to severe hypoxemia and hypercapnia. In one study, 37% of transported ICU patients had significant deterioration in respiratory status, with many requiring an increased level of support.[4] Patients must be carefully evaluated before being transported, and a PEEP valve or transport ventilator must be used for safe transfer in marginal or rapidly deteriorating patients. A ventilator must be set up before the patient's arrival in the ICU so that effective ventilatory support can be reinitiated immediately. The patient's actual compliance and potential for further deterioration must be considered when selecting the type of ventilator to be used.

A small pneumothorax may not be apparent or may be missed on the supine chest radiograph that is usually obtained in the trauma room. As the patient is intubated and receives positive-pressure ventilation, a tension pneumothorax may then develop. A pneumothorax in the mechanically ventilated patient is by definition a tension pneumothorax; it produces not only acute deterioration of respiratory function but profound shock by decreasing venous return to the heart, compromising cardiac output. If a patient is hypotensive with decreased breath sounds, a deviated trachea, distended neck veins, or subcutaneous emphysema in the chest wall, no time can be wasted waiting for a confirmatory chest radiograph; immediate evacuation by large-bore needle thoracentesis, followed by tube thoracostomy, is necessary. Quick relief of hypotension and respiratory embarrassment confirms the diagnosis. The presence of a chest tube does not guarantee that a pneumothorax cannot develop; a tube thoracostomy can become occluded by blood clots or fibrin, or pleural loculations may exist that divide the space into independent compartments.

CIRCULATION

Shock and hypotension in the trauma patient are caused by hypovolemia secondary to hemorrhage until proven otherwise. If hypotension and shock persist despite what should be adequate resuscitation of recognized injuries, another cause must be sought while blood volume restoration is continued. However, the most common cause of continued instability is under-resuscitation. In traumatic shock, the oxygen transport function is compromised at multiple levels: hypoxemia, hypoventilation, hypovolemia, low cardiac output, acute anemia, acidemia, hypothermia, and peripheral hypoperfusion. Altered mentation, peripheral adrenergic discharge, and rapid, thready peripheral pulses are the most evident physical signs. The status of the neck veins is the best clinical indicator of a cardiogenic or cardiac compressive component of shock if more sophisticated modalities of monitoring have not been established.

ECG monitoring is a noninvasive, simple method for detection of arrhythmias suggestive of hypoxia, hypoperfusion, hypothermia, or blunt cardiac injury. Absent central pulses in more than one site while an ECG tracing is present constitute electromechanical dissociation and mandate immediate action to address correctable causes (e.g., profound hypovolemia, tension pneumothorax, cardiac tamponade, hypoxemia, acidosis).

Adequate venous access is necessary for effective resuscitation and must be secured before insertion of monitoring lines. Two large-bore IV lines are the minimum, with 14- or 16-gauge, 5-cm peripheral catheters to allow a flow rate of 300 mL/minute of crystalloids or 150 mL/minute of blood when used with a pressure bag.[5] The flow rate through IV catheters is directly proportional to their diameter and inversely proportional to their length. If central venous access is desired, an 8.5 French introducer is preferred over a multilumen central venous catheter. Flow rates of up to 500 mL/minute of fluid or 250 mL/minute of blood can be obtained through the introducer with pressure bags. Later, it provides a portal for the insertion of a pulmonary artery catheter, if necessary.

All IV catheters placed in the prehospital or emergency department setting should be changed within the first 24 hours in the ICU, because they may have been inserted under less than ideal sterile conditions. Our practice is to change all central catheters over guidewires, culture the intracutaneous segments, and remove the peripheral lines. This should be done only after hemodynamic stability has been established or additional clean IV access has been secured.

The choice of fluid used for resuscitation has been the subject of much debate, and a detailed review of the crystalloid-colloid controversy is beyond the scope of this chapter. We believe that a balanced salt solution, such as Ringer's lactate, is the appropriate choice, both as the initial resuscitation fluid in the trauma room and later in the ICU. Shires and coworkers[6] demonstrated deficits in functional extracellular volume caused by intracellular sequestration of fluid and salt and that the interstitial space must also be resuscitated. Blood and colloids did not improve survival in experimental preparations. Adequate resuscitation of the interstitial space usually results in an unavoidable accumulation of peripheral edema. There should be no attempt to prevent or treat this edema, because it is only a manifestation of the underlying endothelial dysfunction and cannot be prevented if adequate restoration of intravascular and interstitial volumes are to be achieved. The patient mobilizes this fluid later. We do not believe that there is any evidence that colloids are better than crystalloids in terms of outcome or incidence of pulmonary or renal dysfunction. They are equally effective in resuscitation, but a greater amount of salt solution is required to reach the physiologic endpoints of restored tissue perfusion, adequate urine output, and satisfactory oxygen delivery. The cost of fluid resuscitation with crystalloids is dramatically lower; this is most significant, given that colloids offer no advantages.

Ringer's lactate solution can be used in the trauma patient despite the presence of a lactic acidosis resulting from inadequate perfusion. If the patient is properly resuscitated, the liver metabolizes the lactate to bicarbonate. The successfully resuscitated patient, therefore, eventually manifests a metabolic alkalosis. Even head-injured patients should be vigorously fluid resuscitated if they are hemodynamically unsta-

ble. Data from the Trauma Coma Data Bank has suggested that hypotension (<90 mm Hg systolic blood pressure) doubles the mortality and significantly increases the morbidity from traumatic brain injury.[7] Hypotension should never be attributed to head injury without an active search for other causes. Limiting fluid administration in an attempt to avoid cerebral edema allows shock to persist; this leads to inadequate cerebral perfusion pressure, cerebral ischemia, and more severe cerebral edema. The severity of cerebral edema is the same whether the patient is resuscitated with crystalloid or colloid solution.[8]

Unstable trauma patients also require transfusion therapy in addition to crystalloid fluid resuscitation. Trauma patients in hemorrhagic shock initially receive 2 to 3 L of balanced solution rapidly as a fluid challenge. Failure to regain normal and stable vital signs, or stabilization for only a short period of time, indicates the presence of a class III or IV hemorrhage (ATLS criteria), with more than 40% of blood volume lost. In the average patient with a 5-L blood volume, this is a 2-L blood loss. These patients must receive blood, because even with fluid resuscitation and control of external hemorrhage, there may be ongoing internal hemorrhage.

It is crucial to verify that an adequate supply of blood products is available in the blood bank to satisfy the needs of the injured patient in the initial ICU course. A blood sample for type and crossmatching, together with the arterial blood gas sample, are the most important specimens to be obtained from the trauma victim on arrival in the ICU.

It cannot be overemphasized that the trauma patient who has been in hemorrhagic shock and who is still unstable on arrival in the ICU is most likely under-resuscitated. Red blood cells are necessary to provide adequate oxygen-carrying capacity and should continue to be administered to unstable trauma patients. The hematocrit is not a direct measure of blood volume and is not reliable in guiding therapy; the hematocrit may not be a true reflection of the ratio of red cell mass to total blood volume because equilibration may not occur for 24 hours. All blood products and IV fluids must be prewarmed if they are to be administered in massive quantities or at rapid infusion rates to prevent or correct hypothermia.

DISABILITY

A rapid neurologic evaluation, including level of consciousness, mentation, and pupillary size and reaction, must be performed on arrival of the patient at the ICU and the results compared with those of a similar evaluation in the emergency department as reported by the trauma team leader. Any significant deterioration points to the need for a more detailed neurologic examination; reevaluation of oxygenation, ventilation, and perfusion; and investigation of intracranial pathology with immediate brain CT scan without the use of contrast agents. Suspected or measured intracranial hypertension must be treated with hyperventilation and osmotic diuretics while preparations are made for radiologic confirmation and surgical evacuation of intracranial hematomas.

EXPOSURE

Although the patient must have been completely undressed in the trauma room, the MAST applied by the prehospital care team may have been kept inflated because of hemodynamic instability that was poorly responsive to volume administration, the need to proceed with thoracotomy or laparotomy to control hemorrhage, or the presence of an unstable pelvic fracture. In these instances, it is the responsibility of the intensivist to conduct a survey of the abdomen, pelvis, and lower extremities as soon as the garment is temporarily or permanently deflated. The garment must be deflated under careful monitoring of the blood pressure and after restoration of blood volume. Any decrease in blood pressure greater than 5 mm Hg during the deflation process must be followed by administration of a balanced salt solution or blood before further deflation. If more substantial hypotension occurs, the MAST must be reinflated and surgical or radiologic intervention to control hemorrhage considered.

The back is an area that may have been overlooked in the trauma resuscitation room and must be inspected in the ICU by log rolling the trauma victim. After the inspection has been completed, the core temperature should be maintained with blankets, heating lamps, or other devices for the prevention and treatment of hypothermia.

INSERTION OF MONITORING EQUIPMENT

The multiply injured patient is seldom received from the emergency department or operating room without a secured airway, venous access, and continuous ECG monitoring. A nasogastric tube and a urinary Foley catheter are also usually present. If absent, they may be placed before the secondary survey is initiated. However, nasogastric tubes are contraindicated if a cribriform plate fracture is suspected; instead, an orogastric tube should be inserted. Insertion of a urinary catheter is contraindicated in urethral transection, and a suprapubic catheter should be inserted in such cases to measure urine output. This injury must be suspected if there is blood at the meatus, a scrotal hematoma, or a high-riding prostate on digital rectal examination.

ICU monitoring, including continuous ECG monitoring, pulse oximetry, capnography, direct arterial pressure monitoring, pulmonary artery catheterization, cardiovascular and respiratory physiologic monitoring, continuous mixed venous oximetry, and intracranial pressure monitoring, provides the quantum leap of physiologic information necessary to guide and titrate subsequent therapeutic interventions. However, it is crucial not to divert all the nursing and physician attention from reassessing the ABCs and maintaining vital functions while efforts are focused on inserting and calibrating monitoring devices. Resuscitation must continue, guided by whatever methods are available, until more accurate electronic devices are operational. These qualitative physical diagnosis methods (look, listen, and feel) must guide therapy until laboratory or radiologic findings and invasive physiologic measurements provide direct quantitative documentation of the altered physiology to allow appropriate pharmacologic interventions.

COMPLETING THE SECONDARY SURVEY

At this point, the intensivist is ready to complete the secondary survey or detailed topographic examination of the patient (head and face, cervical spine and neck, chest, abdomen, rectum and perineum, pelvis, back, extremities, and nervous system), including placing "tubes and fingers in every orifice," completing other necessary radiologic investigations, and addressing the specific problems discussed in the following sections.

PERSISTENT SHOCK ■

The ICU physician must remember other causes of persistent hypotension after seemingly adequate resuscitation (Table 68-1). Undetected hemorrhage may exist if external blood loss occurred before the patient's arrival at the hospital. Extensive scalp lacerations may result in bleeding significant enough to cause hypotension and shock. This injury is often overlooked because of attention to other, more "serious" injuries. The application of a pressure dressing is usually insufficient and serves only to obscure the ongoing hemorrhage. Early closure of the wound, even if only by temporary stapling, is the best method to control bleeding from scalp wounds.

An abdominal source of hemorrhage should have been addressed in the operating room or excluded before the arrival of the injured patient in the ICU. DPL, CT scan, and ultrasound are the three most common methods used to evaluate abdominal trauma. DPL or ultrasound is preferred for the unstable patient. However, DPL and ultrasound are not reliable to detect pelvic or retroperitoneal hematomas, which can be the source of significant blood loss. Abdominal CT scan can detect these injuries, but it is often reserved for evaluation of hemodynamically stable patients. The still unsurpassed procedure to rule out intraabdominal or retroperitoneal bleeding is exploratory laparotomy, which may be viewed as an extension of the physical examination. (See Chap. 70 for a more detailed discussion on the use of adjuvant techniques in abdominal trauma.)

Tension pneumothorax and massive hemothorax may both present as persistent hypotension. A chest radiograph performed with the patient in the supine position in the emergency room may not detect a small pneumothorax that, under positive-pressure ventilation, may subsequently be-

TABLE 68-1. Causes of Persistent Hypotension

Undetected hemorrhage
Pneumothorax or hemothorax
Cardiac tamponade
Air embolism
Spinal cord injury
Acidosis
Hypothermia
Hypocalcemia
Myocardial contusion

come a tension pneumothorax and present as hemodynamic instability. Although a chest radiograph should be repeated as soon as possible in any unstable trauma patient, the diagnosis of life-threatening tension pneumothorax is clinical and not radiologic, as has already been mentioned. One pleural cavity can easily hold 2 L of blood or more. This accumulation may appear on a supine chest radiograph as only a diffuse haziness over the affected hemithorax. A large-bore chest tube (36 or 40 French) must be inserted for drainage and to assist in the evaluation of the amount and rate of bleeding. It is incorrect to assume that the blood tamponades the bleeding if no chest tube is inserted or that the chest tube should be clamped because the patient can exsanguinate into one hemithorax. The patient may also benefit from autotransfusion of the blood drained. A chest radiograph must be repeated if drainage from the chest stops, because this may signify occlusion of the tube and not cessation of hemorrhage. Patients with significant hemothorax often require a second chest tube; if more than 1500 mL of blood is evacuated through the initial tube thoracostomy or bleeding persists at 200 mL/hour for more than 4 hours, then exploratory thoracotomy is indicated. A common pitfall that may result in undetected hemorrhage is failure to connect a chest tube to suction when the patient is admitted to the ICU. Bleeding from the lung parenchyma increases if the lung is allowed to collapse because suction is not utilized.

Although cardiac tamponade is usually a result of penetrating cardiac injury, it may also be a cause of shock after blunt chest trauma. As blood accumulates in the pericardial sac, pressure increases and prevents diastolic filling, compromising cardiac output. Patients with tamponade may present with hypotension, tachycardia, and an elevated central venous pressure. Beck's triad (distant heart sounds, distended neck veins, and hypotension) is often not present or detectable in acute traumatic tamponade owing to the noise and activity of resuscitation. Pulsus paradoxus and a large cardiac silhouette on chest radiograph are other findings that are frequently absent. Because a low central venous pressure may occur in the presence of hypovolemia even if there is significant tamponade, the absence of distended neck veins does not rule out cardiac tamponade. A cardiac echogram is diagnostic but may be difficult to obtain in a timely fashion. The ICU physician can insert a pulmonary artery catheter to find the characteristic equalization of right- and left-sided atrial pressures and pulmonary artery diastolic pressure. The initial treatment should be the administration of fluids to increase venous return and fill the heart. Volume replacement may allow stabilization of the patient and transportation to the operating room. Pericardiocentesis or subxiphoid pericardial window can be used as a diagnostic and therapeutic maneuver in a patient suspected of having tamponade. They should be considered temporizing measures to be used before definitive operative treatment.

Venous air embolism occurs if a significant volume of air is introduced into the right heart circulation, usually through a central venous pressure catheter.[9] Right ventricle cardiac output becomes ineffective because the heart compresses the air instead of pumping blood. If CPR is not required, the patient must be placed in the left lateral and Trendelenburg position to minimize the amount of air reaching the pulmonary outflow tract. The patient should also be placed on 100% oxygen in an attempt to reduce the size of the air bubble.

Systemic air embolism occurs with much smaller volumes of air and presents as sudden onset of shock in a patient who has sustained a lung injury. This situation is often precipitated by endotracheal intubation and the institution of positive-pressure ventilation. Air enters the pulmonary veins by means of a lung parenchymal injury and travels through the left side of the heart into the systemic circulation. Air entering the coronary arteries causes cardiovascular collapse, whereas air reaching the cerebral circulation causes a sudden neurologic event. Hemoptysis through the endotracheal tube usually precedes the cardiac event and should suggest the potential for air embolism in any patient with blunt chest trauma. Systemic air embolism requires thoracotomy and crossclamping of the pulmonary hilum of the responsible lung to prevent further embolism. Often, air can be observed in the coronary circulation at thoracotomy. Hyperbaric oxygen therapy can be lifesaving or reverse neurologic deficits (see Chap. 51).

A spinal cord injury above the upper thoracic level may produce neurogenic shock as a result of a loss of sympathetic tone. The patient typically presents with signs of autonomic dysfunction such as hypotension, bradycardia, and warm, dry skin. However, the presence of other multisystem injuries often obscures this characteristic presentation. Other findings that suggest the presence of a spinal cord injury are absence of all sensorimotor function below a certain level, flaccidity, absent deep tendon reflexes, and lack of rectal tone. Although the intravascular volume is normal (unless other injuries are present), the consequent fall in peripheral vascular tone creates a relative expansion of the intravascular space. Mild hypotension does not normally need to be treated, but if it results in inadequate perfusion and metabolic acidosis, therapy is required. In this situation, a central venous or pulmonary artery catheter may help to determine treatment, which should consist of cautious volume loading first, followed by administration of α-agonist agents. Because intravascular volume is not depleted, overzealous administration of fluids may cause pulmonary edema. Phenylephrine is most commonly chosen because of its pure α-adrenergic effects and resultant increase in vasomotor tone. Bradycardia may occur because of the predominant parasympathetic influence and can be blocked with atropine.

Acidosis, hypothermia, and hypocalcemia are frequently present in massively injured and resuscitated patients. Acidosis can result in persistent hypotension despite adequate resuscitation. Nonetheless, the primary treatment of lactic acidosis in hypovolemic shock is the restoration of circulating blood volume and oxygen transport. Serial blood gas analyses are useful to appraise the adequacy of resuscitation. As perfusion is restored, the pH reverts toward normal and the base deficit decreases. As long as the patient improves, treatment with sodium bicarbonate is not necessary. Not infrequently, as perfusion improves, lactate is washed out of the periphery, causing a transient worsening of acidemia. This quickly corrects itself if adequate perfusion is maintained.

Myocardial performance may deteriorate if the pH drops below 7.20. Therefore, in the presence of protracted hypotension, shock, and acidosis, the cautious administration of sodium bicarbonate may improve cardiac function. Overcorrection of the pH can be detrimental because the shift in the oxyhemoglobin dissociation curve makes oxygen less available to the tissues. Hypothermia and hypocalcemia are discussed later in the section on massive transfusion.

BLUNT CARDIAC INJURY ■

Myocardial injury caused by blunt trauma may result in arrhythmia, cardiac failure, or valvular or coronary artery damage. However, most patients with a blunt cardiac injury have no identifiable sequelae. Myocardial contusion caused by blunt trauma is frequently produced by a deceleration injury in which the chest strikes the steering wheel in a motor vehicle accident. The anterior wall of the right ventricle is most commonly involved because of its location directly behind the sternum. The presence of blunt chest injuries, such as sternal fractures, multiple rib fractures, pulmonary contusion, hemothorax, or pneumothorax, should alert the physician to the possibility of a myocardial injury. An ECG is obtained to screen for ST- and T-wave ischemic changes consistent with myocardial injury, although significant contusions have been found on autopsy in patients without ECG findings. The pathophysiologic process of myocardial contusion is bleeding into and direct injury to cardiac muscle and not occlusion of coronary vessels. The most common arrhythmia is sinus tachycardia, which, unfortunately, is a common nonspecific finding in the trauma victim. Premature atrial or ventricular contractions are the second most frequent arrhythmia observed. More malignant types of ventricular arrhythmias (i.e., multifocal premature ventricular contractions, triplets, or ventricular tachycardia) can also occur and are treated in the same manner as arrhythmias resulting from other causes. The most common conduction disturbance observed is right bundle branch block, as would be expected from the typical location of the injury in the right ventricle.

The goal for evaluation of patients with suspected myocardial contusion is to separate patients with no or clinically insignificant injuries (grade I and II) from those with increased risk of morbidity and mortality because of significant injuries (grade III and IV). Cardiac isoenzymes such as creatine kinase-MB (CK-MB) have been used to try to identify patients at risk from significant myocardial injury. In one study, patients with both high CK-MB (>5% of total CK) and ECG abnormalities (arrhythmias) had a greater chance of developing cardiac complications.[10] Another study, however, found no relation between CK-MB results and the presence of clinically significant myocardial contusion.[11] Echocardiography has also been used to evaluate patients for abnormal cardiac function, but it also has been inconsistent in identifying patients with greater risk.[12] Echocardiography and radionuclide angiography are sensitive enough to detect segmental areas of abnormal wall motion, indicating the presence of myocardial injury after blunt thoracic trauma. However, these abnormalities are thought to be reversible injuries and do not correlate with morbidity or mortality. We believe that cardiac evaluation beyond ECG and telemetry monitoring should be reserved for patients with grossly abnormal ECG findings, severe arrhythmias, or unexplained hemodynamic instability.

The consensus of the literature is that patients with suspected or diagnosed myocardial contusions can safely undergo emergency surgery for associated injuries.[13,14] Our routine is to place introducer catheters preoperatively in stable patients who are without manifestations of cardiac instability to allow quick intraoperative access for the placement of a pulmonary artery catheter. In patients with strong evidence of a significant blunt cardiac injury, such as hemodynamic instability, we insert invasive hemodynamic monitoring lines as early as possible in the hospital course.

COMPARTMENT SYNDROME ■

A compartment syndrome occurs when tissue pressure rises as a result of interstitial edema or hemorrhage into the soft tissues within a fascial space and exceeds the perfusion pressure, resulting in tissue necrosis. The classic location of the compartment syndrome is in the lower leg, where there are well-defined anterior, lateral, superficial posterior, and deep posterior fascial compartments (Fig. 68-1). A compartment syndrome may also develop in the forearm, upper arm, thigh, or buttock. Intraabdominal compartment syndrome (intraabdominal hypertension) may also occur and is discussed separately.

Compartment syndrome typically occurs in association with orthopedic injuries in which fractures cause bleeding and swelling of the muscle. Crush injuries not associated with fractures can also lead to elevated tissue pressure secondary to edema formation within fascial compartments. Reperfusion after arterial ischemia (traumatic or not) is another cause of severe swelling and compartment syndrome. The use of the MAST for prolonged periods has also been

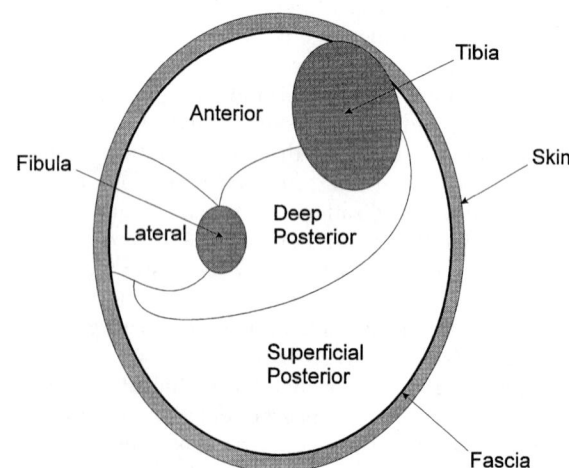

FIGURE 68-1. Schematic drawing of fascial compartments of the left leg.

reported as a cause of compartment syndrome.[15] Other risk factors for the development of compartment syndrome include ischemia for longer than 6 hours and combined arterial and venous injuries.[16]

Early diagnosis before permanent tissue damage has occurred is essential. The five "Ps" described for acute arterial ischemia also appear in association with compartment syndrome: pain, pallor, paresthesia, pulselessness, and paralysis. Pain and paresthesia are usually the earliest signs and are sufficient to suspect the diagnosis. The pain is severe with passive stretching of the muscle groups located within the affected compartment. A tensely swollen extremity found during physical examination may be the first suggestion. The development of any paresthesia should also alert the physician. The patient often describes a "pins and needles" sensation in the affected extremity. The patient can often identify a difference in sensation between the two extremities if both are touched simultaneously. The loss of distal circulation, documented by absent distal pulses, is a late sign and is often associated with some permanent tissue damage. Distal pulses may still be present even if muscle perfusion at the microvascular level has already ceased.

The diagnosis of compartment syndrome is often delayed until the patient is in the ICU because attention was directed toward more life-threatening injuries while the patient was in the emergency room or the operating room. A compartment syndrome may also develop in the ICU slowly over many hours as the patient receives fluid resuscitation.

Confirmation can be made by measurement of compartment pressures. This is especially useful if the clinical examination is unreliable, as is often the case with critically injured patients. Small, portable devices are available that can measure compartment pressures. In the ICU, a needle attached to an arterial line transducer can also accurately measure compartment pressure. The site of needle insertion should be prepared and the needle inserted into the compartment. Measurements of all compartments should be made, because only a single compartment pressure may be elevated. Normal compartment pressure is less than 10 mm Hg. The exact threshold at which tissue damage occurs is not known. If tissue pressure is elevated, it will probably continue to rise with time. It is our practice to perform fasciotomies for compartment pressures of 30 mm Hg or greater. Patients who are hypotensive can develop compartment syndromes at lower tissue pressures.

The treatment of compartment syndrome is decompressive fasciotomy of the affected extremity. A variety of techniques are available, but in general all compartments—four in the lower leg, two in the forearm—should be decompressed. Fasciotomies through small skin incisions should be avoided because further swelling may lead to redevelopment of the compartment syndrome due to the unyielding, swollen dermis.[17] Postoperatively, the wounds are usually treated with wet-to-dry dressings. Most fasciotomies are ultimately covered with a split-thickness skin graft, but occasionally they can be primarily closed if the swelling has sufficiently resolved. Newer devices allow skin approximation so that a surgical procedure is not needed. If ischemia has been significant, the patient is at risk for renal failure secondary to myoglobinuria, which develops as a result of muscle damage. The patient should be kept well hydrated to maintain a brisk urine output. The addition of a mannitol infusion and alkalinization of the urine to produce osmotic diuresis and make the pigment more soluble are additional treatment options, although no scientific studies have established their efficacy.

INTRAABDOMINAL HYPERTENSION (INTRAABDOMINAL COMPARTMENT SYNDROME)

Increased intraabdominal pressure can develop in the trauma patient and lead to multisystem organ failure. The most common cause is hemoperitoneum, which typically occurs postoperatively in patients who develop a coagulopathy during surgery. The most susceptible patients are those with major liver or intraabdominal vascular injuries who received massive transfusion. At the time of abdominal closure, there is a continued capillary ooze because of a multifactorial clotting deficiency and progressive retroperitoneal and visceral swelling. The bleeding continues postoperatively until the patient is adequately rewarmed and the coagulopathy is corrected with the appropriate blood components. By the time this is accomplished, a substantial amount of blood and edema has accumulated in the peritoneal cavity, leading to intraabdominal hypertension. This condition may also occur in patients who are in profound shock and require long operative procedures during which significant bowel and retroperitoneal edema accumulate. The end result is an extremely tight abdominal closure and high intraabdominal pressure. This process can also develop in nonoperated trauma patients who develop large retroperitoneal hematomas.

Elevated intraabdominal pressure carries significant consequences. Cardiac output may decrease dramatically because of decreased venous return and elevated systemic vascular resistance.[18] Peak airway pressure rises to extremely high levels, and there is a marked decrease in tidal volume because of decreased compliance. Patients uniformly require continuous mechanical ventilation and increasing levels of PEEP because functional residual capacity is decreased and intrapulmonary shunt is increased. Renal failure develops precipitously and is thought to be a consequence of decreased cardiac output and direct renal compression.[19]

Intraabdominal pressure can be measured by a long femoral venous catheter. Another simple method uses an indwelling Foley catheter. The tubing of the urinary drainage bag is clamped just distal to the aspiration port. Fifty to 100 mL of sterile saline is injected into the Foley catheter through the aspiration port. The tubing is unclamped just enough to allow the fluid to flow back to the point of the clamp. A 16-gauge needle is used to connect a pressure transducer through the aspiration port. The top of the symphysis pubis is used as the zero point. Intraabdominal pressure greater than 25 mm Hg has been shown to correlate with renal dysfunction. Patients with clinical manifestations of the syndrome and intraabdominal pressures greater than 40 mm Hg should have surgical decompression of the abdomen.[20]

Patients with pressures between 25 and 40 mm Hg should also be considered for surgical decompression if there is clinical evidence of organ dysfunction.

Adequate resuscitation, rewarming, and replacement of coagulation factors are the primary forms of therapy in these patients. After these goals are accomplished, surgical decompression can result in dramatic improvement in cardiac, pulmonary, and renal function while the patient is still on the operating table. Primary closure of the abdomen may not be possible, and a bioprosthetic patch may be necessary. In patients with nonoperative causes of intraabdominal hypertension, invasive monitoring in conjunction with inotropic support is needed to sustain adequate cardiac function. Opening of the abdomen may still be necessary.

DELAYED DIAGNOSES ■

Delayed diagnosis of injuries contributes significantly to the morbidity and mortality of trauma patients. One study revealed a 9% incidence of injuries missed by the initial primary and secondary surveys.[21] Although half of these were extremity injuries, significant spinal fractures, abdominal injuries, and vascular injuries were also missed. The most common reason for overlooking an injury was an altered mental status of the patient secondary to head injury or ingestion of alcohol or drugs. The conclusion of the study was that a tertiary survey should be conducted to search for missed injuries after the patient has been stabilized. Usually, the most suitable location for this tertiary survey in the severely injured patient is the ICU. Spinal cord injury is also frequently associated with missed injuries because of the inability to obtain an optimum physical examination. The most common presentation of missed injury is evidence of hemorrhage.

BONY INJURIES

Routine radiologic survey of the spine, pelvis, and lower extremities has been advocated in obtunded patients with blunt trauma because of their unreliable physical examination.[22] In a group of patients with Glasgow Coma Scale scores of less than 10, there was a 14% incidence of spine injuries, a 10% incidence of pelvic fractures, and a 15% incidence of lower extremity fractures. Musculoskeletal injuries are the most common missed injuries. In patients with hemodynamic instability or head injury, attention is directed away from subtle signs of extremity fractures such as ecchymosis, abrasions, or lacerations in the absence of gross deformity. After patients have been stabilized in the ICU, a tertiary survey searching for these signs should lead to further radiologic evaluation.

Lack of an appropriate level of suspicion, inadequate testing, and misinterpretation of radiographs have been cited as reasons for missing cervical injuries.[23] This is significant because the incidence of secondary deficits is higher in patients with missed spinal injuries. The minimum set of radiographs necessary for adequate evaluation of the cervical spine includes lateral, anteroposterior (AP), and odontoid views.[24] The most common problem encountered is the inability to clear all seven cervical vertebrae, especially the seventh. Instead of spending an extended period repeating films or obtaining additional views, we obtain CT scans with sagittal reconstructions of the specific vertebrae.[25,26]

In stable patients, thoracic and lumbar spine films should be obtained in the trauma room to exclude injuries to these areas. If the presence of other injuries precludes obtaining these films initially, evaluation should be completed in the ICU.

RETROPERITONEAL INJURIES

Retroperitoneal injuries that occur in patients with blunt trauma may be discovered only later. Retroperitoneal hematomas, duodenal injuries, and pancreatic injuries are often discovered at operations performed because of other associated injuries without being suspected preoperatively. Most traumatic retroperitoneal hematomas can be difficult to detect or even missed by DPL if there is no associated intraabdominal injury.[27] CT scan of the abdomen, however, is very sensitive in detecting them. The presence of flank ecchymosis should raise the question of retroperitoneal bleeding, although it may not become visible for 24 to 48 hours after injury. Retroperitoneal hematomas are divided into three types based on location: central, flank, and pelvic.[28] Central hematomas require surgical exploration because of the risk of an associated injury to the pancreas, duodenum, or vascular structures.[27] Injury to a major vessel usually results in rapid deterioration leading to early operative intervention. Flank hematomas are treated nonoperatively unless there is evidence that the hematoma is expanding, or there is a nonfunctioning kidney by CT scan or intravenous pyelography (IVP), or there is extravasation of contrast medium. Pelvic hematomas are also treated nonoperatively.

Patients with pancreatic and duodenal missed injuries may initially have a completely benign abdominal examination and only slowly develop pain and tenderness over the next several days. However, a delay in diagnosis of only 24 hours with a duodenal injury has been reported to carry a mortality rate as high as 40%.[29] DPL may miss isolated injuries of these organs because of their retroperitoneal location.[30,31] Early abdominal CT scanning is no better and can also miss injuries as extensive as a transected pancreas or perforated duodenum. Patients with a history of upper abdominal trauma, even mild epigastric tenderness, and slightly elevated amylase values should be viewed with a high index of suspicion for such injuries. Repetitive physical examinations and serum amylase measurements are most helpful. A repeat CT scan may be useful to detect a developing retroperitoneal inflammatory process. Blunt trauma to the duodenum may result in a hematoma of the wall, which is usually associated with jaundice and signs of a high intestinal obstruction. Although abdominal CT scan can detect the presence of a duodenal hematoma, the classic finding is that of a "coiled spring" appearance on a barium upper gastrointestinal series. Most hematomas resolve within 2 weeks, and operative drainage of the hematoma to relieve obstruction is required only rarely.

INTRAABDOMINAL INJURIES

Blunt intestinal injuries, although uncommon, are easily detected by DPL but may be missed if the patient was evaluated only by abdominal CT. One study collected 10 patients with intestinal injuries who were initially assessed by abdominal CT scan interpreted as negative and subsequently underwent laparotomy because of a missed bowel injury.[32] In addition to perforation, mesenteric tears can occur that lead to intestinal infarction and may not be discovered until several days later, after peritonitis develops. It has been suggested that free fluid in the abdomen on CT scan without evidence of injury to a solid organ should be considered an indication for surgery. The free fluid is presumed to be from a hollow viscus injury until proven otherwise. An alternative approach would be to perform a DPL in any patient with a questionable CT scan and base the decision to operate on the lavage results. It has also been reported that CT scan more often misses intraabdominal injuries than does DPL in obtunded patients.[33]

Most surgeons still routinely perform laparotomy for gunshot wounds to the abdomen, because more often than not there is an injury requiring surgical intervention. Many centers use DPL to evaluate penetrating abdominal stab wounds, although clear criteria for what constitutes a positive lavage result have not been established. Incomplete exploration at laparotomy, especially of a retroperitoneal hematoma, has also been cited as a cause of undetected injuries.[34]

DIAPHRAGMATIC INJURIES

As many as 33% of diaphragmatic injuries from blunt and penetrating trauma are diagnosed late.[35,36] Patients with blunt chest and abdominal trauma often present with multiple abnormalities on chest radiography (e.g., rib fractures, hemothorax, pulmonary contusion, elevated hemidiaphragm) that make it difficult to evaluate the diaphragm.[37] The diaphragm may even appear normal on radiography after it has been ruptured. Abnormal gas patterns and visualization of the nasogastric tube above the diaphragm are signs of left-sided rupture, which is more common than right-sided disruption. Diagnosis of right-sided rupture is more difficult because even if the liver has herniated through the defect, the diaphragm may appear only slightly elevated (Fig. 68-2). Isolated diaphragmatic injuries are the most common injury associated with falsely negative peritoneal lavage, with a missed injury rate of 25% to 33%.[36] CT scanning is helpful only if intraabdominal contents have herniated into the chest.[38] Upper gastrointestinal series and barium enemas are adjunctive radiologic studies of limited value because they, too, are positive only if a visualized viscus has herniated into the chest.[39] Patients who deteriorate suddenly with application of MAST should be suspected of having an undiagnosed diaphragmatic injury. The sudden increase in intraabdominal pressure forces abdominal contents into the chest, compromising cardiac and pulmonary function. Serial chest radiographs are routinely obtained in critically ill patients, and close scrutiny of the diaphragmatic appearance may be the only way to detect the evolution of subtle findings that lead to the diagnosis.

MEDIASTINAL INJURIES

The major difficulty in evaluating patients with a "widened mediastinum" is to decide whether it is real or caused by technical factors.[40] In most situations, a supine AP film is obtained to assess the severely injured patient. The magnification that results may be difficult to differentiate from widening caused by a mediastinal hematoma. If an upright AP chest radiograph can be obtained, the question may easily be answered. Aortography is the primary procedure for the evaluation of possible aortic injuries.[41] Although the most sensitive indicator of an aortic injury is a widened mediastinum, it is not specific because only about 10% of patients with this sign have a positive angiogram. Other causes of widened mediastinum can be contemplated after a negative aortogram has been obtained. These include rupture of mediastinal veins, rib fractures, sternal fractures, vertebral fractures, and aberrant central line placement.

Most patients with an aortic disruption exsanguinate at the time of injury, and only 10% to 20% survive long enough to be transported to the hospital.[42] Of these, 40% die within the first 24 hours if their aortic tear is not repaired. Blunt aortic injury is usually caused by a rapid deceleration injury from a motor vehicle accident or fall from a height. Patients who survive the initial injury do so because there is only a partial tear of the aortic wall, with the adventitia and pleura containing the hematoma. Most of the injuries occur distal to the left subclavian artery at the site of the ligamentum arteriosum. Other radiographic findings associated with aortic injury are listed in Table 68-2. In patients in whom there is a questionable mediastinal shadow and who require head and abdominal CT scanning to evaluate other injuries, a dynamic chest CT scan can be obtained to establish the presence or absence of a mediastinal hematoma. Patients who have an obviously widened mediastinum should proceed directly to aortography. If the presence of a mediastinal hematoma is established, only an aortogram can truly exclude an aortic injury. Transesophageal echography is an alternative screening method to detect injuries and can be used if it can be obtained in a timely fashion.

The stability of the patient determines priorities in management.[43,44] Patients who are unstable because of an intraabdominal injury need laparotomy before aortography. If an aortogram reveals an injury, a necessary abdominal exploration is usually carried out first. Hypertension should be controlled before operative repair by the use of vasodilators and B-blockers such as nitroprusside and esmolol or propanolol. Trimetaphan is an alternative in patients with associated head injuries.

VASCULAR INJURIES

The diagnosis of vascular injuries is difficult in the trauma patient because palpation of peripheral pulses is often unreliable in the presence of associated injuries and shock. The risk of a missed arterial injury is unclear because most studies have had inadequate followup. However, Perry reported on missed arterial injuries in a group of patients who presented with stroke, transient ischemic attack, leg ischemia, and gangrene.[45] The presence of fractures or dislocations or the

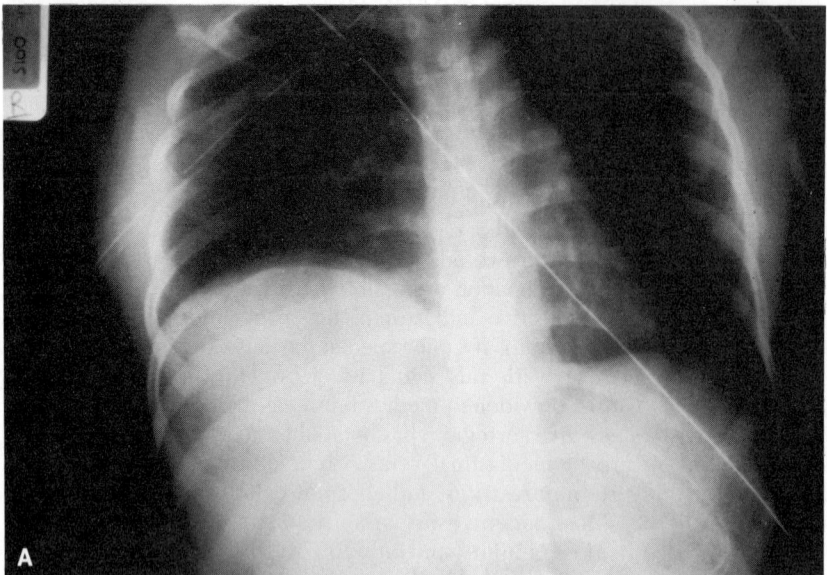

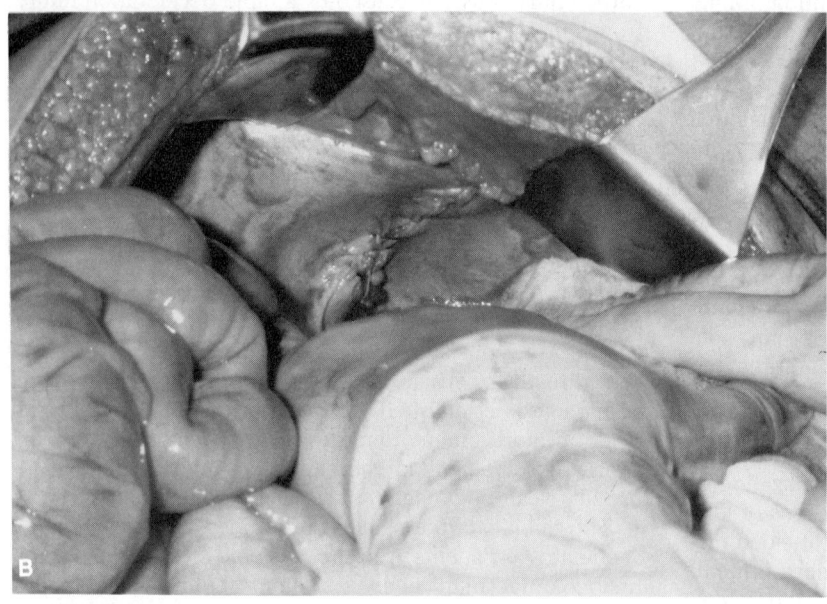

FIGURE 68-2. Diaphragmatic injury. (**A**) Preoperative chest radiograph showing elevated right hemidiaphragm. (**B**) Intraoperative photograph of diaphragm after being repaired. The tear extended from the esophageal hiatus to the lateral chest wall.

proximity of a penetrating wound to the course of a major vessel should raise suspicion of a vascular injury. The five "Ps" associated with acute arterial insufficiency are pain, pallor, pulselessness, paresthesia, and paralysis, all of which can mistakenly be attributed to other causes. Copious bleeding, an expanding or pulsatile hematoma, and absent distal pulses are obvious indications of a vascular injury. Patients with knee dislocations and below-the-knee vascular injuries from blunt trauma are at the highest risk for amputation.[46] Reconstruction delayed more than 6 hours after injury, extensive musculoskeletal injury, crush injuries, and combined

arterial and venous injuries increase the rate of limb loss.[47,48] Complicating factors include extensive soft tissue injury, because of associated infection, and nerve injury, which strongly influences functional recovery. Arteriography is the best method to diagnose vascular injury, but selection of patients for angiography requires a high index of suspicion. The presence of pulses, especially if ascertained only by Doppler examination, does not rule out the possibility of an arterial injury.[48]

Vascular injuries and fractures of the lower extremity are associated with tissue edema and elevated compartment

TABLE 68-2.   Findings Associated With Aortic Injury

Widened mediastinum
Deviation of nasogastric tube
Obscured aortic knob
Apical capping
Deviation of trachea
Depression of left mainstem bronchus
First or second rib fractures
Displaced paraspinal stripe
Thoracic spine fracture
Layering of calcium in the aortic knob

pressure caused by direct trauma and reperfusion of ischemic muscle. Any patient with these injuries is at high risk for development of a compartment syndrome. Prolonged shock and combined arteriovenous injuries put the patient at especially high risk (see earlier discussion).

MASSIVE TRANSFUSION

Uncontrolled hemorrhage associated with devastating traumatic injuries often leads to massive transfusion, which is defined as replacement of more than one blood volume (10 units packed cells). Whole blood is rarely available, and the deficits are treated with blood component therapy (i.e., packed red blood cells, fresh frozen plasma, platelets, and cryoprecipitate). The result may be a variety of hemostatic and metabolic defects. The most immediate goals are to restore circulating blood volume, to assure adequate tissue perfusion and oxygen delivery, and then to correct the other deficits that have occurred. Packed red blood cells and crystalloids are most frequently chosen as initial resuscitation components. Type O blood is administered until crossmatched or type-specific blood becomes available.

The most frequent abnormality observed with massive transfusion is thrombocytopenia, which is caused mostly by dilution but in part by consumption.[49] In actively bleeding trauma patients, the platelet count should be maintained at greater than 100,000 per cubic millimeter (Table 68-3). Lower counts are most often seen after more than 10 units of packed cells have been transfused. Hypothermia-related platelet dysfunction leads to a coagulopathy despite adequate platelet numbers and can be corrected only by rewarming the patient.[50]

Significant decreases in soluble coagulation factors can also be observed secondary to consumption and dilution.[49] Fibrinogen, factor V, and factor VIII are particularly susceptible to depletion in the massively transfused individual because they are the factors most commonly affected by storage. Serial laboratory testing to evaluate the adequacy of coagulation factors and fibrinogen should be performed after transfusion of 10 units of red blood cells.[51] All of the coagulation factors are present in fresh frozen plasma. Highly concentrated amounts of factor VIII and fibrinogen can be administered by using cryoprecipitate. Fibrinogen levels should be maintained higher than 100 mg/dL in bleeding patients (see Table 68-3).

Hyperkalemia is a potential metabolic derangement after massive transfusion because potassium slowly leaks out of red blood cells during liquid storage. This complication is infrequently observed but can be avoided by monitoring of serum potassium levels. Although the plasma in a unit of packed cells has a high potassium concentration, it is usually such a small volume that the potassium is rapidly diluted in the patient's circulation. There is also rapid reuptake of potassium by the red blood cells after transfusion.

Hypothermia is often observed in the severely injured patient who requires massive fluid resuscitation. If room temperature fluids and blood stored at 4°C are administered in large volumes to patients in hypovolemic shock, the body temperature can rapidly reach 32°C or lower.[52] Hypothermia is exacerbated by heat losses from radiation, convection, conduction, and evaporation that occur during surgery when body cavities are open and exposed in a cold operating room for hours. The potential for ventricular arrhythmias increases as the temperature falls. The combination of hypothermia and acidosis lowers the threshold for ventricular fibrillation (which may occur spontaneously and be refractory to treatment at temperatures below 30°C). Hypothermia also shifts the oxyhemoglobin dissociation curve to the left, leading to a decrease in the amount of oxygen available to the tissues.

Monitoring of core temperature is essential and is accurately obtained with pulmonary artery catheter thermistors or Foley catheter thermistors. Other available but less accurate devices include esophageal or rectal probes. Prevention of hypothermia is vital because it is so difficult to reverse. Hypothermia-induced platelet dysfunction may lead to exsanguination in the trauma victim because of diffuse oozing from traumatic and surgical injury sites. The ambient temperature in the operating room must be adjusted to meet the needs of the patient and not the comfort of the caregivers. All fluids and blood products should be warmed before administration. IV fluids can be prewarmed by storing them in a blanket warmer or by microwaving, although the latter technique requires learning appropriate settings and careful monitoring of the final temperature of the fluid infused. Rapid infusion devices act by countercurrent heat exchange to warm fluid, blood, and blood products. Delivery is limited only by the size of the IV catheters used and the personnel available to change bags. Older blood warmers consist of coiled IV tubing immersed in a warm water bath; their major disadvantage is the limited maximal transfusion rate. The addition of warm normal saline to packed red blood cells has been advocated as a safe method of warming blood; this

TABLE 68-3.   Guidelines for Use of Blood Components in Coagulopathy

LABORATORY VALUE	THERAPY
Platelet count <100,000/mm³	Platelets
Prothrombin time >16 sec	Fresh frozen plasma
Partial thromboplastin time >50 sec	Fresh frozen plasma
Fibrinogen <100 mg/dL	Cryoprecipitate

method also increases the rate of administration, because the addition of crystalloid fluid decreases the viscosity of the blood.[53] Warming blankets can be placed underneath and on top of the patient, but surface warming is inefficient because of intense vasoconstriction. Heated, humidified gases at temperatures of 40° to 42°C should be used in intubated patients to assist in warming and to limit heat loss by this route. Gastric and peritoneal lavage can be performed in selected patients, but they are thermodynamically inefficient and are frequently impractical in the postoperative trauma patient because of recent abdominal surgery. The head should be covered, because its high blood flow causes further heat loss. Other, more thermodynamically efficient techniques, such as cardiopulmonary bypass or arteriovenous bypass with a pump, are contraindicated because of the need for systemic heparinization. Continuous arteriovenous rewarming with the use of a modified countercurrent heating mechanism has been reported to be a more efficient method of rewarming.[54]

Citrate is used as an anticoagulant in banked blood and works by binding calcium. There is twice as much citrate present in a unit of blood as is necessary to chelate all of the calcium present. Under normal circumstances, the extra citrate is metabolized by the liver to bicarbonate. However, in patients who have received massive blood transfusions and who become hypothermic, the citrate continues to circulate and binds additional calcium. Decreases in ionized calcium can occur that are significant enough to affect myocardial function and vascular tone. ECG changes consisting of prolonged QT intervals can also be observed. Ionized calcium should be measured in patients who receive more than 8 to 10 units of blood. If persistent hypotension is present, the patient may be treated empirically with calcium chloride while undergoing ECG monitoring for arrhythmias. Additional calcium may be administered as necessary to maintain hemodynamic stability; ionized calcium should be remeasured as well. Coagulation is not affected, because the amount of calcium necessary for clotting is extremely small and tetany occurs before serum ionized calcium is depressed to those levels.

A shift in the oxyhemoglobin dissociation curve as a result of hypothermia and reduced 2,3-diphosphoglyceride (2,3-DPG) levels increases the affinity of hemoglobin for oxygen. The 2,3-DPG levels in banked blood decline during storage, but in stable individuals these levels should be restored to normal after 24 hours. However, in the patient in whom the entire blood volume has been replaced with banked blood, oxygen delivery to the tissues may be impaired by the extremely low 2,3-DPG levels. Because these patients are hypothermic and in shock, they may not be able to restore 2,3-DPG levels until well after the resuscitation period is over. We recommend transfusing these patients to a higher hemoglobin level (10 to 11 g/dL) in order to compensate for the compromised oxygen delivery.

Depending on the age of the stored blood, up to 30% of the red blood cells do not survive the transfusion and are removed from the circulation over a period of 24 hours. In a patient whose entire circulating blood volume has been replaced with banked blood, there is a significant fall in hematocrit even if no further blood loss occurs. This makes assessment of ongoing bleeding difficult to evaluate.

A clinical picture consistent with disseminated intravascular coagulation can often be observed in patients with traumatic brain injury even if they have not been massively transfused.[55] This is thought to be caused by the release of thromboplastin from injured brain tissue. It should be treated with component therapy as suggested earlier.

PELVIC FRACTURES

The overall incidence of pelvic fractures is 37 per 100,000 person-years, with a gradual increase with age and a maximum incidence in elderly women as a result of osteoporosis.[56,57] Pelvic fractures constitute 3% of all fractures, account for 1 in every 1000 hospital admissions, and are the third most frequent injury found in victims of motor vehicle accidents. Approximately 80% represent minor injuries regardless of the severity of trauma. Mortality rates range from 5% (all fractures) to 20% (complex injuries only). Morbidity rates have ranged from 33% to 74%, although many deaths are caused by other system injuries (central nervous system, thorax, abdomen).[58] Mucha and Farrell concluded in 1984 that pelvic fractures were the primary cause of death in 12%, contributory in 53%, and unrelated in 35% of patients in their series.[59]

Pelvic fractures vary in severity from minor injuries that do not require in-hospital treatment to major injuries requiring multidisciplinary efforts to avoid an early death from exsanguination or a late death from multiple system organ failure and sepsis after prolonged traumatic shock. Open pelvic fractures carry an even higher mortality rate (50%) and require operative intervention to prevent the development of sepsis and multiple system organ failure.[60] Pelvic fractures may be classified as open because of a laceration over a bony prominence or, of greater import, because of an extensive perineal laceration or rectal or vaginal involvement.[61] Both the early and the late care of patients with severe pelvic fractures occur in the ICU, and the intensivist must be knowledgeable in the workup and treatment of these serious injuries.

ANATOMY

The pelvis is formed by the sacrum and the innominate bones. The innominate bones are connected posteriorly by strong ligaments (sacroiliac) to the sacrum and anteriorly by a weak joint (pubic symphysis) to each other. The pelvic wall consists of peritoneum, internal iliac vessels, the parietal layer of the pelvic fascia, the sacral plexus and branches, muscles, and bony wall. The pelvic outlet is occluded by the pelvic diaphragm, with a hiatus for the outlet tract of the urinary, genital, and gastrointestinal systems. The visceral contents of the lesser pelvis include the bladder, the urethra, the internal genitalia, and the sigmoid, rectum, and small bowel loops. If a pelvic fracture is being evaluated, damage to other components of the pelvic wall, pelvic diaphragm, and visceral contents must be considered.

DIAGNOSIS OF PELVIC FRACTURE AND ASSOCIATED INJURIES

Numerous classifications of pelvic fractures have been described based on anatomic patterns of pelvic ring disruption or degree of stability.[56,62] Other classification systems are based on the presumed direction of forces applied that resulted in the fracture pattern observed (e.g., AP, lateral, vertical shear, combined).[63,64] A more practical system for the intensivist divides fractures into those that are hemodynamically stable and those that are unstable. The latter group is further divided into those patients who can be maintained in a moderately hypotensive state (systolic blood pressure 60 to 90 mm Hg) and those who are exsanguinating (systolic blood pressure <60 mm Hg). The possibility of a structurally and hemodynamically significant pelvic fracture must be suspected in all victims of major falls, victims of high-speed motor vehicle accidents, ejected occupants of vehicles, victims of motorcycle accidents, and pedestrians struck by motor vehicles. Clinical signs on inspection include ecchymosis and contusions, localized swellings, rotational deformities, limb shortening, perineal wounds, blood at the urethral meatus, labial or scrotal hematoma, and hematuria. Pain or instability on anteroposterior compression (pubis and sacrum) or lateral compression (iliac wings), vaginal lacerations or bleeding on pelvic examination, anorectal lacerations, or high-riding prostate or rectal bleeding on rectal examination are important clinical signs.

An AP pelvic radiograph is the minimal essential workup to establish the presence and nature of a pelvic fracture. More precise radiologic information can be obtained by inlet and outlet Judet views and a CT scan with cuts at 5-mm intervals. The CT scan should be performed after the patient is hemodynamically stable, along with scans of the brain and abdomen in polytraumatized patients. An unstable pelvic ring fracture should alert the clinician to the need for close monitoring and aggressive resuscitation as well as multidisciplinary care from the trauma surgeon, orthopedic surgeon, intensivist, and interventional radiologist.

Pelvic fractures are often associated with significant blood loss and hemodynamic instability as well as equivocal abdominal examinations. It is essential to rule out significant intraabdominal injury as quickly as possible. Abdominal CT with oral and IV contrast media may be used in hemodynamically stable patients. Supraumbilical open DPL (to avoid the pelvic hematoma that is usually confined by the umbilicus) is another valuable technique. There is agreement that a grossly positive tap is an absolute indication for exploratory celiotomy.[65] However, if the lavage is positive by the red blood cell count only, the possibility of a false-positive result caused by diapedesis or a leaking pelvic hematoma leads some clinicians to explore the patient only if a solid viscus injury or large hemoperitoneum is demonstrated on abdominal CT scan. In the hemodynamically unstable patient, we believe that DPL should be performed as soon as possible in the trauma room and that any positive lavage is best

followed by diagnostic celiotomy and then by pelvic stabilization if necessary. It appears particularly risky to send an unstable patient to the CT scanner, further delaying therapeutic celiotomy and orthopedic stabilization. A negative DPL implicates the pelvic fracture as the cause of blood loss.

The diagnosis of pelvic visceral injuries may require other investigations, such as vaginal examination with speculum, proctosigmoidoscopy, retrograde urethrography, and cystography. The presence of blood at the meatus, a scrotal hematoma, or a high-riding prostate suggestive of urethral transection mandates a retrograde urethrogram before the Foley catheter is inserted.[66] In the presence of microscopic or macroscopic hematuria and a pelvic fracture, an IVP or abdominal CT scan and cystogram are indicated to evaluate the urinary tract. Often, the IVP and cystogram must be delayed until after stabilization in the ICU. Although an abdominal CT scan is excellent for evaluation of the upper urinary tract, it may fail to demonstrate bladder rupture. The intensivist must order the radiologic assessment, including a single-film IVP and at least three exposures of a cystogram, including a 100-mL bladder filling, a 400-mL filling, and a postevacuation film (Fig. 68-3).

ASSOCIATED INJURIES

Urethral and bladder injuries are common with fractures of the anterior pelvic ring. Intraperitoneal rupture of the bladder requires surgical repair and suprapubic cystostomy, whereas extraperitoneal rupture is often treated by drainage alone. Urethral transection is managed best by suprapubic cystostomy and delayed repair.

If an anorectal injury is found or an open pelvic fracture secondary to perineal or buttock wound is diagnosed, the patient must have a totally diverting colostomy (either an end colostomy with mucous fistula or a loop colostomy with a stapled distal limb).[67] Irrigation of the distal segment has been recommended to decrease bacterial contamination and septic complications. Vaginal lacerations must be repaired after thorough irrigation and debridement. Injury to the lumbosacral plexus may occur with posterior pelvic ring injury and makes a detailed neurologic examination of the lower extremities essential.[68]

Patients with pelvic fractures are at high risk for thromboembolic complications.[69,70] Thrombus not infrequently occurs in the iliac veins and may not be detectable by noninvasive methods of screening. It has been suggested that subcutaneous heparin and sequential compression devices may be inadequate prophylaxis for patients with severe pelvic trauma.[71] We use warfarin (Coumadin) for prophylaxis against deep venous thrombosis and pulmonary embolism. Prophylactic inferior vena cava filters should be placed in any patient who is not a candidate for anticoagulation.

INITIAL MANAGEMENT

The principal objectives are to avoid hemorrhagic shock and to achieve early control of hemorrhage, reducing the late incidence of sepsis and multiple system organ failure. Early reduction and fixation of many types of pelvic fractures ac-

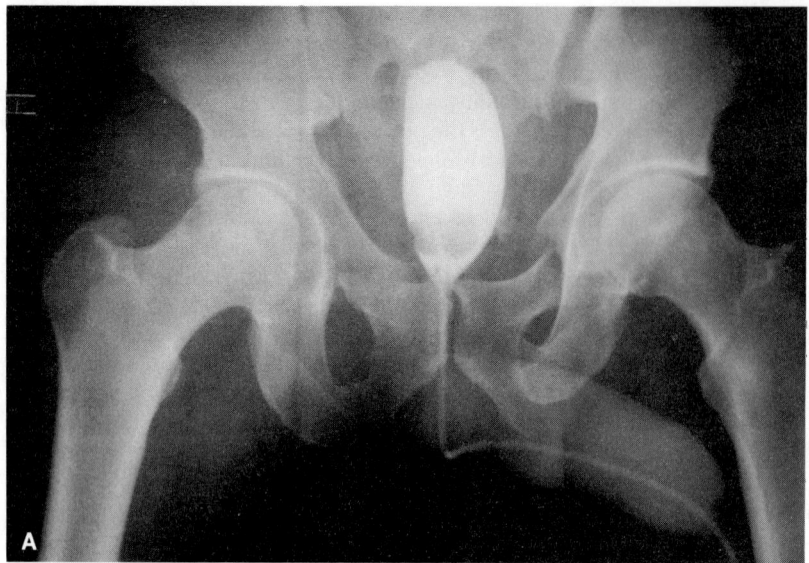

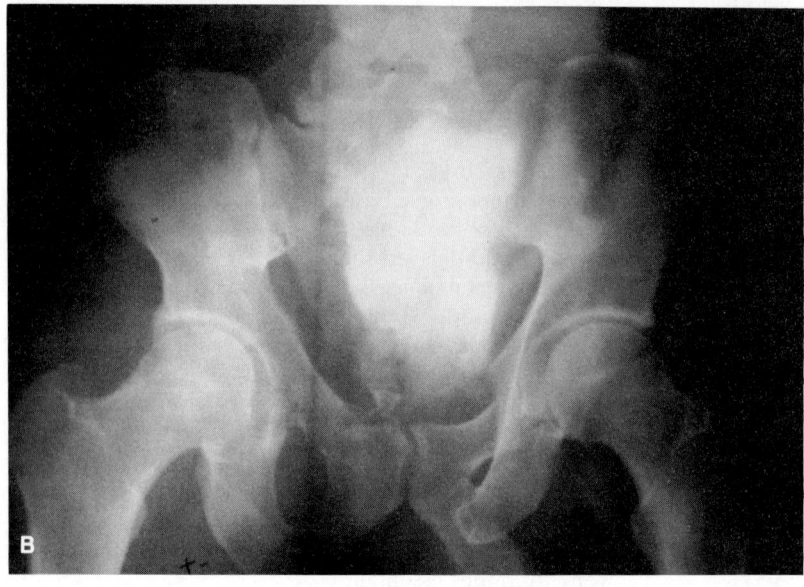

FIGURE 68-3. Pelvic fracture. (**A**) Filling cystogram revealing extensive pelvic hematoma compressing bladder. (**B**) Postevacuation film with extensive extravasation not apparent on the previous film.

complish these goals and also facilitate rehabilitation. The potential sources of hemorrhage in pelvic fractures include fracture sites, pelvic venous plexuses, deep pelvic arterial bleeders, and major arterial injuries. The bleeding may be confined to the soft areolar tissue space of the retroperitoneum, a large potential space with low tissue pressure that accommodates several liters of blood before any tamponade occurs. In the worst-case scenario, bleeding may decompress outside the body through a perineal, vaginal, or rectal laceration or into the peritoneal cavity, producing a large hemoperitoneum.

In general, different therapeutic interventions address different sources. External fixation and the MAST are aimed at fracture site and pelvic venous plexus hemorrhage, whereas angiographic embolization is directed at controlling the deep pelvic arterial bleeders. Major vessel injuries can

be controlled only by direct operative intervention. Pelvic hematomas that decompress into the peritoneal cavity or to the outside through perineal wounds present with exsanguinating hemorrhage and require celiotomy, pelvic packing, perineal wound packing, and application of the MAST.

Protracted hemorrhage must be anticipated, and appropriate preparations must be made for adequate ICU care: several large-bore supradiaphragmatic venous access lines (8-French introducers are best), an ample supply of blood and blood products, a large volume of prewarmed IV fluids, and devices for rapid blood and fluid warming must be made available. Insertion of hemodynamic monitoring equipment must follow and not precede these preparations and the application of the MAST.

Hemodynamically unstable patients may receive as many as 16 to 18 units of packed red blood cells. The hemodynamic status is the most important predictor of outcome—although the mortality rate of stable patients is reported to be 3.4%, the mortality rate of unstable patients reaches 42%.[72,73] Flint,[72] Moreno,[73] and Mucha and Farrell[59] divide the unstable patients into those who can be maintained with aggressive multidisciplinary management and those who are exsanguinating (blood pressure less than 60 mm Hg and minimal or no response to resuscitation), who must be transported to the operating room and explored as a last-resort measure. At celiotomy, the pelvic hematoma is addressed as follows: (1) if a rapidly expanding or pulsatile pelvic hematoma is present or groin pulses are absent, an arterial iliofemoral injury must be considered (incidence <10%) and ruled out by direct exploration; or (2) if the hematoma has decompressed into the peritoneal cavity or to the outside, abdominal or perineal packing is indicated, followed by application of the MAST. Angiography and embolization are necessary if these measures are unsuccessful. If the patient survives, further resuscitation in the ICU is necessary, including correction of shock, acidosis, coagulopathy, and hypothermia, before the packing can be removed in the operating room (usually 48 to 72 hours later).

SKELETAL FIXATION

Patients who have continued bleeding from pelvic fractures should be considered for immediate external fixation of the pelvis.[74] The main goal of applying the external fixator is to control hemorrhage, but it may also provide functional stabilization of the injury. This is accomplished by restoring the pelvic circumference to normal by decreasing anterior widening. The procedure can usually be performed quickly, and if there is no indication for laparotomy, we have, on occasion, had external fixators applied in the ICU. More definitive pelvic stabilization usually involves open reduction and internal fixation of both anterior and posterior elements. This is usually not performed until later in the patient's course, after stability has been achieved, because of the extensive hemorrhage that can be encountered if the initial pelvic hematoma is entered.

ANGIOGRAPHIC EMBOLIZATION

Great success has been achieved in management of selected patients by angiographic localization of bleeding and embolization.[75] Posterior component fractures that do not stabilize after external pelvic fixation or application of the MAST may have lacerated deep pelvic arteries that must be localized angiographically.[76] Embolization or proximal control with detachable balloons stops the arterial bleeding, whereas tamponade controls the venous bleeding. According to Mucha and Welch,[77] the indications for angiography and embolization include (1) more than 6 units of blood transfused in 24 hours; (2) expanding pelvic hematoma visualized at surgery; (3) open pelvic fracture; and (4) major pelvic fracture in a patient undergoing angiography for another reason, such as thoracic aorta or peripheral arterial injury. An arterial bleeding source can be identified in 30% of patients, and, in these patients, an 85% to 90% success rate in controlling hemorrhage can be achieved.

MILITARY ANTISHOCK TROUSERS

Although the role of the MAST in prehospital trauma is controversial, most authors agree that the device is useful in the management of pelvic fractures to achieve temporary stabilization and aid in hemostasis.[62,78] A quick but complete physical examination of the lower abdomen, pelvis, genitalia, and lower extremities must be completed before the garment is applied. It should be applied before moving the patient and makes an ideal splint. The inflation pressure should begin at 40 mm Hg.[79] Prolonged inflation pressure above the diastolic pressure must be avoided to minimize complications.[80] Continuous monitoring must be maintained by an in-line pressure gauge connected to all three compartments, and the inside of the garment must be padded to minimize skin blistering, the most common complication. Angiography and external fixation may be attempted before the MAST is used as the primary mode of treatment. If used as definitive treatment, the MAST can be left inflated for 24 to 48 hours. Compartment syndromes may occur, especially in the presence of lower extremity fractures. The MAST may be used in closed pelvic fractures and after laparotomy for hemostasis and immobilization. Most patients require mechanical ventilation and PEEP because chest compliance and functional residual capacity are reduced and the discomfort produced by the device requires heavy sedation. Deflation of the MAST is accomplished stepwise (10 mm Hg every 6 hours) while hemodynamic stability and changes in hematocrit are carefully assessed. A severely crushed fracture may expand as bleeding continues, even if MAST counterpressure is applied. Angiography or external fixation should be considered.

REFERENCES ■

1. Trunkey DD: A public health problem. In: Moore EE (ed). *Early Care of the Injured Patient.* Ontario, BC Decker, 1990
2. McSwain NE, Butman AM, Coylein B, et al (eds): *Prehospital Trauma Life Support.* St Louis, Mosby Year Book, 1994
3. Committee on Trauma, American College of Surgeons: *Advanced Trauma Life Support Student Manual.* Chicago, American College of Surgeons, 1994
4. Indeck M, Peterson S, Smith J, et al: Risk, cost, and benefit of transporting ICU patients for special studies. *J Trauma* 1988;28:1020
5. Milikan JS, Cain TL, Hansbrough J: Rapid volume replacement for hypovolemic shock: a comparison of techniques and equipment. *J Trauma* 1984;24:428
6. Shires GT, Coln D, Carrico CJ, et al: Fluid therapy in hemorrhagic shock. *Arch Surg* 1964;88:688
7. Chesnut RM, Marshall LF, Klauber MR, et al: The role of secondary brain injury in determining outcome from severe head injury. *J Trauma* 1993;34:216
8. Gunnar W, Jonasson O, Merlotti G, et al: Head injury and hemorrhagic shock: studies of the blood brain barrier and ICP after resuscitation with normal saline, 3% saline solution and dextran 40. *Surgery* 1988;103:398
9. Orebaugh SL: Venous air embolism: clinical and experimental considerations. *Crit Care Med* 1992;20:1169
10. Healy MA, Brown K, Fleiszer D: Blunt cardiac injury: is this diagnosis necessary? *J Trauma* 1990;30:137

11. Biffl WL, Moore FA, Moore EE, et al: Cardiac enzymes are irrelevant in the patient with suspected myocardial contusion. *Am J Surg* 1994;169:523

12. Gunnar WP, Martin M, Smith RF, et al: The utility of cardiac evaluation in the hemodynamically stable patient with suspected myocardial contusion. *Am Surg* 1991;57:373

13. Flancbaum L, Wright J, Siegel JH: Emergency surgery in patients with post-traumatic myocardial contusion. *J Trauma* 1986;26:795

14. Fabian TC, Mangiante EC, Patterson CR, et al: Myocardial contusion in blunt trauma: clinical characteristics, means of diagnosis, and implications for patient management. *J Trauma* 1988;28:50

15. Aprahamian C, Gessert G, Bandyk DF, et al: MAST-associated compartment syndrome: a review. *J Trauma* 1989;29:549

16. Field CK, Senkowsky J, Hollier LH, et al: Fasciotomy in vascular trauma: is it too much, too often? *Am Surg* 1994;60:409

17. Cohen MS, Garfin SR, Hargens AR, et al: Acute compartment syndrome: effect of dermotomy on fascial decompression in the leg. *J Bone Joint Surg Br* 1991;73:287

18. Cullen DJ, Coyle JP, Teplick R, et al: Cardiovascular, pulmonary, and renal effects of massively increased intra-abdominal pressure in critically ill patients. *Crit Care Med* 1989;17:118

19. Harman PK, Kron IL, McLachlan HD, et al: Elevated intraabdominal pressure and renal function. *Ann Surg* 1982;196:594

20. Kron IL, Harman PK, Nolan SP: The measurement of intraabdominal pressure as a criterion for abdominal re-exploration. *Ann Surg* 1984;199:28

21. Enderson BL, Reath DB, Meadors J, et al: The tertiary trauma survey: a prospective study of missed injury. *J Trauma* 1990; 30:666

22. Mackersie RC, Shackford SR, Garfin SR, et al: Major skeletal injuries in the obtunded blunt trauma patient: a case for routine radiologic survey. *J Trauma* 1988;28:1450

23. Reid DC, Henderson R, Saboe L, et al: Etiology and clinical course of missed spine fractures. *J Trauma* 1987;27:980

24. MacDonald RL, Schwartz ML, Mirich D, et al: Diagnosis of cervical spine injury in motor vehicle crash victims: how many x-rays are enough? *J Trauma* 1990;30:392

25. Acheson MB, Livinston RR, Richardson ML, et al: High resolution CT scanning in the evaluation of cervical spine fractures. *Am J Radiol* 1987;148:1179

26. Scalfani SJA: Advances in trauma radiology. *Adv Trauma* 1986;1:71

27. Feliciano DV: Management of traumatic retroperitoneal hematoma. *Ann Surg* 1990;211:109

28. Selivanov V, Chi HS, Alverdy JC, et al: Mortality in retroperitoneal hematoma. *J Trauma* 1984;24:1022

29. Lucas CE, Ledgerwood AM: Factors influencing outcome after blunt duodenal injury. *J Trauma* 1975;15:839

30. Fabian TC, Mangiante EC, Millis M: Duodenal rupture due to blunt trauma. *South Med J* 1984;77:1078

31. Levison MA, Petersen SR, Sheldon GF, et al: Duodenal trauma: experiences of a trauma center. *J Trauma* 1984;24:475

32. Sherck JP, Oakes DD: Intestinal injuries missed by computed tomography. *J Trauma* 1990;30:1

33. Prall JA, Nichols JS, Brennan R, et al: Early definitive abdominal evaluation in the triage of unconscious normotensive trauma patients. *J Trauma* 1994;37:792

34. Scalea TM, Phillips TF, Goldstein AS, et al: Injuries missed at operation: nemesis of the trauma surgeon. *J Trauma* 1988; 28:962

35. Carter JW: Diaphragmatic trauma in southern Saskatchewan: an 11-year review. *J Trauma* 1987;27:987

36. Flancbaum L, Morgan AS, Esposito TJ, et al: Non–left sided diaphragmatic rupture due to blunt trauma. *Surg Gynecol Obstet* 1985;161:266

37. Miller L, Bennett EV, Root HD, et al: Management of penetrating and blunt diaphragmatic injury. *J Trauma* 1984;24:403

38. Voeller GR, Reisser JR, Fabian TC, et al: Blunt diaphragm injuries. *Am Surg* 1990;56:28

39. McElwee TB, Myers RT, Pennell TC: Diaphragmatic rupture from blunt trauma. *Am Surg* 1984;50:143

40. Woodring JH, Dillon ML: Radiographic manifestations of mediastinal hemorrhage from blunt chest trauma. *Ann Thorac Surg* 1984;37:171

41. Gundry SR, Williams S, Burney RE, et al: Indications for aortography in blunt thoracic trauma: a reassessment. *J Trauma* 1982;22:664

42. Parmley LF, Mattingly TW: Non-penetrating traumatic injury of the aorta. *Circulation* 1958;17:1086

43. Townsend RN, Colella JJ, Diamond DL: Traumatic rupture of the aorta: critical decisions for trauma surgeons. *J Trauma* 1990;30:1169

44. Borman KR, Aurbakken CM, Weigelt JA: Treatment priorities in combined blunt abdominal and aortic trauma. *Am J Surg* 1982;144:728

45. Perry MO: Complications of missed arterial injuries. *J Vasc Surg* 1993;17:399

46. Howe HR, Poole GV, Hansen KJ, et al: Salvage of lower extremities following combined orthopedic and vascular trauma: a predictive salvage index. *Am Surg* 1987;53:205

47. Lange RH, Bach AW, Hansen ST, et al: Open tibial fractures with associated vascular injuries: prognosis for limb salvage. *J Trauma* 1985;25:203

48. Keeley SB, Snyder WH, Weigelt JA: Arterial injuries below the knee: fifty-one patients with 82 injuries. *J Trauma* 1983;23:285

49. Rudolph R, Boyd CR: Mass transfusion: complications and their management. *South Med J* 1990;83:1065

50. Ferrara A, MacArthur JD, Wright HK, et al: Hypothermia and acidosis worsen coagulopathy in the patient requiring massive transfusion. *Am J Surg* 1990;160:515

51. Faringer DD, Mullins RJ, Johnson RL, et al: Blood component supplementation during massive transfusion of AS-1 red cells in trauma patients. *J Trauma* 1993;34:481

52. Luna GK, Maier RV, Pavlin EG, et al: Incidence and effects of hypothermia in seriously injured patients. *J Trauma* 1987; 27:1014

53. Wilson EB, Iserson KV: Admixture bloodwarming: a technique for rapid warming of erythrocytes. *Ann Emerg Med* 1987; 16:413

54. Gentilello LM, Cobean RA, Offner PJ, et al: Continuous arteriovenous rewarming: rapid reversal of hypothermia in critically ill patients. *J Trauma* 1992;32:316

55. Kearney TJ, Benlt L, Grote M: Coagulopathy and catecholamines in severe head injury. *J Trauma* 1992;32:698

56. Kane WJ: Fractures of the pelvis. In: Rockwood CA, Green DP (eds). *Fractures in Adults*. Philadelphia, JB Lippincott, 1984

57. Perry JE, McClellan RJ: Autopsy findings in 127 patients following fatal traffic accidents. *Surg Gynecol Obstet* 1964;47:581

58. Mucha P: Recognizing and avoiding complications with pelvic fractures. *Infect Surg* 1985;11:53

59. Mucha P, Farrell MB: Analysis of pelvic fracture management. *J Trauma* 1984;24:379

60. Richardson JD, Harty J, Amin M, et al: Open pelvic fractures. *J Trauma* 1981;22:533

61. Rothenberger DA, Valasco R, Strate R, et al: Open pelvic fracture: a lethal injury. *J Trauma* 1978;18:124

62. Trunkey DD, Chapman MW, Lim RG, et al: Management of

pelvic fractures in blunt trauma injury. *J Trauma* 1974;14:912

63. Pennal GF, Tile M, Waddell JP, et al: Pelvic disruption: assessment and classification. *Clin Orthop* 1980;151:2

64. Tile M: *Fractures of the Pelvis and Acetabulum.* Baltimore, Williams & Wilkins, 1984

65. Mendez C, Gubjer KD, Maier RV: Diagnostic accuracy of peritoneal lavage in patients with pelvic fractures. *Arch Surg* 1994;129:477

66. Rehm CG, Mure AJ, O'Malley KF, et al: Blunt traumatic bladder rupture: the role of retrograde cystogram. *Ann Emerg Med* 1991;20:845

67. Maull KI, Suchelello CR, Ernst CA: The deep perineal laceration—an injury frequently associated with pelvic fracture: a need for aggressive surgical management. *J Trauma* 1977; 17:685

68. Majeed SA: Neurologic deficits in major pelvic injuries. *Clin Orthop* 1992;282:222

69. Buerger PM, Peoples JB, Lemmon GW, et al: Risk of pulmonary emboli in patients with pelvic fractures. *Am Surg* 1993; 59:505

70. White RH, Goulet JA, Bray TJ, et al: Improved outcome with early fixation of skeletally unstable pelvic fractures. *J Trauma* 1991;31:28

71. Poole GV, Ward EF, Griswold JA, et al: Complications of pelvic fractures from blunt trauma. *Am Surg* 1992;58:225

72. Flint L, Brown A, Richardson JA, et al: Definitive control of bleeding from severe pelvic fractures. *Ann Surg* 1979;189: 709

73. Moreno C, Moore EE, Rosenberger A, et al: Hemorrhage associated with major pelvic fracture: a multispecialty challenge. *J Trauma* 1986;26:987

74. Gaffney FA, Thal ER, Taylor WF, et al: Hemodynamic effects of medical antishock trousers (MAST garment). *J Trauma* 1981;21:932

75. Hoffman JR: External counterpressure and the MAST suit: current and future roles. *Ann Emerg Med* 1980;9:419

76. Templeman D, Lange R, Harms B: Lower-extremity compartment syndromes associated with use of pneumatic antishock garments. *J Trauma* 1987;27:79

77. Panetta T, Scalfani SJA, Goldstein AJ, et al: Percutaneous transcatheter embolization for massive bleeding from pelvic fractures. *J Trauma* 1985;25:1021

78. Matalon TS, Athanasoulis CA, Margolies MN, et al: Hemorrhage with pelvic fractures: efficacy of transcatheter embolization. *Am J Med* 1979;133:859

79. Mucha P, Welch TJ: Hemorrhage in major pelvic fractures. *Surg Clin North Am* 1988;68:757

80. Waddell JP: Pelvic ring fractures. *Can J Surg* 1990;33:431

Critical Care, Third Edition, edited by Joseph M. Civetta,
Robert W. Taylor, and Robert R. Kirby.
Lippincott-Raven Publishers, Philadelphia, PA © 1997.

CHAPTER 69

Evaluation of Bleeding in the Surgical Patient

Timothy H. Pohlman
C. James Carrico

IMMEDIATE CONCERNS

MAJOR ISSUES

Postoperative bleeding is either the result of a failure of surgical technique, or the consequence of a disorder of the coagulation mechanism that renders even perfectly executed surgical technique ineffectual. The most common cause of postoperative bleeding is localized (or "surgical bleeding"). Because surgical bleeding may have been caused by unusual events intraoperatively, and because reoperation is frequently required to treat postoperative bleeding, immediate consultation with members of the surgical team is mandatory. Postoperative bleeding also occurs as a result of defects in the hemostatic mechanism, which may develop in critically ill patients rapidly after surgery. The most common causes of coagulopathy in this setting are platelet dysfunction, depletion of coagulation factors, and hypothermia. Furthermore, undiagnosed, preexisting congenital defects in hemostasis, albeit rare, may become manifest under the stress of a surgical procedure. The inherited coagulation defects that could be encountered in a bleeding, postoperative patient are von Willebrand's disease, factor VIII deficiency (classical hemophilia, the disease that disrupted the Imperial Court of Tsar Nicholas II before his abdication), and factor IX deficiency.

STRESS POINTS

1. Postoperative bleeding from failure of surgical hemostasis is a potential complication of any procedure, simple or extensive. Postoperative hemorrhage is recognized by observing symptoms and signs of hypovolemia, including restlessness, anxiety, shortness of breath, pallor, tachycardia, and oliguria. Systemic hypotension indicates significant volume depletion. It is, therefore, a late sign of postoperative bleeding, although measurements of other hemodynamic parameters, such as the central venous pressure, may be more helpful in the diagnosis of postoperative hypovolemia.

2. When a decision to reoperate for postoperative bleeding is required, the variables that are considered include the presence or absence of active bleeding, rate and duration of bleeding, the location and extent of the operative field, and the potential for further complications (for example, a neck wound hematoma may cause airway obstruction). Elderly patients and diabetic patients possess less cardiovascular reserve and, therefore, require diligent observation to recognize postoperative bleeding before hemodynamic instability results.

3. Although all cases of postoperative bleeding should be considered for reoperation, some causes of bleeding should be managed expectantly or by means other than reoperation. For example, severe pelvic fractures are managed by either fracture stabilization or arteriography and embolization in the pelvic vasculature. Conversely, postoperative bleeding that has clearly abated may still require a prompt reexploration. For example, a dehiscence of a vascular anastomosis that is contained and no longer bleeding is likely to evolve

over time into a false aneurysm at that site. To prevent further complications, the anastomosis should be immediately repaired.

4. A coagulopathy resulting from a defect in primary or secondary hemostasis is either inherited and associated with a life-long bleeding tendency, or it is acquired as a complication of one of several pathologic conditions or numerous medications. A defect in the hemostatic mechanism can be recognized by bleeding from the operative site, as well as bleeding from puncture wounds or traumatized tissue outside of the operative field. After deciding whether postoperative bleeding is caused by a failure in the hemostatic mechanism rather than a failure of local hemostasis, the next step should be to differentiate disorders of primary hemostasis from those of secondary hemostasis with a platelet count and template bleeding time.

5. Postoperative bleeding from primary hemostatic failure is classified by conditions of platelet dysfunction, conditions that lower platelet count, or both. Thrombocytopenia is caused by a decrease in production of platelets (chemotherapy or malignancy), sequestration (hypersplenism), an increase in destruction of platelets (disseminated intravascular coagulation), or dilution of circulating platelets (massive transfusion). Acquired disorders of coagulation involving secondary hemostasis are caused by either a decrease in production of clotting factors (cirrhosis) or by an increase in consumption of circulating clotting factors (disseminated intravascular coagulation). Increased consumption of circulating factors, commonly overlaps with increased destruction of platelets for a combined defect in primary and secondary hemostasis.

6. Complex problems of hemostasis that are often encountered in a surgical intensive care unit include obstructive biliary tract disease, chronic liver disease, and massive trauma. Patients admitted to the ICU after cardiopulmonary bypass (CPB) have a tendency to bleed because of transient platelet dysfunction. Also, a specific complication of massive transfusion is the development of a coagulation disorder. Hepatic trauma presents significant technical challenges for the surgeon intraoperatively and can be the basis for the development of severe coagulopathy resulting from multiple factors. Acidosis, hypocalcemia, hypovolemia, and hypothermia, frequent findings in the trauma patient with severe liver injuries, all impair coagulation.

ESSENTIAL DIAGNOSTIC TESTS AND PROCEDURES

1. A thorough history, if time permits, is essential. One should determine if the patient has been anticoagulated or has been placed on medications that interfere with hemostasis. A history of a liver disease portends a deficiency in coagulation factors, as a history of epistaxis, easy bruising, or menorrhagia may suggest von Willebrand's disease or mild classic hemophilia.

2. A careful physical examination should be performed, mostly to determine if postoperative bleeding is caused by the failure of local hemostasis or a defect in coagulation. Coagulopathies can generate prominent systemic findings such as petechia or purpura (for example, the Waterhouse-Friderichsen syndrome after splenectomy).

3. If localized, surgical bleeding has been excluded, one should proceed with a panel of routine laboratory tests of coagulation. A template bleeding time should always be included because it is the only test that identifies a defect in platelet function, one of the most common causes of bleeding postoperatively (caused by ingestion of aspirin). A normal platelet count and template bleeding time essentially eliminate defects in primary hemostasis as the cause of the coagulopathy.

4. Defects in secondary hemostasis are assessed by determining the prothrombin time (PT) and partial thromboplastin time (PTT), which measures activities of factors XII, XI, X, IX, and VIII. Results of these assays are standardized to international reference values. An absolute measure of the fibrinogen level and thrombin coagulation time are useful to differentiate conditions that prolong both the PT and PTT. The fibrinogen level is depressed in coagulopathies produced by consumption, for example, as occurs during sepsis, severe brain injury and obstetric emergencies. The thrombin time is prolonged if the fibrinogen level is less than 100 mg/dL or by abnormal fibrinogen that is associated with liver disease. Its most useful role is in the detection of circulating heparin not detectable by changes in the PTT.

INITIAL THERAPY

1. Whatever the cause of postoperative bleeding, the first action taken in each case is directed to restoring volume to maintain adequate perfusion, after an airway is assured and adequate ventilation verified. Homologous transfusion of red cells is often required, whether completely matched to the patient or as type-compatible blood.

2. A failure of surgical hemostasis intraoperatively causing significant bleeding postoperatively mandates an immediate return to the operating room in most cases. Therapy for defects in coagulation generally involves transfusion of specific components isolated from whole blood. For the more common acquired disorders these include fresh frozen plasma containing all coagulation factors in concentrations approaching those found in normal plasma; cryoprecipitate, which is enriched in factor VIII, von Willebrand factor (vWF), and fibrinogen; and platelet concentrates. Platelets should be given for defects in platelet function, as assessed by the template bleeding time, although the platelet count may be normal. These types of therapies should not be used indiscriminately. Patients transfused with blood components incur substantial risk of complications attributed to transfusion therapy.

EVALUATION OF BLEEDING ∎

After the patient has become hemodynamically stable, a thorough history is an essential part of the evaluation of a bleeding surgical patient, particularly if an abnormality in the coagulation mechanism is suspected. One should determine if the patient has been anticoagulated for any reason or has been placed on medications that interfere with hemostasis (e.g., aspirin, phenylbutazone, or a semisynthetic penicillin). Medications that effect hemostasis frequently cause coagulopathies postoperatively. Severe liver disease impairs coagulation in several ways and should be considered while obtaining the history. Careful attention should be directed to the record of the patient's nutritional status and nutritional therapy. A vitamin K deficiency, occurring during parenteral nutritional therapy, should still be considered as a cause of an acquired coagulopathy despite the attention given to supplementation. Specific information from the patient, family, or prior medical records should be sought concerning past episodes of abnormal bleeding. A history of bleeding gums after brushing, excessive menstrual flow requiring transfusion, frequent epistaxis, melanotic stools, or easy bruising may indicate a preexisting inherited defect in coagulation. Although people with inherited coagulation disorders are usually identified early in life, milder bleeding tendencies may be undetected until the hemostatic mechanism is challenged by a major surgical procedure or trauma. Other predisposing factors that may alter hemostasis include cachexia secondary to malignancy, previous irradiation, and renal failure.

The pattern of bleeding is noted during physical examination, and often distinguishes surgical bleeding from bleeding caused by a coagulopathy. For example, a finding of petechiae suggests a failure of primary hemostasis. Liver failure as a cause of impaired secondary hemostasis can be identified by observing jaundice, ascites, angiomas, and testicular atrophy. The identification of these conditions preoperatively alerts one to the potential for a bleeding problem when the patient returns from the operating room. Postoperatively, a thorough search for infection should always be performed in a bleeding patient because sepsis commonly produces multiple defects in the hemostatic mechanism.

The diagnosis of a disordered coagulation mechanism is based on a panel of routine laboratory studies that are seldom difficult to obtain day or night in most hospitals. These are the template bleeding time, platelet count, PT, PTT, fibrinogen level, and thrombin time. The template bleeding time is the only test that identifies platelet dysfunction, a common cause of abnormal bleeding. The platelet count reveals thrombocytopenia, and a low platelet count also prolongs the bleeding time. If both the bleeding time and platelet count are normal, then it is less likely that the coagulopathy is a result of failure of primary hemostasis. A potential defect in secondary hemostasis is assessed by determining the PT and PTT. The PTT assesses activities of factors XII, XI, X, IX, and VIII, and therefore, identifies many of the inherited disorders of bleeding, usually a deficiency of factor VIII, IX, or vWF. The PT uniquely assesses factor VII. The

PT is prolonged in liver disease or in a hypothermic patient. Anticoagulation therapy with warfarin or heparin, or a reduced level of circulating fibrinogen, affects the PT and the PTT. An absolute measure of the fibrinogen level is useful to differentiate conditions that prolong both the PT and PTT. Fibrinogen is low in coagulation disorders produced by abnormal consumption of coagulation factors, as typically occurs during sepsis. However, fibrinogen may be elevated as an acute-phase reactant during a host response to stress, and a significant decrease caused by a process that consumes fibrinogen may not be detected because the resulting value is still in the "normal" range. The thrombin time will be prolonged if the fibrinogen level is less that 100 mg/dL or by abnormal fibrinogen associated with liver disease.[1] It is also prolonged by circulating fibrin(ogen) products. Its most useful role is in the detection of circulating heparin not detectable by changes in the PTT.

ETIOLOGIES OF POSTOPERATIVE BLEEDING ∎

LOCAL HEMOSTATIC FAILURE

The most common cause of postoperative bleeding is a failure of local hemostasis, also referred to as a failure of "surgical hemostasis," or, euphemistically, as an "acute silk deficiency." Postoperative bleeding is a potential complication of any surgical procedure. When it does occur, it is usually identified within the first 6 to 8 hours postoperatively. Severe hemorrhage is recognized by observing symptoms and signs of hypovolemia, including restlessness, anxiety, shortness of breath, pallor, tachycardia, hypotension, and oliguria. When the rate of postoperative fluid administration is adjusted to restore hemodynamic stability, the only findings will be falling hematocrit associated with increased fluid requirements. This may be mistakenly identified as hemodilution secondary to rewarming, vasodilation, and the administration of large volumes of exsanguine fluid. Extravascular accumulations of blood occasionally produce specific symptoms that aid in the diagnosis of postoperative bleeding. For example, pain caused by irritation of the diaphragm by blood in a subdiaphragmatic collection is referred to the shoulder (Kehr's sign). Postoperative bleeding can be detected and more precisely monitored if it exits by way of a drain placed at the time of surgery. However, absence of blood in a drain should not be taken as evidence that hemorrhage is not occurring, because the drain may clot, and enormous volumes of blood can be sequestered in large body cavities.

The decision to reoperate for postoperative bleeding is largely judgmental. In some instances, it is mandated by exsanguinating, life-threatening hemorrhage. For example, hemorrhage from a leaking coronary artery bypass graft anastomosis usually presents as brisk bleeding of bright red blood from the mediastinal drain. This situation is often catastrophic, and the patient is returned to the operating room urgently. In other situations, the surgeon may choose to treat a disorder of coagulation first and then operate if this fails to control bleeding. Variables to consider when faced with this problem are the presence or absence of active bleeding, rate and duration of bleeding, location, potential for further complications (e.g., a neck wound hematoma causing airway obstruction), and the patient' age and medical condition. Elderly patients and diabetic patients, for example, possess less cardiovascular reserve; therefore, postoperative bleeding in such patients presents additional concerns.

Postoperative bleeding after certain procedures can be particularly dangerous, even if the amount of blood actually lost is minimal. For example, relatively minor bleeding after thyroid or parathyroid surgery may evolve into a life-threatening complication. Routinely, endocrine surgery in the neck is performed with the patient's head and neck slightly elevated, which decreases venous pressure in the operative field (giving a false sense of adequate hemostasis during the procedure). In the postoperative period when the patient is lying flat, increased venous pressure in this position leads to bleeding. Formation of a tense hematoma in the wound tends to impair venous and lymphatic drainage of upper airway mucosa, producing edema and airway obstruction. Simply opening the wound to evacuate the hematoma does not necessarily relieve the airway obstruction, and airway intubation or cricothyroidotomy is required. Many surgeons place small drains, but this does not always prevent formation of a hematoma. In almost all cases, patients who develop large hematomas should be returned to the operating room for control of bleeding. Similarly, wound hematomas develop in 1.4% to 3.0% of patients undergoing carotid endarterectomy, and it is observed more frequently in patients who have received antiplatelet therapy preoperatively or who develop hypertension postoperatively.[2]

When a peripheral vascular anastomotic dehiscence is suspected, the patient should be explored promptly, even if the bleeding has stopped. The anastomosis must be repaired because of the danger of forming a false aneurysm at that site. A contained dehiscence of an anastomosis involving the abdominal aorta may be difficult to recognize if it is small. Postoperatively, an increasing fluid requirement caused by from blood loss must be distinguished from that caused by edema formation in the area of retroperitoneal dissection. An arteriogram should be performed if doubt exists.

Some episodes of bleeding are better managed without operation. After severe pelvic fractures, such as fractures with displacement, severe hemorrhage occurs in the retroperitoneal space. If this hematoma is opened during operation, torrential bleeding, impossible to stop, may develop. If a patient with a pelvic fracture has signs of continuing hemorrhage after hemoperitoneum and hemothorax have been excluded, we reduce the fracture and stabilize the pelvis with an external fixation device, or attempt embolization during arteriography of the pelvic and retroperitoneal vasculature.

DISORDERS OF COAGULATION

Impaired coagulation, resulting from a defect in primary or secondary hemostasis, is either inherited and associated with a life-long bleeding tendency, or it is acquired as a complication of one of several pathologic conditions or numerous medications. If an acquired defect is severe in a postopera-

tive patient, brisk bleeding develops from wounds, as well as from mucous membranes and venipuncture sites. In the acute situation, postoperative blood loss from the surgical field in a coagulopathic patient cannot be controlled with local hemostatic measures. Therefore, diagnosing and treating the underlying condition producing a coagulopathy is paramount. Less severe defects may not completely impair coagulation after minor tissue injury. However, they may lead to severe problems in hemostasis after larger injuries or larger surgical procedures. Coagulopathies are common in the postoperative ICU patient and can involve primary hemostasis, secondary hemostasis, or both.

Postoperative bleeding from a primary hemostatic failure is classified by (1) abnormal platelet function, or (2) an abnormal amount of circulating platelets, resulting from increased destruction of platelets, dilution of platelets, platelet sequestration, or decreased production of platelets.

Disorders of secondary hemostasis are classified by (1) decreased production of clotting factors, (2) coagulation factor dysfunction, or (3) increased consumption of clotting factors.

Primary Hemostatic Failure

PLATELET DYSFUNCTION.   Prior ingestion of aspirin is a common cause of drug-induced coagulopathy leading to abnormal bleeding in the postoperative patient, although spontaneous bleeding caused by preoperative aspirin use is rare.[3] For many reasons, the presence of an aspirin-induced coagulopathy is often unsuspected before surgery, and many over-the-counter medications contain aspirin unknown to the user (e.g., Alka Seltzer). Also, aspirin often is not thought of as a medication and, if not specifically asked, patients do not mention recent ingestion of aspirin while giving a drug history. Aspirin is such a common item in the home that patients may not recall having taken aspirin, even if specifically asked. Furthermore, platelet counts are seldom affected by aspirin, and a template bleeding time, the only common test capable of detecting platelet dysfunction, is often omitted from the preoperative coagulation screen.

Reversible platelet dysfunction is observed in patients who become hypothermic, as a complication of lengthy operations, after massive transfusion of refrigerated blood or room temperature fluids, or with prolonged exposure in the field after trauma. Local wound or general (patient) hypothermia results in decreased platelet thromboxane production and a prolonged bleeding time, reflecting a primary hemostatic failure.[4] Rewarming often is not considered an urgent priority for bleeding, and warming transfused blood or fluids may be omitted. However, rewarming reverses the defect in thromboxane production, and the bleeding time returns promptly to normal. Hypothermia also effects secondary hemostasis (see later).

Acute renal failure, frequently encountered in postoperative ICU patients, can produce a serious bleeding disorder, especially if kidney dysfunction is the result of a pathologic process that also affects coagulation. The mainstay of therapy for hemorrhage in this setting is correction of the underlying etiology and judicious use of peritoneal dialysis or hemodialysis. Peritoneal dialysis, if easily instituted, has been advocated because it does not require the use of heparin in a patient who is bleeding after a surgical procedure.[5] Chronic renal failure is also associated with a bleeding tendency attributed to a functional platelet defect. The bleeding tendency is seldom a problem clinically. Indeed, this mild deficit may have a beneficial effect on the patency of arteriovenous shunts used for vascular access during hemodialysis. Renal transplantation is performed uneventfully in most instances, and bleeding postoperatively usually can be attributed to technical problems with the vascular anastomoses.

THROMBOCYTOPENIA.   The classic presentation of thrombocytopenia is the appearance of petechiae in skin and mucous membranes or microvascular oozing from incised tissue. The risk for significant hemorrhage occurs when platelet counts fall below 20,000/mm[3]. However, if bleeding occurs in the presence of thrombocytopenia, it generally does not stop until the platelet count exceeds 100,000/mm[3]. Thrombocytopenia results from decreased marrow production, sequestration of platelets from the circulation, dilution of circulating platelets, or destruction of circulating platelets.

Chemotherapy and radiation therapy produce thrombocytopenia by suppression of bone marrow megakaryocytes and are the most common cause of bleeding in patients undergoing treatment for neoplastic disorders. Megaloblastic anemia resulting from vitamin B_{12} or folate deficiency is complicated by thrombocytopenia and hemorrhagic complications in a small percentage of cases.[6] Chronic alcoholic patients occasionally are observed to develop severe thrombocytopenia during a period of binge drinking because of a direct toxic effect of alcohol on marrow megakaryocytes in susceptible patients.

Serious infection postoperatively is the most frequent cause of thrombocytopenia caused by increased destruction of circulating platelets in the peripheral circulation.[7] Thrombocytopenia is observed in more than half (56%) of patients with bacteremia, and it is the only abnormality in coagulation that can be detected in a significant number of septic patients.[8] Often, thrombocytopenia is the first indication of infection and impending sepsis.

Unexplained thrombocytopenia in a postoperative patient should, therefore, prompt an immediate search for a septic focus.

Thrombocytopenia caused by increased destruction of platelets in the peripheral circulation occurs as part of thrombotic thrombocytopenia purpura, which includes microangiopathic hemolytic anemia, thrombocytopenia, fluctuating neurologic symptoms, and acute renal failure. The hemolytic-uremic syndrome shares many of the clinical features of thrombocytopenia purpura; however, in the hemolytic-uremic syndrome, children are more commonly affected, the neurologic symptoms are less prominent, and renal dysfunction is more severe. The mainstay of therapy in both is support of renal function.[9]

Posttransfusion purpura occurs approximately 1 week after receiving a blood transfusion in a small number of patients, most of whom are women who previously have been pregnant. These patients lack a specific platelet antigen, P1A[1], that is present on platelets in most others. In response to the foreign antigen, the transfused patient forms anti-P1A[1] antibodies, which cross-react with antigenic determinants on the patient's own platelets, destroying them, producing severe thrombocytopenia. The purpura can last several months. Idiopathic (autoimmune) thrombocytopenic purpura is the classic example of increased destruction of platelets from an immune mechanism. One third of idiopathic thrombocytopenic purpura patients eventually require splenectomy to control the thrombocytopenia. To minimize postoperative bleeding complications, a platelet count above 100,000/mm[3] is necessary. High-dose steroids or plasmapheresis preoperatively occasionally are necessary to achieve this level. Platelets should not be given intraoperatively until the splenic artery is clamped. Several drugs induce thrombocytopenia by an immune mechanism. Quinine (and quinine-containing beverages such as tonic water) is the best example of a substance that produces drug-induced thrombocytopenia and purpura.

Secondary Hemostatic Failure

DECREASED PRODUCTION.   Decreased production of active, circulating coagulation factors occurs secondary to liver failure (where all but one of the coagulation factors are synthesized), to interruption of γ-carboxylation of coagulation factors with coumarin derivatives, or to a vitamin K deficiency, which simulates the effect of coumarin anticoagulation.

IMPAIRED FUNCTION OF COAGULATION FACTORS. Coagulopathy resulting from hypothermia, a common state of the postoperative patient, is partly caused by the effect of temperature on the enzymatic, proteolytic reactions of the coagulation factor cascade. The PT, PTT, and thrombin time do not reflect the suppressive effect of temperature on coagulation because these tests are conducted in the clinical laboratory at 37C. Continuous arteriovenous rewarming, which does not require heparinization of the patient, improves hemostasis more rapidly than any other method not using CPB.[10] Because the levels of coagulation factors are not altered by lower core body temperatures, it is futile to treat a coagulopathy in a hypothermic patient (<34C) with fresh frozen plasma until the patient is warm.

Also, heparin impairs secondary hemostasis through its interaction with antithrombin III and the effect this complex has on the prothrombinase complex.

INCREASED DESTRUCTION OF CLOTTING FACTORS. Depletion of circulating coagulation factors occurs after uncontrolled coagulation is triggered, usually in the intravascular space, by several conditions (Table 69-1). Important clotting factors, notably fibrinogen, are consumed in the process, and it is associated with the fibrinolytic activity from the subsequent action of plasmin. This disorder has been referred to as disseminated intravascular coagulation, defibrination syndrome, fibrinolysis, or consumptive coagulopathy.[11] The term *consumptive coagulopathy* is preferred because this most accurately describes the pathophysiologic characteristics. A hallmark of consumptive coagulopathy is thrombocytopenia caused by trapping of platelets in fibrin mesh. Thus, the findings of hypofibrinogenemia associate with

TABLE 69-1. Syndromes Producing Acute
Consumptive Coagulopathy

DISSEMINATED INTRAVASCULAR COAGULATION

Nonobstetric
    Sepsis
        Gram-negative
        Gram-positive
    Shock
        Cardiogenic
        Hypovolemic
        Anaphylactic
    Head injury
    Burns
    Transfusion reaction
    Drowning
    Pancreatitis
    Hypothermia
    Envenomation
Obstetric
    Premature placental separation
    Amniotic fluid embolism
    Dead fetus
    Septic abortion
    Hydatiform mole
    Eclampsia

LOCALIZED INTRAVASCULAR COAGULATION

Purpura fulminans
Hemangioma
Kasabach-Merritt syndrome
Aneurysm

---

thrombocytopenia in a bleeding patient strongly suggests a consumptive process. Detection of fibrin(ogen) degradation products strengthens the diagnosis. Also, increased destruction of coagulation components causes a prolongation of the thrombin time (as does decreased production of factors).

The critical event in consumptive coagulopathy is the presentation of some element to the intravascular space that initiates coagulation.[9] When this process is fulminant, levels of circulating clotting factors become undetectable, and blood does not clot. In more chronic forms of consumptive coagulopathy, increased production compensates for the increased consumption of factors, and a low-grade consumptive coagulopathy may be paradoxically associated with thromboembolic phenomena. A frequent component of acute or chronic consumptive processes is depletion of platelets and thrombocytopenia (see earlier).

Surgical procedures and trauma (including burns) may produce a consumptive coagulopathy.[12,13] Large areas of damaged tissue release thromboplastic substances that trigger thrombin formation with the subsequent consumption of clotting factors and platelets. Certain types of injuries are more commonly associated with a consumptive coagulopathy. Brain injuries, particularly penetrating injuries, can present with generalized bleeding because brain tissue is an extremely rich source of tissue thromboplastin.[14] Severe burn injuries are frequently complicated by thrombocytopenia, hypofibrinogenemia, low levels of clotting factors, and in-

creased fibrinolysis that can be aggravated by burn wound sepsis. If hemorrhagic shock develops, anoxia and acidosis secondary to inadequate perfusion can produce injury to tissues, contributing to the coagulopathy. Several other mechanisms can disrupt the balance between coagulation and clot dissolution. Antithrombin III levels fall after massive trauma,[15] slowing the inactivation of thrombin formed in the intravascular space. Stasis of blood, as a result of shock, promotes coagulation, as first described by Virchow. Loss of platelets during severe hemorrhage followed by transfusion of stored blood without functional platelets contributes to the bleeding through dilution of platelets in the circulation. A reversible platelet defect has been demonstrated in hypothermic patients[4] that can further aggravate bleeding. Hemolytic reactions during blood transfusions for hemorrhagic shock represent, in effect, an intravascular infusion of tissue thromboplastin, and a consumptive coagulopathy, in addition to acute renal failure, is a prominent feature of this syndrome.

Arguably, infection in the postoperative ICU patient is the predominate cause of consumptive coagulopathies, but the exact mechanism of how coagulation is initiated is not well understood. Bacterial lipopolysaccharide (endotoxin), a component of the bacterial cell wall of gram-negative bacteria, can initiate the intrinsic pathway by direct activation of factor XII. Also, endotoxin may trigger coagulation by inducing expression of a procoagulant activity in circulating leukocytes,[16] hepatic macrophages[17] and endothelial cells.[18] Although endotoxin from gram-negative bacteria is most often implicated as the initiating agent, infections with other organisms, including gram-positive bacteria, protozoa, viruses, and *Rickettsiaceae*, are associated with severe consumptive coagulopathies. Purpura fulminans is an acute disease process involving consumption of coagulation factors that usually develops 2 to 3 weeks after an uneventful bacterial or viral upper respiratory tract infection. Characteristically, platelets and fibrin are deposited in the skin, leading to large areas of hemorrhagic necrosis.

Acute postoperative pancreatitis is a complication of several procedures in the upper abdomen. This results in the release of proteolytic enzymes in to the circulation that can directly activate prothrombin and factor X.[9] In severe cases, potential complications include respiratory, cardiovascular, and renal failure, as well as consumptive coagulopathy.[19] Also, abnormal bleeding can develop with pancreatic abscess as a septic focus.

The more fulminant forms of consumptive coagulopathy are usually associated with obstetric complications such as abruptio placentae, retained dead fetus syndrome, amniotic fluid embolus, and eclampsia.[13] Common to these disorders is the release of a large amount of thromboplastic substance into the intravascular space that initiates widespread massive coagulation.

The laboratory findings of an acute consumptive coagulopathy secondary to any of these conditions are thrombocytopenia associated with hypofibrinogenemia and a prolonged thrombin time. The platelet count is frequently blow 10,000/mm³, and the level of fibrinogen is below 100 mg/dL. In fulminant consumption, as seen in the obstetric complications, fibrinogen may be undetectable. Fibrin(ogen) degradation products may or may not be detectable. The PT, PTT, and the thrombin time also are abnormal. Antithrombin III levels, if measured, are low. Examination of the blood smear occasionally reveals red blood cell fragmentation resulting from mechanical damage of red blood cells by the fibrin mesh. In milder forms, fibrinogen levels may not be significantly depressed. If adequate liver function is present, production of fibrinogen can increase to balance increased fibrinogen consumption. In this instance, radioimmunoassays of fibrinopeptide A, a specific marker of the action of thrombin on fibrinogen, indicates the increased consumption of fibrinogen.[20]

To manage consumptive coagulopathies, attention should be directed early to correction of the specific cause. Drainage of localized abscesses, appropriate antibiotics, and support of failing organ systems should be aggressively pursued. The coagulation system can be supported by replacement of depleted factors with fresh frozen plasma. Platelet units are given until the platelet count exceeds 75,000 to 100,000/ mm^3. Because of a defect in platelet function induced by fibrin(ogen) degradation product, transfusion of platelets to a higher count (than if no defect were present) is necessary. Cryoprecipitate is transfused until the fibrinogen level exceeds 100 mg/dL and the thrombin time is shortened. If whole blood is being transfused, fresh frozen plasma is omitted because stored whole blood is a reasonable source of clotting factors.[21] The use of heparin to interrupt acute intravascular coagulation is controversial,[22] and may be hazardous in the postoperative period. Correcting laboratory abnormalities by administration of components is a temporizing measure while the primary initiating cause is reversed.

COMPLEX POSTOPERATIVE BLEEDING PROBLEMS ■

HEPATOBILIARY DISEASE

Chronic obstructive biliary tract disease and chronic liver disease in the critically ill can lead to defects in the hemostatic mechanism and be the underlying basis of abnormal bleeding after procedures in patients with these problems. Obstruction of the bile duct decrease delivery of bile salts to the intestinal lumen, thereby reducing absorption of lipid-soluble vitamin K. As in other causes of vitamin K deficiency, decreased synthesis of factors II, VII, IX, and X occurs with prolongation of the PT. Liver disease secondary to cirrhosis, chronic active hepatitis, fulminant hepatic failure, or replacement of liver by metastatic tumor disrupts hemostasis in several different ways. Most coagulation factors and several inhibitors are synthesized in the hepatic parenchyma. In addition to decreased synthesis of fibrinogen, the fibrinogen that is synthesized may be abnormal because of abnormal glycosylation of the molecule.[1] This molecular defect in fibrinogen delays aggregation of fibrin monomers. Another important role of the liver in coagulation is clearance of activated coagulation factors. It is suggested that reduced clearance allows circulating activated coagulation factors to precipitate intravascular coagulation, initiating a consumptive coagulopathy. This increased consumption of factors lowers levels already depressed by decreased production. Clearance of fibrin(ogen) degradation products is also reduced in chronic liver disease. These circulate as anticoagulants, inhibiting both fibrin polymerization and platelet function, and thus they contribute to defective coagulation. Thrombocytopenia occurs secondary to the splenomegaly of portal hypertension and marrow suppression from vitamin deficiencies. In alcohol related liver disease, alcohol has a direct toxic effect on megakaryocytes in susceptible people. Liver disease-associated defects in coagulation can make management of other complications, such as bleeding esophageal varices or hemorrhage postoperatively, extremely difficult. Treatment of bleeding in liver failure with vitamin K usually is not successful. Whole blood corrects both the red blood cell deficit and is as effective as fresh frozen plasma in correcting coagulation factor deficits.[21] Platelet transfusions should be used to raise the platelet count above 100,000/ mm^3.

TRANSFUSION-INDUCED BLEEDING

Frequently, patients who sustain major trauma or undergo extensive surgical procedures receive a significant amount of stored blood. Massive transfusion is arbitrarily defined as 10 units (one corporeal blood volume) or more of blood given within a 12-hour period. A specific complication of massive transfusion is the development of a coagulation disorder. Platelet activity is rapidly lost irreversibly at 4C; therefore, units of blood from the blood bank refrigerator have essentially no functional platelets. Previous studies have documented that massive transfusion of stored blood does, in fact, produce a dilutional thrombocytopenia. Furthermore, the degree of dilutional thrombocytopenia correlates directly with the number of units transfused. This degree of thrombocytopenia is not as great in magnitude as would be predicted by simple dilution, and other factors are probably contributing to maintain the platelet count, such as release of platelets from the splenic pool or early release from the bone marrow. Although thrombocytopenia invariably develops during massive transfusion, only about 20% of such patients develop a coagulopathy with generalized oozing from mucous membranes, venipuncture sites, and the operative field. The administration of platelets during massive transfusion to prevent a defect in coagulation has been advocated, but the efficacy of this therapy is doubtful. Reed and colleagues,[23] in a randomized double-blind study, examined the effect of prophylactic platelet transfusion (6 units) after every 12 units transfused of modified whole blood (whole blood from which platelets and cryoprecipitate have been removed). No differences were found between patients transfused with platelets compared with the controls who received fresh frozen plasma. Moreover, the incidence of microvascular bleeding was the same as in a previous study when no prophylactic component treatment was given during massive transfusion.[21] Patients who do develop microvascular bleeding during massive transfusion should receive transfusion of platelet concentrates. Four to 8 units at a time should be given, which will raise the circulation of platelet count by 40,000 to 80,000/mm^3. Additional units should be transfused if necessary to achieve an adequate level for hemostasis, generally greater than 100,000 platelets/mm³. The other labile factors of coagulation lost during cold storage of blood are factors V and VIII. However, dilution of these factors and others below levels needed for hemostasis is rare, and routine administration of fresh frozen plasma after an arbitrary number of transfused units of stored blood is not indicated.[24] Consumptive coagulopathies, however, are associated with conditions such as extensive surgical procedures or trauma that may require treatment with massive transfusion, and in these cases, severe depletion of coagulation factors should be managed with fresh frozen plasma and cryoprecipitate.

Incompatible blood transfusion potentially complicates any transfusion. The exigency and complexity of patients receiving massive transfusion may increase the probability of such a misadventure and make its recognition much more difficult. The subsequent hemolysis produces acute intravascular coagulation and consumptive coagulopathy. The patient develops microvascular oozing from traumatized surfaces, and this is frequently the first indication of a hemolytic transfusion reaction in a patient unable to express any symptoms of such a reaction. A red tinge in the urinary drainage bag from hemoglobinuria strongly suggests the diagnosis. The coagulopathy corrects rapidly after the transfusion is stopped, and therapeutic efforts should be directed to prevention of renal failure secondary to acute tubular necrosis. Mannitol should be given to promote an osmotic diuresis and tubular washout, as well as bicarbonate to alkalinize the urine and to prevent acid precipitation of hemoglobin crystals. Maintaining intravascular volume and renal perfusion is imperative.

LIVER TRAUMA

Severe liver trauma poses significant technical challenges for the surgeon intraoperatively, and it can also lead to the development of severe coagulopathy that persists in to the postoperative period. The basis for the coagulopathy is often multifactorial. Massive transfusion is frequently required during treatment of major liver injury. The thrombocytopenia caused by massive transfusion may be exacerbated by the onset of a consumptive process because of the release of tissue thromboplastin from the damaged tissue. This is particularly true if there is an associated injury to brain tissue that is rich in tissue thromboplastin. Decreased coagulation factor synthesis by the liver in response to injury may prevent repletion of those consumed. Liver injury results in decreased clearance of fibrin(ogen) degradation products, which interfere with fibrin monomer polymerization and normal clot formation. Decreased clearance of plasminogen activators and plasmin contributes to the coagulopathy because of increased fibrinolysis and breakdown of any clot that does form. Acidosis, hypocalcemia, hypovolemia, and hypothermia, frequent findings in the severely traumatized patient, also impede normal coagulation.

A hemostatic defect persists in the postoperative period if significant liver parenchyma has been resected. Also, the development of sepsis aggravates or initiates a consumptive coagulopathy. Management of these difficult cases involves

treating all potential underlying causes of a consumptive process (e.g., localizing and draining an intraabdominal abscess) and transfusing depleted blood components.

CARDIOPULMONARY BYPASS

A tendency to bleed should be expected postoperatively in each patient who undergoes CPB. Difficult surgical hemostasis, extracorporeal circulation, hemodilution, systemic heparinization, and hypothermia, all related to CPB procedures, are predisposing factors for hemorrhagic complications. Furthermore, organ failure, sepsis, and malnutrition are common to patients in the ICU. Numerous medications administered to ICU patients and preexisting coagulation defects may further exacerbate a failing hemostasis system. Reoperation for bleeding after CPB procedures varies by the type of procedure performed but is required for approximately 5% of patients.[25] Reoperation for bleeding is decided on by the surgical team based largely on the rate of blood loss from the mediastinal drains or chest tubes. Criteria for reoperation, as defined by Kirklin and Barratt-Boyes,[26] include losses exceeding 500 mL in the first hour, 440 mL/hour in the first 2 hours, or 300 mL/hour in the first 3 hours. A total blood loss of 1000 mL after 4 hours also mandates reoperation. In addition, a sudden increase in bleeding (>300 mL/hour) in a patient who previously had minimal chest tube drainage, marked widening of the cardiac silhouette on a portable chest radiograph postoperatively, or evidence of cardiac tamponade is an additional indication for reoperation. An isolated site of bleeding is identified in slightly more than half of patients reoperated for bleeding. In the remaining patients, hemostasis results after the evacuation of remaining clot, obliteration of dead space, and correction of coagulopathies. Frequently, a coagulopathy can only be considered after excluding failure of surgical hemostasis during reexploration.

Although there are many potential causes of abnormal coagulation in patients undergoing CPB procedures, the tendency to bleed is, for the most part, secondary to a transient defect in platelet function.[27] Furthermore, aspirin, which is commonly prescribed for patients with coronary artery disease, may exacerbate CPB-induced platelet dysfunction. The cause of platelet dysfunction that develops during CPB procedures is not precisely known but may be related to transient platelet activation during extracorporeal circulation. Some surgeons believe that bubble oxygenators induce a more severe defect than membrane oxygenators, but this has not been completely substantiated. Transient platelet dysfunction does worsen, however, with increasing length of CPB and is exacerbated by hypothermia and by numerous mediations. Platelet dysfunction during and after CPB is associated with a prolongation of the bleeding time and defective ristocetin-induced platelet aggregation, suggesting an abnormality in the interaction of platelets with vWF. This last observation has been the basis of a proposal to treat bleeding by increasing plasma levels of multimeric vWF with vasopressin acetate (DDAVP),[25] although many surgeons believe DDAVP potentiates coronary graft thrombosis. In most cases, the bleeding time normalizes without

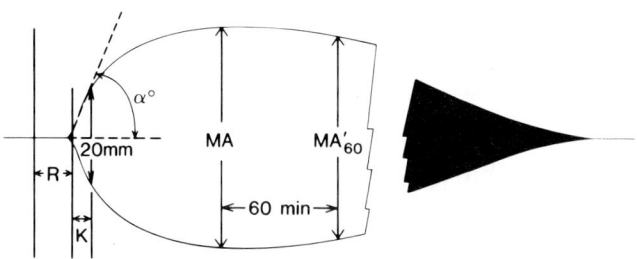

FIGURE 69-1. Parameters of a thromboelastogram tracing. The R value (reaction time) represents the time required for initial clot formation. The K value (coagulation time) measures the time from the R value to the point on the tracing that is 20 mm in amplitude, and the alpha angle ($\alpha°$) measures the slope of the developing amplitude tracing. These two values reflect, in an integrated fashion, the rate of clot formation, fibrin cross-linking, and platelet–fibrin interaction (normal K, 3 to 6 minutes; normal $\alpha°$, 45° to 50°). Both are depressed by hypofibrinogenemia or thrombocytopenia. The maximum amplitude (MA) represents maximum clot strength (normal MA, 50 to 60 mm). The MA′$_{60}$ is the amplitude of the tracing measured at 60 min and reflects clot retraction or lysis. (Reproduced with permission from Spiess BD, Davalle M: Coagulation monitoring in the surgical intensive care unit. *Intensive Care Monit* 1988;4:605.)

TEG Tracings – Examples

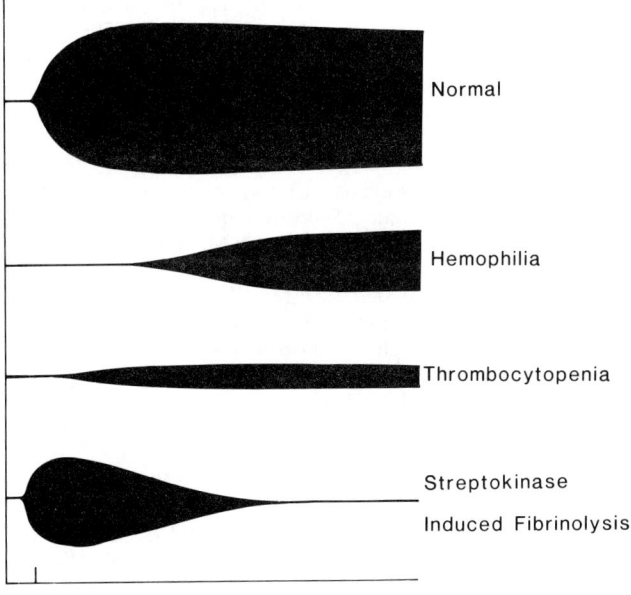

15 min

FIGURE 69-2. Examples of thromboelastogram (TEG) tracing during various coagulopathic states. Also, the maximum amplitude is diminished during disseminated intravascular coagulation, primary fibrinolysis, or uremia. (Reproduced with permission from Spiess BD, Davalle M: Coagulation monitoring in the surgical intensive care. *Intensive Care Monit* 1988;4:605.)

treatment after coming off bypass, usually within 2 to 4 hours. A mild reduction in the platelet count also occurs during CPB procedures, but it is seldom a sole cause of post-CPB bleeding. Postoperative bleeding associated with a persistently prolonged bleeding time may be managed successfully with platelet transfusions (one unit/10 kg body weight).[27] Platelets are transfused as primary therapy for post-CPB bleeding only when the surgical team believes surgical hemostasis has been secured.

Abnormalities in coagulation that occur secondary to CPB can be monitored postoperatively (and intraoperatively) with thromboelastography (TEG).[28] This technique, popular in Europe, is gaining acceptance in the United States. TEG assays various parameters of whole blood clot formation, which are reflected in measurements of the TEG tracing (Fig. 69-1). By measuring different angles and the width of the tracing, an assessment can be made of clot strength and the rates of clot formation, retraction, and lysis. Because this method identifies abnormal platelet function, it is useful in after the changes that occur in coagulation during CPB. Moreover, primary fibrinolysis or consumptive coagulopathy occurring during CPB is readily identified with TEG, as are coagulation disorders caused by preexisting coagulation factor deficiencies or warfarin therapy (Fig. 69-2). Because TEG assesses the various components of coagulation in an integrated fashion, it has become popular with intensivists caring for patients with complex disorders of hemostasis, such as patients receiving liver transplants who also have multifactorial bleeding problems or who are undergoing CPB. In addition, TEG provides an opportunity to assess the effect of hypothermia on a patient's coagulation profile by adjusting the temperature of the apparatus to match the patient's core body temperature.

REFERENCES

1. Martinez J, MacDonald KA, Palascak JE: The role of sialic acid in the dysfibrinogenemia associated with liver disease: distribution of sialic acid on the constituent chains. *Blood* 1983;61:1196
2. Kunkel JM, Gomez ER, Spebar MJ, et al: Wound hematomas after carotid endarterectomy. *Am J Surg* 1984;148:844
3. Mielke CH Jr: Influence of aspirin on platelets and the bleeding time. *Am J Med* 1985;74:72
4. Valeri CR, Feingold H, Cassidy G, et al: Hypothermia-induced reversible platelet dysfunction. *Ann Surg* 1987;205:175
5. Castaldi PA: Hemostasis and kidney disease. In: Ratnoff OD, Forbes CD (eds). *Disorders of Hemostasis*. Orlando, Grune & Stratton, 1984:473
6. Murphy S: Disorders of platelet production. In: Colman RW, Hirsch J, Marder VJ, Salzman EW (eds). *Hemostasis and Thrombosis*. Philadelphia, JB Lippincott, 1982:259
7. Jacobson MA, Young LS, Reed RLD, et al: New developments in the treatment of gram-negative bacteremia. *West J Med* 1986;144:185
8. Neame PB, Kelton JG, Walker IR, et al: Thrombocytopenia in septicemia: role of disseminated intravascular coagulation. *Blood* 1980;56:88
9. Harlan JM: Thrombocytopenia due to non-immune platelet destruction. *Clin Haematol* 1983;12:39
10. Gentilello LM, Cortes V, Moujaes S, et al: Continuous arterio-venous rewarming: experimental results and thermodynamic

model simulation of treatment for hypothermia. *J Trauma* 1990;30:1436

11. Colman RW, Robboy SJ, Minna JD: Disseminated intravascular coagulation: a reappraisal. *Annu Rev Med* 1979;30:359
12. Bennett B, Towler HM: Haemostatic response to trauma. *Br Med Bull* 1985;41:274
13. Hamilton PJ, Stalker Al, Douglas AS: Disseminated intravascular coagulation: a review. *J Clin Pathol* 1978;81:609
14. Kaufman HH, Hui KS, Mattson JC, et al: Clinicopathological correlations of disseminated intravascular coagulation in patients with head injury. *Neurosurgery* 1984;15:34
15. Risberg B, Medegard A, Heideman M, et al: Early activation of humoral proteolytic systems in patients with multiple trauma. *Crit Care Med* 1986;14:917
16. Thiagarajan P, Niemetz J: Procoagulant-tissue factor activity of circulating peripheral blood leukocytes: results of in vivo studies. *Thromb Res* 1980;17:891
17. Maier RV, Ulevitch RJ: The induction of a unique procoagulant activity in rabbit hepatic macrophages by bacterial lipopolysaccharides. *J Immunol* 1981;127:1596
18. Schorer AE, Rick PD, Swaim WR, et al: Structural features of endotoxin required for stimulation of endothelial cell tissue factor production: exposure of preformed tissue factor after oxidant-mediated endothelial cell injury. *J Lab Clin Med* 1985;106:38
19. Lasson A, Ohlsson K: Consumptive coagulopathy, fibrinolysis and protease-antiprotease interactions during acute human pancreatitis. *Thromb Res* 1986;41:167
20. Leeksma OC, Meijer-Huizinga F, Stoepman-van Dalen EA, et al: Fibrinopeptide A and the phosphate content of fibrinogen in venous thromboembolism and disseminated intravascular coagulation. *Blood* 1986;67:1460
21. Counts RB, Haisch C, Simon TL, et al: Hemostasis in massively transfused trauma patients. *Ann Surg* 1979;190:91
22. Feinstein DI: Diagnosis and management of disseminated intravascular coagulation: the role of heparin therapy. *Blood* 1982;60:284
23. Reed RLD, Ciavarella D, Heimbach DM, et al: Prophylactic platelet administration during massive transfusion: a prospective, randomized, double-blind clinical study. *Ann Surg* 1986;203:40
24. Counts RB: Acquired bleeding disorders. In: Menitove JE, McCarthy LJ (eds). *Hemostatic Disorders and the Blood Bank.* Arlington, VA, American Association of Blood Banks, 1984
25. Harker LA: Bleeding after cardiopulmonary bypass [editorial]. *N Engl J Med* 1986;314:1446
26. Kirklin JW, Barratt-Boyes BG: *Postoperative Care in Cardiac Surgery.* New York, Wiley, 1986:139
27. Woodman RC, LA Harker: Bleeding complications associated with cardiopulmonary bypass. *Blood* 1990;76:1680
28. Spiess BD, Davalle M: Coagulation monitoring in the surgical intensive care unit. *Crit Care Clin* 1988;4:605

Critical Care, Third Edition, edited by Joseph M. Civetta,
Robert W. Taylor, and Robert R. Kirby.
Lippincott-Raven Publishers, Philadelphia, PA © 1997.

CHAPTER 70

∎

Abdominal Trauma:
Diagnostic Steps and
Postoperative Considerations

Vicente Cortes
Marc D. Palter
Mark McKenney

IMMEDIATE CONCERNS ∎

MAJOR PROBLEMS

The patient with an actual or a potential abdominal injury
may come to the ICU in a variety of physiologic conditions
that require different responses from the intensivist. Some
typical scenarios include the following:

1. The patient in metabolic failure (shock, hypothermia,
   profound metabolic acidosis, and coagulopathy) after
   having undergone early exploratory laparotomy for hemostasis and damage control: Only an expedited secondary survey may have been done before rushing the
   patient to the operating room. The intensivist must
   complete a secondary survey and plan with the surgeon
   any necessary investigations for life-or limb-threatening extraabdominal injuries. The intensivist assumes
   primary responsibility for the restoration of oxygen
   transport function, normothermia, and hemostatic
   function in preparation for reoperation and definitive surgery.
2. The stable or unstable patient after exploratory laparotomy and definitive treatment of intraabdominal injuries: The intensivist is responsible for maintaining
   or restoring hemodynamic stability, providing postop-

erative care, and watching for missed injuries and postoperative complications.
3. The stable patient with a penetrating abdominal, blunt
   hepatic, or splenic injury admitted for observation and
   nonoperative treatment: The intensivist must watch
   for the development of indications for exploration such
   as hemodynamic instability, a drop in hematocrit, or
   signs of peritoneal irritation.
4. The stable or unstable trauma patient without an overt
   abdominal injury: The intensivist must look for manifestations of abdominal injury keeping in mind that
   associated injuries and drug or alcohol ingestion may
   alter the pain response so that the absence of abdominal physical findings is unreliable to rule out injury.

STRESS POINTS

1. Five abdominal regions are defined using *surface anatomy*: the anterior abdomen, the two flanks, the back,
   and the pelvis. The anatomic location of penetrating
   injuries determines the appropriate diagnostic procedures and imaging studies.
2. The *index of suspicion for injury* is based on the following: mechanism of injury, details of the assault, position
   of the victim and assailant, details of the crash, use

of protective devices, the hemodynamic status of the patient, anatomic location of penetrating injuries, seemingly trivial evidence of blunt trauma, and evolving signs of peritoneal irritation.

3. The primary objective of the evaluation is to *define if an intraabdominal injury is present and whether exploratory laparotomy is indicated*, determined by the potential morbid or lethal effect of the visceral damage without surgical intervention.

4. The *diagnostic modalities* used in abdominal trauma include observation, diagnostic peritoneal lavage (DPL), ultrasonography (US), abdominal computed tomography (CT) scan, angiography, laparoscopy, thoracoscopy, and diagnostic laparotomy.

5. *Exploratory laparotomy is the most definitive diagnostic and therapeutic maneuver* in penetrating and blunt abdominal trauma. It is 99% sensitive; however, a negative result on exploration carries a measurable morbidity and mortality. The mortality rate of abdominal injuries treated by laparotomy is 2% for stab wounds, 12% for gunshot wounds, and 25% for blunt injuries.

6. Laparotomy is indicated for abdominal *gunshot wounds* based on the mechanism of injury alone, because of the high likelihood of intraabdominal injury. Tangential injuries and injuries confined to the back musculoskeletal structures are the exception. Invasive diagnostic procedures (DPL or laparoscopy) or imaging studies (triple-contrast abdominal CT scan) may be used to detect injuries in these cases.

7. Laparotomy is indicated for abdominal *stab wounds* based on the following: clinical findings alone (hemorrhagic shock; signs of peritoneal irritation; evisceration through the wound; blood in the stomach, rectum, or urine; retained stabbing implement; or impalement); intraperitoneal or retroperitoneal air on plain chest or abdominal radiographs; fascial penetration in combination with positive results of invasive diagnostic procedures or imaging studies; or when peritoneal signs developed during observation.

8. Laparotomy is indicated for *blunt abdominal trauma* in the presence of unequivocal signs of peritoneal irritation (generalized tenderness, abdominal wall rigidity, rebound tenderness, and absent bowel sounds); pneumoperitoneum or ruptured diaphragm detected on plain chest radiograph; or abdominal distension and shock unexplained by external hemorrhage, hemothorax, pelvic fracture, long bone fractures, tension pneumothorax, cardiac tamponade, or spinal cord injury.

ESSENTIAL DIAGNOSTIC TESTS AND PROCEDURES

1. *Diaphragm*: Penetrating injuries are usually diagnosed at laparotomy. Stab wounds to the intrathoracic abdomen are best evaluated with thoracoscopy or gasless laparoscopy to rule out diaphragmatic injuries. Findings of blunt diaphragmatic injury may not be evident on the initial chest radiograph and may be recognized only on follow-up films. Definitive diagnosis is made by thoracoscopy, gasless laparoscopy, or laparotomy.

2. *Liver and spleen*: They are the most commonly injured organs in abdominal trauma. Penetrating injuries are staged at laparotomy. Most blunt injuries are diagnosed and staged using abdominal and pelvic CT scan. Blood loss and exsanguination may occur in undiagnosed injuries.

3. *Pancreas and extrahepatic bile ducts*: Intraoperative evaluation in penetrating injuries requires exposure of the pancreas, intraoperative cholangiography through the gallbladder, or on-the-table endoscopic retrograde cholangiopancreatography (ERCP). Blunt injuries are evaluated by an abdominal CT scan and ERCP.

4. *Gastrointestinal tract*: The hollow viscera may be exposed and inspected during exploration for penetrating injuries with the exception of the extraperitoneal rectum, which is examined by rectal digital and endoscopic examination before laparotomy. Blunt injuries are evaluated by physical examination, DPL, and abdominal CT scan for the intraperitoneal portions; radiographic contrast studies for the retroperitoneal segments (esophagography, duodenography); and endoscopy for the extraperitoneal rectum.

5. *Retroperitoneum*: Penetrating retroperitoneal injuries to the major abdominal blood vessels and associated injuries are diagnosed at laparotomy. For blunt retroperitoneal trauma, abdominal and pelvic CT scans are the best diagnostic investigation.

INITIAL THERAPY

1. *Diaphragm*: All diaphragmatic injuries must be repaired surgically. Undiagnosed injuries may result in diaphragmatic hernia, incarceration, and strangulation with high morbidity and mortality rate.

2. *Liver and spleen*: Penetrating hepatic and splenic injuries are treated at laparotomy. Blunt liver and spleen injuries in hemodynamically unstable patients are treated surgically. Blunt injuries in hemodynamically stable patients may be managed nonoperatively and receive close monitoring in the intensive care unit (ICU). In splenic injuries, the goal is to avoid transfusion. Transfusion of 2 to 4 units of packed red blood cells may be acceptable in liver injuries.

3. *Pancreas and extrahepatic bile ducts*: Penetrating injuries require surgery for reconstruction, resection, or drainage. Blunt pancreatic injuries need surgical intervention whenever the main pancreatic duct is involved. Traumatic pancreatitis is treated nonoperatively. Blunt extrahepatic bile duct injuries may be evident only later and require surgical repair.

4. *Gastrointestinal tract*: All perforations of the gastrointestinal tube from blunt or penetrating trauma require surgical intervention. Diversion of the digestive stream may be used to protect duodenal, colonic, and rectal injuries to allow healing.

5. *Retroperitoneum*: Penetrating injuries resulting in hemorrhage or hematoma formation are treated with exploration and surgical repair of vascular and visceral injuries. Blunt injuries resulting in hematoma forma-

tion may need surgical intervention, depending of the location of the hematoma and the likelihood of visceral injury.

6. *The retroperitoneal hemorrhage* associated with pelvic fractures requires multidisciplinary management by the trauma surgeon, intensivist, orthopedic surgeon and interventional radiologist.

Trauma is the leading cause of death from ages 1 to 44 years in the United States. The economic impact of trauma is greater than that of cardiovascular and neoplastic diseases combined; trauma is the leading cause of loss of potential years of productive life. Approximately 153,000 Americans died as a result of injury in 1988; of these deaths, 64% were classified as unintentional, 34% as intentional, and the remaining 2% were unclassified.[1]

Abdominal injuries do not produce most of injury-related fatalities; however, they are commonly the cause of the so-called "preventable trauma deaths." In a retrospective study of 1000 injury-related deaths in England and Wales, 43% of the deaths not related to central nervous system injury were deemed to be potentially preventable. The most commonly missed diagnosis included ruptured liver and ruptured spleen.[2] This British investigation has corroborated the results of many American studies of preventable trauma deaths. Abdominal injuries produce 10% to 13% of all the trauma fatalities and are associated with significant morbidity. Delay in detection or underestimation of the injuries is an important factor in the morbidity and mortality of abdominal injuries. This becomes particularly important in cases of blunt trauma in which few or only subtle signs of internal injury may be present. Therefore, the trauma surgeon and the intensivist must have a high index of suspicion for abdominal visceral injury to detect occult injuries and the early manifestations of complications of injuries already diagnosed.[3]

This chapter outlines the general principles of the workup and management of abdominal trauma and reviews specific organ injuries, including the operative and nonoperative surgical management, early detection, and treatment of complications. We emphasize the implications for the intensivist participating in the care of the injured patient.

GENERAL CONSIDERATIONS IN ABDOMINAL INJURY ■

ANATOMY

The trauma surgeon uses external anatomic landmarks on the torso to define five specific regions which, when traumatized by a blunt or penetrating mechanism, may result in intraabdominal injuries. These regions are the anterior abdomen, the two flanks, the back, and the pelvis, and are defined here in detail.[4,5] The boundaries of the *anterior abdomen* are the fourth intercostal space superiorly (nipple line in males), the anterior axillary lines laterally, and the inguinal ligaments and pubic symphysis inferiorly. Each *flank* is bounded by the anterior and posterior axillary lines, a horizontal line at the level of the sixth intercostal space with midaxillary line superiorly, and the iliac crest inferiorly. The *back* is the region located between the posterior axillary lines from a horizontal line at the level of the tips of the scapulae or seventh intercostal space superiorly, to the iliac wings and the lumbosacral junction inferiorly. The *pelvis* is the region located between the lumbosacral junction, the iliac wings, and the pubis superiorly, and the gluteal folds and the perineum inferiorly.

The superior extent of the anterior abdomen, the two flanks, and the back result from the circumstance that the diaphragm may rise up to that level during maximal expiration. The segment of the torso extending from the superior borders of the anterior abdomen, both flanks and the back, down to the costal margin is known as the *thoracoabdominal region* or *intrathoracic abdomen*. It contains the diaphragm, the liver, the spleen, the distal esophagus, the stomach and duodenum, the pancreas, the adrenals and upper half of the kidneys, the proximal abdominal aorta and its proximal branches, and the suprarenal inferior vena cava (IVC) and its tributaries. Blunt or penetrating trauma to the lower rib cage may, therefore, injure any one of these structures.

The *retroperitoneum* is the space between the posterior abdominopelvic peritoneum and the musculoskeletal structures of the back and flank (psoas major and minor, iliacus and quadratus lumborum muscles, lumbosacral vertebral column, and bony pelvis). The retroperitoneum contains multiple anatomic structures, including the following: (1) portions of the gastrointestinal tract (abdominal esophagus, duodenum except for its first portion, pancreas, ascending and descending colon, and extraperitoneal rectum): (2) the adrenal glands and most of the urinary system (kidneys, ureters and bladder); (3) neural structures (lumbosacral and sympathetic and parasympathetic plexuses); and (4) vascular structures (aorta with visceral and parietal branches, iliac arteries with visceral and parietal branches, IVC with visceral and parietal tributaries and portal vein with its major tributaries). Injury to any of the retroperitoneal structures may result in hematoma formation expanding the space cephalad into the chest, caudad into the thighs, laterally into the flanks, and anteriorly into the small bowel and transverse colon mesenteries. A large volume of blood may be lost in this space without specific symptoms and with minimal physical findings. The retroperitoneum is divided in three zones[3]: (1) *central-medial retroperitoneum*: diaphragm to sacral promontory, renal hilum to renal hilum; (2) *lateral retroperitoneum*: adrenal to the pelvic brim and renal hilum to the paracolic gutter; and (3) *pelvic retroperitoneum*.

The *pelvis* contains the bladder, the distal ureters, the internal genitalia in females, the rectosigmoid, the genitourinary and gastrointestinal tract outlets, small bowel loops, and the iliac vessels. A blunt or penetrating injury to the pelvis may injure any one of these structures.

MECHANISM OF INJURY

Abdominal trauma may result from blunt or penetrating mechanisms. Blunt trauma usually occurs in motor vehicle crashes, affecting occupants or pedestrians. Other causes include falls or jumps from heights, bicycle and motorcycle crashes, interpersonal violence and assaults, and work-related crush injuries. Penetrating injuries are usually the result of firearm wounds (hand guns, rifles, or shot guns) and stab wounds (knives, ice picks, or broken glass fragments) and occasionally from penetration by other sharp objects.

The general principles of primary survey and simultaneous restoration of vital functions, secondary survey, and definitive therapy are followed in blunt trauma and penetrating trauma. However, depending on the mechanism of injury, there is a significant difference in the time used in making the most critical decision: to proceed or not to proceed with exploratory laparotomy. Because blunt abdominal trauma commonly results from motor vehicle crashes and falls, trauma to other anatomic segments such as the head, neck, chest, and extremities may occur simultaneously. In these cases, the symptoms and signs of blunt abdominal injury may be subtle and the diagnosis may require imaging studies or invasive diagnostic procedures. Major injuries to the chest and pelvis, a base deficit exceeding 3 mEq/L, and a history of hypotension are statistically reliable predictors of intraabdominal organ injury.[6] In the presence of multiple injuries, the trauma surgeon must determine the sequence of diagnostic procedures and therapeutic interventions, giving priority to the diagnosis and treatment of life- or limb-threatening injuries. Simultaneous surgical intervention in the head and torso, torso and extremity, or head and extremity may be necessary to treat time-dependent, coexisting life- and limb-threatening injuries.[7,8]

On the other hand, penetrating abdominal trauma is usually confined to the torso and is more amenable to a more rapid and simplified workup before proceeding to abdominal exploration, considering that intraabdominal injury occurs in 88% to 90% of the firearm wounds and in 25% to 33% of the stab wounds.[3,9]

DIAGNOSTIC EVALUATION AND MANAGEMENT

Trauma resuscitation includes the following steps:

1. Assessing and securing airway and breathing
2. Assessing circulatory status
3. Securing two large-bore intravenous lines, preferably in the upper extremities, and initiating the infusion of prewarmed balanced crystalloid solution
4. Obtaining and sending a blood specimen for type and crossmatching for 4 to 6 units of blood
5. Performing a brief neurologic examination (state of consciousness, status of the pupils, and motor function of the extremities)
6. Completely disrobing the patient and inspecting all anatomic segments
7. Preventing hypothermia by maintaining a warm resuscitation room, warming all infused fluids and blood, warming the ventilator inspired gases, and avoiding exposure after the external inspection is completed
8. Conducting a head-to-toe examination, inserting a nasogastric tube, completing a rectal examination, and inserting a Foley catheter
9. Obtaining essential radiographs
10. Obtaining an arterial blood sample for blood gases and serum lactate level and baseline hematology profile, serum chemistries, and blood alcohol level
11. Obtaining a urine sample for immediate dip stick and microscopic examination as well as toxicology screen
12. Administering tetanus toxoid and tetanus immune globulin if indicated
13. Administering an intravenous antibiotic effective against colonic flora whenever exploratory laparotomy is planned[10] (Chap. 67).

Occasionally, trauma patients are admitted to the ICU before a final decision regarding the need for laparotomy has been made. The primary and secondary steps should be confirmed or completed (Chap. 68).

The most important decision in abdominal trauma is to define the need for exploratory laparotomy. Once that decision has been made, the trauma surgeon ought to identify and treat all of the injuries present at the time of exploration. The steps of laparotomy for trauma include the following: (1) obtaining wide exposure through a midline incision; (2) staunching hemorrhage and controlling vascular injuries while allowing the anesthesiologist to complete resuscitation; (3) minimizing soilage by provisional control of gastrointestinal tract perforations; (4) identifying all injuries using specific mobilization maneuvers; and (5) repairing vessels, solid organs, and hollow viscus using conservative techniques to minimize operative time and physiologic abnormalities (shock, transfusion-related coagulopathy, and hypothermia).

The following diagnostic modalities are used in abdominal trauma: (1) observation (serial abdominal examinations by the same surgeon); (2) open or percutaneous DPL; (3) US; (4) abdominal and pelvic CT scan with double contrast (oral and intravenous) or triple contrast (oral, intravenous, and rectal); (5) angiography; (6) diagnostic laparoscopy; (7) diagnostic thoracoscopy; and (8) diagnostic laparotomy.[3,9,10]

Victims of penetrating abdominal trauma with manifestations of hemorrhagic shock should undergo primary survey and expeditious secondary survey with immediate transportation to the operating room for operative control of bleeding (laparotomy for hemostasis within 15 to 30 minutes of arrival to the hospital). Attempts at complete resuscitation in these patients by infusion of massive volumes of blood, colloid, or crystalloid solutions may be detrimental. Obtaining a chest radiograph is necessary only to rule out intrathoracic injury or massive hemothorax. Vigorous infusion of crystalloid solution and blood may be delayed until the skin incision is made.[11]

Victims of blunt trauma with obvious multiple injuries and manifestations of profound hemorrhagic shock at the scene and during transportation should receive rapid infusion of uncrossmatched type O negative blood as well as balanced crystalloid solutions using high-efficiency warmers. Cardiac compressive shock caused by tension pneumothorax, or, less frequently, pericardial tamponade, may be present in these individuals. Distended neck veins and the presence of shock or hypotension unresponsive to blood and fluid administration are the hallmarks of this condition. Blunt trauma patients have multiple potential sites of bleeding. The determination of the site of actual hemorrhage may require the use of the diagnostic modalities listed earlier.

Here we will apply the definition of *hemodynamically stable patient* used by Flint[12]: the patient with a stable, normal arterial blood pressure, adequate ventilation, and clinical evidence of satisfactory peripheral perfusion (palpable radial and pedal pulses, normal capillary refill, and adequate urine output) who has been without additional fluid requirements for more than 30 minutes except for the initial 2 L of balanced crystalloid solution.

PENETRATING INJURIES ■

Bullet wounds to the abdomen cause internal injuries in 88% to 90% of the cases. The incidence of visceral or vascular injuries increases to 96% to 98% if there is evidence that the peritoneal cavity was traversed on physical evaluation or on biplanar radiographic studies.[9] Therefore, the standard approach for gunshot wounds to the anterior abdomen, flanks, and back is exploratory laparotomy to identify and repair all visceral and vascular injuries, unless there is undisputed evidence that the peritoneum was not entered.[9] A chest radiograph to exclude intrathoracic injury or massive hemothorax is the only radiologic workup required for patients in shock. In hemodynamically stable patients, biplanar plain films using radiopaque markers (i.e., paper clips or ECG leads) for entrance or exit wounds are used to help project the pathway of the projectile, keeping in mind that individuals may not have been shot lying in the same position (supine on the radiograph table). In the patient with hematuria but who is not in profound shock, it is prudent to obtain a one-shot double-dose intravenous pyelogram (IVP). The study may identify a renal injury on the involved side, but of greater significance, it will demonstrate the presence or absence of a functional kidney on the opposite side in case nephrectomy is considered. Occasionally, congenital malformations such as a horseshoe kidney or a double ureter and collecting system, which may influence surgical therapy, may be diagnosed as well. In multiple gunshot wounds, the number of bullet wounds should match the number of shots fired. Two holes may be two injuries with retained bullets or a single through-and-through injury. An odd number of holes indicates the presence of single or multiple retained bullets that must be localized using biplanar radiographs to reconstruct their trajectories.[3]

Transpelvic gunshot wounds require immediate exploratory laparotomy if shock, peritoneal signs, hematuria, or rectal bleeding are present and whenever evidence that peritoneum has been entered is clearly demonstrated with biplanar films. Laparotomy is indicated if proctosigmoidoscopy, vaginal examination, DPL, pelvic angiography, and pelvic CT scan with triple-contrast or combination of IVP, or retrograde urethrogram and cystogram demonstrate pelvic vascular, pelvic visceral, or genitourinary or gastrointestinal tract outlet injury.[13]

The following are the only exceptions to the policy of mandatory exploration for abdominal gunshot wounds: (1) hemodynamically stable patients without signs of peritoneal irritation with back wounds confined to the musculature and the vertebral column on biplanar films; and (2) hemodynamically stable patients without signs of peritoneal irritation with clearly tangential or superficial wounds to the anterior abdomen and flanks.

Diagnostic laparoscopy has been useful to rule out peritoneal penetration in the evaluation of tangential gunshot wounds to the anterior abdomen and intrathoracic abdomen.[14] The use of DPL to evaluate actual peritoneal violation by a missile is less accurate. A red blood cell (RBC) count equal or greater than 5000/mm^3 is considered a positive result for peritoneal penetration.[15] However, high-velocity missiles may produce a significant blast injury to intraabdominal organs, even without actual penetration.

Stab wounds to the abdomen produce internal injuries only in 25% to 32% of the cases. Even when peritoneal penetration has occurred, visceral or vascular injury occurs in 50% to 75% of the cases; therefore, a selective approach to exploratory laparotomy is used.[3,9,10] Exploratory laparotomy is indicated immediately for any of the following: shock; signs of peritoneal irritation; evisceration through the wound; evidence of gastric hemorrhage; hematuria or rectal bleeding; a retained stabbing implement; impalement injury; free air in the peritoneal cavity or retroperitoneum on plain radiographs; and a palpable diaphragmatic defect on digital exploration during insertion of a chest tube or extravasation of contrast on radiographic evaluation of the kidney, ureters, or bladder.

In the absence of absolute indications for laparotomy, exploration of the stab wound under local anesthesia (local wound exploration) effectively distinguishes superficial lacerations from potentially penetrating injuries. Local wound exploration is not used in the thoracoabdominal region because a iatrogenic pneumothorax may be induced. The relationships of the multiple fascial and muscular layers of the abdominal wall vary as the individual changes from the position at the time of the injury to the supine position at the time of the evaluation. Following the pathway of the wound through several fascial and muscle layers, especially in obese, muscular, or uncooperative patients, is difficult. We recommend limiting the local wound exploration to determine if the external oblique muscle aponeurosis or rectus sheath has been violated. We believe all wounds that extend beyond the external fascia should be treated as if they penetrated the peritoneal cavity.[3] Blunt probing of stab wounds does not accurately predict peritoneal penetration for the reasons related to anatomy standard earlier. Furthermore, probing may dislodge a clot providing hemostasis or may aggravate an intraabdominal injury; it, therefore, is strongly discouraged. If the anterior abdominal fascia is intact, the wound is irrigated, closed, or left open and packed, and the patient is discharged. If the fascia is violated or the wound is located in the thoracoabdominal region, a workup for visceral or diaphragmatic injury is indicated. DPL may be performed; if the result is positive, laparotomy is performed. If the DPL result is negative, the patient is admitted to the hospital for observation and serial abdominal examinations for at least 24 hours. The RBC count in DPL for abdominal and thoracoabdominal stab wounds is considered a positive result if it is 10,000/mm^3 or greater, to reduce the possibility of missing a significant injury and to maintain an acceptable rate of negative or nontherapeutic laparotomies. The other criteria for a positive DPL results are the same in penetrating and blunt trauma: a white blood cell (WBC) count equal or greater than 500/mm³; amylase level equal or greater than 175 U/mL; bilirubin, bacteria, or intestinal contents in the lavage fluid; and lavage fluid exiting through the chest tube or the Foley catheter.[3,10] The accuracy of DPL in the evaluation of abdominal stab wounds is 94.3%.[15]

Many trauma centers use serial physical examinations by the same physician for at least 24 hours in patients with stab wounds to the anterior abdomen with documented penetration, but without indications for exploration. Delayed operation (false-negative rate) has been reported in 0% to 5.5% of the patients, nontherapeutic laparotomy in 0.9% to 5.8% of the patients, and negative laparotomy in 2.3% to 8.5% of the patients. Narcotics are contraindicated when this approach is used. If signs suggestive of peritoneal irritation are present, delayed surgery may result in significant morbidity and mortality.[9,12] Although patients are seldom admitted to the ICU just for observation after having sustained stab wounds to the abdomen, they may need to have this protocol competently executed by the intensivist to diagnose injuries not evident during the admission evaluation.

Patients with stab wounds to the flank and back also receive selective management. Those without absolute indications for laparotomy undergo local wound exploration to ascertain fascial penetration. Individuals with superficial wounds are discharged from the emergency department, whereas patients with penetrating wounds are admitted for workup with triple-contrast abdominal and pelvic CT scan followed by serial abdominal examinations for 24 hours. Triple-contrast CT scan delineates retroperitoneal injury with a diagnostic accuracy greater than 95%. Patients with pelvic stab wounds may be managed using the protocol outlined for transpelvic gunshot wounds.

Some recommend routine laparotomy for all abdominal stab wounds with peritoneal penetration if an observation protocol is impractical. Diagnostic laparoscopy also has been reported to be an accurate technique to determine peritoneal penetration in stab wounds to the anterior abdomen and flanks.[14] Diagnostic laparoscopy also may be used to diagnose diaphragmatic injuries in stab wounds to the thoracoabdominal region. However, because the creation of a pneumoperitoneum in a patient with a diaphragmatic rent may result in a tension pneumothorax, gasless laparoscopy or thoracoscopy may be preferred. The use of laparoscopy instead of exploratory laparotomy for the diagnosis, staging, and treatment of intraabdominal injuries is not supported in the trauma literature.[14,16,17] A significant number of hollow and solid viscus injuries may be missed at laparoscopy, resulting in significant morbidity and mortality.

BLUNT INJURIES ■

The evaluation of blunt abdominal trauma remains a significant challenge. The initial physical examination in patients without associated head injury has been found to be accurate in only 50% of the cases with a 56% false-positive rate and a 34% to 46% false-negative rate.[18] The combination of absent bowel sounds, diffuse guarding, and rebound tenderness (i.e., peritonitis) remains a valued indication for explora-

tion. An altered pain response resulting from associated head injury, alcohol, or psychotropic drugs, diminished sensation and muscle tone caused by spinal cord injury, and pain from adjacent injuries (rib cage, lumbar spine, pelvis or abdominal wall) may result in unreliable or equivocal physical findings. Furthermore, even the awake and alert patient with negative abdominal findings may need operative treatment of associated injuries under general anesthesia. Adjuvant diagnostic techniques are necessary in these situations.[3,10,15]

Absolute indications for laparotomy include abdominal distention with shock, overt peritonitis, evidence of gastrointestinal tract injury (gastric or rectal bleeding or free air in the peritoneal cavity or retroperitoneum on plain radiographs), or herniation of abdominal viscera into the thorax on chest radiograph. Evidence of intraperitoneal bladder rupture on cystogram and extravasation of contrast on duodenography or IVP are also absolute indications for exploration.[13]

In hemorrhagic shock, determining the source of bleeding is a high priority. Consider (1) external, (2) intrathoracic, (3) pelvic, (4) long bone fractures, or (5) intraperitoneal or (6) retroperitoneal sites. The prehospital report, primary survey, secondary survey, and chest and pelvis radiographs will exclude the first four sites. DPL or US may provide a rapid answer to the question of significant intraabdominal hemorrhage in the resuscitation room.

DPL is the oldest technique in use. It may be easily performed and does not require complex technological equipment to perform, process, or interpret. It has an accuracy rate of 96% to 98%, a false-positive rate of 3%, a false-negative rate of 1.5%, and a complication rate of only 1%.[15] The open and the percutaneous Seldinger techniques are comparable. The percutaneous technique should be avoided in the presence of pelvic fracture, in pregnancy, in a pediatric patient, or in a patient with previous surgery. Aspiration of 10 mL or more of nonclotting blood is considered a grossly positive tap. In blunt trauma, a positive result on DPL is defined as a RBC count of 100,000/mm³ or greater. RBC counts between 50,000/mm³ and 100,000/mm³ are equivocal. In equivocal situations, the abdomen should be examined at frequent intervals to determine if an injury is present, or CT scan of the abdomen and pelvis should be obtained to delineate any solid visceral injuries. The other criteria for a positive DPL finding are the same used for penetrating injuries. However, an isolated WBC equal or greater than 500/mm³ in the DPL effluent in blunt trauma has been shown to have a low positive predictive value for intraabdominal injuries.[3,10,15] In the hemodynamically unstable patient with an associated pelvic fracture, only a grossly positive tap is considered indicative of sufficient bleeding from an intraabdominal organ to require exploratory laparotomy. A DPL finding that is positive only by RBC count criterion is likely to be false positive from diapedesis of red cells from the pelvic hematoma or from a minor solid viscus injury. Attention should be directed to the evaluation and control of the hemorrhage associated with the pelvic fracture (Chap. 68).[19]

DPL is unnecessary if absolute indications for laparotomy are present. It is contraindicated in patients with multiple previous abdominal operations because adhesions may preclude complete distribution of the lavage fluid and increase the risk of complications. DPL may (1) be too sensitive, resulting in negative (so-called nontherapeutic) laparotomy results; or (2) fail to detect retroperitoneal and diaphragmatic injuries. In addition, it cannot be used to stage solid organ injuries.[15]

US is used more frequently in the United States as a diagnostic study in the evaluation of blunt abdominal trauma. US is portable, rapid, and as accurate as DPL but is noninvasive. The US examination may be limited to look for free intraabdominal fluid. Optionally, it can be used to diagnose hepatic, splenic, renal, or pancreatic injuries. In centers with sufficient experience with the technique, it is performed in the resuscitation area; it usually takes about 5 minutes for the detection of hemoperitoneum and 15 minutes to evaluate the liver and the spleen.[15,20–22] For the US to be successfully implemented in the workup of trauma patients, an appropriately trained physician (radiologist, emergency department physician, or preferably, trauma surgeon) must be available immediately to evaluate the real time images. In Europe and Japan, surgeons and surgical residents have been successfully trained in US. An abbreviated US examination is used: the subphrenic spaces bilaterally, subhepatic space, paracolic gutters bilaterally, splenic tip, and pelvis all are evaluated for free fluid. More than 70 mL of free fluid can be detected (a positive result). The liver and spleen may be examined for parenchymal injury.[3,15] Huang and associates[23] examined five areas and assign one or two points, depending on the amount of fluid detected. Patients with three or more points were significantly more likely to require a therapeutic laparotomy.[23] Use of US results is still in a state of flux; however, the following scenarios seem reasonable. In a hemodynamically unstable patient, a positive US finding indicates the need for exploratory laparotomy. If no free fluid is found by US in a hemodynamically unstable patient, the source of bleeding needs further investigation, which may include DPL, CT scan, or repeated US. A positive US finding in a hemodynamically stable patient must be followed by a CT scan of the abdomen and pelvis to stage hepatic or splenic injuries because some may be amenable to nonoperative treatment; US has a 20% to 25% failure rate in detecting spleen or liver injuries.[15] A hemodynamically stable patient with a negative finding on US may be followed with serial abdominal examinations in an evaluable patient or repeated US evaluations if the patient has altered pain response or sensorium, or if the US result is equivocal.

US has numerous advantages. It is fast, inexpensive, noninvasive and accurate; it is also easy to repeat if findings or equivocal or the patient's status changes. The sensitivity of ultrasound ranges from 84% to 99% and the specificity from 97% to 100%.[24] Significant obesity and widespread subcutaneous emphysema are contraindications to abdominal ultrasound.

Diagnostic laparoscopy performed in the emergency department under local anesthesia is difficult to complete and does not offer a significant advantage over DPL or US in the diagnosis of hemoperitoneum. Furthermore, additional costly equipment and trained personnel are necessary.[14,16]

In the hemodynamically stable patient, CT scan is the most widely used technique today to diagnose and stage

intraabdominal injuries accurately. Prerequisites for the CT scan of the abdomen and pelvis to be used effectively are a modern scanner to obtain high-quality studies and in-house, experienced radiologists or trauma surgeons to interpret the studies. CT scan is most useful if DPL is contraindicated in the simultaneous evaluation of concurrent head injuries or pelvic fractures, whenever injuries to the liver or retroperitoneal organs are suspected (i.e., elevated liver or pancreatic enzymes, or microscopic or gross hematuria) or in cases of delayed presentation after blunt abdominal injury. CT scan is a more expensive study. It requires transportation of the patient to the radiology department with the resultant difficulties in monitoring and providing care for critically injured patients. It is frequently described as a "noninvasive" diagnostic technique, but this term is relative because endotracheal intubation, sedation, and neuromuscular blockade may be necessary to obtain a technically satisfactory and interpretable study in the uncooperative, injured patient.[3,10,15] CT scan has an overall accuracy rate of 92% to 98% with false-negative rates as low 1.6% and false-positive rates as low as 3.2%.[15] CT scan is particularly valuable in the followup of ICU patients undergoing nonoperative management of intraabdominal solid viscus injuries, if there are unexplained decreases in the hematocrit, and in the investigation of septic complications of abdominal trauma.

The main disadvantage of CT scan is its inability to detect hollow viscus injuries reliably. Free fluid in the abdomen and pelvis without evidence of solid organ injury is a relative indication for exploratory laparotomy because it may represent a hollow gastrointestinal viscus injury, a mesenteric injury, or a bladder rupture.[3,15,25]

All patients whose trauma was significant enough to warrant investigation but whose DPL, US, or abdominal and pelvic CT scan results were negative must be admitted and examined serially for at least 24 hours to detect evolving signs of peritoneal irritation or intraperitoneal blood loss.

Angiography is both diagnostic and therapeutic in the management of arterial hemorrhage from pelvic fractures. It may also be used in the patient with hematuria and nonvisualization of the kidney on IVP to establish the diagnosis of renovascular injury. Occasionally, arteriography may be used to localize and control solid organ bleeding after exploratory laparotomy. Angiographic studies are expensive, they require additional personnel, and demand transportation of critically injured patients to the radiology suite with the consequent risks.[3,9,10,15]

DIAGNOSTIC LAPAROTOMY

The most sensitive diagnostic test is still exploratory laparotomy performed by a competent surgeon. Specific mobilization maneuvers are necessary to detect injuries to the duodenum, pancreas, and abdominal vasculature, which may be suspected because of injury. A cursory, random or incomplete examination may miss injuries. Exploratory laparotomy is 99% sensitive; however, a negative exploration finding carries measurable morbidity and mortality. A negative laparotomy rate of 7% to 10% is acceptable to avoid missing a life-threatening injury; after all, a negative rate of 15% has been traditionally quoted as acceptable for appendicitis. If

TABLE 70-1. Incidence of Organ Injury in Penetrating
Abdominal Trauma

ORGAN	PERCENTAGE
Small bowel	30
Mesentery, omentum	18
Liver	16
Colon	9
Diaphragm	8
Stomach	7
Spleen	6
Kidney	5
Major blood vessel	4
Pancreas	3
Duodenum	2
Bladder	1
Ureter	1
Biliary tract	1

Reprinted with permission from Blaisdell FW, Trunkey DD:
Abdominal Trauma. New York, Thieme-Stratton, 1982:11.

TABLE 70-2. Incidence of Organ Injury in Blunt
Abdominal Trauma

ORGAN	PERCENTAGE
Spleen	25
Liver	15
Retroperitoneal hematoma	13
Kidney	12
Small bowel	9
Bladder	6
Mesentery	5
Large bowel	4
Pancreas	3
Urethra	2
Diaphragm	2
Major blood vessel	2
Stomach	1
Duodenum	1

Reprinted with permission from Blaisdell FW, Trunkey DD:
Abdominal Trauma. New York, Thieme-Stratton, 1982:13.

the clinical status is deteriorating and there is a high index of suspicion for intraabdominal injury, laparotomy should be performed. Clinical suspicion and physical findings remain the most important factors in decision-making because no adjuvant diagnostic measures are 100% sensitive.

INCIDENCE OF ORGAN INJURY

The incidence of organ injury in abdominal trauma based on penetrating or blunt mechanism is presented in Tables 70-1 and 70-2. The solid viscera (spleen, liver, kidney, and pancreas) account for 55% of the injuries in blunt trauma and for 30% of the injuries in penetrating trauma, whereas the hollow viscera (bowel, stomach, duodenum, and bladder) account for 23% of the injuries in blunt trauma and for 52% of the injuries in penetrating trauma.

MORTALITY AND MORBIDITY IN ABDOMINAL TRAUMA ■

Feliciano and Rozycki[9] report mortality rates of civilian penetrating abdominal trauma treated by laparotomy in a major urban county hospital as 2% for stab wounds and 12% for gunshot wounds. In the absence of major vascular injury, the mortality rate was 2.6%. On the other hand, Cox[26] reports a mortality rate of 25% for blunt abdominal trauma patients treated by laparotomy in a level I urban trauma center. If intraoperative deaths are excluded, the mortality rate was 17%; the causes of death include bleeding, associated head injury, pneumonia, respiratory failure, sepsis, and multiple organ failure. Intensive care plays a significant role in the managing these patients.[26]

The mortality rate of abdominal trauma is proportional to the number of abdominal organs injured. In a series of

300 patients undergoing laparotomy for gunshot wounds, Feliciano and associates[27] report mortality rates of 3.4% for one wound, 5.6% for two, 11.9% for three, 28.6% for four, 33.3% for five, 28.6% for six, and 75% for seven. Burch and associates[28] in a study of 706 laparotomies for colonic injuries report that mortality rates increased with the number of associated injured organs: 0.7% for zero (colon only), 4% for one, 14% for two, 16% for three, 34% for four, 67% for five, 43% for six, 100% for seven or greater. Of 70 deaths, 60% occurred within 48 hours caused by shock and hemorrhage (early deaths), and 40% occurred later because of sepsis, multiple organ failure, shock, and miscellaneous reasons. The complication rate was 44% after the early deaths were excluded. The most common complications included coagulopathies, acidosis, atelectasis, adult respiratory distress syndrome (ARDS), cardiovascular collapse, acute renal failure, pneumonia, phlebitis, small bowel obstruction, and postoperative abdominal hemorrhage. Nine percent of the patients developed an intraabdominal abscess.[28]

These associations constitute the basis of intensive care practice. Patients with major injuries have major physiologic abnormalities soon after operation, including prolonged shock, profound acidosis, hypothermia, coagulopathy, diffuse nonsurgical bleeding, and respiratory failure. Conversely, nonoperated trauma patients who remain unstable or become unstable during their ICU stay should be evaluated for intraabdominal hemorrhage or injury to a solid or hollow viscus. Prompt diagnosis is essential so that immediate laparotomy, staging, and repair can reduce morbidity and mortality.

The decision not to operate is constantly reassessed in the ICU. Look for signs of intraabdominal hemorrhage or peritoneal irritation and laboratory or radiologic manifestations of intraabdominal injury.

SPECIFIC INJURIES ■

The anatomic and technical surgical details are extremely important to the ICU team. The type and severity of the injuries determine the surgical procedures required, the postoperative course, and the likely complications to be expected. Although accurate and complete postoperative notes and diagrams found in the medical record are important, direct communication between the trauma surgeon and the intensivist reveal the intraoperative difficulties encountered and the surgeon's impressions and expectations, as well as details about the surgical tubes, drains, and stomas. The intensivist must know what complications to expect and when they will most likely occur to provide intensive care tailored to the individual patient.

In 1987, the Organ Injury Scaling Committee of the American Association for the Surgery of Trauma began to devise injury severity scores for individual organs or body structures. A grade from I through VI is assigned, depending on a detailed anatomic description. Grades I through V represent increasingly complex injuries and grade VI is considered irreparable damage incompatible with survival. A recently published compilation of the scales is used here to characterize the intraabdominal injuries and to describe the operative and postoperative care[30] (see Organ Injury Scaling Tables in the Critical Care Catalog). The tables for hepatic and splenic injuries are duplicated in this chapter because they are frequently used in the nonoperative management of those injuries (Tables 70-3 and 70-4).

ABDOMINAL WALL AND LOWER CHEST WALL

In firearm wounds, only 10% to 12% of the injuries are tangential (confined to the chest or abdominal walls) without associated intraabdominal visceral or vascular injury. The

TABLE 70-3. Liver Injury Scale (1994 Revision)

	GRADE°	INJURY DESCRIPTION	ICD-9	AIS-90
I	Hematoma	Subcapsular, <10% surface area	864.01 864.11	2
	Laceration	Capsular tear, <1 cm parenchymal depth	864.02 864.12	2
II	Hematoma	Subcapsular, 10–50% surface area; intraparenchymal, <10 cm in diameter	864.01 864.11	2
	Laceration	1–3 cm parenchymal depth, <10 cm in length	864.03 864.13	2
III	Hematoma	Subcapsular, >50% surface area or expanding; ruptured subcapsular or parenchymal hematoma Intraparenchymal hematoma >10 cm or expanding		3
	Laceration	>3 cm parenchymal depth	864.04 864.14	3
IV	Laceration	Parenchymal disruption involving 25–75% of hepatic lobe or 1–3 Couinaud's segments within a single lobe	864.04 864.14	4
V	Laceration	Parenchymal disruption involving >75% of hepatic lobe or >3 Couinaud's segments within a single lobe		5
	Vascular	Juxtahepatic venous injuries; i.e., retrohepatic vena cava/central major hepatic veins		5
VI	Vascular	Hepatic avulsion		6

°Advance one grade for multiple injuries, up to grade III.

ICD-9, International Classification of Diseases, Ninth Revision; AIS-90, Abbreviated Injury Scale, 1990 Version.

Reprinted with permission from Moore EE, Cogbill TH, Jurkovich GJ, et al: Organ injury scaling: spleen and liver (1994 revision). *J Trauma Injury Infection Crit Care* 1995;38:323.

TABLE 70-4. Spleen Injury Scale (1994 Revision)

	GRADE°	INJURY DESCRIPTION	ICD-9	AIS-90
I	Hematoma	Subcapsular, <10% surface area	865.01 865.11	2
	Laceration	Capsular tear, <1 cm parenchymal depth	865.02 865.12	2
II	Hematoma	Subcapsular, 10–50% surface area; intraparenchymal, <5 cm in diameter	865.01 865.11	2
	Laceration	1–3 cm parenchymal depth, which does not involve a trabecular vessel	865.02 865.12	
III	Hematoma	Subcapsular, >50% surface area or expanding; ruptured subcapsular or parenchymal hematoma Intraparenchymal hematoma >5 cm or expanding		3
	Laceration	>3 cm parenchymal depth or involving trabecular vessels	865.03 865.13	3
IV	Laceration	Laceration involving segmental or hilar vessels producing major devascularization (>25% of spleen)		4
V	Laceration	Completely shattered spleen	865.04 864.14	5
	Vascular	Hilar vascular injury which devascularizes spleen		5

°Advance one grade for multiple injuries, up to grade III.

ICD-9, International Classification of Diseases, Ninth Revision; AIS-90, Abbreviated Injury Scale, 1990 Version.

Reprinted with permission from Moore EE, Cogbill TH, Jurkovich GJ, et al: Organ injury scaling: spleen and liver. *J Trauma Injury Infection Crit Care* 1995;38:323.

treatment of the chest or abdominal wall injury is limited to debridement of the skin and subcutaneous rim of contusion followed by dressing changes. High-velocity tangential firearm injuries or short-range shotgun injuries may result in significant destruction of the soft tissues of the abdominal wall. After the intraabdominal injuries have been repaired, the wounds are thoroughly débrided and repaired. Temporary or permanent prosthetic materials may be needed if full-thickness destruction is not amenable to primary repair.[3]

Stab wounds produce intraabdominal visceral or vascular injury in only 25% to 32% of cases. When exploratory laparotomy is indicated, the abdominal wall defect is repaired from inside the abdomen after the intraabdominal injuries have been addressed.[3]

Blunt injuries to the thoracoabdominal region may be associated with splenic, hepatic, and renal injuries. Blaisdell and Trunkey[3] found a 7% incidence rate of intraabdominal disorders in a group of 287 patients with fractures of the lower six ribs. They also found a 20% incidence rate of splenic rupture in patients with fractures of the left ninth and tenth ribs. Lower rib fractures may also cause chest wall pain and splinting that should be controlled with thoracic

epidural analgesia, interpleural anesthesia, or intercostal nerve blocks to avoid atelectasis, pneumonitis, and respiratory failure. Flail chest is often associated with an underlying pulmonary contusion that may require the use of positive end-expiratory pressure with or without intubation (mechanical ventilation, continuous positive airway pressure mask, or bilevel positive airway pressure system). Intraabdominal visceral injury must be ruled out before thoracic epidural analgesia is initiated because abdominal pain and the signs of peritoneal irritation may be obscured.

The abdominal wall is malleable and usually transmits most of the damaging energy to the intraabdominal contents. Therefore, blunt abdominal trauma that results in significant abdominal wall injury such as a contusion indicates high-energy transfer and is likely to be associated with a intraabdominal injury. The epigastric vessels are an exception; they may be injured by low-energy trauma. Lacerations of these vessels result in hematomas confined to the rectus muscle sheaths and present with abdominal pain, a palpable mass that increases in prominence when the patient tenses the abdominal musculature, and findings that simulate peritoneal irritation. Abdominal exploration may be necessary because it is impossible to differentiate between the signs of rectus sheath hematoma and those of intraabdominal visceral injury.[31]

The *seat belt sign* is a skin abrasion or ecchymotic mark on the abdominal wall at the location of the lap belt. It indicates an injury to the abdominal wall varying from contusion or hematoma to complete musculoaponeurotic disruption. Patients with this sign must be carefully evaluated for intraabdominal injury.[32,33]

Shearing injuries to the abdominal wall with separation of the skin and subcutaneous tissue from the underlying fascia with or without skin disruption may be seen in pedestrians run over by motor vehicles or in industrial accidents. If the skin has been violated, exploration, hemostasis, and debridement are indicated followed by local care with dressing changes and delayed reconstruction, depending on the amount of tissue loss. Shearing abdominal wall injuries with intact skin may be diagnosed at the time of laparotomy; they complicate the abdominal wall closure or the placement of ostomies. They may not be diagnosed initially but present as subcutaneous hematomas large enough to result in shock or as areas of skin slough caused by disruption of the cutaneous blood supply.

Blunt injury may also result in traumatic hernias, the protrusion of intraabdominal contents through disrupted musculature, and fascia without skin disruption. The diagnosis is confirmed at exploration by the absence of an identifiable hernia sac.[34,35] They may be caused by a small blunt object (i.e., motorcycle or bicycle handle bar) or by a seat belt. A hernia may also result from avulsion of the muscle fascia in pelvic fractures. US and CT scan are the imaging modalities most helpful in differentiating hematomas, shearing injuries, and traumatic hernias. Hernias should be repaired because bowel and mesenteric injuries may also have occurred and to avoid late incarceration and strangulation.[35]

Evisceration through a stab wound may occur in the ICU if the abdominal wall injury was overlooked at end of laparotomy. Septic complications of abdominal wall shotgun wounds or high-velocity missile wounds vary from simple abscesses to necrotizing soft tissue infections.

DIAPHRAGM

Diaphragmatic injuries are found in 6% and 8% of the patients undergoing laparotomy for blunt and penetrating trauma, respectively.[3] Associated intraabdominal injuries occur in 59% to 88.5% of the patients with blunt diaphragmatic rupture. A study by Boulanger and coworkers[36] showed that in 80 blunt diaphragmatic injuries, 74% were left sided, 20% were right sided, and 6% were bilateral.

In penetrating injuries, associated intraabdominal injuries—primarily to the liver, spleen, and stomach—occur in 89% of the patients.[37]

Most blunt diaphragmatic injuries are grades III and IV, whereas most penetrating diaphragmatic injuries are grade II. Early herniation of abdominal viscera into the thorax is more common in blunt than penetrating diaphragmatic injuries. The stomach, spleen, colon, and small bowel may herniate in left-sided injuries, but usually only the liver and right colon herniate in right-sided injuries.

The diagnosis of diaphragmatic injury is difficult. In 75% to 85% of the cases, the findings on chest radiograph are abnormal but may not be specific. Abnormalities consistent with a diaphragmatic injury include an obscured or abnormal hemidiaphragmatic shadow, a radiolucency or a radiodensity in the lung field, one or more air–fluid levels in the lung field, or the presence of a nasogastric tube in the chest cavity. A contrast study demonstrating displacement of the stomach, small bowel, or colon inside the chest confirms the diagnosis. A normal result on the initial chest radiograph is common; findings may be recognized only in the ICU on follow-up radiographs. DPL fluid exiting through a chest tube is pathognomonic of the injury. A diaphragmatic rent may be palpated during insertion of a chest tube. Other diagnostic methods include direct visualization of the diaphragm by thoracoscopy, laparoscopy, or laparotomy. In the patient with a chest tube, thoracoscopy is the preferred diagnostic procedure.[14,38] During laparoscopy, the posterior portions of the diaphragm may not be visualized, a tension pneumothorax may develop during insufflation, or an air embolism could occur if a hepatic vein injury has occurred.[39] Gasless laparoscopy is, therefore, preferred.[14] Careful inspection and palpation of both hemidiaphragms during laparotomy or thoracotomy are necessary to avoid missing injuries.[37,40]

All grade II to V diaphragmatic lacerations should be repaired to prevent visceral herniation, which may be followed by incarceration and strangulation.[3] The worst complication is missing the diagnosis, resulting in traumatic diaphragmatic hernias that present months to years after blunt or penetrating abdominal trauma. Madden and associates,[40] in a review of delayed diaphragmatic hernias resulting from stab wounds, report a 20% rate of strangulation and a 36% mortality rate.

LIVER

The liver is the most commonly injured organ in abdominal trauma in general. However, hepatic injuries are second in frequency to splenic injuries in blunt abdominal trauma and to small bowel injuries in penetrating abdominal trauma. Liver injuries vary in severity from trivial to lethal and have an overall mortality rate of 10%. Blunt hepatic trauma carries a mortality rate between 20% and 40%.[3] Gunshot wounds have an intermediate mortality rate (8% to 11%), and stab wounds are associated with the lowest mortality rate (2.8% to 5%).[9]

Minor Hepatic Trauma

Grade I and II lacerations and hematomas constitute 90% of penetrating hepatic and 60% of blunt hepatic trauma. Simple surgical techniques suffice, such as temporary packing, application of topical hemostatic agents, high-current electrocautery or the argon beam coagulator, or suture hepatorrhaphy. The mortality rate is less than 10% and is usually related to associated injuries. The use of drains are no longer recommended because bile leaks are rare and they do not evacuate delayed bleeding but increase septic complications.

Major Hepatic Trauma

Grade III, IV, and V injuries constitute 10% of the penetrating trauma cases and 40% of the blunt trauma cases. In a large multicenter series, Cogbill and associates[41] found overall mortality rates of 25%, 46%, and 80%, and mortality rates resulting from the liver injury itself of 6.5%, 30.5%, and 66% for grade III, IV, and V injuries, respectively. Blunt and penetrating trauma were equally represented. Injury to two or more of the eight anatomic segments, described by Hepp and Couinaud, correlated with mortality rates in two reports of liver injuries.[42,43] The leading cause of death in major liver injuries is exsanguinating hemorrhage with transfusion-associated coagulopathy. Late deaths are caused by single or multiple organ failure triggered by sepsis, head injury, or delayed bleeding. Survivors have an overall complication rate of 20%. The specific complications of hepatic injury include intraabdominal abscesses, delayed hemorrhage, biliary fistula, hepatic necrosis, hemobilia and, rarely, hepatic failure. In patients with major hepatic trauma, rapid control of hemorrhage determines the survival. No single technique may be applied in all instances, but general principles include the following:

1. Temporary hemostasis must be secured by manual or pack compression of the organ and cross-clamping of the arterial and portal vascular inflow (Pringle maneuver) while intravascular volume is restored by the anesthesiologist and before definitive repair is undertaken. The Pringle maneuver can be maintained for up to 1 hour. Pachter and associates[44] recommend the use of hepatic protection with high-dosage steroids or topical hypothermia during the use of the Pringle maneuver.
2. The injury must be properly exposed. A xyphopubic laparotomy incision is used with extension into the chest by midsternotomy or right thoracotomy, as necessary. The suspending ligaments are divided for organ mobilization.
3. The anesthesiologist and the circulating nurses must keep the surgeon informed of the blood lost and replaced.
4. Prevention and correction of hypothermia are essential because coagulopathy resulting from platelet dysfunction and prolongation of the prothrombin time occurs when the core temperature falls below 35C. All intravenous solutions, blood, and blood products must be infused through high-efficiency warming devices.
5. Coagulopathy must be aggressively corrected with rewarming and infusion of fresh frozen plasma, cryoprecipitate, and platelets.
6. Automated RBC washing and reinfusion devices should be used to avoid depleting the blood bank.

Advanced surgical techniques to achieve hemostasis include the following:

1. Deep suture hepatorrhaphy
2. Hepatotomy or tractotomy using the finger fracture technique to expose actively bleeding vessels, followed by selective vascular ligation
3. Resectional debridement with selective vascular ligation to remove devitalized parenchyma
4. Selective hepatic artery ligation if bleeding stops with the Pringle maneuver but the vessel cannot be directly controlled
5. Hemostasis of large raw surfaces with argon beam coagulator or application of fibrin glue
6. Viable omental pack to fill large gaping wounds and cover oozing raw surfaces
7. Polyglycolic mesh wrapping
8. Perihepatic packing

Major anatomic resections are associated with a 50% to 60% mortality rate and must be avoided.[3]

Perihepatic packing with laparotomy pads is a life-saving maneuver in the management of major hepatic trauma. The technique allows temporary control of bleeding and transfer of the patient to a higher echelon of care. Perihepatic packing and rapid closure of the abdomen with skin sutures, towel clip skin closure, or prosthetic material is considered when the blood replacement is between 10 and 15 units of blood, the core temperature is less than 32°C, the arterial pH below 7.2, and clinical evidence shows diffuse coagulopathy. Patients with major injuries who undergo perihepatic packing have a 10% to 30% rate of abscess formation and a 29% to 40% mortality rate.[3,9] In contemporary trauma jargon, this procedure is called "damage control."

The use of drains in major liver injuries continues to be debated. The current recommendation is to use closed drainage systems for major liver injuries.[45] Bleeding from stab or missile tracts may be controlled by tamponade with Penrose drains or with balloon catheters. The end of the catheter may be exteriorized through a counter incision so that removal can be done after 72 to 96 hours after hemostasis has taken place.[9,45]

Hepatic Vascular Injuries

Retrohepatic and hepatic vein injuries (grade V vascular injuries) are associated with torrential bleeding and high mortality rates, independent of the associated parenchymal liver injury; these injuries require intraoperative shunting or vascular isolation of the liver followed by repair of the vascular injury. Even perihepatic packing has been used successfully in selected instances.[3,45,46]

Hepatic artery injuries are treated by ligation. Portal vein injuries are treated by venorrhaphy, if feasible; otherwise, ligation is indicated. Combined injuries to the portal vein and hepatic artery are treated by repair of at least the portal vein. Portal vein injuries are associated with a 54% to 71% mortality rate.[47,48]

Hepatic avulsion (grade VI vascular injury) had been uniformly lethal until liver transplantation for liver trauma. These patients tolerate prolonged anhepatic phases in the intensive care while awaiting for a suitable donor.[41,45]

Postoperative Complications

The ICU problems in the immediate postoperative period after severe liver trauma include prolonged shock, metabolic and lactic acidosis, coagulopathy, hypothermia, continued or recurrent bleeding, respiratory failure, and oliguria. These problems are interrelated and must be simultaneously addressed. Resuscitation includes (1) administering prewarmed intravenous fluids, blood, and blood products using high-efficiency fluid warmers; and (2) preventing further heat loss by maintaining high ambient temperature, using heating blankets, completely wrapping the patient with reflective blankets or plastic bags and regular blankets, and heated humidification of inspired gases. The pneumatic antishock garment (PASG) is considered to diminish local bleeding, to limit further consumption of clotting factors, and to prevent perihepatic hematoma formation with an increased likelihood of sepsis. Persistent bleeding is manifested by continued hemodynamic instability, unrelenting lactic acidosis, progressive abdominal distension, and falling hematocrit. If perihepatic packing has not been used, it may be prudent to reexplore the patient to pack the liver. Delayed hemorrhage may present with hemodynamic instability and bleeding through the perihepatic drains. Intraabdominal hypertension with suprarenal vena cava compression and oliguria despite optimization of blood volume, cardiac output, renal perfusion, and diuretics may complicate perihepatic packing. In this circumstance, the intraabdominal pressure should be measured through the Foley catheter and the packing removed if the pressure is greater than 25 mm Hg. Perihepatic packing is removed after correction of shock, acidosis, coagulopathy, and hypothermia; often the patient has achieved cardiovascular, respiratory, and renal stability, usually between 24 and 48 hours.[3,9,43,45]

Portal vein ligation is associated with splanchnic hypertension, sequestration of blood in the portal venous system, and large interstitial losses in the gastrointestinal tract. Early aggressive fluid and blood resuscitation guided by invasive hemodynamic monitoring are necessary.

Hyperpyrexia in the first 3 to 5 days after liver trauma is usually attributed to absorption of devitalized parenchyma; thereafter, pulmonary or intraabdominal sepsis should be suspected. Perihepatic abscess formation is related to the grade of liver injury, the transfusions given, the associated hollow viscus injuries, and the use of open or sump draining systems. The patients harboring intraabdominal abscesses are febrile and may manifest persistent ileus or abdominal distension, right upper quadrant tenderness, frankly purulent perihepatic drainage, leukocytosis, sympathetic pleural effusions, and positive blood cultures. Abdominal CT scan and US may be used to establish the presence of perihepatic or intrahepatic collections, to aspirate the pus or bile by percutaneous tap, and to insert percutaneous drains. If the perihepatic abscess does not resolve with percutaneous drainage and intravenous antibiotics, it should be treated by surgical drainage, preferably through an extraperitoneal approach (subcostal, flank, or posterior incision through the bed of the 12th rib).[3,9,45] If intraabdominal sepsis is considered highly likely despite equivocal or negative results of radiologic studies, reexploration may be undertaken on clinical grounds.

Biliary fistula complicates fewer than 10% of major liver injuries. As healing takes place, most small leaks close. A search for a biloma with CT scan or US and study of the integrity of the biliary tree with hepatobiliary scan are indicated when bilious drainage persists more than 10 days or if the output is greater than 200 mL per day. Bilomas can be drained percutaneously. Major intrahepatic ductal injuries must be further investigated with ERCP and treated with papillotomy to reduce the intraductal pressure and occasionally with internal stenting at the site of injury. In the absence of distal obstruction, most fistulas will close in less than 3 weeks, and reoperation is rarely necessary.

Hemobilia is an uncommon complication of liver trauma. It occurs when an intrahepatic pseudoaneurysm ruptures into the biliary tree. A common presentation is right upper quadrant pain, jaundice, and gastrointestinal hemorrhage. Esophagogastroduodenoscopy is performed to rule out other causes of upper gastrointestinal bleeding and may demonstrate ampullary hemorrhage. Angiography is used to confirm the diagnosis; selective embolization of the injured branch of the hepatic artery can stop bleeding.[3,43,45] Delayed massive bleeding through a drain can be managed in the same manner.

Nonoperative Management of Liver Injuries

With the increased use of CT scan in evaluating blunt abdominal trauma, numerous intermediate- and high-grade liver injuries (II, III and IV) are diagnosed in hemodynamically stable patients. Even if a large amount of free blood is present, stable patients can be managed nonoperatively in the ICU for close observation and serial abdominal examinations, hematocrits, and abdominal CT scans. The amount of blood contained in the peritoneal cavity is estimated on abdomen and pelvis CT scan using a system designed by Federle and Jeffrey.[49] Seven spaces are considered: right subphrenic, left subphrenic, subhepatic, right paracolic, left paracolic, paravesicular (pelvis), and intermesenteric. Blood in fewer than two spaces correlates with less than 250 mL, blood in two to four spaces with 250 to 500 mL, and blood in more than four spaces with more than 500 mL.[49] If hemodynamic instability or generalized peritoneal signs develop, or if transfusion requirements exceed a set limit (usually 3 to 4 units of packed RBCs), observation should be abandoned and either exploratory laparotomy or angiography and embolization performed. Stable patients stay in the ICU or intensive care for 2 to 5 days, depending on the severity of the injury. A follow-up CT scan at 1 week may show a stable injury or early signs of resolution.[50]

SPLEEN

The spleen is the most commonly injured organ in blunt abdominal trauma and a frequently injured organ in penetrating abdominal trauma. Blunt splenic trauma is associated with other injuries: abdominal (25%), skeletal fractures (40%), thoracic injuries (40%), and head injuries (40%). The splenic injuries resulting from penetrating trauma are usually less severe. Early and late postoperative morbidity and mortality from sepsis occur after splenectomy for trauma.[51] The spleen is an important part of the immune system.[51] Preservation of a functioning organ requires conservation of 30% to 40% of the splenic tissue and preservation of the anatomy but does not necessarily depend on the splenic artery as its main blood supply.[52] Accessory spleens, splenosis, or splenic implants do not assume all of the functions of the intact or partially preserved spleen. The asplenic state after trauma carries a risk of developing overwhelming postsplenectomy infection (OPSI), a condition caused not only by capsulated organisms such as *Pneumococcus* (50% of the cases), *Meningococcus*, and *Hemophilus*, but also by *Escherichia coli*, *Staphylococcus*, and *Streptococcus*.[51] The incidence rate of OPSI after trauma varies from 0.17% to 1%, and the mortality rate varies from 50% to 100%.[53]

The treatment of splenic injuries is dictated by the severity of the damage, the presence of associated injuries, and the hemodynamic condition of the patient.[3] There are three modalities of treatment of splenic injuries: splenectomy, operative splenic preservation, and nonoperative management.

Splenectomy remains the treatment of choice when the spleen is severely damaged (grade IV and V splenic injuries), when the patient is in profound shock, when multiple associated injuries demand immediate attention, or when hypothermia, coagulopathy, or preexisting medical conditions contraindicate a prolonged surgical procedure. Drainage of the splenic bed is no substitute for adequate hemostasis and is contraindicated except if there is an associated injury of the tail of the pancreas. In this situation, closed drainage systems are used; if no pancreatic fistula occurs (elevated amylase level in the drainage), they may be removed after 5 days.

Methods of splenic salvage include the following: (1) application of hemostatic agents (grades I and II); (2) hemostasis with high-current electrocautery or argon beam coagulator (grade II); (3) splenorrhaphy by suture repair with pledgets (grades III and IV); (4) wrapping of the spleen with absorbable mesh (grades III and IV), and (5) partial splenectomy. Splenic artery ligation may be used as an adjunct to splenorrhaphy.[52] The rate of operative splenic salvage rate has been reported to be between 15% and 88%, but most of the large series report rates between 45% and 50% with a 1.1% incidence rate of reoperation for bleeding.[53] Repair of the spleen after penetrating injury is possible in 50% to 75% of the cases.[9]

The overall complication rate after splenectomy is 49%, of which 20% are infectious. Splenorrhaphy has a lower rate of complications. Atelectasis, pneumonia, and pleural effusion are the most common complications. Pancreatitis occurs in 2% to 17% of the cases and can be treated conservatively, provided that there was no traumatic or operative injury to the main pancreatic duct in the tail of the gland. ERCP may be performed if there is any doubt. Left subphrenic abscesses are relatively common after splenectomy (3% to 13%) but are rarely seen after splenorrhaphy. Associated gastrointestinal injury and drains increase the incidence. The diagnosis of intraabdominal septic collections is confirmed by CT scan or US, and percutaneous drainage is usually successful. If percutaneous drainage fails, extraperitoneal surgical drainage through the flank or back is preferred because of the posterior location of the collections. Gastric necrosis and gastric fistula may occur if the stomach is injured during ligation of the short gastric vessels. This complication is managed with adequate external drainage and gastric decompression. Postsplenectomy thrombocytosis occurs in more than 50% of the patients but usually

resolves within 2 to 12 weeks. No specific therapy is recommended.[3,51,53]

Nonoperative Management of Splenic Injuries

Nonoperative management of splenic injuries is the standard approach in children: 70% of pediatric splenic injuries are treated nonoperatively, and the success rate is 90%. CT scan enables hemodynamically stable adults without peritoneal signs with isolated grades I to III splenic injuries to be managed in the same fashion. Initial observation, including repeated physical examinations, vital signs, and hematocrits, should take place in an ICU or intermediate care unit. If the patient develops hemodynamic instability or diffuse peritoneal signs, or if the hematocrit falls to a point where transfusion may be necessary, then laparotomy is indicated.[53,54] The goals are to avoid blood transfusion by early laparotomy, to perform splenectomy or splenorrhaphy at operation, and to reinfuse washed scavenged RBCs. Only 12% to 15% of the adult splenic injuries may be managed nonoperatively, but the success rate is 70%. Patients older than 55 years of age should be excluded from nonoperative management.[55]

The reduction in the risk of OPSI by splenic preservation must be balanced against the increased risk of transmission of blood-borne viral diseases associated with transfusions during attempts at operative or nonoperative splenic preservation or when reoperation for postoperative bleeding is necessary. Automated RBC saving devices may decrease the need for homologous transfusion.[56] Transfusions should not be based on hematocrit alone but should be reserved for hemodynamic instability.

OPSI is characterized by a bacteremic shower with malaise, prostration, headache, fever, and gastrointestinal symptoms (i.e., nausea, vomiting, and diarrhea) with rapid progression to coma, cardiovascular collapse, and death within 24 hours of onset. Antibiotics, even when administered early, may fail to arrest the rapid progressive nature of this syndrome. The incidence of OPSI may be reduced with the polyvalent antipneumococcal vaccine. The vaccine is usually administered at the time of discharge. Long-term prophylactic antibiotics seem to be effective in preventing OPSI in children but are impracticable in adults. The patient must be told that his or her immune defenses have been impaired and to seek primary medical care at the first manifestation of an infectious illness in the future.[51]

PANCREAS

Pancreatic injuries occur in 3% to 12% of all cases of severe abdominal trauma.[3] Isolated pancreatic injuries are rare because of the retroperitoneal location of this solid organ. Injuries to the liver, stomach, diaphragm, spleen, kidney, small bowel, major abdominal vessels, colon, or duodenum occur in virtually all cases of penetrating pancreatic trauma. The incidence of associated injuries is also high in blunt trauma; the solid organs (liver, spleen, and kidneys) and the duodenum are the most commonly associated injured organs. The overall mortality rate is as high as 22% for penetrating injuries and 19% for blunt injuries.[57] Death after pancreatic injuries is caused by hemorrhage from major abdominal vessels and liver injuries in 72.1% of the cases. Septic intraabdominal complications cause 15.6% of the deaths, multiple organ failure 8.3%, and central nervous system injury and secondary hemorrhage account for the remaining 4%.[3]

Patients with penetrating pancreatic injuries are explored based on the mechanism of injury (gunshot wounds), the presence of shock, signs of peritoneal irritation, or the results of DPL or abdominal CT scan (stab wounds). Amylase and lipase determinations are not necessary because they are not specific for pancreatic injury.[58] Elevated serum amylase and lipase levels or a progressive rise in serum amylase or lipase levels on serial determinations increase the index of suspicion for pancreatic or proximal enteric perforation and may prompt an abdominal CT scan, contrast duodenography, ERCP, or, less frequently, DPL.[3] Abdominal CT scan is the best study available for the hemodynamically stable patient with a suspected blunt pancreatic injury. If the study result is negative, repeat CT scan 24 hours later may be performed if injury is still suspected on clinical grounds. If the initial or follow-up study reveals traumatic pancreatitis, a possible pancreatic laceration, or gives an equivocal result, then ERCP is performed to visualize the main pancreatic duct. If the main pancreatic duct is injured (ERCP shows extravasation of contrast or duct occlusion), then the patient must undergo laparotomy.[3,59,60]

Pancreatic injuries may be missed during laparotomy if all of the portions of the gland (head, neck, body, and tail) are not exposed and examined. The operative strategy for pancreatic trauma consists of (1) arresting hemorrhage, (2) selective debridement, and (3) controlling the exocrine pancreatic secretions.

Grade I and II injuries are managed by evacuation of hematomas, local hemostasis, and closed drainage. Grade III injuries (distal transection or parenchymal injury with duct injury) are treated by distal pancreatectomy and closed drainage. In hemodynamically stable patients, the spleen may be preserved if it has not been injured.[9,61] Grade IV injuries (proximal transection or parenchymal injury involving the ampulla) are treated with near-total pancreatectomy and closed drainage, preservation of the distal pancreas with Roux-en-Y pancreaticojejunostomy, or, rarely, a pancreaticoduodenectomy (Whipple procedure). The intraoperative diagnosis of pancreatic duct injury is based on the anatomic location of the injury, an intraoperative cholangiogram performed through the gall bladder, or on-the-table ERCP. The duodenum should not be opened because this would convert an isolated pancreatic injury into a combined pancreaticoduodenal injury. Transecting the tail of the pancreas to cannulate the duct is impractical.[3,9] Grade V injuries are usually associated with grade V injuries of the duodenum and distal common bile duct disruption; pancreaticoduodenectomy is usually necessary. The distal pancreas in these resections may be treated by duct ligation and external drainage in hemodynamically unstable patients or by pancreaticojejunostomy or pancreaticogastrostomy.[62,63] In the most severe combined pancreatic, duodenal, and biliary tract injuries associated with other life-threatening vascular injuries and hemodynamic instability, it may be necessary to resort to resection and "damage control" as recommended by Carrillo and associates.[64] The restoration of the ductal and enteric continuity of the gastrointestinal tract is postponed until the patient has been stabilized in the ICU. Pancreatic injuries must be drained. Closed sump drains are the most effective but are associated with increased septic complications; therefore, closed suction drainage systems are preferred.[65] The drains are kept in place until the patient has received a diet that stimulates pancreatic secretion without an increase in the volume or amylase level in the drainage.

The morbidity rate for pancreatic injuries is 30% to 64%. Early hemorrhagic complications are related to associated major vascular and liver injuries. Postoperative hemorrhage may occur in up to 5% to 10% of cases because of erosion of vascular stumps or adjacent vessels by pancreatic drainage or abscess formation. Surgical or angiographic control are necessary. Specific complications include pancreatic fistula (7% to 20%), intraabdominal abscesses (10% to 25%), pancreatic pseudocysts (2%), and postoperative pancreatitis (13%). Severe hemorrhagic pancreatitis occurs in only 2%, but the mortality rate is high. Diabetes and malabsorption are rare except after major resection (greater than 80% of the gland). Most pancreatic fistulas are of low volume (less than 200 mL per day) and close without reoperation. Large output pancreatic fistulas may be initially treated with octreotide (Somatostatin analogue) and, if persistent, should be investigated by fistulogram and ERCP to define the problem, especially to rule out pancreatic duct obstruction. If necessary, an anastomosis of the Roux-en-Y loop to the source of the fistula can be done.

Intraabdominal abscesses are treated by interventional radiologic therapy or surgical drainage and carry a high mortality rate (20% to 25%). Pancreatic abscesses or infected pancreatic necrosis requires surgical debridement and drainage. Percutaneous drainage may be performed initially; if the problem is not corrected, partial clinical improvement may make later surgery safer. Pancreatic pseudocysts may be managed by percutaneous external drainage or surgical internal drainage, if they persist.

Complicated pancreatic injuries frequently require long-term ICU management with mechanical ventilation, parenteral or enteral nutrition, antibiotics, and multisystemic support.

DUODENUM

Duodenal injuries occur in 3% to 5% of the cases of abdominal trauma. A 6.5% to 12.5% mortality rate has been attributed to the duodenal injury alone. Exsanguination from associated major abdominal vascular or liver injuries is the most common cause of death (47.1%). Duodenal fistulae (25%), sepsis (15.5%), and organ failure (10%) are other common causes of death. Penetrating duodenal injuries are usually associated with hepatic, major vascular, enteric, and pancreatic injuries but carry a 14.4% mortality rate, which is lower than the 17.5% mortality rate of blunt duodenal injuries that may be isolated and difficult to diagnose.[3,9,66]

Penetrating duodenal injuries are usually diagnosed early because the patients are explored based on the mechanism of injury (gunshot wounds), the presence of shock, signs of peritoneal irritation, or the results of DPL or abdominal CT scan (stab wounds). The diagnosis of blunt duodenal injuries is based on a suitable mechanism of injury (blow to the upper abdomen with the steering wheel or bicycle handle bar), serial physical examinations, serum amylase levels, plain abdominal films, contrast duodenography, and abdominal CT scan. Complete mobilization and exposure of the duodenum are necessary because a missed duodenal injury has high morbidity and mortality rates resulting from the retroperitoneal extravasation of the highly active enzymatic duodenal contents.

Grade I or Grade II intramural duodenal hematomas are treated nonoperatively unless perforation is present or obstruction persists more than 4 weeks; if discovered at operation, they can be evacuated. Grade I lacerations are imbricated, but grade II lacerations are treated by debridement and repair. Grade III and IV lacerations are treated by debridement and primary repair, duodenal reanastomosis, or Roux-en-Y duodenojejunostomy. The duodenal repairs may be protected with duodenal decompressive tubes (anterograde gastrostomy and retrograde jejunostomy) or methods of duodenal diversion that convert the duodenum into a low-pressure diverticulum. If breakdown of the repair occurs, the end duodenal fistula that is created has a 69% chance of spontaneous closure. Drains are placed close to but not in contact with the duodenal repairs. Grade V injuries are treated by pancreaticoduodenectomy (Whipple procedure) in hemodynamically stable patients or by damage control and staged reconstruction in hemodynamically unstable patients.[3,9,64,66–68]

Snyder and colleagues[69] describe factors related to severity. Injuries are considered mild if they (1) are secondary to stab wounds; (2) involve less than 75% of the duodenal wall circumference; (3) are located in the third or fourth portion of the duodenum; (4) are repaired within 24 hours after injury; and (5) are not associated with injury to the common bile duct. On the other hand, injuries are considered severe if they (1) are secondary to blunt trauma or firearm wound; (2) involve more than 75% of the circumference of the wall; (3) are located in the first or second portion of the duodenum; (4) have an injury-to-repair interval greater than 24 hours; and (5) are associated with injury to the bile duct.

All patients with severe duodenal injuries are candidates for a protective decompressive or diversionary procedures. They must also have a tube or needle jejunostomy catheter placed at the time of surgery so that total enteral nutrition may be provided if duodenal or pancreatic complications arise.

All decompressive tubes (gastrostomy, retrograde jejunostomy, or nasogastric tube) must be patent and functioning (draining fluid and air). These tubes must be periodically irrigated with 10 to 15 mL of normal saline to avoid clogging. Irrigation should also be attempted if drainage ceases. The surgeon must be promptly notified if the tube remains occluded. The tape and sutures fixing the tubes must be inspected frequently. Because these tubes have vital functions for drainage, hollow viscus decompression, and administration of enteral feeding solutions, they should be considered "life lines" for the patient. Tubes "falling out" during position changes and transport reflect a failure to examine, secure, or protect the tubes. This apparently menial task is often ignored or left to staff members who neither appreciate the importance nor understand how to evaluate and secure fixation. Once a tube ostomy is lost, it may be impossible to reinsert. Antacid therapy and Sucralfate should be used with caution, if at all, in the immediate postoperative period after duodenal repair. They may clog the decompression tubes, resulting in duodenal distension, and theoretically, may contribute to creating a duodenal leak. Histamine type 2 (H_2) receptor blockers are preferred to prevent acute erosive gastritis prophylaxis.

Duodenal injuries are associated with a high morbidity rate (average, 63.7%; range, 38% to 125%). The main complications of duodenal injuries are fistula (0% to 16.2%), obstruction (1.1% to 1.8%) intraabdominal abscess (10.9% to 18.4%), recurrent pancreatitis (2.5% to 14.9%), and bile duct fistula (1.3%).[3]

The mortality rate for duodenal fistulae varies from 15% to 40%, resulting from uncontrolled sepsis and multiple organ failure. Duodenal fistulas are of two types. *End duodenal fistulae* occur in the defunctionalized duodenum such as after a Berne diverticularization procedure or a Vaughn pyloric exclusion procedure; because they have been excluded from the gastrointestinal stream, they usually close after 10 to 14 days. On the other hand, *lateral duodenal fistulae* occur if the duodenum is still in continuity with the gastrointestinal tract; they drain profusely, have just a 36% chance of spontaneous closure, and usually require surgical intervention. The management of fistulae includes three phases: (1) stabilization phase: bowel rest, duodenal decompression, adequate drainage, antibiotics, skin protection, H_2 blockers, correction of fluid and electrolyte imbalance, nutritional support, and administration of octreotide; (2) investigation phase: fistulogram and other contrast studies; and (3) repair phase: direct surgical attack after 6 weeks of failed medical management.

EXTRAHEPATIC BILIARY TRACT

Intrahepatic biliary tract injuries are integral part of the liver injuries and have already been discussed earlier. Extrahepatic biliary tract injuries are uncommon. Cox[26] reports no cases of extrahepatic bile duct injury in 870 laparotomies for blunt trauma. Soderstrom and associates[70] report one case of gall bladder rupture (0.07%) and ten cases of gallbladder avulsion (0.7%) in 1449 laparotomies for blunt abdominal trauma. Michelassi and Ranson[71] reviewed the English literature on blunt disruptions of the extrahepatic bile ducts and report a 13% mortality rate. Blunt and penetrating injuries to the porta hepatis have a mortality rate between 24% and 42% related to the vascular injuries, not to the ductal injuries.[47,48]

Penetrating extrahepatic biliary tract injuries are diagnosed at laparotomy. If bile staining of the hepatoduodenal ligament is present but the duodenum and head of the pancreas appear normal, cholangiography through the gall bladder with manual or instrument compression of the distal common bile duct may demonstrate the injury to the biliary tree. Blunt injury to the extrahepatic biliary system may present in an insidious fashion from hours to weeks after injury. Patients usually return 1 to 2 weeks after injury with a syndrome of increasing abdominal distension and pain, nausea, vomiting, jaundice, acholic stools, ascites, and inanition. US or abdominal CT scan may confirm the presence of ascites and, if paracentesis yields bile, the diagnosis of extrahepatic biliary tract injury is almost certain. Hepatobiliary scan can confirm the diagnosis and demonstrate associated hepatic injuries whereas ERCP may define the anatomy of the injury before laparotomy.[72]

Five factors are considered during the surgical management: (1) hemodynamic stability of the patient, (2) associated injuries in the right upper quadrant, (3) location and extent of the injury, (4) the small size of the bile ducts in trauma victims, and (5) tenuous blood supply of the common bile duct. Grade I extrahepatic biliary tract injuries (gallbladder or portal triad contusion or hematoma) are explored and intraoperative cholangiography used to rule out a higher grade injury. Grade II and III injuries require hemostasis or cholecystectomy (complete avulsion, or laceration or perforation of the gallbladder). A transcystic intraoperative cholangiogram may be performed to assess the biliary tract. Grade IV and Grade V hepatic or common bile duct lacerations may be treated with primary repair over a T tube or a ureteral catheter. Most injuries from blunt trauma occur either at the junction of the common bile duct with the pancreas or at the bifurcation of the common hepatic duct.[70] Complete bile duct transection without loss of tissue may be treated by primary anastomosis over a T tube or preferably by biliary enteric anastomosis. Choledochoduodenostomy, Roux-en-Y cholecystojejunostomy, or choledochojejunostomy are necessary in complicated injuries. Ligation of the right or left hepatic duct with or without liver resection is an alternative for proximal injuries.[72]

In hemodynamically unstable patients, external T-tube drainage (hepaticodochostomy or choledochostomy) and staged biliary reconstruction are the proper choice. Even ligation of the common bile duct stump and tube cholecystostomy is a reasonable option if the patient is in shock, is hypothermic and coagulopathic, and if prolongation of the surgical procedure will result in death.[3,47,48]

Specific complications after biliary tract injuries include obstructive jaundice, cholangitis, biliary fistula, hemobilia, pancreatitis, and late biliary cirrhosis. The patency and output of any drainage tube must be carefully monitored. If drainage ceases, the surgeon should be immediately notified so that the tube can be flushed. A cholangiogram may be necessary to document whether the tube has become dislodged.

ESOPHAGUS

Abdominal esophageal injuries are uncommon. Most are caused by penetrating trauma. Rupture of the distal esophagus or avulsion of the gastroesophageal junction rarely occur from a blunt mechanism. In a series of 48 patients with esophageal injuries collected over 15 years, Symbas and colleagues[73] report seven cases (15%) of abdominal esophageal injury. The overall mortality rate of esophageal trauma is approximately 20% to 25%.[74]

In penetrating trauma, in addition to the previously mentioned indications for laparotomy, hematemesis and bright red blood in the nasogastric aspirate are added. Blows to the upper abdomen in the presence of a full stomach may result in rupture of the abdominal esophagus by a mechanism similar to Boerhaave syndrome. Because of its retroperitoneal location, perforation may cause no or only minimal peritoneal signs; superior extension along the periesophageal planes may result in mediastinitis that is also difficult to diagnose. Abdominal CT scan with oral contrast may demonstrate the injury. Hydrosoluble contrast (diatrizoate) esophagography and rigid or flexible esophagoscopy may be used to rule out esophageal injury in these circumstances.

Most abdominal esophageal injuries can be repaired by primary single-layer closure, with a Nissen fundoplication or Thal patch added.[3] A severely injured distal esophagus may be treated by resection and primary esophagogastrostomy.[75] A gastrostomy plus a transgastric jejunal feeding tube is a prudent adjunctive procedure in esophageal injuries to keep the stomach decompressed, to avoid a nasogastric tube passing through the repair site, to diminish reflux, and to provide a route for enteral nutrition. If the patient has other life-threatening injuries, is in shock, and has an extensive esophageal injury, definitive repair may be delayed. In this situation, the distal esophagus is closed with staples and drained, the stomach is closed, and a gastrostomy tube with an indwelling gastrojejunal feeding tube is inserted. The proximal esophagus is decompressed either with a nasogastric sump tube (short term) or a cervical esophagostomy (long term).

The potential complications after esophageal injury include suture line leak, fistula, stenosis, and intraabdominal abscess, but they rarely occur.[73] Infection in the lower mediastinum may produce severe systemic sepsis; therefore, anastomotic leak and mediastinitis as a source of undiagnosed sepsis must be considered after reconstruction of a severe esophageal injury. Chest and abdomen CT scan with oral contrast or a hydrosoluble contrast esophagography can demonstrate leakage or abscess formation so that surgical drainage may be undertaken.

STOMACH

Gastric injuries occur in 7% to 20% of the cases of penetrating trauma and in less than 1% of the blunt abdominal injuries.[3] Cox[26] reports only two gastric perforations in 870 laparotomies for blunt trauma. Durham and associates,[76] in a large series of penetrating gastric injuries, report a delayed mortality rate of 4.5% but only a 0.4% rate of gastric injury related mortality.

Hematemesis and bright red bloody nasogastric drainage suggest gastric injury and are absolute indications for laparotomy in penetrating abdominal trauma. Blunt gastric disruptions may result from a direct force applied to the upper abdomen. In a full stomach, the injury usually occurs along the greater curvature and there may be extensive contamination with gastric contents of high pH and bacterial counts.[67]

Thorough mobilization of the stomach is necessary to avoid missing multiple perforations in penetrating trauma. Gastric injuries are treated by local debridement and primary closure. Extensive repairs may be protected by a gastrostomy tube, which must be kept patent to maintain the decompression and protect the suture lines.

Complications after gastric injury occur in 6% of the cases and include bleeding from the suture line, gastrocutaneous fistula, intraabdominal abscess, gastric outlet obstruction, and empyema.[76] Brunsting and Morton[77] report an abscess rate of 52% and a gastrocutaneous fistula rate of 16% in a series of blunt gastric injuries. A breakdown of the gastric repair is usually treated surgically, although a gastric fistula may close with adequate drainage, gastric decompression, and nutritional support. Simultaneous gastric and diaphragmatic injuries have a 12 times higher incidence of empyema when compared with diaphragmatic injury alone.[3,67,76]

SMALL BOWEL, MESENTERY, AND GREATER OMENTUM

The small intestine, mesentery, and greater omentum are the most commonly injured organs in penetrating abdominal trauma.[3] The small bowel is injured in 49.3% of abdominal gunshot wounds and in 31.6% of abdominal stab wounds.[9] In blunt abdominal trauma, the incidence rate of small bowel injury is approximately 5% to 15%.[3,78] Blunt intestinal injuries occur by three mechanisms: (1) crushing or laceration of the bowel between the spine and a firm object such as a seat belt, steering wheel, boot, or hoof; (2) shearing of the intestine or mesentery at points of relative fixation by sudden deceleration, most commonly the proximal jejunum near the ligament of Treitz or the terminal ileum near the ileocecal valve; and (3) bursting after a sudden increase in pressure in a fluid-filled closed loop of bowel. The mortality rate for blunt small bowel injury has been reported to be as high as 10% to 30% compared with 6% for penetrating injury.[32,33,78,79]

In penetrating injuries, the need for laparotomy is usually easily established and, therefore, the diagnosis is rarely delayed. On the other hand, blunt intestinal injuries have an insidious presentation and the delay in diagnosis is associated with increased morbidity and mortality. A small proximal jejunal perforation may occur without early symptoms or signs. Early diagnosis depends on serial abdominal evaluations, serum amylase levels, and WBC counts, for instance, in nonoperated patients admitted to the ICU for other reasons. Late clinical manifestations include adynamic ileus, abdominal distention, increasing abdominal pain, tenderness, fever, leukocytosis, and occasionally rising serum amylase. Early DPL may yield negative or equivocal results in blunt intestinal trauma; however, a lavage repeated 12 hours later may reveal an elevated WBC count or amylase level, both suggestive of intestinal injury. Abdominal CT scan has not been accurate in the diagnosis of intestinal injury.[25] Peritoneal fluid without solid viscus injury or previous DPL should be considered a sign of a possible small intestine or mesenteric injury and an indication for abdominal exploration.

If the lap seat belt or the seat belt sign is observed, injury of the small intestine should be considered. Seat belt–induced injuries may be divided: complete transections of the proximal jejunum caused by deceleration and associated with mesenteric tears, as well as transverse colon and splenic flexure injuries; shearing or crushing injuries with devascularization and serosal tears, usually in the terminal ileum, associated with cecal, aortic, and caval injuries and lumbar spine fractures; and blow-out perforations, seen in postprandial patients whose small bowel loops are filled with chyle.[80] Perforations may not present for 10 days until there is necrosis of intramural hematomas and may mimic a small bowel obstruction. Penetrating injuries to the greater omentum are characterized by evisceration or hemorrhage, especially in patients with adhesions from previous abdominal operations.

The surgical treatment includes the following: grade I contusions or hematomas, no specific therapy; Grade II injuries, treatment by debridement and primary repair; Grade III injuries, repair or resection and anastomosis may be needed; Grade IV and V injuries, repair or resection and anastomosis are necessary.

In damage control situations, irreparable bowel is resected and the stumps of the remaining intestine are expeditiously closed using stapling devices or umbilical tape; relaparotomy and restoration of the gastrointestinal continuity follow correction of shock, coagulopathy, and hypothermia in the ICU.[3,9,64] Jejunostomies and even ileostomies are best avoided because they are technically difficult to construct in unstable edematous individuals. When multiple small bowel injuries are present, en block resection with a single anastomosis is preferable to multiple suture lines as long as most of the ileum and the ileocecal valve are preserved. Mesenteric rents or defects must be closed to prevent the formation of internal hernias. Mesenteric hematomas are explored to ligate the bleeding vessels.

Proximal injuries to the superior mesenteric artery are treated by debridement, primary repair, patch angioplasty, or vein graft to prevent loss of the entire midgut. Distal injuries cause ischemia of a variable extent; the vessel may be ligated and the compromised bowel resected. Injuries to the superior mesenteric vein should be repaired, but in unstable patients, it may be ligated. Ligation results in significant edema of the small bowel; venous thrombosis and bowel infarction may follow. The viability of the bowel may be ascertained intraoperatively using an ultrasound probe, intravenous fluorescein, or a pulse oximeter. A "second-look" laparotomy is performed when the viability is in doubt.

Specific complications of intestinal injuries include suture line disruption with enterocutaneous fistula formation (0.5% to 1%), wound infection, intraabdominal abscess, sepsis, prolonged ileus, and bowel obstruction. Wound infections become evident around the fourth or fifth postoperative day and require complete opening of the surgical wound. They may be avoided by using the delayed primary closure method in contaminated wounds: the skin and subcutaneous tissue are left open, the wound is treated with dressing changes, and closure is done on postoperative day 4 or 5 using tape or sutures placed at the time of the initial procedure. Intraabdominal abscesses are diagnosed by abdominal CT scan and may be treated by percutaneous drainage or reoperation, depending on their number and location and the presence of associated fistulae.[3]

COLON

The incidence of colonic injury in penetrating abdominal trauma is 9%.[3] The mortality rate of colon trauma since 1985 has been reported to be between 0% and 7% in five prospective series and between 2.6% and 10.5% in eight retrospective series.[67]

Penetrating trauma causes 85% to 96% of the colonic injuries: three quarters of the cases are firearm wounds and one quarter stab wounds. Common associated injuries are small bowel, liver, stomach, kidney, and major vessels.[26] Blunt colonic injuries are less frequent than blunt small bowel injuries and usually result from vehicular crashes, pedestrians struck by motor vehicles, and motorcycle crashes.[80,81] Fifty percent of the blunt colonic injuries are grade I injuries (contusion, hematoma, and partial-thickness laceration), 25% are grade II injuries, and 19% are grade V injuries. Commonly associated organs include the small bowel, spleen, liver, and diaphragm.[81]

Stone and Fabian[82] conducted a prospective randomized study in 1979 that proved the advantages and safety of primary repair in selected patients. Others have liberalized the selection criteria to allow more primary repairs.[83–86] In a prospective study of 100 patients with bullet injuries to the colon, Demetriades and associates[87] performed primary repair in 76% of the cases, reserving colostomy for patients with severe colonic damage requiring resection and for patients with disseminated gross peritoneal contamination. The colostomy group had a higher incidence of intraabdominal septic complications. They concluded that left-sided colonic injuries, multiple colonic perforations, shock on admission, delay greater than 6 hours, more than two associated intraabdominal injuries, a high injury severity score and high penetrating abdominal trauma index were not in themselves contraindications for primary repair.

Currently, all grade I, II, and III colonic injuries are repaired primarily. Grade IV and V right colonic injuries may be treated with resection and ileocolonic anastomosis; grade IV and V left colonic injuries are still treated at most centers with resection, end colostomy, and mucous fistula or the Hartmann procedure (proximal end colostomy and sutured distal end of the bowel left inside the abdomen). Current contraindications for primary repair in blunt or penetrating colonic trauma include massive fecal contamination, need for intraabdominal packing, poor tissue quality or questionable vascularity, severe associated pancreaticoduodenal injury, and associated urinary tract injury with a high potential for urine leak.[67] The intracolonic bypass may increase the safety of colocolonic anastomosis in unprepared bowel.[88] Retained projectiles are associated with abscesses around the missile or in the missile tract; therefore, the bullet should be removed.[89] Short-term (24 hours) perioperative single antibiotic coverage for gram-negative enteric organisms and anaerobes is sufficient.[90] Incisions should be treated by delayed primary closure or allowed to heal by secondary intent.[3]

Complications occur in 15% to 50% of the patients. Specific complications include intraabdominal abscess (9%), peritonitis (4.8%), wound infection (4.7%), and fecal fistula (1.1%).[3] George and coworkers[83] report a 33% incidence rate of septic complications; significant risk factors included transfusion of more than four units of blood, more than two associated injuries, increasing levels of colon injury severity score, and significant contamination. Intraabdominal abscesses are commonly diagnosed using CT scan and treated by percutaneous drainage. Reoperation is occasionally necessary. Peritonitis and peritoneal cellulitis are treated with intravenous antibiotics. Fecal fistulas usually close if there is adequate drainage and bowel rest is provided by elemental low-residue enteral formula or total parenteral nutrition.

RECTUM

Rectal injuries are uncommon. Most result from firearm wounds (82%). An occasional patient is injured by impalement, foreign body, sexual assault, or iatrogenic causes. Pelvic fractures and perineal avulsion injuries may injure the rectum. Burch and coworkers[91] report a 4% mortality in a series of 100 patients with extraperitoneal rectal injury.

Rectal injury should be suspected in any patient with abdominal, pelvic, or perineal trauma. Rectal examination may reveal gross blood or a palpable rectal defect. Although this examination is a fundamental part of the secondary survey and should be performed in male blunt trauma victims before insertion of the Foley catheter, it may have been omitted in a hasty resuscitation. The patient's record should be reviewed in the ICU to detect and then correct inadvertent omissions, such as the rectal examination. Anoscopy and rigid proctosigmoidoscopy should be performed to identify mucosal or full-thickness lacerations if rectal bleeding is present, gross blood is found on rectal examination, or injury is strongly suspected (i.e., significantly displaced anterior element pelvic fracture)—if even the stool is guaiac negative. This is also necessary in the stable patient with penetrating abdominal or transpelvic trauma because the middle and lower thirds of the rectum cannot be evaluated at laparotomy. Associated injuries are common and frequently involve the genitourinary tract, colon, major pelvic vasculature, and small intestine. Preoperative IVP and retrograde urethrogram and cystogram are recommended.[92]

Grade II, III, and IV rectal injuries are treated by (1) complete fecal diversion with loop colostomy with stapled distal limb; (2) debridement and repair of the injuries that communicate with the peritoneal cavity or that are exposed during exploration of other pelvic structures; (3) rectosigmoid washout to remove all the fecal matter and promote healing in the perirectal tissues; and (4) drainage of the presacral space.[67,91–93] Grade V injuries are treated by resection and the Hartmann procedure.

The overall complication rate of rectal trauma is greater than 50%. Rectal injury–related infectious complications occur in 11% of the cases and include intraabdominal and pelvic abscesses, rectocutaneous fistulae, rectovesical fistulae, wound infections, and missile tract infections. The perineum must be inspected daily to detect complications.

Colostomy is indicated for pelvic fractures with associated perineal injuries, all grade II to V rectal injuries, and grade IV and V colonic injuries. Colostomies are contraindicated in unstable patients who are best served by damage control.[94]

Colostomies have a 6.2% rate of complications. Early complications include necrosis, peristomal evisceration or herniation, retraction, and peristomal infection. These are serious and require reoperation. Late diagnosis of these complications may lead to fecal peritonitis and sepsis; therefore, all stomas must be examined on a daily basis to detect complications so that prompt care and reoperation may be provided before systemic effects develop. Renz and associates[95] propose early colostomy closure for rectal injuries if hydrosoluble contrast (diatrizoate) enemas, performed 7 to 10 days after the injury, show that the injury has healed.

RETROPERITONEUM

Patients with penetrating retroperitoneal injuries may have three different presentations: (1) exsanguinating hemorrhage with profound hypovolemic shock; (2) limited blood loss with contained retroperitoneal hematoma and mild to moderate hypotension; and (3) hemodynamically stability with or without physical findings. The hypotensive patient should be transported expeditiously to the operating room. Fluid resuscitation or application of a PASG may result in exacerbating the hemorrhage. Only a chest radiograph and a single-view, double-contrast IVP should be performed in the emergency department or on the operating table.[96]

Exsanguinating hemorrhage is usually found at exploration in the patient in profound shock. Aortic or iliac injuries are repaired primarily or using synthetic grafts, even in the presence of contamination. Infrarenal IVC or iliac vein injuries may be repaired primarily or treated by ligation. Suprarenal IVC injuries should be repaired with synthetic materials without wasting time harvesting large veins or constructing complex vein grafts in unstable patients.[9,96] The damage control operation may be appropriate.

Retroperitoneal hematomas have been classified by Feliciano[97] for the purposes of treatment.

Zone I or Central-Medial Retroperitoneum Hematomas

1. Midline supramesocolic hematomas must be opened after securing proximal and, if possible, distal vascular control because the most commonly injured structures are the proximal abdominal aorta and its branches.
2. Midline inframesocolic hematomas must be opened after obtaining proximal control of the infrarenal abdominal aorta and distal control of the iliac arteries.
3. Portal hematomas are opened after obtaining proximal and distal control of the hepatic artery and the portal vein.
4. Retrohepatic hematomas without bleeding into the peritoneal cavity or through an associated hepatic parenchymal injury should be left alone; experimental studies have proven that spontaneous healing may occur.[98] If active bleeding is present, atriocaval shunt or

hepatic vascular isolation are needed before exposing the injury.

Zone II or Lateral Retroperitoneum Hematomas

1. Perirenal hematomas are explored if they are expanding or pulsatile, if there is extravasation of contrast material, or if loss of renal function has occurred.
2. Paraduodenal hematomas must be opened to rule out injuries to the duodenum, IVC, or right renal pedicle.
3. Pericolonic hematomas must be explored by mobilization of the ascending or descending colon to rule out posterior colonic injuries or injuries to lumbar vessels.

Zone III or Pelvic Retroperitoneum Hematomas

Pelvic hematomas must be explored if they are expanding, after having secured proximal and distal control of the iliac vessels. Rectal or bladder injuries may be present. Preoperative rigid anoscopy and proctosigmoidoscopy should determine the presence of extraperitoneal rectal injuries.

The mortality rate of major vascular retroperitoneal injuries is 67% for the suprarenal abdominal aorta, 58% for the mesenteric abdominal aorta, 50% for the infrarenal abdominal aorta, and 33% for the IVC.[96]

Sixty-seven percent to 80% of the retroperitoneal hematomas result from blunt injuries but occurred in only 2.9% of all victims and 13% of patients in an urban referral trauma center.[99] Fifty percent of the patients had extraabdominal injuries, 52% intraperitoneal injuries, 45% major retroperitoneal visceral and vascular injuries, 34% head injuries, and 55% pelvic fractures. Shock was present on admission in 38% of the patients.

The diagnosis of retroperitoneal hematoma should be considered in the blunt trauma victim admitted to the ICU who has evidence of ongoing blood loss without external bleeding, hemothorax, hemoperitoneum, or pelvic or long bone fractures. The diagnosis is based on physical findings (back or flank soft tissue injuries or Grey Turner's sign—late) radiologic findings (lumbosacral spine fractures or tear drop bladder on cystogram), abdominal and pelvic CT scan results, or operative findings. CT scan is extremely valuable in the hemodynamically stable patient because it demonstrates the location of the hematoma and retroperitoneal visceral injuries. If a large retroperitoneal hematoma without associated musculoskeletal or visceral injury is diagnosed on abdominal and pelvic CT scan, arteriography may define the presence and anatomic location of a retroperitoneal vascular injury before exploration, which facilitates the surgical approach.

The following intraoperative management for retroperitoneal hematomas has been recommended[97,99]:

Management of Zone I or Central-Medial Retroperitoneum Hematomas

1. Midline hematomas may be caused by major vascular injuries or to pancreatic and duodenal injuries and, therefore, must be explored. If a major vascular injury is suspected because of the size or pulsatile

nature of the hematoma, then proximal and distal control should be secured with the appropriate maneuver before entering the hematoma. A central retroperitoneal hematoma that extends up to the esophageal hiatus (parahiatal hematoma) could actually originate in the mediastinum secondary to a blunt aortic injury. Intraoperative transesophageal echocardiogram may confirm the diagnosis; otherwise, a thoracic aortogram should be performed.

2. Retrohepatic hematomas without free bleeding into the peritoneal cavity or through a hepatic parenchymal injury should not be opened.[98] If hepatic parenchymal bleeding is present and a grade V liver injury is suspected, atriocaval shunting or hepatic vascular isolation must be implemented before opening the hematoma.

3. Portal hematomas are opened after proximal and distal control is secured; the extrahepatic biliary tree must be carefully examined for blunt transection.

Management of Zone II or Lateral Retroperitoneum Hematomas

1. Perirenal hematomas (inside Gerota's fascia) should not be opened if preoperative CT scan or intraoperative IVP have excluded grade IV or V renal injuries. A grade IV or V renal injury, an expanding or pulsatile hematoma, or free rupture mandate exploration with prior control of the renal vascular pedicle.

2. Paraduodenal hematomas must be explored to rule out blunt duodenal or pancreatic injuries or right renovascular injuries.

3. Pericolonic hematomas not associated with pelvic fractures and pelvic hematomas must be opened to rule out blunt colonic injury.

Management of Zone III or Pelvic Retroperitoneum Hematomas

Pelvic hematomas usually originate in fracture sites, pelvis venous plexuses, or deep pelvic arterial bleeders. Only the absence of groin pulses—indicating major iliac arterial disruption—requires direct surgical approach. Primary repair or ligation with extraanatomic bypass is recommended if there is contamination. In expanding pelvic hematomas with palpable groin pulses, a rapid closure followed by angiography and embolization is preferred. The management of pelvic fractures and associated hematomas is covered in detail in Chapter 68.

Goins and associates[99] explored 97% of zone I, 41% of zone II, and 16% of zone III hematomas with a 61%, 49%, and 38% incidence rate of visceral and vascular injury, respectively. They report an overall mortality rate of 39%. Shock, associated head injuries, and multiple organ failure caused most of the deaths. Complications occurred in 59% of the patients who survived more than 24 hours. There was a 43% incidence rate of organ failure (ARDS, acute tubular necrosis, liver failure, and disseminated intravascular coagulopathy) and a 24% incidence rate of infectious complications (urinary tract infection, bacteremia, pneumonia, intraabdominal abscess, empyema, and wound infections). Thromboembolism and pancreatitis were rare complications.

Blunt retroperitoneal vascular trauma presents with thrombotic manifestations far more commonly than hemorrhage. Vessel trauma is either a stretch type of injury, disrupting the intima and media but leaving a hemostatic adventitia, or a direct blow or contusion. They may present as absent or weak pulses or lack of motion of the lower extremities resulting from ischemia, mistakenly diagnosed in the trauma resuscitation area or the ICU as a spinal cord lesion. Angiography establishes the nature of the lesion and must be followed by prompt vascular reconstruction.[3,100]

Blunt renovascular injuries have the same stretch-type or direct injury with contusion and thrombosis, and may present without hematuria. The diagnosis is supported by IVP demonstrating nonvisualization and confirmed by poor perfusion on CT scan or complete arterial occlusion on arteriogram. The kidney tolerates 2 to 4 hours of warm ischemia before irreversible dysfunction sets in. Revascularization must be considered only if a short period of ischemia has occurred, the patient is hemodynamically stable without multiple associated injuries, or the other kidney is absent or abnormal.[100] Nephrectomy of a ischemic kidney is indicated only if hypertension or pyogenic infection occurs.

The crude mortality rate of blunt retroperitoneal vascular injuries has been reported as 66% for the aorta, 72% for the IVC, 47% for the iliac vasculature, and 33% for the renal vasculature.[100]

CONCLUSION ◼

Intraabdominal injuries account for 10% to 13% of the injury-related fatalities. Neglected or delayed diagnosis of solid organ injuries may result in early death from exsanguination. These are the preventable trauma deaths that stimulated the creation of regionalized trauma care systems. Similarly, missed or late diagnosis of hollow viscus injuries or retroperitoneal injuries may produce contamination and late death from sepsis and multiple organ failure.[101]

In nonoperated patients admitted to the ICU, an initial abdominal examination by the intensivist after stabilization of vital signs, followed by careful review of the results of the workup and serial reevaluations, may detect subtle or late manifestations of intraabdominal injuries. The intensivist should suspect injury and maintain a dialogue with the surgeon, seeking answers to any doubts and suggesting further diagnostic or therapeutic interventions.

In operated patients, the ICU team must obtain detailed information about the injuries found and the surgical procedures performed to provide care tailored for each patient, because specific injuries are associated with specific constellations of early and late complications. Furthermore, intraabdominal injuries can be missed even during exploratory laparotomy; the ICU team must remain alert to detect this possibility. After celiotomy for trauma, Scalea and colleagues[102] recommend that patients with clinical indications of ongoing bleeding should be investigated or reexplored within 4 hours, and those with early sepsis or multisystem organ failure should undergo abdominal reexploration within 4 days to detect undiagnosed injuries.

REFERENCES ▪

1. Baker SP, O'Neill B, Ginsburg MJ, et al: *The Injury Fact Book*, 2nd ed. New York: Oxford University Press, 1992
2. Anderson ID, Woodford M, De Dombal FT, et al: Restrospective study of 1000 deaths from injury in England and Wales. *Br Med J* 1988;296:1305
3. Blaisdell FW, Trunkey DD (eds): *Abdominal Trauma*, 2nd ed. New York: Thieme Stratton, 1993
4. Gomez GA, Savini MJ Jr: The work-up of the trauma patient. In: Kreis DJ Jr, Gomez GA (eds). *Trauma Management*. Boston: Little, Brown, 1989:47
5. Fildes J: Assessment of abdominal trauma. In: Nyhus LM, Vitello JM, Condon RE (eds). *Abdominal Pain: A Guide to Rapid Diagnosis*. Norwalk, CT: Appleton & Lange, 1995: 167
6. Mackersie RC, Tiwary AD, Shackford, et al: Intrabdominal injury following blunt trauma: identifying the high risk patient using objective risk factors. *Arch Surg* 1989;124:809
7. Trunkey DD: Current concepts: initial treatment of patients with extensive trauma. *N Engl J Med* 1991;324:1259
8. Trunkey DD: Clinical update: decision making in management of critically injured patients. *Surgery* 1992;111:481
9. Feliciano DV, Rozycki GS: The management of penetrating abdominal trauma. In: Cameron JL, Balch CM, Langer B, et al (eds). *Adv Surg* 1995;28:1
10. Moore EE, Ducker TB, Edlich RF, et al (eds): *Early Care of the Injured Patient*, 4th ed. Toronto: BC Decker, 1990
11. Bickell WH, Wall MJ, Pepe PE, et al: Immediate versus delayed fluid resuscitation for hypotensive patients with penetrating torso injuries. *N Engl J Med* 1994;331:1106
12. Flint L: Assessment of abdominal trauma. *Curr Pract Surg* 1994;6:65
13. Duncan AO, Phillips TF, Scalea TM, et al: Management of transpelvic gunshot wounds. *J Trauma* 1989;29:1335
14. Simon RJ, Ivatury RR: Current concepts in the use of cavitary endoscopy in the evaluation and treatment of blunt and penetrating truncal injuries. *Surg Clin North Am* 1995;75:157
15. Feliciano DV: Diagnostic modalities in abdominal trauma: peritoneal lavage, ultrasonography, computed tomography scanning and arteriography. *Surg Clin North Am* 1991;71:241
16. Bergstgein JM, Aprahamian C, Frantzides CT: Diagnostic and therapeutic laparoscopy for trauma. In: Frantzides CT (ed). *Laparoscopic and Thoracoscopic Surgery*. St Louis: Mosby-Year Book, 1995:155
17. Rossi P, Mullins D, Thal ER: Role of laparoscopy in the evaluation of abdominal trauma. *Am J Surg* 1993;166:707
18. Bivens BA, Sachatello CR, Daugherty ME, et al: Diagnostic peritoneal lavage is superior to clinical evaluation in blunt abdominal trauma. *Am Surg* 1978;44:637
19. Mendez C, Gubler KD, Maier RV: Diagnostic accuracy of peritoneal lavage in patients with pelvic fractures. *Arch Surg* 1994;129:477
20. Rozycki GS: Abdominal ultrasonography in trauma. *Surg Clin North Am* 1995;75:175
21. Glaser K, Tschmelitsch J, Klinger P, et al: Ultrasonography in the management of blunt abdominal and thoracic trauma. *Arch Surg* 1994;129:743
22. McKenney M, Lentz K, Nunez D, et al: Can ultrasound replace diagnostic peritoneal lavage in the assesment of blunt trauma. *J Trauma* 1994;37:439
23. Huang M, Liu M, Wu J, et al: Ultrasonography for the evaluation of hemoperitoneum during resuscitation: a simple scoring system. *J Trauma* 1994;36:173
24. McKenney M, Martin L, Lentz K, et al: 1000 consecutive ultrasounds for blunt abdominal trauma. Presentation at the Eastern Association for the Surgery of Trauma, Sanibel, FL, January 1995
25. Sherck JP, Oakes DD: Intestinal injuries missed by computed tomography. *J Trauma* 1990;30:1
26. Cox EF: Blunt abdominal trauma: a 5-year analysis of 870 patients requiring celiotomy. *Ann Surg* 1984;199:467
27. Feliciano DV, Burch JM, Spjut-Patrinely V, et al: Abdominal gunshot wounds: an urban trauma center's experience with 300 consecutive patients. *Ann Surg* 1988;208:362
28. Burch JM, Brock JC, Gevirtzmann L, et al: The injured colon. *Ann Surg* 1986;203:701
29. Renz BM, Feliciano DV: Unnecessary laparotomies for trauma: a prospective study of morbidity. *J Trauma* 1995; 38:350
30. Moore EE, Cogbill TH, Malangoni MA, et al: Organ injury scaling. *Surg Clin North Am* 1995;75:293
31. Zainea GG, Jordan F: Rectus sheath hematomas: their pathogenesis, diagnosis and management. *Am Surg* 1988;54:630
32. Appleby JP, Nagy AG: Abdominal injuries associated with the use of seat belts. *Am J Surg* 1989:157:457
33. Rutledge R, Thomason M, Oller D, et al: The spectrum of abdominal injuries associated with the use of seat belts. *J Trauma* 1991;31:820
34. Damschen DD, Landerscasper J, Cogbill TH, et al: Acute traumatic abdominal wall hernia: case reports. *J Trauma* 1994;36:273
35. Sahdev P, Garramone RR Jr, Desani B, et al: Traumatic abdominal hernia: report of three cases and review of the literature. *Am J Emerg Med* 1992;10:237
36. Boulanger BR, Milzman DP, Rosati C, et al: A comparison of right and left blunt traumatic diaphragmatic rupture. *J Trauma* 1993;35:255
37. Symbas PN, Vlasis SE, Hatcher C Jr: Blunt and penetrating diaphragmatic injuries with or without herniation of organs into the chest. *Ann Thorac Surg* 1986;42:158
38. Uribe RA, Pachon CE, Frame SB, et al: A prospective evaluation of thoracoscopy for the diagnosis of penetrating thoracoabdominal trauma. *J Trauma* 1994;37:650
39. Ivatury RR, Simon RJ, Weksler B, et al: Laparoscopy in the evaluation of the intrathoracic abdomen after penetrating injury. *J Trauma* 1992;33:101
40. Madden MR, Paull DE, Finkelstein JL, et al: Occult diaphragmatic injury from stab wounds to the lower chest and abdomen. *J Trauma* 1989;29:292
41. Cogbill TH, Moore EE, Jurkovich GJ, et al: Severe hepatic trauma: a multicenter experience. *J Trauma* 1988;28: 1433
42. Buechter KJ, Zeppa R, Gomez G: The use of segmental anatomy for an operative classification of liver injuries. *Ann Surg* 1990;211:669
43. Ochsner MG, Jaffin JH, Golocovsky M, et al: Major hepatic trauma. *Surg Clin North Am* 1993;73:337
44. Pachter HL, Spencer FC, Hofstetter SR, et al: Significant trends in the treatment of hepatic trauma: experience with 411 injuries. *Ann Surg* 1992;215:492
45. Gryf-Lowczowski, Benjamin IS: Liver trauma. *Curr Pract Surg* 1994;6:78

46. Buechter KJ, Sereda D, Gomez G, et al: Retrohepatic vein injuries: experience with 20 cases. *J Trauma* 1989;29:1698

47. Sheldon GF, Lim RC, Yee ES, et al: Management of injuries to the porta hepatis. *Ann Surg* 1980;191:703

48. Dawson DL, Johansen KJ, Jurkovich JL: Injuries to the portal triad. *Am J Surg* 1991;161:545

49. Federle MP, Jeffrey RB: Hemoperitoneum studied by computed tomography. *Radiology* 1983;148:187

50. Pachter HL, Hofstetter SR: The current status of nonoperative management of adult blunt hepatic injuries. *Am J Surg* 1995;169:442

51. Lucas CE: Splenic trauma: choice of management. *Ann Surg* 1991;213:98

52. Schwalke MA, Crowley JP, Spencer P, et al: Splenic artery ligation for splenic salvage: clinical experience and immune function. *J Trauma* 1991;31:385

53. Shackford SR: Splenic trauma. *Curr Pract Surg* 1994;6:86

54. Feliciano PD, Mullins RJ, Trunkey DD, et al: A decision analysis of traumatic splenic injuries. *J Trauma* 1992;33:340

55. Smith SJ, Wengrowitz MA, Delong BS: Prospective validation of criteria, including age for safe, non surgical management of the ruptured spleen. *J Trauma* 1992;33:363

56. Witte CI, Esser MJ, Rappaport WD: Updating the management of salvageable splenic injury. *Ann Surg* 1992;215:261

57. Wilson RH, Moorehead RJ: Current management of trauma to the pancreas. *Br J Surg* 1991;78:1196

58. Buechter KJ, Arnold M, Steele B, et al: The use of serum amylase and lipase in evaluating and managing blunt abdominal trauma. *Am Surg* 1990;56:204

59. Jeffrey RB Jr, Federle MP, Crass RA: Computed tomography of pancreatic trauma. *Radiology* 1983;147:491

60. Whittwell AE, Gomez GA, Byers P, et al: Blunt pancreatic trauma: prospective evaluation of early endoscopic retrograde pancreatography. *South Med J* 1989;82:586

61. Cogbill TH, Moore EE, Morris JA, et al: Distal pancreatectomy for trauma: a multicenter experience. *J Trauma* 1991;31:1600

62. Gentilello LM, Cortes V, Buechter KJ, et al: Whipple procedure for trauma: is duct ligation a safe alternative to pancreaticojejunostomy. *J Trauma* 1991;31:661

63. Delcore R, Stauffer JS, Thomas JH: The role of pancreatogastrostomy following pancreatoduodenectomy for trauma. *J Trauma* 1994;37:395

64. Carrillo C, Fogler RJ, Shaftan GW: Delayed gastrointestinal reconstruction following massive abdominal trauma. *J Trauma* 1993;34:233

65. Fabian TC, Kudsk KA, Croce MA, et al: Superiority of closed suction drainage for pancreatic trauma: a randomized, prospective study. *Ann Surg* 1990;211:724

66. Asensio JA, Feliciano DV, Britt LD, et al: Management of duodenal injuries. *Curr Probl Surg* 1993;11:1021

67. Thomson SR, Huizinga KJ, Baker LW: Bowel trauma. *Curr Pract Surg* 1994;6:70

68. Cogbill TH, Moore EE, Feliciano DV, et al: Conservative management of duodenal trauma: a multicenter perspective. *J Trauma* 1990;125:1469

69. Snyder WH, Wegelt JA, Watkyns WL, et al: The surgical management of duodenal trauma: precepts based on a review of 247 cases. *Arch Surg* 1980;115:422

70. Soderstrom CA, Maeedkawan K, Dupreist RW Jr, et al: Gallbladder injuries resulting from blunt abdominal trauma. *Ann Surg* 1981;193:60

71. Michelassi F, Ranson JHC: Bile duct disruption by blunt trauma. *J Trauma* 1985;26:454

72. Feliciano DV: Biliary injuries as a result of blunt and penetrating trauma. *Surg Clin North Am* 1994;74:897

73. Symbas PN, Hachter CR Jr, Vlassis SE: Esophageal gunshout injuries. *Ann Surg* 1980;191:703

74. Glatterer MS Jr, Toon RS, Ellestad C, et al: Managment of blunt and penetrating external esophageal trauma. *J Trauma* 1985;24:784

75. Pate JW: Tracheobronchial and esophageal injuries. *Surg Clin North Am* 1989;69:111

76. Durham RM, Olson S, Weigelt JA: Penetrating injuries to the stomach. *Surg Gynecol Obstet* 1991;172:298

77. Brunsting LA, Morton JH: Gastric rupture from blunt abdominal trauma. *J Trauma* 1987;27:887

78. Stevens SL, Maull KI: Small bowel injuries. *Surg Clin North Am* 1990;70:541

79. Christophi C, McDermott FT, McVey I, et al: Seat belt-induced trauma to the small bowel. *World J Surg* 1985;9:794

80. Dauterive AH, Flancbaum L, Cox EF: Blunt intestinal trauma: a modern-day review. *Ann Surg* 1985;201:198

81. Ross SE, Cobean RA, Hoyt DB, et al: Blunt colonic injury: a multicenter review. *J Trauma* 1992;33:379

82. Stone HH, Fabian TC: Management of perforating colon trauma: randomization between primary closure and exteriorization. *Ann Surg* 1979;190:430

83. George SM, Fabian TC, Voeller GR, et al: Primary repair of colon wounds: a prospective trial in non selected patients. *Ann Surg* 1989;209:728

84. Burch JM, Martin RR, Richardson RJ, et al: Evolution of the treatment of the injured colon in the 1980's. *Arch Surg* 1991;126:979

85. Chappuis CW, Frey DJ, Dietzen CD, et al: Management of penetrating colon injuries: a prospective randomized trial. *Ann Surg* 1991;213:492

86. Martin RR, Burch JM, Richardson R, et al: Outcome for delayed operation of penetrating colon injuries. *J Trauma* 1991;31:1591

87. Demetriades D, Pantanowitz D, Charalambides D: Gunshot wounds of the colon: role of primary repair. *Ann R Coll Surg Engl* 1992;74:381

88. Falcone RE, Wanamaker SR, Santanello SA, et al: Colorectal trauma: primary repair or anastomosis with intracolonic bypass vs. ostomy. *Dis Colon Rectum* 1992;35:957

89. Poret HA, Fabian TC, Croce MA, et al: Analysis of septic morbidity following gunshot wounds to the colon: the missile is and adjuvant for abscess. *J Trauma* 1991;31:1088

90. Fabian TC, Croce MA, Payne LW, et al: Duration of antibiotic therapy for penetrating abdominal trauma: a prospective trial. *Surgery* 1992:112:788

91. Burch JM, Feliciano DV, Mattox KL: Colostomy and drainage for civilian rectal injuries: is that all? *Ann Surg* 1989;209:600

92. Franko ER, Ivatury RR, Schwalb DA: Combined penetrating rectal and genitourinary injuries: a challenge in management. *J Trauma* 1993;34:347

93. Shannon FL, Moore EE, Moore FA, et al: Value of distal colon washout in civilian rectal trauma: reducing gut bacterial translocation. *J Trauma* 1988;28:989

94. Fallon WF Jr: The present role of colostomy in the management of trauma. *Dis Colon Rectum* 1992;35:1094

95. Renz BM, Feliciano DV, Sherman R: Same admission colostomy closure (SACC): a new approach to rectal wounds. A prospective study. *Ann Surg* 1993;218:279

96. Mattox KL, Burch JM, Richardson R, et al: Retroperitoneal vascular injury. *Surg Clin North Am* 1990:70:635

97. Feliciano DV: Management of traumatic retroperitoneal hematoma. *Ann Surg* 1990;211:109

98. Posner MC, Moore EE, Grenholz SK, et al: Natural history of untreated inferior vena cava injury and assessment of venous access. *J Trauma* 1986:26:698

99. Goins WA, Rodriguez A, Lewis J, et al: Retroperitoneal hematoma after blunt trauma. *Surg Gynecol Obstet* 1992;174:281

100. Cooper C, Rodriguez A, Omert L: Blunt vascular trauma. *Curr Probl Surg* 1992;29:283

101. Enderson BL, Maull KI: Missed injuries: the trauma surgeon's nemesis. *Surg Clin North Am* 1991;71:399

102. Scalea TM, Phillips TF, Goldstein AS, et al: Injuries missed at operation: nemesis of the trauma surgeon. *J Trauma* 1988;28:962

Critical Care, Third Edition, edited by Joseph M. Civetta,
Robert W. Taylor, and Robert R. Kirby.
Lippincott-Raven Publishers, Philadelphia, PA © 1997.

CHAPTER 71

■

Evaluating the Acute Abdomen

Jorge Luis Sosa
H. David Reines

IMMEDIATE CONCERNS ■

Patients are admitted for resuscitation and evaluation of an acute abdominal problem preoperatively, have had surgical intervention for an acute abdomen, or will develop an acute abdomen while being treated for other conditions in the intensive care unit (ICU).

Preoperatively, the most important issue is resuscitation to assure organ perfusion and oxygen delivery. Correction of electrolyte and acid–base imbalances is also essential. Some patients may require diagnostic evaluation to determine the cause and need for surgical management.

Postoperative patients should have resuscitation continued, definitive correction of deficits, general supportive care, and close observation for development of complications.

Patients admitted for conditions such as respiratory failure, cardiac dysfunction, renal failure, or trauma can develop acute abdominal complications. These can be catastrophic if unrecognized. Careful attention to the abdominal examination is essential.

STRESS POINTS

1. Appendicitis, cholecystitis, diverticulitis, and other common acute abdominal problems develop in critically ill patients. Patients who are not improving as expected, after adequate treatment of the primary disorder, must be examined for possible intraabdominal complications.
2. Ruptured appendicitis, perforated viscus, gangrenous cholecystitis, strangulated bowel obstruction, and sup-

purative peritonitis are usually treated surgically. Pancreatitis, hepatitis, and sickle cell crisis are often best managed medically. The differentiation is often difficult. An experienced surgeon should be consulted during decision making.
3. One of the most difficult diagnostic problems is the detection of an acute abdomen. Patients are typically intubated, sedated, and receiving multiple medications. The physical examination is often unreliable. They have multiple reasons for fever, leukocytosis, abnormal blood chemistry results, and clinical findings.
4. Common entities include acalculous cholecystitis, perforated ulcer, and intestinal ischemia. Less common problems are appendicitis, diverticulitis, pancreatitis, and missed injuries from trauma. The most important step is to think of them.

ESSENTIAL DIAGNOSTIC TESTS AND PROCEDURES

1. Leukocytosis, including a shift to immature leukocytes, is too nonspecific. Blood chemistry analysis may be helpful, such as hyperamylasemia in pancreatitis or elevated liver enzymes in cholangitis.
2. An abdominal radiograph showing free intraperitoneal air is useful.
3. Abdominal ultrasound can aid in diagnosing cholangitis caused by biliary obstruction, cholecystitis, and occasionally pancreatitis. It can also identify intraperitoneal blood in the setting of abdominal trauma, ectopic pregnancy, and ruptured hepatic lesions.

1099

4. Computed tomographic (CT) scan of the abdomen with contrast enhancement is useful in trauma, diverticulitis, appendicitis, and subphrenic abscess. Gallium and indium scans are of little value.
5. Diagnostic peritoneal lavage (DPL) is particularly helpful in patients with blunt abdominal trauma. An elevated leukocyte count in lavage fluid suggests peritonitis and viscus perforation.
6. Diagnostic laparoscopy (DL) is useful in abdominal trauma, appendicitis, perforated ulcer, and cholecystitis. It can be readily performed at the bedside in the ICU with local anesthesia.

INITIAL THERAPY

1. Intravascular volume deficits are corrected with isotonic fluid administration. In contraction alkalosis, use normal saline. In hemorrhagic shock or metabolic acidosis, Ringer's lactate should be used.
2. Perioperative losses and ongoing third-space losses must be corrected. Adequate urine output, 0.5 to 1 mL/kg/hour, is a useful guide.
3. Osmotic diuresis (from mannitol or glycosuria), polyuric renal failure, or diabetes insipidus may produce adequate or high urine output in the face of depleted intravascular volume.
4. Invasive hemodynamic monitoring may be warranted if urine output alone is an inadequate sole end point.
5. Electrolyte and acid–base disturbances are particularly important in the preoperative patient in whom hypokalemia and other abnormalities may increase the anesthetic risk.

INTRODUCTION ■

An *acute abdomen* is any problem in which the patient's pain or other physical finding originates from an abdominal lesion resulting in serious morbidity or mortality without appropriate therapy.

Acute abdominal problems are frequent sources of admission and complications in ICUs. Early recognition of the acute abdomen and initiation of definitive surgical or medical therapy often determines the ultimate outcome. Therefore, a knowledge of common abdominal problems and appropriate diagnostic modalities, and rapid initiation of therapy are essential parts of the armamentarium of all ICU physicians. A high index of suspicion that an abdominal problem is causing a patient's critical illness is important to stimulate the necessary diagnostic and therapeutic responses.

Searching for a cause of abdominal signs and symptoms is extremely difficult in the critically ill patient. The patient may not be able to give a lucid history, especially if intubated or sedated. Physical findings may be masked by narcotics, steroids, and other therapy administered. Table 71-1 describes a general approach to acute abdominal problems.

Sixteen percent of patients presenting to emergency departments have an acute surgical problem.[1] The most common causes of acute surgical abdominal pain in the outpatient setting are pelvic inflammatory disease, appendicitis,

TABLE 71-1. General Approach to Acute Abdominal Problems

HISTORY

   Pain
   Nausea, vomiting
   Previous surgery
   Previous abdominal symptoms

PHYSICAL

   Tenderness, rebound
   Distention
   Decreased, absent, or hyperactive bowel sounds
   Hypotension, unknown etiology
   Fever, unknown etiology
   Rectal, pelvic examination
   Murphy's, obturator, psoas, Grey-Turner signs
   Peritoneal lavage
   Diagnostic laparoscopy

LABORATORY

   CBC with differential
   Amylase isoenzymes
   Lipase, calcium, phosphorus
   Bilirubin, SGOT, LDH, alkaline phosphatase
   Arterial blood gas, lactate levels

RADIOLOGIC STUDIES

   KUB, upright abdomen, chest, decubitus
   Ultrasound
   CT scan
   Gallium-indium scans

THERAPY

   Nasogastric tube
   Foley catheter
   Fluid resuscitation
   Antacids, sucralfate
   Hemodynamic monitoring
   Antibiotics
   Exploratory laparotomy/laparoscopy
   Chest tube drainage

CBC, complete blood count; SGOT, serum glutamic oxaloacetic transaminase; LDH, lactate dehydrogenase; KUB, kidney–ureter–bladder; CT, computed tomographic.

acute cholecystitis, intestinal obstruction, and duodenal ulcer. Surgical problems also occur frequently in a respiratory care unit. Aranha and Goldberg[2] reported that 32 of 175 (18%) patients on ventilators had an acute abdominal problem. Gastrointestinal bleeding was the most common finding, followed by ileus, bowel obstruction, and peritonitis that required operation.

ANATOMY ■

The peritoneal cavity is a potential space with less than 100 mL of free fluid to lubricate the bowel, liver, and other abdominal organs. Pain sensations from the abdomen are mediated through the somatic sensory and the autonomic nervous systems. Abdominal organs innervated by auto-

TABLE 71-2. Causes of Abdominal Pain by Location

RIGHT UPPER QUADRANT
  Cholecystitis
  Common duct obstruction
  Pancreatitis
  Peptic ulcer disease
  Ureteral obstruction
  Hepatitis
  Right lower lobe pneumonia
  Diverticulitis
  Female genital disease

LEFT UPPER QUADRANT
  Peptic ulcer
  Pancreatitis
  Splenic disease
  Hiatal hernia
  Ureteral obstruction
  Left lower lobe

EPIGASTRIUM
  Peptic ulcer
  Pancreatitis
  Myocardial infarction
  Hiatal hernia

PERIUMBILICUS
  Early appendicitis
  Small bowel obstruction
  Mesenteric artery occlusion
  Expanding/leaking aneurysms

RIGHT LOWER QUADRANT
  Acute appendicitis
  Female genital disease
  Ureteral obstruction
  Diverticulitis
  Enterocolitis
  Colon obstruction

LEFT LOWER QUADRANT
  Sigmoid diverticulitis
  Sigmoid volvulus
  Female genital disease
  Colitis
  Ureteral obstruction

RADIATION TO BACK
  Lower dorsal
  Biliary obstruction
  Pancreatitis
  Ureteral obstruction
  Expanding/leaking aneurysms
  Lower lumbar
  Female genital disease
  Rectal disease

nomic nerves cause visceral pain, especially when stretched or distended. The pain from these organs is transmitted according to developmental patterns: foregut (stomach, liver, biliary tract, spleen, pancreas, and duodenum) radiating to the upper epigastrium; midgut (small bowel, appendix, and right colon) radiating to the periumbilical region; and hindgut (left colon and rectum) radiating to the hypogastrium. Nerves follow the distribution of the blood supply from major splanchnic arteries. This visceral pain is crampy (colicky) in nature and poorly localized; it is often associated with nausea and vomiting.

Somatic pain from peritoneal irritation is well localized over the site of inflammation and is usually a steady, severe pain rather than a paroxysmal cramping type of sensation. Significant peritoneal irritation leads to spasm of the overlying musculature resulting in what is typically described as guarding. Eventually this progresses to rigid abdominal musculature. The pain of peritonitis is significantly aggravated by coughing, deep breathing, increased intraabdominal pressure and motion. Therefore, patients tend typically to lie still. This is in contrast to colicky pain when patients are found thrashing around. The typical distribution of somatic pain for various entities is described in Table 71-2.

Referred pain follows neural pathways. Pain referred to the *epaulet* area of the shoulders may be caused by a ruptured spleen or blood from an ectopic pregnancy irritating the phrenic nerve of the diaphragm, which has a sensory branch in the left shoulder.

HISTORY ■

A detailed review of abdominal symptoms should be obtained from either the patient or a family member. The history should include previous surgery, family history, and a list of medications. It should detail any nausea and vomiting, hematemesis, hematochezia, and constipation. Symptoms of biliary disease, especially pain and jaundice, and a history of ethanol use should be noted.

A careful evaluation of the characteristics of abdominal pain is essential. Its nature, onset, associated symptoms, radiation, and other characteristics are useful in localizing and delineating the etiology.

Abdominal symptoms can be masked by other disease processes. A diabetic patient who presents with diabetic ketoacidosis may have an underlying abdominal catastrophe as a precipitating factor. Syncope is a symptom that can be caused by a ruptured aneurysm, a ruptured spleen, an ectopic pregnancy, or any severe abdominal catastrophe, as well as by neurologic and metabolic problems. Arthritic patients who are taking steroids or nonsteroidal antiinflammatory agents and whose conditions suddenly deteriorate must be suspected of harboring an intraabdominal problem, such as gastrointestinal bleeding or perforation, as a consequence of their medications.

Other diseases that cause abdominal pain include lower lobe pneumonia, renal colic, myocardial infarction, and pericarditis. Although porphyria and sickle cell crises can mimic abdominal catastrophes, they rarely cause admission to ICUs.

PHYSICAL EXAMINATION ■

The initial physical examination of the patient in the ICU is important because it is usually the most complete. The standard routine of inspection, palpation, percussion, and auscultation should be performed. Vital signs, including blood pressure (with the patient sitting if possible), pulse, respiratory rate, and rectal or core temperature, should be taken. Too often, oral or axillary temperatures are normal because of peripheral cooling, nasal oxygen administration, or nasogastric tubes. The presence of hypotension or fever in association with abdominal findings should raise suspicion of an acute intraabdominal process.

Examination of the abdomen in the critically ill patient who may be combative, comatose, narcotized, or paralyzed is difficult. Observation is a technique frequently forgotten in the ICU environment where attention is focused on numerical data. Distention, hematoma, an abdominal scar, and dilated veins are all abnormal findings that should alert the physician to an abdominal problem.

Rebound tenderness is always abnormal and signifies inflammation of the parietal peritoneum. Percussion or pressing gently on the abdomen with sudden release that elicits pain, a grimace, or even movement in a delirious patient suggests an acute problem. Localized tenderness in the right upper quadrant suggests an acute biliary problem, although a tender liver may result from acute right-sided heart failure or hepatitis. Palpation may discern an incarcerated hernia, a distended gallbladder or enlarged spleen, a lower abdominal abscess, or an abdominal aneurysm. Rectal and pelvic examinations are mandatory to discover masses, prostatic infection, and bloody stools.

Auscultation of the abdomen is as important as listening to breath or heart sounds. Absence of bowel sounds is associated with peritonitis, ileus, or severe ischemic disease and is always abnormal. Bowel sounds are frequently absent in paralyzed patients, despite the fact that muscular paralysis should not eliminate the autonomic bowel function. Hyperactive sounds or "rushes" are most common with small bowel obstruction.

The physical examination of the acute abdomen should be performed by an experienced physician. Serial examinations are essential to carefully document any progression of tenderness, muscular rigidity, and the overall trend toward improvement or deterioration. An isolated examination is not nearly as useful as sequential examinations by the same observer. The physician who will ultimately make the decision whether surgical intervention is required should be involved as early as possible.

ADJUNCTIVE PROCEDURES ■

PERITONEAL LAVAGE

When results from the abdominal examination are equivocal and the patient cannot cooperate, DPL may be indicated. It has been useful in differentiating extraalveolar air (barotrauma), presenting as pneumoperitoneum and associated with pneumomediastinum in patients requiring high inspiratory pressures.[3] Lavage can differentiate blood from ascites or an inflammatory exudate caused by pancreatitis. It should be considered when the possibility of ischemic intestine exists or when other causes of peritonitis are suspected. In one series, 23 of 44 critically ill patients with abdominal findings had a positive lavage. There were no false-negative results and three false-positive results. True-positive diagnoses included infarcted bowel, acalculous cholecystitis, perforated bowel, and intraloop abscess.[4] Finding bloody fluid in the patient with suspected ischemic disease usually means severely compromised bowel; bile, bacteria, blood ($>50,000$ cells/mm^3), elevated white blood cell (WBC) count (>250 cells/mm^3), and an elevated amylase level are consistent with ischemia, perforation of a viscus, or hemorrhagic pancreatitis. Other studies reveal similar accuracy rates (95%), with a complication rate of 1% to 5%.[5] The advantage of lavage is the ease with which it can be performed at the bedside to yield information not necessarily gained by more costly and time-consuming tests such as CT scan, angiography, or laparoscopy. Open and closed techniques have been used satisfactorily. Lavage also has been helpful in diagnosing primary peritonitis.

LABORATORY EVALUATION

Laboratory tests should be viewed as adjuncts in the evaluation of patients. They often provide useful data but are rarely diagnostic. Depending excessively on laboratory findings is costly and occasionally misleading. A complete hemogram, including hematocrit, hemoglobin, and complete WBC count, is routine. A decreasing WBC count may give a false sense of improvement, because severe septicemia can cause a leukopenia with a marked shift to the left that will be missed without a differential count. Urinalysis, including specific gravity and analysis for bacteria, bile, and reducing substances, should be performed. Patients with indwelling Foley catheters often have asymptomatic bacteriuria and mild hematuria. If this "benign bacteriuria" prompts a full work-up of the urinary system, it will delay the diagnosis of the true etiology. The serum amylase concentration, especially fractionated into isoenzymes, is helpful in diagnosing intraabdominal catastrophe when it is elevated, but it may be increased in ischemic bowel disease, facial trauma, perforated ulcer, and pancreatitis, or without apparent cause.[6] Calcium, phosphorus, and lipase values are also helpful in determining the severity of pancreatitis. An elevated serum bilirubin level is associated with sepsis, resolving hematoma, hemolysis, and hepatobiliary disease.[7] Likewise, the lactate dehydrogenase concentration may be elevated in numerous disease processes. Liver enzymes, such as serum glutamate oxaloacetic transaminase, serum glutamic pyruvic transaminase, and alkaline phosphatase can be helpful but are rarely diagnostic by themselves.

Laboratory data are most useful in the management and correction of fluids, electrolytes, and acid–base derangements. Persistent acidosis and arterial hypoxemia suggest severe metabolic problems that may be a reflection of unresolved third-space losses from untreated abdominal sepsis or ischemia.

RADIOGRAPHIC STUDIES

Although plain portable radiographs of the abdomen are obtained on most patients with suspicious abdominal findings, their yield is relatively low and their quality is frequently suboptimal. Plain abdominal films are useful to examine abnormal gas patterns intraluminally and extraluminally. The absence of gas may be found with ischemic bowel, whereas small bowel obstruction and colonic volvulus present with massive gaseous distention. An upright abdominal film is desirable; however, many patients in an ICU cannot tolerate this procedure, and, therefore, a left lateral decubitus film to discover air–fluid levels and free air above the liver should be obtained. Free air from a perforated viscus is best seen in an upright chest radiograph, which is usually possible to obtain in the critically ill patient by sitting the patient up in bed and elevating the head of the bed 75 to 90 degrees (Fig. 71-1).

A useful examination for the diagnosis of biliary disease is ultrasonography, which may be rapidly performed at the bedside. It is a fairly inexpensive and noninvasive technique and therefore has gained widespread acceptance. It is often used to evaluate the gallbladder and biliary tree. However, in the critically ill patient who has been taking nothing orally with hyperalimentation for a prolonged period, the gallbladder can be expected to be distended with poor contractility. Thus, the specificity of ultrasound for acalculous cholecystitis is not optimal. It is most often combined with radionuclide scanning in these cases. Ultrasound is useful in demonstrating intraabdominal blood or fluid and to perform percutaneous abscess drainage.

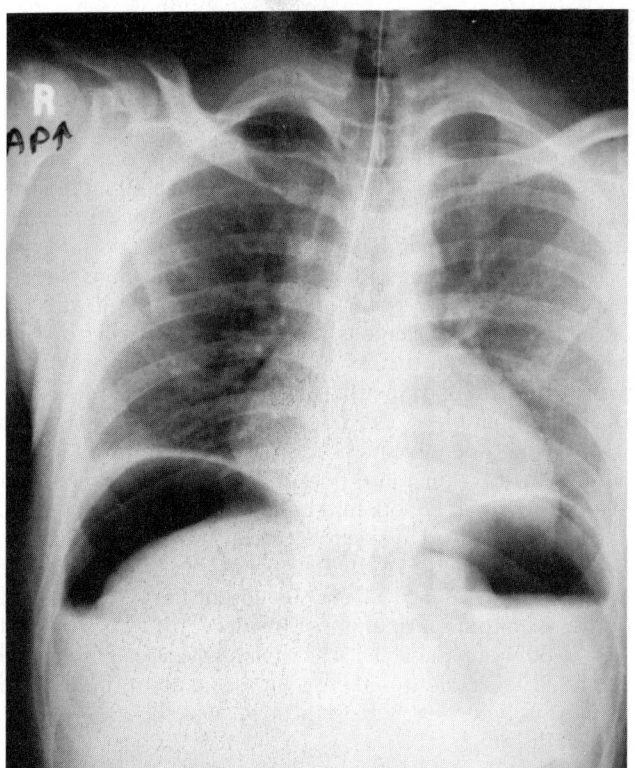

FIGURE 71-1. Pneumoperitoneum secondary to perforated viscus.

The other technique that has played an increasing role in abdominal disease is CT scanning, which is more accurate for diagnosing intraabdominal fluid collections than any other modality.[8] It is especially useful in liver, splenic, renal, and retroperitoneal abscesses but may not be as useful as ultrasound in the diagnosis of right upper quadrant and pelvic masses. Optimal use of CT scan requires oral contrast, which may be difficult for the critically ill patient to ingest and retain. It also requires transporting the patient to the scanner accompanied by a nurse, therapist, and physician, and the possibility exists of an untoward event during transport.

The enthusiasm for CT scanning must be tempered by an evaluation of the efficacy of scans in critically ill patients. In a study by Norwood and Civetta, scans were found to be helpful only in 23% of patients, most of whom had been examined because of postoperative sepsis.[9] These modalities are most useful when used in a focused manner to evaluate physical findings. They are least valuable when used as part of a shotgun approach to sepsis. Gallium scanning has been used to identify intraabdominal abscesses. In one study, gallium scanning was helpful in less than 25% of patients with suspected intraabdominal abscess. The procedure requires transporting the patient to the radiology department on 2 consecutive days. Because of its low specificity, it is not recommended for diagnosing intraabdominal infection in the critically ill.[10]

DL has long been advocated as a tool for abdominal problems. It failed to gain widespread acceptance because of poor optics and instrumentation. With the advent of new videolaparoscopy and instruments specifically developed for laparoscopic use, DL is an effective diagnostic tool.[11]

At the University of Miami-Jackson Memorial Medical Center, DL has been used in the evaluation of the acute abdomen in trauma and nontrauma patients.[11] It has been successfully used in the diagnosis of acalculous and calculous cholecystitis, pelvic inflammatory disease, appendicitis, ischemic bowel, perforated ulcer, and iatrogenic viscus perforation.[12,13]

Bedside laparoscopy can be used in the ICU.[14] An integrated protocol should be developed including a complete instrument cart, trained assistants, experienced surgeons, assistance from anesthesiologists, and an informed and cooperative staff. Intubated patients are temporarily paralyzed after appropriate sedation. Local anesthesia is employed to allow introduction of the Hasson trocar under direct vision. The laparoscope is introduced under low-pressure (5 to 7 mm Hg) carbon dioxide insufflation. Additional trocars are placed as necessary. Extubated patients can benefit from laparoscopy, but the procedure is difficult and requires significant experience with deep sedation and local anesthetic techniques.[14]

THERAPY ∎

The treatment of intraabdominal problems in the acutely ill frequently requires surgical intervention; therefore, consultation should be obtained early in the evaluation. In the preoperative patient, adequate volume resuscitation and electrolyte correction are vital to prepare the patient for surgical repair of the underlying problem. Most fluid losses in preoperative surgical patients are isotonic. Patients who are volume contracted may be hyponatremic, hypochloremic, hypokalemic, and alkalotic because of vomiting, nasogastric suctioning, and third-space losses. These patients require normal saline resuscitation. Only after volume and salt repletion will their chloride-dependent alkalosis resolve. Although hypokalemia may exist, potassium should be administered cautiously until oliguria is resolved.

The specific management of disease entities should be based on well-established surgical principles. Appendicitis, perforated viscus, bowel obstruction, and ruptured aortic aneurysms all require surgical repair. Acute cholecystitis may be treated conservatively for 24 to 48 hours; however, if it does not resolve or if cholangitis or emphysematous cholecystitis is observed, surgery or percutaneous drainage is necessary. Stress ulceration without perforation may be prophylactically treated with antacids, H_2 blockers, and sucralfate, although aggressive pH control may lead to an increase in nosocomial pneumonia.[15-17] Stress ulcer bleeding is rare but is best prevented, and next treated medically because of the high mortality rate (50%) associated with surgery in these critically ill patients.[18,19] If bleeding cannot be contained with conservative measures, however, then operative intervention should be undertaken. Do not wait until multiple transfusions have created dilutional or hypothermic coagulopathies, because mortality rates will approach 100%.

The use of CT scan and ultrasonic-guided drainage and catheter decompression of intraabdominal abscesses has revolutionized care in some postoperative patients. This procedure results in excellent control of the septic source with a low morbidity. It is often preferable to secondary exploratory laparotomy. However, if a patient persists in a downward clinical course, exploration with wide drainage of abscesses may be necessary. In patients with diffuse persistent peritonitis or necrotizing pancreatitis, conversion to an open abdomen with zipper technique may be needed to control the infection (Chap. 72).

Antibiotics are not a panacea for intraabdominal sepsis, and abscesses will form despite adequate coverage. The use of antibiotics in acute abdominal problems is usually adjunctive to prevent systemic sepsis. The prolonged use of antibiotics for localized abscesses instead of surgical or radiologic intervention can lead to morbidity and increased mortality.

Acute abdominal catastrophe may be the first event in the precipitous cascade of multiple organ system failure (MOSF). Unrecognized abdominal sepsis is associated with MOSF in 44% of cases.[20,21] Early aggressive surgical therapy, vigorous fluid replacement, and appropriate antibiotic regimens are necessary to prevent fatal outcome in MOSF.

SPECIAL CONDITIONS

Although appendicitis is the most common abdominal condition requiring surgery, it is rarely seen in the ICU. Pancreatitis and acalculous cholecystitis are more common, especially after open heart surgery. Abdominal distention in elderly patients after orthopedic procedures is frequently caused by ileus and colonic pseudo-obstruction. Patients receiving mechanical ventilation are at high risk for gastrointestinal bleeding, ileus, and unrecognized perforation. Stress ulcer perforation and ileus are insidious causes of respiratory failure and sepsis in any patient with a spinal injury.

The immune-compromised host requires special attention when presenting with abdominal pain. Patients with acquired immunodeficiency syndrome (AIDS) frequently present with abdominal complaints that rarely need surgery. The incidence of abdominal surgical conditions in AIDS patients ranges from 2% to 4%. The common conditions necessitating operation include cholecystitis (60% are acalculous), thrombocytopenia secondary to splenomegaly, and appendicitis, whereas many other processes, including perforation secondary to small bowel ulceration, intussusception, and Kaposi's sarcoma, are encountered. Mortality rates can be extremely high (33% for cholecystectomy when performed for sepsis), whereas the mortality rate for AIDS patients who undergo elective operations (splenectomy for pancytopenia) are the same as for non-AIDS patients.[22]

Neutropenic patients with cancer also present a diagnosis and therapeutic challenge. In patients who underwent emergency celiotomy for suspected intraabdominal disease, the most common disease has been reported to be neutropenic enteropathy (61%) with postoperative mortality up to 32%.[23]

Any stable patient in an ICU developing sudden shock or sepsis must be examined closely for an intraabdominal cause. Several conditions that are common causes of abdominal symptoms in critically ill patients are presented in the following sections.

BILIARY DISEASE

Primary biliary tract disease in critically ill patients appears as calculous or acalculous cholecystitis. Calculous disease may present as acute cholecystitis, cholangitis, or pancreatitis. Acute acalculous biliary disease is a concomitant of critical illness and has been reported in 1% of surgical patients and 0.2% of postoperative cardiac patients.[24]

The differentiation of calculous from acalculous disease can be difficult. Several risk factors are associated with the development of acalculous cholecystitis, including use of narcotics for more than 6 days, gastric suction, prolonged ileus with nothing by mouth, ventilatory support longer than 24 hours, multiple recent operations, more than ten blood transfusions, open wound or abscesses, and intravenous hyperalimentation for more than 3 days.[24,25] The presence of five of these risk factors in a patient with acute abdominal findings should lead to a search for acalculous biliary disease.

The typical picture of right upper quadrant pain, positive Murphy's sign, and fever may be absent in critically ill patients. Symptoms of right upper quadrant pain were present in only 30% of patients with acalculous disease, although all exhibited fever. Peritonitis was an inconsistent finding and present in only 24%. Persistent fever was the most consistent finding.[26]

The laboratory findings of biliary disease are variable. Leukocytosis is common, although nonspecific. Up to 65% of patients with acalculous cholecystitis have elevated bilirubin;

however, a control group of patients receiving multiple transfusions had similar hyperbilirubinemia.[26] Liver enzymes are elevated in less than 50%.[24]

Acute cholecystitis can mimic numerous other disease processes in the abdomen. Conversely, the presence of stones in the gallbladder in patients with nonspecific symptoms is not pathognomonic of acute biliary disease. The discovery of radionucleotide imaging techniques that can distinguish cystic duct obstruction in acute cholecystitis from other causes of abdominal pain have markedly increased our diagnostic acumen.[27] Derivatives of iminodiacetic acid are rapidly taken up by the hepatocytes and excreted into the bile even in patients with elevations of bilirubin up to 6 mg/dL. The test has proved to be 95% accurate in the diagnosis of acute cholecystitis. The presence of fever, mild elevation of bilirubin, sludge on ultrasound, and nonvisualization on DISIDA are accurate indications of acute acalculous cholecystitis in critically ill patients. Caution is urged, however, in patients receiving hyperalimentation, which severely limits the usefulness of the test.[28,29] Furthermore, DISIDA scan requires moving the critically ill patient to the radiology suite for up to 4 hours, and the risk–benefit ratio requires a high degree of clinical suspicion. The treatment of choice has been surgical drainage, either cholecystostomy or cholecystectomy, if the patient is able to tolerate a major procedure. The use of percutaneous cholecystostomy has been reported in severely ill patients.[30] Mortality rate associated with acalculous cholecystitis is as high as 40% secondary to the multiplicity of the patient's problems.[26]

The use of bedside laparoscopy has revolutionized the diagnosis of acalculous cholecystitis. These critically ill patients, who previously were subjected to many diagnostic procedures and trips out of the ICU to confirm the diagnosis, now may have the diagnosis made quickly in their ICU bed. With the advent of videolaparoscopy, DL can be performed at the bedside and definitively rule in or out acalculous cholecystitis.[12,14]

The treatment protocol at the University of Miami-Jackson Memorial Medical Center established three possibilities:

1. If the gallbladder is normal, then the diagnosis is discarded and the search continued for other causes. There is a concerted effort during laparoscopy to evaluate the entire peritoneal cavity and exclude other abdominal disease.
2. If the gallbladder is found to be inflamed or gangrenous, the patient is taken to the operating room for definitive management.
3. If the gallbladder is found to be distended with questionable evidence of inflammation, a cholecystostomy tube is placed.[14]

DL has been performed at the bedside in patients after blunt abdominal trauma and in surgical and medical ICU patients. The results are excellent in acalculous cholecystitis. No false-negative results have occurred, and cholecystitis has been confirmed at surgery and by pathologic examination. A DL has been successfully used to demonstrate ischemic bowel and perforated ulcers, and after percutaneous endoscopically or radiologically placed feeding tubes, to demonstrate tube dislodgment as a cause of abdominal pain.

ABSCESS

The most common causes of primary intraabdominal sepsis are appendicitis, diverticulitis, perforated ulcer, and pelvic inflammatory disease.[31] Postoperative sepsis after abdominal procedures is a frequent cause of acute deterioration in ICU patients.[32,33] Diagnosis of intraabdominal abscess requires astute clinical acumen and proper use of radiographic tools. In a series of 34 patients with postoperative abscess, we found fever intermittent, but present, in all. Only 12% had a palpable mass. Peritonitis was present in 20% and ileus in only 40%. Physical examination was diagnostic in less than 50% of patients. Other organ failure included hepatic failure (10%), adult respiratory distress syndrome (25%), and acute renal failure (20%). Leukocytosis was present in only 85%.[34] Other authors report up to a 75% accuracy of physical findings in the diagnosis of abscess.[35]

Numerous radiographic procedures, including KUB, liver–spleen scan, and gallium scanning, have been performed with only a 50% efficacy rate. In general, gallium scanning is too time consuming and difficult to perform in critically ill patients and is rarely helpful.[10] Ultrasound has been beneficial in diagnosing lesions of the pelvis or right upper quadrant and can be helpful in the diagnosis and drainage of intraabdominal abscesses.[36] The advantage of ultrasound is that it can be performed at the patient's bedside.

CT scanning can be of great value in evaluating and treating localized intraabdominal fluid collections that can be drained and catheters left in place for continuous decompression. This is the most common way to deal with abscesses. Occasionally, an exploratory laparotomy may be required. This is particularly true when there is diffuse abdominal fluid and peritonitis with no discreet abscess. Often these patients have persistent peritonitis and require conversion to an open abdomen.

Antibiotics are adjunctive in treating intraabdominal sepsis. The bacterial flora are related to the organ involved, the host defenses, and the duration of the critical illness. The bacteriologic makeup of peritonitis includes aerobic *Enterobacteriaceae*, *Pseudomonas*, and anaerobes. Broad-spectrum antibiotics, including third-generation cephalosporins, carbepenems, and β-lactamase inhibitors, quinolones, or combinations that contain anaerobic coverage and an aminoglycoside, are drugs of choice.

Mortality from intraabdominal sepsis ranges from 7.5% for single abscess to 43% for patients with multiple abscesses and peritonitis. Overall mortality from intraabdominal infection is 24%.[37] Mortality correlates directly with acute physiology score, malnutrition, age, and shock.[37] Only early recognition, appropriate use of antibiotics, and prompt drainage can improve on these data.

PNEUMOPERITONEUM

The most common cause of pneumoperitoneum is laparotomy or laparoscopy. After abdominal surgery, free air may persist for weeks, although air from laparoscopy is frequently absent at 48 hours. Perforation of abdominal viscus accounts for 90% of the remaining cases.[38] Duodenal ulcers and stress ulceration of the stomach and duodenum are the most common causes of free air, whereas perforated diverticula and distal bowel are less frequent. Gas-producing organisms and peritoneal lavage are also known causes of pneumoperitoneum. The presence of pneumoperitoneum in ventilated patients creates a diagnostic dilemma. In the absence of other signs of an acute abdominal condition, pneumoperitoneum may be secondary to barotrauma (Fig. 71-2). This is usually associated with peak inspiratory pressures greater than 40 cm H_2O pressure. Pneumoperitoneum has been observed in up to 10% of patients who have demonstrated other evidence of extraalveolar air.[38,39] Macklin postulated that air first ruptures through distended alveoli and dissects toward the mediastinum. From there, it dissects down the mediastinum and ruptures into the peritoneal cavity.[40] The diagnosis of perforated viscus may be difficult in paralyzed, mechanically ventilated patients who cannot complain of tenderness and who will have a soft abdomen and absent bowel sounds. Peritoneal lavage has been helpful as a means of differentiating benign pneumoperitoneum from perforated viscus.[5] The presence of bacteria, bile, more than 500 WBCs per mm^3, or any red blood cells can be inferred to indicate an acute abdominal process requiring immediate laparotomy. If the patient deteriorates clinically, emergency laparotomy should also be done immediately. Diagnostic laparoscopy also is a useful adjunct in the evaluation of pneumoperitoneum.[13]

PSEUDO-OBSTRUCTION OF THE COLON

Isolated colonic ileus without mechanical obstruction was first described by Ogilvie.[41] Patients at risk are the elderly and those requiring bedrest, prolonged narcotic use, and mechanical ventilation.[42,43] Massive colonic distention presents a perplexing dilemma in the ICU. Although the cause is unclear, it seems to be a parasympathetic–sympathetic imbalance. The classic physical finding is a rapid onset of a markedly distended, quiet, tympanitic abdomen associated with vomiting and constipation. Laboratory findings are non-specific with normal amylase and WBCs, although hypokalemia and hyponatremia are not uncommon.

Radiographs in the flat and upright positions suggest large bowel obstruction with massive dilatation of the colon and little or no fluid present. Barium enema is frequently used to rule out distal obstruction and volvulus. This should be performed early and under fluoroscopic control to avoid overdistending the colon (Fig. 71-3). Cecal distention can be marked, and a 9- to 12-cm diameter should be considered the upper limits before surgery is contemplated. Beyond this, the risk of perforation is significant.[44]

Treatment consists of nasogastric decompression and the careful placement of a rectal tube. The use of gentle enemas is also advocated. Colonoscopy should be attempted for decompression, although cecal perforation can take place despite colonoscopic decompression.[45,46] Critically ill patients in an ICU should have colonoscopy as early as possible to relieve distention because of the ease of performing this procedure compared with operative cecostomy. Patients with pneumoperitoneum or signs of peritoneal irritation suggesting perforation should undergo immediate surgical exploration.

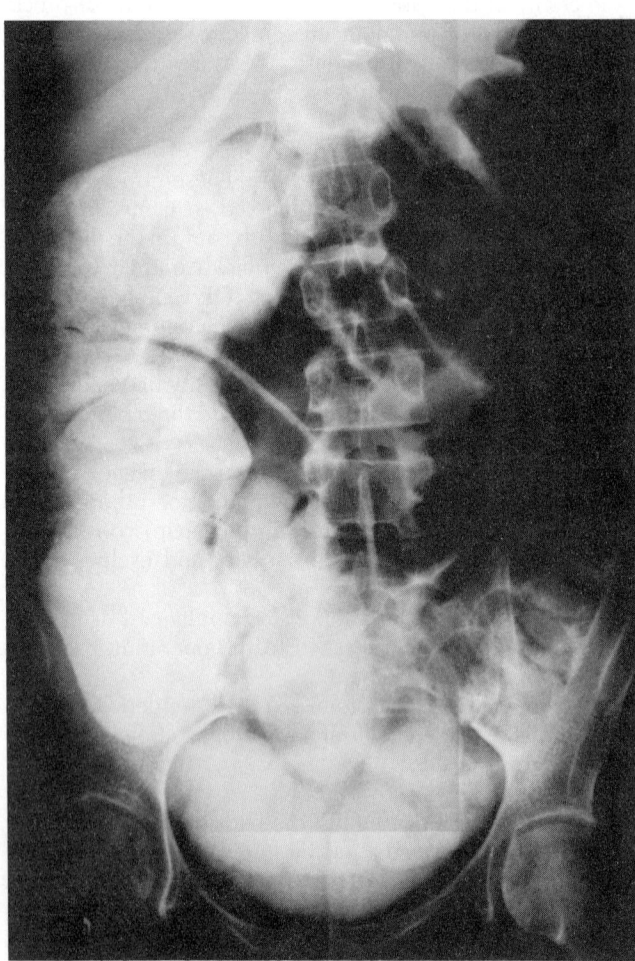

FIGURE 71-3. Barium enema demonstrating colonic ileus without obstruction.

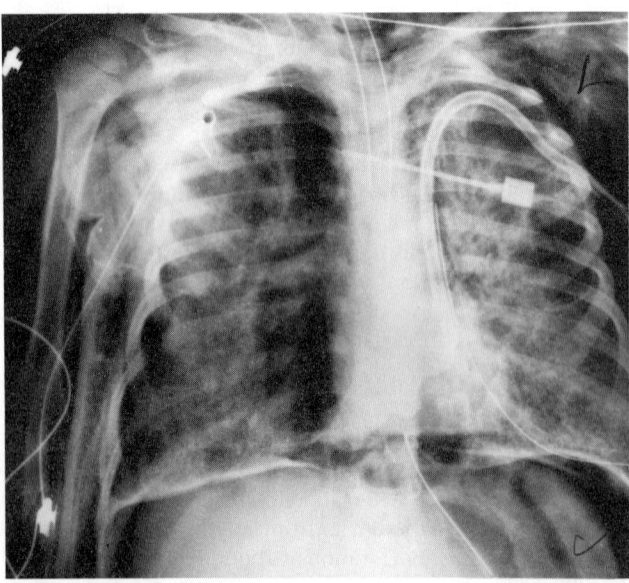

FIGURE 71-2. Pneumoperitoneum secondary to barotrauma.

ACUTE MESENTERIC ISCHEMIA

Numerous causes exist for acute intestinal ischemia. Embolus (50%) or thrombus (25%) of the superior mesenteric artery (SMA) must be differentiated from nonmesenteric thrombosis (20%) and acute mesenteric venous occlusion (5%).[47] Colonic and rectal ischemia have been reported after abdominal aortic aneurysmectomy in which the inferior mesenteric artery was ligated.[48]

A characteristic of gut ischemia is the disparity between the patient's pain and abdominal findings. Pain is found in 75% to 90% of patients. Nausea and vomiting are present in 50% to 60% of patients, whereas upper gastrointestinal bleeding is less common.[48] Abdominal distention is present in 56% to 80%, peritoneal signs in 60%, ileus in 50%, and shock and fever in 30% of patients. Leukocytosis (WBC count of 20,000/mm[3]) is seen in less than 50% of patients. A mild elevation in amylase is common.[49,50]

The presence of physical signs indicating peritoneal irritation is extremely important, because they portend impending or progressive gangrene. Leukocytosis out of proportion to the physical findings, elevated hematocrit, unexplained acidosis, and blood-tinged fluid on peritoneal lavage are all signs of advancing intestinal necrosis.[51]

Plain radiographs are useful to exclude other processes that can stimulate the symptoms. Signs of intestinal ischemia on plain radiographs is a grave prognosticator, with 90% mortality.

Patients at highest risk are those older than 50 years of age with either valvular or atherosclerotic heart disease; congestive heart failure, especially if there is poor control with digitalis and diuretics; hypovolemia or hypotension of any etiology; recent myocardial infarction or cardiogenic shock; or cardiac arrhythmias.[51] Dialysis patients seem to be at added risk for right colon ischemia. The use of sigmoid tonometry also has been suggested to detect colonic ischemia.[52]

Once the diagnosis is suspected, vigorous fluid resuscitation is necessary to maintain adequate blood flow and a pressure head in the mesenteric vessels. Gastrointestinal decompression with a nasogastric tube and proper hemodynamic monitoring are necessary to adequately resuscitate these precarious patients.

Although CT scans may demonstrate clot or ischemia, emergency selective arteriography is the keystone of the diagnostic and therapeutic approach to acute mesenteric ischemia. Arteriography can differentiate occlusive from nonocclusive disease. An acute occlusion is best treated by immediate surgical restoration of circulation by embolectomy or aortosuperior mesenteric artery bypass.

Nonocclusive mesenteric ischemia is diagnosed when mesenteric vasoconstriction on angiogram is seen in the patient with a clinical picture suggestive of intestinal ischemia. Shock and vasopressors make interpretation of the arteriogram difficult. Treatment of this disease is begun in the radiology suite by the administration of papaverine (30 to 60 mg/hour) through a catheter placed selectively in the SMA. If peritoneal signs are present and abdominal exploration is necessary to examine the viability of the bowel, vasodilators and local anesthetics can be injected directly into the base of the mesentery.[47] The role of lytic therapy, such as urokinase or plasminogen activating factor, is unknown.

When papaverine is the primary treatment for nonocclusive ischemia, it is continued for 24 hours and an arteriogram is repeated. Heparin is not used concomitantly.

Maintaining adequate plasma volume and blood pressure is essential to maintain perfusion of the splanchnic vessels. Occasionally, dextran has been used to expand plasma and to decrease sludging.[51] Dopamine is probably the catecholamine of choice if support of blood pressure is necessary because of its theoretical vasodilator effect on the splanchnic vessels, although no clinical data exist to support this. Digitalis should be used cautiously.

Systemic antibiotics are indicated because of the high incidence of positive blood cultures resulting from compromised bowel. Decompression by nasogastric suction can decrease bowel distention.

Mortality rate for acute mesenteric ischemia is 70% to 90%. Embolus in the SMA is still associated with a 44% to 90% mortality rate, whereas nonocclusive ischemia without peritoneal signs has a favorable outcome. Peritonitis is associated with mortality rates of 60% to 90%.[49,51]

The early suspicion of ischemia followed by aggressive and rapid diagnostic workup seems to be the only method for improving this abysmal mortality rate.[52]

CONCLUSION ■

Acute abdominal problems are frequent among ICU patients. The physician must maintain a high level of suspicion that an abdominal problem is present when faced with a deteriorating, critically ill patient. History and physical examination must be used to guide the use of more invasive and expensive tests. Laboratory tests are usually adjunctive and rarely diagnostic. Radiographic procedures, especially ultrasound and CT scans, when appropriately used, can be helpful. Surgical consultation should be obtained early in a patient's course, because treatment frequently requires surgical intervention. Only by maintaining constant vigilance can critical care practitioners guide their patients through the multiple perturbations created by acute abdominal problems.

REFERENCES ■

1. Brewer RJ, Golden GT, Hitch DD, et al: Abdominal pain: an analysis of 1,000 consecutive cases in a university hospital emergency room. *Am J Surg* 1976;131:219
2. Aranha GV, Goldberg NB: Surgical problems in patients on ventilators. *Crit Care Med* 1981;9:478
3. Reines HD: Manifestations of barotrauma in acute respiratory failure. *Am Surg* 1981;47:421
4. Alverdy JC, Saunders J, Chamberlin WH, et al: Diagnostic peritoneal lavage in intra-abdominal sepsis. *Am Surg* 1988;54:456
5. Larson FA, Haller C, Delcore R, et al: Diagnostic peritoneal lavage in acute peritonitis. *Am Surg* 1992;164:449

6. Weaver DW, Busuito MJ, Bouwman DL, et al: Interpretation of serum amylase levels in the critically ill patient. *Crit Care Med* 1985;13:532

7. Miller DJ, Keeton GR, Webber BL, et al: Jaundice in severe bacterial infection. *Gastroenterology* 1976;71:94

8. vanSonnenberg E, Mueller PR, Wittenberg J, et al: Comparative utility of ultrasound and computed body tomography in suspected abdominal abscesses. Presented at the Radiologist Society of North America 66th Scientific Assembly, Dallas, Texas, 1980

9. Norwood SH, Civetta JM: Abdominal CT scanning in critically ill surgical patients. *Ann Surg* 1985;202:166

10. Reines HD, Khoury N, Spicer KM: The efficacy of gallium scanning for diagnosis and treatment of intra-abdominal abscess. *Am Surg* 1982;48:59

11. Sosa JL, Puente I: Laparoscopy in the evaluational management of abdominal trauma. *Int Surg* 1995;79:307

12. Brandt CP, Priebe PP, Jacobs DG: Value of laparoscopy in trauma ICU patients with suspected acalculous cholecystitis. *Surg Endosc* 1994;8:361

13. Forde KA, Treat MR: The role of peritoneoscopy (laparoscopy) in the evaluation of the acute abdomen in critically ill patients. *Surg Endosc* 1992;6:219

14. Sleeman D, Sosa JL, Almeida J et al: Laparoscopy for the diagnosis of acalculous cholecystitis in the critically ill [abstract]. *Clin Invest Med* 1994;17:B18

15. Hastings PR, Skillman JJ, Bushnell LS, et al: Antacid titration in the prevention of acute gastrointestinal bleeding: a controlled, randomized trial in 100 critically ill patients. *N Engl J Med* 1978;298:1041

16. Shuman RN, Schoster DP, Zuckerman GR: Prophylactic therapy for stress ulcer feeding: a reappraisal. *Ann Intern Med* 1987;106:562

17. Tryba M: Risk of acute stress bleeding and nosocomial pneumonia in ventilated intensive care unit patients: sucralfate vs. antacids. *Am J Med* 1987;83:117

18. Cook DJ, Fullder HD, Guyatt et al: Risk factors for gastrointestinal bleeding in critically ill patients. *N Engl J Med* 1994;330:377

19. Hubert JP, Kiernam PD, Wekl JS, et al: The surgical management of bleeding stress ulcers. *Ann Surg* 1980;191:672

20. Fry DE, Pearlstein L, Fulton RL, et al: Multiple system organ failure: The role of uncontrolled infection. *Arch Surg* 1980;115:136

21. Knaus WA, Draper EA, Wagner DP, et al: Prognosis in acute organ-system failure. *Ann Surg* 1985;202:685

22. LaRaja RD, Rothenberg RE, Odom JW, et al: The incidence of intra-abdominal surgery in acquired immunodeficiency syndrome: a statistical review of 904 patients. *Surgery* 1989;105:175

23. Glenn J, Funkhouser WK, Schneider PS: Acute illnesses necessitating urgent abdominal surgery of neutropenic cancer patients: description of 14 cases and review of the literature. *Surgery* 1989;105:778

24. Savino JA, Scalea TM, Del Guercio LRM: Factors encouraging laparotomy in acalculous cholecystitis. *Crit Care Med* 1985;13:377

25. Peterson SR, Sheldon GF: Acute acalculous cholecystitis: a complication of hyperalimentation. *Am J Surg* 1979;138:814

26. Long TN, Heimbach DM, Carrico CJ: Acalculous cholecystitis in critically ill patients. *Am J Surg* 1978;136:31

27. Suarez CA, Black F, Bernstein D, et al: The role of HIDA/PIPIDA scanning in diagnosing cystic duct obstruction. *Ann Surg* 1980;191:391

28. Shuman WP, Gibbs P, Rudd TG, et al: PIPIDA scintigraphy for cholecystitis: false positives in alcoholism and total parenteral nutrition. *Am J Radiol* 1982;138:1

29. Kalff V, Froelich JW, Lloyd R, et al: Predictive value of an abdominal hepatobiliary scan in patients with severe intercurrent illness. *Radiology* 1983;146:191

30. Longmaid HE, Bassett JG, Gottlieb H: Management of gallbladder perforation by percutaneous cholecystostomy. *Crit Care Med* 1985;13:686

31. Altemeier WA, Culbertson WR, Fullen WD, et al: Intra-abdominal abscesses. *Am J Surg* 1973;125:70

32. Sinanan M, Maier RV, Carrico CJ: Laparotomy for intra-abdominal sepsis in patients in an intensive care unit. *Arch Surg* 1984;119:652

33. Hinsdale JG, Jaffe BM: Re-operation for intra-abdominal sepsis: indications and results in modern critical care setting. *Ann Surg* 1984;199:31

34. Reines HD, Gobien RP, Hodges PL, et al: Overcoming difficulties in the diagnosis of postoperative abscess [abstract]. *Crit Care Med* 1983;11:250

35. Wright HK, Dunn E, MacArthur JD, et al: Specific but limited role of new imaging techniques in decision-making about intra-abdominal abscesses. *Am J Surg* 1982;143:456

36. Goletti O, Lippolis PV, Chiarugi M, et al: Percutaneous ultrasound-guided drainage of intra-abdominal abscesses. *Br J Surg* 1993;80:336

37. Dellinger EP, Wertz MJ, Meakins JL, et al: Surgical infection stratification system for intra-abdominal infection: multicenter trial. *Arch Surg* 1985;120:21

38. Hillman KM: Pneumoperitoneum: a review. *Crit Care Med* 1982;10:476

39. Macklin MT, Macklin CC: Malignant interstitial emphysema of the lungs and mediastinum as an important occult complication in many respiratory diseases and other conditions: an interpretation of the clinical literature in the light of laboratory experiment. *Medicine* 1944;23:281

40. Macklin CC: Transport of air along sheaths of pulmonic blood vessels from alveoli to mediastinum: clinical implications. *Arch Intern Med* 1939;64:913

41. Ogilvie H: Large intestine colic due to sympathetic deprivation: a new clinical syndrome. *Br J Med* 1948;2:671

42. Golden GT, Chandler JG: Colonic ileus and cecal perforation in patients requiring mechanical ventilatory support. *Chest* 1975;68:661

43. Wanebo H, Mathewson C, Conolly B: Pseudo-obstruction of the colon. *Surg Gynecol Obstet* 1971;133:44

44. Norton L, Young D, Scribner R: Management of pseudo-obstruction of the colon. *Surg Gynecol Obstet* 1974;138-595

45. Geelhoed GW: Colonic pseudo-obstruction in surgical patients. *Am J Surg* 1985;149:258

46. Strodel WE, Nostrant TT, Eckhauser FE, et al: Therapeutic and diagnostic colonoscopy in nonobstructive colonic dilatation. *Ann Surg* 1983;197:416

47. Stoney RJ, Cunningham CG: Acute mesenteric ischemia. *Surgery* 1993;114:489

48. Birnbaum W, Rudy L, Wylie EJ: Colonic and rectal ischemia following abdominal aneurysmectomy. *Dis Colon Rectum* 1964;7:293

49. Hildebrand HD, Zierler RE: Mesenteric vascular disease. *Am J Surg* 1980;139:188

50. Ottinger LW: The surgical management of acute occlusion of the superior mesenteric artery. *Ann Surg* 1978;188:721

51. Boley SJ, Brandt LJ, Veith FS: Ischemic disorders of the intestine. *Curr Probl Surg* 1978;15

52. Montgomery A, Hartmann M, Jonsson K, et al: Intramucosal pH measurement with tonometers for detecting gastrointestinal ischemia in porcine hemorrhage shock. *Circ Shock* 1989;29:319

53. Bergan JJ: Diagnosis of acute intestinal ischemia. *Semin Vasc Surg* 1990;3:143

Critical Care, Third Edition, edited by Joseph M. Civetta,
Robert W. Taylor, and Robert R. Kirby.
Lippincott-Raven Publishers, Philadelphia, PA © 1997.

CHAPTER 72

■

The Complicated
Postoperative Abdomen

Danny Sleeman
Scott Norwood

IMMEDIATE CONCERNS ■

MAJOR PROBLEMS

The diagnostic evaluation of the postoperative abdomen for complications after surgery is a challenging and difficult problem. The intensive care specialist must have a thorough understanding of the nature of the abdominal disease process and the technical aspects of the surgical procedure that was performed. The intensivist's concerns can be divided into general postoperative problems and problems that are unique for a particular operative procedure. General concerns may also be complicated by chronic medical conditions in our increasing elderly patient population.

A thorough knowledge of the normal postoperative physiologic changes and anticipated findings on physical examination is also important, because only with such knowledge can deviations be identified that may indicate a serious complication or progression of the underlying abdominal disease process.

STRESS POINTS

1. Patients with marginal cardiac and pulmonary reserves may benefit from postoperative monitoring in the ICU.
2. Major complications of liver resections are hemorrhage, hemobilia, liver abscess, vascular compromise of the liver, and liver failure.
3. Major complications of pancreatic surgery are hemorrhage and infection.
4. Specific complications of major aortic surgery are isch-

emia of the sigmoid colon, graft infections, and hemorrhage.
5. Synergistic gangrene and necrotizing fasciitis can be early life-threatening complications of any emergency abdominal operation.
6. Acalculous cholecystitis can be a hidden septic focus that can lead to a high mortality if untreated.
7. The open abdomen technique of daily irrigation is a reliable option in the critically ill patient with diffuse persistent peritonitis.
8. Small bowel fistulas postoperatively can lead to a high morbidity and mortality.
9. A knowledge of commonly used intraabdominal tubes and drains is needed for proper management of the patient.

ESSENTIAL DIAGNOSTIC TESTS
AND PROCEDURES

1. Clinical assessment of the postoperative abdomen is often limited but essential.
2. Abdominal ultrasound can be important for the assessment of the gallbladder and the identification of subphrenic and subhepatic abscesses. Bedside sonography is an important adjunct for diagnosis in the critically ill patient.
3. Computed tomography (CT) is one of the main diagnostic tools to assess the postoperative abdomen. CT can be used to guide percutaneous drainage of abscesses.

1109

4. Angiography (and angiographic control of bleeding) is an important tool.
5. Bedside laparoscopy is a new approach for the diagnosis of intraabdominal problems.

INITIAL THERAPY

1. Prolonged intraabdominal procedures can cause major fluid shifts and hypothermia. This is treated by aggressive fluid therapy and rewarming of the patient.
2. Bleeding complications are usually apparent in the first 24 to 48 hours postoperatively. Blood component therapy, rewarming to correct the coagulopathy, and early reoperation in appropriate cases are the cornerstones of therapy.
3. Sepsis is the most common cause of death. Intraabdominal sepsis, a major problem, is treated by drainage of any purulent intraabdominal fluid collections and antibiotic therapy.
4. The proper use of surgical hardware (tubes and drains), including maintaining proper function postoperatively, is important.

EVALUATING THE ELECTIVE POSTOPERATIVE PATIENT ■

REASONS FOR ICU CARE

Surgical patients frequently receive care in the ICU after elective abdominal operations. The choice of intensive care may be merely a need for close observation, but more often it results from a combination of the potential complications that can occur from the complexity of the operation and the relative risk factors of the patient.

Patients with poor cardiac or respiratory function often are selected for monitoring and careful observation after intraabdominal operations because of the physiologic stress that develops. Pain can significantly restrict respiratory function after abdominal procedures, and vigorous pulmonary toilet and pain relief, without respiratory depression, help prevent postoperative pulmonary complications. Continuous epidural analgesia in the postoperative period may also benefit patients with marginal pulmonary function. Patients with marginal cardiac function benefit from prevention of the adverse effects of sinus tachycardia and other arrhythmias that may develop. Elevated heart rates and minor degrees of hypovolemia from fluid losses may be just enough to precipitate a perioperative myocardial infarction. These patients might benefit from pulmonary artery catheterization.

Morbidly obese patients are at high risk and are labor intensive. Abdominal operations and venous access are more difficult in obese patients; also, the probability of postoperative pulmonary, cardiac, and infectious complications is considered much higher.

Advanced age is no longer a contraindication to major surgery. As our patient population ages, other associated medical problems are encountered. These problems are often better managed in an ICU setting.

Even in the absence of significant patient risk factors, many intraoperative problems, such as "third space" fluid losses and hypothermia, may be more rapidly and effectively treated in the ICU.

COMMON ABDOMINAL PROCEDURES RECEIVING ICU MANAGEMENT

Liver Resections

Major liver resections are often performed for primary or metastatic carcinoma. The extent of resection and the preexisting condition of the liver are the main determinants of morbidity and mortality associated with liver resection. Leaving an adequate amount of functional liver is the key to postoperative survival. Unlike creatinine clearance for renal function, no specific test is available to quantitate hepatocellular function. Standard liver function tests such as lactate dehydrogenase, serum glutamic oxaloacetic transaminase, and serum glutamic pyruvic transaminase levels, alkaline phosphate, and bilirubin are usually elevated postoperatively. Major increases in these tests may signal a catastrophic complication such as hepatic artery or portal vein thrombosis. Prothrombin time (PT) is considered the most sensitive test available to estimate global hepatocellular function. An elevated PT and the inability to correct the coagulopathy with fresh frozen plasma or vitamin K are usually signs of severe liver dysfunction.

Several biochemical derangements can occur after major liver resections. The two most common are hypoglycemia and hypophosphatemia. Serum levels should be monitored closely and treated with glucose and phosphate infusions.

Postoperative complications that are associated with major liver resections include hemorrhage, hemobilia, pyogenic liver abscess, vascular compromise, and liver failure. Hemorrhage is usually diagnosed by cardiovascular instability and increased drainage of fresh blood from the operative site. Frequent fluid boluses and a falling hematocrit are a common ICU presentation, rather than progressive hypotension and tachycardia. Treatment consists of correcting the coagulopathy and reexploration. Hypothermia, if present, should be corrected as it impairs platelet function and prolongs the PT and partial thromboplastin time. Hemobilia can occur in the immediate postoperative period from a communication between a parenchymal branch of the hepatic arterial system and the biliary tree.[1] Hemobilia may initially be unrecognized unless a T tube has been placed into the common bile duct during surgery. Hemobilia generally presents as intermittent gastrointestinal bleeding. The diagnosis is confirmed by endoscopic visualization of blood flowing from the ampulla of Vater. The preferred treatment is selective embolization of the bleeding site. Pyogenic liver abscess after resection has a mortality rate of 50%.[2] Diagnosis is usually confirmed by CT and treatment consists of drainage with CT or ultrasound guidance. Thrombosis of the hepatic artery or the portal vein is a disastrous complication. This usually presents with a rapid rise in liver function tests and PT. The prognosis is usually poor, and treatment is often supportive. Such vascular compromise can lead to liver failure, which is the most lethal complication. Liver failure usually causes an increase in serum bilirubin , liver function tests, and PT. Liver failure is often the first sign of progressive multisystem failure. The prognosis is poor unless a reversible cause such as liver abscess can be found and treated.

Pancreatic Operations

The pancreas lies retroperitoneally, in close association with the duodenum, common bile duct, aorta, inferior vena cava, and the splenic, superior mesenteric, and portal veins. This location, combined with the abundant pancreatic blood supply and its digestive secretions, make pancreatic surgery a treacherous undertaking.

The Whipple procedure, total pancreatectomy, and pancreatic drainage procedures are the most common elective operative procedures. The two major complications after pancreatic surgery are hemorrhage and sepsis. Hemorrhage usually presents with cardiovascular instability and blood emanating from surgical drains. This complication requires immediate reexploration, preferably before six to eight red cell transfusions, the usual number before such a decision is reached.

Septic complications are usually related to ductal or anastomotic disruption. The usual signs and symptoms of sepsis will develop and, if surgical drains are present, a muddy brown effluent may be identified. The key to successful outcome is proper drainage and antibiotic therapy. CT plays an important role in identifying undrained collections. Percutaneous drainage with CT guidance is the drainage procedure of choice.

Pancreatitis and its complications are discussed in Chapter 140.

Major Abdominal Vascular Procedures

Patients undergoing aortic reconstruction for occlusive disease or abdominal aortic aneurysm may benefit from careful postoperative ICU management. The most common cause of death in these patients is myocardial infarction, and perioperative hemodynamic and continuous ST segment may provide early warnings so that treatment may reverse ischemia or a low cardiac output state. Hemorrhage may develop postoperatively, but abdominal distention may not develop if the bleeding is confined to the retroperitoneum. Careful fluid management can maintain a normal arterial blood pressure, and several hours may pass before bleeding is appreciated. Significant hemorrhage requires immediate return to the operating room. The most common cause is technical error, but occasionally no specific bleeding site is found, and hemorrhage may be attributed to prolonged heparin activity or coagulopathy.

Early graft thrombosis can also occur; this should be considered if a decrease in the sequential Doppler pressures of one or both extremities develops. Immediate heparinization and reexploration are needed if graft thrombosis develops.[3]

Early graft infections are first recognized when a wound infection develops in one of the groin incisions.[4] Drainage of the localized abscess may reveal involvement of the distal limb of the graft. Occasionally, bleeding from the groin incision, usually occurring a week to 10 days postoperatively, is the first sign of a graft infection. This dreaded complication is usually associated with a high mortality and difficult reconstructive surgery. Aortoduodenal fistula is a sequela of graft infection, and usually presents with upper gastrointestinal bleeding. The prognosis is poor and treatment consists of removing the graft, oversewing the proximal aortic stump, repairing the duodenum, and extraanatomic bypass to the lower extremities.

Sigmoid ischemia may occur after aortic reconstruction because of interruption of the inferior mesenteric artery. This usually causes abdominal pain and rectal bleeding. Sigmoidoscopy is essential to confirm the diagnosis (treatment depends on the degree of ischemia).

Complicated Gastrointestinal and Biliary Procedures

The most common complications occurring after major gastrointestinal or biliary operations result from bile or intestinal fluid leakage into the peritoneal cavity, infection, or obstruction of the biliary system or a portion of the alimentary tract. After these procedures, ICU care is indicated only if the operation is extensive, prolonged, or if the patient has other significant risk factors or intraoperative complications.

Other than bleeding, few immediate intraabdominal problems develop. Occasionally, a major bile leak can develop and, if not properly drained, severe bile peritonitis and hypotension can rapidly develop.[5] The patient presents with generalized, severe abdominal pain and distention. Bowel necrosis can present in a similar fashion and should be suspected after bowel operations that require transection of one or more bowel loops and mesentery for creation of various anastomoses. Occasionally, the blood supply can be compromised by these maneuvers and necrosis occurs. Check the chart for an operative diagram or discuss the clinical picture with the surgeon to determine if necrosis may have developed.

Most anastomotic leaks are not apparent until 4 to 7 days postoperatively when the patient develops a persistent fever, ileus, or other departure from the normal postoperative course. Gastric surgery can be associated with postoperative pancreatitis, splenic injury, and inadvertent injury to the common bile duct.[6] Delayed gastric emptying caused by "gastric atony" presents as persistent vomiting and increased gastric output past the usual 3- to 7-day period of postoperative ileus. This complication can occur after gastric and pancreatic surgery and is treated by nasogastric drainage. Motility agents such as metoclopramide, cisapride, and erythromycin may be tried, although no definitive studies regarding their efficacy are available.

NORMAL POSTOPERATIVE COURSE ■

Evaluating the abdomen during the first week after laparotomy is more productive if the evaluator has a thorough understanding of the physiologic changes and usual findings of the patient without complications.

There is usually no need to examine the surgical incision during the first 48 hours unless the patient develops signs and symptoms suggesting an early wound infection, such as synergistic gangrene or necrotizing fasciitis. Surgical wound dressings are necessary for 48 hours, after which the incision may remain uncovered unless persistent drainage develops. A normal-appearing abdominal incision shows no significant edema or erythema around the sutures or at the skin edges, which should be completely apposed, with no fluid drainage from the incision. Occasionally, small subcutaneous veins can bleed after skin closure, and a small amount of blood will collect on the initial bandage. This is usually of no consequence, but further bleeding from the incision should be treated with a sterile dry dressing and immediate surgical consultation. Serosanguineous fluid drainage is often the first sign that the fascia beneath the skin has separated (wound dehiscence). This potential complication should *not* be further investigated in the ICU. Specifically, probing the wound to identify defects is not advised. Serosanguineous drainage from an abdominal incision requires immediate attention by the operating surgeon to ensure that wound dehiscence is either ruled out or corrected.

All patients develop some degree of paralytic ileus after laparotomy.[7] This is caused by excitation of the splanchnic sympathetic nerves during the intraoperative manipulation of abdominal viscera. The resulting reflex inhibits peristalsis of the stomach, small bowel, and colon.

Postoperatively, the abdomen may be minimally distended and tympanitic from the inability to move intestinal secretions and gas; however, the abdomen should not be extremely tense. Virtually no normal bowel sounds are audible during the first 24 to 72 hours after major abdominal and retroperitoneal operations, despite the fact that small bowel peristalsis may return as quickly as 6 hours after laparotomy. The rapid return of small bowel function is the basis for early postoperative feeding with a jejunostomy. Stomach function generally does not return to normal for 4 or 5 days. Oral intake is prohibited after major abdominal procedures until the patient either passes flatus or experiences a bowel movement. These signs definitely indicate that the large bowel is functional.

EVALUATING THE POSTOPERATIVE ABDOMEN FOR SEPSIS ■

WARNING SIGNS

Sepsis remains the most common cause of death in critically ill surgery patients.[8] Several warning signs should alert the physician that the patient is not following the normal postoperative course. Although fever and an elevated white blood cell count (>10,000/cm³) are often present, these are not findings specific for infection in an ICU patient.

The first warning sign may be a persistent sinus tachycardia (>120 to 130 beats per minute), despite adequate pain medication and volume resuscitation. Although pain thresholds vary, most patients should not experience severe abdominal discomfort after the fourth or fifth postoperative day (which might explain their tachycardia).

Another warning sign is failure to wean from mechanical ventilation or persistent borderline respiratory dysfunction after extubation. Abdominal surgery significantly restricts respiratory function, and splinting from a painful abdominal incision can contribute to this "respiratory dysfunction," usually treated by ventilatory support. This is expected in patients with poor preoperative respiratory function. However,

by the fourth or fifth day, if tachypnea persists or further attempts at weaning are unsuccessful, the cause may be increased oxygen demands or acute respiratory failure secondary to sepsis.[9]

Some patients are given parenteral nutrition during the perioperative period, depending on the severity of the operative procedure. Increasing difficulty in maintaining normal glucose levels can develop with occult sepsis. The mechanism is similar to the relative insulin resistance that develops at the skeletal muscle level, a physiologic abnormality that is frequently observed in trauma patients.[10]

Persistent tachycardia, hyperglycemia, and respiratory dysfunction are nonspecific for abdominal sepsis; therefore, nonabdominal causes must be eliminated.

Most patients accumulate a positive fluid balance during the first 72 hours after surgery. The degree of positive balance depends on the type and length of the operative procedure. Elective surgical patients are often given 2 to 3 L of intravenous fluid per day in addition to the measured and insensible fluid losses. The pathophysiologic changes resulting in this third space fluid sequestration usually resolve by the third or fourth postoperative day, and fluid balance should approach zero and become negative by the fifth to the seventh day.

A persistent positive fluid balance (past the third or fourth day) is another warning sign that abdominal sepsis may be developing.

Paralytic ileus usually resolves completely by the fifth to seventh postoperative day, but prolonged ileus is common after operations for intraabdominal septic complications. However, in elective surgical patients, a prolonged ileus (>7 days) may signify intraabdominal infection.

Persistent sinus tachycardia, respiratory dysfunction, and hyperglycemia in combination with a continued positive fluid balance and paralytic ileus after the seventh postoperative day should raise the suspicion of intraabdominal sepsis in the elective surgical patient.

AN APPROACH TO EVALUATION

Evaluating sepsis begins with a thorough knowledge of the patient's history, including the type of surgery performed, and an appropriately directed physical examination followed by tests to confirm clinical suspicions. The clinical setting and time course after surgery should also help to direct the evaluation process. Elective surgical patients require few tests other than a good physical examination if fever develops during the first 48 hours postoperatively. A correct diagnosis often can be made based on clinical findings and confirmed by a single appropriate test.[11]

Life-threatening septic complications must be considered, but the evaluation should be clinically relevant so that tests that are of little benefit in directing therapy, such as complete blood cell counts with differential and chest radiographs in the absence of physical findings, are excluded. Further evaluation is indicated if extraabdominal sources for sepsis have been eliminated and the warning signs suggest intraabdominal infection.

The extent of evaluation is partially determined by the elapsed time since surgery and the clinical condition of the patient. Catastrophic complications, such as bowel necrosis or complete anastomotic disruption, usually present in such a dramatic fashion that surgical intervention is immediately required. However, most intraabdominal septic problems do not present in this fashion. The most common presentation is an indolent, gradual onset of multisystem organ failure (MSOF) unless the underlying problem is resolved.

Intraabdominal sepsis rarely is clinically apparent during the first 48 hours after elective abdominal surgery. From 48 hours to 7 days postoperatively, the warning signs begin to develop. Unfortunately, diagnostic tests performed during this period are often unreliable for confirming clinical suspicions. After 1 week, diagnostic tests become more helpful.

An abdominal abscess must develop before it can be detected by CT. Therefore, CT performed in the early postoperative period may be of no benefit, although strong clinical evidence may support this suspicion. This is just one example of the importance of appropriate timing for studies to enhance their sensitivity and specificity.

The First 48 Hours

Temperature elevation within the first 48 hours may, indeed, be a sign of intraabdominal sepsis, but confirmation is unlikely and extraabdominal sources for fever are more common. A careful physical examination should direct testing and therapy. If fever develops, it is crucial that the abdominal incision be examined carefully for early signs of infection (and possibly synergistic gangrene). No specific tests to rule out abdominal sepsis are needed within the first 48 hours.

Days 2 Through 7

Postoperative patients who develop intraabdominal sepsis eventually fall into two categories. The first category includes those patients with infections that can be controlled with antibiotics and supportive care. These patients generally do not show significant organ system dysfunction but exhibit all of the warning signs of abdominal infection. Their immunologic reserves are strong enough to prevent further deterioration.[12] Radiographic studies and scans generally are not helpful during this time, and a period of careful observation, reevaluation, and aggressive support is recommended. Laboratory tests specific for the type of surgery performed (i.e., serum amylase or lipase after pancreatic surgery, liver function studies after biliary or hepatic surgery) may help confirm clinical suspicions.

Further clinical deterioration may place the patient into the second category: patients whose defense mechanisms are not strong enough to prevent MSOF despite vigorous ICU support, antibiotics, and nutritional therapy. Serious consideration should be given to abdominal reexploration before further deterioration develops, because radiographic studies and scans are usually of little benefit in diagnosing the problem or directing therapy during this period.[13,14]

Days 7 Through 14

If warning signs persist after 7 days and reevaluation for extraabdominal sources remains negative, radiographic diagnostic studies should be considered. A chest radiograph and an abdominal series are easy to obtain and are relatively inexpensive. These studies should be reviewed and compared with previous radiographs in consultation with a radiologist before further diagnostic tests are performed. Barium and Gastrografin contrast studies usually are not beneficial in critically ill patients, but they are performed occasionally to identify anastomotic leaks. Similar information is often obtained by abdominal CT with oral contrast, which can demonstrate a leak if contrast material is seen outside the bowel lumen.

Diagnostic sonography is relatively inexpensive when compared with other noninvasive imaging techniques. Sonography can be performed at the bedside, obviating the hazardous and time-consuming patient transfer to the radiology suite. Unfortunately, an accurate study is dependent on the operator and frequently of no benefit when searching for abdominal abscesses.[15] Sonography is the preferred test to confirm acute cholecystitis and intrahepatic abscesses.[16] Nuclear imaging studies of the gallbladder and extrahepatic biliary tract are not helpful in patients without oral intake, and a high false-positive rate is found in patients receiving total parenteral nutrition.[17]

Gallium scans for identification of abscesses are rarely helpful in the critically ill patient.

CT has become the preferred method for diagnosing intraabdominal abscess. Scanners also give precise definition of anatomic detail for successful percutaneous drainage methods that have significantly altered the classic approach to intraabdominal abscess management.

CT scans are not beneficial in critically ill patients during the first week postoperatively, and their use in patients with MSOF is usually without benefit unless a negative scan result strongly supports a decision to discontinue therapy.[18]

Patients with MSOF after elective operations usually do not benefit from CT, and, perhaps, reexploration should be the only diagnostic test in these patients.

A more recent approach in the evaluation of an intraabdominal process in the ICU has been the use of diagnostic laparoscopy at the bedside. This can be especially helpful in the diagnosis of acalculous cholecystitis, and it obviates transfer of the critically ill patient.[19]

SPECIFIC SURGICAL PROBLEMS ■

FISTULAS

A fistula is an abnormal communication between a segment of the alimentary tract and either the external body surface (external fistula) or another hollow internal structure, such as a portion of the alimentary tract, a blood vessel, or a bronchus (internal fistula).

Fistulas can develop after elective or emergency surgical procedures and may cause significant physiologic derangements from fluid and electrolytes bypassing a large portion of the absorptive surface of the alimentary tract.[20] This discussion considers only external fistulas because these are more common and have more physiologic impact on the patient's status.

The metabolic abnormalities depend on the fistula location in the gastrointestinal tract and the electrolyte content of the secretions that are lost. Although electrolyte content can be estimated (Table 72-1), it is a good practice to measure the electrolytes of high-volume fistulas and maintain an accurate record of output to direct replacement therapy and composition.

All alimentary tract secretions are isotonic, and dehydration can develop rapidly if the lost fluid is not replaced. Eight to 10 L of fluid traverse the alimentary tract each day. In general, the higher the fistula's location in the alimentary tract (especially duodenum and jejunum), the more likely it is that a significant fluid and metabolic management problem exists.

Gastric Fistulas

Pathologic fistulas can develop from breakdown of gastrointestinal anastomoses eroding to the skin surface. Most gastric fistulas close spontaneously with bowel rest or parenteral alimentation. Gastric fistulas and prolonged nasogastric suction may produce hypokalemic metabolic alkalosis. This can be avoided by replacing gastric output with 0.9 normal saline with 20 mEq potassium chloride per liter. A nasogastric tube is the most common external "gastric fistula" in elective surgical patients.

Duodenal and Jejunal Fistulas

Secretions from duodenal and proximal jejunal fistulas, which are high in bicarbonate, can cause metabolic acidosis. Large fluid losses (3 to 5 L/day) can occur.

Initial replacement should begin with Ringer's lactate followed by careful titration of bicarbonate as needed to maintain acid–base balance.[20]

Biliary and Pancreatic Fistulas

Biliary and pancreatic fistulas can develop after any major biliary or pancreatic operation. Biliary drainage rarely exceeds 500 to 800 mL/day. The most common "biliary fistula" is the T tube placed into the common bile duct after exploration. Biliary drainage rarely requires replacement unless large volumes (>500 mL/day) persist for more than 7 to 10 days. Because of the high bicarbonate content in bile, metabolic acidosis can develop with prolonged high output. Replacement fluid should be Ringer's lactate, with further addition of bicarbonate as needed to prevent metabolic acidosis.

High-output pancreatic fistulas can also rapidly lead to metabolic acidosis because of the high bicarbonate content (70 to 110 mEq/L) of pancreatic secretions. These fistulas may drain large volumes (1 to 2 L/day) and require aggressive replacement with Ringer's lactate and bicarbonate.[20]

Ileal Fistulas

Ileal fistulas are generally well tolerated, as evidenced by the many patients who are living normally with ileostomies. Sodium, magnesium, and fluid loss can be a problem if the fistula is in the proximal portion of the ileum, but most patients are able to adapt well without significant problems unless underlying bowel disease, such as regional enteritis, has caused the fistula. Replacement fluid for losses is Ringer's lactate. Acid–base abnormalities are uncommon unless large amounts of fluid (2 to 3 L/day) are lost.

Colonic Fistulas

External colonic fistulas are generally of no consequence and close spontaneously unless other conditions such as distal obstruction are present.

Treatment

The mainstay of treatment for any external fistula is local skin management and nutritional support. Local management of the fistula tract is important because secretions, especially from proximal fistulas, can be irritating to the surrounding skin surface. If the tract to the skin surface is well formed, small red rubber catheters can be carefully inserted into the fistula and sutured in place for drainage into a small container such as a bile bag. The skin surrounding a fistula may breakdown from exposure to the fistula drainage. Karaya gum seals can protect the skin surrounding the fistula (Chap. 153). Enterostomal therapists are helpful in developing ways to protect the skin as the fistula is healing.

Patients with external fistulas must receive adequate protein and calorie support for healing. The route of administration depends on the site of the fistulas. High fistulas are usually treated by total parenteral nutrition. Distal ileal and colonic fistulas can be treated by enteral elemental diets.

Most fistulas that will close spontaneously do so in 6 to 8 weeks. If the fistula persists past this time despite correc-

TABLE 72-1. Composition of Alimentary Secretions

TYPE (mEq/L)	VOLUME (mEq/L)	Na⁺ (mEq/L)	K⁺ (mEq/L)	Cl⁻ (mEq/L)	HCO₃⁻ (mEq/L)
Gastric	500–1500	60	10	130	—
Duodenum	—	140	5	80	—
Bile	350–500	145	5	100	35
Pancreas	200–800	140	5	75	115
Ileum	1000–3000	140	5	104	30
Fecal	—	60	30	40	15

tion of protein and calorie deficits, then surgical correction should be considered.

Fistulas and the Open Abdomen

The association of an enterocutaneous fistula and an open abdomen is a difficult surgical problem, with mortality rates up to 60%. Because the fistula is usually located within a bed of granulating tissue covering loops of exposed small bowel, ostomy appliances will not adhere and are usually of no use. A variety of appliances are used to control enteric contents, including drains, tubes, dressings, and skin grafts. However, the key to management of an open abdomen is prevention of fistula formation. Over a 4-year period, we have treated 62 patients with an open abdomen technique.[21] Fistulas occurred in 9 patients (15%). The causal factors were breakdown of feeding jejunostomies (2 patients), an anastomotic leak (1 patient), and gauze dressing changes causing bowel injury (5 patients). One patient developed a fistula with the zipper technique of temporary abdominal closure. The mortality after fistula development was 2 of 9 (22%). Abdominal wall reconstruction and reestablishment of bowel continuity are the goals of treatment and are performed at a later date after the recovery from the critical illness.[22]

Based on our data, several points should be emphasized to avoid fistula development: (1) avoid feeding jejunostomies if an open abdomen technique is anticipated; (2) gauze dressing changes to exposed bowel increases the rate of fistulization and should be avoided; and (3) skin grafts can be used to protect exposed bowel.

ABDOMINAL WOUND INFECTION AND SYNERGISTIC GANGRENE

Abdominal wound infections are usually not life-threatening and treatment consists primarily of opening the skin and subcutaneous space. However, synergistic gangrene is a serious complication with a high mortality rate. Wound infection produced by a combination of gram-positive cocci, gram-negative bacilli, and anaerobes can produce progressive infections of the subcutaneous tissues known collectively as synergistic gangrene or necrotizing fasciitis.[23] Early diagnosis and radical surgical debridement of necrotic tissue in conjunction with high-dose antibiotics are necessary.

A clostridial infection can produce a rapidly progressive life-threatening infection commonly known as *gas gangrene*.[24] Myonecrosis usually begins within a few hours after contamination. Severe pain is often the first sign. Wound inspection may show only mild local edema and irregular blanching at the wound margins. Instead of feeling warm, the skin is usually cool to touch and appears somewhat thickened. Tenderness to palpation is usually minimal considering the severe pain that is present. Crepitation may not be present during the early stages of infection, but a distinctive, putrid odor from volatile aromatic acids and hydrogen sulfide is almost always present. Spread of infection can progress rapidly within hours until the entire abdominal wall is involved. A fulminant septic picture with fever as high as 40°C rapidly develops.

Gas gangrene and necrotizing fasciitis are true surgical emergencies. If these infections are suspected, immediate surgical debridement is required or death will occur within hours of the onset of infection.

ACALCULOUS CHOLECYSTITIS

Acute acalculous cholecystitis is a disease afflicting critically ill patients. The mortality rate may be as high as 70% if left untreated.[25] Difficulty in early diagnosis is the major factor causing this high mortality. The etiology is unclear. Many factors are implicated including biliary stasis, ischemia, and possibly substances toxic to the gallbladder wall. Gallbladder distention secondary to prolonged spasm of the sphincter of Oddi caused by prolonged narcotic administration or developing during total parenteral nutrition may also be a possible cause.

Ultrasound, CT, and cholescintigraphy have a low specificity and high incidence of false-positive results in critically ill patients. Intravenous morphine improves the accuracy of cholescintigraphy.[26] Another approach is to use diagnostic laparoscopy to assess the gallbladder in critically ill patients.[19] Treatment may consist of percutaneous drainage of the gallbladder or laparoscopic cholecystectomy in the operating room.

THE OPEN ABDOMEN

Open management of the abdomen in the critically ill patient is a difficult problem. Steinberg[27] first described an open abdominal technique in 1979.

A review of patients treated at The University of Miami/ Jackson Memorial Medical Center (Miami) revealed four causes that led to treatment by the open abdomen.[28] These are (1) dehiscence of the fascia; (2) necrotizing pancreatitis; (3) inability to close the abdomen because of loss of domain; and (4) diffuse persistent peritonitis.

Dehiscence of the Fascia

Dehiscence of the abdominal fascia after abdominal exploration is common in critically ill patients. Dehiscence ranges from a small fascial separation to bowel evisceration. There are multiple causes, but intraabdominal sepsis is the most important in critically ill patients. Evisceration needs immediate operative correction. Patients with dehiscence from intraabdominal sepsis also should undergo abdominal reexploration.

Surgeons are frequently reluctant to reoperate on critically ill patients because of their often-marginal physiologic condition. As a result, some patients with fascial dehiscence and suspected intraabdominal sepsis undergo CT and are treated nonoperatively ("conservatively") if no abdominal source is identified. Our experience in treating dehiscence conservatively is disappointing[29]: of 7 patients so treated with gauze dressing changes, five patients subsequently developed fistulas. We believed that repetitive gauze dressing changes eventually led to breakdown of the bowel wall. Our primary goal now is early protection of the bowel surface provided by secondary reclosure in the most patients. This also provides an opportunity to explore the abdomen for undiagnosed sepsis. In critically ill patients, bedside skin grafts are applied directly to the exposed bowel; the grafts function as biological protectants.

Necrotizing Pancreatitis

The treatment of necrotizing pancreatitis by marsupialization is discussed in Chapter 140.

Loss of Abdominal Domain

Massive fluid resuscitation can lead to bowel edema, making closure of the abdomen impossible. Fascial closure creates a host of complications including fascial necrosis, cardiovascular and pulmonary complications secondary to increased intraabdominal pressure, and intraabdominal compartment syndrome, which may present as oliguria and occasionally total renal shutdown. This problem, increasingly recognized, was first described after emergency aortic surgery. It is a frequent problem with trauma patients and after liver transplantation; in both situations, massive fluid resuscitation is common.

Several techniques are described to manage this problem, including towel clip closure and a variety of abdominal mesh closures.

Initially, we preferred sialistic mesh attached to the skin or fascia. If the patient survived the initial injury and operation, the abdominal wound was definitively closed at a later date. We have had 15 patients who could not be closed at the initial operation. Secondary closure was attempted in eight patients; four died (50% mortality rate) and seven (87%) became septic.[28] We now attempt secondary closure only in the first 48 hours. Otherwise, the wound is treated with daily irrigation using the mesh and zipper technique (see later).

Bender and others[30] describe a technique in which the intestines are covered with a large sterile rayon cloth placed under the fascial edges. Several retention sutures are used above the cloth to approximate but not close the edges of the wound. The patients are returned to the operating room for closure when the bowel edema subsides. We use this technique preferentially.

Diffuse Persistent Peritonitis

The management of diffuse persistent peritonitis, or "tertiary" peritonitis, has been facilitated by an open technique in the septic critically ill patient. Several techniques have been devised to treat general surgical problems, necrotizing pancreatitis, and trauma and liver transplant patients.

We prefer the propylene mesh and zipper technique described by Heidrich and colleagues[31] and Teichmann and coworkers.[32] Mesh is sutured to the skin or fascia. The mesh is opened in the midline and a zipper is sutured to the cut edges. Daily irrigations are carried out in the ICU. As the peritonitis resolves, the small bowel, the subhepatic, subphrenic, pericolic, and pelvic spaces are all allowed to seal. The mesh and zipper are removed when the bowel loops are adhered; there is no chance for evisceration, and the bowel surface is completely protected by granulating tissue. A skin graft is applied to the granulating bed once maximum contraction of the wound has been achieved.

Patients who survive are left with a large incisional hernia. Abdominal closure and reestablishment of bowel continuity, if an ostomy or fistula has been present, is done much later, when the patient has fully recovered from the critical illness.[22] We have treated 38 general surgery, trauma, and liver transplant patients with the mesh and zipper technique. Survival was best (83%) in the penetrating trauma population. The survival rate for the entire group was 68%. One fistula developed.

TUBE TECHNOLOGY ■

Various tubes and drains are placed during surgery for decompression, feeding, or drainage. This section familiarizes the nonsurgeon with the various types of tubes and drains that a surgical patient may have postoperatively. No tube

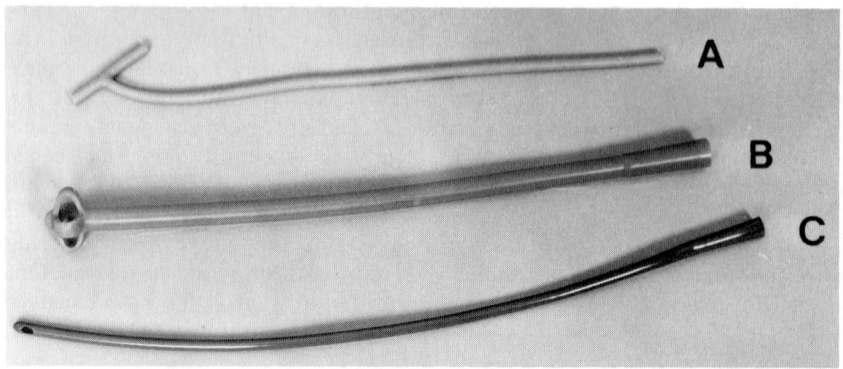

FIGURE 72-1. (**A**) T tube commonly used for stenting and decompressing the biliary tract. (**B**) Mallencott catheter used for gastrostomy, duodenostomy, and cecostomy. (**C**) Red rubber catheter used for abdominal drainage or tube jejunostomy.

should be placed at the time of operation (including nasogastric tubes) or should ever be removed without previously consulting the operating surgeon. Likewise, attempts should never be made to replace a tube or drain that is accidentally removed (including a nasogastric tube) without prior discussion with the operating surgeon.

NASOGASTRIC TUBES

Nasogastric tubes are routinely placed by the anesthesiologist at the beginning of most abdominal operations to maintain gastric decompression. These tubes are usually left in place after surgery if the abdominal procedure is prolonged or complicated. Although these tubes have many uses, the rationale for use postoperatively is to maintain gastric decompression and prevent accumulation of gastric fluid and intestinal gas, which may be a potential source for aspiration and gastric distention during the period of paralytic ileus.

Most agree that a sump nasogastric tube provides the best decompression, and a no. 18 French tube is most effective for postoperative decompression and drainage in adults. A sump nasogastric tube is a double-lumen tube. The larger lumen is connected to continuous low-to-medium pressure wall suction through a container to collect aspirated gastric fluid. The smaller lumen remains open to the atmosphere to allow entrainment of room air into the stomach. The sump maintains stomach pressures near atmospheric during suctioning. This helps prevent tube adherence to the stomach wall, allowing for more effective suction drainage and less "tube trauma" to the stomach wall. To be effective, the smaller sump lumen must be kept patent. The tube is functioning properly if air passage is audible through the smaller sump lumen during continuous suctioning.

LONG INTESTINAL TUBES

Intestinal tubes are placed intraoperatively in patients with recurrent small bowel obstructions. The rationale is to stent the small bowel to prevent acute intestinal angulation while adhesions redevelop. Hopefully, the small bowel then scars into a "position of function" rather than developing areas of angulation that may lead to reobstruction. The two most commonly used long intestinal tubes are the Canter tube and the Baker tube. These tubes have a balloon at the end that can be used as a lead point for placement. The tube can be passed through the nose or mouth into the stomach or through a small lateral abdominal incision into the jejunum or stomach. Generally, suction is not used because the main purpose is stenting and not decompression.

BILIARY TUBES

After common bile duct exploration, T tubes are placed into the duct to prevent stricture, for ductal decompression, and for future biliary access, if necessary (Fig. 72-1A). The T tube is a closed system, always connected to a biliary drainage bag for bile collection. These tubes are sutured securely in place because inadvertent dislodgement within the first 5 days postoperatively would require reoperation for replacement. Drainage is primarily dependent on the degree of

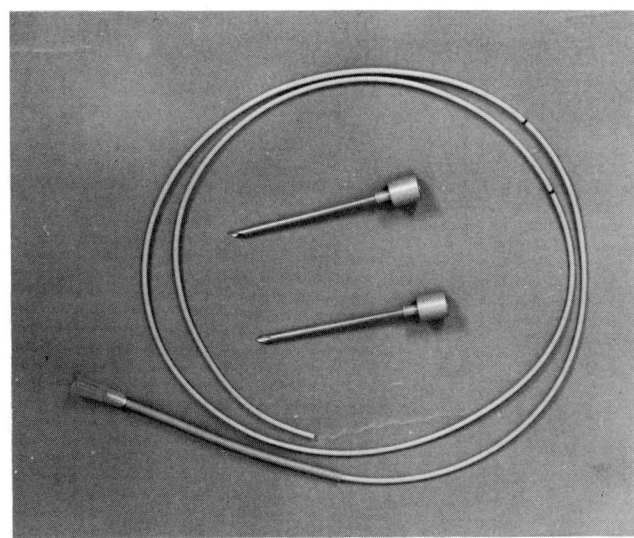

FIGURE 72-2. Needle catheter jejunostomy with needles for insertion into the bowel lumen and through the abdominal cavity.

obstruction distally within the common bile duct. Generally, 100 to 500 mL/day drains from the biliary tract. The amount gradually decreases with time if no distal obstruction is present.

GASTROSTOMY TUBES

Gastrostomy tubes can be placed at the time of surgery or percutaneously with local anesthesia (see Fig. 72-1B). Their function is the same as that of a nasogastric tube. Mushroom-tipped or Mallencott catheters generally are used, although Foley catheters also are used occasionally. No specific maintenance other than frequent irrigation is required for these catheters, which are allowed to drain by gravity. Early dislodgement requires return to the operating room for replacement. A fibrous tract will develop if the tube has been in place for several weeks, allowing for replacement at the bedside, if necessary. If prolonged gastric decompression is anticipated, tube gastrostomy may be indicated to prevent the prolonged discomfort and complications of chronic nasogastric suction tubes.

DUODENOSTOMY TUBES

Duodenostomy tubes are placed at surgery to protect the sutured duodenal stump after gastric resection. Occasionally, a duodenum may be difficult to close after antral resection because of chronic inflammation from peptic ulcer disease. The duodenostomy tube is placed to prevent pressure and fluid buildup in the area of the sutured stump. This essentially creates a "controlled duodenal fistula."

JEJUNOSTOMY TUBES

Jejunostomy tubes are placed at surgery solely to provide enteral nutrition. Many types of tubes can be used, ranging from a smaller version of the gastrostomy tube, to various types of "catheter" jejunostomies (Fig. 72-2) that are in-

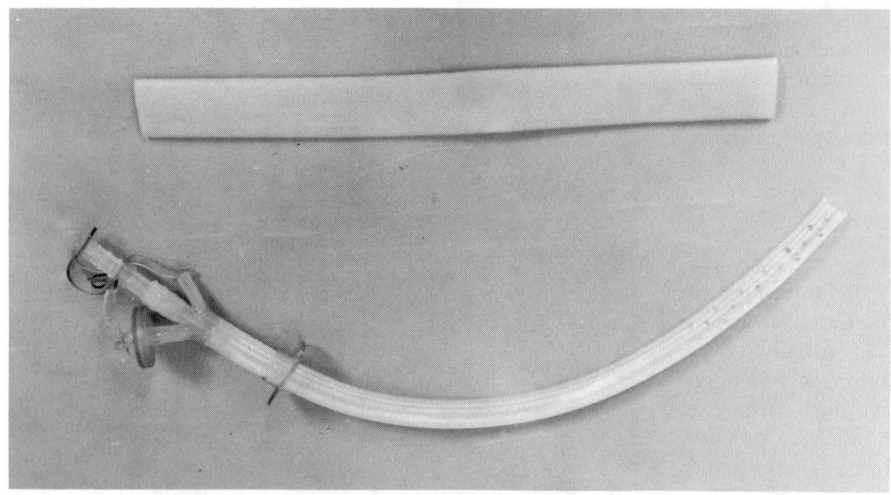

FIGURE 72-3. Penrose drain commonly used for open-system drainage of abscess cavities or potential spaces for fluid collection (*Top*). Davol triple-lumen sump drain used for draining large abscess cavities within the abdomen (*Bottom*).

serted through the antimesenteric border 15 to 20 cm distal to the ligament of Treitz and advanced intraluminally for 10 to 20 cm. Jejunostomies can be used for enteral feedings as soon as small bowel function returns, often obviating or reducing the requirement for total parenteral nutrition. The smaller catheter jejunostomies should be intermittently irrigated with 5 to 10 mL of cranberry juice to maintain patency while not in use.

CECOSTOMY TUBES

Tube cecostomies are used rarely because of the high incidence of cecocutaneous fistulas after removal. The primary use is for decompression of the right colon, although colonoscopic decompression is used more frequently. Tube cecostomy is required occasionally for patients with Ogilvie's syndrome when colonoscopic decompression is contraindicated or unsuccessful. Large (no. 30 French) mushroom catheters are used (see Fig. 72-1B). These tubes require frequent irrigation with 30 to 50 mL of water or saline to prevent tube obstruction with feces.

PERCUTANEOUS DRAINS

Percutaneous drains are inserted by the radiologist for the drainage of abscesses. They are usually no. 8 or 10 French pigtail catheters. They are left to straight drainage and are usually irrigated with 5 mL of saline twice per day. They are followed by "tube checks" done in the radiology suite to assess the size of the abscess cavity. They are removed by the radiologist.

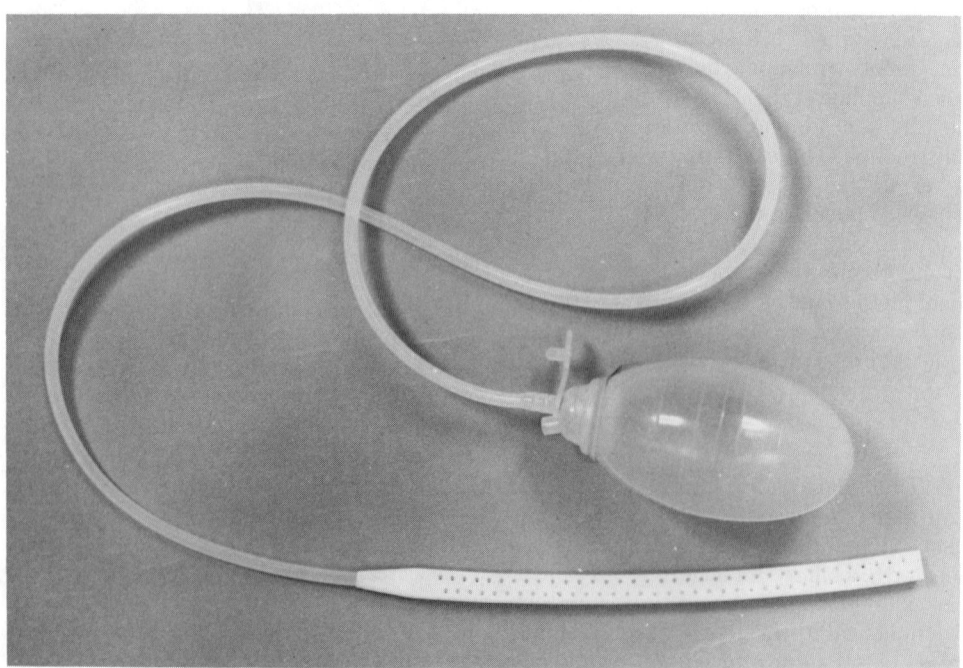

FIGURE 72-4. Jackson-Pratt closed drainage system.

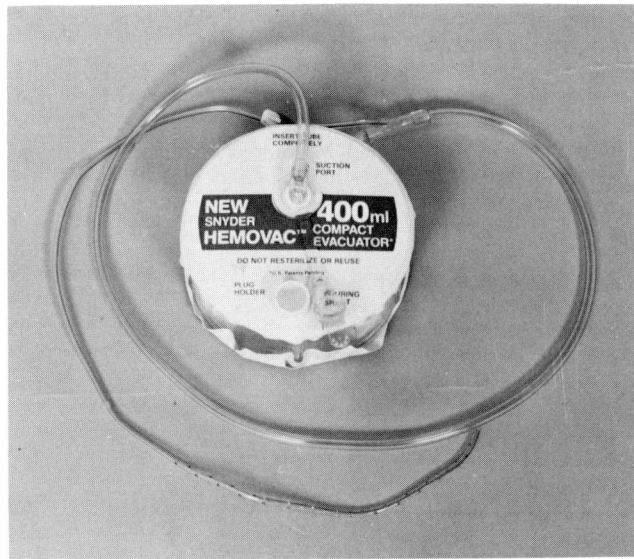

FIGURE 72-5. Snyder Hemovac closed drainage system.

ABDOMINAL DRAINS

Various open and closed drainage systems are used for abdominal abscesses and areas of potential fluid collection that could become a nidus for intraabdominal infection.

Various combinations of Penrose (Fig. 72-3) and red rubber catheter drains (see Fig. 72-1C) are used for passive dependent drainage of infected intraabdominal cavities to prevent further accumulation of purulent material, which may cause reformation of the abscess. These "open system" drainage techniques are considered more hazardous than "closed system" techniques because bacteria may enter the abdomen through the drains unless meticulous drain site care and frequent dressing changes are administered. To prevent this complication, a "semiclosed" triple-lumen sump drain has been developed (see Fig. 72-3). This drain contains two large lumina that can be used for suctioning or instillation of antiseptic solutions. A third smaller lumen is covered by a small air filter and functions as a sump to promote better drainage. These drains are particularly useful for large abscess cavities and pancreatic abscesses that may require irrigation as well as drainage.

Various closed system drains are also available. These systems usually have some type of bulb device that, when deflated, provide continuous closed suction to the area drained. The Jackson-Pratt (Fig. 72-4) and Hemovac (Fig. 72-5) systems are examples. These are used for draining smaller abscess cavities and are frequently placed in areas where a potential fluid collection after surgery could result in serious complications (e.g., in the right subhepatic space after repair of a duodenal perforation). These drains generally require no specific care other than frequent emptying and priming of the bulb or other suction device. Inadvertent removal of any abdominal drain that is vital to surgical outcome may require repeat laparotomy for replacement.

REFERENCES

1. Sondblom P, Saegesser F, Mirkovitch V: Hepatic hemobilia: hemorrhage from the intrahepatic biliary tract. A review. *World J Surg* 1984;8:41
2. Bertel CK, von Heerden JA, Sheedy PF II: Treatment of pyogenic hepatic abscesses: surgical vs. percutaneous drainage. *Arch Surg* 1986;121:554
3. Whittemore AD, Clowes AW, Couch NP, et al: Secondary femoropopliteal construction. *Ann Surg* 1981;193:35
4. Lorentzen J, Nielson OM, Arendrup H, et al: Vascular graft infections. *Surgery* 1985;98:81
5. Rosato EF, Berkowitz HD, Roberts B: Bile ascites. *Surg Gynecol Obstet* 1970;130:494
6. Moody FG, McGreevy JM: Complications of gastric surgery. In: Greenfield LJ (ed). *Complications in Surgery and Trauma*, 2nd ed. Philadelphia, JB Lippincott, 1990:462
7. Grabner JN, Schulte WJ, Condon RE, et al: Relationship of duration of postoperative ileus to extent and site of operative dissection. *Surgery* 1982;31:141
8. Shires GT, Dineen P: Sepsis following burns, trauma, and intra-abdominal infections. *Arch Intern Med* 1982;142:2012
9. Norwood SH, Civetta JM: Ventilatory support in patients with ARDS. *Surg Clin North Am* 1985;65:895
10. Abbott WC, Echenique MM, Bistrian BR, et al: Nutritional care of the trauma patient. *Surg Gynecol Obstet* 1983;142:2012
11. Freischlag J, Busutill RW: The value of postoperative fever evaluation. *Surgery* 1983;94:358
12. Fry DE: The diagnosis of intra-abdominal infection in the postoperative patient. *Probl Gen Surg* 1984;1:558
13. Hinsdale JG, Jaffe BM: Reoperation for intra-abdominal sepsis. *Ann Surg* 1984;199:31
14. Machiedo GW, Tikellis J, Suval W, et al: Reoperation for sepsis. *Am Surg* 1985;51:149
15. Clark RA, Tobin R: Abscess drainage with CT and ultrasound guidance. *Radiol Clin North Am* 1983;21:477
16. Laing FC: Diagnostic evaluation of patients with suspected acute cholecystitis. *Radiol Clin North Am* 1983;21:477
17. Shuman WP, Gibbs P, Rudd TG, et al: PIPIDA scintigraphy for cholecystitis: False positives in alcoholism and total parenteral nutrition. *Am J Radiol* 1982;138:1
18. Norwood SH, Civetta JM: Abdominal CT scanning in critically ill surgical patients. *Ann Surg* 1985;202:166
19. Sleeman D, Sosa JL, Almeida J, et al: Laparoscopy for the diagnosis of acalculous cholecystis in the critically ill. *Clin Invest Med* 1994;17:B18
20. Goodwin CW: Complications of acute fluid loss and replacement. In Greenfield LJ (ed): *Complications in Surgery and Trauma*, 2nd ed. Philadelphia, JB Lippincott, 1990:110
21. Sleeman D, Sosa JL, McKenney M, et al: Intestinal fistulas and the open abdomen. *Can J Surg* 1994;37:340
22. Sleeman D, Sosa JL, Gonzalez A, et al: Reclosure of the open abdomen. *J Am Coll Surg* 1995;180:200
23. Majeski JA, Alexander JW: Early diagnosis, nutritional support and immediate extensive debridement improve survival in necrotizing fasciitis. *Am J Surg* 1983;145:784
24. Hart GB, Lamb RC, Strauss MB: Gas gangrene. *J Trauma* 1983;23:991
25. Cornwell EE, Rodriquez A, Miuisse, et al: Acute acalculous cholecystitis in the critically injured patients. *Ann Surg* 1989;210:52
26. Flancbaum L, Choban P, Sinha R, et al: Morphine cholescintigraphy in the evaluation of hospitalized patients with suspected acute cholecystitis. *Ann Surg* 1994;220:25

27. Steinberg D. On leaving the peritoneal cavity open in acute generalized suppurative peritonitis. *Am J Surg* 1979;137:216
28. Sleeman D, Sosa JL, McKenney M, et al: The multiple causes of the open abdomen in the critically ill. *Clin Intensive Care* 1993;4:38
29. Puente I, Sleeman D, Sosa JL, et al: Management of fascial dehiscence in the critically ill. *Medicina Intensiva* 1993;17:S62
30. Bender J, Bailey C, Saxe J, et al: The technique of visceral packing: recommended management of difficult fascial closure in trauma patients. *J Trauma* 1994;36:182
31. Hedderich G, Wexler M, McLean APH, et al: The septic abdomen: open management with Marlex mesh with a zipper. *Surgery* 1986;99:399
32. Teichmann W, Wittmann DM, Andreone PA: Scheduled reoperations (ettappenlavage) for diffuse peritonitis. *Arch Surg* 1986;121:147

Critical Care, Third Edition, edited by Joseph M. Civetta,
Robert W. Taylor, and Robert R. Kirby.
Lippincott-Raven Publishers, Philadelphia, PA © 1997.

CHAPTER 73

■

Surgical Aspects of Hepatobiliary Disease

Alan S. Livingstone
Jorge Luis Sosa

IMMEDIATE CONCERNS ■

MAJOR PROBLEMS

Cholangitis, acute variceal bleeding, hemobilia, major liver resections, portasystemic shunts for the management of esophageal varices, and other surgical procedures performed in patients with severe hepatic dysfunction are all reasons for admission to the intensive care unit (ICU).

This population has specific problems such as fluid and electrolyte imbalances, coagulopathy, encephalopathy, renal dysfunction, and other metabolic derangements. Resuscitation and supportive care are crucial to prevent hepatic failure in patients with so little hepatic reserve.

STRESS POINTS

1. Preoperative patients with significant hepatic dysfunction often have intravascular volume depletion because of medical management of ascites. Volume resuscitation must be judicious, because sodium loading can increase ascites.
2. Furosemide, spironolactone, other diuretics, and intestinal cathartics may induce many electrolyte abnormalities that need careful correction.
3. Coagulopathy caused by depletion of factors V, VII, and X especially may be corrected by administration of vitamin K over several days. Fresh frozen plasma also may be needed.
4. Patients with portal hypertension–induced gastropathy may be at increased risk of bleeding from gastri-

tis and ulceration. Stress ulceration prophylaxis is warranted.
5. Limited hepatic reserves limit gluconeogenesis, and constant glucose infusions (usually 10%) are usually given to prevent hypoglycemia.
6. Fluid therapy must balance the risks of ascites formation and renal dysfunction. A "marginal" urine output may be accepted, but renal function must be carefully monitored.
7. Infectious complications such as cholangitis and intrahepatic abscess are common after major biliary tract surgery or hepatic resection. Percutaneous biliary decompression and abscess drainage aid in their management.
8. Medical management of variceal bleeding includes vasopressin (with nitroglycerin), beta-blockade, somatostatin, and correction of coagulopathy. Endoscopic sclerotherapy, Sengstaken-Blakemore tubes and transjugular intrahepatic portasystemic shunts can be used in emergency situations. Surgical intervention for acute variceal bleeding is rarely used.

ESSENTIAL DIAGNOSTIC TESTS AND PROCEDURES

1. Hepatic function and reserve is best assessed by parameters of hepatic synthesis, especially prothrombin time (PT) and serum albumin. Other useful parameters include bilirubin, presence of ascites, nutritional status, and encephalopathy.
2. The Childs' classification provides an estimate of he-

1121

patic synthetic ability and reserve. After significant variceal bleeding, the classification may not reflect baseline physiologic status. Before risk assessment for surgery, time should be allowed for return to baseline.

3. Abdominal computed tomography (CT) and ultrasound (US) are useful in evaluating hepatobiliary disorders and complications. Tumors, abscesses, biliary dilatation, and biliary stones are demonstrable on either CT or US. In patients with obstructive jaundice or in those who have undergone dilatation to evaluate stones or masses, US should be the initial screening procedure for evaluation.

4. Radionuclide studies such as PIPIDA scans often are not useful if the patient has been without oral intake or has had an elevated bilirubin for some time.

5. Diagnostic laparoscopy can be used to assess preoperative cirrhosis, liver tumors, or inflammatory processes. Postoperatively, bedside laparoscopy can be used to diagnose acalculous cholecystitis.

INITIAL THERAPY

1. Ascites is easier to prevent than to treat; resuscitation should be less vigorous, especially with respect to crystalloid solutions.

2. Judicious use of diuretics can maintain urinary output in patients who typically have increased total body sodium and water. In patients with renal failure and ascites, paracentesis plus intravenous albumin administration, or peritoneal venous shunting, may be required.

3. Coagulopathy must be corrected using vitamin K and fresh frozen plasma if there is active bleeding.

4. During resuscitation, oncotic pressure should be maintained while minimizing ascites formation. Transfusion with packed red blood cells may be used to maintain adequate intravascular volume without excessive fluid administration.

5. We use 10% dextrose in one half normal saline plus potassium phosphate supplementation at 75 mL/hour as maintenance fluids. If oliguria develops, mannitol (12.5 to 25 g), furosemide (20 to 40 mg), albumin (12.5 g), and small crystalloid boluses usually suffice.

6. Antibiotics for prophylaxis and therapy should cover the typical biliary tract pathogens, *Escherichia coli*, *Enterobacter*, *Klebsiella*, and enterococcus. If possible, aminoglycosides should be avoided in cirrhotic patients, but when their use is deemed appropriate, blood levels should be monitored to avoid renal dysfunction and ototoxicity.

7. Protein intake should be restricted to prevent encephalopathy from nitrogenous waste products. Lactulose should be used to decrease intestinal transit time and limit ammonia absorption, especially with gastrointestinal bleeding.

Contrary to everyone's fervent hopes, surgery has not yet been rendered free from risk, and hepatobiliary procedures are often attended by major problems. Intraoperative US,

the ultrasonic dissector/aspirator, argon beam coagulator, and advanced surgical techniques permit more frequent and greater hepatic resections for neoplastic and benign processes. Portasystemic shunting, whether selective or central, is performed in critically cirrhotic patients with minimal hepatic reserves. Some of the most vexing clinical puzzles relate to the management of these patients. Care of such a person, encircled by the patient's intensivists and surgeons in the ICU, can humble even the most experienced clinician, despite all modern technology. The underlying fluid and electrolyte imbalances, coagulopathy, poor nutritional status, and susceptibility to infection must be addressed in the supportive care of such patients. Although complications cannot always be prevented, many can be minimized or treated at an early stage if an anticipatory attitude is adopted.

MANAGEMENT OF THE CIRRHOTIC PATIENT

Options for managing variceal hemorrhage are enumerated elsewhere, but the impact of the preoperative regimen on the patient's postoperative course must be underscored. It is pure sophistry to treat a cirrhotic patient "conservatively" with 25 units of blood, and, after the patient has developed jaundice, ascites, hepatic coma, and a prolonged PT, to ask a surgeon to perform a shunt for continued bleeding—for a fatal outcome is nearly certain.

AVOIDANCE OF ASCITES

The immediate postoperative management of shunted patients varies, depending on whether it is an elective or emergency procedure, or a central versus a selective distal splenorenal shunt. However, the fundamental principles of fluid therapy remain constant. Fluid management is critical, with efforts being taken to minimize ascites formation while adequately replacing functional extracellular volume. It is much simpler to avoid than to treat tense ascites. Intraoperatively, patients are kept as "dry" as possible, with a urine output of 0.5 mL/kg/hour considered acceptable. This approach is continued postoperatively, with the average adult being given only 75 mL of fluid per hour.

Dilute salt solutions can be used to prevent hyponatremia, but a serum sodium value of 128 to 130 mEq/L is rarely of clinical importance in cirrhotic patients. Invasive monitoring in these patients is often less helpful than in most other circumstances, because the alcoholic patient usually has a high cardiac output and a low pulmonary artery occlusion pressure. Volume loading solely to increase urine output results in disproportionate ascites formation. Clearly, if the patient is hypovolemic and hypotensive, appropriate resuscitation is indicated. However, if the patient has stable vital signs and is only mildly oliguric, the problem is unlikely to be serious or to progress to acute renal failure. The phenomenon is usually transient, resolving within 24 to 48 hours as the effects of surgery and anesthesia abate. Because total body sodium and water are usually elevated, judicious diuresis with 12.5 to 25 g of mannitol or a small dose of loop diuretic usually achieves the desired outcome—reversal of oliguria. If oliguria persists or recurs, colloid in the form of concentrated human albumin rather than large amounts of crystalloid may be used for expansion of the intravascular volume.

Routine use of fresh frozen plasma not only is expensive, but also carries all the risks of blood transfusion and is indicated only for correcting appropriate clotting abnormalities. Blood is transfused as necessary to maintain a hematocrit of greater than 27%.

A notable exception to the relevancy of invasive cardiac monitoring is in the elderly patient who has developed postnecrotic cirrhosis secondary to transfusions during coronary artery bypass surgery. This patient already has established myocardial disease before acquiring cirrhosis, and a pulmonary artery catheter may be essential for this patient's successful management.

Ascites is clearly less of a clinical problem with central than with selective shunts. However, overzealous perioperative sodium administration even to a side-to-side portacaval shunt patient (the best shunt to avoid ascites) predictably produces ascites. In the distal splenorenal shunt patient, the above guidelines are particularly important because the extensive retroperitoneal dissection without portal and liver decompression is a model for ascites formation. Once present, tense ascites may be resistant to standard therapy and may result in leaking ascites, pressure symptoms with loss of appetite and shortness of breath, and azotemia during attempts at diuresis. Simultaneous use of spironolactone and furosemide increases the natriuretic effect of each drug and decreases potassium wasting. A useful parameter to follow during diuresis is the urinary sodium concentration. As long as it is greater than 10 mEq/L, therapy can usually be continued. However, if the urine sodium becomes scant or undetectable, continuing this line of therapy often produces azotemia. Recent studies indicate that large-volume paracentesis with albumin administration is more effective than diuretics in eliminating ascites. It is also associated with less encephalopathy, hyponatremia, and renal impairment.[1]

CHYLOUS ASCITES

In perhaps 1% or 2% of patients with distal splenorenal shunts, chylous ascites supervenes. This is readily diagnosed by paracentesis, which yields the classic milky fluid high in fat. This complication rarely occurs after portacaval shunts. Its significance is that standard therapy is often ineffective, and peritoneovenous shunting is curative.

EARLY POSTSHUNT COMPLICATIONS ■

Certain problems are generic to shunted patients, often centering on the protean manifestations of liver failure. These are hemorrhage, encephalopathy, ascites, and the hepatorenal syndrome.

CONTINUED BLEEDING

After emergency variceal decompression, a patient may return to the ICU with a Sengstaken-Blakemore tube still in place and vasopressin being given. Both of these are rarely needed for long if the shunt has been successful; they can usually be discontinued in less than 24 hours. Portacaval shunting accomplishes an almost instantaneous drop in variceal pressure, whereas a distal splenorenal shunt may take hours or even days to fully achieve this goal. (In fact, varices may persist indefinitely on endoscopic examination after distal splenorenal shunting.) More important, however, is the practical fact that both types of shunts are highly successful in arresting variceal hemorrhage.

If upper gastrointestinal bleeding persists after shunting, a technical problem with the shunt or an alternative bleeding site must be rapidly ruled out. Early endoscopy might pinpoint a missed Mallory-Weiss tear, peptic ulcer, or gastritis, all of which require therapy. If the varices are the source of bleeding, arteriography can identify a technical problem such as a clotted or twisted anastomosis. In certain circumstances, inferior vena caval catheterization with pressure measurements resolves the question of a gradient across an anastomosis.[2] Unfortunately, shunt thrombosis aggravates the already existing splanchnic congestion, exacerbating the diathesis for variceal hemorrhage. Further surgery is warranted and urgently required if the patient is deemed salvageable. Endoscopic sclerotherapy can be a temporizing measure but is unlikely to have long-term success, particularly if failed sclerotherapy was the indication for shunting in the first place.

Occasionally, these patients are in congestive heart failure or are on high levels of positive end-expiratory pressure because of adult respiratory distress syndrome. This may result in elevated right atrial and vena caval pressures being transmitted back across a shunt, preventing immediate variceal decompression. Until these underlying conditions are resolved, complete control of the bleeding may be impossible.

If none of the above circumstances applies, somatostatin, vasopressin, nitroglycerin, beta blockers, endoscopic sclerotherapy, and, occasionally, Blakemore intubation are useful adjuncts. Hematologic parameters should be evaluated, with fresh frozen plasma and platelets transfused when appropriate. Thrombocytopenia is prevalent in portal hypertensives and usually results from splenic sequestration rather than consumption. In elective shunting, platelet levels even as low as 25,000/mm³ rarely require platelet transfusions. After massive blood loss, this may no longer be the case. The problem of hematologic dysfunction in bleeding cirrhotic patients is complex, and the abnormalities in the clotting factors variably represent decreased hepatic synthesis, dilution and depletion caused by hemorrhage and massive volume replacement, and, occasionally, disseminated intravascular coagulation or increased fibrinolysis. Most patients respond well to blood component replacement, but occasionally low-dose heparin and epsilon-aminocaproic acid (Amicar) are administered.

The value of routine gastric acid neutralization or suppression in these postoperative patients is difficult to assess prospectively, but antacids are usually used to keep the gastric pH above 5. Because of possible hepatic dysfunction secondary to some H_2 receptor blockers and proton pump inhibitors, these agents should be used cautiously.

ENCEPHALOPATHY

The pathophysiologic mechanism of hepatic encephalopathy is only beginning to be elucidated. Several toxins, including ammonia, mercaptans, short-chain fatty acids, benzodiazepine-like substances, gamma-aminobutyrate–like substances, and impaired glutamatergic neurotransmission, are suspected causes.[3] When encephalopathy develops in postoperative liver patients, it is of seminal importance to differentiate primary from secondary causes. After a major hepatic resection, fulminant hepatitis, shock, or portosystemic shunting, supportive symptomatic therapy may be all that is needed while the liver regenerates and recuperates. However, it is critical to detect and correct precipitating factors such as sepsis, drugs, electrolyte and pH disturbances, gastrointestinal bleeding, hypoxia, hypercapnia, azotemia, and even a subdural hematoma. Airway protection is critical. Lactulose should be administered, preferably by mouth or rectally if necessary. The oral dose is 30 mL every 6 hours adjusted to produce two to three bowel movements per day. Retention enemas are prepared by mixing 300 mL of lactulose with 700 mL of water and can be repeated every 6 hours. Protein is restricted, but a modified amino acid formula, high in branched-chain amino acids and low in the aromatic amino acids, is well tolerated. This can be administered orally with Hepatic-Aid or parenterally with Hepatamine, and seems to improve neuropsychologic function.[4] Encephalopathy of a mild degree often occurs after portasystemic shunts, and marked encephalopathy after a central shunt may be caused by complete diversion of portal flow to the liver. The incidence and degree can be diminished by limiting the size of the shunt to 8 to 10 mm in diameter. Although much is made of encephalopathy developing after central shunts, coma in the immediate postoperative period is rarely caused by the shunt itself, and other causes must be considered. Early encephalopathy as a consequence of a distal splenorenal shunt is even more exceptional. If it occurs and other causes have been corrected, serious consideration should be given to performing angiography to rule out a missed coronary vein or other collateral that is, in essence, "centralizing" the selective shunt, producing portosystemic encephalopathy. Embolization or surgical interruption of these collaterals may reverse the process.[5]

LEAKING ASCITES

A distressing and dangerous complication of surgery on cirrhotic patients is postoperative leaking ascites. This can be minimized by closing the fascia, subcutaneous tissue, and skin with running sutures, as well as by following the above guidelines for fluid administration. Despite these measures, tense ascites may still leak through the wound, and if left unchecked inexorably results in volume disturbances, hypoalbuminemia, wound and intraabdominal infection, azotemia, and even death. The incision must be carefully inspected for dehiscence, which, if present, should be treated operatively—conservative management rarely has a successful outcome. Fortunately, this is not usually the case, and a slow leak often can be identified from a specific site. A running skin stitch and a layer of collodion, combined with bed rest and aggressive medical management of the ascites, often seals the wound. Severe abdominal distention can be alleviated by paracentesis (at which time a culture specimen should be taken to rule out infected ascites). Rapid reaccumulation of tense, leaking ascites may require placement of a *countersink*, a peritoneal catheter that drains sufficient fluid to take tension off the wound. After 2 or 3 days, if this has been unsuccessful, a peritoneovenous shunt should be seriously considered to avoid continuing fluid and protein losses. A shunt is contraindicated if the ascites is infected.

INFECTED ASCITES

Infected ascites in postoperative cirrhotic patients may have a remarkably benign presentation, with signs of peritonitis, fever, and systemic sepsis being absent. A paracentesis with white blood cell count and culture is essential. A polymorphonuclear leukocyte count of less that 300/mm³ virtually rules out infection. If a solitary organism is identified, this likely represents contamination of the ascites during laparotomy or spontaneous bacterial peritonitis. Intravenous antibiotics and, in more critical patients, peritoneal lavage through dialysis catheters should be instituted. Because of increased susceptibility to nephrotoxicity, aminoglycosides should be avoided, if possible, in cirrhotic patients. A polymicrobial infection often heralds a primary intraabdominal process, requiring celiotomy if the patient is to be salvaged.

HEPATORENAL SYNDROME

As in all surgical patients, renal failure must be avoided, and shunt patients are no different in this objective. However, overenthusiasm in avoiding ascites formation and excessive parsimony in fluid administration can result in oliguria and azotemia. Ascites is eminently more acceptable and treatable than is renal failure, and before the diagnosis of hepatorenal syndrome can be considered, maximum medical therapy, including volume loading and the Galambos cocktail (albumin, mannitol, and furosemide), must be instituted. If the ascites becomes tense, a paracentesis of 5 to 10 L may acutely reduce intraabdominal pressure and promote a brisk diuresis.[6] This is safe as long as intravenous albumin is infused at a rate of 10 g/L of ascites removed.

Occasionally, despite all interventions, oliguria persists in conjunction with a disproportionate rise in blood urea nitrogen and a urine sodium of less than 10 mEq/L. In such patients, if the liver function is reasonably preserved, a peritoneovenous shunt may reverse the hepatorenal syndrome. However, if the patient is deeply encephalopathic and jaundiced and has a prothrombin time prolonged more than 4 seconds, only liver transplantation can avert the inevitable outcome of death.[7]

PANCREATITIS

Because of the extensive dissection and manipulation of the pancreas during the performance of a distal splenorenal shunt, there was initial concern about developing postoperative pancreatitis. Whereas mild hyperamylasemia is common, clinical pancreatitis is rare. If it does occur, even aggressive supportive therapy may be unable to deflect a virulent course.

SURGICAL MANAGEMENT OF ASCITES ■

OPTIONS

Although most patients with ascites can be controlled medically, occasionally a patient is refractory or has other indications for surgical intervention.[8] The usual options are a central shunt (commonly, a side-to-side portacaval) or a peritoneovenous shunt (LeVeen or Denver).[9] A newer option is the transjugular intrahepatic portasystemic shunt procedure. Because of its propensity to stenosis and occlusion, this is particularly useful in patients with a short life expectancy or as a bridge to liver transplantation. If the patient has a history of variceal hemorrhage, stable liver disease, and reasonably preserved hepatic function, a portacaval shunt is a reasonable and more durable choice. If intractable ascites is the only indication for surgery, a peritoneovenous shunt is simpler to perform and can be inserted under local anesthesia.[10] Still, selection of patients is important, because a jaundiced, azotemic patient with markedly abnormal clotting studies will not do well with shunting. Most patients in hepatorenal failure should not undergo operation, because in many it is clearly a brief stage in an irreversible progression to death. If intervention is deemed appropriate in such a patient with advanced hepatic dysfunction, the best results are clearly obtained by liver transplantation.

PREVENTION AND TREATMENT OF COMPLICATIONS

Appropriate perioperative maneuvers can mitigate many of the potentially life-threatening complications associated with peritoneovenous shunting. Patient selection is important, and those with hyperbilirubinemia and a markedly prolonged PT are best avoided. Preoperative cultures of the ascites are always taken, and a short course of prophylactic antibiotics is administered to avoid shunt infection. The coagulopathy that used to be such a problem with this operation can be minimized with heparin, 5000 U injected subcutaneously preoperatively and continued twice daily after surgery for several days. This is greatly abetted by avoiding too rapid an infusion of ascites postoperatively.[11] Accordingly, at surgery, most of the ascites is drained, and in high-risk patients, the abdomen can be irrigated with normal saline before the shunt is inserted.

Although many physicians seem to be concerned by the possibility of hypotension after rapid removal of ascites, this is exceptionally uncommon. An added benefit of ascitic removal is avoidance of volume overload in the immediate postoperative period, obviating the need for routine digitalization and invasive monitoring in these patients. Sodium and fluid intake can be liberalized within reason, but small amounts of diuretics are still usually required. Flow through the shunt is maintained with an abdominal binder and incentive spirometry.

The PT should be monitored postoperatively, but it is unnecessary to follow routinely the thrombin time and fibrin degradation products. (The latter are commonly elevated.) When the PT is prolonged more than several seconds or ecchymoses and incisional bleeding occur, autoinfusion of ascites should be minimized by sitting the patient up, removing the binder, and stopping the breathing exercises. Fresh frozen plasma may correct the coagulopathy. Rarely, a full-blown disseminated intravascular coagulation develops. At this juncture, heparin is administered by constant infusion, and epsilon-aminocaproic acid may be considered. Complete reversal of the coagulopathy may require ligation or removal of the shunt.

Patients who develop shunt infection early in the postoperative period tend to be ill with encephalopathy, systemic sepsis, and a bleeding diathesis. Broad-spectrum antibiotics should be started immediately, but often the shunt has to be removed to clear the infection. The patient then becomes increasingly difficult to manage because the ascites reaccumulates, and oliguria and azotemia ensue. Patients with late shunt infections (weeks or months later) tend to be less sick, more responsive to antibiotics, and more tolerant of shunt removal if it becomes necessary.

A common problem is shunt failure. Early shunt failure is usually technical, such as kinking of the catheter at the clavicle or not placing the tip of the catheter far enough centrally. This can readily be rectified surgically, repositioning the catheter and radiographically verifying its position near or in the right atrium. Late failures usually result from proteinaceous debris in the valve and respond well to valve replacement. Sometimes dietary indiscretion with excessive sodium and fluid ingestion overwhelms the capacity of the valve, or the patient may have stopped wearing the binder and doing the breathing exercises. Occasionally, concomitant coronary artery bypass disease or alcoholic cardiomyopathy results in elevated right atrial pressures that preclude satisfactory shunt function. When this is considered, a pulmonary artery catheter is diagnostically and therapeutically essential.

In evaluating failed shunts, radionuclide scanning is of little value. It confirms what is clinically obvious (that the shunt is not functioning) but does little to elucidate the cause of the problem. A shuntogram is more useful and can be performed by percutaneously injecting contrast material into the shunt tubing as it runs up the chest wall. Although this may specifically localize the level of obstruction, the same information can usually be determined intraoperatively. When shunts repeatedly fail early, venography should be performed to determine whether superior vena caval thrombosis has occurred.

MAJOR HEPATIC RESECTIONS ■

A clear understanding of the segmental anatomy of the liver, in addition to advances in surgical and anesthetic techniques, has permitted more frequent, successful, major hepatic resections. Elective scheduling of these procedures permits routine harvesting of several units of autologous blood. In conjunction with the intraoperative use of a cell saver, this markedly reduces heterologous transfusions. This not only minimizes the risk associated with donor blood, but also may improve survival after resection for malignancies.[12] Even with scrupulous surgical technique, substantial intraoperative hemorrhage cannot always be avoided; therefore, aggressive resuscitation by the anesthesiologist is critical in avoiding the consequences of shock, including ischemic injury to the remaining liver. Whereas 80% hepatectomy is often well tolerated in patients with normal livers, a right hepatic lobectomy in a cirrhotic patient usually results in liver failure and death. Likewise, deeply jaundiced patients have a more complicated postoperative course.

ALBUMIN ADMINISTRATION

Frequently, after a liver resection of greater than 50%, patients develop peripheral edema and even some ascites. However, this is rarely a serious problem. Some authorities advocate routine administration of albumin to these patients, but this rarely corrects the observed hypoalbuminemia. Although this practice is not harmful, it is expensive and is difficult to prove prospectively that it is beneficial.[13] In truth, until the liver regenerates, normal serum albumin levels are unlikely. A similar concern relates to postoperative hypoglycemia, which tends to be a more theoretical than practical problem and is readily controllable with a 5% or 10% glucose infusion. In practice, hyperglycemia is more commonly observed.

NUTRITION

Nutritional support is crucial, and unless the patient quickly resumes eating, enteral or parenteral hyperalimentation should be instituted. Specialized hyperalimentation formulas high in branched-chain and low in aromatic amino acids may be helpful but are not essential in treating most of these patients.

POSTOPERATIVE COAGULOPATHY AND BLEEDING

Substantial operative blood loss in combination with resection of an organ critical for clotting factor synthesis readily explains a postoperative coagulopathy. Administration of fresh frozen plasma and platelets and reversal of hypothermia tend to restore a normal clotting process. Occasionally, cryoprecipitate is necessary. Persistent marked prolongation of the PT and partial thromboplastin time should raise concern about the adequacy and viability of the liver remnant. Some postoperative bleeding is expected, but if more than

4 or 5 units of blood are transfused reexploration should be undertaken. It is imprudent to blame a coagulopathy as the cause until all mechanical causes of bleeding have been excluded. In fact, until surgical hemostasis is obtained and the intraabdominal hematoma (which is acting as a sink for the clotting factors) is evacuated, correction of the coagulopathy may be impossible. Usually, a few bleeding sites can be identified and oversewn, and topical hemostatic agents may be helpful. Electrocautery on a high coagulation setting and the argon beam laser often seal an oozing raw surface. Hepatic artery ligation is occasionally valuable in managing liver bleeding after trauma, but it is dangerous and rarely indicated after major hepatic resection. Further, it precludes the use of hepatic arteriography and embolization, which are sometimes helpful. If all other maneuvers fail, intraabdominal liver packing may be lifesaving. The packs are removed 2 to 3 days later, after the coagulopathy and hypothermia have been corrected and resuscitation has been completed.

JAUNDICE

The sudden removal of more than 50% of hepatic parenchyma of and by itself produces some hyperbilirubinemia. Considering factors such as increased pigment load from transfusions and impaired hepatocellular function from hypotension, medications, and infection, jaundice should be expected after major hepatic resections.[14] However, an inexorable rise or lack of any resolution of the hyperbilirubinemia after 14 days raises the question of a possible operative bile duct injury. A mechanical problem must be distinguished from intrahepatic cholestasis to avoid an unnecessary laparotomy in high-risk patients. If the bilirubin level is not too abnormal and hepatic dysfunction is not too severe, radionuclide scanning may rapidly exclude obstruction. US and CT are noninvasive and may be diagnostic. However, before exploration, direct visualization of the biliary tree is usually desirable. Endoscopic retrograde cholangiopancreatography (ERCP) documents the presence and location of a lesion but, if the obstruction is complete, does not demonstrate the proximal ducts. Percutaneous transhepatic cholangiography is best able to define the proximal anatomy. If the patient is deemed too ill for surgery, percutaneous decompression of the ducts or nasobiliary stenting may be considered as temporizing measures.

BILE FISTULA

Closed suction drains are routinely placed after liver surgery to evacuate bile. Some leaking from the raw, cut surface of the liver is anticipated, but it invariably ceases after a short interval. A persistent biliary fistula usually emanates from a major duct or from an excluded segment of the liver after a nonanatomic resection. Unless jaundice or sepsis develops, there is no urgency to intervene. Precise diagnosis and therapy can await recovery from the original procedure. Before surgical correction, a road map can be obtained by ERCP, transhepatic cholangiography, or contrast material injected through the drain track.

SEPSIS

The large defect left after a hepatic lobectomy often fills with an accumulation of hematoma, bile, and necrotic debris. In a febrile postoperative patient, after the usual extraabdominal sources of fever are ruled out, this locus must be evaluated radiographically for possible abscess formation. US- or CT-guided percutaneous placement of a drain is often therapeutic. If sepsis persists, open drainage should be expeditiously undertaken. The possibility of cholangitis, particularly if an indwelling biliary catheter is present, must be considered and appropriately managed. Often, exchanging, repositioning, or removing the tube resolves this latter problem.

LIVER FAILURE

Major hepatic resections produce an element of liver failure that is predictable, responsive to usual supportive therapy, and usually reversible as the remaining liver regenerates. Occasionally, irreversible liver failure follows over aggressive resection or vascular compromise of the hepatic remnant and is a particular problem in cirrhotic patients. Liver transplantation is the only hope for this group, but it may be difficult to predict exactly when the patient's liver has become nonsalvageable. Because transplantation has become safer, it should be considered earlier before multiple organ system failure develops and worsens prognosis from the liver transplant.[15] A particularly ominous and predictive sign is when the PT is markedly prolonged and fails to respond to vitamin K or fresh frozen plasma.

BUDD-CHIARI SYNDROME ■

A broad spectrum of pathologic processes results in hepatic venous outflow obstruction and postsinusoidal portal hypertension. The end result is the Budd-Chiari Syndrome, which can variably present as an acute abdomen with pain, hepatomegaly, ascites, and liver failure, or more chronically as ascites and bleeding varices. Appropriate therapy is predicated on an accurate diagnosis.[16] Confirmation of the clinical impression is achieved radiographically and pathologically. The caudate lobe, with its separate direct venous drainage into the inferior vena cava may be spared in Budd-Chiari syndrome, and this may be demonstrable on radionuclide scanning as diffuse hepatocellular dysfunction except for the enlarged caudate lobe. Hepatic venography is usually diagnostic, and during this procedure, pressures should be measured in the inferior vena cava below and above the liver, as well as in the right atrium. (This excludes cardiac diagnoses such as constrictive pericarditis.) The venous phase of superior mesenteric arteriography assesses patency and the direction of flow in the portal vein. Liver biopsy, although potentially dangerous, not only confirms the diagnosis of Budd-Chiari syndrome but also can help determine the urgency for surgery. If centrilobular congestion or necrosis is minimal, management can be expectant. However, severe centrilobular congestion and necrosis indicate a failing liver in which rapid hepatic decompression is essential.

The studies may reveal a vena caval web, pulmonary hypertension, or constrictive pericarditis, allowing appropriate therapy. More frequently, the hepatic veins are thrombosed, and the goal is to decompress the liver by converting the portal vein into an outflow tract. If the infrahepatic vena caval pressures are elevated because of compression by the congested caudate lobe, a side-to-side portacaval shunt will be ineffective. A mesoatrial shunt would then be a therapeutic option.[17] In some patients, liver transplantation is clearly the treatment of choice and is curative if successful.[18]

HEMOBILIA ■

An interesting and unusual cause of gastrointestinal bleeding is hemobilia. The classic triad is right upper quadrant pain, jaundice, and melena or hematemesis. As the blood clot accumulates in the bile ducts, it not only produces biliary colic, but also eventually tamponades the source of bleeding. The respite is temporary, because as the clot dissolves, the bleeding resumes, and the classic cycle of intermittent hemorrhage continues. Hemobilia most frequently follows trauma, often by an interval of several weeks. Occasionally, it is a complication of liver biopsy or percutaneous transhepatic instrumentation of the biliary tree.

The diagnosis is often made after other upper gastrointestinal sources are eliminated and requires a high index of suspicion. If the timing is fortuitous, upper endoscopy may visualize blood emanating from the ampulla. Occasionally, a radionuclide bleeding scan is diagnostic. However, the mainstay of diagnosis and therapy is angiography. Most hemobilia is arterial in origin, and hepatic arteriography with selective embolization usually resolves what used to be a difficult surgical challenge. If exploration does become necessary, ipsilateral hepatic artery ligation is not uniformly successful because collaterals may develop, producing recurrent hemobilia. Intraoperative angiography with direct embolization of the appropriate hepatic artery is preferable. The traditional hepatic resection of the involved area is rarely indicated.

POSTOPERATIVE CHOLECYSTITIS ■

Given the high incidence of cholelithiasis in the U.S. population, it is not unexpected that many patients with gall stones (asymptomatic or symptomatic) will undergo major procedures for other reasons. Whether the patient should have an incidental cholecystectomy is a separate issue, but clearly after certain procedures (coronary artery bypass, aortic replacement, trauma) the patient will return to the ICU with the gallbladder in situ. Occasionally, because of biliary stasis, systemic sepsis, and hypotension, the patient develops postoperative cholecystitis, a disease with a high mortality rate.[19] Commonly this is acalculous in nature, perhaps resulting from thrombosis of the cystic artery (an end artery). The major difficulty is establishing the diagnosis, and a high index of suspicion is important.

These patients are often very ill, intubated, and sedated. Their tender incisions and postoperative pain make abdominal examination difficult. If the patient has right upper quadrant tenderness and a palpable mass, the picture is obvious. Unfortunately, this is not usually the case. The patient may not be recovering as quickly as anticipated, may be septic, or may have mild icterus. Once the diagnosis is considered, a radionuclide scan of the biliary tree may show cystic duct obstruction. However, this may be a false-positive result because a fasting patient on hyperalimentation may have sludge in a distended gallbladder, precluding the entrance of radiolabel into the gallbladder. Alternatively, false-negative results can occur because visualization of the gallbladder does not exclude all cases of acalculous, even gangrenous, cholecystitis. US or CT may demonstrate a thickened, inflamed gallbladder with or without stones, perhaps with a pericholecystic collection or even air in the gallbladder wall (emphysematous cholecystitis).[20]

Bedside laparoscopy with direct examination of the gallbladder can be diagnostic and therapeutic. If the gallbladder is normal, cholecystitis is immediately eliminated as a potential cause. If there are ischemic or inflammatory changes, a cholecystostomy tube can be placed or the patient can be transported to the operating room for cholecystectomy by the laparoscopic or open route. Because most patients are already intubated and receiving mechanical ventilation, laparoscopy can be performed using sedation and paralysis in the ICU.[21,22] As a temporizing measure in critically ill patients, a cholecystostomy tube can be placed percutaneously under radiologic guidance.

CHOLANGITIS   ■

Cholangitis is a serious condition secondary to infection in an obstructed biliary tree. Charcot's triad of jaundice, fever and chills, and right upper quadrant pain is classic but not invariably present. The causes include choledocholithiasis, postoperative benign ductal strictures, neoplasms, primary sclerosing cholangitis, and stents.[23]

The course of treatment is dictated by the initial response to antibiotics. Fortunately, most patients rapidly respond to fluids and broad-spectrum antibiotics. Those who remain toxic have a severe syndrome, sometimes referred to as suppurative cholangitis, and may progress to mental stupor and shock. This group must have immediate decompression of the biliary tree. Until recently, this meant emergency surgical placement of a T tube in the common duct. Other options currently available are endoscopic papillotomy with stone removal or placement of a nasobiliary drain, percutaneous cholecystostomy if the cystic duct is patent, and transhepatic biliary decompression. In the critically ill patient, endoscopic retrograde cholangiopancreatography (ERCP) with nasobiliary stenting carries the lowest morbidity and mortality rates and can resolve the septic picture promptly.[24] If the latter interventions are not rapidly therapeutic, surgery should not be delayed.[25]

If conservative management is successful, after the infection has cleared, the biliary tree must be directly visualized by ERCP or percutaneous transhepatic cholangiography (PTHC). Most of these patients have an underlying condition that requires correction to avoid further attacks of cholangitis with its attendant complications.

BILIARY FISTULA AFTER CHOLECYSTECTOMY   ■

Bilious drainage after a cholecystectomy has a different significance and sense of urgency than when it occurs after a major hepatic resection. In this circumstance it is not anticipated, and expectant therapy may not be appropriate.

After cholecystectomy, a small amount of bile may drain from aberrant ducts in the gallbladder bed. This is self-limited and of no consequence. However, any significant bile drainage after 2 or 3 days mandates early investigation to rule out a bile duct injury. A radionuclide biliary scan may give a positive result but is not specific enough to localize an injury. Therefore, either ERCP or transhepatic cholangiography should be performed to assess the integrity of the biliary tree. A blown cystic duct stump may spontaneously seal if there is no distal obstruction requiring treatment. A hepatic or common bile duct injury is ideally treated by early surgical repair. However, if the patient is septic and has an infected subhepatic bile collection, a two-stage approach may be necessary. The interventional radiologist may be able to drain both the abscess and the bile duct, permitting secondary elective reconstruction of the biliary system.

Occasionally, a T tube placed after common bile duct exploration becomes dislodged in the early postoperative period. Bile may come out through a separate drain or around the T tube, the patient may become septic, or bilious ascites may develop. A water-soluble contrast study through the T tube should be obtained immediately. If the tube is only partially out of the duct or is adjacent to it, the interventional radiologist may be able to replace it. If this is unsuccessful but if the duct exploration removed all stones, leaving no distal obstruction, observation can be considered. Otherwise, the duct can be endoscopically stented or the T tube surgically replaced.

REFERENCES   ■

1. Arroyo V, Gines P, Planas R: Treatment of ascites in cirrhosis: diuretics, peritoneovenous shunt, and large volume paracentesis. *Gastroenterol Clin North Am* 1992;21:237
2. Eckhauser FE, Pomerantz RA, Knol JA, et al: Early variceal rebleeding after distal splenorenal shunt. *Arch Surg* 1986; 121:547
3. Munoz SJ, Maddrey WC: Major complications of acute and chronic liver disease. *Gastroenterol Clin North Am* 1988;17: 265
4. Marchesini G, Dioguardi FS, Bianchi GP, et al: Long-term oral branched-chain amino acid treatment in chronic hepatic encephalopathy: a randomized double-blind casein-controlled trial. *J Hepatol* 1990;11:92
5. Hutson DG, Livingstone A, Levi JU, et al: Early hepatic failure

or upper gastrointestinal bleeding following a distal splenorenal shunt. *Surg Gynecol Obstet* 1982;155:46

6. Simon DM, McCain JR, Bonkovsky HL, et al: Effects of therapeutic paracentesis on systemic and hepatic hemodynamics and on renal and hormonal function. *Hepatology* 1987;7:423

7. Iwatsuki S, Starzl TE, Todo S, et al: Liver transplantation in the treatment of bleeding esophageal varices. *Surgery* 1988;104:697

8. Stanley MM, Ochi S, Lee KK, et al: Peritoneovenous shunting as compared with medical treatment in patients with alcoholic cirrhosis and massive ascites. *N Engl J Med* 1989;321:1632

9. Fulenwider TJ, Smith RB, Redd SC, et al: Peritoneovenous shunts: lessons learned from an 8-year experience with 70 patients. *Arch Surg* 1984;119:1133

10. Bechstein WO, Neuhaus P, Steffen R, et al: Peritoneovenous shunting for the treatment of massive ascites [letter]. *N Engl J Med* 1990;322:1750

11. LeVeen HH, Ip M, Ahmed N, et al: Coagulopathy post peritoneovenous shunt. *Ann Surg* 1987;205:305

12. Stephenson KR, Steinberg SM, Hughes KS, et al: Perioperative blood transfusions are associated with decreased time to recurrence and decreased survival after resection of colorectal liver metastases. *Ann Surg* 1988;208:679

13. Akovbiantz A, Schmid M, Schmid E: Postoperative syndromes after liver surgery. *Clin Gastroenterol* 1979;8:471

14. LaMont JT, Isselbacher KJ: Postoperative jaundice. *N Engl J Med* 1973;288:305

15. Spaniert B, Klein RD, Nasrawey SA, et al: Multiple organ failure after liver transplantation. *Crit Care Med* 1995;23:466

16. Millikan WJ, Henderson JM, Sewell CW, et al: Approach to the spectrum of Budd-Chiari syndrome: which patients require portal decompression? *Ann J Surg* 1985;149:167

17. Cameron JL, Herlong HF, Sanfey H, et al: The Budd-Chiari syndrome: treatment by mesenteric–systemic venous shunts. *Ann Surg* 1983;198:335

18. Starzl TE, Demetris AJ, Van Thiel D: Liver transplantation. *N Engl J Med* 1989;321:1014

19. Johnson LB: The importance of early diagnosis of acute acalculous cholecystitis. *Surg Gynecol Obstet* 1987;164:197

20. Mirvis SE, Vainright JR, Nelson AW, et al: The diagnosis of acute acalculous cholecystitis: a comparison of sonography, scintigraphy, and CT. *Am J Radiol* 1986;147:1171

21. Sleeman D, Sosa JL, Almeida J, et al: Bedside laparoscopy in critically ill patients [abstract]. *Crit Care Med* 1994;23:A237

22. Sleeman D, Sosa JL, Almeida J, et al: Laparoscopy for the diagnosis of acalculous cholecystitis in the critically ill [abstract]. *Clin Invest Med* 1994;17:B18.

23. Boey JH, Way LW: Acute cholangitis. *Ann Surg* 1980;191:264

24. Siegel JH, Rodriquez R, Cohen SA, et al: Endoscopic management of cholangitis: critical review of an alternative technique and report of a large series. *Am J Gastroenterol* 1994;89:1142

25. Sievert W, Vakil NB: Emergencies of the biliary tract. *Gastroenterol Clin North Am* 1988;17:245

Critical Care, Third Edition, edited by Joseph M. Civetta,
Robert W. Taylor, and Robert R. Kirby.
Lippincott-Raven Publishers, Philadelphia, PA © 1997.

CHAPTER 74

■

Thoracic Surgery

Eddy H. Carrillo
M. Jack Williams

IMMEDIATE CONCERNS ■

MAJOR PROBLEMS

Initial evaluation and treatment of the thoracic surgical patient involves five categories: (1) support of the respiratory and cardiovascular systems to optimize oxygen delivery, (2) management of fluids, (3) pain control, (4) drainage and obliteration of the pleural cavity, and (5) management of secretions. Orders for mechanical ventilation and cardiovascular medications ("drips") are immediately transcribed and changed as dictated by blood gas determinations and cardiovascular stability. All connections should be checked, secured, and wrapped with tape to prevent leaks. All tubes should be labeled and output documented on arrival to the ICU. An upright chest radiograph should be obtained as soon as possible, to have an accurate estimation of the degree of pneumothorax or fluid that may be present.

Pain control is extremely important. Unless thoracic patients have had intercostal or epidural blocks, they may awaken from general anesthesia with excruciating pain; this leads them to thrash about in bed, to pull on intravenous and monitoring lines, and to fight the ventilator. If they are not intubated, they tend to take shallow, irregular respirations, which lead to poor ventilation and carbon dioxide retention.

Chest tubes should be patent and placed on suction to facilitate drainage. Obliteration of the pleural cavity is best obtained with complete lung expansion. The apical chest tube should be removing air from the thorax, as evidenced by bubbling in the water seal bottle, and the posterior tube should be draining blood; a few clots are inevitable. The early occurrence of large quantities of clot may indicate excessive blood loss because rapid bleeding usually leads to clotting.

Finally, ICU physicians and nurses should have a clear understanding as to the patient's expected medical course and the potential complications. A briefing to the ICU staff by the surgeon usually answers and clarifies all questions. One person or one team needs to coordinate and integrate the overall patient care to prevent unnecessary confusion.

STRESS POINTS

1. Before undertaking any major pulmonary resection, the surgeon must know that the patient's pulmonary reserves are sufficient to tolerate the thoracic incision and any loss of resected tissue.
2. With good anesthesia, the average patient can be extubated in the operating room or soon after admission to the ICU.
3. Because opiate receptors in the spinal cord react to specific endorphins and enkephalin mediators, a continuous epidural infusion with fentanyl provides excellent pain control.
4. All patients who have undergone thoracotomy have large-bore thoracostomy tubes for drainage of air, blood, and other fluids. In the immediate postoperative period, however, the main function of these tubes is to monitor the hourly output from the chest cavity.
5. Acute mediastinal shifts are detrimental, especially in the hypovolemic patient.
6. Suctioning is dangerous! Ventricular extrasystoles are common during suctioning and may progress rapidly to ventricular tachycardia or fibrillation if the suctioning is not limited to 15 seconds.

1131

7. It is normal for the apical tube to bubble vigorously in the immediate postoperative period, and the presence of a small rim of air on the first radiograph is not cause for undue alarm. However, continued pneumothorax or a large pneumothorax may indicate significant atelectasis, malfunctioning tubes, or a leak in the bronchial stump.
8. Tension pneumothorax or cardiac tamponade after trauma may be suggested by the presence of distended neck veins, although associated hypovolemia may minimize this finding or eliminate it altogether.
9. Most thoracic aortic injuries are diagnosed after the injury is suspected, based on the initial supine anteroposterior (AP) view.
10. Cardiac tamponade is a true emergency. A diagnostic pericardiocentesis should be performed. If cardiac tamponade is suspected clinically, transthoracic echocardiography (TTE) or transesophageal echocardiography (TEE) should be performed to confirm or rule out the diagnosis.
11. Cardiac arrhythmias after pneumonectomy occur in approximately 20% to 30% of patients.

ESSENTIAL DIAGNOSTIC TESTS AND PROCEDURES

1. Dyspnea is a predictor of mortality; its presence mandates full pulmonary function evaluation.
2. An upright chest radiograph should be obtained as soon as possible. The radiograph should be carefully evaluated for the following:
   a. position of endotracheal tube
   b. position of chest tubes
   c. position of monitoring lines
   d. presence of pneumothorax
   e. amount of fluid or blood in the thorax
   f. presence of atelectasis or pulmonary infiltrate
   g. degree of mediastinal shift
   h. width of the mediastinum in trauma patients
3. A blood loss of 200 mL/hour for 4 to 6 hours is an indication for reexploration in the postthoracotomy patient and for surgery in the trauma patient.
4. Thoracostomy tube seals should be airtight to maintain an intrapleural vacuum, usually using wall suction of -20 cm H_2O and an underwater seal system.
5. Pulse oximetry is valuable to detect the onset of arterial desaturation so that suctioning can be terminated and oxygen administered.
6. Air leaks will not stop until the lung is fully expanded.
7. Decreased breath sounds and shock may be the only indication of tension pneumothorax, which requires immediate chest decompression.
8. Computed tomography (CT) also is useful to diagnose rib and sternal fractures and parenchymal injuries. Its most important role is the later diagnosis of infected or retained chest collections.
9. Although radiologic signs have been proposed as harbingers of injury to the thoracic aorta, none have enough sensitivity or specificity to replace angiography.

10. Diaphragmatic injuries can be missed initially in trauma patients if the initial chest radiograph is misinterpreted as showing an elevated left diaphragm, a "loculated hemopneumothorax," or extrapulmonary hematoma. The presence of a nasogastric tube in the left chest cavity is confirmatory.
11. Analysis of the waveform of the pulmonary artery (PA) catheter helps to diagnose pericardial tamponade. Usually, there is an elevation and equalization of the right atrial, pulmonary artery diastolic, and pulmonary artery occlusion pressures.

INITIAL THERAPY

1. Smokers should be encouraged to stop smoking before the operation to restore bronchial ciliary function. Patients with chronic bronchitis or active infections should receive appropriate antibiotics.
2. The average elective postoperative patient who needs ventilatory does well starting with an inspired oxygen fraction of 40%, tidal volume of 700 to 800 (10 to 12 mL/kg), an intermittent mandatory ventilation (IMV) rate of 8, and a positive end-expiratory pressure (PEEP) of 4 to 5 cm H_2O.
3. Pressure support (5 cm) can be added to overcome the imposed work of breathing, or patients can be ventilated or weaned using this technique. Starting parameters can be exhaled tidal volume of 7 to 8 mL/kg or the initial level of pressure support estimated by subtracting PEEP from peak inspiratory pressure and dividing by 2.
4. If air is under pressure in the pneumonectomy space, it can be aspirated with a syringe and a three-way stopcock.
5. After each episode of suctioning, the patient should be reoxygenated, by the ventilator, by manual ventilation, or by spontaneous respiration with added oxygen before continuing.
6. In patients undergoing any major thoracic surgical procedure, use a first-generation cephalosporin (cefazolin) for a period of 24 hours postoperatively or longer if there are specific indications. Patients with penetrating injuries to the chest should be treated immediately with therapeutic antibiotics if thoracotomy is performed or if chest tube thoracostomy is done.
7. Pulseless electrical activity may indicate tension pneumothorax, severe hypovolemia, cardiac tamponade, massive pulmonary embolism, or hypothermia.
8. Videothoracoscopy is used for diagnosing diaphragmatic injuries and for evacuating a retained hemothorax.
9. The initial administration of intravenous fluids transiently increases preload and improves cardiac output in tamponade while preparations are made for definitive surgical repair.
10. Prophylactic digitalis has been recommended in elderly patients and in patients with intrapericardial ligation of the pulmonary vessels.
11. Postpneumonectomy pulmonary edema presents as

progressive dyspnea and hypoxia 12 to 24 hours after surgery. Treatment includes controlling fluid administration, morphine, diuretics, and mechanical ventilatory support.

THORACIC SURGERY ■

The thorax often reflects changes or disease in other organ systems. Its physiology is unique, and an understanding of basic cardiopulmonary pathophysiology is essential to the practice of modern surgery. As surgeons ingeniously developed the art of surgery and progressively exploited different organ systems and body cavities during the late nineteenth and early twentieth centuries, it became obvious that a high percentage of surgical failures were not incident to poor surgery but were happening because of an inability to understand or to influence various pathophysiologic changes. Although beautiful technical surgery is the goal of every surgeon, it may well be doomed to failure, or at least mediocrity, if the surgeon is not an accomplished and practicing physiologist. The great surgeon–physiologists of this century, accompanied by the modern pharmacologist–physiologist–anesthesiologist, have established a milieu of understanding and performance that has changed medicine. Despite their achievements, however, it would have been difficult to have arrived at our relative state of perfection without the development of modern critical care units and the coincident emergence of critical care nurses, on whom we rely to perform many daily miracles for which we physicians assume, perhaps, more credit than we deserve.

This chapter is not meant to reiterate long tables, endless algorithms, or a one-two-three method of managing patients, but rather to outline basic principles of care and to provide a pragmatic, simple, and usable approach to thoracic surgical patients.

PREOPERATIVE CONSIDERATIONS ■

Once the surgeon has determined that the patient will tolerate any major pulmonary resection,[1,2] the extent of pulmonary disease and resection dictates the amount of attention focused on the possibility of postoperative pulmonary complications. The presence of dyspnea, hypoxia, and hypercapnia mandates a full pulmonary function evaluation. The need for preoperative cardiac evaluation depends on the expected postoperative stress placed on the heart. Most patients require an electrocardiogram (ECG). If electrocardiographic findings and history are suggestive of underlying cardiac disease, new noninvasive techniques for cardiac evaluation help to determine ventricular function and ejection fractions. For patients with evidence of significant coronary artery disease, coronary arteriography and coronary revascularization may be indicated. Patients at high risk of cardiac events, as determined by the workup, may benefit from invasive monitoring during surgery and the immediate postoperative period.

MANAGEMENT OF THE POSTTHORACOTOMY PATIENT ■

The thoracic surgical patient has, assuming a normal cardiovascular system, at least one outstanding problem: interference with gas exchange. Through surgical, blunt, or penetrating trauma, the patient may have all, or any combination, of the following:

1. Abnormal ventilatory mechanics
2. A restrictive ventilatory defect
3. An obstructive ventilatory defect
4. Defective alveolar gas exchange

Pain and abnormal muscle function secondary to surgery and trauma may severely impair the ability of the patient to ventilate and to clear secretions in a normal manner. This leads to a restrictive ventilatory defect with a significant decrease in the vital capacity (VC) and in the functional residual capacity (FRC). This occurs after abdominal or after thoracic surgery. However, the thoracic surgical patient may have had a preexisting restrictive defect that has been increased by pulmonary resection, and because many thoracic surgical patients are smokers, often a significant degree of chronic obstructive lung disease (COLD) is present. If such a patient develops adult respiratory distress syndrome (ARDS), then oxygenation at the alveolar level is impaired, and a routine postoperative course may rapidly deteriorate into a critical situation.

ROUTINE POSTOPERATIVE CARE

The average thoracic surgical patient arrives in the recovery room or ICU in stable condition, with a normal blood volume, breathing spontaneously, and in a semiawake condition. On some surgical services, it is routine to maintain intubation and artificial ventilation for an arbitrary period after the patient is admitted to a special care unit. This is unnecessary in most instances. With good anesthesia, the average patient can be extubated in the operating room or soon after admission to the recovery room or special care unit. Before the thoracotomy is closed, intercostal nerve blocks with 0.25% bupivacaine with epinephrine in 1:200,000 concentration may be performed. This effectively abolishes the excruciating pain that occurs immediately after surgery and assures that the patient will be able to make a good effort at breathing and coughing, thus preventing or moderating the inevitable decrease in the FRC that occurs from severe pain. This does not block all pain, but it will last from 8 to 12 hours and allows easier control of the remaining pain with judicious use of narcotics.

Narcotics

The use of small intravenous doses of narcotics repeated at frequent intervals is preferable to the traditional administration of large doses intramuscularly every 3 to 4 hours. For example, 1.5 mg of morphine sulfate every 15 to 60 minutes controls pain effectively without oversedating the patient.

One of the most significant recent advances in pain control has been the use of *patient-controlled analgesia*. This involves the use of a small, computerized module into which is inserted a syringe containing a desired concentration of narcotic (e.g., 50 mL of diluent containing 50 mg of morphine). The module is programmed to deliver a predetermined volume of narcotic at a desired time interval, through an intravenous catheter, when the patient pushes a control button. A typical dosage schedule would be to program the module to deliver 1.5 mL (1.5 mg of morphine) every 15 minutes on command by the patient. The programming does not allow the patient to receive more than the ordered amount, regardless of the number of times the button is pushed.

This technique provides excellent pain control in most patients and is especially useful in thoracic and abdominal surgery patients. It can usually be discontinued after 3 days when the patient begins taking oral analgesics. The technique obviates the anxiety and increased pain that occur while awaiting the nurse to draw and administer medication; it is also popular among the nurses because it greatly simplifies pain management. The interaction between the onset of pain and the anxiety that arises during the waiting period for the next dose of intermittent pain medication greatly increases both the perceived intensity of pain and the amount of medication necessary. Patient-controlled analgesia does, however, require that the patients be alert enough to participate in their own care. The patient whose pain is effectively controlled responds in a more positive manner than one who is anxious, fearful, and oversedated; good pain control also allows the achievement of better results from respiratory therapy, physical therapy, and early ambulation.

Epidural Analgesia

We are currently enthusiastic about pain control achieved by continuous thoracic epidural analgesia using synthetic narcotics or local anesthetics. This provides excellent pain management. It is most useful in the first 3 days after surgery. It should not be used, however, unless there is active and continuous participation of the anesthesia department in the postsurgical management of the patient in the ICU. In our hospitals and in many others, a pain management service has been developed by departments of anesthesia. They plan the type of control appropriate and ensure that orders, devices, and all of the details of management are coordinated. The results are impressive: patients are comfortable from the time they awaken and they have near-normal pulmonary function. This salutary combination justifies the efforts necessary to create and coordinate the pain service. Respiratory depression and hypotension occur rapidly in some patients. If epidural analgesia is used, the nursing and the respiratory therapy staffs must be particularly alert to the possibility of atelectasis. Patients with epidural analgesia may feel comfortable, but they may not spontaneously cough and raise secretions unless stimulated to do so. Continuous thoracic epidural analgesia was designed to aid patients in deep respirations and coughing, but it may have the opposite effect unless the attendants are diligent in respiratory care.

Monitoring

The amount of monitoring necessary for patients in the ICU continues to stimulate lively debate. In their excellent review of cardiopulmonary monitoring, Widemann and coworkers[3] state, "In some clinical circumstances, our ability to monitor disease may have outpaced our capacity to intervene therapeutically." In the second part of their review, Widemann and associates[4] discuss the generally accepted indications for peripheral artery and monitoring with the pulmonary artery (PA) catheter, including the following:

1. Myocardial infarction
2. Shock
3. Respiratory failure in COLD
4. Drug overdose
5. After major cardiac and vascular surgery
6. ARDS

In general, the thoracic surgical patient does not require the use of the PA catheter, although it may be necessary in selected patients with major complications or associated diseases, especially myocardial disease, ARDS, and shock.

Monitoring the patient's oxygenation should be routine in thoracic surgery patients. The use of an indwelling peripheral arterial catheter has been standard in recent years because it (1) provides ready access for blood gas determinations during and after surgery; (2) provides accurate and continuous blood pressure monitoring; (3) is inexpensive; and (4) has minimal complications. It is usually discontinued 24 to 48 hours after surgery. A pulse oximeter attached to a finger or toe is a noninvasive way to monitor oxygenation. The oximeter provides continuous monitoring of the arterial oxygen saturation. Because it is continuous, it alerts the ICU staff quickly to changes in the patient's oxygenation. We are using oximeters more commonly in lieu of arterial catheters for the average uncomplicated patient, whereas both are used on severely ill patients.

A central venous catheter also should be used routinely for most thoracic surgical patients. In the absence of severe myocardial dysfunction, it provides a generally accurate estimate of the circulating blood volume, and just as importantly, it provides the most effective route for administering large volumes of fluid or blood.

IMMEDIATE POSTOPERATIVE PERIOD

When the patient is out of surgery and has been settled into the ICU, a complete assessment should be done as a baseline for comparison with later evaluations, accompanied by the following orders:

1. Routine orders are written.
2. Precise ventilator orders are written if the patient is on the ventilator.
3. A chest radiograph is ordered.
4. Fluid orders are written.
5. Pain control is initiated.

In addition, a verbal report is given to the ICU nurse outlining the operative findings, the patient's condition, and the expected postoperative course.

These assessment factors may seem to be routine and unnecessarily reiterated. However, attention to detail is mandatory, and it is common for orders to be written hastily in the operating room with the surgical team then dispersing to other areas, leaving the nurse to decipher illegible orders with no verbal report and with no clear understanding of the expected postoperative course. The anesthesiologist or anesthetist always briefs the nurse on the patient's condition, but this is no substitute for information on expected surgical problems.

Ventilator Orders

In general, patients who are in need of ventilatory support receive positive pressure, and the dependent areas of the lung, which have the smallest airway diameters and are the least compliant, are poorly ventilated. The more compliant and less perfused areas receive the greatest ventilation. This leads to ventilation perfusion mismatching, hypoxemia, and atelectasis. Also, the FRC decreases in almost all anesthetized surgical patients, as in injured patients.[5] These changes are more significant in the initial 48 hours after surgery but usually last for up to a week. Decrease in FRC leads to airway closure and ventilation-perfusion abnormalities with resulting hypoxemia, which may be accentuated in older patients. Alveolar dead space usually increases with mechanical ventilation; therefore, there is a need for increased minute ventilation to maintain a normal $PaCO_2$. It is important to lower either the IMV rate or pressure support quickly as soon as the patient awakens to minimize the adverse effects of mechanical ventilation.

Radiographs: What to Look for

The first postoperative radiograph is an important part of the initial evaluation. The following points should be carefully evaluated:

1. Position of the endotracheal tube
2. Position of central monitoring catheters
3. Presence of a pneumothorax
4. Mediastinal shift
5. Output from chest tubes
6. Amount of fluid or blood in the thorax
7. Presence of atelectasis or pulmonary infiltrate (contusion in the trauma patient)
8. Width of the mediastinum in trauma patients
9. Position of nasogastric tube and gastric distension

POSITION OF THE ENDOTRACHEAL TUBE. Transporting the patient from surgery to the unit occasionally results in dislodgement of the tube despite the utmost care. It may be too high or too low in the trachea; it should be well into the lower portion of the trachea but at least 2 cm above the carina. If it is at, or touching, the carina, it may stimulate continuous coughing, irritate the carina, and if it remains long enough, erode the mucosa at the carina. It is common for tubes to move into the right main stem bronchus. This will result in partial or complete atelectasis of the left lung.

POSITION OF CENTRAL MONITORING CATHETER. The central venous pressure (CVP) catheter should be in the superior vena cava. If it is touching or through the tricuspid valve, it may stimulate arrhythmias. It may also enter the coronary sinus if it is too low. The PA catheter may be too far into the PA, making it hazardous to inflate the balloon. If it is not far enough, it will not wedge. Occasionally, the catheter displace into the right ventricle, where it incites arrhythmias. Malposition of the PA catheter usually can be determined by observation of the pressure tracing, but it is best to ascertain its exact position with radiography.

PRESENCE OF A PNEUMOTHORAX. If the chest tubes are functioning well and if the patient's ventilation is normal, then the lung should be fully expanded. It is normal for the chest tubes, especially the apical tube, to bubble vigorously in the immediate postoperative period, and the presence of a small rim of air is not cause for undue alarm on the first radiograph. However, continued pneumothorax or a large pneumothorax may indicate significant atelectasis, malfunctioning tubes, or a leak in the bronchial anastomosis. Continuous suction with 20 cm H_2O negative pressure clears a small pneumothorax. Automatic stapling devices have decreased the number and amount of postoperative air leaks. *Air leaks will not stop until the lung is fully expanded.* Once the lung is expanded and in apposition to the parietal pleura, the small parenchymal leaks gradually cease; otherwise, they continue to leak into the space and result in a "prolonged air leak" or a bronchopleural fistula.

MEDIASTINAL SHIFT. After a pulmonary resection, the mediastinum shifts toward the resected side and the diaphragm moves upward. This is normal and desirable because it fits the remaining lung to an appropriately sized space. However, an unusual degree of shift may indicate atelectasis and may be a signal that endotracheal suctioning or bronchoscopy is indicated. Small areas of atelectasis, especially discoid atelectasis, are common and almost unavoidable, but they indicate that vigorous pulmonary toilet, increased patient activity, aerosol nebulization, and, often, chest physiotherapy, are needed.

After a pneumonectomy, the mediastinum should be as near the center as possible. Too much air in the pneumonectomy space may compress the remaining lung, making ventilation difficult, and it may impair venous return or incite arrhythmias. Too little air in the immediate postoperative period also may result in an acute mediastinal shift toward the operated side, which can also impair venous return and cause arrhythmias. If there is too much tension in the pneumonectomy space, it can quickly be relieved by aspirating air with a large syringe, a large-bore needle, and a three-way stopcock. It is less common, but occasionally necessary, to have to add air to the space. Acute mediastinal shifts are particularly detrimental to the hypovolemic patient, and they may give false readings from monitoring lines.

OUTPUT FROM CHEST TUBES. It is generally accepted that a blood loss of 200 mL/hour is reasonable in the immediate postoperative or posttrauma period, but for how long? A loss of 200 mL/hour for 24 hours is a major hemorrhage.

A continued blood loss of this magnitude for 4 to 6 hours is an indication for reexploration in the postthoracotomy patient and for surgery in the trauma patient. If the blood loss begins at 200 mL/hour and shows a progressive decrease in volume, cautious observation and blood replacement are all that is necessary.

Pulmonary Toilet and Tracheal Suctioning

Other important factors in the care of postthoracotomy patients include proper positioning, chest physiotherapy, and tracheal suctioning. Positioning of the patient includes using gravity to improve diaphragmatic excursion. The Trendelenburg position facilitates drainage of the lower lobes, and a lateral position facilitates the drainage of the contralateral side. Placing the patient in the prone position facilitates the drainage of the posterior lung segments, where secretions tend to accumulate in the usual supine position. Chest physiotherapy has reduced the incidence rate of postoperative pulmonary complications from 42% to 12% when therapy included preoperative training, diaphragmatic deep breathing, and coughing exercises with postural drainage.[6]

The use of the suction catheter on an "as needed" basis is routine for patients with endotracheal tubes, and the use of nasotracheal suction in patients without tubes is also a useful method to aid patients in clearing their secretions. Like many routine, simple, and frequently repeated maneuvers, suctioning is sometimes performed in a perfunctory and incautious manner. Suctioning is dangerous! We have witnessed fatalities resulting from faulty technique; ventricular extrasystoles are common during suctioning and may progress rapidly to ventricular tachycardia or fibrillation if the suctioning is not limited to 15 seconds. After each episode of suctioning, the patient should be reoxygenated by the ventilator, by manual ventilation, or by normal respiration with added oxygen before continuing. Pulse oximetry is valuable to detect the onset of arterial desaturation so that suctioning can be terminated and oxygen administered. The coughing stimulated by the suction catheter is usually more effective in clearing secretions than is the amount removed by the catheter itself. Once the secretions are brought into the major bronchi or into the trachea, they usually can be removed by quick suctioning. It is not necessary to push the catheter down to the lower lobe bronchi. This is particularly dangerous in patients who have had a pulmonary resection and in whom the bronchial stump is particularly vulnerable to rough suction with stiff catheters. Pushing a catheter through a pneumonectomy stump may result in bronchopleural fistula, infection of the pneumonectomy space, and multiple subsequent operations.

Antibiotics

Prophylactic antibiotics are given in the operating room before the surgical incision is made. For prolonged procedures or in patients undergoing massive resuscitation, another dose is given every 3 hours. There is no benefit from long courses of antibiotic prophylaxis (more than 24 hours). We do not routinely use antibiotics for chest tube thoracostomy after blunt thoracic injuries. However, in patients with penetrating trauma, we do use antibiotics if thoracotomy is performed or with chest tube thoracostomy. The antibiotic of choice is a first-generation cephalosporin.[7]

Body Temperature

Thoracic surgical patients are vulnerable to hypothermia because of the large surface area that is exposed during a thoracotomy in rooms kept cool for the comfort of the operating team, and because of the frequent use of irrigating solutions that are often lower than body temperature. Additionally, the use of blood and intravenous fluids that are not properly warmed aggravates and perpetuates the problem. Even mild hypothermia (core temperature of 34° to 36.5°C) initiates undesirable changes, including the following:

1. Peripheral vasoconstriction and metabolic acidosis
2. Shift of the oxyhemoglobin curve to the left, decreasing the release of bound oxygen from hemoglobin
3. Increase in heart rate, cardiac output, and mean arterial pressure secondary to catecholamine release
4. Progressive and generalized slowing of body enzyme systems
5. "Cold diuresis" secondary to increased central intravascular volume from the severe peripheral vasoconstriction[8]
6. A coagulopathy caused by a reversible depression in platelet production of thromboxane A_2 and release of adenosine diphosphate, which aggregate other platelets in the area and increases the bulk of the platelet plug; hypothermia, therefore, inhibits production of elements necessary for primary hemostasis

Elderly and pediatric patients are particularly susceptible to the detrimental effects of a lowered core temperature. The use of warm irrigating solutions in surgery and the administration of warm blood and fluids are usually enough to prevent or treat mild hypothermia. Although they are commonly used, warming blankets may cause thermal injury; their use should be carefully monitored.

UNUSUAL CIRCUMSTANCES: LESSONS TO BE LEARNED

The following three case reports are examples of occurrences that, because of errors in judgment, rapidly deteriorated into critical situations.

Case 1: A 45-year-old patient had an uncomplicated right upper lobectomy done for carcinoma of the lung; there were no metastases, his prognosis was good, and his immediate postoperative course was uneventful, although he had slightly more than the usual amount of air bubbling from his chest tubes for the first 2 days. On the third postoperative day, his air leak had stopped, and orders were written transferring him to the surgical floor from the ICU. Because of a questionable infiltrate that could not be adequately evaluated on the early morning portable radiograph, the radiologist requested that the patient be sent to the radiology department for a better set of radiographs. This was done. Later, the patient was found in the radiology holding area, radiographs not yet taken, in extremis, with dark cyanosis, semicomatose, and with no palpable pulse. *The chest tubes were clamped*! It was immediately obvious that the patient had a tension pneumothorax. The clamps were removed, the pneumothorax was quickly relieved, and the patient returned to normal.

This case report is an anecdotal example of what can happen when chest tubes are clamped. One author (M.J.W.) has seen several such examples and considers the clamping of chest tubes to be a pernicious and illogical practice. It is often done by the nursing service (and sometimes by physicians) for the transport of patients, and it is the policy on some surgical services to clamp the chest tube for 24 hours after it stops bubbling, whereupon it is removed. To be sure, no harm comes from clamping a nonfunctioning chest tube. But what good can come from it? If a tube is no longer functioning, then a 24-hour period of observation before removal is much safer if the tube is open and ready to resume its normal function in the event of further air leak.

Case 2: A 59-year-old man had a right extrapleural neumonectomy for massive hemoptysis secondary to aspergillosis. Although chronically ill, debilitated, and in negative nitrogen balance, he had done well immediately after surgery and had been extubated 48 hours later. On the seventh postoperative day, the surgery resident elected to insert a subclavian catheter for hyperalimentation because the patient could not eat and refused a feeding tube. A left subclavian catheter was inserted; the postcatheterization chest radiograph showed a 10% pneumothorax. The patient was stable on a 40% ventimask, and a small no. 16 needle catheter was inserted and attached to water seal drainage. Fifteen minutes later, the patient developed a sudden respiratory arrest followed quickly by ventricular fibrillation. He was resuscitated only after insertion of a large no. 36 chest tube. He aspirated gastric contents during this episode and died several weeks later of pneumonia and respiratory insufficiency.

Several errors in judgment are evident on review of this case. The insertion of a subclavian catheter was a poor choice. The patient had two easily accessible internal jugular veins. Under the circumstances, either would have been a safer route for the catheter. Assuming that it was necessary to use the subclavian route, it seems predictable that a pneumothorax on the side of the only remaining lung tissue would be exceedingly dangerous. It would have been safer to have used the opposite side where there was no risk of hitting lung.

It was assumed that the pneumothorax was a "simple" one because the patient was initially asymptomatic. *There is no such thing as a simple pneumothorax.* (This is illustrated dramatically by Case 3.) The use of the small no. 16 catheter for evacuation of the pneumothorax was the poorest judgment of all and directly led to the cardiac arrest. Intravenous-sized catheters are not large enough to evacuate sufficient air in the presence of a significant continuing air leak. A no. 32 chest tube would have been the best choice.

Case 3: On being called to a large hospital emergency department to treat a gunshot wound of the chest, the

author (M.J.W.) encountered the usual frenzied scene: a prostrate, intoxicated, agitated patient was lying in a pool of blood and was attended by the entire staff. Sitting quietly by the door in a wheelchair was a young man who was cyanotic, sweating, and in severe respiratory distress. His blood pressure was 60/40 mm Hg, and he was semicomatose. The blood pressure of the patient with the gunshot wound was 110/70; although he was severely wounded, he was in better condition than the other patient who had been diagnosed by the radiologist, an hour earlier, as having a "simple" 20% pneumothorax. Because of the pressure of multiple patients and, finally, the admission of the trauma patient, the young man's treatment was delayed, and he almost died. Chest tubes were quickly inserted into both patients—the pneumothorax patient first—and both did well.

Because spontaneous pneumothorax is such a common illness and is usually associated with low morbidity, it is easy to forget its potential for developing suddenly into a life-threatening tension pneumothorax. All pneumothoraces should be treated promptly with a chest tube of sufficient size to handle a large air leak. There are many advocates of small catheters, or indeed, no catheters at all, in the management of a small benign-acting pneumothorax. The fact that this is usually successful does not compensate for the unusual circumstances in which it is not.

THORACIC TRAUMA ■

Thoracic trauma is extremely common and accounts for a significant percentage of the morbidity and mortality associated with the management of trauma patients. On the other hand, it is amazing how much trauma the thorax can absorb with only minimal damage to the patient. The flexibility of the chest wall and the lungs often enables these structures to withstand a great deal of blunt force without serious damage to the patient; additionally, the bony thorax often deflects and absorbs the kinetic energy of missiles and knives.[9]

Observation or placement of tube thoracostomy, adequate volume resuscitation, pain control, occasional need for respiratory support, and serial chest radiographs are the only management required in 80% to 85% of patients.[10,11] Less than 10% of blunt chest injuries require an operation, and 15% to 30% of penetrating chest injuries require thoracotomy to control bleeding, repair tracheobronchial disruptions, relieve cardiac tamponade, and control associated injuries. Historically, only a small number of these patients undergo formal pulmonary resections for devastating injuries, and these patients often have a poor outcome.[12]

DIAGNOSIS

Chest Radiograph

Despite some limitations, the initial chest radiograph is the most important diagnostic tool to document or suggest thoracic injuries. Chest radiographs should be deferred in unstable patients. An AP supine radiograph is usually obtained (although upright radiographs are preferred), and it should be adequate to identify the most common thoracic injuries. Later on, lateral or oblique views should be obtained to document sternal or rib fractures. Radiopaque markers should be used to document the entry and exit site of projectiles. Finally, the radiograph is extremely useful to identify the position of tubes and intravascular devices placed during the initial resuscitation.

Computed Tomography

Although there is no doubt that CT is highly accurate in the diagnosis of mediastinal hemorrhage[13,14] and can even detect aortic rupture, there probably are few surgeons who would operate without a thoracic aortogram. It may, however, play a role in the diagnosis of patients undergoing radiographic workup for cranial, abdominal, and pelvic trauma. In some patients, CT-guided drainage of retained intrathoracic collections eliminates major surgical drainage procedures.

Transthoracic Echocardiography and Transesophageal Echocardiography

Both TTE and TEE are safe and rapid techniques for obtaining anatomic and physiologic information about cardiac and vascular structures. They are portable and can be repeated if there are suspicious areas. Their use should be limited to patients who are hemodynamically stable.

Electrocardiography

Electrocardiography is required for monitoring all trauma patients. A 12-lead ECG is obtained specifically to assess ST-T and Q wave changes to document acute myocardial necrosis. In myocardial contusion, typical Q wave findings are not seen in the initial evaluation, but unexplained tachycardia, arrhythmias, premature ventricular contractions, and ST segment changes may be present. Pulseless electrical activity may indicate tension pneumothorax, severe hypovolemia, cardiac tamponade, massive pulmonary embolism, or hypothermia. When bradycardia, premature contractions, and heart block are present, hypoxia, hypoperfusion, or hypothermia should be suspected immediately.

Angiography

Thoracic aortic rupture is found in only a few of the patients in whom it is suspected, yet it is vital to do angiography. Currently, despite its invasive nature, aortography remains the "gold standard" for diagnosis.[13] Its timing must be coordinated with other diagnostic or therapeutic procedures.

Tracheobronchoscopy

Tracheobronchoscopy is the diagnostic test of choice in tracheobronchial trauma. The fiberoptic bronchoscope may be an invaluable tool in resuscitation. Tracheal and selective bronchial intubation may allow ventilation of the normal lung during repair of the contralateral lung. For removal of foreign bodies or in several hemoptysis, the rigid bronchoscope can be more useful.

Thoracoscopy

Videothoracoscopy is used in the diagnosis of diaphragmatic injuries and also in the management of retained hemothoraces, especially after penetrating thoracic trauma.[15]

SPECIFIC INJURIES

Rib Fractures

Usually ribs four through ten are the ones fractured because the scapula and shoulder girdle effectively protect the upper ribs, and the 11th and 12th ribs are so short and flexible that they are uncommonly fractured.[16] One or two rib fractures are usually no cause for alarm and can be treated on an outpatient basis with analgesics and splinting one side of the chest without danger to the patient. However, three or more fractures are better managed by hospitalization and further observation of the patient. One or two rib fractures in an elderly patient, in the patient with COLD, or in the patient with other significant trauma may become important because the decrease in VC and decreased ability to clear secretions, which occur with such fractures, may assume a significance out of proportion to the apparent injury. If the patient's VC exceeds 15 mL/kg, then the patient will probably do well with analgesics or intercostal nerve blocks and continued observation. In the ICU, nerve blocks with 0.25% bupivacaine with epinephrine 1:200,000 are extremely useful in helping the patient to cough, to breathe deeply with an incentive spirometer, and to move around in bed or into a bedside chair. A comfortable patient whose pain is controlled feels better, does better, and is able to cooperate much better than a patient sedated with morphine who continues to have intermittent pain. Pleural catheters, either percutaneously inserted or advanced through an existing chest tube, also may be used to inject bupivacaine. Unilateral injections provide bilateral pain relief in more than half of patients so treated. Inserting a long catheter through the chest tube is easy, requiring no great technical skill or even knowledge of anatomic landmarks. Therefore, it is a useful technique for patients with chest trauma who have had chest tubes inserted for hemothorax or pneumothorax. Management of the medication orders can also be coordinated with a pain service.

Flail Chest

A flail chest occurs when instability of the chest wall produces paradoxical motion with inspiration. This dramatically reduces VC, and efforts by the patient to increase depth of respiration and to increase minute ventilation are inefficient; they increase paradox and increase oxygen consumption because of the increased work of breathing. Fractures or fracture dislocations in two areas are usually necessary to produce significant flail chest. A combination of radiographs and palpation of the chest is necessary to evaluate the injury; it is common for patients to have dislocations of the costochondral junctions, which are not visible on radiograph, associated with posterior rib fractures. If one detects motion or fractures in two locations in three or more ribs, the patient is at high risk for developing significant impairment of ventilation. Lewis[17] emphasizes that patients with rib fractures or flail chest should be evaluated by measuring the VC. Normal VC is 60 to 70 mL/kg; a minimally adequate VC is 15 mL/kg. A decrease in the VC to this level is an indication for intubation and ventilatory support.

A flail chest that was minimal or unnoticed in the emergency department may not become significant or obvious until 8 to 24 hours later, when the splinting afforded by the voluntary and involuntary contractions of chest wall muscles is lost. At this time, the patient may decompensate rapidly. Patients with multiple rib fractures or minimal flail chest should be followed closely in the ICU with serial blood gas determinations. Deterioration in blood gases may be an indication for intubation although the VC may seem to be adequate. If one waits for the VC to reach minimal levels, the first indication of serious trouble may be a respiratory or cardiac arrest.

CONSERVATIVE MANAGEMENT. Patients with a mild to moderate flail chest can often be managed without ventilatory assistance if there is no underlying pulmonary contusion or other significant injury. The patient should be given supplemental oxygen to maintain the PaO_2 at approximately 80 mm Hg, and the pain should be controlled with intercostal blocks and minimal narcotic analgesia. Careful pulmonary toilet with coughing, nasotracheal suction, and chest physiotherapy usually is adequate to clear pulmonary secretions. If chest physiotherapy is used, the patient should have adequate analgesia with nerve blocks or the pain may be intolerable. Pneumothorax is a common complication of intercostal blocks. If one occurs in a patient whose ventilation is already compromised, the patient's condition may deteriorate rapidly.

INTERNAL STABILIZATION WITH VENTILATOR SUPPORT. The use of internal stabilization with ventilator support is the standard by which other methods must be measured. In 1982, James and Moore[18] reviewed the results of treatment of flail chest before and after 1970, when the use of long-term ventilator support became generalized. In six series reported before 1970, the average mortality rate was 33%; in six series reported after 1970, the average mortality rate was 18%. Specific ventilator management must be individualized; however, the use of IMV with approximately 5 cm of PEEP has proven to be an excellent method to maintain the patient's oxygenation, to maintain adequate residual volume, and to allow maximum comfort for the patient. Initially, it is advisable to intubate the patient transorally. After the patient is stabilized, usually a matter of 48 to 72 hours, we prefer to perform a tracheostomy. Most patients require ventilation for 10 to 21 days. They are much easier to manage and are more comfortable with a tracheostomy. A few patients with moderate flail chest improve rapidly after intubation and do not require long-term ventilation;

in these patients, endotracheal intubation for approximately 7 days is sufficient to wean them from the ventilator, and tracheostomy may not be required.

SURGERY. Rarely, a patient has so much chest wall instability that stabilization does not occur with long-term ventilation, and thoracotomy may be necessary to stabilize the ribs with a metal plate. The author (M.J.W) has seen two such cases, and both patients did well after surgery. Although this method of treatment is reported more and more, notice that these are highly selected cases and that this should not be considered standard treatment, at least until some of our large trauma centers can accumulate enough experience to indicate wider use of the technique and can elucidate the criteria for surgery.

Pulmonary Contusion

Pulmonary contusions are extremely common after blunt trauma to the chest. They are usually easy to diagnose in a patient with rib fractures or flail chest, where they are seen as localized infiltrates or opacities on an early chest radiograph. Subsequent chest radiographs show increasing opacification of the areas for 24 to 48 hours and then gradual resolution over the next 7 days. The ICU physician must understand that severe bilateral pulmonary contusions may occur in the absence of rib fractures or flail chest. The admitting chest radiograph may appear normal, and the first sign of pulmonary contusion may be progressive hypoxia. Serial chest radiographs reveal the contusion. One should be particularly alert to the possibility of pulmonary contusion in a patient who has chest wall bruises and contusions in the absence of rib fractures. These patients may require intubation and ventilatory support if they develop progressive hypoxia. In the absence of other indications for mechanical ventilation, they usually can be managed with supplemental oxygen. Administration of oxygen and continuous positive airway pressure using a special face mask can improve ventilatory function sufficiently to obviate the need for intubation and mechanical ventilation.

Although most pulmonary contusions result in localized hematomas that are absorbed and that lead to minimal morbidity, massive trauma may lead to severe generalized pulmonary injury, which may be bilateral and may lead to or coexist with ARDS. Management of these patients remains controversial. The usual admonition is to "keep the patients dry" to decrease or prevent the accumulation of pulmonary water; to use diuretics to remove excess water; and to use plasma, blood, or albumin to maintain the plasma oncotic pressure to decrease the capillary leak that occurs in severely damaged lungs. The latter seems logical but is ineffective. The capillary leak occurs whether or not colloids are given, and if important extracellular fluid deficits are not adequately replenished, the morbidity and mortality may increase. ARDS is the sum total of a complicated series of antecedent physiologic events, and whether incident to pulmonary contusion or resulting from other causes, attention should be directed toward management of the whole patient. It has been demonstrated,[19] and subsequent studies have confirmed, that significant extracellular fluid volume losses occur in surgical patients. Managing these patients requires the judicious replenishment of these losses with a balanced salt solution and replenishment of blood. This may initially require large volumes of crystalloids. The best managed patient is one whose CVP, blood pressure, urine output, and PA occlusion pressure are normal; under these conditions, the patient is less apt to have significant pulmonary failure; if pulmonary failure occurs, it is easier to manage if the cardiovascular function is as near normal as possible.

One author (M.J.W.) once observed a patient with ARDS whose CVP was zero and whose physician was giving him diuretics and vasopressors because his lungs were "wet"; the physician was concerned that the patient was overloaded because of peripheral edema. When the patient died, his lungs were still wet; he died in shock and cardiovascular collapse.

It is certainly wise not to give the patient more fluid than is necessary to maintain a normal cardiovascular and renal function, but the milieu interieur described by Claude Bernard includes the entire body, and it is not probable that the lung can be isolated from the milieu and made selectively "dry."

In summary, the best approach to treating the severely insufficient lung lies in careful fluid and electrolyte management, adequate blood replacement, and the diligent application of modern respiratory support measures in a well-equipped and well-staffed ICU.

Cardiac Contusion

Although cardiac contusion can occur from any direct trauma to the anterior chest wall, it usually occurs when drivers of a vehicle hit the steering wheel with their chest. Bruises or abrasions of the anterior chest or presternal area are usually present, but the patient may complain of nothing more than soreness over the anterior chest. The diagnosis should be suspected in any patient who gives a history of an injury to the anterior chest in a vehicle accident. Fortunately, most cardiac contusions are not serious and require nothing more than supportive treatment.

More money has been spent trying to confirm this diagnosis than any other diagnosis in trauma patients; the yield is low and confirmation usually is unnecessary.

In the absence of significant hemodyamic decompensation, the diagnosis of myocardial contusion rarely affects outcome or management in trauma patients. If patients need to undergo general anesthesia, perioperative invasive monitoring may be initiated. Arrhythmias should be treated as they occur, and inotropic support should be provided as needed.[20] The use of intraaortic balloon pump for treating cardiogenic shock from cardiac contusion is rarely required but may be lifesaving in the occasional patient at the end of the spectrum with this injury.[21]

Currently, we follow the algorithm for the diagnosis and treatment of suspected cardiac contusions proposed by Illig and associates and shown in Figure 74-1. Critically injured patients who require admission to an ICU do not need further workup for cardiac contusion because management will not change. In patients who do not meet criteria for admission to an ICU, clinical suspicion and ECG findings determine the need for further workup. A normal ECG finding usually rules out the need for treatment or observation, and the patient can be discharged or admitted to an unmonitored setting for treatment of associated injuries.

In patients who have significant injury, the most common findings are cardiac arrhythmias, heart block, and tachycardia. Right bundle branch block is common. The diagnosis is established when the MB band of the creatine kinase (CK), expressed as a percentage of the total CK, is elevated. The cardiospecific enzyme, CK-MB, is released from necrotic myocardium, and an elevation of the CK-MB to 5% or more indicates significant damage to the myocardium. Because the right ventricle is anterior and is the most commonly injured portion of the heart, the amount of muscle involved may not be enough to cause an elevation in the CK. Technetium scans have been disappointing in the diagnosis of myocardial injury except in the unusual instance of transmural ventricular damage. The presence of murmurs may indicate septal, valvular, or papillary muscle injury; in these cases, two-dimensional echocardiography may be helpful. Electrocardiographic-gated blood-pool radionuclide an-

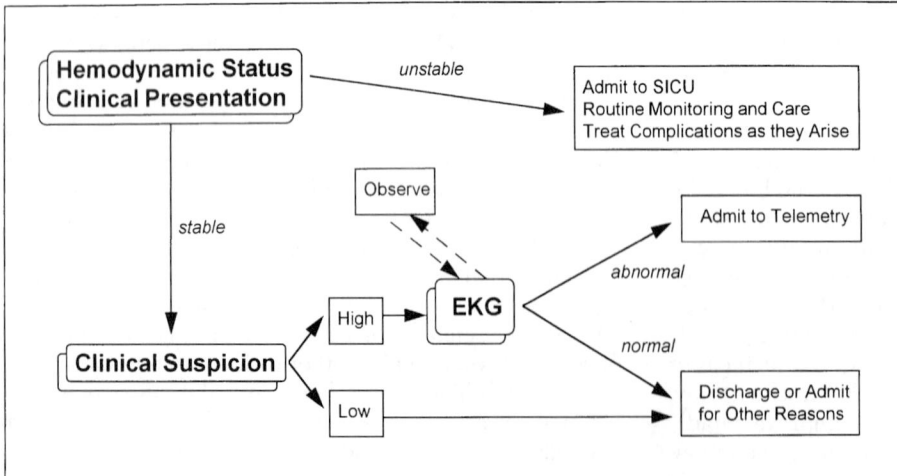

FIGURE 74-1. Protocol for diagnosis and management of suspected myocardial contusion. EKG, electrocardiogram. (From Illig KA, Swierzewski MJ, Feliciano DV, et al: A rational screening and treatment strategy based on the electrocardiogram alone for suspected cardiac contusion. *Am J Surg* 1991;162:537.)

giography has been reported to be an accurate method to evaluate myocardial injury.

Serial electrocardiograms are the best screening method for evaluating patients with myocardial contusion. Usually, the ST elevation, arrhythmias, and heart block subside in several days, occasionally in several weeks, and the patient has no sequelae. The treatment of severe myocardial contusion consists of the measures normally used in managing myocardial infarction.[22] A complete cardiology workup is be necessary for patients who have complications.

Penetrating Chest Trauma

Although penetrating wounds to the chest are a surgical problem and most patients will have had definite treatment before they are admitted to the ICU, it is necessary to monitor them carefully for secondary problems or additional hidden wounds.

When the penetrating wound has damaged only the lung, the patient usually has a hemopneumothorax. In most instances, inserting chest tubes is sufficient treatment. When the lung is expanded by evacuation of the pneumothorax, it usually provides sufficient tamponade to stop the bleeding in the low-pressure pulmonary vessels. The tube also evacuates the blood to allow complete expansion of the lung and provides measurement of the amount of continued bleeding. Although many trauma centers successfully use one posterolateral chest tube, we prefer the use of two chest tubes: one placed posterolaterally to remove blood, and one placed posterolaterally or anteriorly to the apex of the chest to remove air. The apical tube does not remove a significant amount of blood, but it is much more efficient in removing air. In the presence of significant continued bleeding, it is possible for the posterior tube to become plugged with clot; in this event, the air will not be adequately evacuated, and a tension pneumothorax may occur. Most low-velocity gunshot wounds and stab wounds to the pulmonary parenchyma can be managed with chest tubes, and no surgery is necessary. Bleeding may be brisk initially but usually drops below 100 mL/hour within several hours; if the bleeding continues at 200 mL/hour for more than 4 to 6 hours, or if the initial evacuation of blood was 1500 mL or more, then thoracotomy is usually indicated. Such a large hemorrhage usually indicates that a systemic chest wall artery or a major pulmonary vessel is injured.

High-velocity missile wounds present a different set of problems. The cavitation effect produced by absorption of the enormous kinetic energy of the missile may destroy a large amount of lung, may injure larger bronchi, or may produce such large pulmonary hematomas that surgery is indicated early in the management of the injury. One author (M.J.W.) has successfully managed many high-velocity combat injuries, initially with chest tubes alone. However, many of these patients later require thoracotomy for pulmonary resection, decortication, and evacuation of empyema and infected clot. In the civilian setting, the best results are obtained by early thoracotomy, evacuation of blood and clots, and the resection of severely damaged lung to prevent continued air leak, hemorrhage, and empyema.

Patients with high-velocity penetration wounds also are more apt to have air embolism than patients with blunt or low-velocity trauma, although it may occur in any patient who has disruption of the pulmonary parenchyma. Air embolism is more common than was formerly appreciated. It occurs when air from ruptured bronchi is forced into pulmonary veins from which it enters the systemic circulation through the left atrium. It may enter the coronary arteries and cause sudden severe arrhythmias and ventricular fibrillation, or it may enter the cerebral circulation where it causes severe neurologic symptoms. If the air embolus is large enough, it may appear that the patient has had a sudden massive cerebrovascular accident. With smaller emboli, the patients may develop a variety of focal neurologic signs and symptoms. The presence of air embolism often is not appreciated until the patient is intubated and placed on positive-pressure ventilation, which increases the pressure gradient between the open bronchus and the open pulmonary vein. It is commonly associated with significant continued hemoptysis, which, as a diagnostic feature, is not always helpful without other signs because of the frequency with which hemoptysis is seen in pulmonary injury. Nevertheless, any patient who has penetrating chest trauma or a lung laceration from a fractured rib and who develops unexplained neurologic and cardiac symptoms should be carefully evaluated for air embolism. The presence of air in the retinal arteries is diagnostic, but this is not always seen, and in the case of massive embolism, there may be no time to look. If air embolism occurs, positive-pressure ventilation should be stopped and the patient taken immediately to surgery. Massive air embolism may require immediate thoracotomy in the emergency department or in the ICU, in which event the pulmonary hilum should be clamped to prevent further entrance of air into the atrium; positive-pressure ventilation can then be reestablished and the patient taken to the operating room for definitive surgery.

Aortic Rupture

Aortic rupture injuries occur from sudden deceleration, usually from automobile and motorcycle accidents, but occasionally from falls from height. They usually occur at the aortic isthmus just distal to the subclavian artery. Eighty percent of the patients die within a few minutes after injury; of those who survive to reach a hospital, 80% die within 24 hours if the rupture is not surgically repaired. Almost all of the remainder will die within a few weeks, although occasionally a patient will develop a chronic aneurysm. It is important for those working in an ICU to have a high degree of suspicion for aortic rupture because it may not be diagnosed in the early evaluation of severely traumatized patients. Many of the patients, perhaps 35% to 40%, have little external evidence of chest trauma. Most have multiple extrathoracic injuries that demand immediate attention. The most suggestive physical findings are the presence of a systolic murmur, especially over the back, and a pressure differential between the upper and lower extremities that causes a relative hypotension in the lower extremities. These signs are not consistent, however, and their absence does not rule out the injury.

These patients survive to reach the hospital only because the aortic tear is incomplete: the intima and media are torn, leaving the adventitia to contain the blood flow; this results in an expanding adventitial hematoma. Early chest radiographs, especially the hurried AP radiographs taken in most emergency departments, may not suggest the diagnosis. The characteristic findings are widening of the superior mediastinum, blurring or obliteration of the aortic knob, displacement of the trachea to the left, pleural cap, and downward displacement of the left mainstem bronchus. Any patient admitted to the ICU with a history of deceleration injury should be carefully followed with serial chest radiographs; if there is any question as to the possibility of aortic rupture, an aortogram should be performed, and, if the result is positive, the patient should be taken to surgery for definitive repair. Incomplete tears of the subclavian, innominate, and carotid vessels also occasionally occur; they produce similar radiographic findings; an aortogram is diagnostic.

Cardiac Tamponade

Cardiac tamponade most commonly results from penetrating trauma. Blunt cardiac injuries with tamponade can be seen after high-speed motor vehicle accidents, falls from great heights, deceleration injuries, blast injuries, and direct trauma to the chest.[23] Iatrogenic injuries can be seen in the ICU as a result of right heart catheterization, placement of CVP catheters, and endocardial biopsies. Placement of temporary or permanent pacemaker pacing leads in the right ventricle may cause ventricular perforation. Lately, perforations after coronary angioplasty have been reported, with free bleeding into the pericardial sac and cardiac tamponade.[24] Young trauma patients may seem "stable" in the presence of tamponade. However, patients are usually restless and agitated, exhibit air hunger, and may have cyanosis of the upper half of the body. The classic Beck's triad (central venous pressure elevation, systemic hypotension out of proportion to apparent blood loss, and muffled heart tones) is rare and difficult to detect in a noisy ICU. In case of equivocal physical findings of cardiac tamponade in a hypotensive patient, pericardiocentesis should be performed. This can be a lifesaving procedure while preparations are made to transfer the patient to the operating room. However, cardiac injury can be present in as many as two thirds of patients with a negative result on pericardiocentesis.[25] In hemodynamically stable patients in whom the diagnosis is suspected, TTE or TEE can be performed.

Because of diminished cardiac volume during ventricular systole, in patients with PA catheters there is a dominant *x* descent, and the *y* descent is damped or absent because of restricted early ventricular filling (Chap. 57). Our policy is to proceed to immediate pericardial decompression and cardiac exploration in the operating room by subxyphoid pericardial window or mediastinal exploration whenever cardiac injury or tamponade is suspected.

Esophageal Perforation

Most esophageal perforations are secondary to penetrating trauma. Blunt esophageal trauma, although rare, may be lethal if unrecognized. It should be considered in a patient who (1) has a left hemopneumothorax without rib fractures, (2) has sustained a significant blunt injury to the lower chest or epigastrium and presents with pain out of proportion to the clinical findings, (3) has gastric contents in the chest tube drainage, or (4) has significant subcutaneous emphysema or mediastinal air without an obvious source. The diagnosis usually is confirmed by contrast studies with or without endoscopy. Surgery should be performed as quickly as possible. Direct repair of the injury with a thoracotomy is the treatment of choice. If result of the repair is less than desirable, esophageal diversion in the neck and gastrostomy usually is performed.[26]

Diaphragmatic Rupture

Diaphragmatic disruption most commonly occurs on the left side; however, right-sided injury has been observed in 34% of patients.[27] The presence of a nasogastric tube in the left chest cavity is diagnostic. If the diagnosis is not clear, an upper gastrointestinal contrast study should be performed. The treatment is direct surgical repair.

Tracheobronchial Injuries

Tracheobronchial injury incident to penetrating trauma is usually associated with damage to major blood vessels, and the indications for surgery are clear. When tracheobronchial injuries are caused by blunt trauma and deceleration, the diagnosis may not be immediately obvious. Such injury to the trachea usually causes a vertical tear of the membranous portion within a few centimeters of the carina. The major bronchi are usually torn transversely near the take-off of the upper lobe bronchi—these are sometimes missed.

These injuries should be suspected in a patient who has severe mediastinal emphysema; a large, continuing air leak; and continued pneumothorax despite adequate chest tube suction. Massive subcutaneous emphysema may occur over the entire body leading to a grotesque, bloated appearance of the patient, closure of the eyelids, and a characteristic crackling feeling when the skin is indented with the examining finger. The subcutaneous emphysema is not, of itself, dangerous, but it incites great anxiety on the part of the patient and family. If the diagnosis is suspected, bronchoscopy should be performed as soon as the patient is stabilized and, if the diagnosis is confirmed, early surgery is indicated. Partial tracheobronhcial injuries may require only airway maintenance until the leak seals and the acute inflammation and edema resolve. Upper tracheal and laryngeal injuries also are managed by tracheal intubation. The balloon is positioned distal to the injury so that there is no air leak. The injury is stented for 3 to 4 days. If there is partial injury distal to the balloon, high-frequency jet ventilation (HFJV) can be used to minimize airway pressure and inspiratory peak pressures. HFJV also may be used after repairs and resections to decrease the likelihood of suture line dehiscence.[28] If the diagnosis is missed, bronchial stenosis invariably occurs, and late repairs are often unsuccessful. One author (M.J.W.) has performed pneumonectomy on 3 patients in whom bronchial tears were initially missed and in whom late repairs at 6 weeks, 3 months, and 4 months, respectively, were unsuccessful. These patients all developed severe atelectasis and infection.

SPECIAL SITUATIONS AND PROCEDURES ■

POSTTRAUMATIC RETAINED HEMOTHORAX

In the presence of a large hemothorax, chest tube drainage may not drain the chest cavity, usually because of early clot formation and blockage of the chest tubes. An additional concern is the fact that some of these retained hemothoraces can progress to a fibrothorax or empyema. Multiple attempts to drain the chest cavity by placement of more chest tubes or multiple needle thoracentesis increases the risk of contamination of the pleural clot; this is especially true in patients who have sustained penetrating trauma. Early surgical drainage of a retained hemothorax has been shown to reduce hospitalization and the incidence of empyema.[29]

Currently, we obtain a CT scan of the chest if, after 72 hours, the hemothorax has not resolved. Nonloculated and small collections are drained under CT guidance. Large or multiloculated collections are drained thoracoscopically if possible, and if technically it proves to be difficult, we proceed with a formal thoracotomy for drainage and cleaning of the thoracic cavity.[14]

MAJOR PULMONARY RESECTIONS

In a review of 259 patients who underwent urgent thoracotomy after penetrating chest trauma,[30] 43 patients (16%) required major pulmonary resections. The most common complication, pneumonia, was seen in 21 patients (87%). Fifteen patients (62%) developed respiratory failure. Two patients (8%) developed bronchopleural fistulas, which were successfully managed with chest tube thoracostomy and HFJV. Nine pneumonectomies and 34 lobectomies were performed with mortality rates of 66% and 38%, respectively. Ten (53%) deaths occurred in the operating room because of uncontrollable hemorrhage. Six patients died within 48 hours with severe pulmonary edema, cardiogenic shock, and persistent hypoxemia.

TRACHEOESOPHAGEAL FISTULA

Erosion of the membranous wall of the trachea and the anterior esophageal wall by the high-pressure cuff of a tracheostomy tube (usually) or endotracheal tube (less common), often against a rigid nasogastric tube, produces most of the fistulas seen in the ICU. The usual presentation is aspiration of feedings into the tracheobronchial tree or respiratory difficulty while swallowing. Benign acquired tracheoesophageal fistulas are best managed by a single-stage definitive operation that closes the fistula and also removes the associated tracheal disease.[31] In unstable patients, a temporary gastrostomy and feeding jejunostomy may be used until the patient's condition improves.

TRACHEOINNOMINATE FISTULA

Late hemorrhage, around or through the tracheostomy tube, may be secondary to tracheal ulceration, pulmonary parenchymal pathology, or tracheoinnominate artery fistula. Fiberoptic bronchoscopy through the tracheostomy clears the airway and permits evaluation of the distal airway and assessment of the extent of hemorrhage. If hemorrhage continues, the tracheostomy cuff should be hyperinflated and the tube tilted backward, thus pressing the cuff against the anterior tracheal wall. If the bleeding has stopped and no distal disease is apparent, the tracheostomy tube can be removed, and flexible bronchoscopy is performed through the tracheal stoma to visualize an anterior wall ulceration. Persistent hemorrhage requires proximal intubation with an endotracheal tube, removal of the tracheostomy tube, and digital control of the innominate artery, which is obtained by inserting the index finger into the airway and compressing the innominate artery against the right sternoclavicular joint. If the patient can be temporarily stabilized, he should be taken to the operating room for ligation of the innominate artery. Most patients tolerate the ligation of the innominate artery without significant neurologic deficits.[32]

POSTTRAUMATIC EMPYEMA

The American Thoracic Society has classified empyema into three phases based on the natural history of the disease.[33] The first is the exudative or acute phase, characterized by outpouring of sterile fluid in the thoracic cavity in response to inflammation of the pleura. The pleural fluid has low viscosity, a low cellular content, low lactate dehydrogenase, and a normal glucose and pH. The visceral pleura and related lung are mobile.

The fibrinopurulent or transitional phase is characterized by more turbid fluid because of an increment in the number of polymorphonuclear cells. Fibrin is deposited on both pleural surfaces, forming a peel that localizes the empyema but also begins to trap and fix the lung. Also, the pH and glucose levels become progressively lower, and the LDH level becomes progressively higher.

The chronic phase is characterized by the organization of the pleural peel, with ingrowth of capillaries and fibroblasts. This can occur as early as 7 to 10 days but usually occurs at 4 to 6 weeks. The pleural fluid pH is frequently less than 7.0, and the glucose is less than 40 mg/dL.

Empyema should be suspected in any patient with a febrile illness and pleural effusion on a chest radiograph. Thoracentesis, with Gram stain and fluid culture, confirms the diagnosis and guides selection of antibiotics. Pleural fluid with a pH less than 7.20 and glucose less than 40 mg/dL strongly suggests empyema requiring drainage. CT scan of the chest is usually required to distinguish simple empyema from an intraparenchymal process.[34] The goals of treatment of empyema are (1) early diagnosis, (2) appropriate and specific antimicrobial therapy, and (3) obliteration of the pleural space with lung expansion by tube thoracostomy and closed drainage. Percutaneous drainage with CT scan or ultrasound guidance can be extremely useful for multiloculated or small empyemas. In the presence of a bronchopleu-

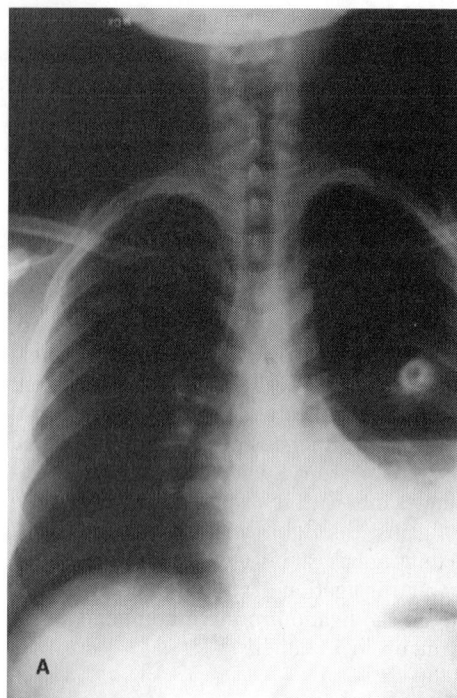 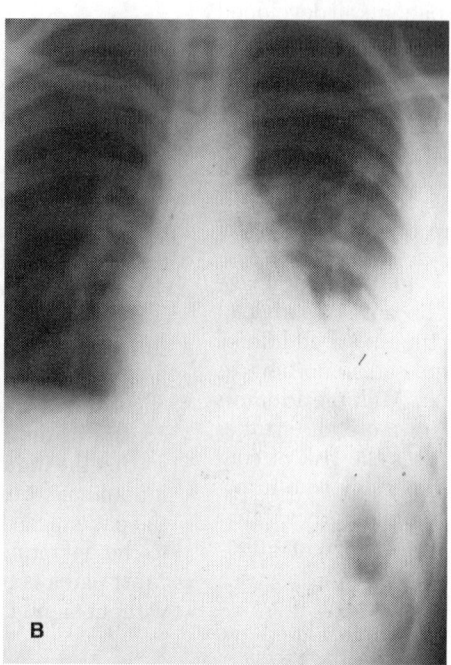

FIGURE 74-2. (A) Traumatic cavitary injury in the left lung with associated hemopneumothorax in a 28-year-old man. The radiograph shows the cavitary effect of the bullet on the lung parenchyma. (B) Insertion of an intercostal tube resulted in drainage of 600 mL of blood and persistent air leak. This radiograph obtained 48 hours later shows increase in parenchymal contusion and a retained hemothorax.

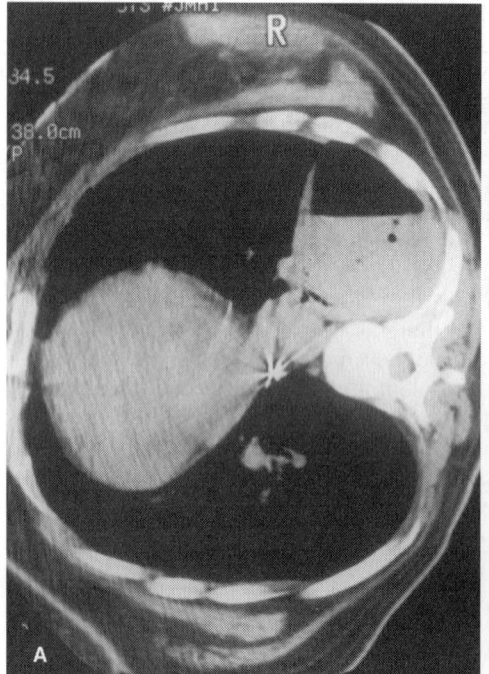 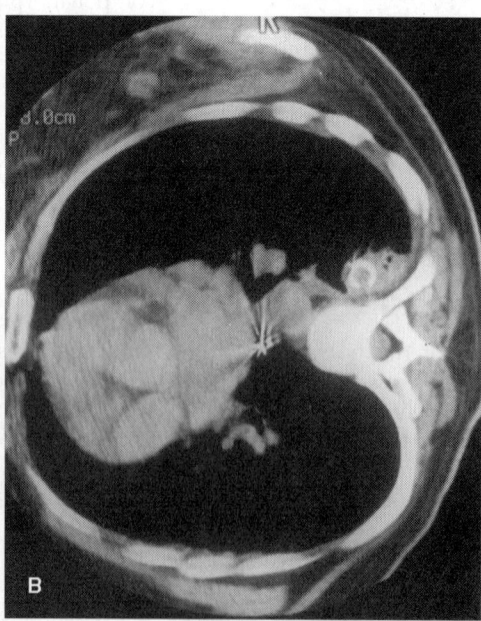

FIGURE 74-3. Same patient as in Figure 74-2. Seven days after admission, a persistent undrained collection is present in the left thoracic cavity. (A) Computed tomography in the right lateral decubitus portion shows extensive contusion with persistent hemopneumothorax. (B) A computed tomography–guided drain is placed in the cavity. Ten days later, there is complete collapse of the cavity with resolution of the hemopneumothorax.

ral fistula, it is extremely important to keep the lung expanded.

Failure of expansion after 4 to 7 days of high-suction drainage is considered an indication for thoracotomy and decortication.

PULMONARY CAVITARY LESIONS

High-velocity gunshot wounds, as seen in wartime and occasionally in civilian life, produce a cavitary injury in addition to bleeding and air leaks secondary to the blast effect (Fig. 74-2).

Even a peripheral bullet may result in irreversible damage to pulmonary tissue, increasing the incidence of lung abscess and empyema.[35] CT helps to delineate the extent of the pulmonary injury and, in selected patients, facilitates guided drainage of retained collections (Fig. 74-3).

POSTTRAUMATIC HEMOPTYSIS

A small group of patients develop delayed life-threatening hemoptysis (more than 600 mL/24 hours) after penetrating chest trauma. The commonest cause is rupture of an abscess into the bronchial tree. If the bleeding stops, prompt bronchoscopy should be performed to determine the source of bleeding.[36]

The most critical problem with massive hemoptysis is asphyxiation caused by blood in the airway. If the origin of the hemorrhage is identified, the appropriate double-lumen endotracheal tube can be placed to isolate the side with bleeding. For bleeding originating in the left bronchi, a large Fogarty catheter can be used to occlude the site of hemorrhage.

CARDIAC ARRHYTHMIAS

Cardiac arrhythmias constitute the most common complication after major thoracic procedures. Most are supraventricular, and of these, atrial fibrillation is the most common.[37] The incidence rate of arrhythmias is 10% to 15% after a lobectomy, but increases to 20% to 25% after a pneumonectomy. They are more common in elderly patients or in patients with underlying cardiac conditions.[38] The prophylactic administration of digitalis is recommended in elderly patients if a major pulmonary resection is contemplated.[39]

REFERENCES ■

1. Miller JI: Thoracic surgery. In: Kaplan JA (ed). *Thoracic Anesthesia*, 2nd ed. New York, Churchill-Livingstone, 1983:25
2. Ali MK, Mountain CF: Predictive loss of pulmonary function after pulmonary resection for bronchogenic carcinoma. *Chest* 1980;77:337
3. Widemann HP, et al: Cardiovascular–pulmonary monitoring in the intensive care unit: I. *Chest* 1984;85:537
4. Widemann HP, et al: Cardiovascular–pulmonary monitoring in the intensive care unit: II. *Chest* 1984;85:656
5. Fiser WB, Friday CD, Read RC: Changes in arterial oxygenation and pulmonary shunt during thoracotomy with endobronchial anesthesia. *J Thorac Cardiovasc Surg* 1982;83:523
6. Braunschweig R: Physical therapy for the thoracic surgical patient. In: Shields TW (ed). *General Thoracic Surgery*, 3rd ed. Philadelphia, Lea & Febiger, 1989:434
7. Grover FL, Richardson JD, Fewell JF: Prophylactic antibiotics in the treatment of penetrating chest wounds. *J Thorac Cardiovasc Surg* 1977;74:528
8. Elder PT: Accidental hypothermia. In: Shoemaker WC, Thompson WL, Holbrook PR (eds). *Textbook of Critical Care*. Philadelphia, WB Saunders, 1984:85
9. Sutherland GR, et al: Anatomic and cardiopulmonary responses to trauma with associated blunt chest injury. *J Trauma* 1981;21:1
10. Washington B, Wilson RF, Steiger Z, et al: Emergency thoracotomy: a four year review. *Ann Thorac Surg* 1985;40:188
11. Pickard LR, Mattox KL: Thoracic trauma: general considerations and indications for thoracotomy. In: Moore EE, Mattox KL, Feliciano DV (eds). *Trauma*, 2nd ed. Norwalk, CT, Appleton & Lange, 1991:319
12. Robinson PD, Harman PK, Trinkle JK: Management of penetrating lung injuries in civilian practice. *J Thorac Cardiovasc Surg* 1988;95:184
13. Miller FB, Richardson JD, Thomas HA, et al: Role of CT in diagnosis of major arterial injury after blunt thoracic trauma. *Surgery* 1989;106:596
14. Raptopoulos V: Chest CT for aortic injury: maybe not for everyone. *AJR* 1994;162:1053
15. Sosa JL, Puente I, Lemasters L, et al: Videothoracoscopy in trauma: early experience. *Surg Laparosc Endosc* 1994;4:295
16. Lewis FR: *Current Therapy of Trauma*. Philadelphia, BC Decker, 1986:235
17. Lewis FR: *Current Therapy of Trauma*. Philadelphia, BC Decker, 1986:236
18. James OF, Moore PG: Respiratory failure after chest injury: the development of effective treatment. *Ann Coll Surg* 1982;64:253
19. Shires T, Williams J, Brown F: Acute changes in extracellular fluids associated with major surgical procedures. *Ann Surg* 1961;154:803
20. Snow N, Richardson JD, Flint LM: Myocardial contusion: implications for patients with multiple traumatic injuries. *Surgery* 1982;92:744
21. Snow N, Lucas AE, Richardson JD: Intra-aortic balloon counterpulsation for cardiogenic shock. *J Trauma* 1982;22:426
22. Mueller HS: Treatment of myocardial infarction. In: Shoemaker WC, Thompson WL, Holbrook PR (eds). *Textbook of Critical Care*. Philadelphia, WB Saunders, 1984:40
23. Liedtke AJ, De Muth WE: Non-penetrating cardiac injuries: a collective review. *Am Heart J* 1973;86:687
24. Murphy DA, Craver JM, Jones EL, et al: Surgical revascularization following unsuccessful percutaneous transluminal coronary angioplasty. *J Thorac Cardiovasc Surg* 1982;84:342
25. Miller F, Polk HC, Richardson JD: Diagnostic pericardial window: a safe alternative to exploratory thoracotomy for suspected heart injuries. *Arch Surg* 1987;122:425
26. Attar S, Hankins JR, Sutter LM, et al: Esophageal perforation: a therapeutic challenge. *Ann Thorac Surg* 1990;50:45
27. Brown G, Richardson JD: Traumatic diaphragmatic hernia: a continuing challenge. *Ann Thorac Surg* 1985;39:170
28. Macneil A, Bisera J, Weil MH: High frequency ventilation: principles of use. *Crit Care Med* 1981;9:190
29. Coselli JS, Mattox KL: Reevaluation of early evacuation of clotted hemothorax. *Am J Surg* 1984;148:786

30. Carrillo EH, Block EFJ, Zeppa R, et al: Urgent lobectomy and pneumonectomy after penetrating thoracic trauma. *Europ J Emerg Med* 1995;1:126

31. Grillo HC, Moncure AC, McEnany T: Repair of inflammatory tracheoesophageal fistula. *Ann Thorac Surg* 1976;22:112

32. Cooper JD: Tracheoinnominate artery fistula: successful management of 3 consecutive patients. *Ann Thorac Surg* 1977;24:439

33. American Thoracic Society: Management of nontuberculous empyema. *Am Rev Respir Dis* 1962;85:93

34. Alexander JC, Wolfe WG: Lung abscess and empyema of the thorax. *Surg Clin North Am* 1980;60:835

35. Brewer LA: Wounds of the chest in war and peace. *Ann Thorac Surg* 1969;7:387

36. Garzon AA, Cerruti MM, Golding ME: Exsanguinating hemoptysis. *J Thorac Cardiovasc Surg* 1982;84:829

37. Beck-Nielsen J, Sorensen HR, Alstup P: Atrial fibrillation following thoracotomy for noncardiac diseases, in particular cancer of the lung. *Acta Med Scand* 1973;193:425

38. Wahi R, McMurtrey MJ, Decaro LF: Determinants of perioperative morbidity and mortality after pneumonectomy. *Ann Thorac Surg* 1989;48:33

39. Shields TW, Ujiki GT: Digitalization for prevention of arrhythmias following pulmonary surgery. *Surg Gynecol Obstet* 1968;126:713

BIBLIOGRAPHY ■

Bitto T, et al: Pneumothorax during positive-pressure mechanical ventilation. *J Thorac Cardiovasc Surg* 1985;89:585

Branthwaite MA: Monitoring respiratory function in the critically ill. *Intensive Care Med* 1982;8:111

Hasembos M, et al: Postoperative analgesia by epidural versus intramuscular nicomorphine after thoracotomy. II. *Acta Anaesthesiol Scand* 1985;29:5787

Hurst JM, DeHaven CB, Branson RD: Use of CPAP mask as the sole mode of ventilatory support in trauma patients with mild to moderate respiratory insufficiency. *J Trauma* 1985;25:1065

Mangano DT: Monitoring pulmonary arterial pressure in coronary artery disease. *Anesthesiology* 1980;53:364

Matthay MA: Invasive hemodynamic monitoring in critically ill patients. *Clin Chest Med* 1983;4:233

Mitchell RR, et al: Oxygen wash-in method for monitoring functional residual capacity. *Crit Care Med* 1982;10:529

Newell JD, Underwood GH, Kelley MJ: The ICU chest film: cardiac versus pulmonary disease. *Cardiol Clin* 1983;1:729

Nyhus LM: Presidential address: Academic surgery—points of view. *Surgery* 1985;98:619

Quinn K, Quebbeman EJ: Pulmonary artery pressure monitoring in the surgical intensive care unit. *Arch Surg* 1981;116:872

Rithalia SV, Ng Y, Tinker J: Measurement of transcutaneous PCO_2 in critically ill patients. *Resuscitation* 1982;10:13

Swan HJC, Ganz W: Hemodynamic measurements in clinical practice: a decade in review. *J Am Coll Cardiol* 1983;1:103

Taylor GA, et al: Symposium on trauma. I. Controversies in the management of pulmonary contusion. *Can J Surg* 1982;25:167

Vicente-Rull JR, et al: Thrombocytopenia induced by pulmonary artery flotation catheters: a prospective study. *Intensive Care Med* 1984;10:29

Watt I, Ledingham IM: Mortality amongst multiple trauma patients admitted to an intensive therapy unit. *Anesthesia* 1984;39:973

Waxman K, Shoemaker WC: Management of postoperative and posttraumatic respiratory failure in the intensive care unit. *Surg Clin North Am* 1980;60:1413

Critical Care, Third Edition, edited by Joseph M. Civetta,
Robert W. Taylor, and Robert R. Kirby.
Lippincott-Raven Publishers, Philadelphia, PA © 1997.

CHAPTER 75

∎

Postoperative Management of the Adult Cardiac Surgical Patient

Daniel J. O'Brien
James A. Alexander

IMMEDIATE CONCERNS ∎

MAJOR PROBLEMS

Irrespective of cardiac function, all patients returning to the intensive care unit (ICU) after open heart surgery are in a state of controlled shock from fluid shifts and varying vascular tone. The physical movement of the patient from the operating table to the bed, together with the endless trip through the corridor to the ICU, may create significant alterations in cardiovascular hemodynamics. This sequence is like the situation in the emergency room after major trauma when cardiovascular collapse is observed with movement. Therefore, the first 30 minutes in the ICU after heart surgery are spent establishing stable state hemodynamics.

STRESS POINTS

1. The first step on the patient's arrival to the ICU should be to transfer arterial pressure monitoring from the portable unit accompanying the patient to the ICU monitor. The systemic arterial pressure waveform allows you to assess adequate systemic perfusion pressure and provides a means to detect arrhythmias while the electrocardiogram (ECG) and other pressure measurement catheters are connected and calibrated.

2. Next, connect the hemodynamic monitoring catheters that provide some measure of central circulatory volume status, including the central venous pressure (CVP) catheter, left atrial pressure (LAP) catheter, or both. The ECG leads are then switched from the transport unit to the ICU system. With these monitors established, others can be connected and calibrated (pulmonary artery pressure, mixed venous oxygen saturation [$S\bar{v}O_2$], and arterial oxygen saturation).

3. Initially, patients should be given 100% oxygen through an endotracheal tube and supported with a mechanical ventilator until stabilized.

4. Patients who experience intravascular volume shifts during transport to the ICU require intravascular volume expansion, bolus dosages of intravenous calcium chloride, or both to maintain adequate systemic pressure and flow during the crucial 15 to 30 minutes required to settle the patient in the ICU.

5. Once stable hemodynamic function is achieved, pressure monitoring can be interrupted to obtain blood samples for various tests, especially arterial and mixed venous blood gas partial pressures and pH, serum potassium, ionized calcium, and serum lactate.

6. Rezeroing of all pressure monitors and calibration of the venous saturation monitor should be performed. For patients with a pulmonary artery catheter, baseline measurements of cardiac output, and calculations of

systemic vascular resistance (SVR) and pulmonary vascular resistance (PVR) are then obtained.

7. Assessment of peripheral pulses in all extremities is extremely important in the first hour and throughout the postoperative period. Although affected sometimes by the presence of severe atherosclerosis, skin temperature, pulse amplitude, and capillary refill time provide essential information about the adequacy of cardiac output. Palpable peripheral pulses are an excellent indicator of systemic perfusion.

ESSENTIAL DIAGNOSTIC TESTS AND PROCEDURES

1. A portable chest radiograph is obtained to determine the proper placement of the endotracheal tube, monitoring catheters, and nasogastric tube. Examine this radiograph closely for evidence of a pneumothorax, hemopneumothorax, and areas of collapse or atelectasis.
2. A word of caution is necessary about obtaining chest radiographs immediately after the patient arrives in the ICU, particularly if the body temperature is below 35.5°C and hemodynamic instability is present. In this situation, postpone the chest radiograph until the temperature rises above 35.5°C to avoid the occurrence of life-threatening arrhythmias during placement of the film cassette. Sudden movement may induce ventricular tachycardia or fibrillation resulting from the reduced fibrillation threshold caused by hypothermia and electrolyte imbalance, especially hypokalemia.
3. In this early period of stabilization, especially when the patient is mildly to moderately hypothermic, serum potassium levels should be assessed rapidly and supplemented to maintain levels in the 4.5- to 5.0-mMol/L range. This assessment helps protect the heart against ventricular irritability. At times, patients arrive to the ICU in an acidotic state.
4. Avoid attempting to correct acidosis with rapid intravenous infusions of sodium bicarbonate. Serum potassium can be acutely lowered, which may enhance ventricular irritability. Once the potassium level is adequate, moderate to severe metabolic acidosis (base deficit > 5 mMol/L) can be corrected with sodium bicarbonate.

INITIAL THERAPY

1. The first hour after transport to the ICU after heart surgery is a critical and unstable time.
2. The goals in this first hour are to maintain adequate systemic perfusion with reasonable cardiac filling pressures, establish adequate oxygenation and respiration, and control cardiac rate and rhythm.
3. During this period of stabilization, major interventions include intravascular volume administration, calcium administration, potassium supplementation, and close observation for excessive blood loss.
4. The principal axiom to bear in mind (see earlier) is that all patients returning to the ICU after cardiac surgery are in a state of controlled shock and must be treated as such.

THE FIRST 8 POSTCARDIOPULMONARY BYPASS HOURS ■

After initial stabilization, a period follows when the heart seems to be performing adequately and the patient is relatively stable. This period of time is designated the *golden period* and lasts for approximately 8 hours after cessation of cardiopulmonary bypass (CPB). Pay careful attention to optimizing cardiac function, because the subsequent 8 to 14 hours are characterized by decreasing cardiac function. The nadir of this decline occurs approximately 12 hours after CPB. Particularly notable is a decrease in ventricular compliance leading to reduced cardiac output at any given filling pressure. This condition generally persists over the next 12 to 24 hours, followed by a gradual improvement in cardiopulmonary performance over the next 48 hours. In the golden period, the goal is to optimize cardiorespiratory performance so that the ensuing decrease in cardiac function from 8 to 24 hours after CPB does not jeopardize end-organ system function.

THE NEXT 16 POST-CPB HOURS ■

The next 16 hours is probably the most challenging time, especially for the patients whose cardiac performance was not optimized during the golden period. Unfortunately, this challenging time often occurs during the late evening and early morning hours.

CHANGES IN HEART COMPLIANCE

The cause of the slump in cardiac performance during this time period is unclear. It can be observed in the "healthiest" heart. Clinically, the heart seems to become noncompliant or "stiff," generally accompanied by decreased compliance of the pulmonary vasculature. In this situation, one usually observes a rise in pulmonary artery pressure and LAP, and a reduction in the systemic arterial pressure, cardiac output, and $S\bar{v}O_2$. If the patient is doing extremely well before the onset of compliance changes, alterations in these parameters may go unnoticed. However, patients with a low output syndrome before the onset of apparent changes in compliance often have significant problems.

Time Course

The usual time course is a steady deterioration in cardiac performance between the 8th to 12th hour. This condition seems to stabilize near the 12th to 13th hour and remains stable for the next 6 to 8 hours. Avoid haphazard manipulations of the determinants of cardiac performance. Once a patient becomes unstable, far more interventions are required to reach a steady state than if the problems were anticipated and appropriate changes made to help maintain stability. Even if these patients remain in a relatively low output state during these 16 hours, they will tolerate this condition better than those who endure marked swings in hemodynamics.

Cardiovascular Changes

As patients enter the stiff period, all parameters of cardiac performance must be evaluated individually. A cogent plan designed to optimize cardiac rate and rhythm, preload, afterload, and contractility is essential. Stroke volume is relatively fixed; therefore, heart rate controls cardiac output. When the ventricle is noncompliant and the heart rate is slow, additional filling time does not improve the ejection fraction to any significant degree, and cardiac output actually falls. Rates of 90 to 110 beats per minute increase cardiac output.

In the stiff period, increasing preload to maintain systemic arterial pressure at the levels achieved during the golden period may result in a marked increase in the left ventricular end-diastolic pressure (LVEDP). This increase in LVEDP may result in pulmonary capillary leakage causing interstitial edema, pulmonary edema, or both. A LVEDP of 10 to 14 mm Hg is desirable. Therefore, once an LVEDP in this range is achieved, attention should be turned elsewhere to look for ways to improve cardiac performance.

Afterload reduction is an efficient way to improve cardiac performance without increasing myocardial oxygen consumption ($M\dot{V}O_2$).[1] However, during this period, a reduction in afterload may result in poorly tolerated hypotension, particularly at mean arterial pressures of 50 to 55 mm Hg. Clearly, afterload reduction should be instituted cautiously.

Patients with a relatively normal cardiac output before surgery often poorly tolerate a cardiac index below 2.0 L/minute/m², a venous PO_2 below 30 mm Hg, or a $S\bar{v}O_2$ below 50% after surgery. Although costly to the heart in terms of $M\dot{V}O_2$, enhancement of cardiac contractility is an effective method to augment performance by improvement of the ejection fraction. In this period, catecholamine support and even multiple drug therapy should be initiated without hesitation because decreased compliance and cardiac performance are finite as long as excessive filling pressures are not achieved.

MYOCARDIAL ISCHEMIA

Increases in heart rate, filling pressures, and contractility to support patients during the stiff period may potentiate myocardial ischemia. ST segments should be monitored closely. In the absence of ischemia, cardiac performance will stabilize by the 12th to 13th post-CPB hour. Then the level of cardiac performance must be evaluated in terms of adequacy for maintaining organ perfusion and survival.

WEANING OF INOTROPIC SUPPORT

A slight but definite improvement in cardiac performance and compliance is usually observed after 24 hours. If catecholamines were started either intraoperatively or in the immediate postoperative period, they should be maintained for at least 24 hours before weaning. As might be expected, if these drugs are weaned too rapidly or too early, patients may return to an unstable state. Moreover, to regain a stable state, far more intervention than previously required is necessary. These patients' compensatory mechanisms of survival generate increased filling pressures and increased peripheral resistance that are difficult to reverse.

THE SECOND 24 POST-CPB HOURS ■

During the second 24 postoperative hours, the amount of active intervention is largely determined by the function of other organ systems such as the lungs, kidneys, liver, and gastrointestinal tract. Cardiac performance generally improves, depending on the amount of cardiac reserve. Small increases in the $S\bar{v}O_2$ and the cardiac output, together with a noticeable decrease in fluid requirements, herald the improvement phase. By the 36th postoperative hour, active diuresis, weaning of catecholamines, and substitution of oral afterload-reducing drugs for intravenous infusions can be considered.

Invasive monitoring with arterial and pulmonary artery catheters should be maintained until minimal pharmacologic support is required. As a general policy, extubation usually is not contemplated until the patient is receiving minimal or no intravenous catecholamine support. The concept behind this approach is that unstable organ systems should be managed one at a time. In many situations, it is advisable to maintain respiratory stability while cardiac parameters improve. No doubt, cardiac performance is enhanced when patients are breathing on their own or with minimal intermittent mandatory ventilation (IMV) rates. However, to clear pulmonary secretions and to minimize ventilation-perfusion mismatch, maintenance of tracheal intubation is advisable. Patients who require maximum support during the first 24 hours after surgery may require an additional 24 hours before any progress is realized.

THE THIRD 24 POST-CPB HOURS ■

The third 24-hour period, 48 to 72 hours after CPB, is characterized by sense of urgency to achieve and maintain cardiac stability without intravenous catecholamine support and to stay ahead of volume shifts from the extracellular compartment to the intravascular space. This sense of urgency comes from the undesirability of maintaining invasive monitoring beyond 72 hours when the likelihood of catheter sepsis increases significantly.

During this period, filling pressures are maintained at reasonable levels, and compliance in the left ventricle should improve rapidly, accompanied by a decrease in interstitial pulmonary water. Lower pulmonary artery pressures and improved cardiac performance at lower filling pressure can be anticipated. Oral afterload-reducing agents, such as prazosin, can be instituted, as can digitalis and oral diuretics.

CATHETERS AND TUBES

The LAP catheter, chest tubes, and pulmonary artery/venous saturation catheter often can be removed. If continuous invasive cardiac monitoring is still considered necessary, a CVP catheter positioned in the superior vena cava will provide a measurement of right ventricular filling pressure and a means to determine the arterial venous oxygen content difference ($C[a - \bar{v}]O_2$). Venous saturation readings from the superior caval–atrial junction correlate closely with the mixed venous saturation readings from the pulmonary artery in the absence of a left-to-right shunt.[2,3] The association of the CVP and LAP will be known by this point, and left heart filling pressures can thus be estimated.

ARRHYTHMIAS

Despite rapid improvements in the third 24-hour period, this is a time when atrial arrhythmias are prominent, including atrial flutter and atrial fibrillation. These are significant problems because the atrial contribution to cardiac output remains high and a rapid heart rate is not well tolerated.

Therapy

Many institutions have their own formula for treating or preventing atrial arrhythmias, and ours is no exception. Patients are usually begun on digitalis as soon as intravenous catecholamines are discontinued; we generally add a β-blocker such as metoprolol, which has less of an adverse effect on the pulmonary bronchomotor tone.

In the past, we avoided combining β-blockers with calcium channel blockers when treating rapid atrial arrhythmias. Currently, we believe that diltiazem is effective in slowing rapid ventricular response to supraventricular tachycardia, especially atrial flutter or fibrillation. Most patients tolerate intravenous diltiazem by either bolus or continuous infusion without significant decreases in blood pressure and $S\bar{v}O_2$. For patients who deteriorate hemodynamically with diltiazem therapy, consider synchronized cardioversion.

In preparation for transfer from the ICU to a hospital ward, adult patients are placed on a drug regimen we call the "Big 5" that includes various dosages of digitalis, furosemide, potassium, prazosin, and metoprolol.

MONITORING AND MANAGING CARDIOVASCULAR PERFORMANCE ■

In the first 8 hours after cessation of CPB, no single physiologic parameter accurately mirrors the patient's clinical status. Therefore, we rely on several physiologic measurements and demonstrable clinical signs to assess the adequacy of cardiovascular performance. Older concepts such as maintaining a "normal" blood pressure at the expense of cardiac output have been difficult to bury. An enormous price is paid for achievement of a normal blood pressure at the expense of myocardial wall tension, $M\dot{V}O_2$, and cardiac output. Sole reliance on the blood pressure, or any other single

parameter, to monitor and judge cardiac performance in the postoperative period can result in significant difficulties.

ARTERIAL BLOOD PRESSURE

For all critically ill patients, a minimum arterial blood pressure is required for overall systemic perfusion and especially for cerebral and renal perfusion. Most adults require a mean arterial pressure of at least 50 to 55 mm Hg.[4] However, patients with severe atherosclerotic disease, particularly in the carotid arteries, require a mean arterial pressure of 60 mm Hg or greater.[5]

Pulse pressure is a useful indicator of systemic perfusion. We recommend display of the arterial waveform at full scale on the pressure monitor. Determination of the systolic, diastolic, and mean pressures as well as the height of the dicrotic notch provides an indication of left ventricular ejection volume. Poorer ventricular ejection is observed when the dicrotic notch is at the base of the arterial pressure trace. Better ventricular output occurs when the dicrotic notch is located midway up the down slope of the tracing, resulting in a greater area under the arterial pressure curve.[6] The arterial pressure waveform also provides an indication of peripheral vascular tone. Harmonic augmentation in peripheral arteries connotes an increase in peripheral vascular tone and is characterized by a sharp, spiked arterial pressure tracing with virtually no dicrotic notch.

Normally, the arterial blood pressure is continuously monitored in a peripheral vessel such as the radial artery. However, any doubt concerning the pressure waveform from a peripheral artery should lead to measurement in a more central vessel, such as the femoral artery. Obviously, a central arterial pressure reading provides better assessment of overall hemodynamic function and cardiac output.

HEART RATE AND RHYTHM

Sinus rhythm is extremely important in the first 24 hours, and efforts should be focused on maintaining sequential atrioventricular (AV) activity for better loading of the ventricles and optimal cardiac output. Normally, the atrial contraction or atrial "kick" contributes approximately 5% of the cardiac output. However, in the postoperative patient, the atrial contribution to cardiac output may be as high as 30%. Maintaining sinus rhythm by atrial pacing or AV sequential pacing with a temporary external pulse generator is advantageous whenever possible.

Pacemakers

Temporary atrial and ventricular pacing wires should be used in every open heart surgical procedure. They are invaluable diagnostically and therapeutically in almost 80% of our patients. For example, some patients in sinus rhythm at rates between 60 to 80 beats per minute who experience premature ventricular contractions may have these arrhythmias abolished by atrial pacing to rates between 100 and 110 beats per minute. Heart rates should be increased to the

100 to 110 range to increase cardiac output, even in patients who have had revascularization procedures.

Newer, temporary AV sequential pacemakers perform in a DDD mode, meaning they will pace the atrium, delay, and then pace the ventricle. The PR interval is adjustable. Remember to evaluate either the right atrial pressure or LAP waveform to help determine the optimal PR interval.

Patients who develop atrial flutter or fibrillation with a rapid ventricular response and hemodynamic instability should be considered candidates for direct-current cardioversion. Whenever possible, rapid atrial pacing should be attempted to overdrive suppress atrial flutter with a 2:1 block. β-Blocking agents can also be used to slow the heart rate and maintain the converted rhythm. Diltiazem therapy, as mentioned earlier, should be monitored carefully, especially for exacerbation of hemodynamic instability.

In certain situations, an atrial pacing wire may be needed to determine the cardiac rhythm and differentiate supraventricular tachycardia. To perform a cardiac atriogram, simply connect the atrial pacing wire to the right arm ECG limb lead and observe the rhythm of leads I, II, or III on the monitor. Observation of the contour of the left and right atrial waveforms is another useful way of determining sinus rhythm.

VENTRICULAR PRELOAD

Ventricular preload, the load on the muscle that determines resting muscle length, is primarily manipulated in the postoperative period by fluid administration. Generally, we try to maintain cardiac preload at an adequate but not excessive level. For the left ventricle, this means maintaining the LVEDP between 8 to 12 mm Hg as assessed by direct LAP measurement. Even for patients who have LVEDP pressures approaching 40 mm Hg before surgery, pressures of 8 to 12 mm Hg should be adequate for postoperative ventricular loading.

Fluid Administration

A difficult tendency for most clinicians to overcome is the desire to increase right and left ventricular filling pressures to their upper limits (22 to 24 mm Hg) to maintain adequate blood pressure. However, attendant to this approach are several problems that are difficult to manage later in the postoperative period, especially pulmonary dysfunction. Remember that immediately after CPB colloid oncotic pressure (COP) is reduced by as much as 50% and returns to normal over a 2-week period of time[7] (Fig. 75-1). Therefore, we caution against trying to achieve maximum cardiac output by moving toward the upper pressure—-volume limits along the Starling curve. Attempts to reach venous pressures between 20 to 22 mm Hg may result in administration of excess fluids accompanied by increased pulmonary interstitial water.

Also, bear in mind that white cell damage caused by CPB leads to the release of lysozymes that disrupt fragile capillary membranes in the lungs. This effect results in a higher leakage rate of intravascular fluids at much lower hydrostatic

pressures and, when combined with a reduction of intravascular proteins (also caused by CPB), tends to promote increased pulmonary interstitial water accumulation and pulmonary edema.[8]

In the first 8 hours after CPB, while the ventricle is relatively compliant, increasing the LVEDP increases the radius of the ventricle. In accordance with the law of Laplace, increasing the ventricular radius results in an increase in wall tension and $M\dot{V}o_2$.[9] Volume requirements during this time are principally determined by changes in SVR, the extent of intravascular volume expansion that occurred during surgery after the cessation of CPB, and the volume of bleeding and urine output.

In our opinion, assessment and manipulation of cardiac filling pressures are best accomplished in conjunction with pulmonary artery and direct LAP monitoring. The LAP catheter provides a continuous approximation of LVEDP in the absence of mitral valve disease. The pulmonary artery occlusion pressure can be substituted for direct LAP assessment of LVEDP.

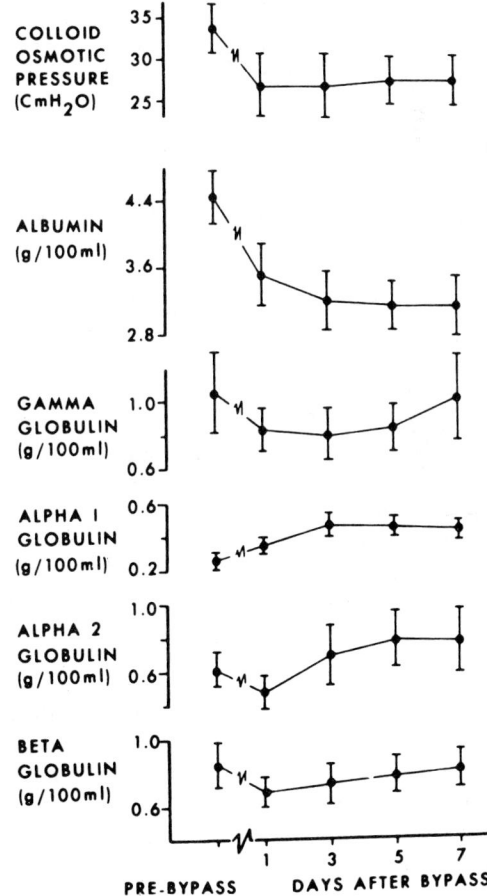

FIGURE 75-1. The relationship between colloid osmotic (oncotic) pressure and plasma proteins during and after cardiopulmonary bypass. (Reproduced with permission from Webber CE, Garnett ES: The relationship between colloid osmotic pressure and plasma proteins during and after cardiopulmonary bypass. *J Thorac Cardiovasc Surg* 1973;65:234.)

CRYSTALLOIDS AND COLLOIDS. Controversy persists concerning which type of fluids to use to maintain postoperative intravascular volume. Specifically, the focus of this debate concerns the administration of crystalloid or colloid (blood products, albumin, or hydroxyethyl starch) solutions.[10] We have employed multiple fluid combinations for maintaining adequate preload, all of which have advantages and disadvantages. Sole reliance on crystalloid solutions such as Ringer's lactate or normal saline for volume expansion may result in an inordinate amount of fluid administration to maintain even minimal levels of adequate preload. Our preference currently is Ringer's lactate, or a combination of 50 to 100 mL of 25% salt poor albumin per liter of Ringer's lactate that yields a solution similar to human plasma protein fraction, such as Plasmanate, but with better protein preservation.

When the hematocrit is low ($< 22\%$) and the patient is bleeding or hemodynamically unstable, blood products are preferred. If red cells are adequate but coagulation factors are abnormal and bleeding continues, fresh frozen plasma and platelets should be considered. Remember, the threshold to give blood is not based solely on whether a patient is bleeding. Maintaining adequate red blood cell mass is essential for achieving optimal tissue oxygenation in terms of oxygen supply and demand for the whole body.

VENTRICULAR AFTERLOAD

Afterload reduction offers the best means for improving cardiac output at little or no expense to the myocardium. Following afterload reduction, ventricular volume, wall tension, and MVO_2 usually are not increased. In some patients, the ejection fraction can be dramatically improved by a reduction in SVR and PVR. To achieve optimal afterload reduction, judicious intravascular volume loading is necessary to maintain adequate blood pressure and improve cardiac output. Once afterload reduction is started, a general guideline is to achieve the cardiac filling pressures observed before the institution of the afterload-reducing agent. We begin afterload-reduction therapy in the operating room before the cessation of CPB at the time of systemic rewarming and continue this therapy throughout the postoperative period. If possible, we attempt to maintain the SVR below 1000 dyne·second·cm^{-5}.

The extent of afterload reduction greatly depends on ventricular performance. Patients with normal or near-normal ventricles who experience minimal side effects from CPB do not require nearly the amount of afterload reduction to augment cardiac output as do patients with poor preoperative ventricular performance.

Reduction

SODIUM NITROPRUSSIDE. Our major afterload-reducing agent for the critically ill patient is sodium nitroprusside (SNP). It increases venous capacitance and directly vasodilates the systemic and pulmonary arterial vessels. It is the ideal drug to use for patients with low cardiac output and unstable hemodynamics because its effect can be controlled rapidly (15 to 20 seconds) after dosage changes. With dosage ranges between 2 to 4 µg/kg/minute, SNP can augment cardiac output by as much as 75% to 100% without increasing MVO_2.

In the operating room, most of our patients are given SNP at 2 µg/kg/minute while they are rewarmed before the cessation of CPB. Dosages are then adjusted after CPB to optimize cardiac output, especially during the 8 post-CPB hours. Dosages of SNP during the golden period range between 2 and 4 µg/kg/minute. With the current emphasis on limiting blood transfusions, afterload-reduction therapy following CPB as a means to optimize cardiac output has decreased because volume requirements are so significant.

NITROGLYCERIN. Patients with relatively normal ventricular function (ejection fraction $> 40\%$) are given nitroglycerin (NTG) in lieu of SNP and NTG or SNP alone. The intravenous dosage of NTG ranges between 0.5 and 2 µg/kg/minute. NTG is primarily a preload-reducing agent, with only a slight effect on the arterioles, but does have the advantage of decreasing coronary artery steal in unrevascularized areas of the heart. For patients who experience low output states postoperatively, we continue to employ a combination of SNP and NTG.

CONTRACTILITY

Some cardiovascular surgical teams empirically administer intravenous catecholamines routinely to all patients who undergo cardiac repair. This intervention has not been our policy, and we individualize decisions concerning the need for catecholamine support during and after surgery. When required, these and other drugs are generally begun in the operating room, in conjunction with weaning from CPB, and are continued into the postoperative period. In the ICU, if cardiac performance is marginal or decreases with time, we quickly exercise the option to improve cardiac contractility pharmacologically and continue to do so throughout the first 24 to 48 hours. Remember that the special conditions of cardiac surgery, CPB, and myocardial preservation (chemical, thermal, or both) profoundly influence postoperative cardiac function.

Drug Choices

Few pharmacologic agents affect only one determinant of cardiac performance. When selecting drugs, individually or in combination, bear in mind that a major goal after CPB is to gain cardiac output with as little increase in MVO_2 as possible.

DOPAMINE. Intravenous dopamine hydrochloride at dosages between 3 and 5 µg/kg/minute can be used to decrease SVR and augment cardiac contractility when a more potent catecholamine is not required. In this dosage range, dopamine also stimulates dopaminergic receptors in the kidney, thereby enhancing renal perfusion. Unless specifically indicated for renal perfusion, dopamine should not be used for patients with pulmonary hypertension because of the possibility of increasing PVR.[11]

A sensitive indicator of changes in the PVR is the difference between pulmonary artery diastolic pressure and LAP. A difference greater than 5 mm Hg indicates a moderate elevation in PVR, enough to impair left heart filling and cardiac output (Fig. 75-2). In patients with pulmonary hypertension we attempt to institute isoproterenol, amrinone, or both to reduce PVR, thereby preventing limitations of right heart function from controlling systemic cardiac output.

DOBUTAMINE. Dobutamine in dosages between 5 and 10 µg/kg/minute is not as effective a drug as isoproterenol, although its chronotropic effects are far less pronounced.

EPINEPHRINE. Epinephrine, 0.01 to 0.05 µg/kg/minute, is our principle choice. These dosage levels are not exceeded unless absolutely necessary to maintain an acceptable mean arterial perfusion pressure.

Often, a combination of drugs such as dopamine, dobutamine, or both, together with epinephrine is chosen. We rarely use levarterenol if the SVR is extremely low (< 600 dyne·second·cm^{-5}) because of the possibility of an allergic response or other unusual circumstance.

COMBINATION THERAPY. The aforementioned catecholamines are always given in combination with some type of afterload- or preload-reducing agent such as SNP or NTG. Most patients who have coronary artery bypass grafting receive 1 to 3 µg/kg/minute of intravenous NTG and, depending on ventricular performance, between 1 to 5 µg/kg/minute of SNP.

When selecting catecholamines, remember that many of these drugs, depending on their dosages, stimulate both beta and alpha receptors. We try to avoid stimulating alpha receptor activity, because our primary goal is to increase contractility, not afterload. In many situations, multiple catecholamines are used synergistically to increase beta receptor activity. For example, if dopamine is started in the early postoperative period, and cardiac performance decreases

significantly 8 to 12 hours after CPB, we add another drug such as dobutamine at 10 µg/kg/minute or epinephrine at 0.01 to 0.05 µg/kg/minute. If the heart rate permits, isoproterenol can be used in dosages between 0.01 and 0.05 µg/kg/minute.

AMRINONE. During the last several years, amrinone lactate has been extremely useful as a second-line drug to augment cardiac contractility and regulate SVR. Amrinone is usually given after a β-agonist has been instituted. The loading dose of amrinone is approximately 1 mg/kg, followed by a second loading dose 15 to 20 minutes later, then an intravenous infusion of 10 µg/kg/minute.

ESMOLOL. In view of the goal to optimize cardiac output without increasing MVo$_2$, be vigilant for myocardial ischemia when catecholamines are used. ST segment changes must be evaluated and treated by increasing NTG dosages and, sometimes, with intravenous β-blocking agents. When rapid-onset β-blockade is necessary, esmolol is a fast-acting drug that can be reversed rapidly if cardiac performance deteriorates.

CARDIAC OUTPUT

A pulmonary artery catheter allows cardiac output measurement by the thermodilution technique. Serial recordings within a ± 10% error margin can be achieved. Additionally, the pulmonary artery catheter facilitates calculation of SVR and PVR, pulmonary and intracardiac shunts, and estimation of LVEDP. Resistance calculations also are subject to measurement errors. Therefore, documentation and analysis of trends are more important than the absolute numbers.

Cardiac output readings should always be converted to a cardiac index (cardiac output divided by the body surface area). The cardiac index takes into account the size of the individual patient and is a better measure for judging the adequacy of tissue perfusion. A cardiac index of 2.0 L/minute/m^2 or greater is usually sufficient to maintain organ performance. However, exceptions exist in certain pathologic conditions. For example, patients who have long-standing mitral stenosis and a preoperative cardiac index of 1.0 L/minute/m^2 may well tolerate a cardiac index of less than 2.0 L/minute/m^2 in the immediate postoperative period. By contrast, higher body temperature and agitation may require a cardiac index greater than 2.0 L/minute/m^2. Bear in mind that these indices are at the lower limits for providing adequate organ function and that postoperative stress normally produces cardiac indices approaching 3.5 to 4.0 L/minute/m^2.

Two major problems are attendant to relying on intermittent measurement of cardiac output. First, cardiac output readings can give a false sense of security, especially when initial values in the normal range between 4 to 5 L/minute are obtained. Generally speaking, the cardiac output should not be the sole criterion used to satisfy concerns about meeting the patient's metabolic demands in terms of tissue oxygen delivery.

The second problem with intermittent measurement of cardiac output is that it *is* intermittent. Even rigid protocols

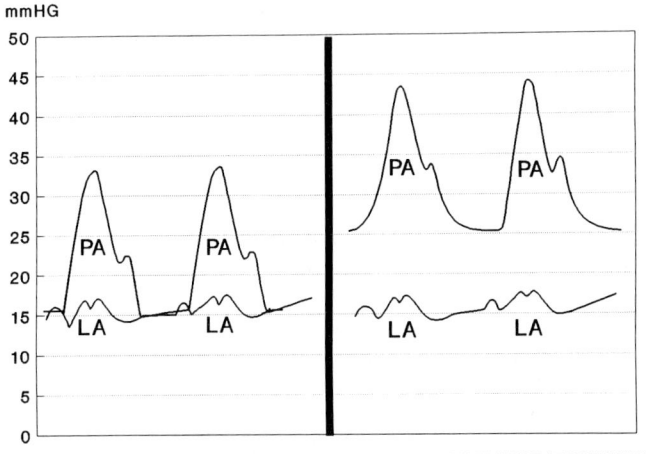

FIGURE 75-2. Instantaneous recognition of increases in pulmonary vascular resistance as pulmonary artery diastolic pressure increases above left atrial pressure.

that call for routine measurement of cardiac output every 2, 4, or 6 hours invariably miss subtle or even more severe changes that occur between measurements. Examples include episodes of agitation and tracheal suctioning. During these events, cardiac output can acutely fall and initiate a rapid downward spiral to hemodynamic instability.

MIXED VENOUS SATURATION

Continuous display of the $S\bar{v}O_2$ affords one the opportunity to observe acute as well as gradual changes in cardiac performance, increasing oxygen consumption ($\dot{V}O_2$), or both. Based on the Fick method of determining cardiac output, changes in the $S\bar{v}O_2$ reflect changes in systemic blood flow as long as $\dot{V}O_2$ remains stable. Acute changes in $\dot{V}O_2$ and cardiac performance are especially demonstrable during episodes of agitation, tracheal suctioning, and rapid extracellular volume shifts. $S\bar{v}O_2$ monitoring is particularly helpful in keeping track of the slow, gradual deterioration of cardiac performance during the second 8-hour period after CPB.

By combining the readings obtained for cardiac output and $S\bar{v}O_2$, one can roughly calculate $\dot{V}O_2$, which should remain within the normal range of 125 to 150 mL/minute/m². Variations in $\dot{V}O_2$ should be assessed; they may be caused by marked alkalosis, agitation, high-dosage narcotics, or catecholamine administration. The product of cardiac output times the $C(a - \bar{v})O_2$ should place $\dot{V}O_2$ within a reasonable range for the patient's condition. Remember that oxygen content depends primarily on the amount of oxygen bound to hemoglobin, the hemoglobin level, and the oxygen saturation according to the equation:

$$\text{Oxygen content} = 1.34 \times \text{hemoglobin} \times \text{\%saturation}$$

Determining the arterial content of oxygen (CaO_2) is particularly important for calculating oxygen delivery to the tissue. Oxygen delivery ($\dot{D}O_2$) is the product of the cardiac output and the CaO_2 according to the following equation:

$$\dot{D}O_2 = \text{cardiac output} \times CaO_2 \times 10$$

The ratio of $\dot{V}O_2$ and $\dot{D}O_2$, or oxygen utilization coefficient (OUC), is the basis of determining overall oxygen supply and demand for the body according to the following equation:

$$\text{OUC} = \frac{\dot{V}O_2 = \text{cardiac output} \times C(a - \bar{v})O_2 \times 10}{\dot{D}O_2 = \text{cardiac output} \times CaO_2 \times 10}$$

The normal range for the OUC is 0.23 to 0.32.

Equipment to measure physiologic parameters such as the arterial pressure and $S\bar{v}O_2$ must be calibrated regularly. $S\bar{v}O_2$ monitors are calibrated in conjunction with venous saturation readings obtained from a mixed venous blood sample from the pulmonary artery. The accuracy of any single measure of cardiac performance should always be evaluated by cross-checking it with another measure. For example, if the arterial pressure waveform is dampened, it may be compared against readings from an oscillometric, Doppler, or return-to-flow technique. Spurious readings should always be evaluated in the context of other parameters and with a suspicion for the accuracy of measurement.

SERUM LACTIC ACID/LACTATE

As a measure of anaerobic metabolism, serum lactate provides invaluable information about the exact status of cardiac performance in meeting the body's oxygen requirement. In the immediate postoperative period, if one had to depend on a single measure to judge the adequacy of cardiac function in meeting the metabolic requirements of the body, lactic acid might be the most useful.

Several problems, however, hamper total reliance on serum lactate as a means to assess cardiac performance. On arrival to the ICU, lactic acid values may range between normal (< 2.0 mMol/L) to as high as 8 to 9 mMol/L. As body temperature rises to normal, serum lactate may actually rise, because underperfused vascular beds open and release large amounts of lactic acid into the systemic circulation. The difficulty in this situation is whether to attribute a rise in serum lactate to a "washout" phenomenon or to a diminution of cardiac performance. Evaluation of the cardiac index, $S\bar{v}O_2$, $C(a - \bar{v})O_2$, SVR, and PVR, in conjunction with *serial* serum lactate determinations, helps to resolve this dilemma. Lactate levels should decrease after 8 hours if perfusion is adequate.

SERUM IONIZED CALCIUM AND POTASSIUM

Rapid access (5 to 10 minutes) to laboratory determinations is essential for guiding therapy, especially in the first 24 hours. In addition to lactic acid, other important serum values include ionized calcium (Ca^{2+}), potassium, hematocrit, glucose, and, at times, sodium.

Serial measurement of Ca^{2+} is especially helpful when solutions containing protein such as blood, fresh frozen plasma, albumin, or plasma protein solutions are administered. Protein binds calcium and may diminish that which is available for cardiac contraction. Clinically, this phenomenon can be recognized during the rapid infusion of protein-containing solutions by noting a rise in cardiac filling pressures, a drop in blood pressure, and a drop in the $S\bar{v}O_2$, all indicative of worsening performance in the face of increasing intravascular volume. In certain situations, particularly in younger patients and more critically ill adults, simultaneous infusion of calcium chloride markedly improves cardiac performance, as observed by a rise in the $S\bar{v}O_2$, lowering of the left atrial filling pressures, and a rise in systemic blood pressure.

Serial measurement of Ca^{2+} affords an opportunity to prevent problems, particularly when the ionized calcium is borderline low, even though the patient is apparently experiencing no ill effects. However, when administering calcium, if you observe a rise in systemic pressure, unchanged or slightly higher filling pressures, and no change or a drop in the $S\bar{v}O_2$, then calcium may be acting as a peripheral vasoconstrictor. In this situation, it should be cautiously withheld. Also remember that despite administration of calcium, serum Ca^{2+} values from whole blood may be low because calcium can be rapidly excreted in the urine, producing a marked increase in urine output.

Postoperative maintenance of adequate serum potassium is crucial, especially after the usually brisk diuresis following

CPB and in conjunction with diuretic therapy. We consider potassium chloride to be a major antiarrhythmic drug after cardiac surgery. Serial serum potassium values should be measured frequently to guide replacement therapy toward a normal to high normal range (4.5 to 5 mMol/L), particularly if the ventricle is irritable.

URINE OUTPUT

In the initial postoperative period, urine output is usually generous but then diminishes dramatically between the 8th to 12th post-CPB hours. It should be measured hourly. Initially, urine output alone should not be heavily relied on to judge cardiac performance, because it is influenced by a host of variables including high serum glucose, denatured plasma protein fractions, and diuretics such as furosemide and mannitol used during CPB. In the latter part of the postoperative period, urine output may be influenced by various hormonal controls mediated by stress (antidiuretic hormone, aldosterone, and cortisol), which generally result in conservation of intravascular volume. Similarly, conservation of intravascular volume occurs in patients who enter surgery with high ventricular end-diastolic filling pressures but return to the ICU after surgery with lower filling pressures. In patients who are accustomed to higher filling pressures, the sudden reduction in atrial pressure usually sets off a strong antidiuretic hormone–mediated response designed to correct what the body perceives as hypovolemia.

Urine output should be maintained at approximately 1 mL/kg/hour if only to wash out the kidneys of various red cell and protein debris caused by CPB. Maintenance of this level of urine output is accomplished using furosemide or mannitol. Diuretic therapy should be guided by the cardiac filling pressures. Low filling pressures with adequate cardiac output may be treated with mannitol, whereas patients with higher filling pressures are treated with furosemide. Diuresis during the early postoperative period should be performed cautiously using the smallest dosages of diuretics necessary to produce urine at 1 mL/kg/hour to avoid hemodynamic instability.

SPECIAL CONCERNS ∎

BLEEDING

Causes

Severe perioperative bleeding (greater than 10 units) occurs in approximately 3% to 5% of patients who undergo CPB. Half of these patients have acquired hemostatic defects.[12] An excellent review of bleeding problems associated with CPB is provided by Woodman and Harker.[12] Approximately 95% to 99% of excessive postoperative bleeding is caused by defective surgical hemostasis, acquired transient platelet dysfunction, and occasionally both.

Bleeding after cardiac operation with CPB is a major destabilizing complication. Controversy, however, persists as to how much can be tolerated and the optimal method of therapy. Despite the more deliberate use of blood recla-

mation and other methods of conservation, therapeutic protocols may influence postoperative bleeding. For example, chronic aspirin therapy for patients with coronary artery disease may contribute to postoperative platelet dysfunction. Obviously, therapeutic decisions are also tempered by concerns regarding antigens and transmissible viruses in blood products.

Treatment

When bleeding does occur, our threshold for returning the patient to the operating room is a blood loss rate through the chest tubes of greater than 3 mL/kg/hour for several consecutive hours. Patients who experience bleeding at this rate cannot be stabilized hemodynamically, irrespective of the amount of volume replacement. If the blood lost through the chest tube is dark, indicative of venous origin, an attempt to control bleeding can be made by increasing positive end-expiratory pressure (PEEP). Arterial bleeding generally is not influenced by elevating PEEP.

Salvage and reinfusion of the autologous blood should be attempted when feasible, especially if the patient has been taking aspirin or is undergoing a second (redo) cardiac operation. This procedure, when performed in the operating room, may influence bleeding in the ICU. Specifically, during the surgical procedure when the prime for the CPB machine is reinfused, attention must be paid to the dosages of protamine used to reverse the heparin and restore activated clotting times to their normal value. In addition, a heparin rebound may occur early postoperatively because of the more rapid metabolism of protamine compared with heparin. In these situations, heparin is unopposed and circulates for several hours.

Given concerns about platelet function after surgery, particularly in patients treated preoperatively with aspirin, the drug desmopressin acetate can be used to enhance overall platelet function. However, caution should be used when giving desmopressin acetate: in several patients, we have observed a severe hypotensive crisis between 5 and 15 minutes after its intravenous administration.

Cardiac Tamponade

Bleeding in the chest after cardiac surgery may not always be expressed in the chest tubes, prompting concern about the possibility of cardiac tamponade. Abrupt cessation of bleeding from the chest tubes warrants close attention to the cardiac filling pressures and to overall cardiac performance.

Two fairly reliable signs of cardiac tamponade are (1) increased or exaggerated cycling of the systolic blood pressure during positive-pressure ventilation, and (2) equalization of right and left atrial and pulmonary artery diastolic pressures. A reduction in $S\bar{v}O_2$ and an increase in $C(a - \bar{v})O_2$ will also be observed. The diagnosis may be confirmed by two-dimensional echocardiography.

In cardiac tamponade, equalization of the atrial pressures does not always occur, despite fastidious attention to calibration of the pressure transducers. Blood clots on the acute margin of the right ventricle may substantially affect cardiac performance without atrial pressure equalization. Additionally, clot formation near the posterior AV groove can simulate supraventricular mitral stenosis, producing a high LAP but no appreciable increase in right atrial pressure.

In severe low-output states, cardiac tamponade must be ruled out by either an exploratory operation in the operating room or a limited opening of the lower portion of the chest incision at the beside. A reasonable maxim for this condition is that patients should not be allowed to die in the ICU from a low-output state without having the chest opened to rule out cardiac tamponade.

VENTILATORY MANAGEMENT

Ventilatory management after cardiac surgery is directed toward optimizing pulmonary function without compromising that of the cardiovascular system. On patient admission to the ICU in our institution, the IMV or synchronous intermittent mandatory ventilation (SIMV) rate is set between 8 and 12 breaths per minute with a tidal volume of approximately 15 mL/kg. Tidal volumes vary according to the individual patient. We do not pressure-limit the ventilator, and we carefully monitor hemodynamic function throughout the period of assisted ventilation. Acute hemodynamic changes may be indicative of the patient distress, a blocked endotracheal tube, the need for suctioning, or a bronchodilator such as albuterol. Most patients have peak airway pressures ranging from 28 to 34 mm Hg. We calculate pulmonary shunts frequently and adjust PEEP to maintain the shunt fraction below 0.15 whenever possible.

Caution is advised when using PEEP above 8 to 10 cm H_2O, because cardiac performance may be altered and cardiac output drop. If higher PEEP is required, we try to compensate by adjusting the IMV/SIMV rate to the lowest level that provides a normal $PaCO_2$ and arterial pH. At an IMV/SIMV rate of 2 to 4 breaths per minute, PEEP of 10 to even 15 cm H_2O usually has little effect on cardiac performance. When high PEEP is used, intravascular volume augmentation may be necessary to raise the effective LVEDP to pre-PEEP levels. As a rule of thumb, one-half the PEEP subtracted from the LAP or pulmonary artery occlusion pressure is the effective LVEDP.

Administration of SNP to patients who are heavy smokers or have severe chronic lung disease may increase the amount of pulmonary shunting and cause extreme hypoxia. Bronchodilators and PEEP as high as 15 to 20 cm H_2O are of little use to correct this problem. In such cases, SNP should be discontinued and substituted with another drug such as NTG (3 to 5 μg/kg/minute) or hydralazine.

The appearance of the acute respiratory distress syndrome (ARDS) after cardiac surgery is much less frequent due, in part, to shorter CPB times and the use of membrane oxygenators. Unfortunately, when ARDS does occur in the postoperative period, it may be accompanied by multiple organ dysfunction syndrome or sepsis.[13]

DIURETIC THERAPY

Diuresis, especially during the improvement period, should always be closely monitored, and excessive urine output is to be avoided. Remember that decreasing fluid accumulation in the extracellular space is a rate-limited process that depends primarily on COP and venous hydrostatic pressure. Excessive diuretic therapy rapidly depletes intravascular volume if the renal response to these drugs is brisk. A dose of 20, 40, or 60 mg of furosemide that results in a urine output of 500 to 1500 mL over several hours may significantly reduce cardiac performance and promote increased SVR.

Smaller and more frequent doses of diuretics produce a more constant diuresis and the ability to maintain a gradual negative fluid balance throughout the second 24-hour postoperative period. A general guideline is to achieve a urine output of approximately 1 to 1.5 mL/kg/hour above the amount of hourly intravenous intake. A sustained diuresis that prevents large hourly urine loss spares the patient rapid volume shifts. To accomplish a stable diuresis, we recommend 1 to 10 mg of furosemide (occasionally slightly higher) every 2 to 4 hours.

The net fluid reduction of a stable, consistent diuresis in a 70-to 80-kg adult is approximately 2 L of fluid over 24 hours. Exceptions to these guidelines occur. High filling pressures resulting from aggressive fluid administration in the first 8 to 12 post-CPB hours that are further exacerbated during the stiff period may require large doses of diuretic to achieve values of 8 to 12 mm Hg. Other exceptions include situations where urine output is low because of poor cardiac performance or preexisting renal dysfunction.

RENAL FAILURE

Patients with a preoperative creatinine clearance of less than 50 mL/minute, who experience an extremely low cardiac output during the first 24 hours after CPB, may develop acute tubular necrosis. Most respond to diuretic therapy and can be maintained in a nonoliguric renal failure. However, some experience oliguric or anuric renal failure. Nonoliguric failure is much easier to manage than is oliguric or anuric failure. In nonoliguric renal failure, volume status and potassium are, generally, less of a problem.

Diuretics

Occasionally, a constant infusion of a furosemide–mannitol or a furosemide–ethacrynic acid–mannitol drip, "dial-a-urine," is indicated. Patients with oliguria should be given a test bolus of both furosemide (80 mg) and mannitol (25 g) and then evaluated for a urine response of greater than 50 mL/hour. An infusion can then be maintained with 5% mannitol, 1 g of furosemide, and possibly 100 mg of ethacrynic acid in a 500-mL solution that is infused at 10 mL/hour. The infusion rate may be increased to as high as 20 mL/hour or maintained as low as 3 mL/hour to reach the target volume of hourly urine output (approximately 100 mL plus the hourly intravenous fluid intake). In our experience, this regimen successfully maintains urine output after surgery, frequently even if acute tubular necrosis is present.

Dialysis

During the first 3 or 4 days after surgery, renal failure resulting from low cardiac output, myoglobinuria, or preexisting dysfunction is best managed with peritoneal dialysis rather than hemodialysis. Hemodialysis creates a more unstable cardiovascular condition than does peritoneal dialysis and requires larger amounts of intravascular volume administration to regain stability after dialysis. In addition, patients generally have a positive fluid balance after hemodialysis.

INDICATIONS.   Intravascular volume overload and elevated serum potassium levels are the principal indications for dialyzing a patient in the immediate postoperative period. For patients without multiple surgical procedures in the abdominal cavity, a single-cuff Tenckhoff catheter can be inserted quickly and dialysis instituted immediately.

TECHNIQUES.   Rapid dialysis infusions with lower volumes and shorter dwell times are generally more effective for removing excess fluid and potassium than larger volumes (1 to 2 L) with dwell times approaching 1 hour. For adult patients, we use 200 to 500 mL of dialysate with dwell times of 20 minutes and a drainage time of 40 minutes. Dialysis runs are made hourly. Effective control of fluid and potassium removal is possible by alternating or combining dialysate solutions of different concentrations (1.5% and 4.5%).

GOAL.   The overall goal during dialysis is to maintain cardiovascular stability. Therefore, fluid removed should only be slightly greater than the hourly amount of fluid intake. When the cardiac filling pressures are high, a more aggressive regimen using a 4.25% dialysate can be used. Remember to monitor the serum glucose frequently when using a higher concentration of dialysate.

Continuous Arterial Venous Hemofiltration

For situations in which peritoneal dialysis is not possible, continuous arterial venous hemofiltration (CAVH) is particularly effective for removing excess fluid volume. The preheparinized CAVH filter can be connected to an arterial catheter placed in the femoral artery and a venous cannula inserted into the femoral or subclavian vein. An advantage of the CAVH filter is that it tends to control potassium, and back pressure on the filter can be varied to help control the amount of fluid removal. Generally, we have not needed systemic anticoagulation. If bleeding is not a problem, however, heparin can be administered, thereby helping to prolong the filter life. Without heparin, the average filter life ranges from 16 to 24 hours.

UNTOWARD CENTRAL NERVOUS SYSTEM SEQUELAE

After cardiac operations with CPB, the incidence rate of stroke is approximately 2% to 5%.[14] Untoward psychologic and cognitive sequelae are more prevalent.[15-17] The precise etiology of neuropsychologic complications remains unclear. However, recent data suggest that microemboli, especially air, are related to both severe and subtle postoperative neuropsychologic deficits.[18] Interestingly, these emboli appear most frequently when the heart and great vessels are surgically manipulated.

During the postoperative period, and especially in the ICU, be vigilant for the appearance of neuropsychologic complications. From the time of their emergence from anesthesia, patients should be assessed for focal motor deficits and the ability to comprehend and follow simple commands.

Delirium

Two types of delirium may develop in the early postoperative period. The first usually is evident as soon as the patient awakens from anesthesia. This organic brain syndrome is characterized by disorientation without aberrations. The second, postcardiotomy delirium, is distinguishable from the early syndrome because it is preceded by a lucid interval, usually 36 to 48 hours in duration, beginning at the time patients awaken from anesthesia. This syndrome is characterized by confusion, disorientation, and disordered thinking and perception. Severe manifestations may include visual and auditory illusions, hallucinations, and paranoid ideation.[19,20] Treatment consists of medication with haloperidol, undisturbed rest, frequent reorientation, assuring patient safety, and reassurance to both the patient and family.

Subtle changes in mentation and thinking processes occur frequently during the first few weeks after surgery. They may be frightening to the patient and may interfere with the immediate recovery process. However, most of these problems are temporary and usually resolve by the sixth postoperative month.[17,21]

SEDATION AND PARALYSIS

In addition to the pain and discomfort characteristic of any major surgical procedure, several conditions occurring after cardiac operation warrant sedation, and, in some cases, complete paralysis. As the patient awakens from anesthesia, a perceived reduction in cardiac performance may result, in part, from shivering, agitation, or both. Shivering can produce a marked increase in $\dot{V}o_2$, a reduction in $S\bar{v}o_2$, and an overall imbalance of oxygen supply and demand in the body, especially in low-output states. Once gross neurologic function is assessed (i.e., movement and sensation in the extremities and the ability to follow simple commands), shivering or agitation is best treated with narcotic agents. If this regimen is ineffective, paralysis should be used.

Our preference is to use a fentanyl infusion to control shivering or agitation, although these conditions can be managed with morphine, a paralytic agent, or both. Meperidine is particularly efficacious, although the mechanism by which it acts is unknown. Among paralytic agents we prefer vecuronium, which has a lesser chronotropic effect than pancuronium. However, if the heart rate is low, pancuronium may be effective in raising it into the 90 to 100 beats per minute range. It is also considerably less expensive than vecuronium. Initial doses for both drugs are the same: 0.1 mg/kg.

When afterload reduction with SNP is employed, fentanyl is probably a more appropriate drug than morphine because it has less effect on the peripheral vasculature. Fentanyl combined with a paralytic agent generally produces a significant increase in $S\bar{v}o_2$ and a decrease in $\dot{V}o_2$. For patients who have pulmonary hypertension as a result of conditions such as mitral valve disease, combined use of fentanyl and a paralytic agent can be useful to reduce PVR. This regimen also prevents the patient from "fighting" the ventilator. Settings can be adjusted to reduce the $PaCO_2$ to 28 to 34 mm Hg and to provide adequate oxygenation, both of which reduce PVR.

NITROPRUSSIDE TOXICITY

Despite its advantages, SNP has the potential side effect of cyanide toxicity. When infusing this drug, remember that each molecule of SNP can release five cyanide ions into the bloodstream. Cyanide is metabolized in the liver by the enzyme rhodanase and converted to thiocyanate. Cyanide metabolism, therefore, is rate-limited and depends on the amount of available rhodanase. Thiocyanate levels in the early postoperative period are meaningless and reflect a *different* toxicity than acute cyanide intoxication. Acute cyanide toxicity can occur as early as 1 to 2 hours after initiation of SNP infusion.

Most patients do not experience cyanide toxicity when receiving SNP in dosages up to 5 µg/kg/minute. However, the incidence of cyanide toxicity increases significantly when dosages exceed 6 µg/kg/minute. Still, some patients are exquisitely sensitive to SNP and may develop cyanide toxicity when receiving as little as 1 µg/kg/minute or less.

Because cyanide has a greater affinity for the cytochrome system, oxygen molecules are not removed from the hemoglobin molecule and cellular oxygen deprivation occurs. Anaerobic cellular metabolism and a buildup of lactic acid produce systemic acidosis. The condition is characterized by a rise in the $S\bar{v}O_2$, a narrowing of $C(a - \bar{v})O_2$, and progressive acidemia.

When the numeric value for lactic acid (mMol/L) rises above that for $C(a - \bar{v})O_2$ (mL/dL), we assume that cyanide toxicity is occurring and substitute another afterload-reduc-

ing agent. By using this method of early detection of cyanide toxicity, we have avoided the need to administer drugs such as amyl nitrite, sodium nitrite, and sodium thiosulfate. When cyanide toxicity is suspected, SNP is weaned rapidly and high-dose NTG, hydralazine, or an angiotensin converting enzyme inhibitor such as captopril is substituted.

If cyanide toxicity is suspected 8 to 10 hours after CPB, prazosin may be administered through the nasogastric tube. Once SNP is stopped, the lactic acid usually returns rapidly to normal with little or no effect on the $C(a - \bar{v})O_2$ and $S\bar{v}O_2$ (Figs. 75-3 and 75-4).

Remember that significant washout of lactic acid from underperfused tissues occurs early after CPB, especially if systemic temperature was reduced below 28°C. A modest rise in the serum lactate should be anticipated during the first 4 to 6 hours after CPB, but should stabilize and then rapidly diminish. Impending cyanide toxicity should be correlated with a decreased $C(a - \bar{v})O_2$ and increased serum lactic acid.

In severe low cardiac output states, $S\bar{v}O_2$ readings in the 40% to low 50% range, a cardiac index below 2.0 L/minute/m^2, and a $C(a - \bar{v})O_2$ in the 6.5 to 8.5 mL/dL range indicate anaerobic cellular metabolism. The cause is a lack of oxygen supply to the tissues, not competitive blocking of oxygen in the cytochrome system. We believe that all patients receiving SNP should have frequent monitoring of their serum lactic acid, $C(a - \bar{v})O_2$, and $S\bar{v}O_2$.

MECHANICAL CARDIAC ASSISTANCE

Mechanical cardiac assist devices include the intraaortic balloon pump (IABP), centrifugal blood pumps, ventricular assist devices, and total artificial hearts. In some cases, extracorporeal membrane oxygenation is indicated for profound cardiorespiratory failure.

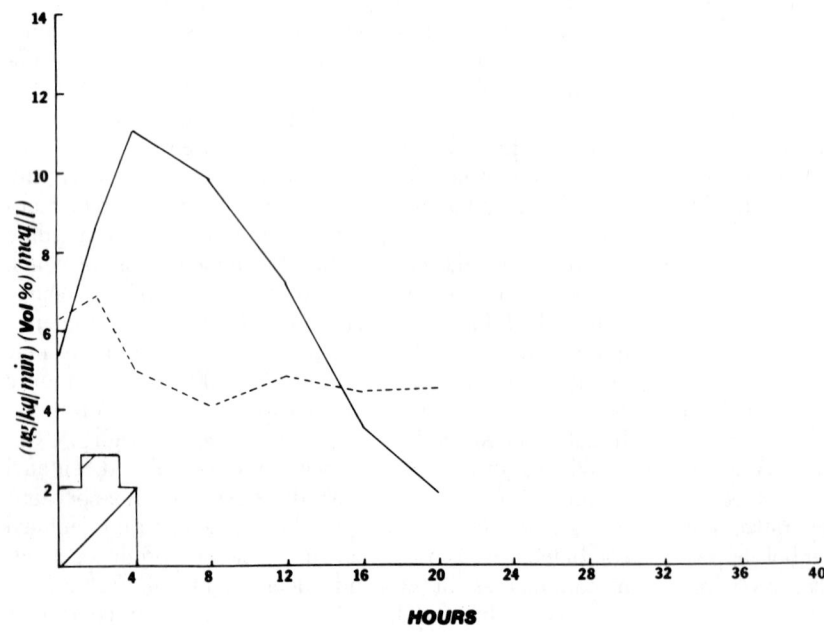

FIGURE 75-3. Representation of lactic acid versus C $(a - \bar{v})O_2$ in presumed cyanide toxicity. Solid line, lactic acid (mEq/L; dashed line, C $(a - \bar{v})O_2$ (mL/dL); hatched area, sodium nitroprusside (µg/kg/minute).

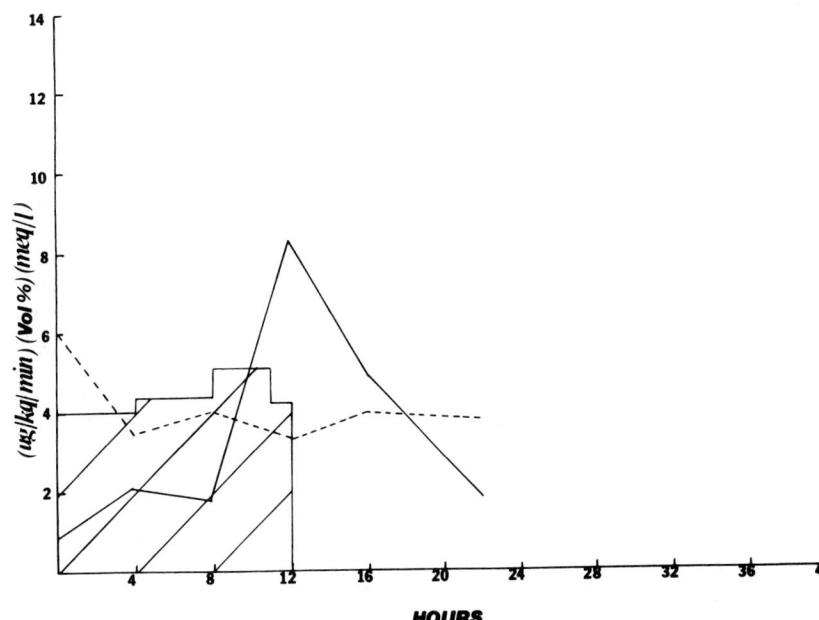

FIGURE 75-4. Representation of lactic acid versus C $(a - \bar{v})O_2$ in presumed cyanide toxicity. Solid line, lactic acid (mEq/L); dashed line, = C $(a -\bar{v})O_2$; hatched area, sodium nitroprusside (μg/kg/minute).

Intraaortic Balloon Pump

The IABP should be considered when patients fail to respond to "pharmacologic pumping" by drug combinations such as epinephrine and SNP. The IABP improves cardiac performance primarily by afterload reduction and augmentation of systemic diastolic pressure, thereby increasing coronary artery perfusion pressure. IABP therapy should be considered early rather than late, and can be instituted quickly using a percutaneous route. All patients with an IABP should receive intravenous dextran (20 mL/hour) or heparin. Patients receiving continuous heparin infusion should have their partial thromboplastin time increased to approximately 60 seconds. When an IABP is inserted through the femoral artery, be vigilant for signs of limb ischemia.

Ventricular Assist Devices and Total Artificial Hearts

Ventricular assist devices, when available, can provide adequate cardiac output for either the right or left ventricle, although biventricular support is probably the most efficacious. Patients can be supported with these devices until the ventricles recover or until cardiac transplantation can be performed. Currently, total artificial heart therapy remains experimental and is limited to patients who are considered viable candidates for cardiac transplantation. A comprehensive review of mechanical cardiac assistance is provided by Staples and O'Brien.[22]

PANCREATITIS

Patients with low cardiac output during CPB or later in the postoperative period may develop acute pancreatitis accompanied by calculous or acalculous cholecystitis. Pancreatitis also may result from diuretic therapy. Watch for signs of abdominal distress 3 to 7 days after surgery. Serum amylase and lipase measurements should be obtained, especially for patients who complain of abdominal distress but have equivocal findings on physical examination.

If left unattended, pancreatitis or a pancreatic abscess can be devastating. Treatment consists of keeping the patient in nil per os status, decompression with a nasogastric tube, and intravenous feedings.

CATHETER SEPSIS

As noted earlier, the incidence of sepsis increases when invasive monitoring catheters are left in place for longer than 72 hours. If a patient remains critically ill and still requires invasive monitoring, we change all catheters to different sites between the third and fourth postoperative day. Avoid rewiring catheters, and, if possible, discontinue the old one for a period of several hours before inserting the new one. However, if the patient is unstable, attempt to insert the new catheter at a different site before removing the old catheter.

ANTIBIOTIC THERAPY

Prophylactic antibiotics are used in virtually all patients who undergo CPB procedures. They are given before the beginning of surgery and are continued for either a set number of dosages or discontinued when the invasive monitoring catheters are removed.

Coverage is generally directed toward staphylococcal organisms, and the usual preference is a broad-spectrum antibiotic such as a first- or second-generation cephalosporin. The epidemiology of the organisms isolated in postoperative patients generally dictates specific prophylactic antibiotic coverage. Examples include protection against methicillin resistant *Staphylococcus aureus* or coagulase-negative *Staphylococcus epidermidis*. For these bacteria, vancomycin is the antibiotic of choice.

If the patient has been hospitalized for a period of time before heart surgery or experienced some other extenuating condition such as prolonged invasive monitoring or tracheal intubation, additional coverage for staphylococcal and gram-negative organisms is advisable. Combinations such as a synthetic penicillin and third-generation cephalosporin or vancomycin and a third-generation cephalosporin or aminoglycoside can be used in the immediate postoperative cardiac patient. For patients with a penicillin allergy, we substitute clindamycin to ensure antistaphylococcal coverage.

When administering antibiotics, watch for fungal overgrowth. For patients who we anticipate will require antibiotics longer than 48 to 72 hours (e.g., prolonged invasive monitoring or intubation), we administer nystatin in large doses (2 million units) in the nasogastric tube or by mouth to suppress gastrointestinal fungal overgrowth. Fluconazole is used for treatment and prophylaxis against fungal sepsis, especially in patients receiving high dosages of broad-spectrum antibiotics.

REFERENCES

1. Kouchoukos N, Karp R: Management of the postoperative cardiovascular surgical patient. *Am Heart J* 1976;92:513
2. Reinhart K, Kersting T, Fohring U, et al: Can central-venous replace mixed venous oxygen saturation measurements during anesthesia? *Adv Exp Med Biol* 1986;200:67
3. Reinhart K, Rudolph T, Bredle D, et al: Comparison of central-venous to mixed-venous oxygen saturation during changes in oxygen supply/demand. *Chest* 1989;95:1216
4. Gutterman D, Marcus M: Advances in understanding the function of the coronary circulation in physiologic and pathologic states. In: Karp R, Laks H, Wechsler A (eds). *Advances in Cardiac Surgery*, vol 2. St Louis, Mosby—Year Book, 1990:1
5. Foster A, Salter D: Cerebral pathophysiologic considerations in patients with coexisting carotid and coronary artery disease. In: Karp R, Laks H, Wechsler A (eds). *Advances in Cardiac Surgery*, vol 2. St Louis, Mosby—Year Book, 1990:203
6. Kouchoukos N, Sheppard L, McDonald D, et al: Estimation of stroke volume from the central arterial pressure contour in postoperative patients. *Surg Forum* 1969;20:180
7. Webber CE, Garnett ES: The relationship between colloid osmotic pressure and plasma proteins during and after cardiopulmonary bypass. *J Thorac Cardiovasc Surg* 1973;65:234
8. Edmunds H, Alexander J: Effect of cardiopulmonary bypass on the lungs. In: Fishman A (ed). *Pulmonary Diseases and Disorders*, vol 2. New York, McGraw-Hill, 1980:1728
9. Kirklin J, Archie J: The cardiovascular subsystem in surgical patients. *Surg Gynecol Obstet* 1974;139:17
10. Gallagher J, Moore R, Kerns D, et al: Effects of colloid or crystalloid administration on pulmonary extravascular water in the postoperative period after coronary artery bypass grafting. *Anesth Analg* 1985;64:753
11. Mentzer R, Alegre C, Nolan S: The effects of dopamine and isoproterenol on the pulmonary circulation. *J Thorac Cardiovasc Surg* 1976;71:807
12. Woodman R, Harker L: Bleeding complications associated with cardiopulmonary bypass. *Blood* 1990;76:1680
13. Alexander JA, Rogers BM: Diagnosis and management of pulmonary insufficiency. *Surg Clin North Am* 1980;60:983
14. Gardner T, Horneffer P, Manolio T, et al: Stroke following coronary artery bypass grafting: a ten year study. *Ann Thorac Surg* 1985;40:574
15. Aberg T: Cerebral injury after open heart surgery: studies using functional biochemical, and morphological methods. In: Hilbermann M (ed). *Brain Injury and Protection During Open Heart Surgery*. Boston, Martinus Nijhoff, 1988:1
16. Taylor K: Pathophysiology of brain damage during open-heart surgery. *Tex Heart Inst J* 1986;13:91
17. O'Brien DJ, Bauer RM, Yarandi, H, et al: Patient memory before and after cardiac operations. *J Thorac Cardiovasc Surg* 1992;104:1116
18. Clark RE, Brillman J, Davis DA, et al: Microemboli during coronary artery bypass grafting: genesis and effect on outcome. *J Thorac Cardiovasc Surg* 1995;109:249
19. Vasquez E, Chitwood W: Postcardiotomy delirium: an overview. *Int J Psychiatr Med* 1975;6:373
20. Blachly P, Starr A: Postcardiotomy delirium. *Am J Psychiatr* 1964;121:371
21. Townes B, Bashein G, Horbein T, at al: Neurobehavioral outcomes in cardiac operations. *J Thorac Cardiovasc Surg* 1989;98:774
22. Staples ED, O'Brien DJ: Cardiac assistance devices and artificial heart. In: Levine B, Copeland EM, Howard RJ, et al (eds). *Current Practice of Surgery*, vol 2, IX, no 6. New York, Churchill Livingstone, 1993:1

Critical Care, Third Edition, edited by Joseph M. Civetta,
Robert W. Taylor, and Robert R. Kirby.
Lippincott-Raven Publishers, Philadelphia, PA © 1997.

CHAPTER 76

Postoperative Management of the Pediatric Cardiac Surgical Patient

Laurie K. Davies
Michael A. Greene

IMMEDIATE CONCERNS

MAJOR PROBLEMS

The interval from completion of cardiac surgery until admission to the intensive care unit (ICU) is one of the most critical times for pediatric patients. To safely and efficiently transport critically ill infants from one locale to another after palliative or reparative heart surgery, the transport must be orderly, all monitoring devices must remain intact and functional, the patient's vital signs must continue to be closely monitored, appropriate ventilation and oxygenation must be maintained, the volume status must remain optimal, and the child must not become hypothermic. Required vasoactive infusions must not be interrupted or the rates inadvertently changed. These goals should be accomplished in as short a period of time to maintain hemodynamic stability.

In the ICU, the transfer of care also must be orderly and expeditious. Teamwork is essential to accomplish this goal, with every member having a specific, defined role. During transport, the patient's heart rate, arterial blood pressure, and oxyhemoglobin saturation (SaO_2) are continuously monitored. If transfer from the transport monitor to the ICU monitor occurs, at least one physiologic variable should be watched at all times. This time period can be one of large volume shifts and hemodynamic instability. Our practice is to connect the left atrial pressure (LAP) catheter first, or

the central venous pressure catheter if a LAP catheter is not present; a quick assessment of intravascular volume is achieved thereby. Next, we connect the arterial catheter, followed by the electrocardiographic (ECG) leads. Leads II and V_5 are continuously monitored, and ST-segment and rhythm analysis is performed. After all monitors have been connected, baseline rhythm strips are acquired to allow comparison during recovery. If the rhythm is other than sinus, intervention with temporary pacing probably will be required.

Oxygen saturation as determined by pulse oximetry is continually monitored. Next, the pulmonary artery pressure and central venous pressure are transduced. We employ continuous monitoring of mixed venous oxygen saturation ($S\bar{v}O_2$) on all complex cases, because this technology provides extraordinarily valuable information for perioperative management. Monitoring of pulmonary artery pressure is especially helpful in patients with problematic pulmonary vascular resistance (PVR). Measurement of oxygen saturation from the central venous and pulmonary artery ports can be useful in determining whether significant residual shunts still exist. Careful measurement of pullback pressures on removal of the pulmonary artery catheter is useful to assess pressure gradients. Continuous mixed venous oximetry can provide an early warning of deteriorating hemodynamic function and may also be helpful in titrating vasoactive infusions.

STRESS POINTS

1. The child undergoing repair of complex cardiac lesions usually remains intubated at the conclusion of surgery. Be sure the patient receives a tidal volume large enough to move the chest.
2. End-tidal carbon dioxide measurement is useful to corroborate tracheal intubation, but it can be misleading with regard to the actual arterial partial pressure of carbon dioxide ($PaCO_2$). Periodic measurement of $PaCO_2$ is essential to document adequate ventilation.
3. The patient almost always has one or more mediastinal tubes, chest tubes, or both connected to a simple closed bottle system or a Pleurovac drainage system. These systems are connected to a "negative" pressure source ranging from -5 to -20 cm H_2O, depending on the patient's size. The tubes must remain patent in order to prevent blood from accumulating around the heart and causing hemodynamic embarrassment.
4. Hourly output from the drainage tubes is carefully monitored and recorded. Excessive drainage (>3 to 5 mL/kg per hour) over several hours may warrant a return to the operating room.
5. Central venous access is necessary for monitoring of superior vena caval pressure and for infusion of vasoactive drugs, potassium, and calcium chloride. We prefer a separate central port for the drugs and another for pressure monitoring. Many introducers have sidearms that work well for this purpose.
6. One or two peripheral intravenous (IV) catheters for volume infusion should be present to provide ready access after the central catheters are discontinued.
7. Crossmatched blood is brought with the patient from the operating room and remains readily available in the ICU for the first several days after surgery.
8. Blood salvaged from the cardiopulmonary bypass machine can be washed free of heparin and packed for reinfusion.

ESSENTIAL DIAGNOSTIC TESTS, PROCEDURES, AND THERAPY

1. Shortly after arrival in the ICU, the patient's temperature is measured. Many pulmonary artery catheters have thermistors that record blood temperature. Some Foley catheters also measure bladder temperature. If neither of these devices is available, our preference is to measure rectal temperature, because skin temperature can be quite misleading if the patient is vasoconstricted or in a low cardiac output state.
2. Warming lights or blankets are used with small infants to prevent hypothermia.
3. Hourly urine output is carefully recorded. Typically, a brisk diuresis occurs for the first few hours after cardiopulmonary bypass.
4. Electrolyte changes can be profound during this time. On the other hand, if the patient's cardiac output is low, renal perfusion and urine output may be compromised.
5. A temporary atrioventricular (AV) sequential pace-maker is available at the patient's bedside. Temporary atrial wires allow more accurate diagnosis of arrhythmias when the right-arm ECG lead is attached to the atrial wire and the obvious atrial deflections in leads I, II, or III are observed. Atrioventricular synchrony is important during this time, because the atrial "kick" contributes far more to cardiac output in the postoperative period than usual.
6. The pacemaker can be useful to establish AV synchrony, to optimize heart rate, to suppress ectopic beats, or, occasionally, with rapid atrial pacing, to break a reentry tachycardia.
7. Before the patient begins to emerge from the anesthetic, restraints are gently applied to prevent injury during awakening. The patient is kept well sedated during this period, particularly as long as mechanical ventilation is required.
8. A chest radiograph is obtained soon after admission to check for position of all tubes and catheters, the presence of significant hemothorax or pneumothorax, and the degree of interstitial edema.
9. A blood gas analysis and "stat" laboratory studies (hematocrit, lactic acid, glucose, potassium, and calcium) are obtained within 15 minutes of the patient's arrival in the ICU. The oximetric pulmonary artery catheter is also calibrated at this time.

HEMODYNAMIC ISSUES ■

PHYSIOLOGIC DIFFERENCES IN CHILDREN

An appreciation of the physiologic differences between infants and adults is essential. Neonates in general tolerate stressful stimuli less well than adults, with resultant rapid changes in pH, lactic acid, glucose, and temperature. They have diminished nutrient stores of fat and carbohydrates. Maintenance of fluid and electrolyte balance in the fasted neonate is a challenge. Neonates and infants have a higher ratio of body surface area to weight than older children and adults and are more prone to hypothermia and dehydration. The newborn child has a higher metabolic rate and increased oxygen consumption ($\dot{V}O_2$). The ratio of alveolar ventilation to functional residual capacity is much higher than in the adult. These factors make the child much more prone to rapid desaturation during airway manipulation. The liver and kidneys are immature, a factor that affects drug disposition and protein synthesis. Diminished glomerular filtration rate and impairment of tubular function make appropriate fluid management critical. The neonate also normally has increased total body water and capillary permeability. Unfortunately, these factors combine to make extracellular fluid overload the norm in neonates after cardiac surgery.

Cardiovascular System

Cardiovascular physiology differs markedly in the newborn child compared with the adult. At birth, both ventricles are approximately equal in size and wall thickness. With the changeover from fetal circulation, the left ventricle (LV) must accommodate a greater pressure and volume workload. It hypertrophies in response to this challenge and becomes roughly twice as heavy as the right ventricle (RV) by about 6 months of age.[1] The neonatal heart is structurally immature. Myofibrils are arranged in a disorderly fashion and have a smaller percentage of contractile proteins than do those in the adult (30% versus 60%).[2]

AUTONOMIC INNERVATION. Autonomic innervation is also incomplete at birth. Sympathetic innervation to the heart is decreased, as are stores of cardiac catecholamines. In contrast, parasympathetic innervation is comparable to that of the adult. These observations are often cited to explain the frequent vagal predominance that occurs in infants compared with adults. Sympathetic innervation also is immature in the peripheral vasculature. Therefore, control of vascular tone and myocardial contractility in infants depends largely on adrenal function and circulating catecholamines.

VENTRICULAR INTERDEPENDENCE. Compliance of the neonatal heart is decreased compared with that of the adult heart. The RV and LV are more intimately interrelated as a result of their decreased compliance and similarity in size. Dysfunction of one ventricle very quickly leads to biventricular failure. Reduced compliance also means that the neonate is less responsive to increases in preload and, in fact, is more sensitive to intravascular volume overload. Through the physiologic range of ventricular filling pressures, stroke volume changes are small. This relatively fixed stroke volume makes the neonate highly dependent on heart rate and sinus rhythm for optimal cardiac performance. Increases in afterload are poorly tolerated by both the right and left sides of the immature heart. Therefore, the neonate responds poorly to either volume or pressure loading, with resting performance on or near the plateau of the cardiac function curve.

PULMONARY VASCULAR RESISTANCE. PVR is high in utero but declines rapidly after birth. Usually, it is lower than systemic levels within 24 hours of birth. Thereafter, it falls at a moderate rate for 5 to 6 weeks, and then more gradually for the next 2 to 3 years. Cardiac defects causing increased blood flow and pressure to the pulmonary arteries delay or prevent normal regression of the pulmonary vessels. Remember that the pulmonary vasculature is highly labile during the first few months of life in children with normal cardiac anatomy. Children with cardiac defects are constantly at risk for pulmonary hypertensive crises, and a marked rise in pulmonary artery pressure can easily result from hypoxemia, hypercarbia, acidosis, or bronchospasm.

ISCHEMIA. Some evidence suggests that neonates respond more resiliently to ischemic injury. They seem to have a greater tolerance of hypoxia, and the central nervous system appears to exhibit a significant degree of plasticity if injury occurs.

These physiologic differences necessitate attentiveness and vigilance that is unparalleled. Care of the critically ill neonate or infant requires close monitoring of as many, if not more, physiologic variables as in adults. Synthesis of all

available data, timely analysis, and appropriate decisionmaking and therapy are mandatory.

APPROACHING THE INDIVIDUAL PATIENT

Complete Repair

Depending on the lesion, appropriate therapy for one child may be ill advised in another. A clear understanding of the pathophysiology and consequences of the lesion is essential to appropriate management. Another aspect of the problem is determination of how complete any previous surgical repair has been. The trend today is to perform complete repairs earlier in infancy than was true previously. This practice necessitates use of cardiopulmonary bypass, the effects of which have been described as a "whole body inflammatory response" because of the generalized activation of complement, neutrophils, cytokines, and other mediators.[3] Expected consequences include an increase in total body water, transient myocardial dysfunction, increased PVR, problems with gas exchange, neurologic morbidity, and abnormal stress responses.

A thoughtful plan must be developed to support the child through the critical first 72 hours of recovery. If cardiac output can be optimized during this time, permanent organ dysfunction can usually be avoided and the patient usually recovers uneventfully. Our philosophy is summarized in Table 76-1. If the patient is not progressing as expected in the recovery phase, the question of a residual anatomic lesion must arise; early echocardiography, cardiac catheterization, or both, should be performed to try to elicit the cause.

Palliative Procedures

Some lesions are not amenable to early repair but, instead, require palliation or a multistaged approach to therapy. If residual lesions are present, we find it helpful to categorize them as involving either (1) increased pulmonary blood flow, (2) decreased pulmonary blood flow, or (3) obstructive lesions. Almost all congenital heart lesions can be categorized in this way. Therapy can then be directed toward ameliorating the abnormality in pulmonary blood flow or toward supporting the failing myocardium (if an obstructive lesion is present).

TABLE 76-1. General Approach to Postoperative Support for the First 72 Hours

Optimize preoperative status (resuscitation as needed, establishment of adequate perfusion, reversal of acidosis, appropriate use of prostaglandin E_1)

Provide aggressive monitoring of physiologic variables in order to develop as clear a picture as possible of the patient's status

Improve cardiac output and oxygen delivery, usually beginning with afterload reduction, followed by early use of low-dose inotropes

Continue mechanical ventilation until the patient's hemodynamic status has been optimized

Provide heavy sedation to blunt the stress response

Aggressively diagnose and treat causes of low cardiac output

Some investigators prefer to classify patients according to whether they are cyanotic or acyanotic and whether they have congestive heart failure. However, those classifications reflect only the manifestations of the disease, not the root cause. Patients can be cyanotic and still have too much pulmonary blood flow if the basis of the cyanosis is inadequate mixing. Therapy for such an individual would be far different than for the patient who is cyanotic because of inadequate pulmonary blood flow.

The expected clinical status of those infants who have been palliated should be known. For example, a neonate who has just undergone the first stage of a Norwood procedure would be expected to be significantly desaturated. An SaO_2 greater than 85% is deleterious in this patient; aggressive therapy must be pursued to limit pulmonary blood flow in order to optimize systemic blood flow.

TISSUE OXYGEN DELIVERY

Optimization of tissue oxygen delivery ($\dot{D}O_2$) in the immediate postoperative period is one of our primary goals. Oxygen delivery is the product of oxygen content and cardiac output. Oxygen content (CaO_2) is determined by hemoglobin (Hgb), SaO_2, and the partial pressure of arterial blood oxygen (PaO_2), as shown in the following equation:

$$CaO_2 = (Hgb \times 1.34 \times SaO_2) + (PaO_2 \times 0.003)$$

In the patient with a tenuous circulatory status, increasing the oxygen-carrying capacity by raising the hemoglobin level to at least 10 to 11 g/dL should be attempted. In the cyanotic child, an even higher hemoglobin level, approaching 14 to 15 g/dL, may be appropriate. Factors that influence cardiac output include heart rate and rhythm, end-diastolic volume (preload), afterload, and myocardial contractility. Marked differences in these factors can exist between the right and the left sides of the heart in children with congenital heart disease. An increase in postoperative $\dot{V}O_2$ can be caused by shivering, anxiety, and hyperthermia, and is to be avoided. Judicious use of sedation and, occasionally, muscle relaxants is imperative.

Mixed Venous Oximetry

Continuous measurement of $S\bar{v}O_2$ is extremely valuable because it reflects the adequacy of $\dot{D}O_2$ when $\dot{V}O_2$ remains constant. Interventions to improve $\dot{D}O_2$ are quickly reflected in the $S\bar{v}O_2$. We often find this information to be more valuable than cardiac output, per se, because it reflects the individual patient's needs. Also, we tend not to do thermodilution cardiac outputs in small children after surgery, because the obligatory water load entailed is significant. However, in the setting of residual intracardiac shunts, the value of measuring pulmonary artery $S\bar{v}O_2$ is limited; measurement from the superior vena cava is more useful.

Mixed venous oxygen saturation data may be misleading in nitroprusside (SNP) toxicity, in which the $S\bar{v}O_2$ is high because cellular oxygen uptake is reduced. The difference between CaO_2 and mixed venous oxygen content ($C\bar{v}O_2$) narrows, serum lactate rises, and the patient often develops a metabolic acidosis. Therapy consists of discontinuing SNP and substituting a different vasodilator if necessary. Intravenous sodium thiosulfate can be used to treat severe SNP toxicity.

Ventricular Function

Patients usually follow a predictable course with regard to ventricular function after cardiac surgery. After initial stabilization, the first 8 hours after surgery are thought of as the "golden" period, during which time the patient's status is critical but reasonably stable. From 8 to 24 hours, ventricular function declines, with a marked decrease in ventricular compliance. In the subsequent 48 hours, compliance and cardiac output gradually improve (see Chap. 75). This sequence is yet another reason to improve cardiac function as much as possible during the first 8 hours, so that subsequent decrements in performance can be tolerated without loss of vital organ function.

FLUID REPLACEMENT

Systemic $\dot{D}O_2$ can be limited by restrictions to left heart filling. Decreased preload may result from hypovolemia, cardiac tamponade, positive airway pressure, or diastolic dysfunction. RV dysfunction or increased PVR sufficient to impede blood flow across the pulmonary bed also diminishes return to the left side of the heart. In these situations, central venous pressure and pulmonary artery pressure are high, but pulmonary artery occlusion pressure and LAP are low. The difference between pulmonary artery diastolic pressure and LAP is a very sensitive measure of PVR.

Preload and Afterload Adjustment

We tend to augment preload until the patient's LAP reaches 10 to 12 mm Hg. As was previously stated, neonates are unable to increase stroke volume significantly further after this level is reached. Patients with predominantly RV dysfunction are exquisitely sensitive to ventilatory maneuvers that affect RV preload and afterload. Another approach to improve systemic oxygen delivery in patients with RV dysfunction creates (or leaves) a right-to-left shunt at the atrial level. This communication allows the right atrium to decompress, blood to be shunted to the left atrium, LV end-diastolic volume to increase, and cardiac output to improve. Some degree of systemic arterial desaturation results, depending on the degree of shunting; usually, however, $\dot{D}O_2$ is improved because cardiac output is increased. As RV function improves, right atrial pressure decreases, the right-to-left shunt is reduced, and SaO_2 rises. Most of these patients do not require any further intervention. During followup catheterization, the atrial septal defect is often undetectable.

Specific Indications

Several factors must be considered in choosing fluid for intravascular volume expansion. If cardiac output is low, $\dot{D}O_2$ must be maximized by increasing the hematocrit. We transfuse packed red blood cells to a target hematocrit of 35% to 40% in the infant with limited cardiac function. Raising the hematocrit past 45% probably is not beneficial because $\dot{D}o_2$ will eventually be limited by elevations in viscosity and decreases in microcirculatory flow.

Another factor to be considered is the patient's coagulation status. If active bleeding is present, the platelet count is low, and the prothrombin time and partial thromboplastin time are abnormal, transfusion of platelets and fresh frozen plasma may be indicated. Abnormalities in clotting capability are more common in the very small child (because of dilutional effects from the pump run) and in the patient with cyanotic heart disease.

For routine postoperative care when the patient is not bleeding, we prefer to limit fluid intake as much as possible, because marked fluid overload results from the surgical experience. In fact, effort is concentrated toward effecting an appropriate diuresis over the first 3 to 4 days after surgery.

DIASTOLIC DYSFUNCTION

In the past few years, the importance of diastolic dysfunction in critical illness has become better appreciated. Diastole is a complex event and is influenced by four phases: (1) active relaxation, (2) passive filling, (3) diastasis (middle phase), and (4) atrial contraction. The active relaxation phase is energy-dependent and, therefore, can be affected by any process that limits $\dot{D}o_2$. Myocardial ischemia, profound anemia, and hypoxemia are deleterious. Diastolic function during the passive filling phase is influenced by the distensibility of the myocardial tissue and the pericardium. Atrial contraction at the end of diastole can be critical, particularly if filling of the ventricle is limited during any of the other diastolic phases.

Because of this complexity, no single therapy is always efficacious in improving diastolic function. If ischemia is a problem, efforts should be directed toward improving myocardial oxygen delivery. If myocardial compliance is an issue (as may commonly be seen with disease states causing myocardial hypertrophy), therapy is more problematic. Unfortunately, few pharmacologic agents have been shown to be efficacious in this situation, although β-adrenergic agonists

(i.e., isoproterenol) and phosphodiesterase inhibitors (e.g., amrinone) have been used with some success.

If the pericardium or chest wall is limiting passive filling, therapy should be directed toward correcting those problems. In some situations, the chest may be left open until myocardial edema has decreased enough so that it can be closed without hemodynamic embarrassment. AV synchrony is essential. The heart rate should be rapid enough so that the limited stroke volume provides the best cardiac output possible, but not so fast as to shorten the diastolic interval and decrease diastolic filling.

CARDIAC RHYTHM AND RATE

From the preceding discussion, the importance of normal sinus rhythm in the infant is apparent. The atrial kick can account for 30% to 40% of the cardiac output. If AV synchrony is absent, a temporary pacemaker should be used to try to mimic normal sinus rhythm as closely as possible. We find examination of the contour of the LAP tracing to be extremely helpful in determining absence or presence of sinus rhythm. Nonsinus rhythms often are characterized by the presence of cannon a waves (Fig. 76-1). This accentuation of the normal a wave occurs when the atrium contracts against a closed AV valve. If the rhythm is still confusing, an atriogram can be performed by connecting one of the temporary atrial leads to the right arm lead of the ECG and observing the obvious atrial deflections on the monitor (Fig. 76-2).

Even if the patient is in sinus rhythm, pacing to a higher rate may be beneficial. As previously noted, the infant's cardiac output is dependent on the heart rate. Stroke volume is relatively fixed, and compliance is low. We prefer to see heart rates between 130 and 160 beats per minute in small children. Heart rates above 180 beats per minute are not beneficial, because diastolic time becomes so short that ventricular filling can be impaired. Some of the most difficult management problems are rapid tachyarrhythmias, especially junctional ectopic tachycardia. Fortunately, many of these rhythms resolve over time if the child's vital organs can be supported during that interval.

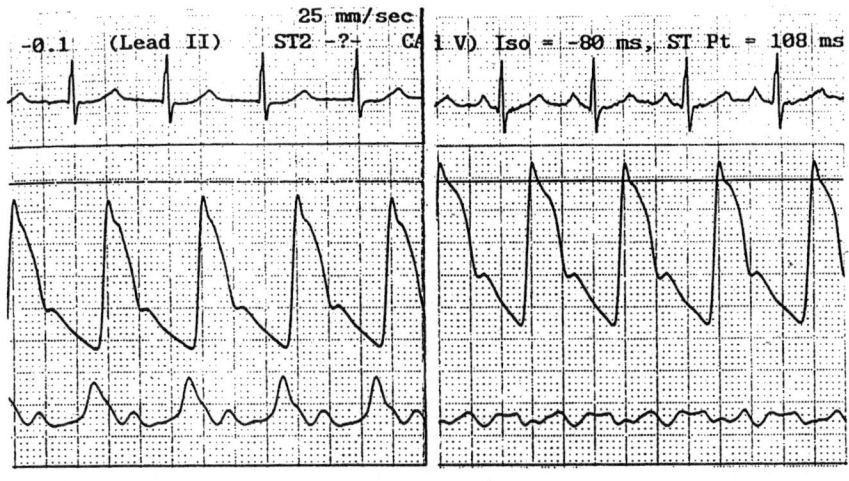

FIGURE 76-1. (**A**) Junctional rhythm showing absence of P waves and cannon a wave in the CVP tracing. (**B**) Sinus rhythm showing obvious P waves and normal CVP tracing. Upper trace, electrocardiogram; middle trace, arterial blood pressure; bottom trace, central venous pressure.

A

B

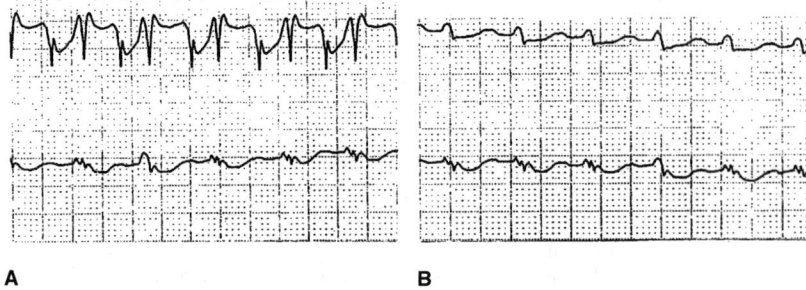

A   **B**

FIGURE 76-2. Electrocardiogram with and without an atriogram. (**A**) The upper trace is an atriogram of lead II with obvious P wave deflection followed by QRS complex. The bottom trace is a standard modified chest lead 1; the P waves are difficult to discern. (**B**) The same patient with standard electrocardiogram of leads II and modified chest lead 1; P waves are difficult to discern.

VASODILATORS

After cardiopulmonary bypass, systemic vascular resistance is usually high in both adults and children because of circulating catecholamines, antidiuretic hormone, and other influences.[4] In the neonate's immature sympathetic nervous system, this response may be amplified by poorly developed sympathetic reflexes, leading to uninhibited vasoconstriction. As previously discussed, the infant's poor myocardial compliance and intolerance of pressure overload make therapy with vasodilators a sensible choice. Afterload reduction is an efficient way to improve cardiac output, because it does not increase myocardial oxygen consumption. In fact, ventricular volume, wall tension, and oxygen consumption may be decreased, with a marked improvement in ejection fraction, systemic vascular resistance, and PVR.

To use vasodilators effectively, fluid volume must be infused simultaneously to maintain adequate filling pressures. We try to keep the LAP constant while titrating the vasodilator. In this fashion, cardiac performance can be improved by as much as twice the level measured before the start of afterload reduction therapy.[5]

INOTROPES

If the cardiac output fails to improve after appropriate volume infusion and vasodilation, addition of an inotropic agent is warranted. This intervention may be necessary especially during the 8 to 24 hours after surgery when ventricular function predictably deteriorates. Table 76-2 lists some commonly used vasoactive drugs and their actions.

Epinephrine

Choice of an inotropic agent is based on the patient's pathophysiology and the hemodynamic goals. Our preference if an agent is needed to improve LV function is to use low-dose epinephrine, starting at 0.01 μg/kg per minute. At this dose, the predominant effect is that of β-receptor stimulation and improvement of cardiac output. Renal perfusion is maintained and often improved, and excessive tachycardia is usually avoided at the lower doses. If increasing doses are required, we add another agent rather than exceeding epinephrine doses of 0.05 μg/kg per minute. Usually we select amrinone or dopamine.

Amrinone

Amrinone offers a different mechanism of action than epinephrine or dopamine. It inhibits the activity of cyclic nucleotide phosphodiesterase (isoenzyme III), which increases the levels of cyclic adenosine monophosphate and increases intracellular ionic calcium concentrations, thereby improving the inotropic state of the heart. The drug appears to act synergistically with low doses of β-adrenergic agonists and has fewer side effects than some of the other catecholamines. It also is a powerful systemic and pulmonary vasodilator. The pulmonary vasodilatory effects of amrinone may depend, in part, on the level of PVR before treatment[6] (Fig. 76-3). Phosphodiesterase inhibitors may be useful in improving compliance and diastolic function.

Dopamine

Dopamine is a useful agent, particularly because of its dopaminergic renal and splanchnic vasodilation effect, which often helps to improve renal perfusion and promote diuresis

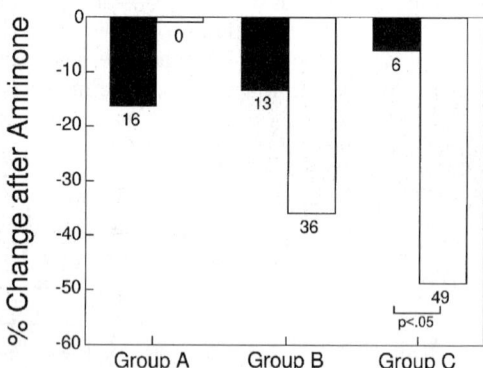

FIGURE 76-3. Percentage decrease in systemic resistance (*solid bars*) and pulmonary vascular resistance (PVR; *open bars*) among three patient groups. Group A, normal pulmonary artery pressure (PAP) and PVR. Group B, increased PAP but normal PVR. Group C, increased PAP and PVR. Amrinone produces the greatest reduction in PVR in group C patients with preexisting pulmonary hypertension and increased PVR. (Robinson BW, Gelband H, Mas MS: Selective pulmonary and systemic vasodilator effects of amrinone in children: new therapeutic implications. *J Am Coll Cardiol* 1993;21:1461.)

TABLE 76-2. Summary of Vasoactive Agents

		CATECHOLAMINES					
		PERIPHERAL VASCULAR EFFECTS			CARDIAC EFFECTS		
AGENT	DOSE RANGE	Alpha	Beta$_2$	Delta	Beta$_1$	Beta$_2$	COMMENTS
Dopamine	2-4 μg/kg/min	0	0	2+	0	0	Splanchnic and renal vasodilator; increasing doses produce increasing alpha effect; may increase pulmonary vascular resistance at higher doses
	4-8 μg/kg/min	0	2+	2+	1-2+	1+	
	>10 μg/kg/min	2-4+	0	0	1-2+	2+	
Dobutamine	2-10 μg/kg/min	1=	2=	0	3-4+	1-2+	Effects vary with dose similar to dopamine; chronotropic advantage probably not apparent in neonates
Epinephrine	0.01-0.05 μg/kg/min	0-1+	1-2+	0	2-3+	2+	Beta$_2$ effect with lower doses; best drug for anaphylaxis
	0.1-0.5 μg/kg/min	4+	0	0	4+	3+	
Norepinephrine	0.01-0.1 μg/kg/min	4+	1+	0	2+	1+	Increases systemic vascular resistance; moderately inotropic; may cause renal ischemia
Isoproterenol	0.01-0.1 μg/kg/min	0	4+	0	4+	4+	Strong inotropic and chronotropic agent; peripheral and pulmonary vasodilator, limited by tachycardia and oxygen consumption
Phenylephrine	0.01-0.5 μg/kg/min	4+	0	0	0	0	Increases systemic vascular resistance, no inotropy; may cause renal ischemia; useful for treatment of TOF spells

		NON-CATECHOLAMINE		
AGENT	DOSES (INTRAVENOUS)	PERIPHERAL VASCULAR EFFECT	CARDIAC EFFECT	CONDUCTION SYSTEM EFFECT
Digoxin	30 μg/kg divided for total digitalizing dose	Increases peripheral vascular resistance 1-2+; acts directly on vascular smooth muscle	Inotropic effect 3-4+; acts directly	Slows sinus node; decreases atrioventricular conduction
Calcium Chloride	10-20 mg/kg/dose (slowly)	Variable; probably depends on serum ionized calcium level	Inotropic effect 3+; depends on ionized calcium	Slows sinus node; decreases atrioventricular conduction
Calcium Gluconate	30-60 mg/kg/dose (slowly)			
Amrinone	1-3 mg/kg loading dose; 5-20 μg/kg/min maintenance	Systemic and pulmonary vasodilator; platelet effects limit long-term use	Increases cardiac output in neonates and infants; may improve diastolic function	Minimal tachycardia

(continued)

TABLE 76-2.   *(continued)*

| | | NON-CATECHOLAMINE | | |
AGENT	DOSES (INTRAVENOUS)	PERIPHERAL VASCULAR EFFECT	CARDIAC EFFECT	CONDUCTION SYSTEM EFFECT
Milrinone	50 μg/kg loading dose; 0.25–0.75 μg/kg/min maintenance	Systemic and pulmonary vasodilator similar to amrinone	Increased cardiac output; may improve diastolic function	Minimal tachycardia; small incidence of arrhythmias
Nitroprusside	0.5–5 μg/kg/min	Donates nitric oxide group to relax smooth muscle and dilate pulmonary and systemic vessels	Indirectly increases cardiac output by decreasing afterload	Reflex tachycardia
Nitroglycerin	0.5–2 μg/kg/min	Similar mechanism to nitroprusside; more preload effect than afterload at usual dose	Little effect on cardiac output if patient is euvolemic	Minimal

Castaneda AR, Jonas RA, Mayer JE Jr, et al: *Cardiac Surgery of the Neonate and Infant.* Philadelphia, WB Saunders, 1994:74.

after surgery. Dopamine's effects are dose dependent, with increased β_1 effects at intermediate doses and increased vascular resistance (α_1 agonism) at higher doses. α-Stimulation can result in unwanted increases in PVR, which may be deleterious in many children with congenital heart disease.

RIGHT-SIDED HEART DYSFUNCTION

Pulmonary Hypertension

RV dysfunction is a frequent postoperative feature in children with congenital heart lesions. Significant increases in PVR after cardiopulmonary bypass are typical and may be poorly tolerated by the immature myocardium (Table 76-3). RV function may be further impaired if a right ventriculotomy was performed during surgery or if aortic crossclamping (with consequent ischemia) was prolonged. If the ventricle was abnormal before repair (e.g., tetralogy of Fallot, pulmonary stenosis) or if it remains volume- or pressure-overloaded, significant RV impairment should be expected.

The child with congenital heart disease may be prone to labile pulmonary hypertension if very young or if the preexisting lesion featured high flow and high pressure to the pulmonary vasculature (e.g., large ventricular septal defect, AV canal, truncus arteriosus). RV dysfunction leads to a decrease in systemic output because the LV can only pump blood that is presented to it. With RV dysfunction, the picture is one of low cardiac output with elevated central venous pressure, elevated pulmonary artery pressure, and low LAP. These increased right-sided pressures lead to hepatic congestion and decreased urine output.

Therapy

Therapy for RV dysfunction is directed toward optimization of preload, reduction of afterload, and control of the hormonal milieu (see Table 76-2). Excessive volume overload tends not to be effective, but leads to venous hypertension and capillary leak. In general, we try to keep the central venous pressure no greater than 12 to 14 mm Hg. The RV seems to be less affected by inotropic agents, but it is exquisitely sensitive to changes in afterload.

VENTILATORY SUPPORT.   Appropriate ventilator strategy is essential because ventricular function is affected by the mechanical effects of ventilation and the biochemical effects of pH and $PaCO_2$. The lungs should be fully expanded; when a normal functional residual capacity is achieved, PVR is at its lowest. Atelectasis or any type of lung compression (e.g., pleural effusion) elevates PVR. On the other hand, hyperinflation causes compression of the septal capillaries and also increases PVR.

Neonates have a closing capacity above functional residual capacity, with some airway closure occurring at the end of each normal tidal breath. A small amount of positive end-expiratory pressure restores functional residual capacity to normal and lowers PVR. Excessive increases in mean intra-

TABLE 76-3. Factors Influencing Pulmonary Vascular Resistance

INCREASED PVR	DECREASED PVR
Lower pH (acidosis or hypercarbia)	Higher pH (bicarbonate or hyperventilation)
High airway pressure	Low airway pressure
Atelectasis or airway closure	Normal FRC
Sympathetic stimulation	Blunted sympathetic response (sedation)
Alveolar hypoxia	Increased F_{IO_2}°
High hematocrit level	Low hematocrit
Drugs (alpha-agonists), humoral influence	Drugs, humoral influence, nitric oxide
Bronchospasm	Bronchodilation

°May not be effective immediately after cardiopulmonary bypass.

F_{IO_2}, fractional inspired oxygen; FRC, functional residual capacity; PVR, pulmonary vascular resistance.

Castaneda AR, Jonas RA, Mayer JE Jr, et al: *Cardiac Surgery of the Neonate and Infant.* Philadelphia, WB Saunders, 1994:76.

thoracic pressure should be avoided, because pulmonary blood flow will be impeded. Hyperventilation with respiratory alkalosis is one of the most powerful tools at our disposal to manipulate PVR. "Stacking" of breaths must be avoided, however, to keep the mean intrathoracic pressure as low as possible. The driving force to lower PVR is the increase in pH rather than the change in $PaCO_2$. Even moderate hypercarbia or metabolic acidosis can profoundly increase PVR and should be avoided if pulmonary hypertension is an issue.

Other factors that may raise PVR include stress and catecholamine surges (see Table 76-3). Heavy sedation can blunt this response and has been shown to be effective during tracheal suctioning.[7] Increases in endogenous production of epinephrine and norepinephrine as $PaCO_2$ rises may explain in part the resultant elevation in PVR from hypercarbia.[8] A high hematocrit also raises PVR. However, oxygen delivery is also influenced by hematocrit, so what the ideal hematocrit is in balancing these factors is unclear. Bronchospasm often causes marked increases in PVR, and aggressive bronchodilator treatment is often necessary.

AFTERLOAD REDUCTION. Pulmonary vascular afterload reduction by pharmacologic agents is only partly successful. The agents most commonly used include SNP and nitroglycerin, isoproterenol, and amrinone or milrinone. These agents have pulmonary and systemic vasodilatory properties. Hence, systemic hypotension often limits their effectiveness in treatment of right-sided heart dysfunction.

NITRIC OXIDE. Preoperatively, oxygen can be a powerful pulmonary vasodilator, but after cardiopulmonary bypass some of the vascular responsiveness seems to be blunted. This effect may occur because of alteration in the vascular endothelium, perhaps as a result of ischemia and impairment of release of endothelium-derived relaxing factor. However, if oxygen is inhaled with nitric oxide, endothelium-derived relaxing factor diffuses to the pulmonary vascular smooth muscle and causes relaxation.[9,10]

Inhaled nitric oxide is quite selective for the pulmonary vascular bed and has few systemic side effects because it avidly binds to hemoglobin in the circulation and is inactivated. Administration of this agent can be extraordinarily helpful if all other measures to decrease PVR have been ineffective. At present, however, it is not readily available in all institutions. It is given in very small concentrations (10 to 80 ppm) and must be closely regulated, because higher concentrations can be toxic to the lungs.

RESPIRATORY MANAGEMENT ■

The cardiovascular and respiratory systems are closely interrelated, anatomically and physiologically; their primary functions are adequate oxygen delivery to meet the tissue metabolic demands and appropriate elimination of carbon dioxide. If $\dot{D}O_2$ is inadequate, anaerobic metabolism and nonrespiratory acidosis result. Acidosis can be associated with further reduction in $\dot{D}O_2$ or maldistribution of flow. Therefore, attention to postoperative respiratory management is critical.

No single ventilatory strategy is appropriate for all patients. Important physiologic differences in the responses of the RV and LV to changes in intrathoracic pressures are well known. RV preload is determined by extrathoracic vessels, whereas RV output traverses intrathoracic vessels. Conversely, LV preload comes from intrathoracic vessels and ejection is largely to extrathoracic vessels. Another confounding variable is ventricular interdependence. Shifts in the ventricular septum can change RV and LV filling markedly and in opposite directions.

Therapeutic respiratory manipulations can significantly affect $\dot{D}O_2$ by altering stroke volume. Patients with right heart dysfunction are particularly sensitive to changes in preload and afterload. Positive-pressure ventilation increases intrathoracic pressure, which is transmitted to the right side of the heart, decreasing venous return to the right atrium. Such patients may benefit from strategies that reduce intrathoracic pressure and improve preload. Therapies directed at reducing right ventricular afterload include increasing pH, lowering $PaCO_2$, optimizing functional residual capacity, increasing alveolar partial pressure of oxygen (PAO_2) and PaO_2, and minimizing intrathoracic pressure. Spontaneous ventilation with low positive end-expiratory pressure and normal to high pH is effective in improving pulmonary blood flow.

LABORATORY VALUES   ■

The frequency and thoroughness of laboratory testing is determined primarily by the complexity of the operative procedure. For simple lesions not requiring cardiopulmonary bypass, such as patent ductus arteriosus ligation or pulmonary artery banding, early postoperative check of the hematocrit, potassium, and arterial blood gas partial pressures is adequate. Further testing is required only if abnormalities require correction or if the SaO_2 is less than satisfactory. Most of these children resume normal dietary and fluid intake within 24 hours of surgery, and further evaluations of cell counts and electrolytes are unnecessary.

Whenever infants and children undergo correction of major defects using cardiopulmonary bypass, the postoperative monitoring of laboratory values becomes crucial. For the first 24 hours, serum potassium, ionized calcium, glucose, arterial blood gas analysis, hematocrit, and lactate are checked at 4-hour intervals. Potassium replacement is given as potassium chloride, 0.33 mMol/kg, over 1 hour through a central catheter to maintain serum potassium at 4.0 to 4.5 mMol/L. Ionized calcium is maintained at a level of 1.25 mMol/L by giving IV calcium chloride by central infusion boluses of about 10 mg/kg over 10 to 15 minutes.

Elevated glucose levels are not treated unless they exceed 400 mg/dL. In neonates and infants, the maintenance venous infusions are made with 10% dextrose in 0.45 normal saline solution to prevent hypoglycemia from inadequate glycogen stores. Sodium bicarbonate ($NaHCO_3$) is used to correct acidosis by the formula:

Required mMol $NaHCO_3$
$$= 0.33 \times \text{Base deficit} \times \text{Body weight in kg}$$

Hematocrit is usually maintained at approximately 40% in the early postoperative period. The appropriate volume of packed red blood cells (PRBCs) to transfuse can be approximated as follows:

PRBC (mL)
$$= (\text{Desired hematocrit} - \text{actual hematocrit}) \times \text{weight (kg)}$$

Lactate is useful as an index of tissue perfusion and $\dot{D}O_2$. Continuous elevation of lactate may signify poor cardiac output, hypoxemia, anemia, or excessive tissue extraction due to agitation. Elevated lactate may also indicate toxicity from IV SNP.

The prothrombin time, partial thromboplastin time, and platelet count are checked immediately and rechecked as necessary based on the amount of bleeding and whether fresh frozen plasma or platelets are transfused to correct a deficit. Additional coagulation studies (e.g., fibrinogen) are ordered as needed. After the initial 24 hours, the laboratory testing frequency is maintained or decreased based on the patient's clinical stability.

A "shunt gas" analysis is obtained the morning after surgery in patients whose intracardiac shunts have been surgically closed. Blood gas measurements from the arterial, superior vena cava, and pulmonary artery catheters are checked, and the partial pressures of oxygen and saturations are compared to determine whether any residual intracardiac shunting is present. Other laboratory values such as digoxin level and aminoglycoside peak and trough levels are checked at the usual indicated intervals.

CARDIAC RHYTHM AND PACING   ■

Although significant rate or rhythm problems uncommonly affect children with congenital heart defects before surgery, most experience at least transient abnormalities of rate or rhythm, or both, afterward. Adequate heart rate and AV conduction are essential to maintain satisfactory cardiac output after major corrective heart surgery. Separation from cardiopulmonary bypass in the operating room often is difficult to impossible until intrinsic or pacemaker-generated AV rhythm is obtained.

TEMPORARY PACING WIRES

Our intraoperative strategy always is to place temporary epicardial atrial and ventricular pacing wires, as well as a skin "ground," before terminating cardiopulmonary bypass. If the patient has an adequate intrinsic rate with intact AV conduction, the native rhythm is undisturbed. If the rate is inadequate, atrial pacing is attempted. If AV conduction abnormalities are present, AV sequential pacing is instituted.

Atrial or AV pacing with the temporary pacing wires is continued in the ICU until the patient has adequate intrinsic heart rate and rhythm. Occasionally, it is difficult to assess whether a patient is in a junctional or sinus rhythm. An atrial pacing wire can be connected to the right limb lead of the ECG to obtain an atriogram and look for atrial P waves (see Fig. 76-1).

POSTOPERATIVE ARRHYTHMIAS

Postoperative arrhythmias are often multifactorial. Electrolyte abnormalities, hypoxemia, and acidosis should all be treated with careful monitoring and correction of potassium, calcium, and magnesium. Administration of excessive dosages of inotropic or chronotropic drugs should be curtailed, and pain and agitation should be treated with morphine and sedatives. An assessment of central and LAP catheters and chest tubes should ensure that they are not in an unusual position that stimulates or irritates the heart.

Premature Ventricular Contractions

Premature ventricular contractions are usually transient and can be suppressed by pacing at a rate 10% to 20% faster than the native heart rate. If rhythm abnormalities persist, a 12-lead ECG is obtained to further define the abnormality and rule out ischemia, particularly in patients who have undergone arterial switch or other procedures requiring coronary transfer or having the potential for coronary injury.

Atrial Flutter and Fibrillation

Atrial flutter may be terminated with a short burst of rapid atrial pacing; after sinus rhythm is achieved, atrial pacing may prevent recurrence. Atrial fibrillation with rapid ventricular response is treated by digitalization. Our practice is to give 15 μg/kg IV, followed by 7.5 μg/kg IV at 8 and 16 hours after the initial dose. We then maintain the patient on 4 μg/kg orally every 12 hours, with monitoring of clinical response as well as digoxin levels.

Supraventricular Tachycardia

If supraventricular tachycardia compromises cardiac output, we occasionally use diltiazem, 0.1 to 0.25 mg/kg IV bolus, followed by an infusion of 0.05 to 0.2 mg/kg per hour. Adenosine, 0.1 to 0.2 mg/kg IV, may terminate supraventricular tachycardia but is usually ineffective for atrial flutter or atrial fibrillation. Synchronous direct current countershock may be necessary if the patient is severely compromised or if the above measures fail.

Bradycardia

After open heart surgery, bradycardia is usually treated with pacing to restore adequate rate. However, in certain circumstances, we also use isoproterenol. Patients undergoing orthotopic heart transplant and patients in whom the beneficial pulmonary vasodilatory effect is desired may improve with isoproterenol at a dose of 0.005 to 0.04 μg/kg per minute. Particularly in transplant patients, low dosages of oral theophylline may help to maintain adequate intrinsic heart rate after the first few days of convalescence.

PERMANENT PACEMAKER IMPLANTATION

The rare child with complete heart block after open heart surgery requires permanent pacemaker implantation. If implantation has been done at the time of the operation, the pacemaker settings must not interfere with the temporary epicardial pacing capability. If the permanent pacemaker is set in a demand mode and pacing through the temporary wires becomes ineffective because of exit block or wire dislodgment, the backup permanent pacemaker may be inhibited by the ineffective pacer spikes from the temporary pacer, resulting in no cardiac mechanical activity. Correction results from turning off the temporary pacemaker, allowing the permanent implanted pacemaker to work uninhibited.

Rarely, transthoracic pacing with a needle or cutaneous patches may be needed if existing pacing wires and drugs cannot restore a rhythm. In the early postoperative period, no patient should be allowed to die from intractable rhythm disturbance without having his or her chest opened to eliminate the chance that tamponade or another correctable factor is present.

TEMPERATURE

Core temperature is monitored early after surgery using a urinary catheter with electronic temperature thermistor. If a urinary catheter is not in place, rectal temperatures are monitored at least hourly. Hypothermia increases the risk of arrhythmias and may contribute to coagulopathy. Attempts to correct low core temperature are initiated as soon as the child arrives in the ICU. Premature neonates and infants are kept in isolettes with overhead warmers, and older children are rewarmed with heated air blankets.

Shivering greatly increases $\dot{V}o_2$. If this problem occurs in mechanically ventilated patients, IV paralytic agents can be given while the patient's temperature is corrected.

High core temperature immediately after surgery may result from severe peripheral vasoconstriction with "conservation" of core temperature. In this setting, pharmacologic vasodilation with SNP usually allows the extremities to warm up and the core temperature to become normal.

SEDATION AND PARALYSIS

Judicious postoperative use of sedative agents may improve hemodynamic stability. If the patient must remain intubated, we are quite liberal in our use of narcotics. IV morphine sulfate in doses of 0.1 to 0.2 mg/kg usually suffices for most children. Occasionally, a fentanyl infusion beginning at 1 to 3 μg/kg per hour may be preferable, particularly in children requiring a constant level of sedation. Blunting of the stress response, especially with maneuvers like tracheal suctioning, is beneficial.

If narcotic sedation is inadequate, additional sedative agents may be required. Addition of a benzodiazepine must be done carefully, because this combination can cause significant myocardial depression. Other agents that may be considered are chloral hydrate or chlorpromazine.

Patients with tenuous hemodynamic function may benefit from a short period of muscle relaxation. We give small bolus doses of either pancuronium or vecuronium (if tachycardia is an issue), allowing the relaxation to wear off periodically in order to assess neurologic function. In patients at risk for seizures, relaxant drugs should be avoided, if possible, or electroencephalographic monitoring should be employed.

INFECTIONS AND ANTIBIOTICS

PROPHYLAXIS

Prophylactic antibiotics are administered to all children undergoing closed cardiac procedures and open heart procedures with cardiopulmonary bypass. The length and complexity of these cases, as well as the frequent use of intracardiac and intravascular prostheses, increase the risk of postoperative wound infection, remote infection, mediastinitis, and endocarditis. Deleterious effects of anesthetic agents and cardiopulmonary bypass on the immune system have been well documented. These effects include decreased concentrations of immunoglobulin and complement, decreased white blood cell counts and impaired phagocytic and chemotactic properties, and decreased ability of the reticuloendothelial system to clear bacteria and endotoxins. The goal of prophylactic antibiotic administration is to provide high bactericidal tissue levels during the procedure and also postoperatively, if invasive intracardiac monitors are used.

Our current regimen is to administer oxacillin, 25 mg/kg, and gentamicin, 2.5 mg/kg IV, on call to the operating room. This regimen is repeated after completion of cardiopulmonary bypass. Subsequently, oxacillin, 25 mg/kg IV every 6 hours, and gentamicin, 2.5 mg/kg IV every 8 to 12 hours, are continued until all invasive catheters are removed, or for at least 48 hours after the procedure. In addition, nystatin (Mycostatin) mouth care is given to prevent fungal infections of the mouth and esophagus. In patients who are allergic to penicillin, the oxacillin is replaced with vancomycin, 15 mg/kg IV, on call to the operating room, followed by 10 mg/kg IV every 12 hours postoperatively.

TREATMENT

For patients operated on for delayed closure of the sternum, mediastinitis, or active endocarditis, we leave a small red rubber catheter in the mediastinum and infuse an antibiotic solution of gentamicin, 8 mg in 100 mL of normal saline solution, at a rate of 1 to 2 mL/kg per hour for 1 week after surgery.

Postoperative fevers exceeding 38.5°C are investigated with appropriate wound checks, chest radiographs, and cultures of urine, blood, and sputum. Antibiotics are adjusted based on culture results. In patients whose cardiac repair includes homograft or bovine pericardial valves or patches, we have noticed a pattern of increased fever persisting up to 2 weeks after surgery. We continue antibiotics in these patients until repetitive cultures fail to demonstrate any infection or bacteremia. Some fevers may be caused by postpericardiotomy syndrome; if exhaustive cultures are negative, these patients are treated with a short dose of oral steroids.

If positive blood cultures follow intracardiac repair, we assume potential endocarditis and obtain an echocardiogram, followed by a minimum of 4 weeks of IV antibiotics with surveillance cultures. An echocardiogram is repeated at the conclusion of therapy, or sooner if fever or positive cultures recur.

After sternotomy or thoracotomy, wound care consists of daily sterile dressing changes. The wound is painted with povidone-iodine solution and allowed to dry before redressing. Steri-Strips are left on until they fall off; if staples are present, they are removed at 7 to 10 days. Staples are left for up to 3 weeks in children undergoing palliative proce-

dures who remain cyanotic after surgery, in malnourished patients, and in patients receiving steroids.

RENAL FAILURE AND DIURETICS ■

Urinary catheters are routinely used, except for relatively minor procedures such as patent ductus arteriosus ligation. Before decannulation after cardiopulmonary bypass, we routinely restore blood volume through the arterial cannula so that patients require very little additional IV fluid in the postoperative period. In the first 24 hours after cardiopulmonary bypass, most patients are allowed to diurese spontaneously without much attempt to force urinary output. During the next 24 hours, an attempt is made to initiate a more vigorous diuresis of at least 1 to 2 mL/kg per hour. IV furosemide is given, up to 2 mg/kg, to maintain this urine output. If circulating blood volume is low, as indicated by low pulmonary artery pressure and LAP, mannitol, 0.5 g/kg, is also given. Dopamine, 3 to 5 µg/kg per minute, is also started if these measures do not provide adequate diuresis.

Acute renal failure develops in 2% to 10% of patients. Usually, it occurs in children with prolonged low cardiac output after correction of a cyanotic lesion. If oliguria persists or anuria develops, all nephrotoxic antibiotics are stopped and careful monitoring of serum potassium is continued. A peritoneal dialysis catheter is then inserted, and dialysis is initiated. Our usual protocol is to dwell and drain in 1-hour cycles, using 15 to 30 mL/kg of peritoneal dialysis solution (1.25% Dianeal). Cell counts and cultures of the dialysate effluent are routinely done. After the child's or infant's general condition improves, kidney function returns and dialysis can be discontinued, usually within 1 to 2 weeks.

LIMB ISCHEMIA ■

Limb ischemia rarely complicates open heart procedures, but it is occasionally seen after subclavian flap repair of coarctation of the aorta or Blalock-Taussig shunting. It usually is identified by pallor or cyanosis, coolness to the touch, edema, absent pulses, and disuse of the arm.

Treatment in this setting must be swift and effective to prevent tissue loss. All invasive central, peripheral, IV, and arterial catheters on the affected side should be removed. The extremity should be elevated on cushions to prevent edema and pressure sores. Circulation is optimized by ensuring adequate cardiac output and blood volume. Anemia is corrected, and all vasoconstrictive drugs are stopped, if possible. Intravenous SNP and diltiazem may provide vasodilation, and a thin layer of nitroglycerin paste may be applied to the skin as well. In extreme cases, consideration should be given to performing a sympathetic block (usually a stellate ganglion block) to promote vasodilation. If surgical bleeding is not a concern, the patient is heparinized.

Ischemia of the lower extremities is almost always caused by the presence of invasive femoral catheters; therefore, the principles listed above are applicable in this situation as well. In most cases, ischemia markedly improves within 24 hours.

BLEEDING ■

CLOTTING ABNORMALITIES

After cardiopulmonary bypass, most patients develop an increased tendency to bleed because of platelet dysfunction and abnormal clotting factors. Hypothermia and some medications also exacerbate this tendency. Bleeding is closely monitored in the early postoperative period, with chest tube outputs recorded at least hourly.

If significant bleeding occurs, prompt reoperation is indicated to avoid the disadvantage of administering large amounts of homologous banked blood products. Most patients bleed only 2 to 3 mL/kg per hour early after surgery; levels of 5 to 10 mL/kg per hour should raise concern. Coagulation studies, platelet count, and fibrinogen level should be checked to analyze the coagulopathy and determine appropriate corrective measures. Desmopressin acetate (DDAVP) or additional protamine may be helpful in some situations.

SURGICAL PROBLEMS

Other indications for reoperation are retained hemothorax or retained large mediastinal hematoma, whether it is causing tamponade or not. Attempts to open chest tubes with suction catheters are usually ineffective and may introduce infection into the chest; therefore, this technique should be avoided. If tamponade with hypotension and pulsus paradoxus occurs, it usually can be relieved in the ICU by opening the subxiphoid portion of the wound. Subsequently, the patient is rapidly transferred to the operating room for definitive control of bleeding and evacuation of residual hematoma.

DONOR-DIRECTED BLOOD TRANSFUSION

If donor-directed blood is used from members of the patient's immediate family, it must be irradiated. If the antigenic makeup is close enough to the recipient's, it is possible for a graft-versus-host reaction to occur. Irradiation of blood products must also be done if the patient has DiGeorge syndrome with absent thymus. If the child is younger than 4 months old, we routinely insist that transfused blood be negative for cytomegalovirus, because these children are more susceptible to infection.

LATER CONCERNS ■

DELAYED CARDIAC TAMPONADE

Delayed cardiac tamponade may present several weeks after open heart surgery, and it occurs most commonly in patients treated with anticoagulants. Physical findings suggesting delayed tamponade are poor feeding, ascites, jugular disten-

tion, pulsus paradoxus, peripheral edema, and pericarditis pain. Chest radiographs demonstrate a widened mediastinum. A transthoracic echocardiogram confirms the diagnosis and helps localize the fluid collection. In most cases, the fluid is thin and serosanguinous. It can readily be evacuated with a 5-Fr, single-lumen, central catheter placed in the pericardium by a subxiphoid approach with echocardiographic guidance. If this approach is unsuccessful, a limited subxiphoid incision can be used.

CHYLOUS COLLECTIONS

If chylothorax or chylopericardium occurs, drainage with a 5-Fr catheter or small chest tube can be used. Almost all chylous collections resolve with drainage, good nutrition, and a fat-limited diet.

NUTRITION

For infants and children who convalesce normally after closed procedures or open heart surgery, nutritional concerns are minimized by early attempts to resume enteral feedings. Nasogastric tubes are used in all patients undergoing heart surgery.

Enteral Feeding

For nonbypass patients, the nasogastric tube can usually be removed at the time of extubation. If gastric distention does not occur, clear liquids are given 4 to 6 hours after surgery, and the diet is advanced to one appropriate for age over the next 12 to 24 hours. One exception to this management protocol for nonbypass patients is the group undergoing repair of coarctation of the aorta.

Nasogastric Drainage

After coarctation repair, elevated epinephrine, norepinephrine, and angiotensin levels may contribute to a paradoxical elevation of blood pressure. Severe arteritis involving the bowel mesentery can lead to bowel ischemia or perforation. In coarctation patients, we continue nasogastric tube drainage for at least 48 to 72 hours, ensuring that abdominal pain, distention, and ileus are not developing. Passage of normal flatus and stool with no abdominal pain or distention is reassuring. At that time, the nasogastric tube is removed and oral feeding is initiated and advanced over 24 hours.

Patients undergoing more complex repair are placed on nasogastric suction while intubated. Gastric pH is checked at 4-hour intervals, and antacids are administered to maintain pH greater than 5. Some carbohydrates are supplied by mixing the IV infusions in 5% or 10% dextrose solutions. If prolonged intubation (>2 or 3 days) is necessary, a small Dobbhoff tube is advanced into the duodenum. After active bowel sounds or bowel movements are present, we begin a constant infusion of half-strength formula. We try to limit the fluids given to 1000 mL/m² per day. If half-strength formula is tolerated for 12 hours, it is changed to full-strength formula with additional glucose polymers (Polycose) and medium-chain triglyceride oil added to provide approximately 100 cal/kg per day.

Hypertrophic Pyloric Stenosis

If a neonate is unable to tolerate feedings, consideration should be given to the diagnosis of hypertrophic pyloric stenosis. We have found this to be a problem in several babies after repair of transposition of the great vessels and total anomalous pulmonary venous return. Pyloromyotomy successfully relieves the pyloric stenosis and allows enteral feeding to begin.

Breast Feeding

Breast feeding is encouraged for the newborn infant, although for a few days immediately after surgery it is not possible. Breast feeding not only promotes special bonding between infant and mother, but also appears to provide a protective effect against respiratory and gastrointestinal illnesses in the baby.[10,11]

Intravenous Hyperalimentation

Central IV hyperalimentation is avoided if at all possible because of the risk of catheter infection and endocarditis. This therapy may be necessary if the patient has evidence of necrotizing enterocolitis or postoperative pancreatitis. In these cases, the central catheter is dedicated to hyperalimentation. Strict precautions to prevent infections are used.

VENTILATOR WEANING AND EXTUBATION

Immediate Extubation

The appropriate time for ventilator weaning and extubation depends on the type of surgery performed and the patient's postoperative course. In general, we extubate children immediately at the end of surgery for most straightforward closed heart procedures (e.g., patent ductus ligation, coarctation of aorta repair, Blalock-Taussig shunt). We also usually extubate patients with simple atrial septal defect repair at the conclusion of surgery. Exceptions to the rule include patients who are bleeding or who are hemodynamically unstable. Children younger than 6 months of age may remain intubated overnight to allow vigorous pulmonary toilet and more gradual awakening.

Delayed Extubation

For more complex repairs, extubation is delayed until the patient's cardiorespiratory status is optimal, excess fluid has been diuresed, and inotropic agents have been weaned. If the course has been prolonged, adequate nutritional status becomes essential for weaning and extubation to be successful. Secretions cannot be excessive. After the patient is judged to be stable enough for extubation, sedative agents are decreased. The intermittent mandatory ventilation rate is decreased, usually two breaths at a time. If the pH remains

acceptable (>7.35) and the respiratory rate and pattern are reasonable, the patient is usually extubated from an intermittent mandatory ventilation rate of 2 to 4 breaths per minute. If the child has been intubated for a period of time, racemic epinephrine is administered by aerosol to help minimize airway and glottic edema.

Circulatory Support

Use of a left ventricular assist device (LVAD) or extracorporeal membrane oxygenation (ECMO) is reserved for patients who have undergone reparative open heart procedures or cardiac transplantation and are unable to be separated from cardiopulmonary bypass owing to severe cardiac dysfunction. Rarely, a patient has been weaned successfully from cardiopulmonary bypass but decompensates in the early postoperative period and requires institution of LVAD or ECMO. In most cases, the existing arterial and venous catheters are connected to a Bio-Medicus centrifugal pump.

For children with poor cardiac ejection who are unlikely to maintain adequate oxygenation with support of LVAD alone, an ECMO circuit provides membrane oxygenation. Heparin is administered to maintain activated clotting time at approximately 200 seconds. The sternum is usually left open, and the skin wound is closed with a polytetrafluoroethylene patch. The patient remains sedated and paralyzed, and the ventilator is placed on minimal settings that maintain alveolar ventilation. Inotropic drugs are minimized, and the patient is maintained in a vasodilated state with the use of SNP. If fluid overload is a problem, an ultrafiltration canister is also placed in-line for removal of excess fluid volume. Patients may be maintained in this state for as long as 7 to 10 days or occasionally even longer; however, infants rarely survive after prolonged periods of circulatory support.

Children who appear to benefit most by postcardiotomy circulatory support are those who have undergone repair of anomalous origin of the left coronary artery from the pulmonary artery. They frequently have profoundly depressed myocardial function that rapidly improves and, in fact, may become normal in the early postoperative period. Children who have undergone orthotopic heart transplantation and who cannot be weaned from bypass may also benefit as the heart recuperates from the prolonged ischemia. In most series, the overall probability of survival after extracorporeal circulatory support following reparative cardiac procedures is approximately 30%.

ECHOCARDIOGRAPHY AND DOPPLER STUDIES

During surgery for correction of major intracardiac defects, we routinely use transesophageal echocardiography even in infants weighing as little as 2.6 kg. This assessment evaluates any significant residual intracardiac shunting, valvular stenosis, or valvular insufficiency; therefore, routine postoperative echocardiography is unnecessary. If, however, a patient has a significant clinical change in the postoperative period, echocardiography is useful to reevaluate for correctable problems. Changes in clinical status may be noted by careful attention to pressure tracing morphology, intracardiac pressures, pulse pressure, and dramatic changes in arterial or venous oxygen saturations.

Early reoperation is indicated if a persistent left-to-right shunt exceeds 1.5/1.0. A residual RV-to-LV pressure ratio greater than 50% after relief of pulmonic stenosis, tetralogy of Fallot repair, or Rastelli operation is associated with a higher morbidity and mortality and may necessitate reoperation to relieve residual LV outflow tract obstruction. If significant mitral, aortic, or tricuspid insufficiency is present in the postoperative sedated patient, it probably will not improve even with afterload reduction and may necessitate reoperation. The goal is to correct the residual defect before a low cardiac output ensues, causing other organ damage.

Another role for postoperative echocardiography is to assess suspected intrapericardial fluid collection and to rule out tamponade. If fluid is present, echocardiography may be helpful to guide placement of a pericardiocentesis catheter for drainage.

TRANSPLANTATION ■

Postoperative management of the neonatal or infant transplant patient requires the collaborative efforts of the surgeon, cardiologist, ICU team, immunologist, and cardiac pathologist.

The transplanted allograft usually requires inotropic and chronotropic support with isoproterenol as well as pulmonary vasodilation with SNP and amrinone. If severe reactive pulmonary hypertension is present, IV prostaglandin E_1 and inhaled nitric oxide may be beneficial.

A combination of IV steroids, cyclosporine, and azathioprine is used for prevention of rejection episodes. Monitoring for acute rejection involves careful daily assessment for changes in clinical condition (e.g., tachycardia, poor feeding, lethargy, arrhythmias, new heart murmurs). Any suspicious change is investigated by an echocardiogram.[12] An increase in LV posterior wall thickness or LV end-diastolic dimension greater than 20%, or a decrease in LV shortening fraction of 20%, is suggestive of rejection. Rejection episodes are treated initially by IV pulsed steroid therapy. Refractory episodes are treated with OKT-3.

If the patient fails to improve or if an elevated plasma renin activity level is identified, endomyocardial biopsy is performed to analyze for humoral or vascular rejection. If immunoglobulin deposits are identified, the immunosuppression therapy may be changed to include cyclophosphamide and plasmapheresis.

REFERENCES ■

1. Keen EN: The postnatal development of the human cardiac ventricles. *J Anat* 1955;89:484
2. Friedman WF: Intrinsic physiological properties of the developing heart. *Prog Cardiovasc Dis* 1972;15:87
3. Butler J, Rocker GM, Westaby S: Inflammatory response to cardiopulmonary bypass. *Ann Thorac Surg* 1993;55:552
4. Gall WE, Clarke WR, Doty DB: Vasomotor dynamics associated with cardiac operations. *J Thorac Cardiovasc Surg* 1982; 83:724
5. Applebaum A, Blackstone E, Kouchoukas N, et al: Afterload reduction and cardiac output in infants early after intracardiac surgery. *Am J Cardiol* 1977;39:445
6. Robinson BW, Gelband H, Mas MS: Selective pulmonary and systemic vasodilator effects of amrinone in children: new therapeutic implications. *J Am Coll Cardiol* 1993;21:1461
7. Hickey PR, Hansen DD, Wessel DL, et al: Blunting of stress responses in the pulmonary circulation of infants by fentanyl. *Anesth Analg* 1985;64:1137
8. Wessel DL, Anand KJS, Hickey PR: Catecholamine and hemodynamic responses to hypercarbia in infants. *Anesthesiology* 1988;69:A780
9. Frostell C, Fratacci MD, Wain JC, et al: Inhaled nitric oxide: a selective pulmonary vasodilator reversing hypoxic pulmonary vasoconstriction. *Circulation* 1991;83:2038
10. Fratacci M, Frostell CG, Chen T, et al: Inhaled nitric oxide: a selective pulmonary vasodilator of heparin-protamine vasoconstriction in sheep. *Anesthesiology* 1991;75:990
11. Beaudry M, Dufour R, Marcoux S: Relation between infant feeding and infections during the first six months of life. *J Pediatr* 1995;126:191
12. Gidding SS, Holzman G, Duffy CE, et al: Usefulness of LV inflow Doppler in predicting rejection in pediatric cardiac transplant patients. *J Am Coll Cardiol* 1992;19(Suppl A): 147A

Critical Care, Third Edition, edited by Joseph M. Civetta,
Robert W. Taylor, and Robert R. Kirby.
Lippincott-Raven Publishers, Philadelphia, PA © 1997.

CHAPTER 77

■

Vascular Surgery and Trauma

Enrique Ginzburg
James M. Hurst
Richard J. Fowl

IMMEDIATE CONCERNS ■

MAJOR PROBLEMS

The major problems involving vascular patients in the ICU
setting can be divided into problems in the acute phase and
chronic phase.

The acute postoperative problems include hypertension,
pain control, bleeding, and graft thrombosis. Chronic phase
problems include wound/graft infections, extremity edema,
and nerve injury with or without neurologic deficits, depending on the type of injuries or reconstruction.

STRESS POINTS

1. The most common causes of postoperative bleeding
   include overdose of anticoagulants and inadequate surgical technique.
2. Common causes of early graft thrombosis are anastomotic stenosis, intimal flap, and twisting or kinking of
   the bypass graft.
3. The most common organisms in skin wound infections
   after vascular reconstruction are *Staphylococcus aureus*
   and *Staphylococcus epidermidis.*
4. Graft infection is a serious condition occurring during
   the time of graft implantation or soon after from hematogenous seeding from a wound or the urinary system,
   or from intravenous catheter sepsis. Early removal of
   catheters is, therefore, encouraged.
5. Pain control is always a problem in postoperative
   patients; however, if patients are given too much analgesia, hypotension can result in thrombosis of an en-
   darterectomized vessel or graft. The use of patient-

controlled analgesia provides an excellent modality for
pain control.
6. Hypertension in postoperative vascular patients should
   be treated because it can aggravate suture line bleeding and cause cardiac decompensation in these patients who often have cardiac compromise.
7. Any change in neurologic status in postoperative patients should be brought to the surgeon's attention
   because this may reflect a stroke after carotid endarterectomy or hemorrhage after anticoagulation.

INITIAL THERAPY

1. *Bleeding*—Correction of anticoagulation or a coagulopathy and reexploration are the only options.
2. *Graft Thrombosis*—Surgical thrombectomy is indicated in the acute phase. Thrombolytic therapy in
   acute arterial thrombosis is therapeutic and diagnostic
   as long as limb-threatening ischemia is not present.
3. *Wound Infection*—Once the diagnosis has been made,
   intravenous antibiotics should be instituted. Failure
   to treat a skin infection can result in graft infection,
   thrombosis, possible limb loss, or even death.
4. *Graft Infection*—For the most part, graft infections
   require removal of the infected graft with need for
   an extraanatomic bypass. Long-term antibiotics with
   replacement of grafts in situ after extensive debridement of the tissues and vessels have proven to be
   effective in selected patients.
5. *Hypertension*—Hypertension should be treated aggressively with nitroprusside, labetalol, or both. They
   offer short half-lives, which permits easy control.
6. *Neurologic Deficit*—The patient should be emergently

reexplored if a neurologic deficit occurs shortly after carotid endarterectomy.

ESSENTIAL DIAGNOSTIC TESTS AND PROCEDURES

1. *Baseline Examination of Extremities*—Baseline examination of extremities distal to reconstruction should be obtained on admission to the ICU. After aortic reconstructions, palpable pulses may not be evident for 6 to 12 hours until the patient becomes normothermic.
2. *Bleeding*—A coagulation profile should be attained; however, persistent tachycardia, hypotension, and low pulmonary artery occlusion pressures that fail to improve with fluid boluses reflect hemorrhage that should be treated surgically.
3. *Graft Thrombosis*—Disappearance of a palpable pulse or audible Doppler signal that was present on arrival to the ICU designates graft thrombosis until proven otherwise. Duplex scan, if available, may demonstrate this finding; however, angiography is the "gold standard."
4. *Wound Infection*—The first sign of infection is expanding erythema, which can proceed to a fluctuant and purulent collection, suggesting a deep infection.
5. *Neurologic Deficit*—A patient who develops a neurologic deficit in the ICU after carotid endarterectomy should be promptly returned to the operating room for immediate reexploration. Valuable time should not be wasted obtaining other unnecessary diagnostic tests.

PRINCIPLES OF INTENSIVE CARE FOR THE VASCULAR PATIENT ■

CLINICAL FEATURES OF PATIENTS WITH ATHEROSCLEROTIC VASCULAR DISEASE

Atherosclerotic vascular disease is usually an affliction of older persons. Many patients have several chronic medical disorders that directly affect the postoperative management. In our experience, the incidence rates of major risk factors are as follows: tobacco use, 57%; hypertension, 52%; cardiac disease, 32%; diabetes, 22%; chronic obstructive pulmonary disease, 10%; renal failure, 6%; and hyperlipidemia, 5%. Careful management of all associated illnesses during the patient's stay in the ICU is mandatory.

CIRCULATION ASSESSMENT

Baseline examination of the extremities distal to the reconstruction should be obtained when the patient arrives in the ICU. The presence or absence of a palpable pulse or audible Doppler signal in the feet or wrists should be noted. If absent, the next higher level should be examined (i.e., popliteal, femoral, and brachial). Using the Doppler, the blood pressure at the ankle should be measured and compared with the brachial pressure as a ratio (ankle–brachial index). This index should be compared with the preoperative value.

In most cases, it is improved immediately after revascularization. Initially, after aortic or extraanatomic reconstructions, palpable distal pulses may be absent because of vasoconstriction from hypothermia. A Doppler signal will be audible in the feet once the patient becomes normothermic (usually within 6 to 8 hours). If pulses or Doppler signals remain absent 4 hours postoperatively, the surgeon should be notified. For upper extremity or infrainguinal reconstructions, a Doppler signal is usually audible in the wrist or foot in the immediate postoperative period. A signal should always be present at the level of the distal anastomosis for all reconstructions. If there is any doubt about the adequacy of the circulation, the surgeon must be informed to determine if further evaluation, such as arteriography, or immediate reoperation is indicated.

CARDIAC MONITORING

Cardiac-related complications are the primary cause of perioperative and late deaths after vascular reconstructive procedures. In a review of data on 1000 patients undergoing routine coronary angiography before peripheral vascular reconstruction, Hertzer and coworkers[1] discovered 92% had coronary artery disease, with 60% demonstrating advanced disease. More importantly, 45% had no clinical symptoms of coronary artery disease before angiography. Eighty-six percent of asymptomatic patients had coronary artery disease. Thirty-seven percent demonstrated advanced disease.

In 1977, Goldman and associates[2] developed a set of risk factors that are helpful in assessing patients for cardiovascular risk (Tables 77-1 and 77-2). We believe that patients who have between 13 and 26 points require perioperative invasive monitoring to undergo a successful surgical procedure.

Because these patients are at high risk for developing cardiac complications, cardiac monitoring assumes a central role in the perioperative management. Patients with compromised ventricular function deserve extensive invasive hemodynamic monitoring, which implies both arterial and pulmonary artery catheter monitoring plus the calculation of direct and derived variables.[3] In so doing, precise fluid management may be undertaken during a difficult procedure. This is particularly important considering that extensive retroperitoneal dissections may cause massive third-space losses of fluid resulting in tremendous volume shifts.

HYPERTENSION MANAGEMENT

Because many patients with extensive cardiovascular disease may be on long-term antihypertensive therapy, their blood pressure must be maintained at a physiologically normal level. Although it is unwise to discontinue beta-blockers or calcium channel blockers in the preoperative period, adequate perfusion to the central nervous system and the coronary arteries must be maintained during anesthesia and the early postoperative period. The most convenient way of managing hypertensive crises is the infusion of drugs that have a rapid onset of action and a short half-life. Sodium nitroprusside meets these requirements. It can be used as a continuous infusion and titrated to the desired physiologic effect. Because the drug is metabolized in the liver and

TABLE 77-1. Computation of the Cardiac Risk Index

CRITERIA	POINTS
1. History	
A. Age >70 y	5
B. MI in previous 6 mo	10
2. Physical examination:	
A. S_3 gallop or JVD	11
B. Important VAS	3
3. Electrocardiogram:	
A. Rhythm other than sinus or PACs on last preoperative ECG	7
B. >5 PVCs/min documented at any time before operation	7
4. General status:	
Po_2 <60 or Pco_2 >50 mm Hg, K <3.0 or HCO_3 <20 mEq/L, BUN >50 or Cr >3.0 mg/dL, abnormal SGOT, signs of chronic liver disease or patient bedridden from noncardiac causes	3
5. Operation:	
A. Intraperitoneal, intrathoracic or aortic operation	3
B. Emergency operation	4
Total possible	53 points

MI, myocardial infarct; JVD, jugular venous distention; VAS, valvular aortic stenosis; PACs, premature atrial contractions; ECG, electrocardiogram; PVCs, premature ventricular contractions; BUN, blood urea nitrogen; Cr, creatinine; SGOT, serum glutamic oxaloacetic transaminase.

Goldman L, Caldera DL, Nussbaum SR, et al: Multifactorial index of cardiac risk in noncardiac surgical procedures. *N Engl J Med* 1977;297:845.

excreted by the kidneys, patients who require prolonged therapy and have abnormal renal or liver function should be monitored for thiocyanate and cyanide toxicity. However, short-term use is safe.

Patients with ischemic coronary artery disease may have the potential for a "coronary steal" phenomenon when given nitroprusside. Therefore, the drug of choice in such patients may be intravenous nitroglycerin. Treatment may be initiated as an intravenous infusion (with special intravenous administration sets to preclude inactivation) with a starting dose of 0.1 μg/kg/minute titrated to physiologic effect. Intravenous nitroglycerin is a drug that has a wide therapeutic margin and has been effective in such cases.

Because of their long half-lives, use of beta-adrenergic blockers may be ill advised. Drugs such as hydralazine, which may cause reflex tachycardia, are not recommended in patients with ischemic heart disease. The drug labetalol is a combined, nonselective antagonist of both alpha- and beta-adrenergic receptors. This drug may be given as either a bolus or continuous intravenous infusion. It is rapidly metabolized by the liver with an elimination time of approximately 3 to 7 hours. Initial doses should begin with the administration of 20 mg infused intravenously over 2 minutes. Repeat injections of 40 to 80 mg may be given every 10 minutes until a maximum dose of 300 mg has been given. Because

of the extended half-life, careful titration is necessary to avoid untoward side effects.

Angiotensin-converting enzyme inhibitors such as enalapril can be safely administered intravenously. In patients with myocardial compromise, enalapril has the added advantage of decreasing systemic vascular resistance. The calcium channel blocker nifedipine is effective in treating not only chronic hypertension but also hypertensive emergencies and angina. In addition to a decrease in systemic vascular resistance (systemic arterial pressure), there is augmentation of cardiac output, stroke volume, and stroke volume index. Another agent that has facilitated the management of hypertensive crises, particularly in patients on chronic beta-blocker therapy, is esmolol. This beta-adrenergic blocker has rapid onset of action, is rapidly metabolized, and, therefore, is quickly cleared from the peripheral circulation when treatment is stopped. The initial dosage guidelines include a loading dose of 500 μg/kg over 1 minute followed by a continuous infusion of 50 μg/kg. The desired physiologic endpoint may be achieved by increasing the infusion by 50 μg/kg every 5 minutes until a maximum dose of 350 μg/kg has been reached or until the desired physiologic endpoint has been reached.

In general, the dosages of drugs metabolized by the liver should be reduced when used with H_2 receptor antagonists, specifically cimetidine. This drug may increase the blood levels of the various antihypertensive agents because of decreased hepatic metabolism. An oral antihypertensive medication should be resumed as soon as possible after gastrointestinal function has returned.

RESPIRATORY MANAGEMENT

Most patients can be extubated in the early postoperative period. Prophylactic ventilatory support does not reduce hospital stay or respiratory complications. Therefore, patients meeting appropriate institutional criteria should be extubated as early as possible. In general, a mode of ventilatory support that provides decreased inspiratory and expiratory work of breathing, as well as the lowest mean airway pressure possible, should be used for these patients.

PAIN MANAGEMENT

Management of pain in elderly patients undergoing vascular reconstructions is of paramount importance. Because these patients may poorly tolerate the alpha-blockade effects of

TABLE 77-2. Assessment of Risk Based on Point Value from the Goldman Index°

POINTS	ASSESSMENT
<13 points	No increased risk
13–26 points	Requires invasive monitoring
>26 points	Correction of life-threatening lesion only
28 of 53 points	Correctable preoperatively

°See Table 77-1.

potent long-acting narcotics such as morphine, short-acting drugs (i.e., fentanyl), which have fewer alpha-blockade side effects than morphine, should be used.

The availability of pain control services in many larger centers has increased the availability of techniques such as continuous epidural analgesia. Use of these modalities will, in many cases, avoid the use of narcotics, particularly in the elderly patient population. These techniques can be safely used in the ICU setting as well as on hospital floors with minimum complications. Patient-controlled analgesia devices permit self-administration of analgesics. Although morphine is often used, doses are usually much smaller so that side effects are less common. Early administration of small doses when pain is just beginning seems to take less drug and to prevent concomitant anxiety caused by delay in obtaining medication, which makes subsequent pain relief more difficult.

PROBLEMS COMMON TO ALL VASCULAR RECONSTRUCTIONS ■

BLEEDING

Incidence

Major bleeding after most types of vascular reconstruction is uncommon.

Etiology

Common causes for postoperative bleeding, regardless of the operative location, include anticoagulant overdose, improperly ligated venous or arterial branches, and leakage from the arterial suture line.[4,5]

Diagnosis

Often, the first manifestation of wound bleeding is a blood-soaked dressing. This should be removed and the wound inspected. If skin edges are the source, there is usually minimal swelling of the wound and the bleeding site can be visualized. If the source is from the deep tissues, there is usually a moderate to massive degree of swelling. Large neck wound hematomas may produce respiratory distress requiring intubation.

Intraabdominal bleeding is suggested by the presence of tachycardia, hypotension, and low pulmonary artery occlusion pressures that fail to improve after fluid boluses. A measurable increase in abdominal girth is a late finding, detectable only after 2 to 3 L of blood have accumulated. Generally, if a patient receives 2 units of packed cells over a 2- to 3-hour period and fails to stabilize, significant bleeding is suggested. Significant bleeding from an anastomosis in the groin may dissect into the retroperitoneum, producing similar findings.

A coagulation profile should be obtained to rule out overdose of anticoagulants as a cause. The surgeon should be notified immediately about any bleeding complication.

Therapy

Skin edge bleeding may be controlled by compression, cautery with a silver nitrate stick, or with nylon sutures. Small wound hematomas may be observed. Large hematomas should be evacuated in the operating room. For intraabdominal bleeding, fluids and blood should be administered to correct hypotension. If profound hypotension and rapid tachycardia develop and there is no evidence for a cardiac cause or hypocoagulability, immediate reexploration is indicated. Anticoagulant overdose of should be treated with protamine sulfate (0.5 to 1 mg protamine per 100 units of heparin given intraoperatively) and fresh frozen plasma.

GRAFT THROMBOSIS

Incidence

The incidence rates of early postoperative graft thrombosis after various arterial reconstructive procedures are as follows: subclavian/vertebral, 2%[6]; aortic, 3%[7]; axillofemoral, 2% to 25%[8]; femorofemoral, 0% to 13%[8]; femoropopliteal, 5% to 15%[9]; and femorotibial, 15% to 30%.[9]

Etiology

The most common cause of early graft thrombosis is technical error. Common errors are anastomotic stenosis, intimal flap, and twisting or kinking of the graft. Other causes include stenosis or occlusion of distal outflow vessels, low cardiac output, graft compression, and a small-diameter vein graft (infrainguinal reconstructions).[5,9,10] A rare cause of early graft failure is a coagulation abnormality producing a hypercoagulable state such as antithrombin III deficiency, protein S or C deficiency, abnormal platelet aggregation, or abnormal plasminogen.[11] For infrainguinal reconstructions, prosthetic grafts are more prone to early thrombosis than vein grafts.[12]

Diagnosis

Disappearance of a distal pulse palpable when the patient first arrives in the ICU suggests graft thrombosis. Disappearance of a previously audible Doppler signal or a change from a biphasic to a monophasic signal also implies graft thrombosis. An ankle–brachial index, which decreases from the initial postoperative value to the preoperative level, is more evidence for graft occlusion. Clinical signs, such as the presence of pallor, mottled skin, and coolness of the extremity, are unreliable in the initial postoperative period. If reoperation for graft limb thrombosis is performed and no cause is discovered, workup for a coagulation abnormality should be performed and should include assay for resistance to activiated protein C, antithrombin III, protein S and C levels, prothrombin time, partial thromboplastin time, fibrinogen level, a platelet aggregation test, and a plasminogen assay.[11]

Therapy

Once the diagnosis of graft occlusion is made, 5000 units of heparin should be given after the surgeon is informed. Thrombectomy and correction of any technical error should then be performed. An additional procedure, such as a distal bypass, may be required to provide adequate outflow.

WOUND INFECTION

Incidence

The incidence rate of this complication is less than 1% after carotid endarterectomy[13] and 4% after aortic reconstructions,[7] with most occurring in the groin incisions.

Etiology

For neck wounds, intraoperative contamination is the most likely cause. For groin infections, possible causes are the presence of *Staphylococcus* in the creases, close proximity of the perineum, and contaminated inguinal lymphatics resulting from infected foot lesions.[14]

Diagnosis

The first sign of infection is expanding erythema around the incision. If untreated, the wound becomes warm, tender, fluctuant, and purulent, which suggests deep infection that may lead to graft infection. The surgeon should be informed when signs of wound infection appear.

Therapy

Once wound erythema appears, treatment should be initiated with intravenous antibiotics effective against *S. aureus*. If a foot infection is present, antibiotic coverage should include agents that are effective against the organisms present in the foot. Oral antibiotics should not be used initially because higher tissue and blood levels are more rapidly obtained with intravenous administration. Failure to treat wound infections aggressively may result in graft infection, which often causes major amputation or death.

GRAFT INFECTION

Incidence

The incidence rates of graft infection for various reconstructions are aortic, less than 1%[7,15]; axillofemoral, 15%[16]; femorofemoral, 5%[17]; and infrainguinal reconstructions, 2.3%.[18] More than three fourths of aortic graft infections occur in the groin.[19,20]

Etiology

Graft contamination generally occurs at the time of implantation. Other factors contributing to graft infection are infected groin lymphatics, wound infection, and hematogenous seeding from a distant infected source such as bladder or soft tissue abscess.[14] Repeat vascular operations for graft thrombosis or false aneurysm repair have also been identified as significant risk factors.[21] A high incidence of *S. epidermidis* contamination of the normal arterial wall has been reported.[22] *S. aureus* and *S. epidermidis* are the most common single organisms found on culture, but often a variety of gram-negative enteric organisms are present.[15,18,23]

Diagnosis

In most cases of infected aortofemoral grafts, clinical findings of infection first appear in the groin. The groin incision may be erythematous, swollen, and tender to palpation; purulent drainage may appear. A false aneurysm was found in 13.5% of patients in one series.[21] If infection is confined to the abdomen, clinical signs are often subtle. The patient may present with malaise, low-grade fever, abdominal or back pain, anorexia, weight loss, and diaphoresis.[15,23] Systemic sepsis, graft occlusion, and septic emboli are less common. Results of laboratory tests such as leukocyte counts and blood cultures are often normal. If a draining sinus is present in a groin incision, contrast sinography is diagnostic for graft infection if the contrast outlines the graft. A computed tomography (CT) scan of the abdomen and pelvis is the most helpful test in diagnosing graft infection. Findings consistent with graft infection include perigraft fluid collections, loss of tissue planes, and perigraft air.[24–27] The major limitation of CT scanning in the early postoperative period is that the presence of perigraft air may be a normal finding up to 6 weeks postoperatively.[28] Indium-111–labeled leukocyte scans have been shown to have an overall accuracy rate of 84% in detecting graft infection but may have up to a 36% false-positive rate.[29]

Infection of extraanatomic (axillofemoral, femorofemoral) and infrainguinal grafts is usually more clinically apparent than that for an aortic graft. Initial signs of infection often appear in an incision and are identical to those for aortofemoral grafts.

Arteriography should be performed in all patients with graft infections to plan further operative therapy. It is not useful diagnostically.

Therapy

Patients with suspected aortic graft infection should be hydrated with intravenous fluids and started on broad-spectrum antibiotics, which should be continued for 10 to 14 days postoperatively. Because these patients often have a prolonged postoperative ileus, we recommend that total parenteral nutrition be started preoperatively or in the immediate postoperative period. Proper operative therapy generally consists of removing the entire infected graft and extraanatomic bypass to revascularize the extremities. If infection is confined to only one groin, then obturator bypass originating from the noninfected graft followed by removal of the infected limb of graft may be appropriate. Postoperatively, these patients are critically ill and require careful ICU monitoring of hemodynamics, fluid status, and ventilation. Prophylaxis against gastrointestinal bleeding is essential, and attention to wound care is important.

For extraanatomic and infrainguinal graft infections, the best treatment is complete graft removal with vascular reconstruction through noninfected tissue planes. If saphenous vein is available, it may be used to replace an infected prosthetic infrainguinal graft. In many cases, vascular reconstruction is impossible and amputation is required.

MANAGEMENT OF SPECIFIC RECONSTRUCTIONS ∎

CAROTID/SUBCLAVIAN RECONSTRUCTIONS

Special Initial Considerations

BLOOD PRESSURE. After carotid endarterectomy, systolic blood pressure should be maintained between 110 and 160 mm Hg. If the patient normally has a low systolic pressure (i.e., 95 to 105 mm Hg), it may be maintained at a lower level. If hypotension develops, this usually responds to a bolus of 500 mL of Ringer's lactate, which may be repeated once. If blood pressure fails to increase, vasopressor agents, such as phenylephrine HCl (Neo-synephrine); initially 0.1 mg/kg/minute may be given as a continuous infusion titrated to an acceptable systolic pressure as long as adequate hydration is maintained.

NEUROLOGIC ASSESSMENT. The patient must have a baseline neurologic examination in the ICU. Narcotic pain medications should be used carefully because they may alter the neurologic examination.

ANTIPLATELET THERAPY. Because endarterectomy creates a rough, thrombogenic surface within the artery, many surgeons prescribe an antiplatelet agent postoperatively. Aspirin, dyprimadole, and low molecular weight dextran are commonly used agents. However, the effectiveness of these agents in preventing postoperative strokes has not been established.

CHEST RADIOGRAPH. After subclavian artery reconstruction, a chest radiograph should be obtained to rule out a pneumothorax. An elevated hemidiaphragm caused by phrenic nerve injury should be noted.

Problems to Be Anticipated

POSTOPERATIVE STROKE/TRANSIENT ISCHEMIC ATTACK
Incidence. The incidence rate of permanent or transient neurologic deficits after carotid endarterectomy in most series is 2% to 3%.[13,30,31] In a community-wide survey of carotid endarterectomy, Kempczinski and associates[32] report a 5.1% stroke rate.

Etiology. Postoperative neurologic complications are most commonly caused by thrombosis of the internal carotid artery or intracerebral embolism presumably originating from the postendarterectomy arterial surface. Other causes include intracerebral hemorrhage, cerebral hypoperfusion resulting from a myocardial infarction, cardiac arrhythmia, severe bleeding (carotid disruption), and overdosage of antihypertensive medication.[33]

Diagnosis. Any change in the neurologic status of the patient must be immediately brought to the attention of the surgeon. Any deficit that persists is best managed by returning the patient to the operating room immediately and reexploring the carotid artery. If a transient ischemic attack occurs that rapidly resolves, an angiogram is appropriate. A duplex scan in the immediate postoperative period has not always been reliable in our experience.

Therapy. If dense hemiplegia or aphasia develops, the surgeon should be notified immediately and a heparin bolus given intravenously (5000 U). The patient should be promptly returned to the operating room for reexploration. If a transient ischemic attack occurs and an angiogram reveals occlusion of the carotid artery, the patient should also be given heparin and returned to the operating room. If the angiography demonstrates a technical error, revision is required. If the arteriogram is normal, the patient should be returned to the ICU for evaluation of other possible causes for a transient ischemic attack. If arteriography is not readily available, the safest course is to reexplore the patient and, if necessary, obtain an intraoperative arteriogram.

HEADACHE. Headache is a common problem that occurs after carotid endarterectomy. A mild headache on the ipsilateral side may be observed. However, if the patient complains of a progressive increase in the severity of the headache or develops visual changes, vomiting, or an altered mental state, the physician should consider the possibility of an intracerebral hemorrhage. Patients with severe headaches should undergo a head CT scan immediately. If there is evidence of intracranial bleeding, a neurosurgeon should be consulted promptly. Mild headaches may be treated with acetaminophen or aspirin.

NERVE INJURIES
Incidence. In a review of data on 450 patients undergoing carotid endarterectomy, the following incidence rates of nerve injury were noted: recurrent laryngeal, 6.7%; hypoglossal, 5.8%; marginal mandibular, 1.8%; and superior laryngeal, 1.8%.[4] Injury to the phrenic nerve and brachial plexus after subclavian reconstructions occurs in about 1% of patients.[6]

Etiology. Nerve injuries rarely result from transection but usually result from traction, inadvertent clamping, or unskilled use of electrocautery.

Diagnosis. Recurrent laryngeal nerve injuries present as prolonged postoperative hoarseness. Visualization of a paralyzed vocal cord during indirect laryngoscopy is diagnostic. Injury of both recurrent nerves after bilateral carotid endarterectomies may result in upper airway obstruction requiring tracheostomy. Tongue deviation toward the injured side is diagnostic of hypoglossal nerve injury. Marginal mandibular nerve injury is manifest by drooping of the ipsilateral corner of the mouth. Phrenic nerve injury produces elevation of the ipsilateral hemidiaphragm, which may lead to postoperative respiratory distress. Injury of the brachial plexus produces motor and sensory dysfunction of the hand and arm.

Therapy. Because over 80% of nerve impairments completely resolve within 3 months,[4] the best therapy is observation. Brachial plexus transections may sometimes be successfully repaired with microsurgical techniques.

THORACIC DUCT INJURY
Incidence. Thoracic duct injury occurs in slightly more than 3% of cases.[6]

Etiology. Duct injury occurs during dissection and exposure of the vessels.

Diagnosis. In thoracic duct injury, clear, light-yellow fluid persistently drains from the neck incision.

Therapy. If the amount of drainage is small, observation is indicated. A large volume of wound drainage requires reexploration for ligation of the thoracic duct.

Operative Mortality

In specialized centers performing carotid endarterectomy frequently, the operative mortality rate is 1% to 2%.[13,30,31] In a report from a community-wide survey, the overall mortality rate was 2.3%.[32] The most common causes of perioperative deaths are strokes and myocardial infarction. The operative mortality rate for subclavian reconstructions is also 1% to 2%.[6]

MESENTERIC AND RENAL RECONSTRUCTIONS

Special Initial Considerations

FLUID MANAGEMENT. Patients undergoing renal artery revascularizations (especially bilateral reconstructions) often have a large volume deficit and may develop high urinary output (>300 mL/hour) in the initial postoperative period. These patients can easily become dehydrated. Therefore, the volume status should be managed with the aid of a pulmonary artery catheter. Patients with cardiac impairment may require higher pulmonary artery occlusion pressures to optimize cardiac output. Patients undergoing mesenteric revascularizations are also at risk for developing dehydration because of large third-space losses that can occur when ischemic bowel is revascularized. Pulmonary artery catheter monitoring is also helpful in these patients.

HYPERTENSION MANAGEMENT. After renal revascularization, labile blood pressure in the immediate postoperative period is common. For hypertension greater than 180 mm Hg systolic, we titrate the blood pressure between 120 and 160 mm Hg systolic with a nitroprusside drip. The rate of nitroprusside must be increased slowly because hypotension can result if it is infused too rapidly.

Problems to Be Anticipated

RENAL ARTERY GRAFT STENOSIS/THROMBOSIS
Incidence. Graft stenosis occurs in about 2% of cases.[34]

Etiology. Causes of renal graft occlusion or stenosis include twisting, kinking, acute angulation, intimal flap, and anastomotic stenosis.[34]

Diagnosis. Signs of graft stenosis or thrombosis are hypertension, renal failure, or flank pain caused by renal infarction. However, these symptoms and signs may be present when the graft is patent. Conversely, the patient may be normotensive with normal renal function, yet have an occluded graft. If anuria occurs in the presence of adequate hydration after bilateral renal revascularization, the surgeon should be notified immediately. A decision must be made regarding the need for arteriography or reoperation for suspected graft occlusion. Intraarterial digital subtraction angiography can be performed with a smaller volume of contrast, thus avoiding further renal damage. However, digital subtraction angiography may only be able to determine if the renal artery graft is patent and may miss a significant technical error such as an intimal flap or stenosis. If renal artery grafts are widely patent, oliguria is likely caused by acute tubular necrosis. All patients who remain severely hypertensive 3 to 5 days postoperatively should undergo conventional angiography to exclude an anatomic lesion as the cause.

Therapy. If graft stenosis or thrombosis is discovered, the patient should be returned immediately to the operating room for a revision. Acute tubular necrosis should be managed in accordance with the principles outlined in Chapter 143.

INTESTINAL INFARCTION AFTER REVASCULARIZATION
Incidence. In a combined series of 116 patients, the incidence rate of intestinal infarction secondary to graft thrombosis was 5.2%.[35–37]

Etiology. Intestinal infarction is usually caused by acute mesenteric graft thrombosis. Reasons for graft occlusion are similar to those for renal artery grafts.

Diagnosis. Because of sequestration, a marked increase in fluid requirement may be one of the earliest signs of bowel infarction. Other findings include tachycardia, hypotension, marked leukocytosis (white blood cell [WBC] count >20,000/mm^3), and unexplained metabolic acidosis.[38] Once the diagnosis of graft thrombosis with intestinal infarction is suspected, the surgeon should be notified immediately. Arteriography should be performed urgently.

Therapy. If graft thrombosis is confirmed by arteriography, urgent reoperation for thrombectomy and revision of the mesenteric arterial graft is indicated. Bowel resection may also be required. If any bowel appears marginally viable, a second reexploration should be performed 24 hours later to reexamine the intestine.

Operative Mortality

For renal revascularizations alone, the operative mortality rate should be less than 2%.[39,40] If combined with an aortic reconstruction, the mortality rate may be as high as 12%.[41] For mesenteric revascularizations, the combined operative mortality rate in 116 patients from three series was 6.9%.[35-37] Three fourths of the deaths resulted from intestinal infarction.

DIRECT AORTIC RECONSTRUCTIONS

Special Initial Considerations

HEMODYNAMICS. Aortic reconstructions produce marked hemodynamic alterations. Large intraperitoneal fluid shifts also occur. Management is further complicated by the frequent occurrence of impaired cardiac function. Therefore, strict attention to vital signs, urine output, and pulmonary artery catheter measurements is the most important aspect in the initial postoperative period. Systolic blood pressure should generally be maintained between 110 and 160 mm Hg but may vary depending on the patient's usual preoperative blood pressure. Pulse rate should be less than 100 beats per minute. Urine output should be at least 40 mL/hour.

Problems to Be Anticipated

DISTAL EMBOLIZATION
Incidence. The incidence rate of this complication after aortic reconstruction ranges from 0.23% to 11%.[42,43] It is much more common after repair of a ruptured aneurysm.[42]

Etiology. Embolization is thought to result from operative manipulation of the aorta during dissection dislodging intraluminal plaque, which is swept distally by blood flow.[5]

Diagnosis. If a large thrombus occludes a major vessel such as the femoral artery, findings are produced that are similar to an acute graft limb occlusion. Microembolization produces mottling and cyanosis of the toes and skin of the lower legs and feet leading to painful gangrene ("trash foot" syndrome).[44] Livedo reticularis of the extremities and rarely of the scrotum and abdominal wall is another sign of microembolization.[45]

Therapy. If a major vessel becomes occluded, a 5000 U bolus of heparin should be given and the patient returned to the operating room for a thrombectomy. Once microembolization has occurred, no effective medical or surgical therapy exists.[44] Lumbar sympathectomy has been advocated

for this condition to improve blood flow to the skin, which may decrease cutaneous tissue loss.[46]

INTESTINAL ISCHEMIA
Incidence. The most common site of intestinal ischemia after aortic repair is the sigmoid and descending colon. If routine postoperative colonoscopy is performed, the incidence rate is 6%.[47] However, the incidence rate of clinically manifest cases is about 2%.[48] This complication may occur in 60% of patients after repair of ruptured abdominal aortic aneurysms,[49] although most cases are not clinically significant. Small bowel ischemia is much less common, occurring in 0.15% of patients undergoing aortic reconstruction.[50]

Etiology. The left colon is supplied by the inferior mesenteric artery (main supply), the superior mesenteric artery through collaterals from the marginal artery of Drummond, and two hypogastric arteries, which supply the rectum through the middle and superior hemorrhoidal arteries. After aortic reconstruction, one or more of these collateral blood supplies may be excluded from flow. This may lead to colonic mucosal ischemia (mild) or to transmural infarction (severe).

Diagnosis. A high index of suspicion is required to make an early diagnosis, which is essential to prevent death. Patients at greatest risk for developing bowel ischemia are those who undergo repair of a ruptured abdominal aortic aneurysm, have a previously patent inferior mesenteric artery that was ligated intraoperatively, and have no mesenteric Doppler signals present after the aortic reconstruction.[48] The most common symptom is diarrhea, which occurs in 75% of patients. This may be bloody or nonbloody and usually occurs 24 to 48 hours postoperatively, but may occur up to 14 days after operation.[48] Bloody diarrhea is more ominous and requires immediate notification of the surgeon. Other clinical findings include a marked increase in abdominal pain, prolonged ileus with abdominal distention, tachycardia over 120 beats per minute, hypotension, increased fluid requirement to maintain urine output (3 L above the 24-hour maintenance requirement), metabolic acidosis, leukocytosis (WBC count over 20,000/mm³), and thrombocytopenia. Any patient who develops bloody diarrhea or persistent nonbloody diarrhea should undergo flexible colonoscopic examination. Adequate examination should include visualization of the splenic flexure (40 to 50 cm from the anus). If superficial mucosal lesions are discovered on the initial examination, repeat examination should be performed every 24 or 48 hours to be certain that they are not progressing.[47] Other diagnostic studies such as arteriography or barium enema are not helpful.

Therapy. Once ischemic lesions are identified on endoscopic examination, a decision must be made regarding observation or operation. If the lesions appear superficial and involve only the mucosa, it is safe to observe the patient with repeat endoscopic examination and assure adequate volume status and cardiac function. If mucosal ischemia progresses, a colectomy should be performed. If the mucosa appears friable, necrotic, and hemorrhagic, then urgent colectomy, Hartmann's pouch, and end colostomy are required.

ACUTE PANCREATITIS

Incidence. The true incidence of postoperative pancreatitis is unknown, but it was found to occur in 2% of survivors of abdominal aortic aneurysm repair.[51]

Etiology. Proposed etiologies are ischemia from pancreatic emboli[52,53] and mechanical trauma during dissection of the proximal aorta near the left renal vein.[54]

Diagnosis. Postoperative pancreatitis should be suspected in any patient who develops prolonged ileus (>5 days) or exacerbation of abdominal pain with nausea and vomiting after oral feedings begin. Screening tests include serum amylase, lipase, and amylase isoenzyme levels. Abdominal CT scan also may be helpful.

Therapy. Once this diagnosis is made, oral intake should be stopped and parenteral nutrition should be administered through a subclavian catheter. A nasogastric tube is not required if the patient is not vomiting and otherwise has mild symptoms. Once the serum amylase level is normal, oral feedings can be resumed slowly.

ACUTE CHOLECYSTITIS

Incidence. Cholelithiasis discovered during aortic procedures ranges from a rate of 4.9% to 20%.[55,56] About 1% of patients may develop acute acalculous cholecystitis after aortic reconstruction.[57]

Etiology. Acute cholecystitis secondary to gallstones is caused by acute obstruction of the cystic duct by a stone. The etiology of acalculous cholecystitis is less certain, but proposed risk factors include a fasting state during hyperalimentation[58]; massive blood transfusions, which produce a large volume of hemoglobin metabolic products[59]; gallbladder ischemia; chronic illness; respiratory failure[60–62]; and the administration of narcotics.[63]

Diagnosis. Acute postoperative cholecystitis, like the other gastrointestinal complications, is a difficult diagnosis to make. Symptoms most commonly occur 2 to 3 weeks postoperatively.[57,64] Clinical signs include fever, leukocytosis (WBC count >10,000/mm^3), elevated bilirubin, right upper quadrant tenderness, nausea, and vomiting.[61] Patients who develop unexplained right upper quadrant pain, fever, and leukocytosis should undergo an ultrasound examination of the gallbladder. Findings consistent with but not specific for cholecystitis are a distended gallbladder with or without stones, a thickened wall, and sludge or stones.[60] Isotope scanning (HIDA) that fails to visualize the gallbladder is also a nonspecific finding because fasting patients frequently

have a nonvisualizing gallbladder. Therefore, these tests must be interpreted in the context of the clinical findings.

Therapy. Once the diagnosis of cholecystitis is made, percutaneous cholecystostomy, with the patient under local anesthesia if critically ill, should be performed.

AORTOENTERIC FISTULA

Incidence. In a one report, the incidence rate of aortoenteric fistula (AEF) as a complication was less than 1%.[15]

Etiology. Proposed causes of AEF are duodenal or small bowel erosion by an inadequately covered graft, proximal aortic anastomotic false aneurysm, primary graft infection with secondary bowel erosion, and local bowel injury during the initial aortic procedure.[65,66]

Diagnosis. Two thirds of patients with AEF have gastrointestinal bleeding as the initial complaint. Of those who present with bleeding, two thirds bleed acutely (half are massive) and the others have signs of chronic blood loss. Patients with AEF who do not bleed initially present with signs of graft infection.[23] An abdominal CT scan should be performed to evaluate for graft infection (see "Graft Infection"). Upper gastrointestinal endoscopic examination should be performed on all patients with a possible AEF to rule out a more common cause for gastrointestinal bleeding, such as an ulcer. It is often difficult to visualize the fistula. Cautious examination of the third and fourth portion of the duodenum is important because massive bleeding may be initiated. Arteriography should be performed in all stable patients before operation to delineate the arterial anatomy because this may affect the type of operation to be performed. Arteriography is usually not useful as a diagnostic test because active bleeding is required to visualize the fistula.

Therapy. Patients with suspected AEF should be hydrated with intravenous fluids and started on broad-spectrum antibiotics. If bleeding from a suspected AEF is massive, the patient should be taken immediately to the operating room. Operative therapy usually consists of removal of the entire graft and extraanatomic bypass to revascularize the extremities. Postoperatively, these patients are gravely ill. Attention should be directed toward replacement of fluids and blood, prevention of systemic infection and stress ulceration, correction of coagulopathies, and continuous assessment of extremity circulation.

Operative Mortality

For elective aortic reconstructions, the recently reported operative mortality rate is approximately 3%.[7,67] Patients who experience rupture of an abdominal aortic aneurysm have a 20% mortality rate if the rupture is contained, but if it is associated with hypotension and renal failure, the mortality rate exceeds 80%.[67] Considerably higher operative mortality rates can be expected with serious complications such as intestinal ischemia (50%),[48] cholecystitis (50%),[57] and graft infection (15% to 28%).[15,21]

EXTRAANATOMIC RECONSTRUCTIONS (FEMOROFEMORAL, AXILLOFEMORAL BYPASS)

Special Initial Considerations

GRAFT TUNNELS.   After the patient arrives in the ICU, the course of the subcutaneous graft tunnels should be inspected. A palpable pulse should usually be present over the graft, except in obese patients and in those in whom a ringed graft was used. Swelling along the course of the tunnel may be a sign of bleeding.

POSITIONING.   Because these grafts are superficial, the patient should not be allowed to lie on the side where an axillofemoral graft is located. Compressive devices, such as abdominal binders, should not be used.

ARM EXAMINATION.   When an axillofemoral graft has been performed, it is important to palpate for a radial or brachial pulse in the donor arm. If an axillofemoral graft occludes, it is equally important to recheck the arm pulses because graft thrombosis may lead to axillary artery thrombosis.[68] Baseline neurologic examination should be performed to rule out a brachial plexus injury.

Problems to Be Anticipated

BRACHIAL PLEXUS INJURY
Incidence.   Brachial plexus injury is an uncommon complication.

Etiology.   Two possible causes of brachial plexus injury are nerve compression because of retraction and direct nerve trauma from sharp instruments or electrocautery.[10]

Diagnosis.   The most obvious finding is a neurologic deficit in the upper extremity that is observed when the patient awakens from anesthesia. Electromyography defines precisely which nerve roots have been injured.

Therapy.   If nerve injury results from compression by a retractor, the deficit may resolve over a few weeks or months.[68] If the nerve is severed or injured with electrocautery, the prognosis is much worse. Neurosurgical consultation should be obtained.

Operative Mortality

In a recent review, the operative mortality rate for axillofemoral grafts ranged from 2% to 17% and for femorofemoral grafts was none to 6%.[8]

INFRAINGUINAL RECONSTRUCTIONS

Special Initial Considerations

LEG ELEVATION.   Because most patients develop leg swelling after an infrainguinal reconstruction, the extremities should be elevated above the level of the heart for 3 days. Bed rest is recommended during this time.

INFECTION.   In patients with foot infections, a prolonged course of antibiotics (7 to 10 days) is recommended, based on culture and sensitivity data. Patients without infections are given prophylactic antibiotics for 24 hours. Antibiotic coverage is especially important when a prosthetic graft is used in the presence of active infection.

ANTIPLATELET AGENTS.   Because vascular grafts below the inguinal ligament generally have low blood flow, they are at a much higher risk for thrombosis. Therefore, we often use antiplatelet agents such as aspirin or low molecular weight dextran. However, the long-term effectiveness of aspirin in improving graft patency remains controversial.[69,70] Low molecular weight dextran has been shown to be effective in reducing the rate of perioperative graft thrombosis.[71]

Problems to Be Anticipated

LEG EDEMA
Incidence.   Postrevascularization leg edema occurs after 70% to 100% of infrainguinal reconstructions.[72]

Etiology.   Leg edema is caused by lymph formation. Etiologic factors after revascularization include increased arterial pressure within the capillary bed, impaired lymph transport resulting from disruption of lymphatics during dissection, and altered capillary permeability, microperfusion, and autoregulation.[73]

Diagnosis.   When a leg becomes swollen after infrainguinal bypass, correct diagnosis is important. Other important causes of leg swelling after revascularization are deep vein thrombosis (DVT), compartment syndrome, and wound hematoma. With postrevascularization edema, the swelling is confined mainly to the calf and is often markedly improved with leg elevation. There is usually no calf tenderness except near the incision. DVT is clinically difficult to differentiate from lymphedema. Because clinical findings are unreliable, the best tests to diagnose DVT are venous ultrasound imaging or venography. Swelling resulting from a wound hematoma is usually apparent on clinical examination. The swelling is mainly confined to the incision, and discoloration and oozing may be present. Diagnosis of compartment syndrome is discussed later in this chapter.

Therapy.   The best therapy for postrevascularization edema is bed rest and leg elevation. Patients with postoperative DVT should be started on continuous intravenous heparin at a rate that elevates the partial thromboplastin time to approximately two times control. Warfarin should be started and continued 3 to 6 months. Large wound hematomas should be evacuated in the operating room; small hematomas may be observed.

Operative Mortality

The operative mortality rate for infrainguinal reconstructions is less than 3%.[74]

VASCULAR TRAUMA ■

COMMON PROBLEMS OF ALL RECONSTRUCTIONS BECAUSE OF TRAUMA

In general, the same complications that occur after elective vascular reconstructions may also occur after reconstruction for traumatic injuries. The incidence of common major complications in both military and civilian series of vascular injuries is summarized in Table 77-3. The major difference between elective vascular reconstructions and posttraumatic reconstructions is that there are often several associated nonvascular injuries in the trauma victim that may have a more profound effect on the overall prognosis. Therefore, the ICU physician must be aware of potential complications that may arise from injured tissues in proximity to a repaired vascular injury.

ROLE OF ARTERIOGRAPHY IN TRAUMA

Thoracic/Neck Injuries

Arteriography is indicated after blunt chest injuries in patients with chest radiograph findings of widened mediastinum, hemothorax, tracheal deviation, pleural cap, or differences in arm blood pressure greater than 20 mm Hg. The most common vascular injury to be concerned about is a tear in the descending thoracic aorta, which can be rapidly fatal if not detected and repaired promptly. Patients who present with any history of a neurologic deficit after blunt neck trauma should undergo arteriography. It may also be appropriate to obtain an arteriogram on patients who have sustained a hyperextension injury to the neck (i.e., head hitting a windshield). These patients may have a carotid dissection, which is often asymptomatic initially but may cause an acute stroke several hours or days after injury.

TABLE 77-3. Incidence of Complications After Vascular Trauma

COMPLICATION	MILITARY[87] (%)	CIVILIAN[88] (%)
Thrombosis	19.3	5.2
Bleeding	4.6	2.0
Graft infection		3.1
Amputation	6.2	1.8
Death	1.7	10.4

Most penetrating injuries to the chest are not amenable to arteriography because patients who have a major vascular injury are often hemodynamically unstable and require urgent operation. However, patients with upper mediastinal injuries may develop false aneurysms, occlusions of the aortic arch vessels, or both, and all hemodynamically stable patients with injury to this area should undergo arteriography. For penetrating neck injuries, we recommend arteriography in all stable patients no matter where the injury is located. However, others believe that penetrating injuries in the area between the clavicle and the angle of the mandible (zone II) that require operative exploration do not always need arteriography, because injuries to the carotid artery in this area can be easily identified during exploration.[75] Injuries at the base of the neck (zone I) and above the angle of the mandible (zone III) require arteriography provided the patient is stable.

Extremity Injuries

The main indication for obtaining an arteriogram after blunt or penetrating extremity trauma is the *absence of a palpable pulse* distal to the injury. It may also be appropriate to obtain an arteriogram, despite the presence of a palpable pulse, with bullet wounds near a major vessel because false aneurysms and intimal injuries may still be present, although they may not require surgical repair. If an arteriogram is not obtained initially, the distal pulses must be carefully monitored. If pulses disappear later, arteriography is mandatory to rule out arterial thrombosis. We have used duplex scanning to evaluate arteries and veins that were near the site of injury in patients with palpable pulses who did not undergo immediate arteriography. We have found this technique to be reliable and believe it may replace arteriography in evaluating proximity injuries, provided there is a state-of-the-art duplex scanner and an experienced vascular technologist available. However, if there is any doubt about the presence of an extremity vascular injury, the safest course is to obtain an arteriogram.

MANAGEMENT OF SPECIFIC VASCULAR INJURIES ■

AORTA AND ITS MAJOR BRANCHES

Great Vessels

Injuries to the brachiocephalic vessels are often associated with injuries to other vital structures such as the trachea and esophagus. The major problem of associated injuries to these structures is that there is an increased risk for developing infection in the mediastinum. If this occurs, a repaired great vessel injury is more susceptible to infection, which may result in arterial disruption and exsanguination. Therefore, the ICU team should watch for signs of mediastinitis, subcutaneous emphysema, and pneumothorax in the postoperative period after repair of a great vessel injury. The surgeon should be notified promptly if such signs develop. Broad-spectrum antibiotics active against both gram-positive and gram-negative aerobes and anaerobes should be started. Drainage of the mediastinum may be required. Patients who sustain injuries to the brachiocephalic arteries may develop other complications, such as neurologic events, hemorrhage, graft infection, and graft thrombosis. Such complications should be managed as previously described for elective carotid and subclavian reconstructions.

Thoracic Aorta

Injuries to the thoracic aorta usually result in massive blood loss. Multiple problems including adult respiratory distress syndrome, renal failure, paraplegia, coagulopathy, and complications of pulmonary and cardiac contusions are common. Postoperative bleeding should be anticipated and is usually diagnosed by increased bloody drainage from the chest tubes. In patients with blunt injury, approximately half will have associated major abdominal, lung, or brain injuries, which are the major cause of morbidity and mortality after successful repair of the aorta.[76] Prolonged ICU support with careful attention to the management of ventilation, fluids, and coagulopathy is required. The mortality rate for those who survive the initial injury and undergo operation is about 20%.[76]

Abdominal Aorta and Branches

Trauma to the abdominal aorta and any of its major intraabdominal branches usually results in massive blood loss. The patient is often taken to the operating room in extremis. These patients are at high risk for developing multisystem organ failure postoperatively. One of the most significant problems is bacterial contamination from concomitant injuries to the gastrointestinal tract. This becomes a critical problem in patients who require a prosthetic graft to repair the aorta or its branch vessels. In general, most surgeons avoid prosthetic vascular grafts in patients with abdominal vascular injuries and bowel contamination because of the risk of infection. In some situations such as an extensive injury to the suprarenal aorta, a prosthetic graft may be the only alternative. Infection of a suprarenal aortic graft is often fatal because graft removal and reconstruction are difficult. Graft infection of the infrarenal aorta is diagnosed and treated, as described previously, for elective aortic reconstructions. Infection of smaller grafts (renal, iliac) should be treated by graft removal and replacement with autogenous vein, extraanatomic bypass, or removal of the end organ (nephrectomy). The overall mortality rate for abdominal aortic injuries is about 60% to 70%.[77,78] The mortality rate for visceral and renal artery injuries is approximately 40%.[79]

EXTREMITY INJURIES

Arteriovenous Fistulas and False Aneurysms

These two complications most commonly occur after a penetrating injury to an extremity.[80] These complications may develop days to years after an injury and may be missed during operative exploration. Therefore, the physician should look for signs of an arteriovenous fistula or false aneurysm while the patient is in the ICU. Clinical findings are the presence of a bruit or thrill over the injured area. A pulsatile mass may also be present. With large arteriovenous fistulas, high-output cardiac failure may result. When these problems are suspected, the best test to confirm the diagnosis is arteriography. Generally, false aneurysms and arteriovenous fistulas should be repaired surgically, provided the patient is stable enough to undergo operation.

Fractures and Arterial Injuries

The incidence rate of fractures associated with arterial injuries ranges from about 10% in the civilian population to nearly 30% for military wounds.[81,82] When the patient with an arterial injury associated with a fracture is admitted to the ICU, care must be taken to keep the limb immobilized. Any forceful movement of the extremity may disrupt the bone alignment and the vascular repair, resulting in arterial thrombosis or possibly severe hemorrhage. The circulation must be assessed hourly, as described previously for elective reconstructions. Any change in the circulation requires notification of the vascular surgeon.

Venous Injuries

The incidence rate of venous injuries associated with arterial injuries in Vietnam was 37.7%.[82] In a civilian series of patients with vascular injuries, the incidence rate of venous injuries was 22%.[83] When a patient returns from the operating room after repair of an extremity with a venous injury, the ICU team must determine how the injury was managed. Careful observation for signs of a compartment syndrome is mandatory if a major deep vein is ligated. If the vein has been repaired, thrombosis may still occur, resulting in a compartment syndrome. Development of marked calf tenderness and swelling are the first signs of this complication. To enhance venous blood flow, the legs should be elevated. Application of pneumatic compression boots over the extremity also facilitates venous return. If the patient has no other serious injuries, we recommend starting heparin as soon as possible after all major venous injuries.

Bullet Embolism

Bullet embolism is an unusual complication that can result from a bullet that penetrates the aorta and is carried distally until it occludes a small artery.[84] Bullet embolism should be considered in any patient who sustains a gunshot wound where no exit wound is present and the bullet cannot be found on radiographs of the injured area. A thorough examination of the extremities is important; a limb with clinical signs of acute arterial thrombosis suggests the location of the bullet. Radiographs of all extremities should be performed until the bullet is located, and an arteriogram should be obtained to identify its location in the arterial tree. The bullet should then be surgically removed.

Compartment Syndrome

Development of this complication occurs after a variety of conditions including arterial emboli (2%), arterial injuries

(32%), venous injuries (14%), and massive soft tissue injury (19%).[85] Compartment syndrome usually occurs when a limb is subjected to an acute ischemic event. Once arterial flow is restored, tissue permeability increases, which results in increased pressure within the fascia-lined muscle compartments of the extremity. Elevated compartment pressure above 30 mm Hg results in nerve and muscle damage. If this pressure is not relieved, nerve damage will occur within minutes and will become permanent within 8 to 12 hours. Muscle death begins within 4 hours and becomes maximal at 12 hours. Early signs of a developing compartment syndrome are fullness over an extremity with pain on palpation, paresthesia, weakness of the involved muscles, and diminished pulses. Paralysis, loss of sensation, and absent pulses are late findings that occur coincident with irreversible muscle necrosis. Patients who show signs of a compartment syndrome should undergo compartment pressure measurements. This involves inserting a catheter into the involved muscle compartment, which is connected to a pressure transducer. If the compartment pressure is over 40 mm Hg, a fasciotomy should be performed. If the pressure remains between 30 to 40 mm Hg for over 4 hours, a fasciotomy should be performed.[86] Fasciotomy should also be considered in patients with pressures less than 30 mm Hg who have clinical signs of compartment syndrome because no absolute critical pressure exists for every patient.[87]

THROMBOLYTIC THERAPY

Although thrombolytic agents have been available for over 100 years, they have not been used extensively until large trials proved their efficacy in venous thrombosis and pulmonary emboli. The current family of approved thrombolytic agents comprises (in order of evolution) streptokinase (SK), urokinase (UK), and tissue plasminogen activator (tPA). The current incentive for their use in peripheral arterial disease stems from the continued high amputation rate (13%)[88] in patients undergoing surgical intervention for acute limb ischemia.

SK is a single-chain polypeptide with a molecular weight of 47,000 Daltons produced by the hemolytic streptococci bacteria and works by its indirect activation of a SK-plasminogen cofactor. This cofactor converts plasminogen to plasmin, which cleaves fibrin and fibrinogen in the circulating and clot-bound forms.

UK is an enzyme found in normal urine. Because it is not a foreign protein as is SK, it produces less allergic reactions. It acts directly on plasminogen, converting it to plasmin.

tPA is an enzyme produced by vascular endothelium. It is clot specific, binding directly to fibrin (unlike SK and UK) and decreases the risks of systemic bleeding.

INDICATIONS AND CONTRAINDICATIONS

Patients with an acute arterial or graft occlusion who do not exhibit progressive neurologic deficits or deterioration on their physical examination (i.e., pain, pallor, and pulselessness) can be considered good candidates for thrombolytic

therapy (Table 77-4). In many respects, the vascular surgeon must judge the risk to limb viability over the 6 to 18 hours for treatment before deciding on thrombolytic therapy. Any patient with loss of motor function, anesthesia, or muscle rigor (critical ischemia) is a poor thrombolytic candidate and should undergo surgical intervention as soon as possible.[89]

Surgical intervention with prompt revascularization by clot extraction alone or in combination with surgical bypass remains the standard for critical ischemia. However, embolectomy catheters, although they are the standard preferred method for clot extraction, rarely accomplish complete thrombectomy and also carry the risk of endothelial injury, complicating and aggravating an already difficult problem.[90]

Lysis time has also been decreased by using pharmacomechanical methods of administration such as pulsed spray catheters, which could increase the usefulness of thrombolysis in patients with rapidly progressive neurologic signs when surgical embolectomy would currently be advocated. Several newer drugs with theoretical advantages over older drugs such as single-chain UK-type plasminogen activator or KIK2PU are currently undergoing trials.[91]

ADMINISTRATION OF THROMBOLYTICS

Recent refinements in intraarterial fibrinolysis have improved overall results. These constitute placement of the infusion catheter directly into the clot, the use of a multihole catheter for rapid infusion, passage of guide wire through

TABLE 77-4. Thrombolytic Therapy

INDICATIONS

Acute deep venous thrombosis <3 d
Pulmonary embolism—massive
Acute arterial occlusion
Acute arterial graft occlusion

CONTRAINDICATIONS—ABSOLUTE

Stroke—within 2 mo
Coagulopathy/active bleeding
Aortic dissection
Allergy to drug
Intracranial tumor/aneurysm
Intracranial/spinal surgery—within 2 mo

CONTRAINDICATIONS—RELATIVE

Surgery—within 10 d
Organ biopsy—within 10 d
Arterial puncture–within 10 d
GI bleeding—within 6 mo
Trauma within 10 d
Recent trauma
Uncontrolled hypertension
Cardiac thrombus
Severe hepatic or renal failure
Pregnancy
Childhood
Hemorrhagic retinopathy
Vascular graft implanted—within 1 mo
Active duodenal ulcer

GI, gastrointestinal.

the clot, use of adjunctive heparin sodium to prevent re-thrombosis or thrombus formation about the catheter, and new dosage strategies employing stepped-down regimens.[92]

Notice that no large randomized prospective studies have compared indications, doses, or agents, and only certain generalizations can be made.

Urokinase Therapy

Once the catheter is placed in the thrombus, the general rule is to infuse 4000 to 5000 units/minute of UK for 2 to 4 hours and follow with an angiogram to determine early clot lysis. If lysis has begun, the rate of infusion is dropped to 100,000 units/hour.[93] This infusion rate is continued up to 72 hours, although most successful lyses occur within 12 to 16 hours. Heparin sodium at rates of 500 to 800 units/hour are used to prevent pericatheter thrombosis.

Tissue Plasminogen Activator

The usual dosage for intraarterial use of tPA is 10 to 20 mg over 6 hours, and it can be repeated up to four times to lyse clot in peripheral vascular cases.[94] One recent study demonstrated the same success rate and decreased bleeding by administering tPA at 1 mg/hour until lysis was achieved; however, the time until lysis occurred was much longer with the low-dosage regimen.[95]

A 100-mg bolus injection of tPA over 2 hours after a pulmonary embolus documented by right heart strain on echocardiography has improved the mortality rate and decreased the rate of recurrent embolization.[96,97]

Intraoperative Use of Thrombolytics

The use of thrombolytics as an adjunct to surgical embolectomy or bypass is promising, but no consensus has been reached as to drug, dosage, method, or patient selection. One recent study demonstrated excellent results (88% success) of UK with adjunctive percutaneous transluminal angioplasty or surgery.[98] Doses of 50,000 to 100,000 units are infused after thrombectomy, and angiography or angioscopy can be used to ascertain completeness of clot lysis.

COMPLICATIONS

Hemorrhage

Streptokinase has the highest rate of bleeding; the other thrombolytics have mostly minor problems, usually located at the site of catheter puncture. This bleeding occurs in up to 30% to 40% of cases. Although death is rare, it has been reported in selected cases of occult retroperitoneal and intracranial hemorrhage.[99] When bleeding occurs, fibrinolytic therapy should be stopped, unless it occurs around a catheter site, which can be easily controlled with compression until fibrinogen levels can be determined. In fact, fibrinogen level is the only relevant laboratory test in lytic-associated hemorrhage. If serum levels are less than 100 mg/dL, then cryoprecipitate should be used. If this maneuver fails, then epsilon-aminocaproic acid should be administered as a 5-g

intravenous loading dose followed by 1 g/hour for 2 to 4 hours.[100]

Although the use of concomitant heparin sodium may inhibit pericatheter clot formation, it may also increase the risk of bleeding complications.

Allergic Reaction

Allergic reaction occurs in about 12% of patients receiving SK,[101] a foreign protein. Symptoms range from a skin rash to anaphylaxis. Mild allergic reactions are treated with antihistamines and steroids. More severe allergic reactions mandate cessation of SK infusion and treatment with large doses of steroids.

Distal Embolization

Distal embolization occurs in about 2% of patients receiving low-dose intraarterial therapy.[102] The limb develops signs of severe ischemia, such as cyanosis, increasing foot pain, coolness diminished sensation, and impaired motor function. However, increasing the infusion dosage twofold over 1 hour has been reported to resolve the "trashing." If clinical signs do not improve, the surgeon involved should be notified and the thrombolytic therapy discontinued.

Thrombosis at the Catheter Site

A thrombus that had formed around the catheter may become dislodged when the catheter is removed, producing acute arterial thrombosis. These patients require operative thrombectomy.

Bleeding Through a Prosthetic Graft

Extravasation of blood through prosthetic vascular grafts during low-dose intraarterial thrombolytic therapy has been reported.[103] In most instances, this has occurred with newly inserted knitted Dacron aortic grafts,[104] but extravasation also has been reported in a graft that had been in place for 4 years.[105] If extravasation through a graft occurs, a decision needs to be made regarding the risks versus benefits of continued therapy.

Contrast-Induced Renal Failure

Because repeated arteriographic studies are required to monitor the progress of intraarterial therapy, the patient is at risk for developing renal failure. To prevent this complication, adequate hydration should be maintained. Arteriograms should be limited to one per day. The total dose of iodinated contrast agent must be recorded during these serial investigations. Fortunately, if renal failure does occur, it usually reverses after about 2 to 3 weeks.

NEW TRENDS IN THROMBOLYTIC THERAPY

The choice of thrombolytic agent should involve risk–benefit ratios concerned with allergenicity, costs, and success rates. Recent studies have shown that UK, although more expen-

TABLE 77-5. Clinical Properties of Current Agents

	SK	UK	tPA
Half-life (min)	23	16	5
Allergy	↑ ↑ ↑	↑	↑
Drug expense	↑	↑ ↑	↑ ↑ ↑
Total expense ($)	25,900	22,200	25,300
Days (Hosp stay)	21.1	11.5	21.3

SK, streptokinase; UK, urokinase; tPA, tissue plasminogen activator.

From Janosik JE, Bettmann MA, Kaul AF, et al: Therapeutic alternatives for subacute peripheral arterial occlusion: comparison by outcome, length of stay, and hospital charges. *Invest Radiol* 1991;26:921; and Perler BA: Fibrinolytic therapy for acutely thrombosed lower extremity arteries and grafts. In: Ernst CB, Stanley JC. *Current Therapy in Vascular Surgery.* 3rd ed. St. Louis, Mosby-Yearbook, 1995:540.

sive than SK, has approximately the same success rate as surgery with less in-hospital days. The overall costs comparing SK, UK, and surgery are similar (Table 77-5). UK's overall costs are slightly lower, and, as previously stated, UK has less allergic potential. Unfortunately, tPA was not investigated in this study but may prove to be the drug of choice.[106] The combined success rates of UK lytic therapy and tPA or surgery is approximately 88%.[107] Excellent results are found in embolic disease whereas half the success rates are found in chronic thrombosis at 2 years.[94]

The use of thrombolytic agents in DVT and its concomitant use with thrombectomy in phlegmasia cerulea syndromes has shown promise in preservation of venous valve competency and venous physiology. It is best instituted within 10 days of venous thrombosis, before the clot becomes adherent. Anticoagulation with heparin sodium followed by oral anticoagulation with warfarin sodium (Coumadin) for a minimum of 3 months is then advocated.

AORTIC DISSECTION ■

Aortic dissection is the most common emergency involving the aorta and is seen two times more frequently than ruptured aortic aneurysm.[108]

The Stanford classification uses the extent of dissection as criteria differentiating the type A and B lesion. Type A involves the ascending aorta, and type B does not. This reflects the increased torsion and traction that occur in the two areas, the origin of the aorta and the proximal descending portion just distal to the ligamentum arteriosum.

Hypertension and cystic degeneration of the media are major predisposing risk factors. Recently, crack cocaine has been associated with this problem.[109] Interventional vascular procedures have caused iatrogenic aortic dissections.[11] Trauma and Marfan's syndrome are other causes.

DIAGNOSTIC METHODS

Transesophageal echocardiography (TEE) has been shown to have 100% sensitivity and specificity for diagnosis. In one study, however, the ability to identify the Stanford type and entry site was correctly predicted 96% and 89% of the time, respectively, when compared with angiography.[111] TEE allowed concomitant diagnosis of aortic regurgitation, pericardial effusion/tamponade, and even suggested myocardial infarction, which alter the overall management of the patient.

TEE also provides quick bedside, intraoperative, and postoperative diagnostic information and can be used to assess repairs. The concomitant use of magnetic resonance imaging or intravascular ultrasound make the noninvasive approach to diagnosis as accurate as angiography.[112]

MANAGEMENT

The optimal management for type A dissections is surgical, because fatal rupture or cardiac tamponade occurs most commonly and unpredictably with this type of dissection. In addition, the results with surgery are superior to medical therapy.[113]

Medical treatment is instituted in type B distal dissections based on the following observations:

1. Drugs that affect ventricular fiber shortening reduce the impulse (dp/dt) and, with control of blood pressure, reduce the major forces that increase dissection.[114]
2. Recent studies have shown a 93% 5-year survival rate with medical management.[115]
3. Initial treatment requires fast-acting agents such as the combination of nitroprusside to control blood pressure and beta-adrenergic blocker to control dp/dt. Trimethaphan camsylate can be used to keep systolic pressure between 100 and 120 mm Hg; however, systolic blood pressure may have to be reduced to 80 or 90 mm Hg to control the patient's pain. Reserpine can be used to control blood pressure and dp/dt.
4. Beta-blockers or calcium channel blockers administered orally are the drugs of choice for long-term management of surgically repaired or medically managed dissections. Experimental self-expandable intraaortic prosthetics have been deployed intraoperatively or by percutaneous catheter sheaths to close the entry sites of the dissection. Endoluminal intravascular prosthetics have been successful in experimental animals and in human subjects with minimal risks and hold great promise.[116,117]

REFERENCES ■

1. Hertzer N, Beven EG, Young JR, et al: Coronary artery disease in peripheral vascular patients: a classification of 1000 coronary angiograms and results of surgical treatment. *Ann Surg* 1984;199:223
2. Goldman L, Caldera DL, Nussbaum SR, et al: Multifactorial

index of cardiac risk in noncardiac surgical procedures. *N Engl J Med* 1977;297:845

3. Rao TLK, Jacobs KH, El-Etr AA: Reinfarction following anesthesia in patients with myocardial infarction. *Anesthesiology* 1983;59:499

4. Hertzer NR: Postoperative management and complications of extracranial carotid reconstruction. In: Rutherford RB (ed). *Vascular Surgery*, 2nd ed. Philadelphia, WB Saunders, 1984:1300

5. Downs AR: Complications of abdominal aortic surgery. In: Bernhard VM, Towne JB (eds). *Complications in Vascular Surgery*, 2nd ed. Orlando, Grune & Stratton, 1985:25

6. Moore WS: Complications of vertebral and subclavian repair. In: Bernhard VM, Towne JB (eds). *Complications in Vascular Surgery*, 2nd ed. Orlando, Grune & Stratton, 1985:753

7. Szilagyi DE, Elliot JP, Smith RF, et al: A 30-year survey of the reconstructive surgical treatment of aortoiliac occlusive disease. *J Vasc Surg* 1986;3:421

8. Ernst CB: Reoperation for occluded extra-anatomic bypass. In: Bergan JJ, Yao JST (eds). *Reoperative Arterial Surgery*. Orlando, Grune & Stratton, 1986:279

9. Brewster DC: Early complications of vascular repair below the inguinal ligament. In: Bernhard VM, Towne JB (eds). *Complications in Vascular Surgery*, 2nd ed. Orlando, Grune & Stratton, 1985:37

10. Bergan JJ: Complications of extra-anatomic bypass grafting to the lower extremity. In: Bernhard VM, Towne JB (eds). *Complications in Vascular Surgery*, 2nd ed. Orlando, Grune & Stratton, 1985:55

11. Towne JB: Hypercoagulable states and unexplained vascular thrombosis. In: Bernhard VM, Towne JB (eds). *Complications in Vascular Surgery*, 2nd ed. Orlando, Grune & Stratton, 1985:381

12. Kempczinski RF: Infrainguinal arterial bypass using prosthetic grafts. In: Kempczinski RF (ed). *The Ischemic Leg*. Chicago, Year Book Medical Publishers, 1985:437

13. Thompson JE: Complications of carotid endarterectomy and their prevention. *World J Surg* 1979;3:155

14. Bandyk DF: Vascular graft infection: epidemiology, bacteriology, and pathogenesis. In: Bernhard VM, Towne JB (eds). *Complications in Vascular Surgery*, 2nd ed. Orlando, Grune & Stratton, 1985:471

15. O'Hara PJ, Hertzer NR, Beven EG, et al: Surgical management of infected abdominal aortic grafts: review of a 25-year experience. *J Vasc Surg* 1986;3:725

16. Livesay JJ, Atkinson JB, Baker JD, et al: Later results of extra-anatomic bypass. *Arch Surg* 1979;114:1260

17. Plecha FR, Plecha FM: Femorofemoral bypass grafts: 10-year experience. *J Vasc Surg* 1984;1:555

18. Durham JR, Rubin JR, Malone JM: Management of infected infrainguinal bypass grafts. In: Bergan JJ, Yao JST (eds). *Reoperative Arterial Surgery*, Orlando, Grune & Stratton, 1986:359

19. Szilagyi DE, Smith RF, Elliot JP, et al: Infection in arterial reconstruction with synthetic grafts. *Ann Surg* 1972;176:321

20. Goldstone J, Moore WS: Infection in vascular prosthesis: clinical manifestation and surgical management. *Am J Surg* 1974;128:225

21. Reilly LM, Altman H, Lusby RJ, et al: Late results following surgical management of vascular graft infection. *J Vasc Surg* 1984;1:36

22. Macbeth GA, Rubin JR, McIntyre KE, et al: The relevance of arterial wall microbiology to the treatment of prosthetic graft infections: graft infection vs. arterial infection. *J Vasc Surg* 1984;1:750

23. Reilly LM, Goldstone J: The infected aortic graft. In: Bergan JJ, Yao JST (eds). *Reoperative Arterial Surgery*. Orlando, Grune & Stratton, 1986:231

24. Brown OW, Stanson AW, Pairolero PC, et al: Computerized tomography following abdominal aortic surgery. *Surgery* 1982;91:716

25. Haaga JR, Baldwin GN, Reich NE, et al: CT detection of infected synthetic grafts: preliminary report of a new sign. *Am J Roentgenol* 1978;131:317

26. Mark A, Moss AA, Lusby R, et al: CT evaluation of complications of abdominal aortic surgery. *Radiology* 1982;145:409

27. Kukora JS, Rushton FW, Cranston PE: New computed tomographic signs of aortoenteric fistula. *Arch Surg* 1984;119:1073

28. O'Hara PJ, Borkowski GP, Hertzer NR, et al: Natural history of periprosthetic air on computerized axial tomographic examination of the abdomen following abdominal aortic aneurysm repair. *J Vasc Surg* 1984;1:429

29. Brunner MC, Mitchell RS, Baldwin JC, et al: Prosthetic graft infection: Limitations of white blood cell scanning. *J Vasc Surg* 1986;3:42

30. Plecha FR, Avellone JC, Beven EG, et al: A computerized vascular registry: experience of the Cleveland Vascular Society. *Surgery* 1979;86:826

31. Sundt TM Jr, Houser OW, Sharbrough FW, et al: Carotid endarterectomy: results, complications, and monitoring techniques. *Adv Neurol* 1977;16:97

32. Kempczinski RF, Brott TG, Labutta RJ: The influence of surgical speciality and caseload on the results of carotid endarterectomy. *J Vasc Surg* 1986;3:911

33. Imparato AM, Riles TS, Lamparello PJ, et al: The management of TIA and acute strokes after carotid endarterectomy. In: Bernhard VM, Towne JB (eds). *Complications in Vascular Surgery*, 2nd ed. Orlando, Grune & Stratton, 1985:725

34. Dean RH: Complications of renal revascularization. In: Bernhard VM, Towne JB (eds). *Complications in Vascular Surgery*, 2nd ed. Orlando, Grune & Stratton, 1985:229

35. Reul GJ Jr, Wukosch DC, Sandiford FM, et al: Surgical treatment of abdominal angina: review of 25 patients. *Surgery* 1974;75:682

36. Stoney RJ, Ehrenfeld WK, Wylie EJ: Revascularization methods in chronic visceral ischemia caused by atherosclerosis. *Ann Surg* 1977;186:468

37. Hollier LH, Bernatz PE, Pairolero PC, et al: Surgical management of chronic intestinal ischemia: a reappraisal. *Surgery* 1981;90:940

38. Stoney RJ, Olcott C IV: Visceral artery syndromes and reconstructions. *Surg Clin North Am* 1979;59:637

39. Lawrie GM, Morris GC Jr, Soussou ID, et al: Late results of reconstructive surgery for renovascular disease. *Ann Surg* 1980;191:528

40. Stanley JC, Whitehouse WM Jr, Graham LM, et al: Operative therapy of renovascular hypertension. *Br J Surg* 1982;69 (Suppl):S63

41. Dean RH, Keyser JE III, Dupont WD, et al: Aortic and renal vascular disease: factors affecting the value of combined procedures. *Ann Surg* 1984;200:336

42. Starr DS, Lawrie GM, Morris GC: Prevention of distal embolization during arterial reconstruction. *Am J Surg* 1979; 138:764

43. May AG, DeWeese JA, Frank I, et al: Surgical treatment of abdominal aortic aneurysms. *Surgery* 1968;63:711

44. Bernhard VM, Towne JB: Complications in vascular surgery. In: Moore WS (ed). *Vascular Surgery: A Comprehensive Review*. New York, Grune & Stratton, 1983:737

45. Kempczinski RF: Atheroembolism. In: Kempczinski RF (ed). *The Ischemic Leg*. Chicago, Year Book Medical Publishers, 1985:81

46. Mehigan JT, Stoney RJ: Lower extremity atheromatous embolization. *Am J Surg* 1976;132:163
47. Ernst CB, Hagihara PF, Daughtery ME, et al: Ischemic colitis incidence following abdominal aortic reconstruction: a prospective study. *Surgery* 1976;80:417
48. Ernst CB: Intestinal ischemia following abdominal aortic reconstruction. In: Bernhard VM, Towne JB (eds). *Complications in Vascular Surgery*, 2nd ed. Orlando, Grune & Stratton, 1985:325
49. Hagihara PF, Ernst CB, Griffen WO Jr: Incidence of ischemic colitis following abdominal aortic reconstruction. *Surg Gynecol Obstet* 1979;149:571
50. Johnson WC, Nabseth DC: Visceral infarction following aortic surgery. *Ann Surg* 1974;180:312
51. Warshaw AL, O'Hara PJ: Susceptibility of the pancreas to ischemic injury in shock. *Ann Surg* 1978;188:197
52. Castleman B, Scully RE, McNeely BU: Case records of the Massachusetts General Hospital. *N Engl J Med* 1967;277:703
53. Castleman B, Scully RE, McNeely BU: Case records of the Masschusetts General Hospital. *N Engl J Med* 1972;286:422
54. McIntyre KE, Bernhard VM: Gastrointestinal problems following aortic surgery. In: Bergan JJ, Yao JST (eds). *Reoperative Arterial Surgery*. Orlando, Grune & Stratton, 1986:207
55. Ouriel K, Ricotta JJ, Adams JT, et al: Management of cholelithiasis in patients with abdominal aortic aneurysm. *Ann Surg* 1983;198:717
56. String ST: Cholelithiasis and aortic reconstruction. *J Vasc Surg* 1984;1:664
57. Ouriel K, Green RM, Ricotta JJ, et al: Acute acalculous cholecystitis complicating abdominal aortic aneurysm resection. *J Vasc Surg* 1984;1:646
58. Peterson SR, Sheldon GF: Acute acalculous cholecystitis: a complication of hyperalimentation. *Am J Surg* 1979;138:814
59. Lindberg EF, Grinnan GLB, Smith L: Acalculous cholecystitis in Vietnam casualties. *Ann Surg* 1970;171:152
60. Gately JF, Thomas EJ: Acute cholecystitis occurring as a complication of other diseases. *Arch Surg* 1983;118:1137
61. Long TN, Heimbach DM, Carrico CJ: Acalculous cholecystitis in critically ill patients. *Am J Surg* 1978;136:31
62. Thompson JW III, Ferris DO, Boggenstoss AH: Acute cholecystitis complicating operation for other disease. *Ann Surg* 1962;155:489
63. Joehl RJ, Koch KL, Nahrwold OL: Opioid drugs cause bile duct obstruction during hepatobiliary scans. *Am J Surg* 1984;147:134
64. Ottinger LW: Acute cholecystitis as a postoperative complication. *Ann Surg* 1976;184:162
65. Bunt TJ: Synthetic vascular graft infections. II. Graft-enteric erosions and graft-enteric fistulas. *Surgery* 1983;94:1
66. Kleinman LH, Towne TB, Bernhard VM: A diagnostic and therapeutic approach to aortoenteric fistulas: clinical experience with 20 patients. *Surgery* 1979;86:868
67. Rutherford RB: Infrarenal aortic aneurysms. In: Rutherford RB (ed). *Vascular Surgery*, 2nd ed. Philadelphia, WB Saunders, 1984:755
68. Kempczinski RF, Penn I: Upper extremity complications of axillofemoral grafts. *Am J Surg* 1978;136:209
69. Kohler TR, Kaufman JL, Kacoyanis G, et al: Effect of aspirin and dipyridamole on the patency of lower extremity bypass grafts. *Surgery* 1984;96:462
70. Green RM, Roedersheimer LR, DeWeese JA: Effects of aspirin and dipyridamole on expanded polytetrafluoroethylene graft patency. *Surgery* 1982;92:1016
71. Rutherford RB, Jones DN, Bergentz S, et al: The efficacy of dextran 40 in preventing early postoperative thrombosis

72. Eickhoff JF, Engell HC: Local regulation of blood flow and the occurrence of edema after arterial reconstruction of the lower limbs. *Ann Surg* 1982;195:474
73. Schubart PJ, Porter JM: Leg edema following femorodistal bypass. In: Bergan JJ, Yao JST (eds). *Reoperative Arterial Surgery*. Orlando, Grune & Stratton, 1986;311
74. Bernhard VM: Bypass to the popliteal and infrapopliteal arteries. In: Rutherford RB (ed). *Vascular Surgery*, 2nd ed. Philadelphia, WB Saunders, 1984:607
75. Perry MO: Vascular trauma. In: Moore WS (ed). *Vascular Surgery: A Comprehensive Review*, 2nd ed. Orlando, Grune and Stratton, 1986:831
76. Watkins L Jr, Gott VL: Blunt and penetrating trauma to the great vessels. In: Glenn WL (ed). *Thoracic and Cardiovascular Surgery*, 4th ed. Norwalk, CT, Appleton-Century-Crofts, 1983:1489
77. Allen TW, Reul GJ, Morton JR, et al: Surgical management of aortic trauma. *J Trauma* 1972;12:862
78. Lim RC Jr, Trunkey DD, Blaisdell FW: Acute abdominal aortic injury: an analysis of operative and postoperative management. *Arch Surg* 1974;109:706
79. Perdue GD Jr, Smith RB: Intra-abdominal vascular injury. *Surgery* 1968;64:562
80. Rich NM, Hobson RW, Collins GJ Jr: Traumatic arteriovenous fistulas and false aneurysms: a review of 558 lesions. *Surgery* 1975;78:817
81. Smith RF, Szilagyi DE, Pfeifer JR: A study of arterial trauma. *Arch Surg* 1963;86:825
82. Rich NM, Baugh JH, Hughes CW: Acute arterial injuries in Vietnam: 1000 cases. *J Trauma* 1970;10:359
83. Gaspar MR, Treiman RL: The management of injuries to major veins. *Am J Surg* 1960;100:171
84. Williams EJ: Embolization of a bullet to the posterior tibial artery following a gunshot wound of the thorax. *J Trauma* 1964;4:258
85. Patman RD: Fasciotomy: indications and technique. In: Rutherford RB (ed). *Vascular Surgery*, 2nd ed. Philadelphia, WB Saunders, 1984:513
86. Porter JM, Taylor LM, Baur GM: Nonatherosclerotic vascular disease. In: Moore WS (ed). *Vascular Surgery: A Comprehensive Review*. New York, Grune & Stratton, 1983:55
87. Rich NM, Spencer FC: Sequelae of acute arterial trauma. In: Rich NM, Spencer FC (eds). *Vascular Trauma*. Philadelphia, WB Saunders, 1978:106
88. Yeager RA, Moneta GL, Taylor LM Jr, et al: Surgical management of severe acute extremity ischemia. *J Vasc Surg* 1992;15:385
89. Lawrence PF, Goodman GR: Thrombolytic therapy. *Clin North Am* 1972;72:4
90. Wasselle JA, Bandyk DF: Intraoperative thrombolysis in peripheral arterial occlusion: review. *Can J Surg* 1993;36:354
91. Andaz S, Shields DA, Scurr JH, et al: Thrombolysis in acute lower limb ischaemia: review. *Eur J Vasc Surg* 1993;7:595
92. Perler, Bruce A: Fibrinolytic therapy for acutely thrombosed lower extremity and grafts. In: Ernst CB, Stanley JC. *Current Therapy in Vascular Surgery*, 3rd ed. St. Louis, Mosby-Yearbook, 1995:540
93. Smith CM, Yellin AE, Weaver FA, et al: Thrombolytic therapy for arterial occlusion: a mixed blessing. *Am Surg* 1994;60:371
94. Decrinis M, Pilger E, Stark G, et al: A simplified procedure or intra-arterial thrombolysis with tissue-type plasminogen activator in peripheral arterial occlusive disease: primary and long term results. *Eur Heart J* 1993;14:297
95. Ward AS, Andaz SK, Bygrave S: Peripheral thrombolysis with

following difficult lower extremity bypass. *J Vasc Surg* 1984;1:765

tissue plasminogen activator: results of two treatment regimens. *Arch Surg* 1994;129:861

96. Mitchell JP, Turlock EP: Tissue-plasminogen activator for pulmonary embolism resulting in shock: two case reports and discussion of literature. *Am J Med* 1991;90:255

97. Goldhaber SZ, Kessler CM, Heit J: Randomized control trial of recombinant tissue plasminogen versus urokinase in the treatment of acute pulmonary embolism. *Lancet* 1988;2:293

98. Schilling JD, Pond GD, Mulcahy MM, et al: Catheter-directed urokinase thrombolysis: an adjunct to PTA/surgery for management of lower extremity thromboembolic disease. *Angiology* 1994;45:851

99. Smith CM, Yellin AE, Weaver FA, et al: Thrombolytic therapy for arterial occlusion: a mixed blessing. *Am Surg* 1994;60:371

100. Bell WR, Meek AG: Guidelines for the use of thrombolytic agents. *N Engl J Med* 1979;301:1266

101. Porter JM, Taylor LM: Current status of thrombolytic therapy. *J Vasc Surg* 1985;2:239

102. Graor RA, Risivs B, Denny KM: Local thrombolysis in the treatment of thrombosed arteries, bypass grafts, and arteriovenous fistulas. *J Vasc Surg* 1985;2:406

103. Comerata AJ: Complications with systemic and localized fibrinolytic therapy. In: Bernhard VM, Towne JB (eds). *Complications in Vascular Surgery*, 2nd ed. Orlando, Grune & Stratton, 1985:421

104. Perler BA, Kinnison M, Halden WJ: Transgraft hemorrhage: a serious complication of low-dose thrombolytic therapy. *J Vasc Surg* 1986;3:936

105. Rabe FE, Becher GJ, Richmond BD, et al: Contrast extravasation through Dacron grafts: a sequelae of low-dose streptokinase therapy. *AJR* 1982;138:917

106. Janosik JE, Bettmann MA, Kaul AF, et al: Therapeutic alternatives for subacute peripheral arterial occlusion: comparison by outcome, length of stay, and hospital charges. *Invest Radiol* 1991;26:921

107. Schilling JD, Pond GD, Mulcahy MM, et al: Catheter-directed urokinase thrombolysis: an adjunct to PTA/surgery for management of lower extremity thromboembolic disease. *Angiology* 1994;5:851

108. Fann-James I, Miller CD: Pathophysiology of aortic dissection. In: Ernst CB, Stanley JC. *Current Therapy in Vascular Surgery*, 3rd ed. St. Louis, Mosby-Yearbook, 1995:206

109. McDermott JC, Schuster MR, Crummy AB, et al: Crack and aortic dissection. *Wis Med J* 1993;92:453

110. Sakamoto I, Hayashi K, Mastunaga N, et al: Aortic dissection caused by angiographic procedures. *Radiology* 1994;191:467

111. Simon P, Owen AN, Havel M, et al: Transesophageal echocardiography in the emergency surgical management of patients with aortic dissection. *J Thorac Cardiovasc Surg* 1992;103:1113, 1117

112. Svensson LG, Labib SB: Aortic dissection and aortic aneurysm surgery. *Curr Opin Cardiol* 1994;9:191

113. Crawford ES: The diagnosis and management of aortic dissection. *JAMA* 1990;264:2537

114. Kirsh MM, Newman C: Medical management of acute aortic dissection. In: Ernst CB, Stanley JC. *Current Therapy in Vascular Surgery*, 3rd ed. St. Louis, Mosby-Yearbook, 1995;206

115. Hara K, Yamaguchi T, Wanibuchi Y, et al: The role of medical treatment of distal type aortic dissection. *Int J Cardiol* 1991;32:231

116. Kato M, Ohnishi K, Kaneko M, et al: Development of an expandable intra-aortic prosthesis for experimental aortic dissection. *ASAIO J* 1993;39:M758

117. Liu DW, Lin PJ, Chang CH: Treatment of acute type A aortic dissection with intraluminal sutureless prosthesis. *Ann Thorac Surg* 1994;57:987

Critical Care, Third Edition, edited by Joseph M. Civetta,
Robert W. Taylor, and Robert R. Kirby.
Lippincott-Raven Publishers, Philadelphia, PA © 1997.

CHAPTER 78

∎

Neurologic Injury: Prevention and Initial Care

Philip A. Villanueva
Bradley H. Ruben
Jonathan Greenberg

IMMEDIATE CONCERNS: HEAD INJURY ∎

MAJOR PROBLEMS

It has been estimated that otherwise avoidable factors potentiate the head injury or its sequelae in up to 75% of head injuries and 54% of head-injury fatalities; these factors include hypoxia or hypercapnia resulting from airway obstruction or hypoventilation, impaired cerebral perfusion from hypovolemia or systemic hypotension, inaccurate diagnosis, inadequate initial management, and delay in transfer for definitive care. According to the Monroe-Kellie doctrine, the total intracranial volume of brain, blood, cerebrospinal fluid (CSF), and any lesion remains a constant. Intracranial pressure (ICP) increases when one component (e.g., a traumatic lesion) increases beyond compensatory reductions in the other components. Normal ICP is less than 15 mm Hg. ICP greater than 15 mm Hg is abnormal; measurements above 20 mm Hg demonstrate unequivocal intracranial hypertension. Effects of head injury are potentiated by hypoxemia and ischemia. The ABCs of resuscitation are critically important because of the frequent association of airway problems and hypotension in head or multiple-trauma patients. Cervical spine injury must be suspected and conclusively ruled out.

STRESS POINTS

1. Guidelines for admission to the intensive care unit (ICU) are as follows:

   a. All patients with significant demonstrable intracranial pathology, including those with effaced basal cisterns or greater than 7 mm pineal (or other midline structure) shift laterally
   b. Patients with a Glasgow Coma Scale (GCS) score less than 13
   c. All patients who have undergone craniotomy for trauma (*exception*: elevation of depressed skull fracture without dural involvement)
   d. Patients requiring ICP monitoring or drainage of CSF by closed ventriculostomy
   e. Patients who evidence significant focal neurologic signs
   f. Head injury associated with significant systemic anatomic or physiologic abnormalities
   g. Probable brain-death patients during confirmation or preparation for organ procurement

2. Persistent ICP elevations above 40 mm Hg are associated with a poor outcome. Outcome is best if ICP remains below 20 mm Hg without treatment; it is improved if ICP can be controlled, even if it was initially elevated, and outcome worsens as control is lost and intracranial hypertension worsens.

3. Hypovolemia may be caused by aggressive administration of diuretics. The rule of thumb for intravenous (IV) fluid therapy (a rate of two thirds' calculated maintenance) should be modified in accordance with right-heart filling pressures, cardiac output, and systemic blood pressure.

4. The syndrome of inappropriate antidiuretic hormone

1195

secretion (SIADH) usually becomes clinically significant when too much free water has been administered; natriuresis may complicate the clinical presentation. Treatment is primarily preventive, by restricting free water in IV fluids. Isotonic or even hypertonic saline solutions, with diuretics, may be necessary if symptoms or neurologic irritability are present. Too rapid correction or over-correction may cause central pontine myelinolysis.

5. Coagulation disorders: Disseminated intravascular coagulation (DIC) or fibrinolysis may occur after penetrating or severe closed head trauma. Clotting elements—particularly platelets, fibrin, and fibrin split products—should be assessed. Clotting factors should be replaced as needed, and the source (injured brain tissue) should be extirpated, if possible.

6. Outcome: The patient's age, best motor response on the GCS, and preservation of pupillary response bilaterally are the best predictors of outcome, although no predictive measure has a high rate of accuracy.

ESSENTIAL DIAGNOSTIC TESTS

1. General parameters: vital signs (especially hypertension with bradycardia, abnormal respiratory patterns)
2. GCS: The three components are eye opening (rated 1 through 4), verbal response (rated 1 through 5), and motor response (rated 1 through 6). Scores range from 3 (no response in all three components) to 15 (spontaneous eye opening, oriented, follows commands; Table 78-1).
3. GCS score 13 to 15: Although injury may exist, ICU admission should not necessarily be based on GCS alone; computed tomography (CT) or other neurologic findings may be a guideline for admission.
4. GCS score 8 to 13: Significant insult has occurred to depress the level of consciousness, and there is a real possibility that a pathologic lesion exists. Intracranial monitoring necessary if the shift of midline structures is significant.
5. GCS score less than 8: ICU admission and ICP monitoring is warranted. Motor examination is the most critical component for neurologic monitoring.
6. Brain stem reflexes: Pupillary size and reactivity, eyelash or corneal reflexes, oculocephalic ("doll's eyes") or oculovestibular reflexes ("ice water calorics"), once cervical spine injury or instability is ruled out
7. Focal neurologic deficit: Strength of upper and lower limbs and comparison of right- and left-sided strength
8. Craniocervical injuries: Scalp or facial trauma with Battle's sign or "raccoon's eyes"; if clear fluid drains from ear or nose, avoid nasal intubation. No response to pain below level of clavicles or bradycardia and *hypotension* may mean cervical spine injury.
9. Serial examinations: Repetitive, consistent, and reproducible evaluations are mandatory for 72 hours. Continuous monitoring is necessary to notice responses to stimulation and medical interventions and to intervene if ICP is increased and sustained. Repeat CT studies should be considered at 24 hours, 72 hours, and 7 days

TABLE 78-1.   Glasgow Coma Scale

VARIABLE	RESPONSE	SCORE
EYES		
Open	Spontaneously	4
	To verbal command	3
	To pain	2
	No response	1
BEST MOTOR RESPONSE		
To verbal command	Obeys	6
To painful stimulus (pressure to nailbeds)	Localizes pain	5
	Flexion—withdrawal	4
	Flexion—abnormal (decorticate rigidity)	3
	Extension (decerebrate rigidity)	2
	No response	1
BEST VERBAL RESPONSE		
(Arouse patient with painful stimulus if necessary)	Oriented and converses	5
	Disoriented and converses	4
	Inappropriate words	3
	Incomprehensible	2
	No response	1
Total		3–15

Jannett B, Teasdale G: Aspects of coma after severe head injury. *Lancet* 1977;i:878.

after injury for severely injured or pharmacologically paralyzed patients.

INITIAL THERAPY

1. Adjunctive supportive measures: Head in midline, with 10-degree elevation; prevention of agitation (sedatives, analgesics, or muscle relaxants may be necessary); prevention of cough reflex with IV lidocaine; prevention of hyperthermia and treatment (including anticonvulsant prophylaxis) of seizure activity, which increases cerebral metabolic demands
2. Treatment of intracranial hypertension and cerebral edema:
   a. Hyperventilation almost immediately decreases ICP by causing vasoconstriction and decreasing intracranial blood volume. Goal of therapy is $PaCO_2$ between 30 and 35 mm Hg.
   b. Osmotic diuretic (mannitol 20% solution, 0.5 to 1.0 g/kg): Maximum effect in approximately 20 minutes; average duration, about 3.5 hours. Repeat doses of 0.25 to 0.50 g/kg every 4 hours. Goal of treatment: serum osmolarity 295 to 310 mOsm.
   c. Loop diuretics (e.g., furosemide) and acetazol-

amide decrease CSF production but can decrease intravascular volume and cause electrolyte and acid-base disturbances. They are considered adjunctive therapy to osmotic diuretics.

d. ICP monitoring and drainage: Monitoring should be performed on postcraniotomy patients in whom cerebral edema is expected, those with nonsurgical intracranial lesions with mass effect (ablation of cisterns or greater than 7 mm shift of midline structures), and those with GCS scores less than 8 (for GCS scores 9 to 13, ICP monitoring is optional). CSF may be vented through a ventriculostomy (occasionally subdural) catheter, if present. Venting may become less effective over time because of additional swelling of brain tissue.

e. Surgical decompression: Significant epidural, subdural, or intraparenchymal clots—as defined by CT scan, GCS score, focal deficits, or neurologic deterioration—should be evacuated. Delayed hemorrhages may occur during the first week after injury, and follow-up CT studies should be obtained. Penetrating injuries should be closed to prevent CSF contamination and infection, which increase ICP.

f. High-dose barbiturate therapy ("barbiturate coma"): A last effort to avert death when all other modalities have failed to reduce intracranial hypertension, it may improve outcome in certain cases. Loading dose: pentobarbital 5 to 10 mg/kg over a 1-hour infusion; then 5 mg/kg over 30 minutes for 3 days. Maintenance dose: 1 to 1.5 mg/kg/hour (monitor by keeping serum levels 3.0 to 5.0 mg/dL or achieving electroencephalogram [EEG] burst suppression). Arterial and pulmonary artery monitoring is indicated. Endpoints of therapy: success (ICP less than 15 to 20 mm Hg for 48 to 72 hours); failure (ICP refractory to maximum doses); or complications (hypotension, low cardiac output unresponsive to therapy) requiring cessation of infusion.

3. ICP measurement should be considered in (1) traumatic injuries requiring a craniotomy, and (2) patients with a GCS of 8 or less.

4. Hyperglycemia should be treated with insulin. Goal of treatment: blood glucose between 100 and 150 mg/dL.

5. Diabetes insipidus (DI) is initially treated with replacement of free water losses. Serum sodium and potassium levels are monitored closely. Aqueous vasopressin (Pitressin), vasopressin tannate in peanut oil, or desmopressin acetate (DDAVP) may be used.

IMMEDIATE CONCERNS: SPINAL INJURY ∎

MAJOR PROBLEMS

1. Injuries to the vertebrae and to the spinal cord may occur separately or together and may or may not have been diagnosed before admission of the patient to the ICU. The development of a spinal cord lesion while the patient is under medical care is such a tragedy that detection and management of spinal cord injury, especially during transport, are necessary skills for the intensivist.

2. Spinal trauma should be considered in the following patients:
   a. All head-injured patients, especially if frontal or facial trauma is present
   b. Patients with penetrating injuries in proximity
   c. Patients who have major crush injuries
   d. All multiple blunt trauma patients
   e. Patients who have sustained major accelerating–decelerating forces

3. Immobilization of the head and neck should be performed until spinal injury can be definitely excluded.

STRESS POINTS

1. The cervical collar is a reminder that cervical injury may be present, *not* a totally effective mechanism to immobilize the cervical spine.

2. Effective immobilization consists of a spinal board, sandbags in proximity to the head, and adhesive strapping, including the board, the sandbags, and the forehead.

3. If the lesion is complete, symmetric, and unchanging, cervical traction or alignment is usually the only initial therapy.

4. If the lesion is incomplete, asymmetric, and, especially, changing, immediate surgery may be required.

5. In cases of penetrating injuries, concomitant tracheal, esophageal, and major vessel injury must be considered. CSF fistulas must be closed or decompressed.

6. Spinal shock encompasses the following: transient reflex depression below the level of injury caused by the abrupt withdrawal of descending excitatory influences from higher centers, as well as persistent inhibition from below the injury.

7. Crycothyroidotomy or tracheostomy may be necessary—it may delay early operations on the cervical spine and should be used only if other methods have failed.

8. Bradycardia and hypotension are common; increased venous capacitance caused by sympathectomy may produce relative hypovolemia.

9. Compensatory tachycardia may be blocked by interruption of cardiac accelerator nerves.

10. Profound bradyarrhythmias and cardiac arrest occur hours to days after injury. Although initial fluid resuscitation may reverse hypotension, inadvertent fluid overload must be avoided. Vasopressor agents may be necessary to increase blood pressure.

11. Gastric hypersecretion is common. Measurement of nasogastric pH and correction are necessary routine measures to prevent perforation or hemorrhage.

ESSENTIAL DIAGNOSTIC TESTS

1. Assessment of baseline function is important; this must be performed at frequent intervals and especially before and after transport.

2. Radiographs of the spine must visualize all vertebrae.
3. Spine CT vertical reconstruction is useful if repeated conventional radiographs do not provide clear views.
4. Continuous electrocardiographic (ECG) and arterial pressure monitoring aids in the prompt detection of bradyarrhythmias and hypotension. Hypoxia-induced effects must be considered and evaluated by frequent measurement of arterial blood gases or continual arterial pulse oximetry.
5. Although fluid therapy may overcome the increased venous capacitance, invasive monitoring should be considered if the desired restoration of blood pressure does not occur.

INITIAL THERAPY

1. Turning, if required, should be done while maintaining alignment ("logrolling") and cervical traction.
2. Conscious patients should be instructed not to sit up or turn the head. Asynchronous breathing pattern is usually present—chest falls with inspiration.
3. To establish an airway, the modified jaw-thrust method without neck extension should be used.
4. Intubation should be performed if respiratory failure is suspected.
5. Blind nasal intubation without movement of the cervical spine is most desirable.
6. Fiberoptic laryngoscopy or bronchoscopy may aid in the passage of the endotracheal tube.
7. In the nonintubated patient, continuous heated aerosols, coughing assisted by the subphrenic thrust, and nasotracheal suctioning may be required. Incentive spirometry may help to maintain lung volumes, and intermittent positive-pressure ventilation may be used to help mobilize pulmonary secretions. If intubation has been performed by the nasotracheal route, maxillary sinusitis may develop.
8. Ventilatory support techniques that encourage spontaneous respiration and maintain functional residual capacity counteract the abnormal physiologic sequelae and maintain diaphragmatic muscle function. Controlled ventilation may promote disuse atrophy of the diaphragm and prolong the period of total mechanical ventilation.
9. Lobar collapse is frequent. Irrigation and suctioning may be effective in aspirating retained secretions. Large tidal volumes (15 to 18 mL/kg) and positive end-expiratory pressure (PEEP) may be necessary to maintain expansion. Fiberoptic bronchoscopy is often necessary.
10. Bradyarrhythmias can be minimized by maintaining arterial oxygen tension and treated by intermittent administration of atropine sulfate. Longer acting sympathomimetics and beta-stimulating cardiac inotropes may be necessary in rare cases. Temporary or permanent cardiac pacing is occasionally necessary.
11. Nasogastric suctioning should be used to prevent abdominal distention, which may further impair pulmonary function.
12. Bladder dysfunction is treated initially with indwelling catheters and later with intermittent catheterization to reduce risks of urinary tract infections. Urine acidification and chronic antimicrobial administration are also useful.

HEAD INJURY ◼

Each year, approximately 500,000 Americans sustain head injuries of sufficient magnitude to warrant medical evaluation and treatment—an incidence of 200 in 100,000.[1,2] One third sustain severe head injuries, and ultimately 50,000 to 60,000 die annually.[1] Motor vehicle accidents (including motorcycle and pedestrian–vehicle accidents) are the most common cause and often are associated with failure to wear seat restraints and alcohol or drug abuse. Other causes include falls, criminal assaults (both blunt and penetrating injuries), and industrial or recreational accidents.[1,2]

It has been estimated in up to 75% of head injuries and 54% of head-injury fatalities that otherwise avoidable factors, including hypoxia or hypercapnia resulting from airway obstruction or hypoventilation, impaired cerebral perfusion from hypovolemia or systemic hypotension, inaccurate diagnosis, inadequate initial management, and delay in transfer for definitive care, potentiate the head injury or its sequelae.[3,4]

Only the accurate, organized, and expeditious assessment and management of head injuries can reduce the significant morbidity and mortality associated with these conditions. Neurosurgical critical care plays an essential part in eliminating or mitigating the central nervous system (CNS) and systemic effects of significant head injury.

PATHOPHYSIOLOGY

Consciousness, the awareness of one's self and environment, requires *arousability*, which depends on the integrity of the ascending reticular activating system (ARAS) of the brain stem; *perception* of environmental stimuli, which requires subcortical and sensory cortical function; and *cognition*, which requires multifocal integration and processing of sensory input by the cerebral cortex. The degree to which consciousness is impaired depends, therefore, on the location and severity of pathophysiologic processes that involve either the ARAS or the cerebral hemispheres.[5]

Intracranial Pressure, Volume, and Blood Flow

The Monro-Kellie doctrine, proposed 150 years ago, states that within the rigid cranial vault, the total volume of the intracranial contents (brain, blood, CSF, and any mass) remains a constant.

Because fluid is incompressible, mass lesions must displace one of the other components for intracranial volume to remain constant. Slowly growing intracranial mass lesions allow for volume compensation by decreased CSF production or displacement, atrophy of brain tissue, or decreased intravascular blood volume. After an acute injury, the rapid development of space-occupying lesions and edema may outstrip normal compensatory mechanisms, resulting in compression of brain tissue and a rise in ICP.

ICP represents resistance to cerebral perfusion pressure (CPP) and cerebral blood flow (CBF). They are related by the following equation:

$$CPP = MAP - ICP$$

where MAP is the mean arterial pressure. The brain's ability to compensate for volume changes within the intracranial compartment is the pressure–volume index (PVI). With progressive loss of compensatory reserves, small changes in intracranial mass lesion volumes can result in dramatic elevations of ICP, causing secondary decrements in CPP and CBF.

Neurologic damage seen after head injury is of two types. The primary injury is that which results from the initial impact, whereas the secondary injury is caused by expansion of mass lesions and brain swelling, and may be significantly aggravated by systemic factors such as hypoxia and hypotension. Normal ICP is between 10 and 15 mm Hg in adults. Above 15 mm Hg, the pressure is considered abnormal; intracranial hypertension is defined as pressures above 20 mm Hg.[6] However, maintenance of an adequate CPP is probably more important. In general, CPP should be maintained between 60 and 120 mm Hg. The poor outcome observed in patients with elevated ICP tends to reflect inadequate CPP resulting in cerebral ischemia.[7,8]

Intracranial Injuries

Intracranial injuries usually result from either direct injuries (blunt or penetrating) to the cortex or from acceleration–deceleration movements of the brain within the calvarial vault; the latter may cause indirect (contrecoup) impacts on bony irregularities and the prominences of the frontal or middle fossae. Cerebral concussions, for example, produce brief loss of consciousness and (retrograde) amnesia in the absence of demonstrable gross cerebral disease, despite evidence of transient ARAS or cortical electrophysiologic dysfunction.

Intracranial hemorrhage occurs in half of head-injured patients with prolonged unconsciousness.[9] Cerebral contusions are a mixture of damaged neuroglial tissue and interstitial hemorrhage, typically appearing as a mixed-density intraparenchymal mass lesion surrounded by a ring of edema. Torsional (angular) acceleration–deceleration injuries produce actual shearing of the subcortical white matter tracts,[10] resulting in diffuse axonal injuries, which are often associated with deep hemorrhages of white matter, corpus callosum, and cerebral and cerebellar peduncles.[11] More violent impacts may produce brain lacerations with secondary intracerebral hemorrhages. Delayed traumatic intracerebral hemorrhages occur in up to 8% of patients sustaining significant head injury and may manifest as late as 7 to 10 days after injury, with the peak incidence occurring within the first 72 hours.[12,13] Serial CT scanning, therefore, should be considered in all patients with significant intracranial disease on admission, failure to improve neurologically, or neurologic deterioration.[12]

Subdural hematomas (SDHs) are the most frequently occurring extraaxial hematomas. They are termed *acute*, *subacute*, or *chronic*, depending on the rate of progression of symptoms and the appearance of the hematoma at surgery. Beneath the inner table of the skull and overlying the cerebral convexity in the subdural space, they typically present as acute or subacute biconcave mass lesions; chronic SDHs may appear as lenticular ("lens-shaped") mass lesions. Subdural bleeding usually results from tearing or avulsion of bridging veins between the cortex and the dural venous sinuses, but SDHs can also occur when small cortical arteriole loops, which protrude through defects in the arachnoid, are torn. SDHs with mass effect on the underlying cortex and progressive neurologic deficit are true surgical emergencies; definitive surgery within 4 hours of injury significantly reduces mortality and morbidity. However, SDHs associated with cortical lacerations, intracerebral hematomas, or edema disproportionate to the SDH carry a much higher mortality risk, largely as a result of the underlying cerebral injury.[14,15]

Epidural ("extradural") hematomas (EDHs) account for about 5% of intracranial hematomas. They mostly arise from lacerations of the middle or accessory meningeal arteries that lie within grooves of the calvarial inner table and supply the dura. Fractures of the skull, usually in the region of the temporal squamosa, are often but not always present. Venous bleeding (from diploic veins after skull fracture) or dural perforating veins also may cause EDH. The hematoma must strip dura away from the inner table of the skull to expand, creating the characteristic lenticular (biconvex) extradural compartment. Nonadherent dura, as occurs in children and young adults, is a prerequisite. Older patients with adherent dura are more prone to SHD formation. Approximately 50% of patients with EDH give a history of a brief loss of consciousness (i.e., a concussion), followed by a "lucid interval" of several hours before the EDH expands sufficiently to compress the brain stem and cause a deterioration in the level of consciousness. Early surgical evacuation usually results in an excellent prognosis, provided irreversible brain stem compression has not occurred.[5,11]

Traumatic hemorrhages of the ventricles may cause direct compression of the rostral ARAS or obstructive hydrocephalus, with increases in ICP. Similarly, traumatic subarachnoid hemorrhage may cause diffuse meningeal irritation, nonfocal clouding of sensorium, and late communicating hydrocephalus.[11]

Herniation Syndromes

Because the cranial vault is only partially compartmentalized by the falx cerebri, tentorium, and foramen magnum, pressure gradients from expanding mass lesions may cause anatomic compression and distortion of brain and its supporting vasculature: a herniation syndrome.[5]

Immediate deficits may result from direct trauma to "eloquent cortex," the cerebral cortex associated with specific functions. Delayed or progressive neurologic dysfunction may represent an ongoing dynamic process, such as an expanding hematoma or worsening cerebral edema, which heralds impending brain herniation. A hemispheric mass lesion may displace the medial cerebral cortex across the midline, termed a *subfalcine* herniation. If the distal anterior cerebral artery is trapped beneath the falx, contralateral monoplegia of the lower extremity will occur. Midconvexity or temporal mass lesions force the medial temporal lobe through the tentorial incisura, forming an *uncal* herniation. It causes compression of the *ipsilateral* oculomotor nerve, resulting in pupillary dilatation and most often compression of the ipsilateral cerebral peduncle, causing *contralateral* hemiparesis. Occasionally, the entire brain stem is pushed across the tentorial incisura, pinning the opposite cerebral peduncle against its adjacent tentorial edge, resulting in *ipsilateral* hemiparesis—the *Kernohan's notch* phenomenon. Mass lesions also cause progressive distortion of the upper brain stem and diencephalon, called a *central* herniation, with progressive deterioration in vegetative functions. Significant distortions may cause evulsion of brain stem vessels, resulting in catastrophic neurologic deterioration and Duret's hemorrhages of the brain stem. Mass lesions of the posterior fossa may produce cerebellar *tonsillar* herniation down through the foramen magnum, causing signs of brain stem dysfunction such as skew gaze deviation, respiratory and cardiovascular dysfunction, arrhythmias, and (terminally) hypotension. *Upward* transtentorial herniation causes catastrophic strangulation of superior cerebellar arteries, with fulminant brain stem dysfunction and bilateral pupillary dilatation from compressed oculomotor nerves.

Other Head Injuries

SCALP LACERATIONS. Scalp lacerations are the most common head injury. Because each side of the scalp is supplied by five major branches of the external carotid artery, significant hemorrhage can occur from a large laceration. Closure of lacerations may not be completed in the emergency department. In these situations, shaving of hair, debridement of the wound, and copious irrigation before suture may prevent a future subgaleal abscess. If a linear nondepressed skull fracture is present, bony and intracranial infection also can be prevented by these procedures.

SKULL FRACTURES. Skull fractures may be linear, diastatic (involving a cranial suture), depressed (if the inner table of bone lies beneath adjacent bone level), or basilar. Basilar skull fractures can involve the anterior, middle, or posterior fossa; they may be associated with periorbital ecchymosis ("raccoon's eyes") or mastoid ecchymosis (Battle's sign), CSF rhinorrhea, otorrhea, or oropharyngeal leakage. Because of the potential of naso–orbito–ethmoidal or cribriform plate injury and risk of transnasal contamination of the subarachnoid space, endotracheal and gastric tubes should not be placed transnasally if CSF rhinorrhea is encountered or basilar skull fracture is suspected. If the patient has been nasally intubated, they should be reintubated orally. Maneuvers that increase ICP (e.g., coughing or Valsalva) should be avoided to decrease CSF flow and so facilitate closure of the dural tear.

PENETRATING INJURIES. Penetrating injuries can create tissue damage beyond the actual tract of injury as a result of kinetic energy dissipation and shock wave effect in the viscoelastic neuroglial tissue.[16]

IMMEDIATE DIAGNOSTIC PROCEDURES

After resuscitative efforts aimed at securing an adequate airway, ensuring adequate ventilation, and establishing adequate systemic perfusion, emergency neuroradiographic examinations may be performed.[11] A cervical spine radiograph series should always be obtained, and a head-injured patient should be presumed to have associated cervical spine injury (because it occurs in 6% to 10% of cases) until spine injury is definitively ruled out. While awaiting clearance of the cervical spine, the neck must be kept immobilized on a spine board with sandbags or in a stiff cervical collar.

CT evaluation of head injury is the current "gold standard" because of speed and its ability to delineate both intracranial and bony disease.[17,18] CT eliminates the need for time-consuming angiography or exploratory surgical explorations for diagnosis. It is also easy to use in serial fashion to diagnose late sequelae of head injury, including delayed traumatic intracerebral hemorrhages and posttraumatic hydrocephalus; to facilitate early therapeutic intervention; and to assess outcome.[13,19] Skull radiographs, in contrast, provide relatively little useful information regarding intracranial disease, although the presence of skull fractures, air–fluid levels in a sinus, pneumocephalus, or a calcified pineal gland shifted to one side on an anteroposterior radiograph may suggest intracranial pathology that warrants further evaluation. Skull radiographs have some usefulness in the evaluation of depressed skull fractures and penetrating injuries; but, as a general rule, they should be considered as ancillary studies *unless* a CT is not readily available. Magnetic resonance imaging (MRI) is usually not suitable for initial assessment of head injury, because MRI cannot image bone and acute hemorrhage cannot be differentiated from brain during the first 72 hours after injury.

GUIDELINES FOR INTENSIVE CARE AND ICU ADMISSION

Patients who have or who are at risk to develop significant neurologic deficit or deterioration are candidates for ICU admission. Assessment is based on neurologic examination, including the GCS (see Table 78-1), neuroradiographic criteria, operative findings, or the need for monitoring. Additionally, patients with multiple injuries or systemic instability also may be candidates for admission despite less severe neurologic involvement. Specifically, patients in the following categories should receive intensive care:

  All patients in coma (GCS less than 8) who are not moribund (GCS of 3)
  All acutely injured nonoperated patients with isolated head trauma with significant demonstrable intracranial disease by CT, regardless of their GCS; this includes patients with small but potentially enlarging lesions such as SDHs, EDHs, contusions (particularly those

involving the temporal lobes), intraparenchymal or intraventricular hemorrhages, cerebral edema, any mass lesion with an associated pineal shift of 7 mm, and effacement of the basal subarachnoid cisterns[19]

All postcraniotomy patients, except for those who had elevation of a depressed skull fracture without dural or cortical involvement

All patients with ICP monitoring or closed ventriculostomy drainage.

Patients with significant focal neurologic deficit, regardless of GCS of 12 or greater, which reflects a significant neurologic insult and possible pathologic lesion (e.g., anoxic brain injury or moderate diffuse axonal injury)

Patients with some degree of neurologic involvement and multisystem trauma with hemodynamic or respiratory instability, need for airway control, risk of coagulopathy, or other major organ system dysfunction

Patients who have probably sustained brain death, for physiologic maintenance in preparation for organ procurement

TREATMENT OF HEAD INJURY

The Airway

Airway obstruction is the primary cause of death in most head trauma victims and a contributing cause in many more. Obstruction may result from direct trauma, such as fractures of facial bones, or from compromise of the airway by edema, blood, or bony intrusion. In the obtunded patient, the tongue may cause upper airway obstruction; laryngeal, pharyngeal, and cough reflexes are depressed or absent. Aspiration of gastric contents is also a frequent occurrence.[11]

Oxygen deprivation and carbon dioxide retention may result from obstruction, leading to cardiorespiratory arrest. These developments compound cerebral edema in the head-injured patient because the resulting cellular hypoxia leads to increased intracranial blood volume and pressure (Fig. 78-1).

Intubation should be performed without hesitation in doubtful cases. It is preferable to intubate a patient with marginal indications and to extubate a few hours later when the condition has improved. If basilar skull fractures are present, with drainage of CSF from the nose or nasal pharynx, nasal intubation should not be performed because of the possibility of intracranial placement of the tube and the increased risk of infection. Preoxygenation should be performed. Yankauer suction should be used rather than pliable and narrow tracheal suction catheters because the semiconscious patient may be agitated and restless, and straining may occur when airway intubation is attempted. Heavy sedation or pharmacologic paralysis may be required to prevent potentially catastrophic increases in ICP, even at the expense of temporarily invalidating the neurologic examination. Transtracheal or IV lidocaine (50 mg) also may suppress tracheal reflexes that can increase ICP by increasing heart rate and blood pressure and, thus, increasing intracranial blood flow and volume.

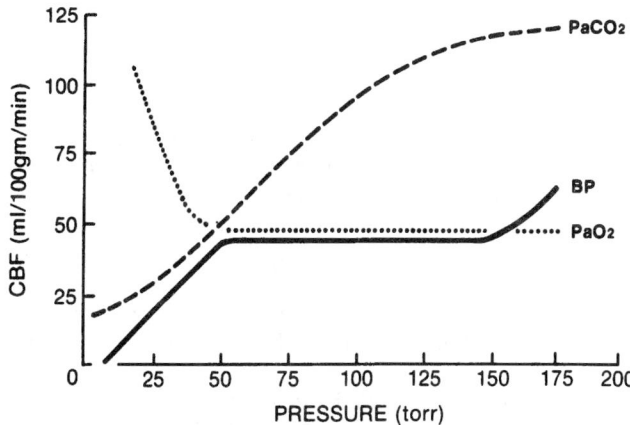

FIGURE 78-1. The effect of blood pressure (BP), PaO_2, and $PaCO_2$ on cerebral blood flow (CBF) in normal brain. (Reproduced with permission from Shapiro HM: Intracranial hypertension: therapeutic and anesthetic considerations. *Anesthesiology* 1975;43:447.)

Considerations Related to Blood Pressure

In patients without head injury and with normal ICP, hypotension may be well tolerated; in head-injured patients, however, this may not be true, especially if ICP is increased. Hypotension in conjunction with increased ICP may reduce CPP (its acceptable range is 60 to 120 mm Hg) and ultimately impair CBF, aggravating the underlying injury. Hypovolemia from hemorrhage or the use of diuretics should be corrected rapidly, and adequate cardiac output must be maintained. In some forms of hypotension (especially spinal shock), an alpha-agonist also may be required. All patients with impaired sensorium secondary to head trauma should be considered to have increased ICP until proven otherwise; maintenance of normal blood pressures in these patients is, therefore, essential. The "two thirds' calculated maintenance" rule of thumb for IV fluid administration must be modified in accordance with right or left heart filling pressures, cardiac output, and systemic blood pressure.

Isolated closed-head injuries rarely cause shock; the normal response to significant head injury includes CNS sympathetic response with significant elevations in serum catecholamine levels.[20] In fact, about 20% of such head-injured patients present with systolic blood pressures over 160 mm Hg.[21] In the absence of preexisting hypertension, elevated systolic pressure (with or without tachycardia) represents an autoregulatory response in an attempt to maintain CPP. Consequently, until the underlying disease has been defined or the ICP measured, the elevated blood pressure should not be treated.

Neurologic Monitoring

On admission to the ICU, the patient should be fully reevaluated. Neurologic monitoring includes the following, at a minimum: serial assessments of the patient's vital signs, with particular attention to such signs of impending herniation or intracranial hypertension as abnormal respiratory patterns (Cheyne-Stokes, central neurogenic hyperventilation, ataxic or apneustic respiration) or bradycardia with hypertension[5]; GCS scoring; the size and responsiveness of the pupils; and movements of the upper and lower extremities and their comparative motor strengths. The head should be rechecked for evidence of overlooked scalp lacerations, facial injuries, or depressed or basilar skull fractures. Adjunctive brain stem reflexes (eyelid, corneal, oculocephalic or oculovestibular, gag) may be assessed, as the situation warrants, once the cervical spine injury or instability has been ruled out by radiographs.

Scores on the GCS (see Table 78-1) are associated with the following clinical findings and management indications:

GCS score 13 to 15: Patients are generally hospitalized, but not in the ICU unless neurologic examination, skull radiographs, or CT scan reveal a lesion or abnormality that warrants consideration for ICU admission.

GCS score 9 to 13: A significant insult has depressed the level of consciousness, with a great likelihood that a pathologic lesion is present. Further workup is necessary, and the patient should be monitored in the ICU.

GCS score below 8: In addition to ICU admission and workup, ICP or other cerebral function monitoring should be initiated. This score defines patients in coma, and the motor examination component of the GCS becomes the most significant aid to monitoring the patient. Prolonged coma (over 24 hours) is associated with greatly increased mortality.[11]

The GCS has definite limitations: eye opening may not be possible with major facial trauma and periorbital edema; the patient with tracheal intubation cannot vocalize; and focal motor deficits on one side may be worse than on the other side (GCS scoring, by convention, scores the better side). Also, brain stem reflexes must be assessed separately. Modifications of the GCS take these limitations into account (Fig. 78-2). Despite these limitations, the simplicity, reproducibility, and interobserver reliability of the GCS are major factors in its almost universal adoption by head injury centers.

Frequent neurologic examination is necessary to detect deterioration or improvement; no other monitoring tools can give this information reliably. Neurologic function can worsen abruptly and without warning, with little time for intervention before permanent injury or death ensues. To achieve continuity of care, members of the critical care team should assess the patient's neurologic status while the neurologist or neurosurgeon is in attendance. The recognized disease and expectations must be discussed, and significant departures from baseline and immediate therapeutic interventions to be undertaken should be specifically articulated. These precautions are designed to minimize discontinuity created by changing personnel and uncertainties caused by assumptions rather than explicit communication. Because brain edema and swelling tend to maximize at 48 to 96 hours after injury, patients should receive at least 72 hours of neurologic monitoring; with significant head trauma, follow-up CT studies should be performed at 24 to 72 hours after injury and again at 1 week after injury to uncover occult delayed hemorrhages, particularly if hemorrhage is present

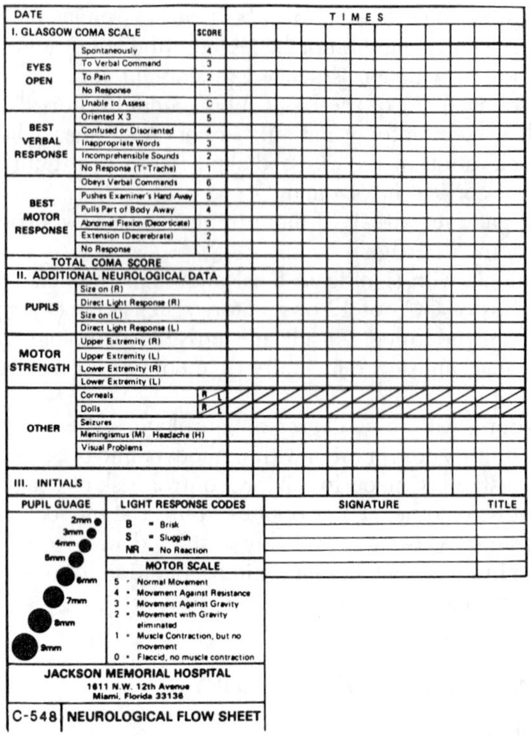

FIGURE 78-2. An example of an ICU flow sheet for serial assessment of neurologic status in head-injured patients, combining the Glasgow Coma Scale, pupillary size and light response, examination of motor strength, and other neurologic signs.

on an initial CT scan. The CNS-compromised patient provides a double challenge. In systemically injured–only patients, the CNS is usually stable and its homeostatic mechanisms preserved. In the case of CNS injury, attention must be paid to treating the injured CNS, but also to its effects on other systems (e.g., cardiac, respiratory, and temperature regulation). CNS insults, as noted previously, may have serious systemic consequences.

Intracranial Pressure Monitoring

Intracranial pressure should be monitored whenever the brain has sustained injuries that have a high likelihood of resulting in hemorrhage, edema, obstruction to flow of CSF, or loss of cerebral autoregulation with vasodilatation. Valid indications for ICP monitoring include the following: an intracranial lesion requiring surgical decompression (postoperative); a nonsurgical mass lesion that obstructs ventricular outflow or produces a significant focal mass effect on adjacent brain tissue; effacement of basal cisterns (even in the presence of moderate head injury); shift of midline structures—particularly the pineal gland—by 7 mm or more; and a GCS score of 8 or less. More subtle signs such as papilledema and loss of retinal venous pulsations may indicate developing intracranial hypertension and be considered as an indication for ICP monitoring. Head-injured patients requiring mechanical ventilation and greater than 15 to 20 cm H_2O PEEP for treatment of pulmonary dysfunction also may require ICP monitoring; similarly, patients treated with pharmacologic paralysis for ventilatory support and a significant head injury can no longer be evaluated neurologically and may be considered for ICP monitoring, even with a high GCS score.[11,19,22]

Increases in ICP may occur without discernible changes in GCS until critical CPP levels are reached or brain stem distortion and dysfunction occur, when sudden, catastrophic decompensation may occur.[23] These insidious changes in ICP may occur particularly in patients with low GCS scores (i.e., GCS less than 8). ICP monitoring may detect early changes and permit therapy to avoid further cerebral edema or neurologic deterioration.

Currently, an intraventricular catheter connected to an external strain gauge remains the most accurate, cheapest, and most reliable means of monitoring ICP. It also permits CSF drainage to assist ICP control, as well as assessment of brain compliance. ICP measurement using fiberoptic or strain gauge transducers within the catheter lumen may provide certain benefits such as CSF drainage and theoretical reduction of infective risk and accuracy in case of ventricular collapse. However, these systems carry a considerably higher cost. Fluid-coupled systems measuring from the epidural, subdural, or subarachnoid spaces may allow for ICP reduction by drainage, but in general may not be as accurate as their intraventricular counterparts.[24] Parenchymal ICP monitoring (using fiberoptic or strain gauge systems) provides several advantages: placement independent of ventricular size or location, and less infective and hemorrhagic risks. However, they may not be recalibrated in vivo, and monitor "drift" may be a significant problem.[25] Antibiotic coverage solely for ICP monitors is usually not indicated and has not been the practice within our institution. Daily aseptic sampling of CSF (when available) allows for monitoring of infective status.

CNS Function Monitoring

In the past, the goal of CNS monitoring was believed to be control of ICP within acceptable levels. As observed previously, such levels were those that allowed for maintaining an adequate CPP.[8] Currently, maintaining CPP is emphasized as the primary goal. However, the recognition of the importance of cerebral ischemia that has come with CPP monitoring has led to the development of other monitoring methods that provide "second-order" information regarding CNS function, for example, circulation, metabolism, and electrical activity.

MONITORING OF CNS CIRCULATION. In general, CNS circulation monitoring is best achieved by monitoring CBF. Although the two terms are not interchangeable, CBF monitoring may provide valuable insight into the CNS circulatory status. Several techniques may be used.

Transcranial Doppler employs the principles of ultrasonography[26] and measures the velocity of flow in the Circle of Willis. The data provided include the velocity of flow, not quantity of flow (i.e., milliliters of blood per 100 g of tissue per second). The major paired vessels are studied. The technique is valuable in identifying cerebral vasospasm (i.e., velocity higher than 200 cm/second). This condition occurs

frequently after trauma and may be associated with worsening of the neurologic state.[27] The technique can also identify hyperemic states after trauma. Low flow or no flow states, as found in brain death, also may be identified. The technique is noninvasive, portable, and reproducible. It does require a competent technician and adequate access to the head.

THERMAL DILUTION MONITORING. Thermal dilution monitoring provides real time monitoring of focal (single gyrus) CBF.[28] It is based on thermal dilution and as such is limited to a small geographic area. The data provided may vary from the "usual" 50 to 55 mL per 100 g tissue per minute. If placed in an area of interest, however, it may provide important information regarding relative changes in CBF. The probe is usually inserted intraoperatively but may be placed in the ICU.

GLOBAL CBF MONITORING. Global CBF monitoring techniques are based on the clearance of inert substances from the brain's circulation. The speed of the clearance correlates with CBF.[29–31] The two conventionally used methods employ nitrous oxide or [133]xenon. The former requires repetitive sampling of arterial and jugular venous blood, and computation of the flow using the "washout" formula. The latter technique uses scintillation counters positioned over the patient's head and measurement of the isotope "count" over a fixed time. A computer is used to analyze the washout curve and determine the CBF. Both techniques provide accurate measurement of global CBF. However, both require a "rest period" between tests to allow complete clearance of the test materials.

Other imaging techniques, such as position emission tomography,[32] single-photon emission computed tomography,[33] and dynamic CT scan,[34] may provide CBF and cerebral metabolic data using tagged tracers. These methods are excellent in showing regional dysfunction but may be technically difficult to perform because they require transport out of the ICU. Like the global CBF techniques, they, too, require a "clearance" time for the tracer.

JUGULAR VENOUS SATURATION MONITORING. The chemical end products of CNS metabolism may be assayed from CSF or jugular venous blood. However, the assay process may be sophisticated and not feasible in many cases. The search for a surrogate parameter resulted in the determination of the cerebral metabolic rate of oxygen utilization ($CMRo_2$).[35]

Because this is a derivation that requires knowledge of the CBF, another indicator has been used. This is the saturation of venous blood in the jugular bulb ($SvJo_2$). In the following equation,

$$CMRo_2 = CBF \times [C(a - v)O_2/100]$$

where $C(a - v)O_2$ is the arteriovenous oxygen content difference of the cerebral circulation. The use of $SvJo_2$ is justified in that it provides at least an indication of CBF. Actual minimal and maximal values for $SvJo_2$ have not been determined, but persistent drops below 50% have been well correlated with poor outcomes.[36] These desaturation episodes usually last at least 15 minutes and frequently are followed by ICP elevations.

Values over 75% are usually associated with hyperemic states or a significant decrease in CNS metabolism. Currently, we prefer a 5.5-French oximetric catheter placed within the jugular bulb; the $SvJo_2$ is measured continuously. The catheter also contains a thermistor, allowing measurement of jugular bulb temperature, which correlates closely with brain temperature (Hayashi N, personal communication, October, 1995). Placement of the catheter may be difficult and requires experience, but its reliability has been good, and currently the systems may provide the best indication of CNS function on a real time basis.[37]

ELECTROPHYSIOLOGIC MONITORING. The electrophysiologic state of the brain also may provide important information regarding cerebral function. The original electrophysiologic technique was EEG monitoring.[38] This has evolved into evoked potential (EP) monitoring.[39] The three commonest techniques used examine the visual, auditory, and somatosensory pathways. They may be monitored continuously and are valuable in assessing changes in the patient's status.[40]

SUMMARY. Monitoring CNS status maintains as normal an intracranial environment as possible. There seems to be a general trend toward less CNS-invasive techniques, such as $SvJo_2$ and CBF monitoring. In addition to reducing the risk to an already compromised CNS, these methods also may provide more in-depth data than that provided by "traditional" ICP monitoring.

General Measures

The management of head injury is based on fundamental physiologic principles. Brain extracellular fluid is only 20% to 30% of the amount found in other tissues. With injury, the normal blood–brain barrier is disrupted, resulting in fluid extravasation into an already small compartment (i.e., vasogenic edema). Also, cerebral arterial vessels lose their autoregulatory capacity (the ability to maintain a constant perfusion pressure over a wide range of systemic blood pressures; see Fig. 78-1). This loss of autoregulation can be focal, regional, or global, depending on the extent of injury. Perfusion of the injured area then becomes passive, that is, directly related to systemic pressure. The goal of therapy is to limit extravasation of fluid while maintaining CBF.

The patient's head should be maintained in a midline position and elevated to 10 degrees. This enhances venous drainage and prevents kinking of the jugular venous system. Prolonged head-down position for cannulation of central veins should be avoided because this position leads to greatly increased intracranial blood volume and ICP.

Agitated behavior, coughing, straining, or anything that may increase intraabdominal or intrathoracic pressure should be prevented because these acts may increase ICP. The use of sedatives (barbiturates, benzodiazepams), analge-

sics (codeine, opiates), or muscle relaxants (pancuronium, vecuronium) may be necessary to control muscle activity. Lidocaine, 25 to 50 mg, administered before endotracheal suctioning, may limit the cough reflex.

Arterial hypertension is a common finding in head-injured patients. It is probably secondary to the Cushing reflex, which is a normal physiologic attempt to maintain perfusion to ischemic brain tissue.[41] This may result in increased intracranial blood volume because of increased flow through nonautoregulated vessels, with resulting increased edema accumulation. Again, the brain-injured patient does not tolerate hypotension as readily as the non–head-injured patient; ischemia is a real possibility. The mean arterial pressure, then, should be maintained in the normal range. The CPP should be maintained above the critical level of 60 mm Hg. In hypertension, vasodilators (trimethaphan), IV antihypertensives (alpha-methyldopa, verapamil, or beta-blockers, if there are no medical contraindications), or sedation should be used. Nitroglycerin and sodium nitroprusside should be avoided because they increase venous capacitance and consequently increase intracranial blood volume.[42,43]

Airway protection and ventilatory support are also of utmost importance. PaO_2 should be maintained near 100 mm Hg. If hypoxia develops (see Fig. 78-1), CBF and intracranial blood volume will increase; also, the hemoglobin-oxygen dissociation curve shifts to the left as the result of hyperventilation-induced hypocapnia and alkalosis. This increases the affinity of hemoglobin for oxygen and may reduce oxygen release to tissues. Supplemental oxygenation by mask may be employed if airway protection is not necessary. If adequate oxygenation cannot be obtained, intubation and PEEP should be used. Although PEEP can raise intrathoracic pressure, obstruct venous inflow, and ultimately increase ICP in a normal patient, in head-injured patients with respiratory failure and decreased pulmonary compliance, PEEP may not be transmitted and ICP may not be affected. If there is any question, ICP may be measured to assess the effect of PEEP.[22]

Respiratory failure also is common in head-injured patients. Hypercapnia must be avoided because CBF and volume increase linearly with carbon dioxide tension (see Fig. 78-1). Airway control may be compromised because of the loss of normal protective reflexes in patients with depressed sensoria. Oral airways and nasal trumpets may work temporarily but do not provide security for airway maintenance or protection from aspiration of oral or gastric secretions. Consequently, intubation should be performed whenever doubt arises.

Neurogenic pulmonary edema and abnormal pulmonary shunting can occur soon after head injury and cause life-threatening hypoxemia similar to noncardiogenic pulmonary edema. The clinical findings and therapy are similar to other forms of respiratory failure.[44]

Seizure activity often follows head injury and greatly increases cerebral metabolism and blood flow. Anticonvulsant prophylaxis should be employed during the first week after injury in patients at high risk to develop posttraumatic seizures. These include depressed skull fractures, penetrating injuries with dural lacerations, cerebral contusions or lacerations, SDHs or intracerebral hematomas, and contaminated or infected wounds contiguous with the subarachnoid space.[45]

Fevers should be controlled and hyperthermia avoided, because each degree Celsius of temperature elevation will increase cerebral metabolic activity by 6% to 8%.

Other monitoring methods may aid management. Arterial catheterization provides for continual measurement of mean arterial pressure for estimating CPP and a route for blood sampling. When diuretics are used to aid in the control of ICP, the pulmonary artery catheter helps to discriminate cardiac from respiratory abnormalities, assess effectiveness of cardiac perfusion by measuring venous oxygenation ($S\bar{v}o_2$), and evaluate the response to treatment. Pulmonary artery catheterization also is helpful when therapy with high-dose barbiturates is used because of their cardiovascular depressive effects.

Management of Intracranial Hypertension

The overriding principle of treating intracranial hypertension is that control of ICP to less than 20 mm Hg improves survival. The specific goals are as follows: (1) to limit edema formation, maintain CPP and CBF, and maintain blood pressure in the normal range to reduce blood flow through nonautoregulated areas; (2) to create an osmotic gradient toward the intravascular compartment; and (3) to eliminate obstruction to normal CSF flow or to prevent acute hydrocephalus. If intracranial hypertension (ICP above 15 to 20 mm Hg) results from a mass lesion, other intracranial components (brain, blood, CSF) must decrease either individually or in combination to attempt to reduce ICP to normal levels.

Whereas intubation may prevent hypercapnia by protecting the airway, hyperventilation has an almost immediate effect in decreasing intracranial blood volume by inducing hypocapnia and cerebral vasoconstriction in the regions of the brain where autoregulation is preserved. Aggressive hyperventilation ($Paco_2 \leq 25$ mm Hg) has formed the cornerstone for ICP management in the past.[46] However, a real danger of severe vasoconstriction with resultant ischemia may result from such a technique.[47] Also, the possibility exists of "rebound" and overshoot if CBF (and hence blood volume) increases with restoration of normocapnia.[47] *Mild to moderate* hyperventilation ($Paco_2$ 30 to 35 mm Hg) does not have a deleterious effect and may be of value, at least early in the course of management.[48] However, the arterial Pco_2 must be followed closely to avoid overshoots and, implicitly, some monitoring of CNS function—whether it be an ICP monitor or a more sophisticated device—should be employed to assess the efficacy of the therapy. For instance, if hyperventilation causes $SvJo_2$ to fall below 50%, it could be stopped.

If hyperventilation fails to decrease ICP to less than 20 mm Hg, an osmotic diuretic is administered while monitoring ICP or level of consciousness. Mannitol, in an initial dose of 0.5 to 1.0 g/kg, is infused in less than 15 minutes; the maximal effect usually takes place in approximately 20 minutes, with an average duration of action of 3.5 hours.[5,49]

The extent and duration of response to mannitol vary; as a rule, the higher the ICP, the shorter the response. Mannitol is then repeated in a dose of 0.25 to 0.5 g/kg intravenously every 4 hours (an alternative, and probably less-effective method, is by continuous IV infusion at an equivalent dose rate). Initially, serum osmolarity is measured every 4 hours. The dose of mannitol should then be adjusted to maintain the serum osmolarity at approximately 10 to 25 mOsm above normal (i.e., between 295 and 310 mOsm). Maximal ICP response to mannitol is achieved at this level; higher levels (i.e., to 315 mOsm) increase the response only minimally, if at all. Doses should be decreased as osmolarity rises to avoid overshooting the upper limit. Rebound swelling (when the osmotically active particles move from the intravascular compartment to brain tissue, thus increasing interstitial fluid) is rarer with mannitol than with other osmotic diuretics.

A solution of 5% urea, another osmotic diuretic, also may be employed, as may oral glycerol (on rare occasions).

Loop diuretics (furosemide, ethacrynic acid, bumetanide) may be effective adjuncts in reducing ICP when administered *after* mannitol has been infused, because a greater fluid load is presented to the proximal and distal tubules and loops of Henle. Furosemide (40 to 80 mg or 0.5 mg/kg) can decrease ICP acutely by reducing intravascular volume. Furosemide, by unknown mechanisms, and acetazolamide (a carbonic anhydrase inhibitor that limits ion exchange across the choroid plexus) decrease the production of CSF. Loop diuretics may promote unwanted serum electrolyte changes, particularly hypokalemia and hyponatremia, that complicate the fluid and electrolyte management of the patient. Compensated hypovolemia in the patient with multiple trauma may be worsened by loop diuretics; the resulting hypotension impairs CPP and CBP; therefore, careful monitoring is necessary.

If ICP remains greater than 20 mm Hg, venting of CSF can be performed if a ventricular catheter has been placed. In younger patients with small ventricles and swollen brains, ventriculostomy placement is difficult, and attempts at drainage often yield only small amounts of CSF. Sufficient CSF is slowly removed to lower ICP to 15 to 20 mm Hg. Occasionally, similar maneuvers may be performed with subdural catheters. The frequency of venting, as well as the amount of CSF vented, is recorded because it varies and is an estimate of the severity of intracranial hypertension or the degree of hydrocephalus. Finally, samples of CSF are taken daily for cells, proteins, glucose, and microbiological studies (Gram stain, culture, and sensitivity); catheter replacement and antibiotic therapy may be required after 5 or more days because of the incidence of nosocomial infection.

In summary, initial management of elevated ICP is treated by hyperventilation, effective within seconds. Osmotic (and loop) diuretics are used to raise serum osmolarity to 295 to 310 mOsm if CSF cannot be vented. CSF may be vented through a ventriculostomy into a closed-drainage system to control abrupt, periodic increases in ICP. Frequently, all three methods are necessary to lower ICP.

Barbiturate Therapy

If intracranial hypertension cannot be controlled, virtually all patients will die.[50] Accordingly, after hyperventilation, osmotic and loop diuretics, sedation, analgesics, muscle relaxants, and CSF drainage have been used, and if there are no surgically accessible mass lesions, high-dose barbiturate therapy should be tried.[51] Barbiturates reduce the cerebral metabolic rate, promote cerebral vasoconstriction (which reduces both cerebral blood volume and flow), promote hypothermia and peripheral vasodilatation, and depress cardiac output; cerebral vasoconstriction is probably the major mechanism of action. Barbiturate therapy has been used in many forms, ranging from seizure prophylaxis to induction of isoelectric EEGs for management of intracranial hypertension; with the latter, it is often viewed as a "last-ditch" effort. Although still controversial,[51,52] it has been reported to be effective in patients without preexisting cardiovascular decompensation.[51]

Induction of barbiturate coma requires commitment to careful monitoring, because myocardial depression, hypotension, sepsis, and hypothermia may occur with high-dose barbiturate therapy. ICP and arterial lines must be in place and functioning reliably. A pulmonary artery catheter should be used to monitor measured and calculated cardiac function. Cardiac inotropic support may be necessary in some instances. Because the neurologic examination (including even pupillary constriction) may be lost at higher serum pentobarbital levels (3 to 4 mg/dL), alternative monitoring modalities must be employed: serial CT scans, brain stem EPs, or bedside transcranial Doppler flow studies. The EEG is used to determine the degree of cerebral activity suppression on pentobarbital.

When used to control ICP, pentobarbital is given as a loading dose of 10 mg/kg over 1 hour, followed by three doses of 5 mg/kg over 30 minutes each. A maintenance dose of 1 mg/kg/hourly is then given. The maintenance dose may be increased to up to 1.5 mg/kg hourly. A serum level of 30 to 50 mg/L is obtained.[53] Occasionally, ICP may be controlled with lesser doses. Once the desired serum level is obtained, further increases in dosage to control ICP tend to be ineffective. High-dose barbiturates were observed to increase the number of patients with a useful recovery,[54] but the prophylactic use of the drug did not improve outcome. Among the complications of their use are hypotension, hypothermia, and sepsis. Because of their cardiovascular effects, a pulmonary artery catheter is placed to monitor and maintain optimal cardiac function. A jugular bulb catheter is frequently placed and used in conjunction with ICP monitoring to "titrate" the drug.

Endpoints for barbiturate therapy should be established at the outset. A successful response is defined as a reduction of ICP to 15 mm Hg or less for 48 to 72 hours. Weaning of pentobarbital should be performed *slowly* (usually halving the daily dose every 24 hours for 3 to 4 days) to prevent rebound intracranial hypertension. Improved intracranial compliance, with an ICP/PVI response of less than 3 mm Hg ICP rise per milliliter of fluid injected intraventricularly, is another criterion for assessing efficacy of the therapy. Failure of therapy includes continued intracranial hypertension in the face of maximal barbiturate therapy (by EEG or serum levels) or the development of refractory cardiac dysfunction that is unresponsive to inotropic or sympathomimetic therapy. Extreme hypothermia should be avoided because this affects lung compliance and coagulation.[51]

Other Treatments

Glucocorticoids are not used in head trauma. Their effect has not been proven,[55,56] and the resulting complications, such as hyperglycemia, immune suppression, and gastrointestinal bleeding, outweigh any potential benefit.[57]

However, the identification of two critical factors in the pathophysiologic mechanisms of head injury has led to the development of several new classes of medications that may be of significant value. The first is the role of excitatory neurotransmitters. These substances, the best known of which are glutamate and aspartate, are released as part of the nonspecific CNS response after head injury. They cause an increase in neuronal activity, which, on a cellular level, results in a massive influx of calcium, resulting in cellular dysfunction and eventually destruction. The class of drugs known as the NMDA (n-methyl-D-aspartate) antagonists block the action of the excitatory neurotransmitter. Laboratory and preliminary clinical studies have shown the efficacy of the NMDA antagonists in protecting the brain from further damage after trauma.[58,59]

The second significant development has been the identification of lipid peroxidation and free radical release as the final stage of cellular destruction.[60] The ischemia to which the traumatized brain is prey results in significant cellular destruction. If reoxygenation (as part of the resuscitative process) occurs, a second insult occurs, the net result being extensive lipid peroxidation and the release of a variety of free radicals, which continue to propagate the destructive cascade. Two classes of drugs seem to be effective in countering this process. The first is the antioxidants (as typified by the 21-aminosteroids), which function as cell membrane protectants by binding the free radicals.[61] The second group, free radical scavengers (represented by superoxide dismutase), terminate the activity of these charged particles by incorporating them into reactions, rendering them neutral and harmless.[62]

All of these medications are currently in the clinical testing phase for head injury. Some have shown distinct efficacy in nontraumatic neural insults. Of critical importance is that they not only increase survival, but also improve the quality of survival.

FLUID AND ELECTROLYTE PROBLEMS

Hypovolemia (from aggressive use of diuretics), hyperosmolarity (from osmotic diuretics, hyperglycemia, or DI), and hyponatremia (from the syndrome of inappropriate secretion of antidiuretic hormone [SIADH]) are common problems encountered in head-injured patients.

Mannitol is used to increase and maintain serum osmolarity rather than to deplete intravascular volume. It can, however, decrease intravascular volume, increase blood urea nitrogen, and impair renal function when used repeatedly.

Loop diuretics compound these detrimental effects. Isotonic solutions should be used to maintain intravascular volume while the mannitol dosage is titrated to achieve the desired serum osmolarity. Invasive cardiovascular monitoring should be used when intravascular depletion is suspected.

Hyperglycemia is often the result of CNS stress responses, which result in the release of growth hormone, catecholamines, and adrenal glucocorticosteroids. Hyperglycemia greater than 150 mg/dL may increase cerebral intracellular lactate levels and worsen prognosis; the use of dextrose-containing fluids and hyperglycemia may worsen cerebral ischemic damage in areas of brain injury.[63] Glycosuria also can cause severe hyperosmolar states, especially in association with mannitol or DI. Hyperglycemia should be controlled by the intermittent administration of insulin or continuous insulin infusion, with frequent checks (at least every 4 hours) of blood glucose levels; the goal is blood glucose levels between 100 and 150 mg/dL.

Diabetes insipidus results from injury to the pituitary stalk or hypothalamus; decreased antidiuretic hormone (ADH) secretion results in polyuria, progressive dehydration and hyperosmolarity, and hyperglycemia. In the absence of excess fluid, diuretic administration, or hyperglycemia, DI should be suspected in cases of polyuria (above 200 to 300 mL/hour) in the presence of increased serum hyperosmolarity or hypernatremia and low urine specific gravity, osmolarity, and sodium. Onset of DI may be abrupt or delayed (often associated with a "paradoxical" early SIADH phase), and it may be self-limited or progressive.

An attempt to correct the hyperosmolar state should be made by replacing calculated free water losses with a hypotonic saline or dextrose and water solution, with appropriate potassium supplementation and insulin administration, at a maintenance rate to which is added the previous hour's urine output. Serum sodium and potassium levels should be checked frequently until the DI is controlled. At times, DI is self-limiting, and aqueous vasopressin can be given intermittently at a dosage adjusted on the basis of urinary output; prolonged DI requires longer-lasting vasopressin tannate in oil. Desmopressin acetate, a synthetic analogue of 8-arginine vasopressin, has decreased vasopressor activity relative to enhanced antidiuretic action and can be administered intranasally at a usual dose range of 0.1 to 0.4 mL daily (sublingual administration requires ten times the intranasal dose). Too rapid correction of the hyperosmolar state may cause cerebral edema and intracranial hypertension; a safe rule is to plan a 50% correction during the first 24 hours and the remainder over the next 48 hours.

ADH secretion is a normal part of the body's response to stress (particularly in children). SIADH occurs frequently in head trauma; it should be suspected if hyponatremia and low serum osmolarity are associated with high urine osmolarity and a high urinary sodium concentration. Because head-injured patients usually receive all of their fluids intravenously, clinically significant SIADH is usually the result of overadministration of free water in IV fluids to patients who cannot excrete free water because of excess ADH. In addition, atrial natriuretic peptide, which is secreted by the heart in response to stress, may mimic SIADH because it may cause urinary sodium loss with hyponatremia, even in the absence of dilutional hypervolemia. Hypoosmolarity and hyponatremia should be corrected by careful free water restriction or diuretics to prevent worsening of cerebral edema. Hypertonic saline solutions may be required if the patient is symptomatic (CNS irritability) or the condition is extreme (serum sodium less than 120). Overly rapid correction of SIADH with increases of serum sodium levels greater than 12 mMol/L/day have been associated with central pontine myelinolysis, with devastating results.[64,65]

COAGULATION DISORDERS

The brain is the organ richest in tissue thromboplastin, with plasminogen activity found in the dura, choroid plexus, and CSF.[66,67] Release of these substances into the systemic vasculature, particularly with penetrating or severe cerebral trauma, may cause fulminant DIC or fibrinolysis. Hypothermia may compound vascular fragility and a primary coagulopathy because of loss of platelet thromboxane release, and catecholamines affect platelet function. Treatment involves replacement of depleted clotting factors and, when possible, extirpation of the source of the coagulopathy. Use of plasminogen inhibitors may worsen the condition, and IV low-dose heparin has been used only in extraordinary circumstances. Close hematologic monitoring (particularly for platelets, fibrinogen, and fibrin split products) is warranted, because DIC and fibrinolysis may present subtly. A high index of suspicion for delayed hemorrhages is a stimulus for follow-up CT scans.[13]

LONG-TERM MANAGEMENT PROBLEMS

Patients with prolonged alterations of sensorium and an inability to protect their airways may require tracheostomy to facilitate pulmonary toilet when the patient is moved from the intensive care area. Atelectasis, pneumonias, arrhythmias, and the metabolic, renal, septic, and nutritional problems associated with any type of major trauma are also present in head-injured patients. The management perspectives rest on the increased susceptibility of the injured brain to further insults. Thus, special efforts are made to maintain normal blood pressure, control body temperature, ensure adequate oxygenation, and promote elimination of carbon dioxide. Problems associated with immobilization and calcium metabolism, including thrombophlebitis and heterotopic calcification, are discussed under the spinal cord injury section.

OUTCOME AFTER HEAD TRAUMA

Regarding outcome after head trauma, Jennett and coworkers noted, "So many factors affect the outcome that it is difficult to predict in the early stages after injury on the basis of clinical evaluation."[7] The Glasgow Outcome Scale, with evaluations performed 6 months after injury, was the result of a multinational and multiinstitutional study to evaluate social capability or dependence with respect to mental and neurologic deficits.[68] The Glasgow Outcome Scale categories are as follows: dead, vegetative, severely disabled (conscious but dependent), moderately disabled (independent but disabled), and good (including mild impairments in neuropsychologic testing).[68]

Outcome must be assessed on the basis of reliable initial categorization and consistent, "standardizable" therapy within a given institution. Within that context, several factors that influence outcome have been identified, including depth of coma, motor response, pupillary reaction, eye movements (Table 78-2), the patient's age, and the presence of an intracranial hematoma. ICP elevations, CT-visualized lesions, impairment of brain stem EP, and reduced CBF impact negatively on outcome.[69–71] More recent work has resulted in the creation of a model based on the patient's age, best motor response on the GCS, and pupillary response in both eyes, with a specific accuracy of 78% and a partial accuracy of an additional 12%.[71] The absence of penetrating injuries or brain death at the time of admission, preservation of pupillary light responses in young patients (younger than 50 years of age), and GCS scores of greater than 4 indicate a better prognosis. For patients younger than 30 years of age with GCS scores of 3 to 4, a good result may occur if bilateral pupillary response is preserved.[71,72] Ultimately, however, no predictor is totally accurate; patients who are expected to live may die from unrelated complications, and some of those who are not expected to survive may do well. Every physician who deals extensively with head-injured patients has been humbled on both accounts, and physicians, therefore, should be cautious in allowing presumptions regarding outcome to influence their management, because they might not take sufficient care to avoid complications and let a negative prediction become a self-fulfilling prophecy.

SPINAL CORD INJURY ■

Acute spinal cord injury is primarily a disease of the young adult male. Most victims are 15 to 40 years of age, with a male : female ratio of at least 2:1.[73] Approximately 10,000 cases occur annually in the United States, a rate of 40.1 per million.[73] Motor vehicle accidents involving alcohol or drug abuse, the failure to use seat belts, motorcycle accidents with failure to wear protective helmets, diving accidents and other contact athletic mishaps, falls, criminal assaults, and home and industrial accidents are the major causes of spinal trauma. Spinal cord injury results in catastrophic medical, socioeconomic, and psychological effects; in decreasing order, pulmonary, cardiovascular, and renal dysfunction are the major causes of death, followed closely by suicide.[73]

TABLE 78-2. Relationship of Best Level of Clinical Function in First 25 Hours After Onset of Coma to Outcome

CLINICAL FEATURE	PATIENTS (no.)	OUTCOME	
		Dead/ Vegetative (%)	Moderate Disability/ Good Recovery (%)
COMA RESPONSE SUM			
>11	57	12	82
8–10	190	27	68
5–7	525	53	34
3–4	176	87	7
PUPILS			
Reactive	748	39	50
Nonreactive	226	91	4
EYE MOVEMENTS			
Intact	463	33	56
Impaired	143	62	25
Absent/bad	186	90	5
MOTOR RESPONSE PATTERN (ANY LIMB)			
Normal or weak	568	36	54
Abnormal	393	74	16
MOTOR RESPONSE PATTERN (BEST LIMB)			
Obeys/localizes	395	31	58
Withdraws/flexes	402	54	35
Extensor/nil	191	85	8

Jennett B, Teasdale G, Braakman R, et al: Prognosis of patients with severe head injury. *Neurosurg* 1979;4:282.

Injury to the vertebrae and stabilizing ligaments can occur without neurologic deficit; conversely, injury to the spinal cord with resulting neurologic deficit can occur without evidence of injury to the spinal column, particularly in children or in the elderly. Failure to recognize the potential for spinal column instability may result in iatrogenic injury during treatment of patients with head injury or multiple trauma. Because a potential traumatic spine injury may not have been identified before ICU admission, intensivists must maintain a high index of suspicion in their initial evaluation. All patients with head trauma, particularly if the frontal or facial regions are involved; patients sustaining penetrating injuries near or with potential trajectories near the vertebral column, particularly in the cervical region; patients sustaining crush injuries or multiple trauma; and patients sustaining acceleration–deceleration injuries, including falls, must be considered likely candidates for potential vertebral column instability or spinal cord injury until definitive diagnostic studies have been obtained. Immobilization of the spinal column—and the head and neck in particular—must be maintained throughout all phases of resuscitation and systemic stabilization until this diagnostic process has been completed.

CERVICAL IMMOBILIZATION

Initial immobilization of the spine is usually performed by emergency medical technicians in the field. This may be done with various spine boards, sandbags, or stiff neck collars. Occasionally, a patient may be transferred from a referring hospital with skeletal traction in place. Intensivists must independently assess the need for and adequacy of prior immobilization, whether the patient is first encountered in the emergency or radiology department or ICU. Because transport of the patient from the ICU to other areas of the hospital for diagnostic and therapeutic interventions is often necessary, adequate spine immobilization must be maintained not only during the initial transportation to the ICU, but also from the ICU. Assuring adequate immobilization during transport from the ICU should be considered the responsibility of the intensive care team, as well as the trauma and neurosurgical teams—a redundant system may offer the patient the best protection.

Patients are usually positioned on a spine board, preferably at the scene of the accident, and this position is maintained throughout the diagnostic workup. The spine is maintained in a "neutral" position (neither flexed or extended) in the sagittal plane; the cervical spine should never be manipulated to reduce deformity until definitive radiologic diagnoses are made. Sandbags are placed on either side of the head to prevent rotation; and continuous adhesive (or Velcro) strapping is placed from the spine board across the sandbags and forehead, and back to the spine board. This is an effective restraint, preventing flexion–extension, rotation, and lateral bending movements of the cervical spine; it also reminds the patient to remain immobile. Conscious and cooperative patients should be instructed to remain supine and not to turn their head. Immobilization with a cervical collar should be considered precautionary only and not viewed as complete protection; even the firmest collars allow some neck movement. It also serves as a reminder that potential cervical spine instability exists. If turning is necessary, however, a collar will help maintain the neck in a "neutral" position; turning patients is performed by "logrolling" their torso and legs while traction and support of the head and neck are maintained.

If spinal injury or instability is disposed, definitive spinal immobilization or stabilization can be instituted.

THE ABCS OF INITIAL MANAGEMENT

Special considerations concerning cardiopulmonary resuscitation, support, and maintenance apply to patients with acute spinal cord injuries. Spinal cord injury produces deficits in motor, sensory, and autonomic nervous system function below the level of injury. Injuries to the low cervical or thoracic spine produce impairment of intercostal muscle function. The diaphragm is innervated by the phrenic nerves, whose neurons arise primarily from the fourth cervical segment, but with contributions from the third and fifth segments. A characteristic respiratory pattern is recognizable: the chest falls paradoxically during inspiration while the abdomen rises. This dyssynchrony will be present if diaphragmatic function is preserved.

Injuries to the middle or upper cervical spine result in loss of diaphragmatic function or intrinsic respiratory drive centers in the cervical spine. Accessory muscles, such as the scalene, sternocleidomastoid, and strap muscles, receive cranial nerve innervation and function to produce tidal volumes of approximately 100 to 150 mL. They also may be used during periods of increased respiratory demand, producing a characteristic extension of the mandible and deepening of the suprasternal notch during inspiration.

Patients who have sustained injuries above the third cervical vertebra usually die before hospitalization unless cardiopulmonary resuscitation is administered at the scene. Despite general public awareness of and training in cardiopulmonary resuscitation techniques, resuscitative efforts may be initiated too late to prevent hypoxic brain injury.

AIRWAY CONTROL

The American Heart Association standards for basic life support and the American College of Surgeons guidelines for advanced trauma life support both recommend that a modified jaw-thrust method be used to establish a natural airway.[74,75] Extension of the cervical spine is avoided by maintaining gentle, in-line manual traction on the head.[75] If respiratory failure is either suspected or confirmed on the basis of dyspnea, tachypnea, or blood gas analysis, an artificial airway must be established. Wherever possible, respiratory insufficiency should be diagnosed as early as possible, so that endotracheal intubation can be performed safely to minimize the risk of inadvertent movement of the cervical spine. If the diagnosis is delayed and the patient progresses to bradycardia, hypotension, or cardiopulmonary arrest, emergency intubation may be more difficult and is associated with a greater risk of additional spinal cord injury.

In the absence of associated facial trauma or a suspected basilar skull fracture, blind nasal intubation is usually considered the procedure of choice because it may be accomplished without movement of the cervical spine. Adequate sedation and mild topical anesthesia both take time, although they can facilitate intubation. A fiberoptic laryngoscope may be used to visualize the larynx; the endotracheal tube also may be passed over the fiberoptic bronchoscope. Oral endotracheal intubation procedures may produce inadvertent hyperextension of the cervical spine; consequently, this route should be employed only when in-line cervical spine traction or firm manual countertraction is applied.

Surgical control of the airway by cricothyroidotomy should be employed in emergency situations only when intubation by other means is not feasible. Tracheostomy is less useful in an emergency situation because of the increased time required to perform the procedure. Because surgical stabilization is often performed on the anterior cervical spine, a contaminated cricothyroidotomy or tracheostomy site may delay definitive spine surgery because of the risk of infection.

If cervical traction is required to reduce or align the spine, the patient may require sedation that, in the presence of impaired or barely compensated respiratory function after spine injury, may precipitate acute ventilatory failure. In these instances, prophylactic intubation before sedation should be considered. With the less common thoracic spine injuries, acute respiratory insufficiency is seldom a problem if the level of injury is below the fourth thoracic vertebra.

CARDIOVASCULAR EFFECTS

Profound depression in cardiac function may occur in patients who have sustained high thoracic or cervical spinal cord injuries. Because sympathetic nervous system outflow begins at the cervicothoracic spine, significant spinal cord injuries rostral to the C8-T1 level may produce a functional sympathectomy. Interruption of the cardiac accelerator nerves (T1-6) results in bradycardia and hypotension. Peripherally, the loss of sympathetic tone produces vasodilation and increased venous capacitance, creating a relative hypovolemia. Because many spine-injured patients are otherwise young and presumed healthy, subtle signs of spinal cord dysfunction may not be appreciated. For example, bradycardia may be considered normal for a young athlete and may not be recognized as a complication of acute spinal cord shock. Similarly, the normal compensatory tachycardia that occurs with hypovolemia secondary to hemorrhage from multisystem trauma may be blocked, masking the clinical presentation.

The essential concept, however, is that the heart itself has been functionally sympathectomized, affecting not only chronotropy but also inotropy. Systemic hypotension can be treated initially with IV fluids, not only to increase the intravascular volume to compensate for the loss of vasomotor tone, but also to improve ejected stroke volume through the Starling mechanism. Because hypovolemia per se is not the direct cause of hypotension, it is prudent to limit resuscitation to prevent overload, ventricular decompensation, or frank ventricular failure. Sinus bradycardia, with rates of 40 to 50 beats per minute, is common after cervical spine injury; if extreme bradycardia, conduction block, or arrhythmia with hypotension occurs, atropine, 0.2 mg to 0.5 mg, can be

administered intravenously. If hypotension persists despite fluid administration, a continuous infusion of a primarily cardiac beta-agonist (e.g., dopamine at 5 to 15 µg/kg/minute or dobutamine at 3 to 20 µg/kg/minute) should be initiated.[73] Isoproterenol hydrochloride (Isuprel) is less useful because its nonselective beta-agonist action may promote peripheral vasodilatation. Although mild sympathomimetic agents such as phenylephrine hydrochloride may be employed, the use of primary alpha-agonists, such as levo-ephedrine bitartrate and metaraminol bitartrate, are not recommended because these agents increase cardiac afterload, impair cardiac output, and may precipitate congestive heart failure. This empirical approach should be considered only as an urgent measure to control profound hypotension; invasive cardiovascular monitoring is usually necessary to differentiate the components of myocardial depression, hypovolemia, and diminished vasomotor tone.[73]

In patients who have sustained multiple trauma, hypotension secondary to spinal shock may conceal hypovolemia from occult blood loss. Because abdominal signs and symptoms may be absent in quadriplegic or high-paraplegic patients, peritoneal lavage or abdominal CT scanning or ultrasound should be considered to determine whether intraabdominal or retroperitoneal injury with occult hemorrhage is present. Similarly, chest radiographs may reveal a hemothorax resulting from a thoracic vascular injury, or hip and pelvis radiographs may demonstrate fractures with associated hemorrhage.

NEUROLOGIC EXAMINATION

The baseline neurologic assessment performed at the time of admission to the hospital must be repeated at frequent intervals, especially if the spinal cord injury is incomplete (Fig. 78-3). This assessment must be repeated before and after each transport. Evaluation should include comparison of motor and sensory function in all extremities. If a conus medullaris or cauda equina injury is suspected, rectal sphincter tone must be assessed. Incomplete or asymmetric spinal cord lesions with evidence of deteriorating neurologic function or spinal column instability may require immediate surgery; complete spinal cord lesions that are bilaterally symmetric and unchanging are usually treated with traction to maintain alignment and either external orthoses or surgical stabilization. Deficits resulting from compression of the inferior conus or cauda equina are treated similarly to peripheral nerve injuries resulting from bony compression: early surgical decompression is performed in the hopes of hastening recovery or improving outcome.

INITIAL DIAGNOSTIC PROCEDURES

Anteroposterior and lateral radiographs of the cervical spine (including the open-mouth view of the odontoid) must adequately demonstrate all seven cervical vertebrae (including the cervicothoracic junction).[75] The seventh cervical vertebra is often difficult to visualize; to improve visualization, the shoulders may be depressed by downward traction on the arms while linear cervical traction is maintained. The "swimmer's view" also may be used to visualize the seventh cervical vertebra. Vertical reconstruction of a CT of the spine may

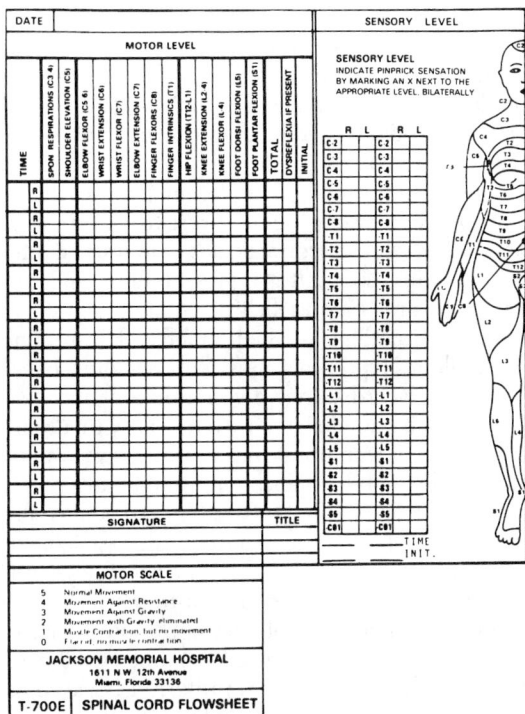

FIGURE 78-3. An example of an ICU flow sheet for serial assessment of neurologic status in spine-injured patients, grading motor strength in all major muscle groups and sensory function.

provide visualization if repeated conventional radiographs fail to demonstrate all cervical vertebrae. Lateral radiographs allow for rapid assessment of the alignment of the cervical spine, presence of fractures, or evidence of prevertebral hemorrhage; degenerative changes such as osteophytes also may be identified. Anteroposterior radiographs demonstrate fractures and may suggest rotatory instability. Dynamic views of spine motion (i.e., flexion–extension radiographs) may be used to assess ligamentous instability or injury when pain is persistent and severe; however, this should be done only if there are no neurologic deficits and no radiographic evidence of fractures or bony instability, and if full patient cooperation is possible. When multilevel injuries could have occurred, thoracic and lumbar spine anteroposterior and lateral radiographs should be performed.

Contrast CT myelography and MRI clearly provide superior visualization of the spinal canal contents, and they should be employed whenever soft tissue lesions, such as extruded intervertebral disc fragments or intraspinal EDHs, or intrinsic spinal cord disease, such as intramedullary hemorrhage, are suspected. Results of these studies may mandate emergency decompressive surgery.

ALIGNMENT OF THE CERVICAL CANAL

The primary goal of early alignment of the vertebral column is the reduction of spinal cord compression and the prevention of further injury; it may also be beneficial in preserving or improving nerve root function at the level of the injury.[73] Diminished pressure on the spinal cord and improved micro-

vascular circulation may reduce spinal cord edema, which can ascend and cause a progressive neurologic deficit.

Alignment is achieved by application of cervical traction, which requires cranial fixation. Tongs, particularly the Gardner-Wells and Crutchfield types, and halo rings are commonly used; all require the insertion of pins into the outer table of the calvarium for stabilization. The Gardner-Wells tongs are technically easier to apply, but the halo rings may be attached immediately to an external cylindrical vest orthosis for immediate skeletal stabilization, once any deformity has been reduced.

Once the tong or ring has been applied, weights are added to a pulley device at the top of the bed. Radiographs of the lateral cervical spine are used to evaluate alignment of the vertebral column. Weights are increased in 2.2-kg (5-lb) increments, with the amount of traction required for reduction estimated at 2.2 to 4.5 kg (5 to 10 lb) per interspace; rarely, more than 22.2 kg (50 lb) of traction are required. Fractures and dislocations generally respond to lesser weights, and even small weights may produce distraction of the spine if ligamentous injury is severe.

Occasionally, facets may be "locked" during injury, preventing reduction even with considerable traction. Cervical paraspinal muscle spasm often is the culprit and may in fact be exacerbated by traction. In this circumstance, muscle relaxants such as diazepam or even pharmacologic paralysis with d-tubocurarine, pancuronium, atracurium, or vecuronium may be necessary to induce muscle relaxation for reduction; on occasion, general anesthesia may be warranted. Because these medications are administered to a patient with already compromised pulmonary and hemodynamic function and stability, elective tracheal intubation should be considered. Mechanical ventilation may be necessary during the period of respiratory depression or total pharmacologic paralysis. Succinylcholine should not be used.

If there is no unstable bony injury, traction is not usually necessary for patients with penetrating cervical injuries, although a cervical collar may be used to provide some support. Tracheal, esophageal, and major vessel injuries also must be considered, and definitive diagnostic procedures completed. Bronchoscopy, esophagoscopy or esophograms, and arteriograms may be necessary, depending on the location of the injury and trajectory of the penetrating agent. Operation on the spinal column is deferred until associated injuries have been ruled out or managed. These patients' spinal cord injuries are managed by observation, with particular attention to monitoring for ascending neurologic deficits or CSF leaks. Entrance wounds are debrided superficially and, if CSF leak is suspected, the wound is closed and a lumbar spinal drain may be placed. Penetrating wounds involving abdominal viscus require surgical repair to prevent CSF contamination with bowel flora.

MANAGEMENT IN THE ICU

Spinal Shock

Spinal shock is caused by the abrupt withdrawal of descending excitatory influences from higher nerve centers to the spine, and by persistent inhibition below the level of injury.[76] Complete interruption of afferent and efferent nerve tracts results in spinal shock below the level of spinal cord injury; this reflex depression is most pronounced close to the area of injury. Reflex depression also may occur cephalad to the level of injury itself because of ascending neuronal edema. It will be expressed by diminished muscular strength, cutaneous sensation, and reflex tendon activity some time after the initial injury. However, the more cephalad impairment is usually transient, even when there is total absence of neuronal function at the level of injury initially, because neuronal transection may not be complete and some dysfunction may be the result of neuronal edema. Some motor or sensory function (pain, light touch, temperature, position, proprioception, or response to vibration) may return later. Return of function generally occurs in a caudad to cephalad direction. The initial flaccid paralysis of spinal shock (paradoxically, an *upper* motor neuron lesion) gives way to spasticity or hyperreflexia as the spinal shock abates.[77] The duration of spinal shock varies considerably, from a few days to many weeks or even months after injury. Infections and other toxic conditions may prolong spinal shock.[78]

Various pharmacotherapies have been tried for treating spinal shock. Recent studies demonstrate a significant response to methylprednisolone when it is administered within 8 hours of injury, in a loading dosage of 30 mg/kg given intravenously over 1 hour, with an IV dosage of 5.4 mg/kg administered hourly over the next 23 hours.[79]

Respiratory Involvement

Even with preservation of spinal cord anterior horn cells of the phrenic nerve, spontaneous respiration may be depressed or absent soon after injury; with spinal shock, it may be weeks or months before phrenic nerve function returns, resulting in prolonged ventilator dependence. During this time, disuse atrophy of the diaphragm may occur during continuous mechanical ventilation.

Respiratory failure is present in virtually all patients with high thoracic or cervical cord injury. Respiratory failure may include hypoxemia, hypercapnia, or diminished mechanics. These injuries often occur in young patients with considerable physiologic reserves; significant deterioration in this reserve may not be detected unless appropriate diagnostic measures are performed. For instance, even if the level of injury is below the fourth cervical vertebra, vital capacity may be as low as 150 to 300 mL during the initial stages of spinal shock. Although most quadriplegic patients have an adequate vital capacity and tidal volume to maintain minute ventilation, they have an ineffective cough because of paralysis of the abdominal and intercostal muscles, and are consequently unable to clear airway secretions. Chest wall compliance is decreased secondary to loss of muscle tone. The supine position, necessary for cervical traction and hemodynamic instability, and the weight of the intraabdominal organs impair function of the diaphragm, the sole remaining respiratory muscle. This may be further complicated by abdominal distention, which may occur with or without associated intraabdominal injuries.

These conditions result in ventilation-perfusion abnormalities, increased intrapulmonary shunt, hypoxemia, and atelectasis. Progression from retained secretions to atelectasis to pneumonitis is also common. Hypercapnia may occur if minute ventilation cannot be maintained.

If the patient is not intubated, continuous heated aerosols with modest oxygen supplementation may aid in thinning pulmonary secretions so that they can be mobilized. The patient's ability to cough, considerably impaired by the paralysis of the thoracic and intraabdominal muscles, may be aided by an assisted subphrenic thrust to help in expelling secretions. However, nasotracheal suctioning is often required in the days soon after injury. Routine suctioning is not necessary, and nasotracheal suctioning should be reserved for the situations in which mobilized secretions cannot be expelled. Hypoxemia must be prevented because it may induce bradycardia. Incentive spirometry may be useful in preventing airway closure. In patients with diminished vital capacities, intermittent positive pressure ventilation may be used to mobilize peripheral pulmonary secretions. Pulmonary secretions may be thick and tenacious, particularly if glycopyrrolate is used to diminish gastric acidity or atropine has been administered to correct bradycardia.

Because intubation in the patient with cervical injury may be difficult and entails special risks, it should be performed before severe compromise or frank respiratory failure develops. Although the nasal route is preferred because of ease of intubation in the emergency situation, there is a high incidence of maxillary sinusitis associated with long-term intubation. The endotracheal tube should be large enough to permit passage of a fiberoptic bronchoscope because of the frequency of recurrent and persistent lung collapse in these patients.

Ventilatory support techniques that encourage spontaneous respiration and maintain functional residual capacity should be considered because they often aid in correcting the abnormal physiology created by the injury. Intermittent mandatory ventilation, synchronized intermittent mandatory ventilation, and pressure support ventilation seem attractive because they all incorporate the patient's contribution to total minute ventilation. Controlled ventilation may result in diaphragmatic atrophy, thus prolonging the period of ventilation. In general, the patient's contribution, however minimal, should be incorporated into the planned formula for total minute ventilation. The loss of functional residual capacity resulting from the supine position, diminished compliance, ventilation-perfusion abnormalities, and the tendency to develop atelectasis should be offset by using PEEP. Large tidal volumes (12 to 15 mL/kg) may foster alveolar recruitment, and PEEP maintains alveolar patency. If compliance is improved by PEEP or pressure support ventilation, in addition to restoration of functional residual capacity and improvement in oxygenation, the work of breathing may be reduced, thus facilitating the weaning process.

Lobar collapse is common and is usually caused by the plugging of segmental bronchi. Saline lavage and endotracheal suctioning may be effective in mobilizing these secretions. Tidal volume may be temporarily increased to 15 to 18 mL/kg and the level of PEEP increased by an additional 5 cm H_2O empirically in an attempt to augment alveolar recruitment and patency. However, fiberoptic bronchoscopy is often necessary for direct aspiration of the affected bronchus. Heated humidification should be provided.

If lobar or total lung collapse recurs and does not respond to increased tidal volumes and PEEP, independent lung ventilation may be considered to avoid overdistention of the normal lung, which may occur if high tidal volumes are employed. A normal tidal volume can be administered to the unaffected lung, and higher tidal volumes and PEEP levels employed only on the affected side.

Tracheostomy

The necessity for, and timing of, tracheostomy in the ventilator-dependent spine-injured patient must be assessed with respect to planned operative intervention, the patient's potential for weaning, and the risks of prolonged intubation. Early operative stabilization of the cervical spine may be considered because it can permit early mobilization or, at least, repositioning to remove the weight of the intraabdominal contents from the diaphragm. A tracheostomy antedating surgery creates a risk of infection, especially if bone grafts are used; 1 to 2 weeks after surgery, however, tracheostomy may be performed with little additional risk. If anterior neck surgery is not contemplated, the major determinant would be the predicted length of ventilator dependence. In the case of more caudal cord lesions with good diaphragmatic function and improving ventilatory mechanics, tracheal intubation should be continued. If diaphragmatic excursions are minimal, if maxillary or sphenoid sinusitis develops, or if operative intervention is not contemplated, tracheostomy can be performed earlier in the hospital course. Nasotracheal and nasogastric intubations should not be used for periods greater than 3 to 4 days. Tubes should be replaced through the mouth when the patient is stable. Tracheostomy devices that permit phonation greatly improve the patient's ability to communicate and should be considered if long-term ventilator dependence is anticipated.

Cardiovascular Impairment

With spinal cord injuries rostral to the fifth thoracic segment, loss of sympathetic outflow during the period of spinal shock can create cardiovascular instability; this instability is more pronounced in cervical lesions. The cardiovascular problems, which can be minor or life-threatening, may last for days or weeks; they occur independent of age or history of cardiac disease and may occur in incomplete as well as complete spine lesions. The young, healthy male patient, a common cervical spinal injury victim, may have surprisingly poor cardiac performance after injury, and even frank left ventricular failure is possible.

Sympathectomy results in dominance of cardiac parasympathetic (vagal) stimuli. Sinus bradycardia occurs in most patients and rates may fall to 20 to 30 beats per minute. Sinus pauses, sinus arrest, or asystole, resulting in escape or junctional rhythms, also occur. These arrhythmias can become more frequent and more pronounced in the presence of hypoxia. The normal response to hypoxia is mediated by the sympathetic nervous system and consists of tachycardia and increased systemic blood pressure. In newly injured quadriplegics, however, parasympathetic effects predominate and profound bradycardia, or even cardiac arrest, may represent the initial response to hypoxia.

Vasomotor Tone

Loss of vasoconstrictor tone resulting from an injury rostral to the fifth thoracic segment results in vasodilation, increased venous capacitance, and (often) hypotension. Venous return is also compromised by the loss of the muscular "pumping" action in the extremities and paralysis of the abdominal musculature, so that the increased intraabdominal pressure found during normal respirations can no longer be created. Relative hypovolemia (revealed by increased intrathoracic pressure during mechanical ventilation or pneumothorax) or actual hypovolemia (hemorrhage or inadequate volume replacement) also may occur. However, the usual reflex sympathetic vasoconstriction and tachycardia are absent. Thus, the clinical presentation of the hypovolemic state will be both accelerated and more profound than might be expected from the degree of hypovolemia actually present. The absence of a premonitory reflex tachycardia as the first usual indication of hypovolemia may allow hypotension to develop before the need for intervention is recognized.

The period of cardiovascular instability persists until vasomotor responsiveness returns. The development of sinus tachycardia after a febrile response or other normal stimuli may be the first sign that cardiovascular instability is abating.

Treatment of Cardiovascular Manifestations

Continuous ECG monitoring is mandatory during acute spinal shock. Arterial pulse oximetry and intermittent arterial blood gas determinations are useful in detecting hypoxemia, which may exacerbate the effects of sympathetic dysfunction. Central venous pressure and monitoring of urinary output are of value in guiding initial fluid administration relative to intravascular volume. Hypotension in the presence of low central venous pressure may indicate increased venous capacitance; however, because spinal shock affects both vasomotor tone and left ventricular performance, pulmonary artery catheterization should be considered when hypotension persists or central venous pressure does not respond despite what is empirically considered to be adequate fluid administration. More accurate titration is possible by monitoring left ventricular filling pressure. Identification of disturbances in vasomotor tone or ventricular failure allows for administration and titration of sympathomimetic agents and inotropic agents, respectively. In patients with multiple injuries or concomitant neurogenic pulmonary edema, pulmonary artery catheterization may be necessary to direct therapeutic modes of ventilatory support.

ARRHYTHMIAS. Asymptomatic bradycardia (i.e., without changes in blood pressure, level of consciousness, or urinary output) should not be treated. IV atropine sulfate in doses of 0.2 to 0.5 mg usually corrects transient symptomatic episodes. Potentiation of bradyarrhythmias by hypoxemia must always be considered, and continuous oximetry may permit early detection before arrhythmias or profound hypotension develops. Endotracheal suctioning and gastric or bladder distension may induce vagal reflex responses causing asystole. Preoxygenation and gentle intermittent suctioning techniques should be used; bladder and gastric drainage catheters should be in place and functioning. Small doses of IV or intratracheal lidocaine or preadministration of medications with mild beta-agonist effects (e.g., terbutaline or metaproterenol) may abort the vagal response. If a bradyarrhythmic episode occurs, assisted manual ventilation with 100% oxygen, a precordial thump, or administration of IV atropine usually restores the heart rate. Occasionally, continuous infusion of dobutamine, isoproterenol, dopamine, or epinephrine may be necessary. Rarely, temporary transvenous pacing may be necessary. Permanent pacing is rarely considered in the ICU, but persistent bradyarrhythmias, when other intensive care problems have resolved, may require pacing to permit safe transfer of the patient to another hospital care area.

NEUROGENIC PULMONARY EDEMA.   Neurogenic pulmonary edema associated with isolated spinal cord injury is rare. Other mechanisms, such as intrinsic cardiac disease, fluid overload, direct chest trauma, or head injury must be considered. The pathophysiologic mechanisms are not clearly understood; the treatment is similar to that for other forms of noncardiogenic pulmonary edema.

Venous Thrombosis and Pulmonary Embolism

The incidence rate of venous thrombosis has been reported to be as high as 22%, with a 10% incidence rate of pulmonary embolism.[80] Hypotension, decreased blood flow (from the flaccid paralysis), and venous stasis (from the loss of vasomotor tone) are considered to be contributing causes. The quadriplegic patient with diminished ability to cough may not demonstrate hemoptysis, or blood may be attributed to irritation caused by endotracheal suctioning; anesthesia of the chest wall may mask pleuritic pain. Increased PR interval, right bundle branch block, or transient sinus tachycardia with right axis deviation of ECG monitoring may be the earliest sign; tachypnea and sudden deterioration in arterial blood gases may be the only clinical manifestations. Thus, a high degree of suspicion must be maintained regarding thrombosis and embolism. Kinetic therapy, using rotating beds to improve peripheral blood flow, decreases the incidence of this complication.[81] Pneumatic venous compression devices, which are thought to increase endothelial production of prostacycline-like substances, also reduce the incidence of venous thrombosis. Eliminating prolonged periods of cervical traction by using halo external orthoses also facilitates earlier mobilization. Prophylaxis with heparin, 5000 to 7000 U subcutaneously every 12 hours has been advocated when prolonged immobility is anticipated.[82]

Gastrointestinal Effects

Spinal shock also affects gastrointestinal function, producing gastric atony and ileus. Nasogastric suction is necessary to prevent gastric dilatation and abdominal distensions, which may further impair pulmonary function or result in regurgitation of gastric contents with subsequent aspiration. Because gastric hypersecretion is common, however, continuous suction can create a hypochloremic metabolic alkalosis because of the loss of hydrochloric acid. Compensatory hypoventilation and the resultant hypercapnia may be interpreted incorrectly as signifying inadequate muscular activity to maintain alveolar ventilation. Careful fluid and electrolyte replacement therapy, therefore, is essential if these additional complications are to be avoided.

Gastric hypersecretion also may result in stress ulceration or hemorrhage, particularly if high-dose corticosteroids are used for more than a short time. Because pain, tenderness, guarding, and other abdominal symptomatology are absent in the quadriplegic patient, and because reflex tachycardia does not occur after sympathectomy, perforation may be silent and present or an abdominal catastrophe because of the difficulty of diagnosis. Fever of unknown origin with leukocytosis may be the only early sign, and recognition of the intraabdominal catastrophe may be delayed until profound shock ensues. Similar considerations pertain to older patients with histories of diverticulitis or diverticulosis. Hyperamylasemia is a common finding, even in the absence of direct abdominal trauma or clinical pancreatitis. It may be the result of gastric reflux through the sphincter of Oddi. Pancreatitis must be considered, however, and ruled out more definitively if hyperamylasemia persists. Gastric hypersecretion must be prevented. Routine monitoring of gastric pH is mandatory until full enteral feedings are possible. Antacids and H_2 blockers (cimetidine, ranitidine, famotidine) used in increasing doses until the pH is consistently maintained above 4.5 are adequate methods of prevention. Sucralfate (Carafate) may be used for prophylaxis as well. Primary gastric acid secretion inhibitors (e.g., misoprostol) also may be of benefit in some cases.

Rarely, spine-injured patients may develop acalculous cholecystitis, either alone or in combination with pancreatitis.[83] Because of the paucity of abdominal symptoms in the quadriplegic patient, this syndrome may present with fever and biliary dysfunction and progress to frank gangrene of the gall bladder with peritonitis if it is not suspected and detected early. Bedside ultrasonography, abdominal CT, or bedside laparoscopy can be used for diagnosis (Chap. 71). Antibiotic therapy and surgical resection are the treatment of choice. Persistent ileus and gastric atony often prevent early enteral feeding, which is clearly preferable to diminish complications associated with IV alimentation and to minimize gastric hypersecretion. If gastric atony persists, direct jejunal feedings may be possible. Tubes can be placed under fluoroscopic guidance, percutaneously, or at laparoscopy. When gastrointestinal function returns and spinal shock abates, patients usually require stool softeners and scheduled laxatives. Fecal impaction or rectal distention may cause severe hypertension secondary to autonomic dysreflexia and even bowel obstruction.

Poikilothermia

The disruption of sympathetic nerve pathways from the hypothalamus to peripheral blood vessels interferes with vasodilatation and sweating in hot environments and with vasoconstriction in cold ones. Thermoregulation mechanisms are, therefore, considerably impaired, and significant hypothermia can occur. In the air-conditioned ICU, the patient must remain covered and body temperature must be maintained; hyperthermia blankets may be necessary. Some degree of hypothermia may persist; in fact, a "normal body temperature" may represent a febrile response and be an early indication of infection.

Genitourinary Problems

Injury to the spinal cord produces initial bladder flaccidity (spinal shock) followed by eventual spasticity; injury to the inferior conus medullaris or cauda equina produces a hypotonic bladder. These conditions predispose to persistent urinary problems over the life span of the quadriplegic or paraplegic patient, including recurrent urinary tract infections, bladder stones, nephrocalcinosis, and life-threatening urosepsis. Bladder catheterization is required to prevent urinary retention and secondary vagal reflex responses during the period of initial management of cardiovascular instability, and also to provide accurate output measurements for calculating fluid balance. Indwelling catheters, which predispose to urinary tract infections, should be removed as soon possible and replaced by intermittent bladder catheterization, which can decrease the incidence of urinary tract infections.[84] After spinal shock resolves, bladder distention can also cause hypertension secondary to dysreflexia, so that a regular schedule of catheterization may be necessary. Chronic urinary tract infection is one of the most frequently encountered problems in patients with spinal cord injury, and it will often cause worsening of spasticity or dysreflexias. When acute renal failure occurs, it usually results from another precipitating event, such as a low flow state or sepsis during the acute phase, or pyelonephritis or renal calculi in long-term patients. Chronic bacterial suppressant therapy, either by urine acidification or antimicrobial, often averts these sequelae.

Problems of Immobilization

Prolonged immobilization predisposes to disorders of calcium metabolism. Heterotopic ossification, painful calcification of muscles, and immobilization of joints may actually worsen the patient's functional status despite recovery or preservation of neurologic function. It may present as a fever of unknown origin with swelling over muscles or joints; a radionuclide bone scan confirms the diagnosis. Treatment with sodium etidronate may be effective if initiated early, but active physical therapy in the ICU is essential for joint mobility preservation. Osteoporosis resulting from inactivity may predispose to hypercalcemia, nephrocalcinosis, and secondary uropathy; late mobilization may risk pathologic fracture. Here too, kinetic therapy and early mobilization remain important goals in ICU management.

Intensive psychological counseling for the spine-injured patient should begin in the ICU; this therapy should be maintained as the patient progresses throughout hospitalization and ultimately rehabilitation.

REFERENCES

1. Bowers SA, Marshall LF: Outcome in 200 consecutive cases of severe head injury treated in San Diego county: a prospective analysis. *Neurosurgery* 1980;6:237
2. Kraus JF: Epidemiology of head injury. In: Cooper PR (ed). *Head Injury,* ed 2. Baltimore, Williams & Wilkins, 1987:1
3. Nuelk DF, Gikas PW: Causes of death in automobile accidents. *JAMA* 1968;203:98
4. Rose J, Valtonen S, Jennett B: Avoidable factors contributing to death after head injury. *Br Med J* 1977;2:615
5. Plum F, Posner JB: *The Diagnosis of Stupor and Coma,* ed 3. Philadelphia, FA Davis, 1980
6. Miller JD, Becker DP, Ward JD, et al: Significance of intracranial hypertension in severe head injury. *J Neurosurg* 1977;47:501
7. Jennett B, Teasdale G, Braakman R, et al: Predicting outcome in individual patients after severe head injury. *Lancet* 1976; i:1031
8. Rosner MJ, Rosner SD, Johnson AH: Cerebral perfusion pressure: management protocol and clinical results. *J Neurosurg* 1995;83:949
9. Roberts JR: Pathophysiology, diagnosis and treatment of head trauma. *Top Emerg Med* 1979;1:41
10. Peerless SJ, Rewcastle NB: Shear injuries to the brain. *Can Med Assoc J* 1967;98:577
11. Geisler FH, Greenberg J: Management of the acute head-injury patient. In: Salcman M (ed). *Neurologic Emergency,* ed 2. New York, Raven Press, 1990:135
12. Diaz GF, Yock DH, Larson D, et al: Early diagnosis of delayed traumatic intracerebral hematoma. *J Neurosurg* 1979;50:217
13. Kaufman HH, Moake JL, Olson JD, et al: Delayed and recurrent intracranial hematomas related to disseminated intravascular clotting and fibrinolysis in head injury. *Neurosurgery* 1980;7:445
14. Jennett B, Teasdale G, Braakman R, et al: Prognosis of patients with severe head injury. *Neurosurgery* 1979;4:282
15. Seelig JM, Becker DP, Miller JD, et al: Traumatic acute subdural hematoma. *N Engl J Med* 1981;304:1511
16. Villanueva PA: Cranial gunshot wounds. In: Ordog G (ed). *Management of Gunshot Wounds.* New York, Elsevier, 1988: 257
17. Masters SJ, McClean PM, Arcarese JS, et al: Skull x-ray examinations after head trauma: recommendations by a multidisciplinary panel and validation study. *N Engl J Med* 1987;316:84
18. Andrews BT, Pitts LH, Lovely MP, et al: Is computed tomographic scanning necessary in patients with tentorial herniation? Results of immediate surgical exploration without computed tomography in 100 patients. *Neurosurgery* 1986;19:408
19. Ropper AH: Lateral displacement of the brain and level of consciousness in patients with an acute hemispheral mass. *N Engl J Med* 1986;314:953
20. Rosner MJ, Newsome HH, Becker DP: Mechanical brain injury: the sympathoadrenal response. *J Neurosurg* 1984;61:76
21. Jennett B, Teasdale G, Galbraith S, et al: Severe head injuries in three countries. *J Neurol Neurosurg Psychiatry* 1977;40: 291
22. Frost EAM: Effects of positive end-expiratory pressure on intracranial pressure and compliance in brain-injured patients. *J Neurosurg* 1977;47:195
23. Andrews BT, Chiles BW, Olsen WE, et al: The effect of intracerebral hematoma location on the risk of brainstem compression and on clinical outcome. *J Neurosurg* 1988;69:518
24. North B, Reilly P: Comparison among three methods of intracranial pressure recording. *Neurosurgery* 1986;18:730
25. Schickner DJ, Young RF: Intracranial pressure monitoring:

fiberoptic monitor compared with the ventricular catheter. *Surg Neurol* 1992;7:251

26. Arnolds BJ, Von Reutern G-M: Transcranial Doppler sonography: examination technique and normal reference values. *Ultrasound Med Biol* 1986;12:115

27. Weber M, Grolimund P, Seiler RW: Evaluation of post-traumatic cerebral blood flow velocities by transcranial Doppler ultrasonography. *J Neurosurg* 1990;27:106

28. Carter LP: Surface monitoring of cerebral cortical blood flow. *Cerebrovasc Brain Metab Rev* 1991;3:246

29. Bell BA: A history of the study of the cerebral circulation and the measurement of cerebral blood flow. *Neurosurgery* 1984;14:238

30. Kety SS, Schmidt CF: the nitrous oxide method for the quantitative determination of cerebral blood flow in man: theory, procedure, and normal values. *J Clin Invest* 1948;27:476

31. Obrist WD, Thompson HK, Wang HS, et al: Regional cerebral blood flow estimated by 133 Xenon inhalation. *Stroke* 1975;6:245

32. Langfitt TW, Obrist WD, Alai A, et al: Computerized tomography, magnetic resonance imaging and positron emission tomography in the study of brain trauma: preliminary observations. *J Neurosurg* 1986;64:760

33. Hill TC, Homan BL: SPECT brain imaging: finding a niche in neurologic diagnosis. *Diagn Imaging* 1985;7:64

34. Yoshino E, Yamaki T, Higuchi T, et al: Acute brain edema in fatal head injury: analysis by dynamic CT scanning. *J Neurosurg* 1985;63:830

35. Robertson CS, Narayan RK, Gokdslan ZL, et al: Cerebral arteriovenous oxygen difference as an estimate of cerebral blood flow in comatose patients. *J Neurosurg* 1989;70:222

36. Sheinbreg M, Kanter M, Robertson CS, et al: Continuous monitoring of jugular venous oxygen saturation in head-injured patients. *J Neurosurg* 1992;76:212

37. Hans P, Franssen C, Damas F, et al: Continuous measurement of jugular venous bulb saturation in neurosurgical patients. *Acta Anesthesiol Belg* 1991;42:213

38. Dow RS, Ulett G, Raaf J: Electroencephalographic studies immediately following head injury. *Am J Psychiatry* 1944;101:174

39. Greenberg RP, Ducker TB: Evoked potentials in the clinical neurosciences. *J Neurosurg* 1982;56:1

40. Greenberg RP, Newlon PG, Hyatt MS, et al: Prognostic implications of early multimodality evoked potentials in severely head-injured patients: a prospective study. *J Neurosurg* 1981;55:227

41. Brown FK: Cardiovascular effects of acutely raised intracranial pressure. *Am J Physiol* 1956;185:510

42. Cottrell JE, Bhagwandas G, Rappaport H, et al: Intracranial pressure during nitroglycerin-induced hypotension. *J Neurosurg* 1980;53:309

43. Cottrell JE, Patel K, Turndorf H, et al: Intracranial pressure changes induced by sodium nitroprusside in patients with intracranial mass lesions. *J Neurosurg* 1978;48:329

44. Berman IR, Ducker TB: Pulmonary, somatic and splanchnic circulatory responses to increased intracranial pressure. *Ann Surg* 1969;169:210

45. Temkin NR, Dimken SS, Wilensky AJ, et al: A randomized, double-blind study of phenytoin for the prevention of posttraumatic seizures. *N Engl J Med* 1990;323:497

46. Paul RL, Polanco O, Tourney SZ, et al: Intracranial pressure responses to alterations in arterial carbon dioxide pressure in patients with head injuries. *J Neurosurg* 1972;36:714

47. Muizelaar JP, Marmarou A, Ward JD, et al: Adverse effects of prolonged hyperventilation in patients with severe head injury: a randomized clinical trial. *J Neurosurg* 1991;75:731

48. Cruz J: An additional therapeutic effect of adequate hyperventilation in severe acute brain trauma: normalization of cerebral glucose uptake. *J Neurosurg* 1995;82:379

49. Marshall LF, Smith RW, Rauscher LA, et al: Mannitol dose requirements in brain injured patients. *J Neurosurg* 1978;48:169

50. Miller JD, Butterworth JF, Guderman SK, et al: Further experiences in the management of severe head injury. *J Neurosurg* 1981;54:289

51. Marshall LF, Marshall SB: Medical management of intracranial pressure. In: Cooper PR (ed). *Head Injury*, ed 2. Baltimore, Williams & Wilkins, 1987:177

52. Ward JD, Becker DP, Miller JD, et al: Failure of prophylactic barbiturate coma in the treatment of severe head injury. *J Neurosurg* 1985;62:383

53. Eisenberg HM, Frankowski RF, Contant C, et al: High-dose barbiturate control of elevated intracranial pressure in patients with severe head injury. *J Neurosurg* 1988;69:15

54. Rockoff MA, Marshall LF, Shapiro HM: High-Dose barbiturate therapy in humans: a clinical review of 60 patients. *Ann Neurol* 1979;6:194

55. Braakman R, Schouten HJA, van Dishoeck MB, et al: Megadose steroids in severe head injury: results of a prospective double-blind clinical trial. *J Neurosurg* 1983;58:326

56. Gudeman SK, Miller JD, Becker DP: Failure of high-dose steroid therapy to influence intracranial pressure in patients with severe head injury. *J Neurosurg* 1979;51:301

57. Marshall LF, King J, Langfitt TW: The complications of high-dose corticosteroid therapy in neurosurgical patients: a prospective study. *Ann Neurol* 1977;1:201

58. Meldrum B, Millan MH, Obrenovitch TP: Excitatory amino-acid release induced by injury. In: Globus NY-T, Dietrich WD (eds). *The Role of Neurotransmitters in Brain Injury*. New York, Plenum Press, 1992

59. Stuart L, Bullock R, Jones M, et al: The cerebral hemodynamic and metabolic effects of the competitive NUDA antagonist CGS19755 in humans with severe head injury. In: *Proceedings of the Second International Neurotrauma Symposium*. Glasgow, 1993

60. Siesjo BK: Pathophysiology and treatment of focal cerebral ischemia. *J Neurosurg* 1992;77:169

61. Hall ED, Yonkers PA, McCall JM, et al: Effects of the 21-aminosteroid U-74,006F on experimental head injury in mice. *J Neurosurg* 1988;68:456

62. Kontos HA, Wei EP: Superoxide production in experimental brain injury. *J Neurosurg* 1986;64:803

63. Lanier WL, Stangland KJ, Scheithauer BW, et al: Effects of intravenous dextrose infusion and head position on neurologic outcome after complete cerebral ischemia (abstract). *Anesthesiology* 1985;63:A110

64. Sterns RH, Riggs JE, Schochet SS Jr: Osmotic demyelination syndrome following correction of hyponatremia. *N Engl J Med* 1986;314:1535

65. Ayus JC, Krothapalli RK, Arieff AI: Treatment of symptomatic hyponatremia and its relation to brain damage. *N Engl J Med* 1987;317:1190

66. Clark JA, Finelli RE, Netsky MG: Disseminated intravascular coagulation following cranial trauma. *J Neurosurg* 1980;52:266

67. Greenberg J, Cohen WA, Cooper PR: The "hyperacute" extraaxial intracranial hematoma: computed tomographic findings and clinical significance. *Neurosurgery* 1985;17:48

68. Jennett B, Bond M: Assessment of outcome after severe brain damage. *Lancet* 1975;i:480

69. Greenberg RP, Newlon PG, Hyatt MS, et al: Prognostic implications of early multimodality evoked potentials in severely head-injured patients. *J Neurosurg* 1981;55:227

70. Clifton GL, Grossman RG, Makela ME, et al: Neurological course and correlated computerized tomography findings after severe closed head injury. *J Neurosurg* 1980;52:611
71. Choi SC, Narayan RK, Anderson RL, et al: Enhanced specificity of prognosis in severe head injury. *J Neurosurg* 1988;69:381
72. Grahm TW, Williams FC Jr, Harrington T, et al: Civilian gunshot wounds to the head: a prospective study. *Neurosurgery* 1990;27:696
73. Greenberg J, Geisler FH: Management of traumatic spine injuries and acute paralysis. In: Salcman M (ed). *Neurologic Emergencies*, ed 2. New York, Raven Press, 1990:167
74. Standards and guidelines for cardiopulmonary resuscitation and emergency cardiac care. II. Basic life support, jaw-thrust maneuver. *JAMA* 1986;255:2916
75. Committee on Trauma: *Advanced Trauma Life Support Manual*, 2nd ed. Chicago, American College of Surgeons, 1989
76. Osterholm JC: The pathophysiological response to spinal cord injury. *J Neurosurg* 1974;40:5
77. Mesard L: Survival after spinal cord trauma. *Arch Neurol* 1978;35:78
78. Guttman L: *Spinal Cord Injuries: Comprehensive Management and Research*. Oxford, Blackwell Scientific Publications, 1976
79. Bracken MB, Shepard MJ, Collins WF, et al: A randomized, controlled trial of methylprednisolone or naloxone in the treatment of acute spinal-cord injury. *N Engl J Med* 1990;322: 1405
80. Perkash A, Prakash V, Perkash I: Experience with the management of thromboembolism in patients with spinal cord injury. I. Incidence, diagnosis, and role of risk factors. *Paraplegia* 1978–1979;16:322
81. Welch GW: Effects of the kinetic bed on venous filling and emptying of the lower extremity. *Crit Care Med* 1981;9:A236
82. Silver JR: The prophylactic use of anticoagulant therapy in the prevention of pulmonary emboli in one hundred consecutive spinal injury patients. *Paraplegia* 1974;12:188
83. Branch CL, Albertson DA, Kelly DL: Post-traumatic acalculous cholecystitis on a neurosurgical service. *Neurosurgery* 1983;12:98
84. O'Flynn JD: Early management of neuropathic bladder in spinal cord injuries. *Paraplegia* 1974;12:83

Critical Care, Third Edition, edited by Joseph M. Civetta,
Robert W. Taylor, and Robert R. Kirby.
Lippincott-Raven Publishers, Philadelphia, PA © 1997.

CHAPTER 79

■

Multiple Fractures

Gregory A. Zych

IMMEDIATE CONCERNS ■

MAJOR PROBLEMS

Patients with musculoskeletal injuries in the critical care unit are often treated with a variety of methods, which may lead to bewilderment as to the proper medical and nursing management of the injured extremities, spine and pelvis. Questions may also arise as to the patient's mobility in and out of bed and transportation for additional diagnostic and therapeutic procedures. The goal for the multiply injured patient with multiple fractures is to mobilize the patient as soon as possible after the initial trauma by early stabilization of all major long bone fractures, pelvic disruptions, and spinal injuries.

Musculoskeletal injuries are often accompanied by soft tissue swelling, which ultimately can lead to compartment syndromes and severe long-term disability if not recognized and treated promptly. The key to this early recognition is a thorough examination of the soft tissues and neurovascular systems of the extremities.

Despite advanced trauma life support protocols, multiply injured patients will have musculoskeletal trauma that is not diagnosed acutely. Careful examination of the musculoskeletal system in all multiple trauma patients within the first 24 to 48 hours detects most of these missed injuries. Appropriate treatment can be given, thus decreasing the chances of a suboptimal outcome.

STRESS POINTS

1. The most common complication of a fracture or dislocation is a neurologic or vascular injury. A comprehensive examination of sensory and motor function must be performed and documented. Patients with altered mental status may not respond appropriately and this

should be considered in the validity of the examination.
2. Extremities immobilized in casts or splints are difficult to examine totally and therefore reliance must be placed on assessment of the exposed parts (e.g., toes or fingers). Swelling should minimized to lessen the pain and decrease soft tissue complications.
3. Skeletal traction is used to immobilize fractures of the cervical spine, pelvis, and femur. Most problems arise when the bed interferes with the traction apparatus or the patient's skin contacts the apparatus, resulting in loss of traction force or pressure points.
4. External fixation devices are used to stabilize fractures of the long bones and pelvis. The pin–skin interfaces must be meticulously maintained to avoid deep soft tissue or bone infection.
5. The most commonly missed areas of injury are the hands and feet, shoulder, knee, and pelvis. With the exception of the pelvis, these are regions that do not routinely undergo radiography acutely unless an obvious sign of local trauma exists.

INITIAL DIAGNOSTIC TESTS AND PROCEDURES

1. Sensation is best evaluated by determining light touch and motor function by observing active voluntary or involuntary motion. Vascular status should be assessed by either palpation or Doppler examination of the peripheral pulses of the wrist or ankle.

   I. *Upper Extremity*
      A. Median nerve
         1. Sensory: volar distal index finger tip
         2. Motor: thumb abduction (movement away from the palm in the horizontal plane)

1219

B. Ulnar nerve
1. Sensory: volar distal small finger tip
2. Motor: index finger abduction (movement toward the thumb in the plane of the palm)
C. Radial nerve
1. Sensory: dorsal first web space between the thumb and index finger
2. Motor: thumb extension at the distal joint
II. *Lower Extremity*
A. Superficial peroneal nerve
1. Sensory: dorsal foot between second and fourth toes
2. Motor: ankle eversion (movement toward outside of the leg)
B. Deep peroneal nerve
1. Sensory: dorsal first web space between great and second toes
2. Motor: ankle dorsiflexion, great toe extension
C. Posterior tibial nerve
1. Sensory: plantar surface of toes and foot
2. Motor: toe flexion

2. If at least one finger cannot be placed between the edge of a cast or splint and the exposed digits, swelling is excessive and measures to decrease it are imperative. The appearance of epidermal blisters is consistent with severe swelling. This problem is often seen in patients with diffuse body edema receiving ventilation with positive end-expiratory pressure.

3. Traction weights are designed to provide a dynamic force in line with the injured extremity. Palpation of the traction line or rope indicates tension proportional to the applied amount of weight. If the line feels slack, something is interfering with the weight.

4. The junction of the external fixation pin and the skin should be clean, with minimal drainage. The skin should be freely movable around the pin without tenting or wrinkling. Gentle tapping of the pin should not produce pain.

5. All joints that are not immobilized should be put through a full range of motion either actively or passively. All long bones should be palpated along their entire length. Any region that has swelling, tenderness, ecchymosis, crepitus, false motion, or restriction of movement requires two radiographs (perpendicular views including the bone and the adjacent joints).

INITIAL THERAPY

1. Any neurologic or pulse deficit must be quantified, documented, and reported to the responsible clinician. If a circumferential cast, splint, or dressing is present, a complete release of any constriction is necessary. Progressive changes may indicate an early compartment syndrome and represent an emergency situation. Distal swelling is best controlled by elevation of the affected extremity above the level of the heart.

2. An obstruction to the skeletal traction force must be eliminated so that the injured skeletal region is ade-

quately immobilized. If any doubt exists, portable radiographs of the affected area will confirm the traction effect.

3. External fixation pin sites should be cleansed at least twice a day with some type of antibacterial solution. Wrinkling or tenting of the skin at the pin site requires surgical release of the skin. All exposed connections of the external fixator should be checked for tightness. No portion of the fixator should touch the patient's skin.

4. Areas of suspected injury should be appropriately splinted or immobilized until the diagnosis is ruled out. The patient's level of activity and physical therapy may also require modification. Fractures of the femoral shaft and some pelvic fractures will need the application of skeletal traction. Neck or back pain should be investigated by examination of perineal sensation, sphincter, and bladder function and proper radiographs. The patient should be kept supine with the neck immobilized.

DIAGNOSIS OF FRACTURES AND DISLOCATIONS

A fracture is defined as any break in the continuity of a cortex of a bone. This includes a broad range from the nondisplaced hairline fracture to a severely displaced and comminuted long bone fracture. Most fractures share certain subjective and objective findings that suggest the diagnosis.

A history should be obtained to determine the mechanism of injury. Automobile passengers have a significant incidence of fractures of the patella, knee, and hip. Automobile drivers, if involved in a lateral collision, often have acetabular or pelvic injuries. Fractures of the tibia and femur are common in motorcycle riders. Pelvic fractures may be seen in patients who have been in frontal collisions in which the air bag deployed but the seat belt was not fastened.

Subjectively, patients complain of localized pain and loss of function of the involved part. Objectively, the fracture has local point tenderness and may have some degree of swelling or ecchymosis, depending on the length of time since injury. If displaced, deformity and false motion will occur at the fracture. Crepitus is an audible and palpable grating that is produced by the fracture ends rubbing against each other. Although crepitus is pathognomonic of fracture, no attempt to move the fracture should be made to elicit this sign.

The diagnosis is confirmed and documented by radiographic examination. In the extremities, radiographs of the entire suspected bone, including the adjacent joints in two perpendicular planes, are necessary. Appropriate similar studies should also be performed for the pelvis and spine, and often computed tomography is used as well.

Joint injuries can be ligamentous sprains, intraarticular fractures, or dislocations. In general, the more severe the trauma, the more likely that associated joint injury will be present. It has been reported that 33% of patients with femur fractures have ipsilateral serious knee injury.[1]

Joint injuries are manifested by local pain and inability to move the joint actively. A traumatic joint effusion usually consists of blood and signifies major ligamentous disruption or intraarticular fracture. There may also be instability or laxity of the joint to stress. Standard joint radiographs should be obtained.

SPECIFIC TREATMENT METHODS

CASTS AND SPLINTS

Casts are rigid circumferential devices made of plaster or various synthetic materials. They are best suited for immobilization of extremity injuries below the shoulder in the upper extremity and below the thigh in the lower extremity. Because of their rigidity, they do not allow for much swelling in the immobilized part. Consequently, it is essential that limbs in casts be elevated to minimize edema. If swelling becomes a problem, it will be necessary to bivalve the cast, that is, split the cast and the padding underneath along the long axis on both sides, from one end to the other. This will relieve the constriction of the part.

Certain injuries may be immobilized in splints that do not encompass the limb circumferentially. These splints accommodate swelling better than casts. This is the preferred immobilization in a patient who may not be able to complain of increasing pain or neurologic deficit because of an altered mental status.

Within the first 48 hours after application, plaster casts or splints are especially susceptible to denting from direct injury or indirect pressure. Indentations may cause localized pressure areas beneath the cast and lead to skin ulcers. A patient complaining of pain under a cast must not be ignored. Plaster casts or splints must be kept dry because wetting causes loss of strength.

TRACTION

Skin

Traction applied directly to the skin is used for hip fractures in the elderly and in young children. In an adult, traction weight greater than 7 lb (3.2 kg) should never be used on the skin. This form of traction is not used for other orthopedic injuries (Fig. 79-1).

Skeletal

Skeletal traction is the application of longitudinal force to an extremity by a metal traction pin placed in a bone. Skeletal traction immobilizes the fracture, maintains fracture reduction, and provides symptomatic relief to the patient. This type of traction is indicated in fractures of the femur, acetabulum, pelvis, and some fractures in the humerus[2] (Fig. 79-2).

KEY POINTS TO CHECK

Traction weights should be free of the floor and bed.

Traction lines should not touch the patient.

The traction splint should be suspended sufficiently to keep the extremity above the bed surface and to allow the patient mobility in bed. The upper end of the splint should not be higher than the gluteal crease and should not impinge on the inner groin. The lower end should not come into contact with any part of the bed.

Care must be taken to avoid pressure points on the skin at the inner groin, knee (especially the fibular head), back of the heel, and toes.

The traction bow should be firmly attached to the traction pin and traction line. It must be clear of the leg. Adequate space should exist between the traction bow and the skin to allow for pin care.

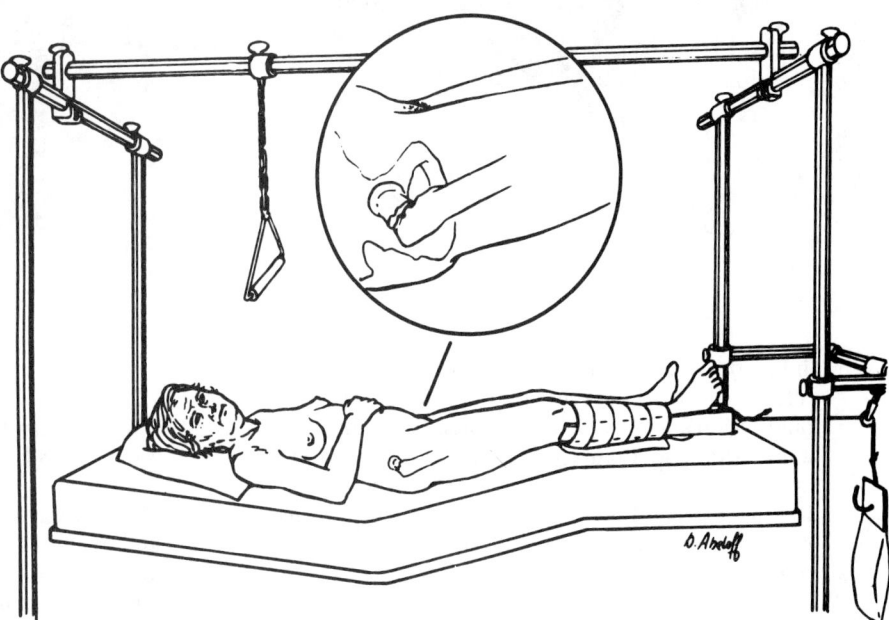

FIGURE 79-1. Skin traction to the lower extremity. This provides minimal immobilization and is used mostly in hip fractures. (Reprinted with permission from Brooker AF, Schmeisser G: *Orthopaedic Traction Manual.* Baltimore, Williams & Wilkins, 1980.)

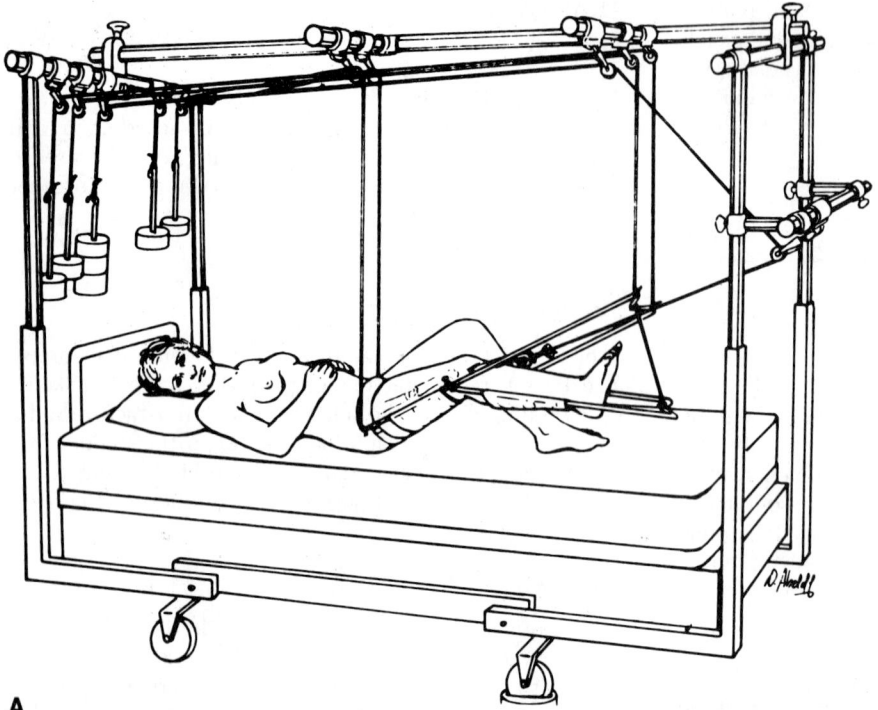

A

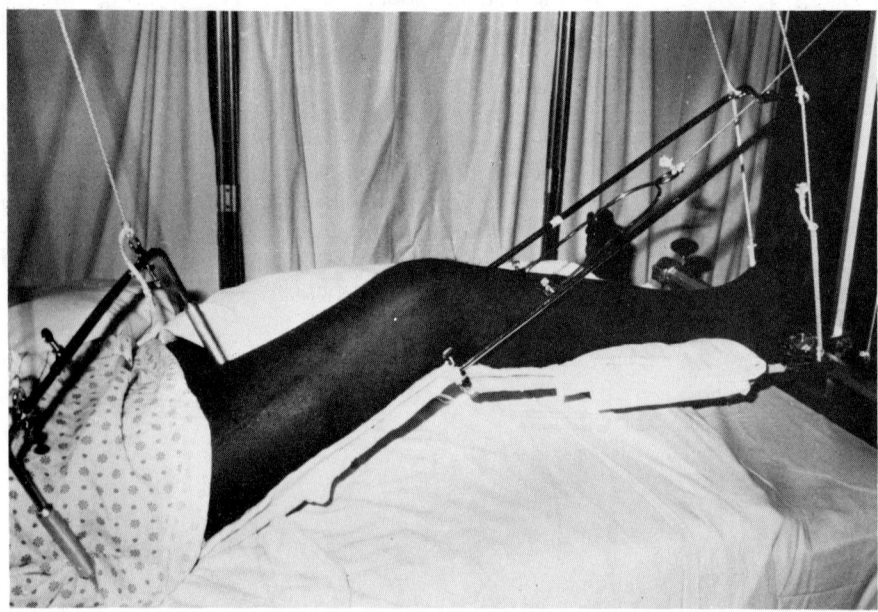

B

FIGURE 79-2. (**A**) Skeletal traction applied through a tibial pin, with the lower extremity supported in the traction splint and a balanced suspension. The weights attached to the splint allow the extremity to "float" above the bed surface; in this manner, limited bed mobility is possible. (Reprinted with permission from Brooker AF, Schmeisser G: *Orthopaedic Traction Manual.* Baltimore, William & Wilkins, 1980.) (**B**) Clinical photograph of a patient with a femoral shaft fracture being treated with skeletal traction and balanced suspension.

Maintain the traction pin–skin interface in optimum condition. The skin edges around the pin should be without tension and kept clean of debris. Normally, a slight amount of daily drainage occurs, but excessive drainage may occur in limbs with thick soft tissues or be indicative of early pin tract infection. Other signs of pin infection are local pain, erythema, and eventual pin loosening.

Most of the time, the patient in traction should be centered in the bed. In some situations when large amounts of weight are used, the patient may be pulled toward the foot of the bed. This can be counteracted by placing the bed in slight Trendelenburg position or, if feasible, decreasing the weight.

DISADVANTAGES. Usually the patient in lower extremity skeletal traction is confined to bed in the horizontal position. For brief periods, the traction can be converted to so-called *field traction* to transport the patient from the intensive care unit (ICU) for procedures. An alternative method, *roller traction*, has been advocated as a means of permitting the patient to get out of bed and still maintain traction force.[3] Field and roller traction should be instituted by or under the direct supervision of a person skilled in orthopedic traction techniques. Bilateral lower extremity traction is difficult to manage and uncomfortable for the patient.

OVERHEAD SKELETAL TRACTION. Overhead traction is indicated in fractures of the shoulder and humerus. The traction pin is placed transversely through the proximal ulna and the shoulder and elbow are at 90-degree flexion, with the forearm supported by a sling (Fig. 79-3).

KEY POINTS TO CHECK

Generally, the traction weight just lifts the shoulder from the bed and weighs no more than 10 lb (4.5 kg). Only a few pounds should be applied to the forearm sling to keep the elbow at 90-degree flexion.

Excess pressure from the sling should be avoided at the wrist and upper forearm.

Other points need to be checked as with lower extremity traction.

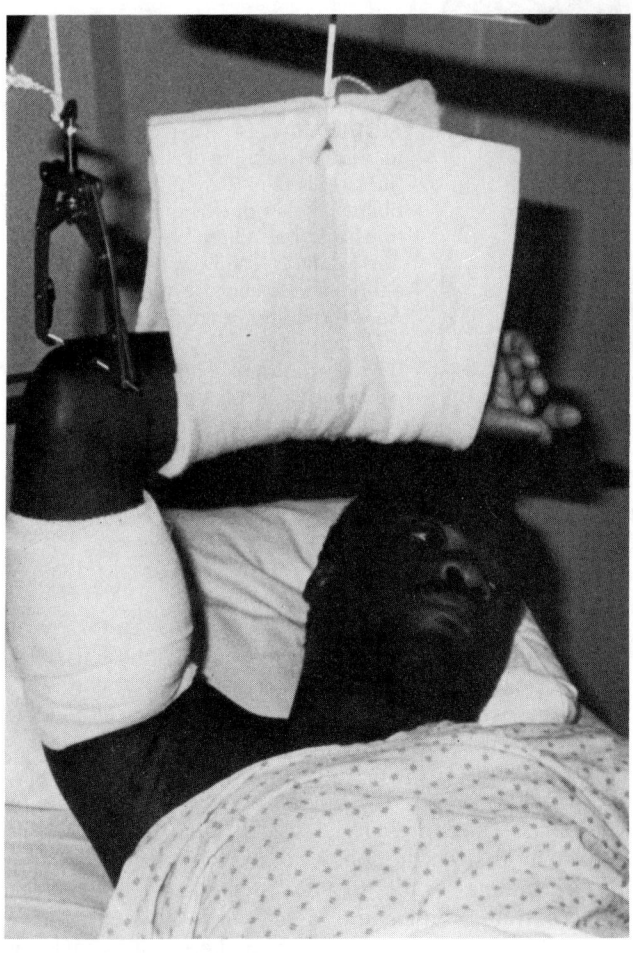

FIGURE 79-3. Overhead skeletal traction for a patient with an open humeral shaft fracture. Excellent access is provided for wound care and pulmonary toilet.

Cervical

Indications for this traction are fractures or dislocations within the cervical spine. Traction is applied to the skull through skeletal tongs (i.e., Gardner-Wells) or, less frequently, a halo. The traction weight is directed over the head of the bed. The patient must be in the supine position.

KEY POINTS TO CHECK

The traction weight must be freely suspended for continuous traction of the spine.

The amount of weight varies from 5 to 50 lb (2.2 to 22.5 kg), depending on the level and type of spine injury. Heavier weights are needed to reduce certain dislocations and are used only temporarily.

The neurologic status must be assessed often to detect the presence of a new deficit or progression of a previous one. This is especially important with any change in traction.

A physician skilled in the management of cervical spine injuries must be present and manually immobilize the neck if traction is to be temporarily discontinued for any reason.

Routine pin care should be done.

The skull should not touch the head of the bed or traction will be negated.

EXTERNAL FIXATION

External fixation is a treatment method that provides stabilization of a fracture or dislocation using pins placed through the skeleton, percutaneously, and attached to some sort of rigid external frame.[4] In this manner, an unstable injury, such as a severe open tibial fracture, can be immobilized without placing a large amount of metallic internal fixation in the contaminated bone. Also, the soft tissue injury is readily accessible for proper care (Fig. 79-4A).

The primary indication for external fixation is the treatment of open fractures, for the reasons stated earlier. Another excellent indication is the unstable pelvic injury. Several studies[5-8] have shown that patients with unstable pelvic fractures treated acutely with external fixation have less morbidity and less nursing demands than those treated with other nonsurgical means. External fixation permits early mobilization of the patient from the horizontal supine position (see Fig. 79-4B).

KEY POINTS TO CHECK

The most important component of an external fixation system is the interface of the bone, pin, and skin. Failure at any one of these points often leads to premature removal of the external fixator. Therefore, the multiple pin sites must be meticulously maintained. The junction of the pin and skin should be free of tension to avoid skin necrosis. If excessive tension is present, the skin requires incision under local anesthesia. The pin sites should also be cleansed at least twice a day to remove any accumulated drainage or debris. Saline solutions are best. After the site is cleansed, an

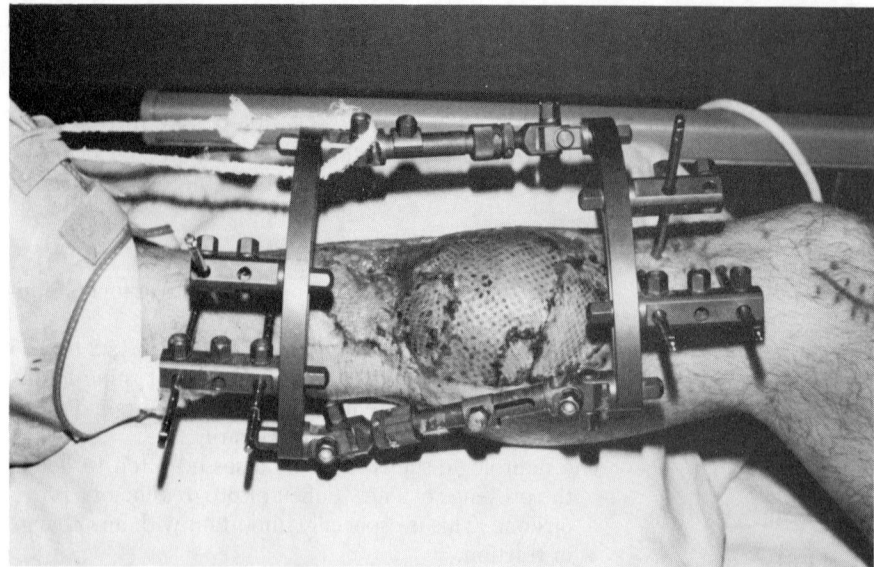

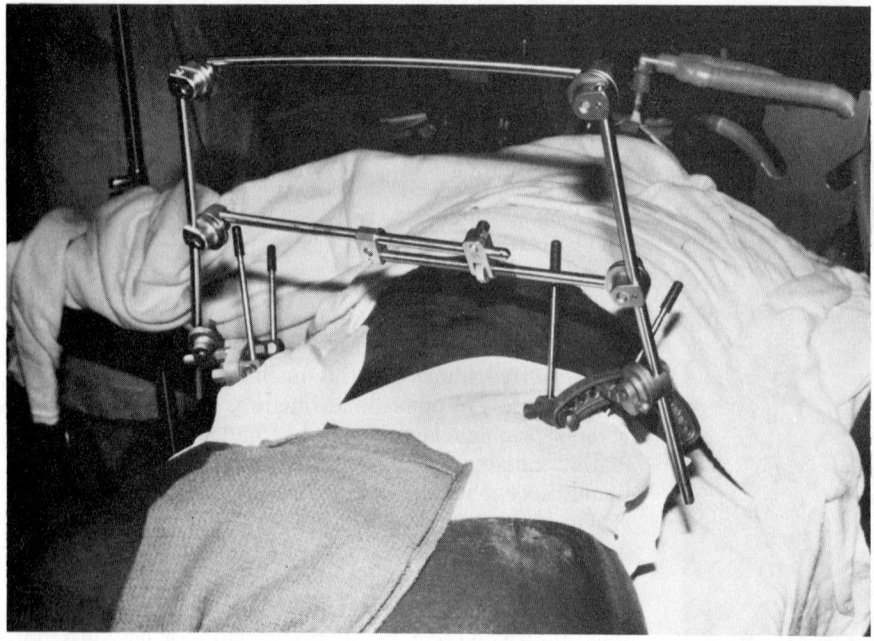

FIGURE 79-4. (**A**) A typical external fixator for the treatment of an open tibial shaft fracture. Half pins are placed through the tibia and below the fracture and connected to a rigid but adjustable external frame. The wound is readily available for surgical debridements and dressing changes. (**B**) An external fixator applied acutely to immobilize an unstable pelvic injury. Pins in the iliac crests are connected to the external frame, which is free of the abdomen. With this treatment method, traction is eliminated and the patient can be mobilized out of bed as required. Nursing management is also facilitated.

antibiotic ointment and a sterile dressing may be applied.

As a rule, no part of the external fixation frame should come into contact with the patient's skin. This contact can cause pressure ulceration and prevent proper wound and pin care.

All types of external fixators have various adjustable parts, nuts, and screws. To immobilize the bone, all of these components need to be tight and should be tightened on a weekly basis. If this is not done, the bone will be unstable and painful.

In the lower leg, open tibial fractures are often treated in external fixation. If the ankle is not included in the frame, the ankle tends to assume the equinus or foot drop position. To prevent this, some type of foot support is necessary to keep the ankle in a neutral position.

This support attaches to the external fixator by an elastic attachment that allows the patient actively to move the ankle if possible. The foot support may apply excessive pressure to the sole and sides of the foot, an inherent danger. In patients with neurologic deficit, pressure sores may develop because pain sensation is not intact. Thus, the foot must be checked frequently for areas of pressure. It is advisable to remove the support from the foot for a few minutes every hour. In some cases, the foot and ankle may be included in the frame construct, bridging the ankle joint with one or more fixation pins in either the tarsal or metatarsal bones.

If not contraindicated, the joints that are not immobilized adjacent to the external fixator should be actively or passively put through a range of motion frequently to eliminate joint stiffness and contractures.

INTERNAL FIXATION

Internal fixation is the stabilization of skeletal injuries by the direct application of metallic implants. These implants include plates, screws, intramedullary nails, pins, and wires (Fig. 79-5).

This fixation requires surgical application of the implants to the bone. After internal fixation, immobilization of the extremity may vary from none to a circumferential cast, depending on the degree of fixation achieved.

This form of fracture treatment probably requires the least nursing care and attention. Rigid internal fixation allows immediate mobilization of the injured part and prevents muscle atrophy. Sound evidence supports that it is important in the early treatment of the multiply injured patient.[3]

KEY POINTS TO CHECK

Usually, the surgical incisions are closed after internal fixation. Wound complications such as hematoma, infection, and wound necrosis may occur. Any unexplained wound swelling, erythema, induration, drainage, or tenderness demands further investigation. Occasionally, the incisions may be left open and either closed later or allowed to heal by secondary intention.

Suction drainage is routinely used after internal fixation and wound closure. Although a good method to avoid wound hematoma, the suction drains provide a direct route to the bone and can be contaminated secondarily by bacteria. Aseptic technique is mandatory in managing these drainage systems. Documenting the output is also important.

The level of activity that the surgeon will permit in the operated extremity must be ascertained. Some types of internal fixation are more rigid than others. In the

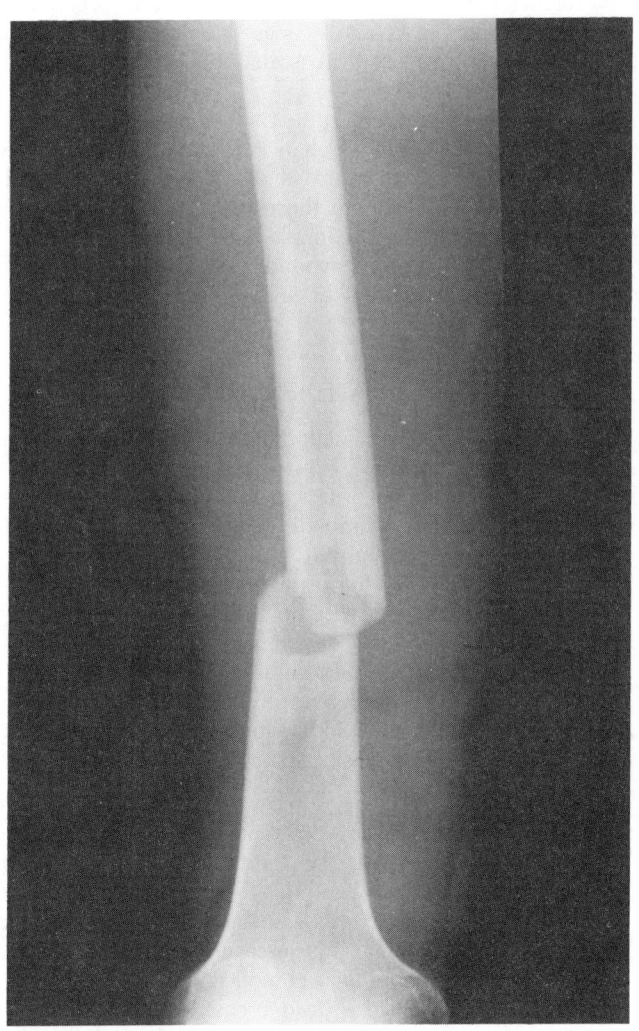
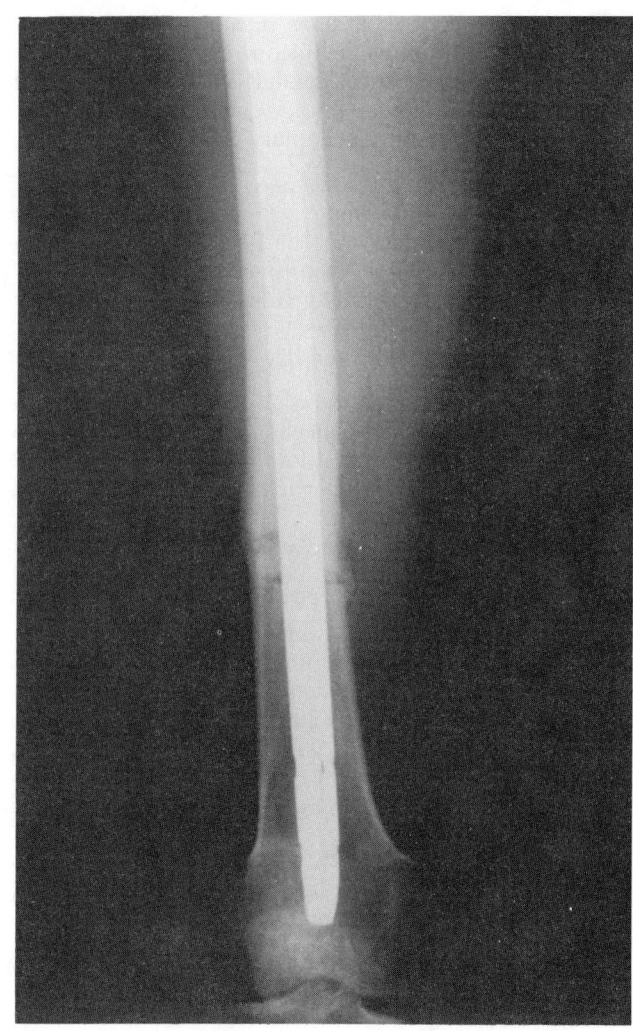

A **B**

FIGURE 79-5. (**A**) Displaced femoral shaft fracture in a patient with multiple injuries. (**B**) After closed intramedullary nailing, the patient can be rapidly mobilized out of bed.

lower extremity, fractures fixed with intramedullary nails can usually be weight bearing, whereas those fixed with plates generally cannot.

Neurovascular compromise may occur after internal fixation resulting from swelling, tourniquet palsy, or direct injury to nerves or blood vessels. The neurovascular status must be checked frequently, documented, and the surgeon notified of any significant finding.

SPECIAL PROBLEMS ■

OPEN FRACTURES

An open fracture is one in which an opening in the skin communicates with the fracture hematoma. This definition includes the entire spectrum of skin wounds, from a minute puncture wound to a severe degloving or crush injury. In most multiply injured patients, open fractures are caused by high-energy trauma with extensive bone and soft tissue involvement.

The great concern about open fractures centers around bacterial contamination of the fracture site through the skin wound and the possible development of deep infection and osteomyelitis. Open fractures have been classified into three types, based on the soft tissue injury[9]:

Type I: a skin wound less than 1 cm generally caused by the fracture from within
Type II: a skin wound more than 1 cm but without significant flaps, degloving, or crushed tissue
Type III: extensive soft tissue injury, crushing, vascular injury, segmental fractures, farm or marine contamination, or high-velocity gunshot wounds.

This classification has important short- and long-term prognostic significance. The infection rate for type I fracture is 0%, for type II is 1.5%, and for type III is 16%.[10] There is also a clear correlation of open fracture types with delayed union and nonunion.

The basic principles of acute treatment of open fractures are the prompt administration of intravenous antibiotics and thorough surgical debridement of the soft tissue and bone. Antibiotics have been demonstrated to lower the infection rate in all types of open fractures.[11] They should be given intravenously when the diagnosis of open fracture is made and continued for 48 to 72 hours. A cephalosporin drug is used for type I fractures and a combination of cephalosporin and aminoglycoside drugs for types II and III (and soil-contaminated) fractures. Appropriate tetanus prophylaxis should also be given. Surgical debridement should be performed within 6 hours of injury; its goal is to decontaminate the fracture site and remove necrotic or damaged bone and soft tissue. Copious irrigation assists in mechanical debridement. Stabilization of the fracture may be accomplished with external fixation, casting, or internal fixation.

KEY POINTS TO CHECK

The proper antibiotic should be administered for the correct amount of time. Tetanus prophylaxis should be checked.

Wound management becomes critical, because after debridement all or part of the original soft tissue wound and surgical incisions are left open acutely. This care is facilitated if the fracture has been stabilized by an external fixator, because ready access is available to the wound. If the fracture has been immobilized in a cast or splint, dressing changes may be ordered by the surgeon. The treatment of open wounds in casts or splints without frequent dressing changes is an established technique. On occasion, wound access may be obtained in casts by cutting a portion of the cast over the wound, thus creating a "window."

Exposed bone in the open fracture wound should be covered with a moist dressing, preferably with normal saline. Wet-to-dry dressings on the bone may cause bone desiccation and subsequent necrosis.

Open fracture wounds are expected to drain. This is the major reason why they are left open. Typically, the drainage is serous or serosanguineous and has no odor. If the drainage is excessive, the dressings should be changed as required to prevent possible secondary contamination. Wounds encased in casts may develop a foul odor because the cast material acts like a sponge and retains secretions.

With proper treatment, infection of open fractures is uncommon. A higher chance of infection should be anticipated in the more severe type II and type III fractures, especially in those with vascular injury. In patients with casts, complaints of increasing wound pain or fever mandate wound inspection. Deep wound cultures should be taken and the surgeon notified.

MULTIPLE TRAUMA AND FRACTURES

The benefits of early stabilization of long bone and unstable pelvic fractures in multiply injured patients are well established.[12] The advantages of this early treatment in patients with isolated or other orthopedic injuries, however, are not so clear. Most multiply injured patients have a sufficiently stable physiologic status to permit acute operative stabilization procedures. Unstable patients should not undergo possibly lengthy surgery if it is believed that the stress of anesthesia and operation cannot be tolerated.

Assuming that the patient's physiologic status permits, the following are primary indications for acute (within 24 hours of injury) operative stabilization, whether external or internal fixation is used:

1. Unstable pelvic injuries (to control acute hemorrhage); pubic symphysis diastasis, 3 cm or greater; vertical or posterior hemipelvis displacement
2. Femoral shaft fractures associated with either head, chest, or abdominal injuries caused by blunt trauma (to decrease pulmonary complications)
3. Major open fractures (to decrease sepsis)
4. Spinal trauma with progressive neurologic deficit.

Most other musculoskeletal trauma can be managed without acute surgical intervention, if no other orthopedic surgical indication exists. In fact, there are several clinical situations when delayed orthopedic surgery is preferable because of soft tissue swelling (juxtaarticular fractures) or other factors.

COMPLICATIONS ■

SWELLING

All musculoskeletal injuries are accompanied by a variable amount of swelling. The degree of swelling is related to the type and magnitude of injury, with the greatest amount seen in displaced fractures and crush injuries. Swelling is secondary to hemorrhage from fractured bones, and tissue edema is a response to injury. Maximal swelling is believed to occur approximately 24 to 48 hours after injury.

Although some swelling is inevitable, excessive swelling should be avoided. If not, local pain may increase and the skin may form *fracture blisters* from rupture of the outer layers of the epidermis. The worst complication is the compartment syndrome, resulting in possible loss of the limb.

All injured extremities, both upper and lower, should be elevated above the heart level. Elevation assists in venous return by gravity drainage. Even marked amounts of swelling can be reduced if the limb is properly elevated. The only contraindications to elevation are reimplantations and suspected compartment syndromes, because elevation may decrease arterial flow in these conditions.

Extremities may be constricted by circumferential casts, dressings, elastic bandages, or braces. These can contribute to swelling by interfering with venous return and acting as tourniquets. The solution is to relieve the constriction by releasing tight dressings or bivalving the cast.

NEUROVASCULAR COMPROMISE

The most common complication of fractures or dislocations is a neurologic or vascular deficit. This deficit may occur at the time of the original trauma and result from blunt or penetrating force. This type is not preventable. Nerve or vessel injury after the initial trauma is largely preventable. The functional outcome of the extremity, in most cases, is directly related to the integrity of the neurovascular systems.

Acute neural injury can be caused by contusion, stretching, or laceration. Most of the time, partial motor and sensory deficits will occur in the injured nerve distribution. Rarely will a complete absence of neural function exist. The recommended treatment is observation for these injuries because most are not lacerations and will recover function. If a nerve laceration is suspected, surgical exploration is indicated with possible repair.

Late neural injury has a variety of etiologies. One cause is direct pressure on a superficial nerve such as the common peroneal at the level of the fibular head, lateral to the knee. This pressure can be secondary to a poorly padded or tight cast or from improper positioning on a traction splint. In operated extremities in which a tourniquet has been used for hemostasis, a nerve palsy can result from prolonged tourniquet time or inappropriate pressure. The extremity will have a circumferential nerve deficit distal to the tourni-

quet site. Recovery is usually complete within a few days to weeks.

The cause of most vascular injuries associated with fractures or dislocations is the original trauma. Vessels may have partial or complete lacerations or intimal damage. An unusual cause is laceration by fracture fragments. The diagnosis of these lesions is typically made at the time of presentation to the hospital and treatment is begun promptly. Musculoskeletal injuries that have a fairly common association with vascular injuries are knee dislocations, supracondylar humeral fractures, and severe crush or open fractures of the tibia or forearm.

COMPARTMENT SYNDROME

One of the most devastating complications of fractures is the compartment syndrome.[13] The pathophysiologic features of this condition begin with swelling within the deep fascial compartments of the extremities. The swelling may be secondary to fractures, crushing, vascular injury, constricting dressings, or several other causes. The deep fascial tissue is dense and unyielding. If swelling continues unabated, the contents of the fascial compartments (nerves, blood vessels, muscles) will be compressed because the fascia cannot accommodate increasing edema, resulting in increasing pressure. Microscopically, the initial event is arteriolar constriction, which produces ischemia. The tissue response to this ischemia is an increase in capillary permeability and extravascular edema. This tissue edema leads to further increases in tissue pressure and compartment swelling with more ischemia. Thus, a vicious cycle is begun, with progressive ischemia producing more swelling. If the pressure is not relieved within hours, irreversible tissue necrosis and permanent neural damage ensues.

Recognition is the key to preventing compartment syndromes. Subjectively, the patient will complain of progressive pain in the extremity that is out of proportion to that expected for the type of injury. Also, the pain usually is not relieved by otherwise adequate doses of analgesics. The patient may also complain of numbness and paresthesia in the distal extremity. In patients with altered mental status, these subjective findings may be absent.

The earliest objective finding is decreased sensation to light touch in the distal extremity. Passive motion of the digits will refer pain to the involved compartment. This phenomenon is believed to be caused by stretching of ischemic muscles. The involved compartments will develop increasing tenseness to palpation. While the syndrome progresses, muscle weakness and anesthesia of the distal skin will occur, followed by total loss of muscle function. A late sign is diminished or absent distal pulses.

The first step in a suspected compartment syndrome is to relieve all constriction around the extremity. Dressings should be released by cutting longitudinally. Circumferential casts must be bivalved, i.e., opened along both long axes, through the cast material, and with the underlying padding cut completely to the skin. If the pain is not immediately eased, the surgeon must be notified.

Methods have been devised to measure the compartment pressures in an extremity.[13,14] A simple one that has been found to be effective and reasonably accurate is to set up the usual equipment to monitor an arterial line. An 18-gauge needle is attached to the tubing and flushed with heparinized saline. The arterial transducer should be at the level of the extremity to be tested and calibrated to zero. A small amount of local anesthesia may be used to infiltrate the skin and subcutaneous tissue only. The needle should then be inserted percutaneously and through the deep fascia into the compartment. A reading is taken to confirm proper placement of the needle. The pressure should fluctuate with active or passive motion of the muscles within the compartment tested. All compartments of the suspected part of the extremity should be measured and the pressures documented.

Pressures up to 30 mm Hg can be normal. Higher values may indicate a compartment syndrome. Conditions that lower the threshold for compartment syndrome are low diastolic pressure, hypovolemia, and anemia. However, do not rely solely on the pressure measurements because the subjective complaints and physical examination are more definitive. Pressure measurements have been most helpful in equivocal cases or in patients with unreliable examinations, such as those with closed-head trauma.

The definitive treatment for compartment syndrome is fasciotomy. The earlier the fasciotomy is done, the better are the chances for complete functional recovery. This condition is a true surgical emergency, and there should be no delay once the diagnosis is made. At operation, all compartments of the involved extremity are released through extensive incisions. The skin incisions are left open. Devices are now available to approximate skin edges once the edema has resolved.

LIMITATION OF JOINT MOTION

A common complication of the treatment of fractures is limitation of joint motion. Factors implicated in this problem are joint immobilization, soft tissue scarring, and muscle adhesion to the fracture site. If the fracture involves the joint surface, loss of motion is seen often. An extremity with a healed fracture but stiff joints will not yield a good functional result.

To a large extent, motion of joints adjacent to a fracture is dependent on the type of treatment of the fracture. Cast immobilization and skeletal traction are associated with a high rate of joint stiffness. Patients in long arm or leg casts should, at the least, be encouraged actively to move the fingers or toes through a full range of motion. Most patients in skeletal traction cannot move the more proximal joints such as the hip and the knee because of the limb position or the traction splints. However, the ankle and toes are free for motion either actively or passively.

Patients in external fixation devices are also prone to loss of joint motion. With the fixator pins placed transversely through the entire width of the extremity, the muscles are impaled. Motion of these muscles can be painful and inhibit joint motion. Devices using half pins, which pass only through the bone, are preferred because they do not cause muscle pain. High-energy open fractures of the tibia are associated with nerve injury and usually are treated with external fixation. Patients may have a foot drop that can develop into a rigid equinus contracture if active measures are not taken to prevent it. Foot supports are useful, especially if they are dynamic and allow the patient to actively plantar flex the ankle while elastically preventing the persistent equinus. These foot supports must be observed carefully, as discussed in the section on external fixation.

Patients with head injuries are susceptible to permanent loss of joint motion. They can have spasticity that must be overcome before the joints can be ranged. Heterotopic ossification is commonly seen and accounts for substantial motion loss. Patients with head injuries should have passive range of motion exercises of all major joints and digits daily or more often.

INFECTION

Sepsis in the musculoskeletal system is a dreaded complication, frequently necessitating multiple surgical procedures and prolonged antibiotic therapy with a poor functional outcome. Clearly, prevention of infection or its prompt treatment assumes paramount importance.

Infection rates differ depending on the type of injury and type of fracture treatment. Infection of a closed fracture is rare, whereas open fractures have had rates as high as 44%.[10] Penetrating wounds to the knee joint carry approximately a 2% sepsis rate. It is axiomatic that the greater the damage to the bone and soft tissue, the greater the likelihood of infection.

Prevention of bone and joint sepsis is crucial in the severely injured patient with multiple fractures. The role of antibiotics in treating open fractures is clearly established. All open fractures have bacterial contamination to a variable degree, depending mostly on the magnitude of injury. Therefore, the administration of antibiotics is therapeutic and not prophylactic. It is recommended that antibiotics be given immediately on hospital admission and continued for 2 to 3 days. Additionally, any further operative procedures on the open fracture should have 24 to 48 hours of perioperative antibiotic coverage. Essentially the same points should be considered for open joint wounds. Wound management for open fractures is controversial, and many different protocols exist.

The diagnosis of an infected open fracture is not always straightforward. Subjectively, the patient may complain of increasing local pain at the fracture, especially with dressing changes or any manipulation of the limb. Objectively, there may be no local wound changes in cases of early infection. Later, increasing tenderness and erythema will occur with some change in the character of the wound drainage. If some signs of inflammation are present, but if the wound drainage appears normal, exploration of the wound is indicated. Pockets of purulent material may be found deep in the extremity, particularly on the dependent side. At this stage, the patient may be febrile with leukocytosis and an elevated sedimentation rate. Deep wound cultures should be obtained and an intravenous cephalosporin antibiotic begun. In the more severe injuries (type III), a high incidence of gram-negative wound infections exists, and an aminoglycoside should be added to the antibiotic regimen.

Any infected open fracture requires thorough surgical debridement. In a certain percentage of cases, retained foreign material or necrotic bone or soft tissue is found. Serial debridements are indicated if the infection is resistant to treatment.

Septic joints can arise from direct penetrating injury and hematogenous seeding. Patients complain of pain and inability to move the joint. Examination reveals a hot, swollen, and tender joint with definite loss of motion. The joint effusion should be aspirated for Gram stain, culture, and synovial analysis. *Staphylococcus aureus* infection is most common, but in a critically ill patient, gram-negative sepsis should be suspected.

In the traumatized patient, the most effective treatment for a septic joint is drainage by surgical arthrotomy with the appropriate intravenous antibiotic. In our experience, treatment by repeated aspiration has had a low rate of success, often requiring surgical drainage secondarily. A good functional result can be expected if the septic joint is treated promptly and aggressively.

CONCLUSION ■

The management of severely traumatized patients with multiple musculoskeletal injuries represents a formidable challenge to the ICU team. Because the presence of long bone or pelvic fractures can significantly affect the morbidity and mortality rates in these patients, the orthopedic surgeon should play a decisive role in decision making. Likewise, the other members of the team must acquire a working knowledge of the basic principles, treatment methods, and possible complications of fractures and dislocations. In this manner, the final outcome of a living patient with healed fractures and normal function should not be an unattainable goal in most cases.

REFERENCES ■

1. Walling AK, Housang S, Spiegel PG: Injuries to the knee ligaments with fractures of the femur. *J Bone Joint Surg [Am]* 1982;64:1324
2. Brooker AF, Schmeisser G: *Orthopaedic Traction Manual.* Baltimore, Williams & Wilkins, 1980:81
3. Mooney V, Claudi BF: Fractures of the shaft of the femur. In: Rockwood CA, Green DP (eds). *Fractures in Adults*, 2nd ed, vol 2. Philadelphia, JB Lippincott, 1984:1367
4. Mears DC: *External Skeletal Fixation.* Baltimore, Williams & Wilkins, 1983:1
5. Saucedo T, Matta J: The treatment of unstable pelvic ring injuries [abstract]. In: *Abstracts of the 53rd Annual Meeting of the American Academy of Orthopaedic Surgeons.* New Orleans, February 1986:40
6. Tile M: *Fractures of Pelvis and Acetabulum.* Baltimore, Williams & Wilkins, 1984:4
7. Wild JJ, Hanson GW, Tullos HS: Unstable fractures of the pelvis treated by external fixation. *J Bone Joint Surg [Am]* 1983;64:1010
8. Johnson KD, Cadambi A, Siebert GB: Incidence of adult respiratory distress syndrome in patients with multiple musculoskeletal injuries: effect of early operative stabilization of fractures. *J Trauma* 1985;25:375
9. Gustilo RB, Anderson JT: Prevention of infection in the treatment of 1,025 open fractures of long bones. *J Bone Joint Surg [Am]* 1976;58:453
10. Gustilo RB: *Management of Open Fractures and Their Complications.* Philadelphia, WB Saunders, 1982:133
11. Patazkis M, Harvey JP, Ivler D: Role of antibiotics in the management of open fractures. *J Bone Joint Surg [Am]* 1974; 56:532
12. Bone LB, Johnson KD, Weigelt J, Scheinberg G: Early versus delayed stabilization of femoral fractures. *J Bone Joint Surg [Am]* 1989:336
13. Murbarak SJ, Hargen AR: Recognition and treatment of compartment syndromes. In: Meyers MH (ed). *The Multiply Injured Patient with Complex Fractures.* Philadelphia, Lea & Febiger, 1984:71
14. Whitesides TE, Haney TC, Morimoto K, et al: Tissue pressure measurements as a determinant for the need of fasciotomy. *Clin Orthop* 1975;113:43

Critical Care, Third Edition, edited by Joseph M. Civetta,
Robert W. Taylor, and Robert R. Kirby.
Lippincott-Raven Publishers, Philadelphia, PA © 1997.

CHAPTER 80

Orthopedic Complications

Jill I. Freedman
F. Kayser Enneking

IMMEDIATE CONCERNS ■

MAJOR PROBLEMS

Orthopedic patients frequently require admission to the intensive care unit (ICU) for management of ongoing blood loss, intraoperative hypovolemia, and postischemia hyperperfusion, all of which contribute to unstable intravascular volume. Patient temperature may be low as a result of tourniquet application, exposure of a large skin surface area, and the use of unheated fluids for volume replacement. Frequently, these patients have underlying cardiovascular disease. Occasionally, this problem has not been appreciated or worked up because exercise intolerance was attributed to arthritis or other underlying orthopedic problems.

Extubation should be carefully considered in these patients, particularly after cervical operative procedures. If a fiberoptic intubation was required because of skeletal deformities or cervical injury, extubation should occur only after the patient's underlying problem (e.g., airway edema) has been controlled. Later problems include fat embolism syndrome (FES), compartment syndrome, deep venous thrombosis (DVT), and pulmonary embolism.

STRESS POINTS

1. Patients undergoing orthopedic surgery often have major intraoperative hemorrhage that can continue into the immediate postoperative period. Ongoing volume resuscitation is frequently the reason for ICU admission.
2. Extubation after spine surgery must be carefully considered. Airway edema, which results from positioning, intraoperative manipulation, and volume resuscita-

tion, must be evaluated before extubation. In addition, other preexisting conditions (e.g., preoperative pulmonary status, neuromuscular disease, abnormal airway anatomy) may complicate the timing of extubation.
3. Cervical collars can impede venous return from the head, decreasing cerebral perfusion pressure in a head-injured patient. Always check the fit of cervical collars to ensure that they are neither too tight nor too loose.
4. Plaster casts emit heat as they harden. Burns and ulcers can develop from poor padding or from covering casts with blankets before they harden.
5. Compartment pressures of more than 30 mm Hg are dangerous. Hourly examinations should be performed on an extremity at risk for compartment syndrome. In an obtunded patient, continuous monitoring of compartment pressures may be indicated.
6. Fat embolism can occur intraoperatively and may be manifested as acute cor pulmonale and cardiac arrest. If the patient survives the initial insult, FES with acute respiratory distress syndrome (ARDS) is likely to follow.
7. FES is usually a diagnosis of exclusion. Neurologic derangement that is not explained by fever, impaired gas exchange, or tachycardia may be present. Physical findings of petechiae and fat in the blood or urine, although classically described, often are not present.
8. Approximately 40% of patients undergoing total hip arthroplasty (THA) and 70% of patients undergoing total knee arthroplasty (TKA) develop DVT in the extremity that has been operated on. Most DVTs form intraoperatively.
9. Pulmonary embolism from proximal migration of a

DVT is most likely to occur when the patient is first mobilized postoperatively.

ESSENTIAL DIAGNOSTIC TESTS AND PROCEDURES

1. Assess intravascular volume status immediately on arrival of the patient at the ICU. Note the drain output that has occurred since the operation was completed and the patient left the operating room. Are the bandages soaked with blood? Obtain baseline hemoglobin and hematocrit values.
2. Check the volume status 1 hour after ICU admission. Frequently, patients drain 500 to 1000 mL in the first hour after surgery. Repeat hemoglobin and hematocrit determination, and obtain coagulation studies if the patient continues to drain at this rate.
3. Keep up with fluid and blood loss. Volume resuscitation is much more difficult if replacement falls behind.
4. The most common sign of FES is neurologic derangement. Initially, patients are restless; later, mental confusion occurs and can progress to coma. Most patients have this picture of global encephalopathy; however, focal signs can develop. Other signs, in order of frequency, are tachycardia, tachypnea, fever, respiratory dysfunction, and petechial rash.
5. Decreased arterial oxygen partial pressure (PaO_2) is the most consistent laboratory finding in FES. Fat globules sometimes are found in the urine, sputum, and retina. However, their absence does not preclude FES. Other abnormalities include unexplained thrombocytopenia, anemia, and increased erythrocyte sedimentation rate.
6. Treatment of FES is supportive. Early steroid administration may be of value, but this fact has not been demonstrated conclusively.
7. Compartment pressures can be measured at the bedside by placing a fluid-filled, hollow needle attached to a pressure transducer into the compartment at risk. Pressures of more than 30 mm Hg warrant close observation; pressures more than 40 mm Hg necessitate fasciotomy. All values must be correlated with clinical observation.

SPINAL SURGERY ■

SCOLIOSIS

Scoliosis is a lateral curvature of the spine that causes vertebral and rib cage deformity. It is sometimes associated with posterior rotation of the spine (kyphoscoliosis). Scoliosis often requires surgical correction because, if untreated, it can cause fatal cardiopulmonary disease. The severity of the curvature is defined by the Cobb angle, with a larger angle describing more severe scoliosis. In general, surgical correction is considered in patients with Cobb angles that exceed 50 degrees, or with smaller curves that have been observed to progress on sequential radiographs. Other indications include trunk deformity, pain, decreased cardiopulmonary sta-

tus, family history of severe scoliosis, and loss of function.[1] Correction usually is achieved by instrumentation of each vertebra in the curve, followed by wiring to rods and resultant distribution of corrective forces.

Types

Idiopathic scoliosis accounts for approximately 75% of all cases.[2] Patients are most commonly females who have no other systemic disease. Congenital scoliosis can result from vertebral anomalies and may be associated with neurologic deficits. These patients commonly have tethered cords, which increases the risk of neurologic damage during corrective surgery.[3] In addition, a high incidence of cardiovascular, gastrointestinal, and urologic anomalies is associated with congenital scoliosis.

Neuromuscular scoliosis can be classified as neuropathic or myopathic. Neuropathic scoliosis is most commonly the result of cerebral palsy. The muscular dystrophies are the cause of most myopathic scoliosis. Curvature worsens as muscular weakness progresses, and postoperative respiratory impairment can be significant.

Cardiopulmonary Effects

Impairment of body growth contributes to decreased functional residual capacity. The thoracic cage is deformed, leading to decreased chest wall compliance, impaired development of the pulmonary vascular bed, and increased pulmonary vascular resistance.[4] The major abnormality in gas exchange is alveolar hypoventilation secondary to ventilation-perfusion mismatch. A long-term study of patients with untreated idiopathic scoliosis showed that the mortality rate was twice that of the general population; average age at death was 46.6 years.[4] Respiratory or right-sided heart failure accounted for 60% of the deaths.

LUNG MECHANICS. A pattern of restrictive lung disease is present, with the greatest decreases in vital capacity (60% of the predicted value), total lung capacity (70% of predicted), and functional residual capacity (80% of predicted), worsening in relation to the degree of curvature.[5,6] Patients with idiopathic scoliosis usually do not have respiratory problems until the Cobb angle is greater than 65 degrees. However, those who have associated neuromuscular disease can have difficulty with angles less than 30 degrees.[7] Vital capacity is a good indicator of postoperative function (Table 80-1). If it is more than 70% of the predicted value, respiratory reserve is probably adequate. If it is less than 40% of that predicted, postoperative mechanical ventilation probably will be required.[2]

Pulmonary function should be expected to worsen acutely after surgery. Vital capacity will decrease by 40% and the alveolar-arterial partial pressure gradient for oxygen ($P[A-a]O_2$) will increase by 50%.[8] Hypoxemia persists for several days, often beyond the duration of intensive care monitoring.[9] These abnormalities usually resolve in 7 to 10 days but can last for weeks. Patients who have muscular weakness, airflow obstruction, or severe decrease in vital capacity before surgery are at higher risk for respiratory

TABLE 80-1. Scoliosis Preoperative Predictors for Postoperative Mechanical Ventilation

Vital capacity <40% predicted
Neuromuscular scoliosis
Decreased airflow on pulmonary function tests
Preoperative hypoxemia
Significant pulmonary hypertension
Right-sided heart failure
Congenital airway anomalies

complications and should be expected to remain intubated postoperatively. Despite surgical correction, only rarely is improvement in vital capacity greater than 10%.[2]

CARDIAC IMPAIRMENT. With prolonged hypoxemia, hypercapnia, and pulmonary vascular constriction, pulmonary hypertension can develop and may lead to cardiac failure. Failure is more often associated with concomitant congenital heart disease, however. Coarctation of the aorta and cyanotic heart disease are frequently seen in association with scoliosis, and occult mitral valve prolapse has been diagnosed in 25% of asymptomatic patients.[2] Electrocardiographic findings of right atrial enlargement and right ventricular hypertrophy are unreliable late findings. Echocardiography is more useful during preoperative evaluation.

BLOOD LOSS. Intraoperatively, the patient is prone. Hypothermia is a constant risk in the exposed patient. Persistent blood loss should be anticipated, with greater losses for increasing numbers of levels instrumented. Losses of half of the total blood volume are not unusual. Induced hypotensive techniques can reduce bleeding and transfusion requirements by an average of 40% and can also decrease operative time.[10-12] Fatal venous air embolism has been reported, because the surgical site is notably higher than the heart.[13,14] This risk is increased by hypovolemia and low right cardiac filling pressure.

Neurologic Damage

Probably the most feared complication after correction of scoliosis is neurologic damage. The incidence of acute neurologic complications during scoliosis surgery is 0.72%.[3] Risk increases with severe deformity, congenital scoliosis, kyphosis, and preexisting neurologic deficit. Injury can occur from direct trauma, compression or stretching of the cord, hematoma, or occlusion of the arterial blood supply during distraction.

Somatosensory evoked potentials measure the cortical or spinal response to a repetitive peripheral sensory stimulus, but anterior cord ischemia can be missed, with resultant motor neuron damage. However, in scoliosis surgery, changes in somatosensory evoked potentials correlate reliably with motor changes. No confirmed false-negative results have occurred with properly conducted monitoring of somatosensory evoked potentials in idiopathic scoliosis, although reports of missed deficits in neuromuscular scoliosis have appeared.[15]

Monitoring of somatosensory evoked potentials in the ICU may be helpful if the patient is oversedated or otherwise unable to follow commands or communicate. A wake-up test is sometimes employed intraoperatively as well. This procedure involves discontinuation of the anesthetic and reversal of neuromuscular blockade after spinal distraction. The patient is asked to move his or her legs to confirm motor function, after which the anesthetic is readministered. A major limitation of this test is that it gives information at only a single time during the operation and poses potential anesthetic risks such as self-extubation. If the patient awakens with a neurologic deficit, the prognosis is variable. Prognosis is better for incomplete rather than complete lesions and can often be improved by removal of rods within 3 hours of diagnosis.[3]

Postoperative Care

NEUROLOGIC. Intense postoperative neurologic observation is essential. In addition, strict attention must be paid to the blood loss that often occurs, with associated changes in vital signs. Venous oozing from bone decortication results in postoperative blood loss that can exceed intraoperative loss. One case report described a revision procedure in which the examination was satisfactory at case conclusion, but several hours later the patient complained of loss of leg sensation and exhibited flaccid paralysis and loss of deep tendon reflexes. Systolic blood pressure was 60 mm Hg, and heart rate was 132 beats per minute. The patient's dressings were noted to be blood-soaked. Within 1 hour of fluid resuscitation, her function had returned to normal, and no permanent sequelae resulted.[16]

PULMONARY. Aggressive pulmonary care is a must. Patients typically are extubated unless they are deemed to be at high risk for postoperative respiratory complications (see Table 80-1). The head of the bed should be elevated to 30 degrees to allow easier lung expansion. Frequent side-to-side log-rolling is recommended. Incentive spirometry is encouraged, as is sitting or standing (or both) by postoperative day 3.[17] Pneumothorax or hemothorax can occur as a result of pleural penetration during establishment of the hook attachment, thoracoplasty, or central venous catheter placement.[17]

VASCULAR. Superior mesenteric artery (SMA) syndrome has been described.[17] Prolonged gastric distention is attributed to either SMA compression of the duodenum or physiologic dysfunction of the stomach and duodenum after a prolonged ileus. It may also occur in association with external compression from placement of a full body cast. The syndrome can be prevented with the use of a nasogastric tube. Elevating the head of the bed to 30 degrees, placing pillows under the knees, and encouraging trunk flexion can help to reduce SMA pressure on the duodenum. An upper gastrointestinal barium study validates the diagnosis. A small catheter should be passed beyond the obstruction for enteral feeding. Clinical signs and symptoms of pancreatitis also have been seen after scoliosis surgery.[18] This problem has been associated with higher intraoperative blood losses.

INFECTION. Wound infection often can be missed. The wound is deep and is closed completely, so the overlying skin appears normal until very late. Because hematoma and fever are normal in these patients, diagnosis can be delayed. Surgical incision and drainage is the definitive treatment.

CERVICAL SPINE SURGERY

The various surgical approaches to correct cervical spine disease directly impact postoperative care. Anterior cervical surgery frequently involves extensive retraction on the trachea and may be associated with large blood loss and large-volume intravenous fluid replacement. This constellation of events can lead to severe edema of the larynx and trachea. In general, patients who undergo cervical corpectomy at two or more levels should remain intubated overnight to allow the edema to resolve.

Transoral and submandibular approaches to the retropharyngeal spine are sometimes employed because of difficulty with patient positioning. Postoperatively, these patients have tremendous retropharyngeal swelling. The endotracheal tube is the only stent in the airway and absolutely should not be removed until the swelling has resolved, often several days after surgery. The patient should be sedated appropriately.

Posterior cervical procedures typically are not associated with airway edema, and extubation at case conclusion is the norm. Those patients with rheumatoid arthritis (RA) undergoing a posterior cervical procedure who initially have a fiberoptic-guided intubation may have less upper airway obstruction after extubation.[19]

JOINT REPLACEMENT ■

Replacement of diseased joints with implantable prosthetic devices is one of the major advances of orthopedic surgery since the early 1960s. Most patients who undergo replacement surgery are older than 60 years of age and generally in good health. Of concern, however, is that these patients may not report symptoms of cardiac or respiratory insufficiency because the adaptive changes that they have made in their lifestyle severely restrict their activity level. These are important considerations in light of the hemodynamic changes that occur during and after surgery.

TOTAL HIP ARTHROPLASTY

THA is usually performed with the patient in the lateral decubitus position. The acetabulum and intramedullary canal of the femur are mechanically reamed and prepared for prosthetic insertion. The femoral component may or may not be cemented in place, depending on the age of the patient and the nature of the disease process. A transient decrease in blood pressure is consistently seen shortly after cementing, owing to decreases in systemic vascular resistance and mean arterial pressure.[20] This effect has been reproduced experimentally by giving parenteral boluses of polymethylmethacrylate monomer to dogs.[21]

Pulmonary Embolization

CEMENTED IMPLANTATION. Occasionally, more profound decreases in blood pressure occur after injection of acrylic monomer and insertion of the prosthetic femoral component. This problem may result from mechanical extrusion of large volumes of air and fat emboli into the venous circulation. In greyhounds, femoral prosthesis cementing caused femoral shaft pressures to rise as high as 900 mm Hg.[22] Marrow elements appeared in the lungs 10 to 120 seconds after the prosthesis was placed. Other studies have found the same results during THA in humans: pulmonary artery blood samples taken 4 minutes after insertion of a femoral prosthesis contained gross and microscopic particles of marrow, platelet, and fibrin aggregates.[23]

In another series, 34 patients undergoing primary THA had fat embolization at the time of placement of the femoral prosthesis.[24] A Doppler ultrasound probe placed over the femoral vein to detect particulate embolization recorded peak sound activity as the prosthesis was firmly seated in the femoral canal. Venous blood analysis confirmed the presence of fat emboli at these peak Doppler recording times. No complications occurred, and no relation seemed to exist between the presence of fat emboli and blood pressure alterations.

Hypoxemia from acute embolism of fat and marrow, coupled with systemic vasodilation from absorption of monomer, may contribute to intraoperative cardiac arrest.[25,26] In the early 1970s, at least ten reports described sudden cardiovascular collapse after placement of acrylic bone cement and prosthetic joint devices. Studies suggest that this complication is exceedingly rare, although certain patient populations and the use of particular instrumentation systems may increase the risk of intraoperative cardiac arrest.[27] THA with long-stem components is associated with substantial risk as well as excessive intramedullary pressurization in a previously undisturbed canal. Advanced age and the use of several batches of polymethylmethacrylate compound the risk. Patients with myelodysplastic disorders, collagen vascular disease, osteoporosis, metastatic cancer, or extremity immobilization have medullary cavity enlargement, an increased liquid marrow fat content, and increased risk for emboli.[28] Those with underlying cardiac and pulmonary disease also are at increased risk.

NONCEMENTED IMPLANTATION. If a noncemented technique is used for femoral prosthesis insertion, these changes occur to a lesser extent. Propst and colleagues studied 20 THA patients undergoing intraoperative transesophageal echocardiography.[29] Segmental wall motion abnormalities occurred more often during insertion of cemented femoral prostheses than during placement of noncemented components. Intracardiac emboli were seen in all patients during surgery; the largest number occurred during reaming of the femur and insertion of the femoral prosthesis. Significantly more emboli were seen if cement was used. No hemodynamic or electrocardiographic changes corresponded with these events.

Ereth and associates prospectively studied 35 patients and also noted greater embolization in cemented arthroplasties compared with noncemented arthroplasties.[30] In addition, they reported decreased cardiac output and increased pulmonary artery pressure in patients receiving cemented prostheses compared with patients receiving noncemented prostheses.

Blood Loss

If a noncemented prosthesis is placed, higher blood loss can be expected during and after the operation. Intraoperative loss for an uncomplicated cemented primary total hip replacement for arthritis is usually between 400 and 800 mL, whereas a noncemented hip replacement may lead to loss of 1000 mL. Anticipated blood loss during arthroplasty for congenital deformities, for cancerous bone lesions, or for revision of a previous joint replacement is much less predictable because of technical difficulties. A blood loss of more than 1500 mL is not uncommon.

A patient undergoing revision of a previous THA is much more likely to require ICU care postoperatively than a patient undergoing a primary procedure. Revision THA is greatly complicated by a previously cemented prosthesis. The old cement must be retrieved, a process that may take minutes to hours; all the while, the patient continues to bleed. Blood loss of many liters is not uncommon during revision hip surgery, and fluid resuscitation frequently is required for many hours afterward.

TOTAL KNEE ARTHROPLASTY

TKA surgery is much like THA with respect to hemodynamic concerns during prosthetic insertion and cementing. Tourniquet use decreases intraoperative blood loss, which ranges from 200 to 400 mL, but adds the risk of hypotension, tachycardia, hypercarbia, and hypoxemia on deflation. During TKA, transesophageal echocardiography has demonstrated emboli in the right heart immediately after tourniquet deflation.[31]

Some surgeons replace both knees during the same operation. This procedure involves reaming, cementing, and prosthetic placement in four long bones, significantly increasing the risk for intraoperative emboli and corresponding hemodynamic changes.[32] In such cases, the knees usually should be replaced sequentially; the second knee replacement should proceed only after uneventful completion of the first. However, if the patient is otherwise healthy and the surgeon has sufficient staff, both knees can be replaced simultaneously. Vigilance is required during tourniquet deflation.[33] The tourniquets should be released at least 10 minutes apart to allow time for recovery before the second insult, thereby minimizing the hemodynamic consequences.

In both TKA and THA, patients who are at high risk for embolization should be identified. Anesthesiologists should consider invasive monitoring in these patients. Intraarterial blood pressure monitoring is critical during insertion of the prosthesis, and central venous access is useful for delivery of vasoactive drugs and assessment of intravascular volume status. Transesophageal echocardiography should also be considered. Postoperatively, the patients are at risk for DVT, pulmonary thromboembolism,[34] and FES. Postoperative

bleeding usually is minimal after THA but can be up to 1000 mL after TKA.

TOTAL SHOULDER ARTHROPLASTY

Total shoulder arthroplasty is not plagued with the catastrophic complications of THA and TKA. The potential for venous air embolism exists because the patient is in the beach chair position (sitting position with hip and knees flexed), rendering the operative site higher than the heart. Nevertheless, this problem rarely is observed. Estimated blood loss is usually not more than 500 mL if the replacement is done for traumatic or degenerative disease. However, if the replacement is related to metastatic cancer, it can be up to 1500 mL. Blood loss is minimal after the prosthesis has been cemented in place.

PATHOLOGIC PROCESSES COMMON TO ORTHOPEDIC PATIENTS ■

COMPARTMENT SYNDROME

Compartment syndrome develops when increased tissue pressure within an osteofascial compartment reduces capillary perfusion below a level necessary to maintain tissue viability.[35] The result is loss of muscle and nerve function and may include infection, gangrene, or myoglobinuria and renal failure.[36] Compartment syndrome can occur in any osteofascial compartment of the body but is most common in the setting of closed fracture of the tibia, for which the incidence is 3% to 17%.[37] It has been described in cases of soft tissue trauma, open fracture, reperfusion after prolonged ischemia, and elective surgery. In addition, the syndrome has been seen with prolonged lithotomy position,[38] spontaneous hemorrhage,[39] intravenous regional anesthesia,[40] and use of pneumatic antishock garments.[41,42]

Military Antishock Trousers

The ICU physician is likely to encounter a patient who has required the military antishock trousers (MAST) for resuscitation. In 1981, a case report described a 21-year-old, multitrauma motor vehicle accident patient who was placed in the MAST for 3½ hours because of persistent shock.[42] Twelve hours after surgery he complained of numbness of the feet and legs and was subsequently observed. On postoperative day 3, he had bilateral fasciotomies for anterior tibial compartment syndromes. The muscle was nonviable and was debrided, and eventually the entire anterior compartment was resected because of necrosis.

Since that first report, severe cases of compartment syndrome have been reported after prolonged (>2 hours) use of the MAST on noninjured extremities.[41,43] If the MAST is used, the minimum pressure possible should be employed, and it should be inflated no longer than absolutely necessary. If the suit is used to control bleeding in severe pelvic fractures, compartment pressures should be monitored and maintained at 40 to 60 mm Hg for no more than 24 to 48 hours. Suit pressures at or above systemic pressures should not be used unless needed to maintain adequate blood pressure. The abdominal compartment pressure must not be significantly higher than leg compartment pressure. Finally, all patients should be monitored closely for development of compartment syndrome after suit removal.

Clinical Presentation

The clinical presentation includes pain out of proportion to the injury or physical findings, sensory changes associated with nerve compression within the compartment (Fig. 80-1), weakness and excessive pain with passive movement of the muscle group within the compartment, loss of voluntary function in those muscles, and tenseness of the fascial boundaries of the compartment.[44] Devices to measure intracompartmental pressure are available. They are particularly useful in patients who are obtunded, sedated, or otherwise unable to communicate.

Diagnosis

The ultimate diagnosis of compartment syndrome is based on the patient's clinical history as well as the signs and symptoms (Table 80-2). High-energy tibial fractures, such as those that occur in a motor vehicle accident, have an incidence of almost 17%.[37] However, low-energy tibial fractures also have potential for compartment syndrome because the compartments have not been disrupted by the fracture itself. A high index of suspicion is essential. Careful serial physical examinations are very helpful, including muscle strength testing, evaluation of pain with passive motion, and sensory assessment of the involved nerves. The results of vascular examination may be normal or only slightly abnormal, even in the most advanced cases. Compartment pressure measurements should be used as an adjunct to clinical assessment,[45] unless the patient is obtunded or uncooperative or residual regional anesthesia is present.

Laboratory abnormalities may indicate that necrosis is already present, but the findings are nonspecific for compartment syndrome. Creatine kinase, lactate dehydrogenase, alanine aminotransferase, potassium, and phosphate may be elevated as a result of muscle cell lysis. Increased creatinine

TABLE 80-2.   Diagnosis of Compartment Syndrome and Fasciotomy Recommendations

CLINICAL SIGNS AND SYMPTOMS

Pain out of proportion to clinical situation
Weakness and pain on passive stretch of muscle
Decreased sensation in distribution of nerves in compartment
Tenseness of fascial boundaries
Vascular examination may be normal or abnormal

TISSUE PRESSURE MEASUREMENT (used as an adjunct to signs and symptoms, unless patient is obtunded)

Fasciotomy recommended if pressures are
   >40 mm Hg
   Within 30 mm Hg of diastolic blood pressure
   30 mm Hg with a high index of suspicion

and blood urea nitrogen may indicate renal failure from myoglobinuria.

Fasciotomy

The level of tissue pressure at which fasciotomy is recommended varies between investigators. Gulli and Templeman recommend fasciotomy if pressures are greater than 40 mm Hg or within 30 mm Hg of the patient's mean arterial pressure.[37] If pressures are between 30 and 40 mm Hg, they operate if the clinical suspicion is high. If pressure is less than 30 mm Hg, they observe the patient with serial examinations and pressure measurements. Pressures should be measured within the fleshy portion of the compartment.

If a commercial device is not available, an arterial pressure transducer may be used with a large (≥16-gauge) needle (Fig. 80-2). A small amount of water (<1 mL) is flushed through the needle, and then the pressure is monitored until it equilibrates. Pressure should be rechecked in a slightly different position to avoid error. Matsen and colleagues recommend continuous pressure monitoring, recognizing that both duration and magnitude of pressure elevation contribute to morbidity.[44] Continuous monitoring is particularly useful in the obtunded patient.

Leg Compartments

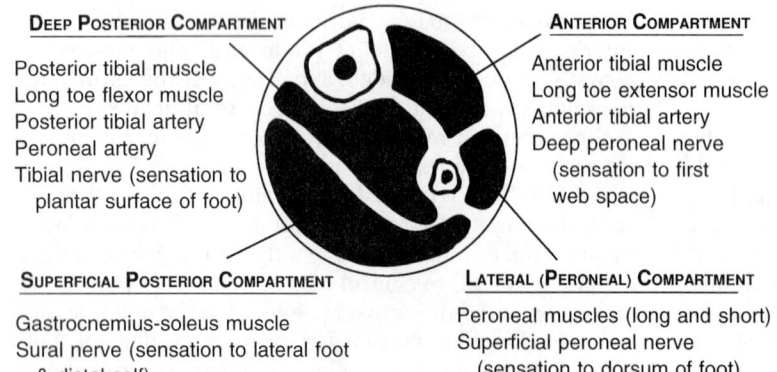

FIGURE 80-1. Leg compartments, showing structures present in the calf.

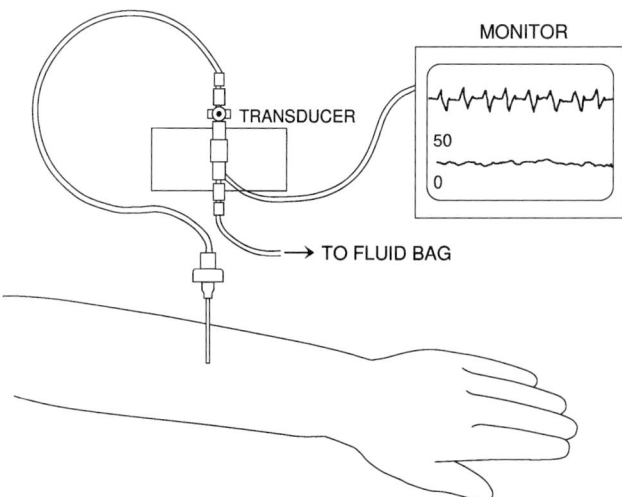

FIGURE 80-2. Measurement of tissue (compartment) pressure after orthopedic extremity trauma. (Enneking FK, Scarborough MT: Anesthesia for orthopedic surgery. In: Kirby RR, Gravenstein N (eds). *Clinical Anesthesia Practice.* Philadelphia, JB Lippincott, 1994:1248)

Fasciotomy is the only treatment that reliably restores normal pressure. In an emergency situation, this procedure can be performed at the bedside if the patient is too unstable for transport to the operating room suite. During fasciotomy, potassium that has been released from the necrotic muscle cells into the central circulation can cause cardiac arrhythmias and arrest.

Postoperative Care

Postoperative hyperkalemia may need to be treated aggressively with hydration, diuresis, and intravenous glucose and insulin. Depending on the degree of injury, an epimysiotomy may be necessary. The wound is debrided carefully, packed with saline-soaked dressings, and splinted. If the compartment syndrome is associated with a fracture, concomitant internal fixation is associated with less morbidity than is closed reduction and cast fixation.[46]

Postfasciotomy care includes continued neurovascular assessment, observation for signs of infection, and maintenance of joint mobility. If muscle injury is extensive, significant amounts of myoglobin may be released as the muscle is reperfused after fasciotomy. The patient must be kept well hydrated and observed closely for myoglobinuria and decreased renal function.[37] Mannitol (1 g/kg) is suggested for prophylaxis against these complications.

In 5 to 7 days, the patient needs to return to surgery for secondary wound closure or split-thickness skin graft. In a study by Sheridan and Matsen, those compartment syndromes that were treated by fasciotomy within 12 hours after diagnosis had normal function in 68% of the extremities.[47] Of those treated with later fasciotomies, only 8% had normal function. The complication rate was much lower for the early group (4.5%) compared with the later group (54%).

Sequelae

Potential sequelae from missed compartment syndrome include prolonged or permanent hypesthesia, dysesthesia, contractures, muscle weakness, renal failure, sepsis, amputation, and death.

FAT EMBOLISM SYNDROME

FES is a subtype of ARDS. It is typically associated with orthopedic trauma.[48,49] The clinical signs and symptoms are seen in 0.5% to 2% of patients with fractures of the long bones, and in up to 10% of patients with multiple skeletal fractures and unstable pelvic injuries.[28] Release of fat emboli as a subclinical event occurs with almost all fractures of long bones and pelvic trauma, although the clinically apparent syndrome is relatively rare.[28] It has been documented after intramedullary reaming and nailing of long bones, during prosthetic knee and hip arthroplasty (previously discussed), and after hip fractures without operation.

Pathogenesis

The pathogenesis of FES is not entirely understood, but most investigators agree that bone trauma leaks fat and marrow elements into the venous circulation[50] (Fig. 80-3). These elements travel to the pulmonary circulation, where an inflammatory reaction ensues. Tissue thromboplastin is released, the complement system is activated, and the extrinsic coagulation cascade produces intravascular fibrin and fibrin degradation products. In combination with leukocytes, platelets, and fat globules, they lead to increased pulmonary vascular permeability and platelet aggregation.

Diagnosis

FES is a diagnosis of exclusion that depends on the clinician's index of suspicion. Signs and symptoms are basically those of ARDS but occur in association with bone trauma. They become evident in 60% of patients by 24 hours and in 85% of patients by 48 hours after fracture.[28]

NEUROLOGIC MANIFESTATIONS. Arterial hypoxemia with fever and neurologic derangements (including drowsiness, restlessness, confusion, disorientation, seizures, stupor, and coma) are hallmarks of this syndrome. Preservation of normal muscle tone and reflexes suggests a favorable prognosis. Nonreactive pupils and depressed deep tendon reflexes usually do not resolve after correction of hypoxemia and are probably caused by ischemia and microscopic hemorrhage in association with emboli in the brain.

Recognition of neurologic manifestations helps to establish the diagnosis. In a retrospective study of 12 patients with FES, 9 initially presented with mild encephalopathy, such as an acute confusional state not attributable to hypoxemia.[51] Four of these patients developed additional focal features with signs of upper motor neuron dysfunction (aphagia, anisocoria, and hemiplegia). Computed tomography scans were normal. In another study of patients with neurologic derangements attributable to FES after bilateral

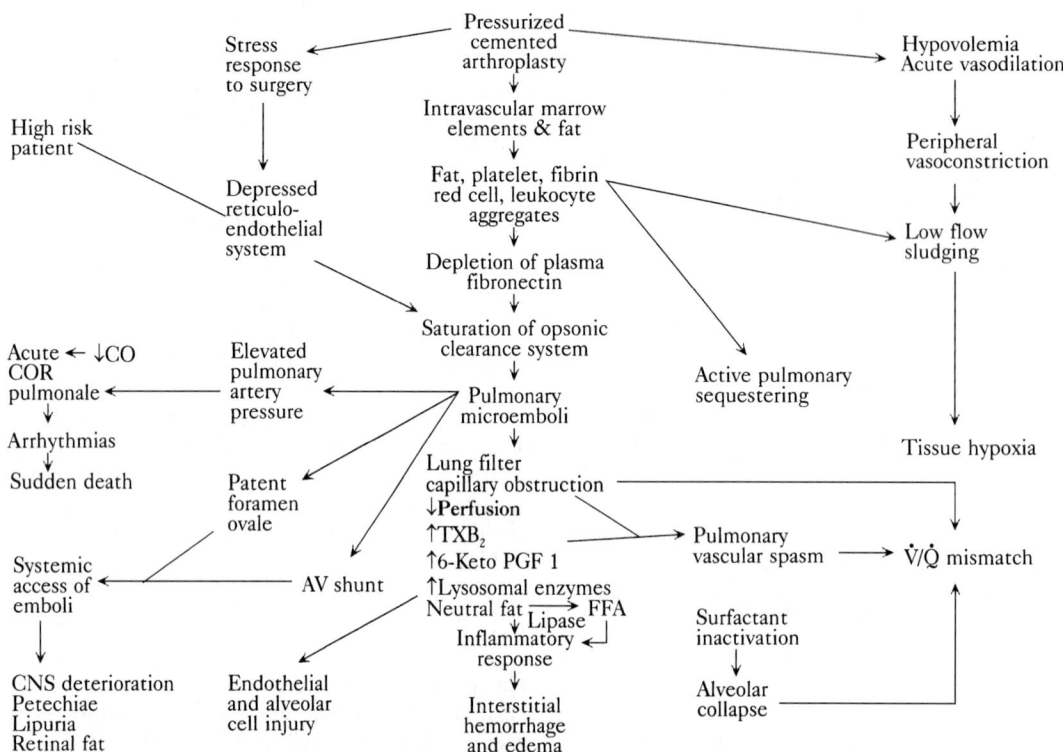

FIGURE 80-3. Pathophysiology of fat embolism syndrome. AV, arteriovenous; CNS, central nervous system; CO, cardiac output; FFA, free fatty acids; 6-Keto-PGF, 6-keto-prostaglandin F_1; TXB_2, thromboxane B_2; $\dot{V}/\dot{Q}$, ventilation-perfusion. (From Enneking FK: Cardiac arrest during total knee replacement using a long-stem prosthesis. Case Conference of the University of Florida. *J Clin Anesth* 1995;7:253)

total knee replacement, agitation, confusion, and lethargy were the most common manifestations.[52] In an elderly patient, differentiation of these postoperative symptoms from those caused by drug effects or senile confusion may be difficult, but FES should be considered.

CARDIOVASCULAR MANIFESTATIONS. In contrast to the subacute onset of respiratory failure, FES can present acutely with right-sided heart failure and arrhythmia. The acute phase is secondary to critical obstruction of the pulmonary circulation by particulate embolization. Acute cor pulmonale in association with bradycardia or cardiac arrhythmia can result. Elderly patients with preexisting lung disease and low pulmonary reserve are most at risk.[53,54] These problems have been observed intraoperatively after cemented THA and TKA procedures and with untreated hip fractures. If the patient survives the initial phase, the classic respiratory and neurologic symptoms of FES ensue.

Petechiae are found in 50% to 60% of patients in a distribution over the anterior chest and neck, axillae, and conjunctivae. The lesions are transient and follow the onset of respiratory distress. Other manifestations of FES are thrombocytopenia, anemia, lipuria, and tachycardia.

Treatment

Hemodynamic and aggressive ventilatory support are the main treatments for FES, because respiratory failure is the leading cause of death. Over the past 20 years, positive-pressure ventilation with continuous positive airway pressure has improved the prognosis dramatically. Other treatments are of more questionable effectiveness. Although infusions of ethanol, heparin, low-molecular-weight dextran, and hypertonic glucose have all been used, none has improved outcome in clinical trials.[55-57]

Some improvement in respiratory function in trauma patients given steroids for FES has been reported, although no dose-response studies have been conducted to determine the appropriate dose.[28,55-57] No studies have investigated steroids for patients in the acute phase of the syndrome. However, a prospective, double-blind, randomized study of trauma patients at high risk for FES found methylprednisolone sodium succinate, 7.5 mg/kg every 6 hours for 12 doses, to be effective prophylaxis in the prevention of FES.[58] Pulmonary hypertension is not improved by methylprednisolone.[59]

FRACTURE STABILIZATION. Growing evidence suggests that early fracture stabilization decreases the incidence of FES. Bone and coworkers randomly assigned 178 patients prospectively to either early or delayed stabilization of their femoral fractures.[60] Some patients had isolated injuries; others had multiple injuries. Those with isolated femoral fractures did equally well with fixation within 24 hours of injury or delayed fixation at 48 hours after injury, although 3 patients in the delayed group developed late pulmonary embolism (after hospital discharge). For those patients who had multiple injuries, early fracture fixation significantly improved pulmonary morbidity, with a corresponding decrease in number of ICU days, number of hospital days, and hospital costs.

Concurrent with Bone's results, Johnson and colleagues published a retrospective analysis of 132 consecutive patients with multiple musculoskeletal injuries that assessed the relation between the time elapsed from injury to operative stabilization of major fractures and the incidence of ARDS.[61] For the overall data set, a delay in orthopedic surgery (>24 hours) was associated with a fivefold increase in ARDS. For the more severely injured patients, only 17% of those in the early stabilization group developed ARDS, but 75% of the delayed group were affected (Table 80-3).

DEEP VENOUS THROMBOSIS AND PULMONARY THROMBOEMBOLISM

DVT remains a critical issue for the orthopedic patient with lower extremity disease. The incidence of DVT is 40% to 50% for THA, 45% to 50% for fractured hip, and 72% for TKA.[62] Fatal pulmonary embolism occurs in 1% to 5% of these patients if no prophylaxis is given. The orthopedic surgical patient is susceptible to venous stasis, intimal injury, and hypercoagulability. Anesthesia and the supine position decrease venous return, anatomic positioning often impairs adequate venous drainage, and tourniquet use contributes to stasis during the procedure. Intimal injury may result from anatomic positioning and tourniquet use, producing a site for clot formation. In addition, hypercoagulability occurs concomitantly. Antithrombin-3 has been shown to decrease for 3 to 5 days after total hip or knee surgery. This deficit impairs modulation of the clotting cascade, increasing the propensity for thrombus formation.

Risk Factors

Risk factors are age, length and type of surgery, previous DVT or embolic episode; secondary risk factors include prolonged immobilization, paralysis, malignancy, obesity, varicose veins, and estrogen. Hull and associates designate as high-risk patients those older than 40 years of age who are undergoing surgery for malignancy or an orthopedic procedure of the lower extremities lasting longer than 30 minutes, and who have hereditary or acquired coagulopathies or secondary risk factors.[63] This group has a 40% to 80% risk of calf vein thrombosis, a 10% to 20% risk of proximal vein thrombosis, and a 1% to 5% risk of fatal pulmonary thromboembolism. All lower extremity orthopedic procedures are thus categorized into this high-risk group.

Prevention

Strategies to prevent thromboembolic disease in orthopedic patients include regional anesthesia, early patient mobilization, mechanical devices (e.g., pneumatic compression stockings), prophylactic drug therapy (Table 80-4), and vascular filters. Multiple studies confirm that prophylactic drug ther-

apy is the most effective means to prevent thromboembolic disease.[64-69] Prophylactic agents include aspirin, dextran, low-dose heparin, low-dose heparin with antithrombin-3, adjusted-dose heparin, adjusted-dose warfarin (Coumadin), low-dose Coumadin, and low-molecular-weight heparin (LMWH).

PROPHYLACTIC ANTICOAGULATION

Coumadin. Coumadin prophylaxis can be administered by several different regimens (see Table 80-4). Low-dose heparin is less frequently employed, although it may be useful in the setting of acute myocardial infarction. All methods recommend therapy until discharge. Postdischarge prophylaxis has been recommended for THA patients to maintain the prothrombin time (PT) at 16 to 18 seconds for 4 to 6 weeks. More recently, some clinicians have adopted the standardized international normalized ratio (INR) in lieu of the PT test, the results of which can vary greatly among institutions because of differences in commercial thromboplastins.[70] The INR should be maintained at 2.0 to 3.0.

In a randomized prospective clinical trial, Wilson and coworkers compared postoperative adjusted, high-dose Coumadin with fixed, low-dose Coumadin (2 mg/day) in 96 patients after lower extremity orthopedic surgery.[71] Before hospital discharge and at a 6-week follow-up, duplex ultrasonography was used to screen for proximal leg DVT, and compression ultrasonography for common femoral, superficial femoral, and popliteal vein thrombosis in both legs. No difference was found between the groups with respect to efficacy or safety. The investigators suggest that although further studies are warranted, low-dose Coumadin may be a more convenient and cost-effective means of prophylaxis.

Antithrombin-3. Antithrombin-3 has been studied because its decrease has been reported after orthopedic surgery, possibly contributing to the increased incidence of DVT. Administration of antithrombin-3 in combination with heparin has been used for DVT prophylaxis in THA patients, although it is not used frequently. Because it is derived from purified human plasma, viral transmission remains a concern.

Low-Molecular-Weight Heparin. A newer method of anticoagulation employs LMWH. These fragments of commercial-grade heparin have reduced ability to catalyze the inactivation of thrombin relative to their ability to inhibit factor Xa. In most comparative studies, standard heparin produced more bleeding for an equivalent antithrombotic effect than did the LMWHs. Stated alternatively, LMWHs have reduced hemorrhagic-to-antithrombotic ratios.

A 1994 critical analysis of LMWH for DVT prophylaxis concluded that it is effective and safe for patients undergoing major orthopedic surgery of the lower extremities.[72] The efficacy and safety profile for patients with THA appears to be similar to that of low-dose Coumadin, but LMWH use was associated with more wound hematomas. For patients with TKA, LMWH was significantly more effective than all other anticoagulant-based prophylaxis methods, and it did not increase bleeding. However, the investigators point out that DVT prevalence was still unacceptably high, and they

TABLE 80-3.   Summary of Studies Showing Association Between Delay in Repair of Long Bone Fracture and Fat Embolism Syndrome

PATIENTS WITH MULTIPLE TRAUMA AND LONG BONE FRACTURE WITH FAT EMBOLISM SYNDROME°		
	Operative Stabilization	*Traction*
384 patients	4.5%	22%
211 patients	1.4%	—

PATIENTS WITH LONG BONE FRACTURE WITH ACUTE RESPIRATORY DISTRESS SYNDROME (n = 132)		
	Early Stabilization (<24 h)	*Late (>24 h)*
	7%	38%
	In Association With Very Severe Injuries	
	17%	75%

PATIENTS WITH LONG BONE FRACTURE (n = 40)		
	Early Stabilization (n = 20)	*Traction for 10 days (n = 20)*
Mechanical ventilation	3.4 d	9.7 d
Intensive care unit	7.5 d	15 d
Hospital stay	23 d	45 d

PATIENTS WITH ISOLATED ACUTE FEMORAL FRACTURE OR FRACTURE ASSOCIATED WITH MULTIPLE INJURIES (n = 178)		
	Early	*Delayed*
ISOLATED FEMUR FRACTURE		
Acute respiratory distress syndrome	0%	0%
Pleural effusion	2.4%	3.7%
Abnormal arterial blood gases	9%	22%
ASSOCIATED WITH MULTIPLE INJURIES		
Acute respiratory distress syndrome	2%	16%
Average time in intensive care unit	2.8 d	7.6 d
Average time in hospital	17.3 d	26.6 d
Average cost	$19,854	$32,915

°Riska EB, Myllynen P: Fat embolism in patients with multiple injuries. *J Trauma* 1982;22:891.

†Johnson KD, Cadamb A, Seibert GB: Incidence of ARDS in patients with multiple musculoskeletal injuries. Effect of early operative stabilization of fractures. *J Trauma* 1985;25:375.

‡Seibel R, LaDuca J, Hassett JM, et al: Blunt multiple trauma, femur traction, and the pulmonary failure–septic state. *Ann Surg* 1985;202:283.

§Bone LB, Johnson KD, Weigelt J, et al: Early versus delayed stabilization of femoral fracture. *J Bone Joint Surg Am* 1989;71:336.

recommend trials including other methods, such as external compression devices.

Summary.   For THA, Coumadin is the single pharmacologic agent of choice; it decreases DVT formation, which usually occurs in 40% to 60% of patients, down to 17% to 30%, with a notable reduction in proximal vein thromboses. For the hip fracture patient, Coumadin or LMWH is employed. For the TKA patient who is at particular risk for proximal thrombosis, the choice of prophylaxis is controver-

TABLE 80-4. Pharmacologic Deep Venous Thrombosis Prophylaxis Techniques

COUMADIN

A. 10 mg po on evening before surgery
   5 mg po on evening of surgery
   Adjust dose thereafter to PT 16–18 s (INR 2–3)
   Continue until discharge

B. Low dose at home 12–14 d before surgery to maintain PT 1.5–3 s longer than control
   POD 1 adjust dose to PT 16–18 s (INR 2–3)
   Continue until discharge

C. 10 mg po on night of surgery
   None of POD 1
   POD 2 adjust dose to PT 16–18 s (INR 2–3)
   Continue until discharge

ADJUSTED LOW-DOSE HEPARIN°

A. 3500 U SQ 2 h before surgery
   3500 U SQ 8 h after surgery
   POD1 and POD2 adjust dose 6 h after morning dose
   Then adjust every other day: after two or three adjustments, start Coumadin or maintain
      patient on last total dose of heparin SQ divided every 12 h

LOW-MOLECULAR-WEIGHT HEPARINS

A. Enoxaparin (Lovinox): 30 mg SQ every 12 h

°Adjustments:
   <36s = +1000 U
   36 − 40s = +500 U
   41 − 45s = ±0
   46 − 50s = −500 U
   >50s = −1000 U

INR, international normalized ratio; po, per os; POD, postoperative day; SQ, subcutaneous; PT, prothrombin time.

From Merli GJ: Deep vein thrombosis and pulmonary embolism in orthopedic surgery. *Med Clin North Am* 1993;77:397.

sial: both LMWH and Coumadin[34] are acceptable, but the risk remains high.

EXTERNAL COMPRESSION DEVICES. External compression devices have gained increased use in orthopedic surgery and are often used in conjunction with pharmacologic interventions to reduce DVT. They reduce stasis in the gastrocnemius-soleus "pump" and may also increase fibrinolysis. Typically, use is begun during surgery with placement on the nonoperated leg and immediately after operation on the operative side. Both calf- and thigh-length external compression sleeves are used; they are worn for 3 to 5 days, with removal only for bathroom use and physical therapy. After the patient is ambulatory, the sleeves can be discontinued.

If the patient has been immobilized for more than 72 hours without any form of prophylaxis, external compression devices are not recommended for fear of disturbing a newly formed clot. In combination with other methods of DVT prophylaxis, they have been shown to decrease the incidence of calf vein DVT. They are not as successful in decreasing proximal vein thrombosis.

ANESTHETIC CHOICES. The type of anesthetic used may have an effect on the development of DVT. Clinical evidence supports regional anesthetic techniques (spinal and epidural) as effective means to minimize venous thromboembolism; they currently are the anesthetics of choice, especially in the higher-risk patients.[73,74]

Diagnosis

Signs and symptoms of DVT include pain, deep tenderness, edema, and rubor. These are nonspecific findings that make clinical diagnosis difficult. The classic Homan's sign of calf discomfort on dorsiflexion of the foot is also unreliable. Therefore, more objective means must be applied. Diagnostic procedures for DVT include impedance plethysmography, fibrinogen scanning (no longer available because of fear of infection on transfusion), contrast venography, ultrasonography, and magnetic resonance venography[75] (Table 80-5).[76-78]

TABLE 80-5. Tests Used in the Diagnosis of Deep Vein Thrombosis°

TEST	SYMPTOMATIC DEEP VEIN THROMBOSIS[†]		ASYMPTOMATIC DEEP VEIN THROMBOSIS[‡]		ANATOMIC AREA	COMMENT
	Sensitivity (%)	Specificity (%)	Sensitivity (%)	Specificity (%)		
Phlebography	Standard for comparison		Standard for comparison		Pelvis, thigh, popliteal area, calf	Invasive; provides equivocal results in cases of recurrent deep vein thrombosis; not easily repeated
Impedance plethysmography	92[§]	95	22	98	Thigh, popliteal area	For provisional diagnosis of primary or recurrent proximal deep vein thrombosis; insensitive to calf thrombi and to nonocclusive proximal thrombi
Ultrasonography (real-time B-mode duplex)	97	97	59	98	Thigh, popliteal area	Most sensitive confirmatory test for symptomatic deep vein thrombosis
Ultrasonography (Doppler flow velocity)	88	88	—	—	Thigh, popliteal area	Can be used on limbs in traction or plaster; interpretation is subjective, requires skill
Magnetic resonance venography[¶]	96	100	—	—	Inferior vena cava, pelvis, thigh	Can distinguish between acute and chronic occlusion; can identify associated abnormalities; noninvasive; expensive; limited availability

°Data were derived from cumulative results summarized by Lensing et al.[76] No data on [^{125}I]-labeled fibrinogen scanning were included, because the test is no longer available.

[†]Testing is mostly used to verify clinical suspicion of deep vein thrombosis.

[‡]Testing is mostly used to screen high-risk patients.

[§]Recent studies have reported lower sensitivity.[77,78]

[¶]Magnetic resonance venography has only been evaluated in small clinical trials.

From Weinmann EE, Salzman EW: Deep vein thrombosis. *N Engl J Med* 1994;331:1631.

CONTRAST VENOGRAPHY. Contrast venography is the diagnostic gold standard. It is an invasive technique that identifies DVT in the lower extremity up to the common iliac vein. Shortcomings include inadequate visualization of proximal veins in 18% of cases and significant variation in interpretation of results.[79] In addition, it puts the patient at risk for allergic reaction, development of DVT, and pain during the procedure.

IMPEDANCE PLETHYSMOGRAPHY. Impedance plethysmography is a noninvasive examination that is highly sensitive to thrombi in the proximal veins but less so in detection of distal occlusion. A pneumatic cuff is placed on the thigh and inflated to 40 mm Hg. Electric impedance is measured between two electrodes. Proximal venous obstruction decreases impedance as the leg becomes engorged with blood. False-positive results have been seen in patients with severe arterial disease or during positive-pressure ventilation. False-negative results are produced if the thrombi are nonocclusive. In general, it is useful for evaluation of the symptomatic patient, and serial studies are reliable.

DUPLEX ULTRASONOGRAPHY. Duplex ultrasonography offers a highly sensitive, noninvasive alternative to more traditional modes of diagnosis. It is particularly good for diagnosis of proximal DVTs (from whence the vast majority of thromboemboli originate) and has become the screening tool of choice for symptomatic DVT.[80]

Treatment

After DVT has been diagnosed, anticoagulants are started immediately to prevent further clot development. Heparin is the mainstay of treatment and should be initiated promptly

TABLE 80-6. Intravenous Heparin for Treatment of Deep Venous Thrombosis

Begin with loading dose of 5000–10,000 U
Follow with infusion of 1000–1400 U/h to maintain a partial prothrombin time of 1.5–2 times the control

(Table 80-6). It may be given intravenously or subcutaneously. Subcutaneous therapy is more convenient for outpatients. Both routes are equally efficacious if the partial thromboplastin time (PTT) is maintained in the therapeutic range (1.5 to 2.5 times the control). LMWH appears to be equally effective. In general, heparin is given for 5 days, after which the patient is switched to Coumadin, to produce a PT of 1.3 to 1.5 times the control (INR between 2 and 3). Oral anticoagulation should continue for at least 3 months.

Less desirable forms of treatment include surgical thrombectomy and thrombolysis. Thrombectomy probably should be reserved for patients whose limb is threatened, because long-term patency is poor. Thrombolysis does not protect better against pulmonary thromboembolism, and it carries a twofold to fourfold increased risk of intracranial hemorrhage.[81] Nonetheless, it is more effective than heparin for opening an occluded vessel and may be considered for iliofemoral DVT in the patient without contraindications for thrombolysis (Table 80-7).[82]

RHEUMATOID ARTHRITIS

Patients with RA frequently require multiple orthopedic interventions in light of their articular disease. They have many associated disease processes. In addition, their pharmacologic interventions have significant side effects that may complicate postoperative care (Table 80-8). Frequently, RA is associated with the presence of serum IgM. This immunoglobulin increases the frequency of vasculitis, nodules, and more severe involvement of foot and hand joints.[83]

TABLE 80-8. Side Effects of Typical Medications Taken by Patients with Rheumatoid Arthritis

MEDICATION	SIDE EFFECTS
Nonsteroidal anti-inflammatory drugs	Gastric irritation, ulceration, renal dysfunction
Salicylates	Gastric erosion, renal toxicity, platelet dysfunction
Corticosteroids	Adrenal suppression
Chloroquine	Retinopathy, neuromyopathy, cardiomyopathy
Gold salts	Mucocutaneous reaction, proteinuria/renal disease, leukopenia, thrombocytopenia, agranulocytosis
D-Penicillamine	As gold salts, rare autoimmune reactions
Sulfasalazine	GI distress, neutropenia, leukopenia, thrombocytopenia, aplastic anemia, eosinophilic pneumonitis, fibrosing alveolitis
Azothioprine	GI distress, leukopenia, thrombocytopenia, anemia, cholestatic hepatitis
Methotrexate	GI distress, bone marrow toxicity, pulmonary toxicity, hepatic fibrosis

Cardiovascular Effects

Patients with RA have a 35% estimated prevalence of cardiovascular disorders, most commonly pericardial disease.[83] Effusions or pericarditis can lead to constrictive pericarditis or, rarely, to tamponade. Granulomatous changes may affect the myocardium and valves, causing conduction defects and valve regurgitation. The mitral valve is most frequently affected, followed in order by the aortic, tricuspid, and pulmonary valves. Focal vasculitis and diffuse arteritis can cause myocardial damage.

TABLE 80-7. Thrombolytic Therapy Dosage Regimens for Treatment of Deep Venous Thrombosis

DRUG	ROUTE	LOADING DOSE	INFUSION DOSE	DURATION
Streptokinase	Peripheral intravenous	250,000 IU	100,000 IU/h	72 h
	Local infusion	No loading	5000–10,000 IU/h Concomitant infusion of heparin at 0.25 U/mL at a rate to keep vein open	72 h
Urokinase	Peripheral intravenous	4400 U/kg over 10 min	4400 units/kg/h	72 h
	Local infusion	No loading	500–2000 units/kg/h	72 h

From Baker WF, Bick RL: Deep vein thrombosis. Diagnosis and management. *Med Clin North Am* 1994;78:697.

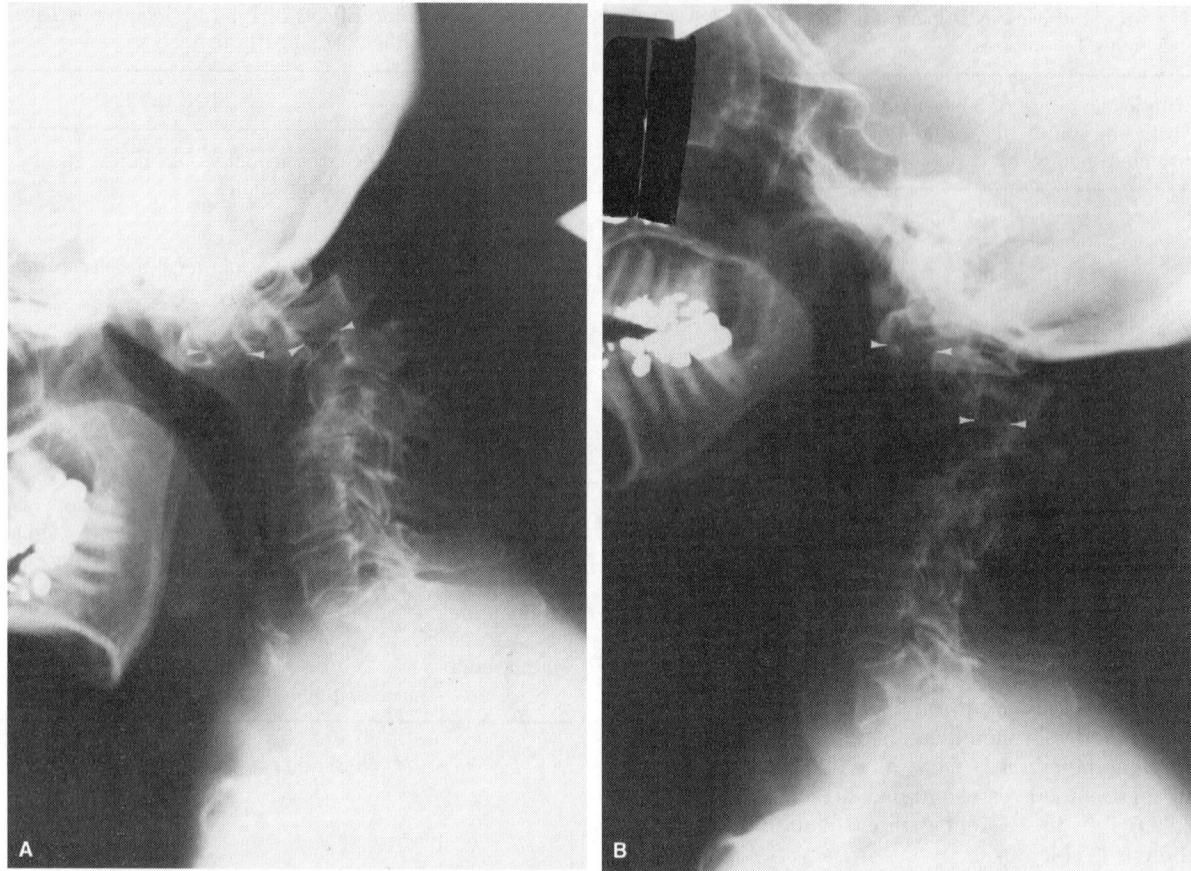

FIGURE 80-4. (**A**) Flexion and (**B**) extension cervical spine radiographs in a 63-year-old woman with severe, longstanding rheumatoid arthritis. Significant anterior atlantoaxial subluxation (10 mm) and C2 on C3 anterior subluxation are demonstrated. Despite the obvious abnormalities, this patient was asymptomatic except for numbness of her right fifth finger. However, attempted awake, translaryngeal intubation was impossible with direct visualization and fiberoptic bronchoscopy. (*Arrows* define the C1-C2 and C2-C3 subluxations.)

Pulmonary Effects

Pulmonary manifestations of RA most often result in restrictive lung disease. Patients may have diffuse interstitial fibrosis or granuloma rheumatoid nodules. In addition, costochondral arthritis and thoracic flexion deformity can decrease chest wall compliance. Other manifestations include pleural effusions (usually small and asymptomatic) and nodules that can cavitate and rupture, leading to pneumothorax, bronchopleural fistula, or infection.

Renal and Hepatic Effects

Renal dysfunction is most often related to drug therapy that causes proteinuria and a nephrotic syndrome. Amyloidosis of the kidneys is found in 20% of patients at autopsy. Clinical hepatomegaly is present in 11% of patients with RA. Biopsies are usually normal.

Anemia

The majority of patients with RA have a mild normocytic, normochromic or hypochromic anemia. The anemia is caused by ineffective erythropoiesis with limitation of iron uptake by maturing erythroblasts. Felty's syndrome, a combination of splenomegaly, leukopenia, and RA, may be present and associated with further anemia and thrombocytopenia.

Cervical Spine and Airway Abnormalities

Rheumatoid involvement of the head and neck may predispose to difficult airway management.[84] Ligamentous involvement results in joint instability with muscle group imbalance leading to joint deformity. If the articular surface of the deformed joint becomes eroded, subluxation often occurs.

Radiologic studies suggest that up to 80% of patients with RA have cervical spine disease.[85] It appears to be more common in males. Patients with juvenile RA do not appear to be at risk. High-risk patients include the elderly and those with neck symptoms, longstanding or erosive disease, or subcutaneous nodules. Atlantoaxial subluxation and subaxial subluxation can progress to cervical cord compression.

ATLANTOAXIAL SUBLUXATION. Atlantoaxial subluxation is the most common radiographic finding in RA, occurring

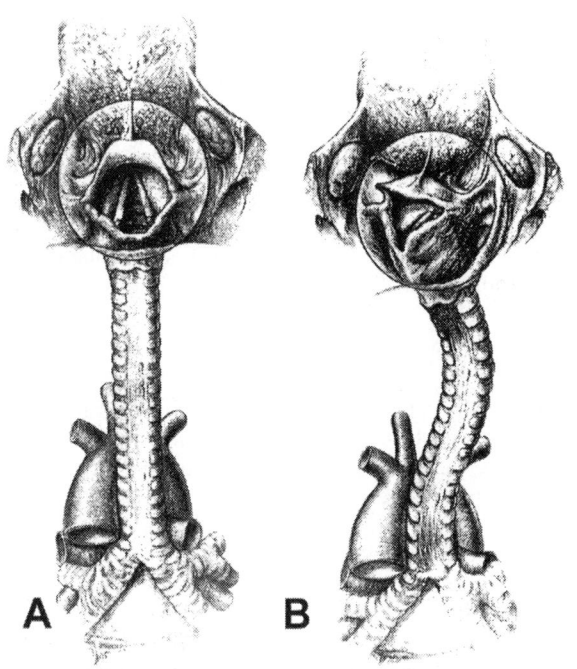

FIGURE 80-5. (**A**) Normal position of the trachea and larynx. Circled area represents the view through a fiberoptic bronchoscope. (**B**) Deviated position of the trachea and larynx associated with severe rheumatoid arthritis. Note the triaxial deviation of the airway and the small glottic opening. (Keenen MA, Siles CM, Kaufman RL: Acquired laryngeal deviation associated with the cervical spinal disease in erosive polyarticular arthritis. *Anesthesiology* 1983; 58:441)

in 25% of patients.[86] Subluxation can occur in the anteroposterior, vertical, lateral, or rotational planes. Anterior atlantoaxial subluxation makes up 80% of all atlantoaxial subluxations.[86] As the atlas shifts anteriorly, the odontoid becomes relatively posterior, reducing the space available for the spinal cord. Subluxation is evaluated by lateral cervical spine films in the flexed position. It is said to be present if the distance from the atlas to the odontoid exceeds 3 mm in patients older than 44 years of age or 4 mm in younger patients (Fig. 80-4). Instability, defined by inability to maintain a relation between vertebrae such that neural structures are not damaged, occurs if the distance exceeds 10 mm.[87]

The most frequent symptom is pain and stiffness in the neck, although many patients are asymptomatic. Patients with anterior atlantoaxial subluxation have a reported 10% incidence of cord compression.[88] Several reports describe sudden death from compression of the upper cervical cord and medulla.[89,90] Vertical subluxation of the odontoid process through the foramen magnum into the posterior fossa occurs in 4% to 35% of patients with RA.[85] It commonly is seen in association with anterior subluxation. Odontoid erosion, which occurs in 20% to 40% of patients with RA, allows posterior subluxation with resultant cord compromise.[86] Subaxial subluxation occurs in 10% to 20% of this population, correlates with disease duration, and most often involves two or more levels, usually at C5-C6. Lateral radiographic views of the spine show a deformity of more than 2 mm.

OTHER DEFORMITIES. Aside from subluxation, fixed flexion deformities commonly affect the lower cervical vertebrae, making direct laryngoscopy difficult or impossible. Temporomandibular disease, which is commonly associated with cervical fixation, limits mouth opening and further hinders intubation.

LARYNGEAL ABNORMALITIES. Laryngeal involvement is present in up to 75% of patients with RA. Patients with erosive polyarticular arthritis affecting the cervical spine can acquire severe tracheal and laryngeal deviation, which looks very much like a scoliosis deformity (Fig. 80-5). Only rarely are symptoms of hoarseness, stridor, or dysphagia seen. Cricoarytenoid arthritis may be recognized by erythema and edema of the vocal cords and decreased size of the glottic inlet. Often, a smaller endotracheal tube can be employed. Exaggerated edema and stridor may occur after extubation.

Airway Management

Airway management is a significant problem. In addition to a careful history and examination for neurologic, cardiac, and pulmonary signs and symptoms, all patients should have periodic cervical spine films for evaluation of subluxation. The cervical spine is quite mobile, and changes in flexion and extension under anesthesia can produce further subluxation and subsequent cord compression. These patients frequently require awake intubation and positioning so that compromised neurologic function can be ascertained. This approach is of even greater concern in the patient with cervical myelopathic symptoms. Intubation under direct visualization with a fiberoptic bronchoscope is usually recommended. Blind nasal techniques can produce trauma to the larynx (e.g., arytenoid dislocation) and contribute to postextubation airway difficulties.

Pain Control

The postoperative period challenges pain management routines to provide effective analgesia while minimizing the risk of depressed ventilation. Regional anesthesia and analgesia can be particularly effective for this patient group. Restrictive lung disease predisposes to respiratory difficulties, and immunosuppressive agents make these patients more susceptible to infection. The timing of extubation must be considered carefully.

MISCELLANEOUS PROBLEMS ■

TOURNIQUETS

Pneumatic tourniquets are frequently used in orthopedic procedures to create a bloodless field and facilitate surgery. Although the benefits are clear, tourniquet use is not without risk and is associated with injuries to muscle and nerve. Based on experimental data, the recommended tourniquet time is $1\frac{1}{2}$ hours to prevent severe irreversible complications.[91,92] Tourniquet paralysis and postoperative electromyographic and functional changes have been seen with shorter times.[93,94]

Acid-Base Changes

If surgery is prolonged, tourniquet deflation is recommended to allow 5 to 15 minutes of reperfusion, the time necessary for the pH and the partial pressures of oxygen and carbon dioxide (Po_2 and Pco_2) to return to normal.[92,95] Subsequent optimal inflation and deflation times are unknown. Transient systemic metabolic acidosis (fall of 0.1 pH unit) should be expected on deflation, as should increased arterial Pco_2 (1 to 8 mm Hg), increased heart rate (10% to 15%), and increased serum potassium. Typically, deflation is well tolerated. However, in head-injured patients, the acute rise in Pco_2 with tourniquet release may have deleterious effects on intracranial pressure (Fig. 80-6).[96]

Venous Embolization and Arterial Thrombosis

McGrath and colleagues noted that 8 of 30 patients undergoing lower extremity surgery had transesophageal echocardiographic evidence of venous embolism with tourniquet deflation, although none was clinically apparent.[97] Several studies indicate that a wider tourniquet should be applied because

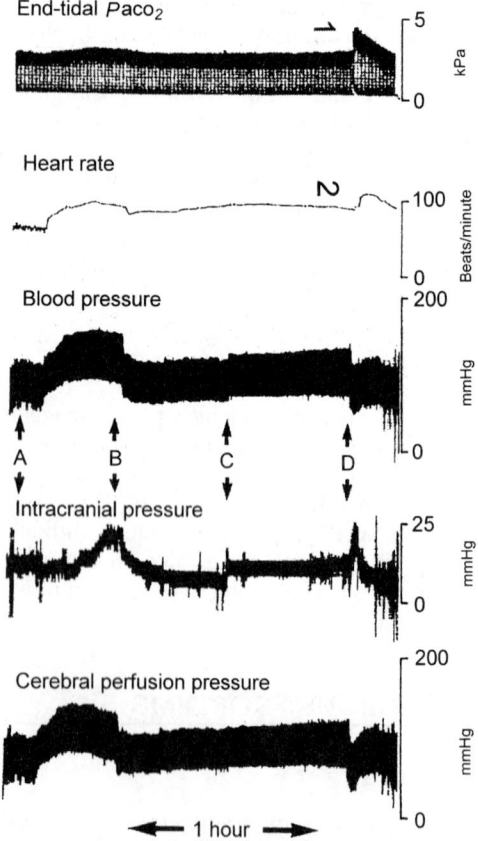

FIGURE 80-6. Recordings of end-tidal partial pressure of carbon dioxide ($Paco_2$), heart rate, blood pressure, intracranial pressure, and cerebral perfusion pressure. Event A, application of tourniquet; B, administration of thiopentone, 250 mg; C, change in height of operating table; D, tourniquet release. (Eldridge PR, Williams SS: Effect of limb tourniquet on cerebral perfusion pressure in a head-injured patient. *Anaesthesia* 1989;44:973)

it reduces the inflation pressures needed for surgical hemostasis.[98,99]

Specific complications of arterial tourniquets are numerous. Intravascular volume overload after extremity exsanguination can occur in patients with poor cardiac reserve. Fatal pulmonary embolus, apparently caused solely by inflation of a tourniquet on a traumatized limb, has been reported.[100,101] Also reported is a case of tibial artery thrombosis caused by disruption of an unrecognized atheromatous plaque after use of a tourniquet.[102]

Skin Damage

Improper padding and placement of the tourniquet can cause minor skin trauma and blisters, and surgical preparation solutions that run under the tourniquet can cause chemical burns. Immediately after deflation, the limb swells by about 10% of its original volume, partially because of reperfusion and partially because of reactive hyperemia.[103] Postischemic edema may not completely resolve until one or more months after surgery. Compartment syndrome has been reported after an 11-hour procedure with intermittent tourniquet use, but it remains a rare complication.[104]

Tourniquet Paralysis

Nerve injury or tourniquet paralysis, which can range from paresthesia to complete paralysis, is the most feared event. Most of these injuries are the result of excessive tourniquet pressures caused by faulty equipment, with duration of application as a secondary influence. The radial nerve is the most common nerve to be injured in the upper extremity because it can be easily compressed against the humerus. Nerves of the lower extremity are better protected by increased muscle bulk. Injury here is much less common, although the peroneal nerve is at particular risk as it winds around the fibular head. Excessive pressure, rather than prolonged tourniquet time, seems to be the mechanism of injury. Fortunately, complete recovery is usually the rule in these nerve lesions, although it may not occur for 6 to 12 months.

Muscle Ischemia

Muscle damage from tourniquet-induced ischemia is less dramatic than nerve damage in its presentation but probably occurs more often. Saunders and associates reported detectable electromyographic deficits in 85% of patients undergoing knee arthrotomy with tourniquet times of 60 minutes or longer. Shorter tourniquet times were associated with fewer electromyographic changes and more rapid clinical recovery.[92]

Posttourniquet Syndrome

A posttourniquet syndrome is characterized by a swollen, stiff, pale limb with weakness but not paralysis, and subjective numbness of the extremity without objective anesthesia. It most likely represents a manifestation of postoperative edema with subsequent compression of vessels, joint capsules, and nerve endings. The syndrome usually resolves within 1 week but can take as long as 6 weeks to clear.

CERVICAL SPINE COLLARS

Advanced trauma life support guidelines advise routine immobilization of the cervical spine for all head-injured patients until a cervical spine injury has been excluded. In addition, patients with multisystem trauma are presumed to have cervical spine injury until proved otherwise. Hence, many orthopedic trauma patients arrive at emergency wards, ICUs, and operating rooms with a hard cervical collar in place. These devices are not entirely benign.

Rigid collars are closely applied to the neck, potentially impeding venous drainage from the head. A small increase in jugular venous pressure is unlikely to have an effect on cerebral blood flow in a normal patient but may be deleterious to a head-injured patient whose intracranial pressure is already elevated. Several case reports support this speculation. Craig and Nielson described a 17-year-old man who sustained a diffuse head injury and small subdural hematoma in a motor vehicle accident.[105] He was sedated, paralyzed, and ventilated and had an ICP monitor in place. After a Stifneck collar was applied according to the manufacturer's instructions, the intracranial pressure rose from 14 to 32 mm Hg within 15 minutes. The collar was removed, and the pressure began to decline. After 20 minutes, it had returned to 14 mm Hg (Fig. 80-7). Pressure elevation was not attributable to other events such as increase in heart rate or blood pressure. Raphael and Chotai measured the effects of cervical collar placement on 9 patients who were scheduled to receive lumbar spinal anesthesia for a surgical procedure.[106] A 22-gauge spinal needle was employed, as was a vertically-held manometer to assess intracranial pressure. In 7 patients, a pronounced trend toward higher values was noted while the collar was in place (Fig. 80-8).

Ferguson and colleagues studied collar-neck interface pressures of six commonly employed cervical collars, both soft and rigid varieties[107] (see Fig. 80-7). The collars that avoided pressure on the neck were the ones that extended their support to the base of the skull, the mandible, and

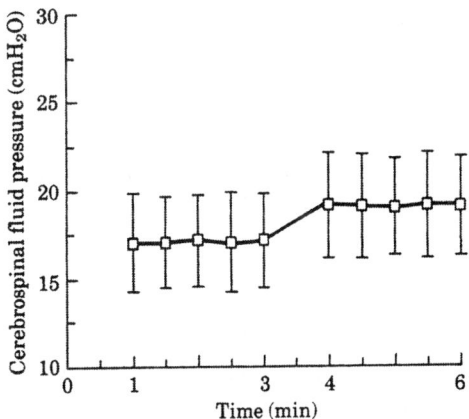

FIGURE 80-8. Mean cerebrospinal fluid pressures with and without the Stifneck collar: minute 1 to 3, collar "off," minutes 4 to 6, collar "on." (Raphael JH, Chotai R: Effects of the cervical collar on CSF pressure. *Anaesthesia* 1994;49:437)

the shoulder girdle. The researchers concluded that these supportive collars probably were most useful in the patient with increased intracranial pressure. An alternative treatment is the use of sandbags, with tape across the forehead to prevent movement.

CASTS

Plaster of Paris casts can cause serious complications if applied improperly. Many of these adverse events also are seen with the newer and more commonly used fiberglass casts.[108] If the underlying skin is compressed, a pressure sore can develop. The patient initially complains of burning pain or discomfort. If the problem is neglected, the discomfort subsides as the skin and nerve endings die. In all cases, the location of the patient's complaint should be evaluated. Another site for skin injury is at the end of a cast that is sharp and causes excoriation. Finally, plaster of Paris hardens by an exothermic process that can produce thermal burns. Temperatures as high as 82°C have been reported.[109]

Tight casts also can play a role in the development of a compartment syndrome. Even if the cast was not tight on application, subsequent limb swelling may produce symptoms (as previously earlier). A "cast syndrome" has been described in the past, predominantly caused by a full body cast that causes duodenal obstruction, subsequent nausea and vomiting, and electrolyte imbalance (SMA syndrome). Infection secondary to cast application is very rare, and allergic reactions are virtually nonexistent.

EPIDURAL CATHETERS IN PATIENTS RECEIVING ANTICOAGULATION THERAPY

Many orthopedic patients receive epidural catheters as part of their anesthetic management. Management of these catheters in the face of active anticoagulation becomes important, because patients are at risk for epidural or spinal hematomas. Hematomas can cause spinal compression and

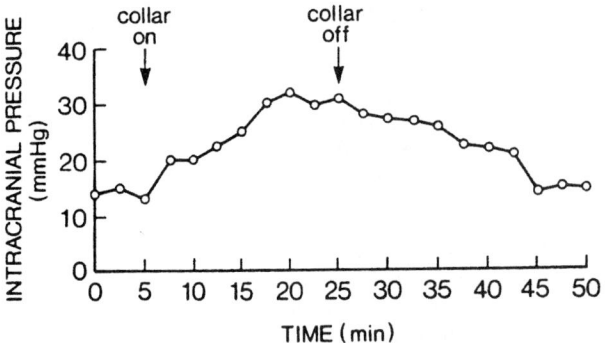

FIGURE 80-7. Changes in intracranial pressure associated with the application of a rigid cervical collar. (Craig GR, Nielson MS: Rigid cervical collars and intracranial pressure. *Intensive Care Med* 1991;17:504)

loss of neurologic function. If they are not surgically decompressed within 12 hours, nerve damage can be permanent.

Numerous case reports describe epidural and spinal hematoma in patients receiving anticoagulants who have had a neuraxial block.[110] Spontaneous epidural hematoma also has been described in patients receiving anticoagulants who never received an epidural catheter. In more than 100 cases of spontaneous hematoma, about one third were associated with anticoagulation.[111]

Clinical Studies and Recommended Guidelines

In general, use of an epidural catheter during anticoagulation is safe if certain guidelines are observed (Table 80-9).[112-137] In 1983, Odoom and Sih reported on 950 patients undergoing 1000 epidural catheter placements for vascular procedures.[132] These patients had been taking oral anticoagulants preoperatively (with documented abnormal clotting studies) and received intravenous heparin intraoperatively. The authors reported no neurologic complications related to spinal cord compression in any of these patients.

In 1981, Rao and El-Etr studied 3164 epidural and 847 subarachnoid catheterizations in patients who subsequently were heparinized during and after surgery.[134] Heparinization was begun at least 1 hour after the catheter was inserted. Blood was freely aspirated from the epidural needle in 4 patients, and their cases subsequently were postponed to the following day. Twenty-four hours after catheter insertion, the catheters were removed 1 hour before the administration of heparin, which then was administered at 6-hour intervals. Fifteen patients complained of low back pain and several had transient paresthesia, but none developed any symptoms or signs of spinal cord compression.

Ruff and Dougherty looked at complications of lumbar puncture followed by heparinization in patients with acute cerebral ischemia.[138] Seven of 342 patients receiving anticoagulants developed significant spinal hematomas or bruises at the site. Analysis concluded that this complication was

TABLE 80-9.   Absence of Hematoma Complication With Combined Use of Anticoagulants and Epidural or Subarachnoid Anesthesia

AUTHORS AND REFERENCE NUMBERS	YEAR	TECHNIQUE	CLOTTING DISORDER AND ANTICOAGULANT	NO. CASES
Horlocker et al[112]	1995	Epidural/spinal	Antiplatelet drugs	386
CLASP[114]	1994	Epidural	Aspirin	1422
Horlocker et al[113]	1994	Epidural	Oral Coumadin	192
Horlocker et al[115]	1994	Epidural/spinal	Antiplatelet drugs	1386
Brent, in de Swiet and Redman[116]	1992	Epidural	Aspirin	2269
Liem et al[117]	1992	Epidural	Systemic heparin	27
Schwander and Bachmann[118]	1991	Epidural/spinal	Unfractionated heparin	5528
Schwander and Bachman[118]	1991	Epidural/spinal	LMWH	13,917
Horlocker et al[119]	1990	Epidural/spinal	Antiplatelet drugs	391
Samama et al[120]	1990	Epidural	Systemic LMWH	10
Blomberg et al[121]	1989	Epidural	Systemic heparin	14
Joachimsson et al[122]	1989	Epidural	Systemic heparin	16
Rosen and Rosen[123]	1989	Caudal/epidural	Systemic heparin	32
Vanstrum et al[124]	1988	Spinal	Systemic heparin	1000
Baron et al[125]	1987	Epidural	Systemic heparin	912
Casey et al[126]	1987	Spinal	Systemic heparin	40
El-Baz and Goldin[127]	1987	Epidural	Systemic heparin	30
Waldman et al[128]	1987	Caudal/epidural	Systemic heparain/ thrombocytopenia/ vitamin K antagonist	336
Aun et al[129]	1985	Spinal	Systemic heparin	40
Benzon et al[91]	1984	Epidural/spinal	Aspirin	246
Fredin et al[130]	1984	Epidural	Unfractionated heparin/ dextran 70	116
Jones et al[131]	1984	Spinal	Systemic heparin	56
Odoom and Sih[128]	1983	Epidural	Vitamin-K antagonist/ systemic heparin	1000
Ellison et al[133]	1981	Epidural	Systemic heparin	700
Rao and El-Etr[134]	1981	Epidural/spinal	Systemic heparin	4011
Mathews and Abrams[135]	1980	Spinal	Systemic heparin	40
Cunningham et al[136]	1980	Epidural	Systemic heparin	100
Lunn et al[137]	1979	Epidural	Systemic heparin	16

LMWH, low-molecular-weight heparin.

Modified from Vandermeulen EP, Van Aken H, Vermylen J: Anticoagulants and spinal-epidural anesthesia. *Anesth Analg* 1994;79:1172.

increased by a traumatic lumbar puncture, by initiation of anticoagulation within 1 hour of the puncture, and by concomitant aspirin therapy. Baron and colleagues reported no complications in a retrospective review of 912 vascular surgery patients who had indwelling epidural catheters and intraoperative total heparinization.[125]

The combination of LMWH, used for DVT prophylaxis, and spinal or epidural anesthesia is not without complication. Despite reports of formal controlled studies in which at least 10,000 patients had no complications,[139] recent case reports of spinal or epidural hematoma exist.[140-143] Rough guidelines, as suggested by Hynson,[140] for LMWH and neuraxial blockade include delaying administration of the block for 10 to 12 hours after the last dose, giving the next dose at least 12 hours after completion of the block, pulling the catheter at least 10 to 12 hours after the last dose, and not redosing for 2 hours after catheter removal. No diagnostic test can determine the degree of anticoagulation with LMWH.

Horlocker and colleagues retrospectively studied 805 patients who received 1013 spinal or epidural anesthetics.[119] Of 391 patients who had routinely taken medications that potentially inhibit platelet function preoperatively, none developed neurologic deficits, although an increased propensity toward "minor" hemorrhagic complications, such as blood aspirated from the catheter, was noted.

Patients who are given thrombolytic therapy after spinal and epidural anesthesia are at risk of developing hematoma and must be monitored carefully. Alternatively, neuraxial block should not be attempted within 24 to 36 hours of thrombolytic therapy. Patients with known coagulopathies or thrombocytopenia should not receive neuraxial block.

Catheter Removal

In the ICU, the epidural catheter should be "pulled" at a time when the coagulation profile is near normal. Removal should occur 4 to 6 hours after the last heparin dose, and anticoagulation should be withheld for at least 1 hour after removal. The PT should be checked for patients receiving low-dose Coumadin, because there is great variability in patient response. Often the catheter is removed before the full Coumadin anticoagulant effect, which takes an average of 7 days, has been achieved.[112,119]

Although normal clotting parameters are desirable before catheter removal, they often are not present. Theoretically, the risk of trauma and hematoma formation is present in the face of abnormal clotting mechanisms, but clinically this problem is not observed. No specific guidelines define what parameters confer reasonably low risk. In one study, PT ranged from 10.9 to 25.8 seconds when the epidural catheters were removed; no neurologic complications occurred.[113]

These patients are at risk for hematoma development and require vigilant postoperative monitoring. We recommend using only narcotic in the epidural infusions (as opposed to local anesthetics) before catheter removal in patients who are receiving anticoagulants. Serial neurologic checks are then made and documented for several hours after catheter removal.

REFERENCES

1. Cucchiara RF, Michenfelder JD: *Clinical Neuroanesthesia.* New York, Churchill Livingstone, 1990:331
2. Gibbons PA, Lee IS: Scoliosis and anesthesia. *Int Anesthesiol Clin* 1985;23:149
3. MacEwen GD, Bunnell WP, Sriram K: Acute neurological complications in the treatment of scoliosis. *J Bone Joint Surg Am* 1975;57:404
4. Kafer ER: Idiopathic scoliosis: Mechanical properties of the respiratory system and the ventilatory response to CO_2. *J Clin Invest* 1985;55:1153
5. Kafer ER: Idiopathic scoliosis: Gas exchange and the age dependence of arterial blood gases. *J Clin Invest* 1976;58:825
6. Kafer ER: Respiratory and cardiovascular functions in scoliosis and principles of anesthetic management. *Anesthesiology* 1980;52:339
7. Smyth RJ, Chapman KR, Wright TA, et al: Pulmonary function in adolescents with mild idiopathic scoliosis. *Thorax* 1984;39:901
8. Lin HY, Nash CL, Herndon CH, et al: The effect of corrective surgery on pulmonary function in scoliosis. *J Bone Joint Surg (Am)* 1974;56:1173
9. Kinnear WJM, Kinnear GC: Pulmonary function after spinal surgery for idiopathic scoliosis. *Spine* 1992;17:708
10. McNeill TW, DeWald RL, Kuo KN, et al: Controlled hypotensive anesthesia in scoliosis surgery. *J Bone Joint Surg Am* 1974;56:1167
11. Lawhorn S, Kahn A: Controlled hypotensive anesthesia during spinal surgery. *Spine* 1982;9:450
12. Smith M, McMaster MJ: The use of induced hypotension to control bleeding during posterior fusion for scoliosis. *J Bone Joint Surg Br* 1983;65:255
13. McCarthy RE, Lonstein JE, Mertz JD, et al: Air embolism in spinal surgery. *J Spinal Disord* 1990;3:1
14. Frankel AS, Holzman RS: Air embolism during posterior spinal fusion. *Can J Anesth* 1988;35:511
15. Ashkenaze D, Mudiyam R, Boachie-Adjei O, et al: Efficacy of spinal cord monitoring in neuromuscular scoliosis. *Spine* 1993;18:1627
16. Taylor BA, Webb PJ, Hetreed M, et al: Delayed postoperative paraplegia with hypotension in adult revision scoliosis surgery. *Spine* 1994;19:470
17. Wenger D, Mubarak S, Leach J: Managing complications of posterior spinal instrumentation and fusion. *Clin Orthop* 1992;284:24
18. Leichtner AM, Banta JV, Etienne N, et al: Pancreatitis following scoliosis surgery in children and young adults. *J Pediatr Orthop* 1991;11:594
19. Wattenmaker I, Concepcion M, Hibberd P, et al: Upper-airway obstruction and perioperative management of the airway in patients managed with posterior operations on the cervical spine for rheumatoid arthritis. *J Bone Joint Surg Am* 1994;76:360
20. Johansen I, Benumof JL: Methylmethacrylate: A myocardial depressant and peripheral dilator. *Anesthesiology* 1979;51:S77
21. Berman AT, Price HL, Hahn JF: The cardiovascular effects of methylmethacrylate in dogs. *Clin Orthop* 1974;100:265
22. Kallos T, Emis JE, Olerud S, et al: Intramedullary pressure and pulmonary embolism of femoral medullary contents in dogs during insertion of bone cement and a prosthesis. *J Bone Joint Surg Am* 1974;56:1363
23. Modig J, Busch C, Olerud S, et al: Arterial hypotension and hypoxemia during total hip replacement: The importance of

thromboplastic products, fat embolism and acrylic monomers. *Acta Anaesthiol Scand* 1975;19:28

24. Herndon JH, Bechtol CO, Crickenberger DB: Fat embolism during total hip replacement. *J Bone Joint Surg Am* 1974; 56:1350

25. Kallos T: Impaired arterial oxygenation associated with use of bone cement in the femoral shaft. *Anesthesiology* 1975;42:210

26. Patterson BM, Healey JH, Cornell CN, et al: Cardiac arrest during hip arthroplasty with a cemented long-stem component. *J Bone Joint Surg Am* 1991;73:271

27. Coventry MB, Beckenbaugh RD, Nolan RD, et al: 2,012 Total hip arthroplasties: A study of postoperative course and early complications. *J Bone Joint Surg (Am)* 1974;56:273.

28. Pellegrini VD, Evarts CM: The fat embolism syndrome. In: Evarts CM (ed). *Surgery of the Musculoskeletal System*, 2nd ed, vol 1. New York, Churchill Livingstone, 1990:37

29. Propst JW, Siegel LC, Schnittger I, et al: Segmental wall motion abnormalities in patients undergoing total hip replacement: Correlations with intraoperative events. *Anesth Analg* 1993;77:743

30. Ereth MH, Weber JG, Abel MD, et al: Cemented versus noncemented total hip arthroplasty: Embolism, hemodynamics, and intrapulmonary shunting. *Mayo Clin Proc* 1992; 67:1066

31. Parmet JL, Horrow JC, Singer R, et al: Echogenic emboli upon tourniquet release during total knee arthroplasty: Pulmonary hemodynamic changes and embolic composition. *Anesth Analg* 1994;79:940

32. Samii K, Elmelik E, Mourtada MB, et al: Intraoperative hemodynamic changes during total knee replacement. *Anesthesiology* 1979;50:239

33. Parmet JL, Berman AT, Horrow JC, et al: Thromboembolism coincident with tourniquet deflation during total knee arthroplasty. *Lancet* 1993;341:1057

34. Vresilovic EJ Jr, Hozack WJ, Booth RE, et al: Incidence of pulmonary embolism after total knee arthroplasty with low-dose Coumadin prophylaxis. *Clin Orthop* 1993;286:27

35. Haljamae H, Enger E: Human skeletal muscle energy metabolism during and after complete tourniquet ischemia. *Ann Surg* 1975;182:9

36. Jorgensen HRI: Myoglobin release after tourniquet ischemia. *Acta Orthop Scand* 1987;58H:554

37. Gulli B, Templeman D: Compartment syndrome of the lower extremity. *Orthop Clin North Am* 1994;25:677

38. Khalil IM: Bilateral compartment syndrome after prolonged surgery in the lithotomy position. *J Vasc Surg* 1987;5:879

39. Brumback RJ: Traumatic rupture of superior gluteal artery without fracture of the pelvis, causing compartment syndrome of the buttock. *J Bone Joint Surg Am* 1990;72:134

40. Hastings H II, Misamore G: Compartment syndrome resulting from intravenous regional anesthesia. *J Hand Surg [Am]* 1987;12:559

41. Taylor DC, Salvian AJ, Shackleton CR: Crush syndrome complicating pneumatic antishock garment (PASG) use. *Injury* 1988;19:43

42. Johnson BE: Anterior tibial compartment syndrome following use of a MAST suit. *Ann Emerg Med* 1981;10:209

43. Bass RR, Allison EJ Jr, Reines HD, et al: Thigh compartment syndrome without lower extremity trauma following application of pneumatic antishock trousers. *Ann Emerg Med* 1983;12:382

44. Matsen FA, Winquist RA, Krugmire RB: Diagnosis and management of compartmental syndromes. *J Bone Joint Surg Am* 1980;62:286

45. Whitesides TE Jr, Haney TC, Morimoto K, et al: Tissue pressure measurements as a determinant for need for fasciotomy. *Clin Orthop* 1975;113:43

46. Gershuni DH, Mubarak SJ, Yaru MC, et al: Fracture of tibia complicated by acute compartment syndrome. *Clin Orthop* 1987;217:221

47. Sheridan GW, Matsen FA: Fasciotomy in the treatment of acute compartment syndrome. *J Bone Joint Surg Am* 1976; 58:112

48. Riska EB, Myllynen P: Fat embolism in patients with multiple injuries. *J Trauma* 1982;22:891

49. Seibel R, LaDuca J, Hassett JM, et al: Blunt multiple trauma, femur traction, and the pulmonary failure–septic state. *Ann Surg* 1985;202:283

50. Enneking FK: Cardiac arrest during total knee replacement using a long-stem prosthesis. Case Conference of the University of Florida. *J Clin Anesth* 1995;7:253

51. Jacobson DM, Terrence CF, Reinmuth OM: The neurological manifestation of fat embolism. *Neurology* 1986;36:847

52. Dorr LD, Merkel C, Melman MF, et al: Fat emboli in bilateral total knee arthroplasty: Predictive factors for neurologic manifestations. *Clin Orthop* 1989;248:112

53. Sevitt S: Fat embolism in patients with fractured hips. *Br Med J* 1972;2:257

54. Williams RP, Makley JT, Carter JR, et al: Fat emboli syndrome in hip replacement for metastatic cancer. In: Brown KLB (ed). *Complications of Limb Salvage Surgery: Prevention, Management, and Outcome*. Montreal, Sixth International Conference, 1991:169

55. Allardyce DB: The adverse effect of heparin in experimental fat embolism. *Surg Forum* 1971;22:203

56. Shier MR, Wilson RF, James RE, et al: Fat embolism prophylaxis: A study of four treatment modalities. *J Trauma* 1977; 17:621

57. Gossling HR, Ellison LH, Degraff AC: Fat embolism. The role of respiratory failure and its treatment. *J Bone Joint Surg Am* 1974;56:1327

58. Schonfeld SA, Ploysongsang Y, DiLisio R, et al: Fat embolism prophylaxis with corticosteroids: A prospective study in high risk patients. *Ann Intern Med* 1983;99:438

59. Byrick RJ, Mullen JB, Wong PY, et al: Prostanoid production and pulmonary hypertension after fat embolism are not modified by methylprednisolone. *Can J Anesth* 1991;38:660

60. Bone LB, Johnson KD, Weigelt J, et al: Early versus delayed stabilization of femoral fracture. *J Bone Joint Surg Am* 1989;71:336

61. Johnson KD, Cadamb A, Seibert GB: Incidence of ARDS in patients with multiple musculoskeletal injuries: Effect of early operative stabilization of fractures. *J Trauma* 1985;25:375

62. Merli GJ: Deep vein thrombosis and pulmonary embolism in orthopedic surgery. *Med Clin North Am* 1993;77:397

63. Hull R, Raskob G, Hirsh J: Prophylaxis of venous thromboembolism: An overview. *Chest* 1986;85:379

64. Francis CW, Pellegrini VD, Marder VJ, et al: Comparison of warfarin and external pneumatic compression in prevention of venous thrombosis after total hip replacement. *JAMA* 1992;267:2911

65. Vresilovic EF, Hozack WJ, Booth RE, et al: Incidence of pulmonary embolism after total knee arthroplasty with low-dose Coumadin prophylaxis. *Clin Orthop* 1993;286:27

66. Hodge WA: Prevention of deep vein thrombosis after total knee arthroplasty: Coumadin versus pneumatic calf compression. *Clin Orthop* 1991;271:101

67. Hull RD, Raskob GE: Current concepts review: Prophylaxis of venous thromboembolic disease following hip and knee surgery. *J Bone Joint Surg Am* 1986;68:146

68. Lotke PA: indications for the treatment of deep venous thrombosis following total knee replacement. *J Bone Joint Surg Am* 1984;66:202

69. Hull RD, Raskob GE, Gent M, et al: Effectiveness of intermittent pneumatic leg compression for preventing deep vein thrombosis after total hip replacement. *JAMA* 1990;263:2313

70. Hirsh J, Dalen JE, Deykin D, et al: Oral anticoagulants: Mechanism of action, clinical effectiveness, and optimal therapeutic range. *Chest* 1992;102:312s

71. Wilson MG, Pei LC, Malone KM, et al: Fixed low-dose versus adjusted higher-dose warfarin following orthopedic surgery. *J Arthroplasty* 1994;9:127

72. Green G, Hirsh J, Heit J, et al: Low molecular weight heparin: A critical analysis of clinical trials. *Pharmacol Rev* 1994;46:89

73. Sorenson RM, Pace NL: Anesthetic techniques during surgical repair of femoral neck fractures. *Anesthesiology* 1992; 77:1095

74. Davis FM, Laurenson VG, Gillespie WJ, et al: Deep vein thrombosis after total hip replacement. *J Bone Joint Surg Br* 1989;71:181

75. Koopman MMW, van Beek EJR, ten Cate JW: Diagnosis of deep vein thrombosis. *Prog Cardiovasc Dis* 1994;37:1

76. Lensing AWA, Hirsh J, Buller HR: Diagnosis of venous thrombosis. In: Colman RW, Hirsh J, Marder VJ, et al (eds). *Hemostasis and Thrombosis*, 3rd ed. Philadelphia, JB Lippincott, 1994:1297

77. Anderson DR, Lensing AW, Wells PS, et al: Limitations of impedance plethysmography in the diagnosis of clinically suspected deep vein thrombosis. *Ann Intern Med* 1993;118:25

78. Heijboer H, Buller HR, Lensing AWA, et al: A comparison of real-time compression ultrasonography with impedance plethysmography for the diagnosis of deep vein thrombosis in symptomatic outpatients. *N Engl J Med* 1993;329:1365

79. Hull RD, Hirsh J, Carter CJ, et al: Pulmonary angiography, ventilation lung scanning, and venography for clinically suspected PE with abnormal perfusion lung scan. *Ann Intern Med* 1983;98:891

80. Mehra MR, Bode FR: Acute deep venous thrombosis. In: Civetta JM, Taylor RW, Kirby RR (eds). *Critical Care*, 2nd ed. Philadelphia, JB Lippincott, 1992:1283

81. Weinmann EE, Salzman EW: Deep-vein thrombosis. *N Engl J Med* 1994;331:1630

82. Baker WF, Bick Rl: Deep vein thrombosis diagnosis and management. *Med Clin North Am* 1994;78:685

83. Skues MA, Welchew EA: Anaesthesia and rheumatoid arthritis. *Anaesthesia* 1993;48:989

84. McArthur A, Kleiman S: Rheumatoid cervical joint disease: A challenge to the anaesthetist. *Can J Anaesth* 1993;40:154

85. Halla JT, Hardin JG, Vitek J, et al: Involvement of the cervical spine in rheumatoid arthritis. *Arthritis Rheum* 1989;32:652

86. Crosby ET, Lui A: The adult cervical spine: Implications for airway management. *Can J Anaesth* 1990;37:77

87. Heywood AW, Learmonth ID, Thomas M: Cervical spine instability in rheumatoid arthritis. *J Bone Joint Surg Br* 1988;70:702

88. Weissman BNW, Aliabadi P, Weinfeld MS, et al: Prognostic features of atlantoaxial subluxation in rheumatoid arthritis patients. *Radiology* 1982;114:745

89. Yaszemski MJ, Shepler TR: Sudden death from cord compression associated with atlanto-axial instability in rheumatoid arthritis. *Spine* 1990;15:338

90. Parish DC, Clark JA, Liebowitz SM, et al: Sudden death in rheumatoid arthritis from vertical subluxation of the odontoid process. *J Natl Med Assoc* 1990;82:297

91. Benzon HT, Brunner EA, Vaisrub N: Bleeding time and nerve blocks after aspirin. *Reg Anesth* 1984;9:86

92. Sapega AA, Heppenstall RB, Chance B, et al: Optimizing tourniquet application and release time in extremity surgery. *J Bone Joint Surg Am* 1985;67:303

93. Saunders KC, Louis DL, Weingarden SI, et al: Effect of tourniquet on postoperative quadriceps function. *Clin Orthop* 1979;143:194

94. Rorabeck CH, Kennedy JC: Tourniquet induced nerve ischemia complicating knee ligament surgery. *Am J Sports Med* 1980;8:98

95. Wilgris EFS: Observations on the effects of tourniquet ischemia. *J Bone Joint Surg Am* 1971;53:1343

96. Bernstein, RL, Rosenberg AD. *Manual of Orthopedic Anesthesia and Related Pain Syndromes*. New York, Churchill Livingstone, 1993:249

97. McGrath BJ, Hsia J, Boyd A, et al: Venous embolization after deflation of lower extremity tourniquets. *Anesth Analg* 1994;78:349

98. Hargens AR, McClure AG, Skyhar MJ, et al: Local compression patterns beneath pneumatic tourniquets applied to arms and thighs of human cadavers. *J Orthop Res* 1987;5:247

99. Moore MR, Garfin SR, Hargens AR: Wide tourniquets eliminate blood flow at low inflation pressures. *J Hand Surg [Am]* 1987;12:1006

100. Pollard BJ, Lovelock HA, Jones RM: Fatal pulmonary embolus secondary to limb exsanguination. *Anesthesiology* 1983; 58:373

101. Hofmann AA, Wyatt RWB: Fatal pulmonary embolus following tourniquet inflation. *J Bone Joint Surg Am* 1985;67:633

102. Giannestras NJ, Cranley JJ, Lentz M: Occlusion of the tibial artery after a foot operation under tourniquet. *J Bone Joint Surg Am* 1977;59:682

103. Monroe MC: The arterial tourniquet. In: Gravenstein N (ed). *Manual of Complications During Anesthesia*. Philadelphia, JB Lippincott, 1991:663

104. Greene TJ, Louis DS: Compartment syndrome of the arm: A complication of the pneumatic tourniquet. *J Bone Joint Surg Am* 1983;63:270

105. Craig GR, Nielson MS: Rigid cervical collars and intracranial pressure. *Intensive Care Med* 1991;17:504

106. Raphael JH, Chotai R: Effects of the cervical collar on CSF pressure. *Anaesthesia* 1994;49:437

107. Ferguson J, Mardel SN, Beattie TF, et al: Cervical collars: A potential risk to the head-injured patient. *Injury* 1993;24:454

108. *3M Scotchcast Casting Products* [product insert]. St Paul, MN, 3M Health Care, 1994

109. Harkess JW, Ramsey WC: Principles of fractures and dislocations. In: Rockwood CA, Green DP, Bucholz RW (eds). *Fractures in Adults*. Philadelphia, JB Lippincott, 1991:49

110. Gustafsson H, Rutberg H, Bengtsson M: Spinal haematoma following epidural analgesia. *Anaesthesia* 1988;43:220

111. Spurny OM, Rubin S: Spinal and epidural hematoma during anticoagulant therapy. *Arch Intern Med* 1964;114:103

112. Horlocker TT, Wedel DJ, Schroder DR, et al: Preoperative antiplatelet therapy does not increase risk of spinal hematoma associated with regional anesthesia. *Anesth Analg* 1995;80:303

113. Horlocker TT, Wedel DJ, Schlichting JL: Postoperative epidural analgesia and oral anticoagulant therapy. *Anesth Analg* 1994;79:89

114. CLASP: A randomized trial of low dose aspirin for the prevention and treatment of pre-eclampsia among 9364 pregnant women. CLASP (Collaborative Low-dose Aspirin Study in Pregnancy) *Lancet* 1994;343:619

115. Horlocker TT, Wedel DJ, Offord KP, et al: Preoperative antiplatelet drugs do not increase the risk of spinal hematoma associated with regional anesthesia [abstract]. *Reg Anesth* 1994;19(Suppl):8

116. de Swiet M, Redman CWG: Aspirin, extradural anaesthesia and the MRC collaborative low-dose aspirin study in pregnancy [letter]. *Br J Anaesth* 1992;69:109

117. Liem TH, Booij LHDJ, Hasenbos MAWM, et al: Coronary artery bypass grafting using two different anesthetic techniques. Part I: Hemodynamic results. *J Cardiothorac Vasc Anesth* 1992; 6:148

118. Schwander D, Bachmann F: Heparin and spinal or epidural anaesthesia: Clinical decision making [in French]. *Ann Fr Anesth Reanim* 1991;10:284

119. Horlocker TT, Wedel DJ, Offord KP: Does preoperative antiplatelet therapy increase the risk of hemorrhagic complications associated with regional anesthesia? *Anesth Analg* 1990;70:631

120. Samama CM, Mouren S, Bridel MP, et al: Use of enoxaparin, a low molecular weight heparin in arterial reconstructive surgery [in French]. *Ann Fr Anesth Reanim* 1990;9:102

121. Blomberg S, Curelaru I, Emanuelsson H, et al: Thoracic epidural anaesthesia in patients with unstable angina pectoris. *Eur Heart J* 1989;10:437

122. Joachimsson PO, Nystrom S-O, Tyden H: Early extubation after coronary surgery in efficiently rewarmed patients: A postoperative comparison of opioid anesthesia versus inhalational anesthesia and thoracic epidural analgesia. *J Cardiothorac Anesth* 1989;3:444

123. Rosen KR, Rosen DA: Caudal epidural morphine for control of pain following open heart surgery in children. *Anesthesiology* 1989;70:418

124. Vanstrum GS, Bjornson KM, Ilko R: Postoperative effects of intrathecal morphine in coronary artery bypass surgery. *Anesth Analg* 1988;67:261

125. Baron HC, LaRaja RD, Rossi G, et al: Continuous epidural analgesia in the heparinized vascular surgical patient: A retrospective review of 912 patients. *J Vasc Surg* 1987;6:144

126. Casey WF, Wynands JE, Ralley FE, et al: The role of intrathecal morphine in the anesthetic management of patients undergoing coronary artery bypass surgery. *J Cardiothorac Anesth* 1987;1:510

127. El Baz N, Goldin M: Continuous epidural infusion of morphine for pain relief after cardiac operations. *J Thorac Cardiovasc Surg* 1987;93:878

128. Waldman SD, Feldstein GS, Waldman HJ, et al: Caudal administration of morphine sulphate in anticoagulated and thrombocytopenic patients. *Anesth Analg* 1987;66:267

129. Aun C, Thomas D, John-Jones SL, et al: Intrathecal morphine in cardiac surgery. *Eur J Anaesthesiol* 1985;2:419

130. Fredin HO, Rosberg B, Arborelius M Jr, et al: On thromboembolism after total hip replacement in epidural analgesia: A controlled study of dextran 70 and low dose heparin combined with dihydroergotamine. *Br J Surg* 1984;71:58

131. Jones SEF, Beasley JM, McFarlane DWR, et al: Intrathecal morphine for postoperative pain relief in children. *Br J Anaesth* 1984;56:137

132. Odoom JA, Sih IL: Epidural analgesia and anticoagulant therapy. *Anaesthesia* 1983;38:254

133. Ellison N, Jobes DR, Schwartz AJ: Implications of anticoagulant therapy. *Int Anesthesiol Clin* 1982;20:121

134. Rao TLS, El-Etr AA: Anticoagulation following placement of epidural and subarachnoid catheters: An evaluation of neurologic sequelae. *Anesthesiology* 1981;55:618

135. Mathews ET, Abrams LD: Intrathecal morphine in open heart surgery. *Lancet* 1980;II:543.

136. Cunningham FO, Egan JM, Inhara T: Continuous epidural anesthesia in abdominal vascular surgery: A review of 100 consecutive cases. *Am J Surg* 1980;139:624

137. Lunn JK, Dannemiller FJ, Stanley TH: Cardiovascular response to clamping of the aorta during epidural and general anesthesia. *Anesth Analg* 1979;58:372

138. Ruff RL, Dougherty JH: Complications of lumbar puncture followed by anticoagulation. *Stroke* 1981;12:879

139. Bergqvist D, Lindblad B, Matzsch T: Low-molecular weight heparin for thromboprophylaxis and epidural/spinal anaesthesia: Is there a risk? *Acta Anaesthesiol Scand* 1992;36:605

140. Hynson JM, Katz JA, Bueff HU: Epidural hematoma associated with Enoxaparin. *Anesth Analg* 1996;82:1072

141. Vandermeulen EP, Van Aken H, Vermylen J: Anticoagulants and spinal-epidural anesthesia. *Anesth Analg* 1994;79:1165

142. Bent U, Gniffke S, Reinbold W: An epidural hematoma following single shot epidural anesthesia (German). *Anaesthesist* 1994;43:245

143. Gerlif C, Myrtue G: Atypical site of epidural hematoma after epidural analgesia (Dutch). *Ugeskr Laeger* 1994;156:7231

Critical Care, Third Edition, edited by Joseph M. Civetta,
Robert W. Taylor, and Robert R. Kirby.
Lippincott-Raven Publishers, Philadelphia, PA © 1997.

CHAPTER 81

Urologic Surgery and Trauma

Thomas E. Ahlering

IMMEDIATE CONCERNS

MAJOR PROBLEMS

Upper abdominal operations include adrenalectomy for benign and frequently hormonally active tumors, radical adrenonephrectomy for adrenal and renal carcinomas, and retroperitoneal lymphadenectomy for testicular carcinoma and retroperitoneal tumors. Cardiovascular problems usually appear as patient unresponsiveness or hypotension. Causes for early cardiovascular instability are unrecognized postoperative hemorrhage, inadequate or excessive fluid replacement, myocardial infarction (MI), and adrenal medullary or cortical insufficiency.

Lower abdominal and pelvic procedures include radical cystectomy, total pelvic exenteration, and radical prostatectomy. An early postoperative complication is urinary drainage obstruction.

Urogenital trauma occurs from either blunt or penetrating injury, which are often managed differently. Proximity injuries warrant evaluation because hematuria is not a sensitive predictor of the presence or severity of urologic injury.

Blunt renal trauma accompanied by gross hematuria or hypotension needs appropriate evaluation radiographically. Nonvascularized renal parenchyma may need excision and renorrhaphy. Ureteral injuries are usually asymptomatic and often without hematuria, but are well defined by intravenous urography with extravasation of contrast. Penetrating bladder injuries need to be surgically repaired. If a ureteral tear extends only part of the way through the urethra, healing probably will obviate an open surgical procedure. With urethral transection, urinary diversion with a suprapubic tube allows resolution of hematoma and facilitates later surgical repair.

Significant genital injuries usually require surgical correction. Injury to the erectile bodies of the penis, whether caused by blunt or penetrating trauma, requires an operation. Similarly, scrotal trauma, when there is bleeding or suspected testicular injury, requires surgical intervention.

STRESS POINTS

1. The most common problems are respiratory, including hypoxemia, malfunction of thoracostomy drainage systems, or unsuspected pneumothorax.
2. Hemorrhage, fluid replacement, and myocardial events require review of medical conditions and sometimes hemodynamic monitoring.
3. After bladder or prostate removal, oliguria can signal cardiovascular problems or urinary obstruction.
4. Penetrating injury to the flank mandates intravenous urogram, even with a clear urinalysis result.
5. Contrast studies provide exquisite detail, without the need for less precise and often meddlesome surgical exploration.
6. Most cases of blunt trauma are managed nonoperatively because these injuries heal with minimal parenchymal loss.
7. Surgery is necessary for gunshot wounds because of blast effect and devitalized tissue.
8. In pelvic fractures, a catheter should not be passed if ureteral injury is suspected until retrograde urethrography is performed.

INITIAL THERAPY

1. Reposition or insert new chest tube for pneumothorax.
2. Provide oxygen or ventilatory support (noninvasive or invasive).
3. Avoid supplemental oxygen greater than 25% to 30% after bleomycin therapy.

1253

4. Consider replacement of adrenal hormones, either catecholamines or glucocorticoids.
5. Use a shunt to release obstruction; when obstruction is ruled out, consider fluid replacement or increasing cardiac output.
6. Manage renal atriovenous fistulae and arterial bleeding with embolization during arteriography.
7. Repair urethral injuries surgically.
8. Repair intraperitoneal bladder ruptures surgically, but catheter drainage and antibiotics suffice for retroperitoneal injuries.
9. Treat urethral injuries initially with suprapubic cystostomy tubes.

ESSENTIAL DIAGNOSTIC TESTS AND PROCEDURES

1. Assess for restlessness or unresponsiveness; check arterial blood gas values and chest radiograph results.
2. Use chest auscultation and examine the thoracostomy drainage system plus the position of the chest tube and connectors.
3. Monitor blood pressure, pulse, and urine output response to fluids; insert a pulmonary artery catheter if necessary.
4. The surgeons should irrigate a urinary shunt to rule out obstruction. A loop-o-gram can be performed after urinary diversion.
5. Use high-dose intravenous pyelography (IVP) with nephrotomography, cystography, urethrography, and computed tomographic scan (CT scan) to outline the urinary tract.
6. Use arteriography for an exact diagnosis in cases of knife wounds with an abnormal finding on IVP.
7. In pelvic fractures, use retrograde urethrography and cystography, especially if there is blood at the meatus.

MAJOR UROLOGIC POSTOPERATIVE MANAGEMENT ■

The most influential factors in a patient's postoperative course are coexisting medical problems and intraoperative complications; attention should quickly focus on these factors. Predisposing cardiac problems include congestive heart failure (CHF), MI within 6 months of surgery, and diastolic hypertension (greater than 110 mm Hg). Respiratory risk factors include smoking, asthma, chronic obstructive lung disease, and bleomycin chemotherapy.[1,2]

UPPER ABDOMINAL PROCEDURES

A discussion of normal postoperative recovery differs according to the incision used, which includes thoracoabdominal, flank, and abdominal incisions. The thoracoabdominal incision involves removing a portion of the 8th, 9th, 10th, or 11th rib and usually requires insertion of a chest tube to reexpand the lung postoperatively. Generally, after 18 to 24 hours, the chest tube can be switched from suction to water seal and removed 24 hours later if there is less than 50 mL of output per 8-hour shift. If temporary mechanical ventilation is needed, the chest tube should not be removed until after extubation. Antibiotics (usually a cephalosporin) are given while the chest tube is in place to prevent empyema. Flank and abdominal incisions generally do not enter the thorax. Atelectasis and fever as high as 39°C (102°F) in the first 3 to 4 postoperative days are common because incisional pain and splinting discourage deep breathing and coughing. Preventive measures include adequate analgesia and incentive spirometry or deep breathing and coughing exercises. If atelectasis develops, it should be managed with aggressive pulmonary toilet or pneumonia may result.

Postoperatively, ileus is normal and can be expected to last for 3 to 6 days. Nasogastric suction is recommended to prevent nausea and vomiting as well as aspiration pneumonia; the tube can be removed after the first 24 to 48 hours if the 24-hour output is less than 500 to 750 mL. Intravenous fluids are adjusted to keep urine output above 50 mL/hour. A Foley catheter may be inserted for more accurate urine output monitoring and for patient convenience for the first 24 to 48 hours. Total fluid output should equal 24-hour urine output plus 500 to 1000 mL of insensible fluid loss. For extensive retroperitoneal dissections, a surprising volume of fluid "third spaces" in the first 36 to 48 hours requires aggressive fluid management (I prefer to administer 150 mL/hour of crystalloid and 50 mL/hour colloid). Daily weights are invaluable if accurate input and output records are not available. Early ambulation aids in return of bowel function, which can be anticipated on the fourth to sixth postoperative day. Liquids are started if bowel sounds are normal. The first 24 hours of diet should be liquid (clear or full), because if a problem arises a nasogastric tube will quickly and completely empty the stomach. When the patient has tolerated a liquid diet for 24 to 48 hours, the diet is advanced to regular. A soft diet may be used if the patient has no teeth or cannot chew, but otherwise it is identical to a regular diet so far as the gastrointestinal tract is concerned. For abdominal distention and cramps, a Harris flush, mini-enema, or suppository will evacuate colon air. The mini-enema is a little more uncomfortable but acts more quickly than the suppository.

Sometimes a Penrose drain may be present in the flank if postoperative drainage is anticipated. If the urinary tract collecting system is entered, it is customary to drain the site and collect the urine in a colostomy bag. Typically, significant amounts of urine drain transiently in the early postoperative period. Monitoring the 24-hour output is important to appreciate whether the amount of drainage is changing. If the drain is placed for serosanguineous or infected fluid, it is kept only as long as there is greater than 50 mL of drainage per 8 hours.

Adrenalectomy

Many adrenal masses are removed because of hormonal overactivity; these patients require special attention. Excision of adrenal cortical tumors that produce steroid-like substances should be managed prophylactically with hydrocortisone because of the risk of acute Addisonian crisis.[3]

The normal stress dose of hydrocortisone is 100 mg given intravenously every 8 hours, which is started in the operating room. The dose is rapidly tailored in the postoperative period to a maintenance dose of 25 to 30 mg hydrocortisone given orally twice a day. A corticotropin stimulation test is given 2 months later to identify patients who need chronic steroidal replacement. It is crucial in patients undergoing adrenalectomy for pheochromocytoma to have adequate preoperative alpha-adrenergic blockade using 10 to 30 mg phenoxybenzamine hydrochloride (four times a day). If blockade is inadequate, the alpha-adrenergic stimulation dramatically contracts volume, and when the tumor is removed the volume contraction is relieved, which frequently leads to severe hypovolemic shock.[3]

Radical Nephrectomy

Radical nephrectomy is performed mostly for renal cell carcinoma but is also used for adrenal cell carcinomas and transitional cell carcinoma of the renal pelvis or ureter. Adrenal cell tumors differ only if there is a hormonally active component. Transitional cell carcinoma of the collecting system differs slightly from renal cell because the entire ureter with a cuff of bladder needs to be removed because of the risk (20% to 30%) of tumor recurrence in the distal ureter. Because the bladder is then repaired, the area is drained in case of urine leak. The most common complication after radical nephrectomy is hemorrhage that manifests as tachycardia, hypotension, a continuously dropping hematocrit, increasing abdominal girth, and respiratory compromise. The most common sites of hemorrhage are lumbar vessels, the spleen, or mesenteric vessels. Pulmonary embolism is fairly unusual. The likelihood of complication is closely linked to the size of the renal mass, but the complication rate generally is low. Excision of renal cell cancer with tumor thrombus involvement of the inferior vena cava (IVC) is the most complicated urologic procedure. These patients are hemodynamically compromised because of partial or total occlusion of venous return from the IVC. The procedure is technically complicated because of the need for temporary occlusion of the blood flow to the bowel, liver, and opposite kidney. Additionally, the procedure may be associated with blood losses between 2 and 24 L (average, 6500 mL).[4] The most common and serious complication is postoperative hemorrhage. Additionally, a deWeese vascular clip may be placed around the IVC at surgery to prevent embolization, which then requires anticoagulation to prevent thrombosis of the IVC.

Retroperitoneal Lymphadenectomy

The primary metastatic sites for testis cancer are paraaortic lymph nodes. Patients with low-volume retroperitoneal disease normally undergo surgery before chemotherapy. These patients do well and have few complications. Patients with substantial retroperitoneal disease or lung metastases are initially treated with cytoreductive intensive combination chemotherapy, usually cisplatin, VP-16, and bleomycin. The operative procedure is arduous, averaging 5 to 8 hours; patients have considerable blood loss (1600 to 1800 mL). Bleo-

mycin-induced pulmonary fibrosis is common and puts the patient at risk for adult respiratory distress syndrome, which is rarely treated successfully in this setting; thus, prevention is critical.[5,6] Two factors are important: the patient should not receive excessive fluid volumes, and the inspired oxygen should be kept below 30% intraoperatively and postoperatively. I support the patient postoperatively with 75 to 100 mL/hour of colloid and 50 to 75 mL/hour of crystalloid.

LOWER ABDOMINAL SURGERY

The emphasis switches from the respiratory system in upper abdominal surgery to the urinary tract in lower abdominal surgery, and includes cystectomy and urinary diversion or radical prostatectomy. When the bladder is removed, a portion of small or large bowel is used as a conduit for the urine, whereas in radical prostatectomy, the bladder remains in continuity with the urethra. For normal postoperative recovery, one should anticipate significant intravenous fluid requirements for the first 36 to 48 hours because of the pelvic node dissection. Vigorous urine output is needed to keep the conduit flushed of mucus. In patients with an ileal conduit, urine output from the stoma is carefully observed and compared with the Penrose output. A sudden decrease in urine output from the stoma and drain is indicative of an intraabdominal collection of urine, a serious complication. Pulmonary complications are avoided by early ambulation, pulmonary toilet, and anticoagulation. Patients undergoing major lower abdominal and pelvic surgeries with node dissections have considerable risk for pulmonary embolism. For prophylaxis, I use warfarin anticoagulation (Table 81-1) and have had no postoperative deaths or symptomatic pulmonary emboli in more than 500 patients.

Radical Cystectomy and Urinary Diversion

Most patients requiring cystectomy have two significant risk factors for perioperative cardiac and pulmonary complications: age and smoking. Most cystectomies are performed for transitional cell cancer of the bladder in patients with an average age of 65 years and a high prevalence of prolonged smoking. Cardiac history is important, and the physician should be aware of a recent MI, CHF, diastolic hypertension greater than 110 mm Hg, and use of β-blockers and antihy-

TABLE 81-1. Schedule for Oral or Nasogastric Administration of Warfarin Anticoagulation[*]

LOADING DOSE	
Postoperatively	10 mg, nasogastric
DAILY SLIDING SCALE	
Patient PT	Warfarin dose (oral)
10–14 sec	5.0 mg
15–17 sec	2.5 mg
18–22 sec	None
>23 sec	Vitamin K 10 mg

[*]As determined by daily prothrombin times (PT).

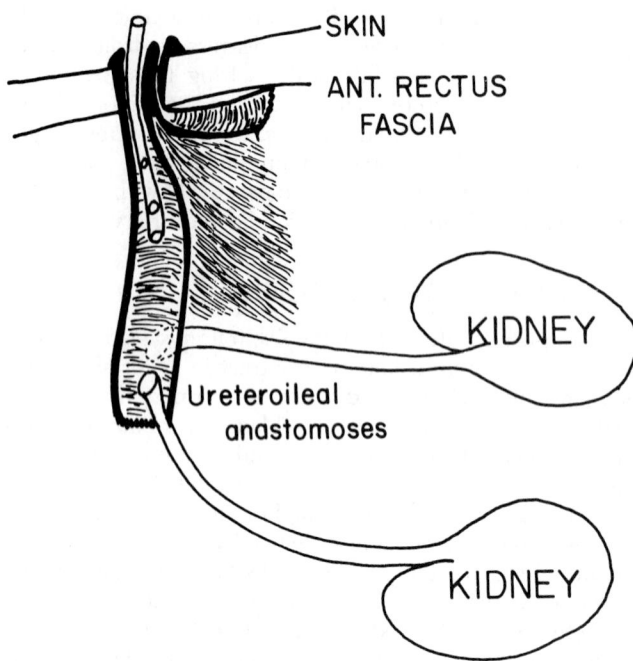

SKIN

ANT. RECTUS
FASCIA

KIDNEY

Ureteroileal
anastomoses

KIDNEY

FIGURE 81-1. Because of mucus production and edema formation where the ileal loop traverses the abdominal wall, obstruction of urine egress may cause urine to leak intraperitoneally from the ureteroileal anastomoses.

pertensives. The two most important factors are MI in the past 6 months and symptomatic CHF.[2] These patients warrant careful fluid status monitoring and prophylactic pulmonary artery and peripheral arterial catheterization with aggressive management of hemodynamic instability using vasoactive drugs.[2] Smoking increases the patient's risk of postoperative atelectasis, pneumonia, and hypoxemia, which are managed with aggressive pulmonary toilet. However, if smoking has been continuously avoided for more than 30 days, most pulmonary functions will have nearly normalized—most important are the forced expiratory volume per second and oxygen exchange.[1]

Management of an ileal loop urostomy requires careful attention because accurate urine output is essential for determining fluid status and preventing a major undrained intraabdominal urine collection. Patients undergoing urinary diversion after high-dose radiation therapy (>5500 rad) have increased risks for ureteroileal anastomotic breakdown because of poor healing from radiation vasculitis and ureteritis. Most ileal loops are constructed as in Figure 81-1, and most leaks occur at the site of anastomosis of the ureter to the ileal loop or the closed proximal end. Because freshly cut bowel produces a lot of mucus and significant edema occurs where it traverses the abdominal fascia, an indwelling stent is placed at surgery through the stoma and into the loop below the rectus fascia. If in the first 48 to 72 hours the urine output is low, the stent should be observed to be appropriately in position and then irrigated gently with 10 mL of normal saline to free any mucus plugs. Most surgeons drain ileal loops so that if inadequate urine output from the

loop is not accompanied with an increased output from the drain, the patient is either not making urine (inadequate fluid replacement, cardiac or renal decompensation) or urine is leaking intraabdominally. Generally, the physical status of the patient indicates inadequate fluids or acute decompensation, but occasionally it is necessary to evaluate for a urine leak. The most consistent early abnormalities experienced are an increase in the blood urea nitrogen level and prolonged ileus. Radiographic studies should begin with a loop-o-gram and then proceed to an IVP to establish bilateral renal function. Urine leaks are best treated conservatively by diverting the urine with percutaneous nephrostomies and by draining undrained urine collections. Primary repair of the leaking anastomosis is difficult and fraught with complications.[7,8]

When a bowel anastomosis is necessary, I routinely use temporary gastrostomy (or nasogastric) drainage to decompress the stomach. Return of bowel function is heralded when bowel sounds and flatus occur. I typically leave the tube in place but clamped for 24 hours to see if the patient tolerates the 1500 mL entering the stomach from normal secretions. When the patient demonstrates tolerance to clamping, the nasogastric tube is removed and the diet advanced (the gastrostomy tube stays in place until a regular diet is tolerated). It is mandatory not to manipulate the rectum (enema or suppository) because of the risk of perforation where the prostate was dissected off the anterior rectal wall.

Radical Prostatectomy

Similar to the radical cystectomy and ileal loop, urine output is most important after a radical prostatectomy. These patients normally have a urethral catheter and a suprapubic Penrose drain. The urethral catheter has two critical functions: it drains the urine, which should not be grossly bloody; and it stents the vesicourethral anastomosis to prevent stricture and preserve continence. It is extremely important that the urethral catheter not come out. The catheter needs to be securely fastened to the patient's penis or thigh to prevent inadvertent removal. Postoperative hemorrhage usually occurs within the first 12 to 24 hours and is observed by increasing lower abdominal girth, dropping hematocrit, and hypotension. Immediate surgical exploration is necessary to control the bleeding, which usually is from the inferior epigastric or middle rectal artery. Also, these patients have increased risk for pulmonary embolism and should be taking anticoagulants. I routinely use warfarin (see Table 81-1).

UROGENITAL TRAUMA ■

Urologic trauma can be divided into two groups according to etiology: blunt and penetrating trauma. Penetrating trauma is usually caused by knives or guns. Careful history and physical examination are critical. Genital examination is essential, noting whether there is blood at the urethral meatus, and a thorough rectal or pelvic examination must not be deferred. A "free-floating" prostate or the presence of a perineal hematoma should alert the examiner to a possible membranous urethral injury. When the patient is sent for radiography, monitoring of vital signs and overall condition must be maintained.

BLUNT TRAUMA

Kidney

Motor vehicle accidents, falls, athletic injuries, and assault are the most common causes of blunt renal trauma. Studies[9,10] have shown that adults with blunt renal trauma that is accompanied by gross hematuria or shock need uroradiographic evaluation. Adult patients who have not been hypotensive (systolic blood pressure <90 mm Hg) and who do not have gross hematuria can be safely observed without uroradiographic evaluation. All pediatric patients (15 years of age or younger) with any degree of hematuria and adult patients with gross hematuria or hypotension need radiographic evaluation. An attempt should be made to resuscitate unstable patients because without adequate radiographic evaluation, retroperitoneal exploration of an undelineated renal injury frequently results in a needless nephrectomy. After the patient is stabilized, radiographic evaluation should consist of a chest radiograph, CT scan with contrast, an IVP with nephrotomograms, and a cystogram. If CT scan is not available, an abdominal scout film, in addition to showing bony injuries, may show loss of the psoas shadow or a shift in the bowel gas pattern caused by a retroperitoneal hematoma (Fig. 81-2). High-dose intravenous contrast (1.5 to 2.0 mL/kg Renografin [meglumine diatrizoate]) should be given as a bolus injection and kidney films exposed at 1, 3, and 5 minutes. Kidney, ureter, bladder (KUB) films should be taken at 10 and 20 minutes with oblique views as well. Nephrotomograms are done from 6 to 12 cm, depending on patient anatomy. The tomograms are essential in the trauma patient because of ileus that so often obscures renal anatomy (Fig. 81-3). A normal study result shows equal bilateral excretion with normal renal outlines and axis as determined by the tomograms, no extravasation of contrast, and well-visualized ureters down to the bladder. A decrease in renal concentration of contrast or a delay in excretion is

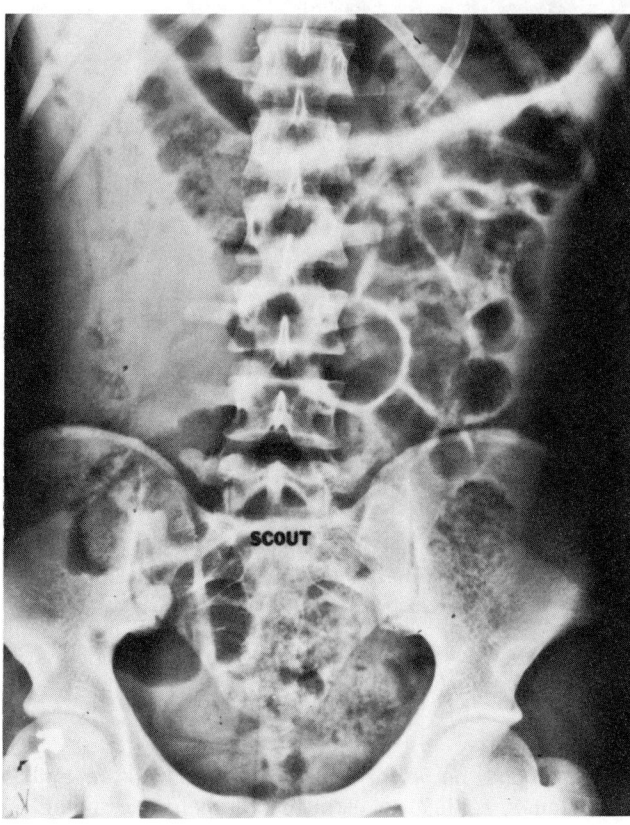

FIGURE 81-2. The scout film should be evaluated carefully for gas pattern, fractures, and free air. This kidney-ureter-bladder study demonstrates shifting of the bowel gas in the right colon, highly suggestive of a large retroperitoneal mass.

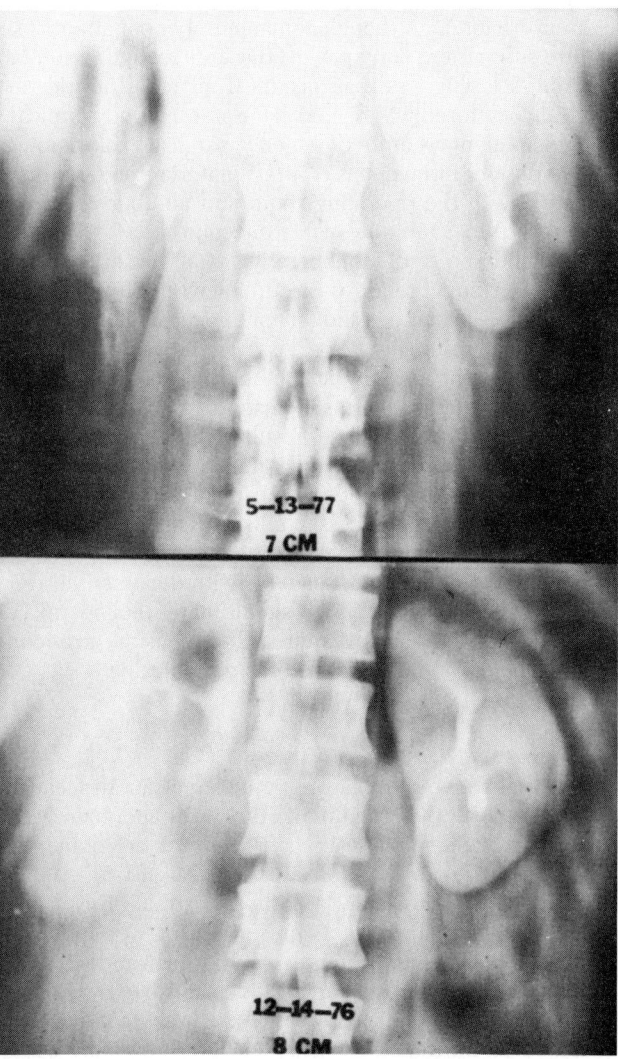

FIGURE 81-3. The kidney-ureter-bladder film in Figure 81-2 had such extensive bowel gas that only nephrotomography could adequately delineate the kidneys. The left kidney is normal because the renal outline is well defined, the renal axis is normal, and excretion of contrast is normal. The right kidney shows poor excretion, abnormal renal axis, and loss of the renal outline.

a renal "contusion." If there is loss of the renal outlines or extravasation of contrast, more severe injuries are present and include perirenal hematomas, cortical lacerations, and major renal fractures with extravasation. An assiduous attempt should be made to demonstrate the integrity of the ureters. Although ureteral injuries from blunt trauma are rare, occasionally a ureter will be avulsed at its junction with the renal pelvis. This is more common in children. Unilateral nonfunction is indicative of renal artery thrombosis. Immediate renal angiography is indicated because prompt surgical correction is the only hope of saving the kidney. If available, the CT scan is the best way to delineate defunctionalized areas of renal parenchyma, demonstrate urinary extravasation, and visualize the location and extent of retroperitoneal hematomas, and may also reveal other intraabdominal injuries.[11] Most renal injuries can be managed nonoperatively, but recent evidence suggests that significant nonvascularized segments of renal parenchyma may need repair by excision and renorrhaphy.[12] Although a small number of patients may require subsequent surgery with this approach, the number of kidneys lost is less than occurs if all renal injuries are surgically explored[13,14] (Fig. 81-4). Some hemodynamically unstable patients require emergency surgical exploration. A double dose of intravenous contrast material can be infused on the way to the operating room and an abdominal film obtained 20 to 30 minutes after injection.

The philosophy of nonoperative management of most blunt renal trauma requires careful follow-up. Frequent hematocrit determinations should continue until the patient is stable, but occasionally blood loss may be fairly persistent. In this case, angiography and embolization of a bleeding vessel is appropriate. If this is unsuccessful, surgical repair can be undertaken. Abscesses resulting from infected urinomas or hematomas are distinctly unusual with conservative management and antibiotics. The diagnosis is best established by CT scan. Abscesses must be surgically drained, but surgical exploration of these delayed events carries a high nephrectomy rate. All patients with documented renal trauma other than a contusion should have a follow-up IVP 4 to 6 weeks and 1 year after injury. Hypertension, an uncommon sequela, should be looked for periodically.

Bladder

There are two types of bladder rupture: intraperitoneal and extraperitoneal. Blunt trauma to the lower abdomen with a distended bladder may cause a rupture at the dome with intraperitoneal extravasation of urine (Fig. 81-5). Alternatively, pelvic fractures may lacerate the extraperitoneal bladder wall (Fig. 81-6). Patients present with lower abdominal pain, inability to void, suprapubic tenderness, and, occasionally, urinary ascites. The diagnosis is established by cystography. If there is a suspicion of a urethral injury because of blood at the meatus, retrograde urethrography should precede catheter insertion.[15] The bladder is filled with 200 to 400 mL of contrast medium infused under gravity, and anteroposterior and postdrainage films are obtained.

Management depends on the location of extravasation. All patients should receive intravenous antibiotics, and intraperitoneal extravasation should be repaired surgically. A cys-

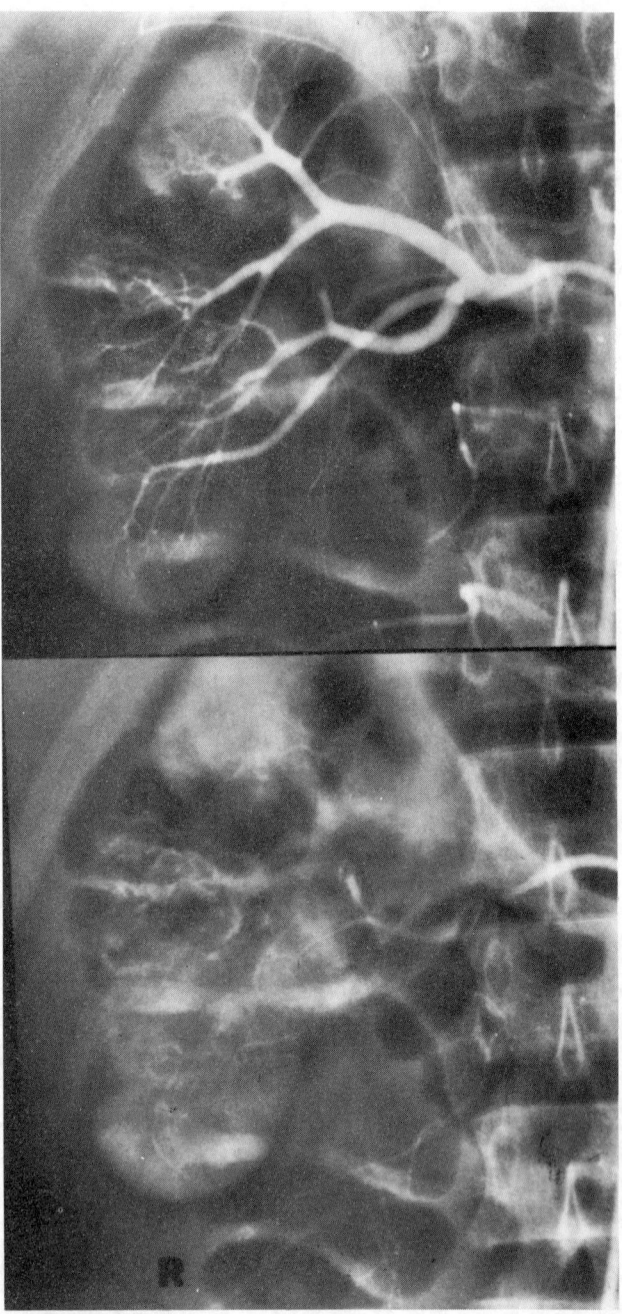

FIGURE 81-4. The angiogram of this kidney is typical of major blunt trauma and shows no major arterial injury. Bleeding is venous and self-limited. The patient was stabilized with fluids and blood and observed at bedrest for 4 days until the gross hematuria subsided. Follow-up consisted of completely normal findings on intravenous pyelography 2 months later.

togram should be performed on the seventh postoperative day, demonstrating no extravasation before catheter removal. Extraperitoneal bladder ruptures are generally small and will heal with catheter drainage alone.[16]

Unrecognized intraperitoneal bladder injuries should be suspected in patients with blunt abdominal trauma who develop uremia, ileus, increasing abdominal girth, and de-

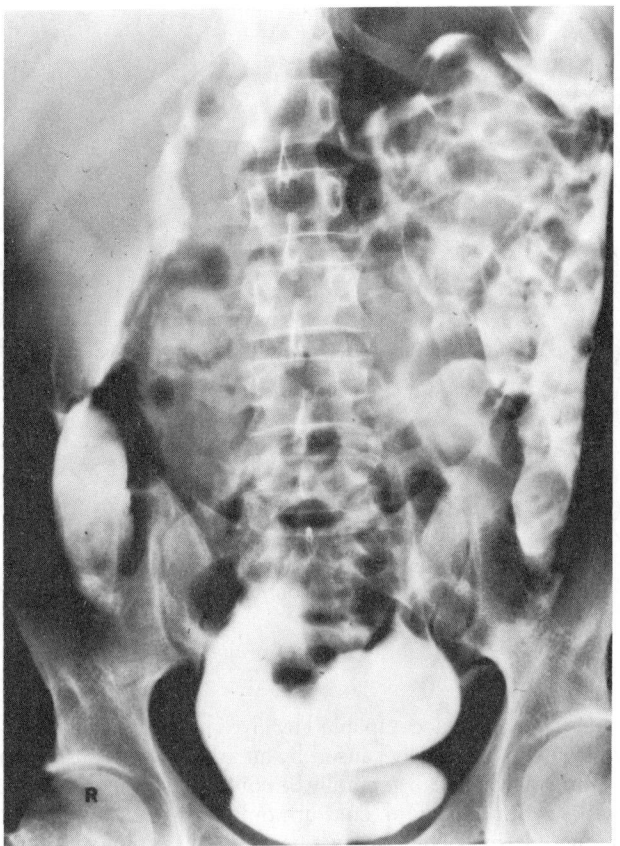

FIGURE 81-5. This patient received blunt trauma to the lower abdomen. The cystogram phase of the intravenous pyelography was normal, emphasizing the need for formal cystography in all of these patients. The contrast material can be seen outlining the small and large bowel, indicative of an intraperitoneal bladder rupture.

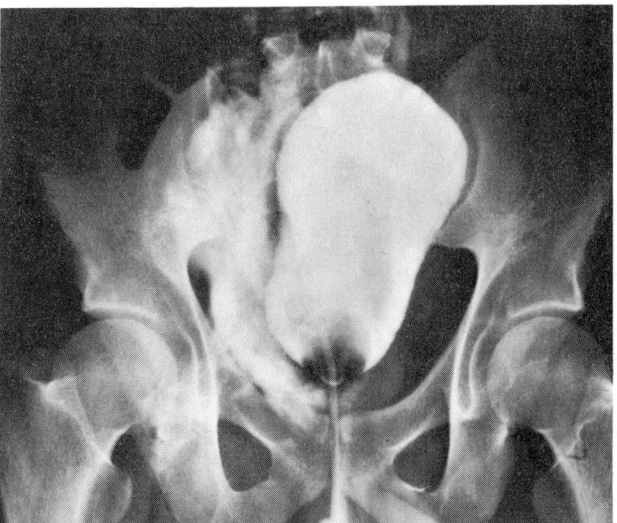

FIGURE 81-6. Cystography reveals a right pubic ramus fracture and a teardrop bladder, which is indicative of significant pelvic hematoma and extraperitoneal extravasation of contrast material.

creased urine output. Sepsis is not a constant finding. A KUB will show a "ground glass" appearance characteristic of ascites. An unrecognized extraperitoneal bladder rupture should be suspected in patients with blunt pelvic injuries, especially with associated pelvic fractures. These patients usually present with fever and sepsis consistent with a pelvic abscess. Intraperitoneal and extraperitoneal injuries are confirmed by cystography and require emergent surgical drainage.

Urethra

The male urethra is divided into two anatomic sections: anterior and posterior. Blunt injury to the posterior urethra occurs when the prostate and pelvis move in different directions, thereby shearing the urethra at the membranous portion; urethral injuries in women are rare. There is usually an associated pelvic fracture. Patients present with gross hematuria, inability to void, blood at the meatus, and a free-floating prostate on rectal examination. If a urethral injury is suspected, retrograde urethrography should precede the cystogram. Attempted catheterization when there has been a partial urethral disruption can extend the tear into a complete urethral disruption, complicating management.[15] Using

a Brodney clamp or an 8-French Foley catheter with the balloon inflated in the fossa navicularis, 20 to 30 mL of contrast is injected. The patient's pelvis should be oblique to examine completely the membranous and prostatic urethra. An adequate urethrogram should show contrast in the proximal urethra and bladder (Fig. 81-7). Membranous urethral injuries are treated with a suprapubic cystostomy tube only (Fig. 81-8). Immediate dissection at the time of injury carries with it an increased risk of incontinence, stricture, major pelvic bleeding, and impotence resulting from disruption of the pelvic nerves.[17] Unrecognized urethral injuries should be suspected in patients with pelvic fractures who become febrile 3 to 7 days after injury. These patients commonly have a urinary tract infection and a perineal hematoma.

PENETRATING TRAUMA

Kidney

Renal injuries are the source of more controversy and confusion than any other area of urogenital trauma. Some trauma surgeons operate on virtually every kidney injury regardless of severity, and others never operate. The key to renal trauma, as in other aspects of urologic trauma, is the accurate definition of the injury. Should the urogram with tomography give a normal result, significant injury most likely has been excluded. An inadequate study does not suffice. An abnormal study result should lead to angiography. I prefer to reserve CT scan for blunt trauma, which is usually treated nonoperatively. Angiography gives information regarding renal arterial anatomy that no other modality can offer.[18] The presence or absence of a hematoma, so beautifully illustrated on CT scan,[19] says nothing about intrarenal anatomy. For anatomy, angiography is the gold standard.

A second significant place for angiography is in the stab wound victim. An arteriovenous fistula or a bleeding segmen-

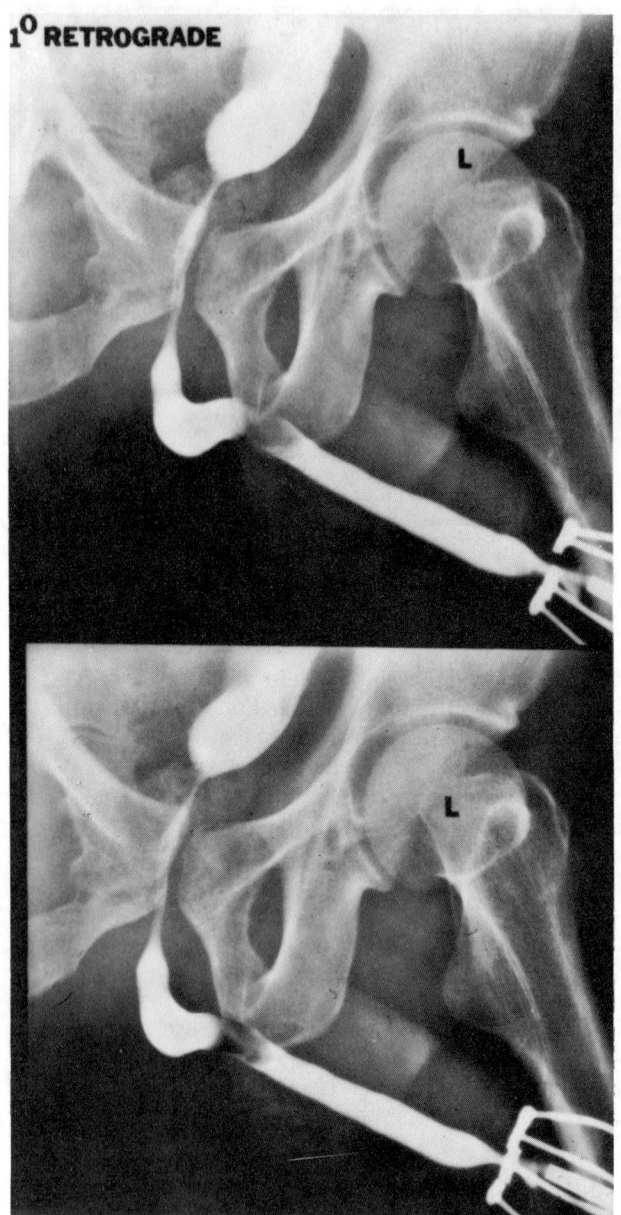

FIGURE 81-7. Normal retrograde urethrography using a Brodney clamp. The pelvis needs to be viewed obliquely, and the most proximal portions of the urethra need to be adequately visualized. Notice the pelvic ramus fracture and the teardrop bladder this time without extravasation.

tal renal artery branch can be identified precisely and effectively embolized[18,20] (Fig. 81-9), occasionally sparing the patient an emergency laparotomy. In my experience, it is unusual that renal stab wounds require surgery. Minor injuries seen on an angiogram are left alone and major injuries embolized. Complications of renal stab wound injuries include renal hemorrhage, urinoma, or abscess formation from an infected urinoma or hematoma. Delayed renal hemorrhage may occur any time and as late as 7 to 10 days after injury. It is usually indicated by a rapid drop in hematocrit

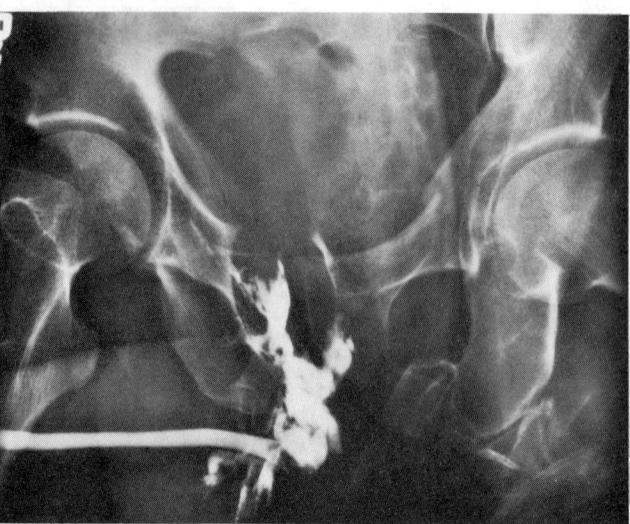

FIGURE 81-8. Urethrogram indicative of complete membranous urethral disruption because no contrast material is seen in the bladder.

and is frequently accompanied by gross hematuria and hypotension. It is generally caused by an arteriovenous fistula or aneurysm, which can generally be controlled by angiographic embolization. A noninfected urinoma is difficult to identify. It may be suspected by an unexpectedly prolonged ileus, nausea, and vomiting. Serum chemistry results, in particular, urea nitrogen and bicarbonate, may be abnormal. An infected urinoma or hematoma is characterized by fever, flank pain, elevated white blood cell count, ileus, nausea, and vomiting. CT scan-guided drainage will establish the diagnosis. If continued urinary extravasation is suggested, an IVP and possibly retrograde pyelography are necessary to identify the location and extent of injury. Surgical intervention is usually required.

Gunshot wounds to the kidney are usually associated with intraabdominal injuries mandating surgery (Fig. 81-10). Postoperative urologic complications include hemorrhage, urinary fistula, and unsuspected urinary tract injuries. Hemorrhage and urinary tract fistula are managed as described for stab wound injuries. Unsuspected associated urinary tract injuries are more common in gunshot injuries because of the projectile nature of the weapon. Gunshot victims who develop gross hematuria postoperatively should be evaluated with an IVP. Patients with any hematuria postoperatively who were not evaluated with an IVP preoperatively or intraoperatively should also be fully examined radiographically if there is a possibility of urologic injury. Delayed identification of urinary tract injuries generally results in emergency surgery. Hypertension on a renovascular basis is rare after partial nephrectomy, but all patients should receive instruction and follow-up postoperatively regarding this possibility.

Ureter

Ureteral injuries are usually identified and well defined by intravenous urography with extravasation seen on the films.

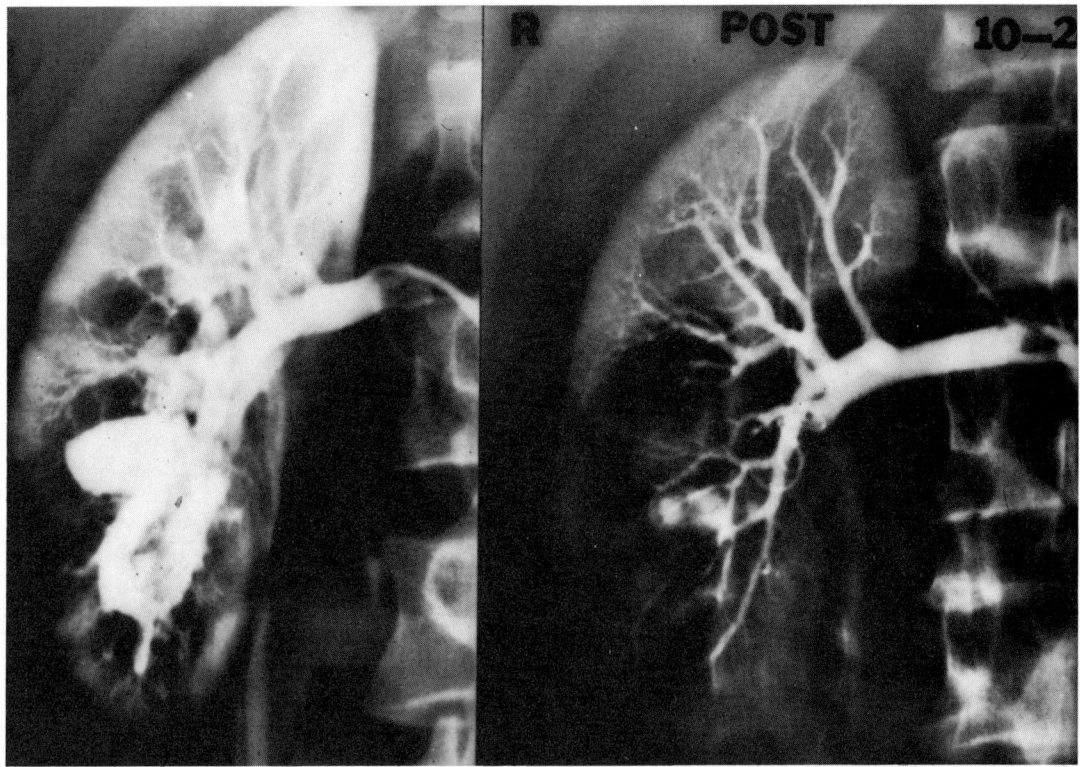

FIGURE 81-9. This patient received a stab wound to the back; his only injury was to the right kidney. Angiography revealed a large arteriovenous fistula that was successfully managed nonoperatively with a vascular coil.

Proximal and middle third ureteral injuries are usually managed by primary repair. Ureteral stents and soft rubber drains are placed and can be evaluated radiographically for position. Even with internal stents, primary end-to-end ureteral repairs commonly leak transiently. Problems arise if a leak is inadequately drained or persistent. Urinary diversion by a percutaneous nephrostomy usually is required to allow the ureter to heal, and drainage of a urinoma is needed if the patient does not improve clinically. Distal third and lower middle third ureteral injuries are handled by ureteral reimplantation into the bladder. Ureteral reimplantation procedures have better results than primary end-to-end ureteral repairs and, although usually drained, they rarely leak.

Bladder

Penetrating bladder wounds are defined by cystography and result in extraperitoneal or intraperitoneal spill of urine. I prefer to perform the necessary intravenous urogram before cystography because extravasation of contrast at the time of cystography may obscure the findings of an associated distal ureteral injury on IVP. All bladder injuries from penetrating trauma are repaired surgically. In a man, a suprapubic cystostomy should be in place to avoid prolonged urethral catheter-ization with the risk of urethral stricture. Missed or delayed bladder injuries are unusual.

EXTERNAL GENITALIA TRAUMA

Skin and Scrotum

Genital tract injury involves trauma (blunt or penetrating) to the scrotum, testicles, and penis. The penis contains the urethra and the paired erectile bodies or corpora cavernosa. Any or all may be injured by blunt trauma, stab wound, gunshot wound, or shotgun wound. Lacerations to the scrotum should be managed by techniques similar to other areas of skin. Appropriate cleaning and debridement are followed by primary repair. Penetrating injuries of the scrotum should lead to suspicion of testicular damage. Often a hematoma is present, preventing accurate palpation of the testicle. If there is a hematocele and an impalpable testicle, exploration is recommended. Occasionally, an ultrasound examination of the scrotum reveals an intact testis when the examiner was unable to palpate one. However, unless this examination is available on an emergency basis, surgery should not be delayed for a test that rarely affects the decision to operate. There is no place for "needling" a hematoma in the scrotum;

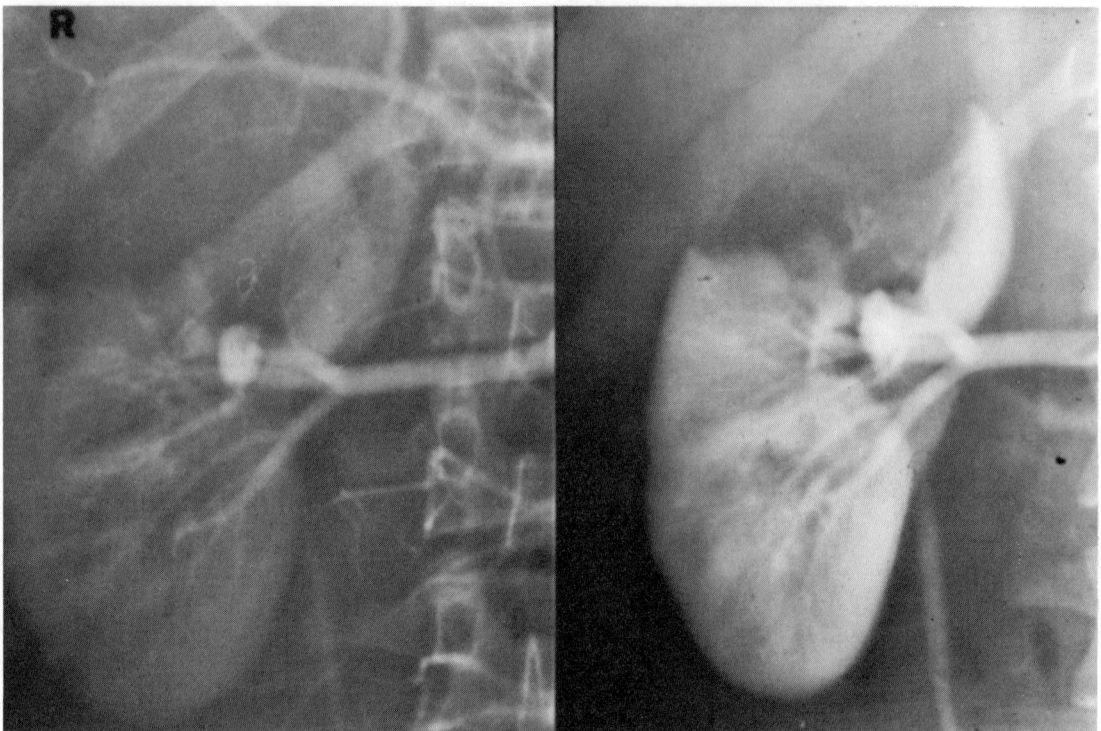

FIGURE 81-10. Angiogram of the right kidney after a gunshot wound showed an arteriovenous fistula of an upper pole artery. The individual artery was ligated, and an upper pole heminephrectomy was performed.

it will become infected. The unoperated fractured testicle will atrophy and become useless after a long period of pain and debility; a repaired testicle will function well and heal rapidly.

Penis

Penile lacerations are treated as any other laceration with one important exception. In an avulsion injury where the skin is removed circumferentially from the proximal penile shaft, surgical intervention for plastic reconstruction is necessary. Otherwise, lymphedema of the remaining distal skin results in an unacceptable cosmetic result. Injury to the urethra should be anticipated with penetrating wounds to the penis, and retrograde urethrography will establish the diagnosis. Erectile tissue injuries should be repaired primarily. Care should be taken preoperatively to document penile sensation because of possible injury to the dorsal neurovascular bundle supplying the penis. If these injuries are managed nonoperatively, there is significant morbidity from pain and swelling as well as the risk of painful penile angulation with erection secondary to scar formation. Shotgun wounds are an exception and can usually be treated nonoperatively with routine wound care. A urethral catheter can be placed after diagnostic urethrography is done. Surgical intervention to remove dozens of pellets often causes more insult than the pellets. In all instances, patients should receive broad-spectrum antibiotics perioperatively to prevent infection.

REFERENCES ■

1. Brown DL, Kirby RR: Operative and perioperative critical care in the surgical patient. *Monogr Urol* 1985;6:1
2. Goldman L: Cardiac risk and complications of non-cardiac surgery. *Ann Surg* 1983;198:780
3. Stewart BH: Adrenal surgery: current state of the art. *J Urol* 1983;129:1
4. Lieskovsky G, Pritchett TR, Skinner DG: Surgical management of renal cell carcinoma. *Monogr Urol* 1984;5:1
5. Huleert JC, Grossman JE, Cummings KB: Risk factors of anesthesia and surgery in bleomycin treated patients. *J Urol* 1983;130:163
6. Donohue JP, Rowland RG: Complications of retroperitoneal lymph node dissection. *J Urol* 1981;125:338
7. Ritchie JP, Skinner DG: Complications of urinary conduit diversion. In: Smith RB, Skinner DG (eds). *Complications of Urologic Surgery: Prevention and Management*. Philadelphia, WB Saunders, 1976:209
8. Libertino JA, Eyre RC: Plan for management of complications after ileal conduit diversion. *AUA Update Series* 1984;3:1
9. Mee SL, McAninch TW, Robinson AL, et al: Radiographic assessment of renal trauma: a 10-year prospective study of patient selection. *J Urol* 1989;141:1095
10. Eastham JA, Wilson TG, Ahlering TE: Radiographic evaluation of adult patients with blunt renal trauma. *J Urol* 1992;148:266
11. McAninch JR, Federle MP: Evaluation of renal injuries with computerized tomography. *J Urol* 1982;128:456
12. Husmann DA, Morris JS: Attempted nonoperative management of blunt renal lacerations extending through the corti-

comedullary junction: the short-term and long-term sequelae. *J Urol* 1990:682

13. Cass AS: Immediate radiologic evaluation and early surgical management of genital urinary injuries from external trauma. *J Urol* 1979;122:772

14. Cass AS, Luxemberg M: Conservative or immediate surgical management of blunt renal trauma. *J Urol* 1983;130:11

15. Fallon B, Wendt JC, Hawtey CE: Urological injury and assessment of patients with fractured pelvis. *J Urol* 1984;131:712

16. Hayes EE, Sandler CM, Corriere JN Jr: Management of the ruptured bladder secondary to blunt abdominal trauma. *J Urol* 1983;129:946

17. Gibson GR: Urologic management and complications of fractured pelvis and ruptured urethra. *J Urol* 1974;111:353

18. Eastham JA, Wilson TG, Larsen DW, Ahlering TE: Angiographic embolization of renal stab wounds. *J Urol* 1992;148: 268

19. Nicolaisen GS, McAninch JR, Marshall GA, et al: Renal trauma: re-evaluation of the indications for radiographic assessment. *J Urol* 1985;133:183

20. Eastham JA, Wilson TG, Ahlering TE: Urologic evaluation and management of renal proximity stab wounds. *J Urol* 1993; 150:1771

Critical Care, Third Edition, edited by Joseph M. Civetta,
Robert W. Taylor, and Robert R. Kirby.
Lippincott-Raven Publishers, Philadelphia, PA © 1997.

CHAPTER 82

∎

Burn Injury

Michael D. Peck
C. Gillon Ward

IMMEDIATE CONCERNS ∎

MAJOR PROBLEMS

The priorities for assessment and treatment of patients with
burn injuries are no different from those of other trauma
patients. The pathophysiology of the injuries is, however,
different, and needs to be understood so that appropriate
treatment decisions can be made. Swelling of the upper
airway can occur rapidly because of direct thermal injury to
the airway and because of accumulation of extravascular
fluid during burn shock. Other deleterious components of
smoke include carbon monoxide and a variety of toxins that
damage the lung parenchyma. The burn injury causes a
release of inflammatory cytokines, leading to increased capillary permeability and cellular swelling. Because of the loss
of the mechanical barrier of the skin and because of the
diffuse suppression of all components of immune response,
burn patients are at high risk for death from invasive bacterial or fungal infection. The burn wound also leads to a
significant increase in the metabolic rate. Removal of the
burned skin and coverage of the wounds ultimately resolves
these problems.

STRESS POINTS

1. Inhalation of smoke can injure a patient in three ways:
   (i) direct thermal damage to the upper airway leading
   to inadequate air exchange, (ii) carbon monoxide poisoning, and (iii) toxic damage to the lung parenchyma.
   Treatment for these problems is the administration
   of humidified oxygen by face mask, or, if necessary,
   nasotracheal intubation and mechanical ventilation
   with positive end-expiratory pressure (PEEP).

2. For approximately the first 24 hours after thermal
   injury, leakage of capillary beds occurs, leading to
   exudation into extravascular tissues. In addition, intracellular sodium regulation is damaged, leading to cellular swelling. Because of these problems, a loss of
   intravascular plasma occurs, which increases in proportion to the size and depth of the burn injury. In
   addition, the requirements for resuscitation fluid increase in a patient with smoke inhalation injury.

3. Infection is a great threat to the burn patient, because
   of loss of the mechanical barrier of the skin, and because of global suppression of the immune response.
   The importance of meticulous infection control policies should be stressed. Early excision of the burn
   wound should be done to remove the dead tissue,
   which harbors bacteria. Burn patients need to be monitored carefully on a daily basis for signs of infection,
   although infection may be subtle and difficult to
   diagnose.

4. Enteral feeding should be instituted in burn patients
   as soon as possible. This reduces the rate of bacteria
   translocation and may, therefore, blunt the hypermetabolic and immunosuppressive responses to
   burn injury.

5. Physical and occupational therapy should begin immediately. Even if patients are obtunded, passive extension of joints prevents muscular and tendon shortening. Active range of motion exercises should be started
   as soon as the patient can cooperate. Contractures of
   burn wounds are the major challenge to recovering
   burn patients during their rehabilitation.

6. Pain from the burn wounds is severe. Combinations
   of narcotic analgesics and sedatives such as benzodiazepines need to be used in high doses for the patient's

comfort during cleaning of the wounds and replications of dressings. Patients also need medication for therapy sessions and to treat background or resting pain.

7. Burn patients and their families require intensive psychological support and counseling.

ESSENTIAL DIAGNOSTIC TESTS AND PROCEDURES

1. If the airway is thought to be compromised, the patient should be intubated immediately because emergency tracheostomy is hazardous.
2. Adequacy of resuscitation is determined by appropriate urine output (600 to 800 mL/m²/day).
3. Invasive monitoring is necessary only in patients with preexisting cardiac disease.
4. Compromise of perfusion of the distal extremities or restriction of respiratory motion may require release of nonelastic burned skin by escharotomies.

INITIAL THERAPY

1. Resuscitation of the burn patient should be done with 0.52 mEq Na$^+$/kg/% burn.
2. Use of lactated Ringer's solution at 4 mL/kg/% burn achieves this goal, but it can also be achieved with less free water if hypertonic sodium solutions are used.
3. Initial wound care involves only the simple debridement of loose tissue at the bedside, followed by application of silver sulfadiazine cream.
4. More extensive surgical debridements are left until the patient is stabilized, at least 3 to 4 days later, unless severe destruction of muscle tissue, by fourth-degree burns or high-voltage electrical current injury, leads to myonecrosis and threatened renal dysfunction.

MANAGEMENT OF RESPIRATORY PROBLEMS ■

MAINTENANCE OF ADEQUATE AIR EXCHANGE THROUGH THE UPPER AIRWAY

Maintenance of adequate air exchange through the upper airway is a high priority, not only during the initial evaluation of the patient, but subsequently throughout the hospital course. Upper airway edema occurs initially because of inflammation resulting from the heat of inspired smoke. The swelling is often exacerbated by accumulation of excess interstitial fluid, which occurs because of capillary leakage and cellular swelling associated with major burns. In most patients with severe burn injuries (>40% total body surface area [TBSA]), the upper airway is compromised even in the absence of smoke inhalation and direct injury to the upper airway.[1] If at any point during the initial evaluation there is any concern about adequacy of the upper airway, the patient should be intubated. There are relatively few complications of short-term intubation, but the loss of an airway in a patient with rapidly swelling face and neck is disastrous, because a tracheostomy is technically difficult to perform under these emergency circumstances.

SMOKE INHALATION

The diagnosis of smoke inhalation injury is sometimes difficult to make. Although routine bronchoscopy is not justified, direct laryngoscopy helps to identify pharyngeal or glottic edema. Signs and symptoms of an inhalation injury such as hoarseness, singed nasal or mustache hair, carbonaceous sputum, facial burns, and a history of being in an enclosed space are all important contributory data, but they are nonspecific. The need for ventilatory support is based on the presence of air hunger, dyspnea, tachypnea, retention of carbon dioxide (CO_2), or hypoxemia. Injury in an enclosed space is always regarded with a high index of suspicion. Respiratory insufficiency secondary to smoke inhalation, however, may not manifest itself until 18 to 36 hours after injury.

CARBON MONOXIDE POISONING

Carbon monoxide poisoning is a significant component of smoke inhalation injury in some patients. Carbon monoxide binds to hemoglobin with an affinity 200 times greater than that of oxygen, thus displacing oxygen. Impairment of oxidative metabolism, especially of the central nervous system, leads to the signs and symptoms of carbon monoxide poisoning: blurred vision or diplopia, nausea, headaches, dizziness, coma, and eventually death in severe cases. The half-life of carbon monoxide bound to hemoglobin is 5 hours when the patient is breathing atmospheric (21%) oxygen. In an intubated patient breathing 100% oxygen, the half-life drops to 1 hour. The diagnosis of carbon monoxide poisoning can be made from the measured carboxyhemoglobin levels from the arterial blood gas, although the severity of carbon monoxide poisoning does not correlate well with these levels. Treatment is straightforward. Patients with mild symptoms can be treated with supplemental oxygen, such as a face mask. Patients with depressed level of consciousness and elevated carboxyhemoglobin levels should be intubated and given 100% inspired oxygen during the first few hours after injury.

INDICATIONS FOR EXTUBATION

Indications for extubation are the resolution of facial and upper airway edema. In a situation uncomplicated by smoke inhalation, infection, or adult respiratory distress syndrome (ARDS), extubation can be accomplished at the end of the postresuscitation diuresis. Simple inspection of the patient's face and neck to see if the generalized tissue swelling has resolved is often adequate. Another useful maneuver is to let down the balloon on the endotracheal cuff, occlude the tube, and see if the patient can breathe around the tube. If the patient can exchange air around the tube, this is a reliable sign that the upper airway edema has diminished.

In some patients, however, extubation cannot be accomplished even after the upper airway edema has resolved. In the early stages of treatment, the most common reason for prolonged intubation is hypoxemia secondary to pulmonary parenchymal damage from the numerous toxins present in smoke, such as aldehydes, hydrochloric acid, and cyanides. The toxic effect of these gases results in a diffusion defect and also predisposes the lungs to pneumonia, ARDS, or both.[2] Pneumonia and ARDS may occur in patients who have not had smoke inhalation injury because the severity of the burn injury results in global immunosuppression. Patients can be managed with endotracheal tubes for up to 3 weeks after injury by using the nasotracheal route. Although there is an increased risk of paranasal sinusitis in such patients,[3] nasotracheal tubes are easier to secure than orotracheal tubes.[4] The size of tube used for this route, however, is usually smaller than orotracheal tubes. An increase in imposed work of breathing occurs; also, narrowing from inspissated secretions is accentuated: both of these factors may be interpreted as "patient failures" during weaning trials (Chap. 15).

INDICATIONS FOR TRACHEOSTOMY

After 3 weeks of intubation, tracheostomy should be considered.[5] Tracheostomies are done primarily to minimize upper airway sequelae and also to facilitate mobilization of the patient. They do so at the expense of an increased rate of tracheal complications. Although patients with nasotracheal tubes can be moved out of bed into a chair, the move risks loss of the airway. Patients with tracheostomies can progress through early stages of rehabilitation, including walking in hallways, while the pulmonary injury is resolving. As is often true in bedside practice, risks and benefits must be balanced in choosing an appropriate route for ventilatory support.

PROBLEMS WITH VENTILATION-PERFUSION RELATIONSHIPS

Problems with ventilation-perfusion relationships are common in critically ill burn patients. Because of the predisposition to pulmonary infections and to multiple organ system failure from sepsis or systemic inflammation, prolonged ventilatory support is common. Treatment is supportive; steroids and prophylactic antibiotics do not ameliorate the lung damage and only increase the risk of infections.[6]

Patients who develop acute pulmonary disease as a result of their burn injury can have difficulty eliminating CO_2. In the initial 24 to 48 hours, this can result from tight, circumferential burns of the trunk that restrict mechanical movement of the chest. These restrictions are reflected in rising inspiratory pressures on the ventilator caused by decreased compliance of the chest wall. The problem can be promptly resolved through escharotomies on the chest.[6] As the flow phase of hypermetabolism begins, CO_2 production increases. Primarily, this can be compensated for by increasing the rate or tidal volume to increase minute ventilation. If compliance decreases, for example, from ARDS, then it may be difficult to prevent respiratory acidosis. Currently, there are many options to provide ventilatory support (Chap. 49). Death rarely is related to an inability to ventilate or oxygenate alone. Closure of the burn wounds is not sufficient to resolve the pulmonary problem once it starts; patients with completely closed burn wounds can die a pulmonary death.

MANAGEMENT OF CARDIOVASCULAR PROBLEMS ■

LOSS OF INTRAVASCULAR VOLUME

Hypovolemia accompanies every burn injury to a degree that is directly proportional to the percentage of the TBSA burned.[7] Burns covering less than 15% to 20% of the TBSA are associated with a relatively minor loss of intravascular volume, which can be replaced easily with oral resuscitation or minimal intravenous fluids. When the burn size exceeds 20% TBSA, however, the loss of intravascular volume can be substantial. Before the importance of adequate fluid resuscitation was appreciated, burns involving more than 30% TBSA were usually fatal.

RESUSCITATION OF BURN SHOCK

Successful resuscitation is now accomplished in most patients. Several formulas have been published, and many variations of these formulas have been practiced in individual burn centers around the world. The formulas hinge on the delivery of three components: sodium, water, and colloid. The simplest formula to use, known either as the *Baxter formula* or *Parkland formula,* was described by Charles Baxter, M.D., when he was Director of the Parkland Memorial Hospital Burn Center, Dallas, Texas. Baxter recommends multiplying four times the patient's weight in kilograms by the percentage of the body surface area burned (4 mL/kg/% burn), to give a total volume of the isotonic electrolyte solution, lactated Ringer's solution, over the first 24 hours after injury. (Glucose-containing solutions are not given to adults in the first 24 hours; early use of glucose may induce an unwanted and dangerous osmotic diuresis.) The formula recommends that half of this volume should be given over the first 8 hours but we believe that it is better to distribute the volume evenly over 24 hours. Colloid solutions, such as 25% salt-poor albumin, are started after the first 24 hours.

Peripheral intravenous catheters are better than central venous catheters because of fewer associated complications. Fluid also can be infused faster through large-bore, short-length catheters than through long, central venous catheters. The best sites for intravenous lines are away from the burn. Catheters can be placed through burn eschar, however, if there are no convenient locations in nonburned areas.

Because the Parkland formula uses measurements of weight and burn size, it is imperative that these parameters be measured accurately as soon as possible after admission. The patient should be weighed before dressings are applied and before edema begins to accumulate. Although the TBSA burned can be calculated using the Rule of Nines, a more exact and preferred determination of the surface area burned can be done by using the Lund-Browder chart (Fig. 82-1). The time of the burn is the starting time for fluid resuscitation, *not* when the patient is first seen in the emergency room.

The attractiveness of the Parkland formula is its simplicity and effectiveness. But the clinical endpoint of this formula, as with any formula used, must be signs of end-organ perfusion reflected by adequate urine output. Pulmonary artery

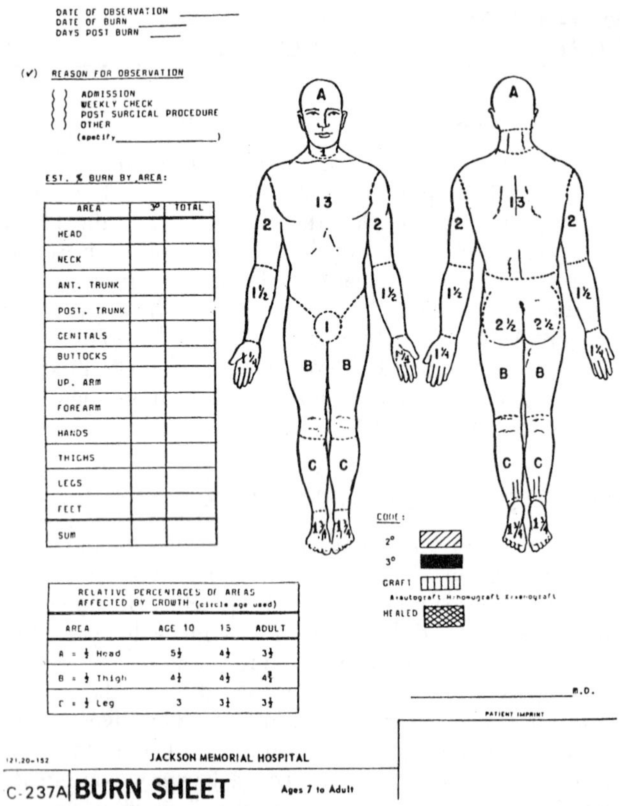

DATE OF OBSERVATION
DATE OF BURN
DAYS POST BURN
(✓) REASON FOR OBSERVATION
ADMISSION
WEEKLY CHECK
POST SURGICAL PROCEDURE
OTHER
(specify)
EST. % BURN BY AREA:
AREA
3°
TOTAL
HEAD
NECK
ANT. TRUNK
POST. TRUNK
GENITALS
BUTTOCKS
UP. ARM
FOREARM
HANDS
THIGHS
LEGS
FEET
SUM
RELATIVE PERCENTAGES OF AREAS AFFECTED BY GROWTH (circle age used)
AREA AGE 10 15 ADULT
A = ½ Head 5½ 4½ 3½
B = ½ Thigh 4¼ 4½ 4¾
C = ½ Leg 3 3¼ 3½
A
13
2
1½
1
2½
B
C
1¾
CODE:
2°
3°
GRAFT
HEALED
M.D.
PATIENT IMPRINT
121.20-152
JACKSON MEMORIAL HOSPITAL
C-237A BURN SHEET
Ages 7 to Adult

FIGURE 82-1. The Lund-Browder chart gives an accurate estimate of burn size. Mapping should be done immediately on admission to calculate fluid resuscitation needs. It should be repeated within 72 hours to ensure that all burned areas are included in the assessment.

catheterization is not needed in most burn patients. If resuscitation is based on the assumption that the filling pressure of the heart, estimated by the pulmonary artery occlusion pressure, should be normal during resuscitation, there will be a risk of fluid overload. In addition, cardiac output decreases immediately after a burn, even with good filling pressures. However, in patients with a prior history of cardiac, pulmonary, or renal disease, a pulmonary artery catheter should be placed to protect the patient from fluid overload.

USE OF HYPERTONIC SALT SOLUTIONS

Burn shock is caused by the systemic response to the inflammatory mediators released by the burn injury, which results in widespread capillary leakage of plasma into interstitial spaces. In addition, impairment in the sodium–potassium exchange pump at the cell membrane leads to intracellular swelling.[8] Sodium in the resuscitation fluid is needed to maintain intravascular volume and to ameliorate cellular edema. Burn patients also may be resuscitated by giving them 0.52 mEq Na^+/kg/% burn. If this is accomplished with a reduction in the amount of free water given, total body swelling may be minimized.[9] Glottic edema requiring intubation and peripheral edema requiring escharotomy can be avoided. An effective solution is a hypertonic salt solution created by adding 100 mEq sodium acetate to each liter of lactated Ringer's solution, giving a total sodium concentration of 230 mEq/L. Lactated Ringer's solution is used as the base solution rather than normal saline to avoid a hyperchloremic metabolic acidosis. The hypertonic resuscitation formula provides exactly the same amount of sodium in the first 24 hours as the classic Parkland formula. The major difference is the volume of water in which the sodium is delivered. The serum sodium needs to be monitored every 6 hours; if it rises above 145 mEq/L, the hypertonic resuscitation should be stopped. Otherwise, this resuscitation is carried out for the first 24 hours after burn injury until there is evidence of diminished capillary leakage, which can be detected by following the hematocrit. The hematocrit begins to rise shortly after burn injury because of hemoconcentration as intravascular plasma is lost. It starts to decline toward the end of the first 24 hours as the capillaries seal. At this point, the hypertonic solution is stopped; thereafter, we prefer to use plain lactated Ringer's solution for maintenance fluids and to start an albumin infusion.[8]

POSTRESUSCITATION DIURESIS

As patients enter the flow phase of burn shock, their fluid demands start to taper off. In the initial hours of the second day after injury, fluid requirements are unpredictable. Some patients clearly stabilize as the capillary leak decreases, which can occur as early as 16 to 18 hours after the burn. Others continue to have intermittently low urine outputs, and they need continued high volumes of fluid resuscitation. Good clinical judgment is required, particularly for the very young and the very old, because the oliguria may not reflect diminished intravascular volume, but rather inability of the kidneys to excrete the increased volume load. Patients at the extremes of ages can develop pulmonary edema within the first few days after burn injury because of inadequate diuresis. Fluid restriction and diuretics are indicated for these patients with oliguria rather than continued intravenous fluid administration. Pulmonary artery catheters or, at least, central venous pressure monitoring, may help guide therapy at this point.

COMPLICATIONS OF RESUSCITATION

The complications of resuscitation of burn patients are related to the components. Aberrations of serum sodium concentration are common, particularly hypernatremia in patients who have received a hypertonic resuscitation. Patients resuscitated with lactated Ringer's solution, especially if sodium acetate or sodium bicarbonate is added to make the solution hypertonic, may develop an alkalemia after resuscitation. These patients hypoventilate to maintain a normal pH. This is a problem in patients with preexisting chronic pulmonary disease because hypoventilation can lead to hypoxemia. Administration of a bicarbonate-wasting diuretic, such as acetazolamide, corrects this imbalance.

The interstitial and intracellular accumulation of resuscitation fluid leads to anasarca, which resolves after 3 to 5 days without sequelae. Unfortunately, patients with smoke inhalation injury probably have the effects of the toxic injury to the lung parenchyma exacerbated by this increase in extravascular fluid. The accumulation of extravascular fluid also threatens perfusion of the extremities. Deeply burned skin loses its elasticity. Extremities can have a large extravascular fluid accumulation, producing tissue pressures that prevent perfusion of capillary beds. Monitoring of adequate perfusion to the distal extremities is mandatory in patients with severe burn injuries, particularly those with circumferential burns of the extremities.[10]

CHEMICAL AND SURGICAL ESCHAROTOMIES

Restriction of respiratory excursions by circumferential burns of the trunk decreases chest wall compliance and is an impediment to adequate ventilation. The treatment is the same as on an extremity. Application of strips of enzymatic debriding agents, such as sutilains ointment, act as a chemical escharotomy. (Precautions must be taken when using enzymatic debriding agents because they will increase fluid losses, which, in turn, increases the difficulty of resuscitating the patient. Enzymatic debriding agents are contraindicated if concern exists about excessive fluid losses.) If the diminished blood flow or respiratory excursions are of an emergent nature, surgical escharotomies are done at the bedside. This is best done by electrocautery, which controls the bleeding vessels. The use of electrocautery requires an anesthetic agent; we prefer to use ketamine. If escharotomy alone does not relieve pressure in the deep compartments, especially with deep burns to the legs, fasciotomy is indicated.

The indication for performing escharotomy may be difficult to judge at times. Peripheral sensory nerves are sensitive to deprivation of oxygen. Symptoms of paresthesia or pain in the digits, hands, or feet should prompt urgent consideration for escharotomies. Because the distal extremities are often discolored by smoke, edema, or erythema, if not burned outright, then determination of capillary refill is essentially useless. Palpation of pulses at the radial, dorsalis pedis, or posterior tibial level is meaningless, because tissue pressures sufficient to prevent venous outflow may not be high enough to impede arterial inflow. An accurate method of assessment is direct measurement of compartmental pressures by use of an 18-gauge needle attached to the pressure transducer used to monitor arterial blood pressure. Pressures in the subcutaneous and intramuscular compartments greater than 30 mm Hg are an indication for escharotomy. Should the compartmental pressures not be relieved after escharotomy, then fasciotomy should be performed.[11]

FLUIDS AND ELECTROLYTES

As patients progress from the postresuscitation phase to wound closure, daily attention must be paid to fluids and electrolytes. The maintenance fluid volume is 1500 mL/m²/day. Insensible losses are increased in burn patients because of the plasma exudate lost through the open wounds. Although the volume of fluid loss cannot be quantified, it can be estimated with the following formula[12]:

$$(25 + \%\text{Body surface area burned}) \times \text{TBSA}$$
$$= \text{Rate of insensible loss (mL/hour)}$$

This estimate can be used to facilitate ordering sufficient additional volumes of fluid that may be required to maintain intravascular volume in patients with large open wounds.

Ironically, burn patients do not seem to have as high a requirement for crystalloid fluid replacement during surgery as do, for example, patients undergoing laparotomy with exposed peritoneal surfaces. In fact, we encourage our anesthesiologists to minimize crystalloid fluid replacement in the operating room, and to concentrate on replacement with packed red blood cells when volume replacement is needed.[13]

SEPTIC SHOCK

Septic burn patients may need volumes of resuscitation fluid close to those required for the initial resuscitation. Whether it is the result of an invasive infection from bacteria or yeast, or whether it is a systemic inflammatory response related to the outpouring of inflammatory cytokines, systemic vascular resistance can drop to extraordinarily low levels for several days. Because the preinjury cardiac status of most of these patients is normal, an increased cardiac output maintains reasonable organ perfusion if adequate intravascular volume is present. To maintain this volume in the face of systemic vascular resistances as low as 200 dyne · second · cm⁻⁵, liters of fluid are required. A normal urine output is a sufficient clinical endpoint. Pulmonary artery catheters are occasionally useful to provide hemodynamic parameters consistent with the diagnosis of sepsis and to guide fluid resuscitation, especially with ARDS or renal failure. We have not found it necessary to use either inotropic or vasoconstrictive pharmacologic agents. Most burn patients who develop a sepsis syndrome so severe that epinephrine is necessary for maintenance of normal blood pressure (low-output septic shock) do not survive.

MAINTENANCE OF ELECTROLYTE HOMEOSTASIS AND ACID–BASE BALANCE ∎

DISTURBANCES OF THE SERUM SODIUM CONCENTRATION

Disturbances of the serum sodium concentration are common in burn patients because of either an iatrogenic deficit or excess of total body sodium or water. The estimated daily sodium requirements for healthy patients is 40 mEq/m²/day. The burn patient with open wounds has additional sodium losses in the exudate from the wounds, similar to the additional insensible losses of water noted above. Judging from the magnitude of the insensible fluid losses from open wounds, sodium losses may be equally as extensive. In patients with large, open burn wounds, more than 3 L of lactated Ringer's solution may be necessary for replacement of insensible losses. Hyponatremia also may be caused by an excess of free water. This problem occurs often in patients whose intravenous medications are prepared using 5% dextrose solutions. Patients receiving two or three different antibiotics may receive 1 or 2 L of free water each day. Most medications can be given in salt solutions, and hyponatremia can be avoided. The burn patient's increased thirst, particularly in children, presents a similar challenge because most fluids such as milk, juices, infant formulas, and nutritional supplements are relatively low in sodium. Oral fluid restriction may be necessary in some patients to avoid hyponatremia.

CHANGES IN SERUM POTASSIUM

Maintenance requirements for potassium are similar to those for sodium. Hypokalemia is not as common, however, as hyponatremia and is usually associated with marked diuresis after the resuscitation period. Hyperkalemia can occur in patients with electrical current injury if a significant amount of skeletal muscle is damaged. The hyperkalemia in these patients may respond to forced diuresis, which is the treatment for the myoglobinuria that accompanies myonecrosis. If hyperkalemia and myoglobinuria are unresponsive to the usual treatments, surgical excision of the injured muscle, including amputation, should be considered.[14]

OTHER ISSUES

Burn patients commonly develop hypocalcemia, hypophosphatemia, and hypomagnesemia in the early postresuscitative period.[15] Disturbances in circulating minerals are usually short lived and do not require intervention. Chronic alcoholics may present with unrecognized depletion of total body magnesium stores, resulting from malnutrition and chronic alcohol intake. Decreased muscle rigidity and difficulty with range of motion exercises may be noticed, and may respond to replacement with intravenous magnesium.

MANAGEMENT OF RENAL FAILURE ■

THE "THIRD KIDNEY"

We have observed that an open burn wound can act as a "third kidney"[16] in that fluids and electrolytes disappear from the circulating blood volume at rates proportional to those cleared by the kidneys themselves. In fact, the presence of large open wounds in patients with acute renal failure has sometimes obviated the need for hemodialysis. When the wounds are closed by skin grafting, azotemia worsens. The third kidney effect has a dramatic impact on the clearance of medications, especially those routinely cleared by the kidneys. Dosing quantities are usually higher and dosing intervals shorter in burn patients[17]; this is particularly true and well known for the aminoglycosides, the levels of which can be measured easily. We measure two to three randomly taken serum levels of aminoglycosides in between the peak and trough levels. This allows construction of a clearance curve.

ACUTE RENAL FAILURE

Acute renal failure may occur as a result of inadequate resuscitation or myoglobinuria. Renal failure later in the hospitalization is often caused by antibiotics, particularly aminoglycosides, or by sepsis. Although controversial, low-dose dopamine may increase urine volume whereas low-dose dobutamine may increase creatinine clearance during these episodes.

Acute renal failure in burn patients is treated the same as for all other patients with renal failure. Fluid administration is adjusted to supply the necessary maintenance and replacements needs without forcing the patient into pulmonary edema. The third kidney effect of the open burn wound often protects patients from fluid overload. Hemodialysis is rarely necessary and may not be tolerated by septic patients who are peripherally vasodilated and borderline hypotensive. Objectives for therapy for the patient with severe burn injuries who develops acute renal failure as a result of sepsis and who does not exhibit resolution of either the sepsis or renal failure should be carefully considered before instituting hemodialysis. Because proven medical treatment may be futile in these patients, hemodialysis may only prolong the dying process.

MANAGEMENT OF BLEEDING DISORDERS ■

COAGULOPATHIES

Except in patients with inherited defects of the coagulation pathway, excessive bleeding from coagulopathy is rare in the first few days after injury. Burn patients tend to have activated thrombolysis because the plasminogen system is activated.[18] For this reason, deep venous thrombosis is a rare clinical entity among burn patients.[19] During operative procedures in which large amounts of blood are lost and replaced, a dilutional coagulopathy may result. If the patient becomes hypothermic, this may be complicated by a reversible defect in platelet function and a prolongation of the prothrombin time. The other setting in which coagulopathy may occur is sepsis, in which disseminated intravascular coagulation may occur as a manifestation of widespread infection. The treatment for disseminated intravascular coagulation is to remove the source of the sepsis, namely the burned wound. This surgery may prove fatal to the patient, however, because of massive exsanguination from the escharectomy sites.

GASTROINTESTINAL HEMORRHAGE

Historically, the most common cause of excessive bleeding in burn patients has been erosive gastritis, known as Curling's ulcers. The incidence of these ulcers has diminished greatly over the years. Although the reasons for this are undoubtedly multifactorial, they probably relate to (1) improved resuscitation and tissue perfusion after injury, (2) increased use of enteral feedings, and (3) meticulous attention to adjusting the gastric pH.[20] Many approaches to the latter can be successful. We use antacids every 2 hours to keep the pH greater than 4.5. In addition, we use vitamin A (10,000 U every other day) to protect the gastric mucosa and cholestyramine to bind bile refluxing from the duodenum. Sucralfate prevents erosive gastritis but is associated with an increased risk of pneumonia in burn patients.[21]

PROVISION OF NUTRITIONAL SUPPORT ■

HYPERMETABOLISM OF BURNS

Before the recognition in late 1970s of the nutritional needs of burn patients, those with severe burn injuries, if they survived, languished in hospital wards with minimal oral intake until they became severely cachectic. Currently it is clear that appropriate nutrition plays a significant role in improving outcome from severe burn injuries.[22]

ENTERAL FEEDING

Although early parenteral feeding has been associated with increased mortality because of an increase in the risk of infections,[23] early enteral feeding has been proposed because it may reduce the translocation of bacteria from the intestinal lumen.[24] Passage of bacteria from the gut into the intestinal lymphatics or portal venous system probably occurs in all healthy individuals. However, the intestinal edema that accompanies the burn resuscitation period and the immunosuppression that follows makes it difficult for the body to clear these microorganisms effectively. Microbial products, either live organisms or cell wall fragments, disseminate through the body prompting the release of cytokines such as tumor necrosis factor (TNF), interleukin-1 (IL-1), and interleukin-6 (IL-6). These cytokines exacerbate the hypermetabolic response and may initiate the systemic inflammatory response syndrome. The rationale for enteral feeding within the first 24 hours of injury is that the presence of food in the gut lumen reduces the rate of microbial translocation. Although not proven definitively in the clinical setting of burn patients, safety and simplicity of early feeding has been demonstrated.[25] One approach is to slowly infuse tube feedings through the nasogastric tube at 10 to 20 mL/hour. Although this clearly does not meet the nutritional needs of adult patients, the small amount of tube feedings is enough to protect the gut mucosa. Long feeding tubes can be placed into the small bowel using endoscopy or fluoroscopy. The advantages of such tubes are higher and earlier rates of infusion, and continuous feeding of patients during surgical procedures requiring general anesthesia.

Despite the theoretical advantages of enteral feeding, difficulties exist. Patients receive, on average, only 80% of the goal rate for enteral feedings because of frequent interruptions for patient care, including radiologic procedures and surgery.[26] This deficit increases when patients develop intestinal ileus, as typically occurs with major infection. Osmotic diarrhea is troublesome, particularly when patients'

feces soil the burn wound dressings. A variety of techniques combat diarrhea, including replacement of intestinal flora with lactobacillus granules and nonpasteurized yogurt, and retardation of small bowel motility with diphenoxylate HCl. Despite the theoretical advantages and need for calories provided by enteral feeding, difficulties exist, and the technique cannot be used in all patients.

PARENTERAL FEEDING

The estimated caloric and protein needs of a patient can be met more reliably with parenteral than enteral feeding. The central venous catheter, which predisposes the patient to invasive infections, particularly the *Candida* species, is a disadvantage. Reports suggest the rate of bacterial translocation is increased with the use of parenteral nutrition compared with enteral nutrition, and that infection rates are higher.[27] Long-term use of parenteral nutrition alone is associated with hepatobiliary dysfunction, including cholestatic hepatitis and acalculous cholecystitis. Nevertheless, parenteral nutrition can be used for patients who do not tolerate enteral feedings because of paralytic ileus of the intestine or diarrhea, and for patients returned to the operating room frequently for serial escharectomies.

ESTIMATION OF CALORIC NEEDS

Burn injury results in an increase in the metabolic expenditure,[28] and initial investigative work performed in the 1970s demonstrates that some burn patients needed as many as 7000 or 8000 kcal/day to maintain weight.[29] Although burn patients still become hypercatabolic after injury, they do not become so to the same degree from changes in management. Because of the effect of earlier enteral feeding and the introduction of procedures that promote early wound closure, the increase in metabolic rate has diminished. Recently, indirect calorimetry has shown that the most severe injuries require no more calories than two times the resting energy expenditure as described by the Harrison-Benedict formula.[30]

Indirect calorimetry is a frequently used tool to estimate caloric needs in these hypermetabolic patients. Studies suggest that this procedure prevents gross underestimation or overestimation of the patient's caloric needs, but in most patients it is probably not superior to estimating their needs from a formula alone.[31] The resting energy expenditure calculated by the Harrison-Benedict formula is multiplied by a stress factor in direct proportion to the size of burn. The stress factor is judged conservatively to avoid overfeeding, which is associated with increased susceptibility to infection (Table 82-1).

PROTEIN REPLETION

Wound repair depends on amino acids, the building blocks. Yet the type of protein used in enteral feedings is also controversial. Evidence suggests partially hydrolyzed proteins are better absorbed and maintain serum proteins better than whole protein or elemental amino acids.[32] The amino acids

TABLE 82-1. Stress Factors for Energy Expenditure Related to Burn Size

TBSA BURN	STRESS FACTOR
0–10%	1.4
11–20%	1.5
21–30%	1.6
31–40%	1.7
41–50%	1.8
51–60%	1.9
>60%	2.0

HARRISON-BENEDICT EQUATIONS[30]

Women:
$$REE = 655 + [4.3 \times Wt\ (lb)] + [4.3 \times Ht\ in)] - [4.7 \times age]$$
Men:
$$REE = 65 + [6.2 \times Wt\ (lb)] + [12.7 \times Ht\ (in)] - [6.8 \times age]$$

TBSA, total body surface area; REE, resting energy expenditure; Wt, weight; Ht, height.

arginine and glutamine have immune-enhancing properties, improve nitrogen retention, and maintain lean body mass. Formulas containing arginine supplements have been reported to reduce infections in trauma patients[33] and to reduce length of stay of critically ill patients.[34]

Judging the amount of protein necessary for recovery from burn injuries is difficult. Massive and unquantified loss of protein from the burn wound exudate precludes nitrogen balance studies based on urine excretion alone. Sequential measurements of serum proteins such as transferrin and prealbumin are a better index of the body's response to the amount and type of dietary protein given, but few clinical studies show a correlation between increase in serum proteins and improved clinical outcome. It is important to avoid overfeeding of protein because it predisposes patients to sepsis.[35] Amounts of protein greater than 3 g/kg/day in adults are usually not tolerated because of azotemia. Dietary protein should be started at an administration rate of 1.5 g/kg/day and should be increased if there is not a subsequent increase in serum protein markers. A patient's diet can also be supplemented with vitamins A and C, and with the trace element zinc, all of which improve wound healing.

TRANSITION TO ORAL FEEDING

Successful weaning of patients from nutritional supplements sometimes occurs earlier than expected. A regular diet with liquid supplements is offered within 24 hours after extubation. The increased thirst of burn patients is used to encourage the intake of protein-containing solutions, either soy- or milk-based supplements, or protein-containing fruit drinks. Using supplements, patients can take up to 2000 kcal each day. It is preferable to feed patients or allow them to feed themselves because of the inherent risks of feeding tubes and central lines.

DIAGNOSIS AND TREATMENT OF SERIOUS INFECTIONS ■

IMMUNOSUPPRESSION OF BURN INJURY

There is no greater problem for the burn patient than infection. Loss of the mechanical barrier between the human body and the environment is the first step in the weakening of defenses. All aspects of the immune system, including phagocytosis, soluble mediators of innate immunity such as complement, antibody production, and cellular (T-cell) defense systems, are compromised by severe burn injury.[36] The most common cause of death in burn patients after the first 48 hours is infection.

INFECTION CONTROL

Actions of the health care team can compromise patient survival. All catheters invading the body, including endotracheal tubes, central venous catheters, and bladder catheters, must be handled with as clean a technique as possible. Although the skin and gut are the source of endogenous bacteria, a greater threat to the patient is colonization with antibiotic-resistant pathogens carried by the burn team from other patients. Washing of hands must be done *without fail* after handling the patient, the patient's bed, or equipment. If dressings are removed and wounds exposed, then sterile gloves must be worn. Compulsive hand-washing alone probably prevents infection more than any other single action. Infection control policies vary from burn center to burn center, but the philosophy remains the same: make every effort to minimize the transmission of bacteria from patient to patient!

DIAGNOSIS OF INFECTIONS

Diagnosis of invasive infection in the burn patient is unusually difficult. All burn patients have elevated core temperatures and white blood cell counts. The significance of these commonly used signs of infection becomes blunted in the burn patient. Helpful signs of infection are the appearance of sugar in the urine, particularly if this appears paradoxically when the blood sugar is within normal limits. Hyperglycemia and increased difficulty in controlling the blood sugars of diabetics are signs of threatening sepsis. A drop in the platelet count, particularly in children, is an early warning sign of sepsis.[37] Qualitative wound cultures done by swabbing the wound yield no new information other than the nature of the bacterial species colonizing the surface of the wound. On the other hand, a biopsy of the burn wound permits a quantitative assay of the number of colony-forming units (CFU) of bacteria per gram of tissue. Burn wound sepsis is likely if the colony count is greater than 10^5 CFU/g, and the quantitative culture also allows isolation and identification of the invading organism. Manifestations of multiple organ dysfunction, such as hypotension, hypoxia, decreased pulmonary compliance, renal failure, or hepatic dysfunction are almost certain signs of septic shock.

TREATMENT OF INFECTIONS

Two questions arise once the diagnosis of infection is suspected. First, does the patient need to be on antibiotics?[238] A sudden change in a patient's condition, such as the onset of high fever in a previously afebrile patient, should prompt serious consideration of initial empiric antibiotic therapy, which can be adjusted later. Although it is preferable to treat known organisms that have known sensitivities, broad-spectrum antibiotics are used until microbial identification is complete. A combination of a penicillin and an aminoglycoside is effective against aerobic gram-positive and gram-negative bacteria; coverage against anaerobic organisms is not necessary. The patient in florid septic shock should be treated with antibiotics, but, unfortunately, the stage is already set for progression to full-blown multiple organ system failure and possibly death. Unfortunately, prophylactic antibiotics have not been shown to improve outcome in burn patients, and widespread empiric use of antibiotics predisposes to the development of antibiotic-resistant strains of bacteria and fungal infections.

The second question to be answered is, do the burn wounds need to be excised?[239] Escharectomy should be done early in the patient's hospital course, because once burn wound infection is established, removal of the eschar may not be sufficient to stop the cascade of events already in motion. In some cases, the systemic reaction to infection is not caused by the widespread proliferation of bacteria throughout the organs of the body but is rather the systemic cytokine response as a result of the outpouring of high levels of inflammatory mediators such as TNF, IL-1, and IL-6. Currently there is no effective treatment for this systemic inflammatory response other than supportive care. Early escharectomy in burn patients is the best preventive measure. Eschar can be conceptualized as an abscess, similar to one sitting inside the peritoneal cavity, except that the pus is on the outside of the body. Removal of the dead, burned skin can have the same effect on the patient's outcome as draining the intraabdominal abscess.

CARE OF THE BURN WOUND ◼

DEPTH OF INJURY

Burn wounds are divided into second- and third-degree wounds, based on the depth of injury. (First-degree burns do not have a significant physiologic effect on the patient, except at the extremes of age, and, therefore, are not typically counted in burn size evaluation.) Second-degree burns penetrate into, but not through, the dermis. Because of the epithelial cells that line the sebaceous glands and the hair follicles, regeneration of epithelium can be accomplished from these discrete islands. The time needed for complete reepithelialization is proportional to the depth of the second-degree burn. Third-degree burns destroy the total depth of the skin, resulting in an open wound with granulation tissue that has no inherent capability of reepithelializing; such wounds close only by contraction. Third-degree burns need

to be closed by split-thickness autografts; this should be done as soon as it is safe.

Superficial second-degree burns reepithelialize within 2 to 3 weeks. Because these shallow burns gain a new layer of skin in time, there is no advantage to the patient in creating a donor site, which will also require 2 weeks to close. Operative debridement of the burns is useful, however, if there is a thick layer of protein exudate adherent to the wound, or if there is cellulitis of the burn wound that does not respond to antibiotic therapy.

Deep second-degree burns require 4 to 6 weeks for reepithelialization. There are disadvantages to allowing these deep second-degree burns to reepithelialize over such a long period of time. First, the patient is at risk of infection throughout the period while the wounds are open. If the area of deep second-degree burns is large enough, the risk may be life-threatening. Second, healing of deep second-degree burns by secondary intention results in poor functional and cosmetic outcomes. Third, the open wounds are painful and interfere with physical therapy.

EXCISION OF BURN WOUNDS

One technique of wound care starts with removal of tenacious protein exudate or burn eschar within the first 5 days after injury in the operating room. Wound excision frequently needs to be done in stages unless the burn is less than 10% of TBSA. Tangential excision can create significant intraoperative blood loss. To minimize the physiologic impact, the initial operations are limited to removal of the burned skin, leaving skin grafting for later dates. The excised wounds are treated with antibiotic creams or covered with skin substitutes. Early escharectomy of the burn wound has probably contributed as much to the better outcome of patients in the last 20 years as any other change in therapy.[40]

TOPICAL TREATMENT OF BURN WOUNDS

Burn wounds are treated from the time of admission with silver sulfadiazine cream. The advantages of silver sulfadiazine cream include a spectrum of antimicrobial activity and a high level of comfort for the patient. The dressings are removed, the wounds debrided, and the silver sulfadiazine reapplied twice a day at the bedside. Silver sulfadiazine cream is not active on the wound for longer than 12 hours.

Mafenide acetate cream is a second topical agent that has the advantage of penetrating the burn eschar better than silver sulfadiazine cream. The disadvantage of mafenide acetate cream is that it causes pain and discomfort, although this discomfort lessens after 15 to 20 minutes. Metabolic acidosis may occur if mafenide acetate is applied to large surface areas because it is a carbonic anhydrase inhibitor. Nonetheless, we occasionally use it on apparently heavily colonized wounds, alternating with silver sulfadiazine. Its application is limited to 25% of the TBSA to prevent or minimize metabolic acidosis. It is also applied to wounds the night before excision to minimize the bacteremia during escharectomy. It is applied to burned ears because it penetrates into the cartilage of the helix.

The simplest and safest method to treat donor sites in critically ill burn patients is to use silver sulfadiazine cream. With this cream, donor sites take 7 to 10 days to close with little chance of becoming infected, but the patient has pain because the wound is cleaned twice a day. Alternatives available are petrolatum-soaked gauze with bismuth, or an elastic nylon mesh impregnated with a surface layer of silicone. The advantage of these synthetic coverings is that patients do not have to undergo dressing changes. The disadvantage is a greater incidence of infection of the donor sites.

THE IMPORTANCE OF PHYSIOTHERAPY ■

PREVENTION OF CONTRACTURES

Physical and occupational therapists visit the patient on the first day after admission. Independent of the patient's general condition, injured upper and lower extremities can be elevated to allow adequate venous drainage and to reduce edema. Passive exercises are begun and, if alert and cooperative, the patient is asked to participate in active exercises. Active and passive exercises to maintain range of motion of the joints are continued throughout hospitalization and the out-patient rehabilitation period.[41]

Two important axioms influence rehabilitation. First, the burn wound will shorten by contraction until it meets an opposing force. Across a flexor surface, this results in a contracture. Second, the position of comfort is the position of contracture. Range-of-motion exercises prevent tendon shortening and restriction of joint motion by burn scar contractures. As patients begin to recover and participate actively in therapy, exercises are designed to increase muscle strength and endurance. A return to activities of daily living frequently takes months.

HETEROTOPIC OSSIFICATION

An abnormal deposition of calcium phosphate crystals in joint spaces or along tendons is a complication of burn injury.[42] Heterotopic ossification restricts the motion of joints, particularly the elbows and knees. Unlike heterotopic ossification seen in spinal cord patients, it does not respond to treatment with etidronate disodium, and early surgical removal is not indicated. Resolution occurs with time in most patients, and few need surgical removal of the ossified crystals in the joints.

THE PSYCHOSOCIAL NEEDS OF THE PATIENT AND FAMILY ■

COUNSELING

Burn injuries are dramatic and are psychologically traumatic for the patient and for those witnessing the accident. Counseling for the patient and family begins the day of admission. Families require support, and burn health care providers should routinely plan meetings. Critically ill burn patients are on a roller coaster ride between life and death that does not stop until the burn wounds are closed, sometimes 2 to 3 months after injury. The family needs to be informed and provided with the means to care for their own physical and psychological needs. It is particularly stressful for families of patients who were transferred from a great distance and who lack nearby support systems. The need to provide support for families can not be overemphasized.

PAIN MANAGEMENT

Patients are preoccupied with pain from the injury and concern about the cosmetic appearance left from the burn scars. Pain management is one of the most challenging issues in burn care.[43] Proper doses of narcotics, such as morphine and sedatives such as benzodiazepines, for both procedural and background pain, are mandatory. Long-acting oral analgesics are given to combat the background pain, but there is no effective substitution in the acute stages for the use of intravenous analgesics.

CHANGES IN LEVEL OF CONSCIOUSNESS

In all patients, awareness and responsiveness decline after the first few days. No neurologic findings accompany this decline to suggest a focal central nervous system lesion. Obtundation may also be related to high doses of narcotics, the outpouring of stress hormones and cytokines after the massive inflammatory response, and to sleep deprivation.[44] Some patients do not regain an alert level of consciousness until the burn wounds are nearly closed. Families need to be reassured that no long-term neurologic sequelae are associated with this depression of mental status.

THE TEAM APPROACH TO BURN CARE ■

Care of burn patients requires a team approach.[45] The primary goal is to keep the patient alive. When a patient's survival is assured, the secondary goal is to ensure that the patient regains the highest quality of life possible. Patients with deep burns of the hands provide a good example. Excision of burn wounds of the hands is done early as part of the overall plan of removing the dead and injured skin to prevent widespread infection. Priority is given to autografting of the hands. Once the skin grafts are adherent and vascularized, physical and occupational therapists can begin to focus on range of motion exercises. As the patient becomes alert and responsive, reassurance and support are provided by the nursing staff while the patient progresses through the painful stages of healing. The patient requires the intervention of a social worker or a psychologist to deal with the overwhelming feelings associated with recovery from the accident, with the pain that accompanies the recovery, and the temporary or permanent loss of function. The team approach is continued throughout outpatient rehabilitation.

REFERENCES

1. Sharar SR, Heimbach DM: Inhalation injury: current concepts and controversies. *Adv Trauma Crit Care* 1991;6:213
2. Demling RH: Smoke inhalation injury. *New Horizons* 1993;1:422
3. Bowers BL, Purdue GF, Hunt JL: Paranasal sinusitis in burn patients following nasotracheal intubation. *Arch Surg* 1991;126:1411
4. Ward CG, Gorham K, Hammond JS, et al: Securing endotracheal tubes on patients with facial burns or trauma. *Am J Surg* 1990;159:339
5. Lund T, Goodwin CW, McManus WF, et al: Upper airway sequelae in burn patients requiring endotracheal intubation or tracheostomy. *Ann Surg* 1985;201:374
6. Clark WR: Smoke inhalation: diagnosis and treatment. *World J Surg* 1992;16:24
7. Youn YK, LaLonde C, Demling R: The role of mediators in the response to thermal injury. *World J Surg* 1992;16:30
8. Baxter C, Shires T: Physiologic response to crystalloid resuscitation of severe burns. *Ann NY Acad Sci* 1968;150:874
9. Monafo WW, Halverson JD, Schechtman K: The role of concentrated sodium solutions in the resuscitation of patients with severe burns. *Surgery* 1984;95:129
10. Moylan JA, Inge WW, Pruitt BA: Circulatory changes following circumferential extremity burns evaluated by the ultrasonic flowmeter: an analysis of 60 thermally injured limbs. *J Trauma* 1971;11:763
11. Saffle JR, Zeluff GR, Warden GD: Intramuscular pressure in the burned arm: measurement and response to escharotomy. *Am J Surg* 1980;140:825
12. Morehouse JD, Finkelstein JL, Marano MA, et al: Resuscitation of the thermally injured patient. *Crit Care Clin* 1992;8:355
13. Heimbach DM: Early burn excision and grafting. *Surg Clin North Am* 1987;67:93
14. Remensnyder JP: Acute electrical injuries. In: Martyn JAJ (ed). *Acute Management of the Burned Patient.* Philadelphia: WB Saunders, 1990:66
15. Szyfeldbein SK, Drop LJ, Martyn JAJ: Persistent ionized hypocalcemia in patients during resuscitation and recovery phases of body burns. *Crit Care Med* 1981;9:454
16. Sosa JL, Ward CG, Hammond JS: The relationship of burn wound fluid to serum creatinine and creatinine clearance. *J Burn Care Rehabil* 1992;13:437
17. Boucher BA, Kuhl DA, Hickerson WL: Pharmacokinetics of systemically administered antibiotics in patients with thermal injury. *Clin Infect Dis* 1992;14:458
18. Neely AN, Warden GD, Rieman M, et al: Components of the increased circulating proteolytic activity in pediatric burn patients. *J Trauma* 1992;33:807
19. Rue LW, Cioffi WG, Rush R, et al: Thromboembolic complications in thermally injured patients. *World J Surg* 1992;16:1151
20. McAlhany JC, Czaja AJ, Pruitt BA: Antacid control of complications from acute gastroduodenal disease after burns. *J Trauma* 1976;16:645
21. Cioffi WG, McManus AT, Rue LW, et al: Comparison of acid neutralizing and non-acid neutralizing stress ulcer prophylaxis in thermally injured patients. *J Trauma* 1994;36:544
22. Alexander JW, MacMillan BG, Stinnett JD, et al: Beneficial effects of aggressive protein feeding in severely burned children. *Ann Surg* 1980;192:505
23. Herndon DN, Barrow RE, Stein M, et al: Increased mortality with intravenous supplemental feeding in severely burned patients. *J Burn Care Rehabil* 1989;10:309
24. Mochizuki H, Trocki O, Dominioni L, et al: Mechanism of prevention of postburn hypermetabolism and catabolism by early enteral feeding. *Ann Surg* 1984;300:297
25. McArdle AH, Palmason C, Brown RA, et al: Early enteral feeding of patients with major burns: prevention of catabolism. *Ann Plast Surg* 1984;13:396
26. Adams S, Dellinger P, Wertz M, et al: Enteral versus parenteral nutritional support following laparotomy for trauma: a randomized prospective trial. *J Trauma* 1986;26:882
27. Kudsk KA, Croce MA, Fabian TC, et al: Enteral versus parenteral feeding. *Ann Surg* 1992;215:503
28. Goodwin CW: Metabolism and nutrition in the thermally injured patient. *Crit Care Clin* 1985;1:97
29. Wilmore DW, Curreri PW, Spitzer KW, et al: Supranormal dietary intake in thermally injured hypermetabolic patients. *Surg Gynecol Obstet* 1971;132:881
30. Cunningham JJ: Factors contributing to increased energy expenditure in thermal injury: a review of studies employing indirect calorimetry. *J Parenter Enter Nutr* 1990;14:649
31. Saffle JR, Larson CM, Sullivan J: A randomized trial of indirect calorimetry-based feedings in thermal injury. *J Trauma* 1990;30:776
32. Trocki O, Mochizuki H, Dominioni L, et al: Intact protein versus free amino acids in the nutritional support of thermally injured animals. *J Parenter Enter Nutr* 1986;10:139
33. Moore FA, Moore EE, Kudsk KA, et al: Clinical benefits of an immune-enhancing diet for early postinjury enteral feeding. *J Trauma* 1994;37:607
34. Bower RH, Cerra FB, Bershadsky B, et al: Early enteral administration of a formula (ImpactRM) supplemented with arginine, nucleotides, and fish oil in intensive care unit patients: results of a multicenter, prospective, randomized, clinical trial. *Crit Care Med* 1995;23:436
35. Peck MD: Sepsis. In: Zaloga GP (ed). *Nutrition in Critical Care.* St Louis: CV Mosby, 1994:599
36. Ninnemann JL: Clinical and immune status of burn patients. *Antibiot Chemother* 1987;39:16
37. Housinger TA, Brinkerhoff C, Warden GD: The relationship between platelet count, sepsis, and survival in pediatric burn patients. *Arch Surg* 1993;128:65
38. Mozingo DW, McManus AT, Pruitt BA: Appropriate use of parenteral antibiotics in managing burns. *Surg Infect Index Rev* 1993;1:16
39. Briggs SE: Rationale for acute surgical approach. In: Martyn JAJ (ed). *Acute Management of the Burned Patient.* Philadelphia: WB Saunders, 1990:118
40. Tompkins RG, Burke JF, Schoenfeld DA, et al: Prompt eschar excision: a treatment system contributing to reduced burn mortality. A statistical evaluation of burn care at the Massachusetts General Hospital (1974–1984). *Ann Surg* 1986;204:272
41. Robson, MD, Barnett RA, Leitch IOW, et al: Prevention and treatment of postburn scars and contracture. *World J Surg* 1992;16:87
42. Tepperman PS, Hilbert L, Peters WJ, et al: Heterotopic ossification in burns. *J Burn Care Rehabil* 1984;5:283
43. Osgood PF, Szyfelbein SK: Management of pain. In: Martyn JAJ (ed). *Acute Management of the Burned Patient.* Philadelphia: WB Saunders, 1990:201
44. Gotschlich MM, Jenkins ME, Mayes T, et al: A prospective clinical study of the polysomnographic stages of sleep after burn injury. *J Burn Care Rehabil* 1994;15:486
45. Ward CG: Burn care: a multidisciplinary specialty. *QRB Qual Rev Bull* 1979;2:2

Critical Care, Third Edition, edited by Joseph M. Civetta,
Robert W. Taylor, and Robert R. Kirby.
Lippincott-Raven Publishers, Philadelphia, PA © 1997.

CHAPTER 83

■

The Obese Surgical Patient

Scott A. Shikora

Jay A. Johannigman

IMMEDIATE CONCERNS ■

MAJOR PROBLEMS

Management of morbidly obese patients in the critical care
setting is challenging and complex. Recent surveys suggest
that 25% of American adults are overweight, and 5% to 10%
qualify as morbidly obese. Morbidly obese patients may
have significant physiologic deficits in cardiac and pulmonary
performance. When this preexisting morbidity is combined
with perioperative changes unique to obese patients, a state
of critical illness often develops. Successful management of
critically ill, morbidly obese patients requires a combination
of preoperative preparation and perioperative interventions.

STRESS POINTS

1. Morbidly obese patients are prone to the development
   of significant cardiovascular disease. These changes
   include the development of left ventricular hypertrophy, chronic systemic hypertension (increased afterload), and pulmonary hypertension. When untreated,
   these factors predispose obese patients to diminished
   cardiac reserve and congestive heart failure (CHF).
2. Obese patients characteristically display alterations in
   pulmonary function. The most common alterations
   include decreases in functional residual capacity
   (FRC) and expiratory reserve volume (ERV). When
   this baseline dysfunction is combined with perioperative changes (i.e., incisional pain, supine position), a
   marked increase in pulmonary morbidity occurs.
3. Sleep apnea is a common occurrence in morbidly
   obese patients. Recognition of sleep apnea and appropriate therapeutic intervention is necessary when managing the obese patient in the ICU.

4. Obesity may be an independent risk factor for the
   development of thromboembolic disease. The diagnosis of a thromboembolic event may be more difficult
   in obese patients. Postoperative stasis and delay in
   ambulation may further increase the risk for thromboembolism in the obese patient.
5. Nutritional support plays a key role in the successful
   management of the obese patient. Early nutritional
   intervention prevents protein wasting and may improve immune response. Use of protein-sparing modified fast (PSMF) may promote the use of endogenous
   fat for energy while maintaining nitrogen homeostasis.

ESSENTIAL DIAGNOSTIC TESTS
AND PROCEDURES

1. Cardiac status should be evaluated by preoperative
   echocardiography. Invasive hemodynamic monitoring
   with a pulmonary artery catheter may allow more accurate determination of ventricular performance.
2. Pulmonary function testing is essential for any morbidly obese patient undergoing major surgery. Early
   mobilization of the obese patient is important, including use of special care beds that allow positioning in
   the upright, sitting positions.
3. Obstructive sleep apnea must be recognized and may
   require evaluation by a pulmonary function laboratory.
4. Pulse oximetry is a useful adjunct in detecting arterial
   hypoxemia in the perioperative period.

INITIAL THERAPY

1. Cardiac monitoring and pulse oximetry should be considered a minimum standard in any obese patient undergoing surgery.

1277

2. Invasive hemodynamic monitoring often allows more precise estimation of ventricular performance. The additional precision provided by use of a pulmonary artery catheter may be of particular benefit in morbidly obese patients with ventricular hypertrophy, pulmonary hypertension, or dilated cardiomyopathy.

3. Mechanical ventilation is often required, with specific attention to preserving or regaining FRC.

OVERVIEW ■

Management of morbidly obese patients poses novel clinical challenges that are often poorly understood. This chapter defines and discusses the unique aspects of critical care in this population.

Obesity is defined as body weight greater than 20% above the ideal weight standard for height and sex. The National Health and Nutrition Examination Surveys 1976–1980 found that 25% of adult Americans, or about 34 million persons, are overweight.[1,2] Of these people, as many as six million are morbidly obese (45 kg [100 lb] or 100% above the ideal weight standard).

Obesity is recognized as a major health concern of western society. Associated with significant obesity are coronary artery disease, diabetes mellitus, hypertension, hepatobiliary disease, endocrine abnormalities, malignancies, degenerative joint disease, cerebral vascular disease, respiratory abnormalities, and sudden death.[3–6] Studies indicate that the relative risks of these conditions have a curvilinear relationship with weight.[3] As weight increases, the prevalence of such illnesses increases disproportionately.[3,7]

In addition to the many medical conditions associated with severe obesity, surgical morbidity is more prevalent in this population.[8] Wound complications, thromboembolic disease, myocardial infarction, respiratory failure requiring mechanical ventilatory support, sepsis, and sudden death may be seen even after minor operative procedures. Therefore, severely obese patients are at risk for complications that may require transfer to an ICU. In addition, these patients can be less likely to respond favorably to therapy, thereby prolonging the ICU stay with its inherent complications. Whereas all critically ill patients warrant excellent, comprehensive care, the unique characteristics of the obese demand a special approach to management.

CARDIOVASCULAR DISEASE ■

Hippocrates was the first to observe that "sudden death is more common in those who are naturally fat than in the lean."[9] In a more contemporary time frame, the first recognition of a possible association between obesity and ventricular dysfunction seems to be the report by Smith and Wilhius in 1933.[10] Since this initial description, a progressive detailing of the physiologic, pathologic, and anatomic changes that occur in the cardiovascular system of the morbidly obese patient has evolved.

CARDIAC FUNCTION

Any increase in body mass must be accompanied by a concomitant expansion of intravascular volume and cardiac output to meet the needs of the added mass. The high-output state of the obese patient is, in part, a reflection of the need to support the metabolic demands of adipose tissue. Fat is an active metabolic tissue; therefore, net oxygen consumption of the morbidly obese patient is often higher than would be predicted from comparison to a lean patient.

Increased cardiac output results from increased stroke volume because heart rate remains relatively unchanged with obesity. Increases in left ventricular filling volume and pressure generate this elevated stroke volume. With time, these changes result in chamber dilatation and increased wall stress (tension). The ventricle's compensation for this increased wall tension is the addition of myocardial contractile units. Thus, patients with moderate to severe obesity characteristically demonstrate some degree of eccentric left ventricular hypertrophy.

HYPERTENSION

Obesity not only generates a state of increased preload and left ventricular hypertrophy, but also predisposes to the development of hypertension.[11,12] The etiology of hypertension is multifactorial and includes elevated levels of catecholamines[13] and mineralocorticoids.[14] If obesity and hypertension are present in the same patient, the left ventricle has to compensate for a double task: the augmented preload/filling volume of obesity and the high afterload produced by hypertension. If this burden persists, it promotes left ventricular dysfunction and predisposes the patient to CHF. Because the degree of ventricular dysfunction may be difficult to assess during a routine preoperative examination, procedures such as echocardiography can be of value.

PULMONARY VASCULAR CHANGES

Hemodynamic changes associated with hypoxemia further complicate the obese patient's cardiac status. The obesity hypoventilation syndrome is associated with chronic hypoxemia, hypercapnia, and respiratory acidosis. It is present in 5% to 10% of extremely obese patients,[15] and may be the result of a series of events triggered by obstructive sleep apnea. This condition results in transient hypoxemia and blunting of the hypoxic ventilatory drive. The increased work of breathing associated with obesity effects a similar diminished ventilatory response to carbon dioxide. A chronic state of hypercapnia and hypoxemia results that promotes pulmonary vasoconstriction and hypotension. The right ventricle is thus exposed to increased flow and pulmonary hypertension; right ventricular hypertrophy ensues.

CLINICAL IMPLICATIONS

The morbidly obese patient has a multiplicity of physiologic events that may promote eccentric left ventricular hypertrophy, right ventricular hypertrophy, combined pulmonary and systemic venous congestion, or a combination of these problems. The significant potential for underlying cardiac dysfunction dictates that a thorough cardiac evaluation be included in the preoperative preparation. The inclusion of two-dimensional (2-D) echocardiography as a requisite component of the preoperative evaluation of the obese patient is prudent to determine the presence and extent of cardiac dysfunction.

Cardiac disease may be difficult to recognize in obesity. Limited exercise tolerance secondary to weight often prevents the manifestations of symptoms such as angina or CHF. In addition, extreme weight may frustrate attempts at exercise tolerance studies or invasive testing. Furthermore, cardiac disease can be occult in younger patients and, therefore, not require treatment before the development of a critical illness.

To minimize the risks of complications, cardiac monitoring is essential. Pulmonary artery catheters are commonly used for monitoring fluid status and cardiac performance. Careful attention must be given to prevent fluid overload. Standard estimations of daily fluid requirements based on body weight are inaccurate. Fluid administration should be titrated by sequential measurement of cardiac filling pressures, urine output, estimates of peripheral perfusion, or all three. Adequate monitoring of oxygenation must be ensured, most commonly by pulse oximetry. Supplemental oxygen and mechanical ventilation may be required more often than in lean individuals.

PULMONARY DISEASE ■

Critically ill obese patients often have associated pulmonary problems. They typically are at greater risk of aspiration pneumonia. For reasons not entirely clear, when compared with the nonobese, the stomachs of overweight patients usually have a larger-than-normal gastric fluid volume and a lower pH.[16] In addition, these patients typically have abnormally high intraabdominal pressure secondary to the large panniculus and increased intraabdominal fat. This problem is exacerbated in the critically ill, who spend most of their time in the supine position. The increase in pressure, coupled with voluminous acidic gastric contents, promote gastroesophageal reflux, pulmonary aspiration, and pneumonia.

The degree to which morbid obesity contributes to respiratory dysfunction has been the subject of numerous investigations. The results of these studies have produced a wide range of conclusions, ranging from no baseline abnormalities to severe dysfunction. This disparity partly results from variation in the definition and age of the population studied. A review of the current literature suggests that a distinct number of respiratory alterations must be considered and evaluated in managing the morbidly obese patient.

CHANGES IN PULMONARY FUNCTION

The most frequently described alterations in the obese patient's pulmonary function are decreased FRC and decreased ERV.[17-19] These changes result from splinting and cephalad displacement of the diaphragm during tidal breath-

ing and predispose obese patients to atelectasis and pulmonary shunting. Ray and coworkers[20] studied 43 otherwise healthy, young (19 to 32 years of age), nonsmoking, morbidly obese patients. This work demonstrated that most obese subjects fell within the 95% confidence limits of normal for the predicted values of pulmonary function tests. Observed changes fell into two general classes: (1) those that changed in proportion to degree of obesity (ERV and diffusing capacity), and (2) those that changed only with extreme obesity (vital capacity, total lung capacity, and maximal voluntary ventilation). These findings suggest that baseline dysfunction is minimal in young, nonsmoking, obese patients.

The loss of FRC and ERV demonstrated in most series of morbidly obese patients has important clinical implications in the perioperative period. As FRC falls, it begins to approach the volume at which airway closure occurs (Fig. 83-1). When FRC falls below closing volume, significant dysfunction ensues as a result of alveolar collapse and alveolar air trapping. The baseline loss of FRC may be further complicated by the physiologic changes effected by surgery. Upper abdominal surgery reduces FRC by as much as 30%.[21] The combination of obesity-induced loss of FRC, coupled with postoperative losses, reduces FRC to such a degree that significant arterial hypoxemia readily occurs. Hypoxemia is further aggravated by supine positioning, the head-down Trendelenburg position, and the placement of subdiaphragmatic laparotomy pads to facilitate exposure.[22]

CLINICAL IMPLICATIONS

Maintenance of FRC

The effects of baseline pulmonary dysfunction combined with the physiologic changes of surgery and perioperative care create a patient who must be aggressively managed to limit or reverse hypoxemia. In the ICU, clinicians must intervene with therapeutic measures demonstrated to be of benefit in recovering FRC and reversing alveolar collapse. Positive end-expiratory pressure remains the mainstay of

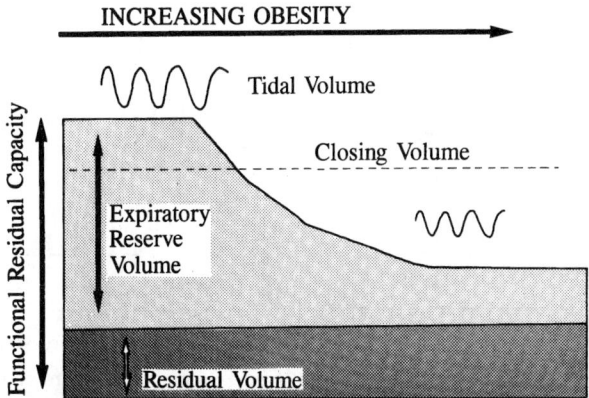

FIGURE 83-1. The progressive decrement in functional residual capacity that occurs with increasing weight results in tidal ventilation occurring at or below closing volume. (From Fox GS: Anaesthesia for intestinal short circuiting in the morbidly obese with reference to the pathophysiology of gross obesity. *Can Anaesth Soc J* 1975;22:307.)

therapy to reestablish FRC and should be used during the intraoperative and perioperative period to recruit collapsed alveolar units.

The hemodynamic implications of positive end-expiratory pressure must be recognized in this group of patients who often display varying degrees of ventricular dysfunction. A simple, yet effective maneuver is the careful use of postoperative positioning (Fig. 83-2). Early mobilization to the upright position results in a significant improvement in FRC during the first 5 postoperative days.[23] Special beds that allow rapid transition to the sitting position facilitate nursing care and, more importantly, are a therapeutic adjunct to reduce postoperative pulmonary morbidity.

Specific Risk Factors

Clinicians must recognize the relationship between obstructive sleep apnea and sudden death. Initial reports of sudden death in the Pickwickian syndrome suggest a pulmonary source,[24,25] which has been confirmed by more recent publications.[26,27] Obese patients who demonstrate hypercapnia (>45 mm Hg), hypoxemia (<60 mm Hg), and a prior history of hospitalization for respiratory disease are more likely to develop respiratory failure that requires intubation.[26]

A high index of suspicion is necessary to provides timely and effective intervention. Evaluation of arterial blood gas values and pulmonary function tests provides valuable information in the preoperative management of obese patients. Those who are identified as having the described risk factors should be maintained in a monitored environment with emphasis on detection of nocturnal hypoxemia and early, aggressive pulmonary support.

Positions

Techniques to minimize respiratory effort can decrease the need for mechanical ventilation. Gravity may be used to improve pulmonary function. When the head of the bed is elevated or the patient is seated in a chair, the intraabdominal contents are displaced downward, allowing greater diaphragmatic excursion. These simple maneuvers may also decrease the incidence of aspiration, whereas nasogastric tube decompression and antacid therapy minimize the risk of reflux.

Support of Gas Exchange

Narcotics and sedatives for pain or anxiety must be used cautiously to prevent respiratory depression. Weaning from mechanical ventilation must be performed carefully using arterial blood gas analysis and pulse oximetry. Hypoxemia or hypercapnia are particularly important signs of fatigue or hypoventilation. Measurement of work of breathing[28] or oxygen cost of breathing may be helpful. Nasal mask continuous positive airway pressure can prevent sleep-related hypoxia. Excellent pulmonary toilet, attention to fluid management, appropriate use of supplemental oxygen, minimal sedation, and mechanical ventilatory support, when necessary, should minimize pulmonary complications.

Operative Interventions

For some patients, prolonged respiratory insufficiency occurs despite the best efforts. Surgical procedures such as tracheotomy or uvulopalatopharyngoplasty[29] may be effective for patients with sleep apnea. However, uvulopalatopharyngoplasty may be less effective in the morbidly obese.[30] Tracheotomy often improves pulmonary toilet, reduces ventilatory effort by relieving soft tissue airway obstruction, and decreases the anatomic dead space. Unfortunately, placement in the obese may be difficult because of abnormal neck anatomy. Some experts recommend specially designed tubes or techniques to overcome the anatomic disadvantages.[31–34]

THROMBOEMBOLIC DISEASE ■

Whether obesity is an independent risk factor for thromboembolism is controversial. In large prospective studies, Quinn and associates[35] and Sigel and coworkers[36] found no association. In contrast, many reports suggest that obesity is a significant risk factor.[37–41] Coon[42] reports that the risk increased one and one half to two times when weight was 20% greater than the standard insurance table values. Bern and coworkers[43] demonstrated that the obese have a deficiency in antithrombin III, a serum protein that inhibits thrombin activity. Unrestricted thrombin activity can lead to an increase in thrombosis. Other conditions that increase the risk of a thrombotic event include sepsis, immobility, increased age, and surgery. Therefore, critically ill, morbidly

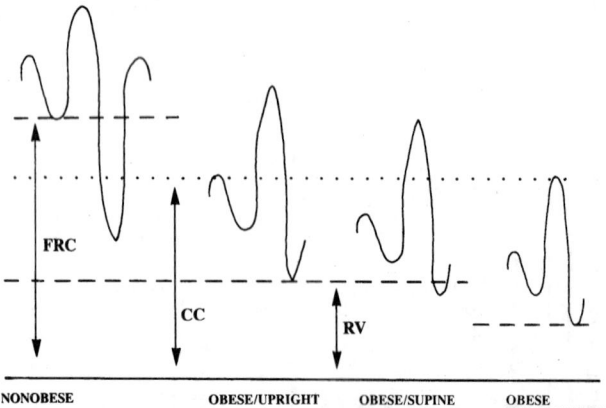

FIGURE 83-2. Effect of position change on lung volumes in obese subjects. Further decline in functional residual capacity (FRC) worsens the relationship between FRC and closing volume or capacity (CC). RV, residual volume. (From Vaughan RW: Pulmonary and cardiovascular derangements in the obese patient. In: Brown BR [ed]. *Anesthesia and the Obese Patient.* Philadelphia, FA Davis, 1982:172.)

obese patients probably are at high risk for thromboembolism.

DIAGNOSIS, PREVENTION, AND TREATMENT

The diagnosis of a thromboembolic event may be difficult. Lower limb venous thrombosis, a common precursor for pulmonary emboli, may be clinically silent, and pulmonary emboli can be asymptomatic or have nonspecific symptoms.[39,44,45] These circumstances are exacerbated in the obese. Physical examination of the lower extremities is usually unreliable, and underlying cardiac and pulmonary disease may mask the symptoms of embolus. Because thromboembolic events can be fatal or severely debilitating, the best treatment is prevention.

Although early ambulation is an excellent preventive measure, it is often impractical in the ICU. For high-risk, critically ill, morbidly obese patients, experts recommend combination therapy.[41,46] Several options are available. For patients at minimal risk for bleeding complications, low-dose heparin is commonly used because several studies report marked reduction in thromboembolic events.[38,39,44,45] Options include twice or three times daily subcutaneous injection or continuous intravenous infusion. Whereas many practitioners administer a larger dose of heparin to compensate for the increase in body mass of obese patients, the goal of treatment is not to achieve true anticoagulation.

In conjunction with heparin therapy, all patients should wear intermittent pneumatic compression sleeves. These devices compress the lower extremities, thereby improving venous flow and stimulating release of prostaglandins that prevent thrombus formation. Other less desirable options for the critically ill include low-dose warfarin and low molecular weight dextran. Warfarin requires oral administration, has too slow an onset of action, and is too unpredictable to be effective. Dextran rarely may cause fluid overload and exacerbate CHF.

SOFT TISSUE PROBLEMS

SKIN CARE AND HYGIENE

Aggressive skin care and hygiene are essential. Increased body weight and immobility exacerbate the risk of skin breakdown and infection. Because of their weight, these patients are difficult to manipulate for bathing and skin inspection. When breakdown does occur, the skin defect usually underestimates the extent of the injury. Necrosis and infection may spread rapidly and widely through the thick subcutaneous fat. Patients may develop extensive infections without manifesting sepsis clinically.

Debridement

Once breakdown is established, proper care dictates aggressive debridement and packing. Often, this approach results in a huge soft tissue defect, usually on the patient's backside, that requires two or three times daily packing changes. These open areas heal with great difficulty and represent an increased risk for sepsis.

Prevention

As is often the case, the best treatment for skin breakdown is prevention. Despite the great efforts needed to turn these patients, daily log rolling for inspection of the back and thorough skin cleaning are essential. Specially constructed beds for the severely obese may be helpful. These beds are designed to facilitate patient movement, thereby improving the ability to provide good skin care. Skin that displays signs of early breakdown must be cared for before further damage is done. The patient must then be positioned to keep body weight off the affected areas.

During the daily skin inspection, all skin folds below the pannus, breasts, groin, and other areas must be spread apart. To minimize the risk of infection, the folds need to be separated, cleaned, dried, and powdered. An antifungal powder is recommended. The covered areas tend to be warm, dark, and moist and, therefore, are an excellent site for bacterial or fungal growth. As with the skin on the patient's dorsum, significant soft tissue infections can develop before the patient becomes clinically septic.

SEPSIS

PREDISPOSING FACTORS

Obese patients are prone to develop sepsis. Wound infections are the most common site. As described earlier, a greater risk of postoperative problems and pneumonia occurs compared with the nonobese because of compromised respiratory mechanics, poor pulmonary toilet, and risk of gastric fluid reflux.

Diabetes Mellitus

Whereas many obese patients have type II diabetes mellitus, others are "silently" glucose intolerant. In either circumstance, hyperglycemia is often found with critical illness because of the insulin resistance associated with the stress response.[47] Hyperglycemia has been shown to adversely affect immunologic function in diabetics and nondiabetic patients,[48-51] thereby increasing the risk of sepsis. Baxter and coworkers[52] demonstrated an increased incidence of sepsis in critically ill diabetic patients whose blood glucose concentration was above 220 mg/dL.

Infections

Other potential sources of sepsis in the obese include catheter infections and decubitus ulcers. Increased body size often obscures anatomic landmarks, greatly increasing the difficulty of central venous or arterial catheter access. Theoretically, the more difficult the access, the more likely the access site is to be contaminated during placement. Decubitus ulcers may develop secondary to immobility and subsequently become infected. Recognition of an infected decubitus ulcer may be delayed by the inability to easily maneuver a heavy patient to assess skin breakdown.

PREVENTION AND TREATMENT

To minimize the risk of sepsis, aggressive pulmonary toilet, early ambulation, and prevention of hyperglycemia should be established goals. In addition, venous and arterial catheters should be placed by the most experienced clinician, not the most junior. Patients should be log-rolled daily and inspected for skin breakdown and other potential sources of sepsis. Operative wounds require frequent examination. A low threshold for exploring a suspicious wound should be maintained. Infected wounds are best treated by opening them widely, establishing drainage, and débriding all nonviable tissue.

DRUG DOSING ■

Obesity causes alterations of normal body composition. Although the lean body tissue compartment is usually enlarged, the adipose tissue mass is increased in a much greater proportion. This relationship significantly alters the bioavailability of medications. Hydrophilic drugs behave similarly in obese and nonobese patients. By contrast, lipophilic drugs have an increased volume of distribution in the abundant fatty tissues.[53] Therefore, larger doses may be required to achieve a serum therapeutic level. In addition, elimination from the serum will be delayed as the medication continues to diffuse out of the fat long after its discontinuation.[53] This phenomenon has potentially adverse effects. Sedatives may have extended activity, thereby preventing ambulation or ventilator weaning.

NUTRITIONAL SUPPORT ■

All critically ill patients, regardless of adiposity, should be nourished in a timely fashion. Hypermetabolism and hypercatabolism of critical illness quickly deplete even abundant nutrient stores. Malnutrition and its consequences are difficult to avoid in the ICU and occur even in the most obese patient. Simply stated, protein-calorie malnutrition is associated with increased morbidity and mortality,[54-56] affecting the respiratory[57] and cardiac systems[58,59] and immune function.[60]

ENTERAL FEEDING

In most cases, feeding should be initiated shortly after hemodynamic stability is achieved, typically within 24 to 48 hours after admission. Enteral nutrition is thought to be superior to total parenteral nutrition (TPN), even for the critically ill. A large body of literature describes benefits in terms of cost, lower complication rate, and favorable effects on metabolic and immune function. The infusion of nutrients intraluminally is important to maintain gut mucosal integrity, a key factor for organism homeostasis and immunologic competence.[61,62] A growing number of studies demonstrate improved nitrogen balance, lower infection rates, improved wound healing, and attenuation of the stress response with early enteral nutrition.[61,63,64]

PARENTERAL FEEDING

Unfortunately, many critically ill patients cannot be adequately nourished by the enteral route, at least initially. Gastrointestinal disease, fluid overload, hyperglycemia, metabolic derangements, formula intolerance, and enteral access difficulty are commonly encountered problems that often mandate parenteral nutrition. In addition, enteral feeding is commonly withheld for surgery and diagnostic tests. Therefore, early in their course, TPN-fed patients tend to receive more nutrients per kilogram of body weight than those given enteral nutrition.[65]

Adverse Effects

Unfortunately for the significantly obese, parenteral nutrition, and to a lesser degree, enteral feeding, can be harmful. This population of patients is susceptible to intravascular volume overload and glucose intolerance. The stress response characteristics of many critically ill patients promotes fluid retention. A close association of obesity and heart disease places the critically ill overweight patient at risk for myocardial infarction, pulmonary edema, and CHF.

Glucose overload associated with feeding has several adverse effects. Concentrated dextrose causes hyperglycemia in both glucose-intolerant and "normal" stressed patients. The administration of excess parenteral glucose enhances lipogenesis, causing hepatic steatosis and subsequent hepatic dysfunction.[66] In addition, excess glucose also increases the production of carbon dioxide, which, in turn, increases respiratory work. For obese individuals with underlying respiratory compromise, this level of respiratory demand can lead to failure.[57,67]

THE PROTEIN-SPARING MODIFIED FAST

The PSMF is a nutritional formulation derived to adequately nourish severely obese patients without adverse effects. It promotes the use of endogenous fat for energy while maintaining nitrogen homeostasis. The PSMF has been widely used for safe, effective weight loss in nonstressed obese patients.[68] This diet relies on the delivery of adequate protein with intentional calorie underfeeding. Typically, it provides approximately 1.5 to 2.0 grams of protein per kilogram of ideal or adjusted body weight (Fig. 83-3). Along with protein, dextrose calories are administered at approximately 60% of the resting energy expenditure. Lipid is usually not provided.

Adjusted BW = .25(ABW - IBW) + IBW

FIGURE 83-3. Equation for calculating adjusted body weight in obesity (body weight >120% of ideal). Adjusted BW, adjusted body weight; ABW, actual body weight; IBW, ideal body weight. (From Wilkens K: Adjustment for obesity. In: *ADA Renal Practice Group Newsletter.* Chicago, American Dietetic Association, 1984.)

Potential Benefits

A protein-sparing, hypocaloric formulation has potential short-term benefits for use in critically ill obese patients.[69] Although experience in this area is limited, the rationale for such a diet is appealing. Potential benefits include the avoidance of glucose-related complications, improved ventilatory mechanics, and increased diuresis. Dickerson and coworkers[70] achieved protein anabolism, increases in serum proteins, and complete wound healing in a group of critically ill obese postoperative patients (Fig. 83-4). Their data also suggest that endogenous fat was oxidized as substrate for energy production.

PREVENTION OF HYPERGLYCEMIA. Despite the exclusive use of dextrose, elevated blood sugar is rarely seen. This finding is unlike the early experience with TPN when formulations provided substantial amounts of dextrose and complications were prevalent. Excessive glucose infusion is associated with lipogenesis. The conversion of glucose into fat increases carbon dioxide production and respiratory demands.[67] The infrequency of hyperglycemia avoids any hyperglycemia-related immune dysfunction.[49-51] Because a smaller amount of glucose is administered with the PSMF, insulin secretion can also be expected to be decreased. Insulin is a potent antinatriuretic hormone; reduced serum levels favor diuresis.[68] By encouraging diuresis and avoiding increased carbon dioxide production, the PSMF may improve respiratory function.[69] For the critically ill obese patient with inherent respiratory dysfunction, this effect can be significant. It may facilitate weaning from mechanical ventilatory support or prevent the need for intubation and mechanical ventilation.

FAT MOBILIZATION AND OXIDATION. Whether the stressed obese patient on hypocaloric feeding can adequately mobilize endogenous fat for oxidation is controversial. In nonstressed patients, decreased insulin secretion and insufficient calorie administration favor fat oxidation. However,

critical illness may alter normal metabolic pathways. Jeevanandam and coworkers[71] demonstrated poor fat oxidation in a population of critically ill obese patients who were not given nutritional support (Fig. 83-5). In contrast, using indirect calorimetry to analyze substrate utilization, Dickerson and coworkers[70] estimated fat oxidation at 68% of nonprotein energy expenditure in a similar population of stressed obese patients who were receiving hypocaloric parenteral nutrition.

PROTEIN SPARING. All of the benefits of the PSMF thus far described can be attributed to the creation of a semistarvation state. In fact, total fasting would also achieve similar results. What differentiates the PSMF from starvation is its protein-sparing effect. This characteristic decreases the negative nitrogen balance generally seen with critical illness.

Infusion of dextrose-free amino acid solutions decreases net nitrogen loss but does not prevent it.[72] Addition of a nonprotein calorie source such as glucose improves protein sparing,[73] partly because of the attenuation of protein catabolism to support gluconeogenesis. After rapid depletion of the glycogen stores, the body relies on gluconeogenesis to support glucose-dependent tissues such as the immune system, the healing wound, and the peripheral nervous system.[74-76] The amount of glucose necessary to achieve maximal protein-sparing is unknown.

ENERGY EXPENDITURE. Nitrogen preservation increases with higher calorie administration, but the effect is blunted as energy delivery increases above 60% of resting energy expenditure[77] (Fig. 83-6). Therefore, the total calories probably need to exceed about 50% of the energy expenditure to be effective. A severely calorie-restricted diet (i.e., providing less than 50% of the energy expenditure) is to be avoided.

The estimation of energy expenditure can be difficult in this population. Energy expenditure in the critically ill is variable.[78] Indirect calorimetry can be accurately used to measure energy expenditure of the critically ill. When esti-

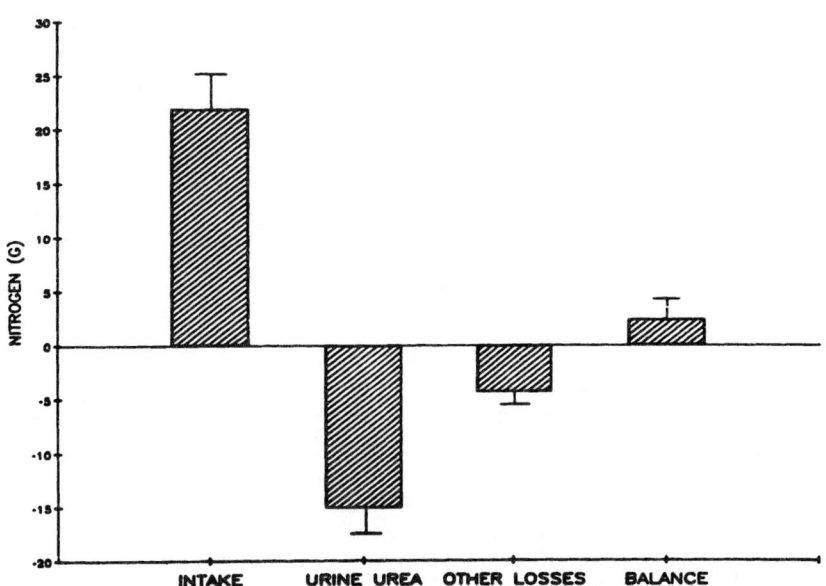

FIGURE 83-4. Nitrogen balance. (From Dickerson RN, Rosato EF, Mullen JL: Net protein anabolism with hypocaloric parenteral nutrition in obese stressed patients. *Am J Clin Nutr* 1986; 44:751.)

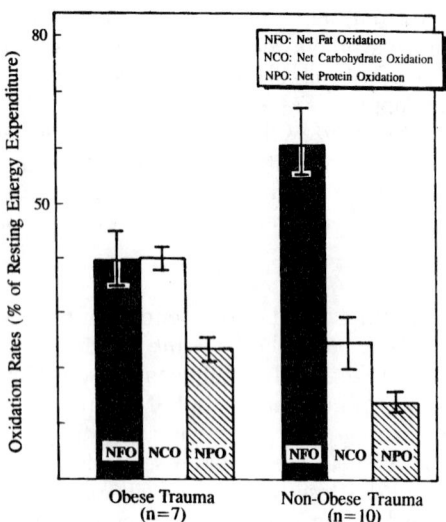

FIGURE 83-5. Net substrate oxidation rates in trauma patients. (From Jeevanandam M, Young DH, Schiller WR: Obesity and the metabolic response to severe multiple trauma in man. *J Clin Invest* 1991;87:268 by copyright permission of the Society for Clinical Investigation.)

mating energy expenditure, use of an adjusted body weight,[79] which essentially ignores adiposity yet assumes a larger than normal lean body mass, prevents overfeeding.

Prevention of Fatty Acid Deficiency

The PSMF is safe and has few contraindications. Despite the use of a lipid-free solution, an essential fatty acid deficiency is unlikely. Linoleic acid, the most important essential fatty

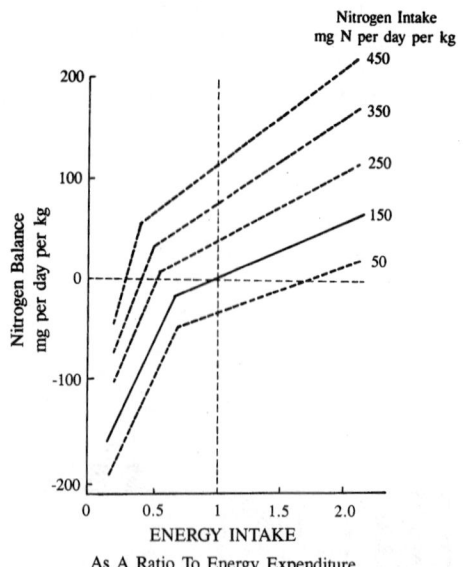

FIGURE 83-6. Relationships between energy intake and nitrogen balance. At any level of nitrogen intake, increasing calorie administration improves nitrogen balance. This effect becomes less prominent when energy provision is increased to greater than half of the energy expenditure. (From Elwyn DH, Kinney JM, Askanazi J: Energy expenditure in surgical patients. *Surg Clin North Am* 1981; 61:545.)

acid, comprises approximately 10% of the stored lipid. Mobilization of this fat releases more than the 2 to 3.5 g of linoleic acid required daily.[80] Even if lipolysis and fat oxidation are poor in the stressed obese patient, most would require this form of nutritional support only for a relatively limited period of time. If a patient requires longer support, an intralipid infusion can be given once a week to prevent an essential fatty acid deficiency.

CONCLUSION ■

Because of the serious medical conditions associated with obesity, significantly overweight patients are at an increased risk to develop complications requiring intensive care. During critical illness, they are more likely than the nonobese to have an unfavorable outcome. For these reasons, the approach to these critically ill patients must differ from other ICU patients. In addition to comprehensive intensive care, treatment strategies must be instituted that recognize the uniqueness of this patient population with regard to cardiovascular, pulmonary, thromboembolic, and septic complications and nutritional support.

The critical care physician must possess a thorough understanding of the significant and wide-ranging physiologic disturbances that occur in the morbidly obese patient. Particular attention must be directed to the recognition and evaluation of organ dysfunction, including eccentric left ventricular hypertrophy, right ventricular hypertrophy, and CHF. Existing changes in pulmonary function (decreased FRC and ERV; baseline hypoxemia and hypercapnia) may be significantly influenced by surgical interventions.

Appropriate care requires a thorough preoperative evaluation, which should include specific consideration of cardiac and pulmonary function. At a minimum, we recommend preoperative pulmonary function testing and arterial blood gas analysis as well as 2-D echocardiography. Consideration should be given to securing special care beds that allow early postoperative mobilization to the upright sitting position. Patients with preoperative hypercapnia or hypoxemia should be maintained in a monitored environment during the perioperative period. Arterial blood gas monitoring and continuous pulse oximetry are essential to their care.

REFERENCES ■

1. Van Itallie TB: Health implications of overweight and obesity in the United States. *Ann Intern Med* 1985;103:983
2. National Institutes of Health Consensus Development Conference statement: health implications of obesity. *Ann Intern Med* 1985;103:147
3. Bray GA: Complications of obesity. *Ann Intern Med* 1985;103:1052
4. Drenick EJ: Sudden cardiac arrest in morbidly obese surgical patients unexplained after autopsy. *Am J Surg* 1988;155:720
5. Van Itallie TB: Obesity adverse effects on health and longevity. *Am J Clin Nutr* 1979;32:2723
6. Fitzgerald FT: The problem of obesity. *Ann Revu Med* 1981;32:221

7. Kral JG: Morbid obesity and related health risks. *Ann Intern Med* 1985;103:1043

8. Pasulka PS, Bistrian BR, Benotti PN, et al: The risks of surgery in obese patients. *Ann Intern Med* 1986;104:504

9. Chadwich J, Mann WN: *Medical Works of Hippocrates*. Oxford, Blackwell Scientific Publications, 1950:154

10. Smith HL, Wilhius FA: Adiposity of the heart. *Arch Intern Med* 1923;152:929

11. Frohlich ED, Messerli FH, Reisen ED, et al: The problem of obesity and hypertension. *Hypertension* 1983;5:71

12. Kannel WB, Brand N, Skinner JJ, et al: Relation of adiposity to blood pressure and development of hypertension: the Framingham study. *Ann Intern Med* 1978;67:48

13. Reisin E, Frohlich ED, Messeili FN, et al: Cardiovascular changes after weight reduction in obesity hypertension. *Ann Intern Med* 1983;98:315

14. Reisin E, Frohlich ED: Obesity: cardiovascular and respiratory pathophysiological alterations. *Arch Intern Med* 1981;141:431

15. Alexander JK: The cardiomyopathy of obesity. *Prog Cardiovasc Dis* 1985;27:325

16. Vaughan RW, Bauer S, Wise L: Volume and pH of gastric juice in obese patients. *Anesthesiology* 1981;55:180

17. Beddell GN, Wilson WR, Seebohm DM: Pulmonary function in obese persons. *J Clin Invest* 1958;37:1049

18. Barrerra F, Reidenberg MM, Winters WL: Pulmonary function in the obese patient. *Am J Med Sci* 1967;32:785

19. Rochester DF, Enson Y: Current concepts in the pathogenesis of the obesity-hypoventilation syndrome. *Am J Med* 1974;57:402

20. Ray CS, Sue DY, Bray G, et al: Effects of obesity on respiratory function. *Am Rev Respir Dis* 1983;128:501

21. Luce JM: Clinical risk factors for postoperative pulmonary complications. *Respir Care* 1984;29:484

22. Vaughan RW, Wise L: Intraoperative arterial oxygenation in obese patients. *Ann Surg* 1976;184:35

23. Forse RA, Tim LK, Marin TJ, et al: The functional residual capacity in the morbidly obese. *Int J Obesity* 1988;12:608

24. MacGregor MI, Block AJ, Ball WC: Serious complications and sudden death in the Pickwickian syndrome. *Hopkins Med J* 1970;126:279

25. Miller A, Granada M: In hospital mortality in the Pickwickian syndrome. *Am J Med* 1975;56:144

26. Fletcher EC, Shah A, Quan W, et al: "Near miss" death in obstructive sleep apnea: a critical care syndrome. *Crit Care Med* 1991;19:1158

27. Rossner S, Lagerstrank L, Persson HE, et al: The sleep apnea syndrome in obesity: risk of sudden death. *J Intern Med* 1991;230:135

28. Banner MJ, Jaeger MJ, Kirby RR: Components of the work of breathing and implications for monitoring ventilator-dependent patients. *Crit Care Med* 1994;22:515

29. Koopmann CF, Moran WB: Surgical management of obstructive sleep apnea. *Otolaryngol Clin North Am* 1990;23:787

30. Svanholm H: Uvulopalatopharyngoplasty in the sleep apnea syndrome. *Arch Otolaryngol Head Neck Surg* 1988;114:45

31. Clayman GL, Adams GL: Permanent tracheostomy with cervical lipectomy. *Laryngoscope* 1990;100:422

32. Headley WB, Rodning CB: Fabricated single lumen tracheal cannula for a morbidly obese patient. *J Otolaryngol* 1993;22:438

33. Ghorayeb BY: Tracheotomy in the morbidly obese patient. *Arch Otolaryngol Head Neck Surg* 1987;113:556

34. McLear PW, Thawley SE: Airway management in obesity hypoventilation syndrome. *Clin Chest Med* 1991;12:585

35. Quinn DA, Thompson BT, Terrin ML, et al: A prospective investigation of pulmonary embolism in women and men. *JAMA* 1992;268:1689

36. Sigel B, Ipsen J, Felix WR: The epidemiology of lower extremity deep venous thrombosis in surgical patients. *Ann Surg* 1974;179:278

37. Anderson FA, Wheeler B, Goldberg RJ, et al: Physician practices in the prevention of venous thromboembolism. *Ann Intern Med* 1991;115:591

38. Greenfield LJ, Proctor MC: Advances in the prophylaxis of venous thrombosis and pulmonary embolism. In: Veith FJ (ed). *Current Critical Problems in Vascular Surgery*, vol 5. St Louis, Quality Medical Publishing, 1993:145

39. NIH consensus conference: prevention of venous thrombosis and pulmonary embolism. *JAMA* 1986;256:744

40. Kakkar VV, Howe CT, Nicolaides AN, et al: Deep vein thrombosis of the leg: is there a "high risk" group? *Am J Surg* 1970;120:527

41. Bajardi G, Ricevuto G, Mastrandrea G, et al: Postoperative venous thromboembolism in bariatric surgery. *Minerva Chir* 1993;48:539

42. Coon WW: Epidemiology of venous thromboembolism. *Ann Surg* 1977;186:149

43. Bern MM, Bothe A Jr, Bistrian B, et al: Effects of low-dose warfarin on antithrombin III levels in morbidly obese patients. *Surgery* 1983;94:78

44. THRIFT Consensus Group: Risk of and prophylaxis for venous thromboembolism in hospitalized patients. *Br Med J* 1992;305:567

45. Coon WW: Venous thromboembolism: prevalence, risk factors, and prevention. *Clin Chest Med* 1984;5:391

46. Wille-Jorgensen P, Ott P: Predicting failure of low-dose prophylactic heparin in general surgical procedures. *Surg Gynecol Obstet* 1990;171:126

47. Cerra FB: Hypermetabolism, organ failure, and metabolic support. *Surgery* 1987;92:1

48. McMurray JF: Wound healing with diabetes mellitus: better glucose control for better wound healing in diabetes. *Surg Clin North Am* 1984;64:769

49. Bagdade JD, Stewart M, Walters E: Impaired granulocyte adherence: a reversible defect in host defense in patients with poorly controlled diabetes. *Diabetes* 1978;27:677

50. Jones RL, Peterson CM: Hematologic alterations in diabetes mellitus. *Am J Med* 1981;70:339

51. Hostetter MK: Handicaps to host defense: effects of hyperglycemia on C3 and Candida Albicans. *Diabetes* 1990;39:271

52. Baxter JK, Babineua TJ, Apovian CM, et al: Perioperative glucose control predicts increased nosocomial infection in diabetics [abstract]. *Crit Care Med* 1990;18:207s

53. Trempy GA, Rock P: Anesthetic management of a morbidly obese woman with a massive ovarian cyst. *J Clin Anesth* 1993;5:62

54. Studley HO: Percentage of weight loss: a basic indicator of surgical risk in patients with chronic peptic ulcer. *JAMA* 1936;166:458

55. Seltzer MH, Slocum BA, Cataldi-Betcher EL, et al: Instant assessment: absolute weight loss and surgical mortality. *J Parenter Enter Nutr* 1982;6:218

56. Dempsey DT, Mullen JL, Buzby GP: The link between nutritional status and clinical outcome: can nutritional intervention modify it? *Am J Clin Nutr* 1988;47:352

57. McMahon MM, Benotti PN, Bistrian BR: A clinical application of exercise physiology and nutritional support for the mechanically ventilated patient. *J Parenter Enter Nutr* 1990;14:538

58. Abel RM, Grimes JB, Alonso D, et al: Adverse hemodynamic and ultrastructural changes in dog hearts subjected to protein-calorie malnutrition. *Am Heart J* 1979;97:733

59. Heymsfield SB, Bethel RA, Ansley JD, et al: Cardiac abnormalities in cachectic patients before and during repletion. *Am Heart J* 1978;95:584

60. Haw MP, Bell SJ, Blackburn GL: Potential of parenteral and enteral nutrition in inflammation and immune dysfunction: a new challenge for dieticians. *J Am Diet Assoc* 1991;91:701

61. Lowry SF: The route of feeding influences injury responses. *J Trauma* 1990;30:S10

62. Alverdy JC: The GI tract as an immunologic organ. *Contemp Surg* 1989;35(Suppl):14

63. Moore EE, Jones TN: Benefits of immediate jejunostomy feeding after major abdominal trauma: a prospective, randomized study. *J Trauma* 1986;26:874

64. Peterson SR, Sheldon GF, Carpenter G: Failure of hyperalimentation to enhance survival in malnourished rats with *E. coli*-hemoglobin adjuvant peritonitis. *Surg Forum* 1979;30:60

65. Kudsk KA, Croce MA, Fabian TC, et al: Enteral versus parenteral feeding: effects on septic morbidity after blunt and penetrating abdominal trauma. *Ann Surg* 1992;215:503

66. Baker AL, Rosenberg IH: Hepatic complications of total parenteral nutrition. *Am J Med* 1987;82:489

67. Askanazi J, Rosenbaum SH, Hyman AI, et al: Respiratory changes induced by the large glucose loads of total parenteral nutrition. *JAMA* 1980;243:1444

68. Bistrian BR: Clinical use of a protein-sparing modified fast. *JAMA* 1972;240:2299

69. Baxter JK, Bistrian BR: Moderate hypocaloric parenteral nutrition in the critically ill, obese patient. *Nutr Clin Pract* 1989;4:133

70. Dickerson RN, Rosato EF, Mullen JL: Net protein anabolism with hypocaloric parenteral nutrition in obese stressed patients. *Am J Clin Nutr* 1986;44:747

71. Jeevanandam J, Young DH, Schiller WR: Obesity and the metabolic response to severe multiple trauma in man. *J Clin Invest* 1991;87:262

72. Greenberg GR, Marliss EB, Anderson GH, et al: Protein sparing therapy in postoperative patients. *N Engl J Med* 1976;294:1411

73. Young GA, Hill GLl: A controlled study of protein-sparing therapy after excision of the rectum. *Ann Surg* 1980;192:183

74. Blackburn GL: Nutrition in surgical patients. In: Hardy JD, Kukora JS, Pass HI (eds). *Hardy's Textbook of Surgery*, 2nd ed. Philadelphia, JB Lippincott, 1988:86

75. Hensle TW, Askanazi J: Metabolism and nutrition in the perioperative period. *J Urol* 1988;139:229

76. Douglas RG, Shaw JHF: Metabolic response to sepsis and trauma. *Br J Surg* 1989;76:115

77. Elwyn DH, Kinney JM, Askanazi J: Energy expenditure in surgical patients. *Surg Clin North Am* 1981;61:545

78. Weissman C, Kemper M, Askanazi J, et al: Resting metabolic rate of the critically ill patient: measured versus predicted. *Anesthesiology* 1986;64:673

79. Wilkens K: Adjustment for obesity. *ADA Renal Practice Group Newsletter*, Winter 1984

80. Mascioli EA, Smith MF, Trerice MS, et al: Effect of total parenteral nutrition with cycling on essential fatty acid deficiency. *J Parenter Enter Nutr* 1979;3:171

Organ Transplantation

Critical Care, Third Edition, edited by Joseph M. Civetta,
Robert W. Taylor, and Robert R. Kirby.
Lippincott-Raven Publishers, Philadelphia, PA © 1997.

CHAPTER 84

◼

Organ Transplantation: An Overview of Problems and Concerns

Ake Grenvik
Joseph M. Darby
Brian A. Broznick

IMMEDIATE CONCERNS ◼

MAJOR PROBLEMS

Developments in organ transplantation over the past 15 years have been nothing short of spectacular. Worldwide, half a million people have received organ transplants. Current results are far superior to other forms of treatment of end-stage single organ failure. As a consequence, the number of people needing and wanting organ transplantation increases every day. In 1995, more than 40,000 potential recipients were waiting for an organ in the United States alone. This number has doubled in the past 5 years. As Table 84-1 shows, the number of brain-dead donors increased by 25% during the 6 years between 1989 and 1994. To a significant degree, this increase was caused by use of older donors; the number of donors older than 50 years of age doubled during the same period. Because the number of patients awaiting transplantation has increased much more rapidly than the number of available donors, the shortage of donor organs has reached almost crisis proportions. Currently, as many as 9 patients awaiting transplantation die each day.

STRESS POINTS

1. Organ transplantation began more than 40 years ago; initially, organs were grafted only from living relatives and non–heart-beating cadavers.
2. Later, the brain death concept made it possible to procure organs from heart-beating cadavers, which provided much better results than the use of organs from cadavers after circulation had stopped.
3. The number of people developing brain death whose families consent to organ donation is insufficient for the current need. Therefore, various categories of non–heart-beating cadavers are again being considered for organ procurement and transplantation, with or without preceding life support of the recipients by artificial organs such as dialysis machines, ventricular assist devices, artificial hearts, and artificial pancreata.
4. Artificial livers and lungs remain in research development. A mechanical ventilator is not an artificial lung but merely a tool to supply oxygen to and remove carbon dioxide from borderline-functioning lungs. On the other hand, extracorporeal lung support devices with oxygenators involve the use of artificial lungs.

TABLE 84-1. Organ Donors in the United States, 1989–1994

YEAR	TOTAL NO. OF DONORS	NO. OF DONORS >50 YEARS OF AGE (%)	KIDNEY	LIVER	HEART	LUNG	PANCREAS
1989	4018	565 (14)	3815	2377	1781	191	799
1990	4513	702 (15)	4311	2875	2169	276	950
1991	4530	796 (18)	4271	3167	2198	395	1066
1992	4521	938 (21)	4277	3335	2247	527	1004
1993	4860	998 (21)	4608	3763	2443	790	1244
1994	5060	1151 (23)	4738	3988	2497	838	1217

5. Direct transplantation of functioning organs without the need for preceding recipient use of artificial organ support is an extremely successful technique. Therefore, solving the donor organ shortage dilemma is of great concern in today's medical community.

6. Use of artificial organs as a bridge to transplantation remains a major problem, with ever-increasing waiting time for a human organ. Permanently replacing major organs with artificial ones is a research project of great potential, although no immediate solution is in sight.

7. Use of animal donors for xenografting is also an unresolved problem, although it probably will provide a future solution to the donor organ shortage.

CURRENT TRANSPLANTATION ACTIVITIES

KIDNEYS

Since the introduction of renal transplantation more than four decades ago, almost 125,000 patients have received such allografts in the United States alone. Worldwide experience exceeds a quarter of a million kidney transplantations.[1] About 11,000 kidneys are transplanted each year in the United States, approximately 20% from living donors and 80% from brain-dead, heart-beating cadavers. One-year graft survival from living donors approaches 95%, and success rates for cadaveric grafts are in the range of 85%. Patient survival reaches 95% to 100% in the predominant centers. Long-term survival after kidney transplantation is also impressive; almost 70% of kidney recipients are alive 10 years later, and more than 50% of their primary grafts are still functioning at that time.[2]

The limiting factor in kidney transplantations is the number of donor organs available. Approximately 22,000 Americans develop end-stage renal disease each year, and 20,000 transplantations could easily be accommodated each year if enough kidneys were available. The quality of life after transplantation is greatly improved, and long-term graft survival is achieved at a lower cost than chronic dialysis.

HEARTS

Barnard reported the first cardiac transplantation in 1967.[3] Since then, heart transplantation has become a routine procedure and is actively performed in more than 170 U.S. medical centers. Almost 2500 such procedures were completed in this country in 1994. The results are excellent, with a 1-year graft survival rate of more than 80% in leading institutions. For comparison, the mortality rate at 1 year among candidates on the waiting list is significantly higher than 50%, and our Pittsburgh experience indicates a death rate of approximately 80% after 2 years of waiting time.

LIVERS

Although it was first performed successfully more than 20 years ago, liver transplantation did not become an accepted, routine procedure until the 1980s, when 1-year graft survival gradually increased to 80%. In 1994, approximately 3600 liver transplantations were performed in the United States.[4]

PANCREATA

Neither total nor segmental pancreas transplantation enjoys the same success rate as the procedures already discussed. The overall 1-year survival rate of pancreas recipients is approximately 80%, but graft survival, defined as lack of insulin dependence, only approaches 50%. More than 1200 pancreas transplantations were performed in the United States in 1994. Centers with the most experience report 90% patient survival and 80% graft survival at 1 year, with the majority of successful procedures having been performed in conjunction with a renal transplantation.[5,6] Islet cell transplantation, once thought promising, has not obtained as good results as the use of solid or segmental grafts.

LUNGS

Although the procedure is considered by some to still be in its infancy, single and double lung transplantations have increased in numbers over the past few years. Initially, only combined heart-lung procedures were carried out in numbers large enough to provide reliable data. However, during 1994, more than 800 lung transplantations were carried out in the United States. Current 1-year survival rates approach 70%.[7]

MULTIPLE ORGANS

The number of patients in need of multiple organ transplantation also has increased. Normally, double organ transplantation is carried out as two separate operations, except for the combination of heart and lungs. The most common procedure is the implantation of both pancreas and kidney in diabetic patients with renal failure.[8,9] Heart-liver,[10] heart-kidney,[11] and liver-kidney[12] transplantations also have been performed. In addition, multiple organs, which may include the liver, pancreas, stomach, small intestine, and colon, have been transplanted en bloc in recent years.

From the immunologic standpoint, transplantation of multiple organs from the same donor is advantageous. However, this approach is not always possible, as in the case of asynchronous transplantation of two organs. In multiple organ transplantation, rejection of one organ but not the other may occur, even if the organs originate from a single donor.

ORGAN NEED VERSUS SUPPLY

Efficient medication to manipulate the immune system has made transplantation more successful than conventional medical therapy for end-stage diseases of some vital organs, particularly the kidney, heart, and liver. The success rates with end-stage pulmonary, pancreatic, and intestinal diseases are not yet equally great. However, advances in all aspects of transplantation are certain to continue.

In 1994, more than 26,000 patients were actively awaiting kidney transplantation in the United States, compared with fewer than 10,000 patients as little as 10 years ago. In January 1995, 3600 individuals were in need of liver transplantation, and almost 3000 were awaiting a new heart. As of June 1995, the number of patients awaiting transplantation had increased to more than 40,000.[13]

POTENTIAL DONORS

Of the 2 million individuals who die each year in the United States, between 12,000 and 27,000 are considered suitable for organ donation, depending on the age limits and medical criteria used. This number would meet the needs of the patients awaiting transplantation if a satisfactory method to bring all such cadavers into a pool of donors were available. However, this goal has not been achieved and probably never will be.[14] Although increased use of available organs has occurred, the size of the potential donor pool has not significantly increased in the United States in the past 5 years.

The actual increase in transplantations performed has resulted from transplant surgeons' willingness to accept older donors and those with a history of hypertension or diabetes. Although these diseases previously were considered to contraindicate organ donation, they do not seriously affect all organs. Therefore, some organs can be recovered that would have been discarded a few years ago. The greatest obstacle in acquiring organs for transplantation remains the refusal by relatives to allow organ donation when the possibility exists.

Categories

Currently, three major categories of organ donors can be identified: living donors; brain-dead, heart-beating cadavers;

and non–heart-beating cadavers. As the demand for organs continues to increase, numerous steps have been taken to enlarge the pool of organ donors. The acceptable age limits have been expanded; particular organs with milder forms of disease and trauma have been less often excluded; and segments of vital organs removed from living donors (e.g., the tail of the pancreas, the left lobe of the liver) have been used for transplantation from a parent to a child. Most recently, transplant surgeons have removed a lobe of a lung of one family member to give to another.

Brain Death

Debate is ongoing concerning the relevance of the brain death concept. In the future, certification of death may include not only conventional heart-beating cadavers who are brain dead but also those with cerebral death (i.e., patients in a permanent vegetative state)[5,15] and those with absent brain (i.e., anencephalic infants).[6] A recent resolution by the American Medical Association has provided an ethical basis for the use of organs from anencephalic babies.[16] However, as long as these infants are alive, it remains illegal to procure their organs.

EVOLUTION OF THE BRAIN DEATH CONCEPT

It has long been appreciated that herniation of a brain lethally injured by trauma or disease leads to death through respiratory and cardiac arrest. However, not until the implementation of intensive care and prolonged mechanical ventilation in the 1950s did brain death, which is caused by increased intracranial pressure above arterial pressure with cessation of all cerebral blood flow, become a condition that could last for days and weeks rather than a few minutes.

Based on criteria published by the Harvard Committee in 1968,[17] the Uniform Determination of Death Act was designed jointly by the American Bar Association, the American Medical Association, and the National Conference of Commissioners on Uniform State Laws, and is now accepted as law in all 50 of the United States. The Act states that "An individual who has sustained either irreversible cessation of circulatory and respiratory functions, or irreversible cessation of all functions of the entire brain, including the brain stem, is dead."

NEUROLOGIC CRITERIA

The neurologic criteria for certification of death vary slightly but essentially include documented cessation of cerebral function and unresponsiveness to stimulation of all cranial nerves. The most important test is to verify that spontaneous breathing is absent in response to strong stimulation of the respiratory center by an arterial carbon dioxide partial pressure greater than 60 mm Hg. Most medical centers require two examinations in order to avoid the possibility of misjudgment. However, the prescribed interval between the two examinations varies greatly, from 2 to 24 hours. If confounding factors are present, such as a drug overdose of sedatives or narcotics, hypothermia, shock or metabolic coma, complete cessation of blood flow to the brain must be documented through four-vessel cerebral arteriography or another acceptable technique.

CONSENT

After death has been certified, consent for organ donation must be obtained before procurement can take place. This process includes cases within the coroner's jurisdiction. Even if consent in writing is available from the deceased, practice in the United States has been to obtain consent from the next of kin as well. However, organ donor cards are increasingly considered legal advance directives, and some states through legislation have indicated that this prior decision by the deceased person cannot be overruled by relatives.

PERSISTENT VEGETATIVE STATE

Although irreversible cessation of all function of the entire brain is required for certification of brain death in the United States, demonstration of cessation of brain stem function is a satisfactory condition in the United Kingdom. There may be no significant difference between these two definitions, because the cerebral hemispheres cannot function independently if the whole brain stem is dead. However, the opposite is not true. In so-called persistent vegetative state (PVS), cortical death is present but the brain stem is more or less intact.

Some ethicists are in favor of defining individuals with PVS as dead, because they have lost consciousness and cognition, and because "personhood," as an indication of human life, is absent. However, patients with PVS have the ability to breathe spontaneously, and large segments of modern society are not ready to decide that life has ceased when the body is still breathing. Furthermore, variable degrees of cerebral death can be present in patients with PVS. Clinically, up to 3 months may be required to determine permanence in medical cases and up to 1 year in those caused by trauma.[18] Some 10,000 patients develop PVS each year in the United States. This large group of patients currently cannot be utilized for organ donation unless treatment is withdrawn and death is certified based on cessation of cardiac function.

ANENCEPHALY

Another category of cerebral death, or rather cerebral absence, is anencephaly. If born alive, anencephalic infants rarely survive longer than 2 weeks without therapy. They have a brain stem with at least some function and may be able to breathe spontaneously. Although they cannot survive, they also cannot be certified dead, unless they stop breathing or the heart ceases to function. Many attempts to use organs from anencephalic donors have been made in different countries, but no acceptable solution to the medicolegal and ethical problems involved in these procedures has evolved.

However, a decreasing number of full-term anencephalic babies are born each year. Hence, this potential donor category is relatively unimportant, although there is a great need for organs by pediatric patients.

PROCEDURAL CONSIDERATIONS ■

DONOR RECOGNITION

The first step in assuring viable organs for transplantation is early recognition of potential donors: patients who, depending on type of injury and clinical status, are likely to progress to brain death despite aggressive life support. The majority of potential donors are patients who have been admitted to an intensive care unit (ICU) with severe blunt or penetrating head trauma or catastrophic intracranial hemorrhage that results in coma, marked impairment of brain stem reflexes, massive brain swelling with compression of basilar cisterns, and refractory intracranial hypertension. Early identification of the potential donor facilitates mobilization of personnel and resources essential to organ procurement. Anticipation, prevention, and aggressive treatment of physiologic instability and other complications associated with brain death result in enhanced organ function after transplantation.

DONOR ASSESSMENT

After the potential donor has been recognized, his or her overall medical eligibility as an actual donor is determined. Because the donor pool remains relatively stable even though demand for organs continues to increase, medical eligibility criteria for organ donation continue to evolve. The physician managing the potential donor in the ICU should involve the local organ procurement organization (OPO) in the determination of medical eligibility while focusing his or her own efforts on maintaining vital organ function.

A thorough patient history and physical examination as well as a general assessment of relevant organ function are the principal factors that determine medical eligibility of the potential donor. The main condition that excludes the potential organ donor from further consideration is the presence of malignancy (except primary brain tumor or localized cutaneous or cervical cancer), active viral infection, acquired immunodeficiency syndrome, tuberculosis, or any other untreated or inadequately treated infectious disease. In the past, extremes of age have also been emphasized as a principal exclusionary factor. However, recent data indicate that age limits can be extended[19-25] and that physiologic function is more important than chronologic age.

After general medical eligibility has been determined and consent for organ donation has been obtained, serologic testing and additional diagnostic testing directed at a more thorough evaluation of individual organ function and suitability are performed according to requirements of the local OPO. Details of individual organ assessment and suitability for organ donation can be found elsewhere.[26]

CERTIFICATION OF DEATH

Before organs can be procured from heart-beating donors, death must be certified and consent for donation must be obtained. In the United States, as noted previously, brain death diagnostic criteria are based on the "whole brain" definition[27] and must be certified in accordance with local state laws. The diagnosis of brain death in pediatric patients (age <5 years) is more complicated than in adults and requires special consideration of age, duration of observation after absent brain function is documented, and additional diagnostic tests.[28]

Confirmatory Tests

The diagnosis of brain death in most potential donors can be made based on clinical criteria alone. However, additional adjunctive testing may be required in circumstances that could potentially mimic brain death (e.g., high blood concentration of barbiturates, pharmacologic neuromuscular blockade, hypothermia). In such circumstances, or if any question regarding the validity of the clinical examination arises, brain death should be confirmed with studies that document absent cerebral blood flow.

Many diagnostic tests can be used,[29] with the conventional bedside cranial radionuclide angiogram having the advantage of being both widely accepted and simple to perform. Another technique increasingly used for confirmation of brain death employs the radionuclide tracer technetium 99m hexamethyl propylenamine oxime (^{99m}Tc-HMPAO). This test can be performed at the bedside and has the advantage of evaluating brain perfusion rather than intracranial blood flow; it can also provide images of the posterior fossa.[30-32]

Some physiologic deterioration of the potential donor may occur during brain death evaluation, particularly with prolonged apnea testing. Worsening hypotension[33] and hypoxemia are the most common problems encountered. Hypotension occurs as hypercarbia and acidosis are produced during apneic oxygenation and may be addressed by the administration of sodium bicarbonate or increased vasopressor administration. Hypoxemia, which can precipitate donor cardiac arrest, is minimized by preoxygenation before apnea testing and by tracheal insufflation of oxygen (e.g., 4 to 6 L/minute) during the apnea test, especially if arterial desaturation occurs.

Documentation

The date and time of death should be documented clearly in the patient's medical record, after certification criteria are met. Physicians who declare brain death in potential donors should not have direct involvement with either organ procurement or transplantation.

DONOR MANAGEMENT

After death of the potential donor is determined to be inevitable, aggressive physiologic support in the ICU must continue up to the time of organ procurement unless medical ineligibility is determined or the family refuses to consent to donation. The principal issues of concern after brain death are hemodynamic instability and other complications that may have occurred as a consequence of brain death, associated injuries, or treatment directed at the primary brain insult. Commonly encountered complications that should be anticipated include hypotension, hypothermia, diabetes mellitus, hypernatremia, hypokalemia, and metabolic acidosis.

Because data are limited regarding donor management that optimizes subsequent allograft function, treatment goals are similar to those of most critically ill patients. Accordingly, support of systemic organ perfusion and prevention of complications related to this management are the main objectives during organ donor maintenance.

General Considerations

General preventive steps are taken to minimize the risk of pulmonary and infectious complications and to preserve the integrity of potentially transplantable tissues such as skin and corneas. Routine nursing practices usually employed in the management of the unconscious patient, such as frequent turning, intermittent manual lung inflation, tracheobronchial suctioning, and lubrication of the eyes with protective closure, are important aspects of donor management. Nasogastric suction minimizes the risk for large-volume gastric aspiration, and exposure to ambient temperature is minimized to prevent excessive decrease in body temperature. Finally, all field resuscitation catheters placed under suboptimal conditions are removed and replaced with aseptic technique as indicated for further resuscitation and monitoring.

Monitoring

Hemodynamic instability and fluctuations in acid-base and electrolyte status necessitate invasive monitoring and frequent blood sampling in the prospective organ donor. Arterial and central venous pressures, arterial oxygen saturation, and hourly urine output are routinely monitored. Pulmonary artery catheterization is occasionally needed if routine resuscitative efforts fail to restore adequate hemodynamic end points or in potential donors with high positive end-expiratory pressure (PEEP) requirements, cardiac tamponade, myocardial contusion, or heart failure. Measurements of core temperature are also required during donor maintenance to facilitate the recognition and treatment of excessive hypothermia. Arterial blood gas partial pressures, serum electrolytes, serum glucose, and hematocrit are measured as clinically indicated. Desirable physiologic end points in the potential organ donor are shown in Table 84-2.

Hemodynamic Support

Hemodynamic instability should be expected in the brain-dead organ donor, and its severity depends in part on the mechanism of brain death development and the therapeutic interventions administered before death. Victims of multisystem trauma with ongoing blood loss and high fluid requirement are more likely to be unstable than donors who

TABLE 84-2. Physiologic End Points in the Organ Donor

Systolic blood pressure	90–120 mm Hg
Central venous pressure	5–10 mm Hg
Urine output	100–250 mL/hr
Core temperature	35°–38°C
Hematocrit	25%
Oxygen saturation	>95%
pH	7.4–7.45

succumb to brain death as a result of isolated, unremitting intracranial hypertension.

Hemodynamic instability occurs in most brain-dead organ donors and is principally manifested as hypotension.[34–37] Hypotension is commonly multifactorial, with loss of vascular tone compounded by fluid losses secondary to diabetes insipidus and the use of osmotic or loop diuretics before death. Because ischemic organ injury is an important factor leading to allograft dysfunction,[38–41] donor hypotension must be aggressively treated.

FLUIDS. Intravascular volume expansion, with the use of crystalloids, colloids, and blood as indicated, is employed initially as the main modality for treating established hypotension and is provided to achieve indicated physiologic end points. Although crystalloids alone can be used, the addition of colloids during donor resuscitation may reduce the total fluid requirement, minimize body cooling, and reduce the potential risk of crystalloid-associated impairment in tissue oxygenation.[42]

Excessive fluid administration is of particular concern for optimal function of donor lungs and heart. Data suggest that fluid resuscitation in potential lung donors should be titrated to achieve a central venous pressure of no more than 6 mm Hg, or a pulmonary artery occlusion pressure of 10 mm Hg, to minimize the adverse effects of fluid administration on lung function.[43] Similarly, high central venous pressure and excessive fluid may result in impaired heart function after brain death.[44,45]

VASOPRESSORS. Vasopressors are usually required at the onset of hypotension and while fluid resuscitation is proceeding. They should be titrated to their minimum effective doses to avoid end-organ damage caused by increased myocardial oxygen consumption or reduced splanchnic and renal blood flow. In this context, dopamine is usually the preferred vasopressor because of its potentially beneficial effect on renal and mesenteric blood flow.[46] Donors in whom hemodynamic stability cannot be achieved or maintained should have a pulmonary artery catheter inserted to better evaluate cardiac function and volume status and to further guide therapy.

THYROID HORMONES. Based on experimental and uncontrolled clinical data, some investigators are now routinely administering thyroid hormones (triiodothyronine or thyroxine) in an attempt to improve hemodynamic stability and organ metabolism in the donor.[47–51] Conflicting data regarding the value of thyroid hormone administration in organ donor management[52–58] have diminished enthusiasm for the use of this novel therapy, especially as an adjunct to hemodynamic support.

URINE OUTPUT. Regarding the assessment of hemodynamic status, urine output cannot be relied on as an indication of the adequacy of fluid volume administration in organ donors because of the frequent occurrence of polyuria caused by diabetes insipidus in brain death. Oliguria usually is not a problem in those donors who receive early and vigorous volume resuscitation. However, because donor urine output appears to be an important determinant of renal graft function,[59] oliguria that is unresponsive to volume expansion should be treated with loop diuretics or mannitol to facilitate the establishment of diuresis.

ARRHYTHMIAS. Cardiac arrhythmias may complicate management of the potential donor, particularly during brain herniation and early after brain death.[26,60] Antiarrhythmics are occasionally required for the control of ventricular or supraventricular tachyarrhythmias and bradyarrhythmias that result in hemodynamic instability. β-Blockers and calcium channel antagonists may cause untoward hypotension[61] and should be used with caution in the brain-dead patient. Because atropine is ineffective in the brain-dead patient, agents such as isoproterenol and epinephrine should be used, if required, for treatment of bradyarrhythmias or in cardiac arrest situations.

CARDIAC ARREST. Cardiac arrest occurs in 4% to 28% of potential organ donors during the maintenance phase.[34,62] Shock, diabetes insipidus, and hypokalemia all appear to predispose the donor to unexpected cardiac arrest.[62] In many cases, organs can be recovered after successful cardiopulmonary resuscitation. Therefore, vigorous resuscitative efforts should be instituted at the onset of cardiac arrest. If consent already has been obtained, the arrested donor can be taken directly to the operating room for organ procurement after death certification based on cessation of cardiac function.

Ventilatory Support

Ventilatory support of the potential organ donor is adjusted to optimize oxygenation, carbon dioxide elimination, and hemodynamic function. Minute ventilation is first adjusted to normalize arterial pH; in most brain-injured patients, this involves a reduction in minute volume and a rise in the partial pressure of carbon dioxide from a hypocapnic to a normocapnic level. Minimal lactic acidosis is commonly present in the potential organ donor[47–49,63,64] and can be managed simply with minor adjustments in minute ventilation.

If severe acidosis is present, sodium bicarbonate or other buffers should be administered to minimize excessive ventilation. This strategy limits the adverse hemodynamic effects of both metabolic acidosis and excessive positive-pressure ventilation. If hypothermia is present, acid-base analysis and correction probably are best approached by using temperature-uncorrected blood gas values to adjust systemic pH. This approach results in higher in vivo pH values, which may ultimately promote better organ function.[65–67]

The fraction of inspired oxygen is titrated with low levels of PEEP to maintain an arterial oxygen saturation of at least 95%. Severe impairments in oxygenation preferentially should be managed with the use of higher concentrations of oxygen rather than high levels of PEEP, to minimize the adverse hemodynamic effects of high PEEP.

Fluid and Electrolyte Management

After the donor has been fluid-resuscitated and stabilized, existing and developing fluid and electrolyte disturbances are specifically addressed. They may be important contributors to instability and premature organ donor loss.[62,68] Hypokalemia and hypernatremia are the most common electrolyte problems and arise mainly as a result of polyuria and excessive solute diuresis associated with diabetes insipidus, hyperglycemia, hypothermia, mobilization of excess body fluids, or administration of mannitol.[26]

In the potential organ donor, polyuria in association with hypernatremia and hypotonic urine is sufficient to support the clinical diagnosis of diabetes insipidus. It often heralds clinical brain death.[69,70] Intravenous desmopressin (DDAVP) is administered in doses of 1 to 2 µg every 8 to 12 hours to minimize ongoing fluid and electrolyte losses after diabetes insipidus is recognized. Prophylactic administration of DDAVP should be avoided, because the polyuria of diabetes insipidus appears to protect against acute tubular necrosis after transplantation.[71] If severe hyperglycemia is present, administration of insulin helps to control fluid and electrolyte losses.

Existing free water deficits and ongoing excess urinary losses should be replaced with hypotonic fluid and added electrolytes as dictated by serum and urine electrolyte measurements. Free water deficit is estimated as follows:

$$\text{Free water deficit in L} = [0.6 \times (\text{Weight in kg})] \\ \times [(\text{Current serum Na}^+/140) - 1]$$

A maintenance intravenous fluid infusion should be initiated, using glucose containing hypotonic salt solution with added electrolytes as indicated, at a rate of 100 to 125 mL/hour. Additional supplements of potassium, phosphate, and magnesium are usually required to maintain normal electrolyte balance. Although excessive hyperglycemia should be avoided, glucose administration does appear to have a favorable effect on posttransplantation liver function.[72,73]

Hypothermia

After brain death, the body becomes poikilothermic and at risk for hypothermia, especially if large volumes of room-temperature fluid and cold blood products have been used during resuscitation. Mean body temperatures range from 31.5° to 34°C[74,75]; values as low as 26°C have been reported. Hypothermia may impair cardiac, renal, and hepatic function,[76,77] and it predisposes the donor to hemodynamic instability and unexpected cardiac arrest.[68]

A reasonable therapeutic end point is the maintenance of core temperature at or above 35°C. To reduce the risk for severe hypothermia, donors should be covered with blankets to minimize environmental exposure. Resuscitation fluids and blood products should be warmed if given in large quantities. If rewarming for hypothermia is required, heated and humidified respiratory gases (37° to 39°C) and external warming devices are usually sufficient.

Miscellaneous Problems

Brain trauma with disseminated intravascular coagulation, hypothermia, hemorrhage, and massive transfusion may predispose the donor to coagulopathy. The frequency of disseminated intravascular coagulation in one study was almost 30%; it occurred largely in those donors with penetrating brain injuries.[78] The impact on organ function, especially on the kidneys, is unclear. However, specific therapy (i.e., heparin) does not appear to be warranted. Donors with evidence of coagulopathy and ongoing hemorrhage should be treated with appropriate blood components to ensure adequate tissue oxygenation and to maintain hemodynamic stability. Antibiotic therapy should be administered to the organ donor who has documented or suspected infection. However, all nephrotoxic antibiotics should be avoided to minimize injury to the kidneys.

ORGAN PROCUREMENT, RECOVERY, AND PRESERVATION ■

ORGAN PROCUREMENT ORGANIZATIONS

The responsibility for identification, recovery, and distribution of cadaveric organs for transplantation has been delegated to the nation's federally certified OPOs. Currently, 65 OPOs exist in the United States, including 48 independent and 17 hospital-based groups.[79] An independent agency is a freestanding, nonprofit organization that normally provides services to more than one transplant center; a hospital-based OPO is usually a subsidiary of a single transplant center.

Responsibilities

One of the primary responsibilities of each OPO is professional and public education. OPOs conduct more than 10,000 teaching programs per year across the United States. Many of these programs are presented to medical and nursing staffs, social service and chaplaincy groups within area hospitals, and so on.[80] However, most are public-oriented programs that, if effectively delivered, result in increased referrals of potential donors, as has been demonstrated in the United Kingdom.

Transplant Coordinators

All OPOs employ nonphysician professionals known as transplant or organ procurement coordinators. These specialists evaluate referred patients regarding suitability for organ or tissue donation. Many times, OPO personnel are the first to discuss the opportunity of organ donation with the family of a dying or brain-dead patient. The coordinators also provide referring physicians and nurses with assistance in the optimal management of the cadaveric donor before and during organ procurement.

Physicians and nurses can expedite the donation process by having readily available all pertinent information, including date of admission, age, height, and weight; medical history and diagnosis; clinical data, such as arterial and central venous pressure; urine output, urinalysis, serum creatinine, and blood urea nitrogen values; results of blood, urine, sputum, and other cultures; ABO blood type; and pertinent social history. With this information, organ procurement or transplant coordinators can usually determine the suitability of a potential donor and whether additional tests need to be performed.

Consent

Probably the most sensitive procedure in the donation process is obtaining consent. Many health care professionals feel uncomfortable approaching families with the request for organ or tissue donation. However, organ procurement specialists are readily available 24 hours a day to provide this service. Whoever discusses donation with the family must be well versed in the entire process of donation and transplantation.

Even more important is that the notification of death and the option of donation be discussed with the family in two separate settings. One of the most unfortunate possible occurrences in the donation request process is for the family to be informed that their loved one is dead and then immediately approached about organ donation.[81] Unless the family of the potential donor previously has discussed and agreed to donation, they will probably refuse if approached in this manner. Studies have shown that coupling of the notification of death with request for organ donation results in a consent rate of 30% or less, whereas 65% of families, or more, may consent if this is not the case.[81] Sensitivity and compassion must be used, and the family must be provided as much time as needed to consider the situation among themselves, ask questions, and finally make an informed decision. Not uncommonly, this process takes more than a day.

After a donor has been identified, suitability determined, and family consent obtained, the next step is to secure permission from the coroner or medical examiner if required by law. This task can also be carried out by the organ procurement specialist. It is not uncommon for potential donor patients to fall under the jurisdiction of a medical examiner or coroner. Cooperation with these professionals is of utmost importance.[82,83] On many occasions, the medical examiner or coroner may have specific requests that must be considered during the procurement process, such as preservation of evidence in homicide cases. A single person should be responsible for coordinating the entire donation process to ensure that all aspects are considered and the procedure is conducted accordingly.

RECOVERY AND PRESERVATION

After all medical and legal aspects of the process have been completed, donated organs are surgically removed. During the recovery of these organs, the process of preservation begins. Depending on which organs are procured, cannulas are introduced into the abdominal aorta, inferior vena cava, portal vein, aortic arch, or pulmonary artery. A hypothermic solution is infused through these cannulas to wash out the donor's blood and cool the organs to a temperature of 4° to 7°C. The most frequently used solution for preservation is Viaspan, which was developed by Belzer and associates[84] and is commonly referred to as the University of Wisconsin, or UW, solution. In some transplant centers, EuroCollins solution,[85,86] a dextrose-based crystalloid, is used for lung preservation. A cardioplegic blood- or plasma-based solution for heart preservation is also used by some specialists.

Heart and lungs continue to have the shortest preservation periods, with a maximum time limit of 6 hours between organ removal from the donor and restoration of circulation in the recipient. Pancreata and livers can be preserved safely for almost 24 hours. Kidneys tolerate the longest ischemic time, up to 72 hours.

After the preservation process has begun and donated organs have been recovered, they are individually packaged in containers or sterilized plastic bags. The procured organs are then placed in a cooler that contains crushed ice and shipped to the selected medical center for transplantation. This type of preservation is known as simple static cold storage.

Another method, which is employed primarily for kidneys, is known as pulsatile perfusion preservation. The initial preservation steps are essentially the same, but instead of being packed in an ice cooler, the donated kidney is placed in a sterile environment with a cannula introduced into the renal artery, and a cold solution is continually pumped through the organ. This process provides oxygen and nutrition to the organ and retains a core temperature of 4° to 7°C. Although such preservation is cumbersome and expensive, it seems to result in better long-term preservation and initial organ function than does simple static cold storage.[87] A number of centers are reviving the method, owing to the time-consuming regulations that must be adhered to regarding organ allocation.

TRANSPLANT ORGANIZATIONS AND ALLOCATION OF ORGANS ■

The list of candidates awaiting transplantation has grown from 10,000 to 40,000 in one decade.[13] Because of this rapid growth, the government, the transplant community, and, most importantly, the public recognized early the need to develop a formal organizational system to ensure high standards of care and equal access to transplantation.

UNITED NETWORK FOR ORGAN SHARING

In 1984, the United States government passed a law, commonly known as the National Organ Transplant Act, which mandated development of the National Organ and Transplantation System.[88] In 1986, the United Network for Organ Sharing (UNOS), located in Richmond, Virginia, was granted the responsibility for this function. The National Organ

Transplant Act requires that transplant centers, organ procurement agencies, and histocompatibility laboratories be members of UNOS. The purpose of UNOS is twofold. The first is to ensure equal access to organs for all patients awaiting transplantation. The second is to establish policies and procedures for standards of operation of all transplant-related organizations.

UNOS is governed by a board of directors made up of no more than 50% physicians. The board includes members of the transplant community and members of the general public, the voluntary health organizations, donor families, patients awaiting transplantation, and transplant recipients. Membership requirements, organ procurement procedures, and histocompatibility standards are designed by UNOS committees and must be approved by the board of directors before implementation. All policy changes are published in the *Federal Register* for public comment. Based on public reaction, new policies may be altered before implementation.

Although a number of problems still exist in the operation of UNOS, this unified front represents the most advanced and best organized approach to transplantation in the world today. Adherence to UNOS policies, for the most part, ensures equal access to transplantable organs for all selected patients.

Allocation

The single most difficult task facing UNOS has been the development of a fair and equitable system to allocate available organs for transplantation.[89] A fairly sophisticated system exists today, but it continues to undergo further refinements.

KIDNEYS AND PANCREATA. Kidneys are allocated by matching ABO blood type, tissue type, percentage of reactive antibodies, and waiting time.[90] Other information regarding the donor is entered into the UNOS computer system, and patients are matched accordingly. Numeric values are assigned, and the eligible patient with the most points is offered the opportunity for transplantation first. A similar system is in place for allocation of pancreata.

HEARTS, LUNGS, AND LIVERS. For the allocation of hearts, lungs, and livers, the selection system varies slightly. Tissue matching is impractical and is not deemed as important in the transplantation of these organs. Lungs are allocated solely on the basis of waiting time and the recipient's distance from the donor site. Most transplantation surgeons agree that if a patient who is awaiting lung transplantation deteriorates to the point of ventilator dependency, transplantation is no longer an option. Therefore, medical criteria, at present, are not used in allocating lungs.

With liver and heart transplantation, the patient's medical condition plays an important role in organ allocation. Numeric status codes are given to patients awaiting heart or liver transplantation. A higher code value is assigned to a recipient who is maintained on mechanical support in an ICU, for example, than to one who is homebound and in fairly healthy condition. The total score is calculated for every waiting patient, and organs are distributed accordingly.

LOCAL PRIMACY. Transplantation surgeons have some leeway to override the allocation system based on specific medical criteria. However, a written explanation must be provided to UNOS for each such case. This possibility was developed to allow individual physician judgment, which must be available in any area of medicine that involves patient selection. With the exception of kidneys, which must be distributed on a national basis, the system has always recognized *local primacy* for organ distribution if a perfect match exists.

This approach has caused a considerable amount of discussion within the transplant community. Organs are allocated to patients waiting within the designated OPO service area before being allocated regionally or nationally. One of the most important reasons for allocating organs on this basis is to stimulate donation. Local primacy allegedly stimulates organ donation for local patients. If all organs were placed into a national pool, health care workers and donor family members might be less eager to work compassionately toward obtaining or providing consent for organ donation.

Because the need for organs has increased significantly in the past decade, local primacy for organ distribution may not be in the best interests of the recipients. Some question the appropriateness of giving an heart or liver to the sickest *local* recipient but not the sickest *national* recipient if the local patient is in a less critical category. The current system of giving priority to local, then regional, and finally national allocation could result in an increased mortality rate for those patients awaiting organs other than kidneys.

LIVING DONORS

The first successful kidney transplantation was performed between identical twins and resulted in a 9-year recipient survival. However, when non-twin siblings or other close relatives were used, the success rate was poor until the development of effective immunosuppression therapy. In 1994, 28% of all transplanted kidneys in the United States came from living relatives. Today, the success rate with such kidneys is significantly better than the results with kidneys transplanted from brain-dead, heart-beating donors. This form of organ donation accounts for 0% to 75% of transplantations in different countries. The highest frequency is reported in Japan, which continues to lack brain death legislation.

In addition to kidneys, the tail of the pancreas has been transplanted from living related donors, but the success rate of this procedure has been less than promising. The high frequency of complications in donors has also resulted in less enthusiasm for this procedure. In recent years, the left liver lobe and even lung lobes have been transplanted from living related donors, usually from parents to children. Although these operations are not yet commonly performed, the results have been encouraging. Living nonrelated donors are also used; in the United States, they are usually spouses or other emotionally-related donors.

In the United States, organs cannot be sold or dealt for profit. However, in developing countries such as India, the selling of a kidney can provide a significant sum to a financially struggling family, sometimes as much as could be earned in a full decade. India has introduced legislation prohibiting organ trade, and recently presented standards for organ donation and transplantation recommend that all countries legislate against organ trade for profit.[91]

NON–HEART-BEATING DONORS

After the first successful organ transplantation in the 1950s, aggressive efforts to use kidneys from just-deceased patients were made, initially with poor results. Use of non–heart-beating cadaver donors all but vanished after heart-beating, brain-dead donors became available in the late 1960s. However, the current shortage of donor organs has led to renewed use of organs from non–heart-beating cadavers. Different types of donors can be identified within this category.

Cardiac Arrest During Evaluation for Brain Death

If consent for organ donation already has been obtained, cardiopulmonary resuscitation may be initiated to maintain some perfusion of donated organs while the donor is brought to the operating room for emergent procurement of organs. Death must first be certified according to traditional cardiac criteria. Because cardiopulmonary resuscitation to save the patient's life in the presence of lethal head injury with evolving brain death is not indicated, it is interrupted in the operating room to permit certification of death after cessation of cardiac function is diagnosed. Kidneys and livers have been transplanted from such donors with good results.

Withdrawal of Life-Sustaining Therapy and Organ Donation After Death

In the 1980s, ICU physicians in the United States were surprised to find patients or their relatives requesting not only withdrawal of life support in hopeless situations but also organ donation after death. After significant problems surrounding transplantation of kidneys from one such donor at the University of Pittsburgh Medical Center in 1992, a policy was designed and approved for this particular situation.[92] If life-sustaining therapy is to be withdrawn, such donors are taken to the operating room for terminal weaning from mechanical ventilation. After cardiac arrest has occurred, death is certified and organ procurement takes place immediately.

A major ethical problem is that family members are not permitted to be present in the operating room during this terminal phase of life. This problem is solved if an adjacent room can be used for this purpose. Nonetheless, no time for prolonged grief and farewell after certification of death is possible, because warm ischemia rapidly reduces the success of graft transplantation. The Universities of Iowa and Pittsburgh have reported successful transplantation of kidneys and livers in this setting.[93,94]

Sudden Cardiac Arrest in Previously Relatively Healthy Patients

Although a technique has been developed for rapid in situ cooling of just-deceased trauma victims or cardiac patients, this possibility for procurement of organs in victims with documented consent (e.g., an organ donor card) is not yet in common use owing to a conflict of interest between efforts to save the patient and those that merely procure organs for transplantation. A potential exists for criticism and lawsuits should family members have the impression that not everything was done to save the life of their relative before organs were removed. Nonetheless, this may become the most common organ donor category in the future.

XENOTRANSPLANTATION

Xenografting was initially attempted more than 25 years ago when primate kidneys were transplanted into humans. Recent advancements in immunosuppression have made further attempts at xenotransplantation more realistic, although not yet successful. Technical difficulties and philosophic concerns surrounding use of higher primates for organ transplantation to humans distinguish this approach. Continued investigation of potential primate donors should answer further questions about control of rejection and may provide an increase in the organ pool available for recipients. However, concern also exists for potential spread of currently unknown zooses.

REFERENCES

1. Ellison M, Daily OP, Breen T, et al: *Annual Report of the U.S. Scientific Registry of Transplant Recipients and the Organ Procurement and Transplantation Network*. Richmond, VA, United Network for Organ Sharing, 1993
2. Held P, Kahan B, Hunsincker L, et al: The impact of HLA mismatches on the survival of first cadaveric kidney transplant. *N Engl J Med* 1994;331:765
3. Barnard CN: A human cardiac transplant: An interim report of a successful operation at Groote Schuur Hospital in Cape Town. *S Afr Med J* 1967;41:1271
4. *UNOS Update* 1995;11:39
5. Kawai A, Paradis IL, Keenan RJ, et al: Lung transplantation at the University of Pittsburgh: 1982–1994. In: Terasaki PI, Cecka JM (eds). *Clinical Transplants, 1994*. Los Angeles, UCLA Tissue Typing Laboratory, 1995
6. Sutherland DER, Moudry-Munns KC: International Pancreas Transplant Registry report. In: Terasaki P (ed). *Clinical Transplants*. Los Angeles, UCLA Tissue Typing Laboratory, 1988
7. Kelly WD, Lillehei RC, Merkel FK, et al: Allotransplantation of the pancreas and duodenum along with the kidney in diabetic nephropathy. *Surgery* 1967;61:827
8. Shaw BW, Bahnson HT, Hardesty RL, et al: Combined transplantation of the heart and liver. *Ann Surg* 1985;220:667
9. Livesey SA, Rolles K, Calne RY, et al: Successful simultaneous heart and kidney transplantation using the same donor. *Clin Transpl* 1988;2:1
10. Margreiter R, Kramar R, Huber C, et al: Combined liver and kidney transplant. *Lancet* 1984;1:1077
11. *UNOS Update* 1995;11:26

12. Mackersie RC, Bronsther OL, Shackford SR: Organ procurement in patients with fatal head injuries. *Ann Surg* 1991; 213:143
13. Veatch R: The whole-brain-oriented concept of death: An outmoded philosophical formulation. *J Thanatol* 1975;13:3
14. Youngner SJ, Bartlett ET: Human death and high technology; The failure of the whole brain formulations. *Ann Intern Med* 1983;99:252
15. Harrison MR: Fetal organ transplantation: Organ procurement for children. The anencephalic fetus as donor. *Lancet* 1986; 2:1383
16. Warren J: AMA adopts resolution approving anencephalic as potential organ donor. *Transplant News* 1994;4:5
17. Beecher H: A definition of irreversible coma: Report of the ad hoc committee of the Harvard Medical School to examine the definition of brain death. *JAMA* 1968;205:337
18. The Multisociety Task Force on PVS: Medical aspects of the persistent vegetative state. *N Engl J Med* 1994;330:1572
19. Schuler S, Parnt R, Warnecke H, et al: Extended donor criteria for heart transplantation. *J Heart Transplant* 1988;7:326
20. Harjula A, Starnes VA, Oyer PE, et al: Proper donor selection for heart-lung transplantation. *J Thorac Cardiovasc Surg* 1987;94:874
21. Szmidt J, Karolak T, Sablinski T, et al: Transplantation of kidneys harvested from donors over sixty years of age. *Transplant Proc* 1988;20:772
22. Klintmalm GB: The liver donor: Special consideration. *Transplant Proc* 1988;20(Suppl 7):9
23. Alexander JW, Vaughn WK: The use of marginal donor for organ transplantation: The influence of donor age on outcome. *Transplantation* 1991;51:135
24. Alexander JW, Bennett LE, Breen TJ: Effect of donor age on outcome of kidney transplantation: A two-year analysis of transplants reported to the United Network for Organ Sharing Registry. *Transplantation* 1994;57:871
25. Marino IR, Doyle HR, Aldrighetti L, et al: Effect of donor age and sex on the outcome of liver transplantation. Submitted for publication, 1995
26. Darby JM, Stein K, Grenvik A, et al: Approach to the management of the heart-beating brain dead organ donor. *JAMA* 1989;261:2222
27. President's Commission for the Study of Ethical Problems in Medicine and Biomedical and Behavioral Research: Guidelines for the determination of death: Report of the medical consultants on the diagnosis of death. *JAMA* 1981;246:2184
28. Task Force for the Determination of Brain Death in Children: Guidelines for the determination of brain death in children. *Ann Neurol* 1987;21:616
29. Powner DJ: The diagnosis of brain death in the adult patient. *J Intensive Care Med* 1987;2:181
30. De al Riva A, Gonzalez FM, Llamas-Elvira JM, et al: Diagnosis of brain death: Superiority of perfusion studies with ^{99m}Tc-HMPAO over conventional radionuclide cerebral angiography. *Br J Radiol* 1992;65:289
31. Schlake H-P, Bottger IH, Grotemeyer K-H, et al: Determination of cerebral perfusion by means of planar brain scintigraphy and ^{99m}Tc-HMPAO in brain death, persistent vegetative state and severe coma. *Intensive Care Med* 1992;18:76
32. Wilson K, Gordon L, Selby JB: The diagnosis of brain death with Tc-99m HMPAO. *Clin Nucl Med* 1993;18:428
33. Jeret JS, Benjamin JL: Risk of hypotension during apnea testing. *Arch Neurol* 1994;51:595
34. Emery RW, Cork RC, Levinson MM, et al: The cardiac donor: A six-year experience. *Ann Thorac Surg* 1986;41:356
35. Robertson KM, Hramiak IM, Gelb AW, et al: Endocrine changes and hemodynamic stability after brain death. *Transplant Proc* 1989;21:1197
36. Powner DJ, Jastremski M, Lagler RG, et al: Continuing care of multiorgan donor patients. *J Intensive Care Med* 1989;4:75
37. Fink MP: In vivo organ preservation in brain dead patients. *J Intensive Care* 1989;4:53
38. Griepp RB, Stinson EB, Clark DA, et al: The cardiac donor. *Surg Gynecol Obstet* 1971;133:792
39. Flanigan WJ, Ardon LF, Brewer TE, et al: Etiology and diagnosis of early post-transplantation oliguria. *Am J Surg* 1976; 132:808
40. Toledo-Pereyra LH, Simmons RL, Olson LC, et al: Cadaver kidney transplantation: Effect of hypotension and donor pretreatment with methylprednisolone and phenoxybenzamine. *Minn Med* 1979;62:159
41. Starzl TE, Demetris AJ, Van Thiel D, et al: Liver transplantation. *N Engl J Med* 1989;321:1014
42. Randell T, Orko R, Hockerstedt K: Perioperative fluid management of the brain-dead multiorgan donor. *Acta Anaesthesiol Scand* 1990;34:592
43. Pennefather SH, Bullock RE, Dark JH: The effect of fluid therapy on alveolar arterial oxygen gradient in brain dead organ donors. *Transplantation* 1993;56:1418
44. Wicomb WN, Cooper DKC, Lanza RP, et al: The effects of brain death and 24 hours storage by hypothermic perfusion on donor heart function in the pig. *J Thorac Cardiovasc Surg* 1986;91:896
45. Mertes PM, el Abassi K, Jaboin Y, et al: Changes in hemodynamic and metabolic parameters following induced brain death in the pig. *Transplantation* 1994;58:414
46. Goldberg LI: Cardiovascular and renal actions of dopamine: Potential clinical applications. *Pharmacol Rev* 1972;24:1
47. Novitsky D, Cooper DKC, Morrell D, et al: Change from aerobic to anaerobic metabolism after brain death, and reversal following triiodothyronine therapy. *Transplant* 1988;45:32
48. Novitsky D, Cooper DKC, Reichart B, et al: Hemodynamic and metabolic responses to hormonal therapy in brain dead potential organ donors. *Transplant* 1987;43:852
49. Novitzky D, Cooper DKC, Human PA, et al: Triiodothyronine therapy for heart donor and recipient. *J Heart Transplant* 1988;7:370
50. Orlowski JP, Spees EK: The use of thyroxine (T-4) to promote hemodynamic stability in the vascular organ donor: A preliminary report on the Colorado experience. *J Transplant Coordination* 1991;1:19
51. Orlowski JP, Spees EK: Eighteen-month graft and patient survival following liver transplantation with organs recovered from cadaveric donors managed with thyroxine: A retrospective study. *J Transplant Coordination* 1991;1:144
52. Howlett TA, Keogh AM, Perry L, et al: Anterior and posterior pituitary function in brain stem–dead donors. *Transplantation* 1989;47:828
53. Robertson KM, Hramiak IM, Gelb AW, et al: Endocrine changes and hemodynamic stability after brain death. *Transplant Proc* 1989;21:1197
54. Macoviak JA, McDougall IR, Bayer MD, et al: Significance of thyroid dysfunction in human cardiac allograft procurement. *Transplant* 1987;43:24
55. Wahlers T, Fieguth HG, Jurmann M, et al: Does hormone depletion of organ donors impair myocardial function after cardiac transplantation? *Transplant Proc* 1988;20(Suppl 1):792
56. Gifford RRM, Weaver AS, Burg JE, et al: Thyroid hormone levels in heart and kidney cadaver donors. *J Heart Transplant* 1986;5:49
57. Koller J, Wieser C, Gottardis M, et al: Thyroid hormones and their impact on the hemodynamic and metabolic stability of

organ donors and on kidney graft function after transplantation. *Transplant Proc* 1990;22:355

58. Garcia-Fages LC, Cabrer C, Valero R, et al: Hemodynamic and metabolic effects of substitute triiodothyronine therapy in organ donors. *Transplant Proc* 1993;25:3038

59. Lucas BA, Baughn WK, Spees EK, Sanfillipo F: Identification of donor factors predisposing to high discard rates of cadaver kidneys and increased graft loss within one year post transplantation: SEOPF 1977–1982. *Transplantation* 1987;43:253

60. Nygaard CE, Townsend RN, Diamond DL: Organ donor management and organ outcome: A 6-year review from a level 1 trauma center. *J Trauma* 1990;30:728

61. Hayek DA, Veremakis C, O'Brien JA, et al: Enhanced vasomotor sensitivity to vasoactive agents during the evolution of brain death. *Chest* 1990;98(Suppl):63S

62. Mallory DL, Nelson JE, Matuschak GM, et al: Risk factors for loss of donor organs in brain-dead ICU patients due to unexpected cardiac arrest. *Chest* 1989;96(Suppl):289S

63. Nishimura N, Miyata Y: Cardiovascular changes in the terminal stage of disease. *Resuscitation* 1984;12:175

64. Powner DJ, Hendrich A, Lagler RG, et al: Hormonal changes in brain dead patients. *Crit Care Med* 1990;18:70

65. Kroncke GM, Nichols RD, Mendenhall JT, et al: Ectothermic philosophy of acid-base balance to prevent fibrillation during hypothermia. *Arch Surg* 1986;121:303

66. Swain JA: Hypothermia and blood pH: A review. *Arch Intern Med* 1988;148:1643

67. White FN: A comparative physiological approach to hypothermia. *J Thorac Cardiovasc Surg* 1981;82:821

68. Hayek DA, Veremakis C, O'Brien JA, et al: Time-dependent characteristics of hemodynamic instability in brain dead organ donors. *Crit Care Med* 1990;18:S204

69. Keren G, Schreiber M, Aladjem M, et al: Diabetes insipidus indicating a dying brain. *Crit Care Med* 1982;10:798

70. Outwater KM, Rockoff MA: Diabetes insipidus accompanying brain death in children. *Neurology* 1984;34:1243

71. Rabanal JM, Teja JL, Quesada A, et al: Does diabetes insipidus in brain dead organ donors protect acute tubular necrosis in the renal grafts? *Transplant Proc* 1993;25:3143

72. Slapak M: The immediate care of potential donors for cadaveric organ transplantation. *Anesthesia* 1978;33:700

73. Palombo JD, Hirschberg Y, Pomposelli JJ, et al: Decreased loss of liver adenosine triphosphate during hypothermic preservation in rats pretreated with glucose: Implications for organ donor management. *Gastroenterology* 1988;95:1043

74. Jastremski M, Powner D, Snyder J, et al: Problems in brain death. *Forensic Sci* 1978;11:201

75. Ouakine GE: Bedside procedures in the diagnosis of brain death. *Resuscitation* 1975;4:159

76. Curley FJ, Irwin RS: Disorders of temperature control: Hypothermia. Part III. *J Intensive Care Med* 1986;1:270

77. Wong KC: Physiology and pharmacology of hypothermia. *West J Med* 1983;138:227

78. Hefty TR, Cotterell LW, Fraser SC, et al: Disseminated intravascular coagulation in cadaveric organ donors: Incidence and effect on renal transplantation. *Transplantation* 1993;55:442

79. Health Care and Finance Administration: *Certified Organ Procurement Organizations, 1990.*

80. Association of Organ Procurement Organizations. *Annual Membership Survey, 1990.*

81. Garrison RN, Bentley FR, Raque GH, et al: There is an answer to the organ donor shortage. *Surg Gynecol Obstet* 1991;173:391

82. Miracle K, Broznick B, Stuart S: Coroner/medical examiner cooperation with the donation process: One OPO's experience. *J Transplant Coordination* 1993;3:23

83. Schafer T, Schkade LL, Warner HE, et al: Impact of medical examiner/coroner practices on organ recovery in the United States. *JAMA* 1994;272:1607

84. Wahlberg JA, Southard JH, Belzer FO: Development of a cold storage solution for pancreas preservation. *Cryobiology* 1986; 23:477

85. Collins GM, Bravo-Sugarman M, Terasaki PI: Kidney preservation for transportation: Initial perfusion and 30 hours' ice storage. *Lancet* 1969;2:1219

86. Dreikorn K, Horsch R, Rohl L: 48 to 96 hour preservation of canine kidneys by initial perfusion and hypothermic storage using the Euro-Collins solution. *Eur Urol* 1980;6:221

87. Barber W, Laskaw D, Deiehoi M, et al: Comparison of simple hypothermic storage, pulsatile perfusion with Belzer's gluconate-albumin solution, and pulsatile perfusion with UW solution for renal allograft preservation. *Transplant Proc* 1993; 25:2394

88. National Organ Transplant Act. Public Law 98-507, October 19, 1984.

89. Stratta R, Taylor R: Kidney allocation in the 1990s: Progress and problems. *Transplant Proc* 1993;25:3065

90. Starzl TE, Shapiro R, Teperman L: The point system for organ distribution. *Transplant Proc* 1989;21:3432

91. *UNOS Update* 1995;11

92. Youngner SJ, Arnold RM: Ethical, psychosocial, and public policy implications of procuring organs from non–heart beating cadaver donors. *JAMA* 1993;269:2769

93. D'Allessandro AM, Hoffmann RM, Knechtle SJ, et al: Controlled non–heart beating donors: A potential source of extrarenal organs. *Transplant Proc* 1995;27:707

94. Casavilla A, Ramirez C, Shapiro R, et al: Liver and kidney transplantation from non–heart beating donors: The Pittsburgh experience. *Transplant Proc* 1996;27:710

Critical Care, Third Edition, edited by Joseph M. Civetta,
Robert W. Taylor, and Robert R. Kirby.
Lippincott-Raven Publishers, Philadelphia, PA © 1997.

CHAPTER 85

∎

Renal Transplantation

Matthew E. Brunson
William W. Pfaff
George W. Burke, III
Gaetano Ciancio

IMMEDIATE CONCERNS ∎

MAJOR PROBLEMS

In the absence of cardiopulmonary risks, the indication for intensive care of the renal allograft patient is monitoring of graft function. Some patients have an obligatory diuresis of several hundred milliliters per hour and can become intravascularly depleted. Others make little urine, requiring judicious fluid therapy that provides optimal graft perfusion while avoiding intravascular volume overload. The most common problem is an inappropriately low urine output. The differential diagnosis includes (1) obstruction of urine flow anywhere between the renal pelvis and the collection bag, (2) graft hypoperfusion, (3) urinary leak, and (4) renal parenchymal disease, usually acute tubular necrosis (ATN). The most important datum is the patient's previous history. End-stage renal failure patients may still make substantial quantities of urine per day. Previously nonoliguric patients with oliguria may have a mechanical blockage to urine flow. A less likely but equally urgent possibility is that cardiac output is markedly diminished. If a brisk diuresis was observed in the operating room or has been recorded in previous hours, a sudden reduction in urine flow should immediately raise suspicion of a mechanical problem.

Frequently, blood clots obstruct the urinary catheter. The patient complains of a sense of fullness and need to urinate. "Milking" the urinary catheter tubing poses no risk of contaminating the closed system and usually dislodges the clots. If catheter irrigation is necessary, meticulously sterile technique is used. Sterile saline, 20 to 30 mL, should be instilled

retrograde to facilitate mechanically breaking up the clot. Avoid overdistention of the bladder, which risks rupture of the ureteroneocystostomy or bladder closure. If irrigation fails to evacuate the clot, remove the Foley catheter and replace it with a larger one (nos. 18 through 20). If clots still accumulate, a triple-lumen urinary catheter permits continuous bladder irrigation. Rarely, cystoscopy is required to evacuate clots.

Other mechanical problems include obstruction of the ureter or urine leak.[1] These should always be suspected when there has been a history of brisk urine flow noted at surgery, but little or none has been noticed since bladder closure. Urine leak can present as severe wound pain, ascites, scrotal or labial edema, and fluid draining from the wound or operative drains with urea nitrogen and creatinine concentrations much higher than serum. Ultrasonography is particularly useful in diagnosing hydroureter or perinephric fluid collections.[2] These problems require immediate operative correction.

After exclusion of outflow problems, determine that the graft is adequately perfused. Norms for "adequate" blood pressure are higher after grafting, especially in children receiving adult kidneys and patients with limited cardiac contractility. To some degree, all transplanted kidneys have sustained predonation procurement and reperfusion injuries.[3] There is an increase in interstitial edema and increased venocapillary resistance, endothelial swelling and denuding, and activation of vasoactive mediators. The resistance of the renal vascular bed is increased. Renal plasma flow requires a higher mean arterial pressure in this setting. The renal transplant recipient usually requires a blood pressure greater

1301

than 120/80 mm Hg. The patient's history of average pretransplant pressures is valuable in targeting perfusion pressure.

Unless there is clear evidence of *intravascular* volume overload, give a bolus of 5 to 10 mL/kg of normal saline to improve urine output. A transient response justifies further volume expansion. Most dialysis-dependent patients have total-body fluid overload. Their "dry weight," used to calculate an endpoint on dialysis, is always in excess of the dry weight they reach with normal renal function. Some specialists advocate routine use of low-dose dopamine to foster renal graft perfusion. Patients with marginal cardiac output often improve renal graft perfusion remarkably with dopamine at 2 to 4 μg/kg/minute.

Rarely, the intrarenal vascular resistance is excessively high, and adequate perfusion pressures do not produce sufficient intrarenal blood flow. This problem dramatically increases the risk of further ischemic injury or even thrombosis. Grafts from pediatric donors, especially those younger than 4 years of age, are prone to thrombosis. As an additional safeguard, we begin all patients on low-dose aspirin therapy (162 mg) immediately after surgery to minimize the risk of thrombosis.

In patients with high titers of preformed antibodies against major histocompatibility antigens, a form of early rejection can occur called *accelerated acute rejection*. This form of rejection is mediated by preexisting antibodies that activate complement and produce progressive thrombosis. Singly or in combination, technical problems, hypoperfusion, and immunologic factors can lead to graft thrombosis. Graft thrombosis is rare, but any hope of graft salvage requires immediate return to the operating room. Graft flow can be documented indirectly by Doppler ultrasonography or radionuclide flow scans, but high suspicion of thrombosis is a contraindication to further immunosuppressive therapy and should be diagnosed early.

STRESS POINTS

1. Acute tubular necrosis is the most common cause of delayed function after renal transplant, but the diagnosis should be accepted only after all the aforementioned problems have been excluded. Living related donor kidneys should *not* have significant ATN unless intraoperative problems are present. Cadaveric kidneys, however, usually have sustained some insult, and a significant incidence of ATN is expected after cadaveric renal grafting.
2. Oliguric ATN rates range from 10% to 30%, depending on donor circumstances, cold ischemic times, and preservation technique.
3. In assessing renal grafts, it is useful to group functions into (1) filtration, (2) secretion, (3) concentration, and (4) systemic metabolism. ATN may impair these functions unequally.
4. If filtration is maintained but there is little secretion or concentration, large volumes of urine output may result without elimination of potassium (K^+), urea, or creatinine.
5. Until full recovery of all elements of renal function

occurs, the patient may require intermittent dialysis for uremia or electrolyte abnormalities.
6. Because of surgical catabolism and the effect of steroids, hyperkalemia and markedly elevated blood urea nitrogen (BUN) may develop soon after transplantation. Plan to dialyze the oliguric patient the next day, temporizing if necessary with K^+-exchange resin enemas, glucose–insulin administration, or bicarbonate infusions.[4]
7. High-output ATN is one cause of polyuria and represents a failure of concentrating ability. But even living related grafts have a polyuric phase because of obligatory osmotic diuresis. Urea and other osmotically active wastes are elevated before transplantation; once filtered in the glomerulus, they produce an obligatory free water loss.
8. Unlike the implication in nontransplant patients, a high hourly urine output may not be a sign of normal or elevated intravascular volume. It is usually necessary to replace most of this volume loss to prevent decreased cardiac output, hypotension, and graft thrombosis.
9. Ideally, urine output begins briskly (e.g., 200 mL/hour) and gradually decreases to 1.0 to 1.5 mL/kg/hour over the next day. The fresh allograft cannot concentrate urine and clear wastes at less than approximately 800 mL/m^2 per day.
10. Renal vein thrombosis often progresses to complete graft infarction, but initially may be manifested by decreasing renal function, hematuria, proteinuria, and leg or graft swelling.[5]
11. Hyperacute or accelerated acute rejection present as rapid, early, and progressive deterioration of urine output and graft blood flow. Graft rupture follows severe rejection and its associated graft swelling. The rupture often begins at a biopsy site or other breach of the renal capsule and presents as pain and hemorrhage. Ureteral necrosis may present after several days or weeks as urine leak, ureteral stenosis, or hydroureter.

ESSENTIAL DIAGNOSTIC TESTS AND PROCEDURES

1. Low urine output can result for several reasons (Table 85-1).
2. BUN and serum creatinine (S_{Cr}) remain the easiest tests to follow. A steady decline in BUN and S_{Cr} suggests improving glomerular and tubular function. The BUN is usually disproportionately elevated as ureogenesis is markedly accelerated by induction steroids, surgical trauma, and bed rest.
3. Blood in the gastrointestinal (GI) tract enhances ureogenesis, and a sharp rise in BUN should heighten suspicion of occult GI bleeding. Drug interactions also confound these tests' interpretation. Cimetidine or trimethoprim/sulfamethoxazole raise S_{Cr} without decreasing glomerular filtration rate.
4. Doppler ultrasonography can demonstrate fluid collections around the kidney, hydroureter, clot in the

TABLE 85-1. Differential Diagnosis of Oliguria

MECHANICAL

    Clots in catheter
    Technical
    Urine leak

VASCULAR

    Technical—arterial or venous thrombosis
    Immunologic (humoral)

PARENCHYMAL

    Drug toxicity (NSAIDs, ACE inhibition, CsA)
    ATN

NSAIDs, nonsteroidal antiinflammatory drugs; ACE, angiotensin converting enzyme; CsA, cyclosporin; ATN, acute tubular necrosis.

ureter or bladder, graft edema, and blurring of the corticomedullary junction and flow to the cortex. Loss of diastolic flow on Doppler ultrasonography suggests increased renal vascular resistance, a condition that has some correlation with acute rejection.

5. Radionuclide scans have become increasingly useful at estimating the quality of flow but are not truly quantitative. These scans can also demonstrate small urine leaks and exclude segmental infarcts.
6. Renal allograft biopsy remains the gold standard for diagnosis of rejection, drug toxicity, and ATN. A core needle biopsy is obtained percutaneously. Ultrasound guidance minimizes the risk of transperitoneal passage or injury to hilar structures, especially in obese patients.

INITIAL THERAPY

1. The patient needs maintenance fluids for respiratory and sweat loss, plus replacement for obligatory urine losses. The urine sodium is usually near 75 mMol/L, and 0.45 normal saline is the replacement fluid of choice.[2]
2. Postgrafting fluid therapy is outlined in Table 85-2. The use of glucose-containing fluids prevents ketosis.

TABLE 85-2. Fluid Therapy After Renal Transplant

$D_5^{1}/4NS$ AT	FOR WEIGHT
3 mL/kg/h	≤10 kg
2 mL/kg/h	10–20 kg
1 mL/kg/h	20–40 kg
0.5 mL/kg/h	>40 kg

Plus replacement of urine loss:
    Replace mL/mL with $^{1}/2$NS up to 400 mL/h maximum
    Above 400 mL/h, replace additional urine output
    $^{1}/2$ mL/mL if CVP <10 cm H_2O

$D_5^{1}/4NS$, 5% dextrose in one fourth normal saline; $^{1}/2$NS, one half normal saline; AT, after transplant; Max, maximum; CVP, central venous pressure.

3. Hetastarch and saline are useful for acutely increasing cardiac preload but are inadequate replacement for the free water loss from diuresis.
4. K^+ and magnesium are elevated by increased tissue breakdown and poor tubular excretion. No supplementation should be given until good clearance is demonstrated.
5. If the patient is volume overloaded, sodium bicarbonate provides an expeditious way to lower K^+ and correct acidosis without the need for dialysis.
6. Phosphate is usually elevated and calcium decreased in renal failure, but these are self-normalizing after transplant and do not require changes in therapy.

IMMUNOSUPPRESSANTS AND THEIR COMPLICATIONS ■

CYCLOSPORINE

Cyclosporine (cyclosporin A [CsA]) is a fungal metabolite that inhibits T-cell production of interleukin-2. It is highly lipophilic and water insoluble. It has only about 30% bioavailability orally, and its absorption is variable, being strongly affected by the immediate milieu of fats and bile in the duodenum. Once absorbed, it is converted by the P450 system to over 17 metabolites of lesser immunosuppressive activity.

CsA may be given orally or intravenously. The oral dose is approximately 8 to 12 mg/kg/day divided into one to four doses. Consistent oral absorption is best achieved by administering CsA with a fatty food in the same manner each day. The intravenous dose is 2 to 4 mg/kg/day, given either as a continuous drip or as boluses administered over 2 hours each three times a day.

There are several important considerations to using the intravenous form. Cyclosporine is solubilized by a cremaphor, which may have its own toxicities. Seizures, beginning as irritability and myoclonic jerks and progressing to generalized major motor events, are the worst complication of the intravenous preparation. These seizures are not dose related and can occur at any time during therapy. They are less common in renal transplant recipients than in liver recipients and may be more likely in patients with a low serum cholesterol level. Patients with sensitivity to the cremaphor or other castor oil products may have allergic reactions characterized by rash and bronchospasm.

In 1995, a new CsA formulation, Neoral, was released for general use.[6] It is a microemulsion that allows more reliable absorption and, therefore, greater bioavailability and individual patient consistency in blood levels. This preparation offers economic advantage by reducing daily dosage by 10% to 20%. There is also a trend toward reduced frequency of acute rejection.

Cyclosporine's major toxicity is arteriolar vasoconstriction, particularly of the renal vessels. This decreases glomerular filtration rate and causes a modest increase in S_{Cr}. At therapeutic CsA levels, the S_{Cr} rises approximately 0.2 mg/dL. This effect is variable, and some patients demonstrate a pronounced sensitivity to the drug. Drug levels in the blood correlate poorly with CsA nephrotoxicity, but it is rare when levels are markedly subtherapeutic. Rejection is less likely than CsA nephrotoxicity when levels are far above the normal therapeutic range.

Defining "therapeutic" blood levels of CsA is dependent on the assay used to measure CsA and the institutional immunosuppressive protocol. Table 85-3 outlines possible ranges of CsA trough levels depending on whether whole blood or serum is tested and whether parent compound only (HPLC), parent-specific monoclonal antibody (MoAb) (in radioimmunoassay or TDx test [Abbott Labs, Abbott Park, IL]), or parent-plus-metabolites (standard radioimmunoassay or TDx) is measured. Institutions that initiate CsA therapy at different times after transplant have different "target" levels and reduce CsA dosage for various indications.

Other CsA side effects include a fine intention tremor, hirsutism, and a moderate elevation in blood pressure. Hyperkalemia and hypomagnesemia are associated with CsA use. Cyclosporine-impaired insulin release is demonstrable experimentally, but is of doubtful clinical importance because previously euglycemic patients remain so. Steroid-induced hyperglycemia is more disturbing to the homeostasis of glucose-intolerant patients than is CsA.

TACROLIMUS

Tacrolimus (FK-506) is a macrolide that, like cyclosporine (CsA), inhibits lymphocyte formation of interleukin-2, although with a different receptor protein. On the basis of multiinstitutional studies[7,8] it has been approved by the Food and Drug Administration for liver transplantation and will likely be used for other organ transplants. This agent is an alternative to cyclosporine, with generally similar features of low water solubility, low bioavailability, cytochrome P450 metabolism, and enhanced metabolism in children. Contrasted with CsA, it has increased frequency of neurologic and GI side effects, renal dysfunction, and hyperkalemia. Tacrolimus is less likely to induce hypertension. The major advantage to this drug is a reduced incidence of acute rejection. The pattern of drug interactions is similar to CsA.

The intravenous solution often used for initial immunosuppression is in a solution of hydrogenated castor oil. This vehicle has been known to cause anaphylaxis and one should be prepared to manage this event with 1:10,000 epinephrine.

STEROIDS

All glucocorticoids suppress immune responses. Prednisone, or methylprednisolone, is almost universally included in induction immunosuppression. Doses are reduced over the first few weeks to "maintenance" levels that are further reduced over the next year. The exact mechanisms of their action are not fully elucidated, but decreased transcription of mRNA encoding for class II major histocompatibility molecules and several cytokines is their major effect. Steroids also impair generation of cyclooxygenase products, which function as secondary signals in rejection. Unlike CsA, steroids depress immune responses broadly. Neutrophils, macrophages, and B lymphocytes all are impaired. The major side effects of steroids are well known. Those of most concern in the transplant recipient are hyperglycemia, decreased mucosal resistance to acid-pepsin, and mood swings.

AZATHIOPRINE

Azathioprine (Imuran) becomes active after conversion to the purine analogue, 6-mercaptopurine. Metabolically active cells such as proliferating lymphocytes are sensitive to its action. Its major toxicity is myelosuppression. It usually takes several days to see a change in white blood count after a change in azathioprine dose, so it is important to begin dose reduction when the white blood cell count is rapidly decreasing or has fallen below 5000/mm^3. Oral and intravenous doses are equivalent. Allopurinol inhibits azathioprine metabolism and should not be used concurrently.

MYCOPHENOLATE MOFETIL

Mycophenolate mofetil, formerly known as RS-61443, was released in 1995 as an immunosuppressant, largely to replace azathioprine. It is currently available only in an oral form and should be started within 48 hours of transplantation. In randomized studies[9,10] it was associated with a decreased frequency of early acute rejection. Adverse events appear more frequently in patients receiving 1.5 g twice daily. Adverse events include GI complaints, leukopenia, and some indications of an increase in immunosuppression-related malignancies.

TABLE 85-3.   Typical Cyclosporin Levels, Depending on Assay Used

	HPLC	RIA OR TDx (PARENT AND METABOLITE)	RIA OR TDx (PARENT ONLY)
Whole blood	150–250 ng/mL	350–500 ng/mL	150–250 ng/dL
Plasma or serum	50–100 ng/mL	50–100 ng/mL	25–75 ng/mL

HPLC, high performance lipid chromotography; RIA, radioimmunoassay; TDx™, Abbott Laboratories, Abbott Park, IL.

ANTILYMPHOCYTE ANTIBODIES

Antilymphocyte antibodies are powerful agents not used for maintenance immunosuppression, but only for induction therapy or for treatment of rejection episodes. There are two general types of preparations: (1) polyvalent, polyclonal sera from inoculated mammals (e.g., equine antithymocyte globulin, equine or caprid Minnesota antilymphoblast globulin, and rabbit antithymocyte sera); and (2) monovalent, MoAbs produced from murine hybridomas (e.g., OKT3).

Polyvalent Sera

The polyvalent sera are historically useful, but are, nonetheless, crude preparations that offer no means by which to monitor their effect. The dosage varies with the preparation and its manufacturing lot, but is approximately 20 to 30 mg of serum per kilogram of body weight, dissolved in a large volume of saline (0.5 mL/mg serum) and administered over 4 to 6 hours. The most common side effect is intravascular volume overload followed by fever, thrombocytopenia, and flu-like symptoms. Patients with previous exposure to animal antibodies should not be treated with sera of the same species for fear of serum sickness or negation of the antilymphocyte effect. Immunity recovers slowly after the last dose of polyclonal ALGs.

Monoclonal (MoAbs)

MoAbs have numerous advantages over polyclonal products. They are an essentially pure preparation in a small volume (5 mL). Efficacy of treatment can be monitored by measuring blood levels of the agent, or flow cytometric counting of the absolute number of circulating lymphocytes bearing the target surface molecule (e.g., the T-cell antigen receptor, CD3). OKT3 is the first MoAb widely used in transplantation. It is a murine hybridoma IgG2a product that recognizes the CD3 marker on T lymphocytes. The CD3 epitope is closely associated with the T-cell antigen recognition site; thus, OKT3 treatment eliminates T lymphocytes capable of recognizing alloantigen and inactivates remaining lymphocytes by making them immunologically "blind."

OKT3 often has dramatic first-dose side effects. These are mediated by the release of tumor necrosis factor and other cytokines from activated lymphocytes or the phagocytes recognizing the antibody-coated cells. Between 30 minutes and 2 hours after the first dose of OKT3, the patient develops a "septic" picture with fever, chills, sweats, myalgia, and tachypnea. Some degree of increased capillary permeability always occurs. Frank pulmonary edema may follow in fluid-overloaded patients. Patients should not receive OKT3 if they are more than 10% above dry body weight; excess fluid should be removed through some form of dialysis first.

Pretreatment with steroids, acetaminophen, and antihistamines minimizes the side effects somewhat but does not eliminate them. Anecdotal reports suggest that indomethacin pretreatment is more effective at blocking side effects, but we have seen failures, and its overall safety in renal

transplantation is a concern. Nonsteroidal antiinflammatory drugs generally should not be used in renal graft recipients. Their inhibition of eicosanoid synthesis causes a loss of intrarenal autoregulation of blood flow, resulting in dramatic increases in S_{Cr}.

Some patients have milder symptoms with the second dose, but most have no further complaints with subsequent OKT3 doses. A small subset of patients may have low-grade fevers throughout their course of OKT3, but this possibility should be accepted only after ruling out an infectious problem. Rarely, a mild, sterile meningitis occurs late in OKT3 therapy; it is manifested as mild headache, with sterile subarachnoid fluid and increased numbers of lymphocytes, but negative results on India ink and crytopcoccal antigen tests. This problem resolves with completion of OKT3 therapy.

MINIMIZING INFECTIONS IN THE IMMUNOCOMPROMISED HOST

Nosocomial infections are the greatest threat to patients immediately after renal transplant.[11] Although opportunistic infections from uncommon pathogens characterize late transplant risks, the patient recovering in the ICU is most likely to develop pneumonia, bacteremia, bladder infection, or wound infection from organisms on the hands of medical caregivers. Contamination of the renal graft from bacteremia is potentially difficult to eradicate. It is imperative that the number of intravenous catheters be kept to a minimum, that rigid attention to hand-washing and gloving be maintained, and that any potentially contaminated catheter, tube, drain, or breathing circuit be changed immediately.

Prophylaxis against later viral and fungal infections begins early. All patients should receive clotrimazole (Mycelex) troches three times daily. Women with indwelling urinary catheters also should receive daily miconazole (Monistat) vaginal suppositories. Begin trimethoprim/sulfamethoxazole as a prophylaxis against *Pneumocystis carinii* pneumonia infection. Recent reports suggest prophylaxis may be effective against viral infections such as cytomegalovirus (CMV).[12,13]

OTHER PROBLEMS

CARDIOVASCULAR DISEASE

There is a high probability for cardiovascular disease to occur in renal transplant candidates. Cardiovascular events are the leading cause of death for patients awaiting transplantation. Most patients coming to renal transplantation are total-body volume overloaded, but their *intravascular* volume status depends on when they last underwent dialysis, on intraoperative volume changes, and on the degree of peripheral vasoconstriction. Most hemodialysis patients have lived in an every-other-day state of intravascular overload for years and have thick, hypertrophic ventricles that are relatively "stiff." They have a narrow range of optimal filling pressures and are at increased risk for subendocardial infarction.

DIABETES MELLITUS

Fifteen percent to 25% of renal graft recipients are diabetic. Their renal failure is the "tip of the iceberg" of their end-organ damage. In managing serum glucose after transplant, hyperglycemia should be expected and, to some degree, tolerated. However, ketosis should be prevented or immediately corrected. Hyperglycemia is fueled by high glucocorticoid doses and the release of epinephrine and other stress mediators by surgical trauma. The patient's preoperative and intraoperative insulin therapy is probably sufficient to prevent ketosis, but not to control hyperglycemia. Other than the markedly increased insulin needs compared with that in pretransplant patients, management of a patient with diabetes is the same as for any postoperative patient. Blood glucose should be monitored frequently until brought under "reasonable" control. We try to keep glucose levels below 350 mg/dL, preferably 150 to 250 mg/dL, but refrain from "tight" control and its inherent risk of hypoglycemia. Ketosis certainly increases insulin resistance and, once manifest, requires much more intensive glucose monitoring and insulin therapy. A continuous infusion insulin drip is indicated.

The kidney metabolizes circulating insulin, so that successful renal engraftment means an increase in insulin needs even after steroids are tapered to maintenance doses. Because some degree of renal dysfunction is always present immediately after transplant, this increase in insulin catabolism has a variable time of onset. In our experience, the greatest increase in insulin needs occurs 7 to 10 days postoperatively. Increased gluconeogenesis and insulin catabolism sometimes tip previously nondiabetic patients into a type II diabetic state. These patients should first be managed by oral hypoglycemics, dietary counseling, and sliding-scale insulin therapy. Many become euglycemic with scheduled reductions in steroid doses and resolution of surgical stress, but a significant subset require long-term insulin injection.

GASTROINTESTINAL PROBLEMS

Constipation is common after renal grafting. Most patients respond to early, preemptory use of mild cathartics, but in some the colonic ileus after retroperitoneal dissection can be severe. Although most patients do best by eating a regular diet as soon as they feel like it, patients complaining of "gas" or constipation should take nothing by mouth until colon activity is established. Distention requires nasogastric suctioning.

Acid-pepsin problems are also common. Approximately two thirds of early transplant patients require H_2 blockers for symptoms of dyspepsia, dysphagia, or "burning." Esophagitis, gastritis, duodenitis, and duodenal ulcer easily develop. Even in the asymptomatic patient, ulcerations should be suspected if the BUN rises out of proportion to S_{Cr}. Regardless of symptoms, a falling hematocrit or guaiac-positive stools should be treated with antacids or ranitidine until confirmed by endoscopy. Cimetidine is *not* used because it raises S_{Cr} levels. Antacids are the next agents of choice. Magnesium-based agents are avoided during periods of renal dysfunction. It seems that gastric mucosal protection with the prostaglandin E_1 analogue, misoprostol, has the salubri-

ous effect of enhanced renal graft survival.[14] Possible mechanisms include less CsA reduction of renal blood flow, additive immunosuppression,[15] decreased use of H_2 blockers (which impair T-suppressor function),[16] or a combination of these.

Enteral perforations and bleeding ulcerations are unusual but dire complications of transplantation. The most common site is the colon, but duodenal bulb ulcers and even small bowel may be involved. Perforations can be alarmingly asymptomatic, being detected first as free air under the diaphragm on routine chest radiographs or air in peritoneal dialysate. The diagnosis should always be entertained, and an upright chest radiograph must be obtained on any patient who "just doesn't look right."

"STABLE" ALLOGRAFT RECIPIENTS READMITTED TO THE ICU ■

Successful transplantation restores patients to an active and useful life, but it does not prevent subsequent occurrence of arteriosclerotic cardiovascular disease, cancer, trauma, and other major problems. The care of transplant patients with other diseases demands an awareness of possible effects on graft function. Because they are immunosuppressed, they must be isolated from and receive prophylaxis against infections with the same diligence as a patient with prosthetic heart valves.

CONVERTING ORAL IMMUNOSUPPRESSANTS TO INTRAVENOUS FORM

Azathioprine may be given in equivalent dose intravenously, but in the presence of sepsis (or other nephrotoxic drugs), its myelosuppressive toxicity may become important and dosage should be reduced. An equal dose of intravenous methylprednisolone can substitute for oral prednisone, although additional "stress" steroids may be needed for trauma when the daily maintenance dosage of prednisone is less than 0.25 mg/kg/day.

Cyclosporine dosing in the ICU is the greatest challenge. Its oral absorption is strongly influenced by the fat content of the meal and amount of bile flow into the duodenum. Fasting, biliary surgery, drug-induced cholestasis, and altered GI motility all can change the "appropriate" dose. It is usually best to rely on intravenous administration. As a rough approximation, the intravenous dose is one third of the total daily dose. This dosage should be 2 to 3 mg/kg day on average. Mix 50% of the total daily dose in 120 mL D_5W to run at 10 mL/hour each 12 hours. CsA levels need to be checked 6 to 12 hours after beginning IV infusion and daily thereafter.

INFECTIONS

Bacterial pathogens are the greatest threat immediately after transplantation, but after 2 to 3 weeks, viral and fungal pathogens increase in frequency as causes of serious illness. CMV infections appear from 2 weeks to several months after transplantation, frequently preceding or following rejection episodes. Low-grade fever, malaise, and lymphopenia characterize mild illness. Life-threatening CMV infections include GI ulcerations, pneumonitis, pancreatitis, hepatitis, and chorioretinitis. Second-pathogen infections are common in the patient with CMV; therefore, herpetic stomatitis, esophagitis, or candidal mucositis may be the first sign of CMV infection. A major advance in the management of CMV infections is the introduction of ganciclovir.[17]

Pneumocystis carinii pneumonia is rare earlier than 1 month after transplant. *Legionella, Aspergillus, Histoplasma,*

and *Cryptococcus* all can be present as nonspecific pulmonary infiltrates. Bronchoalveolar lavage has greatly aided in clarifying these diagnoses. Central nervous system infections with cryptococcus or other fungi, *Toxoplasma,* and mycobacteria are particularly insidious and should be quickly excluded in any transplant patient with persistent headache or mild mental status alterations. The list of possible pathogens is legion and can be compared with that expected in patients with acquired immunodeficiency syndrome. Rubin and Young[18] give a more thorough discussion of these infections.

TABLE 85-4. Drug Interactions Causing a Change in Cyclosporine and Tacrolimus Blood Levels

DRUG	EFFECT	SUGGESTED MECHANISMS
ANTIBIOTICS		
Erythromycin	Very increased levels	Competitive metabolism
Imipenem	?Decreased level	Increased metabolism in animal
	?Increased neurotoxicity	studies
Nafcillin	Decreased levels	Increased metabolism
Sulfamethoxazole trimethoprim (Bactrim/Septra)	Mild decreased levels	Unknown
ANTICONVULSANTS		
Carbamazepine	Decreased levels	Increased metabolism
Phenobarbital	Very decreased levels	Increased metabolism
Phenytoin (Dilantin)	Very decreased levels	Increased metabolism
Valproic acid	No effect	
ANTIFUNGALS		
Intraconazole	Very increased levels	Competitive metabolism
Ketoconazole	Very increased levels	Competitive metabolism
ANTITUBERCULOSUS AGENTS		
Isoniazid	Decreased levels	Increased metabolism
Rifampin	Decreased levels	Increased metabolism and possible T_s elimination
CALCIUM CHANNEL BLOCKERS		
Diltiazem	Very increased levels	Competitive metabolism
Nicardipine	Very increased levels	Competitive metabolism
Nifedipine	No effect	
Verapamil	Very increased levels	Competitive metabolism
GASTROINTESTINAL AGENTS		
Antacids	Variable effect	Altered absorption
Carafate	Variable effect	Altered absorption
Cimetidine	Slightly increased levels	Impaired metabolism
Famotidine	No effect	
Metoclopramide	Increased levels	Increased absorption
Ranitidine	Slightly increased levels	Improved absorption
HORMONES		
Oral contraceptives	Increased levels	Impaired metabolism
Prednisolone	Increased TDx/RIA levels	P-450 inhibition
	Decreased HPLC level	

RIA, radioimmunoassay; TDx™, Abbott Laboratories, Abbott Park, IL; HPLC, High performance lipid chromotography.

TABLE 85-5. Possible Toxicities With Cyclosporine and Tacrolimus in Combination With Other Drugs

ANTIINFECTIVES		
Aminoglycosides	Nephrotoxicity	Decreased renal plasma flow due to CsA
Amphotericin B	Nephrotoxicity	Same
Acyclovir	Nephrotoxicity	Same
Sulfamethoxazole trimethoprim (Septra/Bactrim)	Increased creatinine	Competitive inhibition of creatinine transport
ACE INHIBITORS	Variable effect	Renal flow protection in extrarenal transplants, sporadically worsened corticomedullary distribution of blood flow in renal transplants
ETHANOL	Variable	Increased absorption, variably altered metabolism
NONSTEROIDAL ANTIINFLAMMATORY AGENTS	Nephrotoxicity	Altered corticomedullary blood flow distribution

CsA, cyclosporine.

Epstein-Barr virus infections may manifest as an oligoclonal, lymphoproliferative disorder, which can progress to frank lymphoma. Reduction or withdrawal of pharmacologic immunosuppression is remarkably effective in causing regression of these lymphomas,[19] but additional therapy often is needed. Other neoplasms with unusually increased incidence after transplantation include Kaposi's sarcoma and tumors associated with viral infections such as cervical and vulvar carcinoma. Nonmelanoma skin neoplasms also have a greatly increased incidence compared with that seen in the general population.

MISCELLANEOUS CONCERNS ■

CHRONIC PROBLEMS

Long-term steroid therapy suppresses the hypothalamic-adrenal axis. Steroids raise serum cholesterol and in conjunction with pretransplant disease (e.g., diabetes) may predispose to early atherosclerotic cardiovascular disease. Aseptic necrosis of the femoral heads and cataracts may occur in "young" patients.

Patients taking long-term azathioprine may have little myeloid reserve and are often more likely to develop thrombocytopenia and leukopenia in the face of sepsis, hemorrhage, or myelosuppressive drugs.

Late causes of renal dysfunction still are headed by acute and chronic rejection and CsA toxicity. Additionally, lymphoceles accumulating around the graft impinge on the collecting system, causing obstructive uropathy. Stenosis in the distal ureter or reflux also may occur. All are remedied temporarily by percutaneous drainage. Obtain an ultrasound examination on any patient with late graft dysfunction.

Consider graft renal artery stenosis or native iliac artery stenosis in the long-term graft recipient with hypertension

or declining renal function. These patients are extremely sensitive to angiotensin-converting enzyme inhibitors, making small doses useful with radionuclide renal scans for diagnosis.[20] Stenosis in the aortoiliac inflow is managed by angioplasty or bypass with appropriate protection of renal flow during the procedure. Stenosis at the renal artery anastomosis is sometimes amenable to balloon angioplasty, but this procedure is risky, even for experienced radiologists. These lesions are more "rubbery" than atherosclerotic plaques, and because there is no collateral circulation, the risk of irreparable thrombosis is much greater. Diffuse stenoses and lesions in branch vessels are associated with chronic vascular rejection and have a poor prognosis.

POTENTIAL MEDICATION INTERACTIONS

Tables 85-4 and 85-5 list some known drug interactions pertinent to renal transplantation. In general, because CsA reduces plasma flow, potentially nephrotoxic agents are more likely to cause renal injury. Nonsteroidal antiinflammatory agents impair intrarenal prostaglandin-mediated autoregulation, and angiotensin-converting enzyme inhibitors sometimes cause severe renal dysfunction in renin-sensitive transplant recipients; therefore, these agents should be avoided. Cimetidine does not cause actual renal dysfunction, but competes for creatinine excretion, causing a spurious "worsening" of renal function which is reversible after drug withdrawal.

First-choice agents include those that have shown minimal interactions and have been widely used in transplantation. For hypertension, nifedipine, nitroprusside, and beta-blockers are best choices. Volume overload is the most common cause of hypertension in oliguric patients and is managed with dialysis.

REFERENCES ■

1. Starzl TE, Broth CG, Putnam CW, et al: Urologic complications in 216 human recipients of renal transplants. *Ann Surg* 1973;172:609

2. Petrek J, Tilney NL, Smith EH, et al: Ultrasound in renal transplantation. *Ann Surg* 1977;185:441

3. Maley HT, Bulkley GB, Williams GM: Ablation of free radical-medicated reperfusion injury for the salvage of kidneys taken from non-heartbeating donors. *Transplantation* 1988;45:284

4. Goldszer RC, Lazarus JM: Dialysis support for transplantation. In: Garovoy MR, Guttmann RD (eds). *Renal Transplantation.* New York, Churchill Livingstone, 1986

5. Arnadoltir M, Berganz GE, Berquist D, et al: Thromboembolic complications after renal transplantation: a retrospective analysis. *World J Surg* 1983;7:757

6. Niese D for The International Sandimmune NEORAL Study Group: A double-blind randomized study of Sandimmune Neoral versus Sandimmune in new renal transplant recipients: results after 12 months. *Transplant Proc* 1995;27:1849-56

7. The US Multicenter FK506 Liver Study Group: A comparison of tacrolimus (FK506) and cyclosporine in liver transplantation. *N Engl J Med* 1994;331:1110

8. Todo S, Fung JJ, Starzl TE, et al: Single-center experience with primary orthotopic liver transplantation with FK506 immunosuppression. *Ann Surg* 1994;220:297

9. European Mycophenolate Mofetil Cooperative Study Group: Placebo controlled study of mycophenolate mofetil combined with cyclosporine and corticosteroids for prevention of acute rejection. *Lancet* 1995;345:1321

10. Sollinger HW for the US Renal Transplant Mycophenolate Mofetil Study Group: Mycophenolate mofetil for the prevention of acute rejection in primary cadaveric renal allograft recipients. *Transplantation* 1995;60:225

11. Tilney NL: Transplantation of the kidney: thoughts on decreasing patient hazard and improving graft survival. *Dialysis Transplant* 1979;8:1184

12. Snydman DR, Werner BG, Heinze-Lacey, et al: Use of cytomegalovirus immune globulin to prevent cytomegalovirus disease in renal transplant recipients. *N Engl J Med* 1987;317:1049

13. Balfour HH, Chace BA, Stapleton JT, et al: A randomized, placebo-controlled trial of oral acyclovir for the prevention of cytomegalovirus disease in recipients of renal allografts. *N Engl J Med* 1989;320:1381

14. Moran M, Mozes MF, Maddux MS, et al: Prevention of acute graft rejection by the prostaglandin E_1 analogue misoprostol in renal transplant recipients treated with cyclosporine and prednisone. *N Engl J Med* 1990;322:1183

15. Wiederkehr JC, Dumble L, Pollak R, et al: Immunosuppressive effect of misoprostol: a new synthetic prostaglandin E_1 analogue. *Aust N Z J Surg* 1990;60:121

16. Kim P, Wakefield A, Cohen Z, et al: The reversal of cyclosporin: a mediated suppression of allogeneic induced monocyte procoagulant activity by H_2 antagonists *in vitro. Transplant Proc* 1989;21:844

17. Harbison MA, DeGirolami PC, Jenkins RL, et al: Ganciclovir therapy of severe cytomegalovirus infection in solid-organ transplant recipients. *Transplantation* 1988;46:82

18. Rubin RH, Young LS: *Clinical Approach to Infection in the Immunocompromised Host.* New York, Plenum Press, 1981

19. Penn I, Brunson ME: Cancers after cyclosporine therapy. *Transplant Proc* 1988;20(Suppl 3):885

20. Hrickik DE, Browning PJ, Kopelman R, et al: Captopril-induced functional renal insufficiency in patients with bilateral renal artery stenosis or renal artery stenosis in a solitary kidney. *N Engl J Med* 1983;308:373

Critical Care, Third Edition, edited by Joseph M. Civetta,
Robert W. Taylor, and Robert R. Kirby.
Lippincott-Raven Publishers, Philadelphia, PA © 1997.

CHAPTER 86

■

The Renal and Pancreatic Allograft Recipient

George W. Burke, III
Gaetano Ciancio

IMMEDIATE CONCERNS ■

MAJOR PROBLEMS

On arrival in the ICU, kidney transplant (KT) or simultaneous pancreas/kidney (SPK) transplant recipients require close monitoring of urine output and vital signs, including blood pressure (BP), heart rate, respiratory rate, central venous pressure (CVP), and oxygen (O_2) saturation. If the vital signs are stable and the urine output is acceptable—this may vary from 100 to 1000 mL/hour—then a replacement protocol is used (usually milliliter for milliliter) to maintain hydration, perfusion, and renal filtration. The fall in creatinine is usually commensurate with urine output.

If the urine output should fall dramatically, then the following should be done. Irrigate the Foley catheter gently to dislodge a possible clot, mucous, or other obstruction. If there is no obstruction and no subsequent change in urine output after Foley catheter irrigation, and if the CVP or BP is low (CVP <10 cm H_2O, mean BP <100 mm Hg), then give a bolus with intravenous (IV) fluid: crystalloid, colloid (which is our preference), or blood (if the hematocrit is below 30). This should increase CVP, BP, or both, at which point a diuretic (e.g., furosemide) may further contribute to increasing or restoring urine output. If the CVP and BP are already high (e.g., CVP ≥15 cm H_2O, mean BP 150 mm Hg) then a diuretic (e.g., 50- to 100-mg bolus of furosemide) should be given intravenously. A fall in BP that doesn't respond to volume, or that is accompanied by a fall in hematocrit and O_2 saturation, with or without abdominal dis-

tention, should alert the surgical team to reexplore the patient urgently for bleeding. If urine output doesn't increase after these initial measures (so that the CVP, BP, O_2 saturation, and hematocrit are optimized), then an ultrasound (US)/Doppler study and triple renal scan (nuclear medicine) are indicated to rule out technical problems that may have developed with the artery, vein, or ureterovesical anastomosis postoperatively. The triple renal scan identifies urine extravasation or obstruction and demonstrates flow to the kidney, parenchymal renal uptake, and excretion. The US/Doppler study demonstrates flow within the artery and vein, the degree of hydroureter or hydronephrosis (consistent with obstruction), and fluid collection in the operative site. Obstruction or extravasation or loss of arterial/venous flow requires operative intervention. The most common cause of change in function or delayed renal function is acute tubular necrosis (ATN), which generally resolves with optimization of perfusion parameters over time. Hyperacute rejection seldom occurs because of the crossmatch assay, which identifies antidonor antibody in the recipient (a contraindication to transplantation).

STRESS POINTS

1. After KT or SPK transplantation, the urine output, which is an index of transplant function, depends on the interplay between recipient factors (optimization of perfusion) and donor factors (e.g., quality of organs, preservation/reperfusion injury).

1311

2. Perfusion characteristics are a composite of the following: systemic BP, CVP, or pulmonary artery occlusion pressure (PAOP); cardiac function; O_2 saturation; hematocrit; and heart rate. Each of these parameters can be assessed and modulated by various maneuvers to optimize flow to the transplanted organs.

3. The quality of the allografts and determinants of early function are mostly donor-dependent. Impaired or delayed early graft function can result from hypotension or sepsis occurring preterminally in the donor, prolonged cold ischemia time, or prolonged warm ischemia time in the recipient operation (if there are technical difficulties).

4. A drop in urine output shortly after arrival in the ICU warrants a rapid assessment, including irrigation of the Foley catheter to rule out mechanical obstruction and optimization of perfusion characteristics described earlier.

5. If falling urine output is secondary to delayed graft function, care should be taken to avoid excess fluid administration that might lead to pulmonary edema.

6. Hypotension accompanied by a fall in hematocrit and O_2 saturation with or without abdominal distention should prompt reexploration for bleeding. A fall in hematocrit secondary to dilution with IV fluids is common but should not be accompanied by hypotension, a fall in O_2 saturation, or abdominal distention.

ESSENTIAL DIAGNOSTIC TESTS AND PROCEDURES

1. A complete set of blood tests—including complete blood count; platelet count; electrolytes; blood urea, nitrogen (BUN)/creatinine; glucose; and initial arterial blood gas measurements—are important on admission to the ICU and serially every 6 hours over the first 24 hours. Continuous O_2 saturation monitoring can replace the need for serial arterial blood gas measurements.

2. Urine electrolytes—particularly, potassium but also magnesium and calcium—can be useful in determining the need for potassium, magnesium, or calcium replacement, especially when the urine output is high.

3. US/Doppler study is useful for demonstrating flow in the artery and vein, detecting hydronephrosis or hydroureter (indicating ureteral obstruction), or fluid collections (e.g., hematoma, urinoma, or lymphocele).

4. The nuclear (radioisotope) scan is useful for demonstrating quality of flow to the kidney, as well as uptake and excretion. It is particularly helpful in demonstrating urine extravasation (leak) or obstruction.

INITIAL THERAPY

1. Irrigate the Foley catheter gently to dislodge a possible clot, mucous, or other obstruction. Occasionally, if significant hematuria occurs, the Foley catheter may need to be changed.

2. For SPK transplant recipients, a continuous insulin infusion may be required to maintain the glucose in the normal range. Often, a pancreas transplant will correct the blood glucose after reperfusion, but the glucose may rise secondary to steroid administration, the stress of surgery and anesthesia, or donor characteristics (preservation/reperfusion injury).

3. Optimize perfusion characteristics: if the CVP or BP are low, administer fluids (colloid or crystalloid, as needed).

4. If perfusion characteristics have been optimized and the urine output remains low, then administer a diuretic (50-mg bolus of furosemide).

5. If the urine output does not increase despite optimization of perfusion characteristics, administration of diuretic, and demonstration by US/Doppler study and nuclear scan that the kidney is well perfused without obstruction or leak, then it is important to avoid fluid overload and maintain optimal perfusion parameters.

OVERVIEW

The success rates for KTs and SPK transplants have improved during the last decade, largely because of the availability of new, potent immunosuppressive agents.[1] Ultimately, the cumulative advances in surgical technique, preservation solution and methods, postoperative care, and immunosuppressive regimens have fostered this improvement. Whereas 1-year graft survival is excellent, long-term (>10 years) survival remains a problem.[2,3] The next goal of transplantation is to use immunosuppressive agents or immune modulation to develop tolerance or long-term graft acceptance without immunosuppression.[4]

INITIAL ICU ADMISSION

Candidates for SPK transplantation have type I (insulin dependent) diabetes mellitus (IDDM) with end-stage renal disease. The functioning SPK transplant restores (1) euglycemia, enabling the patient to go off insulin, and (2) normal renal function. The recent landmark Diabetes Control and Complications Trial (DCCT) demonstrated unequivocally the importance of meticulous glycemic control in reducing the long-term complications of *early onset* IDDM.[5] In early onset diabetes mellitus, the autoimmune process and hence glycemic control may be transiently improved with immunosuppression[6]; however, this minor and short-lived effect doesn't justify the toxicity inherent in immunosuppression. Ultimately, hyperglycemia-related abnormalities in the vascular endothelium ensue,[7] contributing to the secondary complications of diabetic triopathy (retinopathy, nephropathy, and neuropathy). Although most SPK transplant candidates already have diabetic triopathy and hypertension (often postural), many also have labile glycemic control. Whereas it is unclear if the results of the DCCT trial may be extrapolated to patients with long-term diabetes mellitus, the restoration of euglycemia unquestionably improves the quality of life[8] and has been demonstrated to improve autonomic neuropathy[8] and cardiac function.[9] Because the maintenance immunosuppression for SPK transplantation is essentially the same as for KT, the application of pancreas transplantation is likely to increase in this group of patients with diabetes mellitus and end-stage renal disease. The most important preoperative issue for these patients is their cardiovascular status. Many have so-called *silent disease*, either resulting from their neuropathy (where they cannot perceive chest pain) or lack of physical activity necessary to bring on cardiac stress. Diabetics who are also hyperlipidemic are at particularly high risk for cardiac dysfunction and coronary artery disease regardless of (young) age. The preoperative workup includes noninvasive stress testing and two-dimensional cardiac echo. If abnormalities are identified in the noninvasive testing, then coronary angiography is performed to define lesions that may be correctable, medically or by angioplasty or surgery. Most recipients have some degree of cardiac compromise[10] but are acceptable candidates if their cardiac status can be optimized.

The SPK transplant operation is significantly larger in scope than a KT alone. It is usually performed in an intraperitoneal fashion, although in a small number of centers a bilateral extraperitoneal approach is used. The dissection is extensive, involving right and left common and external iliac arteries and veins, with mobilization of the large and small bowel cephalad. There is often significant "third space" fluid losses or ascites intraoperatively and postoperatively. This may be enhanced in patients treated with peritoneal dialysis whose peritoneal lining is inflamed or has been infected. The pancreas and duodenum are usually placed on the right side where the iliac vessels are more superficial; the kidney is placed on the left. Anastomosis of the duodenum to the bladder is performed in most centers, although in some centers, enteric drainage is employed. Bladder drainage avoids recipient enteric contamination and allows the monitoring of urine amylase, which may be useful in diagnosing pancreatic rejection.[11] The ureter is anastomosed to the bladder. The pancreas usually tolerates up to 28 to 30 hours of cold ischemia time.[12] It is subject to preservation/reperfusion injury, which manifests as graft pancreatitis. This may be seen as a spectrum from little or no pancreatic edema to severe edema with saponification, a rise in serum amylase and lipase, and full-blown pancreatitis with ensuing respiratory distress. The pancreas transplant historically has had a significant (12% to 20%) thrombosis rate.[13] Often, the blood glucose is corrected in the operating room within 1 hour of pancreas reperfusion, despite the stress of surgery, anesthesia, preservation/reperfusion injury, and steroid bolus therapy generally given during the transplant. If the glucose remains elevated, a continuous insulin infusion is used to maintain the blood glucose between 100 and 120 mg/dL for the theoretical benefit of keeping the pancreatic islet cells at metabolic rest while they recover from the preservation/reperfusion injury.

The duodenum is drained into the bladder, thus draining exocrine secretions into the urine. This results in urine of increased viscosity, increasing the chance of obstructing the Foley catheter; therefore, a fall in urine output should prompt irrigation of the catheter.

A culture of the duodenum is performed to detect yeast and bacteria; findings usually show contamination, although the duodenum is flushed with an antibiotic (polymyxin, bacitracin, and amphotericin) solution before removal from the donor. In some centers, recipients receive prophylactic antibiotics postoperatively to avoid yeast infection. We have had two cases of fungal arteritis involving the Y graft of the donor iliac artery, which resulted in arterial disruption 5 to 7 days after SPK transplantation. We recommend any measure that avoids duodenal contamination: (1) during the donor operation, the duodenum should be flushed with Betadine (providone-iodine) through the nasogastric tube, followed by amphotericin treatment and closing both ends of the duodenum, before placement in Belzer's solution; and (2) in the recipient operation, anastomosis of the duodenum to the bladder should be done as soon as hemostasis of the pancreas has been attained, and the duodenum should be kept closed until the back wall of the bladder anastomosis has been performed—to minimize duodenal spill intraperitoneally. The duodenum is then cultured, and prophylactic amphotericin is begun postoperatively. Amphotericin is discontinued if the duodenal culture is negative for yeast.

In some centers, heparin is routinely used intraoperatively to prevent pancreatic graft thrombosis. We obtain a thromboelastogram and use heparin if there is evidence of hypercoagulability. Some patients have demonstrated a correlation between thrombocythemia (platelet count >500,000/mm³), IDDM, renal failure, historical evidence of hypercoagulopathy (on the venous side, as evidenced by pulmonary embolus; on the arterial side, by advanced atherosclerotic disease), and hypercoagulability by thromboelastogram. Although these patients received heparin intraoperatively, they did not bleed, confirming a tendency toward hypercoagulability.

The most common problem after SPK transplantation is hematuria. Usually self-limited, this occasionally requires cystoscopic intervention. Hematuria may result from activation of pancreatic exocrine enzymes, bleeding from the duodenovesical or ureteral anastomosis, or cytomegalovirus (CMV) infection. Other early urologic or surgical problems include the following: bladder leak, abscess secondary to graft pancreatitis or necrosis, graft thrombosis, and ureteral or urethral stricture. Postural hypotension is a common problem in patients with diabetes mellitus with end-stage renal disease, which occurs frequently after SPK transplantation. This is exacerbated by the obligate pancreatic secretions, which include sodium, bicarbonate, and water, and may cause metabolic acidosis as well as dehydration. Treatment by adding fluids (orally or intravenously, as necessary), dietary salt, bicarbonate, and mineralocorticoids (e.g., fludrocortisone) is usually effective. Acute rejection occurs commonly after SPK transplantation, usually 2 weeks to 1 month after transplantation (earlier than KT); it is often accompanied by fever, tenderness over the kidney or pancreas, and a rise in serum amylase and lipase and BUN and creatinine levels, with a fall in urine amylase. This requires aggressive therapy, usually with steroids, prompt biopsy, and a second course of OKT3, if needed.[14] Recently, the use of FK506-based immunosuppression has resulted in a lesser rate of acute rejection.[14,15]

IMMUNOSUPPRESSION

The addition of CyA in the early 1980s to azathioprine and steroids resulted in a dramatic improvement in graft survival with fewer infectious complications. Currently, quadruple immunosuppression is used in most centers, consisting of the following: (1) an antibody preparation (OKT3 or anti-thymocyte globulin [ATG]) for the early induction period; (2) corticosteroids, high dose initially, tapered over time; (3) azathioprine; and (4) CyA when the serum creatinine is less than 2.0 mg/dL. For KT, the antibody induction is usually 5 to 7 days; for SPK transplantation, it is usually 10 to 14 days. Some centers have recently replaced CyA with FK506, which is used for long-term immunosuppression. Not all centers use antibody induction therapy.[16]

CyA and FK506 have similar mechanisms of action. Both interfere with messenger RNA for certain cytokines, particularly interleukin-2 (IL-2), γ-interferon, and tumor necrosis factor-α. Cyclosporine conversely increases the expression of transforming growth factor-β. Both have pronounced nephrotoxicity and neurotoxicity. The most common symptoms include headache, insomnia and gastrointestinal (GI) disturbances such as nausea, vomiting, diarrhea, constipation, and nonspecific abdominal pain. When used intravenously, cyclosporine has been associated with seizures in liver transplant recipients, particularly those with low serum cholesterol levels. CyA has been associated with hyperkalemia and hypomagnesemia. Both CyA and FK506 are capable of impairing both insulin secretion and insulin utilization in the periphery in liver and KT recipients. We have not observed this in the SPK transplant recipients who remain euglycemic with normal lipid profiles after transplantation.[17]

Because CyA can cause renal arteriolar vasoconstriction, reducing renal arterial flow, the concomitant use of nephrotoxic drugs may exacerbate renal dysfunction. Such nephrotoxic drugs include antibiotics (aminoglycosides, amphotericin B, trimethroprin-sulfamethoxazole, and acyclovir); angiotensin converting enzyme inhibitors; and nonsteroidal antiinflammatory agents. In addition, because CyA is metabolized by the P450 system of the liver, drugs that compete with CyA for P450 will reduce CyA degradation and have the potential to increase CyA levels. Agents that increase CyA serum levels include the following: erythromycin; antifungal agents (ketoconazole, fluconazole, itraconyzole); some calcium channel blockers (diltiazem, nicardipine, and verapamil—but not nifedipine); and others, such as steroids. Metoclopramide also results in increased CyA levels, not by affecting the P450 system, but by increasing absorption through enhancing gastric motility, leading to faster exposure to bile in the duodenum, which is necessary for its absorption. Other agents that enhance P450 activity, leading to greater CyA degradation, and lower CyA levels include the anticonvulsants (phenobarbital, phenytoin, carbamazepine) and antituberculous agents (isoniazid and rifampin). Generally, agents that increase GI motility, reducing time available

for absorption, will reduce CyA levels; contrariwise, those that reduce GI motility, increasing time available for absorption, will increase CyA levels.

Because CyA is dependent on the presence of bile for absorption, measures that divert or reduce bile output or that interfere with the enterohepatic circulation will reduce CyA levels. In contrast, FK506, which shares many of the effects and toxicity of CyA, is not dependent on bile for absorption.

Corticosteroids remain a mainstay of immunosuppression despite well-known side effects. Corticosteroids inhibit multiple immune functions, including the expression of messenger RNA for IL-2 and γ-interferon by mechanisms that are synergistic with CyA. High-dose steroids are used initially and then tapered after transplantation. They are also useful to treat early acute rejection episodes. Unfortunately, the side effects are legion and include the dysregulation of glucose metabolism, gastric mucosal function, bone resorption, and wound healing.

Azathioprine is a thioguanine derivative of mercaptopurine that acts as a purine antagonist and functions as an antiproliferative agent. The T cell seems to be a preferential target, perhaps related to the timing of transplantation and transplant antigen–stimulated proliferative effect. It also affects B cells. Its use is often limited by bone marrow or hepatic toxicity.

Antibody therapy includes ATG (polyclonal—horse, goat, or rabbit) and OKT3 (murine monoclonal anti-CD3). ATG contains antibody to human lymphocytes (T and B cells) and has as an antiplatelet effect. OKT3 binds specifically to the CD3 molecule, which is a five-protein complex, contiguous with the T-cell receptor on the surface of T cells, whose role is to transduce the activation signal across the membrane to the nucleus after recognition by the T-cell receptor of its appropriate target. OKT3 binds to anti-CD3, causing a wave of cytokine release, followed by functional T-cell paralysis.[16,18] The side effects of both antibody preparations are related to the wave of cytokine release and include fevers, chills, diarrhea, hypotension, pulmonary edema—especially in the setting of fluid overload (>3% body weight), or other anaphylactic reactions. Neurologic symptoms, including aseptic meningitis, have been observed after OKT3 therapy. This is usually self-limited and symptoms subside after OKT3 is stopped.

Corticosteroids are usually given 1 hour before and 4 to 6 hours after OKT3 to prevent some of these side effects. This symptom complex is most pronounced after the first dose and often occurs again after the second dose. Generally, symptoms thereafter are significantly less dramatic. Acetaminophen and antihistamines are generally used as "before" and "after" medication as well. Pentoxifylline has been used for its anti–tumor necrosis factor-α effect; however, its utility in controlled clinical trials has been unimpressive.[14]

Several new immunosuppressive agents have shown promise in experimental models of transplantation and are in varying stages of clinical trials. Sirolimus (formally rapamycin), mycophenolate mofetil, deoxyspergualin, and mizoribin are currently undergoing clinical trials. Other experimental drugs showing promise include brequinar sodium, leflunomid, and azaspirane. In addition, monoclonal antibodies to other T-cell markers (e.g., IL-2R, CD4, CD8, and adhesion markers including ICAM-I and LFA-1) are undergoing clinical trials. A possible modification of current murine monoclonal antibodies, called "humanization" would be to incorporate the critical antigen binding portion of the antibody molecule onto a human immunoglobulin backbone. This may prevent the immune response to the foreign immunoglobulin that can inactivate the monoclonal antibody.

SECONDARY ICU ADMISSIONS ■

The pancreas exocrine secretions include bicarbonate, amylase, and other proenzymes, all of which are drained into the bladder. This results in bicarbonate loss, which may cause a metabolic acidosis if insufficient bicarbonate replacement occurs. Occasionally, despite compliant replacement, metabolic acidosis persists. In this case, as in the setting of enzyme activation—which may result in urethritis, severe dysuria, urethral disruption, balanitis, chronic urinary tract infections, or recurrent urinary leak—it may be necessary to convert the bladder drainage of exocrine secretion to enteric drainage.[17] This can be accomplished surgically; if it occurs over 6 months after SPK transplantation, the likelihood of acute rejection (and, therefore, the importance of monitoring urine amylase measurements) is low.[14] The duodenum is also subject to rejection, which may become manifest as a urinary leak. In this case, the duodenovesical anastomosis should be surgically repaired and antirejection therapy started concomitantly. Although the rejection process generally occurs in all three organs—that is, kidney, pancreas, and duodenum concurrently—a discordance rate of up to 20% in each has been reported.

When graft pancreatitis occurs after SPK transplantation, it may result in saponification, exocrine enzyme activation, and fat and pancreatic necrosis. In this setting, localized bacterial or fungal infections may occur.[18] Treatment of peripancreatic infection requires debridement, drainage, and long-term antibiotic therapy.[18,19] Although operative treatment is the mainstay, this can also be achieved with percutaneous placement of drainage catheters when applied in a systematic fashion by irrigation and tube checks through interventional radiologic study. An occasional, although feared complication of localized pancreatic infection is the development of arterial anastomotic pseudoaneurysms. These have been reported and require prompt surgical attention.[20] Thrombosis of the pancreas transplant—early or late—should lead to prompt removal to avoid bladder-derived bacterial or yeast contamination and resulting infection.

REFERENCES ■

1. Ciancio G, Roth D, Burke G, et al: Renal Transplantation in a new immunosuppressive era. *Transplant Proc* 1995;27:812

2. Naimark MJ, Cole E: Determinants of long-term renal allograft survival. *Transplant Rev* 1994;8:93

3. Burke GW, Esquenazi V, Gharagozloo H, et al: Long-term results of kidney transplantation at the University of Miami. In: Terasaki PI (ed). *Clinical Transplant 1989.* Los Angeles, UCLA Tissue Typing Laboratory, 1990:215

4. Miller J, Esquenazi V, Fuller L, et al: The immunologic response to allografts: acute rejection. *Clin Transpl* 1991;5:477

5. Diabetes Control and Complications Trial Research Group: Effect of intensive treatment of diabetes on development and progression of long-term complications in insulin-dependent diabetes mellitus. *N Engl J Med* 1993;329:977

6. Burke GW, Cirocco R, Markou M, et al: Effect of cyclosporine A on serum tumor necrosis factor α in new onset type I insulin-dependent diabetes mellitus. *J Diabet Complications* 1994;8:40

7. King GL, Shiba T, Oliver J, et al: Cellular and molecular abnormalities in the vascular endothelium of diabetes mellitus. *Annu Rev Med* 1994;45:179

8. Hathaway D, Abell T, Cardoso S, et al: Improvement in autonomic function following pancreas-kidney versus kidney-alone transplantation. *Transplant Proc* 1993;25:1306

9. Osama Gaber A, El-Gebely S, Sugathan P, et al: Sustained improvement in cardiac function occurs for diabetic pancreas-kidney recipients but not kidney-alone recipients. *Transplantation* 1994.

10. Gruessner RWG, Dunn DL, Gruessner AC, et al: Recipient risk factors have an impact on technical failure and patient and graft survival rates in bladder-drained pancreas transplants. *Transplantation* 1994;54:1598

11. Burke G, Sutherland D, Najarian J: Intra-abdominal fluid collections in pancreas transplant recipients: T18% versus enteric drainage. *Transplant Proc* 1988;20(Suppl 1):887

12. Sutherland DER, Gruessner WG, Gores PF: Pancreas and islet transplantation: an update. *Transplant Rev* 1994;8:185

13. Sutherland DER, Gores PF, Farney AC, et al: Evolution of kidney, pancreas, and islet transplantation for patients with diabetes at the University of Minnesota. *Am J Surg* 1993;166:456

14. Burke GW, Alejandro R, Nery J, et al: Combined kidney/pancreas transplantation in diabetes mellitus. *J Fla Med Assoc* 1994;81:339

15. Burke GW, Alejandro Dr, Ciancio G, et al: The use of FK506 in simultaneous pancreas/kidney transplantation: rescue, induction and maintenance immunosuppression [abstract]. Submitted to the 5th International Pancreas and Islet Transplant Association (IPITA) Congress, 1995

16. Suthanthiran M, Strom TB: Renal transplantation. *N Engl J Med* 1994;331:365

17. Burke GW, Gruessner R, Dunn DL, et al: Conversion of whole pancreaticoduodenal transplants from bladder to enteric drainage for metabolic acidosis or dysuria. *Transplant Proc* 1990;22:651

18. Everett JE, Wahoff DC, Statz C: Characterization and impact of wound infection after pancreas transplantation. *Arch Surg* 1994;129:1310

19. Douzdjian V, Abecassis MM, Cooper JL, et al: Incidence, management and significance of surgical complication after pancreatic transplantation. *Surg Gynecol Obstet* 1993;177:451

20. Tzakis AG, Carroll PB, Gordon RD, et al: Arterial mycotic aneurysm and rupture: a potentially fatal complication of pancreas transplantation in diabetes mellitus. *Arch Surg* 1989;124:660

Critical Care, Third Edition, edited by Joseph M. Civetta,
Robert W. Taylor, and Robert R. Kirby.
Lippincott-Raven Publishers, Philadelphia, PA © 1997.

CHAPTER 87

∎

Heart-Lung, Double-Lung, and Single-Lung Transplantation

Cesar A. Keller

INDICATIONS ∎

In December 1995, 208 patients were listed for heart-lung transplantation (HLT) and 1,939 for single-lung (SLT) or double-lung transplantation (DLT) in the United States. Because of a limited availability of donors, only 65 heart-lung combinations and 657 lungs were transplanted between January and November of 1994.[1] Indications for each type of transplantation have changed over time. In the early 1980s, HLT was indicated in a large variety of terminal cardiopulmonary conditions. As the demand for organs increased and as the technology of SLT and sequential bibronchial DLT was developed,[2] indications for specific types of transplantation changed. The technology of SLT has been modified. Initially, an end-to-end bronchial anastomosis was done with support derived from an omental wrap dissected from the abdomen, through the diaphragm, and pulled up to the hilum. Currently, the "telescoping" technique is favored to perform the bronchial anastomosis.[3] This procedure provides enough support and microcirculation to the anastomotic site without requiring an omental wrap (Fig. 87-1). Ventilation-perfusion lung scans done before transplantation define which lung will be excised (the one with least perfusion) and substituted by the graft.

DLT was modified from the initial "en block" surgery performed through a medial sternotomy with simultaneous excision of both lungs under cardiopulmonary bypass pump (CBP) support, followed by implantation of the new block of two lungs using an anastomosis in the distal trachea; to the currently used surgery through bilateral thoracotomies with transverse incision of the distal sternum "clam shell technique."[4] This procedure exposes both lungs and mediastinum simultaneously, allowing easier access to areas of pleural and mediastinal bleeding.[3] In DLT, the lung with least function is excised first, followed by implantation of the graft using a telescoping bronchial anastomosis while ventilating and perfusing the opposite (native) lung. Sequentially, ventilation and perfusion are shifted to the newly transplanted lung to implant the opposite lung using a second bronchial anastomosis. This technique seldom requires CBP support. These advances have extended the indications of SLT and DLT, whereas those for HLT are reduced, thus allowing a more efficient use of donated organs. Survival rates for the first year after transplantation have reached 75% to 85% for SLT, 65% to 85% for DLT, and 55% to 65% for HLT; these survival rates continuously improve as transplant technology advances. Table 87-1 describes currently accepted indications for transplantation on psychosocially stable subjects with end-stage lung disease that is refractory to standard medical therapy, without evidence of other organ dysfunction.

INITIAL MANAGEMENT ∎

PREOPERATIVE

Lung transplant recipients preoperatively receive intravenous (IV) azathioprine, 2 mg/kg, and cyclosporine by IV infusion calculated at 2 to 10 mg/kg/day (usually 4 to 6 mg/

1317

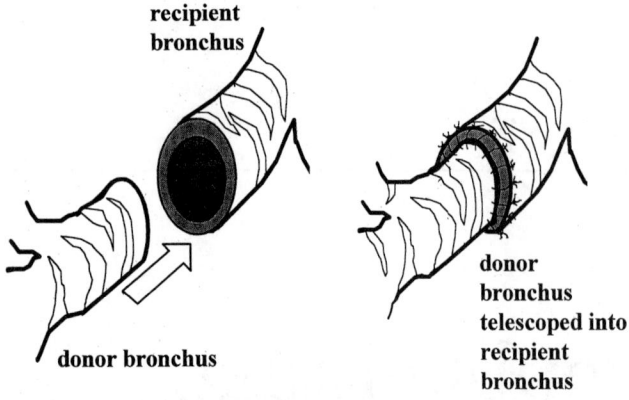

FIGURE 87-1. Telescoping bronchial anastomosis. The donor bronchus is "telescoped" into the recipient bronchus overlapping one or two cartilage rings to provide support and microcirculation to the anastomotic site. This anastomosis can be further supported externally with a vascularized tissue swap obtained from a flap of pericardium.

TABLE 87-1.   Indications for Transplantation

HEART-LUNG TRANSPLANT (age ≤50 y)
 Cyanotic congenital heart disease
 Eisenmenger's complex

DOUBLE-LUNG TRANSPLANT (age ≤50 y)
 Cystic fibrosis
 Bilateral bronchiectasis
 Primary pulmonary hypertension

SINGLE-LUNG TRANSPLANT (age ≤60 y)
 Obstructive lung disease
  Emphysema
  α_1-Antitrypsin deficiency
 Restrictive lung disease
  Idiopathic pulmonary fibrosis
  Occupational lung diseases
  Sarcoidosis
 Pulmonary vascular disease
  Primary pulmonary hypertension
  Eisenmenger's complex with repairable heart defect

hour). Intraoperatively, patients receive a 500-mg IV bolus of methylprednisolone (MPS). Usual postoperative orders on admission to the intensive care unit are shown in Table 87-2.

IMMUNOSUPPRESSION

Cyclosporine, prednisone, and azathioprine constitute the basic triad of immunosuppressive agents that allow the recipient to tolerate a graft obtained from a donor matched only by major blood type.[5] Ideally, the transplant surgery is coordinated to limit the ischemia time to less than 5 hours. This short time does not permit selection of donors matched by tissue typing.

Cyclosporine-A

Cyclosporine-A affects the cellular immune response by blocking the production of interleukin-2 (IL-2), which is followed by a decreased activation of T lymphocytes. Main adverse effects include nephrotoxicity, hypertension, hyperkalemia, hypomagnesemia, hyperlipidemia, and neurotoxicity. Drugs known to increase cyclosporine levels include erythromycin, calcium channel blockers, and ketoconazole.

TABLE 87-2.   Post-operative Orders°

A. NURSING CARE
 Admit to ICU
 Hourly monitoring and charting of ECG, vital signs, hemodynamics, intake and output, daily
  weight; continuous monitoring of Sao_2 and Svo_2
 Nasogastric tube to low suction; check gastric aspirate for pH and hemoccult positive drainage
 Chest tubes: pleural/mediastinal tubes to −20 cm H_2O suction
 Change dressings daily with sterile technique
 Glasgow Coma Scale, check limb strength and pupils until patient is awake
 Strict handwashing technique during patient care
 Chest percussion and postural drainage every 2 h
 Physical therapy consult on postoperative d 2, sit patient in chair. bid
 Laboratory tests:
  Initial 24 h: Hb/Ht, ABGs, Chem 7 every 4 h
  Daily CBC, Chem 7, Ca, Mg, pH, chest radiograph, ABGs
  Every third day: cyclosporin levels, Chem 19

B. IV ORDERS
 D_5.45 NS with _____ mMol KCl at _____ mL/h
 Cardiac output measures every 4 h with 10 mL iced D_5W
 TPN (specific orders for each patient)

(continued)

TABLE 87-2. *(continued)*

C. MEDICATIONS

Immunosuppression:
    Cyclosporine: Continuous infusion (daily dose started at 2–10 mg/kg/d, adjusted to achieve blood levels of 250–350 ng/mL; once patient tolerates PO intake, the total daily IV dose × 3 becomes the daily oral dose, given in two divided doses every 12 h)
      Azathioprine: 2 mg/k/d IV, then changed to PO
      Methylprednisolone: 125 mg IV every 8 h × 3, then MPS or equivalent dose of prednisone
      Prednisone: 1 mg/kg/d tapering down to 0.3 mg/kg/d
      (Some centers include antilymphocytic therapy using OKT3 or ATG in the initial immunosuppressive protocol)

Antibiotics:
    Piperacillin/tazobactam: 3.375 g IV every 6 h; after 72 h, changes are made according to results of cultures obtained from donor and recipient in OR (patients with cystic fibrosis are given antibiotics according to sensitivities from the last sputum culture available from the pretransplant follow-up)
      (Alternatively: Clyndamycin 600 mg IV every 6 h + ceftazidime 1 g IV every 8 h)
    Gancyclovir: All transplants where either donor or recipient have CMV-positive titers (start in postoperative day 7: gancyclovir 5 mg/kg bid for 2 wk, then 5 mg/kg/d up to 90 d after transplant)
    Acyclovir: Transplants where donor and recipient are CMV negative receive 400 mg tid for 8 wk for herpes prophylaxis
    Nystatin: 5 mL swish and swallow qid (oral candidiasis prophylaxis)
    Trimetroprim/sulfamethoxasole: 1 double-strength tablet 3 times/wk to be started 4 wk after transplant for PCP prophylaxis

Vasoactive drugs:
    Dopamine: 200 mg/100 mL D₅W: 2–10 μg/kg/min as required
    Isoproterenol (heart-lung transplants—titrated to heart rate): 1 mg/250 mL D₅W drip as required
    Alprostadil (primary pulmonary hypertension): Titrated to maintain pulmonary hypertension under control (500 μg in 100 mL D₅W, start 0.01 μg/kg/min)

Others:
    Lorazepam: 1–3 mg IV every 2–4 h PRN for sedation
    Morphine sulfate: 2–6 mg IV every 2–4 h for pain
    Ranitidine: 50 mg IVPB every 12 h

ICU, intensive care unit; ECG, electrocardiogram; SaO₂, arterial saturation with oxygen; SvO₂, venous saturation with oxygen; bid, twice daily; Hb/Hct, hemoglobin and hematocrit; ABGs, arterial blood gases; CBC, complete blood cell count; Ca, calcium; Mg, magnesium; IV, intravenous; D₅.45 NS, 5% dextrose in 45% normal saline; TPN, total parenteral nutrition; PO, oral; MPS, methylprednisolone; OR, operating room; CMV, cytomegalovirus; tid, three times daily; qid, four times daily; PCP, *Pneumocystis carinii* pneumonia; D₅W, 5% dextrose in water; PRN, as needed; IVPB, intravenous peripheral bolus; KCl, potassium chloride.
°Protocol currently used at St. Louis University Health Sciences Center, St. Louis.

These drug interactions occasionally can be used specifically to increase the serum level of cyclosporine in patients experiencing difficulties achieving a therapeutic range, as is the case in patients with cystic fibrosis (CF).

Usual dosages are as follows:

Postoperative: 5 to 10 mg/kg/day to achieve 250- to 350-ng/mL serum levels by radioimmunoassay (other techniques are available to establish therapeutic levels in whole blood or serum, with different normal ranges).

Early posttransplant: Usual oral dose, 100 to 300 mg every 12 hours, adjusted to achieve 200- to 300-ng/mL serum levels.

Late posttransplant: Usual oral dose, 50 to 200 mg every 12 hours, adjusted to reach serum levels of 100 to 200 ng/mL.

A new formulation of cyclosporine, Neoral, has better absorption and better pharmacokinetics. Administration of Neoral produces more stable trough levels of cyclosporine. Doses are the same as those for regular cyclosporine.

Corticosteroids

Corticosteroids reduce production of IL-1 and IL-2 from antigen presenting cells and activated lymphocytes, respectively. This is the drug of choice to treat episodes of acute rejection (AR). The most important adverse effects, among many others, are hyperglycemia, delayed wound healing, opportunistic infections, muscle atrophy, osteoporosis, cataracts, and osteonecrosis.

The usual postoperative dosage is methylprednisolone (MPS), 125 mg, given intravenously every 8 hours (three doses), followed by either MPS or prednisone, 1 mg/kg/day, tapering down to 0.3 mg/kg/day over the first month after transplantation. Over the following year, prednisone is tapered to 0.1 mg/kg/day.

Azathioprine

Azathioprine inhibits cellular DNA and RNA synthesis and decreases humoral and cellular immunity. Main adverse effects include pancytopenia and chemical hepatotoxicity.

Usual dosages are as follows:

Early: 2 mg/kg/day
Late: 1 mg/kg/day; doses should be adjusted to maintain white blood cell count between 4000 and 8000/mm³

Antilymphocyte Agents

Antilymphocyte agents have been used either in the initial management of transplantation (induction immunosuppression) or as an alternative to be used only for recurrent rejection, refractory to corticosteroids. Available agents include antithymocyte globulin and Muromonab CD3 (OKT3, a monoclonal antibody). Adverse effects of antithymocyte globulin include formation of antibodies against platelets and red blood cells. Major reactions include anaphylaxis, serum sickness, and respiratory distress. The main adverse effect of OKT3 is a sudden cytokine release syndrome eliciting pyrexia, hypotension, and acute pulmonary edema.[6] This syndrome can be minimized by pretreating OKT3 administration with MPS, acetaminophen, and diphenhydramine.

The usual dosage of OKT3 is 5 mg/day intravenously for 7 to 10 days.

Other Agents

Other agents are used when there is intolerance to the previous ones. They include the following

Methotrexate: 2.5 mg twice a week
Cyclophosphamide: 1 to 2 mg/kg/day
FK506 (tacrolimus): 0.15–0.30 mg/kg twice daily
Mycophemolate mofetil (Cellcept): 1 g/orally twice daily

POSTOPERATIVE MANAGEMENT ■

IMMEDIATE CONCERNS

All transplanted patients initially require ventilatory support while the implanted organ regains function. The emphasis is on integrated management where control of postoperative hemorrhage and maintenance of adequate gas exchange, cardiac output (CO), systemic blood pressure, and adequate renal perfusion are all vital to the preservation of the graft. Common posttransplant problems include bleeding, reimplantation response, airway complications, AR, bacterial and opportunistic infection, diaphragmatic dysfunction, and bronchiolitis obliterans (BO).

Bleeding

Postoperative bleeding usually originates from pleural and mediastinal surfaces, particularly when prolonged cardiopulmonary bypass support is required, or when the removal of the native lung was complicated by presence of pleural adhesions or formation of collateral circulation.[7] Hemorrhage frequently occurs in patients with CF or those with previous thoracic intervention (e.g., pleurodesis, pleural biopsy, chest tube insertion, or previous thoracic surgery). Bleeding also is a frequent complication after HLT, particularly in patients whose cyanotic congenital diseases have favored development of large areas of collateral circulation.

Persistent bleeding is suspected in the patient with a large output of blood through the chest tubes (100 mL/hour or more), when a large infusion of packed red blood cells is required to maintain a normal hemoglobin (Hb) level, or when pleural densities develop in the immediate postoperative time (Fig. 87-2). Occasionally, large intrapleural clots prevent output of blood through the chest tubes; thus, the absence of external bleeding does not rule out the possibility of pleural or mediastinal hemorrhage.

Reimplantation Response (Acute Reperfusion Injury)

Reimplantation response is a posttransplantation noncardiogenic pulmonary edema characterized by an early alveolar infiltrate of the graft, commonly within the first 24 to 48 hours after transplantation.[8] The lung static compliance (CLst) is low, there is progressive decline in the arterial blood saturation with oxygen (SaO$_2$) and, consequently, in the venous blood saturation with oxygen (SvO$_2$). The CO, central venous pressure, and pulmonary artery occlusion pressure (PAOP) are usually normal (Fig. 87-3). The process is likely caused by a combination of ischemic injury and reperfusion injury after explantation of the graft from the donor and reimplantation into the recipient. Prolonged ischemic times (5 hours or longer) favor this process, as does the requirement of large volumes of fluid or blood products during surgery. Although the diagnosis can be suspected by following the parameters mentioned earlier, a lack of improvement after aggressive diuresis and ventilatory support with positive end-expiratory pressure (PEEP) indicates bronchoscopy and transbronchial biopsies to rule out other causes of injury, such as AR or infection.

Airway Complications

Airway complications include the following: ischemia, necrosis, anastomotic dehiscence, bronchial strictures, and mucus plugs. Early after the transplantation, the patient with a denervated organ and poor cough reflex develops thick, tenacious secretions indicating the need for aggressive chest therapy and frequent bronchoscopic toilet. The proximal end of the donor bronchus telescoped into the recipient bronchus undergoes superficial necrosis; enough necrotic

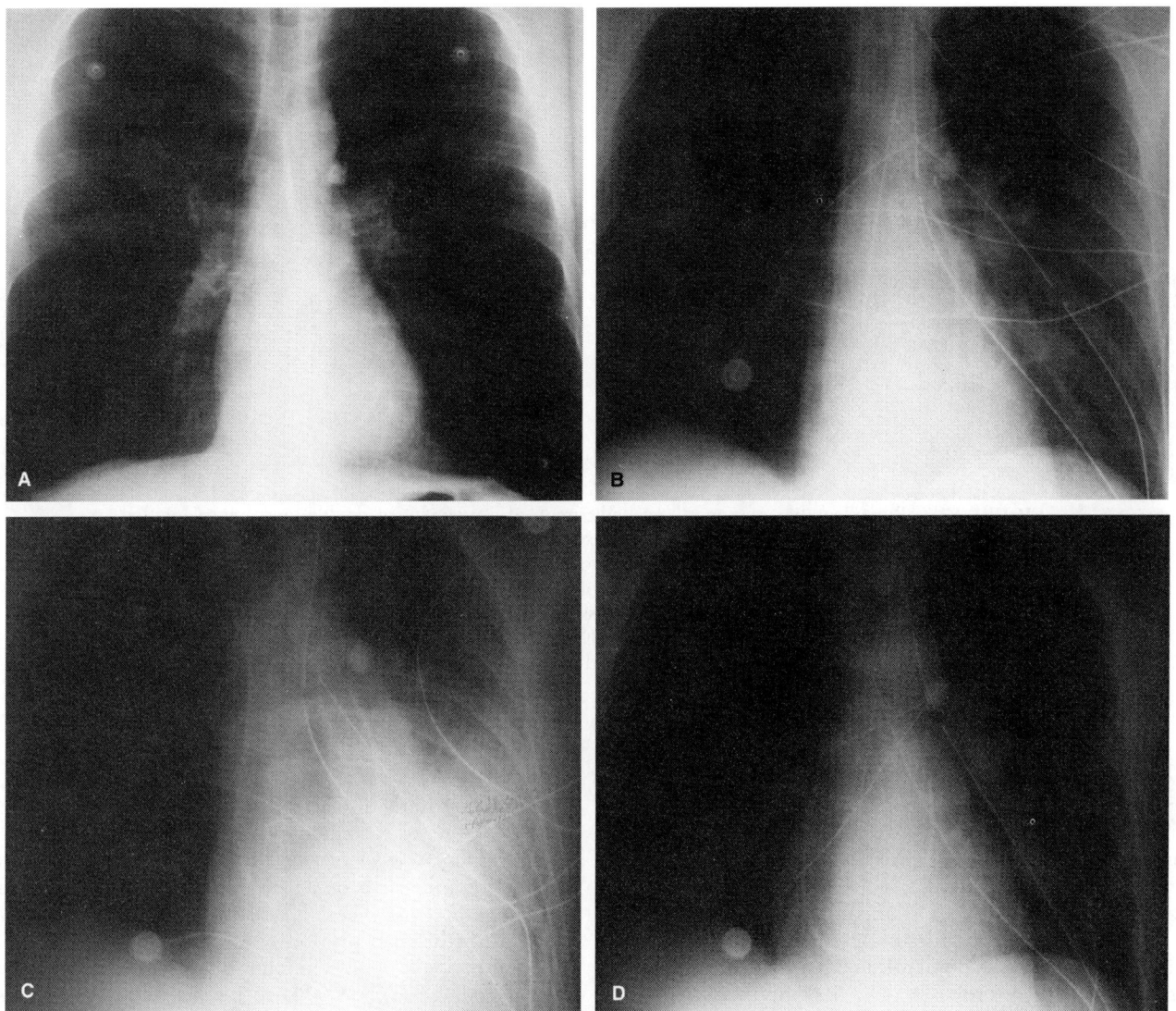

FIGURE 87-2. Postoperative bleeding. (**A**) Radiograph shows a 45-year-old man with end-stage COLD secondary to α_1-antitrypsin deficiency. (**B**) The early postoperative radiograph is shown. Twenty-four hours after surgery, he became tachycardic, hypotensive, and had an acute drop in SvO_2 levels. Output of 400 mL of blood through chest tubes within 1 hour was documented. (**C**) Chest radiograph demonstrated a new pleural density in the left hemithorax. The patient was transfused and taken to surgery. An exploration revealed 1 L of blood in the plural cavity. Once the blood was removed, a small defect was found in the pulmonary artery anastomosis, which was repaired. (**D**) The same patient is shown 24 hours later; bleeding is no longer present.

debris may form as to occlude the airway lumen (Fig. 87-4). Usually, this debris sloughs off by itself or occasionally requires removal by forceps during endoscopy. If the necrosis beyond the suture line is severe, necrotizing ulcers may occur, favoring necrosis and dehiscence. Episodes of severe postoperative anastomotic ischemia or infection commonly are associated with the development of strictures.[9]

Increased airway resistance, localized wheezing, and respiratory distress are all signs suggestive of an airway complication indicating endoscopic review. Prolonged air leak,

pneumothorax, and pneumomediastinum after transplantation suggest the possibility of airway dehiscence (Fig. 87-5). A computed tomography scan of the chest in this event will show necrotizing changes and presence of air around the involved airway.

Acute Rejection

Episodes of AR are common early after transplantation: more than half of transplant patients experience at least one

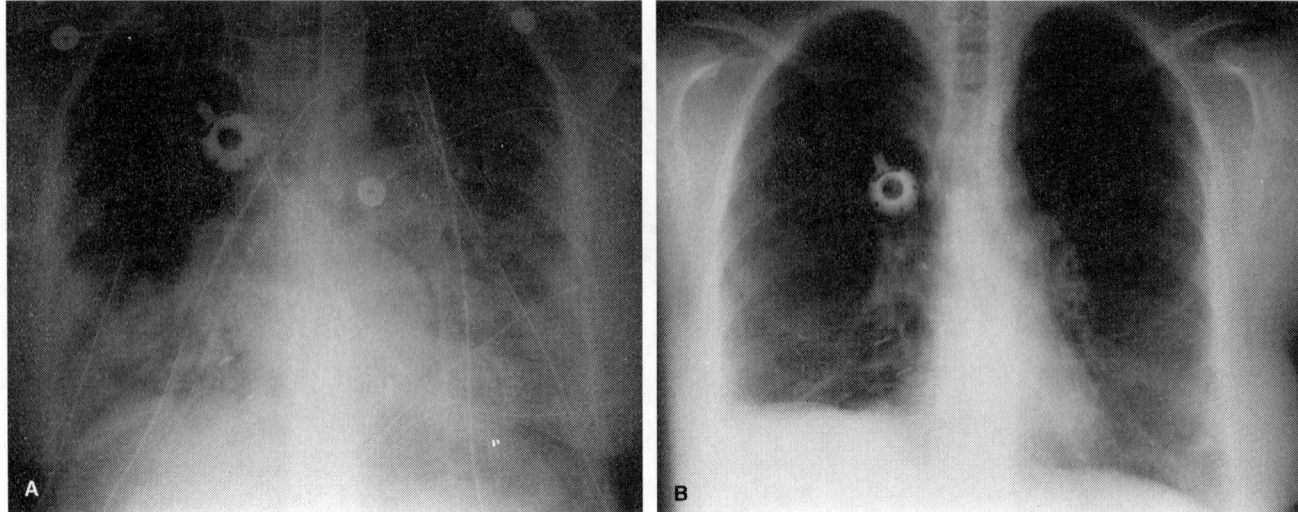

FIGURE 87-3. Reimplantation response. (**A**) Radiograph of a recipient of double-lung transplantation for cystic fibrosis. Because of extensive pleural adhesions and intraopeative bleeding, she required cardiopulmonary bypass pump support. The first lung had 6 hours of ischemia and the second lung, 9 hours. Within 36 hours postoperatively, she developed bilateral interstitial infiltrates and severe hypoxemia requiring high levels of positive end-expiratory pressure (PEEP). Transbronchial biopsies failed to show infection or rejection. With ventilatory support, PEEP, and aggressive diuresis, she improved and was extubated. (**B**) Follow-up film: A transient right diaphragmatic dysfunction remained 3 months later (notice the elevated hemidiaphragm).

episode of AR during the first month after surgery.[5,10] AR should be suspected when the patient shows evidence of oxygen desaturation and develops radiographic lung infiltrates. These events may be associated with a clinical presentation characterized by a "flu-like" syndrome (i.e., fever, malaise). Typically, episodes of AR have a dramatic clinical and radiographic resolution within 24 to 48 hours after treatment with corticosteroids (Fig. 87-6). Empiric treatment of AR should be avoided because the same findings can be caused by infection. Adequate treatment and follow-up of AR is necessary to preserve long-term function of the graft and avoidance of BO.

Repeated measurements of spirometry and pulse oximetry have become routine follow-up for transplant patients immediately after surgery. Even asymptomatic declines in function indicate investigation of possible rejection by bronchoscopy and transbronchial biopsy.[11] Histologic study characteristically shows perivascular lymphocytic infiltrates, which in advanced stages extend into the interstitial space, with or without lymphocytic bronchiolitis. HLT recipients are best monitored with transbronchial biopsies instead of endomyocardial biopsies because AR may be detected in the lung, even in the absence of histologic abnormalities of the heart. Endomyocardial biopsies are done exclusively when clinical or echocardiographic abnormalities suggest pump failure.

Infection

Infection can be categorized as bacterial (early) and opportunistic (late). Infection commonly complicates lung transplantation.[12] Early after transplantation (the first 2 weeks), bacterial processes commonly occur secondary to infections with *Staphylococcus aureus*, *Pseudomonas aeruginosa*, and other gram-negative organisms, as well as infections with *Candida albicans*. These are usually related to nosocomial organisms that had previously colonized the donor during the intubation time. In the following weeks (weeks 2 to 12), cytomegalovirus (CMV),[13] herpes virus, and *Aspergillus* sp. are the most common infectious agents. Late infections (after 3 months) include CMV infection, cryptococcosis, toxoplasmosis, and Epstein-Barr virus (EBV) infection. EBV has been associated with the development of transplant-related lymphoproliferative disease, which at times is indistinguishable from a true lymphoma.

CMV infections are the most frequent and severe in CMV-seronegative recipients of a CMV-seropositive donor (CMV$^+$d/CMV$^-$r). CMV$^+$d/CMV$^+$r and CMV$^-$d/CMV$^+$r also have increased risk of developing CMV disease and pneumonia.

CMV$^-$d/CMV$^-$r may eventually develop CMV disease (10%) if they receive CMV$^+$ blood transfusions or if, subsequently, the lung transplant recipient gets a "de novo" exposure while sexually active. The presence of CMV in the host is defined as follows:

CMV infection: The presence of positive cultures (shell-vial assay or conventional tube cell cultures) in the absence of clinical symptoms without positive inclusions by cytologic or histologic examination.

CMV syndrome: The patient has multisystemic symptoms of infection; CMV cultures yield positive results; there

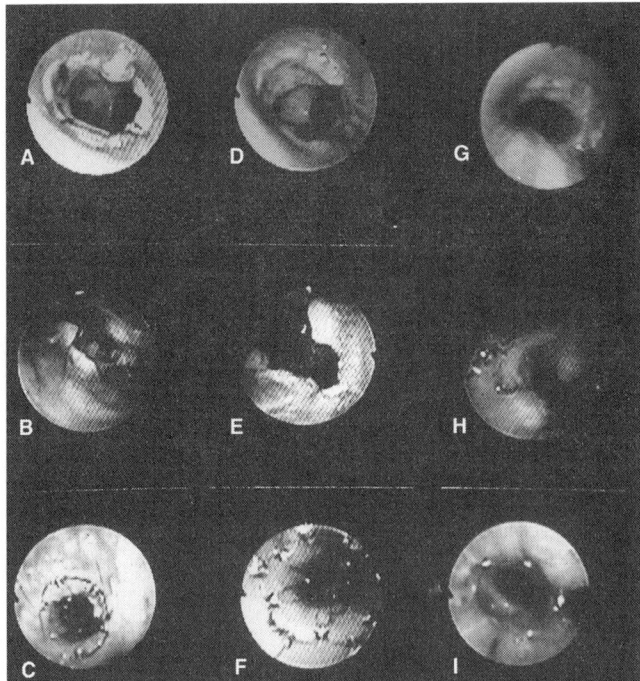

FIGURE 87-4. Bronchoscopic findings in lung transplantation (*top left* to *bottom right*). (**A**) Left main bronchial anastomosis, 1 week after transplant. (**B**) Left main bronchial anastomosis, 1 month after transplant. (**C**) Left main bronchial anastomosis, 1 year after transplant. (**D**) Anastomotic necrosis complicating transplantation (early changes). (**E**) Progressive necrosis, ischemic changes. (**F**) Advanced necrosis eventually producing dehiscence. (**G**) Right lower anastomosis after ballon bronchoplasty and insertion of self-expandable stent (Gianturco). (**H**) Stent in place, bronchoscopy passing through the stent. (**I**) Right main bronchus stent (distal end).

is associated leukopenia, thrombocytopenia, or both; but no viral inclusions are seen by cytologic or histologic study.

CMV disease and pneumonia: The features of CMV syndrome are present and there are typical intracellular inclusions in cells or tissue obtained from any body site. If these inclusions are present in bronchoalveolar lavage (BAL) or lung biopsy specimens, the diagnosis of CMV pneumonia is made.

Aspergillosis commonly complicates transplanted patients who previously experienced chronic lung infections (CF, bronchiectasis); with aspergillosis, previous airway colonization with fungus persists after transplantation. Systemic infections with *Aspergillus* are usually fatal.

Diaphragmatic Dysfunction

Phrenic nerve injury occurs infrequently after transplantation.[14] It is often related to injury created during traction of mediastinal structures while the surgery is performed, and to the use of electrocoagulation for bleeding control near the phrenic nerve region. In most instances, the dysfunction is transitory. Phrenic nerve injury should be suspected when the involved hemidiaphragm remains elevated during spon-

taneous breathing. The patient may show reduced negative inspiratory force (30 cm H_2O or less) and becomes tachypneic when positive-pressure ventilation is discontinued. This process should be suspected in any transplanted patient who has difficulty weaning from the ventilator. Measurement of negative inspiratory force and fluoroscopic evaluation of diaphragmatic motion during spontaneous breathing establishes this diagnosis.

Bronchiolitis Obliterans

Bronchiolitis obliterans is usually a late complication but occasionally occurs as early as 2 months after transplantation. It is characterized by insidious and progressive exertional dyspnea with decline in airflows (forced expiratory volume in 1 second [FEV_1] and forced expiratory flow [$FEF_{25\%-75\%}$]) and the development of a flow–volume curve similar to the one present in emphysema (Fig. 87-7). The chest roentgenogram seldom shows abnormalities, although progressive air trapping will eventually be present. BO is the main cause of long-term morbidity and mortality in transplanted patients, particularly those who had several episodes of AR or CMV pneumonitis early after transplantation.[15] Diagnosis is suspected clinically in patients with slowly progressive dyspnea, associated with a decline in spirometric parameters, and is documented by transbronchial or open lung biopsy specimens showing concentric submucosal fibrosis of bronchioles, which, in advanced stages, may show less cellular fibrous tissue obliterating bronchiolar lumina.[16]

STRESS POINTS

The transplanted lung is subjected to many circumstances that may preclude normal gas exchange after transplantation:

1. Lungs are obtained from brain-dead donors receiving ventilatory and hemodynamic support involving transient intubation and upper airway colonization with nosocomial organisms. They may have periods of hemodynamic instability and usually have received PEEP and positive-pressure ventilation, as well as infusion of large quantities of IV fluids, blood products, and vasopressor agents. All of these factors favor acute lung injury.
2. Donated lungs are subjected to ischemic injury, including the ischemia time (period starting when the donor's aorta is cross-clamped and ending when the bronchial and vascular anastomoses are completed in the recipient and the transplanted lung is ventilated and reperfused). Hypotension and intraoperative or perioperative bleeding may add further ischemic injury.
3. The implanted lung is denervated, the lymphatic drainage is nonfunctional, and bronchial circulation is surgically interrupted. These circumstances favor development of pulmonary edema, early ischemia, and impaired cough reflex with retention of thick, tenacious secretions.
4. The transplant recipient is given combined immunosuppressive therapy to allow tolerance of donor cells;

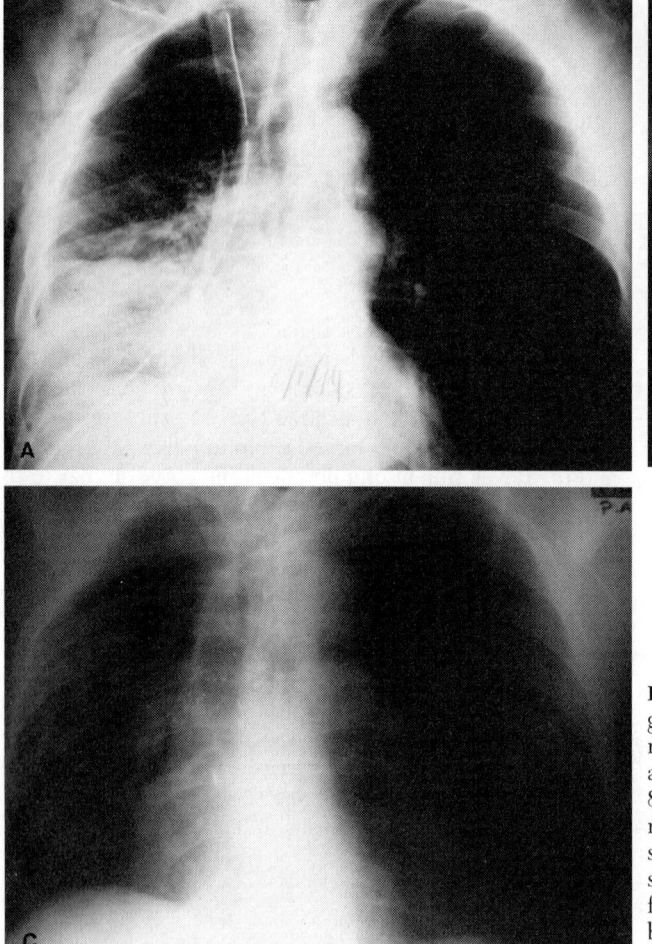

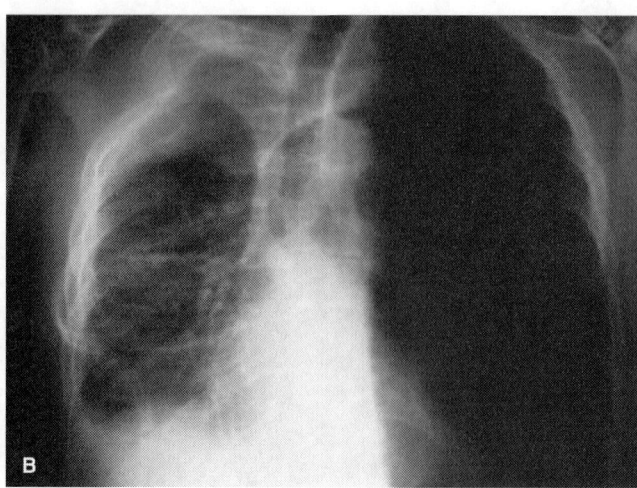

FIGURE 87-5. Anastomotic dehisence: (**A**) Recipient of a right single-lung transplant for emphysema developed persistent pneumothorax and subcutaneous emphysema despite use of chest tube. His anastomosis was necrotic and dehiscent (anastomosis shown in Fig. 87-4). (**B**) Radiograph showing patient after repeated thoracotomy; resection of the necrotic bronchial bordes was done with reanastomosis. A muscle-flap was used to wrap the anastomosis to provide support to the area. (**C**) One year later, the patient is recovered and functional. Because of progressive obstruction of the right main bronchus, this patient received balloon bronchoplasty followed by insertion of a Gianturco stent (seen in figure).

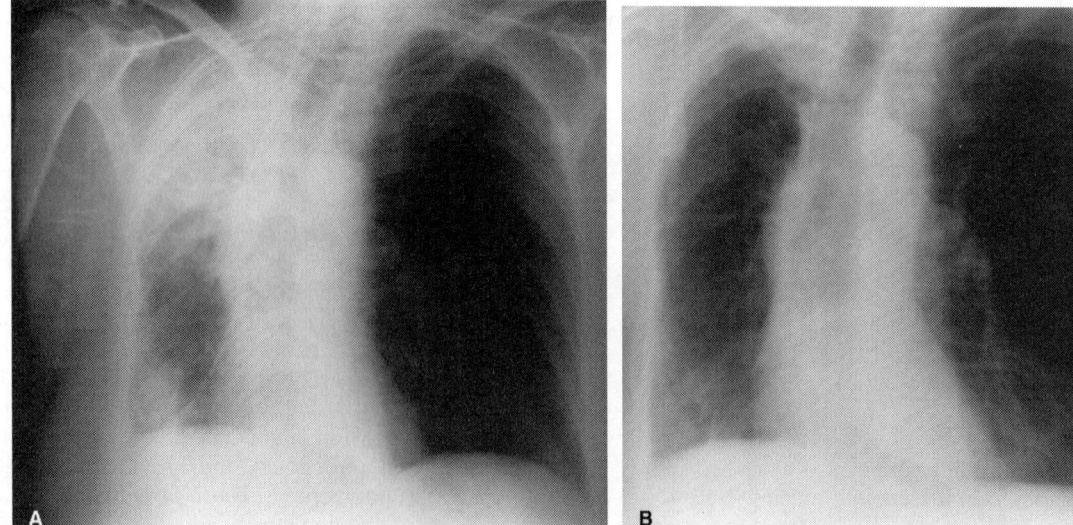

FIGURE 87-6. Acute rejection: (**A**) A recipient of a right single-lung transplant developed fever, shortness of breath, and hypoxemia. Transbronchial biopsies revealed acute rejection, grade 3A. Radiographically, she showed a dense alveolar infiltrate, most prominent in the right upper lobe. (**B**) Same patient 5 days after receiving treatment with 1 daily bolus of methylprednisolone, 15 mg/kg/day for 3 consecutive days. Symptoms reverted within 48 hours.

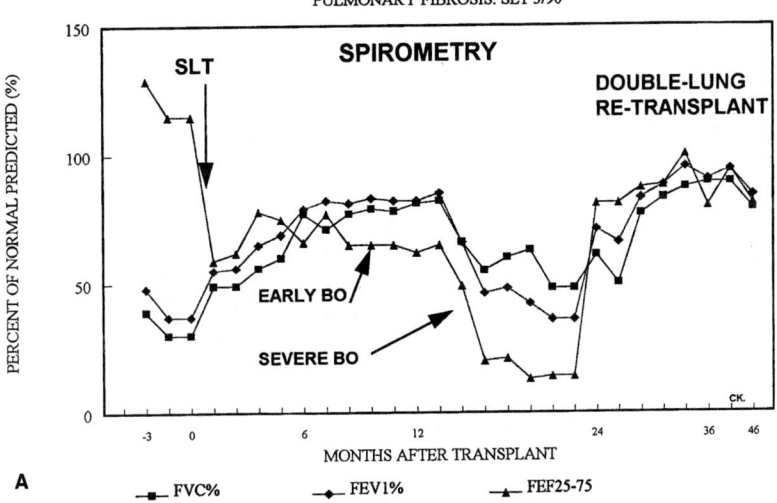

FLOW-VOLUME CURVES

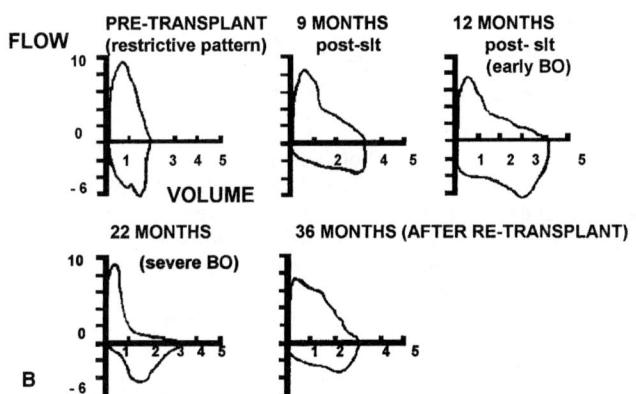

FIGURE 87-7. Bronchiolitis obliterans (BO). (**A**) The progressive changes in forced vital capacity (FVC), forced exhaled volume in 1 second (FEV1%), and forced expiratory flow (FEF$_{25-75}$) before transplant show reduced volumes because of pulmonary fibrosis. After single-lung transplantation (SLT), there is progressive increment in volumes and flows. By 7 months posttransplant, there is progressive drop in FEF$_{25-75}$, followed several months later by drop in FEV$_1$ when the diagnosis was finally proven histologically. Transient slow down of the drop in flow was achieved with enhanced immunosupression, but eventually the patient required a double-lung retransplant to recover function. (**B**) The progressive changes in flow-volume (F-V) curves, starting with the typical restrictive pattern pretransplant, followed by a relatively normal F-V curve. Twelve months posttransplant, he already showed some decline in the midexpiratory curve. By 22 months posttransplant, the F-V curve was consistent with a severe obstructive pattern present mainly in small airways. F-V curve after retransplantation again resembles a normal curve.

in the process, the recipient becomes susceptible to opportunistic infections. Aggressive prophylactic protocols for infection have reduced fatal instances of infection.

5. The telescoping technique for bronchial anastomosis, coupled with a better understanding of the postoperative management of transplanted patients, has reduced instances of anastomotic dehiscence, but telescoping may favor development of strictures with significant airway obstruction.

6. Despite immunosuppressive therapy, AR commonly occurs early after transplantation. When clinically suspected, five to ten transbronchial biopsies are required to establish specific diagnosis and guide therapy.

7. Patients with chronic obstructive lung disease (COLD) who are SLT recipients complicated by severe acute graft injury develop dramatic differences in airway resistance and lung compliance between graft and native lungs. The lung with acute injury shows characteristics of unilateral adult respiratory distress syndrome (ARDS), whereas the native lung is a highly compliant lung with severe airflow obstruction.

8. Of long-term transplant survivors, 25% to 50% will eventually develop graft dysfunction as a result of BO, which is believed to represent chronic rejection. Early recognition and treatment of this process avoids severe dysfunction or death.

ESSENTIAL DIAGNOSTIC TESTS AND PROCEDURES

1. *Lung mechanics and gas exchange*: Effectiveness of ventilatory and hemodynamic support is assessed by calculating adequacy of oxygen delivery to tissues ($\dot{D}o_2$). This concept implies follow-up of Hb, Sao$_2$, Pao$_2$, and CO. Use of an oximetric pulmonary artery catheter (with continuous monitoring of Svo$_2$) and continuous pulse oximetry are of great value to continuously assess the stability of transplant patients. The use of these variables in transplant patients is described in Figure 87-8. Repeated direct measurements of PAOP are avoided to minimize damage to vascular anastomosis. After an initial direct measurement of PAOP, the gradient of PA$_{diastolic}$ minus PAOP is

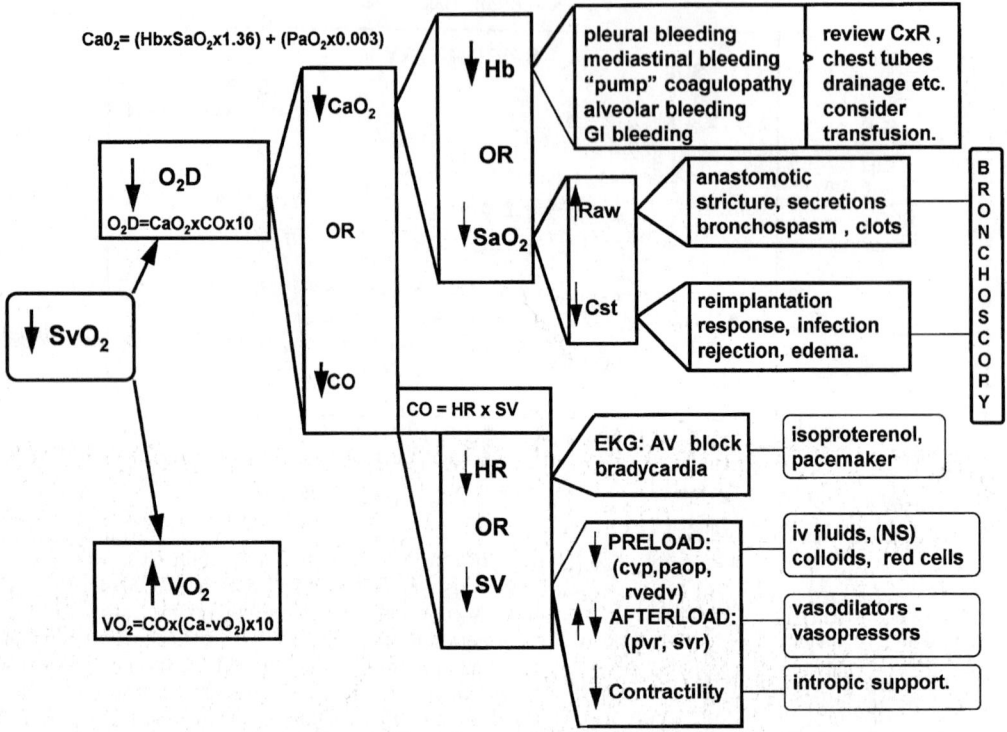

FIGURE 87-8. Use of hemodynamic and gas exchange variables in the management of the lung transplant patient. The lung transplant patient receives close monitoring postoperatively. Oxymetric pulmonary artery catheter and continuous pulse oxymetry allow early recognition of problems. A significant drop in venous saturation with oxygen ($\dot{S}vO_2$) is secondary to either increased oxygen consumption ($\dot{V}O_2$), or most commonly, to a reduction in oxygen delivery to tissues (O_2D). A decreased O_2D is related to either a reduction in arterial oxygen content (CaO_2) or cardiac output (CO). Reduced arterial oxygen results from low hemoglobin (Hb)—from bleeding or anemia—or arterial hypoxemia. If arterial hypoxemia is present, the measurement of airway resistance (Raw) and compliance (Cst) may reveal the potential source of problem; increased Raw occurs in airway problems, whereas low Cst usually reflects parenchymal lung injury. Bronchoscopic revision of airways or sampling of lung parenchyma through transbronchial biopsies reveals the diagnosis. If CaO_2 is normal, then the source of low O_2D will be low cardiac output (CO). Low CO may result from bradycardia (electrocardiogram [EKG] is indicated) or low stroke volume. Assessment of preload (central venous pressure [CVP], pulmonary artery occlusion pressure [PAOP], right ventricular end-diastolic volume [RVEDV]), afterload (pulmonary vascular resistance [PVR], systemic vascular resistance [SVR]) and contractility are indicated to select specific therapy. AV, atrioventricular; $Ca - vO_2$, arterial–venous concentration difference of oxygen; CxR, chest radiograph; HR, heart rate; iv, intravenous; NS, normal saline; stroke volume (SV).

measured and used subsequently to estimate PAOP (where PAOP is $PA_{diastolic}$ minus the known gradient).

2. *Airway resistance (Raw) and static compliance (Cst):* Airway resistance and static compliance can easily be measured on the ventilator at bedside:

$$Raw = \frac{peak\ pressure - plateau\ pressure}{peak\ flow}$$

$$Cst = \frac{tidal\ volume}{plateau\ pressure - PEEP}$$

Normal Raw is less than 5 cm H_2O/L/second; normal Cst is more than 80 mL/cm H_2O.

Trends showing *increased airway resistance* are consistent with airflow obstruction: increased secretions, anastomosis obstruction or stricture, and bronchospasm.

Reduced static compliance suggests interstitial lung processes (in the context of lung transplant); reimplantation response, pulmonary edema, rejection, and infection should all be considered.

3. *Bronchoscopy:* Bronchoscopy plays an important diagnostic and therapeutic role in lung transplantation; the first bronchoscopy is done in the surgical suite immediately after implantation to remove clots and review the anastomosis. Bronchoscopy is repeated be-

fore extubation. Subsequent endoscopies in the immediate postoperative time are usually done when there is a clinical indication: persistent pneumomediastinum or pneumothorax indicates revision of anastomosis to rule out dehiscence (see Figs. 87-4 and 87-5). Any new infiltrate, particularly if associated with hypoxemia, requires bronchoscopy.

After the initial postoperative period, screening procedures are done on a monthly basis for 6 months and subsequently every 3 months for the first year. In addition, any clinical change or any documented reduction in pulmonary function tests warrants endoscopy and biopsy to allow objective and specific therapy. The following diagnostic material is processed with the bronchoscopy specimen for lung transplant recipients in whom infection or rejection is considered:

BAL specimens: Stains for BAL specimens include the following: Gram (bacterial processes), silver stain (*Pneumocystis carinii* pneumonia [PCP], fungi), calcofluor (PCP, fungi), acid-fast bacilli, Papanicolaou (screen for PCP, CMV, or herpetic inclusions). Cultures include the following: protected brush (quantitative bacterial culture) and shell-vial and standard culture for CMV, as well as cultures for herpes, acid-fast bacilli, fungus, and *Legionella*.

Biopsy specimens: Five to ten transbronchial biopsy specimens showing alveolar structures are usually required for adequate reading. Hematoxylin-eosin and silver stains are done routinely; trichrome stains are made when BO is suspected.

When rejection is present, a standardized format to read biopsies is followed[17] to grade the severity of rejection. Documented rejection or infection requires a follow-up biopsy 3 to 4 weeks later to assess the resolution of the process or the need for continued treatment.

4. *Spirometry and pulse oximetry*: FEV_1, $FEF_{25\%-75\%}$, and measurement of SaO_2 by pulse oximetry at rest and exercise constitute the most important parameters to detect AR, infection, and particularly BO. Acute decline of spirometric values and saturation occur in AR and infection. BO should be suspected in any transplant recipient who shows a progressive obstructive pattern, initially characterized by decline in $FEF_{25\%-75\%}$ and eventually in FEV_1(15), with changes in the flow–volume curves (see Fig. 87-7). Currently, a method of grading the severity of BO has been proposed: a score is obtained by calculating the percentage of drop in FEV_1 from the peak achieved after transplantation.[18] Portable devices to measure flows at home or supervised spirometry measured with help of home care personnel facilitates follow-up spirometry to detect early declines in pulmonary function.

INITIAL THERAPY

1. *Mechanical ventilation*: All patients require ventilatory assistance early after transplantation, usually during the first 2 to 7 days. The ventilator is adjusted to provide adequate minute ventilation, and peak flow is regulated to maintain low peak pressures (35 cm H_2O or less). PEEP of 5 to 10 cm H_2O is used. The lowest possible fraction of inspired oxygen is maintained as long as SaO_2 of 92% or higher can be sustained. Modalities such as pressure-controlled ventilation, inverse-ratio ventilation, or high-frequency ventilation may be used in individual cases. SLT may offer challenging ventilatory problems, particularly in recipients with severe COLD complicated by acute graft injury. In these situations, the transplanted lung shows the characteristics of unilateral ARDS (low compliance requiring high levels of PEEP to recruit alveoli), whereas the opposite lung has the characteristics of emphysema (highly compliant lung with increased airway resistance, which develops auto PEEP easily with low peak flows; Fig. 87-9). These patients require manipulations such as positional changes and double-lumen intubation (in severe cases). With positional changes, the lung with the best ventilation/perfusion matching is down and the opposite lung is up. Double-lumen intubation allows differential ventilation using two ventilators: one providing high peak flows, low or no PEEP, and inspiratory-to-expiratory ratios above 1:4 to the emphysema lung; the second ventilator provides low peak flows (to avoid excessive peak pressure) and high PEEP to the transplanted lung with acute injury. The benefits of differential lung ventilation have to be weighed against impaired clearing of secretions while using double-lumen intubation. Once ventilation, oxygenation, and hemodynamics are stabilized, patients can be weaned using modalities associated with continuous positive pressure and pressure support.

2. *Hemodynamic support*: Integrity of bronchial and vascular anastomosis is facilitated by maintaining adequate $\dot{D}O_2$, which depends on maintaining normal arterial oxygen content (CaO_2) and CO.

This concept can be summarized as follows:

$$\dot{D}O_2 = [(Hb \times SaO_2 \times 1.36) + (PaO_2 \times 0.0031)] \times$$
$$[HR \times SV] \times 10$$

where HR is heart rate and SV is stroke volume; a normal value is 800 to 1200 mL of oxygen per minute. We favor monitoring $\dot{D}O_2$ with continuous reading of SvO_2 and SaO_2 as a guide to decide therapeutic manipulations (see Fig. 87-8). Most of these patients have variable degrees of pulmonary hypertension, increased pulmonary vascular resistance, and decreased right ventricular ejection fraction before transplantation. Most of these hemodynamic abnormalities reverse rapidly within the first 24 to 48 hours after transplantation, often preceding improvements in ventilation and gas exchange, which occur later, as the lung recovers from acute lung injury.[19] The transplanted lung is highly susceptible to developing noncardiogenic acute pulmonary edema (reimplantation response). Support of CO seldom requires large infusions of inotropic agents as long as an adequate intravascular volume is preserved. In my institution, central venous pressure, PAOP, and right ventricular end-

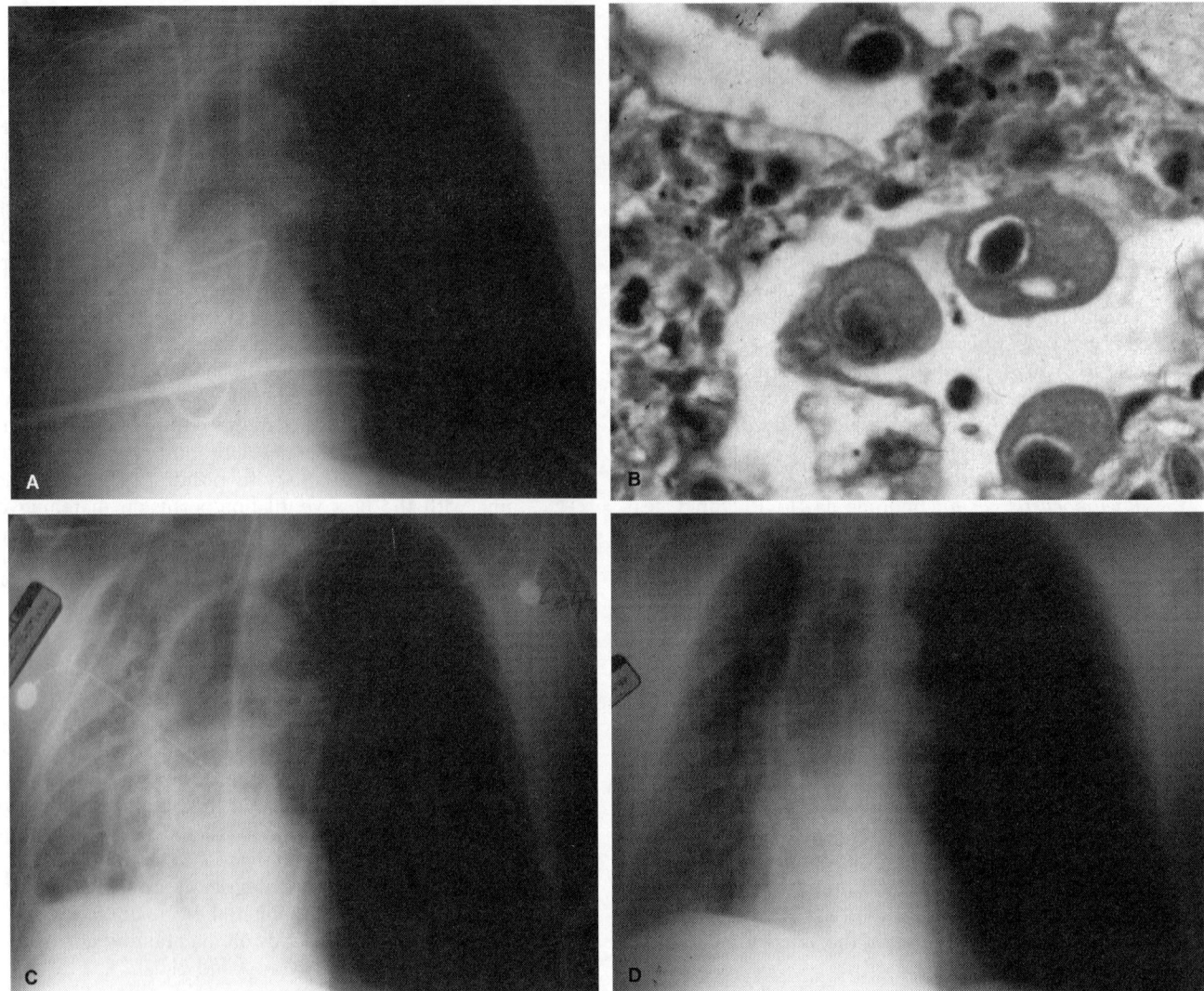

FIGURE 87-9. Severe acute graft injury in COLD: (**A**) Patient with end-stage COLD, recipient of a right single-lung transplantation developed severe respiratory failure, fever, leukopenia, and thrombocytopenia associated with a generalized macular rash. His radiograph revealed complete consolidation of the transplanted organ and hyperinflation of the native lung. (**B**) Transbronchial lung biopsy reveals typical cytomegalovirus inclusions and pneumonitis. Skin biopsy also showed cytomegalovirus infiltration. (**C**) Patient was treated with gancyclovir, 5 mg/kg intravenously every 12 hours for 28 days. He also received ventilatory support, requiring a transient period of differential lung ventilation with two ventilators, which eventually cleared the infiltrates. (**D**) Patient recovered from the insult; 1 year later his radiograph showed typical changes of single-lung transplantation. He remains fully functional despite the severity of the early insult.

diastolic volume are monitored. The goal is to maintain intravascular pressures in the low–normal range to minimize pulmonary edema while providing the patient with enough preload to maintain adequate CO. Low-dose dopamine (2 to 3 μg/kg/min) is maintained to optimize renal perfusion. Systemic hypotension needs to be avoided because it compromises the integrity of the anastomosis as well as the renal function,

which in itself is already compromised by the infusion of cyclosporine.

Maintaining adequate Hb levels is important to preserve adequate CaO_2. The requirement of transfusions to keep Hb levels at 10 g/dL or more suggests active bleeding or bone marrow suppression induced by azathioprine.

3. *Management of bleeding*: Hemorrhagic complications

associated with CBP support are minimized by using the pump for the shortest possible time. Currently, intraoperative bleeding has been significantly reduced with the use of aprotinin (Trasylol), a serine protease inhibitor with the ability not only to inhibit fibrinolysis, but also to preserve platelet function.[20] If significant bleeding occurs early in postoperative time, the patient should be taken back to the operative suite to remove clots from pleural and mediastinal spaces and to surgically reverse the cause of bleeding. Transfusion of blood products (red blood cells, fresh frozen plasma, platelets, and cryoprecipitate) are indicated if there are documented abnormalities measured in the coagulation cascade.

4. *Management of pulmonary reimplantation response:* Pulmonary reimplantation response is best managed by maintaining ventilatory support with PEEP, associated with aggressive diuresis using IV furosemide and renal-dose dopamine infusion. Negative balance is maintained as long as $\dot{D}o_2$ is not compromised. This condition usually reverses in 48 to 72 hours. Cases refractory to standard management may reverse with administration of inhaled nitric oxide.[21]

5. *Management of airway complications:* Bronchoscopy offers an invaluable help to remove thick, tenacious secretions as well as clots and debris commonly present shortly after transplantation. The biopsy forceps can be used to remove thick debris present at the anastomotic site. Aggressive chest therapy is started 4 hours postoperatively and then continued every 2 hours. Patients should be helped to sit in a chair 24 hours after surgery; as soon as they are extubated, physical therapy (ambulation, pedaling in bicycle ergometer, arm exercises) should be started. When significant airway obstruction develops, balloon bronchoplasty can be used.[22] Persistence or recurrence of obstruction may be managed with placement of self-expandable metallic stents through flexible bronchoscopy under fluoroscopic guidance (Fig. 87-10) or silastic stents through a rigid bronchoscope.[23]

6. *Management of AR:* Histologically documented episodes of AR are treated with the following protocol (for rejections grade 1A in symptomatic patients or any grade 2A or higher, regardless of symptoms):
MPS, 15 mg/kg/day (maximum dose, 1 g): one daily dose for 3 consecutive days, followed by
Prednisone, 1 mg/kg/day, tapered to baseline dose over 4 weeks
Repeat biopsy in 3 to 4 weeks if rejection is still present; boluses of MPS are repeated, and follow-up biopsy is repeated.
If rejection persists, OKT3 is used, following the same protocol described for heart transplant recipients.

7. *Management of infection:* Serious infections need specific antibiotic treatment as well as a reduction or even transient discontinuation of immunosuppressive therapy in severe cases. Prophylaxis and early therapy consist of the following:
Bacterial infections: In surgery, the secretions from

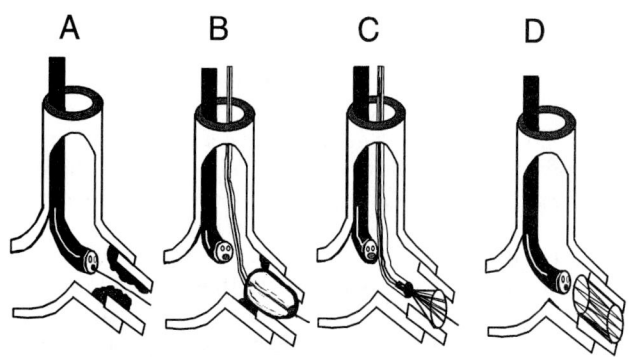

FIGURE 87-10. Balloon bronchoplasty and stent insertion: Procedure involves bronchoscopic visualization of the obstruction and passage of a "J" vascular guidewire distal to the anastomosis (**A**), which subsequently is used to pass a 1- to 1.2-cm wide, 4-cm long angioplasty balloon, which is inflated for 15 to 30 seconds at a time with a LeVeen inflator with pressure gauge up to 4 to 5 atm (**B**). Once the area is dilated, over the same guidewire and with fluoroscopic guidance, a self-expandable stent is pushed out from the introducer (**C**), which, once in the bronchial lumen, will maintain the airway open (**D**).

the donor bronchus are cultured before implantation; this is repeated immediately after surgery. A bronchoscopic aspirate is also submitted for stains and cultures. Wide-spectrum IV antibiotics are started during surgery (piperacillin/tazobactam or association of clindamycin/ceftazidime). Three days later, if the culture results are negative, antimicrobials are discontinued. If there is positive growth in the cultures, specific antimicrobial therapy is started. All suspected episodes of infection should be investigated with bronchoscopy to obtain adequate specimens for culture and histologic study. Empiric therapy should be avoided whenever possible.

Fungal infections: For fungal infections, patients are given oral nystatin to protect against oral candidiasis. If there is evidence of other areas of *Candida* involvement (bronchial lavage, urinary, cutaneous), 200 to 400 mg of IV fluconazole is used; careful adjustment of cyclosporine levels is required because the levels will increase from the interaction with this antifungal. Presence of hyphae in BAL specimens or cultures showing *Aspergillus* in the absence of radiographic infiltrates or histologic abnormalities are consistent with airway colonization by *Aspergillus*. Management includes itraconazole, 200 mg/day, and nebulized amphotericin (5 to 15 mg diluted in 5% dextrose in water nebulized every 8 hours). Systemic fungal infections require the use of IV amphotericin, 25 to 50 mg/day.

Viral infections: CMV disease is common among lung transplant recipients and frequently involves respiratory, gastrointestinal, and hepatic systems. Recurrent CMV infections are associated with AR and possibly with BO.

When either the donor or the recipient are CMV seropositive, the patient should be given prophylactic treatment. On day 7 postoperatively, IV gancyclovir (Cytovene), 5 mg/kg twice daily, is given for 14 days, followed by 5 mg/kg/day from day 21 to 90 postoperatively. This medication needs adjustment if there is renal failure. Gancyclovir may induce renal dysfunction and leukopenia, and requires insertion of a permanent central venous catheter. The introduction of oral gancyclovir may soon resolve these problems. The value of this prophylactic protocol as well as the effect of the addition of CMV-specific immunoglobulin (CytoGam), with or without later addition of oral acyclovir, is being investigated.

Beyond the first 3 months, further CMV prophylactic treatment needs to be restarted if the patient requires enhanced immunosuppression for AR because during these times, the likelihood of active CMV disease increases (it is usually given for 2 weeks after immunosuppression). Some centers add CMV-specific immunoglobulin (CytoGam) to the prophylactic protocol at the following doses: first dose of 150 mg/kg within 48 hours of transplantation; then 100 mg/kg at 2, 4, 6, and 8 weeks after transplantation; followed by 50 mg/kg at 12 and 16 weeks after transplantation. The real effectiveness of different prophylactic protocols is being investigated. The protocols currently used follow guidelines established for bone marrow transplant recipients.[24]

Treatment of documented CMV pneumonitis or disease includes the following: gancyclovir at a dosage of 5 mg/kg every 12 hours for 14 days, followed by 5 mg/kg/day for 14 days. Cases refractory or intolerant to gancyclovir are treated with IV foscarnet (Foscavir) 60 mg/kg/day every 8 hours for 2 weeks followed by a maintenance therapy with 90 mg/kg/day. This therapy follows guidelines investigated in patients with AIDS.[25]

A transplant recipient who is CMV negative with a CMV-negative donor does not require gancyclovir prophylaxis. Acyclovir, 400 mg orally every 8 hours for 4 months may be administered for herpes virus prophylaxis. Patients on gancyclovir are also protected from herpes infections.

EBV and lymphoproliferative disease: Treatment for EBV and lymphoproliferative disease consists of decreasing immunosuppression to the minimum with the addition of acyclovir.

PCP: *Pneumocystis* infections are rarely seen because of the generalized practice of using chronic prophylaxis with trimethoprim/sulfamethoxasole, 1 double-strength tablet three times a week.

8. *Management of diaphragmatic dysfunction*: Diaphragmatic dysfunction occasionally impairs early weaning from the ventilator. Aggressive chest therapy, mobilization, and sitting the patient in a chair as soon as the medical condition is stable are all helpful. Most of these episodes subside partially or completely within few weeks. Occasionally, tracheostomy with prolonged mechanical ventilation is required. In mild cases, the patient can be assisted after extubation using continuous positive airway pressure–pressure support by face or nasal mask.

9. *Management of BO*: The same protocol for treating AR is used for treating BO. Early treatment is important because most patients do not return to baseline function. Therapy occasionally arrests further progression of the syndrome. Cases refractory to boluses of corticosteroids and antilymphocytic therapy could qualify for retransplantation. However, 1-year survival rates are less than 50% in retransplanted patients.[26] The limited availability of donors makes this option controversial.

CONCLUSION ■

In summary, a large group of patients with severe end-stage respiratory failure can be treated with HLT, DLT, or SLT with a reasonably good prognosis and with recovery of adequate pulmonary function. Compulsive management of postoperative complications is required to maintain good long-term function of the graft.

REFERENCES ■

1. United Network of Organ Sharing Administrator of the U.S. Scientific Registry of Transplant Recipients: Preliminary data as of January 12, 1994. In: *Proceedings of the Regional UNOS Meeting*, St. Louis Missouri, March 1995
2. Cooper JD, Pearson FG, Patterson GA, et al: Technique of successful lung transplantation in humans. *J Thorac Cardiovasc Surg* 1987;93:173
3. Calhoun JH, Groover FL, Gibbons WJ, et al: Single lung transplantation. *J Thorac Cardiovasc Surg* 1991;101:816
4. Pasque MK, Cooper JD, Kaiser LR, et al: Improved technique for bilateral lung transplantation: rationale and initial clinical experience. *Ann Thorac Surg* 1990;49:785
5. Judson MA: Clinical aspects of lung transplantation. *Clin Chest Med* 1993;14;2:335
6. Ferran C, Sheehan C, Dy M, et al: Cytokine-related syndrome following injection of anti-CD₃ monoclonal antibody. *Eur J Immunol* 1990;20:509
7. Todd TRJ: Early postoperative management following lung transplantation. *Clin Chest Med* 1990;11:259
8. Bryan CL, Cohen DJ, Gibbons W, et al: Lung transplantation: the reimplantation response. *Crit Care Rep* 1991;2:217
9. Patterson GA, Todd TR, Cooper JD, et al: Airway complications after double lung transplantation. *J Thorac Cardiovasc Surg* 1990;99:14
10. Griffith BP, Paradis IL, Zeevi A, et al: Immunologically mediated disease of the airways after pulmonary transplantation. *Ann Surg* 1988;208:371
11. Marshall SE, Leviston NJ, Kramer MR, et al: Prospective analysis of serial pulmonary function studies and transbronchial biopsies in single lung transplant recipients. *Transplant Proc* 1991;23:1217
12. Dauber JH, Paradis IL, Dummer JS, et al: Infectious complications in pulmonary allograft recipients. *Clin Chest Med* 1990;11:291
13. Ettinger NA, Bailey TC, Trulock EP, et al: Cytomegalovirus infection and pneumonitis: impact after isolated lung transplant. *Am Rev Respir Dis* 1993;147:1017

14. Maurer JR: Therapeutic challenges following lung transplantation. *Clin Chest Med* 1990;11:279

15. Keller CA, Cagle PT, Brown RW, et al: Bronchiolitis obliterans in recipients of single, double and heart-lung transplantation. *Chest* 1995;107:4:973

16. Cagle PT, Brown RW, Frost A, et al: Diagnosis of chronic lung transplant rejection by transbronchial biopsy. *Modern Pathol* 1995;8:137

17. Yousem SA, Berry GJ, Brunt EM, et al: A working formulation for the standardization of nomenclature in the diagnosis of heart and lung rejection: Lung Rejection Study Group. *J Heart Transplant* 1990;9:593

18. International Society for Heart and Lung Transplantation: A working formulation for the standardization of nomenclature and for clinical staging of chronic dysfunction in lung allografts. *J Heart Lung Transplant* 1993;12:713

19. Keller CA, Ohar JA, Baudendistel LJ: Hemodynamics and gas exchange during single lung transplant. *Am J Respir Crit Care Med* 1994;149:A735

20. Royston D: Aprotinin therapy in heart and heart-lung transplantation. *J Heart Lung Transplant* 1993;12:S19

21. Macdonald P, Mundy J, Rogers P, et al: Treatment of severe acute reperfusion injury after lung trasplantation with inhaled nitric oxide. *J Heart Lung Transplant* 1995;14:S88

22. Keller CA, Frost A: Fiberoptic bronchoplasty: description of a simple adjunct technique for the management of bronchial stenosis following lung transplantation. *Chest* 1992;102:995

23. Carre P, Rosseau H, Lombart L, et al: Balloon dilatation and self-expanding metal wallstent insertion for management of bronchostenosis following lung transplantation: The Toulouse Lung Transplantation Group. *Chest* 1994;105:343

24. Schmidt GM, Horak DA, Niland JC, et al: A randomized, controlled trial of prophylactic gancyclovir for cytomegalovirus pulmonary infection in recipients of allogenic bone marrow transplants. *N Engl J Med* 1991;324:1005

25. AIDS Research Group and AIDS Clinical Trials Group: Morbidity and toxic effects associated with ganciclovir or foscarnet therapy in a randomized cytomegalovirus retinitis trial. *Arch Intern Med* 1995;155:65.

26. Novick RJ, Andreassian B, Schafers HJ, et al: Pulmonary retransplantation for obliterative bronchiolitis: intermediate-term results of a North American–European series. *J Thorac Cardiovasc Surg* 1994;107:755

Critical Care, Third Edition, edited by Joseph M. Civetta,
Robert W. Taylor, and Robert R. Kirby.
Lippincott-Raven Publishers, Philadelphia, PA © 1997.

CHAPTER 88

<hr>

Heart Transplantation

Leslie W. Miller

INDICATIONS

Heart transplantation has evolved over the last decade to become the optimal treatment for end-stage heart failure, for selected patients with over 30,000 heart transplants having been performed worldwide (approximately two thirds having been done in the United States) since the initial procedure was performed in 1967 in Capetown, South Africa. Over 100 additional transplants were performed over the following year in approximately 20 institutions, but it quickly became clear that clinicians lacked the understanding of how to control the delicate balance between infection and rejection, and most patients died within weeks to months of the procedure. As a result, the number of procedures decreased to only 10 to 20 per year, largely done at Stanford University, until 1980 when the more selective immunosuppressive drug, cyclosporine, first became available. The improved survival associated with its use led to a dramatic increase in the number of patients undergoing transplantation, which averages approximately 2400 per year.[1] The sine qua non for consideration for heart transplant is refractory congestive heart failure and severe functional limitation despite maximal medical therapy. Ischemic heart disease has become the number one indication (55%), followed by idiopathic cardiomyopathy (48%). More selective immunosuppression[2] and improved patient selection[3,4] have led to the current survival rates of 85% at 1 year, 75% at 3 years, and 65% to 70% at 5 years.

There have been few modifications of the original technical descriptions of orthotopic cardiac transplantation described by Lower and Shumway. Basically, the recipient's native heart is amputated above the atrioventricular valves, leaving only the posterior wall of both atria and normal venous inflow. The donor heart is opened at the atria, which are then anastomosed onto the atrial posterior wall remnant

of the native heart, thereby creating atrial chambers that are nearly twice normal size—a finding that is normal on echocardiogram postoperatively. The aorta and pulmonary artery anastomoses are then completed and the heart reperfused. One new modification is the "bicaval" technique in which the recipient vena cavae are transected 2 to 3 cm above and below the right atrium and then directly anastomosed to the donor vena caval remnant, rather than right atrium. This minimizes trauma to the sinus node during surgery and greatly reduces the need for temporary pacing postoperatively. In addition, the bicaval technique maintains a normal-size atrium, which seems to minimize tricuspid regurgitation postoperatively. Air can become trapped in the pulmonary arteries or in the apex of the heart while it is being sewn in with either technique. Therefore, the apex of the heart is aspirated or vented during rewarming to minimize air embolism, which may go down a coronary artery and be an occult cause of ventricular dysfunction postoperatively.

CANDIDATE SELECTION:
HEMODYNAMIC ASSESSMENT

One of the leading causes of death in the first 5 days after heart transplantation is right ventricular failure in the donor heart because of preexisting, somewhat fixed, pulmonary hypertension in the recipient.[5] Chronic left ventricular failure causes elevation of left ventricular end diastolic pressure, which is reflected back into the left atrium and, finally, the pulmonary capillary bed, resulting in pulmonary hypertension. Over time, this pressure often results in vasoconstriction and a muscularization of the pulmonary veins and arteries, similar to the findings in mitral stenosis, to prevent pulmonary edema and transudation of fluid. The donor right heart fails after transplantation because it is unconditioned

1333

(i.e., unaccustomed to working against a high afterload) as pulmonary vascular compliance prevents normal pulmonary artery systolic pressure from exceeding 15 to 20 mm Hg, despite an increase in flow (cardiac output) of up to fivefold during exercise. Nearly all centers, therefore, obtain a hemodynamic assessment of pulmonary vascular reactivity in the ICU on all patients who are evaluated as candidates for transplantation.[6]

Two hemodynamic variables that have been shown to be risk factors for postoperative right heart failure and correlate with outcome are (1) pulmonary vascular resistance (PVR), which is the difference between pulmonary artery mean pressure and pulmonary artery occlusive pressure (PAOP) divided by the cardiac output (expressed in Wood units), and (2) the transpulmonary gradient (TPG), which is the difference between pulmonary artery mean pressure and PAOP.

$$PVR = \frac{\overline{PA} - \overline{PAOP}}{CO} \quad \text{(Wood units)}$$

$$TPG = \overline{PA} - PAOP$$

Elevations of PVR to over 3 Wood units, or a TPG of more than 15 mm Hg despite vasodilator or inotropic drug infusion, are significant risk factors for right heart failure in the early postoperative period. Data from Stanford[7] show that patients whose PVR is less than 2.5 without drug therapy have a low risk of postoperative right ventricular failure. Patients whose PVR is brought to less than 2.5 with nitroprusside infusion with systolic arterial pressure maintained above 85 mm Hg are at intermediate risk; at higher risk are patients whose PVR goes below 2.5 but with systolic blood pressure below 85 mm Hg. The highest risk patients are those whose PVR cannot be brought below 3.0 Wood units despite infusions of inotropes and dilators. Similar correlations have been reported with TPG above 15 mm Hg. However, patients whose PAOP cannot be brought below 20 mm Hg before transplantation may have further reduction in PVR after transplantation, when left atrial pressure is normalized. Alternatively, a larger donor has been used in an attempt to overcome the pulmonary hypertension after transplantation.[8]

A variety of pharmacologic agents have been used to assess the reactivity of the pulmonary vascular bed and include either vasodilators, most typically sodium nitroprusside, or inotropic drugs, which enhance the flow across the pulmonary bed, causing a reflex dilation of the pulmonary arteries and a lowering of the mean pulmonary artery pressure. Dobutamine, a β_1-agonist type inotrope, has been used primarily for this purpose in many programs; recently, however, the newer phosphodiesterase inhibitor, milrinone,[9] has been shown to not only improve cardiac output, but, because of its potent vasodilating properties, to be at least equally effective and potentially more effective in assessing pulmonary vascular reactivity. Patients may be given a loading dose of milrinone (0.3 to 0.5 µg/kg over 30 minutes), followed by a continuous infusion beginning at 0.1 µg/kg/minute and titrating up as high as 0.8 µg/kg/minute. Many patients may require several hours to even days of chronic infusion of either inotropic drugs or vasodilators plus diuretics to effec-

tively lower the PVR to acceptable levels. This usually can be done without continual hemodynamic monitoring, returning the patient to the ICU after 5 to 7 days of intravenous (IV) therapy to reassess response. Patients who do not respond to these agents, alone or in combination, warrant a trial of the potent vasodilator prostaglandin, PGE-1 (Alprostil). This drug ideally should be given in the morning in a fasting state because of nausea and diarrhea. If hypotension or intolerable symptoms occur, the drip should never be turned off completely, but reduced by 50% every 5 to 10 minutes to prevent serious "rebound" in pulmonary artery pressure. Calcium channel blockers, which are often helpful in treating primary pulmonary hypertension, are rarely used in this setting because of their negative inotropic properties.

STATUS 1 PATIENTS

An increasing number of patients deteriorate while on the waiting list and require chronic inotropic support. Patients with blood type O weighing over 90 kg are at increased risk for prolonged time on the waiting list in most centers because the average donor weighs less than 70 kg and blood group O is the "universal donor" and, therefore, can be used in any potential recipient, regardless of blood type. In addition, patients with a positive antibody screen indicating the presence of preformed circulating antibodies usually require a donor crossmatch and have a significantly increased time on the waiting list. Patients on a transplant list who are admitted to the hospital for refractory heart failure that requires use of IV inotropes are frequently managed in the intensive care unit. They are then elevated to status 1, the highest status on the waiting list (versus status 2, which is for all other patients who are on the list but maintained out of the ICU). In addition to maximal oral heart failure therapy, status 1 patients should be receiving inotropic drugs at dosages of at least 5 µg/kg/minute of dobutamine or its equivalent before warranting status 1 listing. Combinations of milrinone and dobutamine often are additive in improving cardiac output and allow lower doses of both drugs to be used. Dosages of chronic inotropic support should be kept to less than 7.5 µg/kg/minute of dobutamine or 0.6 µg/kg/minute of milrinone to minimize tolerance to the drugs. Attempts should be made at least every 7 to 10 days to wean patients off inotropes because this form of therapy is expensive and this status should be reserved for the sickest patients.

INITIAL POSTOPERATIVE MANAGEMENT ■

IMMUNOSUPPRESSION

There are two basic approaches to perioperative immunosuppression in heart transplantation, much as in other solid organs. The standard approach has evolved to using a triple-drug regimen, which includes *cyclosporine, prednisone,* and *azathioprine* from the time of transplantation.[10] Typically, this includes an oral preoperative dose of cyclosporine (4 to 10 mg/kg) as soon as the patient arrives at the hospital. Alternatively, an IV infusion can be started at a dose of 1 to 2 mg/kg/24 hours (one third of the average oral dose) by mixing 100 mg of cyclosporine in 100 mL of IV fluid. IV cyclosporine can be easily titrated and the infusion decreased if urine output decreases postoperatively, and, conversely, increased if the cyclosporine levels are low and renal function is adequate. Some programs give a smaller oral load in addition to the IV maintenance infusion of cyclosporine. Several potential side effects are associated with its use such as nephrotoxicity and hypertension, which are discussed later.

The second approach to perioperative immunosuppression is to delay the initiation of cyclosporine for several days and to substitute with cytolytic lymphocyte antibody therapy, either OKT3 or ATG. This approach is based on the observation that donor leukocytes remain in the recipient circulation for approximately 10 to 14 days after transplantation. These cells have foreign class 1 and 2 antigens on their surface, and their presence increases the risk of allorecognition and subsequent rejection. These agents are, therefore, given to delete circulating lymphocytes and provide increased immunosuppression during this time period to potentially block allorecognition. If successful, this could lead to potential induction of tolerance or unresponsiveness to the allograft, hence the name "induction therapy."

There are two basic types of lymphocyte antibody preparations, either the polyclonal ATG, or the more commonly used murine monoclonal antibody, OKT3. The monoclonal antibody, OKT3, complexes with the CD3 receptor on the surface of circulating lymphocytes, and although not directly cytotoxic, causes the cells to then be rapidly cleared through the reticuloendothelial system.[11] This complexing with the receptor often triggers a "cytokine release syndrome,"[12] which can be prevented by preadministration of the following four agents given *1 hour before* the OKT3 bolus: (1) 1 g of IV methylprednisolone on day 1, 750 mg day 2, 500 mg on day 3, then 0.3 mg/kg per day during OKT3 administration; (2) 50 to 75 mg of indomethacin (or its equivalent) orally because prostaglandins clearly also mediate some of the cytokine release syndrome; (3) diphenhydramine, 50 to 75 mg orally or intravenously; and (4) two acetaminophen tablets, 325 mg each, also given orally.

OKT3 was initially given for a course of 14 days; however, recent experience suggests that it may be used for as little as 3 to 5 days at a dose of 5 mg/day in an IV push over 30 minutes, or until the patient has cleared the perioperative fluid accumulation and normalized renal function. At that time, cyclosporine can be introduced, and when target levels are achieved, the cytolytic agent can be discontinued without a significant rebound in rejection. Many centers began using lymphocyte antibody preparations in the mid-1980s, but their use in the perioperative period has greatly decreased because of lack of data demonstrating that their use in the perioperative period actually reduces the overall incidence of rejection[13]; also, data showed that using lymphocyte antibody preparations increases the risk of infection and possibility the risk of malignancy. Most programs reserve their use for severe or refractory rejection or in patients with significantly impaired renal function (e.g., creatinine above 2.5 mg/dL) at the time of transplantation.

IV steroids, in the form of methylprednisolone, are generally given in a dose of 500 to 1000 mg intravenously, often before the patient goes on the pump, followed by a dosage of 125 mg every 8 hours for the first day. Oral steroids are then begun at a dose of 1.0 mg/kg orally and decreased by 5 mg/day to a dose of 0.3 mg/kg/day for the first month. If OKT3 or ATG is used perioperatively, the dose of oral steroids is begun at 0.3 mg/kg/day throughout the course of therapy (3 to 14 days) and then increased to 1.0 mg/kg/day and tapered by 5 mg/day to prevent increased rejection when these agents are stopped. Side effects of high-dose steroids include hyperglycemia, psychosis, infection, and elevations in white blood cell count secondary to demargination.

The final component of the "triple therapy" regimen is *azathioprine*. This drug is a nonspecific immunosuppressant that is usually given preoperatively in a dose of 2 to 4 mg/kg/day orally or intravenously and then titrated long term according to the white blood cell count. Side effects include pancytopenia a hepatitis picture with elevated liver function tests, pancreatitis, neutropenia, or megaloblastic anemia.

IMMEDIATE CONCERNS ∎

MAJOR PROBLEMS

Bleeding

Bleeding is a common problem after cardiac surgery, particularly in patients who have had previous sternotomies, because almost all transplant candidates receive oral anticoagulation with warfarin before transplantation. Once the chest is closed, bleeding also can predispose to tamponade because the recipient's native heart is often enlarged and replaced by a small normal heart, thereby creating a large potential pericardial space. It is important to reverse prolonged prothrombin times and other measured alterations in coagulation with specific factors (e.g., vitamin K), platelets, or fresh frozen plasma.

Torsion of Pulmonary Artery

A second technical problem that often precludes getting the patient out of the operating room is torsion of the pulmonary artery anastomosis. Almost all hearts are implanted with a degree of counterclockwise rotation. On occasion, this results in torsion of the pulmonary artery anastomosis, which creates an increased afterload for the right ventricle and is manifest as significant right ventricular dysfunction. The only way to prove this diagnosis is by demonstrating a gradient across the pulmonary artery anastomosis by simultaneous right ventricular and pulmonary artery pressure measurements. This finding usually requires the anastomosis to be redone, but it should be ruled out in patients with high right atrial (RA) pressure after transplantation.

Hyperacute Rejection

A third immediate problem is hyperacute rejection. This entity is relatively uncommon but is usually evident in the operating room soon after the graft is reperfused. Hyper-acute rejection should be anticipated by knowledge of a high preformed antibody titer in the recipient before transplantation, and confirmed by demonstration of a positive donor specific crossmatch with the recipient.[14] Unlike the typical cell-mediated (T-lymphocyte) rejection, this form of rejection is antibody mediated and occurs in patients with pre-formed circulating antibodies that are directed against HLA antigens present on the donor endothelial cells. This antigen–antibody binding results in thrombus formation and vasoconstriction in the coronary arteries because of the significant arteritis and injury to the coronary endothelium, resulting in severe necrosis and hemorrhage into the graft. The graft often turns mottled and is usually unable to be resuscitated in the operating room. Immediate steps to maintain the patient include plasmapheresis,[15] with exchange transfusion of 1–1½ plasma volumes per pheresis, replacing one half of the patient's plasma with type-specific fresh frozen plasma and one half with 5% albumin. This procedure may be required for several days, or until measurement of panel reactive antibodies achieves a low titer or repeat donor-specific crossmatch becomes negative. In addition to plasmapheresis, patients should receive OKT3 in a dosage of 5 mg/day for a minimum of 7 days, and IV cyclophosphamide at a dosage beginning at 750–1000 mg/day for 2 days and then decreasing to 1.0 mg/kg/day titrated to keep the white blood cell count above 4000 cells/mm³. Cyclophosphamide is much more potent than azathioprine and is a more effective anti–B-cell therapy; therefore, azathioprine should be discontinued when cyclophosphamide is used. Finally, high-dose steroids (1 g/day) should be given for a minimum of 3 days. The prognosis of hyperacute rejection is extremely poor and mechanical assistance is often required. The most definitive form of therapy in extreme cases is use of a total artificial heart to remove the source of offending antigens.

INITIAL MANAGEMENT IN THE ICU

Inotropic Support

Most patients require inotropic support for the first 12 to 24 hours after transplantation to help the heart recover from cold preservation. Each program has a favorite regimen that may include a beta-agonist such as isoproterenol, which not only enhances contractility but also helps dilate the pulmonary vascular bed through β₂-agonist properties, as well as being a good positive chronotropic agent. Dosages of 0.01 µg/kg/minute are often started in the operating room and titrated up as needed. Alternatively, dobutamine may be used as a beta-agonist inotrope at dosages of 4 to 8 µg/kg/minute. There is no indication to use isoproterenol and dobutamine simultaneously because their mechanisms of action are identical and their combined use, or use of dosages over 10 µg/kg/minute or 0.1 mg of isoproterenol, hastens the development of down-regulation of beta-receptors and unresponsiveness to these beta-agonists. Another commonly used inotrope is the endogenous catecholamine dopamine, although at doses higher than at 4 to 5 µg/kg/min, a vasodilating agent such as sodium nitroprusside often is required in addition to offset peripheral vasoconstriction while the drug

effectively changes from a β₁-inotrope and low-grade β₂-vasodilator to a vasoconstrictor using both dopaminergic and alpha-receptors. An alternative form of inotropic support that has been shown to be effective both before and after transplantation is the phosphodiesterase inhibitor milrinone.[9] This drug is not only a potent inotrope by virtue of a unique mechanism of inhibition of the phosphodiesterase enzyme, which results in an increase in intracellular cyclic AMP and secondary mobilization of calcium for availability to contractile proteins, but it is also a powerful vasodilator that may have particular benefit in transplant patients with pulmonary hypertension. Milrinone has a fairly prolonged half-life (6 to 10 hours), and the dosage should be started as low as 0.1 µg/kg/minute and titrated up to a maximum of 0.8 to 1.0 µg/kg/minute (with or without a loading dose of approximately 0.5 mg/kg given over 30 minutes). This drug works well in combination with isoproterenol or dobutamine because they have completely different mechanisms of action.

Primary Graft Dysfunction

Most of the early problems after heart transplantation can be anticipated, especially primary graft dysfunction. The risk of this problem is increased by several factors, including the length of cold ischemia time (time between cross-clamping the donor aorta at the time of excising the donor heart until the aortic cross-clamp is removed from the recipient once the heart has been sewn in place). Cold ischemia time beyond 4 hours usually results in increasing systolic and diastolic dysfunction from passive accumulation of preservation fluid and edema in the myocardium. Conversely, problems with infusion of cold cardioplegia or inadequately venting the donor heart during excision may cause warm ischemic injury. Other adverse risk factors include increased donor age (older than 40 years of age), sustained periods of hypotension, or use of high doses of pressor agents to maintain blood pressure in the donor, which may predispose to catechol-induced subendocardial ischemic injury. This injury may be totally unsuspected because many patients on high dosages of pressors (over 15 µg/kg/minute of dopamine or its equivalent) exhibit no problems, whereas patients on lower dosages, especially with episodes of CPR or hypotension, may have extensive subendocardial injury, often with no clear electrocardiographic changes. The decision to use a heart from a potential donor is based on a variety of factors, including the medical status of the potential recipient, with more liberal criteria used for critically ill patients. An echocardiogram has become the minimum to assess the cardiac function of potential donors; however, this study often may be misread and the degree of hypokinesis underestimated or overestimated in patients who may be hemodynamically unstable but whose primary problems are not cardiac in origin, such as hypoxemia or acidosis, and does not impact on the long-term function of the potential donor heart. Mild and even moderate hypokinesis may resolve completely after transplantation, but focal changes are more likely to persist than global hypokinesis. Recently, supplementation of donor hearts with active triiodothyronine has helped to improve donor heart dysfunction.[16]

The clinical presentation of primary graft dysfunction is frequently difficult to separate from hyperacute rejection because the patients often have a high pacing threshold, elevated cardiac filling pressures (usually with near equalization of pressures), and are inotrope- and often pressor-dependent from the initial reperfusion of the graft. On occasion, an intraaortic balloon pump is of benefit to maximize coronary perfusion and decrease requirement for pressors and inotropes. If the heart looks clearly edematous at the time of transplantation and the cold ischemia time has been over 4 hours, it may be that warming and reperfusion for 24 hours will result in substantial improvement. However, if ischemic time was not prolonged and a low output state persists for more than 4 to 6 hours despite pressors, inotropes, and an intraaortic balloon pump, more definitive mechanical circulatory assistance may be required. The outcome with mechanical support in the early transplant period is disappointing; retransplantation should be considered early in these patients, especially if numerous risk factors are present in the donor.

Right Ventricular Failure

One of the leading causes of death in the first 5 days after heart transplantation is right ventricular failure in the donor heart caused by chronic, relatively fixed preexisting pulmonary hypertension in the recipient.[5] Preoperative hemodynamic assessment during transplant evaluation should identify patients who are at risk of developing right ventricular failure secondary to pulmonary hypertension (see earlier). The hemodynamics in these patients after transplantation generally show a mild to extremely elevated mean RA pressure (range, 12 to 20 mm Hg) and pulmonary artery systolic pressure (range, 40 to 70 mm Hg). The PAOP may be mildly elevated, primarily from bowing of the intraventricular septum into the left ventricle (pressure overload) causing an upward shift of the pressure volume curve, which can be mistaken for biventricular failure.

The pulmonary artery pressure may increase in the first 2 to 8 hours after transplantation while the pulmonary vascular bed is exposed to a high–normal cardiac output. If there is little vasoreactivity in the pulmonary resistance bed, pressure becomes flow dependent. A RA pressure above 15 mm Hg in the early posttransplant period is an ominous sign and should be managed with use of vasodilating and inotropic drugs and minimum use of vasopressor agents, using a mean arterial pressure over 65 mm Hg and urine output as the limiting variables. The only important parameter to follow in patients with pulmonary hypertension and right ventricular failure is the mean RA pressure, because it is the best indication of the compensation of the right ventricle. One pitfall in managing these patients is to see the pulmonary artery systolic and mean pressure decrease over the first 12 to 24 hours and to assume that the problem has resolved. If the RA pressure continues to increase while the pulmonary artery pressure decreases, this simply reflects a decrease in flow out of the right ventricle and across the pulmonary vascular bed resulting in lower pulmonary artery pressure, in fact reflecting a worsening condition. RA pressures above 20 mm

Hg are often associated with a significant decline in renal function, and pressures this high that persist longer than 24 hours after transplantation require aggressive drug therapy and, on occasion, mechanical support of the right ventricle for a period of days until the right ventricle can compensate. Vasodilators such as IV prostaglandin are often helpful in this setting.[17] Several centers have reported using direct infusions of prostaglandin through the right atrial or pulmonary artery ports of the right heart catheter combined with the use of a pressor agent through a left atrial infusion line to maximize the delivery of the dilators to the lung and pressors in the systemic circulation, thus offsetting the blood pressure drop mediated by the vasodilators. Patients who require aggressive therapy for right heart failure often remain dependent on these agents for a period of 1 to 3 weeks after transplantation, before the right ventricle fully accommodates to the increased afterload and the normalization of left atrial pressure allows further decline in pulmonary artery resistance. The potential for this problem may be worsened by substantial size mismatch[18] (i.e., using a donor more than 20% to 25% smaller than the recipient) or by gender mismatch, such as a heart from female donor into a male recipient for any given size mismatch.

Temporary Pacing

Approximately 50% to 80% of patients require temporary pacing in the immediate posttransplant period. This is caused by infusion of cardioplegia, prolonged cold preservation, and surgical manipulation of the sinoatrial or atrioventricular node and the intraatrial septum. It is important to identify the pacing "threshold," that is, the minimum amount of milliamperage required to pace the heart. It is not advisable to turn the milliamperage to its maximum (20 mA) while pacing the heart because there may be little warning if the wire loses capture. It is preferable to stay 1 or 2 mA above the threshold, thereby providing a safety margin for a substantial increase in milliamperage should pacing capture become a problem. Patients are often treated with chronotropic agents such as isoproterenol to enhance heart rate response after transplantation, but alternatively, transplanted hearts often can be paced as high as 110 mA per minute without adverse consequences for several days. Denervation, which is created at surgery, makes the transplanted heart dependent on circulating catecholamines for rate response. Patients who spend prolonged periods of time in bed before being able to ambulate after transplantation may remain pacer dependent until they can generate adequate circulating catecholamines to stimulate heart rate. A high-degree heart block with no functional escape mechanism for greater than 4 seconds that persists beyond 3 to 4 days after transplantation may, however, be an indication for permanent pacing. Patients who have been receiving amiodarone before transplantation often have bradycardia, heart block, or both in the early posttransplant period, with a secondary peak of slowing at days 8 to 10 days. A more conservative, watchful approach is indicated in patients who have been on amiodarone before transplantation with regard to permanent pacing, because this is likely to resolve.

Nephrotoxicity

Cyclosporine's mechanism of actions at the cellular level is to inhibit cytokine production by interfering with messenger RNA synthesis.[2] In the kidney, cyclosporine also inhibits the production of the prostacycline (dilator) series of prostaglandins and actually enhances the production of the thromboxane (vasoconstrictor) series; it also increases the synthesis of the vasoconstrictor endothelin, with a net result being vasoconstriction of the afferent arteriole. This glomerular ischemia results in decreased renal function, which may be acute or chronic[19] and is often poorly responsive to, and in fact worsened by, high-dose diuretics. Decreased renal function may warrant significant tapering or discontinuation of cyclosporine for 12 to 24 hours, especially if the levels of cyclosporine are elevated. Use of renal-dosage dopamine (1 µg/kg/minute) may maximize renal blood flow. One potential specific antidote is use of the synthetic vasodilator prostaglandin, misoprostol (in doses of 500 mg twice daily), which may directly offset the effect of cyclosporine at the renal afferent arteriole.[20] Significant, persisting renal dysfunction may require cessation of cyclosporine for a period of days and may warrant use of OKT3 to maintain adequate immunosuppression until cyclosporine can be safely reintroduced.

Hypertension

Hypertension in the immediate posttransplant period may be secondary to volume overload, preexisting renal dysfunction, or the use of cyclosporine. Cyclosporine has been documented to cause hypertension in nontransplant recipients who receive it for treatment of autoimmune disease. One unique feature of hypertension in cardiac transplant patients on cyclosporine is that the blood pressure remains elevated at night. This is caused by sustained increase in systemic vascular resistance (SVR) without the usual nocturnal decrease in cardiac output at night.[21] Whereas a variety of agents have been used to treat this form of hypertension, direct-acting vasodilators such as hydralazine are notoriously ineffective. In contrast, the vasoconstriction mediated at the peripheral vascular level by cyclosporine is often calcium dependent, and the optimal treatment of cyclosporine-associated hypertension is a calcium channel blocker. Use of sublingual or high doses of agents such as nifedipine often result in a precipitous fall in blood pressure, and long-acting (XL) preparations are advised. Alternatively, angiotensin converting enzyme inhibitors have been effective in some patients, although cyclosporine does not seem to effect the renin angiotensin system.

Acute Rejection

Acute cell-mediated (cellular) rejection may occur at any time after transplantation, but 90% of all rejections occur within the first 3 months, and as much as 40% to 45% of all rejection occurs within the first 4 weeks. Data from a registry of over 2000 patients[22] show that several factors are associated with increased risk of rejection: female recipients, female donor (regardless of recipient gender), positive preoperative preformed antibody titer, positive donor-specific crossmatch, cytomegalovirus (CMV) infection, and impaired hepatic or renal function that limits use of standard doses of immunosuppression. Patients usually undergo endocardial biopsy routinely within day 5 to 10 days after transplantation, and then weekly thereafter for 4 weeks. These are predetermined, "surveillance" biopsies, that is, not waiting for a patient to exhibit signs of cardiac dysfunction. Five to seven pieces of endomyocardium are obtained through percutaneous transvenous insertion of a bioptome into the right ventricle. Biopsy specimens are graded 1A, 1B, 2, 3A, and 3B based on the degree of the lymphocytic infiltration and myocardial necrosis.[23] Most centers do not treat grades 1A and 1B, but a grade 2 (focal moderate rejection), particularly early in the posttransplantation period, may warrant intensification of immunosuppression or even low to moderate doses of bolus steroids. Grade 3A rejection indicates diffuse moderate rejection with myocyte damage and is generally treated with 10 to 15 mg/kg of IV methylprednisolone daily for 3 days. If a patient develops hemodynamic compromise in association with proven rejection or if rejection is refractory to steroid therapy, the use of lymphocyte antibody "rescue" therapy is warranted,[24] in particular, the use of OKT3 at a dosage of 5 mg/day IV push over 30 seconds for 7 days. Patients who have evidence of vascular rejection by immunoglobulin deposition on the endothelium of coronary arteries on heart biopsy vessels may benefit from plasmapheresis[18] and the substitution of cyclophosphamide for azathioprine.

Infection

Infection may occur in the early postoperative period.[25] Every attempt should be made to obtain directed cultures of fluid and tissue if fever develops, and the use of computed tomography scans is often helpful to detect the source of infection and guide antimicrobial therapy. The standard antibiotic prophylaxis that is employed in each institution for routine open heart surgery should be the regimen used for heart transplantation, and no prolonged antibiotic exposure should be given to minimize superinfection. Patients who are in the hospital and have IV hemodynamic monitoring catheters or a mechanical assist device in place at the time they are brought to the operating room for transplantation often merit enhanced antibiotic coverage until culture results can be proved to be negative and preexisting lines can be changed or withdrawn entirely. This may include the use of vancomycin and a third-generation cephalosporin for broad coverage for 2 to 3 days. Recognize that most infections within the first 2 weeks after transplantation are nosocomial and are directly related to indwelling catheters. Hemodynamic monitoring is rarely necessary after 24 hours, because drips can be slowly tapered to off by clinical assessment and early mobilization greatly reduces the risk of infection. IV catheters should not be left in place longer than 4 days before they are changed (new location), and every attempt should be made to withdraw urinary or intravascular catheters as early as possible. One exception is chronic indwelling venous access catheters such as the Hickman catheter, which may be kept in place for several weeks after transplantation without increased risk of infection if they are tunnelled subcutaneously and if good attention to sterile technique is used.

In addition to nosocomial infections, there are a variety of early infections for which prophylaxis is commonly employed. Common antimicrobial prophylaxis regimens for treating their respective infections include the following: use of either nystatin or clotrimazole (1 tablet twice daily) for a period of 1 month for *Candida* infection; acyclovir (800 to 1200 mg every day) for 1 month for herpes simplex infection; and 400 mg of sulfamethoxazole with 80 mg of trimethoprim (one oral Septra) three times per week for *Pneumocystis* pneumonia prophylaxis. CMV is a morbid infection in heart and lung transplant recipients.[26] Current strategies include the use of ganciclovir in a dose of (5 mg/kg twice daily, adjusted for renal function) for 14 days, followed by a 1- to 3-month course of high-dose (3200 mg/day) oral acyclovir for anyone who receives a CMV-positive donor. There are over 50 strains of CMV, and evidence of a positive antibody titer against CMV in the recipient before transplantation does not preclude either reactivation of a previous strain or infection with a potentially new strain of CMV from the donor. Patients who are CMV antibody negative who receive a CMV-positive donor are at the highest risk (approximately 40%) of developing active CMV infection in the first 4 weeks after transplantation. CMV infection typically presents with fever, malaise, abdominal cramping, diarrhea, and neutropenia. Suspicion should prompt an IgM antibody titer for CMV infection and blood and urine culture. Toxoplasmosis is a relatively uncommon infection in the United States, and many programs do not even screen the donor or recipient for *Toxoplasma*. Routine use of Septra prophylaxis also may cover *Toxoplasma*, but fever or development of mental status changes within the first 2 to 4 weeks after transplantation should raise the suspicion of *Toxoplasma* infection and prompt culture of the cerebral spinal fluid and IgM titer for *Toxoplasma* to be obtained. Specific therapy includes pyrimethamine.

ESSENTIAL DIAGNOSTIC TESTS AND PROCEDURES

The *electrocardiogram* after transplantation often shows right bundle branch block. In addition, there may be native P waves evident (in addition to donor P waves) in the first 7 to 10 days.

The *echocardiogram* may reveal biatrial enlargement from retention of the posterior half of the native atria plus entire donor atrium. Paradoxic septal motion is often evident. Pericardial effusion may be seen, but is not typically hemodynamically significant.

Hemodynamics may show a restrictive pattern (RA pressure equals pulmonary artery diastolic [PAD] equals PAOP) for up to 8 weeks after transplantation, or RA pressure above PAOP in patients with right ventricular failure secondary to pulmonary hypertension.

STRESS POINTS

1. Many problems in the early posttransplant period can be anticipated by knowledge of several factors in the donor and recipient. It is valuable to know the age, sex, size (height and weight), level of predonation inotropic or pressor support, mechanism of brain injury, periods of hypotension, electrocardiogram and echocardiogram results, plus any problems with warm ischemia and length of cold ischemia.

2. Immediate and early function of the allografted heart may be anticipated by adverse factors in the donor, which include prolonged preservation, advanced age, known coronary disease (which impedes the delivery of cardioplegia), warm ischemia time, high pressor requirement, or significant size disparity.

3. Recipient factors to know include age, height and weight, previous sternotomy, warfarin therapy, preoperative blood urea nitrogen and creatinine, preoperative panel reactive antibody screen, results of donor-specific crossmatch, presence of pulmonary hypertension preoperatively, and best drugs found to reduce pulmonary artery pressure and use of amiodarone.

4. Recipient factors that increase risk of early survival include positive panel reactive antibodies before transplantation, a positive donor specific crossmatch, documented pulmonary hypertension in the recipient before transplantation, significant renal or hepatic dysfunction that may limit the use of adequate doses of immunosuppressive drugs or that is made worse with their use, and infection at the time of transplant.

5. Inotropic drugs are used in most patients early after transplantation to help the heart recover from cold preservation.

6. Temporary pacing is required in up to 80% to 90% of patients for up to 5 days after transplantation and potentially longer in patients on amiodarone before transplantation.

7. Cyclosporine can be given initially (pretransplantation) by either oral or continuous IV infusion. Common early side effects include nephrotoxicity, hypertension, and seizures.

REFERENCES ■

1. Hosenpud JD, Novick RJ, Breen TJ: The Registry of the International Society for Heart and Lung Transplantation: Eleventh Official Report—1994. *J Heart Lung Transplant* 1994;13:561
2. Kahan BD: Drug therapy: cyclosporine. *N Engl J Med* 1989; 321:1725
3. Miller LW: Candidate selection for heart transplantation. *Transplant Proc* 1995;27:1989
4. O'Connell JB, Bourge RC, Costanzo-Nordin MR, et al: Cardiac transplantation: recipient selection, donor procurement, and medical follow-up. *Circulation* 1992;86:1061
5. Greenberg A, Thompson ME, Griffith BJ, et al: Cyclosporine nephrotoxicity in cardiac allograft patients: a 7-year follow-up. *Transplantation* 1990;50:589
6. Stevenson LW, Miller LW: Cardiac transplantation as therapy for heart failure. *Curr Probl Cardiol* 1991;16:219
7. Costard-Jackle A, Fowler MB: Influence of preoperative pulmonary artery pressure on mortality after heart transplantation: testing of potential reversibility of pulmonary hypertension

with nitroprusside is useful in defining a high risk group. *J Am Coll Cardiol* 1992;19:48

8. Yeogh TK, Frist WH, Lagerstrom C, et al: Relationship of cardiac allograft size and pulmonary vascular resistance to long-term cardiopulmonary function. *J Heart Lung Transplant* 1992;11:1168

9. Monrad ES, Baim DS, Smith HS, et al: Milrinone, dobutamine, and nitroprusside: comparative effects on hemodynamics and myocardial energetics in patients with severe congestive heart failure. *Circulation* 1986;73(Suppl 3):168

10. Miller LW: Long-term complications of cardiac transplantation. *Prog Cardiovasc Dis* 1991;33:229

11. Wong JT, Eylath AA, Ghobrial I, et al: The mechanism of anti-CD3 monoclonal antibodies: mediation of cytolysis by inter–T-cell bridging. *Transplantation* 1990;50:683

12. Chatenoud L, Legendre C, Ferran C, et al: Corticosteroid inhibition of the OKT3-induced cytokine-related syndrome: dosage and kinetics prerequisites. *Transplantation* 1991;51:334

13. Renlund DG, O'Connell JB, Bristow MR: Early rejection prophylaxis in heart transplantation: is cytolytic therapy necessary? *J Heart Transplant* 1989;8:191

14. Lavee J, Kormos RL, Duquesnoy R, et al: Influence of panel-reactive antibody and lymphocytoxic crossmatch on survival after heart transplantation. *J Heart Lung Transplant* 1991;10:921

15. Ratkovec RM, Hammond EH, O'Connell JB, et al: Outcome of cardiac transplant recipients with a positive donor-specific crossmatch: preliminary results with plasmapheresis. *Transplantation* 1992;54:651

16. Jeevanandum V, Todd B, Regillo T, et al: Reversal of donor myocardial dysfunction by triiodothyronine replacement therapy. *J Heart Lung Transplant* 1994;13:681

17. Pascual JM, Fiorelli AI, Bellotti GM, et al: Prostacyclin in the management of pulmonary hypertension after heart transplantation. *J Heart Transplant* 1990;9:644

18. Yeogh TK, Frist WH, Lagerstrom C, et al: Relationship of cardiac allograft size and pulmonary vascular resistance to long-term outcome. *J Heart Lung Transplant* 1992;11:1168

19. Bourge RC, Naftel DC, Costanzo-Nordin MR, et al: Pretransplantation risk factors for death after heart transplantation: a multiinstitutional study. *J Heart Lung Transplant* 1993;12:549

20. Paller MS: Effects of the prostaglandin E1 analog misoprostol on cyclosporine nephrotoxicity. *Transplantation* 1988;45:1126

21. Reeves RA, Shapiro AP, Thompson ME, et al: Loss of nocturnal decline in blood pressure after cardiac transplantation. *Circulation* 1986;73:401

22. Kobashigawa JA, Kirklin JK, Naftel DC: Pretransplantation risk factors for acute rejection after heart transplantation: a multiinstitutional study. *J Heart Lung Transplant* 1993;12:355

23. Billingham ME, Cary NR, Hammond E, et al: A working formulation for the standardization of nomenclature in the diagnosis of heart and lung rejection: heart rejection study group. *J Heart Lung Transplant* 1990;9:587

24. Gilbert EM, Dewitt CW, Eiswirth CC, et al: Treatment of refractory cardiac allograft rejection with OKT3 monoclonal antibody. *Am J Med* 1987;82:202

25. Bourge RC, Kirklin JK, Brozena SC, et al: Infection after heart transplantation: a multiinstitutional study. *J Heart Lung Transplant* 1994;13:381

26. Naftel DC, Levine TB, Bourge RC, et al: Cytomegalovirus after heart transplantation: risk factors for infection and death. A multiinstitutional study. *J Heart Lung Transplant* 1994;13:394

Critical Care, Third Edition, edited by Joseph M. Civetta,
Robert W. Taylor, and Robert R. Kirby.
Lippincott-Raven Publishers, Philadelphia, PA © 1997.

CHAPTER 89

■

Orthotopic Liver Transplantation

Mathew E. Brunson
Richard J. Howard

IMMEDIATE CONCERNS ■

MAJOR PROBLEMS

Orthotopic liver transplantation (OLTx) is the preferred treatment for several liver diseases. Management of the liver transplant recipient shares similarities with that of the cirrhotic patient undergoing a major laparotomy[1] in that special attention must be directed to electrolytes, infections, and neurologic status. The patient must not be allowed to become hyponatremic while waiting for OLTx. Because of the high sodium concentration in fresh frozen plasma (FFP) and the rapid rate of fluid infusions during the liver transplant operation, metered increases in serum sodium concentration are impossible; thus, the recipient going into OLTx with a serum sodium less than 125 mMol/dL conceivably is at risk for later pontine myelinolysis from rapid normalization of the serum sodium.[2]

Also, in anticipation of intraoperative events, the serum potassium should be maintained in the low-normal range because rapid flux of potassium at reperfusion of the graft liver can lead to cardiac arrest. In the preoperative patient with renal compromise, potassium *removal* by dialysis or enteral ion-exchange resins is preferred to shifting the potassium concentration with glucose–insulin infusions, which, nevertheless, maintain the total body potassium excess.

Patients with ascites can develop spontaneous bacterial peritonitis and are often maintained on prophylactic antibiotics such as norfloxacin. Bed rest, tense ascites, and muscle wasting contribute to reduced functional residual capacity, decreased clearance of secretions, and potential develop-

ment of pneumonia. Such infections may prevent OLTx. Preoperative prophylactic antibiotic use may select out fungal organisms and resistant bacteria in gut flora. Selective gut decontamination has been advocated to address this issue,[3] but the efficacy of bowel decontamination is uncertain. Because fungal infections significantly increase after gastrointestinal (GI) tract entry during OLTx, prophylaxis with preoperative enteral antifungal agents (nystatin [Mycostatin] or clotrimazole) has the most validity.

STRESS POINTS

1. Hepatic encephalopathy poses dangers of aspiration and cerebral edema. Patients entering stage III coma should be tracheally intubated to protect their airways, to avoid emergency intubation at a later time when coagulopathy may be worse, and to allow hyperventilation, if needed, to control cerebral edema.
2. Use of intracranial pressure monitoring for hepatic coma in fulminant hepatic failure is associated with the risk of intracranial bleeding[4]; however, when used, it demonstrates the extreme lability of intracranial pressure and allows early intervention.
3. Fever, agitation, and arterial hypotension should be controlled to avoid CNS injury.[5] Irreversible intracranial hypertension indicates that the patient cannot be improved by OLTx and should not undergo transplantation.
4. After OLTx, liver functions usually steadily improve to normal; most patients achieve "good" liver function quickly. The injuries from procurement, storage, and

1341

reperfusion are manifested predominantly as an elevation of transaminases.

5. If the new liver graft's physiologic makeup is sufficiently intact to handle basic synthesis and clearance of metabolic wastes, ICU management mainly consists of replacing ongoing fluid losses and avoiding injury to the graft liver during the period of recovery.

6. A small subset of patients have dramatically impaired early graft function. Perhaps from donor instability, suboptimal preservation, or hemodynamic instability after reperfusion, a greater degree of liver injury exists in these patients. They have high transaminase values that increase to the 2000- to 5000-IU/dL range over 24 to 72 hours.

7. Deciding if a particular liver injury is an irreparable, primary nonfunction that can be survived only by retransplantation is critical. Because of the scarcity of organ donors, the decision to "relist" the patient for urgent retransplantation must be made as early as possible.[6]

8. Whenever liver function is unstable, always entertain the possibility of vascular thrombosis or primary nonfunction and move quickly to obtain proof of vessel patency and graft viability.

ESSENTIAL DIAGNOSTIC TESTS AND PROCEDURES

1. The best predictors of graft survival in the initial 24 to 48 hours are bile output, reversal of metabolic acidosis (if present), stabilization of coagulation, and a stable or rising systemic vascular resistance.

2. Immediately after ICU admission, assess prothrombin time (PT), partial thromboplastin time (PTT), platelets, complete blood count (CBC), and D-dimers or fibrin degradation (split) products.

3. Assess hourly fluid requirements to determine plasma losses into the peritoneal cavity and the possibility of continuing bleeding. "Third-space" losses are significant.

4. Hypertension is common, reflecting pain, cold, mineralocorticoid therapy, and other factors. Vasoconstriction also results from cyclosporin A (CsA, Sandimmune).

5. Follow urine output closely to assess possible renal CsA toxicity and preexisting renal dysfunction.

INITIAL THERAPY

1. Calculation of fluid administration requirements must take into account crystalloids, medication carrier fluids, and parenteral nutrition. Fluid boluses frequently are necessary for the first 24 to 36 hours.

2. Low-dose dopamine may be added if signs of low perfusion persist despite fluid infusion.

3. An immunosuppressive state achieved with CsA and FK506 (tacrolimus, Prograf) is essential to graft survival.

4. Observe the patient closely for seizure activity that can be related to cremophor toxicity. If present, immediately stop the CsA infusion. Also consider the possibility of an intracranial hemorrhage, obtain appropriate studies, and treat accordingly.

5. Hypoxemia may be present for several days. No specific therapy is indicated. Maintain oxygenation by standard techniques.

EARLY GRAFT FUNCTION AND PRIMARY NONFUNCTION ■

ASSESSMENT

Because lactate dehydrogenase (LDH), aspartate aminotransferase (AST, SGOT) and alanine aminotransferase (ALT, SGPT) increase with hepatocellular injury, the patient with values greater than about 2000 IU/dL clearly has an allograft that has sustained severe injury. Yet, the important question is the hepatic reserve, because most livers have a remarkable capacity for regeneration, provided there is an adequate residual of functioning tissue. In the first 24 to 48 hours, the best predictors of graft survival are (1) the quality and quantity of bile output, (2) the ability to reverse the metabolic acidosis that has developed during the transplant procedure, (3) the ability to stabilize coagulation parameters with decreasing amounts of platelet and FFP infusion, and (4) a stable or rising systemic vascular resistance, usually with recovery of renal function.[7]

If the patient has a T tube, bile output is directly examined. Excellent graft function produces nearly a liter per day of dark, golden bile. The quantity decreases with less hepatic reserve, but thin, watery bile causes the greatest concern for graft viability.

At the end of the OLTx procedure, the patient should have a citrate load from the administered blood products, plus some degree of lactic acidosis. A well-functioning graft reverses the metabolic acidosis and causes progression to alkalosis, sometimes requiring hydrochloric acid infusion (0.1 N HCl solution). Progressive acidosis is ominous and signals either severe graft dysfunction or grossly impaired cardiac output.

Similarly, intraoperative fibrinolysis, consumption of clotting factors at the extensive operative sites, hypersplenism, and slow graft function usually prevent the patient from having normal clotting study results; however, a working graft clears fibrin split products and reverses fibrinolysis such that the PT should be easily maintained below 20 seconds with minimal FFP infusions. Injured microvasculature consumes platelets, and a persistently dropping platelet count suggests significant graft injury. PGE_1-infusions have been used to prevent further ischemic injury in this setting.[8,9] A clinical picture of ongoing fibrinolysis, PT greater than 25 seconds, and inability to maintain the platelet count greater than 30,000/mm^3 suggest the need for retransplantation.

COAGULATION ABNORMALITIES ■

ASSESSMENT

Initial assessment is outlined in Figure 89-1. When the patient arrives from the operating room, ask about the magnitude of current fluid needs. Include hourly fluid needs with other guidelines to correct the levels of clotting factors. If good perfusion is maintained with little fluid therapy, do not empirically give FFP, platelets, or cryoprecipitate. However, if fluid needs are large, rapid losses of plasma into the peritoneal cavity may be occurring. Both crystalloid and colloid components must be replaced. For optimal graft perfusion, it is better to have the OLTx recipient fully euvolemic, mildly anemic, and hypocoagulable; however, after bleeding starts, the capacity of the newly grafted liver to reverse fibrinolysis may be exceeded. In this setting, more aggressive replacement of blood products is needed.

Next determine whether ongoing blood loss is present. Grossly abnormal clotting studies and diffuse "oozing" must have three questions addressed repeatedly until they are stabilized: (1) What clotting factors are deficient and need to be replaced? (2) Should the patient return to the operating room for hemostasis? (3) Do the clotting problems represent primary nonfunction of the graft?

Immediately send blood specimens for determination of PT, PTT, platelets, CBC, D-dimers or fibrin split products, arterial blood gas values, and pH. Additional specimens must be sent to the blood bank as needed. Maintain an excess of available packed red blood cells, FFP and platelets, usually 10 units of each. Work quickly and aggressively to correct clotting abnormalities until fluid requirements are less than 200 mL/hour or until the PT is less than 20 seconds and the platelet count is greater than 50,000/mm³.

TREATMENT

The opposite extreme of coagulation status is also undesirable. Overcorrection of clotting defect risks vascular thrombosis of the graft and complicates interpretation of clotting studies as a measure of graft function. The goal is a state of mildly abnormal clotting studies rather than complete correction to normal, thus minimizing the risk of vascular thromboses. FFP should be used for active bleeding or when the PT is greater than 20 seconds. Cryoprecipitate is used only to replace fibrinogen deficits. Platelets are not given except for active bleeding or when the platelet count is below 10,000 to 20,000/mm³. Although an obvious risk of bleeding exists when these values are grossly abnormal, there is good evidence that during recovery the patient becomes *hyper*coagulable and is at heightened risk of vascular thrombosis, usually around 7 to 10 days postoperatively.[10]

The patient also needs FFP if a high loss of fluid occurs from peritoneal drains and protein loss exceeds the new liver's synthetic capacity. If the loss is intermediate, 5% albumin solutions are a less-expensive choice. The colloid losses in OLTx always demand some protein replacement in additional to crystalloids.

HEMODYNAMIC FUNCTION AND FLUID THERAPY ■

Portal hypertension is associated with a loss of peripheral and pulmonary vascular tone. A hyperdynamic circulatory state associated with significant microvascular shunting results and persists after OLTx. Because of considerable individual variation, preoperative and intraoperative measures of systemic and pulmonary vascular resistance, arteriovenous oxygen difference, and pulmonary shunt are important "baselines" in interpreting postoperative hemodynamics.

The OLTx recipient has large volumes of third-space sequestration and ongoing protein-rich fluid loss from abdominal drains. Replace these protein-rich fluid losses with 5% albumin in lactated Ringer's solution, Plasmalyte, or another balance salt solution. Full protein replacement is not needed in patients receiving large volumes of FFP or cryoprecipitate (see Fig. 89-1).

Maintenance crystalloid fluids plus intravenous nutrition and carrier fluids for medications all must be considered in determining fluid therapy. Because of the high sodium content of FFP and some medications, maintenance fluids are usually 5% dextrose in 0.5 normal or 0.25 normal saline plus glucose potassium, magnesium, and phosphate, as indicated. Two distinct phases of fluid requirements occur. For approximately 24 to 36 hours after OLTx, the patient requires fluids in excess of calculated maintenance needs because of ongoing third-space losses. A dramatic switch to intravascular volume excess and inappropriate fluid retention then follows, which is signaled by rising central venous pressure (CVP) and mean arterial pressure.

For the first 24 to 36 hours, extra fluid boluses are usually required. Give 10 mL/kg of lactated Ringer's solution for hypotension or urine output less than 0.5 mL/kg/hour if CVP is less than 10 cm H₂O (Fig. 89-2). Although 10 cm

COAGULATION PROBLEMS

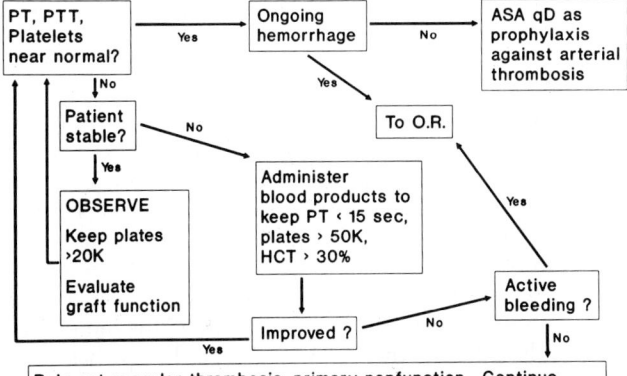

Rule out vascular thrombosis, primary nonfunction. Continue supportive therapy, look for source of necrotic tissue or infection

FIGURE 89-1. Initial assessment and therapy of coagulation problems after orthotopic liver transplantation. PT, prothrombin time; PTT, partial thromboplastin time; ASA, aspirin; qD, every day; O.R., operating room.

FLUID THERAPY
With Consideration of Coagulation Status

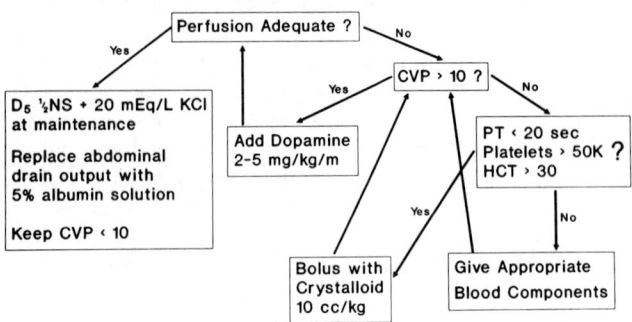

FIGURE 89-2. Early assessment of fluid and electrolyte changes after orthotopic liver transplantation.

H_2O is an arbitrary parameter that should be modified for the individual patient, do not allow excessive increases in CVP and thus hepatic venous pressure. Hepatic venous congestion distends the liver and impairs graft blood flow. In the clinical setting of inadequate perfusion (low urine output, cool extremities, decreased mean arterial pressure), increasing cardiac preload should be limited to the point at which hepatic venous return is impeded. Low-dose dopamine should be added next for its cardiac inotropic effect and visceral flow preservation. Because graft perfusion is critical, it is better to err on the side of liberal fluid administration and adding dopamine early rather than risking hypotension. During this period, the patient is usually maintained on mechanical ventilatory support so oxygenation is rarely compromised.

As third-space losses decrease over 24 to 36 hours, the patient suddenly begins retaining fluid. It is not uncommon to treat a low urine output with a fluid bolus in the morning and yet that evening treat the same problem with diuretics. At this point, be sure to avoid intravascular volume overload, which may require continued mechanical ventilation. Critical clues are CVP, blood pressure, and peripheral perfusion. When CVP is greater than 10 cm H_2O, and hands and feet are warm, give furosemide, 0.5 to 1 mg/kg, intravenously every 6 hours as needed to maintain a brisk diuresis. Restrict total fluids to 1000 to 1500 mL/m². Fluid restriction is important to avoid increasing right pleural effusions, a high CVP, and skin breakdown from peripheral edema. It is usually necessary to concentrate medications and incompletely replace drain losses to maintain a net negative balance, particularly in children.

IMMUNOSUPPRESSION ■

CYCLOSPORIN A AND FK506

The cornerstone of transplant immunosuppression is the selective modulation of cytokine secretion—especially inhibition of interleukin-2 secretion—by T cells. CsA and FK506 are large, lipophilic, cyclic molecules that bind to intracytoplasmic receptors on T cells and alter their cytokine secre-

tion. The dosage range for FK506 is roughly one hundredth that of CsA, it binds to different cytoplasmic receptors, and it shares little structural similarity to CsA; the therapeutic window for both is nearly the same. Both agents have nearly identical side effects, which become problematic within the range of doses needed for effective immunosuppression. Using whole blood and measuring only the parent compound, trough blood levels of roughly 250 to 350 ng/mL for CsA and 10 to 20 ng/mL for FK506 seem to produce effective immunosuppression for both agents while minimizing their toxicities. These ranges are individualized for each patient based on their tolerance of side effects versus risks of rejection.

Administration

Both drugs can be administered in either intravenous or enteral forms, but neurotoxicity is usually worse with the intravenous forms (perhaps resulting from higher concentrations or the cotoxicities of agents used to carry these lipophilic drugs into solution). Enteral absorption of CsA is dependent on bile flow into the intestines and thus can be affected by alterations in graft function, opening or closing of the T tube, and diet. FK506 also has uncertain enteral bioavailability, but it is mainly dependent on gastric emptying. CsA and FK506 are never used simultaneously because their toxicities are additive.

Renal Effects

As a major side effect, both CsA and FK506 produce dose-related, reversible vasoconstriction of the kidneys' afferent arterioles. This produces a decrease in renal plasma flow of roughly 50% at therapeutic doses, but does not decrease glomerular filtration rate as robustly if autoregulation by efferent arteriolar vasoconstriction can maintain glomerular filtration pressure. Nonetheless, patients on CsA or FK506 have compromised renal function, even when their serum creatinine is normal. They are especially susceptible to renal injury from hypovolemia or nephrotoxic drugs. Nonsteroidal antiinflammatory drugs disrupt compensatory renal autoregulation and cannot be used in patients taking CsA or FK506.

POLY- AND MONOCLONAL ANTIBODIES

With pretransplant renal insufficiency or other settings of special concern about the nephrotoxicity of these agents, induction therapy with antibodies directed against T cells is used. Polyclonal preparations such as ALG are giving way to molecularly engineered monoclonal murine antibodies such as OKT3. If adequate OKT3 is administered to eliminate lymphocyte function, rejection is essentially impossible. Patients are not maintained on such drugs for more than 10 to 14 days, but by then CsA or FK506 therapy has been gradually introduced as renal function is returning. Agents such as OKT3 are traditionally used for severe rejection episodes and associated with a "first-dose" syndrome caused by release of cytokines from activated T cells. Fever, arthralgia, myalgia, headache, hypotension, and tachypnea characterize the first-dose syndrome, but are less common during induction therapy because there has been no opportunity for T-cell activation by the graft, and the patient is protected from some of the manifestations by high-dose steroids, intubation, and analgesia. When OKT3 is used, low-dose steroids and azathioprine, with or without CsA, are continued to prevent formation of antimurine antibodies, which would ultimately neutralize OKT3 during its immediate use or prevent later reuse for rejection.

STEROIDS AND AZATHIOPRINE

All patients receive some steroids by a dosing schedule that tapers over the first 7 to 10 days to a maintenance level of 10 to 20 mg/day with further reductions over the next several months. Azathioprine is used as a second-line immunosuppressant at several centers, particularly when CsA is the predominant immunosuppressant. The CsA dosage is limited by myelosuppression. Because thrombocytopenia and leukopenia are common both before and after OLTx, its dose must be reduced or held for a white blood count less than 3000/mm^3, which restricts its ability to act as primary immunosuppression.

MYCOPHENOLATE MOFETIL

Mycophenolate mofetil (RS-61443) should be viewed as a replacement for azathioprine with less myelosuppression. This agent is effective because lymphocytes lack a purine salvage pathway and are thus more sensitive to antimetabolites. By inhibiting lymphocyte proliferation, mycophenolate mofetil promises to be an effective adjunct to CsA or FK506 therapy, which might then allow either lower doses of these agents or elimination of steroids and their side effects.

HYPERTENSION ■

Several factors promote hypertension in the postoperative period. Immediately postoperatively, pain and cold are the most potent and easily correctable stimuli. Corticosteroids, given in high doses to prevent allograft rejection, have significant mineralocorticoid sodium-retaining effect. Cyclosporine causes arteriolar vasoconstriction, particularly in the renal vascular bed. Preexisting hypertension may also contribute.

Sodium nitroprusside is the agent of choice for early control of hypertension. Because of early fluid shifts, the patient can be alternately intravascularly hypovolemic or hypervolemic, making this agent's rapid onset and cessation of action useful. Begin with analgesia and sodium nitroprusside. Nifedipine is also useful in the early postoperative period because it is well absorbed by nasogastric tube or oral administration and has rapid onset of action with good efficacy. Its only problem in this form is the sudden, poorly regulated onset of action and early return of hypertension. As soon as the patient can swallow pills intact, it is much better to administer nifedipine without breaking the capsule, providing a smoother effect. Labetalol, 20 mg, administered intravenously over 2 minutes, can be repeated up to 300 mg.

In general, over the next several days, hypertension can be managed by steady diuresis of excess total body fluids and use of nifedipine as needed. As steroid doses decrease and fluid excess resolves, patients who have been hypertensive may no longer need treatment. On the other hand, some patients who previously had no problems with hypertension may need the introduction of nifedipine by the end of the first week.

As it becomes obvious that the individual patient will need long-term maintenance antihypertensive therapy, long-acting calcium channel blocking agents may be more appropriate. Adults who are still hypertensive on 120 mg/day of controlled-release nifedipine (Procardia XL) or isradipine (DynaCirc), 5 mg twice daily, often respond to the addition of α_2-agonists such as captopril.

The only slow-release form of calcium channel blockers that children can swallow causes profound interactions with CsA.[11] Diltiazem is available in slow-release granules that come in a capsule. The capsule can be opened for dose reduction and the spheres dispersed in foods such as applesauce. CsA dose must be markedly reduced as the competitive inhibition becomes manifested. Although we have used this combination in some children with both difficult-to-manage hypertension and rapid CsA metabolism, the patient is clearly at risk of being underdosed with CsA at some point in the remote future when diltiazem is stopped.

OTHER EARLY PROBLEMS ■

SEIZURES

Twitching, myoclonic jerks, and grand mal seizures after OLTx are usually associated with the cremaphor used to solubilize CsA for intravenous administration. Confusion, white matter edema, and cortical blindness may also occur.[12] Patients with low serum cholesterol levels are thought to be most susceptible, but any patient may have seizures precipitated by intravenous CsA. Immediately stop the infusion if seizures occur. Other contributing factors are swings in sodium concentration, hypomagnesemia, contribution to irritability from other medications (e.g., imipenem), and hypoglycemia. Always include intracranial hemorrhage in the differential diagnosis. Pontine demyelinization after OLTx has been associated with rapid changes in serum sodium concentration.[2]

RIGHT PLEURAL EFFUSION

Pulmonary edema from intravascular volume overload and interstitial infiltrates associated with large transfusions of fluid and blood products can be expected in numerous patients. Because of the subdiaphragmatic dissection, a sympathetic right pleural effusion occurs in most patients. Additionally, preoperative atelectasis and postoperative right phrenic nerve paresis[13] contribute to delayed reexpansion of right lower lung fields. Because of the risk of bleeding from intercostal varices, these effusions should *not* be routinely aspirated. With incentive spirometry and gentle diuresis, these effusions slowly resolve over several weeks.

HYPOXEMIA

Some patients have persistent arterial desaturation while they breathe room air despite complete diuresis of excess fluid, normal work of breathing, and normal liver graft function. Usually, the desaturation is worst in the upright position, so-called *orthodeoxia*. This condition is thought to reflect pulmonary arteriolar dysfunction and shunting that developed with end-stage liver failure.[14] There is no specific therapy beyond oxygen supplementation and the exclusion of other contributing problems.

ASSESSING AND OPTIMIZING GRAFT FUNCTION ■

Orderly assessment of graft viability and recovery addresses four groups of liver function, which form a hierarchy of progressively more severe graft dysfunction: (1) bilirubin conjugation and secretion, (2) elimination of metabolic waste and drugs, (3) protein synthesis, and (4) energy metabolism.

BILIRUBIN SECRETION

Bilirubin secretion is the most sensitive test of liver function. Although its concentration can be artificially high from pre-transplant disease or posttransplant hemolysis, a steady fall in serum bilirubin or the flow of normal quality bile from a T tube requires the brisk flow of substrate to the liver, healthy hepatocytes capable of uptake, conjugation, and secretion, and no mechanical obstruction or leak in the biliary tree. Thus, normal-appearing, viscous, and dark yellow-green bile draining from the T tube or normal brown stools strongly suggest good graft function. Low volume, watery bile, or both suggest graft dysfunction from either ischemia and reperfusion or rejection.

Figure 89-3 shows the usual profile of serum bilirubin concentrations in a patient with good early graft function.

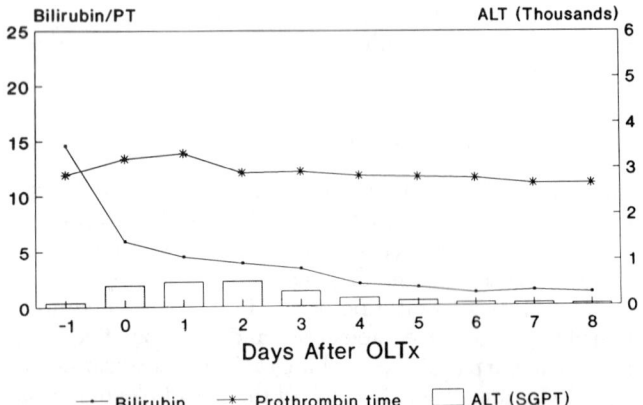

BILIARY ATRESIA

FIGURE 89-3. Usual changes in serum bilirubin, prothrombin time (PT), and alanine aminotransferase (ALT) after orthotopic liver transplantation (OLTx) for biliary atresia.

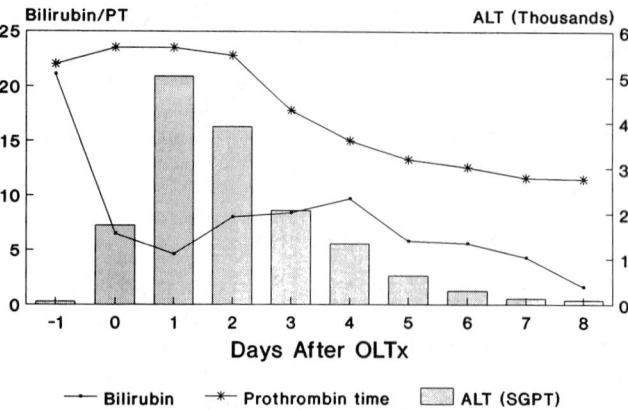

VALPROIC ACID TOXICITY

FIGURE 89-4. Increased ischemic changes indicated by elevated serum bilirubin, prothrombin time (PT), and alanine aminotransferase (ALT) after orthotopic liver transplantation (OLTx) for valproic acid toxicity.

Notice that the immediate posttransplant bilirubin can be especially low because of intraoperative "washout" of the bloodstream. After reequilibration with extravascular bilirubin, the next day's bilirubin is slightly "worse," but falls steadily thereafter. AST and LDH are released by injured hepatocytes; their serum levels rise and fall roughly parallel with bilirubin levels. Figure 89-4 shows the profile of a patient who had a greater degree of ischemic injury to the liver graft but nonetheless recovered steadily.

ELIMINATION OF DRUGS AND METABOLIC WASTE

Elimination of drugs and metabolic waste also show a roughly linear correlation with the degree of graft function. A consumptive coagulopathy from impaired reticuloendothelial removal of fibrinolytic products can cause a prolonged PT and PTT, which confound the determination of clotting factor synthesis. In the absence of necrotic tissue or infection, the graft ultimately corrects the coagulopathy if exogenous clotting factors are given for replacement. One must first assume that bleeding is caused by technical failure at hemostasis. Hoping that ongoing bleeding will stop spontaneously with correction of clotting defects is futile. The patient must be taken back to the operating room to achieve hemostasis while clotting factors are simultaneously corrected.

A severe coagulopathy demands evaluation of graft viability and vessel patency. Coagulopathy from primary nonfunction must be corrected while awaiting retransplantation. In addition to supplying exogenous clotting factors, some success can be anticipated through plasmapheresis. Some patients are desperately ill because of the large volume of necrotic tissue contained in the dead allograft. In such cases, success has sometimes resulted from the grave expediency of removing the graft and leaving the patient anhepatic while awaiting a new donor.

The classic measure of hepatic detoxification is blood ammonia levels, but these add little to the other tests routinely obtained after OLTx. More important is to consider that many drugs may not be normally metabolized either. Compounds removed by biliary excretion may have prolonged half-lives in patients with a picture of centrizonal cholestasis after moderate degrees of ischemia and reperfusion. The P450 system may be less active immediately after transplantation but recovers over 1 to 2 weeks; thus, drugs such as CsA and FK506 may have dramatically longer half-lives early after OLTx.

Considering that any drug with hepatic elimination may have substantial deviation in its pharmacokinetics compared with the non-OLTx population, a safe practice is to use frequent monitoring of drug levels. Daily CsA levels have greatly improved accuracy of dosing, improving the ability to achieve adequate immunosuppression while minimizing toxicity. FK506 levels are becoming more easily obtained and may prove similarly useful.

Because of the afferent arteriole vasoconstriction caused by CsA or FK506, renal elimination of drugs may also be affected. Any patient receiving digoxin, anticonvulsants, vancomycin, or aminoglycosides should have drug levels monitored frequently.

CsA is predominantly eliminated by hepatic conjugation, but because drug levels are monitored daily, there is little risk of toxicity with cautious dosing. Remember that high-pressure liquid chromatography assays measure parent CsA concentrations that may rise with graft dysfunction, but radioimmunoassay or fluorescence-polarization assays generally measure parent and metabolite concentrations and so may not change significantly with graft function decrement and recovery.

A promising new assay of liver function is the monoethylglycine xylidide measure of lidocaine metabolism.[15–17] Conjugation of lidocaine requires brisk blood flow to the liver, drug uptake, and energy-consuming metabolic alteration. This test is sensitive to minor degrees of graft dysfunction, like the secretion of bile.

PROTEIN SYNTHESIS

Hepatic synthesis is more difficult to measure. As is true for pretransplant liver disease, a great amount of hepatic reserve must be lost before the PT, PTT, and albumin values become abnormal. Plasma cholesterol levels, if initially low, show a progressive rise over several days in healthy grafts. Interpretation is less influenced by exogenous administration of proteins and intravenous nutrition. Clotting factors V, VII, and VIII should show a steady rise over the first 3 to 5 days; because they have relatively short half-lives, these proteins are probably the most sensitive to alterations in graft function.

ENERGY METABOLISM

Only with severe graft dysfunction should there be substantial alterations in energy metabolism. Hypoglycemia and lactic acidosis are grave signs. Such severe metabolic derangement usually indicates nearly total graft failure or the concomitant problems of sepsis or cardiogenic shock.

RADIOLOGIC ASSESSMENT

Radiologic assessment of graft function must include Doppler ultrasonography determination of graft vessel patency. With experienced radiologists, the accuracy of this test is excellent, and the false-negative rate (conclusion that vessels are patent when, in fact, they are thrombosed) is essentially zero. Because they are noninvasive, Doppler ultrasonography studies can be repeated at any time of decreased graft function. It is wise to obtain a baseline study early after OLTx. If there is any question of vessel patency, visceral angiography is indicated.

A complementary study to Doppler ultrasonography is a radionuclide scan such as the HIDA scan. With bolus injection and rapid imaging, near-simultaneous imaging of the aorta and the liver strongly suggests hepatic artery patency. The HIDA scan additionally assesses homogeneity of liver uptake, rate of secretion, and possible biliary obstruction or leak.

COMPLICATIONS ∎

PULMONARY

A heightened risk of atelectasis, pulmonary edema, and pleural effusions is present after OLTx. Perioperative defects in clotting probably explain why the incidence of pulmonary emboli is not high. Pain and abdominal distention contribute to atelectasis. Total lung water and pleural effusions are minimized by careful fluid therapy. As noted earlier, an abrupt change from large volume fluid deficits to marked fluid retention usually occurs at about 24 to 36 hours postoperatively. Maintenance of CVP between 6 and 10 cm H_2O is ideal. If tissue perfusion is adequate, as soon as the patient maintains a CVP greater than 10 cm H_2O, we restrict fluids and begin diuretic therapy with furosemide 20 to 60 mg every 6 hours.

RENAL

Preexisting renal disease, hepatorenal syndrome, hypovolemia, intraoperative hypotension, and nephrotoxic drugs all contribute to the fairly frequent rise in blood urea nitrogen (BUN) and creatinine after OLTx, even to the point of needing temporary hemodialysis. CsA and FK506 cause marked reductions in renal plasma flow and accentuate renal injury. It is often necessary to accept creatinine values up to 2.5 mg/dL in adults to achieve therapeutic CsA or FK506 levels and prevent early, severe rejection episodes. For patients with severe early renal dysfunction, some clinicians switch to induction with OKT3 or other antilymphocyte antibody preparations to delay CsA or FK506 for 1 to 2 weeks.

BUN is frequently elevated out of proportion to creatinine. Hypovolemia, CsA or FK506 vasoconstriction, and enhanced catabolism all contribute. A markedly elevated BUN may also signal GI bleeding.

Electrolyte disorders are common. The well-functioning graft that is repairing cellular injury incorporates intracellular ions such as magnesium, potassium, calcium, and phosphate to a degree that usually demands intravenous replacement. An additional interaction is the effect of CsA or FK506 on renal electrolyte handling. Magnesium wasting is common. When magnesium levels are less than 1.5 mg/dL, give 1 g of magnesium sulfate intravenously every 6 to 8 hours until levels are repleted. Potassium levels may be low during a diuresis, but the usual effect of CsA and FK506 is to make the patient somewhat hyperkalemic.

GASTROINTESTINAL

GI bleeding may arise from intestinal suture lines, duodenal ulcers, stress gastritis, nasogastric tube erosions, or viral infections (usually several weeks postoperatively). All OLTx patients need antiulcer prophylaxis. Spontaneous small bowel perforations are a unique event and have been attributed to high-dose steroids, electrocautery injury, or intraluminal fungal ball lesions. Small bowel necrosis from mesenteric vein cannulation should be obvious at the time of surgery but potentially can appear late. Intussusception should be suspected in children with abdominal pain or food intolerance.

Cytomegalovirus (CMV) infections rarely occur before 1 to 2 weeks (usually 6 to 8 weeks) postoperatively, but may present as bleeding ulcerations anywhere along the GI tract. *Candida* colonization leading to candidemia is best prevented by daily enteral antifungal medication.

EARLY INFECTION

The greatest infection threat to the early OLTx patient in the ICU is caused by catheters (intravenous or urinary) and tubes. "Oddball" infections associated with immunosuppressive therapy only arise later; septic deaths early after OLTx result from the same common pathogens found in trauma patients and other ICU inhabitants. Enteric nosocomial organisms are the prime offenders. Risk is amplified by the many catheters and tubes and the level of invasive monitoring. Infection risk is greatly reduced by rapid restoration of homeostasis; early removal of catheters and tubes—especially those that are redundant or marginally needed; orderly nursing care so that time is allowed for careful aseptic technique; limited traffic between the OLTx patient and other patients; and prevention of microbial overgrowth by careful use of antibiotics and bowel decontamination. Although this is the ideal standard of care for all patients, it must be rigorously applied to the OLTx recipient because the immunosuppressed state delays diagnosis and treatment by masking signs of infection. The ability to recover after infection is established is significantly lessened.

In addition to strict aseptic technique in the management of tubes and catheters, prophylactic antimicrobial administration has some usefulness. Preoperative first-generation cephalosporins provide good prophylaxis against wound infections. The gut is a common source of pathogens for later infections, but remember that broad-spectrum antibiotics are likely to promote overgrowth of fungi and resistant organisms rather than prevent infections. Selective gut decontamination preoperatively, antifungal luminal prophylaxis

(clotrimazole [Mycelex] troches four times daily), and enteral feeding best prevent overgrowth with resistant gram-negative aerobes.

Some patients, despite all efforts, develop fever or tachycardia, and a general appearance of being "ill." This picture suggests the possibility of deep infection. The differential diagnosis includes (1) graft rejection, (2) cholangitis, (3) catheter sepsis, (4) intraabdominal abscess or biliary anastomotic leak, (5) viral infections, (6) urinary tract infection, and (7) pneumonia. The most critical distinction is between rejection, which requires increased immunosuppression, and infection, which requires at least no further increase and potentially a decrease in immunosuppression. No algorithm or diagnostic test alone has particularly facilitated this diagnostic dilemma. Some generalities are often useful: Rejection is unlikely before 5 or 6 days after transplantation. Early rejection tends to cause more rapid and dramatic graft dysfunction, whereas late rejection presents as gradually rising bilirubin, AST, ALT, or alkaline phosphatase. Fever is a late sign in rejection rather than its harbinger.

Empiric Antibiotic Therapy

Always collect bacterial, fungal, and viral cultures of sputum, blood, and urine, and drain fluids before initiating antimicrobial treatment. The most likely bacterial pathogens are *Staphylococcus aureus*, *Staphylococcus epidermidis*, and gram-negative aerobes. We frequently use the combination of vancomycin and ceftriaxone. Infection by *Candida* sp. is unlikely without prior aerodigestive or urinary colonization, so empiric antifungal therapy usually is not started early in febrile events. The antifungal agent, fluconazole, is being evaluated as a possible therapeutic and prophylactic agent in immunosuppressed patients; it is the first agent with reasonable antifungal efficacy but low toxicity. Fluconazole mildly inhibits CsA metabolism but does not cause dramatic rises in concentration unless given in high doses or in renal failure. Other antifungal agents such as ketoconazole and itraconazole profoundly inhibit CsA metabolism and also have associated hepatotoxicities. Amphotericin B currently remains the antifungal agent of choice, but it is not used prophylactically because of its nephrotoxicity and the large volume of free water given with its administration. All patients should be given clotrimazole troches four times daily, and female patients should receive antifungal vagina suppositories daily as antifungal prophylaxis.

Antiviral Prophylaxis

Most viral infections present later, but prophylaxis should begin early. Acyclovir is effective against herpes simplex, a common cause of early perioral, perianal, and esophageal lesions. Much research has focused on methods of controlling CMV infections. The CMV-negative recipient of CMV-positive organs is at greatest risk. Many groups either avoid elective OLTx in these combinations or attempt anti-CMV prophylaxis, the latter showing promise but rarely being 100% effective. Administration of immunoglobulin at roughly 500 mg/kg/week, depending on the formulation, is the most common approach. An exciting study by Balfour and coworkers[18] on renal transplant recipients suggests that high-dose acyclovir (not considered effective against CMV disease) may give effective CMV prophylaxis. Gancyclovir is an effective agent for CMV disease but has not been approved for prophylactic use.

LATE INFECTIONS

Whereas early infections are predominantly bacterial and fungal and arise from colonization of the catheter and wounds, late infections include *Pneumocystis carinii*, *Toxoplasma*, fungal infections, and reactivation of latent infections such as viruses and mycobacteria. Routine prophylaxis with trimethoprim/sulfamethaxazole has dramatically reduced the incidence of *Pneumocystis* pneumonia and has probably contributed to the reduction in cases of *Listeria*

monocytogenes sepsis. Patients with sulfa allergies should receive prophylactic pentamidine nebulization.

Because so many odd infections are possible in the immunocompromised host, any OLTx patient with unexplained fever, malaise, headache, or respiratory symptoms should prompt an aggressive search for one of these pathogens. Further studies are chosen based on screening with history and physical examination, chest radiographs, CBC with differential, urinalysis, lumbar puncture (with titers checked for *Cryptococcus* and *Toxoplasma*), and viral cultures. Liver function tests are always obtained as well as an ultrasound study to look for dilated bile ducts, abscesses, and vessel patency. The patient with a pulmonary infiltrate needs bronchoalveolar lavage and transbronchial biopsy to differentiate CMV, fungi, *Legionella*, *Mycoplasma*, and other infectious agents. Abnormal lumbar puncture dictates empiric therapy

TABLE 89-1. Representative Postoperative Orders for Prior Adult OLTx Patients

Admit to ICU, Diagnosis	S/P OLTx
Condition	Critical
Vital signs	q 15 min until stable, then q 1 h; check CVP, UOP hourly; if pulmonary artery catheter present, check PAOP, PAD hourly, and cardiac output q 4 h
Activity	Egg crate foam or air mattress—turn every 1–2 h; out of bed in chair when extubated; warming blanket for temp <35°C; remove when >38.5°
Strict input and output, daily weights	
Drains	NPO; NG to low constant suction; check pH q 1 h, abdominal drains to closed bulb suction, T tube to closed-gravity drainage, Foley catheter to closed gravity drainage
Tests	Upright CXR now and q AM Stat 12-lead ECG Abdominal ultrasonography with Doppler assessment of vessel patency
Blood	CBC, platelets, PT, PTT, ABG, glucose, lactic acid stat and q 4 h Electrolytes, BUN, creatinine, liver profile, Mg, Ca, phosphorus now and q 6 h Differential, amylase, ammonia, cyclosporine level, factors V and VII, now and at 1 AM
Blood bank	Keep 6 units PRBC T&CM available (also 10 units platelets, 6 units FFP if blood loss evident)
Cultures	Blood, urine, throat, sputum, wound for routine bacterial culture today and q 3 d Blood, urine, and sputum for viral cultures weekly, and prn fever
Medications	
Immunosuppression	C₅A 2 mg/kg in 120 mL D₅W: 10 mL/h q 12 h Methylprednisolone (Solu-Medrol 0.5 mg/kg IV q 6 h
Antibiotics	Cefazolin 1.0 g IV q 8 h Mycostatin 5-mL swish and swallow q 6 h until extubated, then clotrimazole (Mycelex) troches qid

SP, after; OLTx, orthotopic liver transplantation; CVP, central venous pressure; UOP, urinary output; PAOP, pulmonary artery occlusion pressure; PAD, pulmonary diastolic pressure; CXR, chest radiograph; PT, prothrombin time; PTT, partial thromboplastin time; PRBC, packed red blood cells; T&CM, type and crossmatch; q, every; NPO, nothing by mouth; FFP, fresh frozen plasma; qid, four times daily; D₅W, 5% dextrose in water; IV, intravenously; prn, as needed; BUN, blood urea nitrogen; NG, nasogastric; stat, immediate; ECG, electrocardiograph; ABG, arterial blood gases; CBC, complete blood cell count.

and further characterization with computed tomography scans and magnetic resonance imaging.

The liver and biliary tree can be sites of infection. Viral hepatitis caused by CMV, herpesvirus or adenovirus, or hepatitis A, B, or C can occur. Any biliary obstruction permits cholangitis with common enteric pathogens; if suspected, empiric antibiotics and stress doses of steroids are initiated as soon as cultures are obtained.

Hepatic artery thrombosis occurring late after OLTx may present as cholangitis, segmental liver infarction with abscess formation, bile duct leak, or multiple bile leaks and strictures. For this reason, any patient with bacterial infections arising in the liver needs definitive evaluation of hepatic artery patency. Like hepatic artery thrombosis in the early postoperative period, these patients need retransplantation, but if liver function is stable, it need not be emergent. Catheter drainage and antibiotic therapy should be used to control the infectious process before retransplantation, if possible.

LATE READMISSIONS TO THE ICU ■

Just as with other solid-organ transplant recipients, OLTx patients return to a normal lifestyle that places them at risk for the "usual" causes of ICU admission such as trauma, myocardial infarction, pneumonia, and so on. In these settings, it is assumed that liver function is normal, but care must be taken that other therapeutic maneuvers do not injure the graft. The most common problem is steroid and CsA dosing. In trauma, infections, or perioperative stress, patients who have chronically taken prednisone may have insufficient reserve in the hypothalamic-adrenal axis to boost endogenous cortisol synthesis. They should be given the equivalent of 3 mg/kg day of cortisol for mild stress (simple operations or mild infections) or 5 mg/kg/day for more severe stress (Table 89-1). In either case, the extra steroids should be rapidly tapered back to baseline immunosuppression. For patients with severe infections, the goal is to reduce steroid use as much as possible, providing only enough to prevent addisonian crisis.

CsA metabolism is affected by several drugs. Daily CsA blood level measurement is necessary whenever the patient is in a rapidly changing state such as ICU admission. Because CsA is so poorly absorbed, the necessary intravenous dose is *approximately* one third of the oral dose. Start with one third of the daily oral dose, give half of this in 120 mL of 5% dextrose in water as a continuous infusion at 10 mL/hour, and renew the mixture every 12 hours. Rate changes of 1 mL/hour thus represent a 10% change in dosing. Intravenous dosing is indicated for situations other than when the patient can take nothing by mouth. External biliary drainage, change in the fat content of meals, giving the drug at a different time relative to meals, frequent antacid therapy, and changes in bowel motility all can dramatically change CsA absorption. In the unstable clinical setting, it is often better simply to convert completely to intravenous CsA pro tempore.

Drug interactions with CsA are legion. Unexpected interactions should be anticipated; thus, daily monitoring of CsA levels and use of common drugs with well-defined interaction profiles are best.

CONSULTATION ■

Although liver transplantation is the preferred treatment for several liver diseases, and the number of transplants performed is steadily increasing, OLTx remains new and complicated. Experience is the most important aid to diagnosis and treatment. Physicians and surgeons who are part of active transplant programs, nonetheless, frequently consult colleagues locally and across the nation. It is the normal standard of care for OLTx patients.

REFERENCES ■

1. Stone MD, Benotti PN: Liver resection. *Surg Clin North Am* 1989;69:383
2. Wszolek ZK, McComb RD, Pfeiffer RF, et al: Pontine and extrapontine myelinolysis following liver transplantation: relationship to serum sodium. *Transplantation* 1989;48:1006
3. Bion JF, Badger I, Crosby HA, et al: Selective decontamination of the digestive tract reduces gram-negative pulmonary colonization but not systemic endotoxemia in patients undergoing elective liver transplantation. *Crit Care Med* 1994;22:40
4. Lidofsky SD, Bass NM, Prager MC, et al: Intracranial monitoring and liver transplantation for fulminant hepatic failure. *Hepatology* 1992;16:1
5. Munoz SJ, Moritz MJ, Bell R, et al: Factors associated with severe intracranial hypertension in candidates for emergency liver transplantation. *Transplantation* 1993;55:1071
6. Gubernatis G, Tusch G, Burckhardt R, et al: Score-aided decision-making in patient with severe liver damage after hepatic transplantation. *World J Surg* 1989;13:259
7. Chazouilleres O, Calmus Y, Vaubourdolle M, et al: Preservation-induced liver injury: clinical aspects, mechanisms, and therapeutic approaches. *J Hepatol* 1993;18:123
8. Greig PD, Woolf GM, Sinclair SB, et al: Treatment of primary liver graft nonfunction with prostaglandin E1. *Transplantation* 1989;48:447
9. Himmelreich G, Hundt K, Neuhaus P, et al: Evidence that intraoperative prostaglandin E_1 infusion reduces impaired platelet aggregation after reperfusion in orthotopic liver transplantation. *Transplantation* 1993;55:819
10. Stahl RL, Duncan A, Hooks MA, et al: A hypercoagulable state follows orthotopic liver transplantation. *Hepatology* 1990;12:553
11. Starzl TE, Demetris AJ: *Liver Transplantation: A 31-Year Perspective.* Chicago, Year Book Medical Publishers, 1990
12. deGroen PC, Aksamit AJ, Rakela J, et al: Central nervous system toxicity after liver transplantation: the role of cyclosporine and cholesterol. *N Engl J Med* 1987;317:861
13. McAlister VC, Grant DR, Roy A, et al: Right phrenic nerve injury in orthotopic liver transplantation. *Transplantation* 1993;55:826
14. Krowka MJ, Cortese DA: Pulmonary aspects of liver disease and liver transplantation. *Clin Chest Med* 1989;10:593
15. Oellerich M, Burdelski M, Ringe B, et al: Lignocaine metabo-

lite formation as a measure of pre-transplant liver function. *Lancet* 1989;1:640

16. Schroeder TJ, Gremse DA, Mansour ME, et al: Lidocaine metabolism as an index of liver function in hepatic transplant donor and recipients. *Transplant Proc* 1989;21:2299

17. Gremse DA, A-Kader HH, Schroeder TJ, et al: Assessment of lidocaine metabolite formation as a quantitative liver function test in children. *Hepatology* 1990;12:656

18. Balfour HH Jr, Chace BA, Stapleton JT, et al: A randomized placebo-controlled trial of oral acyclovir for the prevention of cytomegalovirus disease in recipients of renal allografts. *N Engl J Med* 1989;320:1381

Critical Care, Third Edition, edited by Joseph M. Civetta,
Robert W. Taylor, and Robert R. Kirby.
Lippincott-Raven Publishers, Philadelphia, PA © 1997.

CHAPTER 90

■

Intestinal and Multivisceral Transplantation

Marc G. Webb
Andreas G. Tzakis

IMMEDIATE CONCERNS: PREOPERATIVE CARE ■

MAJOR PROBLEMS

Candidates for intestinal and multivisceral transplantation
are patients with intestinal insufficiency who have developed
life-threatening complications of liver disease or long term
parenteral nutrition. The latter most commonly include liver
failure from total parenteral nutrition (TPN) or inability to
attain vascular access. The preoperative evaluation has two
major goals: (1) to evaluate the condition of all the intraabdominal organs to determine which can be retained and
which must be replaced, and (2) to stabilize and hopefully
improve the patient's general condition so that surgery may
be performed. Each patient has a unique story, and in many
cases, a complicated surgical, medical, and social history.
The preoperative evaluation and management are correspondingly complex.

Preoperative problems of malnutrition, substance abuse,
depleted vascular access, sepsis, and complications of end-
stage liver disease (ESLD) may require that care be rendered in the intensive care unit (ICU) while awaiting a donor
for intestinal or multivisceral transplantation.

STRESS POINTS

1. A detailed history and physical, including details of
   previous operations, is essential. Successful management of complications and preparation of the patient

for transplantation depend on a thorough understanding of the patient's condition and problems.
2. The functional status of the intraabdominal organs
   should be investigated with the aim of determining
   which can be retained and which can be replaced.
   The best—and possibly only—opportunity to also
   transplant a liver, whole pancreas, islet cells, or kidney
   is at the time of the intestinal transplant.
3. Venous vascular insufficiency is a major complication
   of long-standing use of TPN, and represents one of
   the indications for intestinal transplantation. Clotting
   of multiple venous systems may create severe intraoperative problems and can lead to the patient's death.
   Accurate knowledge of the patient's central and mesenteric venous status is mandatory.
4. Nutrition is a major problem in candidates for intestinal and multivisceral transplantation. Preexisting malnutrition from intestinal insufficiency may be compounded by loss of vascular access, catabolism secondary to sepsis, or accompanying liver failure.
5. Cholestatic liver injury is one of the main complications of parenteral nutrition, frequently progressing to
   cirrhosis and ESLD. The consequences of liver failure
   may complicate treatment.
6. Infection is a major problem in this population, and
   a high index of suspicion must be maintained to avoid
   preoperative sepsis.
7. Intestinal failure is a chronic process, and drug dependence is common. Preoperative substance abuse evaluation may simplify postoperative management.

ESSENTIAL DIAGNOSTIC TESTS AND PROCEDURES

1. Baseline laboratory studies for evaluating liver function and nutritional and physiologic status
2. Evaluation of visceral and central venous vascular anatomy by Doppler ultrasonography or venography when vascular thrombosis has been noticed or suspected
3. Evaluation of the gastrointestinal (GI) tract with contrast and radionuclide studies
4. Evaluation of liver anatomy by ultrasound, computed tomography (CT), and possibly biopsy
5. Nutritional evaluation and assessment of growth in pediatric patients
6. Studies evaluating physiologic reserve in cardiac, pulmonary, and renal systems
7. Infectious disease workup and ongoing surveillance
8. Psychiatric, social work, and substance abuse consultations when indicated

INITIAL THERAPY

1. Admitting the patient to an ICU
2. H$_2$ blockers to reduce the risk of GI bleeding
3. Pulmonary care directed against atelectasis, hypoxia, hypercapnia, and the risk of aspiration
4. Blood pressure support with volume replacement and vasopressors
5. Volume overload controlled as indicated with fluid restriction, diuresis, or continuous venovenous hemofiltration (CVVH)
6. Early antibiotic treatment based on clinical suspicion and surveillance cultures
7. Treatment of other specific conditions that led to the ICU admission
8. Maximizing enteral contribution to total nutritional support, then supplying the remaining nutrients necessary through TPN
9. Treatment of complications of concurrent ESLD: coagulopathy, encephalopathy, GI bleeding, hemodynamic instability, and fluid overload

IMMEDIATE CONCERNS: POSTOPERATIVE CARE ■

MAJOR PROBLEMS

The early problems postoperatively include hemodynamic instability, postoperative bleeding and coagulopathy, concerns regarding volume and renal status, and initial graft function if a liver has been transplanted as part of the procedure. Later, rejection, bacterial and viral infections, complications related to technical problems, and nutritional issues become more important.

STRESS POINTS

1. Hemodynamic stability and tissue perfusion should be assessed the moment the patient appears in the ICU, or preferably before—ICU personnel should evaluate the patient in the operating room.
2. When a liver is included in the transplanted graft, its immediate function and viability are critical to the clinical stability and success of the patient. Adequate function can be inferred from hemodynamic stability, good urine output, a dry operative field, and normal-appearing bile.
3. Treatment of volume and renal status is guided by invasive monitoring. The transplanted bowel may sequester a significant amount of fluid. Because graft edema is deleterious to the liver and intestine, the bias is toward caution in fluid administration, the use of colloids in resuscitation, and the use of modest doses of vasopressors if perfusion pressure is too low.
4. Vascular patency is evaluated by early ultrasonography in the ICU. Any abnormal finding should be followed up with graft angiography or reexploration.

ESSENTIAL DIAGNOSTIC TESTS AND PROCEDURES

1. Laboratory studies, including serial hematocrits, prothrombin times (PTs), arterial blood gases, blood sugars, lactic acid levels, electrolytes, and fibrinogen levels
2. Invasive hemodynamic monitoring with close attention to urine output and other fluid losses
3. Chest radiograph and electrocardiogram (ECG)
4. Early Doppler examination of graft vessels

INITIAL THERAPY

1. Optimize oxygen delivery by transfusion, inotropic support, fluid resuscitation, and afterload reduction as needed.
2. Optimize respiratory function with aggressive pulmonary care, modest levels of positive end-expiratory pressure, and respiratory support.
3. Reduce risk of infection with prophylactic antibiotics plus antiviral and antifungal agents. Use selective decontamination of the GI tract.
4. Control fluid overload by volume restriction, diuresis, CVVH, or dialysis.
5. Request cytomegalovirus (CMV)-negative or irradiated blood products.

OVERVIEW ■

Loss of intestinal function historically resulted in the slow starvation of the unfortunate patient.

In 1968, Dudrick introduced TPN, changing the outcome of many patients. Unfortunately, TPN is associated with several complications that render it less than perfect as a long-term solution: line-related sepsis, gradual loss of central venous access, cholestatic liver damage leading to cirrhosis and ESLD,[1] cost, and limitations to lifestyle.

Since the early 1960s, successful intestinal transplantation has been thought to be a possible solution to the limitations of TPN.[2,3] Despite numerous attempts between 1964 and 1990, there were only scattered examples of functioning intestinal grafts.[4-6]

Problems were encountered with rejection, infection, and technical complications, preventing the clinical application of intestinal transplantation from becoming a practical matter. Beginning in 1990, a successful series of intestinal transplantations at the University of Pittsburgh, as well as work in other centers, has shown that the small bowel can be transplanted alone, in combination with a liver, or as part of a multivisceral procedure, although with an elevated risk of mortality and morbidity.[7-11] The ileocecal valve, cecum, and colon also can be included.

Nevertheless, the care of these patients can be a formidable challenge. Preoperative problems of malnutrition, depleted vascular access, sepsis, and complications of ESLD may require care in the ICU while a suitable donor is sought. Postoperative care in the ICU is also necessary. Rejection of the transplanted bowel may present as GI bleeding or sepsis. CMV infection and intraabdominal sepsis remain significant postoperative problems. Squeezing a large mass of viscera into a shrunken space may lead to difficult closure of the abdomen and wound healing problems.

PREOPERATIVE AND OPERATIVE CARE ■

EVALUATION AND TREATMENT OF CANDIDATES FOR INTESTINAL AND MULTIVISCERAL TRANSPLANTATION

There are many and varied conditions (Table 90-1) that may lead to candidacy for isolated intestinal, combined liver–intestinal, or multivisceral transplantation. There must be a complete understanding of the patient's history, previous operations, complications, and concomitant medical problems. The history frequently includes numerous surgical

TABLE 90-1. Indications for Intestinal Transplantation

SHORT GUT SECONDARY TO

Gastroschisis
Jejunoileal atresia
Midgut volvulus
Necrotizing enterocolitis
Status-post resection of bowel for intestinal tumor
Superior mesenteric artery occlusion or mesenteric venous thrombosis
Status-post resection for intestinal trauma or obstruction
Status-post multiple small bowel resections for Crohn's disease

PLANNED RESECTION OF BOWEL OR VISCERA FOR

Gardner's and other multiple polyposis syndromes
Hirshsprung's disease
Microvillous inclusion disease
Intestinal pseudoobstruction
Selected other motility disorders
Extensive but resectable abdominal tumors
Budd-Chiari syndrome with mesenteric venous thrombosis

procedures, complications of intestinal failure, complications of ESLD, problems from loss of vascular access, indication of substance abuse, and multiple infections. Complications must be identified and managed for optimal pretransplant condition. ABO blood type, height, weight, and CMV serology status must be ascertained preoperatively, along with the evaluation of the residual bowel and condition of the liver.

The pretransplant evaluation should answer the following questions: (1) What is the current status of the liver and GI system, and will the patient benefit from an intestinal or combined organ transplant? (2) What kind of graft is likely to be required? (3) What complications of liver–intestinal failure must be treated to optimize the patient's chances of successful transplantation? and (4) Are there any contraindications to transplantation?

The contraindications to transplantation are as follows:

Severe cerebral edema or sustained cerebral hypertension
Evidence of cerebral herniation
Severe preexisting and limiting neurodegenerative disease
Unresectable malignant disease
Uncontrollable sepsis
Active infection outside of the organs to be resected
Human immunodeficiency virus infection
Severe, limiting cardiopulmonary disease
Hemorrhagic pancreatitis

Because cholestatic liver injury is one of the main complications of parenteral nutrition, identification of cirrhosis and possible ESLD and the treatment of any existing complications of liver failure are important. GI bleeding, coagulopathy, encephalopathy, sepsis, hemodynamic instability, and fluid overload may complicate management.

The initial evaluation should include baseline laboratory studies for evaluating liver function and nutritional, infectious, and physiologic status: complete blood cell count, PT and partial thromboplastin time, electrolytes, liver function tests, and arterial blood gases; ammonia, albumin, total protein, transferrin, iron, zinc, and serum vitamin levels; viral serologic workups including human immunodeficiency virus, hepatitis B and C, Epstein-Barr virus (EBV), herpes simplex I and II, and CMV; a hypercoagulable workup (protein S and C, AT3 levels) where indicated, level of panel reactive antibodies, and HLA tissue typing. Many of these tests will have been done recently in other institutions and need not be repeated (serologic workups, for example). Others reflect evolving processes and require frequent monitoring.

A routine chest radiograph is performed. Visceral and central venous vascular anatomy should be evaluated by Doppler ultrasonography or venography when vascular thrombosis has been noticed or suspected. We start with a Doppler ultrasound examination for central, portal, caval, and mesenteric venous patency. This is followed by venography or angiography, including a portal venous phase, when additional information is necessary. A cavagram may be performed if there is evidence for caval obstruction or thrombosis. Magnetic resonance imaging sometimes can be sufficient to establish mesenteric venous or caval patency.

The remaining bowel is evaluated by reviewing previous studies, with additional barium and radionuclide studies ordered as indicated. An idea of the length and functional status of the remnant GI tract is important. Problems with gastric emptying are common in this population,[12] and, if known preoperatively, may lead to modification of the procedure (inclusion of a feeding jejunostomy, for example). All of the information is summarized in a schematic road map that is available at the time of the transplant. Esophagogastroduodenoscopy may be helpful in assessing the result of previous GI surgery or in assessing the degree of portal hypertension.

The liver anatomy can be evaluated using CT of the abdomen and Doppler ultrasound of the liver. These studies are used to assess portal vein patency, determine the presence of varices and ascites, establish splenic and liver size and morphologic features, and to exclude metastatic disease outside of the limits of intended resection in cases in which it is a concern. A liver biopsy may be performed to establish the presence and degree of cirrhosis, or it may be performed at the time of transplantation to help in intraoperative decision-making. If only mild fibrosis is found, an isolated intestinal graft may be performed rather than a larger procedure. The final decision may have to wait until the time of transplantation, because progression of liver failure may occur while the patient is awaiting an appropriate donor. Failure to recognize irreversible liver damage is certain to result in fatal complications.

A physiologic assessment includes evaluation of cardiac, pulmonary, and renal status. An ECG and echocardiogram should be performed in all patients. Cardiac stress testing should be done in patients older than 40 years of age and in those with a positive cardiac history or suggestive symptoms. Coronary angiography may be indicated. Unstable patients may require central venous or pulmonary artery catheterization for evaluation and monitoring. The finding of severe, medically refractive pulmonary hypertension may constitute a contraindication for transplantation because of the risk of intraoperative right heart failure and the high incidence of early mortality in this condition.[13] Pulmonary function testing may be requested, but the presence of pleural effusions or large-volume ascites may obscure the patient's true pulmonary status.

The blood urea nitrogen and creatinine levels may not reflect the true renal status because of sepsis, malnutrition, and muscle wasting; therefore, ultrasonography of the kidneys, examination of urine electrolytes, and a 24-hour creatinine clearance may be necessary. Damage to the kidneys may have occurred from liver failure or nephrotoxic medications. Inasmuch as the immunosuppressive drug regimen also may be nephrotoxic, borderline renal function may evolve into frank renal failure after transplantation.

Insulin dependence or glucose intolerance may deteriorate with steroids and antirejection medication, indicating a need for islet cell or whole pancreas transplantation. Again, the best—and possibly only—opportunity to transplant a liver, pancreas, islet cells, or kidney is at the time of the intestinal transplant.

Malnutrition is a major problem in candidates for intestinal and multivisceral transplantation. Preexisting malnutrition caused by intestinal insufficiency may be compounded by loss of vascular access, catabolism secondary to sepsis, or accompanying liver failure. Electrolyte abnormalities and trace mineral deficiencies may be a result of malabsorption, abnormal intestinal losses, or sepsis. A biochemical evaluation should quantitate the degree of protein malnutrition and vitamin and trace mineral deficiencies so that electrolyte derangements and dietary deficiencies can be corrected preoperatively. Enteral feedings should be used to whatever degree possible, augmented by TPN.

Intestinal transplant candidates are extraordinarily vulnerable to infection for several reasons: intestinal stasis may lead to bacterial and fungal overgrowth in the GI tract, TPN-dependent patients have indwelling venous catheters, and both status in the hospital and concurrent illnesses predispose patients to the acquisition of nosocomial infections. The number of invasive procedures may be a factor. When ESLD is a concurrent problem, there is an impaired immune response resulting partly from failure of the hepatic reticuloendothelial system to clear enteric organisms in the portal venous drainage. The liver has been shown to be the most effective of all human organs in filtering bacteria from the bloodstream,[14] but this function may be compromised by shunting of blood around the liver in portal hypertension, a direct decrease in hepatic reticuloendothelial phagocytic function in liver failure, and decreased synthesis of complement and fibronectin by the diseased liver. The net result is a high incidence of bacterial and fungal infections noticed even in the first week of ICU stay.[15,16]

Fever and leukocytosis may be absent even in the presence of infection, and appropriate cultures should be obtained if infection is suspected. Selective decontamination of the GI tract may be initiated in sick patients. Empiric antibiotic coverage may be indicated in high-risk patients.

Occult infections may be suspected by the appearance of acidosis, disseminated intravascular coagulation, increased encephalopathy, and a decrease in the systemic vascular resistance, urine output, or blood pressure. Any abrupt deterioration in a patient's clinical status should be suspected to be caused by an infection, with initiation of an appropriate workup and empiric treatment. Failure to make an accurate diagnosis may allow an infected patient to undergo transplantation and the necessity for immunosuppression, which portends a poor prognosis. Failure to settle the issue may result in the patient being denied a life-saving procedure.

GI bleeding can be a major problem. Stress ulceration and gastritis are common and are usually treated with H_2 blockers, correction of coagulopathy, and transfusion. When ESLD complicates the picture, portal hypertension, coagulopathy, and thrombocytopenia may be seen. Variceal bleeding may be handled with endoscopic banding and sclerosis, or by correction of coagulopathy and medical treatment with esmolol and somatostatin analogue drips.

A transjugular intrahepatic portasystemic shunt may be effective when other measures fail, but cannot be placed in patients with portal venous thrombosis. The combination of portal, mesenteric, and caval thromboses can lead to an intraoperative bleeding diathesis that is truly untreatable.

Patients with ESLD complicated by mesenteric thrombosis may be candidates for multivisceral transplantation, but if their disease is complicated by caval thrombosis, the chances of intraoperative death from uncontrollable bleeding are extreme, even with preoperative embolization of the superior mesenteric artery (SMA) and celiac trunk.

Encephalopathy may be seen as a complication of ESLD. The contribution of encephalopathy to the risk of other complications, such as respiratory failure and aspiration, depends to a certain degree on the grade of encephalopathy (Table 90-2). Reversible causes of encephalopathy should be identified and treated early; they include the following:

Drugs (sedatives or pain medications)
Electrolyte imbalances and dehydration
Azotemia
Infection
GI bleeding
Dietary protein overload
Constipation
Hypoxia
Hypoglycemia

Electrolyte imbalances should be corrected. Mechanical lavage, enemas or lactulose may be given to reduce the protein load after episodes of GI bleeding, but in cases of short-gut syndrome they are not usually necessary and can be harmful. Hypoxia should be ruled out or treated. Serum glucose may be low, and a continuous intravenous drip should be provided.

Infection can precipitate encephalopathy and should be investigated as a cause. Midazolam can be used in low doses in agitated patients, but in general, sedatives should be used with great caution because they can complicate clinical assessment and precipitate progression of encephalopathy. Opiates should be avoided. Flumazenil treatment may be helpful in reversing the trend into deeper levels of encephalopathy.[17,18]

Coagulopathy may be a result of malnutrition and vitamin K deficiency, or deficiencies in coagulation factor synthesis from ESLD. In addition to providing adequate nutrition, intravenous vitamin K (10 mg infusion) can be given. If the basic deficit is liver failure, the coagulopathy will be generally resistant to vitamin K. An infusion of fresh frozen plasma may be necessary. In addition to coagulopathy from deficiencies in factor production, disseminated intravascular coagulation may result from sepsis or multiorgan system failure, and thrombocytopenia may be an additional factor contributing to the coagulopathy.

Hemodynamic instability may result from sepsis, ongoing volume losses, or loss of vasomotor tone in liver failure.[19] It

may be difficult to differentiate the high-output/low systemic resistance state of advanced liver failure from that of sepsis, particularly because liver failure renders patients vulnerable to infection. A pulmonary artery catheter should be placed early to guide management of the patient's hemodynamic status. Pressor support with low to moderate doses of dopamine, or with renal dose dopamine and norepinephrine, may be necessary.

Attention to respiratory care is critical. Because of progressive encephalopathy, loss of protective reflexes, inanition, loss of immunologic defenses, and prolonged hospital stays, these patients are at extremely high risk for aspiration and nosocomial pneumonia. Hypoxia may be caused by pleural effusions, nonhydrostatic pulmonary edema, intrapulmonary shunting, or simple hypoventilation and atelectasis. For this reason, aggressive pulmonary care is mandatory, and protective intubation may be appropriate. Early intubation and judicious use of positive end-expiratory pressure will improve oxygenation without requiring the increase of inspired oxygen concentrations to potentially toxic levels.

Acute renal dysfunction is seen commonly, and oliguric renal failure is associated with decreased survival. Renal dysfunction may fall into the categories of prerenal azotemia, acute tubular necrosis, or hepatorenal syndrome. Interactive causes include diminished intravascular volume from "third-space" losses and hypoalbuminemia, the effects of sepsis, injudicious diuretic management, diarrhea, and decreased oral intake. Another important contributing factor in cases with concurrent liver failure is loss of vasomotor regulation with inappropriate shunting of blood flow to skeletal muscle, skin, and other areas. Endotoxemia, with reduction of renal perfusion, may be a factor. Fluid overload is frequently seen in ESLD because of hypoproteinemia, hyperdynamic circulation, and, possibly, the superimposed effects of sepsis.

To treat renal dysfunction, filling pressures, cardiac output, and systemic vascular resistance should be monitored. Dopamine or norepinephrine may be useful in counteracting the loss of vasomotor tone and inappropriate shunting. Intravenous fluid may be administered cautiously if filling pressures are low, or diuretics with or without salt-poor albumin may be given if oliguria persists despite normal or high filling pressures. Nephrotoxic drugs should be avoided; if given, dosing should be adjusted carefully using blood levels and pharmacokinetic calculations. Deteriorating renal function may be an indication for early ultrafiltration or dialysis to control azotemia and fluid overload, or to allow for administration of needed blood products. Conventional hemodialysis or CVVH can be used to remove excess volume.

Intestinal failure can be a chronic process, and many of these patients have had multiple operative procedures. Drug dependence is common. Preoperative substance abuse evaluation may simplify postoperative management.

PREPARATION FOR TRANSPLANTATION

Once the patient is found to be a candidate for intestinal or multivisceral transplantation, all remaining issues must be resolved as quickly as possible; optimal supportive and nutritional treatment is continued and complications treated. If there are no contraindications to transplantation, the pa-

TABLE 90-2. Clinical Grade of Hepatic Encephalopathy

1—Confused state with altered mood, sleep habits or behavior; loss of spatial orientation; slowed mentation; asterixis
2—Sleepiness with slow arousability but responsive, inappropriate behavior; incontinence; marked asterixis
3—Stuporous with marked confusion, or coma responsive to painful stimuli
4—Coma unresponsive to painful stimuli

tient is placed on the United Network for Organ Sharing (UNOS) list for transplantation at the earliest possible moment. Donor selection is important because life-threatening complications may be related to a poor donor–recipient match; it may not be possible to close the abdomen after transplantation of a large mass of viscera into a small abdominal cavity; intestinal rejection and the resultant complications of increased immunosuppression may result from use of ABO-nonidentical grafts, or grafts where a positive lymphocytotoxic crossmatch is present between donor and recipient; the frequent occurrence and high morbidity of CMV infections is potentiated by the use of CMV-positive grafts in CMV-negative patients. For this reason, ABO-identical cadaveric donors of the same or smaller size are chosen to minimize complications related to difficult abdominal closure. A preoperative lymphcytotoxic crossmatch and CMV-negative graft are highly desired, even in CMV-seropositive patients. Selective decontamination of the donor intestinal tract is performed whenever possible.

In a recent review of the University of Pittsburgh experience,[20] 59 patients underwent intestinal transplantation. Twenty-two received isolated intestinal grafts, 26 were given combined liver–intestinal grafts, and 11 required multivisceral grafts. Three additional grafts were obtained for isolated intestine, liver–intestine, and multivisceral retransplantation. Intraoperative findings required the planned operative procedure be changed from isolated intestine to liver–intestine in two cases, from liver–intestine to multivisceral in three cases, and from isolated intestine to multivisceral in one case. In addition, changes from liver–intestine to multivisceral transplantation were desired in two cases, but the organs were not available. Three patients originally considered for liver–intestine graft were successfully treated by isolated intestinal graft alone. For these reasons, multivisceral grafts are routinely requested so that any intraoperative requirement may be satisfied.

THE OPERATIVE PROCEDURE

Technical details of intestinal transplantation have been reviewed elsewhere.[21-23] Briefly, arterialization of the graft is achieved with a Carrel patch of donor aorta containing the SMA only, or SMA and celiac trunk together, depending on whether the procedure involves an isolated intestinal, liver–intestine, or multivisceral graft. This may come directly off the aorta or (more commonly) from an extension graft using donor thoracic aorta. In isolated intestinal transplantation, venous outflow is accomplished by a graft-recipient end-to-end or end-to-side portal venous anastomosis. If end-to-end, the native portal vein may be drained by end-to-side anastomosis to donor portal vein or native cava. In liver–intestine or multivisceral grafts, the portal vein is left in continuity between the intestine and liver, with native portal drainage handled as described earlier. In these cases, venous outflow from the graft is by a piggyback donor suprahepatic cava to recipient hepatic vein anastomosis.[24]

Intestinal continuity is reestablished in various ways, depending on the multiple possible combinations of donor and recipient anatomy. Generally, a tube or end feeding jejunostomy and Bishop-Koop ileostomy are required, plus varying combinations of esophagogastrostomy, gastrojejunostomy, duodenojejunostomy, jejunojejunostomy, choledochojejunostomy, colocolostomy, and so on, depending on the exact situation (Figs. 90-1 through 90-3). If stomach is included, a pyloroplasty or gastrojejunostomy is performed for gastric drainage. Details of the posttransplant anatomy, with anastomoses and ostomies, should be drawn schematically in the record at the end of the operation, before memory fades. These details may be invaluable later.

Abdominal closure may be difficult because of intraoperative intestinal fluid sequestration or the problem of trying to use an abdominal cavity that has shrunken. It may be necessary to close skin and subcutaneous tissues only, leaving

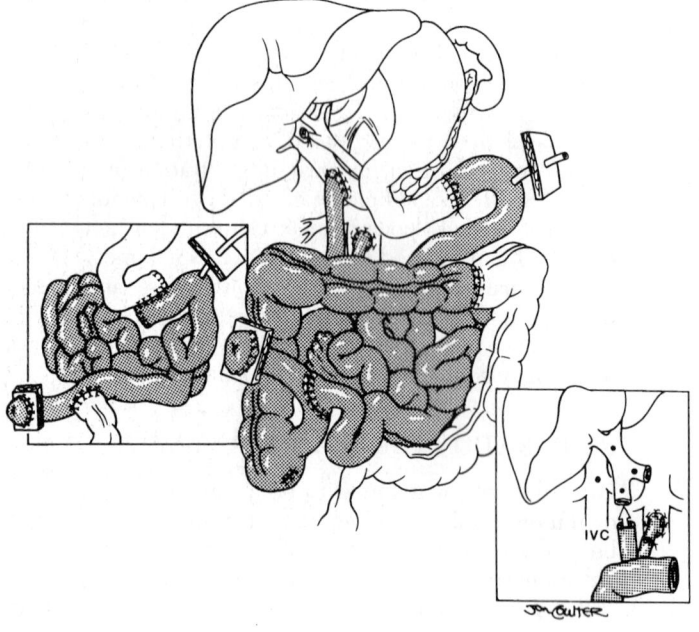

FIGURE 90-1. Isolated intestinal transplantation including half of the colon (*main figure*) or the small bowel only (*left insert*). Graft venous outflow is drained end to side (*main figure*) or end to end (*right insert*) into the portal system. (From Abu-Elmagd K, Todo S, Tzakis A, et al: Three years' clinical experience with intestinal transplant. *J Am Coll Surg* 1994;179:385.)

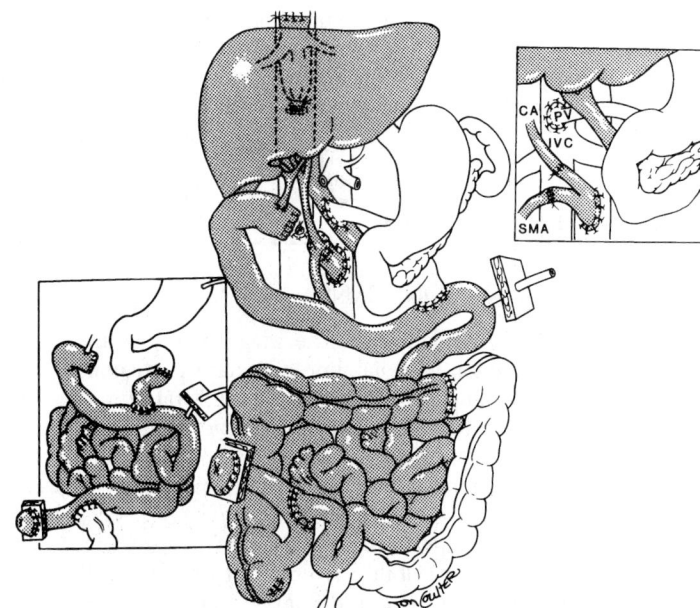

FIGURE 90-2. Liver-intestinal transplantation including part of the colon (*main figure*) or with small bowel only (*left insert*). The host portal vein is drained into the graft portal vein when possible, but in one third of cases this blood was diverted into the vena cava (*right insert*). (From Abu-Elmagd K, Todo S, Tzakis A, et al: Three years' clinical experience with intestinal transplant. *J Am Coll Surg* 1994;179:385.)

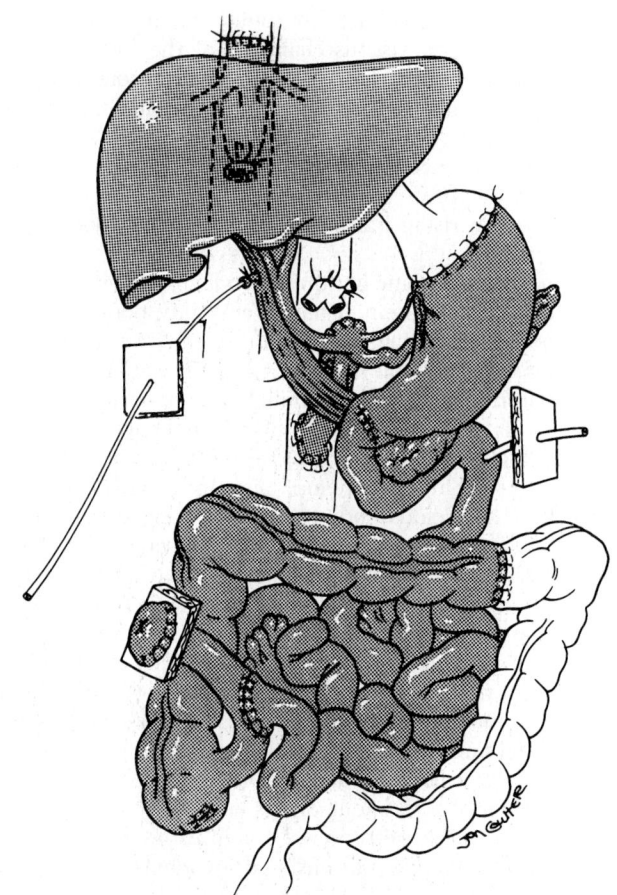

FIGURE 90-3. Full multivisceral operation including the ascending and right transverse colon. Notice that pyloroplasty or pyloromyotomy was performed. (From Abu-Elmagd K, Todo S, Tzakis A, et al: Three years' clinical experience with intestinal transplant. *J Am Coll Surg* 1994;179:385.)

the fascia open, or to use musculocutaneous rotation flaps. Obviously, wound healing problems may occur; it is important not to open, probe, or debride these wounds without the direct knowledge and involvement of the responsible surgeon.

POSTOPERATIVE CARE

POSTTRANSPLANT CONCERNS

Immediately after transplantation, the main concerns are related to liver function and viability, adequate perfusion, the presence of coagulopathy and bleeding, fluid status, and renal function. Later, infection surveillance and treatment, monitoring for rejection, nutrition, intestinal function, and treatment of other complications will become more important.

When a liver is included in the transplant package, its immediate function and viability is critical to the clinical stability and success of the patient. Primary hepatic nonfunction, hyperacute rejection, or vascular thrombosis quickly leads to an unstable clinical course, which may lead to retransplantation or death. Fortunately, the function of the newly transplanted liver can be inferred early from intraoperative findings. Correction of coagulopathy is presaged by the "drying of the field": persistent oozing, an abnormal thromboelastogram, or other evidence of fibrinolysis are not good signs. On the other hand, hemodynamic stability, good tissue perfusion, good urine output, regaining of consciousness, and a dark, viscous character of the bile (observed intraoperatively, or in the T tube) all represent signs that the liver is working. The appearance of the intestinal stomata provides an idea of the perfusion of the bowel and should be satisfactory before moving the patient from the operating room. In the ICU, the clearance of lactate, normalization of PT, and a rising fibrinogen level indicate good hepatic function.

When poor hepatic graft function is suspected from ominous clinical signs (hemodynamic instability, poor renal function, persistent oozing, and lack of arousability) or laboratory findings (markedly elevated or rising PT and lactic acid, or falling fibrinogen level), an immediate search for the cause should be undertaken. A positive lymphocytotoxic crossmatch, high level of panel reactive antibodies, or an autoimmune cause of liver failure may raise suspicion of hyperacute rejection; suspicious findings on ultrasonography or dusky appearing stomata may suggest graft vascular thrombosis. When the issue is unclear, an open biopsy can be done and submitted for routine histologic and immunofluorescent examination. Immediate angiographic examination or reexploration may be indicated.

Hemodynamic status is assessed by examination of the usual parameters—arterial pressure, heart rate and rhythm, filling pressures (including pulmonary artery occlusion pressures), cardiac output, and systemic vascular resistance—and a clinical assessment of tissue perfusion. Continuous mixed venous oximetry may be helpful in addition to the arterial blood gas. Hypertension or hypotension are treated as needed, and cardiac output is augmented as necessary.

Right or left heart failure may be seen after transplantation, and if suspected, transesophageal echocardiography may give additional information with respect to volume status and especially right ventricular function.

Myocardial ischemia or infarction can be evaluated and treatment instituted if they are confirmed.

The status of fluid balance is assessed by examination of the patient's invasive monitoring data, chest radiograph, and clinical examination. Most patients are fluid overloaded as a result of the large amounts of fluid administered in the operating room during the anhepatic phase, while on venovenous bypass, or because of intraoperative hemodynamic instability. Hepatic congestion may retard the liver's recovery from the ischemic insult of transplantation and is dangerous in the early postoperative period. The transplanted and traumatized bowel may develop significant fluid accumulation (third space). Modest pressor support is preferable to over-zealous fluid resuscitation. Acid-base status and electrolytes are monitored and corrected as indicated.

Adequate renal function is an indirect reflection of adequate hepatic function, and directly reflects adequate filling pressures and cardiac output. Nephrotoxic medications should be avoided if possible, or dosed according to drug levels and pharmacokinetic calculations.

Because acute tubular necrosis is a significant and frequent complication of liver and intestinal transplantation, fluid management may require dialysis or CVVH.

Coagulopathy is variably present after transplant procedures that involve replacing the liver, and an elevated PT should be expected; correction may not be necessary in the absence of clinical bleeding. When the PT is markedly elevated (greater than 25 seconds) or is rising, severe hepatic dysfunction should be suspected and a search for a cause instituted.

In this situation or in the presence of bleeding, the PT can be cautiously corrected to less than 20 seconds with factor replacement. Prophylaxis to prevent thrombosis may be withheld, azotemia should be corrected, and platelets should be administered for counts less than 50,000 per mm³.

Immunosuppression is started in the operating room with a steroid bolus and a tacrolimus (FK-506, Prograf) infusion at 0.1 to 0.15 mg/kg/day intravenously, followed by oral dosing at 0.3 mg/kg/day in two divided doses. Subsequent management depends partially on the lymphocytotoxic crossmatch results, which ideally should be negative preoperatively, and will include steroids in either a tapering or maintenance dose.

Intravenously given steroids are changed to an oral route when intestinal function is well established. The ideal tacrolimus blood level of 2 to 3 ng/dL is modified depending on changes in the patient's renal function, graft function, evidence of infection, and evidence of rejection. Because tacrolimus is nephrotoxic in higher doses, it may be necessary to accept decreased renal function to prevent graft rejection. Early hyperacute rejection is a possibility, but the more typical acute cellular rejection (ACR) usually does not develop before the 10th to 14th day after transplantation. Surveillance for rejection by endoscopy and graft biopsy is done routinely (one to two times per week in-house, then weekly for 3 months) or if there are clinical indications of rejection.

Concurrent bone marrow infusion from the donor is being practiced in most of the centers that perform intestinal transplantation as part of an effort to promote chimerism and immunotolerance.

Infection prophylaxis is initiated either before or at the time of the operation, and may continue in some form for weeks or months after the patient leaves the hospital. Intravenous antibiotics with enterococcal and extended gram-negative coverage are given for the first 5 days, and then afterward as indicated, including during episodes of rejection. Intravenous antifungal (amphotericin, 0.2 mg/kg prophylactic dose) and antiviral (gancyclovir, 5 mg/kg twice daily, adjusted for renal clearance) agents are also given. Fungal and gram-positive coverage of permanent intravenous access devices continues until they are removed. Fungal prophylaxis in the form of oral nystatin (Mycostatin, 5 mL orally four times daily) continues until the steroid immunosuppression is discontinued. Pneumocystis prophylaxis in the form of low-dose sulfamethoxazole trimethoprim (Bactrim) is started approximately 1 week after the operation and continued for life. CMV prophylaxis in the form of intravenous gancyclovir and CMV hyperimmune globulin (cytogam) are continued for a variable time postoperatively in "at-risk" patients (either donor or recipient CMV seropositive), depending partly on the intensity of immunosuppression necessary for the patient due to episodes of rejection. Because bacterial translocation is such a problem in intestinal transplant patients, selective decontamination of the GI tract is used. This consists of a mixture of amphotericin or nystatin, an aminoglycoside, and polymyxin E (sometimes known as "Mud"), given enterally four times daily for 4 to 6 weeks after transplantation and during episodes of rejection (Table 90-3).

Prophylaxis against graft thrombosis, particularly in pediatric cases, usually consists of a regimen of minidose heparin (5000 U three times daily for adults; 15 U/kg for children) given subcutaneously, low-dose aspirin (80 mg daily for adults; 2 mg/kg for children), and a low molecular weight dextran infusion (dextran 40 at 40 mL/hour for adults; 1 mL/kg/hour for children). The dextran and heparin are generally begun when the PT is less than 17 seconds. The aspirin is started when the platelet count is greater than 100,000 per mm³. All are discontinued in the face of a severe thrombocytopenia (platelet count less than 40,000 per mm³). Doppler ultrasound surveillance of the graft is performed the first postoperative day and whenever there is clinical suspicion of thrombosis. Unexplained abnormalities on ultrasonography should be investigated by emergent angiography or early reexploration.

In the immediate postoperative period, the patient's nutritional needs can be met with TPN, but assuming the patient is stable, infusions using the feeding jejunostomy or a transgastric small bowel tube can commence at low rates within the first 48 hours. We begin with a 5% dextrose infusion at 10 to 20 mL/hour, which, if tolerated, can be changed to an elemental tube feeding preparation. A low-osmolarity formula should be used to prevent hyperosmolar diarrhea. Once intestinal motility returns, the feedings can be increased by 10 mL/hour every 12 hours as tolerated. The TPN is slowly weaned when enteral caloric intake is greater than 50% of calculated needs. In a review of the Pittsburgh experience, TPN was successfully weaned in 18 to 210 days, with a mean of approximately 2 months.[25] The transplanted bowel has a tendency to lose water, sodium, magnesium, and bicarbonate, leading to predictable electrolyte and volume abnormalities. Bicarbonate and magnesium may be given orally, but intravenous supplementation in dehydrated patients may be necessary.

MANAGEMENT OF LATE PROBLEMS

Intestinal and multivisceral transplant patients require complex medical management and frequently require readmission to the hospital or the ICU.[26]

INFECTION

Despite all efforts to reduce patients' susceptibility to infection, all patients had at least one postoperative infection in several large series.[27-29] Most of these were line related, followed in frequency by wound infections, intraabdominal infections (split evenly between peritonitis and abscesses), and bacterial translocation–associated episodes of septicemia. Review of stool cultures, line status, and clinical examination are important in narrowing the differential, but CT scanning of the abdomen and early reexploration also must be considered.

Along with cultures sent when clinical infection is suspected on clinical grounds, we recommend that quantitative stool cultures be monitored on a twice-weekly basis. It has been observed that single-organism colony counts greater than 10⁹ have been frequently associated with bacteremia of the same organism, presumably from translocation, leading to generalized sepsis if untreated.[30] The incidence of translocation may be modified by selective decontamination of the GI tract, the presence of rejection, the presence or absence of the ileocecal valve, and CMV infection. Along with intravenous antibiotics, these episodes have been treated

TABLE 90-3. Selective Decontamination of the Gastrointestinal Tract

	<5 y	5–12 y	>12 y
Amphotericin B	100 mg	250 mg	500 mg
Gentamycin or tobramycin	10 mg	40 mg	80 mg
Polymyxin	25 mg	50 mg	100 mg

with changes in the selective decontamination mixture suggested by the sensitivity of the organism in the stool or blood. If associated with an episode of rejection, treatment of sepsis may require a paradoxical increase in immunosuppression in addition to antibiotic treatment.

CMV infection has been called the most common infection in transplant patients. The presentation of CMV infection depends largely on specific organ involvement, but a viral syndrome of fever, malaise, nausea, and leukopenia is characteristic, and the diagnosis can be confirmed by isolation of virus in culture or early identification of antigen from blood or tissue specimens, or by identification of viral genome by polymerase chain reaction (PCR). In a review of intestinal and multivisceral transplant patients, 14 of 22 at-risk patients (either donor or recipient CMV seropositive) developed a cytomegaloviral disease: 80% enteritis and 8% hepatitis.[31]

Because weekly monitoring of CMV PCR has been demonstrated to show evidence of active viral replication 2 to 10 days before clinical evidence of disease, routine surveillance may be justified.

Other viral infections seen include EBV infections, adenoviral infections and, less commonly, influenzae, parainfluenzae, respiratory syncytial, varicella zoster, and herpes simplex viral infections.

Treatment of viral infections generally involves some reduction of immunosuppression with the addition of antiviral agents. Intravenous or oral gancyclovir, with or without cytogam, is used for treatment of CMV infection. Resistant strains of CMV may require the addition of foscarnet for treatment. For most other viral infections, acyclovir is used.

In the Kusne series,[27] fungal infections were much less frequent than bacterial and viral infections. The most common fungal infection was *Candida* esophagitis, but line infections, peritonitis, and sinusitis also were seen. These infections usually are successfully treated with amphotericin B and line removal, but surgical drainage also may be necessary. Fluconazole may be used but is generally avoided because of its tendency to raise tacrolimus levels precipitously. More ominous and difficult-to-treat fungal infections include mucormycosis and *Aspergillus* infections; repeated surgical debridement may be required in addition to antifungal agents.[32–37]

REJECTION

The intestine is more immunogenic than most transplanted organs, and rejection is correspondingly a more serious and persistent problem. In a recent review of the Pittsburgh experience,[38] 95% of the intestinal grafts were found to have ACR at one time or another.

The mean time to the first episode of intestinal rejection was 19 days. Twelve of 28 patients whose transplanted graft also included the liver had ACR in the transplanted liver, and 5 of 13 patients with a transplanted colon had biopsy-proven ACR in the colon. One patient with transplanted pancreas had pancreatitis that responded to treatment with elevated immunosuppression. Of seven patients with transplanted stomach, none were demonstrated to have features consistent with ACR. In contrast to another report,[39] the inclusion of a liver with the intestinal graft did not confer protection against rejection in this series.

The transplanted intestine also has the interesting and unique property that rejection may lead to, or present as, a complication of bacterial translocation. Fortunately, there are several clinical indicators of intestinal graft rejection. Fever, increased stomal output, blood in the stomal output, and malabsorption as evidenced by the appearance of a higher percentage of reducing substances in the stool are strongly correlated with rejection. Malaise, nausea, vomiting, and abdominal pain may be present. A picture of septic shock has been seen in several patients.

Endoscopy may reveal patchy erythema, friability, diffuse ulceration, or duskiness of the mucosa, in conjunction with characteristic histologic findings on biopsy. Velvety or glistening mucosa seen on endoscopy argues strongly against intestinal rejection.[40,41] Although stomal biopsies can be done, rejection may exist in a "skip" pattern and may not be apparent unless endoscopy is performed. Cellular infiltration, cryptitis, villous edema, and sloughing of cell surface epithelium are seen microscopically, depending on the severity of the process (Table 90-4).

Treatment of rejection may involve the use of intermittent steroid boluses, reinstitution of intravenous tacrolimus (prograf, FK-506) to boost serum levels quickly, or augmentation of baseline steroid and tacrolimus immunosuppression. Antilymphocyte preparations may be needed for resistant rejection. Azathioprine and cyclophosphamide are used occasionally. Mycophenolate (RS-61443, Cell-cept) also may have an important role in the future of immunosuppression.

Graft-versus-host disease (GVHD) also can be seen; it represents the other side of rejection—an attack on host tissues by immunologic cells derived from the graft.

Manifestations may include unexplained hemolysis, pancytopenia, pneumonitis, diarrhea, mental status changes, and a skin rash. In one patient in the University of Miami series with an isolated intestinal graft, GVHD was seen in a biopsy specimen of the native liver taken when liver function tests rose unexpectedly after transplantation. In addition to the typical histologic picture, the diagnosis can be supported by in situ PCR of HLA antigen markers or karyotyping to distinguish donor from recipient lymphocytes infiltrating the skin and other tissues.

NUTRITION AND INTESTINAL FUNCTION

Intestinal function, as evidenced by intestinal motility, returns 1 to 2 weeks after transplantation. Delayed gastric emptying, on the other hand, is common, can be a prolonged problem, and is seen in one third to one half of intestinal transplant patients. In one series, delays were more prevalent with liquids than with solid foods in the isolated small bowel and liver–intestinal grafts (40% versus 20% in small bowel, 66% versus 33% in liver–small bowel). Patients who have received multivisceral grafts tended to have rapid emptying with liquids (but not with solids), probably because of the pyloroplasty performed on the transplanted stomach.[12]

TABLE 90-4. Indicators of Intestinal Graft Rejection

GRADE OF REJECTION	CLINICAL FINDINGS	ENDOSCOPIC FINDINGS	HISTOLOGIC FEATURES
Acute			
Mild to moderate	Fever Abdominal pain Vomiting Watery diarrhea Ileus Increase of stomal output	Ischemic/dusky mucosa Mucosal edema Hyperemia Decreased peristalsis	Cellular infiltration Villus blunting Cryptitis Mucus/Panethus cell reduction Epithelial cell damage and regeneration
Severe	Severe diarrhea Abdominal pain Abdominal distension Metabolic acidosis Positive blood cultures ARDS	Ulceration Mucosal sluffing Bleeding Loss of peristalsis	Mucosal hemorrhage Mucosal sloughing Microabscesses
Chronic	Chronic diarrhea Malabsorption Progressive weight loss	Pseudomembranes Hypoperistalsis Loss of mucosal folds Oily intestinal contents	Less inflammatory cells Evident cryptitis Regenerative epithelium Submucosal fibrosis

ARDS, adult respiratory distress syndrome.

Adapted from Todo S, Tzakis A, Abu-Elmagd K, et al: Intestinal transplantation in composite visceral grafts or alone. *Ann Surg* 1992;216:223.

Motility problems of the native and transplanted viscera tended to ameliorate with time. Motility is *not* a useful parameter for monitoring rejection because loss of motility is a late sign.[42]

As GI motility returns, enteral feedings are advanced. Low-osmolarity formulas should be used to prevent hyperosmolar diarrhea. Absorptive function is assessed by following stomal output. The volume and water content of the stool give a rough indication of absorption—both are ordinarily increased in intestinal rejection. High stomal output may result from rapid transit time, intestinal infection, or rejection; loperamide (Imodium) or other pharmacologic agents may be used to treat pure hypermotility, but the other possibilities should be ruled out first. Guiaic-positive stools may indicate erosion, ulceration, or frank sloughing of the mucosa. Reducing substances in the stool are measured because they give an indication of the intestine's ability to absorb dietary sugars. The ideal is "no reducing substances detected," but values up to 1% may be seen in the absence of overt rejection. A d-xylose absorption test can be performed for a formal and reproducible assessment.[43] Fat absorption may be abnormal for a more prolonged period, resulting from the interruption of lymphatics during the harvesting and preparation of the graft. Medium chain triglycerides may be added to enteral feedings early because they are not absorbed by the lacteals. As enteral function and feedings improve, TPN is gradually weaned.

Diarrhea and dehydration are frequent problems after intestinal transplantation, particularly when only small bowel is transplanted and enteric drainage is through an ileostomy, or when the length of native or transplanted colon is short. Additional causes of diarrhea are fat malabsorption, rejec-

tion, CMV enteritis, bacterial overgrowth, and *Clostridium difficile* infection. Treatment is supportive, with rehydration, identification of treatable causes, and antidiarrheal drug therapy when rejection and infection are excluded. Acidosis from bicarbonate losses should be treated with oral supplementation.

Speech therapy and dietary consultation may be required after intestinal transplantation, especially in children, many of whom have never learned to eat or to respond to a hunger stimulus appropriately.[44] Training may be necessary, and although the goal of enteral feeding may be met, these children may be resistant to taking an adequate oral intake. Cycling of tube feeding may help in allowing a hunger stimulus and response to develop.

Nutritional status can be monitored by following visceral proteins, weight gain, and dietary intake diaries. Because the frequency of preexisting malnutrition and abnormal fluid retention preoperatively, weight gain is not as reliable a parameter as is an increase in height in children.

POSTTRANSPLANT LYMPHOPROLIFERATIVE DISEASE

Immunosuppressed patients are known to be at elevated risk for development or accelerated growth of neoplasms, the most significant of which may be posttransplant lymphoproliferative disease (PTLD). PTLD occurs in approximately 2% of transplant recipients and represents a spectrum of disease from swollen lymph nodes at one end to a frankly malignant and aggressive lymphoma at the other.

Most cases are found to be associated with EBV infection.

In a series of 54 intestinal and multivisceral transplant patients at the University of Pittsburgh immunosuppressed primarily with tacrolimus, 8 patients (15% of total) developed PTLD. Six patients with PTLD were children (20.6% incidence rate in the pediatric population versus 8% in the adult population).

The time between transplantation and onset of disease ranged between 24 days and 2.3 years, with most of the patients presenting after 10 months.[45] Symptoms and signs included fever, malaise, weight loss, vomiting, diarrhea, lymphadenitis, GI bleeding, intestinal perforation, and ulcerated lesions of the GI tract on endoscopy. Epstein-Barr DNA was detected in all eight specimens.

Any patient presenting with a fever after transplant should be examined carefully for possible lymphadenopathy in cervical, axillary, groin, or tonsillar areas, and EBV infection ruled out. Diagnosis is made histologically by examination of lymph node, tonsillar, or enteric biopsy, and by the demonstration of EBV DNA in the biopsy specimen. A positive EBV PCR from serum may constitute presumptive evidence of early infection and may support a diagnosis of PTLD. EBV-encoded RNA can be demonstrated by in situ hybridization in all cells latently infected with EBV.[46] A chest radiograph should be done on all patients, and CT of the chest and abdomen done in high-risk, recurrent, or proven cases.

Treatment of PTLD consists of reduction of immunosuppression combined with intravenous acyclovir or gancyclovir. Alpha-interferon and foscarnet have been used in advanced, recurrent, or rapidly progressive disease, or where immunosuppression could not be reduced because of recent severe rejection. The mortality in the Pittsburgh experience was three of eight (38.5%). All patients who died were found to have had residual disease at autopsy.

OUTCOME

In a recent review of the Pittsburgh experience,[47] 60 patients had been transplanted since 1990: 28 adults and 32 children. There were 19 deaths (10 of 28 adults and 9/32 children), with 68% overall survivors. Of the survivors, 85% no longer needed TPN, three received TPN because of graft removal, and three were maintained by a combination of TPN and enteral nutrition because of poor graft function.

Indicators of poor outcome included poor nutritional status, a history of significant narcotic abuse, findings of inferior vena caval thrombosis, significant infections of the abdominal wall, and status as an ICU-bound patient with GI bleeding or a total bilirubin of greater than 20 mg/dL.

Intestinal transplantation represents one of the current frontiers in transplantation surgery, and is indicated for a selected group of patients. Significant problems include a high incidence of bacterial, fungal, and cytomegaloviral infections; posttransplant immunoproliferative disease; graft rejection; GVHD; feeding difficulties; and complications related to technical problems. The future of transplantation for the treatment of intestinal insufficiency depends on the development of strategies to eliminate or reduce the morbidity and mortality of these complications.

REFERENCES ■

1. Messing B, Zarka Y, Lemann M, et al: Chronic cholestasis associated with long-term parenteral nutrition. *Transplant Proc* 1994;26:1438
2. Starzl T, Kaupp H, Brock D, et al: Mass homotransplantation of abdominal organs in dogs. *Surg Forum* 1960;30:1128
3. Starzl T, Kaupp H, Brock D, et al: Homotransplantation of multivisceral organs. *Am J Surg* 1962;103:219
4. Clark CI: Recent progress in intestinal transplantation. *Arch Dis Child* 1992;67:976
5. Grant W, Wall R, Zhong R, et al: Experimental clinical intestinal transplantation: initial experience of a Canadian centre. *Transplant Proc* 1990;22:2497
6. Starzl T, Rowe M, Todo S, et al: Transplantation of multiple abdominal viscera. *JAMA* 1989;261:1449
7. Abu-Elmagd K, Todo S, Tzakis A, et al: Three years' clinical experience with intestinal transplant. *J Am Coll Surg* 1994;179:385
8. Reyes J, Tzakis A, Todo S, et al: Small bowel and liver/small bowel transplantation in children. *Semin Pediatr Surg* 1993;2:289
9. Todo S, Tzakis A, Abu-Elmagd K, et al: Intestinal transplantation in composite visceral grafts or alone. *Ann Surg* 1992;216:223
10. Todo S, Tzakis A, Reyes J, et al: Intestinal transplantation at the University of Pittsburgh. *Transplant Proc* 1994;26:1409
11. Tzakis A, Todo S, Reyes J, et al: Clinical intestinal transplantation: focus on complications. *Transplant Proc* 1992;24:1238
12. Furukawa H, Brown M, Abu-Elmagd K: Abnormal gastric emptying after intestinal transplantation. *Transplant Proc* 1994;26:1634
13. Hamdani R, Celluri L, Selby R, et al: Sudden death in patients with pulmonary hypertension undergoing liver transplantation (abstract). *Hepatology* 1991;14(Program issue):282A
14. Beeson P, Brannon E, Warren J: Observations on the sites of removal of bacteria from blood in patients with bacterial endocarditis. *J Exp Med* 1945;81:9
15. Rolando N, Harvey F, Javier B, et al: Prospective study of bacterial infection in acute liver failure: an analysis of 50 patients. *Hepatology* 1990;11:49
16. Rolando N, Harvey F, Brahm J, et al: Fungal infection: a common, recognized complication of acute liver failure. *J Hepatol* 1991;12:1
17. Grimm G, Ferenchi P, Katzenschlager R, et al: Improvement of hepatic encephalopathy treated with flumazenil. *Lancet* 1988;2:1392
18. Howard C: Flumazenil in the treatment of hepatic encephalopathy. *Ann Pharmacother* 1993;27:46
19. Sherlock S: Vasodilatation associated with hepatocellular disease: relation to functional organ failure. *Gut* 1990;31:365
20. Furukawa H, Casavilla A, Abu-Elmagd K, et al: Basic considerations for the procurement of intestinal grafts. *Transplant Proc* 1994;26:1470
21. Todo S, Tzakis AG, Abu-Elmagd K, et al: Cadavearic small bowel-liver transplantation in humans. *Transplantation* 1992;53:369
22. Tzakis AG, Todo S, Reyes J, et al: Liver and small bowel transplantation for short gut syndrome in a child. *Transpl Sci* 1991;27:33
23. Todo S, Tzakis A, Reyes J, et al: Small intestinal transplantation in humans with or without colon. *Transplantation* 1994;57:840
24. Tzakis AG, Todo S, Reyes J, et al: Piggyback orthotopic intestinal transplantation. *Surg Gynecol Obstet* 1993;176:297
25. Nour B, Reyes J, Tzakis AG, et al: Intestinal transplantation

with or without other abdominal organs: nutritional and dietary management of 50 patients. *Transplant Proc* 1994;26:1432

26. Funovits M, Miller S, Kovalak J, et al: Hospitalization and readmission of intestinal transplantation recipients. *Transplant Proc* 1994;26:1419
27. Kusne S, Manez R, Bonet H, et al: Infectious complications after small bowel transplantation in adults. *Transplant Proc* 1994;26:1682
28. Green M, Reyes J, Nour B, et al: Early infectious complications of liver-intestinal transplantation in children: preliminary analysis. *Transplant Proc* 1994;26:1420
29. Reyes J, Abu-Elmagd K, Tzakis A, et al: Infectious complications after human small bowel transplantation. *Transplant Proc* 1992;24:1249
30. Abu-Elmagd K, Todo S, Tzakis A, et al: Intestinal transplantation and bacterial overgrowth in humans. *Transplant Proc* 1994;26:1684
31. Manez R, Kusne S, Abu-Elmagd K, et al: Factors associated with recurrent cytomegalovirus disease after small bowel transplantation. *Transplant Proc* 1994;26:1422
32. Marduchowicz G, Shmueli D, Shapira Z, et al: Rhinocerebral muromycosis in renal transplant recipients: report of three cases and review of the literature. *Rev Infectious Dis* 1986;8:441
33. Morrison VA, McGlave PB: Mucormycosis in the bone marrow tranplant population. *Bone Marrow Transplant* 1993;11:383
34. Kaplan AH, Ponza-Juncal E, Shapiro R, et al: Cure of muromycosis in a renal transplant patient receiving cyclosporin with maintenance of immunosuppression. *Am J Nephrol* 1988;8:139
35. Hay RJ: Liposomal amphotericin B, Ambisome. *J Infection* 1994;28(Suppl 1):35
36. Hall JC, Brewer JH, Reed WA: Cutaneous mucormycosis in a heart transplant patient. *Cutis* 1988;42:183
37. Munckof BW, Jones R, Tosolini FA, et al: Cure of rhizopus sinusitis in a liver transplant recipient with liposomal amphotericin. *Clin Infectious Dis* 1993;16:183
38. Abu-Elmagd K, Todo S, Tzakis A, et al: Rejection of human intestinal allografts: alone or in combination with the liver. *Transplant Proc* 1994;26:1430
39. Calne RY, Sells RA, Pena JR, et al: Induction of immunological tolerance by porcine liver allografts. *Nature* 1969;223:472
40. Hassanein T, Schade R, Soldevilla-Pico C, et al: Endoscopy is essential for early detection of rejection in small bowel transplant recipients. *Transplant Proc* 1994;26:1414
41. Hassanein T, Schade R, Soldevilla-Pico C, et al: Clinical and endoscopic features of rejection in small bowel transplant recipients. *Transplant Proc* 1994;26:1413
42. Ikoma A, Nakada K, Suzuki T, et al: Gastrointestinal motility in the immediate postoperative period after intestinal transplantation, with special reference to acute rejection. *Transplant Proc* 1994;26:1657
43. Kadry Z, Furukawa H, Abu-Elmagd K, et al: Use of the D-xylose absorption test in monitoring intestinal allograft. *Transplant Proc* 1994;26:1645
44. Staschak-Chicko S, Altieri K, Funovits M, et al: Eating difficulties in the pediatric small bowel recipient: the role of the nutritional management team. *Transplant Proc* 1994;26:1434
45. Reyes J, Tzakis A, Bonet H, et al: Lymphoproliferative disease after intestinal transplantation under primary FK-506 immunosuppression. *Transplant Proc* 1994;26:1426
46. Randawa PS, Demetris J, Nalesnik MA: EBER gene expression in Epstein-Barr virus-associated hematologic malignancy. *Leukemia Lymphoma* 1994;13:387
47. Reyes J, Tzakis A, Nour B, et al: Candidates for intestinal transplantation and possible indications of outcome. *Transplant Proc* 1994;26:1447

Critical Care, Third Edition, edited by Joseph M. Civetta,
Robert W. Taylor, and Robert R. Kirby.
Lippincott-Raven Publishers, Philadelphia, PA © 1997.

CHAPTER 91

∎

Bone Marrow Transplantation

Richard K. Burt

In bone marrow transplantation (BMT), morbidity and mortality usually result from regimen-related toxicity, complications of graft-versus-host disease (GVHD), or infection. To minimize toxicity from high-dose chemoradiotherapy, potential candidates should have a normal resting cardiac ejection fraction; pulmonary function indices including diffusing capacity (DLCO), forced expiratory volume in 1 second (FEV$_1$), and forced vital capacity (FVC) greater than 50% to 75% of normal; hepatic transaminases less than twice normal; creatinine less than 2 mg/dL; and a pretransplant performance status that allows the patient to live and function independently.[1–5] The risk of GVHD increases with age, and, therefore, its severity is reduced by usually limiting allogeneic BMT to patients younger than 55 years of age. In contrast, candidates for autologous BMT, which is not complicated by GVHD, may be as old as 65 to 70 years of age.[6] The risk of infection is minimized by various prophylaxis or isolation procedures. Because of the risk of uncontrollable infection after conditioning regimen myeloablation, patients with active infection generally have BMT delayed until the infection is eradicated.[7,8] Despite these precautions, the early mortality rate (first 100 days) of autologous BMT is roughly 5% and in genotypically matched allogeneic transplants, approximately 20%.[7,8]

IMMEDIATE CONCERNS (FIRST 30 DAYS) ∎

CONDITIONING REGIMENS

In the case of allogeneic transplants, conditioning regimens must ablate host immunity to prevent rejection of the graft.[9,10] If the recipient of an allograft has a malignancy,

the conditioning regimen is also designed for tumoricidal activity. The most important immunosuppressive conditioning agents are radiation (e.g., total-body irradiation [TBI]), cyclophosphamide, and antilymphocyte antibodies such as antithymocyte globulin.[10] An exception to the necessity of a conditioning regimen to ensure engraftment is HLA-matched sibling transplantation for severe combined immune deficiency because no host immunity exists.

For autologous BMTs, the selection of conditioning regimen drugs is based on tumor efficacy, a steep dose-response curve, lack of cross-resistance with other drugs, and low extramedullary dose-limiting toxicity. In general, these conditions are most closely approximated by alkylating agents, which are often used in two or more drug combinations. For autologous BMT, immunosuppression is an unnecessary and unwanted side effect of exceeding hematopoietic dose-limiting toxicity. With the exception of hematologic malignancies, TBI generally is not used in autologous marrow transplants because effective tumoricidal doses exceed extramedullary dose-limiting toxicity.

Because the design of conditioning regimens generally has been empirical with few randomized trials, the superiority of one regimen over another has not been clearly established.[11] Therefore, choice of a conditioning regimen depends not only on effectiveness for a particular disease and the need of immunosuppression for engraftment, but also on avoiding toxicity from prior treatment or current organ dysfunction. For example, prior mantle irradiation or exposure to radiosensitizers such as bleomycin or carmustine (BCNU) increases the pulmonary toxicity of TBI, whereas heavy pretreatment of testicular cancer patients with cisplatin increases nephrotoxicity of platinum-based conditioning regimens. The extramedullary dose-limiting toxicity of common conditioning regimen agents is listed in Table 91-1.

TABLE 91-1.   Toxicity of Some Conditioning Regimen Drugs

DRUG/DOSE	EXTRAMEDULLARY DOSE-LIMITING TOXICITY	OTHER TOXICITIES
BCNU (carmustine) (250–600 mg/m^2)	Interstitial pneumonitis	Renal insufficiency, encephalopathy, nausea, vomiting, VOD
Busulphan (12–16 mg/kg)	Mucositis, VOD	Seizures, rash, hyperpigmentation, nausea, vomiting, pneumonitis
CCNU (lomustine) (200–500 mg/m^2)	Interstitial pneumonitis	Renal insufficiency, encephalopathy, nausea, vomiting, VOD
Cyclosphamide (120–200 mg/kg)	Heart failure	Hemorrhagic cystitis, SIADH, nausea, vomiting, pulmonary edema, interstitial pneumonitis
Cytarabine (4–36 g/m^2)	Mucositis, CNS ataxia	Pulmonary edema, conjunctivitis, rash, fever, hepatitis, toxic epidermal necrolysis
Cisplatin (150–180 mg/m^2)	Renal insufficiency, peripheral neuropathy	Nausea, vomiting, renal tubular acidosis, hypomagnesemia
Carboplatin (450 mg/m^2)	Ototoxicity, hepatitis	Renal insufficiency, hypomagnesemia, peripheral neuropathy
Etoposide (450–2000 mg/m^2; 60 mg/kg)	Mucositis	Nausea, vomiting, hemorrhagic cystitis, pneumonia, hepatitis
Ifosfamide (12–16 g/m^2)	CNS—encephalopathy, renal insufficiency	Hemorrhagic cystitis, renal tubular acidosis
Melphalan (120–200 mg/m^2)	Mucositis	Nausea, vomiting, hepatitis, SIADH, pneumonitis, renal insufficiency
Mitoxantrone (30–75 mg/m^2)	Cardiac	Mucositis
Paclitaxel (625 mg/m^2)	Mucositis	Peripheral neuropathy, bradycardia, anaphylaxis
Thiotepa (10 mg/kg)	Mucositis	Intertriginous rash, hyperpigmentation, nausea, vomiting

VOD, venoocclusive disease of the liver; CNS, central nervous system; SIADH, syndrome of inappropriate secretion of antidiuretic hormone.

STEM CELL HARVEST

Stem cells may be collected from the bone marrow, peripheral blood,[12–16] or umbilical cord.[17] The traditional method of collecting stem cells is a bone marrow harvest. This procedure is performed in the operating room under general, epidural, spinal, or caudal anesthesia. The donor may be admitted and discharged the day of the harvest. For an allogeneic BMT donor, an autologous unit of blood may be donated in advance to be available on the day of bone marrow harvest. The complications of bone marrow harvest are rare but include the risk of anesthesia (hypotension, nausea, vomiting, cardiac arrest, and pulmonary emboli) and the procedure itself (pain, hemorrhage, and infection).

Collection of peripheral blood stem cells is an outpatient procedure that is done using an apheresis device. Because of the low number of stem cells normally present in the peripheral blood, chemotherapy, growth factors, or both are used to increase stem cell yield. The timing of apheresis depends on the method of priming stem cells. In general, apheresis is done daily for 1 to 4 days starting 4 days after initiating a growth factor. However, after chemotherapy, apheresis is initiated when the absolute neutrophil count reaches 1000/μL (usually 10 to 16 days after chemotherapy). The advantages of collecting peripheral blood stem cells include the absence of anesthesia; the ability to use it in patients with hypocellular, fibrotic, or disease-infiltrated marrow; and a more rapid myeloid engraftment with a shorter duration of neutropenia. Disadvantages of peripheral blood stem cell collection in allogeneic BMT are exposure of a normal donor to the side effects of growth factors and the possibility of an increased risk to the recipient of acute or chronic GVHD when compared with a bone marrow graft. This is because cells that mediate GVHD are predominately T lymphocytes, and the marrow contains tenfold less T cells compared with peripheral blood. However, in preliminary studies, reinfusion of cryopreserved peripheral blood stem cells has not been associated with an increase in acute GVHD, whereas the risk of chronic GVHD is unknown.[18–20] The cost of a peripheral blood stem cell collection is approximately the same as a bone marrow harvest. Complications of peripheral blood stem cell collection are infrequent and include infection, anaphylaxis, and hypocalcemia, which may cause numbness, parathesia, cramps, nausea, or arrhythmias.

Cord blood stem cells are obtained from the umbilical cord and placental blood at the time of birth. Approximately 2 to 4 × 10⁷ nucleated blood cells per kilogram donor weight are harvested. This is more than tenfold less than than the usual 2 to 4 × 10⁸ nucleated cells per kilogram recipient weight obtained with a marrow harvest. Because of the smaller number of cells that can be collected, cord blood transplants have currently been limited to children. Potential advantages of cord blood are use of a product that would otherwise be discarded, a larger ratio of proliferative progenitor cells per number of cells collected when compared with a marrow harvest, and the possibility of less GVHD from the immature lymphocytes present in cord blood.

STEM CELL INFUSION

Bone marrow or peripheral blood stem cells may be cryopreserved in dimethyl sulfoxide (DMSO).[21] Intracellular contents of lysed cells and DMSO itself may cause hypotension anaphylaxis or arrhythmias, including transient first-, second-, or third-degree heart block.[22] To avoid complications, patients are premedicated with phenhydramine hydrochloride (Benadryl) and methylprednisolone sodium succinate (Solu-Medrol) before infusion. At the time of infusion, intubation equipment and epinephrine should be available at the bedside. If hypotension occurs, the infusion is slowed or temporarily interrupted until the blood pressure stabilizes. If the hematopoietic stem cells have not been cryopreserved, the risk of anaphylaxis is no different than a regular blood transfusion and premedication is not necessary.

Stem cell harvests are routinely analyzed for quality control at various times during collection, processing, storage, or reinfusion. Approximately 0.5% to 3% of cultures obtained during this process are positive for bacterial growth.[23] Most cultures grow gram-positive organisms that colonize the skin; however, pathogenic gram-negative bacteria are occasionally present. Marrow and peripheral blood stem cell collections inconvenience the donor and cost approximately $12,000.00. Thus, despite positive culture results, most centers reinfuse the stem cells after initiating appropriate antibiotic coverage on the recipient.[23] Although controversial, this approach has generally been without adverse side effects.

FLUIDS AND HYPOTENSION

High-dose chemoradiotherapy damages vascular endothelial cells, resulting in extravascular leakage of fluids.[24] Furthermore, GVHD and cytokines such as tumor necrosis factor (TNF), interleukin (IL)-2, and interferon-gamma (IFN γ) contribute to a posttransplant capillary leak phenomenon.[24-27] In addition, patients often receive large volumes of fluids in the form of intravenous medications, parenteral nutrition, and prophylaxis for hemorrhagic cystitis. Therefore, all patients undergoing BMT have a tendency to gain weight. Diuretics are frequently dosed to maintain baseline weight and prevent fluid retention. If hypotension develops, emphasis should be on early invasive cardiovascular monitoring, inotropic support, and red blood cell (RBC) transfusion to maintain intravascular oncotic pressure. Aggressive hydra-

tion may precipitate pulmonary and peripheral edema, even with normal pulmonary artery occlusion pressure (PAOP) and right atrial pressure.

ELECTROLYTES

Electrolyte abnormalities are common in patients undergoing BMT and are secondary to the underlying disease, prophylactic hydration for hemorrhagic cystitis, diarrhea, parenteral nutrition, renal insufficiency, diuretics, and other medications. Ifosfamide, especially in combination with carboplatin, causes a Fanconi's renal tubular acidosis beginning 3 to 7 days after the conditioning regimen.[28] The resulting normal anion gap acidosis may be treated by addition of sodium bicarbonate to intravenous fluids. Other medications associated with renal tubular wasting of electrolytes are amphotericin, foscarnet, and aminoglycosides. The syndrome of inappropriate secretion of antidiuretic hormone may result from high-dose cyclophosphamide and ifosfamide. The immunosuppressive medication, cyclosporine, may cause hypomagnesemia, and hypokalemia or hyperkalemia. Hypomagnesemia increases the risk of cyclosporine-associated seizures. Because most patients undergoing BMT are in a partial or complete remission and are receiving aggressive hydration, tumor lysis syndrome, which causes hyperphosphatemia, hyperkalemia, hypocalcemia, and hyperuricemia, is uncommon. Finally, uric acid, a major antioxidant in blood, is markedly decreased during the early BMT period, independent of allopurinol administration.[29]

BLOOD PRODUCTS

Patients undergoing BMT are immunosuppressed and at risk for developing transfusion-associated GVHD. All blood products except fresh frozen plasma and cryoprecipitate are contaminated by white blood cells (WBCs) and should be irradiated (2500 cGy) before infusion.[30] As a note of caution, hematopoietic progenitor or stem cells (i.e., bone marrow) must be viable to reestablish hematopoiesis and should never be irradiated.

Restriction to cytomegalovirus (CMV)-negative blood products is recommended in allogeneic BMT when both donor and recipient are CMV seronegative and preferred when the recipient is CMV seronegative but the donor is CMV seropositive.[31-33] If CMV-negative blood is not available, removal of WBCs with in-line microfilters (pall filters) may be as effective as CMV-seronegative blood in preventing CMV disease.[34,35] Like all herpes viruses, CMV is a latent virus that is never eradicated from an infected host. Thus, when the allogeneic recipient is CMV seropositive, there is no CMV preference for transfused blood products. Autologous transplants are not complicated by GVHD or posttransplant immunosuppressive medications, and the risk of CMV disease is low.[36] Thus, in autologous transplants, there is no CMV preference for transfused blood products.

In allogeneic transplants, special consideration must be given to ABO incompatibility between the recipient and host.[37-39] As engraftment occurs, the recipient will switch to donor ABO phenotype. However, a transition period exists in which the recipient RBCs and isohemagglutinins remain present. This confusion in terms of blood product support should be viewed in terms of whether a major or minor ABO incompatibility exists between the recipient–donor pair (Table 91-2). A major ABO incompatibility occurs when the recipient has isohemagglutinins to the donor RBC phenotype (e.g., recipient group O, donor group B). To prevent a hemolytic reaction, the donor marrow or peripheral blood stem cells must be depleted of RBCs before infusion. After stem cell infusion, the patient should receive either recipient group RBCs or group O RBCs that are plasma depleted and donor group platelets and plasma. A minor ABO incompatibility occurs when the donor has isohemagglutinins to the recipient RBC blood group (e.g., donor group O, recipient group B). Donor isohemagglutinins are depleted by removing plasma from marrow or peripheral blood stem cells before infusion. After stem cell infusion, the recipient should receive group O RBCs and recipient group plasma and platelets. If the recipient–donor pair have isoagglutinins to each other's ABO phenotype (e.g., recipient group A, donor group B), a combined major/minor ABO incompatibility exists. In this case, infused marrow must be plasma and RBC depleted. After stem cell infusion, the recipient should receive group O RBCs and group AB platelets and plasma. Notice that despite the use of histocompatible platelets (HLA-matched

and crossmatched compatible), patients frequently have platelet refractory thrombocytopenia during the early BMT period. Nonimmune causes include fever, venoocclusive disease (VOD), medications, infection, disseminated intravascular coagulation, and microangiopathic anemia related to cyclosporine or GVHD.[40]

INFECTION PROPHYLAXIS

Bacterial, viral, and fungal infection prophylaxis varies considerably between institutions.[41–46] The risk for infection varies by organism according to the time after BMT and extent of immunosuppression. Prevention of bacterial infections during the early neutropenic interval after BMT is based on two observations: (1) most bacterial gram-negative infections arise from endogenous gastrointestinal flora; and (2) in studies with neutropenic animals, the oral inoculum of gram-negative organisms required to cause death is increased by colonization of the gastrointestinal tract with anaerobes. This has led to selective aerobic gastrointestinal decontamination, initially with nonabsorbable antibiotic regimens such as gentamicin–vancomycin–nystatin, and later with more palatable but also absorbable antimicrobials selective for aerobic organisms such as oral quinolines.[47–49]

TABLE 91-2. Donor–Recipient ABO Incompatibility

MAJOR ABO INCOMPATIBILITY	MINOR ABO INCOMPATIBILITY	MAJOR AND MINOR ABO INCOMPATIBILITY
Recipient has antibody to donor	Donor has antibody to recipient	Recipient has antibody to donor and donor has antibody to recipient
IMMEDIATE HEMOLYSIS		
Prevent by RBC depletion of marrow Some centers use prophylactic recipient plasma exchange before marrow infusion if titer 1:526 or greater	Prevent by plasma depletion of marrow Some centers use prophylactic recipient RBC exchange with group O RBC	Prevent by RBC and plasma depletion of marrow Some centers use prophylactic recipient group O RBC exchange and prophylactic plasma exchange when recipient isohemagglutinin titer 1:526 or greater
DELAYED HEMOLYSIS		
Occurs 2–4 wk after BMT + Direct antiglobulin test Risk increased with high recipient isohemagglutinin titer	Occurs d 9–16 after BMT + Direct antiglobulin test Risk increased with T-cell depleted marrow	+ Direct antiglobulin test
DELAYED ERYTHROPOEISIS		
Plasma exchange, erythropoietin, steroids	—	Plasma exchange, erythropoietin, steroids
TRANSFUSION RECOMMENDATIONS		
RBC: Give recipient type RBC or group O RBC that is plasma depleted, e.g., adsol	RBC: Give group O RBC	RBC: Give group O RBC
Plasma, platelets: Give donor plasma and platelets	Plasma, platelets: Give recipient plasma and platelets	Plasma, platelets: Give AB plasma and platelets

RBC, red blood cell; BMT, bone marrow transplantation; +, positive.

Standards of care for infection prophylaxis vary by institution from strict isolation in laminar airflow (LAF) rooms to ambulation in the BMT unit hallway. In LAF rooms, similar to an operating room, the patient is in a sterile environment; anyone who enters must be gloved and gowned, and the patient's food is sterilized or has a low microbial content (autoclaved or microwaved).[50–54] Prophylactic oral antimicrobial antibiotics are given to destroy enteric pathogens, which not only are reservoirs for infection but also may function as superantigens to increase the severity of GVHD.[55] LAF rooms are becoming obsolete because of questionable cost effectiveness and psychological effects from isolation of the patient. However, certain minimal standards to prevent bacterial infection include the following: a BMT unit set aside from general hospital, patient, and visitor traffic; high-efficiency particulate air (HEPA) filtration to prevent iatrogenic *Aspergillus* infection[56]; meticulous handwashing before entering a patient's room; and a diet without fresh salads, vegetables, or fruits (contaminated with gram-negative bacteria) or pepper (contaminated with *Aspergillus*).[57,58] Other measures such as shoe covers, gloves, masks, gowns, low microbial diets, and anterooms are also commonly used, but their cost-effectiveness is debatable. Bacterial prophylactic measures are generally discontinued when the absolute neutrophil count reaches 500/μL.

Prevention of fungal infections is based on prophylaxis with oral triazoles such as itraconazole or fluconazole, which are usually given orally or intravenously for the first month after BMT.[59] The azole antifungals are effective against most *Candida* sp., but in the immunosuppressed BMT patient, fluconazole has no efficacy and itraconazole has disputable effectiveness against *Aspergillus*. The best prophylaxis of infection by *Aspergillus*, which is iatrogenically spread as an aerosolized spore, is HEPA filtration in each BMT room or ward. For patients with a history of aspergillosis before BMT, the incidence of infection after BMT is 50%.[60] These individuals should receive prophylactic amphotericin intravenously during the early BMT hospitalization.[60]

Herpes simplex reactivation is prevented by prophylaxis of all seropositive recipients with intravenous or oral acyclovir for the first 30 days after BMT.[61] Treatment after the first month results in a high rate of drug-resistant virus and prolongs the development of natural immunity. Therefore, treatment beyond the first 30 BMT days is generally withheld unless clinically indicated by pain, fever, cytopenia from marrow suppression, or interference with nutrition.

FEVER AND NEUTROPENIA

Patients undergoing BMT are immunocompromised from neutropenia, breakdown in mucosal barriers (mucositis), invasive instrumentation (e.g., Foley catheter or central lines), immunosuppressive medications (e.g., cyclosporine, steroids, and methotrexate), and GVHD. Lymphocyte function also is affected with thymic involution, weak proliferative responses to T- or B-cell mitogens, and inverted CD4/CD8 ratios for 6 months after autologous BMT and 1 year after an uncomplicated allogeneic BMT.[62,63] If the allograft is complicated by chronic GVHD, abnormal lymphocyte function persists for as long as the GVHD is present.[64] The risk of

infection depends on the type of graft and correlates with the extent of immunosuppression after transplantation. Phenotypically matched unrelated, related HLA-mismatched, and T-cell–depleted allografts have a greater risk of infection than unmanipulated genotypically matched allografts, which have a greater risk of infection than autograft.

For the neutropenic BMT patient with fever (temperature above 38.0°C), the approach is similar to a non-BMT neutropenic patient.[65] A search for the source should be done, including a chest roentgenogram, blood and urine culture, and physical examination with emphasis on line sites and perineal, oropharyngeal, and sinus regions. Usually no focal source is found, and the patient is started on broad-spectrum antimicrobial antibiotics. The choice of initial antibiotics may be either an antipseudomonal penicillin and aminoglycoside; or antipseudomonal penicillin, aminoglycoside, and vancomycin; or a third-generation antipseudomonal cephalosporin. As a note of caution, autologous and allogeneic BMT patients commonly receive loop diuretics such as furosemide. The ototoxicity of this drug is increased by aminoglycosides and vancomycin. Allogeneic transplant patients are usually on cyclosporine, and the nephrotoxicity of this drug is increased by aminoglycosides. Recurrent or persistent fever for 3 to 5 days without source in a neutropenic patient is an indication for empiric antifungal therapy with amphotericin. The nephrotoxicity of amphotericin is enhanced by cyclosporine and aminoglycosides.

MUCOSITIS

The severity of mucositis depends on the conditioning regimen. The extramedullary dose-limiting toxicity of etoposide, busulfan, cytarabine, thiotepa, and paclitaxel is mucositis. Radiotherapy also contributes to mucositis. Not surprisingly, conditioning regimens containing these agents have a high incidence of severe mucositis. Other factors that increase mucositis are methotrexate and interferon-gamma. A common GVHD prophylaxis regimen is methotrexate on days 1, 3, 6, and 11 combined with daily cyclosporine. Methotrexate should be withheld if severe mucositis develops, whereas interferon-gamma should be discontinued at least 2–4 weeks before initiating TBI.

Management of mucositis includes good oral hygiene (e.g., saline, chlorhexidine, and nystatin rinses) and topical oral analgesics.[66,67] If pain is not controlled with topical analgesia, opioids should be administered by intravenous infusions or patient-controlled analgesia. Severe mucositis may necessitate prophylactic intubation to protect the airway. Ultimately, resolution of mucositis generally correlates with recovery of the neutrophil count. In animal models, myeloid growth factors such as granulocyte colony stimulating factor (G-CSF) protect the oropharyngeal and gastrointestinal mucosa from the cytotoxic effects of high-dose chemoradiotherapy.

DIARRHEA

Diarrhea in the BMT patient may be caused by the high-dose chemoradiotherapy, medications (e.g., antibiotics), infection, or GVHD.[68,69] The conditioning regimen is the most common cause of diarrhea within the first 2 weeks. Nevertheless, an infectious cause should always be suspected. Diarrhea from intestinal mucosal damage due to high-dose chemoradiotherapy generally resolves by posttransplant day 20. Infectious causes of diarrhea include bacterial pathogens (*Clostridium difficile* and *Escherichia coli* 0157:H7) viruses (CMV, herpes simplex, adenovirus, rotavirus, echovirus, astrovirus, Norwalk virus, echovirus, and Coxsackie virus), fungi, bacteria, parasites (*Strongyloides*), and protozoa (*Giardia, Cryptosporidium*). GVHD as a cause of diarrhea may be confirmed by intestinal biopsy, which reveals loss of crypts, vacuolization of crypt epithelium, karyorrhectic apoptotic debris, microabscesses, and, in severe cases, ulceration and complete denuding of the epithelium. Therapy is directed toward appropriate antibiotics for infections and immunosuppression for GVHD. Regimen- and GVHD-associated diarrhea may respond to addition of octreotide, a somatostatin analogue whose mechanism of action is partly through inhibition of secretory hormones.[70] Some viral infections (e.g., from rotavirus) have been reported to respond to oral immunoglobulin.[71]

HEMORRHAGIC CYSTITIS

Hemorrhagic cystitis occurring within 2 weeks of marrow infusion usually results from conditioning regimen agents such as cyclophosphamide, ifosfamide, or etoposide.[72–74] Prophylaxis for hemorrhagic cystitis includes hydration and diuretics to maintain urine output greater than 2.0 mL/kg.[75,76] In addition, mercaptoethane sulfate (Mesna) is often used, especially with high-dose ifosfamide.[77] Mesna is inert in plasma but is hydrolyzed in the urine to reactive monomers that conjugate alkylating agents. It may be infused by many different schedules, but all are based on its short half-life (20 minutes). Consequently, it may be given by continuous infusion or dosed frequently every 2 to 4 hours starting immediately before high-dose chemotherapy and continued until 24 hours after completing cytotoxic drug infusion. Complications of hemorrhagic cystitis are uncontrolled bleeding and clotting of the ureters or urethra, resulting in acute renal failure. Obstruction of the ureters by clots may be asymptomatic or cause renal colic from ureteral spasm. Severe pain may occur in the back or flank and radiate into the groin or genitals.

Treatment of hemorrhagic cystitis consists of placement of a Foley catheter and irrigation of the bladder with an isotonic solution (normal saline) at 250 mL/hour to prevent intravesicular clot formation. Platelet counts should be maintained above 50,000/mL with transfusions, and units of RBCs should be given as necessary to replace blood loss. In uncontrollable bleeding, a 1% solution of alum may be added to the bladder irrigation solution. Discomfort from local bladder spasm may be attenuated with the analgesic phenazopyridine hydrochloride (Pyridium) and an antispasmodic such as oxybutynin chloride (Ditropan). In severe cases, arterial embolization or cystectomy may be necessary.

Hemorrhagic cystitis occurring more than 2 weeks after marrow infusion may result from either the conditioning regimen or virus infection (adenovirus, CMV, and BK) of the vesicular epithelium.[78–80] Except for CMV, no effective antiviral drugs exists for these viruses, and treatment is similar to therapy of hemorrhagic cystitis caused by chemotherapy.

VENOOCCLUSIVE DISEASE OF THE LIVER

Venoocclusive disease of the liver (VOD) is a regimen-related toxicity occurring within the first month after BMT.[81] In contrast to Budd-Chiari syndrome, which involves thrombosis of the large hepatic veins, VOD arises from thrombosis of small terminal hepatic venules (e.g., the central venule). High-dose chemoradiotherapy damages endothelial cells throughout the body. However, metabolism or activation of chemotherapeutic drugs by hepatocytes results in a high local concentration of alkylating or other cytotoxic agents around the central venule endothelial cells. Histologically, the central venule is occluded by concentric fibrosis obliteration. The lesions are best demonstrated by a trichrome-Masson stain and are composed initially of von Willebrand factor, which by day 50 is replaced by collagen.[82] Obliteration of the central venule results in intrahepatic hypertension, elevation or reversal of portal blood flow, and ascites.

VOD is a clinical diagnosis suggested by elevated bilirubin, weight gain, ascites, and tender hepatomegaly[83–85] (Table 91-3). The reported incidence rate of VOD varies from 1.0% to 56%. This variability results partly from different conditioning regimens and slight differences in clinical criteria used to diagnose VOD. For example, although the criteria from Johns Hopkins and Seattle seem to be similar, a retrospective comparison of the two criteria for VOD in the same cohort of transplant patients yields a VOD incidence rate of 32% using Seattle's criteria versus 8% for Johns Hopkins' criteria.[86] Risk factors for VOD are elevation of transaminases before starting the cytoreductive regimen, conditioning regimen intensity, prolonged fever, and patient age.[83] Provided transaminases are normal, a positive result from hepatitis viral serology does not increase the risk of VOD. Altered chemotherapeutic drug metabolism is probably responsible for the decreased incidence of VOD in children and increased risk for VOD in patients with elevated transaminases. Cytokines that cause fever also damage endothelial cells and are probably the cause of an increased risk for VOD

TABLE 91-3. Clinical Criteria for Venoocclusive Disease of the Liver

MCDONALD CRITERIA—SEATTLE	JONES CRITERIA—JOHNS HOPKINS
BEFORE DAY 30 ANY TWO OF THE FOLLOWING:	BEFORE DAY 21 ANY TWO OF THE FOLLOWING:
Bilirubin >27 μmol/L = 1.7 g/dL	Bilirubin >34 μmol/L = 2.0 g/dL
Hepatomegaly	Hepatomegaly
Ascites or weight gain	Ascites
	Weight gain

in patients with prolonged fever. In general, the incidence of VOD has not been significantly different in recipients of allogeneic versus autologous transplants.

The clinical symptoms of VOD may be associated with many common BMT complications. Jaundice may be secondary to hemolysis (e.g., ABO incompatible recipient–donor pair), bacterial sepsis, hepatic candidiasis, parenteral nutrition, drugs (cyclosporine, methotrexate), or GVHD. Initial evaluation should include an ultrasound of the liver with Doppler measurement of portal vein blood flow. Reversal or diminished portal flow is consistent with intrahepatic obstruction of blood flow secondary to VOD.[87] Ultrasonography findings are generally present only when overt clinical disease is present.[88] If the diagnosis remains in doubt, a liver biopsy may be necessary. A percutaneous biopsy is contraindicated because of ascites, coagulopathy of liver insufficiency, and refractory thrombocytopenia. However, a transjugular biopsy may, in general, be performed safely and provides an opportunity to measure the hepatic venous pressure gradient. A gradient greater than 10 mm Hg is consistent with VOD.[89]

Therapy for VOD is predominately supportive. Emphasis should be on avoiding hepatotoxic drugs that will further damage the liver. In severe VOD, patients may develop a hepatorenal syndrome marked by renal insufficiency and a low fractional excretion of sodium. Treatment includes diuretics to maintain baseline weight and oral ursodeoxycholic acid (Ursodiol) to lower the bilirubin and prevent further hepatotoxic injury from free radicals generated by bile acids.[90,91] Some institutions attempt to maintain intravascular volume and renal perfusion with RBC transfusions, aiming to achieve a hemoglobin of 12 to 15 mg/dL. Renal doses of dopamine (0.5 to 2.0 μg/kg/minute) also have been used to maintain renal blood flow.

If the bilirubin rises above 15 to 20 mg/dL, the prognosis without more aggressive intervention is poor. Thrombolytic therapy with infusion of tissue plasminogen activator and heparin has been used with success but may be complicated by life-threatening hemorrhage.[92–96] Once the thrombus has been replaced by fibrin and collagen, thrombolytic therapy is probably ineffective. However, in late VOD, another option is a transjugular intrahepatic portal shunt to decompress the portal vein.[97–99] If the patient has otherwise engrafted without severe GVHD or evidence of disease relapse, consideration also may be given to a liver transplant.[100,101]

RESPIRATORY FAILURE

In the BMT patient, respiratory failure requiring mechanical ventilation has a high mortality.[102] Once intubated, 80% of BMT patients are never extubated. At 6 months, only 3% of patients who required intubation are still alive. Except as an indicated by a surgical procedure, the reason for intubation does not influence survival. The only favorable variables are younger age (younger than 40 years of age) and intubation more than 100 days after transplantation.

Respiratory failure within the first 30 days is usually caused by regimen-related endothelial cell damage, infection, or both.[103–106] In the early transplantation period, radio-

therapy, chemotherapy, free radicals, and cytokines damage pulmonary endothelial cells, leading to blebs in the cell membranes, separation of junctions between cells, and cell necrosis. The end result is pulmonary edema occasionally with focal or diffuse pulmonary alveolar hemorrhage.[107] This may occur without elevation of the PAOP. The median onset of alveolar hemorrhage after BMT is day 12, but it may occur as late as day 50. Symptoms are nonspecific and include dyspnea, hypoxia, and diffuse infiltrates. Although hemoptysis is rare, bronchoalveolar lavage often establishes the diagnosis by demonstrating intrapulmonary hemorrhage. Early in the course of respiratory distress, efforts should be directed toward preventing intubation. Because of diffuse pulmonary capillary leakage, the PAOP should be kept below normal while maintaining intravascular oncotic pressure and oxygen transport. Although not evaluated in prospective studies and, therefore, of unproven benefit, management may include early invasive hemodynamic monitoring, RBC transfusions to maintain the hemoglobin above 12 g/dL, ultrafiltration to decrease intravascular volume, and anticytokine monoclonal antibodies or cytokine receptor antagonists. The use of high-dose steroids is even more controversial but in theory inhibits generation of free radicals, decreases cytokine release, and dampens the inflammatory response.

The repair process after high-dose chemoradiotherapy may further interfere with gas exchange by causing interstitial fibrosis. Infection aggravates parenchymal inflammation and protracts repair of the interstitium. Because of the neutropenia, lymphopenia, immunosuppressive drugs, mucositis, aspiration, and bronchial epithelial cell damage with impaired ciliary motility, patients are susceptible to pulmonary infections. Because of neutropenia, gram-negative and gram-positive pneumonias are common in the first 30 days. Fungal infections of the lung also occur in the early BMT period, and isolation of *Aspergillus* sp. in a nasal or sputum culture mandates initiation of amphotericin. Risk factors for aspergillosis are long-term duration of impaired immunity before starting transplantation (e.g., aplastic anemia or severe combined immune deficiency); transplantations being done in facilities without HEPA filters to prevent inhalation of aerosolized spores; and previous treatment for patients who had a prior episode of invasive fungal infection. During the first BMT month, viral pneumonitis is unusual. The most common etiologic agent is herpes simplex.

HEART FAILURE

Congestive heart failure may arise from volume overload or impairment of left ventricular function secondary to sepsis or toxicity from the conditioning regimen agents such as cyclophosphamide, ifosfamide, or anthracyclines.[108–116] Pretransplant risk factors for congestive heart failure are a previous history of heart failure or a low resting ejection fraction (less than 42%).[3] Prior mediastinal irradiation or anthracycline total dose are not independent risk factors provided the ejection fraction is normal. Cyclophosphamide is a common conditioning agent whose dose-limiting extramedullary toxicity is hemorrhagic myocarditis. Transient ST segment depression and T wave inversions are common during cyclo-phosphamide infusion and should not be viewed as an indication to stop or delay therapy. Cyclophosphamide damages cardiac capillary endothelial cells, leading to hemorrhage between and separation of myocytes. The end result is loss of voltage, congestive heart failure, or pericardial effusion. Unlike doxorubicin (Adriamycin) cardiomyopathy, which arises from myocyte damage, even severe cyclophosphamide-induced left ventricular dysfunction is reversible after an interval of weeks to months.[116]

RENAL FAILURE

Renal insufficiency is usually multifactorial, including the underlying disease (e.g., myeloma paraproteins), a prerenal decrease in glomerular filtration, intrinsic renal dysfunction, or postrenal obstruction. The most common reason for renal insufficiency in the early BMT period is medications, especially amphotericin.[117,118] In the early BMT period, mortality from patients who require dialysis is approximately 85%.[119] Prerenal causes for azotemia include VOD of the liver, diarrhea, diuretics, third spacing from sepsis, hypoalbuminemia, and a capillary leak syndrome from high-dose chemoradiotherapy. VOD of the liver, similar to other causes of prerenal azotemia, is marked by decreased fractional excretion of sodium (FeNa$^+$) in the urine.

Azotemia from intrinsic renal failure may be secondary to acute tubular necrosis (ATN), glomerulonephritis, interstitial nephritis, or renal vascular damage. Causes of ATN in patients undergoing BMT are sepsis, hypovolemia, and medications such as aminoglycosides, amphotericin, platinum compounds, foscarnet, IL-2, cyclosporine, FK506, and imaging contrast dyes. In ATN, the FeNa$^+$ is high, and the urine has muddy hyaline casts. In the BMT patient, renal insufficiency secondary to glomerulonephritis usually results from streptococcal or staphylococcal bacteremia. In glomerulonephritis, the FeNa$^+$ is low, and the urine sediment contains RBC casts and increased protein. Interstitial nephritis arising in the early BMT period is usually drug induced. Causes of allergic interstitial nephritis are penicillins, cephalosporins, sulfamethoxazole–triamterene, and fluoroquinolones. In allergic interstitial nephritis, the urine FeNa$^+$ is high, and the urine sediment contains WBCs, WBC casts, and eosinophils. Renal insufficiency from renal vascular damage in the BMT patient is usually caused by medications such as cyclosporine or FK506 or a hemolytic-uremic syndrome (HUS), which is marked by schistocytes, thrombocytopenia, and azotemia. HUS arises from endothelial cell damage, which may be related to cyclosporine, GVHD, or high-dose chemoradiotherapy.

Postrenal failure in the BMT setting may result from hemorrhagic cystitis with ureteral or urethral obstruction from blood clots, retroperitoneal hemorrhage, urate nephropathy, or drugs that undergo intratubular crystallization and obstruction such as acyclovir, ciprofloxacin, and triamterene. Regardless of the cause, renal insufficiency in the BMT patient may require dose reduction of prophylactic immunosuppressive medications such as cyclopsporine, FK506, or methotrexate, which may result in an increased incidence or severity of GVHD.

ENGRAFTMENT

The definition of graft failure is controversial. However, with a conventional marrow graft, there is usually a rise in peripheral blood WBCs by 3 weeks after BMT. Earlier engraftment occurs using mobilized peripheral blood stem cells with an absolute neutrophil count greater than 500/μL obtained by day 10 to 12. Platelet recovery, defined as greater than 20,000/μL without transfusion, is frequently delayed for an additional 3 to 4 weeks after WBC engraftment. Occasionally, patients remain platelet transfusion dependent for months after BMT. In general, graft failure is defined as failure of the absolute neutrophil count to reach 100/μL by day 28. Causes of graft failure include an inadequate number of normal hematopoietic stem cells or reinfusion of damaged hematopoietic stem cells, damage to the bone marrow stromal cell microenvironment, immunologic rejection, or drug- or viral-mediated immune suppression.[120,121]

The optimal number of stem cells required for engraftment is unknown because no current method exists to identify the true pluripotential stem cell.[122] However, CD34 is a surface membrane marker for immature hematopoietic cells, and retrovirally transduced CD34 cells contribute to long-term engraftment.[123] To ensure adequate engraftment, generally 2 to 4 × 10^8 mononuclear cells/kg recipient weight or 1 to 2 × 10^6 CD34$^+$ cells/kg recipient weight are required. Patients undergoing autologous transplantation who have been heavily pretreated with multiple chemotherapy regimens have lower numbers of CD34$^+$ cells mobilized and generally take longer to engraft either because of decreased functional CD34$^+$ cells or damaged marrow stromal microenvironment. Because hematopoietic cells require marrow stromal support cells to be maintained in long-term culture, damage to the marrow microenvironment stromal cells may be assessed by in vitro long-term marrow cultures. Using this assay, defects in the marrow microenvironment account for approximately less than 5% of graft failure cases.[124-126]

Immune-mediated graft failure is not theoretically possible with autologous transplants, but it is the most common cause of graft failure for allogeneic transplants and correlates with HLA disparity. Graft failure is less than 1.0% for HLA-identical sibling transplants, 6% to 8% for unrelated phenotypically matched transplants, and up to 20% for haploidentical or three antigen-mismatched transplants[127,128] (Table 91-4). Besides donor–recipient histocompatibility differences, other factors that influence the risk of immunologic mediated graft failure are transfusion-induced allosensitization, intensity of the conditioning regimen, donor marrow T-cell depletion, and gender-mismatched transplants. Pretransplant transfusions of RBCs or platelets in patients with aplastic anemia has resulted in a higher rate of graft rejection from sensitization of recipient lymphocytes to alloreactive determinants on donor WBCs. These observations were made before microfilters were available to deplete WBCs, which cause alloimmunization. Therefore, potential allogeneic transplant candidates, especially patients with aplastic anemia, should avoid unnecessary transfusions, especially directed blood donations from a relative, and blood products should be microfiltered to remove WBCs. Removal of donor lymphocytes from the marrow to prevent GVHD increases

TABLE 91-4. Graft-Versus-Host Disease, Graft Failure, and Disease-Free Survival for Transplants With Sibling-Matched or Alternate Donors

DEGREE OF HLA MATCH	ACUTE GVHD GRADE III OR IV (%)	CHRONIC GVHD (%)	GRAFT FAILURE (%)	DFS—AML OR ALL IN REMISSION (%)	DFS—CML IN CHRONIC PHASE (%)	DFS—AML OR ALL RELAPSE (%)	DFS—CML IN TRANSFOR-MATION (%)	DFS—AA (%)
Sibling 6/6	7–15	30–35	<2	50–60	60–80	20	10–35	78–90
Related 5/6	25–30	50	7–9	40–60	60–80	20	10–35	25–40
Related 4/6	45–50	50	21	10–40	—	10	10–30	—
Haplo-identical	50–100	>50	20	10–40	—	10	10–30	—
Unrelated 6/6	45–50	55	6	45	40	20	20	30–40

AA, aplastic anemia; AML, acute myelogenous leukemia; ALL, acute lymphocytic leukemia; CML, chronic myelogenous leukemia; DFS, disease-free survival; GVHD, graft-versus-host disease.

graft failure unless more intense immunosuppressive conditioning regimens are employed.[129] The risk of destruction of donor hematopoietic cells by residual host immunity is also increased when there is a female recipient and a male donor. In this scenario, female recipients previously sensitized by multiparity or transfusion have memory against Y chromosome–specific minor antigens presented on donor hematopoietic cells.[130]

Several medications are myelosuppressive in the early BMT interval and may delay engraftment (e.g., methotrexate, sulfamethoxazole–trimethaprim).[131,132] Viruses, especially herpes simplex and CMV, are myelosuppressive, probably through infection of stromal cells.[133] A decline in peripheral blood counts after initial engraftment should always require a search for a drug or viral culprit. A decline in blood counts after initial engraftment also has been associated with tapering of immunosuppressive medications and responds to reinstitution of full immunosuppression. The effect of GVHD on hematopoiesis is poorly understood, although marrow aplasia and cytopenias are complications of chronic GVHD. Improvement in chronic GVHD with immunosuppression is generally accompanied by improvement in peripheral blood counts.[134,135]

Treatment of graft failure includes hematopoietic growth factors, a second booster graft, or further immunosuppression.[120,136,137] Patients who never engrafted have a poor prognosis. Those with a decline in peripheral blood counts after initial engraftment have a better prognosis. If graft failure—regardless of time interval from transplant—is associated with absence or disappearance of donor hematopoiesis and reemergence of host lymphocytes, then additional conditioning regimen immunosuppression is necessary for a second graft to succeed.

ACUTE GRAFT-VERSUS-HOST DISEASE

The principle manifestations of acute GVHD are rash, diarrhea, and jaundice, individually present or in combination.[138,139] Histologically, the basal cell layer of the skin, biliary ductules of the liver, and crypts of the gastrointestinal tract are involved. Symptoms usually present close to the time of engraftment, but may occur earlier or anytime within the first 100 days. Pathophysiologically, acute GVHD is an allogeneic response mediated by donor T cells, which recognize the recipient as foreign. The incidence and severity of acute GVHD increases with recipient age and HLA disparity between the recipient and host (see Table 91-4).

The major HLA genes are inherited from both paternal and maternal chromosome 6. The classic HLA class I molecules are A, B, and C. However, new HLA class I HLA molecules (e.g., F, G, and H) are being characterized. These molecules are present on the surface of all cells and present small intracellular peptides to T lymphocytes.[140] Of the class I molecules, only HLA-A and HLA-B are currently considered relevant in terms of GVHD. HLA class II molecules are DR, DP, and DQ. These surface molecules present extracellular peptides that are endocytosed, cannibalized, and represented as small peptides on the cell surface in the groove of an HLA class II molecule.[140] Even with a HLA genotypically matched transplant, GVHD may arise from host-derived peptides presented by the HLA molecules and recognized as foreign by the donor T cells.[141]

Clinically, the rash is a maculopapular erythematous lesion often initiating on the palms, soles of the feet, or intertriginous sites, which may then progress to involve the entire integument. Cutaneous GVHD may be pruritic, and in severe cases, bullae may occur. A flare of cutaneous GVHD may be precipitated by exposure to sunlight. Histologically, the dermal epidermal border is disrupted by vacuolar degeneration of epithelial cells, dyskaryotic bodies, acantholysis (separation of cell contract), epidermolysis (separation of the dermal and epidermal layers), and lymphocytic infiltration.[138,139] These clinical and histologic findings are not unique to GVHD and may occur from drug allergies or the high-dose radiochemotherapy used in the conditioning regimen.

Gastrointestinal GVHD causes as diarrhea, often with crampy pain, which in severe cases may be bloody or accompanied by an ileus.[138,139] Histologically, lymphocytes and apoptotic cells are present, and intestinal crypts are lost, which may lead to complete denudation of the epithelium. During the first 2 weeks after BMT, the conditioning regimen may give a similar clinical and histologic picture. Evaluation should include stool cultures for bacteria, fungi, and viruses, especially CMV. Sigmoidoscopy with biopsy is indicated if the diagnosis is in doubt. Hepatic GVHD presents as jaundice and an elevated alkaline phosphatase with or without elevated transaminases. GVHD of the liver may be confused with VOD or infections with CMV or *Candida*. Differentiation may require a transjugular liver biopsy. In GVHD, the liver biopsy specimen shows lymphocytic infiltration of the portal triad with apoptosis of epithelial cells lining the biliary tree.

GVHD and infections secondary to immunosuppressive therapy are the major cause of mortality in allogeneic transplants. Consequently, prophylaxis to decrease the severity of GVHD is necessary for all recipients of an allograft. The most effective method to prevent GVHD is an ex vivo twofold to threefold logarithmic depletion of T cells from the donor graft.[142,143] Using this approach, the decrease in mortality from GVHD is, however, offset by an increase in both graft failure and leukemia relapse. Newer methods of graft engineering to prevent GVHD, improve engraftment, and decrease leukemia relapse are selective depletion or add-back of particular subsets of T cells or natural killer cells to the graft.

Pharmacologic methods of preventing GVHD are technically more simple and more common than T-cell depletion. Initially, methotrexate was given weekly until day 100. Sub-sequently, the combination of daily cyclosporine and methotrexate—given on days 1, 3, 6, and 11 after marrow infusion—was found to be more efficacious in preventing GVHD than either methotrexate or cyclosporine alone.[144] Other pharmacologic prophylactic regimens in use include the combination of cyclosporine and prednisone or a combination of cyclosporine, methotrexate, and prednisone.[145] In HLA-matched sibling transplants, immunoglobulin infused weekly until day 100 results in a lower incidence of acute GVHD.[146] Because GVHD is associated with a lower relapse rate, the goal is not to necessarily eliminate GVHD but rather to balance the risk of GVHD against the risk of leukemia relapse. More immunosuppressive prophylactic regimens are, therefore, employed when the risk of GVHD is highest (HLA mismatched or unrelated donors). Less immunosuppressive regimens may be preferred when there is a higher risk of relapse (e.g., transplant patient in relapse or second or greater remission).

Clinical grading of acute GVHD is scored by individual organ involvement and then combined for an overall grade (Table 91-5). Overall grade I is not clinically significant and does not require a change in therapy. Moderate GVHD is grade II whereas severe GVHD is grade II–IV. If grade II–IV GVHD occurs despite prophylaxis (for patients not already on steroids), first-line therapy is methylprednisolone, usually 1 to 2 mg/kg/day. GVHD resistant to steroids and cyclosporine has a poor prognosis; the cause of death usually is infection.[147] Options include monoclonal or polyclonal antibodies targeted against lymphocytes or cytokines.[148–150] Anti-

TABLE 91-5. Grading Acute Graft-Versus-Host Disease

CLINICAL GRADING OF INDIVIDUAL ORGAN SYSTEMS		
ORGAN	GRADE	DESCRIPTION
Skin	+1	Maculopapular eruption over <25% of body area
	+2	Maculopapular eruption over 25–50% of body area
	+3	Generalized erythroderma
	+4	Generalized erythroderma with bullous formation and often with desquamation
Liver	+1	Bilirubin 2.0–3.0 mg/dL; AST 150–750 IU
	+2	Bilirubin 3.1–6.0 mg/dL
	+3	Bilirubin 6.1–15 mg/dL
	+4	Bilirubin >15 mg/dL
Gut	+1	Diarrhea >30 mL/kg or >500 mL/d
	+2	Diarrhea >60 mL/kg or >1000 mL/d
	+3	Diarrhea >90 mL/kg or >1500 mL/d
	+4	Diarrhea >90 mL/kg or >2000 mL/d; or severe abdominal pain with or without ileus

OVERALL GRADE*					
GRADE	SKIN	LIVER		GUT	ECOG PERFORMANCE
I	+1 to +2	0		0	0
II	+1 to +3	+1	and/or	+1	0–1
III	+2 to +3	+2 to +4	and/or	+2 to +3	2–3
IV	+2 to +4	+2 to +4	and/or	+2 to +4	3–4

ECOG, Eastern Cooperative Oncology Group; AST, aspartate aminotransferase.
*If no skin disease, the overall grade is the higher single organ grade.

thymocyte antibody is a commercially available horse- or rabbit-derived antilymphocyte antibody that is usually infused daily for 7 to 10 days. Trials of anti-CD5 ricin A-chain labeled antibody, anti-TNFα antibody, anti–IL-2α receptor antibody (anti-Tac or BT563), and IL-1 receptor antagonist have resulted in most patients entering a partial or complete remission. However, responses have generally been transient with recurrence of GVHD after stopping antibody infusion. Similar to cyclosporine, FK506 is a macrolide immunosuppressant that inhibits T-cell activation by interfering with IL-2 transcription. FK506 is, however, a more potent immunosuppressant than cyclosporine. Although no prospective controlled trials exist, switching from cyclosporine to FK506 may be useful for GVHD that is resistant to steroids and cyclosporine.[151,152]

INTERMEDIATE CONCERNS (DAYS 30 TO 100)

CMV PROPHYLAXIS

Infection prophylaxis for CMV in autologous transplants is unnecessary. In allogeneic bone marrow transplant recipients, preemptive therapy with ganciclovir is initiated when a surveillance blood or bronchoalveolar lavage (BAL) culture result is positive by shell vial for CMV. CMV viremic patients with lymphocytopenia (CD4 less than 100/μL) are at greatest risk for developing CMV disease.[153] Surveillance shell vials of blood for CMV are usually started after engraftment (absolute neutrophil count above 500/μL) and continued weekly until day 100. A positive shell vial result generally precedes evidence of CMV disease (i.e., tissue involvement) by 7 to 10 days, and preemptive therapy with ganciclovir prevents development of disease.[154–159] Therapy is usually given daily for 10 to 14 days and then three times a week until day 100. A growth factor may be necessary to prevent CMV myelosuppression.

PNEUMONITIS

Thirty to fifty percent of BMT deaths have been reported to be associated with respiratory disease.[160] From BMT day 30 to 100, although bacterial and fungal pulmonary infections occur, the two most common pulmonary disorders are idiopathic and CMV interstitial pneumonitis (IP).

IP is a more frequent complication of allogeneic BMT (40%) than autologous BMT (10%). Risk factors for IP are TBI-based conditioning regimens, severe GVHD, older age, and methotrexate GVHD prophylaxis. The median onset of IP is day 50 to 55. Presentation after 5 to 6 months is unusual. The patient is generally hypoxic and hypocapnic. Physical examination generally reveals basilar crackles, and chest roentgenogram has an interstitial reticular nodular infiltrate. Most interstitial pneumonitis (40% to 65%) is secondary to CMV infection. Diagnosis is generally with BAL. Early intervention with the combination of intravenous γ-globulin and ganciclovir has reduced the mortality of CMV pneumonitis from 100% to approximately 50%.[161–163] Adoptive immunotherapy through infusion of CMV-specific cyto-

toxic lymphocytes holds promise for future therapy.[164] Other opportunistic infectious causes of IP such as *Chlamydia trachomatis* and *Legionella pneumophila* are less common. Because *Pneumocystis carinii* pneumonia has a median onset 2 months after BMT, prophylaxis usually does not begin until after engraftment.

Idiopathic or noninfectious causes of interstitial pneumonia, account for 30% to 50% of post-BMT interstitial pneumonias.[160,165–167] The etiology is not understood but is probably related to conditioning regimen toxicity, GVHD, or some unidentified infectious organism such as human herpes virus-6.[168] As an example of conditioning-drug toxicity, patients who receive high-dose BCNU may develop a drug-induced pneumonitis after hospital discharge that initially presents as decreased exercise tolerance. After BAL to rule out infection, early intervention with steroids usually ameliorates symptoms. Unfortunately, for most cases of idiopathic pneumonia syndrome, steroid therapy has not been proven to be beneficial.

EPSTEIN-BARR VIRUS LYMPHOPROLIFERATIVE DISEASE

Infection of B lymphocytes by Epstein-Barr virus (EBV) results in B-cell proliferation. In the nonimmunocompromised individual, cytotoxic EBV-specific T lymphocytes prevent uncontrolled B-cell proliferation. In immunocompromised allogeneic transplant patients, failure of immune surveillance by EBV-specific T lymphocytes results in a polyclonal or, less often, monoclonal B-cell proliferation.[169,170] The affected lymphocytes may be of donor or host origin. EBV lymphoproliferative syndrome (EBV-LPS) occurs in approximately 0.5% of allogeneic bone marrow transplant recipients. Risk factors for EBV-LPS are a T-cell depleted marrow graft, use of antithymocyte globulin or anti-CD3 antibodies for GVHD, and an HLA-disparate transplant complicated by GVHD. The posttransplant interval for development of EBV-LPS ranges from day 45 to 500, with a median onset between day 70 and 80. Presentation before day 70 is usually associated with fever and aggressive extranodal disease. Onset after day 70 generally has a more indolent course manifest by fever and adenopathy. Antiviral therapy for EBV-LPS is generally ineffective. Intravenous infusion of anti–B-cell antibodies has been effective for polyclonal or oligoclonal proliferations but not monoclonal EBV-LPS.[171] Administration of nonirradiated donor lymphocytes that contain EBV-specific cytotoxic lymphocytes has resulted in remissions of both oligoclonal and monoclonal EBV-LPS within 14 to 30 days of infusion.[172]

LATE CONCERNS (BEYOND DAY 100)

CHRONIC GVHD

Chronic GVHD usually occurs after day 100.[173] In relation to acute GVHD, chronic disease may present de novo in patients without prior acute GVHD; or after a quiescent interval following resolution of acute GVHD; or acute GVHD may progress without remission into chronic

GVHD.[173,174] The most important risk factors for developing chronic GVHD are older recipient age and severity of acute GVHD. Whereas acute GVHD is an alloreactive process that arises from donor lymphocyte recognition of recipient tissue as foreign, chronic GVHD seems to be an autoreactive phenomena, possibly because of aberrant education of the new immune system.

Whereas acute GVHD of the skin manifests as an erythematous rash, chronic cutaneous GVHD is marked by scleroderma-like changes with hypopigmentation and hyperpigmentation, loss of hair follicles, tight firm thickened skin, and joint contractures. Mucosal involvement manifests by dryness, pain, ulceration, and lacy white oral buccosal membranes. Ocular manifestations of chronic GVHD include a sicca conjunctivitis, ectropion, and, in severe cases, ulceration of the cornea. In contrast to acute GVHD of the gastrointestinal tract, which is marked by watery or bloody diarrhea, chronic gastrointestinal GVHD manifests as nausea, anorexia, malabsorption, dysphagia, and weight loss. Ulcerations, strictures, and narrowing may occur at any site along the gastrointestinal tract. Hepatic involvement in chronic GVHD presents similarly to acute GVHD with predominance of cholestasis (elevated bilirubin and alkaline phosphatase).

Chronic GVHD may have a variety of autoreactive aspects including autoantibodies to DNA, mitochondria, smooth muscle, or connective tissue. Autoimmune syndromes associated with chronic GVHD include polymyositis, myasthenia gravis, systemic lupus erythematosus, rheumatoid arthritis, primary biliary sclerosis, and thyroiditis. Chronic GVHD of the lung presents as cough and dyspnea caused by progressive obstructive small airway disease with hyperinflated lungs and reduced midexpiratory flows. Histologically, the process resembles bronchiolitis obliterans. Finally, chronic GVHD resulting from the underlying immune dysregulation causes an immunodeficiency that predisposes to infection independent of the immunosuppressive medications used to treat GVHD.

Chronic GVHD may be limited or extensive (Table 91-6). Limited-stage chronic GVHD has a favorable prognosis and does not require therapy. Extensive-stage GVHD requires therapeutic intervention.[175] For patients with exten-

sive-stage GVHD, poor prognostic indicators are thrombocytopenia (less than 100,000/μL) and a poor performance status. The standard treatment is alternate-day oral cyclosporine and prednisone. Other options include thalidomide, extracorporeal photophoresis, psoralen plus ultraviolet irradiation for chronic cutaneous GVHD, and ursodeoxycholic acid for chronic hepatic GVHD.[175,176] The natural history of chronic GVHD is to "burn out" with time or for the patient to die, usually from an infection.

HERPES ZOSTER

Varicella zoster occurs in 20% of autologous and 20% to 50% of allogeneic bone marrow transplant recipients, usually between day 100 and 360 after BMT.[177,178] It may present with cutaneous or visceral involvement. Occasional patients may have visceral involvement without cutaneous lesions. These patients present with severe acute abdominal pain from virus reactivation in the celiac plexus, which spreads to the pancreas and small bowel. If cutaneous or visceral varicella is suspected, the patient should be hospitalized, placed in isolation, and administered intravenous acyclovir.

SECONDARY MALIGNANCY

In addition to relapse of the original disease, BMT patients are at increased risk for a second malignancy.[179-183] After autologous BMT, there is an increase in clonal karyotypic hematopoietic cell abnormalities characteristic of therapy-related myelodysplastic syndrome, including monosomy 5 or 7 and translocations involving 11q23. These abnormalities have been reported to be as high as 9% in 3 years and are probably related to preharvesting exposure of the marrow to cytoreductive chemotherapy regimens. After allogeneic BMT, the age-adjusted risk of developing a new leukemia, lymphoma, or solid tumor is four to six times higher than the general population. Rarely has leukemia relapse been reported in the donor cells. There appears to be no plateau in the risk of solid tumors after high-dose chemoradiotherapy. Risk factors for developing a second cancer after allogeneic BMT are conditioning with TBI and grade II or greater acute GVHD. The probability of developing a second malignancy within 15 years of an allogeneic transplantation has been estimated at 6% for conditioning regimens without TBI and 20% for TBI-based regimens.

RELAPSE

Relapse more than 1 year after allogeneic BMT may be treated with a second allogeneic transplant.[184-187] If the original allogeneic regimen included TBI, the second transplantation should be a non–TBI-based regimen. If the original transplantation was without TBI, a radiation based regimen should be chosen if effective in that disease. If the original transplant was autologous, it is unlikely that a second autologous transplant would result in a long-term disease-free survival. However, an allogeneic transplant may be offered if indicated.

TABLE 91-6. Chronic Graft-Versus-Host Disease Grades

LIMITED	Disease localized only to skin involvement or hepatic

EXTENSIVE	1. Generalized skin involvement
	2. Limited skin involvement or hepatic involvement and
	   a. Liver histologic features showing chronic progressive hepatits, bridging necrosis, or cirrhosis
	   b. Eye involvement (Schirmer's test with <5 mm wetting)
	   c. Involvement of minor salivary glands or oral mucosa
	   d. Involvement of any other organ

Patients who relapse less than 1 year after allogeneic or autologous transplantation are generally not candidates for a second transplantation because of prohibitive early mortality from the conditioning regimen. However, remission may be reinduced after relapse from allogeneic BMT by withdrawal of immunosuppression with or without addition of a cytokine such as G-CSF or interferon, or infusion of donor peripheral blood leukocytes.[188-192] Donor leukocyte infusions are effective in most (60% to 80%) patients with relapsed chronic myelogenic leukemia. Several cytogenetic and polymerase chain Philadelphia-negative remissions have been reported. In acute myelogenic leukemia, approximately 30% of patients enter remission with administration of donor leukocytes. The time interval to remission after leukocyte infusion is usually 1 to 3 months. Complications of donor leukocyte infusion include bone marrow aplasia and exacerbation of GVHD. If at the time of relapse the patient is a mixed chimera (both host and donor hematopoiesis), marrow aplasia is unlikely because donor hematopoiesis remains after donor leukocyte–mediated ablation of host marrow. If the patient has rejected the donor graft and hematopoiesis is solely host in origin, then the probability of marrow aplasia is high. The risk of GVHD after donor leukocyte infusion is approximately 80% and often has a predilection toward refractory hepatic GVHD. Approaches under development for adoptive immunotherapy of relapsed leukemia after allogeneic BMT include infusion of donor lymphocytes transduced with the herpes simplex thymidine kinase or other suicide genes.[193,194] If severe GVHD occurs, activation of the suicide gene in the infused lymphocytes may terminate GVHD.

HYPOTHYROIDISM

For the first 3 to 6 months after BMT, patients may have a euthyroid sick syndrome with decreased triiodothyronine, decreased thyroxine (T_4), and low thyrotropin (TSH).[195] As in other nonthyroidal diseases associated with the euthyroid sick syndrome, these thyroid hormone abnormalities are reversible and probably are a normal physiologic response to decrease protein catabolism. Hormone replacement therapy is unnecessary.

Primary hypothyroidism after BMT is caused by high-dose radiotherapy in the conditioning regimen.[196-198] Primary hypothyroidism (elevated TSH, low or normal T_4) occurs in less than 2% of non–TBI-containing conditioning regimens and 10% to 60% of TBI-based regimens. Most of these patients have a compensated primary hypothyroidism with elevated TSH but normal T_4. Overt primary hypothyroidism (elevated TSH, low T_4) is rare after chemotherapy conditioning regimens but may develop in 3% to 13% of patients receiving a TBI-based preparatory regimen. The time interval to onset for primary hypothyroidism ranges from 6 to 41 months after BMT with a median of 13 months. The risk of primary hypothyroidism is greater after single-dose TBI than fractionated TBI regimens. Overt hypothyroidism is treated with hormonal replacement therapy. Compensated hypothyroidism may be treated with close follow-up or replacement therapy.

GROWTH AND DEVELOPMENT

For child and adolescent bone marrow transplant recipients, growth and development may be delayed or interrupted, depending on the conditioning regimen.[199-201] Other risk factors for growth retardation are pre-BMT central nervous system radiation, single-dose TBI, chronic GVHD, use of corticosteroid therapy, and patient age. Children treated with single-agent cyclophosphamide do not, in general, experience growth retardation. TBI regimens adversely affect height and growth velocity with single-dose TBI, causing more growth retardation than do fractionated regimens. Radiation also may inhibit normal dental and facial skeletal development, especially in children younger than 6 years of age. Although chemotherapy-only regimens originally were not thought to alter growth, combined busulfan and cyclophosphamide conditioning causes growth retardation comparable with the combination of cyclophosphamide and fractionated TBI.[200] The mechanisms of preparatory regimen growth retardation is incompletely understood but includes direct injury to the growth plates, decreased pituitary and hypothalamic growth hormone production, and primary gonadal failure (decreased estrogens and testosterone; elevated luteinizing hormone and follicle-stimulating hormone). For premenopausal patients, tanner secondary sexual characteristics and menarche are usually delayed.

FERTILITY

Primary gonadal failure (i.e., hypergonadotropic hypogonadism) is common after BMT.[202-204] Recovery of gonadal function is dependent on recipient age and the conditioning regimen. In postmenopausal women treated with cyclophosphamide alone, gonadal dysfunction is generally transitory and return of fertility is common. In patients conditioned with TBI regimens, virtually all develop gonadal failure. The return of menstruation within 10 years of TBI occurs in 90% to 100% of patients younger than 18 years old at the time of BMT, and in 10% to 15% of patients older than 18 years of age at the time of BMT. Results are similar for postmenopausal women conditioned with busulfan and cyclophosphamide. In one study, 50 of 50 patients developed primary gonadal failure, none of whom recovered gonadal function over a 5-year period. Gonadal failure post-BMT is often associated with symptoms of estrogen deficiency including hot flashes, dyspareunia, dysuria, and vaginal dryness, which may be ameliorated by hormonal replacement therapy.[205]

CATARACTS

Steroid therapy and TBI-containing regimens cause cataracts within a median of 2.5 to 5.0 years after BMT.[206-208] The incidence rate of cataracts is 100% for unfractionated TBI, 60% to 80% for fractionated TBI, and 5% for non-TBI regimens. The probability of requiring a cataract operation within 10 years of BMT is 100% for single-dose TBI and 20% for fractionated TBI. Eye shielding would decrease the incidence of cataracts but is generally not done because of concern for leukemia relapse.

LATE RENAL EFFECTS

Reversible renal dysfunction commonly occurs early in the course of BMT and is multifactorial, usually from drugs and sepsis. Long-term renal complications from BMT are rare. However, there are occasional reports of late-onset renal dysfunction consistent with radiation nephropathy occurring after combined multidrug and fractionated TBI regimens.[209] The onset is usually 3 to 7 months after BMT and is characterized by hypertension, edema, uremia, and, occasionally, HUS. Histologic study reveals mesangial proliferation and vascular damage. Cyclosporine used for chronic GVHD, may cause a similar picture of hypertension, renal insufficiency, and HUS.

LATE PULMONARY EFFECTS

Late pulmonary disease generally has a restrictive pulmonary ventilatory pattern with decreased diffusing capacity (DLCO).[210] These abnormalities are thought to be a consequence of the conditioning regimen, especially TBI. Occasionally an obstructive pulmonary function defect occurs, possibly because of recurrent aspirations from GVHD-associated sinus infections or impaired esophageal motility.[211,212] By 6 to 12 months after BMT, pulmonary defects either improve or remain persistent but are generally not progressive. Patients with chronic GVHD are at increased risk for bacterial and fungal infections, bronchiolitis obliterans, and lymphocytic pneumonitis.[213,214] Bronchiolitis obliterans presents as cough, wheezing, and severe obstructive lung disease with hyperinflated diaphragms resulting from obliteration of small bronchioles. It has been reported to occur between 3 and 24 months after transplantation. Although usually associated with allogeneic BMT complicated by chronic GVHD, it has also rarely been seen after autologous BMT. Therapy is generally corticosteroids. Lymphocytic pneumonitis is characterized by a lymphocytic interstitial infiltrate that may progress to fibrosis. The etiology is unclear but thought to be immune mediated and is treated with corticosteroids.

REFERENCES ■

1. Ghalie R, Szidon JP, Thompson L, et al: Evaluation of pulmonary complications after bone marrow transplantation: the role of pretransplant pulmonary function tests. *Bone Marrow Transplant* 1992;10:359
2. Milburn HJ, Prentice HG, du Bois RM, et al: Can lung function measurements be used to predict which patients will be at risk of developing interstitial pneumonitis after bone marrow transplantation? *Thorax* 1992;47:421
3. Hertenstein B, Stefanic M, Schmeiser T, et al: Cardiac toxicity of bone marrow transplantation: predictive value of cardiologic evaluation before transplant. *J Clin Oncol* 1994;12:998
4. Crawford SW, Fisher L, et al: Predictive value of pulmonary function tests before marrow transplantation. *Chest* 1992;101:1257
5. Valls A, Algara M, Marrugat J, et al: Risk factors for early mortality in allogeneic bone marrow transplantation: a multivariate analysis on 174 leukaemia patients. *Eur J Cancer* 1993;29A:1523
6. Ringden O, Horowitz MM, Gale RP, et al: Outcome after allogeneic bone marrow transplant for leukenia in older adults. *JAMA* 1993;270:57
7. Klingemann HG, Shepherd JD, Reece DE, et al: Regimen-related acute toxicities: pathophysiology, risk factors, clinical evaluation and preventive strategies. *Bone Marrow Transplant* 1994;4(Suppl 14):S14
8. Gulati SC, Yahalom J, Whitmarsh K, et al: Factors affecting the outcome of autologous bone marrow transplantation. *Ann Oncol* 1991;1(Suppl 2):51
9. Barrett AJ: Immunosuppressive therapy in bone marrow transplantation. *Immunol Lett* 1991;29:81
10. Storb R: Preparative regimens for patients with leukemias and severe aplastic anemia (overview): biological basis, experimental animal studies and clinical trials at the Fred Hutchinson Cancer Research Center. *Bone Marrow Transplant* 1994;4(Suppl 14):S1
11. Ringden O, Ruutu T, Remberger M, et al: A randomized trial comparing busulfan with total body irradiation as conditioning in allogeneic marrow transplant recipients with leukemia: a report from the Nordic Bone Marrow Transplantation Group. *Blood* 1994;83:2723
12. Kessinger A: Autologous and allogeneic transplantation with peripheral blood stem cells. *Prog Clin Biol Res* 1992;377:603
13. Nemunaitis J, Rosenfeld C: Mobilization of peripheral stem cells for transplantation. *J Hematother* 1993;2:351
14. Lowry PA, Tabbara IA: Peripheral hematopoietic stem cell transplantation: current concepts. *Exp Hematol* 1992;20:937
15. Janssen WE: Peripheral blood and bone marrow hematopoietic stem cells: are they the same? *Semin Oncol* 1993;20(Suppl 6):19
16. Craig JI, Turner ML, Parker AC: Peripheral blood stem cell transplantation. *Blood Rev* 1992;6:59
17. Flomenberg N, Keever CA: Cord blood transplants: potential utility and potential limitations. *Bone Marrow Transplant* 1992;1(Suppl 10):115
18. Korbling M, Przepiorka D, Huh YO, et al: Allogeneic blood stem cell transplantation for refractory leukemia and lymphoma: potential advantage of blood over marrow allografts. *Blood* 1995;85:1659
19. Bensinger WI, Weaver CH, Appelbaum FR, et al: Transplantation of allogeneic peripheral blood stem cells mobilized by recombinant human granulocyte colony-stimulating factor. *Blood* 1995;85:1655
20. Schmitz N, Dreger P, Suttorp M, et al: Primary transplantation of allogeneic peripheral blood progenitor cells mobilized by filgrastim (granulocyte colony-stimulating factor). *Blood* 1995;85:1666
21. Rowley SD, Bensinger WI, Gooley TA, et al: Effect of cell concentration on bone marrow and peripheral blood stem cell cryopreservation. *Blood* 1994;83:2731
22. Styler MJ, Topolsky DL, Crilley PA, et al: Transient high grade heart block following autologous bone marrow infusion. *Bone Marrow Transplant* 1992;10:435
23. Prince HM, Page SR, Keating A, et al: Microbial contamination of harvested bone marrow and peripheral blood. *Bone Marrow Transplant* 1995;15:87
24. Peters AM, Vassilarou DS, Hows JM, et al: Bone marrow transplantation: effects of conditioning and cyclosporin prophylaxis on microvascular permeability to a small solute (tech-

netium 99m diethylene triamine penta-acetic acid). *Eur J Nucl Med* 1991;18:199

25. Cahill RA, Zhao Y, Murphy R, et al: High urinary leukotriene E4 (LTE4) and thromboxane 2 (TXB2) levels are associated with capillary leak syndrome in bone marrow transplant patients. *Adv Prostaglandin Thromboxane Leukot Res* 1991; 21B:525

26. Oeda E, Shinohara K, Kamei S, et al: Capillary leak syndrome likely the result of granulocyte colony-stimulating factor after high-dose chemotherapy. *Intern Med* 1994;33:115

27. Funke I, Prummer O, Schrezenmeier H, et al: Capillary leak syndrome associated with elevated IL-2 serum levels after allogeneic bone marrow transplantation. *Ann Hematol* 1994; 68:49

28. Beckwith C, Flaharty KK, Cheung AK, et al: Fanconi's syndrome due to ifosfamide. *Bone Marrow Transplant* 1993; 11:71

29. Durken M, Agbenu J, Finckh B, et al: Deteriorating free radical-trapping capacity and antioxidant status in plasma during bone marrow transplantation. *Bone Marrow Transplant* 1995;15:757

30. Leitman SF, Holland PV: Irradiation of blood products: indications and guidelines. *Transfusion.* 1985;25:293

31. Rubie H, Attal M, Campardou AM, et al: Risk factors for cytomegalovirus infection in BMT recipients transfused exclusively with seronegative blood products. *Bone Marrow Transplant* 1993;11:209

32. Bowden RA: Cytomegalovirus infections in transplant patients: methods of prevention of primary cytomegalovirus. *Transplant Proc* 1991;23:136

33. Miller WJ, McCullough J, Balfour HH, et al: Prevention of cytomegalovirus infection following bone marrow transplantation: a randomized trial of blood product screening. *Bone Marrow Transplant* 1991;7:227

34. De Witte T, Schattenberg A, Van Dijk BA, et al: Prevention of primary cytomegalovirus infection after allogeneic bone marrow transplantation by using leukocyte-poor random blood products from cytomegalovirus-unscreened blood-bank donors. *Transplantation* 1990;50:964

35. van Prooijen HC, Visser JJ, van Oostendorp WR, et al: Prevention of primary transfusion-associated cytomegalovirus infection in bone marrow transplant recipients by the removal of white cells from blood components with high-affinity filters. *Br J Haematol* 1994;87:144

36. Wingard JR, Chen DY, Burns WH, et al: Cytomegalovirus infection after autologous bone marrow transplantation with comparison to infection after allogeneic bone marrow transplantation. *Blood* 1988;71:1432

37. Pihlstedt P, Paulin T, Sundberg B, et al: Blood transfusion in marrow graft recipients. *Ann Hematol* 1992;65:66

38. Gale RP, Feig S, Ho W, et al: ABO blood group system and bone marrow transplantation. *Blood* 1977;50:185

39. Buckner CD, Clitt RA, Sanders JE, et al: ABO incompatible marrow transplants. *Transplantation* 1978;26:233

40. Benson K, Fields K, Hiemenz J, et al: The platelet-refractory bone marrow transplant patient: prophylaxis and treatment of bleeding. *Semin Oncol* 1993;20(Suppl 6):102

41. Wimperis JZ, Baglin TP, Marcus RE, et al: An assessment of the efficacy of antimicrobial prophylaxis in bone marrow autografts. *Bone Marrow Transplant* 1991;8:363

42. Momin F, Chandrasekar PH: Antimicrobial prophylaxis in bone marrow transplantation. *Ann Intern Med* 1995;123:205

43. Dekker AW, Verdonck LF, Rozenberg-Arska M: Infection prevention in autologous bone marrow transplantation and the role of protective isolation. *Bone Marrow Transplant* 1994;14:89

44. Rowe JM, Ciobanu N, Ascensao J, et al: Recommended guidelines for the management of autologous and allogeneic bone marrow transplantation. *Ann Intern Med* 1994;120:143

45. Wingard JR: Advances in the management of infectious complications after bone marrow transplantation. *Bone Marrow Transplant* 1990;6:371

46. Karp JE, Merz WG, Dick JD, et al: Strategies to prevent or control infections after bone marrow transplants. *Bone Marrow Transplantation* 1991;8:1

47. Winston DJ, Ho WG, Nakao SL, et al: Norfloxacin versus vancomycin/polymyxin for prevention of infections in granulocytopenic patients. *Am J Med* 1986;80:884

48. Schmeiser T, Kern WV, Hay B, et al: Single-drug oral antibacterial prophylaxis with ofloxacin in BMT recipients. *Bone Marrow Transplantation* 1993;12:57

49. Winston DJ, Ho WG, Bruckner DA, et al: Ofloxaxin versus vancomycin/polymyxin for prevention of infections in granulocytopenic patients. *Am J Med* 1990;88):36

50. Russell JA, Poon M, Jones AR, et al: Allogeneic bone-marrow transplantation without protective isolation in adults with malignant disease. *Lancet* 1992;339:38

51. Buckner CD, Clift RA, Sanders JE, et al: Protective environment for marrow transplant recipients. *Ann Intern Med* 1978;89:893

52. Nauseef WM, Maki DG: A study of the value of simple protective isolation in patients with granulocytopenia. *N Engl J Med* 1981;304:448

53. Schimpff SC, Hahn DM, Brouillet MD, et al: Comparison of basic infection prevention techiques, with standard room reverse isolation or with reverse isolation plus added air filtration. *Leukemia Res* 1978;2:231

54. Mahmoud HK, Schaefer UW, Schuning F, et al: Laminar air flow versus barrier nursing in marrow transplant recipients. *Blut* 1984;49:375

55. Beelen DW, Haralambie E, Brandt H, et al: Evidence that sustained growth suppression of intestinal anaerobic bacteria reduces the risk of acute graft-versus-host disease after sibling marrow transplantation. *Blood* 1992;80:2668

56. Sherertz RJ, Belani A, Kramer BS, et al: Impact of air filtration on nosocomial *Aspergillus* infections: unique risk of bone marrow transplant recipients. *Am J Med* 1987;83:709

57. Shooter RA, Gaya H, Cooke EM, et al: Food and medicaments as possible sources of hospital strains of *Pseudomonas aeruginosa. Lancet* 1969;1:1227

58. Remington JS, Schimpff SC: Please don't eat the salads. *N Engl J Med* 1981;304:433

59. Goodman JL, Winston DJ, Greenfield RA, et al: A controlled trial of fluconzaole to prevent fungal infections in patients undergoing bone marrow transplantation. *N Engl J Med* 1992;326:845

60. Richard C, Romon I, Baro J, et al: Invasive pulmonary aspergillosis prior to BMT in acute leukemia patients does not predict a poor outcome. *Bone Marrow Transplant* 1993; 12:237

61. Saral R, Burns WH, Laskin OL, et al: Acyclovir prophylaxis of herpes-simplex-virus infections. *N Engl J Med* 1981;305: 63

62. Atkinson K: Reconstruction of the haemopoietic and immune systems after marrow transplantation. *Bone Marrow Transplant* 1990;5:209

63. Storek J, Saxon A: Reconstruction of B cell immunity following bone marrow transplantation. *Bone Marrow Transplant* 1992;9:395

64. Friedrich W, O'Reilly RJ, Koziner B, et al: T-lymphocyte reconstitution in recipients of bone marrow transplants with and without GVHD: imbalances of T-cell subpopulations hav-

ing unique regulatory and cognitive functions. *Blood* 1982; 59:696

65. Hughes WT, Armstrong D, Bodey GP, et al: Guidelines for the use of antimicrobial agents in neutropenic patients with unexplained fever. *J Infect Dis* 1990;161:381

66. Woo S, Sonis ST, Monopoli MM, et al: A longitudinal study of oral ulcerative mucositis in bone marrow transplant recipients. *Cancer* 1993;72:1612

67. Epstein JB, Vickars L, Spinelli J, et al: Efficacy of chlorhexidine and nystatin rinses in prevention of oral complications in leukemia and bone marrow transplantation. *Oral Surg Oral Med Oral Pathol* 1992;73:682

68. Yolken RH, Bishop CA, Townsend TR, et al: Infectious gastroenteritis in bone marrow transplant recipients. *N Engl J Med* 1982;306:1010

69. Cox GJ, Matsui SM, Lo RS, et al: Etiology and outcome of diarrhea after marrow transplantation: a prospective study. *Gastroenterology* 1994;107:1398

70. Ely P, Dunitz J, Rogoscheske J, et al: Use of a somatostatin analogue, octreotide acetate, in the management of acute gastrointestinal graft-versus-host disease. *Am J Med* 1991; 90:707

71. Kanfer EJ, Abrahamson G, Taylor J, et al: Severe rotavirus-associated diarrhoea following bone marrow transplantation: treatment with oral immunoglobin. *Bone Marrow Transplant* 1994;14:651

72. Yang CC, Hurd DD, Case LD, et al: Hemorrhagic cystitis in bone marrow transplantation. *Urology* 1994;44:322

73. Russell SJ, Vowels MR, Vale T: Haemorrhagic cystitis in paediatric bone marrow transplant patients: an association with infective agents, GVHD and prior cyclophosphamide. *Bone Marrow Transplant* 1994;13:533

74. Sabau DM: Hematuria in bone marrow transplant patients. *J Am Soc Nephrol* 1992;3:916

75. Turkeri LN, Lum LG, Uberti JP, et al: Prevention of hemorrhagic cystitis following allogeneic bone marrow transplant preparative regimens with cyclophosphamide and busulfan: role of continous bladder irrigation. *J Urol* 1995;153:637

76. Meisenberg B, Lassiter M, Hussein A, et al: Prevention of hemorrhagic cystitis after high-dose alkylating agent chemotherapy and autologous bone marrow support. *Bone Marrow Transplant* 1994;14:287

77. Hows JM, Mehta A, Ward L, et al: Comparison of Mesna with forced diuresis to prevent cyclophosphamide-induced hemorrhagic cystitis in marrow transplantation: a prospective randomized study. *Br J Cancer* 1984;50:753

78. Bedi A, Miller CB, Hanson JL, et al: Association of BK virus with failure of prophylaxis against hemorrhagic cystitis following bone marrow transplantation. *J Clin Oncol* 1995;13:1103

79. Liles WC, Cushing H, Holt S, et al: Severe adenoviral nephritis following bone marrow transplantation: successful treatment with intravenous ribavirin. *Bone Marrow Transplant* 1993;12:409

80. Spach DH, Bauwens JE, Myerson D, et al: Cytomegalovirus-induced hemorrhagic cystitis following bone marrow transplantation. *Clin Infect Dis* 1993;16:142

81. Bearman SI: The syndrome of hepatic veno-occlusive disease after marrow transplantation. *Blood* 1995;85:3005

82. McDonald GB, Hinds MS, Fisher LD, et al: Veno-occlusive disease of the liver and multiorgan failure after bone marrow transplantation: a cohort study of 355 patients. *Ann Intern Med* 1993;118:255

83. McDonald GB, Sharma P, Matthews DE, et al: Veno-occlusive disease of the liver after bone marrow transplantation: diagnosis, incidence, and predisposing factors. *Hepatology* 1984;4:16

84. Jones RJ, Lee KSK, Beschorner WE, et al: Venoocclusive disease of the liver following bone marrow transplantation. *Transplantation* 1987;44:778

85. Shulman HM, Gown AM, Nugent DJ: Hepatic veno-occlusive disease after bone marrow transplantation: immunohistochemical identification of the material within occluded central venules. *Am J Pathol* 1987;127:549

86. Blostein MD, Paltiel OB, Thibault A, et al: A comparison of clinical criteria for the diagnosis of veno-occlusive disease of the liver after bone marrow transplantation. *Bone Marrow Transplant* 1992;10:439

87. Herbetko J, Grigg AP, Buckley AR, et al: Veno-occlusive liver disease after bone marrow transplantation: findings at duplex sonography. *AJR* 1992;158:1001

88. Hommeyer SC, Teefey SA, Jacobson AF, et al: Veno-occlusive disease of the liver: prospective study of US evaluation. *Radiology* 1992;184:683

89. Shurman HM, McDonald GB: Tranvenoces liver biopsies and pressure measurement in bone marrow transplant recipients. *Hepatology* 1992;16:148

90. Essell JH, Thompson JM, Harman GS, et al: Pilot trial of prophylactic ursodiol to decrease the incidence of veno-occlusive disease of the liver in allogeneic bone marrow transplant patients. *Bone Marrow Transplant* 1992;10:367

91. Essell J, Schroeder M, Thompson J, et al: A randomized double-blind trial of prophylactic ursodeoxycholic acid vs. placebo to prevent veno-occlusive disease of the liver in patients undergoing allogeneic bone marrow transplantation. *Blood* 1994;84(Suppl 1):250a

92. Baglin TP, Harper P, Marcus RE, et al: Veno-occlusive disease of the liver complicating ABMT successfully treated with recombinant tissue plasminogen activator. *Bone Marrow Transplant* 1990;5:439

93. Bearman SI, Shuhart MC, Hinds MS, et al: Recombinant human tissue plasminogen activator for the treatment of established severe venocclusive disease of the liver after bone marrow transplantation. *Blood* 1992;80:2458

94. Laporte JP, Lesage S, Tilleul P, et al: Alteplase for hepatic veno-occlusive disease complicating bone marrow transplantation. *Lancet* 1992;339:1057

95. Rosti G, Bandini G, Belardinelli A, et al: Alteplase for hepatic veno-occlusive disease after bone-marrow transplantation. *Lancet* 1992;339:1481

96. Ringden O, Wennberg L, Ericzon BG, et al: Alteplase for hepatic veno-occlusive disease after bone marrow transplantation. *Lancet* 1992;340:546

97. Murray JA, LaBrecque DR, Gingrich RD, et al: Successful treatment of hepatic venocclusive disease in a bone marrow transplant patient with side-to-side portacaval shunt. *Gastroenterology* 1987;92:1073

98. Jacobson BK, Kalayoglu M: Effective early treatment of hepatic venocclusive disease with a central splenorenal shunt in an infant. *J Pediatr Surg* 1992;27:531

99. Ochs A, Sellinger M, Haag K, et al: Transjugular intrahepatic portosystemic stent-shunt (TIPS) in the treatment of Budd-Chiari syndrome. *J Hepatol* 1993;18:217

100. Nimer SD, Milewicz AL, Champlin RE, et al: Successful treatment of hepatic venocclusive disease in a bone marrow transplant patient with orthotopic liver transplantation. *Transplantation* 1990;49:819

101. Rapoport AP, Doyle HR, Starzl T, et al: Orthotopic liver transplantation for life-threatening venocclusive disease of the liver after allogeneic bone marrow transplant. *Bone Marrow Transplant* 1991;8:421

102. Faber-Langendown K, Caplan AL, McGlave PB: Survival of adult bone marrow transplant patients receiving mechanical

ventilation: a case for restricted use. *Bone Marrow Transplant* 1993;12:501

103. Seiden MV, Elias A, Ayash L, et al: Pulmonary toxicity associated with high dose chemotherapy in the treatment of solid tumors with autologous marrow transplant: an analysis of four chemotherapy regimens. *Bone Marrow Transplant* 1992; 10:57

104. Carlson K, Backlund L, Smedmyr B, et al: Pulmonary function and complications subsequent to autologous bone marrow transplantation. *Bone Marrow Transplant* 1994;14:805

105. Jules-Elysee K, Stover DE, Yahalom J, et al: Pulmonary complications in lymphona patients treated with high-dose therapy and autologous bone marrow transplantation. *Am Rev Respir Dis* 1992;146:485

106. Breuer R, Lossos IS, Berkman N, et al: Pulmonary complications of bone marrow transplantation. *Respir Med* 1993; 87:571

107. Agusti C, Ramirez J, Picado C, et al: Diffuse alveolar hemorrhage in allogeneic bone marrow transplantation. *Am J Respir Crit Care Med* 1995;151:1006

108. Quezado ZM, Wilson WH, Cunnion RE, et al: High-dose ifosfamide is associated with severe, reversible cardiac dysfunction. *Ann Intern Med* 1993;118:31

109. Pihkala J, Saarinen UM, Lundstrom U, et al: Effects of bone marrow transplantation on myocardial function in children. *Bone Marrow Transplant* 1994;13:149

110. Lewkow L, Hooker J, Movahed A: Cardiac complications of intensive dose mitoxantrone and cyclophosphamide with autologous bone marrow transplantation in metastatic breast cancer. *Int J Cardiol* 1992;34:273

111. Cazin B, Gorin NC, LaPorte JP, et al: Cardiac complications after bone marrow transplantation. *Cancer* 1986;57:2061

112. Braverman AC, Antin JH, Plappert MT, et al: Cyclophosphamide cardiotoxicity in bone marrow transplantation: a prospective evaluation of new dosing regimens. *J Clin Oncol* 1991;9:1215

113. Ayash LJ, Wright JE, Tretyakov O, et al: Cyclophosphamide pharmacokeinetics: correlation with cardiac toxicity and tumor response. *J Clin Oncol* 1992;10:995

114. Goldberg MA, Antin JH, Guinan EC, et al: Cyclophosphamide cardiotoxicity: an analysis of dosing as a risk factor. *Blood* 1986;68:1114

115. Steinherz LJ, Steinherz PG, Mangiacasale D, et al: Cardiac changes with cyclophosphamide. *Med Pediatr Oncol* 1981; 9:417

116. Gottdiener JS, Appelbaum FR, Ferrans VJ, et al: Cardiotoxicity associated with high-dose cyclophosphamide therapy. *Arch Intern Med* 1981;141:758

117. Zager RA, O'Quigley J, Zager BK, et al: Acute renal failure following bone marrow transplantation: a retrospective study of 272 patients. *Am J Kidney Dis* 1989;13:210

118. Zager RA: Acute renal failure in the setting of bone marrow transplantation. *Kidney Int* 1994;46:1443

119. Lane PH, Mauer SM, Blazer BR, et al: Outcome of dialysis for acute renal failure in pediatric bone marrow transplant patients. *Bone Marrow Transplant* 1994;13:613

120. Quinones RR: Hematopoietic engraftment and graft failure after bone marrow transplantation. *Am J Pediatr Hematol Oncol* 1993;15:3

121. Berthou C, Devergie A, Esperou-Bourdeau H, et al: Late marrow failure occuring after HLA identical bone marrow transplant. *Bone Marrow Transplant* 1991;7(Suppl 2):50

122. Orlic D, Bodine DM: What defines a pluripotent hematopoietic stem cell (PHSC): will the real PHSC please stand up! *Blood* 1994;84:3991

123. Dunbar CE, Cottler-Fox M, O'Shaughnessy JA, et al: Retrovirally marked CD34-enriched peripheral blood and bone marrow cells contribute to long-term engraftment after autologous transplantation. *Blood* 1995;85:3048

124. O'Flaherty E, Sparrow R, Szer J: Bone marrow stromal function from patients after bone marrow transplantation. *Bone Marrow Transplantation* 1995;15:207

125. Torok-Strob B, Holmberg L: Role of marrow microenvironment in engraftment and maintenance of allogeneic hematopoietic stem cells. *Bone Marrow Transplant* 1994;14(Suppl 4):S71

126. Holmberg L, Seidel K, Leisenring W, et al: Aplastic anemia analysis of stromal cell function in long-term marrow cultures. *Blood* 1994;84:3685

127. Davies SM, Ramsay NKC, Haake RJ, et al: Comparison of engraftment in recipients of matched sibling or unrelated donor marrow allografts. *Bone Marrow Transplant* 1994;13: 51

128. Bearman SI, Mori M, Beatty PG, et al: Comparison of morbidity and mortality after marrow transplantation form HLA-genotypically identical siblings and HLA-phenotypically identical unrelated donors. *Bone Marrow Transplant* 1994;13:31

129. Champlin R: T-cell depletion for allogeneic bone marrow transplantation: impact on graft-versus-host disease, engraftment, and graft-versus-leukemia. *J Hematother* 1993; 2:27

130. Goulmy E, Termijtelen A, Bradley BA, et al: Y-antigen killing by T cells of women is restricted by HLA. *Nature* 1977; 266:544

131. Domenech J, Linassier C, Gihana E, et al: Prolonged impairment of hematopoiesis after high-dose therapy followed by autologous bone marrow transplantation. *Blood* 1995;85:3320

132. Canals C, Marti JM, Martinez E, et al: Hematological recovery after autologous bone marrow transplantation in acute leukemia: predictive factors. *J Hematother* 1993;2:75

133. Bilgrami S, Almeida GD, Quinn JJ, et al: Pancytopenia in allogeneic marrow tranplant recipients: role of cytomegalovirus. *Br J Haematol* 1994;87:357

134. Nakao S, Nakatsumi T, Chuhjo T, et al: Analysis of late graft failure after allogeneic bone marrow transplantation: detection of residual host cells using amplification of variable number of tandem repeats loci. *Bone Marrow Transplant* 1992;9:107

135. Atkinson K, Dodds A, Concannon A, et al: Late onset transfusion-dependent anaemia with thrombocytopenia secondary to marrow fibrosis and hypoplasia associated with chronic graft-versus-host disease. *Bone Marrow Transplant* 1987; 2:445

136. Weisdorf DJ, Verfaillie CM, Davies SM, et al: Hematopoietic growth factors for graft failure after bone marrow transplantation: a randomized trial of granulocyte-macrophage colony-stimulating factor (GM-CSF) versus sequential GM-CSF plus granulocyte-CSF. *Blood* 1995;85:3452

137. Stroncek DF, McGlave P, Ramsey N, et al: Effects on donors of second bone marrow collections. *Transfusion* 1991;31:819

138. Ferrara JLM, Deeg HJ: Graft-versus-host disease. *N Engl J Med* 1991;324:667

139. Deeg HJ, Storb R: Graft-versus-host disease: pathophysiological and clinical aspects. *Annu Rev Med* 1984;35:11

140. Barber LD, Parham P: Peptide binding to major histocompatibility complex molecules. *Annu Rev Cell Biol* 1993;9:163

141. Brochu S, Baron C, Belanger R, et al: Graft–host tolerance in bone marrow transplant chimers: absence of graft-versus-host disease is associated with unresponsiveness to minor histocompatibility antigens expressed by all tissues. *Blood* 1994;84:3221

142. Martin PJ, Hansen JA, Buckner CD, et al: Effects of in

vitro depletion of T cells in HLA-identical allogeneic marrow grafts. *Blood* 1985;66:664

143. Ringden O, Pihlstedt P, Markling L, et al: Prevention of graft-versus-host disease with T cell depletion or cyclosporin and methotrexate: a randomized trial in adult leukemic marrow recipients. *Bone Marrow Transplant* 1991;7:221

144. Storb R, Deeg HJ, Whitehead J, et al: Methotrexate and cyclosporine compared with cyclosporine alone for prophylaxis of acute graft versus host disease after marrow transplantation for leukemia. *N Engl J Med* 1986;314:729

145. Leelasiri A, Greer JP, Stein RS, et al: Graft-versus-host disease prophylaxis for matched unrelated donor bone marrow transplantation: comparison between cyclosporine-methotrexate and cyclosporine-methotrexate-methylprednisolone. *Bone Marrow Transplant* 1995;15:401

146. Sullivan KM, Kopecky KJ, Jocom J, et al: Immunomodulatory and antimicrobial efficacy of intravenous immunoglobulin in bone marrow transplantation. *N Engl J Med* 1990;323:705

147. Sayer HG, Longton G, Bowden R, et al: Increased risk of infection in marrow transplant patients receiving methylprednisolone for graft-versus-host disease prevention. *Blood* 1994;84:1328

148. Belanger C, Esperou-Bourdeau H, Bordigoni P, et al: Use of an anti–interleukin-2 receptor monoclonal antibody for GVHD prophylaxis in unrelated donor BMT. *Bone Marrow Transplant* 1993;11:293

149. Antin JH, Ferrara JL: Cytokine dysregulation and acute graft-versus-host disease. *Blood* 1992;80:2964

150. Herve P, Flesch M, Tiberghien P, et al: Phase I-II trial of a monoclonal anti-tumor necrosis factor and antibody for the treatment of refractory severe acute graft-versus-host disease. *Blood* 1992;79:3362

151. Nash RA, Etzioni R, Storb R, et al: Tacrolimus (FK506) alone or in combination with methotrexate or methylprednisolone for the prevention of acute graft-versus-host disease after marrow transplantation from HLA-matched siblings: a single-center study. *Blood* 1995;85:3746

152. Koehler MT, Howrie D, Mirro J, et al: FK506 (tacrolimus) in the treatment of steroid resistant acute graft-versus-host disease in children undergoing bone marrow transplantation. *Bone Marrow Transplant* 1995;15:895

153. Einsele H, Ehninger G, Steidle M, et al: Lymphocytopenia as an unfavorable prognostic factor in patients with cytomegalovirus infection after bone marrow transplantation. *Blood* 1993;82:1672

154. The TH, van der Ploeg M, van den Berg AP, et al: Direct detection of cytomegalovirus in peripheral blood leukocytes: a review of the antigenemia assay and polymerase chain reacton. *Transplantation* 1992;54:193

155. Boeckh M, Bowden RA, Goodrich JM, et al: Cytomegalovirus antigen detection in peripheral blood leukocytes after allogeneic marrow transplantation. *Blood* 1992;80:1358

156. Goodrich JM, Mori M, Gleaves CA, et al: Early treatment with ganciclovir to prevent cytomegalovirus disease after allogeneic bone marrow transplantion. *N Engl J Med* 1991;325:1601

157. Schmidt GM, Horak DA, Niland JC, et al: A randomized, controlled trial of prophylactic ganciclover for cytomegalovirus pulmonary infection in recipients of allogeneic bone marrow transplantation. *N Engl J Med* 1991;324:1005

158. Ljungman P, De Bock R, Cordonnier C, et al: Practices for cytomegalovirus diagnosis, prophylaxis, and treatment in allogeneic bone marrow transplant recipients: a report from the Working Party for Infectious Disease of the EBMT. *Bone Marrow Transplant* 1993;12:399

159. Webster A, Blizzard B, Pillay D, et al: Value of routine surveil-lance cultures for detection of CMV pneumonitis following bone marrow transplantation. *Bone Marrow Transplant* 1993;12:477

160. Clark TG, Hansen JA, Hertz MI, et al: Idiopathic pneumonia after bone marrow transplantation: NHLBI workshop summary. *Am Rev Respir Dis* 1993;147:1601

161. Emanuel D, Cunningham I, Jules-Elysee K, et al: Cytomegalovirus pneumonia after bone marrow transplant successfully treated with the combination of ganciclovir and high-dose intravenous immune globulin. *Ann Intern Med* 1988;109:777

162. Reed EC, Bowden RA, Dandliker PS, et al: Treatment of cytomegalovirus pneumonia with ganciclovir and intravenous cytomegalovirus immunoglobulin in patients with bone marrow transplants. *Ann Intern Med* 1988;109:783

163. Ljungman P, Engelhard D, Link H, et al: Treatment of interstitial pneumonitis due to cytomegalovirus with ganciclovir and intravenous immune globulin: experience of European Bone Marrow Transplant Group. *Clini Infect Dis* 1992;14:831

164. Riddell SR, Watanabe KS, Goodrich JM, et al: Restoration of viral immunity in immunodeficient humans by the adoptive transfer of T cell clones. *Science* 1992;257:238

165. Granena A, Carreras E, Rozman C, et al: Interstital pneumonitis after BMT: 15 years' experience in a single institution. *Bone Marrow Transplant* 1993;11:453

166. Crawford SW, Hackman RC: Clinical course of idiopathic pneumonia after bone marrow transplantation. *Am Rev Respir Dis* 1993;147:1393

167. Kaplan EB, Pietra GG, August CS: Intersititial pneumonitis, pulmonary fibrosis, and chronic graft-versus-host disease. *Bone Marrow Transplant* 1992;9:71

168. Cone RW, Hackman RC, Huang ML, et al: Human herpes virus 6 in lung tissue from patients with pneumonitis after bone marrow transplantation. *N Engl J Med* 1993;329:156

169. Zutter MM, Martin PJ, Sale GE, et al: Epstein-Barr virus lymphoproliferation after bone marrow transplantation. *Blood* 1988;72:520

170. Shapiro RS, McClain K, Frizzera G, et al: Epstein-Barr virus associated B cell lymphoproliferative disorders following bone marrow transplantation. *Blood* 1988;71:1234

171. Fischer A, Blanche S, Le Bidois J, et al: Anti–B-cell monoclonal antibodies in the treatment of severe B-cell lymphoproliferative syndrome following bone marrow and organ transplantation. *N Engl J Med* 1991;324:1451

172. Papadopoulos EB, Ladanyi M, Emanuel D, et al: Infusions of donor leukocytes to treat Epstein-Barr virus–associated lymphoproliferative disorders after allogeneic bone marrow transplantation. *N Engl J Med* 1994;330:1185

173. Atkinson K: Chronic grarft-versus-host disease. *Bone Marrow Transplant* 1990;5:69

174. Sullivan KM, Shulman HM, Storb R, et al: Chronic graft-versus-host disease in 52 patients: adverse natural course and successful treatment with combination immunosuppression. *Blood* 1981;57:267

175. Siadek M, Sullivan KM: The management of chronic graft-versus-host disease. *Blood Rev* 1994;8:154

176. Vogelsang GB, Farmer ER, Hess AD, et al: Thalidomide for the treatment of chronic graft-versus-host disease. *N Engl J Med* 1992;326:1055

177. Atkinson K, Storb R, Prentice RL, et al: Analysis of late infections in 89 long-term survivors of bone marrow transplantation. *Blood* 1979;53:720

178. Han CS, Miller W, Haake R, et al: Varicella zoster infection after bone marrow transplantation: incidence, risk factors and complications. *Bone Marrow Transplant* 1994;13:277

179. Socie G, Henry-Amar M, Bacigalupo A, et al: Malignant

tumors occuring after treatment of aplastic anemia. *N Engl J Med* 1993;329:1152

180. Deeg HJ, Witherspoon RP: Risk factors for the development of secondary malignancies after marrow transplantation. *Hematol Oncol Clin North Ame* 1993;7:417

181. Traweek ST, Slovak ML, Nademanee AP, et al: Clonal karyotypic hematopoietic cell abnormalities occuring after autologous bone marrow transplantation for Hodgkin's disease and non-Hodgkin's lymphoma. *Blood* 1994;84:957

182. Lowsky R, Lipton J, Fyles G, et al: Secondary malignancies after bone marrow transplantation in Adults. *J Clin Oncol* 1994;12:2187

183. Witherspoon RP, Deeg HJ, Storb R: Secondary malignancies after marrow transplantation for leukemia or aplastic anemia. *Transplantation Science* 1994;4:33

184. Boiron JM, Cony-Makhoul P, Mahon FX, et al: Treatment of hematological malignancies relapsing after allogeneic bone marrow transplantation. *Blood Rev* 1994;8:234

185. Barrett AJ, Locatelli F, Treleaven JG, et al: Second transplants for leukaemic relapse after bone marrow transplantation: high early mortality but favourable effect of chronic GVHD on continued remission. A report by the EBMT Leukaemia Working Party. *Br J Haematol* 1991;79:567

186. Mrsic M, Horowitz MM, Atkinson K, et al: Second HLA-identical sibling transplants for leukemia recurrence. *Bone Marrow Transplant* 1992;9:269

187. Wagner JE, Vogelsang GB, Zehnbauer BA, et al: Relapse of leukemia after bone marrow transplantation: effect of second myeloablative therapy. *Bone Marrow Transplant* 1992;9:205

188. Kumar L: Leukemia: management of relapse after allogeneic bone marrow transplantation. *J Clin Oncol* 1994;12:1710

189. Drobyski WR, Keever CA, Roth MS, et al: Salvage immunotherapy using donor leukocyte infusions as treatment for relapsed chronic myelogenous leukemia after allogeneic bone marrow transplantation: efficacy and toxicity of a defined T-cell dose. *Blood* 1993;82:2310

190. Drobyski WR, Roth MS, Thibodeau SN, et al: Molecular remission occuring after donor leukocyte infusions for the treatment of relapsed chronic myelogenous leukemia after allogeneic bone marrow transplantation. *Bone Marrow Transplant* 1992;10:301

191. Giralt S, Escudier S, Kantarjian H, et al: Preliminary results of treatment with filgrastim for relapse of leukemia and myelodysplasia after allogeneic bone marrow transplantation. *N Engl J Med* 1993;329:757

192. Giralt SA, Champlin RE: Leukemia relapse after allogeneic bone marrow transplantation: a review. *Blood* 1994;84:3603

193. Bordignon C, Bonini C, et al: Transfer of HSV-tk gene into donor peripheral blood lymphocytes for in vivo modulation of donor anti-tumor immunity after allogeneic bone marrow transplantation. *Hum Gene Ther* 1995;6:813

194. Tiberghien P, et al: Ganciclovir treatment of herpes simplex thymidine kinase-transduced lymphocytes: an approach for specfic in vivo donor T-cell depletion after bone marrow transplantation. *Blood* 1994;84:1333

195. Vexiau P, Perez-Castiglioni P, Socie G, et al: The euthyroid sick syndrome: incidence risk factors and prognostic value soon after allogeneic bone marrow transplantation. *Br J Haematol* 1993;85:778

196. Lio S, Arcese W, Papa G, et al: Thyroid and pituitary function following allogeneic bone marrow transplantation. *Arch Intern Med* 1988;148:1066

197. Carlson K, Lonnerholm G, Smedmyr B, et al: Thyroid function after autologous bone marrow transplantation. *Bone Marrow Transplant* 1992;10:123

198. Sklar CA, Kim TH, Ramsey NK: Thyroid dysfunction among long-term survivors of bone marrow transplantation. *Am J Med* 1982;73:688

199. Sanders JE, Seattle Marrow Transplant Team: The impact of marrow transplant preparative regimens on subsequent growth and development. *Semin Hematol* 1991;28:244

200. Wingard JR, Plotnick LP, Freemer CS, et al: Growth in children after bone marrow transplantation: busulfan plus cyclophosphsphamide versus cyclophosphamide plus total body irradiation. *Blood* 1992;79:1068

201. Sanders JE, Pritchard S, Mahoney P, et al: Growth and development following marrow transplantation for leukemia. *Blood* 1986;68:1129

202. Hinterberger-Fischer M, Kier P, Kalhs P, et al: Fertility, pregnancies and offspring complications after bone marrow transplantation. *Bone Marrow Transplant* 1991;7:5

203. Cust MP, Whitehead MI, Powles R, et al: Consequences and treatment of ovarian failure after total body irradiation for leukaemia. *Br Med J* 1989;299:1494

204. Spinelli S, Chiodi S, Bacigalupo A, et al: Ovarian recovery after total body irradiation and allogeneic bone marrow transplantation: long-term follow up of 79 females. *Bone Marrow Transplant* 1994;14:373

205. Schubert MA, Sullivan KM, Schubert MM, et al: Gynecological abnormalities following allogeneic bone marrow transplantation. *Bone Marrow Transplant* 1990;5:425

206. Tichelli A, Gratwohl A, Egger T, et al: Cataract formation after bone marrow transplantation. *Ann Intern Med* 1993;119:1175

207. Dunn JP, Jabs DA, Wingard J, et al: Bone marrow transplantation and cataract development. *Arch Opthalmol* 1993;111:1367

208. Bray LC, Carey PJ, Proctor SJ, et al: Ocular complications of bone marrow transplantation. *Br J Ophthalmol* 1991;75:611

209. Tarbell N, Guinan EC, Niemeyer C, et al: Late onset of renal dysfunction in survivors of bone marrow transplantation. *Int J Radiat Oncol Biol Phys* 1988;15:99

210. Depledge M, Hons B, Biol MI, et al: Lung function after bone marrow grafting. *J Radiat Oncol Biol Phys* 1983;9:145

211. Schultz KR, Green GJ, Wensley D, et al: Obstructive lung disease in children after allogeneic bone marrow transplantation. *Blood* 1994;84:3212

212. Sisson JH, Reed EC, Robbins RA, et al: Impairment of nasal mucociliary clearance during bone marrow transplantation. *Bone Marrow Transplant* 1994;13:631

213. Schwarer AP, Hughes JMB, Trotman-Dickerson B, et al: A chronic pulmonary syndrome associated with graft-versus-host disease after allogeneic marrow transplanation. *Transplantation* 1992;54:1002

214. Yousem SA: The histological spectrum of pulmonary graft-versus-host disease in bone marrow transplant recipients. *Hum Pathol* 1995;26:668

SECTION VIII

The Obstetric Patient

Critical Care, Third Edition, edited by Joseph M. Civetta,
Robert W. Taylor, and Robert R. Kirby.
Lippincott-Raven Publishers, Philadelphia, PA © 1997.

CHAPTER 92

■

Cardiac Disease and Hypertensive Disorders in Pregnancy

Christopher F. James

IMMEDIATE CONCERNS ■

MAJOR PROBLEMS

Pregnancy, labor, delivery, and the immediate postpartum period cause profound physiologic changes that may result in exacerbations of chronic illnesses or death from an acute obstetric pathologic process. Major obstetric conditions include hypertensive disorders; amniotic fluid embolism; peripartum cardiomyopathy; and hemorrhagic or septic shock from placenta previa, abruptio placentae, uterine atony, inversion or rupture, and chorioamnionitis. The major nonobstetric conditions during pregnancy include respiratory disorders—mainly asthma, pneumonia, pulmonary embolus, and pulmonary aspiration (see Chap. 94)—and cardiac disease, including rheumatic and congenital abnormalities.

STRESS POINTS

1. Significant hemodynamic changes occur in pregnancy (Table 92-1). Maternal blood volume increases throughout pregnancy and peaks to about 40% above nonpregnant levels at term.[1] The increase in plasma volume (45% to 55%) is greater than the increase in red blood cell volume (20% to 30%), resulting in a relative anemia of pregnancy. This increase in blood volume is associated with an increase in cardiac output, which begins early in gestation and peaks at levels 30% to 40% over nonpregnant values between

20 and 30 weeks.[1,2] The increase then plateaus until term.

2. The enlarging uterus in the third trimester predisposes to aortocaval compression and decreased cardiac output in supine patients. However, in the lateral position, cardiac output is maintained in the latter part of pregnancy. Turning from the supine to the lateral decubitus position increases cardiac output from 8% at 20 to 24 weeks to as much as 30% near term.[3]

3. Inferior vena cava compression occurs in up to 90% of near-term parturients in the supine position. However, only about 10% to 15% of patients manifest the supine hypotensive syndrome because of shunting of venous blood away from the caval system to the azygous system by the intervertebral plexus of veins. Patients most susceptible to supine hypotension are those with polyhydramnios and multiple gestation.

4. The increase in cardiac output with gestation is dependent on heart rate and stroke volume. Heart rate gradually increases throughout pregnancy, starting as early as 4 weeks' gestation, with a 10% to 15% increase by term. Stroke volume, in contrast, peaks during the second trimester with a 20% to 40% increase over the nonpregnant state.

5. During labor, cardiac output rises another 15% to 45% above prelabor values with an additional increase of 10% to 25% during uterine contractions (Fig. 92-1). The increase in cardiac output in labor

1389

TABLE 92-1. Hemodynamic Changes in Pregnancy

	% CHANGE*		
	Pregnancy	*Labor and Delivery*	*Postpartum*
Cardiac output	+30–50	+50–65†	+60–80
Heart rate	+10–15	+10–30†	−10–15
Stroke volume	+20–30	+40–70	+60–80
Blood volume	+20–80	—	+0–10
Plasma volume	+44–55	—	+0–30
Red cell volume	+20–30	—	−10
Oxygen consumption	+20	+40–100†	−10–15
Systemic vascular resistance	−10–25	—	—
Systemic blood pressure			
Systolic	−5	+10–30†	+10
Diastolic	−10	+10–30†	+10
Pulmonary vascular resistance	−30	—	—
Pulmonary artery occlusion pressure (PAOP)	0	—	—
Colloid oncotic pressure (COP)	−10	—	—
COP–PAOP	−25	—	—

*Percent change from nonpregnant state.

†Percent change without regional anesthesia (local anesthetic).

during contractions versus that seen between contractions is greater late in the first stage (34%) versus early in the first stage (16%)[4] (see Fig. 92-1).

6. Oxygen consumption increases 20% during pregnancy and may increase as much as 40% to 100% during active labor. In the immediate postpartum period, cardiac output increases 30% to 40% over the labor period or 60% to 80% over the nonpregnant state, with the increased blood volume to the central circulation from the contracted uterus, alleviation of aortocaval compression, and slight decrease in total peripheral resistance.

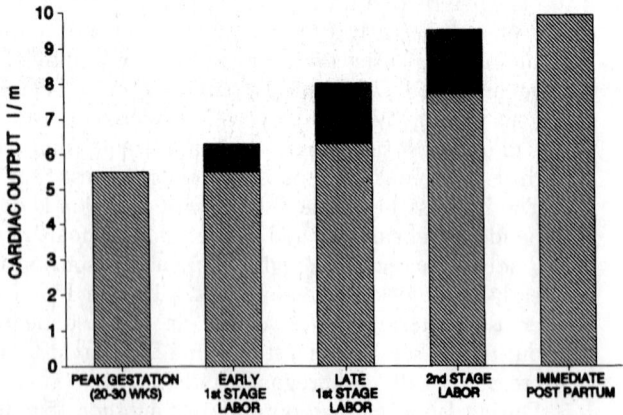

FIGURE 92-1. Cardiac output (CO) during pregnancy, labor, and delivery. (Estimated values without regional anesthesia, because CO may vary dramatically among individuals. Solid bars represent CO increases during contractions.)

7. Cardiac output and other hemodynamic parameters have been thought to return to their baseline, prepregnant state by 6 weeks after delivery. However, cardiac output may remain elevated for at least 12 weeks.[5]

8. Systemic arterial pressure changes minimally during pregnancy. There is a slight decrease in systolic and diastolic pressures, the latter more than the former, resulting in an increase in pulse pressure. Systemic vascular resistance decreases 10% to 20% during pregnancy. Moreover, systemic vascular resistance may remain decreased for at least 12 weeks.

9. Venous pressure in the lower extremities increases and peaks near term as the gravid uterus compresses the inferior vena cava, especially when the patient is supine, while central venous pressure remains unchanged. Total body water increases by about 2 kg throughout pregnancy.

10. Invasive pulmonary artery (PA) catheterization in low-risk, near-term pregnant patients (36 to 38 weeks) reveals a significant decrease in pulmonary vascular resistance, colloid oncotic pressure (COP), and COP–pulmonary artery occlusion pressure (PAOP) gradient with no change in PAOP or left ventricular stroke work index.[6]

11. Until recently, we did not appreciate that significant changes in maternal body composition and cardiopulmonary and metabolic functions occur by 7 weeks of gestation. These changes include increases in body fat (2%), plasma volume (11%), heart rate (16%), minute ventilation (24%), and oxygen consumption (10%).[7]

ESSENTIAL DIAGNOSTIC TESTS, PROCEDURES, AND THERAPY

1. With significant increase in oxygen consumption, especially during labor, along with a decrease in functional residual capacity, the importance of adequacy of preoxygenation and denitrogenation before rapid sequence induction of anesthesia cannot be overemphasized.
2. Morbidity and mortality statistics from England and Wales reveal that anesthetic-related maternal mortality is predominantly caused by inability to intubate the trachea or by pulmonary aspiration during general anesthesia.[8,9] Thus, an awake orotracheal intubation should be considered when airway patency is suspect.
3. Despite an average 200- to 500-mL blood loss for routine, uncomplicated vaginal deliveries and an 800- to 1000-mL blood loss for cesarean section deliveries, blood transfusions are seldom necessary because of the increased blood volume and the autotransfusion of approximately 500 mL of blood from the contracted uterus in the postpartum period. Although this increase in blood volume protects against blood loss at delivery, pulmonary congestion and cardiac failure can result in patients with underlying cardiac dysfunction.
4. Normal factors in pregnancy that favor the development of pulmonary edema include an increase in intravascular volume, decreased blood viscosity ("physiologic anemia of pregnancy"), decreased COP, and fluid shifts, especially in the immediate postpartum period.
5. Patients with minimal cardiac reserve may tolerate early pregnancy and subsequently decompensate from increasing blood volume and cardiac output in the late second trimester and early third trimester.
6. Patients with moderate cardiac reserve may tolerate pregnancy well until labor and delivery or the puerperium. Thus, cardiac patients should continue to be closely monitored in the postpartum period because cardiac decompensation most frequently occurs during this time; the prepregnant baseline state may not be reached for as long as 12 weeks after delivery.
7. Uterine displacement by maternal position (lateral decubitus), bed position (left lateral tilt), or uterine displacement devices is imperative, especially in the last trimester, to avoid aortocaval compression. Moreover, maternal hypotension and placental hypoperfusion from aortocaval compression can be compounded by regional anesthesia that interferes with compensatory sympathetic nervous system mechanisms.
8. Earlier studies in elective cesarean section patients revealed up to a 90% incidence rate of hypotension under spinal anesthesia without pretreatment with intravenous fluid bolus and with the patient in the supine position.[10] Recently, despite attention to intravenous fluid augmentation and patient position, the incidence rate of hypotension in elective cesarean

section patients with epidural anesthesia, with or without prophylactic ephedrine, approached 30%.[11]
9. As a consequence of some of these cardiovascular changes, normal symptoms during pregnancy include fatigue, dyspnea, decreased exercise capacity, and light-headedness (Table 92-2). Cardiac signs are distended neck veins, peripheral edema, loud first heart sound, loud third heart sound, systolic ejection murmurs, and continuous murmurs (cervical venous hums and mammary souffle). Fourth heart sounds and diastolic murmurs occur rarely in normal pregnancy and should be considered pathologic unless proven otherwise.
10. Normal chest radiographic findings demonstrate increased lung markings (prominent pulmonary vasculature from the decreased lung volume and a horizontal position of the heart caused by diaphragmatic elevation). Electrocardiographic (ECG) changes may include a left QRS axis deviation and nonspecific ST segment and T wave changes.
11. In summation, the normal signs and symptoms of pregnancy may simulate pathologic disease states, thereby rendering the diagnosis of heart disease difficult. Problems of more invasive diagnostic methods during pregnancy make echocardiography a valuable and safe diagnostic tool. Specifically, transesophageal echocardiography has been used recently for anesthetic management in the perioperative period in New York Heart Association (NYHA) class IV patients with a cardiomyopathy.[12]

TABLE 92-2. Normal Cardiac Symptoms and Signs in Pregnancy

SYMPTOMS
  Fatigue
  Dyspnea
  Decreased exercise tolerance
  Light-headedness
  Syncope

SIGNS
  General
    Distended neck veins
    Peripheral edema
    Hyperventilation
  Heart
    Loud S_1; increased split S_1
    Loud S_3
    Systolic ejection murmur
    Continuous murmurs (venous hum, mammary souffle)
  Chest radiograph
    Increased pulmonary vasculature
    Horizontal position of heart
  Electrocardiogram
    Left axis deviation
    Nonspecific ST-T wave changes
    NSR, sinus tachycardia, SVT

NSR, normal sinus rhythm; SVT, supraventricular tachycardia.

HYPERTENSIVE DISORDERS ■

Hypertension during pregnancy has been classified with difficulty by the American College of Obstetricians and Gynecologists. Simply, hypertension in pregnancy can be divided into four categories: (1) pregnancy-induced hypertension made up of mild and severe preeclampsia and eclampsia; (2) chronic hypertension (hypertension that presents before pregnancy); (3) chronic hypertension with superimposed preeclampsia or eclampsia; and (4) latent or transient hypertension of the third trimester. Most chronic hypertensive pregnant patients have essential hypertension, which has no appreciable effect during pregnancy unless end-organ damage is present. Similarly, latent or transient hypertension is also relatively benign, occurring in the last trimester or the immediate postpartum period with a return of normotension by the first 2 weeks after delivery.

PREECLAMPSIA/ECLAMPSIA

Etiology

Preeclampsia is defined as hypertension occurring after 20 weeks' gestation (unless a hydatidiform mole is present). It is accompanied by proteinuria (>300 mg/24 hours) and peripheral edema. The etiology is unknown but may be related to the following: uteroplacental ischemia, resulting in increased vascular resistance and decreased uteroplacental blood flow; an immunologic disorder resulting in a vascular endothelial injury; or a prostaglandin imbalance with greater levels of thromboxane than prostacyclin, resulting in vasoconstriction and platelet aggregation.

Recently, an early marker of preeclampsia in the first trimester has been demonstrated by an exaggerated response of platelet intracellular calcium when exposed to arginine vasopressin[12] and increased plasma fibronectin levels.[13] Severe preeclampsia is defined by one or more of the following: systolic blood pressure greater than 160 mm Hg; diastolic blood pressure greater than 110 mm Hg; mean arterial pressure greater than 120 mm Hg; proteinuria greater than 5 g in 24 hours; oliguria less than 500 mL in 24 hours; and headaches, visual disturbances, epigastric pain, pulmonary edema, or cyanosis. Eclampsia results when seizures occur that are not related to other underlying disorders.

Pathophysiology

Preeclampsia is characterized by decreased plasma volume, decreased albumin levels, and increased blood viscosity. Generalized arteriolar vasospasm accounts for the hypertension in preeclampsia,[14] which is labile because of intensive sensitivity of the vasculature to endogenous and exogenous pressor peptides and catecholamines. Despite an increase in total body water from salt and water retention, intravascular volume is decreased below that of a normal pregnancy but may be slightly higher than in the nonpregnant state. Albumin and COP are further decreased from normal pregnancy and markedly lower than in the nonpregnant state.[15]

Renal function impairment is reflected by decreased renal blood flow and glomerular filtration rate secondary to swelling of intracapillary glomerular cells, fibrin deposition along the basement membranes, and afferent arteriolar spasm. The central nervous system (CNS) changes are characterized by irritability and hyperreflexia. Eclampsia consists of grand mal seizures with tonic and clonic phases. The etiology is unknown but may be attributed to cerebral microcirculatory obstruction, platelet–fibrin clots, or intense cerebral vasoconstriction.

Although disseminated intravascular coagulation is rare in preeclampsia/eclampsia, other coagulation abnormalities are common. Thrombocytopenia occurs in up to 15% of severe preeclamptics and 30% of eclamptics, along with increased fibrin split products and slightly prolonged partial thromboplastin times.[16]

Management

The definitive treatment of preeclampsia/eclampsia is delivery of the fetus and placenta. Otherwise, management includes prevention of convulsions, decrease of CNS hyperactivity, and control of hypertension. Magnesium sulfate is the most commonly used anticonvulsant for this purpose in the United States. It is usually administered as a slow intravenous bolus of 2 to 4 g, followed by a continuous infusion of 1 to 3 g/hour to maintain therapeutic levels of 4 to 6 mEq/L. Greater serum levels can lead to progressive disappearance of deep tendon reflexes and respiratory or cardiac arrest. Magnesium sulfate also produces mild sedation, peripheral vasodilation, and decreased uterine tone and potentiates both depolarizing and nondepolarizing muscle relaxants.

In addition to bed rest and magnesium sulfate administration, antihypertensive agents such as hydralazine are used. For an acute hypertensive crisis, a continuous infusion of trimethaphan, nitroglycerin (NTG), or sodium nitroprusside (SNP) should be used with intraarterial monitoring of blood pressure. Nitroprusside should be used only for short-term management of severe hypertension (the perioperative or peridelivery period) to diminish the risk of fetal cyanide toxicity. Moreover, SNP and NTG should be used cautiously in patients with severe CNS manifestations. The drugs may contribute to increases of intracranial pressure by diminishing cerebral blood flow autoregulation. Despite the potential drawbacks of SNP, it is the most effective of the agents for acute control of severe hypertension, that is, before anesthesia induction for delivery by cesarean section. NTG may not adequately lower blood pressure because its main effect is venodilation, and trimethaphan has a high incidence of tachyphylaxis.

Clinical Considerations

Most severe preeclamptic patients have normal or hyperdynamic left ventricular function with normal PA pressure. Thus, a CVP monitor usually is adequate to assess volume status and left ventricular function. However, severely preeclamptic patients may develop cardiac failure, progressive and marked oliguria, or pulmonary edema. In such cases, a PA catheter is indicated for proper diagnosis and treatment, because right and left ventricular pressures may not correlate.[17,18] Systemic blood pressure should be monitored at least with an automatic blood pressure device. An intraarterial catheter monitor is indicated for protracted severe hypertension and therapy with potent antihypertensive agents. Spinal anesthesia is not recommended in severe preeclampsia/eclampsia. Systemic blood pressure cannot be as well controlled because of the more rapid onset of action and more profound block with spinal anesthesia than can occur with a slowly titrated lumbar epidural anesthetic.

After vaginal or cesarean delivery, the severe preeclamptic patient should be placed in an ICU for continued hemodynamic monitoring, blood pressure control, and CNS observation. The risk for pulmonary edema and eclampsia is greater in the early postpartum period because fluid shifts are significant. Moreover, the lower COP may predispose these patients to pulmonary edema.

HELLP Syndrome

A subset and rare group of severe preeclamptic/eclamptic patients manifest hemolytic anemia, increased levels of liver enzymes, and thrombocytopenia (HELLP syndrome).[19] These patients may not present with severe hypertension, thereby delaying the diagnosis and treatment. Aggressive supportive care and expeditious delivery are necessary to diminish maternal and perinatal morbidity and mortality.

CARDIAC DISEASE ■

The incidence rate of cardiac disease during pregnancy ranges from 0.4% to 4%, with the maternal mortality rate ranging from 0.4% to 6.8%, depending on the lesion and the NYHA functional classification.[20] Patients with NYHA class I and II cardiac disease generally have a good prognosis during pregnancy. However, the patient's status may change with the progression of pregnancy and during labor, delivery, and the postpartum period considering that over 40% of women with cardiac disease first develop pulmonary edema in the third trimester.

Rheumatic heart disease is still the most common form of heart disease in pregnancy, despite its declining incidence and the increased incidence of congenital heart disease with palliative or corrective surgery. The most common valvular lesion with a rheumatic origin in pregnancy is mitral stenosis (aortic involvement more commonly occurs after the childbearing years). Major complications of rheumatic heart disease in pregnancy include ventricular failure, atrial arrhythmia, pulmonary embolism, and infective endocarditis. Table 92-3 classifies cardiac disease as high-risk or lower-risk disorders.

VALVULAR LESIONS

Mitral Stenosis

Mitral stenosis accounts for approximately 90% of the rheumatic valvular lesions in pregnancy.[21] Clinical symptoms are nonspecific and include fatigue and dyspnea. Physical examination of the heart includes a mid-diastolic–presystolic murmur heard best in the left lateral decubitus position. Results

TABLE 92-3. Heart Disease in Pregnancy

HIGH-RISK DISORDERS
Rheumatic heart disease
  Mitral stenosis
  Aortic stenosis
Congenital heart disease
  Eisenmenger's syndrome
  Tetralogy of Fallot
  Marfan's syndrome
  Aortic coarctation
Other
  Peripartum cardiomyopathy
  Primary pulmonary hypertension
  NYHA class III or IV
  Myocardial infarction

LOWER-RISK DISORDERS
Rheumatic heart disease
  Mitral insufficiency
  Aortic insufficiency
Congenital heart disease
  Atrial septal defect
  Ventricular septal defect
  Patent ductus arteriosus
  Corrected tetralogy of Fallot
Other
  Mitral valve prolapse
  Asymmetric septal hypertrophy

NYHA, New York Heart Association.

from chest radiographs and ECG monitoring may be normal early in the course of the disease; however, signs of chamber enlargement and pulmonary congestion are present with progression. Mitral stenosis is characterized by left ventricular filling impairment. Avoidance of tachycardia, increased PA pressure, decreased systemic vascular resistance, and increased central blood volume therefore are essential in patient management.

CLINICAL CONSIDERATIONS.   Pregnancy aggravates mitral stenosis because of the increased blood volume and heart rate, leading to a high incidence of pulmonary edema and atrial fibrillation. Because of the hemodynamic changes and demands with the progression of pregnancy, surgical correction may be advisable in the second trimester if medical therapy is inadequate. Less-invasive surgical procedures than mitral valve replacement should be considered if possible because they may prove to have a lower morbidity and mortality for mother and fetus (see below).

For labor and for vaginal delivery, intravenous sedation and perineal analgesia with pudendal nerve blocks may be adequate. Excessive sedation may lead to hypoventilation, resulting in high PA pressures, which would be detrimental. Moreover, inadequate analgesia can lead to higher systemic and pulmonary pressures and to arrhythmias. However, the pain and stress of labor predisposes to tachycardia. Because these patients are dependent on diastolic filling time, increases in heart rate may lead to cardiac decompensation. A conservatively dosed lumbar epidural anesthetic with special attention to fluid status, left uterine displacement, and careful use of α-adrenergic agents to treat hypotension is often helpful: these patients are dependent on high left ventricular filling pressures and cardiac output. Although not as effective as neuraxial local anesthetics for labor pain relief, epidural intrathecal narcotics may be a reasonable compromise and superior to parental drugs because the hemodynamic consequences of local anesthetics are avoided.

For cesarean section delivery, lumbar epidural anesthesia is indicated for patients with mild mitral stenosis. General anesthesia may be the preferred method for patients with severe mitral stenosis as long as drugs that induce tachycardia (ketamine, pancuronium, and anticholinergics) are avoided. A narcotic–relaxant technique should be used without nitrous oxide, which may further increase PA pressure.

Patients with moderate to severe mitral stenosis who are in labor or undergoing vaginal or cesarean deliveries should be managed with intraarterial and central venous or PA catheters. Remember that the PAOP may overestimate left ventricular end-diastolic pressure. Even patients with class III or class IV mitral stenosis should be allowed to labor, and cesarean section should be performed for obstetric indications. However, to properly manage these patients during labor and delivery, a PA catheter should be placed at the start or before the induction of labor. Central venous pressure monitoring may fail to correlate with measurements of PA pressure.[22] When significant pulmonary hypertension is present, epidural local anesthetics should be avoided or used sparingly as an adjunct to neuraxial narcotics.

Aortic Stenosis

Aortic stenosis is a valvular lesion rarely seen during pregnancy. It can be of rheumatic or congenital origin. Clinical manifestations include congestive failure, syncope, angina, and a systolic ejection murmur, which is heard best at the second right intercostal space and radiating to the neck. The pathophysiologic makeup of aortic stenosis includes left ventricular systolic pressure overload. As in mitral stenosis, a decrease in systemic vascular resistance is poorly tolerated. Moreover, because of the fixed stroke volume, a decrease in heart rate and venous return is also detrimental. The overall mortality rate associated with aortic stenosis in pregnancy is 17%, with the greatest risk in patients with shunt gradients over 100 mm Hg.

CLINICAL CONSIDERATIONS.   Aortic stenosis is poorly tolerated during pregnancy because of the increased physiologic demands. In severe lesions, regional anesthesia has been avoided because of the resulting local anesthetic-induced sympathectomy, which can lead to bradycardia and decreased venous return. However, a recent study demonstrated good results in patients with severe aortic stenosis managed during labor with a carefully titrated epidural anesthetic.[23] Moreover, lumbar epidural or intrathecal narcotics, as in the combined spinal epidural technique, can be used as the sole agent with careful supplementation by lumbar epidural local anesthetics, if needed. For milder cases, careful and conservative lumbar epidural analgesia can be administered for labor and delivery. Otherwise, management includes systemic medication and pudendal nerve blocks.

For cesarean section, general anesthesia with a narcotic–relaxant technique is indicated rather than potent inhalation agents, which may further depress the compromised heart. Severe lesions benefit from intraarterial and central venous or PA catheterization and monitoring. However, PAOP may actually underestimate left ventricular end-diastolic pressure, depending on the compliance of the left ventricle. Moreover, placement of a PA catheter in a patient with severe aortic stenosis can lead to major arrhythmias. These seem to be related to the increase in endogenous catecholamine levels required to maintain an adequate cardiac output.

Mitral Insufficiency

Mitral insufficiency is the second most common valvular lesion in pregnancy and is manifested by left ventricular volume overload.[21] Severe mitral insufficiency is associated with left ventricular failure and a pansystolic murmur at the apex of the heart that radiates to the axilla. Increases in systemic vascular resistance, decreased heart rate, atrial arrhythmias, and myocardial depressants are poorly tolerated.

CLINICAL CONSIDERATIONS.   Mitral insufficiency is better tolerated during pregnancy than are stenotic lesions. Lumbar epidural anesthesia is preferred for labor and delivery and cesarean section because it prevents increases in systemic vascular resistance. If general anesthesia is used for cesarean section delivery, potent inhalation agents should be avoided because of their myocardial depressant effects. In patients with severe mitral regurgitation, intraarterial, central venous, and PA catheterization are recommended. The mean PAOP in chronic mitral insufficiency overestimates left ventricular end-diastolic pressure because of the compliant left atrium and the presence of prominent V waves.

Aortic Insufficiency

Aortic insufficiency also is relatively rare in pregnancy and is manifested by left ventricular volume overload. Symptoms are related to left ventricular failure. Clinical signs include an early diastolic murmur along the left sternal border. As in mitral regurgitation, increases in systemic vascular resistance, decreased heart rate, and myocardial depressants are poorly tolerated.

CLINICAL CONSIDERATIONS.   Aortic insufficiency also is reasonably well tolerated during pregnancy. Anesthetic considerations are the same as for mitral regurgitation. If general anesthesia is required for cesarean section, a narcotic–relaxant technique should be used in severe cases. Patients with aortic insufficiency manifested by pulmonary congestion and a decrease in diastolic blood pressure may require intraarterial, central venous, or PA catheterization. The PAOP may underestimate left ventricular end-diastolic pressure significantly.

CONGENITAL HEART DISEASE

Approximately 25% of heart disease in pregnancy is congenital. It can be categorized as left-to-right shunt, right-to-left shunt, and aortic lesions.

Left-to-Right Shunt

The most common congenital heart lesions are atrial septal defects (ASDs) and ventricular septal defects (VSDs), which are usually well tolerated in pregnancy. Nevertheless, the risk of left ventricular failure in pregnancy is increased. Major considerations include avoidance of increase in systemic vascular resistance and heart rate and supraventricular arrhythmias.

CLINICAL CONSIDERATIONS. Lumbar epidural anesthesia is indicated for labor, vaginal delivery, and delivery by cesarean section because it lowers systemic vascular resistance. In the presence of pulmonary hypertension, with atrial or VSDs, regional anesthesia with local anesthetics should be used with caution to prevent decreases in systemic vascular resistance that may promote right-to-left shunting. Neuraxial narcotics are a viable alternative, especially during the earlier stages of labor. They may have to be supplemented conservatively with local anesthetics. When general anesthesia is required for cesarean section, inhalation agents or narcotics, or combinations of the two, can be used.

Right-to-Left Shunt

The high-risk congenital disorders in pregnancy include right-to-left shunts, as seen in tetralogy of Fallot and Eisenmenger's syndrome (any congenital heart lesion with a bidirectional or right-to-left shunt at the atrial, ventricular, or aortic level). Patients with uncorrected cyanotic heart disease have increased spontaneous abortion rates, pulmonary embolization, congestive heart failure, and incidence for congenital heart defects in the fetus. A high hematocrit (≥65%) is not only an indication of the severity of the cardiac disease, but also in itself has a poorer prognosis secondary to complications from hyperviscosity (decreased cardiac output, organ hypoperfusion, and thrombosis).

CLINICAL CONSIDERATIONS. During pregnancy, right-to-left shunting is increased because of decreased systemic vascular resistance, resulting in decreased PA perfusion and hypoxia. A recent review on maternal and fetal outcome in patients with Eisenmenger's syndrome reveals maternal and fetal mortality rates of 26% and 44%, respectively.[24] Because only 26% of pregnancies reached term, the authors suggest that these patients should be hospitalized from 20 weeks onward. During hospitalization, oxygen administration and PA vasodilation should be considered. Decreased systemic vascular resistance, blood volume, and venous return should be avoided. Increased pulmonary vascular resistance promotes right-to-left shunting; therefore, hypercapnia and hypoxia also are to be avoided. Moreover, oxytocin for induction of labor should be avoided or used with caution because even transient decreases in peripheral resistance may increase right-to-left shunting and result in further cardiopulmonary decompensation.

Patients should be monitored with intraarterial and CVP catheters. For labor and delivery, systemic medication or pericervical and pudendal nerve blocks should be used. Lumbar epidural anesthesia should be used with extreme caution during labor and delivery. Again, neuraxial narcotics

may be a reasonable choice in these patients to partially control their pain. For cesarean section, general anesthesia is recommended.

Although primary pulmonary hypertension is not a right-to-left disorder, it does fall in the category of high-risk congenital disorders in pregnancy. The high mortality rate (40% to 60%) with primary pulmonary hypertension may be related to the absence of a shunt (as seen with Eisenmenger's syndrome), which decompresses the PA pressures and increases left ventricular filling. Similar guidelines apply for primary pulmonary hypertension as for right-to-left shunt lesions. Increased pulmonary vascular resistance, decreased venous return, and decreased systemic vascular resistance should be avoided.

Aortic Disease

Coarctation of the aorta and aortic manifestations of Marfan's syndrome pose significant problems in pregnancy. Although histologic changes involving the aortic intima and media are controversial (loss of elastic fibers and other connective tissue changes), physiologic changes during pregnancy, including increased blood volume and increased blood pressure during labor and delivery, may promote aortic dissection. Regional anesthesia for labor, delivery, and cesarean section may be indicated to avoid hypertension and tachycardia. However, decreased systemic vascular resistance and bradycardia may be harmful in coarctation of the aorta. If general anesthesia is used for cesarean section, halothane seems indicated to avoid the hypertensive and tachycardic effects of other agents.

Postsurgical Correction

Patients who have had corrected ASDs and VSDs and simple coarctation repair tolerate pregnancy well. Barring any residual sequelae, patients with corrected tetralogy of Fallot[25] also tolerate pregnancy. Residual problems include conduction disturbances, ventricular dysfunction, patch leaks, and postvalvulotomy regurgitation.[26]

PERIPARTUM CARDIOMYOPATHY

Peripartum cardiomyopathy is an uncommon form of heart disease affecting pregnant patients in the last month of pregnancy or more commonly from 2 to 6 months postpartum. The etiology is unknown, and the disease is either pregnancy related or represents an exacerbation of an underlying latent cardiac disorder. It is most commonly found in women who have twins, preeclampsia/eclampsia, older multiparous women, blacks, and in the presence of viral infections. The mortality rate is high (up to 84%) in the subset of patients with persistent cardiomegaly beyond 6 months.[27]

Pathologic findings include four-chamber enlargement with normal coronary arteries and valves. Light microscopic findings include myocardial hypertrophy and fibrosis with scattered mononuclear infiltrates. Clinical signs include symptoms of ventricular failure with possible associated pulmonary emboli and myocardial infarction. Before delivery, treatment includes bed rest, diuresis, digitalization, and preload/afterload reduction.

Clinical Considerations

For labor and vaginal and cesarean delivery, lumbar epidural anesthesia is preferable to counter some of the effects of increased venous return, heart rate, and stroke volume with uterine contractions. A PA catheter aids the management of these patients because right and left ventricular pressures often do not correlate. If general anesthesia is used for cesarean section delivery, a narcotic muscle relaxation technique should be used to avoid the myocardial depressant effects of potent inhalation agents. Perioperative management of these patients can be further evaluated by transesophageal echocardiography, which aids in management.[12] If inotropic support is needed for peripartum cardiomyopathy or heart failure from other causes, amrinone or low-dose epinephrine (0.02 to 0.03 μg/kg/minute) decrease uterine blood flow less than high-dose dopamine.[28]

MITRAL VALVE PROLAPSE

Mitral valve prolapse is a common valvular lesion occurring in 5% of the general population and up to 17% of young women of child-bearing-age.[29] A wide range of clinical and echocardiographic manifestations is possible. It is characterized by floppy mitral valve leaflets and may result from mucinous changes in the connective tissues of the valve leaflets. It also may involve regional dysfunction of the mitral annulus fibrosus.[30] Auscultatory findings include a mid-to-late systolic click, which is often accompanied by a mid-to-late systolic murmur.

Most patients with mitral valve prolapse are asymptomatic, and such patients tolerate pregnancy well, with no evidence of cardiac complications. Moreover, the incidence of antepartum and intrapartum complications or signs of fetal distress are no different when compared with pregnant patients with no known cardiac disorders.[31] These patients should be treated in a routine fashion, except for possible bacterial endocarditis prophylaxis during labor and delivery if an accompanying systolic murmur of mitral regurgitation is present.

A small subset of patients, especially with severe redundant mitral valve leaflets, may develop the known complications of mitral valve prolapse, which include arrhythmias, mitral insufficiency, infective endocarditis, and sudden death. As in mitral regurgitation, increases in systemic vascular resistance and decreased preload are not well tolerated in patients with associated mitral valvular incompetence.

Clinical Considerations

During labor and vaginal delivery, continuous ECG monitoring should be instituted in symptomatic patients. Lumbar epidural anesthesia is preferred for labor, vaginal delivery, and cesarean section delivery. Preload must be maintained by adequate administration of intravenous fluids to minimize the degree of prolapse.

ASYMMETRIC SEPTAL HYPERTROPHY

During pregnancy, the course of asymmetric septal hypertrophy (ASH)—also termed idiopathic hypertrophic subvalvular stenosis or hypertrophic obstructive cardiomyopathy—is

variable because the normal increase of blood volume is beneficial, whereas the decrease in systemic vascular resistance and the increase in heart rate may be detrimental. Complications seem to arise late in pregnancy, often appearing during labor as a result of stress, pain, and increased circulating catecholamines. Moreover, the immediate postpartum period results in blood loss and decrease in systemic vascular resistance. Atrial fibrillation and supraventricular tachycardias are a common feature of this cardiac anomaly; thus, β-blockers are indicated. Unfortunately, the latter are not without significant sequelae, including intrauterine growth retardation with chronic use, and neonatal bradycardia and hypoglycemia with acute use. However, sudden onset tachycardia and ventricular compromise indicate the need for drugs such as propranolol or esmolol, despite these potential problems. Oxytocin postdelivery should be used with caution and only as an infusion (not a bolus) and may be substituted for methylergonovine maleate (Methergine).

Appropriate management includes maintenance of adequate blood volume and insertion of a PA catheter. Although regional anesthesia is relatively contraindicated in this setting, a carefully titrated lumbar epidural cannot be ruled out for labor to avoid increases in myocardial contractility. However, spinal anesthesia should be avoided. Epidural narcotics alleviate the side effects of epidural local anesthetics.

MYOCARDIAL INFARCTION

Although the incidence of myocardial infarction in pregnancy is uncommon (older reports estimate 1 in 10,000), it may be increasing with older parturients, and other risk factors such as smoking and cocaine use. Most infarcts occur during the third trimester. Maternal mortality rate is approximately 35% at the time of or within 2 weeks of infarction.[32] During the first two trimesters, the mortality rate is 23% compared with 45% in the third trimester. Postmortem coronary artery studies have revealed a spectrum of findings, including atherosclerosis, thrombus, dissection, and normal vessels, suggestive of spasm or lysed thrombi or emboli.

Clinical Considerations

Patients with known ischemic heart disease should have their medications continued (i.e., nitrates, β-blockers) with ECG monitoring (V_5 or without V_4 leads).

Those with unstable angina, recent infarction, or heart failure should be monitored with an arterial cannula and PA catheter. Vaginal delivery should be allowed with epidural anesthesia to relieve the stress of labor. Although elective cesarean section also may relieve the stress of labor and vaginal delivery, the mortality rate in one review was higher in cesarean section patients (23%) than in vaginal delivery patients (14%).[32] However, the decision on mode of delivery should be determined by the technique that provides the least hemodynamic compromise and is dependent on the patient's gestational and labor status.

Regional anesthesia is the anesthetic of choice for vaginal delivery and cesarean section, but remember that hypotension can decrease coronary perfusion. Ephedrine, with its increase in heart rate, is not the pressor agent of choice despite its relatively benign effects on uteroplacental perfusion. Although α-adrenergic agonists such as phenylephrine are less favorable for uteroplacental perfusion, they do not seem to have adverse effects at low rates of infusion. For general anesthesia, narcotic–relaxant technique, with or without potent inhalation agents and nitrous oxide, is recommended.

CARDIAC ARRHYTHMIAS IN PREGNANCY

Arrhythmias during gestation, and especially labor and delivery, are common. Hormonal changes, stress, and anxiety are contributing factors; however, most arrhythmias are not serious unless they are associated with organic heart disease.

Atrial Fibrillation

Atrial fibrillation associated with mitral stenosis results in a high incidence of heart failure and high maternal mortality rate. It also is associated with peripartum cardiomyopathy, hypertensive heart disease, and ASDs. Patients with acute atrial fibrillation and significant hemodynamic changes require direct current cardioversion. Cardioversion with 20 to 100 J reportedly has no adverse effects on the fetus, remainder of gestation, or subsequent delivery. In hemodynamically stable patients, digitalis can be administered, also with no significant adverse effects in the fetus despite placental transfer. β-Adrenergic blockers such as propranolol or labetalol and a calcium channel blocker such as verapamil may be required. Despite sporadic reports of intrauterine growth retardation with or without fetal hypoglycemia, bradycardia, or hyperbilirubinemia after chronic maternal propranolol administration, the incidence of these complications is low. Recent data suggest that the fetal β-blockade is less with maternally administered labetalol compared with that seen with esmolol. Moreover, fetal hypoxia was also present with maternally administered esmolol.[33] Calcium channel blockers should be used with caution because hypotension and decreased placental perfusion can occur, especially when nifedipine is used instead of verapamil.

Supraventricular Tachycardia

Supraventricular tachycardias during pregnancy can occur with or without organic heart disease. In the absence of underlying cardiac disease, these tachycardias are not associated with increased morbidity. However, in patients with rheumatic mitral disease, supraventricular tachycardia increases the incidence of heart failure, which peaks in the third trimester and is associated with a mortality rate of 5%. Treatment includes direct current cardioversion, carotid sinus massage, verapamil, edrophonium, β-blockers, or digoxin, or adenosine.

Wolff-Parkinson-White Syndrome

The incidence of Wolff-Parkinson-White (WPW) syndrome in pregnancy is probably increased. Previously asymptomatic patients with preexcitation are predisposed to supraventricular tachyarrhythmias during pregnancy, and patients with

TABLE 92-4. Cardiovascular Drugs to Avoid in Pregnancy

Phenytoin	Fetal hydantoin syndrome
	Cardiopulmonary and genital anomalies
	Hemorrhage
	Tumors
Disopyramide	Uterotonic
Phenylephrine, methoxamine°	↓ Uterine blood flow
Warfarin (Coumadin)	Warfarin embryonic syndrome
	Fetal and neonatal hemorrhage
Dopamine°	↓ Uterine blood flow
	↑ Uterine vascular resistance

°Decreased uterine blood flow with high doses. Low doses may be tolerated.

known WPW syndrome have an increased incidence of tachyarrhythmias during pregnancy.[34] Adenosine has been shown to be effective in terminating supraventricular tachyarrhythmias in the peripartum period.[35]

Ventricular Arrhythmias

Ventricular arrhythmia during pregnancy may be associated with mitral valve prolapse, peripartum cardiomyopathy, ischemic heart disease, and digitalis toxicity. Antiarrhythmic agents of choice are lidocaine and procainamide.

Bradycardia

Bradyarrhythmias during pregnancy are rare and may result from hypothyroidism, myocarditis, and drug-induced or congenital or acquired heart blocks. Permanent pacemakers are indicated for hemodynamically significant bradycardia.

Antiarrhythmic Drugs

Relatively safe antiarrhythmic drugs during pregnancy include digitalis, quinidine, lidocaine, procainamide, β-adrenergic blockers (labetalol), and calcium channel blockers (verapamil). Drugs that are less safe in pregnancy are phenytoin (birth defects, bleeding), disopyramide (uterotonic), and calcium channel blockers (nifedipine—hypotension, fetal hypoxia; Table 92-4).

CARDIAC SURGERY DURING PREGNANCY ■

As in other nonobstetric surgery during pregnancy, if cardiac surgery is necessary, it should take place during the early part of the second trimester to avoid the embryonic stage of the first trimester and the more marked hemodynamic changes of the third trimester. If medical management can ameliorate the disease process, surgery should be postponed until the patient has recovered at least 4 to 6 weeks postpartum.

Cardiac procedures during pregnancy are mitral and aortic valve replacements secondary to rheumatic heart disease, congenital anomalies, or bacterial endocarditis. Mitral balloon valvuloplasty recently has been used as a safer alternative to mother and fetus than open mitral valve commissurotomy or replacement, or even closed commissurotomy for short- and intermediate-term results.[36] Other procedures include removal of atrial myxomas, ASD and VSD repairs, and repair of tetralogy of Fallot.

Special intraoperative considerations in pregnant patients include (1) fetal monitoring during and after surgery; (2) maintenance of high flow and systemic mean arterial pressure during cardiopulmonary bypass, and (3) uterine displacement devices if the patient is in the supine position for a median sternotomy. Although the pregnant patient has fared well with open heart procedures, fetal mortality rate can be high. Generally, better results are seen in closed heart procedures. Postoperatively, fetal monitoring should be continued and maternal analgesia maintained to avoid precipitating labor from accelerated postoperative pain.

PREGNANCY AFTER CARDIAC SURGERY

Pregnancy and outcome in patients after cardiac surgery are similar to the general population.[37] Patients with nontissue heart valve prostheses pose a greater risk during pregnancy as a result of their coagulation status. Fewer maternal and fetal complications occurred after porcine valve replacement than mechanical valves, although reoperation for degenerative changes were greater with tissue valves.[38]

Heparin is the anticoagulant agent of choice during pregnancy because its high molecular weight prevents placental crossover and it is not teratogenic. Unfortunately, it can be administered only parenterally and has been associated with maternal bleeding, thrombocytopenia, and fetal and neonatal hemorrhage.[39] Warfarin and its derivatives are contraindicated during conception and the first trimester because it has a high incidence of CNS anomalies or warfarin embryopathy.[39] Maternal, fetal, and neonatal hemorrhage has been described. Thus, anticoagulant management includes heparin (intravenous, subcutaneous) in the first trimester, and either maintaining heparin in the second and third trimesters or switching to warfarin during the latter two trimesters.

Approximately 2 weeks before delivery, warfarin should be discontinued to diminish the risk of fetal hemorrhage during labor and delivery, and the patient should be started back on heparin. Heparin should be discontinued approximately 4 to 6 hours before delivery and resumed within 12 to 24 hours after delivery.

With the increasing number (>12,600) and survival (5-year, 72%) of heart transplant recipients, some women of child-bearing age who have undergone this procedure may become pregnant.[40,41] Potential problems include limited cardiac responses of the denervated heart to the marked hemodynamic changes of pregnancy, along with the absence of chest pain, which can make the detection of ischemia more difficult. Infections and gastrointestinal disorders are exacerbated in these patients because of the immunosuppressive therapy. One case report described a heart transplant patient who delivered a normal but premature infant at 31 weeks' gestation.

CARDIOPULMONARY RESUSCITATION ■

Pregnancy poses further problems during cardiopulmonary resuscitation (CPR). In the third trimester and near term, particularly, the gravid uterus impairs venous return. Thus, during CPR, the uterus should be displaced (i.e., left uterine tilt). Moreover, if defibrillation is required, the left breast needs to be displaced, because of marked enlargement during pregnancy.

Despite previous recommendations to perform an emergency cesarean section only for fetal survival after maternal resuscitation has failed, more aggressive management, such as prompt cesarean delivery, may be advantageous not only for fetal survival, but also may increase maternal survival.[42] Obviously, the blood loss accompanying a cesarean delivery during an arrest should be addressed by aggressive fluid and blood replacement as needed.

SUMMARY ■

The early prenatal course of the pregnant cardiac patient should include restriction of physical activity; optimization of cardiac medication, including the appropriate use of anticoagulants when necessary; and early diagnosis and treatment of anemia and infection. If indicated, closed or open heart surgery should not be withheld because of pregnancy, but should be scheduled in the second trimester, if possible.

Labor and delivery considerations include bacterial endocarditis prophylaxis, avoidance of the supine position, supplemental oxygen, a second intravenous infusion route, continuous electrocardiography, automated blood pressure measurement, and pulse oximetry. Invasive monitoring may be indicated.

The choice between spontaneous labor, elective induction of labor, and elective cesarean section should be made on an individual basis, depending on the patient's cardiac lesion, overall medical condition during pregnancy and labor, obstetric history, gestational age, and stage of labor. Obviously, this decision should involve the input of the obstetrician, anesthesiologist, cardiologist, and intensive care specialist.

In general, anesthetic considerations include regional anesthesia (epidural preferable to spinal) for most regurgitant valvular lesions, cardiomyopathy, ischemic heart disease, left-to-right shunts, mild-to-moderate stenotic valvular lesions, and possibly severe stenotic lesions if it is carefully titrated. Systemic medications and general anesthesia are indicated for right-to-left shunts, pulmonary hypertension, severe asymmetric septal hypertrophy, and severe stenotic valvular lesions. Epidural or intrathecal narcotics may be used in these cases without the addition of local anesthetics, thus avoiding the hemodynamic responses of regional anesthesia with local anesthetics.

REFERENCES ■

1. Ueland K: Maternal cardiovascular dynamics. VII. Intrapartum blood volume changes. *Am J Obstet Gynecol* 1976;126:671

2. James CF, Banner T, Levelle JP, et al: Noninvasive determination of cardiac output throughout pregnancy. *Anesthesiology* 1985;63(Suppl 3A):A434

3. Ueland K, Hansen JM: Maternal cardiovascular dynamics. II. Posture and uterine contractions. *Am J Obstet Gynecol* 1969;103:1

4. Robson SC, Dunlop W, Boys RJ, et al: Cardiac output during labour. *Br Med J* 1987;295:1169

5. Capeless EL, Clapp JF: When do cardiovascular parameters return to their preconception values? *Am J Obstet Gynecol* 1991;165:883

6. Clark SL, Cotton DG, Lee W, et al: Central hemodynamic assessment. *Am J Obstet Gynecol* 1989;161:1439

7. Clapp JF, Seaward BL, Sleamaker RH, et al: Maternal physiologic adaptations to early pregnancy. *Am J Obstet Gynecol* 1988;159:1456

8. Morgan M: Anesthetic contribution to maternal mortality. *Br J Anaesth* 1987;59:842

9. Davies JM, Weeks S: Difficult intubation in the parturient. *Can J Anaesth* 1989;36:668

10. Clark RB, Thompson DS, Thompson CH: Prevention of spinal hypotension associated with cesarean section. *Anesthesiology* 1976;45:670

11. Brizgys RV, Dailey PA, Shnider SM, et al: The incidence and neonatal effects of maternal hypotension during epidural anesthesia for cesarean section. *Anesthesiology* 1987;67:782

12. Zemel MB, Zemel PC, Berry S, et al: Altered platelet calcium metabolism as an early predictor of increased peripheral vascular resistance and preeclampsia in urban black women. *N Engl J Med* 1990;323:434

13. Lockwood CJ, Peters JH: Increased cellular fibrinonectin precede the clinical signs of preeclampsia. *Am J Obstet Gynecol* 1990;168:352

14. Symonds EM: Aetiology of preeclampsia: a review. *J R Soc Med* 1980;73:871

15. Bletka M, Hlavatj V, Tenkova M, et al: Volume of whole blood and absolute amount of serum proteins in the early stages of late toxemia of pregnancy. *Am J Obstet Gynecol* 1970;106:10

16. Pritchard JA, Cunningham FG, Mason RA: Coagulation changes in eclampsia: their frequency and pathogenesis. *Am J Obstet Gynecol* 1976;124:855

17. Strauss RG, Keefer JR, Burke T, et al: Hemodynamic monitoring of cardiogenic pulmonary edema complicating toxemia of pregnancy. *Obstet Gynecol* 1980;55:170

18. Benedetti TJ, Cotton DB, Read JC, et al: Hemodynamic observations in severe preeclampsia with a flow-directed pulmonary artery catheter. *Am J Obstet Gynecol* 1980;136:465

19. Weinstein L: Syndrome of hemolysis, elevated liver enzymes, and low platelet count: a severe consequence of hypertension in pregnancy. *Am J Obstet Gynecol* 1982;142:159

20. Sullivan JM, Ramanathan KB: Management of medical problems in pregnancy: severe cardiac disease. *N Engl J Med* 1985;313:304

21. Szekely P, Snaith L: *Heart Disease and Pregnancy*. Edinburgh, Churchill Livingstone, 1974

22. Clark SL, Phelan JP, Greenspoon J, et al: Labor and delivery in the presence of mitral stenosis: central hemodynamic observations. *Am J Obstet Gynecol* 1985;152:984

23. Easterling TR, Chadwick HS, Otto CM, et al: Aortic stenosis in pregnancy. *Obstet Gynecol* 1988;72:113

24. Stoddart P, O'Sullivan G: Eisenmenger's syndrome in pregnancy: a case report and review. *Int J Obstet Anesthesia* 1993;2:159

25. Singh H, Bolton PJ, Oakley CM: Pregnancy after surgical correction of tetralogy of Fallot. *Br Med J* 1982;285:168

26. Graham TP: Ventricular performance in adults after operation for congenital heart disease. *Am J Cardiol* 1982;50:612

27. Demakis JG, Rahimtoola SH, Sutton GC, et al: Natural course of peripartum cardiomyopathy. *Circulation* 1971;44:1053

28. Fishburne JI Jr, Dormer KJ, Payne GG, et al: Effects of amrinone and dopamine on uterine blood flow and vascular responses in the gravid baboon. *Am J Obstet Gynecol* 1988;158:829

29. Nishimura RA, McGoon MD, Shub C, et al: Echocardiographically documented mitral-valve prolapse: long-term follow-up of 237 patients. *N Engl J Med* 1985;313:1305

30. Hutchins GM, Moore GW, Skoog DK: The association of floppy mitral valve with disjunction of the mitral annulus fibrosus. *N Engl J Med* 1986;314:535

31. Rayburn WF, Fontana ME: Mitral valve prolapse and pregnancy. *Am J Obstet Gynecol* 1981;141:9

32. Hankins GDV, Wendel GD, Leveno KJ, et al: Myocardial infarction during pregnancy: a review. *Obstet Gynecol* 1985;65:139

33. Castro MI, Eisenach JC: Maternally administered esmolol produces fetal blockade and hypoxemia [abstract]. *Anesthesiology* 1988;69:A708

34. Widerhorn J, Widerhorn ALM, Rahimtoola SH, et al: WPW syndrome during pregnancy: increased incidence of supraventricular arrhythmias. *Am Heart J* 1992;123:796

35. Afridi I, Moise KI, Rokey R: Termination of supraventricular tachycardia with intravenous adenosine in a pregnant woman with Wolff-Parkinson-White syndrome. *Obstet Gynecol* 1992;80:481

36. Esteves CA, Ramos AIO, Braga SLN, et al: Effectiveness of percutaneous balloon mitral valvotomy during pregnancy. *Am J Cardiol* 1991;68:930

37. Nunley WC, Kolp LA, Dabinett LN, et al: Subsequent fertility in women who undergo cardiac surgery. *Am J Obstet Gynecol* 1989;161:573

38. Lee C-N, Wu C-C, Lin P-Y, et al: Pregnancy following cardiac prosthetic valve replacement. *Obstet Gynecol* 1994;83:353

39. Hall JB, Pauli RM, Wilson KM: Maternal and fetal sequelae of anticoagulation during pregnancy. *Am J Med* 1980;68:122

40. Kriett JM, Kaye MP: The registry of the International Society for Heart Transplantation: 7th official report, 1990. *J Heart Lung Transplant* 1990;9:323

41. Lowenstein BR, Vain NW, Perrone SV, et al: Successful pregnancy and vaginal delivery after heart transplantation. *Am J Obstet Gynecol* 1988;158:589

42. O'Connor RL, Sevarino FB: Cardiopulmonary arrest in the pregnant patient: a report of a successful resuscitation. *J Clin Anesth* 1994;6:66

Critical Care, Third Edition, edited by Joseph M. Civetta,
Robert W. Taylor, and Robert R. Kirby.
Lippincott-Raven Publishers, Philadelphia, PA © 1997.

CHAPTER 93

■

Hemorrhagic Disorders

Connie E. Taylor

IMMEDIATE CONCERNS ■

MAJOR PROBLEMS

Hemorrhage remains a major cause of morbidity and mortality in the obstetric patient.[1,2] The parturient is at the same risk for all the medical and surgical hemorrhagic disorders as any patient presenting to the critical care unit but, in addition, she must sustain a highly vascular organ on whose adequate perfusion the life of the fetus depends. Appropriate care requires understanding of the cardiovascular and hematologic changes of pregnancy and the special complications associated with the gravid uterus.

STRESS POINTS

1. Pregnancy is attended by profound alterations in maternal blood volume, red blood cell mass, and hemodynamic parameters. These changes enable the parturient to cope with the circulatory and metabolic demands of the enlarging uterus, placenta, and fetus, and to withstand the significant blood loss associated with even an uncomplicated delivery (Fig. 93-1).
2. Blood volume at term is 40% to 50% above that seen in the nonpregnant state. Changes in individual parturients range from 20% to 100%. Circulating blood volume undergoes a moderate expansion in the first trimester, becomes more marked in the second, and continues to rise slightly throughout the third trimester. At term, blood volume is 74 mL/kg, an increase of greater than 1.5 L over that seen in the nonpregnant state.[3-5]
3. The increase in plasma volume is proportionately greater than the increase in red blood cell mass, resulting in a slight, dilutional "anemia of pregnancy." However, values of less than 11.0 g/dL or a hemato-

crit of 33% or less should be considered abnormal. The most common etiology of anemia in pregnancy is iron deficiency, but adequate prenatal iron supplementation should maintain a relatively normal hematocrit.[6]

4. Cardiac output increases significantly during the first trimester and remains elevated throughout gestation, returning to normal shortly after delivery. This 30% to 50% increase is a result of an increase in heart rate and stroke volume.[7-10]
5. Pulmonary and systemic vascular resistances fall, allowing the parturient to accommodate the increased intravascular volume without hemodynamic decompensation, and central venous pressures remain normal.
6. The left ventricle undergoes eccentric enlargement, maintaining normal left ventricular function and pulmonary capillary wedge pressures in the face of increased filling volumes.[8,9] Most investigators report a decrease of mean arterial pressure.[7-10]
7. Circulatory compromise to the parturient and her fetus ensues when she is placed supine with the weight of the gravid uterus impinging on the abdominal aorta and vena cava.
8. Brachial artery pressure does not reliably reflect perfusion pressure in the lower extremities and uterus.
9. Radiologic studies document arterial occlusion and venous congestion, severely compromising uterine perfusion pressure when the parturient is supine.[11,12] Changing position from supine to lateral is associated with a rise in cardiac output of greater than 20%.[10,13]
10. Many pregnant women experience signs and symptoms of circulatory compromise—hypotension, diaphoresis, nausea, vomiting, and light-headedness—when placed supine. It is an easy, but often forgotten matter to place a rolled-up blanket, foam wedge, or

1401

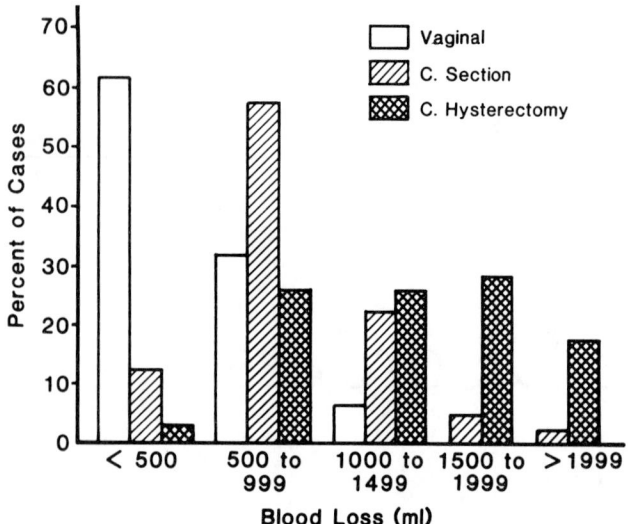

FIGURE 93-1. Blood loss after vaginal delivery, cesarean section, and cesarean hysterectomy. (Prichard JA, Baldwin RM, Dickey JC, et al.: Blood volume changes in pregnancy and the puerperium. *Am J Obstet Gynecol* 1962;84:1271.)

pillow under the right hip so that the weight of the uterus is not on the great vessels.

ESSENTIAL DIAGNOSTIC TESTS, PROCEDURES, AND THERAPY

1. Cardiopulmonary resuscitation of the near-term patient is complicated by the gravid uterus. Normally, adequate chest compression requires that the patient be placed on a hard, flat surface with the direction of the thoracic thrust exactly perpendicular to the torso.

2. In this setting, this position is tantamount to attempting resuscitation with aortocaval cross-clamping. Manual displacement of the uterus off the vena cava may be of limited use, but in the absence of immediate improvement the patient must be delivered by cesarean section within 4 minutes of arrest to maximize successful maternal and fetal outcome.[14,15]

3. If rapid fluid resuscitation is unsuccessful, and more aggressive pharmacologic support of the circulation is undertaken as a temporizing measure pending emergent delivery, ephedrine in 10- to 20-mg boluses should be the initial pressor given.

4. If additional treatment is necessary, combined α- and β-agonists are preferred. Remember that at higher doses, α activity predominates. Delivery is the only option for successful fetal and maternal resuscitation.

5. The therapy for hemorrhage in the pregnant patient is no different from appropriate therapy in any patient population: crystalloid resuscitation, blood component replacement as indicated, and expeditious identification of the etiology and initiation of definitive intervention.

6. If the fetus is immature and not in distress, and maternal hemodynamic function is stable, chronic

transfusion therapy may be indicated. Reliable, large-bore cannula venous access and rapid volume replacement are the first lines of therapy.

7. In life-threatening hemorrhage, before emergent operative delivery, maternal perfusion pressures must be maintained to ensure major organ and fetal viability.

8. Ephedrine with indirect β-agonist and direct vaso-constricting properties, as noted earlier, is the pressor agent of choice in obstetrics. It can be administered in 10- to 20-mg boluses or as a continuous infusion. In experimental models, ephedrine does not cause a decrease in uterine blood flow at doses sufficient to raise maternal blood pressure, whereas α-agonists were associated with a decrease in uterine blood flow.[16]

9. Recent studies have reevaluated phenylephrine, a pure α-agonist. When this agent is used in healthy women undergoing elective cesarean section under spinal or epidural anesthesia, intermittent boluses of 40 to 100 μg cause no untoward effects in mother or fetus.[17,18] Notice that these data are from studies in healthy parturients and uncompromised fetuses, and the findings may not hold true in hemorrhagic shock.

10. One should not withhold necessary therapy for maternal resuscitation for fear of compromising uterine perfusion. Until the mother is hemodynamically stable, uterine perfusion remains in jeopardy.

CARDIOVASCULAR CHANGES WITH OBSTETRIC DRUGS ■

DRUGS USED TO ARREST LABOR

Because prematurity is associated with increased perinatal morbidity and mortality, if the mother and fetus are stable, the obstetrician will attempt to arrest labor. Magnesium sulfate and the β-mimetic agents, ritodrine and terbutaline, all provide uterine relaxation. These therapies, however, are associated with cardiovascular changes that may affect accurate evaluation and successful resuscitation of the hemorrhaging patient.

β-Sympathomimetic agents used for tocolysis are predominantly β₂ selective, but all possess some β₁ activity that stimulates increases in heart rate. Pulmonary edema, which can be either cardiogenic or noncardiogenic; fluid overload from iatrogenic fluid administration or secondary to direct effects of these agents on salt and water retention; myocardial ischemia; cardiac arrhythmias; and maternal death all are complications of therapy. Peripheral vasodilatation may result in hypotension resistant to fluid resuscitation and ephedrine, particularly in the bleeding patient.[19,20] Obstetric hemorrhage may be chronic and relatively unimpressive at any given point in terms of volume, but significant in terms of a compromise in hemodynamic reserves.

Magnesium sulfate, while causing an initial transient decrease in blood pressure, has few maternal side effects when given in appropriate clinical doses. However, with inappropriate therapy or decreased renal excretion, toxic levels may occur. At 10 mEq/L, the patellar reflex is ablated; at higher levels, respiratory and cardiovascular collapse may ensue. Calcium chloride, 1 g, should be titrated intravenously for life-threatening complications.

Nifedipine, a calcium channel blocker, has been shown to be as effective for tocolysis as the β-mimetic agents, with better patient tolerance. It causes a decrease in systemic and pulmonary vascular resistances with a resultant increase in cardiac output. It has minimal effect on the cardiac conduction system. Hypotension may occur when the drug is administered to the hypovolemic patient and there may be potentiation of the cardiovascular side effects of magnesium sulfate with concurrent administration.[21]

DRUGS USED TO INCREASE UTERINE TONE

Pharmacologic therapy to enhance uterine tone is routine at the time of delivery. Initial treatment is with oxytocin; rapid infusion of large doses is associated with a drop in blood pressure and an increase in heart rate, which may be associated with electrocardiographic changes suggestive of myocardial ischemia. The drop in pressure usually occurs within several minutes of drug administration and is proportionate in magnitude and duration to the dose.[22] Unhappily, bolus administration often occurs in the setting of decreased uterine tone and blood loss, further enhancing hypotension. The drug should be given in dilute solution by intravenous infusion, commonly 20 units per liter of balanced salt solution.

If uterine tone does not respond promptly to external massage and oxytocin, methylergonovine is often used. Hypertension is the primary complication, and the drug should be avoided in the setting of preeclampsia, chronic hypertension, or cardiac disease. It should only be given intramuscularly. The standard dose is 0.2 mg.

If postpartum uterine bleeding does not respond to oxytocin or ergot preparations, prostaglandin $F_{2\alpha}$, may be effective. It can be given intramuscularly or intramyometrially and has been shown to increase uterine tone and arrest hemorrhage in numerous patients with uterine atony, thereby avoiding the need for surgical intervention.[23,24] Marked maternal oxygen desaturation 5 to 10 minutes after administration, secondary to intrapulmonary shunting, has been reported in some patients. Other cardiovascular side effects have been reported as minimal.

COAGULATION CHANGES ■

Uncomplicated pregnancy is associated with an increase in the concentration of circulating coagulation factors. Most significant are factors I (fibrinogen), VII, VIII, IX, and X. Clinically, hemostasis is normal. In laboratory tests, usually performed to evaluate bleeding and guide appropriate transfusion therapy, the most striking alteration is an increase in plasma fibrinogen. This elevation is seen by the third month and rises steadily from an initial average level of 235 mg/dL to value of 385 mg/dL before delivery at term.

The coagulation changes of pregnancy are postulated to be induced by subclinical intravascular coagulation, primarily in the uteroplacental circulation.[25] In support of this theory is the observation that platelet counts drop in the last 8 weeks of gestation in association with a significant rise in mean platelet volume. These changes are consistent with a process of consumption and hyperdestruction and the release of newer, larger platelets into the circulation.[26] Although the alterations are significant, platelet counts remain within normal limits. Prothrombin, partial thromboplastin, and bleeding times also remain within normal limits.

HEMORRHAGIC COMPLICATIONS ■

PLACENTAL ABRUPTION

Separation of the placenta from the uterus normally occurs after delivery of the fetus. The uterus, emptied of the products of conception, contracts vigorously, achieving hemostasis at the implantation site, even in the face of systemic coagulopathy. When the placenta separates prematurely before fetal delivery, life-threatening hemorrhage may ensue because the myometrium is unable to contract adequately to reestablish vascular integrity.

Placental abruption complicates between 0.05% and 1.0% of all deliveries, with an associated perinatal mortality rate between 20% and 35%.[27,28] It begins with hemorrhage into the decidua basalis; clot forms, and the placenta separates. The process can be chronic and self-limiting, with adequate functional placenta remaining intact to sustain fetal life support, or it may be paroxysmal and catastrophic, with complete separation and fetal demise. Hemorrhage may present vaginally or may be concealed (Fig. 93-2). Concealed hemorrhage poses a far greater risk because the extent of hemorrhage is easily underestimated and resuscitation may be delayed. In addition, placental abruption, particularly abruption extensive enough to result in fetal demise, may be associated with a consumptive coagulopathy as thromboplastic products enter the maternal circulation. Grading of abruptio placentae is summarized in Table 93-1.

Diagnosis

The exact etiology of abruptio placentae remains unknown. Maternal hypertension, either pregnancy-aggravated or pregnancy-induced, grand multiparity, and a prior history of placental abruption seem to confer a higher risk for its occurrence.[29,30] It is seen with increasing frequency as a result of crack and cocaine use. Placental abruption may also complicate maternal trauma.[31]

Vaginal bleeding, uterine irritability and tenderness, back pain, and fetal distress all are associated with abruption of the placenta. Classically, abruption is associated with painful vaginal bleeding, in contrast to placenta previa, in which vaginal bleeding is painless. Ultrasonography is not a useful diagnostic tool for placental abruption, beyond ruling out an abnormally positioned placenta. Large retroplacental clot may not be appreciated; the diagnosis of abruption should be made on the basis of clinical signs and symptoms.

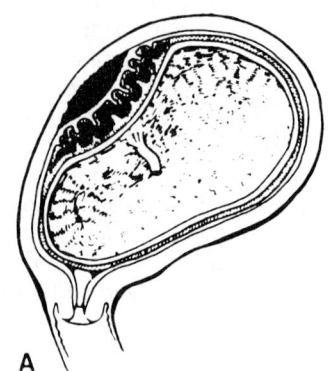 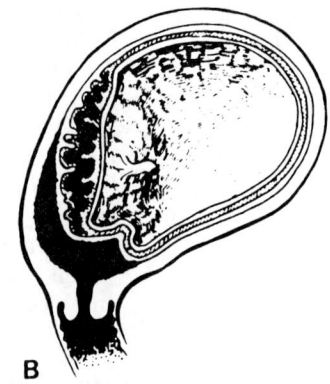 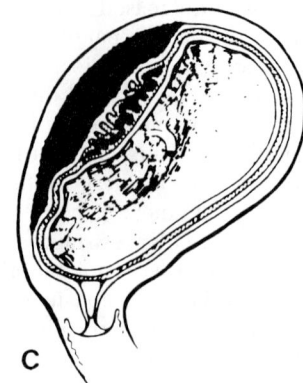

FIGURE 93-2. Types of abruptio placentae. (**A**) Mild abruption with some concealed hemorrhage. (**B**) Severe abruption with external hemorrhage. (**C**) Severe abruption with concealed hemorrhage. (Hayashi RH, Castillo MS: Bleeding in pregnancy. In: Knoeppel R, Drukker J [eds]. *High-Risk Pregnancy: A Team Approach.* Philadelphia, WB Saunders, 1986:428.)

Treatment

Significant maternal or fetal stress requires emergent operative delivery. If a preexisting condition does not mandate operative delivery, if the mother and fetus are stable, and if delivery is indicated (mature fetus, onset of labor, rupture of membranes), the vaginal route may be undertaken with continuous fetal monitoring. Because placental abruption may be associated with disseminated intravascular coagulation (DIC), vaginal delivery is preferable whenever possible. Once the clinical suspicion of placental abruption is entertained, supplemental oxygen, good venous access, evaluation of bleeding and clotting parameters, and typing and crossmatching of blood should be undertaken in a setting in which emergent operative intervention is available.

PLACENTA PREVIA

When the placenta is implanted in the lower uterine segment or is impinging on the cervical os, it is referred to as placenta previa. Four grades are described: *class I*, complete previa, in which the placenta covers the os; *class II*, partial previa, in which the placenta partially overlaps the os; *class III*, marginal previa, in which the edge of the placenta lies at the margin of the internal os; and *class IV*, low-lying placenta, in which the placenta is implanted in the lower uterine segment (Fig. 93-3).[27]

TABLE 93-1. Categories for Placenta Previa

Low lying placenta (type 1)—The placenta is implanted in the lower uterine segment, but placental tissue does not encroach upon or cover the internal os of the cervix.

Marginal placenta previa (type II)—The placenta lies low in the lower uterine segment and actually impinges on the internal os.

Partial placenta previa (type III)—The internal os is partially but not completely covered by placental tissue.

Total placental previa (type IV)—Placental tissue covers the entire cervical os.

In the second trimester, placenta previa may be a normal variant, which, with differential growth, moves away from the os and comes to lie within the body of the uterus at term.[32] When the abnormal position persists, however, it poses the risk of life-threatening hemorrhage.

The incidence of placenta previa ranges from 0.3% to 1.9%, with an associated perinatal mortality rate of 8% to 24%.[33-35] It is associated with multiparity, advanced maternal age, and prior cesarean section; the incidence rate with four or more prior abdominal deliveries increases to 10%. Placenta previa is associated with an increased risk of placenta accreta, a condition in which the placenta grows into the myometrium and becomes abnormally adherent. In an unscarred uterus, the presence of placenta previa is associated with a 5% risk of placenta accreta; placenta previa occurring when the patient has undergone four or more prior cesarean deliveries carries a 67% risk of associated placenta accreta. Placenta accreta may result in overwhelming hemorrhage with attempted delivery of the placenta in more severe cases requiring aortic cross-clamping and hysterectomy.

Diagnosis

A pregnant woman who presents with vaginal bleeding in the second half of pregnancy should be considered to have a placenta previa until proven otherwise. The parturient with a complete previa is more likely to present earlier in pregnancy with vaginal bleeding, whereas those with lesser grades usually present in labor when cervical dilation results in disruption of the vascular attachment.[34]

Because vaginal examination of the parturient with placenta previa can induce hemorrhage, it should be performed only if this condition has been excluded by ultrasound examination or in the cesarean section operating room with the personnel and setup necessary to perform emergency abdominal delivery. Adequate venous access, the availability of blood products, and a setup for infant resuscitation must be established. If the infant is preterm, the examination should be deferred unless fetal or maternal distress man-

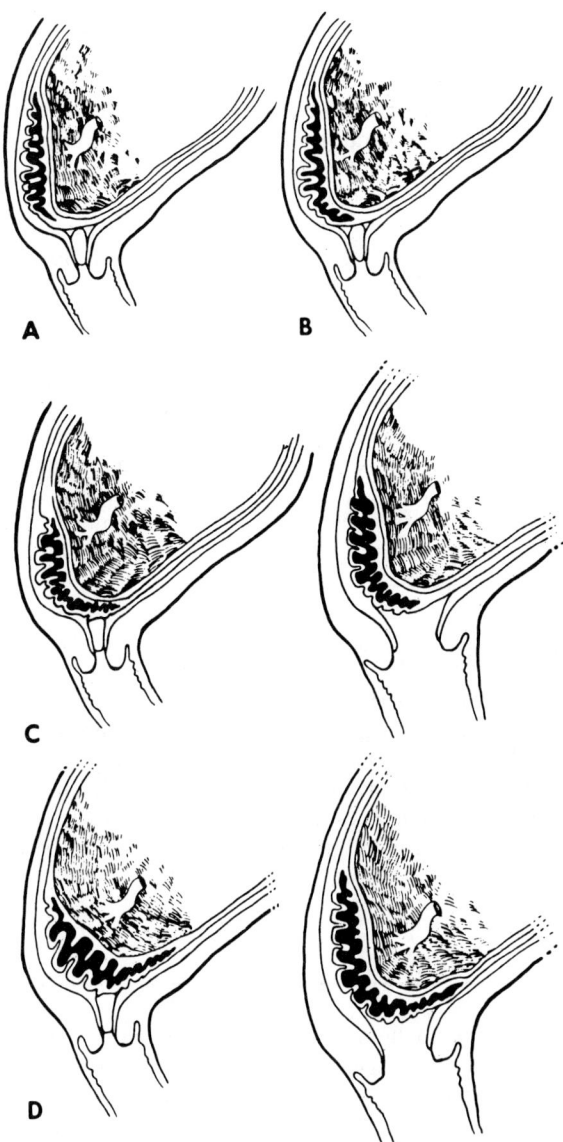

FIGURE 93-3. Classification of placenta previa. (**A**) Class I. (**B**) Class II. (**C**) Class III with closed and partially open cervix. (**D**) Class IV with closed and partially open cervix. (Hayashi RH, Castillo MS: Bleeding in pregnancy. In: Knoeppel R, Drukker J [eds]. *High-Risk Pregnancy: A Team Approach.* Philadelphia, WB Saunders, 1986:426.)

dates delivery.

Unlike placental abruption, where DIC may be induced by thromboplastic substances forced into the maternal circulation, placenta previa rarely requires blood products other than red blood cells unless the resuscitation is extensive enough to cause a dilutional coagulopathy.

Treatment

If the parturient presents with vaginal bleeding before term and mother and fetus are stable, she can be managed with transfusion therapy and bed rest. Immediate access to opera-

tive delivery and neonatal resuscitation is essential in the event that more vigorous bleeding requires intervention. The goal is to continue the pregnancy until fetal maturity can be documented by a mature lecithin:sphingomyelin ratio (>2.0), at which time cesarean delivery is performed.[36] In spite of improvement in maternal and neonatal outcome with this "expectant" management, both premature and mature infants born of patients with placenta previa have an increased incidence of perinatal hypoxia with resultant neurologic compromise.[33]

Cesarean section for placenta previa is associated with an increased risk of intraoperative hemorrhage. The uterine incision may involve the placental bed with resulting maternal and fetal blood loss. Lower uterine segment contractility is poor, bleeding may be difficult to control after delivery of the placenta, and the placenta may be abnormally adherent. Thus, even if the patient is not bleeding actively at the time of operation, the risk for hemorrhage is significantly increased and an appropriate degree of preparedness is indicated.

UTERINE RUPTURE

In addition to abnormalities of the placenta and its implantation, the integrity of the uterus itself may be interrupted, resulting in profound maternal hemorrhage with significant impact on maternal and perinatal morbidity and mortality. It must be considered in the differential diagnosis of obstetric hemorrhage.

Data regarding the incidence rate of uterine rupture vary widely from series to series; a recent review cites 0.02% to 0.08%.[37] It may occur in a previously scarred uterus or de novo, but separation of a previous cesarean section scar remains the most common cause. An extensive number of clinical conditions allegedly are associated with uterine rupture, essentially including any situation in which mechanical weakening occurs or an undue force is exerted on the uterus. Although rupture may occur without identifiable risk factors, those that should heighten one's suspicion are summarized in Table 93-2. Although rare, rupture may also occur in the setting of maternal trauma.

Diagnosis

In its classic presentation, uterine rupture occurs in the laboring patient who, at the height of a contraction, experiences a "ripping" or "tearing" pain. Effective uterine contractions cease, vaginal bleeding ensues, the presenting fetal

TABLE 93-2. Risk Factors Predisposing to Uterine Rupture

Prior cesarean section
Prior myometrial resection or other gynecologic surgery
Grand multiparity
Injudicious use of oxytocin
Internal version
Breech extraction
Midforceps delivery
Overly vigorous fundal pressure to facilitate vaginal delivery

part is no longer palpable, and an odd abdominal mass is present where the fetus has been extruded into the peritoneal cavity. As with other clinical entities, the patient often does not exhibit the classic signs and symptoms.

The pain ascribed to uterine rupture may actually result from associated placental abruption and localized uterine hypertonus.[37] However, the parturient may not complain of abdominal pain, and bleeding into the peritoneal cavity will result in an unimpressive vaginal show. Labor may continue unimpeded. Loss of station (level of the fetus in the birth canal) and change in uterine contour, if present, should assist in making the diagnosis. The most consistent finding associated with uterine rupture is the sudden appearance of fetal distress, most frequently the onset of variable decelerations at a point in labor when their appearance would not be anticipated.[38]

Treatment

As with the other clinical entities discussed, hemorrhage with interruption of the placental circulation is a true emergency, and outcome is dependent on an appropriate high index of suspicion, rapid diagnosis, aggressive transfusion therapy, and definitive operative intervention. Fetal mortality rate ranges from 50% to 75%.[27]

If the presentation is not catastrophic, paracentesis or culdocentesis with ultrasonic guidance may aid in the diagnosis of hemoperitoneum. In the setting of maternal or fetal distress, prompt surgical intervention is indicated. Adequate resuscitation and hemodynamic stability before operation may be impossible in the face of arterial bleeding at the rupture site, and operation should not be delayed. Good venous access cephalad to the surgical site and prompt replacement therapy are mandatory. Cesarean hysterectomy may be necessary, but if hemodynamic parameters permit, repair and salvage of the uterus are often feasible.

POSTPARTUM HEMORRHAGE

Bleeding after fetal delivery can occur from the placenta site, from trauma to the reproductive tract, or from systemic coagulopathy. Most often the cause is uterine atony, because hemostasis is dependent on complete separation of the placenta from its implantation site and compression of the intrauterine vessels by contraction of the myometrium. Retained products of conception must be evacuated either manually or by curettage. If uterine tone cannot then be induced by uterine massage or with pharmacologic agents, ligation of the vascular supply to the uterus or, in extreme cases, hysterectomy must be performed to control bleeding. Inspection of the birth canal should reveal those cervical or vaginal lacerations that are responsible for bleeding.

Postpartum transfusion therapy should be guided by the maternal hemodynamic status. If the mother is stable, as evidenced by blood pressure, pulse, and urine output, I replace blood loss with crystalloid and delay transfusion of blood products until the hematocrit falls below 20%. Blood may be given at a later point in the mother's hospital course if she is symptomatic from the anemia.

COAGULOPATHIES ▪

INTRAUTERINE FETAL DEMISE

Although it is taught that intrauterine fetal demise is a potent stimulus to DIC, it is rarely of clinical concern if the demise is of less than 1 month's duration. Labor usually occurs spontaneously before that time. When coagulopathy does occur, delivery of the fetus, complete evacuation of the products of conception, and transfusion of red blood cells and coagulation factors are indicated.

AMNIOTIC FLUID EMBOLISM

At cesarean section or during vaginal delivery, if a sufficient quantity of amniotic fluid, especially when contaminated with meconium, gains access to the maternal circulation, respiratory embarrassment, circulatory collapse, and DIC may occur. The treatment is directed at ventilatory and circulatory support and transfusion of red blood cells and coagulation factors.

SEPSIS

The parturient is at risk for infection from the urinary tract and the uterine bed. Endotoxemia is a well-known trigger for DIC. Therapy consists of appropriate ventilatory and hemodynamic support, together with transfusion of red blood cells and coagulation factors as directed by laboratory evaluation of coagulation parameters, microbiologic studies, and antibiotics.

CONCLUSIONS ▪

The approach to hemorrhage in the pregnant patient is basically the same as in any patient with bleeding.[39] The focus of therapy is to maintain adequate oxygenation and perfusion to major organs, including the gravid uterus. It is always better to be overly aggressive. Administer supplemental oxygen; establish reliable, large-bore intravenous cannulas with blood administration sets; type and crossmatch blood products, obtain a complete blood count and coagulation panel, and displace the uterus from the great vessels. Diagnosis and intervention are determined in consultation with the attending obstetric staff.

There is no question as to which patient—mother or fetus—demands the focus of resuscitation, because without adequate maternal oxygenation and perfusion, the fetus will not survive in utero. If possible, resuscitation should be attempted with means that have been shown to spare the uterine circulation, but necessary therapy should not be withheld from the mother for fear of its effects on the fetus.

REFERENCES ▪

1. Gibb D: Confidential enquiry into maternal death. *Br J Obstet Gynaecol* 1990;97:97

2. Rochat RW, Koonin LM, Atrash HK, et al: The maternal mortality collaborative: maternal mortality in the United States. Report from the maternal mortality collaborative. *Obstet Gynecol* 1988;72:91

3. Pritchard JA, Baldwin RM, Dickey JC, et al: Blood volume changes in pregnancy and the puerperium. *Am J Obstet Gynecol* 1962;84:1271

4. Pritchard JA: Changes in the blood volume during pregnancy and delivery. *Anesthesiology* 1965;26:393

5. Ueland K: Maternal cardiovascular dynamics. VII. Intrapartum blood volume changes. *Am J Obstet Gynecol* 1976;126:671

6. McFee JG: Anemia in pregnancy: a reappraisal. *Obstet Gynecol Surv* 1973;28:769

7. Ueland K, Metcalfe J: Circulatory changes in pregnancy. *Clin Obstet Gynecol* 1975;18:41

8. Clark SL, Cotton DB, Lee W, et al: Central hemodynamic assessment of normal term pregnancy. *Am J Obstet Gynecol* 1989;161:1439

9. Katz R, Karliner JS, Resnik R: Effects of a natural volume overload state (pregnancy) on left ventricular performance in normal human subjects. *Circulation* 1978;58:434

10. Ueland K, Novy M, Peterson EN, et al: Maternal cardiovascular dynamics. IV. The influence of gestational age on the maternal cardiovascular response to posture and exercise. *Am J Obstet Gynecol* 1969;104:856

11. Bienarz J, Branda LA, Maqueda E, et al: Aortocaval compression by the uterus in late pregnancy. III. Unreliability of the sphygmomanometric method in estimating uterine artery pressure. *Am J Obstet Gynecol* 1968;102:1106

12. Bienarz J, Crottogini JJ, Curuchet E, et al: Aortocaval compression by the uterus in late human pregnancy. II. An arteriographic study. *Am J Obstet Gynecol* 1968;100:203

13. Ueland K, Hansen J: Maternal cardiovascular dynamics. II. Posture and uterine contractions. *Am J Obstet Gynecol* 1969;103:1

14. Katz VL, Dotters DJ, Droegemueller W: Perimortem cesarean delivery. *Obstet Gynecol* 1986;68:571

15. Marx GF: Cardiopulmonary resuscitation of late-pregnant women. *Anesthesiology* 1982;56:156

16. Ralston DH, Shnider SM, deLorimier AA: Effects of equipotent ephedrine, metaraminol, mephenteramine, and methoxamine on uterine blood flow in the pregnant ewe. *Anesthesiology* 1974;40:354

17. Moran DH, Perillo M, LaPorta RF, et al: Phenylephrine in the treatment of hypotension following spinal anesthesia for cesarean delivery. *J Clin Anesth* 1991;3:301

18. Ramanathan S, Grant GJ: Vasopressor therapy for hypotension due to epidural anesthesia for caesarean section. *Acta Anaesthesiol Scand* 1988;32:559

19. Benedetti TJ: Maternal complications of parenteral β-sympathomimetic therapy for premature labor. *Am J Obstet Gynecol* 1983;145:1

20. Gross TL: How tocolytics affect mother, fetus, and neonate. *Contemp Obstet Gynecol* 1982;20:195

21. Childress CH, Katz VL: Nifedipine and its indications in obstetrics and gynecology. *Obstet Gynecol* 1994;83:616

22. Hendricks CH, Brenner WE: Cardiovascular effects of oxytocic drugs used postpartum. *Am J Obstet Gynecol* 1970;108:751

23. Bruce SL, Paul RH, Dorsten JP: Control of postpartum uterine atony by intramyometrial prostaglandin. *Obstet Gynecol* 1982;59:475

24. Hankins GV, Berryman GK, Scott RT, et al: Maternal arterial desaturation with 15-methyl prostaglandin F_2 alpha for uterine atony. *Obstet Gynecol* 1988;72:367

25. Fletcher AP, Alkjaersig NK, Burstein R: The influence of pregnancy upon blood coagulation and plasma fibrinolytic enzyme function. *Am J Obstet Gynecol* 1979;134:743

26. Fay RA, Hughes AO, Farron NT: Platelets in pregnancy: hyperdestruction in pregnancy. *Obstet Gynecol* 1983;61:238

27. Cunningham FG, MacDonald PC, Gant NF (eds): *Williams Obstetrics*, 18th ed. Norwalk, CT, Appleton & Lange, 1989:695

28. Hurd WW, Miodovnik M, Hertzberg V, et al: Selective management of abruptio placentae: a prospective study. *Obstet Gynecol* 1983;61:467

29. Pritchard JA: Genesis of severe placental abruption. *Am J Obstet Gynecol* 1970;108:22

30. Sholl JS: Abruptio placentae: Clinical management in nonacute cases. *Am J Obstet Gynecol* 1987;156:40

31. Pearlman MD, Tintinall JE, Lorenz AP: Blunt trauma during pregnancy. *N Engl J Med* 1990;323:1609

32. Wexler P, Gottesfeld KR: Second trimester placenta previa: an apparently normal presentation. *Obstet Gynecol* 1977;50:706

33. Brenner WE, Edelman DA, Hendricks CH: Characteristics of patients with placenta previa and results of "expectant management." *Am J Obstet Gynecol* 1978;132:180

34. Crenshaw C, Jones DED, Parker RT: Placental previa: a survey of twenty years experience with improved perinatal survival by expectant therapy and cesarean delivery. *Obstet Gynecol Surv* 1973;28:461

35. Singh PM, Rodrigues C, Gupta AN: Placenta previa and previous cesarean section. *Acta Obstet Gynecol Scand* 1981;60:367

36. Clark SL, Koonings PP, Phelan JP: Placenta previa/accreta and prior cesarean section. *Obstet Gynecol* 1985;66:89

37. Phelan JP: Uterine rupture. *Clin Obstet Gynecol* 1990;33:432

38. Rodriguez MH, Masaki DI, Phelan JP, et al: Uterine rupture: are intrauterine pressure catheters useful in the diagnosis? *Am J Obstet Gynecol* 1989;161:666

39. Schneider JM: Hemorrhage: related obstetric and medical disorders. In: Bonica JJ, McDonald JS (eds). *Principles and Practice of Obstetric Analgesia and Anesthesia*. Batimore, Williams & Wilkins, 1995:865

Critical Care, Third Edition, edited by Joseph M. Civetta,
Robert W. Taylor, and Robert R. Kirby.
Lippincott-Raven Publishers, Philadelphia, PA © 1997.

CHAPTER 94

■

Pulmonary Abnormalities

Robert R. Kirby

IMMEDIATE CONCERNS ■

MAJOR PROBLEMS

Intensive respiratory care of the obstetric patient should be undertaken only in the ICU where specialized equipment and personnel are concentrated. Causes of acute respiratory failure during pregnancy include aspiration of gastric contents, pulmonary infection, asthma, beta-adrenergic tocolytic therapy, air embolism, amniotic fluid embolism, and thromboembolism. Indications for intubation and mechanical ventilation are similar for pregnant and nonpregnant patients.

A PaO_2 of 60 mm Hg normally represents an arterial oxyhemoglobin saturation (SaO_2) of 90%. Substantial increases in PaO_2 above 60 mm Hg effect a maximal 10% increase in SaO_2 if arterial pH stays constant. Conversely, a PaO_2 less than 60 mm Hg produces a significant reduction in saturation.

The maximal fraction of inspired oxygen (FIO_2) generally achieved with nasal cannulae at an oxygen flow rate of 6 L/minute is 0.40. Increasing flow to higher levels does not increase the tracheal FIO_2. A FIO_2 of 0.6 usually can be provided with a simple face mask. Higher FIO_2 requires non-rebreather or partial rebreather masks. However, a patient who requires a FIO_2 greater than 0.6 with a mask to achieve a SaO_2 of 90% is at constant risk of significant hypoxemia. Should the mask be removed for only a short period of time, an obstetric patient with a pregnancy-induced reduction of functional residual capacity (FRC) will desaturate faster than a nonpregnant patient. Fetal hypoxia, with possible catastrophic results, will quickly follow.

Failure of ventilation is defined by respiratory acidemia, as the partial pressure of arterial carbon dioxide ($PaCO_2$) rises and the pH decreases. Normal $PaCO_2$ in the pregnant patient is approximately 30 to 34 mm Hg beginning in the first trimester. Thus, a *seemingly* normal $PaCO_2$ of 40 mm Hg in a pregnant patient is elevated and must be thoroughly assessed as a possible indicator of acute respiratory failure.

Therapeutic options beyond supplemental oxygen include continuous positive airway pressure (CPAP) and mechanical ventilation with positive end-expiratory pressure (PEEP). Positive-pressure ventilation maintains the FRC and decreases the work of breathing.

STRESS POINTS

1. A decision to intubate the trachea should not be taken lightly. Nasotracheal intubation is relatively contraindicated during pregnancy. The nasal mucosa is engorged, hyperemic, and friable. Bleeding is easily started and difficult to stop. Even if successful, the tube size that passes the turbinates is often so small as to make spontaneous breathing difficult and may even compromise mechanical support.
2. Orotracheal intubation, even in the best of circumstances, is problematic. Mechanical difficulties include manipulation of a standard laryngoscope handle between the patient's chin and enlarged breasts. Visualization of the larynx is rendered difficult by the frequent presence of oropharyngeal and supraglottic edema. Fiberoptic bronchoscopy can be used to aid tube placement but requires skill and experience.
3. The predisposition to vomiting increases the risk of pulmonary aspiration of gastric contents even in an awake individual.
4. Significant hypertension may result from laryngoscopy and is particularly marked in patients with hypertensive disorders of pregnancy. Cerebral edema and intracranial hemorrhage can result in severely preeclamptic patients.

1409

5. As with nasotracheal intubation, a small-diameter tube may be needed because of laryngeal or tracheal edema. However, work of breathing is increased significantly, and occult PEEP may occur because of the increased expiratory resistance in a small-diameter tube.

6. Endotracheal tube cuff design affects pressure transmitted to the mucosa. A larger tube size means that a smaller volume of air needs to be injected into the pilot tube to effect a cuff seal. Hence, pressure necrosis is less likely to result from the cuff's approximation to the edematous tracheal mucosa.

7. A CPAP system may be used if the patient's problem is primarily hypoxemia, not hypercapnia; central respiratory control mechanisms are intact; and the work of breathing is not excessive.

8. Obstetric patients have a naturally occurring reduction of FRC. Superimposed further reduction of FRC in acute respiratory failure increases intrapulmonary shunting and hypoxemia. Fetal compromise is a real possibility.

9. When excessive maternal hyperventilation results from inappropriate ventilator support, adverse fetal effects may be profound. Careful titration is indicated with observation for beneficial and adverse effects on mother and fetus.

ESSENTIAL DIAGNOSTIC TESTS AND PROCEDURES

1. A high index of suspicion for respiratory complications is necessary. Pregnancy presents some unique problems (2 patients, amniotic fluid embolism) and increases others (rapid desaturation, aspiration of gastric contents).

2. Standard monitors (including pulse oximeters) should be used routinely. Invasive monitors (e.g., pulmonary artery catheters) can be useful to differentiate cardiogenic and noncardiogenic pulmonary edema.

3. Don't forget fetal monitoring! Everything that is done to the mother potentially affects the baby.

4. Beware of a normal $PaCO_2$ in a patient with suspected respiratory compromise. Such a value represents respiratory failure until proven otherwise.

5. Sudden cardiovascular collapse should elicit an immediate search for an embolic episode (thrombus, air, or amniotic fluid).

INITIAL THERAPY

1. Provide oxygen and secure the airway if necessary. Pregnant patients desaturate rapidly.

2. Be gentle with tracheal intubation. The airway from the nose distally is edematous, friable, and easily damaged.

3. Anticipate intubation difficulties, and be prepared with optional approaches.

4. Think about the drugs you give and their possible effects on the fetus, particularly in the first trimester or if delivery is imminent.

5. Keep the compromised patient in the ICU. Obstetric wards generally are ill-equipped to care for acutely ill patients with problems outside those related to the pregnancy per se.

PHYSIOLOGIC CONSIDERATIONS ■

Pregnant women undergo significant changes in cardiopulmonary function, the normal extremes of which must be appreciated by anyone who cares for them. Minute ventilation increases, and $PaCO_2$ values of 30 to 32 mm Hg are common. The FRC is reduced by upward diaphragmatic and rib cage displacement. Bronchial smooth muscle is more reactive; pharyngeal and airway mucosal edema are often prominent; and salivary gland activity is increased.

Obstetric patients are prone to aspiration of gastric contents, amniotic fluid embolism, and bronchospasm; wheezing is one of the earliest, yet nonspecific, signs in many cases.[1] Pulmonary edema associated with preeclampsia, drug reactions, congenital heart disease, or aspiration may provoke wheezing as a result of partial small airways obstruction. Respiratory problems are the basis for a significant percentage of obstetric ICU admissions (Table 94-1).

These changes are exacerbated by abnormal conditions such as preeclampsia. Pulmonary edema, in combination with the normally reduced FRC, predisposes to an even more rapid decrease in PaO_2. Mucosal edema and hyperemia

TABLE 94-1. Antepartum and Postpartum ICU Admitting Diagnoses

ICU ADMITTING DIAGNOSIS	ANTEPARTUM		POSTPARTUM	
	No. of Patients	*Ventilated*	*No. of Patients*	*Ventilated*
Respiratory failure	7	5	6	5
Hemodynamic instability	2	0	11	5
Neurologic dysfunction	2	2	4	2
Total	11	7 (66%)	21	12 (57%)

From Kirkpatrick SJ, Matthay MA: Obstetric patients requiring critical care: a five year review. *Chest* 1992;101:1407.

contribute to airway bleeding and potentially rapid obstruction during tracheal intubation. Increased pulmonary microvascular pressure, coupled with decreased colloid oncotic pressure, can trigger pulmonary edema. The condition is worsened by a variety of other factors, including embolization syndromes, sepsis, shock, aspiration of gastric contents, and abruptio placentae.

VENTILATION AND PERFUSION ■

LUNG VOLUME AND ALVEOLAR VENTILATION

When a normal adult lies supine, the FRC decreases by 500 mL because of cephalad displacement of the diaphragm. This change is accentuated by the gravid uterus, further reducing FRC. As a result, hemoglobin desaturation is more rapid when ventilation is impaired or interrupted.

Both tidal volume and respiratory rate increase at term.[1] These changes are associated with a 50% increase of minute ventilation and a 70% increase of alveolar ventilation (Table 94-2). The reduction of $PaCO_2$ is significant ($\leq 25\%$), but not so great as would be predicted from the increase in ventilation. Widespread ventilation/perfusion ($\dot{V}/\dot{Q}$) changes may occur, but dead space is reportedly unchanged. Increased carbon dioxide production, in association with increased oxygen consumption, must be invoked to explain this phenomenon. These variations result from altered metabolic activity (e.g., normal metabolic rate of the mother, products of conception, work of carrying the fetus). Respiratory muscle work during labor can augment 300%.

PULMONARY BLOOD FLOW

Maternal blood volume at term is approximately 40% above nonpregnant levels. Cardiac output increases by 30% to 40% between 20 and 30 weeks of gestation. Both heart rate and stroke volume are increased (see Table 94-2). An increase in cardiac output of 15% to 45% above prelabor values occurs during labor, and even more so during uterine contractions. In the immediate postpartum period, it increases yet another 30% to 40% above labor values as blood previously directed to the placenta is returned to the maternal systemic circulation.

Tachypnea-induced decrease in pleural pressure augments right ventricular filling and is associated with interventricular septal displacement.[2] Increased transmural pulmonary vascular pressure may occur. In pregnancy, high peripheral venous pressure results from the gravid uterus. Venous return (in the absence of vena caval obstruction) is enhanced, further increasing transmural pulmonary vascular pressure. These changes often are reflected by an engorged pulmonary vascular bed observed on chest radiographs. The possibility of pulmonary edema, particularly in cases of preexisting cardiopulmonary disease, is a real threat.

Position Changes

In the supine position, spontaneous ventilation predominantly involves dependent lung areas.[3] Relatively little venti-

TABLE 94-2. Cardiopulmonary Changes in Normal Pregnancy

CARDIOVASCULAR FEATURES

Cardiac output	↑ 30–40% at 20–30 wk
	↑ Additional 15–45% during labor
	↑ Additional 10–25% during uterine contraction
Erythrocytes	↑ 20–30% at term
Plasma volume	↑ 45–55% at term

RESPIRATORY FEATURES

Minute ventilation	↑ 50% at term
Alveolar ventilation	↑ 70% at term
$PaCO_2$	30–32 mm Hg
PaO_2	Unchanged or slightly decreased
Oxygen consumption	Increased
Carbon dioxide production	Increased
Functional residual capacity	Decreased

lation occurs in nondependent lung fields. Pulmonary blood flow is distributed similarly, and passive $\dot{V}/\dot{Q}$ matching results.

If the patient is paralyzed and manually or mechanically ventilated during anesthesia, significant $\dot{V}/\dot{Q}$ alterations occur. The flaccid diaphragm moves passively but is impeded in its posterior descent by the abdominal contents, an effect that is accentuated by the gravid uterus.[3] In this circumstance, most ventilation is nondependent. Pulmonary perfusion, however, remains largely dependent because of the relatively low-pressure characteristics of the pulmonary circulation. The high cardiac output of pregnancy may partially offset this $\dot{V}/\dot{Q}$ imbalance. On the other hand, if vena caval compression significantly reduces venous return, as it does in 10% or more of supine pregnant patients, the imbalance may be increased. The effect of reduced cardiac output and shunting on PaO_2 is shown in Table 94-3 and Figure 94-1.

Central Control of Respiration

Although much of the central nervous system's activity is depressed during pregnancy, respiratory control mechanisms are activated. By the sixth week of gestation, reductions of alveolar and arterial PCO_2 occur and persist throughout pregnancy. This response is enhanced at high altitude, and $PaCO_2$ values between 20 and 27 mm Hg have been reported. Chronic hypocapnia is associated with renal excretion of bicarbonate, resulting in a return of arterial pH toward normal. Serum bicarbonate levels as low as 12 to 14 mMol/L may occur during hypoxia-induced hypocapnia in pregnancy, leading an inexperienced observer to diagnose a significant nonrespiratory (metabolic) acidosis. In reality, this change is a normal compensatory response to chronic hypoxia and hypocapnia. The decreased buffering capacity, however, may contribute to the dyspnea experienced by many women during pregnancy.

TABLE 94-3. Effects of Shunt and Cardiac Output on PaO_2

CONDITIONS	CO (L/min)	$P\bar{v}O_2$ (mm Hg)	$C\bar{v}O_2$ (mL/100 mL)	CaO_2 (mL/100 mL)	$C(a - \bar{v})O_2$ (mL/100 mL)	$\dot{Q}s/\dot{Q}t$	PaO_2 (mm Hg)
Normal	5	47	14.8	19.8	5	0.02	600
Shunt	5	42	13.8	18.8	5	0.20	250
Decreased cardiac output	2.5	18	7.5	17.5	10	0.20	90

CO, cardiac output; $P\bar{v}O_2$, partial pressure of oxygen venous blood; $C\bar{v}O_2$, mixed venous oxygen content; CaO_2, arterial oxygen content; $C(a - \bar{v})O_2$, arterial–mixed venous oxygen content difference.

DIAGNOSIS AND TREATMENT OF RESPIRATORY FAILURE ■

Diagnostic and therapeutic modalities in pregnancy-associated respiratory failure are usually the same as in nonpregnant patients. Pulse oximetry enhances monitoring capabilities and management.[4] Combined with appropriately used fetal monitoring, the incidence and severity of maternal and fetal hypoxemia should be diminished.

Mechanical or manual ventilation with PEEP and CPAP are effective in the treatment of many forms of acute respiratory failure. However, their potentially adverse effects on venous return, particularly if aortocaval compression is significant, can present major maternal and fetal problems. Conversely, noncardiogenic pulmonary edema can be acutely exacerbated by increased pulmonary arterial blood flow and pressure. Sudden changes in the patient's condition, of an even greater magnitude than in the nonpregnant individual, are therefore to be expected.

Obstetric patients are often managed on the ward far too long before consultation is sought for respiratory and other basically nonobstetric conditions. If any patient should receive the benefits of critical care, it is the pregnant woman with serious or life-threatening disease. Unfortunately, many intensivists have little or no experience in the management of sick obstetric patients. Increased interaction between specialists is essential to reduce maternal and fetal morbidity and mortality. Advances in this area should be no less progressive than in perinatology.

PULMONARY EMBOLIZATION SYNDROMES

Thromboembolism

Pulmonary thromboembolization is the third leading cause of death in the United States, accounting for approximately 200,000 deaths annually.[5] Pregnancy predisposes women to dependent venous stasis. Most clots form in pelvic, iliofemoral, and popliteal vessels. Antepartum pulmonary embolization is rare, but the incidence increases dramatically in the postpartum period.[6]

Symptoms and signs are nonspecific and depend on the size of the embolus[5] (Table 94-4). Of major importance is fixed splitting of the second heart sound (i.e., right ventricular overload) and a flow murmur over the lung fields. A chest radiograph may show focal oligemia (Westermark's

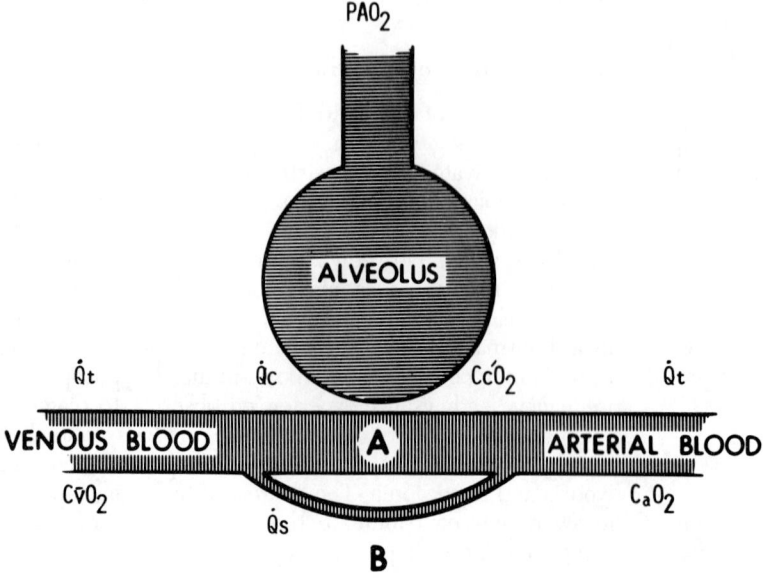

FIGURE 94-1. Venous blood in the pulmonary circulation may pass through areas that are well ventilated (**A**) or hypoventilated or nonventilated (**B**). If the cardiac output decreases and systemic extraction of oxygen increases, the venous oxygen content will be less than normal. Any portion of the reduced cardiac output passing through *B* will cause a greater decrease in the resultant CaO_2 and PaO_2 than if cardiac output is normal. $\dot{Q}t$, total cardiac output; $\dot{Q}s$, shunted portion of cardiac output; $\dot{Q}c$, capillary flow; CaO_2, arterial oxygen content; $C\bar{v}O_2$, mixed venous oxygen content; $Cc'O_2$, end-capillary oxygen content (after equilibrating with ideal alveolus); PaO_2, alveolar PO_2 in "ideal" alveoli.

TABLE 94-4. Signs and Symptoms of Pulmonary Thromboembolization

INDICATION	PATIENTS AFFECTED (%)
SIGNS	
Tachypnea	90
Tachycardia	45
Increased P$_2$	53
Localized crackles	58
Fever	45
Thrombophlebitis	40
Supraventricular dysrhythmias	15
SYMPTOMS	
Dyspnea	84
Chest pain	88
Apprehension	59
Cough	53
Hemoptysis	30

sign) and the ECG occasionally reveals P pulmonale and right axis deviation. Definitive diagnosis requires pulmonary angiographic studies. In severe cases, cardiovascular collapse can rapidly supervene.

Initial therapy is entirely supportive and includes oxygen, sometimes in conjunction with tracheal intubation and positive-pressure ventilation, fluid infusion, and cardiovascular support with inotropic agents. In severe cases, right ventricular failure (acute cor pulmonale) may be life-threatening, and infusions must be carefully monitored. Although the classic $\dot{V}/\dot{Q}$ abnormality is an increase in dead space, intrapulmonary shunting and hypoxemia also may be increased by the development of interstitial pulmonary edema. Improvement with PEEP and CPAP often is dramatic.

Heparin therapy for documented pulmonary thromboembolism is the preferred treatment, but it can produce bleeding in obstetric patients. Initial doses are 5000 to 10,000 USP units intravenously, followed by a continuous infusion of 500 to 1000 USP units/hour. A partial thromboplastin time of one and one half to two times normal is the desired end point. Thrombolytic therapy with streptokinase, urokinase, or thromboplastinogen activator is associated with a high incidence of bleeding, but may be lifesaving in the worst cases. Vena caval plication and insertion of caval filters have decreased in popularity.[5]

Amniotic Fluid Embolism

Amniotic fluid embolism occurs in 1 patient in 10,000 deliveries. It is most commonly seen with multiparity, prolonged and difficult labor, cephalopelvic disproportion, placenta previa, polyhydramnios, uterine tetany, precipitate delivery, after cesarean section, and with intrauterine fetal demise.[7] Its onset may be heralded by cardiovascular collapse and frequently entails dyspnea, cyanosis, shock, seizures, and coma.[3] The maternal mortality rate is as high as 86%. It does not seem to be related to induction of labor.

Differential diagnoses include other pulmonary embolic events, eclampsia, intracranial hemorrhage, and heart failure. Fetal squamous cells and other elements have been aspirated through central venous or pulmonary artery catheters.[8] However, because most patients do not have such catheters in place, diagnosis by this method is of limited value.

Therapy is supportive and includes oxygen, positive-pressure ventilation, fluids, vasopressors, and expeditious uterine evacuation. Uterine evacuation enhances venous return and allows closure of uteroplacental sinusoids and endocervical veins.

Venous Air Embolization

Although commonly associated with sitting neurosurgical procedures, venous air embolization has been reported in pregnant patients during or after cesarean section and during orogenital sex when the sexual partner blows air forcefully into the vagina.[9–11] Placental separation followed by entry of air into the venous sinuses may be fatal in these circumstances. Air blown into the vagina should be considered as a possible factor in pregnant patients brought to the emergency room in extremis for whom no other cause can be ascertained.

After percutaneous vascular cannulation, significant venous air embolization can occur through large-bore needles or cannula introducers in spontaneously breathing patients. Up to 100 mL of air each second can be entrained through a 14-gauge catheter in the subclavian or internal jugular vein during a deep and rapid inspiration. If these techniques are used, patients should be placed in a head-down position and instructed to hold their breath any time the needle or cannula hub is open to air.

Treatment includes aspiration of air if a central catheter is in situ and placement of the patient in a left lateral decubitus position. Based on a study in dogs, this classic positioning recently has been questioned.[12] However, the preponderance of data in animals and humans supports its use.[13–15] Vasopressors are desirable for hypotensive patients. Oxygen should be administered, with positive-pressure ventilation if necessary. Paradoxic air embolism to the arterial circulation has been reported as a risk if pulmonary artery pressure is greatly increased. Some investigators debate the merits of manual or mechanical ventilation and PEEP during resuscitation, because both modes of therapy can increase pulmonary vascular resistance.[16] However, such therapy clearly is necessary in cases of cardiopulmonary collapse.

Fat Embolization

Fat embolization is likely only after trauma and fractures of the pelvis and long bones. Early stabilization and fixation of fractures is indicated in most cases. Treatment is largely supportive. Evidence does not support the prophylactic use of heparin or steroids. Prevention of hypoxia is essential to maternal and fetal well-being and is best achieved by oxygen administration and PEEP and CPAP, with or without mechanical ventilation.

PULMONARY ASPIRATION OF GASTRIC CONTENTS

Of all the respiratory disorders in pregnancy, pulmonary aspiration of gastric contents is best known and perhaps most feared. Described by Curtis Mendelson[1] in 1945, it has been studied extensively since. The reported mortality is high, although in my experience the outcome is usually good. Parturients are at particular risk because of delayed gastric emptying, relaxed cardioesophageal sphincter tone, increased abdominal pressure, and the inevitably full stomach. Vomiting normally is increased during the first trimester of pregnancy, but it sometimes persists as hyperemesis gravidarum.

Physical characteristics of aspiration syndromes depend on what is aspirated and how much[17] (Table 94-5). With acid aspiration (i.e., associated volume of 25 mL or greater at a pH of 2.5 or less), wheezing, cyanosis, dyspnea, and tachypnea occur. With particulate matter aspiration (e.g., food chunks), airway obstruction with stridor, tachypnea, wheezing, and coughing predominate.

In severe cases, pulmonary edema may result from sudden increases of pulmonary capillary endothelial permeability. Hypoxemia, hypercapnia, and nonrespiratory acidosis are prominent features and can be life-threatening. A chest radiograph is positive in approximately 90% of cases, although a delay in radiographic manifestation of as long as 24 hours sometimes occurs. Most commonly involved is the right lower lobe, followed by the left lower and right middle lobes. Widespread and confluent infiltrates may be indistinguishable from other forms of the acute respiratory distress syndrome (ARDS).

Therapy is supportive and includes oxygen, establishment of an artificial airway in most cases, and positive airway pressure (i.e., PEEP and CPAP with or without mechanical ventilation). Except for the removal of food or other solid particles, do not waste time trying to suction the aspirated material. The damage is done immediately. Similarly, do not bother to neutralize a suspected acid aspiration with sodium bicarbonate or other alkali. The damage will only be made worse.

No valid evidence supports the use of corticosteroids in ameliorating aspiration. Antibiotics may be useful if the

TABLE 94-5. Findings in Pulmonary Aspiration

ACID

Cyanosis
Tachypnea
Dyspnea
Wheezing
Bloody sputum (severe cases)
Suprasternal or intercostal retractions
Hypotension

PARTICULATE

Stridor
Tachypnea
Wheezing
Coughing

aspirated material is known to be infected. Otherwise, they should be withheld until culture results document the source of infection. Aerosolized β_2-selective agents, such as terbutaline, albuterol, or metaproterenol can be of value in alleviating bronchospasm. Mucosal and submucosal edema often are responsive to the nebulization of racemic epinephrine.

Prevention of aspiration is desirable but often difficult in pregnancy because patients usually are not in nil per os status. Remember that the time from which to consider that the stomach was full is not when the last meal was eaten, but when labor began (often several hours later). Assume every pregnant woman has a full stomach.

ACUTE RESPIRATORY FAILURE

Differentiation of acute respiratory failure from embolization and aspiration syndromes is arbitrary, because the latter conditions can produce life-threatening pulmonary insufficiency. However, because mechanisms of damage and pathophysiologic changes vary somewhat, the division into separate categories is reasonable.

A variety of lesions predispose the patient to ARDS[18] (Table 94-6). In many cases, polymorphonuclear leukocytes seem to play a key role.[19] Leukoembolization and leukoag-

TABLE 94-6. Etiologic Factors in Adult Respiratory Distress Syndrome

CONDITION	CAUSES
Obstetric	Eclampsia, amniotic fluid embolism
Sepsis	
Trauma	Burns, fat emboli, pulmonary contusion, nonthoracic trauma, near drowning
Infection	Viral, bacterial, fungal, pneumonia, tuberculosis
Toxic gas inhalation	Oxygen, smoke, NO_2, NH_3, Cl_2, phosgene
Aspiration of gastric contents	
Drug injection	Heroin, methadone, barbiturates, thiazides, propoxyphene, salicylates, colchicine
Metabolic	Uremia, diabetic ketoacidosis
Miscellaneous	Pancreatitis, disseminated intravascular coagulation, bowel infarction, cacinomatosis, paraquat poisoning

glutination within the pulmonary microvasculature, followed by neutrophil release of toxic-free radicals of oxygen, produce increased endothelial permeability, increased interstitial lung water, terminal airway closure, atelectasis, and right-to-left intrapulmonic shunting. The hallmark of this syndrome is hypoxemia, which is often severe and frequently refractory to the administration of oxygen and manual or mechanical ventilation.[18,20]

Because trauma tends to be a disease of young people (i.e., leading cause of death in persons younger than 40 years age), we see an increasing number of pregnant victims. Because the FRC is already reduced during pregnancy, the additional loss of FRC characteristics with ARDS is probably less well tolerated in pregnancy than in the nonpregnant state.

The $PaCO_2$ in ARDS and pregnancy characteristically is low. Hence, a normal value (>35 mm Hg) is cause for alarm. In view of the propensity for severe hypoxemia, all pregnant patients with ARDS or any form of respiratory failure should be continuously monitored with a pulse oximeter. An oxyhemoglobin saturation below 90% (i.e., PaO_2 of 55 to 60 mm Hg during pregnancy) represents a serious threat to the fetus and indicates major impairment of lung function. Frequent arterial blood gas analysis is essential.

Treatment is supportive. A few patients respond to oxygen therapy, clearance of secretions, and chest physiotherapy. Most require tracheal intubation, PEEP or CPAP, and mechanical ventilation.[21] Because of the tendency in late pregnancy for compression of the inferior vena cava and a reduction of venous return, positive airway pressure may be poorly tolerated. A recent study showed that demand-flow airway pressure release ventilation (APRV) provides effective partial ventilatory support at lower peak pressure than pressure support ventilation and synchronized intermittent mandatory ventilation.[22] Hence, APRV may result in less circulatory compromise to the pregnant patient. The cardiovascular effects of mechanical ventilation, many of which are accentuated in pregnancy, have been comprehensively summarized by Pinsky.[23] Permissive hypercapnia, carefully regulated by low-rate low–tidal volume mechanical ventilation,[24] has theoretical appeal, not only to reduce problems such as barotrauma and air embolization, but also to lessen the circulatory impact.

Specific treatment is limited. All infectious processes (e.g., pneumonia, sepsis) should be aggressively treated with appropriate antibiotics. Steroids are of no proven benefit and should not be used in established ARDS. Some evidence suggests that they may be beneficial if administered prophylactically. However, because we usually do not have the luxury of knowing which patient will develop respiratory failure, prophylactic treatment is unlikely to be of much value.

ASTHMA

The overall incidence and severity of asthma seems to be unaffected by pregnancy. Patients receiving long-term bronchodilator therapy should be continued on their established drug regimen. The importance of early medical intervention and aggressive treatment of severe asthmatic attacks cannot be overemphasized in view of the risk of fetal asphyxia. Commonly employed drugs are associated with a negligible risk of first-trimester teratogenicity.

Pregnancy has a mixed effect on asthma: 49% of patients are unchanged, 29% improve, and 22% become worse. Improvement may result from the increased release of progesterone and cortisol in pregnancy, but upper airway edema, increased oxygen consumption, and decreased pulmonary reserve can exacerbate the condition. Patients who are chronically symptomatic should continue effective drug therapy, including theophylline, corticosteroids, beta-adrenergic agonists, and cromolyn.

Intravenous aminophylline may be used during acute exacerbations. If a patient is receiving chronic theophylline therapy, the intravenous dose of aminophylline should be limited to 0.5 to 0.9 mg/kg. For each 1.0 mg/kg administered, the serum theophylline level will increase an average of 2 μg/mL.[25] Toxicity is a real problem and a baseline serum measurement should be obtained before beginning treatment. Oxygen therapy (i.e., nasal cannula, catheter, face mask) may be necessary during labor and delivery. Constant monitoring with a pulse oximeter is essential during this period, supplemented if necessary by arterial blood gas analysis.

TUBERCULOSIS

Tuberculosis, which once was thought to have been largely eradicated, is again on the rise, and increasing numbers of cases are to be expected during pregnancy. Drug therapy with isoniazid and rifampin usually is effective and subjects the fetus to minimal risk. Appropriate isolation procedures during labor and delivery should be employed. Disposable ventilator circuits make patient management and infection control easier than was previously true.

Since 1990, nosocomial and correctional system transmission of multidrug-resistant tuberculosis has been reported to the Centers for Disease Control.[26] Most cases were in HIV-positive patients. Multidrug-resistant tuberculosis reportedly is resistant to isoniazid, rifampin, pyrazinamide, ethambutol, streptomycin, kanamycin, and ethionamide. Patients with this disease die rapidly. Its significance in obstetrics is yet to be determined.

CHRONIC LUNG DISEASE

Bronchiectasis

In the 1950s and 1960s, bronchiectasis received major attention. It can still present severe problems, but its incidence in the United States since 1970 has diminished, presumably as a result of better antibiotic therapy. When a patient with bronchiectasis is encountered, aggressive antibiotic and chest physiotherapy are indicated. Tracheobronchial toiletry is important, particularly if an endotracheal tube is inserted during general inhalation anesthesia.

Emphysema and Chronic Bronchitis

Emphysema and chronic bronchitis in the childbearing age group are rare. Because the basic conditions are irreversible, they cannot be cured. Nevertheless, any reversible component (e.g., airway edema, bronchospasm) should be treated aggressively with aerosolized topical vasoconstrictors and bronchodilators, respectively. Prevention of hypoxemia or hypercapnia beyond baseline levels requires hospitalization and careful observation in an ICU.

Cystic Fibrosis

Cystic fibrosis in pregnancy once was a rarely encountered problem because few patients lived until their childbearing years. Today, longer survival is common, and reports of successful completion of pregnancy in women with cystic fibrosis have been published.[27] Worsening of baseline pulmonary function often does not occur with pregnancy. Careful evaluation and close monitoring during gestation are essential, and hospitalization, vigorous pulmonary toilet, and aggressive antibiotic therapy are indicated at the first sign of pulmonary complications.

Kyphoscoliosis

Chronic restrictive lung disease (e.g., pulmonary interstitial fibrosis, kyphoscoliosis) in pregnancy is rare. If severe, successful conclusion of the pregnancy represents a major threat to maternal survival. Termination of pregnancy should be considered in advanced kyphoscoliotic lung disease. The best ventilator support therapy is largely ineffective in acute cor pulmonale, a real risk with the superimposed cardiopulmonary stress of pregnancy.

PULMONARY EDEMA

Pulmonary edema indicates a predisposing factor[28] (Table 94-7). Major concerns are management of the effects (predominantly hypoxemia) and establishment of the causes. Management is reasonably easy to address, because therapy is usually the same as for other forms of ARDS, the characteristic finding of which is pulmonary edema. However, in pregnant patients, particularly those with congenital heart disease, the problem may be cardiovascular in origin and considerably more difficult to treat.

Pulmonary artery catheterization is indicated in selected patients if the origin during pregnancy is not clear.[29] A low pulmonary artery occlusion pressure, for practical purposes, eliminates left ventricular failure as an etiologic factor. A high pulmonary artery pressure may reflect preeclampsia or other forms of noncardiogenic pulmonary edema. The distinction between these disease categories is significant. Diuresis, which may be indicated for left ventricular failure, is an obvious threat to both maternal and fetal well-being in a mother who is hypovolemic and has noncardiogenic pulmonary edema. Sequential measurements of cardiac output, central venous pressure, pulmonary artery occlusion pressure, and mixed venous oxygen saturation, together with calculated values of systemic and pulmonary vascular resistance, can guide therapy based on physiologic end points.

In severe preeclampsia, inappropriate fluid therapy can precipitate significant elevation of pulmonary artery pressure and an increase of fluid deposition in the pulmonary intersti-

TABLE 94-7. Causes of Pulmonary Edema

CARDIOGENIC (HIGH PRESSURES)

Cardiac dysfunction
    Decreased left ventricular contractility
    Mitral stenoses
    Mitral regurgitation
    Intravascular volume overload
    Arrhythmias
Pulmonary venous dysfunction
    Venous occlusive disease
    Neurogenic pulmonary vasoconstriction
Pulmonary embolization
    Amniotic fluid
    Thrombus
    Fat
    Air
Airway obstruction
    Edema
    Asthma
    Foreign body
Preeclampsia
    Pulmonary hypertension
Miscellaneous
    Pneumothorax
    Tumor
    One-lung anesthesia (down lung syndrome)

NONCARDIOGENIC (PERMEABILITY)

Acute respiratory distress syndrome
Aspiration syndromes
Pulmonary embolization
Abruptio placentae
Dead fetus syndrome
Sepsis

---

tium. A lowering of plasma oncotic pressure after delivery may exacerbate this problem, although the data are not convincing. If preeclampsia progresses to eclamptic seizures, pulmonary aspiration of gastric contents can make the differential diagnosis problematic.

If airway obstruction occurs after a failed intubation or after extubation, the patient's inspiratory efforts against a closed glottis may produce negative-pressure pulmonary edema.[30,31] This condition sometimes generates severe hypoxemia and a radiographic picture similar to diffuse aspiration. The multifactorial origins of noncardiac (permeability) pulmonary edema are difficult to differentiate. Even if a permeability problem leads to initial manifestations of pulmonary edema, pulmonary hypertension from any cause will make it worse. Careful fluid management during labor, anesthesia, delivery, and in the postpartum period is mandatory.

SHOCK

Hemorrhage leading to cardiovascular insufficiency and shock is a common problem in obstetrics. Causes include placenta previa, abruptio placentae, obstetric injuries (e.g., lacerations), retained products of conception, uterine atony, and major trauma. Historically, it was thought that shock could lead to acute pulmonary insufficiency. This view was so prevalent that the term "shock lung" frequently was applied. Recent studies suggest that, in the absence of sepsis or direct thoracic trauma, shock does not lead to lung dysfunction. Conditions that produce shock, however, may produce concurrent lung damage. Respiratory and multiorgan system failure in sepsis and septic shock are serious problems associated with high mortality.

REFERENCES ◼

1. Mendelson CL: The aspiration of stomach contents into the lungs during anesthesia. *Am J Obstet Gynecol* 1946;52:191
2. Robotham JL, Scharf SM: Effects of positive and negative pressure ventilation on cardiac performance. *Clin Chest Med* 1983;4:161
3. Freese AB, Bryan AC: Effects of anesthesia and paralysis on diaphragmatic mechanics in man. *Anesthesiology* 1974;41:242
4. Coté CJ, Goldstein EA, Coté MA, et al: A single-blind study of pulse oximetry in children. *Anesthesiology* 1988;68:184
5. Currie RB: Pulmonary embolism. In: Kirby RR, Taylor RW (eds). *Respiratory Failure*. Chicago, Year Book Medical Publishers, 1986:335
6. Cheney FW, Taylor JV: Pulmonary disorders. In: Bonica JJ (ed). *Principles and Practice of Obstetric Analgesia and Anesthesia*. Philadelphia, FA Davis, 1969:990.
7. Morgan M: Amniotic fluid embolism. *Anaesthesia* 1979;34:20
8. Scharf RHM, de Campo T, Civetta JM: Hemodynamic alterations and rapid diagnosis in a case of amniotic-fluid embolus. *Anesthesiology* 1977;46:155
9. Pashayan AG: Monitoring the neurosurgical patient. In: Gravenstein N (ed). *Problems in Anesthesia: Monitoring*. Philadelphia, JB Lippincott, 1987:104
10. Aronson ME, Nelson PK: Fatal air embolism in pregnancy resulting from an unusual sex act. *Obstet Gynecol* 1967;30:127
11. Kaufman BS, Kaminsky SJ, Rackow EC, et al: Adult respiratory distress syndrome following orogenital sex during pregnancy. *Crit Care Med* 1987;15:703
12. Mehlhorn U, Burke EJ, Butler BD, et al: Body position does not affect the hemodynamic response to venous air embolism in dogs. *Anesth Analg* 1994;79:734
13. Orebaugh SL: Venous air embolism: clinical and experimental considerations. *Crit Care Med* 1992;20:1169
14. Pitts JS, Presson RG Jr: A review of the pathophysiology of venous air embolism. *Anesthesiol Rev* 1991;18:29
15. Shupak RC: Air embolism and its effect on anesthetic management. *Curr Rev Clin Anesth* 1991;14:113
16. Lucas WJ: How to manage air embolism. In: Vaughan RW (ed). *Problems in Anesthesia: Perioperative Problems/Catastrophes*. Philadelphia, JB Lippincott, 1987:288
17. James CF: Pulmonary aspiration of gastric contents. In: Gravenstein N, Kirby RR (eds). *Complications in Anesthesiology*, 2nd ed. Philadelphia, Lippincott-Raven, 1996:175
18. Petty TL, Ashbaugh DG: The adult respiratory distress syndrome: clinical features, factors influencing prognosis and principles of management. *Chest* 1971;60:233
19. Tate RM, Pepine JE: Neutrophils and the adult respiratory distress syndrome. *Am Rev Respir Dis* 1983;128:552
20. Ashbaugh DG, Bigelow DB, Petty TL, et al: Acute respiratory distress in adults. *Lancet* 1967;2:319
21. Taylor RW: The adult respiratory distress syndrome. In: Kirby RR, Taylor RW (eds). *Respiratory Failure*. Chicago, Year Book Medical Publishers, 1987:208
22. Chiang AA, Steinfeld A, Gropper C, et al: Demand-flow airway pressure release ventilation as a partial ventilatory support mode: comparison with synchronized intermittent mandatory ventilation and pressure support ventilation. *Crit Care Med* 1994;22:1431
23. Pinsky MR: Cardiovascular effects of ventilatory support and withdrawal. *Anesth Analg* 1994;79:567
24. Hickling KG, Walsh J, Henderson S, et al: Low mortality rate in adult respiratory distress syndrome using low-volume, pressure-limited ventilation with permissive hypercapnia: a prospective study. *Crit Care Med* 1994;22:1568
25. Kirby RR: Respiratory system. In: Gravenstein N (ed). *Manual of Complications During Anesthesia*. Philadelphia, JB Lippincott, 1991:325
26. Centers for Disease Control: Transmission of multidrug-resistant tuberculosis among immunocompromised persons in a correctional system: New York, 1991. *MMWR CDC Surveill Summ* 1992;41:507
27. Brown MA, Taussig LM: Fertility, birth control and pregnancy in adult patients with cystic fibrosis. *Pulmonary Perspect* 1988;5:1
28. Mecca RS: Clinical aspects of pulmonary edema. In: Kirby RR, Taylor RW (eds). *Respiratory Failure*. Chicago, Year Book Medical Publishers, 1986:193
29. Keefer JR, Strauss RG, Civetta JM, et al: Noncardiogenic pulmonary edema and invasive cardiovascular monitoring. *Obstet Gynecol* 1981;58:46
30. Wilms D, Shure D: Pulmonary edema due to upper airway obstruction in adults. *Chest* 1988;94:1090
31. Sulek C: Negative-pressure pulmonary edema. In: Gravenstein N, Kirby RR (eds). *Complications in Anesthesiology*, 2nd ed. Philadelphia, Lippincott-Raven, 1996:191.

Critical Care, Third Edition, edited by Joseph M. Civetta,
Robert W. Taylor, and Robert R. Kirby.
Lippincott-Raven Publishers, Philadelphia, PA © 1997.

CHAPTER 95

■

Trauma and the Acute Abdomen

Sharon Salamat
Anthony Lai

IMMEDIATE CONCERNS ■

MAJOR PROBLEMS

The physiologic changes associated with pregnancy alter the maternal response to trauma and acute abdominal pathologies. Mother and fetus are best served by rapid diagnosis and aggressive treatment of all maternal injuries and disease processes. Both acute and continued management of these patients necessitate a multispecialty team cognizant of the utility and interpretation of diagnostic studies, medication effects, and timing and implications of delivery.

STRESS POINTS

1. Physical trauma in pregnancy is a relatively common occurrence. Initial assessment and resuscitation is identical to that of the nonpregnant patient.
2. Maternal management takes priority over fetal assessment until stability is assured. If maternal cardiopulmonary arrest occurs, however, emergency cesarean delivery should be commenced within 4 minutes for a fetus assessed to be potentially viable (≥26 weeks' gestation after antenatal hypoxia). The success of this therapy may depend on capabilities of neonatal care in hospital or region.
3. No diagnostic or therapeutic intervention should be withheld if it is deemed necessary for maternal well-being, regardless of potential fetal effects. Documentation of intentions is crucial, as is recognition that association does not prove causation (e.g., high rates

of fetal loss in first trimester occur because of congenital anomalies, regardless of maternal trauma). Underlying maternal medical conditions should be kept in mind.
4. Fetal assessment after maternal stabilization includes establishing and dating the pregnancy, assuring fetal well-being, and determining whether labor is occurring.
5. The most clinically significant consequence of blunt abdominal trauma in pregnancy is abruptio placentae, which is best detected by continuous monitoring of contractions and fetal heart rate. Penetrating abdominal trauma is usually detrimental to the fetus, but the enlarged uterus protects the gravida compared with her nonpregnant counterpart.
6. Although the incidences of appendicitis, cholecystitis, and bowel obstruction are all similar in pregnant and nonpregnant patients, the incidence of diffuse peritonitis and the rate of mortality are greater because of diagnostic and surgical delays.
7. In the intraoperative and postoperative periods, adequate maternal oxygenation and volume replacement are most important for prevention of preterm labor and fetal distress. Pregnant patients are at greater risk of developing pulmonary and thrombotic complications.
8. With some exceptions, medications required in the intensive care unit (ICU) may be used safely and effectively during pregnancy. Additional medications include tocolytics, corticosteroids for fetal lung maturity, and anti-D globulin in the unsensitized Rh-nega-

1419

tive patient.

9. In the absence of unstable pelvic fracture or outlet obstruction, vertical (classic) uterine scar, or other obstetric contraindications, vaginal delivery after spontaneous labor is the goal of every pregnancy. Personnel and equipment should be available in the event that an emergency cesarean delivery is required for fetal distress that is unresponsive to intrauterine resuscitative measures.

10. Maternal brain death before fetal viability is reached poses a unique set of ethical, economic, and medical challenges.

ESSENTIAL DIAGNOSTIC TESTS AND PROCEDURES

Maternal

1. Immediate assessment is unaltered for pregnant trauma victims. Pregnancy-associated changes in vital signs, laboratory values, and radiographic studies must be kept in mind. A high index of clinical suspicion is required for the diagnosis of gastrointestinal tract causes of acute abdomen.

2. Additional laboratory studies include coagulation indices, Rh-factor status, atypical antibody identification, and the Kleihauer-Betke test.

3. Imaging studies to evaluate maternal injuries include all necessary radiographs, computed tomography, magnetic resonance imaging, and, more recently, ultrasound. Peritoneal lavage is reliable and safe in pregnancy.

Fetal

1. In viable gestations, continuous monitoring of fetal heart rate and uterine contractions should be performed for at least 4 hours after any blunt abdominal trauma and in all patients who are intubated or otherwise unable to communicate.

2. Adjunct fetal assessment techniques include ultrasound for pregnancy dating, documentation of viability, and determination of well-being.

INITIAL THERAPY

1. Maternal resuscitation should focus on protection of the airway, lateral uterine displacement, adequate oxygenation and volume resuscitation, and serial assessment of urine output, blood oxygen, acid-base status, and coagulation indices.

2. Abruptio placentae should be managed by fluid and blood replacement, correction of coagulopathy, and delivery. Uterine rupture requires immediate laparotomy.

3. Surgical management of the acute abdomen is similar to that in the nonpregnant patient. Consideration may be given to performing laparoscopy for diagnosis or therapy, depending on gestational age and the surgeon's experience.

4. Cesarean delivery at the time of exploratory laparotomy is indicated only in instances of fetal distress and, possibly, if peritonitis occurs after viability or if the gravid uterus interferes with proper surgical therapy regardless of viability. Viability depends as much on neonatal care capabilities as fetal age.

The acutely ill or injured gravida presents the challenges of managing 2 patients simultaneously and recognizing that pregnancy-related physiologic changes alter the assessment of maternal stability. Physical trauma complicates 1 pregnancy in 12 and is the leading cause of nonobstetric maternal death.[1] This high incidence reflects the reproductive age range (high incidence of trauma); pregnancy-specific risk factors, including a greater likelihood for being a victim of domestic violence; and center-of-gravity changes in late gestation.

Management of acute abdomen resulting from nonobstetric pathology in pregnancy is often delayed because presentation is altered and the physician may not be suspect the true problem. Preoccupation with the pregnancy has occasionally interfered with expedient diagnosis and therapy, resulting in detriment to both mother and fetus. This chapter addresses the management of the acutely ill pregnant patient who arrives in the ICU after sustaining a condition (e.g., trauma, acute abdomen, surgery) in which the pregnancy is coincidental.

INITIAL ASSESSMENT AND MANAGEMENT ■

Initial assessment and treatment (ABCs) of the posttraumatic or acutely-ill pregnant patient are similar to those of the nonpregnant patient, with the exception that pregnancy-related physiologic changes should be kept in mind when interpreting vital signs and laboratory results (Table 95-1). Supplemental 100% oxygen by mask should be administered until maternal and fetal conditions are completely assessed. Endotracheal intubation should be performed early, rather than after problems have developed. In securing the airway, it should be realized that pregnant women are at increased risk for vomiting and aspiration secondary to decreased gastrointestinal motility and sphincter competency. Placement of a nasogastric tube is therefore prudent, and if intubation is required, it should be performed using rapid sequence induction with cricoid pressure. Decreased residual lung capacity and ventilatory reserve caused by diaphragmatic elevation also render the pregnant patient more susceptible to the hypoxic effects of apnea and hypoventilation. Oxygenation should be assessed by continuous pulse oximetry and overall gas exchange and acid-base balance by arterial blood gas determination. Needle or closed tube thoracostomy should be performed promptly if pneumothorax is suspected. The tube should be placed slightly higher than normal (at the third or fourth intercostal space) in later gestation.

Cardiovascular changes include decreased systolic and diastolic blood pressures, with nadirs at midtrimester that are 10 mm Hg below nonpregnant values; heart rate increases to

TABLE 95-1. Relevant Anatomic and Physiologic Changes During Pregnancy

SYSTEM	CHANGE
Cardiovascular	↑ Cardiac output by 40-50% ↑ Heart rate by 15 bpm ↓ Blood pressure by 10 mm Hg midtrimester, then ↑ to normal ↑ Plasma volume by 50%
Respiratory	↓ Residual lung capacity ↓ Arterial Pco_2 to 28-31 mm Hg ↓ Arterial HCO_3 to 18-22 mMol/L ↑ Arterial pH to 7.44
Gastrointestinal	↓ Motility ↓ Sphincter competency Intestinal displacement into the upper abdomen in later gestation Blunting of peritoneal sensation
Hematologic	↓ Hemoglobin 1-3 g/dL ↑ Leukocytes to 5-14 × 10⁹/L ↑ Fibrinogen to 350-400 mg/100 mL

approximately 15 beats per minute (bpm) above nonpregnant rates in the third trimester; and hemoglobin decreases of about 1 to 3 g/dL secondary to hemodilution. These physiologic changes in combination should not be interpreted as reactions to blood loss, and patients should not be transfused on the basis of these changes. Assessment of intravascular volume status is further complicated by both a 50% increase in cardiac output, leading to delayed signs of shock, and supine vena caval compression, possibly leading to hypotension unrelated to blood loss. Sensitive indicators of maternal hypoperfusion include relative acidosis, decreased bicarbonate values, increased lactate levels, and decreased urine output after bladder catheterization.

If cardiopulmonary arrest occurs, resuscitation should be begun immediately, with the uterus displaced laterally. If a strong pulse is not obtained after several thoracic compressions and the fetus is assessed to be potentially viable, a cesarean delivery should be started within 4 minutes and the infant delivered within 5 minutes of maternal cardiac arrest. This timing is based on survival rates for neurologically intact infants.[2] Although, in the management of obstetric conditions, 24 weeks is considered the lower limit of viability, the dual insults of antenatal hypoxia and immaturity make survival of a fetus of less than 26 weeks' gestation unlikely. No absolute limit should be set; rather, the capability of the hospital's neonatal ICU or regionalization of neonatal care may modify the gestational age at which the fetus should be considered viable, not just in maternal arrest but all situations considered in this chapter. Cardiopulmonary resuscitation should be carried out during and after the cesarean delivery, which is done without wasting precious minutes to prepare a sterile field or to have the patient moved to an operating room. There may be maternal benefit from evacuation of the uterus, as relief of caval compression improves cardiac output.

Placement of intravenous lines for resuscitation in the lower extremities and groin should be avoided, if possible, because fluid delivery by these routes may be inadequate in advanced gestation and deep vein thrombosis is more likely to occur. Normal saline or lactated Ringer's solution should be given, 3 mL for each mL estimated blood lost, during the first 30 to 60 minutes of resuscitation. To avoid isoimmunization in Rh-negative mothers, only Rh-negative blood should be transfused until the maternal Rh-factor status is known. Peripherally-selective vasopressors such as norepinephrine bitartrate should be avoided, if possible, because they reduce uterine blood flow. As with other interventions, they should not be withheld if required for maternal stability. Centrally-acting agents such as ephedrine restore both maternal blood pressure and uterine blood flow. Finally, the pneumatic antishock garment may be used in pregnant patients, but the abdominal compartment should not be inflated, because the increased intraabdominal pressure may compromise placental perfusion and force the already-elevated maternal diaphragm further into the chest.

DIAGNOSTIC STUDIES ■

ASSESSING THE MOTHER

After the initial care, additional diagnostic studies may be subdivided into those assessing maternal morbidity and those evaluating fetal well-being. Because the majority of clinical situations do not involve conflicting maternal and fetal interests, expedient maternal evaluation benefits both patients and therefore is reviewed first. Additional maternal laboratory studies include a complete blood cell count and coagulation indices—platelet count, prothrombin time, partial thromboplastin time, and fibrinogen level. It should be remembered that pregnancy is accompanied by both leukocytosis and hyperfibrinogenemia (see Table 95-1). Rh-factor status should be determined as soon as possible. Any other atypical antibodies to blood group antigens should also be identified, because they may result in hemolytic disease of the newborn. Especially in Rh-negative patients, a Kleihauer-Betke test is helpful in determining the presence and degree of fetomaternal hemorrhage, which can lead to both fetal compromise and maternal decompensation.

Radiographic studies should not be withheld if they are considered necessary.[3] Fetal effects (e.g., pregnancy loss, teratogenesis, microcephaly, mental retardation, childhood cancers) depend on the dose of radiation and the gestational age. It is unlikely that effects occur at a fetal dose of less than 10 rads[4] (Table 95-2). It should be realized that the rate of congenital anomalies in the general population is 3% to 6%, and the estimated overall pregnancy loss rate is 50% to 60% from conception. General guidelines for performing radiographic studies in pregnancy include abdominal shielding, elimination of duplicate and unnecessary films by involving the most experienced radiologist, and documentation of medical need for the study despite the known potential risks. Certain radiographic findings are considered physiologic in pregnancy, including diaphragm elevation, variable cardiac size and axis, dilation of the renal pelvices and ure-

TABLE 95-2. Approximate Fetal Dosage From Diagnostic Radiation Exposure

EXAMINATION	DOSE (RADS)
Chest radiograph	0.008
Kidney, ureter, and bladder	0.3
Lumbosacral spine	0.3
Upper gastrointestinal series	0.6
Barium enema	0.8
Intravenous pyelogram	0.5-1.0
Abdominal or pelvic computed tomography	5-10

ters, bladder positional changes, and widening of the symphysis pubis and sacroiliac joints in later gestation.

Magnetic resonance imaging has been used in pregnancy without any identifiable risks to the fetus.[5] Problems with interpretation of these studies may result, however, especially if excessive fetal movement is present.

Diagnosis of intraperitoneal hemorrhage by peritoneal lavage may be safely performed during pregnancy using the same indications and interpretation as for the nonpregnant patient.[6] An open technique should be performed, above the umbilicus if the pregnancy is advanced. Recently, abdominal ultrasound has been shown to be an effective alternative method for diagnosis of intraperitoneal hemorrhage.[7] Because the American Institute of Ultrasound in Medicine has concluded that there are no confirmed biologic effects at intensities used in present diagnostic ultrasound instruments, this method has obvious advantages over peritoneal lavage and computed tomography in pregnancy.[8]

Finally, underlying maternal medical conditions should be excluded. Eclamptic seizures and severe metabolic derangements associated with poorly controlled diabetes mellitus have been known to precipitate trauma.

FETAL ASSESSMENT

Obstetric assessment is performed only after maternal stability has been assured. Studies include establishing and dating the pregnancy, assessing fetal well-being, and determining whether labor has begun. Measurement of the β subunit of human chorionic gonadotropin, produced by the placenta, is specific for pregnancy and is positive as early after conception as 1 to 2 weeks in the blood and 2 to 4 weeks in the urine.[9] The presence of fetal heart activity by real-time ultrasound definitively establishes the diagnosis of pregnancy. Fetal heartbeat may be detected as early as 6 to 8 weeks after the last menstrual period. Doppler technology may also be used to detect fetal heart activity at approximately 10 to 14 weeks, although with less sensitivity and specificity. Normally, the fetal heart rate is greater than 120 bpm, but maternal tachycardia or fetal bradycardia may lead to a false-positive or false-negative diagnosis of pregnancy, respectively. Maternal obesity or excessive fetal movement may also impede detection of the fetal heart rate, and the absence of fetal heart sounds cannot immediately be interpreted as proof of fetal death. Auscultation of fetal heart

activity with a stethoscope may be possible by 20 weeks, although maternal obesity may again make this difficult and it may be detectable only in later gestation.

Dating of the pregnancy is best accomplished by ultrasonographic determination of crown-rump length in the first trimester, and by fetal femur length or biparietal diameter thereafter. Charts compiled from uncomplicated pregnancies are used to date the pregnancy.[10,11] The accuracy of ultrasound in dating the pregnancy decreases with gestational age; measurements obtained in the third trimester are only accurate to within ±3 weeks of the actual age. Maternal obesity may technically hinder accurate sonographic dating. An attempt to elicit historical information from the patient, family, or prenatal care provider is therefore important. After 20 weeks' gestation, the fundal height, measured in centimeters from the symphysis pubis, roughly correlates with gestational age. This method of dating the pregnancy may provide inaccurate information in the settings of multiple gestation, uterine fibroids, or maternal obesity, and it should be used only as a last resort.

After the pregnancy has been established and dated, fetal well-being should be assessed. Before viability, this entails only detection of fetal heart activity, or lack of it, and intermittent monitoring if the fetus is alive. If fetal death in utero is confirmed by real-time ultrasound, attempts at delivery may be delayed for up to 4 weeks. In most women, spontaneous delivery usually occurs before this time. After 3 to 4 weeks, a coagulopathy related to the retained fetus occasionally develops; it may be detected by a fall in serial fibrinogen levels before any clinical manifestation. Maternal fibrinogen levels are normally significantly greater than nonpregnant values (see Table 95-1). Uterine evacuation after fetal death in utero may be accomplished with the use of prostaglandins or oxytocin.[12] Even if laparotomy is undertaken for other indications, it is not advisable to perform a hysterotomy unless evacuation of the uterus is required for surgical therapy.

For potentially viable fetuses, continuous external monitoring of both fetal heart rate and uterine activity is recommended. Signs of fetal well-being include a normal baseline heart rate (120 to 160 bpm), good beat-to-beat variability (5 to 25 bpm), and acceleration without deceleration (Fig. 95-1). Decreased variability in the absence of decelerations may be the result of immaturity of the fetal autonomic nervous system if the period of gestation is less than 32 weeks, or it may reflect maternal medications.

Decreased beat-to-beat variability, fetal tachycardia (>160 bpm) or bradycardia (<120 bpm), and decelerations occurring after the peak of a uterine contraction (late decelerations) may all be indicative of fetal distress. Efforts should be made to correct maternal hypoxia and maintain uterine perfusion. Maternal hemoglobin oxygen saturation should be maintained at 90% or greater. The patient should be repositioned to decrease vena caval compression, and volume replacement should be instituted. If evidence of fetal distress persists despite these measures, cesarean delivery should be performed if the fetus is viable. A neonatologist and neonatal respiratory therapist should be present, and all necessary resuscitative equipment should be available at the time of delivery.

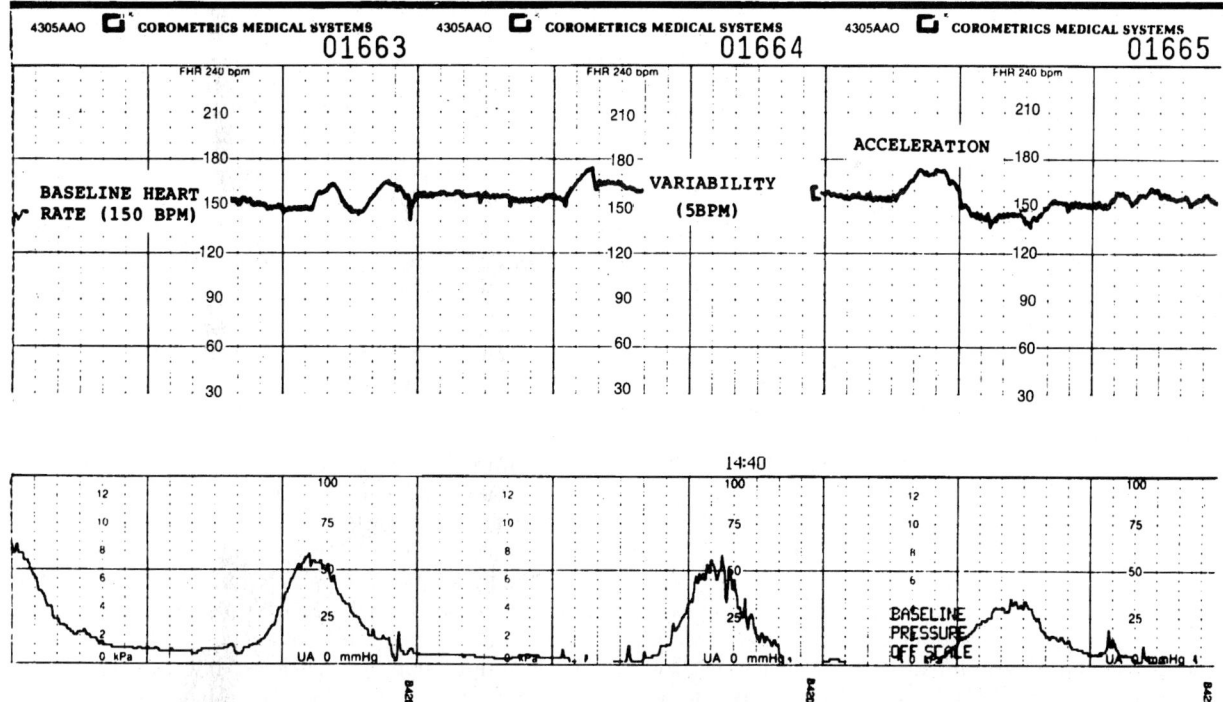

FIGURE 95-1. Fetal heart tracing showing normal baseline (120–160 beats per minute [BPM]), normal variability (5–25 BPM), and acceleration without deceleration.

Ultrasound may also be used to assess signs of fetal well-being, including breathing movements, flexion and extension of the limbs, general body movement and tone, and normal amniotic fluid volume.

Finally, a pelvic examination should be performed to determine whether cervical dilatation or rupture of membranes has occurred, and to exclude vaginal bleeding. Ideally, this should be performed by an obstetrician after fractures of the pelvic, spine, and femur have been excluded.

SPECIFIC MANAGEMENT ■

BLUNT TRAUMA

Blunt abdominal trauma in pregnancy is caused most often by motor vehicle accidents, followed by falls and direct assaults.[13] One study demonstrated that in an inner-city population, 1 of every 12 women was battered during pregnancy.[14] Assault should be suspected if the patient has facial, breast, or abdominal bruises or abnormal affect.

Maternal death after blunt trauma is most commonly caused by head injury. Significant morbidity also occurs as the result of intraabdominal injuries. The markedly increased blood flow to pelvic viscera predisposes the pregnant woman to serious retroperitoneal hemorrhage after lower abdominal and pelvic trauma. Bladder injuries are more common after the first trimester because of abdominal displacement of this organ. Bowel injuries occur less frequently owing to protection of the bowel by the enlarged uterus. Exploratory laparotomy to evaluate and treat maternal inju-

ries should be performed for the same indications as for the nonpregnant patient. Concurrent cesarean delivery should be performed for a viable fetus demonstrating evidence of distress or if the gravid uterus interferes with adequate surgical therapy, regardless of gestational age.

Injuries to the uterus and its contents are unusual before 12 weeks' gestation in the absence of pelvic fracture. After this time, when the uterus becomes an abdominal organ, blunt trauma may result in placental separation (abruptio placentae) or laceration, uterine rupture, or direct fetal injury. Abruptio placentae occurs after 1% to 5% of minor and 40% to 50% of life-threatening injuries.[13,15] Placental separation of greater than 50% usually results in fetal death and consumptive coagulopathy. Frequent findings include uterine tenderness or contractions, fetal distress, and vaginal bleeding. Because the latter may not occur until after a significant amount of blood has been sequestered in the myometrium, monitoring of fetal heart rate and contractions should be continued for at least 4 hours after even minor abdominal trauma.[15] Although ultrasound may detect retroplacental blood clots and amniocentesis may yield bloody amniotic fluid, these tests are not as sensitive as cardiotocographic monitoring in detecting abruptio placentae. Uterine contractions secondary to abruptio placentae may be difficult to differentiate from those of preterm labor unrelated to placental separation. β-Mimetic tocolytic agents should not be used until the latter has been ruled out, because they can produce fetal or maternal tachycardia, adding to confusion concerning the diagnosis.

Uterine rupture occurs less frequently than abruptio placentae after severe blunt abdominal trauma, complicating less than 1% of all injuries.[16] Fetal survival is rare. Direct fetal injuries are also infrequent, but the most common are fetal skull and brain injuries after maternal pelvic fracture. Ultrasound may occasionally detect fetal intracranial hemorrhage, but most fetal injuries remain undetected until after delivery.

PENETRATING TRAUMA

Penetrating abdominal trauma in pregnancy results in very disparate outcomes for mother and fetus because, in later gestation, the enlarged uterus usually sustains the brunt of the injury. Perinatal mortality therefore ranges from 41% to 71%, and maternal mortality occurs in less than 5% of penetrating injuries.[17] The low incidence of maternal visceral injuries has led some authors to consider selective laparotomy in these patients, if they are hemodynamically stable.[18,19] Otherwise, the management is the same as for nonpregnant victims of penetrating trauma.

ACUTE ABDOMEN

When assessing the pregnant patient with an acute abdomen, it is important to consider obstetric, gynecologic and gastrointestinal (general surgical) conditions. Obstetric conditions include abruptio placentae and uterine rupture, both reviewed earlier. Abruptio placentae is associated with hypertension, preeclampsia, and ingestion of cocaine. Management includes fluid and blood resuscitation, correction of coagulopathy, and delivery. Vaginal delivery is preferable in the absence of obstetric contraindications or fetal distress. Occasionally, uterine rupture may occur in pregnant patients with prior cesarean delivery with or without labor. The patient may complain of a sudden onset of severe, "tearing" pain and she may demonstrate anxiety; her condition may progress to shock. Management includes immediate laparotomy, delivery, and either uterine repair or hysterectomy, depending on the extent of damage and the estimated time interval between rupture and exploration.

The most common nonobstetric pelvic pathologies are adnexal torsion and fibroid degeneration. The former is associated with acute, crampy or continuous pain. Management is laparotomy or, more recently, laparoscopy. Red degeneration, or hemorrhagic infarction, of uterine fibroids may occur during pregnancy or puerperium and frequently causes localized pain that is acute, sharp or aching. Mild-to-moderate leukocytosis and low-grade fever may also occur. The treatment is nonoperative and includes rest, hydration, and analgesia.

The most common gastrointestinal disorders include appendicitis, cholecystitis, and bowel obstruction. Approximately 0.1% of pregnant women undergo an appendectomy.[20] This is the same rate as for the nonpregnant population; however, an increased mortality rate results from delay before surgery, approaching 5% in the third trimester.[21] Diagnosis is hindered by the common occurrence of nausea, vomiting, and leukocytosis in pregnancy, the blunted peritoneal sensation, and the upward and lateral displacement of the appendix with advancing gestation.[22] Although nausea and vomiting are common in the first trimester, they

should arouse suspicion in the second or third trimester. Surgical management is similar to that of the nonpregnant patient.

The incidence of acute cholecystitis has been reported to be approximately 1 in 1000 deliveries.[23] Surgical management should be considered if initial medical treatment is unsuccessful or if cholecystitis is recurrent. The optimal time for cholecystectomy is during the early second trimester, when the uterus is still too small to impinge on the surgical field but the risk of spontaneous abortion is low.

Bowel obstruction occurs in 1 in 2500 to 3500 deliveries, approximately the same incidence as in the general population.[24] The most common causes are adhesions from prior surgery and volvulus, and abdominal pain is the most common symptom.[25] The high maternal (6% to 20%) and fetal (26%) mortality rates are again attributed mainly to diagnostic difficulties and delay before surgery. Continuous or colicky abdominal pain occurring in an obstetric patient with a history of prior surgery, especially if it occurs when the uterus is a dynamic abdominal organ (i.e., midpregnancy, term, and immediately after delivery), should alert the physician to the possibility of this diagnosis. Surgical decompression should be performed as soon as possible after nasogastric decompression, intravenous fluid resuscitation, and broad-spectrum antibiotic coverage have been instituted.

Diffuse peritonitis secondary to a perforated viscus is more common in pregnant than in nonpregnant patients. In addition to the previously discussed reasons, the normal abdominal compartmentalization is lacking. A pregnancy loss rate of 35% has been reported, including preterm delivery and fetal death.[26] Because of this high fetal mortality, severe diffuse peritonitis may be one indication for cesarean delivery at the time of surgery for a viable fetus.

POSTOPERATIVE PERIOD ■

Return of gastrointestinal function may be delayed, and oral feeding should therefore not occur until adequate motility has been documented. Because of associated physiologic changes, pregnant women are at increased risk for development of pulmonary and thrombotic complications after surgery or serious injury. Atelectasis and pulmonary infections occur more commonly in pregnant patients because of decreased respiratory excursion. Pregnant and, especially, postpartum patients are at increased risk for development of venous thrombosis because of their hypercoagulable state and mechanical factors that promote stasis. Prophylactic heparin treatment should be considered, especially in patients who have sustained orthopedic injuries and in those in whom prolonged immobilization is anticipated.

Preterm labor (i.e., before 37 weeks' gestation) may occur in postoperative patients. In the intubated and unaware patient, external tocodynamometric monitoring is the preferred method to detect uterine contractions. Pelvic examination can be used as necessary to assess cervical change. In hemodynamically stable patients without uteroplacental injury, tocolytic agents may be indicated if uterine activity continues despite adequate maternal oxygenation and hydration and if cervical change is documented. Magnesium sulfate is the agent of choice in this setting. β-Sympathomimetics have more cardiovascular side effects.[27] The prostaglandin inhibitor, indomethacin, which has recently been used for tocolysis before 32 weeks' gestation, should not be used in this setting, because recent evidence suggests a greater likelihood of postoperative maternal pulmonary injury.[28]

MEDICATIONS

Medications include those used commonly in the ICU and those required for obstetric care. The former include analgesics, antibiotics, antihypertensives, diuretics, anticoagulants, and vasopressors (previously reviewed).

Morphine and meperidine have been used in pregnancy without associated fetal malformations. Prolonged use may lead to neonatal withdrawal, and use in the immediate perinatal period may cause respiratory depression in the newborn infant. Codeine should not be used, especially in the first trimester, because of its association with congenital anomalies.[29]

Penicillin derivatives, cephalosporins, erythromycin, clindamycin, metronidazole, and antifungal agents have all been used during pregnancy without adverse fetal effects. Aminoglycosides have been associated with fetal nephrotoxicity and ototoxicity and should be used cautiously. Nitrofurantoin may precipitate hemolysis in individuals with glucose-6-phosphate dehydrogenase deficiency. Sulfonamides used near the time of delivery carry the theoretical risk of causing kernicterus in the newborn, as a result of displacement of bilirubin from albumin. The new quinolones are not approved in pregnancy because of adverse effects on bone and cartilage growth. Tetracycline use is contraindicated during pregnancy because of adverse effects on developing bones and teeth. Tetanus prophylaxis should be administered for the same indications as for the nonpregnant patient.

Several antihypertensive agents have been used safely and effectively in pregnant patients. The most experience has been accumulated with nifedipine, hydralazine, and methyldopa. Sodium nitroprusside may cause fetal thiocyanate toxicity after prolonged use, and it is therefore best used only as an alternative agent in the management of acute, severe and unresponsive hypertension.[30] Labetalol has recently been used in the management of hypertension and preeclampsia in pregnancy, with encouraging results.[31] Angiotensin converting enzyme inhibitors, agents of choice in treating type I diabetics with hypertension, are contraindicated after the first trimester because of the associated effects on fetal and neonatal renal function as well as oligohydramnios.[32]

If diuretic medications are required to treat pulmonary edema, furosemide may be administered. Thiazide diuretics have been associated with neonatal thrombocytopenia, jaundice, and severe electrolyte disturbances.[29]

Anticoagulation should be accomplished with the use of heparin, because it does not cross the placenta. Oral anticoagulants cross the placenta and are contraindicated throughout pregnancy.[29]

The obstetric medications commonly used in critically ill gravidas include tocolytic agents (reviewed earlier), anti-D globulin, and medications to enhance fetal lung maturity. Administration of hyperimmune anti-D globulin is recommended for all Rh-negative pregnant women with any abdominal trauma, in hope of preventing sensitization.[15] The Kleihauer-Betke assay for quantitation of fetomaternal hemorrhage is useful in determining the amount of this medication that is necessary. Most patients are protected by one ampule (300 μg).

Critically ill pregnant patients may deliver before term. Recently, a National Institutes of Health Consensus Development Panel reported that antenatal corticosteroids administered between 24 and 34 weeks' gestation substantially decreased neonatal mortality and morbidity, not only in terms of respiratory distress syndrome but also with respect to intraventricular hemorrhage and necrotizing enterocolitis.[33] Two doses of 12 mg betamethasone should be given intramuscularly 24 hours apart, and then this regimen should be repeated weekly. The major adverse maternal effects—impaired glucose control in diabetic patients and pulmonary edema—if the drug is used in combination with tocolytic agents, should be considered.

TOTAL PARENTERAL NUTRITION

Total parenteral nutrition can meet the nutritional needs of the critically ill patient and her growing fetus. It has been employed safely and effectively; previous concerns regarding an association with preterm labor and preeclampsia have not been substantiated.[34,35] Plasma glucose levels should be kept below 120 mg/dL if parenteral nutrition is used while the patient is pregnant.

DELIVERY CONCERNS ■

Vaginal delivery after spontaneous labor should be anticipated in the majority of postoperative and posttraumatic patients, barring an obstetric contraindication. Exceptions include women with unstable pelvic fractures or injuries obstructing the birth canal. Patients undergoing hysterotomy by a vertical uterine incision should be counseled as to the need for elective cesarean delivery in all future pregnancies, because of the high incidence of uterine rupture.

Spinal cord injury has important implications with respect to labor and delivery. In parturients with lesions above T10, uterine contractions are usually painless but may manifest as spasticity, clonus, or shoulder pain. Autonomic hyperreflexia, a rare but life-threatening complication in patients with a lesion at T7 or above, can be precipitated by uterine contractions or even by bladder distention. This condition may be prevented and abolished by the use of epidural anesthesia during labor.[36]

MATERNAL BRAIN DEATH ■

Brain death during pregnancy, a rare occurrence, presents a unique set of circumstances. Apart from the many ethical and economic issues involved, management of the inevitable multiple organ system failure in gravidas remote from term necessitates close interaction and participation of all members of a multispecialty team. Such intensive management has on occasion been successful at carrying a previable gestation to one in which only mild neonatal morbidity has resulted.[37] Accurate assessment of gestational age is crucial, as is determination of the timing of delivery based on the capabilities of the hospital's neonatal unit or regionalization of neonatal care. Family members should be integrally involved in decisionmaking through substituted judgment, and resort to the courts should be avoided if possible. Some previous court decisions may have been made too rapidly, because not only did they contradict both family members' desires and medical judgment by prioritizing fetal concerns, but they still resulted in adverse fetal outcome.[38]

CONCLUSION

Successful management of trauma and critical illness during pregnancy depends on a team approach involving the disciplines of emergency and critical care medicine, general surgery, obstetrics, and neonatology. Successful diagnosis and treatment of the mother also benefits her fetus. Care providers should recognize, but resist, any emotional urge to focus on the fetus before maternal stability is achieved. They must also prepare for heightened and unusual stress associated with adverse outcome for either the mother or the fetus.

REFERENCES

1. Peckman CH, King RA: A study of intercurrent conditions observed during pregnancy. *Am J Obstet Gynecol* 1963;87:609
2. Katz VL, Dotters DJ, Droegemueller W: Perimortem cesarean delivery. *Obstet Gynecol* 1986;68:571
3. National Council on Radiation Protection and Measurements: *Medical Radiation Exposure in Pregnant or Potentially Pregnant Women.* NCRP Report No. 54. Washington, DC: NCRP, 1977
4. Brent PL: The effects of embryonic and fetal exposure to x-ray, microwaves, and ultrasound. In: Smith MK (ed). *Clinics in Perinatology.* Philadelphia, WB Saunders, 1986:615
5. Johnson IR, Symonds EM, Kean OM, et al: Imaging of the pregnant human uterus with nuclear magnetic resonance. *Am J Obstet Gynecol* 1984;148:1136
6. Esposito TJ, Gens DR, Smith LG, et al: Evaluation of blunt abdominal trauma occurring during pregnancy. *J Trauma* 1989;29:1628
7. McKenney M, Lentz K, Nunez D, et al: Can ultrasound replace diagnostic peritoneal lavage in the assessment of blunt trauma. *J Trauma* 1994;37:439
8. American Institute of Ultrasound in Medicine: AIUM statement on clinical safety. *J Ultrasound Med* 1984;3:R10
9. Speroff L, Glass RH, Kase NG (eds): Clinical assays. In: *Clinical Gynecologic Endocrinology and Infertility,* 5th ed. Baltimore, Williams & Wilkins, 1994
10. O'Brien GD, Queenan JT: Dating gestation in the first 20 weeks. In: Saunders RC, James AE (eds). *Ultrasonography in Obstetrics and Gynecology,* 3rd ed. Norwalk, Appleton-Century-Crofts, 1985
11. Graham D, Saunders RC: Assessment of gestational in the second and third trimesters. In: Saunders RC, James AE (eds). *Ultrasonography in Obstetrics and Gynecology,* 3rd ed. Norwalk, Appleton-Century-Crofts, 1985.
12. American College of Obstetricians and Gynecologists: *Diagnosis and Management of Fetal Death.* ACOG Technical Bulletin No. 176. Washington, DC, American College of Obstetrics and Gynecologists, 1993
13. Rothenberger D, Quattlebaum FW, Perry JF Jr, et al: Blunt maternal trauma: a review of 103 cases. *J Trauma* 1978;18:173
14. Helton AS, McFarlane J, Anderson ET: Battered and pregnant: a prevalence study. *Am J Public Health* 1987;77:1337
15. American College of Obstetricians and Gynecologists: *Trauma During Pregnancy.* ACOG Technical Bulletin No. 161. Washington, DC, American College of Obstetricians and Gynecologists, 1991
16. Crosby WM: Traumatic injuries during pregnancy. *Clin Obstet Gynecol* 1986;26:902
17. Buchsbaum HJ: Penetrating injury of the abdomen. In: Buchsbaum HJ (ed). *Trauma in Pregnancy.* Philadelphia: WB Saunders, 1979;82
18. Franger AL, Buchsbaum HJ, Peaceman AM: Abdominal gunshot wounds in pregnancy. *Am J Obstet Gynecol* 1989;160:1124
19. Awwad JT, Azar GB, Seoud MA, et al: High-velocity penetrating wounds of the gravid uterus: review of 16 years of civil war. *Obstet Gynecol* 1994;83:259
20. Marre RI, Kallen B: Appendectomy during pregnancy: a Swedish registry of 778 cases. *Obstet Gynecol* 1991;77:835
21. DeVore GR: Acute abdominal pain in the pregnant patient due to pancreatitis, acute appendicitis, cholecystitis, or peptic ulcer disease. *Clin Perinatol* 1980;7:349
22. Cunningham FG: *Gastrointestinal Disorders.* Williams Obstetrics Supplement No. 7. Norwalk, CT, Appleton & Lange, 1994.
23. Landers D, Carmona R, Crombleholme W, et al: Acute cholecystitis in pregnancy. *Obstet Gynecol* 1987;69:131
24. Davis MR, Bohon CJ: Intestinal obstruction in pregnancy. *Clin Obstet Gynecol* 1983;26:832
25. Perdue PW, Johnson HW Jr, Stafford PW: Intestinal obstruction complicating pregnancy. *Am J Surg* 1992;164:384
26. Cooperman M. Complications of appendectomy. *Surg Clin North Am* 1983;65:1233
27. Besinger RE, Niebyl JR: The safety and efficacy of tocolytic agents in the treatment of preterm labor. *Obstet Gynecol Surv* 1990;45:415
28. de Veciana M, Towers CV, Major CA, et al: Pulmonary injury associated with appendicitis in pregnancy: who is at risk? *Am J Obstet Gynecol* 1994;171:1008
29. Briggs GG, Freeman RK, Yaffe SJ (eds): *Drugs in Pregnancy and Lactation,* 4th ed. Baltimore, Williams & Wilkins, 1994
30. Nelson DM: Think of sodium nitroprusside for severe preeclampsia. *Contemp Obstet Gynecol* 1985;27:103
31. Mabie WC, Gonzalez AR, Sibai BM, et al: A comparative trial of labetalol and hydralazine in the acute management of severe hypertension complicating pregnancy. *Obstet Gynecol* 1987;70:328
32. Rosa FW, Bosco LA, Graham CF, et al: Neonatal anemia with maternal angiotension-converting enzyme inhibition. *Obstet Gynecol* 1989;74:371

33. National Institutes of Health, Consensus Development Panel: Effect of corticosteroids for fetal maturation on perinatal outcomes. *JAMA* 1995;273:413
34. Kirby DF, Fiorenza V, Craig RM: Intravenous nutritional support during pregnancy. *J Parenter Enteral Nutr* 1988;12:72
35. Greenspoon JS, Safarik RH, Hayashi JT, et al: Parenteral nutrition during pregnancy: lack of association with idiopathic preterm labor or preeclampsia. *J Reprod Med* 1994;39:87

36. Baraka A: Epidural meperidine for control of autonomic hyperreflexia in a paraplegic parturient. *Anesthesiology* 1985;62: 688
37. Field DR, Gates EA, Creasy RK, et al: Maternal brain death during pregnancy: medical and ethical issues. *JAMA* 1988; 260:816
38. University Health Services, Inc. v. Piazzi, No. CV86-RCCV-464, Superior Court of Richmond County, Georgia, 1986.

Critical Care, Third Edition, edited by Joseph M. Civetta,
Robert W. Taylor, and Robert R. Kirby.
Lippincott-Raven Publishers, Philadelphia, PA © 1997.

CHAPTER 96

■

Fetal Monitoring Concerns

Donald Caton

IMMEDIATE CONCERNS ■

MAJOR PROBLEMS

Although physicians know a great deal about fetal life, we use only a small part of the information available for clinical management. Problems stem from the persistence of an old and pervasive idea that the placenta has only a limited capacity to transfer nutrients. This concept, in its most extreme form, implies that the fetus exhausts the capacity of the placenta by term, exposing it to the fearsome option of death in utero or birth. According to this view, the metabolite in shortest supply is oxygen, a conviction that continues to have tremendous impact on patient management today.

Care of a critically ill pregnant patient creates special problems. The physician must consider the effect of therapy on the child as well as on the mother. Unfortunately, evaluation of the clinical condition of the child is difficult. Tests available for this purpose are neither precise not specific.

STRESS POINTS

1. Most tests of fetal well-being have been designed for use during labor and consist of measurements of fetal heart rate and acid base balance. These tests assume that the primary stress during labor is oxygen deprivation, imposed by abnormalities in uterine or umbilical blood flow or placental transfer.
2. In recent years, other tests have been developed to assess fetal well-being during the prepartum period. These include estimates of fetal weight and growth by ultrasound, the frequency of spontaneous fetal movements, changes in heart rate in relation to spontaneous fetal movements, changes in fetal heart rate in relation to spontaneous or induced uterine contractions, and measurements of uterine or umbilical blood flow ve-

locity with Doppler devices.
3. None of the aforementioned tests are designed for evaluation of the fetus of an acutely ill woman. Their use for this purpose is limited.
4. Drugs often used in the management of critically ill patients—narcotics, tranquilizers and sedatives, for example—rapidly cross the placenta and alter the frequency of fetal movements and the normal patterns of variation of fetal heart rate. This response alters the interpretations of these observations.
5. Many of the tests assume that oxygen deprivation is the critical factor in most situations. The intensivist, however, may be dealing with abnormalities of electrolytes, glucose, or temperature variables not evaluated by current tests of fetal well-being.
6. Most important, however, the fetus has better means to cope with acute stress than we originally thought. In other words, we may have worried more about fetal problems than was warranted.

ESSENTIAL DIAGNOSTIC TESTS AND PROCEDURES

1. The physician dealing with an acutely ill pregnant patient should ask several questions:
   • Is the fetus alive?
   • If alive, is the fetus old enough to survive if delivered prematurely?
   • Would early delivery of the child help the mother's condition?
   • What are the feelings of the family about the survival of the child?
   • What is the risk of the medical or surgical problem precipitating early labor?
   • Will labor and delivery help or hinder the management of the underlying problem?

1429

- If the patient is in labor, should it be stopped and how?
- Is the condition of the fetus related to labor or to the acute medical problem of the mother?

2. Many of these questions can be best answered by specialists. For this reason, an important first step in management is to obtain early evaluations of the mother and fetus by a perinatologist and neonatologist.

3. It may be useful to obtain baseline measurements of heart rate, fetal size and activity, and uterine blood flow velocity. Although these measurements may not help with acute management decisions, they will establish the viability of the child (which may be important for medicolegal reasons) and may be of help in the management of the patient if the acute care extends for several weeks or months.

INITIAL THERAPY

1. With respect to specific management questions, it is important to recognize the limitations of methods available to evaluate the fetus.

2. Clinicians have to treat the mother without knowing the effect on the fetus. Fortunately, in most instances, it is safe to assume that therapy that helps the mother probably helps the child.

SPECIAL CONSIDERATIONS ■

When using any test or monitors, clinicians must make judgments. They must know the sensitivity and specificity of the test, the incidence of false-negative and false-positive results, the situations in which the test will be accurate, and those in which it may be misleading. Finally, they must understand the implications of a truly positive test result. For these reasons, it is appropriate to review pertinent points concerning the development and application of fetal monitoring.

BACKGROUND

Based in part on outdated information, tradition demands that every term infant be considered in a precarious position and that maternal management should proceed accordingly. In today's litigious society, this viewpoint constitutes a heavy burden and also goes against recent information that suggests the fetus has reserves enabling it to cope with all but the most serious conditions.

The difficulty lies in our inability to evaluate fetal status precisely. Currently, we deal fairly well with the normal fetus and the one already severely stressed. Problems come with infants between these extremes: those that may be stressed to the point that they have invoked but not yet exhausted their adaptive mechanisms. Current methods lack the sensitivity and specificity to detect these circumstances. As a result, we deal with our uncertainty by treating all infants as if they are on the edge of disaster. If this approach poses no problems for mother and infant, it can be justified.

In many circumstances, however, it does. Accordingly, we must ask if we can do better. How can we avoid being rushed into an unwise course of action?

Oxygen Deprivation and Hypoglycemia

Part of the clinical dilemma stems from our rigid adherence to oxygen deprivation as an explanation for intrauterine stress. Virtually all methods for evaluating and treating the unborn child assume that this molecule is the metabolic substrate in shortest supply. Given the multitude of factors that affect fetal condition and viability, no justification exists for such a myopic approach. Unless fetal physiology differs greatly from that of adults, we must assume that severe hypoglycemia wreaks no less havoc on the brain than does acute hypoxia. Do observations of fetal heart rate or measurements of scalp pH detect acute hypoglycemia? Unlikely! Yet, we continue to rely on these measurements to evaluate fetal condition and, in so doing, fail to develop a substitute technology that takes into account all that we already know about fetal glucose metabolism. Throughout adult and pediatric medicine, batteries of tests are used to evaluate each organ system; clinical skills include the selection of appropriate measurements. In no other specialty do physicians assume that one or two tests, in this case electrocardiography (ECG) and scalp pH, are sufficient to identify the various clinical problems threatening their patients.

Fetal Electrocardiographic Monitoring

At the same time, we do not use fetal ECG monitoring to its full extent. The possibility exists that acute electrolyte abnormalities cause problems, perhaps even death. We have considerable insight concerning the effects of high and low concentrations of potassium and ionized calcium on various components of the ECG. Yet, we have not used this information in the management of obstetric patients. These circumstances would simply be curiosities if the clinician were not forced to act. Unfortunately, many common problems require the physician to weigh the risks to the mother against those to the fetus when deciding on a course of action or therapy.

Maternal–Fetal Interactions

Any physician dealing with pregnant women has experienced a situation in which the care of the mother had to be modified because of concern for the presumed effect on the child. For example, vasopressors with pure alpha-adrenergic action may be the therapy of choice when treating hypotension. Nevertheless, the clinician hesitates for fear that vasoconstriction of the uterine vasculature may place the infant at some unreasonable, yet undefined, risk. Or, because of a diagnosis of "acute fetal bradycardia," an anesthesiologist may feel pressured to induce anesthesia by a rapid-sequence technique in a woman for whom prudence dictates a slower but safer awake intubation because of some anatomic peculiarities of the upper airway.

Both examples illustrate situations in which the preferred mode of management of the mother may be modified out of concern for its effect on the infant. Usually, such decisions are strongly influenced by the assumption that the term fetus is at risk, even in the best of circumstances, or that the fetal ECG or scalp pH is sensitive and specific enough to detect problems. Laboratory data and clinical experience suggest that both assumptions are open to question. The time is ripe to develop a new perspective on the management of the pregnant patient and her passenger.

FETAL OXYGENATION ■

Preoccupation with fetal oxygenation developed only during the last century. Before 1880, clinicians questioned whether the fetus even required oxygen. Clinical observations by two 19th century obstetricians, Adolph Gusserow and his student, Paul Zweifel, demonstrated otherwise.[1] Prompted by Gusserow, Zweifel used newly developed analytic techniques of light absorption to demonstrate that umbilical arterial blood contained less oxygen than that in the umbilical vein, implying that oxygen crossed the placenta and was consumed by the fetus. (It is noteworthy that Zweifel was also the person who unequivocally demonstrated that drugs, including inhalational anesthetics, cross the placenta[2]).

OXYGEN CONSUMPTION

Although investigators accepted Zweifel's demonstration that the fetus consumed oxygen, they argued about the amount. In early experiments, they used measurements of umbilical blood flow and cord gases to calculate fetal oxygen consumption, an approach carried out during surgery with anesthetized animals. The rates they measured were low, far less than those obtained on awake newborns of the same species. On the basis of this evidence, they compared the fetus with a metabolic parasite, responsible neither for warming itself nor for synthesizing its own metabolites. Maternal tissues, they claimed, performed virtually all essential processes for the fetus.

The low rates of measured fetal oxygen consumption had important clinical implications, particularly with respect to the character of fetal metabolism and whether it conformed to the rules carefully worked out for free-living animals. If not, clinicians and scientists had to develop a new set of rules to describe fetal metabolism. Furthermore, a low rate of oxygen consumption diminished the significance of periods of fetal hypoxia. Deprivation had no significance for an organism reputed to use no oxygen.

Ironically, the data from the laboratory disagreed with clinical observations. For example, investigators who measured the mother's metabolic rate before and after delivery believed that the oxygen consumption of the fetus and newborn were nearly the same. The discrepancy between laboratory and clinical data remained unresolved for almost a century, but the latter eventually prevailed, probably because

they were direct measurements although they were less accurate.[3]

OXYGEN SUPPLY AND AVAILABILITY

Coincident with the controversy about amounts of oxygen consumed was the debate about its availability. After investigators ascertained that oxygen crossed the placenta and the fetus used it, attention focused on whether the amounts available were adequate to satisfy fetal needs. The preponderance of evidence, they believed, suggested that the answer was no. For example, they knew that the placenta achieved its maximum weight early in pregnancy, whereas the fetus grew most rapidly toward term. Correctly, they equated the weight of the fetus with its requirements for oxygen. With equal conviction, they equated the weight of the placenta with its functional capacity or, to be more precise, with its capacity to transfer oxygen, although in this case they eventually were proven wrong.

Existing clinical and experimental data seemed to support the idea that the fetus outgrew the capacity of the placenta. Cord blood drawn from exteriorized fetuses of anesthetized animals closer to term had lower saturations and higher hematocrits. Similarly, cord blood of infants delivered vaginally also tended to be hypoxemic and acidemic with high hematocrit. Low oxygen levels suggested decompensation, and high hematocrits suggested a compensatory response. Physicians assumed measurements at delivery were representative of fetal gases in utero before labor, although they were cautioned against this interpretation by Nicholas Eastman, who was one of the first to study fetal oxygenation.[4,5]

STRESS OF LABOR

Even as these issues were debated, investigators understood something of the stress imposed by labor. For example, they knew that each contraction of the myometrium exerts sufficient lateral pressure on the spiral arteries to slow and even stop placental blood flow, and thereby cause fetal oxygen values to fall. They also knew that every fetus, no matter how normal, develops a metabolic acidosis and an elevated hematocrit during labor, even in the absence of catastrophic events such as a prolapsed cord, placental abruptio, maternal shock, or hypoxemia.

Aortocaval Compression

Inappropriate clinical management would aggravate any of these problems. For example, compression of the inferior vena cava with the patient in the supine position had two effects. By diminishing venous return, it lowered arterial blood pressure and cardiac output and thereby limited placental perfusion. Elevated venous pressure, transmitted to the intervillous space by uterine veins, also increased the risk of premature placental separation. Maternal hemorrhage, hypovolemia, dehydration, metabolic imbalance, infection, respiratory insufficiency, or the inappropriate use of drugs imposed additional problems.

SUMMARY

Prevailing perceptions of the fetal condition presented a bleak prospect to physicians responsible for the care and management of patients. They believed the *normal* fetal environment had deteriorated by term to the point of invoking and perhaps exhausting fetal adaptive mechanisms. On the edge of survival, the fetus then had to negotiate the stress of normal labor and still find reserves to deal with the devastation of a catastrophic event, if one occurs. Given such a condition, it seemed remarkable that any newborn survived, much less thrived.

Clinical lore and principles of patient management reflect this preoccupation with intrauterine hypoxia. For example, meconium in the amniotic fluid was attributed to hypoxic stimulation of bowel contractions and evacuation into the amniotic fluid. Faith in this clinical sign was so strong at one time that fresh meconium in the amniotic fluid was considered sufficient indication for immediate cesarean section delivery. Even now people interchange phrases such as "neonatal depression," "low Apgar score," and "fetal hypoxia" despite the known fact that drugs, trauma, prematurity, and a host of other factors may cause a similar picture.

MONITORING

Given this historical background, we can understand that physicians sought to improve patient management by finding ways to measure fetal oxygen. Generally, their attempts were disappointing. Efforts to relate the condition of the neonate to saturations, partial pressures, or concentrations of oxygen in umbilical cord blood were unsuccessful. Simply, the Apgar score of any given newborn bore no predictable relationship to any of these measurements. A healthy, vigorous infant was as likely to have an extremely low umbilical cord oxygen as was a severely depressed child to have a high value. The explanation for this seemingly paradoxic observation probably lies in the character of oxygen metabolism. Total body oxygen stores are low and are quickly exhausted with any disruption of supply, even before physical damage is detected. By the same token, oxygen stores also rise quickly when the supply is reestablished. Consequently, normal blood values may coexist with physical damage from previous deprivation. Despite the discrepancies, physicians continued to focus on oxygenation rather than to reexamine their perceived notions and to search for alternate ways to attack the problem.

FETAL HEART RATE

The fetal heart rate had long been used to evaluate fetal well-being, but a technologic development in the 1960s facilitated its increased use. At that time, Edward Hon developed methods to detect the fetal ECG and to make continuous electronic measurements of the beat-to-beat interval. His innovation replaced cumbersome, intermittent, auscultatory measurements. Subsequently, he described the now-familiar patterns of heart rate deceleration as they occurred in relation to uterine contractions: early, late, and variable.

Limitations

With experience, the limitations of fetal heart rate measurements became clear. Other patterns appeared, for example, tachycardia and sinusoidal variation, that did not fit prevailing theory. Also, although the monitoring was highly sensitive, the predictability of such monitoring was poor. Many infants believed to be in distress from examination of heart rate tracings and delivered by cesarean section appeared normal after birth. The incidence of cesarean sections rose dramatically, but there was no evidence for a concomitant fall in fetal mortality rate.[6]

In fact, with respect to fetal outcome, recent studies show *no* advantage of electronic monitoring over auscultation. On the surface, this finding might prompt a physician to discard fetal monitoring altogether. I think this would be a mistake.[7–13] Keep in mind that these data applied only to laboring patients and that the methods of clinical auscultation were rigorous and carried out by highly trained people. Most important, the patient management problems that confront the critical care specialist are different from those facing the obstetrician.

Modifications

Response to this diagnostic dilemma was twofold. Attempts were made to refine the ECG measurement by examining such characteristics as the PR interval and the beat-to-beat variability or by defining, with some precision, how much slowing over what period of time actually constituted bradycardia. More recently, measurement of heart rate changes during spontaneous or induced uterine contractions in non-laboring, high-risk patients has been used as a diagnostic test of "fetal well-being" (a term unencumbered with a scientific definition). Other investigators measure fluctuations of beat-to-beat variability occurring with a frequency of 40 to 60 Hz ("vagal tone"), which are synchronous with and presumably caused by in utero fetal respiratory activity. Beat-to-beat variability is diminished or abolished by atropine or hypoxia. Variation of this sort is too small to be detected by visual inspection and can be evaluated only by mathematical analysis. The usefulness of beat-to-beat variability, which has a good theoretical basis, has yet to be tested.[14,15]

SCALP PH

Other investigators attempted to supplement information from heart rate tracings with measurements of fetal scalp pH.[16–18] The approach had a sound basis. Limitations of oxygen measurements included the rapid increase of oxygen even after prolonged deprivation. Presumably, pH measurements avoided this problem because the value reflected the amount of fixed acids accumulated during periods of anaerobic metabolism. Because fetal scalp sampling was cumbersome and time-consuming, it was performed only when heart rate tracings were sufficiently worrisome to promote concern for fetal well-being. Although pH offered advantages in predictability, the test required that a major change in acid–base status occur to be useful (i.e., a decrease of pH to 7.25 or less from a normal value of 7.4). Considering that pH measures hydrogen ions on a logarithmic scale, this change represents a tremendous accumulation of hydrogen ions. Although widely used by obstetricians, chances are that measurements of fetal pH will not be available to the critical care specialist.

TRANSITION CHANGES

If concepts pertaining to fetal oxygenation were correct as originally promulgated, no further comment would be necessary. Many proved incorrect, however, or at best were misleading. As is often the case in medicine and in science, interpretations of the facts, not the facts themselves, were in error. For example, fetal oxygen and pH were low when investigators analyzed the cord blood from anesthetized animals or newly delivered infants. However, the assumptions that these values typified conditions in utero were incorrect. Manipulation during surgery stimulated the uterus, causing constriction of its arteries and a diminished uterine blood flow, a response that increased in severity the closer the subject was to term. Thus, the observed deterioration of oxygenation and pH resulted from increased sensitivity to handling, and not from any inherent deterioration of utero-placental function.

CHRONIC ADAPTATIONS ■

With better methods of study, investigators learned that the environment of the unstressed fetus is remarkably stable with respect to oxygen, glucose, and every metabolite tested during the last part of gestation (Table 96-1). Oxygen does not decrease, nor does hematocrit rise, as was previously thought. The stability even exists at high altitude, where the mother is chronically hypoxic, an observation that prompted more detailed studies of placental function. Subsequently, the functional capacity of the placenta was found to be increased throughout pregnancy, although its weight remained constant. Structural and functional changes within the placenta cause a systemic increase in its *diffusion capacity* (DC) for oxygen, urea, and other components that keep pace with the fetal weight and, pari passu, metabolic activity.[19–21]

PLACENTAL DIFFUSION CAPACITY

Individual factors governing placental DC are the same as those affecting this measurement in the lung; they include surface area (SA), mean diffusion distance (d), the physiochemical characteristics of intervening tissue, and the transplacental concentration gradient of the substance in question (Table 96-2). Surface area, normally measured in square meters, refers to the total area of all microscopic villi, similar to the alveolar surface area of the lungs. Diffusion distance refers to the mean distance that substances must traverse when they move between maternal and fetal blood. Factors governing the concentration gradient include the mean concentration of substances on either side of the placenta (or partial pressure in the case of gases) and the rate of delivery of the substance to and from either side of the placenta. Rate of delivery is determined by the rates of flow of uterine and umbilical blood and by the carrying capacity of the blood, which, in the case of oxygen, is related directly to hemoglobin concentration.

The close relationship between fetal weight (and metabolic activity) and DC throughout pregnancy reflects adjustments in each of these components. For example, as pregnancy advances, fetal capillaries in placental villi move toward the surface, decreasing the diffusion distance; microvilli become convoluted, increasing the surface area; and uterine blood flow increases, maintaining the concentration gradients. These placental characteristics also affect the movement of drugs.[22,23]

COMPENSATORY CHANGES

The delivery system for essential substrates shows remarkable flexibility. In the event of any inadequacy, compensatory changes occur elsewhere. An experimentally induced fall in maternal hemoglobin stimulates increased rates of uterine blood flow so that oxygen delivery, the product of flow and oxygen concentration, remains stable. Limitation of placental growth induces higher rates of uterine blood flow and overdevelopment of the remaining placental tissue. Similar adaptations occur clinically in women with anemia and heart disease and in infants afflicted with anemia from a hemolytic disorder.[24,25]

Far from representing the inflexible system originally conceived by clinicians, the placenta clearly shows a consider-

---

TABLE 96-1. Evidence for Stability of the Intrauterine Environment Until Onset of Labor

1. Stable concentration of blood constituents (e.g., hematocrit, Po_2, glucose concentrations)

2. A consistent relationship between weight of the fetus and various structural and functional characteristics of the placenta (e.g., surface area, diffusion capacity)

3. A consistent relationship between weight of the fetus and flow/kg tissue of umbilical and uterine circulations

4. Appropriate adaptive changes in the event of maternal or fetal stress, which may involve either structural or functional change

---

TABLE 96-2. Diffusion Capacity

Defining the amount of material transferred per unit time per unit difference of concentration gradient (DC):

$$DC = \frac{k(SA)(\Delta C_1 - C_2)}{d}$$

k = constant that varies with the physiochemical properties of the intervening tissue
SA = surface area of the membrane
d = mean diffusion distance
$\Delta C_1 - C_2$ = mean concentration gradient between maternal and fetal blood

able ability to adapt to special circumstances. Perhaps the most remarkable examples of this adaptability are cases in which the placenta implants on the omentum, the liver, or other abdominal organs, rather than on the uterine mucosa. Despite the unfavorable site, the fetus often achieves normal weight, apparently because it has the capacity to extract the necessary nutrients from whatever maternal tissues are available.

Clinical observations suggest that factors limiting the delivery of oxygen to the fetus stimulate, by mechanisms not yet identified, compensatory change in placental morphology or physiology. Placental size, relative to the fetus, tends to be greater when some maternal factor, hypoxemia, or anemia limits availability of oxygen to the fetus. Placental surface area also is greater than normal in proportion to the severity of anemia in cases of erythroblastosis fetalis. In other instances, higher than normal rates of uterine blood flow compensate for disruptions of placental development or decreased maternal oxygen-carrying capacity, maintaining fetal homeostasis in the face of disruption from within or without.

It is difficult to appreciate the extent to which the aforementioned observations contradict prevailing thought or the extent to which they have been ignored in clinical practice. Current clinical literature is rife with allusions to the developmental incompetence of the placenta. For example, we ascribe morphologic changes in the placenta during pregnancy to *aging* or *senescence* and not to *maturation*. We assume, de rigueur, that placental infarcts compromise function, although we lack the evidence necessary to prove this thesis. We interchange words such as *neonatal depression* and *hypoxia*, although we know the former may be caused by many factors completely unrelated to the availability of oxygen.

ACUTE ADAPTATIONS ■

The forgoing examples illustrate adaptations to chronic stress. Clinicians may rejoin saying that they must also consider the capacity of the fetus to deal with acute stress, as encountered in pregnant women who are trauma victims, acutely ill with a medical disease, or in labor. But even here, clinical concepts contradict current information. The normal fetus has several mechanisms that enable it to survive acute stress (Table 96-3).

METABOLIC RATE

Fluctuation of metabolic rate constitutes an important acute adaptive response.[26] Whereas the normal rate of oxygen consumption of the unstressed fetus varies from 10 to 15 mL/kg/minute, it may decrease to 4 mL/kg/minute or less during acute stress. In fact, the low rate that early investigators mistook for normal metabolic activity probably exemplifies this response. Presumably, this change occurs when the fetus stops growing (growth being a process that requires high rates of energy consumption) and uses only the energy necessary to sustain body homeostasis. Rates of 4 mL/kg/minute

TABLE 96-3.   Adaptations of Hypoxia

1. Structural changes within the placenta (e.g., increased surface area, decreased diffusion distance)
2. Increased flow/kg of uterine or umbilical blood flow
3. Increased fetal hematocrit
4. Decreased growth rate decreasing fetal requirements
5. Decreased fetal movement
6. Placental metabolism of lactate
7. Redistribution of fetal cardiac output to the brain and heart
8. Premature labor

are typical for a nongrowing adult. Viewed in this light, infants who fail to grow in utero evince an effective adaptive response. They keep their metabolic requirements low by two mechanisms: (1) by virtue of their total size, and (2) by the cessation of growth. Acute stress may evoke this response rapidly.

LACTATE METABOLISM

The placenta metabolizes lactate as another response to stress.[27,28] During periods of hypoxia, the fetus may revert to anaerobic metabolism. If lactate is produced, it is metabolized by the placenta, traverses the placenta to be metabolized by the mother, or remains in the fetal circulation. The route taken seems to depend on the severity of hypoxia. Two of the three pathways are protective; only in the latter circumstance is there a tendency for development of a metabolic acidosis.

FETAL BRADYCARDIA

Fetal bradycardia also may be a manifestation of an adaptive response and not hypoxic myocardial depression.[29] A *diving reflex* in human neonates and in adult aquatic birds and mammals consists of bradycardia and peripheral vasoconstriction. This reflex preserves circulation to the heart and brain at the expense of peripheral tissue perfusion during water immersion and prolongs the time that these two essential organs can survive without damage. It is especially prominent in premature infants; in term infants, it tends to disappear during the first 2 days of life. It may be elicited by vagal stimulation as well as by hypoxia.

Presumably, this reflex is no less protective for human infants in utero than for free-living diving animals, but it does create a diagnostic problem. The clinician reading fetal heart rate tracings cannot distinguish with certainty the bradycardia of severe myocardial depression from reflex bradycardia. The one may warrant immediate cesarean section; the other may simply be a sign of a healthy response to stress.

SPONTANEOUS MOVEMENT

The tendency to decrease spontaneous movements during hypoxia is related to the diving reflex and is seen in fetuses and some newborns. This response is exactly the opposite to that which occurs in hypoxic adults who respond by struggling and attempting to escape. The flaccid response diminishes fetal oxygen requirements during periods of deprivation, thus prolonging the time of survival without damage to the brain and heart. Some evidence suggests that the fetal central nervous system of many species seems to have greater capacity than the adult central nervous system to withstand periods of oxygen deprivation.[30]

SUMMARY ■

In summation, current techniques of fetal monitoring should be used by the critical care specialist. Their primary use lies in the documentation of the infant's status on admission of the mother to the intensive care area. Secondarily, fetal monitoring may be used to identify drugs or therapy for the mother that may be harmful to the fetus. In using fetal monitoring technology, however, the critical care physician should be mindful of its limitations. In view of the high probability of false-positive tests during labor, it seems unwarranted to withhold therapy essential for the well-being of the mother simply on the basis of these tests.

Obstetricians have become increasingly conservative in the interpretation of the data. In a recent position paper, the American College of Obstetrics and Gynecology expressed concern about the use of the terms *fetal distress* and *birth asphyxia*.[31] Fetal distress, they suggest, is imprecise and nonspecific. It has little predictive value "even in high risk populations." Similarly, they suggest that the term *asphyxia* be reserved for those situations in which objective measurements of oxygen deprivation are documented, including a profound metabolic or mixed acidemia, an Apgar Score of 3 or less for 5 minutes, or evidence of neonatal neurologic sequelae. The intensivist should notice that most of these conditions can be established only *after delivery*. They will, therefore, have little impact on maternal management in an intensive care unit.

REFERENCES ■

1. Doderlein A: Zum gedachtnis P. Zweifel. *Arch Gynakol* 1927;131:1
2. Caton D: Obstetric anesthesia and concepts of placental transport: a historical review of the nineteenth century. *Anesthesiology* 1977;46:132
3. Carpenter TM, Murlin JR: The energy metabolism of mother and child just before and just after birth. *Arch Intern Med* 1911;7:184
4. Eastman NJ: Fetal blood studies: the oxygen relationships of umbilical cord at birth. *Bull Johns Hopkins Hosp* 1930;47:221
5. Eastman NJ, McLane CM: Fetal blood studies: the lactic acid content of umbilical cord blood at birth. *Bull Johns Hopkins Hosp* 1931;48:261
6. Haverkamp AD, Orleans M: A controlled trial of the differential effects of intrapartum fetal monitoring. *Am J Obstet Gynecol* 1979;134:399
7. Painter MJ, Depp R, O'Donoghue PD: Fetal heart rate patterns and development in the first year of life. *Am J Obstet Gynecol* 1978;132:271
8. Low JA, Galbraith RS, Muir D, et al: Intrapartum fetal asphyxia: a preliminary report in regard to long-term morbidity. *Am J Obstet Gynecol* 1978;130:525
9. Banta HD, Thacker SB: Assessing the costs and benefits of electronic fetal monitoring. *Obstet Gynecol Surv* 1979;34:627
10. Paneth N, Stark RI: Cerebral palsy and mental retardation in relation to indicators of perinatal asphyxia: an epidemiologic overview. *Am J Obstet Gynecol* 1983;147:960
11. Leveno KJ, Gunningham GF, Nelson S, et al: A prospective comparison of selective and universal electronic fetal monitoring in 34,995 pregnancies. *N Engl J Med* 1986;315:615
12. Rosen MG, Dickinson JC: The paradox of electronic fetal monitoring: more data may not enable us to predict or prevent infant neurologic morbidity. *Am J Obstet Gynecol* 1993;168:745
13. Shy KK, Luthy DA, Bennett FC, et al: Effects of electronic fetal heart rate monitoring, as compared with periodic auscultation, on the neurologic development of premature infants. *N Engl J Med* 1990;322:588
14. Donchin Y, Caton D, Porges SW: Spectral analysis of fetal heart rate in sheep: the occurrence of respiratory sinus arrhythmia. *Am J Obstet Gynecol* 1984;148:1130
15. Snijders RJM, Ribbert LSM, Visser HA, et al: Numeric analysis of heart rate variation in intrauterine growth-retarded fetuses: a longitudinal study. *Am J Obstet Gynecol* 1992;166:22
16. Kubli FW, Hon EH, Khazin AF, et al: Observations on heart rate and pH in the human fetus during labor. *Am J Obstet Gynecol* 1969;104:1190
17. Wood C, Newman W, Lumley J, et al: Classification of fetal heart rate in relation to fetal scalp blood measurements and Apgar score. *Am J Obstet Gynecol* 1969;105:942
18. Caldwell BM, Graham FK, Penoyer MM, et al: The utility of blood oxygenation as an indicator of postnatal condition. *J Pediatr* 1957;50:434
19. Comline RS, Silver M: Daily changes in foetal and maternal blood of conscious umbilical and uterine vessels. *J Physiol (Paris)* 1970;209:567
20. Barron DH, Metcalfe J, Meschia G, et al: *Adaptations of Pregnant Ewes and Their Fetuses to High Altitude.* Oxford, Pergamon Press, 1963:115
21. Makowski EL, Battaglia FC, Meschia G, et al: Effect of maternal exposure to high altitude upon fetal oxygenation. *Am J Obstet Gynecol* 1968;100:852
22. Meschia G, Cotter JR, Breathmach CS, et al: The diffusibility of oxygen across the sheep placenta. *Q J Exp Physiol* 1965;50:466
23. Clavero JA, Botilla Llusia J: Measurement of the villous surface in normal and pathologic placentas. *J Obstet Gynaecol Br Commonw* 1963;86:234
24. Beischer NA, Sivasamboo R, Vohra S, et al: Placental hypertrophy in severe pregnancy anaemia. *Am J Obstet Gynecol* 1970;77:398
25. Caton D, Crenshaw C, Wilcox CJ, et al: O_2 delivery to the pregnant uterus: its relationship to O_2 consumption. *Am J Physiol* 1979;237:R52

26. Caton D, Henderson J, Wilcox J, et al: Oxygen consumption of the uterus and its contents and weight at birth of lambs. In: Longo LD, Reneau DD (eds). *Fetal and Newborn Cardiovascular Physiology*. New York, London, Garland STPM Press, 1976:123

27. Huckabee WE, Metcalfe J, Prystowsky H, et al: Insufficiency of O_2 supply to pregnant uterus. *Am J Physiol* 1962;202:198

28. Huckabee WE, Metcalfe J, Prystowsky H, et al: Movements of lactate and pyruvate in pregnant uterus. *Am J Physiol* 1962;202:193

29. Irving L: Respiratory reflexes in diving mammals. *Physiol Rev* 1939;19:112

30. Himwich HE, Bernstein AO, Herrlich H, et al: Mechanisms for the maintenance of life in the newborn during anoxia. *Am J Physiol* 1942;135:387

31. ACOG Committee Opinion, Committee on Obstetric Practice. *Fetal Distress and Birth Asphyxia*, No. 137 April, 1994

Environmental Hazards

Critical Care, Third Edition, edited by Joseph M. Civetta,
Robert W. Taylor, and Robert R. Kirby.
Lippincott-Raven Publishers, Philadelphia, PA © 1997.

CHAPTER 97

■

Protecting the Practitioner: Acquired Immunodeficiency Syndrome and Hepatitis

Salvatore Lopalo
A. Joseph Layon

ACQUIRED IMMUNODEFICIENCY SYNDROME ■

HISTORICAL CONSIDERATIONS

The acquired immunodeficiency syndrome (AIDS) is thought to have been present on the African continent for several decades. Antibodies to the human immunodeficiency virus (HIV) have been identified in sera obtained and stored from patients seen there in the 1950s, although there has been some controversy as to the fidelity of data obtained from this stored material[1] and the damaged national pride related to this suggestion.[2] Nonetheless, approximately two thirds of the world's 3 million cases of AIDS have occurred in Africa. In some African special-risk populations, such as prostitutes, the HIV infection rate approximates 30%; it is thought that about 9 million sub-Saharan Africans are infected with HIV.[3]

AIDS was recognized in the United States in San Francisco and New York in 1981 after increasing numbers of young, previously healthy male homosexuals and drug abusers presented with disease constellations that included Kaposi's sarcoma and *Pneumocystis carinii* pneumonia. Kaposi's sarcoma had been, until then, a rare and usually benign form of cancer,[1] seldom seen even in large metropolitan hospitals. *P. carinii* pneumonia had previously been seen in immunocompromised cancer patients or those receiving high-dose steroids, although it had also been described in newborns.

The new disorder, initially and unfortunately termed the "gay plague" and gay-related immunodeficiency (GRID) syndrome, was characterized by profound cellular immunodeficiency resulting in the development of unusual opportunistic infections, unusual manifestations of more common infections, and malignancy. Because most of the cases of the clinical syndrome involved homosexual men, it was initially thought that the disease was related to lifestyle habits of that population, such as recurrent rectal exposure to sperm or use of amyl nitrate "poppers." Because AIDS increasingly thereafter was seen in other populations, such as intravenous drug abusers and hemophiliacs, this theory was abandoned by the mainstream scientific community in favor of an infectious agent theory.

In 1983, a suspected causative agent of AIDS, termed lymphadenopathy-associated virus or human T-cell lymphotropic virus (HTLV-III), was identified simultaneously in France and the United States.[4] The virus was later renamed HIV. At least two related versions of HIV exist: HIV-1 and HIV-2. HIV-1 is thought to be the primary causative agent of human immunodeficiency virus disease (HIVD) and AIDS throughout the world. HIV-2 is largely confined to western Africa and appears to be less virulent than HIV-1,[7,8] taking an average of 25 instead of 10 years to progress to AIDS. HIV-1 and HIV-2 have the same modes of transmission, but the latter agent appears to be transmitted less efficiently than HIV-1, both perinatally and sexually. A related retrovirus, the simian immunodeficiency virus, which is more closely related to HIV-2 than HIV-1, causes disease of varying clinical severity in monkeys and has been rarely reported in humans.[5,6]

EPIDEMIOLOGY

The operating room and critical care environments are hazardous. Risks include transmission of infection. The central issue with regard to HIV infection and health care workers involves two specific points: (1) Should different techniques (e.g., anesthetic) be used for patients who are HIV infected? and (2) What are the risks of HIV transmission from patient to worker, and from worker to patient?

As of April 1995, 461,234 cases of AIDS had been reported in the United States; approximately 60% (282,220) of these afflicted individuals have died.[9] By August 1995, 42,294 new cases of AIDS had been reported for the year[10]; each week, 1000 to 2000 new cases are reported to the Centers for Disease Control and Prevention (CDCP). Those affected continue to be predominately in homosexual and bisexual men (55%); heterosexual intravenous drug abusers (24%); and other heterosexuals adults (7%). The remaining cases are pediatric, transfusion-related, or of indeterminate cause. It is *high-risk behavior*, rather than status as a *group member*, that puts an individual in harm's way. A homosexual intravenous drug abuser who uses clean injection apparatus and unadulterated drugs and practices monogamy with a long-term partner is unlikely to become infected with HIV. Conversely, a promiscuous heterosexual practicing unsafe sex is at significant risk.

In the United States, HIV infection is the sixth leading cause of death among women 25 to 44 years of age and the second leading cause of death among men of the same age group.[11] Further, in 1989 AIDS became the sixth leading cause of death for adolescents and young adults aged 15 to 24 of both sexes.[12] The HIV-infected person who presents for medical care today was probably infected 8 to 10 years ago; prevention is thus of paramount importance.

HIVD/AIDS AND "OTHERNESS"

HIV/AIDS is an extraordinary disease because society views it prejudicially and irrationally. Even among health care workers, such attitudes often accompany discussion about HIVD/AIDS or the treatment of potentially afflicted patients. Emotional responses probably result because the first cases identified in the United States occurred among socially marginalized persons (i.e., members of the gay community and intravenous drug abusers). The "otherness" of these first victims led to a flood of hate mongering, some from representatives of organized religion and other self-appointed watchdogs of public morality.[13] Maltreatment often was justified on the ground that the disease was divine punishment for personal behavior.

Because those with HIVD/AIDS in the United States may be so categorized, the mainstream medical population as well as the general population have portrayed the victims of HIVD/AIDS as somehow different from the rest of us, implying that HIVD/AIDS is something that could never happen to us. This type of presumption has occurred frequently, and just as often incorrectly, throughout history. Syphilis initially was called the Neapolitan disease because it was first described in Italians. Later, after it infected the French, it was termed the French pox. This sexually transmitted disease, however, eventually infected persons of diverse ethnic groups, even though historical documents show that contemporary officials hoped it would be restricted to others. Tuberculosis in the 19th century and cancer early in the 20th century were also viewed as diseases of others.[14,15] In each of these examples, the language used to refer to the disease implies at least two basic concepts: (1) victims are responsible for their suffering, and (2) sufferers are different in some fundamental way from those who are unafflicted. That such thinking still exists near the second millennium is as remarkable as it is disheartening.

The undeniable bias against people with HIVD/AIDS adversely affects the entire community. Until recently, attempts to combat HIV disease were met with glib statements about abstinence; other means of prevention, needle exchange programs, and education about safer sex were neglected. The problematic nature of these education and preventive measures stems from political rather than medical forces. Under the Reagan and Bush administrations, even the CDCP, an organization purportedly protected from political pressures, was forced to follow political dogma rather than sound health principles.[16] CDCP programs, according to the former head of its AIDS group, often were dictated by what those in the administration thought was politically correct, rather than what was best for the American people from a medical and public health point of view. Again, we would do well to recall that HIVD first presented on the African continent in heterosexuals; the disease is not, as suggested by some, a special punishment sent from God to gays and drug abusers. Limitation of HIV education and prevention measures puts each of us at risk.

HEALTH CARE WORKERS AND HIV TRANSMISSION ■

INCIDENCE

Transmission From Health Care Workers to Patients

The popular press has emphasized HIV transmission by health care workers. However, extensive testing of more than 3000 patients cared for by HIV-positive physicians and dentists has been identified HIV transmission in only one cluster of 5 patients.[17-22] Compared with the transmission of hepatitis B by infected health care workers to more than 300 patients in the early 1970s, transmission of HIV to 5 patients, although unacceptable, is quite low.

Transmission From Patients to Health Care Workers

The reverse risk, that of HIV transmission to a health care worker from an infected patient after percutaneous exposure, is about 0.5% (see next section), also significantly lower than the risk of similar transmission of hepatitis B, which is about 30%. This risk differential of approximately 1 to 60 presumably holds in the opposite direction as well. Therefore, if HIVD/AIDS were an "ordinary" disease, we could expect a major effort to immunize health care workers against hepatitis B, while concerns about transmission of HIV from health care workers to patients would fade away. Unfortunately, HIVD/AIDS is not ordinary.

Seroconversion

Several series suggest an approximate 0.5% risk of HIV seroconversion after a single puncture with a blood- or secretion-contaminated instrument.[23-26] Because of the frequency of blood contamination by needle sticks, however, the cumulative lifetime risk of occupationally acquired HIV may range from less than 1% to as much as 10%. Data from the CDCP show that, in health care workers with no known risk factors, the current prevalence of HIV infection is not greater than in the general population. From 1981 to June 1994, occupationally transmitted HIV infection was documented in 42 health care workers. Thirty-six (86%) of these cases resulted from percutaneous exposure, 4 (9.5%) from mucocutaneous exposure, and 1 (2.4%) from both.[27] These numbers almost certainly represent underestimates; only about 12% of surgical needle-puncture injuries are reported.[28]

IMPLICATIONS

With the exception of the five previously-mentioned cases of HIV transmission from a dentist to his patients, no case of transmission from a health care worker to a patient has been documented.[17] Precisely how this dental-related transmission occurred remains a mystery. The involved dentist died, and his office records are unclear concerning the precise technique he used to sterilize instruments. Although these cases suggest to some that all health care workers should be tested for HIV seropositivity, such a strategy has found little support among those who provide health care. Five transmissions, although clearly not inconsequential for the infected patients, represent a very slight risk to the general population. Analysis of the available data suggests essentially no risk to a patient from HIV-seropositive workers;[29] requiring all health care workers to be tested for HIV would represent a high-cost, low-benefit political maneuver.

Two recent analyses of HIV testing of medical personnel using standard cost-effectiveness methods yielded, at best, indeterminate results because of the unclear data regarding HIV seroprevalence and transmission risk.[30] At worst, expenditures for each life saved by prevention of HIV infection were in excess of those usually accepted ($700,000 to $1.1 million).[31] These analyses did not take into account the admittedly difficult-to-determine social costs of HIV seropositivity to medical personnel regarding employment, disability, and social stigma.

TESTING OF HEALTH CARE WORKERS AFTER POSSIBLE EXPOSURE ■

Although the risk of exposure to blood and bodily fluids is high, the risk of HIV transmission to health care workers has been the subject of some controversy.[23-26,28,32,33] Based on our understanding of the epidemiologic aspects of HIV, we think that the lifetime risk of the health care worker is higher than is usually appreciated.

RISK OF SEROCONVERSION IN HEALTH CARE WORKERS

Assume an HIV seroprevalence of 1% (the present range is 0.02% to 5.2%), a frequency of puncture wounds of 1% (this is conservative; it ranges as high as 2.5%[24]), and an overall risk of seroconversion of 1% (presently estimated at approximately 0.5%) after a needle-stick injury from a patient who is HIV positive. The overall risk of HIV infection after one needle-stick injury is 1 in 1,000,000:

$$.01 \times .01 \times .01 = .000001, \text{ or } 10^{-6}$$

If an anesthesiologist cares for 4 patients per day for 250 workdays per year, the risk over a 1-year period increases to 1 in 1000:

$$4 \times 250 = 1000, \text{ or } 10^3$$

$$10^3 \times 10^{-6} = 10^{-3}$$

Over an average career of 40 years, the risk becomes 1 in 25:

$$40 \times 10^{-3} = 4 \times 10^{-2}, \text{ or } 0.04$$

In a program with 80 residents, therefore, three can be expected eventually to die of occupationally acquired HIV disease (assuming they all work for 40 years).

Even if one assumes the current, lower rate of seroconversion (0.5%), the lifetime risk for one health care worker would be 1 in 50:

$$0.01 \times 0.01 \times 0.005 = 0.0000005, \text{ or } 5 \times 10^{-7}$$

$$10^3 \times 5 \times 10^{-7} = 5 \times 10^{-4}$$

$$40 \times 5 \times 10^{-4} = 2 \times 10^{-2}, \text{ or } 0.02$$

This translates into 1 death from occupationally acquired HIV disease over the 40-year careers of 80 residents.

This risk does not belong to health care workers alone; it also extends to their spouses and children. This latter consideration may be the best, if not the only, reason to test health care workers for HIV (as well as for hepatitis B). Unfortunately, because of the politicization noted earlier, HIV seropositivity may affect employability as well as health status.

THE IDEAL WORLD

The question of HIV testing after possible exposure must be considered carefully. At least two answers can be provided. The first response would apply in an ideal world; in such a place, although fear of many diseases exists, no special bias is held against persons with HIV infection. Rational health care and disability systems are in place so that health care workers who become HIV positive do not become destitute because of job loss. In this ideal world, routine testing of health care workers who are at moderate to high risk for infection may be reasonable every 6 to 12 months. Certainly, after traumatic exposure to a patient who is or may be HIV positive, testing is sensible immediately and at 6 weeks, 3 months, 6 months, and 1 year.[34]

The patient in question would be tested in the same manner. Even if the patient tests HIV positive, the health care worker would have some sense of security in knowing that only about 0.5% of traumatic exposures to HIV-positive material result in seroconversion. Whether the HIV-exposed health care worker would be given therapy with zidovudine or another antiviral agent is unclear, because seroconversion has occurred even with zidovudine treatment.[34,35] In any case, information on the use of antiviral agents would be available to health care workers and their personal physicians. This mode of diagnostic surveillance is similar to that currently used for tuberculosis, varicella, and hepatitis B in health care workers.

THE REAL WORLD

In our real world, two concerns are paramount after exposure to a possibly infected patient: (1) Will health care workers who test positive lose their jobs?[36] and (2) Will disability insurance be provided to house officers and medical students? At our institution, medical students are not covered by disability insurance because they have no income, and house officers have very limited coverage. Furthermore, insurance companies conceivably could attempt to minimize financial risk by denying benefits to health care workers whose claims were based on occupational exposure to HIV.

We believe that a health care worker exposed to a patient potentially infected with HIV should be tested anonymously. This form of testing is available throughout the United States and should be used whenever job security may be at risk. This approach may affect insurance coverage. However, if the health care worker later seroconverts, he or she will have no documentation of testing. Therefore, an on-the-job incident report should be filed even if HIV testing is carried out anonymously.

The patient should also be tested. In Florida, this testing is done in one of two ways. Either informed consent is obtained, the patient is offered pretest and posttest counseling, and the test result is entered on the patient's chart, or, if consent is not possible (e.g., with a comatose patient), the test may be performed on a blood specimen obtained for another reason. In that case, the result is not entered on the patient's chart. The first option is the best. According to Florida statute, a health care worker who chooses the second option must be tested at the same time as the patient

or must provide the results of an HIV test performed within 6 months of exposure.[37]

Situations arise in which a competent patient may refuse to be tested, perhaps out of fear of the result or a sense of privacy. This example is yet another result of the unique politicization of HIVD/AIDS. Precedents abound for sacrificing personal choice in the face of public health concerns. Uncooperative patients with active pulmonary tuberculosis can be incarcerated. If the rights of the health care worker and the patient conflict in this type of situation, it is not clear that the demands of the latter necessarily should prevail. To allow such a view routinely is tantamount to saying that, with regard to HIVD, rights are universal except for health care workers.

The situation of potential HIV transmission needs to be handled with care, compassion, and perhaps legislation. Having asserted that testing is the appropriate course of action to follow after possible exposure, we leave the precise means unspecified, given the medical, emotional, political, and financial implications of seroconversion.

PREVENTION ■

Most occupational HIV exposures are preventable if reasonable precautions are taken. However, the nature of invasive procedures is such that accidental punctures caused by scalpel blades, unseen needles, or other devices will inevitably occur. The best we can do is strive to minimize these incidents.[38-43] This approach becomes critically important because there apparently is an asymptomatic pool of HIV-positive individuals that comprises 16% to 18% of the populations studied.[44-46]

Such information should make us more compulsive in our attention to detail in order to prevent inadvertent inoculation with HIV-positive material in the emergency department, operating room, or intensive care unit (ICU). Health care workers may be at highest risk for inoculation with HIV-positive material not from an individual known to have AIDS but from a young trauma victim or routine elective surgical patient for whom care is being provided.

METHODS

All patients and all blood or body fluid specimens must be considered to be infectious at all times. The CDCP has promulgated precautions to be taken while caring for all patients. Although these approaches have been repeated to the point that they have almost become "background noise," their importance is undiminished.[47]

Universal Precautions

Universal precautions (Table 97-1) are those taken with *all* patients, because HIV-infected individuals frequently cannot be identified by history or physical examination. Of particular significance are cases in emergency care settings such as trauma and resuscitation, in which exposure to blood or body fluids is likely and the patient's infectious status is

TABLE 97-1. Universal Precautions

Barriers	Gloves, masks, eyewear as appropriate
Decontamination	Hand washing
Needles	Do not bend, break, resheathe
Ventilation devices	
Dermatologic considerations	Protect weeping, exudative lesions
Pregnant health care workers	Take extra care

TABLE 97-3. Laboratory Precautions

All universal precautions	
Waste	Well-constructed containers with tops
Droplet/Mist	Use biological safety hood
Pipetting	Mechanical pipetters
Clean-up	Decontaminate after spills and before transportation or repair of equipment; dispose of contaminated clothing

unknown. Universal precautions include gloves, eye protection, and protection for any abraded or open skin.

Invasive Precautions

Invasive precautions (Table 97-2) are those taken in addition to the universal precautions if an invasive procedure is to be performed. An invasive procedure is defined by the CDCP as any surgical entry into tissue cavities or any organ, or repair of any traumatically induced lesion. This category includes cardiac catheterization and other angiographic procedures, vaginal or cesarean delivery, intravascular catheter placement, and dental surgical procedures. We also consider nasogastric intubation to be invasive because of the possibility of blood contamination. Liquid-impermeable gowns and, in some circumstances, shoe covers are added to universal precautions.

Laboratory Precautions

Laboratory precautions (Table 97-3) are those recommended for healthcare workers in clinical laboratories. Blood and body fluids from all patients, regardless of known HIV status, must be considered infectious until proven otherwise. The precautions noted supplement universal precautions and include minimization of needle use, exclusively mechanical pipetting, and, depending on the circumstance, use of liquid-impermeable gowns.

Areas of integumentary contamination with a patient's blood or secretions must be washed with germicidal soap as soon as it is practical and safe to do so. Gloves must be worn whenever care is administered to patients. This practice does not include the initial portion of the patient encounter, in which one greets and shakes the patient's hand, nor external contact made in the operating room before conduction of anesthetic.

TABLE 97-2. Invasive Precautions

All universal precautions	
Barriers	Gowns, watch for glove tears

TYPES OF INJURIES

Different types of exposures carry different risks. Cutaneous contamination, barring breaks in the skin, is usually without great risk. It should nonetheless be handled with the precautions noted.

Needle Punctures

Exposure through hollow-tip needles such as those used to start intravenous infusions is recognized to be responsible for approximately 61% of contamination events occurring in operating room personnel. In the operating room, these exposures occur more commonly in anesthesiologists than in surgeons. In the ICU, any person employing such devices is at risk.

Sharp Injuries

Among surgical personnel, sharp injuries are most often inflicted by a solid instrument such as a scalpel or a sharp clamp. Wright and colleagues[39] noted that three types of sharp injuries account for almost 60% of occurrences: (1) injuries caused by instruments left on the surgical field when not in use (24%), (2) injuries to hands used in direct retraction of tissue (17%), (3) injuries to stationary hands holding instruments and injured by a second instrument (16%). Only 6% of sharp injuries occurred during passage of instruments between a scrub nurse and a surgeon. Such sharp instruments are less commonly used in the ICU, but they are present in central vascular access trays, thoracotomy and tracheotomy sets, and ventriculostomy trays, among others.

Needles should never be resheathed; this practice may lead to puncture wounds. All sharp objects should be discarded in a puncture-proof container immediately after use. This container should be placed as close to the procedure site as possible. Instruments not in use must be removed from the field; the use of hands as retractors must be minimized, and double gloving should be the norm. Data suggest that preventative measures are too frequently ignored by health care workers during patient care.[41,42] Of even more significance, up to 84% of blood contacts are preventable by barriers such as face masks, shields, and fluid-resistant gowns and gloves.[40,43]

RESPONSIBILITY TO PATIENTS

One may argue that the patient, under a strictly defined concept of autonomy, has the right to know the HIV status of workers providing health care. Under the principle of nonmalfeasance, physicians should not put their patients at risk. A careful and responsible HIV-positive health care worker, we think, does not do so. We also believe that mandating HIV testing would, in the long term, worsen rather than enhance both patient rights and medical care. With only 5 cases of HIV dental transmission documented, mandated HIV testing of health care workers would in no way alter the progression of HIVD in our society. The only likely effect would be to destroy the careers of those testing positive or refusing on principle to be tested. The false peace of mind obtained for society at large would have been purchased with precious coin, indeed.

RESPONSIBILITY TO HEALTH CARE WORKERS

It is strict duty of the health care worker to look after any patient who requires care, regardless of the patient's HIV status.[14,48] Taking this position requires full realization of the possible, although unlikely, risk that the health care worker may become HIV positive through accidental exposure to contaminated material. This small risk is part of the responsibility taken when the physician's mantle is assumed.

Demanding that physicians care for all patients needing their assistance, including those who are HIV positive, is reasonable; further demanding that physicians put their livelihood and family at risk is not. To do so would result in physicians' turning away patients who in any way "appear" to be at risk. Our opinion is that health care workers who are at risk to become HIV positive in the course of their work should be afforded a degree of protection beyond that normally thought to be the responsibility of either the employer or society.

We envision a joint public-private venture with voluntary participation. If the rate of HIV seroconversion among health care workers remains in proportion to that seen in society in general, this plan would cost no more than we collectively pay today. If, on the other hand, an increase in the proportion of health care workers who develop HIVD occurs, a plan such as we describe will ensure that those who put themselves at risk need not have concern, at least, for their families' economic well-being.

The essential parts of our proposed plan are as follows:

1. As a matter of safety and concern for the patient's well-being, health care workers will undergo HIV testing at 6- to 12-month intervals.
2. Any health care worker who seroconverts to HIV positive will remain on the job until his or her chief of service and a committee of colleagues (agreed on by both the infected health care worker and the administration, and including a lay person) determine that it is no longer in the best interests of the institution, the health care worker, or the patient for the infected worker to do so.
3. At that time, the health care worker will be moved to a new job at the same salary and, as often as possible, within the same department or health center. The transfer must be agreed to by all concerned.
4. After the health care worker becomes no longer able to work, disability insurance will continue to pay the salary previously earned, and any shortfall in departmental funds will be made up by disability insurance payments or by federal or state funds derived from a special tax.

Attempts to determine whether the infection was contracted as a result of occupational exposure or in some other way are inappropriate and could lead to abuse of an ill colleague.

These suggestions are neither radical nor unworkable. They attempt to address the concerns of our frightened citizenry as well as those of health care workers who must provide care to both HIV-positive and HIV-negative patients. The keys to success of this proposal are consistency, fairness, and the trust of our fellow citizens that their welfare, as well as ours, is being looked after.

THE HEPATITIDES ■

RELEVANT EPIDEMIOLOGY

If we are concerned about the possibility of HIV infection in the health care setting, we must be even more vigilant with regard to the hepatitides. Although there is no increased prevalence of HIV among healthcare workers, the same is not true regarding hepatitis B virus (HBV).[49] HIV infects only with great difficulty; HBV is approximately 60 times more infectious than HIV when blood borne.

According to the CDCP, 49,551 cases of hepatitis occurred in the United States in 1994. Of these, 23,507 were hepatitis A; 11,402 were hepatitis B; 4233 were hepatitis non-A, non-B (NANB), including hepatitis C (NANB/C); and 409 were unspecified.[50] These data are significantly different from those of 1988, when approximately 57,000 cases of hepatitis occurred, of which 28,000 were hepatitis A, 23,200 hepatitis B, 2600 hepatitis NANB/C, and 2500 unspecified.[51] The decline in hepatitis B and unspecified hepatitis and the increased classification of NANB/C hepatitis are striking. As of September 1, 1995, 17,358 cases of hepatitis A, 6411 cases of hepatitis B, and 2799 cases of NANB/C hepatitis had been reported for the year.[52]

Hepatitides may be divided into two main groups, those considered primary and those that are secondary. The primary hepatitides account for approximately 95% of the cases of hepatitis encountered in clinical practice. As the name suggests, these organisms primarily affect the liver. Secondary hepatitides account for only about 5% of hepatitis encountered in clinical practice and only secondarily affect the liver.

HEPATITIS A

Hepatitis A virus (HAV) is found in the stool of acutely infected individuals. In the United States, seroprevalence increases with age, so that at 50 years of age approximately

50% of individuals are seropositive.[53] A specific IgG immunoglobulin is found in the plasma of previously infected individuals.

Clinical and Serologic Features

Symptoms of infection caused by HAV are seen 2 to 6 weeks after inoculation. For this reason, it has been termed short-incubation hepatitis. During the symptomatic period, elevated serum levels of transaminases are noted. Jaundice may follow several days after the onset of symptoms, but anicteric disease is common. Just before the onset of symptoms, viral particles are noted in the stool and serum; shedding of the virion, as well as infectiousness, starts with the onset of jaundice.[53]

Transmission

HAV is transmitted by the fecal-oral route, although parenteral transmission does occur uncommonly.[54] This agent is not thought to be of any significance in posttransfusion hepatitis, and it rarely causes fulminant hepatitis. Chronic carrier states and chronic hepatitis do not occur with HAV. The reservoir for the infectious process is thought to consist of the large number of persons with clinically inapparent disease, from whom the organism is transmitted to uninfected individuals. An increase in hepatitis A among homosexual men has been noted.[55] This observation may indicate a return to less safe sexual practices that result in fecal contamination.

Prevention

A vaccine to prevent hepatitis A is now available in the United States; this agent was previously licensed in 40 countries including Canada.[56] The vaccine is prepared in human cell culture, purified, and inactivated in formalin; each milliliter of the agent contains 1440 EL.U. (ELISA units) of viral antigen. The recommended dose is 1 mL into the deltoid muscle, followed by another 1-mL injection 6 to 12 months later; the pediatric (2 to 18 years) dose is two 0.5-mL intramuscular injections (720 EL.U./mL) 1 month apart, followed by a booster injection 6 to 12 months later.[56] Protective antibody levels are detectable in 80% to 98% of adults within 15 days of the initial injection, and in 96% within 30 days; protection is expected to last 10 years after the booster.[56] The vaccine and hepatitis A immune globulin may be given at the same time if immediate protection is needed; the vaccine is recommended for travelers to endemic areas and for members of high-risk groups.

HEPATITIS B

HBV infection is a major cause of acute and chronic hepatitis, cirrhosis, and primary hepatocellular carcinoma in the United States, Western Europe, and Australia.[57-59] The disease occurs primarily in adults, and approximately 0.1% to 0.5% of the general population are chronic viral carriers. This low incidence of viral carriage, in contrast to the approximately 10% incidence of individuals in the same population

who are positive for hepatitis B surface-antigen antibody (HBsAb), implies that most HBV infection is self-limited and followed by immunity. Only occasionally does the chronic carrier state result. However, these chronic carriers appear to be the reservoir that perpetuates the virus.

Composition

HBV is a DNA virus consisting of a core region containing viral DNA, DNA polymerase, and core antigen. The viral outer coat consists of the surface antigen (HBsAg). The complete infectious virion is termed the Dane particle. Another antigen, termed the "e" antigen (HBeAg), is present only in serum containing the Dane particle. Although the biologic significance of this finding has not been entirely clear, the presence of HBeAg correlates well with infectivity.

Risk of Infection

The risk of infection with HBV depends on one's activity. Health care workers with frequent blood contact (e.g., anesthesiologists) are considered to be at intermediate risk for HBV. One percent to 2% of that population are positive for HBsAg, and approximately 10% to 20% are positive for some serologic marker of HBV infection.[49,60] Because HBV can be transmitted sexually, individuals with multiple sexual partners increase their risk for HBV infection.[59]

Clinical and Serologic Features

The incubation period of HBV ranges between 6 and 24 weeks, depending on both the size of the inoculum and its portal of entry. For example, an infusion of 50 mL of infected blood may result in a patient becoming HBsAg positive in only a few weeks; a 50-μL inoculation most often results in detectable surface antigen only after 3 to 4 months.

Serologic features[58] are important in the diagnosis of viral infection: HBsAg is noted before any other clinical or laboratory finding is observable. The Dane particle marker, HBeAg, and DNA polymerase parallel the rise of HBsAg. Approximately 2 weeks after the appearance of these markers, liver enzymes, including aspartate transaminase, begin to rise. Symptoms may be noted approximately 6 weeks after the onset of antigenemia.

Antibody Formation

As HBV-associated DNA polymerase becomes detectable, HBsAg levels peak. The first antibody against HBV, noted within 2 to 4 weeks after initiation of antigenemia, is the IgM core antibody (HBcAb). The IgG isotype of HBcAb may persist for months to years after the antigenemia has cleared. Except in those patients who eventually develop chronic viral disease, HBsAb is noted for several weeks after clearing of viral antigen. The presence of HBsAg indicates unequivocally either acute or chronic HBV infection. Conversely, the presence of HBsAb usually implies a successful response to HBV and confers lifelong protection against further infection. A small group of individuals with HBV infection are negative for both HBsAg and HBsAb but positive for HBcAb. These individuals are capable of transmitting HBV until HBsAb is produced. Most infected individuals, however, clear the viral antigen, resulting in ultimate recovery.

Chronic Carriers

Approximately 5% to 10% of HBV-infected individuals become chronic carriers[60]; a subgroup of those with HBV-induced chronic liver disease go on to develop cirrhosis, hepatocellular carcinoma, or both. Carriers are most frequently patients who developed mild, anicteric, acute hepatitis followed by gradual return of normal results of liver function studies. Despite these normalizing biochemical parameters, patients are unable to clear the antigen, and no HBsAb is detected. Chronic carriers are frequently asymptomatic and are thus in a position to infect others unknowingly. Approximately 10% of HBV-infected patients have clinical manifestations for longer than 6 months; these individuals are classified as having chronic hepatitis.

Recently, a strain of HBV has been identified in which a mutation in the precore/core promoter region exists (G-to-A point mutation at nucleotide 1896, also termed A1896), such that translation of HBeAg is aborted.[61] Patients with this mutated HBV have been noted to have fulminant disease, although not all fulminant disease is associated with HBV-A1896. The mutated virus strain is infrequently found in the United States or France but has been seen in Japan, Israel, southern Mediterranean countries, and Australia.[62]

Transmission

Fecal-oral or urine-oral transmission of HBV is thought unlikely, because HBV particles are usually not found in stool and urine. However, viral particles have been found in saliva, semen, vaginal secretions, tears, and breast milk. The major routes of transmission are thought to be parenteral and mucosal (sexual). The parenteral route is most frequently identified in cases that are acquired in the hospital or by intravenous drug abusers. Only 10% of cases of posttransfusion hepatitis are caused by HBV. In these cases, the viral antigen is present in such low titer that the immunoassay used to screen donated blood cannot detect it. The blood donor may also be part of that small group with undetectable HBsAg and HBsAb but a positive titer for HBcAb.

Health care workers are put at risk for HBV infection from accidental needle sticks. That the infection rate is only 10% seems to be a result of the small amount of inoculum present on the sharp objects. Transmission can occur if inapparent cuts or abrasions are inoculated with infectious material; conjunctival contamination followed by infection can also occur.

In contrast to HIV infection, an excess incidence of HBV infection occurs among health care workers.[49,60] One study, in which the serum of patients presenting to an inner-city emergency room were tested for HBV, hepatitis C virus (HCV), and HIV-1, showed that the seroprevalence of HBsAg was 5%.[63] This figure is more than ten times that quoted for healthy adult, first-time blood donors.

NON-A, NON-B HEPATITIS

Non-A, non-B hepatitis is caused by HCV,[64-67] hepatitis E virus (HEV),[66-68] and GB viruses[69]; other viral agents probably are involved as well. Because several viral agents are responsible for NANB hepatitis, it is now termed non–A-E hepatitis.[64]

Clinical Features

Hepatitis non–A-E is the major cause of posttransfusion hepatitis, and, at least until recently, it occurred in approximately 7% to 12% of patients who received blood transfusions.[70] With our ability to test for the anti-HCV antibody[70,71] and for surrogate markers,[72-74] the incidence appears to be decreasing and is now in the range of 0.57% to 6%.[70,71]

Until the discovery of HCV and the development of an assay for antibody to this viral agent, no clinical serologic test for the direct detection of infected blood was available. Assays for HBcAb and serum alanine aminotransferase served as indirect markers for NANB infectivity and therefore were used as surrogates to screen blood.[72-74] If the presence of these markers was determined for equal numbers of units transfused, recipients of HBcAb-positive blood had an approximately twofold higher incidence of posttransfusion hepatitis. Specifically, the incidence ranged from 4% to 6% in recipients of HBcAb-negative blood, and from 8% to 14% in recipients of HBcAb-positive blood.

Elimination from the donor pool of blood positive for HBcAb removed about 5% of the donated units and resulted in the decrement of 20% to 40% of cases of NANB hepatitis. However, exclusion of blood positive for anti-HCV could have prevented about 80% of posttransfusion hepatitis.[70] Although HCV is only one of the responsible agents, it is thought to account for approximately 80% of transfusion-associated non–A-E hepatitis.[71] The serologic assays (an enzyme-linked immunosorbent assay and a confirmatory recombinant immunoblot) used in screening detect HCV with a sensitivity of 80% to 85% and a specificity of 89% to 97%.[70] (In this case, sensitivity refers to the percentage of patients developing non–A-E hepatitis after receiving at least 1 unit of blood product with a positive test result, and specificity is the percentage of patients not developing non–A-E hepatitis who received only blood products with a negative test result.)

Transmission

Hepatitis non–A-E rarely may be transmitted by the oral-fecal route. It has an epidemiologic pattern more resembling HBV than HAV; specifically, it is most commonly transmitted through needle sticks and transfusions. The period between inoculation and onset of symptoms ranges from 2 to 20 weeks and averages 8 weeks. Although symptoms range from mild to fulminant, HCV hepatitis is milder than HBV during the acute stage. Up to 50% of cases are anicteric and show only moderate biochemical abnormalities. Spontaneous resolution occurs approximately 12 weeks after infection in most patients. In 20% to 70% of both transfusion- and community-acquired cases, biochemical and pathologic abnormalities suggest chronic disease.[75]

Serologic Features

Until the development of assays for HCV, the diagnosis of non–A-E hepatitis was by exclusion. Access to analytic materials has resulted in some intriguing findings. For example, Akahane and colleagues[76] showed that anti-HCV was present in up to 27% of spouses (52 men and 102 women) of patients with chronic HCV infection (66 with chronic hepatitis, 49 with cirrhosis, and 39 with hepatocellular carcinoma). The relatively low infection rate of the spouses, and the fact that infection was not found in any of the seven spouses who had been married for less than 10 years, suggest that HCV is less transmissible sexually than HBV.

Therapy

Therapeutic options for HCV are limited, but approximately 25% of patients placed on long-term therapy with interferon-α, 3×10^6 U three times weekly, have been shown to have prolonged and complete normalization of aminotransferase activity and perhaps even eradication of infection.[77] Seeff and colleagues,[78] in an elaborate and long-term (18 years average follow-up) study, found no increased all-cause mortality in patients after transfusion-associated NANB hepatitis. However, a significant increase in the number of deaths related to liver disease was noted in the NANB group, as opposed to the control group.

Some controversy exists as to whether vertical transmission of HCV from mother to infant occurs and the efficiency of this mode of transmission. Wejstal[79] and Ohto[80] and their associates found that transmission occurred in a small proportion of patients studied (1 of 21 in the former study, 3 of 54 in the latter). Ohto noted that transmission seemed to occur when the mother had relatively high titers of serum HCV RNA.[80] Conversely, Reinus and colleagues[81] were unable to document transmission in any of 24 infants (including 1 set of twins) of mothers with HCV infection, even though 16 of the 23 mothers were positive for HCV RNA by polymerase chain reaction.

HEPATITIS D

Hepatitis D (delta hepatitis) occurs only with HBV infection. The agent, hepatitis D virus (HDV) is an incomplete RNA virus requiring antecedent or concomitant infection with HBV in order to infect the host.[57,66] It is sometimes considered a complication of HBV infection. Delta hepatitis is most frequently encountered in intravenous drug abusers or patients who are recipients of multiple transfusions.[82] A chronic carrier state and chronic hepatitis are known to occur, as is massive hepatic necrosis. Anti-HDV antibody is similar to HBcAb in that it signifies that infection has occurred but is not protective. Prevention is most important with regard to this disease.

HEPATITIS E

HEV is an RNA virus that was formerly called enterically transmitted non-A, non-B hepatitis.[66,68] Although it is similar in mode of transmission to HAV, the two viral agents are unrelated in structure, stability, and genome. HEV has been associated with large outbreaks of hepatitis during floods and other catastrophes in which sewage handling becomes suboptimal. Disease caused by the viral agent is usually self-limited and mild, but 10% to 20% of women infected during their third trimester of pregnancy sicken and die from fulminant hepatic failure. HEV has been seen in transplant centers in patients with fulminant hepatic failure.

PROTECTIVE AND THERAPEUTIC MEASURES ■

IMMUNIZATION

Based on the foregoing data, all health care workers should be immunized with hepatitis B vaccine. It is given as 20 μg intramuscularly three times, with the second and third dose given 1 and 6 months after the first.[83,84] After blood exposure has occurred, the series of events that should be followed depends on the source of the exposure and the immunization status of the health care worker exposed.[83]

Known Low-Risk Source

If the source is an individual at low risk of being HBsAg positive, an unvaccinated health care worker should have the vaccine series initiated. A vaccinated person requires no treatment.

Known High-Risk Source

If the source is an individual at high risk of being HBsAg positive, several things should be done. If the exposed health care worker is unvaccinated, the hepatitis B vaccine series should be initiated. Further, the person who was the source of the exposure should be tested for HBsAg and, if the result is positive, a dose of hepatitis B immune globulin (HBIG) should be given immediately to the exposed health care worker. The dose is 0.06 mL/kg intramuscularly.[83] If the exposed individual had been vaccinated in the past and was a vaccine nonresponder, the source should be tested for HBsAg status. If the source is indeed HBsAg positive, the HBIG and a booster dose of hepatitis B vaccine should be given immediately.

Known Serologic-Positive Source

If the source is known to be HBsAg positive, the unvaccinated individual should be given HBIG immediately, and the series of HBV vaccine immunizations should be started. If the exposed individual was previously vaccinated, the level of antibody should be tested. An inadequate antibody concentration (<10 sample ratio units by radioimmunoassay or negative by enzyme immunoassay) should lead to administration of a dose of HBIG and a hepatitis B vaccine booster dose.[83]

SECONDARY HEPATITIDES

In the differential diagnosis of viral hepatitis, one must consider the possibility of an agent that affects the liver secondarily rather than primarily. Such agents include cytomegalovirus, disseminated herpes simplex virus, Coxsackie virus A and B, Epstein-Barr virus, and yellow fever virus. These infectious agents account for approximately 5% of clinical hepatitis. No further discussion of these agents is offered here.

REFERENCES ▪

1. Katner HP, Pankey GA: Evidence for a Euro-american origin of human immunodeficiency virus. *J Natl Med Assoc* 1987; 79:1068
2. Bennett FJ: AIDS as social phenomenon. *Soc Sci Med* 1987;25:529
3. De Cock KM, Ekpini E, Gnaore E, et al: The public health implications of AIDS research in Africa. *JAMA* 1994;272:481
4. Ho DD, Pomerantz RJ, Kaplan JC: Pathogenesis of infection with human immunodeficiency virus. *N Engl J Med* 1987; 317:278
5. Khabbaz RF, Heneine W, George JR, et al: Brief report: Infection of a laboratory worker with simian immunodeficiency virus. *N Engl J Med* 1994;330:172
6. Essex M: Simian immunodeficiency virus in people. *N Engl J Med* 1994;330:209
7. Travers K, Mboup S, Marlink R, et al: Natural protection against HIV-1 infection provided by HIV-2. *Science* 1995; 268:1612
8. Cohen J: Can one type of HIV protect against another type? [research news]. *Science* 1995;268:1566
9. Case watch. *AIDS Clin Care* 1995;7:53
10. Cases of specified notifiable diseases: United States, weeks ending August 26, 1995, and August 27, 1994. *MMWR Morb Mortal Wkly Rep* 1995;44:631
11. Selik RM, Chu SY, Buehler JW: HIV infection as leading cause of death among young adults in US cities and states. *JAMA* 1993;269:2991
12. Selected behaviors that increase risk for HIV infection among high school students—United States, 1990. *MMWR Morb Mortal Wkly Rep* 1992;41:231
13. Selby GR: AIDS and the moral law. *N C Med J* 1983;44:275
14. D'Amico R, Layon AJ: AIDS and the politics of morbidity. *Telos* 1988;76:115
15. Osler W, McCrae T: *The Principles and Practice of Medicine.* New York: Appleton, 1920:269
16. Francis DP: Toward a comprehensive HIV prevention program for the CDC and the nation. *JAMA* 1992;268:1444
17. Recommendations for preventing transmission of human immunodeficiency virus and hepatitis B virus to patients during exposure-prone invasive procedures. *MMWR Morb Mortal Wkly Rep* 1991;40(RR-8):1
18. Rogers AS, Froggatt JW III, Townsend T, et al: Investigation of potential HIV transmission to the patients of an HIV-infected surgeon. *JAMA* 1993;269:1795
19. Dickinson GM, Morhart RE, Klimas NG, et al: Absence of HIV transmission from an infected dentist to his patients: An epidemiologic and DNA sequence analysis. *JAMA* 1993;269: 1802
20. von Reyn CF, Gilbert TT, Shaw FE Jr, et al: Absence of HIV transmission from an infected orthopedic surgeon: A 13-year look-back study. *JAMA* 1993;269:1807
21. Update: Transmission of HIV infection during an invasive dental procedure—Florida. *MMWR Morb Mortal Wkly Rep* 1991;40:21
22. Update: Transmission of HIV infection during invasive dental procedures—Florida. *MMWR Morb Mortal Wkly Rep* 1991; 40:377
23. Lifson AR, Castro KG, McCray E: National surveillance of AIDS in health care workers. *JAMA* 1986;256:3231
24. McCray E: Occupational risk of the acquired immunodeficiency syndrome among health workers. *N Engl J Med* 1986; 314:1127
25. Update: Acquired immunodeficiency syndrome and human immunodeficiency virus infection among health care workers. *MMWR Morb Mortal Wkly Rep* 1988;37:229
26. Henderson DK, Fahey BJ, Willy M, et al: Risk for occupational transmission of human immunodeficiency virus type 1 (HIV-1) associated with clinical exposures: A prospective evaluation. *Ann Intern Med* 1990;113:740
27. Centers for Disease Control and Prevention: *HIVD/AIDS surveillance report, 1994.* Atlanta: Centers for Disease Control and Prevention 1994:6(#1):15.
28. Lowenfels AB, Wormser GP, Jain R: Frequency of puncture injuries in surgeons and estimated risk of HIV infection. *Arch Surg* 1989;124:1284
29. Robert LM, Chamberland ME, Cleveland JL, et al: Investigations of patients of health care workers infected with HIV: The Centers for Disease Control and Prevention database. *Ann Intern Med* 1995;122:653
30. Phillips KA, Lowe RA, Kahn JG, et al: The cost-effectiveness of HIV testing of physicians and dentists in the United States. *JAMA* 1994;271;851
31. Owens DK, Harris RA, Scott PMcJ, et al: Screening surgeons for HIV infection: A cost-effectiveness analysis. *Ann Intern Med* 1995;122:641
32. Jones ME: A thing about AIDS. *Anaesth Intensive Care* 1989;17:253
33. McKinney WP, Young MJ: The cumulative probability of occupationally-acquired HIV infection: The risks of repeated exposures during a surgical career. *Infect Control Hosp Epidemiol* 1990;11:243
34. Tokars JI, Marcus R, Culver DH, et al: Surveillance of HIV infection and zidovudine use among health care workers after occupational exposure to HIV-infected blood. *Ann Intern Med* 1993;118:913
35. McLeod GX, Hammer SM: Zidovudine: Five years later. *Ann Intern Med* 1992;117:487
36. Aoun H: When a house officer gets AIDS. *N Engl J Med* 1989;321:693
37. 381.004 Florida Statutes (1992 Supp).
38. Harrison CA, Rogers DW, Rosen M: Blood contamination of anaesthetic and related staff. *Anaesthesia* 1990;45:831
39. Wright JG, McGeer AJ, Chyatte D, et al: Mechanisms of glove tears and sharp injuries among surgical personnel. *JAMA* 1991;266:1668
40. Matta H, Thompson AM, Rainey JB: Does wearing two pairs of gloves protect operating theatre staff from skin contamination? *Br Med J* 1988;297:597
41. Hammond JS, Eckes JM, Gomez GA, et al: HIV, trauma, and infection control: Universal precautions are universally ignored. *J Trauma* 1990;30:555
42. Gerberding JL, Schecter WP: Surgery and AIDS: Reducing the risk [editorial]. *JAMA* 1991;265:1572
43. Panlilio AL, Foy DR, Edwards JR, et al: Blood contacts during surgical procedures. *JAMA* 1991;265:1533
44. Baker JL, Kelen GD, Sivertson KT, et al: Unsuspected human immunodeficiency virus in critically ill emergency patients. *JAMA* 1987;257:2609

45. Kelen GB, Fritz S, Qaqish B, et al: Unrecognized human immunodeficiency virus infection in emergency department patients. *N Engl J Med* 1988;318:1645
46. St. Louis ME, Rauch KJ, Petersen LR, et al: The Sentinel Hospital Surveillance Group: Seroprevalence rates of human immunodeficiency virus infection at sentinel hospitals in the United States. *N Engl J Med* 1990;323:213
47. Mullan RJ, Baker EL, Bell DM, et al: Guidelines for prevention of transmission of human immunodeficiency virus and hepatitis B virus to health-care and public-safety workers. *MMWR Morb Mortal Wkly Rep* 1989;38(S-6):1
48. Layon AJ, D'Amico R: Intensive care for patients with acquired immunodeficiency syndrome: Medicine versus ideology. *Crit Care Med* 1990;18:1297
49. Berry AJ, Isaacson IJ, Kane MA, et al: A multicenter study of the prevalence of hepatitis B viral serologic markers in anesthesia personnel. *Anesth Analg* 1984;63:738
50. Centers for Disease Control: Cases of selected notifiable diseases: United States, weeks ending December 31, 1994, and January 1, 1994 (52nd week). *MMWR Morb Mortal Wkly Rep* 1995;43:968
51. Centers for Disease Control: Summary of notifiable diseases—United States 1988. *MMWR Morb Mortal Wkly Rep* 1988;37:3
52. Centers for Disease Control: Cases of selected notifiable diseases: United States, weeks ending August 26, 1995, and August 27, 1994 (34th week). *MMWR Morb Mortal Wkly Rep* 1995;44:631
53. Centers for Disease Control: Recommendations for protection against viral hepatitis. *Ann Intern Med* 1985;103:391
54. Lemon SM: Type A viral hepatitis. *N Engl J Med* 1985;313:1059
55. Centers for Disease Control: Hepatitis A among homosexual men: United States, Canada, Australia. *MMWR Morb Mortal Wkly Rep* 1992;42:15
56. Hepatitis A vaccine. *Med Lett Drugs Ther* 1995;37:51
57. Ockner RK. Acute viral hepatitis. In: Wyngaarden JB, Smith LH (eds). *Cecil's Textbook of Medicine*, 18th ed. Philadelphia, WB Saunders 1988:818
58. Czaja AJ: Serologic markers of hepatitis A and B in acute and chronic liver disease. *Mayo Clin Proc* 1979;54:721
59. Alter MJ, Ahtone J, Weisfuse I, et al: Hepatitis B virus transmission between heterosexuals. *JAMA* 1986;256:1307
60. Thomas DL, Factor SH, Kelen GD, et al: Viral hepatitis in health care personnel at the Johns Hopkins Hospital. *Arch Intern Med* 1993;153:1705
61. Sato S, Suzuki K, Akahane Y, et al: Hepatitis B strains with mutations in the core promoter in patients with fulminant hepatitis. *Ann Intern Med* 1995;122:241
62. McIvor C, Morton J, Bryant A, et al: Fatal reactivation of precore mutant hepatitis B virus associated with fibrosing cholestatic hepatitis after bone marrow transplantation. *Ann Intern Med* 1994;121:274
63. Kelen GD, Green GB, Purcell RH, et al: Hepatitis B and hepatitis C in emergency department patients. *N Engl J Med* 1992;326:1399
64. Choo QL, Kuo G, Weiner AJ, et al: Isolation of a cDNA clone derived from a blood-borne non-A non-B viral hepatitis genome. *Science* 1989;244:359
65. Kuo G, Choo QL, Alter HJ, et al: An assay for circulating antibodies to a major etiologic virus of human non-A, non-B hepatitis. *Science* 1989;244:362
66. Purcell RH: The discovery of the hepatitis viruses. *Gastroenterology* 1993;104:955
67. Hayashi PH, Zeldis JB: Molecular biology of viral hepatitis and hepatocellular carcinoma. *Compr Ther* 1993;19:188
68. Krawczynski K: Hepatitis E. *Hepatology* 1993;17:932
69. Simons JN, Leary TP, Dawson GJ, et al: Isolation of novel virus-like sequences associated with human hepatitis. *Nature Medicine* 1995;6:564
70. Barrera JM, Bruguera M, Ercilla G, et al: Incidence of non-A, non-B hepatitis after screening blood donors for antibodies to hepatitis C virus and surrogate markers. *Ann Intern Med* 1991;115:596
71. Donahue JG, Munoz A, Ness PM, et al: The declining risk of post-transfusion hepatitis C virus infection. *N Engl J Med* 1992;327:369
72. Koziol DE, Holland PV, Alling DW, et al: Antibody to hepatitis B core antigen as a paradoxical marker for non-A non-B hepatitis agent in donated blood. *Ann Intern Med* 1986;104:488
73. Stevens CE, Aach RD, Hollinger FB, et al: Hepatitis B virus antibody in blood donors and the occurrence of non-A non-B hepatitis in transfusion recipients. *Ann Intern Med* 1984;101:733
74. Czaja AJ, Davis GL: Hepatitis non-A non-B. *Mayo Clin Proc* 1982;57:639
75. Alter MJ, Margolis HS, Krawczynski K, et al: The natural history of community-acquired hepatitis C in the United States. *N Engl J Med* 1992;327:1899
76. Akahane Y, Kojima M, Sugai Y, et al: Hepatitis C virus infection in spouses of patients with type C chronic liver disease. *Ann Intern Med* 1994;120:748
77. Romeo R, Pol S, Berthelot P, et al: Eradication of hepatitis C virus RNA after alpha-interferon therapy. *Ann Intern Med* 1994;121:276
78. Seeff LB, Buskell-Bales Z, Wright EC, et al: Long-term mortality after transfusion-associated non-A, non-B hepatitis. *N Engl J Med* 1992;327:1906
79. Wejstal R, Widell A, Mansson A-S, et al: Mother-to-infant transmission of hepatitis C virus. *Ann Intern Med* 1992;117:887
80. Ohto H, Terazawa S, Sasaki N, et al: Transmission of hepatitis C virus from mothers to infants. *N Engl J Med* 1994;330:744
81. Reinus JF, Leikin EL, Alter HJ, et al: Failure to detect vertical transmission of hepatitis C virus. *Ann Intern Med* 1992;117:881
82. Lettau LA, McCarthy JG, Smith MH, et al: Outbreak of severe hepatitis due to delta and hepatitis B viruses in parenteral drug abusers and their contacts. *N Engl J Med* 1987;317:1256
83. Centers for Disease Control: Recommendations for protection against viral hepatitis. *Ann Intern Med* 1985;103:391
84. Olin BR (ed). *Drug Facts and Comparisons 1990*. Philadelphia, JB Lippincott, 1990:467.

Critical Care, Third Edition, edited by Joseph M. Civetta,
Robert W. Taylor, and Robert R. Kirby.
Lippincott-Raven Publishers, Philadelphia, PA © 1997.

CHAPTER 98

∎

Temperature-Related Injuries

J. Christopher Farmer

IMMEDIATE CONCERNS ∎

MAJOR PROBLEMS

Extremes of body temperature are life-threatening conditions that depend on prompt recognition and return of body temperature toward normal.

STRESS POINTS

1. Extremes of body temperature are most commonly diseases of the elderly and chronically ill.
2. Diagnosis becomes problematic when other medical conditions confuse the clinician and further delay the initiation of life-saving therapy (e.g., sepsis and primary central nervous system events in the elderly).
4. Dysfunction or failure of major organ systems follows when therapeutic interventions are delayed.
5. In addition to normalizing body temperature, other important concerns include immediate assessment of airway patency and confirmation of ventilatory and circulatory status.
6. After resuscitation of vital functions, the patient should be rapidly removed from the severe environment and potentially offending drugs should be discontinued.

HYPOTHERMIA ∎

Hypothermia is defined as a core body temperature of less than 35°C (95°F).[1-3] Unintentional or accidental hypothermia may be precipitated by a variety of acute and chronic medical conditions, environmental exposure, or drugs. Table 98-1 outlines clinical causes and disorders associated with hypothermia. Hypothermia may be further classified as mild, moderate, or severe. The clinical severity usually defines the duration and aggressiveness of the required therapy as well as the prospect for a successful outcome.[4]

Hypothermia impacts recovery and survival from other important medical conditions. Mortality of major trauma victims is reportedly increased in some centers when significant hypothermia coexists at presentation. Other adverse influences include increased surgical blood loss and cardiovascular complications, such as clinically significant myocardial ischemia.[5-7] Patients with sepsis have a markedly worse mortality when they present with hypothermia as opposed to fever.[8]

The exact incidence of hypothermia is unknown. However, it is thought to be an underrecognized condition, particularly in the elderly.[2,3,9,10] In the United States, 9362 hypothermia-related deaths were reported between 1979 and 1990.[11] Elderly patients who develop hypothermia are more likely to live alone, to have other intercurrent illnesses, to have their home heating turned off, and to wear inappropriately light clothing for actual indoor ambient temperatures.[12] Sepsis syndrome is significantly more common in elderly patients initially presenting with accidental hypothermia.[13] To underscore this serious problem, 11% of elderly patients with hypothermia have a recurrence within 1 year, and 90% of all elderly patients are dead within 1 year of their initial hospitalization for hypothermia.[14] In the United States, however, clinically significant hypothermia is most commonly seen in alcoholic patients.[15,16]

Any clinical history suggesting the disorders or perturbations listed in Table 98-1 mandates an accurate assessment of body temperature. Many of the hospital thermometers are not calibrated below 35°C and may contribute to underdiagnosis. Accidental hypothermia associated with major operative procedures is also probably underdiagnosed.[17,18] A

TABLE 98-1.   Causes of Accidental Hypothermia

CLINICAL CAUSE	ASSOCIATED DISORDERS
Central nervous system	Head trauma, tumor, stroke, Wernicke's encephalopathy, Shapiro's syndrome, Parkinson's disease, multiple sclerosis, sarcoidosis, acute spinal cord transection/ paraplegia
Metabolism	Hypoglycemia, hypothyroidism, hypoadrenalism, panhypopituitarism, diabetic ketoacidosis, anorexia nervosa (protein–calorie malnutrition)
Dermal insult	Burns, erythroderma, ichthyosis, psoriasis, other exfoliative dermatitides
Infection	Generalized sepsis
Other chronic diseases	Advanced age (impaired thermoregulatory mechanisms), chronic heart failure, chronic renal failure, chronic hepatic insufficiency
Environmental exposure	Outdoor activities and physical/metabolic exhaustion, cold water immersion, inadequate indoor heating (particularly in the elderly)
Drugs	Ethanol, muscle relaxant drugs (paralytics), phenothiazines, barbiturates, tricyclic antidepressants, toxic dose lithium, clonidine, anticholinergic drugs

recent study concluded when the air-to-skin temperature gradient in an operating room exceeds 4°C, net patient heat loss occurs unless a heating blanket is employed.[19]

TEMPERATURE REGULATION

Hypothermia represents a loss of balance between heat generation and heat dissipation. At rest, most heat is produced by energy-consuming metabolic processes in the body viscera. During exercise, heat is primarily generated by skeletal muscle metabolism. Shivering, an example of this metabolic shift, is aimed at increased heat production to maintain body temperature. In contrast, heat loss is predominantly mediated by sweating, cutaneous vasoconstriction, or vasodilatation. Voluntary mechanisms include seeking appropriate shelter, adding clothing, and altering the activity level.

Patients who develop hypothermia have inadequate voluntary and involuntary heat-generating and heat-preserving mechanisms. For example, shivering may not provide enough heat to overcome the ambient temperature gradient, or energy supplies eventually become depleted and thermogenesis declines. Adequate protective clothing or warm shelter may not be available. Elderly patients present a particularly difficult problem, because voluntary and involuntary thermoregulatory mechanisms may be impaired at their baselines. The capacity of normal physiologic thermoregulatory mechanisms to produce and conserve heat declines as age increases. Because the ability to perceive temperature changes is also deranged in the elderly, exposure to adverse temperature gradients may occur without attempts to alter their environment. Other chronic underlying disorders also may impair thermoregulation in the elderly. Alcoholics have impaired perception of their environment and altered thermoregulatory mechanisms.

CLINICAL SYNDROME

Patients with mild hypothermia have core body temperatures of 32° to 35°C. Blood pressure, heart rate, and respiratory rate are initially increased, but they may decline as the syndrome progresses. Muscle tone is increased and is frequently accompanied by active shivering. The level of consciousness may be depressed, typically manifested as stupor or confusion. There is evidence of peripheral vasoconstriction (i.e., diminished pulses, pallor, acrocyanosis, and coolness to touch of the extremities). Cardiac output falls as the heart cools and myocardial contractility decreases. As hypothermia worsens (moderate hypothermia) patients become more obtunded and are often incoherent, if they are capable of verbal expression. The core temperature is between 28° and 32°C. Coma usually supervenes at body temperatures less than 30°C, and all vital signs are invariably subnormal. Compensatory mechanisms (e.g., shivering) are absent, and muscle tone is rigid. Bowel sounds are absent. This combination of physical findings (i.e., stiff or board-like abdominal musculature and a dropping blood pressure) may mimic intraabdominal sepsis if body temperature is not accurately measured. Hypothermia is considered severe at body temperatures less than 28°C. In addition to the apparent absence of higher neurologic function, brain stem and deep tendon reflexes usually cannot be demonstrated. The patient is either apneic or has an agonal respiratory pattern. Pulselessness most frequently results from spontaneous ventricular fibrillation and less frequently from an agonal rhythm or asystole.

As core body temperature falls, the renal cellular basal metabolic rate decreases to a respiratory quotient as low as 0.65 at 32°C.[2] This results in decreased renal tubular cell reabsorptive function and "cold diuresis," which usually persists until intravascular volume depletion occurs. Overall hepatic function also decreases, as does adrenal cortical activity; measured cortisol levels may actually rise as a result of decreased hepatic clearance. Pancreatic function remains undisturbed until body temperature drops below 32°C. Most patients develop an adynamic ileus.

Common laboratory findings include hemoconcentration (i.e., elevated hemoglobin and hematocrit), elevated serum glucose concentration (particularly as pancreatic function waivers), decreased serum potassium concentration, elevated serum transaminase levels, and elevated serum amylase levels. Cold-induced granulocytopenia does not correlate with the severity of illness in hypothermic patients. Prothrombin and activated partial thromboplastin times are prolonged as body temperature falls, but may be missed as in vitro assays are performed at 37°C by default.[20] Metabolic acidosis develops as a result of extremity hypoperfusion and increased energy consumption with shivering, both of which contribute to lactate generation. The oxyhemoglobin dissociation curve shifts to the left as body temperature decreases. Blood gas measurement of pH is falsely depressed and PaO_2 is falsely increased if arterial gas solubility coefficients are not corrected for temperature. Progressive prolongation of the PR, QRS, and QT electrocardiographic (ECG) intervals is common as hypothermia worsens. The Osborn J-wave (Fig. 98-1) after the QRS complex is pathognomonic of hypothermia, but it is frequently absent.[3,21] Ventricular and supraventricular ectopy are commonly seen. The threshold for ventricular fibrillation is decreased, and ventricular fibrillation may be precipitated by excessive handling of a patient or by attempts to place a pulmonary arterial catheter or transvenous pacemaker.

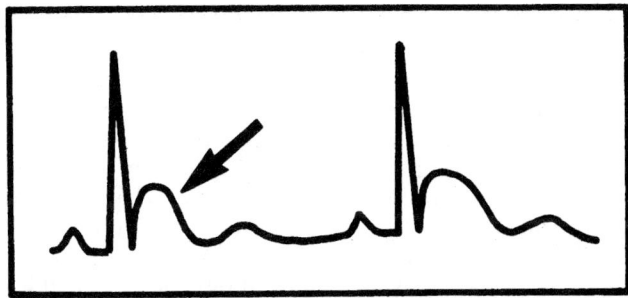

FIGURE 98-1. Osborn J-wave (*arrow*) after the QRS complex, pathognomonic of hypothermia.

THERAPEUTIC APPROACH

The mainstay of clinical therapy is the return of core body temperature to normal, although there is controversy about how this is best achieved. Other means of supportive therapy should aggressively continue until normothermia (or near-normal body temperature) is attained. All methods of clinical assessment, particularly regarding the permanence of organ dysfunction and even death, are highly inaccurate until the patient is adequately rewarmed. Figure 98-2 is an algorithm summarizing the initial management of these patients.

Techniques of rewarming include active and passive methods and external and internal (core) methods. *Passive external rewarming* consists of adding an insulating layer (e.g., a blanket or sleeping bag) to the patient and allowing the patient's own heat-generating mechanisms to restore body temperature. *Active external warming* techniques use devices (e.g, hot water bottles, submersion in a tank of warm

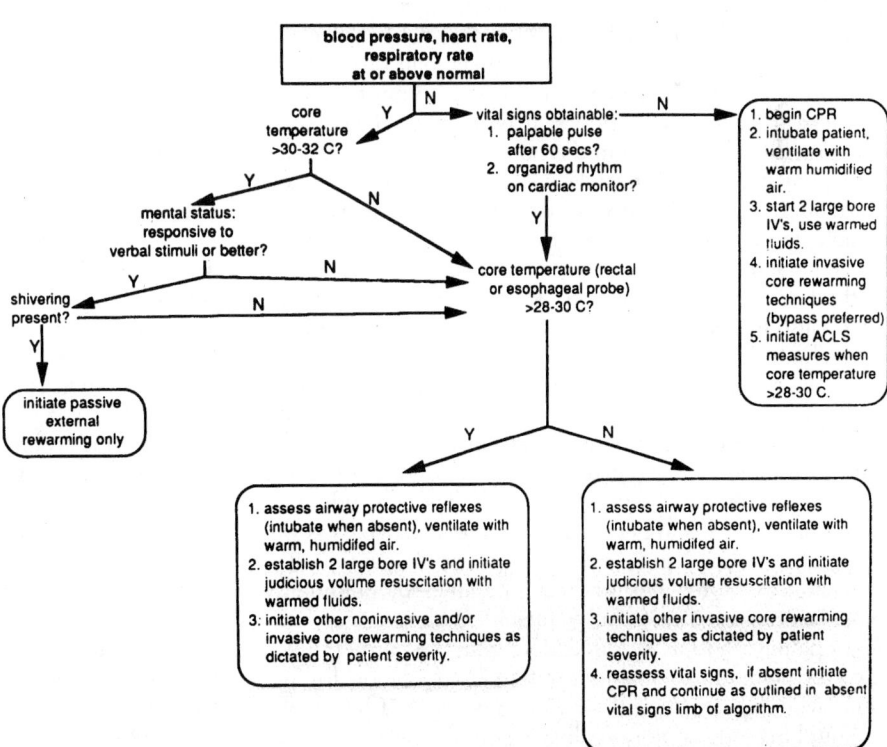

FIGURE 98-2. Therapeutic algorithm for patients with hypothermia. Y, yes; No, no; ACLS, advanced cardiac life support; IVs, intravenous lines; CPR, cardiopulmonary resuscitation.

water, heating blankets), which are placed in contact with a hypothermic patient, generate their own heat. Passive techniques are adequate in selected situations of mild hypothermia in which complications of the disorder are not yet evident and rapid rewarming is not required. Active external and core-rewarming techniques are necessary for resuscitation from severe forms of hypothermia. The definitive method in humans is not clear, however. Early reports using active external rewarming describe hypotension or "rewarming shock" associated with peripheral vasodilatation and intravascular volume depletion as rewarming is accomplished. These problems are mostly obviated if volume repletion is promptly established and maintained during rewarming.[22] Giesbrecht and others[23] report the use forced-air warming as an active external rewarming method for mild immersion hypothermia. In their study, a warmed air source was blown into warming covers over volunteers with cold-water immersion-induced hypothermia ranging from 34.5° to 35.5°C. In comparison with passive external warming, forced-air external rewarming attenuated the afterdrop and metabolic stress/shivering (measured as oxygen consumption) associated with hypothermia.

Invasive core-rewarming methods include peritoneal dialysis, hemodialysis, partial cardiopulmonary bypass, thoracotomy with mediastinal irrigation, rectal and gastric lavage, and mechanical ventilation with warm humidified air. Intravenous fluids may be administered at surprisingly hot temperatures. Fildes and others[24] report the safe use of fluids as hot as 65°C (149°F) in an animal model. Theoretically, these techniques rewarm core structures in parallel with the heart. As a result, cardiac output and tissue perfusion should be reestablished in proportion to peripheral cellular metabolic demands as the respiratory quotient rises toward normal. In contrast, active external rewarming may increase peripheral cellular metabolic activity before the heart is able to adequately distribute oxygen and metabolic substrate to these areas, potentiating an existing ischemic injury or metabolic disturbance. Furthermore, if partially warmed blood is returned to the core from the periphery, the rate of core rewarming may actually be delayed. Despite these purported shortcomings, no difference in survival and clinical or histopathologic morbidity has been prospectively demonstrated between active external rewarming and core-rewarming methods.[22,25] Hemodialysis with warmed dialysate solutions (40°C) also has been reported as an effective "core rewarming technique."[26]

In one study, core rewarming shortened the duration of cardiopulmonary resuscitation for patients who had cardiopulmonary arrest and decreased volume of crystalloid fluids used to replete intravascular volume, but it did not affect outcome.[25] However, several other studies conclude that percutaneous or open-chest cardiopulmonary bypass is the treatment of choice in pulseless, hypothermic patients if it is available.[27-31] Most authors recommend cardiopulmonary bypass as the most calorically efficient method available to warm patients and as an effective adjunct to cardiopulmonary resuscitation to maintain artificial circulation for patients who experience cardiopulmonary arrest. If available, it should be used preferentially.

As body temperature falls below 30°C, cardiac ventricular arrhythmias are likely to ensue. Attempts to restore a perfusing cardiac rhythm are unlikely to succeed until core temperature is raised above this level; bretylium seems to be the drug of choice to modulate ventricular fibrillatory threshold.[32-34] The role of cardiac transvenous pacemakers, as with other forms of refractory asystole, seems to be of limited additional value. Similarly, attempts to place a transvenous pacemaker in patients with hemodynamically unstable bradycardia may irritate the heart and lead to deterioration of the rhythm to asystole or ventricular fibrillation.

Prompt repletion of intravascular volume is mandatory, especially if active external rewarming techniques are used in a severely hypothermic patient. However, insertion of a central venous monitoring device, such as a pulmonary arterial catheter, is not routinely recommended because it may also induce ventricular fibrillation or asystole. Bronchopneumonia is a frequent complication of hypothermia, typically secondary to aspiration. Obtunded, hypothermic patients may have altered airway protective mechanisms (e.g., cough and gag reflexes). Early intubation should be performed if any doubt exists about the adequacy of these reflexes. Other measures aimed at prophylaxis, such as empiric antibiotics or continuous heparin infusion to prevent deep venous thrombosis, are generally ineffective and should be avoided. Heparin was anecdotally unhelpful for 1 patient with disseminated intravascular coagulation (DIC).[35] Soft tissue infarction may occur as a result of cell freezing, particularly in areas most prone to exposure, such as the nose, ears, face, and digits. Rewarming of these areas should not be attempted until it is clear that renewed exposure to the cold will not occur, because soft tissue damage may be extended.

HYPERTHERMIA ■

HEATSTROKE SYNDROME

Heatstroke is a heat-related illness with documented body temperatures of 41.1°C (106°F) or more. Alternatively, it may be considered a syndrome with body temperatures of 40.6°C (105°F) or greater, plus anhidrosis, altered mental status, or both.[36,37] Heatstroke may be further classified as exertional or nonexertional (i.e, classic heatstroke). Exertional heatstroke syndrome is typically seen in healthy young adults who overexert themselves during times of unusually high ambient temperatures or in an environment to which they are not acclimatized. Their thermoregulatory mechanisms are intact, at least initially, but endogenous heat production outstrips heat dissipating mechanisms. Nonexertional heatstroke afflicts elderly and debilitated individuals with chronic underlying diseases. These patients present during times of increased ambient temperatures, but their thermoregulatory mechanisms are already impaired. In urban populations, cocaine-associated heatstroke is becoming the most common cause. A variety of conditions and drugs that are associated with heatstroke syndrome are listed in Table 98-2.[39-43]

TABLE 98-2. Causes of Heat Stroke Syndrome

CLINICAL CAUSE	ASSOCIATED DISORDERS
EXERTION	
Environmental	Supranormal ambient temperatures, increased humidity levels
Physiologic	Lack of physical conditioning or overexertion (e.g., military recruits), lack of acclimatization
NONEXERTION	
Environmental	Supranormal ambient temperatures, increased humidity levels, lack of air conditioning, lack of shrubbery or trees around dwelling, height of home floor above ground level
Physiologic	Advanced age, alcoholism, congestive heart failure, renal insufficiency, diabetes mellitus, chronic obstructive pulmonary disease, dementia or schizophrenia, cystic fibrosis, thyrotoxicosis, hypokalemia, dehydration
Drugs	Alcohol, diuretics, phenothiazines, anti-parkinsonians, anticholinergics, beta-blockers, tricyclic antidepressants, amphetamines, hallucinogens, butyrophenones

Like hypothermia, the incidence, morbidity, and mortality of heatstroke are difficult to quantitate because of misidentification of patients with other clinical disorders. From 1979 to 1991, 5224 deaths were ascribed to heat injury as the primary cause.[44] During a several-day June heat wave in the northeast, the medical examiner's office of Philadelphia reported 118 deaths related to heat injury. More recently, in July of 1995, the medical examiner's office of Chicago reported over 500 heatstroke-related deaths within a several-day period.

TEMPERATURE REGULATION

Incremental skeletal muscle metabolic activity, such as strenuous exercise, increases total body heat production. At basal metabolic levels, skeletal muscle heat production ranges from 65 to 85 kcal/hour, but it may increase to as high as 900 kcal/hour in situations of progressive exertion.[42] Mechanisms to dissipate this additional heat include sweating (with attendant evaporative heat losses) and cutaneous vasodilatation, which results in heat loss through radiation, conduction, and convection. If the ambient temperature exceeds body temperature, heat may be lost only through evaporation associated with sweating. Even at maximal efficiency, sweating produces only 400 to 650 kcal/hour of heat dissipation. Increasing levels of humidity and pooling of sweat further decrease the efficiency of evaporation as an adequate means of heat loss. In a poorly acclimatized person, heatstroke syndrome occurs if exercise levels are sustained or if means of lowering the body temperature are not sought.

Acclimatization is a physiologic process whereby an individual adapts to work in a hot environment.[42] These adaptations include decreased sweat production each hour (which develops only over extended periods of time), decreased sweat sodium concentrations, increased aldosterone secretion, increased maximal cardiac output and stroke volume), and decreased maximal heart rate. Acclimatized people

drink greater quantities of water spontaneously and have baseline increases in calculated extracellular fluid volumes. The metabolic efficiency of these individuals seems to increase, and net heat production for a given unit of work performed decreases. All of these factors substantially reduce the risk of exertional heatstroke developing as a result of demanding physical work in ambient temperatures that approach or exceed body temperature.

Hydration status independently influences the development of heatstroke. Sawka and associates demonstrated that inadequate hydration reduces the maximum tolerated core temperature.[38] Furthermore, this was not influenced by aerobic fitness (maximum tolerated core temperature), per se.

Nonexertional heatstroke syndrome also develops if ambient temperatures are increased and thermoregulatory mechanisms are impaired from the outset. Advancing age decreases the ability to produce sweat and impairs perception of changes in body or ambient temperatures. Underlying chronic diseases, most notably cardiovascular disease with diminished cardiac reserve, impair the body's ability to respond to volume and temperature changes. Many commonly prescribed medications for elderly or debilitated patients (e.g., beta-blockers, diuretics, anticholinergics, major tranquilizers) may contribute to impaired responsiveness to these changes.

CLINICAL SYNDROME

Although the typical history for patients with exertional heatstroke syndrome seems self-evident, usually little or no clinical warning presages the onset of classic heatstroke. As thermoregulatory mechanisms fail, body temperature climbs rapidly; a patient can quickly lapse from the apparent baseline health status to coma or obtundation with a high core temperature. Several environmental factors are associated with the development of nonexertional heatstroke.[37,39,45] These include habitation of substandard housing (particularly upper floors of multistory buildings) and absence of air conditioning. Trees or shrubbery around a residential dwelling lower ambient temperatures, decreasing the risk of developing heatstroke. Irritability or irrationality may precede the development of either form of heatstroke. Heatstroke syndrome should therefore be suspected in any patient, but particularly in the elderly and debilitated, who present with unexplained mental status changes during times of increased ambient temperatures.

Uncompensable heatstress develops in people who exert themselves in hot or humid environments while wearing clothing that does not allow them to achieve a thermal steady state.[41] Examples include firefighters in protective clothing, soldiers who don biological/chemical protective gear, and others. These individuals may develop heatstroke because of an inability to utilize evaporative body heat dissipation methods at relatively lower ambient temperatures.

Significant dehydration is most common in patients with exertional heatstroke syndrome and may be reflected as elevated blood urea nitrogen and creatinine levels or hemoconcentration. Sodium, potassium, phosphate, calcium, and magnesium serum concentrations are frequently low early in the clinical course of the syndrome.[37,40,42,46-48] Sodium, potassium, and magnesium losses occur primarily through increased sweating and can be massive. Hypokalemia decreases sweat secretions and skeletal muscle blood flow, further impairing heat dissipation.[37] Hyperkalemia may ensue if significant skeletal muscle damage and cellular lysis develops.[40] Hypocalcemia is seen in patients with significant rhabdomyolysis and is primarily a result of calcium salt precipitation and deposition in injured skeletal muscle. Creatine kinase elevation is invariably present and is considered by some to be a necessary diagnostic feature for heatstroke.[42] Elevations may be extreme in cases of severe rhabdomyolysis.

DIC is uncommon, and it is a poor prognostic marker if present. A mixed acid-base disorder (i.e., metabolic acidosis/respiratory alkalosis) is most common. Hyperthermia alone may cause primary hyperventilation and respiratory alkalosis. Hypoperfusion, tissue hypoxia, and anaerobic metabolism may lead to lactic acidosis with respiratory compensation, depending on systemic metabolic demands. Of these, primary respiratory alkalosis is less frequently seen.

Temperature affects the solubility of oxygen and carbon dioxide. The values returned on a blood gas report will be inaccurate unless the coefficients are corrected for temperature. The $PaCO_2$ and PaO_2 will be falsely low and the pH falsely elevated.

COMPLICATIONS

Myocardial pump failure, arrhythmias, acute renal failure, rhabdomyolysis, seizures, hepatic failure, respiratory failure in adult respiratory distress syndrome (ARDS), and DIC may develop in association with heatstroke. The laboratory findings generally suggest their presence. Cardiac muscle damage and frank tissue infarction occur frequently in patients with exertional or classic heatstroke and are related to the toxic effects of heat on myocytes and to coronary artery hypoperfusion if hypovolemia coexists.[49] This may occur even

in the absence of significant coronary artery disease. Patients with depressed myocardial function usually demonstrate hypotension as a prominent feature. However, even patients who do not sustain significant myocardial damage may present initially with hypotension. Conversely, hypovolemia and peripheral vasodilatation secondary to the effects of heat may lead to high-output cardiac failure. Tachyarrhythmias, particularly those of ventricular origin, may be life-threatening.

Multifactorial renal damage is seen to a greater or lesser extent in almost all patients with hyperthermic injury. Acute renal failure develops five to six times more commonly in patients with exertional heatstroke (30%-35%). Dehydration, renal hypoperfusion, and pigmenturia (rhabdomyolysis) appear to be casual. Uric acid nephropathy may also develop as a result of strenuous muscular activity. Concomitant hypokalemia may exacerbate renal insufficiency by further decreasing glomerular filtration rate and renal blood flow.[37]

Rhabdomyolysis is common in patients with exertional heatstroke and may be severe. Rapid development of profound hyperkalemia may impose an immediate threat to survival, mandating emergency institution of life-saving therapeutic measures. Severe hypocalcemia often develops in patients with rhabdomyolysis, but exogenous calcium should not be administered unless serious ventricular ectopy secondary to hyperkalemia supervenes, because the calcium may worsen rhabdomyolysis. Anterior compartment syndromes of the distal lower extremity may develop in conjunction with rhabdomyolysis; appropriate patient monitoring should be performed.[50]

The central nervous system is particularly sensitive to the damaging effects of hyperpyrexia. Widespread cell death occurs, with the Purkinje cells of the cerebellum being most affected. Cerebral edema and petechial hemorrhages are also seen. The clinical correlates of these histopathologic changes include marked depression of mental status and, less frequently, generalized seizure activity. Survivors of severe heatstroke syndrome often have residual evidence of cerebellar dysfunction on physical examination.

Reversible hepatic damage occurs in most patients with heatstroke; the liver is sensitive to the toxic effects of heat. During strenuous exercise, hepatic venous blood temperature is often as much as 3°C to 4°C warmer than measured core body temperature and may increase the risk of hepatic cellular injury. Cholestasis and centrilobular necrosis elevate bilirubin and serum transaminases.[48] Severe or fulminant hepatic necrosis leading to the demise of a patient is a rare event; these changes are typically self-limited and without long-term morbidity.

ECG abnormalities noted in this patient population are common.[51] Sinus tachycardia and QT prolongation are most frequently seen (40-60 % of all patients), followed by nonspecific ST-T wave changes and ST-T wave changes suggestive of cardiac ischemia.

DIC ranges from an observed but asymptomatic laboratory finding of hypofibrinogenemia and thrombocytopenia to severe clinical bleeding. Patients with DIC are more likely to develop ARDS; in one study, the association was greater than 90%. Patients with DIC and ARDS had a 75% mortality rate.[43] Assays of coagulation factors and plasminogen are normal in most patients, including those with prolonged coagulation studies, suggesting that qualitative function of the coagulation system may be affected by heat exposure. Furthermore, heat enhances plasma fibrinolytic activity and directly activates platelets and may specifically trigger DIC in patients with heatstroke.[52]

In pediatric patients (usually infants), heatstroke can mimic hemorrhagic shock and encephalopathy syndrome (HSE).[53] This syndrome is characterized by acute onset encephalopathy, fever (≥39°C), shock (BP < 50 mm Hg), watery diarrhea, severe DIC, and renal/hepatic dysfunction. The cause of this syndrome remains unknown, but it is suspected to be infectious in origin. Some argue that HSE and heatstroke are merely variations of the same disorder, but this remains undecided at this time.

THERAPEUTIC APPROACH

Survival is inversely related to the intensity and duration of hyperpyrexia; duration is of greater significance.[37,54] Effective lowering of the core body temperature usually requires only external techniques. These include immersion in an ice water bath or wetting the skin with tepid water or alcohol, followed by the use of fans to facilitate evaporation and heat dissipation. Gastric or peritoneal lavage with iced saline is only rarely required in cases of refractory temperature elevation or if thermogenesis is ongoing, as in malignant hyperthermia. Otherwise, it does not offer any advantage over evaporative techniques.[55] Vigorous skin massage should accompany immersion cooling techniques to prevent dermal stasis of cooled blood as local cutaneous vasoconstriction occurs. As the temperature approaches 39°C, efforts to cool a patient should be terminated, because the body temperature will continue to fall 1°C to 2°C. From a practical perspective, immersion techniques are unsatisfactory if monitoring, specific therapy for other complications (e.g., seizures), or airway protection are needed. Evaporative methods allow placement on a bed with treatment as the usual intensive care patient and are equally effective.

Intravenous administration of chlorpromazine (10-50 mg every 6 hours) may prove useful in preventing shivering and associated thermogenesis. Dantrolene has not been shown to be efficacious in humans with heatstroke.[56] However, other research has failed to demonstrate (in an animal model) a significant difference in cooling time or survival rate.[57] Therefore, dantrolene is not recommended for routine use at this time.

Intravascular volume repletion should be individualized. Dehydration may not be a prominent feature of classic heatstroke syndrome. It is much more common in patients with exertional heat injury. Hypotension may reflect volume depletion, peripheral vascular vasodilatation, or primary myocardial dysfunction, in which case little volume resuscitation is needed. Early placement of a pulmonary arterial catheter is recommended in circumstances in which uncertainty about volume status or myocardial performance exists. Oxygen delivery is often less than normal and pulmonary shunt fraction is increased in these patients.[58] Isoproterenol is the traditional inotropic drug of choice for heatstroke patients with myocardial dysfunction and inadequate cardiac output, because it has little or no agonist influence on peripheral alpha receptors, which cause vasoconstriction and impaired heat dissipation. I think this purported advantage is overshadowed by myocardial irritant properties of the drug. Dobutamine is a more logical choice for isolated cardiac pump dysfunction.

Seizures occur commonly in heatstroke victims and should be treated with intravenous diazepam or other similar benzodiazepines. Endotracheal intubation should be considered for patients with significant mental status changes and impaired cough and gag reflexes. The efficacy and clinical role of dehydrating agents (e.g., mannitol, furosemide) for the management of cerebral edema in these patients is uncertain. However, these drugs may potentially benefit some patients at risk for developing acute renal failure secondary to rhabdomyolysis.

Acute renal failure in association with rhabdomyolysis can be a major source of patient morbidity. Prevention measures include prompt re-establishment of intravascular volume and blood pressure to adequate perfusing levels, maintenance of an adequate urine flow, and correction of other concomitant metabolic abnormalities. An initial dose of mannitol may benefit a small subset of patients with rhabdomyolysis and early oliguria. The serum potassium level should be closely monitored for development of life-threatening hyperkalemia. Glucose, insulin, and calcium solutions should be given emergently to patients with ECG changes or increasing ventricular ectopy. Hemodialysis may be required to manage these metabolic perturbations.

Coagulation disorders in heatstroke syndrome are relatively common. Anecdotal evidence and small series clinical trails suggest that some benefit may be achieved with continuous-infusion heparin therapy in patients with severe DIC.[37,46,48] Dextran administration for intravascular volume repletion and maintenance of blood pressure is usually discouraged, because it may contribute to development of a clinical bleeding disorder.

MALIGNANT HYPERTHERMIA AND THE NEUROLEPTIC MALIGNANT SYNDROME ■

Malignant hyperthermia and the neuroleptic malignant syndrome are disorders of body temperature related to an inequity between heat generation and heat dissipation. Unlike heatstroke, endogenous heat production (without influence from ambient temperatures) is responsible for elevation in core body temperature. Physiologic heat-dissipating mechanisms and hypothalamic regulation of temperature may also become impaired, particularly in the neuroleptic malignant syndrome. In addition to hyperpyrexia, both of these conditions share profound muscular rigidity as a common feature. Malignant hyperthermia and the neuroleptic malignant syndrome are uniquely characterized by their association with an assortment of drugs. Although other predisposing conditions have been described, these drugs are usually essential for development of these syndromes. A complete listing is included for review in Table 98-3.[59-64]

TABLE 98-3. Drugs Associated With Malignant Hyperthermia and the Neuroleptic Malignant Syndrome

CONDITION	ASSOCIATED DRUGS
MALIGNANT HYPERTHERMIA	
Volatile anesthetics	Halothane, cyclopropane, enflurane, methoxyflurane, isoflurane, sevoflurane, desflurane, diethyl ether
Depolarizing muscle relaxants	Succinylcholine, decamethonium
Antiarrhythmics	Lidocaine
NEUROLEPTIC MALIGNANT SYNDROME	
Phenothiazines	Fluphenazine, chlorpromazine, levomepromazine, thioridazine, trimeprazine, trifluoperazine, prochlorperazine
Butyrophenones	Haloperidol, bromoperidol
Thioxanthenes	Thiothixene
Dibenzozepines	Loxapine
Dopamine-depleting drugs	Alpha-methyltyrosine, tetrabenazine
Dopamine agonist withdrawal	Levodopa, levodopa/carbidopa, amantadine

The in vitro muscle contraction test is the gold standard for identification of individuals susceptible to malignant hyperthermia. A segment of biopsied skeletal muscle is exposed to halothane or caffeine. Development of sustained muscle contracture specifically identifies individuals at risk for malignant hyperthermia.[65] Other authors have espoused increased in vitro specificity with ryanodine to stimulate contracture response instead of caffiene or halothane.[66]

TEMPERATURE REGULATION

People who develop malignant hyperthermia have a genetically inherited predisposition for this disorder. A gene for malignant hyperthermia has been identified on chromosome 19.[67,68] This gene most likely codes for calcium channels on the sarcolemmal membrane. As a result, skeletal muscle membrane permeability to calcium may be abnormal under certain circumstances. When permeability decreases, free, unbound, ionized calcium can be released from muscle storage sites. These storage sites normally maintain skeletal muscle relaxation by sequestering calcium from the muscle contractile apparatus.[64] Administration of the anesthetic drugs outlined in Table 98-3 may unpredictably result in rapid release of calcium into the myoplasm, followed by development of vigorous muscle contracture, rigidity, and increased muscle metabolic activity. The resultant surge in thermogenesis can cause core body temperature to soar at an overwhelming rate of 1°C every 5 minutes. Hypothalamic regulation of body temperature and normal heat dissipation mechanisms usually appear intact.[64] Unfortunately, they are inadequate to deal with the magnitude of the problem.

Several other medical conditions predispose patients to the development of malignant hyperthermia. Most notably, Duchenne's muscular dystrophy, Becker's muscular dystrophy, and central core disease are primary muscle diseases that are associated with malignant hyperthermia. Succinylcholine appears to be a particularly dangerous drug in this patient population.

Administration of certain neuroleptic drugs (see Table 98-3) may instigate a similar, although usually less intense, elevation in core body temperature. Caroff and colleagues suggest that patients with a genetic predisposition for malignant hyperthermia may also be at risk for developing the neuroleptic malignant syndrome.[69] However, Adnet and others[70] feel that abnormal sarcolemmal calcium permeability is not shared in the pathogenesis of these two disorders. Patients with the neuroleptic malignant syndrome do develop muscle rigidity and hyperthermia, the mechanism of which is not yet defined. Hypothalamic temperature set–point regulation may be additionally affected by drug-induced dopamine receptor blockade.[63] Subsequent heat-dissipating mechanisms may be impaired by this altered set point.

CLINICAL SYNDROME

During anesthesia, malignant hyperthermia is characterized by development of trismus, which is the initial event in 50% of patients, followed by whole-body rigidity and marked increase in core body temperature. This process may begin at any time during anesthetic induction or thereafter, and it proceeds with frightening rapidity. The metabolic consequences of this syndrome include combined respiratory and metabolic acidosis and elevated serum potassium, sodium, and calcium levels. If significant myonecrosis follows, the serum potassium concentration may rapidly rise to life-threatening levels, and the serum calcium concentration may fall as calcium salts are deposited in injured muscle. Early harbingers of a malignant hyperthermic crisis include masseter muscle contraction after succinylcholine administration, cyanosis, increasing CO_2 production, tachycardia, tachypnea, and unstable blood pressure.[71,72] Anesthesia should be aborted if these findings appear or if malignant hyperthermia is otherwise suspected. Continuous measurement of end-tidal CO_2 levels (i.e., capnography) may be of additional value.[73] Capnography provides an early warning, because CO_2 production increases dramatically while malignant hyperthermia is still in its initial phases and not otherwise clinically detectable. As the syndrome progresses, profound increases in core body temperature usually leave little doubt about their cause.

Neuroleptic malignant syndrome should be suspected in patients given any neuroleptic drug who subsequently develop signs of muscular rigidity, dystonia, or unexplained catatonic behavior, followed by hyperpyrexia. Diaphoresis, tachycardia, hypertension or hypotension, and increased respiratory rate also accompany the syndrome as markers of underlying autonomic instability. Laboratory data are variable in this syndrome, with the notable exception of consistent creatine kinase elevation in patients who develop rhabdomyolysis.

TABLE 98-4. Scoring Rules for the Malignant Hyperthermia Clinical Grading Scale

PROCESS	INDICATOR	POINTS
PROCESS I: RIGIDITY	Generalized muscular rigidity (in absence of shivering from hypothermia, or during or immediately after emergence from inhalational general anesthesia)	15
	Masseter spasm shortly after succinylcholine administration	15
PROCESS II: MUSCLE BREAKDOWN	Elevated creatine kinase >20,000 IU after anesthetic that included succinylcholine	15
	Elevate creatine kinase >10,000 IU after anesthetic without succinylcholine	15
	Cola-colored urine in perioperative period	10
	Myoglobin in urine >60 μg/L	5
	Myoglobin in serum >170 μg/L	5
	Blood/plasma/serum K^+ >6 mMol/L (in absence of renal failure)	3
PROCESS III: RESPIRATORY ACIDOSIS	P_{ETCO_2} >55 mm Hg with appropriately controlled ventilation	15
	Pa_{CO_2} >60 mm Hg with appropriately controlled ventilation	15
	P_{ETCO_2} >60 mm Hg with spontaneous ventilation	15
	Pa_{CO_2} >65 mm Hg with spontaneous ventilation	15
	Inappropriate hypercapnia (in anesthesiologist's judgment)	15
	Inappropriate tachypnea	10
PROCESS IV: TEMP INCREASE	Inappropriately rapid increase in temperature (in anesthesiologist's judgment)	15
	Inappropriately increased temperature >38.8°C (101.8°F) in the perioperative period (in anesthesiologist's judgment)	10
PROCESS V: CARDIAC INVOLVEMENT	Inappropriate sinus tachycardia	3
	Ventricular tachycardia or ventricular fibrillation	3
PROCESS VI: FAMILY HISTORY (USED TO DETERMINE MH SUSCEPTIBILITY ONLY)	Positive MH family history in relative of first degree°	15
	Positive MH family history in relative not of first degree°	5
OTHER INDICATORS THAT ARE NOT PART OF A SINGLE PROCESS†	Arterial base excess more negative than −8 mMol/L	10
	Arterial pH <7.25	10
	Rapid reversal of MH signs of metabolic or respiratory acidosis with IV dantrolene	5
	Positive MH family history together with another indicator from the patient's own anesthetic experience other than elevated resting serum creatine kinase°	10
	Resting elevated serum creatine kinase° (in patient with a family history of MH)	10

K^+, potassium; P_{ETCO_2}, end-tidal pressure of carbon dioxide; IV, intravenous; MH, malignant hyperthermia; Temp, temperature.
°These indicators should be used only for determining MH susceptibility.
†These should be added without regard to double-counting.

(continued)

TABLE 98-4.   *(continued)*

Instructions for Use: Scoring Rules for the Malignant Hyperthermia Clinical Grading Scale

I. MH indicators

    a. Review the list of clinical indicators. If any indicator is present, add the points applicable for each indicator while observing the double-counting rule below, which applies to multiple indicators representing a single process.

    b. If no indicator is present, the patient's MH score is zero.

II. Double-counting

    a. If more than one indicator represents a single process, *count only the indicator with the highest score.* Application of this rule prevents double-counting when one clinical process has more than one clinical manifestation.

    Exception: The score for any relevant indicators in the final category of Table 98-4 ("Other Indicators") *should* be added to the total score without regard to double-counting.

III. MH susceptibility indicators

    a. The italicized indicators listed below apply only to MH susceptibility. Do not use these indicators to score an MH event. To calculate the score for MH susceptibility, add the score of the italicized indicators below to score for the highest ranking MH event.

        Positive family history of MH in relative of first degree
        Positive family history of MH in relative not of first degree
        Resting elevated creatine kinase
        Positive family history of MH together with another indicator from the patient's own anesthetic experience other than serum creatine kinase

Interpreting the Raw Score: MH Rank and Qualitative Likelihood

RAW SCORE RANGE	MH RANK	DESCRIPTION OF LIKELIHOOD
0	1	Almost never
3–9	2	Unlikely
10–19	3	Somewhat less than likely
20–34	4	Somewhat greater than likely
35–49	5	Very likely
50+	6	Certain

In 1994, several recognized experts published a clinical grading scale for the prediction of malignant hyperthermia.[74] These criteria and instructions for their use are summarized in Table 98-4. This work represents the most significant efforts to date from the anesthesia community to prospectively quantitate and objectify the risk of developing malignant hyperthermia in individual patients. Additional validating data from various patient populations/clinical centers are expected to follow.

COMPLICATIONS

Complications arising from malignant hyperthermia and neuroleptic malignant syndrome generally parallel those of heatstroke syndrome. However, complications associated with malignant hyperthermia may be more severe because temperature elevations are more extreme. For example, rhabdomyolysis and hepatic necrosis may be particularly fulminant. DIC is more common, although it does not appear to correlate with outcome as it does in heatstroke syndrome.[64] Renal failure is seen almost exclusively in patients with severe rhabdomyolysis, but primary myocardial damage caused by direct thermal injury occurs less frequently than

in heatstroke syndrome. Development of ventricular tachyarrhythmias seems to parallel the degree of metabolic perturbation (e.g., hyperkalemia). Seizures are an uncommon complication of either syndrome. Patients with the neuroleptic malignant syndrome may also be at increased risk for aspiration pneumonia, because of dystonia and impaired ability to handle secretions.[75]

THERAPEUTIC APPROACH

Successful treatment of malignant hyperthermia and neuroleptic malignant syndrome depends on early clinical recognition and prompt withdrawal of the suspected inciting agent. In malignant hyperthermia, discontinuation alone is often adequate therapy if the syndrome is not well established.[64] Recovery from the neuroleptic malignant syndrome may similarly occur with discontinuation of the drug; however, 5 to 7 days may be needed for return to the patient's baseline.[74]

Sodium dantrolene, the drug of choice for malignant hyperthermia, should be administered emergently to patients if hyperpyrexia continues progressively despite anesthetic removal. The recommended dose is 2 mg/kg given intravenously. This dose may be repeated every 5 to 10 minutes, to a total dose of 10 mg/kg. This takes precedence over all other supportive therapeutic measures. Sodium dantrolene inhibits calcium release from the sarcoplasmic reticulum, decreasing available calcium for ongoing muscle contraction. Muscle weakness may develop after sodium dantrolene administration, but respiratory muscle function and airway protective measures typically remain intact. Several animal studies have investigated the effects of various calcium channel blockers on muscle contracture with malignant hyperthermia.[76–78] In general, these drugs are not effective after the syndrome is established, but they may obviate or moderate the muscle contracture response if used prophylactically before anesthetic exposure. Clinical use of these drugs is not recommended at this time. Similarly, pretreatment of swine susceptible to malignant hyperthermia with magnesium sulfate before anesthetic exposure may also moderate the contracture response.[79]

The role of sodium dantrolene for the neuroleptic malignant syndrome is less well defined, although it has reduced thermogenesis in multiple case reports.[60,61,63] Recommended doses are similar to those used for malignant hyperthermia. Administration of greater than 10 mg/kg is associated with hepatic toxicity. Scattered, anecdotal reports suggest a variety of other drugs may be used to manipulate thermogenesis. These include bromocriptine, amantadine, and levodopa/carbidopa.[60,61,63,74] All of these drugs increase central neurologic dopaminergic tone, mediating the hypothalamic and peripheral mechanisms that increase core body temperature. Their efficacy varies.

Other supportive measures to ameliorate hyperpyrexia in malignant hyperthermia and the neuroleptic malignant syndrome should be undertaken after pharmacologic manipulation has been initiated or perhaps simultaneously if additional manpower is available. These therapeutic modalities are outlined under therapy for heatstroke syndrome. Specific emphasis should be placed on assessing the adequacy of airway protection in patients with the neuroleptic malignant syndrome; liberal endotracheal intubation is recommended.

REFERENCES ■

1. Moss J: Accidental severe hypothermia. *Surg Gynecol Obstet* 1986;162:501
2. Larach MG: Accidental hypothermia. *Lancet* 1995;345:493
3. Danzl DF, Pozos RS: Accidental hypothermia. *N Engl J Med* 1994;331:1756
4. Medical aspects of mountain climbing: roundtable discussion *Physician Sports Med* 1977;5:45
5. Bernabei AF, Levison MA, Bender JS: The effects of hypothermia and injury severity on blood loss during trauma laparotomy. *J Trauma* 1992;33:835
6. Frank SM, Higgins MS, Breslow MJ, et al: The catecholamine, cortisol, and hemodynamic responses to mild perioperative hypothermia: a randomized clinical trial. *Anesthesiology* 1995;82:83
7. Gubler KD, Gentilello LM, Hassantash SA, et al: The impact of hypothermia on dilutional coagulopathy. *J Trauma* 1994;36:847
8. Clemmer TP, Fisher CJ Jr, Bone RC, et al: Hypothermia in the sepsis syndrome and clinical outcome: the methylprednisolone severe sepsis study group. *Crit Care Med* 1992;20:1395
9. Hypothermia-related deaths. *MMWR* 1994;43:849, 855
10. Danzl DF, Pozos RS, Auerbach PS, et al: Multicenter hypothermia study. *Ann Emerg Med* 1987;16:1042
11. Hypothermia-related deaths. *MMWR Morb Mortal Wkly Rep* 1993;42:917
12. Woodhouse P, Keatinge WR, Coleshaw SR: Factors associated with hypothermia in patients admitted to a group of inner city hospitals. *Lancet* 1989;ii:1201
13. Kramer MR, Vandijk J, Rosin AJ: Mortality in elderly patients with thermoregulatory failure. *Arch Intern Med* 1989;149:1521
14. Brody GM: Hyperthermia and hypothermia in the elderly. *Clin Geriatr Med* 1994;10:213
15. Weyman AE, Greenbaum DM, Grace WJ: Accidental hypothermia in an alcoholic population. *Am J Med* 1974;56:13
16. Fitzgerald FT: Hypoglycemia and accidental hypothermia in an alcoholic population. *West J Med* 1980;133:105
17. Marelli D, Chui RC, Fleiszer DM, et al: Residual hypothermia in patients recovering in the intensive care unit from cardiac surgery. *Can J Surg* 1988;31:434
18. Medley JR: Incidental hypothermia during surgery for peripheral vascular disease. *Br J Anaesth* 1990;46:713
19. English MJ, Farmer C, Scott WA: Heat loss in exposed volunteers. *J Trauma* 1990;30:422
20. Rohrer MJ, Natale AM: Effect of hypothermia on the coagulation cascade. *Crit Care Med* 1992;20:1402
21. Solomon A, Barish RA, Browne B, et al: The electrocardiographic features of hypothermia. *J Emerg Med* 1989;7:169
22. Ledingham IM, Mone JG: Treatment of accidental hypothermia: a prospective clinical study. *Br Med J* 1980;280:1102
23. Giesbrecht GG, Schroeder M, Bristow GK: Treatment of mild-immersion hypothermia by forced-air warming. *Aviat Space Environ Med* 1994;65:803
24. Fildes J, Sheaff C, Barrett J: Very hot intravenous fluid in the treatment of hypothermia. *J Trauma* 1993;35:686
25. Moss JF, Haklin M, Southwick HW, et al: A model for the treatment of accidental severe hypothermia. *J Trauma* 1986;26:68
26. Hernandez E, Praga M, Alcazar JM, et al: Hemodialysis for treatment of accidental hypothermia. *Nephron* 1993;63:214
27. Vretenar DF, Urschel JD, Parrott JC, et al: Cardiopulmonary bypass resuscitation for accidental hypothermia *Ann Thorac Surg* 1994;58:895
28. Gregory JS, Bergstein JM, Aprahamian C, et al: Comparison of three methods of rewarming from hypothermia: advantages of extracorporeal blood warming. *J Trauma* 1991;31:1251
29. Gentilello LM, Cobean RA, Offner PJ, et al: Continuous arteriovenous rewarming: rapid reversal of hypothermia in critically ill patients. *J Trauma* 1992;32:325
30. Antretter H, Dapunt OE, Mueller LC: Portable cardiopulmonary bypass: resuscitation from prolonged ice-water submersion and asystole. *Ann Thorac Surg* 1994;58:1786
31. Wong PS, Pugsley WB: Partial cardiopulmonary bypass for the treatment of profound accidental hypothermic circulatory collapse. *J Royal Soc Med* 1992;85:640
32. Dronen S, Nowak RM, Tomalanovich MC: Bretylium tosylate and hypothermic ventricular fibrillation. *Ann Emerg Med* 1980;9:335
33. Kochar G, Kahn SE, Kotler MN: Bretylium tosylate and ventricular fibrillation in hypothermia. *Ann Intern Med* 1986;105:624
34. Orts A, Alcaraz C, Delaney KA, et al: Bretylium tosylate and electrically induced cardiac arrhythmias during hypovolemia in dogs. *Am J Emerg Med* 1992;10:311
35. Carr ME, Wolfert AI: Rewarming by hemodialysis for hypothermia: failure of heparin to prevent DIC. *J Emerg Med* 1988;6:277

36. Jones TS, Liang AP, Kilbourne EM, et al: Morbidity and mortality associated with the July 1980 heat wave in St. Louis and Kansas City, Mo. *JAMA* 1982;247:3327
37. Knochel JP: Environmental heat illness: an eclectic review. *Arch Intern Med* 1974;133:841
38. Sawka MN, Young AJ, Latzka WA, et al: Human tolerance to heat strain during exercise: influence of hydration. *J Appl Physiol* 1992;73:368
39. Kilbourne EM, Choi K, Jones TS, et al: Risk factors for heatstroke: a case control study. *JAMA* 1982;247:3332
40. Hart GR, Anderson RJ, Crumpler CP, et al: Epidemic classical heat stroke: clinical characteristics and course of 28 patients. *Medicine* (Baltimore) 1982;61:189
41. Montain SJ, Sawka MN, Cadarette BS, et al: Physiological tolerance to uncompensable heat stress: effects of exercise intensity, protective clothing, and climate. *J Applied Physiol* 1994;77:216
42. Porter AM: Heat illness and soldiers. *Mil Med* 1993;158:606
43. Jimenez-Mejias ME, Montano-Diaz M, Villalonga J: Classical heatstroke in Spain: analysis of 78 cases. *Medicina Clin* (Barc) 1990;94:481
44. Heat-related deaths: Philadelphia and United States, 1993–1994. *MMWR Morbid Mortal Wkly Rep* 1994;43:453
45. Heatstroke. *MMWR Morbid Mortal Wkly Rep* 1981;30:277
46. O'Donnell TF: Acute heat stroke: epidemiologic, biochemical, renal, and coagulation studies. *JAMA* 1975;234:824
47. Tucker LE, Stanford J, Graves B, et al: Classical heatstroke: clinical and laboratory assessment. *South Med J* 1985;78:20
48. Hassanein T, Razack A, Gavaler JS, et al: Heatstroke: its clinical and pathological presentation, with particular attention to the liver. *Am J Gastroenterol* 1992;87:1382
49. Zahger D, Moses A, Weiss AT: Evidence of prolonged myocardial dysfunction in heat stroke. *Chest* 1989;95:1089
50. Amundson DE: The spectrum of heat related injury with compartment syndrome. *Mil Med* 1989;154:450
51. Akhtar MJ, Al-Nozha M, Al-Harti S, et al: Electrocardiographic abnormalities in patients with heat stroke. *Chest* 1993;104:411
52. Gader AM, Al-Mashhadani SA, Al-Harthy SS: Direct activation of platelets by heat is the possible trigger of the coagulopathy of heat stroke. *Br J Haematol* 1990;74:86
53. Zuckerman GB, Conway EE, Singer L: Hemorrhagic shock and encephalopathy syndrome and heatstroke: a physiologic comparison of two entities. *Pediatr Emerg Care* 1994;10:172
54. Tom PA, Garmel GM, Auerbach PS: Environment-dependent sports emergencies. *Med Clin North Am* 1994;78:305
55. White JD, Kamath R, Nucci R, et al: Evaporation versus iced peritoneal lavage treatment of heatstroke: comparitive efficacy in a canine model. *Am J Emerg Med* 1993;11:1
56. Bouchama A, Cafege A, Devol EB, et al: Ineffectiveness of dantolene sodium in the treatment of heatstroke. *Crit Care Med* 1991;19:176
57. Amsterdam JT, Syverud SA, Barker WJ, et al: Dantrolene sodium for treatment of heatstroke victims: lack of efficacy in a canine model. *Am J Emerg Med* 1986;4:399
58. Dahmash NS, Al-Harthi SS, Akhtar J: Invasive evaluation of patients with heat stroke. *Chest* 1994;103:1210
59. Gronert GA: Malignant hyperthermia. *Anesthesiology* 1980; 53:395
60. Neuroleptic malignant syndrome. *Lancet* 1984;i:545
61. Smego RA, Durack DT: The neuroleptic malignant syndrome. *Arch Intern Med* 1982;142:1183
62. Morris HH III, McCormick WF, Reinarz JA: Neuroleptic malignant syndrome. *Arch Neurol* 1980;37:462
63. Guze BH, Baxter LR: Neuroleptic malignant syndrome. *N Engl J Med* 1985;313:163
64. Urwyler A, Censier K, Kaufmann MA, et al: Genetic effects on the variability of the halothane and caffiene muscle contracture tests. *Anesthesiology* 1994;80:1287
65. Hackl W, Mauritz W, Schemper M, et al: Prediction of malignant hyperthermia susceptibility: statistical evaluation of clinical signs. *Br J Anaesth* 1990;64:425
66. Hopkins PM, Ellis FR, Halsall PJ: Ryanodine contracture: a potentially specific in vitro diagnostic test for malignant hyperthermia. *Br J Anaesth* 1991;66:611
67. Heffron JJ, McCarthy, TV: Current views of the molecular basis of the malignant hyperthermia syndrome. *Acta Anaesthesiol Belg* 1990;41:73
68. McCarthy TV, Healy JM, Lehane M, et al: Recent developments in the molecular genetics of malignant hyperthermia: implications for future diagnosis at the DNA level. *Acta Anaesthesiol Belg* 1990;41:107
69. Caroff SN, Rosenburg H, Fletcher JE: Malignant hyperthermia susceptibility in the neuroleptic malignant syndrome. *Anesthesiology* 1987;67:20
70. Adnet PJ, Krivosic-Horber RM, Adamantidis MM, et al: The association between the neuroleptic malignant syndrome and malignant hyperthermia. *Acta Anaesthesiol Scand* 1989;33:676
71. Kaus SJ, Rockoff MA: Malignant hyperthermia. *Pediatr Clin North Am* 1994;41:221
72. O'Flynn RP, Shutack JG, Rosenberg H, et al: Masseter muscle rigidity and malignant hyperthermia susceptibility in pediatric patients: an update on management and diagnosis. *Anesthesiology* 1994;80:1228
73. Meier-Hellman A, Romer M, Mannemann L, et al: Early recognition of malignant hyperthermia using capnography. *Anaesthesist* 1990;39:41
74. Larach MG, Localio AR, Allen GC, et al: A clinical grading scale to predict malignant hyperthermia susceptibility. *Anesthesiology* 1994;80:771
75. Wedel DJ, Quinlan JG, Iaizzo PA: Clinical effects of intravenously administered dantrolene. *Mayo Clin Proc* 1995;70:241
76. Harrison GG, Wright IG, Morrell DF: The effects of calcium channel blocking drugs on halothane initiation of malignant hyperthermia in MHS swine and on the established syndrome. *Anaesth Intensive Care* 1988;16:197
77. Foster PS, Hopkinson KC, Denborough MA: Effect of diltiazem, verapamil and dantrolene on the contractility of isolated malignant hyperpyrexia-susceptible human skeletal muscle. *Clin Exp Pharmacol Physiol* 1989;16:799
78. Adnet PJ, Krivosic-Horber RM, Haudecoeur G, et al: Diltiazem and nifedipine reduce the in vitro contracture response to halothane in malignant hyperthermia-susceptible muscle. *Can J Anaesth* 1990;37:556
79. Lopez JR, Sanchez V, Lopez I, et al: The effects of extracellular magnesium on myoplasmic calcium ion concentrations in malignant hyperthermia in susceptible swine. *Anesthesiology* 1990;73:109

Critical Care, Third Edition, edited by Joseph M. Civetta,
Robert W. Taylor, and Robert R. Kirby.
Lippincott-Raven Publishers, Philadelphia, PA © 1997.

CHAPTER 99

Toxicology: General Approach

Jeffrey A. Sadowsky

IMMEDIATE CONCERNS ■

MAJOR PROBLEMS

Patients present in a variety of ways after a drug overdose or poisoning. The patient may appear relatively normal, may be highly aggressive and agitated, or may present with frank coma. The history provides important information, although it is often unreliable in the depressed or suicidal patient. The initial concern is to stabilize the patient and to apply the basic principles of advanced cardiac life support: airway, breathing, and circulation. Seizures should be treated. The initial treatment of hypothermia or hyperthermia may make the difference between life and death. Patients with a depressed level of consciousness should receive thiamine, glucose, and naloxone. Signs of trauma or focal neurologic deficits should be evaluated with the appropriate imaging studies. A detailed history may pinpoint the specific toxin ingested or inhaled. A complete toxicologic examination is imperative. Psychiatric consultation is advisable in all suicide attempts.

STRESS POINTS

1. Emergency management implies stabilization of the patient (airway, breathing, and circulation).
2. A detailed history is essential in the poisoned patient. The history can provide information regarding identification of the toxic agent, timing of ingestion, and onset of symptoms. Toxidromes are symptom complexes specific for a toxin or a group of toxins.
3. The physical examination can distinguish between structural versus metabolic causes of altered mental status. Focal neurologic deficits may require immediate surgical intervention. Metabolic causes of altered

mental status require supportive care and further evaluation.
4. To prevent further absorption, the toxic agent should be distanced from the patient or the patient should be removed from the environment of exposure. Enhancing poison elimination can be nonspecific (e.g., provoking emesis, using gastric lavage or activated charcoal), relatively specific (e.g., hemodialysis), or poison specific (e.g., antidotes).
5. Appropriate supportive care clearly decreases morbidity and mortality.

ESSENTIAL DIAGNOSTIC TESTS AND PROCEDURES

1. The poisoned patient needs to be monitored with a continuous electrocardiogram and frequent vital signs.
2. Basic blood tests, including chemistry, hemogram, arterial blood gases, and a focused toxicologic screen, are essential.
3. Imaging studies such as computed tomography of the head are frequently used to exclude the possibility of structural neurologic lesions.

INITIAL THERAPY

1. Adequacy of airway, breathing, and circulation is first addressed and treated as necessary (Fig. 99-1).
2. Patients with altered mental status should receive thiamine, glucose, and naloxone.
3. The patient should be distanced from the toxic agent. This is followed by induction of emesis, gastric lavage, and administration of activated charcoal, as indicated.
4. Antidotes used for specific toxic agents are shown in Table 99-1.

1463

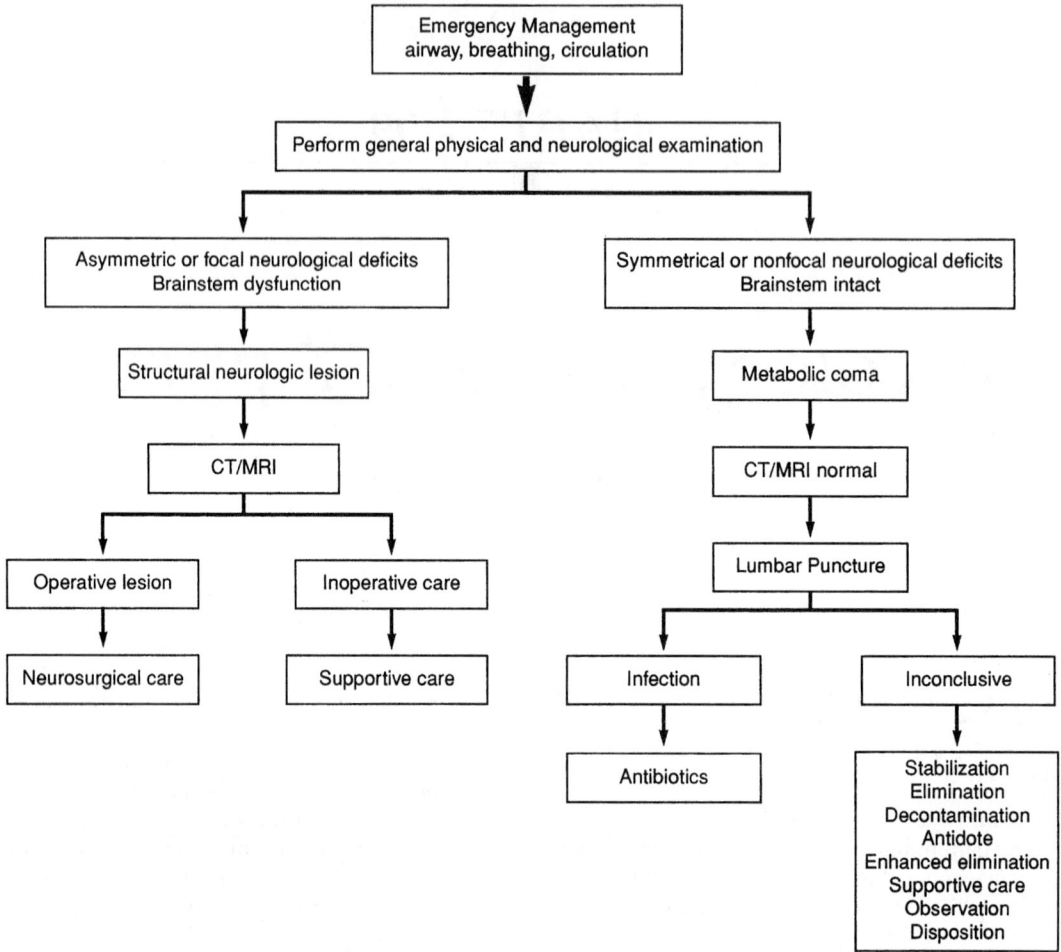

FIGURE 99-1. Algorithm for evaluation of altered mental status in the patient with a presumed poisoning or drug overdose. CT, computed tomography; MRI, magnetic resonance imaging.

5. Admission to an appropriate care unit and continued supportive care are essential.
6. Institution of suicide precautions and psychiatric consultation are often warranted.
7. Sources for toxicologic information are shown in the appendix at the end of this chapter.

HISTORY ■

Poisons date back to antiquity and had many different applications. They were used as "potions" by magicians and priests, and given to potential criminals because it was thought that such potions were benign to the innocent and lethal to the guilty.[1] Poisons were also used for hunting, being placed on the head of arrows. This is actually how the term *toxicology* came about. It is derived from two Greek terms: toxikos, which means "bow," and toxikon, which means "poison into which arrowheads are dipped."[2,3] Poisons were subsequently used for murder or official executions, hemlock being a popular poison for these occasions.

Frequently abused substances also can be traced throughout history. These substances were used much in the same fashion as today, the only difference being that the harmful consequences were not know until recently. Opium and alcohol have been used for over 5000 years. Relatively recently (late 1800s to present), cocaine, heroin, and marijuana have come in and out of popularity.

Poisoning is a major worldwide health problem, causing up to 3% of emergency department (ED) visits per year. The incidence has been increasing throughout this century, and although it is difficult to extract an accurate number, it is currently estimated to be between 2 to 10 million events annually in the United States.

There are many types of poisonings with varying presentations, each raising different concerns and requiring specific management strategies:

1. *Accidental poisoning* is most frequently encountered in children but also occurs in adults.
2. *Deliberate self-poisoning* is the most common form in adults and is also referred to as attempted suicide.
3. *Homicidal poisoning* is uncommon in contemporary

TABLE 99-1. Antidotes

POISON/DRUG	ANTIDOTE	INDICATIONS	DOSAGE	COMMENTS
Acetaminophen	Acetylcysteine (Mucomyst)	Unknown quantity ingested <24 h elapsed Ingested dose >140 mg/kg Serum acetaminophen level >140 mg/kg	140 mg/kg orally once, then 70 mg/kg for 17 doses	Activated charcoal has been shown to absorb acetylcysteine in vitro and may do so in patients
Arsenic, lead, mercury	Dimercaprol (BAL in oil)	Any symptoms from arsenic exposure Asymptomatic children with blood levels >70μg/dL Any symptoms from mercury and the patient is unable to take D-penicillamine	3–5 mg/kg deep IM every 4 h until GI symptoms subside and the patient can be switched to D-penicillamine or 3–5 mg/kg deep IM q 4 h for 2 d, then every 4–12 h for up to 7 additional d or 3–5 mg/kg deep IM q 4 h for 2 d, then 3 mg/kg/dose q 6 h, then 3 mg/kg/dose q 12 h for 7 more d	Used in conjunction with calcium EDTA in lead poisoning
	D-penicillamine (Cuprimine)	After BAL therapy or in asymptomatic patients with excess lead burden or in any symptomatic patient	100 mg/kg/day po up to 2 g in 4 divided doses for 5 d	Possible contraindication for penicillin allergic patients
Lead, ?arsenic, ?mercury	Succimer (Chemet)	Asymptomatic children with blood lead 45–69 μg/dL; not FDA approved for adult lead exposure or other metals	10 mg/kg or 350 mg/m² orally q 8 h for 5 d Reduce to 10 mg/kg or 350 mg/m² q 12 h for an additional 2 w	Monitor liver function Emits "rotten egg" sulfur odor
Lead	Calcium edetat (EDTA)	Symptomatic patients or asymptomatic children with blood levels >50μg/dL	50–70 mg/kg/day deep IM or slow IV infusion in 3–6 divided doses for up to 5 d	If urine flow is not established, hemodialysis must accompany calcium EDTA dosing
Atropine anticholinergics, tricyclic antidepressants	Physostigmine salicylate (Antilirium)	Myoclonic seizures, severe arrhythmias	Adult: 0.5–2 mg slow IV push Children: 0.5 mg slow IV push; repeat as required for life-threatening symptoms	Extreme caution is advised—it should be considered only in the presence of life-threatening anticholinergic symptoms
Intrathecal baclofen		Refractory seizures or arrhythmias unresponsive to conventional therapies		
Benzodiazepine	Flumazenil (Romazicon)	As adjunct to conventional management of benzodiazepine overdose	0.2 mg IV over 30 s; wait 30 s, then give an additional 0.3 mg IV over 30 s; additional doses of 0.5 mg over 30 s at 1-min intervals up to a cumulative dose of 3 mg	Onset of reversal usually within 1–2 min Contraindicated in patients with epilepsy, increased intracranial pressure, or coingestion of a seizuregenic agent (e.g., tricyclic antidepressants)
Beta-blocking agents Hypoglycemic agents	Glucagon	Beta-blocker–induced cardiac dysfunction Treatment of hypoglycemia	0.5–1 mg SC, IM, or IV; may repeat after 15 min	Require liver glycogen stores IV glucose must also be given to treat hypoglycemia
Coumarin derivatives, acrylamide, indanedione derivatives	Vitamin K/ phytonadione	Large ingestions (e.g., warfarin rodenticides) or chromic exposure or greater than normal prothrombin time	5–15 mg SC, IM, or IV	If given IV, it must be given slowly, can produce cardiovascular collapse

(continued)

TABLE 99-1. *(continued)*

POISON/DRUG	ANTIDOTE	INDICATIONS	DOSAGE	COMMENTS
Cyanide	Amyl nitrate, sodium nitrate, sodium thiosulfate (cyanide antidote package)	Begin treatment at first sign of toxicity if exposure is known or strongly suspected	Break ampule of amyle nitrate and allow patient to inhale for 15 s, then remove for 15 s; use a fresh ampule every 3 min. Continue until sodium nitrate (31 solution) 300 mg (0.15 to 0.33 mL/kg over 5 min in children) can be injected at 2.5–5 mL/min, then immediately inject 12.5 g of 25% sodium thiosulfate, slow IV (1.65 mL/kg in children)	If symptoms return, treatment may be repeated at half of the normal dosages (see package insert for pediatric doses). Do not use methylene blue to reduce elevated methemoglobin levels. Oxygen therapy may be useful when combined with sodium thiosulfate therapy
Digitalis	Digoxin immune fab (Digibind)	Life-threatening cardiac arrhythmias, serum levels > 5 ng/mL or ingestion of more than 10 mg (or 4 mg in children)	Multiply serum digitoxin concentration by 5.6 and multiply the result by the patient's weight in kilograms; divide this by 1000 and divide the result by 0.6. This gives the dose in number of vials to use. For other dosing methods, see package insert	Monitor potassium levels, continuous ECG
Pit viper bites (rattlesnakes, cottonmouths, copperheads)	Antivenin (Crotalidae) polyvalent (equine origin)	Mild, moderate, or severe symptoms and history of envenomation by a pit viper	3–10 vials of antivenom in 250–1000 mL NS over 4–6 h	
Ethylene glycol or methanol	Ethanol	Ethylene glycol or methanol blood levels >20 mg/dL or blood levels not readily available and suspected ingestion of toxic amounts, or any symptomatic patient with a history of ethylene glycol or methanol ingestion	Loading dose: 7.5–10 mL/kg IV 10% ethanol in D_5W over 1 h Maintenance dose: 1.4 mL/kg/h IV of 10% ethanol in D_5W; maintain blood ethanol level of 100–200 mg/dL	If dialysis is performed, adjustment of ethanol dosing is required
Heparin	Protamine sulfate	Severe hemorrhage	Maximum rate of 5 mg/min up to a total dose of 200 mg in 2 h; 1 mg of protamine neutralizes 90 U of beef lung heparin or 115 U of pork intestinal heparin	Monitor PTT or ACT
Hydrofluoric acid	Calcium gluconate	Calcium gluconate gel 2.5% for dermal exposures of 20% concentration SC injections of calcium gluconate for dermal exposures of 20% concentration or failure to respond to calcium gluconate gel	Massage 2.5% gel into exposed area for 15 min Infiltrate each square centemeter of exposed area with 0.5 mL of 10% calcium gluconate SC using a 30-gauge needle	Calcium gluconate gel currently is not available; contact regional poison control center for compounding instructions
Iron	Deferoxamine (Desferal)	TIBC, SI > 350 µ/dL, inability to obtain SI in a reasonable time and patient is symptomatic	Mild symptoms: 10 mg/kg IM up to 1 g every 48 h Severe symptoms: 10–15 mg/kg/h IV, not to exceed 6 g in 24 h; rates up to 35 mg/kg have been given	
Isoniazid, monomethyl-hydrazine–containing mushrooms (*Gyromitra*)	Pyridoxine (vitamin B_6)	Unknown overdose or ingested amount >80 mg/kg	Pyridoxine IV in the amount of INH ingested or 5 g if the amount is unknown given over 30–60 min	Cumulative dose is arbitrarily limited to 40 g (20 g in children)

(continued)

TABLE 99-1. *(continued)*

POISON/DRUG	ANTIDOTE	INDICATIONS	DOSAGE	COMMENTS
Methemoglobin inducers (e.g., nitrites, phenaxopyridine)	Methylene blue	Cyanosis, methemoglobin level >30% in an asymptomatic patient	1–2 mg/kg per dose IV over 2–3 min; may repeat doses as needed clinically. Injection can be given as 1% solution or diluted in NS	Treatment can result in falsely elevated methemoglobin levels when measured by a cooximeter; large doses may cause hemolysis
Methotrexate	Leucovorin (citrovorum factor, folinic acid)	Methotrexate-induced bone marrow depression; also may be useful in pyrimethamine-trimethoprim bone marrow depression	The dose should be ≥dose of methotrexate ingested; usually 15–100 mg/m² is given IV or po q 6 h for 8 doses	Most effective if given withn 1 h after exposure; may not prevent liver toxicity; monitor levels, may enhance toxicity of fluorouracil
Opiates	Naloxone (Narcan)	Coma or respiratory depression from unknown cause or from opiate overdose	0.4–2 mg IV bolus; doses may be repeated if there is no response, up to 10 mg	For prolonged intoxication, a continuous infusion may be used
Organophosphate and carbamate insecticides, mushrooms containing muscarine (*Inocybe* or *Clitocybe*)	Atropine	Myoclonic seizures, severe hallucinations, weakness, arrhythmias, excessive salivation, involuntary urination and defecation	Adult: 2 mg IV Child: 0.05 mg/kg IV Adult: 0.6 mg/dose IV Child: 10–30 μg/kg/dose up to 0.4 mg/dose IV	
Organophosphate insecticides	Pralidoxime (2-Pam, Protopam)	An adjunct to atropine therapy for the treatment of profound muscle weakness, respiratory depression, muscle twitching	Adult: 2 g IV at 0.5 g/min or infused in 250 ml NS over 30 min Child: 25–50 mg/kg in 250 mL saline over 30 min	Most effective when used in the first 24–36 h after exposure; dosage may be repeated in 1 h followed by q 8 h if indicated

EDTA, ethylene diamine tetraacetic acid; FDA, Food and Drug Administration; deep IM, deeply intramuscularly; GI, gastrointestinal; po, orally; q, every; IV, intravenously; SC, subcutaneously; NS, normal saline; ECG, electrocardiographic monitoring; TIBC, total iron-binding capacity; SI, saturation index; INH, isoniazid; D₅W, 5% dextrose in water, PTT, prothrombin time; ACT, activated clotting time; BAL, bronchoalveolar lavage.

society, although several cases involving cyanide-laced analgesic capsules have occurred.

4. *Therapeutic poisoning* results from the over-prescription of pharmacologic agents.

Many serious adverse reactions started to be noticed and reported in the early to mid-1900s. In 1937, more than 100 deaths occurred from a preparation of sulfa called Elixir of Sulfanilamide-Massengill. This preparation contained 72% diethylene glycol, which was used as a vehicle for its delivery. Little was then known about ethylene glycol toxicity, therefore resulting in many cases of renal failure and death.[4] In the 1960s, the use of thalidomide resulted in about 5000 cases of severe congenital anomalies.[5] In 1981, a "gasping syndrome" was seen in several premature neonates, causing their demise. The syndrome manifested itself by a severe metabolic acidosis, respiratory depression with gasping, and encephalopathy.[6] High blood levels of benzyl alcohol and its metabolite benzoic acids were found and were traced to heparinized bacteriostatic sodium chloride solution (which was used to flush indwelling catheters) and bacteriostatic water (used to mix medications). In 1989 to 1990, eosinophilia-myalgia syndrome appeared, affecting more than 1500 people who had ingested large amounts of L-tryptophan.[7]

DIAGNOSIS AND THE GENERAL APPROACH TO THE POISONED PATIENT ■

The clinician needs to maintain a high index of suspicion to diagnose a poisoning because the presentation can be subtle and highly variable. Poisoning should be suspected in a patient presenting with multiple organ dysfunction syndrome until proven otherwise. Poisoning is an important consideration in anyone with a change in baseline mental status, in any head injury or trauma victim, or in a young patient complaining of chest pain or presenting with a potentially lethal arrhythmia. Poisoning also should be suspected in patients coming from a fire scene or chemical plant accident, and especially in any patient with an unexplained metabolic acidosis.

This chapter outlines the approach to the patient in whom poisoning is suspected. Emergency management is first begun, followed by a clinical evaluation, including a history, a physical examination, and evaluation of laboratory results. Elimination and decontamination measures follow. Antidotes are given if indicated. Through all of these steps, the patient receives careful observation and supportive therapy.

EMERGENCY MANAGEMENT

A patient who arrives in the ED with a presumed poisoning or drug overdose should be given high priority and provided with continuous monitoring and close observation. Under critical circumstances, immediate physician evaluation is necessary.

Airway

The initial step is to secure the airway without improperly manipulating the cervical spine. The neck should be immobilized in the comatose patient if there is any question about the status of the cervical spine. Cervical spine trauma should be excluded radiographically and clinically.

Breathing

The clinician should establish that breathing is present and that it is adequate to sustain life. The respiratory pattern should be evaluated. The presence of respiratory irregularity, such as Cheyne-Stokes, Biot's, or agonal respirations, signals impending respiratory failure and respiratory arrest. The patient in this case should be ventilated with 100% oxygen with a bag-valve-mask and tracheally intubated as quickly as possible. The patient who presents with a depressed level of consciousness should also be intubated. Intubation under these circumstances secures and protects the airway, an important procedure before gastric lavage.

Circulation

The pulse is used to evaluate the heart rate and rhythm and volume status. Assessment of skin perfusion adds additional information about the patient's hemodynamic status. Electrocardiograph monitoring should be continuous, and intravenous (IV) access should be established and blood drawn for full chemical evaluation, complete blood cell counts, coagulation panel, and cultures as dictated by the clinical presentation. Qualitative and quantitative drug levels, including illicit drugs as well as prescribed drugs, are selectively obtained, depending on the patient's clinical presentation (toxidrome). Commonly assayed drugs include acetaminophen, aspirin, benzodiazepines, opioids, cannabis, barbiturates, theophylline, and digoxin. Tricyclic levels are occasionally helpful in the qualitative sense but do not correlate well with the level of poisoning. Obtaining arterial blood gas measurements is essential. An immediate fingerstick glucose level also should be obtained and is more advantageous than waiting for the blood glucose level from the chemistry panel.

All comatose patients—even those without pinpoint pupils and those with focal neurologic findings—should be treated with naloxone, thiamine, and dextrose. Dextrose is given as an IV bolus of 1 mL/kg of a 50% glucose solution. The only patients who should not receive dextrose are those who are clearly in diabetic ketoacidosis. Hypoglycemia is exceedingly dangerous and may be the cause of unexplained coma. Even if the patient is subsequently found to be normoglycemic or even hyperglycemic, no harm has been done by administering glucose.

Thiamine is given as a 100-mg IV bolus to adults who have been given or are to receive 50% dextrose in water, in order to prevent the precipitation of Wernicke's encephalopathy.

Naloxone is given as a 2-mg bolus that can be administered intravenously, intramuscularly, or endotracheally. A dose of 2 mg is the usual starting dose, rather than 0.4 to 0.8 mg, because some common opioids, such as codeine and propoxyphene, require a larger dose of naloxone to be effective. Naloxone is given at the same dose, independent of age or weight. This large dose is benign in most comatose patients. An exception to this guideline is the chronic opioid user. Large doses of naloxone can precipitate opioid withdrawal symptoms under these circumstances. The chronic opioid user who is apneic should receive the full 2-mg dose of naloxone and observed for withdrawal symptoms. If the patient is suspected of being opioid dependent and is not apneic, small doses of naloxone should be given to avoid serious opioid withdrawal. If repeated doses are needed, a continuous IV drip of naloxone can be beneficial. Patients who are frequent abusers of illicit fentanyl derivatives, the so-called "designer drugs," usually require large amounts of naloxone.

If there is suspicion of potentiating a withdrawal syndrome, the patient should be restrained before naloxone is administered, for protection of the patient and the clinical staff. The onset of action of naloxone given intravenously is about 2 minutes. If opioid withdrawal is precipitated by naloxone, the effects begin to dissipate in about 15 to 20 minutes and are gone after 30 minutes. The withdrawal syndrome produced by the administration of naloxone should not be treated with opioids. Rather, supportive care is rendered because the effect of the naloxone is brief.

CLINICAL EVALUATION

A thorough history and physical examination are crucial to the diagnosis in the potentially poisoned patient. Laboratory tests are helpful to delineate the substances, quantitate their absorption, and monitor their end-organ effects. The toxic patient can present in many different ways, and a high grade of suspicion is warranted. Poisoned patients commonly present with coma, cardiac arrhythmias, metabolic acidosis, seizures, nausea, and vomiting. Poisoning should be suspected in all patients involved in trauma and in those with acute mental status changes. Patients sometimes present with symptom complexes, or toxidromes, which may give clues to the unknown poisoning (Table 99-2).

Medical History

A properly conducted medical history can provide useful information, although it is notoriously unreliable in patients who intentionally overdose. The simple questions of who, what, when, how much, where, and why should be asked. All treatment from the time of ingestion until the time of presentation should be documented.

SATS. The acronym *SATS* (*S*, substance [the brand name and its ingredients]; *A*, amount ingested; *T*, time ingested;

TABLE 99-2. Toxidromes

TOXIDROME	CHARACTERISTIC FINDINGS	POSSIBLE TOXIC AGENT
Anticholinergic	Agitated, hallucination, tachycardia, tachypneic, flushing, dry skin and mucus membranes, urinary retention, blurred vision, myoclonus, choreoathetosis, seizures	Atropine, antihistamine, tricyclic antidepressants, baclofen, benztropine, Jimson weed
Cholinergic	Salivation, lacrimation, urination, defecation, gastrointestinal cramps, emesis (SLUDGE); wheezing, bradycardia, coma, pin-point pupils	Organophosphate insecticides, pilocarpine, carbamates, nicotine
Extrapyramidal	Awake, trismus, hyperreflexia, choreoathetosis, and tremor	Phenothiazine, diphenhydramine, haloperidol, benztropine
Hallucinogenic	Derealization, depersonalization, perception distortions	Cannabinoids, cocaine, amphetamines, phencyclidine
Narcotic	Altered mental status, unresponsiveness, shallow respirations, slow respiratory rate, pin-point pupils, bradycardia, hypothermia, hypotension, track marks	Opiates, propoxphene, lomotil, pentzocine
Sedative-hypnotic	Altered mental status progressing to frank coma, delirium or hallucinations, slow and shallow respirations, mydriasis, hypothermia, hypotension, diminished reflexes	ETOH, opiates, barbiturates, tricyclic antidepressants, fentanyl, benzodiazepines, methadone, meprobamate, glutethimide, propoxy anticonvulsants and antipsychotics
Seizuregenic	Agitated, hyperthermic, hyperreflexic	Cocaine, xanthines, anticholinergics, phencyclidine, isoniazid, strychnine, lidocaine, nicotine, camphor
Stimulant	Agitated, excessive speech and motor activity, euphoria, paranoia, mydriasis, tachycardia, hypertension, hyperreflexia, tremor, seizures, diaphoresis, metabolic acidosis	Amphetamines, cocaine, xanthines, ephedrine/pseudoephedrine, phencyclidine, methylphenidate, nicotine
Salicylate	Semicomatose or agitated, tachypnea, fever, diaphoresis, tinnitus, alkalosis then acidosis	Salicylates, oil of wintergreen
Serotonin	Confusion, facial flushing, diaphoresis, myoclonus, hyperreflexia, diarrhea	Fluoxetine, sertraline, phenelzine, tranylcypromine, clomipramine, tryptophan, isoniazid
Solvent	Altered mental status, dizziness, restlessness, headache, incoordination, derealization and depersonalization	Acetone, toluene, hydrocarbons, naphthalene, chlorinated hydrocarbons
Tricyclic antidepressants	Initially agitated with progression to coma, shallow and slow respirations, cardiac arrhythmia, seizure, hypotension, prolongation of the OT interval	

ETOH, ethanol.

S, symptoms) is useful in obtaining the basic information about the drug or poison. Try to relate the time of ingestion to the time of the onset of symptoms and note what interventions have taken place.

WHO. How is the patient acting? Obtain *AMPLE* information: *A*, age and allergies; *M*, current medications; *P*, past medical history, incidents of substance abuse or intentional ingestion; *L*, time of last meal (which may influence absorption); and *E*, events leading to the present condition. Emergency medical service personnel can furnish considerable information about how the patient was found and the patient's original and ongoing status. Female patients of childbearing age should assumed to be pregnant until proven

otherwise. Medical alert bracelets and other indicators of important clinical conditions should be sought because they also furnish necessary information.

WHAT. Obtain the trade and generic name of the substance or its ingredients and the route of exposure. Sometimes it is beneficial to call the pharmacy noted on the label to inquire about other drugs purchased by the patient that might have been ingested.

WHEN. Document the time of exposure and the time the patient was last seen. The timing is important because it can be used to estimate the onset of symptoms (if they have not manifested), when the peak action is expected to occur, and duration of effect. Quantitative serum drug concentrations are difficult to properly interpret without knowing the time of ingestion.

HOW MUCH.   The amount and the strength of the agent taken should be sought. A child's swallow equals 0.3 mL/kg, or approximately 1 teaspoonful; an adult swallows approximately 15 mL, or about 1 tablespoonful.[8] Where and what the patient was doing can elicit helpful clues. A child found in the kitchen may have ingested a common household cleaner such as detergent. If the child was found lethargic or unresponsive in the bedroom, one might suspect the ingestion of perfumes containing ethanol. Hydrocarbons are found in the garage. Recreational substances, for instance, marijuana and cocaine, are usually used in groups, in contrast to heroin, which is usually used alone. Of course, environmental hazards and occupational toxins should always be sought.

WHY.   Try to ascertain the patient's intent. Was the ingestion accidental, intentional, or the result of a therapeutic error?

Physical Examination

A thorough physical examination helps to corroborate the suspected diagnosis and to detect other unsuspected problems. The comatose patient should be completely undressed and examined thoroughly. Telltale signs of trauma should be sought by examining every inch of the patient, because trauma could be the sole cause of coma.

Vital Signs

Rigorous and frequent documentation of vital signs is essential when dealing with an unstable, comatose patient. Vital signs can create and also narrow a list of differential diagnosis while also contributing information about the substances ingested.

The core body temperature must be evaluated and managed appropriately in the early stages of poisoning. Life-threatening hyperthermia can easily be appreciated by touch; hypothermia is much easier to miss, especially in winter months when most of the patients presenting in the ED feel cold to the touch. Life-threatening hyperthermia (40.5°C [105°F] or higher), regardless of the etiology, must be addressed immediately. Most investigators agree that lowering the core temperature to about 38.5°C (101°F) is adequate. The important issue is to bring down the temperature immediately, using a fan and cool mist treatment and, if needed, ice.[9] Care should be taken to prevent shivering. Significant, life-threatening temperature elevation occurring during a toxicologic emergency may result from a variety of causes, including direct stimulation of the central nervous system (CNS), impaired thermoregulation, excessive muscle activity, impaired dissipation of heat, and impaired thermoregulation.[10,11] Hyperthermia can lead to massive muscle breakdown causing myoglobinuria and, consequently, renal failure. Toxicologic emergencies seen with hyperthermia include the following: cocaine and other sympathomimetic

overdoses, alcohol withdrawal, malignant hyperthermia, neuroleptic malignant syndrome, anticholinergics, sedative-hypnotic withdrawal, salicylates, and thyroid storm. A complete discussion of hyperthermia, its causes, and its management is found in Chapter 98.

Hypothermia may mimic death; therefore, resuscitative measures should continue until the patient is rewarmed and patients should not be pronounced dead until they are rewarmed. Hypothermia may be associated with exposure, cold water immersion, CNS trauma, transection of the spinal cord, barbiturates, benzodiazepines, ethanol, beta-adrenergic blockers, hypoglycemia, opioids, tricyclic antidepressants, carbon monoxide, chloral hydrate, and CNS depressants. Hypothermia can render some medications ineffective while the patient is hypothermic, and as the patient becomes euthermic, these previously inactive medications can achieve toxic blood levels, resulting in iatrogenic toxicity. A complete discussion of hypothermia, its causes, and its management is also found in Chapter 98.

Pulses can be used to evaluate heart rate, rhythm, stroke volume, blood pressure, systemic vascular resistance, and overall peripheral perfusion. Hypotension should be aggressively treated with volume replacement if the lungs are clear on auscultation. Vasoactive pressors should be used as a last resort because of their arrhythmogenic potential, especially in patients at high risk of arrhythmias. If there is no evidence of hemodynamic compromise, infusion of large amounts of IV fluids should be discouraged. Volume loading with forced diuresis is only marginally effective in eliminating drugs and poisons and may be associated with significant complications such as pulmonary and cerebral edema. Lung auscultation should be repeated every 5 to 10 minutes if the patient requires continued fluid resuscitation. Persistent hypotension after a fluid challenge of 500 mL to 1 L of isotonic fluid suggests a few possibilities. Is the toxin ingested by the patient a myocardial depressant? Is the substance producing vasodilation? Has there been concomitant trauma (e.g., intraabdominal hemorrhage, spinal shock)? Other catastrophes need to be considered, such as an acute myocardial infarction with cardiogenic shock, pulmonary embolism, sepsis, ruptured aortic aneurysm, and severe acidemia. Persistent hypotension with associated pulmonary crackles mandates placement of a pulmonary artery catheter to guide management of vasoactive and inotropic agents.

Hypotension-associated poisoning is seen frequently with antihypertensive agents, especially beta-adrenergic blockers, calcium channel blockers, barbiturates, carbon monoxide, monoamine oxidase (MAO) inhibitors, opioids, tricyclic antidepressants, and the organophosphate insecticides. If hypotension is associated with bradycardia, then agents such as clonidine, beta-adrenergic blockers, calcium channel blockers, cardiac glycosides, and the organophosphates should be considered.[12]

Hypertension also can be associated with tachycardia or bradycardia. When hypertension is seen with tachycardia, agents such as anticholinergics, CNS stimulants (e.g., cocaine, amphetamines), hallucinogens, phencyclidine, MAO inhibitors, nicotine, organophosphates, sympathomimetics (e.g., theophylline), thyroid hormones, and withdrawal from sedative-hypnotics constitute a list of possibilities. Hypertension and bradycardia are associated with any substance that increases the intracranial pressure, hypervitaminosis A, nalidixic acid, tetracycline, and chronic lead poisoning.[13]

Bradycardia is commonly seen with beta-adrenergic blockers, calcium channel blockers, cardiac glycosides, cholinergic agents, and CNS depressants. Tachycardias are seen with alcohol, anticholinergics, cardiac glycosides, CNS stimulants, phencyclidine, phenothiazines, salicylates, sympathomimetics, thyroid hormones, and the tricyclic antidepressants.

SKIN. Skin findings can be helpful, especially in a patient who is comatose and when the history is sketchy. Signs of trauma such as needle tracks, bruises, burns, lacerations, or surgical scars can be helpful in determining the route of administration as well as a possible diagnosis. For example, a patient with a thyroidectomy scar should be suspected of myxedema or hypocalcemia. Skin color may be pale, blue, pink, red, yellow, or even spotted. A pink color of the skin with flushing suggests an allergic reaction, niacin ingestion, toxic shock syndrome, an alcohol-disulfiram reaction, anticholinergic poisoning, or fever. A bright red "boiled lobster" appearance is seen in borate poisoning, usually in children who have ingested roach insecticide. A petechial rash and ecchymoses are commonly seen in coagulopathies, warfarin overdose, salicylate overdose, or in fulminant meningococcemia. Jaundice and hepatic failure can result from a delayed reaction to acetaminophen overdose or arsenic or carbon tetrachloride ingestion. Bullous skin lesions are seen with prolonged pressure or hypoxia to an area of skin. These lesions are often seen after ingestion of sedative-hypnotic agents, with carbon monoxide poisoning, and with thermal burns. Diaphoresis is associated with hypoglycemia, salicylate intoxication, acetaminophen overdose, organophosphate poisoning, cocaine use, thyroid storm, and in any withdrawal syndrome.

BREATH. Attempting to identify odors on the patient's breath may be important in the poisoned patient. Alcohol is a common odor. Ethanol is often consumed along with other toxic agents, and it is frequently associated with trauma. Therefore, it is not prudent to attribute a patient's coma or altered mental state to alcohol alone. The patient with diabetic ketoacidosis has a fruity odor. Arsenic poisoning usually presents with a garlic odor. A cleaning fluid smell suggests carbon tetrachloride.

LUNGS. Early and accurate assessment of the airway and breathing, described previously, is important for the recognition and management of impending respiratory failure, and it may prevent its evolution to cardiopulmonary arrest. "Quiet tachypnea," or tachypnea without respiratory distress, is seen in acidemia with respiratory compensation. Aspiration pneumonitis, irritant fumes, inhaled gases, CNS stimulants, withdrawal states, or ingested substances (that interfere with oxygen transport or tissue utilization of oxygen) are associated with an increased work of breathing, therefore producing tachypnea with respiratory distress.[14]

Shallow, ineffective respirations may be caused by poisoning with agents that interfere with performance of the respiratory muscles. Curare, botulism, snake bites, tick paralysis, paralytic shell fish poisoning, and organophosphate insecticides can cause dysfunction of muscle contraction, leading to paralysis and respiratory arrest.

Bradypnea and apnea may be caused by CNS depressants such as alcohol, opioids, benzodiazepines, barbiturates, clonidine, neuroleptics, and the anticonvulsants.

Wheezing is not only associated with reactive airways disease, but can be seen with beta-adrenergic blockers, cholinergic medications, and organophosphates. Bronchospasm can be induced in atopic individuals by acetylsalicylic acid and sulfites.[15]

Auscultation can identify a pneumothorax or even a pneumomediastinum, which can be seen in individuals who snort cocaine or smoke marijuana. Excessive negative intrathoracic pressure generated during a snorting or deep inhaling maneuver causes rupture of alveoli and predisposes to the development of pneumothorax and pneumomediastinum.

Pulmonary edema can be classified as cardiogenic and noncardiogenic. Cardiogenic pulmonary edema is associated with beta-adrenergic blockers, calcium channel blockers, and antiarrhythmics because their negative inotropic action. Noncardiogenic pulmonary edema can be precipitated by opioids, cocaine, barbiturates, organophosphate insecticides, and the salicylates. The exact mechanism is not well understood. The direct noxious effects of inhaled gases also can precipitate pulmonary edema.[16,17]

HEART. Physical examination of the heart reveals information regarding the state of chronotropism, as seen by rate and rhythm, inotropy, and vascular tone. A 12-lead electrocardiogram is important in all seriously poisoned patients and might suggest and narrow a differential diagnosis. A wide QRS complex and supraventricular arrhythmias suggest tricyclic antidepressant intoxication, whereas a narrow QRS complex is seen with hypocalcemia and ethylene glycol poisoning.[18,19] Torsade de pointes is caused by a prolonged QT interval, usually after ingestion of phenothiazines, quinidine, procainamide, or organophosphates, or it may be seen with hypocalcemia and hypomagnesemia.[20] An arrhythmia in any young person should suggest the possibility of cocaine use.

ABDOMEN AND EXTREMITIES. The abdomen is examined for any signs of trauma or intraabdominal catastrophe. Likewise, the extremities are examined for trauma, fractures, vascular insufficiency, or a compartment syndrome.

NEUROLOGIC. The responsiveness scale *AVPU* rates the patient's neurologic status according to the following: *A*, awake and alert; *V*, response to verbal stimuli; *P*, response to pain; and *U*, unresponsive. If the patient is awake and alert, the cognitive function can be evaluated by using the full mini-mental status examination or an abbreviated version.

The pupils should be assessed for size, shape, reactivity to light, consensual reflex, and corneal reflex. Nystagmus, ocular movements, or deviation of the eyes should be noted.

Fundoscopy is performed looking for retinal hemorrhages and papilledema.

Mydriasis is produced by *SAW*: *S*, sympathetic agents; *A*, anticholinergic agents; or *W*, withdrawal. A unilateral dilated pupil can be seen with glutethimide intoxication or with mydriatic drops and, therefore, does not always constitute a neurosurgical emergency. However, a unilateral dilated pupil with a downgoing, outwardly deviated eye is consistent with a structural lesion and needs immediate attention.

Mydriasis can be further classified as nonreactive, reactive, and delayed. A pure anticholinergic poisoning can cause a nonreactive mydriasis. A reactive mydriasis is produced by sympathomimetics or MAO inhibitors, or withdrawal from opioids, ethanol, or carbon monoxide.

Miosis (pinpoint pupils) is significant for overdose of opioids, clonidine, organophosphate insecticides, nicotine, and phencyclidine. Miosis unresponsive to naloxone indicates pontine damage.

Nystagmus is most frequently seen with anticonvulsants but also can be seen with opioids, ethanol, phencyclidine, and sedative-hypnotics.

In the comatose patient, extraocular movements are tested by the ice water caloric test or the doll's eye reflex. Do not attempt to perform an ice water caloric test on an awake patient because it is uncomfortable. The doll's eye reflex can be safely performed only after the cervical spine has been cleared for any injury. Therefore, in patients with a suspected cervical spine injury, the test of choice is ice water calorics. Performance of the ice water caloric and doll's eye tests are described in Chapter 133.

Muscle strength in a cooperative patient can be graded on a scale of 0 to 5, where 0 is no muscular contraction detected, 1 is a barely detectable flicker, 2 is active movement with gravity eliminated, 3 is active movement against gravity, 4 is active movement against gravity and some resistance, 5 is normal.[21]

If the patient is comatose, the response to noxious stimulus is used to evaluate motor function. Noxious stimuli can be applied by pressing on the supraorbital ridge or to the nail beds or with a sternal rub. The motor response to these stimuli in a comatose patient can be described as localization, flexion, extension, or no response (flaccid).[22,23]

Other motor abnormalities should be investigated such as focal weakness, flaccidity, spasticity, fasciculations, or involuntary movements. Deep tendon reflexes can alert the physician to structural neurologic abnormalities.

The information obtained by the neurologic examination allows differentiation of coma into toxic-metabolic causes versus structural defects[23]:

Toxic-metabolic causes: The pupillary light reflex retains its integrity and remains intact. Pupillary light reflexes are usually preserved until the terminal stages of coma.
Structural neurologic disease: Usually is manifest as asymmetric or focal deficits.

Of course, exceptions occur; for example, a mass lesion may cause compression of the brain stem bilaterally or conversely, or a toxic-metabolic disorder such as hyperosmolar nonketotic hyperglycemia[23] or hypoglycemia may produce focal deficits.[24]

Seizures

Almost any drug or toxin in large doses can cause seizures. Simple seizures can be managed by ABC principles (airway, breathing, and circulation) followed by observation. However, if the seizures are repetitive or status epilepticus, constituting a medical emergency, then appropriate aggressive management with benzodiazepines followed by phenytoin is needed (Chap. 134). Seizures from theophylline or amoxapine toxicity are notoriously difficult to treat. Other drug-induced seizures require specific management, such as the use of pyridoxine for isoniazid-induced seizures or naloxone for propoxyphene-induced seizures. Hypoglycemia, eclampsia, hypoxia, meningitis, or malignant hypertension should be considered in the differential diagnosis of any seizure.

Gastrointestinal Disturbance

Iron poisoning may manifest as abdominal pain, nausea, and vomiting. These patients are at high risk for massive gastrointestinal hemorrhage. Arsenic poisoning characteristically causes severe diarrhea, whereas theophylline causes nausea and vomiting. Marked salivation and a mucous diarrhea are seen in mercury intoxication. This may develop into a hemorrhagic colitis.[25]

Laboratory Evaluation

The laboratory is an adjunct to the history and physical examination and should be used to confirm the clinician's suspicions. If the physical examination discloses a focal neurologic deficit, a computed tomography scan of the head should be performed without delay. As mentioned previously, toxicologic screens can be helpful but should be ordered selectively. Quantitative drug concentrations are essential for management in the patient poisoned with acetaminophen, digoxin, ethanol, methanol, ethylene glycol, carbon monoxide, salicylate, iron, lead, and lithium because they predict outcome and guide specific therapy.

The presence (or absence) of a metabolic acidosis is important to determine. If metabolic acidosis is present, an anion gap should be calculated:

$$\text{Anion gap} = \text{Na}^+ - (\text{Cl}^- + \text{HCO}_3^-) \text{ mMol/L}$$

A normal (or negative) anion gap varies between 3 and 11 mMol/L. A value higher than this is termed a positive anion gap. The variables determining the differential diagnoses of anion gap–positive versus anion gap–negative metabolic acidosis are different. An anion gap–positive metabolic acidosis occurs with ethylene glycol, methanol, and salicylate poisoning. Lactic acidosis associated with tissue hypoxia (hypoperfusion, cyanide, carbon monoxide poisoning), diabetic and alcoholic ketoacidosis, and renal failure are other common causes of anion gap–positive metabolic acidosis. Anion gap–negative metabolic acidosis is seen in intoxication with bromide, iodine, and lithium; hypercalcemia and hypermagnesemia also are often associated with anion gap–negative metabolic acidosis.

The presence of ketosis in the absence of acidosis suggests isopropyl alcohol intoxication.

Normal serum osmolality is 280 to 295 mOsm. The osmolality should be measured and calculated. Serum osmolality may be calculated using the following equation:

Calculated serum osmolality mOsm/L

$$= 2(Na) + BUN/3 + Glucose/20$$

Normally, the measured serum osmolality is no greater than 10 mOsm/L more than the calculated serum osmolality. A difference of 10 mOsm/L or greater between the measured osmolality and the calculated serum osmolality is called an osmolar gap. This is important in that it suggests the presence of osmotically active substances that are not accounted for by the calculated osmolality such as ethyl alcohol, methanol, isopropyl alcohol, ethylene glycol, glycerol, or mannitol.

Specific imaging tests should be obtained to evaluate any suspicion of trauma or to follow-up any evidence of trauma on physical examination.

ELIMINATION OF THE POISON

An important concept in toxicology is to distance the patient from the toxic agent. This can be achieved by removing the patient from an area of a toxic inhalant, such as carbon monoxide, chlorine gas, or hydrogen sulfide. The initial treatment under these circumstances is the administration of 100% oxygen. Aggressive removal of toxic agents from the eyes, skin, or gastrointestinal tract may limit their toxic effects.

The eyes can come into contact with many substances such as caustic acids or bases. This type of exposure should be treated with abundant irrigation with water for at least 30 minutes. All patients should undergo a complete ophthalmologic examination, including visual acuity and slit-lamp examination. Ophthalmologic consultation is indicated in cases of serious exposures.

Toxic exposure to the skin warrants removal of the clothing around the area of exposure followed by copious irrigation with water for 15 to 30 minutes. Patients exposed to insecticides should remove all clothing and shower for 30 minutes because residual insecticide can be continuously absorbed.

The gastrointestinal tract is the most common port of entry for toxic agents. Many methods have been used to block toxin absorption, inactivate the toxin, or to enhance its elimination. No single method can be defined as the "gold standard," and controversy surrounds this topic. Current therapies include induction of emesis, gastric lavage, charcoal administration, cathartics administration, and use of whole-bowel irrigation. Although the role of ipecac[26] and the routine use of gastric lavage[27,28] have been questioned, activated charcoal does have an important role in emergency management of poisoning.[29] Multiple-dose administration of activated charcoal is indicated for significant poisoning with tricyclic antidepressants,[30] digoxin,[31] phenobarbital,[32] and theophylline.[33]

When considering gastric emptying, one needs to determine the risk of the ingestion to the patient versus the risk of possible aspiration during the gastric emptying procedure. The questions to be considered are: "How much time has elapsed since the ingestion?" and "Will gastric emptying remove a significant amount of the ingested substance?"

Gastric emptying should not be performed if the drugs or poisons ingested pose little true risk to the patient or if the ingestion occurred many hours before medical attention. Drugs or poisons that pose high potential risk to the patient (e.g., cyanide) should be treated with gastric emptying if clinically indicated.

The time interval from the ingestion to the initiation of gastric emptying is an important determining factor in the utility of the procedure. Some substances are rapidly absorbed (e.g., alcohol, acetaminophen) and gastric emptying therefore must be initiated almost immediately for adequate results. Even for the many drugs that are absorbed more slowly, the yield of gastric emptying is unimpressive.

Studies have demonstrated that under ideal circumstances, some drugs and poisons can be removed from the stomach.[34] It also has been shown that gastric emptying decreases absorption.[35] It remains to be proven, however, that clinical outcome is altered by gastric emptying. Most experts recommend that an attempt to empty the stomach be made if a patient presents relatively early and if the ingested substance is of high toxic potential such as cyanide, colchicine, podophyllin, or tricyclic antidepressants.

Gastric emptying can be accomplished by inducing emesis with a substance such as syrup of ipecac or by gastric lavage. Syrup of ipecac has been available over the counter since 1966. It has an excellent safety record. Syrup of ipecac produces vomiting by stimulating the chemoreceptor trigger zone of the CNS. Its emetic effect remains intact independent of fluid ingestion[36] or even with concomitant antiemetic ingestion. Prolonged emesis is rare but has been reported, and can delay the initiation of more definitive therapy such as administration of activated charcoal. Contraindications to induced emesis include a depressed level of consciousness, seizures, and ingestion of caustics or petroleum distillates.

Gastric lavage is performed by passing a large-bore tube (Ewald) through the nose or mouth into the stomach. Tap water is sufficient for lavage in adults, but children are more susceptible to electrolyte imbalances and therefore saline solution is used. Lavage is performed until the fluid is clear, and then activated charcoal is administered through the tube. The tube can then be removed in the awake patient or replaced with an nasogastric tube in the comatose patient. Caustic alkali ingestion is a contraindication to gastric lavage.

Complications are relatively rare and largely preventable by appropriate patient selection and by using the proper technique. Emesis induced by ipecac can cause protracted vomiting,[37] aspiration,[38] Mallory-Weiss syndrome,[39] intracerebral hemorrhage,[40] pneumomediastinum, pneumoretroperitoneum,[41] and even diaphragmatic rupture.[42] Gastric lavage potentially can cause nasal, oral, and pharyngeal injury, esophageal tears or perforation, and aspiration.[43–45]

Activated charcoal has an important role in management of the poisoned patient. Charcoal is the residue from various organic materials produced by burning substances such as wood, bone starch, lactulose, sucrose, and coconut shells.[46] The absorptive capacity is increased, or "activated," by treating it with steam at extremely high temperatures (600° to 900°C). The activated charcoal to drug ratio optimally should be 10:1. Activated charcoal often is premixed with a cathartic such as sorbitol and can be used in most poisonings, even if the toxic agent is unknown initially. The agents listed in Table 99-3 are not effectively absorbed by activated charcoal. Serial administration of activated charcoal is indicated as the initial treatment of poisoning with digoxin,[31] tricyclic antidepressants,[30] glutethimide,[47] phenobarbital,[32] and theophylline.[33] There are no absolute contraindications to the use of activated charcoal.

Cathartics are used to facilitate the passage of toxic substances from the body. Agents used as cathartics include sorbitol, magnesium sulfate, and magnesium citrate. Recently, polyethylene glycol, a nonabsorbable, osmotically active compound, has been used for whole-bowel irrigation. Use of polyethylene glycol is especially useful with sustained-release capsules and iron tablets and in cases of cocaine body packing.

Enhanced Elimination of Absorbed Substances

Once absorption of a toxic agent has been decreased, the next step is to enhance its elimination. Methods for enhancing elimination of toxic compounds are specific for individual drugs or poisons. Methods currently available include the following: forced diuresis, manipulation of the pH, peritoneal dialysis, hemodialysis, hemofiltration, hemoperfusion, plasmapheresis, and toxin-specific antibodies. Intensive supportive care has kept the mortality relatively low in poisoned patients who reach the hospital alive.[48,49] Each elimination technique carries a risk of complications.[50-52] When deciding, therefore, to initiate an elimination technique, the risks and benefits need to be examined carefully.

Forced diuresis was popular when barbiturates were one of the most common overdoses, but because of its unproven efficacy and the associated complications of pulmonary and cerebral edema, most centers have abandoned its use.

Acidification of the urine to enhance elimination of weak acids such as phencyclidine and amphetamine is not used anymore. This technique as been associated with serious metabolic acidosis and renal damage, and may impair the elimination of other drugs such as phenobarbital and salicylates.

Alkalinization of the blood and urine is advantageous for certain drug overdoses. Alkalinization of the urine enhances the elimination of salicylates,[53] phenobarbital,[54] and herbicide 2,4-dichlorophenoxyacetic acid.[55] The goal of alkalinizing the urine is to achieve a urine pH of 7 to 8. Systemic alkalinization is useful on toxic overdoses of tricyclic antidepressants and quinidine, and also to maintain renal elimination of methotrexate in patients given high-dose folinic acid rescue therapy.[56] Administration of sodium bicarbonate also has been advocated to protect the kidneys from myoglobinuria seen in rhabdomyolysis (Chap. 152). The complications seen with sodium bicarbonate administration result from the sodium load, alkalosis, and hypokalemia.

Peritoneal dialysis is a relatively simple but slow method to enhance drug elimination. It also is less effective than hemodialysis or hemoperfusion, although it may be used during transport of a patient to a facility with hemodialysis or hemoperfusion capability. Peritoneal dialysis can enhance the elimination of water-soluble, low molecular weight, poorly protein bound substance with a low volume of distribution. Examples include alcohols, lithium, salicylates, and theophylline.

Hemodialysis can be performed relatively rapidly and also enhances the elimination of water-soluble substances of low molecular weight that are poorly protein bound and have a low volume of distribution. Hemodialysis is associated with potential serious complications. It should be used with caution to enhance poison elimination in the hemodynamically or thermally unstable patient, in the presence of renal dysfunction, and in the presence of prolonged coma. Hemodialysis is preferred to hemoperfusion for the removal of methanol,[57] ethylene glycol,[58] salicylates,[59] and lithium.[60] Hemodialysis is contraindicated if the toxic substance is not effectively dialyzable (Table 99-4), if effective antidotes are available, and in the presence of shock or serious coagulopathy.

Hemoperfusion is the parenteral analogue of oral-activated charcoal. Its indications and contraindications are similar to those mentioned for hemodialysis. Hemoperfusion is not limited by low water solubility, high molecular weight, or increased protein binding. Hemoperfusion has been used effectively to enhance the elimination of carbamazepine, phenobarbital, phenytoin, and theophylline.

OBSERVATION AND DISPOSITION

Selected overdose patients need in-hospital observation if the substance ingested has the potential for delayed or prolonged complications. Drugs such as iron, acetaminophen, and mercury have a latent phase and show evidence of organ dysfunction 48 to 72 hours after ingestion. Some agents have prolonged effects, such as hemorrhagic colitis after a mercury overdose or disseminated intravascular coagulation after snake bites.

The disposition of a poisoned patient is usually a team effort, including a primary care physician, a psychiatrist, and a social worker. Continued follow-up is usually necessary and should be arranged. Patient education is an important

TABLE 99-3. Toxins Not Adsorbed by Charcoal

Acids	Ipecac
Alkalis	Lithium
Bromide	Malathion
Cyanide	Methanol
DDT	N-Methylcarbamate
Ethanol	Potassium
Ethylene glycol	Tobramycin
Ferrous sulfate	Tolbutamide
Iodide	

DDT, chlorophenothane.

TABLE 99-4. Agents Not Eliminated by Dialysis

Aluminum	Magnesium
Benzodiazepines	Mercury
Carbon tetrachloride	Methaqualone
Chlordiazepoxide	Methotrexate
Chlorpropamide	Narcotics
Cocaine	Organophosphates
Cyanide	PCP
Cyclophosphamide	Phenothiazines
Digoxin	Procainamide
Hallucinogens	Quinidine
Iron	Secobarbital
Isoniazid	Tricyclic antidepressants

PCP, phencyclidine.

adjunct for primary prevention of repeated episodes. Clinicians must maintain a high level of suspicion for child abuse, child neglect, and even elder's abuse and neglect.

PREGNANCY

The physiologic changes of pregnancy should be taken into account when treating the pregnant female patient. Total blood volume and cardiac output are increased through most of the second trimester and throughout the third trimester; this may mask the early signs of hypoperfusion and hypotension associated with some poisonings. When hypotension becomes apparent, the uterine blood supply has already been compromised. Therefore, blood pressure should be continuously monitored and aggressively treated. The tidal volume in pregnancy is increased, thereby lowering the $PaCO_2$. This needs to be taken into account when interpreting arterial blood gas measurements. Antidotes should be used if available and if there is evidence of a serious intoxication. Carbon monoxide is particularly toxic to the fetus; therefore, many recommend aggressive use of hyperbaric oxygenation (Chap. 131). Status epilepticus is life-threatening to the pregnant female and requires the rapid treatment. Consultation with the obstetrician is essential for the best possible results.

TREATMENT REFUSAL: THE UNCOOPERATIVE PATIENT

Any patient who has intentionally ingested a potentially harmful or lethal substance is not rational and cannot refuse treatment. There are several ways to deal with the uncooperative patient. One is to wait until the patient becomes unable to resist. This method is not appropriate in a patient who has ingested large amounts of acetaminophen, which would result in a delay in treatment. Patients who have ingested an immediately life-threatening substance should be restrained, preferably by physical means or by pharmacologic means if necessary, and should then be treated appropriately for the poisoning.

APPENDIX 99-1

TOXICOLOGY INFORMATION

INTERNET TOXICOLOGY RESOURCES

American Association of Poison Control Centers
http://www.nlu.edu/~pharmacy/aapcc.html

California Department of Health Services
http://www.parentsplace.com/readroom/lead/index.html

Drug Abuse Resource
http://www.edu/~martint/pages/drugsabus.htm

Environmental Toxicology Resources
http://www.pitt.edu/~martint/pages/envtox.htm

HyperDOC The National Library of Medicine
http://www.nlm.nih.gov

Medconnect: Medical education for physicians
http://www.medconnect.com/h

Medical, Clinical and Occupational Toxicology Resource Home Page
http://www.pitt.edu/~martini/welcome.htm

National Toxicology Program
http://NTP-server.niehs.nih.gov/

Occupational Medicine and Toxicology Resources
http://www.pitt.edu/~martint/pages/omtoxres.htm

Pharmacy and Pharmacology Resources
http:www.pitt.edu/~martint/pages/pharmres.htm

Poison Control Centre Database
http:aabiomed.nus.sq/PID/PCC/centre.html

The Virtual Medical Center
http:www-sci.lib.uci.edu/~martindale/Medical.html

ToxFAQs/ Agency for Toxic Substances and Disease Registry
http://atsdr

Toxicology Internet Resources
http://www.pitt.edu/~martint/toxres.htm

Toxicology Internet URLs
http://tigger.unic.edu/~crockett/toxlinks.html

Toxicon:Medical Toxicology On-Line
http://www.uic.edu/~crockett/default.html

TriService Toxicology Consortium
http://excalibur.aamrl.wpafb.af.mil/

COMPUTER DATABASES

Chemline, Medline, Toxline, Toxnet
National Library of Medicine
301-496-6193
1-800-638-8480

National Technical Information Service (NTIS)
703-487-4600

Registry of Toxic Effects of Chemicals (RTELS)
(NIO5H)
301-496-6193
1-800-638-8480

Database Vendors With Databases Searchable On-Line by Individuals, Research Institutions, or Medical Libraries

BRS
1200 Route 7
Latham, NY 12110
518-783-1161, 1-800-553-5566, 1-800-833-4707
CA Search (Chemical Abstracts), Biomedical Literature, NTIS (National Technical Information Services), Hazardline, Medline, IRCS Medical Science (full medical paper texts)

Chemical Information Systems, Inc.
7215 York RD
Baltimore, MD 21212
1-800-CIS-USER, 301-321-8440

CTCP (Clinical Toxicology of Commercial Products), RTECS, SPHERE (Medical Aspects of Cutaneously Absorbed Substances)

CompuServe, Inc.
5000 Arlington Centre Blvd
Columbus, OH 43220
614-457-8600, 1-800-848-8900
Hazardline

DIALOG Information Services, Inc.
3460 Hillview Ave
Palo Alto, CA 94304
415-858-3785, 1-800-227-1927, 1-800-982-5838
CA Search (Chemical Abstracts), CRGS—Chemical Regulations and Guidelines System,
EMBAE (Biomedical Literature), Environmental Bibliography, NTIS, OSHA, SCI-
SEARCH (Science Citation Index Current Contents, Medline)

MEDIS
Mead Data Center
9333 Springboro Pk
Dayton, OH 45401
1-800-227-4908
Medline

National Library of Medicine
MEDLARS Management Section
8600 Rockville Pk
Bethesda, MD 20209
301-496-6193
Toxline (Toxicology Literature), Medline (Biomedical Literature), RTECS, Toxnet

NIOSH Mailing List
Publications Officer
NIOSH
5555 Ridge Ave
Cincinnati, OH 45213
513-841-4287

Oak Ridge National Laboratory
P.O. Box 2008
Oak Ridge, TN 37831
615-576-1743
ICE database (Radioisotopes—Health Effects)

SDC Information Services
2500 Colorado Avenue
Santa Monica, CA 90406
213-453-6194, 1-800-352-6689
CA Search, NTIS

Seafood Safety Line (Food and Drug Administration)
Rockville, MD
1-800-332-4010

STN International
c/o Chemical Abstracts Service
P.O. Box 3012
Columbus, OH 43210
614-421-3600, 1-800-848-6533
CA Search

National Occupational Hazard Survey
513-841-4491

"Turkey Talk" Line
(Butterball Turkey Company)
1-800-323-4848 November–December only

Toxicology Information and Scientific Evaluation Group
National Toxicology Program
301-496-1152

NIOSH Information System
Cincinnati, OH
1-800-356-4674

Rapid-Response Literature Searches (Fee for Service)

Toxicology Information Response Center (TIRC)
Oak Ridge National Laboratory (ORNL)
615-576-1743

GENERAL

American Medical Association
Department of Drugs (Identification of Foreign Drugs)
Chicago, IL 60610
312-464-4572

Poisindex-Micromedex Inc.
660 Baccock St, Suite 350
Denver, CO 80204
1-800-525-9083

View Data System–Scottish Poisons Information Bureau
Royal Infirmary
Edinburgh
EH3, 9YW, Scotland

INFORMATION RESOURCE AGENCIES

Agency for Toxic Substances and Disease Registry (ATSDR)
Emergency Response Coordinators—24 hours
404-452-4100 days
404-329-2888 nights, weekends

Cancer Information Service (National Cancer Institute)
Office of Cancer Communication
NCI Building 31, Room 10A18
Bethesda, MD 20205
1-800-4-CANCER
5:00 AM to 9:00 PM PST

Center for Occupational Hazards (Art Hazards Information Center)
5 Beekman St
New York, NY 10038
212-227-6220
10:00 AM to 5:00 PM Monday–Friday

Chemical Transportation Emergency Center
(CHEMTREC)
2501 M St, NW
Washington, DC 20037
1-800-424-9300, 202-887-110—24 h

Chevron/Ortho Emergency Information Center
415-233-3737 (collect)—24 h

Drug Abuse Warning Network (DAWN)
8905 Fairview Rd
Silver Spring, MD 20910
1-800-FYI-DAWN

National Animal Poison Control Center
University of Illinois
College of Veterinary Medicine
2001 S. Lincoln

Urbana, IL 61801
900-680-0000 $0.20 first 5 min/$2.95 each additional min
1-800-548-2423 $30 flat fee

National Center for Drugs and Biologics
HFN-310
Food and Drug Administration
5600 Fishers Ln
Rockville, MD 20857
301-443-2895

National Institute for Environmental Health Sciences (NIEHS)
Dr. Edward Gardner Jr, Program Director
Research Grants Programs
Extramural Program
NIEHS
P.O. Box 12233
Research Triangle Park, NC 27709
919-541-3345
8:30 AM to 5:00 PM

National Pesticide Telecommunications Network
Department of Preventive Medicine, School of Medicine
Texas Technical University Health Sciences Center
Lubbock, TX 79430
1-800-858-7378 (toll-free in U.S.)—24 h
1-806-743-3091 (outside of U.S., non–toll-free)—24 h

National Response Center (Oil and Chemical Spills)
U.S. Coast Guard Headquarters
2100 2nd St, SW, Room 2611
Washington, DC 20590
1-800-424-8802, 202-426-2675—24 h

Office of Toxic Substances (Environmental Protection Agency)
401 M St, SW
Washington, DC 20460
202-382-3813

Office of Consumer Affairs, HFE-88
Food and Drug Administration
5600 Fishers Ln
Rockville, MD 20857

U.S. Agency for Toxic Substances and Disease Registry
Atlanta, GA 30333
Emergency Response
404-452-4100, 404-329-2888—24 h
415-974-8927 PST

GOVERNMENT AGENCIES

Washington, DC Area

Animal and Plant Health Inspection Service (Animal Vaccines)
U.S. Department of Agriculture
Washington, DC 20250
202-436-8633

Bureau of Alcohol, Tobacco, and Firearms
Room 4402
Ariel Rios Federal Building
1200 Pennsylvania Ave, NW
Washington, DC 20226
202-566-7135

Consumer Product Safety Commission
Washington, DC 20207
1-800-638-CPSC

Drug Enforcement Administration
U.S. Department of Justice
1405 Eye St, NW
Washington, DC 20537
202-633-1000

Environmental Protection Agency
401 M St, SW
Washington, DC 20460
202-829-3535

Federal Trade Commission
6th St and Pennsylvania Ave, NE
Washington, DC 20580
202-523-3598

Food and Drug Administration
Office of Consumer Affairs (HFE-88)
5600 Fishers Ln
Rockville, MD 20857
301-443-3170

Food and Safety Inspection Service
U.S. Department of Agriculture
Meat and Poultry Hotline, Room 1163S
Washington, DC 20250
1-800-535-4555
10 AM–4 PM EDT

National Institute for Occupational Safety and Health
NIOSH Regional Offices
513-533-8236

National Institute on Drug Abuse
5600 Fishers Ln, Room 10A43
Rockville, MD 20857
301-443-6500

National Marine Fisheries Service
U.S. Department of Commerce
Washington, DC 20235
202-634-7111

Nuclear Regulatory Commission
Office of Public Affairs
Washington, DC 20555
202-492-7715

Atlanta

Centers for Disease Control
Atlanta, GA
404-639-2888

HHS, PHS, CDC, NIOSH
101 Marietta Tower, Suite 1007
Atlanta, GA 30323
404-221-2396

Boston

HHS, PHS, CDC, NIOSH, Region I
JFK Federal Building, Room 1401
Boston, MA 02203
617-223-4045

Denver

HHS, PHS, CDC, NIOSH, Region VIII
1194 Federal Office Building
Denver, CO 80294
303-837-6382, 703-487-4600

NTIS (National Technical Information Service)
703-487-4600

RTELS (Registry of Toxic Effects of Chemicals)
(NIOSH)
301-496-6193, 1-800-638-8480

Canada

Canadian Transportation Emergency Center (C.A.N.V.T.E.C.)
Ottawa, Canada
613-996-6666

Canadian Chemical Referred Center
Ottawa, Canada
613-237-6215

INFORMATION CENTERS

Chemicals 615-574-7797
Environmental Mutagens 615-574-7871
Environmental Teratology 615-574-7871
Toxicology Data 615-574-7587

Information Response to Chemical Concerns (IRCC)
IRCC Project Coordinating Officer
National Institute of Environmental Health Sciences
P.O. Box 12233
Research Triangle Park, NC 27709

Modified from Eilers MA, Garrison TE: Toxicologic problems: general management principles. In: Rosen P, Barkin RM (eds). Emergency Medicine: Concepts and Clinical Practices, ed 3, vol 3. St Louis, Mosby–Year Book, 1992:2476.

REFERENCES ■

1. Mann J: *Murder, Magic and Medicine.* New York, Oxford University Press, 1992
2. American Heritage Dictionary, ed 2. Boston, Houghton Mifflin, 1991
3. Timbrell JA: Introduction to toxicology. London, Taylor & Francis, 1989
4. Geiling EHK, Cannon PR: Pathological effects of elixir of sulfanilamide (diethylene glycol) poisoning: a clinical and experimental correlation—final report. *JAMA* 1938;111:919
5. Modell W: Mass drug catastrophes and the roles of science and technology. *Science* 1967;156:346
6. Gershanik J, Boecler B, Ensley H, et al: The gasping syndrome and benzyl alcohol poisoning. *N Engl J Med* 1982;307:1384
7. Vorgas J, Uitto J, Jimenez SA: The cause and pathogenesis of eosinophilia-myalgia syndrome associated with tryptophan use. *N Engl J Med* 1990;323:357
8. Jones DV, Work CE: Volume of a swallow. *Am J Dis Child* 1964;102:427
9. Flomenbaum NE: General management of the poisoned or overdosed patient. In: Goldfrank LR (ed). *Toxicologic Emergencies.* Norwalk, CT, Appleton and Lange, 1994:25
10. Corin MI: *The Febrile Child: Clinical Management of Fever and Other Types of Pyrexia.* New York, Wiley, 1982
11. Tomarken JL, Britt BA: Malignant hyperthermia. *Ann Emerg Med* 1987;16:1253
12. Benowitz NL, Goldschalger N: Cardiac disturbances in toxicologic patient. In: Haddad LM, Winchester FJ (eds). *Clinical*

Management of Poisoning and Drug Overdose. Philadelphia, WB Saunders, 1983:65

13. Mofenson HC, Caraccio TR: *Initial Evaluation and Management of the Poisoned Patient.* Viccellio, Pleds, Little, Brown 1993

14. DaSilvia AMT: Management of respiratory complications. In: Haddad LM, Wincherster JF (eds). *Clinical Management of Poisoning and Drug Overdose.* Philadelphia, WB Saunders, 1990:198

15. Menzel DB, McCellan RO: Toxic responses of the respiratory system. In: Cassaret JL, Doull J, Klaasen CD (eds). *Cassaret and Doull's Toxicology: The Basic Science of Poisons.* New York, Macmillan, 1986:330

16. Garay SM: Pulmonary principles. In: LK Goldfrank (ed). *Toxicologic Emergencies.* New York, Appleton-Century-Crofts, 1985:80

17. Shanies HM: Noncardiac pulmonary edema. *Med Clin North Am* 1977;61:1319

18. Benowitz NL, Goldschalger N: Cardiac disturbances. In: Haddad LM, Winchester FJ (eds). *Clinical Management of Poisoning and Drug Overdose.* Philadelphia, WB Saunders, 1990:63

19. Hessler R: Cardiovascular principles. In: Goldfrank LR (ed). *Toxicologic Emergencies.* Norwalk, CT, Appleton & Lange, 1994:181

20. Stratmann HGG, Kennedy HL: Torsades de pointes associated with drugs and toxins: recognition and management. *Am Heart J* 1987;113:1470

21. Bates B: *A Guide to Physical Examination and History Taking,* ed 6. Philadelphia, JB Lippincott, 1995

22. Teasdale G, Knill-Jones R, Van Der Sande J: Observer variability in assessing impaired consciousness and coma. *J Neurol Neurosurg Psychiatry* 1978;41:603

23. Plum F, Posner J: *The Diagnosis of Stupor and Coma,* ed 3. Philadelphia, FA Davis, 1982

24. Montgomery BM, Pinner CA: Transient hypoglycemic hemiplegia. *Arch Intern Med* 1964;114:680

25. Haddad LM, Roberts JR: A general approach to the emergency management of poisoning. In: Haddad LM, Winchester JF (eds). *Clinical Management of Poisoning and Drug Overdose.* Philadelphia, WB Saunders, 1990:2

26. Curtis RA, Barone J, Giacona N: Efficacy of ipecac and activated charcoal/cathartic. *Arch Intern Med* 1984;144:48

27. Kulig K, Bar-Or D, Cantrill SV, et al: Management of acutely poisoned patients without gasrtic emptying. *Ann Emerg Med* 1985;14:562

28. Blake DR, Bramble MG, Evans JG: Is there excessive use of gastric lavage in the treatment of self poisoning? *Lancet* 1978;ii:1362

29. Park GD, Spector R, Goldberg MJ, et al: Expanded role of charcoal therapy in the poison and drug overdose patient. *Arch Intern Med* 1986;146:969

30. Crome P, Dawling S, Braithwaite RA, et al: Effect of activated charcoal on absorption of nortriptyline. *Lancet* 1977;ii:1203

31. Pond S, Jacobs M, Marks J, et al: Treatment of digitoxin overdose with oral activated charcoal. *Lancet* 1981;ii:1177

32. Berg MJ, Berlinger WG, Goldberg MJ, et al: Acceleration of the body clearance of phenobarbital by oral activated charcoal. *N Engl J Med* 1982;307:642

33. Berlinger WG, Spector R, Goldberg MJ, et al: Theophylline clearance by oral activated charcoal. *Clin Pharmacol Ther* 1983;33:351

34. Comstock EG, Faulkner TP, Boisaubin E, et al: Studies on the efficacy of gastric emptying as practiced in a large metropolitan hospital. *Clin Toxicol* 1981;18:581

35. Tanberg D, Driven BG, McLeod JW: Ipecac-induced emesis

verses gastric lavage: a controlled study in normal adults. *Am J Emerg Med* 1986;4:205

36. Gorbcich PA, Lacouture PG, Lovejoy FH: Effect of fluid volume on ipecac-induced emesis. *J Pediatr* 1987;110:970

37. Chafec-Bahamon C, Lacouture PG, Lovejoy FH Jr: Risk assessment of ipecac in the home. *Pediatrics* 1985;75:1105

38. Pollack MM, Dunbar BS, Holbrook PR et al: Aspiration of activated charcoal and gastric contents. *Ann Emerg Med* 1981;10:528

39. Tandberg D, Liechty EJ, Fishbein D: Mallory-Weiss syndrome: an unusual complication of ipecac-induced emesis. *Ann Emerg Med* 1981;10:521

40. Klein-Schwartz W, Gorman RL, Oderda GM et al: Ipecac use in the elderly: the unanswered question. *Ann Emerg Med* 1984;13:1152

41. Wolowodiuk OJ, McMicken DB, O'Brien P: Pneumomediastinum and retropneumoperitoneum: an unusual complication of syrup of ipecac-induced emesis. *Ann Emerg Med* 1984;13:1148

42. Robertson WO: Syrup of ipecac associated fatality. *Vet Hum Toxicol* 1979;21:87

43. Kulig KW, Bar-Or D, Cantrill SV, et al: Management of acutely poisoned patients without gastric emptying. *Ann Emerg Med* 1985;14:562

44. Wald P, Stern J ,Weiner B, et al: Esophageal tear following forceful removal of an impacted oral-gastric lavage tube. *Ann Emerg Med* 1986;15:80

45. Askenasi R, Abramowicz M, Jeanmart J, et al: Esophageal perforation: an unusual complication of gastirc lavage. *Ann Emerg Med* 1984;13:146

46. Park GD, Spector R, Goldberg MJ, et al: Expanded role of charcoal therapy in the poison and drug overdose patient. *Arch Intern Med* 1986;146:969

47. Fiser RH, Maetz HM, Treuting JJ, et al: Activated charcoal in barbiturate and glutethimide poisoning. *J Pediatr* 1971;78:1045

48. Henderson A, Wright DM, Pond SM: Experience with 732 acute overdose patients admitted to an intensive care unit over 6 years. *Med J Aust* 1993;158:28

49. Litovitz TL, Holm KC, Bailey KM, et al: 1991 Annual Report of the American Association of Poison Control Centers National Data Collection System. *Am J Emerg Med* 1992;10:452

50. Cherskov M: Extracorporeal detoxification: still debatable. *JAMA* 1982;247:3047

51. Lorch JA, Garella S: Hemoperfusion to treat intoxications. *Ann Intern Med* 1978;19:301

52. Winchester JF: Evolution of artificial organs: extracorporeal removal of drugs. *Artif Organ* 1986;10:316

53. Morgan AG, Polak A: The excretion of salicylate in salicylate poisoning. *Clin Sci* 1971;41:475

54. Linton AL, Luke RG, Briggs JD: Methods of forced diuresis and its application in barbiturate poisoning. *Lancet* 1967;ii:377

55. Prescott LF, Park J, Darrien I: Treatment of severe 2,4-D and mecoprop intoxication with alkaline diuresis. *J Clin Pharmacol* 1979;7:110

56. Chan H, Evans WE, Pratt CB: Recovery from toxicity associated with high-dose methotrexate: prognostic factors. *Cancer Treat Rep* 1977;61:797

57. McCoy HG, Cipolle RY, Ehlers SM, et al: Severe methanol poisoning: application of pharmacokinetic model for ethanol therapy and hemodialysis. *Am J Med* 1979;67:804

58. Parry MF, Wallach R: Ethylene glycol poisoning. *Am J Med* 1974;57:143

59. Hill JB: Salicylate intoxication. *N Engl J Med* 1973;21:1110

60. Clendeninn NJ, Pond SM, Kaysen G, et al: Potential pitfalls in the evaluation of the usefulness of hemodialysis for the removal of lithium. *J Toxicol Clin Toxicol* 1982;19:341

Critical Care, Third Edition, edited by Joseph M. Civetta,
Robert W. Taylor, and Robert R. Kirby.
Lippincott-Raven Publishers, Philadelphia, PA © 1997.

CHAPTER 100

∎

Toxicology: Specific Drugs and Poisons

Richard P. Ryskamp
Robert W. Taylor

This chapter focuses on the care of patients with common drug overdoses and poisonings. A complete toxicologic work is beyond the scope of this chapter. Therefore, the most common and problematic drugs and toxins are presented in a detailed fashion, whereas less common or serious poisonings receive less emphasis. The general approach to the poisoned patient is presented in Chapter 99. Substance abuse and withdrawal from alcohol, cocaine, and opioids is covered in Chapter 101.

ACETAMINOPHEN ∎

N-acetyl-p-aminophenol, or APAP, known as acetaminophen in the United States and as paracetamol in many other countries, is probably the most popular antipyretic and analgesic in the world. It is also an ingredient in numerous "cold" and "flu" medications and in many prescription analgesics. It is a remarkably safe drug at standard doses, but because of its wide availability, overdoses are common. The initial clinical presentation in overdose is usually bland, but without prompt antidote therapy, untreated patients are at risk to develop potentially fatal hepatic necrosis 1 to 4 days later.

TOXICOLOGY

Acetaminophen is metabolized primarily in the liver, where most is converted to inactive compounds by conjugation with sulfate and glucuronide, and then excreted by the kidney. A minor metabolite of acetaminophen is responsible for toxic-

ity in overdose, not acetaminophen itself or its principal metabolites. A small portion, usually less than 5%, is metabolized by the hepatic cytochrome P-450 mixed-function oxidase enzyme system to a toxic metabolite believed to be *N*-acetyl-benzoquinoneimine. This toxic metabolite has a propensity to react with sulfhydryl groups. At usual doses, it is quickly detoxified by combining irreversibly with the sulfhydryl group of glutathione to produce a nontoxic conjugate that is then uneventfully excreted by the kidney. However, in an overdose situation, hepatocellular supplies of glutathione become exhausted and the toxic metabolite is free to react with cellular membrane molecules, resulting in widespread hepatocyte damage and death, apparent clinically as acute hepatic necrosis. The antidote to acetaminophen overdose, *N*-acetylcysteine (NAC), presumably works primarily by supplying sulfhydryl groups to react with the toxic metabolite so that it does not damage cells. Other mechanisms of action also may come into play. If given within 8 hours of ingestion, NAC reliably prevents toxicity. Beyond 8 hours after ingestion, there is a sharp decline in its effectiveness because the cascade of toxic events in the liver has already begun.

Damage generally occurs preferentially in hepatocytes because this is where acetaminophen is metabolized and where the toxic metabolite is produced. However, acute renal failure also may occur. In some cases, this is secondary to the hepatic failure, for instance, in hepatorenal syndrome or multiple organ system failure. But in other cases, acute renal failure may be the primary clinical manifestation of toxicity. It is thought that in these cases, for some reason, a significant amount of toxic metabolite is produced in the kidney and less is produced in the liver. Considerable toxicity also can occur in myocytes and pancreatic cells, manifested clinically as myocarditis and pancreatitis.

The susceptibility to toxicity from acetaminophen overdose is highly variable. In adults, single doses above 10 g or 140 mg/kg have a reasonable likelihood of causing toxicity. Single doses above 25 g have a high risk of lethality.[1] Toxicity also can occur with multiple smaller doses when the total dose within 24 hours exceeds these levels. Toxicity may occur with smaller doses when taken repeatedly.

Some patients demonstrate an increased susceptibility to toxicity, which has occurred in adults with doses reported as low as 4 g/day. Death has occurred after overdoses as small as 6 g. Fasting seems to be a risk factor,[2] probably because of depleted glutathione stores. Chronic ingestion of barbiturates or antituberculous medications,[3] especially isoniazid,[4] also increase the susceptibility for toxicity, presumably because of stimulation of the P-450 oxidase system. Chronic alcohol ingestion also may be a risk factor.

CLINICAL MANIFESTATIONS

Patients generally have nonspecific symptoms, or even no symptoms, during the first 12 to 24 hours. Anorexia, nausea, vomiting, and diaphoresis are common initially but often resolve after several hours. Only in massive overdoses have life-threatening clinical manifestations (coma and metabolic acidosis) been observed early, before the onset of hepatic failure.[5]

Evidence of liver toxicity may develop in 1 to 4 days, although in severe cases evidence may appear in 12 hours. Right upper quadrant pain and tenderness may be present. Laboratory studies may show evidence of massive hepatic necrosis with markedly elevated transaminase values, elevated bilirubin, and prolonged coagulation times. When transaminase levels exceed 1000 IU/L, acetaminophen-induced hepatotoxicity can be diagnosed, although levels may exceed 10,000 IU/L. Generally, the aspartate aminotransferase is somewhat higher than the alanine aminotransferase.

In some cases, massive hepatic necrosis leads to fulminant hepatic failure with complications of bleeding, hypoglycemia, renal failure, hepatic encephalopathy, cerebral edema, sepsis, multiple organ failure, and death. In many cases, the hepatic necrosis may run its course, hepatic function may return, and the patient may survive with liver function returning to normal in a few weeks.

TREATMENT

Uncomplicated overdoses are managed with gastrointestinal decontamination and NAC administration. The efficacy of NAC depends on the promptness of its administration. The sooner it is given the better, but a reliably good outcome is secured if it is administered within 8 hours of acetaminophen ingestion. After 8 hours, the risk of acute hepatic necrosis and death starts to rise. The guidelines for NAC administration are clearly defined, but there is considerable room for the physician's own judgment regarding gastric lavage and activated charcoal administration.

Circumstances determine whether the potential benefits of gastric lavage or activated charcoal outweigh the risks and disadvantages. Acetaminophen absorption from the gastrointestinal tract is complete within 2 hours under normal circumstances, although this can be somewhat slowed when ingested with food and markedly slowed when ingested in massive amounts or together with drugs that slow gastrointestinal motility. Ipecac has no role because it is not effective at removing ingested drug and because the vomiting that it induces delays administering activated charcoal and NAC.

Gastric lavage is routinely helpful only within 2 or perhaps 4 hours of ingestion. Coingestion of food or drugs that reduce gastric motility may make lavage worthwhile for 24 hours after ingestion.

Activated charcoal is more often potentially helpful than gastric lavage. Activated charcoal adsorbs acetaminophen well and thus reduces its gastrointestinal absorption if given soon enough after an ingestion. It carries much less risk of pulmonary complications than gastric lavage. Formerly, there has been reluctance to give charcoal in acetaminophen ingestion because of concern that the charcoal might also adsorb the NAC. It is doubtful that this concern is justified. Studies have shown that the amount of NAC adsorbed by charcoal is no more than 39% when both are given together,[6] and other studies have shown less or no significant difference.[7] Spiller and others[8] found no adverse effect on clinical outcome when both charcoal and NAC were administered. In fact, charcoal seemed to be beneficial to the clinical outcome.

There is fairly uniform agreement in favor of charcoal administration up to 4 hours after ingestion. Charcoal can be administered beyond 4 hours after ingestion at the clinician's discretion; it is generally a benign therapy. Certainly, if concern exists that there may be coingestion of other drugs for which charcoal is indicated, then charcoal should be given.

There are conflicting recommendations regarding whether or how to modify the NAC regimen after charcoal is given. One option is to use lavage to remove the charcoal after an hour and then administer the NAC, but it is questionable whether removal of the charcoal is so important that it is worth the risk of an extra gastric lavage. It is probably better to leave the charcoal in the stomach and to proceed with the usual *N*-acylcysteine regimen either immediately or after waiting an hour, or to increase the loading dose of NAC by 40%.[9] The problem with increasing the dose of NAC is that this may aggravate nausea and vomiting, which already can be a problem at lower doses of NAC because of the combined effects of acetaminophen toxicity, NAC, and charcoal; giving even more NAC may not be realistic or necessary.

In actual practice, the issue is not usually too difficult to resolve. If almost 8 hours or more have elapsed since a potentially toxic ingestion, then charcoal is probably not useful, and NAC should be given as soon as possible. In fresher ingestions, one can give charcoal as soon as the patient arrives, wait until the acetaminophen level returns from the laboratory, and still give NAC within the 8-hour period during which it is maximally effective. If repeat doses of charcoal are indicated because of another ingested drug, then the subsequent doses of charcoal and NAC can each be given staggered every 2 hours.

Serum acetaminophen level is used to help assess the risk of potential toxicity of an overdose. When the time of ingestion is known, the acetaminophen toxicity nomogram depicted in Figure 100-1 is used to assess the likelihood of toxicity.[10] If ingestion occurred more than 4 hours before admission, the level should be drawn on arrival and run immediately. An acetaminophen level drawn within 4 hours of ingestion cannot be used to estimate risk because absorption may not be complete. If time of ingestion is not known but may have been within 4 hours, an acetaminophen level should be drawn immediately and then repeated in 2 or 4 hours to ensure that the peak level has been found. When using the nomogram, remember that the history of the time of ingestion may be inaccurate, and also keep in mind the factors that may increase the susceptibility of some patients to toxicity.

If clinical suspicion of a toxic overdose is high, if laboratory turnaround time for acetaminophen level is not rapid, or if it is almost 8 hours or more since ingestion, it is prudent to begin NAC administration immediately. Therapy may be stopped later only if the acetaminophen level documents a nontoxic overdose. It may also be prudent to initiate therapy, based on a reliable history of ingestion of a potentially toxic quantity of acetaminophen, even if the serum level falls in

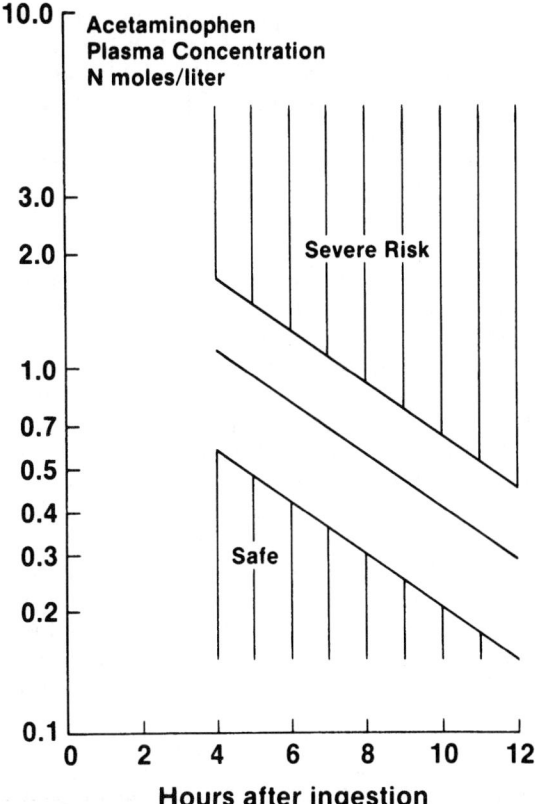

FIGURE 100-1. Semilogarithmic plot of plasma acetaminophen level versus time modified from Rumack and Matthews.[10] A single plasma acetaminophen level drawn 4 hours after ingestion is useful in predicting hepatotoxicity. Serum levels drawn before 4 hours may not represent peak levels. The graph is useful only for a single ingestion.

the safe range initially; there may be delayed absorption or a laboratory error.

NAC is given enterally as a 140 mg/kg loading dose, and then 70 mg/kg every 4 hours for 17 more doses. It can be a difficult medication to administer because of its taste and its tendency to cause nausea and vomiting. To maximize tolerance, it should be diluted down to a 5% solution from the commercially available 10% or 20% solution. It can be diluted with fruit juice or soda to improve taste. To minimize the smell, it should be served ice cold in a cup with a lid and a straw.

If patients refuse or are unable to drink it, it must be given through a tube. Giving the initial loading dose through the gastric lavage tube often is convenient. If the NAC is vomited, consider administering an antiemetic such as droperidol, metoclopramide, or ondansetron and then readminister the dose, perhaps more diluted or more slowly. It can also be given through a nasogastric or nasoduodenal tube, even as a slow infusion.

NAC is an extremely safe drug. The enteral preparation has problems with taste, odor, and gastric tolerance, and occasionally skin rash occurs, but life-threatening adverse reactions do not occur. It is also indicated for pregnant patients with acetaminophen toxicity. The manufacturer's recommendation is avoidance of administration if an encephalopathy is present because of the theoretical concerns that it may worsen encephalopathy. However, studies have shown that it is safe even under these circumstances.[11,12]

Intravenous NAC is used routinely outside of the United States and is available within the United States as an investigational drug. It is an option for patients who cannot tolerate enteral NAC or for whom enteral intake is contraindicated. It has occasionally been associated with allergic reactions such as anaphylaxis and bronchospasm. If it is needed, the physician may call the Rocky Mountain Poison and Drug Center at 1-800-525-6115. The usual regimen for intravenous administration has been 300 mg/kg over 20 hours, but a new regimen of 980 mg/kg over 48 hours seems to more effective, especially when administration is delayed.[13]

Baseline liver laboratory studies should be obtained initially in a patient with a potentially toxic acetaminophen overdose. Studies should include bilirubin, aspartate aminotransaminase, alanine aminotransaminase, and prothrombin time. Studies should be repeated daily.

NAC is most effective when given within 8 hours of ingestion. Under these circumstances, serious hepatotoxicity has been rare. Prognosis is also excellent if liver study results are normal at the time that the first dose of NAC is given; there have been no reported fatalities in this group.

NAC is still efficacious when started beyond 8 hours after toxic ingestion and clearly should be given,[12] although risk of hepatic failure and death rises as delay increases. Patients with liver toxicity from subacute or chronic acetaminophen overdose also may benefit and should also receive NAC.[14] The same is true even if fulminant hepatic failure and multiple organ system failure are already present.[15] There are apparently other mechanisms by which NAC works besides providing sulfhydryl groups during the metabolism of acetaminophen. Possible mechanisms include an antioxidant action, improved oxygen delivery through microcirculatory changes, a modulation of the immune response, or enhancement of cells' ability to survive by helping them repair damage. Once it has been determined that a potentially toxic overdose has occurred, NAC must be continued for the entire 18-dose, 72-hour course, even after acetaminophen becomes undetectable in the blood. Patients do not necessarily have to remain in the intensive care unit (ICU), although they should remain under close medical supervision.

If hepatic failure develops, NAC should be continued beyond the standard 18 doses until hepatic function improves or until the patient dies or has a liver transplant.[11,12]

Most patients with acetaminophen-induced fulminant hepatic failure survive, but there is significant mortality. The mortality rate starts to climb on day 2 after the ingestion, reaches a maximum on day 4, and then gradually decreases. Patients with a poor prognosis must be identified early and transferred expeditiously to a center capable of liver transplantation. Timeliness is crucial. Often there is only a window of 1 to 2 days between the onset of fulminant hepatic failure and the onset of complications that make the patient unfit for receipt of a transplant. Such complications include cerebral edema, shock, and infection.

Acidemia is the most ominous indicator of probable mortality and thus of the need for transplant. A mortality rate of 95% without transplant was reported in patients who had a documented serum pH of less than 7.30.[16] Other indicators of a poor prognosis include renal insufficiency, grade 3 or worse hepatic encephalopathy, a markedly elevated prothrombin time, or a rise in prothrombin time from day 3 to day 4.[17] Pereira and coworkers[18] found that a factor V level less than 10% of normal indicated a bad prognosis (91% mortality), and a ratio of factor VIII to factor V of less than 30 indicated a good prognosis (100% survival).

Although liver transplant can give a second chance to some who would otherwise have died, many others die awaiting donor livers, and there is significant mortality even in those who do receive livers. Prevention of acetaminophen toxicity is clearly preferable, and physicians must be diligent to help prevent such outcomes. Because of the ubiquity of acetaminophen, the blandness of the early clinical manifestations, and the effectiveness of antidote therapy, it is prudent to check an acetaminophen level on all patients presenting with intentional overdose of any drug. If a potentially toxic quantity of acetaminophen has been ingested, treatment must be prompt and adequate. Acetaminophen poisoning also should be considered in the differential diagnosis of patients presenting with fulminant hepatic failure or acute hepatitis, and NAC administration is probably beneficial even when the diagnosis is made beyond 48 hours after ingestion.

SALICYLATES ■

Salicylates are available in a wide variety of prescription and nonprescription preparations. By far the most popular, aspirin (acetylsalicylic acid) has been available as a medication since 1899. Aspirin also is an ingredient in several popular prescription medications such as Norgesic, Percodan and Fiorinal. Other salicylates include the following: bismuth subsalicylate, an ingredient in Pepto-Bismol, recently popularized for its role in treating *Helicobacter pylori* infections and traveler's diarrhea; choline magnesium trisalicylate (Trilisate); choline salicylate (Arthropan); magnesium salicylate (Doan's caplets); and salicylsalicylic acid or salsalate (Disalcid). Bismuth subsalicylate ingestion can be suspected by the presence of radiopaque densities seen on plain radiographs of the abdomen.[19,20]

Poisoning also can occur from topical exposure to salicylates, which are found in products such as Ben-Gay, Aspercreme, and various keratolytics and sunscreens. Oil of wintergreen is a particularly potent source of salicylate, each teaspoon containing the same amount of salicylate as 7 g of aspirin.[21] Oil of wintergreen ingestion may be detected by the characteristic odor.

TOXICOLOGY

After ingestion, aspirin and most other salicylates are rapidly converted to salicylic acid, the biologically active salicylate. Salicylic acid exerts its therapeutic action by inhibiting prostaglandin synthesis. After single therapeutic doses, salicylic acid is metabolized by the liver and eliminated within 2 to 3 hours. However, after repeated or toxic doses, hepatic enzymes become saturated and serum half-life can become prolonged to more than 24 hours. At such high levels, renal excretion increases significantly and becomes the predominant route of elimination, although renal function itself may become a casualty of severe or prolonged salicylate toxicity.

At toxic levels, salicylate is a metabolic poison, interfering with glucose metabolism by uncoupling oxidative phosphorylation. Mitochondria become unable to produce sufficient amounts of adenosine triphosphate (ATP), the vital intracellular energy source, despite excessive consumption of glucose and excessive production of carbon dioxide. Cellular dysfunction and injury occur. The brain, being exquisitely dependent on glucose metabolism, is particularly vulnerable to salicylate-induced toxicity and damage.

Salicylic acid's acid-base behavior contributes to its deadliness at toxic doses, and an important factor in the course of salicylate poisoning is the presence or absence of acidosis. Salicylic acid is a weak acid with a pKa of 3.0. At a normal physiologic pH of 7.4, 99% of it is ionized as salicylate and unable to diffuse into the intracellular compartment. However, as acidemia develops, more and more of the salicylate becomes nonionized and able to diffuse into cells. At a pH of 7.2, twice as much salicylate is nonionized as at a pH of 7.4, greatly increasing its tendency to penetrate into and accumulate in tissues such as brain, and greatly increasing the subsequent toxicity.[22]

Salicylic acid has its own impact on the body's acid-base balance. In mild to moderate salicylate toxicity, there is a stimulation of the medullary respiratory center, apparent clinically first as increased depth of respiration and then also as increased respiratory rate. A respiratory alkalosis results. The kidneys' response to the respiratory alkalosis is a bicarbonate diuresis, creating a compensatory metabolic acidosis.

Severe toxicity is associated with the development of a primary metabolic acidosis, usually of the increased anion gap variety.[23] Its etiology is incompletely understood. The acidity of salicylate itself contributes only a small part of the acidosis. Much of the rest can be explained by the production of ketoacids and lactic acid secondary to the uncoupling of oxidative phosphorylation. The onset of a metabolic acidosis is ominous: it not only is a sign of cellular metabolic distress, but it begets even greater toxicity as more and more salicylate becomes nonionized and enters cells—a deadly positive feedback process. Acidosis is a marker of severe salicylate toxicity and is usually associated with evidence of cellular dysfunction, especially brain dysfunction.[24] Correction of acidosis is therefore fundamental in treating salicylate toxicity.

When only salicylate is involved in a poisoning, respiratory acidosis does not occur until late in the course of severe toxicity. It occurs in part because of a hypermetabolic state and the marked increase in carbon dioxide production. It is also associated with severe depression of the entire brain, including the respiratory center.

A multidrug overdose may alter the clinical presentation. Many intentional overdoses include sedatives, hypnotics, or other respiratory depressants, which may depress the central nervous system and the respiratory center. The classic early respiratory alkalosis may not occur.[23] Instead, a respiratory acidosis may be seen early in the course. When this occurs, salicylate toxicity is potentiated as diffusion of salicylic acid is facilitated.[22]

CLINICAL MANIFESTATIONS AND DIAGNOSIS

It is important to differentiate between an acute overdose and chronic toxicity. Diagnosis of an acute overdose is relatively easy, and the associated mortality rate is extremely low. Diagnosis of chronic toxicity may be difficult, and mortality rate has been found to be around 15% with many of the survivors having extremely complicated courses.

Salicylate toxicity can occur with an acute ingestion of 150 mg/kg. An ingestion of 500 mg/kg is potentially lethal.[21] Diagnosis of an acute intentional overdose is usually not difficult because a history is generally available; even if the clinician is not told that salicylates were taken, at least it is usually known that some type of drug ingestion has occurred. After an acute oral ingestion, the first symptoms may be gastrointestinal and related to the irritant effects of salicylates on the gastric mucosa; even gastrointestinal bleeding and perforation have occurred. Subsequent symptoms are generally caused by the initially stimulant and then toxic effects of salicylate on the central nervous system: tinnitus, hearing impairment, dizziness, diaphoresis, irritability, and hyperventilation, frequently with complaints of dyspnea. Even if no history is obtainable, the acid-base disturbances often provide a clue that should prompt the performance of a serum salicylate level. As mentioned earlier, the classic initial disturbance is a respiratory alkalosis. In the later stages, a metabolic acidosis, usually with an elevated anion gap, is present. The most frequent presentation is a combination of respiratory alkalosis and metabolic acidosis.[23]

Chronic toxicity is more deadly because of the elevated tissue levels of salicylate, which generally are already causing the cellular, especially central nervous system, dysfunction that led to the patient's presentation for medical care.

Prompt diagnosis of chronic salicylate toxicity is vital; a delay in diagnosis is associated with a significantly worsened prognosis.[24,25] But diagnosis is often delayed or missed for various reasons. Because of altered mental status, a history often is not obtainable; even when patients are capable of giving a history, intoxications are usually accidental; the patient may not think to mention analgesic over-the-counter or topical medications, and the physician may not specifically ask. Acute gastrointestinal symptoms are generally absent, although the presence of abdominal pain and vomiting have led to unwarranted laparotomy.[26] The presentation may mimic other conditions. Hyperventilation, anxiety, agitation, and hallucinations may mimic psychiatric disorders.[27] Seizures and encephalopathy progressing to coma may suggest a primary neurologic problem. Temperature elevations are not uncommon, and the clinical presentation can suggest heat stroke, neuroleptic malignant syndrome, or severe hyperthyroidism. A metabolic acidosis associated with the presence of ketones in the serum may lead to a misdiagnosis of diabetic or alcoholic ketoacidosis; however, the titer of ketones is much lower in salicylate intoxication. The clinical course may resemble sepsis with fever, leukocytosis, immature neutrophils in the peripheral smear, pulmonary infiltrates, encephalopathy, coagulopathy and hypotension with low systemic vascular resistance.[28] Salicylate poisoning must be considered in the differential diagnosis of all of the above presentations, especially when the classic acid-base disturbances are present.

The diagnosis of salicylate overdose or toxicity is usually easily confirmed or ruled out with timely serum salicylate levels. However, the level itself must be interpreted cautiously. A therapeutic level is generally considered to be between 10 and 20 mg/dL. A level above 25 may be well tolerated in an acute overdose, but in chronic overdose the same level may be associated with severe clinical manifestations. This is because after prolonged exposure to persistently high levels of salicylate, the intracellular salicylate level eventually equilibrates with the extracellular level. And, as discussed earlier, in the presence of acidemia this equilibration process is accelerated. Thus, a falling salicylate level in the presence of acidemia may be not a good sign, signaling the diffusion of salicylate into cells rather than clearance out of the body. Thus, a salicylate level must be interpreted in the context of the serum pH and the patient's clinical status.

TREATMENT

The management of salicylate toxicity consists of (1) prevention of further absorption of salicylate; (2) supportive measures, including resuscitation with volume and sodium bicarbonate; and (3) promotion of salicylate clearance by urinary excretion, repeated doses of activated charcoal, or extracorporeal methods.

In acute salicylate ingestion, administration of activated charcoal is the most effective measure to prevent further salicylate absorption and has little associated risk. Activated charcoal binds salicylate in the gut well. The usual dose is 50 to 100 g, or 1 g/kg. Sorbitol is generally added to the initial dose of activated charcoal, and this may reduce gastrointestinal salicylate absorption further,[29] presumably by reducing gut transit time and preventing desorption of salicylate from the charcoal.[30] Repeated doses of activated charcoal are valuable in ensuring complete and continued adsorption of salicylate and also in enhancing salicylate elimination (discussed later).

If performed sufficiently soon after acute ingestion, gastric lavage may be an important adjunct to activated charcoal administration in the prevention of salicylate absorption. The greatest benefit is provided when gastric lavage is both preceded by and followed by activated charcoal.[31] The clinician must use judgment as to whether the anticipated benefit of lavage is worth the associated risk of aspiration. Most salicylates are usually completely absorbed within 3 hours after a therapeutic dose; methylsalicylate can take up to 6 hours to be absorbed. However, absorption may be delayed by 12 hours or more after an acute overdose. Situations favoring delayed absorption include ingestion of enterically coated aspirin and coingestion of food or of drugs that slow gastric motility, such as narcotics or anticholinergics.

Ipecac administration has fallen out of favor because of evidence showing that aspirin absorption is more effectively prevented by activated charcoal administration alone than with ipecac alone or in combination with activated charcoal.[32]

In moderate to severe intoxications, whether acute or chronic, supportive measures must be taken before, during, and after gastrointestinal decontamination. Stabilization of airway, ventilation, and vital signs are the initial top priorities. Common life-threatening complications requiring appropriate management include hyperthermia and hypothermia, hypovolemia, acidosis, hypokalemia, hypoglycemia, hypocalcemia, coagulopathy, hypotension, noncardiogenic pulmonary edema, respiratory failure, coma, and seizures.

Dangerous extremes of temperature should be corrected by external cooling or warming. Hyperpyrexia is common in chronic intoxication because of the marked increase in metabolic rate; temperature should not be allowed to exceed 40C. Hypothermia is especially encountered in acute intoxication.[24] This may be caused by environmental exposure or coingestion of another drug that promotes vasodilation and heat loss, such as alcohol.

Vigorous rehydration is generally necessary because fluid deficits may be large, especially in chronic intoxication. There is often a 2- to 4-L fluid deficit. During the phase of respiratory alkalosis, an osmotic diuresis occurs as the kidneys compensate by wasting bicarbonate, sodium, and potassium. The presence of ketosis also promotes osmotic diuresis. Meanwhile, intake of fluids and electrolytes is usually impaired because of neurologic dysfunction or gastrointestinal symptoms. Hypernatremia may be seen as a result of disproportionately large free water deficits from diaphoresis and hyperventilation.

Oliguria is usually prerenal and responds to correction of hypovolemia. Varying degrees of resistant oliguria may occur, ranging from a transient sodium-avid state to acute tubular necrosis.

Close monitoring of arterial blood gases is essential because of the supreme importance of the prevention or correction of acidemia. The serum pH should be kept around 7.45 to 7.50, and acidemia must be scrupulously avoided. A bolus of sodium bicarbonate over several minutes, 1 to 2 mMol/kg, often is indicated. Subsequent bicarbonate can be added in appropriate amounts to intravenous fluid to maintain the desired mild alkalemia. In most cases, it is reasonable to start with a rate of administration of 1 to 2 mMol/kg/hour.

Spontaneous or iatrogenic hyperventilation may be useful for immediate correction of metabolic acidosis. However, bicarbonate administration is more beneficial, and even patients moderately alkalotic from spontaneous hyperventilation should receive judicious amounts of intravenous bicarbonate. Acetazolamide has been used to alkalinize urine and facilitate salicylate excretion. However, this occurs at the expense of creating a metabolic acidosis and is therefore dangerous and not recommended.

Patients generally present with marked potassium deficits. This is usually primarily from renal potassium wasting during the period of respiratory alkalosis characteristic of the earlier course of salicylate toxicity. If later a metabolic acidosis supervenes, a normal serum potassium may disguise severe depletion, which becomes evident as the acidemia is corrected and potassium reenters cells. Depending on the potassium level, the degree of acidosis, and the degree of oliguria, up to 20 mMol of potassium chloride per hour may have to be given initially. Serum potassium levels must be monitored frequently, especially when serum pH is rising.

Glucose requirements are markedly increased because of reliance on glycolysis rather than oxidative phosphorylation for cellular energy production. In the early stages of salicylate intoxication, gluconeogenesis and glycogenolysis are stimulated, and hyperglycemia may be observed. Later, gluconeogenesis becomes impaired, glycogen stores are exhausted, and severe hypoglycemia can ensue.[33] Therefore, serum glucose level must be monitored closely. Hypoglycemia must be dealt with aggressively, especially because glucose concentrations in the brain can be markedly lower than in the blood.[34] Generally it is wise to be generous with dextrose administration and to ensure a continuous supply of glucose[22]; if needed, insulin can be administered judiciously. Intravenous fluids with 5% or 10% dextrose are recommended. A regimen to consider is to add 100 to 150 mMol of sodium bicarbonate (2 to 3 ampules) to each liter of 5% dextrose in water (D_5W) and use this as the hydration fluid.

The calcium level also should be monitored. Tetany can occur, caused by hypocalcemia aggravated by alkalemia from either salicylate-induced respiratory alkalosis or iatrogenic administration of bicarbonate. Treatment consists of calcium replacement and avoidance of excessive alkalemia.

Coagulopathy can occur, so coagulation studies should be checked. Chronic salicylate toxicity can be associated with deficiency of the vitamin K–dependent coagulation factors. The coagulopathy may respond to vitamin K administration. In severe toxicity, coagulopathy can occur secondary to hepatic dysfunction or disseminated intravascular coagulation, and fresh frozen plasma administration may be needed.

Hypotension is usually caused principally by hypovolemia. In some cases, low systemic vascular resistance may require vasopressors.

Pulmonary edema may complicate the clinical course in more than a third of cases of severe toxicity.[35] Older patient age and chronic intoxication are major risk factors. Most of these cases appear to be noncardiogenic, caused by a capillary leak syndrome.[36] However, myocardial dysfunction and overvigorous hydration can lead to hydrostatic pulmonary edema, and pulmonary artery catheter insertion may be useful.

Intubation and mechanical ventilation may be required for a variety of reasons, including hypoxemia, impending respiratory acidosis, and altered mental status. Cardiac arrests are liable to occur during intubation, perhaps because of transient worsening of acidosis as ventilatory drive is suppressed with sedatives.[37] Ventilation requirements may be increased because of increased carbon dioxide production. Hyperventilation can be used to optimize serum pH initially, and then reduced as serum bicarbonate deficit is replenished.

Stupor, coma, and seizures may be caused directly by salicylate toxicity, but other correctable causes should be considered, especially hypoglycemia and severe acid-base disturbance. Generous dextrose administration may be prudent, even if serum glucose level is normal. Seizures should be aggressively treated, not only to prevent brain injury, but also to prevent worsened acidosis and the associated increase in salicylate toxicity.

In all but the mildest intoxications, it is imperative to enhance salicylate elimination from the body. Extracorporeal removal is the most reliable and rapid way to eliminate salicylates and should be employed immediately in severe intoxications. In mild to moderate intoxications, it is indicated to enhance renal excretion through urinary alkalinization, or to stimulate gastrointestinal elimination by repeated doses of activated charcoal, or both.

Extracorporeal methods of removing salicylate consist of charcoal hemoperfusion and hemodialysis. They are both effective. Charcoal hemoperfusion is simpler and more efficient than hemodialysis, but hemodialysis often is preferable because it can simultaneously correct metabolic derangements such as acidosis. Peritoneal dialysis does remove salicylate but is much less effective than hemodialysis or hemoperfusion and generally is not indicated.

Extracorporeal removal should be employed without delay in cases of severe intoxication or when adequate excretion cannot be obtained through the urine or gastrointestinal tract. Markers for severe toxicity include seizures, coma, and a salicylate level of greater than around 50 mg/dL in chronic toxicity or greater than around 100 mg/dL in acute overdoses. Other indications include renal failure, cerebral edema, and pulmonary edema.

Alkalinization of the urine can be effective in hastening salicylate clearance in cases of mild to moderate salicylate toxicity. Under normal circumstances, urine within the renal tubules is acid, favoring conversion of ionized salicylate to nonionized salicylic acid, which is then reabsorbed rather than excreted. If urine is alkalinized, more salicylate remains trapped in its ionized form within the tubules and cannot

be reabsorbed. Studies show that for each one-unit rise in urinary pH, urinary salicylate clearance increases more than fourfold.[38]

However desirable, alkalinizing the urine is easier said than done. First, enough sodium bicarbonate must be administered to alkalinize the serum to the optimal pH of about 7.5, being careful not to cause tetany or excessive hypervolemia, alkalemia, hypernatremia, or hypokalemia. The large potassium deficits must be corrected before the kidneys will produce alkaline urine. Finally, hypovolemia must be corrected before adequate amounts of urine are produced. All of this may take at least several hours to accomplish. Even then, persistent renal dysfunction can undermine the production of adequate amounts of urine. Contraindications to attempted urinary alkalinization include renal failure, cardiac dysfunction, pulmonary edema, and cerebral edema; in such situations, extracorporeal removal is indicated.

Forced diuresis has been advocated as a way to increase salicylate clearance. However, this provides little or no benefit beyond that provided by alkalinization of the urine, and is probably not worth the associated risks of volume overload and pulmonary and cerebral edema. Although adequate amounts of urine are needed, a copious diuresis adds little to salicylate clearance; certainly, a urine output of 150 mL/hour is adequate.[39]

Salicylate clearance also may be enhanced by administration of repeated doses of activated charcoal.[40,41] Efficacy may exceed that of urinary alkalinization.[40] The two methods seem to have an additive effect.[42] Repeated doses of activated charcoal probably is also effective even in chronic intoxication in which no salicylates are in the gut. The charcoal is believed to work by performing a sort of gastrointestinal dialysis. A dosage of 1 mg/kg every 4 hours can be used. Ileus or gastric distention is a contraindication.

When successful, alkalinization of the urine and repeated doses of activated charcoal can reduce the serum half-life of toxic levels of salicylate from more than 24 hours down to less than 6 hours. However, these methods do have their shortcomings: persistent oliguria or aciduria or ileus may render these methods ineffective, and precious hours may be lost before the lack of effectiveness is appreciated. Thus, when these methods are used, improvements in clinical status must be documented, particularly an improving neurologic status, improving acidemia, and a falling salicylate level. If improvement is shown, these methods should be continued at least until serum salicylate level has fallen to around 30 mg/dL in chronic toxicity or somewhat higher in acute overdoses, depending on the clinical situation. If deterioration occurs or if these methods are not working, extracorporeal methods must be employed.

CYCLIC ANTIDEPRESSANTS

It is helpful to consider the cyclic antidepressants in two separate categories: the first-generation agents and the second-generation agents. The first-generation cyclic antidepressants have been in widespread use since the 1960s and are characterized by their tricyclic structure. Because of their troublesome side effects and their lethality in overdose, considerable effort has been expended in developing cyclic antidepressants with fewer side effects and less toxicity in overdose. These newer, or second-generation, cyclic antidepressants started appearing on the market in the 1980s and form a heterogeneous group. They are generally not tricyclic in structure.

The first-generation cyclic antidepressants (tricyclic antidepressants [TCAs]) available in the United States consist of the following: amitriptyline (Elavil, Endep), desipramine (Norpramin, Pertofrane), doxepin (Sinequan, Adapin), imipramine (Janimine, Tofranil), nortriptyline (Pamelor), protriptyline (Vivactil), and trimipramine (Surmontil). Clomipramine (Anafranil) also is a member of this class of drugs but is used primarily for treatment of obsessive-compulsive disorders rather than depression. The TCAs are believed to combat depression by blocking reuptake of norepinephrine and serotonin, causing accumulation of these neurotransmitters in the brain. At therapeutic doses, frequent adverse effects include sedation, anticholinergic effects, and hypotension secondary to alpha-adrenergic blockade. In overdose, these effects are exaggerated, but the lethality of the tricyclics lies primarily in their cardiac toxicity, including refractory cardiac arrhythmias. The second-generation cyclic antidepressants were released with the hope that they would be less toxic when taken in overdose. This hope has not been uniformly realized. But rather than begin a discussion of the individual second-generation cyclic antidepressants, we first discuss poisoning with the first-generation (tricyclic) agents and then briefly mention how poisoning with the individual second-generation agents differs.

TOXICOLOGY

Tricyclic antidepressants are readily absorbed from the gastrointestinal tract, although in overdose absorption may be incomplete or delayed because of reduced gastrointestinal motility from anticholinergic effects. Only small amounts remain in circulation; most is rapidly taken up in tissues, and most of the circulating drug is bound to plasma proteins. The binding to plasma proteins is influenced by serum pH. In acidemia, more drug becomes dissociated from plasma protein, increasing toxicity. In alkalemia, there is increased protein binding, reducing the concentration of free drug and reducing toxicity. Metabolism to inactive metabolites occurs in the liver at rates that vary greatly among individuals, with half-lives varying from hours to more than 3 days.

Toxicity usually occurs after ingestion of 10 mg/kg or more. Clinical manifestations of overdose are caused by the anticholinergic effects, by the blockade of biogenic amine (especially norepinephrine) uptake resulting in cardiovascular instability, by alpha-adrenergic blockade, and by the quinidine-like effects.

The anticholinergic effects are most apparent in mild overdoses and in the early stages of more severe overdoses. Manifestations include mydriasis, blurred vision, dry mouth, sinus tachycardia, ileus, urinary retention, agitation, psychosis, and hyperpyrexia. More severe signs of toxicity, including

hypotension, lethal cardiac arrhythmias, coma, and seizures, usually result from the other properties of tricyclics.

Because of their blockade of norepinephrine uptake, TCAs often initially have an adrenergic effect. Levels of circulating catecholamines have been shown to be elevated during the first few hours after ingestion.[43] This, combined with the anticholinergic effects, usually results in sinus tachycardia. Hypertension also may be seen early in the course. Hypotension develops later as norepinephrine supplies become exhausted and sympathetic tone is lost.

Alpha-adrenergic blockade causes venous and arterial dilation. This is a second factor contributing to hypotension.

A third factor contributing to hypotension is myocardial depression from quinidine-like actions on the heart. Similar to quinidine, the TCAs have type 1A antiarrhythmic properties, sometimes referred to as "membrane stabilizing." Effects are seen primarily in the His-Purkinje conduction system and in the ventricular myocardium. Phase 4 depolarization is slowed, reducing automaticity, and phase 0 inward flow through the fast sodium channels is slowed, slowing conduction and reducing contractility. Electrocardiographically, a prolongation of the PR, QRS, and QT intervals can be seen. The widened QRS complex tends to develop a rightward axis, especially during the terminal 0.04 seconds of the complex, and a right bundle branch block may be seen. ST segment and T wave abnormalities also occur. The impaired cardiac conduction manifests itself clinically as conduction blocks and bradyarrhythmias of varying severity: first-degree atrioventricular (AV) block, Mobitz II second-degree block, complete heart block, and asystole. Ventricular tachycardia also is commonly seen and can degenerate rapidly into ventricular fibrillation. Ventricular tachycardia has been theorized to be caused by unidirectional intraventricular conduction blocks that permit sustained reentry circuits.

Other cardiac arrhythmias can occur from the interaction of anticholinergic, adrenergic, and quinidine-like effects on the heart. Acidosis and myocardial ischemia secondary to hypoperfusion also may contribute. Sinus tachycardia is common. Torsade de pointes, reentrant supraventricular tachycardia, and atrial fibrillation occur uncommonly. When QRS complexes are wide, it may be difficult to distinguish between ventricular rhythms and supraventricular rhythms with conduction block.

It may be quinidine-like effects in the central nervous system that cause the seizures that are frequently seen. Seizures are generally short-lived, but status epilepticus can occur. Coma is common but generally resolves in 12 to 24 hours. Generalized myoclonus is frequently seen and may be difficult to differentiate from seizure activity unless the patient is awake. Marked or prolonged motor hyperactivity can result in hyperthermia. Other neurologic manifestations include dysarthria, ataxia, nystagmus, hyperreflexia, choreoathetosis, and delirium.

TREATMENT

Initial Management

Sudden dramatic deterioration in the first hours after toxic ingestion is characteristic. A patient with minimal symptoms can have a life-threatening arrhythmia, start seizing, or become abruptly comatose with a compromised airway. For this reason, all patients with a history suspicious for possible toxic ingestion must be closely observed with monitoring of cardiac rhythm and must have immediate establishment of venous access.

The electrocardiogram (ECG) is a useful indicator of tricyclic toxicity. One should be performed as part of the initial assessment and repeated any time that the clinical status changes. According to multiple studies[44,45] but not without exception,[46] when the maximal limb-lead QRS interval is equal to or greater than 100 milliseconds, there is an increased likelihood of subsequent major complications. As is discussed later, this can aid in the determination of disposition of stable patients.

Gastrointestinal decontamination is vital and consists of administration of activated charcoal with a cathartic and, in most cases, gastric lavage. Gastric lavage is probably more useful in tricyclic overdose than in any other type of ingestion. It is certainly indicated within the first 2 hours after ingestion and may worthwhile for several hours after ingestion. Administration of activated charcoal is the most valuable intervention and should be done regardless of how many hours have elapsed since ingestion. Multiple doses at intervals of between 1 to 6 hours may be even better. However, enthusiasm for charcoal must be tempered with respect for the TCAs anticholinergic properties and concern for gastric distention and subsequent aspiration. The first dose should be given together with a cathartic. Administration of syrup of ipecac even to an alert patient is contraindicated because it delays charcoal administration and because of the possibility of abrupt worsening of mental status leading to risk of aspiration.

Management of Complications

Lacking any specific antidote, further care of the patient primarily consists of close observation with immediate supportive measures as the anticipated complication occur. The most common life-threatening complications consist of compromise of airway or ventilation, circulatory compromise from ventricular tachycardia, bradyarrhythmias or hypotension, and seizures.

Compromise of the airway and ventilation is common, is often abrupt, and can occur because of circulatory compromise, seizure activity, or coma. Immediate tracheal intubation and mechanical ventilation is indicated in these cases. But even in awake patients, adequacy of oxygenation and ventilation must be assured. Pulse oximetry and close observation are indicated. Arterial blood gas measurements should be obtained in any patient with impaired level of consciousness; any respiratory acidosis is an indication for tracheal intubation and mechanical ventilation.

Circulatory compromise from hypotension or life-threatening arrhythmias demands immediate measures that are somewhat different than in other situations. First of all, hypotension must be treated especially aggressively because it is often a predecessor of cardiac arrest. Secondly, the administration of sodium bicarbonate (50 to 100 mMol intra-

venously [IV]) is indicated as an initial measure in managing acute circulatory compromise, whether it be from hypotension or arrhythmias. The usefulness of alkalinization is only partly explained by the increased binding of TCAs to plasma proteins that occurs with alkalosis. There appear to be other mechanisms too. Both the sodium[47] and the bicarbonate may directly antagonize the tricyclic's quinidine-like effect on myocardial conduction.

Patients manifesting major cardiovascular toxicity such as hypotension, ventricular arrhythmias, conduction blocks, or markedly widened QRS should have their serum pH maintained at around 7.5.[48] There is debate as to whether this is best achieved by hyperventilation or by bicarbonate administration. Potassium may have to be supplemented because alkalinization may induce hypokalemia. In all patients, acidosis should be scrupulously avoided.

In the past, phenytoin has been proposed as an antidote for the quinidine-like effects of TCAs. There have been anecdotal reports of occasional dramatic narrowing of widened QRS complexes and of conversion of ventricular tachycardia after phenytoin administration. When interpreting these reports, bear in mind that these abnormalities also can resolve spontaneously without treatment. Recent controlled studies in animals do not support the use of phenytoin either as prophylaxis or as reliable effective therapy of arrhythmias or conduction abnormalities. The studies show either no benefit[49] or worsened frequency and duration of ventricular tachycardia.[50] Therefore, routine use of phenytoin cannot be recommended.

As mentioned earlier, first-line treatment of ventricular tachycardia is sodium bicarbonate administration, possibly combined with electrical cardioversion or defibrillation with cardiopulmonary resuscitation (CPR) when indicated. In many cases, alkalinization alone results in resolution of the arrhythmia. Lidocaine is the next drug of choice and is also frequently effective.[51] Beyond this, options are limited, and pharmocologic intervention may be more deleterious than the arrhythmia itself. All class 1A antiarrhythmics (quinidine, procainamide, and disopyramide) are contraindicated, as are members of class 1C (encainide, flecainide, and propafenone). Overdrive pacing, magnesium, and bretylium may potentially be useful, but a major drawback to bretylium is its sympathetic ganglionic blockade, which would severely aggravate the hypotensive effects of the tricyclics. Beta-blockers have been used and have helped tachyarrhythmias and even improved conduction, but have resulted in severe hypotension.

Heart block and bradyrrhythmias usually do not respond to atropine because the site of the conduction block is usually distal to the AV node. Temporary ventricular pacing is indicated in high-grade block. Isoproterenol can be used to maintain a rhythm while pacing is being established. When all else fails, prolonged CPR exceeding an hour has been reported to be successful.[52]

Hypotension must be treated aggressively, first with alkalinization of the serum and then with judicious crystalloid administration. In some cases, both can be provided simultaneously with an infusion of 100 to 150 mMol of sodium bicarbonate in 1 L of D$_5$W. If there is not an adequate response to 2 or 3 L, vasopressors are probably needed. Norepinephrine is most commonly recommended, although phenylephrine also is acceptable. Dopamine may be ineffective and deleterious if the body's stores of norepinephrine are depleted. Dobutamine may be useful in treating myocardial depression. Both fluids and inotropic agents must be administered judiciously, because patients with myocardial depression are susceptible to pulmonary edema from volume overload, and ventricular irritability may be aggravated by inotropic agents. Therefore, a pulmonary artery catheter may be useful to guide therapy, although the possibility of catheter passage inducing ventricular arrhythmias also must be weighed. In refractory cases, an intraaortic balloon pump may be helpful.

Seizures are usually brief and may not require anticonvulsant treatment, but prolonged seizures can lead to lethal arrhythmias as lactic acidosis develops. Benzodiazepines are recommended as initial therapy to terminate seizures. Diazepam, 5 to 10 mg IV, can be repeated about every 15 minutes up to a maximum dose of 40 mg. Lorazepam, 1 to 2 mg IV also can be given repetitively; it has a slower onset of action but offers the advantage of a longer duration of action. It is not always necessary to follow the benzodiazepine with an additional anticonvulsant unless the seizure persists. Phenytoin has traditionally been the standard first-line anticonvulsant to be used, but the recent studies (see earlier) showing a proarrhythmic effect have convinced some authorities to recommend phenobarbital or pentobarbital instead. Other animal studies cast doubt on phenytoin's effectiveness against seizures.

Prevention of acidosis from developing during seizures is a higher priority than during seizures under other circumstances. During periods of generalized motor seizure activity, sodium bicarbonate should be given early and often. In persistent cases, one should consider short-term neuromuscular blockade while awaiting completion of the administration of the loading dose of anticonvulsant. A single dose of an agent like vecuronium does well.

Management of coma is supportive. Hypoglycemia should be ruled out. Empiric administration of glucose, thiamine, and naloxone should be considered. Flumazenil should not be given to patients who may have ingested tricyclics because seizures may be precipitated.

Physostigmine administration has been advocated for the treatment of the anticholinergic toxicity of TCAs. Indeed, physostigmine has the potential to transiently improve delirium and other anticholinergic effects. Physostigmine administration recently has being discouraged because of reports of adverse events, including seizures, severe bradycardia, asystole, and vomiting.

Other complications can occur with TCA overdose. These include noncardiogenic pulmonary edema, aspiration pneumonia, rhabdomyolysis, syndrome of inappropriate secretion of antidiuretic hormone, and neuroleptic malignant syndrome. These may be managed in standard fashion.

Because little TCA remains free in the circulation, there is no role for forced diuresis, dialysis, or hemoperfusion. Cimetidine, haloperidol, and morphine should be avoided because these compete with TCAs for hepatic metabolism.

TRIAGE

Because TCAs are toxic in overdose and are frequently prescribed to depressed patients who may be or may become suicidal, they are implicated in more successful suicidal drug ingestions than any other class of prescription drug. On the other hand, TCA ingestions are extremely common and most have a benign course, and not every TCA overdose needs to be admitted to an ICU.

Callaham and Kassel[53] found in a retrospective study that in more than 80% of the fatal tricyclic ingestions, the patients were pronounced dead at the scene or dead on arrival at the hospital. Of the in-hospital fatalities, half of the patients presented critically ill with coma, seizure, respiratory depression, or hypotension. The other half presented with minimal signs of poisoning but had marked deterioration during the first hour after arrival. This study and others have shown that patients who remain stable for the first hours after admission and who receive proper initial management have an excellent prognosis.

On initial presentation, a decision regarding admission can be made on the basis of the presence of major signs of toxicity on physical examination, on the cardiac monitor, and on the ECG. Major signs of toxicity include the following: impaired level of consciousness; respiratory depression, either clinically or on arterial blood gases; seizures; hypotension; arrhythmias or conduction blocks; and limb-lead QRS duration greater than or equal to 100 milliseconds.

Any patient with a major sign of toxicity should receive aggressive gastrointestinal decontamination and be admitted to an ICU for close observation and management. Patients without any major signs of toxicity should receive immediate gastrointestinal decontamination including activated charcoal and cathartic and should then be observed closely for 6 hours. If there are no major signs of toxicity in 6 hours, if minor signs of toxicity (such as sinus tachycardia less than 120 beats per minute) are decreasing rather than increasing, and if bowel sounds are active, these patients then can generally be discharged to psychiatric care after a final dose of charcoal.[53,54] Absent or diminished bowel sounds should be grounds for admission, because it suggests an ileus and the likelihood that the charcoal may not effectively adsorb the drug.

There has been uncertainty about how long to observe patients in an ICU. In the 1960s and 1970s, there were reports of sudden death late in the course of TCA poisoning, up to 6 days after ingestion. These have generally occurred in patients who did not receive activated charcoal or who were recovering from poisoning with major signs of toxicity. It seems that delayed fatalities can be avoided by administering activated charcoal in all cases and by close observation in an intensive care setting for 24 hours after resolution of all major toxicity.

In some patients, QRS prolongation can persist for up to 3 days beyond resolution of all other clinical signs of toxicity. In these patients, the risk of complications resolves earlier than the QRS prolongation.[55] It is reasonable that these patients who have been observed in an ICU for 24 hours beyond resolution of all other signs of toxicity subsequently can be observed in a telemetry unit until their QRS complex returns to baseline.

Plasma levels may be of value diagnostically, but they provide no additional prognostic information beyond that provided by the patient's clinical status and ECG.[44] Generally, a level of TCA plus active metabolite greater than 1000 μg/L correlates with toxicity.

SECOND-GENERATION AGENTS

Management of overdoses with second-generation cyclic antidepressants must be individualized, depending on the toxicity of the particular drug. Certain aspects of management can be cautiously extrapolated from those for the first-generation agents. Clinical experience with these poisonings is limited, and detailed management guidelines do not appear in the literature. Gastrointestinal decontamination and period of close observation of at least 6 to 12 hours should be minimal precautions in the stable patient with a potentially toxic ingestion. A poison control center can give more detailed and current recommendations.

Amoxapine (Asendin) and maprotiline (Ludiomil) have considerable toxicity in overdose. Maprotiline has cardiotoxicity similar to the tricyclics and an increased propensity to induce seizures.[56] Amoxapine generally causes cardiotoxicity only at large doses (2 g)[57] but has marked neurotoxicity, being associated with intractable seizures leading to death and brain damage.[58] Bupropion (Wellbutrin) has been associated with seizures both at therapeutic doses and in overdose; however, the clinical course in overdose has been mild.

The four newest second-generation cyclic antidepressants selectively inhibit serotonin reuptake and do not cause anticholinergic effects. These four are fluoxetine (Prozac), trazodone (Desyrel), sertraline (Zoloft), and paroxetine (Paxil). Toxicity in overdose generally has been mild, with serious cardiotoxicity being seen only in massive overdose or in susceptible patients. Manifestations generally have consisted of sedation, gastrointestinal disturbances, and sinus tachycardia. Notice that fluoxetine, which together with its active metabolite has a half-life of several days, and can cause prolonged but usually mild sedation.

LITHIUM ◼

Lithium was discovered in 1817 by Ardedsson and was used in the nineteenth century for a variety of ailments, including rheumatism, renal calculi, and gout.[59] It is currently an important drug in the psychiatrist's armamentarium because it is highly effective in controlling mania and in preventing manic episodes in patients with manic-depressive illness. Because of its high level of use in a potentially depressed population and because of a narrow toxic-to-therapeutic window, lithium overdose is a moderately common and potentially life-threatening toxicologic problem in critical care.

TOXICOLOGY

Lithium is a group IA alkali metal, a position it shares with sodium, and potassium. It is a smaller molecule than either sodium or potassium, which accounts for some of its intracellular effectiveness. Lithium carbonate is typically prescribed as a 300-mg capsule (8.12 mMol of lithium ion) as an immediate-release preparation, or as a 450-mg sustained-release capsule (12.8 mMol of lithium ion). Most patients on maintenance therapy require approximately 900 to 1200 mg/day to maintain the desired effect at a blood level of 0.6 to 1.2 mMol/L. Treatment of acute mania may require as much as 1800 mg/day. Because serious side effects occur at a level close to the therapeutic range, serum levels should be followed closely. After administration of the immediate-release preparation, lithium is absorbed completely from the gastrointestinal tract within 8 hours. Peak serum levels occur at approximately 2 to 4 hours with the immediate-release preparations and at 4 to 12 hours with the sustained-release preparation. Lithium is not protein bound and distributes freely in total body water (except in the cerebrospinal fluid). It has a volume of distribution of 0.7 to 0.9 L/kg. Lithium is actively transported out of the cerebrospinal fluid where the level is approximately 40% of the blood level.[60] Six to 10 days are required to reach a steady state concentration and see the desired clinical effect. The mechanism by which lithium achieves its beneficial effect is not known. Lithium is concentrated in liver, bone, muscle, brain, kidney, and thyroid. The drug's elimination half-life varies with the duration of therapy and is approximately 29 hours initially, but may be as long as 58 hours in chronic users.[61] Lithium is freely filtered by the glomerulus and over 95% of a dose is excreted in the urine. Clearance of lithium is reduced in patients with renal failure and dose adjustments must be made accordingly.

A variety of factors influence a patient's risk of lithium toxicity including old age, prior history of brain injury, schizophrenia, volume depletion, and diuretic use.[62] Increased lithium levels and toxicity have been reported in patients using a variety of nonsteroidal antiinflammatory drugs.[63] Indomethacin and diclofenac seem to be the most important drugs in this class. Angiotensin converting inhibitors also have been reported to increase lithium levels after 3 to 4 weeks of use.[64,65]

CLINICAL MANIFESTATIONS

In the individual patient, lithium levels correlate poorly with clinical toxicity; however, moderate symptoms are typically seen when serum lithium levels are 1.5 to 2.5 mMol/L, serious symptoms are seen at levels of 2.5 to 3.5 mMol/L, and life-threatening symptoms are seen at levels above 3.5 mMol/L. The serum lithium level is a more reliable indicator of intracellular lithium and toxicity in the patient receiving chronic lithium therapy than in the patient with an acute ingestion.

Neurologic

Whereas a variety of organ systems are affected by lithium intoxication, neurologic symptoms predominate. Tremors occur in up to 80% of patients receiving lithium. Fatigue, muscle weakness, slowed reaction time, and difficulty concentrating are common. Cerebellar symptoms including dysarthria,[66] ataxia, nystagmus, and discoordination appear as levels rise. Choreiform movements and Parkinsonian movements also are seen. As lithium levels rise, hyperreflexia, hypertonia, and myoclonus may be seen. Lithium intoxication induces seizures in some patients. A depressed level of consciousness progressing to coma is seen in severe intoxications.[67] Some patients develop permanent neurologic abnormalities related to lithium ingestion.

Renal

Renal tubular dysfunction is commonly altered with lithium therapy. Lithium inhibits antidiuretic hormone's effect on the renal tubule, causing polyuria, an impaired renal concentrating defect, and diabetes insipidus. The defect correlates with the lithium dose, serum level, and duration of treatment. Most cases resolve within 3 weeks after lithium has been discontinued, although a persistent defect has been observed.[68,69]

Metabolic/Endocrine

Lithium blunts calcium feedback inhibition of parathyroid hormone, resulting in a mild hypercalcemia and mild elevation in parathyroid hormone level in some patients.[70,71] Parathyroid hyperplasia and parathyroid adenomas have been described.[72,73]

Hypermagnesemia has been reported.[74] Blood glucose levels may be elevated in patients receiving lithium. This has been attributed to an increase in glucose absorption from the gut and reduced insulin production and secretion.[75]

Lithium antagonizes thyroid function. Of patients taking lithium, 5% to 10% develop hypothyroidism and goiter.[76,77] This may be treated by discontinuing lithium or by administering thyroid hormone.

Gastrointestinal

Transient nausea, vomiting, diarrhea, and abdominal pain occur with the initiation of lithium in some patients.[78] These symptoms also may herald lithium toxicity.[79]

Cardiovascular

Serious cardiac complications are unusual. ST segment depression and T wave flattening or inversion are the most characteristic ECG abnormalities. Prolongation of the QT interval and U waves also are seen.[80,81] Conduction and rhythm abnormalities are rare but do occur. Sinus node dysfunction leading to syncope occurs in some patients.[82] Serious ventricular rhythm disturbances are unusual in the absence of underlying cardiac disease.[83] Cardiovascular collapse has been reported in severe lithium overdose.[84]

Miscellaneous

Many patients gain weight while taking lithium. Neutrophilia is common, usually at about 1.5 times normal. Neutrophil function appears normal. Eosinophil counts may be also elevated. A variety of skin manifestations have been reported. Burning, itching, and tearing of the eyes have been reported.[85]

TREATMENT

The patient's clinical presentation rather than the serum lithium level determines management. Lithium should be discontinued. Airway management and intravenous access are the first treatment issues. Cardiac monitoring is indicated. Because most lithium-intoxicated patients are sodium and water depleted, intravascular volume should be repleted with isotonic saline solutions. Gastric emptying is the next step for an acute intoxication. In the setting of subacute or chronic lithium intoxication, gastric emptying is less important. Activated charcoal does not bind lithium but should be used if multidrug ingestion is suspected. Polyethylene glycol (Colyte, GoLytely) given as whole-bowel irrigation (10 L over 5 hours) has been effective, especially with the sustained-release lithium preparation.[86] Forced diuresis and alkalization of the urine have yielded disappointing results.

Hemodialysis is the treatment of choice for serious lithium toxicity because it most effectively increases lithium ion clearance. Most patients with lithium levels above 3.5 mMol/L require hemodialysis. Unstable patients with severe neurologic findings who have lithium levels above 2 mMol/L benefit from dialysis.[87,88] Prolonged and repeated dialysis often is necessary because of the wide volume of distribution of this drug. Repeat dialysis should be guided by serum levels and clinical course.

ANTIPSYCHOTIC DRUGS ■

Antipsychotic drugs are primarily used in treating psychoses such as schizophrenia, the manic phase of manic-depressive illness, and severe agitated behavior. They are also used in managing nausea and occasionally hiccups. Antipsychotic drugs also are referred to as neuroleptic agents. The descriptive term *neuroleptic* initially was introduced to denote the calming affects that chlorpromazine had on psychotic patients. These patients had a suppression of spontaneous movement, a reduced interest in the environment, and reduced displays of emotion. These agents are a diverse group of drugs, the major classes of which include phenothiazines, butyrophenones, indoles, dibenzoxazepines, and diphenylbutylpiperidines. The precise mechanism of action of the neuroleptic agents is not known but probably involves alteration in dopaminergic neurotransmission in the cortex, limbic system, and basal ganglia. The antiemetic effect results from inhibition of dopaminergic receptors in the medullary chemoreceptor trigger zone.[89]

TOXICOLOGY AND CLINICAL MANIFESTATIONS

Six types of neurologic side effects involving the extrapyramidal system occur with these drugs:

1. Acute dystonia—spasms of the muscles of the tongue, face neck and back
2. Akathisia—motor restlessness
3. Parkinsonism—bradykinesia, rigidity, mask facies, shuffling gait, tremor

4. Neuroleptic malignant syndrome—fever, rigidity, unstable blood pressure
5. Perioral tremor—rare, late finding
6. Tardive dyskinesia—rare, late finding, oral–facial dyskinesia, choreoathetosis[89]

Other side effects include anticholinergic toxicity (dry mucus membranes, tachycardia, ileus, mydriasis, urinary retention and hypotension), priapism, agranulocytosis, photosensitivity, cholestatic jaundice, lowered seizure threshold, and tachyarrhythmias.[90-94]

When taken in overdose, toxicity can be life threatening, with central nervous system and cardiovascular system effects predominating. Symptoms from an ingested overdose are apparent within 2 to 6 hours. The central nervous system can be involved with delirium, obtundation, stupor, and coma. Cerebral edema can occur. Status epilepticus has been reported and may lead to rhabdomyolysis. Respiratory depression can occur. Tachyarrhythmias and bradyarrhythmias are seen. Because QRS and QT intervals are typically prolonged, torsade de points may occur.[95] Hypotension is often seen. Pulmonary edema, renal failure, hypothermia, and coagulation defects are included on the list of serious toxicities.[1,95]

TREATMENT

Acute dystonic reactions are treated by discontinuation of the drug and administration of diphenhydramine, 25 to 50 mg IV or intramuscularly (IM), or benztropine mesylate, 1 to 2 mg IV or IM. This is typically followed with the same medication (enteral or parenteral) for several days.

Treatment of neuroleptic malignant syndrome is covered in Chapter 98.

Treatment of the patient who has overdosed on antipsychotic medication is largely supportive. Standard measures such as tracheal intubation, mechanical ventilation, gastric emptying, and activated charcoal administration should be employed as the clinical circumstance dictates. The hypotensive patient should receive intravascular volume expansion with isotonic colloid solutions. Ventricular tachyarrhythmias should be treated with lidocaine and electrical cardioversion as indicated. In the presence of prolonged QRS and QT intervals, type 1a antiarrhythmic agents (quinidine, procainamide, disopyramide) should be avoided, as should beta-blocking agents. Torsade de points often responds to magnesium sulfate, 2 to 4 g IV. Bradycardia usually responds to atropine, isoproterenol, or cardiac pacing. Seizures should be treated with benzodiazepines and phenytoin, as outlined in Chapter 134.

BENZODIAZEPINES ■

Since their introduction more than three decades ago, benzodiazepines have become widely used for a variety of purposes including sedation, anxiolysis, and muscle relaxation. Members of this class currently available in the United States consist of alprazolam (Xanax), chlorazepate (Tranxene), chlordiazepoxide (Librium), clonazepam (Klonopin), diazepam (Valium), flurazepam (Dalmane), lorazepam (Ativan), midazolam (Versed), oxazepam (Serax), prazepam (Centrax), temazepam (Restoril), and triazolam (Halcion).

TOXICOLOGY AND CLINICAL MANIFESTATIONS

Benzodiazepines are rapidly absorbed from the gastrointestinal tract. Metabolism is primarily hepatic, and half-life is highly variable, ranging from a couple hours to several days. However, the duration of their effect in an acute overdose is much shorter, because initial distribution to highly perfused tissues like brain is followed by redistribution of drug into less perfused tissues like muscle and fat.

Because of their widespread use, benzodiazepines are frequently involved in drug overdoses. The clinical manifestations of overdose of benzodiazepines as a single agent are generally mild, consisting usually of dizziness, weakness, disorientation, and somnolence. Evidence of cerebellar dysfunction with ataxia, diplopia, and dysarthria may be seen. Paradoxical tremulousness and agitation have been reported. Although impaired level of consciousness is common, it is rare to see deep coma with unresponsiveness to pain, loss of deep tendon reflexes, or life-threatening respiratory and cardiovascular depression.

TREATMENT

Patients with pure benzodiazepine ingestion often are not admitted to the ICU. More commonly seen in the ICU is the scenario of benzodiazepine ingestion in the context of multidrug overdose. When ingested in combination with agents that impair consciousness, such as alcohol, narcotics, tricyclic antidepressants (TCAs), and sedative–hypnotic agents, a benzodiazepine potentiates the depressant effects of these agents, resulting in more profound central nervous system and respiratory depression and commonly leading to respiratory failure.

When a patient presents with impaired level of consciousness and it seems likely that this is because of ingestion of a benzodiazepine or other central nervous system depressant, the clinician nevertheless must remain alert to the possibility of alternative causes. Thiamine and naloxone probably should be administered to all patients, and hypoxemia and hypoglycemia should be promptly ruled out. While awaiting test results, empiric administration of oxygen and glucose may be prudent. Even a history of benzodiazepine ingestion or a positive result on the urine toxicology screen for benzodiazepines does not rule out another more menacing pathologic process.

Flumazenil

Although administration of flumazenil (Romazicon), a benzodiazepine antagonist, can be both a diagnostic and therapeutic intervention in benzodiazepine overdose, it has associated risks. It can reliably reverse the central nervous system depression of benzodiazepines, producing dramatic improvement in level of consciousness.[96] In mixed overdoses, the response may be less complete, depending on how large a role other agents are playing in the clinical picture. A clear improvement in consciousness after flumazenil administration is strong evidence that a benzodiazepine is contributing to the central nervous system depression. However, a response to flumazenil is not completely specific for benzodiazepine ingestion; some patients who have not ingested benzodiazepines may appear to respond. This may be coincidental in some cases, but there is evidence that flumazenil may oppose the central nervous system depression seen in other conditions such as promethazine intoxication,[97] ethanol intoxication, and hepatic encephalopathy.[98] Nevertheless, even a nonspecific response to flumazenil may permit the clinician to obtain a history from the patient or may obviate the need for urgent computed tomography of the brain or lumbar puncture.

Therapeutically, a good response to flumazenil can obviate the need for tracheal intubation and mechanical ventilation in cases where a benzodiazepine is contributing significantly to respiratory depression.[99] However, this has not been shown to decrease the time to ICU discharge, and its use is associated with several problems. First, the flumazenil dose required is highly variable, ranging from 0.3 to 5 mg or more.[98] Second, resedation is common because its half-life, about an hour, is shorter than the half-life of most benzodiazepines. A continuous infusion of flumazenil may prevent this.[100] Third, it has some of its own adverse effects, including nausea, vomiting, and pain at the site of injection. Finally, in some patients, the ingested benzodiazepine may provide protection against problems that can become manifest once flumazenil removes the benzodiazepine's protective effect. These problems may include the following:

1. Benzodiazepine withdrawal in chronic users
2. Seizures in patients who have epilepsy or who have ingested other drugs that can cause seizures, such as TCAs,[101–103] propoxyphene,[98] and cocaine.[104] (The clinical presentation and ECG should be examined closely for signs of TCA toxicity before flumazenil is administered.[102])
3. Ventricular tachycardia in patients who have also ingested drugs such as chloral hydrate[105] and TCAs[106]
4. Catecholamine surge with hypertension and tachyarrhythmias in patients who have these conditions chronically or in those who have ingested stimulant drugs
5. Sudden aggression in patients with baseline behavioral problems or in patients who have ingested other drugs, such as hallucinogens, that cause behavioral problems[107]
6. Agitation, which may be a direct adverse effect of flumazenil

Because of these possible adverse events, flumazenil is not recommended as standard therapy for benzodiazepine overdose.

Standard Treatment Measures

Standard therapy consists of gastrointestinal decontamination and supportive measures.

The mainstay of gastrointestinal decontamination is the administration of activated charcoal, which results in good adsorption of residual benzodiazepine in the gut and prevents further systemic uptake. The first dose is usually given together with a cathartic. Repeat doses of charcoal should be given if symptoms of benzodiazepine toxicity persist. Gastric lavage in the first 2 hours after ingestion is commonly recommended, but in a pure benzodiazepine overdose its utility is questionable; because the clinical course is usually benign, the risk of aspiration may outweigh any likely benefit.

Airway or ventilatory compromise is best managed with tracheal intubation and mechanical ventilation. Hypotension usually responds to moderate quantities of intravenous crystalloid. If deep coma, respiratory failure, or shock are present, the clinician must search for another etiology for these problems; it is more likely that there has been ingestion of another agent or that there is some other pathologic process.

BETA-BLOCKERS ■

Beta-blockers are commonly used for cardiovascular and noncardiovascular disorders, making them one of the most prescribed classes of drugs. Because of their common use, toxic exposure is on the rise. More than 20 beta-blockers are available, each with slightly different pharmacologic properties. Pharmacologic differences between the agents may influence the clinical presentation of the poisoned patient.[108,109]

TOXICOLOGY

Understanding the physiologic mechanisms of the beta-adrenergic receptor is important in understanding the therapeutic and toxic properties of these drugs. Catecholamines bind to beta-receptors at the cell membrane, resulting in phosphorylation of the G-protein complex. The phosphorylated G-protein provides energy for synthesis of cyclic adenosine monophosphate (cAMP) through the enzyme adenyl cyclase. As an intracellular messenger, cAMP stimulates protein kinase, causing an increase of intracellular calcium. cAMP is then metabolized by phosphodiesterase.[110]

The cellular expression of beta-adrenergic stimulation depends on the type of cell and the type of receptor. At least two beta-receptors exist: β_1-receptors are located predominantly in myocardial cells, the kidney, and the eye; and β_2-receptors are widely scattered in vascular, bronchial, and other smooth muscle, skeletal muscle, adipose tissue, pancreas, and liver. Stimulation of β_1-receptors causes and increase in the inotropic and chronotropic state of the heart, causes increased renin secretion, and increases aqueous humor production in the anterior chamber of the eye. Stimulation of β_2-receptors causes bronchial, vascular, intestinal and uterine smooth muscle relaxation. In addition, β_2-receptor stimulation increases lipolysis, gluconeogenesis, and insulin release. Blockage of beta-receptors results in a decreased intracellular production of cAMP and a blunting of the previously described responses.

Beta-blocking drugs also may have a myocardial membrane–stabilizing effect independent of intracellular cAMP. Here they are thought to decrease sodium entry into the cell through fast sodium channels, slowing phase zero of the action potential. This membrane "stabilizing" effect may be important when these drugs are taken in overdose.

CLINICAL MANIFESTATIONS

The severity of the clinical presentation vary greatly, depending on the underlying health of the patient, the specific drug ingested, the amount ingested, and the timing of ingestion. Propranolol in the most frequently reported beta-blocking drug involved in poisoning.

Bradycardia and delay in myocardial conduction and decreased myocardial contractility occur in most beta-blocker overdoses. First-degree AV block, intraventricular conduction delays, bundle branch block, and AV dissociation may occur.[111] Hypotension may occur and is thought to be caused primarily by decreased contractility rather than slow heart rate, because in animal models the hypotension has persisted despite cardiac pacing at normal heart rates.[112] Hypertension has been reported with pindolol, which has a partial agonist effect.[113] Congestive heart failure and pulmonary edema have been reported, typically occurring in patients with underlying heart disease.

A variety of central nervous system symptoms may be seen, including lethargy, stupor, coma, and seizures. The membrane stabilizing effect of beta-blockers taken in overdose is likely operative here. Respiratory symptoms are few. Respiratory depression is centrally mediated. Bronchospasm is reported only occasionally. Renal failure has been reported from ingestion of a large quantity of labetalol.[114] Hypoglycemia and hyperkalemia have been reported but are unusual. Other complications are rare.

TREATMENT

Standard measures should be employed such as airway protection, gastric emptying, and activated charcoal. Repeated doses of activated charcoal have been recommended.

Glucagon is the most effective agent for reversal of bradycardia and myocardial depression. It acts by stimulating a specific glucagon receptor independent of beta-receptors. Activation of the glucagon-specific receptor enhances adenyl cyclase activity and increases intracellular cAMP, thus improving both the inotropic and chronotropic state of the heart. Glucagon is given as a bolus of approximately 5 mg IV, then as a continuous infusion at approximately 1 to 5 mg/hour. There is no defined maximum dose. Doses as high as 10 mg/hour have been reported. A diluent provided by the manufacturer contains 2 mg of phenol per 1-mg vial of glucagon. When using glucagon to treat beta-blocker overdose, the manufacturer's diluent should not be used; rather, glucagon should be prepared in 5% dextrose or 0.9% saline solutions. Phenol may produce seizures, hypotension, and arrythmias.[115,116]

Atropine has been used to treat the bradycardia associated with beta-blocker overdose but is rarely effective with large overdoses. Other agents such as epinephrine, norepinephrine, dopamine, dobutamine, and isoproterenol have been used alone or in combination with glucagon with varying degrees of success. Cardiac pacing may be effective for bradycardia resistant to pharmacologic management.[117] Cardiovascular support using intraaortic balloon counterpulsation also has been used successfully.[118] Seizures should be treated in the standard fashion with benzodiazepines and phenytoin (Chap. 134).

CALCIUM CHANNEL BLOCKERS ■

Calcium channel blockers are commonly used in managing hypertension, myocardial ischemia, and cardiac arrhythmias. Because of this common use, intentional and unintentional overdose has become increasingly common.

These agents decrease the transport of calcium across myocardial cell and vascular smooth muscle membranes, thereby decreasing cardiac contractility and promoting vasodilation. The conduction system is also affected so that sinoatrial and AV conduction is delayed.[119]

TOXICOLOGY

When calcium channel blockers are taken in overdose, the cardiovascular system, central nervous system, gastrointestinal system, and glucose metabolism are most deranged. Clinical effects occur within 30 to 60 minutes of ingestion. An overdose of 5 to 10 times the therapeutic dose is problematic.[120]

The therapeutic effects of different calcium channel blockers vary; however, when taken in overdose, the problems created are similar. Hypotension and cardiac arrhythmias occur with equal frequency with verapamil and nifedipine. Conduction defects are most common with verapamil. Nifedipine has little effect on conduction.[121]

CLINICAL MANIFESTATIONS

Hypotension is the most common cardiovascular feature. It is caused primarily by peripheral vasodilation and to some extent by myocardial depression. Cardiogenic and noncardiogenic pulmonary edema may occur. Cardiac rhythm disturbances include sinus bradycardia, second- and third-degree heart block, sinus arrest with escape rhythms, and asystole. These complications can be worsened in the presence of significant underlying cardiac disease and in the presence of concomitant beta-blockade.[122]

Lethargy, confusion, and, rarely, seizures can be seen. If coma occurs, it is most likely secondary to cerebral hypoperfusion from hypotension. Nausea and vomiting are common. Hyperglycemia occurs because insulin secretion is suppressed. Lactic acidosis can occur from global tissue hypoperfusion.[123]

TREATMENT

Standard measures such as airway protection and gastric emptying should be employed based on the clinical presentation. Activated charcoal should be used. Some recommend use of repeated charcoal administration, particularly in the presence of sustained-release calcium channel preparations.

Whole-bowel lavage with polyethylene glycol has been used effectively and is recommended by some.[124] Patients with serious overdoses should be admitted to the ICU for continued supportive care and ECG monitoring.

Hypotension should be managed by administering isotonic saline solutions and intravenous calcium. Calcium improves myocardial contractility in many patients but has minimal effect on vasodilation or heart rate. The amount of calcium required depends on the dose ingested. A usual dosage is 0.2 mL/kg of 10% calcium chloride IV over 5 minutes. This can be repeated every 15 to 20 minutes to a total of 4 dosages.[123] Alternatively, calcium chloride in normal saline may be given as a continuous infusion with a starting rate of 20 to 50 mg/kg/hour.[122] The infusion rate is titrated to effect. Serum calcium levels should be measured after 30 minutes of infusion and every 2 hours thereafter. Some investigators recommend larger calcium doses.[125] Not all patients respond to calcium; however, clinical improvement is seen in most cases.[121]

Glucagon increases the intracellular cAMP level and has positive inotropic and chronotropic effects. It is given as an initial dose of 3.5 to 5 mg IV. This may be repeated. A constant infusion of 1 to 5 mg/hour may be needed.[126]

Refractory hypotension may require administration of agents such as epinephrine, norepinephrine, dopamine, or dobutamine. Amrinone has improved cardiac performance in case reports.[127] Patient management is facilitated by placing a pulmonary artery catheter under these circumstances.

Bradycardia may be treated with atropine, although this proves to be ineffective in many patients. Isoproterenol has been used to increase heart rate. Patients with symptomatic bradycardia may require cardiac pacing. Intraaortic balloon counter pulsation has been effectively used in severely toxic patients. Hyperglycemia, although common, rarely requires treatment.

Overdose with verapamil and diltiazem carries a worse prognosis than the other calcium channel blockers.[125] Verapamil is more commonly associated with life-threatening complications than diltiazem.[121] Little experience has been had with the newer calcium channel blockers taken in overdose.

DIGITALIS ■

The incidence of digitalis toxicity is on the decline. Largely because of a the introduction of new classes of cardiac drugs to treat heart failure and supraventricular tachyarrhythmias, fewer patients are taking digitalis glycosides. Studies published in the 1960s and 1970s suggest that up to 20% of patients taking digoxin experienced signs or symptoms of toxicity at some time during their clinical course.[128,129] The development of a reliable assay for serum digoxin concentrations in 1969 aided in the conformation of toxicity. The reported incidence rate of death secondary to digoxin toxicity has varied greatly from 1%[130,131] to as high as 41%.[129] These differences might be explained by differences in practice patterns between the 1960s and the 1980s. Absence of digoxin blood levels in the older studies make direct comparisons difficult. The mortality associated with digitalis toxicity today is most likely on the low rather than the high side.

TOXICOLOGY AND CLINICAL MANIFESTATIONS

Digoxin decreases activity of the sodium–potassium ATPase pump, leading to increased intracellular calcium.[132] This accounts for its therapeutic effectiveness. When taken in overdose, the effects seen are an exaggeration of its normal therapeutic action. Poisoning with digoxin may occur with acute or chronic ingestion. Many coexisting factors predispose to toxicity with digoxin.[133] Renal insufficiency and electrolyte abnormalities lead the list. Patients with hypothyroidism also are at risk, as are those with advanced pulmonary disease. Digoxin levels are increased in the presence of quinidine, verapamil, and amiodarone.

Renal Insufficiency

In advanced renal insufficiency, digoxin's volume of distribution is decreased so that lower doses of digoxin should be used. Furthermore, a reduced glomerular filtration rate decreases clearance of digoxin, predisposing to digoxin toxicity.

Electrolyte Abnormalities

Digoxin binding to the sodium–potassium ATPase pump is affected by the plasma potassium concentration. Hypokalemia decreases the rate of the pump, and this is accentuated in the presence of digoxin toxicity.

Hypomagnesemia also predisposes to digoxin toxicity. A poor correlation exists between serum and tissue magnesium levels; however, some digoxin-associated arrhythmias are suppressed by empiric administration of magnesium.

Hypercalcemia increases ventricular automaticity, and its presence in association with digoxin may act synergistically in provoking ventricular arrythmias.

Thyroid Disease

Hypothyroid patients do not clear digoxin normally and are at risk for toxicity at "normal doses." Hyperthyroidism increases the volume of distribution of digoxin.

Respiratory Disease

Patients with severe respiratory disease are likely to experience episodes of hypoxemia and hypercapnia. These, in association with digoxin excess, may predispose to cardiac arrhythmias. Also, the beta-adrenergic agents often used in patients with obstructive airways disease increase the possibility of digoxin-related arrhythmias.

Cardiac Manifestations

Virtually any cardiac rhythm disturbance can be seen with digoxin toxicity. AV junctional block of varying degrees and an increased ventricular automaticity are the most common manifestations of digoxin toxicity. At toxic levels, digoxin acts directly to prolong the AV nodal refractory period. This is often seen clinically as a regularization of the ventricular response rate in patients with atrial fibrillation. Paroxysmal atrial tachycardia with block also has been associated with digoxin toxicity. Sinus arrest or sinus exit block caused by a direct effect of the drug on the sinoatrial node are seen. Premature ventricular beats, bigeminy, trigeminy, ventricular tachycardia, and ventricular fibrillation also occur.

Particularly suggestive of digoxin toxicity are the rare rhythm disturbances such as fascicular tachycardia, biventricular bigeminy with alternating right and left axis deviation, and bidirectional ventricular tachycardia.

Extracardiac Manifestations

Fatigue and anorexia are common complaints. Visual disturbances are reported, such as halos around bright objects and changes in color perception. Headache, confusion, and neuralgic pain also are reported.

TREATMENT

The clinician should have a high degree of clinical suspicion when considering the possibility of digoxin toxicity. Minor rhythm disturbances such as more frequent ventricular ectopy, first-degree AV block, or an accelerated junctional pacemaker in the setting of atrial fibrillation simply require temporary withdrawal of the drug followed by dosage adjustment.

Sinus bradycardia, sinoatrial arrest, and AV block sometimes respond to treatment with atropine. Temporary cardiac pacing may be necessary in some patients.

Potassium administration is indicated for ectopic ventricular arrhythmias and induced AV block and can be life-saving under these circumstances in some patients. It should be used even if the serum potassium level is in the normal range.

Digoxin-Specific Fab Fragments

Fab fragments of high-affinity, digoxin-specific, polyclonal antibodies are widely available for treatment of digoxin toxicity. This agent is sheep protein, so that use of the Fab fragment rather than the whole antibody reduces the antigenicity and increases the clearance of the Fab–digoxin complex. Fab fragments have a large volume of distribution and effectively remove digoxin from the myocardium and other tissue binding site. Few adverse effects have been reported in large trials.

Fab fragments are indicated in severely intoxicated patients (particularly the hyperkalemic patient) with serious cardiac rhythm disturbances who do not immediately respond to other therapies. The package insert gives careful instructions for estimating the appropriate dose to give for acute and chronic ingestion. With massive digoxin overdose and severe toxicity, administration of 800 mg IV is recommended over 30 minutes. If cardiac arrest is imminent, the agent may be given as a bolus. Serum digoxin levels are unreliable for several days after administration of Fab fragments.[134]

THEOPHYLLINE

Although less popular in its primary use as a bronchodilator, theophylline remains a leading cause of fatal poisoning. It is available in a variety of forms, both by prescription and over-the-counter; as a single drug and as a combination drug product; and as a parenteral solution, rectal suppository, and oral preparations. Oral preparations are made in liquid and powder formulations and both non–sustained-release and sustained-release tablets and capsules. Peak serum levels are produced within 2 hours after ingestion of liquids and within 4 hours after ingestion of non–sustained-release tablets or capsules. Sustained-release theophylline preparations usually yield a peak level within 4 to 12 hours after a therapeutic dose; but after an overdose, absorption is erratic and the level may not peak until more than 24 hours after ingestion.

TOXICOLOGY AND CLINICAL MANIFESTATIONS

Theophylline is cleared primarily by the liver through the cytochrome P-450 mixed-function oxidase system. At high therapeutic levels, this enzyme system becomes saturated and half-life can be prolonged from the usual 4 to 8 hours to up to 12 hours. There are other factors that slow hepatic metabolism and contribute to accidental chronic poisoning: viral infection; worsened hepatic function of any etiology, including passive venous congestion from congestive heart failure; and coadministration of various drugs, including cimetidine, erythromycin, and the quinolone class of antibiotics.

Theophylline causes catecholamine release and stimulation of β_1- and β_2-adrenergic receptors. The β_1-stimulation causes inotropic and chronotropic cardiac stimulation, manifested clinically as tachycardia and myocardial irritability with atrial and ventricular arrhythmias. The β_2-stimulation, causing bronchodilation and peripheral vasodilation, often is not apparent clinically but is believed to be responsible for resistant hypotension that is occasionally encountered.

Manifestations and prognosis differ, depending on whether poisoning is acute or chronic. Acute poisoning refers to a patient not previously taking theophylline who then takes a single large dose. Chronic poisoning refers to a patient who becomes intoxicated after repeated doses over a period of time.

In acute poisoning, initial symptoms often are gastrointestinal, including nausea, vomiting, diarrhea, and abdominal pain. There is evidence of adrenergic hyperstimulation. Tachycardia is nearly universal and can be extreme. Diaphoresis and tremors are common. Signs of central nervous system hyperstimulation develop, including irritability, agitation, and confusion. Respiratory stimulation may be manifest as dyspnea and respiratory alkalosis. Leukocytosis can be marked; when associated with abdominal pain, a misdiagnosis of a surgical abdomen is possible. Biochemical abnormalities occur, including hypokalemia, hypophosphatemia, hypomagnesemia, and hyperglycemia.[135] Lactic acidosis can occur and may be marked.[136] Occasionally, cardiovascular collapse is seen secondary to loss of peripheral vascular tone. Cardiac arrhythmias are extremely common and include sinus tachycardia, atrial fibrillation, paroxysmal supraventricular tachycardia, multifocal atrial tachycardia, multifocal premature ventricular contractions, ventricular tachycardia, and ventricular fibrillation.[137] Besides malignant cardiac arrhythmias, the other major cause of morbidity and mortality is seizure activity, which often is resistant to therapy and may proceed to status epilepticus. Coma, hypoventilatory respiratory failure, rhabdomyolysis, and compartment syndrome occur occasionally, usually as sequelae of seizure activity.[138]

In chronic poisoning, potentially lethal manifestations occur at lower serum levels than in acute poisoning. Chronic poisoning may be more difficult to recognize because nausea, vomiting, and sinus tachycardia are less likely to be present. In some cases, patients may have no warning symptoms before developing a potentially lethal problem such as a cardiac arrhythmia or seizure activity. In chronic poisoning, patients are unlikely to develop hypotension, biochemical disorders,[139] or rhabdomyolysis.

Because of its narrow therapeutic index, theophylline is a common cause of poisoning. Therapeutic range is generally accepted as 10 to 20 mg/L. Most people manifest some degree of toxicity at a level of 25 mg/L. In acute poisoning, severe toxic manifestations (seizures, malignant cardiac arrhythmias, hypotension) are likely to occur at levels of 80 to 100 mg/L. In chronic poisoning, there is poor correlation between the level and the risk of severe toxicity,[140] with severe toxicity potentially occurring at levels anywhere above the therapeutic range.

TREATMENT

The basics of treatment consist of gastrointestinal decontamination, accelerated removal of theophylline, and supportive measures. Throughout treatment, it is important to follow the clinical condition closely and to monitor serum theophylline levels frequently. The level should be checked every couple of hours until it is clearly falling. Thereafter, the level should be checked periodically, especially after ingestion of sustained-release theophylline, to ensure that there is no reintoxication from a bezoar.

Standard gastrointestinal decontamination is indicated after acute toxic ingestion. Prompt gastric lavage should be performed if the patient presents within a few hours of ingestion. When sustained-release preparations have been ingested, lavage is probably useful even 24 hours after ingestion. Activated charcoal should be given; it adsorbs theophylline in the gut well. A cathartic is administered to speed the evacuation of the charcoal–theophylline complex and any unabsorbed sustained-release theophylline remaining in the gut.

In cases of mild to moderate toxicity, administration of multiple doses of activated charcoal has become standard therapy. There is ample evidence that charcoal can perform gastrointestinal dialysis to remove theophylline even after it has been absorbed systemically,[141] potentially shortening theophylline half-life by 50% or more, yielding a half-life of less than 4 hours. A dosage of 20 to 40 g should be given every 2 hours until the serum theophylline level has fallen

to less than 20 to 25 mg/L.[142] Additional cathartic should be given if charcoal stools have not yet been passed.

Persistent vomiting commonly presents a problem, particularly when trying to administer multiple-dose activated charcoal therapy. Antiemetics such as droperidol and metoclopramide can be used. Recently, ondansetron has been reported to be dramatically effective in cases where other antiemetics have failed.[143–145] Another approach is deep sedation with endotracheal intubation and mechanical ventilation.[146]

Multiple-dose activated charcoal therapy may fail because of ileus or delayed gastric emptying. Lack of bowel sounds is a clue that gastrointestinal dialysis is not likely to succeed. A theophylline level rising toward the severely toxic range or a deteriorating clinical condition are strong indications for more aggressive intervention, namely extracorporeal removal of theophylline.

Extracorporeal removal of theophylline is indicated in severe poisoning. Certainly, such intervention is urgent when there are life-threatening events such as malignant cardiac arrhythmias, recalcitrant hypotension, and seizures. But one must not wait for such complications to occur. Once they occur, it may be too late; the prognosis has already markedly worsened. For example, about one third of patients with seizures will die, and many of the rest will have permanent disability. For this reason, relatively liberal use of extracorporeal removal is justified in patients who have not yet manifested life-threatening complications but who are believed to be at high risk.[142] The clinician must weigh the risks of extracorporeal removal against the risks of developing a life-threatening complication. Lacking dependable clinical warning signs of impending complications, it is prudent to proceed with extracorporeal removal if the theophylline level exceeds 60 to 100 mg/L in acute poisoning or 30 to 60 mg/L in chronic poisoning. A major factor in determining whether to perform extracorporeal removal is the actual or likely rate of theophylline clearance without the procedure[147] (i.e., efficiency of hepatic clearance and multiple-dose activated charcoal). Extracorporeal removal should be continued until the theophylline is less than 20 to 25 mg/L. After termination of the procedure, theophylline level should continue to be monitored. Sometimes a rebound in the level can occur as theophylline is released from tissue stores or, more significantly, as it continues to absorbed from the gut.

Hemoperfusion is the standard method of extracorporeal removal of theophylline. It is extremely efficient, reducing serum half-life of theophylline to about 2 hours. Dramatic clinical improvement can result. It is relatively safe, the most common adverse events being hypotension, hypocalcemia, and thrombocytopenia. Hemodialysis is an effective and acceptable alternative if hemoperfusion is not readily available. It is less efficient, reducing the serum half-life of theophylline to about 4 hours. It is worthwhile to continue multiple-dose activated charcoal and hemodialysis concomitantly, if possible.

Serious complications also must be treated supportively. Beta-blockers play an important role in the management of the cardiovascular toxicity of theophylline. They are generally well tolerated but may occasionally precipitate bronchospasm in asthmatic patients. Short-acting agents such as propranolol or esmolol are preferred. Symptomatic supraventricular arrhythmias usually respond well to beta-blockers alone. Ventricular tachycardia should be treated with standard antiarrhythmics such as lidocaine, although beta-blockers also should be administered as tolerated.

Hypotension should generally be treated initially with judicious volume expansion. Propranolol is useful in reversing hypotension, presumably by blocking the excessive β_2-adrenergic–mediated peripheral vasodilation. Esmolol, a selective β_1-blocker, theoretically should be less effective for this purpose, although it has been used successfully.[148] An alpha-adrenergic agent such as norepinephrine or phenylephrine can be helpful for persistent hypotension.

Seizures can be focal or generalized. They tend to be prolonged, recurrent, and resistant to therapy. As phenobarbital is being loaded IV, generous doses of benzodiazepines should be given to terminate seizure activity. More than 20 mg of diazepam may be necessary. Allowance must be made for the accelerated removal of phenobarbital by multiple-dose activated charcoal, hemoperfusion, and hemodialysis. Phenytoin is not recommended because of lack of efficacy in clinical reports[149] and in animal studies.[150] Benzodiazepines and barbiturates also are the preferred agents to use if sedation is needed because they lower the seizure threshold.

Electrolyte disturbances such as hypokalemia should be treated conservatively. It must be remembered that the low serum level may not reflect a true deficit, but rather an intracellular shift. Over-aggressive replacement can lead to rebound excess as theophylline toxicity resolves. If coma or seizures occur, relevant biochemical disorders, especially hypoglycemia, should be ruled out.

ALCOHOLS ■

The most widely used and abused alcohol is ethanol; clinical problems related to its abuse are discussed in Chapter 101. Isopropanol, methanol, and ethylene glycol poisoning are discussed here. These alcohols are widely available in households and garages and are frequently ingested by accident, as a suicide attempt, or by alcoholics desperate because of interruption of their ethanol supply.

Among these low molecular weight aliphatic alcohols there are certain similarities but also some marked differences. All cause gastric irritation, inebriation, and central nervous system depression. All are relatively weak toxins of themselves but are metabolized by the hepatic enzyme alcohol dehydrogenase to metabolites of varying toxicity. Isopropanol is a more potent inebriant and central nervous system depressant than ethanol and tends to cause more gastrointestinal irritation than ethanol; it is metabolized to acetone, which is also a central nervous system depressant but does not usually cause irreversible damage of itself. Methanol and ethylene glycol also cause a degree of inebriation and are weak toxins, but ingestion of these agents is most significant because of severe delayed toxicity resulting from the production of toxic metabolites.

Treatment of inebriation is largely supportive, but diagnosis and treatment of methanol and ethylene glycol ingestion must be prompt and aggressive to prevent the formation of the toxic metabolites. Dialysis can be definitively lifesaving by removing both the alcohol as well as the toxic metabolites. Ethanol administration is another crucial intervention. Alcohol dehydrogenase, the rate-limiting enzyme in the breakdown of methanol and ethylene glycol and in the formation of the toxic metabolites, has markedly greater preference for ethanol than these other alcohols. An ethanol level of greater than 100 mg/dL virtually turns off their metabolism, allowing elimination of the methanol or ethylene glycol by nonhepatic routes. In mild poisoning, renal excretion is sufficient once toxin production has been turned off. In severe poisoning, ethanol administration limits toxin production while awaiting accomplishment of dialysis.

The alcohols also have varying tendencies to cause a high anion gap metabolic acidosis. Methanol and ethylene glycol cause marked degrees of it, but isopropanol does not. Methanol is metabolized to formic acid, and ethylene glycol is metabolized to oxalic and glycolic acids; these acids account for most of the high anion gap acidosis as well as for most of the toxicity; thus, there is a good correlation between the presence of acidosis and the degree of toxicity. The remainder of the acidosis is accounted for by lactic acid. Isopropanol is metabolized by alcohol dehydrogenase to acetone and then to carbon dioxide and water. Considerable levels of acetone may accumulate, but acidosis usually does not occur.

Although the presence of a high anion gap acidosis is often the clue that leads to the diagnosis of methanol or ethylene glycol poisoning, this finding is variable, especially early in the course. An earlier clue for ingestion of any alcohol may be the presence of an osmolal gap. This refers to the difference between measured osmolality, determined by freezing point depression, and calculated osmolality, estimated (in mOsm/L) by the following formula:

$$2[\text{Na (mMol/L)}] + \text{glucose (mg/dL)}/18$$
$$+ \text{BUN (mg/dL)}/2.8$$

where BUN is blood urea nitrogen. The difference, the osmolal gap, is supposed to be less than 10 mOsm/L. The differential diagnosis of an elevated osmolal gap includes alcohol ingestion, ketotic states, hyperlipidemia, and hyperproteinemia.

METHANOL

Methanol is found in paint removers and a variety of other solvents and is used as an antifreeze, especially in windshield washing solutions. It may also be an ingredient in Sterno canned heat, shellacs, paints, duplicating fluid, gasoline additives, and nail polish remover. Small amounts sometimes are intentionally added to industrial ethanol to render it nonpotable. Homemade alcoholic beverages contaminated by small amounts of methanol have led to epidemics of methanol toxicity. Small quantities, as little as 30 mL or 0.4 mL/kg, can result in significant morbidity and mortality because of its toxic metabolites, formaldehyde and formic acid. There has been occasional toxicity from absorption through the skin and through the lungs.

Absorption from the gastrointestinal tract is rapid. Renal and pulmonary excretion occur, but meanwhile significant amounts are metabolized in the liver first by alcohol dehydrogenase to formaldehyde and then by aldehyde dehydrogenase to formic acid. The former reaction is the rate-limiting step. Formic acid is metabolized, in turn, to carbon dioxide in a reaction in which folic acid is a cofactor. Folic acid deficiency may cause slowing of this step, causing increased formic acid levels and toxicity.

Methanol causes a high anion gap metabolic acidosis. Formic acid accounts for most of it; lactic acid from tissue hypoxia and formate-induced mitochondrial dysfunction accounts for the rest. As acidemia develops, formic acid tends to concentrate in the central nervous system and eyes, which do not become acidotic as quickly.

Initial manifestations of methanol poisoning result from the effects of methanol itself and may be minimal or absent. If present, early symptoms may include nausea, vomiting, abdominal pain, headache, and vertigo. Abdominal pain may be severe enough to mimic a surgical emergency. Although methanol is a significantly less potent inebriant than ethanol, high levels can produce stupor, coma, and respiratory arrest.

Serious manifestations may be delayed up to 12 to 24 hours after the ingestion. Despite minimal initial manifestations, late toxicity can occur as the toxic metabolites and concomitant acidosis are produced. The most serious damage usually occurs in the eyes and in the central nervous system.

The ocular damage is thought to be caused by formaldehyde produced in the retina giving rise to edema and inflammation. Patients may complain of blurred vision or of "snowstorms" or "flashes" obscuring their vision. Funduscopic examination may reveal retinal edema and hyperemia of the optic disk. Physical findings may include diminished visual acuity, visual field deficits, and fixed or dilated pupils. These pathologic features may be reversible in some cases if intervention is prompt and aggressive, but permanent blindness is a common sequelae.

Central nervous system dysfunction can be a sign of cerebral edema. Seizures also may occur. Central nervous damage also may be irreversible.

Other potential complications include hypophosphatemia and pancreatitis. Hyperamylasemia can occur without pancreatitis because of increased plasma salivary activity.

Diagnosis of methanol intoxication is confirmed by a serum methanol level. A high index of suspicion for the diagnosis must be maintained to prevent irreparable organ damage. Suspicion should be raised by the history or the presence of a metabolic acidosis. Late in the course, a serum formate level may be helpful.

In addition to the usual measures for any poisoned patient, specific treatment of methanol ingestion consists of (1) correcting metabolic acidosis, (2) slowing the metabolism of methanol into formic acid through ethanol administration, and (3) accelerating the removal of methanol by hemodialysis. Gastrointestinal decontamination is effective only when done early because methanol is rapidly absorbed.

Hemodialysis is the definitive means of removing methanol from the body and markedly improves prognosis in serious ingestion. Indications for dialysis include serum methanol level above 50 mg/dL, ingestion of a potentially lethal amount of methanol, presence of significant or refractory metabolic acidosis, or evidence of neurologic or ocular dysfunction.[151] Dialysis should be continued until the metabolic acidosis has cleared and the methanol level is less than 25 mg/dL, because methanol level may rebound after dialysis as intracellular methanol redistributes. Some authorities measure a formic acid level and dialyze if this is greater than 20 mg/dL. Peritoneal dialysis is much less effective than hemodialysis.

The presence of significant metabolic acidosis is an indication for dialysis. But even as preparations for dialysis are being made, it is prudent to administer sodium bicarbonate to correct the metabolic acidosis. This helps to decrease toxicity, presumably by encouraging the redistribution of formic acid out of tissues. Large amounts of sodium bicarbonate may be necessary. Fluid and electrolyte disturbances may result, but hemodialysis can be used to correct these disturbances also.

At blood ethanol levels of 13 to 30 mg/dL, ethanol fully saturates alcohol dehydrogenase, effectively turning off production of toxic metabolites. Ethanol administration is indicated immediately in both mild and severe methanol ingestion. In all potentially toxic ingestion, it can be started while the methanol level is pending. It should be continued if the level is above 20 mg/dL. In cases where dialysis will be done, it limits toxicity while arrangements for dialysis are being made, and should then be continued during and after dialysis. It is generally recommended to try to maintain a serum ethanol level of 100 to 200 mg/dL. At these levels, the patient will be inebriated but not stuporous. The recommended dosage is 0.6 to 0.8 g/kg as a bolus over 30 to 60 minutes, followed by maintenance administration of 0.08 to 0.15 g/kg/hour. Ethanol is preferably given IV as a 10% solution, but enteral administration of a 20% to 40% solution is acceptable if no parenteral preparation is available. Dialysis also removes ethanol, so during dialysis measures must be taken to maintain ethanol levels. This can be done by adding 100 to 200 mg/dL of ethanol to the dialysate or by increasing the maintenance rate to .25 to .35/kg/hour. Even after dialysis, ethanol should be continued until the methanol level is undetectable. Ethanol levels must be monitored frequently.

Some authorities recommend folic acid administration, especially if an acidosis is present. This may assist in the breakdown of formic acid (discussed earlier). Doses as high as 30 mg IV every 4 hours have been suggested. Alternatively, leucovorin folinic acid can be given instead.

An investigative drug, 4-methylpyrazole, has been shown to inhibit alcohol dehydrogenase, preventing toxicity if given sufficiently early. This drug has been used extensively in Europe in place of ethanol for both methanol and ethylene glycol poisoning.

ETHYLENE GLYCOL

Ethylene glycol is most frequently encountered as a major component of antifreeze but is also found in various solvents, paints, lacquers, and cosmetics. It has a sweet and pleasant taste, which encourages its ingestion. Like methanol, it is not toxic of itself but is metabolized by alcohol dehydrogenase to several extremely toxic metabolites, including glycoaldehyde, glycolic acid, glyoxylic acid, and oxalic acid. Ingestion of as little as 100 mL, or 1 to 1.5 mL/kg, can be fatal to an adult.

It is rapidly absorbed from the gastrointestinal tract, reaching peak levels at about 2 hours. There is some renal but no significant pulmonary excretion. Most of an ingested dose is metabolized hepatically. The first step, conversion by alcohol dehydrogenase to glycoaldehyde, is the rate-limiting step in its metabolism. Glycoaldehyde is potent in causing central nervous system dysfunction, accounting for the deterioration in mental status seen within several hours after an ingestion. Glycoaldehyde is further metabolized to other toxins, including glycolic acid, glyoxylic acid, and oxalic acid. A high anion gap metabolic acidosis is produced. This mostly results from accumulation of glycolic acid, and, to a lesser extent, lactic acid.

Initial clinical manifestations are generally inebriation and gastrointestinal irritation. Subsequently, usually within the first 12 to 18 hours, there may be development of metabolic acidosis and evidence of progressive central nervous system dysfunction, including hallucinations, encephalopathy, seizures, and coma.[152] Ocular motility is occasionally affected by cranial nerve deficits or nystagmus, and papilledema and diminished visual acuity may occur. Somewhat later, cardiopulmonary problems are seen such as hypertension, tachycardia, arrhythmias, myocardial dysfunction, and then shock and adult respiratory distress syndrome. After 24 to 72 hours, acute renal failure commonly develops, which is usually oliguric and often associated with back pain. Renal failure may be permanent or may resolve after days or weeks. Urinalysis usually reveals calcium oxalate crystals and red blood cells. The precipitation of calcium oxalate crystals in body tissues can give rise to ectopic calcification and hypocalcemia. The latter can cause tetany and hypotension, requiring intravenous calcium administration. Cranial nerve palsies can be a late sequelae, occurring 6 to 18 days after ingestion.[153]

As is the case with methanol, intoxication must be diagnosed early to prevent irreversible organ damage. Clinical suspicion can be confirmed by a serum ethylene glycol level. If ethylene glycol levels cannot be run in a timely fashion, as is the case at many hospitals, a preliminary diagnosis may be based on an appropriate history and physical findings, including inebriation without the odor of alcoholic beverages or an appropriately elevated alcohol level, an elevated serum osmolar gap, a high anion gap acidosis, hypocalcemia, and calcium oxalate crystals in the urine. A simple way to confirm an ethylene glycol ingestion involving automobile antifreeze involves the use of a Wood's lamp to detect fluorescence of the patient's skin, gastric contents, or urine[154]; many brands of antifreeze contain sodium fluorescein to aid mechanics in the detection of cooling system leaks. In large overdoses, the magnitude of the increased osmolal gap can be used to estimate the ethylene glycol level, once other causes of increased osmolal gap have been excluded, including ethanol and methanol ingestion. Late in the course, serum glycolic acid levels may be helpful.

Treatment is similar to that for methanol ingestion. This includes gastrointestinal decontamination within the first couple of hours, bicarbonate administration to correct acidosis, ethanol administration to halt production of toxic metabolites, and dialysis to remove both ethylene glycol and the toxic metabolites. Correction of acidosis greatly reduces toxicity and should be done immediately; large amounts of sodium bicarbonate may be necessary. Ethanol administration is indicated immediately in both mild and severe ingestion[155] unless it is known that the quantity ingested is nontoxic, if the serum ethylene glycol level is less than 20 mg/dL, and if there are no symptoms or metabolic derangements such as acidosis. Indications for dialysis include an ethylene glycol level greater than 20 to 50 mg/dL, significant metabolic acidosis, renal failure, and cardiovascular deterioration. Dialysis should be continued until ethylene glycol is nearly undetectable and metabolic acidosis is resolved; this may take more than 12 hours of continuous dialysis.[156] Peritoneal dialysis does aid in removal but is much less effective than hemodialysis.

Pyridoxine and thiamine are cofactors in the metabolism of some of the toxic metabolites and should be supplemented. A suggested regimen is 50 mg of pyridoxine IM and thiamine 100 mg IM, both given every 4 hours for 2 days. Magnesium also is a cofactor, and supplementation should also be considered, especially in alcoholic patients.

ISOPROPANOL

Rubbing alcohol is the most common source of significant ingestion of isopropanol. But isopropanol is found in a variety of household products such as skin lotions, aftershave lotions, rubbing alcohol, and window cleaner. Sometimes it is used in solvents and antifreeze preparations where it may be associated with ethanol, methanol, or propylene glycol. An ingestion of 2 to 4 mL/kg or 200 mL of a 70% solution is potentially lethal. Toxicity also may occur from extensive dermal contact and perhaps also from inhalation.

Gastrointestinal absorption is rapid; most of an ingested dose is absorbed within 30 minutes. Some is excreted renally but most is metabolized in the liver by alcohol dehydrogenase to acetone. Acetone is removed slowly through the urine and the breath and through hepatic metabolism; it has a half-life of 8 to 26 hours.[157]

Isopropanol is about twice as potent as ethanol in causing central nervous system depression. In addition, the more slowly metabolized acetone also is a potent central nervous system depressant; thus, the effects of isopropanol ingestion are more profound and prolonged than ingestion of the same amount of ethanol. Clinical manifestations are similar to those of ethanol ingestion.

Early symptoms include nausea, vomiting, and abdominal pain. Hemorrhagic gastritis and tracheobronchitis have been reported. Patients may present with evidence of central nervous system dysfunction, including headache, dizziness, blurred vision, weakness, ataxia, nystagmus, dysarthria, areflexia or hyperreflexia, cognitive defects, and confusion. Seizures, coma, and respiratory arrest occur quickly with large ingestions.[158] In larger ingestions, hypotension is common, caused by hypovolemia from fluid loss, vasodilation, and myocardial depression. Arrhythmias and myocardial necrosis may occur. One must also watch for hypoglycemia, because, as in ethanol ingestion, gluconeogenesis is inhibited. Hemolytic anemia has been reported. In contrast to methanol and ethylene glycol poisoning, acidosis is not present unless there is lactic acidosis from hypoperfusion or alcoholic ketoacidosis from concomitant starvation. High levels of acetone can interfere with serum creatinine measurements, giving falsely elevated results.

Diagnosis is based on clinical suspicion confirmed by serum isopropanol level. Besides an appropriate history, clues include the presence of inebriation, the odor of isopropanol or acetone on the breath, ketones in the blood or urine, and an osmolal gap. Acetone level may be useful late in the course.

Ingestion of isopropanol is much more benign than ingestion of methanol or propylene glycol, and the prognosis is excellent if other agents have not been ingested. Supportive treatment is usually sufficient. Gastrointestinal lavage may be worthwhile within the first hour or two of ingestion, but charcoal is not helpful. It does bind isopropanol, but such large quantities of charcoal would have to be given that it is not practical. Hemodialysis or, less preferably, peritoneal dialysis should be strongly considered in cases of severe intoxication associated with coma, refractory hypotension, or isopropanol levels greater than 400 mg/dL.

INSECTICIDES: CHOLINERGIC AGENTS ■

Most insecticides used currently are either organophosphates or carbamates. These two classes of insecticides are discussed together because they are both cholinergic agents and give rise to similar clinical manifestations in poisoning. Recently, their popularity has increased because they have the advantage of being rapidly degraded in the environment and thus cause much less ecological havoc. Unfortunately, exposure of humans to these agents can lead to severe poisoning, although morbidity and mortality can be greatly reduced with prompt recognition and appropriate therapy.

Poisoning most commonly occurs as intentional suicidal ingestion, but is also frequently seen in adults as accidental topical or inhalational exposure during agricultural or industrial work. Poisoning in children is seen from ingestion of consumer products or from topical or inhalational exposure while playing in contaminated areas. In some developing countries, organophosphate insecticides are the most popular agent for suicidal ingestions and cause more deaths than any other class of poison.

The organophosphate and carbamate insecticides exert their acute toxic effects through the inactivation of acetylcholinesterase, the enzyme responsible for the hydrolysis of the neurotransmitter acetylcholine into the inert chemicals acetic acid and choline. The subsequent accumulation of acetylcholine at synapses results in the cholinergic syndrome that is characteristic of organophosphate and carbamate poisoning.

A major distinction between organophosphates and carbamates is the reversibility of their binding (and inactivation) of acetylcholinesterase. The binding between carbamate and acetylcholinesterase reverses spontaneously; acetylcholinesterase is only temporarily inactivated, and recovery occurs within 1 or 2 days with no specific antidote therapy being required. In contrast, the binding between organophosphates and acetylcholinesterase does not reverse spontaneously, although initially it can potentially be reversed by specific antidotes called oximes. If the antidote is not given, the bond between the organophosphate and acetylcholinesterase undergoes a process called aging. This occurs progressively over a period of time that varies according to the specific agent, usually a day or so. After aging is completed, acetylcholinesterase is permanently inactivated, and subsequent recovery must proceed slowly over weeks as replacement enzyme is synthesized.

The oxime antidote used in the United States is pralidoxime, or 2-PAM. Administration of the antidote pralidoxime before aging has occurred dramatically ameliorates the cholinergic syndrome in organophosphate poisoning. Pralidoxime combines irreversibly with organophosphate molecules. As long as the organophosphate–acetylcholinesterase complex has not aged, pralidoxime combines permanently with the organophosphate, breaking the organophosphate–acetylcholinesterase bond, freeing acetylcholinesterase and regenerating its enzymatic activity.

THE CHOLINERGIC SYNDROME

Acetylcholine is a vital neurotransmitter at the neuromuscular junction, within the autonomic nervous system and within the central nervous system. The cholinergic syndrome is a result of pathologic accumulation of acetylcholine within the synapses, the response of acetylcholine receptors to over stimulation by acetylcholine, and the subsequent effects on effector cells.

Acetylcholine receptors are classified as either muscarinic or nicotinic. Muscarinic receptors are found at the synapses between postganglionic parasympathetic nerve fibers and effector cells. Nicotinic receptors are found at the synapses between preganglionic and postganglionic nerve fibers of both the parasympathetic and sympathetic autonomic nervous systems, as well as at the neuromuscular junction.

Acetylcholine accumulation within synapses initially causes marked stimulation of the effector organ. At muscarinic receptors this effect tends to be sustained, but at nicotinic receptors there is subsequent depression. Therefore, the two major features of the cholinergic syndrome are marked parasympathetic stimulation (sustained muscarinic stimulation) and muscular weakness with fasciculations progressing to flaccid paralysis (transient nicotinic stimulation with subsequent depression). Sympathetic stimulation is a variable feature of the cholinergic syndrome; often it is not apparent because of its tendency to be transient and because its manifestations are usually overwhelmed by the opposing parasympathetic stimulation.

Acetylcholine also is an important neurotransmitter within the central nervous system, where most of its receptors are muscarinic. Organophosphates penetrate the blood–

brain barrier well and cause prominent brain dysfunction; carbamates generally do not.

Atropine is a competitive inhibitor of acetylcholine at muscarinic but not at nicotinic receptors. It is useful in the cholinergic syndrome because it ameliorates parasympathetic excess and may help central nervous system dysfunction, but it has no effect on muscular weakness.

CLINICAL MANIFESTATIONS

Excess stimulation of the muscarinic receptors and parasympathetic nervous system is responsible for many of the most obvious and characteristic manifestations of organophosphate and carbamate poisoning. This includes hypersecretion of all exocrine glands, causing lacrimation, hypersalivation, bronchorrhea, diaphoresis, and watery diarrhea. Other manifestations of excessive parasympathetic activity include bradycardia, bronchospasm, miosis, nausea, vomiting, abdominal cramping, and occasionally involuntary urination and defecation.

The most clinically significant manifestation of the cholinergic stimulation of nicotinic receptors is muscular weakness. Initially fasciculations are evident, then there is progression to a flaccid paralysis.

The cholinergic stimulation of the nicotinic receptors of the sympathetic nervous system is evident to a variable degree. Sympathetic tone contributes to the sinus tachycardia that is actually more frequent than bradycardia. Patients occasionally have mydriasis instead of miosis, which hopefully does not lead the clinician away from the proper diagnosis of cholinergic syndrome. Other effects caused by the stimulation of the sympathetic nervous system include hypertension and hyperglycemia.

Manifestations of cholinergic syndrome within the central nervous system include headache, insomnia, irritability, emotional lability, decreased ability to concentrate, psychosis, dysarthria, ataxia, choreoathetosis, delirium, coma, seizures, and focal motor deficits.

Toxicity can occur within 5 minutes in cases of massive ingestion or inhalation but may be delayed up to 12 to 24 hours,[159] especially in cases of dermal exposure or after exposure to highly fat-soluble organophosphates. In cases of delayed symptoms, patients may not offer a history of exposure, not appreciating its relevance to their symptoms. A further obstacle to diagnosis of mild or early organophosphate toxicity is the nonspecific nature of the initial symptoms, which may include headache, dizziness, mild generalized weakness, chest tightness, dyspnea, abdominal cramping, and nausea.

As toxicity progresses, the characteristic signs of the cholinergic syndrome become more prominent. Muscle fasciculations are extremely specific for the cholinergic syndrome. The findings of hypersalivation and miosis are usually present and helpful diagnostically. Lacrimation, bronchospasm, and bradycardia usually are not observed, but when present also are helpful. Other signs of toxicity, such as generalized weakness and encephalopathy, are frequently present but are nonspecific and not helpful in coming to the specific diagnosis. Bronchorrhea is a helpful sign, but before tracheal intu-

bation it may be evident only nonspecifically as rhonchi, rales, or hypoxemia.

Severe intoxications are characterized by major compromise of central nervous system, respiratory or cardiovascular status. Patients may present with seizures, coma, or severe respiratory distress. In these cases, life-threatening situations may distract the physician's attentions away from diagnostic clues of cholinergic toxicity. Cholinergic toxicity must remain in the differential diagnosis of the patient presenting with such problems.

In most cases, diagnosis is facilitated by a history of possible exposure. Sometimes the petroleum-based carrier of the insecticide causes an odor that may be a clue to the diagnosis, and a garlic-like odor has been associated with some organophosphate poisonings.

Synaptic acetylcholinesterase activity cannot itself be directly measured, but diagnosis of toxicity can be confirmed or excluded by measurement of cholinesterase enzyme activity in the red blood cells or in the plasma, because both of these enzymes also are inactivated by cholinergic insecticides. Erythrocyte (true) cholinesterase is the identical enzyme as the acetylcholinesterase found in synapses; measurement of its activity is specific and closely reflects the status of acetylcholinesterase at the synapses. Plasma (pseudo-) cholinesterase is a different enzyme and thus provides a less direct indication of the degree of poisoning; its measurement is more easily performed and thus more widely and more rapidly available, and in early poisoning it is a more sensitive indicator of poisoning. Some patients have chronic depression of plasma cholinesterase levels and may have results falsely indicative of poisoning; this occurs in patients with liver disease, anemia, malnutrition, and familial succinylcholine sensitivity.

Levels should be drawn as soon as the diagnosis is suspected. Results are usually expressed as a percentage activity compared with control. Results have high degrees of intrapatient variability, which sometimes makes interpretation difficult.[160] In severe poisoning, the level is predictably low, less than 20% to 50%. However, levels may even exceed 100% in mild poisoning,[161] and levels considerably less than 100% can be seen in patients that are not poisoned. Intermediate results are more valuable when followed serially as a patient convalesces, enabling a retrospective diagnosis to be made.[161] In carbamate poisoning levels rebound quickly, and levels already may be normal if they are drawn too late.[162] In organophosphate poisoning, the erythrocyte cholinesterase level rebounds quickly after pralidoxime administration, but the plasma cholinesterase level remains unaffected.

Although anticholinesterase levels can provide specific evidence of poisoning, therapy of the poisoning, including atropine administration, must proceed based on a clinical diagnosis. The response to atropine should be observed closely because it may provide valuable diagnostic information to support or refute the diagnosis. The diagnosis is supported by a beneficial clinical response, especially if bradycardia resolves and copious secretions diminish. The diagnosis also is supported by the lack of anticholinergic signs, such as mydriasis and drying of secretions, after administration of a 2-mg dose.

TREATMENT

Decontamination is indicated in acute intoxications and even in acute asymptomatic exposures. If no symptoms appear within 12 hours, then subsequent development of symptoms is not likely. If symptoms do develop, then appropriate antidote therapy and supportive measures are indicated.

The goal of decontamination is to prevent further absorption of toxin. Procedures are adapted to the patient's route of exposure. To prevent becoming exposed themselves, caregivers must take appropriate precautions including gowns, gloves, masks, and goggles.

Gastric decontamination consists of gastric lavage and administration of activated charcoal. It may be wise to withhold cathartic in patients already having diarrhea. Ipecac should not be given because of the likelihood of sudden onset of coma and subsequent aspiration. If the vehicle of the insecticide is a volatile hydrocarbon, consideration should be given to tracheal intubation before gastric lavage.

Skin decontamination consists of removal of all clothing and jewelry, all if which should be placed in a plastic bag. Then skin should be washed with an alkaline soap or a solution of 5% hypochlorite, which can be made by diluting household bleach with tap water. Care must be taken not to abrade skin, which increases absorption.

Conjunctival exposure occurs from vapors and aerosols. This usually is associated with miosis. Copious irrigation of the eyes should be performed in these cases.

If clinically significant signs of poisoning are present, atropine should be given as soon as the diagnosis is suspected and as soon as reasonable oxygenation has been ensured. (In severe hypoxemia, atropine can precipitate ventricular fibrillation.) Large doses of atropine may be needed to oppose the muscarinic over stimulation. An initial dose of 1 to 2 mg can be given. Based on clinical response, the dose can be increased to 2 to 5 mg and repeated every 10 to 15 minutes as needed. The goal is to dry the secretions from the tracheobronchial tree. Normal breath sounds may be a good indicator that enough atropinization has been accomplished. Dilated pupils occur early and may not necessarily be a sign of adequate atropinization. Neither is moderate sinus tachycardia an endpoint for atropine administration.

Once adequate atropinization is accomplished, maintenance atropine must be administered. Continuous infusion may be helpful. Doses of hundreds of milligrams per day may be needed. Once cholinergic toxicity starts resolving, the atropine dose should be tapered to avoid anticholinergic toxicity.

Atropine itself can cause central nervous system toxicity including delirium, coma, seizures, and weakness; this may be indistinguishable from the cholinergic syndrome itself.[163] If such toxicity is suspected but yet more anticholinergic effect is needed for bronchorrhea or other signs of parasympathetic stimulation, consider substituting atropine with glycopyrrolate, an anticholinergic that does not cross the blood–brain barrier and tends to cause less tachycardia.[164]

Atropine often provides dramatic clinical benefit by improving the muscarinic manifestations of the cholinergic syndrome. However, it should be remembered that atropine has no effect on the nicotinic syndrome; atropine has no effect on the generalized muscular weakness that may com-

promise ventilation. In carbamate poisoning, the nicotinic manifestations can be treated only supportively and atropine is the only antidote therapy indicated; fortunately, carbamate toxicity is usually short-lived. In clinically significant acute organophosphate poisoning, both the nicotinic and muscarinic manifestations may respond to subsequent administration of pralidoxime. If a patient is ill enough to have benefited from atropine, then the administration of pralidoxime also is indicated. If there is doubt about whether the illness is caused by organophosphate poisoning versus carbamate poisoning or some other process, it is best to proceed immediately with pralidoxime administration; it is usually well tolerated,[165] and the potential benefits far exceed the risks. Pralidoxime works well for poisoning with many organophosphate agents and poorly for poisoning with some other agents, but administration is nonetheless indicated for all of them.

Early administration of pralidoxime is crucial; greatest benefit is derived if it is given within 6 hours of poisoning, although administration up to 24 to 48 hours and beyond can be beneficial and is worthwhile. Patients most likely to benefit even from late administration are those who have gradual release of organophosphate from depots in body fat (especially in the case of highly lipid soluble organophosphates) or in the gastrointestinal tract.

The initial dose of pralidoxime for an adult is 1 g. It is mixed in 0.9% normal saline and infused IV over 20 or more minutes. In about 30 minutes, a clinical response should be seen consisting of resolution of fasciculations, improved muscle strength, and less parasympathetic hyperstimulation (reflected in reduced atropine requirements). If clinical response is inadequate, the dose can be repeated after an hour.

In mild poisoning, the loading dose should be followed by 0.5 to 1 g IV every 6 to 8 hours for 24 to 48 hours. In severe poisoning, the loading dose should be followed by a continuous infusion starting at up to 500 mg/hour. Dosage may have to be modified in renal insufficiency. Pralidoxime levels may be helpful.

Supportive measures also are extremely important throughout treatment. Potential life-threatening complications to be managed include respiratory failure, coma, seizures, hypotension, and cardiac arrhythmias.

It is especially important to be vigilant in observing the patient's respiratory status and in ensuring adequate airway, ventilation, and oxygenation. Many patients are in respiratory distress at initial presentation, and respiratory failure is the most frequent cause of death in untreated or undertreated patients; it is usually multifactorial in etiology. Ventilation may be impaired by bronchospasm, respiratory muscle weakness, and direct depression of ventilatory drive in the medullary respiratory center. The integrity of the airway may be compromised from hypersalivation, bronchorrhea, inhibition of cough reflexes, and impaired consciousness. Secretions can block airways and compromise oxygenation. Aspiration of gastric contents is a major concern. When a volatile hydrocarbon is the insecticide solvent, chemical pneumonitis can result from inhalation of the fumes. Finally, noncardiogenic pulmonary edema is frequently seen in severe poisonings.[162] For all of these reasons, tracheal intubation and mechanical ventilation is required in severe intoxications.

In less severe intoxications, prompt atropine administration may improve oxygenation by decreasing bronchorrhea and should be given until secretions are dried. In severe intoxications, atropine should also be given promptly but only after oxygenation has been addressed. Atropine also helps bronchospasm; aminophylline should not be used, although inhaled beta-agonists are acceptable. Ipratropium also may be helpful.

Severe brain dysfunction, including coma, seizures, and status epilepticus, is not generally seen with carbamate poisoning but is common in severe organophosphate poisoning. Sometimes these problems improve after administration of atropine and pralidoxime; otherwise, treatment is standard. Seizures should be terminated promptly to avoid brain damage, hyperthermia, and rhabdomyolysis. Diazepam is the drug of first choice for seizures; phenytoin and phenobarbital also may be used.

Hypotension is best managed with appropriate volume administration. Occasionally, pressors may be needed.

Cardiac rhythm must be monitored because lethal arrhythmias can occur. Initially, these tend to be tachyarrhythmias caused by increased sympathetic tone, then followed by bradyarrhythmias and heart block caused by increased parasympathetic tone. Patients are also at risk for ventricular tachycardia and torsade de pointes in organophosphate poisoning, sometimes 5 days or more after poisoning. Prolonged QT intervals are commonly seen and probably play a role in arrhythmogenesis. These arrhythmias may respond to ventricular pacing or isoproterenol infusion. Cardiac rhythm should be monitored until the QT interval has normalized.[166]

Sedation is best accomplished with benzodiazepines. Opioids should be avoided. Succinylcholine is also best avoided; because it is metabolized by pseudocholinesterase, it is likely to have a prolonged action. Glucose levels should be closely monitored, because both hypoglycemia and hyperglycemia can occur.

Persistent abdominal tenderness after the resolution of the acute cholinergic syndrome should raise suspicions for pancreatitis. This complication may be a sequela of hyperstimulation of pancreatic exocrine secretion and spasm of the sphincter of Oddi.[167]

Carbamate poisoning usually resolves in a day or so. Organophosphate poisoning takes considerably longer, resolving in about 10 days in cases of successful antidote treatment, and longer if treatment was delayed or unsuccessful. Recovery is often characterized by relapses, especially with highly lipid soluble agents, and in these cases pralidoxime may have to be continued for many days.

Pulmonary problems such as adult respiratory distress syndrome and pneumonia are frequent, late major complications.[162] Hepatotoxicity can be seen in poisoning with certain organophosphates that are hepatically metabolized. Neuropsychiatric problems may be observed for weeks after recovery but often resolve. Peripheral polyneuropathy is seen as a delayed and often permanent sequela.

ACKNOWLEDGMENT ■

The authors thank Drs. R.F. Raper and M. McD. Fisher who provided the material for this chapter for the first two editions of this book.

REFERENCES ■

1. Koch-Weser J: Acetaminophen. *N Engl J Med* 1976;295:1297
2. Whitcomb DC, Block GD: Association of acetaminophen hepatotoxicity with fasting and ethanol use. *JAMA* 1994; 272:1845
3. Nolan CM, Sandblom RE, Thummel KE, et al: Hepatotoxicity associated with acetaminophen usage in patients reciving multiple drug therapy for tuberculosis. *Chest* 1994;105:408
4. Murphy R, Swartz R, Watkins PB: Severe acetaminophen toxicity in a patient receiving isoniazid. *Ann Intern Med* 1990;113:799 and 1991;114:253(erratum)
5. Flanagan RJ, Mani TGK: Coma and metabolic acidosis early in severe acute paracetamol poisoning. *Hum Toxicol* 1986;5:179
6. Elkins BR, Ford DC, Thompson MB, et al: The effect of activated charcoal on *N*-acetylcysteine absorption in normal subjects. *Am J Emerg Med* 1987;5:483
7. Renzi FP, Donovan JW, Martin TG, et al: Concomitant use of activated charcoal and *N*-acetylcysteine. *Ann Emerg Med* 1985;14:568
8. Spiller HA, Krenzelok EP, Grande GA, et al: A prospective evaluation of the effect of activated charcoal before oral *N*-acetylcysteine in acetaminophen overdose. *Ann Emerg Med* 1994;23:519
9. Chamberlain JM, Gorman RL, Oderda GM, et al: Use of activated charcoal in a simulated poisoning with acetaminophen: a new loading dose for *N*-acetylcysteine? *Ann Emerg Med* 1993;22:1398
10. Rumack BH, Matthews H: Acetaminophen poisoning and toxicity. *Pedatrics* 1975;55:871
11. Harrison P, Wendon J, Gimson A, et al: Improvement by acetylcysteine of hemodynamics and oxygen transport in fulminant hepatic failure. *N Engl J Med* 1991;324:1852
12. Harrison P, Keays R, Bray G, et al: Improved outcome of paracetamol-induced fulminant hepatic failure by late administration of acetylcysteine. *Lancet* 1990;1:1572
13. Smilkstein MJ, Bronstein AC, Linden C, et al: Acetaminophen overdose: a 48-hour intravenous *N*-acetylcysteine treatment protocol. *Ann Emerg Med* 1991;20:1058
14. Howland MA, Smilkstein MJ, Weisman RS: Acetaminophen. In: Goldfrank LR, Flomenbaum NE, Lewin NA, et al (eds). *Goldfrank's Toxicologic Emergencies*, ed 5. Norwalk, CT, Appleton & Lange, 1994:487
15. Keays R, Harrison P, Wendon J, et al: Intravenous acetylcysteine in paracetamol induced fulminant hepatic failure: a prospective controlled trial. *Br Med J* 1991;303:1026
16. O'Grady JG, Alexander G, Hayllar K, et al: Early indicators of prognosis in fulminant hepatic failure. *Gastroenterology* 1989;97:439
17. Harrison P, O'Grady J, Keays R, et al: Serial prothrombin time as prognostic indicator in paracetamol induced fulmnant haepatic failure. *Br Med J* 1990;301:964
18. Pereira L, Langley P, Hayllar K, et al: Coagulation factor V and VII/V ratio as predictors of outcome in paracetamol induced fulminant hepatic failure: relation to other prognostic indicators. *Gut* 1992;33:98
19. Sainsbury SJ: Fatal salicylate toxicity from bismuth subsalicylate. *West J Med* 1991;155:637
20. Vernacc MA, Belucci AG, Wilkes BM: Chronic salicylate toxicity due to consumption of over-the-counter bismuth subsalicylate. *Am J Med* 1994;97:308
21. Flomenbaum NE, Goldfrank LR: Salicylates. In: Goldfrank LR, Flomenbaum NE, Lewin NA (eds). *Goldfrank's Toxicologic Emergencies*, ed 5. Norwalk, CT, Appleton & Lange, 1994:501

22. Hill JB: Salicylate intoxication. *N Engl J Med* 1973;288:1110
23. Gabow PA, Anderson RJ, Potts DE, et al: Acid-base disturbances in salicylate poisoning in adults. *Arch Intern Med* 1979;138:1481
24. Thisted B, Krantz T, Strom J, et al: Acute salicylate self-poisoning in 177 consecutive patients treated in the ICU. *Acta Anaesthesiol Scand* 1987;31:312
25. Anderson RJ, Potts DE, Gabow PA, et al: Unrecognized adult salicylate intoxication. *Ann Intern Med* 1976;85:745
26. Pond SM, Armstrong JG, Henderson A: Late diagnosis of chronic salicylate intoxication. *Lancet* 1993;342:687
27. Gittelman DK: Chronic salicylate intoxication. *South J Med* 1993;86:683
28. Leatherman JW, Schmitz PG: Fever, hyperdynamic shock and multiple-system organ failure: a pseudo-sepsis syndrome associated with chronic salicylate intoxication. *Chest* 1991; 100:1391
29. Keller RE, Schwab RA, Krenzelok EP: Contribution of sorbitol combined with actitivated charcoal in prevention of salicylate absorption. *Ann Emerg Med* 1990;19:654
30. Filippone GA, Fish SS, Lacouture PG, et al: Reversible adsorption (desorption) of aspirin from activated charcoal. *Arch Intern Med* 1987;147:1390
31. Burton BT, Bayer MJ, Barron L, et al: Comparison of activated charcoal and gastric lavage in the prevention of aspirin absorption. *J Emerg Med* 1984;1:411
32. Curtis RA, Barone J, Giacona N: Efficacy of ipecac and activated charcoal/cathartic. *Arch Intern Med* 1984;144:48
33. Raschke R, Arnold-Capell PA, Richeson R, et al: Refractory hypoglycemia secondary to topical salicylate intoxication. *Arch Intern Med* 1991;151:591
34. Thurston JH, Pollock PG, Warren SK, Jones EM: Reduced brain glucose with normal plasma glucose in salicylate poisoning. *Clin Invest* 1970;49:2139
35. Walters JS, Woodring JH, Stelling CB, et al: Salicylate-induced pulmonary edema. *Radiology* 1983;146:289
36. Hormaechea E, Carlson RW, Rogove H, et al: Hypovolemia, pulmonary edema and protein changes in severe salicylate poisoning. *Am J Med* 1979;66:1046
37. Berk WA, Andersen JC: Salicylate-associated asystole: report of two cases. *Am J Med* 1989;86:505
38. Morgan AG, Polak A: The excretion of salicylate in salicylate poisoning. *Clin Sci* 1971;41:475
39. Prescott LF, Balali-Mood M, Critchley JAJH, et al: Diuresis or urinary alkalinisation for salicylate poisoning? *Br Med J* 1982;285:1983
40. Hillman RJ, Prescott LF: Treatment of salicylate poisoning with repeated oral charcoal. *Br Med J* 1985;291:1472
41. Mofenson HC, Caraccio TR, Greensher J: Gastrointestinal dialysis with activated charcoal and cathartic in the treatment of adolescent intoxications. *Clin Pediatr* 1985;24:678
42. Vertrees JE, McWilliams BC, Kelley HW: Repeated oral administration of activated charcoal for treating aspirin overdose in young children. *Pediatrics* 1990;85:594
43. Merigian KS, Hedges JR, Kaplan LA, et al: Plasma catecholamine levels in cyclic antidepressant overdose. *Clin Toxicol* 1991;29:177
44. Hulten BA, Adams R, Askenasi R, et al: Predicting severity of tricyclic antidepressant overdose. *Clin Toxicol* 1992;30:161
45. Boehnert MT, Lovejoy FH: Value of the QRS duration versus the serum drug level in predicting seizures and ventricular arrhythmias after an acute overdose of tricyclic antidepressants. *N Engl J Med* 1985;313:474
46. Foulke GE, Albertson TE: QRS interval in tricyclic antidepressant overdosage: inaccuracy as a toxicity indicator in emergency settings. *Ann Emerg Med* 1987;16:16
47. Hoegholm A, Clementsen P: Hypertonic sodium chloride in severe antidepressant overdosage. *Clin Toxicol* 1991;29:297
48. Haddad LM: Managing tricyclic antidepressant overdose. *Am Fam Physician* 1992;46:153
49. Mayron R, Ruiz E: Phenytoin: does it reverse tricyclic antidepressant induced cardiac conduction abnormalities? *Ann Emerg Med* 1986;15:876
50. Callaham M, Schumaker H, Pentel P: Phenytoin prophylaxis of cardiotoxicity in experimental amitriptylene poisoning. *J Pharmacol Exp Ther* 1988;245:216
51. Frommer DA, Kulig KW, Marx JA, et al: Tricyclic antidepressant overdose: a review. *JAMA* 1987;257:521
52. Orr DA, Bramble MG: Tricyclic antidepressant poisoning and prolonged external cardiac massage during asystole. *Br Med J* 1981;283:1107
53. Callaham M, Kassel D: Epidemiology of fatal tricyclic antidepressant ingestion: implications for management. *Ann Emerg Med* 1985;14:1
54. Tokarski GF, Young MJ: Criteria for admitting patients with tricyclic antidepressant overdose. *J Emerg Med* 1988;6:121
55. Shannon MW: Duration of QRS disturbances after severe tricyclic antidepressant intoxication. *Clin Toxicol* 1992;30:377
56. Wedin GP, Oderda GM, Klein-Schwartz W, et al: Relative toxicity of cyclic antidepressants. *Ann Emerg Med* 1986; 15:797
57. Munger MA, Effron BA: Amoxapine cardiotoxicity. *Ann Emerg Med* 1988;17:274
58. Litovitz TL, Troutman WG: Amoxapine overdose: seizures and fatalities. *JAMA* 1983;250:1069
59. Strobusch AD, Jefferson JW: The checkered history of lithium in medicine. *Pharmacy History* 1980;22:72
60. Terhaag B, Scherber A, Schaps P, et al: The distribution of lithium into the cerebrospinal fluid, brain tissue and bile in man. *Int J Clin Pharmacol Biopharmacol* 1978;16:333
61. Goodnick PJ, Fieve RR, Meltzer HL, et al: Lithium elimination half-life and duration of therapy. *Clin Pharmacol Ther* 1981;29:47
62. Schou M: Pharmacology and toxicology of lithium. *Ann Rev Pharmacol* 1976;16:231
63. Rageb MA: The clinical significance of lithium-nonsteroidal antiinflammatory drug interactions. *J Clin Psychopharmacol* 1990;10:350
64. Correa F, Eiser A: Angiotensin converting enzyme inhibitors and lithium toxicity. *Am J Med* 1992;93:108
65. Groleau G: Lithium toxicity. *Emerg Med Clin North Am* 1994;12:511
66. Solomon K, Vickers R: Dysarthria resulting from lithim carbonate: a case report. *JAMA* 1975;231:280
67. Depaulo J, Folstein MF, Correa EI: The course of delirum due to lithium intoxication. *J Clin Psychiatry* 1982;43:447
68. Baldessarini RJ: Lithium salts: 1970–1975. *Ann Intern Med* 1975;83:527
69. Simiard M, Gumbimer B, Lee A, et al: Lithium carbonate intoxication: a case report and review of the literature. *Arch Intern Med* 1989;149:36
70. Hall RCW, Perl M, Pfefferbaum B: Lithium therapy and toxictiy. *Am Fam Physician* 1979;19:133
71. Christenson TAT: Lithium hypercalcemia and hyperparathyroidism. *Lancet* 1976;ii:144
72. Graze KK: Hyperparathyroidism in association with lithium therapy. *J Clin Psychiatry* 1981;41:38
73. Garfinkle N, Exrin C, Stancer HC: Hypothyroidism and hyperparathyroidism associated with lithium. *Lancet* 1973;ii:331
74. Christiansen C, Baastrup PC, Transbol I: Development of "primary" hyperparathyroidism during lithium therapy: longitudinal study. *Neuropsychobiology* 1980;2:280

75. Shopsin D, Stern S, Gershon S: Altered carbohydrate metabolism during treatment with lithium carbonate. *Arch Gen Psychiatry* 1972;26:366

76. Schou M, Amdisen A, Jensen SE, et al: Occurrence of goitre during lithium treatment. *Br Med J* 1968;3:710

77. Wolff J: Lithium interactions with the thyroid gland. In: Cooper TB, Gershon S, Kline N, et al (eds). *Lithium: Controversies and Unresolved Issues*. Amsterdam, Exerpta Medica, 1979:552

78. Lydiard RB, Gelenberg AJ: Hazards and adverse effects of lithium. *Ann Rev Med* 1982;33:327

79. Reisberg B, Gershon S: Toxicology and side effects of lithium therapy. In: Cooper TB, Gershon S, Kline N, et al (eds). *Lithium: Controversies and Unresolved Issues*. Amsterdam, Exerpta Medica, 1979:449

80. Bucht G, Smigan L, Wahlin A, et al: ECG changes during lithium therapy: a prospective study. *Acta Med Scand* 1984; 216:101

81. Mateer JR, Clark MR: Lithium toxicity with rarely reported ECG manifestations. *Ann Emerg Med* 1982;11:208

82. Palileo EV, Coelho A, Westveer D, et al: Persistent sinus node dysfunction secondary to lithium therapy. *Am Heart J* 1983;106:1443

83. Tilikian AG, Schroeder JS, Kao JJ, et al: The cardiovascular effects of lithium on man: a review of the literature. *Am J Med* 1976;61:655

84. Wellens HJ, Cats VM, Düren DR: Symptomatic sinus node abnormalities following lithium carbonate therapy. *Am J Med* 1975;59:285

85. Lydiard RB, Gelenberg AJ: Hazards and adverse effects of lithium. *Ann Rev Med* 1982;33:327

86. Smith SW, Ling L, Halstenson CE: Whole-bowel irrigation as a treatment for acute lithium overdose. *Ann Emerg Med* 1991;20:536

87. Hansen HE, Amdisen A: Lithium intoxication. *Am J Med* 1978;47:123

88. DePaulo JR: Lithium. *Psychiatr Clin North Am* 1984;7:587

89. Baldessarini RJ: Drugs and the treatment of psychiatric disorders. In: Gilman AG, Rall TW, Neis AS, et al (eds). *The Pharmacologic Basis of Therapeutics*, ed 8. New York, Macmillan, 1990:393

90. McGuigan MA: Phenothiazines. *Clin Toxicol Rev* 1981;3:4

91. Trayle WH: Phenothiazine-induced agranulocytosis. *JAMA* 1986;256:1957

92. Fishbain DA: Priapism resulting from fulphenazine hydrochloride trestment reversed by diphenhydramine. *Ann Emerg Med* 1985;14:600

93. Fowler ND, McCall D, Chou T, et al: Electrocardiographic changes and cardiac arrhythmias in patients receiving psychotic drugs. *Am J Cardiol* 1981;37:223

94. Peterson C: Seizures induced by acute loxapine overdose. *Am J Psychiatry* 1981;138:1089

95. Zee-Cheng CS, Mueller CE, Seifert CF, et al: Haloperidol and *torsades de pointes. Ann Intern Med* 1980;140:975

96. Höjer J, Baehrendtz S: The effect of flumazenil (Ro-15-1788) in the management of self-induced benzodiazepine poisoning. *Acta Med Scand* 1988;224:357

97. Plant JR, MacLeod DB: Response of a promethazine-induced coma to flumazenil. *Ann Emerg Med* 1994;24:979

98. Spivey WH, Roberts JR, Derlet RW: A clinical trial of escalating doses of flumazenil for reversal of suspected benzodiazepine overdose in the emergency department. *Ann Emerg Med* 1993;22:1813

99. Chern TL, Hu SC, Lee CH, Deng JF: Diagnostic and therapeutic utility of flumazenil in comatose patients with drug overdose. *Am J Emerg Med* 1993;11:122

100. Winkler E, Almog S, Kriger D, et al: Use of flumazenil in the diagnosis and treatment of patients with coma of unknown etiology. *Crit Care Med* 1993;21:538

101. Mordel A, Winkler E, Almog S, et al: Seizures after flumazenil administration in a case of combined benzodiazepine and tricyclic antidepressant overdose. *Crit Care Med* 1992;20:1733

102. Hodgkinson DW, Driscoll P: Diagnostic utility of flumazenil in coma with suspected poisoning. *Br Med J* 1991;302:238

103. Burr W, Sandham P, Judd A: Death after flumazenil. *Br Med J* 1989;298:1713

104. Derlet RW, Albertson TE: Flumazenil induces seizures and death in mixed cocaine–diazepam ingestions. *Ann Emerg Med* 1994;23:494

105. Short TG, Maling T, Galletly DC: Ventricular arrhythmia precipitated by flumazenil. *Br Med J* 1988;296:1070

106. Marchant B, Wray R, Leach A, et al: Flumazenil causing convulsions and ventricular tachycardia. *Br Med J* 1989;299:860

107. Lopez A, Rebollo J: Benzodiazepine withdrawal syndrome after a benzodiazepine antagonist. *Crit Care Med* 1990;18:1480

108. Prichard B, Battersby L, Cruickshank JM: Overdosage with beta-adrenergic blocking agents. *Adv Drug React Poison Rev* 1984;3:91

109. Frishman WH: Beta-adrenergic blockers. *Med Clin North Am* 1988;72:37

110. Toraason B: Biochemical principles of cardiac toxicology. In: Baskin SI (ed). *Principles of Cardiac Toxicology*. Boca Raton, CRC Press, 1991:39

111. Weinstein RS: Recognition and management of poisoning with beta-adrenergic blocking agents. *Ann Emerg Med* 1984;13:1123

112. de Wildt D, Sangster B, Langemeijer J, et al: Different toxicological profiles for various beta-blocking agents on cardiac function in isolated rat hearts. *J Toxicol Clin Toxicol* 1984;22:115

113. Thorpe P: Pindolol in hypertension. *Med J Aust* 1971;135:1242

114. Smit AJ, Mulder POM, de Jong PE, et al: Short reports: acute renal failure after overdose of labetolol. *Br Med J* 1986;293:1142

115. Smith RC, Wilkenson J, Hull RL: Glucogon for propranolol overdose. *JAMA* 1985;254:2412

116. Critchley JA, Ungar A: The management of acute poisoning due to beat-adrenoceptor antagonists. *Med Toxicol Adverse Drug Exp* 1989;4:32

117. Kenyon CJ, Aldinger GE, Joshipura P, et al: Successful resuscitation using external cardiac pacing in beta adrenergic antagonist-induced bradysystolic arrest. *Ann Emerg Med* 1988;17:711

118. Lane AS, Woodward AC, Goldman MR: Massive propranolol overdose poorly responsive to pharmacologic therapy: use of an intra-aortic balloon pump. *Ann Emerg Med* 1987;16:1381

119. Sperelakis N: Cyclic AMP and phosphorylation in regulation of calcium infulx into myocardial cells and blockade by calcium antagonist drugs. *Am Heart J* 1984;107:347

120. Kenny J. Calcium channel blocking agents and the heart. *Br Med J* 1985;291:1150

121. Ramoska EA, Spiller HA, Winter M, et al: A 1-year evaluation of calcium channel blocker overdoses: toxicity and treatment. *Ann Emerg Med* 1993;22:196

122. Kerns W, Kline J, Ford MD: β-Blocker and calcium channel blocker toxicity. *Emerg Med Clin North Am* 1994;12:365

123. Kenny J: Treating overdose with calcium channel blockers. *Br Med J* 1994;308:992

124. Buckley NA, Dawson AH, Howarth DM, et al: Slow release verapamil poisoning: use of polyethylene glycol whole-bowel lavage and high-dose calcium. *Med J Aust* 1993;158:202

125. Buckley NA, Whyte IM, Dawson AH: Overdose with calcium channel blockers. *Br Med J* 1994;308:1639

126. Doyon S, Roberts JR: The use of glucagon in a case of calcium channel blocker overdose. *Ann Emerg Med* 1993;22:1229

127. Goenen M, Col J, Compere A, et al: Treatment of severe verapamil poisoning with combined amrinone-isoproterenol therapy. *Am J Cardiol* 1986;58:1142

128. Hurwitz N, Wade OL: Intensive hospital monitoring of adverse reaction to drugs. *Br Med J* 1969;1:531

129. Beller GA, Smith TW, Abelmann WH, et al: Digitalis intoxication: a prospective clinical study with serum level correlations. *N Engl J Med* 1971;284:989

130. Mahdyoon H, Battilana G, Rosman H, et al: The evolving pattern of digoxin intoxication: observations at a large urban hospital from 1980 to 1988. *Am Heart J* 1990;120:1189

131. Litovitz TT, Schmitz BF, Holm KC: 1988 Annual Report of the American Medical Association of Poison Control Centers Data Collection System. *Am J Emerg Med* 1989;7:479

132. Smith TW: Digitalis: mechanisms of action and clinical use. *N Engl J Med* 1988;318:358

133. Kelly RA, Smith TW: Recognition and management of digitalis toxicity. *Am J Cardiol* 1992;69:108G

134. Antman EM, Wenger TL, Butler VP, et al: Treatment of 150 cases of life-threatening digitalis intoxication with digoxin-specific Fab antibody fragments: final report of a multicenter study. *Circulation* 1990;81:1744

135. Hall KW, Dobson KE, Dalton JG: Metabolic abnormalities associated with intentional theophylline overdose. *Ann Intern Med* 1993;119:1161

136. Bernard S: Severe lactic acidosis following theophylline overdose. *Ann Emerg Med* 1991;20:1135

137. Sessler CN: Theophylline toxicity. *Am J Med* 1990;88:567

138. Titley OG, Williams N: Theophylline toxicity causing rhabdomyolosis and acute compartment syndrome. *Intensive Care Med* 1992;18:129

139. Shannon M: Hypokalemia, hyperglycemia and plasma catecholamine activity after severe theophylline intoxication. *Clin Toxicol* 1994;32:41

140. Shannon M: Predictors of major toxicity after theophylline overdose. *Ann Intern Med* 1993;119:1161

141. Kulig KW, Bar-Or D, Rukmack BH: Intravenous theophylline poisoning and multiple-dose charcoal in an animal model. *Ann Emerg Med* 1987;16:842

142. Cooling DS: Theophylline toxicity. *J Emerg Med* 1993;11:415

143. Brown SGA, Prentice DA: Ondasetron in the treatment of theophylline overdose. *Med J Aust* 1992:156:512

144. Sage TA, Jones WN, Clark RF: Ondansetron in the treatment of intractable nausea associated with theophylline toxicity. *Ann Pharmacother* 1993;27:584

145. Roberts JR, Carney S, Boyle SM, et al: Ondansetron quells drug-resistant emesis in theophylline poisoning. *Am J Emerg Med* 1993;11:609

146. Henderson A, Wright DM, Pond SM: Management of theophylline overdose patients in the intensive care unit. *Anaesth Intensive Care* 1992;20:56

147. Park GD, Spector R, Roberts RJ: Use of hemoperfusion for treatment of theophylline intoxication. *Am J Med* 1983;74:961

148. Seneff M, Scott J, Friedman B, et al: Acute theophylline toxicity and the use of esmolol to reverse cardiovascular instability. *Ann Emerg Med* 1990;19:671

149. Paloucek FP, Rodvold KA: Evaluation of theophylline overdoses and toxicities. *Ann Emerg Med* 1988;17:135

150. Hoffman A, Pinto ED, Gilhar D: Effect of pretreatment with anticonvulsants on theophylline-induced seizures in the rat. *J Crit Care* 1993;8:198

151. Gonda A, Gault H, Churchill D, et al: Hemodialysis for methanol intoxication. *Am J Med* 1978;64:749

152. Parry MF, Wallach R: Ethylene glycol poisoning. *Am J Med* 1974;57:143

153. Spillane L, Roberts JR, Meyer AE: Multiple cranial nerve deficits after ethylene glycol poisoning. *Ann Emerg Med* 1991;20:208

154. Winter ML, Ellis MD, Snodgrass WR: Urine fluorescence using a Wood's lamp to detect the antifreeze additive sodium fluorescein: a qualitative adjunctive test in suspected ethylene glycol ingestions. *Ann Emerg Med* 1990;19:663

155. Jacobsen D, Ostby N, Bredesen JE: Studies on ethylene glycol poisoning. *Acta Med Scand* 1982;212:11

156. Curtin L, Kraner J, Wine H, et al: Complete recovery after massive ethylene glycol ingestion. *Arch Intern Med* 1992;152:1311

157. Pappas AA, Ackerman BH, Olsen KM, et al: Isopropanol ingestion: a report of six episodes with isopropanol and acetone serum concentration time data. *Clin Toxicol* 1991;29:11

158. Rich J, Scheife RT, Katz N, et al: Isopropyl alcohol intoxication. *Arch Neurol* 1990;47:322

159. Namba T, Nolte CT, Jackrel J, et al: Poisoning due to organophosphate insecticide. *Am J Med* 1971;50:475

160. Nouira S, Abroug F, Elatrous S, et al: Prognostic value of serum cholinesterase in oganophosphate poisoning. *Chest* 1994;106:1811

161. Coye MJ, Barnett PG, Midtling JE: Clinical confirmation of organophosphate poisoning by serial cholinesterase analyses. *Arch Intern Med* 1987;147:438

162. Goswamy R, Chadhuri A, Mashur AA: Study of respiratory failure in organophosphate and carbamate poisoning. *Heart Lung* 1994;23:466

163. Bardin PG, van Eeden SF, Moolman JA, et al: Organophosphate and carbamate poisoning. *Arch Intern Med* 1994;154:1433

164. Bardin PG, van Eeden SF: Organophosphate poisoning: grading the severity and comparing treatment between atropine and glycopyrrolate. *Crit Care Med* 1990;18:956

165. Tafuri J, Roberts J: Organophosphate poisoning. *Ann Emerg Med* 1987;16:193

166. Ludiomirsky A, Klein HO, Sarelli P, et al: Q-T prolongation and polymorphous ("tordades de pointes") ventricular arrhythmias associated with organophosphate insecticide poisoning. *Am J Cardiol* 1982;49:1654

167. Dressel TD, Goodale RL, Arneson MA, et al: Pancreatitis as a complication of anticholinesterase insecticide intoxication. *Ann Surg* 1979;189:199

Critical Care, Third Edition, edited by Joseph M. Civetta,
Robert W. Taylor, and Robert R. Kirby.
Lippincott-Raven Publishers, Philadelphia, PA © 1997.

CHAPTER 101

■

Substance Abuse and Withdrawal: Alcohol, Cocaine, and Opioids

Joan Shaffer

IMMEDIATE CONCERNS ■

MAJOR PROBLEMS

More than 9 million Americans are thought to be alcoholics.[1] Over 30 million Americans have experimented with cocaine, and approximately 5 million are regular users.[2,3] Over 500,000 people in this country are addicted to opioids.[4] Casual or habitual use of these drugs contributes to acute and chronic illness. Substance use underlies many forms of injury, including vehicular accidents, falls, near drownings, thermal injury, homicide, and suicide.[5-7] Over 10% of patients evaluated medically for acute drug intoxication require admission to an ICU. At least one half of these patients have used more than one drug.[8]

STRESS POINTS

1. The patient acutely intoxicated with ethanol may be hyperventilating, therefore airway management is a high priority.
2. Chronic alcohol users tend to have depleted thiamine, phosphate, magnesium, and glycogen stores.
3. Seizure, subarachnoid hemorrhage, and stroke should be considered in the cocaine abuser who presents with altered mental status.
4. Cocaine-related chest pain or myocardial infarction (MI) can occur up to 96 hours after cocaine use.

5. The patient who is comatose secondary to opioid overdose typically presents with miotic pupils and shallow respirations.

ESSENTIAL DIAGNOSTIC TESTS AND PROCEDURES

In addition to a careful medical history and physical examination, the following additional studies may be considered in the substance-abuse patient with altered mental status.

1. Stat blood glucose
2. Toxicology screen
3. Arterial blood gas
4. Electrocardiogram and cardiac enzymes (cocaine intoxication, chest pain)
5. Computed tomography scan of the head

INITIAL THERAPY

1. Give 50 mg of thiamine followed by 25 g of dextrose to the patient who presents with an altered mental status believed to be secondary to alcohol intoxication. If the patient becomes more responsive, follow with a constant infusion of 10% dextrose in water and monitor blood glucose levels. If the patient does not respond, administer 0.4 to 2 mg of intravenous (IV) naloxone.

2. Treat the patient in alcohol withdrawal with benzodiazepines while carefully monitoring respiratory and hemodynamic status.
3. Benzodiazepines are the initial anticonvulsant of choice for cocaine-related seizures.
4. Treat cocaine-related cardiac ischemia with oxygen, aspirin, and nitrates. Thrombolytic agents can be used in the setting of cocaine-associated acute MI if no contraindications exist.
5. Phentolamine may be useful in cocaine-related myocardial ischemia.
6. Avoid type 1a antiarrhythmic agents in patients with cocaine intoxication because they decrease the seizure threshold.
7. Avoid beta-adrenergic blockers in the cocaine user because they may exacerbate coronary vasoconstriction caused by unopposed alpha-adrenergic stimulation.
8. Treat acute agitation secondary to cocaine use with IV benzodiazepines, being aware of airway and hemodynamic implications.
9. Avoid neuromuscular blockade, if possible, in the cocaine-intoxicated patient because it may mask seizure activity.
10. Treat acute hypertension secondary to cocaine toxicity with nitroprusside or labetalol.
11. After ensuring an adequate airway, the patient with an opioid overdose should receive naloxone. Be mindful that naloxone can precipitate acute withdrawal symptoms in the chronic opioid abuser. Naloxone can be given in a dosage of 2 mg intravenously every 4 minutes to a total of 20 mg. If central nervous system (CNS) depression is not reversed at this point, other causes of coma must be considered. If the patient becomes more responsive after naloxone, the dose that was required to reverse sedation can be given hourly by continuous infusion.
12. Methadone (20 to 30 mg), buprenorphine (2 to 4 mg), or clonidine (15 to 20 µg/kg) can be used to treat acute opioid withdrawal. Buprenorphine itself can be addictive. Hypotension and bradycardia can limit clonidine use for acute opioid withdrawal.

ETHANOL ■

Red red wine, you make me feel so fine
Red red wine, I can't get you off my mind
Red red wine, I loved you right from the start
Right from the start with all my heart
Red red wine, I'm gonna love you till I die...
—UB-40, "Red Red Wine"

Ethanol (ethyl alcohol) is the most abused drug in this country and is, therefore, a major medical and social problem. (Other alcohols, such as methanol, isopropyl, and ethylene glycol, are discussed in Chap. 100.)

Ethanol is rapidly absorbed in unaltered form from the stomach and small intestine. The presence of food (especially milk and fatty foods) in the stomach delays absorption, whereas the presence of water enhances absorption. Ethanol diffuses freely into body tissues. It is chiefly degraded in the liver. Less than 10% is excreted by the lungs or kidneys or through the skin. Several hepatic enzyme systems independently metabolize ethanol to acetaldehyde. The primary degradation pathway is in the hepatic cytosol by alcohol dehydrogenase, with nicotinamide adenine dinucleotide as a cofactor. Acetaldehyde generated by this process is in turn metabolized through the Krebs cycle to carbon dioxide and water: 7/kcal/g is liberated in this process. Most persons can metabolize about 150 mg of ethanol per kilogram body weight per hour. This is equivalent to about 12 ounces of beer or 1 ounce of 90-proof whiskey.

ACUTE TOXICITY

Common features of ethanol intoxication are shown in Table 101-1. Ethanol is a sedative-hypnotic drug and exerts its primary effects on the CNS. Intoxication depends on the rate of rise of the blood alcohol level and the length of time over which it is maintained. Blood alcohol levels of 20 to

TABLE 101-1. Clinical Manifestations of Alcohol Intoxication

Central nervous system
  Decreased inhibition
  Slowed reaction time
  Visual disturbance
  Incoordination
  Slurred speech
  Diplopia
  Nystagmus
  Lethargy, stupor, coma
Cardiovascular
  Vasodilation
  Cardiac dysrhythmias
  Myocardial depression
Respiratory
  Hypoventilation
  Aspiration
Metabolic
  Electrolyte abnormalities
    Hypoglycemia
    Hypophosphatemia
    Hypomagnesemia
  Acid-base disturbance
    Respiratory acidosis
    Metabolic alkalosis (vomiting)
    Metabolic acidosis (alcoholic ketoacidosis)
Gastrointestinal
  Gastritis
  Increased incidence of peptic ulcer
  Pancreatitis
  Alcoholic hepatitis
Hematologic
  Suppression of all bone marrow cell lines
Other
  Suppression of ADH (diuresis)
  Increased sweating
  Altered temperature regulation

ADH, antidiuretic hormone.

30 mg/dL are often associated with a mild euphoria, delayed reaction time, decreased inhibition, and alteration in judgment. Most persons exhibit gross intoxication at levels above 150 mg/dL. Obtundation develops at levels above 300 mg/dL, and death may result from respiratory depression or cardiovascular collapse when levels exceed 400 to 500 mg/dL.[9,10]

Acute ethanol intoxication is often associated with an increased heart rate and cardiac output, whereas prolonged intoxication may be associated with depressed myocardial contractility.[11] Acute intoxication is also associated in some persons with a variety of cardiac arrhythmias, especially atrial fibrillation ("holiday heart" syndrome). Cutaneous vessels dilate whereas splanchnic vessels constrict. Increased sweating associated with cutaneous vasodilation may account for the decrease in core temperature often associated with acute ethanol intoxication.

Metabolic problems related to alcohol ingestion can be life threatening and are often difficult to manage. Alcohol enhances the urinary excretion of phosphate and magnesium and can cause clinically significant hypophosphatemia and hypomagnesemia. The alcoholic patient often has marginal glycogen stores. Because alcohol also inhibits hepatic gluconeogenesis, it may precipitate profound hypoglycemia. A variety of acid-base disturbances are seen in acute alcoholic intoxication. Depression of the respiratory center in the severely intoxicated person may be associated with hypoventilation and a respiratory acidosis. Nausea and vomiting may cause hypokalemia and metabolic alkalosis. The chronic alcoholic may develop alcoholic ketoacidosis. This syndrome usually follows acute intoxication coupled with insufficient nutrient intake. The liver produces excessive ketones in response to starvation. Pancreatitis is frequently present in these patients. The blood glucose may be low or high in this setting but is rarely above 300 mg/dL. The condition usually responds to volume replacement and administration of glucose. Thiamine should be administered before glucose to avoid precipitation of acute beriberi and Wernicke-Korsakoff syndrome (Table 101-2).

Ethanol ingestion may cause acute gastritis and gastrointestinal bleeding. Alcoholics have an increased incidence of peptic ulcer disease and pancreatitis. Acute alcohol intoxication may precipitate alcoholic hepatitis in the chronic user. All bone marrow cell lines are suppressed by alcohol ingestion. Suppression of antidiuretic hormone by ethanol causes diuresis and may lead to profound hypovolemia, especially if there is associated nausea, vomiting, or diarrhea.

TREATMENT OF ACUTE INTOXICATION

Treatment of acute ethanol intoxication is largely supportive. If the patient presents with an altered mental status, 50 to 100 mg of thiamine, 25 g of glucose, and 2 mg of naloxone should be administered intravenously. If the patient responds to the administration of glucose or if blood glucose levels are depressed, a continuous infusion of 10% glucose should be given. The airway should be intubated in the obtunded or comatose patient. Positive-pressure ventilation should be instituted if alveolar hypoventilation is present. Gastric lavage is useful only if performed within 1 hour of

TABLE 101-2. Disorders Associated With Chronic Alcoholism

Nervous system
  Wernicke-Korsakoff syndrome
  Dementia
  Cerebral atrophy
  Cerebellar degeneration
  Marchiafava-Bignami disease
  Central pontine myelinolysis
  Peripheral neuropathy
Cardiovascular
  Alcoholic cardiomyopathy
  Arrhythmias
  Conduction disturbances
  Hypertension
Gastrointestinal
  Increased incidence of oropharyngeal, laryngeal, and
    esophageal cancer
  Nausea and vomiting
  Gastritis
  Peptic ulcer disease
  Esophageal varices
  Mallory-Weiss syndrome
  Hemorrhoids
  Pancreatitis
  Liver disease
    Fatty degeneration
    Cirrhosis
    Alcoholic hepatitis
    Hepatic cancer
  Decreased ileal absorption of vitamin B_{12} and folate
Hematologic
  Bleeding diathesis
  Thrombocytopenia
  Anemia
  Pancytopenia
Metabolic
  Abnormal glucose, protein, and lipid metabolism
  Hypophosphatemia, hypomagnesemia, hyperuricemia
  Ketoacidosis
Malnutrition
Increased risk of infection
Interaction with other drugs

ingestion or if a multidrug ingestion is suspected. As previously mentioned, alcoholic ketoacidosis is treated with IV administration of glucose and saline. Insulin is not indicated. Hypothermia should be corrected. Fluid, electrolyte, and acid-base disturbances are corrected, depending on the clinical presentation. Hemodialysis has been used in cases of massive ethanol ingestion.[12]

ALCOHOL WITHDRAWAL

Chronic excessive alcohol ingestion depresses central alpha- and beta-receptors and potentiates the inhibitory neurotransmitter γ-aminobutyric acid. The CNS increases neuronal activity to compensate. When alcohol consumption stops, this enhanced neuronal activity leads to the hyperadrenergic state that causes the symptoms seen in alcohol withdrawal (tachycardia, hypertension, hyperreflexia, tremor).[13] And, indeed, Abraham and Shoemaker[14] have shown that cardiac index increases by 36% during delirium tremens (DTs), and the oxygen delivery and oxygen consumption are each 25% higher during DTs when compared with the control or recovery phases.

Central α₂-adrenergic agonists such as clonidine and lofexidine ameliorate these adrenergically mediated signs and symptoms of alcohol withdrawal. When Baumgartner and Rowen[15] compared clonidine to chlordiazepoxide in the management of acute alcohol withdrawal, they found that patients treated with clonidine had lower blood pressures, heart rates, and respiratory rates and less tremor, diaphoresis, and restlessness when compared with patients treated with chlordiazepoxide. Clonidine did not cause clinically significant hypotension. Cognitive scores were comparable between the two groups, and clonidine was as effective as chlordiazepoxide in relieving subjective complaints of alcohol withdrawal.[15]

Excessive doses of benzodiazepines have been used in the treatment of DTs. Indeed, Nolop and Natow report using 2640 mg of diazepam over 48 hours in one patient without ill effect.[16] But, benzodiazepines bind at the γ-aminobutyric acid–benzodiazepine receptor, and once these receptors are saturated, additional drug cannot bind. Patients may tolerate high doses of benzodiazepines but do not necessarily benefit from them.[17]

DTs usually last 2 to 5 days, but in 5% to 10% of cases, DTs last greater than a week. A small percentage of patients remain delirious for several weeks and require continuing treatment. Be aware, however, that after head trauma, a subdural hematoma can evolve subacutely in the alcoholic patient. A repeat computed tomography scan of the head or a magnetic resonance imaging scan may be warranted 7 to 10 days into a course of protracted delirium to rule out a slowly accumulating subdural hematoma.[17]

Approximately 3% to 5% of untreated alcohol withdrawal patients progress to grand mal seizures. Patients who have been drinking heavily for only a few years but have undergone several detoxification admissions are at higher risk of alcohol withdrawal seizures than patients who have long drinking histories but have undergone fewer detoxification admissions. Previous nonalcohol-related admissions also increase the risk of alcohol withdrawal seizures. This association has been termed the "kindling effect." According to the kindling hypothesis, each withdrawal episode is an irritative phenomenon to the brain. The accumulation of multiple episodes lowers the seizure threshold.[18] The accumulation of multiple prior withdrawals also leads to more severe DTs with each episode.[19]

Elderly alcoholics have a longer alcohol withdrawal with more withdrawal symptoms than younger alcoholics. This is believed to represent more than just the kindling effect, because the elderly alcoholics studied did not have significantly more prior admissions.[20]

ALCOHOL AND CHRONIC DISEASE

Chronic alcoholism is associated with many disorders encountered in the ICU (see Table 101-2).

COCAINE

There were lines on the mirror
There were lines on her face
She pretended not to notice
She was caught up in the race...
—Eagles, "Life in the Fast Lane"

Cocaine is an alkaloid prepared from leaves of *Erythroxylon coca*. It is related in chemical structure to the psychoactive drugs atropine and scopolamine, but is often misclassified with the sympathetic amines because many of its effects are similar to those of amphetamines. Colombia and Peru are the main countries supplying cocaine to the United States.

Cocaine hydrochloride is prepared by dissolving alkaloidal cocaine in hydrochloric acid. A water-soluble salt that is 89% cocaine by weight is formed. Cocaine hydrochloride is most commonly distributed as white powder, crystals, or granules. It decomposes on heating and melts at 195°C.[21,22] Cocaine alkaloid ("free base," "crack") is made from cocaine hydrochloride by many users. The cocaine base can be extracted by a potentially dangerous and explosive method using ether or by a simpler and safer method using baking soda and water. Free-base cocaine is heat stable, melts at 98C, and vaporizes at higher temperatures.

The powdered form of cocaine is frequently used intranasally (snorting). Because the drug causes intense vasoconstriction, its absorption by this route becomes limited over time. It is common practice to snort 30 to 60 mg of cocaine or more in each nostril and to repeat the process several times an hour over several hours.[23] Used this way, the euphoric effect lasts 1 to 5 hours beyond the last administration.

Smoking free-base cocaine has become a widespread practice. This is usually done with a water pipe or by mixing free-base cocaine with tobacco and rolling the mixture into a cigarette. Vaporized cocaine is then presented to vascular-rich pulmonary bed, and the levels rise rapidly. This way the euphoria lasts only up to 20 to 30 minutes. Because cocaine hydrochloride decomposes when heated, it cannot be used by this route.

Cocaine is often injected intravenously, usually 16 to 32 mg, as a straight agent or mixed with other drugs such as heroin ("speedball").[24] Subcutaneous or intramuscular injections are also occasionally seen. Cocaine is readily absorbed from most mucosal surfaces; hence, although done less often, it is administered orally, sublingually, vaginally, or rectally.

Cocaine is extensively metabolized by deesterification (plasma esterases) and N-demethylation, and the urinary excretion of unchanged cocaine ranges from 1% to 15%. Two major metabolites, ecgonine methyl ester and benzoylecgonine, account for 18% to 60% and 20% to 55%, respectively, of the urinary excretion of a dose. The route of administration doesn't affect metabolic excretion patterns appreciably: half-lives of most metabolites range from 45 to 90 minutes with a total body clearance of 1.7 to 2.1 L/minute.[25] Subjective rating of euphoria declines within minutes after constant concentrations are achieved, demonstrating rapid desensitization and acute tolerance.[26,27] Duration of positive urinary metabolites is somewhat dependent on the assay technique and also on the activity of plasma cholinesterases, which are of primary importance in the metabolism of cocaine.[21]

Cocaine has a steady-state volume of distribution of 2 L/kg, which reflects the high lipid solubility of this drug, resulting in a fourfold to tenfold brain-to-plasma ratio.[26,27] Cocaine's lipophilic nature, compounded with rapid distribution into and out of the CNS, suggests a highly abusive profile (rush and crash) and increased incidence of kindling. The major neurochemical actions of cocaine are (1) CNS stimulation with release of dopamine; (2) inhibition of neuronal catechol uptake, resulting in generalized sympathetic nervous system stimulation; (3) release or blockade of serotonin reuptake; and (4) inhibition of sodium current in neuronal tissue, resulting in local anesthetic effect.[28]

TOXICITY

A multitude of disorders have been associated with cocaine intoxication (Table 101-3). Cocaine hydrochloride is bitter to taste, and because of its properties as a local anesthetic, it numbs the tongue, lips, nose, and other mucosal surfaces. In large doses, cocaine may cause a generalized impairment of neuronal impulse transmission leading to CNS depression,

coma, respiratory depression, and respiratory arrest. At low doses, stimulation is the common feature of cocaine use. The euphoria produced by cocaine is the principal reason for its abuse. Excessive CNS stimulation can occur and is manifested by tremulousness, agitation, sleeplessness, paranoia, and frank psychosis. Aggressive and assaultive behavior is common in cocaine overdose.

Seizures can be induced, even on the first exposure, because cocaine lowers the threshold for seizures.[29–31] Cocaine-related seizures are mostly brief and self-limited, occurring soon after taking cocaine, although the interval between last use of cocaine and onset of seizures can be several hours.[32] Sustained or repeated seizure activity suggests hyperthermia, intracranial hemorrhage, metabolic abnormality, or massive intake of cocaine, as in the case of cocaine body packers. Recreational drug use, especially with cocaine, seems to be a prominent and growing risk factor for strokes of all kinds in young adults.[33,34] Also, cerebral atrophy, predominantly in the temporofrontal regions, has been noticed in patients with chronic cocaine abuse.[35] Subarachnoid hemorrhage may occur within moments of drug use, possibly related to hypertension, both in people with anatomic abnormalities and without.[32,36–38] Cerebral infarctions have been reported.[33,34] Transient ischemic attacks and ischemic cerebrovascular accidents also have been reported.[32,34]

TABLE 101-3. Clinical Manifestations of Cocaine Use

ANESTHETIC EFFECTS	**RESPIRATORY**
Localized numbness	Pulmonary edema
Central neuronal depression	Pulmonary hypertension
Coma	Respiratory arrest
	Septic pulmonary emboli
CENTRAL NERVOUS SYSTEM	Pulmonary vascular occlusion
Euphoria	Pneumothorax
Alertness	Pneumomediastinum
Tremor	Hemoptysis
Sleeplessness	
Paranoia	**GASTROINTESTINAL**
Psychosis	Acute mucosal ischemia
Headache	GI perforations
Seizures	
Cerebrovascular	**METABOLIC**
Transient ischemic events	Weight loss
Intracerebral hemorrhages	Hyperthermia
Subarachnoid bleeds	Rhabdomyolysis
Cerebritis	Local and systemic infections
	Endocarditis
CARDIOVASCULAR	Nasal mucosal injury
Tachycardia	Nasal septal perforation
Arrhythmias	Chronic rhinitis
Hypertension	Deep venous thrombosis of upper
Myocardial infarction	extremity
Myocarditis	
Aortic dissection, rupture	**OBSTETRIC COMPLICATIONS**
Sudden death	Spontaneous abortions
Cardiomyopathy	Abruptio placentae
	Intrauterine growth retardation
	Prematurity

GI, gastrointestinal.

Cocaine inhibits the neuronal uptake of catecholamines, causing enhanced sympathetic stimulation. This in turn is associated with intense vasoconstriction, which can lead to end-organ ischemia. Intestinal ischemia and infarction have been reported, as have renal infarction and limb ischemia.[24,39,40] Also, the ischemic episodes have been implicated in acute gastroduodenal perforations associated with the use of crack cocaine.[41]

Chest pain is the most common presentation of cocaine-induced MI. The onset of chest pain often occurs within 30 minutes of the use of IV cocaine. With the use of crack cocaine, the onset of chest pain is usually $1^1/2$ hours after use; with intranasal cocaine, the chest pain usually occurs greater than 2 hours after use. But, cocaine-related chest pain has occurred as late as 96 hours after use.[42,43]

Acute MI results not only from the primary effect of cocaine, but also from its secondary effects (i.e., on platelets, coagulation cascade, vascular endothelium, or combinations of these), leading to thrombus formation.[44–46]

Periods of silent ischemia are common in chronic users of cocaine, as shown by Holter tests and during periods of withdrawal.[47] Apart from structural changes in epimyocardial vessels, Majid and Patel[48] describe considerable wall thickening in the intramyocardial small coronary arteries in people with cocaine-induced chest pains. Dilated cardiomyopathy and congestive heart failure can occur secondary to chronic cocaine use.[49,50]

Cocaine-induced MIs have been documented in patients with normal and abnormal electrocardiograms. Lange and colleagues[51,52] have shown that cocaine reduces myocardial oxygen supply by decreasing coronary blood flow. This coronary vasoconstriction is caused by alpha-adrenergic stimulation; it is exacerbated by beta-adrenergic blockers and improved by the alpha-adrenergic blocking agent phentolamine. Therefore, beta-adrenergic blockers such as propranolol may increase cocaine-induced myocardial ischemia. Also, phentolamine may be useful in decreasing cocaine-induced myocardial ischemia.[51,52]

Cocaine is intensely arrhythmogenic when taken in large quantities because of its effects on catecholamines. Sinus tachycardia, supraventricular tachycardia, premature ventricular beats, ventricular tachycardia, ventricular fibrillation, or asystole may occur.

Whereas lidocaine can control cocaine-induced arrhythmias, animal studies have shown that lidocaine decreases the seizure threshold in cocaine-treated animals.[53]

Early therapy for cocaine-induced MI should consist of oxygen, aspirin, and nitroglycerin as required for pain relief. If pain persists, patients with cocaine-induced MI are candidates for thrombolytic therapy, unless they have standard contraindications such as severe hypertension or bleeding.[42,43] Beta-adrenergic blockers should be avoided, and type 1a antiarrhythmics should be used with caution. Phentolamine may be useful in this situation.

Dramatic elevations of blood pressure may be seen and are partly responsible for subarachnoid hemorrhage, stroke, intracerebral bleed, and MI. Rupture of the ascending aorta in previously healthy men has been reported.[54] Pulmonary edema[55,56] and pulmonary hypertension are also seen. Hypo-

ventilation leading to respiratory arrest may occur because of respiratory depression. Septic pulmonary emboli and pulmonary vascular obstruction resulting from foreign body granulomas or angiothrombosis may develop as a consequence of IV use.[57] Pneumothorax and pneumomediastinum are reported secondary to cocaine snorting and crack inhalation.[58] Massive hemoptysis with diffuse alveolar hemorrhage is a reported complication of smoking free-base cocaine.[59–61] Crack lung, a condition of pulmonary infiltrates and bronchospasm, and bronchiolitis obliterans also have been reported after cocaine abuse.[62,63]

Hyperpyrexia may result from muscle hyperactivity or as a direct effect of cocaine on temperature regulatory centers. Rhabdomyolysis is common in this setting and in my experience often is associated with guarded outcome. Also, recently a possible variant of neuroleptic malignant syndrome with rapid death has been described with cocaine use.[64] Seizures, hypotension or hypertension, arrhythmia, coma, and cardiac arrest may point to a subgroup of patients who are prone to severe rhabdomyolysis and may need close monitoring and aggressive therapy.[65,66]

The IV substance abuser is prone to a variety of local and systemic infections, including infective endocarditis and acquired immunodeficiency syndrome (Chaps. 109 and 120).

DIAGNOSIS OF ACUTE INTOXICATION

Patients with cocaine intoxication may present with a variety of primary complaints such as altered mental status, chest pain, syncope, palpitations, seizures, or attempted suicide.[67] This is usually recognized by characteristic findings of CNS stimulation such as agitation, mydriasis, sweating, hypertension, and tachycardia. However, the effects of other drugs such as amphetamines, phencyclidine, and anticholinergics and some medical conditions such as meningitis, encephalopathy, epilepsy with status, and thyrotoxicosis may mimic cocaine intoxication.[28]

TREATMENT FOR ACUTE INTOXICATION

The agitation and psychosis of cocaine overdose usually can be managed with titrated doses of IV diazepam, 5 to 20 mg, lorazepam, 2 to 4 mg, or midazolam, 5 to 10 mg slowly. Caution should be exercised with all because these agents can cause CNS depression and respiratory depression or arrest if given too rapidly or in too high a dose. Haloperidol is not recommended because of the lack of experimental support[27,68,69] and significant clinical difficulties in sedative hypnotic withdrawal in humans and animal studies, particularly when treatment is initiated in the presence of agitation and hyperthermia. Paralysis with pancuronium bromide (0.1 mg/kg) may be required in patients with persistent muscular activity and hyperthermia. Vecuronium bromide (0.1 mg/kg) may be a better choice in the phase of unstable cardiac status or tachyarrhythmias. Tracheal intubation and mechanical ventilation are required in this setting. Seizures are controlled in the usual manner with IV diazepam or other standard antiepileptics (Chap. 134). If neuromuscular paralysis is used to control hyperthermia or muscular hyperactivity caused by seizures, brain seizure activity may persist unrecognized and hence warrants continuous electroencephalographic monitoring.[28]

Hyperthermia should be treated aggressively by rapid cooling with cool water, fanning, and other measures (Chap. 98). Conduction and evaporation prove rapidly efficacious. Control of associated agitation, psychosis, or seizures is essential to achieve and maintain cooling while avoiding brain, hepatic, and muscle cell destruction.[68] There is no evidence that other pharmacologic agents like dantrolene play a role in enhancing the cooling process in these patients with life-threatening hyperthermia.[70]

Hypertension can be effectively treated with nitroprusside, 0.5 to 10 µg/kg/min, or IV labetalol, 20 to 40 mg, followed by a titrated dose (Chap. 122). Cocaine-intoxicated patients should be considered to have acute elevations in blood pressure, and unless there is documentation or clinical evidence of longstanding hypertension, there should be no concern about cerebral hypoperfusion with immediate lowering of blood pressure to normal levels.[68]

CLINICAL MANIFESTATIONS OF WITHDRAWAL

Psychological and biochemical dependency on cocaine may be intense. Cocaine causes unusual activation of the dopamine system and blocks the dopamine uptake, especially in the pleasure centers of the brain.[71] Dopamine is trapped in the synapse, where it is metabolized rather than reused, and dopamine resources become depleted. The result is that normal basic needs like hunger, thirst, and sex drive cannot be met without cocaine. The brain becomes dopamine deficient, and even a short period of cocaine abstinence results in a real withdrawal state.

The clinical effects of cocaine withdrawal include depression, irritability, sleep and appetite dysfunction, and, worst of all, intense desire and craving for more cocaine. To the addict, cocaine often is no longer used to feel good but to avoid feeling bad. Various phases of cocaine abstinence and its symptomatology are discussed in detail by Talbert and coworkers.[25] The dopamine agonist bromocriptine mesylate has been administered to cocaine addicts in several studies with good results.[25,72–74] A supportive environment and professional drug counseling are clearly warranted.

OPIOIDS ■

> It makes me feel like a man,
> When I put a spike into my vein,
> Then I'll tell you things aren't quite the same
> —Lou Reed, "Heroin"

Opioids include all drugs—synthetic as well as natural—that have morphine-like properties. Overdose of these compounds is often associated with life-threatening hypoventilation that must be quickly recognized and rapidly reversed.[75] Opioids act through integrated CNS opioid receptors, which was discovered in 1971.[76] There are at least

five opioid receptors with various physiologic roles including analgesia, ventilatory depression, drug dependence, bradycardia, dysphoria, hallucinations, sedation, and miosis. Opioids are classified as receptor agonists or antagonists. Some have combined properties: they stimulate one type of receptor and antagonize another. A classification of opioids is given in Table 101-4.

TOXICITY

The purity of illicit heroin in the United States has improved over recent years and the price has fallen. This has led to increased snorting (intranasal administration) and smoking of heroin. Whereas these routes of administration deliver heroin less efficiently than the traditional IV route, the avoidance of needles decreases the risk of human immunodeficiency virus infection.

However, heroin is still most commonly self-administered intravenously ("mainlining"), intramuscularly, subcutaneously, and intradermally ("skin popping").

The primary toxic manifestations of opioids are mediated by the mu- and kappa-receptors in the CNS. The typical patient with opioid intoxication presents in coma, with miotic

TABLE 101-4. Classification of Opiate Drugs

Opioid agonists
  Natural opium derivatives
    Morphine
    Codeine
  Semisynthetic opioids
    Heroin
    Hydromophone (Dilaudid)
    Oxymorphine (Numorphan)
    Oxycodone (Percodan, Perocet)
  Synthetic opioids
    Meperidine (Demerol)
    Methadone (Dolophine)
    Levorphanol tartrate (Levo-Dromoran)
    Paregoric (Parepectolin, tincture of opium)
    Diphenoxlate (Lomotil)
    Fentanyl (Sublimaze)
    Propoxyphone (Darvon)
Pure opioid antagonists
  Naloxone (Narcan)
  Naltrexone (Trexan)
Agonists–antagonists
  Nalorphine (Nalline)
  Levallorphan (Lorfan)
  Pentazocine (Talwin)
  Butorphanol (Stadol)
  Nalbuphine (Nubain)
  Cyclazocine
  Propiram
  Profadol

From Bickel WH, O'Benar JD: Life-threatening opioid toxicity. In: Dellinger RP (ed). *The Substance Abuser: Problems in Critical Care.* Philadelphia, JB Lippincott, 1987:106.

pupils and shallow respirations. Common clinical effects of these drugs are shown in Table 101-5.

The CNS effects range from apathy to coma. Seizures may occur. The most worrisome feature of CNS depression is hypoventilation. Tidal volume decreases first, and then at higher doses respiratory rate falls. Seizures can occur, perhaps related to hypoventilation and hypoxemia.

An opioid-induced release of histamine from mast cells can precipitate bronchospasm, urticaria, and pruritus. Other respiratory complications include aspiration of gastric contents, pulmonary edema, pulmonary hypertension, adult respiratory distress syndrome, and septic pulmonary emboli.[57,77,78] Intravenously injected illicit opioids are rarely pure, and often are mixed with microcrystalline cellulose, talc, or cellulose. These fillers are capable of producing angiothrombosis and a foreign body granulomatous reaction.

Venous capacitance dilatation occurs with opioid use. This may precipitate preload reduction, a fall in cardiac output, and hypotension. A pronounced decrease in gastrointestinal peristalsis and increased ileocecal and anal sphincter tone are responsible for the constipation frequently seen with opioid use. Urinary retention may be caused by increased detrusor muscle tone. Local infections, endocarditis, and other systemic infections are especially common in the IV user.

TREATMENT FOR ACUTE INTOXICATION

Because the usual cause of death from opioid overdose is ventilatory failure, the most urgent intervention in the case of acute opioid intoxication is airway management and ventilation (Chap. 50). IV access should be obtained as soon as

TABLE 101-5.   Clinical Manifestations of Opioid Intoxication

Central nervous system
  Analgesia
  Apathy
  Lethargy
  Seizures
  Coma
  Ventilatory depression
  Nausea
  Emesis
  Miosis
Respiratory
  Histamine release—bronchospasm
  Pulmonary edema
Cardiovascular
  Venous dilation
  Preload reduction
  Hypotension
Gastrointestinal
  Decreased peristalsis
  Decreased hydrochloric acid secretion
  Constipation
Genitourinary
  Urinary retention
Integument
  Histamine release—urticaria, pruritis

possible. This may be a difficult task because IV drug addicts go to extreme lengths to obtain access. Peripheral veins may not be accessible, requiring central venous cannulation. Titrated volume expansion should be administered to the hypotensive patient.

Naloxone, a pure opioid antagonist, reverses all of the opioid-induced CNS and ventilatory depressant effects. The dose required to reverse opioid effects depends on the amount and type of opioid administered. IV naloxone in a dose of 0.4 to 0.8 mg is recommended for the obtunded patient without signs of ventilatory depression. An initial dose of 2 mg is recommended in patients with ventilatory depression. Larger doses may be required in patients who have administered large quantities of opioids. Some opioids (codeine, propoxyphene, diphenoxylate, pentazocine, butorphanol, and nalbuphine) require more naloxone than others for reversal of depressant effects. If the altered mental status is not reversed in several minutes, larger doses of naloxone are indicated.[75] Naloxone can be given in dosages of 2 mg intravenously every 4 minutes as necessary, to a total dose of 20 mg. If CNS depression is not reversed by 20 mg of naloxone, alternate causes should be aggressively addressed (e.g., hypoglycemia, hypothermia, head trauma). Close observation of the patient after naloxone administration is warranted because of its short half-life. After 20 to 30 minutes, toxic opioid side effects often reappear. The patient may require repeated bolus injections of naloxone or a continuous infusion may be started. The initial amount of naloxone required to reverse the CNS effects is given each hour as a continuous infusion. Additional boluses may be required as the infusion is started.

TREATMENT FOR OPIOID WITHDRAWAL

The chronic administration of exogenous opiates is thought to lead to diminished endogenous opioid peptides. When these exogenous opiates are discontinued, the patient often goes into opioid withdrawal. The clinical manifestations of opioid withdrawal are outlined in Table 101-6. Methadone and buprenorphine have been used to treat opioid withdrawal acutely and opioid addiction chronically.

Buprenorphine is a semisynthetic partial opioid agonist or mixed agonist antagonist. Buprenorphine has high affinity, but low activity at the mu-opioid receptor. It has low toxicity in high doses, partly because its mu-antagonistic effects limit the opioid effects of sedation, respiratory depression, and hypotension. With chronic administration, buprenorphine produces less physical dependence than do pure agonists (such as methadone), but patients can become addicted to buprenorphine. A 2- to 4- mg dose of buprenorphine is roughly equivalent to 20 to 30 mg of methadone in preventing opioid withdrawal symptoms. The features of buprenorphine withdrawal are similar of the features of heroin withdrawal but are more prolonged (8 to 10 days) and less intense.[79]

Adrenergic agonists such as clonidine and guanfacine also have been used to suppress opiate withdrawal reactions. Clonidine alone in high doses (15 to 20 µg/kg) can suppress the signs and symptoms of opiate withdrawal within 24 hours and shorten acute withdrawal reactions by 3 to 4 days.[80]

TABLE 101-6. Clinical Manifestations of Opioid Withdrawal

Early (4–10 h)
  Yawning
  Lacrimation
  Rhinorrhea
  Sneezing
  Sweating
Intermediate (12–18 h)
  Restless sleep
  Piloerection
  Restlessness
  Irritability
  Anorexia
  Flushing
  Tachycardia
  Tremor
  Hyperthermia
Late (>24 h)
  Fever
  Nausea
  Vomiting
  Abdominal pain
  Diarrhea
  Difficulty sleeping
  Muscle spasm
  Joint pain
  Involuntary ejaculation
  Suicidal ideation

However, systolic hypotension and bradycardia sometimes limit clonidine usage. Guanfacine is at least as effective as clonidine in controlling withdrawal symptoms and has fewer cardiovascular problems.[81,82]

HEROIN BODY PACKERS

Heroin body packers are individuals who transport concentrated heroin by swallowing wrapped packages or inserting them into their vaginas or rectums. These packages are subsequently removed from the gastrointestinal tract using cathartics, suppositories, or enemas. Packages that are swallowed are sometimes placed in toy balloons to allow easier swallowing. Body packers usually take antidiarrheal drugs to prevent premature passage of the packages.[83]

Abdominal radiographs usually show the location of the packages and allow tracking of the packages as they move through the gastrointestinal tract. But, a negative result on plain abdominal radiograph does not rule out body packing. A water-soluble contrast study of the bowel may visualize packages in this situation.[83] Body packers should receive activated charcoal. If the heroin packages are in the colon, enemas or whole-bowel irrigation with polyethylene glycol should be used to facilitate elimination. However, polyethylene glycol binds to activated charcoal and decreases its effectiveness.

If there is evidence of systemic absorption from leaking packages, opioid toxicity should be treated with a continuous infusion of naloxone. Determine the amount of naloxone required to reverse the initial signs of toxicity and give that amount hourly in a continuous infusion. If the urine is positive for narcotics, the patient either used opioid recently or the packages are leaking.[83]

Surgical intervention is indicated to remove remaining packages in the patient who has radiologic evidence of retained packages in the stomach or evidence of bowel obstruction. Surgical intervention also may be indicated if there is evidence of ongoing opioid absorption.

REFERENCES ■

1. Arena JM: *Poisoning: Toxicology, Symptoms, Treatments*, ed. 4. Springfield, IL, Charles C Thomas, 1979
2. Abelson HI, Miller JD: A decade of trends in cocaine use in the household population. *Natl Inst Drug Abuse Res Monogr Ser* 1985;61:35
3. Fishburn PM: *National Survey on Drug Abuse: Main Findings, 1979.* DHHS publication (ADM) 80-976. Rockville, MD, National Institute of Drug Abuse, 1980
4. Bickell WH, O'Benar JD: Life-threatening opioid toxicity. In: Dellinger RP (ed). *The Substance Abuser: Problems in Critical Care.* Philadelphia, JB Lippincott, 1987:106
5. Lowenfels AB, Miller TT: Alcohol and trauma. *Ann Emerg Med* 1984;13:1056
6. Zuska JJ: Wounds without a cause. *Bull Am Coll Surg* 1981;66:5
7. Peterson B, Krantz P, Kristensson H, et al: Alcohol-related death: a major contributor to mortality in urban middle-aged men. *Lancet* 1982₀₀:1088
8. Stewart RB, Forgnone M, May FE, et al: Epidemiology of acute drug intoxication: patient characteristics, drugs and medical complications. *Clin Toxicol* 1974;7:513
9. Fazekas JF, Alman RW: *Coma: Biochemistry, Physiology and Therapeutic Principles.* Springfield, IL, Charles C Thomas, 1962
10. Johnston RE, Reier CE: Acute respiratory effects of ethanol in man. *Clin Pharmacol Ther* 1973;14:503
11. Friedman HS, Lieber CS: Cardiotoxicity of alcohol. *Cardiovasc Med* 1977;2:111
12. Marc Aurcle J, Schreier GE: The dialysance of ethanol and methanol: a proposed method of treatment for massive intoxication by ethyl or methyl alcohol. *J Clin Invest* 1960;39:802
13. Bartrug B, Fullwood J: Delirium tremens in acute myocardial infarction. *Heart Lung* 1994;23:21
14. Abraham E, Shoemaker W: Cardiorespiratory patterns in severe delirium tremens. *Arch Intern Med* 1985;145:1057
15. Baumgartner GR, Rowen RC: Clonidine vs chlordiazepoxide in the management of acute alcohol withdrawal syndrome. *Arch Intern Med* 1987;147:1223
16. Nolop KB, Natow A: Unprecedented sedative requirements during delirium tremens. *Crit Care Med* 1985;13:246
17. Miller FT, Protracted alcohol withdrawal delirium. *J Subst Abuse Treat* 1994;11:127
18. Lechtenberg R, Worner TM: Total ethanol consumption as a seizure risk factor in alcoholics. *Acta Neurol Scand* 1992;85:90
19. Lechtenberg R, Worner TM: Relative kindling effect of detoxification and non-detoxification admissions in alcoholics. *Alcohol Alcohol* 1991;26:221
20. Brower KJ, Mudd S: Severity and treatment of alcohol withdrawal in elderly vs younger patients. *Alcohol Clin Exp Res* 1994;18:196
21. Cregler LL, Mark H: Medical complications of cocaine abuse. *N Engl J Med* 1986;315:1495

22. Siegel RK: Cocaine smoking. *J Psychoactive Drugs* 1982;14:271
23. Olson KR, Benowitz NL: Life-threatening cocaine intoxication. In: Dellinger RP (ed). *The Substance Abuser: Problems in Critical Care.* Philadelphia, JB Lippincott, 1987:95
24. Fischman MW, Schuster CR, Resnekov L, et al: Cardiovascular and subjective effects of intravenous cocaine administration in humans. *Arch Gen Psychiatry* 1976;33:983
25. Hall WC, Talbert RL: Cocaine abuse and its treatment. *Pharmacotherapy* 1990;10:47
26. Chow MJ, Ambre JJ: Kinetics of cocaine distribution, elimination and chronotropic effects. *Clin Pharmacol Ther* 1985;38:318
27. Ambre JJ, Belknap SM, Nelson J: Acute tolerance to cocaine in humans. *Clin Pharmacol Ther* 1988;44:1
28. Mueller PD, Olson KR: Cocaine. *Emerg Med Clin North Am* 1990;8:481
29. Cohen S: Cocaine: acute medical and psychiatric complications. *Psychiatr Ann* 1984;14:747
30. Jonsson S, O'Meara M, Young JB: Acute cocaine poisoning importance of treating seizures and acidosis. *Am J Med* 1983;75:1061
31. Van Dyke C, Byck R: Cocaine. *Sci Am* 1982;246:128
32. Lowenstein DH, Massa SM, Rowbothem MC: Acute neurological and psychological complications associated with cocaine. *Am J Med* 1987;87:841
33. Kaku DA: Emergence of recreational drug use as a risk factor for stroke in young adults. *Ann Intern Med* 1990;113:821
34. Levine SR, Brust J CM: Cerebrovascular complications of the use of crack form of alkaloidal cocaine. *N Engl J Med* 1990;323:699
35. Leone AP, Dhuna A: Cerebral atrophy in habitual cocaine abusers: a planimetric CT study. *Neurology* 1991;41:34
36. Schwartz KA, Cohen JA: Subarachnoid hemorrhage precipitated by cocaine snorting. *Arch Neurol* 1984;41:705
37. Cregler LL, Mark H: Relation of stroke to cocaine abuse. *N Y State J Med* 1987;87:128
38. Green RM: Multiple intracerebral hemorrhages after smoking cocaine. *Stroke* 1990;21:957
39. Nalbandian H, Sheth N, Dietrich R, et al: Intestinal ischemia caused by cocaine ingestion: report of two cases. *Surgery* 1985;97:374
40. Sharff JA: Renal infarction associated with intravenous cocaine abuse. *Ann Emerg Med* 1984;13:1145
41. Lee H, LaMante HR: Acute gastroduodenal perforations associated with crack. *Ann Surg* 1990;211:15
42. Hollander JE, Hoffman RS: Cocaine-induced myocardial infarction: an analysis and review of the literature. *J Emerg Med* 1992;10:169
43. Hollander JE: Use of phentolamine for cocaine-induced myocardial ischemia. *N Engl J Med* 1992;327:361
44. Amin M, Gaselman G: Acute MI and chest pain syndromes after cocaine use. *Am J Cardiol* 1990;66:1434
45. Tonga G, Tempesta E, Tonga AR: Platelet responsiveness and biosynthesis of thromboxane and prostacycline in response to in vitro cocaine treatment. *Hemostasis* 1985;15:100
46. Isner JM, Chokshi SK: Cardiovascular complications of cocaine. *Curr Probl Cardiol* 1991eb:95
47. Nadamanee K, Gorelick DA: Myocardial ischemia during withdrawal. *Ann Intern Med* 1989;111:876
48. Majid PA, Patel B: An angiographic and histologic study of cocaine induced chest pain. *Am J Cardiol* 1990;65:812
49. Weiner RS, Lockhart JT: Dilated cardiomyopathy and cocaine abuse. *Am J Med* 1986;81:699
50. Shereif H, Rajkalla M, Hall S: Cocaine induced heart disease. *Am Heart J* 1990;120:1403
51. Lange RA, Cigarroa RG: Cocaine-induced coronary-artery vasoconstriction. *N Engl J Med* 1989;321:1557
52. Lange RA, Cigarroa RG: Potentiation of cocaine-induced coronary vasoconstriction by beta-adrenergic blockade. *Ann Intern Med* 1990;112:897
53. Derlet RW, Albertson TE: Lidocaine potentiation of cocaine toxicity. *Ann Emerg Med* 1991;20:135
54. Barth CW III, Bray M, Roberts WC: Rupture of the ascending aorta during cocaine intoxication. *Am J Cardiol* 1986;57:496
55. Cucco RA, Yoo OH: Nonfatal pulmonary edema after freebase smoking. *Am Rev Respir Dis* 1987;136:1250
56. Kline JN: Pulmonary edema after freebase cocaine smoking. *Chest* 1990;97:1009
57. Zimmerman JL, Dellinger RP: Septic pulmonary emboli in the intravenous substance abuser. In: Dellinger RP (ed). *The Substance Abuser: Problems in Critical Care.* Philadelphia, JB Lippincott, 1987
58. Matthew E, Seaman M: Barotrauma related to inhalational drug abuse. *J Emerg Med* 1990;8:141
59. Ettinger NA, Albin RJ: Review of respiratory effects of cocaine. *Am J Med* 1989;87:664
60. Goodwin JE, Harle RA: Cocaine, pulmonary hemorrhage and hemoptysis. *Ann Intern Med* 1989;110:843
61. Murray RJ, Albin RJ: Diffuse alveolar hemorrhage temporally related to cocaine smoking. *Chest* 1988;93:427
62. Forrester JM, Steele AW: Crack lung: an acute pulmonary syndrome with a sprectrum of clinical and histological findings. *Am Rev Respir Dis* 1990;142:462
63. Kissner DG, Lawrence WD: Crack lung: pulmonary disease caused by cocaine abuse. *Am Rev Respir Dis* 1987;136:1250
64. Kosten TR, Kleber HD: Rapid death during cocaine abuse: a variant of neuroleptic malignant syndrome? *Am J Drug Alcohol Abuse* 1988;14:335
65. Dwelch R, Todd K: Incidence of cocaine associated rhabdomyolysis. *Ann Emerg Med* 1991;20:154
66. Brody S, Wrenn KD: Predicting the severity of cocaine associated rhabdomyolysis. *Ann Emerg Med* 1990;19:1137
67. Darlet RN, Albertson TE: ED presentation of cocaine intoxication. *Ann Emerg Med* 1989;18:182
68. Goldfrank LR, Hoffman RS: The cardiovascular effects of cocaine. *Ann Emerg Med* 1991;20:165
69. Darlett RN, Albertson TE, Rice P: Effect of haloperidol in cocaine and amphetamine intoxication. *J Emerg Med* 1989;7:633
70. Fox AN: More on rhabdomyolysis associated with cocaine intoxication. *N Engl J Med* 321:1271
71. Dackis CA, Gold MS: New concepts in cocaine addiction: the dopamine depletion hypothesis. *Neurosci Biobehav Rev* 1985;9:469
72. Taylor WA, Gold MS: Pharmacological approaches to treatment of cocaine dependence. *West J Med* 1990;152;572
73. Giannini AJ, Banngartel P: Bromocryptine therapy in cocaine withdrawals. *J Clin Pharmacol* 1987;27:267
74. Dackis CA, Gold MS: Pharmacological approaches to cocaine addiction. *J Subst Abuse Treat* 1985;2:139
75. Goldfrank LR, Eddy A: Opioids. In: Goldfrank LR, Flomenbaum NE, Lewin NA, et al (eds). *Goldfrank's Toxicologic Emergencies,* ed 3. Norwalk, CT, Appleton-Century-Crofts, 1986:404
76. Goldstein A, Lowney LI, Pal BK: Stereospecific and nonspecific interactions of the morphine narcotic congener levorphanol in subcellular fractions of mouse brain. *Proc Natl Acad Sci USA* 1971;68:1742
77. Duberstein JL, Kaufman DM: A clinical study of an epidemic of heroin intoxication and heroin-induced pulmonary edema. *Am J Med* 1971;51:704

78. Gottlieb LS, Boylen TC: Pulmonary complications of drug abuse. *West J Med* 1974;120:8

79. San L, Cami J: Assessment and management of opioid withdrawal symptoms in buprenorphine-dependent subjects. *Br J Addict* 1992;87:55

80. Cuthill JD, Beroniade V: Evaluation of clonidine suppression of opiate withdrawal reactions: a multidisciplinary approach. *Can J Psychiatry* 1990;35:377

81. San L, Tato J: Flunitrazepam consumption among heroin addicts admitted for inpatient detoxification. *Drug Alcohol Depend* 1993;32:281

82. San L, Cami J: Efficacy of clonidine, guanfacine and methadone in the rapid detoxification of heroin addicts: a controlled clinical trial. *Br J Addict* 1990;85:141

83. Utecht MJ, Stone AF: Heroin body packers. *J Emerg Med* 1993;11:33

Critical Care, Third Edition, edited by Joseph M. Civetta,
Robert W. Taylor, and Robert R. Kirby.
Lippincott-Raven Publishers, Philadelphia, PA © 1997.

CHAPTER 102

Envenomation

Charles L. Bryan
Charles A. Weber
Kenneth A. Perret

IMMEDIATE CONCERNS ■

MAJOR PROBLEMS

The severity of illness exhibited by envenomation victims
varies widely. A small percentage of persons may develop
life-threatening conditions. Precise identification of the
snake, spider, scorpion, or jellyfish is important and can help
direct further specific therapy. Antivenin is available for the
most serious envenomations in this country, including those
from rattlesnake, coral snake, water moccasin, and black
widow spider bites. Therapy is otherwise summarized for
all envenomations by the rapid application of first aid without
mutilation and supportive care.

STRESS POINTS

1. Compared with other etiologies of critical illness,
venomous snake bites account for a few intensive
care unit (ICU) admissions per year.
2. Proper diagnosis of snake envenomation depends
heavily on a description of the snake or examination
of the snake itself.
3. The identification of poisonous snakes is based on
characteristics of dentition, head shields, pupils, and
tail, and the presence or absence of a heat-sensing pit.
4. Most medically significant envenomations are caused
by pit vipers. Rattlesnake bites are the most serious,
cottonmouth (water moccasin) bites are of intermediate severity, and copperhead bites usually produce
no major systemic injury.
5. Systemic effects of rattlesnake venom involve hematologic abnormalities and effects on the cardiovascu-

lar, respiratory, and neurologic systems. Systemic poisoning by coral snake venom produces drowsiness,
euphoria, weakness, nausea, vomiting, fasciculations,
excessive salivation, extraocular muscle paresis, hypotension, delayed general paresis, and cardiopulmonary failure.
6. Knowledge of the black widow spider's morphologic
features is important in establishing a diagnosis. The
female adult body is 0.5 cm with a leg spread up to
40 mm and red markings on the ventral surface.
7. Black widow spider venom contains the most potent
neurotoxins per volume found in nature.
8. The clinical presentation of widow spider envenomation can be characterized as an ascending wave of
painful muscle spasm accompanied by varying degrees of adrenergic and cholinergic excitation.
9. The most common cardiovascular manifestations of
widow spider envenomations are tachycardia and hypertension, but congestive heart failure and myocardial ischemia have been reported in patients with
preexisting heart disease.
10. Brown recluse spiders have a leg span of up to 5 cm.
The body surface is dark brown to light tan. On the
dorsal aspect of the cephalothorax is a midline band
of darker color shaped like a violin.
11. The brown recluse spider injects a venom into its
host, which produces endothelial and platelet damage
resulting in edema, thrombosis, and local ischemic
necrosis.
12. Viscerocutaneous or systemic recluse spider envenomation may occur suddenly, particularly in children.
Fever, chills, nausea, vomiting, arthralgias, and a variable rash develop within 24 to 48 hours. The rash

may be macular, morbilliform, petechial, generalized, or localized to the trunk and flexural areas.

13. As in other types of envenomation, the clinical picture produced by a scorpion sting is determined by the size and susceptibility of the victim, the amount of venom injected, and the virulence of the venom.

14. Other than scorpion envenomations from southern Arizona and northern Mexico, most scorpion stings in this country are similar in content and presentation to wasp stings.

15. The victim of scorpion envenomation may manifest tachycardia, hypertension, hyperglycemia, mydriasis, piloerection, and perspiration caused by sympathetic mediators.

16. Laboratory manifestations of scorpion envenomation include hyperglycemia, hypernatremia, and leukocytosis.

17. The severity of jellyfish stings depends on the number of successful discharges and on the composition of the venom.

18. The main effects of all of the toxins are pain, paralysis, and urticaria, often localized to the contact area. Pain is usually the earliest symptom, ranging from a mild stinging sensation to an intense burning.

INITIAL THERAPY

1. When treating rattlesnake bites, tourniquets may predispose to greater local necrosis and early limb loss. Tourniquets may be used in the prehospital management of elapid envenomations only if placed tight enough to restrict venous and lymphatic flow, yet loose enough to allow arterial flow.

2. Incision and suction should be done only if the victim is more than 30 minutes from medical care and if it can be performed within 5 minutes of the snake bite. The incision should be less than 1 cm in length and 3 mm in depth, placed directly through the fang punctures.

3. Proper use of antivenin is the most important aspect of hospital care of rattlesnake envenomation victims. The bite can be graded as no envenomation, minimal, moderate, or severe, based on the local appearance and clinical presentation requiring 0, 4, 7, or 15 or more units of antivenin, respectively. Antivenin should be diluted in 500 to 1000 mL of normal saline or 5% dextrose in water and administered intravenously (IV) over 2 to 4 hours.

4. Fasciotomy should be undertaken in patients with objective evidence of a compartment syndrome, that is, those with decreased blood flow in the absence of thrombosis and those with increased intracompartmental pressure.

5. Specific therapy for black widow spider bites involves parenteral administration of specific. Antivenin is an equine derivative of *Latrodectus mactans* but offers cross-protection to the other *Latrodectus* species. It provides prompt dramatic relief of symptoms when administered within 2 hours of the bite.

6. Supportive therapy for black widow spider bites consists of analgesics and muscle relaxants.

7. Most brown recluse spider bite lesions heal spontaneously; therefore, delayed elective surgery should be performed only to close a refractory ulcer or to correct disabling or disfiguring scars.

8. The treatment of scorpion stings is primarily supportive. Propranolol and phentolamine can be used to reverse hemodynamic changes. Intravenous calcium and phenobarbital have been effective in relieving muscle spasms and convulsions, respectively.

9. Jellyfish nematocysts on the skin should be removed and the affected area inactivated with household vinegar. For inactivating nematocysts from sea nettle, a slurry of baking soda should be used.

VENOMOUS SNAKE BITES ■

Compared with other etiologies of critical illness, venomous snake bites account for few ICU admissions per year. The case fatality rate of untreated or improperly treated envenomations is significant enough to warrant scrutiny by the critical care physician. To properly diagnose a case of snake envenomation, the clinician must be acquainted with the epidemiologic and morphologic features of the organism, the appearance of the envenomation puncture site, and the sequence of morbid events that may follow. Folklore surrounding snake envenomations as well as controversial treatment regimens often misdirect and complicate treatment of the victim. Therefore, the critical care physician must also be familiar with various first aid procedures as well as conventional and controversial treatment regimens that may have been invoked by the referring physician or the good Samaritan. Consequently, this section summarizes the epidemiology, diagnosis, and treatment of snake envenomations indigenous to the United States and Canada.

There are about 3000 snake species in the world, of which 300 are dangerous to humans.[1] Likewise 20 poisonous species from a total of 120 species residing in the United States are potential human menaces. Close contact with domestic and imported snakes results in 45,000 snake bites per year in this country, of which 8000 are venomous. Approximately 12 deaths occur per year as a result of these envenomations. Equally significant is the suffering, limb loss, loss of function, and loss of economic productivity that result from nonfatal envenomations. Before the advent of antivenin, morbidity in the form of scarring, contractures, or amputations affected 75% of victims, and mortality occurred in 10% to 35%.[2]

Venomous reptiles are found in temperate and tropical areas around the world. These reptiles include the Colubridae, Elapidae, Hydrophyidae, Crotalidae, and Helodermatidae.[3] Ninety percent to 99% of venomous snake bites in the United States are produced by pit vipers (Crotalidae) and most of the remainder are produced by coral snakes (Elapidae).

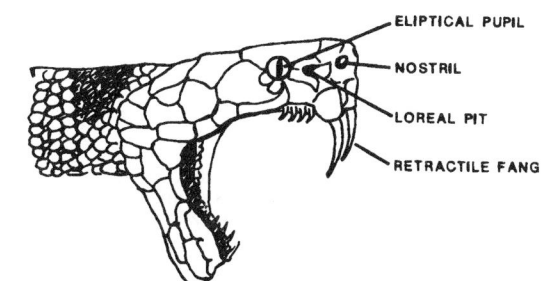

MORPHOLOGY OF THE PIT VIPER (CROTALIDAE)

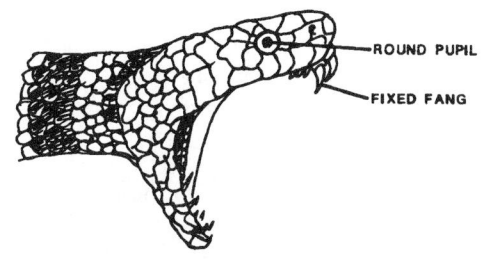

MORPHOLOGY OF THE CORAL SNAKE (ELAPIDAE)

FIGURE 102-1. Identification of poisonous snakes.

Precise species identification of a particular snake is difficult for the untrained physician. However, with careful attention to several key morphologic points, one should be able to differentiate snakes that are poisonous from those that are harmless[4] (Fig. 102-1). The identification of poisonous snakes is based on characteristics of dentition, head shields, pupils, and tail, and the presence or absence of a heat-sensing pit. All pit vipers (rattlesnakes, cottonmouths, copperheads) have large anterior retractile fangs that are easily recognized and contain a venom channel. Careful inspection of a pit viper reveals a small depression on the side of its head midway and slightly below a line connecting the eye and nostril. This depression is a heat-sensing pit used by the snake for location of prey. The pupils of pit vipers are elliptical and vertical, whereas those of most nonvenomous snakes are round (although venomous coral snakes also have round pupils). The tail of 30 species of American pit vipers is modified into several loosely interlocking horny segments that produce a threatening "rattle" when shaken, hence the name "rattlesnake." The ventral plates caudal to the anus in pit vipers are arranged in a single row, whereas those in the coral snake are arranged in a double row similar to most nonpoisonous snakes.

Coral snakes have shorter, permanently erect anterior fangs that also contain a venom channel or groove. On the lateral aspect of the head, the presence of a shield (loreal shield) separating those shields bordering the eyes from those bordering the nostril excludes coral snake identification. Coral snakes have no loreal shield. The coral snake also has characteristic tricolor bands of black, red, and yellow or white. The red bands are bordered by yellow or white bands and the bands encircle its body. Nonvenomous mimics of the coral snake also are enveloped by tricolor bands, but

the red borders the black, and the bands do not totally encircle the body ("red on black, venom lack; red on yellow, kill a fellow").

The venom glands of poisonous snakes are modifications of salivary glands.[5] The venom of a single snake may contain 5 to 15 enzymes, 3 to 12 nonenzymatic proteins and peptides, and six or more other substances.[6–8] These substances exert simultaneous toxic or lethal effects on the integumentary, hematologic, nervous, respiratory, and cardiovascular systems. The clinical picture also can be complicated by the effects of other endogenous mediator release, such as histamine, bradykinin, and adenosine. Therefore, snake venoms cannot be classified purely as "neurotoxic" or "cardiotoxic." The most important deleterious components of snake venom are shown in Table 102-1. Hyaluronidase is found in all venoms and produces hydrolysis of connective tissue stroma, allowing the dispersion of other toxic components. Crotalid venom is rich in proteinases, amino acidases, and phospholipases; therefore, it produces clinical changes related to cellular destruction, membrane permeability, and coagulation. Elapid venoms vary widely among species but contain more neurotoxins and cardiotoxins, resulting in various expressions of nerve and heart toxicity.

The clinical spectrum of abnormalities produced in a single victim by a given snake venom varies with the size and species of snake, the quantity of venom injected, the number and location of bites, the presence of bacteria in the snake's mouth, the age and health of the victim, and any treatment previously rendered. As many as 30% of crotalid bites and 50% of elapid bites may result in no envenomation.[8] The venom channel is recessed above the tip of the fang, and the venom injected may be reduced by poor penetration or glancing blows, causing venom to be lost over the skin and clothing surface. The volume of venom available to a particular snake may be reduced by previous feedings.

Most medically significant envenomations are caused by pit vipers. Rattlesnake bites are the most serious, cottonmouth (water moccasin) bites are of intermediate severity, and copperhead bites usually produce no major systemic injury.[9] Many snakebites are experienced by individuals who do not attempt to move away from the snake; many of these persons are under the influence of alcohol. The manifestations of snake envenomations can be divided into local and systemic effects. Rattlesnake venom causes local pain, swelling, erythema, ecchymosis, and occasional bleb formation at the puncture site. Later, the increased membrane permeability and cellular destruction produced by various proteases result in spreading edema and tissue sloughing. If the bite is on an extremity, a compartment syndrome may result.

Systemic effects of rattlesnake venom involve hematologic abnormalities and effects on the cardiovascular, respiratory, and neurologic systems. The coagulation alterations result from several proteases acting on various parts of the coagulation cascade. Fibrin degradation products increase whereas fibrinogen and circulating platelets decrease. Simon and Grace[10] studied the coagulation defects produced by rattlesnake venom in dogs. They believed that the predominant effect was caused by an increase in thrombin-like activity. Recently, other investigators have produced evidence

TABLE 102-1. Contents of Snake Venom

COMPONENT	CROTALID	ELAPID	EFFECT
Proteinases	Heavy	Minimal coagulation, anticoagulation	Tissue destruction
Hyaluronidase (spreading factor)	Moderate	Moderate	Hydrolyzes connective tissue stroma
Cholinesterase	Minimal	Heavy	Catalyzes hydrolysis of acetylcholine
Phospholipase A	Heavy		Hemolysis may potentiate neurotoxins
Phosphodiesterase	Minimal	Heavy	Unknown
Neurotoxins	Minimal	Heavy	Flaccid paralysis
Cardiotoxins	Minimal	Heavy	Depolarizing

supporting primary fibrinogenolysis as the mechanism of afibrinogenemia rather than consumption of fibrinogen from thrombin activity.[11,12] The coagulation defects may result in local bleeding, epistaxis, hemoptysis, hematuria, and gastrointestinal bleeding. Also, intravascular hemolysis may occur.

Neurologic sequelae affecting rattlesnake envenomations are weakness, sweating, numbness, paresthesias, fasciculations, convulsions, and coma. The coma may be secondary to hypovolemia or to a direct effect of the toxin.[13] Other findings are nausea, vomiting, respiratory depression, and pulmonary edema, especially in more severe cases. Elapid bites account for the largest number of worldwide deaths but only a small percentage of deaths in the United States.

Coral snake bites produce predominantly systemic effects. Local findings are minimal and the puncture site may be missed. The victim may have numbness or weakness in the bitten extremity. Systemic poisoning by coral snake venom produces drowsiness, euphoria, weakness, nausea, vomiting, fasciculations, excessive salivation, extraocular muscle paresis, hypotension, delayed general paresis, and cardiopulmonary failure.[8]

Proper diagnosis of snake envenomation depends heavily on a description of the snake or examination of the snake itself. The site of envenomation also provides important visual clues. Potentially morbid crotalid bite sites demonstrate early local swelling and erythema. Therefore, if after a known crotalid bite the victim demonstrates no local changes over several hours of observation, the person can be released from the hospital. Elapid or coral snake bites are associated with minimal local changes and systemic complications may be delayed. Therefore, specific antivenin therapy may need to be initiated in these victims before any local or clinical signs appear. The diagnosis of any significant envenomation is supported by the clinical manifestations mentioned earlier. Most victims of snake bite can relate some information about the attacker. Immunoassays and bioassays have been used experimentally to identify various snake venoms in tissue.[14] Minton and colleagues[15] prepared an enzyme-linked immunosorbent assay against the venoms of the Western diamondback rattlesnake, the Mojave rattlesnake, and the copperhead. They were able to detect venom levels of 0.1 to 0.01

μg/mL in tissue fluid removed from the bite site of several species of rattlesnakes. These assays may be helpful in the future to identify specific venoms in victims from endemic snakebite areas, especially if historical information is limited.

The treatment of clinically significant snake envenomations is shrouded in controversy. It can be divided into first aid, specific antivenin therapy, and supportive therapy (Table 102-2).

By the time most snake bite victims reach a hospital, first aid measures may have already been undertaken and additional first aid measures are too late to be of any value. In the past, these measures have included tourniquets, cryotherapy, and incision and suction.

Advocates of constricting tourniquets believe they may reduce the systemic distribution of venoms by obstructing superficial venous and lymphatic return. Opponents think tourniquets may predispose to greater local necrosis and early limb loss.[16] The consensus of most authors is that tourniquets may be used in the prehospital management of elapid envenomations only with certain precautions. The tourniquet should be placed proximal to the bite and only tightly enough to occlude lymphatics and superficial veins. It should be loose enough to allow a finger to be placed underneath, and it should be slowly and sequentially released only after antivenin has been initiated at the hospital. Limited systemic morbidity may occur at the risk of increasing local morbidity. The use of tourniquets in crotalid envenomations remains speculative.[12]

Advocates of cryotherapy believe that cooling the bitten extremity may inactivate the enzymatic components of venom. Cryotherapy use is condemned in the current literature. There are many nonenzymatic toxic components of venom, and doubt exists as to whether the temperature can be lowered enough to decrease enzyme activity. In addition, cryotherapy undertaken as packing the bitten extremity in ice has been shown to increase the risk of amputation and tissue necrosis.[17] A local ice pack applied for less than 30 minutes in the prehospital period may afford some pain relief without increasing the risk of tissue damage.[18]

Incision and suction also were recommended in the past as means of removing local reservoirs of deposited venom.

TABLE 102-2.   Treatment for Snake Envenomations

FIRST AID

    Tourniquets—mildly occlusive proximal to bite
    Cryotherapy—local ice pack for symptom relief
    Incision and suction—within 5 min of bite,
        —if over 30 min from hospital, incision through puncture, 30 min of suction

SPECIFIC

Crotalid°	
Severity	Antivenin Crotalidae Polyvalent
No envenomation	0 vials IV
Mild envenomation	1–4 vials IV
Moderate envenomation	4–7 vials IV
Severe envenomation	15 or more vials IV
Elapid°	
Severity	Micrurus fulvius antivenin
Historical exposure	3–5 vials IV
Onset of symptoms	3–5 vials IV q 4 h prn

SUPPORTIVE

    Debride necrotic tissue
    Fasciotomy for compartment syndrome
    Immobilize in position of function
    Replace consumed coagulation factors
    Oxygen, ventilation, hemodialysis prn

IV, intravenously; q, every; prn, as needed.
°Skin test for allergy to horse serum first.

When improperly administered, this technique can increase local injury. Russell and Picchioni[19] suggest that incision and suction should be done only within 5 minutes of the snake bite if the victim is more than 30 minutes from medical care. The incision should be less than 1 cm in length and 3 mm in depth, placed directly through the fang punctures. Suction should be applied for 30 minutes.

Other first aid measures are cleansing the wound area, immobilizing the bitten extremity in a position of function below the heart, and transporting the victim to the nearest medical care facility as soon as possible. An awareness of the first aid measures applied to a particular snake bite victim in the prehospital period assists the critical care physician in care of the victim.

Two kinds of antivenin, made by Wyeth-Ayerst Laboratories, are commercially available in the United States: one for pit viper bites and one for Eastern coral bites. There is no antivenin for the toxin of the Arizona coral snake; however, envenomation by this species usually produces self-limiting illness. Proper use of antivenin is the most important aspect of hospital care of crotalid envenomation victims. Antivenin decreases local tissue damage as well as hematologic and other systemic aberrations. There is an unfortunate lack of prospective trials looking at indications and dosages of antivenin.[20-23] Based on empiric trials, the clinician should begin antivenin as soon as possible, depending on the clinical severity of the bite. The victim should first be skin-tested for sensitivity to horse serum protein. An immediate wheal-and-flare response signals a potential immediate hypersensi-tivity response to antivenin; however, a negative reaction does not mean the patient is immune to anaphylaxis.[24] Therefore, proceed with caution. The conjunctival sensitivity test advocated in the package literature is even less reliable than the skin test. If the victim's skin test gives a negative result, antivenin administration is guided by the severity of envenomation.

Rattlesnake victims can be graded as no envenomation, minimal, moderate, or severe. No envenomation is apparent in the absence of local or systemic reactions, in which case antivenin should not be given. Minimal envenomation is marked by mild local swelling without systemic symptoms; victims should receive 1 to 4 units of antivenin. Moderate envenomation is associated with local ecchymosis and swelling and systemic weakness, sweating, syncope, nausea, vomiting, anemia, or thrombocytopenia. Victims graded as moderate should receive 4 to 7 units of antivenin. Severe envenomation is heralded by marked local necrosis and systemic signs of hypotension, paresthesias, coma, pulmonary edema, or respiratory failure. These patients should be given 15 or more units of antivenin.[1] Less antivenin is needed for water moccasin envenomations, and antivenin is rarely needed for copperhead bites except in children and elderly victims.

Antivenin should be diluted in 500 to 1000 mL of normal saline or 5% dextrose in water and administered IV over 2 to 4 hours. The volume of diluent should be reduced in pediatric patients and patients with limited cardiac reserve. The patient should be evaluated at least every 15 minutes during antivenin administration and every 4 hours thereafter. Evaluation should consist of vital signs, urine output, appearance and circumference of the involved extremities, coagulation parameters, and hemoglobin, hematocrit, and serum electrolyte determinations. The patient's clinical condition should be periodically evaluated and antivenin should be administered for up to 24 hours as long as abnormalities are progressing. If a hypersensitivity reaction develops or if the initial skin test demonstrates sensitivity to horse serum, the patient should be given diphenhydramine (Benadryl), 50 mg IV, and an epinephrine infusion should be started.[25] Antivenin should be held for 5 minutes, and the infusion should be started slowly. Antivenin is most effective if given within 4 hours of the bite, less valuable after 8 hours, and questionable after 24 hours.[19] If coagulation defects occur after the first 24 hours, antivenin still may be beneficial.[26]

If historical evidence strongly supports coral snake envenomation, the victim should be given three to five vials of *Micrurus fulvius* antivenom initially after the appropriate skin test. Three to five vials of additional antivenin should be given after symptoms develop and every 4 hours, depending on the clinical severity.

Delayed serum sickness may occur in any patient who has received antivenin; the frequency of occurrence is proportional to the amount of antivenin administered. Therefore, all patients receiving antivenin should be observed for several days.

Early debridement and fasciotomy are advocated by some authors, based on the premise that debridement removes venom and toxic mediators and that fasciotomy aborts an inevitable compartment syndrome.[18] Unfortunately, a compartment syndrome is difficult to diagnose by clinical means, and early surgical intervention often leads to prolonged convalescence, increased tissue damage, and greater scarring. Russell and coworkers[1] believe that fasciotomy is never necessary if antivenin treatment has been adequate, based on a series of 500 patients treated with antivenin. The consensus is that debridement should be delayed and used to remove necrotic tissue. Fasciotomy should be undertaken in patients with objective evidence of a compartment syndrome, that is, those with decreased blood flow in the absence of thrombosis and those with increased intracompartmental pressure.[27] Noninvasive vascular studies may identify patients at risk for ischemia.[28]

Supportive measures for maintaining victims of snake envenomation have been partially covered. The wound should be thoroughly cleaned and the extremity maintained in a slightly dependent functional position. Coagulopathies should be corrected with fresh frozen plasma and platelets. Blood transfusions should be given to replace blood loss from hemolysis and bleeding. Oxygen ventilatory support and hemodialysis may be necessary for pulmonary and renal complications of severe envenomation. Tetanus toxoid or tetanus immune globulin should be administered based on the victim's previous immunization history. Corticosteroids are of no proven value for envenomation and may interfere with the action of antivenin. However, corticosteroids may be used for hypersensitivity reactions to antivenin. Prophylactic antibiotics also are of no proven value.

BLACK WIDOW SPIDER BITES ■

Various species of the widow spider *Latrodectus* are distributed throughout the temperate and subtropical zones of the world. They are found in every state of the continental United States.[29,30] Human envenomation by these female spiders is referred to as latrodectism. *L mactans*, indigenous to the southeastern United States, is commonly referred to as the "black widow" and accounts for most deaths from latrodectism in this country. *Latrodectus hesperus* is another species frequently associated with latrodectism and resides in the western United States. Other species less often associated with latrodectism are included in Table 102-3.

Knowledge of the widow spider's morphologic features is important in establishing a diagnosis (Fig. 102-2). The female adult body is 0.5 cm with a leg spread of up to 40 mm. The surface topography is shiny black with a red marking on the ventral aspect of the spider's abdomen. The red marking may vary because of regional adaptations from a typical hourglass configuration (*L mactans*) to red triangles (*L variolus*) or spots (*L bishopi*). The male *Latrodectus* is much smaller

TABLE 102-3. Worldwide Causes of Latrodectism

SPECIES	LOCATION
Latrodectus bishopi	Florida
Latrodectus geometricus	California, Florida
Latrodectus hesperus	Western U.S.
Latrodectus mactans	Southeastern U.S.
Latrodectus variolus	Eastern U.S., Canada
Latrodectus curariensis	Brazil, Argentina
Latrodectus hasseltii	Australia, New Zealand
Latrodectus lugubris	Russia
Latrodectus maculatus	South Africa
Latrodectus malmigniatus	Europe
Latrodectus tredecimguttatus	Europe

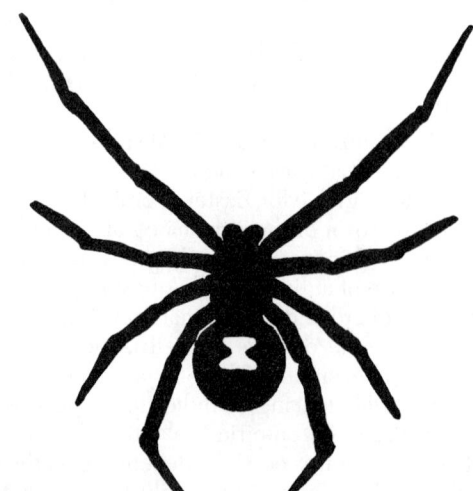

FIGURE 102-2. Morphologic features of *Latrodectus mactans*, ventral aspect.

with white abdominal stripes and does not possess enough venom to be toxic for humans. The black widow gets its name from past rare observations in which the female was seen consuming its mate. In most cases, the female experiences a period of lassitude after copulation, which allows the male to escape.

Reports of latrodectism suggest that these spiders have migrated from a rural to an urban existence.[29–31] They reside in dark areas such as between rocks, within sheaves of wheat, within seldom-used clothing, or in corners of basements and garages. Earlier in this century, epidemics were more common. Black widow spider bites of the buttock and genitalia were hazards of outdoor lavatory use in the United States and Australia.[32,33] Epidemics of latrodectism were reviewed by Bettini[31] and were believed to be caused by importation and meteorologic conditions favoring proliferation of the organism in various geographic areas. Recently, sporadic cases have been more common. Reports of black widow spider envenomations peak during warmer periods because of several factors. First, spiders and humans are more active during warm weather, thereby increasing the chance of contact. Second, the venom may be more potent at higher temperatures because of pH changes, therefore increasing the clinical severity of the illness and thus the likelihood of being reported.

Latrodectus spiders are nonaggressive; human envenomation occurs as a result of casual contact in which the spider is inadvertently threatened. The venom is extruded from paired glands in its cephalothorax through modified chelicerae into the victim. A case was recently reported in which a woman became ill after conjunctival contact with crushed black widow spider debris.[34] The victim experienced typical symptoms of latrodectism.

Black widow spider venom contains the most potent neurotoxins per volume found in nature. The major component is a 130,000-dalton protein known as alpha-latrotoxin.[35] The toxin binds to specific receptors located on vertebrate presynaptic membranes, causing selective release of various neurotransmitters including glutamate, epinephrine, and acetylcholine.[36–38] The action of the venom is partially dependent on intracellular calcium, but it is not inhibited by calcium or sodium channel blocking drugs (e.g., verapamil).[30,38] On the other hand, excess extracellular calcium or magnesium inhibits the initial exocytosis of neurotransmitter vesicles, and parenteral calcium has been used clinically to relieve symptoms of latrodectism.[39]

The clinical presentation can be characterized as an ascending wave of painful muscle spasm accompanied by varying degrees of adrenergic and cholinergic excitation. Initially the bite, if noticed, is described as a pin-prick sensation followed by a variable asymptomatic period of 10 to 30 minutes. Painful muscle spasms first develop in the large muscle groups closest to the bite site and then spread to the trunk, resulting in spasm of abdominal, pelvic, and back muscles. Involvement of the abdominal muscles has led to a misdiagnosis of "acute abdomen" in the past. Severe abdominal muscle spasm may compromise breathing and produce respiratory failure. The victim cannot sit still and exhibits a form of anesthesia. The victim may demonstrate increases in body secretions such as sweating, lacrimation,

excess salivation, and bronchorrhea. Skin manifestations vary from a target lesion at the bite site to any type of generalized rash, the most common being scarlatiniform.

The most common cardiovascular manifestations are tachycardia and hypertension, but congestive heart failure and myocardial ischemia have been reported in patients with preexisting heart disease. Involvement of the central nervous system causes headache, delirium, psychosis, convulsions, and, rarely, coma. Laboratory tests reveal concentrated urine, albuminuria, leukocytosis, and an elevated creatine kinase level. High-risk patients may experience complications of shock, coma, stroke, myocardial infarction, acute renal failure, respiratory failure, and death. Patients at risk include children younger than 16 years of age, adults older than 60 years, and any person with preexisting heart disease. In most cases, the syndrome abates within 48 hours, but aches and malaise may persist for up to 1 week.

The diagnosis of latrodectism is based on strong historical evidence of contact with a black widow spider along with the typical syndrome. The victim should be encouraged to bring in the spider or its parts for proper identification, and the local poison control center should be notified.

Treatment for latrodectism can be divided into specific and supportive therapy (Table 102-4). Specific therapy involves parenteral administration of specific antivenin. Antivenin is an equine derivative of *L mactans* but offers crossprotection to the other *Latrodectus* species. It has been used extensively in Australia and provides prompt dramatic relief of symptoms when administered within 2 hours of the bite. Antivenom is contraindicated in the patient with a history of allergy to horse serum. If time allows, a test dose of horse serum protein (0.02 mL of 1:10 dilution of test material in saline injected intracutaneously) should be administered. If the patient does not develop a wheal at the test site, the serum may be given. If time does not permit a skin test, the patient can be given diphenhydramine (1 mg/kg IV) and epinephrine (1:1000, 0.25 mL subcutaneously) while the antivenin is prepared. One ampule of lyophilized antivenin is reconstituted in 2.5 mL diluent and administered intramuscularly or diluted in 50 mL of saline and administered IV over 15 minutes. The route of administration depends on the condition of the victim. The use of antivenin should be reserved for high-risk patients, particularly children, elderly patients with preexisting heart disease, and patients with a severe initial presentation.

Supportive therapy consists of analgesics and muscle relaxants. Narcotic analgesics such as morphine have been used frequently and are most effective when given parenterally. Muscle relaxants include calcium gluconate, methocarbamol, benzodiazepines, and dantrolene sodium. Key[39] compares parenteral calcium gluconate treatment with methocarbamol treatment for the relief of painful muscle spasm secondary to latrodectism. He found that 6 of 13 patients were cured of symptoms by calcium gluconate, but only 1 of 10 patients treated with methocarbamol achieved significant symptomatic relief. Relief from calcium treatment is rapidly attenuated, and multiple doses are usually necessary. Ryan[40] reports protracted and pronounced symptom relief in 5 of 8 patients treated with dantrolene sodium when compared

TABLE 102-4. Treatment for Latrodectism

	DOSE
TYPE SPECIFIC	
Antivenin*	1 amp IM
	1 amp/50 mL IV NS 10 min
SUPPORTIVE	
Calcium gluconate 10%	1–2 mL/kg up to 10 mL over 10 min q 4 h prn
or	1 mg/kg IV initially then 25 mg PO q 4 h for
Dantrolene sodium	maximum of 6 doses
or	
Methocarbamol	Adults: 10 mL IV over 10 min
	Then 10 ml/250 ml D$_5$W over 3–4 h not to exceed
	30 mL/day
	Children: 60 mg/kg/24 h in 4 doses IV
Valium	Adults: 5–10 mg IV q 4 h prn
OTHER	
Morphine	4 mg IV q 5 min titrated to desired effect
IV fluids	
Hospitalization	
Antihypertensive medications	

amp, ampule; IM, intramuscularly; NS, normal saline; IV, intravenous; prn, as needed; PO, orally; q, every; D$_5$W, 5% dextrose in water.
*Pretest for allergy to horse serum.

with patients treated with centrally acting muscle relaxants. Valium also produces significant relief of muscle spasm, but has not been compared prospectively with the other drugs and is limited by sedation. Therefore, risk–benefit analysis suggests calcium gluconate as the initial agent, followed by dantrolene sodium, methocarbamol, or diazepam. Recommended doses are given in Table 102-4.

All patients with documented black widow spider bites should be observed for at least several hours. If symptoms are minor, the patient can be sent home with a responsible adult. Victims with severe symptoms and those at risk for complications should be hospitalized for observation treatment.

BROWN RECLUSE SPIDER BITES ■

Loxoscelism refers to human disease caused by various species of the genus *Loxosceles*. *Loxosceles laeta* is responsible for loxoscelism in Central and South America, whereas *L reclusa* causes the disease in the United States. In addition to producing a painful gangrenous ulcer, the bite of *L reclusa* is occasionally complicated by systemic toxicosis referred to as *viscerocutaneous loxoscelism*.

The first case of illness in the United States caused by a brown spider bite was reported by Schmaus in 1929.[41] The patient was a 24-year-old woman who developed local pain, rash, fever, leukocytosis, and a local erythematous pustule at the bite site. No description of necrosis was recorded. In 1940, Gotten and MacGowan[42] described *blackwater fever*

in a 3-year-old Mississippi girl with a necrotizing skin lesion. This was probably the first reported case of intravascular hemolysis associated with a brown spider bite.[42] In 1957, *L reclusa* was definitely connected with necrotic arachnidism.[43] Since then, several cases of brown recluse spider bites have been reported in North America, South America, and Israel. Reports of *L reclusa* were once limited to the Mississippi and Ohio River valleys and are increasing in other parts of the United States.

The spider's body is 1.0 to 1.5 cm in length and 5 to 7 mm across (Fig. 102-3). It has a leg span of up to 5 cm. The body surface is dark brown to light tan. On the dorsal aspect of the cephalothorax is a midline band of a darker color shaped like a violin. The base of this violin configuration begins at the spider's three pairs of eyes and the neck of the violin extends back toward the abdomen.

Loxosceles spiders prefer to live indoors in storage sheds, closets, and stored clothes. They also can be found outdoors under rocks or in any dark crevice. Most cases of loxoscelism result from contact with inhabited clothing.[41,44]

The venom contains necrotizing and spreading factors. The harmless spreading factor hyaluronidase accounts for most of the venom. Toxicity is mainly caused by sphingomyelinase D, which is a phospholipase rarely found in other venoms. Most venoms of snakes, bees, and arthropods contain phospholipase A$_2$. Sphingomyelinase D cleaves choline from substances such as phosphatidylcholine and sphingomyelin found in platelet and vascular endothelial membranes. This process produces increased membrane permeability and thrombosis. Rees and coworkers[45] injected

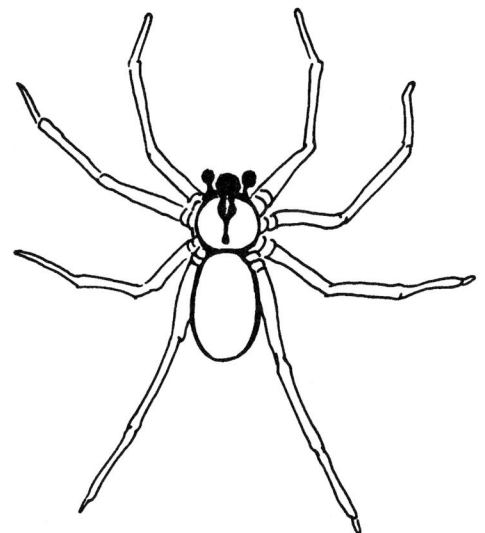

FIGURE 102-3. Morphologic features of *Loxosceles reclusa*, dorsal aspect.

purified sphingomyelinase D into the skin of rabbits and produced a typical dermonecrotic lesion. They concluded that membrane damage activated inflammatory mediators, which provoked an intense inflammatory response. Smith and Micks[46] also investigated *Loxosceles* venom in rabbits and guinea pigs. They described an infiltration of polymorphonuclear cells followed by edema and hemorrhage. They were able to decrease the inflammation and damage by inhibiting the polymorphonuclear cells or complement with nitrogen mustard and zymosan-aggregated human globulin.

In summation, the brown recluse spider injects a venom into its host, which produces endothelial and platelet damage resulting in edema, thrombosis, and ischemic necrosis. This process is accelerated by complement and other inflammatory mediators that incite an intense polymorphonuclear response.

The intravascular hemolysis associated with viscerocutaneous loxoscelism is less well described. Nance[47] reviews hemolytic anemia associated with necrotic arachnidism and proposes three mechanisms, none of which have been proven. Direct action of the venom and glucose 6 phosphate dehydrogenase (G6PD) deficiency have been virtually ruled out in animal studies. Coombs'-positive antibodies have been identified in five cases of viscerocutaneous loxoscelism, but other cases have been Coombs' negative.[48]

The clinical presentation of loxoscelism is variable. Minor bites may resolve or progress to necrosis or systemic involvement, depending on the susceptibility of the host, the amount of venom, and possible immunization from previous envenomations. Cutaneous or necrotizing loxoscelism begins as tiny puncture marks or a bluish spot at the bite site. After 2 to 8 hours, a large erythematous halo and blister develop along with pain. Within 24 hours, ischemic necrosis and intracutaneous hemorrhage occur. After 3 to 4 days, the lesion takes on a stellate violaceous appearance. At 7 to 14 days, the central part of the lesion becomes depressed and sharply demarcated, leading to eschar formation. The eschar eventually sloughs, leaving a 1- to 10-cm open ulcer. Most

of the ulcers heal within 3 weeks by secondary intention. Seven cases of necrotizing *Loxosceles* spider bites in Israel were reported by Efrati.[44] In six cases, the ulcer healed spontaneously whereas one required suturing to close a 4 × 6 cm defect.

Viscerocutaneous or systemic loxoscelism may occur suddenly, particularly in children. Fever, chills, nausea, vomiting, arthralgias, and a variable rash develop within 24 to 48 hours. The rash may be macular, morbilliform, petechial, generalized, or localized to the trunk and flexural areas. Complications include seizures, vasculitis, and a severe intravascular hemolysis that may bring on acute renal failure and death. Eichner[48] reviews 200 brown spider bite cases reported between 1958 and 1984. He found 25 cases of spider bite hemolysis and six deaths (five were children). The most significant laboratory finding relating to systemic loxoscelism is a rapidly dropping hemoglobin value with hematuria, hemoglobinuria, and proteinuria. All patients with significant cutaneous or viscerocutaneous loxoscelism develop leukocytosis, averaging white blood cell counts of 20,000 to 30,000. Signs of a consumptive coagulopathy and Coombs' positivity are variably present. Elevated liver enzymes and pulmonary infarction also have been reported.

Definitive diagnosis usually rests with specific identification of the spider and a compatible clinical picture.

Treatment for most brown recluse spider bites is unnecessary because most produce no significant sequelae. For those cases that progress to cutaneous or viscerocutaneous loxoscelism, treatment is entirely supportive because no specific therapy is available for clinical use (Table 102-5). Antivenin has been developed but is restricted to experimental trials. In the past, treatment of the necrotizing cutaneous form has included steroids, antihistamines, alpha-blockers, low molecular weight dextrans, wide surgical excision,[43,49,50] antibiotics, and dapsone. Steroids have been given systemically and injected directly into the bite site without any effect. Likewise, steroids mixed with brown recluse spider venom and injected into laboratory animals have demonstrated no protection.[51] Antihistamines, alpha-blockers, and low molecular weight dextrans are also of no benefit.[50] Early, wide surgical excision with grafting has been advocated but has

TABLE 102-5. Treatment of Brown Recluse Spider Bites

CUTANEOUS

Delayed surgery for debridement
Dapsone (see text)
Splint involved extremity
Analgesics
Antibiotics for secondary infection
Tetanus toxoid for patients at risk

VISCERAL

Maintain hydration
IV steroids for early hemolysis
Transfusions for hemolysis
Dialysis for renal failure

IV, intravenous.

never been demonstrated prospectively to offer less disability or disfiguring than the natural history of the lesion.[51]

Most brown spider bite lesions heal spontaneously; therefore, delayed elective surgery should be performed only to close a refractory ulcer or to correct disabling or disfiguring scars. Recently, dapsone has shown some promise in treating cutaneous loxoscelism. Rees and coworkers[52] compare early surgical excision with dapsone and elective delayed surgical excision in 31 patients who presented with necrotizing skin lesions within 1 to 9 days of a brown recluse spider bite (most presented less than 5 days after the bite). Of 14 patients who underwent early surgical excision, 5 developed delayed wound healing (more than 3 weeks) and 7 developed objectionable scarring. Of 17 patients treated with dapsone, 1 developed a wound complication, 1 developed objectionable scarring, and 1 required a delayed skin graft. More experience with dapsone is needed before it can be readily recommended.[53] However, because nothing better is available, it can be used with caution in patients who develop necrosis and bullae formation within the first 24 hours after the spider bite. Most patients should be treated conservatively, with reassurance, splinting of the involved extremity, cold patches, analgesics, and tetanus toxoid for patients at risk. Antibiotics should be reserved for patients whose lesions become secondarily infected.

Treatment of viscerocutaneous loxoscelism also is supportive. Victims should be hospitalized in a critical care setting. Hydration should be maintained. Systemic steroids, 1 mg/kg/day, may decrease hemolysis if given early. Blood transfusion should be given to maintain adequate oxygen delivery because the hemolytic process has not been shown to be increased by transfusions. Dialysis may be necessary if acute renal failure develops.

SCORPION ENVENOMATION ■

There are 650 existing species of scorpions, and only a few are lethal.[54] Many others produce envenomations similar to Hymenoptera stings (wasps, hornets) and therefore are potentially lethal only if the victim is allergic to the venom. The only lethal form found in the United States is *Centruroides exilicauda*, which resides predominantly in Arizona. Before the 1950s, deaths were attributed to scorpion stings more often than the sting of any other venomous animal. Mortality has been decreased by better scorpion control.[55] In Brazil, *Tityus serrulatus* has been associated with a 12% overall mortality rate and 60% mortality rate in small children. Other lethal species include *Centruroides suffusus* in Mexico and *Leiurus quinquestriatus* in North Africa and Israel. The manifestations of envenomations by most of these species are similar and, therefore, treatment is similar.

The scorpion is 1.5 to 2.0 cm in length with two claws and a long segmented tail known as a telson (Fig. 102-4). The telson bears a pair of poison glands and tapers to a sting. The scorpion's color varies from yellowish to black. The composition of venom varies with the species, season, age, and nutritional state of the scorpion.[56,57] *C exilicauda* contain two classes of toxins.[55] The first class (Ia, IIa, IIIa,

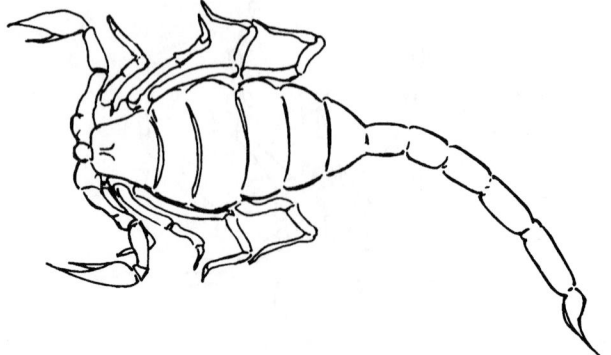

FIGURE 102-4. Morphologic features of *Centruroides sculpturatus,* dorsal aspect.

and IIIb) affects the activation process of sodium channels such that spontaneous and repetitive action potentials occur. The second class of toxins (IVa) prevents complete inactivation through their effect on sodium channels. The end result is a release of norepinephrine, epinephrine, and acetylcholine from adrenergic neurons, neuromuscular areas, and the adrenal glands. The juxtaglomerular apparatus releases excess renin.

As in other types of envenomation, the clinical picture produced by a scorpion sting is determined by the size and susceptibility of the victim, the amount of venom injected, and the virulence of the venom. The sting of nonlethal scorpions in the United States produces a significant local reaction manifest as immediate erythema, induration, and pain. Lethal species of scorpions produce a mild local reaction with hyperesthesia followed by hypoesthesia and a noticeable lack of swelling. The absence of swelling after a scorpion sting therefore may be considered a danger signal.

Clinically, the massive release of neurotransmitters produces a variety of adrenergic and cholinergic manifestations. The victim may manifest tachycardia, hypertension, hyperglycemia, mydriasis, piloerection, and perspiration caused by sympathetic mediators. The victim also may experience salivation, lacrimation, urination, defecation, and gastric distention. The most common findings in 51 victims younger than 13 years of age reported by Amitai and colleagues[58] included tachycardia, irritability, profuse sweating, priapism, and vomiting. Two of the patients in that series died. Other signs include laryngospasm, opisthotonus, or emprosthotonos. Severe envenomation may produce pulmonary edema, arrhythmias, focal myocardial necrosis, coma, and death. Symptoms may last from 24 to 48 hours. If the victim survives the first 3 hours without severe respiratory or circulatory effect, the prognosis usually is good.

Laboratory manifestations of scorpion envenomation include hyperglycemia, hypernatremia, and leukocytosis. The treatment of scorpion stings is primarily supportive (Table 102-6). Specific antivenom is available for most of the lethal varieties including *C exilicauda* in Arizona and *C suffusus* in Mexico. Gueron and coworkers[59] studied the benefit of various vasoactive drugs in preventing cardiovascular side effects in dogs envenomated by *L quinquestriatus*. Propranolol and phentolamine were most effective in reversing he-

TABLE 102-6. Treatment of Lethal Scorpion Envenomation

MEDICATION	DOSE°
Hemodynamic changes	
Propranolol	0.5–1 mg/kg PO
Phentolamine	Adults, 5 mg IV or IM
	Children, I mg IV or IM
Cholinergic	0.2 mg/kg IV up to 2 mg
change—atropine	
Muscle spasm—calcium (IV)	10 mg/kg IV
Convulsions—phenobarbital	10 mg/kg IV

PO, orally; IV, intravenously; IM, intramuscularly.
°Titrated to desired effect.

modynamic changes. Hexamethonium was ineffective and atropine was effective only for dominant cholinergic effects. Bawashar and Bawashar[60] report similar beneficial effects with prazocin in patients stung by *Buthus tamulus*. Intravenous calcium and phenobarbital have been effective in relieving muscle spasms and convulsions, respectively.

In summation, scorpion bite patients may require hospitalization in a critical care setting with generous respiratory and cardiovascular support.

MARINE ENVENOMATIONS ■

Organisms of the phylum Coelenterata, including jellyfish (class Scyphozoa), the Portuguese man-of-war and sea hydroids (class Hydrozoa), and the anemones and fire corals (class Anthozoa), possess nematocysts[61,62] (Fig. 102-5). The adult jellyfish consists of an umbrella-shaped head or medusa tailed by tentacles. The tentacles are actually modified polyps that serve as feeding or reproductive structures or as nematocysts. Each nematocyst contains a spiral-coiled thread tipped with a toxin-bearing barb that can be ejected into the skin. The severity of the sting depends on the number of successful discharges and on the composition of the venom. Contact in the water with the tentacles is the most common means of exposure to the nematocysts.

The Portuguese man-of-war (*Physalia physalis*) consists of a complex colony of floating polyps and medusae. The intense pain and occasional paralysis caused by many stings from this jellyfish can result in drowning. Dead Portuguese man-of-war, dead jellyfish, and free nematocysts or fragments of tentacles that bear nematocysts, which may be washed onto the shore after storms, still may be capable of discharging venom. The popularity of scuba diving and snorkeling has increased the chances of contact with the nematocysts of sessile coelenterates, such as sea anemones.

The Scyphozoa contain the larger jellyfish, including the deadly box-jellyfish (*Chironex fleckeri*), which is not a problem in the United States. It is usually found in tropical climates of the Indian and Pacific oceans including the coastal waters of Australia. The box-jellyfish is so named because of its four translucent panels that roughly form a box. The sting of the box-jellyfish is painful and it can cause death within minutes. The mortality rate is 15% to 20%; for that reason, a Chironex antivenin is available in endemic areas. The Scyphozoa also include sea nettles (*Dactylometra quinquecirrha*), which pose a greater chance of exposure to swimmers of this country, but the sting in most cases is a minor annoyance.

CLINICAL MANIFESTATIONS

The clinical response depends on the nature of the venom and on the number of nematocyst envenomations.[63,64] The main effects of all of the toxins are pain, paralysis, and

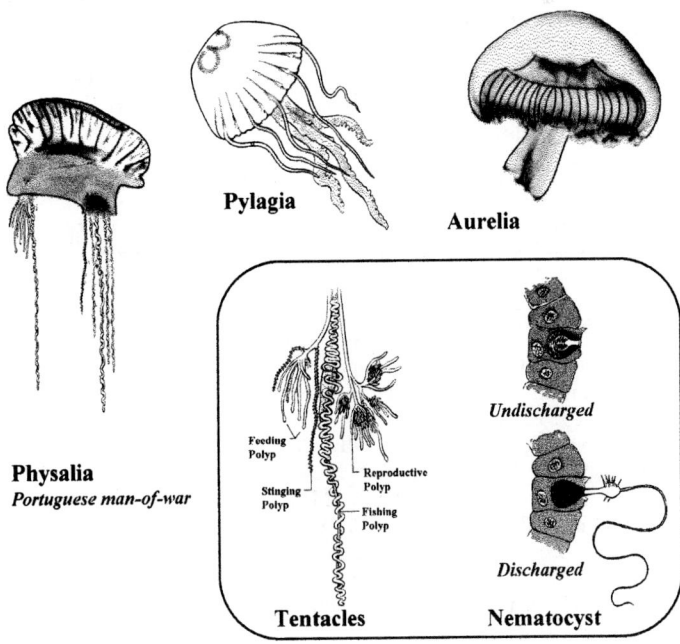

FIGURE 102-5. Morphologic features of colenterates toxic to man.

urticaria often localized to the contact area. Pain is usually the earliest symptom, ranging from a mild stinging sensation to an intense burning. Stings from jellyfish or the Portuguese man-of-war usually cause linear, elevated, edematous, erythematous cutaneous eruptions; anemone and fire coral stings are usually punctate. Urticarial eruptions and systemic anaphylactic reactions may occur. Muscle pain, dyspnea, and vomiting also may be prominent. Hypotension and death may occur in individuals of all ages, but most commonly in children, after stings by the box-jellyfish.

TREATMENT

Tentacles adhering to the skin should be removed immediately with a gloved or protected hand to prevent further envenomation by nematocysts. Nematocysts on the skin should be inactivated with household vinegar; for inactivating nematocysts from sea nettle, a slurry of baking soda should be used.[65,66] Rubbing the affected area should be avoided as should the application of alcohol or of fresh (but not salt) water because these actions cause nematocysts to discharge. Antihistamines may relieve pruritus. If hypotension or systemic anaphylaxis develops, epinephrine should be administered.

Other marine animals may cause serious, and at times fatal, envenomations. The bite of the blue-ringed octopus introduces tetrodotoxin, a potent neurotoxin also found in the puffer fish. No antivenin is available, and supportive therapy, especially to prevent respiratory failure, is indicated. Some species of cone shells also contain toxins that cause neuromuscular blockade; therapy is supportive to prevent respiratory failure.

Fish in the family Scorpaenidae envenomate by spines located on their dorsal, anal, or pelvic fins. Intense local pain develops at the site of envenomation. For stings by lionfish and scorpion fish, immersion of the affected site in nonscalding hot water for 30 to 90 minutes relieves the pain, presumably by destroying the heat-labile toxin.[67] The wound should be cleansed, and tetanus prophylaxis and other supportive care should be provided as necessary. An antivenin is available for scorpaenids but is generally needed only for envenomations by stonefish, which are indigenous to the Indo-Pacific region.

REFERENCES ■

Venomous Snake Bites

1. Russell FE, Carlson RW, Wainschel J, et al: Snake venom poisoning in the United States: experiences with 550 cases. *JAMA* 1975;233:341
2. Christopher DG, Rodning CB: Crotalidae envenomation. *South Med J* 1986;79:159
3. Kunkel DB, Curry SC, Vance MV, et al: Reptile envenomations. *J Toxicol Clin Toxicol* 1983–84;21:503
4. Minton SA: Identification of poisonous snakes. *Clin Toxicol* 1970;3:347
5. Kochva E, Gans C: Salivary glands of snakes. *Clin Toxicol* 1970;3:363

6. Jimenez-Porras JM: Biochemistry of snake venoms. *Clin Toxicol* 1970;3:389
7. Russel FE, Puffer HW: Pharmacology of snake venoms. *Clin Toxicol* 1970;3:433
8. Kunkel DB, Curry SC, Vance MV, et al: Reptile envenomations. *J Toxicol Clin Toxicol* 1983–84;21:503
9. Abramowicz M (ed): Treatment of snakebite in the USA. *Med Lett* 1982;24:87
10. Simon TL, Grace TG: Envenomation coagulopathy in wounds from pit vipers. *N Engl J Med* 1981;305:443
11. Budrynski AZ, Pandya BV, Rubin RN, et al: Fibrinogenolytic afibrinogenemia after envenomation by western diamondback rattlesnake (*Crotalus atrox*). *Blood* 1984;63:1
12. Russel FE: Pressure and immobilization for snakebite remains speculative [letter]. *Ann Emerg Med* 1982;11:702
13. Ekenback K, Hulting J, Persson H, et al: Unusual neurological symptoms in a case of severe crotalid envenomation. *Clin Toxicol* 1985;23:357
14. Frethewie ER: Detection of snake venom in tissue. *Clin Toxicol* 1970;3:445
15. Minton SA, Weinstein SA, Wilde CE: An enzyme-linked immunoassay for detection of North American pit viper venoms. *Clin Toxicol* 1984;22:303
16. Stewart ME, Greenland S, Hoffman JR: First aid treatment of poisonous snakebite: are currently recommeded proocedures justified? *Ann Emerg Med* 1981;10:331
17. McCollough NC, Gennare JF: Treatment of venomous snakebite in the United States. *Clin Toxicol* 1970;3(3):483
18. Glass TG: *Management of Poisonous Snakebite.* San Antonio, TX: Thomas G. Glass, 1976
19. Russel FE, Picchioni AL: Snake venom poisoning. *Clin Toxicol Consultant* 1983;5:73
20. Buntain WL: Successful venomous snakebite neutralization with massive antivenin infusion in a child. *J Trauma* 1983;23:1013
21. Lindsey D: Controversy in snake bite: time for a controlled appraisal. *J Trauma* 1985;25:462
22. Minton SA, Bailey WJ: Letter to the editor. *J Trauma* 1985;25:464
23. Mogelvang LC: Snakebite treatment [letter]. *South Med J* 1984;77:279
24. Malasit P, Warrel DA, Chanthavanich P, et al: Prediction, prevention, and mechanism of early (anaphylactic) antivenom reactions in victims of snake bites. *Br Med J* 1986;292:17
25. Otten EJ, McKimm D: Venomous snakebite in a patient allergic to horse serum. *Ann Emerg Med* 1983;12:624
26. Tiwari I, Johnston WJ: Blood coagulability and viper envenomation. *Lancet* 1986;i:613
27. Whitesides TE, Haney TC, Morimoto K, et al: Tissue pressure measurements as a determinant for the need of fasciotomy. *Clin Orthop* 1975;113:43
28. Curry SC, Kraner JC, Kunkel DB, et al: Noninvasive vascular studies in management of rattlesnake envenomations to extremities. *Ann Emerg Med* 1985;14:1081

Black Widow Spider Bites

29. Kobernick M: Black widow spider bites. *AFP* 1984;29:241
30. Rauber A: Black widow spider bites. *J Toxicol Clin Toxicol* 1983–84;21:473
31. Bettini S: Epidemiology of latrodectism. *Toxicology* 1964;2:93
32. Bogen E: Arachnidism: a study in spider poisoning. *JAMA* 1926;86:1894
33. Sutherland SK, Trinca JC: Survey of 2144 cases of red–black spider bites. *Med J Aust* 1978;2:620

34. Fuller GK: Spider (*Latrodectus hesperus*) poisoning through the conjunctiva. *Am J Trop Med Hyg* 1984;33:1037
35. Mallart A, Haimann C: Differential effects of alpha-latrotoxin on mouse nerve endings and fibers. *Muscle Nerve* 1985;8:151
36. Valtorta F, Madeddu L, Meldolesi J, et al: Specific localization of the alpha-latrotoxin receptor in the nerve terminal plasma membrane. *J Cell Biol* 1984;99:124
37. Kawagoe R, Onodera K, Takeuchi A: On the quantal release of endogenous glutamate from the crayfish neuromuscular junction. *J Physiol* 1982;322:529
38. Yamamoto C, Matsui H: Black widow spider venom: excitatory action on hippocampal neurons. *Brain Res* 1982;244:382
39. Key GF: A comparison of calcium gluconate and methocarbamol (Robaxin) in the treatment of latrodectism (black widow spider envenomation). *J Trop Med Hyg* 1981;30:273
40. Ryan PJ: Preliminary report: experience with the use of dantrolene sodium in the treatment of bites by the black widow spider *Latrodectus hesperus*. *J Toxicol Clin Toxicol* 1983–84;21:487

Brown Recluse Spider Bites

41. Schmaus LF: Case of arachnoidism (spider bite). *JAMA* 1929;92:1265
42. Gotten HB, MacGowan JJ: Blackwater fever (hemoglobinuria) caused by spider bite. *JAMA* 1940;114:1547
43. Madrigal GC, Ercolani RL, Wenzl JE: Toxicity from a bite of the brown spider (*Loxosceles reclusus*). *Clin Pediatr* 1972;11:641
44. Efrati P: Bites by *Loxosceles* spiders in Israel. *Toxicology* 1969;6:239
45. Rees RS, Nanney LB, Yates RA, et al: Interaction of brown recluse spider venom on cell membranes: the inciting mechanism? *J Invest Dermatol* 1984;83:270
46. Smith WC, Micks DW: The role of polymorphonuclear leukocytes in the lesion caused by the venom of the brown spider. *Loxosceles reclusa*. *Lab Invest* 1970;22:90
47. Nance WE: Hemolytic anemia of necrotic arachnidism. *Am J Med* 1961;31:801
48. Eichner ER: Spider bite hemolytic anemia: positive Coombs' test, erythophagocytoses, and leukoerythroblastic smear. *Am J Clin Pathol* 1984;81:683
49. Zeligowski AA, Peled IJ, Wexler MR: Eyelid necrosis after spider bite. *Am J Ophthalmol* 1986;101:254

50. Fardon DW, Wingo CW, Robinson DW, et al: The treatment of brown spider bite. *Plast Reconstr Surg* 1967;40:482
51. Rees RS, Shack RB, Withers EH, et al: Management of the brown recluse spider bite. *Plast Reconstr Surg* 1981;68:768
52. Rees RS, Altenbern DP, Lynch JB, et al: Brown recluse spider bites. *Ann Surg* 1985;202:659
53. Berger RS: Management of brown recluse spider bite [letter]. *JAMA* 1984;251:889
54. Yarom R: Scorpion venom: a tutorial review of its effect in men and experimental animals. *Clin Toxicol* 1970;3:561
55. Rachesky IJ, Banner W, Dansky J, et al: Treatments for *Centruroides exilicauda* envenomation. *AJDC* 1984;138:1136
56. Shulov A: Venom of the scorpion *B. quinquestriatus* and the preparation of antiserum. *Trans R Soc Trop Med Hyg* 1939;33:253
57. Shulov A, Weissmann R, Ginsburg H: Experimental estimation of the toxic strength of the lyophized venom of the scorpion. *Harefuah* 1957;53:309
58. Amitai Y, Mines Y, Aker M, et al: Scorpion sting in children. *Clin Pediatr* 1985:24:136
59. Gueron M, Adolph RJ, Grupp IL, et al: Hemodynamic and myocardial consequences of scorpion venom. *Am J Cardiol* 1980;45:979
60. Bawashar HS, Bawashar PH: Prazosin in management of cardiovascular manifestations of scorpion sting. *Lancet* 1986;i:510
61. Halstead BW: *Coelenterata: Poisonous and Venomous Marine Animals of the World*. Princeton, NJ, Darwin Press, 1978:87
62. Fisher AA: Water-related dermatoses. II. Nematocyst dermatitis. *Cutis* 1980;25:242
63. Burnett JW, Calton GJ: Jellyfish envenomation syndromes updated. *Ann Emerg Med* 1987;16:1000
64. Fisher AA: Toxic and allergic cutaneous reactions to jellyfish with special reference to delayed reactions. *Cutis* 1987;40:303
65. Williamson JA, Le Ray LE, Wohlfahrt M, et al: Acute management of serious envenomation by box-jellyfish (*Chironex fleckeri*). *Med J Aust* 1984;141:851
66. Burnett JW, Rubinstein H, Calton GJ: First aid for jellyfish envenomation. *South Med J* 1983;76:870
67. Kizer KW, McKinney HE, Auerbach PS: Scorpaenidae envenomation: a 5-year poison center experience. *JAMA* 1985;253:807

Critical Care, Third Edition, edited by Joseph M. Civetta,
Robert W. Taylor, and Robert R. Kirby.
Lippincott-Raven Publishers, Philadelphia, PA © 1997.

CHAPTER 103

■

Electrical Injuries

Kenneth A. Perret
Charles A. Weber
Charles L. Bryan

IMMEDIATE CONCERNS ■

MAJOR PROBLEMS

Electrical injuries are relatively uncommon events, accounting for about 3% of admissions to burn units.[1] Their manifestations are frequently devastating in scope and require an intensive approach to evaluation, monitoring, and management. The immediate and early management of such victims clearly has a critical effect on survival, so that a basic understanding of the classification, pathophysiologic mechanisms, and management of the clinical manifestations is essential to the critical care physician. Manifestations and treatment of electrical injuries are outlined in Tables 103-1 and 103-2.

STRESS POINTS

1. Alternating-current injuries are more dangerous than direct-current injuries because of the tetanizing effect of alternating current that "locks" the victim's grasp to the current source and prolongs contact time.
2. Alternating current most commonly induces ventricular fibrillation.
3. Subfascial edema in the extremities can lead to a compartment syndrome.
4. Low-voltage exposure may result in massive necrosis if the duration of contact is sufficient.
5. The heart is particularly sensitive to alternating current. A current of 100 mA is sufficient to produce ventricular fibrillation. Nonspecific electrocardiographic (ECG) changes are seen in 50% of electrical

injury victims. Creatinine kinase-MB (CK-MB) isoenzyme elevations have been seen in 56% of victims without other evidence of myocardial infarction. Significant arrhythmias seem to be uncommon. Surgical procedures should not be delayed based on questionable cardiac findings.

6. Renal toxicity results from volume depletion and pigment-induced acute tubular necrosis. Because of minimal cutaneous damage, traditional formulas based on total-body surface area burned are of no value.
7. Up to 70% of victims experience loss of consciousness or transient paralysis followed by recovery within 5 to 10 minutes. Aside from the medical treatment of seizures, nervous system manifestations have limited impact on management.
8. Musculoskeletal and cutaneous injuries secondary to trauma frequently dominate the clinical picture. Injuries such as long bone fractures, spinal fractures, joint dislocation, or splenic rupture should be excluded.
9. Almost all lightning strike victims survive if they do not sustain a cardiac or respiratory arrest. Dilated and fixed pupils do not necessarily mean that brain death has occurred. These patients should undergo prolonged cardiopulmonary resuscitation. The most common rhythm is asystole.
10. Marked autonomic dysfunction is a unique occurrence.
11. Volume resuscitation is not normally warranted in lightning injury because significant underlying tissue destruction seldom occurs.

TABLE 103-1. Manifestations of Electrical Injuries

CARDIOVASCULAR

Cardiorespiratory arrest, ventricular fibrillation, arrhythmias, myocardial infarction, nonspecific ECG

RENAL

Pigmenturia, acute tubular necrosis

NERVOUS SYSTEM

Cerebral—transient loss of consciousness, confusion, headache, amnesia, seizures, coma
Spinal cord—paralysis, transection, ALS, causalgia
Peripheral—compartment syndromes, delayed injury

MUSCULOSKELETAL AND CUTANEOUS

Long bone and spinal fractures, myonecrosis, compartment syndromes, thermal burns

ALS, amyotrophic lateral sclerosis; ECG, electrocardiographic.

TABLE 103-2. Treatment for Electrical Injuries

Prolonged cardiopulmonary resuscitation
ECG monitoring (see text)
Intravenous crystalloid fluid replacement; titrate fluids to maintain 50 to 100 mL urine output/h
Monitor urine for myoglobin; if present push urine output to 100–150 mL/h; add manitol, alkalinization; eliminate myoglobin source
Serial neurovascular exams of limbs; early radical debridement for grossly involved extremities, compartment syndrome, markedly elevated serum CK levels, or as guided by ^{99m}Tc scanning
Search for skeletal, spinal trauma; cervical immobilization of unconscious victim

ECG, electrocardiographic; CK, creatine kinase.

ESSENTIAL DIAGNOSTIC TESTS AND PROCEDURES

1. All patients who have sustained loss of consciousness, cardiac arrest, arrhythmias, or ECG changes should undergo ECG monitoring.
2. Urine output should be followed closely and monitored for myoglobinuria.
3. Computed tomographic (CT) scanning of the head is recommended for persistent or late-onset coma.
4. Detailed radiographic examination is warranted to search for traumatic injuries. Cervical immobilization should be used until cervical fractures are ruled out.

INITIAL THERAPY

1. Cardiopulmonary resuscitation should be attempted even if prolonged arrest has occurred.
2. Administer crystalloid solution to maintain a urine output of 50 to 100 mL/hour. Increase urine output to 100 to 150 mL/hour if myoglobinuria occurs. Urine alkalization is also recommended.
3. Early, extensive debridement of necrotic muscle is recommended to decrease myoglobinuria and relieve heightened compartmental pressures.
4. Prophylaxis for *Clostridia* infection with high-dose penicillin and serial quantitative wound cultures should be considered.
5. Avoid overhydration in victims of lightning strike.

CLASSIFICATION ■

Exposure to electrical current can be categorized according to the type of current (alternating or direct) and the voltage level of the source. Most electrical injuries occur as the result of contact with alternating current, whereas injury from direct current is primarily limited to the uncommon lightning injury victim. The electrical source is considered low tension if the voltage potential is less than 1000 V and high tension when the voltage exceeds this value. Alternating-current injuries are thought to be more dangerous than a direct-current injury of comparable voltage,[2] primarily because of the tetanizing effect of alternating current, which often locks the victim's grasping hand to the current source and prolongs contact time. This tends to occur less frequently in high-voltage injuries in which the victim is often literally thrown clear from the electrical source.[3] Alternating current also has a definite propensity to induce ventricular fibrillation, an effect not usually seen in victims of direct-current injury.[4]

BASIC MECHANISMS IN ELECTRICAL INJURY ■

There are several mechanisms by which contact with an electrical source may indirectly injure the victim, such as burn injuries caused by ignition of the victim's clothing by the arcing current or the skeletal trauma from violent tetanic muscular contraction. The most striking aspect of electrical injury is the damage produced directly from the interaction of electrical current as it passes through the victim's tissues.

This current–tissue interaction produces a thermal injury in the cutaneous and deep tissues. Heat energy is produced as electrical energy is dissipated in tissues. The amount of heat produced by an electric current is described by a modification of Ohm's Law:

$$J = I^2RT$$

where J is joules of energy, I is the current, R is tissue resistance to current flow, and T is time over which the current is applied.

Heat-induced damage increases as a function of the square of the current as well as in direct proportion to the tissue resistance and duration of contact.[5] The high resistance of skin to electrical current and the resultant heat production account for much of the cutaneous burn injury seen at the entrance and exit wounds of electrical victims. Bone is another tissue with high electrical resistance[6] and is associated with thermal injury in the form of coagulation necrosis of the surrounding tissues, predominantly skeletal muscle. This explains the characteristic noncutaneous pathologic lesion seen in electrical injuries. The resultant pattern of electrical damage resembles a crush injury because of the extensive myonecrosis. This deep tissue injury occurs most prominently near sites of cutaneous electrical contact,[7] although the superficial tissue layers are often spared.[8] The damage is most severe in extremities, primarily because the body acts as a volume conductor. The low cross-sectional area of a limb allows for an increase in current density and, therefore, greater thermal damage.[9,10] Likewise, there is less thermal damage internally as the current traverses the torso with its larger cross-sectional area.

Several other points deserve emphasis in describing the pathophysiologic mechanisms of electrical injury. As described earlier, the muscle tissue adjacent to bone is often severely affected by thermal myonecrosis. In the limbs, these areas are bound by rigid fascial compartments. The subfascial edema that results from the current injury leads to a compartment syndrome that compounds the tissue damage by disrupting vascular and neural structures.[8] The second point is that some tissues, despite low electrical resistances, are more sensitive to electrical injury than others. These tissues include neural and vascular structures.[10] Damage to the vascular intima is well described and is believed to result in thrombosis. Progressive or delayed tissue necrosis has been postulated to occur by thrombosis at these sites of intimal damage.[11] Hunt and associates[9] refute this concept, however, based on their animal model of electrical injury. Damage to the medial vascular layer is believed to account for the frequent clinical occurrence of small vessel aneurysmal dilatation and delayed hemorrhage.

Another form of electrical injury occurs when current arcs from a high-tension source to the victim despite lack of direct physical contact with the source itself. The temperature in such arcs can exceed 2500°C and can be associated with extensive localized skin and deep tissue injury.[12]

A final point relates to the equation $J = I^2RT$. Although extensive deep tissue damage is usually associated with high-voltage contact, even low-voltage exposure may result in massive necrosis if the duration of contact is sufficient.

CLINICAL MANIFESTATIONS AND MANAGEMENT ■

Because of the complex nature of electrical injury, the clinical manifestations are presented on a system-by-system basis, and specific management points are addressed therein (see Tables 103-1 and 103-2).

CARDIOPULMONARY

The cardiopulmonary system is particularly sensitive to the acute effects of alternating current. As little as 100 mA of alternating current is sufficient to produce ventricular fibrillation.[2] Relatively low levels of current across the chest also are capable of inducing tetanic contractions of the respiratory muscles, leading to respiratory arrest. An effect on the central respiratory center has been postulated but not proven.[5] Institution of cardiopulmonary resuscitation is critically important and should be performed even if prolonged arrest has occurred, because complete recovery in this situation has been documented.[13,14] The usual advanced cardiac life support measures should be followed. After resuscitation and transfer to a medical facility, all patients who have sustained loss of consciousness, cardiac arrest, arrhythmias, or ECG changes of acute myocardial infarction, or who have been subjected to a trans-chest current should undergo ECG monitoring. Nonspecific ECG changes have been seen in up to 50% of electrical injury victims.[15] Housinger and co-workers,[16] in a study of electrical injury victims, found CK-MB isoenzyme elevation in 56%, although technetium Tc 99m pyrophosphate scans and serial electrcardiograms showed no other evidence of myocardial infarction. Furthermore, although cases of well-documented myocardial infarction with acute electrical injury exist,[13,17,18] review of several large series since 1969 reveals this to be an uncommon event. Cardiac isoenzymes apparently do not reflect actual myocardial damage (the elevation of CK-MB has been soundly traced to skeletal muscle origin by the work of McBride and associates[17]). Late cardiac complications, including repetitive or hemodynamically significant arrhythmias, also appear to be uncommon. These are important points in that multiple surgical procedures are usually necessary in the electrically injured patient and should not be delayed on the basis of questionable cardiac findings, because these procedures appear to be well tolerated.[1,8,11,13,16,17]

Other cardiac findings include right bundle branch block[1] and transient global hypokinesis.[19]

RENAL

Little evidence supports the occurrence of direct renal injury from electric current. Instead, renal toxicity in electrical injury victims occurs as a result of volume depletion and shock, and most importantly from acute tubular necrosis secondary to pigmenturia. The source of these hemochromogens is primarily necrotic muscle and occasionally hemolysis. Aggressive fluid management is key in preventing this occasionally fatal complication. The cutaneous burns of the electrical victim are often minimal, leading to an underestimation of the deep tissue damage and associated third-space fluid loss. Traditional fluid formulas based on total-body surface area burns are of no value. Current fluid management techniques based on urine output seem to be successful in that the incidence of acute renal failure in recent series is close to zero[13] compared with a higher incidence in older series[1,15] and the current incidence reported in underdeveloped countries.[20] When acute renal failure occurs, it is associated with a high mortality rate.

Recommended management includes administering crystalloid solution to maintain a urine output of 50 to 100 mL/hour and monitoring the urine for myoglobin. If myoglobinuria occurs, a higher urine output of 100 to 150 mL/hour should be the goal of fluid replacement. Alkalization of the urine and the use of mannitol is also advocated. To reduce the filtered pigment load, many favor early extensive debridement of necrotic muscle and even the use of plasmapheresis.[13] If acute renal failure ensues, hemodialysis is preferred over peritoneal dialysis because of a high incidence of peritoneal complications.[15]

High-output renal failure also has been described in electrical injury.[3]

NERVOUS SYSTEM

Numerous neurologic sequelae have been described in victims of electrical injury and may take the form of cerebral, spinal cord, or peripheral nerve injury. Immediately after electrical exposure, up to 70% of victims experience loss of consciousness or transient paralysis[11] followed by recovery within 5 to 10 minutes. Confusion, agitation, headache, mood disturbance, and retrograde amnesia are common sequelae, whereas seizures and autonomic disturbances occur less often within the first several days.[12]

Aside from the medical treatment of seizures, these manifestations of electrical injury have limited impact on management. Persistent or late-onset coma is likely to be related to cerebral edema, closed-head trauma, or cerebral thrombosis and generally portends a poor prognosis.[21] A search for potentially reversible conditions with the use of CT scanning of the head seems to be reasonable. An aggressive approach to monitor and control intracranial pressure is advocated by some.[12]

Delayed neurologic complications occur unpredictably. They consist of partial or complete spinal cord transection, transverse myelitis, ascending paralysis, causalgia, amyotrophic lateral sclerosis, and spastic paraplegia. These events may occur many months after the initial injury and are poorly explained, often localizing neuroanatomically to areas distant from the site of electrical injury.[22,23]

In contrast to these phenomena are the commonly occurring peripheral nerve injuries that are directly associated with electrical injury and have important management implications. The mechanisms of injury include direct trauma from the flow of current and secondary compressive phenomena caused by the tourniquet effect of subfascial edema. Direct neural injury from current flow usually is limited to motor fibers and is readily reversible.[24] The neurologic injury resulting from compartment syndromes is variable, depending on the degree to which early surgical intervention relieves the heightened compartment pressures.[24] This emphasizes the need for detailed serial neurologic examinations and an aggressive surgical approach to save neurologically intact limbs.

The most commonly injured peripheral neural structures are the ulnar and median nerves.[24] Delayed nerve injury may occur because of scarring.[23]

MUSCULOSKELETAL AND CUTANEOUS INJURIES

Musculoskeletal and cutaneous injuries frequently dominate the clinical picture in these patients and may consist of

injuries not directly related to current flow. Examples include trauma as a result of the victim falling or being thrown by the current source, or injury as a result of the violent tetanic contractions frequently encountered in electrical injury. The end results may include long bone fractures, spinal fracture, joint dislocations, or splenic rupture. The frequency with which these events occur warrants a careful search for underlying traumatic injury by physical and radiographic examination. Unconscious victims should be treated with cervical immobilization until cervical fractures have been ruled out.[25] The direct tissue damage produced by electric current consists primarily of deep tissue coagulation necrosis. The goals of management are twofold. First, every attempt is made to salvage affected limbs. The second goal is to limit the systemic effects of necrotic muscle. The untoward effects of undebrided tissues include pyomyositis, sepsis, renal injury, and hypotension (several anecdotes attest to the reversal of hypotension after debridement of necrotic muscle, which is believed to be a result of the elimination of undefined "toxins"). Fortunately, both of these goals are realized simultaneously by the early exploratory surgery of affected limbs. Indications for early fasciotomy are a charred, mummified distal limb, a grossly swollen extremity, or evidence of a compartment syndrome.[8,13] In other patients, findings are much more subtle and are apparent only on close clinical follow-up. In that setting, marked elevation of serum CK enzyme levels should prompt further search for occult devitalized muscle.

Further studies that have been used to assess the extent of deep tissue injury are angiography (generally believed to be of little value), wick catheters (to monitor compartmental pressures), and ^{99m}Tc stannous pyrophosphate scans. Scanning with ^{99m}Tc has been used to identify occult necrotic muscle not apparent on surgical exploration. It is reliable enough to guide the level of amputation and to spare the patient surgery when results are negative.[22] The short half-life of the isotope also allows serial scanning to assess adequacy of debridement.[7] Others favor the use of serial exploration and frozen section muscle biopsy to assess tissue viability.[26] Early radical fasciotomy and debridement have allowed better salvage rates of functional limbs and a reduction in the systemic effects of electrical injuries.

The cutaneous sequelae of electrical injury vary from the focal, full-thickness burns at the entry and exit sites to more extensive flame burns. In general, burns in electrical victims average less than 20% of the total body surface area. At times, the extent of cutaneous injury may obscure underlying deep tissue damage. When this possibility exists, exploratory surgery of the involved limbs should be considered. The management of the cutaneous burns should follow standard therapies for thermal injuries.

GENERAL

Many of the published series reveal infections to be fairly common occurrences with sepsis, pyomyositis, wound cellulitis, and bronchopneumonia dominating. Treatment regimens including aggressive debridement of necrotic tissues, prophylaxis for *Clostridia* infection (with high-dose intravenous penicillin), and serial quantitative wound cultures (followed by appropriate antibiotics) have markedly reduced infectious complications in recent series of electrically injured patients.[10,13] When sepsis occurs in these patients, [99mTc] scanning may reveal an area of inadequately debrided muscle that may be the focus of infection.[7]

Overall, the mortality rate for victims of electrical injury is approximately 2%, usually attributed to closed-head trauma, infection, or acute renal failure. Late complications include vascular aneurysms with hemorrhage[3] and cataracts.[27]

PREVENTION

An estimated 1200 deaths occur annually in the United States from electrical injury; about 20% occur in children. These accidents fall into several unrelated epidemiologic patterns. Household electrical injuries account for 1% of all deaths occurring in the home and are usually related to appliances.[28] Additionally, over 4000 emergency room visits in the United States annually are related to appliance and extension cord injuries. Extension cords seem to be particularly dangerous to young children in whom mouth burns are common from sucking the female end of the cord.[29] Hopefully these injuries and fatalities might be prevented through better public awareness and passive devices such as ground–fault circuit interrupters or immersion detectors.[28]

Two distinct groups of patients are severely injured by high-voltage lines. One is a subset of adolescent men who are involved in mischievous activities when electrocution occurs.[26] The other major subset is occupationally related high-voltage injuries. These account for more than 90% of electrical injury victims in most series and are nearly always male utility company employees.[11,30] Although these injuries are often caused by fatigue, inattentiveness, or carelessness, immediate solutions to the problem do not seem apparent.

LIGHTNING INJURIES

The discussion of lightning strike injuries often includes aspects that are somewhat unusual if not mystical. Examples of this include descriptions of "glowing" victims or of complete recovery after prolonged cardiopulmonary arrest.

Approximately 150 to 300 fatalities and 1000 to 1500 serious lightning-related injuries occur each year in the United States. Up to 74% of these victims sustain significant permanent sequelae. Seventy percent of lightning strikes involve single victims, 15% involve two victims, and 15% involve three or more victims.[31] Almost all lightning strike victims survive if they do not sustain a cardiac or a respiratory arrest.[32] Dilated and fixed pupils do not mean that death has occurred.[33] Because of these observations, it is commonly recommended that triage priority be reversed and attention be given to the apparently "dead" victims rather than the wakeful but confused victims.

Lightning strike injury leads to paralysis of the respiratory centers that may outlast the return to normal cardiac electrical activity.[34] Because of this, it is important to administer aggressive cardiopulmonary resuscitation and continue to ventilate the patient for at least several hours or until the recovery of spontaneous respiration. Most victims develop spontaneous respiratory efforts within 30 minutes after a lightning-induced respiratory arrest, and the results of artificial respiration are good.[33]

The direct current of a lightning strike differs from the more common alternating current injury in several ways. The most common rhythm after lightning strike is asystole, unlike the propensity toward ventricular fibrillation seen in alternating-current victims. However, there have been numerous case reports of ventricular fibrillation in lightning victims. This may occur as a result of prolonged respiratory arrest and its attendant hypoxia and acidosis. Repetitive ventricular arrhythmias also may occur in lightning injury.[35] Myocardial necrosis has been well documented in lightning injury but seems to be uncommon.[36,37]

A unique occurrence in lightning injury is marked autonomic dysfunction. This includes labile hypertension and bronchospasm and findings of cyanotic, pulseless limbs that spontaneously revert to normal. This latter phenomena allows for a somewhat expectant approach to the cyanotic limb in lightning victims, with delay of any attempt at fasciotomy for several hours.[38] Table 103-3 lists the clinical manifestations of lightning injury.

Deep tissue necrosis and its complications occur distinctly less often in lightning injury victims, but should still be suspected during evaluation. The cutaneous burns often take unusual arborizing or spider-like configurations. These patterns reflect an external path of the direct current on the victim's skin[39] resulting in a "flash" burn. Cataracts are the most common ophthalmic injury noticed after lightning strike and can occur from a few days to many years after the event.[40] Corneal lesions, hyphema, iritis, vitreous hemorrhage, retinal detachment, and optic nerve injury have been reported.[41] More than half of victims are found to have ruptured tympanic membranes, and a temporary sensorineural hearing loss is common.[32,42]

Initially, the lightning strike victim should be handled as any trauma patient, following the ABCs and evaluating for cervical spine injury along with other potential secondary injuries. Aggressive cardiopulmonary resuscitation should be initiated as already mentioned. Volume resuscitation is not normally warranted because the victims seldom have sustained significant underlying tissue destruction as in electrical burns.[34] Overhydration can also exacerbate cerebral edema, which is commonly seen in lightning-related injuries.[31]

Once the patient arrives in an emergency room, the same guidelines as for all severely ill or injured patients should be followed. An electrocardiogram and radiographs of suspected injuries should be obtained. Hypotension should lead

TABLE 103-3. Manifestations of Lightning Injury

Prolonged cardiorespiratory arrest (asystole) followed by complete recovery
Repetitive ventricular arrhythmias
Myocardial necrosis
Autonomic dysfunction—labile hypertension, bronchospasm, spontaneous normalization of pulseless, cyanotic limbs
Arborizing, "spider-like" cutaneous burns
Deep tissue injury uncommon

to consideration of intraabdominal or intrathoracic hemorrhage as well as neurogenic shock from spinal cord injury. Burns may need local debridement, and a tetanus booster should be given. Mental status changes should be evaluated with CT scanning of the head to look for evidence of intracerebral hemorrhage or edema.

The most common abnormality after recovery of consciousness is paralysis. Most patients improve spontaneously within 24 hours after the injury. Some authors suggest that corticosteroids may help the recovery of electrically injured nerves and muscle. Whereas many of the abnormalities resolve, permanent deficits have been recorded.[33] Retrograde amnesia is common. Many peculiar psychological states occur that may reflect a psychological reaction to the injury. Reappearance of symptoms during a thunderstorm has been called *lightning psychorecidividism*.[43]

Because lightning is responsible for more fatalities than any other natural phenomenon, the general public must be educated as to how to avoid a lightning strike.[44] Stay indoors during an electrical storm. A closed automobile offers protection to those who are inside and not in contact with metal surfaces. Leaning on the outside of a car can be especially hazardous. The rubber tires of a car offer no particular protection. If caught in an open field, avoid tall trees, hilltops, and telephone poles. It is best to find the most depressed area of ground and curl up with hands close together or squat down with feet together to decrease contact points. If outdoors, discard all metal objects such as rifles, golf clubs, hearing aids, and jewelry. The use of a telephone should be avoided during an electrical storm.[33]

The key to management of the lightning strike victim is prolonged cardiopulmonary resuscitation. After thorough evaluation for secondary injuries, good supportive care generally leads to a good prognosis.

REFERENCES ■

1. Divincenti FC, Moncrief JA, Pruitt BA: Electrical injuries: a review of 65 cases. *J Trauma* 1969;9:497
2. Artz CP: Changing concepts of electrical injury. *Am J Surg* 1974;128:600
3. Dixon GR: The evaluation and management of electrical injuries. *Crit Care Med* 1983;11:384
4. Craig SR: When lightning strikes. *Postgrad Med* 1986;79:109
5. Sances A, Larson SJ, Myklebast J, et al: Electrical injuries. *Surg Gynecol Obstet* 1979;149:97
6. Davies DM: Burns. *Br Med J* 1985;290:989
7. Hunt J, Lewis S, Parkey R, et al: The use of technetium-99m stannous pyrophosphate scintigraphy to identify muscle damage in acute electric burns. *J Trauma* 1979;19:409
8. Parshley PF: Aggressive approach to the extremity damaged by electric current. *Am J Surg* 1985;150:78
9. Hunt JL, Mason AD, Masterson TS, et al: The pathophysiology of acute electrical injuries. *J Trauma* 1976;16:335
10. Solem L, Fischer RP, Strate RG: The natural history of electrical injury. *J Trauma* 1977;17:487
11. Butler ED, Gant TD: Electrical injuries with special reference to the upper extremities. *Am J Surg* 1977;134:95
12. Thompson JC, Ashwal S: Electrical injuries in children. *Am J Dis Child* 1983;137:231
13. Holliman CJ, Saffle JR, Kravitz M, et al: Early surgical decompression in the management of electrical injuries. *Am J Surg* 1982;144:733
14. Taussig HB: "Death" from lightning—and the possibility of living again. *Ann Intern Med* 1968;68:1345
15. Hartford CE, Ziffren SE: Electrical injury. *J Trauma* 1971; 11:331
16. Housinger TA, Green L, Shahangian S, et al: A prospective study of myocardial damage in electrical injuries. *J Trauma* 1985;25:122
17. McBride JW, Labrosse KR, McCoy HG, et al: Is serum creatinine kinase-MB in electrically injured patients predictive of myocardial injury? *JAMA* 1986;255:764
18. Purdue GF, Hunt JL: Electrocardiographic monitoring after electrical injury: necessity or luxury. *J Trauma* 1986;26:166
19. Lewin RF, Arditti A, Sclarovsky S: Non-invasive evaluation of electrical cardiac injury. *Br Heart J* 1983;49:190
20. Haberal M: Electrical burns: a 5-year experience: 1985 Evans Lecture. *J Trauma* 1986;26:103
21. Skoog T: Electrical injuries. *J Trauma* 1970;10:816
22. Hunt JL, Sato RM, Baxter CR: Acute electrical burns. *Arch Surg* 1980;115:434
23. Farrell DF, Staff A: Delayed neurological sequelae of electrical injuries. *Neurology* 1968;18:601
24. Salisbury RE, Dingeldein GP: Peripheral nerve complications following burn injury. *Clin Orthoped Rel Res* 1982;163:92
25. Saffle JR, Schnelby A, Hofmann A, et al: The management of fractures in thermally injured patients. *J Trauma* 1983;23:902
26. Burke JF, Quinby WC, Bondoc C, et al: Patterns of high tension electrical injury in children and adolescents and their management. *Am J Surg* 1977;133:492
27. Saffle JR, Crandall A, Warden GD: Cataracts: A long-term complication of electrical injury. *J Trauma* 1985;25:17
28. Budnick LD: Bathtub-related electrocutions in the United States, 1979–1982. *JAMA* 1984;252:918
29. McLoughlin E, Crawford JD: Burns. *Pediatr Clin North Am* 1984;32:61
30. Rouse RG, Dimick AR: The treatment of electrical injury compared to burn injury: a review of pathophysiology and comparison of patient management protocols. *J Trauma* 1978;18:43
31. Cooper MA: Lightning injuries. In: Auerbach PS, Geehr EC (eds). *Management of Wilderness and Environmental Emergencies*, ed 2. St Louis, CV Mosby, 1989:173
32. Cooper MA: Lightning injuries: prognostic signs for death. *Ann Emerg Med* 1980;9:134
33. Patten BM: Lightning and electrical Injuries. *Neurol Clin* 1992;10(4).
34. Fontanorosa PB: *Ann Emerg Med* 1993;22:378
35. Kotagal S, Rawlings CA, Chen S, et al: Neurologic, psychiatric, and cardiovascular complications in children struck by lightning. *Pediatrics* 1982;70:190
36. Kleiner JP, Wilkin JH: Cardiac effects of lightning stroke. *JAMA* 1978;240:2757
37. Jackson SHD, Parry DJ: Lightning and the heart. *Br Heart J* 1980;43:454
38. Peters WJ: Lightning injury. *Can Med Assoc J* 1983;128:148
39. Amy BW, McManus WF, Goodwin CW, et al: Lightning injury with survival in five patients. *JAMA* 1985;253:243
40. Strasser EJ, Davis RM, Menchey MJ: Lightning injuries. *J Trauma* 1977;17:315
41. Casten JA, Kytilia J: Eye symptoms caused by lightning. *Acta Opthalmol* 1963;41:139
42. Ghezzi KT: Lightning injuries. *PGM* 1989;86:197
43. Critchley M: Neurological effects of lightning and of electricity. *Lancet* 1934;i:68
44. Weigel E: Lightning: the underrated killer. *NOAA* 1986;16:2

Critical Care, Third Edition, edited by Joseph M. Civetta,
Robert W. Taylor, and Robert R. Kirby.
Lippincott-Raven Publishers, Philadelphia, PA © 1997.

CHAPTER 104

∎

Anaphylaxis

Stewart J. Levine
R. Dwaine Rieves
James H. Shelhamer

IMMEDIATE CONCERNS ∎

MAJOR PROBLEMS

Anaphylactic and anaphylactoid reactions represent acute
medical emergencies requiring rapid recognition and effective intervention to prevent potentially life-threatening sequelae. Activation of mast cell and basophil populations by
either IgE-dependent (i.e., anaphylactic reactions) or IgE-
independent (i.e., anaphylactoid reactions) mechanisms results in the release of multiple mediators capable of altering
vascular permeability, vascular and bronchial smooth muscle
tone, as well as recruiting and activating inflammatory cell
cascades. Initial sequelae, which may occur within seconds
or as much as 1 hour after exposure to an inciting stimulus,
include tachycardia, flushing, pruritus, faintness, and a sensation of impending doom. Dermatologic (i.e., urticaria and
angioedema) and gastrointestinal (i.e., abdominal distension,
nausea, emesis, and diarrhea) manifestations are common.
Involvement of the cardiovascular and respiratory systems
may result in potentially life-threatening manifestations,
such as cardiovascular collapse caused by vasodilation and
capillary leak, myocardial depression, myocardial ischemia
and infarction, and atrial fibrillation, as well as upper airway
obstruction, bronchospasm, intraalveolar hemorrhage, and
noncardiogenic, high-permeability pulmonary edema. Without prompt recognition and effective intervention, the manifestations of anaphylactic and anaphylactoid reactions can
be fatal.

STRESS POINTS

1. Anaphylactic reactions represent type I immune responses mediated by IgE bound to mast cells or basophils. Common inciting agents include β-lactam antibiotics and Hymenoptera stings. Other common
   causes include other antibiotics, local anesthetics, serum products, and foods.
2. Anaphylactoid reactions represent IgE-independent
   activation of mast cells or basophils with resultant degranulation and mediator release. Common inciting
   agents include iodinated radiocontrast media, neuromuscular depolarizing agents, and opiates, all of which
   induce direct mast cell activation; nonsteroidal antiinflammatory agents acting through cyclooxygenase inhibition; and blood products acting through complement activation.
3. The differential diagnosis of anaphylactic and anaphylactoid reactions includes cardiac arrhythmias, myocardial infarction, distributive or hypovolemic shock,
   vasovagal syncope, asthma, pulmonary embolism, upper airway obstruction secondary to a foreign body,
   hypoglycemia, carcinoid syndrome, systemic mastocytosis, and hereditary angioedema.
4. Epinephrine is the initial drug of choice for the management of anaphylactic or anaphylactoid reactions. H_1
   and H_2 blocking agents also should be administered.
   Corticosteroids are not effective for the acute management of anaphylactic or anaphylactoid reactions, but

may prevent biphasic anaphylaxis or attenuate prolonged reactions.

INITIAL THERAPY

1. Remove the inciting agent (i.e., remove Hymenoptera stinger) and follow with a local epinephrine injection and proximal tourniquet placement; discontinue intravenous medication; consider gastric lavage and administration of activated charcoal if the inciting agent was ingested.
2. Administer epinephrine. For mild to moderate reactions, give 0.3 mL of a 1:1000 solution subcutaneously and repeat every 15 minutes as needed; for severe life-threatening reactions, give 3 mL of a 1:10,000 solution intravenously (IV) in an adult or 0.01 to 0.05 mL/kg of a 1:10,000 epinephrine solution to a child (this also may be administered through an endotracheal tube: 3 to 5 mL of a 1:10,000 solution to an adult).
3. Establish intravenous access for hydration and provide supplemental oxygen.
4. Administer histamine antagonists to block vasodilation, capillary leak, and shock (H_1 blockade, 50 mg of diphenhydramine IV; H_2 blockade, 50 mg of ranitidine IV).
5. Administer vasopressors for persistent hypotension (epinephrine, 0.1 µg/kg/minute; dopamine, 5 µg/kg/minute; or norepinephrine [Levophed], 2 to 3 µg/minute and titrate to mean arterial pressure of 60 mm Hg).
6. Establish and maintain upper airway patency. Consider a trial of nebulized racemic epinephrine (0.3 mL in 3 mL normal saline). If airway obstruction is imminent, perform endotracheal intubation or, if unsuccessful, consider needle-catheter cricothyroid ventilation, cricothyrotomy, or tracheostomy.
7. Administer inhaled β_2-agonists for bronchospasm. Consider addition of aminophylline as second-line therapy.
8. Consider corticosteroid therapy for prolonged anaphylaxis or to prevent biphasic anaphylaxis (100 to 250 mg of hydrocortisone IV every 6 hours). Corticosteroids are not effective therapy for the acute manifestations of anaphylactic or anaphylactoid reactions.
9. Consider glucagon administration (1 to 5 mg IV over 1 minute, then 1 to 5 mg/hour in a continuous infusion) in the setting of prior beta-blockade because of its positive inotropic and chronotropic effects mediated by a beta-receptor–independent mechanism.
10. Prevent recurrent episodes by avoidance of the inciting agent, desensitization, or premedication with corticosteroids and H_1 and H_2 blockade. For prophylaxis of radiocontrast reactions, use low-osmolar radiocontrast media and premedicate with corticosteroids and H_1 antagonists. Ephedrine also may be useful in this setting if not contraindicated (i.e., in patients with cardiac disease, hypertension, hyperthyroidism, or advanced age).

CLINICAL MANIFESTATIONS

The clinical syndromes associated with systemic anaphylactic and anaphylactoid reactions represent potential acute medical emergencies because they are associated with a rapid, critical destabilization of the cardiovascular and respiratory systems. These syndromes, which are clinically indistinguishable, may be rapidly fatal if appropriate therapy is not instituted immediately. Initial symptoms, which can appear within seconds to minutes but may be delayed by as much as 1 hour after exposure to an inciting agent, are often nonspecific.[1] These symptoms include tachycardia, faintness, cutaneous flushing, diffuse or palmar pruritus, and a sensation of impending doom.[2,3] Subsequent manifestations indicate involvement of the cutaneous, gastrointestinal, respiratory, and cardiovascular systems (Table 104-1). Common dermatologic manifestations include urticaria and angioedema, whereas abdominal distention, nausea, emesis, and diarrhea suggest involvement of the gastrointestinal system.

It is the involvement of the cardiovascular and respiratory systems, however, that is responsible for the fatal complications of anaphylactic and anaphylactoid reactions. A sensation of a "lump in the throat," hoarseness, dysphonia, or dyspnea may precede acute upper airway obstruction secondary to laryngeal edema. Other pulmonary manifestations include acute bronchospasm, intraalveolar pulmonary hemorrhage, bronchorrhea, and a noncardiogenic, high-permeability–type pulmonary edema.[4,5] Tachycardia and syncope may precede the development of hypotension and frank cardiovascular collapse.[6,7] Anaphylactic shock occurs as a consequence of diminished venous return secondary to systemic vasodilation and intravascular volume contraction caused by capillary leak. Although transient increases in cardiac output may occur at the onset of anaphylaxis, hemodynamic parameters later reveal decreases in cardiac output, systemic vascular resistance, stroke volume, and pulmonary artery occlusion and central venous pressures.[7-12] In addition, the acute onset of a lactic acidosis and diminished oxygen consumption have been noticed after an anaphylactoid reaction.[13]

Other potentially serious cardiovascular manifestations are myocardial ischemia and acute myocardial infarction, atrioventricular and intraventricular conduction abnormalities (prolonged PR interval, transient left bundle branch block), and supraventricular arrhythmias (atrial fibrillation).[1] Severe but reversible myocardial depression also has been reported.[6] Hematologic manifestations, such as disseminated intravascular coagulation and hemoconcentration secondary to volume contraction, also may complicate anaphylactic and anaphylactoid reactions.[3]

The diagnosis of systemic anaphylactic and anaphylactoid reactions are mostly established on the basis of clinical grounds alone because expedient institution of appropriate therapy is mandatory. These diagnoses should be considered when typical multisystem manifestations (flushing, urticaria, pruritus, angioedema, hypotension, acute upper airway obstruction, bronchospasm) occur in a direct temporal relationship with exposure to an inciting agent. Laboratory tests, such as the presence of elevated serum mast cell tryptase

TABLE 104-1. Clinical Manifestations of Anaphylactic and Anaphylactoid Reactions

SYSTEM	SYMPTOM	SIGN/CLINICAL MANIFESTATION
RESPIRATORY		
Upper	Dyspnea, dysphonia, hoarseness, cough, lump in throat	Upper airway obstruction caused by laryngeal edema and spasm, bronchorrhea
Lower	Dyspnea, cyanosis	Noncardiogenic pulmonary edema, bronchospasm, acute hyperinflation, alveolar hemorrhage
CARDIOVASCULAR	Palpitations, faintness, weakness	Shock, tachycardia, capillary leak, syncope, supraventricular arrhythmias, conduction disturbances, myocardial ischemia and infarction
CUTANEOUS	Flushing, pruritus	Urticaria, angioedema, diaphoresis
GASTROINTESTINAL	Abdominal pain, bloating, cramps, nausea	Emesis, diarrhea, hepatosplenic congestion; rarely hematemesis and bloody diarrhea
NEUROLOGIC	Dizziness, disorientation, hallucinations, headache, feeling of impending doom	Syncope, lethargy, seizures
OCULAR	Conjunctival pruritus	Conjunctival suffusion, lacrimation
NASAL	Pruritus, sneezing	Rhinorrhea, nasal congestion
HEMATOLOGIC		Hemoconcentration, DIC

DIC, disseminated intravascular coagulation.
Modified from Kaliner M: Anaphylaxis. *NER Allergy Proc* 1984;5:324.

levels, may be useful in confirming the clinical diagnosis retrospectively.[14] Because of the multisystem nature of anaphylactic and anaphylactoid reactions, the list of differential diagnoses that must be considered is extensive. Diagnostic possibilities include cardiac arrhythmias, myocardial infarction, distributive or hypovolemic shock, vasovagal syncope, asthma, pulmonary embolism, upper airway obstruction secondary to ingestion of a foreign body, hypoglycemia, and the carcinoid syndrome.[2,15,16] Clinical signs suggesting one of these alternative diagnoses include pallor, bradycardia, and normal sinus rhythm (which are more suggestive of a primary arrhythmia, conduction disturbance, or vasovagal syncope), as well as the absence of pruritus, urticaria, and angioedema.[2] Other disorders that should be included in the differential diagnosis include systemic mastocytosis, which rarely causes acute systemic manifestations identical to those of anaphylactic reactions, and hereditary angioedema, which should be suspected when laryngeal edema is present in the absence of hypotension, asthma, urticaria, and flushing.[2]

The clinical manifestations of systemic anaphylactic and anaphylactoid reactions represent the sequelae of the sudden release of numerous activated mediators from tissue mast cells and circulating basophils. Iodinated radiocontrast media, β-lactam antibiotics, and Hymenoptera stings represent the most common etiologic agents responsible for anaphylactic and anaphylactoid reactions (Table 104-2). True anaphylactic reactions are classified as type I immune responses, in which an inciting antigen to which the person has previously been sensitized enters the body (commonly through the skin, lungs, or gastrointestinal tract) and interacts with IgE that is bound to mast cells or basophils, thereby causing release of preformed, as well as newly synthesized, mediators.[10] A list of antigens commonly associated with anaphylactic reactions is presented in Table 104-3. Furthermore, drugs that are routinely used in the intensive care unit (ICU) that can precipitate anaphylactic reactions include the following: propofol (although a nonspecific histamine-releasing effect also has been postulated); aprotinin-con-

TABLE 104-2.   Frequency of Anaphylactic Events and Deaths

AGENT	FREQUENCY OF EVENTS		DEATHS/y (U.S.)
	Mild (%)	*Severe (%)*	
Penicillin	0.5–1	0.04	400–800
Hymenoptera	0.5	0.05	≥100
Contrast media	5	0.10	250–1000

Kaliner M: Anaphylaxis. *NER Allergy Proc* 1984;5:324.

taining topical fibrin glue; and latex, which is found in gloves, intravenous tubing, barium enema balloons, bladder catheterization catheters, and ventriculoperitoneal shunts.[17–19] In addition, IgE-mediated anaphylaxis is an infrequent sequelae of thrombolytic therapy with streptokinase and anisoylated plasminogen streptokinase activator complex, occurring in 0.1% to 0.4% of cases, respectively.[20,21]

In contrast, anaphylactoid reactions occur as a result of an IgE-independent reaction between a causative agent and the mast cell or basophil, which results in degranulation and release of mediators. Anaphylactoid reactions are precipitated by several different mechanisms, including the follow-ing: direct mast cell degranulating agents (radiocontrast media, opiates, muscle depolarizing agents); complement-mediated reactions (immune complex formation secondary to transfusion of IgA-positive blood products to an IgA-deficient recipient with IgG anti-IgA antibodies); nonsteroidal antiinflammatory agents (which block the cyclooxygenase pathway and thereby favor conversion of arachidonic acid into lipoxygenase mediators); and unclassified mechanisms (exercise-induced and idiopathic recurrent anaphylaxis)[1,2] (Table 104-4). Notice that direct mast cell degranulating agents, such as iodinated radiocontrast agents, produce anaphylactoid reactions in up to 10% of persons.[1] In addition, anaphylactoid reactions occur in up to 35% of persons with prior reactions to iodinated radiocontrast agents on reexposure to these agents.

MANAGEMENT

The clinician must have a high index of suspicion for anaphylactic and anaphylactoid reactions because they require a prompt clinical diagnosis and a rapid therapeutic response. Because anaphylactic and anaphylactoid reactions both represent sequelae of mast cell and basophil degranulation, the therapeutic approaches to these disorders are identical.

TABLE 104-3.   Etiologic Agents for Anaphylaxis (IgE Mediated)

HAPTENS

   β-lactam antibiotics
   Sulfonamides
   Nitrofurantoin
   Demethylchlorotetracycline
   Streptomycin
   Vancomycin
   Local anesthetics
   Others

SERUM PRODUCTS

   γ-Globulin
   Immunotherapy for allergic diseases
   Heterologous serum

FOODS

   Nuts
   Shellfish
   Buckwheat
   Egg white
   Cottonseed
   Milk
   Corn
   Potato
   Rice
   Legumes
   Citrus fruits
   Chocolate
   Others

VENOM

   Stinging insects, particularly
      Hymenoptera, fire ants

HORMONES

   Insulin
   Adrenocorticotropic hormone
   Thyroid-stimulating hormone

ENZYMES

   Chymopapain
   L-Asparaginase

MISCELLANEOUS

   Seminal fluid
   Others

Modified from Austen KF: Systemic anaphylaxis in man. *JAMA* 1965;192:108; and Kaliner M: Anaphylaxis. *NER Allergy Proc* 1984;5:324.

TABLE 104-4.   Etiologic Agents for Anaphylactoid Reactions

COMPLEMENT-MEDIATED REACTIONS	ARACHIDONIC ACID MODULATORS
Blood	Nonsteroidal antiinflammatory drugs
Serum	Tartrazine (possible)
Plasma	
Plasmate (but not albumin)	IDIOPATHIC
Immunoglobins	Most common conclusion after thorough evaluation
NONIMMUNOLOGIC MAST CELL ACTIVATORS	UNKNOWN
Opiates and narcotics	Sulfites
Radiocontrast media	Others
Dextrans	
Neuromuscular blocking agents	THERMOREGULATORY MECHANISM
Others	Exercise

Adapted from Kaliner M: Anaphylaxis. *NER Allergy Proc* 1984;5:324.

Therapeutic interventions are divided into three main categories: (1) emergency basic life-support measures, (2) specific therapy directed at ameliorating the acute physiologic effects of mast cell–derived mediators, and (3) identification and removal of the inciting agent. Because of the potentially life-threatening nature of the complications of anaphylactic and anaphylactoid reactions, all three major therapeutic interventions must be instituted simultaneously (Table 104-5).

Initial attention should be given to assessment and stabilization of the pulmonary and cardiovascular manifestations of anaphylaxis, because these are the major causes of death. Epinephrine is the mainstay of initial management and

TABLE 104-5.   Acute Management of Anaphylactic and Anaphylactoid Reactions

1. Discontinue infusion of possible offending agents, remove Hymenoptera stingers, inject epinephrine (0.1–0.2 mL of a 1:1000 solution) SC or IM at site of anaphylatoxin and place tourniquet proximal to site to interrupt venous blood flow.
2. Epinephrine: In mild to moderate anaphylaxis, administer 0.3 mL of a 1:1000 solution subcutaneously; may repeat at 15-min intervals as needed. In severe anaphylaxis, administer up to 3 mL of a 1:10,000 solution IV to an adult (less if potential cardiac toxicity is a concern) or 0.01–0.05 mL/kg to a child. If intravenous access is not available, may administer 3–5 mL of a 1:10,000 solution through an endotracheal tube to an adult.
3. Establish intravenous access, provide supplemental oxygen; place patient in Trendelenburg position if hypotensive.
4. Antihistamines: H₁ blockade—diphenhydramine 50 mg IM or IV
                      H₂ blockade—ranitidine 50 mg IV
5. Institute fluid resuscitation with colloid or crystalloid for hypotension. If hypotension persists after fluid resuscitation, administer either epinephrine 0.1 μg/kg/min, dopamine 5 μg/kg/min or L-norepinephrine 2 to 3 μg/min IV and titrate to mean arterial pressure of 60 mm Hg. Consider glucagon administration (1–5 mg IV over 1 min, followed by 1–5 mg/h by continuous infusion) if patient had previously received beta-antagonist medications. May also consider naloxone and MAST if hypotension persists.
6. Maintain airway patency. Administer racemic epinephrine nebulizer (0.3 mL in 3 mL of saline) for evidence of upper airway obstruction. If upper airway obstruction prevents adequate ventilation, perform orotracheal intubation. If orotracheal intubation is unsuccessful, perform needle catheter transcricothyroid ventilation, cricothyrotomy, or tracheostomy.
7. Treat bronchospasm. Administer epinephrine (see step 3), H₁ antihistamines (see step 4), and selective β₂-agonists (albuterol 2.5 mg (0.5 ml of a 0.5% solution) in 3 mL saline through a nebulizer). Aminophylline (5 mg/kg loading dose over 30 min IV, followed by infusion of 0.3 to 0.9 mg/kg/h) may be administered as second-line therapy.
8. Hydrocortisone 100 to 250 mg IV every 6 h to prevent biphasic anaphylaxis and for therapy of prolonged anaphylactic reactions.
9. Transfer patient to ICU for observation with continuous electrocardiography, pulse oximetry, and, if required, arterial and pulmonary arterial catheter placement.

SC, subcutaneously; IM, intramuscularly; IV, intravenously; ICU, intensive care unit; MAST, military antishock trousers.

should be immediately administered subcutaneously at a dose of 0.3 to 0.5 mL of a 1:1000 solution. Doses may be repeated at 5- to 10-minute intervals as needed. Epinephrine decreases mediator synthesis and release by increasing intracellular concentrations of cAMP and antagonizes many of the adverse actions of the mediators of anaphylaxis.[2,10,22] In cases of severe laryngospasm or frank cardiovascular collapse, or when there is an inadequate response to subcutaneous epinephrine administration, up to 3 to 5 mL of a 1:10,000 epinephrine solution may be given IV to an adult (less if potential cardiac toxicity is a concern) or 0.01 to 0.05 mL/kg of a 1:10,000 epinephrine solution may be given IV to a child.[23]

When epinephrine is administered IV, the clinician should be aware of the potential adverse consequences of severe tachycardia, myocardial ischemia, hypertension, severe vasospasm, and gangrene (when infused by peripheral venous access).[24] If intravascular access cannot be immediately established, then 0.5 mL of a 1:1000 solution may be administered intramuscularly or 3 to 5 mL of a 1:10,000 solution may be instilled into the airways using an endotracheal tube.

Initial assessment and management of patients with anaphylactic or anaphylactoid reactions should focus on the potential for cardiovascular collapse and shock, which is largely mediated by the systemic release of histamine from mast cells and basophils. Blood pressure measurements should be obtained frequently, and an indwelling arterial catheter should be inserted in cases of moderate to severe anaphylaxis. Both H_1 and H_2 antagonists are required to reverse these manifestations.[25] Diphenhydramine hydrochloride (25 to 50 mg IV or intramuscularly) and ranitidine (50 mg IV over 5 minutes) are commonly used in this setting. If intravenous cimetidine is administered IV, it must be given slowly because of its potential to cause hypotension or asystole.[24,26] If hypotension persists despite administration of epinephrine and H_1 and H_2 blockers, aggressive volume resuscitation should be instituted.

Admission to the ICU is warranted for invasive monitoring with arterial and pulmonary artery catheters, electrocardiography, pulse oximetry, and frequent arterial blood gas measurements. If hypotension persists despite aggressive volume resuscitation, vasopressor therapy with continuous infusions of epinephrine (0.1 μg/kg/minute), dopamine (5 μg/kg/minute), or L-norepinephrine (2 to 3 μg/minute) should be instituted and titrated to a mean arterial pressure of 60 mm Hg. Several reports suggest that in cases of anaphylactic shock resistant to vasopressor therapy, the use of naloxone and military antishock trousers may be helpful.[1,27]

If impending upper airway obstruction secondary to laryngeal edema is suspected, racemic epinephrine (0.3 mL in 3 mL of saline through a nebulizer) should be administered in addition to systemic epinephrine. Use of selective beta-agonists is not recommended in this setting because vasodilation may worsen the severity of the laryngeal edema.[24] Supplemental oxygen should be supplied, and the physician should be prepared to maintain a patent airway if progressive laryngeal edema occurs. Orotracheal intubation may be attempted if the airway obstruction compromises effective ventilation despite pharmacologic intervention; however, attempts may be unsuccessful if laryngeal edema is severe. If

endotracheal intubation is unsuccessful, then either needle-catheter cricothyroid ventilation (Fig. 104-1), cricothyrotomy, or surgical tracheostomy is required to maintain an adequate airway. Commercial kits are available that contain all of the equipment required for establishing an airway after puncture of the cricothyroid membrane by an angiocatheter. A guidewire is then passed into the trachea and an airway is established after successive dilatations with over-the-wire catheters. Clinicians must be familiar with at least one of these techniques in the event that endotracheal intubation cannot be accomplished.

In addition to laryngeal edema, the airway may be compromised by bronchospasm and bronchorrhea during anaphylaxis. Therapy should consist of supplemental oxygen, epinephrine administration, H_1 antagonists, and inhaled β_2-adrenergic agonists and aminophylline (listed in order of administration). In case of severe bronchospasm, the patient should be observed in the ICU where continuous pulse oximetry and frequent arterial blood gas measurements can be obtained by an indwelling arterial catheter.

An emergent evaluation for the inciting etiologic agent must accompany initial therapeutic interventions. After the etiologic agent is identified, the clinician should attempt to prevent further access to the circulation or to limit further absorption. Infusions of possible etiologic agents should be stopped and the contents saved for analysis. If a Hymenoptera sting is responsible, the stinger should be removed. Small amounts of local epinephrine (0.1 to 0.2 mL of a 1:1000 solution) should be injected next to a subcutaneous or intramuscular injection site that is dispersing the inciting agent. A tourniquet also should be placed proximal to the injection site and pressure applied to occlude venous return. After successful pharmacologic therapy, the tourniquet may be cautiously removed and the patient carefully observed for recurrent adverse sequelae. In cases in which the offending agent was ingested, consideration may be given to insertion of a nasogastric tube to perform gastric lavage and gastric instillation of activated charcoal.

After initial successful therapy for anaphylactic or anaphylactoid reactions, continued observation for at least 24 hours in a monitored setting for recurrent manifestations is prudent. Biphasic anaphylaxis occurs in 25% of patients in whom potentially life-threatening manifestations may recur after an asymptomatic period of up to 8 hours following an initially successful therapy.[15] Although corticosteroids have no immediate effect on the signs and symptoms of anaphylaxis, they can be used to prevent the late manifestations of biphasic anaphylaxis. The usual dose is 100 to 250 mg of hydrocortisone IV every 6 hours.[11]

The management of anaphylaxis in a patient receiving beta-antagonist medications represents a special circumstance in which the manifestations of anaphylaxis may be exceptionally severe.[28] Beta-blockade increases mediator synthesis and release, as well as end-organ sensitivity. In addition, beta-blockade antagonizes the beneficial beta-mediated effects of epinephrine therapy, thereby resulting in unopposed alpha-adrenergic and reflex vagotonic effects (vasoconstriction, bronchoconstriction, bradycardia). Therapy of anaphylaxis occurring in patients receiving beta-antagonist drugs, however, is similar to that of other patients. In addition, atropine may be useful for heart block and refractory

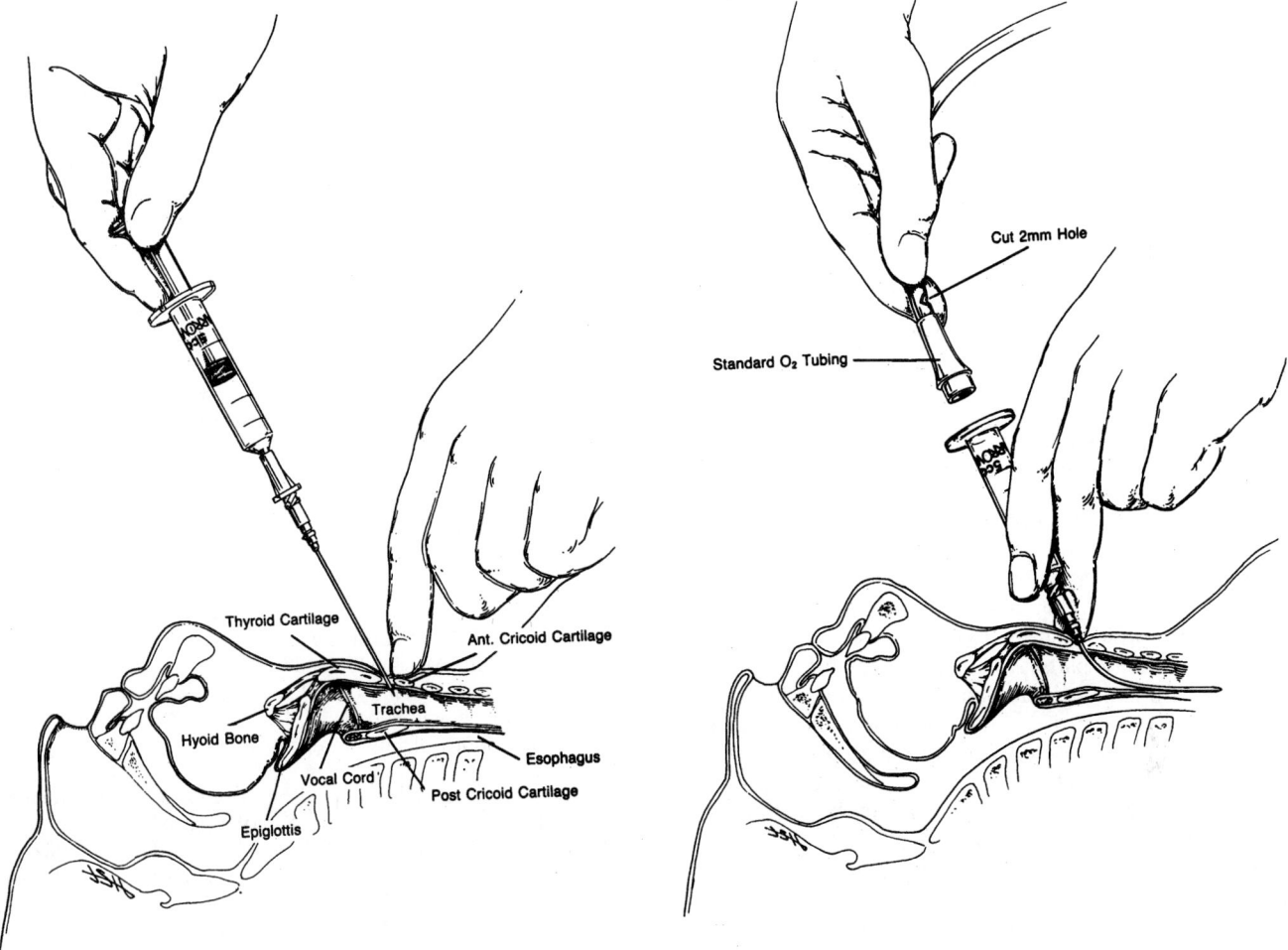

FIGURE 104-1. Needle catheter transcricothyroid ventilation. The trachea is cannulated between the thyroid cartilage and the cricoid ring, the needle is withdrawn, placement is confirmed by withdrawing air through the catheter, and a syringe barrel-oxygen tubing assembly is inserted into the catheter hub. Oxygen is administered at rate of at least 15 L/minute and the lungs are insufflated by briefly occluding the hole in the oxygen tubing. Exhalation occurs through the larynx, which is obstructed to inspiration. This procedure is a temporizing measure that must be emergently followed by incisional cricothyrotomy or tracheostomy.

bronchospasm, whereas glucagon (which increases cAMP levels through a beta-receptor–independent mechanism) has been reported to reverse the cardiovascular manifestations of anaphylaxis in patients receiving beta-antagonists.[28,29] Glucagon can be administered as a 1- to 5-mg intravenous infusion over 1 minute, followed by a continuous infusion at 1 to 5 mg/hour.[30] Furthermore, these patients may require extended periods of observation because of the long duration of action of many beta-antagonist medications.

PREVENTION ■

The ideal method of managing severe, systemic anaphylactic and anaphylactoid reactions is by preventing their occurrence. Persons with a known sensitivity should avoid reexposure to inciting etiologic agents. In addition, administration of beta-antagonist medications should be avoided.

For patients who must be reexposed to antigens that have caused reactions previously, desensitization can be instituted using standard regimens.[2] Those who are at risk for for shock from Hymenoptera stings should carry an emergency kit containing epinephrine in a spring-loaded syringe that facilitates self-administration, as well as a rapidly absorbed antihistamine. Patients with a history of adverse reactions to intravenous radiocontrast material should receive prophylaxis before repeat exposure. Pretreatment regimens must contain corticosteroids, which may be given as oral prednisone, 50 mg every 6 hours for 24 hours before administration of radiocontrast media.[24,31,32] Adjunctive therapy with H_1 antihistamines (diphenhydramine, 50 mg every 6 hours by mouth) is also recommended.[24,31,33] Although combination H_1 and H_2 antihistamine therapy has been reported to prevent the cardiopulmonary response to histamine and decrease the frequency of urticaria, angioedema, and respiratory symptoms after administration of radiocontrast media,[14,31] a prior prospective study has found that the addition of cimetidine to a pretreatment regimen of prednisone, diphenhydramine, and ephedrine was associated with an increased incidence of cutaneous reactions to radiocontrast media.[34]

The addition of ephedrine to corticosteroids and H_1 antihistamines has been shown to further decrease the frequency of radiocontrast media reactions; however, it should be used cautiously in patients with heart disease, hypertension, or hyperthyroidism, as well as in the elderly.[31,34,35] In addition, the use of low-osmolar radiocontrast media has been associated with one third to one fourth the incidence of serious reactions compared with reactions seen with higher osmolar contrast media.[36]

PATHOGENESIS ■

The systemic manifestations of anaphylactic and anaphylactoid reactions represent sequelae that result from release of inflammatory mediators by mast cells and basophils by IgE-dependent or IgE-independent mechanisms. Release of histamine from preformed mast cell granules seems to be the principal primary pathophysiologic mediator, resulting in systemic vasodilation, increased vascular permeability, bronchoconstriction, pruritus, and increased mucus production.[10,22,37] Other preformed mediators include eosinophil and neutrophil chemotactic factors and mast cell proteases, which may increase vascular permeability by degrading the blood vessel basement membrane.[37]

Other important mediators of anaphylaxis are generated by the metabolism of membrane phospholipids after the activation of quiescent mast cells and basophils.[37] Activation of the 5-lipoxygenase pathway results in synthesis of leukotrienes, including leukotrienes C4, D4, and E4 (formerly termed the slow-reacting substance of anaphylaxis), as well as LTB4. Leukotrienes C4, D4, and E4, along with the intermediary products 5-hydroxyeicosatetraenoic acid and 5-hydroperoxyeicosatetraenoic, elicit increases in vascular permeability and bronchoconstriction, whereas leukotriene B4 possesses eosinophil and neutrophil chemotactic properties.[10,37] Activation of the cyclooxygenase pathway leads to the production of prostaglandin D_2, which produces bronchoconstriction. Platelet-activating factor is also newly synthesized by activated mast cells and can result in bronchoconstriction, increased vascular permeability, platelet aggregation, and neutrophil chemotaxis.[22,37] These primary mediators then facilitate the production of a diverse number of secondary mediators by platelets, neutrophils, eosinophils, and other cells with resultant activation of the complement, coagulation, and fibrinolytic pathways.[10]

IMPLICATIONS AND OUTCOME ■

Anaphylactic and anaphylactoid reactions represent important potentially reversible, acute respiratory and cardiovascular emergencies. Although the optimal management method is that of prevention, prompt diagnosis and institution of therapy are crucial after these reactions have been initiated to prevent the fatal cardiovascular and pulmonary manifestations. Factors associated with improved survival include the sensitivity of the person to the inciting agent, the duration between the exposure and the onset of symptoms (short latency periods are associated with more severe manifestations), the route and dose of the offending agent (larger doses and parenteral administration are associated with more severe manifestations), and the interval between onset of symptoms and subsequent diagnosis and institution of appropriate therapy.[1,38] Optimal management of acute systemic reactions includes appropriate pharmacologic intervention, support of pulmonary and cardiovascular function, and removal of the offending agent. Expeditious institution of these measures helps to reduce the morbidity and mortality associated with these potentially life-threatening syndromes.

REFERENCES ■

1. Wasserman SI, Marquardt DL: Anaphylaxis. In: Middleton E, Reed CE, Ellis EF, et al (eds). *Allergy: Principles and Practice.* St Louis, CV Mosby, 1988:1365
2. Kaliner MA: Anaphylaxis. *NER Allergy Proc* 1984;5:324
3. Smith PL, Kagey-Sobotka A, Bleecker ER, et al: Physiologic manifestations of human anaphylaxis. *J Clin Invest* 1980;66:1072
4. Delage C, Irey NS: Anaphylactic deaths: a clinicopathologic study of 43 cases. *J Forensic Sci* 1972;17:525
5. Carlson RW, Schaeffer RC, Pun VK, et al: Hypovolemia and permeability pulmonary edema associated with anaphylaxis. *Crit Care Med* 1981;9:883
6. Raper RF, Fisher MM: Profound reversible myocardial depression after anaphylaxis. *Lancet* 1988;i:386
7. Hanashiro PK, Weil MH: Anaphylactic shock in man: report of two cases with detailed hemodynamic and metabolic studies. *Arch Intern Med* 1967;119:129
8. Moss J, Fahmy NR, Sunder N, et al: Hormonal and hemodynamic profile of an anaphylactic reaction in man. *Circulation* 1981;63:210
9. Silverman HJ, Van Hook C, Haponik EF: Hemodynamic changes in human anaphylaxis. *Am J Med* 1984;77:341
10. Haupt MT, Carlson RW: Anaphylactic and anaphylactoid reactions. In: Shoemaker WC, Holbrook PR, Thompson WL (eds). *The Society of Critical Care Medicine: Textbook of Critical Care,* ed 2. Philadelphia, WB Saunders, 1989:993
11. Nicolas F, Villers D, Blanloeil Y: Hemodynamic pattern in anaphylactic shock with cardiac arrest. *Crit Care Med* 1984;12:144
12. Wasserman SI: The heart in anaphylaxis. *J Allergy Clin Immunol* 1986;77:663
13. Fawcett WJ, Shephard JN, Soni NC, et al: Oxygen transport and haemodynamic changes during an anaphylactoid reaction. *Anaesth Intensive Care* 1994;22:300
14. Schwartz LB, Metcalfe DD, Miler JS, et al: Tryptase levels as an indicator of mast cell activation in systemic anaphylaxis and mastocystosis. *N Engl J Med* 1987;316:1622
15. Sullivan TJ: Systemic anaphylaxis. In: Lichenstein LM, Fauci AS (eds). *Current Therapy in Allergy, Immunology, and Rheumatology,* ed 3. Toronto, BC Decker, 1988:91
16. Haupt MT: Anaphylaxis and anaphylactic shock. In: Parrillo JE (ed). *Current Therapy in Critical Care Medicine,* ed 2. Philadelphia, BC Decker, 1991:5862

17. Laxenaire MC, Mata-Bermejo E, Moneret-Vautrin DA, et al: Life-threatening anaphylactoid reactions to propofol (Diprivan). *Anesthesiology* 1992;77:275

18. Mitsuhata H, Horiguchi Y, Saithoh J, et al: An anaphylactic reaction to topical fibrin glue. *Anesthesiology* 1994;81:1074

19. Schwartz HA, Zurowski D: Anaphylaxis to latex in intravenous fluids. *J Allergy Clin Immunol* 1993;92:358

20. Tisdale JE, Stringer KA, Antalek M, et al: Streptokinase-induced anaphylaxis. *DICP* 1989;23:984

21. Massel D, Gill JB, Cairns JA: Anaphylactoid reaction during an infusion of recombinant tissue-type plasminogen activator for acute myocardial infarction. *Can J Cardiol* 1991;7:298

22. Perkin RM, Anas NG: Mechanisms and management of anaphylactic shock not responding to traditional therapy. *Ann Allergy* 1985;54:202

23. Yunginger JW: Anaphylaxis. *Curr Probl Pediatr* 1992;22:130

24. Shelhamer JH, Kaliner MA: Anaphylaxis and anaphylactic shock. In: Parrillo JE (ed). *Current Therapy in Critical Care Medicine*. Toronto, BC Decker, 1987:47

25. Kaliner M, Sigler R, Summers R, et al: Effects of infused histamine: analysis of the effects of H-1 and H-2 histamine receptor antagonists on cardiovascular and pulmonary responses. *J Allergy Clin Immunol* 1981;68:365

26. Parrillo JE: Intravenous cimetidine administration commonly produces a decrease in arterial pressure in critically ill patients. *Update Crit Care Med* 1986;1:5

27. Gullo A, Romano E: Naloxone and anaphylactic shock. *Lancet* 1983;i:819

28. Toogood JH: Risk of anaphylaxis in patients receiving betablocker drugs. *J Allergy Clin Immunol* 1988;81:1

29. Zaloga GP, Delacey W, Holmboe E, et al: Glucagon reversal of hypotension in a case of anaphylactoid shock. *Ann Intern Med* 1986;105:65

30. Raby RB, Blaiss MS: Anaphylaxis and serum sickness. In: Rakel RE (ed). *Conn's Current Therapy*. Philadelphia, WB Saunders, 1995:675

31. Cohan RH, Dunnick NR, Bashore TM: Treatment of reactions to radiographic contrast material. *AJR* 1988;15:263

32. Lasser EC, Berry CC, Talner LB, et al: Pretreatment with corticosteroids to alleviate reactions to intravenous contrast material. *N Engl J Med* 1987;317:845

33. Patterson R, DeSwarte RD, Greenberger PA, et al: Drug allergy and protocols for management of drug allergies. *NER Allergy Proc* 1986;7:325

34. Greenberger PA, Patterson R, Tapio CM: Prophylaxis against repeated radiocontrast media reactions in 857 cases: adverse experience with cimetidine and safety of beta-adrenergic antagonists. *Arch Intern Med* 1985;145:2197

35. Greenberger PA, Patterson R, Radin RC: Two pretreatment regimens for high-risk patients receiving radiographic contrast media. *J Allergy Clin Immunol* 1984;74:540

36. Fischer HW: Cost vs. safety: the use of low-osmolar contrast media. *JAMA* 1988;260:1614

37. Serafin WE, Austen KF: Mediators of immediate hypersensitivity reactions. *N Engl J Med* 1987;317:30

38. Sheffer AL: Anaphylaxis. *J Allergy Clin Immunol* 1985;75:227

SECTION X

Infectious Disease

Critical Care, Third Edition, edited by Joseph M. Civetta,
Robert W. Taylor, and Robert R. Kirby.
Lippincott-Raven Publishers, Philadelphia, PA © 1997.

CHAPTER 105

An Approach to the Use
of Antimicrobial Agents

George E. Crawford
Mimi Emig

IMMEDIATE CONCERNS ∎

MAJOR PROBLEMS

The clinician in the intensive care unit (ICU), faced with
patient with a potentially life-threatening infection, must
choose appropriate antimicrobial therapy from the cornucopia of agents currently available. The ideal agent would
be nontoxic, inexpensive, and capable of selectively killing
pathogenic organisms while leaving the host's normal flora
intact. Unfortunately, the ideal antimicrobial agent does not
exist. We usually must choose between agents that have a
narrow spectrum of activity and those with a broader spectrum of activity that eliminate the normal flora, predisposing
to colonization and infection by resistant or opportunistic
organisms. Therapy in critically ill patients must often be
initiated before a specific pathogen is identified, dictating
the use of broader spectrum antibiotics or combinations
of antibiotics.

STRESS POINTS

1. Host factors influence likely pathogens and potential
   antibiotic toxicities.
2. Efforts should be made to identify a source and site
   of infection and to obtain specimens for culture and
   rapid diagnostic tests before starting empiric therapy.
3. Familiarity with the spectrum of activity and toxicities
   of antimicrobial agents is required to choose empiric
   agents that are likely to be effective.

ESSENTIAL DIAGNOSTIC TESTS
AND PROCEDURES

1. Perform a directed medical history and physical examination to identify potential sources and sites of
   infection.
2. For all patients with suspected infection, culture urine
   and blood and obtain a chest radiograph.
3. Sputum, if any, should undergo Gram staining and
   culture.
4. Further diagnostic testing should be directed at suspected sites of infection.

INITIAL THERAPY

1. In a critically ill patient, initial antibiotics should be
   effective against all pathogens likely be responsible for
   the illness.
2. Initial intravenous therapy is preferable to ensure
   rapid and reliable achievement of therapeutic levels
   at the site of infection.
3. Patients should be reassessed frequently for therapeutic response and toxicity, and to identify the need for
   adjunctive therapy such as surgery.
4. The choice of antibiotics should be reassessed after a
   pathogen is identified and the patient's response to
   therapy is determined.
5. Failure of empiric therapy should prompt a reevaluation of the patient to identify the reason for failure.

PRINCIPLES OF ANTIBIOTIC SELECTION ■

The clinician must follow several basic principles when choosing antimicrobial therapy. First, relevant host factors (which influence not only which pathogens are more likely but also what toxicities may occur with therapy) should be reviewed. Second, efforts should be directed at identifying the source and site of infection and isolating a pathogen. Finally, antimicrobial agents should be chosen that are effective against the most likely pathogens. Each of these principles is discussed in the following sections.

HOST FACTORS

The clinician should carefully review the relevant historic and clinical factors before initiating empiric antimicrobial therapy.

Acquisition of Infection

Historical factors can indicate which pathogens are the most likely to cause disease in a given patient. Aspects of the patient's history that should be reviewed include the following:

1. Is the infection community acquired (occurring before or within 72 hours of admission) or nosocomial? Pathogens causing community-acquired infections are often more sensitive to antibiotics; these infections may be treated with less toxic (and often less expensive) antibiotics. Conversely, bacteria causing nosocomial infections are more likely to be multiply resistant and may require more toxic antibiotics. As an example, pathogens commonly seen in community-acquired pneumonia include *Streptococcus pneumoniae, Haemophilus influenzae,* and *Mycoplasma;* nosocomial pathogens include *Staphylococcus aureus* and gram-negative bacteria.

2. If the infection was community acquired, did the patient have exposures that influence the likely pathogens? Sources of outpatient exposure include infectious diseases circulating in the community, travel to an area of endemic disease, exposure to ill family members, exposure to unusual pathogens through work or hobbies (e.g., psittacosis in owners of birds), and common-source outbreaks. Recognition of potential exposures helps to guide diagnostic evaluation and may require modification of empiric therapy to treat unusual pathogens not covered by typical broad-spectrum antibiotics.

3. If the infection was nosocomial, what therapy and procedures has the patient already had? Prior antimicrobial therapy, invasive or surgical procedures, and hospitalization in an ICU may predispose to infection by altering the host's normal flora, bypassing normal host defenses, or exposing the patient to resistant pathogens.[1] Information on the local prevalence of organisms and sensitivity patterns is of great value. Chapter 106 discusses nosocomial infections in further detail.

4. Does the patient have an underlying illness? Certain conditions and immune defects carry an increased risk for specific pathogens.[2–6] Table 105-1 gives examples of immune defects and associated pathogens. Current corticosteroid therapy may mask signs or symptoms of infection; these patients may not mount a fever or have localizing signs despite ongoing infection. Chapter 107 discusses infections in patients with the acquired immunodeficiency syndrome (AIDS); Chapter 109 addresses infections in patients with other immunocompromising conditions.[7]

5. What is the suspected site of infection? The importance of the physical examination is discussed later in "Diagnosis of Infection." Determining the probable site of infection can guide antibiotic selection by suggesting likely pathogens. For example, agents effective against gram-negative pathogens should be used in

TABLE 105-1. Pathogens Associated With Immune Deficits

IMMUNE DEFICIT	USUAL PATHOGENS	TYPICAL SETTINGS
Granulocytopenia	Aerobic gram-negative bacilli, *Staphylococcus aureus,* *Candida, Aspergillus*	Hematologic malignancy, postchemotherapy
Cell-mediated immunosuppression	*Cytomegalovirus,* *neumocystis,* herpes zoster, *Nocardia, Listeria, Cryptococcus, Legionella, Strongyloides*	AIDS, renal transplantation, Hodgkin's disease
Hypogammaglobulinemia or dysgammaglobulinemia	*Streptococcus pneumoniae, Haemophilus influenzae*	Chronic lymphocytic leukemia, multiple myeloma, congenital hypogammaglobulinemia
Asplenia	*S. pneumoniae, Capnocytophaga* (DF-2), *Neisseria meningitidis, Klebsiella*	Posttrauma, sickle cell anemia, poststaging laparotomy for Hodgkin's disease

AIDS, acquired immunodeficiency syndrome.

urinary tract infections, whereas antibiotics for a suspected catheter infection should be directed against *Staphylococcus* and *Enterococcus*. More specific information on particular sites of infection is given in the following chapters: central nervous system (CNS), Chapter 110; urinary tract infections, Chapter 111; endocarditis and catheter infections, Chapter 110; and pneumonia, Chapter 124.

6. Has the patient received recent antibiotic therapy? If so, a new infection is likely to be resistant to those drugs. The yield of bacterial cultures is lower in patients with recent or current antibiotic therapy; this is particularly important when diagnosing endovascular infections (e.g., endocarditis). If diarrhea is present, stool should be sent for *Clostridium difficile* toxin assay.

Drug Metabolism and Toxicity

The logical selection of empiric antimicrobial therapy also requires an understanding of host factors that influence drug metabolism and potential toxicities. The spectrum of activity, appropriate dosage and dosage intervals, and costs of antimicrobial agents are covered later. Host factors that influence the pharmacokinetics and toxicities include the following:

1. Does the patient have impaired hepatic or renal function? If possible, agents that may induce further hepatic or renal dysfunction should be avoided if equally efficacious nontoxic agents are available. Potentially life-saving antibiotics (e.g., aminoglycosides) should not be withheld in the setting of renal failure, but may require dose adjustment to avoid potential toxicity. Dose adjustments of antibiotics in hepatic and renal failure are listed in Critical Care Catalogue, Appendix F, respectively.

2. Does the patient have a history of hypersensitivity to an antibiotic? The most common antibiotics causing allergic reactions are penicillins, cephalosporins, and sulfonamides.

   In a patient with a history of penicillin allergy, the overall risk of reaction to a penicillin is about 25%. The greatest risk is in patients with a history of recent anaphylactic reaction. Negative skin test results to benzylpenicilloyl-polylysine and minor determinant mixture predict a low risk of anaphylactic reaction with penicillin therapy. All penicillins may cross-react; documented reaction to penicillin skin testing is a contraindication to the use of any penicillin. In rare instances where penicillins are the drug of choice for severe infections (e.g., group A streptococcal infection), oral or parenteral desensitization can be used.[8,9]

   The use of cephalosporins in patients with documented penicillin allergy remains controversial. The risk of allergic reaction in these patients is usually less than 5%.[10] Many clinicians use cephalosporins in penicillin-allergic patients who have a remote history of nonanaphylactic reactions, but avoid cephalosporins in those with a recent history of anaphylactic reaction. Carbapenems may also cross-react. Monobactams may

be used in penicillin-allergic patients without cross-reactivity.

3. Does the patient have severe glucose-6-phosphate dehydrogenase deficiency? This deficiency is more common in African-Americans; patients may experience severe hemolytic anemia with the administration of sulfonamides, chloramphenicol, or primaquine.

4. Is the patient pregnant? Pregnancy alters the metabolism of drugs in the mother, and drugs may cross the placenta and cause side effects in the fetus. Maternal volume of distribution, hepatic metabolism, and glomerular filtration rate increase in pregnancy, resulting in lower drug levels. If a serious infection that requires antibiotics is present, the older classes of antibiotics (e.g., β-lactams) are generally used. Table 105-2 can be used to guide the selection of antibiotic agents in pregnant patients. Because of the risk of liver disease

TABLE 105-2. Antibiotic Use in Pregnancy

ANTIMICROBIAL	FETAL TOXICITY
CONTRAINDICATED OR SAFER ALTERNATIVES AVAILABLE	
Amantadine	Embryotoxic, teratogenic
Azoles	Embryotoxic, teratogenic in animals
Clarithromycin	Teratogenic in animals
Erythromycin estolate°	None
Metronidazole	Fetotoxicity in animals
Nitrofurantoin	Hemolysis at term
Tetracycline°	Tooth staining and dysplasia
Trimethoprim	Teratogenicity in rats
Trimethoprim-sulfamethoxazole	Kernicterus, teratogenicity, skeletal growth retardation
CAUTION: USE ONLY FOR STRONG INDICATION AND LACK OF SUITABLE ALTERNATIVES	
Acyclovir	None known
Aminoglycosides	Eight-nerve toxicity
Amphotericin B	Azotemia, hypokalemia
Azithromycin	None known
Clindamycin	None known
Flucytosine	Potentially teratogenic
Isoniazid°	Possible neuropathy and seizures
Quinolones	Arthropathy in immature animals
Rifampin°	None known
Sulfonamides	Kernicterus, hemolysis
Vancomycin	None known
PROBABLY SAFE	
Cephalosporins	None known
Erythromycin base	None known
Paromomycin	None known
Penicillins	None known

°Avoid if possible because of the risk of maternal hepatoxocity.

in pregnancy, potentially hepatotoxic agents should be avoided.

DIAGNOSIS OF INFECTION

When infection is suspected in a patient, the clinician should attempt to isolate the responsible pathogen. Empiric broad-spectrum antibiotics never negate the need for an evaluation for the source of infection. The identification of a site of infection and the isolation of a specific pathogen (and accompanying antibiotic sensitivities) permit directed antimicrobial therapy, often with lower toxicity than that seen with broad-spectrum antibiotics. Table 105-3 lists the drug of choice and alternative drugs for many infectious agents[11]; importantly, sensitivity data (when available) should further direct antibiotic therapy.

The severity of illness of the patient dictates the urgency of identifying a pathogen and initiating therapy. In an otherwise stable patient, the initiation of antimicrobial therapy can await the microbiologic identification of a pathogen. In a critically ill or immunocompromised patient, antimicrobial therapy should be initiated after obtaining appropriate cultures.

Physical Examination

The physical examination often reveals a likely focus of infection. Localizing signs may be minimal in the elderly, in neutropenic patients, and in those on corticosteroids. Besides routine examination, particular attention should be focused on sites that can harbor infection in the critically ill patient, which include the following:

1. Head and neck: Check for meningeal signs, particularly if the patient has had a neurosurgical procedure, has pneumonia, or is immunocompromised. If the patient has (or recently had) a nasogastric or nasal endotracheal tube, check for sinusitis.
2. Chest: Listen carefully for a new or changing murmur, suggestive of endocarditis.
3. Rectal: Neutropenic patients may develop a perirectal abscess; erythema and induration may be minimal, but tenderness is usually present. (Notice: Because of the risk of bacteremia, a digital rectal examination should be done atraumatically, if at all, in neutropenic patients.)
4. Intravascular catheter sites: Carefully check for erythema, tenderness, or exudate at all catheter sites. If

TABLE 105-3.   Drugs of Choice in Serious Infections°

ORGANISM	DRUG OF CHOICE	ALTERNATIVE DRUGS
GRAM-POSITIVE COCCI		
Staphylococcus aureus[†] or *Staphylococcus epidermidis*		
Penicillin-sensitive	Penicillin G	Cephalosporin,[†] vancomycin, or clindamycin
Penicillinase-producing[§]	Oxacillin or nafcillin	Cephalosporin, vancomycin, or clindamycin
Methicillin-resistant[ǁ]	Vancomycin	Quinolone, TMP/SMZ, minocycline
Nonenterococcal streptococci[+]	Penicillin G	Cephalosporin, vancomycin, or clindamycin
Enterococcus	Penicillin or ampicillin + gentamicin	Vancomycin + gentamicin
Streptococcus pneumoniae[¶]	Pencillin G	Cephalosporin, vancomycin, macrolide, or clindamycin
GRAM-POSITIVE BACILLI		
Actinomyces israelii	Penicillin G	Tetracycline
Bacillus anthracis	Penicillin G	Tetracycline, macrolide
Clostridium difficile	Metronidazole	Oral vancomycin
Clostridium perfringens	Penicillin[#]	Clindamycin, metronidazole, tetracycline, imipenem
Clostridium tetani	Penicillin°°	Tetracycline
Corynebacterium diphtheriae	Macrolide[#]	Penicillin
Corynebacterium JK	Vancomycin	Penicillin G + gentamicin, erythromycin
Listeria monocytogenes	Ampicillin gentamicin	TMP/SMZ
Nocardia asteroides	Sulfonamide	TMP/SMZ, minocycline, ampicillin + erythromycin
Proprionobacterium sp.	Penicillin	Clindamycin, erythromycin
GRAM-NEGATIVE COCCI		
Moraxella catarrhalis	TMP/SMZ	Amox-clavulanic acid, ceftriaxone, macrolid, tetracycline
Neisseria gonorrhea	Ceftriaxone	Penicillin G, quinolone
Neisseria meningitidis	Penicillin G	Ceftriaxone

TABLE 105-3. *(continued)*

ORGANISM	DRUG OF CHOICE	ALTERNATIVE DRUGS
ENTERIC GRAM NEGATIVE BACILLI		
Bacteroides		
Oral source	Penicillin	Clindamycin, cefoxitin, metronidazole, cefotetan
Bowel source	Metronidazole	Cefoxitin, cefotetan, imipenem, amp-sulbactam ticar-clavulanate, pip-tazobactam, clindamycin
Citrobacter	Imipenem gentamicin	Aminoglycoside, quinolone, piperacillin, aztreonam
Enterobacter sp.[++]	Quinolone	Aminoglycoside, piperacillin, carbenicillin, aztreonam
Escherichia coli	3rd-generation cephalosporin	Gentamicin, tobramycin, imipenem, quinolone aztreonam, piperacillin, tazobactam, TMP/SMZ
Klebsiella	3rd-generation cephalosporin	As for *E. coli*
Proteus mirabilis	Ampicillin	Aminoglycoside, quinolone, cephalosporin, piperacillin, ticarcillin, TMP/SMZ
Proteus, nonmirabilis	3rd-generation cephalosporin	Aminoglycoside, quinolone, piperacillin, aztreonam, imipenem
Providencia	2nd- or 3rd-generation cephalosporin	Gentamicin, amikacin, piperacillin, aztreonam imipenem, ticarcillin, mezlocillin, TMP/SMZ
Salmonella typhi	Ceftriaxone or quinolone	Ampicillin, TMP/SMZ
Salmonella, nontyphi[††]	Cefotaxime, ceftriaxone, or quinolone	Ampicillin, TMP/SMZ
Serratia	3rd-generation cephalosporin	Gentamicin, amikacin, imipenem, aztreonam piperacillin, TMP/SMZ, quinolone
Shigella	Quinolone	Ampicillin, TMP/SMZ, ceftriaxone, cefixime
Yersinia enterocolitica	TMP/SMZ	Aminoglycoside, tetracycline, 3rd-generation cephalosporin, quinolone
OTHER GRAM-NEGATIVE BACILLI		
Acinetobacter	Imipenem	Aminoglycoside, piperacillin, ticarcillin, TMP/SMZ, minocycline, doxycycline
Eikenella corrodens	Ampicillin	Penicillin G, erythromycin, tetracycline, ceftriaxone
Francisella tularensis	Streptomycin, gentamicin	Tetracycline
Fusobacterium	Penicillin	Clindamycin, metronidazole, cefoxitin
Haemophilus influenzae	3rd-generation cephalosporin	Ampicillin, imipenem, quinolone, cefuroxime[§§], quinolone, macrolide, TMP/SMZ
Legionella	Erythromycin (1 g q 6 h) + rifampin	
Pasturella multocida	Penicillin G	Tetracycline, cephalosporin, amps-sulbactam
Pseudomonas aeruginosa	Anti-pseudomonal penicillin[‖] + tobramycin	Aztreonam, ceftazidime, amikacin, imipenem, quinolone
Pseudomonas cepacia	TMP/SMZ	Ceftazidime
Spirillum minus	Penicillin G	Tetracycline, streptomycin
Streptobacillus moniliforms	Penicillin G	Tetracycline, streptomycin
Vibrio cholerae[¶]	Tetracycline	TMP/SMZ, quinolone
Vibrio vulnificus	Tetracycline	Cefotaxime
Xanthomonas maltophilia	TMP/SMZ	Quinolone, minocycline, ceftazidime
Yersinia pestis	Streptomycin	Tetracycline, gentamicin
CHLAMYDIAE		
Chlamydia pneumoniae (TWAR)	Tetracycline	Macrolide
Chlamydia psittaci	Tetracycline	Chloramphenicol
Chlamydia trachomatis	Macrolide	Sulfonamide, tetracycline
MYCOPLASMA sp.	Macrolide	Tetracycline
RICKETTSIAE	Tetracycline	Quinolone
SPIROCHETES		
Borrelia burgdorferi	Doxycycline, amoxicillin	Penicillin G, macrolide, cefuroxime, ceftriaxone, cefotaxime

(continued)

TABLE 105-3. *(continued)*

ORGANISM	DRUG OF CHOICE	ALTERNATIVE DRUGS
Borrelia sp.	Tetracycline	Penicillin G
Treponema pallidum	Penicillin	Tetracycline, ceftriaxone
VIRUSES		
Cytomegalovirus	Ganciclovir##	Foscarnet
Herpes simplex	Acyclovir	Foscarnet
HIV	Zidovudine (AZT)	Didanosine (DDI), Lamivudine (#TC), ††† Ritonavir†††
Influenza	Amantadine	Rimantadine
Respiratory syncytial	Ribavirin	
Varicella zoster	Acyclovir	Famciclovir°°°
FUNGI		
Aspergillus	Amphotericin B	Itraconazole
Blastomyces	Amphotericin B or itraconazole	Ketoconazole
Candida+++		
Mucosal	Fluconazole	Ketoconazole, itraconazole
Systemic	Fluconazole	Amphotericin B
Coccidioides	Amphotericin B or fluconazole	Itraconazole, ketoconazole
Cryptococcus	Amphotericin	Fluconazole, itraconazole
Histoplasma	Itraconazole or Amphotericin B	
Pseudallescheria	Ketoconazole or itraconazole	
Zygomycosis ("mucor")	Amphotericin B+++	

°This tables does not consider minor infections that may be treated with oral agents, single-agent therapy, or less toxic drugs. Sensitivity testing must be done on bacterial isolates to confirm the sensitivity pattern.

†Some authorities recommend clindamycin as the first choice for toxin-producing staphylococci, streptococci, or clostridia.

‡First-generation cephalosporins are most active. If endocarditis is suspected, do not use clindamycin. Some authorities recommend the addition of gentamicin for endocarditis caused by nonenterococcal streptococci or tolerant staphylococci.

§Penicillinase-producing staphylococci are also resistant to ampicillin, amoxicillin, carbenicillin, ticarcillin, mezlocillin, and piperacillin

‖Methicillin-resistant staphylococci should be assumed to be resistant to all cephalosporins and penicillins, even if disk testing suggests sensitivity.

¶Some stains show intermediate- or high-level pencillin resistance. Highly resistant strains are treated with vancomycin, or rifampin, or both. In regions with high prevalence of resistant pneumococcus, ceftriaxone or vancomycin should be considered until sensitivity is known.

#Use as an adjunct to debridement of infected tissues.

°°Use as an adjunct to active and passive immunization.

++Because of rapid development of resistance, cephalosporins not recommended even if initial tests indicate susceptibility.

††Uncomplicated *Salmonella* enteritis should not be treated with antibiotics.

§§Should not be used in meningitis because of poor CNS penetration.

‖‖Anti-pseudomonal penicillins include ticarcillin, mezlocillin, and piperacillin.

¶¶Primary therapy is fluid and electrolyte repletion.

##Oral form should be used only in maintenance therapy of retinal cytomegalovirus.

°°°Approved only for mild herpes zoster in immunocompetent hosts.

+++*Candida kruseii* and *Torulopsis glabrata* may be resistant to azole therapy.

†††In multidrug combinations.

a vascular access device does demonstrate signs of infection, it should be cultured and removed.

5. Wounds: Surgical wounds should be closely examined for signs of wound infection or abscess.

6. Skin: The skin may be the site of infection, and infections may have cutaneous manifestations. Decubitus ulcers can become superinfected and can result in underlying osteomyelitis; infection of a decubitus ulcer

may require drainage or debridement along with antibiotic therapy. Diffuse erythroderma suggests toxic shock syndrome from *S aureus* or group A streptococci. Peripheral embolic phenomena (Janeway lesions, Osler nodes, and splinter hemorrhages) can occur in endocarditis. *Pseudomonas* infection can produce ecthyma gangrenosum. Petechial and purpuric lesions suggest overwhelming sepsis or *Neisseria men-*

ingitidis infection. Disseminated *Neisseria gonorrhea* infection can produce pustular lesions, usually on the distal extremities. Digital ischemia in an asplenic patient with sepsis can occur with *Capnocytophaga* (DF-2) infection.

Laboratory Evaluation

Gram staining and culture of potentially infected sites should always be performed. As a routine, sputum and urine should be examined and cultured, as appropriate. Blood cultures should be drawn before the initiation of antimicrobial therapy.[12] In asplenic patients with overwhelming bacteremia, Gram staining of the buffy coat may demonstrate the etiologic organism. A chest radiograph should be obtained to check for new or persistent infiltrates that suggest pneumonia. The clinical setting guides further diagnostic evaluation with culture of other fluids (cerebrospinal fluid [CSF], pleural fluid, or ascites) or additional radiographic studies. Specialized laboratory studies (e.g., *Legionella* DFA, serologic studies for diagnosis of rickettsial illnesses) may be indicated and should be requested based on the clinical suspicion for particular pathogens.

Gram staining of material from potentially infected sites can suggest a particular pathogen. If the Gram stain shows a predominant morphologic type of bacteria, more specific antibiotic therapy can be directed against the likely pathogen. Gram-positive cocci in clusters are likely to be staphylococci. Gram-positive cocci in chains often represent streptococci or *Enterococcus*; gram-positive diplococci are present in pneumococcal infection. Small gram-negative coccobacillary forms are seen in *Haemophilus* infections. A Gram stain showing multiple morphologic types of bacteria can indicate a polymicrobial infection (as occurs in an abscess) or may represent contamination of the specimen by colonizing flora.

ANTIBIOTIC THERAPY ∎

After reviewing host factors and attempting to identify a site of infection, the clinician must choose an initial empiric regimen. The antibiotics chosen should be effective against the pathogens that are most likely to be causing the patient's illness. Drug characteristics that influence antibiotic selection include spectrum of activity, route of administration, potential toxicities, and cost of therapy. Therapy must be reevaluated after its initiation to determine efficacy, toxicity, and anticipated duration of treatment.

SPECTRUM OF ACTIVITY

Individual agents and their efficacy against particular organisms are detailed in the section "Antimicrobials Useful in the Critical Care Unit." Drugs are *bactericidal* if their main mechanism of action is irreversible inhibition of growth. These agents include the β-lactams, vancomycin, metronidazole, aminoglycosides, rifampin, and the quinolones. *Bacteriostatic* drugs, such as the tetracyclines, macrolides, and clindamycin, inhibit bacterial growth in a reversible fashion. Growth resumes when the agent is removed. These agents require the assistance of host defenses to be effective.

With few exceptions, there is no clinical difference in the response to bacteriostatic and bactericidal drugs. The distinction is clinically relevant in infective endocarditis,[13] bacterial meningitis,[14] and infections in neutropenic patient[15]; these infections require therapy with bactericidal agents. The use of bacteriostatic agents in any of these three settings carries a high incidence of relapse or primary failure of therapy.

The penetration of an antimicrobial agent into infected tissue must be considered. This is particularly important when choosing agents for the treatment of bacterial meningitis and biliary tract disease. Antibiotics may penetrate poorly into undrained abscesses and obstructed urinary or biliary tracts. Tissue penetration by antibiotics is also relevant in the treatment of pneumonia (where higher levels of drugs are needed) and urinary tract infections (where lower levels are effective because of the urinary concentration of many agents).

DOSAGE AND ROUTE OF ADMINISTRATION

Antibiotics can be given orally, intramuscularly (IM), or intravenously (IV). Intravenous therapy is generally used in critically ill patients because it is a reliable route of administration. There is no clear-cut difference in toxicity or efficacy between intermittent and continuous intravenous administration of antibiotics. Intramuscular injection may be used for drugs designed to be absorbed slowly from a depot (e.g., benzathine penicillin). Patient discomfort, local complications, and unreliable absorption of some drugs limit the intramuscular route. Oral administration is convenient and less costly than parenteral therapy; absorption may be unreliable, and blood levels may be lower than those seen with intravenous administration.

The initial recommended dosages and estimated purchase costs[16,17] of common antibiotic agents are listed in Table 105-4. Local costs may vary, and administration costs (e.g., intravenous tubing) are not included. In general, higher dosages are used for severe infections and for infections where drug penetration is limited (e.g., meningitis); lower dosages are used for urinary tract infections.

ANTIBIOTIC TOXICITY

All commonly prescribed antimicrobial agents have potential side effects. Table 105-5 lists toxicities caused by various antimicrobial agents. Antibiotic toxicity can be idiosyncratic or can be caused by allergic reactions, direct dose-related toxicity, or alteration in the host's normal flora. Dose-related toxicity of particular antimicrobial agents is described in "Antimicrobial Agents Useful in the Critical Care Unit."

Allergic reaction to an antimicrobial agent is one of the most common antimicrobial toxicities. The first line of defense against allergic reactions is a good history, focusing on previous drug reactions and allergic problems. The classic IgE-mediated anaphylactic reaction can be seen with any drug; anaphylaxis to penicillin is the prototype of this type of reaction.[18] Allergic reactions to penicillins are discussed in more detail in the section on host factors influencing drug metabolism and toxicity (discussed earlier). More frequently, drug allergy presents as a rash; the spectrum of rashes extends from nonspecific maculopapular rashes to life-threatening exfoliative dermatitis.

Fever can be an important manifestation of antimicrobial toxicity, and should be suspected if the patient develops recrudescent fever despite apparently successful treatment of the primary infection. If the patient has been sensitized by previous therapy, drug fever may occur early in therapy. More typically, drug fever occurs after 1 or more weeks of therapy. Patients with drug fever may appear surprisingly well, despite high fever. Eosinophilia can be a clue to the occurrence of drug fever, but it is not universally present.

Antimicrobial agents alter the host's normal flora. A significant side effect of broad-spectrum antimicrobial agents is secondary superinfection or subsequent infection. The risk of a second infection increases with longer duration of therapy and with broad-spectrum combinations that suppress normal flora. Secondary infections are most commonly caused by *C difficile*, yeast, filamentous fungi, and antibiotic-

resistant bacteria. Shifts in flora are minimized by (1) using a single agent with a narrow spectrum that is directed at the etiologic organism, and (2) discontinuing antibiotic therapy after the infection has been adequately treated.

MONOTHERAPY VERSUS COMBINATION THERAPY

Infections in patients with normal immune defenses can usually be treated adequately with a single antimicrobial agent. Despite this, the administration of multiple antibiotics to treat a seriously ill patient remains commonplace.

Combination therapy has several disadvantages when compared with monotherapy. The cost of treating a patient's illness is greatly increased by the inappropriate use of combination therapy when a single antimicrobial agent would suffice. The chance of adverse reactions to antimicrobial agents is increased with combination therapy. Indeed, certain agents may potentiate the risk of toxicity; for example, concomitant therapy with vancomycin increases the risk of neph-

TABLE 105-4.   Cost and Initial Dosage of Selected Parenteral Antimicrobial Agents°

ANTIBIOTIC	USUAL DOSE	COST/ d ($)
Ampicillin	2 g q 6 h	27.40
Ampicillin/sulbactam	3 g q 6 h	46.58
Penicillin G	2 million U q 4 h	10.40
Piperacillin—non-*Pseudomonas*	3 g q 6 h	68.44
Piperacillin—*Pseudomonas*	3 g q 4 h	102.66
Piperacillin/tazobactam	3.375 g q 6 h	57.45
Ticarcillin/clavulanate	3.1 g q 6 h	51.40
Nafcillin	2 g q 6 h	51.28
Cefazolin	1 g q 8 h	10.65
Cefotetan	2 g q 12 h	42.52
Cefotaxime	2 g q 8 h	63.58
Cefoxitin	2 g q 8 h	70.85
Ceftazidime	2 g q 8 h	85.36
Ceftizoxime	2 g q 8 h	63.42
Ceftriaxone	2 g q 24 h	61.45
Cefuroxime	1.5 g q 8 h	40.38
Aztreonam	1 g q 8 h	45.30
Imipenem	500 mg q 6 h	89.60
Amikacin	7.5 mg/kg q 12 h or 15 mg/kg q 24 h	128.97
Gentamicin	2 mg/kg q 12 h or 5 mg/kg q 24 h	8.84
Tobramycin	2 mg/kg q 12 h or 5 mg/kg q 24 h	36.80
Vancomycin	1 g q 12 h	37.62
Erythromycin	1 g q 6 h	71.18
Clindamycin	600 mg q 8 h	49.20
Metronidazole	500 mg q 6 h	31.48
Ciprofloxacin	400 mg q 12 h	57.60
Ofloxacin	400 mg q 12 h	50.08
Trimethoprim-sulfamethoxazole	5 mg/kg trimethoprim q 6 h	40.01
Pentamidine	300 mg q 24 h	98.75
Ganciclovir	5 mg/kg q 12 h	69.60
Foscarnet	60 mg/kg q 8 h	146.50

°Doses and costs are based on a 20 kg adult with normal renal and hepatic function. Cost is average wholesale pharmacy cost and may vary.
q, every.

TABLE 105-5. Side Effects of Antibiotics

ORGAN SYSTEM	TOXICITY	DRUG
Nervous system	Seizures, tremors	Amantadine
	Seizures	Imipenem
	Sleep disorder	Isoniazid, quinolones
	Myoclonic seizures	Penicillins
	Hearing loss	Aminoglycosides (irreversible), erythromycin (reversible)
	Vestibulopathy	Aminoglycosides (irreversible)
	Retinopathy	Ethambutol
	Neuromuscular blockade	Aminoglycosides
	Peripheral neuropathy	ddI, ddC, aminoglycosides
Pulmonary	Interstitial lung disease	Macrodantin
Gastrointestinal	Nausea, vomiting, diarrhea	Macrolides, tetracyclines, clindamycin
	Cholestatic jaundice	Erythromycin
	Hepatitis	Isoniazid, rifampin, tetracyclines, ddI, nitrofurantoin, azoles (especially ketoconazole)
	Pancreatitis	Pentamidine, ddC
Hematologic	Marrow suppression	Chloramphenicol, pentamidine, sulfonamides, ganciclovir, vancomycin
	Hemolysis	Sulfonamides, nitrofurantoin, primaquine
Renal	Renal insufficiency	Aminoglycosides, pentamidine, penicillins, amphotericin, sulfonamides, acyclovir
Fluids/electrolytes	Hypokalemia, hypomagnesemia	Amphotericin, foscarnet
	Hypophosphatemia	Foscarnet
	Hypoglycemia or hyperglycemia	Pentamidine
	High sodium load	Ticarcillin, piperacillin, ddI
Cardiovascular	Hypotension	Foscarnet, amphotericin
	Arrhythmias	Amantadine, pentamidine
	Phlebitis	Erythromycin, penicillins, cephalosporins, vancomycin, aztreonam, imipenem, acyclovir (if extravasates)
Skin	Rash	Any, but especially penicillins, cephalosporins, sulfonamides
	Stevens-Johnson syndrome	Sulfonamides, penicillins
	"Red-man" syndrome	Vancomycin
Miscellaneous	Fever	Amphotericin, penicillins, cephalosporins

rotoxicity from aminoglycosides. Lastly, antagonism between antimicrobial agents may occur with combination therapy; in vitro antagonism seems to be more common than in vivo antagonism. Clinically relevant antagonism is best documented in the treatment of pneumococcal meningitis; patients treated with penicillin alone had a 21% mortality rate, whereas those treated with penicillin plus a tetracycline had a 79% mortality rate.[19]

Monotherapy in Specific Clinical Settings

CRITICALLY ILL PATIENTS. Adequate diagnostic specimens should be collected before initiating or changing antimicrobial therapy. As discussed earlier, a thorough history and examination are irreplaceable in guiding antimicrobial therapy. Newer agents with broad spectra of activity often cover the likely pathogens in many clinical settings. If no single agent can provide reliable activity against the suspected infectious agents in a critically ill patient, combination therapy may be appropriate until microbiologic results are available. In this situation, therapy should be narrowed after sensitivity data are available. This is addressed later in "Reassessment of Therapy."

FEBRILE NEUTROPENIA.   In general, monotherapy with ceftazidime is appropriate if the patient is hemodynamically stable and has no localizing signs of infection.[20] Single-agent therapy in these patients has reduced toxicity and is as effective as combination therapy in most trials. Importantly, monotherapy with ceftazidime has minimal activity against anaerobes and reduced activity against gram-positive cocci. Experience with monotherapy in severe *Pseudomonas* infections is limited. The clinician must closely monitor the patient for nonresponse and for the emergence of resistance or secondary infection. As with all other empiric regimens, therapy should be tailored based on clinical response and microbiologic data. Chapter 108 discusses the management of fever in neutropenic patients in more detail.

Combination Therapy

Combination therapy is superior to monotherapy in several settings. In treating severely immunocompromised hosts (e.g., patients undergoing organ transplantation or patients with human immunodeficiency virus [HIV]), clinicians may have to resort to initial polypharmacy to treat possible bacterial, fungal, and viral infections. Indications for ongoing combination therapy in immunocompetent hosts include the following:

1. Tuberculosis: Combination therapy is clearly effective in preventing the emergence of resistance in tuberculosis[21]; active tuberculosis must never be treated with monotherapy. Chapter 112 describes the therapy of tuberculosis.
2. Intraperitoneal and pelvic infections: Bowel flora (particularly gram-negative and anaerobic organisms) cause these infections; adequate antibiotic regimens may need to include an aminoglycoside and clindamycin. Newer carbapenems and β-lactam plus β-lactamase inhibitors (e.g., ticarcillin plus clavulanate) have adequate spectra of activity against intraabdominal pathogens and may be adequate as monotherapy.
3. Endocarditis: Endocarditis caused by *Enterococcus* or viridans streptococci should be treated with penicillin plus an aminoglycoside.[22] In the treatment of methicillin-sensitive *S aureus* endocarditis, the addition of gentamicin to nafcillin or oxacillin results in a shorter duration of bacteremia and fever. For left-sided *S aureus* endocarditis (which requires 4 to 6 weeks of antibiotics), gentamicin should be stopped after 5 days to minimize the risk of nephrotoxicity. For uncomplicated right-sided *S aureus* in injection drug users, the combination of gentamicin plus oxacillin or nafcillin may be used for a total course of 2 weeks with good cure rates.[23]
4. *Pseudomonas aeruginosa* infections: Combination therapy with a β-lactam plus an aminoglycoside in documented *P aeruginosa* infections results in improved survival when compared with monotherapy.[24]

REASSESSMENT OF THERAPY

After the initiation of empiric antimicrobial therapy, the patient should be closely watched for clinical evidence of progression or improvement of infection. The clinician must carefully reassess the patient who is failing on initial empiric therapy. Clinical worsening may occur despite the use of appropriate antibiotics. Alternatively, clinical deterioration may result from inappropriate initial therapy. If the patient is worsening, the clinician should reexamine the patient, review available data, and repeat the laboratory evaluation. The likelihood of unusual or resistant pathogens must be reassessed, with adjustments in therapy if needed.

Identification and susceptibility testing of the responsible pathogen are critical in guiding antibiotic therapy. If an isolated pathogen is resistant to the current agents, sensitivity data should direct changes in therapy. If the laboratory data suggest that the current therapy should be effective, the usual causes of failure of "appropriate therapy" must be considered (Table 105-6).

If the patient appears to be clinically responding, the least toxic and most narrow-spectrum antibiotic regimen effective against the identified pathogen should be selected. The susceptibility testing of an isolated pathogen should be reviewed; therapy can be changed to less toxic or less costly agents based on results of such testing. Clinical improvement can occur despite laboratory testing showing resistance to initial therapy. If this is the case, one must evaluate whether the isolated organism is truly the etiologic agent, whether the sensitivity testing is relevant, or whether the patient is spontaneously improving. A change in therapy may be indicated. If no etiologic agent has been identified but the patient is improving, initial therapy generally should be continued. Even in these situations, the clinician should consider discontinuing toxic agents directed against organisms unlikely to be causing the patient's illness.

TABLE 105-6.   Failure of Appropriate Therapy

CAUSE	EXAMPLE
Site of infection	Undrained abscess, obstruction
Drug pharmacology	Poor absorption, increased excretion
Drug penetration	Meningitis, biliary tract infection
Concomitant therapy	Antibiotic antagonism; antacids and tetracycline
Compliance	Failure to take drug
Immunocompetence	Steroids, granulocytopenia, HIV
Misleading laboratory data	Identification of nonpathogens
Acquired resistance	Single agent INH therapy in active TB
Superinfection	Nosocomial pneumonia

HIV, human immunodeficiency virus; INH, isoniazid; TB, tuberculosis.

After a site of infection and etiologic agent are identified, the clinician should determine the anticipated length of therapy. If the anticipated duration of therapy is clear, an order can be written for the antibiotic to be automatically stopped (e.g., "vancomycin 1 g IV q 12 hours × 14 days"). This avoids the inadvertent continuation of therapy after an adequate course of treatment. Adjustments in the duration of therapy may be needed based on the patient's clinical response and complications of infection. As an example, treatment for infection of an intravenous catheter needs to be extended beyond 10 days if the patient develops endocarditis or fails to promptly clear bacteremia.

PROPHYLACTIC ANTIBIOTICS ∎

Antibiotic prophylaxis is designed to prevent overt illness by preventing acquisition of exogenous organisms (malaria prophylaxis), preventing the spread of normal flora to a normally sterile site (urinary tract infection prophylaxis), or preventing the development of overt disease from asymptomatic infection (isoniazid tuberculosis prophylaxis). Prophylaxis is generally limited in terms of the etiologic agent (as in the case of rheumatic fever prophylaxis) or in duration (surgical prophylaxis). Attempts to prevent infection by a broad range of organisms for a protracted period are generally fruitless because of changes in host flora under antimicrobial selection pressure.

The decision to give prophylactic antibiotics should be based on an analysis indicating that the benefits outweigh the costs and risks of therapy. Consideration of the cost of prophylactic therapy is particularly important because the patients treated are usually asymptomatic, and often many must be treated for each one who actually benefits. The benefits of therapy depend on the likelihood of infection, the seriousness of the infection if it occurs, and the effectiveness of the proposed prophylactic therapy in preventing the infection. The costs of prophylaxis include not only the actual expense of treatment but also the costs of toxicity, allergic reactions, superinfection, and changes in host and hospital flora. In situations in which the risk of serious infection is small, it may be preferable to allow some infections to occur and to treat infected patients specifically.

Ideally, prophylactic regimens should be based on demonstrated efficacy in a controlled trial. In the absence of such data, prophylaxis is usually based on a narrow-spectrum, nontoxic antibiotic demonstrated to be effective against the etiologic agent, given for a brief period that includes the period of maximum risk. Limiting administration of the drug to the period of risk minimizes the cost of prophylaxis.

Surgical prophylaxis is generally accepted when contamination of the operative field is unavoidable (e.g., surgery on the upper airway or large bowel, or vaginal hysterectomy) or for cases in which infection of a prosthesis (prosthetic joint, blood vessel, or heart valve) would be disastrous.[25] The risk of infection is increased and prophylaxis may be warranted in patients older than 70 years of age undergoing biliary tract surgery for acute cholecystitis, obstructive jaundice, and common duct stones, and in patients undergoing gastric surgery who have obstruction, hemorrhage, gastric ulcer, gastric malignancy, or achlorhydria. Typically, the drug is initiated immediately before operation so that tissue levels are present at the beginning of the procedure, and is continued for only 12 to 24 hours postoperatively.[26] Use of second- and third-generation cephalosporins has not been shown to be superior to the less costly first-generation drugs in most circumstances.

The role of antibiotic prophylaxis in the neutropenic host continues to be controversial because of problems with toxicity, patient tolerance, and colonization with resistant organisms. Studies with quinolone antimicrobials such as norfloxacin and ciprofloxacin suggest that they may be of value in preventing infections in neutropenic hosts in selected settings.[27] Accepted nonsurgical chemoprophylactic regimens pertinent to the ICU include the following:

Bacterial endocarditis—For patients at increased risk of intravascular infection, prophylaxis is indicated before procedures that are likely to produce a bacteremia. Chapter 118 discusses which patients should be receive prophylactic antibiotics and what regimens are recommended to reduce the risk of endocarditis.

H influenzae—For household contacts of children with invasive *H influenzae* disease and children attending day care centers with *H influenzae* outbreaks: rifampin, 20 mg/kg/day (not to exceed 600 mg) for 4 days.

Meningococcal disease—Prophylaxis is used to prevent carriage of the organism in the oropharynx and the development of meningococcal disease, and is indicated for household contacts of patients with meningococcal disease (meningitis or meningococcemia). Medical personnel are at low risk of contracting the disease through performance of routine duties; prophylaxis is recommended if mouth-to-mouth resuscitation was given. Three regimens are available: (1) rifampin, 600 mg by mouth every 12 hours for four doses; (2) ciprofloxacin, 250 mg by mouth once; or (3) ceftriaxone, 1 g IM once.

Plague pneumonia—For persons with respiratory exposure to a patient with *Yersinia pestis* pneumonia: tetracycline, 15–30 mg/kg in four divided doses (250–500 mg qid).

Urinary tract infection—Prophylaxis is not indicated for prevention of urinary tract infections in patients with indwelling urinary catheters.

Tuberculosis—For individuals with a positive tuberculin test result and no evidence of active disease who are either younger than 35 years of age or (1) are recent skin test converters, (2) have had recent contact with active tuberculosis, (3) have an underlying predisposition caused by immunosuppressive disease or therapy, or (4) show evidence of inactive disease on chest radiographs: isoniazid, 300 mg/day by mouth for 6 months.

HIV—The risk of HIV transmission after exposure to infected body fluids varies with the route of exposure and the type of body fluid. Infectivity is greatest in percutaneous injury with a hollow-bore needle, and is less in injuries with suture needles or mucocutaneous splash injuries. Blood contact carries the highest risk of infection; the risk is less with contact with semen or cervical secretions, and is negligible with urine, sputum, saliva, and tears. Postexposure prophylaxis has not been studied in a randomized fashion, and HIV conversion has occurred after occupational exposure despite immediate initiation of prophylaxis. For workers sustaining an injury that carries a substantial risk of infection (e.g., HIV-positive blood inoculation through a hollow-bore needle), consideration can be given to postexposure prophylaxis using 200 mg of zidovudine (AZT) by mouth five times daily for 4 to 6 weeks. Other regimens have been suggested, especially if the source is likely to be zidovudine resistant.

Influenza—For high-risk persons during influenza A outbreaks who have not been immunized: immunization followed by either amantadine, 200 mg/day orally, or rimantadine, 200 mg/day orally, for 2 weeks. If a high-risk individual is unable to receive vaccination and has been exposed to influenza, prophylaxis with amantadine or rimantadine should be extended to 6 weeks.

Varicella-zoster virus (VZV)—Postexposure prophylaxis should be considered in individuals at risk of complications from VZV who have no history of chickenpox. Antibody-negative persons at risk for complications of VZV include the following: (1) those with congenital cellular immunodeficiency; (2) persons with AIDS; (3) persons receiving cytoreductive chemotherapy or radiation therapy; (4) persons on steroids (at doses greater than 1 mg/kg/day of prednisone); and (5) pregnant women. High-risk individuals exposed to VZV may be treated with 800 mg of acyclovir three times a day for 7 days. If exposure has occurred within approximately the last 4 days, varicella-zoster immune globulin also may be given to reduce the risk of development of varicella.

Pneumocystis carinii—For immunosuppressed patients at high risk for Pneumocystis infections: 5 mg/kg of trimethoprim (TMP) plus 25 mg/kg of sulfamethoxazole (SMZ) daily in two divided doses. This therapy in AIDS patients is associated with a high rate of drug reactions. Giving 50 mg of dapsone by mouth daily or 300 mg of pentamidine by inhalation every 4 weeks are alternatives for AIDS patients.

ANTIMICROBIALS USEFUL IN THE CRITICAL CARE UNIT ■

PENICILLINS

The first and still one of the most widely used groups of antibiotics is the penicillins. Penicillins are generally well-tolerated and are bactericidal against a broad range of pathogens. The usefulness of the prototype drug, penicillin G, has been extended by the advent of new classes of penicillins with extended activity. The most important problem with the penicillins is allergic reactions, which occur in 1% to 10% of patients and include skin rashes (more common with ampicillin), drug fever, and anaphylaxis. A patient allergic to one penicillin should be considered allergic to all penicillins. These drugs penetrate well into all body tissues except unin-

flamed meninges. The high ratio of toxic-to-therapeutic dose and improved penetration in the presence of inflammation makes treatment of even CNS infection possible with high doses. The main pathway of excretion of the penicillins is by the kidneys, with dose-related CNS excitability (myoclonic jerks and seizures) seen only in patients given high doses in the presence of renal failure. High-dose penicillin also may cause platelet dysfunction (carbenicillin and ticarcillin), interstitial nephritis (methicillin), hepatitis (oxacillin), neutropenia (nafcillin), hyperkalemia (potassium penicillin G), hypokalemia or sodium overload (carbenicillin), or antibiotic-associated colitis (ampicillin).

PENICILLIN G. Penicillin G (parenteral) is the drug of choice for group A streptococci, pneumococci, *Neisseria*, and penicillin-sensitive staphylococcal infections.

PENICILLINASE-RESISTANT PENICILLINS. Penicillinase-resistant penicillins (oxacillin, nafcillin) are the drugs of choice for penicillinase-producing staphylococci. They are also effective against penicillin-sensitive streptococci and pneumococci. Methicillin is rarely used because of the risk of interstitial nephritis. Staphylococci resistant to these agents ("methicillin-resistant") also are resistant to the cephalosporins and should be treated with vancomycin.

EXTENDED SPECTRUM PENICILLINS. Extended spectrum penicillins (ampicillin) has activity similar to penicillin G, with additional activity against many strains of *H influenzae*, *Escherichia coli*, *Proteus mirabilis*, *Salmonella*, and *Shigella*. They are not active against penicillin-resistant staphylococci. Skin rash is common with ampicillin, especially in patients with mononucleosis.

ANTI-PSEUDOMONAL PENICILLINS. Anti-pseudomonal penicillins (carbenicillin, ticarcillin, piperacillin, azlocillin, mezlocillin) have a spectrum that includes the organisms sensitive to ampicillin. They are also active against some anaerobes, indole-positive *Proteus*, *Enterobacter*, and *Pseudomonas*. Piperacillin, mezlocillin, and azlocillin are more active than carbenicillin and ticarcillin, particularly against *Klebsiella* and *Pseudomonas*, with piperacillin being the most active of the three. Sodium overload and hypokalemia are problems with carbenicillin and ticarcillin. Platelet dysfunction may occur with any of this group, with mezlocillin having some advantages in this regard. If these agents are used alone, resistance may emerge during therapy. Serious infections are generally treated with a combination of one of these agents with an aminoglycoside. None of these agents is active against penicillin-resistant staphylococci.

β-LACTAM INHIBITOR–PENICILLIN COMBINATIONS. Combinations of a β-lactam inhibitor plus a penicillin (sulbactam plus ampicillin, clavulanic acid plus ticarcillin, tazobactam plus piperacillin) amplify the spectrum of effectiveness of the parent penicillin against some β-lactamase–producing organisms such as *Klebsiella*, *H influenzae*, methicillin-sensitive *S aureus*, and some *Proteus* strains. They have excellent activity against anaerobes, including *Bacteroides fragilis*. Notice that the usual dose of piperacillin-tazobactam (3.375 g every 6 hours) is not adequate to treat serious *Pseudomonas* infections.[28]

CEPHALOSPORINS

The cephalosporins share many of the properties of the penicillins, including bactericidal activity based on the presence of a β-lactam ring. They are generally well tolerated and are predominantly excreted by the kidneys. They may also cause allergic reactions, and a patient allergic to one cephalosporin should be considered allergic to all. Cephalosporins are frequently used as an alternative drug in patients with penicillin allergy, but patients allergic to penicillin may be at increased risk for cephalosporin allergy. Cephalosporins are relatively contraindicated in patients with a history of an immediate anaphylactic reaction to penicillin. Disulfiram reactions are seen with cefamandole and cefoperazone. Cephalosporins may potentiate nephrotoxicity of other agents, including aminoglycosides and loop diuretics.

Cephalosporins are usually divided into three generations, based on differences in antibacterial spectrum. In general, second- and third-generation cephalosporins have superior activity against gram-negative rods, with some loss of activity against gram-positive cocci, especially *Staphylococcus*. Cephalosporins also differ in pharmacologic makeup; some are suitable for oral administration, and there are differences in dose and half-life. None of the first- or second-generation cephalosporins are effective in the treatment of meningitis, but the third-generation agents have good CSF activity. The clinician's confusion and hospital costs may be minimized by the recognition that the drugs within each generation are similar. The hospital may choose to stock only one drug from each generation (perhaps two of the second-generation group) and test that drug in the microbiology laboratory. The choice among otherwise equivalent drugs may be made on the basis of cost.

FIRST-GENERATION CEPHALOSPORINS. First-generation cephalosporins (cephalothin, cephapirin, cephradine, cefazolin) show good activity against methicillin-sensitive staphylococci, streptococci (other than enterococci), *E coli*, *P mirabilis*, and *Klebsiella pneumoniae*. Cephalothin frequently causes phlebitis. Cefazolin is better tolerated IM, has a longer half-life, and requires lower doses at longer intervals.

SECOND-GENERATION CEPHALOSPORINS. Second-generation cephalosporins include cefoxitin, cefmetazole, cefotetan, cefamandole, cefonicid, ceforanide, and cefuroxime. They have increased activity against gram-negative organisms, with some loss of gram-positive activity. Cefoxitin and cefotetan have improved activity against anaerobes, including *B fragilis*. The other drugs are more active against *H influenzae* and some gram-negative organisms. Cephamandole may be associated with prolonged prothrombin times. Cefonicid and ceforanide have longer half-lives. Cefuroxime is the only second-generation drug to provide good activity in CSF.

THIRD-GENERATION CEPHALOSPORINS. The third-generation cephalosporins include cefotaxime, cefepime, cefoperazone, ceftizoxime, ceftriaxone, and ceftazidime. They have an even broader spectrum of activity against gram-negative organisms, including some multidrug-resistant nos-

ocomial organisms and some strains of *P aeruginosa*, with further loss of gram-positive activity. They also have excellent activity against the penicillinase-producing gonococci and *H influenzae* and moderate activity against anaerobes, including *B fragilis*. Cefotaxime, ceftizoxime, and ceftriaxone have the best gram-positive activity and are particularly useful in meningitis caused by enteric gram-negative rods; they are acceptable alternatives for meningitis caused by *H influenzae* and *Neisseria*. Ceftazidime and cefepime are the most active against *P aeruginosa*. Ceftriaxone has a longer half-life but decreased activity against *Pseudomonas* and *Bacteroides*. Cefoperazone has been associated with increased bleeding and prolonged prothrombin time. Resistant strains, especially of *Pseudomonas* and *Enterobacter*, may emerge during therapy and continue to be a problem.

OTHER β-LACTAM ANTIBIOTICS

The broadest spectrum antibiotic to appear is imipenem, the first of the carbapenems. The drug is given in fixed combination with cilastatin, which inhibits a renal peptidase, improves urinary levels of active drug, and prevents formation of a toxic metabolite. The spectrum of activity includes gram-positive cocci (except methicillin-resistant staphylococci and some enterococci), anaerobic bacteria (including *B fragilis*), and gram-negative rods (except *Xanthomonas*, *Flavobacterium*, and some *Pseudomonas* species), although resistant *Pseudomonas* has emerged during therapy, particularly of pneumonia. Addition of an aminoglycoside should be considered in this situation. Imipenem is not effective against *Mycoplasma* or *Chlamydia*. Clinical experience is still limited, and there is insufficient evidence to assess efficacy in meningitis. Side effects are similar to the other β-lactam antibiotics, including allergy, thrombophlebitis, and superinfections. Allergic reactions may be more common in patients allergic to penicillin or cephalosporins. Seizures occur in up to 1% of patients. Old age, renal insufficiency, previous neurologic injury, and a high dose of imipenem increase this risk. Rapid infusions have been associated with nausea, vomiting, and occasional hypotension, which was reversible with slowing of the infusion rate. Meropenem (not yet released) seems to have a spectrum of activity similar to that of imipenem, but may have less risk of seizures.

Aztreonam, a monobactam, has a spectrum similar to the aminoglycosides. It is active against gram-negative bacteria, including *P aeruginosa*, but is inactive against gram-positive cocci and anaerobes. The toxicity is similar to other β-lactams, including local reactions at the site of injection, allergic reactions, diarrhea, nausea, and vomiting. Aztreonam seems to be safe to use in patients allergic to other β-lactams.

AMINOGLYCOSIDES

Aminoglycosides (gentamicin, tobramycin, amikacin, streptomycin) must be given parenterally and are renally excreted. Their spectrum of activity includes aerobic and facultative gram-negative rods, including most strains of *P aeruginosa*. They have poor activity against anaerobes and some gram-positive cocci such as the pneumococcus. They do not penetrate the CNS well, and do not work well in an acid environment (e.g., in abscesses). The usual mechanism of resistance is inactivation by a variety of bacterial enzymes. All aminoglycosides require dose modification and serum level monitoring in patients with renal insufficiency. In renal insufficiency, the initial dose is unchanged, and subsequently the same dose is given at adjusted intervals. Inadequate drug levels are associated with treatment failure. In critically ill patients, the first dose may be doubled to ensure adequate initial therapy.

The aminoglycosides are similar in terms of metabolism and toxicity; ototoxicity (both auditory and vestibular) and nephrotoxicity are the main problems. Ototoxicity and nephrotoxicity are uncommon until the patient has been on aminoglycosides for more than 1 week. Ototoxicity may be irreversible even if therapy is stopped, and the resultant vestibulotoxicity may be particularly disabling. The risk of ototoxicity and nephrotoxicity increases if aminoglycosides fail to reach a low trough. Thus, frequent monitoring of aminoglycoside levels is indicated. In patients with renal insufficiency, aminoglycosides should not be withheld in potentially life-threatening gram-negative infections; dosing by trough can minimize the risk of toxicity. Less common toxic effects include increased neuromuscular blockade and neuropathy; aminoglycosides should be used with caution (if at all) in patients with myasthenia gravis.

Gentamicin and tobramycin are almost indistinguishable clinically, with the same recommended dosages, similar spectra of activity, and the same optimal serum levels. Gentamicin can be used for synergy against *Enterococcus faecium*; tobramycin and amikacin are ineffective against *E faecium*. Tobramycin has marginally better activity against *Pseudomonas*, and gentamicin has marginally better activity against *Serratia*.

Amikacin is similar to gentamicin except that the milligram per kilogram per day dose is three times greater, and amikacin is active against some gram-negative rods that are resistant to gentamicin. This broader activity results from the greater resistance of amikacin to enzyme inactivation.

Streptomycin is not commonly used because of a high incidence of ototoxicity but may have a role in the treatment of multidrug-resistant tuberculosis.

Dosing of Aminoglycosides

Aminoglycosides can be dosed one to three times daily. Once daily aminoglycoside dosing is less nephrotoxic than more frequent dosing and is efficacious in gram-negative infections.[29] Daily dosing of aminoglycosides has not been studied in infective endocarditis; until further data are available, aminoglycosides should be dosed every 8 to 12 hours for endocarditis therapy.

Target aminoglycoside levels are shown in Table 105-7. The peak levels of an aminoglycosides correlate with efficacy. Optimal levels vary with the dosing frequency and the type of infection being treated. Higher peak levels are achieved if the aminoglycoside is being dosed only once daily. Lower levels are required if the drug is being used for synergy (e.g., *Enterococcus*, coagulase-negative *Staphylococcus*), whereas higher levels are needed to treat pneumonia. Aminoglycoside peaks should be drawn 30 minutes after a dose finishes infusing.

Aminoglycosides are renally cleared, and small decrements in creatinine clearance allow the accumulation of aminoglycosides (and thus increase the risk of nephrotoxicity from these agents). Thus, a small rise in creatinine should prompt the checking of aminoglycoside levels and appropriate dosage adjustment. In patients with acute or chronic renal insufficiency, aminoglycosides should be dosed less frequently to allow the trough to reach adequately low levels. Dosing of aminoglycosides in renal failure is discussed in Chapter 143.

A recommended initial dosage in patients with normal renal function (for tobramycin or gentamicin) is 5 to 6 mg/kg IV every 24 hours or 2 to 3 mg/kg IV every 12 hours. For amikacin, a starting dose of 15 mg/kg every 24 hours or 7.5 mg/kg every 12 hours can be used. Patients with cystic fibrosis have increased clearance of aminoglycosides; tobramycin or gentamicin should be dosed at 7.5 to 10 mg/kg/day to achieve therapeutic levels.

TETRACYCLINES

The tetracyclines (tetracycline, doxycycline, minocycline) are available for parenteral and oral use. Parenteral tetracyclines may cause severe liver toxicity, especially in pregnant women. Except for doxycycline, tetracyclines cause increased catabolism with elevations of blood urea nitrogen in patients with renal insufficiency. Tetracyclines are relatively contraindicated in children younger than 8 years of age because of tooth staining. Doxycycline is often used in patients with renal failure because it is excreted by the liver and no dose adjustment is needed. Oral absorption is decreased by antacids. Tetracyclines are bacteriostatic but have

TABLE 105-7. Optimal Aminoglycoside Levels

SITUATION	GENTAMICIN OR TOBRAMYCIN	AMIKACIN
Trough	<2	<8
Peak—every 12-h therapy		
Synergy	4	12
Primary therapy	6	18
Pneumonia	8	24
Peak—every 24-h therapy	15	45

a broad range of activity against gram-positive and gram-negative bacteria, as well as *Chlamydia* and *Rickettsia*. They are primarily indicated in a variety of uncommon infections including Rocky Mountain spotted fever, plague, psittacosis, lymphogranuloma venereum, cholera, and brucellosis.

MACROLIDES

The macrolides include erythromycin, azithromycin, and clarithromycin. Erythromycin is available in oral and parenteral forms, whereas the other two macrolides are available only in oral forms. The spectrum of activity includes most gram-positive bacteria, including *S aureus*, nonenterococcal streptococci, pneumococci, *Corynebacterium diphtheriae*, *Legionella*, *Bordetella pertussis*, *Campylobacter*; *Mycoplasma pneumoniae*, and *Chlamydia*. Erythromycin's status as the drug of choice against *Legionella* has earned it a role in the empirical therapy of overwhelming pneumonia. Resistant strains of staphylococci are relatively common in the hospital environment, and this drug should not be relied on for coverage in serious infections. Serious infections should be treated IV. Erythromycin (given orally or IV) often causes abdominal distress, including nausea, vomiting, and diarrhea. These side effects are less common with azithromycin and clarithromycin. With intravenous administration, local phlebitis is common and may be severe. Phlebitis can be decreased by mixing the dose in 250 to 500 mL of normal saline with 10 mg of hydrocortisone and infusing over 2 to 3 hours. Erythromycin estolate and, less commonly, other erythromycins may cause cholestatic jaundice. High doses of erythromycin (4 g/day) can cause reversible hearing loss, which may be profound. Hearing generally returns within several days of the cessation of treatment.

CLINDAMYCIN

Clindamycin can be given orally or parenterally and is generally well tolerated. It is bacteriostatic and is active against gram-positive cocci, including *S aureus*, streptococci, pneumococci, but not enterococci. Its main niche is found in the treatment of anaerobic infection, including *B fragilis*. It is not active against clostridia other than *Clostridium perfringens* and *Clostridium tetani*. It penetrates well into all tissues other than the CNS and the meninges. The main side effect is diarrhea, which is usually nonspecific but may include antibiotic-associated colitis caused by *C difficile*.

VANCOMYCIN

Vancomycin is a bactericidal antibiotic that interferes with cell wall synthesis. It is active against gram-positive bacteria, including *S aureus*, streptococci (including the enterococcus), pneumococcus, *Clostridium*, and *Corynebacterium*. It is excreted almost entirely by the kidneys. The dosage must be modified in patients with renal insufficiency by multiplying the dosage interval by the creatinine. In patients on dialysis, 1 g IV per week has been effective in treating staphylococcal infections. Toxicity includes local phlebitis, allergic reactions, drug fever, ototoxicity, and nephrotoxicity. The risks of nephrotoxicity and ototoxicity are increased by the concomitant use of an aminoglycoside. Rapid intravenous infusion can cause flushing of the face, neck, and trunk with hypotension, termed the *red man syndrome*. This reaction is not an allergic one, and can be decreased by giving the drug over 2 to 3 hours. Vancomycin given orally is not well absorbed, and its oral use is limited to antibiotic-associated colitis caused by *C difficile* that has failed metronidazole treatment. The dose for *C difficile* is 250 mg by mouth every 6 hours; intravenous administration is generally inadequate for the treatment of colitis. Parenteral vancomycin is useful for serious infections with gram-positive organisms in penicillin-allergic patients and for infections with methicillin-resistant staphylococci or penicillin-resistant corynebacteria. It is also useful in prophylaxis for endocarditis in cardiovascular surgery.

TRIMETHOPRIM/SULFAMETHOXAZOLE

A fixed-dose combination of TMP, a folic acid antagonist, and a SMZ (TMP/SMZ) has activity against pneumococci and some gram-negative rods, including *H influenzae* and *Legionella*. It may be given orally or parenterally and penetrates all body spaces well. The principal use for TMP/SMZ is in the treatment of urinary tract infections, bronchitis, otitis, and enteric infections such as shigellosis. In the ICU, it is often given for treatment of *P carinii* pneumonia. Toxicity includes allergic reactions, crystalluria, hemolytic anemia, megaloblastic anemia, and thrombocytopenia. The dose must be adjusted for renal insufficiency. Serum levels may be useful for severe disease.

METRONIDAZOLE

Metronidazole is available for oral and parenteral administration. It is a bactericidal agent with activity essentially limited to anaerobic bacteria. Microaerophilic streptococci may be resistant, and failures have been reported in pleuropulmonary infections. It is used to treat serious anaerobic infections and may have a special advantage in brain abscesses. It is also effective in colitis caused by *C difficile*. Toxicity includes nausea, a metallic taste in the mouth, disulfiram reactions, stomatitis, and paresthesias. Metronidazole is teratogenic and carcinogenic in animals, but these effects have not been shown in humans.

QUINOLONES

Quinolones (ciprofloxacin, ofloxacin, lomefloxacin) inhibit DNA gyrase, which controls the supercoiling of bacterial DNA. Quinolones are bactericidal against many gram-negative rods (including *P aeruginosa*), with lesser activity against staphylococci. The quinolones have little activity against anaerobes and streptococci. Ciprofloxacin and ofloxacin are available for oral or intravenous use. Most clinical experience exists with ciprofloxacin, which also is the most active against *P aeruginosa*. Ciprofloxacin is effective against urinary, enteric, and systemic infections. The quinolones should be used with caution in respiratory infections because they have unreliable activity against streptococci. Quinolones may be useful for prophylaxis of infection in neutropenic patients.[27]

Some quinolones undergo liver metabolism, and all are excreted in the urine. Toxicity seems to be modest, consisting of nausea, dizziness, rash, insomnia, diarrhea, and allergic reactions. Although the quinolones seem to be useful, their cost is high compared with that of other urinary tract drugs; also, resistance can emerge. Their greatest value may be in providing oral alternatives for therapy, lessening the risks and costs of parenteral treatment.

ANTIFUNGAL AGENTS

Amphotericin B

Amphotericin B remains the most effective therapy for serious fungal infection.[30] It is the drug of choice for most systemic fungal infections (except chromoblastomycosis, *Candida lusitaniae*, and *Pseudallescheria boydii*) in seriously ill patients.[31] In nonneutropenic patients with candidemia, fluconazole is a safe alternative to systemic amphotericin.[32] Amphotericin must be given IV, where it binds to cell membranes and body proteins, with slow excretion over a period of weeks to months. The drug must be diluted in 5% dextrose in water (because salt-containing solutions cause precipitation) and infused over 2 to 6 hours. The spectrum of activity includes almost all pathogenic fungi, with uncommon resistant isolates. Toxicity is common with fever, chills, malaise, anemia, and thrombophlebitis in most patients. Prior administration of antipyretics, an antihistamine, meperidine, or hydrocortisone (25 to 50 mg) may help mitigate chills and fever. The most important toxicity is azotemia,[33] which is usually reversible on discontinuation of the drug or lowering of the dose. Most clinicians use a creatinine of 3.0 mg% or a blood urea nitrogen level of 30 mg/dL as an indication to discontinue the drug briefly or to lower the dose if possible. In patients with preexisting renal failure, no dose adjustment is needed. Anemia and hypokalemia are common, and transfusion or potassium supplementation may be required. Patients also frequently complain of malaise, headache, nausea, vomiting, and weight loss.

The dose and duration of amphotericin B therapy is not well defined for most infections. In indolent infections, patients are treated with incremental doses, beginning with 1 mg over 20 to 30 minutes. On successive days, the dose is increased by 5 to 10 mg/day until a desired dose of 0.3 to 0.6 mg/kg/day is reached. In critically ill patients, escalating doses may be given immediately after each other, and doses as high as 1.2 mg/kg/day may be required in serious fungal infections. Patients with serious fungal infections are usually treated for 6 to 12 weeks to a total dose of 2 to 3 g. *Candida* infections, especially of mucous membranes, may be treated with smaller doses on the order of 500 mg. Meningeal infections, especially meningeal *Coccidioidomycosis*, may require supplemental intrathecal administration because of the poor penetration of amphotericin B into CSF.

Azoles

Azoles (ketoconazole, itraconazole, fluconazole) are a group of antifungal drugs that inhibit the demethylase enzyme in the biosynthetic pathway of of ergosterol, one of the constituents of the fungal cell membrane. Fluconazole is available for intravenous or oral use; ketoconazole and itraconazole are only available in oral form. The combination of high doses of azoles with antihistamines can cause torsades de pointes.

Ketoconazole is active against mucocutaneous candidiasis, dermatophytes, histoplasmosis, blastomycosis, paracoccidioidomycosis, and coccidioidomycosis. Absorption of ketoconazole and itraconazole requires stomach acid and is impaired by antacids or H_2 receptor blockers (e.g., cimetidine). Ketoconazole is not a first-line drug for acute systemic infections because of the usual slow clinical response. It is primarily of value in less serious infections; treatment must be prolonged, and relapses occur after discontinuation. Nausea, vomiting, and toxic hepatitis are the usual dose-limiting toxicities. Decreased steroid synthesis with decreased testosterone and adrenal function may occur.

Oral fluconazole is better tolerated than ketoconazole, and absorption is not dependent on stomach acid. Its spectrum of activity is similar to ketoconazole.[34] Because CSF levels are 80% of serum levels, it may also play a role in the treatment of cryptococcal meningitis.[35] It seems to be effective in oral and esophageal candidiasis. Fluconazole seems to be safe and effective in treating candidemia in nonneutropenic patients; *Torulopsis glabrata* and *Candida kruseii* may be resistant to fluconazole,[36] and fungemia with these organisms should probably be treated with systemic amphotericin. A trial comparing amphotericin and fluconazole in cryptococcal meningitis showed equivalent overall results, but an excess of early deaths in the fluconazole group suggests that initial treatment with amphotericin may be preferable. Fluconazole is useful in the chronic suppression of *Cryptococcus* in patients with AIDS.

Itraconazole is available for oral use and is absorbed better with food. It is useful for treatment of histoplasmosis and blastomycosis and for the prevention of relapse of disseminated histoplasmosis in AIDS patients.[37] Data on the use of itraconazole in the treatment of other fungal infections are limited.

ANTIVIRAL AGENTS

Agents effective against acute and chronic viral infections are becoming available. Use of these agents is often limited by high cost, toxicity, limited efficacy, limited availability of viral culture and sensitivity studies, and emergence of resistance. Despite this, in some situations, antiviral chemotherapy can be lifesaving. Except for foscarnet and amantadine, all of the following drugs are nucleoside analogues. Because of this, they are known or suspected to be mutagenic and teratogenic. They are relatively contraindicated in pregnant women. The use of gloves and safety hoods is prudent in handling these drugs to prevent exposure of caregivers.

Acyclovir

Acyclovir is available for oral and intravenous use. It is active against herpes simplex virus and VZV infections. Intravenous acyclovir is effective against these infections in compromised hosts,[38] primary herpetic infections in normal hosts, and herpes encephalitis. Oral acyclovir is incompletely absorbed, but is effective in preventing recurrences of genital and labial herpes,[39] and is of modest benefit in treating herpes zoster or recurrent herpesvirus infections in normal hosts. Toxicity includes crystalluria with renal impairment and encephalopathic changes,[40] particularly with high doses or in patients with renal insufficiency. Emergence of resistant strains of herpes simplex virus has been associated with clinical failure in some immunocompromised patients.[41] Famciclovir has been licensed for use in treating herpes zoster in normal hosts, but is not recommended in immunocompromised hosts or those with primary chickenpox.[42]

Amantadine and Rimantadine

The spectrum of amantadine and rimantadine is limited to influenza A viruses. It is effective in preventing clinical infection[43] and is of modest benefit in shortening the duration and severity of infection if begun within 48 hours of the onset of clinical illness. It is of particular benefit when a strain-specific vaccine is not available or has not been administered. These drugs can be used in immunocompromised persons who may not respond to the vaccine.[44] Toxicity includes mild CNS excitability, which is seen more often with amantadine than with rimantadine. Amantadine and rimantadine are teratogenic in animals and should not be given to pregnant women. Rimantadine seems to have less CNS toxicity, but is more expensive than amantadine.

Foscarnet

Foscarnet is used in selected settings in the treatment of cytomegalovirus (CMV) and herpes simplex virus infections in AIDS. The most important toxicity is renal insufficiency, but seizures and electrolyte disturbances may occur.

Ganciclovir

Ganciclovir is active against CMV. It is available for intravenous administration and is primarily excreted in the urine. It is clearly effective against CMV retinitis in AIDS patients. Its role in other CMV infections such as gastrointestinal infection in AIDS patients and pneumonia in bone marrow transplant patients is less certain. Ganciclovir is teratogenic and carcinogenic in animals. In humans, the primary toxicities are neutropenia and thrombocytopenia. Its myelosuppressive effects are additive to zidovudine,[45] and the combination is often poorly tolerated. The oral form of ganciclovir is poorly absorbed and seems to be useful only in the chronic suppression of CMV retinitis.

Ribavirin

Ribavirin is a synthetic nucleoside that has been demonstrated to be clinically effective against respiratory syncytial virus when administered by aerosol, and Lassa fever by intravenous route. The aerosol may cause bronchospasm in patients with hyperreactive airways. Use of ribavirin is problematic in view of cost, uncertainty of long-term benefit, and environmental contamination.

Nucleoside Analogues

The nucleoside analogues (zidovudine, dideoxyinosine, dideoxycytidine) are active against HIV. AZT is most commonly used in the treatment of HIV. Postexposure prophylaxis with AZT may decrease the risk of transmission of HIV, although failures do occur. The most serious toxicities of AZT are anemia and neutropenia; these are dose related and are more common in patients with advanced disease or those who are treated with other myelosuppressive drugs. A myopathy may occur related to the drug or the HIV infection.

Dideoxyinosine (ddI) is available for HIV-infected patients who have failed treatment or do not tolerate AZT. Dideoxycytidine is reserved for ddI failures. Neither causes bone marrow toxicity. Both can cause peripheral neuropathy. ddI is associated with pancreatitis, which may be severe.

REFERENCES ■

1. Jauregui L, Cushing RD, Lerner AM: Gentamicin/amikacin resistant gram-negative bacilli at Detroit General Hospital. *Am J Med* 1977;62:882
2. Adams HG, Jordan C: Infections in the alcoholic. *Med Clin North Am* 1984;68:179
3. Mezzano S, Pesce AJ, Pollak VE, et al: Analysis of humoral and cellular factors that contribute to impaired immune responsiveness in experimental uremia. *Nephron* 1984;36:15
4. Crespo J: Dialysis related infections. *Heart Lung* 1982;11:111
5. Rayfield EJ, Ault MJ, Keusch GT, et al: Infection and diabetes: the case for glucose control. *Am J Med* 1982;72:439
6. Gordon JE, Scrimshaw NS: Infectious disease in the malnourished. *Med Clin North Am* 1970;54:1495
7. Armstrong D: Empiric therapy for the immunocompromised host. *Rev Infect Dis* 1991;13(Suppl 9):S763
8. Green GR, Peters GA, Geraci JE: Treatment of bacterial endocarditis in patients with penicillin hypersensitivity. *Ann Intern Med* 1967;67:235
9. Sullivan TJ: In: Middleton E, et al (eds). *Allergy: Principles and Practice.* St Louis, CV Mosby, 1989:1523
10. Rohr, Saxon: *Ann Intern Med* 1987;107:204
11. The choice of antimicrobials. *Med Lett* 1994;36:53
12. Aronson M, Bor D: Blood cultures. *Ann Intern Med* 1987; 106:246
13. Tompsett R, Pizette M: Enterococcal endocarditis: lack of correlation between therapeutic results and antibiotic sensitivity tests. *Arch Intern Med* 1962;109:146
14. McCracken GH: Management of bacterial meningitis: current status and future prospects. *Am J Med* 1984;76:215
15. Klasterski J, Cappel R, Daneau D: Clinical significance of in vitro synergism between antibiotics in gram negative infections. *Antimicrob Agents Chemother* 1972;2:470
16. Cost of some parenteral antibiotics. *Med Lett* 1994;36:8
17. Finkel AS, Hammond JM, Karlin DS, et al: 1995 Drug Topics Red Book. Montvale, NJ: Medical Economics, 1995
18. Rudolph AH, Price EV: Penicillin reactions among patients in venereal disease clinics: a national survey. *JAMA* 1973;223: 449
19. Lepper MH, Dowling HF: Treatment of pneumococcic meningitis with penicillin compared with penicillin plus aureomycin. *Arch Intern Med* 1951;88:489
20. Pizzo PA: Management of fever in patients with cancer and treatment-induced neutropenia. *N Engl J Med* 1993;328:1323

21. Initial therapy for tuberculosis in the era of multidrug resistance. *MMWR* 1993;42 RR-7:1

22. Bisno AL, et al: Antimicrobial treatment of infective endocarditis due to viridans streptococci, enterococci, and staphylococci. *JAMA* 1989;261:1471

23. Chambers, et al: Right-sided *Staphylococcus aureus* endocarditis in intravenous drug abusers: two-week combination therapy. *Ann Intern Med* 1989;109:619

24. Simon GL, et al: Clinical trial of piperacillin with acquisition of resistance by *Pseudomonas* and clinical relapse. *Antimicrob Agents Chemother* 1980;18:167

25. Antimicrobial prophylaxis in surgery. *Med Lett* 1993;35:91

26. Simmons BP: Guideline for the prevention of surgical and wound infections. *Am J Infect Control* 1984;11:133

27. Winston DJ, Winston GH, Nakao SL, et al: Norfloxacin versus vancomycin/polymyxin for prevention of infections in granulocytopenic patients. *Am J Med* 1986;80:884

28. A reminder: piperacillin/tazobactam is not for *Pseudomonas*. *Med Lett* 1994;36:110

29. Gilbert DW: Once-daily aminoglycoside dosing. *Antimicrob Agents Chemother* 1991;35:399

30. Armstrong D: Treatment of opportunistic fungal infections. *Clin Infect Dis* 1993;16:1

31. Systemic antifungal drugs. *Med Lett* 1994;36:16

32. Rex JH, et al: A randomized trial comparing fluconazole with amphotericin B for the treatment of candidemia in patients without neutropenia. *N Engl J Med* 1994;331:1325

33. Perfect JA, et al: Adverse drug reactions to systemic antifungals: prevention and management. *Drug Safety* 1992;7:323

34. Zervos, et al: Fluconazole in fungal infections: a review. *Infect Dis Clin Practice* 1994;3:94

35. Saag, et al: Comparison of amphotericin B with fluconazole in the treatment of acute AIDS-associated cryptococcal meningitis. *N Engl J Med* 1992;326:83

36. Hitchcock CA, et al: Fluconazole resistance in *Candida glabrata*. *Antimicrob Agents Chemother* 1993;37:1962

37. Como JA, Dismukes WE: Oral azole drugs as systemic antifungal therapy. *N Engl J Med* 1994;330:263

38. Wagstaff AJ, et al: Acyclovir: a reappraisal of its antiviral activity, pharmacokinetic properties and therapeutic value. *Drugs* 1994;47:153

39. Goldberg LH, et al: Long-term suppression of recurrent genital herpes with acyclovir. *Arch Dermatol* 1993;129:582

40. Eck P, et al: Acute renal failure and coma after a high dose of oral acyclovir. *N Engl J Med* 1991;325:1178

41. Kost RG, et al: Brief report: recurrent acyclovir-resistant genital herpes in an immunocompetent host. *N Engl J Med* 1993;329:1777

42. Famciclovir for herpes zoster. *Med Lett* 1994;36:97

43. *Med Lett* 1993;35:109

44. Prevention and control of influenza: recommendations of the advisory committee on immunization practices (ACIP). *MMWR* 1995;Apr 21:44(RR-3):1

45. Hochster H, et al: Toxicity of combined ganciclovir and zidovudine for cytomegalovirus disease associated with AIDS. *Ann Intern Med* 1990;113:111

Critical Care, Third Edition, edited by Joseph M. Civetta,
Robert W. Taylor, and Robert R. Kirby.
Lippincott-Raven Publishers, Philadelphia, PA © 1997.

CHAPTER 106

■

The Prevalence and Importance of Nosocomial Infections in the Intensive Care Unit

Mark G. McKenney
Scott Norwood

IMMEDIATE CONCERNS ■

MAJOR PROBLEMS

The emergence of critical care units and advances in managing single organ system failure have created the potential for recovery in patients who otherwise would not have survived. However, prolonged survival in critical care units has created a unique and equally deadly problem: multiple organ system failure (MOSF), which usually results from the metabolic and immunologic responses to infection.

Centralization of care for critically ill patients, although advantageous from a care delivery standpoint, creates significant problems for physicians and nurses charged with the prevention of hospital-acquired (nosocomial) infection. Nosocomial infection is defined as an infection that occurs in the hospital that was not present or incubating at the time of admission.[1] Nosocomial infections are endemic and epidemic in intensive care units (ICUs) and represent a significant source of morbidity, mortality, and cost.[2-8] Infections that develop in the critical care environment account for 25% of all nosocomial infections and rates are five to ten times higher than on general wards.[2,9] Hospital-wide

epidemiologic data may not accurately describe the ICU population.[10,11]

STRESS POINTS

1. The ICU patient is at risk for eight types of nosocomial infection:
   Pneumonia
   Intravascular catheter-related infections
   Wound infections
   Urinary tract infections (UTIs)
   Invasive fungal infections
   Sinusitis
   Antibiotic associated colitis
   Ventriculitis or meningitis from intracranial pressure (ICP) monitors
2. Prolonged mechanical ventilation, invasive monitoring, and antibiotic therapy are associated with a much higher incidence of nosocomial infection in the ICU.
3. Although positive cultures from various sites in septic ICU patients are frequently obtained, it is not clear whether these cultures represent true nosocomial infections, a fact that may be obscured in large epide-

miologic studies based solely on the presence or absence of positive cultures.

4. Pneumonia has the highest mortality rate of the nosocomial infections. Differentiating pneumonia from colonization is difficult because of early, rapid upper airway colonization with gram-negative bacteria.

5. High mortality rates may reflect inaccurate nosocomial infection diagnoses in patients with hypermetabolism and altered immune defenses rather than failed antimicrobial therapy.

6. Evaluation of catheter-related infection is confusing because of a variety of important clinical questions and the misinterpretation of the available data specific to critical care patients.

7. The diagnosis of "catheter-related infection," therefore, is made either by obvious clinical signs of local infection (which should be infrequent, because such signs occur relatively late in the course of catheterization) or by positive semiquantitative culture of a removed intracutaneous catheter segment.

8. Postoperative patients are also at risk for wound infections.

9. Infections from gram-positive and gram-negative organisms usually present within different time frames with different clinical scenarios.

10. Although urosepsis is a common problem epidemiologically, the urinary tract is not a common source of systemic sepsis in critically ill ICU patients.

11. Urosepsis is much more common in patients with urinary tract obstruction or instrumentation.

12. Patients who are intubated or have nasogastric tubes may develop sinusitis. Facial trauma is also a risk factor. Sinusitis may be the cause of fever in an ICU patient but rarely leads to life-threatening infection.

13. Head-injured patients with ICP monitors are at risk for ventriculitis and meningitis.

ESSENTIAL DIAGNOSTIC TESTS AND PROCEDURES

1. Fever, leukocytosis, purulent secretions, and radiographic demonstration of pulmonary infiltrates are nonspecific in the ICU population; interventions that provide a true diagnosis should be applied.

2. Quantitative cultures obtained bronchoscopically, using the protected specimen brush (PSB) or bronchoalveolar lavage (BAL), may be more accurate tests for diagnosing nosocomial pneumonia.

3. Consider catheter-related infections in terms of the interacting factors of the host, the organisms causing the infection, and the surrounding environment.

4. Obtain semiquantitative cultures of the intracutaneous segment of the catheter to diagnose catheter-related nosocomial infection. If 15 or more colonies of organisms are identified, remove the catheter to prevent subsequent bacteremia.[12]

5. All wounds should be examined for signs of infection. Such infections may develop after clean and clean-contaminated surgical procedures.

6. Bacteriuria and pyuria on urinalysis should signal the possibility of urosepsis, and only then should urine cultures be obtained.

7. Fungal infections seem to be increasing in ICUs.[13] Risk factors for developing invasive fungal infections are common in the critically ill patient and include antibiotic administration, parenteral nutrition, steroids, and organ transplantation.

8. Diagnosing fungal infection remains difficult because blood or urine culture results are positive in less than half the patients with disseminated disease.

9. A high index of suspicion for sinusitis should be reserved for any intubated patient with fever or foul-smelling nasal discharge. Diagnosis is confirmed with either ultrasound or computed tomographic scan. Infections are usually bacterial.

10. The "wonder drugs" given to so many ICU patients increase the risk of antibiotic-associated colitis, leading to an increased rate of infection.[14]

11. Diagnosis of antibiotic-associated colitis is suspected in patients who develop diarrhea and is confirmed by fecal assay for *Clostridium difficile* toxin.

12. Ventriculostomy infection rates up to 27% have been reported.[15] Infections have been related to length of ICP monitor use and contamination during insertion. Different diagnostic and treatment plans have been offered to provide early diagnosis and to limit infections.

INITIAL THERAPY

1. Empiric antibiotic therapy should be reserved for patients who are clinically septic, with signs of cardiovascular instability or persistent metabolic acidosis.

2. Also, consider antibiotic therapy when the consequences of bacteremia outweigh the risk of host colonization by pathogenic, antibiotic-resistant, or opportunistic microorganisms, such as in patients with prosthetic grafts.

3. Based on current definitions and considerations, replacement of an indwelling central venous or arterial catheter using a guidewire exchange (GWX) method and semiquantitative culture of the intracutaneous segment of the removed catheter is an appropriate diagnostic measure.

4. If the catheter segment culture is positive, remove the exchanged (new) catheter and insert another catheter at a different anatomic site.

5. Frequent bladder catheter changes and routine microbiologic monitoring of the urine usually are not helpful.

6. Amphotericin B has many side effects, making the decision to treat without clear evidence of an invasive fungal infection more complex.

7. Treatment of sinusitis consists of decongestants, nasal sprays, and broad-spectrum antibiotics. If this fails, drainage is indicated.

8. Vancomycin, metronidazole, and bacitracin have been used as treatment for antibiotic-associated colitis. With

the recent emergence of vancomycin-resistant entero-cocci, vancomycin should not be used to treat colitis. Relapses are common and careful follow-up is necessary.

RISK FACTORS AND SCOPE OF NOSOCOMIAL INFECTIONS IN CRITICAL ILLNESS ■

Developing an infection is a function of the virulence of the organism and the resistance of patient defense mechanisms. Common ICU isolates causing nosocomial infections usually are endogenous organisms with low intrinsic pathogenesis.[16] The risk factors for developing these infections are invasive procedures and altered host immunity, both of which are prevalent in the critically ill patient.

Invasive devices used in the critical care patient are inde-pendent risk factors for the development of nosocomial in-fections.[4,16] ICU patients who develop a nosocomial infection have an increased mortality rate, but cause and effect are unclear. Infections are usually minor or controlled. The ICU nosocomial infection is more likely to be another manifesta-tion of the underlying critical illness and not necessarily the cause. Marshall and Sweeney[8] studied infection and the septic response in 211 surgical intensive care unit (SICU) patients. Infection was established with microbiologic and radiographic results. A septic response score was also estab-lished based on core temperature, white blood cell count, Glasgow Coma Score, insulin requirements, and cardiac out-put. Infection was associated with an increased mortality, but the critical factor was the magnitude of the septic re-sponse and not the nature of the infection.

Immune function is dramatically altered in the critically ill patient.[17] Loss of delayed type hypersensitivity reaction is evident by inability to mount a response to skin testing with common antigens.[18] Impaired lymphocyte activation has been demonstrated in vitro in traumatized patients and is associated with increased infection and death.[19]

The overall mortality rate in patients with nosocomial infections approaches 44%,[4] but such epidemiologic data may be misleading because there is no good method for distinguishing between the impact of the patient's underly-ing disease and the offending pathogen in determining out-come. Analysis becomes more difficult when the nosocomial infection occurs in the ICU, where therapy is often begun before identifying a source or site of infection. Routine blood and sputum cultures are often nondiagnostic because of widespread antimicrobial use. Thus, existing epidemiologic data may not be relevant.

The definition of nosocomial infection may be somewhat artificial. To simplify data collection, many studies consider infections to be hospital acquired if the first samples from which isolated microorganisms are obtained were collected on or after the third hospital day.[21] The true definition is an infection that is neither present nor incubating at the time of admission to the hospital.[22] Unfortunately, this can be difficult to establish.

Patients who are treated in critical care units have a dramatically higher incidence of nosocomial infection than non-ICU hospitalized patients.[2,9,22–28] Sepsis and multiple or-gan system failure (MOSF) are the most common causes of late death in ICU patients.[22–26] The invasive devices designed to improve the chances for survival tend to increase coloniza-tion by nosocomial organisms and greatly increase the risk of infection in this vulnerable population.[25] Although surgical and trauma patients are less likely to have chronic underlying diseases than medical patients, surgical patients have twice the incidence of nosocomial infection because of greater exposure to invasive devices and multiple invasive proce-dures.[26,27] Chronic underlying disease states are more im-portant cofactors in predicting survival, but the frequent use of invasive devices more accurately predicts the risk of nosocomial infection.[27]

Large reviews attribute 30% to 40% of hospital-wide nosocomial infections to urinary tract sources. Surgical wounds account for 20%, pneumonia accounts for 15%, bacteremia for 7%, and various other sites for the remain-der.[22] The most common nosocomial infections in ICU pa-tients are attributed to the respiratory tract and intravascular catheter infections. Wound infections are common in SICUs but less common in medical ICUs. UTIs make up a smaller percentage of nosocomial infections in the ICU than on the general wards. CNS infections are unusual in the general wards but common in the subgroup of ICU patients with ICP monitors or after CNS surgery. Sinusitis, although not life threatening, is especially common in the intubated ICU patient. Although positive cultures are often obtained from various sites in most ICU patients, it is often unclear whether these positive cultures represent invasive infections.

Epidemiologic trends show not only an increase in differ-ent types of organisms, but also an increased frequency of polymicrobial infections.[29] At least 20% of nosocomial infections are caused by multiple pathogens, and the likeli-hood of isolating multiple organisms is particularly high for ICU patients, diabetic patients, and patients with altered host defenses.[30] It is not surprising that multiple organisms can be isolated from skin wounds, the respiratory tract, urine, and vascular devices in critically ill patients. It is not clear, however, whether organisms cultured from ICU patients represent true nosocomial infections, because "colonization" may be misrepresented as "infection" in large epidemiologic series. Therefore, nosocomial infection data that are not specific to ICU patients, although influencing standards of care, may not accurately reflect the true incidence of infec-tion in critically ill patients.

HOSPITAL-ACQUIRED RESPIRATORY INFECTIONS ■

Pneumonia is the most common fatal hospital-acquired in-fection, occurring in 9% to 21% of patients requiring me-chanical ventilation, with an associated mortality rate of 20% to 80%.[31–35] Gram-negative bacilli are the pathogens usually responsible for nosocomial infections (75% to 90% of cases), contributing significantly to the mortality rate of critically ill patients. The upper respiratory tracts of most patients intubated for more than 48 hours become colonized with gram-negative bacteria.[31,36] Others have estimated that 10% to 25% of critically ill surgical patients develop a true nosocomial pneumonia.[37] The percentage of true pneumonias seems to be high in patients with acute respiratory failure or direct thoracic trauma. This high mortality rate from theoretically reversible infections may be a function more of diagnostic inaccuracy and altered immune defenses in the critically ill ICU patient rather than antimicrobial therapeutic failure.

Making a diagnosis of nosocomial pneumonia in critically ill patients is not as straightforward as diagnosing community-acquired pneumonia. Most patients requiring mechanical ventilation for respiratory failure have, or will soon develop, fever, infiltrates, leukocytosis, and purulent secretions if intubated for more than 48 hours. Autopsy studies in patients with adult respiratory distress syndrome (ARDS) show that these clinical signs do not accurately predict the presence of pneumonia.[38,39] Other investigators have shown that less than 50% of intubated patients who develop these clinical signs have significant infections, as indicated by their clinical improvement *without* antibiotics.[40,41]

Because of rapid airway colonization, conventional bacteriologic methods for diagnosis often provide misleading information.[31] Organisms responsible for nosocomial pneumonia originate in the oropharynx[32] and intestinal tract.[42] Stress ulcer prophylaxis with gastric alkalinization contributes to upper gastrointestinal tract colonization and creates a source of organisms that may be silently aspirated into the respiratory tract.[43,44] In fact, altering the bacterial flora of the oropharynx and gastrointestinal tract may be the most important factor contributing to the increased incidence of pneumonia in critically ill patients.

One animal study showed that 9 of 11 nonhuman primates had gram-negative oropharyngeal colonization before the onset of gram-negative pneumonia.[45] Other studies show that up to 90% of ICU patients who develop pneumonia have prior oropharyngeal colonization with the same gram-negative bacterial species.[46,47] Oropharyngeal colonization with gram-negative bacteria is also related to the patient's general state of health and nutritional status.[48] Most clinicians, regrettably, have given up attempts to diagnose pneumonia in critically ill patients, electing instead to use broad-spectrum antimicrobial agents liberally.[41] Such therapy may be unnecessary, expensive, and harmful to the patient by potentiating upper airway and gut colonization with gram-negative and fungal organisms. It also seriously compromises efforts to diagnose future nonrespiratory infections precisely.[41]

Gram-negative bacterial adherence to epithelial cells is important in the pathogenesis of oropharyngeal colonization. Gram-positive organisms normally colonize the oropharynx and help to prevent adherence and colonization by gram-negative bacilli. "Colonized" patients have fewer gram-positive cocci and more gram-negative bacilli adherent per epithelial cell.[49] Although direct clinical evidence is lacking, fibronectin depletion may play a role in this colonization phenomenon: in vitro gram-positive cocci bind well to cells

rich in fibronectin, whereas gram-negative bacilli bind well only to epithelial cells that are deficient in this glycoprotein.[50,51] Regardless of the colonization mechanism, bacterial entry and proliferation into the lower respiratory tract must occur before invasive pneumonia develops.

Features important to the clinical diagnosis of nosocomial pneumonia are listed in Table 106-1. Unfortunately, these findings are often found in the ICU patient without pneumonia, too. Fever and leukocytosis may result from any cause of inflammation; purulent secretions may be produced in association with tracheal intubation and repeated suctioning[32]; infiltrates occur (not necessarily with associated infection) in all patients who develop ARDS; and, finally, pathogenic bacteria are cultured from the bronchi of 75% to 100% of critically ill patients.[46] In fact, none of the usual criteria for diagnosing pneumonia is significantly predictive in patients with ARDS.[38]

A patient demonstrating the systemic inflammatory response syndrome (SIRS) should have a thorough evaluation performed to look for possible infections. Initial diagnostic interventions are performed to obtain culture specimens from sites that are most likely to provide a true diagnosis. A peripheral blood specimen should be obtained for culture. If pleural fluid is present in sufficient quantity to be safely aspirated, this should also be examined by Gram stain and culture.[48] Therapy can be specifically directed if organisms are identified from one of these sources.

Routine sputum cultures, obtained with suction catheters through endotracheal or tracheostomy tubes, are often performed to guide antimicrobial therapy, despite their reported unreliability in mechanically ventilated patients.[31,36] Rigorous sputum surveillance with multiple Gram stains and serial sputum cultures may eventually identify a predominant organism, improve diagnostic accuracy, and guide antimicrobial therapy in the appropriate direction. However, upper airway and endotracheal tube colonization can be responsible for misinterpretation.

The PSB, introduced in 1979, is considered a more reliable technique to improve culture accuracy.[40] Optimal results are achieved only with careful attention to minor details, and quantitative cultures are recommended, with 10^3 colony-forming units per milliliter (CFU/mL) considered diagnostic for pneumonia.[31]

Bronchoalveolar lavage is the established method for diagnosing opportunistic pneumonia in immunosuppressed patients because contamination of the bronchoscopic suction channel does not seem to create a diagnostic dilemma in these patients.[31,52] Animal[53] and human[54] studies suggest that quantitative cultures of BAL fluid, in combination with Giemsa stains and Gram stains, provide the most accurate

TABLE 106-1. Clinical Diagnosis of Nosocomial Pneumonia

Fever
Leukocytosis
Purulent secretions
New or progressive chest radiograph infiltrates
Pathogenic bacteria in tracheobronchial secretions

and rapid diagnosis for pneumonia in mechanically ventilated patients.

Meduri and associates[31] recommend the following approach to diagnosing and treating respiratory infections in mechanically ventilated patients, with the assumption that initiating broad-spectrum antibiotics in the absence of pneumonia can be potentially harmful. First, if physical examination is unrewarding and the patient has no cardiovascular instability or contraindications to bronchoscopy, obtain PBS and BAL cultures.[31] Identifying organisms with greater than 7% of alveolar cells recovered by BAL may be helpful in diagnosing pneumonia earlier, and Gram stain of BAL-recovered cells aids in selecting the appropriate antimicrobial therapy.[54] Negative stains, confirmed by the absence of significant growth on quantitative culture of PSB ($<10^3$CFU/mL) or BAL ($<10^4$ CFU/mL), should direct attention to other possible causes for fever and pulmonary infiltration.[31]

Transthoracic needle aspiration may be the most accurate method for diagnosing nosocomial pneumonia, especially in immunocompromised patients,[55] but this procedure may be hazardous in mechanically ventilated patients.

Initiate empiric antibiotic therapy only in patients who are clinically septic, with signs of cardiovascular instability or persistent metabolic acidosis. Antibiotics are also started in situations in which the consequences of bacteremia outweigh the risk of antibiotic therapy (i.e., patients with vascular prosthetic grafts), causing host colonization with potentially pathogenic antibiotic-resistant organisms.

CATHETER-RELATED NOSOCOMIAL INFECTIONS

CLINICAL SIGNIFICANCE

Catheter-related infections leading to bacteremia occur in less than 1% of hospitalized patients, but most of these infections occur in ICU patients.[56] Ten percent of patients hospitalized in SICUs for more than 72 hours develop nosocomial bacteremia, many of which develop from catheter-related infections.[25] This figure extrapolates to over 50,000 cases of catheter-related bacteremia yearly.[56] Some of these infections are preventable if appropriate infection control measures are used, but the study of catheter-related nosocomial infections is characterized by considerable confusion because of a variety of important clinical questions and misinterpretation of what little specific data are available. Definitions are diverse and often used incorrectly, resulting in misapplication and misunderstanding of concepts.

Catheter-related or "line" sepsis must be considered in terms of three interacting factors: the host, the organism, and the environment. Often, attention is directed only toward the catheter or foreign body breaking the integrity of the skin barrier (thus providing an easy pathway for organisms to gain access to vulnerable areas). Other environmental factors must be considered. These include the type of dressing, the frequency of dressing changes and materials used, the type of systemic or topical antimicrobial selected, and the indications for antimicrobials. The external components of the pressure monitoring or infusion system can be a source of

organisms being introduced by caregivers. Breaks in sterile technique can be minimized in many ways: continuous mixed venous oximetry catheters eliminate the need for frequent mixed venous blood sampling; closed injectate systems for measuring cardiac output also reduce the frequency of pulmonary artery (PA) catheter manipulations.[57] Finally, surgical cutdowns should be avoided because the risk of catheter-related complications is probably much higher than that of percutaneous catheter insertion.[58]

Traditional concepts must be updated with respect to the type of infecting organisms. *Staphylococcus epidermidis* is the most common organism isolated in line sepsis. Gram-negative organisms, *Pseudomonas* species, and various fungal species are also common. Host factors are difficult to quantitate. Few data support what seems to be a common-sense principle: the sicker the patient, the more likely that catheter-related sepsis will occur. A recent prospective study compares critically ill septic SICU patients with nonseptic SICU patients. The incidence of bacteremia from triple-lumen catheters was 9.6% in the septic (sicker) group compared with 0% in the nonseptic group of patients.[59] No local site (catheter-related) infections developed in the nonseptic patients, compared with 22.6% of positive catheter site infections in the septic group. The interpretation and relevance of catheter-related infections is determined by understanding the incidence and interplay of several factors: the severity of illness, which determines the duration of monitoring; elective and clean surgical procedures versus emergency procedures for septic diagnoses; and short-term versus long-term hospitalization. Coexisting MOSF and sepsis occur in the longest term ICU patients with the highest risk of sepsis and, ultimately, the highest mortality rate.

Long-term broad-spectrum antimicrobials, common in this subgroup of patients, might be expected to increase the risk of "superinfection," which may account for the predominance of typically nonpathogenic or opportunistic organisms in these situations.

DEFINITION

Erroneous delineation of contamination, colonization, and true infection has led to confusion and incorrect interpretation of earlier clinical investigations. Table 106-2 incorporates definitions that are generally accepted and used in most of the recent studies addressing the problem of "catheter infection."

Catheter infection is an imprecise term. Although it is clear that inanimate objects do not become infected, evidence suggests that bacteria may be able to live and multiply on catheter surfaces, deriving nutrients from catheter polymers, the deposited glycocalyx of certain bacterial species, and other nonviable bacteria.[60]

Confusion from these various terms arises from earlier erroneous interpretations of clinical investigations. Catheter infection was diagnosed in the past when blood culture specimens obtained through the catheter (TTC cultures) were positive.[12] Interpretations that these cultures indicated catheter-related nosocomial infection were published in the late 1970s and early 1980s. Maki and colleagues[12] subsequently popularized the concept of semiquantitative cathe-

TABLE 106-2. Definitions of Catheter-Related
Nosocomial Infections

CATHETER-RELATED INFECTION

A term frequently used for a positive catheter segment culture.
If semiquantitative cultures are used, the presence of ≥15
colonies on a blood agar plate is considered positive.[3]
Although true infection should ideally be defined by more
than just a specific number of organisms recovered from a
catheter segment (i.e., presence of local inflammation,
purulence, or systemic signs of infection such as fever or
elevated white blood cell count), the objective finding of a
positive catheter segment culture has been frequently used
to define a catheter-related infection. The term *catheter-
related infection* does not necessarily imply that a locally
invasive infection is present, nor does it justify antibiotic
therapy.

CATHETER-RELATED SEPTICEMIA

(or bacteremia): Criteria for making this diagnosis are
simultaneous isolation of the same microorganism from a
catheter segment quantitative or semiquantitative culture and
a peripheral blood culture.

CONTAMINATION

The presence, in a specimen taken for culture, of organisms
introduced by the person collecting the specimen during the
course of obtaining the sample.

COLONIZATION

Organisms within a host without producing either a local or
systemic response. The skin and gastrointestinal tract are
often colonized with pathogenic bacteria in hospitalized
patients. This concept is also applied to the subcutaneous
skin tract produced by introducing a vascular catheter. The
skin tract is considered colonized if there are <15 colonies
present on semiquantitative catheter culture and there are
no signs of local infection or systemic bacteremia.

ter segment cultures, using a technique whereby a 5-cm
portion of the removed catheter was rolled on a blood agar
plate. If more than 15 colonies of organisms were identified,
there was a 16% incidence rate of peripheral bacteremia or
local infection. If fewer than 15 colonies were found, no
associated cases of bacteremia or local infection were identified. Most specimens cultured in the original study were
short peripheral intravenous catheters.[12] Thus, the "tip" and
"intracutaneous segment" were exactly the same specimen.
In fact, when only long catheters were studied, the intracutaneous segment (the 5-cm portion residing in the subcutaneous tract) actually gave the important information. The catheter tip, which resided in vivo in the bloodstream, usually
had fewer organisms (<15 or a nondiagnostic number) or
was actually sterile.

Thus, confusion results from the following factors: interpretation of TTC cultures as evidence of "catheter infection"; the mistaken substitution of a tip culture for long
catheters instead of the more appropriate intracutaneous
segment, which traverses the anatomic area whereby organ-

isms gain access; and the use of broth cultures that may be
positive even if only a few organisms are present.

PATHOGENESIS

Bacterial colonization within or around any type of catheter
begins almost immediately after catheter insertion,[60] and the
final determinant of whether such colonization ultimately
leads to clinical infection is multifactorial. Three theories
regarding the pathogenesis of catheter-related septicemia
have been proposed.

The prevailing hypothesis is that bacterial colonization
and subsequent infection begins at the interface of the catheter and the skin insertion site.[61] Bacteria either advance or
multiply distally along the external catheter surface within
the subcutaneous tract, and ultimately gain access to the
venous circulation causing bacteremia. The skin is the most
common source for organisms causing catheter-related infection and bacteremia.[62] Most data suggest that virtually all
catheter-related infections and bacteremia caused by coagulase-negative staphylococci[63] (the most common organisms
isolated) and *Staphylococcus aureus* originate from the skin.
Approximately 50% of all yeast infections also develop from
the skin.[62,63]

In vitro electronic microscopic examination of catheter
segments show that coagulase-negative staphylococci adhere
to catheter surfaces within 30 minutes at areas of catheter
surface irregularities.[60] Microcolonies develop within 1 hour,
with heavy colonization occurring within 6 to 12 hours, first
in singular, then in multiple layers. These colonies eventually
become covered with a glycocalyx coating, which may form
a barrier against antibiotics, phagocytic neutrophils, and
macrophages.[60,64,65] In vitro studies show that bacteria can
grow on catheter surfaces, even when externally supplied
nutrients are absent.[60] This characteristic seems possible only
when bacteria are capable of using catheter components as
nutrient sources. Catheter surface erosion in vitro does occur, suggesting that catheter components or added anti-
thrombogenic layers are nutritional sources for bacteria.
Lysed bacterial cells may also supply nutrients to other viable
bacteria.[60] Infections beginning at the skin–catheter interface (insertion site) are the most common sources of catheter-related bacteremia.[66]

A second theory suggests that the catheter hub may be
a source of catheter-related bacteremia.[67] Bacteria are introduced through the hub from frequent manipulations, migrating down the inner lumen surface to the venous circulation.
Sitges-Serra and coworkers[67,68] believe this to be the most
common route for catheter-related bacteremia. These investigators have condemned the insertion site theory, emphasizing that none of the studies using intracutaneous segment
cultures speciated the coagulase-negative staphylococci.
Thus, they believe that no good evidence implicates *Staphylococcus epidermidis* organisms isolated from intracutaneous
catheter segments as the same organisms that cause peripheral bacteremia.[68]

A third possibility suggests that reservoirs of remote infections in the host produce bacteremia and subsequent catheter seeding. This mechanism may occur, particularly in septic

patients with abscesses, drains, and wounds, but is much less common than external sources for infection.[69] Factors facilitating catheter seeding include organism type, degree and duration of bacteremia, the patient's clinical status, and time of catheter use.[69] Fungal[62] and enteric organisms such as enterococci, *Escherichia coli*, and *Klebsiella* may cause catheter infections by hematogenous spread.[70,71]

Infusate contamination also has been implicated in the pathogenesis of catheter-related bacteremia in the past.[72] Parenteral nutrition solutions[73] and lipid emulsions[74] (including propofol, a sedative suspended in a liquid emulsion) can support bacterial and fungal growth, but the risk of developing catheter-related septicemia from infusate contamination currently is low.

RISK FACTORS

Risk factors for catheter-related infection and septicemia can be grouped into patient-related and hospital-related categories. Many of these environmental risk factors are difficult to quantitate.

Duration of catheter site use is one of the most important hospital-related risk factors for catheter-related infection and septicemia.[56,59,69] It may be a cofactor in the severity of underlying illness, with septic patients being at a much higher risk than nonseptic patients. Length of hospitalization before catheter insertion also is a possible risk factor[59] but is difficult to distinguish from the severity of illness factor; it may represent a quantitation of this more important patient-related risk.

Hampton and Sheretz[56] recently reviewed all prospective studies of vascular-access infection that used quantitative culture techniques to estimate the risk of infection per day of catheterization. These studies vary from a low risk of 0.7% per day in catheters dedicated for total parenteral nutrition to 3.3% per day for central venous catheters. Many studies cited in this review do not separate critically ill patients from other patients, nor do they separate septic from nonseptic patients. In a recent study examining triple-lumen catheter infection rates in critically ill patients, no infections were reported in nonseptic patients, but a 22.6% incidence rate of catheter-related infection and a 9.6% incidence rate of bacteremia were reported from catheter sites in septic patients.[59]

Catheter sites were used much longer in the septic group (15.1 ± 12.6 days) than in the nonseptic group (8.12 ± 4.1 days), but the catheter infection rate per 100 site-days was only 1.47% in the septic group. The number of hospital days before catheter insertion was much higher in the septic (14.52 ± 12.83 days) than in the nonseptic group (1.38 ± 2.23 days), possibly quantitating the severity of the underlying disease process. Hospital days before insertion may be more important than time of site use, because five of the seven cases of catheter-related bacteremia occurred within the first 7 days of site use. These infections occurred despite strict daily site care and GWXs every 4 to 6 days.[59] The experience of the individual performing the insertion procedure[75,76] may also be an important risk factor.

CATHETER MAINTENANCE

Site

Site care is a crucial factor in preventing catheter-related septicemia. Three different site care regimens are compared in a study of 827 peripheral and central venous catheters: iodophor ointment, polymyxin-neomycin-bacitracin (PNB) ointment, or no antibiotic ointment.[77] All dressings were changed every 48 hours. There was no difference in the incidence of catheter-related septicemia, but the rate of catheter-related infection (considered a precursor to septicemia) was significantly lower in the PNB group (2.2%) compared with that of the control group (6.5%; $p = 0.02$). The group receiving iodophor ointment had 50% of the infection rate (3.6%; $p =$ ns) of that of the control group. Three of four patients with fungal infections, including one with *Candida fungemia*, were treated with PNB. The authors conclude that topical antimicrobial agents conferred only modest protection against catheter-related infection. If ointment is used, then topical PNB for peripheral venous catheters, and iodophor ointment for central venous catheters and arterial catheters, are recommended.[77]

Dressings

Dressing change regimens also have been extensively studied. Peripheral intravenous catheters should be removed at 72 hours with one dressing change at 48 hours. One large study of over 2000 peripheral Teflon catheters showed no difference in skin site colonization, catheter-related infection, or bacteremia between catheter sites treated with dry gauze compared with transparent polyurethane or iodophor-transparent dressings.[78] These investigators believe that either sterile gauze or a transparent dressing can remain in place until the catheter is removed.[78] Others report that bacterial colonization for peripheral catheters is increased, correlating transparent dressings with increased catheter tip colonization and hospital cost.[79] Two recent studies implicate transparent dressings for central venous catheters, with a much higher incidence of catheter-related infection and septicemia when compared with dry gauze dressings.[80,81] Skin insertion site colonization is associated with higher rates of subcutaneous tunnel colonization and subsequent bacteremia.[80] Transparent dressings impede moisture evaporation from the insertion site[79–81] and may, therefore, enhance bacterial colonization, especially in critically ill or diaphoretic patients. Daily dressing changes are recommended when diaphoresis is a problem.

Duration of Insertion

Length of catheter site use is an unresolved issue. In nonhospitalized patients, Broviac and Hickman catheters are used almost indefinitely, and certain types of catheter-related bacteremia are treated with antibiotics rather than by catheter removal.[82] Such practice in the ICU probably would lead to disastrous consequences. A recent study investigates the infection risk associated with different long-term catheter maintenance methods in SICU patients.[83] Three methods of site management were evaluated: (1) catheters changed to a new site every 7 days, (2) no predetermined interval change with change to a new site only when clinically indicated, and (3) GWX every 7 days. A catheter change was mandatory in the presence of a positive blood culture, skin site infection (defined as purulent drainage, expanding erythema or cellulitis, or a positive qualitative swab culture), or sepsis without a likely source in all three groups. No difference in infection risk among the three methods of long-term catheter care was found. Therefore, the method with the least complications and expense should be used. This study supports the general guidelines of not routinely changing catheters at a predetermined time interval; exchanging by guidewire when a new catheter is needed or when catheter-associated septicemia is suspected (because this is safer); and, when there is evidence of skin site infection, removing the catheter and placing another catheter at a new site.[83]

Guidewire Exchange

GWX is a safe and effective method for diagnosing catheter-related infection and prolonging catheter site use.[59,71,84] It is more effective when every attempt is made to sterilize the entire external portion of the catheter and the surrounding skin before exchange. This technique not only prevents contamination of the new catheter during GWX, but should also yield a more accurate semiquantitative culture of the intracutaneous catheter segment because the catheter is removed through a "sterile field."[71] If bacteria are capable of living, growing, and multiplying on catheter surfaces without external nutrient sources, as suggested by in vitro studies,[60,64,65] GWX may help to prevent infection by removing externally and internally adherent bacteria before a "critical mass" develops that may cause bacteremia.

One criticism is that intracutaneous tract contamination, which may occur while performing the GWX, may perpetuate local infection or create subsequent infection of the new catheter. A recent study suggests that this occurrence is unlikely because 12 culture-positive catheters (defined as more than 15 colonies by semiquantitative culture) were replaced with new catheters by GWX, and subsequent catheter cultures showed no growth in eight, contamination in one, and subsequent positive cultures in only three.[83] These results suggest that GWX may confer some protection against catheter-related infection.

DIAGNOSTIC TECHNIQUES

A positive local (site) infection is considered the most common precursor to catheter septicemia. Therefore, if localized infection can be controlled, or aborted at an early stage, most bacteremic episodes can be avoided. Most investigators would agree that a positive catheter broth culture is too sensitive for the diagnosis of catheter-related infection,[56] because false-positive rates up to 50% are reported.[12] Swab cultures may also be too sensitive. As a result, various quantitative culture techniques were developed to better delineate infection from colonization.[56] The semiquantitative technique developed by Maki and associates[12] is used extensively and provides reliable results. The culture is performed by rolling a 5-cm catheter segment (tip or intracutaneous) across a blood agar plate in a reproducible, defined manner. A positive culture was defined in the initial study as 15 or more colonies per plate,[12] although most culture-positive catheters in that study yielded confluent growth. A positive catheter segment culture resulted in a 16% risk of catheter bacteremia. There was no local infection or bacteremia if there were less than 15 CFUs on culture.

Other more complex methods include gram-staining techniques[85] and broth quantitative cultures,[86] which have not gained the wide acceptance of the semiquantitative culture. Moyer and coworkers[87] compare various culture techniques and recommend semiquantitative cultures as the best and simplest test for diagnosing catheter-related sepsis. However, quantitative blood cultures withdrawn through permanent (Hickman or Broviac) indwelling catheters also may be an acceptable approach in patients with difficult venous access.[87]

A recurring question concerns the value of routine broth TTC blood cultures to diagnose catheter-related infection. A recent study by Wormser and coworkers[88] advocates TTC cultures for diagnosing peripheral bacteremia. These investigators examined 200 blood cultures in ICU or oncology patients and determined that cultures taken by arterial, pulmonary artery, and central venous pressure catheters were 96% sensitive and 98% specific in correctly diagnosing bacteremia when compared with cultures obtained simultaneously from peripheral venipuncture. The authors emphasize that catheter site duration was relatively short when most of the cultures were withdrawn (<4 days), and strict stopcock disinfection by the same phlebotomist may have decreased the incidence of false-positive results.[88] Microbial catheter colonization may still contaminate TTC blood specimens, and more data are needed before this practice can be routinely recommended.

Although others have also advocated TTC cultures,[89] unless the clinician knows precisely how these cultures are obtained and the length of catheter use, TTC cultures should be reserved for only those situations in which peripheral venipuncture is not possible. Routine TTC cultures should never be used to diagnose catheter-related infection unless some form of quantitative culture is performed.

SPECIFIC CATHETER TYPES

Pulmonary Artery Catheters

Various investigators report a higher rate of catheter septicemia with PA catheters when compared with other catheter types.[90] Myers and colleagues[91] report a catheter-related infection rate of 5.8% when the mean duration of catheterization was 4.2 ± 1.8 days. Hudson-Civetta and associates[92] report a 10% rate of positive catheter segment cultures at 3 days in a large group of patients with documented abdominal sepsis. In a follow-up study, a GWX protocol was used to determine whether PA catheter (and other types of central venous catheters) sites could be used for longer periods to avoid the risk of repeated central venipunctures.[93] An increased rate of catheter-related infection was identified in nonseptic patients at 6 versus 4 days of catheter use (33% versus 12%, p <0.05). There was also a striking relationship between the ICU day of catheter placement and the likelihood of subsequent catheter-related infection, including catheters placed at 6 days or earlier compared with those placed after 7 days (p <0.005). Both studies[92,93] report no episodes of catheter-related bacteremia from positive catheter segment cultures at 4 days or less, but the rate of catheter-related bacteremia from positive segment cultures continued to rise with the ICU day of catheterization in both clean and septic patients. This observation strongly supports the concept that infections from PA and other types of central venous catheters are directly related to the length and severity of illness in clean and septic patients.

A recent study of 152 PA catheters comparing three methods of long-term catheter maintenance reports a 6% incidence rate of bacteremia when catheters remained in place up to 11.5 ± 1.7 days (mean ± sem). Guidewire exchange of the catheter or change to a new site at 7 days did not decrease the risk of catheter-related sepsis.[83] Whether more frequent GWXs may decrease the incidence of catheter-related infection and subsequent sepsis is unclear, although frequent exchanges at 4- to 6-day intervals do not seem to decrease the risk.[59]

Multilumen Central Venous Catheters

Some investigators condemn using multilumen central venous catheters because of higher infection rates when compared with single-lumen catheters.[94] Most of them use total parenteral nutrition as the entry criterion for patient selection; others have included PA catheter data. Such criteria and comparisons may bias these studies, because patients with multilumen or PA catheters are usually sicker than patients receiving single-lumen catheters. Thus, the perceived higher infection rate may not be related to the type of catheter, but to the difficulty in maintaining sterility, to more frequent catheter manipulations, and to the patient's immune status. A recent study[83] in critically ill SICU patients reports a 3.4% rate of catheter colonization (which we have defined as catheter-related infection; see Table 106-1) and only a 2.1% incidence rate of catheter-related sepsis (bacteremia) in triple-lumen catheters used for an average of 22.6 days.

Another study separated triple-lumen catheter infections in septic and nonseptic critically ill surgical patients. No catheter-related infection or bacteremia occurred in the nonseptic patients, but the incidence rate of catheter-related infection in the septic group was 22.6%, with a 9.6% incidence rate of associated bacteremia.[59] The catheter infection rate per 100 site-days, however, was only 0.9% for both septic and nonseptic patients combined, which is similar to rates published for single-lumen catheters.[59] Therefore, the risk of triple-lumen catheter infections is no higher than that for single-lumen catheters; however, septic patients are at higher risk, regardless of catheter type.[59]

To determine appropriate reasons for GWX of central venous catheters, Ball and associates[95] prospectively studied 146 ICU patients with 387 catheters. They found that there was a significant increase in the rate of positive catheter segment semiquantitative cultures if GWX was performed for local inflammation at the site, when compared with catheters changed for technical problems or those removed because they were no longer needed. Interestingly, they found that catheters changed for fever spike of 2°F above highest temperature in prior two days did not have an increased infection rate. They conclude that fever spike alone should be rejected as an automatic indication for catheter exchange. In its place, GWX should be performed when the catheter remains as the likely source of fever spike after other sources have been considered. In a follow-up study, Ball[96] compares the infection rate of antimicrobial impregnated catheters to regular catheters. She found that protected catheters had a significantly decreased overall infection rate. Also, protected catheters did not have a significant increase in the rate of intracutaneous segment semiquantitative cultures after 10 days compared with the unprotected catheters. This allowed for a significantly longer duration of catheter use and for fewer catheters to be used per patient.

Arterial Catheters

In 1979, Band and Maki[97] studied catheter-related infections from arterial catheters and determined that the main variables for infection risk were percutaneous versus cutdown insertion (ninefold increase in catheter-related bacteremia with cutdowns) and length of arterial cannulation time. The overall rate of catheter-related infection was 18%, with 70% of infections occurring in catheters used over 96 hours; all five cases of catheter-related bacteremia occurred in patients with catheter sites for more than 96 hours. Another study also supports time of site use as an important factor, reemphasizing that the risk of infection is low for catheter sites used for less than 96 hours.[98] In the latter study, 27% of sites used more than 96 hours became colonized, as evidenced by a positive swab culture of the entry site. Catheter-related infection developed in 9.5% of radial and femoral artery sites used up to 14 days (mean 6.4 days). Forty-four percent of axillary sites were infected after 96 hours of use.[98] Radial and femoral artery sites can be used for prolonged periods if skin site colonization is controlled with good site care.[98] GWX can also be used to confirm the presence of arterial catheter-related infection.[98] The low risk of arterial catheter-related infection and bacteremia is supported by other recent studies.[83,99]

SURGICAL WOUND INFECTIONS ■

Accurate diagnosis of wound infection depends on a thorough knowledge of the patient's history, physical examination, and bacteriologic information from Gram stain and wound culture. Nosocomial wound infections can develop after both clean and clean-contaminated surgical procedures.[100] Physical examination must always include the surgical incision to rule out occult infection and the occasional catastrophic, rapidly progressive infections that can lead to death if not immediately treated. Most nosocomial wound infections can be diagnosed by careful inspection of the wound to identify the typical signs of erythema, edema, and tenderness.[101] The incubation period for wound infections from *S aureus* is usually 4 to 6 days.[101] These infections are usually well localized and characterized by the presence of thick, creamy, odorless pus. Infected wounds are usually erythematous, edematous, and painful, and almost always respond to local drainage procedures. Antibiotics are not necessary unless extensive cellulitis is present or bacteremia is documented by positive peripheral blood cultures.

Gram-negative wound infections usually result from contamination with enteric contents and, therefore, may be accompanied by anaerobic streptococci or *Bacteroides fragilis* if the large bowel was the target of operation or injury. The incubation period for most of these organisms is 7 to 14 days.[101] Systemic signs of infection, such as fever, tachycardia, and hyperglycemia, often outweigh local signs of infection, but erythema, edema, and pain are often present. Wound infections caused by gram-negative enteric organisms are treated with surgical drainage, debridement of devitalized tissue, and antibiotic coverage for gram-negative enteric organisms and anaerobes.

HOSPITAL-ACQUIRED URINARY TRACT INFECTIONS

The urinary tract is the most common origin of gram-negative bacteremia in large epidemiologic studies.[102] Pyuria and bacteriuria are identified in approximately 50% of patients with urinary catheters within 2 weeks and virtually 100% of patients at 6 weeks after catheter insertion.[103] Approximately 80% of nosocomial UTIs are associated with urinary catheters.[104] One study of 40,718 patients admitted to a large university hospital identified 1233 nosocomial UTIs (3.0% over 23 months).[105] Diagnosis of UTIs was made in symptomatic patients by either one mixed culture of 100,000 CFU/mL or more, or a single pure culture of 100,000 CFU/mL or more. Only 12 patients (1.0% of UTIs; 0.1% of entire hospital population) developed bacteremia. In the same study, men with hospital-acquired UTIs developed bacteremia twice as often as women. This may be because bacteremia from a UTI in men develops primarily from the area of the prostatic urethra, where the rich venous plexus, with the absence of a muscularis layer, invites bacterial seeding.

Three main pathways allow bacteria to enter the urinary tract. The most common pathway is through the anterior (external) urethra during bladder catheterization.[106] Medical personnel may also contaminate the external collecting system during urine specimen collections. Bacteria can then gain access to the urinary tract through the catheter lumen, especially if drained urine is allowed to reflux into the bladder. Finally, bacteria from the patient's perineum, or from the hands of medical personnel, may migrate or become deposited at the urethral meatus and enter the urinary tract by the thin film of fluid between the urethral mucosa and external catheter surface.[107]

Incomplete bladder emptying in catheterized patients allows microorganisms to proliferate to high concentrations,

defeating the protective effect of "bladder flushing," which is provided by a normal voiding pattern.[108] Excessive catheter manipulations (bladder lavage, catheter exchanges, pulling the catheter by an agitated patient), or a blocked catheter causing bladder distention may cause excessive mucosal damage that promotes bacterial adherence and invasive infection.[103] Routine catheter cultures, prophylactic antibiotics, frequent catheter exchanges, daily meatal care, bladder irrigations, instillation of hydrogen peroxide and other products into collection systems, and treatment of asymptomatic bacteriuria in a normal host are not helpful in preventing UTIs and urosepsis.[103,109]

The hallmark of diagnosis of urinary infections remains urinalysis and urine culture. Bacteriuria and pyuria should alert the physician to the possibility of a urinary source for sepsis. Unfortunately, correlation of symptoms with these findings in ICU patients is often impossible, and antibiotics may be started when the urinary tract is not the true source for sepsis. Epidemiologic studies show that catheter-acquired bacteriuria is more common in orthopedic and urology patients, in patients who are catheterized after the sixth hospital day, and in patients who require catheterization for 7 days or longer.[109]

Enteric organisms are predominantly responsible for UTIs. *E coli*, *Klebsiella*, *Enterobacter*, *Proteus*, enterococci, and *Pseudomonas* are most often cultured.[110] Various *Candida* species are also frequently identified, with *C albicans* the cause of most fungal infections.[111] The incidence of fungal UTIs has increased in recent years because of the widespread use of broad-spectrum antibiotics in patients with indwelling bladder catheters.[111] Other risk factors include diabetes mellitus, immunosuppressive agents, parenteral nutrition, disturbances causing decreased urine flow, and radiation therapy.[102] The pathogenesis is similar to that of nosocomial bacterial UTIs,[112] and the diagnosis is confirmed by quantitative urine culture showing 100,000 CFU/mL.[112,113]

Asymptomatic bladder colonization does not usually require therapy. Modifying risk factors leading to its development, such as discontinuing antibiotics or removing the bladder catheter, may be the only treatment necessary.[112] In critically ill patients, such practice is not always possible, and therapy directed toward eradicating fungal colonization (such as bladder irrigations with amphotericin B) may be helpful.[114] Bladder irrigation is controversial and probably not necessary in most patients.[112,115] Disseminated candidiasis requires therapy with either amphotericin B or fluconazole, one of the class of triazole antifungal agents.[116]

Given the fact that enteric organisms are the predominant agents of infection, it is surprising that *B fragilis* is not a common infectious agent. *B fragilis* and other enteric anaerobes do not proliferate well in the acidic urine environment.[110] This characteristic, combined with the fact that the usual mode of infection results in exposure to aerobic conditions, accounts for the paucity of anaerobic UTIs. Anaerobic UTIs, primarily from clostridial species, however, do occur in critically ill surgical patients.[117] Anaerobes should be suspected if Gram stain of the urine shows gram-positive rods or gram-negative rods with subsequent negative aerobic cultures. The rare finding of cystitis emphysematosa (gas-filled vesicles and cysts in the bladder mucosa and musculature) on abdominal radiographs should also alert you to the possibility of anaerobic UTI.[117] The diagnosis is confirmed by obtaining a suprapubic needle aspirate urine specimen for culture to ensure anaerobic collection.

One consequence of large epidemiologic studies is the adoption of specific guidelines for preventing catheter associated UTIs in noncritically ill hospitalized patients. This broad information has also been applied to specific groups, such as renal transplant patients.[118,119] A recent prospective urinary microbiologic evaluation in 100 SICU patients showed that early microbiologic urine monitoring was unnecessary.[120] Initial urine catheter cultures were negative in 92 patients, and both urine and reservoir bag specimens were evaluated daily. The mean duration of catheterization was 4 days, and only 2.5% of urine specimens yielded microorganisms. Of 20 patients with any positive culture, six had microorganisms in the reservoir bag alone. The remaining 14 patients had organisms in both the bladder and the bag urine. The urine reservoir bag was the apparent source of microorganisms in the bladder urine in only three cases. The daily incidence of new cases and the cumulative rate of bladder bacteriuria remained below 7% and 22%, respectively, during the first week of catheterization.

Life-table analysis showed that the probability of remaining free of bacteriuria after 1 week was 0.77, by which time 74% of patients were no longer at risk. These rates are similar to those previously reported for various patient groups outside the ICU. No documented cases of bacteremia were associated with bacteriuria in this study. Although epidemiologic studies of nosocomial UTIs identify urosepsis as the cause of over 3000 deaths per year[102] and as being responsible for significant increases in hospital costs,[105] the urinary tract is not a common source of systemic sepsis in critically ill patients unless obstruction or urinary tract instrumentation has occurred.

FUNGAL INFECTIONS ■

Fungal infections are occurring more frequently in ICUs[121] and fungi are isolated in as many as 42% of patients with nosocomial infections.[7] *Candida* is the most common fungal agent in nosocomial infection. There are seven species in the *Candida* genus: *C albicans, C guilliermondi, C krusei, C parakrusei (parapsilosis), C pseudotropicalis, C stellatoidea,* and *C tropicalis.* All seven species can cause infection in humans, but *C albicans* is the most common isolate and, in animal studies, the most virulent.[15]

Candida is not a normal isolate from the stomach but in 55% to 65% of normal volunteers, it was isolated from the small bowel and colon.[122] Risk factors for developing invasive *Candida* infections are prior antibiotic administration, parenteral nutrition, steroids, and organ transplantation.[15,123,124]

The risk associated with antibiotics is proportional to the number of different antibiotics administered.[123]

Disseminated candidiasis is difficult to reliably diagnosis and prophylactic treatment is controversial because of the toxicity of amphotericin B.[125] Criteria for diagnosis and systemic treatment include positive blood cultures after re-

moval of intravascular catheters, culture of *Candida* from three or more sites, or endophthalmitis.[126,127] Blood or urine cultures are positive in less than half the patients with disseminated candidiasis, making the decision to treat even more complex.

Treatment of disseminated candidiasis is with systemic amphotericin B. Fluconizole has been offered as an alternative. Preventive measures of intravascular catheter monitoring, early discontinuance of Foley catheters, and avoidance of long-term broad-spectrum antibiotics. Prophylactic use of oral ketoconizole, oral fluconizole, or oral amphotericin B may be of help.[128]

SINUSITIS ■

Sinusitis accounts for at least 5% of ICU nosocomial infections.[129] The incidence could be higher because infections can be missed if the index of suspicion is not high. Acute sinusitis occurs from impaired drainage of the maxillary sinuses. Risk factors include intubation, nasogastric tubes, and facial trauma.[130] Michelson and others[131] report that nasotracheal intubation led to sinusitis in 95% of ICU patients, whereas orotracheal intubation led to sinusitis in 63%. Nasostracheal patients also had an earlier onset of sinusitis and a significantly higher incidence of bilateral sinusitis.[131] Fassoulaki and Pamouktsoglou[132] regard the nasotracheal tube as the major factor in the development of nosocomial sinusitis. Acute sinusitis is usually a bacterial infection.[133] An awake patient may complain of severe head cold, nasal congestion, purulent rhinorrhea, headache, and fever.[134] Patients with altered mental status may only have fever and possibly foul-smelling nasal discharge. To confirm the diagnosis, several options are available. Plain radiographs require multiple views to obtain a confidence level of 85%.[135,136] In addition, these examinations are difficult in intubated patients.[131] Computed tomographic scanning of the sinuses reveals the most detail, but transport in the critically ill patient is not always feasible.[137] Ultrasound has also been suggested to evaluate sinusitis.[138–141] A high correlation exists between ultrasound and antral puncture. Ultrasound has the added advantages of bedside use and patient safety. Decongestants and nasal spray may be used for symptomatic relief along with broad-spectrum antibiotics.[142] If this fails, then surgical drainage is indicated.

ANTIBIOTIC-ASSOCIATED PSEUDOMEMBRANOUS COLITIS ■

C difficile can be cultured in up to 21% of hospitalized patients.[143] The incidence of nosocomial infection is increasing.[144–146] Antibiotics suppress the endogenous flora and the *C difficile* proliferate.[147] Symptoms range from mild diarrhea to fulminant sepsis with megacolon. The diagnosis should be investigated in hospitalized patients who develop diarrhea, regardless of whether they are receiving tube feedings. In patients receiving enteral feedings who develop diarrhea, *C difficile* was responsible in 17% to 22%.[148,149] Diagnosis is confirmed by fecal assay for *C difficile* toxin and possibly sigmoidoscopy, although rectal sparing is common.[144] Treatment consists of discontinuing offending antibiotics, fluid resuscitation, and antibiotic therapy against *C difficile*.[149] Vancomycin, metronidazole, and bacitracin have been used as treatment. To curtail the emergence of vancomycin-resistant enterococci, vancomycin should not be used as the primary treatment in ICUs. Relapses occur in up to 25% of patients.[150] Repeat stool specimens can be obtained 2 weeks after a course of antibiotics to document eradication of the *C difficile*.[148]

HOSPITAL-ACQUIRED VENTRICULITIS AND MENINGITIS ■

Ventricular catheters are commonly placed to diagnose and aid in the management of increased intracranial pressure. The nosocomial infection rate for ventriculostomies is reported between 0% and 27%.[151–166] The overall risk of infection has been estimated at 1.5 infections per 100 monitoring days.[167]

Etiology of infection is believed to be either contamination at time of insertion or catheter contamination after insertion. Mayhall and coworkers[156] in 1984 performed a prospective epidemiologic study of ventriculostomy-related infections in 172 consecutive neurosurgical patients. They defined infection as culture-proven ventriculitis or meningitis. They determined that the risk factors for ventriculostomy-related infections were (1) duration of ventricular catheter of more than 5 days, (2) irrigation of the system, (3) intracranial pressure over 20 mm Hg, (4) intracerebral hemorrhage with intraventricular hemorrhage, and (5) neurosurgical operations. In another study, Clark and others[168] retrospectively reviewed the records of 140 trauma patients with ICP monitors. They conclude that duration of catheter insertion was a risk factor. In addition, Clark and associates found that concurrent infection at another site and requirement for serial monitors increased the infection rate. They also determined that prophylactic use of antibiotics did not decrease the rate of ventriculostomy infection. Clark and colleagues recommend that catheters be removed or replaced by 72 hours. Mayhall and others[156] recommend catheter removal by the fifth day. Kanter and coworkers[167] studied 65 children with acute brain injury and ICP monitors. They determined that the infection risk actually decreased after day 6. The declining risk of infection over time led Kanter and others to conclude that infection was introduced at the time of insertion. They recommend using a single ventriculostomy as long as required, reinserting a new monitor only for malfunction. Kanter and others also advise daily surveillance cultures to identify an infection of the system.

REFERENCES ■

1. Donowitz LG (ed): *Hospital acquired infection in the pediatric patient*. Baltimore, Williams & Wilkins, 1988

2. Wenzel RP, Thompson RL, Landry SM, et al: Hospital-acquired infections in intensive care unit patients: an overview with emphasis on epidemics. *Infect Control* 1983;5:371

3. Chandrasekar PH, Kruse JA, Mathews MF: Nosocomial infection among patients in different types of intensive care units at a city hospital. *Crit Care Med* 1986;14:508

4. Craven DE, Kunches LM, Lichtenberg DA, et al: Nosocomial infection and fatality in medical and surgical intensive care unit patients. *Arch Intern Med* 1988;148:161

5. Daschner FD, Frey P, Wolff G, et al: Nosocomial infections in intensive care wards: a multicenter prospective study. *Intensive Care Med* 1982;8:5

6. Donowitz LG, Wenzel RP, Hoyt JW: High risk of hospital-acquired infection in the ICU patient. *Crit Care Med* 1982;10:355

7. Marshall JC, Christou NV, Horn R, et al: The microbiology of multiple organ failure: the proximal GI tract as an occult reservoir of pathogens. *Arch Surg* 1988;123:309

8. Marshall JC, Sweeney D: Microbial infection and the septic response in critical surgical illness: sepsis, not infection, determines outcome. *Arch Surg* 1990;125:17

9. Massanari PM, Hierholzer WJ: The intensive care unit. In: Bennett JV, Brachman PS (eds). *Hospital infections*. Boston: Little, Brown, 1986:285

10. Velimirovic B: Hospital infections from the WHO perspective. *Infect Control* 1983;4:364

11. Platt R, Polk BF, Murdouk B, et al: Mortality associated with nosocomial urinary tract infection. *N Engl J Med* 1982;307:637

12. Maki DG, Weise CE, Sarafin HW: A semiquantitative culture method for identifying intravenous catheter-related infections. *N Engl J Med* 1977;296:1305

13. Louria DB, Stiff DP, Bennett B: Disseminated moniliasis in the adult. *Medicine (Baltimore)* 1962;41:307

14. Kofshy P, Rosen L, Reed J, et al: Clostridium difficile: a common and costly colitis. *Dis Colon Rectum* 1991;34:244

15. Paramore CG, Turner DA: Relative risks of ventriculostomy infection and morbidity. *Acta Neurochirurgica* 1994;127:79

16. Nathens AB, Chu PTY, Marshall JC: Nosocomial infection in the surgical intensive care unit. *Surgical Infections* 1992;6:657

17. Abraham E: Host defense abnormalities after hemorrhage, trauma, and burns. *Crit Care Med* 1989;17:934

18. Christou NV: Host defence mechanisms in surgical patients: a correlative study of the delayed hypersensitivity skin-test response, granulocyte function and sepsis. *Can J Surg* 1985;28:39

19. Keane RM, Birmingham W, Shatney CM, et al: Prediction of sepsis in the multitraumatized patient by assays of lymphocyte responsiveness. *Surg Gynecol Obstet* 1983;156:163

20. Bryan CS, Reynolds KL, Brenner ER: Analysis of 1,186 episodes of gram-negative bacteremia in non-university hospitals: the effects of antimicrobial therapy. *Rev Infect Dis* 1983;5:629

21. Klastersky J: Nosocomial infections due to gram-negative bacilli in compromised hosts: considerations for prevention and therapy. *Rev Infect Dis* 1985;7(Suppl 4):552

22. Gardner P, Arrow PM: Hospital-acquired infections. In: Braunwald E, Isselbacher KG, Petersdorf RG, et al (eds): *Harrison's Principles of Internal Medicine*, 11th ed. New York, McGraw-Hill, 1988:470

23. Caplan ES, Hoyt N: Infection surveillance and control in the severely traumatized patient. *Am J Med* 1981;144:449

24. Donowitz LG: High risk of nosocomial infection in the pediatric critical care patient. *Crit Care Med* 1986;14:26

25. Maki DG: Risk factors for nosocomial infection in intensive care. *Arch Intern Med* 1989;149:30

26. Fry DE, Pearlstein L, Fulton RL, et al: Multiple system organ failure: the role of uncontrolled infection. *Arch Surg* 1980; 115:136

27. Craven DE, Kunches LM, Lichtenberg DA, et al: Nosocomial infection and fatality in medical surgical intensive care patients. *Arch Intern Med* 1988;148:161

28. Goldmann DA, Freeman J, Durbin WA Jr: Nosocomial infection and death in a neonatal intensive care unit. *J Infect Dis* 1983;147:635

29. McGowan JE: Changing etiology of nosocomial bacteremia and fungemia and other hospital-acquired infections. *Rev Infect Dis* 1985;7(Suppl 3):357

30. Kiani D, Quinn EL, Burch KH, et al: The increasing importance of polymicrobial bacteremia. *JAMA* 1979;242:1044

31. Meduri GU: Ventilator-associated pneumonia in patients with respiratory failure. *Chest* 1990;97:1208

32. Tobin MJ, Grenvik A: Nosocomial lung infection and its diagnosis. *Crit Care Med* 1984;12:191

33. Craven DE, Steger KA, Barber TW: Preventing nosocomial pneumonia: state of the art and perspectives for the 1990's. *Am J Med* 1991;91(Suppl 3B):44S

34. Inglis TJJ: Pulmonary infection in intensive care units. *Br J Anaesth* 1990;65:94

35. Niederman MS, Fein AM: The interaction of infection and the adult respiratory distress syndrome. *Crit Care Clin* 1986;2:471

36. Wanner A, Amikam B, Robinson MJ, et al: Comparison between the bacteriologic flora of different segments of the airways. *Respiration* 1973;30:561

37. Shires GT, Dineen P: Sepsis following burns, trauma, and intra-abdominal infections. *Arch Intern Med* 1982;142:2012

38. Andrews CP, Coalson JJ, Smith JD, et al: Diagnosis of nosocomial bacterial pneumonia in acute, diffuse lung injury. *Chest* 1981;80:254

39. Bell RC, Coalson JJ, Smith JD, et al: Multiple organ system failure and infection in adult respiratory distress syndrome. *Ann Intern Med* 1983;99:293

40. Fagon JY, Chastre J, Hance AJ, et al: Detection of nosocomial lung infection in ventilated patients. *Am Rev Respir Dis* 1988;138:110

41. Johanson WG Jr: Ventilator-associated pneumonia: light at the end of the tunnel? *Chest* 1990;97:1026

42. Johanson WG Jr, Pierce AK, Sanford JP, et al: Nosocomial respiratory infections with gram-negative bacilli. *Ann Intern Med* 1972;77:701

43. Palmer DL: Microbiology of pneumonia in the patient at risk. *Am J Med* 1984;76(Suppl):53

44. Driks MR, Craven DE, Celli BA, et al: Nosocomial pneumonia in intubated patients randomized to sucralfate versus antacids and/or histamine type 2 blockers: the role of gastric colonization. *N Engl J Med* 1987;317:1376

45. Crouch TW, Higuchi JH, Coalson JJ, et al: Pathogenesis and preventation of nosocomial pneumonia in a non-human primate model of acute respiratory failure. *Am Rev Respir Dis* 1984;130:502

46. Selden R, Lees S, Wang WLL, et al: Nosocomial *Klebsiella* infections: intestinal colonization as a reservoir. *Ann Intern Med* 1971;74:657

47. Dumoulin GC, Paterson DC, Hedley-White J, et al: Aspiration of gastric bacteria in antacid-treated patients: a frequent cause of postoperative colonization of the airway. *Lancet* 1982;i:242

48. Podnos SD, Toews GB, Pierce AK: Nosocomial pneumonia in patients in intensive care units. *West J Med* 1985;143:622

49. Johanson WG Jr, Hugushi JH, Chaudhuri TR, et al: Bacterial adherence to epithelial cells in bacillary colonization of the respiratory tract. *Am Rev Respir Dis* 1980;121:55

50. Abraham SN, Beachey EH, Simpson WA: Adherence of *Streptococcus pyogenes*, *Eschericia coli*, and *Pseudomonas aeruginosa* to fibronectin-coated and uncoated epithelial cells. *Infect Immun* 1983;41:1261

51. Woods DE, Bass JA, Johanson WG Jr, et al: Role of adherence in the pathogenesis of *Pseudomonas aeruginosa* lung infection in cystic fibrosis patients. *Infect Immun* 1980;30:694

52. Bartlett JG, Alexander J, Mayhew J, et al: Should fiberoptic bronchoscopy aspirates be cultured? *Am Rev Respir Dis* 1976;114:73

53. Johanson WG Jr, Seidenfield JJ, Gomez P, et al: Bacterial diagnosis of nosocomial pneumonia following prolonged mechanical ventilation. *Am Rev Respir Dis* 1988;137:259

54. Chastre J, Fagon JY, Soler P, et al: Quantification of BAL cells containing intracellular bacteria rapidly identified ventilated patients with nosocomial pneumonia. *Chest* 1989;95:190S

55. Castellino RA, Blank N: Etiologic diagnosis of focal pulmonary infection in immunocompromised patients by fluoroscopically guided percutaneous needle aspiration. *Radiology* 1979;132:563

56. Hampton AA, Sheretz RJ: Vascular access infections in hospitalized patients. *Surg Clin North Am* 1988;68:57

57. Nelson LD, Martinez O, Anderson H: The incidence of positive cultures in open versus closed thermodilution injectate delivery systems. *Crit Care Med* 1986;14:291

58. Moran JM, Atwood RP, Rowe MI: A clinical and bacteriologic study of infections associated with venous cutdowns. *N Engl J Med* 1965;272:554

59. Norwood SH, Jenkins G: An evaluation of triple-lumen catheter infections using a guidewire exchange technique. *J Trauma* 1990;30:706

60. Peters G, Loui R, Pulverer G: Adherence and growth of coagulase-negative staphylococci on surfaces of intravenous catheters. *J Infect Dis* 1982;146:479

61. Beam TR: Vascular access catheters and infections. *Infect Surg* 1989;5:156

62. Bjornson HS, Colley R, Bower RH, et al: Association between microorganism growth at the catheter insertion site and colonization of the catheter in patients receiving total parenteral nutrition. *Surgery* 1982;92:720

63. Martin MA, Pfaller MA, Wenzel RP: Coagulase-negative staphylococcal bacteremia. *Ann Intern Med* 1989;110:9

64. Gristina AG: Biomaterial-centered infection: microbial adhesion versus tissue integration. *Science* 1987;237:1588

65. Gilsdorg JR, Wilson K, Beals TF: Bacterial colonization of intravenous catheter materials in vitro and in vivo. *Surgery* 1989;106:37

66. Franceschi D, Gerding RL, Phillips G, et al: Risk factors associated with intravascular catheter infections in burned patients: a prospective randomized study. *J Trauma* 1989; 29:811

67. Linares J, Sitges-Serra A, Garan J, et al: Pathogenesis of catheter sepsis: a prospective study with quantitative and semiquantitative cultures of catheter hub and segments. *J Clin Microbiol* 1985;21:357

68. Sitges-Serra A, Linares J, Garan J: Catheter sepsis: the clue is the hub. *Surgery* 1985;97:355

69. Henderson DK: Intravascular device-associated infection: current concepts and controversies. *Infect Surg* 1988;7:365

70. Kovacevich DS, Faubion WC, Bender JM, et al: Association of parenteral nutrition catheter sepsis with urinary tract infections. *J Parenter Enter Nutr* 1986;10:639

71. Pettigrew RA, Lang SDR, Haydock DA, et al: Catheter-related sepsis in patients on intravenous nutrition: a prospective study of quantitative catheter cultures and guidewire changes for suspected sepsis. *Br J Surg* 1985;72:52

72. Maki DG, Rhame FS, Mackel DC, et al: Nationwide epidemic of septicemia caused by contaminated intravenous products. I. Epidemiologic and clinical features. *Am J Med* 1976;60:471

73. Goldmann DG, Martin WT, Worthington JW: Growth of bacteria and fungi in total parenteral nutrition solutions. *Am J Surg* 1973;126:314

74. Crocker KS, Noga R, Filibeck DG, et al: Microbial growth comparisons of five commercial parenteral lipid emulsions. *J Parenter Enter Nutr* 1984;8:391

75. Armstrong CW, Mayhall CG, Miller KB, et al: Prospective study of catheter replacement and other risk factors for infection of hyperalimentation catheters. *J Infect Dis* 1986;154:808

76. Sitzmann JV, Townsend TR, Siler MC, et al: Septic and technical complications of central venous catheterization: a prospective study of 200 consecutive patients. *Ann Surg* 1985;202:766

77. Maki DG, Band JD: A comparative study of polyantibiotic and iodophor ointments in prevention of vascular catheter-related infection. *Am J Med* 1981;70:739

78. Maki DG, Ringer M: Evaluation of dressing regimens for prevention of infection with peripheral intravenous catheters. *JAMA* 1987;258:2396

79. Craven DE, Lichtenberg DA, Kunches IM, et al: A randomized study comparing a transparent polyurethane dressing to a dry gauze dressing for peripheral intravenous catheter sites. *Infect Control* 1985;6:361

80. Conly JM, Grieves K, Peters B: A prospective randomized study comparing transparent and dry gauze dressings for central venous catheters. *J Infect Dis* 1989;159:310

81. Dickerson N, Horton P, Smith S, et al: Clinically significant central venous catheter infections in a community hospital: association with type of dressing. *J Infect Dis* 1989;160:720

82. Clarke DE, Raffin TA: Infectious complications of indwelling long-term central venous catheters. *Chest* 1990;97:966

83. Eyer S, Brummitt C, Crossley K, et al: Catheter-related sepsis: a prospective, randomized study of three methods of long-term catheter maintenance (unpublished data)

84. Snyder RH, Archer FJ, Endy T, et al: Catheter infection: a comparison of two catheter maintenance techniques. *Ann Surg* 1988;208:651

85. Cooper GL, Hopkins GC: Rapid diagnosis of intravascular catheter-associated infection by direct gram staining of catheter segments. *N Engl J Med* 1985;312:1142

86. Cleri DJ, Corrado ML, Seligman SJ: Quantitative culture of intravenous catheters and other intravascular inserts. *J Infect Dis* 1980;141:781

87. Moyer MA, Edwards LD, Farley L: Comparative culture methods on 101 intravenous catheters. *Arch Intern Med* 1983;143:66

88. Wormser GP, Onorato IM, Preminger TJ, et al: Sensitivity and specificity of blood cultures obtained through intravascular catheters. *Crit Care Med* 1990;18:152

89. Tafuro P, Colbourn D, Gurevich I, et al: Comparison of blood cultures obtained simultaneously by venipuncture and from vascular lines. *J Hosp Infect* 1986;7:283

90. Damen J: The microbiologic risk of invasive hemodynamic monitoring in open-heart patients requiring prolonged ICU treatment. *Intensive Care Med* 1988;14:156

91. Myers ML, Austin TW, Sibbald WJ: Pulmonary artery catheter infections. *Ann Surg* 1985;201:237

92. Hudson-Civetta JA, Civetta JM, Martinez OV, et al: Risk and detection of pulmonary artery catheter-related infection in septic surgical patients. *Crit Care Med* 1987;15:29

93. Civetta JM, Hudson-Civetta JA, Dion L: Duration of illness affects catheter-related infection and bacteremia [abstract]. In: *Program and Abstracts of the 27th Interscience Conference on Antimicrobial Agents and Chemotherapy*, vol 60, 1987: 1141

94. Hilton E, Haslett TM, Borenstein MT, et al: Central catheter infections: single- versus triple-lumen catheters. *Am J Med* 1988;84:667

95. Ball S, Hudson-Civetta J, Civetta J: Re-evaluation of insertion and guidewire exchange (GWX) protocols effectiveness and validity. *Crit Care Med* 1995;23(Suppl):A250

96. Ball S, Hudson-Civetta J, Civetta JM: Decreasing catheter-related infection, patient risk and hospital costs by continuous quality improvement. *Crit Care Med* 1996;A24:24

97. Band JD, Maki DG: Infections caused by arterial catheters used for hemodynamic monitoring. *Am J Med* 1979;67:735

98. Norwood SH, Cormier B, McMahon NG, et al: Prospective study of catheter-related infection during prolonged arterial catheterization. *Crit Care Med* 1988;16:836

99. Leroy O, Beuscart C, Santre C, et al: Nosocomial infections associated with long-term artery cannulation. *Intensive Care Med* 1989;15:241

100. Olson MM, Lee JT: Continuous 10-year wound infection surveillance. *Arch Surg* 1990;125:794

101. Lively JC, Pruitt BA: Infection-related complications. In: Greenfield LJ (ed). *Complications in Surgery and Trauma*, 2nd ed. Philadelphia, JB Lippincott, 1990:96

102. Bahnson RR: Urosepsis. *Urol Clin North Am* 1986;13:627

103. Seiler WO, Stahelin HB: Practical management of catheter-associated UTIs. *Geriatrics* 1988;43:43

104. Warren JW: Nosocomial urinary tract infections. In: Mandell GL, Douglas RG, Bennet JE (eds). *Principles and Practice of Infectious Diseases*, 3rd ed. New York, Churchill Livingstone, 1990:2205

105. Krieger JN, Kaiser DL, Wenzel RP: Urinary tract etiology of bloodstream infections in hospitalized patients. *J Infect Dis* 1983;148:57

106. Carson CC: Nosocomial urinary tract infections. *Surg Clin North Am* 1988;68:1147

107. Kass EH, Schneiderman LJ: Entry of bacteria into the urinary tract of patients with inlying catheters. *N Engl J Med* 1970; 282:33

108. Lipsky BA: Urinary tract infections in men. *Ann Intern Med* 1989;110:138

109. Shapiro M, Simchen E, Izraeli S, et al: A multivariate analysis of risk factors for acquiring bacteriuria in patients with indwelling urinary catheters for longer than 24 hours. *Infect Control* 1984;5:525

110. Cuhna BA: Nosocomial urinary tract infections. *Heart Lung* 1982;11:545

111. Fisher JF, Chew WH, Shadomy S, et al: Urinary tract infections due to *Candida albicans. Rev Infect Dis* 1982;4:1107

112. Pierone G: Candiduria in hospitalized patients. *Infect Surg* 1990;9:19

113. Kozinn PJ, Taschdjian CL, Goldberg PK, et al: Advances in the diagnosis of renal candidiasis. *J Urol* 1978;119:184

114. Wise GJ, Kozinin PJ, Goldberg P: Amphotericin B as a urologic irrigant in the management of noninvasive candiduria. *U Urol* 1981;128:82

115. Rivett AG, Perry JA, Cohen J: Urinary candidiasis: a prospective study in hospitalized patients. *Urol Res* 1986;14:183

116. Galgiani JN: Fluconazole: a new antifungal agent. *Ann Intern Med* 1990;113:177

117. Bromberg K, Gleich S, Ginsberg MB: Clostridia in urinary tract infections. *South Med J* 1981;75:1298

118. Schaeffer AJ: Catheter-associated bacteriuria in patients in reverse isolation. *J Urol* 1982;128:752

119. Lobo PI, Rodolph LE, Krieger JN: Wound infections in renal transplant recipients: a complication of urinary tract infections during allograft malfunction. *Surgery* 1982;92:491

120. Martinez OV, Civetta JM, Anderson K, et al: Bacteriuria in the catheterized surgical intensive care patient: a prospective survey of 100 patients. *Crit Care Med* 1986;14:188

121. Wey SB, Motomi Mori MS, Pfaller MA, et al: Hospital-acquired candidemia. *Arch Intern Med* 1988;148:2642

122. Cohen R, Roth F, Delgrado E, et al: Fungal flora of the normal human small and large intestines. *Engl J Med* 1969;280:638

123. Wey SB, Motomi Mori MS, Pfaller MA, et al: Risk factors for hospital-acquired candidemia. *Arch Intern Med* 1989; 149:2349

124. Sobel JD: *Candida* infections in the intensive care unit. *Crit Care Clin* 1988;4:325

125. Hughes JM, Remington JS: Systemic candidiasis: a diagnostic challenge. *Calif Med* 1972;116:8

126. Burchard KW, Minor LB, Slotman GJ, et al: Fungal sepsis in surgical patients. *Arch Surg* 1983;118:217

127. Solomkin JS, Flohr AB, Simmons RL: *Candida* infections in surgical patients: dose requirements and toxicity of amphotericin B. *Ann Surg* 1982;195:177

128. Slotman GJ, Burchard KW: Ketoconazole prevents *Candida* sepsis in critically ill surgical patients. *Arch Surg* 1987;122:147

129. Caplan ES, Hoyt NJ: Nosocomial sinusitis. *JAMA* 1982; 247:639

130. Linden BE, Aguilar EA, Allen S: Sinusitis in the nasotracheally intubated patient. *Arch Otolaryngol Head Neck Surg* 1988;144:860

131. Michelson A, Schuster B, Kamp D: Paranasal sinusitis associated with nasotracheal and orotracheal long-term intubation. *Arch Otolaryngol Head Neck Surg* 1992;118:937

132. Fassoulaki A, Pamouktsoglou P: Prolonged nasotracheal intubation and its association with inflammation of paranasal sinuses. *Anesth Analg* 1989;69:50

133. Druce HM: Emerging techniques in the diagnosis of sinusitis. *Ann Allergy* 1991;66:132

134. DeWeese DD, Saunders WH: Acute and chronic sinusitis. In: *Textbook of Otolaryngology*, 6th ed. St Louis: CV Mosby, 1982:223

135. O'Reilly MJ, Reddick EJ, Black W, et al: Sepsis from sinusitis in nasotracheally intubated patients. *Am J Surg* 1984;147:601

136. Chidekel N, Jensen C, Axelsson A, et al: Diagnosis of fluid in the maxillary sinus. *Acta Radiol Diagn* 1970;10:433

137. Hansen M, Poulsen MR, Bendixen DK, et al: Incidence of sinusitis in patients with nasotracheal intubation. *Br J Anaesth* 1988;61:231

138. Gianoli GJ, Mann W, Miller RH: B-Mode ultrasonography of the paranasal sinuses compared with CT findings. *Otolaryngol Head Neck Surg* 1992;107:713

139. Druce HM: Diagnosis of sinusitis in adults: history, physical examination, nasal cytology, echo, and rhinoscope. *J Allergy Clin Immunol* 1992;90:436

140. Revonta M: Ultrasound in the diagnosis of maxillary and frontal sinusitis. *Acta Otolaryngol* 1980;370(Suppl):1

141. Jannert M, Andreasson L, Holmer N-G, et al: Ultrasonic examination of the paranasal sinuses. *Acta Otolaryngol* 1982; 389(Suppl):1

142. Hansen M, Poulsen MR, Bendixen DK, et al: Incidence of sinusitis in patients with nasotracheal intubation. *Br J Anaesth* 1988;61:231

143. Tedesco FJ: Pseudomembranous colitis: pathogenesis and therapy. *Med Clin North Am* 1982;66:655

144. Talbot RW, Walker RC, Beart RW Jr: Changing epidemiology, diagnosis, and treatment of *Clostridium dificile* toxin–associated colitis. *Br J Surg* 1986;73:457

145. Mulligan ME: Epidemiology of *Clostridium dificile*–induced intestinal disease. *Rev Infect Dis* 1984;6:222

146. Kaatz GW, Gitlin SD, Schaberg DR, et al: Acquisition of *Clostridium difficile* from the hospital environment. *Am J Epidemiol* 1988;127:1289

147. Tedesco FJ: Pseudomembranous colitis: pathogenesis and therapy. *Med Clin North Am* 1982;66:655

148. Kofsky P, Rosen L, Reed J, et al: *Clostridium difficile*: a common and costly colitis. *Dis Colon Rectum* 1991;34:244

149. Edes TE, Walk BE, Austin JL: Diarrhea in tube-fed patients: feeding formula not necessarily the cause. *Am J Med* 1990; 88:91

150. McFarland LV, Mulligan ME, Kwok RY, et al: Nosocomial acquisition of *Clostridium difficile* infection. *N Engl J Med* 1989;320:204

151. Aucoin PJ, Kotilainen HR, Gantz NM, et al: Intracranial pressure monitors: epidemiologic study of risk factors and infections. *Am J Med* 1986;80:369

152. Blomstedt G: Results of trimethoprim-sulfamethoxazole prophylaxis in ventriculostomy and shunting. *J Neurosurg* 1985;62:649

153. Friedman W, Vries J: Percutaneous tunnel ventriculostomy: summary of 100 procedures. *J Neurosurg* 1980;53:662

154. Kusske JA, Turner PT, Ojemann GA, et al: Ventriculostomy for the treatment of acute hydrocephalus following subarachnoid hemorrhage. *J Neurosurg* 1973;38:591

155. Lundberg N: Continuous recording and control of ventricular fluid pressure in neurosurgical practice. *Acta Psychol Neurol Scand* 1960;149(Suppl):45

156. Mayhall CG, Archer NH, Archer-Lamb V, et al: Ventriculostomy-related infections. *N Engl J Med* 1984;310:553

157. Mollman HD, Roskswold GL, Ford SE: A clinical comparison of subarachnoid catheters to ventriculostomy and subarachnoid bolts: a prospective study. *J Neurosurg* 1988;68:737

158. Narayan RK, Kishore PRS, Becker DP, et al: Intracranial pressure to monitor or not to monitor? *J Neurosurg* 1982; 56:650

159. Ohrstrom JK, Skou JK, Ejlertsen T, et al: Infected ventriculostomy: bacteriology and treatment. *Acta Neurochir (Wien)* 1989;100:67

160. Powell MP, Crockard HA: Behavior of an extradural pressure monitor in clinical use. *J Neurosurg* 1985;63:745

161. Smith RW, Alksne JF: Infections complicating the use of external ventriculostomy. *J Neurosurg* 1976;44:567

162. Stenager E, Gerner-Smidt P, Kock-Jensen C: Ventriculostomy-related infections: an epidemiological study. *Acta Neurochir (Wien)* 1986;83:20

163. Sundbarg G, Kjallquist A, Lundberg N, et al: Complications due to prolonged ventricular fluid pressure recording in clinical practice. In: Brock M, Dietz H (eds). *Intracranial Pressure*. Berlin, Heidelberg, New York, Springer-Verlag, 1972: 348

164. Sundbarg G, Nordstrom C, Soderstrom S: Complications due to prolonged ventricular fluid pressure recording. *Br J Neurosurg* 1988;2:485

165. Winfield JA, Rosenthal P, Kanter RK, et al: Duration of intracranial pressure monitoring does not predict daily risk of infectious complications. *Neurosurgery* 1993;33:424

166. Wyler AR, Kelly WA: Use of antibiotics with external ventriculostomies. *Neurosurgery* 1972;37:185

167. Kanter RK, Weiner LB, Patti AM, et al: Infectious complications and duration of intracranial pressure monitoring. *Crit Care Med* 1985;13:837

168. Clark WC, Muhlbauer MS, Lowrey R, et al: Complications of intracranial pressure monitoring in trauma patients. *Neurosurgery* 1989;25:20

Critical Care, Third Edition, edited by Joseph M. Civetta,
Robert W. Taylor, and Robert R. Kirby.
Lippincott-Raven Publishers, Philadelphia, PA © 1997.

CHAPTER 107

An Approach to the Febrile ICU Patient

David V. Shatz
Scott Norwood

IMMEDIATE CONCERNS ■

MAJOR PROBLEMS

With the mortality from sepsis still approaching 50%, fever in critically ill surgical and medical patients elicits a sense of urgency in identifying the etiology. Although infection is commonly the source of fever, other possibilities must be included in the differential diagnosis, and a logical, deliberate approach should be followed to localize the source, avoiding rote ordering of expensive and nonspecific laboratory tests and radiographs. An exhaustive treatise on every cause of fever is beyond any single textbook chapter. A rational clinical approach to evaluating fever in critically ill patients is presented here.

The evaluation process should be "therapy directed" so that tests that have no major impact on clinical management are avoided. The initial febrile episode should be evaluated with a careful review of the patient's history and a thorough physical examination. If this approach fails to identify a source, no further procedures are necessary unless the patient is severely immunocompromised or a high probability of bacteremia exists. If a second febrile episode occurs, further testing should be performed. Figure 107-1 provides guidelines for evaluation.

STRESS POINTS

1. Catheter-related infection is virtually nonexistent for the first 48 hours after insertion, and central venous catheters are infrequent sources of fever if strict protocols for insertion and maintenance are followed.

2. Central venous catheters impregnated with silver sulfadiazine-chlorhexadine (ARROWgard) further reduce the chances of catheter sepsis and allow these lines to safely remain in place for longer periods of time.

3. Fever in the immediate postoperative period requires careful inspection of all surgical or traumatic wounds.

4. Crush injury syndrome, and occasionally tetanus, can cause fever in the postoperative trauma patient.

5. Because of limitations with conventional radiographs, sonography, and radionuclide scanning, computed tomography (CT) has become the preferred method for diagnosing intraabdominal abscess.

6. Sources of fever other than infection must be considered under certain clinical conditions. Up to 30% of hospitalized patients experience some type of adverse drug reaction.

7. Approximately 90% of blood transfusion reactions are allergic or febrile.

8. Malignant hyperthermia (MH) is usually observed during general anesthesia but may not develop until the patient reaches the ICU. Early symptoms can be confused with thyrotoxicosis, undiagnosed pheochromocytoma, or neuroleptic malignant syndrome.

9. Acute adrenocortical insufficiency is rare, but can occur in patients who are being weaned from steroids and suddenly develop fever and hypotension.

1589

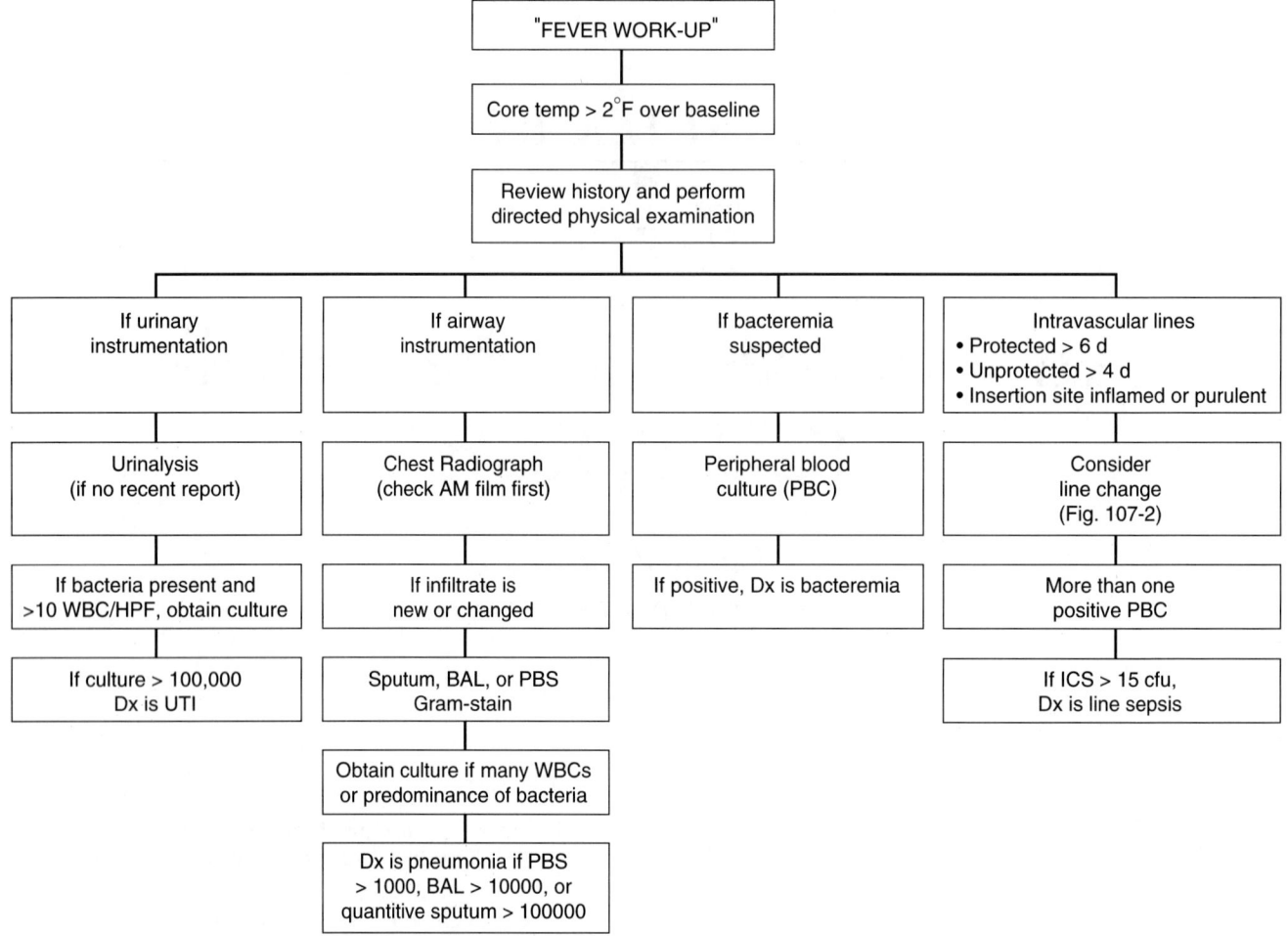

FIGURE 107-1. Guidelines for evaluating infectious sources of fever. BAL, bronchoalveolar lavage; PBS, protected brush specimen; Protected, silver sulfadiazine-chlorhexidine impregnated catheters; Dx, diagnosis; PBC, peripheral blood culture; ICS, intracutaneous catheter segment; CFU, colony forming units; Baseline temp, highest level on previous day; WBCs, white blood cells; HPF, high-power field; UTI, urinary tract infection.

ESSENTIAL DIAGNOSTIC TESTS AND PROCEDURES

1. Sputum Gram stain should precede any cultures when pneumonia is suspected.
2. Urinalysis should always precede urine culture, which is obtained only when bacteria and more than 10 white blood cells per high-powered field are present on urinalysis.
3. Meningitis is an uncommon cause of fever in surgical ICU patients, but must be considered in any critically ill patient who develops altered mental status associated with high fever.
4. CT is not as reliable in critically ill patients when compared with scanning in hospital populations in general; it can be helpful but should not be used to search blindly for a source of sepsis as part of a fever workup.
5. Fever may be an isolated symptom (drug fever) or the first sign of anaphylaxis or serum sickness.

6. Fever may accompany acute hemolytic reactions, with the first manifestation being sudden diffuse bleeding from multiple sites. This potential life-threatening complication must be considered if fever develops within 30 minutes after beginning a blood product transfusion.

INITIAL THERAPY

1. An approach to managing potential catheter-related febrile episodes is outlined in Figure 107-2.
2. Gas gangrene and necrotizing fasciitis from clostridial or streptococcal organisms can occur within the first 48 hours postoperatively. Other types of infections occur later, but most can be diagnosed with careful inspection and palpation of the wound.
3. Intraabdominal infectious processes are not likely to be detected by CT in the first 5 to 7 days postoperatively. Abdominal reexploration may be necessary in

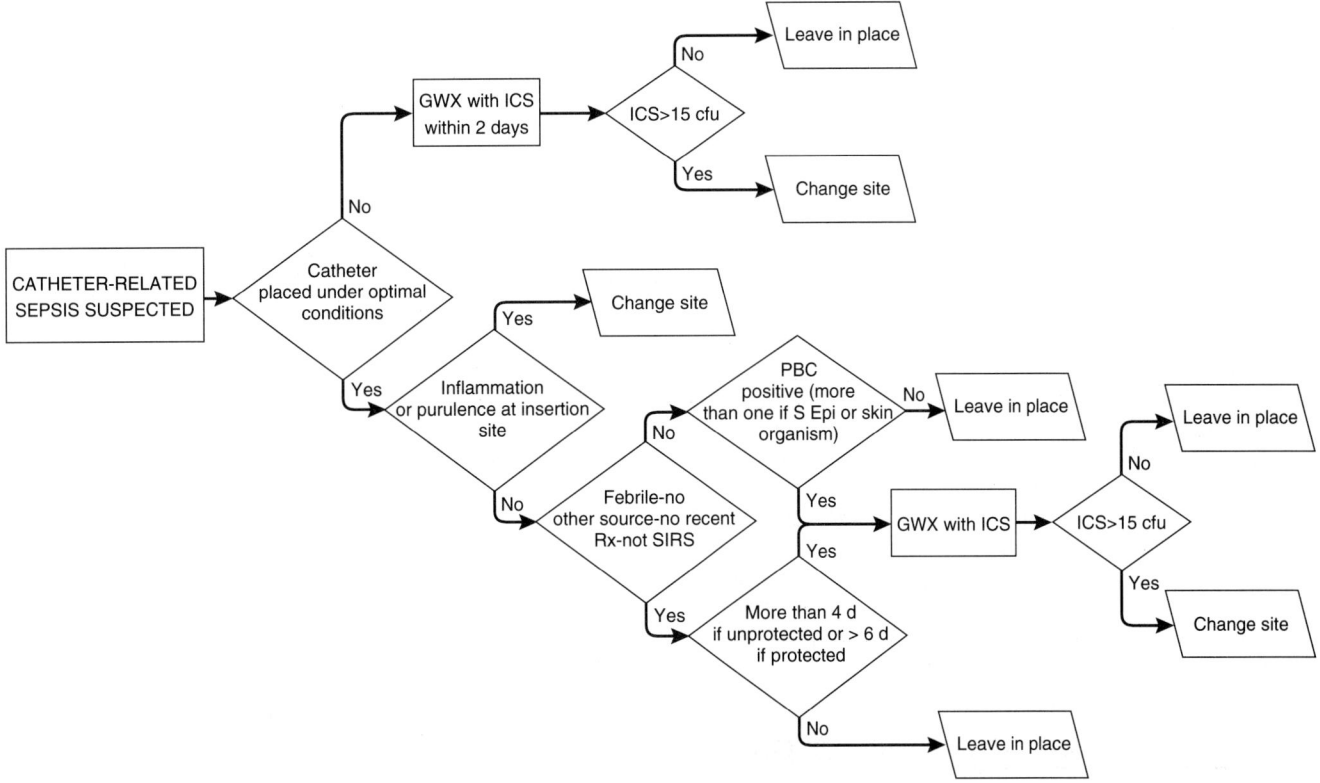

FIGURE 107-2. An approach to the management of potential catheter-related febrile episodes. GWX, guidewire exchange; ICS, intracutaneous catheter segment; Protected, silver sulfadiazine-chlorhexidine impregnated catheters; CFU, colony forming units; PBC, peripheral blood culture; S Epi, staphlococcal epidermatis; Rx, therapy; SIRS, systemic inflammatory response system.

some patients and should be considered before the onset of multiple organ system failure (MOSF).

4. Drugs with a high probability of allergic reactions should be discontinued or replaced, if possible.
5. Fever causes major alterations in oxygen consumption and may be detrimental to elderly patients or those with limited ability to increase oxygen delivery, and should therefore be treated aggressively in these patients.
6. Metabolic responses to increased body temperature make fever detrimental in patients sustaining intracranial trauma and should be aggressively controlled.

DEFINITION, PATHOPHYSIOLOGY, AND PURPOSE ■

Fever is a disorder of normal body thermoregulation that is controlled in the anterior hypothalamus. This ancient mechanism may have evolved as a means to combat infection. Certain organisms, such as those producing syphilis and gonorrhea, are heat sensitive and can be destroyed in vivo by artificially inducing fever. In the ICU patient, however, the detrimental aspects of fever usually outweigh any potential benefits. The most important role for fever in critically

ill patients is to provide an early warning sign for infection or inflammation.[1]

Thermoregulatory mechanisms are precisely balanced over a narrow range during health so that body temperature is usually maintained at $37° ± 1°C$, with values lowest in early morning and highest in late afternoon.[2] Adverse physiologic side effects include vasoconstriction and shivering, which can dramatically increase oxygen consumption. Negative feedback mechanisms usually maintain temperatures below $41°C$ clinically.[2] However, with disorders such as MH, these feedback mechanisms are lost, and body temperatures above $41°C$ are common.

Various pathophysiologic mechanisms cause fever. Substances called *pyrogens* are often responsible in humans and various laboratory models. In addition to infectious pyrogens (viruses, bacteria, fungi), antigen–antibody complexes,[3] steroids,[4] and other inorganic substances can produce experimental fevers.[5] Depending on the causative agent, the characteristics vary with respect to time of onset, duration, and character of the fever curve.[2] All pyrogens evoke a common mediator, *endogenous pyrogen*, or interleukin-1, a monokine produced by leukocytes.[6] Interleukin-1 elicits fever by altering the activity of temperature-sensitive neurons located in the anterior hypothalamus. This monokine is an extremely sensitive hormone; as little as 35 ng produces clinical fevers up to 0.6C above baseline in experimental animals.[7]

COMMON CAUSES OF FEVER ■

Febrile ICU patients are classified into four groups: (1) patients who are incubating an infection when admitted; (2) patients whose fevers are an expression of their underlying disease (granulomatous infections, tumors of the reticuloendothelial system, connective tissues diseases, and others); (3) patients who develop an endogenous febrile process after admission (perforated ulcer, appendicitis, gout); and (4) patients who develop fever from medical or surgical therapy or from nosocomial infections.[8] Common causes of fever in medical and surgical ICU patients are listed in Tables 107-1 and 107-2. Many of these causes are common to both groups of patients, and some are diagnoses of exclusion. A rational diagnostic approach must be developed to direct therapy and eliminate needless laboratory tests and radiographs.

Infection is the most common cause of fever in medical and surgical ICU patients. Sepsis remains one of the leading causes of death in critically ill patients,[9] and therefore infection must always be considered; it must be actively but rationally eliminated as the cause of fever before other less common causes are considered.

FEVER AS A PREDICTOR OF INFECTION ■

Fever can be classified as intermittent, remittent, sustained, and relapsing.[8] Intermittent fever, in which the body temperature returns to normal each day, is characteristic of pyogenic

TABLE 107-1. Potential Causes of Fever in Medical ICU Patients

Infections
  Bacterial
  Fungal
  Viral
Thromboembolism
Drug fevers
Transfusion-related causes
Skin-related problems/decubiti
Neoplasms
  Lymphoma, leukemia
  Pancreatic cancer
  Hypernephroma
  Hepatoma
Central nervous system disorders
  Cerebrovascular accidents
  Tumors
  Hemorrhage
  Hematopoietic disorders
  Connective tissue/immunologic disorders
Metabolic disorders
  Adrenocortical insufficiency
  Thyroid crisis (storm)
  Gout
  Porphyria
Alcohol and drug withdrawal

TABLE 107-2. Potential Causes of Fever in Surgical ICU Patients

Infections related to surgery or trauma
  Wound infection
  Intraabdominal abscess
  Crush syndrome
  Tetanus
Nonsurgically related infections
  Pneumonia
  Urinary tract infection
  Catheter-related infection
  Neurologic sources
Adrenocortical insufficiency
Pheochromocytoma (undiagnosed)
Drug fevers
Transfusion-related fevers
Malignant hyperthermia

infection. It is the most common type of fever observed in ICU patients, partly because antipyretics are aggressively used. Remittent fevers, in which the temperature falls but does not return to normal, is considered the most common febrile response to diseases not specific to ICU patients.[8] Fever usually occurs abruptly under most clinical ICU situations and can vary significantly in degree of elevation per individual.

The primary goal of diagnosis is to separate infection from other causes of fever (many of which require no specific therapy). In young, previously healthy patients, fever may not cause significant harm or discomfort. However, in older patients, elevated body temperatures can significantly increase oxygen consumption, altering the balance between oxygen delivery and utilization. Fever should therefore be treated aggressively in these patients. Acetaminophen or indomethacin can be given rectally to minimize these adverse effects. Indomethacin may be contraindicated in patients at risk for ulcer disease because this agent may exacerbate or initiate an acute bleed. Similarly, the antiplatelet effects of indomethacin must be considered in the critically ill patient. Occasionally, antipyretic agents may cause a sharp decrease in temperature followed by involuntary muscle contractions (a chill).[8] Chills also produce increased oxygen consumption. A sharp reduction in temperature can be avoided by administering antipyretic agents at least every 3 hours around the clock rather than prescribing these agents only for temperature elevations above a certain level. For higher fevers that produce violent muscular contractions, small doses of parenteral morphine sulfate (or meperidine) with or without chlorpromazine, may be helpful.

The approach to evaluating patients with community-acquired causes of fever and sepsis is different from the approach in ICU patients. For ruling out infection, the evaluation process in the medical and surgical patient (with the exception of wound infections and intraabdominal sepsis) is similar.

Galicier and Richet[10] studied 693 postoperative patients to determine the etiology of postoperative fever (defined as >38°C). The overall rate of fever was 14% for clean, 13.4%

for clean contaminated, and 13.1% for contaminated surgical procedures. Similar postoperative fever rates are found in gynecologic[11] and pediatric surgical patients.[12] After elective, uncontaminated surgery, fever from infectious origins began significantly later (2.7 versus 1.6 days) and lasted significantly longer (5.4 versus 3.5 days) than fever for which no infectious source was determined. Only 50% of infections in the study group caused fever. Therefore, if fever were used as the only criterion to diagnose infection, sensitivity and specificity for this clinical sign would be 0.53 and 0.62, respectively. Of the febrile patients in this study for whom no source of infection was found, 94.1% had only one episode of temperature elevation. Although not all patients were critically ill, this study suggests that a reasonable approach to evaluating a patient after an initial febrile episode is a thorough physical examination only. If the physical examination reveals an abnormality, appropriate tests can be ordered to confirm clinical suspicions.

Other investigators have attempted to quantify fever as a diagnostic or screening sign for postoperative pulmonary complications.[13] Fever and chest radiographs were evaluated in 270 patients after elective intraabdominal surgery. The incidence of fever (temperature $\geq 38°C$) was 40%, with positive findings on chest radiographs in 57% of these patients. Sensitivity and negative predictive value for fever were just below 50%, and the specificity and positive predictive values were 68% and 66%, respectively.[13] The authors concluded that fever was not a reliable indicator of the presence or absence of postoperative pulmonary complications. Fever may actually be unreliable in predicting the presence of any type of infection during the immediate postoperative period.[14]

In another study of patients after abdominal operations, 71 of 464 patients (15%) had rectal temperatures above 38.5°C on two consecutive measurements. Infection was discovered in 19 of 71 patients (27%), and a correct diagnosis could have been made on clinical findings with confirmation by one appropriate test in 14 patients (74%).[15] A history and directed physical examination would have revealed the source of fever in most cases, but this fact did not prevent the usual response of ordering a battery of tests, including complete blood cell count, chest radiograph, and "pancultures" (urine, blood, sputum, and wound cultures). The only test with a high positive yield was the nondiagnostic and relatively unimportant complete blood cell count (44% positive). Frequently used tests had low positive rates in this study. For example, urine cultures were obtained in 86% of patients but were positive in only 10%; chest radiographs were performed in 75% of patients with only one positive result; two blood cultures (only 5% positive) were obtained in 60% of the patients. Most tests are ordered to detect the most common causes of postoperative infection. From this perspective, all the postoperative infections were correctly identified by rote ordering of tests or cultures, except for infection in one patient with a subdiaphragmatic abscess, which was ultimately confirmed by CT. However, 3.8 tests were ordered per febrile patient; only 18% (49 of 268) of tests were positive and only 7% (19 of 268) were useful in diagnosing the infection ultimately determined to be the cause of fever.[15] This study clearly demonstrates that a

more rational and clinically oriented approach should be considered.

RECOMMENDED APPROACH TO FEVER EVALUATION ■

Rather than using a purely diagnosis-directed approach to fever, the evaluation should also be therapy directed. Tests that have no significant impact on therapeutic interventions should be avoided, or at least postponed, until further clinical changes increase their true usefulness. "Low-yield" or non-specific tests should not be ordered early in the evaluation process. A "shotgun" approach to evaluation is discouraged.

The most important reason for evaluating a febrile episode is to determine whether fever is an early warning sign of sepsis, a part of the disease, or a developing nosocomial infection. The prevalence of nosocomial infections in ICU patients is discussed in Chapter 106.

EVALUATING INFECTIOUS SOURCES OF FEVER

The first febrile episode (defined as more than 1.3°C [2°F] above baseline temperature) should be evaluated with a careful review of the patient's history and a thorough physical examination. If this approach fails to identify a source, no further evaluation is necessary. Exceptions to this rule are severely immunocompromised patients or patients with a high probability of bacteremia, where a positive blood culture would significantly alter therapy. A thorough physical examination should always precede any laboratory or radiographic test. If a second febrile episode occurs, further testing should be considered. Figure 107-1 provides guidelines for diagnosing nosocomial infections.

Respiratory Infections

Pneumonia is one of the most common hospital-acquired infections leading to death and occurs in approximately 20% of patients requiring mechanical ventilation.[16] Nosocomial respiratory infections are discussed in detail in Chapter 106. If the clinical setting and physical examination are consistent with pneumonia, a portable chest radiograph should be obtained (upright if possible). The presence of new or significantly different infiltrates suggests pneumonia. If the patient's trachea has been intubated for more than 48 hours, upper airway colonization has already occurred.[17] A specimen should be obtained for Gram stain. If the Gram stain reveals numerous white blood cells or a predominant type of organism, appropriate specimens for culture should be obtained.

The methods for obtaining a valid culture are notoriously inaccurate in the intubated critically ill patient.[16] Quantitative analysis of endotracheal aspirates improves the diagnostic accuracy when a count of more than 10^5 colony-forming units (CFU) per milliliter is used. Presence of elastin fibers on potassium hydroxide stains of sputum samples is a specific, although not sensitive, test for the presence of necrotizing lung infections (gram-negative bacilli, *Staphylococcus aureus*).

The protected specimen brush, introduced in 1979, is considered a more reliable technique to improve culture accuracy.[18] Optimal results are achieved only with careful attention to minor details, and quantitative cultures are recommended with 10^3 CFU/mL considered diagnostic for infection.[16]

Bronchoalveolar lavage (BAL) has become the established method of diagnosing opportunistic pneumonia in immunosuppressed patients because contamination of the bronchoscopic suction channel does not seem to create a diagnostic dilemma in these patients.[16] Animal[19] and human[20] studies suggest that quantitative cultures of BAL fluid (considered positive if more than 10^4 CFU/mL are present), in combination with Giemsa stains and Gram stains, provide the most accurate and rapid diagnosis for pneumonia in mechanically ventilated patients.

Leeper[16] recommends the following approach to diagnosing and treating respiratory infections in mechanically ventilated patients with the adult respiratory distress syndrome. When the diagnosis of pneumonia is suspected, hemodynamically stable patients not receiving antibiotic therapy and with no contraindication to bronchoscopy should undergo lower respiratory tract sampling (bilateral protected specimen brushing and BAL). Patients receiving antibiotics for extrapulmonary infections should continue with these agents, but patients receiving empiric antibiotics for fever may have their antibiotics discontinued for 48 hours before bronchoscopy. Antibiotics should then be adjusted according to culture sensitivities in patients with pneumonia documented by bronchoscopic specimen. If equivocal cultures result, follow-up bronchoscopic examination is done. If no infection is documented by bronchoscopic cultures, diagnostic evaluation for the fever is continued.

Empiric antibiotic therapy should be initiated in patients who are clinically septic. Antibiotics should also be started in patients in whom the consequences of bacteremia outweigh the risks of antibiotic therapy (i.e., patients with vascular prosthetic grafts). Empiric antibiotics should be based on bacteria that historically predominate in each individual ICU. For example, if methicillin-resistant staphylococcus aureus is an organism historically present, infections believed likely to be caused by a gram-positive organism should be empirically covered with vancomycin, which should be adjusted when bacterial sensitivities become available. Similarly, if gram-negative organisms are likely to be the etiology of an infectious process, broad-spectrum antibiotics used to treat gram-negative organisms (e.g., imipenem–cilastatin, ticarcillin–clavulanate, piperacillin, or ceftazidime) should be started empirically. Because of the rapid rise of resistant strains of *Pseudomonas*, ICUs with even a low incidence of *Pseudomonas* infections should consider employing two empiric agents for suspected infections with gram-negative organisms. These antibiotics should both possess potent antipseudomonal properties and act at different sites within the bacteria. For example, the combination of a cell wall antibiotic (penicillin, cephalosporin, or carbapenem) with an antiribosomal agent (aminoglycoside) provides strong coverage against gram-negative organisms and synergistic action against *Pseudomonas*.

Urinary Tract Sources of Fever

Although nosocomial urinary tract infections are a common cause of fever in the hospital population collectively, urosepsis is not a common source of systemic sepsis in critically ill patients unless significant obstruction or urinary tract instrumentation has occurred (Chap. 106). If the urinary tract is suspected and no recent urinalysis has been reported, a urinalysis should be obtained. A urine culture is necessary only when bacteriuria and at least 10 white blood cells per high-powered field are present.[21]

Catheter-Related Febrile Episodes

Strict guidelines concerning the use and maintenance of central venous access catheters, pulmonary artery catheters, and arterial catheters should be developed based on available data specific to ICU patients (Chap. 106), individual institution populations, and individual patient risks. If strict aseptic technique and catheter maintenance guidelines are followed, catheter-related infection as a source of fever will be infrequent. Civetta and others[22] showed that positive culture results from central catheters accounted for unexplained fever spikes in only 5% of catheters removed from both "clean" and septic patients. These catheter-related infections occurred after the sixth ICU day in 75% of cases in both groups.[22] Central venous catheters placed under strict sterile techniques may be left in position indefinitely until (1) the insertion site becomes inflamed or purulent, (2) new systemic signs of infection are believed to be caused by the catheter, or (3) the catheter is no longer needed. Using the culture technique described by Maki and others,[23] guidewire exchanges of catheters and culturing of the intracutaneous segment directs the diagnosis and treatment of catheter-related sepsis. Ball and associates[24] have shown a 28% incidence rate of contamination on the first exchange (mean 4.1 days), with contamination of subsequent catheters exchanged over a guidewire decreasing in frequency to 6% by the fourth exchange. Detailed records of catheter microbiologic history are necessary to ensure catheters are changed appropriately. Catheters impregnated with silver sulfadiazine-chlorhexidine seem to decrease the incidence of catheter contamination,[25] using chlorhexidine to alter cell membrane permeability with the subsequent entry and binding of silver ion to the bacterial DNA helix.[26] Thus, the use of these catheters should even further reduce the incidence of catheter-related infections, which has been demonstrated clinically.[27] Unprotected catheters have a significantly higher rate of infection of the intracutaneous segment after 10 days, whereas the rate of positive intracutaneous segment cultures in protected catheters in place for longer than 10 days is equal to those in place for fewer than 10 days. With the ability to leave central venous catheters in position longer, the added risk and expense of multiple guidewire exchanges can be significantly reduced.

Likewise, arterial catheters are an uncommon source of sepsis. In a study of arterial catheter-related infection, no positive semiquantitative arterial catheter cultures occurred within less than 96 hours of site use.[28] The positive culture rate increased to 9.5% at 97 to 120 hours, but did not increase thereafter up to 340 hours. No associated episodes of bacteremia were attributed to the arterial catheter sites.[28] One exception is arterial catheters placed in the axillary artery, and to a lesser degree, in the femoral artery. Presumably because of skin folds and dermal sweat glands and the relative inability to keep the insertion site clean, catheters in these sites have a higher incidence of contamination and should be changed weekly. Figure 107-2 outlines the management of potential catheter-related infection.

Surgical and Traumatic Wounds

High fever in the immediate postoperative period (within 48 hours) mandates careful inspection of all surgical or traumatic wounds. Surgical dressings should be completely removed and wounds carefully inspected and palpated for signs of infection. In addition to wound infections, fever can be associated with crush injury syndrome and tetanus.

The crush injury syndrome was first described by German authors in 1914 and later discussed in-depth during World War II in victims of aerial bombings who were trapped for prolonged periods under collapsed buildings.[29] Crushed extremities appear pale and edematous. The skin overlying the crushed muscle is usually pale and tense, often with vesicles. Fluid extravasates from the intravascular space into the osteofascial muscle compartments, resulting in a significant rise in hemoglobin and hematocrit despite profound hypovolemia. High levels of myoglobin are excreted, which can cause acute renal failure. These injuries may be associated with higher fevers in the postinjury period despite the relatively benign external appearance of the injured limb.[30]

Tetanus, the clinical syndrome resulting from infection by the anaerobic bacillus *Clostridium tetani*, is relatively uncommon in western countries.[31] Clinical symptoms develop from a potent neurotoxin produced by the bacillus. This high molecular weight protein is taken up by the ganglia of the central nervous system. From the site of the wound, the toxin travels directly up the motor network of the peripheral nerves to the spinal cord and the medulla, ultimately producing excessive discharge from motor neurons resulting in the characteristic tetanic spasms. Trismus and dysphagia are the initial features in most cases.[31] In severe cases, muscular spasms of increasing frequency and duration are superimposed on the muscular hypertonicity, resulting in crush fractures of vertebrae and death from respiratory failure.

Any wound may be a nidus for the bacteria, but a specific wound is identified in only 60% of reported tetanus cases.[31] Deep penetrating injuries with a focus of necrotic tissue place patients at particularly high risk. Elevated temperatures may be an early sign, and the interval between the first symptoms and the first severe spasms may vary from less than 24 hours to over 10 days.[31] Patients with a history of parenteral substance abuse, puncture injury, or other contaminated traumatic injuries are at risk for developing this rare but lethal disease. Treatment includes large doses of human antitetanus serum and penicillin. Supportive care

with mechanical ventilation and complete muscle paralysis may be necessary for as long as 6 to 8 weeks.[31]

Neurologic Sources

Meningitis should be considered in any patient who develops altered mental status associated with excessively high fever. The prevalence of meningeal infections is higher in medical ICU patients and is an uncommon but potentially lethal complication, after neurosurgery or closed head injury. The reported incidence rate of bacterial meningitis is approximately 0.03% after spinal injury, 0.3% after craniotomy,[32,33] and 0% to 9% after transphenoidal hypophysectomies.[34–36] Bacteria gain entrance to the meningeal space from contiguous sites of colonization or infection, most commonly the nasal mucosa or skin incision site if intraoperative contamination develops.[34] Postoperatively, skin incisions, indwelling drains, and cerebrospinal fluid (CSF) leaks may predispose to infection.[35,36] Hematogenous spread from a distant site of infection is rare but occasionally may develop.

Approximately 50% of cases of meningitis after craniotomy or spinal surgery occur during the first postoperative week. Twenty-five percent occur during the second week, and the remainder occur thereafter.[34] About 85% of cases after transphenoidal hypophysectomy develop in the first 7 days.

Clinical features of meningitis such as headache, nuchal rigidity, and decreased mentation commonly accompany uncomplicated elective cranial surgery. These symptoms are also difficult to identify after head trauma or emergency surgical procedures. Therefore, the presence or absence of these findings is not reliable for diagnosing meningitis.

Meningitis after head or spinal cord injury seems to be an uncommon problem, possibly because many of these patients are treated with broad-spectrum antibiotics for other associated injuries. The most important diagnostic procedure is lumbar puncture for CSF examination and culture. CT should first be performed to exclude brain abscess and radiographic signs of elevated intracranial pressure (if intracranial pressure monitoring is not in use), because lumbar puncture in this situation may cause brain herniation.

In most cases of postoperative or posttraumatic meningitis, CSF protein is 100 to 500 mg/dL. The white blood cell count usually exceeds 1000/mm³ with over 75% neutrophils, and glucose concentration is less than 40 mg/dL in 85% of cases. Gram stain demonstrates organisms in over 50% of cases.[30,33] The infecting organisms are usually enteric gram-negative bacilli, primarily *Klebsiella, Enterobacter,* and *Pseudomonas aeruginosa.*[8,34,37] The third-generation cephalosporin, ceftazidime, in combination with an aminoglycoside, provides the best empiric antibacterial coverage.[38]

Bacterial meningitis develops in about 1% of patients with closed head injuries after blunt trauma.[34] Patients at risk are those with basilar skull fractures in which a dural tear creates a communication between the subarachnoid space and the nasal cavity, paranasal sinuses, or the ear canal, allowing bacteria to enter the meninges.[34] CSF rhinorrhea may be clinically evident, depending on the size and number of dural tears (40% are associated with multiple tears). It develops in only 10% to 15% of patients. Periorbital ecchymoses (anterior fossa fractures), unilateral or bilateral anosmia (ethmoid region), hemotympanum, bloody ear drainage, and ecchymoses behind the ear (middle cranial fossa) are clinical signs of basilar skull fracture. The most useful test to distinguish CSF from nasal secretions is the glucose concentration, which exceeds 30 mg/dL in CSF fluid unless an infection is already present.[34] Nasal secretions have lower values.

The true risk of developing meningitis with closed head injuries and dural fistulas is not known because many fistulas probably close spontaneously. Among closed head injuries severe enough to require medical attention, recognized basilar skull fractures occur in about 25%, with meningitis developing in 2% to 9% of these patients.[34]

No evidence supports the use of prophylactic antibiotics to prevent meningitis in patients with basilar skull fractures and CSF leaks.[39,40] By generating resistance and encouraging overgrowth of gram-negative organisms, prophylactic antibiotics may actually be harmful[34]; any infection that subsequently develops can be more difficult to treat and is associated with a higher mortality rate. Most dural fistulas after trauma close spontaneously within 2 weeks, and neurosurgical repair is necessary only for large fistulas or those complicated by recurrent episodes of meningitis.[34]

Intraabdominal Sources

Intraabdominal sepsis, which persists after surgical procedures performed to eradicate a septic focus or as a complication of elective surgery, is a common contributing cause of MOSF.[41-44] The diagnosis may be completely overlooked or its recognition significantly delayed in many situations. Early localization and drainage of septic foci are keys to a successful outcome. In critically ill patients, diagnosis may be delayed because of minimal localizing physical signs and the logistical difficulty of transporting patients from the relative safety of the ICU for diagnostic testing.

Limitations with physical examination and conventional radiography have led to the frequent use of sonography, nuclear scans, and CT. An evaluation process that is therapy directed should be developed so that tests that have no major impact on clinical management are avoided. Likewise, abdominal reexploration should be considered under certain clinical situations if systemic sepsis persists. Although aggressive fluid resuscitation, antibiotic therapy, and nutritional and metabolic support are important contributors to prolonged survival in patients with intraabdominal sepsis, ultimate outcome requires drainage of septic foci before host defenses are overwhelmed and MOSF develops. Early diagnosis and abscess drainage are essential for improved survival.[43-45]

Intraabdominal sepsis begins with the introduction of bacteria into the peritoneal cavity. Fry[46] describes three possibilities: (1) a mass of bacteria overwhelms the host's immunologic defense mechanisms, resulting in death; (2) host defense mechanisms are so strong, or the size of the inoculum is so small, that complete resolution occurs; and (3) a "biologic standoff" exists between bacteria and the host, resulting in an abdominal abscess. A thorough knowledge

of the patient's history and a complete physical examination should precede direct testing to confirm clinical suspicions. Examination may identify an obvious extraabdominal source such as septic phlebitis from an old intravenous catheter site, sinusitis caused by a nasotracheal or nasogastric tube,[47] a palpable perirectal abscess, epididymitis induced by prolonged bladder catheterization, an infected decubitus ulcer, or an infected surgical wound. If physical examination fails to reveal a source, the abdomen, particularly in surgical patients, must be strongly suspected.

ABDOMINAL RADIOGRAPHS. Abdominal radiographs are reported to identify an abscess in up to 50% of patients,[48,49] but these studies are often not useful postoperatively because paralytic ileus may obscure details. The classic feature of abscess on plain radiograph is the presence of extraluminal gas as either a single bubble, a mottled pattern, or extraluminal air-fluid levels.[50,51] Other common but nonspecific findings are reactive pleural effusion, hemidiaphragm elevation, and the presence of an intraabdominal mass causing bowel loop displacement.[51] In critically ill patients, such findings are usually obscured, and plain abdominal radiographs are infrequently used for diagnosis.

Barium or Gastrografin contrast studies are also infrequently used. Postoperative paralytic ileus and the ready availability of more sensitive studies, such as sonography and CT, make contrast studies less useful for diagnosing intraabdominal septic foci. However, they may be helpful in patients with prolonged postoperative ileus to diagnose small bowel obstruction or breakdown of gastroenteric anastomoses.

Acalculous cholecystitis is a disease most frequently seen in critically ill patients, particularly those not receiving enteral alimentation. Because of the patients' inability to relate symptoms of right upper quadrant pain, this source of fever may be overlooked. However, careful physical examination will elicit tenderness and guarding in the right upper quadrant of the abdomen and suggest the gallbladder as the source of the fever. Although liver function tests may be abnormal, these are fairly nonspecific in the critical care setting. Ultrasound may reveal pericholecystic fluid or subserosal edema without ascites, intramural gas, and wall thickening, suggesting acute cholecystitis. Echogenic foci are absent, and gallbladder distention is likely to be present, although this is a normal finding in most ICU patients, with and without gallbladder disease. Abdominal CT results may also suggest cholecystitis. Although sonography can be conducted at the bedside, CT requires transporting potentially unstable patients to the radiology suite, and as such, may not be a viable option. And although both examinations may reveal findings consistent with acute acalculous cholecystitis, neither examination nor percutaneous drainage is able to discern gallbladder necrosis. For these reasons, bedside diagnostic laparoscopy has been introduced using local anesthesia, limited sedation, and minimal pneumoperitoneum. If the gallbladder appears only inflamed, a percutaneous drainage catheter can be placed immediately and under direct vision. If the gallbladder is necrotic, the patient is taken to the operating room for urgent cholecystectomy.[52]

ULTRASONOGRAPHY. Ultrasonography is a sensitive tool for detecting fluid collections in the abdomen and pelvis. The flexibility, speed, and portability of currently available real-time equipment allow rapid examination in the ICU.[53] Anatomic areas best suited for ultrasonography are the right upper quadrant, the pelvis, and the left upper quadrant (if the spleen is present) because of the intrinsic acoustic windows created by liver, spleen, and bladder. Consequently, sonography is highly successful in these areas.[53] Visceral abscesses can also be demonstrated in the liver, kidney, and spleen as irregular, encapsulated areas of lower sonodensity.[54] Ultrasonography is the procedure of choice for diagnosing postoperative or posttraumatic acute cholecystitis. As mentioned above, ultrasonography can be useful in the diagnosis of acalculous cholecystitis but is limited in regards to necrosis.

Considerable overlap occurs in the sonographic appearance of hematomas, loculated ascitic fluid, seromas, bilomas, and abscesses, often making the diagnosis of intraabdominal abscess difficult based on ultrasonography alone.[53] Ultrasonography is also operator dependent and difficult to use in patients with open abdominal wounds, stomas, and bulky abdominal dressings. Interpretation is difficult when large amounts of bowel gas are present, a common finding in postoperative patients.[53]

Ultrasound-directed percutaneous drainage of intraabdominal fluid collections is often a good alternative to the more expensive CT-guided technique, and can be done at the bedside, obviating the need for transport out of the ICU.

RADIONUCLIDE SCANNING. Whereas anatomic changes can be detected by radiograph, CT, sonography, and magnetic resonance imaging (MRI), scintigraphy (SCINT) is based on functional changes such as protein sequestration or leukocyte migration and may provide specific information for infection. Imaging of an organ or a body region is performed when clinical symptoms and findings localize the process to a particular area. When localizing symptoms or signs are not present, or organ/region imaging is not diagnostic, total body SCINT can be performed to identify an elusive focus of infection.

Radiopharmaceuticals used for infection-localizing scans are gallium citrate Ga 67, indium chloride In 111, and technetium Tc 99m. [67]Gallium citrate and ^{111}In-leukocyte SCINT have been effectively used in clinical practice,[55] whereas radiolabeled IgG,[56] antigranulocyte antibodies, chemotactic oligopeptides, and quinolones are still under evaluation.

Gallium Scintigraphy. Gallium accumulates in inflammatory sites; any abnormal activity must be differentiated from physiologic activity at sites of gallium accretion or excretion. In addition to bowel and early renal activity, a normal gallium scintigram has activity in the liver, bone marrow and skeleton, lacrimal glands, salivary glands, nasopharynx, thymus, breasts, testicles, and sometimes, spleen. Gallium is also a tumorophilic radiopharmaceutical. Despite these shortcomings in specificity, gallium SCINT is reasonably sensitive (sensitivity higher than 95%, specificity varies between 65 and 95%), readily available and easy to perform.

Leukocyte Scintigraphy. The most widely used marker for leukocyte labeling used to be [111]In. Recently, technetium Tc 99m carried by the lipophilic agent HMPAO has been introduced for leukocyte labeling. The time-consuming process of cell harvesting and labeling requires 50 to 80 mL of blood and an incubation period of 30 minutes. The labeled leukocytes are resuspended in plasma and slowly injected intravenously. Imaging is performed at 24 hours for ^{111}In, but may be done at 2 hours for [99m]Tc. Leukocyte SCINT is performed as a total body study. Sensitivity varies with rates of 90% to 95% for acute intraabdominal infections, less for indolent processes (70% to 90%). Specificity is thought to be relatively high (>95%).

Acute infections (abdominal abscesses or phlegmon) with intense accumulation of leukocytes into body areas that are devoid of physiologic leukocyte migration are the most likely to be visualized by leukocyte SCINT studies. In acute infections of the abdomen, leukocyte SCINT is more advantageous than gallium because physiologic bowel activity and prominent healing wounds do not interfere with ^{111}In–leukocyte scintigrams as they normally do with gallium SCINT. Gallium is preferable to leukocyte imaging in some infections that do not evoke a prominent acute inflammatory response (chronic encapsulated abscesses, old empyemas) and is preferable for early detection of *Pneumocystis carinii* pneumonia. Because of limitations of blood availability, ^{67}Ga SCINT is also preferable in small children.

COMPUTED TOMOGRAPHIC SCANNING. Because of limitations associated with conventional radiographic tests, sonography, and nuclear scans, CT has become the preferred method for diagnosing intraabdominal abscess.[52,53,57,58] CT signs of abscess include a well-defined, low-attenuated, round or oval mass with a density (attenuation coefficient) usually between water (0 to 20 Hounsfield units) and solid tissue (40 to 60 Hounsfield units).[53] Intracavitary gas is seen in 40% to 50% of abscesses,[57] presenting as either air-fluid levels or small, finely dispersed air bubbles throughout the fluid collection. Obliteration of surrounding fat planes, displacement of surrounding viscera, and a "rind sign" resulting from hypervascularity of the surrounding inflammatory wall after intravenous contrast enhancement also are reported findings.[52,53] Infection or inflammation without abscess formation creates only higher attenuation edema of surrounding fat with no fluid density and, when focal, is consistent with phlegmon formation. This is often the only sign of diverticulitis or appendicitis when no abscess has formed.[52]

Results of CT are reported to be uniformly excellent, with both sensitivity and specificity over 90% to 95%.[52,53,58-60] Most studies report accuracies from a broad category of patients and do not describe the temporal relationship to intervention, nor do they examine the usefulness in arriving at a clinical decision to drain the abscess. Furthermore, the accuracy in critically ill patients with suspected intraabdominal sepsis is not usually addressed.

Roche[61] reviews 135 CT scan findings in 111 patients and showed that CT aided or altered the medical management in only 55% of patients. Another study determined the impact of CT in 53 critically ill surgical patients at risk for developing intraabdominal abscess.[62] Of the 72 scans obtained, only 17 (23%) provided beneficial information, whereas 55 (77%) provided information that either was not used or actually detrimental to patient care. Sensitivity and specificity were defined to extend beyond just accuracy of the test and included the impact of the information obtained on therapy. Sensitivity in this study was only 48% with a specificity of 64%.[62]

Several suggestions can be made to improve the accuracy of CT in critically ill patients:

1. Abdominal CT should not be performed before the eighth postoperative day.
2. CT should not be done as a final effort to detect a correctable source of sepsis in patients with MOSF, unless a negative scan finding would strongly support a decision to discontinue therapy.
3. Patients with solid malignant tumors and postoperative sepsis have a high mortality rate, and close evaluation of their overall status and prognosis should take precedence over efforts limited to diagnosis (such as CT).
4. CT rarely provides useful information in patients with established MOSF related to sepsis, and outcome is not improved with this method.
5. CT should be used to search for intraabdominal abscess *only* if there is a reasonable probability that the information will affect treatment decisions.
6. As the difficulty in making a clinical diagnosis increases, the probability that CT will be useful diminishes in critically ill patients.

Variations in the accuracy of CT and other tests are often a function of the expertise and experience of each particular institution.[57] Physicians who regularly treat critically ill patients with suspected intraabdominal sepsis should evaluate their institutions' experiences and base their clinical practice on each institution's pattern of accuracy.[57]

MAGNETIC RESONANCE IMAGING.   MRI can be used for detecting intraabdominal abscess[63,64] but there are limitations in severely ill patients.[52] Respiratory motion, abdominal scan time (up to 3 hours), and the need for nonmagnetic monitoring equipment, ventilators, and intravenous pumps make routine use of MRI impractical. As technology improves and scan times decrease, MRI may become more practical, but currently CT remains the most practical and accurate radiologic test for evaluating critically ill patients.[52]

LAPAROTOMY.   Abdominal reexploration may be the only definitive diagnostic and therapeutic maneuver in many cases. Sinanan and associates[65] reviewed 100 abdominal explorations in 71 patients with suspected intraabdominal sepsis and determined that 81% of explorations detected an intraabdominal process that completely explained or contributed to the septic condition. Fifty-six percent of laparotomies revealed one or more abscesses. The importance of this study is that in patients with no direct evidence of an intraabdominal focus, 67% had positive laparotomy results. However, the 81% mortality rate in this group was high, regardless of the determined cause of sepsis. Septic shock or

documented bacteremia before empiric laparotomy was associated with a 90% mortality rate.

A retrospective study of 50 patients who had relaparotomy for sepsis evaluated the reliability of clinical and laboratory tests for predicting findings at reoperation and ultimate outcome.[66] Diagnosis leading to primary operation, time interval since first operation, onset of fever, highest white blood cell count, serum albumin level, and other demographic data were not predictive for positive findings. Seventy-eight percent of these patients had positive findings at laparotomy and the overall mortality rate was only 26%. Seventy-two percent of patients had one or no organ system dysfunction, and 88% survived. The 16 patients with MOSF had a 56% mortality rate.[65] The authors concluded that patients should be reexplored before the onset of MOSF because the mortality rate in those with negative reexploration was only 18.2%.

Other investigators have also studied empiric laparotomy.[37,67,68] The primary concern with reoperation is determining the relative risk of a negative laparotomy finding. Reports range from 18% to 71%,[37,65,67,68] raising the question of whether these patients are too sick to undergo a major operative procedure, particularly if the procedure fails to identify a surgically correctable lesion. The primary determinant of mortality in patients with negative laparotomy findings seems to be the preoperative presence of MOSF. If a negative finding on exploration occurs before MOSF development, mortality rates in the range of 18% to 30% can be expected.[57] Therefore, in the critically ill septic patient with no identifiable source and the potential for an intraabdominal abscess despite negative diagnostic test results, the question is not whether reexploration increases the mortality rate after the onset of MOSF, but whether it increases survival potential. If reexploration is attempted in patients with MOSF, the resulting high mortality rate should not be attributed to the operation but to the systemic effects of undiagnosed infection[57] or the sepsis syndrome.

OTHER CRITICAL ETIOLOGIES OF FEVER

Drug Allergies

Up to 30% of hospitalized patients are estimated to experience at least one adverse drug reaction.[69] Various drugs produce allergic reactions by virtue of their ability to combine with endogenous micromolecules, primarily proteins, polysaccharides, and polynucleotides. Serum antibodies can also develop to drug metabolites.[70]

Fever may be the first sign of the two most serious types of allergic drug reactions: anaphylaxis and serum sickness.[70] Anaphylactic drug reactions are rare but potentially fatal, developing rapidly and reaching a maximum allergic response within 5 to 30 minutes.[70] Anaphylactic reactions are type I, IgE-mediated reactions characterized by itching, urticaria, angioedema, dyspnea, and abdominal pain.[71] These early symptoms may be masked or may go unrecognized in the ICU until bronchospasm and hypotension develop. Various drugs have been reported to produce fatal anaphylactic reactions (Table 107-3).

Serum sickness is a type III, or immune complex reaction, that develops 6 to 21 days after drug administration.[69] It is

TABLE 107-3. Drugs Associated With Fatal
Anaphylactic Reactions

Penicillins
Organic mercurials
Opiates
Organic iodides (radiopaque dyes)
Local anesthetics
Streptomycin
Sulfobromophthalein (BSP)
Dehydrocholate sodium (decholin)
Fluorescein
Congo red
Dextran
Aspirin
Heparin
Vitamin B$_{12}$
Tetracyclines
Cephalosporins
Insulin

TABLE 107-5. Other Drugs Implicated in Drug Fevers

Allopurinol	Methyldopa
Antihistamines	Nitrofurantoin
Azathioprine	Pentazocine
Barbiturates	Phenytoin
Cimetidine	Procainamide
Diazoxide	Procarbazine
Folic acid	Propylthiouracil
Hydralazine	Sulindac
Ibuprofen	Triamterine
Isoniazid	

characterized by fever, rash, lymphadenopathy, arthralgia
or arthritis, nephritis, edema, and neuritis. Urticarial and
maculopapular rashes are particularly common and may occur locally at an earlier drug injection site. This syndrome
develops from antigens that remain in the circulation for
prolonged periods so that when antibody is first formed,
intravascular antigen is still present, permitting circulating
antigen–antibody complex formation.[70] Drugs known to
cause serum sickness are listed in Table 107-4. In addition
to these two allergic responses, fever can occur as an isolated
manifestation of drug allergy.[72] Other drugs known to cause
fever are listed in Table 107-5.

TABLE 107-4. Drugs Associated With Serum Sickness
and Other Cytotoxic Reactions

SERUM SICKNESS	HEMOLYTIC ANEMIA
Penicillins	Quinine
Sulfonamides	Quinidine
Thiouracils	Dipyrone
Cholecystographic dyes	Aminosalicylic acid
Diphenylhydantoin	Mephenytoin
Aminosalicylic acid	Stibophen
Streptomycin	Cephalothin
Antivenin	Phenacetin
Cephalosporins	Methyldopa
Dextrans	Mefenamic acid
Hydantoins	

THROMBOCYTOPENIA
Quinine
Quinidine
Meprobamate
Chlorthiazide
Thiouracils
Chloramphenicol
Sulfonamides

If drug allergy is the suspected source of fever in a critically ill patient, all drugs should be carefully reviewed, and
those known to be associated with a high incidence of allergic
reactions should be discontinued or replaced with another
suitable drug, if possible. Determining the exact drug that
is causing a drug allergy in patients who are on multiple
medications can be difficult. The likelihood of an allergic
reaction to any drug increases with the duration and number
of courses of therapy.[73] There is no single test for drug
allergy, because several different pathogenic mechanisms
lead to allergic symptoms.[74] Most allergic reactions can be
simply managed by withdrawing the drug. However, if the
patient develops severe systemic side effects, such as vasculitis, interstitial nephritis, severe dermatitis, or hepatitis, high-
dose corticosteroid therapy may be necessary.[75]

Blood Transfusion Reactions

Approximately 90% of blood product reactions are allergic
or febrile.[76] Allergic reactions may also produce a febrile
response, with reactions varying from hives to acute anaphylaxis.[77] Most allergic reactions are mild and self-limited.
Treatment consists of stopping the blood product infusion
and administration of antihistamines, usually diphenhydramine hydrochloride.

Febrile reactions are usually caused by antibodies to white
blood cells. These reactions are often harmless and self-
limited, but further evaluation is mandatory because fever
may also accompany hemolysis or may be caused by blood
products that have been contaminated with bacteria.[77] Febrile reactions generally begin within 30 minutes to 2 hours
after a blood product transfusion is begun. The fever generally lasts between 2 and 24 hours and may be preceded
by chills.[77]

Hemolytic transfusion reactions are estimated to occur in
1 of every 6000 units of blood transfused.[78] Acute hemolytic
transfusion reactions occur when red blood cells are given
to patients with preexisting alloantibody.[79] Approximately
80% of these reactions are a result of clerical identification
errors, resulting in the patient receiving ABO incompatible
blood. Most hemolytic transfusion reactions are accompanied by early minor symptoms of chills, fever, chest pain,
nausea, dyspnea, pain at the infusion site, and back pain. In
alert, or noncritically ill patients, these symptoms often can
be recognized early enough so that prompt attention limits
the amount of incompatible blood transfused and hemolysis

is minimized. However, patients who receive blood in the operating room or ICU often are not be able to report these early symptoms, and fever, hypotension, diffuse bleeding, oliguria, or hemoglobinuria are the first signs.[79] The blood transfusion must be immediately discontinued because the severity of the reaction is related directly to the number of incompatible red blood cells transfused.[79] The suspected blood unit and all attached tubing and solutions should be returned to the laboratory for verification of all clerical work. Blood should be withdrawn from a site remote to the infusion site and checked for free hemoglobin. A direct antiglobulin (direct Coombs') test should be performed. The urine is checked for hemoglobin and, if positive, a brisk diuresis is maintained.

Hemolytic transfusion reactions may be delayed up to 2 weeks.[79] In these situations, patients with no detectable antibody to red blood cell antigens at the time of transfusion develop antibodies sufficient to destroy transfused red blood cells several days after transfusion. If enough donor red blood cells are still in circulation and if the antibody titer rises rapidly, clinically significant hemolysis can occur. The symptoms of delayed hemolysis include fever, jaundice, and an unexplained fall in hematocrit. Antibodies against antigens in the Rh, Kidd, Duffy, and Kell blood groups are involved with this type of reaction.[79] The direct antiglobulin test is usually positive with these reactions.

Malignant Hyperthermia

MH is a clinical syndrome in which skeletal muscle activity suddenly and unexpectedly increases, causing increased oxygen consumption, lactic acid and heat production, and severe respiratory and metabolic acidosis. Body temperature rapidly increases, often as high as 1°C per 5 minutes.[80] The syndrome is triggered by a decrease in the control of intracellular calcium within the skeletal muscle, resulting in the release of free, unbound, ionized calcium from sites in the skeletal muscle that normally maintain relaxation.[81] MH usually develops in the operating room after the induction of general anesthesia. However, it is not unusual for the onset to be delayed for several hours; therefore, the symptoms may not develop until the patient has reached the recovery room or the ICU. Anesthetics and muscle relaxants that trigger MH include halothane, enflurane, isoflurane, sevoflurane, methoxyflurane, cyclopropane, ether, succinylcholine, and decamethonium.[80] Other anesthetic agents and muscle relaxants also have been implicated in various case reports.

Early diagnosis is more difficult than the treatment. Signs of increasing metabolism may be subtle. Other clinical signs develop before the rise in temperature, which may be as high as 43°C (109.4°F). Onset of symptoms may be delayed until the patient begins to emerge from general anesthesia,[82] and early symptoms can mimic thyrotoxicosis[83] (Chap. 149), pheochromocytoma (Chap. 148), or the neuroleptic malignant syndrome.[84]

MH should be suspected if there is sudden onset of sinus tachycardia, tachypnea, dysrhythmia, cyanosis, muscle rigidity, and an unstable blood pressure. These symptoms can develop before the onset of fever. Arterial blood gases

show a severe mixed metabolic and respiratory acidosis. Mixed venous oxygen tension ($P\bar{v}O_2$) and carbon dioxide tension ($P\bar{v}CO_2$) generally change more dramatically than arterial blood gases.[80] Normally, $P\bar{v}CO_2$ should be only about 5 mm Hg higher than $PaCO_2$. If $PaCO_2$ is greater than 60 mmHg and the patient has an acute fall in serum HCO_3^- of 5 to 7 mEq/L, the diagnosis is made (assuming that hypoventilation as a cause for hypercapnia has been eliminated). $PaCO_2$ may rise as high as 100 mm Hg with pH decreasing to 7.00. Treatment must be immediate to offset the rapid development of fever and death. Early mortality rates were reportedly as high as 70%.[75] However, with dantrolene therapy, mortality rates have decreased to less than 10%.[80]

Treatment includes discontinuance of all anesthetic agents, and hyperventilation with 100% oxygen. Dantrolene is administered in 2 mg/kg boluses every 5 minutes for a total dose of 10 mg/kg. The dose may be repeated every 4 to 8 hours for a total of three doses.[80] Sodium bicarbonate is initially given at a rate of 2 to 4 mEq/kg and titrated to maintain normal acid–base balance. Fever should be controlled with surface cooling blankets and iced intravenous saline, if necessary. Cooling is stopped at 38° to 39°C to prevent hypothermia.

Patients can develop myoglobinuria, and a brisk diuresis should be maintained to avoid acute renal failure. Continued therapy is dictated by the clinical course. If ventricular dysrhythmia develops, procainamide is the drug of choice.[80]

MH is discussed in greater detail in Chapter 98.

Neuroleptic Malignant Syndrome

Neuroleptic malignant syndrome (NMS) also produces hyperthermia, but differs from MH in that the former is presumably a disorder of central or presynaptic origin while MH is a muscular disorder. Because haloperidol is used more frequently in the ICU setting, NMS may be encountered more often, its etiology being associated with most antipsychotic agents. Like MH, NMS presents with hyperthermia and skeletal muscular rigidity. Besides withdrawal of the offending agent, treatment with sodium dantrolene relieves muscle contraction and the resulting hyperthermia.

Neuroleptic malignant syndrome is discussed in-depth in Chapter 98.

Adrenocortical Insufficiency

Acute adrenocortical insufficiency is a rare cause of fever in the critically ill patient. The availability and effective use of steroid replacement therapy have virtually eliminated hypotensive crises caused by lack of corticosteroids after most elective surgical procedures.[85] However, adrenocortical crisis can still occasionally develop in the ICU patient, usually manifested by a sharp rise in body temperature and hypotension.

Adrenocortical crisis should be considered in patients who suddenly develop fever while being weaned from high steroid dosages, especially those who may have abdominal abscesses or other remote infections in which more than just a maintenance dose of hydrocortisone is required. In elective surgical patients, acute adrenal insufficiency usually develops within the first 72 hours postoperatively. The syndrome includes sinus tachycardia, fever, and hypotension.[85] Acute adrenocortical crisis results from an abrupt disparity between the metabolic need for glucocorticoids and the amount of these hormones available. Thus, severe metabolic stress, which can result from systemic sepsis or MOSF, may produce acute adrenocortical insufficiency, even when the hormone supply that is available is adequate during the patient's normal basal state.[85]

If the diagnosis of adrenocortical insufficiency is suspected, the patient should receive immediate therapy. Hydrocortisone (200 mg) is administered intravenously, followed by 50 to 100 mg every 6 hours, unless there is a question of underlying sepsis or the patient has MOSF. Higher doses may be necessary in these situations. Dramatic clinical improvement within minutes of steroid administration occurs when adrenocortical insufficiency is the cause of fever and hypotension.

Pulmonary Embolization Syndromes

Pulmonary embolism can cause fever in critically ill patients and should be considered in patients who are at risk for developing deep venous thrombosis and pulmonary thromboembolism.[86] This subject is discussed in greater detail in Chapter 125.

REFERENCES ■

1. Lively JC, Pruitt BA: Infection-related complications. In: Greenfield LJ (ed). *Complications in Surgery and Trauma*, 2nd ed. Philadelphia, JB Lippincott, 1990:81
2. Bernheim HA, Block LH, Atkins E: Fever: Pathogenesis, pathophysiology, and purpose. *Ann Intern Med* 1979;91:261
3. Root RK, Wolff SM: Pathogenetic mechanisms in experimental immune fever. *J Exp Med* 1968;128:309
4. Bodel P, Dillard M: Steroids and steroid fever. I. Production of leukocyte pyrogen in vitro etiocholanolene. *J Clin Invest* 1968;47:107
5. Petersdorf RG, Bennett IL: Studies on the pathogenesis of fever. VIII. Fever-producing substance in the serum of dogs. *J Exp Med* 1957;106:293
6. Dinarello CA: Interleukin-1. *Rev Infect Dis* 1984;6:51
7. Dinarello CA, Golden NP, Wolff SM: Demonstration and characterization of two distinct human leukocytic pyrogens. *J Exp Med* 1974;139:1369
8. Petersdorf RG, Root RK: Chills and fever. In: Braunwald E, Isselbacher KG, Petersdorf RG, et al (eds). *Harrison's Principles of Internal Medicine*, 11th ed. New York, McGraw-Hill, 1988:470
9. Shires GT, Dineen P: Sepsis following burns, trauma, and intra-abdominal infections. *Arch Intern Med* 1981;142:2012
10. Galicier L, Richet H: A prospective study of postoperative fever in a general surgery department. *Infect Control Hosp Epidemiol* 1985;6:487
11. Ledger WJ, Child MA: The hospital care of patients undergoing hysterectomy: an analysis of 12,026 patients from the professional activity study. *Am J Obstet Gynecol* 1973;117:423
12. Young RSW, Buck JR, Filler RM: The significance of fever following operations in children. *J Pediatr Surg* 1982;17:347
13. Roberts J, Barnes W, Pennock M, et al: Diagnostic accuracy of fever as a measure of postoperative pulmonary complications. *Heart Lung* 1988;17:166
14. Bell DM, Goldmann DA, Hopkins CC, et al: Unreliability of fever and leukocytosis in the diagnosis of infection after cardiac valve surgery. *J Thorac Cardiovasc Surg* 1978;75:87
15. Freischlag J, Busuttil RW: The value of postoperative fever evaluation. *Surgery* 1983;94:358
16. Leeper KV: Diagnosis and treatment of pulmonary infections in adult respiratory distress syndrome. *New Horizons* 1993;1:550
17. Wanner A, Amikam B, Robinson MJ, et al: Comparison between the bacteriologic flora of different segments of the airways. *Respiration* 1973;30:561
18. Fagon JY, Chastre J, Hance AJ, et al: Detection of nosocomial lung infection in ventilated patients: use of a protected specimen brush and quantitative culture technique in 147 patients. *Am Rev Respir Dis* 1988;138:110
19. Johanson WG Jr, Seidenfield JJ, Gomez P, et al: Bacterial diagnosis of nosocomial pneumonia following prolonged mechanical ventilation. *Am Rev Respir Dis* 1988;137:259
20. Chastre J, Fagon JY, Soler P, et al: Quantification of BAL cells containing intracellular bacteria rapidly identifies ventilated patients with nosocomial pneumonia. *Chest* 1989;95:190S
21. Martinez OV, Civetta JM, Anderson K, et al: Bacteriuria in the catheterized surgical intensive care patient: a prospective study of 100 patients. *Crit Care Med* 1986;75:1298
22. Civetta JM, Hudson-Civetta JA, Dion L: Duration of illness effects catheter-related infection and bacteremia [abstract]. *Program and Abstracts of the 27th Interscience Conference on Antimicrobial Agents and Chemotherapy*, 1987;69:1141
23. Maki DG, Weise CE, Sarafin HW: A semiquantitative culture method for identifying intravenous-catheter-related infection. *N Engl J Med* 1977;296:1305
24. Ball ES, Hudson-Civetta J, Civetta JM: Re-evaluation of insertion and guidewire exchange (GWX) protocols' effectiveness and validity. *Crit Care Med* 1995;23:A250
25. Clemence MA, Jernigan JA, Titus MA, et al: A study of an antiseptic impregnated central venous catheter for prevention of bloodstream infection [abstract]. *Program and Abstract Proceedings of the 33rd Interscience Conference on Antimicrobial Agents and Chemotherapy*, 1993
26. Modak SM, Fox CL: Binding of silver sulfadiazine to the cellular components of *Pseudomonas aeruginosa*. *Biochem Pharmacol* 1973;22:2391
27. Ball S, Hudson-Civetta J, Civetta JM: Decreasing catheter-related infection, patient risk and hospital costs by continuous quality improvement. *Crit Care Med* 1996;A24:24
28. Norwood SH, Cormier BA, Moss AM, et al: Prospective study of catheter-related infection during prolonged arterial catheterization. *Crit Care Med* 1988;16:836
29. Bywaters EGL: War medicine series: crushing injury. *Br Med J* 1942;2:643
30. Weiner SL, Barrett J: Explosions and explosive device-related injuries. In: Weiner SL, Barrett J (eds). *Trauma Management for Civilian and Military Physicians*. Philadelphia, WB Saunders, 1986:23
31. Westaby S: Tetanus and antibiotic prophylaxis. In: Westaby S (ed). *Wound Care*. St Louis, CV Mosby, 1986:91
32. Buckwold FH, Hand R, Hansebout RR: Hospital acquired bacterial meningitis in neurosurgical patients. *J Neurosurg* 1977;46:494
33. Mombelli G, Klastersky J, Coppens L, et al: Gram-negative bacillary meningitis in neurosurgical patients. *J Neurosurg* 1983;58:634
34. Hirschmann JV: Meningitis following neurosurgery and blunt head trauma. *Infect Surg* 1990;9:13

35. Romanowski B, Tyrell DLJ, Weir BKA, et al: Meningitis complicating transphenoidal hypophysectomy. *Can Med Assoc J* 1981;124:1172

36. Gransden WR, Wickstead M, Eykyn SJ: Meningitis after transphenoidal excision of pituitary tumors. *J Laryngol Otol* 1988; 102:33

37. Mancebo J, Domingo P, Blanch L, et al: Post-neurosurgical and spontaneous gram-negative bacillary meningitis in adults. *Scand J Infect Dis* 1986;18:533

38. New HC: Cephalosporins in the treatment of meningitis. *Drugs* 1987;34(Suppl):135

39. Frazee RC, Mucha P, Farnell MB, et al: Meningitis after basilar skull fracture: does antibiotic prophylaxis help? *Postgrad Med* 1988;83:267

40. Klastersky J, Sadaghi M, Brihaye J: Antimicrobial prophylaxis in patients with rhinorrhea or otorrhea: a double-blind study. *Surg Neurol* 1976;6:111

41. Hinsdale JG, Jaffe BM: Re-operation for intra-abdominal sepsis. *Ann Surg* 1984;199:31

42. Bohnen J, Boulanger M, Meakins JL, et al: Prognosis in generalized peritonitis: relation to cause and risk factors. *Arch Surg* 1983;118:285

43. Pitcher WD, Musler DM: Critical importance of early diagnosis and treatment of intra-abdominal infection. *Arch Surg* 1982;117:328

44. Rogers PN, Wright RH: Postoperative intra-abdominal sepsis. *Br J Surg* 1987;74:973

45. Doberneck RC, Mittelman J: Reappraisal of the problems of intra-abdominal abscess. *Surg Gynecol Obstet* 1982;154:875

46. Fry DE: The diagnosis of intra-abdominal infection in the postoperative patient. *Probl Gen Surg* 1984;1:558

47. Deutschman CS, Wilton P, Sinow J, et al: Paranasal sinusitis associated with nasotracheal intubation: a frequently unrecognized and treatable source of sepsis. *Crit Care Med* 1986; 14:111

48. Connell TR, Stephens DH, Carlson HC, et al: Upper abdominal abscesses: a continuing and deadly problem. *AJR* 1980; 134:759

49. Halber MD, Daffner FH, Morgan CL, et al: Intra-abdominal abscesses: Current concepts in radiologic evaluation. *AJR* 1979;133:9

50. Woodard S, Kelvin FM, Rice RP, et al: Pancreatic abscess: importance of conventional radiology. *AJR* 1981;136:871

51. Gerzof SG, Oates ME: Imaging techniques for infections in the surgical patient. *Surg Clin North Am* 1988;68:147

52. Sleeman D, Sosa JL, Almeida J, et al: Laparoscopy for the diagnosis of acalculous chole-cystitis in the critically ill. *Clin Invest Med* 1994;19(Suppl):B18

53. Mueller PR, Simeone JF: Intra-abdominal abscesses: diagnosis by sonography and computed tomography. *Radiol Clin North Am* 1983;21:425

54. Kuligowska E, Connors S, Shapiro J: Liver abscess: sonography in diagnosis and treatment. *AJR* 1982;138:253

55. Sfakianakis GN, Al-Sheikh W, Heal A, et al: a prospective comparative clinical study of the sensitivity and specificity of In-111–leukocyte and gallium-67 scintigraphy in the diagnosis of occult sepsis. *J Nucl Med* 1982;23:618

56. Serafini AN, Garty I, Vargas-Cuba R, et al: Clinical evaluation of a scintigraphic method for diagnosing inflammations/infections using indium-111–labeled nonspecific human IgG. *J Nucl Med* 1991;32:2227

57. Haaga J, Alfidi R, Havrilla T, et al: CT detection and aspiration of abdominal abscesses. *AJR* 1977;128:465

58. Saini S, Kellum JM, O'Leary MP, et al: Improved localization and survival in patients with intra-abdominal abscesses. *Am J Surg* 1983;145:136

59. Trunet P, LeGall JR, Fagniez PL, et al: Computed tomography and post-laparotomy intra-abdominal abscesses. *Intensive Care Med* 1982;8:193

60. Whitley NO, Shatney CH: Diagnosis of abdominal abscesses in patients with major trauma: the use of computed tomography. *Radiology* 1982;147:179

61. Roche J: Effectiveness of computed tomography in the diagnosis of intra-abdominal abscess. *Med J Aust* 1981;25:85

62. Norwood SH, Civetta JM: Abdominal CT scanning in critically ill surgical patients. *Ann Surg* 1985;202:166

63. Cohen JM, Weinreb JC, Maravilla KR: Fluid collections in the intraperitoneal and extraperitoneal spaces: comparison of MR and CT. *Radiology* 1985;155:705

64. Wall SD, Fisher MR, Amparo EG, et al: Magnetic resonance imaging in the evaluation of abscesses. *AJR* 1985;144:1217

65. Sinanan M, Maier R, Carrico J: Laparotomy for intra-abdominal sepsis in patients in an intensive care unit. *Arch Surg* 1984;119:652

66. Machiedo GW, Tikellia J, Suval W, et al: Re-operation for sepsis. *Am Surg* 1985;51:149

67. Ferraris VA: Exploratory laparotomy for potential abdominal sepsis in patients with multiple organ failure. *Arch Surg* 1983;118:1130

68. Driver T, Kelly GL, Eiseman B: Re-operation after abdominal trauma. *Am J Surg* 1978;135:747

69. Blaiss MS, deShazo RD: Drug allergy. *Pediatr Clin North Am* 1988;35:1131

70. Parker CW: Drug allergy. Part I. *N Engl J Med* 1975;292:511

71. Anderson JA, Adkinson NF: Allergic reactions to drugs and biologic agents. *JAMA* 1987;258:2891

72. Tabor PA: Drug induced fever. *Drug Intell Clin Pharmacol* 1986;20:413

73. Parker CW: Drug allergy. Part II. *N Engl J Med* 1975;292:732

74. Parker CW: Drug allergy. Part III. *N Engl J Med* 1975;292:957

75. Sheffer AL, Pennoyer DS: Management of adverse drug reactions. *J Allergy Clin Immunol* 1984;74:580

76. Rush B, Lee N: Clinical presentation of nonhemolytic transfusion reactions. *Anaesth Intensive Care* 1980;8:125

77. Rutledge R, Sheldon GF, Collins ML: Massive transfusion. *Crit Care Clin* 1986;2:791

78. Pineda A, Brzica S, Taswell H: Hemolytic transfusion reaction: recent experience in a large blood bank. *Mayo Clin Proc* 1978; 53:378

79. Gregory SA, McKenna R, Sassetti RJ, et al: Hematologic emergencies. *Med Clin North Am* 1986;70:1129

80. Gronert GA: Malignant hyperthermia. In: Miller RD (ed). *Anesthesia.* New York, Churchill Livingstone, 1986:1971

81. Gronert GA: Malignant hyperthermia. *Semin Anesth* 1983;2: 197

82. Schulte-Sasse U, Hess W, Eberlein HJ: Postoperative malignant hyperthermia and dantrolene therapy. *Can Anaesth Soc J* 1983;30:635

83. Stevens JJ: A case of thyrotoxic crisis that mimicked malignant hyperthermia. *Anesthesiology* 1983;59:263

84. Guze BH, Baxter LR Jr: Current concepts: neuroleptic malignant syndrome. *N Engl J Med* 1985;313:163

85. Bergland RM, Gann DS, DeMaria EJ: Pituitary and adrenal. In: Schwartz SI, Shires GT, Spencer FC (eds). *Principles of Surgery,* 5th ed. New York, McGraw-Hill, 1989:1576

86. Hyers TM, Hull RD, Weg JG: Antithrombotic therapy for venous thromboembolic disease. *Chest* 1986;89(Suppl):26S

Critical Care, Third Edition, edited by Joseph M. Civetta,
Robert W. Taylor, and Robert R. Kirby.
Lippincott-Raven Publishers, Philadelphia, PA © 1997.

CHAPTER 108

■

Infections in the Immunocompromised Host

Gregory P. Melcher
Douglas R. Leigh

IMMEDIATE CONCERNS ■

MAJOR PROBLEMS

One of the most difficult clinical challenges for critical care physicians is the immunocompromised patient. Owing to advances in the treatment of previously fatal or untreatable chronic illnesses, the numbers of immunocompromised patients have increased dramatically. Infection is a frequent complication of immunosuppression, occurring either as a manifestation of the underlying disease or the therapy used to treat it. Familiarity with the presentation of immunocompromised patients and the infectious complications they may experience is a necessity for the critical care physician. As a result of immunosuppression, the patient may offer little in terms of symptoms or examination findings, though their infections are often more severe or fulminant. The differential diagnosis for each clinical syndrome is typically extended significantly beyond that for the immunocompetent patient. Understanding the immune deficits of the patient (granulocytes, humoral or cellular immune function) will allow the clinician to develop a hierarchical differential diagnosis. The list of potential pathogens for a particular disease process may be long, and the therapies used to treat these organisms often diverse or toxic. Multisystem disease is common, complicating diagnostic efforts necessary to pinpoint the cause or causes of disease so that specific therapy can be instituted. Some subsets of immunocompromised patients often seen in the intensive care unit may have unique or common infectious problems based on the nature of the injuries to their immune defense: the granulocytopenic patient, the

corticosteriod-treated patient, and renal and bone marrow transplant recipients are discussed with regard to these problems.

STRESS POINTS

1. Despite a frequent lack of an obvious source for fever in the immunocompromised patient, a thorough history and careful physical exam remain the most powerful diagnostic tools available in the care of these patients.
2. Fever may be the sole indicator of a potentially life-threatening infection in a granulocytopenic patient. The duration and severity of the granulocytopenia increases the risk for infection. Early initiation of empirical broad spectrum antimicrobial therapy is mandatory in this setting.
3. Prolonged (4–7 days) or recurrent fever in a patient with granulocytopenia on broad spectrum empiric antibacterial therapy should prompt consideration of a fungal etiology.
4. Bacterial organisms important to consider in the differential diagnosis of infectious processes involving the corticosteriod-treated patient include *Pneumocystis carinii, Nocardia, Listeria,* and *Legionella.* Suspicion for these organisms may also be increased based on a lack of clinical response to initial empiric β-lactam antimicrobial therapy.
5. In formulation of a differential diagnosis for infectious problems following solid organ or bone marrow transplantation one should evaluate the current primary

1603

host defense defects, with reference to the time elapsed since transplant, to aid in identification of major infectious risks.

6. Cytomegalovirus is the single most important infectious organism in renal allograft recipients, causing the majority of febrile episodes in the period of 1 to 6 months post-transplant. Additionally, cytomegalovirus is the most commonly identified infectious etiology of interstitial pneumonitis in the bone marrow transplant patient.

ESSENTIAL DIAGNOSTIC TESTS AND PROCEDURES

1. Careful investigation of even minor complaints in the febrile immunosuppressed patient is warranted, as the typical signs and symptoms of infection may be lacking.

2. An aggressive initial diagnostic approach with a goal of obtaining a rapid microbiologic etiology is necessary. Delays in diagnosis due to a desire to approach the patient less invasively or due to degree of illness often leads to the eventual performance of a diagnostic procedure, out of necessity, in a patient with perhaps even greater clinical instability as a result of well-intended, but inadequate or ineffective, empiric therapy. Procedures as quickly and easily obtained as a skin biopsy for the presence of skin lesions may commonly lead to an infectious diagnosis, particularly for fungemia with opportunistic molds.

3. When procedures are performed and tissue or body fluids are obtained, it is essential that the appropriate cultures, histopathologic studies, and available rapid diagnostic studies (including the Gram stain) are requested, encompassing the infectious organisms in the differential. Discussion with the microbiology laboratory, the pathology department, or a consultant in infectious diseases may be helpful in obtaining the most information from clinical specimens.

4. The possibility of a wound infection should be considered and evaluated in the febrile renal transplant patient by means of a sterile needle aspiration of the wound and radiographic evaluation of the deep perinephric space.

INITIAL THERAPY

1. A variety of strategies are currently acceptable for initial empiric therapy in the febrile granulocytopenic patient (e.g. monotherapy with ceftazidime), though modification of the initial coverage is often necessary based upon the results of initial cultures obtained in evaluation of the febrile episode.

2. Despite undesirable toxicities, amphotericin B therapy becomes necessary for patients in the setting of prolonged or recurrent fever while receiving broad spectrum antibacterial therapy.

3. Sulfamethoxazole and trimethoprim (SMZ/TMP) is effective therapy for both *P carinii* and *Nocardia asteroides* related illnesses. Erythromycin is the drug of choice for treatment of *Legionella*. Combination ther-

apy with ampicillin and gentamicin is beneficial for severe listeriosis.

4. Acyclovir is effective in the treatment and prophylaxis against illness caused by herpes simplex virus in immunocompromised patients. Due to the poor prognosis associated with cytomegalovirus disease in transplant recipients, there is increasing interest in earlier treatment with ganciclovir-based regimens.

5. Although empiric antimicrobial therapy may be warranted in specific instances (e.g. fever and granulocytopenia), specific therapy directed by microbiologic and pathologic specimens or a strong clinical suspicion based on epidemiological or clinical data will limit toxicity and improve patient outcome.

APPROACH TO THE IMMUNOCOMPROMISED HOST ■

The evaluation of an immunocompromised patient with a suspected infectious complication is similar to the approach to any febrile patient (see Chap. 107). Certain aspects of the evaluation deserve special emphasis for immunocompromised hosts. Historical data should include underlying diseases and medications, particularly recent corticosteroid or cytotoxic chemotherapy, which may have an impact on the severity or type(s) of immune defects. A thorough epidemiologic history, including travel, exposure to ill persons, pet or animal contact, occupation, avocations, and environment at onset of infectious process (community or hospital), may provide useful clues to possible etiologies. Often, infectious diseases present with a paucity of symptoms and signs in immunocompromised patients. Thus, particular importance must be placed on any symptoms reported or elicited, particularly headache, localized pain or irritation, and dyspnea. These subtle complaints may be the only evidence localizing an occult infectious process.

The physical examination should emphasize the organ systems most frequently involved with infectious complications, such as the central nervous system (CNS), the urinary tract, the integument, and the lungs. A fundoscopic examination should be performed to look for retinal changes that may suggest candidal endophthalmitis or cytomegalovirus and toxoplasmic chorioretinitis. The sinuses should be assessed, particularly in nasally intubated patients, for occult infection. The perirectal area should be examined carefully for local erythema or tenderness, often an occult source of fever and bacteremia in granulocytopenic patients. Special attention should be given to the skin examination, as dermatologic lesions are frequently the first manifestation of a systemic infection and are often of fungal etiology. Demonstration of the pathogen through skin biopsy and potentially microbiologic identification by culture may lead to improved survival with the prompt initiation of directed therapy.

Certain laboratory tests can be useful in evaluating the extent of immunosuppression and providing evidence of multisystem involvement. The absolute granulocyte count (polymorphonuclear cells and bands) is easily obtained from the complete blood count and is important in defining the extent of immunodeficiency. Liver function tests, such as aspartate transaminase, alkaline phosphatase, and bilirubin, may reflect a systemic rather than a localized process. The serum creatinine is important as a marker of renal function. Many antimicrobial agents are metabolized or excreted by the kidneys and require dosage adjustments based on the creatinine clearance. A chest radiograph is an indispensable diagnostic tool for the immunocompromised host due to the frequent lack of symptoms in patients with active pulmonary processes.

After the patient has been assessed for the immune defects, organ system involvement, and epidemiologic background, a differential diagnosis of the likely etiologies can be constructed. A diagnostic plan can then be initiated to confirm or rule out these possibilities. This database will help the clinician decide whether to begin empirical therapy for the most likely pathogens while awaiting diagnostic procedures, or to defer therapy until more information is available. The diagnostic pathway leading to the choice of therapy should be pursued aggressively for several reasons. First, immunocompromised patients as a group are less tolerant of delays in diagnosis because of their tenuous clinical status. Second, the differential diagnosis often includes several pathogens with totally different therapeutic options (e.g., cytomegalovirus, *Aspergillus*, *Pneumocystis*) and a diagnostic procedure may be able to direct specific therapy, avoiding toxicity from nonessential therapy. Finally, in some cases there are multiple pathogens involved in the infectious process, and optimal outcome depends on the proper treatment regimen. Thus, it is important to make a microbiologic or tissue diagnosis.

Biopsy of involved tissue for culture, special staining, and histopathology should be considered for each patient individually. The importance of a thorough evaluation of any body fluid or tissue specimen obtained from an immunocompromised host must not be overlooked. The microbiology laboratory should be alerted to the specimen's arrival so that it can be Gram stained and processed for bacterial, mycobacterial, viral, and fungal cultures. At this time, if a fastidious organism such as *Legionella* is suspected, special media can be requested and the cultures can be held for an extended duration. Also, rapid diagnostic tests such as direct immunofluoresence for *Legionella* can be performed. It is important that part of the specimen be sent for cytology or histopathology. Coordination with the pathologist allows the preparation of special stains that may detect pathogens not recovered in culture. Discussions with a consultant in infectious diseases are useful to determine what rapid diagnostic tests are available and also to provide guidance for specimen collection and transportation.

THE GRANULOCYTOPENIC PATIENT

The granulocytopenic patient is probably the most frequently encountered immunocompromised host, generally as a result of myelotoxic chemotherapy for hematologic malignancies and solid tumors. The primary immune defect is a decreased number of the phagocytic cells responsible for

defense against bacterial and some fungal pathogens. Absolute granulocytopenia is defined as <500/mm³ polymorphonuclear cells and bands. If the leukocyte count is falling because of recent chemotherapy, many would consider 1000 cells/mm³ or less as indicative of granulocytopenia. The likelihood of infection increases in relationship to both the severity (particularly with granulocyte counts <100/mm³) and the duration of the granulocytopenia.[1]

PRESENTATION

The most important and often the sole predictor of infection in the granulocytopenic patient is fever, commonly defined as a single oral temperature of 38.3°C or greater, or several temperatures of 38°C or greater. Other typical signs and symptoms of infection may be entirely lacking. Erythema and pain may be the only evidence of a localized process such as pharyngitis, cellulitis, or catheter infection. Clinical symptoms of a urinary tract infection (dysuria, frequency) or pneumonia (cough, purulent sputum production) are not reliable.[2] Thus, clinical suspicion of infection in the febrile granulocytopenic patient must be very high, and a thorough examination is essential.

The most common sites of infection are the sinopulmonary, perioral, and gastrointestinal systems,[3] though any mucosal barrier whose integrity has been violated is suspect. Cytotoxic drugs often cause mucosal sloughing throughout the gastrointestinal tract. This predisposes to local invasion by the colonizing microflora, resulting in pharyngitis, esophagitis, anorectal cellulitis or abscess, and bacteremia. It is the granulocytopenic patient who is most likely to have occult anorectal infection without fluctuance or ulceration because of the inability to form an acute inflammatory response. Patients may have peripheral, or more commonly, central intravenous catheters for chemotherapy, hyperalimentation, and medication administration. All catheters breach the natural barrier to microbial invasion provided by the skin. These sites are a frequent source of localized infection and bacteremia. A complete skin examination is very important, and prompt biopsy of any new lesions, particularly those that are discolored or necrotic, is essential.

Historically, the most common organisms causing bacteremia in granulocytopenic patients were gram-negative rods, notably *Escherichia coli*, *Klebsiella pneumoniae*, and *Pseudomonas aeruginosa*. However, in recent years there has been a significant rise in the isolation of gram-positive pathogens in cases of bacteremia and serious infections, particularly *Corynebacterium jeikeium*, viridans streptococci, *Staphylococcus aureus*, and *Staphylococcus epidermidis*. Granulocytopenic patients are also at risk for opportunistic fungal infections, particularly when the duration of neutropenia has been prolonged. The most common isolates are *Candida*, *Aspergillus*, *Zygomycetes* (e.g., *Mucor*, *Rhizopus*), and *Cryptococcus*. Any fungus isolated from a sterile site or biopsy culture in these patients should be considered a pathogen. Reactivation of latent herpes simplex virus is the most frequent viral infection, particularly in patients with oral mucosal damage from cytotoxic chemotherapy.

DIAGNOSIS

The diagnosis of infection in granulocytopenic patients requires a high index of suspicion combined with a willingness to perform procedures that may provide useful information. At the onset of fever, the basic laboratory evaluation should include a complete blood count with differential, a urinalysis, a urine Gram stain and culture, blood cultures, and cultures with Gram stains of any site of suspected infection based on the presentation. The clinician should fully evaluate any area in which the patient has pain. Oral ulcerations should be swabbed for viral culture. Sinus radiographs may detect occult disease. A chest radiograph may identify an infiltrate when the patient has minimal or no pulmonary symptoms. Pulmonary infiltrates should be evaluated systematically yet aggressively, including consideration of transbronchoscopic lavage and biopsy or open lung biopsy if indicated. Any suspicious skin lesions should be biopsied for histopathology and culture. The symptom complex of fever, right upper quadrant pain, and an increasing alkaline phosphatase level during recovery from a prolonged granulocytopenia suggests hepatosplenic candidiasis.

THERAPY

Experience with febrile granulocytopenic patients has demonstrated that the 48-hour mortality of untreated cases may be dramatically high and can be significantly reduced through the use of empirical therapy. After the patient is evaluated and cultures have been obtained, antibacterial therapy should be promptly initiated. If a source of the fever is discovered and a Gram stain or other procedure has indicated a likely pathogen, specific therapy directed against the organism can be started. However, more often the source of fever is occult and empirical therapy must be initiated.

The antibacterial choices for empirical therapy in the febrile granulocytopenic patient has changed in response to alterations in the frequencies with which the various pathogens cause infection (see earlier). At present, the acceptable options for treatment are appropriately more varied, and ideally should be tailored to the prevailing pathogens and their susceptibility patterns within each treating facility. Monotherapy with a third generation cephalosporin (ceftazidime 2 grams IV every 8 hours) or a carbapenem (imipenem-cilastatin 0.5–1 gram IV every 6 hours) is an effective initial approach, comparing favorably with more complex regimens.[4,5] Historically, the combination of a semisynthetic antipseudomonal penicillin and an aminoglycoside was felt to be the therapy of choice. Double β-lactam combinations (an antipseudomonal penicillin or monobactam and a third-generation cephalosporin) have shown equal efficacy to the β-lactam and aminoglycoside combination in some studies. An important caveat to all empirical therapy is that modifications may often be necessary based upon close observation of the patient's clinical response to treatment and the results of the initial and subsequent cultures. Due to the lack of a demonstrable survival advantage and the risk of promoting colonization or infection with vancomycin-resistant organisms, vancomycin therapy is included in the initial regimen only when gram-positive bacterial infection is suggested by catheter infection, gram stain, or culture, or a high institutional prevalence of MRSA infection.[6]

Though there have been significant advances in antifungal therapies, the drug of choice for empiric treatment of fungal infections in the granulocytopenic patient is intravenous amphotericin B (AMB). The question of when to initiate empirical AMB for suspected fungal superinfection is troublesome, particularly in a critical care setting where any increased toxicity impacts adversely on other organ systems. Yet it is the persistently febrile granulocytopenic patient on broad-spectrum antibacterial therapy who is at highest risk for fungal infection. The diagnosis of systemic fungal infection is difficult to make and blood cultures are infrequently positive in disseminated mycoses other than *Candida*. Most fungal infections are not diagnosed until autopsy.[7] Thus, the use of empirical AMB is advocated if there is continued granulocytopenia and fever unresponsive to more than 4 to 7 days of antibacterial therapy.[8,9]

The hematopoietic growth factors are new agents being investigated as both preventative and adjunctive treatment in the granulocytopenic patient. Both granulocyte colony-stimulating factor (G-CSF) and granulocyte-macrophage colony-stimulating factor (GM-CSF) are capable of reducing the incidence, severity, and duration of chemotherapy-induced granulocytopenia. Additional benefits of significant reductions in granulocytopenic fever, culture-confirmed infections, antibiotic use, and days of hospitalization have been seen.[10] Though the precise role of these agents is currently under active investigation, use of these agents currently appears appropriate in patients with prolonged granulocytopenia resulting from chemotherapy.[9,11]

THE CORTICOSTEROID-TREATED PATIENT ∎

The number of patients treated with corticosteroids is constantly rising and includes those with malignancies, collagen vascular diseases, autoimmune disorders, and various forms of pulmonary disease. The number of immunosuppressed hosts at risk for infection has similarly expanded. Corticosteroids predominantly affect the mononuclear cell population, causing monocytopenia and relative lymphopenia by redistributing the T cells from the circulation, thus impairing their access to inflammatory sites.[12] Additionally, steriods inhibit cytokine secretion from macrophages or may inhibit their activation. Various effects on the polymorphonuclear cell, such as decreased adherence, phagocytosis, and killing activity, have been attributed to corticosteroids in vitro; however, in vivo prednisone has less discernible effects on polymorphonuclear function except at pharmacologic doses.[13] The predominant immune defect induced by corticosteroids is an impairment of cellular immunity, thus placing the host at risk for fungal, viral, and protozoal infection as well as several otherwise uncommon bacterial infections. Corticosteroids can also reactivate dormant mycobacterial and fungal infections by impairing the cellular immunity responsible for their control. Several common pathogens important to remember when dealing with the steroid-treated patient are *P carinii*, *Nocardia*, *Listeria*, and *Legionella*. Each of these is discussed separately, emphasizing the key points in presentation, diagnosis, and therapy. Fungal infections are addressed later.

PNEUMOCYSTIS CARINII

Now felt to be more closely related to fungi than to protozoa,[14] *P carinii* has a global distribution with a unique tropism for the alveolar walls of the immunocompromised, leading to a potentially life-threatening pneumonia. Though overshadowed by the occurrence of *P carinii* pneumonia (PCP) in relationship to HIV infection (see also Chap. 109), PCP may also be seen in patients with malignancy, the severely malnourished, transplant patients, and others receiving immunosuppressive therapy, particularly corticosteriods.

Presentation

The onset of symptoms is often associated with recent tapering or discontinuation of steroid therapy. The onset may be indolent, with progressive dyspnea and dry cough over several weeks, or it may be fulminant, with ventilatory failure requiring mechanical ventilation. Immunocompromised patients without HIV infection tend to have a less insidious illness. Associated fever is a frequent finding; dyspnea is nearly universal. Physical examination findings depend on the stage of infection and may be uninformative or may reveal diffuse or localized crackles on lung auscultation associated with other signs of ventilatory distress. The PaO_2 is often low but may be normal in the early stages. The chest radiograph is usually abnormal but highly variable, the spectrum extending from a unilateral perihilar infiltrate to the more common pattern of diffuse bilateral interstitial infiltrates. Pleural effusions or mediastinal lymphadenopathy are not typical.

Diagnosis

Indirect tests suggestive of but lacking specificity for PCP include an elevated lactic dehydrogenase level and erythrocyte sedimentation rate, exercise desaturation, and diffuse lung uptake on gallium scanning. Since *Pneumocystis* cannot be reliably cultured, the diagnosis requires demonstration of the organism in pulmonary secretions or tissue. In labs with carefully controlled sputum induction methods, the diagnosis may sometimes be made by staining induced sputum. Usually, transbronchoscopic lavage and biopsy are required. Lavage alone may be positive in 80% of cases, and both procedures combined have a yield approaching 95%.[15] A rapid diagnosis may be made by examination of the lavage specimen or touch preps of the biopsy with Gomori methenamine-silver (GMS), calcofluor white, or toluidine blue O stains. An increased level of sensitivity and high specificity may be provided by commercially available indirect or direct immunofluorescent stains of bronchial lavage or induced sputum specimens for *Pneumocystis* using monoclonal antibodies.[16]

Therapy

Effective therapy is available to treat *P carinii* pneumonia. SMZ/TMP at a dosage of 20 mg/kg/day of the TMP component, given in divided doses every 6 hours, has advantages of both intravenous (IV) and oral forms of treatment and less toxicity than alternative therapies for those without HIV infection, making it the drug of choice. Pentamidine (4 mg/kg/day IV or, less preferably, intramuscularly) can serve as an alternative therapy for patients who fail SMZ/TMP, are allergic to sulfa drugs, or develop toxicity requiring discontinuation of therapy. Intravenous trimetrexate at 45 mg/m² day along with leucovorin at 20mg/m² IV or PO every six hours is an additional potential second line agent. Early adjunctive corticosteriod therapy for moderately severe PCP should be considered in immunosuppressed patients without HIV infection under similar circumstances to those with HIV infection.[17] If a patient has not had significant subjective and objective improvement within 72 to 96 hours after therapy is initiated, the clinician must consider either clinical failure or a concomitant pulmonary process that may or may not be infectious. After 14 to 21 days of high-dose therapy, prophylaxis should be instituted to prevent relapse in those patients who remain at risk through continued immunosuppression.

NOCARDIA

Associated with the increasing number of immunosuppressed patients over the past 20 to 30 years are the reports of systemic infection with *Nocardia*. The most common isolates are from the *N asteroides* complex, but there are additionally reported cases of serious infection with *N brasiliensis*, *N otitidiscaviarum*, and *N transvalensis*. Up to 85% of *Nocardia* infections occur in those with underlying immunosuppression, with corticosteroid or antineoplastic therapy most commonly associated.[18]

Presentation

Nocardia causes primarily a pulmonary infection but has a significant propensity to disseminate. The onset of illness due to nocardiosis is frequently subacute to chronic, with associated fever, moderately productive cough, and malaise. Findings on chest radiograph are variable, ranging from nodular infiltrates, consolidation, and frank abscesses to diffuse infiltrates. Pleural effusions are commonly found ipsilateral to parenchymal disease.[18] Hematogenous dissemination from a primary pulmonary focus results most often in formation of brain abscesses. The skin, kidneys, liver, and spleen are less common sites of dissemination. *Nocardia* can cause a primary cutaneous infection without preceding pulmonary involvement; however, the presence of branching, filamentous gram-positive rods grown aerobically from culture, or staining weakly acid-fast on a skin biopsy in an immunocompromised host should lead to a search for disseminated nocardiosis. Similarly, symptoms such as headaches, dizziness, and alterations in mental status, or signs of focal neurologic deficits in an immunocompromised patient with a pulmonary infiltrate should immediately bring to mind the possibility of nocardiosis or aspergillosis.

Diagnosis

Sputum smear and culture for *Nocardia* has a relatively low yield in most centers, even in patients with advanced pulmonary disease. The prompt establishment of a diagnosis of pulmonary or systemic nocardiosis usually requires an invasive procedure such as a biopsy from clinically involved sites.[18] *Nocardia* may be identified on Gram stain or modified acid-fast stains of sputum or wound drainage, Brown-Brenn tissue Gram stains, or GMS stains of biopsy specimens. Recovery of *Nocardia* may be enhanced by ensuring that cultures are held long enough to allow for slow growth. Controversy remains regarding the ability of *Nocardia* to colonize the bronchopulmonary tree without causing disease.[19] Despite the arguments favoring this position, the presence of *Nocardia* species in the sputum of an immuno-suppressed patient, particularly in the setting of prior corti-costeriod therapy, requires further investigation and consid-eration of early treatment.[18,20] Determination of the full extent of disease once *Nocardia* is identified is important, as it impacts on the choice of therapy, the treatment dura-tion, and prognosis. If pulmonary nocardial infection is docu-mented, the patient should have a computed tomography (CT) scan of the brain to exclude an occult brain abscess.

Therapy

Because of the relative infrequency of *Nocardia* infection, controlled trials of therapy have not been performed to firmly establish optimal treatment. The wealth of clinical experience has been with sulfonamides such as sulfadiazine (in oral doses ranging from 6 to 8 g/day), sulfisoxazole (4 to 12 g/day), or the combination of sulfamethoxazole and trimethoprim (5–20 mg/kg/day of TMP equivalent IV or PO, in divided doses every 12 hours). For severe nocardial infections, serum sulfonamide levels should be measured 2 hours after an oral dose with the goal of a level between 10 and 15 mg/dL. Other alternatives on the basis of sulfa allergy, toxicity, clinical failure, or demonstration of drug resistance include minocycline (200–300 mg PO b.i.d.), cilastatin-imi-penem (0.5 g IV every 6 hours), and amikacin (5–7.5 mg/kg every 12 hours).[18,21] Antimicrobial susceptibility testing at specialized reference laboratories may be of benefit in selecting among these or additional alternative therapies and in identification of drug resistance. Medical therapy for nocardiosis should be continued for a minimum of 12 months in immunosuppressed patients. Surgical drainage of soft tis-sue abscesses, empyemas, and complicated pleural effusions is required. Surgical decompression of brain abscesses, par-ticularly those of large size, and clinically progressing or enlarging by serial CT while on medical therapy results in mortality reduction and should also be considered.[18,21] If the underlying disease state allows, a reasonable adjunct, though

of unproven benefit, is the reduction of immunosuppressive therapy to the lowest possible dose.

LISTERIA MONOCYTOGENES

Though capable of causing illness in the immunocompetent, *L monocytogenes* is a gram-positive bacteria which acts pre-dominately as an opportunistic organism. *Listeria* infection is most commonly seen in those with an underlying malig-nancy, during pregnancy, in the neonate or the elderly, and in those receiving immunosuppressive therapy, particularly renal transplant recipients.

Presentation

The most common clinical presentations are meningitis or primary bacteremia, together comprising 80% to 90% of cases. Parenchymal CNS involvement may also occur, with or without meningitis. Initial symptoms are often acute, with fever being nearly universal. Headache, nuchal rigidity, and an altered level of consciousness may be seen in approxi-mately 50% or more of meningitis cases.[22,23] Focal neurologic signs in those with CNS involvement, particularly cranial nerve palsies, and gastrointestinal complaints in those with primary bacteremias, occur in a significant though lesser proportion of patients.

Diagnosis

The index of suspicion for *Listeria* must be high in immuno-compromised hosts. The diagnosis is typically made through culture of the cerebrospinal fluid (CSF) or blood, though caution must be exercised not to dismiss the gram-positive rods initially isolated as diptheroid contaminants. Central nervous system listeriosis is frequently associated with bac-teremia (~75%).[24] The presence of *L monocytogenes* in a blood culture should prompt an examination of the CSF. Examination of the spinal fluid is nonspecific and variable, but most commonly demonstrates a polymorphonuclear pre-dominant pleocytosis, a mildly elevated protein, and a nor-mal glucose level. The Gram stain is positive in a minority of cases. If meningitis is suspected in a patient on corticosteroid therapy but the Gram stain is unrevealing, therapy should be initiated to include *Listeria* while awaiting the results of the culture.

Therapy

The optimal treatment of *Listeria* infection has not been established through controlled clinical studies. Ampicillin (2 g IV every 4 hours) or penicillin G (2–4 million units IV every 4 hours) has been felt to be the drug of choice for listeriosis. In vitro data has demonstrated synergistic bacteri-cidal activity for the combination of ampicillin and gentami-cin, suggesting combined therapy may be warranted, partic-ularly in severe infections. SMZ/TMP (5 mg/kg IV every 8 hours) is an alternative agent with bactericidal activity against *Listeria* and good CNS penetration. Tetracyline, erythromy-cin, and chloramphenicol may be less effective, bacteriostatic alternatives. Due to the risk of relapse with shorter courses of therapy, a minimum of 3 to 4 weeks of treatment is recommended for nonperinatal listeriosis.[24] Reduction of immunosuppressive therapy is a prudent adjunctive measure, if possible. Additionally, enteric precautions are indicated to prevent nosocomial transmission to other patients.

LEGIONELLA

Legionella species are a group of related, yet antigenically distinctive, gram-negative rods that are capable of causing severe pneumonitis in both community and nosocomial settings. The organism is widely distributed in nature and can be recovered from many freshwater environments. Despite this widespread distribution, outbreaks tend to be associated with circumscribed geographic areas; nosocomial outbreaks are often associated with contaminated water sources.[25] *Legionella* species are intracellular organisms and cellular immunity is the major host defense mechanism. Thus, if *Legionella* species are endemic in a community or hospital, the patients at highest risk for development of infection and the more severely affected will be those with altered cellular immunity.[26,27]

Presentation

There is little in the way of physical, laboratory, or radiographic findings which can be said to be specific for *Legionella* pneumonia.[26] Unlike the prominent multisystem complaints initially reported with *Legionella pneumophila*, immunosuppressed patients frequently present only with fever and a scanty productive cough. Chest radiographs are almost always abnormal, but the pattern varies from unilateral consolidation to bilateral diffuse infiltrates.[26,28] *Legionella* must always be considered in the immunocompromised patient with pneumonia, particularly those with a poor clinical response to initial empiric β-lactam antimicrobial therapy with or without aminoglycosides.

Diagnosis

Though isolation of the organism in culture from respiratory tract specimens or blood remains the most definitive, albeit delayed, method of establishing a diagnosis, several rapid diagnostic tests are now commercially available. Sputum, bronchoalveolar lavage, and biopsy specimens can be submitted for detection of *Legionella* antigen using a direct fluorescent antibody (DFA) technique.[28] Monoclonal DFA tests with enhanced sensitivity (50–60%) and specificity (94–99%) improve the ability to make a rapid diagnosis. An additional rapid detection method, applicable to respiratory tract specimens, is a commercially produced DNA probe for *Legionella* species, with a reported specificity similar to that of the DFA test.[29] A less direct method of diagnosis, using a radioimmunoassay (RIA) detecting *L pneumophila* antigen in the urine, is also available, with a reported sensitivity of 80% to 99% and a specificity of 99%.[26] An enzyme immunoassay (EIA) is now commercially available, with a reported sensitivity of 97.7% and a specificity of 100%. The urinary antigen assay detects antigen only from *L pneumo-*

phila serogroup 1, the serogroup accounting for approximately 70% to 90% of infections. It offers the advantage of noninvasiveness, but may also increase the potential for missing a co-infecting agent if a more direct diagnostic evaluation is not additionally undertaken.

Isolation of *Legionella* species requires a special culture medium and buffered charcoal yeast extract agar, and may require up to 5 days to grow. Thus, it is important to inform the microbiology laboratory that you suspect legionellosis when the specimen is submitted. An indirect fluorescent antibody or enzyme-linked immunosorbent assay is available in many laboratories to establish a serologic diagnosis, but has limited use in the critical care setting. A fourfold rise in titer is considered diagnostic, but may take over 8 weeks for the fourfold rise to occur.

Therapy

Though not established through controlled clinical trials, the drug of choice for infection due to *Legionella* species is erythromycin (1 g q.i.d.). Intravenous therapy is the preferred route of administration in those with severe illness. There are no controlled studies comparing single-drug with combination therapy. However, benefit from the addition of rifampin has been reported, possibly by providing more rapid reduction in bacterial numbers and reducing lung damage.[30] Our recommendation for initial treatment is to use erythromycin along with rifampin (600 mg IV or PO) for the first 5 to 7 days of treatment, followed by erythromycin alone. Immunocompromised patients should complete three weeks of treatment to prevent relapses. The newer macrolides, azithromycin and clarithromycin, preliminarily appear to be reasonable alternatives to erythromycin when oral therapy is appropriate. The quinolone agents, SMZ/TMP, or doxycycline have also been suggested as alternatives, perhaps particularly useful when drug interactions with cyclosporine are a concern.

THE RENAL TRANSPLANT RECIPIENT

Renal allograft recipients are dependent on the chronic administration of drugs such as prednisone, azathioprine, cyclophosphamide, cyclosporine, and tacrolimus (FK506) for the maintenance of graft function. During periods of acute rejection, significant increases in dosage of some of these agents are required in an effort to reverse the rejection process. The combined effect of these drugs is one of constant immunosuppression, particularly of cellular-mediated immunity. As a result, infection is a frequent complication for renal transplant recipients. Certain infectious syndromes can be expected to occur at different time periods after renal transplantation (Fig. 108-1). Chronologic division of likely infectious complications for liver[31] and heart transplant recipients[32] have also been devised. The early post-transplant period is complicated predominantly by the typical bacterial pathogens and *Candida* species commonly seen in the postoperative surgical patient as well as herpes simplex virus. Generally, the period after the first post-transplant month is

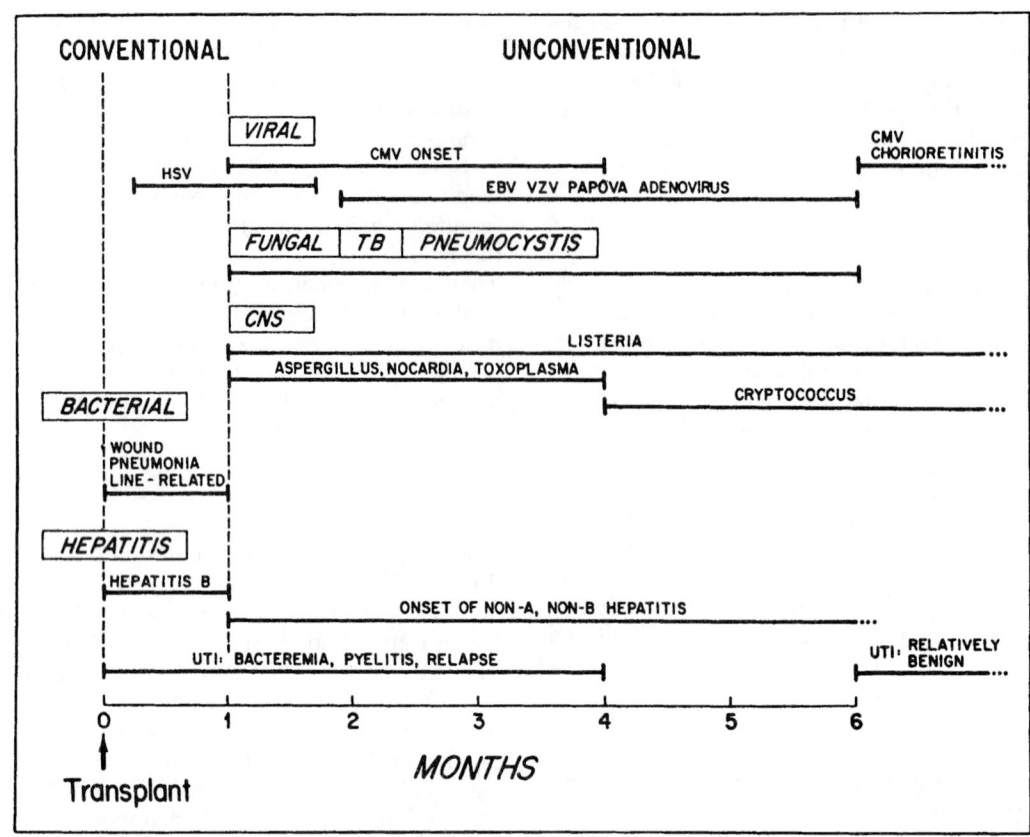

FIGURE 108-1. Timetable for the occurrence of infection in the the renal transplant patient. (From Rubin RH, Wolfson JS, Cosimi AB, et al: Infection in the renal transplant recipient. *Am J Med* 1981;70:406. Used with permission.)

associated with opportunistic fungal and bacterial infections. Central nervous system infection is rare in the first month after transplant but is significant in the following months. Certain factors can determine to some degree which infectious complications are likely to be encountered, including the types of immunosuppression employed, the underlying disease of the transplant population, and the epidemiology of various microbial agents (e.g., *Legionella* or *Aspergillus* species) unique to a given region or institution.

INFECTIONS IN THE FIRST MONTH

Wound Infections

Wound infection and related sepsis can be a significant cause of morbidity and mortality, particularly with involvement of the deep perinephric spaces. Flawless surgical technique is required for prevention of anastomotic leaks, hematomas, or lymphoceles. With advances in surgical technique and the use of closed suction drainage, the incidence of wound infection is currently expected to be low. Diagnosis of a wound infection requires a high index of suspicion. Patients with unexplained fever should undergo either ultrasound or CT scanning to evaluate for deep collections of perinephric fluid and sterile needle aspiration of the wound. Any fluid collection identified should be drained by closed suction and

antimicrobial therapy based on the culture results administered for 10 to 14 days.

Urinary Tract Infection

The incidence of urinary tract infections (UTIs) and urosepsis in the early post-transplant period has significantly diminished to less than 10% with the use of prophylactic SMZ/TMP.[33] However, the urinary tract remains a significant source of infection at any time after transplant. Infections acquired within the first 3 months are frequently associated with pyelonephritis, bacteremia, and a high relapse rate when treated with a typical 14 day course of therapy. Urinary tract infections occurring after 6 months generally are benign and can be treated with conventional therapy. The finding of candiduria is a common concern in the renal transplant patient and fluconazole treatment is recommended in an effort to prevent complications from arising.[33]

Other Infections

The other major infections occurring in the first 30 days after renal transplant are catheter sepsis, pneumonia, and reactivation of latent herpes simplex oralis or genitalis. Candidal infections are of particular concern because of a greater propensity to disseminate in immunocompromised hosts. Thus, it is important to limit the number of intravenous lines and to change them frequently. After intravenous access is no longer required, lines should be removed. Pneumonia is usually nosocomial and is most frequently caused by the resistant gram-negative rods indigenous to a given institution. As noted in the previous section, *Legionella* species, if present in the environment, are more commonly isolated in immunosuppressed patients. Herpes simplex virus reactivation is discussed later in the section on bone marrow transplant recipients.

Uncommonly, a patient may become severely affected post-transplant as a result of either an unrecognized and untreated infection prior to transplant or an unrecognized infection involving the donor organ. One example of the former problem is that of a transplant recipient with a previously unrecognized and perhaps asymptomatic *Strongyloides* infection who may develop a hyperinfection syndrome with pulmonary and gastrointestinal hemorrhagic complications and gram-negative sepsis post-transplant. The latter problem is exemplified by the transmission of hepatitis B or C or the HIV virus from the donor organ.

INFECTIONS 1 TO 6 MONTHS AFTER TRANSPLANT

The cumulative effect of immunosuppressive therapy is usually greatest in the first 6 months after transplant. Cell-mediated immunity is ablated and not allowed to recover until the patient is tapered to a maintenance immunosuppressive therapy regimen. Even at this time cell-mediated immunity is impaired by the antirejection regimen. Episodes of acute and chronic rejection are treated with increased doses of these drugs, which further impair host defenses. Immunomodulatory effects related to herpes group viral infections, particularly cytomegalovirus, also contribute to the degree of immunosuppression beyond that of drug therapy alone. Thus, it is during this time frame that the transplant patient is generally at most risk for life-threatening opportunistic infections (see Fig. 108-1).

Cytomegalovirus

Cytomegalovirus (CMV) is the most important organism in renal allograft recipients, with evidence of infection in 60% to 90% of patients. CMV is responsible for the majority of febrile episodes during the period of one to six months post transplant. Infection usually occurs within 4 months but can be seen up to 2 years after transplant.[33,34] Most infections are the result of reactivation of latent virus; a smaller number are primary infections associated with acquisition of CMV from the allograft of a seropositive donor or from blood transfusion. A major risk factor for reactivation of latent CMV infection in the host or the donor organ is the high level of cellular immunosuppression induced by monoclonal antibodies to T cells (OKT3) or anti-lymphocyte globulin therapy used to reverse acute rejection. CMV infection impacts on renal transplant recipients in three distinct ways: the infectious disease syndromes produced by the virus; increased viral-induced immunosuppression with subsequently increased propensity to develop opportunistic infections, and viral-induced renal allograft dysfunction.[33]

PRESENTATION. The clinical presentation of CMV disease is diverse in terms of organ system involvement and range of severity. The most common form of CMV infection, usually associated with reactivation of latent CMV in seropositive transplant recipients, is a subacute febrile illness associated with leukopenia, mild hepatitis, constitutional symptoms, and allograft dysfunction. CMV pneumonitis may occur after one to two weeks of milder illness with fever, dyspnea, a nonproductive cough, and hypoxemia. The chest radiograph most commonly demonstrates diffuse interstitial and alveolar infiltrates, though many other patterns have been described.[35] The radiographic appearance may be further influenced by coinfection or superinfection by other pathogens. Gastrointestinal manifestations of CMV infection, including nausea, vomiting, transaminitis, abdominal pain, and gastrointestinal bleeding from mucosal ulcerations, usually occur in the setting of widespread CMV infection.[36] However, on rare occasions it may be seen without other organ system involvement, making it essential that CMV be included in the differential diagnosis and evaluation of these signs and symptoms. A potentially lethal CMV syndrome has been described that begins with the typical fever and leukopenia but is followed by severe prostration, hypoxemia, and the development of severe hepatic and pulmonary dysfunction. Associated complications include muscle wasting, gastrointestinal hemorrhage, CNS depression, and often superinfection.[37] Early diagnosis and initiation of effective therapy diminish the risk of severe manifestations.

DIAGNOSIS. The duration of time required and the low predictive value of serologic studies for CMV disease makes these forms of testing unacceptable for clinical evaluation of renal transplant patients. Diagnostic efforts have become focused on identifying the virus itself in clinical specimens (body fluids or tissues) through the use of monoclonal antibodies to detect CMV antigens. The shell vial assay, involving centrifugation of clinical specimens onto fibroblast monolayers followed by indirect immunofluorescent staining using monoclonal antibodies, allows for results within 24 to 48 hours. CMV viremia correlates highly with the presence or potential development of CMV-related disease. Additionally, CMV antigenemia assays of buffy coat preparations using monoclonal antibodies against specific CMV proteins provide results within 24 hours and have shown quantitative correlation with CMV disease activity.[38] Tissue biopsy specimens should be evaluated histopathologically for typical viral inclusion bodies or by immunohistochemical stains for CMV.

THERAPY. Ganciclovir, an analogue of acyclovir, demonstrates anti-CMV activity in vitro, and has been efficacious in treating established CMV disease in solid organ and bone marrow transplant (BMT) recipients.[39,40] Use of ganciclovir for CMV-associated pneumonitis, hepatitis, and gastrointestinal disease has become standard of care. The recommended dosage is 5 mg/kg IV every 12 hours for 14 to 21 days followed by a maintenance dose of 5 mg/kg once daily or Monday through Friday. Dosage adjustment for renal dysfunction is required. Since CMV disease frequently complicates the treatment for organ rejection or graft-versus-host disease in BMT recipients, maintenance ganciclovir therapy is usually continued until the immunosuppressive regimen used has been reduced to maintenance levels. The major toxicity associated with ganciclovir is granulocytopenia which, combined with the cellular immune deficiency, places the patient at risk for superinfection by opportunistic fungi and bacteria. It is essential to monitor the granulocyte count frequently and to interrupt therapy if the absolute granulocyte count falls below 1000/mm³. Use of G-CSF to aid in neutrophil recovery should additionally be considered and may allow for uninterrupted therapy with ganciclovir. In the setting of severe CMV disease, consideration should be given to combination therapy with intravenous immunoglobulin (500 mg/kg IV every other day for 10 doses) along with ganciclovir based on the experience in BMT recipients,[41] though studies confirming the benefit are lacking in renal transplant recipients.

Due to the severe morbidity and mortality associated with CMV disease, emphasis has been placed on preventing acquisition or reactivation of CMV infection. Organ transplant recipients who are CMV-negative and receive organs from CMV-seronegative donors should receive only CMV-negative blood products. Intravenous CMV immunoglobulin and oral acyclovir have both demonstrated effectiveness in preventing primary and reactivation CMV disease.[42,43] Increasing interest has developed in early preemptive therapy with ganciclovir for those patients at greatest risk for CMV disease such as those requiring anti-lymphocyte antibody therapy or in those with CMV viremia without other evidence of disease, based on extrapolations from BMT treatment strategies.

Central Nervous System Infections

Renal allograft recipients appear to have a propensity for developing CNS infections, which are a major cause of morbidity and mortality. *L monocytogenes* (discussed earlier) is the most common bacterial cause of meningitis. A typical setting in which it may be seen is shortly after immunosuppressive therapy is bolstered for treatment of rejection.[23] It is important to remember that the only sign of CNS infection may be a mild headache; this complaint alone, associated with fever, mandates an evaluation of the CSF to rule out meningitis.

Cryptococcus neoformans is the most common fungal CNS infection in renal transplant recipients, with an onset usually at more than 6 months after transplantation. The typical presentation is a subacute or chronic meningitis, often with weeks of intermittent headaches and fever. The portal of entry is the lungs, with subsequent fungemia leading to CNS metastasis. Cryptococcal meningitis may be seen in isolation or concurrent with cryptococcal involvement at other sites, such as the lungs, urinary tract, and skin. The finding of cryptococcal disease at these sites warrants a lumbar puncture to rule out early CNS involvement. A serum cryptococcal antigen test is helpful as a sensitive indicator of cryptococcal disease. Evaluation of the CSF should include tests for the presence of cryptococcal antigen, an India ink preparation for encapsulated yeast, and fungal cultures. Controversy exists regarding optimal treatment of cryptococcal meningitis in renal transplant patients, due to an absence of comparative data in this population. In the critical care patient, however, initial therapy with AMB (0.5–0.8 mg/kg/day) and flucytosine (25–37.5 mg/kg every 6 hours) is suggested to maximize rapidity of clinical control over the infection. Levels of flucytosine should be monitored and maintained in the range of 40 to 60 μg/mL to avoid the toxicities of granulocytopenia and thrombocytopenia. Fluconazole (400–800 mg/day), which has significantly less side effects than AMB or flucytosine, is often substituted once clinical stability is clearly established. Treatment is usually continued until there is no further evidence of disease by CSF culture and cryptococcal antigen testing. Careful follow up for relapse over the next 6 to 12 months is essential.

Other less common etiologies of CNS infections are *Toxoplasma gondii*, *N asteroides*, and *Aspergillus fumigatus*, usually seen within the first 4 months post-transplant. These organisms tend to cause focal brain infection, frequently associated with focal neurologic signs. *Aspergillus* and *Nocardia* brain abscesses usually result from metastatic spread from pulmonary foci. Thus, identifying and treating pulmonary infection may prevent CNS metastasis. Whenever pulmonary *Aspergillus* and *Nocardia* are present, a search for disseminated disease should be initiated. *Toxoplasma* infections, on the other hand, are usually the result of reactivation of previously dormant foci. The waning of cellular immunity associated with the immunosuppressive regimen allows the infection to reactivate and replicate, causing focal abscesses. The initial clinical and radiographic appearance of these infections may be quite similar, although the treatments are widely divergent. In the absence of a pulmonary focus, a brain biopsy may be required to establish a tissue diagnosis to guide therapy.

Other Infections

P carinii, discussed earlier, is an important cause of opportunistic pneumonia, with an incidence of approximately 10% in renal transplant patients.[42] Additional etiologies of pulmonary and sinus infections in renal transplant recipients are opportunistic fungal infections with *Aspergillus*, *Zygomycetes*, or *Cryptococcus*. In addition, because of their prolonged immunosuppression, these patients are at increasing risk for reactivation of a former infection with the endemic fungi (histoplasmosis, coccidioidomycosis, and blastomycosis). A thorough epidemiologic history is useful to identify those at risk so that once a pulmonary or systemic illness begins, an early evaluation for reactivation can be initiated. Though reactivation of tuberculosis is more common in transplant patients than in the general population, most patients with positive purified protein derivative (PPD) skin tests prior to transplant and with no other risk factors do not develop active disease. Tuberculosis should be considered in the evaluation of pulmonary infiltrates in these patients but is a less likely causal agent than are opportunistic pathogens.

BONE MARROW TRANSPLANT RECIPIENT ■

Recipients of allogeneic BMT are the epitome of the immunosuppressed host. As a result of the preconditioning therapy, which involves high-dose cytotoxic chemotherapy and frequently total body irradiation, bone marrow elements are ablated and both humoral and cellular immunity are eradicated. Thus, in the period immediately after the BMT, the patient is devoid of most host defenses. The natural mucosal barriers also are interrupted by the effects of the preparative therapy. It is not surprising that these patients are at high risk for infectious complications. Like renal transplant recipients, patients undergoing bone marrow transplants have characteristic infectious complications that reflect the immune defects present at each stage of the process (Table 108-1). Though some degree of overlap between stages must be recognized, chronologic separation of potential infections throughout the BMT process serves as a useful guide in formulation of a differential diagnosis.

PRETRANSPLANT TO ENGRAFTMENT INFECTION

The predominant infections manifested in the pretransplant, conditioning, and pre-engraftment stages are those associated with the underlying disease and granulocytopenia. (See earlier discussion of the granulocytopenic patient.) Additionally, reactivation of herpes simplex virus (HSV types I and II) early in the post-transplant period is common (40–80% of recipients). The typical presentation is painful mucocutaneous lesions of the oral cavity or genital area, which may be confused with chemotherapy-induced mucositis. HSV pneumonia is an uncommon complication, causing only 5% of nonbacterial pneumonias. Pneumonia usually results from contiguous spread of oropharyngeal lesions, but also may spread hematogenously.[44] The diagnosis of HSV pneumonia has typically been made postmortem, and therefore it is an important complication to prevent. Oral or genital lesions should be swabbed and submitted for culture. HSV typically produces characteristic cytopathologic effects within 24 to 72 hours. Immunofluorescent stains for HSV should be obtained on lung biopsy specimens in addition to culture and histopathologic examination. Acyclovir is effective in the treatment of active HSV disease in a variety of dosing strategies (200–400 mg PO five times a day or 5 mg/kg IV every 8 hours).[45] Additionally, acyclovir has been shown to be beneficial in prevention of reactivation of latent HSV infection. Patients who are seropositive for HSV before transplant should be treated with acyclovir (250 mg/m^2 IV two or three times daily or 800 mg PO twice daily) for the first 30 to 45 days after the procedure.

INTERSTITIAL PNEUMONITIS PERIOD (POST-ENGRAFTMENT INFECTION)

After engraftment of the donor marrow, the BMT recipient remains immunosuppressed because of defects in humoral and cellular immunity. Graft-versus-host disease (GVHD) is a complication which may arise in this time frame and, along with the drugs used to treat this complication, further adds to the cellular immune defects.

The predominant infectious complication in the first 4 months after engraftment is interstitial pneumonitis, a clinical syndrome classically characterized by fever, dyspnea, a non-productive cough, and malaise. This occurs in approximately 40% of allogeneic grafts and 15% to 20% of syngeneic grafts. The onset is usually subacute, but a fulminant phase leading to ventilatory failure requiring mechanical ventilation can develop. The chest radiograph most often reveals diffuse bilateral interstitial infiltrates, but there may be areas of focal consolidation. The differential diagnosis for this clinical picture is extensive and includes many noninfectious causes, such as drug toxicity, recurrent malignancy, radiation pneumonitis, pulmonary veno-occlusive disease, pulmonary edema syndromes, pulmonary hemorrhage, and, most commonly, idiopathic interstitial pneumonitis. In patients under-

TABLE 108-1. Timetable for the Occurrence of Infection in the Bone Marrow Transplant Recipient

PRETRANSPLANT TO ENGRAFTMENT PRETRANSPLANT TO ~30 DAYS	INTERSTITIAL PNEUMONITIS PERIOD ~30–100 DAYS	LATE POST-TRANSPLANT 100 DAYS OR LATER
Major Pathogens • Bacteria (gram-negative enterics and increasingly gram-positive organisms) • Fungi (*Candida, Aspergillus*) • HSV	• CMV pneumonitis (~40%) • *Aspergillus, Candida,* others • PCP (5–15%) • HSV or VZV pneumonitis (<10%) • Toxoplasmosis (uncommon) • Adenovirus (uncommon)	• Varicella-zoster virus (>40%) • Bacteria-encapsulated organisms (~33%) • Fungi (20%)
Primary Host Defense Defects • Skin barrier breach (mucositis, central catheters) • Decreased phagocytes	• Abnormal cell mediated immunity • Skin barrier breach (with acute GVHD) • Decreased humoral immunity	• Delayed recovery of cell medicated and humoral immunity • Skin breach (in chronic GVHD)

Adapted from Van der Meer JWM, Guiot HFL, van der Broek PJ, et al: *Semin Hematol* 1984;21:124.

going syngeneic transplants more than 50% of cases are idiopathic. Among infectious etiologies, CMV is the most common, causing nearly 50% of cases in allogeneic grafts. In both transplant groups, a smaller percentage of pneumonitis is caused by *P carinii* and viruses such as herpes simplex, varicella-zoster, and adenoviruses.[46] GVHD is a very significant risk factor for the development of CMV pneumonitis. Due to high mortality rates once CMV disease is evident, current emphasis in allogeneic transplant patients is toward surveillance of blood, urine, and throat cultures for CMV and early preemptive treatment with ganciclovir and intravenous gammaglobulin (IVIG). The recommended treatment for CMV interstitial pneumonitis is ganciclovir 5 mg/kg iv every 12 hours, along with IVIG 500 mg/kg iv every other day for 21 days.[47]

The broad differential and diverse therapies for the various potential causes of interstitial pneumonitis, along with high mortality rates for untreated infections (90% for CMV pneumonia), make it important to establish a tissue diagnosis. Various groups debate whether to perform transbronchoscopic biopsy and lavage or to pursue an open procedure initially. Each case should be individualized, keeping in mind the clinical status of the patient, the progression of the pneumonitis, possible complications associated with the procedure, and perhaps most important, whether the clinicians think they can afford the 24-hour delay for an open lung biopsy while awaiting results of the transbronchoscopic biopsy. If a diagnostic procedure is imminent (within 4–6 hours), and the patient has engrafted their marrow (absolute granulocyte count >500/mm³), then antimicrobial therapy can await the results of the rapid diagnostic tests performed on the biopsy specimen. If the procedure or the necessary results will be delayed one should initiate therapy based on the most likely pathogens (CMV, *P carinii*, HSV).

Invasive mycoses and fungemia caused by *Candida*, *Aspergillus*, and other opportunistic molds may occur in the period of granulocytopenia, but perhaps more often manifest themselves following engraftment. As with CMV infection, the risk of fungal infections in this time frame is related to the occurrence of GVHD, which may continue to compromise the integrity of both mucosal and skin barriers. Corticosteroids used for treatment of GVHD impair alveolar macrophage function allowing inhaled fungal spores of *Aspergillus* to become invasive. Furthermore, neutrophil function is impaired resulting in a suboptimal host response and an inability to prevent progression of the infection. Pulmonary infiltrates must be aggressively pursued diagnostically for histopathology and cultures because the likelihood of a successful therapeutic outcome may depend upon the delay imposed between onset of the disease process and initiation of treatment. Isolation of an opportunistic mold such as *Aspergillus* from sputum or bronchoalveolar lavage fluid in a febrile, compromised host should be regarded as an invasive disease and treatment begun immediately with amphotericin B (1.0–1.5 mg/kg/day). It should be emphasized that a microbiologic diagnosis for invasive mycoses is important, since many fungi with a histopathologic appearance similar to *Aspergillus*, such as *Fusarium* or *Trichosporon*, may be resistant to amphotericin B. In these cases, triazole compounds are sometimes beneficial as an alternative therapy for am-

photericin B-resistant organisms. Consultation with an infectious diseases specialist is appropriate for suspected invasive mycoses in immunocompromised hosts.

LATE INFECTIONS

Varicella-zoster virus (VZV) is a source of cutaneous eruptions in nearly 30% of BMT recipients within the first year, with a median time to onset of 5 months. Of these infections, approximately 45% disseminate and 12% result in death. The majority of VZV infections (84%) represent reactivation of latent zoster virus; of those that disseminate and are fatal, however, nearly 40% are from primary varicella.[48] The presence of localized or disseminated zosteriform lesions in a BMT patient should prompt therapy with acyclovir (12.5 mg/kg or 500mg/m² of body surface area, IV every 8 hours).[45] On rare occasions a patient may present with the confusing picture of severe abdominal pain as a manifestation of visceral VZV prior to development of any characteristic skin lesions or other signs of dissemination.

Among long-term survivors (>6 months), recurrent sinopulmonary infections are the predominant bacterial complications, resulting particularly from encapsulated organisms such as *Streptococcus pneumoniae* and *Hemophilius influenzae*. The predilection to pyogenic infections, seen particularly in the patient with chronic GVHD, can be correlated to defects in opsonic activity[49] and continued impairments in neutrophil function,[50] reflecting the delayed reconstitution of the immune system. For this reason, it is recommended that prophylaxis with SMZ/TMP or a penicillin be used in patients with chronic GVHD. A late-onset interstitial pneumonitis may also occur, due to pathogens similar to those found in the first 100 days after transplant.[51] An aggressive diagnostic workup remains necessary to evaluate for treatable causes, including *P carinii*, CMV, and VZV.

REFERENCES

1. Bodey GP, Buckley M, Sathe YS, et al: Quantitative relationships between circulating leukocytes and infection in patients with acute leukemia. *Ann Intern Med* 1966;64:328
2. Sickles EA, Greene WH, Wiernik PH: Clinical presentation of infection in granulocytopenic patients. *Arch Intern Med* 1975;35:715
3. Lee JW, Pizzo PA: Management of the cancer patient with fever and prolonged neutropenia. *Hematol Oncol Clin North Am* 1993;7:919
4. Bodey GP: Empirical antibiotic therapy for fever in neutropenic patients. *Clin Infect Dis* 1993;17(Suppl 2):S378
5. Hughes WT, Armstrong D, Bodey GP, et al: Guidelines for the use of antimicrobial agents in neutropenic patients with unexplained fever. *J Infect Dis* 1990;161:381
6. Centers for Disease Control and Prevention: Recommendations for preventing the spread of vancomycin resistance. *MMWR* 1995;44:3–4
7. DeGregorio MW, Lee WMF, Linker CA, et al: Fungal infections in patients with acute leukemia. *Am J Med* 1982;73:543
8. EORTC International Antimicrobial Therapy Cooperative Group: Empiric antifungal therapy in febrile granulocytopenic patients. *Am J Med* 1989;86:668
9. Pizzo PA: Management of fever in patients with cancer and

treatment-induced neutropenia. *N Engl J Med* 1993;328:1323

10. Crawford J, Ozer H, Stoller R, et al: Reduction by granulocyte colony-stimulating factor of fever and neutropenia induced by chemotherapy in patients with small-cell lung cancer. *N Engl J Med* 1991;325:164

11. Dale DC: Potential role of colony-stimulating factors in the prevention and treatment of infectious diseases. *Clin Infect Dis* 1994;18(Suppl 2):S180

12. Fauci AS, Dale DC, Balow JE: Glucocorticoid therapy: mechanisms of action and clinical considerations. *Ann Intern Med* 1976;84:304

13. Losito A, Williams DG, Cooke G, et al: The effects on polymorphonuclear leukocyte function of prednisolone and azathioprine in vivo and prednisolone, azathioprine and 6-mercaptopurine in vitro. *Clin Exp Immunol* 1978;32:423

14. Edman JC, Kovacs JA, Masur H, et al: Ribosomal RNA sequence shows *Pneumocystis carinii* to be a member of the Fungi. *Nature* 1988;334:519

15. Stover DE, Zaman MB, Hadju SI, et al: Bronchoalveolar lavage in the diagnosis of diffuse pulmonary infiltrates in the immunosuppressed host. *Ann Intern Med* 1984;101:1

16. Kovacs JA, Ng VL, Masur H, et al: Diagnosis of *Pneumocystis carinii* pneumonia: improved detection in sputum with use of monoclonal antibodies. *N Engl J Med* 1988;318:589

17. NIH-UC Expert Panel for Corticosteriods as Adjunctive Therapy for *Pneumocystis* Pneumonia: consensus statement on the use of corticosteriods as adjunctive therapy for *pneumocystis* pneumonia in the acquired immunodeficiency syndrome. *N Engl J Med* 1990;323:1500

18. Rolfe MW, Strieter RM, Lynch JP: Nocardiosis. *Semin Respir Med* 1992;13:216

19. Young LS, Armstrong D, Blevins A, et al: *Nocardia asteroides* infection complicating neoplastic disease. *Am J Med* 1971; 50:356

20. Simpson GL, Stinson EB, Egger MJ, et al: Nocardial infections in the immunocompromised host: a detailed study in a defined population. *Rev Infect Dis* 1981;3:492

21. Filice GA, Simpson GL: Management of Nocardia infections. In: Remington JS, Swartz MN (eds). *Current Clinical Topics in Infectious Diseases*, Vol 5. New York, McGraw-Hill, 1984:49

22. Nieman RE, Lorber B: Listeriosis in adults: a changing pattern. Report of eight cases and review of the literature, 1968–1978. *Rev Infect Dis* 1981;2:207

23. Stamm AM, Dismukes WE, Simmons BP, et al: Listeriosis in renal transplant recipients: report of an outbreak and review of 102 cases. *Rev Infect Dis* 1982;4:665

24. Gellin BG, Broome CV: Listeriosis. *JAMA* 1989;261:1313

25. Blatt SP, Parkinson MD, Pace E, et al: Nosocomial Legionnaires' disease: aspiration as a primary mode of disease acquisition. *Am J Med* 1993;95:16

26. Edelstein PH: Legionnaires' disease. *Clin Infect Dis* 1993; 16:741

27. Saravolatz LD, Burch KH, Fisher E, et al: The compromised host and Legionnaires' disease. *Ann Intern Med* 1979;90:533

28. Edelstein PH, Meyer RD, Finegold SM: Laboratory diagnosis of Legionnaires' disease. *Am Rev Respir Dis* 1980;121:317

29. Pasculle AW, Veto GE, Krystofiak S, et al: Laboratory and clinical evaluation of a commercial DNA probe for the detection of *Legionella* spp. *J Clin Micro* 1989;27:2350

30. Roig J, Carreres A, Domingo C: Treatment of Legionnaires' disease: current recommendations. *Drugs* 1993;46:63

31. Winston DJ, Emmanouilides C, Busuttil RW: Infections in liver transplant recipients. *Clin Infect Dis* 1995;21:1077

32. Petri WA Jr: Infections in heart transplant recipients. *Clin Infect Dis* 1994;18:141

33. Rubin RH: Infection in organ transplant recipients. In Rubin RH, Young LS (eds). *Clinical Approach to Infection in the Compromised Host.* New York, Plenum, 1994:629

34. Rubin RH, Wolfson JS, Cosimi AB, et al: Infection in the renal transplant recipient. *Am J Med* 1981;70:405

35. Ettinger NA, Trulock EP: Pulmonary considerations of organ transplantation. *Am Rev Respir Dis* 1991;143:1386

36. Buckner FS, Pomeroy C: Cytomegalovirus disease of the gastrointestinal tract in patients without AIDS. *Clin Infect Dis* 1993;17:644

37. Simmons RL, Lopez C, Balfour HH Jr, et al: Cytomegalovirus: clinical virological correlations in renal transplant recipients. *Ann Surg* 1974;180:623

38. Smith TF, Wold AD, Espy MJ, et al: New developments in the diagnosis of viral diseases. *Infect Dis Clin North Am* 1993;7:183

39. Erice A, Jordan MC, Chace BA, et al: Ganciclovir treatment of cytomegalovirus disease in transplant recipients and other immunocompromised hosts. *JAMA* 1987;257:3082

40. Paya CV, Hermans PE, Smith TF, et al: Efficacy of ganciclovir in liver and kidney transplant recipients with severe cytomegalovirus infection. *Transplantation* 1988;46:299

41. Emanuel D, Cunningham I, Jules-Elysee K, et al: Cytomegalovirus pneumonia after bone marrow transplantation successfully treated with the combination of ganciclovir and high-dose intravenous immune globulin. *Ann Intern Med* 1988;109:777

42. Rubin RH: Infectious disease complications of renal transplantation. *Kidney Int* 1993;44:221

43. Rubin RH, Tolkoff-Rubin NE: Antimicrobial strategies in the care of organ transplant recipients. *Antimicrob Agents Chemother* 1993;37:619

44. Ramsey PG, Fife KH, Hackman RC, et al: Herpes simplex virus pneumonia: clinical, virologic, and pathologic features in 20 patients. *Ann Intern Med* 1982;97:813

45. Whitley RJ, Gnann JW: Acyclovir: a decade later. *N Engl J Med* 1992;327:782

46. Meyers JD, Flournoy N, Thomas ED: Nonbacterial pneumonia after allogeneic marrow transplantation: a review of ten years' experience. *Rev Infect Dis* 1982;4:1119

47. Zaia JA: Prevention and treatment of cytomegalovirus pneumonia in transplant recipients. *Clin Infect Dis* 1993;17(Suppl 2):S392

48. Locksley RM, Flournoy N, Sullivan KM, et al: Infection with varicella-zoster virus after marrow transplantation. *J Infect Dis* 1985;152:1172

49. Winston DJ, Schiffman G, Wang DC, et al: Pneumococcal infections after human bone-marrow transplantation. *Ann Intern Med* 1979;91:835

50. Zimmerli W, Zarth A, Gratwohl A, et al: Neutrophil function and pyogenic infections in bone marrow transplant recipients. *Blood* 1991;77:393

51. Wingard JR, Santos GW, Saral R: Late onset interstitial pneumonia following allogeneic bone marrow transplantation. *Transplantation* 1985;39:21

Critical Care, Third Edition, edited by Joseph M. Civetta,
Robert W. Taylor, and Robert R. Kirby.
Lippincott-Raven Publishers, Philadelphia, PA © 1997.

CHAPTER 109

■

Human Immunodeficiency Virus in the Intensive Care Unit

Loretta M. O'Brien
Richard E. Winn

IMMEDIATE CONCERNS ■

MAJOR PROBLEMS

This chapter focuses on human immunodeficiency virus (HIV) infection in the intensive care unit (ICU) setting. After a brief review of the pathogenesis and progression of HIV infection, important clinical syndromes seen in HIV-infected patients are discussed, emphasizing clinical presentation, diagnostic modalities, and therapeutic management. Ethical issues such as utilization of ICU and "do-not-resuscitate" orders are discussed as they apply to HIV-infected patients. Finally, infection control procedures are reviewed. A comprehensive review of the HIV epidemic and the acquired immunodeficiency syndrome (AIDS) is beyond the scope of this chapter, and the reader is referred to other sources for further information.[1-2]

STRESS POINTS

1. HIV causes progressive immune system impairment that eventually leads to immune compromise as seen with AIDS.

The views expressed in this chapter are those of the authors and do not reflect official policy of the Department of Defense or other departments of the United States government.

2. The primary immune defect results from the infection of $CD4^+$ T lymphocytes, or $CD4^+$ cells.
3. The hallmark of this defect is a decreased cellular immunity proportional to the decreasing $CD4^+$ count.
4. The $CD4^+$ defect also creates a cascade of immune disregulation, causing marked abnormalities of humoral immunity and neutrophil function.
5. By these defects, HIV-infected patients are predisposed to bacterial infections at any $CD4^+$ count.
6. Overall, the $CD4^+$ count can be used with fair accuracy to predict both the degree of dysfunction and the potential infectious complications seen with HIV infection (Table 109-1).
7. The prognosis of HIV infection and AIDS has been altered considerably with the use of antiretroviral therapy, prophylactic antibiotic therapy for opportunistic infections, and improved treatment for the infections once they occur.
8. General statements about survival based on a patient's $CD4^+$ count criteria or duration of infection are problematic because patient survival can vary widely.
9. Survival is best predicted by the patient's complications of HIV infection.
10. For instance, the median survival of a patient with an AIDS-defining diagnosis of systemic lymphoma is 3.3 months compared with the 18.8 months for a

1617

TABLE 109-1. Complications of HIV Infection by CD4$^+$ Count

CD4$^+$ COUNT (cells/mm^3)	DIAGNOSIS
Any	*Hemophilus influenzae* infections *Mycobacterium tuberculosis* *Pseudomonas aeruginosa* infection *Streptococcus pneumoniae* infections
<250	*Coccidioides immitis* infections
<200	*Cryptococcus neoformans* meningitis *Pneumocystis carinii* pneumonia *Toxoplasma gondii* encephalitis
<100	*Mycobacterium avium* complex *Rhodococcus equi* infections Norcardiosis
<50	Cytomegalovirus disease Disseminated *Histoplasma capsulatum*

HIV, human immunodeficiency virus.

TABLE 109-2. Reasons for Admission to a Medical ICU in 133 HIV-Infected Patients

ADMITTING DIAGNOSIS	NO.	PERCENT
Respiratory failure	90	67.7
From PCP	68	51.0
Neurologic problems	16	12.0
Sepsis	10	7.5
Renal/metabolic disease	6	5.0
Other	11	8.0
Drug toxicity	3	2.0
Cardiac	4	3.0

PCP, *Pneumocystis carinii* pneumonia; ICU, intensive care unit; HIV, human immunodeficiency virus.

From Smith RL, Levine SM, Lewis ML: Prognosis of patients with AIDS requiring intensive care. *Chest* 1989;96:857.

patient with an AIDS-defining diagnosis of Kaposi's sarcoma (KS).[3]

ESSENTIAL DIAGNOSTIC TESTS AND PROCEDURES

1. Because routine laboratory tests do not provide much information about HIV staging, the total lymphocyte count can be used to predict the CD4$^+$ count. If the absolute lymphocyte count is less than 2000 cells/dL, then the patient's CD4$^+$ count can be presumed to be less than 200 cells/mm^3 until confirmed.[4]
2. HIV-infected patients should be approached in a systematic and thorough manner, as for any other immunocompromised host.
3. The diagnostic approach can be modified to reflect the unique medical problems that occur with HIV infection.
4. Patients occasionally present for medical care who are unable to provide any medical history. Use the available information as clues to both the patient's risk of HIV infection as well as the complications of a known HIV infection. The possibility of HIV infection needs to be considered in every patient, but especially with a patient with the following risk factors: sexual intercourse with a person with a known HIV infection; sexual intercourse with a person who is at risk for HIV infection, such as injection drug users, commercial sex workers, or persons with multiple sex partners; use of contaminated, unsterilized needles for any skin-piercing procedure such as acupuncture, use of illicit drugs, steroid injections, ear piercing, and tattooing; and use of blood products or clotting factors, especially before November 1985. In addition, the medication list of the HIV-infected patient can provide important information. Just as the use of nitroglycerin implies

that a patient has coronary artery disease, the use of gancyclovir implies that an HIV-infected patient has cytomegalovirus (CMV) disease and therefore a CD4$^+$ count of less than 50 cells/mm^3.

INITIAL THERAPY

1. Patients with HIV infection are admitted to ICUs primarily for respiratory failure from *Pneumocystis carinii* pneumonia (PCP) (Table 109-2).
2. Although the other complications of HIV only occasionally require treatment in the ICU setting, they may coexist with respiratory failure and complicate an ICU admission.
3. Infections are the most common serious problem in HIV-infected patients. Table 109-3 shows the important pathogens and recommended therapies.
4. Because the medications used with HIV infection may be unfamiliar to a provider, Table 109-4 reviews the medications frequently prescribed, the indications for their use, and the associated side effects.

PULMONARY MANIFESTATIONS OF HIV ■

Pulmonary manifestations of HIV infections are common. Respiratory failure from PCP is the leading reason for ICU admission in HIV-infected patients.[5] Because of the abnormal immune responses seen even with early HIV infection, these patients can present with unusual or atypical radiographic findings. It is also common for an HIV-infected patient to present with more than one pulmonary process, including a noninfectious process. With these caveats, the pulmonary complications of HIV infection can be considered by radiographic patterns (Table 109-5).

TABLE 109-3. Treatment for Infections in HIV-Infected Patients

ORGANISM	PREFERRED REGIMENS	ALTERNATIVE REGIMENS
Candida species		
Thrush	Nystatin 500,000 U gargled 5×/d Clotrimazole oral troches 10 mg 5×/d Ketoconazole 200–400 mg PO qd Fluconazole 50–100 mg PO qd	Ampho B 0.3–0.5 mg/kg/d IV Itraconazole 200 mg PO qd
Esophagitis	Fluconazole 100–400 mg PO qd for 2–3 wk	Ampho B 0.3–0.5 mg/kg/d IV for 7 d; may use 5FC 100 mg/kg/d IV
Coccidioidomycosis		
Initial therapy	Ampho B 0.5–1.0 mg/kg/d IV for 8+ wk; total dose 2.0–2.5 g	Fluconazole 400 mg PO qd Itraconazole 200 mg PO bid
Meningitis	Intrathecal Ampho B	Fluconazole 400 mg PO qd
Maintenance	Fluconazole 400 mg PO qd Ampho B 1.0 mg/kg/wk	Itraconazole 200 mg PO qd
Cryptococcosis		
Meningitis	Ampho B 0.5–1.0 mg/kg/d IV; may use 5FC 100 mg kg/d Ampho B 0.7 mg/kg/d for 10–14 d, then Fluconazole 400 mg PO qd for 8–10 wk	Fluconazole 400 mg PO qd for 6–10 wk
Without meningitis	Treat as if meningitis Fluconazole 400 mg PO qd for 6–10 wk	
Maintenance	Fluconazole 200–400 mg PO qd	Ampho B 1.0 mg/kg/wk
Cytomegalovirus		
Retinis	Foscarnet 60 mg/kg IV q 8 h for 14–21 d Gancyclovir 5 mg/kg IV q 12 h for 14–21 d	Alternating or combining foscarnet and gancyclovir
Esophogitis, colitis, pneumonitis	Gancyclovir 5 mg/kg IV q 12 h for 14–21 d Foscarnet 60 mg/kg IV q 8 h for 14–21 d	
Maintenance	Foscarnet 90–120 mg/kg/d IV Gancyclovir 5 mg/kg/d IV	
Herpes simplex virus		
Mild	Acyclovir 200 mg PO 5×/d for 10 d	Give dose IV
Severe	Acyclovir 5 mg/kg IV q 8 h for 10 d Acyclovir 800 mg PO 5×/d for 10 d	Foscarnet 40 mg/kg IV q 8 h for 3 wk
Visceral	Acyclovir 10 mg/kg IV q 8 h for 10 d	Foscarnet 40 mg/kg IV q 8 h for 3 wk
Maintenance	Acyclovir 400 mg PO bid	Foscarnet 40 mg/kg/d IV
Histoplasmosis, disseminated		
Initial therapy	Ampho B 0.5–1.0 mg/kg/d IV to 500 mg	Itraconazole 300 mg PO bid for 3 d, then 200 mg PO bid
Maintenance	Itraconazole 200 mg PO bid	Ampho B 1.0–1.5 mg/kg/wk
Mycobacterium avium complex		
Treatment	Clarithromycin 500 mg PO bid plus Ethambutol 15–25 mg/kg/d PO	Use 3- or 4-drug regimen (add to clarithromycin and ethambutol): Ciprofloxacin 750 mg PO bid Rifampin 600 mg PO qd Clofazamine 100 mg PO qd Amikacin 7.5–17 mg/kg/d IV
Prophylaxis	Rifabutin 300 mg PO qd	
Mycobacterium tuberculosis		
Empiric therapy	4-Drug regimen: Isoniazid 300 mg PO qd Rifiampin 600 mg PO qd Pyrazinamide 15–30 mg/kg/d PO Ethambutol 15–25 mg/kg/d PO	4-Drug regimen: Isoniazid 300 mg PO qd Rifiampin 600 mg PO qd Pyrazinamide 15–30 mg/kg/d PO Streptomycin 15 mg/kg/d IM

(continued)

TABLE 109-3. *(continued)*

ORGANISM	PREFERRED REGIMENS	ALTERNATIVE REGIMENS
	5-Drug regimen (add to above regimen): Streptomycin 15 mg/kg/d IM, Ethionamide 15–20 mg/kg/d PO PAS 150 mg/kg/d PO, Capreomycin 15–30 mg/kg/d IV, Cycloserine 15–20 mg/kg/d PO	
Prophylaxis	Isoniazid 300 mg PO qd for 12 mo	Rifampin 600 mg PO qd
Nocardia sp.	Sulfadiazine 4–8 g PO or IV qd; maintain sulfa level 15–20 μg/mL	TMP-SXT DS tablets, 4–6 PO qd Imipenem ± amikacin
Pneumocystis carinii Mild–moderate infection	TMP-SXT (dosed by TMP) 5 mg/kg PO or IV q 6–8 h for 21 d	Pentamidine 4 mg/kg/d IV for 21 d Clindamycin 600 mg PO or IV q 6 h plus Primaquine 15 mg base PO qd for 21 d Atovaquone 750 mg PO tid for 21 d
Moderate–severe infection	TMP-SXT (dosed by TMP) 5 mg/kg IV q 6–8 h for 21 d All should also receive: Prednisone 40 mg PO bid for 5 d, then 40 mg PO qd for 5 d, then 20 mg PO qd for 11 d	Pentamidine 4 mg/kg/d IV for 21 d
Prophylaxis	TMP-SXT DS tablet, 1 PO qd	Aerosolized pentamidine 300 mg q mo Dapsone 25–100 mg PO qd
Rhodococcus equi	Vancomycin 2 g IV qd with/without Rifampin 600 mg PO qd Ciprofloxacin 750 mg PO bid or Imipenem 500 mg IV q 6 h for 2–4 wk	Erythromycin 0.5–1.0 g IV q 6 h
Toxoplasma encephalitis Initial therapy	Pyrimethamine 200 mg load, then 50–100 mg PO qd plus sulfadiazine 4–8 g PO qd for 4–8 wk plus folinic acid 10 mg PO qd	Pyrimethamine 200 mg load, then 50–100 mg PO qd plus clindamycin 600 mg IV or PO q 6 h for 4–8 wk plus folinic acid 10 mg PO qd
Maintenance	Pyrimethamine 25–50 mg PO qd plus sulfadiazine 2–4 g PO qd All should get folinic acid 5 mg PO qd while on pyrimethamine	Pyrimethamine 25–50 mg PO qd plus clindamycin 300 mg PO q 6 h

Ampho B, amphotericin B; PO, orally; qd, every day; IV, intravenously; q, every; 5FC, 5-Fluorocytosine; bid, twice daily; PAS, Para-aminosalicylic acid; TMP-SXT, trimethoprim-sulfamethoxazole; DS, double strength; tid, three times daily; IM, intramuscularly.

Adapted from Bartlett JG, Fienberg, J: Management of opportunistic infections in patients with HIV infection. *Infect Dis Clin Pract* 1994;3:423.

.

The diagnostic approach to pulmonary manifestations must be based on an understanding of HIV infection and its complications. Although HIV-infected patients are predisposed to numerous pulmonary complications, a logical approach can be made using the patient's clinical history, the degree of immunosuppression as indicated by the CD4$^+$ count, and the chest radiograph. Using this information, a provider can create a reasonable differential diagnosis for the patient's problems. For both the HIV-infected patient and the normal host with a pulmonary process, there is a progression from noninvasive tests to invasive tests directed by severity of illness and response to therapy. However, the diagnostic algorithm for the HIV-infected patient has been modified to evaluate the patient with a normal radiograph as seen with early PCP (Fig. 109-1). Resting and exercise arterial blood gas measurements are 91% sensitive in these patients.[6] Gallium scanning also can be used to help evaluate patients with pulmonary symptoms. However, the time required to complete the test (48 hours) decreases its utility, especially in the ICU.[6] It is essential that the appropriate diagnostic tests are performed on the specimens. At a minimum, the evaluation should include Gram stain and bacterial culture, acid-fast smear and culture, and fungal stain and culture. In addition, specialized testing procedures may be

TABLE 109-4. Indications for Use and Side Effects of Medications Used in HIV Infection

GENERIC NAME	INDICATIONS FOR USE	SIDE EFFECTS
Acyclovir	Herpes simplex virus Varicella-zoster virus	N/V, headache, increased creatinine
Amikacin	*Mycobacterium avium* complex *Nocardia* sp.	Ototoxicity, increased creatinine
Atovaquone	*Pneumocystis carinii*	Diarrhea
Azithromycin	*M. avium* complex	N/V, diarrhea
Ciprofloxacin	*M. avium* complex	N/V, diarrhea, restlessness
Clarithromycin	*M. avium* complex	N/V, abnormal taste
Clindamycin	Toxoplasmosis *Pneumocystis carinii*	N/V, diarrhea
Clofazamine	*M. avium* complex *Mycobacterium tuberculosis*	N/V, diarrhea, skin discoloration
Cycloserine	*M. tuberculosis*	Convulsions, psychoses, confusion
Dapsone	*P. carinii* Toxoplasmosis	Hemolysis in G6PD, rash
Didanosine	HIV infection	Pancreatitis, peripheral neuropathy
Ethambutol	*M. avium* complex *M. tuberculosis*	Optic neuritis
Fluconazole	Candidiasis Cryptococcosis Coccidioidomycosis Histoplasmosis	Nausea, elevated AST/ALT
Flucytosine	Cryptococcosis	Leukopenia
Foscarnet	Cytomegalovirus Herpes simplex virus	Renal failure, hypocalcemia, hypophosphatemia
Gancyclovir	Cytomegalovirus	Neutropenia
Isoniazid	*M. tuberculosis*	Elevated AST/ALT, hepatic failure, peripheral neuropathy
Itraconazole	Histoplasmosis	N/V, headache, rash, edema
Ketoconazole	*Candida* mucositis	Elevated AST/ALT, gynecomastia
Pentamidine	*P. carinii*	Hypoglycemia, renal failure leukopenia, pancreatitis, orthostatic hypotension
Primaquine	*P. carinii*	Hemolysis in G6PD deficiency
Pyrazinamide	*M. tuberculosis*	Elevated AST/ALT
Pyrimethamine	Toxoplasmosis	Anorexia, N/V, pancytopenia
Rifampin	*M. tuberculosis* *M. avium* complex	Elevated AST/ALT
Rifabutin	*M. avium* complex	Rash, N/V, neutropenia
Streptomycin	*M. tuberculosis*	Ototoxicity, renal failure
Sulfadiazine	Toxoplasmosis	Fever, rash
Trimethoprim-sulfamethoxazole	*P. carinii* *Nocardia* sp.	Rash, fever, anemia, leukopenia
Zalcitabine	HIV infection	Peripheral neuropathy, pancreatitis
Zidovudine	HIV infection	Anemia, leukopenia, headache, N/V

ALT, alanine aminotransferase; AST, aspartate aminotransferase; N, nausea; V, vomiting; HIV, human immunodeficiency virus; G6PD, glucose-6-phosphatase deficiency.

Adapted from Drugs for AIDS and associated infections. *Med Lett* 1993;35:79.

necessary to make a diagnosis. Both the microbiology and pathology departments must be aware of your diagnostic concerns and needs so that the appropriate diagnostic tests are performed.

The initial concern in treating the HIV-infected patient with a pulmonary process is to consider public health issues. Given the increased incidence of tuberculosis in this population, any HIV-infected patient with a pulmonary infiltrate should be placed in respiratory isolation until tuberculosis has been ruled out. The next concern is usually the choice

of antimicrobial therapy. As for all patients, antimicrobial therapy is best directed by confirmatory diagnostic tests. Every effort should be made to make a diagnosis in these patients, given their tendency to have atypical presentations and infections with unusual organisms. However, it may be necessary to begin the HIV-infected patient on empirical antimicrobial therapy before the diagnostic evaluation is complete. In this instance, the choice of antibiotics should cover the organisms likely to cause the patient's signs and symptoms. If a patient does not respond to the chosen antibi-

TABLE 109-5. Radiographic Findings and Associated Diseases in HIV Infection

RADIOGRAPHIC FINDINGS	DISEASE
Diffuse reticulonodular infiltration	*Pneumocystis carinii* pneumonia Disseminated tuberculosis *Cryptococcus neoformans* Disseminated histoplasmosis Disseminated coccidioidomycosis Interstitial pneumonitis Lymphoma
Focal alveolar consolidation	Bacterial pneumonia Disseminated coccidioidomycosis Kaposi's sarcoma
Normal	*P. carinii* pneumonia Disseminated tuberculosis Disseminated histoplasmosis Disseminated *Mycobacterium avium* complex
Cavitation	*P. carinii* pneumonia Tuberculosis *Rhodococcus equi* *Nocardia* sp.
Pleural effusion	Kaposi's sarcoma Bacterial pneumonia *R. equi*
Adenopathy	Disseminated *M. avium* complex Disseminated tuberculosis Disseminated histoplasmosis Disseminated coccidioidomycosis *C. neoformans*

From Meduri GU, Stein DS: Pulmonary manifestations of acquired immunodeficiency syndrome. *Clin Infect Dis* 1992;14:98; Cadranel JL, Chouaid C, Denis M: Causes of pleural effusions in 75 HIV-infected patients. *Chest* 1993;104:655; and Joseph J, Strange C, Sahn SA: Pleural effusions in hospitalized patients with AIDS. *Ann Intern Med* 1993;118:856.

otics, the diagnosis should be reconsidered. The failure may indicate that the presumptive diagnosis is incorrect or that there is more than one disease process present.

Occasionally, HIV-infected patients with a pulmonary processes progress to respiratory failure. With the improved diagnostic and therapeutic modalities, the HIV-infected patient requiring mechanical ventilation has a markedly improved outcome compared with 10 years ago. The usual means of ventilating a patient with respiratory failure has been endotracheal intubation with positive-pressure ventilation. Recently, interest has been renewed in the use of continuous positive airway pressure (CPAP). The physiologic actions of CPAP decrease intrapulmonary shunting, which is the primary pathologic abnormality with PCP. CPAP has the additional advantage of being able to be delivered by mask (MCPAP), thus avoiding endotracheal intubation. MCPAP allows better titration of care to patients with do-not-resuscitate orders. In addition, as the health care system

is further strained by the HIV epidemic, MCPAP may allow better use of limited ICU resources. With respiratory failure from PCP, MCPAP was as effective as endotracheal intubation and positive-pressure ventilation. MCPAP should be considered an option for properly selected HIV-infected patients with respiratory failure.[7]

PNEUMOCYSTIS CARINII PNEUMONIA

Since the advent of the HIV epidemic in 1981, PCP remains the overall leading AIDS-defining diagnosis in the United States. The use of prophylactic therapy has been shown to decrease the incidence of PCP threefold, but the incidence of PCP remains high in HIV-infected patients receiving little or no medical care. Using the revised 1993 Centers for Disease Control Surveillance Case Definition for AIDS, 16% of the AIDS-defining diagnoses in 1993 were PCP.[8] In addition, over 67% of the ICU admissions in HIV-infected patients are for respiratory failure from PCP.[5] Therefore, PCP remains an important infection in HIV-infected patients.

The incidence of PCP is affected by a couple of variables. First, the HIV-infected patient is at risk to develop PCP when the CD4$^+$ count decreases to less than 200 cells/mm^3. Also, as mentioned previously, the incidence of PCP is decreased with prophylactic therapy. Trimethoprim-sulfamethoxazole (TMP-SMX) is more effective in preventing PCP than the alternative agents, including inhaled pentamidine and dapsone. Although there are prophylaxis failures, the use of TMP-SMX prophylaxis in a compliant patient makes the diagnosis of PCP much less likely.

Clinically, the patient with PCP presents with a history of fever, dyspnea, and nonproductive cough. The symptoms are subacute, often progressing over 1 to 4 weeks. High fever, rigors, and pleuritic chest pain are uncommon and, if present, should suggest a different infectious agent. The classic chest radiographic finding is bilateral interstitial infiltrates with a lower lobe predominance. However, the chest radiograph also can show normal or unchanged lungs, apical infiltrates (especially in patients on inhaled pentamidine therapy), spontaneous pneumothorax, and cystic lesions. Additional evaluation may reveal an increased alveolar-to-arteriole oxygen gradient difference [P(A − a)O$_2$] or hypoxemia on arterial blood gas measurement and an elevated serum lactate dehydrogenase level (LDH).[8]

The diagnosis of PCP is made by demonstrating the organism in induced sputum, bronchoalveolar lavage (BAL) fluid, or lung tissue. The diagnostic yield of induced sputum is 77% and of bronchoscopy with BAL, 86% to 97%.[9] Because lung tissue is rarely needed to make the diagnosis in the HIV-infected patient, transbronchial biopsy and open lung biopsy are reserved for patients whose initial evaluation is nondiagnostic (see Fig. 109-1). The organisms are identified in these specimens by special stains (modified Giemsa or Gomori-methenamine silver) or immunofluorescence with monoclonal antibody.[8]

TMP-SMX is the drug of choice and should be given to all patients with PCP if possible. Alternative agents exist for patients who cannot tolerate the TMP-SMX (see Table 109-3). The severity of PCP, as defined by the degree of hypoxia, also impacts the therapy. Mild-to-moderate PCP is defined by a room air PaO$_2$ greater than 70 mm Hg and moderate-

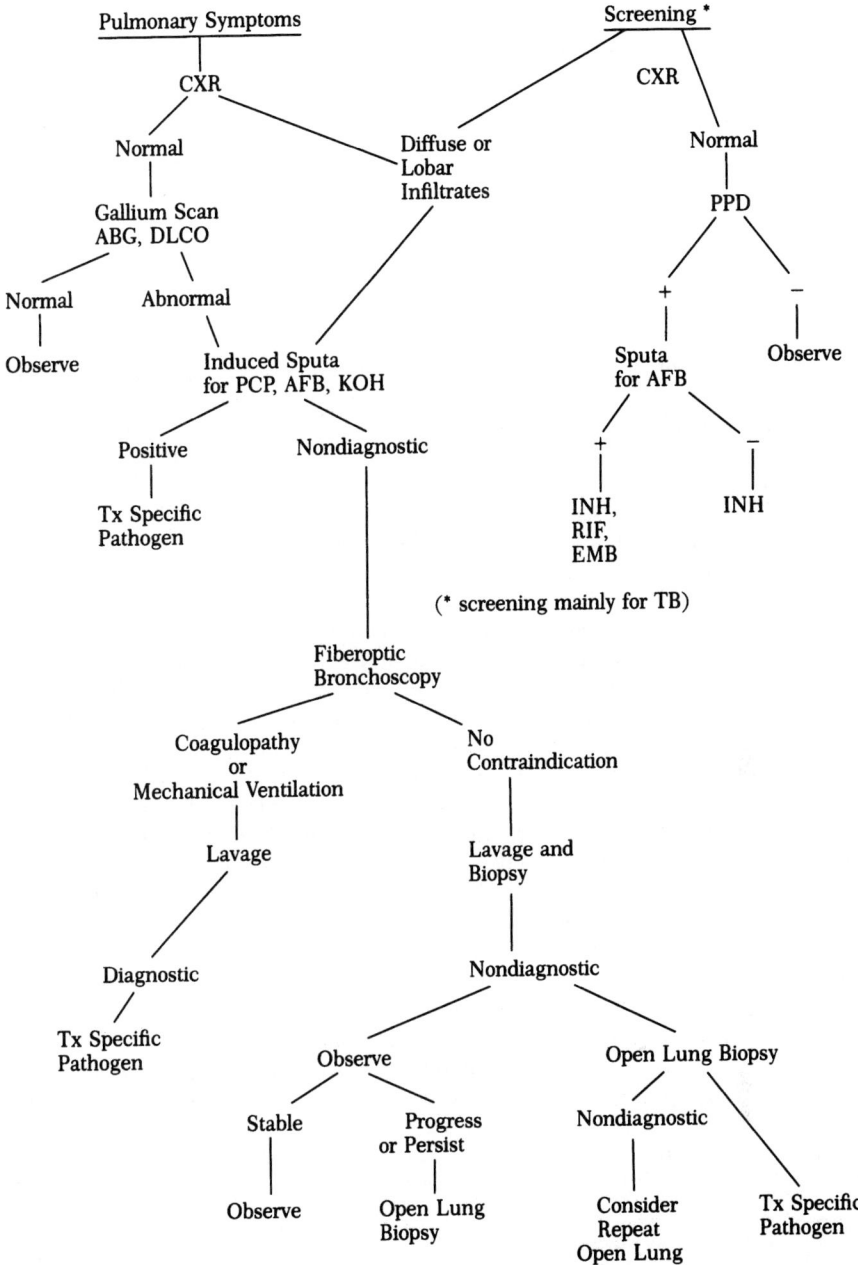

FIGURE 109-1. Diagnostic evaluation for diffuse pneumonia in patients with AIDS. (Adapted from Murray JF, Felton CP, Garay SM: *N Engl J Med* 1984;310:25; and Masur H, Kovacs JA, Ognibene F, et al: Infectious complications of AIDS. In: DeVita VT Jr, Hellman S, Rosenberg SA [eds]. *AIDS: Etiology, Diagnosis, Treatment and Prevention.* Philadelphia, JB Lippincott, 1985:161.)

to-severe PCP by a room air PaO_2 less than 70 mm Hg or a $P(A - a)O_2$ greater than 35. Patients with mild-to-moderate PCP may be treated with oral medication and do not benefit from corticosteroids. However, patients with moderate-to-severe should be treated with both intravenous medication and corticosteroids (see Table 109-3). A response to therapy is generally seen within 5 to 7 days.[8]

The prognosis of PCP has improved since the beginning of the HIV epidemic. The mortality of PCP varies with the severity of infection, with estimates of overall mortality rate ranging from 2% to 39%. Poor prognostic signs include LDH greater than 450 IU at time of diagnosis, increasing LDH with PCP therapy, greater degree of hypoxia at presentation, and pneumothorax.[9] Although data from 1984 to 1987 re-

vealed an uniformly poor prognosis, HIV-infected patients with respiratory failure from PCP have a survival rate to hospital discharge of 38% to 55%.[5] In addition, once discharged from the hospital, the long-term survival of PCP patients requiring intubation is similar to patients who survive mild PCP.[8]

BACTERIAL PNEUMONIA

In some institutions, bacterial pneumonia has replaced PCP as the most common pneumonia requiring hospitalization in HIV-infected patients.[10] Bacterial pneumonia in this setting can be caused by numerous bacteria. However, the bacterial pneumonias can be divided into three clinical categories: community-acquired pneumonia, most commonly caused by the encapsulated organisms *Streptococcus pneumoniae* and *Hemophilus influenzae*; nosocomial pneumonia; and infections with unusual pathogens such as *Rhodococcus equi* and *Norcardia* species. Interestingly, infections caused by *Legionella* species and *Mycoplasma* species are infrequently reported.

The signs and symptoms of pneumonia caused by encapsulated organisms are similar for the HIV-infected patient and the normal host. Fever, productive cough, and, frequently, pleuritic chest pain occur. Although infections with these organisms occur throughout the course of HIV infection, they frequently occur early and may be the initial manifestation of HIV infection. The chest radiograph shows segmental or lobar homogenous opacities in 76% of the cases with infrequent pleural effusions and cavitation. Additional laboratory data may include leukocytosis with a left shift and hypoxia. The diagnosis is made by isolating the organism from sputum or blood. Blood cultures should always be performed in HIV-infected patients suspected of having bacterial pneumonia because the incidence of bacteremia is higher than in the normal hosts. Most HIV-infected patients are treated with parenteral broad-spectrum antibiotics, followed by appropriate antibacterial susceptibility testing of the isolate. Most patients are afebrile and clinically improved by the fifth day of therapy. The mortality rate seems to be comparable with that seen in HIV-seronegative patients.[10]

Nosocomial pneumonia occurs late in the course of HIV infection, frequently after an AIDS-defining diagnosis has been made. The causative organisms are reported to be staphylococci and aerobic gram-negative rods, although little data are available.[11] Importantly, the frequency of *Pseudomonas aeruginosa* nosocomial pneumonia seems to be increasing. Risk factors for developing these infections include indwelling venous catheters, myelosuppressive therapy, steroid use, and neutropenia. The clinical signs and symptoms are similar to the community-acquired pneumonia with the radiograph typically showing lobar consolidation. The diagnosis is made by isolating the organism in sputum or blood. Antibiotic therapy should be based on susceptibility testing, but empirical therapy should include an antipseudomonal β-lactam antibiotic and an aminoglycoside for possibility of *P. aeruginosa* infection. The mortality rate of *P. aeruginosa* pneumonia is over 33%.[10]

Although it is impossible to discuss every cause of pneumonia, two bacteria that warrant further discussion are *R. equi* and *Nocardia* species. These bacteria have distinct clinical presentations and are being reported with increasing frequency in HIV-infected patients. In addition, because both are gram-positive bacteria that are partially acid-fast, they can be confused with other pathogens such as mycobacteria. These infections occur late in the course of HIV infection, with most patients having AIDS or CD4$^+$ counts less than 100 cells/mm^3.[12,13] The symptoms for both infections commonly include fever, cough, fatigue, and dyspnea. Chest radiographs show infiltrates in over 80% of patients that are predominately unilobar but may involve multiple lobes as the pneumonia progresses. Approximately 20% of the patients with nocardiosis have coincidental brain abscesses and may present with headache and mental status changes.[12]

Pleural effusion and cavitation occur with both infections but are more common with *R. equi*. Diagnosis is made by isolating the organism from an involved site. Cultures of sputum, pleural fluid, and BAL fluid have yielded the organism. In addition, blood cultures often give positive results in *R. equi* infections.[13] Antibiotic therapy is best directed by susceptibility testing, but recommendations for empirical therapy are given in Table 109-3. The optimal duration of therapy is unknown, but life-long therapy is often necessary to prevent relapses. The prognosis of these infections is poor, with a mortality rate of over 40%.[12,13]

FUNGAL PNEUMONIA

The lung is the portal of entry for most of the opportunistic fungal infections that occur in HIV-infected persons. Because these infections rapidly disseminate, the patient typically presents with a systemic infection and is coincidentally found to have pulmonary involvement. A pulmonary syndrome can precede the development of disseminated disease, however. In addition, patients with systemic fungal infection can present with pulmonary complaints and an abnormal result on chest radiograph. In either of these settings, the provider must consider fungal etiologies to appropriately evaluate and treat the HIV-infected patient.

Cryptococcus neoformans is best known as a cause of meningitis. However, the development of cryptococcal meningitis is commonly preceded by a spontaneously resolving pneumonia. Approximately one third of patients with cryptococcal disease also present with respiratory complaints that include cough, dyspnea, and pleuritic chest pain. The chest radiograph typically shows diffuse interstitial infiltrates that are indistinguishable from PCP. Diagnosis is made by isolation of the organism in blood, sputum, or BAL fluid. The diagnosis is also suggested by a positive, specific cryptococcal antigen test result of blood or pleural fluid. Given the propensity of this organism to disseminate, isolated pulmonary cryptococcal infection should be treated as if cryptococcal meningitis is present[14] (see Table 109-3).

Coccidioides immitis, a systemic fungal infection endemic to the southwestern United States, is a frequent cause of life-threatening infection in HIV-infected patients with CD4$^+$ counts less than 250 cells/mm^3.[15] The clinical presentation and course of the infection is variable, dependent in part on the patient's underlying immune status. The typical clinical history is a protracted illness with symptoms of fatigue, fever, cough, chest pain, headache, and dyspnea.[16] The most common radiographic presentation, occurring in 40% of HIV-infected patients, is diffuse bilateral reticulonodular pulmonary infiltrates.[15] Approximately 30% of HIV-infected patients have focal radiographic findings such as alveolar infiltrates, nodules, and mediastinal adenopathy. Extrathoracic involvement, present in 25% of patients, includes the skin, lymph nodes, liver, and meninges. Laboratory data are nonspecific, but the patients may have an eosinophilia. The diagnosis of coccidioidomycosis needs to be considered in any patient who traveled to an endemic area, regardless of the duration or extent of this travel. Diagnosis is made by isolating the organism from an involved site. Both sputum and BAL fluid examination and culture are good diagnostic tests for patients with pulmonary involvement.[14] The classic spherule is readily identifiable in specimens and the cultures usually yield positive results in 3 to 5 days. Serologic testing, specifically the complement fixation and tube precipitin, may suggest the diagnosis and provide some information about the extent of disease as well as the response to therapy. Any patient diagnosed with coccidioidomycosis should have a thorough evaluation for extrathoracic disease, including a lumbar puncture (LP) when headache, nausea, or nuchal rigidity are present. The outcome of coccidioidomycosis in HIV-infected patients is variable. The median survival for patients with diffuse infiltrates is only 1 month, but many patients with focal pulmonary disease have a clinical course that is indistinguishable from HIV-seronegative patients.[15] Treatment is recommended for HIV-infected patients with CD4[+] counts less than 250 cells/mm³, extrathoracic disease, or diffuse pulmonary infection. Therapy should include induction therapy followed by life-long suppressive antifungal therapy (see Table 109-3).

Histoplasma capsulatum, a systemic fungal infection endemic to the Mississippi and Ohio river valleys, generally causes disseminated disease in HIV-infected patients with low CD4[+] counts (see "Sepsis and Bacteremia"). Like cryptococcal disease, many of the patients with disseminated disease have the pulmonary symptoms of cough and dyspnea at presentation. Patients with CD4[+] counts greater than 300 cells/mm³ also present with localized pulmonary infections. Subacute presentation with 1 to 2 months of symptoms is usual. The chest radiograph typically reveals miliary reticulonodular infiltrates but also may reveal mediastinal adenopathy and nodules. The diagnosis of histoplasmosis needs to be considered in any patient with travel to an endemic area. The diagnosis is made by isolating the organism in a specimen from a involved site or by detection of antigen in the blood and urine. The best culture results are obtained from blood and bone marrow cultures, but bronchoscopy cultures give positive results in approximately 50% of the cases. The organism also can be identified using special stains (Gomorimethenamine silver and periodic acid–Schiff), but care needs to be given to distinguish this organism from *Torulopsis glabrata* and *P. carinii*. The medical management of histoplasmosis consists of induction therapy followed by life-long suppressive therapy with an antifungal agent[16] (see Table 109-3).

MYCOBACTERIAL PNEUMONIA

The prevalence of tuberculosis in HIV-infected persons is increased more than 300-fold.[6] Although the HIV infection itself does not predispose the patient to develop tuberculosis, these patients tend to have additional risk factors for exposure to tuberculosis, such as injection drug use, immigration from an endemic region, and ethnic background.[11] However, the HIV-infected patient's level of immune dysfunction does impact the presentation of the *Mycobacterium tuberculosis* infection. Early in the HIV infection, the patients present with tuberculosis that is confined to the lungs. The radiograph reveals the typical radiographic findings for tuberculosis, the localized infiltrates, and cavitation with an upper lobe predominance. With decreasing CD4[+] count and increasing

anergy, the patients have increased evidence of extrapulmonary involvement.[6] The chest radiograph often has the atypical findings of interstitial infiltrates, lower lobe predominance, and adenopathy but also can be normal.[11] The diagnosis is made by the culture identification of *M. tuberculosis* in sputum, BAL fluid, transbronchial biopsy, or lymph node biopsy specimen. Blood cultures infrequently give positive results, even with miliary tuberculosis.[17] Positive acid-fast smear results suggest a mycobacterial infection, but only culture can differentiate *M. tuberculosis* from the atypical mycobacteria. Antituberculous therapy should be started in any HIV-infected patient with pulmonary infiltrates and acid-fast bacilli in pulmonary specimens until the final identification is made. The initial therapy consists of a four- or five-drug regimen, depending on the patient's risk for multidrug-resistant tuberculosis (see Table 109-3). Respiratory isolation should be continued until the patient is no longer at risk for transmission of *M. tuberculosis*. The prognosis of tuberculosis in HIV-infected patients poor but is partly dependent on the stage of the underlying HIV infection.[11] One study showed that HIV-infected patients who required ICU monitoring or intubation had an in-hospital mortality rate of more than 50%.[18]

Although disease has been reported with every atypical mycobacteria, over 90% of these cases are caused by *Mycobacterium avium* complex (MAC).[6] MAC infection occurs late in the course of HIV infection, when the CD4[+] count is less that 100 cells/mm³. The patient usually presents with disseminated disease and the coincidental finding of an abnormal chest radiograph. Pulmonary symptoms are rare, as is the occurrence of localized pulmonary infection. The most common symptoms are 2 to 6 weeks of fever, weight loss, anorexia, and weakness. Abdominal adenopathy and hepatosplenomegaly are common. Chest radiographic findings of MAC infection vary widely and include a normal radiograph result, interstitial infiltrates, reticulonodular infiltrates, and adenopathy.[17] The diagnosis is made by isolating the organism from blood, bone marrow, or lymph node specimens. As with tuberculosis, the presence of acid-fast bacilli on a smear suggests the diagnosis of mycobacterial disease without distinguishing between the different mycobacteria. Because MAC can colonize the bronchial tree, the isolation of MAC from sputum or BAL fluid is not diagnostic of MAC infection. However, this finding should prompt a search for other evidence of disseminated disease.[6] The optimal therapy for MAC is unclear, and several regimens have been used (see Table 109-3). Most patients have a symptomatic improvement with treatment of the MAC infection, but the therapy is only suppressive.

VIRAL INFECTIONS

The incidence of pneumonitis from CMV is uncertain because this virus is often shed asymptomatically in the oropharyngeal secretions of immunocompromised patients, including HIV-infected patients. The isolation of these viruses from sputum or BAL fluid may represent lower respiratory tract contamination. The diagnosis is certain only if there is evidence of viral cytopathic effect on lung tissue. In patients with tissue-proven viral pneumonitis, the clinical presentation is subacute onset of dyspnea and nonproductive cough and the chest radiographs have diffuse interstitial infiltrates. Often, the signs and symptoms of CMV pneumonitis are obscured by the presence of another opportunistic infection. Intravenous gancyclovir is the therapy of choice (see Table 109-3) with a response rate of 40% to 50%.[19]

NONINFECTIOUS PULMONARY PROCESSES

HIV-infected patients also present with pulmonary symptoms and findings that result from noninfectious processes. Interstitial pneumonitis is a frequent finding in HIV-infected patients with pulmonary symptoms. The patients present with cough, dyspnea, fever, and diffuse reticulonodular infiltrates on the radiograph. Pulmonary involvement of KS is also common, occurring in up to 40% of the patients with KS. These patients present with dyspnea, cough, wheezing, pleuritic chest pain, and hemoptysis. The chest radiographic findings are variable. There may be interstitial infiltrates, nodules, pleural-based lesions, and pleural effusions.[6] In contrast, pulmonary involvement in AIDS-related lymphoma is uncommon.[20] The patients can have interstitial or reticulonodular infiltrates, but mediastinal adenopathy is rare.[6] The presence of mediastinal adenopathy in a patient with AIDS-related lymphoma should prompt further evaluation. These noninfectious diagnoses are made by examination of lung tissue obtained by transbronchial biopsy or open-lung biopsy. It is important to ensure that the patient does not have a coincidental second infectious process.

NEUROLOGIC MANIFESTATIONS OF HIV INFECTION ∎

HIV-infected patients occasionally require ICU monitoring for neurologic problems (see Table 109-2). The neurologic diseases may be categorized by clinical presentation and etiologic agent. Although helpful in organizing an approach to these patients, these categories can be used to oversimplify the differential diagnosis. HIV-infected patients also get the neurologic complications seen in normal hosts, such as bacterial meningitis and brain abscesses. Therefore, the differential diagnosis of a neurologic process in HIV-infected patients must include both the HIV-associated complications and age-appropriate disease processes. The diagnostic algorithm for patients with a neurologic process has been modified primarily to manage the increased incidence of focal central nervous system (CNS) lesions (Fig. 109-2). Because these lesions occur frequently and may only produce nonfocal findings, a head imaging study is recommended before a LP. This section emphasizes the processes seen with HIV infection.

MENINGITIS

Meningitis from *C. neoformans* is a frequent complication of HIV infection, occurring in at least 5% of the AIDS patients in the United States. The patient is at risk for this infection when the CD4$^+$ count drops to 200 cells/mm³. The almost universal symptom is headache, but other common symptoms are fever and malaise.[21] Examination can reveal lethargy, confusion, and cranial nerve palsies.[22] Focal findings are unusual, and computed tomography (CT) studies of the head are usually normal. The cerebrospinal fluid (CSF) studies can be normal in up to 50% of patients but often show increased opening pressure, increased protein, and decreased glucose. CSF pleocytosis, when present, is always mononuclear.[23] Cryptococcal meningitis is diagnosed by a positive result of a CSF India ink stain, a CSF cryptococcal antigen titer greater than 1:8, or a positive CSF culture.[22] Isolation of the organism in blood culture or increased serum cryptococcal antigen is suggestive of meningitis because this organism rapidly disseminates to the central nervous system. Optimal medical management is uncertain, but most recommend intravenous amphotericin B induction therapy followed by maintenance therapy with fluconazole (see Table 109-3). Patients with increased intracranial pressure may require mechanical drainage with LP or intraventricular shunt for pressure relief. The use of corticosteroids in patients with increased intracranial pressure is not routinely recommended. The mortality rate of cryptococcal meningitis in the first 2 weeks of therapy is significant at 10% to 25%. The characteristics that predict a poor outcome include any alteration in patient's mental status, CSF cryptococcal antigen greater than 1:1024, a CSF leukocyte count less than 20 cells/mm³, and age older than 35 years.[21]

Given the extrapulmonary nature of *M. tuberculosis* in HIV-infected patients, they have an increased risk of tuberculous meningitis. Common clinical symptoms include fever, headache, and mental status changes.[24] In patients admitted to ICU with tuberculosis, 25% had CNS involvement manifested by coma.[18] CT of the head commonly gives abnormal result, showing hydrocephalus, enhancing or nonenhancing lesions, or meningeal enhancement. CSF studies are rarely normal and typically reveal a lymphocytic pleocytosis and low glucose. The acid-fast stains of CSF are positive in approximately 22% of the cases. The detection of acid-fast bacilli on CSF stains is presumed to be of *M. tuberculosis* because the atypical mycobacteria are an infrequent cause of central nervous system disease. Once the diagnosis is suspected, the patient is begun on four- or five-drug regimen until susceptibility testing is available (see Table 109-3). The prognosis of tuberculous meningitis is poor with an in-hospital mortality rate of 33%.[24]

FOCAL LESIONS OF THE CENTRAL NERVOUS SYSTEM

The incidence of encephalitis from *Toxoplasma gondii* varies by geographic region, but it is estimated that approximately 10% of HIV-infected patients in the United States will develop this infection. In HIV-infected patients, toxoplasmic encephalitis occurs with a CD4$^+$ count less than 200 cells/mm³. Patients generally present with a mixture of focal and generalized neurologic dysfunction, depending on the location, size, and number of lesions. In 50% to 89% of patients, focal findings that correspond to the anatomic location of the lesions predominate. Patients most commonly present with hemiparesis and speech disorders but can also have headache, seizures, mental status changes, personality changes, and psychosis. The onset of symptoms is usually subacute with a few patients presenting with a fulminant encephalitis. The laboratory studies, including CSF examination, are nonspecific and unhelpful except to rule out other processes. Because over 95% of cases are caused by reactivated disease, serologic testing is helpful only to determine patients at risk to develop toxoplasmic encephalitis. The diagnosis is suggested by CT or magnetic resonance imaging (MRI) studies that show multiple ring-enhancing lesions. Definitive diagnosis can be made only by demonstrating the organism in clinical specimens. However, given the inability to biopsy all brain lesions, an algorithm has been developed to allow for clinical diagnosis (see Fig. 109-2). If CT or MRI findings are consistent with toxoplasmic encephalitis and a positive serology for *T. gondii*, empirical therapy for toxoplasmosis is started (see Table 109-3). The presumptive diagnosis is correct if the patient's baseline abnormalities, except headache and seizure, improve after 10 to 14 days of therapy. If the patient fails to respond or deteriorates, a brain biopsy for diagnosis should be performed. HIV-infected patients with toxoplasmosis require maintenance therapy to prevent relapse.[25]

Primary CNS lymphoma, another important cause of focal lesions in HIV-infected patients, is a disease of late HIV infection. Patients have $CD4^+$ counts less than 100 cell/mm^3 and often have multiple coincidental opportunistic infections, including those of the CNS. The presenting symptoms are similar to toxoplasmosis with focal neurologic deficits, seizures, headache, altered mental status, and personality changes. Examination of the CSF shows lymphomatous involvement in up to 25% of the cases. Head CT or MRI shows lesions that are larger (over 3 cm) and fewer in number (one or two) than expected with toxoplasmosis. The diagnosis is made by brain biopsy as indicated in Figure 109-2. The optimal therapy for these patients is undefined but currently includes cranial irradiation. Prognosis is dismal, with a median survival of 2.5 months despite therapy. The patient's course is frequently complicated by opportunistic infections.[20]

SEPSIS AND BACTEREMIA

Sepsis syndrome is an important reason for ICU admission in HIV-infected patients (see Table 109-3). As in HIV-seronegative patients, sepsis syndrome is most commonly caused by bacteria. The HIV-infected patient also can develop sepsis with opportunistic infections, especially disseminated histoplasmosis. In addition, these patients are at risk to develop adrenal insufficiency, which can mimic sepsis.

BACTEREMIA

Patients with HIV infection have an increased risk of bacteremia caused by the immune dysregulation that occurs with HIV infection. Many patients have the additional risk factors of disruption of the integument barrier, immunosuppressive therapy, and neutropenia. The risk from neutropenia seems to be less in HIV-infected patients than in other patient groups. With HIV infection, only severe neutropenia (less than 500 cells/dL) is associated with a high risk of bacterial infections and warrants empirical antibiotic coverage for a febrile episode.[26]

Over 20% of the bacteremic patients have normal examinations without an apparent source for the bacteremia. However, the remainder of the bacteremic episodes are associated with specific clinical syndromes. As previously mentioned, pneumococcal pneumonia is associated with bacteremia in up to 50% of patients with HIV infection. HIV-infected patient with pneumococcal bacteremia respond well to appropriate antibiotics except for a possible increased incidence of relapse.[26]

Bacteremia associated with gastroenteritis is another common clinical syndrome in the HIV-infected patient. The bacteremia results from the gastrointestinal infection itself. The nontyphoidal *Salmonella* species cause bacteremia in 45% of HIV-infected patients with salmonellosis compared with the 9% bacteremia in the HIV-seronegative patients. The enteritis caused by *Campylobacter* species also is associated with an increased incidence of bacteremia. The patient generally presents with fever and watery diarrhea. Laboratory evaluation reveals leukocytosis with a left shift (immature neutrophils) and anemia that may be Coombs' test positive in patients with salmonellosis. HIV-infected patients respond well to appropriate antibiotic therapy, but relapse commonly occurs after therapy. The patients with relapse may require chronic suppressive therapy.[26]

Bacteremia also has been associated with the use of central venous catheters in HIV-infected patients. Studies suggest that the risk of catheter-related infection is increased in patients with HIV infection versus in patients with other immunocompromising diseases. Over 20% of the catheter-related infections in HIV-infected patients are associated with bacteremia. The *Staphylococcus* species are the causative agents in 81% of these infections. The standard treatment of catheter-related infections and bacteremia are effective in HIV-infected patients. There is a tendency for *Staphylococcus aureus* bacteremia to have late metastatic infections develop.[26]

P. aeruginosa is increasingly associated with bacteremia in HIV-infected patients and warrants further discussion. The risk factors for developing *P. aeruginosa* infection in HIV-infected patients are similar to the HIV-seronegative patient and include previous antibiotic therapy, use of immunosuppressive agents, and recent hospitalization. However, approximately 55% of the *P. aeruginosa* bacteremia in HIV-infected patients is community acquired. *P. aeruginosa* bacteremia is commonly associated with pulmonary or catheter-related infections, and the patients frequently present with sepsis. The best therapeutic outcome is seen with the use of double coverage with an antipseudomonal β-lactam or monobactam antibiotic plus aminoglycoside. However, one third of the patients experienced a relapse of infection, and the overall mortality rate is 40%. Given the predisposition for this infection, empirical antibiotic therapy for a severely ill HIV-infected patient should include adequate coverage for *P. aeruginosa*.[27]

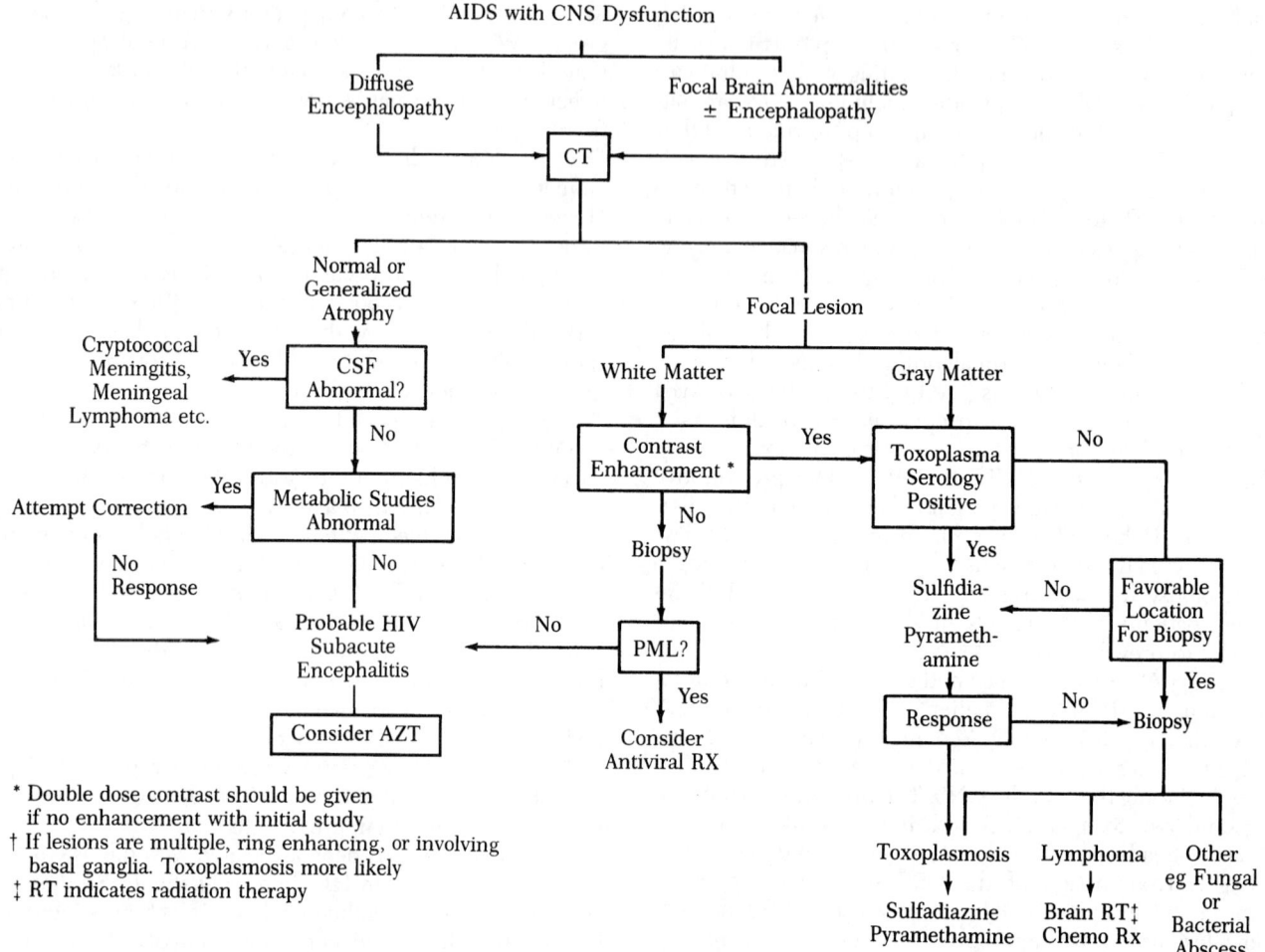

FIGURE 109-2. Approach to the patient with AIDS who has central nervous system dysfunction. CT, computed tomography; CFS, cerebrospinal fluid; HIV, human immunodeficiency virus; Rx, therapy; RT, radiation therapy; PML, progressive multifocal leukoencephalopathy; AZT, zidovudine. (Adapted from Snider W, Simpson DM, Nielsen S: Neurological implications of acquired immune deficiency syndrome: analysis of 50 patients. *Ann Neurol* 1983;14:403.)

DISSEMINATED HISTOPLASMOSIS

Disseminated infection caused by *H. capsulatum* can cause a sepsis syndrome in HIV-infected patients. Histoplasmosis generally presents with 1 to 2 months of fever, fatigue, and weight loss. Pulmonary manifestations are common, as previously discussed. This pathogen can also disseminate widely and cause meningitis presenting with headache, mental status changes, and seizures; gastrointestinal infection presenting with diarrhea, abdominal pain, and intestinal obstruction; and skin lesions of virtually every description. The sepsis syndrome, found in 10% to 20% of the HIV-infected patients, is associated with shock, respiratory failure, hepatic and renal failure, and rhabdomyolysis. The laboratory evaluation reveals a pancytopenia and coagulopathy. The diagnosis is made by isolating the organism from an involved site. The cultures with the highest yield are blood and bone marrow cultures. Unfortunately, the culture results may take up to 4 weeks, limiting the usefulness of this diagnostic test

in a severely ill patient. Rapid diagnosis of disseminated histoplasmosis can be made by finding the antigen in urine or serum. The medical management of disseminated histoplasmosis includes timely institution of antifungal therapy followed by life-long suppressive therapy (see Table 109-3). The outcome depends on the severity of the infection, but the sepsis syndrome caused by disseminated histoplasmosis in HIV-infected patients has a high mortality.[16]

ADRENAL INSUFFICIENCY

Up to 80% of HIV-infected patients have abnormal adrenal glands at autopsy. The most common abnormality is CMV adrenalitis, but MAC, KS, lymphoma, and *Toxoplasma* and *Cryptococcus* infections also have been associated with adrenal disease. Few HIV-infected patients have clinically apparent adrenal insufficiency. However, many do have an abnormal response to corticotropin stimulation indicating subclinical adrenal dysfunction. These patients with border-line adrenal function may be predisposed to adrenal insufficiency at times of stress. In addition, certain medications can precipitate adrenal crisis by either interfering with steroid synthesis or increasing steroid metabolism in the liver. These medications, such as rifampin, ketoconazole, and fluconazole, are frequently used in the treatment of HIV infection. Therefore, adrenal dysfunction should be considered as a cause of hypotension in any HIV-infected patient.[28]

GASTROINTESTINAL MANIFESTATIONS OF HIV ■

Although infrequent causes of ICU admission, the gastrointestinal manifestations of HIV infection can complicate any hospitalization. Infections are the most common cause of gastrointestinal problems, but malignancies also can present with abdominal symptoms. Patients with HIV infection also get diseases that occur in the HIV-seronegative patients, such as peptic ulcer disease and appendicitis. The problems are often grouped by clinical symptoms to assist in a diagnostic approach.

DIARRHEA

Diarrhea is the most common gastrointestinal symptom in patients with AIDS, reported in 50% to 90% of patients. The causes are numerous but are primarily infectious. In addition to the organisms that cause infections in immunocompetent hosts, the possible pathogens include opportunistic infections such as CMV, *Isospora belli*, MAC, and *Microsporidia*. The clinical presentation is variable, but fever and weight loss are often seen. The presence of tenesmus suggests distal colon or rectal involvement and the presence of voluminous watery diarrhea suggests small bowel involvement.[29]

A stepwise evaluation of the HIV-infected patient with diarrhea results in a diagnosis in approximately 85% of the patients. The first step is up to three stool specimens for bacterial culture, *Clostridium difficile* toxin, and parasite studies. The parasitologic evaluation should include saline, iodine, trichrome, and acid-fast preparations. If these test results are negative, the second step is endoscopic examination and biopsy. All patients generally receive an esophagogastroduodenoscopy with small bowel biopsy. If the patient also has symptoms attributable to the large bowel or rectum, the endoscopic examination includes a colonoscopy. All biopsy specimens are sent for the appropriate culture and stains to evaluate for CMV, MAC, and fungi. In addition, any colonic specimens should be evaluated for herpes simplex virus (HSV).[30]

The first issue of treatment is supportive care. These patients can have significant volume and electrolyte abnormalities because of the unremitting nature of their diarrhea. Given the numerous diagnostic possibilities, therapy is best directed by test results and not empiricism. Finally, many of the patients require antimotility agents for control of their diarrhea. If possible, these antimotility agents should be initiated after a diagnosis is established, especially if the patient has fever. This may help prevent exacerbation of an infection such as *C. difficile* colitis and pathogenic bacterial infection. The antimotility agents that have been used include loperamide and diphenoxylate hydrochloride.[30]

DYSPHAGIA AND ODYNOPHAGIA

Dysphagia and odynophagia are common symptoms in HIV-infected patients with esophageal infections caused by *Candida albicans*, HSV, and CMV. In addition, HIV-infected patients can develop idiopathic or aphthous ulcerations that are clinically indistinguishable from HSV and CMV. The diagnosis is made by an endoscopic biopsy that reveals no evidence of infection by cytopathic appearance or culture. Aphthous ulcerations may respond to oral, intravenous, or intralesional steroid therapy.[29]

Patients with *Candida* esophagitis typically present with oral thrush and dysphagia. These findings are sufficient for a presumptive diagnosis of esophageal candidiasis. The diagnosis is confirmed by endoscopy that reveals white plaque-like lesions throughout the esophagus. Initial therapy is an oral azole with intravenous amphotericin B reserved for persistent candidiasis (see Table 109-3). With proper therapy, the patient has improved symptoms within 2 weeks. Treatment with an oral azole is often used as a diagnostic trial in patients with dysphagia and oral thrush.[29]

HSV and CMV cause an ulcerative disease in the esophagus. Patients with these infections present with odynophagia with or without dysphagia. HSV esophagitis also can cause retrosternal pain caused by esophageal spasm. Because the ulcerations have no characteristic appearance, endoscopy with biopsy is essential for diagnosis. The specific diagnosis is made by finding the characteristic cytopathic changes in biopsy specimens. The initial therapy consists of acyclovir for HSV and gancyclovir for CMV (see Table 109-3). Foscarnet therapy may be used for infections that fail initial therapy. The role of suppression therapy is uncertain.[29]

ABDOMINAL PAIN

The causes of abdominal pain in the HIV-infected patient include the HIV-associated diseases and the diseases seen in immunocompetent hosts. The clinical presentation of abdominal processes, such as an acute abdomen or obstruction, are not altered by HIV infection. However, the differential diagnosis must be broadened to include the CD4⁺ appropriate diseases that affect gastrointestinal tract in HIV-infected patients (see Table 109-1). The treatment for the infections are outlined in Table 109-3.

Pancreatitis can occur in HIV-infected patients. It is often caused by medications, such as pentamidine, didanosine, and TMP-SMX, or infections, such as CMV. The clinical presentation is similar for HIV-infected patients and normal hosts except that HIV-infected patients tend to have greater anemia and leukopenia. In the HIV-infected patient, the pancreatitis is associated with a prolonged hospital course and a higher mortality.[31]

Appendicitis also occurs in HIV-infected patients. In approximately one fourth of HIV-infected patients, the appendicitis is associated with an AIDS-related etiology such as CMV. The presenting symptoms are the same as for normal hosts, but the leukocyte count is frequently normal. In recent reviews, no perioperative deaths occurred and the postoperative complication rate was less than 20%. There is often a delay in surgical intervention caused by error in diagnosis or concerns about excessive morbidity and mortality.[32]

The HIV-associated causes of chronic abdominal pain include CMV, MAC, KS, and lymphoma. Most of these diseases have systemic symptoms or evidence of involvement outside of the gastrointestinal tract. The diagnosis is generally made by demonstrating the pathogen or malignancy on biopsy specimens obtained by endoscopic examination. Occasionally, intestinal perforation occurs because of these disease processes. Surgical intervention should be considered, but the operative mortality is unfortunately high.[29]

Hepatobiliary disease also can result from an HIV-associated process. Acalculous cholecystitis, sclerosing cholangitis, and AIDS cholangiopathy can be caused by CMV and *Cryptosporidium* species. The patient presents with right upper quadrant abdominal pain and serum alkaline phosphatase elevation. Often, an ultrasound may reveal an abnormal biliary system. Endoscopic retrograde cholangiopancreatography is indicated in these patients for diagnosis and therapeutic intervention. The liver also can become involved with MAC, KS, and lymphoma. Although the patient may present with focal right upper quadrant fullness or pain, systemic symptoms and an elevated serum alkaline phosphatase may be witnessed. The diagnosis is usually made without a liver biopsy, given the systemic nature of these process.[29]

FEVER OF UNKNOWN ORIGIN ■

Fever is a common finding in HIV-infected patients, occurring in approximately 50% of patients each year. Although many HIV-infected patients with fever have localizing findings, there may be only nonspecific signs or symptoms such as weight loss or malaise. A diagnosis is usually made using diagnostic tests directed by patient history and physical examination. Occasionally, despite efforts to make a diagnosis, the HIV-infected patient remains febrile without an apparent source for over 2 weeks. In this setting, the most common diagnoses are MAC, PCP in patients receiving aerosolized pentamidine prophylaxis, and lymphoma. Therefore, in the persistently febrile HIV-infected patient, diagnostic considerations should be include an appropriate evaluation for these diseases. With a thorough evaluation, the cause of the fever can be found for most HIV-infected patients. The fever rarely results from the HIV infection itself.[33]

ICU UTILIZATION IN HIV INFECTION ■

In this time of increasing demands on the dwindling health care resources, the utility of ICU admissions in patients with a systemic illness is being reevaluated. This scrutiny is particularly true for HIV infection because the ongoing epidemic places continued demands on all aspects of health care. In addition, there may be social and medical biases against the HIV-infected patient. The diagnosis of AIDS is often inaccurately perceived as more terminal than other systemic illnesses. However, the in-hospital mortality for the HIV-infected patient with PCP requiring ICU treatment is similar to that of the patient with cancer, neutropenia, renal failure, or cardiomyopathy who requires ICU treatment.[34] Despite these survival statistics, HIV-infected patients may be directed away from limited ICU resources. This problem could be avoided if standards for ICU utilization were equally applied to all patients. The allocation of medical resources should rely on rational, objective criteria that assesses medical need, not perceived social worth; the balance of risk versus benefit; and the patient's desires.[35]

When considering an ICU admission, determine whether the patient believes that this treatment will result in a reasonable quality of life.[34] Many HIV-infected patients have well-defined desires about the recommended diagnostic and therapeutic measures. Many also have a "living will" outlining their desires for intensive care and life-sustaining treatments. Interestingly, the HIV-infected patient's preferences and physicians' attitudes result in a rate of do-not-resuscitate orders that exceeds the rate for other systemic diseases such as metastatic lung cancer.[36] Therefore, many treatment issues are easily resolved by discussing the options with the HIV-infected patient.

Health care providers also need to have an understanding of the patient's overall ICU survival.[34] Although the prediction of survival is difficult for the HIV-infected patient, the presence of an AIDS-defining illness can help estimate the patient's survival for the HIV infection itself. In addition, survival data may be available for the acute process prompting the ICU admission. This allows the provider to predict both the in-hospital mortality and long-term survival. In addition, the Acute Physiologic Assessment and Chronic Health Evaluation system can prognostically stratify acutely ill patients. Although this system has been used in HIV, the predictive value of the system may be decreased for these patients.[35]

CONTROL OF HIV INFECTION IN THE ICU ■

Although there have always been occupational hazards, such as hepatitis B, the advent of the HIV epidemic increased the concern for transmission of infection from patient to health care worker. In 1985, the concept of "universal precautions" was established to protect the health care worker. If properly implemented, these infection control measures prevent the transmission of the blood-borne pathogens such as HIV and hepatitis B.[37]

Although HIV has been isolated in almost every body fluid, blood is the most important source of HIV in the work place. As a result of numerous studies, much is known about the risk of infection after exposure to body fluids of HIV-infected patients. First, the highest rates of transmission occur after injection of HIV-infected blood. The risk of infection with HIV after a needle-stick exposure with blood from a patient known to be HIV-seropositive is approximately 0.5%. This is compared with the 6% to 30% risk of hepatitis B infection after a needle-stick injury.[37] Second, transmission can occur if HIV-infected blood comes into contact with damaged skin, such as skin affected by acne or lacerations.[38] Third, there have been no cases of seroconversion after intact cutaneous or mucous membrane exposure to HIV-infected blood or body fluids.[37] Finally, there have not been any seroconversions after exposure to an HIV-infected patient's saliva. This has been documented in the nonsexual household contacts of HIV-infected patients and in health care workers who gave mouth-to-mouth resuscitation to an HIV-infected patient.[38] This information is the basis for infection control measures and the postexposure recommendations for HIV.

INFECTION CONTROL GUIDELINES

Because the risk of transmission varies widely based on the type and extent of exposure, infection control measures could be implemented in a stepwise manner dependent on the risk of exposure. However, several aspects of the transmission of HIV infection must be remembered. Any noninfectious body fluid, such as saliva, can become infectious if contaminated with blood. Also, in emergency settings such as in the ICU, it may be difficult to differentiate between body fluids.[37] Finally, many patients have asymptomatic and undiagnosed HIV infection. Because of these concerns, many institutions and health care workers use a standard set of precautions for each contact with every patient.[39]

Barrier protection is an important part of these infection control measures. Gloves should always be worn when touching any body fluid, mucous membranes, or nonintact skin or when handling the items soiled by body fluids. Gloves should be changed after each patient contact and the hands washed immediately. Any health care worker with open sores or exudative skin lesions should avoid direct patient contact. Protective eyewear and masks also should be worn during procedures prone to the splattering of body fluids. If soiling of clothes is expected, then gowns or protective clothing should be used. To minimize the need for mouth-to-mouth resuscitation, mouthpieces, resuscitation bags, and other ventilation equipment should be readily available. Also, there should be strict adherence to needle and sharp item safety protocols to avoid needle-stick injuries.[39]

Current recommendations for disinfection and sterilization are adequate for decontamination of instruments and equipment used on HIV-infected patients. Potentially contaminated equipment should not be used on multiple patients unless the equipment has been properly decontaminated. Environmental exposures with blood should be cleaned with an Environmental Protection Agency—approved hospital disinfectant. Gloves should be worn during the cleaning process and any cleaning cloths should be considered potentially infectious.[40]

HIV infection itself is not a reason to place a patient into isolation. HIV-infected patients may require isolation for other reasons, such as concern for pulmonary tuberculosis or infection with varicella-zoster virus. However, if the HIV-infected patient is too ill to observe good hygiene, as seen in patients with profuse diarrhea or altered mental status, they should be in a single room. Because HIV-infected patients often asymptomatically shed the herpesviruses, contact with severely immunocompromised patients, such as those with leukemia or transplant recipients, should be avoided.

TRANSMISSION FROM THE HEALTH CARE WORKER TO PATIENTS

Despite strict adherence to the principles of universal precautions, certain invasive surgical and dental procedures have been implicated in the transmission of blood-borne pathogens from health care workers to their patients. The characteristics of these exposure-prone procedures include the digital palpation of a needle tip in a body cavity as well as the simultaneous presence of a health care worker's fingers and a sharp instrument in a poorly visualized or highly confined anatomic site. Examples of these procedures include certain oral, cardiothoracic, colorectal, obstetric, and gynecologic procedures. Invasive procedures that do not have these characteristics have a substantially lower risk of transmitting blood-borne pathogens.[41]

Transmission HIV from a health care worker to a patient can be minimized if a few guidelines are followed. All health care workers should follow universal precautions. Exposure-prone procedures should be identified by medical, surgical, and dental organizations and the institutions where the procedures are being performed. If an invasive procedure is not identified as exposure prone, the HIV-infected health care worker may perform the procedure, provided they are maintaining good technique and infection control practices. If a procedure is identified as exposure prone, the HIV-infected health care worker should not perform the procedure until counsel has been sought from an expert review panel. At this time, mandatory testing of health care workers for HIV infection is not recommended.[41]

MANAGING EXPOSURES TO HIV

If a needle-stick or splash exposure does occur, the area should be washed immediately if possible. The type and extent of exposure should be determined to define the risk of transmission to the health care worker. If the HIV status of the patient is unknown, the patient is counseled and asked to consent to testing. If the patient declines to have the HIV test performed, their risk of HIV infection should be assessed by clinical and epidemiologic data.[39]

It is essential that the exposed health care worker be evaluated by providers experienced in handling this situation. If the exposure source is infected or potentially infected with HIV, the health care worker should have baseline HIV testing performed and, if results are negative, follow-up testing should be performed at 6 weeks, 3 months, and 6 months. An exposed health care worker should be counseled about behavior modifications, such as "safer" sexual practices and avoidance of blood donation until transmission of infec-

TABLE 109-6. Zidovudine Prophylaxis for Occupationally Exposed Health Care Workers

EXPOSURE	TREATMENT
Massive (transfusion)	Recommended
Definite parenteral (intramuscular injection)	Endorsed
Possible parenteral (subcutaneous or mucosal)	Not encouraged
Doubtful parenteral (nonbloody)	Discouraged
Nonparenteral (cutaneous)	Not provided
Zidovudine prophylaxis: 200 mg PO q 4 h for 72 h, then 200 mg PO q 4 h 5× daily for 4 wk	

PO, orally; q, every.

From Gerberding JL: Limiting the risks of health care workers. In: Sande MA, Volberding PA (eds). *The Medical Management of AIDS*. Philadelphia, WB Saunders, 1995.

tion has been ruled out. Also, the use of zidovudine prophylaxis should be discussed with the health care worker. The overall efficacy of zidovudine prophylaxis is unknown, and there have been documented failures of this regimen. However, the prophylaxis may be recommended based on the type of exposure (Table 109-6). If this prophylaxis is given, it should be started within 1 hour of the exposure, if possible. The health care worker must then be referred to an experienced provider for the proper follow-up.[39]

REFERENCES   ◼

1. Cohen PT, Sande MA, Volberding PA (eds): *The AIDS Knowledge Base: A Textbook on HIV Infection from the University of California, San Francisco and the San Francisco General Hospital*. Boston, Little Brown, 1994
2. Broder S, Merigan TC, Bolognesi D (eds): *Testbook of AIDS Medicine*. Baltimore, Williams and Wilkins, 1994
3. Jacobson LP et al: Changes in Survival after Acquired Immunodeficiency Syndrome (AIDS): 1984-1991. *Am J Epidemiol* 1993;138:952
4. Blatt SP, et al: Total lymphocyte count as a predictor of absolute CD4+ count and CD4+ percentage in HIV-infected persons. *JAMA* 1993;269:622
5. Wachter RM, Luce JM, Hopewell PC: Critical care of patients with AIDS. *JAMA* 1992;267:541
6. Meduri GU, Stein DS: Pulmonary manifestations of acquired immunodeficiency syndrome. *Clin Infect Dis* 1992;14:98
7. DeVita MA, Friedman Y, Petrella V: Mask continuous positive pressure in AIDS. *Crit Care Clin* 1993;9:137
8. Moe AA, Hardy WD: *Pneumocystis carinii* infection in the HIV-seropositive patient. *Infect Dis Clin N Am* 1994;8:331
9. Safrin S: *Pneumocystis carinii* pneumonia in patients with the acquired immunodeficiency syndrome. *Sem Respir Dis* 1993;8:96
10. Daley CL: Bacterial pneumonia in HIV-infected patients. *Sem Respir Dis* 1993;8:104
11. Murray JF, Mills J: Pulmonary infectious complications of human immunodeficiency virus infection. *Am Rev Respir Dis* 1990;141:1356
12. Javaly K, Horowitz HW, Wormser GP: Nocardiosis in patients
with human immunodeficiency virus infection: report of 2 cases and review of the literature. *Medicine* 1992;71:128
13. Harvey RL, Sunstrum JC: *Rhodococcus equi* infection in patients with and without human immunodeficiency virus infection. *Rev Infect Dis* 1991;13:139
14. Stansell JD: Pulmonary fungal infection in HIV-infected persons. *Sem Respir Dis* 1993;8:116
15. Galgiani JN: Coccidioidomycosis. *West J Med* 1993;159:153
16. Wheat J: Histoplasmosis and coccidioidomycosis in individuals with AIDS: a clinical review. *Infect Dis Clin N Am* 1994;8:467
17. Inderlied CB, Kemper CA, Bermudez LE: The *Mycobacterium avium* complex. *Clin Micriobiol Rev* 1993;6:266
18. Gachot B, Wolff M, Regnier B: Severe tuberculosis in patients with human immunodeficiency virus infection. *Intensive Care Med* 1990;16491
19. Drew WL: Cytomegalovirus infection in patients with AIDS. *Clin Infect Dis* 1992;14:608
20. Levine AM: Acquired immunodeficiency syndrome-related lymphoma. *Blood* 1992;80:8
21. Powederly WG: Cryptococcal meningitis and AIDS. *Clin Infect Dis* 1993;17:837
22. Simpson DM, Tagliati M: Neurologic manifestations of HIV infection. *Ann Intern Med* 1994;121:769
23. Berger JR, Levy RM: The neurologic complications of human immunodeficiency virus infection. *Med Clin N Am* 1993;77:1
24. Mariuz P, Bosler EM, Luft BJ: Toxoplasmosis in individuals with AIDS. *Infect Dis Clin N Am* 1994;8:365
25. Berenguer J et al: Tuberculous meningitis in patients infected with the human immunodeficiency virus. *N Engl J Med* 1992;326:668
26. Northfelt DW, Polsky B: Bacteremia in persons with HIV infection. *AIDS Clin Rev* 1991;58
27. Mendelson MH et al: *Pseudomonas aeruginosa* bacteremia in patients with AIDS. *Clin Infect Dis* 1994;18:886
28. Masharana U, Schambelan M: The endocrine complications of acquired immunodeficiency syndrome. *Adv Intern Med* 1993;38:323
29. Chui DW, Owen RL: AIDS and the Gut. *J Gastroenter Hepatol* 1994;9:291
30. Smith PD, et al: Gastrointestinal infections in AIDS. *Ann Intern Med* 1992;116:63
31. Cappell MS, Marks M: Acute pancreatitis in HIV-seropositive patients: a case control study of 44 patients. *Am J Med* 1995;98:243
32. Whitney TM, et al: Appendicitis in acquired immunodeficiency syndrome. *Am J Surg* 1992;164:467
33. Sepkowitz, et al: Fever among outpatients with advanced human immunodeficiency virus infection. *Arch Intern Med* 1993;153:1909
34. Raffin TA: Intensive care unit survival of patients with systemic illness. *Am Rev Respir Dis* 1989;140:S2841
35. Zoloth-Dorfman L, Carney B: The AIDS patient and the last ICU bed: scarcity, medical futility, and ethics. *QRB* 1991;17:175
36. Wachter RM et al: Life-sustaining treatment for patients with AIDS. *Chest* 1989;95:647
37. Guidelines for prevention of transmission of human immunodeficiency virus and hepatitis B virus to health-care and public-safety workers. *MMWR.* 1989;38(S-6):1
38. Gurevich I: Acquired immunodeficiency syndrome: realistic concerns and appropriate precautions. *Heart and Lung.* 1989;18107
39. Gerberding JL: Limiting the risks of health care workers. In: Sande MA, Volberding PA (eds). *The Medical Management of*

AIDS. Philadelphia, WB Saunders, 1995

40. Taylor J: Reducing the risk of chance infection: infection control specific to HIV and the intensive care unit. *Prof Nurse* 1991;6:582

41. Centers for Disease Control: Recommendations for preventing transmission of human immunodeficiency virus and hepatitis B virus to patients during exposure-prone invasive procedures. *AORN J* 54:576

Critical Care, Third Edition, edited by Joseph M. Civetta,
Robert W. Taylor, and Robert R. Kirby.
Lippincott-Raven Publishers, Philadelphia, PA © 1997.

CHAPTER 110

Neurologic Infections

David H. Gremillion

IMMEDIATE CONCERNS

Infections of the central nervous system (CNS) are often rapidly fatal or debilitating when undiagnosed but are almost invariably treatable when suspected and diagnosed early. This presents the clinician with a challenge for rapid diagnosis and treatment. Recently developed diagnostic techniques, such as computed tomography (CT) and cerebrospinal fluid (CSF) antigen assays, have supplemented the traditional CSF examination. The possibility of safely arriving at an accurate diagnosis has improved dramatically. Similarly, the introduction of new therapeutic agents directed at bacteria, viruses, and fungi has greatly improved our opportunity for effecting a cure with minimal complications.

When evaluating a patient with suspected CNS infection, an important first step is to determine whether or not focal neurologic signs are present. If focal neurologic findings or papilledema cannot be detected on initial examination, lumbar puncture should be performed. In such cases, the likelihood of intracranial mass lesions is greatly reduced and lumbar puncture is safe.

CLINICAL PRESENTATION AND INITIAL DIAGNOSTIC MEASURES

SUSPECTED CNS INFECTION WITH NO FOCAL NEUROLOGIC SIGNS

The absence of focal neurologic signs is reassuring but not absolute in ruling out mass lesions or dangerous cerebral edema. Even though mass lesions may be present without focal signs, the absence of such signs reduces the risk of lumbar puncture. In general, proceeding directly to CSF examination is justified in the setting of suspected CNS infection with no focal signs.

Bacterial Meningitis

Neurologic infection may be difficult to recognize at the extremes of life. In young infants and in the aged, the typical signs of meningeal irritation may be attenuated or absent. Subtle clues, such as irritability and poor feeding, may be the only indications of infection in infants. In elderly patients, clinical signs of bacterial meningitis may be limited to confusion, lethargy, fever, or hypothermia. Concurrent disease or immunosuppression may increase the risk of opportunistic pathogens in the elderly with subtle clinical presentation.[1]

In normal hosts, signs of meningitis are more typical (Table 110-1). Meningeal irritation and altered mental status are frequent, with headache, nausea, vomiting, and photophobia often present. Involuntary rigidity of the neck muscles resulting from meningeal irritation is a classic sign of bacterial meningitis. The Brudzinski sign is involuntary knee and hip flexion with flexion of the neck. Pain and difficulty in extending the knee in a supine patient in a 90 thigh flexion at the hip is the classic Kernig sign and a strong clinical clue to meningeal irritation. Nuchal rigidity may be difficult to elicit in comatose or immunosuppressed patients and in those with diffuse neurologic impairment.

Meningism may occur without meningeal irritation in lobar pneumonia, septicemia, mastoiditis, cervical adenitis, cervical osteoarthritis, and peritonsillar abscess. Similarly, cervical osteoarthritis may manifest pain and suggestive neck stiffness in the elderly in the absence of meningeal irritation. Convulsions or coma occur on presentation in up to one third of patients with bacterial meningitis. Cranial neuropathies may occur without necessarily reflecting increased intracranial pressure (ICP) or poor prognosis, particularly when present early. Head CT should be performed in all such cases to reduce the risk of post-lumbar puncture complications.

Nonneurologic signs may be useful during the examination of patients with suspected neurologic infection. Patients

TABLE 110-1. Frequency of Clinical Signs in Bacterial Meningitis, by Pathogen*

CLINICAL SIGN	PATHOGEN			
	Meningococcus (53 cases)	*Pneumococcus* (63 cases)	*Haemophilus* (35 cases)	*Other* (58 cases)
Fever	85%	46%	83%	66%
Vomiting	70	25	54	43
Headache	47	25	17	38
Confusion	38	56	49	50
Chills	38	21	3	19
Stiff neck	28	11	49	24
Sore throat	25	5	9	3
Rhinorrhea	21	14	40	17
Earache	4	10	11	10
Myalgia	4	2	0	2
Photophobia	4	0	0	0
Arthralgia	8	0	0	2

*All numbers are percentage of total cases for each pathogen.

Adapted from Carpenter RR, Petersdorf RG: The clinical spectrum of bacterial meningitis. *Am J Med* 1962;33:262

with meningococcal meningitis commonly have pleomorphic petechial lesions and large purpuric or ecchymotic lesions. Erythema nodosum and bullous disease, as well as an evanescent morbilliform rash, may also be seen in meningococcal disease but are less specific. In addition to a careful examination of the skin, the clinician should direct attention to potential primary sites of nonneurologic infections, such as pneumonia, endocarditis, otitis media, suppurative sinusitis, pyoderma, or joint infections. These foci of infection may be secondary or predisposing to bacterial meningitis and occur in up to one third of patients with bacterial meningitis.

Epidemiologic and Clinical Clues to Specific Pathogens

Rapid institution of antimicrobials may be life- or function-sparing when managing neurologic infections. Unfortunately, Gram stain and cultures of the CSF are not always successful in the presumptive identification of pathogens. A careful assessment of epidemiologic and clinical clues may help to narrow the field of potential pathogens and allow a rational selection of antimicrobials.

HAEMOPHILUS INFLUENZAE. *H influenzae*, which accounts for 10,000 cases in the United States each year, is the most frequent cause of bacterial meningitis under age six. Passively acquired maternal antibodies protect the neonate until immunity begins to wane at approximately 3 months of age. Exceptions may exist when additional risk factors are superimposed upon the age factor. *H influenzae* meningitis may occur in adults, but is rarely in epidemic form and usually preceded by a defect in humoral immunity, asplenia, or suppurative sinus disease.[2] Higher incidence has been reported in Eskimos, Navajo Indians, blacks and crowded populations of low socioeconomic status. Peak incidence of the disease follows a spring and fall distribution.

NEISSERIA MENINGITIDIS. *N meningitidis* infection is most common in the young and decreases in incidence through young adulthood; by age 45, it causes less than 10% of meningitis. Although large epidemics continue to occur in other parts of the world, only sporadic and small clusters have been reported in the United States over the past four decades. The majority of cases are caused by serogroup B, which is not well-covered by available vaccines. Each serogroup has characteristic, although loosely overlapping, clinical patterns, with serogroups A and C associated with epidemic disease and meningococcemia, serogroup B with sporadic disease, and serogroup Y with pulmonary disease. Studies in military recruit populations have proven that crowding and pharyngeal carriage rates are not related to epidemics. The presence of petechiae should alert the clinician to the possibility of *N meningitidis*, since these lesions are present in 50% of such cases, but are unusual with other pathogens. Similar rashes occur infrequently in patients with enteroviral disease, and if meningism is present, they may justify antibiotic therapy while awaiting cultures.

Approximately 5% of patients present with fulminant meningococcemia, often progressing to shock and death before CSF abnormalities are detected. *N meningitidis* meningitis may provoke stimulated, manic behavior. A high incidence of joint involvement is reported, and serositis is common with articular, pericardial, and tendon sheath inflammation appearing after the first week of disease. Unlike pneumococcus, recurrent disease due to *N meningitidis* is extremely uncommon. Patients with a deficiency of the terminal components of complement (C5–C8) and immunoglobulin A deficiency are susceptible to meningitis and fulminant meningococcemia.[3] The high-reported frequency of complement deficiency in patients with meningococcal disease (30%) suggests that all such patients should be studied for complement deficiency.[4]

STREPTOCOCCUS PNEUMONIAE. *S pneumoniae* (pneumococcus) usually causes meningitis in the normal host only at the extremes of life. The peak incidence occurs under age 1 and over age 50. Over 50% of patients have an antecedent suppurative focus of infection of the sinuses, ear, or lung. Risk factors include asplenia, humoral immunity deficit, and dural tears, particularly those contiguous to a sinus. Because of the intense inflammation and dense exudative process associated with infections caused by this organism, coma, seizure, and focal neurologic signs are more common early in the disease and may result in a higher rate of morbid sequelae[5] and mortality.[6]

GRAM-NEGATIVE ROD. Gram-negative rod (GNR) meningitis is often hospital acquired and may occur in the setting of head trauma, recent neurosurgery, or other procedures involving breach of the dura. Nosocomial bacterial meningitis has increased with 40% of all cases being hospital acquired in one study [7]. Neonates and granulocytopenic patients are at particular risk of GNR meningitis, as are patients with ventricular shunts and other remote sites of GNR infection such as pyelonephritis [8]. Other risk factors are parameningeal foci of infection, trauma, chronic debilitated status, and advanced age. The clinical presentation of GNR meningitis is different from that associated with other pathogens. Meningeal signs may be minimal in the debilitated, chronically ill, and elderly or very young patients who are more frequently affected. These factors have led to an aggressive approach to lumbar puncture in patients with neurologic signs and the above risk factors.

Aseptic Meningitis Syndrome

Presenting symptoms and signs of nonbacterial meningitis may be indistinguishable from those of bacterial meningitis. In general, however, patients are less ill, with lower fever and a less toxic appearance. Headache is often severe in adults, whereas confusion, lethargy, and lassitude may dominate the clinical picture in children. Many infectious and noninfectious diseases may present with aseptic meningitis syndrome. Notable among these are partially treated bacterial meningitis, leptospirosis, Lyme disease, lymphogranuloma venereum, syphilis, tuberculosis, fungal disease, and collagen vascular diseases.

Acute HIV infection should be considered in patients with risk factors. Neurosarcoidosis may cause a chronic granulomatous meningitis and mimic tuberculosis or fungal meningitis.[9] Viral meningitis occurs throughout the year but is more common during the summer and fall months, thus mimicking the seasonality of the enteroviruses. Bacterial meningitis is more common during the winter and spring months but either may occur throughout the year. Viral prodrome often precedes the aseptic meningitis complication and may provide valuable clues to the specific cause. Antecedent parotitis may suggest mumps, or a morbilliform rash during a measles epidemic may presage a complicating meningitis or encephalitis. In some cases, even the best clinical and epidemiologic clues are insufficient to distinguish bacterial meningitis from septic meningitis, and the clinician must resort to CSF examination and culture.

SUSPECTED CNS INFECTION WITH FOCAL NEUROLOGIC SIGNS

The presence of focal neurologic signs or papilledema suggests that an intracranial mass lesion is present. In such cases the clinician should consider delaying lumbar puncture until a CT scan can be performed to rule out cerebral edema or mass effect and thus eliminate the possibility of uncal herniation. Rapid neurologic deterioration and even death may occur following lumbar puncture in 25% of patients with intracranial abscess. When meningeal signs are present and neurodiagnostic studies are judged necessary, therapy should not be delayed for the performance of CT scans or lumbar punctures. A single dose of a well-selected antibiotic may be lifesaving and should not be delayed beyond the first hour after presentation. Cultures of the CSF are not substantially affected by a single dose of intravenous antibiotic. Careful examination should be performed to detect remote foci of infection that may have seeded a brain abscess or subdural empyema. Examination of the sinuses and ear canal may disclose infection contiguous to intracranial suppuration.

Spinal Epidural Abscess

Epidural abscess is an uncommon process and the diagnosis is often delayed or missed entirely. A high index of suspicion is essential because fewer than 25% of cases are suspected on admission. Typical presenting findings are fever, malaise, and back pain. The vague and nonspecific nature of these early clues often leads the clinician to consider a viral or self-limited process. Progression of the infection is followed by persistent spinal pain, nerve root pain, and eventually weakness and anesthesia, with sphincter control deficits. The duration of back pain before diagnosis is highly variable but averages 16 days (range, 2–42 days).[10] Nerve root pain is present in more than 90% of patients and, although it may be a presenting finding, it usually follows the onset of persistent spinal ache by 2 to 3 days.

Spread of epidural abscess may occur from local contiguous foci such as decubiti or vertebral osteomyelitis, or may be a local consequence of recent spinal surgery. In such cases, gram-negative pathogens are somewhat more common. The mode of spread in 25% to 50% of cases is hematogenous from a remote suppurative focus. Cutaneous infections are most common, followed by urinary tract infections, sepsis, pneumonia, and infected intravenous lines. Approximately 75% of patients have clinical or historical evidence of an antecedent infection when spinal epidural abscess is diagnosed. *Staphylococcus aureus* is overwhelmingly the most common cause of spinal epidural abscess, accounting for 69% to 90% of cases. Gram-negative pathogens and a variety of opportunistic pathogens occur but are much less likely.[11] In some parts of the world, *Mycobacterium tuberculosis* is very common, but it accounts for less than 25% of epidural abscesses in the United States. The indolent nature of tuberculous disease renders it less of a surgical emergency.[12] Alternate diagnostic possibilities to be considered include disk herniation, acute transverse myelitis, inflammatory joint disease, and neoplasm.

When the typical clinical picture suggests the diagnosis, immediate evaluation is necessary. Plain radiographs of the affected area may show evidence of vertebral osteomyelitis, which is accompanied by epidural abscess in approximately 20% of cases. A study with negative results is not helpful since delayed evidence of osteomyelitis is characteristic and paravertebral mass is often not apparent. MRI is almost always abnormal and is the procedure of choice to document the process.[13] Myelography continues to be useful in some cases. Cerebrospinal fluid typically shows increased protein, mild polymorphonuclear pleocytosis (often less than 150), and normal glucose.

Once documented, a spinal epidural abscess is considered a neurosurgical emergency. Antibiotic therapy without drainage is ineffective. Presumptive antistaphylococcal therapy should be initiated preoperatively with nafcillin or vancomycin and maintained for 3 to 4 weeks or longer, if appropriate to the management of any associated infection. When vertebral osteomyelitis or endocarditis is present, 6 to 8 weeks of parenteral therapy should be given. Antibiotics should be altered for optimal coverage when the definitive microbiologic diagnosis is made.

Cranial Epidural Abscess

This process is similar to spinal epidural abscess but is less common. Infection may result from infected sinuses, orbital infection, trauma, neurosurgery, or other CNS infection. Subdural empyema is commonly present and usually accounts for any observed neurologic deficits. The role of CT scanning is better documented in cranial epidural abscess and is the diagnostic procedure of choice.

Subdural Empyema

Accumulation of pus in the space between the dura and the arachnoid often arises by direct extension from infections of the paranasal sinuses or middle ear, or from osteomyelitis. Frontal sinusitis with or without cranial osteomyelitis is a predisposing factor in as many as 75% of cases of nontraumatic subdural empyema. Presenting signs and symptoms result from increased intracranial pressure, meningeal irritation, or surrounding cortical inflammation at the site of the empyema. Meningeal signs are present in 80% of patients and focal neurologic findings in 80% to 90%. The clinical presentation may be dominated by complications such as brain abscess or cortical vein thrombosis. The technique of choice for documenting subdural empyema is CT scanning, but false-negative CT scans have been reported. The microbiology is similar to that of chronic sinusitis or brain abscess, with streptococci, staphylococci, anaerobic streptococci, and gram-negative rods commonly present.

A combination of medical and surgical therapy is required for a successful outcome in patients with subdural empyema. Craniotomy results in a higher success rate than drainage through burr holes.[14] Empirical antibiotic coverage may be instituted with a penicillinase-stable penicillin or with chloramphenicol, but is adjusted to specific therapy based on culture and sensitivity reports when available.

Brain Abscess

Brain abscess is an uncommon infection that occurs about one fifth as often as bacterial meningitis. Diagnosis can be challenging because many patients are afebrile and have an indolent clinical course that may not be suggestive. Mortality rate from brain abscess was once high, and even into the antibiotic era death rates of 40% to 60% were reported. Dramatic reductions in mortality rates, however, have resulted since the introduction of better imaging techniques for intracranial disease[15]. Drainage procedures guided by CT have provided earlier microbiologic diagnosis and more effective drainage of intracranial suppuration.[16]

Brain abscess may arise from direct contiguous spread from nearby infection or from hematogenous spread from a remote site of infection. Direct spread is often from a nearby extracerebral site of infection, such as frontal sinusitis or mastoiditis, and these lesions are commonly located in the frontal or temporal lobes. In contrast, brain abscess arising from hematogenous spread is often in the distribution of the middle cerebral artery. Typical underlying infections for hematogenous spread include endocarditis, pneumonia, or skin and soft tissue infections. Patients with congenital heart disease and right-to-left shunting or pulmonary arteriovenous fistulae are more likely to have brain abscesses from hematogenous spread.

Increased recognition of brain abscess in the immunocompromised host over the past two decades is a result of better imaging techniques and higher prevalence resulting from immunosuppression. In these patients, *Nocardia asteroides,* phycomycoses, *Cryptococcus neoformans, Toxoplasma gondii, Candida* species, and other opportunistic pathogens should be considered in addition to the usual brain abscess pathogens. Because of an increased likelihood of brain abscess in immunocompromised patients with meningitis, these patients should receive early consideration for brain imaging studies.

Patients with brain abscess often have a short duration of symptoms. The most common presentation is severe headache, alterations of mood or consciousness, irritability, confusion, and nausea and vomiting of less than 2 weeks' duration. Fever is present in approximately 50% of patients with brain abscess and is less common in the elderly. In about two thirds of patients, a clue to the origin is apparent at the time of initial diagnosis.

When the diagnosis of brain abscess is suspected, a brain imaging technique such as MRI or CT scan should be performed to determine the extent of cerebral edema and the size and position of the lesion. Cerebrospinal fluid examination by lumbar puncture should not be done because of an enhanced risk of complications with increased ICP. Furthermore, CSF is not generally helpful in the diagnosis of brain abscess because it merely reflects changes characteristic of a parameningeal focus of infection and often does not contain the causative pathogens. Only after midline shifts, large lesions, and cerebral edema have been excluded by CT scanning should a lumbar puncture be performed. The CT scan may become positive early in the course of brain abscess, before the development of encapsulated suppuration. This "cerebritis" stage of brain abscess may be amenable to antibiotic therapy and may not require surgical drainage.[17]

Surgical or CT-guided drainage of the necrotic and purulent material is essential for an effective cure of brain abscess. In carefully selected patients who pose a high surgical risk, antibiotics alone may be curative when given in high doses over long periods.[18] Antibiotic therapy should include coverage for anaerobes as well as aerobes, since anaerobes are present in approximately 50% of cases of brain abscess. Intravenous penicillin and chloramphenicol should be administered in divided doses when brain abscess is documented. The combination of cefotaxime and metronidazole has proven effective in recent studies [19]. If *S aureus* is suspected because of a penetrating head injury or occurrence of brain abscess following craniotomy, vancomycin or a penicillinase-resistant penicillin such as oxacillin or nafcillin should be substituted for penicillin G. *S aureus* CNS disease continues to have a high rate of neurologic sequellae and mortality.[20]

Antibiotic therapy should be maintained for a minimum of 3 to 4 weeks unless management of an underlying infection, such as endocarditis or osteomyelitis, requires longer treatment.

Prognosis is determined partly by the extent of underlying disease, delay in diagnosis and drainage, and age of the patient. Mortality has declined from 60% in the 1960s and earlier to under 20% during the present era of high suspicion and early diagnosis.

Herpes Encephalitis

Herpes encephalitis is caused by herpesvirus hominis (HVH) type I (rarely type II) and is the most common fatal encephalitis in the United States. Neonatal encephalitis is most often caused by type II HVH acquired during passage through an infected birth canal. Adults typically present with a subacute febrile syndrome characterized by headache and altered mentation. Focal neurologic findings and seizure are present in 70% of cases.

Presumptive diagnosis can be made with a combination of CT scan or MRI, EEG, and CSF examinations, but definitive diagnosis requires biopsy of affected brain tissue. Typically, CSF shows elevated opening pressures, moderate pleocytosis (50–500 lymphocytes), normal glucose, and elevated protein. Some reports have suggested that the presence of red cells in the CSF, in the right clinical setting, indicates herpes encephalitis. Completely normal CSF is seen in a small number of cases. Serology for herpes antibodies in CSF is too insensitive and results are too long delayed to be clinically useful. The EEG and CT scan are abnormal in 80% and 60% of cases, respectively, but alone are insufficient to establish a definitive diagnosis. The combination of clinical findings and neurodiagnostic studies was correct and only 57% of cases entered into a large cooperative study.[21] Brain biopsy has proven to be an effective method of establishing the diagnosis but the need for biopsy in the current era of safe and relatively effective therapy has been questioned.

Acyclovir in a dose of 10 mg/kg every 8 hours for 10 days is now the treatment of choice. A mortality rate of less than 20% and a morbid sequelae rate of less than 50% can now be expected from a disease that was once fatal in 70% of cases, with high survivor morbidity rate. Acyclovir resistant strains have been reported but remain uncommon.

ESTABLISHING THE DIAGNOSIS ■

Definitive diagnosis of neurologic infections depends on the clinician's working knowledge of the microbiology laboratory and judicious use of ancillary diagnostic information provided by radiologic, serologic, and chemical tests. Recent major advances have improved accuracy and speed in all of these areas. Pathogens are cultured in more than 90% of cases of acute meningitis, 50% of brain abscesses, 70% of tuberculous meningitis, and 65% of fungal meningitis. These yields are not affected by single doses of potentially lifesaving antibiotics, and therapy should not be delayed to obtain CSF cultures. As soon as possible after collection, CSF should be plated on blood and chocolate agar—preferably at the bedside where feasible. When GNR meningitis is likely, MacConkey agar should be inoculated. Culture for fungi and tuberculosis is justified only when clinical or epidemiologic clues suggest these pathogens. Definitive diagnosis by culture is always delayed by 24 hours to as much as 6 weeks (mycobacteria), so its major usefulness is not to select initial therapy but to alter initial therapy when pathogens and their sensitivities are known. Cultures of concurrent nonneurologic sites of infection are frequently useful. Bacteremia is detected in 30% to 60% of *N meningitidis* meningitis, 40% of pneumococcal meningitis, and 80% of *H influenzae* meningitis.

CEREBROSPINAL FLUID EXAMINATION

Examination of the CSF is the single most important determination in the management of neurologic infections. Such examinations often provide critical information on diagnosis, prognosis, and response to therapy. Although essential in the evaluation of neurologic infection, it is not without risk or diagnostic pitfalls. The reported complications should not be a deterrent to performing a lumbar puncture when clinically indicated to evaluate neurologic infection. When focal neurologic signs exist or evidence of increased ICP is present, a noninvasive test, such as CT or brain scan, should be performed to identify possible mass lesions or evidence of cerebral edema and increased ICP, which allow for a more careful determination of the need for lumbar puncture. The actual rate of risk of serious complication in the presence of papilledema is between 1% and 8%; this necessitates consideration of less invasive tests when possible.[22] Spinal hematoma may occur in as many as 6% to 7% of patients with coagulation defects, including immunocompromised hosts with thrombocytopenia.

Cerebrospinal fluid supplies both general and, in many cases, specific etiologic information.[23] Among the routine tests performed (Table 110-2), the association of a low glucose level and elevated polymorphonuclear leukocyte count are the most important because they may establish a "purulent profile." When present, this profile often represents justification for empirical antibiotic therapy pending the re-

TABLE 110-2.   Typical Cerebrospinal Fluid Findings in Neurologic Infection

FINDING	Normal	Bacterial	Viral	Parameningeal	Fungal
Cell count (cells/mm^3)	0–5	100–5000	10–500	<500	0–1000
Protein (mg/dL)	15–40	>100	50–100	>60	>60
Glucose (mg/dL)	50–75	<40	Normal	Normal	<40
Specific stain for pathogen		Positive in $^3/_4$		Negative	Positive in <$^1/_4$

sults of more specific diagnostic tests. Identification of a casual organism on culture or Gram stain is useful when positive. When results are negative, antigen detection assays may be useful.

Specialized tests may speed the specific etiologic diagnosis by detection of pathogens or their byproducts in CSF (Table 110-3). Counterimmunoelectrophoresis (CIE) has been generally abandoned in favor of latex particle agglutination (LPA) and coagglutination techniques, which adapt well to routine laboratory use. Commercial development of LPA has led to almost universal availability of kits for most of the common pathogens. By using CSF bacterial antigen tests only when other tests are negative costs can be reduced greatly with no detrimental effect on patients.[24] Gram stain and culture establish the cause of bacterial meningitis in over 90% of cases and, for these, antigen detection is unnecessary. The latex cryptococcal antigen test has become the standard for early diagnosis of cryptococcal meningitis.[25] Enzyme-linked immunoassays for CSF antigen detection have been promising in limited trials for diagnosing infection caused by *H influenzae*, pneumococcus, meningococcus, and *Streptococcus agalactiae*. Quantitation of CSF bacterial antigen has been reported to provide important prognostic information as well as aiding in the diagnosis because the quantity of antigen present on initial lumbar puncture correlates with outcome.

TABLE 110-3.   Cerebrospinal Fluid Tests in Suspected Neurologic Infection

ROUTINE TESTS°	SPECIALIZED TESTS[†]
Cell count with differential	India ink stain
Glucose	VDRL
Protein	Bacterial antigen assay
Gram stain	Counterimmunoelectrophoresis
Culture and sensitivity	Latex agglutination
	Endotoxin assay
	Limulus lysate assay
	Acid-fast smear
	Viral serology
	Fungal antigen assay
	Cytology for malignancy

°Should be ordered on all CSF specimens.
[†]Request should be restricted to specimens from patients with suggestive epidemiologic or clinical findings.

Monoclonal antibody techniques may improve sensitivity and specificity of antigen detection in the future. These specialized tests have shown greatest usefulness in pediatrics, neonatal meningitis, and partially treated bacterial meningitis.

Cerebrospinal fluid is almost always abnormal in tuberculous and fungal meningitis. Very low glucose concentrations are characteristic and low-to-moderately elevated white cell counts with lymphocytic predominance are the rule. Specific stains are positive in 80% of cases when large volumes (over 10 mL) of CSF are centrifuged and the precipitate stained.[26]

RADIOLOGIC TESTS

Rapid developments in the field of neuroradiology have provided great advantages to the clinician in managing CNS infection.[27] Computed tomography has proven sensitive and specific in the diagnosis of a broad range of infections characterized by mass lesions[28] and is now the procedure of choice for subdural empyema, brain abscess, tuberculoma, and cerebral cysticercosis; CT is also very useful in herpes encephalitis, progressive multifocal leukoencephalopathy (PML), and Jakob–Creutzfeldt disease. Magnetic resonance imaging, where available, is proving to be useful and may eventually replace CT scanning for many of its current indications. Particular advantage has been demonstrated in diseases with abnormal myelination, such as PML and other diffuse encephalitides, and MRI has proven superior in detecting cerebral edema near a necrotic focus, cavernous sinus thrombosis, and posterior fossa lesions. Cerebral angiography is currently limited to infections in which demonstration of a clinically significant arteritis is important.

SEROLOGIC DIAGNOSIS

Because of the inherent delay and imprecision in diagnosing neurologic infections by paired serologies, their use is often limited to the research setting or epidemiologic studies. Paired serologic techniques are most often employed in viral infections of the CNS because other diagnostic modalities and treatment implications are limited in these infections. A serum specimen should be collected early in the course and preserved until a convalescent serum specimen can be obtained and sent "paired" with the acute specimen to a reference laboratory. Single or sequential serologies are useful for both diagnosis and assessment of treatment in patients with fungal meningitis, syphilis, toxoplasmosis, leptospirosis,

TABLE 110-4. Serologic Tests in the Diagnosis of Neurologic Infection

---

Paired Serology
  Viral aseptic meningitis syndrome
  Viral encephalitis
Single or Sequential Serology
  Coccidioidal meningitis
  Cryptococcal meningitis
  Histoplasmosis
  Toxoplasmosis
  Syphilis
  Leptospirosis
  Mononucleosis
  Cysticercosis
  Amebiases

---

mononucleosis, cysticercosis, and amebiasis, and to rule out many of the noninfectious etiologies of acute and chronic meningitis, such as collagen vascular diseases (Table 110-4).

MANAGEMENT ■

EMPIRICAL SELECTION OF ANTIBIOTICS

Many patients with a neurologic infection have a presumptive pathogen identified within 1 hour and a definitive pathogen identified within the first 24 hours of hospitalization. Because of the potential seriousness of neurologic infections, however, antibiotics must often be started earlier on empirical grounds. The principles that apply to the selection of empirical antibiotics in other categories of infection are identical with those in neurologic infections,[29] that is, a knowledge of the most likely etiologic pathogens, the antibiotic sensitivities of those pathogens, and the antimicrobial spectrum and pharmacokinetic properties of the antibiotics. In neurologic infections, the clinician must also consider penetration of the antibiotic into the CSF. The latter two factors—penetration into CSF and antimicrobial sensitivities of the likely pathogens—are well known. Selection of the agent of choice, therefore, depends on identification of the likely pathogen.

Two categories of clinical information help the clinician to predict potential pathogens: age and clinical status. Table 110-5 lists likely pathogens and antibiotics of choice for given age and clinical criteria. It is important to alter the empirically selected antibiotics when definitive identification of the pathogen is available. The possibility of penicillin resistance in *S pneumoniae* has led to routine sensitivity screening for this pathogen. In some areas where penicillin resistance is common, empiric vancomycin and cefotaxime empiric therapy have become the therapy of choice.

Bactericidal antibiotics are necessary in the management of neurologic infections because of impaired host defenses at the infection site. Upon entering CSF, bacteria enjoy unrestricted growth. Normal CSF contains no phagocytic cells, immunoglobulin M, or complement.[30] Host defenses thus cannot be relied on to assist bacteriostatic drugs in eradicating the infection. The importance of bactericidal antibiotics has been documented in animal models. Antibiotics selected for management of neurologic infections must penetrate the CSF. The blood–brain barrier efficiently excludes most drugs, and even when penetration into the CSF occurs, it is relatively inefficient. Many of the third-generation cephalosporins have relatively good penetration and are gaining increasing acceptance in the management of meningitis.[31] Poor penetration into the CSF has also required physicians to use high doses of antibiotics administered intravenously so that serum concentration can produce an effective gradient to aid diffusion into CSF. Although frequent dosing schedules for antibiotics in meningitis have been traditional, animal studies have shown that less frequent dosing intervals are equally effective. Experimental studies

TABLE 110-5. Empirical Antibiotics for Neurologic Infection by Age and Clinical Situation

	LIKELY PATHOGEN	ANTIBIOTIC OF CHOICE
AGE		
Neonate (0–6 weeks)	*E Coli*; GBP streptococci°	Ampicillin and cefotaxime
Child (6 weeks–10 years)	*H Influenzae*; *N Meningitidis*	Ampicillin and chloramphenicol
Adult (10–50 years)	*N Meningitidis*	Cefotaxime
Adult (>50 years)	*S Pneumoniae*; *N Meningitidis* *Listeria monocytogenes*	Cefotaxime and Ampicillin
CLINICAL SITUATION		
Immunocompromised host	Many	Ampicillin and cefotaxime
Penetrating head injury	*S Aureus*	Nafcillin
CSF rhinorrhea	*S Pneumoniae*	Aqueous penicillin G

°Group B streptococci.

indicate that it is more important to achieve high peak CSF concentrations of antibiotics than to maintain continuous levels.

The use of combinations of antibiotics to manage meningitis is most often a result of the clinician's desire to cover potentially resistant pathogens. The use of chloramphenicol and ampicillin to manage *H influenzae* meningitis is an example. Pathogens for which combinations are commonly used are *M tuberculosis* and enterococcus. Enterococcal meningitis may require intrathecal therapy for eradication.[32] Treatment should be maintained for 10 to 14 days when treating *N meningitidis* or *S pneumoniae* meningitis. Longer courses may be required in *Listeria* meningitis. Avoid the urge to reduce dosage as the patient improves. Reduced inflammation of the meninges decreases CSF penetration and justifies high doses, even with improvement.

Nonantibiotic therapy in neurologic infections is primarily directed at complications. Cerebral edema may require mannitol infusion or decadron administration. Cerebral edema is the only proven indication for decadron when managing bacterial meningitis. In the setting of bacterial meningitis under adequate antibiotic therapy, corticosteroids do not pose a clinically significant immunosuppression problem. Fluid restriction may be useful to reduce cerebral edema and minimize effects of possible development of the syndrome of inappropriate antidiuretic hormone secretion (SIADH). No more than two thirds of the calculated fluid requirement should be given during the first 3 days. When fluids are required for septic shock management, they should be given cautiously and with monitoring. Appropriate fluid management in meningitis can minimize cerebral edema and reduce morbidity and mortality.[33] Seizures may occur early in the course of bacterial meningitis and should be treated vigorously with intravenous diazepam or phenytoin. Prophylactic use of analeptics is not generally recommended.

Corticosteroids have now been proven to be of benefit in infants and children with meningitis. Reduction of cerebral edema early in the course is accompanied by fewer neurologic complications and improved survival. Dexamethasone should be given for the first 3 to 4 days of therapy and rapidly tapered thereafter.[34] Adjunctive decadron therapy improves outcome in infants and children with meningitis.[35] The evidence is less compelling in adults.

Monitoring therapy is best accomplished with clinical parameters. Fever usually responds by the fourth treatment day, but neurologic deficits may persist and are a poor gauge of response. Repeat lumbar puncture on the second treatment day is sometimes done in difficult or complicated cases. If the right empirical antibiotic was chosen, viable organisms will almost invariably be absent at 36 hours. Intracranial pressure monitoring devices have been used only infrequently, and most authorities consider them to be relatively contraindicated during CNS infection.

PREVENTION OF BACTERIAL MENINGITIS   ■

Preventive measures for bacterial meningitis are often directed against *N meningitidis*, *H influenzae* type B, and occasionally *S pneumoniae*. The frequent occurrence of these pathogens as causes of meningitis, the public panic that is often caused by their occurrence, and the availability of adequate preventive measures for these pathogens are the primary reasons for the attention. Two forms of prophylaxis are available: immunization and antibiotics.

Secondary cases of meningitis, defined as those occurring within 30 days of an index case, are between 200 and 1000 times more frequent than sporadic cases. For *H influenzae* type B, secondary cases beyond the age of 6 years are rare and prophylaxis is not justified.[36] For meningococcal disease, all ages are at risk, although young children appear to be more so. To be at sufficient risk to warrant prophylaxis, a contact must have relatively close exposure to an index case. In general, this requires residence in the same household or shared sleeping quarters. Classmates of affected primary or secondary school children are not considered to be high-

TABLE 110-6.   Preventive Measures for Bacterial Meningitis

	DRUG	DOSE	COMMENT
CHEMOPROPHYLAXIS			
N. meningitidis	Rifampin	600 mg b.i.d. for 2 days	
Alternate	Minocycline	100 mg b.i.d. for 2 days	Vestibular toxicity
Alternate	Sulfadiazine	500 mg b.i.d. for 2 days	When sulfa-sensitive
H. influenzae B	Rifampin	600 mg every 24 hours for 4 days (Child)—20 mg/kg/day for 4 days	
IMMUNOPROPHYLAXIS			
N. meningitidis	Quadrivalent vaccine	1 dose (adult) 2 dose (<10 years)	Protective effect delayed 14 days
H. influenzae B	Monovalent vaccine	1 dose age 2–6 years°	Protective effect delayed 14 days
S. pneumoniae†	23 strains covered	Single dose	Protective effect delayed 14 days

°Children vaccinated at less than 24 months of age may require a second dose.
†Optimal period for reimmunization has not been established

risk exposures. On the other hand, residents of nursing homes and children in day care centers are at a substantial risk and generally deserve prophylaxis. Hospital personnel in contact with a patient with meningitis are considered to be at very low risk and should receive prophylaxis only when intimate contact with respiratory secretions occurs.

Antimicrobial prophylaxis has as its goal the eradication of colonization in contacts. It is noteworthy that many antibiotic regimens that are effective in the therapy of bacterial meningitis are ineffective in its prophylaxis and do not eradicate the carrier state. Intramuscular penicillin has been shown to be ineffective in prophylaxis for meningococcal meningitis. Suggested chemoprophylactic regimens are shown in Table 110-6 for the given pathogens and age. It is important to institute antimicrobial prophylaxis as soon as possible after the exposure to bacterial meningitis and to ensure patient compliance with the prophylactic regimen. Sensitivity of the infecting agent to sulfadiazine should be established before its prophylactic use. Minocycline is effective but is often associated with significant vestibular toxicity and should be used as a second-choice agent to rifampin.[37]

Pneumococcal meningitis does not require prophylaxis of even close contacts since pneumococcal carriage is very common. Persons at high risk for the development of pneumococcal meningitis include those with specific host immunity defects, such as splenectomy or sickle cell disease, or those with dural tears from surgery or trauma. Some authorities advocate the administration of penicillin to reduce the risk of pneumococcal meningitis in these patients. The futility of maintaining antibiotics over a long period and the attendant risk of resistance and side effects have limited the usefulness of this approach.

In the case of asplenia, the patient should be instructed to maintain a starter supply of oral antibiotics (oral penicillin-VK or sulfamethoxazole and trimethoprim) at home, to begin therapy as soon as toxic symptoms occur, and to report to his or her physician as soon as possible.

Another strategy for prevention of bacterial meningitis is immunization. The protective effect of immunization is delayed for 10 to 14 days and should never be used as an alternative to antimicrobial prophylaxis, but as a complementary regimen that is generally applied to larger populations. Vaccine for *N meningitidis* is limited to serogroups A, C, Y, and WI-35. An adequate vaccine to group B is not generally available. A recently licensed vaccine to *H influenzae* type B (HIB) should be limited to high-risk patients under the age of 6.[38] Widespread use of the new HIB polysaccharide-conjugate vaccine has dramatically reduced the incidence of *H influenzae* meningitis.[39] Pneumococcal vaccine contains antibiotics against 23 of the most common serogroups of *S pneumoniae*. Its use is best documented for pneumonia prevention, but it is probably also useful for recurrent meningitis in high-risk patients.

INFECTION CONTROL CONSIDERATIONS

Strict isolation is generally required only for patients with meningococcal meningitis and *H influenzae* B meningitis and is necessary only during the first 24 hours of antibiotic coverage. Risk to hospital personnel and nearby patients is extremely low in the absence of intimate contact with respiratory secretions. Other forms of meningitis do not require isolation. Patients with meningococcal and *H influenzae* meningitis should be reported to state health authorities to ensure that small epidemics can be recognized quickly and that public health measures can be undertaken.

Hospital-acquired meningitis is increasing in frequency and is generally limited to neurosurgery patients, patients with ventricular shunts, and neonates.[40,41] All procedures that result in a puncture of the meninges for dye instillation or removal of CSF are associated with a very small risk of nosocomial bacterial meningitis. The most common pathogens involved in hospital-acquired meningitis are *Staphylococcus* species and gram-negative rods. These account for over 50% of reported cases. *Listeria monocytogenes* has been associated with rare instances of hospital outbreaks of meningitis secondary to consumption of contaminated vegetables or imported cheeses.

The use of an ICP monitoring device may be complicated by GNR meningitis. The lowest infection rate is associated with the subarachnoid screw (7%), followed by the subdural cup catheter (15%), and the ventriculostomy catheter (20%).[42] Risk of infection drops the longer the device is in place, suggesting that infection occurs during implantation. Unlike intravenous catheters, routine reinsertion of ICP monitoring devices may increase the risk of infection, and a single device should be used as long as monitoring is necessary.[32]

Reports of spurious bacterial meningitis should alert the clinician to the potential for inappropriate diagnosis and treatment. These cases have most often been related to nonviable gram-negative rods present in specimen collection tubes. Since initial management of meningitis often depends on Gram stains of the CSF, patients may inappropriately receive antimicrobials based on spurious microorganisms in commercial lumbar puncture kits.

COMPLICATIONS OF BACTERIAL MENINGITIS ■

Complications of bacterial meningitis are very common and can be divided into neurologic and nonneurologic categories (Table 110-7).[43] Severe morbidity and mortality have not declined appreciably over the past three decades.[44] Close observation of patients with meningitis and frequent repetition of the examination are important because detection of subtle clues suggesting a neurologic or systemic complication may be lifesaving. Cranial nerve abnormalities appear in 10% to 20% of patients with bacterial meningitis and principally involve the third, fourth, sixth, or seventh cranial nerve.[45] Hearing deficit may be permanent and occurs more commonly with meningococcal meningitis. Long-term neurologic deficit occurs in 10% to 20% of patients who recover from bacterial meningitis. A significant but uncertain proportion suffer subtle changes of behavior or cognitive function; this is more prevalent in infants and young children. Hemiparesis or quadriparesis occurs in 11% of patients and may appear either early, due to occlusive vascular inflammation, or late when the patient's clinical status is improving. Persistent focal cerebral signs suggest subdural empyema, cerebral abscess, or cortical vein thrombosis.

TABLE 110-7. Complications of Central
Nervous System Infections

NEUROLOGIC COMPLICATIONS

  Seizure
  Cerebral edema°
  Coma[†]
  Cranial neuropathy
  Cortical vein thrombosis[†]
  Brain abscess[†]
  Subdural empyema[†]
  Encephalopathy°

NON-NEUROLOGIC COMPLICATIONS

  Shock[†]
  Coagulation disorders[†]
  Septic complications[†]
  Prolonged fever
  SIADH
  Volume overload

°Implies negative prognosis only late in course.
[†]May convey important negative prognostic information.

Specific clinical syndromes are associated with septic thrombosis of each of the major cerebral veins. Cavernous sinus thrombosis presents with exophthalmos, periorbital edema, and decreased pupillary reflexes. Lateral sinus thrombosis manifests sixth cranial nerve deficit, facial pain or loss of sensation, and papilledema. Superior sagittal sinus thrombosis presents with bilateral motor weakness and papilledema. Petrosal sinus thrombosis presents with pain and sensory deficit.

One fourth of patients with bacterial meningitis experience a focal or generalized seizure disorder, which may be followed by transient paralysis (Todd paralysis). This should be differentiated from a more persistent paresis, which implies a focal suppurative or thrombotic complication. Seizures are most frequently due to cerebral inflammation but may be related to accompanying physiologic events, such as electrolyte disturbance, hypoglycemia, hyperpyrexia, or penicillin neurotoxicity. The latter occurs with very large penicillin doses given in the presence of renal failure. Altered mental status and coma occur in all forms of bacterial meningitis. Meningococcal infections are occasionally associated with a hyperactive manic state that can be difficult to control with sedation. Acute cerebral edema frequently complicates bacterial meningitis and can produce a variety of secondary neurologic findings, such as cranial neuropathies, altered mental status, seizure disorder, or one of the herniation syndromes. The risk of cerebellar herniation increases with lumbar puncture; if elevated pressures are documented during a lumbar puncture, immediate therapeutic measures should be directed at reducing cerebral edema. Papilledema is distinctly uncommon early in bacterial meningitis and, when present, suggests a mass lesion such as brain abscess or subdural empyema.

Non-neurologic complications may overshadow the clinical course of a patient with bacterial meningitis. Bacteremia occurs in 60% of patients with meningococcal meningitis and may be accompanied by an acute or chronic meningococcemia syndrome. Disseminated intravascular coagulopathy and shock occur frequently in the course of meningococcal infection and have a high mortality rate. Petechiae are an important harbinger of meningococcemia but are not specific, having been reported in patients with pneumococcal sepsis with splenectomy, *H influenzae* bacteremia, and, less commonly, in other bacteremias. These may progress to ecchymoses and severe microvascular compromise, with the loss of digits and renal function. Persistent or recurrent fever beyond the fourth treatment day may be drug related or due to suppurative complication. It is rare for thermoregulatory deficit to follow meningitis; this should be an exclusion diagnosis of last resort. Digit and skin necrosis following meningococcemia is commonly accompanied by fever. Bacteremia occurs in 40% of patients with pneumococcal meningitis and may result from or cause a secondary site of infection. Bacteremia is unusual in staphylococcal meningitis and suggests concurrent staphylococcal endocarditis. Hypothalamic inflammation during bacterial meningitis may lead to SIADH, which requires careful fluid and electrolyte management. Remote suppurative foci of infection in the course of bacterial meningitis are hard to distinguish from underlying infections that may have preceded the meningitis. These may require drainage, alternate antibiotics, or longer antibiotic courses for cure. Meningococcal arthritis and synovitis are relatively common and may require drainage.

SPECIAL CLINICAL CONSIDERATIONS ■

THE IMMUNOCOMPROMISED HOST

Central nervous system infections in patients with immune deficits are common, occurring in 5% to 10% of transplant recipients and patients with lymphoma. Fewer data are available for patients with leukemia and those receiving steroids on a chronic basis, but clinical experience has shown that these patients also have frequent CNS infections. Mortality rate is inordinately high, with 44% to 77% of patients dying of their infection. Early diagnosis and treatment are therefore imperative.[46]

Management of CNS infection in the immunocompromised host is complicated by three important factors. First, the list of potential pathogens is large and includes organisms not ordinarily considered or difficult to diagnose (Table 110-8). Lowered host resistance adds unusual and generally avirulent pathogens to the list of possibilities. Second, the clinical and laboratory findings as well as the course of infection are often modified by the underlying disease or its therapy. Recent antibiotic therapy is common and may interfere with culture, Gram stain, or other potentially helpful CSF studies. Steroids or other immunosuppressants may lessen meningism and obscure other traditionally helpful clues. Third, multiple pathogens may be present simultaneously or sequentially.

Three important differences in management principles distinguish the immunocompromised group from nonimmunocompromised patients with CNS infection. First, the threshold for obtaining CSF for examination is much lower.

TABLE 110-8. Central Nervous System Infection and Specific Host Immunity Deficit

DEFICIT	PATHOGEN	CLINICAL SYNDROMES°
Defective cell-mediated immunity	*Listeria monocytogenes*	AM, CM, E
	Nocardia asteroides	AM, CM, M
	Cryptococcus neoformans	CM, M
	Aspergillus species	M, AM
	Papovavirus JC	E
	Toxoplasma gondii	E, M
	Herpesvirus group	E
Neutropenia	*Pseudomonas aeruginosa*	AM
	Candida species	CM, AM, M, E
	Aspergillus species	AM, M
	Phycomycoses	M, AM
Defective humoral immunity (splenectomy)	*Streptococcus pneumoniae*	AM
	Haemophilus influenzae	AM
	Neisseria meningitidis	AM

°AM, acute meningitis; CM, chronic meningitis; M, mass lesion; E, encephalitis.

Clinical findings are often more subtle because of the moderating effect of neutropenia and reduced inflammation caused by the disease or its treatment. A slight change in personality or persistent headache or back pain in the presence of unexplained fever may thus be sufficient justification for a lumbar puncture. Second, immunocompromised patients deserve earlier use of diagnostic modalities directed at detecting mass lesions. Reduced inflammation because of the disease or its treatment renders the clinical clues suggesting mass effect less reliable. Also, many of the unusual pathogens associated with immunocompromised patients are characterized by mass formation (e.g., *Nocardia* species, phycomycoses, *Toxoplasma*, *Aspergillus* species, tuberculosis). Indications for a brain scan, CT scan, or MRI are thus not necessarily limited to patients with focal neurologic signs but should also be considered in slow responders. Unfortunately, these tests are less effective when edema and inflammation are reduced, and they may need to be repeated frequently. Third, empirical antibiotic therapy often invites multiple rather than single agents to accommodate the uncertainty associated with a large group of potential pathogens and to ensure adequate coverage of gram-negative pathogens.

Patients with acquired immunodeficiency syndrome (AIDS) have a high incidence of neurologic complications, including infection.[47] Approximately 95% of patients have abnormal CNS findings at autopsy. A partial listing of CNS infections in AIDS patients is presented in Table 110-9. Because of the subtleties of early presentation, clinicians should consider early lumbar puncture and CT in patients with suggestive findings. A majority of patients with AIDS may have AIDS encephalopathy. Progressive intellectual and motor dysfunction eventually lead to global dementia and severe motor deficits. Evidence is mounting that the AIDS encephalopathy syndrome is caused by direct infection by the human immunodeficiency virus (HIV) rather than one of the candidate etiologies commonly associated with AIDS (cytomegalovirus, herpesvirus).[48] Noninfectious causes of

CNS abnormality include Kaposi's sarcoma, primary CNS lymphoma, and vascular myelopathy.

A practical approach to the immunocompromised host with suspected CNS infection is to first take an inventory of other concurrent sites of infection. Seeding from these sites occurs more frequently in the presence of lowered host resistance. Pulmonary tuberculosis may be an important clue to the etiology of meningitis; a pathogen responsible for bacterial endocarditis may have seeded the meninges and *Candida* sepsis indicates particular susceptibility to this pathogen and may be the harbinger or sequela of *Candida* meningitis. Next, examination of the CSF should be accomplished. Spuriously low pleocytosis may be expected in neutropenic patients. Whether or not to perform a CT scan of the head first depends on clinical judgment, presence of focal neurologic deficits, and availability. If preliminary CSF

TABLE 110-9. Central Nervous System Infection in AIDS Patients

Toxoplasma gondii
Cytomegalovirus
Fungal abscesses
    Candida species
    Aspergillus species
    Cryptococcus neoformans
Varicella-zoster virus
Herpes simplex virus
Mycobacterium tuberculosis
Atypical *mycobacterium* species
Progressive multifocal encephalopathy
Cryptococcal meningitis
Aseptic meningitis
Viral transverse myelitis
Human immunodeficiency virus
Syphilis

tests suggest a particular pathogen, specific coverage for that pathogen should be instituted. Because a second unsuspected pathogen may be present in the immunocompromised patient, an additional spectrum-broadening agent should be employed until culture results are known. Third-generation cephalosporins have found particular utility in this clinical setting.[49] A reasonable initial regimen is the combination of ampicillin and cefotaxime. If a remote focus of infection with *Pseudomonas* species is present or other clinical clues suggest this pathogen, an intrathecal aminoglycoside should be given until the etiologic agents are identified.

GRAM-NEGATIVE ROD MENINGITIS

Gram-negative rods are the fourth most common cause of bacterial meningitis, and the incidence of GNR meningitis has been increasing in the last two decades.[50] Mortality rate has declined from a high of 40% to 80% to 10% to 20% with the introduction of third-generation cephalosporins. Risk factors for GNR meningitis are primarily those associated with a breach of the anatomic barriers for the CNS. Cranial trauma and neurosurgical complications account for the majority of cases: 60% to 70% of postneurosurgical meningitis is caused by GNRs. Other risk factors are congenital dermal sinuses to the CNS and conditions predisposing to gram-negative bacteremias, such as pyelonephritis, diabetes, urinary tract infection, and immunosuppression. *Escherichia coli* and *Klebsiella pneumoniae* account for two thirds of the reported cases.[51] Virtually any GNR has the potential to produce meningitis, and most have been reported to do so. Clinical manifestations and CSF findings are not distinctive and are generally identical with those found in other types of bacterial meningitis. Gram stain of the CSF is somewhat less efficient, with 60% to 70% positive. Counterimmuno-electrophoresis and latex fixation tests for detecting antigens are more valuable in GNR meningitis. Limulus lysate assay may be of particular value in GNR meningitis because high sensitivity has been reported.

Management of GNR meningitis has been compromised by the poor penetration into CSF of antibiotics useful for gram-negative rods. Thus, aminoglycosides have limited usefulness when given peripherally, although they may be critical in the management of concurrent gram-negative sepsis. To obtain useful CSF levels, intrathecal or intraventricular injections are required. Direct instillation of aminoglycosides into ventricular reservoirs may improve outcome by placing the antibiotic in the region of the invariably present ventriculitis. The technique of intrathecal or intrareservoir instillation of aminoglycosides is not without difficulty. Patient acceptance has been poor and arachnoiditis is not uncommon. If the organism is known to be sensitive to chloramphenicol, ampicillin, or third-generation cephalosporins, these become the drugs of choice. Empirically, however, these agents should not be relied on because many pathogens will be resistant. Only 30% of GNRs causing meningitis are sensitive to ampicillin. Chloramphenicol is bacteriostatic and thus theoretically less acceptable in GNR meningitis. For patients with GNR meningitis, third-generation cephalosporins such as cefotaxime have been shown to be very effective when *Pseudomonas aeruginosa* and *Acinetobacter calcoaceticus* are not involved. Ceftazidime may be more useful in the management of *P aeruginosa* infections. Sulfamethoxazole and trimethoprim achieve useful penetration into the CSF and, when sensitive organisms are recovered, may be a second-choice consideration.[52]

CENTRAL NERVOUS SYSTEM MANIFESTATIONS OF TUBERCULOSIS

Tuberculosis of the CNS is a rare infection in the United States. Therefore, unfortunate delays often occur in the recognition and treatment of those few cases. Clinical forms of CNS tuberculosis include acute tuberculous meningitis, tuberculoma, and tuberculous spondylitis (Pott disease).[53] Patients at risk are those with AIDS, the elderly in nursing homes, and patients with intercurrent conditions that compromise cell-mediated immunity (e.g., malignancy, certain viral infections, and chronic abuse of drugs, including alcohol). Evidence of tuberculosis is often found elsewhere in the body, but 40% of patients with tuberculous meningitis have no other evidence of disease. This finding is more common in children than in adults. Tuberculin skin tests may be falsely negative in a significant minority of patients and are therefore of little use in excluding the diagnosis. Cerebrospinal fluid in tuberculous meningitis characteristically is lymphocytic, with fewer than 500 cells/mm^3 in 80% of cases. The remainder have between 500 and 1500 cells/mm^3. Acid-fast bacilli are not commonly present on single-stained specimens of the CSF, but repeated examinations from serial spinal taps dramatically improve the diagnostic yield to over 75% of proven cases. Protein is elevated and glucose reduced in the typical case. Treatment for tuberculous meningitis should be initiated when the disease is suspected, because proof that *M tuberculosis* is present may require weeks of culture. Isoniazid and rifampin both penetrate the CSF and, used together, are the treatment of choice for tuberculous CNS disease.

PARTIALLY TREATED BACTERIAL MENINGITIS

Patients with bacterial meningitis often have a "viral" prodrome and many have been started on antibiotics prior to clinical manifestations of meningeal irritation. Partial treatment commonly confuses the diagnostic picture and requires special management. If the duration of prior antibiotic therapy exceeds 24 hours, interference with Gram stains and culture should be expected. Other CSF parameters, such as protein, glucose, and cell count, are not generally affected by a brief course of oral antibiotics. Patients presenting with a history of prior treatment and signs suggesting meningeal irritation should have a lumbar puncture performed. If a purulent CSF is detected, empirical parenteral antibiotic therapy should be instituted. With a nondiagnostic CSF with a very low pleocytosis or near-normal glucose, the clinician may elect to withhold antibiotic therapy and repeat the lumbar puncture after an interval of approximately 12 hours or sooner if clinical deterioration occurs.

CHRONIC MENINGITIS

Chronic meningitis may be caused by a broad array of infectious and noninfectious etiologies (Table 110-10).[54] This broad syndrome is said to exist when meningeal signs occur in the presence of persistent CSF abnormalities for at least 4 weeks. The patient's history is particularly valuable in determining the etiology of chronic meningitis. Careful inquiry for past neurologic disease or signs suggesting vasculitis, toxin exposure, or other epidemiologic clues is necessary. Careful attention to the history of compromised host status, other known systemic disease, and travel history provides valuable information.

VIRAL MENINGOENCEPHALITIS

With fewer than 4300 cases reported to the Center for Disease Control and Prevention (CDC) each year, viral meningoencephalitis is an uncommon infection. However, this statistic probably underestimates the true incidence because of inefficient reporting. Often, mild cases are unrecognized or mistaken for noninfectious diseases such as toxic or metabolic encephalopathies.

Arboviruses are the most common cause of encephalitis in the United States, accounting for 10% to 50% of all reported cases. All are vectored by mosquitoes or ticks and therefore show typical seasonality with summer epidemics (Table 110-11). The mortality rate varies with age and with the specific virus. St. Louis encephalitis has a 20% mortality rate in persons over age 50. California equine encephalitis and western equine encephalitis have the lowest mortality rate (2%) and a high incidence of mild or unapparent infection. Eastern equine encephalitis has an abrupt onset and fulminant course, with mortality rates in the 50% to 60% range. Neurologic sequelae are common in survivors.

Other viruses are uncommon causes of encephalitis. Enteroviruses are a common cause of aseptic meningitis but an uncommon cause of encephalitis, accounting for only 2% of reported cases. Other causes are Epstein–Barr virus and cytomegalovirus, the latter being common in patients with AIDS. Parainfectious encephalitis is a noninfectious inflammation of the brain that is presumed to be due to a delayed hypersensitivity reaction. Clinical signs are identical

TABLE 110-11. Etiologies of Viral Meningoencephalitis

AGENT	SEASONAL OCCURRENCE	MORTALITY RATES (%)
Arboviruses		
Eastern equine	Summer	50–60
St. Louis	Summer	5–20
Western equine	Summer	2–3
California	Summer	2–3
Others		
Enteroviruses*	Summer/fall	Rare
Cytomegalovirus	All year	
Epstein-Barr	All year	Rare
Mumps virus	Winter/spring	Rare
Human immunodeficiency virus		

*Echovirus, coxsackievirus, poliomyelitis virus.

Centers for Disease Control: Encephalitis surveillance, 1978.

with infectious encephalitis and follow the inciting vaccination or viral infection by 4 to 14 days.[55]

Most patients with encephalitis have concurrent meningeal involvement. Alterations of mental status with fever, nuchal rigidity, and headache are characteristic presenting signs. Epidemiologic history and presenting signs provide important clues to diagnosis. State health authorities should be contacted to determine patterns of disease in the area. Cerebrospinal fluid typically shows a low cell count with lymphocytic predominance, normal glucose, and elevated protein. Definitive diagnosis depends on viral culture and paired serologies. With the exception of herpesvirus encephalitis (discussed earlier) there is no available therapy for viral meningoencephalitis other than supportive and rehabilitative care.

REFERENCES ■

1. Behrman RE, Meyers BR, Mendelson MH, et al: Central nervous system infections in the elderly. *Arch Intern Med* 1989;149:1596
2. Spagnuolo PJ, Elnor JJ, Lerner PI, et al: Hemophilus influenzae meningitis: the spectrum of disease in adults. *Medicine* 1982;61:741
3. Veeder MH, Folds JD, Yount WJ, et al: Recurrent bacterial meningitis associated with C8 and IgA deficiency. *J Infect Dis* 1981;144:399
4. Fijen CA, Kuijper EJ, Tjia HG, et al: Complement deficiency predisposes for meningitis due to nongroupable meningococci and Neisseria related bacteria. *Clin Infect Dis* 1994;18:780
5. Boor V, Paulson OB, Rasmussen N: Pneumococcal meningitis: late neurologic sequelae and features of prognostic impact. *Arch Neurol* 1984;41:1045
6. Phister HW, Feiden W, Einhaupl KM: Spectrum of complications during bacterial meningitis in adults. Results of a prospective clinical study. *Arch Neurol* 1993;50:575
7. Durand ML, Calderwood SB, Weber DJ, et al: Acute bacterial meningitis in adults. A review of 493 episodes. *N Engl J Med* 1993;328:21

TABLE 110-10. Etiologies of Chronic Meningitis

INFECTIOUS CAUSES	NONINFECTIOUS CAUSES
Mycobacterium tuberculosis	Meningeal carcinomatosis
Cryptococcus neoformans	Vasculitis
Nocardia asteroides	Sarcoidosis
Coccidioides immitus	Systemic lupus erythematosus
Histoplasma capsulatum	Behçet disease
Treponema pallidum	Mollaret meningitis
Candida species	Heavy metal poisoning
Aspergillus species	Toxin exposure
Toxoplasma gondii	
Human immunodeficiency virus	

8. Unhanand M, Mustafa MM, McCracken GHJ, et al: Gram-negative enteric bacillary meningitis: a twenty-one-year experience. *J Peds* 1993;122:15

9. Chapelon C, Ziza JM, Piette JC, et al: Neurosarcoidosis: signs, course and treatment in 35 confirmed cases. *Medicine* 1990; 69:261

10. Baker AS, Ojemann RG, Swartz MN, et al: Spinal epidural abscess. *N Engl J Med* 1975;293:463

11. Calthman DM, Caplan JG, Littman N: Infectious agents in spinal epidural abscesses. *Neurology* 1980;30:844

12. Riska E: Spinal tuberculosis treated by antituberculous chemotherapy and radical operation. *Clin Orthop* 1976;119:148

13. Hlavin ML, Kaminski HJ, Fenstermaker RA, et al: Intracranial suppuration: a modern decade of postoperative subdural empyema and epidural abscess. *Neurosurgery* 1994;34:974

14. Bannister G, Williams B, Smith S: Treatment of subdural empyema. *J Neurosurg* 1970;32:35

15. Yang SY, Zhao CS: Review of 140 patients with brain abscess. *Surg Neurol* 1993;39:290

16. Kaplan K: Brain abscess. *Med Clin North Am* 1985;69:345

17. Whelan MA, Hilal SK: Computed tomography as a guide in the diagnosis and followup of brain abscess. *Radiology* 1980; 135:663

18. Yang SY, Zhao CS. Review of 140 patients with brain abscess. *Surg Neurol* 1993;39:290

19. Sjolin J, Lilja A, Eriksson N, et al: Treatment of brain abscess with cefotaxime and metronidazole: prospective study on 15 consecutive patients. Clin Infect Dis 1993;17:857

20. Jensen AG, Espersen F, Skinhoj P, et al: Staphylococcus aresus meningitis: a review of 104 nationwide, consecutive cases. *Arch Intern Med* 1993;153:1902

21. Whitley RJ, Soong SJ, Linnemann C, et al: Herpes simplex encephalitis: clinical assessment. *JAMA* 1982;274:317

22. Marton KI, Jean AD: The spinal tap: a new look at an old test. *Ann Intern Med* 1986;104:840

23. Conley JM, Ronald AR: Cerebrospinal fluid as a diagnostic body fluid. *Am J Med* 1983; 75:102

24. Maxson S, Lewno MJ, Schutze GE: Clinical usefulness of cerebrospinal fluid bacterial antigen studies. *J Peds* 1994;18:91

25. McGinnis MR: Detection of fungi in the CSF. *Am J Med* 1983;28:129

26. Kennedy DH, Fallon RJ: Tuberculous meningitis. *JAMA* 1979;241:264

27. Sarwar M, Falcof G, Naseem M: Radiologic techniques in the diagnosis of CNS infections. *Neurol Clin* 1986;4:41

28. Neu PFJ, Davis KRI: The role of CT scanning in diagnosis of infections of the CNS. *Curr Top Clin Infect Dis* 1980;1:21

29. McCabe WR: Empiric therapy for bacterial meningitis. *Rev Infect Dis* 1983;5:S74

30. Tauber MG, Sande MA: Principles in the treatment of bacterial meningitis. *Am J Med* 1984;76:224

31. Cherubin CE, Corrado M, Nair SR, et al: Treatment of gram negative bacillary meningitis: role of the new cephalosporin antibiotics. *Rev Infect Dis* 1982;4:S453

32. Stevenson KB, Murray EW, Sarubbi FA: Enterococcal meningitis: report of four cases and review. *Clin Infect Dis* 1994; 18:233

33. Brown LW, Feigin RD: Bacterial meningitis: fluid balance andtherapy. *Pediatr Ann* 1994;23:82

34. Havens PL, Wendelberger KJ, Hoffman GM, et al: Corticosteroids as adjunctive therapy in bacterial meningitis: a meta-analysis of clinical trials. *Am J Dis Child* 1989;143:1051

35. Schaad UB, Lips U, Gbehm HE, et al: Dexamethasone therapy for bacterial meningitis in children. *Lancet* 1993;342:457

36. Fleming DW, Cochi SL, Hull HF, et al: Prevention of Hemophilus influenzae infections in day care: a public health prospective. *Rev Infect Dis* 1986;8:568

37. Cuevas LE, Hart CA: Chemoprophylaxis of bacterial meningitis. *J Antimicrob Chemother* 1993;31(Suppl B):79

38. Update: Prevention of *Hemophilus influenzae* type B disease. *MMWR* 1986;35:170

39. Wenger JD: Impact of Haemophilus influenzae type b vaccines on the epidemiology of bacterial menigitis. *Infect Agents Dis* 1993;2:324

40. Hodges GR, Perkins RL: Hospital associated bacterial meningitis. *Am J Med Sci* 1976;271:335

41. Aucoin PJ, Kotilainen HR, Gonz NM, et al: Intracranial pressure monitors: epidemiologic study of risk factors and infections. *Am J Med* 1986;80:369

42. Sell SH: Longterm sequelae of bacterial meningitis in children. *Pediatr Infect Dis* 1983;2:90

43. Phister HW, Feiden W, Einhaupl KM: Spectrum of complications during bacterial meningitis in adults. Results of a prospective clinical study. Arch Neurol 1993;50:575

44. Hooper DC, Pruitt AA, Rubin RH: CNS infection in the chronically immunosuppressed. *Medicine* 1982;61:166

45. Levy RM, Bredesen DE, Rosenbloom ML: Neurological manifestations of AIDS: experience at UCSF and review of the literature. *J Neurosurg* 1985;62:475

46. Price RW, Bradford AN, Eun-sook C: AIDS encephalopathy. *Neurol Clin* 1986;4:285

47. Cherubin CE, Eng RHK: Experience with the use of cefotaxime in the treatment of bacterial meningitis. *Am J Med* 1986;80:398

48. Cherubin CE, Mar JS, Sierra MF, et al: Listeria and gram negative bacillary meningitis in New York City, 1972–1979: frequent cases of meningitis in adults. *Am J Med* 1981;71: 199

49. Landesmann SH, Cherubin CE, Corado ML: Gram negative bacillary meningitis: new therapy and changing concepts. *Arch Intern Med* 1982;142:939

50. Levitz RE, Quintaliani R: Trimethoprim sulfamethoxazole for bacterial meningitis. *Ann Intern Med* 1984;100:881

51. Sheller JR, Desprez RM: CNS tuberculosis. *Neurol Clin* 1986; 4:143

52. Ellner JJ, Bennett JE: Chronic meningitis. *Medicine* 1976;55: 341

53. Kennard C, Swash M: Acute viral encephalitis: its diagnosis and outcome. *Brain* 1981;104:129

54. Ellner JJ, Bennett JE: Chronic meningitis. *Medicine* 1976;55:341

55. Kennard C, Swash M: Acute viral encephalitis: its diagnosis and outcome. *Brain* 1981;104:129

Critical Care, Third Edition, edited by Joseph M. Civetta,
Robert W. Taylor, and Robert R. Kirby.
Lippincott-Raven Publishers, Philadelphia, PA © 1997.

CHAPTER 111

Urinary Tract Infections

Mark E. Appleman
Richard E. Winn

IMMEDIATE CONCERNS

MAJOR PROBLEMS

Urinary tract infections (UTIs) occur frequently in intensive care unit (ICU) patients. These infections range from incidental findings on admission to life-threatening pyelonephritis with gram-negative sepsis and shock. Hospitalized non-ICU patients with UTIs have increased mortality compared with hospitalized patients without UTI. A similar increase in mortality has not been found in ICU patients.[1] The reasons for this observation are not clear. This chapter examines the following conditions as they relate to the ICU: symptomatic and asymptomatic uncomplicated cystitis, pyelonephritis with its attendant complications, indwelling catheter-related issues, and bacterial and fungal nosocomial infections.

STRESS POINTS

1. Many ICU patients have asymptomatic bacteriuria.
2. *Escherichia coli* is the most common microbial cause of UTI.
3. Pyelonephritis is characterized by bacterial invasion of the renal interstitium resulting in an acute inflammatory response and suppurative necrosis.
4. The most common mechanism of acquiring pyelonephritis is by the ascending route.
5. Functional or mechanical obstruction of urine flow is a major predisposing risk factor for pyelonephritis.
6. Patients with pyelonephritis are almost always febrile, often with a temperature above 40°C (104°F).
7. Acute focal bacterial nephritis is defined as a renal mass caused by an acute focal parenchymal infection without the formation of pus.

8. If left untreated, acute focal bacterial nephritis progresses to renal abscess.
9. Perinephric abscess is defined as a collection of purulent material material located between the kidney and Gerota's fascia.
10. Pyonephrosis implies an obstructed urinary tract filled with pus.
11. Acute papillary necrosis is a condition that is seen only in severe bacterial interstitial nephritis.
12. Acute bacterial prostatitis can be severe and may lead to septic shock.
13. Approximately 80% of nosocomial UTIs are caused by urinary catheters.
14. The presence of yeast (*Candida* sp and *Torulopsis glabrata*) in the urine is common in ICU patients.

ESSENTIAL DIAGNOSTIC TESTS AND PROCEDURES

1. The urine Gram stain result is probably the most important clue in tentatively identifying the suspected pathogen.
2. Urine culture colony counts of more than 10^5 microorganisms per milliliter are usually significant.
3. Significantly lower colony counts may be important in patients with urinary catheters.
4. Antibody-coated bacteria tests are relatively specific for upper tract disease.
5. Excretory urography, ultrasonography, and computed tomography (CT) scans may demonstrate hydronephrosis, acute focal parenchymal nephritis, renal and perinephric abscess, and acute papillary necrosis.

INITIAL THERAPY

1. Several key factors must be considered in choosing antimicrobial agents for treatment of UTIs, including the suspected pathogens, epidemiology, hospital antibiotic resistance patterns, the antibiotic's potential adverse effects, costs, pharmacokinetics, and spectrum of activity of specific antibiotics.
2. The effectiveness of therapy can be reassessed clinically and by repeating the urine Gram stain 24 hours after the institution of therapy.
3. Acute focal bacterial nephritis often resolves with antibiotic therapy alone.
4. Renal abscesses and perinephric abscesses should be drained. This can often be accomplished percutaneously.
5. Percutaneous nephrostomy is the preferred initial treatment for pyonephrosis.
6. Removal of the urinary catheter, amphotericin B bladder washes, and fluconazole are used to treat funguria.

CYSTITIS

The presence of bacteria in the urine requires differentiating between asymptomatic bacteriuria and a true UTI. Many patients admitted to the ICU have asymptomatic bacteriuria as an incidental finding. This is particularly common in the elderly, in whom pyuria may be absent.[2] The presence of pyuria may have more to do with the technique of analysis in the laboratory. Pyuria is defined as the presence of ten or more leukocytes per high-power field in a urine sediment. Bacteriuria is found in about 10% of elderly men and 20% of women living at home; it can be found in up to 25% of patients in nursing homes. Hospitalized elderly patients have an even higher probability of acquiring bacteriuria or true infection.[3] This increased risk occurs even when urinary catheterization is not done. Many patients in the ICU have urinary catheters for at least some period of time, further increasing the risk of infection.[4]

Most authorities consider urine culture colony counts of more than 10^5 microorganisms per milliliter to be significant, that is, a high likelihood of a true infection being present. In an asymptomatic patient, this colony count has an 80% chance of being a true infection. If a repeated culture yields the same results, the probability increases to 95%.[5] Significantly lower colony counts may be important in patients with urinary catheters.

E coli is the most common microbial cause of UTI, although in older patients it is less common than in young women. A 20% incidence rate of resistance to ampicillin may be expected in community-acquired infections with *E coli*.[6] Infections with gram-positive organisms are most commonly caused by coagulase-negative staphylococci in young women (*Staphylococcus saprophyticus*), but in older patients of both sexes enterococci are more likely to be present. *Staphylococcus aureus* accounts for only about 1% of all UTIs and is most common in elderly men who have had urinary tract manipulations.[7]

Symptomatic UTIs require antimicrobial therapy, and commonly an empiric regimen is necessary pending the results of the urine culture. The urine Gram stain may be helpful and should be performed routinely. Female patients with cystitis alone may be treated with single-dose oral therapy with 3.0 g amoxicillin, or trimethoprim-sulfamethoxazole (two double-strength tablets), provided that none of the following conditions exists: renal stones, prior infections with resistant organisms, and known urologic abnormalities (including urinary catheters). Three days of oral therapy may be more effective than the single-dose regimen. Treatment of immunocompromised patients or those with complicated UTI depends on the physician's clinical judgment. Choices range from oral ampicillin, fluoroquinolones, or trimethoprim-sulfamethoxazole to intravenous therapy with a third-generation β-lactam antimicrobial, or the latter combined with an aminoglycoside. Patients requiring intravenous antimicrobial drugs should have blood cultures done before therapy is started. If single-dose therapy is given, a urine culture should be repeated in 48 to 72 hours; if infection persists, more prolonged therapy is indicated.

Asymptomatic UTIs should be confirmed with a repeat culture before treatment. In general, antimicrobial therapy is not indicated because these infections tend to be benign and there is a high incidence of recurrence after therapy; in addition, older patients have a higher incidence of adverse drug reactions.[3] However, ICU physicians must consider each case carefully. Immunocompromised patients should receive treatment.

PYELONEPHRITIS

Pyelonephritis is characterized by bacterial invasion of the renal interstitium resulting in an acute inflammatory response and suppurative necrosis. Pathologically, multiple areas of suppurative inflammation in the parenchyma, which are well demarcated from surrounding areas of uninvolved kidney, are seen. The areas of inflammation may be discrete focal abscesses or large, wedge-shaped areas of coalescent suppuration.[8]

PATHOPHYSIOLOGY

The most common mechanism of acquiring pyelonephritis is by the ascending route.[9] Bacteria enter the urethra and migrate to the bladder and then to the kidneys. The renal medulla seems to have a greater susceptibility to infection than does the cortex because of impaired leukocyte function secondary to hypertonicity. Ascending bacteria can cause infection in the kidney after they reach the renal pelvis and medulla. Bacterial seeding of the renal cortex also may occur by the hematogenous route during bacteremia, but in experimental models this seems to occur only in the presence of renal outflow obstruction. The hematogenous route is considered less important in the pathogenesis of pyelonephritis. Prior renal damage secondary to trauma, ischemia, or analgesic abuse predisposes the kidney to infection. Functional or mechanical obstruction of urine flow is a major predisposing risk factor for pyelonephritis. Obstruction results in disruption of the normal peristaltic activity of the ureters, preventing the urine from "washing away" the bacteria. Functional obstruction can be induced by some gram-negative bacterial toxins that seem to cause decreased peristalsis.

Anatomic defects such as a diverticulum also may predispose to infection. Microbial factors have a major role in the development of pyelonephritis. Some motile bacteria can ascend in the ureters despite normal peristaltic activity and urine flow. Specific strains of gram-negative bacilli can cause pyelonephritis, whereas other strains of the same species cannot. These pyelonephritogenic strains have been best studied using *E coli* and produce virulence factors that can increase resistance to the bactericidal activity of serum, increase bacterial adherence to uroepithelial cells, and cause hemolysin activity.[5] Host defense factors[10] include peristalsis and urine flow in the ureters, intrinsic bactericidal activity of the urine, and the production of IgM and IgA antibodies secreted into the urine during upper tract infection. The actual importance of this humoral immunity is not clear. Other host factors such as advanced age, alcoholism, diabetes mellitus, and malignancy also predispose to infection.

MICROBIOLOGY

Gram-negative bacilli cause most cases of pyelonephritis; *E coli* leads the list. However, an elderly man or woman with a history of multiple UTIs is less likely to have an *E coli* infection than is an otherwise healthy young woman. *Proteus mirabilis, Klebsiella pneumoniae, Enterobacter, Serratia, Pseudomonas aeruginosa,* and *Citrobacter* all are common causes of pyelonephritis. Anaerobic bacteria are distinctly unusual and should not be considered in empiric therapy except in unusual circumstances. Coagulase-negative *Staphylococcus* is a common cause of cystitis but is uncommon in pyelonephritis, and most gram-positive infections are caused by an enterococcus, *Enterococcus faecalis. S aureus,* a rare cause of cystitis, is a rarer cause of pyelonephritis, but it can cause a secondary bacteremia.[7] Most cases of *S aureus* bacteriuria in toxic patients are secondary to bacteremia from another source (e.g., an infected central intravenous catheter or endocarditis).

DIAGNOSIS

The diagnosis of pyelonephritis is usually not difficult, particularly in a young woman. Patients are almost always febrile, often with a temperature above 40°C (104°F); they frequently appear "toxic" and complain of flank or low back pain. Nausea and vomiting, chills or rigors, and dysuria are frequently present. Some patients, especially the elderly, may be asymptomatic or have nonspecific complaints.[11] Abdominal ileus may occur, but peritoneal signs are unusual. Other conditions such as renal infarction can mimic pyelonephritis.

A marked leukocytosis is common, although with sepsis the leukocyte count may be low with a significant shift toward immature cells. The blood urea nitrogen and creatinine values are normal unless shock or underlying renal disease is present. Urinalysis most frequently reveals pyuria and bacteriuria; white blood cell casts indicate upper tract infection.[12-14] Elderly patients may have an entirely normal urine sediment.[15] Complete ureteral obstruction of the affected kidney also may result in a normal urinalysis. The urine culture usually reveals the causative organism, but, in one study of bacteremia secondary to UTI, 19% of patients had fewer than 10^5 organisms on culture.[16] The laboratory should be alerted to identify any isolated organisms when pyelonephritis is suspected.

In the ICU, pyelonephritis can usually be diagnosed with little difficulty. Ureteral catheterization can definitively prove the diagnosis but may be difficult and time consuming, especially in a critically ill patient. Antibody-coated bacteria tests are relatively specific for upper tract disease but are available only at specialized laboratories and have not been standardized. Contrast studies (e.g., excretory urograms) are not helpful in diagnosing acute pyelonephritis; ultrasonography and CT scans also are nonspecific. Gallium scans are abnormal but cannot be interpreted until 48 to 72 hours after injection. Indium 111–labeled autologous leukocyte scans are more helpful.[17] Renal scanning with technetium 99-DMSA (^{99}Tc-DMSA) is sensitive for pyelonephritis and shows a specific pattern of striated or flare-diminished renal uptake.[17] In addition, it is readily available and requires little time to perform. Thus, in a critically ill patient in whom the diagnosis of pyelonephritis is suspected but not proven, the ^{99}Tc-DMSA study is the preferred procedure.

UROSEPSIS

Bacteremia with or without sepsis is the most serious immediate sequela of acute pyelonephritis. This condition is commonly referred to as urosepsis, although the actual definition of this term is "sepsis resulting from the decomposition of extravasated urine."[18] Pyelonephritis is the leading cause of bacteremia in elderly patients admitted to community hospitals.[19] A 5-year study of community-acquired bacteremia reveals that 21% were secondary to UTIs, and the overall mortality rate in these patients was 4.8%.[20] Ten percent of patients presented in shock; this group had a 32% mortality rate compared with 1.8% for those not in shock. The initial empiric antibiotic regimen selected had no effect on the patient's outcome, whether or not it was appropriate. In a larger study of gram-negative bacteremia, this was reaffirmed, although appropriate therapy begun after the results of the blood cultures clearly improved survival.[21]

TREATMENT

The patient admitted to the ICU for a UTI is often seriously ill and requires aggressive empiric antibiotic therapy. Although the physician should keep in mind Bryan and Reynolds' data[20] that the initial empiric antimicrobial regimen has no effect on prognosis, it seems reasonable that using the proper drugs initially for a serious infection should be beneficial. Several key factors must be considered in choosing the antimicrobial agents: suspected pathogens, epidemiology, hospital antibiotic resistance patterns, potential adverse effects, costs, pharmacokinetics, and spectrum of activity of specific antibiotics. These factors are considered in turn.

The use of the urine Gram stain is probably the most important clue in tentatively identifying the suspected pathogen. A drop of unspun urine is allowed to air dry on a slide, then is heat fixed and Gram stained. The presence of a single organism per high-power field correlates with greater than 10^5 colonies of bacterial microorganisms per milliliter in the urine. Also, one should be able to distinguish between gram-negative rods as a group, gram-positive cocci in chains (enterococcus) or clusters (*Staphylococcus* sp.), and yeast.

The setting in which the infection occurs is important in determining both the possible pathogen and its likely susceptibilities. A previously healthy young female patient is most likely to be infected with *E coli*, whereas a hospitalized elderly patient could have one of many pathogens present.

Knowing antibiotic resistance patterns for bacterial microorganisms in each hospital is important; these are usually summarized monthly or yearly by the microbiology laboratory or infection control service. Physicians should have this information available. There may be considerable variation in the susceptibility of an organism to a particular antimicrobial from one hospital to another (e.g., *P aeruginosa* to the aminoglycosides). Up to 20% of community-acquired *E coli* infections are resistant to ampicillin, and 30% of hospital-acquired strains are resistant to ampicillin and cefazolin; 20% to 30% of hospital-acquired *K pneumoniae* organisms are resistant to cefazolin.[6]

Potential adverse effects of antimicrobial agents must be considered, including drug allergies. Penicillins such as carbenicillin and ticarcillin, including ticarcillin-clavulanate, have a high sodium content and might be unsuitable in a patient with severe heart failure. Third-generation cephalosporins may cause coagulopathies; most are not clinically significant. Trimethoprim-sulfamethoxazole is associated with leukopenia and may not be appropriate in an already neutropenic cancer patient.

The third-generation cephalosporins and penicillins are considerably more expensive than ampicillin, as is vancomycin compared with oxacillin. However, one should always opt for the most appropriate drug; cost must be a secondary consideration. Likewise, pharmacokinetics are less likely to be important in the initial regimen (except in the case of renal or liver failure), because the commonly used drugs all attain excellent serum and urine levels.

Knowledge of the antimicrobial spectrum of activity against the common urinary tract pathogens is crucial.[22] Of the penicillins, ampicillin is the most commonly used and the least expensive. Because of increasing resistance, it cannot be relied on for treatment of most gram-negative bacteria, and its use empirically in the ICU should be limited to suspected enterococcal infections. Carbenicillin and ticarcillin have essentially been replaced with newer penicillins such as azlocillin, mezlocillin, and piperacillin, which have a much wider spectrum of activity and significantly lower sodium content. These antimicrobial agents are effective against most gram-negative bacteria, including *P aeruginosa*. In vitro, piperacillin seems to be best for this organism, although the difference may not be clinically important. These antimicrobial drugs are also good against enterococci, but not *S aureus*. Imipenem is also a good choice because coverage against *Pseudomonas* is excellent. Alternatively, aztreo-

nam may be considered and is particularly useful when penicillin allergy is present or renal dysfunction is a concern mitigating against aminoglycosides. The development of resistance also has markedly diminished the role of first-generation cephalosporins. Second-generation drugs such as cefamandole and cefuroxime have somewhat better gram-negative coverage against *E coli* or *K pneumoniae* and are probably adequate initial coverage for *S aureus*. However, they have no activity against enterococci. The third-generation cephalosporins have broad-spectrum activity against gram-negative bacteria but are not reliable against *S aureus* and enterococci. Ceftazidime and cefoperazone are active against *P aeruginosa*, with the former having better in vitro data. Aztreonam has a spectrum of activity similar to ceftazidime but seems to be safe in patients with significant allergies to β-lactam antibiotics.[23]

The aminoglycosides are excellent antimicrobial agents in ICU patients, despite the risks of ototoxicity and nephrotoxicity. In most cases, they should not be used alone, especially with enterococci or *P aeruginosa*. Considerable variation in susceptibility within this group may exist among hospitals, but in general gentamicin remains commonly effective and significantly less expensive.

Trimethoprim-sulfamethoxazole also has an excellent spectrum of activity and is useful in patients with penicillin allergies. It is not effective against *P aeruginosa* and enterococci. Imipenem has extremely broad coverage against gram-negative and gram-positive organisms and should cover essentially all potential urinary tract pathogens. However, the drug is expensive, and some concerns have been raised about its ability to induce bacterial resistance.

Quinolone agents such as ofloxacin and ciprofloxacin have excellent activity against gram-negative organisms, but they are only borderline against enterococci and *S aureus*. Ciprofloxacin is more active for *P aeruginosa* infections than ofloxacin, but there may be considerable resistance to these agents in individual hospitals.

If the urine Gram stain suggests an enterococcal infection, appropriate therapy is ampicillin or piperacillin combined with an aminoglycoside. In the penicillin-allergic patient, vancomycin may be substituted. If *S aureus* infection is strongly suspected, oxacillin or nafcillin alone or combined with an aminoglycoside is effective. If this organism is considered a somewhat less likely pathogen, cefuroxime is reasonable therapy. Gram-negative bacilli seen on Gram stain are somewhat less helpful because a specific organism cannot be identified. The antibiotic regimen chosen depends on the clinical circumstances but in general includes either piperacillin-mezlocillin or a third-generation cephalosporin coupled with an aminoglycoside. Trimethoprim-sulfamethoxazole along with gentamicin is an excellent choice for a community-acquired infection. If *P aeruginosa* infection is strongly suspected, the cephalosporin used should be ceftazidime or cefoperazone. If the urine Gram stain does not reveal an organism, the combination of piperacillin and an aminoglycoside is best because it is effective against enterococci as well.

Although some authorities use single-drug therapy, we believe that the critically ill ICU patient should receive an aminoglycoside also in the empiric regimen. If the patient is less critically ill and not immunocompromised, single-drug therapy might be considered.

The effectiveness of therapy can be reassessed clinically and by repeating the urine Gram stain in 24 hours. No organisms should be seen, and the culture should be negative. If bacteria are still present, the antimicrobial agents might need to be adjusted pending the initial culture results. After the organism has been identified and susceptibilities are available, a cheaper or less toxic drug should be substituted if possible. If the patient has improved considerably, the aminoglycoside also might be withdrawn at this time. However, enterococci and *P aeruginosa* infections do considerably better with the synergy provided by an aminoglycoside. Ten to 14 days of intravenous antibiotics for pyelonephritis are usually recommended, but, if the patient has had a prompt clinical response, switching to an appropriate oral antibiotic after 5 to 7 days of therapy is acceptable.

COMPLICATIONS

The patient with uncomplicated pyelonephritis should show a definite clinical response within 72 hours after the initiation of appropriate antimicrobial therapy; most patients are better in 48 hours. If the patient has not improved considerably or certainly if the patient's course deteriorates, it is highly probable that one or more complications exist, and further diagnostic evaluation is required. In addition, any patient who has had recurrent infections, is a male patient, or has abnormal renal function requires evaluation, even if there is clinical improvement.

Uncomplicated pyelonephritis is a focal suppurative process in the renal parenchyma. As the disease progresses, a spectrum of conditions may occur, from acute focal bacterial nephritis to renal abscess to perinephric abscess. Other complications are pyonephrosis and acute papillary necrosis. Clinically, these conditions are indistinguishable.

Acute Focal Bacterial Nephritis

Acute focal bacterial nephritis, also called *acute lobar nephronia*, is defined as a renal mass caused by an acute focal parenchymal infection without the formation of pus (liquefaction). It can mimic a renal abscess or tumor, but unlike these conditions it resolves completely with antimicrobial agents alone.

Although acute pyelonephritis is a focal process, radiologic studies do not demonstrate a discrete lesion. In acute focal bacterial nephritis, a definite mass is present. Ultrasonography has excellent sensitivity and is usually specific for this condition; CT scans are specific but not as sensitive.[24] The sensitivity of the excretory urogram is variable, ranging from 100%[25] to 56%,[24] and abnormal findings are nonspecific and require further evaluation.

Occasionally, renal abscess and acute focal bacterial nephritis cannot be distinguished; therefore, a diagnostic percutaneous aspiration is required. In the latter condition, no pus is obtained. The treatment of acute focal bacterial nephritis is antimicrobial agents and time. If the diagnosis is certain and the patient clinically improves, further imaging studies are not necessary.[24]

Renal Abscess

If untreated, acute focal bacterial nephritis progresses to central liquefaction, resulting in the formation of an abscess (or carbuncle). In the past, most renal abscesses were believed to be secondary to hematogenous seeding of the kidney during a bacteremia, usually with *S aureus*. Such infections currently represent a much lower percentage of cases, and most are caused by gram-negative rods that infect the kidney by the ascending route.

Excretory urograms show a mass or filling defect in most cases but are not specific for renal abscess. Ultrasound and CT scans are highly sensitive; in most instances, the findings are suggestive but not diagnostic of an abscess, and therefore diagnostic percutaneous aspiration is necessary. This is performed with the aid of CT or ultrasound guidance through a flank (posterior) approach and is a safe procedure. The finding of pus establishes the diagnosis.

Medical therapy with antimicrobial agents alone may cure some patients with renal abscess, even in the presence of large lesions.[26] However, the presence of calculi in the same kidney invariably requires surgery. Percutaneous drainage of the abscess is the safest and most economical initial therapy.[24,27] A pigtail or trocar catheter is inserted into the abscess cavity, usually at the same time the diagnostic tap is done, and left in place for drainage. The urologist should be consulted before treatment in the event of complications, but these are unusual. Even if loculation of the abscess is visible on scans, this treatment may be successful. Patients usually respond with defervescence within 1 to 2 days, and if no response has occurred by 3 days, a repeat CT scan should be obtained. Drainage usually lasts 10 to 14 days, and the catheter can be removed 1 to 2 days later, after a follow-up scan has been done to ensure adequate drainage. If there is a strong contraindication for a percutaneous procedure, it may be reasonable to continue to treat the patient with antimicrobial agents and close observation alone, recognizing that a certain percentage of these patients develop perinephric extension.

Perinephric Abscess

Perinephric abscess is defined as a collection of purulent material located primarily in the area between the kidney and Gerota's fascia, although it may extend a considerable distance. In a study done before CT scanners were available, almost two thirds of the patients had a palpable abdominal or flank mass, and 80% of the patients with positive blood cultures died.[28] The mortality rate in a more recent study was still 27%; thus, aggressive management is crucial.[29]

Excretory urograms are frequently abnormal but nonspecific. Ultrasonography results may be nonspecific, and the full extent of disease is often not well described. CT is the most sensitive procedure available but also may be nonspecific.[27]

Treatment for perinephric abscess is the same as that for a renal abscess—percutaneous drainage. However, a perinephric abscess cannot be treated with antibiotics alone, and affected patients require frequent reevaluation in light of the high mortality rate.

Pyonephrosis

In the presence of obstruction of the renal outflow tract, dilatation of the collecting system occurs. When this system is filled with pus, it is called pyonephrosis. Patients with this condition are at increased risk for extension of the infection into the perinephric tissues.[30] Excretory urograms reveal urinary obstruction, and CT scanning reveals a dilated renal pelvis, which may be diagnostic if layering of contrast dye above the purulent fluid is seen. Ultrasonography is probably the best test, revealing the dilated renal pelvis along with low-level internal echoes.[24] If any of these studies suggests the presence of hydronephrosis in a patient not responding to therapy, the diagnosis of pyonephrosis must be excluded. This is done by antegrade pyelography, which is performed similarly to a percutaneous aspiration. If purulent urine is obtained, the diagnosis is confirmed.

Percutaneous nephrostomy is the preferred treatment and involves placing a drain in the renal pelvis. The clinical response is usually prompt, and most patients become afebrile within 24 hours. However, unlike percutaneous drainage of renal abscesses, significant morbidity can occur from this procedure, with up to 9% of patients developing septic or hemorrhagic shock.[30] The drainage tube remains in place until the underlying cause of obstruction (50% are secondary to stones) is corrected.

Acute Papillary Necrosis

Acute papillary necrosis is a condition that is seen only in severe bacterial interstitial nephritis. Patients may fail to respond to antimicrobial therapy or may deteriorate into shock. The urine may be sterile at this stage, although pyuria and fragments of sloughed papillae may be seen. It is usually a bilateral condition, which can result in anuria secondary to ureteral obstruction from sloughed papillae or azotemia from loss of nephrons. The diagnosis is best made with excretory urograms and nephrotomograms showing haziness or ulceration of papillae or sinus formation. Treatment is directed toward the bacterial infection and support of the cardiovascular status. This condition should be suspected in a diabetic patient who deteriorates despite therapy.

DIAGNOSTIC APPROACH

In each of the aforementioned conditions, the different diagnostic procedures have varying degrees of sensitivity and specificity. Nuclear resonance imaging is not specific and probably has little role in evaluating these patients. Excretory urograms are best for identifying acute papillary necrosis and defining the anatomy of the lower urinary tract (ureters and bladder) but lack specificity for the other conditions. Ultrasonography is best for identifying pyonephrosis, and CT scanning is best for renal and perinephric abscesses. Because some concern has been raised about the sensitivity of the excretory urogram, we favor a modification of the approach suggested by Zaontz and others.[25] All patients unresponsive to antimicrobial therapy after 72 hours should undergo an excretory urogram with nephrotomograms. This should be immediately followed by a CT scan, whether or not the urogram result is normal. This identifies all of the potential renal inflammatory conditions with minimum contrast injection and in a short time. If contrast material is contraindicated, an ultrasound study should be obtained.

PROSTATITIS ■

Acute bacterial prostatitis can be severe and lead to septic shock. Patients often complain of low back and perineal pain, along with symptoms of bladder irritability and varying degrees of outflow obstruction. Rigors are common, and patients seem to be in severe distress. Rectal examination reveals a swollen, boggy, and extremely tender prostate. Prostatic massage should not be performed because of the risk of potential bacteremia. Urine culture does not always reveal the responsible organism, which is a gram-negative rod in most cases; 80% are caused by *E coli*.[31] Treatment for prostatitis is similar to that for acute pyelonephritis. If urinary retention occurs, suprapubic needle aspiration of the bladder is preferred over urethral catheterization.

NOSOCOMIAL INFECTIONS ■

Nosocomial UTIs are common and potentially serious problems in the ICU. Approximately 80% of nosocomial UTIs are caused by urinary catheters.[32,33] By definition, these infections are considered "complicated" (the presence of an abnormality in the urinary outflow tract) and are often not properly managed. By the tenth day of catheterization, 50% of patients have a UTI.[34] In general, ICU patients have the same risk of acquiring these infections as do other patients.[34] It has been found that 40% of UTIs could have been prevented if the catheter had been removed at the appropriate time and that more than one third of the total catheterization days were unnecessary.[35]

Using the usual cutoff point of more than 10^5 organisms to define a UTI is not appropriate in the catheterized patient. *Any* amount of bacteria in a cultured urine specimen will progress to more than 10^5 organisms, usually within 3 days.[36] The microbiology laboratory must be made aware of the importance of identifying any bacteria present in amounts equal to or greater than 10^2 in a patient with a urinary catheter.

Eighty-four percent of nosocomial UTIs are caused by gram-negative rods, with *E coli* causing less than 50% of these.[32] *Proteus, Klebsiella, Pseudomonas, Enterobacter,* and *Serratia* are the other most common isolates. Most gram-positive infections are caused by enterococci, followed by coagulase-negative staphylococci and *S aureus;* the latter causes less than 2% of nosocomial UTIs.[37]

Of importance to the ICU physician is that between 1% and 4% of patients with these infections get a secondary bacteremia.[32,37,38] *Serratia* and *Klebsiella* are the two organisms most often responsible and, along with *P aeruginosa,* have the highest mortality rate.[32] A study of 221 bacteremias secondary to nosocomial UTIs reveals an overall direct mortality rate of 12.7%; all deaths occurred in patients with chronic or progressive underlying disease.[38] If shock was present, the mortality rate was 35%. Thus, although many patients with asymptomatic nosocomial UTIs do not need antimicrobial therapy, those in an ICU usually often need aggressive treatment.

Nosocomial catheter-related UTIs are common in chronically instrumented patients, particularly those with spinal cord injuries.[39–42] It is critically important that strictly maintained closed systems be used. Catheters should be changed at reasonable intervals, at least 30 days. This is important in nursing home patients as well. Urinary asepsis occasionally can be maintained by using urinary acidification techniques. Dysuria limits this method in those with normal sensation; however, in those with spinal cord injury, urine pH can be reduced to minimize bacterial and fungal growth. Mandelamine or hippurate with ascorbic acid can be titrated to low pH; patients need to be informed about dysuria from the therapy so they do not think the method is failing. When dysuria occurs, the dose of medication can be reduced while maintaining the lowered pH. When true infection occurs, antimicrobial agents can be used intercurrently with reinstitution of preventatives after resolution of infection.[43]

FUNGAL INFECTIONS ■

The presence of yeast in the urine is a relatively common finding in hospitalized patients, particularly in those in the ICU for any prolonged period.[44] These infections are often a source of considerable debate as to their importance and proper therapy. Most are caused by members of the genus *Candida*, along with *T glabrata*. Several factors place a patient at risk for developing candiduria: antibiotic therapy, presence of a Foley catheter, especially for more than 10 days, diabetes mellitus, cirrhosis, steroids or other immunosuppressants, and an abnormal genitourinary anatomy. In general, the presence of low levels (less than 10,000 colonies/mL) of yeast is not significant. However, in the ICU, these patients should be closely watched and the urine recultured. Colony counts of over 10,000 organisms strongly suggest candidiasis, and patients require therapy if the diagnosis is confirmed on subsequent culture.[45]

It is often difficult to localize the site of the yeast infection in the urinary tract, but this is critical in determining the appropriate therapy. Testing for antibody coating is not helpful because it is positive in both upper and lower tract disease. Clinical signs and symptoms are also nonspecific. Excretory urograms can identify a fungus ball if present (upper tract disease). Serum precipitins to the yeast may become positive in renal disease and are used by some clinicians to make therapeutic decisions.[46] However, others believe that the high incidence of false-negative results and a borderline acceptable specificity make this test less helpful.[47] The presence of pseudohyphae in the urine as being an indicator of tissue invasion is not universally accepted.

Asymptomatic patients with no predisposing factors for candiduria or patients in whom the risk factors can be modified (e.g., removing the catheter) have a benign prognosis and need not be treated; few patients in the ICU fall into this category. Symptomatic patients and those at high risk for dissemination should have an excretory urogram to look for fungus balls or obstruction and can then be treated in one of several ways. A triple-lumen catheter can be placed into the bladder and amphotericin B instilled for 5 to 7 days. This can be either a continuous irrigation with 15 mg in 1 L of 5% dextrose in water solution or recurrent boluses of 200 to 300 mL of the same solution, clamping the catheter for 60 to 90 minutes. The latter method has the theoretic advantage of treating the bladder more uniformly. If funguria persists, systemic amphotericin B therapy is indicated. Alternatively, oral flucytosine (5-FC) or fluconazole can be given.[48] 5-FC is well absorbed orally and excreted unchanged in the urine. However, a significant percentage of *Candida* isolates are resistant to 5-FC, and therefore susceptibility testing should be done first. If bone marrow production is impaired or there is renal dysfunction, 5-FC should be used with caution and with measurement of blood levels. In addition, drug resistance can develop during therapy. Therapy is continued for 1 week after cultures are negative.[46] Ketoconazole is no longer indicated for UTI. A newer agent, fluconazole, does reach therapeutic levels in urine and avoids the potential renal toxicity of amphotericin B. This may be of critical importance in treating fungal UTI in renal transplant patients.

If systemic candidiasis is present or renal involvement is strongly suspected, systemic therapy with amphotericin B, with or without 5-FC, is indicated. However, some cases of renal candidiasis can be successfully treated with a prolonged course of 5-FC alone[47] or fluconazole. Some strains of *Candida* exhibit resistance to fluconazole, including *T glabrata*.

REFERENCES ■

1. Fagon JY, Novara A, Stephan F, et al: Mortality attributable to nosocomial infections in the ICU. *Infect Cont Hosp Epidemiol* 1994;15:428
2. Baldassarre JS, Kaye D: Special problems of urinary tract infection in the elderly. *Med Clin North Am* 1991;75:375
3. Kaye D: Urinary tract infections in the elderly. *Bull NY Acad Med* 1980;56:209
4. Stamm WE: Catheter-associated urinary tract infections: epidemiology, pathogenesis, and prevention. *Am J Med* 1991; 91:65S
5. Sobel JD, Kaye D: Urinary tract infections. In: Mandell GL, Douglas RG, Bennett JE (eds). *Principles and Practice of Infectious Diseases*. New York, John Wiley & Sons, 1990:582
6. Neu HC: The emergence of bacterial resistance and its influence on empiric therapy. *Rev Infect Dis* 1983;5(Suppl):S9
7. Demuth PJ, Gerding DN, Crossley K: *Staphylococcus aureus* bacteriuria. *Arch Intern Med* 1979;139:78
8. Robbins SS, Cotran RS, Kumar V: *Pathologic Basis of Disease*. Philadelphia, WB Saunders, 1984:1032
9. Sobel JD: Bacterial etiologic agents in the pathogenesis of urinary tract infection. *Med Clin North Am* 1991;75:253
10. Measley RE Jr, Levison ME: Host defense mechanisms in the pathogenesis of urinary tract infection. *Med Clin North Am* 1991;75:275
11. Nicolle LE: Urinary tract infection in the elderly. *J Antimicrobiol Chemther* 1994;33:S99

12. Blaufox MD: Current concepts in the diagnosis of urinary tract infection. *Curr Opinion Neprol Hyper* 1994;3:629

13. Pappas PG: Laboratory in the diagnosis and management of urinary tract infections. *Med Clin North Am* 1991;75:313

14. Sodeman TM: A practical strategy for diagnosis of urinary tract infections. *Contemp Issues Clin Microbiol* 1995;15:235

15. Yoshikawa TT, Norman DC: Treatment of infections in elderly patients. *Med Clin North Am* 1995;79:651

16. Strand CL, Bryant JK, Sutton KH: Septicemia secondary to urinary tract infections with colony counts less than 10^5 CFU/ml. *Am J Clin Pathol* 1985;83:619

17. Handmaker H: Nuclear renal imaging in acute pyelonephritis. *Semin Nucl Med* 1982;12:246

18. *Stedman's Medical Dictionary*. Baltimore, Williams & Wilkins, 1982:1522

19. Esposito AL, Gleckman RA, Cram S, et al: Community-acquired bacteremia in the elderly: an analysis of one hundred consecutive episodes. *J Am Geriatr Soc* 1980;28:315

20. Bryan CS, Reynolds KL: Community-acquired bacteremic urinary tract infection: epidemiology and outcome. *J Urol* 1984;132:490

21. Bryan CS, Reynolds KL, Brenner CR: Analysis of 1186 episodes of gram-negative bacteremia in non-university hospitals: the effects of antimicrobial therapy. *Rev Infect Dis* 1983;5:629

22. Kim ED, Schaeffer AJ: Antimicrobial therapy for urinary tract infections. *Sem Nephrol* 1994;14:551

23. Stamm WE, Hooton TM: Management of urinary tract infections in adults. *N Engl J Med* 1993;329:1328

24. Kuligowska E, Newman B, White SJ, et al: Interventional ultrasound in detection and treatment of renal inflammatory disease. *Radiology* 1983;147:521

25. Zaontz MR, Pahira JJ, Wolfman M, et al: Acute focal bacterial nephritis: a systematic approach to diagnosis and treatment. *J Urol* 1985;133:752

26. Hoverman IV, Gentry LO, Jones DW, et al: Intrarenal abscess: report of 14 cases. *Arch Intern Med* 1980;140:914

27. Gerzof SG, Gale ME: Computed tomography and ultrasonography for diagnosis and treatment of renal and retroperitoneal abscesses. *Urol Clin North Am* 1982;9:185

28. Thorley JD, Jones SR, Sanford JP: Perinephric abscess. *Medicine* 1974;53:441

29. Bova JG, Potter JL, Arevalos E, et al: Renal and perirenal infection: the role of computerized tomography. *J Urol* 1985;133:375

30. Yoder IC, Lindfors KK, Pfister RC: Diagnosis and treatment of pyonephrosis. *Radiol Clin North Am* 1984;22:407

31. Meares EM: Prostatitis: a review. *Urol Clin North Am* 1975;2:3

32. Stamm WE, Martin SM, Bennett JV: Epidemiology of nosocomial infections due to gram-negative bacilli: aspects relevant to development and use of vaccines. *J Infect Dis* 1977;136 (Suppl):S151

33. Warren JW: The catheter and urinary tract infection. *Med Clin North Am* 1991;75:481

34. Garibaldi RA, Burke JP, Dickman ML, et al: Factors predisposing to bacteriuria during indwelling urethral catheterization. *N Engl J Med* 1974;291:215

35. Hartstein AI, Garber SB, Ward TT, et al: Nosocomial urinary tract infection: a prospective evaluation of 108 catheterized patients. *Infect Control* 1981;2:380

36. Stark RP, Maki DG: Bacteriuria in the catheterized patient: what quantitative level of bacteriuria is relevant? *N Engl J Med* 1984;311:560

37. Krieger JN, Kaiser DL, Wenzel RP: Urinary tract etiology of bloodstream infections in hospitalized patients. *J Infect Dis* 1983;148:57

38. Bryan CS, Reynolds KL: Hospital-acquired bacteremic urinary tract infection: epidemiology and outcome. *J Urol* 1984;132:494

39. Kamitsuka PF: The pathogenesis, prevention and management of urinary tract infection in patients with spinal cord injury. *Curr Clin Top Infect Dis* 1993;13:1

40. Cardenas DD, Hooton TM: Urinary tract infection in persons with spinal cord injury. *Arch Phys Med Rehab* 1995;76:272

41. Stover SL, Lloyd LK, Waites KB, et al: Neurogenic urinary tract infection. *Neurol Clin* 1991;9:741

42. Perkash I: Long-term urologic management of the patient with spinal cord injury. *Urol Clin North Am* 1993;20:423

43. Carson CC III: Antimicrobial agents in urinary tract infections in patients with spinal cord injury. *Urol Clin North Am* 1993;20:443

44. Wong-Beringer A, Jacobs RA, Guglielmo BJ: Treatment of funguria. *JAMA* 1992;267:2780

45. Goldberg PK, Kozinn PJ, Wise GJ, et al: Incidence and significance of candiduria. *JAMA* 1979;241:582

46. Janosko EO, McRoberts JW: Evaluation and treatment of urinary candidiasis. *South Med J* 1979;72:1578

47. Fisher JF, Chew WH, Shadomy S, et al: Urinary tract infections due to *Candida albicans*. *Rev Infect Dis* 1982;4:1107

48. Voss A, Meis JF, Hoogkamp-Korstanje JA: Fluconazole in the management of fungal urinary tract infection. *Infection* 1994;22:247

Critical Care, Third Edition, edited by Joseph M. Civetta,
Robert W. Taylor, and Robert R. Kirby.
Lippincott-Raven Publishers, Philadelphia, PA © 1997.

CHAPTER 112

Bacterial Infections

Judith R. Anderson
Ferric C. Fang

Bacterial infections are among the leading causes of morbidity and mortality in the intensive care unit.[1] Patients may be admitted with bacterial infections or acquire infections while in the ICU. Infections that develop in the ICU are among the most difficult to treat because they are often caused by organisms resistant to most antimicrobial agents. The nosocomial pathogens most commonly encountered in the ICU are Gram-negative bacilli and staphylococci; these agents are responsible for many additional days of hospitalization and substantial increases in the cost of treatment. Many nosocomial infections can be avoided by proper aseptic technique, isolation procedures, and good handwashing practices (see Chap. 106).

This chapter presents a survey of bacterial infections that may be encountered by the intensive care specialist. Infections are grouped by organism to facilitate exposition; common pathogens are described in greater detail. Bacterial infections specific to the immunocompromised patient are discussed in Chapter 108. Table 112-1 outlines bacterial organisms most often encountered in critical care settings.

STAPHYLOCOCCUS AUREUS ■

There are more than 20 species of the genus *Staphylococcus* now recognized.[2] These organisms are Gram-positive, non-motile cocci occurring singly or in pairs, tetrads, clusters, and occasionally short chains. They are easily recovered on conventional culture media. *S aureus* colonies may appear gray-white, pale yellow, or golden, and most strains are β-hemolytic. *S aureus* produces coagulase, which is helpful in identification since it is the only *Staphylococcus* of clinical importance possessing this characteristic. A rapid test for bound coagulase is useful for preliminary identification, but

the more reliable detection of free coagulase may take 18 to 24 hours. Most coagulase-negative staphylococci (e.g., *Staphylococcus epidermidis*) have white colonies and are non-hemolytic on blood agar. *Staphylococcus saprophyticus* may be pigmented, and is presumptively identified by its resistance to novobiocin.

STAPHYLOCOCCAL BACTEREMIA

Staphylococcus aureus bacteremia usually arises from an obvious local source, commonly a skin or soft tissue infection, trauma, operative wound, or intravascular line. It also occurs frequently in intravenous drug abusers. Occasionally, *S aureus* bacteremia complicates pneumonia or osteomyelitis. Trivial skin infections may result in bacteremia and sometimes a source is never found, particularly in children, elderly adults, and immunocompromised hosts. In these instances, the possibility of endocarditis must be strongly entertained. Affected patients are often acutely ill, with high fever, chills, and marked leukocytosis; others present with symptoms principally referable to localized foci of infection, such as osteomyelitis or septic arthritis.

Removal of contaminated lines, surgical removal of suppurated veins, or drainage of abscesses should be performed in addition to the prompt institution of antimicrobial therapy. Removal of infected prosthetic devices such as orthopedic pins or nails, prosthetic joints or heart valves, and ventricular shunts should be performed in the vast majority of cases. Anticoagulation should be strongly considered for septic central vein thrombophlebitis.[3]

A major dilemma in the management of some patients is the distinction between transient bacteremia and endocarditis. A full discussion of this issue may be found in Chapter 120. In general, endocarditis is less likely if an obvious re-

TABLE 112-1. Pathogenic Bacteria Encountered in Critical Care Settings

AEROBIC BACTERIA	Pasteurella
	Pseudomonads
Gram-positive Cocci	P aeruginosa
Staphylococci	P (Burkholderia) cepacia
S aureus	Stenotrophomonas
Coagulase-Negative	maltophilia
Staphylococci	Vibrionaceae
Streptococci	Aeromonas
S pyogenes (group A)	Plesiomonas
S agalactiae (group B)	Vibrio cholerae
S pneumoniae	Halophilic Vibrios
viridans Streptococci	
S milleri/intermedius	**ANAEROBIC BACTERIA**
group	
Enterococci	*Gram-positive Cocci*
	Gram-negative Cocci
Gram-negative Cocci	*Gram-positive Bacilli*
Moraxella catarrhalis	Actinomyces
Neisseria	Clostridia
N meningitidis	C botulinum
N gonorrhoeae	C difficile
	C perfringens
Gram-positive Bacilli	C tetani
Bacillus	Other
B anthracis	Propionibacterium acnes
Other	
Corynebacteria	*Gram-negative Bacilli*
C diphtheriae	Bacterioides
C jeikeium	Fusobacterium
Other	Pigmented anaerobic bacilli
Listeria	
Nocardia	**MISCELLANEOUS BACTERIA**
	Bartonella (Rochalimaea)
Gram-negative Bacilli	Capnocytophaga
Acinetobacter	Chlamydia
Campylobacter	Mycobacteria
C fetus ssp. fetus	M avium-intracellulare
C jejuni	M kansasii
Helicobacter	M tuberculosis
Enterobacteriaceae	Mycoplasma
Enterobacter	Rickettsia
Escherichia	Coxiella burnetii
Klebsiella	Ehrlichia
Proteus	R prowazekii
Salmonella	R rickettsii
Shigella	Spirochetes
Yersinia	Borrelia
Other	Leptospira
Flavobacterium	Treponema
Francisella	
HACEK Organisms	
Haemophilus influenzae	
Other	
Legionella	

movable source of bacteremia is identified and there is no evidence of abnormal heart valves, circulating immune complexes, metastatic foci of infection, or a history of intravenous drug abuse.[4] Hospital acquisition and a low intensity or brief duration of *S aureus* bacteremia also make endocarditis less likely. If endocarditis cannot be excluded with confidence, treatment for presumed endocarditis would be prudent.[5]

STAPHYLOCOCCAL ENDOCARDITIS

Recent data indicate that *S aureus* is responsible for approximately one quarter of native valve endocarditis,[6] and generally presents as an acute process with high fever and chills (see Chap. 120). A heart murmur or the classic signs of subacute endocarditis may be absent. Central nervous system complications occur in about 25% of patients, and metastatic involvement of joints, brain, kidney, spleen, pericardium, bone, or lung is seen in nearly 50% of cases. Careful frequent auscultation is indicated because a murmur may develop during the course of treatment. Although a normal echocardiogram does not rule-out infective endocarditis, demonstration of vegetations can help to confirm the diagnosis and correlates with a somewhat higher incidence of adverse events such as emboli, valvular disruption, and congestive heart failure. Transesophageal echocardiography (TEE) is more sensitive than transthoracic echocardiography for the detection of valvular vegetations.[7]

Annular myocardial abscesses are particularly serious complications of infective endocarditis. Serial electrocardiograms (ECGs) or cardiac monitoring should be considered, although conduction disturbances are neither sensitive nor completely specific for the presence of perivalvular extension. Transesophageal echocardiography appears to be the most sensitive method of detecting a perivalvular abscess.[8] Pulmonary findings such as pleural friction rub or effusion are often seen in right-sided endocarditis, and chest radiographs may reveal multiple pulmonary infiltrates or cavitary nodular lesions. Renal involvement may include infarction, perinephric abscess, pyelonephritis, or glomerulonephritis resulting from immune complex deposition. Acute renal failure from glomerulonephritis usually resolves on antimicrobial therapy in this setting, although recovery may take several months.

Staphylococcus aureus is the predominant pathogen causing endocarditis in intravenous drug abusers. The tricuspid valve is most frequently involved, but other valves may be involved as well. Patients with *S aureus* endocarditis often fail to defervesce immediately upon initiation of treatment, but usually are afebrile by the end of the first week. Persistent fever warrants a search for an extravalvular focus of infection, such as splenic or perivalvular abscess.

Staphylococcus aureus is responsible for 10% to 20% of prosthetic valve endocarditis. The diagnosis of early prosthetic valve endocarditis (within the first 2 months after surgery) may be confounded by the presence of concomitant pneumonia or urinary tract infection. New or changing murmurs are highly suspicious findings, but are not invariably present. New conduction abnormalities, shock, or peripheral embolic signs are only present in a minority of patients. The presentation of late prosthetic valve endocarditis closely resembles that of native valve endocarditis.

In all types of staphylococcal endocarditis, blood cultures are nearly always positive. Arterial blood cultures offer no advantage over venous samples, even when right-sided endocarditis is suspected.

The preferred treatment of *S aureus* native valve endocarditis consists of nafcillin or oxacillin, 2 g intravenously (IV) every 4 hours. Cefazolin 1 g IV every 6 hours may be used in penicillin-allergic patients. Vancomycin 1 g IV every 12 hours may be used in patients allergic to both penicillins and cephalosporins, but is probably somewhat inferior in activity.[9] Standard treatment duration is a minimum of 4 weeks. Recent studies suggest that 2 weeks of nafcillin or oxacillin plus an aminoglycoside are effective in carefully selected intravenous drug abusers with isolated right-sided *S aureus* endocarditis who lack evidence of hemodynamic compromise, left-sided emboli, extravalvular foci, large (>2 cm) vegetations, or a delayed (>96 hours) response to therapy.[10] Valve replacement is indicated for patients whose cardiac function deteriorates despite appropriate antimicrobial therapy. It has also been recommended for patients with recurrent systemic emboli, uncontrolled septicemia, or cardiac abscesses.[11]

Staphylococcus aureus prosthetic valve endocarditis should be treated with nafcillin or oxacillin for 6 to 8 weeks, and the addition of an aminoglycoside during the first 2 weeks of therapy should be considered.[12] Early valve replacement is advocated by many authorities, and most patients with staphylococcal prosthetic valve endocarditis ultimately require valve replacement for complete resolution of infection. Anticoagulant therapy should be continued in patients whose prosthetic valves require anticoagulation.

TOXIC SHOCK SYNDROME

Although toxic shock syndrome (TSS) was first described in children, it became the focus of public attention in 1980 when cases involving young menstruating women were reported. Tampon use was implicated and a higher incidence was seen with high-absorbency products. The majority of TSS cases still occur in young menstruating women but cases are also seen in both men and women with staphylococcal surgical wound and other skin infections, pulmonary infections, osteomyelitis, and various other non-tampon-related conditions.[13]

Staphylococcus aureus is the etiologic agent in classic TSS, although a similar clinical syndrome may occur in association with group A streptococcal (*Streptococcus pyogenes*) infections (see later). Vaginal *S aureus* isolation rates exceed 90% in menstruating women with TSS. Specific phage types of *S aureus* (types 1, 29, 52) are more frequently isolated. Elaboration of bacterial exotoxins in hosts lacking protective antibody is believed to be responsible for the characteristic systemic manifestations of the syndrome. The onset of illness is usually acute, with high fevers, chills, nausea, vomiting, diarrhea, and myalgias. A diffuse blanching erythema is seen over the trunk, and conjunctival injection and oropharyngeal hyperemia are present. Syncope, confusion, hypotension, renal failure, and thrombocytopenia occur as the illness progresses. More than 50% of patients have an elevated serum creatinine, and approximately half have leukocytosis and elevated liver enzymes. Other laboratory findings may include hypocalcemia and an elevated serum creatine kinase.

Toxic shock syndrome should be considered in any illness of sudden onset characterized by multisystem involvement in a menstruating woman or patient with recent surgery, skin infection, abscess, or other suspected staphylococcal infection. Women suspected of having TSS should have a pelvic examination; tampons should be removed and cultured and vaginal and cervical cultures should be obtained. Cultures from blood and infected sites should be obtained from any patient with symptoms suggesting TSS. Aggressive fluid replacement and antistaphylococcal antimicrobial therapy such as oxacillin, nafcillin, or cefazolin should be administered as soon as appropriate cultures are obtained. Vancomycin can be used in patients allergic to penicillin. Suppurative foci should be drained. Patients may require the entire spectrum of intensive care, including ventilatory support, vasopressors, and hemodynamic monitoring. Renal failure, severe thrombocytopenia, digital gangrene, respiratory distress syndrome (RDS), and cardiac complications may occur. Desquamation of palms and soles, usually beginning around the nails, is characteristically seen during the recovery period.

The use of antibiotics during TSS reduces the rate of recurrence, as does discontinuation of tampon use. Although patients with TSS may not develop antibodies to staphylococcal toxin, recurrences seem to be clinically milder than the original episode.

STAPHYLOCOCCAL PNEUMONIA

Although about 80% of the adult population carry *S aureus* in their upper respiratory tracts at some time during their lives (most often in the anterior nares and posterior pharynx), community acquired *S aureus* pneumonia is not particularly common except in certain circumstances (see Chap. 124). It can be seen following or concomitant with influenza, in intravenous drug abusers with septic phlebitis or endocarditis, and in dialysis patients with shunt infections. Hospitalized patients following aspiration or intubation, patients with intravascular line sepsis, children, elderly patients, and patients with cystic fibrosis or bronchiectasis are also at increased risk for *S aureus* pneumonia.

The clinical presentation typically consists of high fever, chills, productive cough, dyspnea, and chest pain. In a patient with antecedent influenza, an abrupt respiratory deterioration may be noted as *S aureus* infection supervenes. Patients with hematogenous *S aureus* pneumonia generally have predominantly constitutional symptoms referable to the septicemia, and multiple pulmonary infiltrates on the chest radiograph are often the first indication of lung involvement.

The roentgenographic findings vary from multiple small nodules or patchy infiltrates to isolated consolidation or rapidly cavitating disease. Pneumatocoeles are commonly seen in children. Pleural effusions are common, and empyemas, which tend to loculate, are seen in about 10% of cases.

Isolation of *S aureus* from blood cultures or pleural fluid is the most definitive diagnostic test, but therapy must often be initiated on the basis of the sputum Gram stain. High-risk patients with increased sputum polymorphonuclear cells and Gram-positive cocci in clusters should receive empiric antistaphylococcal treatment until a definitive diagnosis is made. A positive sputum culture without predominance of staphylococci on Gram stain is more difficult to interpret, since many individuals may asymptomatically harbor *S aureus* in their upper respiratory tract.

STAPHYLOCOCCAL MENINGITIS

Although *S aureus* is not a common cause of meningitis, it can occasionally cause meningitis in persons with sinusitis, bacteremia, endocarditis, or brain abscess. It is most frequently seen in the setting of neurosurgery or trauma, including patients with placement of intraventricular shunts (see Chap. 110). Although staphylococcal endocarditis and bacteremia can be treated with first-generation cephalosporins in penicillin-allergic patients, staphylococcal meningitis cannot be treated in this manner because of the poor penetration of these agents into cerebrospinal fluid (CSF). Nafcillin or oxacillin, 2 g IV every 4 hours, should be used. If the organism is methicillin-resistant or the patient is allergic to penicillin, vancomycin 1 g IV every 12 hours should be used with monitoring of serum and CSF levels. In certain instances, the addition of rifampin or intrathecal vancomycin may be beneficial.

STAPHYLOCOCCAL PERICARDITIS

Purulent pericarditis can be hematogenous, resulting from bacteremia associated with septic phlebitis, endocarditis, or infected vascular catheters. Pericarditis may also result from chest trauma, surgery, or a contiguous focus of infection such as myocardial abscess, osteomyelitis, or mediastinitis. Clinical suspicion of purulent pericarditis should be aroused when any patient with one of the aforementioned risk factors deteriorates hemodynamically, develops a pericardial friction rub, or is noted to have an increasing cardiac silhouette on chest radiograph or other signs of pericardial effusion. Immediate evaluation by echocardiogram is mandatory. Aspiration or open drainage is required in addition to antistaphylococcal antibiotics. Pericardial stripping may be indicated.

STAPHYLOCOCCAL ORBITAL CELLULITIS

Orbital cellulitis in adults may result from contiguous infection involving the sinuses or following surgery or trauma. The presentation is characterized by orbital pain and swelling and erythema of the eyelid. Fever, rhinorrhea, headache, and proptosis are followed by conjunctival inflammation, chemosis, and in extreme cases, panophthalmitis. Progressive pain, ophthalmoplegia, and increased intraocular pressure are seen. It is important to distinguish orbital cellulitis from the less serious condition of preseptal cellulitis, involving only the space anterior to the orbital septum.[14] In preseptal cellulitis, signs of orbital disease (e.g., proptosis, ophthalmoplegia, visual loss) are not present.

Unless the etiology of the infection is obvious (e.g., a foreign body), sinus studies should be obtained. Computed tomography (CT) scanning is useful in demonstrating the extent of orbital involvement as well as associated sinus abnormalities. The involved sinus should be drained and cultured and blood cultures should be obtained. *S aureus* is the most common cause of orbital cellulitis in older children and adults. Antistaphylococcal therapy, such as nafcillin or oxacillin, 2 g IV every 4 hours, or cefazolin, 1 g IV every 6 to 8 hours, should be used. If other organisms are suspected, or in children where *Haemophilus influenzae* is a possibility, a third-generation cephalosporin such as cefotaxime may be added. *H influenzae* has previously been the most common cause of orbital cellulitis in young children, although the efficacy of the HIB vaccine has significantly reduced the incidence of this condition.

STAPHYLOCOCCAL OSTEOMYELITIS

Staphylococcus aureus is the most common cause of hematogenous osteomyelitis in adults and older children. It is frequently associated with staphylococcal infections of the skin, bacteremia, antecedent trauma, or IV drug abuse. The axial skeleton is most commonly affected. Symptoms may be restricted to localized pain and low-grade fever or may be more severe. Palpation or percussion over the affected area—typically a vertebral body—may cause an intensification of pain. Bone radiographs are not helpful in acute osteomyelitis but bone scans are usually abnormal. Magnetic resonance (MR) imaging may demonstrate marrow edema.[15] The erythrocyte sedimentation rate (ESR) is generally elevated and blood cultures may be positive. The suspected area of involvement should be aspirated or a bone biopsy should be obtained for culture. In all cases of vertebral osteomyelitis, serial neurologic examinations are indicated for early detection of cord compression from an associated epidural abscess. This complication generally requires expeditious surgical exploration, although some epidural abscesses without neurologic compromise may resolve with medical therapy alone.[16] Antistaphylococcal therapy such as nafcillin or oxacillin, 2 g IV every 4 hours, should be administered. Vancomycin may be substituted if methicillin-resistant *S aureus* (MRSA) is involved or if the patient is intolerant to penicillins. Therapy should be continued for 6 weeks or longer, depending upon the response.

Staphylococcus aureus is a major pathogen in postoperative osteomyelitis as well. Management depends upon the nature of the operative procedure, presence of foreign bodies, vascular supply, and stability of the union. Staphylococcal osteomyelitis from a contiguous focus is seen following puncture wounds, retained foreign bodies, adjacent septic arthritis, soft tissue abscesses, or other infections. Debridement is necessary in addition to adequate antimicrobial therapy.

STAPHYLOCOCCAL SEPTIC ARTHRITIS

Staphylococcus aureus is by far the most common cause of septic arthritis in children and older adults, often occurring as a consequence of bacteremia, endocarditis, orthopedic procedures, arthroscopy, or trauma. It may also be seen following joint aspiration or due to extension of contiguous osteomyelitis. In drug addicts with bacteremia, sacroiliac or sternoclavicular joints are frequently involved whereas in other bacteremic patients, the knee, hip, elbow, or shoulder joints are more commonly affected.

The patient usually presents with fever, leukocytosis, and an elevated ESR. The involved joint is swollen, warm, tender, and painful on movement. Limited range of motion helps to differentiate septic arthritis from the more benign condition of septic bursitis. Joint aspiration yields cloudy fluid with a poor mucin clot. The glucose content may be less than half the serum value, and there are usually more than 50,000 granulocytes/mm³. Gram-positive cocci are evident on smear in about three fourths of cases and cultures are nearly always positive.[17] Repeated aspiration should be performed in addition to antimicrobial therapy and surgical drainage may be required. Open drainage is probably advisable in all cases involving the hip joint. Antimicrobial therapy should be continued for a minimum of 3 weeks, with longer courses indicated when osteomyelitis is present.

STAPHYLOCOCCAL WOUND INFECTIONS

Postoperative staphylococcal wound infections typically present 2 to 6 days after a surgical procedure with low-grade fever, wound tenderness, and mild constitutional symptoms. Examination may show a small amount of drainage and erythema. Removal of suture material may reveal pockets of purulent material and further exploration may demonstrate a hematoma. Infected wounds should be explored and debrided and the extent of infection determined. The length of antistaphylococcal therapy is determined by the extent of infection and clinical course, but 7 to 10 days are usually sufficient unless osteomyelitis or retained foreign materials are present.

STAPHYLOCOCCAL CELLULITIS

Staphylococcus aureus and β-hemolytic streptococci are the most common causes of cellulitis in adults. They are often difficult to distinguish clinically and both can infect areas of trauma. Patients present with a warm, tender, erythematous, swollen area of skin, frequently located over an extremity. Blood cultures should be obtained and the edge of the affected region may be aspirated for culture, but the diagnostic yield of this procedure is low. A punch biopsy is more likely to provide a microbiologic diagnosis but is seldom required except in immunocompromised hosts. Empiric therapy in adults should consist of nafcillin or oxacillin, 2 g IV every 4 hours, or cefazolin, 1 g IV every 6 to 8 hours. These agents will treat both *S aureus* and streptococci adequately until the results of cultures are known. Vancomycin may be used in patients allergic to β-lactam antibiotics. Antimicrobial coverage in young children should also cover *H influenzae*. Elevation of the affected extremity is an important component of management.

METHICILLIN-RESISTANT STAPHYLOCOCCUS AUREUS

Since its initial description in 1961, MRSA has emerged as a major clinical problem worldwide, particularly in the hospital setting. MRSA strains are resistant to all β-lactam antibiotics and frequently are resistant to other agents as well, including aminoglycosides, erythromycin, and fluoroquinolones. Experimental and clinical data indicate that MRSA is equivalent in virulence to methicillin-susceptible strains. The identification of MRSA in the clinical laboratory can sometimes be difficult, and special methods have been recommended to avoid misidentification.[18] Vancomycin or teicoplanin are the agents of choice in the treatment of MRSA infections. However, neither of these agents is effective in eradicating MRSA colonization. Combination therapy with agents such as minocycline 100 mg every 12 hours, rifampin 600 mg every 12 to 24 hours, and mupirocin applied topically to the nares twice a day is often effective in patients with persistent colonization.

COAGULASE-NEGATIVE STAPHYLOCOCCI ■

There are more than 20 recognized species of coagulase-negative staphylococci, many of which constitute part of the normal human flora. *S epidermidis* is the species most often associated with human infection. All are gram-positive, catalase-positive, and occur principally in pairs, tetrads, or clusters. Most, but not all, lack hemolytic activity on blood agar.

Although they are common culture contaminants, coagulase-negative staphylococci have been increasingly recognized as important nosocomial pathogens. Patients with prosthetic devices including intravascular catheters are at great risk for infection with these organisms. Coagulase-negative staphylococci produce a mucoid exopolysaccharide substance that enables them to adhere to foreign surfaces. Once embedded in this sticky glycocalyx, these organisms are very difficult to eradicate from implanted foreign bodies.

COAGULASE-NEGATIVE STAPHYLOCOCCAL ENDOCARDITIS

Coagulase-negative staphylococci are not common causes of native valve endocarditis, but can cause significant valvular destruction when such infection does occur. The initial clinical presentation is subacute and mimics valvular infection with viridans streptococci. In particular, native valve coagulase-negative staphylococcal endocarditis may complicate line-associated bacteremia (see Chapter 105).

In contrast, coagulase-negative staphylococci are very common causes of prosthetic valve endocarditis (PVE). Early PVE, occurring within the first 2 months of surgery, is thought to result from contamination at surgery or during the immediate post-operative period when multiple lines are in place. Later cases of PVE are associated with a somewhat better outcome but still are associated with substantial morbidity and mortality.

Valvular dysfunction or fever in a patient with a prosthetic valve should alert the clinician to the possibility of PVE. The onset may be acute or subacute. Often, none of the classic peripheral stigmata of subacute endocarditis, such as splinter hemorrhages or other embolic signs, are seen. Infection of the cloth ring is generally present, which may result in partial valvular dehiscence or extension into the septum with involvement of the conduction system. Electrocardiograms should be obtained to look for the presence of new conduction blocks or other dysrhythmias. A new regurgitant murmur, suggestive of a paravalvular leak, may be audible. An echocardiogram, preferably a transesophageal study, should be obtained to assess valvular function and perivalvular extension.

Multiple blood cultures should be obtained. It has been suggested that perivalvular abscesses may not produce a continuous bacteremia, and not all of the blood cultures will be positive in some cases. Since coagulase-negative staphylococci are common skin contaminants, it may be difficult to evaluate the significance of a single positive culture in a patient presenting with fever. Proper collection technique is important in minimizing the risk of contamination.

The treatment of PVE due to coagulase-negative staphylococci includes vancomycin as the primary antimicrobial agent. Regardless of in vitro susceptibility testing results, coagulase-negative staphylococci causing serious infections should be presumed to be methicillin-resistant because heteroresistance is very common and may not be detected by routine studies in the clinical laboratory. Vancomycin, rifampin, and gentamicin are often given in combination.[12] Serum bactericidal titers may be obtained to determine whether this regimen enhances bacterial killing in vitro. Patients should defervesce by the end of the first week of therapy. Persistent fever beyond ten days should prompt consideration of myocardial abscess or valve replacement, as should hemodynamic deterioration, new murmurs, or persistent bacteremia. In fact, successful management of staphylococcal PVE usually requires valve replacement.

STAPHYLOCOCCAL CATHETER INFECTIONS

Coagulase-negative staphylococci are the most common etiologic agents in line sepsis (see Chap. 34). Patients with coagulase-negative staphylococcal bacteremia generally have central venous or arterial lines. The emergence of coagulase-negative staphylococci as a common cause of bacteremia in granulocytopenic patients is primarily attributable to the long-term use of central venous catheters in these patients. The adherence properties of coagulase-negative staphylococci explain the tendency of these organisms to infect catheters and the difficulty in sterilizing infected lines with antimicrobial therapy alone.

Patients with positive blood cultures for coagulase-negative staphylococci and vascular catheters should be recultured, even if the physician believes that no sepsis exists. In some cases, culture may demonstrate heavy catheter colonization prior to the development of clinical signs of infection. A comparison of semiquantitative blood cultures (e.g., pour plates, lysis-centrifugation) obtained from lines and peripheral phlebotomy sites may help to confirm the presence of an infected line. Optimally, infected catheters should be removed and replaced at new vascular sites because new catheters replaced over a guide wire become quickly colonized with the same organism.

With infected surgically-tunneled catheters (e.g., Hickman and Groshong catheters) it is sometimes possible to eradicate coagulase-negative staphylococcal infection with 2 weeks of antimicrobial therapy alone in selected cases.[19] Such infected catheters should not be left in place if tunnel infection is evident, patients are severely ill, or septic central venous thrombophlebitis is present. Moreover, if fever and bacteremia do not respond rapidly to the institution of antimicrobial therapy, the infected catheter should be removed. Vancomycin is the agent of choice.

STAPHYLOCOCCAL CEREBROSPINAL FLUID SHUNT INFECTIONS

Coagulase-negative staphylococci are the most frequent causes of CSF shunt and ventriculostomy infections. Symptoms include fever, variable meningeal signs, shunt malfunction, or signs of local inflammation around placement sites. The CSF may show a mild-to-marked pleocytosis. CSF glucose may be normal or low. Patients with ventriculoperitoneal shunts frequently have peritonitis. In some instances, infections may be satisfactorily treated without complete removal of the shunt, usually with a combination of systemic and intrashunt administration, and distal shunt revision.[20] However, shunt removal is required for a satisfactory outcome in most cases.

STAPHYLOCOCCAL PROSTHETIC VASCULAR GRAFT INFECTIONS

Staphylococcal species are very common pathogens in prosthetic vascular graft infections and the incidence of coagulase-negative staphylococci may be increased by the widespread use of β-lactam agents for prophylaxis.

The presentation depends upon the location of the involved graft. In superficial areas, wound drainage and fever, pain, and graft limb dysfunction may be seen. Symptoms may be insidious in deeper grafts, and patients may complain only of non-specific symptoms such as vague back or abdominal pain, anorexia, low-grade fever, and malaise. At times, the major symptom is bleeding or graft dysfunction. Aortoenteric fistulas may present with massive gastrointestinal hemorrhage and occasionally result in unilateral clubbing in the involved lower extremity. Fever in a patient with a prosthetic vascular graft is always of concern and physicians should suspect indolent infection in any cases of graft failure or dysfunction.

Blood cultures are not always positive. The infection may be localized around the external surface of the graft and the lumen may be uninvolved. The white blood count may be normal or elevated and the ESR is usually elevated. Angiography, ultrasound, CT scanning, magnetic resonance imaging (MRI),[21] and gallium or indium-labeled leukocyte scans have all been reported to be useful in clarifying the diagnosis in some cases. Vancomycin alone or in combination with rifampin should be administered. Usually graft replacement is required; only in very unusual circumstances should an attempt be made to sterilize the graft or suppress infection in situ.

STAPHYLOCOCCAL PERITONEAL DIALYSIS CATHETER INFECTIONS

Coagulase-negative staphylococci are the most common pathogens isolated from continuous ambulatory peritoneal dialysis (CAPD) patients with peritonitis. The patient usually presents with abdominal tenderness, particularly upon drainage of the dialysate, and nausea may occur. The dialysate typically appears cloudy; fever may not be present. The peritoneal fluid usually contains more than 100 polymorphonuclear cells/mm^3. Gram stains may reveal organisms and cultures are usually positive. However, the infecting organisms may be highly diluted by the large volumes of dialysis fluid. Filtration or concentration of dialysate is sometimes performed.

Treatment for CAPD-associated coagulase-negative staphylococcal peritonitis may be given intravenously or intraperitoneally with vancomycin, which can be given at 5 to 7 day intervals because of its long half-life in anuric patients. Many cases may be managed without catheter removal.[22] The duration of treatment is controversial; because of a high relapse rate, some authorities advocate continuing treatment for 1 month.

STREPTOCOCCAL AND ENTEROCOCCAL INFECTIONS ■

Streptococci and enterococci are catalase-negative Gram-positive cocci typically visualized in primary clinical specimens in pairs or chains. Streptococci may be phenotypically classified by their effects on culture medium containing sheep blood: α-hemolytic organisms produce green pigments from hemoglobin, β-hemolytic organisms cause complete erythrocyte lysis, and non-hemolytic organisms have no effect on sheep red blood cells. Most streptococcal infections encountered in critical care settings are caused by *S pyogenes* (β-hemolytic, Lancefield group A), *Streptococcus agalactiae* (β-hemolytic, Lancefield group B), *Streptococcus pneumoniae* (α-hemolytic), viridans streptococci (usually α-hemolytic), and the *Streptococcus milleri/intermedius* group (variable hemolysis, variable Lancefield group antigen). Most enterococcal infections are caused by *Enterococcus faecalis* or *Enterococcus faecium* (both usually non-hemolytic, Lancefield group D). *Streptococcus* infections are most often community-acquired, whereas many *Enterococcus* infections are nosocomial in origin.

STREPTOCOCCUS PYOGENES (GROUP A STREPTOCOCCUS) ■

Streptococcus pyogenes (group A, β-hemolytic Streptococcus) is a pathogen of major medical significance. Important suppurative infections associated with *S pyogenes* include pharyngitis, skin and soft tissue infections (impetigo, erysipelas, cellulitis, lymphangitis, necrotizing fasciitis, myositis), pneumonia, bacteremia, and meningitis. Streptococcal pharyngitis may be associated with local complications such as otitis, sinusitis, and peritonsillar or retropharyngeal abscess. Elaboration of exotoxins by *S pyogenes* may produce scarlet fever or a syndrome resembling TSS. *S pyogenes* infections may also be complicated by the non-suppurative complications of acute rheumatic fever or post-streptococcal glomerulonephritis occurring weeks later.

Streptococcal pharyngitis is suggested by the presence of purulent tonsillar exudate, tender submandibular lymphadenopathy, and prominent constitutional symptoms, but there is significant clinical overlap with pharyngitis of other etiologies. Although rapid tests to detect pharyngeal *S pyogenes*

are now widely available, the throat culture has been established as the most sensitive diagnostic method. Penicillin VK 250 mg PO q.i.d. for 10 days is standard therapy, with erythromycin used in penicillin-allergic individuals (although some strains are erythromycin-resistant). Despite decades of penicillin use, no penicillin-resistance has ever been detected in a clinical isolate of *S pyogenes*. The primary goal of therapy is the prevention of suppurative and non-suppurative complications, although there is some evidence that the duration of pharyngitis symptoms may be slightly shortened by antimicrobial therapy. Patients with peritonsillar or retropharyngeal abscesses complicating streptococcal pharyngitis require prompt drainage.

Streptococcus pyogenes skin and soft-tissue infections are often characterized by rapid spread, a tendency to involve lymphatics, and systemic toxicity. However, impetigo, the most superficial streptococcal skin infection, causes honey-like crusting lesions in the absence of significant constitutional signs. Impetigo is most frequently seen in young children and responds readily to penicillin. Erysipelas is a deeper *S pyogenes* infection involving the dermis and cutaneous lymphatics. The presence of a raised, erythematous margin clearly demarcating involved and uninvolved areas is a hallmark of erysipelas. Cellulitis, in contrast, has a flat margin which may blend almost imperceptibly with uninvolved skin. As streptococcal cellulitis evolves, watery blisters frequently appear as a consequence of lymphatic obstruction. Lymphangitis and lymphadenitis manifested as linear red streaks leading toward swollen tender regional lymph nodes are highly suggestive of a streptococcal etiology. Necrotizing fasciitis or myositis are the most feared forms of streptococcal soft tissue infection. In contrast to similar syndromes caused by mixed aerobic and anaerobic bacteria, necrotizing streptococcal infections typically lack crepitus or malodorous drainage. Small areas of cutaneous anesthesia or necrosis are suggestive, but are not invariably present. Necrotizing fasciitis is best diagnosed by direct surgical exploration, and examination of tissue by frozen section may be helpful in selected cases.[23] An elevated serum creatine phosphokinase (CPK) may be the only clue to the presence of myonecrosis. Aggressive debridement is critical in the management of necrotizing streptococcal soft tissue infections.

Streptococcus pyogenes pneumonia is relatively uncommon but clinically distinctive. Invasion of lymphatics typically results in the early development of a large pleural effusion out of proportion to the parenchymal infiltrate. Organisms are usually present in the pleural fluid, which is serosanguinous rather than frankly purulent. Tube thoracostomy drainage of infected effusions is indicated and decortication may be required. *S pyogenes* meningitis is quite uncommon, and generally arises by direct extension from an adjacent suppurative focus.

Group A streptococcal infections may be associated with shock and extreme systemic toxicity. Production of pyrogenic exotoxins is believed to be responsible for many of the most severe manifestations. Fulminant clinical presentations with hypotension, thrombocytopenia, electrolyte disturbances, renal impairment, and respiratory distress are referred to as streptococcal toxic shock.[24] Aggressive supportive care and debridement of necrotic tissue are critical aspects of the management of this condition. Because of the purported role of toxin production and suggestive observations from animal models, some authorities advocate the addition or substitution of clindamycin for penicillin in severely ill patients.

The "pyogenes-like" β-hemolytic streptococci (groups C and G streptococci) occasionally cause clinical syndromes similar to those associated with *S pyogenes*. These streptococci are also associated with cellulitis in patients with vascular insufficiency. Penicillin is regarded as the antimicrobial agent of choice in groups C and G streptococcal infections, with the addition of an aminoglycoside in patients with endocarditis.

STREPTOCOCCUS AGALACTIAE (GROUP B STREPTOCOCCUS) ■

Streptococcus agalactiae is weakly β-hemolytic and expresses the Lancefield group B antigen. This organism is most notable as a cause of infection in neonates and peripartum women. More than 20% of pregnant women are colonized in the lower gastrointestinal and genital tracts. Acquisition of *S agalactiae* by the newborn infant during parturition can lead to sepsis, pneumonia, meningitis, or other suppurative complications. The mother may develop chorioamnionitis, endometritis, wound infection, or bacteremia. Maternal mortality is low in this setting, but neonatal morbidity and mortality are substantial.

In non-pregnant adults, *S agalactiae* is an important cause of bacteremia and an occasional cause of localized infections including cellulitis, pneumonia, endocarditis, urinary tract infection, arthritis, and osteomyelitis. Major risk factors for *S agalactiae* colonization and infection are diabetes mellitus, cancer, liver or renal failure, advanced age, and AIDS.[25] Mortality in non-pregnant adults with bacteremia exceeds 40 %. Although all *S agalactiae* strains are susceptible to penicillin, relatively high minimal inhibitory concentrations (MICs) warrant the use of high antimicrobial doses (penicillin G, 12–24 million units per day in divided doses). The addition of an aminoglycoside should be considered in patients with endocarditis.

STREPTOCOCCUS PNEUMONIAE ■

Streptococcus pneumoniae, the pneumococcus, is the most common cause of community acquired pneumonia, the second most common cause of bacterial meningitis, and a leading cause of mortality in the United States. Individuals at greatest risk for serious pneumococcal infections include patients with alcoholism, HIV infection, sickle-cell disease, chronic obstructive lung disease, splenectomy, hypogammaglobulinemia, or multiple myeloma. Pneumococci are readily recognized on sputum or cerebrospinal fluid Gram stains as Gram-positive lancet-shaped diplococci, often surrounded by a capsular halo. Since *S pneumoniae* is sensitive to drying and competes poorly with normal flora in culture,

a significant percentage of sputum cultures from patients with pneumococcal pneumonia may fail to demonstrate the organism. This underscores the importance of prompt handling of specimens for culture, careful examination of Gram stains, and collection of blood cultures in patients with suspected pneumococcal pneumonia.

Streptococcus pnemoniae can be a constituent of the normal flora, so a positive sputum culture must be interpreted in the context of clinical and radiographic findings. Typically, patients with pneumococcal pneumonia have an illness of acute onset beginning with a shaking chill and fever. An antecedent viral upper respiratory syndrome is frequently noted. A cough productive of greenish or rust-colored sputum, dyspnea, and pleuritic chest pain are usually present. However, elderly patients may present with little more than altered mental status. Physical examination reveals evidence of localized consolidation and fine crackles. Occasionally, lower lobe pneumonia may mimic an acute abdominal process. Mild jaundice may be seen in association with lobar pneumonia, further confounding the diagnostic assessment. Laboratory studies typically show leukocytosis and arterial hypoxemia resulting from ventilation-perfusion mismatch. The chest radiograph in pneumococcal pneumonia may demonstrate segmental or lobar consolidation or multiple patchy infiltrates. Pleural effusions are not uncommon. The standard treatment of pneumococcal pneumonia remains penicillin or ceftriaxone, although the emergence of β-lactam-resistant *S pneumoniae* is clearly a concern (see later). Despite appropriate antimicrobial therapy, some patients will succumb to pneumococcal pneumonia, often within the initial days of illness. Recovering patients will usually defervesce in response to antimicrobial therapy within a few days, but chest x-rays may take weeks to months for resolution. Screening studies for HIV infection or multiple myeloma should be considered in patients lacking obvious risk factors for serious pneumococcal disease.

The most important pulmonary complications of pneumococcal pneumonia are parapneumonic effusion, empyema, and lung abscess. Thoracentesis should be performed if pleural effusions are loculated or greater than 10 cm on a lateral decubitus radiograph. Tube thoracostomy is recommended if organisms are seen on Gram stain, pH is <7.0, glucose is <50, or frank pus is obtained. Even patients with sterile parapneumonic effusions may benefit from drainage if persistent fever or chest pain are present. Lung abscesses are very uncommon complications of pneumococcal pneumonia and appear to be particularly associated with the highly mucoid type 3 capsular serotype.

Pneumococcal meningitis may occur by hematogenous spread or by direct extension from an intracranial suppurative focus. Patients with skull fractures are at increased risk. The clinical features of pneumococcal meningitis are not distinct from other acute meningitis. The cerebrospinal fluid Gram stain demonstrates organisms in roughly two thirds of cases. Occasionally, bacteria may be found in cerebrospinal fluid before the development of a pleocytosis and hypoglycorrhachia. Counterimmunoelectrophoresis (CIE) or latex methods to detect pneumococcal antigen are not much more sensitive than Gram stain, but may be useful in partially-treated cases. The mortality in patients with pneumococcal meningitis is substantial and many survivors are left with residual sequelae due to inflammatory neurologic injury. Experimental and clinical observations suggest that the initial bacterial lysis induced by antimicrobial therapy exacerbates inflammatory events in the central nervous system. Some animal model and preliminary clinical data indicate that early administration of corticosteroids (e.g., dexamethasone 10 mg every 6 hours for 4 days) as part of the initial therapy of acute bacterial meningitis can reduce the incidence of neurologic complications,[26] but other studies have failed to demonstrate such benefit.[27] If corticosteroid therapy is used, it should be initiated concomitantly with the initiation of antimicrobial therapy.

Other infections caused by *S pneumoniae* include otitis, sinusitis, mastoiditis, endocarditis, septic arthritis, purulent pericarditis, and peritonitis. Pneumococcal endocarditis is uncommon but tends to be highly destructive. Pneumococcal pericarditis usually occurs as a complication of pneumonia or empyema, and progresses rapidly to cause tamponade unless a drainage procedure is performed.

S pneumoniae strains resistant to penicillin and other antimicrobial agents such as cephalosporins, tetracyclines, chloramphenicol, erythromycin, clindamycin, sulfamethoxazole/trimethoprim, and aminoglycosides are an increasing problem in many regions throughout the world.[28] Although pneumococcal respiratory infections caused by most of these resistant strains will still respond satisfactorily to penicillin, this agent cannot be used for the treatment of meningitis caused by a resistant strain. Unfortunately, the optimal therapeutic regimen for drug-resistant pneumococcal meningitis remains to be established. Ceftriaxone may be useful in this setting, but some penicillin-resistant strains are also highly-resistant to ceftriaxone. Vancomycin is active in vitro against drug-resistant *S pneumoniae*, but has been variably effective in clinical experience. In cases in which drug-resistant pneumococcal meningitis is strongly suspected, an initial combination of vancomycin and ceftriaxone may be the best choice at present. It is important that all isolates of *S pneumoniae* from blood or cerebrospinal fluid be tested for resistance to penicillin and third-generation cephalosporins, in order to guide therapy.

VIRIDANS STREPTOCOCI

The viridans streptococci are a heterogenous group of organisms which normally inhabit the oral cavity, upper respiratory tract, female genital tract, and gastrointestinal tract. The term "viridans" means "green," and most viridans streptococci produce green α-hemolysis on blood agar. However, some viridans streptococci are non-hemolytic or even β-hemolytic. The most commonly encountered viridans streptococcal species are *Streptococcus sanguis*, *Streptococcus mitis*, *Streptococcus mutans*, and *Streptococcus salivarius*. Organisms belonging to the *S milleri/intermedius* group are included under the general category of viridans streptococci, but the distinctinve phenotypes and clinical manifestations of

TABLE 112-2. In Vitro Minimal Inhibitory Concentration for the Isolate

PENICILLIN MIC (μg/mL)	THERAPY
≤0.1	Penicillin × 4 wks **or** Penicillin + aminoglycoside × 2 wks
>0.1, <0.5	Penicillin × 4 wks **and** aminoglycoside × 2 wks
≥0.5	Penicillin + aminoglycoside × 4–6 wks

this group warrants their separate consideration (see later).

The most important clinical syndrome caused by viridans streptococci is endocarditis. Approximately one third of infective endocarditis is caused by viridans streptococci. These organisms have specific mechanisms of adherence which enhance their ability to colonize the oral cavity and also their binding to cardiac valves. The clinical presentation of viridans streptococcal endocarditis is usually subacute. Treatment should be dictated according to the in vitro penicillin MIC for the isolate (Table 112-2).

Preliminary clinical experience suggests that ceftriaxone may provide an effective alternative to penicillin in the treatment of viridans streptococcal endocarditis.[29]

Viridans streptococci are considered to be of low pathogenicity and ordinarily are not encountered frequently in the critical care setting. However, patients with granulocytopenia are at risk for overwhelming viridans streptococcal bacteremia.[30] In this specific setting, cardiovascular collapse and acute respiratory distress may be seen, with an attendant mortality of approximately 10%. Significant risk factors for this syndrome include mucositis, prophylactic use of sulfamethoxazole and trimethoprim or fluoroquinolones, and use of antacids or histamine (H_2) receptor antagonists.

STREPTOCOCCUS MILLERI/ INTERMEDIUS GROUP ■

The *S milleri/intermedius* group are taxonomically heterogenous and confusing, having undergone many nomenclature revisions.[31] These organisms are sometimes otherwise referred to as microaerophilic streptococci, capnophilic streptococci, *Streptococcus anginosus*, or *Streptococcus constellatus*. They are distinctive and clinically important principally because of their association with localized suppurative infections. Some confusion arises from the phenotypic variability of the *S milleri/intermedius* group: isolates may be α-, β-, or non-hemolytic, and may group as Lancefield A, C, F, or G (or are non-groupable). However, they are clearly microbiologically and clinically distinct from conventional β-hemolytic group A, C, or G streptococci. Members of the *S milleri/intermedius* group form tiny colonies compared with other streptococci, and colonial growth is enhanced by the presence of CO_2. Isolates often have a "butterscotch" odor, attributed to the elaboration of diacetyl. Specific biochemical tests enable clinical laboratories to identify the *S milleri/intermedius* group with good accuracy.

The *S milleri/intermedius* group are the major streptococci found in lung abscess, pleural empyema, brain abscess, and liver abscess. Other frequent infections include odontogenic abscess, endocarditis, appendiceal or other intraabdominal abscess, osteomyelitis, arthritis, and cutaneous abscess. Penicillin therapy, along with surgical drainage, is usually effective, but penicillin resistance has been increasingly reported. Vancomycin, clindamycin, or the combination of penicillin and an aminoglycoside may be required in specific cases.

ENTEROCOCCI ■

With advancing medical progress, the enterococcus has emerged from the normal gastrointestinal flora to become one of the leading nosocomial pathogens in the United States. Most enterococcal infections are caused by *E faecalis*. However, 5% to 10% of enterococcal infections are caused by *E faecium*, which is important for its antimicrobial resistance patterns. Enterococci are readily identified in the clinical laboratory by their ability to grow in 6.5% NaCl, resistance to bile, and ability to hydrolyze esculin and L-pyrrolidonyl-β-naphthylamide (PYR).

The most important infections caused by enterococci are urinary tract infections, endocarditis, infections of vascular catheters, abdominal and pelvic infections, and wound infections. Rare cases of meningitis, pneumonia, or other localized infections have been reported. In abdominal, pelvic, and wound infections, enterococci are often mixed with other aerobic and anaerobic flora, leaving uncertainty as to their pathogenic role. The resistance of enterococci to widely-used prophylactic antimicrobial agents, such as cephalosporins, is undoubtedly responsible for much of their emergence as important pathogens. Molecular strain typing methods have demonstrated the ability of resistant enterococci to be transmitted from person-to-person in the hospital setting. The most useful currently-available drugs in the treatment of enterococcal infections are ampicillin, vancomycin, streptomycin, and gentamicin. However, isolates resistant to each of these antimicrobial agents have been reported with increasing frequency.[32] Infections localized to the urinary tract generally respond well to ampicillin, vancomycin, or nitrofurantoin. Treatment of more serious infections should be guided by in vitro susceptibility testing. Successful therapy of endocarditis or meningitis requires bactericidal therapy, which can only readily be achieved by the combination of ampicillin or vancomycin with an aminoglycoside. The treatment of infections caused by enterococci resistant to both ampicillin and vancomycin is currently unsatisfactory; aminoglycosides are of no use in the absence of an active cell-wall agent. The treatment of endocarditis caused by enterococci with high-level resistance to all aminoglycosides is also problematic. Fluoroquinolones and other experimental regimens are currently being investigated.

MORAXELLA (BRANHAMELLA) CATARRHALIS ■

Moraxella catarrhalis (formerly *Branhamella*) is an aerobic Gram-negative diplococcus now recognized as a common cause of respiratory infections.[33] Most isolates produce β-lactamases. *M catarrhalis* may cause sinopulmonary infections, bronchitis, otitis media in children, and bronchopneumonia in adults, particularly in individuals with underlying pulmonary disease. Patients typically present with mild-to-moderate fever, cough, sputum production, and leukocytosis. The chest x-ray may show lobar or interstitial infiltrates with patchy consolidation. Bacteremia is extremely uncommon. Useful agents in the treatment of *M catarrhalis* infections include amoxicillin/clavulanate, ampicillin/sulbactam, sulfamethoxazole/trimethoprim, fluoroquinolones, and third generation cephalosporins.

NEISSERIA MENINGITIDIS ■

Neisseria meningitidis is a Gram-negative, coffee bean–shaped diplococcus. Clinically important serogroups include A, B, C, and Y. Tetravalent vaccines are available for groups A, C, Y, and W-135, but the B capsule is not sufficiently immunogenic. Although the meningococcus is carried in the nasopharynx by some healthy adults, comparatively few individuals develop disease. This seems to be related at least in part to the level of circulating antimeningococcal antibody. The carrier state seems to confer group-specific as well as some cross-protective immunity against subsequent disease.

Meningococcal meningitis is seen most frequently in children and the incidence declines progressively with age. However, it remains the second most common cause of meningitis in persons over 10 years of age. Patients usually present with fever, headache, variable mental status changes, myalgias, and meningeal signs. Young children and elderly individuals may initially present without neurologic signs or symptoms. The petechial rash frequently seen with this disease helps to differentiate it from other causes of purulent meningitis, but is not invariably present. A similar rash may occasionally occur with pneumococcal meningitis, particularly in asplenic patients. The meningococcal rash is seen most often on the trunk and lower extremities or in areas under pressure from clothing. It may also be seen on mucous membranes. Larger, ecchymotic lesions can develop. Empiric therapy of patients with purulent meningitis should always account for the possibility of meningococcal disease, unless a different organism is evident on the Gram stain of cerebrospinal fluid. Patients with recurrent meningococcal meningitis should be evaluated for possible complement deficiency or hypoglobulinemia.

The cerebrospinal fluid is usually turbid with a predominance of polymorphonuclear cells, and the glucose is generally less than 50% of the serum level. However, these characteristic changes may be absent very early in the course of disease. The Gram stain demonstrates organisms in about

75% of cases, and the blood cultures are positive in 50%. Latex agglutination or CIE methods may detect meningococcal antigen in the cerebrospinal fluid or urine, but false-negative results are common. These studies are particularly useful in patients who may have been partially treated prior to obtaining a lumbar puncture.

The severe thrombocytopenia, disseminated intravascular coagulation (DIC), shock, and heart failure that can occur in meningococcal meningitis are thought to result from bacterial endotoxin. Renal and adrenal infarction can occur, as well as myocarditis, hemorrhagic pulmonary edema, and adult respiratory distress syndrome (ARDS). Treatment consists of penicillin G 240,000 units/kg/day in divided doses (up to a total of 24 million units/day). For patients allergic to penicillin, chloramphenicol or third generation cephalosporins such as ceftriaxone or cefotaxime may be substituted. Treatment with any of these agents should be continued for 10 to 14 days.

Respiratory isolation is required for the first 24 hours after initiation of treatment in patients with invasive meningococcal infections, and chemoprophylaxis is recommended for household or intimate contacts, for unprotected medical personnel who have performed cardiopulmonary resuscitation or intubation, and for day care or other contacts within a closed population. The standard prophylactic regimen for adults is rifampin 600 mg every 12 hours for two days. In recent studies, single doses of ciprofloxacin, ofloxacin,[34] or ceftriaxone also appear to be effective alternatives.

Neisseria meningitidis is spread via a respiratory route, and close physical contact or crowding appear to increase the incidence of colonization and infection. Group Y is the serotype most commonly associated with pneumonia. Patients with meningococcal pneumonia usually present with a sore throat, chills, fever, chest pain, and rales. Pleuritic chest pain may occur. Bronchopneumonia is usually evident radiographically, and small pleural effusions may be seen in about 20% of cases.

Because *N meningitidis* may be present in the posterior nasopharynx of healthy people, isolation of the organism from expectorated sputum does not necessarily indicate that it is responsible for illness. Recovery of *N meningitidis* from pleural fluid, blood, or from protected bronchoscopic or transtracheal specimens are more likely to be significant. Secondary hematogenous meningococcal pneumonia may be seen in patients with bacteremia or meningitis. Penicillin, third-generation cephalosporins, or fluoroquinolones may be used in the treatment of primary meningococcal pneumonia in adults. Penicillin or a cephalosporin would be preferable in patients with concomitant meningitis.

Meningococcemia may be chronic, acute, or fulminant. In chronic cases, intermittent fever, headache, and a transient maculopapular or petechial rash may be seen. Myalgias are common, and joint involvement occurs in about 20% of patients. This clinical presentation may be mistaken for disseminated gonococcal infection. Patients may feel well between episodes of transient bacteremia, and blood cultures during these periods may be negative. All patients with chronic meningococcemia should be evaluated for possible complement deficiency.[35] Treatment is important, because approximately one fifth may progress to develop meningitis.

More frequently, meningococcemia presents as an acute illness, often following an upper respiratory infection. Patients typically complain of fever, chills, arthralgias, and myalgias. Tachycardia and tachypnea are common, as is a characteristic petechial rash. Cough, sore throat, prostration, gastrointestinal complaints, and mild hypotension may be present. Headache, a stiff neck, or confusion may indicate the presence of meningitis. Penicillin 12 million units/day in divided doses should be administered, with higher doses if meningeal involvement is suspected. Antimicrobial therapy should be continued at least 5 days after the patient is afebrile.

Fulminant illness (Waterhouse-Friderichsen syndrome) occurs in about 10% of patients with meningococcemia and is associated with a very high mortality rate. This syndrome is characterized by the sudden onset of chills, high fever, prostration, headache, and the development of petechial or ecchymotic lesions. Fulminant meningococcemia may progress in a matter of hours with evolution of diffuse skin involvement, coma, DIC, and cardiovascular collapse. Appropriate antimicrobial therapy must be instituted immediately. Penicillin, third-generation cephalosporins, or chloramphenicol may be used as described for meningococcal meningitis. Aggressive supportive care including cardiopulmonary support is frequently required. Recent reports suggest that plasmapheresis or plasma exchange may reduce mortality in fulminant meningococcal sepsis.[36] Prophylaxis of contacts and patient isolation are indicated as for meningococcal meningitis.

NEISSERIA GONORRHOEAE

Neisseria gonorrhoeae, the gonococcus, is an oxidase-positive Gram-negative diplococcus transmitted by sexual contact. Although *N gonorrhoeae* is an unusual pathogen in the ICU, extragenital infection involving the bloodstream, joints, meninges, or heart may occasionally produce severe illness. Disseminated gonococcal infection (DGI) is typically manifested as fever and tenosynovitis and is associated with a small number of pustular, hemorrhagic, or frankly necrotic skin lesions scattered over the extremities. The clinical presentation may be mistaken for chronic meningococcemia. Alternatively, patients may present with septic arthritis involving a single joint. Culture specimens from normally sterile body fluids should be plated onto chocolate medium with enhanced humidity and CO_2, while cultures of the oropharynx, urethra, cervix, or anus should be plated onto selective media (e.g., modified Thayer-Martin medium) to inhibit the growth of normal flora. Third generation cephalosporins are the currently preferred agents for the treatment of disseminated gonococcal infection.[37]

BACILLUS INFECTIONS ■

Infection with these spore-forming Gram-positive rods may be seen occasionally in immunocompromised hosts or intravenous drug abusers. Endocarditis, bacteremia, dialysis access and other catheter-associated infections, and endophthalmitis have been reported.[38] More frequently, however, *Bacillus* species are isolated as environmental contaminants. Susceptibility to penicillin and cephalosporins is variable. Treatment alternatives include clindamycin, vancomycin, erythromycin, tetracycline, and aminoglycosides.

Bacillus anthracis, the causative agent of anthrax, is usually transmitted by contact with infected animals or contaminated animal products. Anthrax is very rare in the United States. Clinical manifestations may include a necrotic and edematous ulcer at the site of inoculation, fulminant sepsis, pneumonia, mediastinitis, gastrointestinal distress, and meningitis. *B anthracis* organisms are non-motile and non-hemolytic, distinguishing them from many non-pathogenic *Bacillus* species. Penicillin is the antimicrobial agent of choice, with erythromycin, tetracycline, or chloramphenicol as alternatives.

CORYNEBACTERIA (DIPHTHEROIDS) ■

Corynebacteria are nonmotile, pleomorphic Gram-positive bacilli. *Corynebacterium diphtheriae* is the causative agent of diphtheria, a serious infection with respiratory, cardiac, and neurologic manifestations. Partly as a consequence of mass immunization, diphtheria has become extremely rare in the United States. Other *Corynebacterium* species ("diphtheroids") cause infections in immunocompromised hosts and patients with indwelling foreign bodies.[39] Infections of intravascular catheters, ventricular shunts, and orthopedic hardware are particularly frequent. The urease-positive *Corynebacterium* group D2 can cause alkaline-encrusted cystitis, a notoriously difficult management problem.[40] Because diphtheroids are commonly isolated as skin contaminants, single isolates from blood cultures must be interpreted with caution. Although the majority of *Corynebacterium* species are susceptible to erythromycin or penicillin, *Corynebacterium jeikeium* and *Corynebacterium* group D2 are usually resistant to most antimicrobial agents except vancomycin.

LISTERIA MONOCYTOGENES ■

Listeria monocytogenes is a β-hemolytic Gram-positive bacillus which may be isolated from a wide range of plant, animal, and environmental sources. On direct smears, *Listeria* may appear as cocci, coccobacilli, or rods, leading to misidentification as streptococci or diphtheroids. In adults, *Listeria* are most important as agents of meningitis and septicemia. Patients with advanced age, lymphoproliferative disorders or other T-cell defects, organ transplants or other immunosuppressive therapy, pregnancy, and cirrhosis are at increased risk of listeriosis.

The presentation of listerial meningitis may be acute or subacute and is clinically indistinguishable from meningitis of other cause. Stiff neck, fever, and altered mental status are commonly present. Focal CNS findings may be indicative of brain abscess or rhombencephalitis. CSF findings are extremely variable and nonspecific; either mononuclear or polymorphonuclear cell predominance may be seen.[41] The protein is usually, but not invariably, elevated and the glucose may be low or normal. Although CSF cultures are usually positive, Gram stains are insensitive. Patients with *Listeria* brain abscess frequently have positive blood cultures and negative CSF cultures. *Listeria* meningitis is treated with high-dose intravenous penicillin or ampicillin, and gentamicin may be added intravenously or intrathecally. In the penicillin-allergic patient, sulfamethoxazole/trimethoprim appears to be the best alternative.[42] Third-generation cephalosporins lack sufficient activity and should not be used. A course of treatment of at least 3 weeks is advisable because of a substantial relapse rate associated with shorter regimens. The mortality and incidence of neurologic sequelae are considerable and increase with a delay in therapy. *Listeria* should be considered in the selection of empiric antimicrobial therapy for any elderly or otherwise compromised host with meningitis, until a specific microbiologic diagnosis is confirmed.

Listeria septicemia occurs principally in immunocompromised patients. Patients may range from mildly to severely symptomatic, with fever, weakness, nausea, and vomiting. Hypotension or coagulopathy may be present. The course may be complicated by abscesses of the brain or liver. Blood cultures are usually positive. In pregnant women, listeriosis often presents as a flu-like illness without localizing signs or symptoms. A gastrointestinal prodrome may be elicited from the history. Meningitis, respiratory distress syndrome, or endocarditis may occasionally occur, but the greatest risk is to the fetus. Untreated maternal listeriosis may result in premature labor, intrauterine death, or neonatal listeriosis (granulomatosis infantiseptica). Treatment should be initiated with penicillin or ampicillin, perhaps accompanied by an aminoglycoside.

NOCARDIA ■

Nocardia are aerobic, branching, filamentous Gram-positive bacilli which are capable of causing serious human infections, particularly in hosts with impaired cellular immunity. *Nocardia* are acid-fast, but do not retain carbolfuchsin as avidly as mycobacteria; hence, a modified "partial acid-fast" protocol with less vigorous decolorization is required to demonstrate their acid-fastness. Although *Nocardia* have been recovered from a wide range of infections, the majority of clinical isolates are obtained from the respiratory tract, skin lesions, lymph nodes, or brain abscesses. The roentgenographic appearance of pulmonary nocardiosis is quite variable, ranging from bronchopneumonia to multiple abscesses. Prolonged therapy for several months, usually with sulfamethoxazole/trimethoprim, is required. Serum sulfa levels of 100 to 150 μg/mL are desirable. Alternative agents include imipenem, minocycline, third-generation cephalosporins, amikacin, amoxicillin/clavulanate, and clarithromycin. However, individual strain susceptibilities vary, so in vitro susceptibility testing should be performed to guide therapy.[43]

ACINETOBACTER ▪

Acinetobacter baumannii (formerly *Acinetobacter calcoaceticus* variant *anitratus*) has emerged as an important nosocomial pathogen, particularly in the ICU setting. *A baumannii* typically appears as a large Gram-negative diplococcus on Gram stains of primary material, but may be initially misidentified as a pneumococcus on occasion because of its tendency to retain crystal violet. *Acinetobacter* may also be mistaken initially for *Neisseria* or *Moraxella*. Risk factors for serious *Acinetobacter* infection include intravenous catheters or other instrumentation, broad spectrum antimicrobial use, and admission to an ICU. Bacteremia, pneumonia, and urinary tract infection are the most frequent clinical manifestations, but virtually any body site may be infected with *A baumannii*. Most nosocomial strains are resistant to many antimicrobial agents, including penicillins, cephalosporins, and gentamicin. The most active agents are generally regarded to be imipenem and amikacin, although resistance to either of these agents has been reported with increasing frequency.[44,45] Some strains are susceptible to ceftazidime, ampicillin/sulbactam, fluoroquinolones, sulfamethoxazole/trimethoprim, and doxycycline. Polymyxin B is active in vitro, but is unlikely to be effective in the treatment of systemic infections for reasons related to its mechanism of action.[46] In view of the great difficulty encountered in treating nosocomial *Acinetobacter* infections, aggressive attempts to control the transmission of this pathogen in the hospital setting are warranted.

CAMPYLOBACTER AND HELICOBACTER ▪

Campylobacter are motile, curved, fastidious Gram-negative bacilli which require special media for cultivation. *Campylobacter* may be found in the intestinal tracts of many wild and domesticated animals, and may be transmitted to humans by raw poultry, beef, lamb, pork, or unpasteurized dairy products. Water supplies may be contaminated by *Campylobacter* in animal feces. Both animal-to-human and human-to-human transmission have been documented.

Patients with *Campylobacter jejuni* infections typically present with abdominal pain, fever, and diarrhea which may be bloody. Bacteremia is uncommon. Guillain-Barré syndrome[47] or reactive arthritis may occur as late complications. Erythromycin appears to ameliorate the course of infection. Newer macrolides such as azithromycin also appear to have good activity. Fluoroquinolones have been used in the treatment of *C jejuni* enteritis and have the advantage of providing coverage against other common enteric bacterial pathogens. However, resistance to fluoroquinolones has emerged

rapidly among *C jejuni* and approaches 50% in some regions.[48] Third-generation cephalosporins, chloramphenicol, or aminoglycosides may be useful in the treatment of extraintestinal infections.

Campylobacter fetus subspecies *fetus* is more likely than *C jejuni* to cause bacteremia and less likely to cause gastrointestinal disease. This species exhibits a propensity to infect vascular endothelium, which can result in thrombophlebitis, endocarditis, pericarditis, and mycotic aneurysms. Cellulitis, osteomyelitis, pneumonia, arthritis, and meningoencephalitis have been reported. Prolonged or relapsing bacteremia may occur in immunocompromised hosts. Treatment alternatives include third-generation cephalosporins, chloramphenicol, aminoglycosides, and imipenem.

Helicobacter pylori is a motile, curved Gram-negative bacillus[49] which has recently been established as the major etiologic agent in gastritis and peptic ulcer disease. *H pylori* infection is associated with a significant subsequent risk of developing gastric cancer. In the ICU setting, *H pylori* infection is usually an incidental diagnosis made during diagnostic or therapeutic esophagogastroduodenoscopy (EGD).[14] C-urea breath testing or serologic studies may also help to establish the diagnosis. Treatment may be deferred until the patient is stable and can tolerate an oral combination regimen. *Helicobacter cinaedi* and *Helicobacter fennelliae* can cause enteric infection and sustained bacteremia in patients with AIDS.

ENTEROBACTERIACEAE ▪

The Enterobacteriaceae family of Gram-negative bacilli encompasses important human pathogens as well as constituents of the normal gastrointestinal tract flora. All are oxidase-negative facultative anaerobes capable of fermenting glucose to acid. Nearly one half of significant nosocomial bacterial isolates are members of the Enterobacteriaceae. Several of the most important genera will be discussed below.

ENTEROBACTER ▪

Enterobacter species are opportunistic pathogens principally associated with hospital infections. Urinary tract, wound, respiratory, and catheter-associated infections are most frequently seen. Because of the presence of an inducible chromosomal β-lactamase, the use of cephalosporins or penicillins is not recommended for the treatment of serious infections caused by *Enterobacter* species. Even strains which initially appear to be susceptible to these antibiotics in vitro may subsequently develop resistance during the course of therapy.[50] Imipenem and amikacin are the most reliably active agents against resistant nosocomial strains, and fluoroquinolones or sulfamethoxazole/trimethoprim are also active against some isolates.

ESCHERICHIA ■

Escherichia coli is the most commonly isolated enteric organism. In outpatients, *E coli* is most important as a cause of urinary tract infections and gastroenteritis. Although most *E coli*-associated diarrhea is a self-limited illness, some enterohemorrhagic strains which produce Shiga-like toxin (e.g., serotype O157:H7) can cause severe hemorrhagic colitis or hemolytic-uremic syndrome.[51]

Common nosocomial *E coli* infections include urinary tract infections, primary or secondary intraabdominal infections, and bacteremia. Intraabdominal infections may arise spontaneously (usually in patients with hepatic cirrhosis) or result from suppurative foci such as cholecystitis, cholangitis, appendicitis, peridiverticular abscess, or bowel perforation. Bloodstream invasion may result in the sepsis syndrome (see Chap. 28) and its attendant multisystem complications. Less common *E coli* infections include pneumonia, wound infections, septic arthritis, meningitis, osteomyelitis, line infections, and prosthetic valve endocarditis. Treatment of *E coli* infections generally involves both antimicrobial agents and drainage or resection of suppurative foci. Ampicillin resistance is now observed in approximately one third of strains, and resistance to antipseudomonal penicillins such as piperacillin is not unusual. Cephalosporins are more reliable, although extended-spectrum *E coli* β-lactamases which hydrolyze third-generation cephalosporins are being reported with increasing frequency. Most strains are susceptible to sulfamethoxazole/trimethoprim, ampicillin/sulbactam, fluoroquinolones, imipenem, aztreonam, and aminoglycosides. Antimicrobial therapy of O157:H7 infections may precipitate hemolytic-enemic syndrome, and is not recommended.

KLEBSIELLA ■

Klebsiella is an important cause of nosocomial urinary tract, biliary, wound, respiratory, and intravascular catheter-associated infections. These organisms may be distinguished from many other enteric bacilli by their non-motility and highly mucoid colonial morphology. As with *E coli*, bloodstream invasion with *Klebsiella* may result in life-threatening sepsis. Necrotizing community acquired *Klebsiella* pneumonia (Friedländer pneumonia) classically occurs in alcoholic patients, often with an underlying history of chronic lung disease. The illness is acute and rapidly progressive, with fever, chills, prostration, pleuritic pain, and cough productive of bloody sputum. A bulging fissure is sometimes evident on chest x-ray. Lung abscess and empyema are common complications. *Klebsiella* infections are usually treated with a third-generation cephalosporin, and an aminoglycoside may be added if the patient is severely ill. However, extended-spectrum β-lactamases have been described in *Klebsiella*[52] as in *E coli*. Selection of alternative agents should be guided by in vitro susceptibility testing.

PROTEUS ■

The principal *Proteus* species causing human infection are indole-negative *Proteus mirabilis* and indole-positive *Proteus vulgaris*. *Proteus* are notable for their ability to swarm on some agar media. The urinary tract is by far the most common site of *Proteus* infection, and these organisms facilitate the persistence of infection by their ability to split urea and promote formation of struvite urinary tract stones. Less common *Proteus* infections include wound infections, chronic otitis media, keratitis, meningitis, bacteremia, pneumonia, and intraabdominal infections. Most *P mirabilis* are susceptible to β-lactam antibiotics and aminoglycosides, but *P vulgaris* infections are more difficult to treat.

SALMONELLA ■

Most individuals infected with the Gram-negative bacillus *Salmonella* have subclinical or mild self-limited gastrointestinal illness. However, life-threatening enteric fever, bacteremia, or focal suppurative infection may also result. The syndrome of enteric fever is most commonly associated with *Salmonella typhi*, but may also be caused by *Salmonella paratyphi* and occasionally by other *Salmonella* serotypes as well. Most cases in the United States are associated with foreign travel. Affected patients typically have fever without localizing symptoms. The classic clinical signs of "rose spots" and relative bradycardia occur only in a minority of cases. The white blood count may be low, normal, or elevated, but a "shift to the left" is common. A specific diagnosis usually results from culture of blood, stool, or bone marrow. Serologic tests are not recommended because of both poor sensitivity and specificity. Neuropsychiatric abnormalities and intestinal hemorrhage or perforation may be particularly troublesome complications. The mortality in untreated patients is approximately 15%. Fluoroquinolones appear to be the antimicrobial therapy of choice, and the adjunctive use of dexamethasone has been found to be beneficial in severely ill patients.[53] Third-generation cephalosporins are an effective alternative to fluoroquinolones. Ampicillin, sulfamethoxazole/trimethoprim, and chloramphenicol remain useful for susceptible strains, but emerging resistance has been a problem in many parts of the world.

In the developed world, infection with nontyphoidal *Salmonella* is much more common than typhoid fever. Infection may be acquired from a variety of animals and food products, particularly poultry and eggs. While most of the nontyphoidal *Salmonella* serovars cause only gastroenteritis, a few serovars (e.g., *Salmonella typhimurium*, *Salmonella dublin*, *Salmonella enteritidis*, *Salmonella choleraesuis*) are associated with invasive disease.[54] Patients with underlying illnesses such as malignancy, sickle cell disease, and AIDS are at especially high risk for extraintestinal salmonellosis. Sustained bacteremia, endovascular infection, and focal infections (e.g., splenic abscess, brain abscess, empyema) are among the more serious complications. Although antimicrobial therapy is not routinely recommended for *Salmonella*

gastroenteritis because it may prolong the carrier state,[55] it should be considered in immunocompromised hosts or patients with extraintestinal disease. Third-generation cephalosporins, fluoroquinolones, or sulfamethoxazole/trimethoprim are among the most useful agents. Susceptibility testing should be performed, because resistance to each of these drugs has been reported in nontyphoidal *Salmonella* isolates.

SERRATIA

Serratia are generally associated with nosocomially acquired infections. Detection of DNAse production is useful in distinguishing *Serratia* from other Enterobacteriaceae. Some strains also produce a red pigment. *Serratia marcescens* cause the majority of *Serratia* infections, although *Serratia rubidaea*, *Serratia odorifera*, *Serratia plymuthica*, and members of the *Serratia liquefaciens* group are occasionally isolated from clinical specimens. Respiratory infections, urinary tract infections, and bacteremia are the *Serratia* infections most often encountered in the ICU. Endocarditis, osteomyelitis, cellulitis, and keratitis are seen less frequently. *Serratia* infections are often associated with intravascular catheters or other foreign bodies, as well as contaminated disinfectant solutions. *Serratia* is variably susceptible to second and third generation cephalosporins, monobactams, quinolones, aminoglycosides, and sulfonamides. Resistance may develop during prolonged monotherapy, so the combination of a β-lactam antibiotic and an aminoglycoside is often recommended for serious infections requiring an extended period of treatment.

SHIGELLA

Shigella are non-motile, non-lactose fermenting members of the Enterobacteriaceae. Shigellosis may be caused by *Shigella dysenteriae*, *Shigella flexneri*, *Shigella boydii*, and *Shigella sonnei*; *S sonnei* is responsible for most of the *Shigella* infections in the United States. Although patients of any age may acquire *Shigella*, children are most frequently afflicted. Fever is often the initial symptom, followed rapidly by the development of abdominal pain, myalgias, and watery diarrhea. Subsequent colonic involvement results in the syndrome of dysentery, with bloody diarrhea, mucus, and tenesmus. The clinical course may be complicated by dehydration, electrolyte derangements, and neurologic abnormalities including seizures.

A stool exam usually demonstrates neutrophils and red blood cells. The peripheral white blood count is often elevated, in contrast to typical cases of salmonellosis. Endoscopy may reveal superficial ulceration with mucosal friability, but is not essential for diagnosis. Blood cultures are seldom positive. Treatment is recommended for highly symptomatic patients with shigellosis. Ampicillin, sulfamethoxazole and trimethoprim, or nalidixic acid have been most widely used, but resistance to each of these agents has been a problem

in some geographic areas. If antimicrobial resistance is a problem in local strains of *Shigella*, fluoroquinolones may provide an alternative. These agents have the additional advantage of good activity against some strains of *Campylobacter*. However, fluoroquinolones may carry some risk of cartilage toxicity when used in children. Antimicrobial therapy appears to decrease fecal shedding of the organism and duration of illness, but is not necessary in patients who are only mildly symptomatic.

YERSINIA

Yersinia pestis, the causative agent of plague, is a nonmotile, aerobic, Gram-negative bacillus with marked bipolar staining characteristics. Enzootic plague occurs in small mammals, especially rodents, and is transmitted by fleas. Wild or domesticated carnivores can contract plague by consuming rodents, or by contact with infected fleas. Humans may acquire plague from flea bites or direct contact with infected animal tissue. Infected cats have also been recognized as important vectors of transmission from enzootic foci to humans. Rarely, plague may be spread from person-to-person by a respiratory route, but this mode of transmission has not occurred in the United States since 1924.

Bubonic plague is the most common form of plague in humans. Fever, prostration, headache, and other nonspecific symptoms occur with, or are followed shortly by, a localized area of exquisitely painful, enlarged lymph nodes (buboes). The buboes are usually oval or round and warm, with surrounding edema; they are most often found in the inguinal, femoral, axillary, or cervical nodes. The disease may progress rapidly, with the development of nausea, vomiting, diarrhea, altered mental status, and shock.

Primary septicemic plague is manifested by a sepsis syndrome without lymphadenopathy. Primary plague pneumonia is rare and results from inhalation of organisms. Patients with primary pneumonia present with acute fever, chills, headache, and cough productive of bloody sputum along with signs of respiratory insufficiency. Any form of plague may be complicated by meningitis, DIC, and secondary hematogenous pneumonia.

When plague is suspected, Gram and Wayson stains should be immediately performed on material aspirated from buboes, CSF, or sputum. Blood and other material should be cultured. Since *Yersinia* grows more slowly than other Enterobacteriaceae, plates should be held for 72 hours. Microbiology laboratories should be notified whenever plague is suspected, so that appropriate precautions may be taken to minimize the risk to technical personnel. Sera should be obtained during acute and convalescent phases.

Antimicrobial therapy should be initiated as soon as plague is suspected. Streptomycin 30 mg per kg per day IM or IV in 2 divided doses is the standard treatment, and should be administered for 10 days. Tetracycline 30 to 50 mg per kg per day divided every 6 hours or doxycycline 100 mg every 12 hours are alternative agents. Chloramphenicol is preferred in cases of meningitis, and a loading dose of 25 mg per kg IV is followed by 50 to 75 mg per kg per day divided every 6 hours. Recent animal studies suggest that third-generation cephalosporins or fluoroquinolones may be effective in the treatment of *Y pestis* infection,[56] but human data are lacking.

Plague is a reportable infection, and the appropriate health department should be notified when plague is suspected. All patients with plague should be placed in strict isolation for the first 72 hours of treatment. Wound and skin precautions should be continued for patients with buboes. Persons known to have regular or close contact with patients prior to treatment should receive tetracycline prophylaxis.

Yersinia enterocolitica most commonly causes enterocolitis with watery diarrhea, abdominal pain, and fever. Mesenteric adenitis may be caused by either *Y enterocolitica* or *Yersinia pseudotuberculosis*. When mesenteric adenitis presents with right lower quadrant pain, fever, and leukocytosis, it is easily mistaken for acute appendicitis. *Y enterocolitica* septicemia is uncommon and most often associated with an underlying illness such as cancer, diabetes mellitus, hepatic cirrhosis, and iron overload. Transfusion-acquired *Y enterocolitica* sepsis has also been reported. Some patients with yersiniosis may develop reactive polyarthritis or erythema nodosum.

The diagnosis of *Y enterocolitica* infection is generally made from culture of stool, blood, or lymph nodes. The laboratory should be notified when yersiniosis is suspected, so that selective media may be employed.

Fluoroquinolones appear to be the agents of choice in the treatment of *Y enterocolitica* infections.[57] Third-generation cephalosporins, aminoglycosides, chloramphenicol, tetracycline, and sulfamethoxazole/trimethoprim are also active.

OTHER ENTEROBACTERIACEAE ■

Other enteric bacteria occasionally associated with nosocomial infection include *Citrobacter, Hafnia, Morganella,* and *Providencia.* Most of these infections involve the respiratory or urinary tracts. Resistance to multiple antimicrobial agents is common among these organisms, so treatment should be guided by susceptibility testing.

FLAVOBACTERIUM ■

Flavobacterium species are non-motile aerobic Gram-negative rods which grow well on blood and chocolate agar, but often poorly or not at all on enteric media. Colonies are usually yellow-pigmented, which provide a clue to identification. Flavobacteria are multiply-resistant to antimicrobial agents and most strains produce β-lactamases. *Flavobacterium meningosepticum* is highly associated with infection in newborn infants. The most common clinical syndrome is meningitis. Nosocomial waterborne infections with *Flavobacterium* species may be seen in all age groups, and include bacteremia, endocarditis, wound infections, and pneumonia. In adults, *Flavobacterium* infections frequently occur in patients with underlying medical disorders. A variety of drugs

have been recommended for the treatment of neonatal *F meningosepticum* infections, including sulfamethoxazole/trimethoprim, vancomycin, clindamycin, rifampin, and occasionally the fluoroquinolones. The use of fluoroquinolones in children must be tempered by concern about possible cartilage toxicity. In the seriously ill adult patient, empiric therapy with both sulfamethoxazole/trimethoprim and ofloxacin may be advisable until the results of susceptibility testing are available.

FRANCISELLA ■

Francisella tularensis is a fastidious small aerobic Gram-negative coccobacillus which grows poorly or not at all on many common culture media. Unanticipated growth of this organism represents a significant hazard to laboratory personnel. Therefore, the clinical laboratory should be alerted when tularemia is suspected, to insure appropriate media selection and handling precautions. Contact with infected ticks, rodents, lagomorphs, felines, or, occasionally, birds is responsible for most cases of tularemia. Although local and regional tularemia involving mucous membranes, lymphatics, or skin are most commonly encountered, typhoidal or pneumonic tularemia can cause significant morbidity and mortality. Typhoidal tularemia presents most often as generalized sepsis with fever, chills, myalgias, abdominal pain, nausea, and vomiting. Diarrhea and pulmonary infiltrates frequently occur. Skin lesions are variably seen. Pneumonic tularemia may be clinically indistinguishable from other causes of atypical pneumonia. Streptomycin remains the antimicrobial agent of choice in nonmeningeal tularemia, with gentamicin an acceptable alternative.[58] Relapse rates are higher in cases treated with bacteriostatic drugs such as tetracycline or chloramphenicol, although the latter agent is typically added when treating *F tularensis* meningitis. Imipenem and fluoroquinolones such as ciprofloxacin have been used successfully, but published experience is limited. Ceftriaxone failure has been reported, so the use of third generation cephalosporins is not recommended.

HAEMOPHILUS INFLUENZAE ■

Haemophilus species are small, pleomorphic Gram-negative bacilli. *H influenzae* is the most pathogenic species for man and most adult *H influenzae* infections are caused by nonencapsulated organisms. Respiratory infections such as otitis, conjunctivitis, sinusitis, bronchitis, and bronchopneumonia are common, but more invasive infections or bacteremia are rare.

Serotype b *H influenzae* is principally a pathogen of early childhood. The HIB vaccine has dramatically reduced the incidence of type B *H influenzae* infection in the United States.[59] Occasionally, this organism causes serious disease in adults, especially in patients with impaired humoral immunity (e.g., splenectomy, AIDS). Important clinical syndromes associated with type B *H influenzae* include meningitis, epiglottitis, pneumonia, and cellulitis. With ampicillin-resistant organisms now commonly isolated, third-generation cephalosporins are preferred as the initial therapeutic agents in patients with serious infections.

OTHER HACEK ORGANISMS ■

HACEK is an acronym for *Haemophilus, Actinobacillus, Cardiobacterium, Eikenella,* and *Kingella.* These small pleomorphic fastidious Gram-negative bacilli can be found in the upper respiratory tract. Each of the HACEK species can cause a variety of infections including arthritis, diskitis, empyema, and bite wound infections, and each is capable of infecting native or prosthetic heart valves. HACEK organisms are fastidious, somewhat slow-growing, and may fail to trigger some semi-automated blood culture systems. Their growth in blood culture is easily suppressed by the presence of antibiotics, and they may be overgrown by more rapidly multiplying organisms when present in mixed infections. HACEK organisms are occasionally responsible for "culture negative endocarditis." The microbiology laboratory should be notified when culture-negative endocarditis is suspected, so that blind subcultures and prolonged incubation of blood culture bottles may be performed. The HACEK organisms are uniformly susceptible to third generation cephalosporins, which are probably the therapeutic agents of choice. Aminoglycosides are often added during the initial treatment course for endocarditis.

LEGIONELLA ■

Legionella are aerobic Gram-negative bacilli which normally inhabit a variety of aquatic environments. The diagnosis of *Legionella* infections is complicated by the inability of these organisms to grow on routine culture media. Respiratory infection most commonly presents as one of two distinct syndromes: Pontiac fever and Legionnaires' disease.

Pontiac fever is a flulike illness lasting 2 to 7 days, which presents with fever, headache, malaise, and myalgias. Pneumonia does not occur. This syndrome is self-limiting, and antimicrobial therapy is not required.

Legionnaires' disease is a more serious condition, particularly in immunocompromised hosts. *Legionella pneumophila* accounts for the majority of human infection. However, more than 50 *Legionella* species have now been identified, and many of these have occasionally been associated with pneumonia. The incubation period varies from 2 to 10 days. Fever, malaise, anorexia, and myalgias are noted initially, followed by cough, chills, and headache. Pleuritic chest pain and gastrointestinal symptoms are reported by a sizable percentage of patients. Mental status abnormalities such as confusion, lethargy, and hallucinations may be present.

Bilateral patchy infiltrates are usually noted early in the course of Legionnaires' disease and may progress to consolidation. Nodules may be seen on chest x-ray, particularly in infections with *Legionella* species other than *L pneumophila.* Multiple studies are indicated in an attempt to confirm the diagnosis of *Legionella* infection, since no single test is completely sensitive. Culture on buffered charcoal yeast extract medium (BCYE), direct fluorescent antibody (DFA) staining of clinical specimens, serologic tests, and urinary antigen detection are most often employed.

Erythromycin 1 g IV every 6 hours is the initial therapeutic agent of choice, and rifampin 600 mg PO every 12 hours may be added in severe cases. Possible alternative agents include ciprofloxacin, sulfamethoxazole/trimethoprim, doxycycline, and clarithromycin. A minimum course of 3 weeks is recommended for Legionnaires' disease.

PASTEURELLA ■

Pasteurella multocida is a non-motile Gram-negative coccobacillus, possessing a characteristic "mousey" odor on culture media. Infections with *P multocida* usually result from animal bites or other animal contact, although in some cases an animal exposure cannot be identified. Cellulitis, lymphadenitis, tenosynovitis, septic arthritis, and osteomyelitis can follow bite wounds. Less commonly, pneumonia, bacteremia, meningitis, or peritonitis can be seen.[60] Pneumonia is more common in patients with underlying chronic obstructive lung disease. Amoxicillin/clavulanic acid is effective in less severe cases, and ampicillin/sulbactam may be used in more severe infections. These agents will also provide coverage for other bite-associated pathogens such as *S aureus,* streptococci, *Eikenella corrodens,* and anaerobes. Ceftriaxone may be used for the treatment of meningitis, as well as for long-term therapy of septic arthritis and osteomyelitis.

PSEUDOMONAS AERUGINOSA ■

Pseudomonas aeruginosa is a motile, aerobic, oxidase-positive, non-lactose-fermenting Gram-negative bacillus. *P aeruginosa* is a serious opportunistic pathogen in the hospital setting, causing more than 10% of nosocomial bacterial infections. Neutropenic patients, burn or trauma patients, patients with cystic fibrosis, patients receiving broad-spectrum antimicrobial therapy, and patients with AIDS[61] are at particular risk. In addition to generalized sepsis, *P aeruginosa* can cause an enormous spectrum of local infections, involving the respiratory tract, central nervous system, skin, heart, urinary tract, eye, musculoskeletal system, and gastrointestinal tract.[62] Some of these will be discussed in further detail.

PSEUDOMONAL PNEUMONIA

Necrotizing pneumonia due to *P aeruginosa* is most often seen in intensive care settings, in which underlying lung disease, widespread antibiotic use, and respiratory equipment increase the risk of disease. The clinical presentation is usually acute and severe, with toxicity, fever, chills, productive cough, dyspnea, and altered mental status. Hypotension is a frequent finding and may be among the initial clinical manifestations. Diffuse bronchopneumonia is often seen, typically involving the posterior segments preferentially. Small pleural effusions are common. A Gram stain of the respiratory secretions demonstrates slender Gram-negative bacilli and neutrophils. Optimal therapy consists of an aminoglycoside and antipseudomonal penicillin (e.g., piperacillin) or cephalosporin (e.g., ceftazidime). Imipenem-cilastatin may be used in place of the β-lactam agent.

Patients with cystic fibrosis (CF) have a quite different clinical presentation. Most CF patients develop chronic respiratory infection with mucoid *P aeruginosa*, which is associated with acute exacerbations and chronic progression of respiratory impairment. Patients may complain of low-grade fever, persistent cough, anorexia, dyspnea, and wheezing. The chest radiograph usually shows patchy infiltrates with peribronchial thickening. Intermittent courses of combination antimicrobial therapy with agents such as piperacillin, ceftazidime, imipenem, aminoglycosides, and fluoroquinolones can help to ameliorate acute respiratory exacerbations. However, such therapy is almost inevitably associated with the eventual development of antibiotic-resistant strains.

PSEUDOMONAL MENINGITIS

Hematogenous spread of organisms from a distant site of infection, contiguous spread from an intracranial focus, or introduction during trauma or neurosurgery may result in *P aeruginosa* meningitis. Ommaya reservoirs, ventriculostomies, and CSF shunts are also prone to infection. Patients usually present with fever, headache, altered mental status, and meningeal signs, but immunocompromised hosts may lack symptoms directly referable to the central nervous system. Ceftazidime appears to be the antimicrobial agent of choice, unless in vitro testing demonstrates the organism to be resistant. The addition of an intraventricular or intrathecal aminoglycoside may be warranted in severe cases. Imipenem and ciprofloxacin may be useful alternative agents, but experience is limited. Drainage of suppurative foci and removal of prosthetic material are important aspects of therapy.

PSEUDOMONAS IN BURN PATIENTS

Pseudomonas aeruginosa is a major cause of burn wound sepsis. Colonization of burn patients usually occurs shortly after admission to the burn unit. These organisms have the ability to proliferate rapidly in necrotic tissue, from which they can spread to underlying viable areas. Early excision of necrotic tissue, use of wound coverings, stringent isolation practice, and topical therapies may help to limit the incidence of this problem. Wounds should be examined at least every 24 hours, and frequent debridement may be required.

Topical agents such as silver sulfadiazine or silver nitrate may be used initially prior to heavy wound colonization, but these agents do not penetrate eschars. Mafenide acetate, which does penetrate eschars, is preferred once colonization is established.

Pseudomonas aeruginosa infection may extend from burned areas to involve normal skin. Dark brown, black, or green discoloration, hemorrhage, or rapid eschar separation may occur. Fever, leukocytosis or leukopenia, mental status changes, oliguria, hypotension, and ileus may precede or occur concurrently with the skin findings. A wound biopsy including an area of unburned tissue should be obtained expeditiously when *Pseudomonas* infection is suspected. Histologic evidence of bacterial invasion into normal tissue or quantitative cultures demonstrating $>10^5$ organisms per gram of tissue should be considered indicative of burn wound sepsis. Systemic combination antimicrobial therapy (antipseudomonal penicillin or cephalosporin plus an aminoglycoside), debridement, and penetrating topical therapy should be employed. Antibiotic coverage prior to manipulation of the wound is preferable. Initial selection of antimicrobial agents should take the prevailing susceptibility patterns of organisms isolated from the burn unit into account.

PSEUDOMONAL ENDOCARDITIS

Pseudomonal endocarditis can occur on native or prosthetic heart valves (see Chap. 105). Intravenous drug abusers constitute the majority of patients with native valve infections, which frequently involve the tricuspid valve.

Patients with right-sided native valve *P aeruginosa* endocarditis may present subacutely, with fever, cough, and pleuritic chest pain. Most patients have an evident right-sided murmur. The chest radiograph may reveal patchy pulmonary infiltrates and pleural effusions. The echocardiogram demonstrates tricuspid insufficiency or other abnormalities in the majority of cases. Serial echocardiograms may be indicated in patients with initially normal studies, when endocarditis is strongly suspected.

Left-sided pseudomonal endocarditis generally presents acutely, with fever, evidence of systemic embolization, and heart failure. Metastatic foci of infection may develop in the brain, spleen, and other organs. Treatment of pseudomonal endocarditis consists of a β-lactam antibiotic to which the isolate is susceptible in vitro, as well as an aminoglycoside. Therapy should be administered for at least 6 weeks.

Left-sided infection generally requires valve replacement in addition to antimicrobial therapy. A thorough investigation to rule out metastatic foci of infection should be undertaken prior to surgery, if possible. Tricuspid valve endocarditis may require valve replacement or repair in refractory cases with recurrent or persistent bacteremia. Some authorities have advocated valvulectomy without replacement in intravenous drug abusers with tricuspid valvular endocarditis. However, this procedure is not infrequently complicated by the late development of right-sided heart failure and cannot be recommended.

PSEUDOMONAS (BURKHOLDERIA) CEPACIA ■

Pseudomonas (Burkholderia) cepacia is a pigmented, nonfermentative Gram-negative bacillus principally known as a plant pathogen. Although *P cepacia* has low intrinsic pathogenicity for humans, its resistance to most antimicrobial agents and its ability to grow in diverse environmental sources (including distilled water, povidone-iodine, and chlorhexidine) have led to its emergence as a significant nosocomial pathogen. Reported clinical manifestations include pneumonia, urinary tract infections, line infections, endocarditis, arthritis, and meningitis.

In addition, *P cepacia* can be a serious respiratory pathogen in patients with cystic fibrosis.[63] *P cepacia* respiratory infection in this setting is associated with respiratory deterioration and increased mortality, especially following lung transplantation. Selective media may enhance the recovery of *P cepacia* from respiratory specimens. Epidemiologic evidence indicates that *P cepacia* may be spread from person-to-person, as well as by contaminated fluids or respiratory equipment. Some strains are susceptible in vitro to fluoroquinolones, sulfamethoxazole/trimethoprim, minocycline, chloramphenicol, third-generation cephalosporins, or antipseudomonal penicillins, but resistance to any or all of these agents may develop.

STENOTROPHOMONAS (XANTHOMONAS) MALTOPHILIA ■

Stenotrophomonas (Xanthomonas) maltophilia is a non-fermentative Gram-negative bacillus of uncertain taxonomic status. Intrinsic resistance to many antimicrobial agents and an ability to grow in a variety of hospital environments has resulted in the emergence of *S maltophilia* as an important nosocomial pathogen. Underlying malignancy, instrumentation, and prior broad-spectrum antimicrobial therapy are the major predisposing factors for infection. Pneumonia, bacteremia, skin infections, and urinary tract infections account for the majority of clinical isolates. Many infections are associated with foreign bodies, such as intravascular catheters, endotracheal tubes, genitourinary catheters, prosthetic heart valves, peritoneal dialysis catheters, and ventriculoperitoneal shunts. Removal of foreign material is a critical aspect of the management of *S maltophilia* infections.[64] Sulfamethoxazole/trimethoprim is usually the antimicrobial agent of choice, although resistant strains have been reported. Minocycline and ticarcillin/clavulanic acid (Timentin) are useful alternative agents. Strains are uniformly resistant to imipenem, and are typically resistant to all aminoglycosides. The activity of third-generation cephalosporins, antipseudomonal penicillins, and fluoroquinolones is highly variable.

VIBRIOS AND RELATED ORGANISMS ■

The genus *Vibrio* includes several species of pathogenic curved Gram-negative bacilli. All are motile and most are oxidase-positive. *Vibrio cholerae*, the notorious cholera bacillus, causes fulminant dehydrating diarrhea which can be fatal within hours of onset. Although pandemic cholera has not reached the United States since the nineteenth century, the seventh cholera pandemic has spread extensively thoughout Latin America, including Mexico. Isolated U.S. cases have occurred in travelers or from ingestion of imported food. An eighth cholera pandemic is now believed to be underway in South Asia.[65] Confirmatory diagnostic culture of *V cholerae* from stool or rectal swabs is best performed on selective medium (e.g., thiosulfate citrate bile salts sucrose agar). The mainstay of cholera treatment is oral or intravenous correction of fluid and electrolyte imbalances. Tetracycline is also administered to shorten the duration of illness.

The halophilic (salt-loving) vibrios, including *Vibrio vulnificus*, *Vibrio alginolyticus*, and *Vibrio damsela*, are principally important as causes of soft-tissue infection and septicemia. These organisms constitute part of the normal marine flora and may be acquired by contact with seawater or ingestion of uncooked seafood. Patients with hepatic cirrhosis or iron overload are particularly susceptible to the most severe complications of halophilic *vibria* infections, which include primary or metastatic necrotizing soft-tissue infection and overwhelming sepsis. Hemorrhagic bullous cutaneous lesions are a distinctive clinical feature.[66] Tetracycline appears to be the antimicrobial agent of choice.

Aeromonas and *Plesiomonas*, two other waterborne members of the family Vibrionaceae, have also been associated with diarrhea and extraintestinal infection. Necrotizing *Aeromonas* soft tissue infection may clinically mimic infection with halophilic vibrios. Medicinal leeches are symbiotically colonized with *Aeromonas hydrophila* and may provide a source of infection in surgical patients.[67] Susceptibility testing of *Aeromonas* and *Plesiomonas* isolates is recommended because considerable strain variability has been observed.

ANAEROBIC COCCI ■

Anaerobic Gram-positive cocci, mostly belonging to the genus *Peptostreptococcus*, and anaerobic Gram-negative cocci belonging to the genus *Veillonella* are not infrequently isolated from clinical sites, including blood and other body fluids, bones and joints, abscesses, and wounds. Their intrinsic pathogenicity is low, but experimental models indicate that the anaerobic cocci may act in synergy with other organisms. Consequently, these organisms are usually isolated in mixed culture along with aerobic or other anaerobic flora. Most anaerobic cocci are susceptible to β-lactams, imipenem, clindamycin, and chloramphenicol, although resistance to penicillin or clindamycin is occasionally encountered. Anaerobic Gram-positive cocci are also susceptible to vancomycin. Susceptibility to metronidazole is variable.

ACTINOMYCOSIS ■

Actinomycosis is an indolent, chronic suppurative infection caused by *Actinomyces israelii* and other faculative or anaerobic filamentous Gram-positive bacilli. These organisms constitute part of the normal endogenous flora of the oral cavity, gastrointestinal tract, and female genital tract. Trauma or surgery, poor dentition, and intrauterine device (IUD) use are important risk factors for the development of actinomycosis. Typical actinomycotic lesions are characterized by multiple sinus tracts, "sulfur granules" containing masses of organisms, and invasion of adjacent structures without regard to normal tissue planes. Culture methods are insensitive and histologic examination is often essential for a definitive diagnosis. Cervicofacial actinomycosis ("lumpy jaw") is the most common form of illness, but actinomycosis may also involve the chest, abdomen, pelvis, or brain. Mixed infection with other anaerobes or fastidious Gram-negative bacilli such as *Actinobacillus actinomycetemcomitans* is frequently seen. A prolonged course of penicillin, tetracycline, erythromycin, or clindamycin is usually effective. The choice of antimicrobial agents should probably take "associate" organisms into account when mixed infection is present. Surgical debridement or drainage may be useful in selected cases.

CLOSTRIDIAL INFECTIONS ■

Clostridium are spore-forming anaerobic Gram-positive bacilli. The major pathogenic clostridia are *Clostridium botulinum*, *Clostridium difficile*, *Clostridium perfringens*, and *Clostridium tetani*.

CLOSTRIDIUM BOTULINUM

Clostridium botulinum elaborates the most potent toxin in nature. The action of botulinum toxin is localized at cholinergic nerve endings, impairing transmission at ganglionic synapses, postganglionic parasympathetic synapses, and neuromuscular junctions. After irreversible binding of the toxin in the presynaptic cleft, recovery can occur only following the development of new neuromuscular junctions and terminal axons. Seven types of *C botulinum* have been described; types A, B, E, and F are the most common causes of human botulism.

The three most common types of botulism are food-borne, wound, and neonatal, with food-borne the most frequently seen. The incubation of food-borne botulism is usually from 12 to 36 hours, while the incubation of wound botulism is usually 4 to 14 days. Botulism is characterized by a descending paralysis, with the highest cranial nerves affected first. Intra- or extraocular ophthalmoplegia is typically the initial neurologic manifestation. Diplopia may be the first symptom, followed by other bulbar complaints such as dysarthria, dry mouth, and dysphagia. Nystagmus and ptosis are more common with type A botulism. Descending weakness of the neck, shoulders, diaphragm, upper extremities, and lower extremities follows. Gastrointestinal symptoms, such as nausea, vomiting, diarrhea, and abdominal pain are seen early in food-borne botulism; these symptoms are rare in wound botulism. Sensation remains intact and consciousness is unimpaired unless the patient is hypoventilating. Patients are usually afebrile on presentation, except patients with wound botulism who have fever secondary to the infected wound. Deep tendon reflexes are variable and pupils may be normal, sluggishly reactive, or fixed. The CSF is typically normal, although mildly elevated protein may be noted.

Electromyographic (EMG) studies show decreased amplitude of the muscle action potential in response to a single supramaximal stimulus,[68] but facilitation is seen with repetitive stimuli at rates of 25 to 50 per second. These changes are not seen early in botulism but appear later in the course of illness. Definitive diagnosis of botulism requires detection of the toxin in stool, gastric contents, serum, or food. The organism may be cultured from infected wounds, but fewer than half of patients with wound botulism have positive wound cultures.

In suspected cases of botulism, health authorities must be immediately contacted to assist with diagnosis and epidemiologic considerations, as well as with the acquisition of antitoxin. State health departments have a designated authority to receive such calls at any hour, as do the Centers for Disease Control and Prevention (404-329-2888).

Administration of trivalent equine antitoxin may reduce mortality and shorten the clinical course. Administration of 1 vial IM and 1 vial IV is currently recommended, but patients should first be tested for immediate hypersensitivity to horse serum. Desensitizaton is advised in patients with severe reactions. Patients must be monitored carefully after administration of antitoxin because acute reactions may even occur in patients with negative skin testing.

Other important aspects of therapy include supportive care and ventilatory support. Patients with wound botulism should have wound debridement and removal of foreign bodies; penicillin is often administered to eradicate wound colonization but is of unproven benefit. Ventilatory failure is a common cause of death in patients with botulism. Respiratory function and vital capacity should be carefully followed; intubation is usually required if the vital capacity falls below 30% of the predicted value. Aspiration pneumonia is a significant risk. The clinical course is prolonged, with slow recovery. Some patients who recover from botulism have persistent impairment in respiratory function for up to a year.

CLOSTRIDIUM DIFFICILE

Clostridium difficile is the major causative agent of antibiotic-associated enteric disease ranging from mild diarrhea to pseudomembranous colitis. Clindamycin, ampicillin, and cephalosporins are frequently associated with *C difficile*-associated diarrhea, while erythromycin, tetracycline, and chloramphenicol are rarely associated and aminoglycosides are almost never implicated. The disease may occur during or up to a few weeks following a course of antimicrobial therapy.

Patients typically present with fever, abdominal pain, and non-bloody diarrhea. Occasionally, fever is the initial manifestation in the absence of gastrointestinal signs or symptoms. Colonic thickening may be apparent on abdominal CT studies. Sigmoidoscopic examination may reveal small raised yellow-white plaques interspersed with areas of normal-appearing mucosa. Removal of overlying mucus may demonstrate pseudomembranes. In 20% to 30% of cases, involvement is limited to the right colon.

Diagnostic evaluation should include both cytotoxin assay and *C difficile* culture.[69] Tissue culture or enzyme immunoassay (EIA) methods may be used to detect the presence of cytotoxin. However, direct stool toxin assays are negative in as many as a third of affected patients. Diagnostic sensitivity is increased by the inclusion of culture using selective media. However, since patients may be colonized with nontoxigenic *C difficile*, culture isolates should be tested for the ability to elaborate toxin. Either a positive direct cytotoxin assay or a culture demonstrating a toxigenic strain of *C difficile* is consistent with the diagnosis of *C difficile*-associated diarrhea.

Treatment of *C difficile* colitis consists of discontinuing the offending antibiotics if possible and administering either oral metronidazole 500 mg three times a day or oral vancomycin 125 mg four times a day, for about 10 days. Relapses are common and should be retreated. In patients unable to take oral medications, intravenous metronidazole may be combined with vancomycin administered by retention enema.

CLOSTRIDIUM PERFRINGENS

Food poisoning caused by *C perfringens* usually occurs 8 to 12 hours after the ingestion of contaminated food (such as recooked meat) and presents with watery diarrhea, abdominal pain, and nausea. Bloody diarrhea, vomiting, or systemic signs such as fever are unusual. Fecal leukocytes are absent in this toxin-mediated disease. Definitive diagnosis depends upon isolation of *C perfringens* from contaminated food. The illness is self-limiting. In some areas of the world, type C strains of *C perfringens* may also be associated with the highly lethal syndrome of necrotizing enteritis (pigbel).

Necrotizing *C perfringens* soft tissue infection and myonecrosis (gas gangrene) most often follow traumatic or surgical wounds. Grossly contaminated or poorly perfused deep wounds carry the greatest risk. A spectrum of illness ranging from cellulitis to fasciitis to myonecrosis may be seen. Myonecrosis is generally limited to skeletal or myometrial muscle. Toxins elaborated by *C perfringens* contribute to local necrosis and intravascular hemolysis. A minority of cases may be caused by other clostridia, including *Clostridium novyi*, *Clostridium septicum*, and *Clostridium histolyticum*. *C septicum* infections should prompt a search for an underlying bowel malignancy. Since *Clostridium* species frequently colonize well-healing wounds, simple culture isolation in the absence of clinical signs is not diagnostic of infection.

Clostridial myonecrosis presents with severe and progressive pain in the affected area. In contrast to other skin infections, the affected area is initially pale, swollen, tense, and cool. The skin gradually becomes discolored and bullae may appear. A thin, foul-smelling discharge may seep from the wound. In cases due to *C perfringens*, Gram stain reveals large "boxcar" Gram-positive rods without spores, but few polymorphonuclear cells are present.

The patient appears toxic and anxious, with tachycardia, low-grade fever, and diaphoresis. Illness progresses rapidly, with hypotension, renal failure, and circulatory collapse. Crepitation may be present in the involved area or gas may be seen radiographically, but these are late findings. At exploration, the involved muscle appears beefy red, pale, or necrotic, and does not contract with stimulus. Blood cultures are positive in about 15% of patients.

Wide early debridement of all involved tissues is essential in clostridial myonecrosis. Prompt aggressive exploration is indicated as soon as the illness is suspected. In uterine gas gangrene, complete hysterectomy is required.

Penicillin G 16 to 24 million units/day IV in divided doses is the standard antimicrobial therapy, but animal models suggest that the addition or substitution of metronidazole or clindamycin might be preferable.[70] Chloramphenicol is another alternative. Hyperbaric oxygen therapy has been anecdotally reported to be a useful adjunctive measure, but should not supplant prompt surgical debridement.

A variety of clostridial species including *C perfringens* may occasionally be associated with bacteremia, emphysematous cholecystitis, intraabdominal abscess, empyema, and other infections.

CLOSTRIDIUM TETANI

Clostridium tetani is widely distributed in soil and in the intestines of man and other animals. Immunization is completely effective in preventing illness and tetanus is uncommon in the United States. It usually occurs in incompletely immunized individuals and in drug abusers who self-administer subcutaneous injections. It is rarely seen in neonates in this country.

The most common form of the disease is generalized tetanus, which typically presents with trismus, dysphagia, and hypertonia of the skeletal musculature, resulting in progressive rigidity. Painful muscle spasms occur with increasing frequency and may be provoked by sudden stimuli such as light, noise, or movement. High fevers are seen in severe cases. Some patients exhibit disturbances of the autonomic nervous system, manifested by wide variations in blood pressure ranging from hypotension to systolic pressures of 300 mm Hg. Cardiac dysrhythmias, tachycardia, diaphoresis, or hyperpyrexia can also be seen in these cases. Muscle spasms and rigidity may compromise respiratory function and respiratory failure, atelectasis, or pneumonia are frequently seen.

Localized tetanus consists of muscle rigidity occurring in the same anatomic region as the original wound—usually on one of the extremities. Localized tetanus may precede the generalized form of the disease.

The diagnosis of tetanus is usually made from the history and clinical assessment. Gram stain and anaerobic cultures of the suspect wound should be performed at the time of debridement, but these studies are frequently negative. Blood cultures are not useful, and the CSF should be normal.

Treatment of *C tetani* infection consists of 500 IU human tetanus immunoglobulin (hTIg) given intramuscularly or intravenously. Doses of up to 10,000 IU have been used in some cases. Intrathecal doses of 250 to 1000 IU, with or without corticosteroids, have also been tried; horse serum antitoxin is not used in the United States. The wound must be carefully debrided, and some authorities recommend infiltration of the wound with hTIg before debridement, while others recommend systemic hTIg prior to the procedure.

Sedation and muscle relaxation with benzodiazepines or barbiturates are useful, along with airway protection and a frequent assessment of ventilatory function.[71] All patients with tetanus should be treated in an ICU, and stringent efforts should be made to minimize environmental stimuli. The use of drugs such as pancuronium or dantrolene, and mechanical ventilation may be required. Aggressive pulmonary care and nutritional support are mainstays of therapy. Intravenous penicillin or erythromycin should be given to eradicate residual *C tetani*. Drugs such as propranolol or labetalol may be required to control autonomic disturbances.

Because tetanus does not confer immunity, a full course of immunization should be instituted during the recovery period in unvaccinated or incompletely vaccinated patients.

PROPIONIBACTERIUM ACNES ■

Propionibacterium acnes is an obligately anaerobic, pleomorphic Gram-positive bacillus which normally resides on the skin. *P acnes* has been implicated as a contributory agent in inflammatory acne. In the hospital setting, *P acnes* is most often encountered as a blood culture contaminant. However, *P acnes* can also be an important pathogen in infections of implanted foreign materials, such as ventriculostomy catheters, ventriculoperitoneal shunts, and orthopedic hardware. Vancomycin is the antimicrobial agent most often employed in these situations.

ANAEROBIC GRAM-NEGATIVE BACILLI ■

The anaerobic Gram-negative bacilli of clinical importance have undergone recent taxonomic revision and now include members of the genera *Bacteroides, Prevotella, Porphyromonas, Fusobacterium,* and *Bilophila.* These organisms are prevalent constituents of the normal flora of the oral cavity, gastrointestinal tract, skin, and female genital tract. Oral anaerobes play an important role in head and neck infections such as Ludwig's angina, chronic sinusitis, odontogenic infections, aspiration pneumonia, lung abscess, and brain abscess. Gastrointestinal anaerobes are extremely important contributors in the pathogenesis of intraabdominal abscess. Cutaneous anaerobes are frequently involved in infected decubitus ulcers, diabetic foot infections, and necrotizing fasciitis. Serious female genital tract infections such as endometritis, tubo-ovarian abscess, and septic abortion usually involve anaerobes.

Fastidious anaerobes are poorly recovered from swab specimens. Optimal recovery of anaerobic bacteria requires collection of purulent material in a sterile syringe, evacuation of air, and prompt transport to the microbiology laboratory. Anaerobic bacteria generally grow more slowly than facultative organisms and may not be detected for several days. Therefore, empiric antimicrobial therapy in the aforementioned clinical settings should include anaerobic coverage until the anaerobic cultures have been incubated for a sufficient duration of time.

BACTEREMIA

The clinical presentation of anaerobic bacteremia is extremely variable, ranging from a virtually asymptomatic patient to one with fulminant sepsis. Bacteremia with *Fusobacterium necrophorum* has been specifically associated with septic jugular vein thrombophlebitis (Lemierre's syndrome) occurring as a complication of head and neck infection.[72] In the management of anaerobic infections, drainage is of even greater importance than antimicrobial therapy. An aggressive diagnostic work-up to identify the underlying source of undrained infection is indicated whenever anaerobic bacteremia is detected. Metastatic foci of infection at contiguous or distant sites may continue to pose therapeutic problems even after the primary site has been adequately drained.

INTRA-ABDOMINAL INFECTIONS

Abdominal abscesses most frequently occur when the peritoneal cavity is contaminated with gastrointestinal tract contents following surgery, trauma, or visceral perforation. Anaerobes are associated with intra-abdominal abscesses and secondary peritonitis in the majority of cases. Most of these infections are polymicrobial, with coliforms and streptococci participating as well. The diagnosis of an intra-abdominal infection depends upon careful physical examination supported by diagnostic studies such as ultrasound, CT scan, and indium-labelled leukocyte scan. However, in some cases the focus of infection can be identified only at exploratory laparotomy. Bacteremia, septic phlebitis, and metastatic infection are serious complications. Management requires percutaneous or surgical drainage in addition to antimicrobial therapy.

Useful agents in the management of intra-abdominal infections include ampicillin/sulbactam, imipenem-cilastatin, and some second-generation cephalosporins such as cefoxitin or cefotetan. Clindamycin or metronidazole have excellent activity against abdominal anaerobes but should be combined with other agents with better activity against enteric Gram-negative bacilli or streptococci.

HEAD AND NECK INFECTIONS

Head and neck infections usually involve anaerobes, often in mixed culture with streptococci and fastidious oral Gram-negative bacilli.[73] Ludwig's angina is one example of a deep space infection of the head and neck. In this condition, cellulitis of the sublingual and submaxillary spaces arises from dental infection and rapidly spreads to cause massive neck swelling and protrusion of the tongue. The patient complains of difficulty swallowing or talking and may exhibit signs of airway compromise.

Airway protection, along with ampicillin/sulbactam or clindamycin, are the most important elements of therapy. Drainage may be beneficial if CT scans demonstrate a discrete abscess, but diffuse edema without focal liquefaction is more typically seen.

ASPIRATION PNEUMONIA

Aspiration of oropharyngeal contents because of altered consciousness or loss of gag reflexes can cause pneumonia (see Chap. 125). Aspiration pneumonia typically occurs in the posterior segments of the upper lobes or the superior or basilar segments of the lower lobes. The pneumonitis resulting from aspiration may initially be sterile, but subsequent suppuration due to infection with mixed anaerobic and facultative oral bacteria commonly develops. In the hospital setting, enteric Gram-negative bacilli and *S aureus* may also be involved. Patients with aspiration pneumonia present with fever and a pulmonary infiltrate on x-ray, which may be cavitary. The sputum demonstrates polymorphonuclear leukocytes and mixed bacteria and is often fetid. Frank abscess formation warrants a prolonged course of therapy and empyema is a frequent complication in this setting. Mixed aerobic-anaerobic empyemas usually require open drainage for definitive management. Penicillin has been traditionally used in the treatment of aspiration pneumonia and is usually effective. However, penicillin-resistant oral anaerobes have been isolated with increasing frequency, possibly explaining some treatment failures. Alternative agents include clindamycin, ampicillin/sulbactam, or the combination of penicillin plus metronidazole. Third-generation cephalosporins are less desirable because of reduced activity against anaerobic bacteria. The therapeutic regimen should be modified if a predominance of enteric bacilli or staphylococci are noted on Gram stain.

BRAIN ABSCESS

Anaerobic bacteria are well-recognized pathogens in brain abscess (see Chap. 110), which can result from hematogenous or contiguous spread. Otitis, mastoiditis, sinusitis, dental infection, lung abscess, and trauma or neurosurgery are the most important risk factors for brain abscess involving anaerobes.[74] Patients typically present with the subacute development of headache, fever, focal neurologic deficits, lethargy, nausea, and vomiting. However, any of these signs or symptoms may be absent, making the diagnosis a challenging one. Seizures, meningismus, or papilledema are noted in a minority of cases. CT or MRI scans with contrast are the most useful diagnostic studies. Lumbar puncture is contraindicated. Whenever feasible, aspiration is indicated for both diagnostic and therapeutic reasons. Brain abscesses involving anaerobes are generally treated with the combination of high-dose penicillin and metronidazole for an average of 4 to 6 weeks. Limited clinical observations suggest that third-generation cephalosporins may be substituted for penicillin. Nafcillin should be added when *S aureus* is suspected.

BARTONELLA (ROCHALIMAEA) INFECTIONS ■

Four species of the pleomorphic Gram-negative bacillus *Bartonella* have been recognized as human pathogens. *Bartonella henselae* (formerly *Rochalimaea henselae*) is probably

the species most likely to be encountered in the critical care setting. Recent evidence strongly implicates *B henselae* as a causative agent in the majority of cases of cat scratch disease.[75] Although most immunocompetent patients with cat scratch disease experience regional lymphadenopathy which regresses spontaneously over one or more months, a few experience complications including involvement of liver, bone, or the central nervous system. More than 90% of patients with cat scratch disease report an antecedant cat scratch or bite. Diagnosis may be confirmed by modified Warthin-Starry staining of bacteria on lymph node biopsy (with negative staining by Gram and acid-fast protocols) and specific serologic tests. Antimicrobial therapy of cat scratch disease is often unnecessary and responses to most agents are quite variable. In one retrospective review, ciprofloxacin, gentamicin, and sulfamethoxazole/trimethoprim were most often associated with apparent benefit.[76]

Bartonella henselae infection has dramatically different clinical manifestations in HIV-infected or other severely immunocompromised hosts, causing the syndrome of "bacillary angiomatosis."[77] Initially, infected patients may demonstrate undifferentiated fever without evidence of focal infection. Subsequently, raised red or violaceous cutaneous lesions are frequently noted, which may be mistaken for Kaposi's sarcoma on casual inspection. Involvement of extracutaneous sites including lymph nodes, bone, mucosal surfaces, lung, liver, spleen, bone marrow, heart, and central nervous system can occur. The diagnosis of bacillary angiomatosis is imperative because of its excellent response to antimicrobial therapy, in contrast to most cases of cat scratch disease. The reasons for the different responsiveness of these conditions to antimicrobial therapy are unknown. Erythromycin has been recommended as the agent of choice for bacillary angiomatosis, with doxycycline a good alternative. Newer macrolides may have even better activity.

The other pathogenic *Bartonella* species included *Bartonella bacilliformis*, *Bartonella elizabethae*, and *Bartonella quintana*. *B bacilliformis* is the etiologic agent of acute Oroya fever and chronic verruga peruana, two diseases occurring exclusively in high altitude river valleys of Peru, Ecuador, and Colombia. *B elizabethae* has been recently reported as an unusual cause of endocarditis. *B quintana* is principally of interest as the cause of trench fever, a louse-borne illness which afflicted more than one million soldiers during World War I. Recently, *B quintana* also has been implicated as a cause of cutaneous bacillary angiomatosis, bacteremia, or endocarditis in HIV-infected or other debilitated patients.[78] The relative importance of *B quintana* and *B henselae* as causes of bacillary angiomatosis is not well-established, but *B henselae* has been reported much more frequently in this context.

CAPNOCYTOPHAGA ■

Capnocytophaga are long, filamentous, fastidious Gram-negative bacilli with a characteristic gliding motility. Some *Capnocytophaga* species (previously designated DF-1) are part of the normal human oral flora, while others (previously known as DF-2) may be found in the mouths of normal dogs (and to a lesser extent, cats). *Capnocytophaga* may cause severe and sometimes fatal infections in immunocompromised patients. Bacteremia with human *Capnocytophaga* species is particularly associated with patients undergoing chemotherapy for malignant disease. Bacteremia with animal-associated species is particularly fulminant in asplenic patients and may mimic meningococcemia with DIC.[79] Imipenem, ampicillin/sulbactam, clindamycin, erythromycin, and doxycycline are highly active against *Capnocytophaga* species. Susceptibility to fluoroquinolones and third-generation cephalosporins is variable.

CHLAMYDIA   ■

There are three recognized *Chlamydia* species: *Chlamydia trachomatis*, *Chlamydia psittaci*, and *Chlamydia pneumoniae*. *C trachomatis* is an important cause of sexually transmitted disease, trachoma, and perinatal infection, but is seldom of concern in the critical care setting. *C psittaci* is the etiologic agent of psittacosis, a pneumonitis of birds which may be transmitted to humans. Psittacosis characteristically presents with fever, non-productive cough, and prominent headache. Pulmonary findings are often subtle and underestimate the extent of pneumonitis demonstrated on x-ray. Roentgenographic findings are variable, but frank consolidation is generally absent. There is considerable clinical overlap with Q fever, mycoplasmic pneumonia, *C pneumoniae* pneumonia (see later), legionellosis, fungal pneumonia, and viral pneumonia. The diagnosis of psittacosis is most readily confirmed serologically. Tetracyclines are the preferred therapeutic agents, and erythromycin is an acceptable alternative. Although most patients recover uneventfully, illness can be severe and even fatal, especially if untreated.[80]

Chlamydia pneumoniae (originally designated TWAR) is an important cause of upper respiratory tract illness and pneumonia.[81] Unlike *C psittaci*, *C pneumoniae* does not have an avian reservoir. Serologic studies suggest that *C pneumoniae* is responsible for about 10% of community acquired pneumonia. Although *C pneumoniae* respiratory illness is usually mild, severe or persistent illness has been reported, most often in elderly or immunocompromised hosts. Laboratory confirmation requires isolation of *C pneumoniae* in tissue culture, a rise in specific antibody, or polymerase chain reaction (PCR) detection of *C. pneumoniae* DNA. Since these studies are not widely available, the diagnosis of *C pneumoniae* infection is often presumptive. Tetracycline, erythromycin, or newer macrolides (azithromycin, clarithromycin) are recommended as therapy. Some patients appear to require retreatment.

MYCOBACTERIUM AVIUM-INTRACELLULARE   ■

Mycobacterium avium-intracellulare (M avium complex, MAI,MAC) are ubiquitous acid-fast bacilli which can be isolated from a variety of environmental and animal sources. The lungs are the most important site of localized MAI infection. Lung infection may bear some clinical and roentgenographic resemblance to pulmonary tuberculosis, but typically occurs in patients with underlying chronic lung disease. Other focal sites of MAI infection include lymph nodes, bone, and skin. Disseminated MAI infection is a frequent and serious infectious complication in patients with AIDS. Disseminated infection may develop from primary foci in the lungs or gastrointestinal tract. Nearly all patients with AIDS and disseminated MAI have advanced levels of immunocompromise, with less than 100 CD4 cells/μL blood.[82] Enormous microbial burdens (up to 10^{10} organisms per gram tissue) result in severe constitutional symptoms, including fever and weight loss. Multiple peripheral cytopenias are common. Involvement of the small intestine may produce a Whipple's-like malabsorption syndrome. The diagnosis of disseminated MAI infection is most often made by isolation of organisms from blood or bone marrow. Nucleic acid probes can provide rapid diagnostic confirmation. Antimicrobial treatment of MAI infection should include multiple agents; clarithromycin, ethambutol, rifampin, rifabutin, ciprofloxacin, clofazimine, streptomycin, or amikacin are among the agents most often used.

MYCOBACTERIUM KANSASII   ■

Mycobacterium kansasii is a photochromogenic (yellow-pigmented in the presence of light) non-tuberculous mycobacterium which causes pulmonary and occasionally extrapulmonary disease in immunocompromised hosts. Pneumoconiosis, chronic obstructive lung disease, and HIV infection are the most important predisposing factors. Patients with *M kansasii* infection usually respond well to a combination of isoniazid, rifampin, and ethambutol, despite only intermediate in vitro susceptibility of the organism to isoniazid.

MYCOBACTERIUM TUBERCULOSIS   ■

Mycobacterium tuberculosis is an acid-fast, aerobic, slow growing bacillus. Tuberculosis seen in the intensive care setting includes severe pulmonary disease, miliary TB, pericarditis, and CNS infections. Tuberculous bone and joint, skin, lymph node, renal, or gastrointestinal infections do not usually require intensive care.

PULMONARY TUBERCULOSIS

Primary tuberculous infection is usually controlled by host responses but may leave a residual calcified lung nodule and hilar lymph node (Ghon complex). Subsequent reactivation of quiescent infection occurs insidiously, with development of fatigue, weight loss, intermittent fever, and night sweats. Progressive destructive pneumonitis results in cough and dyspnea, frequently accompanied by hemoptysis or chest pain. Reactivated pulmonary foci most often occur in the apical posterior segments of upper lobes and superior segments of lower lobes. Chest radiographs may reveal cavitary infiltrates, fibrosis, hilar adenopathy, or pleural effusions. Changes may occur so gradually that x-rays are misinterpreted as stable, unless serial films over several months are examined; ICU patients receiving daily chest radiographs are particularly susceptible to this pitfall. Roentgenographic changes are often atypical in patients with HIV infection.[83]

Cultures and acid-fast smears should be obtained when tuberculosis is suspected. Because these organisms divide slowly, positive culture results generally take from 10 to 21 days in the BACTEC system, or from 21 to 48 days on conventional solid medium.

A purified protein derivative (PPD) skin test (5 TU) should be placed unless the patient is previously documented to have a positive tuberculin test. Induration $\geq$10 mm at 48 to 72 hours is generally considered to be positive, although tests $\geq$5 mm may be considered positive in high-risk patients, and any induration may be considered positive in HIV-infected individuals. A negative PPD does not rule out active tuberculosis. Additional skin tests using mumps or candidal antigens may be placed concomitantly in an attempt to assess a patient's overall immune responsiveness, but are of limited value.

MILIARY TUBERCULOSIS

Miliary or disseminated tuberculosis may occur during the primary episode of infection, or more frequently, following reactivation. Patients with impaired immunity due to aging, immunosuppressive drugs, or other intercurrent illness are at greatest risk. Non-specific in its presentation, miliary tuberculosis may be easily missed unless specifically sought by respiratory cultures and biopsies of bone marrow, liver, or lymph nodes. Skin tests are frequently negative, and the classic fine nodular densities on chest radiograph may be initially absent. Miliary tuberculosis responds well to antimicrobial therapy when recognized early, underscoring the importance of timely diagnosis.[84]

TUBERCULOUS PERICARDITIS

Tuberculous infection of the pericardium usually results from contiguous spread of infection from caseating lymph nodes.[85] Patients present with pleural effusion and may lack fever or evidence of tuberculosis at other sites. Chest pain, dyspnea, a pericardial friction rub, or physical findings suggesting cardiac tamponade may be present. Pericardiocentesis may be required if hemodynamic compromise is present, or if pyogenic infection is suspected. However, pericardial biopsy may be required to establish the diagnosis of tuberculous pericarditis. Constrictive pericarditis may occur as a late complication.

TUBERCULOUS MENINGITIS

Tuberculous meningitis may occur in association with other foci of active disease or as an isolated clinical entity. A predilection for basilar involvement is seen, with the frequent occurrence of cranial nerve palsies. Hydrocephalus may be noted on CT or MRI scans.

Patients may present with headache, fever, confusion, and vomiting. Some may exhibit vague personality disturbances, perhaps accompanied by fever and flu-like symptoms. A careful clinical evaluation may reveal evidence of extrameningeal tuberculosis in the lungs, genitourinary tract, or bone. Laboratory abnormalities are non-specific, with the exception of hyponatremia resulting from syndrome of inappropriate antidiuretic hormone (SIADH). Lumbar puncture is the most important diagnostic procedure. Lymphocyte-predominant CSF pleocytosis (usually more than 100 cells/mm^3 but rarely greater than 1500 cells/mm^3), elevated protein, and low or normal glucose are characteristic findings.[86] Mycobacterial cultures of CSF are usually positive, but smears are generally negative. Rapid diagnostic studies utilizing the polymerase chain reaction (PCR) are currently in development.

TREATMENT OF TUBERCULOSIS

In response to the recent surge in drug-resistant tuberculosis in the United States, new guidelines for the treatment of tuberculosis have been issued recently.[87] In settings where the prevalence of drug-resistance disease is below 4%, patients may be treated initially with isoniazid (INH), rifampin, and pyrazinamide (PZA). If drug-susceptibility is confirmed by in vitro testing after the first 2 months of treatment, the regimen may be changed to INH and rifampin 2 or 3 times a week for an additional 4 months. In areas with greater than 4% prevalence of resistant tuberculosis, initial therapy should consist of isoniazid, rifampin, PZA, and either ethambutol or streptomycin. Second- or third-line agents such as ofloxacin, cycloserine, and ethionamide are sometimes required in the treatment of multi-drug resistant *M tuberculosis*. Longer courses of therapy may be warranted in patients with AIDS and patients with tuberculous vertebral osteomyelitis. Corticosteroids are usually administered as adjunctive therapy in patients with tuberculous pericarditis and in those with tuberculous meningitis if neurologic deficits are present.

MYCOPLASMAL INFECTIONS ■

Mycoplasma are ubiquitous bacteria which lack a cell wall. Of the mycoplasmas, *Mycoplasma pneumoniae*, *Mycoplasma hominis*, and *Ureaplasma urealyticum* are best established as human pathogens. *M pneumoniae* most frequently causes an "atypical" pneumonia syndrome in young adults, which is generally self-limited unless unusual complications such as ARDS occur. Serology, culture, and a variety of rapid testing methods may be employed to establish the diagnosis of *M pneumoniae* infection. The presence of high cold agglutinin titers are consistent with *M pneumoniae* pneumonia, but are non-specific. Erythromycin, newer macrolides, or tetracyclines are effective in ameliorating symptoms. *M hominis* is associated with genitourinary, post-partum, and post-surgical infections. Tetracycline, ciprofloxacin, or clindamycin are usually active against *M hominis*, but erythromycin is ineffective. *Ureaplasma* is associated with genitourinary infections.

RICKETTSIAL INFECTIONS ■

The most serious rickettsial illness occurring in the United States is Rocky Mountain spotted fever (RMSF). RMSF is a tick-borne illness caused by *Rickettsia rickettsii*, a small intracellular bacterium. Despite its name, RMSF is most common along the south and north atlantic states, with the exception of Montana and South Dakota, where it is endemic. RMSF typically presents with fever, headache, myalgia, and a petechial rash. General signs of sepsis, nausea, vomiting, and abdominal pain may also be seen. The rash usually begins on the extremities after a few days of illness. In a minority of patients, the rash may be found within the first 24 hours of illness, or not at all. Palms and soles are typically but not invariably involved. Untreated, RMSF can follow a fulminant course with hypotension, renal failure, CNS dysfunction, pulmonary edema, and death. Doxycycline and tetracycline are the therapeutic agents of choice, but chloramphenicol may be substituted in pregnant women or children. In vitro studies support the possible use of fluoroquinolones,[88] but there are insufficient clinical data to support the use of these drugs as first-line agents.

BORRELIA ■

Borrelia are spirochetal organisms which include the etiologic agents of relapsing fever and Lyme disease. Relapsing fever may be louse-borne or tick-borne. Pyrexial episodes lasting several days are punctuated by periods of afebrility. Neurologic, cardiac, and hematologic complications may occur. The diagnosis of relapsing fever is best established by observing the spiral organisms on peripheral blood smears obtained during febrile periods. Tetracycline is the treatment of choice and appears to significantly reduce both morbidity and mortality associated with this disease.

Borrelia burgdorferi is the causative agent of Lyme disease. This condition is characterized by the appearance of a skin lesion, erythema chronicum migrans (ECM), which appears at the site of a tick bite. Beginning as a small papule, ECM expands outward with an erythematous border and central clearing. Secondary lesions are common. ECM lesions are warm and tender, resolving over weeks to months. Constitutional symptoms such as malaise, headache, fatigue, and myalgias may be present. Following the early cutaneous phase of Lyme disease, patients may develop evidence of cardiac, neurologic, or rheumatologic involvement. Myocarditis with AV block may result in ICU hospitalization.

Serologic testing is the most useful means of confirming the diagnosis of Lyme disease, but is insensitive in the early ECM stage of illness. Doxycycline or cefuroxime are administered to patients with ECM, and ceftriaxone is usually recommended for the treatment of late complications.[89]

LEPTOSPIROSIS ■

Leptospira are motile spirochetes which grow only on special media. Therefore, most leptospirosis is diagnosed by serologic testing. Leptospirosis develops through contact with infected domestic or wild animals or their urine. Rats are the most common source of human leptospirosis, but dogs, livestock, and cats are also recognized sources. The illness usually presents with chills, fever, severe headache, pronounced conjunctival suffusion, and myalgias lasting from 3 to 7 days. A second brief (1–3 days) immune phase of illness frequently follows. This phase typically presents with a severe headache (often with meningeal signs), myalgias, abdominal pain, nausea, vomiting, adenopathy, and variable pulmonary findings. Fever is low-grade or absent at this time. Both the initial and immune phases of illness are usually self-limited. A minority of patients with leptospirosis develop a severe form of illness (Weil's disease), characterized by renal failure and jaundice; hemorrhagic manifestations and myocarditis may also be seen. Therapy with penicillin, ampicillin, tetracycline, or doxycycline is thought to shorten the course of illness in leptospirosis,[90] and is likely to reduce morbidity and mortality in Weil's disease.

SYPHILIS ■

Treponema pallidum, the causative agent of syphilis, is a sexually-transmitted pathogen infrequently encountered by critical care specialists; however, neurosyphilis is occasionally seen in the ICU. Neurosyphilis may be manifest as asymptomatic CSF abnormalities, syphilitic meningitis, meningovascular syphilis, tabes dorsalis, or paretic neurosyphilis. In asymptomatic neurosyphilis, the CSF typically demonstrates a lymphocytic pleocytosis and elevated protein. However, CSF studies can be completely normal despite the presence of viable spirochetes. Serologic testing is crucial in diagnosis, since *T pallidum* cannot be cultivated in vitro. The serum fluorescent treponemal antibody absorption (FTA-Abs) is almost always positive, and the CSF venereal disease research laboratory (VDRL) test may be positive, but is relatively insensitive. Syphilitic meningitis usually occurs within the first two years of infection and resembles aseptic meningitis of other causes. Meningovascular syphilis may present from 1 to 10 years or more after infection with focal neurologic deficits, seizures, or personality changes. Focal arterial narrowing may be demonstrated on cerebral angiography. Tabes dorsalis is uncommon and causes posterior column and dorsal root signs, such as ataxic wide-based gait and loss of propioceptive, deep pain, and temperature sensation. Paretic neurosyphilis is also rare and should be considered in an evaluation of unexplained dementia. Concomitant HIV infection can be associated with unusually rapid progression of *T pallidum* infection to neurosyphilis, as well as with a suboptimal response to therapy.[91] The standard recommended therapy for neurosyphilis consists of penicillin G 12 to 24 million units/day IV in divided doses for a minimum of 10 days.

REFERENCES ■

1. Nathens AB, Chu PTY, Marshall JC: Nosocomial infection in the surgical intensive care unit. *Infect Dis Clin North Am* 1992;6:657

2. Koneman EW (ed): *Color Atlas and Textbook of Diagnostic Microbiology*, 4th ed. Philadelphia, JB Lippincott, 1993
3. Verghese A, Widrich WC, Arbeit RD: Central venous septic thrombophlebitis: the role of medical therapy. *Medicine* 1985;64:394
4. Bayer AS, Lam K, Ginzton L: *Staphylococcus aureus* bacteremia: clinical, serologic, and echocardiographic findings in patients with and without endocarditis. *Arch Intern Med* 1987;147:457
5. Jernigan JA, Farr BM: Short-course therapy of catheter-related *Staphylococcus aureus* bacteremia: a meta-analysis. *Ann Intern Med* 1993;119:304.
6. Bayer AS: Infective endocarditis. *Clin Infect Dis* 1993;17:313
7. Birmingham GD, Rahko PS, Ballantyne F: Improved detection of infective endocarditis with transesophageal echocardiography. *Am Heart J* 1992;123:774
8. Carpenter JL: Perivalvular extension of infection in patients with infectious endocarditis. *Rev Infect Dis* 1991;13:127
9. Karchmer AW: *Staphylococcus aureus* and vancomycin: the sequel. *Ann Intern Med* 1991;115:739
10. DiNubile MJ: Short-course antibiotic therapy for right-sided endocarditis caused by *Staphylococcus aureus* in injection drug users. *Ann Intern Med* 1994;121:873
11. Alsip SG, Blackstone EH, Kirklin JW: Indications for cardiac surgery in patients with active infective endocarditis. *Am J Med* 1985;78(Suppl 6B):138
12. Heimberger TS, Duma RJ: Infections of prosthetic heart valves and cardiac pacemakers. *Infect Dis Clin North Am* 1989;3:221
13. Arbuthnott J, et al: International symposium on toxic shock syndrome. *Rev Infect Dis* 1989;11(Suppl 1):S1
14. Lessner A, Stern GA: Preseptal and orbital cellulitis. *Infect Dis Clin North Am* 1992;6:933
15. Schauwecker DS, Braunstein EM, Wheat LJ: Diagnostic imaging of osteomyelitis. *Infect Dis Clin North Am* 1990;4:441
16. Wheeler D, Keiser P, Rigamonti D: Medical management of spinal epidural abscesses: Case report and review. *Clin Infect Dis* 1992;15:22
17. Goldenberg DL, Reed JI: Bacterial arthritis. *New Engl J Med* 1985;312:764
18. Mulligan ME, Murray-Leisure KA, Ribner BS: Methicillin-resistant *Staphylococcus aureus*: a consensus review of the microbiology, pathogenesis, and epidemiology with implications for prevention and management. *Am J Med* 1993;94:313
19. Mayhall CG: Diagnosis and management of infections of implantable devices used for prolonged venous access. *Curr Clin Topics Infect Dis* 1992;12:83
20. McLaurine RL, Frame PT: Treatment of infections of cerebrospinal fluid shunts. *Rev Infect Dis* 1987;9:595
21. Justich E, Amparo EG, Hricak H: Infected aortoiliofemoral grafts: magnetic resonance imaging. *Radiol* 1985;154:133
22. Rubin J, Ray R, Barnes T: Peritonitis in continuous ambulatory peritoneal dialysis. *Am J Kidney Dis* 1983;2:602
23. Stamenkovic I, Lew PD: Early recognition of potentially fatal necrotizing fasciitis: use of frozen-section biopsy. *New Engl J Med* 1984;310:1689
24. Stevens DL: Invasive group A streptococcal infections. *Clin Infect Dis* 1992;14:2
25. Farley MM, Harvey RC, Stull T: A population-based assessment of invasive disease due to group B *Streptococcus* in nonpregnant adults. *New Engl J Med* 1993;328:1807
26. Lebel MH, Freij BJ, Syrogiannopoulos GA: Dexamethasone therapy for bacterial meningitis: results of two double-blind, placebo-controlled trials. *New Engl J Med* 1988;319:964
27. Wald ER, Kaplan SL, Mason EO Jr.: Dexamethasone therapy for children with bacterial meningitis. *Pediatrics* 1995;95:21
28. Applebaum PC: Antimicrobial resistance in *Streptococcus pneumoniae*: an overview. *Clin Infect Dis* 1992;15:77
29. Francioli P, Etienne J, Hoigne R: Treatment of streptococcal endocarditis with a single daily dose of ceftriaxone sodium for 4 weeks: efficacy and outpatient treatment feasibility. *JAMA* 1992;267:264
30. Elting LS, Godey GP, Keefe BH: Septicemia and shock syndrome due to viridans streptococci: a case-control study of predisposing factors. *Clin Infect Dis* 1992;14:1201
31. Gossling J: Occurrence and pathogenicity of the *Streptococcus milleri* group. *Rev Infect Dis* 1988;10:257
32. Leclercq R, Dutka-Malen S, Brisson-Noel A: Resistance of enterococci to aminoglycosides and glycopeptides. *Clin Infect Dis* 1992;15:495
33. Hager H, Verghese A, Alvarez S: *Branhamella catarrhalis* respiratory infections. *Rev Infect Dis* 1987;9:1140
34. Gilja HO, Halstensen A, Digranes A: Single-dose ofloxacin to eradicate tonsillopharyngeal carriage of *Neisseria meningitidis*. *Antimicrob Agents Chemother* 1993;37:2024
35. Ellison RT, Kohler PF, Curd JG: Prevalence of congenital or acquired complement deficiency in patients with sporadic meningococcal disease. *New Engl J Med* 1983;308:913
36. vanDeuren M, Santman FW, van Dalen R: Plasma and whole blood exchange in meningococcal sepsis. *Clin Infect Dis* 1992;15:424
37. Centers for Disease Control and Prevention: 1993 Sexually transmitted diseases treatment guidelines. *MMWR* 1993;42 (Suppl RR-14):47
38. Sliman R, Rehm S, Shlaes DM: Serious infections caused by *Bacillus* species. *Medicine* 1987;66:218
39. Coyle MB, Lipsky BA: Coryneform bacteria in infectious diseases: clinical and laboratory aspects. *Clin Microbiol Rev* 1990;3:227
40. Soriano F, Aguado JM, Ponte C: Urinary tract infection caused by *Corynebacterium* group D2: report of 82 cases and review. *Rev Infect Dis* 1990;12:1019
41. Nieman RE, Lorber B: Listeriosis in adults: a changing pattern. Report of eight cases and review of the literature. *Rev Infect Dis* 1980;2:207
42. Spitzer PG, Hammer AM, Karchmer AW: Treatment of *Listeria monocytogenes* infection with trimethoprim-sulfamethoxazole: case report and review of literature. *Rev Infect Dis* 1986;8:427
43. Wallace RJ, Steele LC: Susceptibility testing of *Nocardia asteroides* for the clinical laboratory. *Diagn Microbiol Infect Dis* 1988;9:155
44. Lambert T, Gerbaud G, Bouvet P: Dissemination of amikacin resistance gene *aphA6* in *Acinetobacter* spp. *Antimicrob Agents Chemother* 1990;34:1244
45. Urban C, Go E, Mariano N: Effect of sulbactam on infections caused by imipenem-resistant *Acinetobacter calcoaceticus* biotype *anitratus*. *J Infect Dis* 1993;167:448
46. Tunkel AR: Topical antibacterials. In: Mandell GL, Bennett JE, Dolin R (eds). *Principles and Practice of Infectious Diseases*. New York, Churchill Livingstone, 1995:381
47. Mishu B, Blaser MJ: The role of *Campylobacter jejuni* infection in the initiation of Guillain-Barre syndrome. *Clin Infect Dis* 1993;17:104
48. Sanchez R, Fernandez-Baca V, Diaz MD: Evolution of susceptibilities of *Campylobacter* spp. to quinolones and macrolides. *Antimicrob Agents Chemother* 1994;38:1879
49. Marshall BJ, Warren JR: Unidentified curved bacilli in the stomach of patients with gastritis and peptic ulceration. *Lancet* 1984;1:1311
50. Chow JW, Fine MJ, Shlaes DM: *Enterobacter* bacteremia: clinical features and emergence of antibiotic resistance during therapy. *Ann Intern Med* 1991;115:585
51. Karmali MA, Petric M, Lim C: The association between idiopathic hemolytic uremic syndrome and infection by verotoxin-

producing *Escherichia coli. J Infect Dis* 1985;151:775

52. Sirot J, Chanal C, Petit A: *Klebsiella pneumoniae* and other *Enterobacteriaceae* producing novel plasmid-mediated β-lactamases markedly active against third-generation cephalosporins: epidemiologic studies. *Rev Infect Dis* 1988;10:850

53. Hoffman S, Punjabi NH, Kumala S: Reduction of mortality in chloramphenicol-treated severe typhoid fever by high-dose dexamethasone. *New Engl J Med* 1984;310:82

54. Fang FC, Fierer J: Human infection with *Salmonella dublin. Medicine* 1991;70:198

55. Neill MA, Opal SM, Heelan J: Failure of ciprofloxacin to eradicate convalescent fecal excretion after acute salmonellosis: experience during an outbreak in health care workers. *Ann Intern Med* 1991;114:195

56. Bonacorsi SP, Scavizzi MR, Guiyoule A: Assessment of a fluoroquinolone, three β-lactams, two aminoglycosides, and a cycline in treatment of murine *Yersinia pestis* infection. *Antimicrob Agents Chemother* 1994;38:481

57. Gayraud M, Scavizzi MR, Mollaret HH: Antibiotic treatment of *Yersinia enterocolitica* septicemia: a retrospective review of 43 cases. *Clin Infect Dis* 1993;17:405

58. Enderlin G, Morales L, Jacobs RF: Streptomycin and alternative agents for the treatment of tularemia in the literature. *Clin Infect Dis* 1994;19:42

59. Adams G, Deaver KA, Cochi SL: Decline of childhood *Haemophilus influenzae* type b (Hib) disease in the Hib vaccine era. *JAMA* 1993;269:221

60. Weber DJ, Wolfson JS, Swartz MN: *Pasteurella multocida* infections: report of 32 cases and review of the literature. *Medicine* 1984;63:133

61. Kielhofner M, Atmar RL, Hamill RJ: Life-threatening *Pseudomonas aeruginosa* infections in patients with human immunodeficiency virus infection. *Clin Infect Dis* 1992;14:403

62. Bodey GP, Bolivar R, Fainstein V, et al: Infections caused by *Pseudomonas aeruginosa. Rev Infect Dis* 1983;5:279

63. Goldmann DA, Klinger JD: *Pseudomonas cepacia*: biology, mechanisms of virulence, epidemiology. *J Pediatr* 1986;108:106

64. Elting LS, Bodey GP: Septicemia due to *Xanthomonas* species and non-*aeruginosa Pseudomonas* species: increasing incidence of catheter-related infections. *Medicine* 1990;69:296

65. Gorbach SL: The eighth cholera pandemic. *Infect Dis Clin Pract* 1994;3:212

66. Hill MK, Sanders CV: Localized and systemic infections due to *Vibrio* species. *Infect Dis Clin North Am* 1987;1:687

67. Lineaweaver WC, Hill MK, Buncke GM: *Aeromonas hydrophila* infections following use of medicinal leeches in reimplantation and flap surgery. *Ann Plast Surg* 1992;29:238

68. Cherington M: Botulism. *Sem Neurol* 1990;10:27

69. Peterson LR, Kelly PJ: The role of the clinical microbiology laboratory in the management of *Clostridium difficile*-associated diarrhea. *Infect Dis Clin North Am* 1993;7:277

70. Stevens DL, Bryant AE, Adams K: Evaluation of therapy with hyperbaric oxygen for experimental infection with *Clostridium perfringens. Clin Infect Dis* 1993;17:231

71. Bleck TP: Tetanus: pathophysiology, management, and prophylaxis. *Dis Mon* 1991;37:545

72. Moreno S, et al: Lemierre's disease: postanginal bacteremia and pulmonary involvement caused by *Fusobacterium necrophorum. Rev Infect Dis* 1989;11:319

73. Blomquist IK, Bayer AS: Life-threatening deep fascial space infection of the head and neck. *Infect Dis Clin North Am* 1988;2:237

74. Yoshikawa TT, Quinn W: The aching head: intracranial suppuration due to head and neck infections. *Infect Dis Clin North Am* 1988;2:265

75. Regnery RL, Martin M, Olson J: Serologic response to "*Rochalimaea henselae*" antigen in suspected cat scratch disease. *Lancet* 1992;340:557

76. Margileth AM: Antibiotic therapy for cat-scratch disease: clinical study of therapeutic outcome in 268 patients and a review of the literature. *Pediatr Infect Dis J* 1992;11:474

77. Relman DA, Loutit JS, Schmidt TM: An approach to the identification of uncultured pathogens: the agent of bacillary angiomatosis. *New Engl J Med* 1990;323:1573

78. Relman DA: Has trench fever returned? *New Engl J Med* 1995;332:461

79. Kullberg JB, Westendorp RG, van 't Wout JW: Purpura fulminans and symmetrical peripheral gangrene caused by *Capnocytophaga canimorsus* (formerly DF-2) septicemia: a complication of dog bite. *Medicine* 1991;70:287

80. Verweij PE, Meis JF, Eijk R: Severe human psittacosis requiring artificial ventilation: Case report and review. *Clin Infect Dis* 1995;20:440

81. Grayston JT: Infections caused by *Chlamydia pneumoniae* strain TWAR. *Clin Infect Dis* 1992;15:757

82. Ellner JJ, Goldberger MJ, Parenti DM: *Mycobacterium avium* infection and AIDS. *J Infect Dis* 1991;163:1326

83. Hopewell PC: Tuberculosis and the human immunodeficiency virus infection. *Sem Respir Infect* 1991;4:111

84. Kim JH, Langston AA, Gallis HA: Miliary tuberculosis: epidemiology, clinical manifestations, diagnosis, and outcome. *Rev Infect Dis* 1990;12:583

85. Fowler NO: Tuberculous pericarditis. *JAMA* 1991;266:99

86. Klein NC, Damsker B, Hirschman SZ: Mycobacterial meningitis: retrospective analysis from 1970 to 1983. *Am J Med* 1985;79:29

87. Centers for Disease Control and Prevention: Recommendations of the advisory council for the elimination of tuberculosis: initial therapy for tuberculosis in the era of multidrug resistance. *MMWR* 1993;42(RR-7):1

88. Raoult D, Drancourt M: Antimicrobial therapy of rickettsial diseases. *Antimicrob Agents Chemother* 1991;35:2457

89. Steere AC: Lyme disease. *New Engl J Med* 1989;321:586

90. Watt G, Padre LP, Tuazon ML: Placebo-controlled trial of intravenous penicillin for severe and late leptospirosis. *Lancet* 1988;1:433

91. Musher DM, Hamill RJ, Baughn RE: Effect of human immunodeficiency virus (HIV) infection on the course of syphilis and on the response to treatment. *Ann Intern Med* 1992;113:872

Critical Care, Third Edition, edited by Joseph M. Civetta,
Robert W. Taylor, and Robert R. Kirby.
Lippincott-Raven Publishers, Philadelphia, PA © 1997.

CHAPTER 113

∎

Fungal and Viral Infections

Stephen B. Greenberg

There is an increasing awareness of fungal and viral pathogens in the intensive care patient population. Patients in the
intensive care unit (ICU) are often immunosuppressed, with
defects in humoral or cell-mediated immunity. Underlying
diseases (e.g., lymphoproliferative malignancies) or procedures that alter immune mechanisms are common. Fungi
and viruses are often secondary infectious agents in these
patients. Because of the increased number of patients being
admitted to ICUs, physicians must become familiar with the
pathogenesis, clinical presentation, and treatment of these
nonbacterial agents. This chapter reviews the relevant fungal
and viral pathogens and the associated syndromes that may
be seen in ICU patients.

FUNGAL INFECTIONS ∎

CLINICAL EPIDEMIOLOGY

Opportunistic infections with fungi are increasing in frequency, especially in immunosuppressed patients with acquired immunodeficiency syndrome (AIDS) or malignancy,
after major surgery or major burns, and in bone marrow
and solid organ transplantation patients.[1] Cofactors contributing to these fungal infections are use of broad-spectrum
antimicrobial agents, corticosteroids, cytotoxic chemotherapy, and long-term indwelling catheters (Table 113-1). In
addition to *Candida albicans*, Aspergillus species, and the
Zygomycetes, newly recognized fungal pathogens now include non-albicans species of *Candida*, yeasts other than
Candida, *Fusarium* species, and agents of phaeohyphomy-
cosis.

   Neutrophil phagocytosis is a primary host defense mechanism against tissue invasion and dissemination with fungi.[2]
Normal host defense mechanisms are also altered by use of
adrenal corticosteroids, which appear to enhance the estab-

lishment of several different infections, including fungi.
Some studies have suggested that antibiotics are a factor
predisposing to systemic fungal infection, but others have
failed to demonstrate an increase in antibiotic use among
patients with fungal infections. Nevertheless, colonization
of the gastrointestinal tract by *Candida* species appears to
be increased with the administration of broad-spectrum antimicrobial agents. Indwelling vascular catheters and total
parenteral nutrition have been associated with an increased
frequency of fungemia. Patients who have had extensive
surgery, are diabetic, have chronic acidosis, are chronically
malnourished or debilitated, or are alcohol and drug abusers
also appear to have an increased likelihood of developing
fungal infections. These are the groups that are likely to
develop disseminated fungal infection and to require intensive care during their hospitalization.

CANDIDIASIS

Microbiology and Pathogenesis

Candida species are usually found on mucocutaneous surfaces but can overgrow and invade tissue if there are alterations in host defenses.[3] Although the most common manifestations of candidal infections involve superficial skin
diseases and vaginitis, disseminated forms are important
causes of morbidity and mortality in many hospitalized
patients.

   Candida species, especially *C albicans*, are significant
nosocomial pathogens. Patients at high risk have leukemia
or solid tumors and leukopenia. Bone marrow transplant
recipients, burn patients, and premature infants are also
prone to these fungal infections. Approximately 10% to 15%
of all hospital-acquired bloodstream infections are due to
nosocomial candidemia. Primary candidemia rates have increased dramatically during the past 10 years in both small
and large hospitals.

TABLE 113-1. Clinical Epidemiology of Fungal Infections

NORMAL HOST

    Extensive surgery
    Antibiotic therapy
    Intravenous catheters

COMPROMISED HOST

    Adrenal corticosteroid therapy
    Malignancy, hematologic
    Neutrophil dysfunction
    Alcohol and drug abuse
    Diabetes mellitus
    Acquired immunodeficiency syndrome
    Total parenteral nutrition
    Malnutrition

Candida species can be cultured on blood and Sabouraud agar within 1 to 2 days. Simple laboratory tests can be performed within 1 to 3 hours to identify *C albicans*, but the other species of *Candida* require additional tests for specific identification.[4]

Candida are often part of the microflora of the oropharynx and gastrointestinal tracts of normal hosts. This commensal status may change to invasion if there are alterations in the host. Diabetic patients have increased serum glucose available as a substrate for growth of the fungus. Steroids, antibiotics, and mucosal surface damage with decreased host defenses can lead to a change from noninvasive infection of *Candida* to one of disease. Most recently, published studies have suggested that the polymorphonuclear leukocyte is the important cellular defense against *Candida*; when defects in leukocyte function exist, the incidence of *Candida* suprainfection is increased.

Although *C albicans* is the most frequent isolate from hematogenously disseminated candidiasis, *Candida tropicalis*, *Candida parapsilosis*, *Candida krusei*, and *Candida lusitaniae* have been reported in increasing frequency.[5] *C tropicalis* accounts for approximately 30% of all fungal infections in patients with bone marrow transplants or hematologic malignancies. Persistent colorization with *C tropicalis* has been associated with hematogenous dissemination. *C parapsilosis* infections have been found following invasive procedures, hyperalimentation, or prosthetic devices. Unlike *C tropicalis*, *C parapsilosis* bloodstream infections are not associated with prior colorization but due to injection of the organisms directly into the bloodstream.[6] In granulocytopenia patients with malignancy, fungemia due to *C krusei* has been reported with increasing frequency. *C krusei* is resistant to fluconazole and bloodstream infections with this yeast have a high mortality rate.[7] Recent reports with *C lusitaniae*, a pathogenic yeast in immunocompromised hosts, demonstrate infection of the respiratory tract, urine, or blood. Development of resistance to amphotericin B has been reported frequently with *C lusitaniae*.[5]

Clinical Disease

The most common clinical presentations of candidal infections are involvement of the oropharynx or gastrointestinal tract and disseminated infection (Table 113-2).[8] There may also be involvement of the heart with endocarditis, primary infection of the kidney, lung, and brain, and suppurative infection of central veins as a complication of parenteral nutrition.[9] In addition, in infants or children with defects in cell-mediated immunity, mucocutaneous candidiasis is seen occasionally.

The most frequent presentation of oropharyngeal infection with *Candida* is thrush or evidence of candidal infection on the mucous membranes of the mouth. Thrush is frequently found in persons who have altered immune defenses but can also occur in normal persons. These lesions can be asymptomatic or quite painful. They are raised white patches found along the gums, tongue, and buccal mucosa. To make a diagnosis, one can either culture the lesions or look for budding yeast with pseudohyphae under light microscopy.

Although the gastrointestinal tracts of normal people frequently culture positive for *Candida*, significant infection usually occurs in people who have had prolonged intraabdominal surgical procedures or are immunosuppressed. If the esophagus is involved, erosions and ulcerations in the distal esophagus are seen. Patients with esophagitis secondary to candidal infection complain of retrosternal pain, dysphagia, and odynophagia; however, a significant subgroup of patients have no clinical symptoms that point to the diagnosis. It is common to find esophageal infection in association with oropharyngeal lesions. To make a definitive diagnosis, one must recover *Candida* from localized ulcerations or demonstrate tissue invasion by biopsy. Esophagrams may be normal despite severe esophagitis in a significant subgroup of patients.

Disseminated candidiasis usually occurs in either immunosuppressed hosts or as a nosocomial infection in patients who have been made susceptible by an underlying disease or associated treatment.[10] Clinically, patients with disseminated candidiasis may present with a fever of unknown origin or in septic shock. Involvement of the kidneys or heart is not infrequent in disseminated disease, and other organ systems may be involved as well. Observing macronodular skin lesions or detecting endophthalmitis may be helpful in indicating disseminated candidiasis in an individual patient. These clinical findings, however, are seen in a minority of patients, so that definitive diagnosis is possible only by demonstrating that fungus has invaded tissue or by isolating *Candida* from normally sterile body sites.

A positive blood culture for *Candida* may represent either transient fungemia or disseminated candidiasis. In addition, several studies have demonstrated that blood cultures may be negative in patients subsequently found to have invasive candidiasis either at postmortem or by tissue diagnosis. Serologic tests are not helpful because of their low sensitivity and specificity.

Patients with transient candidemia often have intravenous catheters for parenteral hyperalimentation. If a patient has a positive blood culture for *Candida* associated with intrave-

TABLE 113-2.   Common Fungal Infections

HOST/FUNGUS	MAJOR CLINICAL PRESENTATIONS	DIAGNOSTIC METHODS
NORMAL HOST		
Aspergillus	Allergic bronchopulmonary	Serum IgE, precipitins
Blastomyces	Acute pneumonitis: chronic lung or skin	Culture, tissue
Candida	Vaginitis; thrush; candidemia; intravenous catheter	Culture/smear
Coccidioides	Acute pneumonitis; chronic cavitary; pulmonary nodule	Precipitins, complement fixation
Cryptococcus	Pulmonary; meningitis	Culture, latex agglutination
Histoplasma	Acute pulmonary; progressive dissemination in infants and elderly; chronic cavitary in chronic airway obstruction	Culture
COMPROMISED HOST		
Diabetes mellitus		
Candida	Disseminated; pyelonephritis; vaginitis	Culture/smear
Mucorales	Rhinocerebral; pulmonary	Culture, tissue
Torulopsis	Pyelonephritis	Culture
Malignancy or corticosteroids		
Aspergillus	Invasive/lung	Culture, preciptin antibody
Candida	Esophagitis; disseminated; transient fungemia	Culture
Coccidioides	Disseminated	Culture
Cryptococcus	Pulmonary; disseminated	Culture, latex agglutination
Histoplasma	Progressive; disseminated	Culture
Mucorales	Rhinocerebral; pulmonary; disseminated	Culture, tissue
Torulopsis	Disseminated; fungemia	Culture
Prior antibiotics or intravenous catheters		
Candida	Vaginitis; thrush; esophagitis; disseminated	Culture
Torulopsis	Disseminated	Culture

nous catheterization, it is appropriate to remove the catheter and to observe the patient for evidence of disseminated disease.[11] Repeat blood cultures are important; if the fungemia continues to be present 72 hours after removal of the catheter, dissemination should be suspected. In some severely ill patients, institution of antifungal therapy and removal of the catheter should be performed immediately after a report of positive blood cultures.

Candidal endocarditis, although uncommon, should be suspected in intravenous drug abusers, in patients who have had intravenous catheterization for a prolonged period, and in those recovering from recent cardiac surgery. The aortic valve is the most frequently affected site, but any valve may be involved. The manifestations are similar to those of bacterial endocarditis except that patients with candidal endocarditis tend to have large valvular vegetations, associated with embolic episodes to medium-sized arteries throughout the body.

One should suspect the possibility of candidal endocarditis if there are major embolic episodes, large vegetations by echocardiography, or endophthalmitis in patients who have a predilection for this fungal infection. Negative blood cultures do not exclude the possibility of candidal endocarditis. Candidal involvement of central veins may occur as a complication of intravenous hyperalimentation. Patients with this

complication often have fever, soft-tissue abscess, and positive blood cultures despite removal of the intravenous lines.

Candida also infects the genitourinary tract and is a frequent colonizer of the urine in patients receiving antibiotics, in diabetic patients, or in association with indwelling catheters. If *Candida* colonizes the urine, patients are usually asymptomatic and no therapy is needed. However, involvement of the upper tract and pyelonephritis may occur. Frequently, if the bladder catheter is removed or antibiotics are discontinued, or if control of diabetes is improved, no specific antifungal therapy will be required for asymptomatic candiduria. However, distinguishing between colonization and infection of the lower urinary tract with cystitis is often difficult.[12] In patients with chronic indwelling catheters, candidal infection often disappears spontaneously. If colony counts persist after correcting underlying factors, then therapy should be considered. Making a diagnosis of primary infection of renal parenchyma with *Candida* is often difficult. Patients who have been described as having candidal pyelonephritis are usually female, have diabetes mellitus or some other underlying disease, or have had a recent surgical procedure. To diagnose candidal pyelonephritis, one should demonstrate repeated evidence of candidal infection of the urinary tract with serial cultures. The intravenous pyelogram may be abnormal, and fungus balls may be seen. *Candida* serologic tests are probably not too useful in this condition. Hyphae or pseudohyphae in the urine are not sufficient to establish the diagnosis of candidal pyelonephritis.

Renal involvement is common in disseminated candidiasis because of the hematogenous spread of the organism, with the subsequent formation of renal abscesses. The diagnosis of renal involvement in disseminated candidiasis depends on both positive urine and blood cultures. Definitive diagnosis, however, can be made only if tissue is obtained and appropriately sectioned.

ASPERGILLOSIS

Aspergillus species can cause asymptomatic infection, hypersensitivity pneumonitis, or disseminated, overwhelming infection in immunocompromised hosts.[13] This fungus grows easily on routine fungal culture media, and it is a common colonizer of both sputum and mucous membranes. Infections in humans are most commonly caused by *Aspergillus fumigatus, Aspergillus flavus,* or *Aspergillus niger.*

Clinically, isolation of *Aspergillus* species from sputum may represent colonization or a possible manifestation of allergic bronchopulmonary aspergillosis, aspergilloma, or invasive aspergillosis (see Table 113-2). Allergic bronchopulmonary aspergillosis is a hypersensitivity reaction to *Aspergillus* antigens. In this disorder, bronchospastic symptoms with episodic wheezing and cough are common and are associated with pulmonary infiltrates, fever, and peripheral eosinophilia. The diagnosis of this syndrome depends on detection of peripheral blood eosinophilia, a positive skin test to *Aspergillus* antigenic extract, a serum precipitating antibody, an elevated total serum IgE, and positive sputum cultures (in more than two thirds of patients).[14] Chest radiographs in this disorder may show small infiltrates with hilar adenopathy or chronic lobar consolidation.

Patients with aspergillomas usually have underlying tuberculosis or sarcoidosis. They are often asymptomatic, and the aspergillomas are saprophytic colonizers without clinical significance. In some instances, hemoptysis may occur, manifested either by blood-streaked sputum or by massive bleeding. The chest radiograph is usually characteristic, demonstrating an intracavitary mass lesion surrounded by a crescent of air. Sputum cultures and serum precipitins are usually positive, but skin tests against *Aspergillus* antigens are negative.

In patients with leukemia and lymphomas and in transplant recipients, *Aspergillus* is an increasingly important opportunistic pathogen.[15] Patients with other malignant diseases and those receiving immunosuppressant agents are also at increased risk of invasive aspergillosis. Most of these patients develop a necrotizing pneumonia and present with unremitting fever and widely disseminated pulmonary infiltrates while receiving broad-spectrum antibiotic therapy. Involvement of the sinuses or orbits with *Aspergillus* is not uncommon. Approximately one fourth of patients with invasive aspergillosis have associated brain, liver, renal, or myocardial abscesses and gastrointestinal bleeding. The definitive diagnosis of disseminated, invasive pulmonary aspergillosis depends on detection of tissue invasion. Skin tests, blood cultures, and serology are usually not helpful. Lung biopsy may be necessary for definitive diagnosis because of the potential for multiple and unusual pathogens in the immunocompromised host.

Rarely, aspergillosis can affect the heart and cause endocarditis. In these cases, the patient may appear clinically to have large vegetations, although blood cultures are negative. As in candidal endocarditis, early valve replacement and aggressive chemotherapy are needed to increase survival.

Involvement of the eye by *Aspergillus* may occur after surgery or injury to the eye. Endophthalmitis due to *Aspergillus* may manifest as conjunctivitis or hypopyon.

FUNGAL PNEUMONIA

The fungi most commonly associated with pneumonias are *Histoplasma capsulatum, Coccidioides immitis,* and *Blastomyces dermatitidis* (see Table 113-2). Histoplasmosis is a common cause of infection in more than 30 states in the United States.[16] The organism, although commonly isolated from soil, has been associated with bats and birds. Inhalation of airborne fungi appears to be the route of pulmonary infection. Most people are asymptomatic because of their host defense mechanisms. Symptomatic infection may range from mild malaise to severe, life-threatening pneumonia. The majority of patients have either a normal chest radiograph or patchy pneumonia, while one fourth have a diffuse miliary pattern. Risk factors associated with dissemination are increasing age and immunosuppression. To detect the organism histologically, lymph node biopsy or transbronchial biopsy may be necessary. Skin testing is neither sensitive nor specific. A recently described radioimmunoassay for the detection of *H capsulatum* in urine and serum may prove to be useful in the rapid diagnosis of disseminated histoplasmosis.[17]

Coccidioides immitis is commonly found in the southwestern United States, with more than 100,000 new cases reported each year.[18] Only 40% of infected people are symptomatic, with manifestations ranging from an influenza-like syndrome to acute respiratory distress syndrome (ARDS). Most patients have a self-limited disease, with improvement and resolution in 6 to 8 weeks. In patients who are diabetic or immunocompromised, cavitary lesions may develop on radiographs. In healthy people, chronic pulmonary disease tends to be indolent. Less than 1% of patients develop disseminated infection to extrapulmonary sites such as bone, meninges, and skin. A sputum or culture demonstrating *C immitis* is diagnostic because nasopharyngeal contamination is not known to occur. Diagnosis can be made serologically by detecting elevated serum IgM precipitins or elevated titers of complement-fixing antibodies. In patients with disseminated disease or persistent symptoms, in pregnant women, and in those with severe underlying disease, treatment is usually necessary.

Blastomyces dermatitidis is found in the southeastern and south-central United States and in the Midwest along the Great Lakes.[19] Inhalation of organisms leads to infection, with dissemination occurring hematogenously to organs throughout the body. As is the case in coccidioidomycosis, pulmonary disease may be self-limited or manifest as widespread pneumonia. Acute respiratory failure has been reported with miliary spread and following endobronchial spread of the disease. Diagnosis requires growth of the organism because serologic and skin tests are not sensitive or specific. Mortality in patients with ARDS secondary to blastomycosis is quite high, and these patients should receive adequate antifungal chemotherapy as quickly as possible.

OTHER FUNGAL INFECTIONS

Torulopsis (Candida) glabrata Infections

Although there are many *Torulopsis* species, only *T glabrata* is pathogenic for humans. It causes disease similar to *Candida*, with which it can be confused both in isolation and disease manifestations (see Table 113-2).[20] In fact, some texts refer to *T glabrata* as *Candida glabrata*. Normally, *Torulopsis* species are saprophytic inhabitants of the skin, mucous membranes, and intestinal tract. In patients who are immunosuppressed, this fungus may become an opportunistic pathogen. Clinically, *Torulopsis* may be associated with sepsis, renal infection, endocarditis, or meningitis. In patients with blood cultures positive for *Torulopsis*, the clinical findings may be similar to gram-negative endotoxic shock. *Torulopsis* species can colonize the urine and also may invade the kidney by hematogenous dissemination, especially in diabetic patients or patients on antibiotics. Renal infection with *Torulopsis* produces a clinical presentation similar to pyelonephritis, although the blood cultures may be negative.

Infections Due to Yeasts Other Than Candida

Yeasts of the genera *Trichosporon*, *Malassezia*, *Rhodotorula*, and *Saccharomyces* cause an increasing number of serious infections, especially in immunocompromised hosts.[5] Catheter-associated infections have been reported due to *Malassezia* species, *Rhodotorula rubra*, and *Saccharomyces cerevisiae*. Trichosporonosis is an opportunistic infection in immunocompromised hosts. The clinical manifestations are similar to disseminated candidiasis. Amphotericin B is the drug of choice, although mortality is high if granulocytopenia continues.

Cryptococcosis

Cryptococcus neoformans causes disease in many organs of the body in both immunocompetent and immunocompromised hosts.[21] The organism can be cultured in the laboratory on selective fungal media, and growth usually occurs within several days. The most common area of disease with cryptococcus is the lungs; infection may be asymptomatic or symptomatic (see Table 113-2). Disseminated disease may involve the central nervous system (CNS), skin, bone, or other organs.

Pulmonary cryptococcosis is usually mild and transient. Illness may be manifested by nonspecific respiratory symptoms such as cough, chest pain, sputum production, and low-grade fever. With pulmonary involvement, dissemination to other organ systems can occur. Culturing cryptococci from respiratory secretions does not prove infection; this may only represent colonization. Evidence of tissue invasion by biopsy

of the lung is necessary for definitive diagnosis. Cryptococcal antigen is diagnostic in only 50% of cases. Findings on chest radiographs are variable and nondiagnostic. Any patient with pulmonary cryptococcosis should have cultures for *Cryptococcus* from other body fluids, such as spinal fluid, urine, and secretions, to rule out disseminated disease.

With dissemination, cryptococci can infect almost any organ of the body. The CNS is a common site of disseminated disease, and infection may manifest as meningitis or as a space-occupying lesion (a cryptococcoma). Approximately half of patients with cryptococcal meningitis are immunosuppressed, and in these patients the clinical course is more severe. The disease usually presents as a subacute or chronic meningoencephalitis with headache, altered mental status, meningeal signs, cranial nerve palsy, and increased intracranial pressure. Diagnosis depends on detection of cryptococci in the cerebrospinal fluid (CSF). India ink stains for evidence of *Cryptococcus* are only positive in 50% of patients with meningitis. There is an increased possibility of isolation when multiple samples are obtained with large volumes of fluid. If the cryptococcal antigen is positive in the CSF, it is diagnostic. However, only 70% of patients with cryptococcal meningitis have positive CSF antigen tests. When both serum and CSF cryptococcal antigen tests are performed, the sensitivity increases to 90%.

In 5% to 15% of cases with disseminated disease, skin or bone is involved. Skin manifestations can include ulcerations, subcutaneous swellings, abscesses, draining sinuses, nodules, papules, or plaques. Diagnosis is made by skin biopsy and appropriate culture. Destructive lesions of bones can occur if fungi are lodged there and grow. Radiographically, these appear as lytic lesions without sclerosis, most commonly involving long bones, cranial bones, and vertebrae. Because of the possibility of widespread dissemination, finding cryptococci in any body fluid requires a search for evidence of cryptococcal infection in other parts of the body.

MUCORMYCOSIS

Mucormycosis, or phycomycosis, is an infection caused by the fungi of the order Mucorales. These fungi produce local infections and severe disease in patients with diabetes or leukemia as well as in normal hosts (see Table 113-2).[22] These fungi can be cultured on routine fungal media and detected on microscopic examination of scrapings or biopsy material.

Mucormycosis can present in a rhinocerebral, pulmonary, gastrointestinal, or disseminated form. Rhinocerebral mucormycosis is most commonly associated with diabetes, especially when ketoacidosis is present. The fungi enter the upper respiratory tract through inhalation and produce infection in the nasal mucosa or palate. With invasion of the organism, the ophthalmic and internal carotid arteries may be affected, resulting in thrombosis of contiguous vessels. Symptoms include sinusitis and orbital cellulitis. Neurologically, the patient may present with ophthalmoplegia, cranial nerve palsies, and hemiplegia. The nasal turbinates may be black and necrotic, and ptosis and proptosis of the affected eye may be present. Biopsy of necrotic areas shows the characteristic nonseptate hyphae on smear or pathologic staining of tissue.

With combined antifungal chemotherapy and surgery, the mortality rate approximates 50%; neurologic sequelae occur in a significant number of survivors.

Involvement of the lungs occurs most often in patients with leukemia, lymphoma, or severe leukopenia. Most commonly, the person presents with fever and pulmonary infiltrates that progress during antibiotic therapy. Gastrointestinal mucormycosis occurs in patients with severe malnutrition, kwashiorkor, or colitis. The lower small intestine and colon are infected, with ulcerations and penetration of the bowel wall. Patients may present with abdominal pain and bloody diarrhea and eventually develop peritonitis. The disseminated form of mucormycosis occurs in patients with severe underlying disease such as leukemia. Patients are acutely ill and present a septic picture. Abscess formation and infarcts may occur in organs throughout the body. There may be skin lesions, similar to ecthyma gangrenosum, which characteristically show nonseptate hyphae on biopsy. Occasionally, patients with mucormycosis may present with endocarditis, encephalitis, or local wound infections.

ANTIFUNGAL THERAPY

Several antifungal agents are available to treat systemic fungal infections (Table 113-3). The main drug for treatment of systemic fungal disease remains amphotericin B,[23] which works by interacting with cellular membranes of fungi so that membrane function is disrupted. The drug's distribution throughout the body is poor; it is eliminated through the biliary tract and is not affected by renal dysfunction. Some believe that the total dose of amphotericin B is the most crucial determinant of effective therapy, whereas others believe that it is the *duration* rather than total dose that is important for recovery.

Amphotericin B is the standard by which other anti-fungal agents are measured in the treatment of life-threatening infections. This polyene antifungal agent remains the drug of choice for the treatment of aspergillosis, disseminated candidiasis, cryptococcosis and zygomycosis. Mortality rates for nosocomial candidemia range from 30% to 50% despite amphotericin B therapy, and may reach 85% for invasive aspergillosis.

The dose of amphotericin B is increased gradually until a full intravenous dose is eventually reached (0.5 mg/kg/day). At the highest level of intravenous administration, the daily dose is infused slowly over several hours to decrease the possibility of side effects. The maximum dose is usually up to 0.7 to 1 mg/kg/day, especially if an alternate-day dose regimen is employed.

Several side effects and toxicities are associated with the administration of amphotericin B. Nephrotoxicity is a major problem and must be carefully watched for. When the serum creatinine exceeds 3 mg/100 mL, many think that a dose adjustment is necessary until kidney function improves. Others prefer trying an alternate-day, rather than a daily regimen, to decrease the possibility of nephrotoxicity. The nephrotoxicity that is found early after amphotericin B administration is usually related to the daily dose, whereas later nephrotoxicity is related to the total dose administered. In most patients, renal function returns to near-normal levels after therapy is stopped, but occasionally renal failure will require dialysis. A rare complication in patients receiving amphotericin and white blood cell transfusions includes a pulmonary reaction manifested by dyspnea, hypoxemia, and interstitial infiltrates.

Toxicity from amphotericin B may be prevented by antipyretics, antihistamines, and sodium repletion. Medications such as aminoglycosides, cyclosporin A or diuretics should not be used if possible. Pentoxifylline is being studied as a possible agent to reduce amphotericin B nephotoxicity. Other formulations of amphotericin B that employ liposomes, lipid complexes, or cholesterol dispersion are being tested in the hopes of finding a less toxic preparation.

Amphotericin B is useful for several fungal infections and has shown synergistic activity with 5-fluorocytosine, especially for cryptococcal infections. 5-Fluorocytosine (5-FC)

TABLE 113-3. Antifungal Chemotherapy

DRUG	INDICATIONS	ROUTE OF ADMINISTRATION	MAJOR SIDE EFFECTS
Amphotericin B	Aspergillosis, blastomycosis, candidiasis, coccidioidomycosis, cryptococcosis, histoplasmosis	Intravenous, intrathecal	Anorexia, anemia, fever, nausea, renal dysfunction, hypokalemia, phlebitis
5-Fluorocytosine	Candidiasis, cryptococcosis	Oral	Leukopenia, thrombocytopenia, liver dysfunction, diarrhea
Ketoconazole	Candidiasis, coccidioidomycosis, histoplasmosis, paracoccidioidomycosis	Oral	Nausea, itching, hepatitis, suppression of testosterone and adrenal cortisol production
Clotrimazole/miconazole	Candidiasis	Oral/topical	
Fluconazole	Candidiasis, cryptococcosis	Oral, intravenous	Anorexia, nausea, vomiting, skin rash, drug interactions
Itraconazole	Aspergillosis blastomycosis, chromomycosis, histoplasmosis	Oral	

is an oral antifungal drug that is rarely used alone.[24] It works by interfering with the synthesis of pyrimidines and is distributed throughout the body, including the CNS. It is well absorbed from the gastrointestinal tract. The daily dose in patients with normal kidney function is 100 to 150 mg/kg. Side effects include hepatic dysfunction, leukopenia, thrombocytopenia, and gastrointestinal disorders. Because drug resistance has been detected when 5-fluorocytosine is used alone, it has been combined with amphotericin B and has been found effective, especially in candidal and cryptococcal infections.[25]

The azole antifungal compounds include the imidazoles (miconazole and ketoconazole) and the triazoles (fluconazole and itraconazole).[26] Miconazole is the agent of choice for *Pseudallescheria boydii* infections. Ketoconazole may be useful in blastomycosis, paracoccidioidomycosis, cavitary histoplasmosis, and nonmeningeal coccidioidomycosis, but is not to be used for severe fungal infections in immunosuppressed or neutropenic patients. Life-threatening cardiac arrhythmias, a newly recognized side effect of ketoconazole, occur in patients taking concurrent terfenadine or astemizole.

Ketoconazole has activity against *Candida* species, *C immitis*, *H capsulatum*, *B dermatitidis*, and Paracoccidioides brasiliensis. It is absorbed orally but can be inhibited by administration of antacids and H_2 antagonists. In higher doses, ketoconazole has been associated with nausea and vomiting, suppression of testosterone synthesis with resulting decreased libido, gynecomastia, menstrual irregularities, and, rarely, hepatic dysfunction. It is recommended for use in all forms of histoplasmosis and in blastomycosis. It has some activity in chronic mucocutaneous candidiasis and oral thrush.

Fluconazole and intraconazole are broad-spectrum triazoles with less toxicity than the imidazoles. Fluconazole can be administered orally or parenterally.[27] It has good activity against Candida species and *Cryptococcus neoformans*, but not against Aspergillus, Zygomycetes or *H capsulatum*.

Fluconazole is a broad-spectrum antifungal drug approved for the treatment of oropharyngeal and esophageal candidiasis and cryptococcal meningitis.[28] Fluconazole may be an alternative to amphotericin B in patients unable to tolerate serious side effects. Unlike ketoconazole, fluconazole does not interact with P-450 enzyme systems and, therefore, should have fewer interactions with other drugs. Although the initial in vivo studies look promising, fluconazole should be restricted until additional studies support its use as a first-line antifungal drug.

Itraconazole, unlike fluconazole, has high protein binding and low serum concentration.[29] It is considered the agent of choice for the treatment of blastomycosis, histoplasmosis, paracoccidioidomycosis, sporotrichosis, and chromomycosis. Itraconazole may prove to be useful in acute and chronic aspergillosis and *P boydii*.

The only antifungal combination with proven efficacy is amphotericin B and 5-FC in cryptococcal meningitis. In vitro benefits of combination antifungal agents has been shown with amphotericin B and rifampin, amphotericin B and azoles, and azoles plus 5-FC. However, documentation of enhanced clinical response awaits further controlled clinical trials.

VIRAL INFECTIONS   ■

CLINICAL EPIDEMIOLOGY

Viruses can cause either acute, nonpersistent, or persistent infections.[30] In acute viral infections, host defenses help eliminate the virus from the body, and reinfection is usually prevented by the development of specific antibodies. Persistent viral infections can be chronic or latent, with disease recurrences over several years. An important example of an acute viral infection is influenza. Latent infections are typified by the herpesviruses.

The status of the host can determine clinical responses to the viral infection. Patients with heart and lung disease may have serious influenza infections. Chronic infections with enteroviruses are seen in patients who are hypogammaglobulinemic. Patients with secondary immunodeficiencies due to malignancies, organ transplants, or cytotoxic agents are prone to herpesvirus infections.

Unlike bacterial infections, viral infections in the ICU are not readily transmissible between patients. However, certain exotic viruses, such as Ebola and Marburg viruses, are highly contagious in a hospital setting. Susceptible adult personnel can be infected from patients and should be warned about this possibility. Guidelines for isolation precautions have been published by the Centers for Disease Control and Prevention (CDC) (Table 113-4).[31] Specific instructions are given concerning the infectious material that is present and whether masks, gowns, gloves, and private rooms are necessary. In those viral infections transmitted by respiratory secretions, airflow patterns between rooms should comply with federal regulations.

VIRAL PNEUMONIA

Viruses are etiologic agents in 10% of all cases of community acquired pneumonia.[32] In adults, the most common cause of viral pneumonia is the influenza virus. Although most cases of influenza are not associated with pneumonia, pulmonary involvement is found in more than 75% of patients over 70 years of age. Pulmonary complications of influenza are more common in patients with chronic heart and lung disease, but they can develop in otherwise healthy young adults.

Influenza A characteristically occurs in winter epidemics. Typically, fever, headache, myalgias, and cough are present.[33] During this acute illness, primary influenza pneumonia may develop. It has a rapid course, diffuse infiltrates, and a high mortality rate. Secondary bacterial pneumonias usually develop as the patient appears to be improving from an uncomplicated influenza illness. Although the frequency of pneumonia due to *Staphylococcus aureus* increases after influenza, *Streptococcus pneumoniae* is still the most common cause of this pulmonary complication. Localized or segmental influenza pneumonia may occur in normal hosts, without the high mortality rate or secondary bacterial infection being present. Rales are heard on physical examination several days after the onset of symptoms. Antibiotics are not needed, and mortality is low in these patients with localized viral pneumonia.

TABLE 113-4. Viral Disease-Specific Isolation Precautions

DISEASE	PRECAUTIONS INDICATED	INFECTIOUS MATERIAL
AIDS	PR, G, Gl	Blood and body fluids
Adenovirus	PR, G	Respiratory secretions and feces
Arthropod-borne encephalitis	None	None
Arthropod-borne viral fever	Gl	Blood
Bronchiolitis—unknown etiology	PR, G	Respiratory secretions
Bronchitis		
Adults	None	Respiratory secretions
Infants	PR, G	Respiratory secretions
Conjunctivitis—viral or unknown etiology	PR, Gl	Purulent exudate
Creutzfeldt–Jakob disease	Gl	Blood, brain tissue, and spinal fluid
Croup	PR, G	Respiratory secretions
Cytomegalovirus	None, except pregnant personnel need to be counseled	Urine and respiratory secretions
Dengue fever	Gl	Blood
Encephalitis—unknown etiology	PR, G, Gl	Feces
Enterovirus (echovirus, coxsackie, and poliovirus)	PR, G, Gl	Feces
Epstein-Barr virus (infectious mononucleosis)	None	Respiratory secretions
Erythema infectiosum	PR, M	Respiratory secretions
Gastroenteritis, viral	PR, G, Gl	Feces
Guillain–Barré syndrome	None	
Hemorrhagic fevers (e.g., Lassa fever)	PR, M, G, Gl	Blood, body fluids, and respiratory secretions
Hepatitis	PR, G, Gl	Blood and body fluids, feces
Herpes simplex		
Mucocutaneous	PR, Gl	Lesion secretions from infected site
Neonatal	PR, G, Gl	Lesion secretions
Herpes zoster		
Immunocompromised host	PR, M, G, Gl	Lesion secretions and respiratory secretions
Normal host	PR, Gl	Lesion secretions
Influenza		
Adults	None	Respiratory secretions
Infants	PR, G	Respiratory secretions
Lymphocytic choriomeningitis	None	
Measles (rubeola)	PR, M	Respiratory secretions
Meningitis, aseptic	PR, G, Gl	Feces
Mumps	PR, M	Respiratory secretions
Pharyngitis		
Adults	None	Respiratory secretions
Infants	PR, G	Respiratory secretions
Pneumonia, viral		
Adults	None	Respiratory secretions
Infants	PR, G	Respiratory secretions
Rabies	PR, M, G, Gl	Respiratory secretions
Respiratory syncytial virus	PR, G	Respiratory secretions
Rubella (German measles)	PR, M	Respiratory secretions
Smallpox	PR, M, G, Gl	Respiratory secretions and lesion secretions
Varicella (chickenpox)	PR, M, G, Gl	Respiratory secretions and lesion secretions

PR, private room; M, masks; G, gowns, if soiling is likely; Gl, gloves for touching infectious material.

Adapted from CDC guidelines for isolation precautions in hospitals. *Infect Control* 1983;4:249

Diagnosis of influenza infection can be made by viral culture or by one of several serologic tests. Rapid methods for detecting viral antigens in clinical specimens are becoming more available in diagnostic laboratories. Throat or nose swab specimens are best for recovery of virus in uncomplicated cases; sputum is probably better in patients with tracheobronchitis or pneumonia. The virus grows well in tissue culture or embryonated chicken eggs, so that positive isolates can often be detected within 48 hours.

Other common respiratory viruses can cause severe respiratory illness requiring hospitalization. These occur most commonly in infants and children, but adults occasionally are affected. Influenza B virus can cause epidemics, but this virus does not appear to cause as much primary pneumonia as influenza A strains. Respiratory syncytial virus is associated with severe lower respiratory tract infections in infants. Respiratory syncytial virus has been shown to cause protracted illness in nursing home patients and exacerbations of lung disease in patients with chronic obstructive pulmonary disease.[34] Infections with respiratory syncytial virus in nursing homes may be epidemic and indistinguishable from influenza A.

Viral pneumonia in adults can occasionally be caused by adenoviruses and measles virus. In children and military recruits, adenoviruses are important causes of respiratory disease and, in rare cases, cause a fulminant necrotizing pneumonia.[35] Atypical measles in adolescents and young adults may be associated with mild pneumonia or acute respiratory failure.[36]

In adults who develop chickenpox (varicella), the illness may be severe and involve the lung in up to 15% of cases. The pneumonia in adults may be fulminant and rapidly fatal if not treated early and appropriately. Pregnant women and patients receiving steroids who develop varicella pneumonia have had high mortality rates reported in older studies.[37,38]

VIRAL MENINGITIS AND ENCEPHALITIS

Between 10,000 and 15,000 cases of viral ("aseptic") meningitis and encephalitis are reported each year in the United States.[39] With viral meningitis, signs and symptoms and meningeal inflammation associated with pleocytosis in the CSF are usually present (Table 113-5). Patients with encephalitis have brain inflammation, manifested clinically by fever, headache, and alteration in mental status.

Viruses can invade the CNS by hematogenous route or by nerve tissue. In the case of rabies and poliomyelitis, entry by the neural route is the most important. Invasion of the brain by herpes simplex viruses can occur through the olfactory bulb; the most likely mode of spread, as with other viruses infecting the CNS, is hematogenous dissemination.

The terms *viral meningitis* and *aseptic meningitis* have been used to denote the same process; however, they should be separated because there are important bacterial agents associated with the aseptic meningitis syndrome. The patient's age and the season of the year are important clues to the viral etiology of meningitis. Onset of clinical symptoms is usually gradual, with fever, malaise, anorexia, myalgias,

TABLE 113-5. Viral Encephalitis in the United States

EPIDEMIOLOGY	VIRUS	DIAGNOSTIC TEST	ISOLATION PRECAUTION
EPIDEMIC			
Arthropod borne	Eastern equine	Serology	None
	Western equine		
	Venezuelan equine		
	St. Louis		
	Powassan		
	California		
	Colorado tick fever		
Enterovirus	Echoviruses	Virus isolation	Enteric
	Coxsackie A and B		
	Polioviruses		
SPORADIC			
Herpesviruses	Herpes simplex types 1 and 2	Virus isolation	None
	Varicella-zoster		Lesion and respiratory secretions
	Epstein-Barr		None
	Cytomegalovirus		None
Rabies	Rabies	Serology, virus detection	Respiratory secretions
Associated with respiratory disease	Influenza A and B	Serology, virus isolation	None
	Adenovirus		None
Others	Lymphocytic choriomeningitis	Serology, virus isolation	Respiratory secretions
	Measles		Respiratory secretions
	Mumps		
POSTINFECTIOUS			
Herpesviruses	Varicella-zoster	Serology (?)	None
	Epstein-Barr		
Associated with respiratory disease	Influenza A and B	Serology	None
Others	Rubella	Serology	None
	Mumps		
	Measles		
	Vaccinia		

and sore throat being common complaints. Physical findings include fever and nuchal rigidity, with or without a positive Kernig's or Brudzinski's sign.

Few laboratory studies help in the diagnosis of viral meningitis and encephalitis. CSF findings include elevation of the opening pressure, mononuclear cell pleocytosis, and moderately elevated protein. Glucose levels are commonly normal, but 10% of patients with mumps meningitis and occasional patients with herpes simplex virus types 1 and 2 have hypoglycorrhachia. CSF, throat washings, and stool specimens from suspected cases can be sent for virus culture. Some viruses (e.g., enteroviruses) are relatively easy to recover from specimens, whereas others are rarely recovered. If a viral etiology of the meningitis or encephalitis is suspected, appropriate serologic tests need to be done on acute and convalescent sera.

Over 50% of viral meningitis cases are probably caused by enteroviruses.[40] With the widespread use of polio vaccines, coxsackieviruses and echoviruses are now responsible for most viral meningitis epidemics during the early summer and fall. An uncommon cause of viral meningitis is the mumps virus. Parotitis is not specific or sensitive for diagnosis of mumps, and half of patients with mumps meningitis never develop parotitis.

Lymphocytic choriomeningitis is caused by contact with infected rodents.[41] Meningitis and pneumonitis have been reported in infected persons. Outbreaks have been reported in people who work with laboratory animals and in family members who have infected pet hamsters.

Primary infection with herpes simplex virus type 2 has been associated with meningitis in 0.5% to 5% of all infected patients.[42] Recovery is usually without sequelae, and recurrent attacks of meningitis are rarely reported.

Encephalitis cases can be either epidemic or sporadic. The most common causes of epidemic encephalitis in the United States are the arboviruses.[43] They comprise a group of viruses that are transmitted by arthropod vectors. The seven arboviruses isolated in North America account for more than 50% of all encephalitis cases during epidemics. Most cases are caused by the St. Louis, California, eastern equine, and western equine encephalitis viruses. Because these viruses present similar clinical pictures, specific virologic diagnosis requires serologic tests in conjunction with clinical and epidemiologic information. Virus cultures are not helpful in diagnosis, and acute and convalescent serum samples must be sent to the appropriate laboratories for antibody determinations.

The most common cause of sporadic cases of encephalitis in the United States is herpes simplex virus type 1.[44] Reactivation of latent herpes simplex virus probably contributes to 70% of the cases of herpes simplex encephalitis. Patients usually have signs and symptoms of fever, headache, and obtundation. Many have a history of personality changes, seizures, or autonomic dysfunction and focal neurologic changes. The CSF may demonstrate lymphocyte pleocytosis and increased numbers of red blood cells. The virus is rarely cultured from CSF of infected patients. No noninvasive tests are readily available that can diagnose this infection in a high percentage of patients. Computed tomography scans, electroencephalograms, and brain scans may demonstrate

focal abnormalities, but they are not specific for herpes simplex encephalitis. The only sensitive and specific test for herpes simplex encephalitis is the brain biopsy. This procedure has few complications and can aid in diagnosing non-herpesvirus infections that are treatable (e.g., tuberculosis).

Less common causes of sporadic encephalitis include the other herpesviruses (varicella-zoster, cytomegalovirus, and Epstein-Barr virus) and rabies. Varicella or herpes zoster has caused encephalitis in addition to other neurologic complications such as Guillain–Barré syndrome, transverse myelitis, and Reye syndrome. Varicella encephalitis has a worse prognosis than herpes zoster–associated encephalitis.[45] Cytomegalovirus and Epstein-Barr virus are rare causes of encephalitis. Cytomegalovirus encephalitis occurs in immunocompromised patients, and Epstein-Barr virus encephalitis occurs in less than 1% of patients with mononucleosis.

In rabies, a history of an animal bite is important but is not always available or known (Table 113-6). The incubation period is usually 3 to 7 weeks after exposure but may be as short as 10 days or as long as 2 years.[46] Encephalitis is a late stage of the disease and is associated with convulsions. Recovery is extremely rare.

IMMUNOCOMPROMISED HOSTS

Immunodeficiency can be either congenital or acquired. Congenital immunodeficiencies can involve neutrophil dysfunction, complement deficiencies, or deficiencies in humoral and cell-mediated immunity. Infections related to congenital defects in host defense mechanisms occur predominantly in children. Viruses, fungi, and intracellular bacteria are common pathogens in patients with defective cell-mediated immunity. Herpesviruses are the major cause of serious morbidity and mortality in this group, although severe infections with measles and adenovirus have been reported.[47,48]

TABLE 113-6. Rabies Diagnosis and Prevention

DIAGNOSTIC CLUES

Animal bite: dogs, cats, bats, skunks, raccoons, and foxes are most common
Paresthesias, hydrophobia, and restlessness
Convulsions

PREVENTION

Immunize all household pets
Treat animal bites and scratches immediately
Cleanse thoroughly
Apply 50% rabies immune globulin around wound
Do not suture
Suspected domestic animal should be captured and observed (7–10 days); wild animals should be captured and sacrificed for laboratory diagnosis
Postexposure immunization includes human rabies immune globulin (20 IU/kg) and five intramuscular injections of human diploid cell rabies vaccine (days 0, 3, 7, 14, and 21)

Acquired immunodeficiencies are more common than congenital ones and can be mild or severe, depending on the type and degree of immunosuppression. Nonspecific host defense mechanisms can be impaired as a result of burns, trauma, foreign bodies, or malnutrition. Specific host defense mechanisms are impaired with burns, exfoliative dermatitis, nephrotic syndrome, protein-losing enteropathy, malignancies, collagen–vascular disease, corticosteroid therapy, and cancer chemotherapy. In addition, problems with acquired immunodeficiency are observed in patients with intravenous drug abuse or organ transplants (heart, renal, and bone marrow).

The herpesviruses are the most important family of viruses that cause serious infections in immunodeficient patients. Because of their capacity for latency, these viruses can produce both acute and recurrent disease. Endogenous reactivation can occur after primary infection and cause disease. Cell-mediated immune mechanisms are thought to be of major importance in maintaining the latent state and clearing virus during an acute episode.

Herpes Simplex Virus

Immunocompromised patients are at increased risk for more frequent and severe herpes simplex virus infections.[49] These infections are characterized by progressive extension of local disease rather than hematogenous dissemination. Mucocutaneous lesions may extend and progress to large ulcerations in the orofacial and genital areas. Visceral involvement is seen most frequently with tracheitis, esophagitis, or pneumonia. Transplant recipients are particularly susceptible to these infections.

In burn patients, herpes simplex virus infections can involve not only the skin but also visceral organs. Cutaneous dissemination of herpes simplex virus can be observed in patients with eczema, pemphigus, or Sézary syndrome.[50] Before the availability of antiviral agents for herpes simplex virus, these skin infections were associated with extensive morbidity and a low but significant mortality. Newer agents have made treatment relatively easy and effective.

Hepatitis caused by herpes simplex virus is more common in the pediatric population than in adults.[51] In all age groups, the disease is usually seen in an immunocompromised host; in adults, the most frequent underlying conditions are renal transplantation, pregnancy, and steroid administration. The mortality rate of herpes simplex virus hepatitis is greater than 80%, with rapid progression to fulminant hepatic necrosis. Few patients have received adequate emergency antiviral therapy prior to death.

Pneumonitis secondary to herpes simplex virus occurs predominantly in immunocompromised transplant recipients.[52] Interstitial pneumonitis can develop either by local extension from herpetic tracheobronchitis or by hematogenous dissemination. Mixed infection with bacteria, fungi, or parasitic organisms is common. Although herpes simplex virus has been isolated from the lower respiratory tract of 40% of ARDS patients, the relationship between herpes simplex virus isolation and ARDS is unknown. Mortality from untreated herpes simplex virus pneumonitis approaches 80%, so that in suspected cases antiviral therapy should be started as quickly as possible.

Esophagitis can occur by direct extension from oropharyngeal herpes simplex virus infection or by reactivation and spread to esophageal mucosa through the vagus nerve.[53] The symptoms of odynophagia, dysphagia, and substernal chest discomfort are not specific for herpes simplex virus esophagitis. Neither barium swallow nor endoscopy can differentiate herpes simplex virus from other causes of esophageal ulceration; biopsy and culture are needed for definitive diagnosis.

Varicella-Zoster Virus

Varicella (chickenpox) can cause severe infections in immunocompromised infants, children, and adults.[54] Complications of pneumonia, encephalitis, and secondary bacterial infection are the most common causes of death. Transplant recipients have a high mortality from untreated varicella.

Herpes zoster (shingles) is the recurrent form of varicella. This infection increases in prevalence with increasing age and is seen more frequently in certain malignancies, such as Hodgkin's disease and lymphoma.[55] Transplant patients are also at increased risk. The infection is usually confined to a dermatome distribution, but dissemination is more frequent in the immunosuppressed host. Dissemination is defined by more than 10 vesicles appearing outside the primary dermatome and implies that viremia has occurred. Herpes zoster will disseminate beyond the initial dermatome in approximately 25% of affected Hodgkin's disease patients if no early antiviral therapy is given. Dissemination usually occurs within 1 week of the onset of skin lesions, even in the presence of serum-neutralizing antibodies.

Morbidity from herpes zoster can be severe if postherpetic neuralgia develops. This complication is seen most commonly in the elderly and in immunosuppressed patients. The pain may last for months to years and is difficult to treat. Mortality, although rare, is more likely to occur in infected marrow transplant patients. Complications of herpes zoster that can be fatal include encephalitis, hepatitis, and pneumonia.[56] No controlled studies have demonstrated benefit from antiviral therapies once these complications are present, but they probably should be attempted in selected cases.

Epstein-Barr Virus

Infectious mononucleosis caused by Epstein-Barr virus is common in otherwise healthy children and young adults. Although most people recover from the infection, unusual complications have been reported. The most severe of these include splenic rupture, aplastic anemia, upper airway obstruction, and encephalitis. Causes of death, which occurs rarely, include hepatic failure, myocarditis, and hemorrhage.

In the recently delineated X-linked lymphoproliferative syndrome, affected male family members have difficulty with Epstein-Barr virus infections.[57] Once infected, they die of overwhelming infectious mononucleosis, with or without aplastic anemia, and lymphoproliferative malignancies. These patients have deficits in both their humoral immunity and natural killer cells.

Cytomegalovirus

The prevalence of cytomegalovirus infections in transplant recipients is very high.[58] In renal transplant patients, the infection rate ranges from 60% to 90%. Approximately 50% of bone marrow or heart transplant patients become infected. Immunosuppressed patients with malignancy and collagen–vascular disease also have a high prevalence rate.

In allograft organ recipients, the source of cytomegalovirus is either exogenous (blood transfusion, donor organ, or environment) or endogenous (latent virus). Reactivation of latent state is associated with cytotoxic agents and the graft-versus-host reaction that often accompanies transplantation.[59] The frequency of cytomegalovirus infection is much higher in cytomegalovirus-seropositive kidney transplant recipients than in seronegative recipients. However, seronegative recipients who receive kidneys from seropositive donors have higher infection rates than those whose allografts are from seronegative donors.

Asymptomatic cytomegalovirus infection is often found in immunocompromised patients. Most symptomatic infections in renal or bone marrow transplant patients occur in the first few months of immunosuppressive treatment. The most common syndrome is fever associated with malaise, fatigue, myalgias, and night sweats. Pneumonia is second in frequency and can lead to respiratory failure and death. In bone marrow recipients, cytomegalovirus pneumonia has a 70% mortality rate. Diagnosis of pneumonia in these patients often requires lung biopsy because cytomegalovirus often coexists with other pathogens such as *Pneumocystis carinii*, fungi, and other viruses.[60]

Other manifestations of cytomegalovirus infection in immunocompromised hosts include chorioretinitis, hepatitis, and gastrointestinal syndromes.[61–63] Cytomegalovirus has been reported to cause esophagitis, gastritis, pancreatitis, and colitis and can be fatal in these situations. Cytomegalovirus retinitis is indicative of disseminated disease and can lead to blindness if it is not treated early or if immunosuppression is not reversed.

All of the herpesviruses except Epstein-Barr virus can be cultured in selective tissue culture cells. Recent or past Epstein-Barr virus infection can be diagnosed only by serology. Herpes simplex and varicella-zoster skin lesions have characteristic multinucleated giant cells when stained and examined under the microscope. Acute and convalescent sera can be obtained for specific antibody tests if a retrospective diagnosis is needed.

EXOTIC VIRAL INFECTIONS

In the mid-1970s, with the eradication of smallpox, several new viruses that were highly contagious and produced lethal infections were identified in Africa.[64] Because of the relatively long incubation period (up to 3 weeks) and the long periods of virus excretion, these viruses can be imported into nonendemic countries by means of air travel.

The viruses associated with nosocomial transmission include Lassa, Marburg, Ebola, and Congo-Crimean hemorrhagic fever viruses. Person-to-person transmission occurs through contaminated secretions or body fluids. Lassa fever, an arenavirus related to lymphocytic choriomeningitis, is transmitted to humans by contact with an infected rat species or with an infected human. Clinically, the patient has a mild febrile illness with sore throat, cough, and retrosternal or epigastric pain. Shock is the major manifestation associated with death. Diagnosis requires the documentation of an antibody rise or virus isolation. Marburg and Ebola viruses have 3- to 10-day incubation periods and similar clinical manifestations. Both diseases begin with fever, headache, malaise, and prostration. Four to six days after the onset of illness, hemorrhagic manifestations appear. All three of these viruses (Lassa, Ebola, and Marburg) are endemic to Central Africa.

Congo-Crimean hemorrhagic fever has been documented to occur from Eastern Europe to Central Asia and Africa. The virus is a member of the Bunyaviridae family and is transmitted by ticks. Symptoms of fever, headache, and myalgias are often accompanied by hemorrhagic signs. Thrombocytopenia is common and can be associated with disseminated intravascular coagulation.

If a suspected case is admitted to a hospital in a nonendemic country, immediate patient isolation, with adequate ventilation, is necessary. Guidelines for hospital care and appropriate infection control have been developed (Table 113-7).[65] Additional information concerning diagnosis, treatment, and care of these suspected cases can be obtained from the CDC.

Hantavirus Infection

A recently described acute illness in the Southwestern states caused by a newly isolated Hantavirus (Muerto Canyon virus) can present as an unexplained ARDS.[66] Other Hantaviruses have been identified as the cause of Korean hemorrhagic fever and Epidemic Neuropathica. Similar viruses have been isolated from rodents in the United States but no clinical illness in humans had been documented prior to the 1993 outbreak.

The clinical illness in the four-corners area (border of Arizona, New Mexico, Colorado, and Utah) has been manifested by rapidly progressive respiratory failure with hypoxemia, leukocytosis and lactic acidosis.[67] Although no specific therapy has been identified, ribavirin is being considered because of its activity in Korean hemorrhagic fever.

ANTIVIRAL THERAPY

Six antiviral drugs are currently approved in the United States (Table 113-8). They are ganciclovir, vidarabine, trifluorothymidine, amantadine, acyclovir, and ribavirin. Interferon is only approved for the treatment of specific cancers, although it has broad-spectrum antiviral activity. Several of these agents have limited use and are mentioned only briefly.

Acyclovir, a nucleoside analog of guanosine, has potent antiviral activity against herpesviruses.[68] Inhibition of virus

Text continues on p. 1699

TABLE 113-7. Management of Suspected Exotic Communicable Diseases (ECD)

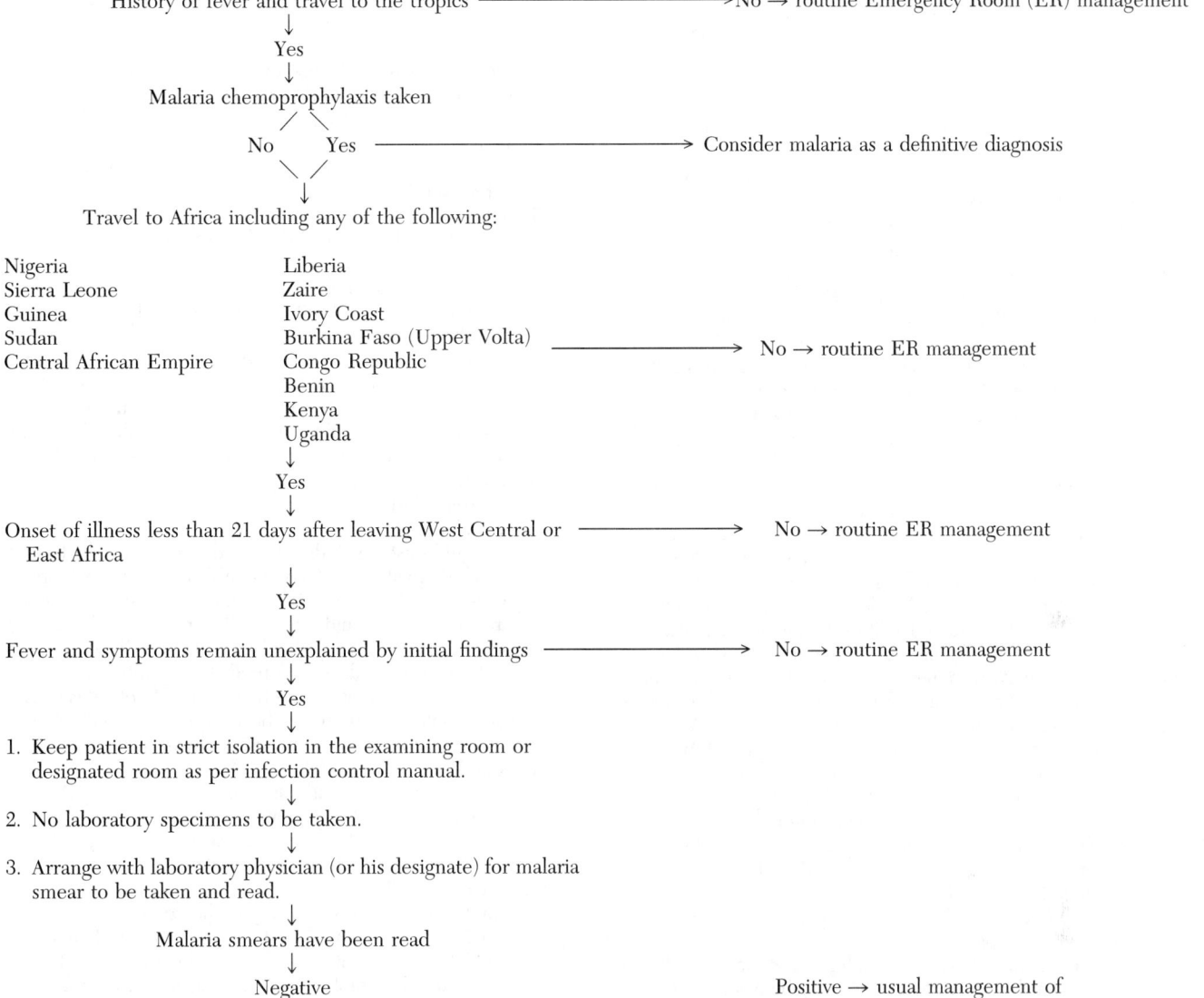

History of fever and travel to the tropics ⟶ No → routine Emergency Room (ER) management
↓
Yes
↓
Malaria chemoprophylaxis taken
No   Yes ⟶ Consider malaria as a definitive diagnosis
↓
Travel to Africa including any of the following:

Nigeria	Liberia
Sierra Leone	Zaire
Guinea	Ivory Coast
Sudan	Burkina Faso (Upper Volta)
Central African Empire	Congo Republic
	Benin
	Kenya
	Uganda

⟶ No → routine ER management
↓
Yes
↓
Onset of illness less than 21 days after leaving West Central or East Africa ⟶ No → routine ER management
↓
Yes
↓
Fever and symptoms remain unexplained by initial findings ⟶ No → routine ER management
↓
Yes
↓
1. Keep patient in strict isolation in the examining room or designated room as per infection control manual.
↓
2. No laboratory specimens to be taken.
↓
3. Arrange with laboratory physician (or his designate) for malaria smear to be taken and read.
↓
Malaria smears have been read
↓
Negative

Positive → usual management of malaria patient

STEPS 1–9 (BELOW) MUST NOW BE UNDERTAKEN.

At this point, the patient is considered a possible ECD case until proven otherwise, and the following steps should be taken:
1. Do not admit the patient.
2. Immediate consultation with a physician who has been designated within the hospital for these types of events or an infection control practitioner.
3. Advise the Medical Director of the hospital (or his designate) or other administrative personnel as appropriate.
4. It is essential to advise the Medical Office of Health of a possible case of ECD at this point.
5. Instruct laboratories to retrieve all specimens that they have received and place in plastic bags in a segregated area of the laboratory. Retain all laboratory specimens in a dedicated ice chest (similar to a portable cooler).
6. Initiate and maintain a list of all contacts including staff, patients and visitors, in cooperation with Emergency Supervisor. (Contact during the 3-week infective period in

following ways: face-to-face; sharing the same residence; close exposure during travel, or exposure to infected biologic specimens.)
7. Restrict contacts by using one-to-one nursing.
8. For disinfection of the detention area refer to management of transfer and terminal clean-up.
9. Following exposure, all staff should remove contaminated clothing, don clean attire, and proceed to a secluded shower area for showering and a complete change of clothing.

ADMITTED PATIENTS

Should a patient who has already been admitted to the hospital be diagnosed as having an ECD, the following specifications are recommended for inclusion in the hospital contingency plan for high-security isolation. It should be noted that isolation for these cases must be strictly enforced until the

(continued)

TABLE 113-7. *(continued)*

patient is no longer excreting virus. For example, Lassa virus has been identified in the urine for 3 weeks or up to 60 days.

SPECIFICATIONS

1. Room
   The hospital contingency plan should specify a previously identified area in the hospital that will conform closely to the Canadian Contingency Plan. Some additional points to remember in choosing this room are:
   a. Other patients already admitted to this area must be transferred to other areas of the hospital for their own protection.
   b. Preferably the room selected should be at the highest level of the building and in as remote an area as possible. The room must have directional air flow at all times and be under negative pressure to the rest of the facility. When a mechanical air system is provided, the ventilation must be designed to prevent reversal of air flow, and the air must be filtered before being vented to the outside. If no mechanical ventilation exists in the facility, some alternative method must be designed to evacuate the room air without recirculation within the facility.
   c. When an area is chosen for isolating these patients, sufficient room must be allocated to provide an anteroom, male and female change rooms, as well as showering and toilet facilities. Clean and dirty utility rooms for storage of appropriate items must be made available. Arrangements also should be made for the removal of contaminated wastes in such a way as to limit exposure to these items as much as possible. After doublebagging, these items should be placed in rigid, unbreakable, sealed containers for transport. This material must be transported under supervision to the autoclave and then to the incinerator.
   d. The room should be segregated as much as possible from other patient care areas, and traffic to the room should be restricted.
   e. A daily log must be kept of all persons entering and leaving the patient's room.
   f. A list of those who may be admitted to the room should be available. A security guard may be posted at the entrance to the isolated area.
   g. The surfaces of walls, ceilings, and floors should be impervious to liquids and readily cleanable. The rooms should also be capable of being sealed to permit fumigation during terminal cleaning.
   h. Before the room is put into use, it should be emptied of all items except those necessary to care for the patient.
2. Gowns and Other Protective Clothing
   Good quality disposable clothing, similar to that worn in the operating room, is necessary. This should be purchased and stored in sufficient quantity to maintain adequate protection until further supplies can be received. Plastic aprons worn over the gowns are optional but may provide additional protection. Protective clothing should be donned before entering the designated isolation area.
3. Masks
   For added protection, two high-efficiency masks with safety goggles should be worn. These should be stored where they can be obtained quickly. Attending personnel can wear full face respirators with high-efficiency particulate air (HEPA) filters or nose and mouth respirators with HEPA filters and safety goggles.

4. Caps and Boots
   Balaclava type hoods and disposable shoe covers similar to those worn by operating room staff should be worn at all times.
5. Gloves
   Double gloving with good quality surgical gloves must also be put on before entering the isolation area. Wearing of gloves does not negate the use of good handwashing.
6. Discarded Protective Clothing
   These articles must be doublebagged in autoclavable bags, autoclaved,° and then incinerated.
7. Sphygmomanometer and Stethoscope
   These should be retained in the patient's room until confirmation of diagnosis. If the diagnosis is a confirmed ECD, then this equipment should be doublebagged in plastic bags and sterilized with ethylene oxide before reuse.†
8. Needles and Syringes
   Disposable needles and syringes should be used. These should be placed in puncture-resistant containers. All needles and syringes must be doublebagged in autoclavable bags, autoclaved, and then incinerated.‡ Needles should not be recapped or bent after use to prevent self-inoculation.
9. Dressings and Tissues
   See solid waste.
10. Liquid Waste
    All liquid waste, including bed bath water, must be treated by diluting with 5.25% commercial sodium hypochlorite (Chlorox or Javex) to a 1:5 solution (for example, 1 part Javex to 4 parts liquid waste). Let stand 24 hours and pour into wide mouth polypropylene containers. These should next be autoclaved, then poured directly into the sewer system. The patient should be instructed *not* to use the toilet facilities until he has been declared noninfectious. An ambulatory patient may use a chemical toilet.
11. Solid Waste
    All discarded solid material such as clothing, disposable linen, excreta, and disposable bed pans removed from the patient's room and anteroom must be doublebagged in autoclavable bags, then incinerated.
12. Instruments, Trays
    Nondisposable items of this type should be fully sterilized in a 2% glutaraldehyde solution for at least 10 hours then doublebagged in autoclavable bags and autoclaved before reuse. Any disposable devices should be autoclaved and incinerated.§
13. Thermometer
    This should be kept in the patient's room until isolation is terminated then discarded as solid waste. The thermometer should be stored dry and wiped with an alcohol swab between use.
14. Linen
    All linen should be disposable. If a supply of old linen is on hand and no disposable material available, this may be utilized. It should be removed from the isolation area as solid waste.
15. Dishes
    These should be disposable and disposed of as solid waste.
16. Clothing and Personal Effects
    All the patient's clothing and personal effects should be doublebagged in plastic bags and sterilized with ethylene oxide.†
17. Laboratory Specimens
    No specimens should be taken without consultation with the laboratory director and other medical authorities. As

(continued)

TABLE 113-7. *(continued)*

soon as the patient is suspected of having an ECD, it must be determined what laboratory work is necessary. Because of the danger involved to those exposed in taking specimens, these should be limited to those essential for immediate clinical diagnosis and management of the patient. Policies and procedures for the handling of laboratory specimens and equipment should be developed by the director of laboratory services.

18. Patient's Chart
    This must be kept outside the isolation area at all times.
19. Visitors
    Visitors should not be permitted. If the isolation room is under construction, a viewing window for visitors may be considered.
20. Transporting of Patients
    Patients will be transported to the designated isolation area using the following procedures, unless a Contaminant Transport Isolator is available.
    a. All personnel transporting the patient must be attired in protective clothing as previously described.
    b. The corridor and elevator must be vacated. Where the physical facility permits, doors will be closed.
    c. All the patient's clothing and personal effects will be doublebagged in autoclavable bags and taken with the patient via stretcher to the isolation area. The bags will then be stored in the dirty utility room until such time as the diagnosis is confirmed or denied.
    d. All procedures that are not essential to the immediate care of the patient should be postponed or carried out in the designated isolation area. Patient transfer should be undertaken as quickly as possible using the patient's bed or stretcher. The patient should wear a high-efficiency mask. Bed cradles covered with sheets may be placed over patient, for transport. Disinfection of the transfer route is not necessary.
    e. The patient's initial room should be disinfected after transfer as indicated in terminal cleaning (item 22).

21. Concurrent Cleaning
    This should be kept to a minimum and carried out by nursing staff when necessary. All cleaning material will be disposable where possible and will be retained in the patient's room until isolation is terminated. A suitable disinfectant will be used for contaminated surfaces. A 5.25% sodium hypochlorite solution may be used.
22.. Terminal Cleaning
    Cleaning personnel must wear all protective clothing as previously described, with the addition of rubber boots. All removable items should be doublebagged, autoclaved, then incinerated.

    After isolation is terminated, all openings in the room, such as windows and doors, should be sealed with tape. The entire room must be decontaminated by fumigation with formaldehyde gas and left for up to 6 hours.

    Appropriate respiratory protection is essential if personnel need to enter fumigated areas for any purpose before the gas is exhausted. All room surfaces and furniture must be washed with a 5.25% sodium hypochlorite solution. All cleaning cloths and mop heads should be doublebagged and incinerated.
23. Handling and Disposal of Corpses
    Before an autopsy is performed, it is important to consider if the information obtained will outweigh the risks involved. It is suggested that the isolation room be used for autopsy if one is performed. Autopsy personnel will wear the same protective clothing as previously described. No personal clothing will be worn. After autopsy, the body should be placed in three large commercial type plastic bags after removing as much air as possible and then sprayed with 10% formalin. The body should be placed in a coffin, then filled with sawdust impregnated with 10% formalin, and the body should not be handled further by undertakers or embalmers. The body must be cremated or buried in accordance with provincial or state regulations.

°Autoclave time and pressure should be adjusted appropriately to the load. Autoclavable bags should be used to obviate the need for further handling by personnel before autoclaving.
†If an ethylene oxide sterilizer is not available, reusable equipment should be autoclaved and then incinerated.
‡It is highly recommended that disposable items be used whenever possible.
§If an ethylene oxide sterilizer is not available and the diagnosis has been confirmed as an ECD, this material should be autoclaved in autoclavable bags and then incinerated.

Campbell BA, Pequegna, MD, Clayton AJ: A hospital contingency plan for exotic communicable diseases. *Infect Control* 1984;5:49.

replication occurs by inhibiting the incorporation of deoxynucleotide triphosphates into herpesvirus DNA and by termination of the DNA chain. The drug is most active against herpes simplex virus types 1 and 2 and is less active against the varicella-zoster virus. Acyclovir has no activity against cytomegalovirus and little activity against Epstein-Barr virus. The drug is converted to its active form in herpes-infected cells by the virus-coded thymidine kinase.

Distribution of acyclovir is throughout all tissues. The drug is excreted unchanged in the urine. In patients with renal insufficiency, the drug must be given in reduced doses. Acyclovir can be given orally, intravenously, or by topical ointment. Phlebitis at the site of intravenous administration may occur. Other side effects include crystalluria with renal failure, liver enzyme elevation, and, possibly, CNS toxicity.

Indications for use in immunocompromised patients include orofacial, esophageal, genital, and other localized herpes simplex infections. Several studies have shown the effectiveness of prophylaxis for varicella-zoster infections in bone marrow recipients and in immunocompromised hosts. In immunocompetent and immunocompromised patients, acyclovir is effective for herpetic keratoconjunctivitis (topical ointment), herpes simplex encephalitis (10 mg/kg IV every 8 hours), and the first episode of herpes genitalis (response

TABLE 113-8. Antiviral Chemotherapy

DRUG	INDICATIONS	ADMINISTRATION	MAJOR SIDE EFFECTS

Acyclovir	Herpes simplex virus
	  Genital
	  Keratoconjunctivitis
	  Mucocutaneous/
	    immunocompromised host
	  Encephalitis
	  Neonatal infection
		Intravenous/oral/topical	Mild local pain with topicals, phlebitis with intravenous use, elevated liver enzymes, reversible elevation in serum creatinine, ? CNS toxicity

	Varicella-zoster virus
	  Immunocompromised host
	  Normal host
	  Keratoconjunctivitis
		Intravenous/oral/topical	

Vidarabine (adenine arabinoside)	Herpes simplex virus
	  Encephalitis
	  Neonatal
	  Keratoconjunctivitis
		Intravenous/topical	Nausea and vomiting, CNS disturbances

	Varicella zoster virus	Intravenous/topical (ophthalmic)	
Ganciclovir	Cytomegalovirus Retinitis	Intravenous	Neutropenia, ? decreased spermatogenesis, phlebitis

Amantadine/ rimantadine	Influenza A virus
	  Prophylaxis
	  Early treatment
		Oral	CNS disturbances, sleep disturbance, loss of appetite, nausea

Ribavirin	Respiratory synctial virus Bronchitis and/or pneumonia	Aerosol	Hepatic dysfunction
	Influenza A and B°	Aerosol/oral	
	Lassa fever	Intravenous	
Interferon	Rhinovirus/coronavirus° HSV/VZV, mucocutaneous°	Topical Intravenous/intramuscular	Local irritation, leukopenia, fatigue and myalgias, fever
	Hepatitis B, chronic	Intramuscular	
	Hepatitis C, chronic	Intramuscular	
	Papillomavirus (venereal warts)	Intralesional/Intramuscular	

°Not approved for use.

with intravenous more than oral more than topical).[69] Treatment of recurrent herpes genitalis is not as effective as prophylaxis. For treatment of severe herpesvirus infection, early acyclovir administration is recommended. For herpes zoster, treatment success is increased if acyclovir is begun within 72 hours of the onset of skin lesions. Whether steroids are effective in decreasing the incidence of postherpetic neuralgia is unclear.

Vidarabine (adenine arabinoside) has activity against many DNA viruses, especially herpes simplex virus types 1 and 2, varicella-zoster, and Epstein-Barr virus.[70] It has much less activity against cytomegalovirus. The mechanism of action is not well-defined. Much of the drug is deaminated to the less active hypoxanthine derivative following intravenous administration. Dosages of vidarabine need to be reduced in patients with renal insufficiency.

Vidarabine is approved for use in herpes simplex encephalitis (15 mg/kg/day IV over 12–24 hours) and herpes zoster (10 mg/kg/day IV over 12–24 hours). The ophthalmic ointment is approved for use in herpes keratoconjunctivitis and

is given five times each day. Because intravenous administration of vidarabine increases fluid requirements and because acyclovir is more effective in herpes simplex encephalitis, vidarabine is now used infrequently.

An antiviral drug similar to acyclovir in structure and mechanism of action but with good activity against cytomegalovirus is 9-(1,3-dihydroxy-2-propoxymethyl) guanine triphosphate (DHPG or ganciclovir).[71] Although its pharmacokinetics are similar to acyclovir, ganciclovir has more bone marrow depressive activity. Significant neutropenia has been an important side effect in immunocompromised hosts treated for cytomegalovirus disease. Clinical evaluations are being conducted in immunosuppressed patients with life-threatening cytomegalovirus disease to see if ganciclovir can reduce the extremely high mortality in these patients.

Amantadine and an analog, rimantadine, have in vitro and in vivo effectiveness against influenza A viruses.[72,73] Although the exact mechanism of action is debated, several investigators believe these drugs interfere with virus uncoating. They are well-absorbed after oral administration and are slowly excreted by the kidney. In patients with renal insufficiency and in the elderly, the dose should be reduced. Side effects include CNS toxicity, loss of appetite, and, occasionally, dry mouth and urinary retention.

During influenza A epidemics, amantadine and rimantadine have been shown to be about 70% effective in prevention of illness.[74] The drug is only effective for prophylaxis as long as it is taken daily. As a therapeutic agent, amantadine has been shown to reduce the duration of fever and systemic symptoms by 50% if begun within 48 hours of symptom onset. No controlled trials are available on the effectiveness of oral amantadine or rimantadine for influenza pneumonia.

Ribavirin has activity against influenza A and B viruses, respiratory syncytial virus, and several other viruses.[75] Its mechanism of action is incompletely understood, and its pharmacokinetics are not completely defined. Red blood cells concentrate phosphorylated nucleotides of the drug, so that it is not completely eliminated from the body for days. Ribavirin can be given orally, by aerosol, or intravenously. Oral administration has been associated with hepatic dysfunction. Aerosolized ribavirin has been shown to be effective for respiratory syncytial virus infection in infants and young children.[76] It also has activity against influenza A and B infections when given in aerosol form within the first 24 hours of illness. When given intravenously, it has been shown to be effective against Lassa fever.

Although they are still experimental, recombinant and purified human interferons have been found to be effective against several common viral diseases.[77] Serious herpesvirus and chronic hepatitis B and C infections have shown some response to high-dose parenteral interferon. Because of the local and systemic side effects, additional studies are needed before interferon's potential clinical usefulness can be realized. Interferon alpha is now approved for condyloma acuminata and chronic hepatitis B and hepatitis C infections.

REFERENCES ■

1. Bodey GP: Fungal infection and fever of unknown origin in neutropenic patients. *Am J Med* 1986;80:112
2. Degregorio MW, Lee WM, Linker CA, et al: Infections in patients with acute leukemia. *Am J Med* 1982;73:543
3. de Repentigny L, Reiss E: Current trends in immunodiagnosis of candidiasis and aspergillosis. *Rev Infect Dis* 1984;6:301
4. Hopwood V, Warnock DW: New developments in the diagnosis of opportunistic fungal infection. *Eur J Clin Microbiol* 1986;5:379
5. Anaissie EJ, Bodey GP, Rinaldi MG: Emerging fungal pathogens. *Eur J Clin Microbiol Infect Dis.* 1989;8:323
6. Weems JJ Jr: *Candida parapsilosis*: epidemiology, pathogenicity, clinical manifestations, and antimicrobial susceptibility. *Clin Infect Dis.* 1992;14:756
7. Wingard JR, Merz WG, Rinaldi MG, et al: Increase in *Candida krusei* infection among patients with bone marrow transplantation and neutropenia treated prophylactically with fluconazole. *N Engl J Med* 1991;325:1274
8. Crislip MA, Edwards JE Jr: Candidiasis. *Inf Dis Clin North Amercia* 1989;3:103
9. Torres–Rojas JR, Stratton CW, Sanders CV, et al: Candidal suppurative peripheral thrombophlebitis. *Ann Intern Med* 1982;96:431
10. Edwards JE Jr, Lehrer RI, Stiehm ER, et al: Severe candidal infections: clinical perspective, immune defense mechanisms, and current concepts of therapy. *Ann Intern Med* 1978;89:91
11. Walsh TJ, Bustamente CI, Vlahov D: Candidal suppurative peripheral thrombophlebitis: recognition, prevention, and management. *Infect Control* 1986;7:16
12. Frangos DN, Nyberg LM: Genitourinary fungal infections. *South Med J* 1986;79:455
13. Rinaldi MG: Invasive aspergillosis. *Rev Infect Dis* 1983;5:1061
14. Glimp RA: Fungal pneumonias: III. Allergic bronchopulmonary aspergillosis. *Chest* 1981;80:85
15. Meyer RD, Rosen P, Armstrong D: Phycomycosis complicating leukemia and lymphoma. *Ann Intern Med* 1972;77:871
16. Williams DM, Krick JA, Remington JS: Pulmonary infection in the compromised host. I. *Am Rev Respir Dis* 1976;114:359
17. Wheat J, French MLC, Kamel S, et al: Evaluation of crossreactions in *Histoplasma capsulatum* serologic tests. *J Clin Microbiol* 1986;23:493
18. Bayer AS: Fungal pneumonias: pulmonary coccidioidal syndromes. I. Primary and progressive primary coccidioidal pneumonias: diagnostic, therapeutic, and prognostic considerations. *Chest* 1981;79:575
19. Sarosi GA, Hammerman KJ, Tosh FE, et al: Clinical features of acute pulmonary blastomycosis. *N Engl J Med* 1974;290:540
20. Kauffman CA, Tan JS: *Torulopsis glabrata* renal infection. *Am J Med* 1974;57:217
21. Lewis JL, Rabinovich S: The wide spectrum of cryptococcal infections. *Am J Med* 1972;53:315
22. Lehrer RI, Howard DH, Sypherd PS, et al: Mucormycosis. *Ann Intern Med* 1980;93:93
23. Norris SM: Amphotericin—How safe and effective? *Infect Control* 1985;6:243
24. Bennett JE: Antifungal agents. In: Mandell GL, Douglas RG Jr, Bennett JE (eds). *Principles and Practice of Infectious Diseases*, 3rd ed. New York, Wiley, 1990:361
25. Bennett JE, Dismukes WE, Duma RJ, et al: Comparison of amphotericin B alone and combined with flucytosine in the treatment of cryptococcal meningitis. *N Engl J Med* 1979;301:126
26. Bodey GP: Azole antifungal agents. *Clin Infect Dis.* 1992;14(Suppl 1):S161
27. Goodman JL, Winston DJ, Greenfield RA, et al: A controlled trial of fluconazole to prevent fungal infections in patients undergoing bone marrow transplantation. *N Engl J Med* 1992;326:845
28. Powderly WG: Therapy for cryptococcal meningitis in patients with AIDS. *Clin Infect Dis* 1992;14(Suppl 1):S54
29. Pfaller MA, Rinaldi MG: Antifungal susceptibility testing: current state of technology, limitations, and standardization. *Infect Dis Clin North Am* 1993;7:435
30. Notkins A, Oldstone MBA (eds): *Concepts in Viral Pathogenesis*. New York, Springer-Verlag, 1984
31. Centers for Disease Control and Prevention: Guidelines for isolation precautions. *Infect Control* 1983;4:249
32. Greenberg SB: Viral pneumonia. *Infect Dis Clin North Am* 1991;5:603
33. Louria DB, Blumenfield HL, Ellis JT, et al: Studies on influenza in the pandemic of 1957–58. *J Clin Invest* 1959;38:213
34. Garvie DO, Gray J: Outbreak of respiratory syncytial virus infection in the elderly. *Br Med J* 1980;281:1253
35. Myerowitz RL, Stalder H, Oxman MN, et al: Fatal disseminated adenovirus infection in a renal transplant recipient. *Am J Med* 1975;59:591
36. Rand KH, Emmons RW, Merigan TC: Measles in adults: an unforeseen consequence of immunization. *JAMA* 1976;236:1028

37. Harris RE, Rhodes ER: Varicella pneumonia complicating pregnancy: report of a case and review of literature. *Obstet Gynecol* 1985;25:734

38. Weinstein L, Meade RH: Respiratory manifestations of chickenpox: special consideration of the features of primary varicella pneumonia. *Arch Intern Med* 1956;98:91

39. Greenberg SB: Viral meningitis and encephalitis. *Textbook of Internal Medicine* 1992;2211:2216

40. Ratzan KR: Viral meningitis. *Med Clin North Am* 1985;69:399

41. Vanzee BE, Douglas RG Jr, Betts RF, et al: Lymphocytic choriomeningitis in university hospital personnel. *Am J Med* 1975;58:803

42. Hevron JE Jr: Herpes simplex type 2 meningitis. *Obstet Gynecol* 1977;49:622

43. Johnson RT: *Viral Infections of the Nervous System.* New York, Raven Press, 1982

44. Nahmias AJ, Whitley RJ, Visintine AN, et al: Herpes simplex virus encephalitis: laboratory evaluations and their diagnostic significance. *J Infect Dis* 1982;145:829

45. Jemsek J, Greenberg SB, Taber L, et al: Herpes zoster–associated encephalitis: clinicopathologic report of 12 cases and review of the literature. *Medicine* 1983;62:81

46. Maton PN, Pollard JD, Davis JN: Human rabies encephalomyelitis. *Br Med J* 1976;1:1038

47. Siegel MM, Walter TK, Ablin AR: Measles pneumonia in childhood leukemia. *Pediatrics* 1977;60:38

48. Muller SA, Herrmann EC Jr, Winkelmann RK: Herpes simplex infections in hematologic malignancies. *Am J Med* 1972;52:102

49. Corey L, Spear PG: Infections with herpes simplex viruses. *N Engl J Med* 1986;314:686

50. Swart RNJ, Vermeer BJ, Van Der Meer JWN, et al: Treatment of eczema herpeticum with acyclovir. *Arch Dermatol* 1983;119:13

51. Chase RA, Pottage JC Jr, Haber MH, et al: Herpes simplex viral hepatitis in adults: two case reports and review of literature. *Rev Infect Dis* 1987;9:329

52. Graham BS, Snell JD: Herpes simplex virus infection of the adult lower respiratory tract. *Medicine* 1983;62:384

53. Shortsleeve MJ, Gauvin GP, Gardner RC, et al: Herpetic esophagitis. *Radiology* 1981;141:611

54. Dolin R, Reichman RC, Mazur MH, et al: Herpes zoster-varicella infections in immunosuppressed patients. *Ann Intern Med* 1978;89:375

55. Goffinet DR, Glatstein EJ, Merigan TC: Herpes zoster-varicella infections and lymphoma. *Ann Intern Med* 1972;76:235

56. Triebwasser JH, Harris RE, Bryant RE, et al: Varicella pneumonia in adults. *Medicine* 1967;46:409

57. Purtilo DT: Fatal infectious mononucleosis in familial lymphohistiocytosis. *N Engl J Med* 1974;291:736

58. Glenn J: Cytomegalovirus infections following renal transplantation. *Rev Infect Dis* 1981;3:1151

59. Winston DJ, Gale RP, Meyer DV, et al: Infectious complications of human bone marrow transplantation. *Medicine* 1979;58:1

60. Meyers JD, Flournoy N, Thomas ED: Nonbacterial pneumonia after allogeneic marrow transplantation: a review of ten years' experience. *Rev Infect Dis* 1982;4:1119

61. Murray HW, Knox DL, Green WR, et al: Cytomegalovirus retinitis in adults: a manifestation of disseminated viral infection. *Am J Med* 1977;63:574

62. Clarke J, Craig RM, Safro R, et al: Cytomegalovirus granulomatous hepatitis. *Am J Med* 1979;66:264

63. Betts RF: *Syndromes of Cytomegalovirus Infections.* Chicago, Year Book Medical Publishers, 1980:447

64. Hopkins CC, McCormick JB: Isolation and management of contagious, highly lethal diseases. In: Remington JS, Swartz MN (eds): *Current Clinical Topics in Infectious Diseases.* New York, McGraw-Hill, 1984:86

65. Campbell BA, Pequegna MD, Clayton AJ: A hospital contingency plan for exotic communicable diseases. *Infect Control* 1984;5:565

66. Centers for Disease Control and Prevention: Hantavirus disease: southwestern United States, 1993. *Morb Mortal Wkly Rep.* 1993;42:570

67. Centers for Disease Control and Prevention: Outbreak of hantavirus infection:-southwestern United States, 1993. *Morb Mortal Wkly Rep.* 1993;42:477

68. Fiddian AP, Brigden D, Yeo JM, et al: Acyclovir: an update of the clinical applications of this antiherpes agent. *Antiviral Res* 1984;4:99

69. Meyers JD, Wade JC, Mitchell CD, et al: Multicenter collaborative trial of intravenous acyclovir for treatment of mucocutaneous herpes simplex virus infection in the immunocompromised host. *Am J Med* 1982;73:229

70. Hirsch MS, Schooley RT: Treatment of herpesvirus infections. I. *N Engl J Med* 1983;309:963

71. Collaborative DHPG Treatment Study Group: Treatment of serious cytomegalovirus infections with 9-(1,3-dihydroxy-2-propoxymethyl)guanine in patients with AIDS and other immunodeficiencies. *N Engl J Med* 1986;314:801

72. Oxford JS, Galbraith A: Antiviral activity of amantadine: a review of laboratory and clinical data. *Pharmacol Ther* 1980;11:181

73. Hayden FG, Hall WJ, Douglas RG Jr: Therapeutic effects of aerosolized amantadine in naturally acquired infection due to influenza A virus. *J Infect Dis* 1980;141:535

74. Dolin R, Reichman RC, Madore HP, et al: A controlled trial of amantadine and rimantadine in the prophylaxis in influenza A infection. *N Engl J Med* 1982;307:580

75. Knight V, Wilson SZ, Alling DW: Ribavirin small particle aerosol treatment of influenza. *Lancet* 1981;2:945

76. Hall CB, McBride JT, Walsh EE: Aerosolized ribavirin treatment of infants with respiratory syncytial viral infections. *N Engl J Med* 1983;308:1443

77. Greenberg SB: Human interferon in viral diseases. *Infect Dis Clin North Am* 1987;2:383

Critical Care, Third Edition, edited by Joseph M. Civetta,
Robert W. Taylor, and Robert R. Kirby.
Lippincott-Raven Publishers, Philadelphia, PA © 1997.

CHAPTER 114

Unusual Infections

Richard E. Winn

Infectious diseases make a significant contribution to the practitioner's experience encountered in the intensive care unit (ICU). Previous chapters have documented the variable presentation and etiology of these infections. Infections may occur, resulting in admission to the ICU or resulting from such admission. Morbidity and mortality may be profound, and clinical management may tax the outer limits of medical technologic advancement.

Many of the general approaches to infectious diseases have already been discussed as part of an organ system approach in this text. This chapter touches on a potpourri of infectious-related entities that may be encountered in the ICU other than those already described. Although they are not seen with the frequency of most hospital-related diseases, the morbidity and mortality may be high because of nonrecognition, difficulty in diagnosis, and less-than-ideal treatment modalities.

Discussed in this chapter are zoonoses, including rickettsiae and *Ehrlichia*; borrelia (relapsing fever) and Lyme disease; tularemia; brucellosis; plague; hantavirus pulmonary syndrome; hemorrhagic fever; infections of the head and neck; and, finally, malaria (cerebral), which may present as perhaps the only parasitic medical emergency.

RICKETTSIAL DISEASES ▪

Rickettsiae are small obligate, intracellular microorganisms that are coccobacillary and weakly gram negative. Rickettsiae are easily divided into four major groups, three of which are arthropod borne (Q fever is inhaled): the spotted fever group, typhus group, scrub typhus group, and Q fever group. Many rickettsial infections are found only in parts of the world other than the United States, and these are not dis-

cussed; however, the ease and speed of travel may allow these unusual infections into the United States. The remaining important rickettsial diseases for the ICU physician are Rocky Mountain spotted fever, typhus of the endemic and epidemic form, and Q fever. *Ehrlichia* has been recently added to the list of human rickettsial pathogens. They are also obligate intracellular organisms.

Rickettsiae are acquired by inhalation or through intermediary arthropod vectors. The arthropod vector varies (mites, fleas, ticks). Arthropod saliva, feces, or body fluids are introduced through percutaneous inoculation or by scratching excretions into the wound. The rickettsiae multiply locally and then invade the bloodstream and disseminate throughout the body. The basic pathologic mechanism of the rickettsioses is nearly identical. Infection of endothelial cells occurs and results in vasculitis. Endothelial cells swell, and thrombus formation occludes small blood vessels. Perivascular hemorrhage occurs through extravasation of plasma. Third spacing of fluid may cause hemoconcentration and shock. These vascular changes are responsible for the rash and systemic signs. Subsequent disease is mild in endemic typhus and is most severe in epidemic typhus and Rocky Mountain spotted fever. Intracerebral lesions are especially common in severe rickettsial disease and may account for the prominence of encephalopathic manifestations in some patients. In contrast, *Ehrlichia* infection does not result in endothelial infection, rash is uncommon, and vasculitis is rare.

The most common rickettsial disease encountered in the United States today is Rocky Mountain spotted fever. Endemic (murine) typhus is uncommon but underdiagnosed, especially in Texas and the southeastern United States. Epidemic typhus, once thought to have been eradicated from the United States, is known to be present in flying squirrels and is transmitted to humans primarily on the East Coast.

ROCKY MOUNTAIN SPOTTED FEVER

Although Rocky Mountain spotted fever was originally described in the Rocky Mountains, it is more commonly seen in the southeastern and mid-Atlantic states. A case ratio of 4.5:100,000 population was reported in 1935 to 1939 in the Rocky Mountain area and made up 50% of the total reported cases.[1] In contrast, southcentral, east southcentral, and south Atlantic states had 80% of cases reported in 1970 through 1974. Two thirds of reported cases today occur in North Carolina, South Carolina, Virginia, Maryland, Georgia, Tennessee, and Oklahoma,[2] with Oklahoma reporting the most cases in the United States as well as the highest rate.[3]

Rocky Mountain spotted fever is caused by *Rickettsia rickettsii* and is transmitted by various species of Ixodid ticks, especially *Dermacentor andersoni*, the wood tick, *Dermacentor variabilis*, the dog tick, and possibly *Amblyomma americanum*, the Lone Star tick. Ticks themselves are actually resistant to rickettsial infection. In infected ticks, the rickettsia exists in latent form, requiring feeding for 4 to 10 hours before reactivation of rickettsia. This is important in human transmission because early, careful removal of ticks without crushing may prevent the acquisition of rickettsiae. Rocky Mountain spotted fever is distinctly seasonal, with most cases occurring between April and mid-September, and is usually acquired in rural or wooded areas. The disease is especially common in children and young adults. Sixty-three percent of patients are younger than 20 years of age.

After a variable incubation period of 2 to 14 days, the illness begins abruptly with fever, chills, intractable headache, myalgia, abdominal pain, sweating, photophobia, bone pain, and malaise or frank prostration. Gastrointestinal symptoms may be prominent, including nausea, vomiting, diarrhea, and pain. The major clinical manifestations, however, are fever, rash, and edema. Up to 50% of patients have palpable splenomegaly. Additional manifestations include periorbital edema, conjunctival infection, and extreme behavioral irritability. A rash appears at day 2 to 6 of illness; it may be difficult to detect in blacks and may not always appear, even in lighter skinned races.[4] The rash is the most dependable and characteristic physical finding. The exanthem of the spotted fever group usually begins peripherally and involves the wrists, ankles, palms, and soles and moves centripetally toward the trunk. It is initially macular, becomes maculopapular, and progresses to petechiae, purpura, or frankly hemorrhagic lesions. Up to 50% of patients have decreased platelets or coagulation abnormalities.[5] Elevated fibrin split products are frequently seen with elevated plasma proteins. Rickettsiae are demonstrable at all sites of disease. Cyanosis and skin necrosis from thrombotic vascular occlusion occur at pressure points or end arteries and elsewhere, including earlobes, scrotum, nose, fingers, toes, buttocks, and soft palate. Application of a tourniquet produces showers of petechiae, reflecting increased capillary fragility. Accompanying severe skin hyperesthesia may be seen. As the disease progresses, central nervous system (CNS) manifestations become prominent, including tremor, rigidity, delirium, seizures, coma, meningismus, optic fundus changes, or central blindness and other manifestations of encephalop-

athy.[3] Lumbar puncture is generally performed and, when done, results are almost invariably within normal limits. The electroencephalogram result is abnormal in 30%, although serial tests may reveal universal abnormalities.

Most complications of the illness relate to local rickettsial invasion and include myocarditis with electrocardiographic changes, myositis with increase in creatine kinase, jaundice, hyponatremia, interstitial pneumonitis, renal failure, and circulatory collapse.[6-8] Edema is prominent late in the illness, presumably reflecting increased vascular permeability. There has been an increase in both morbidity and mortality of the disease since 1960. The mortality rate is highest in patients older than 40 years of age. The diagnosis of Rocky Mountain spotted fever must be made on clinical grounds with prompt initiation of therapy.[9] Clinical suspicion is aroused when a person presents with a febrile illness from an endemic area, particularly after vacationing or camping. In general, a highly suspicious physician should consider this disease in anyone with obscure fever occurring in an endemic region during tick seasons. Other helpful information includes whether the patient's family dog has been in an area where tick infestation is likely.[10] History of tick bite is usually elicited with careful questioning in some 75% of patients. Delays in the prompt initiation of therapy result in increased mortality. A mean of 7 days elapsed from onset of illness to initiation of effective antimicrobial therapy in one study.[3] Without treatment, 20% to 80% of patients die, generally between days 8 and 11. Even with treatment, 5% to 10% of patients die if the onset of therapy is delayed.[11]

As with cerebrospinal fluid (CSF), routine laboratory information is usually not helpful in interpreting the etiology of the illness. Skin biopsy for immunofluorescent staining[12] or indirect peroxidase staining[13] and serologic techniques are useful. Fluorescent antibody testing yields positive results in about 50% of patients. Immunoperoxidase staining may increase sensitivity and decrease interpretation errors. Diagnostic yield decreases once treatment has begun. Culture is difficult and also is potentially hazardous to laboratory personnel, usually requiring tissue culture or animal inoculation. Serologic tests are helpful but are not diagnostically useful in the acute phase. A fourfold antibody rise is usually diagnostic of Rocky Mountain spotted fever. Latex agglutination is a useful screening test. When positive, microimmunofluorescent antibody tests are performed for confirmation. Microimmunofluorescence tests of serum can measure IgG or IgM responses. Diagnostic titers are considered to be greater than or equal to 1:128 with a compatible illness. A fourfold titer rise is preferable. A complement fixation titer of 1:8 to 1:16 is considered to be significant in someone with compatible disease. Some authors consider a single titer greater than or equal to 1:16 to be diagnostic. The Weil-Felix test, which is based on the fortuitous cross-reactivity of certain rickettsiae with *Proteus vulgaris* antigens, has fallen into disfavor for diagnosis because of cross-reactivity with other infectious agents, including leptospira and borrelia, and with severe liver disease and pregnancy. Cross-reactivity also occurs among the different rickettsiae. To be considered diagnostic, *Proteus* OX titers must increase at least fourfold from the acute to convalescent serum. A promising technique needing further evaluation is the use of enzymatic amplification employing the polymerase chain reaction (PCR).[14,15]

Treatment is with tetracycline, 50 to 100 mg/kg/day (usual maximum of 2 g/day in children and 4 g/day in adults in divided doses), doxycycline, or chloramphenicol (4 g/day in divided dose). The advent of β-lactam antibiotics and their widespread empiric use has led to a resurgence in rickettsial infections.[16] Sulfonamides are probably contraindicated because they seem to stimulate the growth of rickettsiae. Although in vitro data suggest efficacy for the spotted fevers, clinical data are lacking for the use of fluoroquinolones. Among the macrolides, roxithromycin and josamycin are effective against Rocky Mountain spotted fever.[17] Supportive management is crucial (parenteral fluids, transfusions, sedation, and oxygen). Fluid overload must be avoided. Although corticosteroids may reduce toxicity, particularly in severe cases, the true efficacy of steroids has never been demonstrated. Heparin is not of proven efficacy.

With prompt antibiotic therapy, patients generally improve dramatically in 3 to 4 days. The treatment duration is usually 1 week or 3 to 4 days beyond the crest of clinical improvement, which may be a duration of 9 days to 2 weeks.

ENDEMIC TYPHUS

The peak of murine or endemic typhus (*Rickettsia mooseri* or *Rickettsia typhi*) occurred in the United States in 1944 with more than 5000 cases. Today only 30 to 50 cases are reported yearly, many of them from southern Texas,[18] particularly along the Gulf of Mexico. There has been an increase in cases reported since 1976.[19] Endemic typhus is usually much milder than Rocky Mountain spotted fever or classic epidemic typhus but shares clinical features with both. Symptoms are indistinguishable from mild epidemic typhus. Onset is abrupt with fever, chills, and malaise progressing to prostration, severe headache, conjunctival injection, nausea, vomiting, diarrhea, myalgia, confusion, lethargy, delirium, stupor, or coma. Cardiac, CNS, renal manifestations, and edema are uncommon. Rash is apparent only in 25% to 66% of patients and is difficult to identify in dark-skinned races. The rash generally begins, in contrast to the spotted fever group, on the trunk and spreads peripherally, usually sparing the face, palms, and soles. The rash may be hidden in the axillae or on the inner surface of the arms. The rash may be confused with viral or drug exanthems. As with the spotted fever group, early lesions are macular and blanch with pressure; older ones do not. Occasionally the rash becomes hemorrhagic.

Endemic typhus is transmitted by the rat flea and outbreaks are usually associated with rat-infested buildings. The disease is transmitted not by salivary inoculation but by introduction of rat fecal material into bite wounds by persons scratching the skin irritation. Dried feces also may be spread by aerosol inhalation. Laboratory workers have become infected.[20] As with Rocky Mountain spotted fever, there are no diagnostic laboratory abnormalities. CSF is usually normal, and recovery is usually spontaneous. Severe disease may be rarely encountered. Patients also may have fever of unknown origin, which may last up to 4 weeks. Diagnostically, increases in *Proteus* OX-19 titers are seen using Weil-Felix tests. Discrimination from other rickettsial diseases requires complement fixation or immunofluorescence. The PCR may prove useful over time with typhus as well as Rocky Mountain spotted fever.[21] The effect of antibiotics on the assay are unknown. Rickettsiae again may be identified in skin biopsy specimens as with Rocky Mountain spotted fever. The treatment is similar to that of Rocky Mountain spotted fever, with tetracycline or chloramphenicol. Fluoroquinolones have demonstrated clinical efficacy against typhus.[17]

EPIDEMIC TYPHUS

Louse-borne or classic typhus is the most important historically of the rickettsioses and has been associated with wars and famines. It is, however, a distinctly unusual infectious entity in the United States,[22] with the last known cases, until recently, reported in 1950 and having been acquired in Mexico. This rickettsial infection was thought to have been eradicated until recent studies established its presence on the East Coast in ground squirrels and their ectoparasites,[23] with occasional transmission to humans. Flying squirrels have been found in many eastern states to have both bacteriologic and serologic evidence of infection. Both their fleas and lice harbor the organism. Data on approximately 10 patients with *Rickettsia prowazekii*, the etiologic rickettsia, have been reported since 1977. The incubation period is 10 to 14 days but may be shorter if the inoculum is large. Epidemic typhus is characterized clinically by the abrupt onset of chills, fever, headache, malaise, photophobia, weakness, and generalized backache and myalgia. These symptoms are similar to endemic typhus but are more severe. As with other typhus group infections, the rash usually begins on the chest (more apparent laterally in the axillae) and spreads to the abdomen and then to the rest of the body except the face, palms, and soles. Lesions are macules or maculopapules that initially blanch but later become purpuric and form groups without becoming confluent. A brownish pigmentation follows the purpuric lesions. Encephalopathic phenomena are common, including hallucinations and psychoses, delirium, stupor, and extrapyramidal phenomena. Relative bradycardia and hypotension are usually present. Gangrene of the toes, feet, earlobes, nose, penis, scrotum, or vulva may occur. Bronchopneumonia and renal failure are common complications. Aside from severity, it may be extremely difficult to differentiate epidemic from endemic typhus on clinical grounds. From 8% to 40% of epidemic typhus patients die without treatment. Diagnostic tests and therapy are the same as for Rocky Mountain spotted fever and endemic typhus. Agglutinins to *Proteus* OX-19 are seen using Weil-Felix tests.

Q FEVER

Cases of Q fever encountered in the ICU are distinctly unusual with the exception of Q fever endocarditis and atypical pneumonia. This infection is associated primarily with animals, including sheep and cattle, and is caused by *Coxiella burnetii*. Human Q fever is distinct from the other rickettsioses in having no arthropod vector and is transmitted primarily through the inhalation of contaminated dust arising from domesticated animal secretions and excretions, such as placenta, milk, wool, hides, and soil. The incubation period is usually 9 to 20 days, and the fever may last from 1 to 3 weeks. In contrast with the other rickettsial infections, there is classically no rash with Q fever. In addition to endocarditis, this organism may cause atypical pneumonia. Adult respiratory distress syndrome as a complication of atypical pneumonia has been reported. Hepatitis also may be seen. The overall mortality rate is approximately 1%. The diagnosis is made on clinical and serologic grounds. Weil-Felix agglutinins are negative in Q fever, and diagnosis is usually based on a complement-fixing antibody or specific agglutinins.[24] Antibodies to *C burnetii* do not crossreact with other pathogenic rickettsiae, and a rise in agglutination titers is considered convincing evidence of Q fever infection. Phase 1 complement-fixing antibodies appear, usually in high titer in Q fever endocarditis. A diagnosis of uncomplicated Q fever may be based on a rise in phase 1 or phase 2 agglutinins or phase 2 complement-fixing antibodies. Sixty-five percent of patients have significant complement-fixing antibodies within 2 weeks of onset, and 90% are positive by 30 days.

When Q fever is suspected or documented, treatment with tetracycline or doxycycline should be initiated. Chloramphenicol may also be used in lieu of the tetracycline drugs. Tetracycline in four equally divided doses is given (25 mg/kg/day), usually equivalent to 2 g/day in adults. For doxycycline, 100 mg orally twice daily should be used. Chloramphenicol is also administered orally at 50 mg/kg/day in four equally divided doses. Duration of treatment should be 2 weeks. Q fever endocarditis requires prolonged therapy with antimicrobial agents. Bactericidal antimicrobial agents are not available for Q fever, so valve replacement is frequently necessary for hemodynamic reasons or cure. Additional antimicrobial agents may be necessary for effective treatment, including clindamycin, lincomycin, trimethoprim-sulfamethoxazole, and rifampin. For Q fever endocarditis, a falling antibody titer to phase 1 antigen is a useful indicator of response to therapy.

EHRLICHIA

Human infection caused by *Ehrlichia* was first described in 1986 in an individual thought to have Rocky Mountain spotted fever. Since then, over 360 cases have been identified through the Centers for Disease Control, Atlanta, Ga.[25–27] Most cases are encountered in the southcentral and southeastern United States. There is a high association with tick exposure. The annual incidence has been estimated at 3 to 5 cases per 100,000 at risk. Two forms of disease have been described, monocytic ehrlichiosis (HME) and granulocytic ehrlichiosis (HGE).[28] HME has been found to be caused by *Ehrlichia chafeensis*, named for Ft. Chaffee, Ark, where the

soldier/patient was infected. Army maneuvers there place humans into significant contact with ticks (seroconversion approximately 1.3%).[29] A related *Ehrlichia* is responsible for HGE. The symptoms of both infections are nonspecific: headache, fever, and myalgia; however, progressive leukopenia, anemia, and thrombocytopenia develop and may occur with other organ involvement, particularly the liver. Rash is uncommon, resulting in the appellation of "spotless" fever. Most reported cases have been severely ill with more than 60% being hospitalized, but serologic surveys indicate a high proportion of symptomless infections. Men are infected more often, probably representing exposure risk; female patients have severe infection and are hospitalized as frequently as male patients. The complication rate is also high (15.9%), manifesting as disseminated intravascular coagulation (DIC), CNS disease mimicking encephalitis or meningitis, and renal failure.[26] The fatality rate ranges from 2% to 5% for HME and 7% to 10% for HGE. The diagnosis may be made using serologic techniques; an indirect fluorescent antibody titer of 1:80 is necessary to establish a diagnosis or a fourfold titer rise.[26] There are cross-reactions with other rickettsiae. Peripheral blood can be examined for the presence of morulae in circulating cells but is low yield with HME and laborious in HGE. The PCR seems sensitive and specific (87%) but availability is a problem.[30] In vitro susceptibility testing suggests that chloramphenicol, ciprofloxacin, erythromycin, and trimethoprim-sulfa will not be efficacious but supports clinical evidence of the utility of doxycycline and possible utility of rifampin.[31] A persistent infection with *E chaffeensis* has been reported despite the use of doxycycline and chloramphenicol.[32]

BRUCELLOSIS

Brucellosis is a zoonosis caused by small, nonmotile, nonencapsulated, gram-negative coccobacilli. They are grown with difficulty in the microbiology laboratory and frequently are a cause of culture-negative endocarditis. They can cause significant systemic disease, ranging from bacteremia and fever of unknown origin to localized complicated disease such as osteomyelitis.[33] The brucellae are characteristically associated with several animal species, including cattle, swine, goats, sheep, and dogs. Infections are commonly encountered along border states of Mexico. Ingestion of goat milk or soft cheese from Mexico may increase risk of acquisition.[34] Laboratory cases also may be seen. Approximately 500,000 cases are reported annually in the world; *Brucella abortus* is the most common organism encountered in the United States.[35] Clinically, brucellosis can be divided into subclinical, acute, subacute, relapsing, and chronic illness. The most important forms of disease pertinent to the ICU are the acute and subacute diseases and the localized disease with complications.

The incubation period of acute brucellosis is several weeks to months. Symptoms are nonspecific, including malaise, chills, drenching sweats, fatigue, and weakness in more than 90% of patients. Myalgia, anorexia, weight loss, arthralgia, and nonproductive cough also may be seen. Few localizing physical signs develop: fever occurs in more than 95%, splenomegaly is detectable in 10% to 15%, lymphadenopathy in 14%, and hepatomegaly less frequently. More than 5% of patients with brucellosis have a relapse usually within 2 to 3 months, but some have had relapses as long as 2 years after illness. Localization of *Brucella* is dependent on infection of macrophages and has been reported from almost any organ of the body. The most common site is the skeletal system, primarily the vertebral bodies of the lumbosacral spine, and the joints, particularly weight-bearing joints such as the knee. Correct diagnosis is often delayed. Neurologic complications may occur, including meningitis and encephalitis. CSF protein is usually mildly elevated, and the glucose, although usually normal, also may be slightly depressed. Adenosine deaminase may be elevated similar to tuberculous meningitis.[36] *Brucella* infection also can result in "culture-negative" endocarditis, myocarditis with acute pulmonary edema,[37] and pericarditis. Other sites of involvement include the genitourinary tract, lungs, hepatobiliary tract, spleen, skin and soft tissue, eyes, and the bone marrow.

The diagnosis of brucellosis is made by a positive result on culture of sterile body fluids or tissues or by fourfold or greater rise in antibody titer. Serologic information is obtained from the standard agglutination test. The agglutination titer is greater than or equal to 1:160 in presumptive cases (96%).[38] Culture establishes the diagnosis definitively; however, culture positivity may vary from as low as 10% to 30% to as high as 75% to 85%. It is also dependent on the culture medium used. Bone marrow biopsy for culture enhances the yield. Blood culture may be superior to bone marrow for *Brucella melitensis*. Therapy of brucellosis is provided by tetracycline. The number of relapses with tetracycline alone, however, may be unacceptably high, and the combination of streptomycin with tetracycline decreases the relapse rate.[39] Seven weeks of therapy with tetracycline or doxycycline followed by streptomycin for 3 weeks has been reported to eliminate relapse.[34] Other single drugs used effectively have included chloramphenicol or fluoroquinolones. The use of trimethoprim-sulfamethoxazole alone has been discontinued because of the high relapse rate of approximately 30%. The combination of trimethoprim-sulfamethoxazole with rifampin is an excellent combination for use in children. Disturbingly, resistance to ciprofloxacin has been observed during treatment of *Brucella* osteomyelitis despite minimum inhibitory concentration data showing good activity. Tetracycline has been successfully used in combination with rifampin, but relapse rates are higher than with streptomycin. Tetracycline dosage is usually 2 g/day for at least 21 days with the addition of streptomycin 1 g/day intramuscularly for the first 14 days of tetracycline therapy. Gentamicin in combination also has been clinically effective with few relapses. In localized brucellosis, surgical drainage of abscesses should be performed when indicated in combination with antimicrobial therapy. Removal of infected heart valves is probably necessary for cure of endocarditis,[40] although one published report demonstrated medical cure using pefloxacin, a fluoroquinolone.[41]

TULAREMIA

Tularemia is a bacterial infection caused by *Francisella tularensis*, a small gram-negative nonmotile coccobacillus. Although widely distributed in nature and infecting several mammalian animal hosts, predominantly rabbits, rodents, and ticks in the United States, infection of humans is relatively uncommon. Men are infected much more frequently than women. The disease seems to occur year-round; however, it is more frequently reported in endemic areas in the summer months. Reporting of this disease reached a peak in the 1930s.[42] Human acquisition depends on exposure to rabbit or rodent secretions or the bite of the infected tick. Cats have become more important as transmitters of disease through bites. Approximately 51 cases have been reported in association with cats since 1928.[43] Less than 300 cases per year are reported in the United States for all years but one since 1970.[44] Despite reported disease from the entire United States, most cases have occurred in the southcentral region, including Texas, Oklahoma, Missouri, Arkansas, and Utah. Clinical disease is characterized by the abrupt onset of myalgia, malaise, headache, and fatigue. The most common accompanying physical finding is the development of regional, painful lymphadenopathy. Tularemia should be considered in any person from an endemic area with outdoor exposure, especially hunters. Atypical pneumonia may be observed and is characterized by nonproductive to minimally productive cough and upper respiratory symptoms.[45,46] Rigors may be seen infrequently in addition to diarrhea. Hepatosplenomegaly, rash, and ocular findings also occur. Findings on chest radiographs are characteristic of atypical pneumonia, including interstitial pneumonia or diffuse bronchial or lobar pneumonia. Hilar adenopathy is usually present, as is pleural effusion. Cavitation and calcification are rare. Severe complications of tularemia, including pericarditis, peritonitis, meningitis, and osteomyelitis, remain rare. Therefore, in the absence of pulmonary disease, tularemia may be uncommonly observed in the ICU. Hepatitis with hepatomegaly and also renal failure may be seen. Routine laboratory findings are usually not helpful in diagnosis. Leukocytosis may be seen with white blood cell counts in the 15,000 to 20,000/mm³ range. Diagnosis is made on the basis of culture or serologic macrotube or microtube agglutination. A single convalescent titer of greater than or equal to 1:160 is diagnostic. Ideally, serial acute and convalescent sera should be tested. Initial negative agglutination becomes positive within 2 weeks of illness in most patients. Serologic titers reach a maximum in 4 to 8 weeks and are usually sustained for long periods. The mortality rate of tularemia in the preantibiotic era was 5% to 40%. This mortality rate has recently been reduced to less than 1% because of treatment regimens. Streptomycin (15 to 20 mg/kg/day intramuscularly in divided dose) is efficacious and should be used for 7 to 10 days. This regimen is recommended for all forms of the infection. Larger initial doses in severe cases (30 mg/kg/day) may be considered for a brief time, 3 days or less, followed by the lower dose mentioned. Gentamicin or other aminoglycosides seem to be equally efficacious and may have lesser toxicities than streptomycin. Relapse after the use of gentamicin has been reported with subsequent treatment success with ciprofloxacin.[47] Close posttreatment monitoring seems warranted. Tetracycline and chloramphenicol have unacceptable relapse rates (as high as 30%), but retreatment with the same drug is usually effective. Rifampin has excellent in vitro activity and bears further investigation, particularly in combination. No data are currently available to suggest that corticosteroids have efficacy in this illness. General supportive measures are extremely important in the critically ill patient.

PLAGUE ■

Plague is a severe, usually acute illness caused by *Yersinia pestis*, a nonspore-forming, nonmotile, bipolar-staining, gram-negative coccobacillus. Endemic areas for this microorganism exist throughout the world; in the United States, however, endemic areas are confined primarily to the western states, including Arizona, New Mexico, and parts of southern California, where it is endemic among rodent species.[48] Because of the restricted locale of infected rodent populations, this infection has become unusual in the United States. However, occasional importation of unrecognized cases or travel from endemic areas to nonendemic areas results in cases outside of the usual geographic locations. Human infection still occurs (California 1988, Colorado 1992 to 1993),[49] and a death resulting from by plague occurred in Arizona in 1987. Forty-six cases of plague from the United States were reported to the World Health Organization in the 15-year period from 1961 to 1976. The overall mortality rate during that interval was 7%. Despite a diminution in case reporting from the early 1960s, there has been a subsequent increase in the reporting of cases over the last 15 to 20 years. This is perhaps reflected by an increase in the incidence in rodent plague population or increased exposure to infected animal populations.[50]

Infection occurs usually by either direct inoculation or from inhaled aerosol from human to human or from the animal host. The incubation period is variable, usually being 2 to 3 days in pneumonic plague and 2 to 10 days in bubonic or septicemic plague. The most common clinical presentation is that of bubonic plague. The bubo or lymph node enlargement, usually in a regional distribution, occurs as a result of proliferation of organisms with subsequent lymphatic migration. An eschar develops at the site of the bite followed by tender, palpable, regional lymphadenopathy. After incubation, tachycardia, headache, generalized aching, prostration, and severe malaise may be seen, and in addition, abdominal pain, gastroenteritis, and diarrhea also may be present. Spontaneous drainage of lymph nodes is not common in treated cases; however, surgical incision with drainage may be necessary in isolated instances. Septicemic plague, which is unusual, accounts for a small portion of cases; most are rapidly fatal.[51] Lymphadenopathy is usually absent. Because septicemic and pneumonic plague have little to distinguish them from other infectious diseases, they hold the highest mortality in this illness. Primary plague

pneumonia is fulminating and highly contagious and is virtually always fatal if untreated. DIC (elevated fibrin split products), hemodynamic shock, secondary plague pneumonia, and meningitis are the principal complications of plague; however, multiple abscesses, cardiac failure, and gangrene may be seen. Gangrene involving the distal digits, nose, penis, or other body parts may result from DIC.

Diagnosis can usually be made by aspiration of a lymph node through uninvolved skin with Gram stain and culture. Bipolar staining gram-negative bacilli, which are the sine qua non of plague, are seen in two thirds of aspirates. Needle aspiration should be performed with care because aerosolization of aspirated fluid may result in secondary cases. Giemsa stain may be better than Gram stain for showing bipolar staining. Immunofluorescent staining is highly specific as a diagnostic method. Aspirated fluid and cultures of blood are usually positive in bubonic plague, with the organism growing well but slowly on solid media. Cultural recovery may be delayed by prior antimicrobial therapy. Blood cultures are always positive in septicemic plague. Strict infection control procedures should be used when persons are diagnosed or suspected of having plague. In addition, they should be reported to public health officials. Streptomycin, tetracycline, chloramphenicol, or sulfonamides seem to be beneficial in the treatment of plague; trimethoprim-sulfamethoxazole also seems to be effective. Streptomycin, 30 mg/kg/day, should be given intramuscularly in divided doses every 6 to 12 hours for 7 to 10 days together with tetracycline, 30 to 50 mg/kg/day. Tetracycline therapy is continued for 2 weeks. Substitution of alternative aminoglycosides seems premature on the basis of available evidence. In the event of pregnancy or plague meningitis, chloramphenicol in a dose of 50 to 75 mg/kg/day in divided doses every 6 hours should be substituted for tetracycline. Antibiotic resistance has never been reported de novo or during therapy; therefore, there is no rationale for combination therapy and, in addition, efficacy is excellent with single drugs.[52] Intensive supportive critical care measures may be needed for tissue hypoxia, shock, third spacing, DIC, and other complications. Prophylaxis with tetracycline or trimethoprim-sulfamethoxazole should be strongly considered for 7 days in close contacts of victims of pneumonic plague. Drainage of buboes is unnecessary in most instances, unless impending spontaneous drainage is anticipated. The mortality rate from untreated bubonic plague has been reduced from the 50% to 60% range to 15% with appropriate antimicrobial therapy.

BORRELIOSIS ■

Borreliosis and Lyme disease are caused by spirochetal organisms distantly related to the spirochetes of syphilis. Most borrelia-related disease is transmitted by arthropod vectors such as lice or ticks.[53] Reservoirs in the tick-associated disease include wild mammal populations. Because of international travel, cases may be imported.[54,55] Louse-borne disease is strictly transmitted from human to human. Louse-borne disease also is normally seen only in cases of interdiction of normal hygienic practices, as in wartime or in close crowding.

Tick-borne disease is seen frequently in the western United States where exposure to the vector occurs, primarily in isolated cabins and camping situations. The disease is transmitted by the soft-bodied tick, *Ornithodoros*. A history of a bite is seldom elicited because the bite is painless. After a variable incubation period (difficult to establish), the patient usually acutely develops malaise, fever, severe headache, myalgia, and arthralgia. The diagnosis is not usually suspected until the patient recovers and then develops several relapsing courses of fever. The diagnosis of borrelia is made on the basis of a Wright or Giemsa stain of the peripheral blood smear showing the characteristic spirochete in the plasma. Although penicillin has activity against borrelia, the preferred drug is tetracycline, which has been shown to cause predictably less severe manifestations of the Jarisch-Herxheimer reaction and which produces fewer relapses. Oral doxycycline may be used if the patient is not toxic and is less expensive.[56] Chloramphenicol and erythromycin also have been used successfully.

Lyme disease is a relatively newly described disease caused by *Borrelia burgdorferi*, which is transmitted by the *Ixodes* tick.[57] This disease, first recognized in Lyme, Connecticut, is transmitted by the tick and results in a skin lesion (erythema chronicum migrans). If the infection is treated at this point, no further complications may occur; however, in the event of late or no treatment, patients may develop meningitis or other neurologic symptomatology as well as carditis or arthritis. Diagnosis is made on the basis of skin biopsy with silver stain or skin biopsy culture as well as culture of other sterile body fluids. However, diagnosis is more commonly made from the combination of clinical suspicion *and* serologic techniques. Serologic test results alone have been shown to be affected by interlaboratory and intralaboratory variability and reproducibility.[58] Both IgM and IgG antibodies are produced. The IgG antibody is highest when arthritis is present. In early, mild Lyme disease, there was no difference in response between penicillin, tetracycline, or ceftriaxone, but prevention of major late sequelae was higher using tetracycline over penicillin,[59] and ceftriaxone was superior to penicillin in more severe, early disease.[60] Other oral agents used in early disease have included amoxicillin and azithromycin.[61] Cefotaxime (2 g three times daily or 3 g twice daily) and ceftriaxone (2 g once daily) are considered the drugs of choice for late disease.[62] Prophylaxis with antimicrobial agents is not indicated because the risk of acquisition is low.

HANTAVIRUS PULMONARY SYNDROME ■

Hantavirus pulmonary disease is an infection that was unknown until 1993 when an outbreak of acute illness was described in the Four Corners area of Arizona, New Mexico, and Colorado.[63] A prodromal illness characterized by fever, myalgia, and headache with progression to cough followed over an interval of hours to days by the rapid development of respiratory failure or the adult respiratory distress syndrome was observed. In the initial outbreak, there were seven confirmed cases with four deaths (1993). Since then, there have been greater than 106 cases confirmed in 20 states, and 54 in the Four Corners area. The overall mortality rate is 52%.[64,65] Preliminary laboratory evidence suggesting a hantavirus has been confirmed using PCR from blood and autopsy tissue. The virus has been named the Sin Nombre virus. Rodent testing in the initial outbreak incriminated the deer mouse (*Peromyscus*), a peridomestic mouse, as the vector (29% of these rodents were serologically positive for the new hantavirus). Cases have been described in Rhode Island, Florida, and other sites outside of the geographic distribution of the deer mouse, suggesting more than one vector. Voles also have been found to harbor the virus.[66] The Centers for Disease Control has shown other related viruses (Black Creek Canal virus) capable of producing the same constellation of symptoms and signs.[67]

Previously, hantaviruses have been shown to cause hemorrhagic fever with renal syndrome (HFRS) in the the Orient and Korean hemorrhagic fever. Disease also has been described in the former Soviet Union, the Far East, China, Japan, and Scandinavia. Spread of this particular infection is through rodent secretions and excretions to humans. The clinical illness is characterized by presence or absence of fever, hypotension, and oliguria followed by a diuresis and a convalescent phase. Individuals develop an erythematous petechial rash of the face, neck, shoulders, and upper trunk. Most individuals experience a slow and uneventful recovery.

Diagnosis of pulmonary hantavirus infection depends on serologic findings: IgM antibodies can be demonstrated to hantavirus antigens; otherwise, individuals must show a fourfold or greater increase in IgG antibody in paired specimens. Immunoblasts may be observed in the peripheral circulation.[68] Immunohistochemical stains can be performed on tissue for hantavirus and PCRs may be used to amplify antigen material from tissue specimens. Efficacious treatment of pulmonary hantavirus infection is essentially unknown. Ribavirin, which has been useful for HFRS, has not proven to be efficacious in hantavirus pulmonary syndrome. Aggressive supportive measures, including mechanical ventilation and pressor agents to maintain blood pressure, should be seriously considered because there have been survivors where these measures have been used. As with most infectious diseases as time has passed, the mortality rate, which was originally upward of 80% to 90%, has declined to 52%.[65]

HEMORRHAGIC FEVER ■

The recent reemergence of Ebola virus in central Africa, with its unknown ecology, epidemiology, and treatment, coupled with an extraordinarily high mortality rate, has focused research efforts into the arena of the hemorrhagic fever viruses. The clinical syndrome of hemorrhagic fever may be caused by members of the arenaviruses, Bunyaviruses, and filoviridae. Although several viral organisms can cause hemorrhagic fever, the clinical features among them are similar, despite variable mortality rates. An insidious prodromal illness characterized as malaise, myalgia, conjunctival suffusion, and progressive fever occurs and lasts for a variable period before the onset of vascular disease manifested as petechial or purpuric skin lesions (cutaneous hemorrhages). Chest pain and cough are frequently seen with Ebola virus infections but do not allow for discrimination from other hemorrhagic fevers. Clinical shock ensues accompanied by multiple organ system failure. A frightening constellation of signs of CNS deterioration and vascular dissolution with rapid death is observed with Ebola virus. The mortality rates are lower with Marburg, Lassa, and other hemorrhagic fever viruses. Diagnosis depends on clinical suspicion in sporadic cases and serologic tests. Treatment is supportive; ribavirin has efficacy in HFRS hantavirus disease. Specific treatment recommendations are lacking; interferon may reduce viral burden but has been disappointing clinically. Further research is needed for more precise recommendations.

HEAD AND NECK INFECTIONS ■

Infections of the head and neck may be potentially devastating because of consequences of impairment of vital organs such as the eye and the airway. Infections of the head and neck that may be seen in the ICU include orbital cellulitis; endophthalmitis; malignant external otitis; epiglottitis; and infections of the deep spaces of the neck, including Ludwig's angina, laryngeal abscess, and suppurative thrombophlebitis. Discussions of the etiologies and treatments of orbital cellulitis, endophthalmitis, and malignant otitis are beyond the scope of this chapter.

EPIGLOTTITIS

Epiglottitis is an infection of the epiglottis, usually caused by *Hemophilus influenzae*, a small gram-negative, pleomorphic bacillus.[69] This particular microorganism primarily causes infection in infants and children, meningitis being common. However, it also may be responsible for epiglottitis in these persons as well as in adult patients. The annual incidence has been estimated at 9.7 per million with a mortality rate of 7.1%.[70] Most recent reports stress the reduction of cases of epiglottitis in children and the increase in adults.[71] There has also been an increase in organisms other than *H influenzae* causing disease in adults.[70] The host response to the infection of the epiglottis results in significant edema of the epiglottis with a characteristic cherry-red appearance. The aryepiglottic folds and prevertebral soft tissue also may be affected. The pharynx and true vocal cords are rarely affected. In adults, these characteristic findings are seen with lesser frequency.[72] The patient may die of asphyxiation caused by sudden respiratory obstruction, particularly when this disease is not recognized or the patient is treated without regard for the potential for subsequent airway obstruction. Diagnosis of epiglottitis may be made clinically on the basis of a markedly inflamed epiglottis and evidence for edema of the epiglottis as seen on a soft tissue radiograph of the lateral neck. Radiograph results may be negative in some patients.[70] Fibrolaryngopharyngoscopy can be performed, although care must be used to prevent laryngeal obstruction.[73] Fever (up to 40°C [105°F]) and severe throat pain

are seen. The course is usually fairly rapid. Treatment is directed toward prevention of edema, including the adjunctive use of corticosteroids in addition to definitive treatment with antimicrobial agents directed against *H influenzae* and gram-positive microorganisms. However, primary attention to airway integrity should be maintained up to and including tracheostomy for prevention of airway obstruction.[74] Not all patients need be tracheally intubated immediately but need to be watched closely.[71] If tracheal intubation is required, this is best accomplished in the operating room by the physician most experienced in airway management. The patient should immediately be begun on intravenous antibiotic therapy directed toward *H influenzae* and gram-positive organisms after appropriate cultures of blood and the epiglottis are made. Cefuroxime or a third-generation cephalosporin is usually recommended until susceptibility test results return because of the high rate of resistance of *H influenzae* to ampicillin. Augmented penicillins (ampicillin-sulbactam, ticarcillin-clavulanate) may be considered, and chloramphenicol, 100 mg/kg/day, can still be used as initial therapy. In the event of penicillin hypersensitivity, chloramphenicol may be used alone (anaphylaxis history, IgE allergy) or cefuroxime or other third-generation cephalosporins (possibly ceftriaxone, 2 g/day) (IgG allergy) may be used. Humidity with oxygen administration and avoidance of dehydration are important adjunctive measures. The artificial airway can usually be removed within 48 hours because patients generally improve within 36 to 48 hours after initiation of appropriate antibiotic therapy. However, antimicrobial agents should be continued for a total of 7 to 10 days.

DEEP-SPACE INFECTIONS OF THE NECK

Ludwig's angina and other deep-space infections of the neck are usually aggressive infections that involve the submandibular, sublingual, lateropharyngeal, and submental fascial spaces.[75] The infections are usually caused by combinations of aerobic streptococci, staphylococci, and anaerobic bacteria.[76] Clinically, the fever and pharyngitis precede the onset of neck swelling. A toxic appearance is variable. Ultimately, difficulty with oral secretions is observed and drooling may be present.[77] Swelling in the submental area causes superior displacement of the tongue and floor of the mouth (double-tongue sign). Typically, the neck exhibits brawny induration without fluctuance. Diagnosis is made on clinical grounds. Sonography or computed tomography may be helpful in localizing collections of purulent material.[78] Treatment is directed toward surgical drainage in conjunction with appropriate antimicrobial agents.[79] Of primary importance is maintenance of the airway, which must be secured by cricothyrotomy or tracheostomy. Tracheal intubation may result in rupture of a lateral pharyngeal abscess with aspiration of purulent material. Because an expanding abscess occurs in the area of a closed space, particularly around the airway, the potential disastrous results from the progressing infection can be appreciated. Other complications of Ludwig's angina include mediastinitis, bacteremia, suppurative thrombophlebitis, and shock. Surgical intervention in the instance of nonfluctuant brawny induration is usually left up to the discretion of the surgeon, once the airway is secure.

However, most cases (68%) have required an incision and drainage procedure. Antimicrobial agents chosen usually include those with activity against most organisms of the oral airway, including aerobic and anaerobic bacteria; therefore, penicillin, cephalosporins, and clindamycin or metronidazole should be considered. Gram-negative organisms also may be seen infrequently, including anaerobes and *Pseudomonas aeruginosa*. Therefore, aminoglycosides or third-generation cephalosporins also should be considered.

CEREBRAL MALARIA ■

Malaria is the first or second most common infectious disease in the world. Infections with *Plasmodium falciparum*, caused by infection of all ages of red blood cells with subsequent lysis, may result in encephalopathy directly caused by occlusion of small blood vessels in the brain and indirectly caused by local hypoxemia. "Cerebral malaria" occurs as a direct complication of *P falciparum*, as mentioned, although tissue hypoxia resulting from any malarial infection can pose a risk of cerebral ischemia and infarction. Cerebral abnormalities range from mild confusion to overt coma. Organic brain symptoms, psychoses, and meningismus may be observed. Focal neurologic symptoms are rare. Lumbar punctures should be performed but are usually not diagnostic. Alterations in CSF cell counts and chemistries are not common, although an increased opening pressure may be seen. Hypoglycemia is an important cause of reversible neurologic changes. Hypoglycemia can develop within hours to days of beginning therapy and occurs in as many as 11% of patients with coma.[80] *Plasmodium* species other than *P falciparum* infect either young or senescent red blood cells, so that if greater than 5% of erythrocytes are affected, *P falciparum* should be suspected. Complications from stasis by lysed or affected erythrocytes include black water fever (pigmenturia), which involves acute tubular necrosis, renal failure, and pulmonary dysfunction caused by altered pulmonary capillary dynamics and tissue hypoxia. When death occurs from CNS disease, occlusion of cerebral blood vessels with parasitized erythrocytes, edema, and secondary hemorrhage are witnessed histopathologically. The overall mortality rate from cerebral malaria ranges from 5% to 50%.

Distinction of *P falciparum* from other species is critically important in therapy for two reasons: chloroquine or quinine resistance, and presence or absence of extra erythrocytic infection. Areas of chloroquine resistance include parts of South and Central America, East and West Africa, and Southeast Asia. Quinine resistance appears significantly limited to Southeast Asia only. References should be consulted for determining prevalence of chloroquine resistance. Empiric therapy with either chloroquine (infection acquired in areas where chloroquine resistance is not seen) or the combination of quinine with sulfasoxazole and pyrimethamine or tetracycline (areas of chloroquine resistance) is used.[81,82] Quinidine, an isomer of quinine that is the only parenteral form currently available in the United States, is used in place of quinine. Cardiac monitoring is essential because hypotension, QT abnormalities and arrhythmias,

altered sensorium, and blindness have been observed from quinidine administration.[80] In addition to specific antimicrobial chemotherapy, aggressive supportive management, including fluid resuscitation for dehydration and shock or peritoneal or hemodialysis for fluid overload or pulmonary edema, may be required. Corticosteroids, previously thought to improve outcome in cerebral malaria, have been shown to be deleterious (increased mortality rate) and are no longer recommended. Aspirin, heparin, and aminocaproic acid also are detrimental and no longer used. Deferoxamine has been shown to decrease coma in children.[83] Whole-body red blood cell exchange may be performed to eliminate the parasite load (parasitemia more than 10% with signs of organ dysfunction).[82,84] No treatment with primaquine or other antimalaria drugs for extraerythrocytic disease is indicated for *P falciparum*, because there is no extraerythrocytic form of infection.

REFERENCES ■

1. Riley HD Jr: Rickettsial diseases and Rocky Mountain spotted fever: I. *Curr Probl Pediatr* 1981;11:1
2. D'Angelo LJ: Rocky Mountain spotted fever in the United States: 1975–1977. *J Infect Dis* 1978;138:273
3. Kirk JL, Fine DP, Sexton DJ, et al: Rocky Mountain spotted fever: a clinical review based on 48 confirmed cases, 1943–1986. *Medicine* 1990;69:35
4. Westerman EL: Rocky Mountain spotted fever. *Arch Intern Med* 1982;142:1106
5. Fine D, Mosher D, Yamada T, et al: Coagulation and complement studies in Rocky Mountain spotted fever. *Arch Intern Med* 1978;138:735
6. Riley HD Jr: Rocky Mountain spotted fever. *Hosp Pract* 1977;12:51
7. Walker DH, Mattern WD: Acute renal failure in Rocky Mountain spotted fever. *Arch Intern Med* 1979;139:443
8. Donohue JF: Lower respiratory tract involvement in Rocky Mountain spotted fever. *Arch Intern Med* 1980;140:223
9. Oster CN: Early diagnosis of Rocky Mountain spotted fever. *Arch Intern Med* 1979;139:400
10. Gordon JC, Gordon SW, Peterson E, et al: Rocky Mountain spotted fever in dogs associated with human patients in Ohio. *J Infect Dis* 1983;148:1123
11. Hattwick MAW, Retailliau H, O'Brien RJ: Fatal Rocky Mountain spotted fever. *JAMA* 1978;240:1499
12. Woodward TE, Pedersen CE Jr, Oster CN, et al: Prompt confirmation of Rocky Mountain spotted fever: identification of rickettsiae in skin tissues. *J Infect Dis* 1976;134:297
13. Dumler JS, Gage WR, Pettis GL, et al: Rapid immunoperoxidase demonstration of *Rickettsia rickettsii* in fixed cutaneous specimens from patients with Rocky Mountain spotted fever. *Am J Clin Pathol* 1990;93:410
14. Tzianabos T, Anderson BE, McDade JE: Detection of *Rickettsia rickettsii* DNA in clinical specimens by enzymatic amplification using polymerase chain reaction technology. *Ann NY Acad Sci* 1990;590:553
15. Dumler JS, Walker DH: Diagnostic tests for Rocky Mountain spotted fever and other rickettsial diseases. *Dermatol Clin* 1994;12:25
16. Marrie TJ, Raoult D: Rickettsial infections of the central nervous system. *Semin Neurol* 1992;12:213

17. Raoult D, Drancourt M: Antimicrobial therapy of rickettsial diseases. *Antimicrob Agents Chemother* 1991;35:2457

18. Elliott LB, Fournier PV, Teltow GJ: Rickettsia in Texas. *Ann NY Acad Sci* 1990;590:221

19. Riley HD Jr: Typhus fevers: II. *Curr Probl Pediatr* 1981;11:1

20. Bellanca J, Iannin P, Hamory B, et al: Laboratory-acquired endemic typhus: Maryland. *MMWR* 1978;27:1

21. Carl M, Tibbs CW, Dobson ME, et al: Diagnosis of acute typhus infection using the polymerase chain reaction. *J Infect Dis* 1990;161:791

22. McDade JE, Shepard CC, Redus MA, et al: Evidence of *Rickettsia prowazeckii* infections in the United States. *Am J Trop Med Hyg* 1980;29:277

23. Russo PK, Mendelson DC, Etkind PH, et al: Epidemic typhus (*Rickettsia prowazekii*) in Massachusetts: evidence of infection. *N Engl J Med* 1981;304:1167

24. Rose NR, Friedman H, Fahey JL (eds): *ASM Manual of Clinical Laboratory Immunology*, ed 3. Washington, DC, 1986:593

25. Walker DH, Dumler JS: Emerging and reemerging rickettsial diseases. *N Engl J Med* 1994;331:1651

26. Dumler JS, Bakken JS: Ehrlichial diseases of humans: emerging tick-borne infections. *Clin Infect Dis* 1995;20:1102

27. Harkess JR: Ehrlichiosis. *Infect Dis Clin North Am* 1991;5:37

28. Standaert SM, Dawson JE, Schaffner W, et al: Ehrlichiosis in a golf-oriented retirement community. *N Eng J Med* 1995;333:420

29. Yevich SJ, Sanchez JL, DeFraites RF, et al: Seroepidemiology of infections due to spotted fever group rickettsiae and *Ehrlichia* species in military personnel exposed in areas of the United States where such infections are endemic. *J Infect Dis* 1995;171:1266

30. Everett ED, Evans KA, Henry RB, et al: Human ehrlichiosis in adults after tick exposure: diagnosis using polymerase chain reaction. *Ann Intern Med* 1994;120:730

31. Brouqi P, Raoult D: In vitro antibiotic susceptibility of the newly recognized agent of ehrlichiosis in humans, *Ehrlichia chaffeensis*. *Antimicrob Agents Chemother* 1992;36:2799

32. Dumler JS, Sutker WL, Walker DH: Persistent infection with *Ehrlichia chaffeensis*. *Clin Infect Dis* 1993;17:903

33. Shehabi A, Shakir K, El-Khateeb M, et al: Diagnosis and treatment of 106 cases of human brucellosis. *J Infect* 1990;20:5

34. Radolf JD: Brucellosis: don't let it get your goat. *Am J Med Sci* 1994;307:54

35. Trujillo IZ, Zavala AN, Caceres JG, et al: Brucellosis. *Infect Dis Clin North Am* 1994;8:225

36. daCunha S, Gaspar E, Melico-Silvestre A, et al: Neurobrucellosis: another cause of increased adenosine deaminase activity in cerebrospinal fluid. *J Infect Dis* 1990;161:156

37. Jubber AS, Gunawardana DRL, Lulu AR: Acute pulmonary edema in *Brucella* myocarditis and interstitial pneumonitis. *Chest* 1990;97:1008

38. Young EJ: Serologic diagnosis of human brucellosis: analysis of 214 cases by agglutination tests and review of the literature. *Rev Infect Dis* 1991;13:359

39. Cisneros JM, Viciana P, Colmenero J, et al: Multicenter prospective study of treatment of *Brucella melitensis* brucellosis with doxycycline for 6 weeks plus streptomycin for 2 weeks. *Antimicrob Agents Chemother* 1990;34:881

40. Winn RE: Brucellosis. In: Doern G (ed). *Diagnostic Procedures for Bacterial, Mycotic and Parasitic Infections*, ed 7. Washington, DC, American Public Health Assoc, 1988:183

41. Micozzi A, Vendetti M, Gentile G, et al: Successful treatment of *Brucella melitensis* endocarditis with pefloxacin. *Eur J Clin Microbiol Infect Dis* 1990;9:440

42. Evans ME, Gregory DW, Schaffner W, et al: Tularemia: a 30-year experience with 88 cases. *Medicine* 1985;64:251

43. Capellin J, Fong IW: Tularemia from a cat bite: case report and review of feline-associated tularemia. *Clin Infect Dis* 1993;16:472

44. Craven RB, Barnes AM: Plague and tularemia. *Infect Dis Clin North Am* 1991;5:165

45. Weinberg AN: Respiratory infections transmitted from animals. *Infect Dis Clin North Am* 1991;5:649

46. Martin RE, Bates JH: Atypical pneumonia. *Infect Dis Clin North Am* 1991;5:585

47. Risi GF, Pombo DJ: Relapse of tularemia after aminoglycoside therapy. *Clin Infect Dis* 1995;20:174

48. Kaufman AF, Boyce JM, Martone WJ: Trends in human plague in the United States. *J Infect Dis* 1980;141:522

49. Morris JT, McAllister CK: Bubonic plague. *South Med J* 1992;85:326

50. von Reyn CF, Weber NS, Tempest B, et al: Epidemiologic and clinical features of an outbreak of bubonic plague in New Mexico. *J Infect Dis* 1977;136:489

51. Migden D: Bubonic plague in a child presenting with fever and altered mental status. *Ann Emerg Med* 1990;19:207

52. Butler T: Yersinia infections: centennial of the discovery of the plague bacillus. *Clin Infect Dis* 1994;19:655

53. Southern PM Jr, Sanford JP: Relapsing fever: a clinical and microbiological review. *Medicine* 1969;48:129

54. Colebunders R, DeSerrano P, VanGompel A, et al: Imported relapsing fever in European tourists. *Scand J Infect Dis* 1993;25:533

55. Trape JF, Duplantier JM, Bouganali H, et al: Tick-borne borreliosis in West Africa. *Lancet* 1991;337:473

56. Karlsson M, Hammers-Berggen S, Lindquist L, et al: Comparison of intravenous penicillin G and oral doxycycline for treatment of Lyme neuroborreliosis. *Neurology* 1994;44:1203

57. Nadelman RB, Wormser GP: A clinical approach to Lyme disease. *Mt Sinai J Med* 1990;57:144

58. Luger SW, Krauss E: Serologic tests for Lyme disease. *Arch Intern Med* 1990;150:761

59. Weber K, Preac-Mursic V, Neubert U, et al: Antibiotic therapy of early European Lyme borreliosis and acrodermatitis chronica atrophicans. *Ann NY Acad Sci* 1990;539:324

60. Weber K, Preac-Mursic V, Wilske B, et al: A randomized trial of ceftriaxone versus oral penicillin for the treatment of early European Lyme borreliosis. *Infection* 1990;18:91

61. Spach DH, Liles WC, Campbell GL, et al: Tick-borne diseases in the United States. *N Engl J Med* 1993;329:936

62. Hassler D, Zoller L, Haude M, et al: Cefotaxime versus penicillin in the late stage of Lyme disease: a prospective randomized therapeutic study. *Infection* 1990;18:16

63. Hjelle B, Jenison S, Mertz G, et al: Emergence of hantaviral disease in the southwestern United States. *West J Med* 1994;161:467

64. Simonsen L, Dalton MJ, Breiman RF, et al: Evaluation of the magnitude of the 1993 hantavirus outbreak in the southwestern United States. *J Infect Dis* 1995;172:729

65. Zeitz PS, Butler JC, Cheek JE, et al: A case–control study of hantavirus pulmonary syndrome during an outbreak in the southwestern United States. *J Infect Dis* 1995;171:864

66. Mackow ER, Luft BJ, Bosler E, et al: More on hantavirus in New England and New York. *N Engl J Med* 1995;332:337

67. Ravkov EV, Rollin PE, Ksiazek TG, et al: Genetic and serologic analysis of Black Creek Canal virus and its association with human disease and *Sigmodon hispidus* infection. *Virology* 1995;210:482

68. Nolte KB, Fedderson RM, Foucar K, et al: Hantavirus pulmonary syndrome in the United States: a pathological description of a disease caused by a new agent. *Human Pathol* 1995;26:110

69. Branefois-Helander P, Jeppson PH: Acute epiglottitis: a clinical, bacteriological and serologic study. *Scand J Infect Dis* 1975;7:103

70. Glock JL, Morales WJ: Acute epiglottitis during pregnancy. *South Med J* 1993;86:836

71. Mayo-Smith MF, Spinale JW, Donskey CJ, et al: Acute epiglottitis: an 18-year experience in Rhode Island. *Chest* 1995;108:1640

72. Mayo-Smith MF, Hirsch PJ, Woodzinski SF, et al: Acute epiglottitis in adults: an eight year experience in the state of Rhode Island. *N Engl J Med* 1986;314:1133

73. Rundcrantz H, Karlsson G: Acute epiglottis treated by intubation. *Int J Pediatr Otorhinolaryngol* 1983;5:261

74. Battaglia JD, Lockhart CH: Management of acute epiglottitis by nasotracheal intubation. *Am J Dis Child* 1975;129:334

75. Hought RT, Fitzgerald BE, Latta JE, et al: Ludwig's angina: report of two cases and review of the literature from 1945 to January 1979. *J Oral Surg* 1980;38:849

76. Geiseler PJ, Wheat P, Williams RA, et al: Isolation of anaerobes in Ludwig's angina. *J Oral Surg* 1979;37:60

77. Meyers BR, Lawson W, Hirschman SZ: Ludwig's angina case report, with review of bacteriology and current therapy. *Am J Med* 1972;53:257

78. van der Brempt X, Derue G, Severin F, et al: Ludwig's angina and mediastinitis due to *Streptococcus milleri*: usefulness of computed tomography. *Eur Respir J* 1990;3:728

79. Levitt GW: Cervical fascia and deep neck infections. *Otolaryngol Clin North Am* 1976;9:703

80. Hamer DH, Wyler DJ: Cerebral malaria. *Semin Neurol* 1993;13:180

81. Wyler DJ: Malaria: resurgence, resistance, and research. *N Engl J Med* 1983;308:875

82. Panisco DM, Keystone JS: Treatment of malaria: 1990. *Drugs* 1990;39:160

83. Gordeuk V, Thuma P, Brittenham G, et al: Effect of iron chelatin therapy on recovery from deep coma in children with cerebral malaria. *N Eng J Med* 1992;327:1473

84. Melcher GP, Winn RE, Greenberg A: Treatment of cerebral malaria (CM) using red cell exchange (RCE) and intravenous (IV) quinidine (QUIN). Presented at the 86th Annual Meeting American Society for Microbiology, Washington, DC, March 23–28, 1986

Cardiovascular Disease and Dysfunction

Critical Care, Third Edition, edited by Joseph M. Civetta,
Robert W. Taylor, and Robert R. Kirby.
Lippincott-Raven Publishers, Philadelphia, PA © 1997.

CHAPTER 115

◾

Evaluation of Chest Pain

Stephen P. Taylor

IMMEDIATE CONCERNS ◾

MAJOR PROBLEMS

Chest pain can be a harbinger of life-threatening illness. Cardiovascular, pulmonary, and gastrointestinal causes of chest pain may be life threatening. The symptoms of chest pain may be classic or atypical. Classic symptoms usually point to an obvious diagnosis. Atypical symptoms are more problematic because of considerable overlap of symptoms between many disease processes. Patients with chest pain in the ICU should undergo a rapid and focused evaluation.

The success of this evaluation is dependent on having a complete differential diagnosis (Table 115-1) and assuring that the workup proceeds in a logical sequence (Fig. 115-1). This chapter assists the clinician in obtaining an etiologic diagnosis for the cause of chest pain.

STRESS POINTS

1. First, exclude life-threatening processes. Fortunately, the differential diagnosis of life-threatening processes presenting with chest pain is limited.
2. The "classic symptoms" of myocardial infarction (chest pressure, squeezing sensation), pericarditis (sharp, catch-like pain), and aortic dissection (excruciating, knife-like pain) should be sought.
3. Atypical chest pain is common in the ICU, and obtaining a specific etiologic diagnosis can be difficult. Nevertheless, the clinician can narrow the differential by obtaining a careful history and performing a meticulous physical examination.
4. This information can subsequently be used to select the most appropriate tests or procedures needed to prove or disprove the suspected diagnosis.

ESSENTIAL DIAGNOSTIC TESTS AND PROCEDURES

History

1. *Chief complaint and history of the present illness*: The clinician should allow the patient to describe the character (pressure, sharp, burning, pleuritic), duration (minutes, hours, days), intensity (scale of 0 to 10), location, radiation, and onset (sudden, gradual) of the pain. Associated symptoms and signs such as nausea, vomiting, diaphoresis, dyspnea, presyncope, and syncope should be noted. Factors that worsen or relieve the symptoms should be obtained.
2. *Past medical history*: Patients should be thoroughly evaluated for a history of cardiopulmonary and gastrointestinal disease. Coronary artery disease, obstructive lung diseases, hypertension, peripheral vascular disease, diabetes, hypercholesterolemia, Marfan's syndrome, connective tissue diseases, gastroesophageal reflux, and peptic ulcer disease all are associated with acute chest pain.
3. *Family history*: A family history of glucose intolerance, coronary artery disease, and sudden or premature death should be investigated.
4. *Social history*: A history of alcohol, cigarette, cocaine, or other drug use should be sought.

Physical Examination

1. *Vital signs*: Changes in heart rate, blood pressure, pulse pressure, pulmonary artery waveforms and pressure, ventilatory parameters, temperature, and urine output should be noted.
2. *Inspection and palpation*: Examination of the head, neck, chest, and abdomen may reveal significant disease. Disrobe the patient and visually inspect for obvi-

TABLE 115-1. Differential Diagnosis of Chest Pain

CARDIOVASCULAR

   Myocardial infarction
   Angina pectoris
   Aortic valve disease
   Hypertrophic cardiomyopathy
   Myocarditis
   Pericarditis
   Dressler's syndrome
   Pulmonary embolism
   Pulmonary hypertension
   Aortic dissection
   Thoracic aneurysm
   Pericardial effusion
   Mitral valve prolapse

PULMONARY

   Pulmonary embolism
   Pneumothorax
   Asthma
   Pleuritis
   Pneumonia
   Chronic obstructive pulmonary disease
   Intrathoracic tumor
   Tracheitis and tracheobronchitis

GASTROINTESTINAL

   Esophageal spasm
   Esophageal reflux
   Esophagitis
   Esophageal rupture
   Foreign bodies (food, pills)
   Peptic ulcer disease
   Nasogastric tube erosions
   Gastritis
   Colonic distention
   Biliary disease

MUSCULOSKELETAL

   Costochondritis
   Intercostal muscle cramps
   Rib fractures
   Trauma

OTHER

   Herpes zoster
   Mediastinitis
   Diaphragmatic flutter
   Psychoneurosis

ous deformities and asymmetry. Significant point tenderness and crepitations should be sought by applying firm pressure to the anterior, lateral, and posterior chest wall. Cardiac impulses my reveal significant underlying disease. Palpate and note the symmetry of all upper and lower extremity pulses. Palpation of the abdomen for tenderness and pulsatile masses is vital in making the diagnosis of thoracic and intraabdominal disease. Note the presence of nasogastric, orogastric, and endotracheal tubes.

3. *Auscultation*: The neck should be auscultated to evaluate for the presence of significant upper airway obstruction (stridor). Careful auscultation of the chest should assess symmetry of breath sounds. Abnormal sounds (i.e., rales, wheezing, rhonchi, friction rubs) and their location should be noted. Heart sounds should be carefully studied. The cardiac rate and rhythm should be noted. Close attention to findings suggestive of valvular heart disease is important. The abdomen should be auscultated, and the presence and quality of bowel sounds should be noted.

The Use of Diagnostic Tests in Chest Pain

1. *Electrocardiogram (ECG)*: A normal ECG practically excludes cardiac ischemia. A pattern of myocardial ischemia or infarction usually provides an etiologic diagnosis. Aortic dissection as a cause of myocardial infarction, ischemia, or both must be considered. Nondiagnostic ECG changes (i.e., old left bundle branch block) neither prove nor disprove significant cardiac ischemia.
2. *Echocardiography*: The echocardiogram plays an important role in evaluating chest pain and is frequently used to diagnose regional wall motion abnormalities, aortic stenosis, dissecting aortic aneurysm, pericardial effusion, and cardiac tamponade. Preserved regional wall motion occasionally occurs early in the process of significant cardiac ischemia. Transesophageal echocardiography (TEE) has a sensitivity approaching 100% for aortic dissection.
3. *Chest radiography*: The chest radiograph may provide important clues regarding the cause of chest pain. The presence or absence of the following radiographic abnormalities should be determined: subcutaneous air, rib fractures, pneumothorax, pulmonary infiltrates, widened mediastinum, pleural effusions, and intraperitoneal free air.
4. *Radionuclide perfusion lung scan*: Intubated patients or patients too ill for transport who are believed to have pulmonary embolism (PE) may undergo bedside perfusion lung scanning. Whereas this test is often nondiagnostic, a normal scan result is a sensitive negative predictor for the presence of pulmonary emboli.
5. *Radionuclide ventilation/perfusion ($\dot{V}/\dot{Q}$) lung scan*: Patients who are not intubated and who are stable for transport to the nuclear medicine department may undergo a $\dot{V}/\dot{Q}$ scan to determine the probability of PE. Normal- and high-probability findings on $\dot{V}/\dot{Q}$ scan often are sensitive enough to dictate therapy without further evaluation. Patients with low- and intermediate-probability $\dot{V}/\dot{Q}$ scan results, depending on the level of clinical suspicion, frequently require pulmonary angiography (Chap. 127).
6. *Duplex ultrasound of the lower extremities*: Although the diagnosis of a deep vein thrombosis (DVT) may eliminate the need for $\dot{V}/\dot{Q}$ scan or pulmonary angiogram, other causes of chest pain should be considered and disproved as necessary.

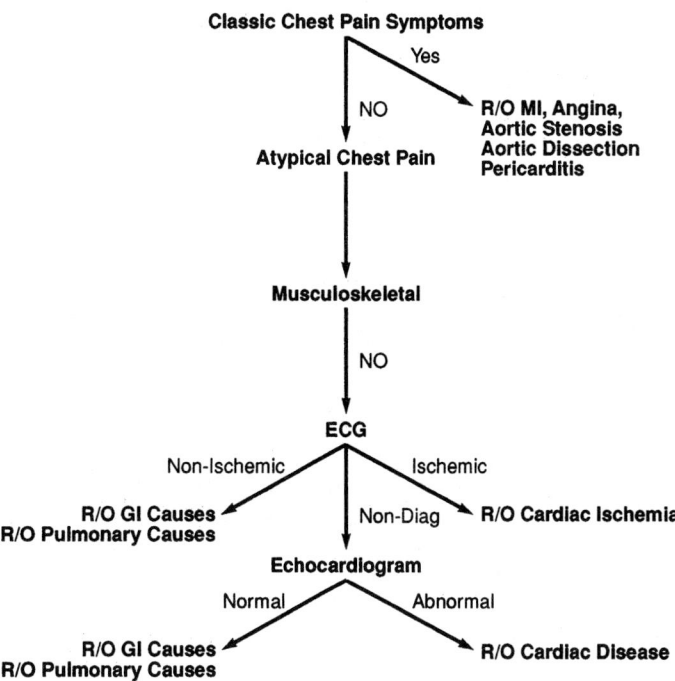

FIGURE 115-1. Algorithm for evaluation of chest pain. ECG, electrocardiogram; R/O, rule out; MI, myocardial infarction; GI, gastrointestinal; Non-Diag, nondiagnostic.

DIFFERENTIATION OF CHEST PAIN SYNDROMES ■

Pinpointing the origin of chest pain is often problematic because nociceptors from within the myocardium, aorta, pleura, lungs, and esophagus traverse a common neuronal pathway to the cortex.[1]

Structures within the thorax that are relatively insensitive to pain include the lung parenchyma and visceral pleura. The parietal pleura, upper airways, musculoskeletal structures of the upper torso, diaphragm, and mediastinal structures often generate pain in disease states. Diabetic neuropathy, differing pain thresholds, medications, and varying levels of consciousness all may greatly influence a patient's description of the chest pain.

CLASSIC CHEST PAIN

Certain disease processes are associated with characteristic pain patterns. For example, an inflammatory process involving the pleural surfaces of the lungs or heart may produce pleuritic chest pain. This type of pain is described as a sharp, scratchy, or catch-like discomfort. Pneumonia, PE, and pericarditis produce inflammatory processes with this type of pain. Patients who describe their chest discomfort as retrosternal, squeezing, pressure-like, or heavy in nature often are diagnosed with myocardial ischemia.[2,3] One of the most dramatic presentations of chest pain is that of acute aortic dissection. Patients frequently describe an excruciating, sharp, knife-like retrosternal pain radiating to the back. The evaluation of patients presenting with classic chest pain syn-

dromes should be directed to specifically confirm or exclude the suspected diagnosis.

ATYPICAL CHEST PAIN

As shown in Figure 115-1, the approach to patients with chest pain can be systematic and organized. Musculoskeletal or cutaneous causes of atypical chest pain should be excluded. An ECG is then obtained. If the ECG result is normal, cardiac ischemia is possible but less likely.[4] If the index of suspicion for cardiac ischemia is high, irrespective of the ECG, one should proceed with further studies to either confirm or negate the suspected diagnosis. If the index of suspicion for cardiac ischemia is low, causes of chest pain such as PE, aortic dissection, pleural inflammation, pneumothorax, and gastroesophageal disease should be considered. If the ECG reveals new ischemic changes, one may assume that this is the primary cause of the patient's discomfort. Patients with abnormal ECG results at baseline may or may not have obvious ischemic changes. In some circumstances (i.e., cardiopulmonary stability), it is reasonable to attempt to quickly remedy the discomfort by giving therapeutic trials such as "GI cocktail" or sublingual nitroglycerin, or by removing the nasogastric tube. If there is a significant index of suspicion for myocardial ischemia, irrespective of the response to this "therapeutic trial," one should proceed with further evaluation (i.e., echocardiogram) to confirm the diagnosis. Many patients in the adult ICU have significant undiagnosed coronary artery disease. An echocardiogram, unless the result is totally normal, usually is not sensitive enough to exclude acute and significant cardiac ischemia. Stress echocardiography, nuclear medicine studies, or cardiac catheterization may be necessary under these circumstances. The urgency with which to pursue these tests depends on the acuity of illness. Patients who are fragile and have significant underlying disease or trauma are less tolerant of physical insults and therefore warrant an aggressive approach. This is particularly true if the suspected diagnosis changes the current therapy.

DIFFERENTIAL DIAGNOSIS OF LIFE-THREATENING CAUSES OF CHEST PAIN ■

PULMONARY CAUSES OF CHEST PAIN

Pulmonary Embolism

Approximately 200,000 patients die each year of PE. The mortality of untreated PE is five times greater than treated cases.[5] Patients at risk for the development of PE are those with low-flow and hypercoagulable states, such as the following:

Congestive heart failure
Pregnancy
Prior DVT
Advanced age
Orthopedic injuries
Orthopedic surgery
Pelvic surgery
Stroke
Prolonged bedrest

The signs and symptoms of PE have been well described.[6] The clinical presentation of acute PE includes the following:

Abrupt onset of dyspnea
Chest pain unrelieved with nitroglycerin
Apprehension
Tachypnea
Diaphoresis
Fever
Tachycardia
Increased P2
Dyspnea at rest
Thrombophlebitis of the lower extremity
Decreasing PaO_2

The most common complaint is the sudden onset of pleuritic chest pain. Nonpleuritic discomfort occurs less frequently. Approximately 84% of patients complain of dyspnea. Apprehension, cough, and hemoptysis occur in 50% of patients. Some patients present with syncope.

On physical examination, most patients have tachycardia and tachypnea. Fever is seen in nearly half of affected patients. Patients with large or multiple emboli often have evidence of hypoperfusion. A narrowed pulse pressure, poor peripheral perfusion, hypotension, low urine output, and mental status changes are common signs of hypoperfusion. Patients may demonstrate a widened alveolar–arterial pressure gradient. Acute PE with a 25% to 50% occlusion of the cross-sectional area of the pulmonary circulation often

results in an abrupt rise in the right atrial, right ventricular, and pulmonary artery pressures. A decrease in the cardiac output with a concurrent widening in the arterial–venous difference in the partial pressure of oxygen and a decrease in the venous saturation with oxygen may be seen. The resultant increase in impedance to blood flow through the pulmonary vasculature may be reflected by an increase in the difference between the pulmonary artery diastolic and the pulmonary artery occlusion pressure.

Once a strong suspicion of PE is entertained, one should proceed with further diagnostic studies, such as $\dot{V}/\dot{Q}$ lung scan and pulmonary angiography. Diagnostic findings in acute PE include an enlarged pulmonary artery on chest radiograph and localized decrease in vascular lung markings. Many patients who are thought to have PE undergo noninvasive duplex ultrasound studies of the lower extremities. If the duplex ultrasound is positive for DVT and anticoagulation is the sole treatment of choice, the distinction between DVT and PE becomes moot. It should be recognized, however, that many ICU patients who have had femoral vein catheters may develop a "catheter-related clot" in the traumatized vein. The natural history of these clots is unclear at this time. Patients who are at high risk for complications associated with anticoagulation or those who require an inferior vena caval filter, lytic therapy, or surgery often require a more invasive evaluation (Chap. 127).

Patients too unstable for transport may undergo a lung perfusion scan at the bedside. During this procedure, technetium 99m–labeled human macroaggregated albumin is injected intravenously and lodges in the pulmonary capillary bed. A gamma-camera then maps the distribution of blood flow through the pulmonary arteries. Although perfusion defects as small a 2 cm in diameter can be detected, such defects are nonspecific. Disturbances in pulmonary blood flow can be caused by regional hypoxia, emphysema, atelectasis, hypovolemia, asthma, bronchitis, pleural effusions, and pneumonia. Thus, the virtue of a lung perfusion scan is in its high sensitivity. A normal scan finding practically excludes PE.

In the more stable patient, a $\dot{V}/\dot{Q}$ lung scan should be performed. This test is particularly helpful when the results yield either normal or high probability for PE.[7] Low- or intermediate-probability findings on $\dot{V}/\dot{Q}$ scans in patients for whom a high index of suspicion for PE is held by the clinician warrant further diagnostic evaluation.

The pulmonary angiogram is the diagnostic reference standard for PE.[8,9] Angiograms are typically reserved for patients with low- or intermediate-probability $\dot{V}/\dot{Q}$ scan results in whom a high index of suspicion for PE is held by the clinician.

The risk versus benefit of the pulmonary angiogram should be considered. Sudden cardiac decompensation from the contrast material, causing a severe elevation in the pulmonary artery pressure, is a feared complication in patients with severe pulmonary hypertension. A recent study documents that a pulmonary artery pressure above 70 mm Hg or severe right ventricular dysfunction, as represented by a right ventricular end-diastolic pressure over 30 mm Hg, was associated with a 2% to 3% risk of death during pulmonary angiography. In a facility with experienced radiologists, pulmonary angiography is, therefore, a relatively safe procedure. Its risk must be weighed against the risk of missing the diagnosis or making an incorrect diagnosis.

Pneumothorax

Pneumothorax is an abnormal collection of air between the parietal and visceral pleurae. It is a common entity in the ICU setting. If undiagnosed, it can be rapidly fatal. Pneumothoraces are either spontaneous, traumatic, or iatrogenic. Irrespective of the etiology, a pneumothorax can have a significant impact on oxygenation and hemodynamics. The array of clinical presentations ranges from mild pleuritic chest pain with the sensation of shortness of breath to full cardiac arrest. The clinician should look for the following signs and symptoms when pneumothorax is suspected:

Tachypnea
Dyspnea at rest
Dyspnea with exertion
Localized decrease in breath sounds
Unilateral hyperresonance to chest percussion
Dyspnea of abrupt onset
Increased peak airway pressure
Sudden hemodynamic instability
Arterial desaturation

Patients are often apprehensive and demonstrate tachypnea and tachycardia. Auscultation and percussion of the chest often reveal decreased breath sounds, hyperresonance, and tympany of the affected side. Tracheal deviation, jugular venous distention, hypotension, and shock are indicators of an immediate life-threatening process (tension pneumothorax).

A chest radiograph should be obtained in the relatively stable patient believed to have a pneumothorax. Expiratory radiographs increase the likelihood of visualizing a small pneumothorax. Chest radiographs are usually diagnostic when the lung parenchyma is normal. The diagnosis of tension pneumothorax should ideally be made clinically, and the pneumothorax evacuated without waiting for results of a chest radiograph.

Patients who are critically ill and undergoing mechanical ventilation are at risk of developing a pneumothorax. Such patents may have increased peak airway pressures, arterial desaturation, and increased oxygen extraction. Despite sedation, some patients may become agitated and diaphoretic. Compression of the mediastinal structures with a subsequent decrease in preload may result in a significant decrease in the cardiac output and hemodynamic instability. If a ball-valve mechanism occurs during positive-pressure ventilation, a life-threatening tension pneumothorax may rapidly develop.

A pneumothorax in a patient with severe underlying pulmonary disease may be extremely difficult to diagnose.[10,11] Loculated pneumothoraces are frequently missed on portable radiographs of critically ill patients. Once suspected, this diagnosis must be confirmed or negated because nearly half of all untreated pneumothoraces progress to tension pneumothorax. In these circumstances, a computed tomography (CT) scan of the chest often is necessary to make the diagnosis.

CARDIOVASCULAR CAUSES OF CHEST PAIN

Aortic Dissection

Aortic dissection is the result of blood flowing through an intimal tear that subsequently causes a longitudinal separation within the media. Untreated acute aortic dissection is associated with a 50% mortality within the first 48 hours. Clinical manifestations, etiology, and treatment can be readily differentiated by using the Standford classification of aortic dissection. The Standford classification divides dissections into two major anatomic locations: (1) proximal, where the aorta and its branches proximal to the left subclavian artery (type A); and (2) distal, where the aorta and its branches distal to the left subclavian artery (type B).

Ninety percent of the patients with either type A or B acute aortic dissections present with chest pain representative of active intimal tearing. Patients complain of the sudden onset of excruciating chest discomfort. This discomfort is sharp and tearing in nature, radiating to the back, abdomen, and extremities. Syncope, diaphoresis, and generalized weakness frequently occur. Patients may have evidence of shock with mental status changes, cool clammy skin, low urine output, hypertension or hypotension, and lactic acidosis (Chap. 121). The clinical presentation of aortic dissection includes the following signs and symptoms:

Abrupt onset
Maximal severity at onset
Knife-like or tearing substernal chest pain
Severe back pain
Chest pain unrelieved by nitroglycerin
Apprehension
Fever
Tachycardia
Elevated diastolic blood pressure
Diaphoresis

Type A dissections are most often seen in young patients with Marfan's syndrome or cystic medial necrosis. Upper extremity weakness, diminished or loss of upper extremity pulses, asymmetric upper extremity blood pressure, hemiplegia, Horner's syndrome, recurrent laryngeal nerve damage, hemopericardium, and cardiac tamponade all are associated with type A dissections. Acute aortic valvular insufficiency and dissection of the coronary artery ostium resulting in an acute myocardial infarction may occur. A prominent diastolic murmur of aortic insufficiency and congestive heart failure may be present.

Type B aortic dissections are usually seen in older patients with a history of hypertension and atherosclerosis. Paresthesia, weakness, and pain of the lower extremities may result from compromised blood flow to the spinal arteries, iliac arteries, or both. Diminished or unequal lower extremity pulses and pressures relative to the upper extremities also are suggestive of distal dissection of the aorta. Manifestation of mesenteric and renal ischemia may occur.[12] The radiographic data suggestive of a type A dissection include a widened superior mediastinum and left pleural effusion. Chest radiographs of type B dissections are usually unrevealing. One may, however, see a widened descending aorta relative to the ascending aorta.

When a dissection is suspected, immediate surgical consultation is required and a rapid diagnosis is warranted. Although aortography is the reference standard, the CT scan, magnetic resonance imaging, and TEE are sensitive and specific.[13-15] The specific tests used to make the diagnosis depend on local expertise and practice patterns.

Acute Pericarditis

Acute pericarditis is an inflammatory process of the pericardium caused by a variety of disorders. It is the most common disease of the pericardium. Pericarditis is commonly caused by infection, trauma, autoimmune disease, or neoplasm (Chap. 121).

The diagnosis of acute pericarditis is established by the presence of chest pain, pericardial friction rub, and ECG abnormalities. A more complete list of the clinical features of acute pericarditis is as follows:

Chest pain at rest
Exacerbation of chest pain with breathing
Chest pain lasting longer than 20 minutes
Chest pain unrelieved with nitroglycerin
Fever
Sinus tachycardia
ST segment elevation without reciprocal depression
Inverted T waves
Pericardial friction rub
Leukocytosis

Pericardial effusions of various sizes are seen by echocardiography.[16]

The pain of acute pericarditis is pleuritic in nature and often is described as a sharp, retrosternal discomfort radiating to the back and shoulders. This pain is relieved by leaning forward and worsened by recumbency, inspiration, and cough. The chest pain of acute pericarditis may be band-like with radiation to the arms. Similar to that of a myocardial infarction.

Pathognomonic for acute pericarditis is a three-component friction rub. This rub is heard best over the left sternal border with the patient sitting upright and leaning forward. It is high pitched and scratching in nature. The rub is often transitory and may be confused with aortic stenosis or mitral regurgitation. Careful auscultation of the early diastolic component makes the distinction.

In the absence of a large pericardial effusion, subepicardial inflammation often yields a classic triphasic ECG. In the acute stages, one may see diffuse ST segment elevation

with concurrent PR depression in the limb and precordial leads. In 24 to 48 hours, ST and PR segments normalize; however, diffuse T wave inversion occurs. The T wave abnormalities subsequently resolve with time.

The distinction between myocardial infarction and pericarditis may be difficult initially. Sequential ECGs demonstrating concave morphologic features of the ST segments and absence of Q waves are suggestive of pericarditis. With the development of a large pericardial effusion, reduced QRS voltage, oscillatory voltage pattern, and atrial arrhythmias are sometimes present.[17,18]

Most patients who are diagnosed with acute pericarditis have an uneventful recovery with bedrest and antiinflammatory drug therapy. However, a substantial number of patients have persistent chest discomfort, fever, leukocytosis, generalized illness, or hemodynamically significant pericardial effusions.

In these patients, aggressive diagnostic strategies including pericardiocentesis are warranted (Table 115-2). Despite an aggressive search, a diagnosis is obtained in only approximately 20% of cases.[19,20]

Cardiac Ischemia

An imbalance between myocardial oxygen supply and demand is the basic pathophysiologic process for a variety of disease entities. Myocardial infarction, myocardial ischemia, aortic stenosis, hypertrophic cardiomyopathy, right ventricular hypertension, and severe anemia all are associated with the development of such an imbalance. The distinction between these disease processes is made by medical history, review of systems, physical examination, ECG, chest radiographs, and other related studies.

TABLE 115-2. Diagnostic Tests for Acute Pericarditis

Echocardiogram
Pericardiocentesis
Evaluation of pericardial fluid
  the following suggests bacterial pericarditis
    >2000 WBCs
    Purulent pericardial fluid
    Positive Gram stain/culture
CBC with differential
Serum urea and creatinine
Blood cultures
Tuberculin skin test
Antinuclear antibodies
Rheumatoid factor
Serologic tests for brucella
Salmonella
Toxoplasma
Mycoplasma
Human immunodeficiency virus
Thyrotropin

WBCs, white blood cells; CBC, complete blood cell count.

CLASSIC ANGINA PECTORIS. Angina pectoris is defined as a recurrent chest discomfort lasting less than 15 minutes precipitated by stress and relieved by nitroglycerin or rest. The discomfort typically radiates to the left shoulder and medial aspect of the left arm. Such discomfort is often but not invariably associated with diaphoresis, nausea, and vomiting. The usual clinical presentation of angina pectoris includes the following:

Exertional substernal chest pain
Chest pain lasting less than 20 minutes
Chest pain relieved with nitroglycerin
Crushing chest pain
Radiation of pain to the neck, upper extremities, or both
Diaphoresis
Arrhythmia

Physical examination and ECG analysis are often normal between attacks. During attacks, however, increased heart rate, distant heart sounds, and a diffuse apical impulse may develop. Localized papillary muscle dysfunction may cause the late systolic murmur of mitral regurgitation. Typical ST segment depression, hyperacute T waves, or arrhythmias may develop during ischemia. The diagnosis of angina is based on clinical suspicion with ECG confirmation of ischemic changes during episodes of chest pain. The tools for diagnosing myocardial ischemia include the following: ECG changes during attacks; stress echocardiography; nuclear medicine scan; exercise stress testing; and cardiac catheterization.

CLASSIC MYOCARDIAL INFARCTION. Myocardial infarction is usually caused by acute coronary thrombosis (Chap. 115). Symptoms of myocardial infarction are similar but more intense than angina pectoris. Unlike angina, pain from myocardial infarction is rarely relieved with nitroglycerin. Many patients develop an overwhelming sense of doom. Apprehension, diaphoresis, and peripheral cyanosis are often seen. Left ventricular failure as manifested by pulmonary edema and shock may occur. The clinical presentation of acute myocardial infarction includes the following:

Increasing substernal chest pain
Chest pain of greater than 20 minutes' duration
Chest pain unrelieved by nitroglycerin
Chest pain at rest
Apprehension
Fever
Narrow pulse pressure
Diaphoresis
ST segment elevation with reciprocal depression
Q wave formation

A completely normal ECG is rarely found with an acute myocardial infarction. The ECG frequently shows elevated ST segments in at least two contiguous leads with simultaneous Q wave formation. Nontransmural infarction is associated with subendocardial damage and is not associated with the formation of Q waves. The diagnosis of acute myocardial infarction presenting as atypical chest pain and an equivocal ECG reading is difficult. Diagnosing myocardial infarction requires an aggressive approach under these circumstances. Simply ordering cardiac enzymes is not sufficient because results are usually delayed beyond the window of opportunity for intervention. An untreated myocardial infarction places the patient at high risk for significant morbidity and mortality. Patients with persistent atypical chest pain and equivocal ECG findings should proceed to coronary angiography unless an echocardiogram result is normal. Urgent coronary angiography and ascending aortography is especially warranted if lytic therapy is considered because patients with undiagnosed pericarditis or aortic dissection often have fatal outcomes.[21] The diagnostic tools for acute myocardial infarction are medical history and physical examination, ECG, nuclear scan, echocardiogram, cardiac catheterization, and cardiac enzymes.

AORTIC STENOSIS. Aortic stenosis is a narrowing of the aortic valve orifice secondary to congenital abnormality, valvular degeneration (calcific), or rheumatic heart disease (Chap. 118). Discomfort associated with aortic stenosis mimics typical angina pectoris. The clinical presentation of aortic stenosis includes the following:

Exertional dyspnea
Chest pain at rest
Heart gallop
Forceful localized apical impulse
Murmur of aortic stenosis
Decreased aortic component of S2
S4
Left axis deviation on ECG
Left ventricular hypertrophy on ECG

Although the syndrome of chest pain in patients with aortic stenosis is anginal, only 40% of such patients have coronary artery disease. The remaining patients develop ischemia secondary to altered perfusion pressures within a hypertrophied ventricle.[22] The diagnosis of aortic stenosis is based on symptoms with confirmation by echocardiography, coronary angiography, or both; heart catheterization with left ventricular and aortic pressure gradient is also a diagnostic tool. Patients with severe aortic stenosis (less than 1.0 cm^3 valve area) who develop chest pain and hypotension are at a high risk of immediate death and require aggressive management.

GASTROINTESTINAL CAUSES OF CHEST PAIN

Unless chest pain is related to obvious life-threatening gastrointestinal disease, many patients initially undergo an evaluation for myocardial ischemia. Most patients with severe gastrointestinal disease have a prior history of gastroesophageal reflux, peptic ulcer disease, caustic ingestion, forceful vomiting, or recent instrumentation.

Esophageal Injury and Rupture

Most causes of esophageal injury are suggested by history. Patients who attempt suicide by ingesting lye or other caustic agents may have obvious injury to the oropharynx. In this circumstance, emergency endoscopy may be warranted. Less obvious causes of chest pain related to esophageal injury include mucosal damage by ingested pills or the presence of pill fragments lodged in the distal esophagus. Occasionally, nasogastric tubes have been found to be the culprit of significant esophageal trauma with resultant chest pain.

Acute increases in intraabdominal pressure secondary to vomiting, heavy lifting, trauma, or straining during defecation have been associated with esophageal wall tear and rupture. Without a preceding event, making the diagnosis is extremely difficult because this process may easily mimic myocardial infarction, pneumothorax, or esophageal spasm. Undiagnosed esophageal rupture may result in life-threatening mediastinitis. The diagnosis of a nonperforating esophageal injury is frequently obtained by upper endoscopy. The presence of subcutaneous emphysema, pleural effusion, or mediastinal air on chest radiograph is suggestive of esophageal perforation. This may be confirmed by barium or water-soluble contrast studies of the entire esophagus (Chap. 142).

Esophageal Spasm

Esophageal spasm is a motility disorder characterized by abnormal lower esophageal sphincter tone. Phasic propulsive contractions cause diffuse spasm of the esophagus. These spasms are associated with substernal chest pain that is squeezing in nature and may occur with exercise, thus making this disorder difficult to distinguish from angina pectoris. Unlike angina pectoris, the discomfort is often induced by very hot or cold liquids. Dysphagia with liquid and solid food may accompany the discomfort.

Once this disease entity is considered, a variety of tests can aid the clinician in establishing the diagnosis. Esophageal scintigraphy, esophageal manometry, and provocative tests all have been used.

DIFFERENTIAL DIAGNOSIS OF NON–LIFE-THREATENING CAUSES OF CHEST PAIN

COSTOCHONDRITIS

Inflammation of the costochondral joints frequently results in chest wall pain. This pain is exacerbated by applying pressure over the affected area, by deep breathing, or by coughing. Often patients can point to the exact area of inflammation.

HERPES ZOSTER

Reactivation of latent varicella-zoster virus with subsequent posterior root neuronal viral replication and inflammation can result in severe chest pain. This process can be triggered by trauma, surgery, immunosuppression, and a multitude of other immunologic stresses. The distribution of pain is usually along a particular dermatome with eventual eruption of vesiculopustules on an erythematous base. The Tzanck

test demonstrating multinucleated giant epidermal cells is diagnostic.

ASTHMA AND CHRONIC OBSTRUCTIVE LUNG DISEASE

A well-known association exists between between atypical chest pain and obstructive lung disease. Patients describe a variety of symptoms ranging from sharp stabbing discomfort to pressure-like sensations. Bronchodilators may provide relief in some patients.

PSYCHOSOMATIC CHEST PAIN

Psychosomatic chest pain is a diagnosis of exclusion. Patients may present with either classic or atypical symptoms. Significant coronary artery disease is frequently excluded by coronary angiography. Many of these patients have clinical depression and need aggressive intervention.

CONCLUSION

The evaluation of patients with chest pain should be organized and proceed rapidly in logical sequence. The evaluation should include a review of the patient's past medical history, history of present illness, risk factors, and a detailed physical examination. This initial evaluation should narrow the differential diagnosis and direct the clinician so that appropriate tests or procedures are performed.

REFERENCES

1. Richter JE: Overview of diagnostic testing for chest pain of unknown origin. *Am J Med* 1992;92:41S
2. Levine HJ: Difficult problems in the diagnosis of chest pain. *Am Heart J* 1980;100:108
3. Christie LG Jr, Conti CR: Systematic approach to evaluation of angina-like chest pain: pathophysiology and clinical testing with emphasis on objective documentation of myocardial ischemia. *Am Heart J* 1981;102:897
4. Rude RE, Poole WK, Muller JE, et al: Electrocardiographic and clinical criteria for recognition of acute myocardial infarction based on analysis of 3,697 patients. *Am J Cardiol* 1983;52:936
5. Dalen JE, Alpert JS: Natural history of pulmonary embolism. *Prog Cardiovasc Dis* 1975;17:259
6. Bell WR, Simon TL, DeMets DL: The clinical features of submassive and massive pulmonary emboli. *Am J Med* 1977; 62:355
7. PIOPED Investigators: Value of ventilation/perfusion scan in acute pulmonary embolism: results of the Prospective Investigation of Pulmonary Embolism Diagnosis (PIOPED). *JAMA* 1990;263:2753
8. Goldhaber SZ, Norpurgo M: Diagnosis, treatment and prevention of pulmonary embolism. *JAMA* 1972;268:1727
9. Perlumutt LM, Braun SD, Newman GE, et al: Pulmonary angiography in the high-risk patient. *Radiology* 1980;136:295

10. Tocino IM, Miller MH, Fairfax WR: Distribution of pneumothorax in the suprine and semirecumbent critically ill adult. *AJR* 1981;137:699

11. Ziter FMH, Westcott JL: Supine subpulmonic pneumothorax. *AJR* 1981;137:699

12. Cambria RP, Brewster DC, Gertler J, et al: Vascular complications associated with spontaneous aortic dissection. *J Vasc Surg* 1988;7:199

13. Chan K: Impact of transesophageal echocardiography on the treatment of patients with aortic dissection. *Chest* 1992;101:406

14. Cigarroa JE, Isselbacher EM, DESanctis RW, et al: Diagnostic imaging in the evaluation of suspected aortic dissection: old standards and new directions. *N Engl J Med* 1993;328:35

15. Nienaber CA, Spielmann RP, von Kodolitsch Y, et al: Diagnosis of thoracic aortic dissection: magnetic resonance imaging versus transesophageal echocardiography. *Circulation* 1991;85:434

16. Horowitz MS, Schults CS, Stinson EB, et al: Sensitivity and specificity of echocardiographic diagnosis of pericardial effusion. *Circluation* 1974;50:239

17. Spodick DH: Arrhythmias during acute pericarditis (100) cases. *JAMA* 1976;235:39

18. Spodick DH: Diagnostic electrocardiographic sequences in acute pericarditis. *Circulation* 1973;48:575

19. Zayas R, Anguita M, Torres F, et al: Incidence of specific etiology and role of methods for specific diagnosis of primary acute pericarditis. *Am J Cardiol* 1995;75:378

20. Permanyer-Miralda G, Sagrista-Sauleda J, Soler-Soler J: Primary acute pericardial disease: a prospective series of 231 consecutive patients. *Am J Cardiol* 1985;56:623

21. Heymann TD, Culling W: Cardiac tamponade after thrombolysis. *Postgrad Med J* 1994;70:455

22. Marcus ML, Doty DB, Hiratzka LF, et al: Decreased coronary reserve: a mechanism for angina pectoris in patients with aortic stenosis and normal coronary arteries. *N Engl J Med* 1982;307:1362

Critical Care, Third Edition, edited by Joseph M. Civetta,
Robert W. Taylor, and Robert R. Kirby.
Lippincott-Raven Publishers, Philadelphia, PA © 1997.

CHAPTER 116

■

Acute Myocardial Infarction: Contemporary Management Strategies

Normand Racine

Atherosclerotic coronary heart disease continues to be the leading cause of death in North America. Approximately 1,500,000 patients suffer acute myocardial infarction (AMI) annually in the United States, and 50% die within 1 hour of the onset of symptoms.[1,2] The mortality rate of hospitalized patients before thrombolytic therapy was 10% to 13%.[3–5] Because infarct size is a strong prognostic indicator of morbidity and mortality, it is imperative that therapy be immediately directed toward limitation of infarct size.[6–9] This chapter summarizes the current knowledge and addresses the evolving issues in the management of AMI.

In the 1970s, emphasis was placed on therapies designed to decrease myocardial oxygen requirements. In 1980, De-Wood and associates[10] showed an 87% occlusion rate of the infarct-related vessel. These results confirmed that intracoronary thrombus is the primary event in patients presenting with AMI. The importance of rapid interventions to achieve coronary reperfusion, improve myocardial salvage, and enhance survival in patients with AMI is well established.[11–19]

IMMEDIATE CONCERNS

■

Various combined therapies are available to maximize myocardial salvage, and it is accepted that rapid treatment conveys greater benefit. Confronted with a patient with AMI, the physician must decide which therapy is most beneficial and answer a series of questions.

1. Should the patient receive aspirin?
2. Is the patient a candidate for thrombolytic therapy?
3. Is the patient a candidate for coronary angioplasty?
4. Should the patient be heparinized?
5. Should the patient receive intravenous beta-blockers?
6. Would the patient benefit from intravenous nitroglycerin?
7. Should the patient receive calcium blockers?
8. Should the patient receive lidocaine?
9. Should the patient receive angiotensin-converting enzyme (ACE) inhibitors?

ROLE OF ASPIRIN IN ACUTE MYOCARDIAL INFARCTION

■

SHOULD THE PATIENT RECEIVE ASPIRIN?

Yes, the patient should receive 160 to 325 mg of chewable aspirin (ASA) as soon as possible after suspected AMI, then 325 mg daily indefinitely unless he is allergic to ASA. This approach should be done regardless of the presence of electrocardiographic ST elevation and the patient receiving thrombolytic therapy. Aspirin is now recognized as an essential part of medical management of AMI and the earlier you administer it the greater the benefit.

The Second International Study of Infarct Survival (ISIS-2) trial marked a new era in the use of aspirin in patients with AMI.[12] This study evaluated 17,187 patients who received aspirin alone, streptokinase alone, both aspirin and streptokinase, or placebo within the first 24 hours of the onset of suspected AMI. ASA was given at a dose of 162.5 mg on the day of infarction and daily thereafter for 1 month. ASA therapy alone showed a 23% reduction of vascular mortality at 5 weeks compared with placebo (2p<0.00001), and a significant reduction similar to streptokinase therapy alone (25% reduction). Interestingly, ASA combined with streptokinase showed a significant additive benefit compared with each agent alone, with an astonishing overall 42% reduction of vascular mortality (Fig. 116-1). Aspirin with successful lysis also appeared to reduce the risk of reocclusion and in-hospital reinfarction by approximately 50%.[12,20–22]

Meta-analysis from ten trials of patients after myocardial infarction evaluated the secondary prevention of vascular disease using long-term therapy with antiplatelet agents. The analysis showed a reduction of nonfatal myocardial infarction by 31% (p<0.0001), nonfatal stroke by 42% (p<0.0001) and vascular death by 13% (p<0.01).[23]

The prevention of major vascular events in the acute and late postmyocardial infarction trials render aspirin a very cost-effective therapy in the short- and long-term management of these patients.

WHAT IF THE PATIENT IS ALLERGIC TO ASPIRIN?

Then I recommend that you give ticlopidine 250 mg p.o. STAT, then 250 mg b.i.d. You need to remember that use of ticlopidine has been limited by side effects, including potentially significant neutropenia. However, in an AMI situation the potential benefits outweigh the risks. Ticlopidine is an antiplatelet agent acting at the platelet membrane to alter and reduce platelet reactivity to a number of substances including adenosine diphosphate (ADP), von Willebrand factor, fibrinogen, thromboxane A_2, and serotonin, and by possibly acting by inhibiting membrane-bound adenylate cyclase activity. It has been shown to be clinically useful in prevention of stroke and reinfarction.[24]

THROMBOLYSIS ■

The emergence of intravenous thrombolytic therapy during the 1980s is one of the most significant advances in the therapy of AMI. With the overwhelming evidence of improved survival, the early use of thrombolysis is now conventional therapy.[11–19] Thrombolysis may also prevent infarct expansion and promote healing.[25,26]

You should determine as soon as possible: Is the patient a candidate for thrombolytic therapy? Before administering thrombolytic therapy, the following criteria for thrombolysis in acute myocardial infarction must be considered:

Indications:

1. Chest pain more than 30 minutes consistent with AMI
2. ECG changes showing:
   a. New or presumed new ST-segment elevation >1 mm in at least 2 contiguous frontal leads (leads I, aVL, II, III, aVF) or >2 mm in at least 2 contiguous precordial leads (the V leads), or
   b. New or presumed new left bundle-branch block

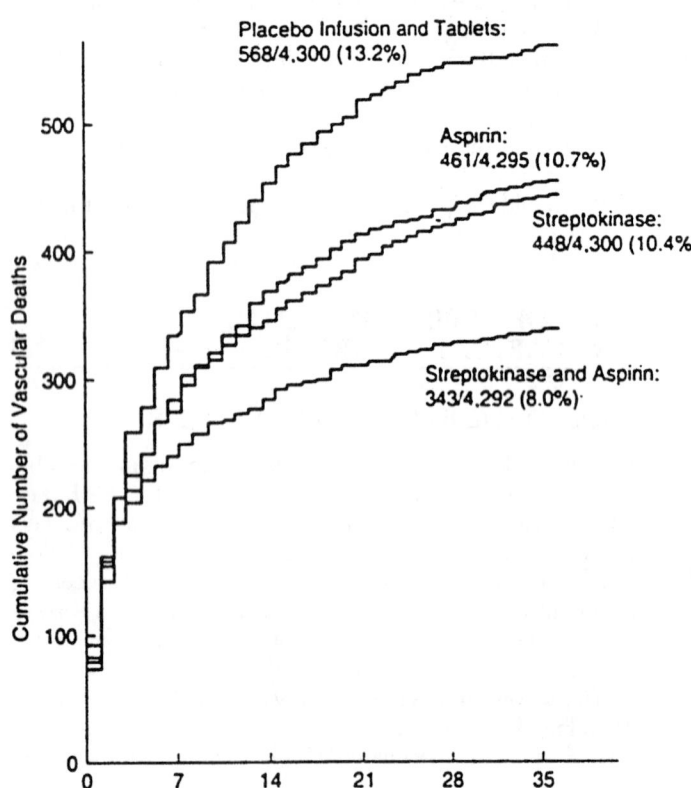

FIGURE 116-1. Cumulative 5-week vascular mortality after suspected myocardial infarction. Mortality was reduced by 23% for aspirin alone, 25% for streptokinase alone, and 42% for combined streptokinase and aspirin compared to neither. (From ISIS-2 Collaborative Group: Randomized trial of intravenous streptokinase, oral aspirin, both, or neither among 17,187 cases of suspected acute myocardial infarction. *Lancet* 1988;2:349, with permission.)

3. Time to administration from onset of symptoms:
   a. <6 hours: most beneficial
   b. 6 to 12 hours: lesser but still beneficial
   c. >12 hours: diminishing benefits but potentially useful if patient has residual pain.

Absolute Contraindications

1. Active bleeding
2. Suspected aortic dissection
3. Recent major surgery or trauma <2 weeks
4. Recent head trauma
5. Intracranial hemorrhage or aneurysm, arteriovenous malformation, neoplasm
6. History of hemorrhagic stroke
7. Pregnancy
8. Diabetic hemorrhagic retinopathy or other hemorrhagic ophthalmic condition
9. Treatment not initiated within 24 hours of the onset of symptom
10. Acute pericarditis
11. Suspected ventricular rupture
12. Previous allergic reaction to streptokinase or anisoylated plasminogen streptokinase activator complex (APSAC)
13. Hypertension >200/120 mm Hg
14. Prolonged or traumatic cardiopulmonary resuscitation.

Relative Contraindications

1. Cardiogenic shock
2. Gastrointestinal or genitourinary hemorrhage in the previous 6 months
3. Stroke in the previous 6 months (may consider this to be an absolute contraindication)
4. Major surgery, organ biopsy, major trauma in the previous 2 to 4 weeks
5. Women during menstruating period
6. Significant hepatic or renal dysfunction
7. Early post-partum period
8. Known bleeding diathesis.

I would like to draw your attention to broad recommendations in the management of AMI, including the role of thrombolytic therapy.[27–32] The following guidelines in the setting of AMI are to be considered:

1. Hospitals routinely caring for patients with AMI could administer thrombolytic therapy if monitoring facilities are available and if the staff are experienced in the treatment of cardiac arrhythmias.
2. Before initiating thrombolytic therapy for each patient, the physician must evaluate the patient for relative and absolute contraindications.
3. To ensure rapid response if an adverse event occurred, a physician must be clearly identified as responsible for the care of the patient designated to receive a thrombolytic agent.
4. Thrombolytic agents should be considered in all patients with suspected AMI who meet the criteria for thrombolysis described earlier.

5. Patients who have previously received streptokinase or APSAC should not be rechallenged with these two agents because of the possibility of resistance from antistreptokinase antibody and the increased risk of allergic reactions. Instead they should receive recombinant tissue-type plasminogen activator (rt-PA).
6. Patients not responding to a thrombolytic agent or patients who are hemodynamically compromised should be considered for emergency coronary angiography to assess the feasibility of an emergency coronary dilatation.

WHICH THROMBOLYTIC AGENT SHOULD YOU USE?

Recombinant tissue-type plasminogen activator appears to have an edge advantage over streptokinase and APSAC. Although the first large trials (ISIS-3, GISSI-2, International Study Group) to compare these thrombolytic agents directly showed no significant difference in efficacy, there was some variation in the rates of reinfarction, cerebral hemorrhage, and allergic reaction.[17,18,33] The most recent trial GUSTO (Global Utilization of Streptokinase and rt-PA for Occluded Coronary Arteries) demonstrated that, in comparison with conventional treatment with streptokinase, a regimen of accelerated-dose rt-PA "front-loaded" regimen (given over 90 minutes instead of 180 minutes) achieved an additional 14% reduction in 30-day mortality.[19]

Unfortunately, in an era of cost containment, there has been heated debate as to the most appropriate choice of thrombolytic agent in various clinical settings, since the administration of rt-PA results in an excess cost of $29,000 per year of life saved when costs are averaged for a ten-year period.[32,34]

When rt-PA is used wisely this greater cost appears acceptable, particularly when used early (less than 4 hours from symptom onset) in the "specific" subgroups, which include:

age <75 years
anterior MI
new bundle branch block
diabetes
Killip class III
heart rate >100 beats/min
previous myocardial infarction.

The conventional dosages of the three most commonly used thrombolytic agents are:

1. Front-loaded tissue-type plasminogen activator (t-PA): 1 mg/Kg (maximum of 100 mg) given intravenously as follows:
   a. 15 mg IV bolus
   b. followed by 0.75 mg/Kg IV over 30 minutes (maximum of 50 mg)
   c. followed by 0.50 mg/Kg IV over 60 minutes (maximum of 35 mg)
2. Streptokinase: 1.5 million IU intravenous infusion over 60 minutes
3. APSAC: 30 U by intravenous infusion over 2 to 5 minutes.

Originally, intracoronary thrombolysis was compared with that of placebo.[35–37] The reperfusion rates reported by these studies ranged between 70% and 75%. However, the inevitable delay between the time of onset of symptoms and administration of intracoronary streptokinase limits its value. The potential complications, the lack of availability of this procedure in community hospitals, and the costs involved renders the widespread application of intracoronary thrombolytic therapy impractical and expensive.

Therefore, the role of intravenous thrombolytic agents was evaluated. The reperfusion rates of 31% to 62% achieved with intravenous streptokinase were not as impressive as with the intracoronary route.[38,39] These disappointing results motivated the evaluation of the second-generation thrombolytic agents, such as rt-PA and APSAC.[40–42] Table 116-1 illustrates some characteristics and clinical effects of the three most commonly used thrombolytic agents in AMI.

The reduction in mortality achieved with thrombolytic therapy compared with placebo in the first few hours of AMI has been demonstrated by five large studies (Table 116-2).[11,12,14,15,43] The GISSI-I study, assessing IV streptokinase, showed a significant reduction in mortality of 18% (p=0.0002).[11] The ISIS-2 study, using IV streptokinase, reflected a 25% reduction in mortality at 5 weeks (p<0.00001).[12] The ISAM (Intravenous Streptokinase in Acute Myocardial Infarction) trial, evaluating IV streptokinase, showed a non-significant 11% reduction in mortality compared with the conventional group.[43] The ISAM results may be related to an insufficient number of patients enrolled to demonstrate a significant difference.

Concerns about the use of intravenous streptokinase are the nonselectivity for fresh thrombus and lower early reperfusion rate compared with intravenous t-PA as shown in the TIMI-I (First Thrombolysis in Myocardial Infarction) trial (reperfusion rates of 31% and 62%, respectively; p<0.001).[44] Therefore, two large trials using second-generation thrombolytic agents were compared with placebo to assess their efficacy. The ASSET (Anglo-Scandinavian Study of Early Thrombolysis) trial, using IV t-PA, showed a mortality reduction of 27% at 4 weeks (p=0.0011). The AIMS (Acute Myocardial Infarction Study) trial, using APSAC, showed a 47% reduction in mortality rate at 30 days (p=0.0016).[15]

Pooled analysis of these five large mortality end-point trials, using intravenous thrombolytic agents compared with placebo for patients enrolled within 6 hours of the onset of symptoms, demonstrated a 22 ± 3% reduction of the risk of mortality. Although these five trials indirectly show that intravenous streptokinase appear to have similar efficacy as t-PA, there came the need to compare these various thrombolytic therapies directly to determine if they are really clinically comparable.

To determine which thrombolytic agent is superior three large trials have been developed. First, the GISSI-2 trial randomized 12,490 patients to four treatment groups (i.e., streptokinase alone, streptokinase plus heparin, t-PA alone, and t-PA with heparin).[18] There was no statistically significant difference in mortality rates between the two thrombolytic agents (9.0% for t-PA versus 8.6% for streptokinase). The clinical relevance of the GISSI-2 results have been questioned because subcutaneous heparin, rather than intravenous heparin, was used and started late, that is, 12 hours after thrombolysis. The major concerns were that the route and time of administration of heparin may not have been ideal nor early enough after the administration of t-PA due to its short half-life. Therefore, reocclusion may occur more easily with t-PA requiring that IV heparin be given early to help maintain a continuous antithrombotic effect.

The ISIS-3 trial, involving 41,299 patients, directly compared three thrombolytic agents (i.e., streptokinase, t-PA, APSAC). This trial showed no difference in the 35-day mortality rates among these agents: 10.6%, 10.3%, and 10.5% in the streptokinase, t-PA, and APSAC groups, respectively. The reinfarction rate was slightly less with t-PA than with streptokinase or APSAC (2.9%, 3.5%, and 3.6%, respectively; 2p<0.02). The total incidence of any strokes was

TABLE 116-1. Characteristics and Clinical Effects of Three Commonly Used Thrombolytic Agents for Acute Myocardial Infarction

CHARACTERISTICS	SK°	t-PA°	APSAC°
Half-life (min)	18–20	4–6	95–100
Fibrinogen depletion	Extensive	Moderate	Extensive
Vessel patency at 90 min	40–50%	80–85%[#]	60–65%
Vessel patency at 24 hr	85%	85%	85%
Reinfarction	3.5%	3%	3.5%
Hypotension	5–7%	3–4%	5–7%
Allergic reactions with persistent shock	0.3%	0.1%	0.5%
Intracranial hemorrhage	0.3%	0.6%	0.6%
Major bleeds (ie, transfusions)	1.0%	1.0%	1.0%

°APSAC, anisoylated plasminogen streptokinase activator complex; SK, streptokinase; t-PA, tissue plasminogen activator.
[#]Based on the accelerated t-PA regimen.

TABLE 116-2. Mortality Rates of Large Trials of Intravenous Thrombolytic Agents

| | | | | MORTALITY (%) | | |
TRIAL°	AGENT#	TIME (hr)	NO. OF PATIENTS	*Treatment*	*Control*	*Reduction (%)*
GISSI-1[11]	SK	<12	11806	10.7	13	18
ISIS-2[12]	SK	<24	17187	9.2	12	25
ISAM[43]	SK	<5	1741	6.3	7.1	11
ASSET[14]	t-PA	<5	5011	7.2	9.8	27
AIMS[15]	APSAC	<6	1258	6.4	12.1	47
Pooled analysis			37003	9.2	11.8	22 ± 3

°AIMS, APSAC Intervention mortality study; APSAC, anisoylated plasminogen streptokinase activator complex; ASSET, Anglo-Scandinavian study of early thrombolysis; GISSI-I, Gruppo Italiano per lo Studio della Streptochinasi nell'Infarto miocardico; ISAM, intravenous streptokinase and myocardial infarction; ISIS, International study of infarct survival.
#SK, streptokinase; t-PA, tissue plasminogen activator

lower in the streptokinase group than in the t-PA or APSAC groups (1.04%, 1.39%, and 1.26%, respectively; 2p<0.01); similarly, the cumulative incidence of cerebral bleeds was significantly lower in the streptokinase group than in the t-PA or APSAC groups (0.24%, 0.66%, and 0.55%, respectively; 2p<0.0001). However, the clinical relevance of these differences is controversial considering the low absolute incidence of total strokes or cerebral bleeds.[17]

In order to evaluate if the regular t-PA regimen used in the GISSI-2 and ISIS-3 trials could be improved further, the GUSTO trial used an accelerated t-PA administration (so-called front-loaded regimen) with concomitant intravenous heparin. Since t-PA has a very short half-life it was postulated that the administration of IV heparin would help reduce the reocclusion rate by providing a continuous antithrombotic effect. In this GUSTO trial, 41,021 patients were assigned to one of four different thrombolytic strategies (streptokinase and subcutaneous heparin, streptokinase and IV heparin, accelerated t-PA, and IV heparin, or a combination of streptokinase plus t-PA with IV heparin). The mortality rates in these four groups were respectively 7.2%, 7.4%, 6.3%, and 7.0%. This represented a 14% reduction in mortality for accelerated t-PA as compared with the two streptokinase strategies (p=0.001).[19]

These results tend to confer a slight advantage in favor of the accelerated t-PA strategy. As we mentioned earlier, in an era of cost containment, and using the GUSTO subgroup analysis, it appears reasonable to consider t-PA as the agent of choice in the following conditions: myocardial infarction (MI) less than 4 hours from onset of symptom, anterior MI, new bundle branch block, diabetes, Killip 3, heart rate >100 beats/min, patients less than 75 years old, and previous MI.

I would like to emphasize a few other aspects concerning thrombolytic therapy. First, a paradoxic increase in death was observed for the streptokinase group compared with the conventional therapy on the first hospital day, although the overall in-hospital benefit of streptokinase is well-shown (Fig. 116-2).[12,45] The mechanisms for this early increase in

mortality in the streptokinase group is probably cardiac rupture and reperfusion injury.[45]

Second, only a minority of AMI patients (approximately 33%) actually receive thrombolytic therapy.[46] Despite the impressive survival benefits obtained with thrombolytic therapy this therapy may be underused. To optimize its use, physicians must be informed about the potential benefits, and the community must be educated to seek medical attention promptly after the onset of ischemic cardiac symptoms. Contraindications to therapy must also be assessed in each patient.

Third, Cragg and associates[47] showed that in-hospital mortality was significantly higher among patients either excluded from thrombolytic therapy because of age (>76 years) or presenting more than 4 hours after the onset of symptoms. Approximately 15% of the patients with AMI are 75 years or older. The limited data available for this group shows a significant reduction in mortality of 33% if treated with a thrombolytic agent (Fig. 116-3).[12]

Fourth, the benefits of thrombolytic therapy for patients who present more than 6 hours after the onset of AMI symptoms is less impressive. The ISIS-2 trial showed a modest reduction of 13.5% in mortality among patients randomized to streptokinase 5 to 24 hours after the onset of symptoms.[12] Meanwhile the Late Assessment of Thrombolytic Efficacy (LATE) and Estudio Multicentrico Estreptoquinasa Republicas de America del Sur (EMERAS) trials evaluating the role of t-PA and streptokinase respectively showed a significant mortality reduction of approximately 10% to 20% when administered within 6 to 12 hours from symptom onset.[48,49] It is reasonable to consider thrombolytic therapy for patients presenting within 6 to 12 hours from onset of symptoms, particularly if they manifest recurrent or ongoing symptoms.

Fifth, AMI presenting with cardiogenic shock do not appear to benefit substantially from thrombolytic therapy.[50] The literature related to this group is limited since clinical trials have frequently excluded them. Kennedy and col-

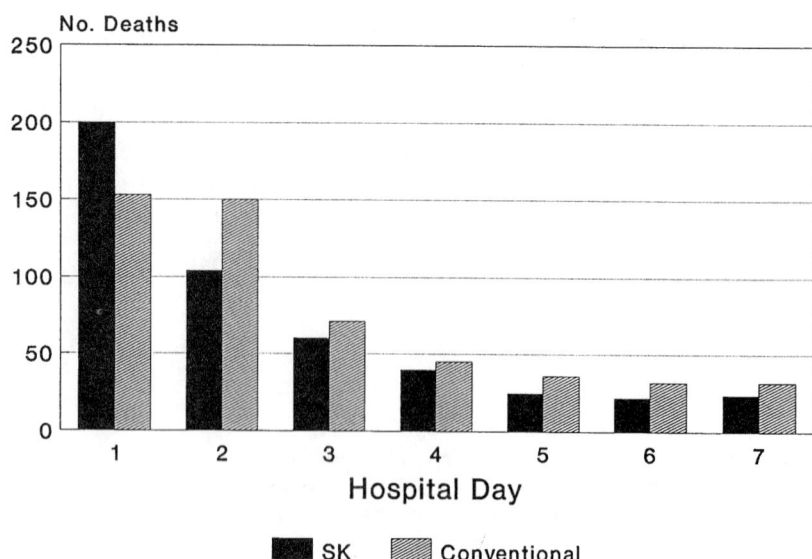

FIGURE 116-2. The GISSI-1 trial demonstrated a paradoxical worsening of mortality in the first hospital day for patients receiving intravenous streptokinase (SK) compared with conventional therapy, although subsequently the overriding in-hospital benefit of streptokinase was shown. A significant proportion of these patients were found to have cardiac rupture at autopsy.

leagues showed that reperfusion with lytic therapy is less likely in cardiogenic shock than for those not in shock (43 versus 71%). However, if reperfusion was successful the survival rate was higher than those in whom reperfusion was not achieved (58% versus 16%).[51] Unfortunately, the same groups of patients that are frequently excluded from thrombolytic trials are less likely to receive lytic therapy in the community setting.[52] I would recommend that if you have access to a catheterization laboratory you proceed immediately to an angiogram and potentially an angioplasty. In the absence of such facilities you should attempt thrombolytic therapy.

Sixth, uncontrolled hypertension (i.e., systolic blood pressure>200 mm Hg or diastolic blood pressure>120 mm Hg) should be treated aggressively in the setting of AMI to reduce the myocardial workload and enable the initiation of thrombolytic therapy.

Seventh, the decision to withhold a potentially life-saving therapy based on arbitrary cut-off periods occurring after major surgery, gastrointestinal bleed, past cerebrovascular events, organ biopsy, bundle branch block, or cardiogenic shock must be assessed on an individual basis according to the benefit-risk profile in each patient.

A few observations can summarize the vast literature on intravenous and intracoronary streptokinase. The studies that described an improvement in regional or global left ventricular function were generally limited to patients in whom thrombolytic therapy was successfully delivered within 4 hours.[53–58] The earlier the administration, the more likely that reperfusion was achieved and the better the survival rate.[13,59] Clinical reinfarction occurred frequently in the early months after successful thrombolysis, suggesting that a significant proportion of the patients may need additional or adjuvant therapy.

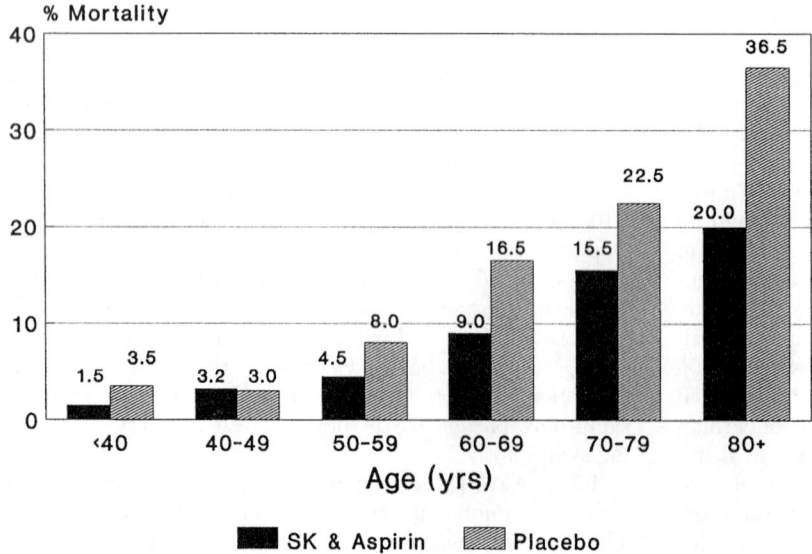

FIGURE 116-3. The 5-week vascular mortality as a function of age for patients receiving intravenous streptokinase for suspected acute myocardial infarction in the ISIS-2 trial. The graph demonstrates the relatively greater odds reduction in mortality obtained in the elderly patients—particularly for those older than 80, in whom a 45% reduction in mortality is shown.

PERCUTANEOUS TRANSLUMINAL CORONARY ANGIOPLASTY ■

IS THE PATIENT A CANDIDATE FOR CORONARY ANGIOPLASTY?

Percutaneous transluminal coronary angioplasty (PTCA) is an excellent alternative to thrombolytic therapy and should be considered in the following settings:

1. Patients not eligible for thrombolysis
2. Patients not responding to thrombolytic therapy and persistent symptoms
3. Patients hemodynamically unstable (e.g., cardiogenic shock)
4. Patients with documented significant recurrent ischemia, which was spontaneous or provoked by predischarge exercise testing.

The lack of widespread availability of PTCA in community hospitals and its related costs renders the choice of primary thrombolytic therapy a more readily applicable option. However, primary PTCA is an attractive option if you have rapid access to a catheterization laboratory and experienced personnel.

Most patients who undergo successful thrombolysis of the infarct-related artery have a residual tight stenosis, and reocclusion may occur in one third of these patients despite full heparinization.[60] Because only 33% of patients with AMI are considered eligible for thrombolytic therapy, we need to develop alternatives. Patients not eligible for thrombolysis therapy should be considered for PTCA. Approximately 50% to 70% of patients catheterized in the acute phase of myocardial infarction are candidates for PTCA.[61-63]

Furthermore, the growing evidence in the area of thrombolysis in AMI supports the concept of an open artery as the best predictor of long-term patient benefit. Figure 116-4 demonstrates that TIMI flow grade 3 at 90-minute angiography is an excellent predictor of 30-day mortality. Several randomized trials have shown superior TIMI grade 3 flow reperfusion rates (>90%), and a higher likelihood of sustaining this level of flow with direct angioplasty compared to the most effective thrombolytic regimen in GUSTO (approximately 54%).[19,63-66] It is therefore not surprising that primary PTCA has become an attractive option. It also allows visual assessment of the patient's coronary anatomy early in the course of the infarction, thereby facilitating decision making.

Percutaneous transluminal coronary angioplasty can be performed as a primary or adjuvant therapy to thrombolysis. The various PTCA modalities available consist of primary, immediate, rescue, delayed, and elective PTCA. Primary PTCA is defined by angioplasty performed as the primary therapy in patients with AMI. Immediate and delayed PTCA represent angioplasty performed either 2 hours or 18 to 48 hours, respectively, after thrombolytic therapy, irrespective of the clinical response to thrombolysis. Rescue PTCA is generally defined as angioplasty performed in a patient who failed thrombolytic therapy, remains clinically symptomatic, and may still benefit from urgent salvage mechanical reperfusion. Elective PTCA is defined as angioplasty performed

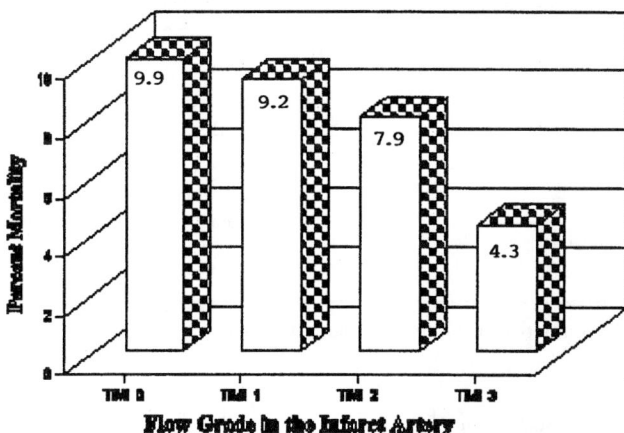

FIGURE 116-4. The relationship between the mortality rate according to TIMI flow grade at 90-minute angiography in the GUSTO trial. Data are taken according to flow grade regardless of the thrombolytic agent used. (TIMI grade 0, no perfusion, no flow beyond the occlusion; TIMI grade 1, flow penetrates beyond the area of obstruction but fails to opacify the entire coronary artery bed distal to the obstruction; TIMI grade 2, flow penetrates beyond the area of obstruction and opacifies with delay the entire coronary artery; TIMI-3, flow beyond the area of obstruction and opacification without delay of the entire coronary bed distal to the obstruction.)

only if there is spontaneous recurrence of ischemia after initial successful medical therapy or significant ischemia provoked by predischarge exercise test.

The reported 6 weeks hospital mortality rate for patients who underwent primary, immediate, delayed, or elective PTCA are 3.7%, 7.2%, 3.6%, and 4.8% respectively.[67]

It remains unclear whether thrombolysis or primary angioplasty is superior due to the absence of large trials directly comparing both modalities in AMI.

The limited data available in patients presenting with cardiogenic shock appear to indicate a twofold to threefold increase in survival if treated with primary PTCA.[68]

Currently, only 15% to 20% of the American hospitals taking care of patients with AMI are equipped and staffed to readily supply a 24-hour coverage for emergency angioplasty. There is no need for the routine transfer of all patients after thrombolysis and for routine predischarge catheterization.[69] However, it is advisable for these patients to undergo objective assessment to detect residual myocardial ischemia by the use of exercise testing, with or without thallium imaging. Patients with significantly abnormal noninvasive evaluation should then be investigated invasively.

ROLE OF HEPARIN IN ACUTE MYOCARDIAL INFARCTION ■

SHOULD THE PATIENT BE HEPARINIZED?

The following guidelines should be considered for the use of heparin in AMI:

TABLE 116-3.   Mortality Rate of Three Large-Scale Acute Intravenous Beta-Blocker Trials Compared to Placebo in Acute Myocardial Infarction

TRIAL	NO. PTS.	AGENTS	DOSE	MORTALITY (%)* B-blockers	Placebo	Mortality Reduction
Goteborg[77]	1395	metoprolol	15 mg i.v. + 100 mg po bid	5.7	8.9	36%
MIAMI[75]	5778	metoprolol	15 mg i.v. + 100 mg po bid	4.3	4.9	12%
ISIS-1[79]	16027	atenolol	5–10 mg i.v.	4.6	3.9	15%
Pooled analysis				4.1	4.9	16%

*At 3 months for Goteborg trial, 15 days for MIAMI, and 0–7 days for ISIS-1.

1. Aspirin for all patients, unless allergic
2. Thrombolysis therapy, if clinically indicated
   a. *If rt-PA is used*: initiate heparin simultaneously in a 5000 U bolus followed by an IV infusion of 1000 U/hr
   b. *If streptokinase is used*: initiate within 4 hours of ending lysis therapy heparin 5000 U bolus followed by an IV infusion of 1000 U/hr (note that the use of IV heparin with streptokinase is controversial; I use it in most cases)
3. If thrombolysis therapy is not utilized: initiate heparin in a 5000 U bolus followed by an intravenous infusion of 1000 U/hr as soon as possible.

If the patient has an uncomplicated course, heparin can be discontinued within the next four to five days.

The role of intravenous heparin is to improve infarct-artery patency. There is a discrepancy between the potential benefits of heparin depending on the type of thrombolytic agent utilized. Presently we believe that the combination of rt-PA with heparin is beneficial in reducing the incidence of reocclusion and recurrent myocardial ischemia.[70] Similar benefit of heparin with streptokinase or APSAC is suggested but not as firmly established.[12,17,18,33,71] Therefore, the use of IV heparin with streptokinase or APSAC should be determined on an individual basis.

Adequate anticoagulation is influenced by the dose and the method of administration of heparin. It seems that adjuvant intravenous heparin is most beneficial when the degree of prolongation of activated partial thromboplastin time (aPTT) values are >1.5 times control and inversely correlates with the incidence of reocclusion. Subcutaneous heparin (12,500 U every 12 hours) has previously been shown to produce inadequate anticoagulation during the first 24 hours of administration and therefore should not be avoided.[72]

ROLE OF INTRAVENOUS β-ADRENERGIC BLOCKING AGENTS   ■

SHOULD THE PATIENT RECEIVE A β-ADRENERGIC BLOCKING AGENT?

Yes, you should use a beta-blocker in the absence of contraindications. Exclusion criteria are:

1. Heart rate <65 beats/minute
2. Second- or third-degree AV block
3. Congestive heart failure (Killip class III or shock)
4. Systolic pressure <105 mm Hg
5. History of asthma or significant chronic obstructive lung disease
6. History of allergy to a beta-blocker
7. More than 6 hours from onset of AMI and absence of chest pain.

To optimize the benefits I recommend that you initiate therapy intravenously and as early as possible. Familiarize yourself with two of the various beta-blockers to be at ease with their clinical effects and side effects:

1. Propanolol IV 1 mg/minute to a total dose of 7 to 10 mg or until you achieve a heart rate of 65 to 70 beats/minute. You should also immediately initiate a beta-blocker orally such as metoprolol, 25 to 75 mg b.i.d., or Atenolol, 25 to 50 mg daily, or
2. Metoprolol 5 mg IV over 5 minutes (1 mg/min). Repeat every 5 minutes to a total dose of 15 mg or until you achieve a heart rate which remains above 65 to 70 beats/minute, followed immediately by a beta-blocker orally, or
3. Atenolol 5 mg IV over 5 minutes (1 mg/min). Repeat once 10 minutes later to a total dose of 10 mg or until you achieve a heart rate which remains above 65 to 70 beats/minute, followed immediately by a beta-blocker orally.

Large trials involving more than 30,000 patients have shown that intravenous beta-blockers in the early hours of AMI provide various benefits. Beta-blockers may help relieve the chest pains as well as reduce infarct size, the recurrence of post-infarction angina, reinfarction, ventricular arrhythmias, myocardial rupture, myocardial remodeling, and mortality (Table 116-3).[73–77]

Those patients more likely to benefit from intravenous and oral beta-blockade are those with anterior wall infarction, large MI, persistence of chest pain presenting very early in the course of AMI (<6 hours), or a previous myocardial infarction.[78] The additive mortality benefit of acute intravenous beta-blockers over oral therapy is probably modest and is best characterized by the ISIS-1 study. The benefit of early intravenous beta-blockade occurs within the first 24 hours after AMI and appears mainly related to the reduction of early cardiac rupture.[79]

All of these trials have been done with populations not receiving early thrombolytic therapy or angioplasty. A subgroup of patients in the Thrombolysis In acute Myocardial Infarction (TIMI-1) study were also assigned to receive intravenous beta-blockers and showed a reduction of myocardial ischemic events.[44] Beta-blockade therapy may be a particularly useful adjunctive therapy in the setting of thrombolytic therapy because intravenous streptokinase has shown an early paradoxic increase in death, partly due to cardiac rupture, on the first day of hospitalization.[12,45]

Whether mortality reduction is related to antiarrhythmic effects, anti-ischemic effects, or a reduction in myocardial rupture remains unclear. In view of its pharmacologic profile, beta-blockers likely reduce clinical events by all three mechanisms. They reduce oxygen demand which, in turn, lessens ischemia and protects against electrical instability. The fall in heart rate and decrease in contractility may reduce myocardial wall tension and may protect against myocardial expansion and rupture.

Before hospital discharge, oral beta-blockers should be considered for a period of 1 to 2 years, particularly in patients at intermediate or high risk for recurrent events.

ROLE OF INTRAVENOUS NITROGLYCERIN ■

WOULD THE PATIENT BENEFIT FROM INTRAVENOUS NITROGLYCERIN?

A significant proportion of patients appear to benefit from IV nitroglycerin. Therefore, unless there are contraindications to its administration (such as systolic pressure <100 mm Hg or cardiogenic shock), I recommend that you initiate intravenous nitroglycerin for a period of 24 to 72 hours in the following conditions:

1. Evidence of ST segment elevation (transmural infarction) or extensive ST segment depression
2. Persistent chest pain or associated dyspnea
3. Associated congestive heart failure (Killip II or III)
4. Early presentation of AMI (<6 hours from onset of symptoms)
5. Contraindications to thrombolysis
6. Systolic blood pressure above 180 mm Hg despite medical therapy.

How should you administer nitroglycerin?

1. Mix nitroglycerin 50 mg in dextrose 5% 250 cm³
2. Monitor blood pressure and clinical response closely
3. Initiate nitroglycerin infusion at 3 cm³/hr (10 μg/min)
4. Increase the infusion by 3 to 6 cm³/hr (10 to 20 μg increments) every 5 to 10 minutes
5. Titrate the infusion to:
   a. decrease the mean blood pressure by 10% for normotensive patients or by 30% for hypertensive patients (BP>140/90)

b. maintain systolic blood pressure >100 mm Hg
   c. obtain symptomatic relief
6. Caution with in inferior wall or right ventricular infarction.

These patients are more sensitive to nitroglycerin and may develop severe hypotension. If hypotension develops, stop the IV nitroglycerin infusion, transfer the patient in Trendelenburg position, and, if there is no rapid response, give rapid crystalloid IV infusion (i.e. 250–750 cm³ of 0.9 % NaCl solution).

Intravenous nitrates improve myocardial ischemia primarily by affecting preload and afterload, which can reduce oxygen requirements, myocardial wall stress, and expansion of the infarcted region, resulting in a long-term improvement in clinical outcome.[80–82] Nitrates also improve blood flow by increasing the collateral flow and dilating the stenosed coronary arteries.[83,84]

Ten randomized trials evaluated intravenous nitroglycerin or nitroprusside in AMI. Although three of them showed a reduction in mortality, the trials taken individually are too small to provide convincing evidence of improved survival. Yusuf and associates[85] evaluated these trials collectively to obtain more reliable data on mortality. The overall mortality from intravenous nitrate treatment was reduced by 35%, compared with control therapy: 13.3% and 18.9%, respectively (p<0.001). However, these results were obtained prior to the thrombolytic era.

Although the rationale for the use of intravenous nitrates remains, it is unknown if they are as effective in reducing mortality in patients receiving thrombolytic therapy. I currently recommend continued use of intravenous nitroglycerin for a period of 24 to 72 hours in patients with the criteria mentioned earlier.

ROLE OF CALCIUM CHANNEL BLOCKERS ■

SHOULD THE PATIENT RECEIVE CALCIUM CHANNEL BLOCKERS?

In most patients calcium-blockers will not be necessary. However we may consider using calcium-blockers in the following conditions:

1. Poor, or absence of, clinical response to nitrates and beta-blockers
2. Side effects or contraindications to beta-blockers

Although clinical trials have been performed with nifedipine, verapamil, and diltiazem, only the Diltiazem Reinfarction Study showed a reduction in nonfatal reinfarction. However, there was no effect on mortality during evolving infarction at 14 days.[86]

A recent review from Helad,[87] which includes 23 randomized trials using calcium channel blockers in AMI, allows us to evaluate the benefits of this class of medication. These data show a nonsignificant decrease in mortality in the calcium blocker-treated group in short- and long-term studies, compared with the placebo group. There was no detectable difference between the various calcium channel blockers used, although verapamil and diltiazem appear to be the calcium-blockers with the greatest confidence after myocardial infarction in patients who have never had overt evidence of heart failure.

Although the benefits from calcium channel blockers during the very early phase of AMI have not yet being demonstrated, we may use these agents appropriately in the management of postinfarction angina in patients not responding to nitrates or beta-blockers.

LIDOCAINE ■

SHOULD THE PATIENTS RECEIVE LIDOCAINE?

Most patients will not require lidocaine. You should consider using intravenous lidocaine in patients with suspected AMI or ischemia in the following settings:

1. Associated ventricular premature beats that are frequent (>6/min), closely coupled (R on T phenomenon), multiform in configuration, or occurring in short bursts of three or more in succession
2. Patients with ventricular tachycardia or ventricular fibrillation who require defibrillation or cardiopulmonary resuscitation
3. Prophylactic lidocaine to patients 70-years-old or younger with uncomplicated AMI or ischemia, without ventricular premature beats, and within the first 6 hours of the onset of symptoms, particularly if not yet continuously monitored in a coronary care unit.

The conventional dosages of intravenous lidocaine are as follow:

1. Initiate lidocaine with a bolus of 1 mg/kg (not to exceed 100 mg), to be given at a rate of approximately 20 to 50 mg/min, followed by a second intravenous bolus of 0.5 mg/kg 10 to 15 minutes later
2. Then continue with a maintenance infusion rate of 1 to 4 mg/kg.

Based on the pharmacokinetics of lidocaine, it is usually recommended that a second bolus be administered to prevent transient subtherapeutic plasma concentrations that otherwise tend to occur 30 to 120 minutes after the initial bolus.[88] The maintenance infusion usually provides steady-state plasma levels between 1 and 5 μg/mL. However, in patients with heart failure or shock it is usually safer to administer a lower maintenance rate (i.e. 1 to 2 mg/kg). This avoids toxic levels that may be created due to reduced hepatic blood flow and metabolism.[89]

The incidence of bradyarrhythmia and ventricular arrhythmia is high during the first hour of AMI.[90] Approximately 60% of patients with AMI die within 1 to 2 hours of the onset of symptoms.[91] Most of these deaths are sudden and a significant proportion of them are secondary to malignant arrhythmias, such as ventricular fibrillation.[92]

To reduce early mortality, physicians often treat prophylactically with an antiarrhythmic agent (e.g., lidocaine) to prevent complex ventricular ectopy. At least 14 randomized trials consisting of 9,155 patients have assessed the potential benefit of this practice.[93] Analyzed individually, most did not show significant benefit from prophylactic treatment, although the lack of statistical significance may be related to the small number of subjects in each study. However, a meta-analysis from these trials indicate a 35% reduction in the incidence of ventricular fibrillation, with borderline statistical significance (p< 0.04) and without a significant reduction of overall mortality, and indicated a trend toward an increased incidence of asystole.[93] The role of prophylactic lidocaine during the first 12 to 24 hours remains a controversial issue, but we believe that there is a subgroup of patients for whom lidocaine prophylaxis should be considered.

The role of prophylactic intravenous infusions of lidocaine remains controversial and should be limited to less than 24 hours. Prophylactic lidocaine should be particularly considered in small community hospitals without 24-hour in-house staff physician coverage. The administration of intramuscular lidocaine should be avoided in the evolving era of early intervention and the increasing use of intravenous heparin and thrombolytic agents.

The most commonly reported adverse effects occur in 7% to 39% of patients, are dose-related, and involve primarily the central nervous system (e.g., drowsiness, confusion, seizures, dizziness, paresthesias).[94] Cardiovascular effects, such as bradycardia, asystole, and hypotension, are also observed. Although the incidence of asystole is low (0.6% of patients in the treatment group versus 0.3% in the control group), it is still of some concern. Close clinical observation is advisable to detect them promptly.

ANGIOTENSINE-CONVERTING ENZYME INHIBITORS (ACE-I) ■

SHOULD THE PATIENT RECEIVE ANGIOTENSINE-CONVERTING ENZYME INHIBITORS?

The literature has shown a favorable role of oral ACE-i early in AMI which appears in the presence and in the absence of beta-blockers and thrombolytic therapy.[95-98] It appears reasonable to administer an oral ACE-i to patients at high risk of death during the early phase post-infarction. ACE-i therapy in the appropriate patient should be started within a few days but not necessary immediately after hospital admission. The subgroups more likely to benefit are patients, hemodynamically stable, with:

1. Clinical evidence of heart failure (Killip class 2 or 3)
2. Echocardiographic evidence of left ventricular ejection fraction (LVEF) <40 %
3. Anterior wall myocardial infarction
4. Large myocardial infarction
5. History of a previous infarction
6. Tachycardia.

The ACE-i should be administered orally with a proper initiation dose and stepwise titration in a monitored setting due to the potential precipitation of symptomatic hypotension. Intravenous ACE-i seems unnecessary and possibly harmful. Once started, the therapy should be continued indefinitely, unless the LVEF after the first year is >40 % and the patient is asymptomatic or in the presence of undesirable side effects. A multitude of agents are now introduced on the market. I have only included four of the most commonly used ACE-i proven to be effective in AMI at the present time. The recommended ascending dosage is usually as follows:

1. Captopril: initiate at 6.25 mg orally. If the patient remains hemodynamically stable over the next 6 to 8 hours you could increase the dosage to 12.5 mg, 18.75 mg, and then 25 mg every 6 hours, or
2. Lisinopril: initiate at 2.5 mg orally. If well-tolerated, titrate daily to 5.0 mg, 7.5 mg, and then 10.0 mg, or
3. Enalapril: initiate at 2.5 mg orally. If well-tolerated, titrate every 12 hours to 5.0 mg, 7.5mg, and then 10.0 mg b.i.d., or
4. Ramipril: initiate at 2.5 mg orally. If well-tolerated, titrate every 12 hours to 5.0 mg b.i.d. if hemodynamically tolerated. In the elderly, consider initiating at 1.25 mg.

Remember, if the patient does not tolerate a particular dosage it is recommended that the next dosage be modified to a lower concentration, which was previously tolerated. Furthermore, it is advisable to be more conservative in the dosage of the elderly or patients with carotid disease or history of previous cerebrovascular disease, such that a higher systolic blood pressure cutpoint be used in order to avoid "relative" hypotension. You should aim to lower the mean systolic blood pressure by approximately 10% in normotensive patients and 30% in hypertensive patients.

Various studies have shown echocardiographically that ACE-i attenuate infarct expansion and remodeling. Once started, ACE-i should be continued indefinitely in patients with heart failure or left ventricular dysfunction (LVEF<40%), unless there are undesirable side effects. Avoid immediate intravenous administration of an ACE-i since it carries a non-negligeable risk for hypotension.

HEART FAILURE AND CARDIOGENIC SHOCK ▪

It is not surprising that myocardial ischemia severe enough to cause muscle necrosis can create hemodynamic alterations that precipitate heart failure and cardiogenic shock, with subsequent high mortality. Clinical heart failure in this setting can be caused by a variety of events, and it is important to understand the pathophysiologic processes associated with left ventricular dysfunction in patients with AMI.

You must remember that the mortality related to cardiogenic shock from a mechanical cause is very high. These patients merit a very rapid and aggressive approach which may include mechanical ventilation, coronary angiography, PTCA, intra-aortic balloon pump, or emergency cardiac surgery. The limited data available in patients presenting with cardiogenic shock appear to indicate a two- to threefold increase in survival if treated with primary PTCA.[68]

TABLE 116-4. Causes of Heart Failure During Acute Myocardial Infarction

---

Massive muscle necrosis
Severe muscle ischemia with dysfunction ("stunning")
Ventricular free wall rupture
Acute mitral regurgitation
   Papillary muscle dysfunction from ischemia
   Papillary muscle rupture from necrosis
Formation of ventricular septal defect
Pericardial effusion with cardiac tamponade
Right ventricular involvement in infarction
Unstable rhythms (i.e. sustained ventricular tachycardia, rapid atrial fibrillation)

DIFFERENTIATION FROM CHRONIC HEART FAILURE ▪

The development of acute heart failure is quite different from chronic heart failure unaccompanied by sudden ischemic events. If left ventricular dysfunction develops gradually, there is a progressive ventricular dilation that allows time for better hemodynamic compensation of the left ventricular wall stress. Heart failure during infarction is accompanied by an increase in end-systolic and end-diastolic left ventricular volumes. The ventricular diastolic pressure tends to develop more rapidly than in chronic heart failure. These changes increase left ventricular wall stress and worsen ischemia, precipitating a downward spiral of events that may lead to worse left ventricular dysfunction, severe pulmonary edema, and shock.

Table 116-4 lists the common etiologies of congestive heart failure associated with AMI. Generally, these difficulties develop because of ischemic injury to the ventricles.

MECHANICAL COMPLICATIONS ▪

In addition to extensive muscle necrosis, lack of structural integrity may also cause acute heart failure. Papillary muscle dysfunction or rupture due to ischemia or necrosis can cause acute mitral regurgitation. This can produce heart failure of varying severity evolving to sudden pulmonary edema, subsequent shock, and death.[99] The murmur accompanying papillary muscle rupture or dysfunction varies in relation to duration of systole, and its radiation depends on the leaflet involved and the extent of regurgitation. If the patient has profound pulmonary edema and is in cardiogenic shock, a new systolic murmur may not be appreciated. If this complication is suspected, an immediate bedside echocardiography is very useful to establish rapidly the correct diagnosis. If echocardiography is unavailable, a pulmonary artery catheter can be inserted. The pulmonary artery occlusion pressure (PAOP) tracing may show an increased V wave, which is a nonspecific finding seen in conditions leading to a noncompliant, infarcted ventricle. An elevated wedge pressure with pulmonary hypertension and a large V wave with a new systolic murmur and low forward output strongly suggest papillary muscle dysfunction or an acute ventricular septal defect. Echocardiography can be helpful by demonstrating flailing motion of the mitral leaflet during systole, and Doppler echocardiographic techniques can diagnose and quantify regurgitation into the left atrium.

Rupture of the ventricular septum also may cause severe heart failure and shock. These ventricular communications most frequently occur at the junction of the septum and the anterior or posterior left ventricular free wall, where collateral blood flow is sometimes attenuated. This explains why septal rupture occurs most often in patients experiencing their first transmural myocardial infarction. These patients generally have less collateral blood flow than those who have had prior infarcts.[100] Like papillary muscle rupture or severe papillary muscle dysfunction, rupture of the interventricular septum produces dramatic clinical deterioration, characterized by new systolic murmur, heart failure, and cardiogenic shock. Right heart failure becomes apparent early, with subsequent pulmonary edema. The quality of the murmur varies, with or without a systolic thrill, and is clinically indistinguishable from acute papillary muscle rupture or dysfunction.[101] This condition must be differentiated from acute mitral regurgitation by echocardiography or right heart catheterization; an inappropriate increase in oxygen saturation is observed when passing the catheter from the right atrium through the right ventricle to the pulmonary artery.

Ventricular free wall rupture during myocardial infarction generally occurs several days after the acute event, is more common in women, and is seen in patients with extensive anterior or inferoposterior wall infarcts. Hemodynamic deterioration usually occurs suddenly but may present progressively. Blood leaks into the pericardial space, and cardiac tamponade can rapidly occur. We have seen a few cases of subacute ventricular wall rupture within the first 24 hours of AMI. Mesa and associates[102] demonstrated impressive short- and long-term survival in patients undergoing emergency surgical repair for subacute ventricular wall rupture. A fibrinous exudate sometimes forms over the defect and blood clots (i.e., pseudoaneurysm formation) without subsequent tamponade. Two-dimensional echocardiography is helpful in making a correct diagnosis.[103]

Pericardial effusion and cardiac tamponade can be seen independently of cardiac rupture in patients with AMI. When an infarct extends to the pericardial surface, it may produce pericarditis. Significant effusions sometimes occur several days after infarction, with the peak incidence at 1 week. If a large effusion develops, hemodynamic compromise may ensue. Effusions are usually small, and the pericarditis is associated with transient, but at times severe, chest pain, atelectasis, and electrocardiographic changes. Therapy consists of aspirin, indomethacin, or oral corticosteroids.

RIGHT VENTRICULAR INFARCTION DIAGNOSIS AND THERAPY

The diagnosis of significant right ventricular involvement carries important implications. An acute inferior or inferoposterior wall myocardial infarction, elevated neck veins with systemic hypotension, and clear lung fields suggest right ventricular infarction. Although the incidence of right ventricular infarction assessed by noninvasive methods is high (30–60%), full clinical expression of the syndrome is less frequent.[104,105]

The classical hemodynamic findings of right ventricular infarction include a normal pulmonary artery pressure with low left ventricular filling pressure, low cardiac output, and elevated right ventricular end-diastolic and right atrial pressures. Although acute and chronic cor pulmonale or pericardial disease can produce a similar clinical picture, the hemodynamic abnormalities of right ventricular infarction are improved with rapid volume expansion. Inotropic agents may be required if hypoperfusion due to hypotension persists despite adequate restoration of left ventricular filling pressure; this suggests concomitant left ventricular dysfunction.[106] Hemodynamically significant bradyarrhythmias may necessitate dual-chamber temporary pacing. Echocardiography and radionuclide blood pool scans are helpful in diagnosing these patients, revealing right ventricular dilation, wall motion abnormalities, and left ventricular dysfunction.

If hypotension can be corrected, the prognosis in right ventricular infarction is good because the left ventricle often has adequately preserved function. The prognosis worsens with concomitant left ventricular dysfunction.

CARDIOGENIC SHOCK

The clinical syndrome of cardiogenic shock is characterized by decreased mentation, peripheral signs of hypoperfusion and high adrenergic tone (i.e., sweating, vasoconstriction), oliguria, hypotension, and tachycardia. Hemodynamic evaluation demonstrates a depressed cardiac index and high pulmonary artery pressures. Patients without mechanical complications, such as papillary muscle dysfunction or rupture, free wall cardiac rupture, or ventricular septal defect formation, usually have extensive infarction involving more than 40% of the left ventricle. The mechanical complications may be improved with surgical intervention. Alternatively, the patient can be stabilized with intravenous vasodilator or inotropic infusions; intra-aortic balloon counterpulsation may also be considered. Invasive hemodynamic monitoring is mandatory for pharmacotherapeutic intervention and titration before decisions are made about definitive surgical therapy.

CLINICAL GUIDELINES FOR HEMODYNAMIC MONITORING

It is important to accurately assess the severity of left ventricular dysfunction because maneuvers performed in the coronary care unit may worsen this state. More than half of the patients with a moderate reduction in resting cardiac output and an increase in left ventricular filling pressure have no clinical signs of left ventricular dysfunction. Clinical evaluation frequently does not identify patients with low cardiac output who have normal chest radiographs and physical examinations. However, correlation of the chest radiograph

TABLE 116-5. Circumstances Prompting
Hemodynamic Monitoring

Sustained hypotension (systolic blood pressure <90 mm Hg)
Persistent, unexplained resting tachycardia (4 hours of heart rate
> 100 beats/minute)
Anuria/oliguria > 12 hours
Metabolic acidosis
Inappropriate agitation, confusion, coma
Unexplained hypoxemia (room air (Pa_{O2} < 70 mm Hg)
Shock
Severe pulmonary disease if the contribution of congestive heart
failure to the degree of dyspnea is unclear

---

and clinical evaluation with hemodynamic measurements has demonstrated that the presence of cardiomegaly, gallop rhythms, and pulmonary edema may help predict which patients with myocardial infarction will develop shock.[107,108]

There is an unfortunate tendency to institute potent therapeutic measures in patients with myocardial infarction before precise hemodynamic indices are known. Intravenous furosemide, for example, may create a decline in PAOP without compromising the cardiac output if ventricular filling pressures are elevated and there is pulmonary congestion. However, if the clinical diagnosis of heart failure is incorrect and the PAOP is normal, diuretic therapy may actually decrease the cardiac output and cause deterioration of an already compromised myocardial flow reserve. This can be particularly detrimental in patients who present with right ventricular infarction.

The clinical situations outlined in Table 116-5 are potential indications for invasive hemodynamic monitoring because physical examination may not correlate well with the extent of left ventricular dysfunction. Table 116-6 summarizes the formulae used to calculate hemodynamic information after right heart catheterization and lists normative data used to guide therapeutic interventions.

RECOMMENDED APPROACH TO CONGESTIVE HEART FAILURE ■

In patients with shock and heart failure in the face of AMI, it is important to restore adequate tissue perfusion as quickly as possible by optimizing left ventricular performance. One should always consider the possibility of correctable mechanical abnormalities. Complementary goals include maintenance of adequate oxygenation, correction of acid-base abnormalities, and optimization of cardiac filling pressure, outflow impedance, and contractility. The general measures to consider are:

1. Maintain adequate oxygenation: this may require facial O_2 support or intubation and mechanical ventilation. It is extremely important to ensure adequate oxygenation rapidly.
2. Correct acid-base abnormalities: hyperventilation may be required to compensate for a metabolic acidosis due to a low output state.
3. Aspirin which reduces mortality and reinfarction in AMI should be given routinely.

TABLE 116-6. Relevant Hemodynamic Variables

HEMODYNAMIC PARAMETERS	NAME/FORMULA	UNITS	NORMAL VALUE	PREFERRED VALUE
MEASURED PARAMETERS				
HR	Heart rate	Beats/min	60–100	<99
BP	Blood pressure	mm Hg	120/80	mean, <80
CVP	Central venous pressure	mm Hg	1–6	>3
PAP	Pulmonary artery pressure	mm Hg	25/10	mean, <18
PAOP	Pulmonary artery occlusion pressure	mm Hg	6/12	>6; <15
CO	Cardiac output	L/min	4–6	>5.0
DERIVED PARAMETERS				
CI	Cardiac index = CO/body surface area	L/min/m²	2.6–4.2	>3.0
SVI	Stroke volume index = (CI)(1000)/HR	ml/beat/m²	33–47	>35
PVRI	Pulmonary vascular resistance index = 80 (PAP mean–PAOP mean)	dynes-sec-cm5/m2	45–225	<226
VSWI	Right ventricular stroke work index = (SVI)(PAP mean)(.0144)	(g)(m)/(beat)(m2)	4–8	
RCWI	Right cardiac work index = (CI)(PAP mean)(.0144)	(kg)(mg)/m²	0.4–0.6	
SVRI	Systemic vascular resistance index = 80 (PAP mean − CVP)/CI	dynes-sec-cm5/m2	1700–2750	<2500
LVSWI	Left ventricular stroke work index = (SVI)(BPM)(.0144)	(g)(m)(beat)	44–68	>55
LCWI	Left cardiac work index = (CI)(BP mean)(.0144)	(kg)(m)/m²	3–5	>5

4. Adequate intravenous heparinization to reduce the risk of left ventricular thrombus, deep vein thrombosis, and coronary artery thrombus formation and propagation in low flow state.
5. Hemodynamic monitoring with a pulmonary artery catheter in severe cases, mainly to determine the cardiac index, pulmonary artery pressure, PAOP, and systemic vascular resistance and to determine the response to therapy.
6. Reduce left ventricular afterload: nitroprusside IV may be useful in patients with low cardiac index ($<$ 2.0–2.5 L/min/m^2), high PAOP, and high systemic vascular resistance.
7. Reduce myocardial ischemia: nitroglycerin IV may be helpful if there is suspicion of ongoing ischemia, mitral regurgitation, or elevated PAOP.
8. Inotropic support with dobutamine to maintain a cardiac index above 2.0 L/min/m^2.
9. Vasopressors to reverse hypotension such as norepinephrine.
10. Diuretics such as furosemide. It is critical to determine right and left ventricular filling pressure before administering diuretic therapy to avoid hypotensive episodes.
11. Low left ventricular filling pressure (low PAOP): left and right ventricular pressure may be adjusted to an optimal level by volume expansion with saline solution, albumin, dextran, or if appropriate, blood infusion. This is particularly important in patients with right ventricular infarction.

When left ventricular pump function is altered, stroke volume and cardiac output can be increased, improving distal tissue perfusion, by reducing impedance to ejection. This can be accomplished with intravenous or oral vasodilator drugs, particularly those with afterload-reducing effects, such as nitroprusside and nitroglycerin.[109] Sodium nitroprusside can be titrated in increasing doses (20–400 μg/min) while observing arterial pressure, pulmonary capillary wedge pressure, and signs of peripheral perfusion. With similar monitoring, nitroglycerin may be given in doses ranging from 5 to 200 μg/min. Both nitroprusside and nitroglycerin have profound venodilatory effects and may significantly lower preload.

In severely hypotensive patients, vasopressors that increase systemic vascular resistance (i.e., phenylephrine, high-dose dopamine, norepinephrine) may be required. Restoration of arterial pressure may improve hemodynamics and increase cardiac output. However, these drugs also constrict the renal and splanchnic vascular beds, and prolonged infusion is ultimately detrimental.

Predominantly inotropic agents, such as dopamine, may raise arterial pressure in hypotensive individuals. However, inotropic agents augment myocardial oxygen consumption and therefore should be used cautiously in cases of ischemic heart disease. Agents that exert a positive inotropic effect on the cardiovascular system include phenylephrine, epinephrine, and high doses of dopamine. Inotropic agents that have a net vasodilatory effect on the periphery and that may decrease systemic pressure despite positive inotropy include

isoproterenol, dobutamine, and low-dose dopamine. Amrinone is a phosphodiesterase inhibitor that has positive inotropic and peripheral vasodilatory properties and produces a response similar to that seen with dobutamine infusion. Combinations of inotropic and vasodilator drugs may be beneficial. Combined therapy with dobutamine or dopamine plus nitroprusside or nitroglycerin frequently provide optimal hemodynamics, with the greatest augmentation of left ventricular function. Digitalis have minimal inotropic effect in AMI and may increase systemic vascular resistance.[110] Patients with acute infarcts do not benefit from these agents unless they are used to control the ventricular response in atrial fibrillation or convert atrial dysrhythmias to more stable rhythms.

NONINVASIVE IMAGING TECHNIQUES ◼

THALLIUM-201 SCINTIGRAPHY

The myocardial uptake of thallium-201(^{201}Tl) depends upon coronary blood flow and normal myocardial cell function. Thallium defects are therefore seen with acute necrosis, myocardial ischemia, or scar. Thallium-201 scintigraphy is highly sensitive in detecting the presence of myocardial infarction, with 83% of patients showing defects during acute imaging.[111] With early imaging ($<$6 hours), biochemically small and non-Q wave myocardial infarcts demonstrate perfusion defects. Sensitivity diminishes if imaging is performed more than 24 hours after the onset of anginal symptoms.

The extent of ^{201}Tl perfusion defects has prognostic importance. Becker and associates[112] prospectively studied 91 patients with suspected myocardial infarction (Killip class I or II) using ^{201}Tl scintigraphy and radionuclide ventriculography sequentially within 15 hours of chest pain. A thallium defect involving 40% or more of the ventricle or an ejection fraction of less than 35% identified high-risk patients with mortality rates of 64% and 60%, respectively, at 6 months. Conversely, if the thallium defect was less than 40% or the ejection fraction greater than 35%, 6-month mortality rates were only 8% and 11%, respectively.

Thallium-201 single-photon emission computed tomography (SPECT) allows visualization of the heart from a three-dimensional perspective, unlike conventional two-dimensional planar imaging. Multiple transaxial 6-mm-thick tomographic slices can be seen in three separate planes perpendicular and parallel to the long axis of the heart, permitting quantification of the left ventricular volume. Quantification of infarct size with ^{201}Tl SPECT may complement (if not supplant) radionuclide ventriculography as the most important prognostic tool for evaluating patients during myocardial infarction.[113]

TECHNETIUM 99M ISONITRILES

Technetium 99m (^{99m}Tc) isonitrils are radionuclide agents used for the detection of myocardial perfusion defects at rest.[114] These agents accumulate proportionally to the myocardial distribution of coronary blood flow. Unlike ^{201}Tl, these agents do not redistribute and require separate injections of the radionuclide during ischemia and rest to differentiate between reversible and irreversible myocardial injury. ^{99m}Tc isonitrils have a relatively slow myocardial clearance, thereby favoring SPECT image acquisition. The imaging, which can be obtained several hours later, reflects the myocardial perfusion status during each injection.

The images allow assessment of the amount of myocardium at risk during AMI and evaluate the patency rate obtained spontaneously, after thrombolytic therapy, or after angioplasty. A study evaluated the efficacy of ^{99m}Tc isonitril in 30 patients with first AMI, of which 23 patients had received t-PA within 4 hours of the onset of symptoms.[115] ^{99m}Tc isonitril was injected before thrombolytic therapy, and data acquisition was performed hours later with repeat imaging at 18 to 48 hours and at 6 to 14 days after the AMI. The patients who demonstrated a patent infarct-related artery had more than 30% reduction in defect size using SPECT imaging, compared with patients with persistent occlusion. This new noninvasive technique for assessing myocardium at risk during AMI is promising.

GATED RADIONUCLIDE ANGIOGRAPHY

Gated radionuclide angiography is useful for assessing regional and global left ventricular function by a convenient and accurate count-based method. Given the prognostic importance of left ventricular function and the poor correlation between clinical signs and LVEF, radionuclide angiography provides a reliable, noninvasive way of assessing global function.[116,117]

Patients with anterior myocardial infarction have a lower global LVEF than those with inferior infarction and more marked regional wall motion abnormalities.[116,118] Gated radionuclide angiography can play an important role in establishing concomitant right ventricular infarction in patients with acute inferior myocardial infarction.[105]

A normal LVEF in the postinfarction patient generally predicts a good clinical outcome; many patients with compromised left ventricular function (ejection fraction <40%) develop future complications or die.[112,117,118]

TECHNETIUM 99M SCANNING

Technetium 99m pyrophosphate (^{99m}Tc-PYP) is a radiopharmaceutical that labels acutely necrotic myocardium. It is particularly helpful in diagnosing myocardial infarction in patients who present 24 hours after the onset of symptoms when creatine kinase myocardial muscle (MB) isoenzymes may no longer be elevated. Clinical reinfarction can also be confirmed through serial scanning. Scintigraphy is ideally performed within 24 to 72 hours of suspected infarction in the absence of thrombolytic therapy, but may become negative within 2 to 3 days if thrombolytic therapy was used and reperfusion achieved.[119]

The intensity and pattern of myocardial tracer uptake serve as prognostic indicators. Holman and colleagues[120] reported that in patients with suspected myocardial infarction and a normal ^{99m}Tc-PYP scan, the 6-month complication rate was negligible, with no mortality. Likewise, no complications were observed in postinfarction patients who had small scin-

tigraphic uptake (<16 cm^2), but morbidity and mortality rose sharply as the extent and intensity of myocardial uptake increased. Patients with massive uptake (>40 cm^2) had an 88% in-hospital complication rate, with only 37% surviving into the late follow-up period.

The doughnut scintigraphic pattern predicts a poor clinical outcome and is exemplified by intense tracer uptake in the peripheral area of infarction, with less central uptake. This is probably due to severely diminished blood flow to the central zone of infarction, with minimal or no myocardial calcium deposition. In one retrospective study, 67% of patients demonstrating the doughnut pattern developed left ventricular failure with infarction.[121] In infarct patients followed prospectively after hospital discharge, 100% of those with the doughnut pattern suffered complications, compared with 43% and 12% of patients with focal and diffuse tracer uptake, respectively.[122] Mortality was 83% with the doughnut pattern but minimal for the focal or diffuse patterns (6% and 0%, respectively). Patients who have persistently positive scans after infarction are another high-risk group for the development of congestive heart failure, angina, and ventricular dyssynergy.[123] Despite the prognostic value of ^{99m}Tc-PYP scintigraphy, its practical clinical use remains primarily the confirmation of suspected myocardial infarction when MB-CK isoenzyme and ECG criteria are lacking.

ECHOCARDIOGRAPHY

Two-dimensional echocardiographic evaluation provides information about systolic left ventricular performance, regional wall motion abnormalities, cardiac chamber size, pericardial effusion, concomitant valvular pathology, and complications like flail mitral valve leaflet. Doppler echocardiographic techniques can detect shunts and diagnose the degree of valvular insufficiency. Because echocardiographic systems are portable, relatively easy to use, and do not require radioisotope administration, they are an ideal tool in the intensive care setting. Echocardiography has additional advantages over most radionuclide and angiographic techniques in that it can produce images of the heart from multiple planes, provide clear definition of cardiac valves and papillary muscles, and direct views of regional wall motion and thickening. Echocardiography can be serially repeated with minimal inconvenience for better understanding of the clinical evolution.

Doppler echocardiography allows measurement of blood flow velocity and identifies disturbances of normal flow patterns caused by valvular lesions or intracardiac defects.[124] The clinical use of two-dimensional and pulsed Doppler echocardiography in AMI are listed in Table 116-7.

Two-dimensional echocardiography is a sensitive means of detecting wall motion abnormalities, the development of abnormal endocardial motion, and the loss of thickening in myocardial segments supplied by occluded coronary vessels. The extent of infarct can be determined from a two-dimensional echocardiographic study using wall motion indexes.[125,126]

Like radionuclide angiography, two-dimensional echocardiographic assessment of ejection fraction has long-term

TABLE 116-7.   Clinical Uses of Echocardiography in Acute Myocardial Infarction

TWO-DIMENSIONAL STUDY	PULSED DOPPLER STUDY
Determination of ejection fraction	Detection of septal defect
Detection of wall motion abnormalities	Calculation of shunt quantity
Detection of pericardial effusion	Detection of mitral regurgitation
Detection of right ventricular dysfunction	Calculation of cardiac output
Detection of papillary muscle rupture	
Detection of aneurysm formation	
Detection of mural thrombi	
Determination of clinical prognosis	

prognostic importance. VanReet and associates[127] echocardiographically evaluated patients after AMI. They determined that an ejection fraction above 35% was associated with a hospital mortality rate of 2% and a 1-year mortality rate of 8%; patients with ejection fractions below 35% had a 37% hospital mortality rate and a 56% 1-year mortality rate. The predictive value of echocardiographic determination of ejection fraction appears similar to that provided by radionuclide determination, but the procedure is less expensive, widely available, and can be performed repetitively in the coronary care unit at bedside in many hospitals.

Thrombi can be diagnosed by two-dimensional echocardiography and the incidence is reported to be as high as 32%.[72] Most patients with mural thrombi have ECG evidence of anterior myocardial infarction. It is possible that the incidence of mural thrombus will decrease with thrombolytic therapy.

Echocardiography can also differentiate at the bedside rupture of the ventricular septum after myocardial infarction from acute mitral regurgitation due to papillary muscle rupture or dysfunction in patients becoming rapidly unstable.[128] In these conditions, echocardiography can accelerate medical diagnosis, intervention, and potentially enhance survival.

Formation of a left ventricular aneurysm is a late complication of myocardial infarction and can be detected by echocardiography. Pseudoaneurysm formation with left ventricular free wall rupture and pericardial effusion with involvement can be diagnosed expeditiously.

A limitation of echocardiography in AMI is difficulty in imaging, particularly if the patient is unstable and mechanically ventilated. However, at least one or two views can be obtained for more than 90% of patients. The greatest limitation of echocardiography is the operator's expertise. With experienced operators, this technique can provide a rapid diagnosis, stratify patients into low- or high-risk categories, monitor serial changes, and diagnose complications related to the infarction at the bedside for optimal management.

Q WAVE AND NON-Q WAVE MYOCARDIAL INFARCTIONS ■

APPROPRIATE DIAGNOSIS

The diagnosis of AMI includes the presence of elevated MB-CK. If there is only a single sample, diagnosis must be based on at least a twofold elevation above normal. Patients admitted more than 72 hours after the onset of chest pain should have lactate dehydrogenase isoenzymes analyzed or pyrophosphate scintigraphy, because MB-CK may have normalized.[129]

The clinical relevance of ECG diagnosis of Q wave or non-Q wave infarction remains controversial. Although the development of a Q wave pattern on the ECG is highly specific for AMI (albeit somewhat insensitive), no such reliable ECG criterion has evolved for confirmation of a non-Q wave infarction. The only agreement on the diagnosis of non-Q wave infarction is that changes must be restricted to the ST-T segment without evolution of a Q wave. Because these repolarization changes are nonspecific, the diagnosis of non-Q wave infarction can only be made with the corroboration of positive isoenzyme studies.

PROGNOSIS

Pooled data from 25 short-term studies confirm that Q wave infarction is associated with approximately twice the in-hospital mortality of non-Q wave infarction (19.9% and 10.2%, respectively; p<0.0001).[130] However, the long-term mortality of non-Q wave infarction at 1 to 3 years is similar to or higher than that of Q wave infarcts.[130–132] These results indicate that the early survival advantage of the non-Q wave infarct group is lost over the months after hospital discharge.

Most studies have demonstrated a significantly higher rate of reinfarction among patients with non-Q wave infarction compared with the Q wave group (approximately 15% and 5%, respectively; p<0.001).[130] These observations may explain the loss of initial survival advantage in the non-Q wave group.

Observations from early trials have helped elucidate the pathogenesis of non-Q wave infarction. Several angiographic studies have shown no difference in the number of diseased vessels, the distribution of stenoses, or the amount of myocardium at risk between Q wave and non-Q wave infarctions. However, complete obstruction of the infarct-related artery occurred in fewer patients with non-Q wave infarction.[130,133] Moreover, 30% to 40% of the non-Q wave infarctions demonstrate ST elevation initially and an earlier and lower peak creatine phosphokinase activity. Contraction band necrosis, the hallmark of reperfusion, is a common postmortem observation in patients with non-Q wave infarction. Therefore, non-Q wave infarction appears associated with transient thrombotic occlusion and intermittent increased vasomotor tone, resulting in lysis of the clot and earlier reperfusion than Q wave infarction.

NONINVASIVE PREDISCHARGE ASSESSMENT OF UNCOMPLICATED MYOCARDIAL INFARCTION

Risk stratification of patients convalescing from uncomplicated AMI requires two noninvasive and readily available tests with which the clinician can establish risk, plan for additional testing, and develop rational therapy. For the purpose of this discussion, the uncomplicated patient is defined as ambulatory, free of chest pain, and without overt heart failure during the latter phase of hospitalization. A more aggressive approach is recommended for patients with angina pectoris after AMI and those with decompensated congestive heart failure, for whom early cardiac catheterization with consideration of intervention (e.g., angioplasty, bypass surgery) is indicated.

Two assessments are recommended for uncomplicated patients in whom the tests are feasible. The first is a quantitative evaluation of left ventricular function by radionuclide angiography or two-dimensional echocardiography (day 3–14). The second is a predischarge submaximal exercise testing to detect significant residual clinical or silent ischemia.

The results of these two tests permit the clinician to estimate the risk of future cardiac events and mortality. This approach allows the physician to provide important advice to the patient about return to work and monitored exercise program.

ASSESSMENT OF LEFT VENTRICULAR FUNCTION

Noninvasive quantitative assessment of left ventricular function can be effectively carried out using radionuclide angiography or two-dimensional echocardiography with comparable results of global LVEF.[134] Bigger and colleagues[135] performed radionuclide ventriculograms in 766 patients with AMI before hospital discharge. The 1-year mortality in patients with LVEF<50% was less than 7%, in contrast to patients with LVEF< 30%, who had a mortality greater than 30%.

SUBMAXIMAL EXERCISE TESTING

Submaximal exercise testing for carefully selected patients (i.e., no evidence of clinical congestive heart failure or unstable angina pectoris) can be performed safely after myocardial infarction. Théroux and colleagues[136] exercised 210 selected patients to a modest workload (5 units of basal metabolic oxygen consumption [METS]) without any complications. According to the absence or presence of angina or ST-segment depression, Théroux could stratify patients into two prognostic groups. Approximately two thirds of the patients had a negative exercise test. A positive exercise test identified patients with a 16% incidence of sudden death and a 27% 1-year total cardiac mortality, compared with rates of 0.7% and 2.1%, respectively, for those with a negative test.

Fuller and colleagues[137] showed that coronary angiography in infarct patients with a positive exercise test almost always correlates with multivessel coronary artery disease. Starling and colleagues[138] documented the utility of a 6-week maximal exercise test that identifies additional patients at risk for myocardial infarction in whom predischarge submaximal tests were negative.

Exercise testing at a safe, modest workload before hospital discharge identifies a high-risk group who merit consideration of prophylactic therapy, more aggressive monitoring and follow-up, and early cardiac catheterization.

THALLIUM-201 SCINTIGRAPHY

A review by Kotler and Diamond[139] demonstrated that exercise thallium scintigraphy compares favorably to submaximal exercise testing in uncomplicated myocardial infarction before hospital discharge. Thallium scintigraphy is performed after intravenous injection of 2 to 3 mCi of ^{201}Tl at peak exercise. Redistribution images are taken 3 to 4 hours later. An exercise perfusion defect that resolves indicates ischemia, and lack of tracer redistribution may indicate scarring but does not exclude viable jeopardized myocardium.[140]

Gibson and associates[141,142] showed that predischarge exercise ^{201}Tl scintigraphy was more accurate in detecting multivessel disease and identifying high- and low-risk groups for cardiac events than exercise ST-segment depression alone after uncomplicated AMI. An increase in exercise ^{201}Tl lung uptake also predicts more extensive coronary artery disease, cardiac events, and left ventricular dysfunction.[142,143]

Dilsizian and associates[140] demonstrated that exercise thallium scintigraphy can be imprecise in cases of perfusion defects that are "fixed" on the redistribution images 3 to 4 hours later. These images may falsely indicate nonviable myocardium. They enrolled 100 patients and identified 33% of the exercise-induced defects to be irreversible on the initial redistribution images. However, 49% of these "fixed" defects improved or showed a normal thallium uptake after an injection of thallium at rest. Eighty-seven percent of these lesions subsequently showed normal thallium uptake and improved regional wall motion after coronary angioplasty. These results indicate that a second thallium injection at rest could enhance the detection of ischemic but viable jeopardized myocardium.

Exercise ^{201}Tl scintigraphy is useful for the stratification of low- and high-risk patients with uncomplicated AMI. It is most cost effective in patients with abnormal resting electrocardiograms compared with exercise electrocardiography.

RADIONUCLIDE ANGIOGRAPHY

An alternative to ^{201}Tl exercise scintigraphy is the radionuclide angiography exercise test. The exercise performed is usually supine bicycling. Abnormal tests predict multivessel disease and a poor 1-year prognosis.[144,145] The exercise ejection fraction provides additional prognostic information over the resting value alone, particularly in patients who have greater residual myocardial ischemia but preserved resting left ventricular function. This is frequently observed after non-Q wave and inferior myocardial infarction, but it is less common after anterior infarction, in which there is generally greater resting left ventricular dysfunction. Abnormal responses consist of a fall in global ejection fraction or the development of new left ventricular regional wall motion abnormalities.

Radionuclear techniques should be used if rest conduction or ST abnormalities, left ventricular hypertrophy, or drug-induced ST-segment changes are present on the 12-lead ECG.

IMPLICATIONS FOR THERAPY

The primary physician caring for a patient with uncomplicated myocardial infarction can use the results of LVEF determination and exercise testing to guide further workup and medical therapy. Although only general guidelines can be given, several recommendations seem appropriate.

Patients with a positive exercise test before hospital discharge should be considered for coronary angiography. Those with an LVEF less than 40%, ventricular dysrhythmia, and a positive exercise test are at high risk ($\geq$30% 1-year mortality) and should have longer hospitalization, early cardiac catheterization, and further medical or surgical therapy. Many patients fall into the lowest risk group: LVEF>40%, no ventricular dysrhythmia, and a negative exercise test. In these patients, early discharge, rapid ambulation, and early return to work are preferable to a more aggressive approach. Maximal exercise testing should be considered at 6 weeks to uncover residual ischemia.

Finally, appropriate risk factor education and intervention (e.g., smoking cessation, weight loss, lipid profiling, blood pressure control) are always part of the optimal care of patients with coronary artery disease.

REFERENCES ■

1. American Heart Association: *1987 Heart Facts.* Dallas, American Heart Association National Center, 1987
2. Braunwald E: *Heart Disease: A Textbook of Cardiovascular Medicine,* vol 2. Philadelphia, WB Saunders, 1988:1222
3. Gillum, RF, Folsom A, Luepker RV, et al: Sudden death and acute myocardial infarction in a metropolitan area, 1970–1980. *N Engl J Med* 1983;309:1353
4. Pryor DB, Harrell FE Jr, Lee KL, et al: An improving prognosis over time in medically treated patients with coronary artery disease. *Am J Cardiol* 1983;52:444
5. Peli S, Fayerweather WE: Trends in the incidence of myocardial infarction and in associated mortality and morbidity in a large employed population, 1957–1983. *N Engl J Med* 1985;312:1005
6. Sobel BE, Bresnahan GF, Shell WE, et al: Estimation of infarct size in man and its relation to prognosis. *Circulation* 1972;46:640
7. Rogers WJ, McDaniel HG, Smith LR, et al: Correlation of angiographic estimates of myocardial infarct size and accumulated release of creatine kinase MB isoenzyme in man. *Circulation* 1977;56:199

8. Holman BL, Chisholm RJ, Braunwald E: The prognostic implications of acute myocardial infarct scintigraphy with ^{99m}Tcpyrophosphate. *Circulation* 1978;57:320
9. Geltman EM, Ehsani AA, Campbell MK, et al: The influence of location and extent of myocardial infarction on long-term ventricular dysrhythmia and mortality. *Circulation* 1979;60:805
10. DeWood A, Spores CRNA, Notske R, et al: Prevalence of total coronary occlusion during the early hours of myocardial Infarction. *N Engl J Med* 1980;303:897
11. Gruppo Italiano per lo Studio della Streptochinasi nell' Infarto Miocardico (GISSI): Effectiveness of intravenous thrombolytic treatment in acute myocardial infarction. *Lancet* 1986;1:397
12. ISIS-2 (Second Inernational Study of Infarct Survival) Collaborative Group: Randomised trial of intravenous streptokinase, oral aspirin, both, or neither among 17,187 cases of suspected acute myocardial infarction. *Lancet* 1988;2:349
13. Van de Werf F, Arnold AER, for the European Cooperative Study Group for recombinant tissue type plasminogen activator: Intravenous tissue plasminogen activator and size of infarct, left ventricular function, and survival in acute myocardial infarction. *Br Med J* 1988;297:1374
14. Wilcox RG, von der Lippe B, Olsson CG, et al for the ASSET Study Group: Trial of tissue plasminogen activator for mortality reduction in acute myocardial infarction. *Lancet* 1988;2:525
15. AIMS Trial Study Group: Effect of intravenous APSAC on mortality after acute myocardial infarction: preliminary report of a placebo-controlled clinical trial. *Lancet* 1988;1:545
16. White HD, Norris RM, Brown MA, et al: Effect of intravenous streptokinase on left ventricular function and early survival after acute myocardial infarction. *N Engl J Med* 1987;317:850
17. ISIS-3 (Third International Study of Infarct Survival) Collaborative Group: A randomised comparison of streptokinase vs tissue plasminogen activator vs anistreplase and of aspirin plus heparin vs aspirin alone among 41,299 cases of suspected acute myocardial infarction. *Lancet* 1992;339:753
18. Gruppo Italiano per lo Studio della Sopravvivenza nell' Infarto Miocardico: GISSI-2: a factorial randomised trial of alteplase versus streptokinase and heparin versus no heparin among 12,490 patients with acute myocardial infarction. *Lancet* 1990;336:65
19. GUSTO (Global Utilization of Streptokinase and rt-PA for Occluded Coronary Arteries): An international randomized trial comparing four thrombolytic strategies for acute myocardial infarction. *N Engl J Med* 1993;329:673
20. Fuster V, Dyken ML, Vokonas PS, et al for the Special Writing Group: Aspirin as a therapeutic agent in cardiovascular disease. *Circulation* 1993;87:659
21. Verheugt FWA, van der Laarse A, Funke-Kupper AJ, et al: Effects of early intervention with low-dose aspirin (100 mg) on infarct size, reinfarction and mortality in anterior wall acute myocardial infarction. *Am J Carciol* 1990;66:267
22. Roux S, Christeller S, Ludin E: Effects of aspirin on coronary reocclusion and recurrent ischemia after thrombolysis: a meta-analysis. *J Am Coll Cardiol* 1992;19:671
23. Antiplatelet Trialists' Collaboration: Secondary prevention of vascular disease by prolonged antiplatelet treatment. *Br Med J* 1988;296:320
24. Haynes RB, Sandler RS, Larson EB, et al: A critical appraisal of ticlopidine, a new antiplatelet agent: effectiveness and clinical indications for prophylaxis of atherosclerotic events. *Arch Intern Med* 1992;152:1376
25. Hockman JS, Chew H: Limitation of infarct expansion by

reperfusion independent of myocardial salvage. *Circulation* 1987;75:299

26. Lavie CJ, O'Keefe Jr, Chesebro JH, et al: Prevention of late ventricular dilatation after acute myocardial infarction by successful thrombolytic reperfusion. *Am J Cardiol* 1990;66:31

27. Naylor CD, Armstrong PW, for the Ontario Medical Association Consensus Group on Thrombolytic Therapy: Guidelines for the use of intravenous thrombolytic agents in acute myocardial infarction. *Can Med Assoc J* 1989;140:1289

28. Collen D: Coronary thrombolysis: streptokinase or recombinant tissue-type plasminogen activator? *Ann Intern Med* 1990;112:529

29. Yusuf S, Sleight P, Held P, McMahon S: Routine medical management of acute myocardial infarction: lessons from overviews of recent randomized controlled trials. *Circulation* 1990;82(Suppl II):117

30. Guidelines for the early management of patients with acute myocardial infarction: A report of the American College of Cardiology/American Heart Association Task Force on assessment of diagnostic and therapeutic cardiovascular procedures (subcommittee to develop guidelines for the early management of patients with acute myocardial infarction). *Circulation* 1990;82:664

31. Le traitement thrombolytique de l'infarctus du myocarde, Conseil consultatif de pharmacologie, Ministère de la Santé et des Services sociaux, Gouvernement du Québec, février 1995

32. Cairns J, Armstrong P, Belenkie I, et al: The Canadian consensus conference on coronary thrombolysis: 1994 update. *Can J Cardiol* 1994;10:517

33. The International Study Group: In-hospital mortality and clinical course of 20,891 patients with suspected acute myocardial infarction randomised between alteplase and streptokinase with or without heparin. *Lancet* 1990;336:71

34. Naylor CD, Bronskill S, Goel V: Cost-effectiveness of intravenous thrombolytic drugs for acute myocardial infarction. *Can J Cardiol* 1993;9:553

35. Anderson JL, Marshall HW, Bray BE, et al: A randomized trial of intracoronary streptokinase in the treatment of acute myocardial infarction. *N Engl J Med* 1983;308:1312

36. Khaja F, Walton JA Jr, Brymer JF, et al: Intracoronary fibrinolytic therapy in acute myocardial infarction: report of a prospective randomized trial. *N Engl J Med* 1983;308:1305

37. Kennedy JW, Ritchie JL, Davis KB, et al: Western Washington randomized trial of intracoronary streptokinase in acute myocardial infarction. *N Engl J Med* 1983;309:1477

38. Spann JF, Sherry S, Carabello BA, et al: Coronary thrombolysis by intravenous streptokinase in acute myocardial infarction: acute and follow-up studies. *Am J Cardiol* 1984;53:655

39. Alderman EL, Jutzy KR, Berte LE, et al: Randomized comparison of intravenous versus intracoronary streptokinase for myocardial infarction. *Am J Cardiol* 1984;54:14

40. Collen D, Topol EJ, Tiefenbrunn AJ, et al: Coronary thrombolysis with recombinant human tissue-type plasminogen activator: a prospective, randomized, placebo-controlled trial. *Circulation* 1984;70:1012

41. Timmis AD, Griffin B, Crick JCP, Sowton E: Anisoylated plasminogen streptokinase activator complex in acute myocardial infarction: a placebo-controlled arteriographic coronary recanalization study. *J Am Coll Cardiol* 1987;10:205

42. Anderson JL, Rothbard RL, Hackworthy RA, et al for the APSAC Multicenter Investigators: Multicenter reperfusion trial of intravenous anisoylated plasminogen streptokinase activator complex (APSAC) in acute myocardial infarction: controlled comparison with intracoronary streptokinase. *J Am Coll Cardiol* 1988;11:1153

43. The I.S.A.M. Study Group: A prospective trial of intravenous streptokinase in acute myocardial infarction (I.S.A.M.). *N Engl J Med* 1986;314:1465

44. TIMI-I: Phase I findings: the thrombolysis in myocardial infarction (TIMI) trial. *N Engl J Med* 1985;312:932

45. Mauri F, DeBiase AM, Franzosi MG, et al: G.I.S.S.I.: analisi delle cause di morte intraospedaliera. *G Ital Cardiol* 1987; 1711:37

46. Muller DWM, Topol EJ: Selection of patients with acute myocardial infarction for thrombolytic therapy. *Ann Intern Med* 1990;113:949

47. Cragg DR, Bonema JD, Ramos RG, et al: Ineligibility for intravenous thrombolytic therapy predicts high mortality after acute myocardial infarction [abstract]. *Circulation* 1989; 80(Suppl II):522

48. LATE Study Group: Late assessment of thrombolytic efficacy study with alteplase 6–24 hours after onset of acute myocardial infarction. *Lancet* 1993;342:759

49. EMERAS (Estudio Multicentrico Estreptoquinasa Republicas de America del Sur) Collaborative Group: Randomised trial of late thrombolysis in patients with suspected acute myocardial infarction. *Lancet* 1993:342:767

50. Col NF, Gurwitz JH, Alpert JS, et al.: Frequency of inclusion of patients with cardiogenic shock in trials of thrombolytic therapy. *Am J Cardiol* 1994;73:149

51. Kennedy JW, Gensini GG, Timmis GC, et al.: Acute myocardial infarction treated with intracoronary streptokinase: a report of the society for cardiac angiography. *Am J Cardiol* 1985;55:871

52. Goldberg RJ, Gore JM, Alpert JS, et al: Cardiogenic shock after acute myocardial infarction. *N Engl J Med* 1991;325:1117

53. Rentrop KP, Feit F, Blanke H, et al: Effects of intracoronary streptokinase and intracoronary nitroglycerin infusion on coronary angiographic patterns and mortality in patients with acute myocardial infarction. *N Engl J Med* 1984:311:1457

54. Raizner AE, Tortoledo FA, Verani MS, et al: Intracoronary thrombolytic therapy in acute myocardial infarction: a prospective, randomized, controlled trial. *Am J Cardiol* 1985; 55:301

55. Simoons ML, Serruys PW, Van Den Bran M, et al: Early thrombolysis in acute myocardial infarction: limitation of infarct size and improved survival. *J Am Coll Cardiol* 1986;7:717

56. Topol EJ, O'Neill WW, Langburd AB, et al: A randomized, placebo-controlled trial of intravenous recombinant tissue-type plasminogen activator and emergency coronary angioplasty in patients with acute myocardial infarction. *Circulation* 1987;75:420

57. White HD, Norris RM, Brown MA, et al: Effect of intravenous streptokinase on left ventricular function and early survival after acute myocardial infarction. *N Engl J Med* 1987;317:850

58. National Heart Foundation of Australia Coronary Thrombolysis Group: Coronary thrombolysis and myocardial salvage by tissue plasminogen activator given up to four hours after onset of myocardial infarction. *Lancet* 1988;1:203

59. Sherry S: Appraisal of various thrombolytic agents in the treatment of acute myocardial infarction. *Am J Med* 1988; (Suppl 2A):31

60. Meyer J, Mery W, Schmitz H, et al: Percutaneous transluminal coronary angioplasty immediately after intracoronary streptolysis of transmural myocardial infarction. *Circulation* 1982;66:905

61. Bates ER, Califf RM, Stack RS, et al for The Thrombolysis and Angioplasty in Myocardial Infarction Study Group: Thrombolysis and angioplasty in myocardial infarction (TAMI-1) trial: influence of infarct location on arterial pat-

ency, left ventricular function and mortality. *J Am Coll Cardiol* 1989;13:12

62. The TIMI Research Group: Immediate vs delayed catheterization and angioplasty after thrombolytic therapy for acute myocardial infarction: TIMI II A results. *JAMA* 1988;260:2849

63. The TIMI Study Group: Comparison of invasive and conservative strategies after treatment with intravenous tissue plasminogen activator in acute myocardial infarction: results of the thrombolysis in myocardial infarction (TIMI) phase II trial. *N Engl J Med* 1989;320:618

64. Grines CL, Browne KF, Marco J, et al for The Primary Angioplasty in Myocardial Infarction Study Group: A comparison of immediate angioplasty with trhombolytic therapy for acute myocardial infarction. *N Engl J Med* 1993;328:673

65. O'Keefe JH, Rutherford BD, McConahay DR, et al: Early and late results of coronary angioplasty without antecedent thrombolytic therapy for acute myocardial infarction. *Am J Cardiol* 1989;64:1221

66. O'Neill W, Timmis GC, Bourdillon PD, et al: A prospective randomized clinical trial of intracoronary streptokinase versus coronary angioplasty for acute myocardial infarction. *N Engl J Med* 1986;314:812

67. Michels KB, Yusuf S: Does PTCA in acute myocardial infarction affect mortality and reinfarction rates? A quantitative overview (meta-analysis) of the randomized clinical trials. *Circulation* 1995;91:476

68. Lee L, Bates ER, Pitt B, et al: Percutaneous transluminal coronary angioplasty improves survival in acute myocardial infarction complicated by cardiogenic shock. *Circulation* 1988;78:1345

69. Rogers WJ, Babb JD, Baim DS, et al: Is predischarge coronary arteriography beneficial in patients with myocardial infarction treated with thrombolytic therapy [astract]? *J Am Coll Cardiol* 1990;15(Suppl A):64A

70. Hsai J, Hamilton WP, Kleiman N, et al: Heparin-induced prolongation of partial thromboplastin time after thrombolysis: relation to coronary artery patency. *J Am Coll Cardiol* 1992;20:31

71. The SCATI (Studio sulla Calciparina nell'Thrombosi Ventriculare nell'Infarto) group: Randomized controlled trial of subcutaneous calcium-heparin in acute myocardial infarction. *Lancet* 1989;2:182

72. Turpie AGG, Robinson JG, Doyle DJ, et al: Comparison of high-dose with low-dose subcutaneous heparin to prevent left ventricular mural thrombosis in patients with acute transmural anterior myocardial infarction. *N Engl J Med* 1989;320:352

73. Yusuf S, Sleight P, Rossi P, et al: Reduction in infarct size, arrhythmias and chest pain by early intravenous beta blockade in suspected acute myocardial infarction. *Circulation* 1983;67(Suppl I):32

74. Roberts R, Rogers WJ, Mueller HS, et al for the TIMI Investigators: Immediate versus deferred β-blockade following thrombolytic therapy in patients with acute myocardial infarction: results of the thrombolysis in myocardial infarction (TIMI) II-B study. *Circulation* 1991;83:422

75. The MIAMI Trial Research Group: Metoprolol in acute myocardial infarction (MIAMI). *Am J Cardiol* 1985;56:1G

76. First International Study Group on Infarct Survival Collaborative Group (ISIS-I): Randomized trial of intravenous atenolol among 16,027 cases of suspected acute myocardial infarction: ISIS-I. *Lancet* 1986;2:57

77. Herlitz J, Holmberg S, Pennert K, et al: The Goteborg metoprolol trial in acute myocardial infarction. *Am J Cardiol* 1984;53:1D

78. The Beta-Blocker Pooling Project Research Group (BBPP): Subgroup findings from randomized trials in post infarction patients *Eur Heart J* 1988;9:8

79. ISIS-1 (First International Study of Infarct Survival) Collaborative Group: Mechanisms for the early mortality reduction produced by beta-blockade started early in acute myocardial infarction: ISIS-1. *Lancet* 1988;1:921

80. McGregor M: Pathogenesis of angina pectoris and role of nitrates in relief of myocardial ischemia. *Am J Med* 1983;74(Suppl 6B):21

81. Jugdutt BI, Warnica JW: Intravenous nitroglycerin therapy to limit myocardial infarct size, expansion, and complications: effect of timing, dosage, and infarct location. *Circulation* 1988;78:906

82. Jugdutt BI, Wortman C, Warnica WJ: Does nitroglycerin therapy in acute myocardial infarction reduce the incidence of infarct expansion? *J Am Coll Cardiol* 1985;5:447

83. Horwitz LD, Gorlin R, Taylor WJ, et al: Effect of nitroglycerin on regional myocardial blood flow in coronary artery disease. *J Clin Invest* 1971;50:1578

84. Brown BG, Bolson E, Petersen RB, et al: The mechanisms of nitroglycerin action: stenosis vasodilation as a major component of drug response. *Circulation* 1981;64:1089

85. Yusuf S, Collins R, MacMahon S, et al: Effect of intravenous nitrates on mortality in acute myocardial infarction: an overview of the randomized trials. *Lancet* 1988;1:1088

86. Gibson R, Boden WE, Theroux P, et al for the Diltiazem Reinfarction Study Group: Diltiazem and reinfarction in patients with non-Q wave myocardial infarction. *N Engl J Med* 1986;315:423

87. Helad PH, Yusuf S: Effects of β-blockers and calcium channel blockers in acute myocardial infarction. *Eur Heart J* 1993;14:(Suppl F):18

88. Nattel S, Zipes DP: Clinical pharmacology of old and new antiarrhythmic drugs. *Cardiovasc Res* 1980;11:221

89. Heger JJ, Prystowsky EN, Zipes DP: Clinical choice of antiarrhythmic drugs. In: Josephson ME (ed). *Ventricular Tachycardia—Mechanisms and Management.* Mt. Kisco, NY, Futura Publishing, 1982

90. Pantridge JF, Webb SW, Adgey AA: Arrhythmias in the first hours of acute myocardial infarction. *Prog Cardiovasc Dis* 1981;23:265

91. Braunwald E: *Heart Disease: A Textbook of Cardiovascular Medicine,* vol 2. Philadelphia, WB Saunders, 1992:1200

92. Fulton M, Julian DG, Oliver MF: Sudden death and myocardial infarction. *Circulation* 1969;40(Suppl 4):182

93. MacMahon S, Collins R, Peto R, et al: Effects of prophylactic lidocaine in suspected acute myocardial infarction: an overview of results from the randomized, controlled trials. *JAMA* 1988;260:1910

94. Bleifeld W, Merx W, Henrich KW, et al: Controlled trial of prophylactic treatment with lidocaine in acute myocardial infarction. *Eur J Clin Pharmacol* 1973;6:119

95. Pfeffer JM, Pfeffer MA, Braunwald E: Influence of captopril on mortality and morbidity in patients with left ventricular dysfunction after myocardial infarction–results of the Survival and Ventricular Enlargement Trial (SAVE). *N Engl J Med* 1992;327:669

96. The Acute Infarction Ramipril Efficacy (AIRE) Study Investigators: Effect of ramipril on mortality and morbidity of survivors of acute myocardial infarctionwith clinical evidence of heart failure. *Lancet* 1993;342:821

97. Gruppo Italiano per lo Studio della Sopravvivenza nell'infarto Miocardico. GISSI-3: effects of lisinopril and transdermal glyceryl trinitrate singly and together on 6-week mortality and ventricular function after acute myocardial infarction. Lancet 1994;343:1115.

98. ISIS-4 (Fourth International Study of Infarct Survival) Collaborative Group: A randomised factorial trial assessing early oral captopril, oral mononitrate, and intravenous magnesium sulphate in 58,050 patients with suspected acute myocardial infartion. Lancet 1995;345:669.

99. Vlodaver Z, Edwards JE: Rupture of ventricular septum of papillary muscle complicating myocardial infarction. *Circulation* 1977; 55:815

100. Hutchins GM: Rupture of the intraventricular septum complicating myocardial infarction: Pathological analysis of ten patients with clinically diagnosed perforations. *Am Heart J* 1979; 97:165

101. Meister SG, Helfant RH: Rapid bedside differentiation of ruptured intraventricular septum from acute mitral insufficiency. *N Engl J Med* 1972; 287:1024

102. Mesa JM, L„pez-Send„n J, Larrea J, et al: Surgical treatment of subacute ventricular rupture after myocardial infarction. Long-term follow-up [abstract]. *Circulation* 1990;82:(Suppl III):296

103. Bates RJ, Beutler S, Resnekov L, et al: Cardiac rupture—challenge in diagnosis and managment. *Am J Cardiol* 1977;40:429

104. Wackers JF, Lie KI, Sokale EB: Prevalence of right ventricular involvement and inferior wall infarction assessed with myocardial imaging with thallium 201, technetium 99m pyrophosphate. *Am J Cardiol* 1978:42:358

105. Sharpe DM, Botvinick EH, Shames DM: Noninvasive diagnosis of right ventricular infarction. *Circulation* 1978;57:483

106. Lorell B, Leimbach RC, Pohost GM, et al: Right ventricular infarction: clinical diagnosis and differentiation from cardiac tamponade and pericardial restriction. *Am J Cardiol* 1979; 43:465

107. Forrester JS, Diamond GA, Swan HJC: Correlative classification of clinical and hemodynamic function after acute myocardial infarction. *Am J Cardiol* 1977;39:137

108. Kupper W, Bleifelt W, Hanrath P, et al: Left ventricular hemodynamic and function in acute myocardial infarction: studies during the acute phase, convalescence and late recovery. *Am J Cardiol* 1977;40:900

109. Cohn JN, Mathew KJ, Franciso JA, et al: Chronic vasodilator therapy in the management of cardiogenic shock in intractable left ventricular failure. *Ann Intern Med* 1974;81:777

110. Marcus FI: Use of digitalis in acute myocardial infarction. *Circulation* 1980;62:17

111. Wackers FJT, Sokole EB, Samson G, et al: Value and limitations of thallium-201 scintigraphy in the acute phase of myocardial infarction. *N Engl J Med* 1976;295:1

112. Becker LC, Silverman KJ, Bulkley BH, et al: Comparison of early thallium-201 scintigraphy and gated blood pool imaging for predicting mortality in patients with acute myocardial infarction. *Circulation* 1983;67:1272

113. Mahmarian JJ, Verani MS, Pratt CM, et al: Quantification of acute myocardial infarct size using thallium-201 single photon emission computed tomography: comparison with CK-MB sizing. *J Am Coll Cardiol* 1987;9:174A

114. Kiat H, Maddahi J, Roy LT, et al: Comparison of technetium-99m methoxy isobutyl isonitrile and thallium-201 for evaluation of coronary artery disease by planar and tomographic methods. *Am Heart J* 1989;117:1

115. Wackers FJT, Gibbons RJ, Verani MS, et al: Serial quantitative planar technetium-99m isonitrile imaging in acute myocardial infarction: efficacy for noninvasive assessment of thrombolytic therapy. *J Am Coll Cardiol* 1989;14:861

116. Battler A, Slutsky R, Karliner J, et al: Left ventricular ejection fraction and first third ejection fraction early after acute myocardial infarction: value for predicting mortality and morbidity. *Am J Cardiol* 1980;45:197

117. Schelbert HR, Henning H, Ashburn WL, et al: Serial measurements of left ventricular ejection fraction by radionuclide angiography early and late after myocardial infarction. *Am J Cardiol* 1976;38:407

118. Shah PK, Pichler M, Berman DS, et al: Left ventricular ejection fraction determined by radionuclide ventriculography in early stages of first transmural myocardial infarction. *Am J Cardiol* 1980;45:542

119. Wheelan K, Wolfe C, Corbett JR, et al: Early positive technicium-99m stannous pyrophosphate images as a marker of reperfusion in patients receiving thrombolytic therapy for acute myocardial infarction. *Am J Cardiol* 1985;56:252

120. Holman BL, Chisholm RJ, Braunwald E: The prognostic implications of acute myocardial infarct scintigraphy with ⁹⁹ᵐTcpyrophosphate. *Circulation* 1978;57:320

121. Rude RE, Parkey RW, Bonte FJ, et al: Clinical implications of the technetium-99m stannous pyrophosphate myocardial scintigraphic "doughnut" pattern in patients with acute myocardial infarcts. *Circulation* 1979;59:721

122. Ahmad M, Logan KW, Martin RH: Doughnut pattern of technetium-99m pyrophosphate myocardial uptake in patients with acute myocardial infarction: a sign of poor long-term prognosis. *Am J Cardiol* 1979;44:13

123. Olson HG, Lyons KP, Aronow WS, et al: Follow-up technetium-99m stannous pyrophosphate myocardial scintigrams after acute myocardial infarction. *Circulation* 1977;56:181

124. Quinones MA: Echocardiography in acute myocardial infarction. *Cardiol Clin* 1984;2:123

125. Hager JJ, Weyman AE, Wann SD, et al: Cross-sectional echocardiographic analysis of the extent of left ventricular synergy in acute myocardial infarction. *Circulation* 1980;61:113

126. Gibson RS, Bishop HL, Stramm RB, et al: Value of early two-dimensional echocardiography in patients with acute myocardial infarction. *Am J Cardiol* 1982;49:110

127. VanReet RE, Quinones MA, Poliner LR, et al: Comparison of two-dimensional echocardiography with gated radionuclide ventriculography in the evaluation of global and regional left ventricular function in acute myocardial infarction. *J Am Coll Cardiol* 1984;3:243

128. Dropac M, Gilbert B, Howard R, et al: Ventricular septal defect after myocardial infarction: diagnosis by two-dimensional echocardiography. *Circulation* 1983;67:335

129. Pratt CM, Roberts R: Non-Q-wave myocardial infarction: recognition, pathogenesis, prognosis, and management. *Baylor Coll Med Cardiol Series* 1985;8:5

130. Gibson RS: Non-Q-wave myocardial infarction: diagnosis, prognosis, and management. *Curr Probl Cardiol* 1988;13:9

131. Maisel AS, Ahnve S, Gilpin E, et al: Prognosis after extension of myocardial infarction: the role of Q-wave or non-Q-wave infarction. *Circulation* 1985;71:211

132. Goldberg RJ, Gore JM, Alpert JS, et al: Non-Q-wave myocardial infarction: recent changes in occurrence and prognosis—a community wide perspective. *Am Heart J* 1987;113:273

133. DeWood MA, Stifter WF, Simpson CS, et al: Coronary arteriographic findings soon after non-Q-wave myocardial infarction. *N Engl J Med* 1986;315:417

134. Quinones MA, Waggoner AD, Reduto LA, et al: A new, simplified and accurate method for determining ejection fraction with two-dimensional echocardiography. *Circulation* 1981;64:744

135. Bigger JT, Fleiss JL, Kleiger R, et al: The Multicenter Post-Infarction Research Group: the relationships among ventricular arrhythmias, left ventricular dysfunction, and mortality in the 2 years after myocardial infarction. *Circulation* 1984;69:250

136. Théroux P, Waters DD, Halphen C, et al: Prognostic value

of exercise testing soon after myocardial infarction. *N Engl J Med* 1979;301:341

137. Fuller CM, RAizner AE, Verani MS, et al: Early postmyocardial infarction treadmill stress testing: an accurate predictor of multivessel coronary disease and subsequent cardiac events. *Ann Intern Med* 1981;94:734

138. Starling MR, Crawford MH, Kennedy GT, et al: Treadmill exercise tests predischarge and six weeks post-myocardial infarction to detect abnormalities of known prognostic value. *Ann Intern Med* 1981;94:721

139. Kotler TS, Diamond GA: Exercise thallium-201 scintigraphy in the diagnosis and prognosis of coronary artery disease. *Ann Intern Med* 1990;113:684

140. Dilsizian V, Rocco TP, Freedman NMT, et al: Enhanced detection of ischemic but viable myocardium by the reinjection of thallium after stress-redistribution imaging. *N Engl J Med* 1990;323:141

141. Gibson RS, Taylor GJ, Watson DD, et al: Predicting the extent and location of coronary artery disease during the early postinfarction period by quantitative thallium-201 scintigraphy. *Am J Cardiol* 1981;47:1010

142. Gibson RS, Watson DD, Craddock GB, et al: Prediction of cardiac events after uncomplicated myocardial infarction: A prospective study comparing predischarge exercise thallium-201 scintigraphy and coronary angiography. *Circulation* 1983; 68:321

143. Gibson RS, Watson DD, Carabello BA, et al: Clinical implications of increased lung uptake of thallium-201 during exercise scintigraphy 2 weeks after myocardial infarction. *Am J Cardiol* 1982;49:1586

144. Corbett JR, Dehmer GJ, Lewis SE, et al: The prognostic value of submaximal exercise testing with radionuclide ventriculography before hospital discharge in patients with recent myocardial infarction. *Circulation* 1981;64:535

145. Dewhurst NG, Muir AL: Comparative prognostic value of radionuclide ventriculography at rest and during exercise in 100 patients after first myocardial infarction. *Br Heart J* 1983; 49:111

Critical Care, Third Edition, edited by Joseph M. Civetta,
Robert W. Taylor, and Robert R. Kirby.
Lippincott-Raven Publishers, Philadelphia, PA © 1997.

CHAPTER 117

Heart Failure

Mandeep R. Mehra
Hector O. Ventura

IMMEDIATE CONCERNS

MAJOR PROBLEMS

Advanced heart failure continues to be a clinical dilemma with increasing incidence and prevalence. Left ventricular ejection fraction remains the single most valuable measurement that not only contributes to diagnostic segregation into systolic heart failure and diastolic heart failure, but also provides important prognostic insights.

STRESS POINTS

1. While treatment of advanced heart failure with reduction in symptoms should be the immediate therapeutic goal, the population-based goal of management of patients with left ventricular dysfunction lies in prevention of left ventricular dysfunction.
2. If left ventricular dysfunction develops, then prevention of the transition of the state asymptomatic ventricular dysfunction to symptomatic overt heart failure is the therapeutic goal.
3. The alarming presence of high residual mortality even in the treatment groups of large scale clinical trials of advanced failure suggest a substantial need for the continued development of novel treatment strategies.

ESSENTIAL DIAGNOSTIC TESTS AND PROCEDURES

1. Once a diagnosis of systolic heart failure has been established by assessment of left ventricular ejection fraction, preferably by echocardiographic techniques, the clinician should attempt to establish the presence of signs and symptoms that would assist evaluation of

the hemodynamic perturbations which can then be targeted by pharmacologic therapy.
2. The presence of orthopnea is a reliable indicator of an elevated pulmonary artery occlusion pressure.
3. Similarly, clinical evidence of hepatosplanchnic congestion is provided by the presence of abdominal pain, anorexia, and early satiety. This is generally indicative of severe tricuspid regurgitation and elevated right-sided filling pressures.
4. The most reliable clinical indicator of a reduction in cardiac output is a proportional pulse pressure (systolic blood pressure [SBP]−diastolic blood pressure [DBP]/SBP) that is <25%.
5. These three cardinal manifestations of advanced heart failure assist a clinician in designing therapeutic goals by the use of intravenous diuretics, intravenous vasodilators, and intravenous inotropic therapy.
6. While invasive monitoring using pulmonary artery catheterization is not indicated for the mere diagnosis of advanced heart failure, it may provide valuable guidance in achieving hemodynamic goals that are associated with improved symptom relief as well as improved survival characteristics.

INITIAL THERAPY

1. Effective therapy in the advanced heart failure patient includes a reduction of right atrial pressures to <7 mm Hg, reduction of pulmonary artery occlusion pressure to <16 mm Hg, and a reduction of systemic vascular resistance to 1220 dynes/sec/cm^{-5} at a systolic blood pressure >80 mm Hg.
2. Once these hemodynamic parameters are obtained, every effort should be made to wean intravenous ther-

1749

apy while upwardly titrating oral vasodilators, particularly converting-enzyme inhibitors.

3. It has been demonstrated that use of angiotensin-converting enzyme (ACE) inhibitors in advanced heart failure are not only associated with improvement in morbid parameters, but also provide a mortality benefit.

4. To date, oral inotropic therapy has proved to be disappointing by the demonstration of enhanced mortality. However, use of intravenous inotropic therapy is very effective in the acute critical care setting where temporary hemodynamic restoration of the failed ventricle is necessary.

5. The two most effective intravenous inotropic agents include dobutamine and milrinone. The advantages of milrinone include a greater pulmonary vasodilating property and a lesser taxation on myocardial oxygen demand.

6. The patient with heart failure refractory to diuretic therapy should be considered for extrarenal fluid removal by ultrafiltration techniques.

7. When all pharmacologic measures have been exhausted and the patient remains symptomatic, prompt consideration for mechanical assistance with intra-aortic balloon pump must be initiated.

8. If a patient is deemed to be a candidate for heart transplantation and appears to demonstrate systemic clinical deterioration, consideration should be given for placement of a mechanical ventricular assist device.

9. Novel emerging therapies in systolic heart failure relate to the beneficial role of beta-blockers and the emergence of angiotensin II receptor blocking agents, as well as the potential survival benefit accorded by the use of the oral intropic agent, vesnarinone. The use of these agents should be limited to an experimental monitored setting at this time, and are not recommended for general clinical use.

INTRODUCTION ∎

The widely accepted dogma of considering the clinical syndrome of heart failure as a mere manifestation of hemodynamic perturbations has been recently challenged. Central to this cardinal concept is the revelation that the major abnormality that characterizes heart failure is not simply that of altered cardiac physiology, but encompasses the more important problem of a markedly diminished life expectancy that surpasses aggressive malignant states. This is further emphasized by the fact that many recent observations in the management of heart failure, such as the beneficial role of beta-blocking agents and the deleterious impact of inotropic therapy, have yielded findings that are clearly not explained by conventional wisdom. Therefore, the emphasis for investigating therapeutic approaches has now centered upon viewing the long-term consequences of heart failure by examining abnormalities of cell proliferation and growth, genetic abnormalities, and systemic neurohormonal aberrations that are responsible for the more global manifestations of chronic heart failure.[1]

A PRIMER IN MYOCARDIAL CELLULAR ABNORMALITIES

It is well recognized that myocardial cell populations are heterogeneous and include not only myocytes, but also fibroblasts, vascular smooth muscle, and endothelial cells. In fact, myocytes comprise only one third of the total myocardial cell population, while the remaining two thirds are dominated by the non-myocyte compartment, particularly the interstitial fibroblasts.[2] Whereas the myocyte is all important in determining the actual process of cell contraction, the scaffolding provided by the interstitium is seminal in the coordination of simultaneous force generation in an energy-efficient manner that eventually leads to the contraction and relaxation of the heart as a whole. Therefore, it should become obvious that abnormalities in cardiac contraction can result from disease not only in the myocyte compartment, but also in the non-myocyte compartment. This concept is of importance in developing a framework to understand myocardial remodeling, the overall end result of cellular aberrations that determine eventual prognosis in heart failure. It has been convincingly established that the ratio of myocardial mass to chamber volume and their surrogates of wall thickness and chamber diameter are an important determinant of survival in heart failure.[3]

Abnormalities of Calcium Handling

In the healthy heart, the low concentrations of myoplasm calcium are maintained by ion exchange carriers (sarcolemmal sodium calcium exchanger), pumps (sarcoplasmic reticulum calcium pump), and by binding to cellular protein components (myofilaments, calmodulin, sarcolemmal phospholipids).[4] Myocardial cell calcium flux by L-type channels that are maximally activated by depolarization remain activated throughout the plateau phase of the action potential. This influx triggers sarcoplasmic reticulum calcium release into the cytosol, which in turn results in interaction of the myofilament proteins actin and myosin by cross bridges that emanate from the myosin head. This composite process is called "excitation-contraction coupling", and variations in the amount of cytosolic calcium are important in determining the contraction strength. The actions of myofilaments, pumps, and ion channels are an ATP energy consuming process, the energy being derived from oxidative phosphorylation within mitochondria. The myofilament energy reserve is in the form of phosphocreatine, with this substance being converted to ATP for energy use and back to its native form from mitochondrial generated ATP to maintaining energy reserves. It has also been demonstrated that changes in cytosolic calcium determine the overall ATP supply and consumption, thus alluding to the role of cellular calcium in maintaining energy balances.[5]

In cardiac muscle derived from the failing heart, contraction time is prolonged in intracellular calcium transients, and these exhibit marked abnormality.[6] Furthermore, failing hearts have an inability to restore a low resting calcium concentration during diastole.[7] The cellular consequence of these aberrations is a resultant state of "energy starvation" and cytosolic calcium overload. Thus, abnormalities in "calcium cycling" from the sarcoplasmic reticulum to the cytosol and back, termed as calcium oscillations, are known to occur spontaneously, rather than in an organized and synchronous manner as is normally seen in the heart.[8] In fact, the functional consequences of abnormal spontaneous calcium oscillations can be summarized as the three cardinal manifestations of heart failure: dysrhythmia, systolic dysfunction and enhanced diastolic tone leading to diastolic dysfunction. Asynchronous spontaneous calcium oscillations can result in high cytosolic calcium loads during diastole and cause impaired relaxation of the ventricle. Similarly, lack of homogeneity of diastolic sarcolemmal lengths leads to a poorly coordinated systolic contraction with resultant systolic dysfunction. Lastly, asynchronous calcium oscillations can result in focal areas of cytosolic calcium overload, which can then trigger a spontaneous action potential and thus lead to triggered dysrhythmias.

Myocardial Remodeling

Myocardial remodeling is the name given to the term that denotes an alteration in myocardial architecture with its expression of altered ventricular chamber geometry that accompanies the state of hypertrophy. As alluded to earlier, it is important to emphasize that wall thickness is determined not only by myocyte size, but also more importantly by the alignment of the myocytes relative to one another. This myocyte alignment is determined by the interstitial fibrillar collagen network that provides scaffolding for myocardial contraction. The interstitium of the failing heart is characterized by degradation of the collagenase scaffolding that is no longer strong enough to preserve myocyte alignment, thereby leading to myocardial cell slippage.[9] This results in wall thinning, despite an increase in overall mass and myocyte hypertrophy, and leads to the eventual pathologic expression of the "big baggy heart" of dilated cardiomyopathy. Thus it is important in understanding the concept of myocardial remodeling to bear in mind that ventricular geometry in pathologic hypertrophy is not only a result of a change in the myocyte size, but also a change in the alignment of the myocytes as a result of changes in the interstitial scaffolding.

Ventricular Hypertrophy:Physiological or Pathological?

It is important to recognize that all ventricular hypertrophy is not pathological. The representative example of this is seen in the ventricular hypertrophy that accompanies exercise training in an effort to normalize wall stress, as in the athletic heart. This "physiologic" hypertrophy is not associated with a reduction in the life-span of the patient. On the other hand, left ventricular hypertrophy that accompanies chronic hypertension, or chronic dilated cardiomyopathy is most certainly "pathologic" because it is associated with an increased incidence of sudden death in this patient population.[10] What then is the difference between physiologic and pathologic ventricular hypertrophy? In ventricular hypertrophy that accompanies severe exercise training, the overall myocardial architecture remains normal. Myocyte as well as non-myocyte compartment growth is balanced with resultant

maintenance of the alignment of the myocytes with respect to each other, as well as maintenance of the support structure and interstitium. In striking contradistinction to this, ventricular hypertrophy that follows pathologic states is accompanied by a marked alteration in the fibrous tissue response in the interstitium which is expressed as an accumulation of type I fibrillar collagen in the interstitium as well as adventitia of the intramyocardial coronary vessels.[11] Interstitial fibroblast growth and enhanced collagen synthesis relative to degradation determines the overall abnormality in myocardial structure and is the hallmark of pathologic ventricular hypertrophy.

Neurohormonal Determinants of Myocardial Hypertrophy

Unlike "physiologic" ventricular hypertrophy, the stimulus to the development of "pathologic" ventricular hypertrophy is not simply an imposed hemodynamic load but is in fact an interplay of neural, endocrine, and hormonal factors that influence the metabolism of the non-myocyte compartment of the myocardium. These factors can adversely alter structure by deviating from what might otherwise be an adaptive growth of myocytes. It has been increasingly recognized that elevations in plasma angiotensin II and aldosterone are associated with abnormal fibrous tissue response in the non-myocyte myocardial compartment.[12]

EPIDEMIOLOGY OF HEART FAILURE ■

INCIDENCE AND PREVALENCE

Systolic heart failure is a major clinical and public health problem in western countries. Heart failure is currently the only cardiovascular disorder with an increasing population prevalence.[13] It is conservatively estimated that heart failure accounts for more than 400,000 cases occurring annually with 900,000 hospitalizations.[14] It is further estimated that more than 2,000,000 to 3,000,000 Americans are affected with this disease entity.[15] Not only does the incidence of heart failure more than double in the general population with each decade after age 45, but heart failure is also the leading and most expensive cause of hospitalization after age 64.[16] Furthermore, the prevalence of heart failure is relatively similar by gender as well. There is a high prevalence in males in the age group of 55 to 64; however, by age 65 the differences between males and females are too small to be significant.[17]

MORTALITY

More alarming is the revelation of new age-adjusted survival data from patients with heart failure in the Framingham Heart Study that indicates persisting high lethality without significant prognostic improvement during the 40-year period of 1948 to 1988.[18] Furthermore, the National Health and Nutrition Examination Survey showed that mortality for heart failure increases in a graded fashion with advancing age, and with men more likely to die than women.[19] The ten-year mortality for those age 55 to 64 was 15% in women and 64% in men. For those age 65 to 74, ten-year mortality was 50% in women and 73.5% in men. Thus, because of the increased risk of heart failure in the elderly, more aggressive diagnostic and therapeutic strategies are deemed necessary for this patient cohort.

ETIOPATHOGENESIS ■

ETIOLOGIES

Heart failure can result from either impaired systolic or altered diastolic function. There are three major causes of systolic dysfunction that lead to heart failure. First, loss of viable muscle (as seen in acute myocardial infarction). Second, a primary abnormality of cardiac muscle such as a cardiomyopathy due to viral, metabolic, infiltrative, toxic, or idiopathic etiologies. Third, mechanical abnormalities such as valvular dysfunction, hypertension, or congenital malformations can lead to states of pressure or volume overload with consequent ventricular dysfunction. In an overview of contemporary etiologies of congestive heart failure, Teerlink and colleagues[20] reported that ischemic heart disease comprises 50% of all cases of systolic heart failure, and in approximately 20% of such patients the diagnosis of exclusion of idiopathic dilated cardiomyopathy is most appropriate. Other identifiable causes of systolic dysfunction include valvular heart disease, hypertension and alcoholic cardiomyopathy. Before a patient is labeled to have idiopathic dilated cardiomyopathy they must be evaluated for occult endocrine abnormalities such as pheochromocytoma and thyroid dysfunction, metabolic abnormalities such as hemochromotosis, nutritional deficiency states, and collagen vascular abnormalities such as lupus erythematosus, polyarteritis nodosa, and scleroderma. Moreover, it should also be emphasized that approximately 10% of the patients with new onset of dilated cardiomyopathy without any identifiable cause are found to suffer from myocarditis (Fig. 117-1).[21]

Whereas the majority of patients with advanced heart failure suffer from systolic dysfunction, a significant proportion of patients will suffer from pure diastolic dysfunction with impaired ventricular filling. Its recognition is of paramount importance in determining appropriate therapeutic strategies. For the most part, the discussion to follow will primarily focus on advanced heart failure resulting from left ventricular systolic dysfunction. A brief discussion of diastolic dysfunction is provided towards the end of this chapter.

NEUROHORMONAL ACTIVATION IN ADVANCED HEART FAILURE ■

A number of hemodynamic and neurohormonal alterations are present in advanced heart failure. Thus, it has been shown that neurohormonal systems such as the sympathetic nervous system and the renin-angiotensin-aldosterone system are activated in patients with heart failure.

SYMPATHETIC NERVOUS SYSTEM ACTIVATION

The activation of the sympathetic nervous system plays two distinct roles. First, it is initially adaptive and results in an increase in heart rate and myocardial contractility which leads to an enhanced cardiac output. Second, an increase in sympathetic tone maintains peripheral vascular resistance and perfusion pressure gradients of the peripheral systemic organ beds. However, it has been postulated that the chronic increase in sympathetic drive and catecholamines results in circulatory effects that are maladaptive.[22] Catecholamines have been shown to stimulate protein synthesis and to produce collagen deposition and myocardial fibrosis, leading to pathologic ventricular hypertrophy and remodeling. In addition, high doses of norepinephrine can cause myocarditis, myocardial necrosis, and cardiomyopathy. More importantly, the clinical validation of the concept of maladaption has emerged from the demonstration of elevated plasma norepinephrine as an important predictor of mortality in heart failure patients. This hypothesis has been tested in a multi-center clinical trial where plasma norepinephrine levels in excess of 600 pg/mL were found to predict a poor prognosis in symptomatic patients with heart failure.[23]

RENIN-ANGIOTENSIN-ALDOSTERONE ACTIVATION

Angiotensin II has been proposed as the conductor of the orchestra[12] that determines maladaptive peripheral and central neurohormonal mechanisms in heart failure. The activation of the renin-angiotensin system in heart failure leads to venous and arterial vasoconstriction in the peripheral circulation. Angiotensin II also functions as a growth factor by stimulating smooth muscle proliferation, as well as left ventricular hypertrophy, leading to adverse ventricular remodeling.[24] Another consequence of activation of this neurohormonal system is an elevated aldosterone activity which results in sodium and water retention. The net result is an increase in ventricular filling pressures and peripheral perfusion pressure. More recently, the existence of a tissue neurohormonal system distinct from the systemic renin-angiotensin system has been proposed.[25] In support of this, it

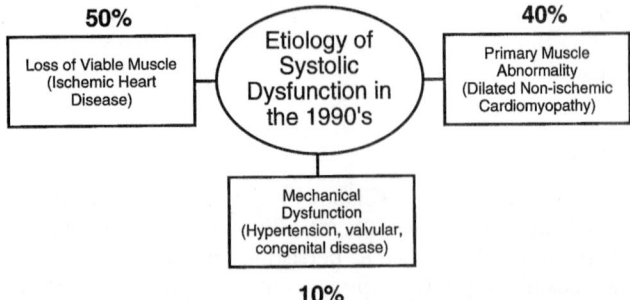

FIGURE 117-1. Schema illustrating the type and frequency of commonly encountered primary etiologies of advanced systolic heart failure.

has been demonstrated in both animal and human experimental conditions that ACE is present in myocardial tissue, a demonstration of the presence of tissue renin-angiotensin systems operating at a local level.

ATRIAL NATRIURETIC PEPTIDE

Another compensatory neurohormonal mechanism in patients with heart failure relates to the elucidation of atrial natriuretic peptide factors in response to cardiac chamber stretch.[26] The physiologic effects of atrial natriuretic peptide include sodium excretion, vasodilatation, and inhibition of renin and aldosterone release. Although the secretion of atrial natriuretic factor is higher, it may not be adequate to negate opposing sympathetic activity, but may nevertheless contribute to the maintenance of fluid balance in patients with heart failure. Thus, the activation of atrial natriuretic peptide in response to atrial distention is in fact an attempt to counter balance the effects of the renin-angiotensin-aldosterone system activation. However, it has been suggested that the effects of atrial natriuretic factor on diuresis are diminished in patients with heart failure due to decreased renal responsiveness to atrial natriuretic peptide as the syndrome of heart failure progresses. Furthermore, in a recent investigation, heart failure patients with an atrial natriuretic peptide level in excess of 125 pg/mL were found to have a significantly increased mortality, even when adjusted for other prognostic variables.[27]

NEUROHORMONAL ACTIVATION: ADAPTATION OR MALADAPTION? ■

Although activation of neurohormonal mechanisms is an effort to maintain hemodynamic parameters and perfusion pressure to vital organ beds, they eventually become maladaptive.[28] For example, the increase in vascular tone, as a result of neurohormonal activation, eventually results in increased impedance to left ventricular emptying as well as a further compromise of systolic ventricular function. Furthermore, angiotensin II is also known to be arrhythmo-

genic and might promote ischemia as well. Salt and water retention eventually result in pulmonary and venous congestive and peripheral edema. These maladaptive effects are also expressed in peripheral changes that occur in patients with heart failure and can account for several of their clinical manifestations. There is a decrease in blood flow to skeletal muscle, skin, splanchnic, and renal vascular beds, as well as an inability to increase blood flow to skeletal muscles in response to vasodilator stimuli such as exercise.[29] These changes lead to exercise intolerance and physical deconditioning, which further impairs vasodilatation due to reduced vascular release of endothelium derived relaxing factor. In summary, the neurohormonal mechanisms involve not only the heart but the peripheral circulation as well and it is the confluence of these abnormalities in the periphery and center that determine the eventual elaboration of the clinical syndrome in patients with heart failure (Fig. 117-2).

PROGNOSTIC FACTORS IN ADVANCED HEART FAILURE ■

A number of clinical variables have been used to predict survival in this complex clinical syndrome. These factors, which are interactive, can be deduced from laboratory investigations and can assist the clinician to establish prognosis with a reasonable clinical preciseness. Table 117-1 lists factors that have been proven to have relevance in predicting survival in heart failure.

LEFT VENTRICULAR FUNCTION

Measurement of the systolic performance of the heart is commonly obtained by estimation of left ventricular ejection fraction by radiographic, radionuclide or echocardiographic techniques. Most studies to date have identified left ventricular ejection fraction as an important independent predictor of survival in heart failure. A curvilinear relationship exists between survival and left ventricular ejection fraction, with a sharp increase in mortality once the ejection fraction declines below 20%.[30] However, it is important to emphasize

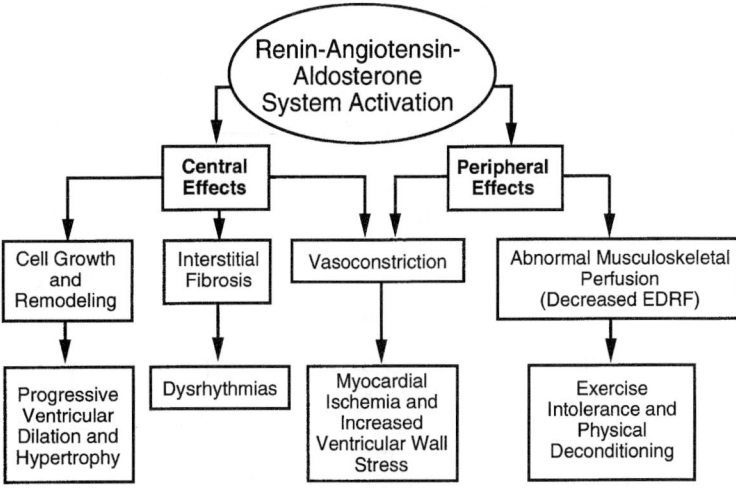

FIGURE 117-2. Schema depicting the impact of neurohormonal activation at the target central (cardiac) and peripheral (musculoskeletal) sites. The global pathologic confluence of maladaptive neurohormonal activation determines the elucidation of the cardinal clinical manifestations of heart failure.

TABLE 117-1.   Predictors of Survival in Heart Failure

VARIABLE	CLINICAL PARAMETER
Ventricular Function	Left ventricular ejection Fraction < 30% Right ventricular ejection Fraction < 35%
Exercise Tolerance	NYHA class IV symptoms Peak oxygen consumption <14mL/kg/min 6 minute walk test < 300 meters
Cardiac Size	Cardiomegaly by radiography Left ventricular end diastolic diameter >7 cm Left ventricular end diastolic volume >130 mL
Electrolytes	Serum Sodium <134 meq/L
Hemodynamics	Left ventricular stroke work index < 20 g/m² Cardiac index < 2,25 l/min/m² Pulmonary artery occlusion pressure >27 mm Hg
Contractile Reserve	Lack of hemodynamic response to dobutamine
Dysrhythmias	Ventricular tachycardia Atrial fibrillation
Neurohormones	Norepinephrine >600 pg/mL Atrial nitriuretic peptide >125 pg/mL

that all patients with a depressed left ventricular ejection fraction do not manifest congestive symptoms and may not have a decline in exercise tolerance.

EXERCISE TOLERANCE

The assessment of functional class by the New York Heart Association (NYHA) criteria is also of prognostic relevance. Those patients with NYHA class IV category symptomatology (symptoms at rest) are known to have a mortality of 50% at one year.[31] Maximal exercise testing has also been used to predict prognosis in patients with heart failure. Thus, it has been previously shown that patients who can exercise at a peak aerobic capacity of 14 mL/kg/min or less have a significantly worse prognosis than patients who retain a more normal exercise capacity.[32] It is important to point out that measurement of peak aerobic capacity by assessing oxygen consumption needs to be adjusted for age, sex, and size of the patient, which may thus refine the prognostic implications of exercise testing.[33] Furthermore, measurements of peak oxygen consumption can improve or decline over the natural course of the disease process. A more simple and prognostically relevant exercise test, the six-minute walk test, has been recently demonstrated to predict a poor survival in patients with heart failure who are self paced and walk for less than 300 meters in a six-minute period.[34]

CARDIAC SIZE

The simplest roentgenographic measurement of an increased cardiothoracic ratio is known to be a useful parameter for prognostic assessment.[35] Echocardiographic measurements of end-diastolic left ventricular diameter greater than 7 cm, as well as end-systolic volumes greater than 130 mL have been reported as adverse predictors of survival.[36]

HEMODYNAMIC ABNORMALITIES

A cardiac index of less than 2.25 L/min/m², a pulmonary artery occlusion pressure of more than 25 mm Hg, and a right atrial pressure greater than 10 mm Hg are also indicators of a poor prognosis in patients with heart failure.[37] While hemodynamics do appear to segregate prognosis in heart failure patients, it is important to realize that the clinical conditions of some patients do not change even after near normalization of ventricular filling pressures and cardiac output. Moreover, hemodynamic parameters appear to lose their prognostic ability in the presence of chronic refractory symptoms. These observations further emphasize the complexity of the syndrome of heart failure, and underscore the importance of peripheral changes in determining symptomatic syndrome elucidation.

CONTRACTILE RESERVE

Patients with heart failure who do not respond to beta-adrenergic stimulating drugs such as dobutamine have a decreased survival rate.[38] The underlying relevance of this finding may relate to a reduction in beta-receptor density or a possible uncoupling between the beta-adrenergic receptor and the G proteins that are ultimately responsible for cyclic adenosine 5'-monophosphate (AMP) activation.

ELECTROLYTE ABNORMALITIES

A serum sodium less than 134 mEq/L is known to be a poor prognostic indicator.[39] Hyponatremia is a reflection of hyperreninemia, and is a surrogate marker of the degree of activation of the renin-angiotensin-aldosterone system. It has also been demonstrated that a change in serum sodium is more reflective of an acute change in the clinical situation of the patient rather than being a chronic marker of prognosis.[40] In addition, patients with the lowest serum sodium are likely to suffer the greatest hypotension during initiation of ACE inhibitor therapy.

NEUROHORMONAL ACTIVATION

Plasma norepinephrine has been found to be a powerful prognostic indicator. Indeed, Cohn and colleagues[23] have tested this hypothesis in a large multi-center clinical trial and found that a progressive rise in plasma norepinephrine appears to identify patients who are more likely to die from progressive left ventricular dysfunction. Plasma atrial natriuretic peptide has also been found to be increased in patients with ventricular dysfunction, even before the onset of overt congestive heart failure.[41] It has been found that the higher the plasma atrial natriuretic peptide, the more likely the patient is to have biventricular failure and thus a further poor outcome.[27]

ATRIAL AND VENTRICULAR DYSRHYTHMIAS

Sudden death, presumably dysrhythmic, accounts for 50% of all mortality in patients with heart failure. The majority of patients with systolic heart failure have complex ventricular arrhythmias.[42] Thus the presence of complex ventricular arrhythmias is not, by itself, an indication for treatment in patients with heart failure, but appears to identify patients with a poorer prognosis. Similarly, the presence of atrial fibrillation, particularly in the presence of left bundle branch block, is known to identify patients with heart failure that are likely to have a worse outcome.[43]

ETIOLOGY OF HEART FAILURE

An earlier study by Franciosa and colleagues[44] suggested that patients with ischemic cardiomyopathy had a worse prognosis than patients with non-ischemic idiopathic dilated cardiomyopathy. This may be due to intrinsic characteristics that differentiate non-ischemic cardiomyopathy from its ischemic counterpart. Thus, non-ischemic dilated cardiomyopathy is often related to several etiologic factors, particularly those that can be reversed. Certain patients with non-ischemic dilated cardiomyopathy may have myocarditis, a syndrome that is known to manifest spontaneous ventricular recovery. Furthermore, toxic cardiomyopathy, such as those that occur in chronic alcoholic states, or nutritional cardiomyopathy as in beri-beri, may be reversible by removal of the offending factor or by nutritional supplementation.

MISCELLANEOUS PROGNOSTIC FACTORS

Two factors of prognostic importance relate to the presence of severe mitral regurgitation, as well as involvement of the right ventricle in left ventricular cardiomyopathic states. Thus, patients with severe mitral regurgitation and biventricular dysfunction have a worse outcome than patients with univentricular dysfunction in the absence of mitral regurgitation.[45,46]

CLINICAL TRIALS IN THE MEDICAL MANAGEMENT OF HEART FAILURE ■

COOPERATIVE NORTH SCANDINAVIAN ENALAPRIL SURVIVAL STUDY (CONSENSUS)

The Scandinavian Study[47] investigated the use of the ACE inhibitor enalapril in patients with severe (NYHA class IV) symptomatic heart failure. This study demonstrated a 40% reduction in the six-month mortality in the treated patient group. This was the first study that demonstrated a beneficial impact of ACE inhibitors in favorably modulating the natural history of severe heart failure resulting from systolic dysfunction.

VETERANS ADMINISTRATION HEART FAILURE TRIAL (V-HEFT)

The V-HeFT Study[48] was the first trial to demonstrate a survival improvement from any medical regimen utilized for the treatment of mild-to-moderate congestive heart failure. This trial investigated the hypothesis that the addition of a vasodilator to conventional therapy would alter prognosis in heart failure patients and demonstrated that the addition of a combination of hydralazine and isosorbide dinitrate to patients with mild-to-moderate heart failure who remain symptomatic, despite the use of digitalis and a diuretic, leads to a 34% reduction in two-year mortality.

THE STUDIES OF LEFT VENTRICULAR DYSFUNCTION (SOLVD)

Following the foot steps of the CONSENSUS Study, the SOLVD Treatment Trial[49] extended the benefits of ACE inhibitor therapy to patients with mild-to-moderate symptoms of heart failure. Heart failure patients who received conventional therapy with diuretics and digitalis had a 16% reduction in the risk of death when treated with the ACE inhibitor, enalapril, for an average of 40 months, with few side effects. This trial also demonstrated that ACE inhibitor-treated patients were less likely to be hospitalized with heart failure, thereby lessening morbidity.

THE SECOND VETERANS ADMINISTRATION HEART FAILURE TRIAL (V-HEFT-II)

Since the earlier V-HeFT Study had demonstrated a beneficial effect of the vasodilator regimen of hydralazine and isosorbide dinitrate, the investigators designed the second V-HeFT Study[50] to compare this previously proven regimen to enalapril in symptomatic patients with mild-to-moderate heart failure. This study found a survival advantage with the use of the ACE inhibitor enalapril, compared to the vasodilator combination. Interestingly, although mortality was reduced more substantially in the ACE inhibitor group, it was the hydralazine isosorbide-vasodilator combination treated group that experienced the greatest symptomatic relief and hemodynamic improvement. These findings further emphasize the importance of modulation of the neuro-endocrine axis in patients with heart failure and its importance in determining eventual prognosis, and point out that hemodynamic improvement does not necessarily result in a better prognosis.

STUDIES OF LEFT VENTRICULAR DYSFUNCTION PREVENTION ARM (SOLVD-PREVENTION)

The clinical evidence that ACE inhibition may be beneficial in delaying the transition from a state of asymptomatic left ventricular dysfunction to overt clinical heart failure was portrayed in the SOLVD-Prevention Study.[51] This trial examined in excess of 4000 patients with left ventricular ejection fractions of less than 0.35 who were asymptomatic and not receiving any medical therapy for heart failure. This patient group was then randomly assigned to treatment with enalapril or placebo, and demonstrated that the ACE inhibitor-treated group was associated with a greater trend toward reduction in mortality and greater reduction in cardiovascular deaths. This study did not achieve statistical significance in terms of a mortality benefit; however, the reduction in the combined endpoint of development of heart failure and death was statistically significant in patients randomized to receive the drug enalapril.

THE SURVIVAL AND VENTRICULAR ENLARGEMENT TRIAL (SAVE)

The SAVE Study[52] investigated the hypothesis that ACE inhibitors could prevent adverse left ventricular remodeling following myocardial infarction. The clinical rational for the study was obtained from animal studies of myocardial infarction that demonstrated a beneficial influence of ACE inhibitors in attenuating ventricular enlargement. The SAVE Study enrolled patients between day 3 to day 16 following myocardial infarction, who also had evidence of a left ventricular ejection of <0.40. All such patients were asymptomatic from a heart failure a standpoint. The patient group was randomized to receive either a placebo or the ACE inhibitor captopril titrated to a dose range of 50 mg three times daily. This study demonstrated that long-term treatment with captopril lead to reduction in not only all cause mortality, but also cardiovascular deaths as well as the development of clinical heart failure. More surprising was the demonstration of the reduction in the incidence of recurrent myocardial infarctions in the ACE inhibitor-treated group. Furthermore, the benefits of captopril persisted even when examined in relation to other proven therapeutic measures including beta-blockers, aspirin, and the use of thrombolytic therapy.

THE ACUTE INFARCTION RAMIPRIL EFFICACY STUDY (AIRE)

In the AIRE Study,[53] patients with transient signs and symptoms of heart failure following the acute phase of myocardial infarction were randomly assigned to placebo or the ACE inhibitor ramipril. The active therapy group experienced a near 30% reduction in the risk of death. As in the SAVE Trial,

this reduction in mortality was, once again, independent of the use of thrombolytic agents, aspirin, or beta-blockers.

POOLED STUDIES OF ACE INHIBITORS ■

More recently, Garg and Yusuf,[54] on behalf of the ACE inhibitor pooling project, have combined all known placebo-controlled trials of ACE inhibition in symptomatic heart failure patients. This meta-analysis included data from 32 studies, with a total of 7000 patients, and found the overall risk reduction with the use of ACE inhibitors to be 24% for mortality and 37% for a combined endpoint of mortality or hospital admission. It also became evident from this study that the effect of ACE inhibition was seen within three months of therapy, and was most pronounced in the patients with the worst left ventricular function. This meta-analysis also alluded to the possible evidence of a class effect from all various ACE inhibitors.[55] However, it should be emphasized that the majority of patients in this pooled meta-analysis were treated with the drug enalapril.

CLINICAL USE OF ACE INHIBITORS ■

With such clear evidence that ACE inhibitors are beneficial in influencing the natural history of congestive heart failure resulting from systolic dysfunction, it is obvious that the clinician is faced with the mandatory responsibility of initiating ACE inhibitors in all such patients. Therefore, it is important to outline some clinical caveats in the use of ACE inhibition. Dosing of ACE inhibitors in the trials previously mentioned have generally exceeded the doses that are typically used by physicians. Thus, when using enalapril, the dose should be started at 2.5 mg twice per day, and titrated to a tolerated dose of 20 mg twice per day. The mean dose at which benefit has been demonstrated in the clinical trials is a dose of 15 to 17 mg per day. Captopril should be started at 6.25 mg three times per day, and titrated upward to 50% three times daily as tolerated. ACE inhibitors are known to raise serum potassium as well as serum creatinine levels. Other important side effects include symptomatic hypotension, particularly in hyponatremic patients, dry cough, taste alteration and angioedema, which are thought to be related to lack of degradation of bradykinin. It is important to emphasize, however, that in general most trials of ACE inhibitors have demonstrated good patient tolerance, with most side effects being reversible following discontinuation of medication.

ORAL INOTROPIC THERAPY–HOPELESS OR A GLIMMER OF HOPE? ■

The long-term use of oral inotropic support in left ventricular systolic dysfunction has remained controversial because it has been demonstrated that patients receiving certain classes of oral inotropic therapies suffer an adverse outcome. A discussion of major published trials ensues.

RANDOMIZED ASSESSMENT OF DIGOXIN ON INHIBITORS OF THE ANGIOTENSIN-CONVERTING ENZYME (RADIANCE)

In the RADIANCE Study,[56] 178 symptomatic patients with mild-to-moderate congestive heart failure, who were in normal sinus rhythm and receiving digoxin, diuretics, and an ACE inhibitor, were randomly assigned in a double-blind fashion to withdraw or continue with digoxin. This study demonstrated that the patient group in which digoxin was withdrawn suffered a six-fold higher increase in morbidity as assessed by a necessity for change in background therapy, emergency room visits, or hospital admissions.

DIGITALIS INVESTIGATORS GROUP TRIAL (DIG)

The DIG Trial is investigating the hypothesis that the use of digoxin confers a survival benefit in patients with heart failure. This National Institute of Health-sponsored study, dubbed the DIG Trial, is enrolling nearly 7000 patients with ejection fractions less than 0.45 who remain symptomatic on diuretics and ACE inhibitors. Preliminary results of the DIG trial, reported at the American College of Cardiology (March 1996, Orlando, FL), did not find evidence for a survival benefit by the use of digoxin. However, investigators noticed a trend toward decreased hospitalizations. The use of digoxin for systolic dysfunction will remain a controversial matter until final publication of the trial data. However, long-term studies have demonstrated that therapy with digoxin improves left ventricular function in heart failure.[57] Meta-analytical studies have suggested that patients most likely to benefit from the use of digoxin are those with severe systolic dysfunction (left ventricular ejection fraction less than 20%), those that manifest a S_3 gallop and those who are not in sinus rhythm.

PROSPECTIVE RANDOMIZED MILRINONE SURVIVAL EVALUATION (PROMISE)

The oral phosphodiesterase inhibitors, of which oral milrinone is a prototype agent, was studied in the PROMISE Trial[58] by enrolling 1088 patients with moderate-to-severe congestive heart failure. These patients were randomly assigned to oral milrinone over a median period of six months. Unfortunately, this study was terminated early because of a near 30% increase in all cause mortality associated with the use of oral milrinone. This adverse effect was felt to be related to a proarrhythmic effect of phosphodiesterase inhibition. It should, however, be emphasized that the intravenous form of this phosphodiesterase inhibitor continues to play an important role in salvage of the failing heart in acute critical care settings.

PROSPECTIVE RANDOMIZED FLOSEQUINAN LONGEVITY EVALUATION (PROFILE)

Flosequinan, an agent with vasodilator properties, was found to cause an increase in mortality associated with the 100 mg daily dose in the PROFILE Study,[59] a randomized placebo-controlled investigation. Although this drug had been approved by the U.S. Food and Drug Administration in March, 1993 for use in patients who remain symptomatic despite conventional therapy, this drug was withdrawn by the manufacturer after revelation of the study results and is currently unavailable for routine use in the United States.

VESNARINONE

Vesnarinone is a quinolone derivative with effects on sodium channels as well as cardiac potassium channels. In addition, this agent has mild phosphodiesterase inhibition properties, and holds promise as a second-line inotropic drug in addition to digitalis. A recent preliminary study of vesnarinone has demonstrated that patients receiving a 60 mg daily dose of this drug have a survival advantage, with a 60% reduction in all cause mortality by six months.[60] It was interesting to note that in this same trial, the higher 120 mg daily dose administrated was associated with an increased mortality, and that arm had to be terminated early. At this time, the use of this drug remains confined to clinical trials. The results of this drug study demonstrate that non-digitalis inotropic agents have a narrow therapeutic toxic window. Therefore, the appropriate clinical role of these agents awaits more definitive establishment by clinical trials.

PIMOBENDAN MULTI-CENTER RESEARCH GROUP STUDY

Pimobendan is a unique inotropic agent that appears to act by calcium sensitization. This drug is currently the subject of investigation in a clinical trial. To date, this inotropic drug has been shown to increase exercise duration as well as quality of life in patients with heart failure who are already receiving digitalis, diuretics and vasodilators. An initial report from the pimobendan Multi-Center Research Group Study[61] of 198 patients with moderate-to-severe heart failure for three months demonstrated no obvious increase in mortality or adverse outcome.

A SUMMARY OF CLINICAL TRIALS IN ADVANCED HEART FAILURE ■

The clinical trials enumerated above demonstrate that today, the pharmacologic treatment of systolic dysfunction is associated with a beneficial impact on the natural history of congestive heart failure. To that end, the most important revelation has been in the finding of favorable neurohormonal modulation by the use of ACE inhibitors. On the other hand, the story regarding inotropic agents, particularly digoxin, remains unwritten. Most non-digitalis inotropic agents evaluated thus far have demonstrated an adverse outcome in the natural history of heart failure. Vesnarinone appears to be a promising inotropic agent that might provide a second-line inotropic drug, in addition to digitalis. The ongoing challenge is to prevent, limit, or treat the initial insult to the heart, thereby aborting the development of ventricular dysfunction. This has become increasingly obvious by the demonstration that heart failure can be prevented by the use of ACE inhibitors. This interruption in the progressive cycle of ventricular enlargement following an insult is today the most important advance in medical therapeutics in heart failure. The possible mechanisms to explain worse outcomes with inotropic therapy have not yet been explored. However, several hypotheses abound. The enhanced contractility might be accompanied by increased myocardial energy requirements and precipitation of ischemia. Cytosolic calcium overload may have a direct toxic effect upon the myocyte and initiate programmed cell death or necrosis. In addition, accompanying increases in sodium, potassium, and calcium oscillations may trigger arrhythmias. Finally, inotropic agents may impair diastolic relaxation and thus worsen pump function. While several strides have been made in our evolution into an era in the prevention of heart failure, we need to devise other safe therapeutic strategies that can enhance cardiac performance and simultaneously improve survival (Table 117-2).

THE UNIQUE MANAGEMENT OF REFRACTORY ADVANCED SYSTOLIC HEART FAILURE ∎

DEFINITION

Refractory advanced systolic heart failure can be defined as a clinical situation of the persistence of signs and symptoms despite maximal medical therapy. This is an unique patient group that will be frequently encountered by physicians caring for patients in the critical care setting. It is therefore important to compare and contrast the features in the clinical recognition as well as response to therapy that characterize refractory advanced systolic heart failure.

CLINICAL FEATURES

Dyspnea

Dyspnea that follows moderate exertion generally results from anaerobic metabolism and its consequent effect of an activation in the respiratory drive to eliminate carbon dioxide. On the contrary, dyspnea that occurs at rest in patients with refractory heart failure results from elevated intrapulmonary pressures at rest, which become intolerable with any increase in venous return or systemic vascular resistance. Yet, the patients with chronic severe advanced heart failure may demonstrate confirmatory physical evidence of severe congestion only by subtle physical findings. When therapy is targeted to relieve congestion in such patients, they often demonstrate dramatic improvement in exercise tolerance.

Orthopnea, Anorexia, and Gastrointestinal Distress

Orthopnea, anorexia, and *gastrointestinal distress* are often related to systemic venous congestion and also can be usually relieved by therapy targeted at systemic fluid reduction. The most common error in the management of the advanced heart failure patient is in an underestimation of the degree of fluid overload. Orthopnea is a most sensitive clinical indicator of elevated left sided filling pressures, even in the absence of other signs of fluid overload. Many patients who are breathless at rest are told that they do not have heart failure because their lung fields are clear. It is a well-recognized fact that the vast majority of patients with severe symptoms do not demonstrate pulmonary rales even when pulmonary artery occlusion pressures exceed 30 mm Hg. This occurs because of the compensatory effect of pulmonary lymphatics, which can adapt chronically to increase fluid removal almost twenty-fold.[62] Thus, they can relieve congestion in the air spaces that are responsible for rales, but not in the interstitial areas which compromise compliance and diffusion, as well as ventilatory reserve in these patients.

Jugular Venous Distension

Jugular venous distension is often the only physical evidence that a patient's dyspnea is related to elevated intracardiac filling pressures. In fact, peripheral edema is present in

TABLE 117-2. Benefits of Therapy in Heart Failure Due to Systolic Dysfunction

CLINICAL STATUS	ACE INHIBITORS	HYDRALAZINE-ISOSORBIDE	DIGOXIN
Asymptomatic LV dysfunction (EF <40%)	Beneficial	Unknown	Unknown
Mild-moderate heart failure	Beneficial	Beneficial	Under investigation
Severe heart failure	Beneficial	Unknown	Probably beneficial

TABLE 117-3. Reliability of Clinical Signs and Symptoms in Predicting Elevated Left-sided Filling Pressures

MOST SENSITIVE	Orthopnea (90%) Abdominojugular test (90%) Elevated jugular venous pressure (80%)
LEAST SENSITIVE	Pulmonary rales (15%) Peripheral edema (25%)

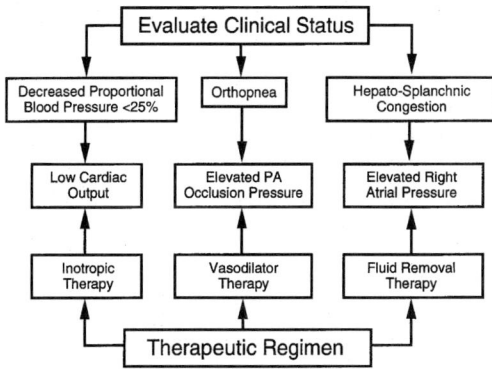

FIGURE 117-3. The clinician must establish the goals of therapy by evaluating the three principle symptoms and signs of cardiac decompensation. Once the clinical status has been established, the clinician must move to structure an individual therapeutic regimen tailored to the patient's needs.

less than one fourth of patients with decompensated heart failure. Table 117-3 demonstrates the clinically established values of physical findings for congestion in advanced chronic heart failure.

Proportional Blood Pressure

Proportional blood pressure is an important physical finding in the patient with advanced heart failure in the presence of sinus rhythm. An arterial pulse pressure of less than 25% of the systolic pressure has been shown to be a reliable indicator of a markedly reduced cardiac index of less than 2 L/min/m^2.[62]

THERAPEUTIC GOALS

Before the clinician plans a therapeutic course for the patient with refractory heart failure, the targets of any therapeutic approach need to be established. As illustrated in Fig. 117-3, the clinician must seek to establish three cardinal findings. First, a patient with orthopnea is most likely to have a pulmonary artery occlusion pressure above 22 mm Hg, thus indicating elevated left ventricular filling pressures. Second, the clinician should seek to establish the presence of hepato-splanchnic congestion as evidenced by the presence of abdominal discomfort, anorexia, and early satiety. Such patients also often have evidence of hepatomegaly on palpation. The third sign that the clinician should seek to establish is that of a reduction in the proportional pulse pressure. As indicated early, patients with a proportional pulse pressure of less than or equal to 25% often manifest a cardiac index of less than 2.2 L/min/m^2. Improvement in these three clinical parameters can often be an effective guide to appropriate therapy and lead to long-term patient symptom relief. Less obvious but equally important clinical benefits include improvement of sleep patterns with a reduction in the incidence of nighttime sleep apnea, as well as an improvement in parameters of nutrition.[63,64]

TAILORED MEDICAL THERAPY ■

As suggested previously, since most of the cardinal symptoms of advanced heart failure result from elevated filling pressures, the most effective therapies are those that target a

reduction in filling pressures. At the outset, it is important to emphasize that it has been inappropriately assumed that the patient with advanced dilated cardiomyopathy may require a higher filling pressure in order to maintain an optimal cardiac output. Experience with treating this distinct patient population has in fact demonstrated that the cardiac output is not only maintained, but frequently maximized by aggressive reduction of ventricular filling pressures largely attributable to the forward redistribution of mitral and tricuspid regurgitant stroke volumes.[65]

HEMODYNAMIC GOALS

Patients with chronic severe heart failure achieve their best cardiac outputs at near normal ventricular filling pressures. A study by Stevenson and Tillisch[66] examined 25 patients with advanced heart failure with an average left ventricular ejection fraction of 0.18, and demonstrated maintenance of stroke volume in relation to pulmonary capillary wedge pressures at near normal ranges. The beneficial influence of lower filling pressures in this patient population is multifactorial: first, it may relate to an improvement in sub-endocardial perfusion resulting from reduction in wall stress; second, a decrease in the filling pressure may occur without an appreciable change in the left ventricular volume, suggesting that the beneficial influence may reflect a decrease in right ventricular distension; and third, a reduction in right atrial and consequent decrease in coronary sinus pressures can result in an improvement in myocardial venous drainage leading to an improved left ventricular compliance and decreased wall stress. In addition, Stevenson and colleagues[67] have demonstrated that the major cause for the higher stroke volume and lower filling pressures appears to be the forward redistribution of regurgitant flow, which often consumes more than 50% of the total left ventricular ejected volume. These observations quite effectively counter an existing myth for the maintenance of higher filling pressures to maintain cardiac outputs in patients with dilated hearts.

TABLE 117-4.   Hemodynamic Goals of Therapy
in Advanced Heart Failure

HEMODYNAMIC PARAMETER	TARGET GOAL
Right atrial pressure	< 8 mm Hg
Pulmonary artery occlusion pressure	< 16 mm Hg
Systolic blood pressure	> 80 mm Hg
Systemic vascular resistance	< 1200 dynes-sec-cm^{-5}

HEMODYNAMIC RESPONSES TO THERAPY AND SURVIVAL

The achievement of precise hemodynamic goals that have been correlated with demonstration of an improved survival in patients with advanced heart failure has been termed tailored medical therapy. The principles underlying tailored medical therapy are illustrated in Table 117-4. In a study that evaluated the importance of hemodynamic response to therapy in predicting survival in patients with advanced left ventricular dysfunction it was demonstrated that the achievement of pulmonary artery occlusion pressures to less than 16 mm Hg was associated with a 50% lower one-year mortality in the patient group despite comparable initial filling pressures at presentation.[68] Indeed, patients who achieved this hemodynamic goal had a one-year survival that was equivalent to that obtained from heart transplantation.

In brief, the hemodynamic goals relate to optimal hemodynamic stabilization by 24 to 48 hours through the use of intravenous diuretics and intravenous vasodilators. The pulmonary artery occlusion pressure should be lowered to less than or equal to 15 mm Hg with a right atrial pressure reduced to less than or equal to 7 mm Hg at a systolic blood pressure of greater than or equal to 80 mm Hg. Once these hemodynamic goals are attained, a titration of high dose oral vasodilators should begin while intravenous therapy is weaned down.

CARDIAC OUTPUT: HOW MUCH IS SUFFICIENT?

It is important to note that a direct increase in cardiac output is not the final goal of therapy for heart failure. In a study of over 600 patients with severe chronic heart failure, the achievement of a cardiac index of above 2.2 L/min/m^2 was not an important predictor of survival.[69] In the same study, however, the achievement of lower filling pressures below the median value of 16 mm Hg was clearly associated with a better survival. This is not meant to de-emphasize the importance of cardiac output for survival and exercise capacity maintenance, as well as maintaining vital organ function. Most recent experience with pharmacologic agents that directly increase cardiac output also suggests that this target results in an increased mortality in patients with advanced heart failure.[58,59] Therefore, it is recommended that the goal for cardiac output should be to maintain a cardiac index of

above 2.2 L/min/m^2; however, it is unclear whether interventions that increase the cardiac output to greater levels produce any greater clinical benefit. It maybe of greater importance to target improvement in exercise cardiac output augmentation rather than rest cardiac output augmentation.

IMPORTANCE OF SYSTEMIC VASCULAR RESISTANCE

One other caveat in the treatment of advanced heart failure patients relates to the presence of severely elevated systemic vascular resistance. Such patients cannot attain normal left ventricular filling pressures even with aggressive diuretics until and unless effective vasodilatation has been initiated. Most patients can achieve targets of improved systemic vascular resistance of 1200 dynes/sec/.cm^{-5}. Thus, therapy aimed at reduction of ventricular filling pressures should not ignore an equal emphasis on reducing systemic vascular resistance to these levels.

PRACTICAL ASPECTS OF INTRAVENOUS INOTROPIC THERAPY ■

The principle use of intravenous inotropic support is in the patient with advanced heart failure who has decompensated with evidence of reduction in systemic blood pressures and a marked reduction in cardiac output that threatens vital organ perfusion. In such clinical situations, intravenous inotropic support can often temporarily improve ventricular performance and achieve clinical stabilization.

MECHANISM OF ACTION

Two major classes of intravenous inotropic therapy are currently approved and available. These include beta-adrenergic agonists such as dobutamine, and phosphodiestrase inhibitors, such as amrinone and milrinone. Both beta-adrenergic stimulation and phosphodiestrase inhibition share a common final pathway in leading to an increase in intracellular cyclic AMP (Fig. 117-4). Cyclic AMP augments

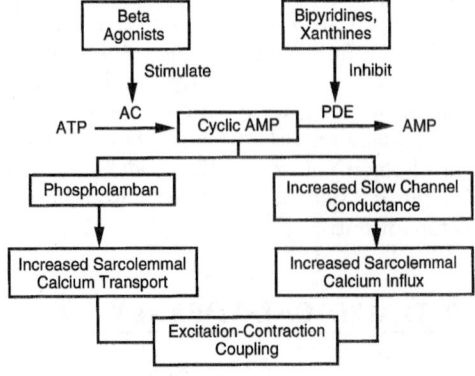

FIGURE 117-4. Simplified schema of the pathways leading to cellular effects of inotropic agents. AC, adenylate cyclase; PDE, phosphodiesterase.

intracellular concentration of calcium via subsequent phosphorylation of several proteins. These actions enhance myocardial contractility, as well as improve diastolic relaxation.

DOBUTAMINE

Dobutamine, a predominant β_1-agonist synthetic catecholamine, produces an increased contractility and reduced aortic impedance, and thereby serves to augment stroke volume and cardiac output while decreasing left ventricular filling pressures. The use of dobutamine in the treatment of advanced heart failure gained widespread acceptance after Leier and colleagues[70] reported symptomatic and hemodynamic improvement by the use of a continuous infusion of intravenous dobutamine. Moreover, these investigators demonstrated that symptomatic relief persisted in 68% of patients for at least one week after therapy with this agent.[71] The precise reasons why persistent clinical improvement occurs in symptoms in exercise performance with intermittent dobutamine infusions have remained a clinical enigma. Unverferth and colleagues[71] assessed ultra-structural changes in 11 patients with heart failure treated with dobutamine by performing an endomyocardial biopsy. These investigators demonstrated a decreased mitochondrial size on electron microscopy, as well as evidence of an improved cristae-to-matrix ratio of mitochondria suggesting improvement in myocardial energetics. However, a careful analysis of the data reveals that these changes probably reflect increases in subendocardial blood flow as well as improvement in chamber size. It has also been suggested that the long-term symptomatic relief may in fact result from improvement in diastolic indices and not just systolic myocardial performance.

Mode of Administration

Dobutamine is generally initiated in a dose of 2.5 µg/kg/min, and titrated upwards to clinical or hemodynamic goals. Some untoward effects such as precipitation or exacerbation of myocardial ischemia are likely related to the metabolic cost of increasing myocardial contractility, which leads to an increase in myocardial oxygen consumption. Other important side effects of this drug, such as ventricular dysrhythmias and myocardial necrosis, may, in part, be related to

cytosolic overloading with calcium. Therefore, it is important to monitor the patients' rhythm when using intravenous inotropic therapy with dobutamine. The development of desensitization of myocardial beta-receptors, which results in the progressive loss of receptor responsiveness to their agonist, represents a major limitation to the long-term persistent use of beta-agonist. To prevent de-sensitization, it has been clinically suggested that dobutamine be used in an intermittent infusion protocol. This can then allow the down-regulated beta-receptors to be up-regulated during periods of lack of exposure to dobutamine.

MILRINONE

The phosphodiesterase inhibitor, milrinone, is usually administered in a loading of dose of 50 µg/kg given over a 20 minute period. A maintenance dose of 0.375-0.75 µg/kg/min is then initiated to achieve hemodynamic and clinical targets. The vasodilatory properties of milrinone are more likely to cause hypotension, particularly in patients with underlying renal insufficiency. Moreover, it is also important to point out that unlike dobutamine, which has a short half-life, milrinone has an average elimination half-life of 108 minutes in moderate-to-severe heart failure.

An important clinical attribute to milrinone is its ability to achieve potent pulmonary vasodilatation, which can be exploited in the presence of severe pulmonary hypertension.[72] An unique side effect related to milrinone is that of thrombocytopenia. However, this is rather uncommon and has been reported to occur only in 0.4% of the patients treated with this agent. Table 117-5 establishes a clinical algorithm for the disparate use of dobutamine, milrinone, or its combination in patients with advanced heart failure.

FLUID REMOVAL IN REFRACTORY HEART FAILURE

DIURETICS

Fluid removal by the use of diuretics remains an integral part of the management of advanced heart failure. Several reports have suggested that continuous intravenous adminis-

TABLE 117-5. Suggested Guidelines for the Selection of Inotropic Agents

	DOBUTAMINE	MILRINONE
Systolic blood pressure <80 mm Hg	First choice in case of cardiogenic hypotension	Usually in combination with another pressor agent
Pulmonary hypertension	Not a good pulmonary vasodilator	First choice; lowers pulmonary vascular resistance
Myocardial ischemia	More taxing on myocardial oxygen demand	First choice; least taxing on myocardial oxygen demand

tration of loop diuretics may be superior to intermittent administration. In a study by Lahav and colleagues,[73] patients with severe heart failure who received a continuous infusion of furosemide, produced a significantly greater diuresis and natriuresis than intermittent bolus infusion of the drug. The mechanisms by which a continuous infusion of diuretics is more effective may be related to the decrease in rapid fluctuations of intravascular volume, thereby causing a relatively constant hourly urine output. In addition, it may also prevent an accumulation of toxic levels of the drug, resulting in fewer and less severe side effects.

In our clinical experience, we have found success with the use of intravenous continuous infusion of the diuretic bumetanide administered over 12 to 24 hours. Of particular clinical importance is the ability to titrate the hourly rate of diuresis in advanced heart failure patients by changing infusion rates. However, a significant number of patients become refractory to intravenous diuretic therapy, and require extra renal removal of fluid by a variety of methods. In fact, extra renal means of fluid removal in advanced heart failure patients have been shown to provide both short- and long-term benefits.

EXTRA-RENAL FLUID REMOVAL

Clinically available modalities for extra renal fluid removal include peritoneal dialysis, chronic ambulatory peritoneal dialysis, isolated ultrafiltration, continuous arterial venous hemofiltration, and intermittent veno-venous hemofiltration. Of these techniques, the latter two have been found to be of the greatest applicability in the refractory patient with advanced heart failure. Several reports have provided insight about the pathophysiologic responses to extra-renal fluid removal in patients with advanced heart failure. Marenzi and coworkers[74] studied the effects of isolated ultrafiltration on 32 consecutive patients. These authors demonstrated that patients refractory to intravenous diuretics who underwent isolated ultrafiltration had a five-fold increase in their post ultrafiltration urinary outputs and a reduction in neurohormonal abnormalities evidenced by a decrease in plasma norepinepherine, renin, and aldosterone levels. Agostini and colleagues[75] investigated long-term effects of isolated ultrafiltration and demonstrated evidence of sustained improvement in exercise capacity with evidence of an improved diuretic sensitivity which could be maintained for up to three months after the initial treatment. In addition, Dileo and coworkers[76] investigated 19 patients with diuretic-resistant advanced heart failure, treated them with machine-driven or arterial pressure-driven hemofiltration and demonstrated a restoration of response to diuretics in 12 of 19 study patients. Misler and Nidus[77] described the use of repeated outpatient intermittent ultrafiltration treatments and demonstrated that weekly treatments of approximately 4 liters of fluid removal were associated with clinical stability in the outpatient setting up to one year. These studies demonstrate that both short- and long-term clinical improvement can be attained with a variety of extra renal fluid removal techniques, and this approach should be utilized in the critical care setting for patients with advanced heart failure who demonstrate diuretic resistance.

NON-PHARMACOLOGICAL CARDIAC ASSISTANCE   ■

Whereas the majority of patients with advanced heart failure may be stabilized with a combination of oral and intravenous pharmacologic therapies, a sizable number of patients, particularly those awaiting heart transplantation, become refractory to such therapeutic support. Therefore, mechanical ventricular assist systems that can effectively bridge patients to heart transplantation have been developed.

BIOLOGIC-ASSIST SYSTEMS

Heterotopic Heart Transplantation

Heterotopic heart transplantation involves use of a donor heart in a parallel circuit to the recipient heart in order to sustain a life-preserving cardiac output. This procedure pioneered by Novitzky and Barnard currently is used principally in patients with severe pulmonary hypertension or large body habitus who would otherwise not qualify for orthotopic cardiac transplantation.[78] The major problem that limits the use of this technique is the fact that problems with the native heart, such as persistence of angina, ischemia and arrhythmic death still can occur.

Cardiomyoplasty

Cardiomyoplasty is a technique that involves using one of the large muscles of the body, usually the latissimus dorsi, to augment cardiac output and support the failing left ventricle.[79] The procedure first requires a prolonged-paced training (12 weeks) of the skeletal muscle to adapt to continuous contractions without fatigue, and once this muscle is adequately trained, it is then wrapped around the heart in order to obtain an increase in ventricular function. Special pacing leads are then attached at multiple points so that synchronized contraction of this muscle can occur in a coordinated fashion with that of the left ventricle. Although this technique has gained widespread use in South America and Europe, it is currently limited to experimental protocols that are investigating its utility in class III advanced heart failure in the United States.

MECHANICAL-ASSIST SYSTEMS

Intraaortic Balloon Counter Pulsation

Intraaortic balloon counter pulsation affords diastolic augmentation of blood pressure with systolic afterload reduction and is the most commonly used mechanical assistance system. It is inserted as a percutaneous system through the femoral artery. The major limitations are a lack of mobility of the patient and predisposition to infection, as well as a high incidence of embolic events causing limb ischemia. In general, the maximum improvement in cardiac index expected by use of this device is of the order of 0.8 L/min/m^2.[80] While this level of augmentation may sound insufficient, it is sometimes enough to stabilize patients until a donor heart can be obtained.

Left Ventricular Assist Devices

Left ventricular assist devices, particularly those that can be implanted into the body are the next level of mechanical support. Several of these are available including the Thoratec device, the Norvacor device, and the Thermocardio Systems Heartmate (Thermocardiosystems, Inc., Woburn, MA). The last of these devices, dubbed the Heartmate, is a pneumatically triggered dual pusher-plate type pump. The distinct advantage of this pump over others is that the blood device interface is such as to cause endothelial cell growth and endothelialization of the pumping chamber. Thus, thrombo-embolic complications from this device have been kept to a minimum. Yet, infection is the major risk with this type of an assistance, since the drive lines disrupt the natural barrier of the skin.

SELECTION CRITERIA FOR IMPLANTABLE VENTRICULAR ASSIST DEVICES

Patients suitable for implantation of the Heartmate left ventricular assist device should have failed conventional medical management and support with an intra-aortic balloon pump. Hemodynamically, these patients should have evidence of systemic hypotension with a reduced cardiac index and chronically elevated pulmonary capillary wedge pressures. Furthermore, patients who also demonstrate evidence of systemic deterioration with evidence of worsening renal and hepatic function should also be considered for mechanical assistance. It should be noted that patients with chronic irreversible renal failure, chronic irreversible liver failure, respiratory failure, severe blood dyscrasias, severe right ventricular dysfunction, and small body surface area are not candidates for implantation of permanent left ventricular assist devices.

After implantation of a left ventricular assist device, early ambulation is begun with initiation of a full-scale rehabilitation program with most patients able to resume normal activity levels within 3 to 4 weeks. Since a relatively normal cardiac output, as well as systemic, renal, and hepatic function are restored, such patients can then be prepared for a safe waiting period until heart transplantation is undertaken. It usually requires 3 to 4 weeks of ventricular assist support to effect systemic restoration of metabolic aberrations and to restore physical conditioning. In essence, patients undergoing such extended ventricular assist device support may become better transplant candidates.[81]

EMERGING PHARMACOLOGIC THERAPEUTICS IN HEART FAILURE

THE USE OF BETA-BLOCKERS IN DILATED CARDIOMYOPATHY

In 1979, Swedberg and colleagues[82] demonstrated a trend towards prolongation of survival in dilated cardiomyopathy by use of beta-receptor blockade. The same group has since reported symptomatic and possible prognostic benefit from the use of beta-blockers in patients with impaired systolic function. It should be noted that the beneficial influence of beta-blockers in heart failure has been reported to have been confined to patients with predominantly dilated non-ischemic cardiomyopathy. The exact mechanism by which beta-adrenergic blockade improves ejection fraction in patients with dilated cardiomyopathy remains a clinical enigma. A recent investigation by Eichhorn and coworkers[83] attempted to elucidate the mechanisms of beta-blocker benefit. These investigators demonstrated that treatment of patients with dilated cardiomyopathy with metoprolol improves myocardial performance and energetics, and favorably alters substrate use. Not only did these authors demonstrate an increase in ejection fraction and left ventricular performance in the metoprolol-treated group, but they also found evidence for a positive relationship between coronary sinus norepinepherine and the myocardial respiratory quotient which suggested that adrenergic deactivation had an important, favorable effect on substrate use. In using beta-blockers in heart failure, the clinician should begin with a very low dose of 6.25 mg twice per day of metoprolol, and gradually titrate weekly up to a dose of 50 mg twice daily. It should be emphasized that, at this time, beta-blockers and patients being contemplated should be selected very carefully; the latter should be well-compensated, and, at least initially, closely monitored. Recent evidence has also pointed to the beneficial impact of the vasodilatory beta-blockers carvedilol and bucindolol in improving survival beyond that provided by ACE inhibitors.[84,85]

ANGIOTENSIN II RECEPTOR ANTAGONISTS

A new class of pharmacological agents that are specific blockers of the angiotensin II receptor have recently become clinically available. All the beneficial hemodynamic effects of ACE inhibitors are well-known, and usually ascribed to the prevention or formation of angiotensin II by these agents. ACE inhibitors affect other neurohormonal systems as well, particularly those involved with bradykinin and substance P. These latter effects are believed to produce deleterious consequences of ACE inhibition including the side effects of cough and angioedema. Thus there is an appealing clinical rationale for considering the use of angiotensin II receptor blockers in heart failure.

First, angiotensin II antagonists may provide an equivalent beneficial effect in hemodynamics in advanced heart failure without the potentially deleterious side effects. Second, it is conceivable that an angiotensin II antagonist could be combined with an ACE inhibitor to yield a synergistic response. A recent study by Gottlieb and colleagues[86] evaluated the hemodynamic and neurohormonal effects of the angiotensin II receptor blocking agent, losartan. It was found that losartan caused vasodilatation in a dose-dependant fashion. Of interest, the reduction in the mean arterial pressure and systemic vascular resistance grew larger to a dose of 25 mg, but the higher doses of the agent did not produce additional vasodilatation. It was noted that in the 24 hours following lorsatan administration, a compensatory increase in the plasma concentration of angiotensin II and plasma renin activity occurred. A recent study by Dickstein and coworkers[87] has demonstrated that the short-term (12 weeks) hemodynamic and neurohormonal influences of losartan compare favorably with the ACE inhibitor enalapril in moderate-to-severe systolic heart failure.

While losartan and its active metabolites represent an exciting new therapeutic class that may have relevance in treating patients who are intolerant to ACE inhibitors because of adverse effects, there is insufficient scientific evidence at this time to recommend their general use as first line agents.

DIASTOLIC DYSFUNCTION: THE OTHER SIDE OF THE COIN ∎

DEFINITION

The term diastolic dysfunction refers to the inability of the ventricle to accept blood at a low ventricular pressure, with an accompanying delay in filling. In order to compensate for these pathologic consequences, the atrial pressure must increase. This leads to diastolic heart failure evidenced by pulmonary or systemic congestion even in the absence of an abnormality in the systolic function of the left ventricle.

ETIOLOGY

There are three major mechanical and physical factors that play a role in determining systolic function of the left ventricle. These include properties of the relaxed ventricle, dynamic properties intrinsic to the myocardium, and factors extrinsic to the myocardium. These three entities are summarized in Table 117-6. Infiltrative myopathies, hypertrophic states, and ischemia typically result in impaired dynamic relaxation of the ventricle. On the other hand, abbreviated filling time, increased wall stiffness, and reduced filling are abnormalities that relate to passive properties of a relaxed ventricle. Similarly, extrinsic factors including pericardial restraint or right ventricular diseases that influence the inter-

TABLE 117-6. Etiology of Pure Diastolic Dysfunction

ABNORMALITIES OF DYNAMIC RELAXATION

Hypertrophic states: aortic stenosis, systemic hypertension, hypertrophic cardiomyopathy
Ischemic states: unstable angina, infarction, exercise related ischemia
Cardiomyopathy: diabetes mellitus

ABNORMALITIES OF A RELAXED VENTRICLE

Reduced filling time: atrial fibrillation
Reduced filling capacity: mitral stenosis
Increased stiffness: amyloidosis, hemochromatosis, endomyocardial fibrosis

EXTRINSIC ABNORMALITIES

Pericardial restraint: constriction, tamponade
Interventricular interaction: right ventricular overload or infarction

action of the right ventricle with the left ventricle by septal function can result in diastolic dysfunction.

PREVALENCE OF ISOLATED DIASTOLIC DYSFUNCTION

In the 1980s, several investigations alluded to the presence of pure isolated diastolic dysfunction. Dougherty and colleagues,[88] as well as Soufer and associates,[89] reported that 30% of patients referred to their nuclear laboratories with the diagnosis of congestive heart failure demonstrated preserved systolic function on radionuclide ventriculography. In the same year, Kunis and colleagues[90] reported a cohort of elderly patients with ischemic heart disease and recurrent pulmonary edema despite normal left ventricular systolic function. These same observations ushered in studies emphasizing the role of diastolic heart failure, particularly in elderly patients, in patients with hypertension, and in those with renal failure undergoing dialysis. Indeed, Topol and colleagues[91] described a syndrome of hypertensive, hypertrophic cardiomyopathy in elderly patients with dyspnea or chest pain.

PROGNOSIS OF DIASTOLIC HEART FAILURE

The natural history of isolated left ventricular diastolic heart failure has not been well defined. In the Veterans Administrative Cooperative Study of patients with congestive heart failure, patients with predominant diastolic dysfunction were found to have a better short-term prognosis than those with systolic dysfunction. The annual mortality was 8% for the cohort with diastolic heart failure, whereas the group with predominantly systolic heart failure had a mortality of 19% during an average follow-up of 2.3 years.[92] In a separate investigation, Brogan and colleagues[93] examined the long-term clinical course of 53 patients with hemodynamic and angiographic evidence of isolated left ventricular dysfunction followed over a period of six years. New onset of heart failure was diagnosed in up to 40% of the patients, while 20% required recurrent hospital admissions. However, only 7.6% of the study group died from cardiovascular causes, alluding to an overall favorable prognosis for this disease entity. Thus, when compared with systolic heart failure, diastolic heart failure appears to be less morbid, and is associated with substantially lower mortality. However, it is important to keep in mind that these investigations do not focus on the transition of diastolic heart failure to systolic heart failure. Furthermore, these data do not apply to diastolic heart failure related to specific causal entity such as aortic stenosis or hypertrophic cardiomyopathy; both of which are associated with substantial morbidity and mortality.

PITFALLS IN THE DIAGNOSIS OF DIASTOLIC HEART FAILURE

Diastolic heart failure is difficult to diagnose. The burden of proof lies on the clinician, and he or she must exclude the possibility of another disorder that might mimic this syndrome. A study by Remes and colleagues[94] suggested that almost half of all diagnoses of heart failure might be explained by etiologic imitations which include underlying pulmonary disease, obesity and reversible ischemia. Thus it is important to note that if the diagnosis is in doubt, other objective tests such as pulmonary function tests and cardiopulmonary exercise testing may help in differentiating noncardiac causes of dyspnea. In a patient presenting with a clinical history of heart failure, it is important to note that these symptoms may occur as a result of intermittent reversible systolic dysfunction. Characteristic situations in which this may be the case include accelerated hypertension and severe coronary disease, both of which can produce transient flash pulmonary edema from profound diminution in systolic performance. In such situations, ventricular function measured after the acute episode may have resolved and may reveal essentially no functional abnormality of performance.[95] With ischemia as a culprit in this situation, it usually represents substantive coronary disease that tends to jeopardize a large part of the myocardium. Furthermore, intermittent and severe mitral regurgitation caused by papillary muscle dysfunction resulting from ischemia can also produce pulmonary edema.

THERAPEUTIC GOALS

The preeminent goal of the clinician in treating diastolic heart failure is first to identify and treat the underlying etiologic disorders. Thereafter, the clinician should concentrate on reduction of systemic and pulmonary congestion, and on maintaining a heart rate and ventricular filling time that is adequate for cardiac performance. In addition, clinicians should attempt to restore atrial booster pump dysfunction if it exists.[96]

CONCLUSION ∎

The past several decades have yielded an increased understanding of the pathophysiologic mechanisms underlying the development of heart failure. This has lead to a more precise and effective treatment of this disease entity and has resulted in a favorable impact in the natural history of this disease. Yet, despite the enormous explosion in our knowledge concerning treatment opportunity of heart failure, we continue to remain oblivious of many aspects of the syndrome. To this end, new approaches that are rigorously tested and derived from sound laboratory principles will be required if future advances are to be made. Whereas the immediate challenge is in the effective recognition and improved therapeutics of patients with advanced heart failure, the challenge for the future lies in preventing the syndrome from ever evolving to its morbid state.

REFERENCES ∎

1. Katz AM: The cardiomyopathy of overload: an unnatural growth response in the hypertrophied heart. *Ann Intern Med* 1994;121:363
2. Weber KT: Cardiac interstitium in health and disease: the fibrillar collagen network. *J Am Coll Cardiol* 1989;13:1637
3. Lee TH, Hamilton MA, Stevenson LW, et al: Impact of left ventricular cavity size on survival in advanced heart failure. *Am J Cardiol* 1993;72:672
4. Wier WG: Cytoplasmic calcium in mammalian ventricle: dynamic control by cellular processes. *Annu Rev Physiol* 1990; 52:467
5. Morgan JP: Abnormal intracellular modulation of calcium as a major cause of cardiac contractile dysfunction. *N Engl J Med* 1991;325:625
6. Siri FM, Krueger J, Nordin C, et al: Depressed intracellular calcium transients and contraction in myocytes from hypertrophied and failing guinea pig hearts. *Am J Physiol* 1991;261: H514
7. Breuckelmann DJ, Nabauer M, Erdman E: Intracellular calcium handling in isolated ventricular myocytes from patients with terminal heart failure. *Circulation* 1992;85:1046
8. Lakatta EG, Talo A, Capogrossi MC, et al: Spontaneous sarcoplasmic reticulum calcium release leads to heterogeneity of contractile and electrical properties of the heart. *Basic Res Cardiol* 1992;87(Suppl 2):93
9. Schaper J, Hein S: The structural correlate of reduced cardiac function in human dilated cardiomyopathy. *Heart Failure* 1993;9:95
10. Levy D, Garrison RJ, Savage DD: Prognostic implications of echocardiographically determined left ventricular mass in the Framingham Heart Study. *N Engl J Med* 1990;322:1561
11. Chapman D, Weber KT, Eghbali M: Regulation of fibrillar collagen types I and III and basement membrane type IV collagen gene expression in hypertrophied rat myocardium. *Circ Res* 1990;67:787
12. Morgan HE, Baker KM: Cardiac hypertrophy: mechanical, neural, and endocrine dependence. *Circulation* 1991;83:13
13. Ghali JK, Cooper R, Ford E: Trends in hospitalization rates for heart failure in the United States—1973–1986: evidence for increasing population prevalence. *Arch Intern Med* 1990; 150:769
14. Kannel WB, Belanger AJ: Epidemiology of heart failure. *Am Heart J* 1991;121:951
15. National Center for Health Statistics: *Health, United States 1990*. U.S. Department of Health and Human Services, DHHS Publication No. (PHS)91-1232. Washington, D.C., U.S. Government Printing Office, 1991
16. Parmley WW: Pathophysiology and current therapy of congestive heart failure. *J Am Coll Cardiol* 1989;13:771
17. McKee PA, Castelli WP, McNamara PM, et al: The natural history of congestive heart failure: the Framingham Heart Study. *N Engl J Med* 1971;285:1441
18. Ho KKL, Anderson KM, Kannel WB, et al: Survival after the onset of congestive heart failure in Framingham Heart Study subjects. *Circulation* 1993;88:107
19. Schocken DD, Arrieta MI, Leaverton PE, et al: Prevalence and mortality rate of congestive heart failure in the United States. *J Am Coll Cardiol* 1992;20:301
20. Teerlink JR, Goldhaber SZ, Pfeffer MA: An overview of contemorary etiologies of congestive heart failure. *Am Heart J* 1991;121:1852
21. Leiberman EB, Hutchins GM, Herskowitz A, et al: Clinicopathologic description of myocarditis. *J Am Coll Cardiol* 1991;18:1617
22. Levine TB, Francis GS, Goldsmith SR, et al: Activity of the sympathetic nervous system and renin-angiotensin system assessed by plasma hormone levels and their relationship to hemodynamic abnormalities in congestive heart failure. *Am J Cardiol* 1983;49:1659
23. Cohn JN, Levine TB, Olivari MT, et al: Plasma norepinephrine as a guide to prognosis in patients with chronic congestive heart failure. *N Engl J Med* 1984;311:819

24. Crawford DC, Chobanian AV, Brecher P: Angiotensin II induces fibronectin expression associated with cardiac fibrosis in the rat. *Circ Res* 1994;74:727
25. Dzau VJ, Re R: Tissue angiotensin system in cardiovascular medicine: a paradigm shift? *Circulation* 1994;89:493
26. Raine AEG, Erne P, Burgisser E, et al: Atrial natriuretic peptide and atrial pressure in patients with congestive heart failure. *N Engl J Med* 1986;315:533
27. Gottleib SS, Kukin ML, Ahern D, et al: Prognostic importance of atrial natriuretic peptide in patients with chronic heart failure. *J Am Coll Cardiol* 1989;13:1534
28. Goldsmith SR, Francis GS, Levine TB, et al: Regional blood flow response to orthostasis in patients with congestive heart failure. *J Am Coll Cardiol* 1983;1:1391
29. Zelis R, Mason DT, Braunwald E: A comparison of the effects of vasodilator stimuli on peripheral resistance vessels in normal subjects and in patients with congestive heart failure. *J Clin Invest* 1968;47:960
30. Cohn JN, Johnson GR, Shabetai R, et al: Ejection fraction, peak oxygen consumption, cardiothoracic ratio, ventricular arrhythmias, and plasma norepinephrine as determinants of prognosis in heart failure. *Circulation* 1993;87(Suppl VI):5
31. Parameshwar J, Keegan J, Sparrow J, et al: Predictors of prognosis in severe chronic heart failure. *Am Heart J* 1992;123:421
32. Mancini DM, Eisen H, Kussmaul W, et al: Value of peak oxygen consumption for optimal timing of cardiac transplantation in ambulatory patients with heart failure. *Circulation* 1991;83:778
33. Richards DR, Mehra MR, Ventura HO, et al: Can maximal oxygen consumption predict outcome of heart failure in women as well as in men: evidence for a gender mismatch. *Circulation* 1995;92(Suppl 1):I402
34. Bittner V, Weiner DH, Yusuf S, et al: Prediction of mortality and morbidity with a 6-minute walk test in patients with left ventricular dysfunction. *JAMA* 1993;270:1702
35. Gradman A, Deedwania P, Cody R, et al: Predictors of total mortality and sudden death in mild to moderate heart failure. *J Am Coll Cardiol* 1989;14:464
36. White HD, Norris RM, Brown MA, et al: Left ventricular end-systolic volume as the major determinant of survival after recovery from myocardial infarction. *Circulation* 1987;76:44
37. Unverferth DV, Majorien RD, Moeschberger ML, et al: Factors influencing the one-year mortality of dilated cardiomyopathy. *Am J Cardiol* 1984;54:147
38. Dubois-Rande J-L, Merlet P, Roudot F, et al: Beta adrenergic contractile reserve as a predictor of clinical outcome in patients with idiopathic dilated cardiomyopathy. *Am Heart J* 1992;124:679
39. Lee WH, Packer M: Prognostic importance of serum sodium concentration and its modification by converting-enzyme inhibition in patients with severe chronic heart failure. *Circulation* 1986;73:257
40. Saxon LA, Stevenson WG, Middlekauff HR, et al: Predicting death from progressive heart failure secondary to ischemic or idiopathic dilated cardiomyopathy. *Am J Cardiol* 1993;73:62
41. Francis GS: Determinants of prognosis in patients with heart failure. *J Heart Lung Transplant* 1994;13:S113
42. Stevenson WG, Stevenson LW, Middlekauff HR, et al: Sudden death prevention in patients with advanced ventricular dysfunction. *Circulation* 1993;88:2953
43. Middlekauff HR, Stevenson WG, Stevenson LW: Prognostic significance of atrial fibrillation in advanced heart failure. *Circulation* 1991;84:40
44. Franciosca JA, Wilen M, Ziesche S, et al: Survival in men with severe chronic left ventricular failure due to either coronary artery disease or idiopathic dilated cardiomyopathy. *Am J Cardiol* 1983;51:831
45. Ventura HO, Murgo JP, Smart FW, et al: Current issues in advanced heart failure. *Med Clin North Am* 1992;76:1057
46. Polak JF, Holman BL, Wynne J, et al: Right ventricular ejection fraction: an indicator of increased mortality in patients with congestive heart failure associated with coronary artery disease. *J Am Coll Cardiol* 1983;2:217
47. The CONSENSUS Trial Study Group: Effects of enalapril on mortality in severe congestive heart failure: results of the Cooperative North Scandinavian Enalapril Survival Study (CONSENSUS). *N Engl J Med* 1987;314:1429
48. Cohn JN, Archibald DG, Ziesche S, et al: Effect of vasodilator therapy on mortality in chronic congestive heart failure: results of a Veterans Administration Co-operative Study. *N Engl J Med* 1986;314:1547
49. The SOLVD investigators: Effect of enalapril on survival in patients with reduced left ventricular ejection fractions and congestive heart failure. *N Engl J Med* 1992;325:293
50. Cohn JN, Johnson G, Ziesche S, et al: A comparison of enalapril with hydralazine-isosorbide dinitrate in the treatment of chronic congestive heart failure. *N Engl J Med* 1992;325:303
51. The SOLVD investigators: Effect of enalapril on mortality and the development of heart failure in asymptomatic patients with reduced left ventricular ejection fractions. *N Engl J Med* 1992;327:685
52. Pfeffer MA, Braunwald E, Moye LA, et al: Effect of captopril on mortality and morbidity in patients with left ventricular dysfunction after myocardial infarction: results of the survival and ventricular enlargement trial. *N Engl J Med* 1992;327:669
53. The Acute Infarction Ramipril Efficacy (AIRE) Study Investigators: Effect of ramipril on mortality and morbidity of survivors of acute myocardial infarction with clinical evidence of heart failure. *Lancet* 1993;342:821
54. Garg R, Yusuf S, for the Collaborative Group on ACE Inhibitor Trials: Overview of randomized trials of angiotensin-converting enzyme inhibitors on mortality and morbidity in patients with heart failure. *JAMA* 1995;273:1450
55. Mehra MR, Ventura HO: Commentary on "ace inhibitors reduce mortality and hospitalization in congestive heart failure." *ACP J Club* 1995;123:62
56. Packer M, Gheorghiade M, Young JB, et al: Withdrawal of digoxin from patients with chronic heart failure treated with angiotensin-converting-enzyme inhibitors. *N Engl J Med* 1993;329:1
57. Arnord SB, Byrd RC, Meister W, et al: Long-term digitalis therapy improves left ventricular function in heart failure. *N Engl J Med* 1980;303:1443
58. Packer M, Carver JR, Rodeheffer RJ, et al: Effect of oral milrinone on mortality in severe chronic heart failure. *N Engl J Med* 1991;325:1468
59. Packer M, Rouleau J, Swedberg K, et al: Effect of flosequinan on survival in chronic heart failure: preliminary results of the PROFILE study [abstract]. *Circulation* 1993;88(Suppl 1):I301
60. Feldman AM, Bristow MR, Parmley WW, et al: Effects of vesnarinone on morbidity and mortality in patients with heart failure. *N Engl J Med* 1993;329:149
61. Kubo SH, Gollub S, Bourge R, et al: Beneficial effects of pimobendan on exercise tolerance and quality of life in patients with heart failure: results of a multi-center trial. *Circulation* 1992;85:942
62. Stevenson LW, Perloff JK: The limited reliability of physical signs for the estimation of hemodynamics in chronic heart failure. *JAMA* 1989;261:884
63. Ribero JP, Knutzen A, Rocco MB, et al: Periodic breathing during exercise in severe heart failure. *Chest* 1987;92:555
64. Carr JS, Stevenson LW, Heber D, et al: Prevalence and hemodynamic correlates of malnutrition in severe heart failure sec-

ondary to ischemic or idiopathic dilated cardiomyopathy. *Am J Cardiol* 1989;63:709

65. Hamilton MA, Stevenson LW, Child JS, et al: Sustained reduction in valvular regurgitation and atrial volumes with tailored vasodilator therapy in advanced congestive heart failure secondary to dilated cardiomyopathy. *Am J Cardiol* 1991;67:259

66. Stevenson LW, Tillisch JH: Maintenance of cardiac output with normal filling pressures in dilated heart failure. *Circulation* 1986;74:1303

67. Stevenson LW, Brunken RC, Belil D, et al: Afterload reduction with vasodilators and diuretics decreases mitral valve regurgitation during upright exercise in advanced heart failure. *J Am Coll Cardiol* 1990;15:174

68. Stevenson LW, Tillisch JH, Hamilton MA, et al: Importance of hemodynamic response to therapy in predicting survival with ejction fraction <20% secondary to ischemic or non-ischemic dilated cardiomyopathy. *Am J Cardiol* 1990;66:1348

69. Stevenson LW, Fonarow G, Hamilton MA, et al: Why cardiac output is not a good hemodynamic target for therapy in advanced heart failure. *Circulation* 1994;90:I611

70. Leier CJ, Webel J, Bush CA: The cardiovascular effects of the continuous infusion of dobutamine in patients with severe cardiac failure. *Circulation* 1977;56:468

71. Unverferth DV, Magorien RD, Altschuld R, et al: The hemodynamic and metabolic advantages gained by a three-day infusion of dobutamine in patients with congestive cardiomyopathy. *Am Heart J* 1983;106:29

72. Colucci WS, Wright RS, Jaski BE, et al: Milrinone and dobutamine in severe heart failure: differing hemodynamic effects and individual patient responsiveness. *Circulation* 1986;73 (Suppl 3):175

73. Lahav M, Regev A, Ra'anani P, et al: Intermittent administration of furosemide vs continuous infusion preceded by a loading dose for congestive heart failure. *Chest* 1992;102:725

74. Marenzi G, Grazi S, Giraldi F, et al: Interrelation of humoral factors, hemodynamics and fluid and salt metabolism in congestive heart failure: effects of extracorporeal ultrafiltration. *Am J Med* 1993;94:49

75. Agostini P, Marenzi G, Laurie G, et al: Sustained improvement in functional capacity after removal of body fluid with isolated ultrafiltration in chronic cardiac insufficiency: failure of furosemide to provide the same result. *Am J Med* 1994;96:191

76. DiLeo M, Pacitti A, Bergerone A, et al: Ultrafiltration in the treatment of refractory congestive heart failure. *Clin Cardiol* 1988;11:449

77. Misler S, Nidus BD: Long term ultrafiltration as a treatment of refractory congestive heart failure. *NYS J Med* 1984;518

78. Novitsky D, Cooper D, Barnard C: The surgical technique of heterotopic heart transplantation. *Ann Thorac Surg* 1983;36:476

79. Carpentier A, Chachques JC, Ascar C, et al: Dynamic cardiomyoplasty at seven years. *J Thorac Cardiovasc Surg* 1993;106:42

80. Birovljev S, Radovancevic B, Burnett CM, et al: Heart transplantation after mechanical circulatory support: four years' experience. *J Heart Lung Transplant* 1992;11:240

81. Oz MC, Rose EA, Levin HR: Selection criteria for placement of left ventricular assist devices. *Am Heart J* 1995;129:173

82. Swedberg K, Waagstein F, Hjalmarson A, et al: Prolongation of survival in congestive cardiomyopathy by beta-receptor blockade. *Lancet* 1979;1:1374

83. Eichhorn EJ, Heesch CM, Barnett JH, et al: Effect of metoprolol on myocardial function and energetics in patients with non-ischemic dilated cardiomyopathy: a randomized, double blind, placebo-controlled study. *J Am Coll Cardiol* 1994;24:1310

84. McTavish D, Campoli-Richards D, Sorkin EM: Carvedilol: a review of its pharmacodynamic and pharmacokinetic properties and therapeutic efficacy. *Drugs* 1993;45:232

85. Woodley SL, Gilbert EM, Anderson JL, et al: Beta-blockade with bucindolol in heart failure caused by ischemic versus idiopathic dilated cardiomyopathy. *Circulation* 1992;84:2426

86. Gottlieb S, Dickstein K, Fleck E, et al: Hemodynamic and neurohormonal effects of the angiotensin II antagonist losartan in patients with congestive heart failure. *Circulation* 1993;88:1602

87. Dickstein K, Chang P, Willenheimer R, et al: Comparison of the effects of losartan and enalapril on clinical and exercise performance in patients with moderate or severe chronic heart failure. *J Am Coll Cardiol* 1995;26:438

88. Dougherty AH, Naccarelli GV, Gray EL, et al: Congestive heart failure with normal systolic function. *Am J Cardiol* 1984;54:778

89. Soufer R, Wohlgelernter D, Vita NA, et al: Intact systolic left ventricular function in clinical congestive heart failure. *Am J Cardiol* 1985;55:1032

90. Kunis R, Greenberg H, Yeoh CB, et al: Coronary revascularization for recurrent pulmonary edema in elderly patients with ischemic heart disease and preserved ventricular function. *N Engl J Med* 1985;313:1207

91. Topol EJ, Traill TA, Fortuin NJ: Hypertensive hypertrophic cardiomyopathy of the elderly. *N Engl J Med* 1985;312:277

92. Cohn JN, Johnson G, Veterans Administration Cooperative Study Group: Heart failure with normal ejection fraction: the V-HeFT study. *Circulation* 1990;81(Suppl III):48

93. Brogan WC, Hillis LD, Flores ED, et al: The natural history of isolated left ventricular diastolic dysfunction. *Am J Med* 1992;92:627

94. Remes J, Miettinen H, Reunanen A, et al: Validity of clinical diagnosis of heart failure in primary health care. *Eur Heart J* 1991;12:315

95. Dodek A, Kassebaum DG, Bristow JD: Pulmonary edema without cardiomegaly: ischemic cardiomyopathy and the small stiff heart. *Am Heart J* 1972;85:281

96. Mehra MR, Lavie CJ, Ventura HO: Diastolic dysfunction. What role does it play in heart failure? *Intern Med* 1995;16:12

Critical Care, Third Edition, edited by Joseph M. Civetta,
Robert W. Taylor, and Robert R. Kirby.
Lippincott-Raven Publishers, Philadelphia, PA © 1997.

CHAPTER 118

∎

Valvular Heart Disease

W. Ross Davis

IMMEDIATE CONCERNS ∎

Valvular disease in the critically ill can be considered in two primary categories: patients who are critically ill as a result of valvular heart disease, and patients who are critically ill from other causes but have concomitant valvular disease. Of greatest concern is left heart valvular disease, although in selected patients right heart valvular lesions can be important. Hemodynamic consequences of decompensated valvular lesions include pulmonary venous hypertension with pulmonary edema or diminished cardiac output with tissue hypoperfusion. Management is determined by the type of lesion and its hemodynamic consequences and is modified by coexisting derangements. Determination of the hemodynamic derangement by invasive monitoring and continuous measurement of mixed venous oxygen saturation, transcutaneous estimation of arterial oxygen saturation, and calculated cardiovascular variables such as left ventricular stroke-work index, systemic vascular resistance, and pulmonary vascular resistance can be useful.

Patients with life-threatening valvular disease generally present to the critical care unit with one or more manifestations of congestive heart failure that must be stabilized (see Chap. 117) before proceeding further. Two levels of diagnosis must then be established. The first level involves defining the type and degree of valvular heart disease. The second level of diagnosis involves determination of acute precipitating events in the patient's deterioration. These can include uncontrolled hypertension, noncompliance with diet or medication regimens, infection, pulmonary embolism, myocardial infarction, cardiac dysrhythmia, abrupt changes in the valvular lesion, endocrine abnormalities (particularly diabetic ketoacidosis or hyperthyroid crisis), and acute renal failure.

Critically ill patients with valvular heart disease must receive infectious endocarditis prophylaxis when procedures having high risk for bacteremia are performed (Chap. 120).

CRITICAL ILLNESS CAUSED BY VALVULAR HEART DISEASE ∎

Although valvular disease is often apparent on physical examination, detection may be made difficult by environmental noise, pulmonary rhonchi, or other factors. Further, with severe aortic or mitral stenosis and a failing left ventricle, cardiac murmurs may be unimpressive or even absent. Early performance of echocardiography is imperative in patients with unexplained heart failure. If the quality of the transthoracic echo is not optimal, transesophageal echocardiography should be performed. Electrocardiography frequently reveals the existence of concomitant ischemic heart disease, left ventricular hypertrophy, atrial abnormalities, arrhythmias, or right ventricular hypertrophy. Portable plain film chest radiography can be invaluable in revealing pulmonary venous or arterial hypertension, pulmonary edema, and lung parenchymal abnormalities and in allowing evaluation of the cardiac contour. Because of the distortion produced by anteroposterior supine radiographs, every effort should be made to obtain sitting 183-cm (72-inch) posteroanterior radiographs when the patient's condition allows.

Once both levels of diagnosis have been made, an estimate of the reversibility of the hemodynamic defect is possible and plans for management can be developed. Specific management decisions depend on the lesion present, its inherent physiology, and the presence of complicating factors.

It is common for patients to be critically ill from other causes and have concomitant valvular disease. The effect on the management plan made by the valvular disease is determined by the resultant hemodynamic burden, the presence of other cardiac abnormalities, and the degree of other physiologic derangements.

COMPLICATING CARDIAC VALVULAR DISEASE IN CRITICALLY ILL PATIENTS ■

Because these patients present with other illnesses, valvular disease is often detected only by the discovery of cardiac murmurs on physical examination, valve calcification or cardiac contour abnormalities on chest radiograph, or unexplained evidence of left ventricular hypertrophy or atrial abnormality on electrocardiogram (ECG). When abnormalities are suspected, Doppler echocardiography is the most useful diagnostic tool for defining the extent of valvular abnormality.

Once the valvular abnormality is defined, its impact on the management plan can be determined by consideration of its severity and specific hemodynamic characteristics (see later sections). All valve lesions have several common considerations, however. Many procedures undertaken in the intensive care unit (ICU) are indications for infectious endocarditis prophylaxis. Fever and other abnormalities that increase peripheral oxygen demand may not be well tolerated and should be treated vigorously. Paroxysmal tachycardia, sinus tachycardia, and atrial fibrillation, which can adversely affect left ventricular filling times and lead to hemodynamic deterioration, should be aggressively treated. Definitive treatment of arrhythmias might include the judicious use of digoxin, intermittent or constant infusion of verapamil or other antiarrhythmic drugs, or, in extreme cases, urgent cardioversion.

CONSIDERATIONS IN SPECIFIC VALVULAR ABNORMALITIES ■

The delivery of care to the critically ill patient is a challenging endeavor that does not lend itself to the development of standard approaches. Rather, appropriate therapy is most effectively delivered when care is individualized on the basis of a careful analysis of specific abnormalities and a good understanding of the physiology, possible causes, natural history, and differential diagnosis. Because abnormalities of the cardiac valves are common, an understanding of these aspects of each valvular lesion is imperative.[1,2]

MITRAL STENOSIS

ETIOLOGY.   Almost all mitral stenosis in adults is of rheumatic origin. Uncommon causes include congenital mitral stenosis, carcinoid syndrome, rheumatoid arthritis, systemic lupus erythematosus, and the mucopolysaccharidases.

PATHOPHYSIOLOGY.   Mitral stenosis produces a resistance to flow from the left atrium into the left ventricle, resulting in increased left atrial and pulmonary venous pressures. Resting mitral flow rates remain normal until the resistance becomes extremely elevated, but flows can be maintained with exercise or stress only by an increased left atrial–left ventricular pressure gradient. Any physiologic state that causes an increase in cardiac output (e.g., exercise, fever, anxiety, pain) or a decrease in diastolic filling time (e.g., tachycardia, atrial fibrillation) increases mitral valve flow rates and left atrial pressure. Some patients with severe mitral stenosis also develop an abnormally high pulmonary vascular resistance. Pulmonary arterial hypertension occurs in severe disease. In advanced cases, pulmonary hypertension causes right ventricular dysfunction. Cardiac output at rest is generally preserved until the disease is far advanced, but cardiac output response to exercise or other stresses may be blunted. As the disease progresses, resting cardiac output is also reduced. Left ventricular function is generally normal in patients with pure mitral stenosis. The presence of cardiogenic pulmonary edema or low cardiac output does *not* imply left ventricular dysfunction.

PRESENTATION.   Patients with decompensated mitral stenosis generally present with pulmonary edema. Findings of low cardiac output are uncommon and, in the absence of pulmonary edema, suggest coexisting disease. Any of the precipitating causes discussed previously can cause decompensation in patients with mitral stenosis; however, atrial fibrillation, pregnancy, and infectious endocarditis are likely to cause decompensation. Physical findings of mitral stenosis include a loud first heart sound, an opening snap, and a typical diastolic low-frequency rumbling murmur. Auscultatory findings of mitral stenosis may be minimal in low-flow states.

DIAGNOSTIC STUDIES.   There are no specific ECG findings for mitral stenosis. Atrial fibrillation is present in 40% to 50% of patients. If the patient remains in sinus rhythm, P-mitral and left atrial abnormalities are common. Right axis deviation and right ventricular hypertrophy, when present, suggest pulmonary hypertension and are ominous signs. If left ventricular hypertrophy is present, additional cardiac lesions are likely.

Radiographic findings include pulmonary venous hypertension and left atrial enlargement. In uncomplicated mitral stenosis, the left ventricle and right heart are normal. Right heart enlargement implies pulmonary arterial hypertension. Left ventricular enlargement implies additional cardiac lesions, such as mitral regurgitation or ischemic heart disease.

Echocardiography is diagnostic for mitral stenosis. Pulmonary hypertension may be evident by Doppler study. When well visualized, the area of the mitral orifice can be determined during the two-dimensional study or by Doppler study.

THERAPEUTIC CONSIDERATIONS.   In the absence of additional cardiac lesions, left ventricular function should be normal. Therefore, if patients are hypotensive or have inadequate peripheral perfusion, treatments that augment left ventricular performance are not likely to be helpful. Early invasive testing to define measures of cardiovascular function may be helpful. Pulmonary artery occlusion pressures in mitral stenosis do not correlate with left ventricular diastolic pressure but do provide information about the patient's pulmonary venous pressures and propensity to develop pulmonary edema.

Patients with mitral stenosis are extremely sensitive to changes affecting mitral valve flow rates. Conditions that increase cardiac output such as fever, pain, anxiety, tachycardia, and atrial fibrillation should be aggressively treated. Emergency surgery or valvuloplasty is rarely, if ever, required. Indeed, if the precipitating event is one that can be controlled well (e.g., atrial fibrillation, pregnancy, hyperthyroidism), surgical intervention may not be required for several years.

Thromboembolic events are common, and anticoagulation should be established when possible. Patients with thromboembolic events should be considered for early surgical intervention, once stabilized, because the risk of recurrent embolization is high.

MITRAL REGURGITATION

Mitral regurgitation is common in the critically ill. Most patients have chronic mitral regurgitation as one of several problems. Occasional patients have acute mitral regurgitation as a cause of hemodynamic decompensation.

Chronic Mitral Regurgitation

ETIOLOGY. Patency of the mitral apparatus depends on structural and functional integrity of the mitral leaflets, the mitral annulus, the chordae tendineae, the papillary muscles, the left atrium, and the left ventricle.[3] Disruption of anatomy or abnormalities of function of any of these structures can result in regurgitation. There are, therefore, many potential causes for mitral regurgitation. Chronic rheumatic heart disease, isolated rupture of chordae tendineae, mitral valve prolapse, ischemic papillary muscle dysfunction, and infectious endocarditis account for most cases.[4]

PATHOPHYSIOLOGY. Mitral regurgitation causes a reduction in left ventricular afterload and an increase in left ventricular preload. The reduction in afterload results from reduced resistance to ventricular emptying because the low-pressure, high-compliance left atrium is in parallel with the high-pressure, low-compliance aorta. The increase in preload results from the increased volume presented to the ventricle in diastole. This ventricular volume overload is symptomatically well tolerated because of the reduction in wall stress afforded by mitral regurgitation for any given aortic pressure and left ventricular diastolic volume. Significant loss of myocardial function may occur before the onset of symptoms. A gradual increase in severity allows the left atrium to increase in size and compliance so that the pulmonary vascular bed is usually spared any increases in pressure until late in the course of the disease. The degree of regurgi-

tant flow depends on orifice size and on the ventricular–atrial pressure gradient. Both of these may change significantly with changes in systolic blood pressure, contractility, and preload. Because of the interaction of decreased wall stress and reduced afterload in severe mitral regurgitation, clinical indices of systolic function, such as the ejection fraction (EF), used to estimate the contractile state of the left ventricle, are unreliable. For example, the EF in mitral regurgitation is generally increased when contractility is normal; a normal EF usually indicates a significant loss of myocardial function, and by the time the EF is reduced to 50% or less, advanced myocardial dysfunction is generally present.

Chronic mitral regurgitation can be subdivided into two groups, with different physiologic origins and management needs. The primary form is caused by anatomic or functional disruption of the mitral apparatus. Secondary mitral regurgitation results from severe left ventricular dysfunction from other causes. The differentiation is often difficult, but several factors are useful. In primary cases, the degree of regurgitation is severe, with regurgitant fractions greater than 0.5. Indices of left ventricular function such as the EF are usually high, normal, or modestly reduced, and the left atrium tends to be massively enlarged. In secondary cases, the degree of regurgitation tends to be moderate, with regurgitant fractions less than 0.4. Left ventricular EF is severely decreased, and left atrial enlargement tends to be moderate.

PRESENTATION. In the absence of a precipitating event or a second hemodynamic abnormality, patients with chronic primary mitral regurgitation are rarely critically ill on presentation. Patients with secondary mitral regurgitation frequently present with pulmonary edema or cardiogenic shock caused by decompensation of left ventricular function.

The cardiac rhythm is frequently irregularly irregular. The peripheral pulses have a collapsing quality. The apical impulse is sustained and enlarged. An apical systolic thrill may be present. A left parasternal lift is more likely related to the enlarged left atrium than to right ventricular involvement. Auscultation may reveal a soft first heart sound and a widely split second sound. A third heart sound is common. The murmur of mitral regurgitation is pansystolic and radiates toward the left axilla. Louder murmurs imply more severe regurgitation. The intensity of the murmur does not change greatly with varying cardiac cycle lengths.

DIAGNOSTIC STUDIES. The ECG frequently reveals atrial fibrillation. If normal sinus rhythm is present, a left atrial abnormality in lead V_1 is common. Findings of left ventricular hypertrophy or enlargement are usually present.

Chest radiography reveals pulmonary venous hypertension late in the course of primary disease; this finding is frequent in secondary disease. The left atrium is enlarged, as is the left ventricle. Right heart enlargement is common in secondary disease and unusual in primary disease.

Echocardiography is useful in differentiating primary and secondary disease because left ventricular function and anatomic features of the mitral apparatus are readily defined. Doppler studies not only detect the presence of mitral regurgitation but also give quantitative data. In secondary disease, the mitral leaflets are normal or mildly thickened and typically have a reduced excursion. The left ventricle is enlarged, and left ventricular function is markedly reduced. Findings in primary mitral regurgitation may include leaflet thickening, mitral valve prolapse, flail leaflet, or papillary muscle dysfunction; left ventricular function is generally normal, and the pattern of contraction is that of left ventricular enlargement with vigorous contraction.

THERAPEUTIC CONSIDERATIONS. In critically ill patients, the differentiation of primary from secondary mitral regurgitation is important because management may be different. The critically ill patient with secondary mitral regurgitation requires treatment of the underlying left ventricular failure (Chap. 117).

Management of the decompensated patient with primary mitral regurgitation includes a careful evaluation for precipitating causes, because abrupt decompensation is not an expected part of the natural history of the disease. Hypertensive crisis, infectious endocarditis, and chordae tendineae, or papillary muscle rupture, are of particular concern. Vasodilators and diuretics play a central role in treating decompensated patients with primary disease[5]; positive inotropic agents also may be useful because of the inherent myocardial dysfunction. Digoxin may play a role in intermediate to long-term management. Because of their undesirable effects on afterload, agents that primarily increase peripheral vascular resistance, such as norepinephrine and metaraminol, should be avoided if possible.

The patient who is critically ill from other causes requires careful control of blood pressure and volume status: increases can lead to a disproportionate increase in regurgitant volume and left ventricular preload.

Acute surgical intervention is rarely required to stabilize patients with either primary or secondary mitral regurgitation. Only if there is superimposition of severe, acute mitral regurgitation should surgery be required (see the following section). Mitral valve replacement or repair is not expected to be beneficial in patients with secondary disease and is rarely indicated. Patients with primary mitral regurgitation who present with decompensation should be considered for elective valve surgery after stabilization.

Acute Mitral Regurgitation

Acute mitral regurgitation is frequently unrecognized on initial presentation. When appropriately diagnosed, medical stabilization is usually possible, but early surgical intervention is usually necessary.[6]

ETIOLOGY. The cause of acute mitral regurgitation is abrupt disruption of part of the mitral apparatus, with resultant significant valvular insufficiency. Although there are many possible etiologies, the most common is rupture of the chordae tendineae, resulting in a flail leaflet. Such disruption can be spontaneous or can result from infectious endocarditis or mitral valve prolapse. Papillary muscle rupture or dysfunction is less common. Of particular concern is rupture of a papillary muscle head after myocardial in-

farction (usually 2 to 7 days). Rarely, perforation of the mitral valve leaflets causes acute mitral regurgitation.

PATHOPHYSIOLOGY. The incompetent mitral valve causes ejection of a significant portion of the left ventricular stroke volume into the left atrium; however, because the chambers are not dilated, the increases in volume are accompanied by significant increases in systolic left atrial and diastolic left ventricular pressures. These pressure abnormalities affect the pulmonary vascular bed, with resultant pulmonary venous hypertension and, in severe cases, pulmonary edema and pulmonary arterial hypertension.

PRESENTATION. Most patients are in good health before the abrupt onset of symptoms. The intensity of symptoms is related to the severity of regurgitation, and symptoms can range from cardiogenic shock to pulmonary edema (most common) to exertional dyspnea. Patients with papillary muscle rupture frequently describe recent chest discomfort consistent with a myocardial infarction. Occasionally, patients may present with acute onset of fatigue, dyspnea, and chest pain.

Physical examination reveals a triad of findings that strongly suggests acute mitral regurgitation. Sinus tachycardia is the expected rhythm. The presence of atrial fibrillation suggests preexisting disease. A new or changed apical systolic murmur is present. The murmur of acute mitral regurgitation is early systolic or systolic-decrescendo in quality because of equalization of left ventricular and left atrial pressures in mid-systole to late systole. A prominent fourth heart sound is usually heard and excludes chronic mitral regurgitation because the dilated left atrium of the chronic form has poor contractility and cannot produce an audible fourth heart sound. The carotid impulse generally has a rapid upstroke and decline. The apical impulse is hyperdynamic but not displaced. Early closure of the aortic valve leads to a widely split second heart sound. A third heart sound is typical. Because of the increased flow through the mitral valve, a diastolic rumble similar to that of mitral stenosis is common.

DIAGNOSTIC STUDIES. There are no diagnostic ECG changes, but once the diagnosis is established, the ECG may be helpful in determining the cause. Atrial fibrillation or left ventricular hypertrophy suggests preexisting cardiac disease. Right ventricular strain or enlargement suggests pulmonary hypertension. Papillary muscle dysfunction is suggested by Q waves of myocardial infarction.

The chest radiograph is usually striking, revealing marked pulmonary venous hypertension and pulmonary edema in the presence of a normal cardiac contour.

Echocardiography is useful in defining the anatomic abnormality and in excluding several conditions that may mimic acute mitral regurgitation. Flail leaflets are easily visualized, as is the typical wall motion abnormality and valve leaflet motion of papillary muscle dysfunction. Vegetations caused by infectious endocarditis are occasionally seen. Doppler studies can identify regurgitant flow and demonstrate the typical flow pattern of acute mitral regurgitation.

Pulmonary artery catheterization reveals a typical large V wave in the pulmonary artery occlusion trace.

THERAPEUTIC CONSIDERATIONS.   Vasodilators such as nitroprusside are the principal pharmacologic agents useful in treating acute mitral regurgitation. Inotropic agents are generally not useful unless systemic resistance is low and hypotension is present. Sinus tachycardia is a physiologic response to the hemodynamic lesion and should not be treated in most circumstances. Monitoring of systemic and pulmonary artery pressures is usually required. Patients who do not stabilize with vasodilators should have intraaortic balloon counterpulsation established. Early valve surgery is lifesaving in many patients, including those with papillary muscle disruption after myocardial infarction. Delay of surgical intervention is inadvisable.

AORTIC STENOSIS

Obstruction to left ventricular outflow can be valvular, subvalvular, or supravalvular.[7] Supravalvular lesions are rarely encountered in adults. Subvalvular discrete lesions are uncommon but important when present. Subvalvular dynamic lesions (idiopathic hypertrophic subaaortic stenosis [IHSS] and other hypertrophic obstructive cardiomyopathies) rarely present with symptoms limited to outflow obstruction and are best considered a type of cardiomyopathy (see Chap. 117). Valvular aortic stenosis is the cause of left ventricular outflow tract obstruction in most patients seen in the ICU.

ETIOLOGY.   Most patients with congenitally abnormal and inherently stenotic aortic valves are discovered in childhood, adolescence, or young adulthood during routine physical examination. Patients who present later in life have usually acquired aortic stenosis as a result of traumatic heart disease, calcific degeneration of a bicuspid valve, or senile calcific degeneration of a normal valve. Uncommon causes include atherosclerosis, rheumatoid valvulitis, and ochronosis.

PATHOPHYSIOLOGY.   Aortic stenosis produces an increase in systolic left ventricular pressures. Concentric left ventricular hypertrophy results, allowing the wall stress to remain normal.[8] The less compliant, thickened left ventricle becomes more dependent on the atrial contribution to diastolic filling, such that left ventricular performance can deteriorate when atrial contraction is lost during atrial fibrillation or atrial–ventricular dissociation. Cardiac output is usually normal at rest but may not increase normally with exercise or stress. Myocardial oxygen consumption increases because of the increased myocardial mass and left ventricular afterload. Oxygen delivery is limited by relative shortening of diastole and the effects of high intracavitary pressures. Acute imbalances can result in angina pectoris, pump failure, or paroxysmal arrhythmias. Relatively early in the course, right ventricular compliance may decrease because of hypertrophy of the septum.

Late in the course, the ability of the ventricle to compensate by concentric hypertrophy is exceeded. The ventricle then dilates and cardiac function is maintained by Frank-Starling mechanisms. Myocardial contractility, however, declines rapidly, and the patient is at risk for decompensation. As the left ventricle fails, pulmonary venous hypertension, reduced cardiac output, and pulmonary arterial hypertension develop.

PRESENTATION.   Symptomatic patients typically present with congestive heart failure, angina pectoris, syncope, or, uncommonly, systemic embolization. Patients may occasionally present with infectious endocarditis. Rarely, patients present with cardiogenic shock; these patients represent a particularly difficult management challenge.

Physical examination typically reveals pulses with a delayed rise and small amplitude (pulsus parvus et tardus). A shudder may be appreciated in the carotid pulse. A systolic thrill may be present at the base of the heart. Examination of the jugular venous wave typically reveals prominent A waves. Palpation of the precordium discloses a sustained apical impulse and may demonstrate a presystolic impulse. With the onset of left ventricular failure, the apical impulse becomes displaced inferiorly and laterally. Auscultation reveals a normal or soft first heart sound and a prominent fourth heart sound. The second heart sound is typically single. Aortic stenosis produces a crescendo-decrescendo murmur that ends before the second heart sound. Increased duration and intensity of the murmur as well as late peaking of intensity are indicators of severe stenosis. If the valve is mobile, an early systolic opening click may be present, localizing the outflow obstruction to the valve. As the left ventricle fails, the intensity and duration of the murmur declines because of diminished aortic valve flow. For this reason, the presence of congestive heart failure, low-amplitude carotid impulses, and a systolic basilar heart murmur of any intensity should alert the intensivist to the possibility of critical, life-threatening aortic stenosis.

DIAGNOSTIC STUDIES.   The ECG is helpful in diagnosing aortic stenosis. Sinus rhythm is typical. Atrial fibrillation, in the absence of heart failure, is frequently a clue to the coexistence of other abnormalities. Left atrial enlargement may be present and does not imply concomitant mitral valve disease or other disorders. Most patients have left ventricular hypertrophy, although its absence does not exclude severe aortic stenosis. Left ventricular strain is less common but indicates severe aortic stenosis. Abnormalities in conduction, such as incomplete atrioventricular block, bundle branch block, and intraventricular conduction delay are common.

Chest radiography before the onset of left ventricular failure typically demonstrates a left ventricular configuration without cardiomegaly, a dilated ascending aorta, and, on careful analysis of the lateral radiograph, calcification of the valve cusps. Once the left ventricle begins to decompensate, cardiomegaly and pulmonary venous hypertension become apparent.

Echocardiography is most useful in localizing left ventricular outflow obstruction. Thickening and calcification of the aortic valve are apparent in cases of valvular disease, and typical findings of discrete subvalvular, supravalvular, or dynamic subvalvular stenosis are easily appreciated. Routine studies cannot accurately estimate the degree of stenosis, but Doppler studies can frequently quantitate the degree of stenosis and also allow the detection of associated valve lesions, such as aortic insufficiency or mitral regurgitation.[9]

THERAPEUTIC CONSIDERATIONS. Because of changes in compliance with left ventricular hypertrophy, patients with aortic stenosis are extremely volume sensitive and can develop pulmonary edema secondary to diastolic dysfunction before systolic function deteriorates. For this reason, quantification of systolic function is important in patients with aortic stenosis and pulmonary edema. Cardiogenic pulmonary edema does *not* imply that systolic left ventricular dysfunction is present. Similarly, volume requirements in patients with aortic stenosis who are critically ill from other causes should be carefully assessed. When one is unsure, hemodynamic monitoring is advisable. If the left ventricle is dilated and has reduced systolic function, inotropic agents can be helpful in improving cardiac output.

Initial modalities for treating pulmonary edema are diuretics and sodium restriction. Predominantly venous vasodilators, such as nitroglycerin, may be helpful but should be used with caution after systemic and pulmonary arterial pressure monitoring is established. Balanced or predominantly arterial vasodilators such as nitroprusside should be used carefully. In the patient with moderate aortic stenosis and cardiac dysfunction from other causes, these agents may augment cardiac output by reducing left ventricular afterload. Arterial pressure monitoring and extreme caution are imperative with the use of these drugs.[10]

Any patient who is admitted to an ICU for care of the sequelae of aortic stenosis should be strongly considered for early elective valve surgery because of the unfavorable natural history of unoperated symptomatic aortic stenosis.[11] Patients presenting with cardiogenic shock from critical aortic stenosis have an extremely high hospital mortality. Most of these patients can be stabilized with medical therapy but generally remain critically ill. Once the acute decompensation has been controlled and the patient is stabilized, urgent valve replacement should be considered.

A significant amount of effort recently has been placed into the development of nonsurgical means of relieving aortic obstruction. In the cardiac catheterization laboratory, most patients with symptomatic aortic stenosis, including those who are critically ill, can receive aortic valvuloplasty with initial mortality and morbidity comparable with a traditional surgical approach. Unfortunately, the degree of improvement in the valvular obstruction is often minimal, although adequate to acutely relieve symptoms. Further, most patients (approximately 60%) who have initial success with valvuloplasty re-stenose over the first 6 months to 1 year. Currently, aortic valvuloplasty should be reserved for patients who have a short anticipated life span from other disease, for those who are elderly and in poor health, or for patients with severe decompensation who may benefit from an emergency valvuloplasty, allowing surgery to be performed more safely after initial improvement.

Significant aortic stenosis is a major determinant of cardiovascular risk for noncardiac surgery. Careful evaluation of risk is required for critically ill patients with aortic stenosis for whom noncardiac surgical procedures are indicated.

AORTIC REGURGITATION

Patients presenting to the ICU with decompensated aortic regurgitation or with compensated aortic regurgitation and other critical illness can be subgrouped as having chronic or acute aortic regurgitation; most have the chronic form.

Chronic Aortic Regurgitation

Patients with chronic aortic regurgitation are well compensated for long periods before decompensation and occasionally are aware of their disorder. When decompensation occurs, an acute precipitating factor is probably responsible.[12]

ETIOLOGY. Aortic regurgitation can arise from a plethora of causes that produce distortion or perforation of the valve leaflets or distortion of the aortic root. Common causes of valve leaflet damage include rheumatic fever, infectious endocarditis, trauma, degeneration of a bicuspid valve, or rheumatoid disease. Diseases that cause aortic regurgitation by dilatation of the ascending aorta include annuloaortic ectasia, cystic medial necrosis (frequently associated with Marfan's syndrome), syphilitic aortitis, ankylosing spondylitis, and aortic dissection.

PATHOPHYSIOLOGY. The amount of regurgitation is determined by three factors: the area of the regurgitation valve orifice, the duration of diastole, and the diastolic pressure gradient between the aorta and left ventricle. Aortic regurgitation results in volume overload of the left ventricle. The ventricle compensates by dilatation and eccentric hypertrophy. Stroke volume increases so that forward output is maintained. Left ventricular diastolic pressures remain normal until late in the disease. After a period of years, left ventricular compliance decreases and ventricular diastolic pressures increase, myocardial contractility declines, and pulmonary venous hypertension develops. Eventually, cardiac output falls and pulmonary arterial hypertension and right ventricular failure develop.

PRESENTATION. Patients with the chronic form may present with decompensation or with another critical illness complicated by aortic regurgitation. In decompensated patients, pulmonary edema is common, but decreased cardiac output, peripheral hypoperfusion, and hypotension are sometimes found. Angina pectoris may be present because of either coronary artery disease or imbalances in myocardial oxygen delivery and demand.

Examination typically reveals a wide pulse pressure and a low diastolic blood pressure. Systolic pressure may be normal or elevated. There are several possible peripheral findings, including a to-and-fro motion of the head synchronous with the cardiac cycle, cyclic change in pupil size, pulsations in the liver or uvula, and enlarged spleen. A rapidly rising and collapsing peripheral pulse is typical. Carotid pulsations may be bisferious, with a palpable thrill even in the absence of aortic stenosis. Palpation of the precordium reveals the apical impulse to be sustained, enlarged, and displaced. Auscultation reveals a normal or soft first heart sound. The second heart sound is typically normal. A fourth sound is common and indicates left ventricular hypertrophy. When heart failure develops, a third sound is present. The murmur of aortic regurgitation, best heard at the left upper sternal border, is a decrescendo high-pitched diastolic murmur that is normally relatively soft. The duration of the murmur correlates with the severity of aortic regurgitation. A systolic ejection murmur caused by an increased stroke volume is commonly heard. Occasionally, patients have the Austin-Flint murmur, a low-frequency diastolic murmur similar to that of mitral stenosis.

DIAGNOSTIC STUDIES. The ECG typically reveals left axis deviation and left ventricular diastolic volume overload pattern (prominent Q waves in leads I, aVL, and V_3 through V_6, with tall peaked T waves). Later in the disease, ST segments are depressed, with inverted T waves. Conduction abnormalities are more common when aortic regurgitation is caused by calcific valve disease or inflammatory processes.

Chest radiography typically reveals left ventricular enlargement. Pulmonary venous hypertension is seen late in the disease. The ascending aorta is typically prominent, but significant enlargement or widening of the mediastinum may be clues to the presence of aortic dissection. Calcification may be present in the aortic valve.

Echocardiography reveals a left ventricular volume-overload pattern in compensated disease and an enlarged, poorly contracting ventricle in decompensated disease. Anatomic information may be gained about the aortic valve and aortic root. High-frequency diastolic oscillations are frequently seen on the anterior leaflet of the mitral valve. Doppler studies can quantitate the amount of aortic regurgitation and document the existence of other valve lesions.[13]

THERAPEUTIC CONSIDERATIONS. For pulmonary edema, diuretics are most useful, but venous or arterial vasodilators are also helpful. Patients with reduced cardiac output frequently respond to vasodilators, inotropic agents, or a combination thereof. In patients with chronic aortic regurgitation who present with acute decompensation, there should be an aggressive search for a precipitating cause, with particular attention to possible infectious endocarditis. Intraaortic balloon counterpulsation is absolutely contraindicated because aortic regurgitation is increased by the device.

Most patients stabilize with medical therapy, but early elective valve surgery should be considered because the outlook for medically treated symptomatic disease is poor. Decompensated patients who do not improve with aggressive medical therapy should undergo emergency valve replacement. Mortality with medical therapy alone in this group approaches 100%, and many moribund patients survive with surgery.[12]

Maneuvers that increase afterload also increase the regurgitant fraction and should be avoided if possible.

Acute Aortic Regurgitation

Acute aortic regurgitation is an uncommon cause of critical illness. Recognition is important because the physical findings may be subtle and early surgical intervention is imperative for a good outcome.[14]

ETIOLOGY. Acute aortic regurgitation most frequently results from infection of a bicuspid aortic valve.[15] Rupture of the valve as a result of chest trauma is infrequent. Aortic dissection, spontaneous rupture of a valve with myxomatous degeneration, and fenestrations are uncommon causes of acute aortic regurgitation.

PATHOPHYSIOLOGY. In acute aortic regurgitation, the left ventricle does not have time to compensate for the diastolic volume overload. As a result, ventricular dilatation is limited and left ventricular diastolic pressures are extremely high. Left atrial and pulmonary venous pressures also rise, but partial protection is afforded by early diastolic closure of the mitral valve if it is competent. Pulmonary edema commonly results. Because the stroke volume does not increase in proportion to the regurgitant volume, a hypoperfusion state is common. Reflex sinus tachycardia results. Aortic and ventricular pressures equilibrate early in diastole, so there is little decrease in aortic diastolic pressures. Because forward stroke volume is changed only slightly, aortic systolic pressures do not rise. The net result is that aortic pulse pressure does not widen. Peripheral vascular resistance increases.

PRESENTATION. These patients are usually extremely ill on presentation; many are moribund. There are gradations of severity, however, and occasional patients are not extremely ill. The onset is typically the abrupt, catastrophic deterioration of a previously healthy person. Almost all have pulmonary edema. Many have evidence for diminished cardiac output. Patients with closed chest trauma may present several days after the event and may have little other evidence of significant chest injury. Patients with aortic dissection may have associated findings such as asymmetric pulses, stroke, myocardial infarction, or pericardial tamponade.

The patient with severe acute aortic regurgitation appears extremely ill. Careful attention should be given to stigmata of Marfan's syndrome, which strongly suggest the presence of a ruptured valve or aortic dissection. The heart rate is rapid, and differentiation of systole and diastole may be difficult. The pulse pressure is not widened. The peripheral findings of chronic aortic regurgitation are typically absent. Palpation of the precordium may be unremarkable. An abrupt, mid-diastolic bulge coinciding with a third heart sound is sometimes present. The auscultatory findings are usually subtle. The first heart sound is soft or absent because of early closure of the mitral valve. The second sound is variable. Atrial contraction may not open the mitral valve, so a fourth sound may not be present. A third heart sound is typical. The diastolic murmur is short, ending when aortic and ventricular diastolic pressures equalize, and is often surprisingly soft. A soft aortic systolic flow murmur may be present. The Austin-Flint murmur is a frequent finding.

DIAGNOSTIC STUDIES. The ECG is often normal except for sinus tachycardia. Evidence for left ventricular hypertrophy implies a preexisting cardiac abnormality. Nonspecific ST and T wave abnormalities are common.[16]

The chest radiograph can exclude other possible diagnoses and provide anatomic data useful in establishing an etiology. The cardiac silhouette in acute aortic regurgitation is not usually enlarged; cardiomegaly implies a preexisting abnormality or a different diagnosis. A dilated ascending aorta suggests the presence of aortic dissection. Pulmonary venous hypertension and pulmonary edema are expected.

Echocardiography can demonstrate the physiology of acute aortic regurgitation nicely, showing the early closure and late opening of the mitral valve. Important information is gained about the etiology if valve vegetations, leaflet redundancy, or evidence of aortic dissection are seen. Perhaps the most important use of echocardiography, however, is to suggest or exclude other diagnoses. For example, a dilated left ventricle or left ventricular hypokinesis makes isolated acute aortic regurgitation unlikely.

THERAPEUTIC CONSIDERATIONS. By far the most common cause of acute aortic regurgitation is infectious endocarditis. The possibility of aortic dissection is significant enough to warrant thoracic computed tomography or transthoracic echocardiography. Pulmonary edema should be treated with diuretics. Some authors think that digitalis use is warranted.[17] Inotropic agents may be useful in treating inadequate cardiac output, but vasodilators are more likely to be effective. Careful monitoring of arterial and pulmonary artery pressures is important. Inotropic agents should be avoided in patients with aortic dissection.

Medical interventions should be used only to stabilize the patient's condition in preparation for definitive emergency surgery. Although consideration is often given to delaying surgery to allow longer antibiotic therapy in patients with infectious endocarditis, this approach carries a significant risk of sudden decompensation because these patients can seldom be stabilized long enough for a full course of antibiotic therapy.

TRICUSPID VALVE DISEASE

Tricuspid valve disease is common among patients presenting to the ICU but rarely requires specific treatment.

Tricuspid Regurgitation

Tricuspid regurgitation is common in critically ill patients but is often unrecognized.

ETIOLOGY. Tricuspid regurgitation is most often a consequence of pulmonary hypertension or right ventricular dysfunction and is designated functional or secondary in such cases. Disruption of the tricuspid valve and resultant incompetence (primary tricuspid regurgitation) is less common and can result from an array of causes, including rheumatic fever, trauma,[18] tricuspid valve prolapse, and, particularly in drug addicts, infectious endocarditis.

PATHOPHYSIOLOGY. Tricuspid regurgitation results in a volume overload of the right atrium and ventricle. In the absence of preexisting right ventricular failure or pulmonary hypertension, the condition is often asymptomatic. Such patients may develop progressive right heart failure after many years. Tricuspid regurgitation worsens the hemodynamic effects of pulmonary hypertension and right ventricular dysfunction, resulting in diminished cardiac output and peripheral congestion.[19]

PRESENTATION. Patients with the secondary form typically present with findings of their primary disease in addition to the findings of tricuspid regurgitation, which include weakness and fatigue, ascites, peripheral edema, hepatic congestion with mild jaundice, anorexia, and wasting. In addition, patients with primary tricuspid regurgitation from infectious endocarditis frequently have evidence for multiple pulmonary septic infarctions. When the underlying cause is rheumatic fever, rheumatic mitral valve disease is invariably the predominant lesion.

Physical examination is usually dominated by findings specific for the primary disorder. Findings associated with the tricuspid regurgitation itself are typically unimpressive and include increased jugular venous pressure with a prominent V wave and loss of the x descent. The liver may be pulsatile. The pansystolic murmur is typically located at the lower left sternal border but may occasionally be heard better over the xiphoid. The murmur classically increases with maneuvers that increase venous return, such as inspiration. A left parasternal presystolic or systolic lift is common.

DIAGNOSTIC STUDIES. There are no specific ECG findings for tricuspid regurgitation, although an increased frequency of atrial fibrillation and incomplete or complete right bundle branch block have been noted.

The results of the chest radiography may vary widely, depending on the effects of the underlying primary disease. Findings typical of tricuspid regurgitation include increased systemic venous pressure (demonstrated by a dilated azygous vein) and an enlarged right heart.

Doppler echocardiography is the best diagnostic tool. Associated cardiac lesions, pulmonary hypertension, and right heart chamber enlargement also can be detected.

THERAPEUTIC CONSIDERATIONS. Tricuspid regurgitation rarely requires specific treatment. In the secondary form, treatment should be geared toward the primary lesion. In the primary type, treatment is directed toward the immediate cause. Decompensated patients with primary tricuspid regurgitation are so rare that the diagnosis should always be questioned. When it is confirmed, gentle diuresis to relieve peripheral congestion may be helpful. Patients with infectious endocarditis of the tricuspid valve and persistent infection despite adequate antimicrobial therapy can, in the absence of pulmonary hypertension, tolerate removal of the valve and delayed replacement.

Tricuspid Stenosis

Tricuspid stenosis is extremely uncommon, occurring almost exclusively in association with rheumatic mitral stenosis.[20,21]

ETIOLOGY. For all practical purposes, the condition is always rheumatic in origin.

PATHOPHYSIOLOGY. Obstruction to right atrial outflow caused by tricuspid stenosis results in elevated systemic venous pressures and in right atrial enlargement. In advanced cases, cardiac output may be low. Systemic venous hypertension may result in peripheral edema, hepatic congestion, and ascites. The obstruction to atrial emptying may moderate the effects of mitral stenosis on the pulmonary vasculature.

PRESENTATION. These patients usually present with findings attributable to their concomitant mitral stenosis but have systemic venous hypertension disproportionate to the degree of pulmonary congestion. Peripheral edema, ascites, and hepatomegaly are common. An accentuated A wave is present in the jugular venous contour. The murmur is usually presystolic when sinus rhythm is present but may be mid-diastolic in atrial fibrillation. It is most prominent at the lower left sternal border and characteristically increases dramatically in intensity with inspiration.

DIAGNOSTIC STUDIES. The ECG is nonspecific. Most patients have sinus rhythm. Findings of right ventricular hypertrophy are typically absent, but right atrial enlargement, with tall P waves in the inferior leads (leads II, III, and aVF) is common. The typical chest radiography reveals an enlarged right atrium without evidence for pulmonary hypertension. Echocardiography is usually confirmatory by demonstrating the typical anatomic findings of tricuspid stenosis in addition to mitral stenosis.

THERAPEUTIC CONSIDERATIONS. Specific treatment is rarely required. Therapy is directed toward the associated mitral stenosis, which usually is the cause of acute decompensation. Atrial fibrillation may be particularly poorly tolerated. Peripheral edema can be treated with gentle diuresis and sodium restriction, but caution is necessary because right and left ventricular filling characteristics may be adversely affected and cardiac output may fall. Definitive treatment is surgical, combined with mitral valve surgery.

PULMONIC VALVE DISEASE

Pulmonic valve disease is an extremely rare cause of admission to an adult ICU. Management considerations are usually directed toward other disorders.

Pulmonic Stenosis

ETIOLOGY. Pulmonic stenosis is usually congenital. Severe forms or those associated with other cardiac anomalies are generally identified and treated in childhood. Subvalvular and supravalvular obstructions to right ventricular outflow are usually congenital; an exception is acquired infundibular stenosis from pulmonary hypertension.

PATHOPHYSIOLOGY. Pulmonic stenosis causes obstruction to right ventricular outflow. Right ventricular hypertrophy results, and, if right ventricular failure or tricuspid regurgitation develops, systemic venous hypertension can result.

The degree of stenosis, once established, tends to be stable; if decompensation does not occur in childhood, subsequent deterioration is unlikely.[22] Occasionally, patients manifest increasing right ventricular outflow obstruction, perhaps caused by secondary infundibular hypertrophy.

PRESENTATION. Fatigue, atypical chest pain, and syncope are the usual presenting complaints of patients who have severe pulmonic stenosis. When right ventricular failure or tricuspid regurgitation occurs, systemic venous hypertension may be present. Elevated right atrial pressures in the presence of a patent foramen ovale or atrial septal defect can result in a right-to-left shunt at the atrial level.

Physical examination typically reveals a large jugular venous A wave. In the absence of right ventricular failure or tricuspid regurgitation, jugular venous pressure remains normal. A left parasternal systolic lift is common with significant pulmonic stenosis. The murmur is best heard at the left upper sternal border and typically radiates to the left clavicle. A palpable thrill may be present. The intensity of the murmur does not correlate well with severity, but increasing duration and late systolic peaking are indicators of significant stenosis. An ejection click is usually present. As severity increases, the pulmonic component of the second heart sound is increasingly delayed; thus, wide splitting of the second sound indicates more severe stenosis.

DIAGNOSTIC STUDIES. The ECG is normal in mild pulmonic stenosis. With increasing severity, findings of right ventricular hypertrophy are common. The presence of criteria for right atrial enlargement indicates severe stenosis.

The chest radiograph does not correlate well with severity of disease but does display several typical findings. The most characteristic is an enlargement of the pulmonary trunk and left pulmonary artery, with a relatively normal right pulmonary artery. An increased heart size indicates end-stage disease or a concomitant disorder.

Echocardiography is particularly useful because characteristic changes in the pulmonic valve pattern can be documented by the M-mode study; a typical anatomic deformity can be seen on the two-dimensional study; and Doppler evaluation of blood flow can document turbulent, high-velocity flow. Right heart chamber sizes and wall thickness also can be documented.

THERAPEUTIC CONSIDERATIONS. Pulmonic stenosis rarely requires specific therapy, even in critically ill patients. Patients presenting with right heart failure, chest discomfort, or syncope should be considered for surgical intervention, usually on an elective basis.

Pulmonic Insufficiency

Pulmonic insufficiency generally has a benign course as an isolated abnormality.[23] The natural history is that of the associated lesions.

ETIOLOGY. Insufficiency may be secondary to pulmonary hypertension or, rarely, to leaflet damage caused by infectious endocarditis, rheumatic fever, or carcinoid syndrome. Occasionally, pulmonic insufficiency is congenital.

PATHOPHYSIOLOGY.   In the absence of pulmonary hypertension, the volume overload of the right ventricle is well tolerated. Decompensation with resulting right ventricular failure can occur when pulmonary hypertension develops from other causes.

PRESENTATION.   Pulmonic insufficiency is usually an incidental auscultatory finding in patients admitted to the ICU for other reasons. Physical findings include the typical decrescendo diastolic murmur along the upper left sternal border. The intensity of the murmur does not correlate well with the severity of regurgitation.

DIAGNOSTIC STUDIES.   The ECG is usually normal. The presence of right ventricular hypertrophy suggests pulmonary hypertension.

The chest radiograph is normal in mild insufficiency. The pulmonary trunk may be prominent when the insufficiency is moderate to severe. Pulmonary hypertension may be present.

Echocardiography with Doppler study can be useful for differentiating pulmonic from aortic insufficiency and for establishing right heart chamber sizes and associated abnormalities.

THERAPEUTIC CONSIDERATIONS.   Specific treatment is rarely required. Therapy should be directed toward control of pulmonary hypertension, when present. When the right heart fails, diuretics and sodium restriction are useful. Some authors suggest that cardiac glycosides are helpful.

MULTIVALVULAR DISEASE

Combined valve disease is common.[24] As previously mentioned, tricuspid regurgitation, mitral regurgitation, and pulmonic insufficiency can be secondary to other cardiac lesions, including diseases of other valves. In these circumstances, management is generally directed toward the primary lesion. Primary multivalvular disease is common in rheumatic disease. The effect of several lesions is a combination of the effects of each lesion.

Mitral Stenosis Plus Aortic Regurgitation

Approximately two thirds of patients with mitral stenosis have a diastolic murmur at the upper sternal border; 90% of these murmurs are caused by aortic regurgitation. Only about 5% to 10% are associated with clinically significant left ventricular volume overload.

Aortic Stenosis Plus Mitral Stenosis

Obstruction to left atrial emptying from mitral stenosis may mask some of the effects of aortic stenosis. Augmentation of ventricular filling by atrial contraction is impaired, and thus an important compensatory mechanism for maintenance of cardiac output by the hypertrophied ventricle is blunted or lost. Pulmonary venous congestion, atrial fibrillation, and systemic embolization, all predominantly manifestations of mitral stenosis, tend to be accentuated.

Aortic Regurgitation Plus Mitral Regurgitation

The combination of aortic and mitral regurgitation is relatively common. Both lesions result in left ventricular volume overload. Findings referable to aortic insufficiency usually predominate. Severe regurgitation through both valves is poorly tolerated because of severe pulmonary venous hypertension.

Mitral Regurgitation Plus Aortic Stenosis

Aortic stenosis is not often seen with mitral regurgitation, but the combination, when present, has particularly deleterious hemodynamic consequences. The resistance to left ventricular outflow worsens the mitral regurgitation, with resultant loss of effective stroke volume and severe pulmonary venous hypertension. Physical findings with this combination of abnormalities may be particularly confusing, because the effects on the peripheral pulses are diametrically opposed and the murmurs both occur in systole.

REFERENCES ∎

1. Hungenholtz PG, Ryan TJ, Stein SW, et al: The spectrum of pure mitral stenosis: hemodynamic studies in relation to clinical disability. *Am J Cardiol* 1962;10:773
2. Dalen JE: Mitral stenosis. In: Dalen JE, Alpert JS (eds). *Valvular Heart Disease*. Boston, Little, Brown, 1981:41
3. Roberts WC, Perloff JK: Mitral valvular disease: a clinicopathologic survey of the conditions causing the mitral valve to function abnormally. *Ann Intern Med* 1972;77:939
4. Waller BF, Morrow AG, Maron BJ, et al: Etiology of clinically isolated severe, chronic, pure mitral regurgitation: analysis of 97 patients over 30 years of age having mitral valve replacement. *Am Heart J* 1982;104:276
5. Harshaw CW, Grossman W, Munroe AB, et al: Reduced systemic vascular resistance as therapy for severe mitral regurgitation of valvular origin. *Ann Intern Med* 1975;83:312
6. DePace NL, Nestico PF, Morganroth J: Acute severe mitral regurgitation: pathophysiology, clinical recognition and management. *Am J Med* 1985;78:293
7. Roberts WC: Valvular, subvalvular and supravalvular aortic stenosis: morphologic features. *Cardiovasc Clin* 1973;5:97
8. Sassayama S, Ross J Jr, Franklin D, et al: Adaptations of the left ventricle to chronic pressure overload. *Circ Res* 1976;38:172
9. Hatle L: Noninvasive assessment and differentiation of left ventricular outflow tract obstruction with Doppler ultrasound. *Circulation* 1981;64:381
10. Greenberge BH, Massie BM: Beneficial effects of afterload reduction therapy in patients with congestive heart failure and moderate aortic stenosis. *Circulation* 1980;61:1212
11. Carabello BA, Green LH, Grossman W, et al: Hemodynamic determinants of prognosis of aortic valve replacement in critical aortic stenosis and advanced congestive heart failure. *Circulation* 1980;62:42
12. Alpert JS: Chronic aortic regurgitation. In: Dalen JE, Alpert JS (eds). *Valvular Heart Disease*. Boston, Little, Brown, 1981:231
13. Grayburn PA, Smith MD, Handshoe R, et al: Detection of aortic insufficiency by standard echocardiography, pulsed doppler echocardiography and auscultation. *Ann Intern Med* 1986;104:599

14. Perloff JK: Acute severe aortic regurgitation: recognition and management. *J Cardiovasc Med* 1983;8:209

15. Weinstein L, Rubin RH: Infective endocarditis. *Prog Cardiovasc Dis* 1973;16:239

16. Perloff JK, Singer D: Electrocardiogram of free aortic insufficiency. *Circulation* 1962;26:786

17. Walsh RA, O'Rourke RA: The present therapeutic role of digitalis. *Drug Ther* 1978;8:61

18. Morgan JR, Forker AD: Isolated tricuspid insufficiency. *Circulation* 1971;43:559

19. McCord MC, Blount SG Jr: The hemodynamic pattern in tricuspid valve disease. *Am Heart J* 1952;44:671

20. Wooley CF, Fontana ME, Kilman JW, et al: Tricuspid stenosis: atrial systolic murmur, tricuspid opening snap and right atrial pressure pulse. *Am J Med* 1985;78:375

21. Yousof AM, Shafei MZ, Endrys G, et al: Tricuspid stenosis and regurgitation in rheumatic heart disease: a prospective cardiac catheterization study in 525 patients. *Am Heart J* 1985;110:60

22. Johnson LW, Grossman W, Dalen JE, et al: Pulmonic stenosis in the adult: long term follow-up results. *N Engl J Med* 1972;287:1159

23. Kirshenbaum HD: Pulmonic valve disease. In: Dalen JE, Alpert JS (eds). *Valvular Heart Disease.* Boston, Little, Brown, 1981:329

24. Braunwald E: Multivalvular disease. In: Braunwald E (ed). *Heart Disease.* Philadelphia, WB Saunders, 1984:1123

Critical Care, Third Edition, edited by Joseph M. Civetta,
Robert W. Taylor, and Robert R. Kirby.
Lippincott-Raven Publishers, Philadelphia, PA © 1997.

CHAPTER 119

Cardiac Arrhythmias

W. Ross Davis

Cardiac arrhythmias are commonly seen in the ICU. They are conveniently grouped as supraventricular or ventricular, and as bradycardic or tachycardic. Arrhythmias may result from several causes, including enhanced automaticity, reentry, triggered automaticity, and abnormal conduction.

IMMEDIATE CONCERNS

The ability to diagnose an arrhythmia is based on determination of the basic rhythmic pattern; each pattern has a specific differential diagnosis.[1] The eight basic patterns are listed in Table 119-1; Table 119-2 presents a partial differential diagnostic list for each pattern.

An outline for analyzing arrhythmias is presented in Table 119-3. Once the rhythm pattern is determined ("get a gestalt"), one should proceed to evaluate the QRS complex to determine whether it is initiated by a supraventricular impulse or is ectopic ("quiz the QRS"). In general, this reduces to an analysis of the QRS duration because ventricular complexes less than or equal to 120 milliseconds are virtually always caused by supraventricular mechanisms. Wider QRS complexes may be ventricular ectopics or may be caused by supraventricular beats with aberrant ventricular conduction. Several criteria may be used to decide whether wide ventricular complexes are more likely to be aberrantly conducted or ectopic (Table 119-4). In the ICU, however, one should initially treat wide complex arrhythmias as ventricular in origin. Occasionally, invasive monitoring techniques may be required for definitive diagnosis.

Once the origin of the QRS is determined, the P waves should be identified and their sites of origin established if possible ("cherchez le P"). Next, the relationship between the P wave and QRS should be examined to determine which site is controlling cardiac activity ("who's driving the bus?"). Finally, one should identify the *primary* underlying arrhythmia ("sight the target"), because several arrhythmias may be present, for example, atrial flutter with complete heart block or atrial fibrillation with ventricular tachycardia. Failure to determine the primary problem could lead to difficulties in treatment.

DIAGNOSTIC MANEUVERS

In addition to the electrocardiogram (ECG), several diagnostic techniques are helpful in defining arrhythmias. Most can be rapidly performed at the bedside, and they often allow rapid diagnosis when ECG analysis has been inconclusive.

PHYSICAL EXAMINATION

Physical examination can be helpful but often is not considered in the diagnosis of arrhythmias. Attention to the jugular venous wave may demonstrate flutter waves in atrial flutter or fibrillation waves in atrial fibrillation. Intermittent cannon A waves may be seen with ventricular premature beats (VPBs), complete heart block, or atrioventricular (AV) dissociation. Auscultation may reveal a variable first heart sound in AV dissociation, complete heart block, or atrial fibrillation.

VAGAL MANEUVERS

Vagal maneuvers, such as the Valsalva maneuver or carotid sinus massage, may be diagnostic in patients with difficult tachycardias. Table 119-5 lists common responses of several arrhythmias to vagal maneuvers.

TABLE 119-1.   Eight Basic Rhythm Patterns

Regular rhythm at normal rates	Early beats
Unexpected pauses	Regular bradycardia
Regular tachycardia	Bigeminal rhythms
Group beating	Chaotic irregularity

Adapted from Marriott HJL: *Practical Electrocardiography*, ed 7. Baltimore, Williams & Wilkins, 1983.

TABLE 119-2.   Causes of the Eight Basic Rhythm Patterns

Regular rhythm at normal rates
  Normal sinus rhythm
  Accelerated junctional rhythm
  Accelerated idioventricular rhythm
  Atrial flutter with 4:1 conduction
  Atrial tachycardia with block
Early beats
  Extrasystole
  Parasystole
  Capture beats
  Intermittent improved conduction during heart block
  Rhythm resumption after inapparent bigeminy
Pauses
  Nonconducted PACs (most common)
  Second-degree AV block (types I and II)
  Second-degree SA exit block
  Concealed conduction
  Concealed junctional extrasystoles
Bradycardia
  Sinus bradycardia
  Nonconducted atrial bigeminy
  Second- and third-degree AV block
  Second- and third-degree SA block
Bigeminy
  PACs and PVCs
  3:2 SA and AV block
  Atrial tachycardia or flutter with alternate 4:1 and 2:1 conduction
  Nonconducted atrial trigeminy
  Reciprocal beating
  Concealed junctional extrasystoles
Chaos
  Atrial fibrillation
  Atrial flutter with variable conduction
  Multifocal atrial tachycardia
  Wandering pacemaker
  Multifocal PVCs
  Parasystoles
  Combinations of the above
Regular tachycardia
  Sinus tachycardia
  Paroxysmal atrial tachycardia
  Atrial flutter
  Ectopic atrial tachycardia
  Junctional tachycardia
  Ventricular tachycardia
Group beating
  Nonconducted extrasystoles
  SA nodal Wenckebach exit block
  AV nodal Wenckebach block

PACs, premature atrial contractions; AV, atrioventricular; SA, sinoatrial; PVCs, premature ventricular contractions.

Adapted from Marriott HJL: *Practical Electrocardiography*, ed 7. Baltimore, Williams & Wilkins, 1983.

TABLE 119-3.   Principles of Arrhythmia Analysis

Get a gestalt
Quiz the QRS
Cherchez le P
Who's driving the bus?
Sight the target

Adapted from Marriott HJL: *Practical Electrocardiography*, ed 7. Baltimore, Williams & Wilkins, 1983.

TABLE 119-4.   Differentiation of Aberrant Ventricular Condition From Ventricular Ectopy

CHARACTERISTICS FAVORING ABERRANT VENTRICULAR CONDUCTION
  Right bundle branch block with R' >R
  Rate >170
  Initial QRS vector same as conducted QRS
  QRS duration <140 msec
  Normal axis
  Preceding P'
  Ashman's phenomenon

CHARACTERISTICS FAVORING VENTRICULAR ECTOPY
  Left axis deviation
  QRS >140 msec
  Monophasic or diphasic in V_1
  Fusion or capture beats
  Rate <170
  AV dissociation
  R > R' in V_1
  Concordant precordial pattern
  ! NOTHING IS ABSOLUTE !

AV, atrioventricular.

TABLE 119-5.   Response of Arrhythmias to Vagal Maneuvers

Sinus tachycardia	Slows gradually, returns to intrinsic rate when maneuver is ended
Ectopic atrial tachycardia	Stepwise decrease in AV conduction, may develop 2:1 or 3:1 conduction
PAT	No response or breaks suddenly to sinus rhythm
Atrial flutter	Decrease in AV conduction, may go from 2:1 to 3:1 or 4:1 conduction
Atrial fibrillation	Gradual decrease in ventricular rate, returns to original rate after termination of maneuver
MAT	No response or may cause some P waves to be nonconducted
Ventricular tachycardia	No response

PAT, Paroxysmal atrial tachycardia; MAT, multifocal atrial tachycardia; AV, atrioventricular.

SPECIAL RECORDING TECHNIQUES

Special surface leads, such as the Lewis lead, may be useful in delineating atrial activity in selected patients but rarely yield more information than might be obtained by standard leads II and V₁. Recording of simultaneous atrial electrograms and ECG can be useful in demonstrating atrial and ventricular rhythms and their relationships. Atrial electrograms can be recorded from epicardial leads after cardiovascular surgery, from esophageal electrodes, or from transvenous intraatrial electrodes.

PACING TECHNIQUES

Occasionally, although adequate ECG tracings or atrial electrograms can be obtained, an arrhythmia remains undiagnosed. For example, if a patient has a narrow complex supraventricular tachycardia (SVT) at 150 bpm, the ECG and atrial recording may show simultaneous activation of the atrium and ventricle without revealing whether the arrhythmia is sinus tachycardia, paroxysmal atrial tachycardia (PAT), ectopic atrial tachycardia (EAT), or nonparoxysmal junctional tachycardia. By pacing the atrium at a rate faster than the arrhythmia, information can be gained that may make the diagnosis. If the arrhythmia is sinus tachycardia, the sinus node will likely return at an initially slower rate (overdrive suppression), and the first spontaneous activity after cessation of pacing will be atrial. If the arrhythmia is PAT, it will either be terminated by pacing or be unchanged after the cessation of pacing. EATs still may be difficult to delineate from sinus tachycardia but may occasionally be successfully interrupted. With nonparoxysmal junctional tachycardia, the junctional pacemaker also displays overdrive suppression, but the first spontaneous beat after cessation of pacing will be a QRS complex.

SUPRAVENTRICULAR ARRHYTHMIAS ■

ABNORMALITIES OF RATE

Sinus rates above 100 bpm are *sinus tachycardia*. The rate may exceed 200 bpm. Critically ill patients may have sinus tachycardia for a variety of reasons, including fever, pain, hypoxemia, volume depletion, emotion, thyrotoxicosis, drugs, and shock. Sinus rates of less than 60/minute are *sinus bradycardia* and may be caused by carotid sinus massage, drugs, increased intracranial pressure, sinus node dysfunction, inferior myocardial infarction, obstructive jaundice, and other conditions.[2]

ABNORMALITIES OF RHYTHM

Premature atrial contractions (PACs) are characterized by a premature abnormal P wave. Conduction to the ventricle may be variable and create pauses or an early, widened QRS. A compensatory pause is not generally seen. Nonconducted PACs are the most common cause of unexpected pauses.

PAT is a regular, generally narrow complex, reentry arrhythmia with rates usually between 160 and 250 bpm. The reentry circuit may be in the atrium and AV node, or it may involve an accessory pathway. When PAT resolves, it ends abruptly.

EAT is a regular tachycardia with rates between 160 and 250 bpm. The electrophysiology of this arrhythmia is not well understood, but it does not involve the AV node as a part of a reentry pathway and may well be caused by an abnormal automatic site. Many patients with EAT demonstrate 2:1 AV conduction. EAT is commonly caused by digitalis toxicity but also may be seen in patients with severe heart disease in the absence of digitalis toxicity. Occasionally, EAT is seen in patients with otherwise normal hearts.

The diagnosis of *chaotic* or *multifocal atrial tachycardia* (MAT) is made when multiple forms of P waves and an irregular tachycardia are present. This pattern is most commonly seen in patients with pulmonary disease. Aberrantly conducted QRS complexes are frequently present in MAT.

Atrial flutter usually demonstrates an atrial rate between 250 and 350 bpm and is usually accompanied by 2:1, 3:1, or 4:1 AV conduction. The classical P wave morphologic picture in atrial flutter consists of a "sawtooth" pattern in the inferior leads and a train of P waves in lead V₁. Most patients with atrial flutter have organic heart disease; rheumatic heart disease or coronary disease predominate, but atrial flutter is also seen with hypertensive heart disease, cardiomyopathy, pulmonary disease, hyperthyroidism, pericarditis, and other conditions.

Atrial fibrillation is completely chaotic atrial activity. Ventricular activation is irregular. If the ventricular rate is greater than 200/minute, an accessory pathway may be present. Ventricular rates below 70 bpm in the absence of drugs known to slow AV conduction strongly suggest high-degree AV block. Many patients with atrial fibrillation have organic heart disease, but many have otherwise normal hearts.

Junctional arrhythmias important in critical care are limited to premature junctional contractions (PJCs), paroxysmal junctional tachycardia, and nonparoxysmal junctional tachycardia.

PJCs often are impossible to distinguish from PACs unless one can clearly demonstrate that there is no preceding P wave or that the PR interval is too short for conduction. The implications of PJCs are the same as those of PACs.

Paroxysmal junctional tachycardia is clinically identical to PAT, except in the rare occurrence of double tachycardia—simultaneous and independent junctional and atrial tachycardia.

Nonparoxysmal junctional tachycardia occurs when there is abnormal enhancement of the automatic cells of the AV junction. The rate is usually 70 to 130 bpm. This arrhythmia is typically the result of digitalis intoxication.[2-5]

VENTRICULAR ARRHYTHMIAS ■

VPBs are wide complex ventricular systoles that occur before the anticipated beat, are not preceded by a PAC, have a fixed coupling interval, and are followed by a fully compensatory pause. Retrograde conduction to the atrium may be present. VPBs may be monomorphic or polymorphic. If they occur in pairs, VPBs are termed *ventricular couplets*. Three or more sequential VPBs constitute *paroxysmal ventricular tachycardia*. All degrees of VPBs may be seen in normal people as well as patients with cardiac disease. Causes of ventricular ectopy in the intensive care unit include, among others, digitalis intoxication, hypoxemia, myocardial infarction, hypokalemia, antiarrhythmic drugs, and other drugs.

Accelerated idioventricular rhythm is a type of nonparoxysmal ventricular tachycardia with rates of 70 to 100 bpm. This rhythm is usually seen in the setting of inferior myocardial infarction with sinus bradycardia and is readily abolished by an increased sinus rate.

Ventricular flutter is an extremely rapid form of ventricular tachycardia with rates greater than 200 bpm. *Ventricular fibrillation* is chaotic ventricular activity. *Asystole* is absence of cardiac activity. Each of these three arrhythmias leads to sudden death if not terminated promptly.[3,5]

WIDE COMPLEX TACHYCARDIA

Occasionally, a patient may develop an arrhythmia with a rate in the range of 140 to 180 bpm with a QRS complex greater than 120 msec that cannot be delineated as being either primarily supraventricular with aberrancy or ventricular in origin with the techniques available. These are best described as *wide complex tachycardias*. Any attempt to further diagnose the rhythm disturbance without compelling evidence may lead to inappropriate treatment.

ATRIOVENTRICULAR BLOCK

Atrioventricular block is classically grouped by measurement of the PR interval and by observation of the frequency of nonconducted supraventricular impulses.[2,5]

First-degree AV block exists when the PR interval is greater than 200 milliseconds and each P wave is followed by a QRS. In patients with a narrow complex QRS, the conduction delay is usually localized to the AV node. In patients with bundle branch block, however, the conduction delay may be at any level. More than half of patients with left bundle branch block and first-degree AV block have prolonged His bundle conduction.

In *second-degree AV block*, there is an intermittent failure of the supraventricular impulse to reach the ventricles. The PR interval may be normal or abnormal in the complexes that are conducted. Second-degree block is divided into *Mobitz types I and II AV block*. Mobitz type I (Wenckebach phenomenon) is more common and is diagnosed when three criteria are met: (1) the PR interval is progressively lengthened until a P wave is blocked; (2) the RR interval is progressively shortened until a P wave is blocked; and (3) the RR interval containing the blocked P wave is shorter than the sum of two PP intervals. Because of the periodic pauses, a "gestalt" of grouped beating is created. The presence of type I second-degree AV block strongly suggests that the level of block is the AV node. This type of AV block is common with digitalis intoxication, inferior myocardial infarction, and rheumatic fever.

Mobitz type II second-degree AV block is less common and is diagnosed when there are intermittent blocked P waves but the PR interval remains constant. Type II second-degree AV block is usually at the infranodal level and is often associated with bundle branch block.

High degree AV block is diagnosed when two or more consecutive atrial impulses fail to conduct, the atrial rate is reasonable (less than 140 bpm), and there is no intervening escape rhythm.

Complete or *third-degree heart block* is present when supraventricular impulses completely fail to reach the ventricles. Ventricular excitation is initiated by subsidiary pacemakers distal to the site of block. The diagnosis can be made only if the atrial rate is faster than the ventricular rate. In about 60% of patients, the level of block is below the His bundle and the QRS complexes are wide. Patients with block at or above the His bundle commonly, but not predictably, have narrow QRS complexes.

MANAGEMENT

GENERAL PRINCIPLES

The initial step in determining appropriate management after an arrhythmia is recognized is to determine the hemodynamic consequences and the patient's tolerance of the arrhythmia.[6] In addition, a careful search for reversible causes of arrhythmias (e.g., hypoxemia, hypokalemia, digitalis toxicity, myocardial infarction) must be made. Too often, arrhythmias in the critically ill patient are treated with antiarrhythmic drugs when the patient is not at any particular risk from the arrhythmia or when correction of a related threatening problem would be preferable. Given that the incidence rate of serious adverse reactions—including life-threatening proarrhythmic effects—with antiarrhythmic drugs is 8% to 20%, and that patients can die from unrecognized reversible causes of arrhythmias, the need to search thoroughly for such abnormalities is apparent.

MANAGEMENT OF SPECIFIC ARRHYTHMIAS

Sinus tachycardia is usually an indicator of an underlying problem and rarely requires specific treatment. Occasionally, hyperadrenergic patients with accelerated hypertension, myocardial infarction, or thyrotoxicosis may benefit from specific therapy. The drugs of choice in these cases are beta-blockers, which may be given intravenously (propranolol, 1 to 3 mg every 5 minutes to a total of 0.1 mg/kg) or orally. Care must be taken not to treat patients with poor left ventricular function with beta-blockers. Pulmonary disorders with airflow obstruction are strong relative contraindications to beta-blockers.

The treatment of bradycardias, including sinus bradycardia and AV block, has been addressed by the American Heart Association as outlined in the Appendix to this book. Sinus bradycardia, first-degree AV block, and type I second-degree AV block require treatment only when hemodynamically significant. Type II second-degree AV block, high degree AV block, and third-degree AV block always should be treated. Pharmacologic treatment, when appropriate, can include atropine, 0.5 to 1 mg intravenously (IV), which can be repeated as needed to a maximum of 3 mg. When pharmacologic therapy is ineffective for sinus or junctional bradycardias or for type I second-degree AV block, external or transvenous pacing may be instituted. Even if pharmacologic interventions result in improvement, patients with type II second-degree AV block, high-degree AV block, or complete heart block should have transvenous temporary pacing established. Because the currently available external pacemakers are effective and are well tolerated, they can be helpful in stabilizing a patient so that placement of a transvenous pacemaker can be done under controlled circumstances.

Premature atrial beats and PJCs are seldom an independent indication for drug therapy but frequently mark the emergence of an underlying problem. PAT, paroxysmal junctional tachycardia, and reciprocating tachycardias using an accessory pathway can be considered under the general heading of *SVT*. In the critical care setting, these should virtually always be treated. Unstable SVT (e.g., with hypotension, angina, or congestive heart failure) requires emergency synchronized cardioversion with 50 to 200 J. The drug of choice for stable SVT is adenosine, 6 mg IV using rapid push followed in 2 to 3 minutes by a 12-mg rapid intravenous push if needed. This drug produces AV block and often converts reentry arrhythmias that use the AV node as part of the reentry circuit to sinus rhythm. Automatic atrial arrhythmias do not convert, but the transiently produced AV block frequently facilitates definitive diagnosis. Verapamil is an alternative intravenous drug, and a 5-mg dose can be given followed in 15 to 20 minutes by 10 mg IV if needed. Remember that verapamil can shorten the refractory period of accessory pathways, leading to increases in ventricular rates and possible ventricular fibrillation if the patient should develop atrial fibrillation. Therefore, immediate availability of a defibrillator is imperative. If therapy with adenosine or verapamil is unsuccessful, elective cardioversion, digoxin, beta-blockers, and therapeutic pacing can be considered.

Fortunately, EAT is relatively rare, because it can be particularly difficult to treat. If EAT is caused by digoxin toxicity and the patient is stable, one can discontinue the digitalis preparation and give support. Unstable patients with digitalis toxicity may respond to treatment with Fab fragments of digoxin-specific antibody. When the arrhythmia results from heart failure, it may respond to treatment of the failure. In idiopathic EAT, little seems to work well, although some reports indicate that flecainide is useful. I have had good short-term success with atrial overdrive pacing at a rate higher than the intrinsic atrial rate. This generally produces 2:1 or 3:1 AV conduction at pacing rates of 200 to 250 bpm, effectively slowing the ventricular rate from 150 to 200 bpm down to 75 to 100 bpm. This is only a short-term treatment. Some patients with EAT have been paced into atrial fibrillation, with better control of ventricular rates. Occasional patients respond only to surgical therapy with excision of the atrial focus or ablation of the AV node and placement of a VVI pacemaker.

MAT is more common than EAT, but treatment also can be difficult. The mainstay of treatment is aggressive therapy of the underlying, usually pulmonary, disease. Verapamil works well in many patients, not only controlling the ventricular response but occasionally reducing the frequency of the atrial activity. Verapamil should be avoided in patients who have significant left ventricular systolic dysfunction.

Atrial flutter should be treated by cardioversion if the patient is unstable. When the patient is stable, the treatment proceeds in two stages. First, control of the ventricular response is obtained with verapamil, digoxin, or beta-blockers. Once this is accomplished, treatment with a type 1a antiarrhythmic (quinidine or procainamide) can be started to effect conversion to sinus rhythm. Alternatively, elective cardioversion can be performed. Another option that can be used at any time is atrial overdrive pacing.

Atrial fibrillation should be treated with cardioversion when the patient is unstable. Patients with a rapid (more than 200 bpm) wide complex ventricular response to atrial fibrillation should be assumed to have a participating accessory pathway. Drug therapy can be two staged, identical to that used with atrial flutter to attempt conversion to sinus rhythm, or can be directed only toward control of the ventricular rate if conversion to sinus rhythm is not desired. Heart rate can be controlled with intermittent therapy with verapamil, beta-blockers, or digoxin, or with continuous-infusion verapamil (5 to 10 mg intravenous bolus followed by a 5- to 10-mg/hour infusion), diltiazem (0.25 mg/kg IV over 2 minutes followed by a 5- to 15-mg/hour intravenous infusion), or esmolol (500 µg/kg over 1 minute followed by an infusion of 50 to 200 µg/kg/minute).

Nonparoxysmal junctional tachycardia is most commonly seen in the critically ill as a manifestation of digitalis toxicity and should be treated as such. Attempts at cardioversion should be avoided because patients with digitalis toxicity who are cardioverted have a tendency to develop unresponsive ventricular fibrillation.

The American Heart Association has developed protocols addressing the treatment of ventricular arrhythmias.[6] Although these are certainly not the only acceptable methods for treatment, they represent the best understanding of the physiology of ventricular arrhythmias and must be considered the standard for comparison. These protocols are reproduced in the Appendix and form the basis for subsequent discussion.

Isolated VPBs require treatment only if they are frequent enough to cause a significant effective bradycardia. For example, if the sinus rate is 80 bpm and the patient develops ventricular bigeminy, the effective rate may be 40 bpm. Evidence that increasing numbers of VPBs are an independent cause of more complex ventricular arrhythmias is unconvincing. Rather, the patient with increasing VPB frequency should be considered to have an underlying unstable condition that is likely to cause more complex arrhythmias. Therapy, therefore, should ideally be directed toward the underlying cause. Specific treatment for VPBs, when appropriate, could include lidocaine or procainamide.

Ventricular couplets may be considered as a more pressing example of ventricular ectopy. A search for the precipitating cause is still imperative, but most authorities recommend that suppressive therapy with lidocaine or procainamide be started.

Sustained and nonsustained ventricular tachycardia should always be treated by the American Heart Association protocol.

Ventricular fibrillation and ventricular flutter should be treated with emergency defibrillation.

Asystole is particularly difficult to treat. Success is often predicated not on specific cardiac therapy, but on the discovery and correction of a severe underlying physiologic abnormality, such as profound acidosis or hypoxemia.

Wide complex tachycardia of unknown cause should first be treated as ventricular tachycardia with lidocaine, 1 mg/kg intravenous push every 5 to 10 minutes to a maximum dose of 3 mg/kg. If there is no response, adenosine (as discussed earlier) should be used. If the arrhythmia persists, procainamide, 20 to 30 mg/minute to a total of 17 mg/minute can be used. Although bretylium could be tried next, if lidocaine, adenosine, and procainamide fail to convert the rhythm, synchronized cardioversion should be strongly considered.

REFERENCES ■

1. Marriott HJL: *Practical Electrocardiography*, ed 8. Baltimore, Williams & Wilkins, 1981
2. Baker JT: Recognition and management of arrhythmias. In: Bone RC (ed). *Critical Care: A Comprehensive Approach*. Park Ridge, IL, ACCP, 1984:304
3. Jackson LK: Sustained and nonsustained ventricular tachycardia: genesis, significance and management. In: Rackley CE (ed). *Advances in Critical Care Cardiology*. Philadelphia, FA Davis, 1986:83
4. Del Negro AA, Fletcher RD: Supraventricular tachycardia emergencies: diagnosis and management. In: Rackley CE (ed). *Advances in Critical Care Cardiology*. Philadelphia, FA Davis, 1986:101
5. Chou TC: The cardiac arrhythmias. In: Chou TC (ed). *Electrocardiography in Clinical Practice*. Philadelphia, WB Saunders, 1991
6. Guidelines for Cardiopulmonary Resuscitation and Emergency Cardiac Care: Recommendations of the 1992 National Conference. *JAMA* 1992;268:2171

Critical Care, Third Edition, edited by Joseph M. Civetta,
Robert W. Taylor, and Robert R. Kirby.
Lippincott-Raven Publishers, Philadelphia, PA © 1997.

CHAPTER 120

■

Infective Endocarditis

Stephen B. Greenberg

IMMEDIATE CONCERNS ■

MAJOR PROBLEMS

Infective endocarditis is an infection of the endothelial surface of the heart, usually involving heart valves. As such, it is a potentially disabling and life-threatening condition.

STRESS POINTS

1. Acute and subacute forms of infective endocarditis occur. Organisms of high virulence such as *Staphylococcus aureus* cause acute endocarditis. Organisms of low virulence such as *Streptococcus viridans* cause subacute endocarditis. Gram-positive bacteria predominate in most forms of endocarditis. Gram-negative bacteria are rare causes of endocarditis and are predominantly reported in the setting of intravenous drug abuse.
2. Risk factors for endocarditis include rheumatic heart disease, congenital heart disease, degenerative heart disease, and mitral valve prolapse.
3. The mitral valve is most commonly involved, with the aortic valve a close second.
4. The tricuspid valve is most commonly involved in intravenous drug abusers.
5. Degeneration of heart valves leading to heart failure and systemic embolization are two of the major complications of infective endocarditis.

ESSENTIAL DIAGNOSTIC TESTS
AND PROCEDURES

1. History and physical examination are primary.
2. Fever, new or changing cardiac murmurs, evidence of systemic embolization, petechiae, glomerulonephritis,

Janeway lesions, Roth's spots, and Osler's nodes may be seen.
3. Echocardiography is helpful in diagnosis and monitoring. The sensitivity rate of transesophageal echocardiography is above 95%.
4. Blood culture results are usually positive in patients with bacterial endocarditis.
5. Anemia and an elevated erythrocyte sedimentation rate are found in over 75% of patients with endocarditis.

INITIAL THERAPY

1. Prophylactic antibiotics are recommended for prevention of infective endocarditis for patients at risk who are having procedures likely to cause bacteremia.
2. Treatment of infective endocarditis requires bactericidal antibiotics given parenterally for several weeks.
3. Combinations of antibiotics that rapidly kill bacteria have been shown to increase recovery.
4. The choice of antibiotics is based on antimicrobial susceptibility tests.
5. Progressive or significant heart failure is a leading cause of death and is the number one reason for early surgery. Patients with gram-negative bacterial endocarditis and fungal endocarditis do particularly poorly with medical management alone.

OVERVIEW ■

Infective endocarditis is defined as an infection of the endothelial surface of the heart with microorganisms present in the lesion. The usual site of infection is the heart valve, although vegetations can be found with mural thrombi or around septal defects in rare cases. The term *infective endo-*

carditis has replaced the previous designation of *bacterial endocarditis* because fungi, chlamydiae, and rickettsiae are known to be causative organisms in addition to bacteria.[1]

Two forms of infective endocarditis were described in the earlier literature. The term *subacute* denoted a more insidious onset, less toxicity, and a longer clinical course; previous heart damage was present in a high percentage of patients.[2] The *acute* form was associated with a more rapid onset, increased toxicity, and shorter duration of clinical findings and was seen in patients who often lacked a history of heart disease.[3] In addition, the microbiology differed between the two forms. Organisms of low virulence (i.e., S viridans) were most frequently found in cultures from patients with subacute endocarditis. In acute forms, more pathogenic organisms (i.e., S aureus) were commonly isolated.[4] Although the bacteriologic distinctions remain helpful, there is sufficient overlap of the syndromes to make the clinical separation less important.

With the introduction of penicillin therapy, the mortality rate from infective endocarditis decreased from almost 100% to as low as 30% to 40%. Since that time, however, there has been no further significant decrease in the mortality rate.[5,6] The frequency of occurrence of this relatively uncommon infection has not changed appreciably since before the antibiotic era.[7] Nevertheless, the morbidity in those who survive and the impact on health costs remain sufficient to warrant continued studies of improved prophylaxis and therapy.

In the last decades, there have been changes in the target populations, the clinical presentation, the microbiology, and therapeutic interventions associated with infective endocarditis. An increased frequency of endocarditis has been observed in intravenous drug abusers, after procedures performed in the hospital, after prosthetic valve placement, and in the elderly.[8,9] The decrease in rheumatic heart disease underlying infective endocarditis has been documented.[10] An increase in more virulent organisms, especially among intravenous drug abusers, has become important over the last 15 to 20 years.[11] Combination therapies, a shortened total course of antibiotics, and increasing surgical intervention are recognized as necessary in managing these patients.[12] These changes are discussed in detail in the following sections.

EPIDEMIOLOGY

Although the true incidence of infective endocarditis is not easily determined, the number of cases per hospital admission has remained the same (approximately 1 in 1000) for the last 30 years.[11] However, changes have occurred in the mean age of patients, the percentage of cases of acute disease, the distribution of valve involvement, and the frequency and etiology of heart disease.

Before the advent of penicillin therapy, infective endocarditis was a disease of young people. In the report by Thayer in 1926, the median age was younger than 30 years.[3] Recent studies have shown most patients to be older than 50 years of age.[6] Men are more likely than women to have infective endocarditis and also to be older when they acquire it.

Today, 30% to 40% of all cases of infective endocarditis can be classified as acute[13] compared with only 20% in the preantibiotic era. This may reflect the decline in underlying heart disease and the increase in nosocomial endocarditis associated with catheters, pacemakers, and shunts.

In most series, the mitral valve is the most commonly involved; the aortic valve is involved almost as often. The tricuspid valve is involved mainly in intravenous drug abusers and is otherwise rarely infected.[14] Infection of the pulmonary valve has rarely been documented. Simultaneous involvement of both left- and right-sided disease also is unusual.

The underlying heart diseases associated with infective endocarditis include rheumatic heart disease, congenital heart disease, degenerative disease, and mitral valve prolapse. Half of the reported cases in the last 20 years have been secondary to rheumatic heart disease. Most of these cases involve the mitral valve; women are more often affected than men. Several congenital defects have been associated with 5% to 25% of endocarditis cases. These defects are predominantly patent ductus arteriosus, ventricular septal defect, bicuspid aortic valve, and Fallot's tetralogy.[15] Degenerative disease, such as calcified mitral annulus, has been reported in a high percentage of elderly patients with infective endocarditis and may be an important factor contributing to the increased incidence of endocarditis in this age group.[16] Mitral valve prolapse associated with infective endocarditis was reviewed recently.[17] Recognition of this common condition as a precursor of infective endocarditis is a result of its high prevalence in the population and the increased availability of echocardiographic diagnostic techniques. Nevertheless, no underlying cardiac disease is found in over 50% of acute cases of infective endocarditis.[10]

PATHOLOGY AND PATHOGENESIS

For infective endocarditis to occur, several events must take place in a fairly uniform sequence. Platelet-fibrin deposits on the valvular endothelium occur if there is local trauma or turbulent blood flow. Recent animal studies have shown that when bacteria enter the bloodstream, they adhere more readily to the platelet-fibrin deposits.[18] Earlier studies explained why the vegetations occur most commonly on the atrial surface of the mitral valve and the ventricular surface of the aortic valve.[19] Stenotic lesions or septal defects with a jet lesion are associated with increased turbulence and increased likelihood of bacterial colonization. The bacteremia that is needed to complete the sequence is usually transient and accompanies dental, gastrointestinal, urologic, or gynecologic procedures.[20] With colonization of the damaged valve, the vegetation continues to enlarge. Bacteria grow below the surface of the vegetation and are sequestered from normal heart defense mechanisms.

Pathologically, the vegetation is composed of platelet aggregates, fibrin, and colonies of bacteria. Neutrophils and red blood cells are rarely found. If the infection spreads, one can see perforation of the valve leaflet, chordae tendineae rupture, or valve ring abscesses. In cases of acute endocarditis, involvement of the myocardium by abscesses or infarction is common.

In the preantibiotic era, embolic phenomena were clinically evident in most patients. By contrast, less than half of patients now have clinically demonstrable peripheral emboli. When emboli occur, they frequently involve the kidney, spleen, or cerebral circulation.[21]

When the kidneys are involved, abscesses, infarction, or glomerulonephritis can be found. The glomerulonephritis is usually diffuse or focal; membranoproliferative glomerulonephritis is the least common. Immune complexes are thought to mediate the glomerulonephritis associated with infective endocarditis.[22]

Cerebral emboli are commonly found in cases of infective endocarditis. Mycotic aneurysms may occur in cerebral vessels and go undetected in many cases, although they are found in approximately 10% of autopsy series. Microabscesses in the brain can occur in staphylococcal endocarditis, but acute purulent meningitis is rare.

Other pathologic involvement with emboli has been documented in the lung, skin, spleen, and eye. Right-sided endocarditis is commonly associated with pulmonary emboli, with or without infarction. The skin manifestations of emboli (i.e., petechiae, Osler's nodes, and Janeway lesions) are found less often than they were in the preantibiotic era. Osler's nodes are thought to be associated with immune complexes, whereas recent studies suggest that Janeway lesions are subcutaneous abscesses.[23] Hemorrhage in the nerve fiber layer of the retina, or Roth's spot, can be found in many cases of infective endocarditis.[24]

DIAGNOSTIC CRITERIA   ▪

The diagnosis of infective endocarditis is made in most patients on the basis of clinical findings and often results in many "probable" and "possible" cases. A newly described set of criteria for the diagnosis of infective endocarditis has been published.[11] The definitive diagnosis can be based on pathologic or clinical criteria (Tables 120-1 and 120-2). Major clinical criteria require positive blood culture results with typical microorganisms, or persistently positive blood culture results and evidence of endocardial involvement by positive echocardiogram or new valvular regurgitation.

TABLE 120-1. New Criteria for the Diagnosis of Infective Endocarditis

Definite infective endocarditis
  Pathologic Criteria:
    Microorganisms: Demonstrated by culture or histologic evaluation in a vegetation, or in a vegetation that has embolized, or in an intracardiac abscess, *or*
    Pathologic lesions: Vegetation or intracardiac abscess present, confirmed by histologic study showing active endocarditis
  Clinical criteria (see definitions below):
    2 Major criteria, *or*
    1 Major and 3 minor criteria, *or*
    5 Minor criteria
Possible infective endocarditis: Findings consistent with infective endocarditis that fall short of "definite," but not "rejected"
Rejected: Firm alternate diagnosis explaining evidence of infective endocarditis, *or* resolution of infective endocarditis syndrome, with antibiotic therapy for 4 d or less, *or* no pathologic evidence of infectious endocarditis at surgery or autopsy, with antibiotic therapy for 4 d or less

Durack D, Lukes AS, Bright DK, et al: New criteria for diagnosis of infective endocarditis: utilization of specific echocardiographic criteria. *Am J Med* 1994;96:200.

TABLE 120-2. Definitions of Terminology Used in the Proposed New Criteria for Diagnosis of Infective Endocarditis

MAJOR CRITERIA
  1. Positive blood culture for infective endocarditis: typical microorganism for infective endocarditis from 2 separate blood cultures:
     a. Viridans streptococci, *Streptococcus bovis*, HACEK group, *or*
     b. Community-acquired *Staphylococcus aureus* or enterococci, in the absence of a primary focus, *or*
     Persistently positive blood culture, defined as microorganism consistent with infective endocarditis from:
     a. Blood cultures drawn more than 12 h apart, *or*
     b. All of 3, or majority of 4 or more separate blood cultures, with first and last drawn at least 1 h apart
  2. Evidence of endocardial involvement:
     Positive echocardiogram for infective endocarditis:
     a. Oscillating intracardiac mass, on valve or supporting structures, or in the path of regurgitant jets, or on iatrogenic devices, in the absence of an alternative anatomic explanation, *or*
     b. Abscess, *or*
     c. New partial dehiscence of prosthetic valve, *or*
     New valvular regurgitation (worsening or changing of preexisting murmur not sufficient)

MINOR CRITERIA
  1. Predisposition: Predisposing heart condition or intravenous drug use
  2. Fever: ≥38.0°C (100.4°F)
  3. Vascular phenomena: Arterial embolism, septic pulmonary infarcts, mycotic aneurysm, intracranial hemorrhage, Janeway lesions
  4. Immunologic phenomena: Glomerulonephritis, Osler's nodes, Roth's spots, rheumatoid factor
  5. Echocardiogram: Consistent with infective endocarditis but not meeting major criterion above
  6. Microbiologic evidence: Positive blood culture but not meeting major criterion above, *or* serologic evidence of active infection with organism consistent with infective endocarditis

Durack D, Lukes AS, Bright DK, et al: New criteria for diagnosis of infective endocarditis: utilization of specific echocardiographic criteria. *Am J Med* 1994;96:200.

TABLE 120-3. Incidence of Clinical Features in Infective Endocarditis

>75%	50–75%	25–50%	<25%
Fever	Embolic phenomena	Chills Weakness	Weight loss Anorexia
Heart murmur	Previous heart disease	Splenomegaly	Arthralgias Back pain

Based on published data.[2,4,10,25]

CLINICAL MANIFESTATIONS ■

The signs and symptoms of infective endocarditis can involve any organ system and often are confused with other medical conditions.[25] Fever and heart murmur are the most frequently detected symptom and sign, respectively (Table 120-3). With renal failure, congestive heart failure, or advanced age, fever may be absent. No specific pattern of fever is pathognomonic, but temperatures rarely exceed 39.4°C (103°F). With right-sided endocarditis, a heart murmur may not be heard. Only in a few cases is a changing murmur or onset of a new murmur described.

Peripheral manifestations are present in approximately 50% of cases. Splinter hemorrhages are uncommon and may be secondary to trauma. If the disease is of long duration, clubbing may be found. Petechiae are common and occur secondary to the local vasculitis or emboli. Detailed examination of the conjunctivae, extremities, and mucus membranes of the mouth usually reveals these petechiae. In addition, a close examination may disclose the less common Osler's nodes and Janeway lesions. Osler's nodes may be found in patients with nonbacterial thrombotic endocarditis, gonococcal infections, and hemolytic anemia. Unlike the painless macular Janeway lesions of embolic origin, Osler's nodes are usually painful and nodular. Roth's spots are hemorrhagic retinal lesions that occur in a small percentage of endocarditis patients and also have been described with severe anemia, leukemia, and systemic lupus erythematosus.

The frequency of nonspecific symptoms such as chills, weakness, weight loss, and fatigue may cause the physician to consider other systemic problems or chronic diseases. Symptoms and signs referable to the musculoskeletal system are common as an initial or concomitant complaint. Arthralgia, arthritis, low back pain, and diffuse myalgia are reported to be common.[26]

A wide variety of neurologic conditions are associated with infective endocarditis. These neurologic manifestations may be the initial presentation or may occur among the complications seen in these infections.[27] Cerebral emboli may lead to hemiplegia, ataxia, aphasia, or change in mental status. A young person with an acute stroke should be evaluated for possible endocarditis. Subarachnoid hemorrhage secondary to mycotic aneurysms is unusual and is correlated with a high mortality rate.

Patients with right-sided endocarditis usually have signs and symptoms referable to the pulmonary system.[8] Intravenous drug addicts have an increased incidence of tricuspid valve endocarditis. Pleuritic chest pain and dyspnea are common complaints. Chest radiographs may reveal infiltrates compatible with septic pulmonary emboli.

LABORATORY TESTS ■

Although abnormalities in laboratory test results are commonly found in cases of endocarditis, most are not diagnostic. Anemia and elevated erythrocyte sedimentation rates are found in more than 75% of cases (Table 120-4). Other hematologic abnormalities, such as thrombocytopenia and leukocytosis, are detected less often. Monocytosis has been reported in cases of endocarditis but is also found in other infectious diseases such as tuberculosis and typhoid fever. Less frequent abnormalities include microscopic hematuria, proteinuria, hypergammaglobulinemia, hypocomplementemia, and positive rheumatoid factor.

The detection of circulating immune complexes may be helpful in diagnosis and management.[28,29] Although a third of patients with septicemia and 10% of normal controls have circulating immune complexes, these are present in high

TABLE 120-4. Incidence of Laboratory Test Abnormalities in Infective Endocarditis

>75%	50–75%	25–75%	<25%
Anemia Elevated erythrocyte sedimentation rate	Proteinuria	Hematuria Rheumatoid factor Hypergammaglobulinemia	Decreased complement Thrombocytopenia Leukocytosis

Based on published data.[2,4,6]

titers in most patients with definite infective endocarditis. With appropriate treatment, the levels decrease.

Blood culture results are usually positive in patients with bacterial endocarditis. The bacteremia is continuous, with low colony counts.[30] Most cultures contain 1 to 30 bacteria per milliliter. Most studies demonstrate the usefulness of obtaining at least three blood culture sets in the first 24 hours. Blood should be injected into trypticase soy and thioglycolate broth. If the patient has recently received antibiotics, additional blood cultures should be done. Cultures should be kept by the laboratory for 3 weeks; subcultures should be plated on days 1 and 3.

In patients who have not received antibiotics, the incidence rate of culture-negative endocarditis should be less than 5%.[31] If the patient has received antibiotics recently, the microbiology laboratory should be contacted so that hypertonic or supplemented media is used in testing. This may help in detecting cell wall–defective or nutritionally deficient organisms. To detect certain anaerobes or *Brucella* species, cultures may have to be kept longer than 3 weeks.

Special cultures or serologic tests are necessary to detect nonbacterial infective endocarditis. Fungal endocarditis is associated with negative blood culture results in most cases, and special media often are required to increase recovery.[32,33] Although several serologic tests are available for detecting *Candida* antigen and antibodies, these should be used to support and not to diagnose cases of *Candida* endocarditis. However, only serologic tests are available to diagnose unusual cases of endocarditis secondary to chlamydiae or rickettsiae.[34–36]

The usefulness of tests detecting teichoic acid antibodies in cases of staphylococcal endocarditis is controversial. Although more than 95% of patients with *S aureus* endocarditis have positive antibody titers, there are false-positive results in a significant minority of patients with bacteremia.[37] If the test result is positive in a patient with clinical evidence of endocarditis, therapy should be continued for a longer total course (4 to 6 weeks). If the test result is negative in a patient with *S aureus* bacteremia who lacks evidence of endocarditis, the duration of therapy may be shorter (2 to 4 weeks). If the test result is negative but there is clinical evidence of *S aureus* endocarditis, the patient should be treated for endocarditis.

With improvements in echocardiography, vegetations no larger than 2 mm in size can be detected. Sensitivity rate for detecting vegetations was approximately 50% with single-dimension (M-mode) echocardiography.[38] With transesophageal imaging, the sensitivity rate of two-dimensional echocardiograms is greater than 95%. Transesophageal echocardiography is three times more sensitive than transthoracic echocardiography for detecting abscesses and valvular perforations. There are cases, however, in which echocardiography cannot distinguish between vegetations and other findings such as thickened or ruptured leaflets and chordae tendineae. Thus, the diagnosis of infective endocarditis should not be made on echocardiographic findings alone.

Vegetations are larger on tricuspid than aortic or mitral valves. With vegetations larger than 10 mm in diameter, embolization is more likely. Nevertheless, the size of vegetations does not correlate with likelihood of heart failure, risk of death, or final outcome.[39]

If a vegetation is found, there is an increased risk of systemic emboli and congestive heart failure, and the need for surgical intervention is greater. In aortic valve involvement, a positive finding on echocardiogram usually suggests that emergency surgery is necessary.[39]

Although quantitative blood cultures have been obtained for diagnosis at the time of cardiac catheterization in a few published reports, the most common use for this invasive procedure has been to define the hemodynamic and anatomic status of the patient before surgery.[40] Cardiac catheterization is not associated with increased risk if performed properly, and it can provide information concerning the degree of valvular insufficiency and document the involvement of more than one valve. Cardiac catheterization should only be performed in patients who are candidates for immediate surgery.

MICROBIOLOGY ■

The etiology of infective endocarditis is predominantly bacterial. Over the last 40 years, the relative frequencies of bacterial isolates in endocarditis cases have changed.[2,4,6,11,41–44] Approximately one third of current cases are caused by the ungroupable streptococci, *S viridans* (Table 120-5). The incidence of endocarditis caused by streptococci has not changed over this span of time. However, there have been increases in the percentage of cases caused by staphylococci, gram-negative bacilli, and fungi. The distribution of organisms varies considerably, depending on specific host factors, such as age, history of intravenous drug abuse, or prosthetic valve placement.

S viridans are alpha-hemolytic and usually untypeable by the Lancefield system. When their presence is associated with endocarditis, there is often a subacute course and underlying heart disease. The source of the *S viridans* is

TABLE 120-5. Changes in the Etiology of Bacterial Endocarditis Over the Last 40 Years[°]

CAUSE	INCIDENCE[†]	PERCENTAGE OF TOTAL[‡]
Streptococcus viridans	Unchanged	20–40
Staphylococcus aureus	Increased	15–25
Blood culture negative	Decreased	5–10
Gram-negative bacilli	Increased	5–10
Other streptococci[§]	Unchanged	5–10
Fungi	Increased	1–5
Staphylococcus epidermidis	Increased	1–5

[°]Based on published data.[2,4,6,41–44]
[†]Change in reported incidence from 1940s to 1980s.
[‡]Ranges based on reported cases.
[§]Including enterococcus.

thought to be the mouth. Other streptococci associated with endocarditis are often recovered from the gastrointestinal tract. *Streptococcus bovis* and *Streptococcus faecalis* (enterococcus) are important causes of endocarditis and belong to group D streptococci by the Lancefield system. Distinguishing between these two streptococci is important because of the therapeutic and underlying disease implications. *S bovis* bacteremia has been associated with carcinoma of the colon.[45] Enterococcal endocarditis is more difficult to treat, and its frequency is increasing in intravenous drug abusers.[46,47] Other typeable streptococci have been associated with rare cases of endocarditis in diabetic patients or pregnant women.[48,49] More common nontypeable strains such as *Streptococcus mutans* and *Streptococcus milleri* have been recovered in 15% to 20% of endocarditis patients infected by streptococci.

S aureus is the coagulase-positive staphylococcus recovered in most cases of acute infective endocarditis. This virulent bacterium can destroy normal valves and lead to complications such as myocardial abscesses, valve ring abscesses, and purulent pericarditis.[50] Distinguishing *S aureus* bacteremia from endocarditis can be difficult, but the distinction is important for therapy (Table 120-6). Community-acquired bacteremia is more likely to be associated with endocarditis than hospital-acquired bacteremia. Nonetheless, the clinical distinction may not be clear. *Staphylococcal epidermidis*, or coagulase-negative staphylococcal endocarditis, is predominantly found in association with prosthetic valves.

Endocarditis caused by aerobic gram-negative bacilli remains uncommon, although the incidence of septicemia from these bacteria is increasing. The most common gram-negative bacilli reported to cause endocarditis are *Salmonella* species, *Escherichia coli*, *Serratia marcescens*, and *Pseudomonas aeruginosa*. The latter two gram-negative bacteria have been reported predominantly in intravenous drug abusers from certain areas.[51,52] The mortality rate of these cases ranges from 60% to 80%.

Unusual aerobic gram-negative, gram-positive, and anaerobic bacteria have been reported to cause infective endo-

TABLE 120-7.   Differential Diagnosis of Culture-Negative Endocarditis

---

Recent antibiotic treatment prior to blood cultures
"Fastidious" bacteria with special growth requirements
Fungi that grow poorly in blood cultures
Nonbacterial causes
   Q fever
   Chlamydia infection
   Viruses (?)

---

carditis, but the total number of cases is small compared with those caused by streptococci and staphylococci.

A group of fastidious gram-negative organisms with a predilection to cause infective endocarditis is the "HACEK" microorganisms: *Hemophilus* species, *Actinobacillus actinomycetemcomitans*, *Cardiobacterium hominis*, *Eikenella*, and *Kingella* species. When they cause prosthetic valve endocarditis, there is a better chance of achieving a cure with antibiotics alone than with infection by other gram-negative bacteria.

Fungi are increasing in frequency as a cause of endocarditis because of their increase among intravenous drug abusers and patients who have had cardiovascular surgery or prolonged intravenous therapy through a central venous catheter.[53] Most cases are caused by *Candida* or *Aspergillus* species. Clinically, fungal endocarditis is associated with peripheral emboli to major vessels. In intravenous drug abusers, *Candida parapsilosis* and *Candida tropicalis* are the usual organisms isolated. In other patients, *Candida albicans* and *Aspergillus* species predominate.

Culture-negative endocarditis is decreasing in incidence[31] (Tables 120-5 and 120-7). Improvements in blood culture bottles and microbiologic techniques have helped to detect slow-growing fastidious bacteria and fungi. Culture-negative endocarditis, when it occurs, continues to be most frequently associated with right-sided endocarditis, renal insufficiency, and mural endocarditis. Prior administration of antibiotics

TABLE 120-6.   Distinguishing *Staphylococcus aureus* Endocarditis from Bacteremia

SUGGESTIVE OF ENDOCARDITIS	SUGGESTIVE OF BACTEREMIA	SEEN IN BOTH
New pathologic or changing heart murmur	Hospital acquired	Disorders of mentation
Major embolic events	Promptly treated bacteremia related to wounds or use of intravenous devices	Metastatic abscesses
New splenomegaly (rare)		Shock
Peripheral microembolic signs (rare)		Delayed response to treatment, persistent fever, blood cultures positive on treatment
Rheumatic valvular heart murmur		
Community-acquired bacteremia, delayed treatment, no primary site of infection		

and endocarditis caused by chlamydiae, rickettsiae, fungi, and, perhaps, viruses are associated with negative blood culture results.

THERAPY ■

Treatment of infective endocarditis requires bactericidal antibiotics given parenterally for several weeks. Because of the location of the infection in an area of impaired host resistance and the numerous bacteria present in the vegetation, eradication takes weeks of therapy and relapse is common. Combinations of antibiotics that rapidly kill the bacteria have been shown to increase recovery.[12] The choice of antibiotics is based on antimicrobial susceptibility tests. Whether monitoring of serum bactericidal concentrations and antimicrobial blood levels alters the outcome of treated infective endocarditis remains controversial.[54]

Organisms associated with endocarditis may be separated by minimum inhibitory concentrations (MICs) into those extremely sensitive to penicillin (MIC less than 0.2 µg/mL) and those more resistant to penicillin therapy (MIC greater than 0.2 µg/mL). *S viridans, S bovis,* and *Streptococcus pneumoniae* are in the sensitive group; *S faecalis* (enterococcus) is more resistant to penicillin.

Several regimens are available and efficacious in treating *S viridans* (Table 120-8). The cure rate is over 90% when penicillin is used alone (12 to 20 million U/day) for 4 weeks or with gentamicin (1.0 mg/kg IV every 8 hours) for 2 weeks.[55] Vancomycin (0.5 g intravenously [IV] every 6 hours) for 4 weeks can be used in the penicillin-allergic patient. Other regimens recommended for penicillin-allergic patients include a first-generation cephalosporin such as cefazolin for 4 weeks, combined with streptomycin for the initial 2 weeks.

The optimal treatment of enterococcal endocarditis has been debated.[56,57] Most investigators support combination therapy with high-dose penicillin (20 million U/day IV) plus an aminoglycoside. Because high-level streptomycin resistance has been found in 25% to 50% of enterococcal isolates from recent endocarditis patients, initial aminoglycoside therapy should include gentamicin (1 mg/kg IV every 8 hours) until complete sensitivity studies are available. If the duration of symptoms before initiating antibiotic therapy is more than 3 months or if the mitral valve is infected, the patient should receive a full 6 weeks of antibiotics.[57] If the patient is penicillin allergic, vancomycin (0.5 g IV every 6 hours) should be given; an aminoglycoside can be given concomitantly.[58] However, this combination has the potential for increased nephrotoxicity, and no definitive clinical data demonstrate its superiority over vancomycin alone.

S aureus endocarditis should be treated with a penicillinase-resistant penicillin such as nafcillin or oxacillin (2 g IV every 4 hours) for 4 to 6 weeks. Recent studies have failed to demonstrate significant clinical benefit with the addition of an aminoglycoside to nafcillin.[59] However, this organism is associated with high mortality and increased morbidity, so some investigators contend that the addition of an aminoglycoside for the first week of therapy may be justified. If the patient is penicillin allergic or the strain is methicillin resistant, then vancomycin (0.5 g IV every 6 hours) for 4 to 6 weeks is the recommended alternative regimen.

The mortality rate from endocarditis associated with gram-negative bacilli is high with medical management alone. Several studies demonstrate the necessity of valve replacement in conjunction with antibiotic therapy.[60,61] Combination therapy for *Pseudomonas* endocarditis includes a broad-spectrum penicillin, such as carbenicillin, ticarcillin, or azlocillin, along with high-dose aminoglycoside therapy, such as gentamicin or tobramycin, 7 to 9 mg/kg/day IV. Although medical therapy is sometimes successful in tricuspid endocarditis caused by *P aeruginosa*, investigators recommend that surgical intervention be used when the aortic or mitral valves are involved.[52]

Endocarditis caused by *S pneumoniae, Neisseria gonorrhoeae,* or anaerobic bacilli usually is responsive to parenteral penicillin (20 million U/day IV) for 4 weeks. *Bacteroides fragilis* is the major anaerobe that is not sensitive to penicillin. For this anaerobe, metronidazole, clindamycin, or chloramphenicol should be used.

Surgical intervention is recommended to treat fungal endocarditis, although no data are available to document its improved efficacy. Mortality rates with amphotericin B therapy alone have been greater than 80%. Nevertheless, this agent remains the first choice for antifungal drug therapy. Side effects from amphotericin B include fever, chills, phlebitis, anemia, hypokalemia, and renal insufficiency. Dosage schedules vary, but most investigators agree the total dose and duration of treatment are important. Valve replacement for aortic or mitral valve involvement is performed 1 or 2 weeks after amphotericin B has been instituted.[33] After surgery, the drug is continued for an additional 6 to 8 weeks to reach a total dose approximating 2 to 3 g. Whether the addition of other antifungal agents such as 5-fluorocytosine or rifampin increases survival is not known.

Treatment of Q fever or chlamydial endocarditis requires both antimicrobial agents and surgery for cure.[34,35] Tetracycline should be given for prolonged periods (6 to 12 months) after valve replacement. Failures have been reported after therapy, so that careful clinical follow-up is essential in these rare cases.

The indications for surgery in infective endocarditis have been described by Dinubile[62] (Table 120-9): major and minor criteria are proposed for surgical intervention in active endocarditis. Progressive or significant heart failure is a leading cause of death and is the primary reason for early surgery. Multiple emboli, bacteremia that continues despite appropriate antibiotics, and fungal endocarditis are additional indications. Other situations that may warrant surgery include congestive heart failure that improves with medical therapy, vegetations on the aortic valve detected by M-mode echocardiography, gram-negative bacillus tricuspid endocarditis, and early (less than 30 days) prosthetic valve endocarditis. Thus, the use of surgery as an adjunct to antimicrobial ther-

(text continues on page 1796)

TABLE 120-8. Regimens for Treating Infective Endocarditis

ANATOMIC SITE/ DIAGNOSIS/ MODIFYING CIRCUMSTANCES	ETIOLOGIES (usual)	SUGGESTED REGIMENS	
		Primary	*Alternative*
INFECTIVE ENDOCARDITIS—NATIVE VALVE—EMPIRICAL RX AWAITING CULTURES			
Valvular or congenital heart disease including mitral valve prolapse but no modifying circumstances	*Streptococcus viridans* (30–40%), "Other" strep (15–25%), Enterococci (5–18%), Staphylococci (20–35%)	Penicillin G 20 million U qd IV (continuous or divide q4h) or ampicillin 3.0 gm q4h IV + nafcillin or oxacillin 2.0 gm q4h IV + gentamicin 1.0 mg/kg q8h IM or IV (not once daily dosing)	Vancomycin 1.0 g° q12h IV + gentamicin 1.0 mg/kg° q8h IM or IV
Heart failure, new valvular insufficiency murmur, "toxic" patient, associated pneumonitis or meningeal signs			
Suspected injection drug use	*Staphylococcus aureus, Pseudomonas* sp., enterococci		
INFECTIVE ENDOCARDITIS—NATIVE VALVE—CULTURE POSITIVE[†]			
Age <65 y + normal auditory & renal function	*S. viridans, Streptococcus bovis* (MIC ≤0.1 µg/ mL)	Penicillin G 10–20 million U/d IV × 2 wk + gentamicin 1.0 mg/kg q8h IV or IM (not to exceed 80 mg, not once daily dosing!) × 2 wk	Ceftriaxone 2.0 g IV q24h × 4 wk or vancomycin (15 mg/kg IV [not to exceed 1.0 g] q12h for 4 wk)
	"Nutritionally variant" or "tolerant" strep (MIC >0.1–<0.5 µg/mL)	Penicillin G 20 million U/d IV × 4 wk + gentamicin 1.0 mg/ kg q8h IV or IM × 2 wk	
INFECTIVE ENDOCARDITIS—NATIVE VALVE—CULTURE POSITIVE			
Age >65 y or ↓ auditory or renal function	*S. viridans* (MIC ≤0.1 µg/mL)	Penicillin G 10–20 million U/d IV × 4 wk	As for age <65
Symptoms <3 mo	Enterococci, nutritionally variant strep, *S. viridans* (MIC >0.1 µg/mL)	Penicillin G 20–30 million U qd IV × 4 wk + gentamicin 1.0 mg/kg° q8h IV or IM (not single daily dosing) × 4 wk	Vancomycin 1.0 g° q12h IV × 6 wk + gentamicin 1.0 mg/kg° q8h IV or IM × 4–6 wk (4 vs 6 wk not established)
Symptoms >3 mo		Penicillin G (6 wk) + gentamicin (4 wk) (dosage: see above)	
	S. aureus	PRSP[‡] (nafcillin or oxacillin 2.0 g q4h IV for 4–6 wk (see comments) + gentamicin 1.0 mg/kg q8h IV or IM × 3–5 d	Cephalothin 2.0 g q4h IV or cefazolin 2.0 g q8h IV (is preferable to vancomycin) + gentamicin or vancomycin. In the UK, regimens are flucloxacillin 2.0 g q4h IV + either fusidic acid 500 mg q8h po (or IV) or gentamicin[∥]
	HACEK group (see comments)	Usually (penicillin G [HD] or ampicillin) + gentamicin while awaiting blood culture results. Definitive regimen determined by in vitro susceptibilities. Alternative: ceftriaxone 2.0 gm IV qd (4 wk).	

ADJUNCT DIAGNOSTIC OR THERAPEUTIC MEASURES AND COMMENTS

If patient not acutely ill and not in heart failure, we prefer to await blood culture results, obtaining more if required because treatment must be tailored to organism & susceptibilities. PRSP[j] + gentamicin coverage of enterococci may not be adequate, hence addition of penicillin G pending cultures. If cultures remain negative ("culture negative endocarditis") consider rare possibilities such as fungal, Q fever, psittacosis, brucellosis, but if tests are negative rx penicillin G (HD) or ampicillin + gentamicin for 6 wk. When blood cultures are positive, modify regimen from empiric to specific based on organism, in vitro susceptibilities, clinical experience

If heart failure (pulmonary edema, hypotension) progresses on medical rx, need valve replacement

Aqueous crystalline pen G 10–20 million U/d IV + gentamicin 1.0 mg/kg (not to exceed 80 mg) IM or IV q8h for 2 wk. (Procaine penicillin G 1.2 million U IM q6h + strep; less experience but equally effective,[§] not recommended in children.) Cure rates >99% with ceftriaxone. If *S. bovis*, investigate for bowel disease

Penicillin G 10–20 million U/d IV for 4 wk. Cure rate >99%[¶]

Penicillin G 20 million U/d IV × 6 wk + gentamicin 1.0 mg/kg IV q8h × 6 wk
Relapse rate 10–20%.[#] Tobramycin, amikacin *NOT* synergistic vs *Enterococcus faecium*. 1/6 of HLGR enterococci may show synergy with streptomycin. Test enterococci for high level (>1000 μg/mL) resistance to gentamicin (HLGR) β-lactamase production (nitrocephin disc) and vancomycin resistance[°°]

Gentamicin (peak serum levels 3 μg/mL). If abscesses suspected after gentamicin, begin rifampin (rifampin 600 mg qd po). If uncomplicated rx 4 wk, if clinical response slow or abscesses rx 6 wk. IDUs with right-sided endocarditis respond to 2 wk rx (nafcillin + tobramycin for 2 wk).[††] A 4-wk course of rifampin (600 mg qd) + cipro (750 mg bid po) for right-sided endocarditis has been successful. Response to vancomycin or vancomycin-rifampin for MRSA (median 9 d) is slower than response of MSSA to nafcillin (2–5 d).[‡‡] TMP/SMX (320/1600 mg IV q12h) has been used successfully in some patients with right-sided MRSA endocarditis.[§§]

HACEK (acronym for slow-growing fastidious gram-negative organisms: *Hemophilus parainfluenzae, Hemophilus aphrophilus, Actinobacillus, Cardiobacterium, Eikenella, Kingella*). *H. aphrophilus* resistant to vancomycin, clindamycin, methicillin, and often ampicillin

(continued)

TABLE 120-8.   *(continued)*

ANATOMIC SITE/ DIAGNOSIS/ MODIFYING CIRCUMSTANCES	ETIOLOGIES (usual)	SUGGESTED REGIMENS	
		Primary	*Alternative*
INFECTIVE ENDOCARDITIS—PROSTHETIC VALVE—CULTURE POSITIVE			
Early (<2 mo postop in U.S., <4 mo postop in Europe)	*S. aureus, Enterobacteriaceae, S. epidermidis,* diphtheroids	Vancomycin + gentamicin + rifampin (6 wk) (see comments) (dosage: see above)	Depends on specific organism. For *S. aureus, S. epidermidis* (methicillin-resistant) choices include TMP/SMX, ciprofloxacin-rifampin—experience limited, consultation required. *Enterobacteriaceae* or *Pseudomonas:* tobramycin (high dose) + AP Pen or P Ceph 3 AP
	Candida, Aspergillus	Amphotericin B + flucytosine	
Late (>2 mo postop in US., >4 mo in Europe)	*S. viridans*	Same as viridans strep, MIC >0.1–<0.5 μg/mL	
	Enterococci	Same as enterococci, symptoms >3 mo	
	S. aureus *S. epidermidis*	PRSP[‡] + gentamicin + rifampin	Vancomycin + gentamicin + rifampin
	Enterobacteriaceae	Depends on organism and in vitro sensitivities	

rx, therapy; *Staph aureus,* strep, streptococci; MIC, minimum inhibitory concentration; qd, every day; IV, intravenously; IM, intramuscularly; po, orally; bid, twice daily; HD, high density; postop, postoperative; TMP/SMX, trimethoprim-sulfamethoxalone.
°Assumes estimated creatinine clearance ≥80 mL/min.
[†]See *JAMA* 1989;261:1471.
[‡]PRSP (nafcillin or oxacillin 2.0 g q4h IV), PRSP oral (dicloxacillin 500 mg q6h po), APAG, IMP 0.5 g q6h IV, TC/CL 3.1 g q6h IV, PIP/TZ 3.375 g q6h IV, AM/SB 3.0 g q6h IV, P Ceph 1 (cephalothin 2.0 g q4h IV or cefazolin 2.0 g q8h IV), ciprofloxacin 750 mg bid po or 400 mg bid IV, vancomycin 1.0 g q12h IV, rifampin 600 mg qd po, aztreonam 2.0 g q8h IV.
[§]See *JAMA* 1992;267:246.
[‖]See *Lancet* 1985;2:815.
[¶]See *JAMA* 1979;241:1801.
[#]See *Rev Infect Dis* 1987;9:908.
°°Enterococci, esp. *E. faecium,* becoming increasingly resistant to available drugs (*Lancet* 1993;342:76). For infections other than endocarditis, enterococcal infections, if susceptible, can

apy for these infections seems to be increasing in importance.

Surgical removal of the infected prosthetic valve in conjunction with appropriate antimicrobial therapy increases the survival rate in patients with these difficult infections.[63-65] Surgery should be performed before the course of antibiotics is completed and as soon as the patient is clinically stable. Antimicrobial regimens for these infections are similar to those used in native valve endocarditis.

The increased incidence of *S epidermidis* as a cause of prosthetic valve endocarditis needs to be considered when empirical therapy for presumed endocarditis is instituted. Most investigators support the combined use of vancomycin (0.5 g IV every 6 hours), rifampin (300 mg orally every 12 hours), and gentamicin (1 mg/kg IV every 8 hours) for treating *S epidermidis* endocarditis. The duration of therapy once the valve is replaced also is controversial. If no evidence of extravalvular infection is found at the time of surgery, antimicrobial agents should be continued for an additional 2 to 4 weeks after surgery. If valve ring abscess or annular infection is observed, then antimicrobial agents should be given for 6 to 8 weeks from the time of surgery.

Recommendations for prophylactic antibiotics in the prevention of bacterial endocarditis have been a source of confusion for many years. Although there are no data from controlled clinical trials, prophylactic antibiotics are recommended for patients who are at risk and who are having procedures likely to cause bacteremia. Both the patient's underlying heart disease and the likelihood that the procedure will initiate bacteremia must be considered in deciding when prophylaxis is to be used.

Endocarditis prophylaxis is recommended for patients with prosthetic heart valves, most congenital cardiac malfor-

ADJUNCT DIAGNOSTIC OR THERAPEUTIC MEASURES AND COMMENTS

S. aureus: gentamicin for only 5 d (peak serum levels 3 μgmL). Start rifampin on d 6. If no clinical response in 7–10 d, consider early surgery. *S. epidermidis*: 75% resistant to PRSP and all PRSP-resistant are clinically resistant to P Ceph 1 even if "sensitive" in vitro. Treat with vancomycin + gentamicin + rifampin for 1st 14 d, then continue vancomycin + rifampin to complete 6 wk. Removal of prosthesis often required

Early surgery required. *Aspergillus* endocarditis often presents as embolus to major artery. With surgery + medical rx, mortality with *Aspergillus* still >90%

See early PVE, above

be cured by ampicillin or vancomycin alone. In endocarditis, cidal activity is required for cure. β-lactams and vancomycin are only static and require an aminoglycoside for cidal activity. With ↑ resistance this poses serious problems. In endocarditis: (1) if high-level resistance to gentamicin and streptomycin, β-lactamase negative—ampicillin 12 g/d IV for long course (8–12 wk). (2) β-lactamase + but aminoglycosidic susceptible—vancomycin + gentamicin for 6 wk. (3) Vancomycin resistant + β-lactamase positive + aminoglycoside resistant—consider teicoplanin and probable surgical removal of valve. Rifampin + ciprofloxacin + gentamicin used successfully in 2 patients (*Ann Intern Med* 1992;117:112). Infectious Disease consultation indicated (ampicillin + ciprofloxacin cidal in vitro for many strains of *E. faecium* [AAC 1993;37:1904]).
††See *Ann Intern Med* 1988;109:619.
‡‡See *Ann Intern Med* 1991;115:674.
§§See *Ann Intern Med* 1992;117:390.

Adapted from Stanford JP, Gilbert DN, Sande MA, et al: Antimicrobial Therapy, Inc, Dallas, Texas, Guide to Antimicrobial Therapy, 1995:18.

mations, rheumatic and other acquired valvular dysfunction, idiopathic hypertrophic subaortic stenosis, mitral valve prolapse with insufficiency, and previous history of bacterial endocarditis.[66] No endocarditis prophylaxis currently is recommended for isolated secundum atrial septal defect, ligated patent ductus arteriosus, repaired secundum atrial septal defect, or postoperative coronary artery bypass graft surgery.

Manipulation of teeth and gums or of genitourinary and gastrointestinal tracts is associated with significant bacteremia. Therefore, endocarditis prophylaxis is recommended for these procedures. In addition, surgical procedures or biopsy involving respiratory mucosa, bronchoscopy with a rigid bronchoscope, and incision and drainage of infected tissue require endocarditis prophylaxis.

Recent recommendations on antibiotic coverage include both standard and special regimens with dental, respiratory, genitourinary, and gastrointestinal procedures (Tables 120-10 through 120-12). Prophylaxis is given before and for a few hours (6 to 8) after the procedure. Most regimens include a penicillin with or without an aminoglycoside. Vancomycin is recommended for the penicillin-allergic patient.

Patients undergoing cardiac surgery should receive antibiotics that cover staphylococci at the time of surgery. Penicillinase-resistant penicillin or first-generation cephalosporins often are recommended. Prophylaxis should start immediately before the operative procedure and continue for no more than 2 days after surgery. Prophylactic antibiotics are not required in cardiac catheterization and angiography, but should be considered in patients undergoing

(text continues on page 1800)

TABLE 120-9. Surgical Intervention in Active Endocarditis: Criteria and Indications

Major criteria: Any single criterion requires early operation
  Progressive heart failure
  Significant heart failure°
  Multiple embolic episodes
  Persistent bacteremia despite appropriate antibiotics
  Fungal endocarditis
  Extravalvular foreign body
  Development of heart block, bundle branch block, or purulent pericarditis†
  Prosthetic valve dehiscence or obstruction
  Relapse following "adequate" trial‡

Minor criteria: Any three criteria predict a high rate of antibiotic failure with resultant
    (often sudden and major) complications: surgery should be considered in certain
    patients if only two criteria are met.
  Congestive heart failure resolved with medical therapy
  Single embolus
  Definite left-sided vegetations seen on M-mode echocardiography
  Early mitral valve closure or flail valve leaflets
  Early prosthetic endocarditis caused by other than highly penicillin-sensitive streptococci
  Gram-negative rod tricuspid endocarditis
  Persistent fever without other identifiable cause
  New regurgitant murmur in aortic prosthetic endocarditis
  Lack of appropriate cell wall antibiotic

°Symptoms and signs of heart failure fail to resolve after "simple" medical therapy. If heart failure predated endocarditis, "resolution" would imply a return to baseline.
†Conduction defects should be persistent and unrelated to drug therapy or ischemic cardiac disease; these should occur in the setting of aortic valve involvement.
‡"Adequate" implies the use of the best available antibiotics in the maximum tolerated dosage for a minimum of 6–8 w.

Dinubile MJ: Surgery in active endocarditis. *Ann Intern Med* 1982;96:656.

TABLE 120-10. Recommended Standard Prophylactic Regimen for Dental, Oral, or Upper Respiratory Tract Procedures in Patients Who Are at Risk°

DRUG	DOSING REGIMEN†
STANDARD REGIMEN	
Amoxicillin	3 g orally in 1 h before procedure; then 1.5 g 6 hr after initial dose
AMOXICILLIN/PENICILLIN-ALLERGIC PATIENTS	
Erythromycin	Erythromycin ethylsuccinate, 800 mg, or erythromycin stearate, 1 g, orally 2 h before procedure; then half the dose 6 h after initial dose
or	
Clindamycin	300 mg orally 1 h before procedure and 150 mg 6 h after initial dose

°Includes those with prosthetic heart valves and other high-risk patients.
†Initial pediatric doses are as follows: amoxicillin, 50 mg/kg; erythromycin stearate, 20 mg/kg; and clindamycin, 10 mg/kg. Follow-up doses should be one half the initial dose. *Total pediatric dose should not exceed total adult dose.* The following weight ranges also may be used for the initial pediatric dose of amoxicillin: <15 kg, 750 mg; 15–30 kg, 1500 mg; and >30 kg, 3000 mg (full adult dose).

TABLE 120-11. Alternate Prophylactic Regimens for Dental, Oral, or Upper Respiratory Tract Procedures in Patients Who Are at Risk

DRUG	DOSING REGIMEN*
PATIENTS UNABLE TO TAKE ORAL MEDICATIONS	
Ampicillin	Intravenous or intramuscular administration of ampicillin, 2 g, 30 min before procedure; then intravenous or intramuscular administration of ampicillin, 1 g, or oral administration of amoxicillin, 1.5 g, 6 h after initial dose
AMPICILLIN/AMOXICILLIN-ALLERGIC PATIENTS UNABLE TO TAKE ORAL MEDICATION	
Clindamycin	Intravenous administration of 300 mg 30 min before procedure and an intravenous or oral administration of 150 mg 6 h after initial dose
PATIENTS CONSIDERED HIGH RISK AND NOT CANDIDATES FOR STANDARD REGIMEN	
Ampicillin, gentamicin, and amoxicillin	Intravenous or intramuscular administration of ampicillin, 2 g, plus gentamicin, 1.5 mg/kg (not to exceed 80 mg), 30 min before procedure; followed by amoxicillin, 1.5 g, orally 6 h after initial dose; alternatively, the parenteral regimen may be repeated 8 h after initial dose
AMPICILLIN/AMOXICILLIN/PENICILLIN-ALLERGIC PATIENTS CONSIDERED HIGH RISK	
Vancomycin	Intravenous administration of 1 g over 1 h, starting 1 h before procedure; no repeated dose necessary

*Initial pediatric doses are as follows: ampicillin, 50 mg/kg; clindamycin, 10 mg/kg; gentamicin, 2 mg/kg; and vancomycin, 20 mg/kg. Follow-up doses should be one half the initial dose. *Total pediatric dose should not exceed total adult dose.* No initial dose is recommended in this table for amoxicillin (25 mg/kg is the follow-up dose).

TABLE 120-12. Regimens for Genitourinary and Gastrointestinal Procedures

DRUG	DOSING REGIMEN*
STANDARD REGIMEN	
Ampicillin, gentamicin, and amoxicillin	Intravenous or intramuscular administration of ampicillin, 2 g, plus gentamicin, 1.5 mg/kg (not to exceed 80 mg), 30 min before procedure; followed by amoxicillin, 1.5 g, orally 6 h after initial dose; alternatively, the parenteral regimen may be repeated once 8 h after initial dose
AMPICILLIN/AMOXICILLIN/PENICILLIN-ALLERGIC PATIENT REGIMEN	
Vancomycin and gentamicin	Intravenous administration of vancomycin, 1 g, over 1 h plus intravenous or intramuscular administration of gentamicin, 1.5 mg/kg (not to exceed 80 mg), 1 h before procedure; may be repeated once 8 h after initial dose
ALTERNATE LOW-RISK PATIENT REGIMEN	
Amoxicillin	3 g orally 1 h before procedure; then 1.5 g 6 h after initial dose

*Initial pediatric doses are as follows: ampicillin, 50 mg/kg; amoxicillin, 50 mg/kg; gentamicin, 2 mg/kg; and vancomycin, 20 mg/kg. Follow-up doses should be half the initial dose. *Total pediatric dose should not exceed total adult dose.*

procedures who have indwelling transvenous pacemakers, arteriovenous shunts for dialysis, or ventriculoatrial shunts.

REFERENCES ■

1. Bayer AS: Infective Endocarditis. *CID* 1993;17:313
2. Lerner PI, Weinstein L: Infective endocarditis in the antibiotic era. *N Engl J Med* 1966;274:199
3. Thayer WS: Studies on bacterial (infective) endocarditis. *Johns Hopkins Hosp Rep* 1926;22:1
4. Pelletier LL, Petersdorf RG: Infective endocarditis: a review of 125 cases from the University of Washington Hospitals, 1963–1972. *Medicine* 1977;56:287
5. Cherubin CE, Neu HC: Infective endocarditis at the Presbyterian Hospital in New York City from 1938–1967. *Am J Med* 1971;51:83
6. Garvey GJ, Neu HC: Infective endocarditis: an evolving disease. *Medicine* 1978;57:105
7. Watanakunakorn C, Burkert T: Infective endocarditis at a large community teaching hospital, 1980–1990. *Medicine* 1993;72:90
8. Chambers HF, Korzeniowski OM, Sande MA, et al: *Staphylococcus aureus* endocarditis: clinical manifestations in addicts and nonaddicts. *Medicine* 1983;62:170
9. Masur H: Prosthetic valve endocarditis. *J Thorac Cardiovasc Surg* 1980;80:31
10. Venezio FR, Westenfelder GO, Cook PV, et al: Infective endocarditis in a community hospital. *Arch Intern Med* 1982;142:789
11. Durack D, Lukes AS, Bright DK, et al: New criteria for diagnosis of infective endocarditis: utilization of specific echocardiographic criteria. *Am J Med* 1994;96:200
12. Sande MA, Scheld WM: Combination antibiotic therapy of bacterial endocarditis. *Ann Intern Med* 1980;92:390
13. Moulsdale MT, Eykyn SJ, Phillips I: Infective endocarditis, 1970–1979: a study of culture-positive cases in St. Thomas' Hospital. *Q J Med* 1980;49:315
14. Roberts WC, Buchbinder NA: Right-sided valvular infective endocarditis: a clinicopathologic study of 12 necropsy patients. *Am J Med* 1972;53:7
15. Kaye D: Definitions and demographic characteristics. In: Kaye D (ed). *Infective Endocarditis.* Baltimore, University Park Press, 1976:1
16. Lowes JA, Hamer J, Williams G, et al: Ten years of infective endocarditis at St. Bartholomew's Hospital: analysis of clinical features and treatment in relation to prognosis and mortality. *Lancet* 1980;i:133
17. Baddour LM, Bisno AL: Infective endocarditis complicating mitral valve prolapse: epidemiologic, clinical, and microbiologic aspects. *Rev Infect Dis* 1986;8:117
18. Durack DT, Beeson PB: Experimental bacterial endocarditis. I. Colonization of a sterile vegetation. *Br J Exp Pathol* 1972;53:44
19. Rodbard S: Blood velocity and endocarditis. *Circulation* 1963;27:18
20. Everett ED, Hirschmann JV: Transient bacteremia and endocarditis prophylaxis: a review. *Medicine* 1977;56:61
21. Weinstein L, Schlesinger JJ: Pathoanatomic, pathophysiologic, and clinical correlations in endocarditis. Part I. *N Engl J Med* 1974;291:832
22. Gutman RA, Striker GE, Gilliland BC, et al: The immune complex glomerulonephritis of bacterial endocarditis. *Medicine* 1972;51:1
23. Kerr A Jr, Tan JS: Biopsies of the Janeway lesion of infective endocarditis. *J Cutan Pathol* 1979;6:124
24. Silverberg HH: Roth spots. *Mt Sinai J Med* 1970;37:77
25. Weinstein L, Rubin RH: Infective endocarditis: 1973. *Prog Cardiovasc Dis* 1973;16:239
26. Churchill MA, Geraci JE, Hundar GG: Musculoskeletal manifestations of bacterial endocarditis. *Ann Intern Med* 1977;87:754
27. Pruitt AA, Rubin RH, Karchmer AW, et al: Neurologic complications of bacterial endocarditis. *Medicine* 1978;57:329
28. Bayer AS, Theofilopoulos AN, Eisenberg R, et al: Circulating immune complexes in infective endocarditis. *N Engl J Med* 1976;295:1500
29. Kauffman RH, Thompson J, Valentijn RM, et al: The clinical implications and the pathogenetic significance of circulating immune complexes in infective endocarditis. *Am J Med* 1981;71:17
30. Werner AS, Cobbs CG, Kaye D, et al: Studies on the bacteremia of bacterial endocarditis. *JAMA* 1967;202:199
31. Pesanti EL, Smith IM: Infective endocarditis with negative blood cultures: an analysis of 52 cases. *Am J Med* 1979;66:43
32. Washington JA II: The role of the microbiology laboratory in the diagnosis and antimicrobial treatment of infective endocarditis. *Mayo Clin Proc* 1982;57:22
33. Rubenstein E, Noreiga ER, Simberkoff MS, et al: Fungal endocarditis: analysis of 24 cases and review of the literature. *Medicine* 1975;54:331
34. Jones RB, Priest JB, Kuo CC: Subacute chlamydial endocarditis. *JAMA* 1982;247:655
35. Tobin MJ, Cahill N, Gearty G, et al: Q fever endocarditis. *Am J Med* 1982;72:396
36. Applefeld MM, Billingsley LJ, Tucker HJ, et al: Q fever endocarditis: a case occurring in the United States. *Am Heart J* 1977;93:669
37. Kaplan JE, Palmer DL, Tung KSK: Teichoic acid antibody and circulating immune complexes in the management of *Staphylococcus aureus* bacteremia. *Am J Med* 1981;70:769
38. Mugge A, Daniel WG, Frank G, et al: Echocardiography in infective endocarditis: assessment of prognostic implications of vegetation size determined by the transthoracic and the transesophageal approach. *J Am Coll Cardiol* 1989;14:631
39. Steckelberg JM, Murphy JG, Ballard D: Emboli in infective endocarditis: the prognostic value of echocardiography. *Ann Intern Med* 1991;114:635
40. Welton DE, Young JB, Raizner AE, et al: Value and safety of cardiac catheterization during active infective endocarditis. *Am J Cardiol* 1979;44:1306
41. Finland M, Barnes MW: Changing etiology of bacterial endocarditis in the antibacterial era. *Ann Intern Med* 1970;72:341
42. Rabinovich S, Evans J, Smith IM, et al: A long-term view of bacterial endocarditis, 337 cases: 1924–1963. *Ann Intern Med* 1965;63:185
43. Uwaydah MM, Weinberg AN: Bacterial endocarditis: a changing pattern. *N Engl J Med* 1965;273:1231
44. Kaplan EL, Rich H, Gersony W, et al: A collaborative study of infective endocarditis in the 1970's: emphasis on infections in patients who have undergone cardiovascular surgery. *Circulation* 1979;59:327
45. Steinberg D, Naggar CZ: *Streptococcus bovis* endocarditis with carcinoma of the colon. *N Engl J Med* 1977;297:1354
46. Serra P, Brandimarte C, Martino P, et al: Synergistic treatment of enterococcal endocarditis. *Arch Intern Med* 1977;137:1562
47. Reiner NE, Gopalakrishna KV, Lerner PI: Enterococcal endocarditis in heroin addicts. *JAMA* 1976;235:1861
48. Jemsek JG, Gentry LO, Greenberg SB: Malignant group B

streptococcal endocarditis associated with saline-induced abortion. *Chest* 1979;76:695

49. Shlaes DM, Lerner PI, Wolinsky E, et al: Infections due to Lancefield group F and related streptococci (*S milleri, S anginosus*). *Medicine* 1981;60:197
50. Bayer AS: Staphylococcal bacteremia and endocarditis: state of the art. *Arch Intern Med* 1982;142:1169
51. Cooper R, Mills J: Serratia endocarditis: a follow-up report. *Arch Intern Med* 1980;140:199
52. Reyes MP, Lerner AM: Current problems in the treatment of infective endocarditis due to *Pseudomonas aeruginosa*. *Rev Infect Dis* 1983;5:314
53. Tsao MMP, Katz D: Central venous catheter–induced endocarditis: human correlate of the animal experimental model of endocarditis. *Rev Infect Dis* 1984;6:783
54. Coleman DL, Horwitz RI, Andriole VT: Association between serum inhibitory and bactericidal concentrations and therapeutic outcome in bacterial endocarditis. *Am J Med* 1982;73:260
55. Wilson WR, Guiliani R, Geraci JE: Treatment of penicillin-sensitive streptococcal infective endocarditis. *Mayo Clin Proc* 1982;57:95
56. Herzstein J, Ryan JL, Mangi RJ, et al: Optimal therapy for enterococcal endocarditis. *Am J Med* 1984;76:186
57. Wilson WR, Wilkowske CJ, Wright AJ, et al: Treatment of streptomycin-susceptible and streptomycin-resistant enterococcal endocarditis. *Ann Intern Med* 1984;100:816

58. Bisno AL, Dismukes WE, Durack DT, et al: Antimicrobial treatment of infective endocarditis due to viridans streptococci, enterococci, and staphylococci. *JAMA* 1989;261:1471
59. Korzeniowski OM, Sande MA, The National Collaborative Endocarditis Study Group: Combination antimicrobial therapy of *Staphylococcus aureus* endocarditis in patients addicted to parenteral drugs and in nonaddicts: a prospective study. *Ann Intern Med* 1982;97:496
60. Noriega ER, Rubinstein E, Simberkoff M, et al: Subacute and acute endocarditis due to *Pseudomonas cepacia* in heroin addicts. *Am J Med* 1975;59:29
61. Reyes MP, Palutke WA, Wylin RF, et al: *Pseudomonas* endocarditis in the Detroit Medical Center 1969–1972. *Medicine* 1973;52:173
62. Dinubile MJ: Surgery in active endocarditis. *Ann Intern Med* 1980;96:650
63. Dismukes WE, Karchmer AW, Buckley MJ, et al: Prosthetic valve endocarditis: analysis of 38 cases. *Circulation* 1973;48:365
64. Wilson WR, Jaumin PM, Danielson GK, et al: Prosthetic valve endocarditis. *Ann Intern Med* 1975;82:751
65. Karchmer AW, Dismukes WE, Buckley MJ, et al: Late prosthetic valve endocarditis. *Am J Med* 1978;64:199
66. Dajani AS, Bisno AL, Chung KJ, et al: Prevention of bacterial endocarditis: Recommendations by the American Heart Association. *JAMA* 1990;264:2919

Critical Care, Third Edition, edited by Joseph M. Civetta,
Robert W. Taylor, and Robert R. Kirby.
Lippincott-Raven Publishers, Philadelphia, PA © 1997.

CHAPTER 121

∎

The Pericardium

Thomas L. McKiernan

The pericardium is a serous membrane envelope with a visceral layer that closely adheres to the epicardial surface and an outer parietal layer; together, these layers form a potential space that surrounds the heart in the mediastinum.

The pericardium's mechanical functions include limiting excessive myocardial dilatation as well as maintaining normal ventricular compliance and the functionally optimal cardiac shape. The membranous functions of the pericardium include reducing external friction and acting as a barrier to inflammation from contiguous structures.

The pericardium primarily affects diastolic function; it can secondarily affect systolic function.

The intrapericardial pressure is usually negative; it is approximately equal to and varies with the pleural pressure at the same hydrostatic level. Pericardial pressure affects myocardial transmural pressure by the following relationship: transmural pressure equals cavitary pressure minus adjacent intrapericardial pressure. Because the intrapericardial pressure is normally negative, this usually adds to the normal transmural pressure gradient.[1]

The pericardial pressure–volume curve is generally flat as pericardial volume increases, and when further distention is impossible, a sharp rise in the intrapericardial pressure occurs (Fig. 121-1). This exponential curve accounts for the rapid clinical response when even small amounts of fluid are removed in cardiac tamponade.[2] The pericardium is highly resistant to acute stretching but adapts and expands to great dimension when subjected to a chronic stretching process.

These characteristics of the pericardium can be altered significantly by pathologic processes common in critical care medicine. This chapter deals with the most common clinical problems, which include acute pericarditis, pericardial tamponade, pericardial constriction, effusive-constrictive pericarditis, and the postpericardiotomy syndrome.

ACUTE PERICARDITIS ∎

Inflammation of the pericardial sac results in acute pericarditis. Exudation of inflammatory fluid into the pericardial space can increase the fluid content to a greater than normal level and results in pericardial effusion. This effusion is caused by an inflammatory exudation and occlusion of the normal drainage of epicardial venous and lymphatic systems by the inflammatory process. Pericardial effusion also can occur in the absence of pericardial inflammation, for example, in a hemorrhagic effusion. Common causes of acute pericarditis are shown in Table 121-1. Most often, clinically recognizable pericarditis in the adult is idiopathic. In these cases, a variety of viruses are often suspected causes; an etiologic agent is infrequently demonstrated. The most commonly demonstrated virus is the Coxsackie B group, which tends to elicit myopericarditis in children and pleuropericarditis in adults (also called Bornholm disease).[3] Influenza, Epstein-Barr, varicella, hepatitis, mumps, and human immunodeficiency viruses also cause pericarditis.

Pericarditis caused by infectious organisms other than viruses is less frequent now than it was in the preantibiotic era. Bacterial and tuberculous pericarditis are now more frequent in children and in immunocompromised patients. In adults, *Staphylococcus aureus* is still the most common organism, and there is an apparent decline in streptococcal and pneumococcal infections. Pus should be evacuated promptly from the pericardium, usually by operative intervention, because of the need to establish a definitive diagnosis, eradicate the infection, and prevent constrictive pericarditis. *Borrelia burgdorferi,* the organism responsible for Lyme's disease, also causes myopericarditis. Tuberculous pericarditis was once a common cause of acute and constrictive pericarditis but is rare in the United States. Mycobacterial infection must be ruled out in any case of suspected

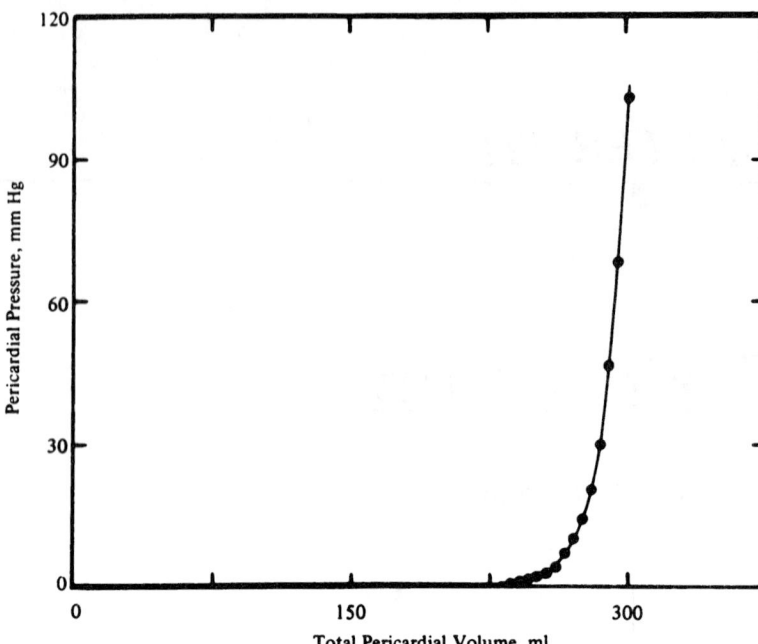

FIGURE 121-1. Pericardial pressure-volume curve (canine). Notice the rapid rise of the pericardial pressure after intrapericardial volume reaches approximately 225 mL. (Shabetai R: Function of the pericardium. In: Fowler NO [ed]. *The Pericardium in Health and Disease.* Mount Kisco, NY, Future, 1985:19.)

purulent pericarditis. A constellation of fever, small to moderate pericardial effusion, and pericardial rub suggests infection with gram-negative organisms in the immunocompromised host and with *Haemophilus influenzae* in children. Antibiotics have influenced purulent pericarditis in the following ways: the incidence has decreased, survival has increased, drainage is still necessary, resistant organisms have appeared, some cases are masked, more hospital-acquired cases have occurred, and there is a greater incidence after cardiac surgery.[4]

Pericarditis also can be caused by lymphoma, leukemia, melanoma, and breast, lung, and renal cell carcinoma when the offending neoplasm directly invades the pericardium. The prognosis with neoplastic pericarditis and effusion is poor. Pericarditis also is seen in systemic lupus erythematosus, rheumatoid arthritis, and scleroderma. Renal failure can induce acute pericarditis that can be refractory to the treatment. Renal failure–induced pericarditis usually disappears after beginning dialysis and is not related to serum blood urea nitrogen level. Renal failure–associated constrictive pericarditis is a real problem because of the prolonged survival of patients receiving dialysis. Radiation pericarditis often follows a mediastinal dose of 4000 rad or more and also can lead to acute cardiac tamponade. The long-term effects of radiation also can lead to constrictive pericarditis.

Iatrogenic pericarditis is primarily drug related. Procainamide, through the drug-induced "lupus syndrome," can produce acute pericarditis. Hydralazine and other therapeutic agents also can cause acute pericarditis.

Acute pericarditis after acute transmural myocardial infarction can mimic recurrent angina pectoris and, if the patient is receiving anticoagulants, can lead to cardiac tamponade. This condition is directly associated with myocardial infarction and is thought to be caused by visceral epicardial irritation.

CLINICAL FINDINGS

Symptoms of acute pericarditis are characteristic and include sharp and usually persistent chest pain that is generally pleuritic. The pain is severe so that only the most shallow breathing is tolerated. The pain is somewhat improved by sitting upright. Dyspnea also may be present. Signs of acute pericarditis include fever and a three-component friction rub that is evanescent. This friction rub component occurs in early diastole, presystole, and systole. A pleuropericardial rub also may be heard. The laboratory may report positive acute-phase reactants (especially the erythrocyte sedimentation rate) and an elevated white blood cell count. The chest radiograph shows an enlarged cardiac silhouette when over 200 mL of fluid has accumulated in the pericardial sac. Acute pericarditis also can present silently or with any combination of the signs and symptoms mentioned earlier. Thus, a high index of suspicion is needed to avoid missing the diagnosis.

The electrocardiogram (ECG) has been characterized as having four different stages in acute pericarditis; these stages can evolve over hours to days and weeks. Stage I includes classic and diffuse ST elevations with a concave ST segment and significant PR segment depression. Stage II is normalization of the ECG. Stage III is the development of diffuse T wave inversion that may persist or normalize; normalization of the ECG defines Stage IV[5] (Fig. 121-2). The ECG may include all stages or none in the evolution of acute pericarditis. Electrocardiographic differential diagnosis includes unstable angina, acute myocardial infarction, variant angina, hypertrophic cardiomyopathy, and pulmonary embolism— all of which can mimic the ECG changes described earlier. The key to diagnosis is the diffuse nature of these changes, the absence of localization to a particular ECG anatomic area, PR segment depression, and the absence of ST depression except in lead aVR.

TABLE 121-1. Common Causes of Pericarditis

Idiopathic
Viral
Tuberculous
Bacterial
Mycotic
Parasitic
Acquired immune deficiency syndrome
Neoplastic
    Primary
    Metastatic
    Contiguous spread
Myxedema
Uremia
Rheumatologic diseases
    Rheumatoid arthritis
    Systemic lupus erythematosus
    Scleroderma
Postmyocardial infarction
Postpericardiotomy
Trauma
Aortic dissection and rupture of the heart
Radiation
Drug-induced
    Procainamide
    Hydralazine
    Quinidine
    Isoniazid
    Methysergide
    Daunorubicin
    Penicillin
    Streptomycin
    Phenylbutazone
    Minoxidil
Miscellaneous
    Sarcoid
    Amyloidosis
    Acute pancreatitis
    Chylopericardium

The triad of typical chest pain, pericardial friction rub, and the aforementioned ECG changes confirms the diagnosis of acute pericarditis. This diagnosis must be differentiated from acute myocardial infarction and pulmonary embolism. The use of creatinine kinase isoenzymes (CK-MB), lactate dehydrogenase isoenzymes, and nuclear scanning helps to rule out myocardial infarction. However, CK-MB isoenzymes can be positive in acute myopericarditis and may confuse the diagnosis. The ECG and history should also support myocardial infarction before this diagnosis is made. Pulmonary embolism can be diagnosed with arterial blood gases, ventilation/perfusion lung scan, and, if indicated, pulmonary angiography.

Several studies demonstrate that arrhythmias are rare but do occur in acute pericarditis.[6] Atrial arrhythmia, in particular, can occur as a first manifestation of acute pericarditis. Frequent and significant arrhythmias should suggest myocardial or valvular involvement in addition to a pericardial disease process.

TREATMENT

Acute pericarditis is usually treated with antiinflammatory drugs. These include high-dose salicylates (300 to 900 mg of aspirin four times daily) and all of the nonsteroidal antiinflammatory agents, especially indomethacin (25 to 50 mg four times daily). These drugs should be given on a full stomach to prevent adverse gastrointestinal effects. Some patients may be refractory to these agents and may require a course of corticosteroids. Corticosteroid therapy should be reserved for aspirin and nonsteroidal drug nonresponders. The side effects of corticosteroid treatment include peptic ulcer disease, sodium retention, hypokalemia, hypoglycemia, Cushing's syndrome, suppression of the adrenal axis, and reactivation of infection. When an acute bacterial infection has been excluded and the patient's gastrointestinal status and cardiovascular status have been properly assessed, corticosteroids can be given. Prednisone is usually given in a dose of 60 mg/day for 5 days, then 40 mg/day for 5 days, then 20 mg/day for 5 days, with a continued tapering of the dose by 5 mg/week until the drug is withdrawn. Many variations on this dosing regimen exist.

The presence of acute pericarditis in acute myocardial infarction requires caution with the use of intravenous heparin. This drug is not, however, absolutely contraindicated. Thrombolytic agents have been reported to lead to cardiac tamponade and should be used with caution in the patient with acute myocardial infarction and acute pericarditis.

Recurrence of acute pericarditis is also common and often requires long-term corticosteroid therapy along with other antiinflammatory drugs. Colchicine has been used to treat chronic pericarditis with some success.[7] This aggressive therapy relieves symptoms and may prevent chronic scarring and constriction of the pericardium. In general, pericarditis symptoms subside in several days to weeks. The major complication is tamponade, which occurs in less than 5% of patients.

CARDIAC TAMPONADE ∎

Cardiac tamponade is a serious problem that can be rapidly fatal. If the correct diagnosis is made in a timely fashion, treatment may be lifesaving.

The pericardium resists sudden stretching but gradually expands in response to a chronic distending force. This allows the separation of cardiac tamponade into acute and chronic syndromes. Fowler[8] describes tamponade as the accumulation of pericardial contents to the extent that hemodynamically significant cardiac chamber compression occurs. Shabetai[9] defines it as the equalization of the intrapericardial pressure and the right ventricular diastolic pressure. Acutely, this occurs with rapid fluid entrance into the pericardium, causing a marked and rapid elevation of intrapericardial pressure. The causes of such an event are diverse. Intrapericardial hemorrhage may occur from trauma, ischemic myocardial rupture, or aortic dissection and rupture. This may happen in the postoperative patient, especially when anticoagulants are used. In this acute syndrome, the triad of increased central and pulmonary venous pressure, systemic

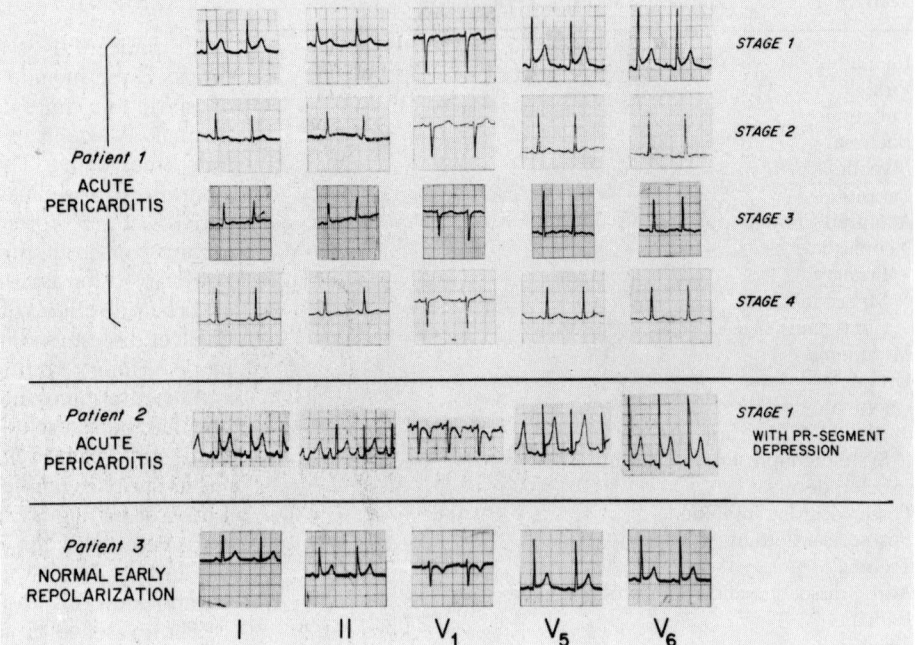

FIGURE 121-2. Three patients' electrocardiograms (ECGs). Patient 1 has acute pericarditis and demonstrates the four ECG stages in the evolution of acute pericarditis. Patient 2 has pericarditis and demonstrates significant PR depression. Patient 3 does not have pericarditis but has early repolarization. Notice the striking similarity to patients 1 and 2. (Vignola P, Johnson RA, Scannell G: Pericardial disease. In: Johnson RA [ed]. *The Practice of Cardiology.* Boston, Little, Brown, 1980:668.)

hypotension, and a normal heart contour is present. Pulsus paradoxus and pericardial effusion also can be appreciated.

CLINICAL FINDINGS

The patient with pericardial tamponade often is confused, agitated, and restless. Tachycardia and tachypnea are present. Breathing may become labored as accessory muscles are activated for respiration. The chronic condition may be more occult: the patient presents with a low-output state, right upper quadrant pain caused by swelling of the hepatic capsule, or even ascites and edema. Other symptoms may relate to the underlying etiology of the acute tamponade. In this acute setting, it usually takes less than 200 mL of fluid to compromise the heart, and the intrapericardial pressure rises from a normal of −3 mm Hg to 15 mm Hg or greater.

Classic clinical signs include an increased jugular venous pulse demonstrating a rapid x descent but no y descent because of the inability of the heart to fill in early diastole. Compression of the heart throughout the entire diastolic cycle explains this sign and characterizes acute tamponade. An accentuated pulsus paradoxus also is present and can be ascertained by inspection of the arterial pressure tracing, by palpation of an artery, or with a sphygmomanometer. This finding represents an accentuation of the normal fluctuation of the arterial pressure caused by changes in intrathoracic pressure and cardiac output. Normally, arterial pressure falls with inspiration and rises with expiration. The amount of paradox is gauged by measuring the systolic blood pressure and observing the difference in the level at which the Korotkoff sounds are heard only during expiration and the level at which they are heard throughout the respiratory cycle. A paradoxical pulse greater than 10 mm Hg is abnormal but may not be seen in tamponade when severe aortic insuffi-

ciency or atrial septal defect are present. Pulsus paradoxus can be seen with severe chronic obstructive pulmonary disease and asthma, however, and is rarely present with constrictive pericarditis.[10] In acute cardiac tamponade, hypotension often is present and the pulse may be unobtainable or may disappear completely with inspiration.

Other clinical signs of acute cardiac tamponade are distant and muffled heart sounds and an often-quiet precordium. Compensatory catecholamine release, caused by a decreased cardiac output, leads to sinus tachycardia and often to peripheral vasoconstriction. The ECG usually shows signs of acute pericarditis, including sinus tachycardia, PR depression, and abnormal T wave changes. Electrical alternans involving the P, QRS, and T vectors of the ECG is almost pathognomonic of pericardial tamponade. However, QRS alternans alone is the most common finding[11] and probably results from the movement of the heart in a large volume of fluid. It is not always present in cardiac tamponade (Fig. 121-3).

Cardiac tamponade is a clinical diagnosis based on the previously described symptoms and findings. However, the best adjunctive test is the echocardiogram.[12] When a moderate to large pericardial effusion is demonstrated echocardiographically, the probability of tamponade is increased (Fig. 121-4). Effusions seen with acute tamponade are usually smaller than those seen with chronic tamponade. Inadequate time often exists in acute tamponade to perform the echocardiogram because of circulatory collapse. If it can be completed, decrease in the right ventricular end-diastolic dimensions (less than 8 mm) during inspiration often is found. This is often accompanied by a shift of the intraventricular septum toward the left ventricular cavity and by paradoxical septal motion. One of the more sensitive echocardiographic indicators of acute cardiac tamponade is early diastole collapse of the right ventricle.[13] The large anterior and posterior

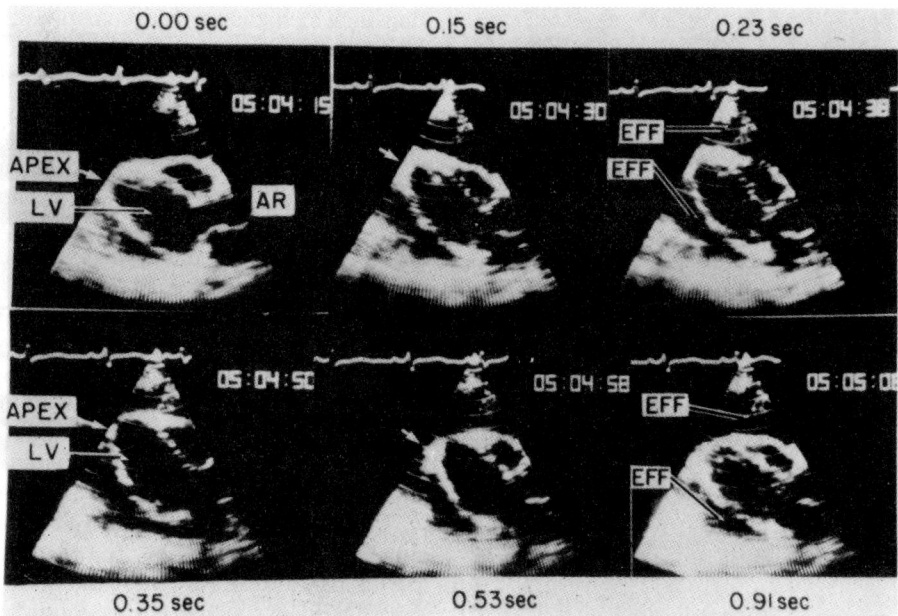

FIGURE 121-3. Six successive echocardiographic frames in the long axis from a patient with a large pericardial effusion. The electrocardiogram shows QRS alternans. Each upper frame corresponds approximately to the frame below at the same stage of the cardiac cycle; the cardiac cycle of the upper frames immediately precedes the cycle of the lower frames. Notice that the ventricular position and apex (*arrows*) are different in two succeeding cardiac cycles. This explains the alternation in QRS amplitude. (D'Cruz DA: Pericardial disease. In: Talano JV, Gardin JM [eds]. *Textbook of Two-Dimensional Echocardiography.* New York, Grune & Stratton, 1983:227.)

pericardial effusion that allows the heart to "swing" in the fluid and that produces QRS alternans is more common when the effusion has accumulated over a long period of time.

The hemodynamic profile of acute cardiac tamponade is characteristic and can be assessed by placement of a pulmonary artery catheter. The right-sided cardiac pressures are elevated and the diastolic pressures equilibrate. The right atrial mean pressure, right ventricular diastolic pressure, pulmonary artery diastolic pressure, and the left ventricular pressure are elevated and are measured within 2 to 3 mm Hg of each other. The pressure contour does not show a "dip plateau" sign, and pulsus paradoxus can be seen on an arterial pressure tracing. The pressures in chronic congestive heart failure are elevated but do not equilibrate in diastole. These measurements often can be made in the ICU setting to confirm the diagnosis of cardiac tamponade. Chronic tamponade develops more slowly and, therefore, passively stretches the pericardium to large volumes before significant compression of the heart chamber occurs. The patient's underlying illness may be symptomatically manifest. The most common causes of chronic tamponade include bronchogenic carcinoma, carcinoma of the breast, lymphoma, renal failure, tuberculosis, and idiopathic pericarditis.[14]

The physical findings in chronic tamponade include an accentuated pulsus paradoxus, an absent y descent, and decreased heart sounds; the systemic blood pressure is usually maintained, and the cardiac silhouette is enlarged on chest radiograph.

TREATMENT

Pericardiocentesis should be performed in any patient with acute tamponade and a reduction in systolic pressure of more than 30 mm Hg from the baseline level. The patient should be placed in a supine position at a 45-degree angle, and the area between the xiphoid and the left costal arch should be sterilized. A 7.6-cm (3-inch) aspiratory needle (16 to 18 gauge) with a short bevel should be directly attached to a three-way stopcock and a 50-mL syringe, and the needle advanced at an angle of 45 degrees to the abdominal wall and oriented in a posterocephalad direction.[15] Once the needle enters the subcutaneous tissue, it should be connected to the V lead of the ECG. As the needle punctures the pericardium, gentle suction usually yields freely flowing fluid.

If the tip of the needle contacts the epicardium, the ECG suddenly demonstrates ST segment elevation. The needle should then be withdrawn until the changes disappear. Complications of this procedure include pneumothorax, myocardial laceration, and coronary artery laceration. Many authors have pointed out the high risk of this procedure, which should be approached with experience and caution.

If the patient in acute cardiac tamponade can be stabilized by volume expansion and vasopressor support, then a safer and equally effective drainage of pericardial fluid can be accomplished by surgical subxiphoid pericardial resection and drainage. Subxiphoid resection can be performed in a sterile environment under local anesthesia; pericardial fluid can be removed and pericardial tissue obtained for biopsy

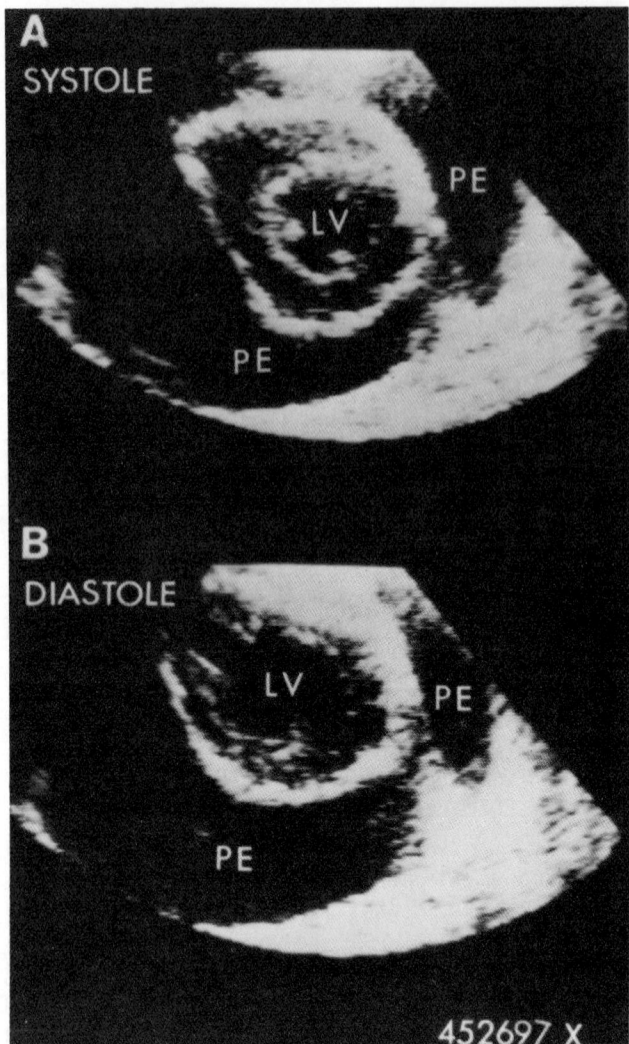

FIGURE 121-4. Short-axis, two-dimensional echocardiogram of a patient with a large pericardial effusion demonstrating the shift in cardiac position from systole to diastole. PE, pericardial effusion; LV, left ventricle. (Feigenbaum H: *Echocardiography*, ed. 3. Philadelphia, Lea & Febiger, 1981:494.)

and culture.[16] Percutaneous balloon pericardiotomy is being developed as another nonsurgical means to drain large pericardial effusions. Initial trials have been successful, but studies remain to be completed.

CONSTRICTIVE PERICARDITIS

Constrictive pericarditis is a chronic pericardial condition. Patients with this condition have a fixed decrease in chamber compliance. Constrictive pericarditis most commonly results from neoplasia, radiation, previous surgery, and idiopathic causes. Shabetai[17] defines constrictive pericarditis as a condition in which the pericardium becomes scarred, thereby losing its compliance and restricting diastolic volume. All chambers of the heart are restricted equally. The signs and symptoms of constrictive pericarditis generally occur over a prolonged period and are similar to those of biventricular congestive heart failure and cor pulmonale. Swelling of the lower extremities, increase in weight, and increasing abdominal girth from ascites are common. Fatigue and increasing shortness of breath are also noticed, and occult constriction is common.

Physical findings include increased jugular venous pressure with a prominent x and y descent. A loud early diastolic sound (pericardial knock) also may be appreciated on auscultation. The abdominal examination often reveals an enlarged liver secondary to congestion, along with ascites and splenomegaly. Significant lower extremity edema also can be demonstrated.

Unlike the situation in cardiac tamponade, blood pressure is maintained and less than 20% of patients have a significant pulsus paradoxus. The chest radiograph may show an enlarged cardiac silhouette. Calcium in the pericardium may be found, especially if the patient is examined by fluoroscopy.

The classic ECG findings of chronic constrictive pericarditis are nonspecific but include T wave inversions and atrial fibrillation. Echocardiography does not play a major role in the diagnosis of constrictive pericarditis, although many subtle diagnostic points have been described in the literature. The echocardiogram may show a thickened pericardium, but in the absence of a large pericardial effusion, this is often hard to differentiate from the myocardium and epicardium.

Cardiac catheterization pressure tracings are the key to diagnosis. In contrast to cardiac tamponade, the early phase of diastole occurs with a normal filling pressure, resulting in the classic dip and plateau on the right ventricular pressure traces. Occult constrictive pericarditis may be evaluated by performing volume loading at catheterization; the normal right and left heart pressures elevate and equilibrate in diastole.

Constrictive pericarditis may be treated with diuretics if symptoms are mild. Moderate to severe disease, however, requires removal of the pericardium by surgical stripping.

Features of cardiac tamponade and constrictive pericarditis often occur simultaneously, referred to as *effusive-constrictive pericarditis*. This may occur in a patient with neoplasia who develops a malignant pericardial effusion and who has previously received thoracic radiation that has scarred the pericardium. The patient usually presents a history similar to that given earlier. Accurate diagnosis requires hemodynamic studies both before and after treatment (Fig. 121-5).

Patients with restrictive cardiomyopathy have a clinical presentation almost identical to constrictive pericarditis. This condition is most commonly caused by amyloidosis in this country. The best tool to exclude cardiac amyloidosis is echocardiography and myocardial biopsy using amyloid-specific stains. Hemosiderosis also may cause restrictive cardiomyopathy.

POSTPERICARDIOTOMY SYNDROME ■

The postpericardiotomy syndrome was originally described as postmyocardial infarction pericarditis. It was thought to be a reaction to the injury of the epicardium in a myocardial infarct. Later, Engle and Ito[18] noted the same clinical syndrome in children and adults who experienced an opening of the pericardium. The syndrome occurs in 10% to 30% of patients who have undergone pericardiotomy and is thought to be an immune complex reaction to the patient's own pericardium.[19] The patient usually has symptoms of chest pain and fever beginning 2 weeks to 3 months after surgery. Malaise, night sweats, and myalgia are often present. Pericardial effusion is generally small or absent, but cardiac tamponade can occur, especially in patients who are receiving anticoagulants. The physical examination may or may not reveal a friction rub; a low-grade fever is often reported. The ECG generally demonstrates nonspecific changes similar to those of pericarditis. The erythrocyte sedimentation rate is usually elevated to greater than 50 mm/hour. The white blood cell count most often is normal, and the chest radiograph may demonstrate an infiltrate. The postpericardiotomy syndrome may increase the risk of early coronary artery bypass graft closure, and aggressive treatment has been recommended.[20] The disease is usually self-limited if left untreated; however, salicylates and nonsteroidal antiinflammatory drugs often decrease symptoms and speed recovery. Refractory cases may occur but usually respond rapidly to corticosteroids. High doses are given initially (short term), and doses are then tapered over 1 month to 6 weeks. Advocates of corticosteroid therapy claim that this treatment reduces the incidence of later constrictive pericarditis. Treatment with corticosteroids requires the exclusion of infection before initiation of therapy.

REFERENCES ■

1. Morgan BC, Guntheroth WG, Dillard DH: Relationship of pericardial to pleural pressure during quiet respiration and cardiac tamponade. *Cir Res* 1965;16:493
2. Shabetai R: Function of the pericardium. In: Fowler NO (ed). *The Pericardium in Health and Disease.* Mount Kisco, NY, Futura Publishing, 1985:19
3. Shabetai R: Acute viral and idiopathic pericarditis. In: Shabetai R (ed). *The Pericardium.* New York, Grune & Stratton, 1981:348
4. Spodick DH: The normal and diseased pericardium: current concepts of pericardial physiology, diagnosis, and treatment. *J Am Coll Cardiol* 1983;1:240
5. Spodick DH: Diagnostic electrocardiographic sequences in acute pericarditis. *Circulation* 1973;48:575
6. Spodick DH: Arrhythmias during acute pericarditis (100 cases). *JAMA* 1976;235:39
7. Guindo J, de la Serna AR, Ramio J, et al: Recurrent pericarditis: relief with colchicine. *Circulation* 1990;82:1117
8. Fowler NO: Physiology of cardiac tamponade and pulsus paradoxus. *Mod Concept Cardiovasc Dis* 1978;48:115
9. Shabetai R: Cardiac tamponade. In: Shabetai R (ed). *The Pericardium.* New York, Grune & Stratton, 1981:224
10. Fowler NO: The paradoxical pulse (pulses paradoxus). In: Fowler NO (ed). *The Pericardium in Health and Disease.* Mount Kisco, NY, Futura Publishing, 1985:235
11. Spodick DH: Electric alternation of the heart. *Am J Cardiol* 1962;10:155
12. Horowitz MS, Schultz CS, Stinson EB, et al: Sensitivity and specificity of echocardiographic diagnosis of pericardial effusion. *Circulation* 1974;50:239
13. Armstrong WF, Schilt BF, Helper DJ, et al: Diastolic collapse of the right ventricle with cardiac tamponade: an echocardiographic study. *Circulation* 1982;65:1491
14. Guberman BA, Fowler NO, Engel PJ, et al: Cardiac tamponade in medical patients. *Circulation* 1981;64:633

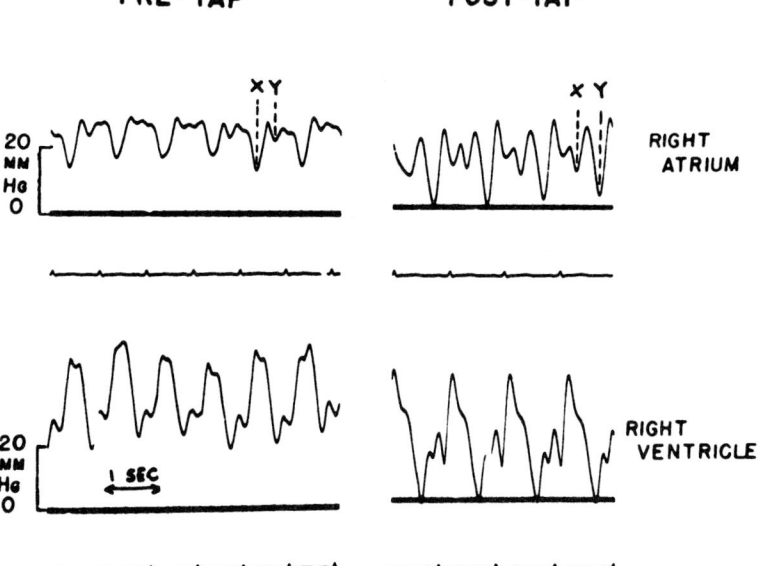

FIGURE 121-5. Right atrial and right ventricular pressures, before and after removal of pericardial fluid, in a patient with subacute effusive-constrictive pericarditis that followed radiotherapy. The right atrial pulse shows a prominent systolic descent (X >Y) initially and a predominantly diastolic descent (X <Y) after removal of the fluid. The diastolic "dip-plateau" pattern in the right ventricle pulse is prominent only after removal of the fluid, in association with the X <Y right atrial pulse. (Fowler NO: Constrictive pericarditis. In: Fowler NO [ed]: *The Pericardium in Health and Disease.* Mount Kisco, NY, Futura, 1985:317.)

15. Lorell BH, Braunwald E: Pericardial disease. In: Braunwald E (ed). *Heart Disease: A Textbook of Cardiovascular Medicine.* Philadelphia, WB Saunders, 1984:1487

16. Santos GH, Frater RW: The subxiphoid approach in the treatment of pericardial effusion. *Ann Thorac Surg* 1977;23:468

17. Shabetai R: Constrictive pericarditis. In: Shabetai R (ed). *The Pericardium.* New York, Grune & Stratton, 1981:154

18. Engle MA, Ito T: The post-pericardiotomy syndrome. *Am J Cardiol* 1961;7:73

19. Engle MA, McCabe JC, Ebert PA: The post-pericardiotomy syndrome and antiheart antibodies. *Circulation* 1974;49:401

20. Urschel HC, Razzuk MA, Gardner M: Coronary artery bypass occlusion secondary to postpericardiotomy syndrome. *Ann Thorac Surg* 1976;22:528

Critical Care, Third Edition, edited by Joseph M. Civetta,
Robert W. Taylor, and Robert R. Kirby.
Lippincott-Raven Publishers, Philadelphia, PA © 1997.

CHAPTER 122

■

Hypertensive Emergencies and Urgencies

Patrick C. McKillion
R. Phillip Dellinger

IMMEDIATE CONCERNS ■

MAJOR PROBLEMS

Hypertension affects up to 60 million Americans and is
a major risk factor for the development of cardiovascular,
cerebrovascular, and chronic renal diseases. Control of hypertension has a major impact on the course of these diseases. In the vast majority of these patients, hypertension
is not immediately life-threatening, and the goal of therapy
is to prevent long-term sequelae. In a small percentage of
patients with essential hypertension, and in some patients
with severe hypertension associated with specific disease
states (secondary hypertension), acute organ injury is ongoing or likely to occur and rapid reduction of blood pressure
is mandatory.

Situations requiring rapid reduction of blood pressure
may be divided into emergencies—those situations requiring
reduction of blood pressure to target level within 1 hour—-
and urgencies—those situations requiring reduction of blood
pressure to a target level within 24 hours (Table 122-1).[1]

STRESS POINTS

1. Initial concerns in patients with hypertensive emergencies should be oriented toward identification of
   end-organ damage and choice of appropriate pharmacotherapy, as well as toward the appropriate degree
   of blood pressure lowering.

2. The initial screening evaluation should include the
   following:
   a. Careful evaluation of the central nervous system
      (CNS)
   b. Cardiopulmonary evaluation to detect acute left
      ventricular failure or myocardial ischemia, or both
   c. Blood urea nitrogen (BUN) and creatinine mea-
      surement to ascertain new or worsening renal in-
      sufficiency
   d. Screening for dissecting thoracic aortic aneurysm
      in the appropriate clinical setting.
3. Although infrequently present, it is important to diagnose and respond to secondary causes of hypertensive
   emergency, which may include an acute CNS vascular
   event (need for early computed tomography [CT] of
   the brain), eclampsia (need for magnesium sulfate and
   delivery as soon as possible), renal failure (need for
   examination of urine sediment for evidence of glomerulonephritis and consideration, if appropriate, for hemodialysis), pheochromocytoma (need for diagnosis
   and treatment with phentolamine), renal vascular
   causes, and drug-induced causes (such as cocaine or
   tyramine consumption in the presence of monoamine
   oxidation inhibitors).

ESSENTIAL DIAGNOSTIC TESTS AND PROCEDURES

Physical Examination

1. Most patients with a hypertensive emergency have a
   history of hypertension. African-Americans, men, and

1811

TABLE 122-1. Situations Requiring Blood Pressure Reduction

Hypertensive emergencies
  Severe hypertension° with acute end-organ damage
    Central nervous system
    Myocardial ischemia
    Left ventricular failure
    Renal insufficiency
  Severe hypertension with:
    Eclampsia
    Head trauma
    Extensive burns
    Postoperative bleeding
    Pheochromocytoma
    Intracranial hemorrhage
  Any degree of hypertension with dissecting aortic aneurysm
Hypertensive urgencies
  Accelerated hypertension
  Perioperative hypertension

°Diastolic blood pressure >120 mm Hg.

patients with chronic renal disease appear to be at higher risk than others. CNS damage is suggested by symptoms of headache, visual disturbances, confusion, or seizures. Headaches are steady, anterior, and most severe in the morning. Substernal chest pain suggests hypertension-induced myocardial ischemia or infarction. It may be difficult at times to differentiate between myocardial ischemia-induced hypertension and hypertension-induced myocardial ischemia. However, in reality the treatments are similar and differentiation is not absolutely necessary. The sudden onset of severe tearing chest pain is reported by more than 90% of patients with acute dissection of the thoracic aorta.

2. Blood pressure must be interpreted in context. Although a diastolic blood pressure greater than 140 mm Hg is seen in most patients requiring acute reduction, children or patients who were previously normotensive may have CNS damage at diastolic blood pressures as low as 110 mm Hg. Any diastolic blood pressures greater than 90 mm Hg are of concern in a patient with aortic dissection. Many patients with chronic hypertension may have diastolic blood pressures greater than 120 mm Hg without evidence of acute end-organ damage or symptoms.

3. Grade IV (papilledema) retinal changes, if present, are diagnostic of increased intracranial pressure in patients with severe hypertension and hypertensive emergency. Grade III retinal changes (cotton-wool exudates and flame-shaped hemorrhages) represent ischemic injury to retinal nerve fibers and rupture of retinal blood vessels, which indicate a diagnosis of hypertensive urgency. Other fundus changes, such as arteriolar narrowing and arteriovenous nicking, are not specific for acute CNS damage. Mental status changes and a myriad of neurologic findings (often transient) may be present with hypertension-induced CNS in-

jury, including nystagmus, weakness, Babinski sign, and lateralizing defects.

4. Inspiratory crackles, a third heart sound, and tachycardia suggest acute left ventricular failure, whereas pulse deficits, paraplegia, aortic insufficiency, and pericardial friction rub suggest acute aortic dissection.

5. Renal dysfunction is associated with minimal physical examination abnormalities.

Laboratory Evaluation

1. The cardinal sign of acute hypertensive nephropathy is a previously unrecognized elevation of serum creatinine in the presence of severe hypertension. The urinalysis may show an active sediment with microscopic or gross hematuria. Anemia suggests preexisting renal disease. Mild hypokalemia is frequently seen and is usually secondary to high renin levels. Red blood cell casts suggest acute glomerulonephritis and renal-induced hypertension.

2. Many chronically hypertensive patients have evidence of left ventricular hypertrophy on the electrocardiogram (EKG). The EKG is most useful in ruling out acute myocardial ischemia or infarction.

3. The chest radiograph is best compared to previous films. Acute pulmonary edema (perihilar acinar filling pattern) in association with a severely elevated diastolic pressure is the hallmark of acute cardiac end-organ damage. A widened mediastinum is suggestive of aortic dissection, but contrast angiography or CT scanning is required to confirm this diagnosis.

INITIAL THERAPY

1. The ideal management of a hypertensive emergency includes admission to an ICU and continuous arterial pressure monitoring. This allows titration of medication and close observation of the patient for development of new symptoms and medication side effects. If ICU admission must be delayed, it is acceptable to monitor patients with frequent cuff pressures, but certain drugs with rapid onset of action (sodium nitroprusside and trimethaphan camsylate) should probably be avoided.

2. The goal of therapy is to arrest and hopefully reverse the progression of end-organ damage. Agents used must lower blood pressure quickly to acceptable levels yet have few deleterious effects. Rapid reduction of blood pressure is not without risk.

3. Mean arterial blood pressure is obtained either directly from an arterial catheter or calculated as diastolic pressure plus one third the pulse pressure. In normotensive patients, autoregulation prevents cerebral blood flow from falling until the mean arterial blood pressure drops below 60 mm Hg. In chronically hypertensive patients, autoregulation is altered. Cerebral blood flow may fall at mean blood pressures as high as 120 mm Hg with resultant cerebral ischemia (Figure 122-1).[2,3] Indeed, many cases of cerebral and cardiac damage due to excessive blood pressure low-

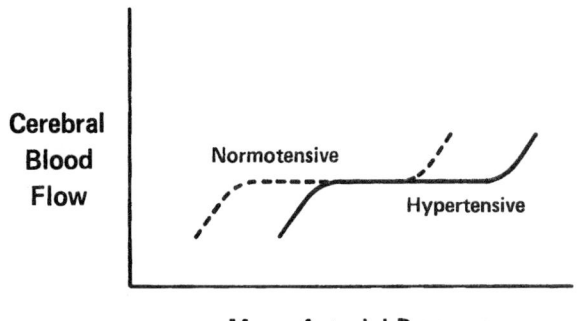

Mean Arterial Pressure

FIGURE 122-1. Cerebral blood flow decreases at a higher mean arterial pressure in hypertensive patients than in normal patients because of alterations in autoregulation.

ering have been documented. When blood pressure is lowered acutely in patients with or without acute CNS events, and results in deterioration of CNS status, the aggressiveness of hypotensive therapy should be decreased. Although renal function may transiently deteriorate during treatment, this should not deter the clinician. Long-term renal function is better maintained with aggressive antihypertensive treatment.

4. Parenteral therapy is preferred for hypertensive emergencies (Table 122-2). Reducing blood pressure over 1 to 2 hours to a mean of 120 mm Hg or a 15% to 25% reduction in mean arterial pressure is a reasonable goal. Oral medications are begun after 12 to 24 hours, and the blood pressure is reduced to the normal range over the next several days.

DRUGS USED IN HYPERTENSIVE EMERGENCIES

Sodium Nitroprusside

Sodium nitroprusside is the drug of choice for most hypertensive emergencies. Many characteristics make it ideal, including its rapid onset of action, immediate reversibility, and minimal side effects.[4] In addition it is the most potent of the parenteral hypotensive agents. The mechanism of action is direct dilatation of arterioles and veins. Its main effect comes from the decrease in systemic vascular resistance and resultant lowering of mean arterial pressure. The reduction in venous tone leads to a decrease in preload and a fall in cardiac output (except in patients with left ventricular failure, where it may not change or may rise).

Sodium nitroprusside should be administered in the ICU with an infusion pump. Continuous intra-arterial pressure monitoring is suggested. The initial infusion rate is 0.5 to 1.0 μg/kg/min. The desired blood pressure may then be "dialed in" by adjusting the infusion rate. The drug should be shielded from light to prevent degradation. In the blood, nitroprusside decomposes to cyanide, which is then converted to thiocyanate, primarily in the liver. Thiocyanate is excreted in the urine. Cyanide or thiocyanate toxicity rarely occurs unless infusion is longer than 72 hours or the infusion rate is high (greater than 3 μg/kg/min).[5] At a maximum

dose rate of 10 μg/kg/min, infusion should not exceed ten minutes.[6] Renal insufficiency increases the incidence of toxicity. Cyanide toxicity is heralded by metabolic acidosis; altered mental status, nausea, and hyperreflexia suggest thiocyanate toxicity. If toxicity is suspected, the drug should be discontinued. Treatment with amyl nitrate, thiosulfate, and hydroxocobalamin may be helpful in cases of cyanide toxicity[7]; dialysis is necessary in cases of severe thiocyanate toxicity. If prolonged infusion or high infusion rates are used, daily thiocyanate levels should be determined. If levels exceed 10 mg/dL, the infusion should be stopped.

Diazoxide

Diazoxide is a potent arteriolar-dilating agent. Reduction of blood pressure occurs almost immediately and is accompanied by a reduction in systemic vascular resistance with an increase in cardiac output and heart rate. Because the drug is avidly bound to albumin, it was initially believed that large bolus administration (300 mg) would be required to provide adequate concentrations of the free drug. This method of administration is associated with an unacceptable incidence of hypotension, stroke, and myocardial ischemia.[8] Minibolus administration is preferred because it is effective and associated with fewer side effects. Diazoxide is administered intravenously in multiple doses of 100 mg spaced 5 minutes apart until the desired blood pressure is reached. Diazoxide may also be slowly infused at a rate of 30 mg/min.[9] The most common side effect is tachycardia, which can be counterbalanced with small doses of intravenous propranolol. Fluid retention, nausea, vomiting, mild hyperglycemia, and arrest of labor may also be seen. Although ICU admission and intra-arterial pressure monitoring are desired, they are not mandatory when diazoxide is administered. Diazoxide is contraindicated in treatment of hypertension associated with myocardial ischemia and dissecting thoracic aortic aneurysms.

Labetalol

Labetalol competitively inhibits both alpha- and beta-adrenergic receptors. The intravenous form is ideally suited for treatment of hypertensive urgencies and emergencies. The beta-blockade is noncardioselective and one fifth the potency of propranolol. The alpha-blocking properties predominate clinically in the treatment of hypertensive emergency. Blood pressure reduction is accompanied by a marked reduction in systemic vascular resistance with little change in cardiac output or heart rate. For loading purposes the drug may be given intravenously in boluses of 20 to 80 mg every 10–15 minutes based on effect following a test dose of 20 mg.[10] Loading by continuous infusion at 2 mg/min is also effective and is less likely to produce unwanted hypotension. In some patients loading with continuous infusion rates of 0.5 to 1.5 mg/min may be more appropriate.[11] Side effects include headache, pain at the injection site, nausea, and flushing. During loading, the dosing of labetalol is discontinued when target blood pressure is reached. An oral agent is then instituted.

Even though the beta-blockade of labetalol is considerably less potent than propranolol, the drug should be avoided

TABLE 122-2. Parenteral Antihypertensive Agents

DRUG	ADULT DOSE AND ROUTE OF ADMINISTRATION	MECHANISM	ONSET OF ACTION	DURATION OF EFFECT	COMMENTS
Sodium nitroprusside (Nipride)	Continuous IV infusion Initial rate: 0.5–1.0 μg/kg/min Titrate to desired blood pressure Maximum 10 μg/kg/min for no more than 10 min	Direct vasodilation	Immediate	Minutes	Requires ICU and arterial pressure monitoring Side effects: hypotension, cyanide and thiocyanate toxicity, nausea Concentration of continuous infusion: 0.2 mg/mL
Trimethaphan camsylate	Continuous IV infusion 0.5–5 mg/min	Ganglionic blockade	Immediate	Minutes	Requires ICU and arterial pressure monitoring Side effects: urinary retention, ileus, orthostatic hypotension, cycloplegia Concentration of continuous infusion 1 mg/mL
Diazoxide (Hyperstat)	Minibolus 50–100 mg every 5 min Continuous IV infusion 7.5–30 mg/min	Direct arteriolar dilation	2–5 min	4–12 h	ICU, arterial line optional Variable duration of action Side effects: tachycardia, angina, vomiting, hypotension, hyperglycemia
Labetalol	20-mg test dose then 20–80 mg every 10–15 min Maximum 300 mg Continuous IV infusion 0.5–2.0 mg/min (up to total of 300 mg)	Combined alpha- and beta-blockade	5–15 min	2–12 h	ICU, arterial line optional Avoid in uncompensated heart failure and hypertension secondary to a low output state Contraindicated in heart block, severe sinus bradycardia, and asthma Concentration of continuous infusion: 1 mg/mL
Phentolamine mesylate	IV bolus 2.5–10 mg Report as needed	Alpha-blockade	Immediate	2–10 min	ICU, arterial line optional Side effects: hypotension, tachycardia, vomiting, angina, nausea
Hydralazine	IM or IV injection 5–20 mg	Direct arteriolar dilation	15–30 min	2–4 h	ICU, arterial line optional Side effects: tachycardia, flushing, angina
Esmolol	Loading dose infusion of 500 μg/kg/min over 1 min followed by a 4-min maintenance infusion of 50 μg/kg/min. If desired effect not achieved after 5 min, may repeat the loading dose and increase maintenance infusion to 100 μg/kg/min. Maximum dose of maintenance infusion is 250–300 μg/kg/min.	β₁-selective adrenergic blocker	Immediate	Minutes	Contraindicated in asthma and second- or third-degree atrial ventricular block Use with caution in the presence of systolic cardiac dysfunction

TABLE 122-2.   *(continued)*

DRUG	DOSE AND ROUTE OF ADMINISTRATION	MECHANISM	ONSET OF ACTION	DURATION OF EFFECT	COMMENTS
Enalaprilat	IV injection 0.625–1.25 mg every 6 h	Angiotensin converting enzyme inhibitor	15 min	12–24 h	Useful in cardiac failure or high renin states
Nitroglycerin	Continuous IV infusion 5–200 μg/min	Direct vasodilatation	1–2 min	1–3 min	Particularly useful in treating severe hypertension in the presence of symptomatic coronary artery disease
Nicardipine hydrochloride	Continuous IV infusion 5–15 mg/hr	Calcium channel blocker	1–3 min	15–40 min	Effective agent for postoperative hypertension and has the least potential cardiac contractility suppression of currently available calcium channel blockers; may produce tachycardia

IV, intravenous; IM, intramuscular; ICU, intensive care unit.

in certain situations, including severe sinus bradycardia, heart block greater than first degree, and asthma. In pheochromocytoma its use is controversial, although it has been shown to be effective in other states of adrenergic excess.[12] Several considerations need to be addressed when using labetalol in patients with heart failure. As a general rule, beta blockade is avoided in patients with "heart failure." In patients with hypertensive crisis, where a high systemic vascular resistance exists in the presence of an hypertrophied left ventricle, a combination alpha- and beta-adrenergic blocker such as labetalol may be very effective. Labetalol has not been studied in pregnancy and should be avoided in that setting. We have found labetalol effective in selected patients with hypertensive emergencies and consider it the drug of choice in situations where ICU monitoring is not immediately available or practical. It is particularly useful in patients with CNS and renal end-organ damage.

Trimethaphan Camsylate

Trimethaphan is a ganglionic blocking agent and like labetalol is an option (after intravenous nitroprusside plus intravenous propranolol) for blood pressure reduction in patients with dissecting aortic aneurysms (DAA). Trimethaphan produces orthostatic blood pressure reduction by decreasing cardiac output and peripheral vascular resistance. The head of the bed must be elevated for optimal blood pressure control. The rate of rise of arterial pressure with each cardiac contraction (dP/dT) is reduced, a desired effect in DAA. The lack of reflex tachycardia allows it to be used in DAA without beta-blockade. The pronounced side effects of gan-

glionic blockade include dry mouth, visual changes, paralytic ileus, and urinary retention, which have limited its use in recent years.

Hydralazine

Hydralazine, like diazoxide, is a direct arteriolar dilator that is also associated with an undesirable reflex tachycardia. This reflex tachycardia is associated with increased myocardial oxygen demand and makes both diazoxide and hydralazine poor choices in patients with coronary artery disease. It has a delayed onset of action (15–30 minutes) and a variable duration of effect (2–4 hours). Although hydralazine is consistently effective in lowering severe elevations of blood pressure in patients with renal insufficiency and eclampsia, it has little role in other hypertensive emergencies.

Clonidine and Nifedipine

Although parenteral agents are the drugs of choice in hypertensive emergencies, the literature supports potential successful treatment of these states with orally administered clonidine or sublingual nifedipine.[13,14] Clonidine and nifedipine are more typically used in hypertensive urgencies, and are further discussed later in the chapter.

Phentolamine Mesylate

Phentolamine is a parenteral alpha-adrenergic blocking agent with a rapid onset of action and a short duration of effect. It is the drug of choice for treatment of a hypertensive emergency in patients with pheochromocytoma and mono-amine oxidase inhibitor–tyramine interaction. It is also useful in patients with severe hypertension after discontinuance of clonidine therapy. The antihypertensive effects are short lived, and repeated boluses may be needed. Hypotension may occur; other potential side effects include tachycardia, vomiting, and headache. Angina and myocardial ischemia can be provoked.

Diuretics

Although diuretics are useful adjuncts in the treatment of chronic hypertension, their role in the management of hypertensive emergencies is not as clear. In the management of chronic hypertension, they increase the effectiveness of vasodilating antihypertensive agents and prevent secondary fluid retention. Volume status may, however, be difficult to assess in patients with a hypertensive emergency. To assume that all patients with severe hypertension have expanded intravascular volume is incorrect. In addition, salt repletion may actually lower blood pressure by decreasing renin release in certain patients.

Patients with acute congestive heart failure may have a high pulmonary capillary pressure in the absence of an increased intravascular volume. Successful treatment of acute pulmonary edema may be associated with an increase or no change in intravascular volume, and furosemide probably exerts its primary beneficial effect in this circumstance acutely through afterload reduction.[15] It would seem that the use of a second afterload reducing agent in the management of hypertensive emergency is rarely indicated because potent single agents are available. The clinician markedly reduces the incidence of overtreatment and resultant hypotension by using a single therapeutic agent.

We have observed precipitous drops in blood pressure in patients treated with both sodium nitroprusside and furosemide, presumably from additive effects on arteriolar tone. Furosemide and other loop diuretics should be used cautiously in patients with a hypertensive emergency and should not be considered first-line drugs in this situation.

Esmolol

Although esmolol has been used as an antihypertensive, primarily in the postoperative cardiac surgery patient, it is primarily beneficial as a heart rate controller and is not FDA approved for treatment of hypertension. It should be used with caution in patients with systolic cardiac dysfunction and is contraindicated in second or third atrial ventricular block as well as asthma.[16]

Nicardipine

Nicardipine is a dihydropyridine-derivative calcium channel blocker that is 100 times more water soluble than nifedipine. It is an intravenously administered titratable calcium channel blocker, and has been shown to be effective in the management of severe postoperative hypertension.[17–19] It may be particularly useful in patients with cardiac or cerebral ischemia. The dose is independent of patient weight, and can

be begun at 5 mg per hour and the infusion increased by 2.5 mg per hour every five minutes to a maximum of 15 mg per hour to achieve blood pressure control. It is the least likely of the currently available channel blockers to be associated with negative inotropy. It may on occasions be associated with tachycardia.

Enalaprilat

Enalaprilat, an intravenous angiotensin converting enzyme (ACE) inhibitor, is useful for treating hypertension, particularly when associated with high renin states.[20,21] Inhibition of angiotensin converting enzyme results in vasodilatation by decreasing angiotensin II vasopressor activity and decreasing aldosterone secretion. Excessive hypotension may occur, particularly in sodium or volume depleted patients. Like other ACE inhibitors, edema is a potential complication. Enalaprilat should be considered a second-line drug for treating hypertensive emergencies.

Fenoldopam Mesylate

Fenoldopam is a new antihypertensive available for use by intravenous route.[22,23] It exerts its effect through postsynaptic dopamine-1 receptor agonism. It lowers blood pressure by decreasing peripheral vascular resistance with minimal change in heart rate and an increase in renal blood flow. It has rapid onset of action and short duration of effect with a half life of approximately ten minutes. It may prove to be particularly useful in patients with jeopardized renal function in the presence of severe hypertension.

SPECIFIC CONSIDERATIONS ■

CENTRAL NERVOUS SYSTEM DAMAGE

A strong relationship exists between severe hypertension and cerebrovascular disease. Severe hypertension may be associated with altered mental status, headache, and transient neurologic findings. If treated quickly and effectively these symptoms resolve; if not, they may progress to coma and death. If mean arterial pressure has been lowered to 120 mm Hg and neurologic findings persist, other diagnoses must be considered. The differential diagnosis includes acute thrombotic stroke, intracerebral or subarachnoid hemorrhage, CNS mass lesions, cerebral embolus, and encephalitis. Careful clinical assessment over time is required to establish the diagnosis. A CT scan is usually helpful. Lumbar puncture should be avoided in those patients without definitive diagnosis who may have increased intracranial pressure unless bacterial meningitis is suspected.

Maintaining adequate cerebral blood flow is critical in patients with CNS hemorrhage or stroke. The effect of blood pressure lowering on cerebral blood flow is not predictable.[24] If blood pressure is excessively high (diastolic 130 or greater), we will lower blood pressure to a diastolic of 110 to 120 mm Hg. Others might use a higher threshold. Our choice for lowering blood pressure in these circumstances is labetalol. Nitroprusside is a reasonable alternative but usually requires placement of arterial line to monitor blood pressure. Diazoxide is less desirable due to its long duration of action and frequency of side effects. It is also recommended that blood pressure be gradually lowered to a mean of 120 mm Hg when severe hypertension accompanies head trauma. The clinician should be prepared to stop the infusion if neurologic deterioration accompanies therapy. Decisions to lower blood pressure following intracranial hemorrhage in attempts to decrease the incidence of rebleeding are controversial and must be counterbalanced against potential to lower cerebral blood flow.

If blood pressure remains severely elevated in ischemic stroke, direct vascular damage and increased cerebral edema may lead to expansion of the infarct. On the other hand, if blood pressure falls excessively, perfusion in the peri-infarction zone may be inadequate, leading to progressive infarction. If diastolic blood pressure is 130 mm Hg or greater, we will lower diastolic to 110 to 120 mm Hg. This should be done in the ICU. Nitroprusside, again, is the drug of choice. Labetalol is a reasonable alternative, particularly if intensive monitoring capability is not available. Although it is thought that antihypertensive agents such as labetalol have no effect on cerebral blood flow, whereas clonidine, for example, lowers cerebral blood flow, it is not known which of these effects is desirable in patients with hypertensive emergency, increased intracranial pressure, and CNS end-organ damage. Nitroprusside with balanced vasodilatation throughout the circulation could increase cerebral blood flow. In patients in whom elevated intracranial pressure is the primary determinant of morbidity this could be deleterious. However, nitroprusside has passed the "test of time" and does not appear to be deleterious in this patient population. When nitroprusside is used in patients with hypertension as the inciting factor for cerebral edema, lowering the blood pressure is the single most important action in decreasing cerebral edema. The advantage or disadvantage of an antihypertensive drug that decreases cerebral blood flow (such as clonidine), however, is not as clear. On one hand, we are concerned about decreasing cerebral blood flow because it may increase the incidence of a cerebral ischemia, whereas on the other hand decreasing cerebral blood flow is one of the main treatment modalities in patients with primary cerebral edema (e.g., the head injury patient who is hyperventilated). A recent study supports decreases of mean arterial pressure of greater than 16% from baseline as putting the patient with stroke at jeopardy by decreasing cerebral perfusion.[25]

DISSECTING AORTIC ANEURYSM

Dissecting aortic aneurysm occurs in patients with chronic hypertension and in those with congenital malformations of the aorta, such as Marfan's syndrome. Dissection is initiated by an intimal tear and is potentiated by an expanding hematoma. Death occurs secondary to rupture of the hematoma into the pleural, pericardial, or peritoneal spaces or by occlusion of major vessels such as the carotid or renal arteries. Mortality of untreated DAA exceeds 90%.

Aortic aneurysms may be divided into those involving the aortic arch and those involving the descending aorta only.

Aortic dissection is suggested by the occurrence of sudden, severe, tearing chest pain in a patient with a history of hypertension. The patient may be dyspneic, confused, and exhibit focal neurologic signs. Proximal dissection may be associated with signs of cardiac tamponade or aortic insufficiency; distal dissection may lead to pulse deficits, hemothorax, and an acute abdomen if abdominal extension occurs. Rupture of the aneurysm is a surgical emergency associated with cardiovascular collapse. Angiography is the gold standard to establish the diagnosis and to determine the extent of dissection in anticipation of surgical repair. Although CT scanning has always been an excellent mode for diagnosing DAA, new-generation CT scanners in the hands of an experienced radiologist may also allow adequate definition of anatomy to guide surgery.

Surgical repair is recommended for DAA involving the ascending aorta after the blood pressure is reduced. Medical therapy is favored by most for uncomplicated dissection of the descending aorta.[26] Surgery is reserved in distal dissection for patients who show evidence of progression of the dissecting hematoma despite intensive medical therapy.

Medical therapy includes alleviation of pain and reduction of blood pressure to the lowest level that allows adequate organ perfusion. Trimetaphan camsylate has desirable hemodynamic properties in the management of hypertension in acute dissection. It immediately reduces blood pressure and reduces cardiac output, and decreases the steepness of the pulse wave contour (dP/dT), but bothersome side effects and the necessity to keep the head of the bed elevated are disadvantages. Sodium nitroprusside is more frequently used, but when used alone, it may have the undesired effect of increasing dP/dT. If nitroprusside is used, the patient should be treated with propranolol (1 mg IV every 5 min) until beta-blockade is obtained prior to starting nitroprusside infusion. Beta-blockade should then be maintained with oral or intravenous propranolol. Drugs that produce tachycardia, such as diazoxide and hydralazine, are contraindicated.

RENAL INSUFFICIENCY

Prior to the advent of antihypertensive therapy, survival in hypertensive emergency was short, and renal failure was a major cause of mortality. Although it is clear that renal function may transiently deteriorate during vigorous antihypertensive therapy, long-term renal function is improved.[27,28] Indeed, many patients with oliguric acute renal failure have significant recovery of renal function with a combination of blood pressure control and supporting dialysis.[29]

No clear data suggest a target blood pressure that allows for healing of renal lesions without leading to some degree of tubular necrosis. We generally reduce blood pressure over several hours with labetalol until a mean arterial pressure of 120 mm Hg is achieved. Some authors prefer diazoxide or hydralazine because these agents are reported to enhance renal blood flow.[30] After 24 hours the patient is given oral medications to maintain diastolic blood pressures below 90 mm Hg. Pulmonary artery pressure monitoring may be required if the patient's volume status is questionable. Patients who are obviously volume overloaded may require either high doses of loop diuretics or acute dialysis to lower blood pressure. Treatment of severe hypertension associated with oliguric renal failure is dialysis.

MYOCARDIAL ISCHEMIA

Hypertension frequently accompanies cardiac ischemia.[31] Hypertension is usually mild and transitory but, if sustained, it may lead to increased ventricular wall tension, increased myocardial oxygen demand, and a poor prognosis.[32,33] Occasionally, cardiac ischemia is accompanied by severe hypertension, the treatment of which may reduce infarct size.[34] Many of the agents used to treat ischemic chest pain (nitrates, morphine, beta-adrenergic blockers, calcium-channel blockers) also reduce blood pressure. Our approach to patients with myocardial ischemia and severe hypertension is initially to use sublingual nitrates and morphine followed by intravenous nitroglycerin if unsuccessful. If blood pressure cannot be controlled with intravenous nitroglycerin, sodium nitroprusside may be used. This agent is effective at reducing blood pressure and has been shown to improve left ventricular performance and reduce myocardial oxygen demand in acute myocardial infarction.[35] Although a "cardiac steal" phenomenon has been described, we have not found it to be a clinical problem. Labetalol may also reduce blood pressure during cardiac ischemia. By reducing heart rate, systemic vascular resistance, and blood pressure, myocardial oxygen demand is reduced. Labetalol should be used with caution in patients with significant systolic cardiac dysfunction. Nifedipine as a calcium channel blocker lowers blood pressure and offers the additional benefit of increase in myocardial blood flow to areas of ischemia. Potential disadvantages include reflex tachycardia as well as a possibility of a precipitous drop in aortic diastolic pressure and coronary artery perfusion pressure. Diazoxide and hydralazine should not be used because of predictable occurrence of reflex tachycardia and associated increases in oxygen demand.

ACUTE LEFT VENTRICULAR FAILURE

Hypertension may either be the cause of left ventricular failure or a secondary phenomenon. We consider hypertension to be the primary cause of left acute ventricular failure if the diastolic blood pressure is greater than 130 mm Hg. Other factors favoring hypertension as the underlying problem include a near normal-sized heart on chest radiograph and a history of hypertension. These patients typically present with very high blood pressure, chest radiograph with minimally enlarged cardiac silhouette, and pulmonary edema. Severe hypoxemia is present with or without CO_2 retention. Pink frothy sputum is a hallmark of this potentially life-threatening situation. These patients are best treated in the ICU with sodium nitroprusside. Nitroprusside is ideal because of its short half-life and its ability to reduce afterload and preload with little increase in heart rate. Nitroglycerin is an alternative that has less afterload reducing capability when compared with nitroprusside but offers the advantage of a potential increase in myocardial blood flow to ischemic areas in patients with coronary artery disease and acute myocardial ischemia. Intravenous loop diuretics may be useful as an immediate venous and arteriolar vasodilator pend-

ing institution of continuous intravenous afterload reduction. The subsequent diuretic effect may or may not be desirable depending on intravascular volume status. Morphine may also be used as a temporizing measure prior to institution of nitroprusside when severe hypertension is the primary cause of cardiac failure.

Trimethaphan is also useful but has unpleasant side effects. Diazoxide and hydralazine reduce peripheral resistance and improve left ventricular performance but are associated with a reflex increase in heart rate and myocardial oxygen demand and should be avoided in this setting.

If the underlying problem is considered to be heart failure (less severe elevations of blood pressure, no evidence of noncardiac hypertensive end-organ damage, and an enlarged cardiac silhouette) conventional therapy for heart failure is indicated. Generally, the acute administration of nitrates, diuretics, morphine, and other afterload-reducing agents results in decrease of blood pressure, but more importantly improvement in cardiac output.

PREECLAMPSIA AND ECLAMPSIA

Preeclampsia occurring in pregnancy is the syndrome of hypertension, edema, and proteinuria. Preeclampsia generally appears in nulliparous women after the 20th gestational week. Preexisting essential hypertension is common. Some of these patients may progress to eclampsia, a hypertensive emergency. These patients may develop seizures and end-organ damage typical of other hypertensive emergencies (cerebral hemorrhage, heart failure and renal failure, and microangiopathic hemolytic anemia). Delivery of the fetus is the treatment of choice.[36]

Patients with eclampsia should be hospitalized in the ICU and the blood pressure lowered to a diastolic of 90 to 100 mm Hg.[37,38] No medical treatment is ideal. Hydralazine has traditionally been the drug of choice. It is particularly effective in preeclamptic and eclamptic women and does not decrease placental blood flow. Potential problems include tachycardia and side effects that mimic symptoms of eclampsia (nausea, vomiting, headaches, and anxiety). Hydralazine may be associated with fetal distress in some patients; diazoxide is an alternative. The labor arresting potential of diazoxide may be overcome with oxytocin. The primary concern is excessive hypotension, which can be dangerous to both mother and fetus. Sodium nitroprusside is effective and safe for the mother. The fetus, however, may be at risk for cyanide toxicity, and this drug is therefore not recommended. Labetalol is a promising agent for treatment.[39,40] Fetal monitoring is recommended.

PHEOCHROMOCYTOMA

Pheochromocytomas are catecholamine-secreting tumors associated either with sustained hypertension or paroxysms of extremely high blood pressure. Other symptoms include diaphoresis, weight loss, palpitations, headache, and dyspnea. Acute pulmonary edema, encephalopathy, and intracranial hemorrhage may occur. Pheochromocytoma crisis is treated with intravenous phentolamine mesylate, 2.5 to 5 mg given every 5 minutes as necessary. If the crisis persists, sodium nitroprusside may be substituted. A few patients have been resistant to alpha-blockade and have required administration of alpha-methyl-paratyrosine, an inhibitor of catecholamine synthesis.[41] Beta-blockers (including labetalol) may lead to paradoxical hypertension in pheochromocytoma if used alone.[42] After their blood pressure is controlled, these patients may be maintained on phenoxybenzamine or prazosin.

ANTIHYPERTENSIVE WITHDRAWAL

Abrupt discontinuation of antihypertensive therapy may be associated with an abrupt rise in blood pressure. Blood pressure rarely if ever exceeds pretreatment levels, and reinstitution of therapy is adequate in most cases.[43] Intravenous phentolamine mesylate, sodium nitroprusside, or labetalol may be used in severe cases.

PEDIATRIC HYPERTENSIVE EMERGENCIES

The occurrence of severe hypertension in pediatric patients is infrequent, but potentially organ system and life threatening. Presentation includes severe headache, blurred vision, and seizures. Facial palsy is a neurologic abnormality that may be noted in pediatric patients. Hypertensive retinopathy and congestive heart failure associated with left ventricular hypertrophy may be present. Unlike adults, the causes of hypertensive emergencies are limited and include primarily renal parenchymal disorders with or without severe renal dysfunction. Renal causes include reflex nephropathy, unilateral atrophic renal disorders, and renovascular disorders. End-stage renal disease of any cause should also be considered. Renal disorders can be detected by utilizing a combination of BUN and creatinine determination, routine urinalysis, and routine renal ultrasonography. Renal vascular disease may manifest with proteinuria only. Less likely causes of severe hypertension are pheochromocytoma and renin-secreting tumors. Treatment of hypertensive emergencies in pediatric patients includes nitroprusside as the drug of choice delivered at 1–10 μg per kilogram per minute. This necessitates admission to the intensive care unit in most circumstances. Labetalol hydrochloride is an option to nitroprusside. In the absence of availability of treatment with intravenous short-acting drug therapy, nifedipine may be given in an initial dose of .25 mg per kg. ACE inhibitor therapy may be of particular benefit in renal vascular causes; a captopril dose for infants is 0.01 to 0.25 mg/kg per dose and for children is 0.1 to 0.2 mg/kg per dose. Captopril may be associated with abrupt decreases in blood pressure. Intravenous phentolamine mesylate is recommended in the presence of pheochromocytoma.[44]

PERIOPERATIVE HYPERTENSION

Poorly controlled hypertension, defined as a diastolic blood pressure above 110 mm Hg or a systolic blood pressure above 200 mm Hg, is associated with an increased operative risk and the development of arrhythmias,[45] myocardial ischemia or infarction,[45,46] neurologic complications,[47] and perioperative blood pressure lability.[46] Adequate blood pressure

control before surgery has been shown to reduce the risk of intracranial hemorrhage[48] and postoperative myocardial reinfarction.[49] A reasonable goal for blood pressure control before elective surgery is a systolic pressure under 170 mm Hg and a diastolic under 110 mm Hg.[50] Oral or parenteral agents can be considered in the preoperative setting.

Severe burns, pheochromocytoma, hyperthyroidism, stroke, aortic dissection and amphetamine or cocaine overdose are just some of the medical conditions associated with severe perioperative hypertension.[51] A careful history and physical examination may help to prevent the development of severe hypertensive episodes.

Prolonged periods of intraoperative hypertension are associated with an increased risk of postoperative complications including renal insufficiency, myocardial ischemia, and hemorrhage.[52,53] The parenteral vasodilators, nitroprusside and nitroglycerin, have the advantage of being short-acting and titratable, thus reducing the risk of prolonged periods of hypotension. Other parenteral agents shown to be effective in treating intraoperative hypertension include labetalol[54] and nicardipine. Rectal nifedipine was used to manage intraoperative hypertension in neurosurgical procedures and found to be effective, safe, and easy to administer.[55]

The type of surgical procedure has been shown to increase the risk of postoperative hypertension: for example, abdominal aortic aneurysm repair (57%), carotid endarterectomy (20% to 80%) and coronary artery bypass graft (33% to 61%).[56,57] Complications include rupture of vascular suture lines, intracerebral hemorrhage, arrhythmias, pulmonary edema, and myocardial ischemia.[45,46,56,58] Postoperative hypertension can also be caused by pain, hypoxemia, hypercarbia, hypothermia, excessive fluid administration, and anxiety due to the presence of an endotracheal tube or emergence from general anesthesia.[50,51] The patient should be evaluated and treated for these conditions prior to the initiation of antihypertensive therapy.

Nitroprusside and nitroglycerin are commonly used to control postoperative hypertension. Caution is advised when using nitroprusside after cardiac surgery due to the possibility of inducing tachycardia which may increase myocardial oxygen demand and a coronary artery steal phenomenon.[59,60] Parenteral labetalol, esmolol, nicardipine and isradipine have also been shown to be effective in treating postoperative hypertension.[61,62,63]

BURNS

Severe hypertension may accompany extensive burns; the reasons are unclear. Some cases may require treatment with sodium nitroprusside; labetalol and diazoxide are acceptable alternatives.

HYPERTENSIVE URGENCIES ■

Accelerated hypertension, traditionally defined as severe hypertension and grade III retinopathy (flame-shaped hemorrhages but no papilledema), may progress to hypertensive emergency if untreated but does not require immediate

TABLE 122-3.   Oral Antihypertensive Agents

DRUG	DOSE AND ROUTE OF ADMINISTRATION	MECHANISM	ONSET OF ACTION	DURATION OF EFFECT	COMMENTS
Clonidine	Initial dose 0.2 mg then 0.1 mg every h to a total of 0.7 mg if needed. Maximum dose 0.7 mg	Central alpha-agonist	30–60 min	12–20 h	Side effects: hypotension, sedation, dry mouth. Monitor blood pressure for 4 h after last dose
Nifedipine	10 mg oral or sublingual. May repeat in 10 min if needed	Calcium antagonist	10 min	3–8 h	Side effects: tachycardia, fluid retention, dizziness, angina (rare)
Minoxidil	Initial dose 20 mg then 10–20 mg every 4 h as needed	Direct arteriolar dilation	30–120 min	12–24 h	Side effects: tachycardia, fluid retention. Diuretics and beta-blockers used to counter fluid retention and reflex tachycardia, respectively
Captopril	6.25–25 mg oral	Angiotensin converting enzyme inhibitor	15 min	2–8 h	Side effects: rash, proteinuria, acute renal failure

lowering or parenteral therapy. Hypertension in the preoperative patient should also be lowered gradually with oral agents if the diastolic blood pressure exceeds 110 mm Hg. There is no evidence that severe hypertension in the asymptomatic patient who has no end-organ damage need be treated urgently. These patients are best treated with conventional antihypertensive regimens with close follow-up (Table 122-3).

DRUGS USED IN HYPERTENSIVE URGENCY

Clonidine

Clonidine is a centrally acting alpha-agonist that reduces blood pressure by decreasing central sympathetic outflow, vascular tone, and blood pressure. The main advantage of clonidine is that it is not associated with secondary increases in heart rate or cardiac output. An initial dose of 0.2 mg orally is given followed by 0.1 mg/hr until the desired blood pressure is achieved or a total dose of 0.7 mg is given.[64] Patients should then be observed for an additional 4 hours to monitor for overmedication. Clonidine may then be continued, or the patient may be switched to another regimen. "Clonidine loading" has been used extensively to treat severe hypertension over the past 5 years with success, even in patients with hypertensive emergencies. We have also found clonidine useful in patients who present to the emergency department with symptoms attributable to diastolic blood pressure elevations of 120 mm Hg or greater but yet have no end-organ damage. These patients cannot be classified as having a hypertensive urgency or emergency. We use clonidine to acutely lower blood pressure in this patient group, being careful to avoid excessive reductions in blood pressure.

Our target, when using clonidine in patients with hypertensive urgencies, is to lower diastolic blood pressure to between 110 and 120 mm Hg. All patients have their blood pressure monitored for at least 4 hours after their last dose of clonidine.

Nifedipine

Nifedipine is a calcium antagonist that has been used for acute lowering of blood pressure.[15] The capsule is punctured or chewed, facilitating drug absorption in the gastrointestinal tract. The onset of effect is seen in minutes, and the maximal effect occurs in 30 to 40 minutes. A single dose of 10 mg is effective in most patients. This may be repeated if needed. Tachycardia and precipitous drops in blood pressure, especially with repetitive doses, is a concern.

Minoxidil

Minoxidil is the most potent of the oral antihypertensive agents. Like hydralazine and diazoxide, it acts by dilating systemic arterioles leading to reductions in blood pressure, reflex tachycardia, and fluid retention. The onset of action is 2 hours, with the maximum effect seen in 4 hours. Concomitant administration of diuretics and beta-blockers may be required. Minoxidil is the best oral agent for treating patients with uncontrolled hypertension and renal insufficiency.[65] Diuretics are added for associated fluid retention. Beta-blockers may be necessary to combat reflex tachycardia.

Captopril

Captopril is an orally active inhibitor of the formation of angiotensin II, a potent vasoconstrictor. A single dose of 25 mg of captopril usually lowers blood pressure to reasonable levels in 90 minutes.[66] Onset of action is in five minutes and duration of effect is four hours. Unlike nifedipine, captopril is unlikely to produce a rise in heart rate. Use of angiotensin converting enzyme inhibitors over days may be associated with rise in BUN and creatinine, necessitating discontinuation of therapy in some instances. We use captopril only in treating hypertensive urgencies that accompany scleroderma, renal artery stenosis,[67] and other high-renin states.

REFERENCES ■

1. Joint National Committee on Detection, Evaluation and Treatment of High Blood Pressure: The 1984 report of the Joint National Committee. *Arch Intern Med* 1984;144:1045

2. Strangaard S, Olesen J, Skinhoj E, et al: Autoregulation of brain circulation in severe arterial hypertension. *Br Med J* 1973;1:507

3. Ram CV, Kaplan NM: Hypertensive emergencies. In: Shoemaker WC, Thompson WC, Holbrook PR (eds). *Textbook of Critical Care.* Philadelphia, WB Saunders, 1984:460

4. Palmer RF, Lasseter KC: Sodium nitroprusside. *N Engl J Med* 1975;292:294

5. Cohn JN, Burke LP: Nitroprusside. *Ann Intern Med* 1979; 91:752

6. New labeling for sodium nitroprusside emphasizes risk of cyanide toxicity. *FDA Med Bull* 1991;Mar:3

7. Cottrell JE, Casthely P, Brodie JD, et al: Prevention of nitroprusside-induced cyanide toxicity with hydroxocobalamin. *N Engl J Med* 1978;298:809

8. Kanada SA, Kanada DJ, Hutchinson RA, et al: Angina-like syndrome with diazoxide therapy for hypertensive crisis. *Ann Intern Med* 1976;84:696

9. Ram CV, Kaplan NM: Individual titration of diazoxide dosage in the treatment of severe hypertension. *Am J Cardiol* 1979; 43:627

10. Cressman MD, Vidt DO, Gifford RW, et al: Intravenous labetalol in the management of severe hypertension and hypertensive emergencies. *Am Heart J* 1984;107:980

11. Wright JT, Wilson DJ, Goodman RP, et al: Labetalol by continuous intravenous infusion in severe hypertension. *J Clin Hypertension* 1986;1:39

12. Rosenthal T, Rabinowitz B, Boichis H: Use of labetalol in hypertensive patients during discontinuation of clonidine therapy. *Eur J Clin Pharmacol* 1981;20:237

13. Cohen IM, Katz MA: Oral clonidine loading for rapid control of hypertension. *Clin Pharmacol Ther* 1978;24:11

14. Ram CV: Calcium antagonists in the treatment of hypertension. *Am J Med Sci* 1985;290:118

15. Wilson JR, Reichek N, Dunkman WB, et al: Effect of diuresis on the performance of the failing left ventricle in man. *Am J Med* 1981;70:234

16. Gray RJ: Managing critically ill patients with esmolol. *Chest* 1988;93:398

17. Wallin JD, Fletcher E, Ram CVS, et al: Intravenous nicardipine for the treatment of severe hypertension. *Arch Intern Med* 1989;149:2662

18. Wallin JD, Cook ME, Blanski L, et al: Intravenous nicardipine for the treatment of severe hypertension. *Am J Med* 1988; 85:331

19. Begon C, Dartayet B, Edouard A, et al: Intravenous nicardipine for treatment of intraoperative hypertension during abdominal surgery. *J Cardiothorac Anesth* 1989;3:707

20. Evans RR, Henzler MA, Weber EM, et al: The effect of intravenous enalaprilat (MK-422) administration in patients with mild to moderate essential hypertension. *J Clin Pharmacol* 1987; 27:415

21. Rutledge J, Ayers C, Davidson R, et al: Effect of intravenous enalaprilat in moderate and severe systemic hypertension. *Am J Cardiol* 1988;62:1062

22. Weber RR, McCoy CE, Ziemniak JA, et al: Pharmacokinetic and pharmacodynamic properties of intravenous fenoldopam, a dopamine$_1$-receptor agonist, in hypertensive patients. *Br J Clin Pharmacol* 1988;25:17

23. Holcslaw TL, Beck TR: Clinical experience with intravenous fenoldopam. *Am J Hypertens* 1990;3:120S

24. Calhoun DA, Oparil S: Treatment of hypertensive crisis. *N Engl J Med* 1990;323:1177

25. Lisk DR, Grotta JC, Lamki LM, Tran HD, et al: Should hypertension be treated after acute stroke? a randomized controlled trial using single photon emission computed tomography. *Arch Neurol* 1993;50:855-862

26. Wheat MW: Current status of medical therapy of acute dissecting aneurysms of the aorta. *World J Surg* 1980;4:563

27. Lawton WJ: The short-term course of renal function in malignant hypertension with renal insufficiency. *Clin Nephrol* 1982;17:277

28. Pohl JE, Thurston H, Swales JD: Hypertension with renal impairment: influence of intensive therapy. *Q J Med* 1974; 18:569

29. Barcenas CG, Eigenbrodt E, Long DL, et al: Recovery from malignant hypertension with anuria after prolonged hemodialysis. *South Med J* 1976;69:1230

30. Alpert MA, Bauer JH: Hypertensive emergencies: management. *Cardiovasc Rev Rep* 1985;6:602

31. Littler WA, Honour AJ, Sleight P, et al: Direct arterial pressure and the electrocardiogram in unrestricted patients with angina pectoris. *Circulation* 1973;98:125

32. Gibson TC: Blood pressure levels in acute myocardial infarction. *Am Heart J* 1987;96:475

33. Fox KM, Tomlinson IW, Portal RW: Prognostic significance of acute systolic hypertension after myocardial infarction. *Br Med J* 1975;3:128

34. Shell WE, Sobel BE: Protection of jeopardized ischemic myocardium by reduction of ventricular afterload. *N Engl J Med* 1974;291:481

35. Renard M, Riviere A, Jacobs P, et al: Treatment of hypertension in acute stage of myocardial infarction. *Br Heart J* 1983;49:522

36. Lindheimer MD, Katz AI: Hypertension in pregnancy. *N Engl J Med* 1985;313:675

37. Barron WM: Hypertension. In: Barron WM, Lindheimer MD (eds). *Medical Disorders During Pregnancy.* St. Louis: Mosby-Yearbook, 1991:1

38. Mabie WC, Gonzalez AR, Sibai BM, et al: A comparative trial of labetalol and hydralazine in the acute management of severe hypertension complicating pregnancy. *Obstet Gynecol* 1987; 70:328

39. Mabie WC, Ratts TE, Sibai BM: The central hemodynamics of severe preeclampsia. *Am J Obstet Gynecol* 1989;161:1443

40. Pickles CJ, Symonds EM, Pipkin FB: The fetal outcome in a randomized double-blind controlled trial of labetalol versus placebo in pregnancy-induced hypertension. *Br J Obstet Gynecol* 1989;96:38

41. Hauptman JB, Modlinger RS, Ertel NH: Pheochromocytoma resistant to alpha adrenergic blockade. *Arch Intern Med* 1983;143:2321

42. Navaratnarajah M, White DC: Labetalol and pheochromocytoma. *Br J Anaesth* 1984;56:1179
43. Ram CV, Engelman K: Abrupt discontinuation of clonidine therapy. *JAMA* 1979;242:2104
44. Lieberman E: Pediatric Hypertension: Clinical Perspective. *Mayo Clin Proc* 1994;69:1098
45. Prys-Roberts c, Greene LT, Meloche R, et al: Studies in relation to hypertension: II. Haemodynamic consequences of induction and endotracheal intubation. *Br J Anaesth* 1971;43:531
46. Prys-Roberts, Meloche R, Foex P: Studies of anaesthesia in relation to hypertension. I: Cardiovascular responses of treated and untreated patients. *Br J Anaesth* 1971;42:122
47. Assidao CB, Donegan JH, Whitesell RC, Kalbfleisch JH. et al: Factors associated with perioperative complications during carotid endarterectomy. *Anesth Analg* 1982;61:631
48. Cafferata HT, Merchant RF, DePalma RG: Avoidance of post carotid endarterectomy hypertension. *Ann Surg* 1982;196:465
49. Rao TLK, Jacobs KH,Et-Etr AA: Reinfraction following anesthesia in patients with myocardial infarction. *Anesthesiology* 1983;59:499
50. Wolfsthal SD: Is blood pressure control necessary before surgery? *Med Clin North Am* 1993;77:349
51. Leslie JB: Incidence and aetiology of perioperative hypertension. *Acta Anaesthesiol Scand Suppl* 1993;99:5
52. Charlson ME, MacKenzie R, Gold JP, et al: Postoperative renal dysfunction can be predicted. *Surg Gynecol Obstet* 1989;169:303
53. Roy LW, Edelist G, Gilbert B: Myocardial ischemia during non-cardiac surgical procedures in patients with coronary artery disease. *Anesthesiology* 1979;51:393
54. Zimmerman JL: Hypertensive Crisis: emergencies and urgencies. In: Ayres SM, Grenvik A, Holbrook PR, et al (eds). *Textbook of Critical Care*, 3rd ed. Philadelphia: WB Saunders Company, 1995:522
55. Gaur A, Pande RK, Kaushik S: Rectal nifedipine for the management of intraoperative hypertension. *J Neurosurg Anesthesiol* 1993;5:237
56. Gal TJ, Cooperman LH: Hypertension in the immediate postoperative period. *Br J Anaesth* 1975;47:70
57. Goldman L, Caldera DL: Risks of general anesthesia and elective operation in the hypertensive patient. *Anesthesiology* 1979;50:285
58. Towne JB, Berchard VM: The relationship of postoperative hypertension to complications following carotid endarterectomy. *Surgery* 1980;88:575
59. Flaherty JT: Comparison of intravenous nitroglycerin and sodium nitroprusside in acute myocardial infarction. *Am J Med* 1983;74(Suppl 6B):53
60. Mann T, Cohn PF, Holman BL, et al: Effect of nitroprusside on regional myocardial blood flow in coronary artery disease. *Circulation* 1978;57:732
61. Marty J. Role of isradipine and other antihypertensive agents in the treatment of peri- and postoperative hypertension. *Acta Anaesthesiol Scand Suppl* 1993;99:53
62. Singh PP, Dimicm I, Sampson I, Sonnenklar N, et al: A comparison of esmolol and labetalol for the treatment of perioperative hypertension in geriatric ambulatory surgical patients. *Can J Anaesth* 1992;39:559
63. Halpren NA, Goldberg M, Neely C, et al: Postoperative hypertension: A multicenter, prospective, randomized comparison between intravenous nicardipine and sodium nitroprusside, *Crit Care Med* 1992;20:1637
64. Anderson RJ, Hart GR, Crumpler CP, et al: Oral clonidine loading in hypertensive emergencies. *JAMA* 1981;246:848
65. Mitchell HC, Graham RM, Pettinger WA: Renal function during long term treatment of hypertension with minoxidil. *Ann Intern Med* 1980;93:676
66. Case DB, Atlas SA, Sullivan PA, et al: Acute and chronic treatment of severe and malignant hypertension with the oral angiotensin converting enzyme inhibitor captopril. *Circulation* 1981;64:765
67. Hricik DE, Browning PJ, Kopelman R, et al: Captopril-induced functional renal insufficiency in patients with bilateral renal artery stenoses or renal-artery stenosis in a solitary kidney. *N Engl J Med* 1983;308:373

Pulmonary Disease and Dysfunction

Critical Care, Third Edition, edited by Joseph M. Civetta,
Robert W. Taylor, and Robert R. Kirby.
Lippincott-Raven Publishers, Philadelphia, PA © 1997.

CHAPTER 123

■

The Acute Respiratory Distress Syndrome

Barbara J. Foner
Scott H. Norwood
Robert W. Taylor

IMMEDIATE CONCERNS ■

MAJOR PROBLEMS

The acute respiratory distress syndrome (ARDS) is characterized by nonhydrostatic pulmonary edema and hypoxemia associated with a variety of etiologies causing both direct and indirect insults to the lungs. The process develops acutely (usually within 72 hours of the precipitating event), requires immediate recognition, and often leads to death despite maximal medical support. Therapeutic goals in the setting of ARDS are to provide appropriate resuscitation measures and to quickly identify the underlying precipitating event and address or eliminate it, if possible. Adequate tissue perfusion and oxygenation must be maintained to support vital organs. Prevention of complications and the prompt recognition of their presence is critical to prevent late deaths.[1]

STRESS POINTS

1. The term *acute respiratory distress syndrome* rather than *adult respiratory distress syndrome* is preferred because the syndrome clearly is not limited to adults.
2. ARDS is commonly seen with the systemic inflammatory response syndrome (SIRS) and the multiple organ dysfunction syndrome (MODS).
3. Risks factors for developing ARDS include SIRS,

pulmonary contusion, aspiration, inhalation of toxic substances, near-drowning, long bone fractures, pancreatitis, diffuse pneumonia, and multiple blood transfusions.
4. Most patients with ARDS demonstrate similar clinical and pathologic features, irrespective of the cause of the acute lung injury (ALI).
5. The lung's response to injury can be divided into an exudative phase, an early proliferative phase, and a late proliferative phase.
6. A variety of inflammatory mediators have been implicated in the pathogenesis of ALI.
7. The neutrophil plays a central role in ALI.
8. The severe hypoxemia associated with this syndrome is caused by intrapulmonary shunting that occurs with alveolar flooding.
9. A reduction in functional residual capacity (FRC) and lung compliance are hallmarks of ARDS.
10. Radiographic changes seen in patients with ARDS are characteristic but nonspecific and rarely reveal the etiology of the syndrome.

ESSENTIAL DIAGNOSTIC TESTS AND PROCEDURES

1. History and physical examination
2. Chest radiograph

1825

3. Arterial blood gas measurements
4. Further diagnostic tests, based on the clinical circumstances

INITIAL THERAPY

1. Most patients require early endotracheal intubation and positive-pressure ventilation.
2. The goal of mechanical ventilation is to provide adequate oxygenation and carbon dioxide elimination while keeping to a minimum complications such as oxygen toxicity, barotrauma, volutrauma, and hemodynamic compromise.
3. Several experimental therapies are under investigation.

OVERVIEW

The syndrome that is known as ARDS was observed many years before Ashbaugh and coworkers'[2] initial description, and has been known by a variety of other names (Table 123-1). These investigators describe a heterogeneous group of patients with acute onset of tachypnea, hypoxemia, and stiff lungs. The underlying precipitating events included trauma, fat embolism, pancreatitis, pneumonia, aspiration, and drug ingestion. The mortality rate in the series was 58%. Since then, the list of inciting events has grown, the pathophysiologic mechanism is better understood, and data accumulate, but there has not been a substantial change in mortality.[3–5]

ARDS is most commonly seen with the SIRS[6] and MODS, highlighting the fact that this is a localized response to a systemic process. The published annual incidence in the United States is 150,000 cases. This number is suspect, how-

TABLE 123-1. Synonyms of ARDS

Adult hyaline membrane disease
Adult respiratory insufficiency syndrome
Congestive atelectasis
DaNang lung
Hemorrhagic atelectasis
Hemorrhagic lung syndrome
Hypoxic hyperventilation
Postperfusion lung
Posttraumatic atelectasis
Posttraumatic pulmonary insufficiency
Progressive pulmonary consolidation
Progressive respiratory distress
Pump lung
Shock lung
Traumatic wet lung
Transplant lung
White lung
Wet lung

ARDS, acute respiratory distress syndrome.
Taylor RW, Duncan CA: The adult respiratory distress syndrome. *Res Medica* 1983;1:17.

ever, because of the difficulty in defining and tracking cases. The process is initiated by an inciting event followed by a series of clinical and pathologic occurrences. Mortality depends on the underlying etiology. The definite risk factors for the development of ARDS include SIRS, pulmonary contusion, aspiration, inhalation of toxic substances, near-drowning, and long bone fractures. Probable risk factors include severe pancreatitis, diffuse pneumonia, and multiple blood transfusions.[7] Risk factors are additive: in one series, one risk factor led to a 25% incidence rate of ARDS; two risk factors, 42%; and three risk factors, 85%.[8]

Until recently, there has been a lack of uniformity in the definition of ARDS. The American Thoracic Society and the European Society of Intensive Care Medicine held a series of meetings in 1992, from which the American–European Consensus Committee on ARDS was formed.[9] The first word of the acronym has reverted back to *acute* rather than *adult* because the syndrome itself is clearly not limited to adults. The ARDS is on a continuum with ALI, which is a less severe form of impairment. ALI is defined as a syndrome of inflammation and increased pulmonary capillary permeability that is associated with a constellation of clinical, radiologic, and physiologic abnormalities that cannot be explained by, but may coexist with, left atrial or pulmonary capillary hypertension. It is associated with numerous conditions, most often sepsis syndrome, aspiration, primary pneumonia, or multiple trauma. The technical difference between ALI and ARDS is the degree of hypoxemia. ALI is present when the PaO_2 divided by the fraction of inspired oxygen (FIO_2) is 300 mm Hg or less, regardless of the level of positive end-expiratory pressure (PEEP), whereas ARDS is present when the PaO_2 divided by FIO_2 is 200 mm Hg or less, regardless of the level of PEEP. Although PEEP may have a significant influence on the shunt fraction, its effects are variable and time dependent. For this reason, it was deleted from the oxygenation requirement. The onset of hypoxemia in these conditions is acute, excluding chronic underlying pulmonary conditions. The pulmonary artery occlusion pressure measurement is helpful but not essential for diagnosis.

ETIOLOGY

Although ARDS may be caused by or associated with many conditions or diseases (Table 123-2), most patients demonstrate similar clinical and pathologic features, irrespective of the cause of the ALI. Most therapy for ARDS is supportive; however, in some instances, specific treatment for the inciting cause is necessary. Why one person with an acute illness develops ARDS and another with the same apparent illness does not remains unexplained. Risk factors for developing ARDS have been identified[7,8] (Table 123-3). Age does not seem to be an important risk factor. Aspiration of gastric contents and sepsis are highly associated with ARDS.

Pulmonary aspiration is one of the most common associated factors in the development of ARDS. In one study, 34% of patients witnessed to aspirate gastric contents subsequently developed ARDS.[7] Aspiration of material with a pH less than 2.5 is especially likely to cause ALI.[10–12] Particulate

TABLE 123-2. Conditions Associated With ARDS

SHOCK

Hemorrhagic	Cardiogenic
Septic	Anaphylactic

TRAUMA

Burns	Nonthoracic trauma
Fat emboli	(especially head trauma)
Lung contusion	Near-drowning

INFECTION

Viral pneumonia	Gram-negative sepsis
Bacterial pneumonia	Tuberculosis
Fungal pneumonia	

INHALATION OF TOXIC GASES

Oxygen	Cadmium
Smoke	Phosgene
NO_2, NH_3, Cl_2	

ASPIRATION OF GASTRIC CONTENTS (ESPECIALLY WITH A pH <2.5)

DRUG INGESTION

Cocaine	Fluorescein
Heroin	Propoxyphene
Methadone	Salicylates
Barbiturates	Chlordiazepoxide
Ethchlorvynol	Colchicine
Thiazides	Dextran 40

METABOLIC

Uremia	Diabetic ketoacidosis

MISCELLANEOUS

Pancreatitis	Leukoagglutinin reaction
Postcardiopulmonary	Eclampsia
bypass	Air or amniotic fluid emboli
Postcardioversion	Bowel infarction
Multiple transfusions	Carcinomatosis
DIC	

ARDS, acute respiratory distress syndrome; NO_2, nitrogen dioxide; NH_3, ammonia; Cl_2, chlorine; DIC, disseminated intravascular coagulation.

Taylor RW, Duncan CA: The adult respiratory distress syndrome. *Res Medica* 1983;1:17.

matter, even in the absence of severe acidity, may cause ARDS. Aspiration also may lead to bacterial pneumonia.

Pulmonary and systemic infections are associated with development of ARDS. Bacterial, fungal, viral, and protozoan organisms have been implicated. Gram-negative septic shock has an especially strong association with ARDS, and the mortality rate may be as high as 90%.

All forms of shock have been linked with ARDS. The syndrome has previously been called "shock lung" by many investigators, highlighting the importance of shock in the development of ALI. However, ascertaining the relative importance of shock as a single risk factor in the development of ARDS is difficult. Only 2% to 7% of patients presenting with hemorrhagic shock as a single risk factor subsequently develop ARDS.[7,13,14] Most patients with hemorrhagic shock also have sustained trauma and received multiple transfusions, so that it is difficult to isolate hemorrhagic shock as an independent, major risk factor.

Multiple risk factors for development of ARDS may exist in the traumatized patient. Causative factors include long bone fractures, fat embolism, pulmonary contusion, hemorrhage, multiple transfusions, and increased risk of infection. Fulton and Jones[15] report posttraumatic pulmonary insufficiency in 22% of patients with multiple traumatic injuries, which included primary chest trauma. Fourteen percent of patients with multiple trauma who had no primary chest trauma subsequently developed respiratory failure. Head injury has been associated with ARDS. The exact mechanism is not certain but seems to involve an intense central sympathetic outflow, resulting in a shift of blood from systemic to low-resistance pulmonary vascular beds. Pulmonary hypertension and hypervolemia may follow and alter pulmonary capillary permeability.

Near-drowning victims often develop ARDS. Approximately 90% of fresh or salt water near-drowning accidents involve alveolar flooding. Surfactant is washed out by salt water or destroyed by fresh water, and a direct osmotic alveolar injury can occur.[16]

Inhalation of toxic gases such as nitrogen dioxide (NO_2), ammonia, chlorine, and sulfur dioxide can cause ARDS.[17-20] Smoke inhalation may lead to ALI, especially when associated with burning plastic or other synthetic materials that liberate toxic fumes. High-concentration oxygen is toxic to the alveolar capillary membrane. Oxygen free radicals (O_2^-,

TABLE 123-3. Risk Factors Associated With Development of ARDS

MAIN

Sepsis	Multiple transfusions
Aspiration	Pulmonary contusion

TRAUMA PATIENTS

Age >70 y	APACHE II score ≥20
Female gender	

OTHERS

DIC	Burns
Pneumonia	Cardiopulmonary bypass
Long bone fractures	
Bacteremia	

ARDS, acute respiratory distress syndrome; APACHE, Acute Physiology Score and Chronic Health Evaluation; DIC, disseminated intravascular coagulation.

Pepe PE, Potkin RT, Reus DH, et al: Clinical predictors of the adult respiratory distress syndrome. *Am J Surg* 1982;144:124; Hudson LD, Milberg JA, Anardi DJ, et al: Clinical risks for development of the acute respiratory distress syndrome. *Am J Respir Crit Care Med* 1995;151:293; and Fowler AA, Hamman RF, Good JT, et al: Adult respiratory distress syndrome: risk with common predispositions. *Ann Intern Med* 1983;98:593.

·OH) and hydrogen peroxide are thought to be the responsible agents.

ALI also has been associated with ingestion of a variety of drugs (see Table 123-2). The drug usually has been taken in massive overdose. Cocaine and heroin use is strongly linked to development of pulmonary edema.

Multiple blood transfusions have been implicated in the development of ARDS; however, recent studies question their importance as an isolated risk factor. It is clear that on rare occasion, leukoagglutinins may precipitate pulmonary edema and ARDS during blood transfusion.[21,22] Disseminated intravascular coagulation (DIC) seems to be associated with ARDS. Bone and associates[23] report DIC in 7 of 30 patients with the syndrome. A relationship between pulmonary capillary endothelial damage and DIC is likely; however, direct cause and effect has not been established.

PATHOPHYSIOLOGY ■

STRUCTURAL RESPONSE TO INJURY

Under normal circumstances, gas is separated from the capillary blood by the ultrathin alveolar-capillary membrane (Fig. 123-1). The membrane has a thickness of about 0.5 μm, which allows for efficient gas exchange. The alveolar epithelium and the capillary endothelium rest on basement membranes. The interstitial space lies between the membranes and contains interstitial fluid, connective tissue, and scattered fibroblasts. The membranes fuse at the capillary-alveolar interface.

Pulmonary capillary endothelial cells are similar to endothelial cells found in other vascular beds. These cells produce and degrade prostaglandins, metabolize vasoactive amines, convert angiotensin I to angiotensin II, and produce, in part, coagulation factor VIII. Vasoactive agents synthesized by these cells may be partially responsible for regulation of ventilation and perfusion relationships. Endothelial cells are joined by loose intercellular junctions.

The type I pneumocyte is a flattened cell with thin cytoplasmic extensions. These cells are highly differentiated and, when damaged, cannot replicate. The cells join one another tightly and are normally impermeable to water.[24] The type II pneumocyte is usually found at the junction of the alveolar septa. These cuboidal cells are covered with microvilli. Surfactant is produced in the abundant cytoplasmic lamellar bodies and in the cytoplasmic microsomes of the type II pneumocyte.[25]

The lung's response to injury occurs in a predictable fashion, irrespective of the etiology of acute respiratory failure. It can be divided into an exudative phase, an early proliferative phase, and a late proliferative phase.[26] Histologic study of this acute alveolar damage reveals that it is diffuse and nonspecific and rarely reveals the etiology of the original insult (Table 123-4). Interstitial and then alveolar edema develops within 24 hours of the acute insult. Inflammatory cells and erythrocytes spill into the interstitium and the alveolus. Type I alveolar cells are sensitive to this type of injury and are soon destroyed, leaving a denuded basement membrane. Alveolar epithelial damage seems to be more significant at this stage than endothelial damage.

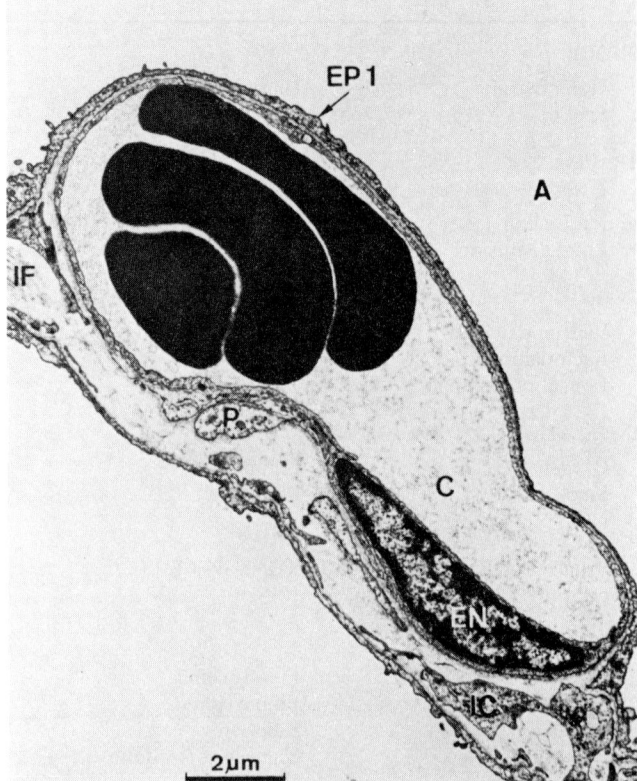

FIGURE 123-1. Electron micrograph of a normal interalveolar septum. EP1, cytoplasm of a normal alveolar cell; EN, pulmonary capillary endothelial cell nucleus; C, capillary lumen; P, pericyte; IF, interstitial fibers; IC, interstitial cell. (Bachofen M, Weibel ER: *Clin Chest Med* 1982;3:35.)

Edema fluid that collects in the interstitial space is initially drained by the pulmonary lymphatics. When the capacity of the lymphatics is exceeded, edema fluid accumulates around terminal bronchioles and larger vessels. As the process continues, fluid accumulates in the interstitial space adjacent to the alveoli and subsequently pours into the alveoli themselves. The alveolar-capillary membrane is often thickened at this stage.

Alveolar type II cells seem to be resistant to injury in the early stages of acute alveolar damage. Within about 72 hours of injury, these cells begin to proliferate, covering the previously denuded basement membrane.

Aggregates of plasma proteins, cellular debris, fibrin, and remnants of surfactant condense and adhere to the denuded alveolar surface, forming hyaline membranes. These are characteristically seen lining alveolar ducts and respiratory bronchioles (Fig. 123-2).

The alveolar septum thickens markedly over the next 3 to 10 days as it is infiltrated by proliferating fibroblasts, plasma cells, leukocytes, and histiocytes. Capillary injury becomes apparent at this stage. Hyaline membranes organize, and microatelectasis is seen. Fibrotic changes may develop by the end of the first week. This often occurs first in alveolar septa and hyaline membranes. Fibrosis becomes most apparent in the respiratory ducts and bronchioles, and alveolar structure may become virtually unrecognizable.

TABLE 123-4. Structural Response to Injury

EXUDATIVE PHASE (24–96 h)

Alveolar and interstitial edema
Capillary congestion
Destruction of type I alveolar cells
Early hyaline membrane formation

EARLY PROLIFERATIVE PHASE (3–10 d)

Increased type II alveolar cells
Cellular infiltration of the alveolar septum
Organization of hyaline membranes

LATE PROLIFERATIVE PHASE (7–10 d)

Fibrosis of hyaline membranes and alveolar septum
Alveolar duct fibrosis

Connors AF, McCaffree DR, Rogers RM: The adult respiratory distress syndrome. *Dis Mon* 1981;27:1.

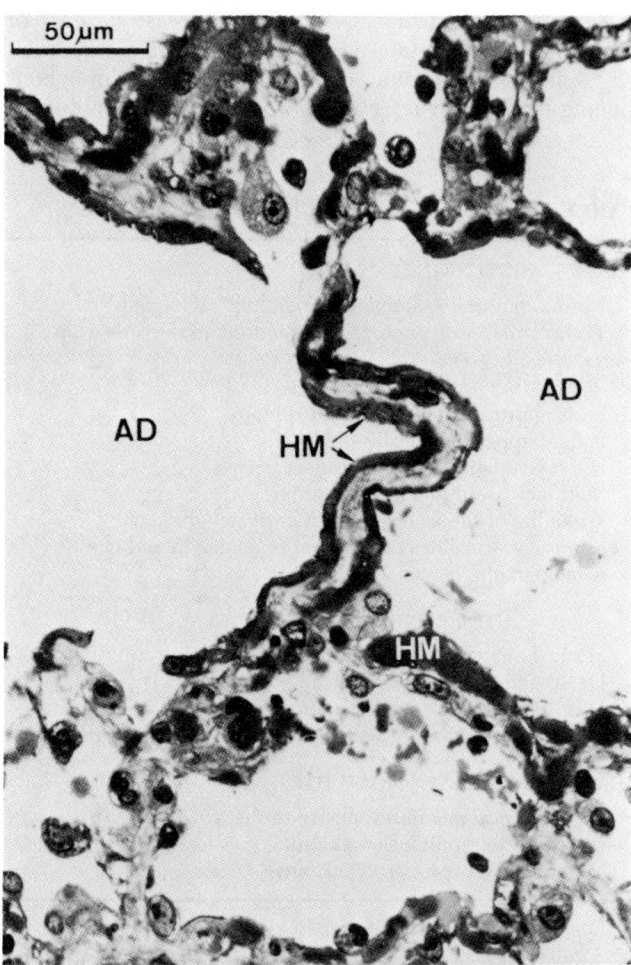

FIGURE 123-2. Light microscopic view of hyaline membranes (HM) lining alveolar ducts (AD). (Bachofen M, Weibel ER: *Clin Chest Med* 1982;3:35.)

Not all patients with ARDS progress through the entire pathologic process described earlier. Some patients recover within several days and never develop fibrosis, whereas others progress to end-stage fibrosing alveolitis. Even the extensively involved lung may resolve pulmonary fibrosis.[27]

NONCARDIOGENIC PULMONARY EDEMA

The total weight of the normal lung at autopsy is less than 700 g. However, in patients dying of ARDS, lung weight is uniformly more than 1000 g. Much of this increased weight results from increased extravascular lung water (EVLW). This "noncardiogenic" pulmonary edema is a central feature of ARDS.

The movement of water across biologic membranes is determined by the balance of hydrostatic and osmotic pressures that oppose one another across the membrane. The Starling equation quantitating fluid filtration also can be written as follows:

$$\dot{Q}_f = K(P_{CAP} - P_{INT}) - \sigma(\pi_{CAP} - \pi_{INT})$$

where $\dot{Q}_f$ equals net transvascular fluid flow, K equals filtration coefficient, P_{CAP} equals pulmonary capillary hydrostatic pressure, P_{INT} equals pulmonary perivascular interstitial space hydrostatic pressure, σ equals reflection coefficient (a measure of the effectiveness of the membrane in preventing flow of solute as compared to flow of water), P_{CAP} equals pulmonary capillary oncotic pressure, and P_{INT} equals pulmonary perivascular interstitial space oncotic pressure.

The increase in EVLW that occurs in ARDS is secondary to a derangement of alveolar capillary permeability.[28] The endothelial and epithelial intercellular junctions are probably the foci of fluid flow. Increases in both fluid and protein flux occur from the capillary space to the interstitial and intraalveolar spaces at normal to low hydrostatic pressures. We have little understanding of the exact mechanisms that lead to intercellular junctional changes. Furthermore, it is not clear whether all permeability changes act through a common pathway.

MECHANISMS OF ACUTE LUNG INJURY

The exact mechanisms of ALI are currently under intense investigation. Although clearing, the water surrounding this story remains a bit murky. When it is finally settled, perhaps it will lead to specific therapy that will allow us to neutralize the capillary leak phenomenon and fibrotic response. A variety of inflammatory mediators have been implicated in the pathogenesis of ALI (Chaps. 20 and 25).[29] The macrophage is thought to play an important role in release of cytokines and modulation of the inflammatory response.[29,30]

A central role in lung damage is played by the neutrophil. Kaplan and Goffinet[31] report the rapid onset of leukopenia during hemodialysis in 4 patients with chronic renal failure. The decrease in the white blood cell count began within minutes of the onset of dialysis and disappeared within an hour. Craddock and associates[32] established the pulmonary vascular bed as the hiding place of the disappearing leukocytes. Aggregation of leukocytes occurs in this setting because complement is activated by the cellophane coil and

C5a is generated. C5a is known to cause leukocyte aggregation and margination and to promote embolization to the pulmonary microvasculature. Other chemotaxins that may lure the neutrophil to the pulmonary microvasculature include bacterial factors, other complement components, lymphokines, prostaglandins, leukotrienes, and immunoglobulin fragments.[33]

Neutrophils accumulate in great numbers in the pulmonary microvasculature in patients with ARDS, and a large body of evidence implicates the granulocyte as a central figure in ALI.[34] Neutrophils are capable of releasing at least three groups of substances that can destroy lung tissue and alter lung function. These substances include granular substances, products of arachidonic acid metabolism, and species of reduced oxygen.

Neutrophil granules contain proteases, elastase, collagenase, cathepsins, cationic proteins, lysozyme, lactoferrin, and myeloperoxidase. Elastase and collagenase destroy basement membrane, elastic tissue in arterial walls, and lung tissue. Proteases digest enzymes, and structural proteins activate complement and Hageman factor and cleave fibrinogen.

Species of reduced oxygen include superoxide anion, hydrogen peroxide, and hydroxyl radical, all of which can damage lipid membranes, lung fibroblasts, parenchymal cells, endothelial cells, and a variety of enzymes. Normal lung defense mechanisms such as α_1-antitrypsin may be inactivated by superoxide radicals and oxygen.

Neutrophils produce and release a variety of arachidonic acid metabolites, which include prostaglandins, thromboxane, and leukotrienes. Each may have major effects on vascular permeability, vascular tone, and airway reactivity. Products of arachidonic acid metabolism coupled with mechanical obstruction of pulmonary capillaries by leukocytes, platelets, and fibrin thrombi probably account for the pulmonary artery hypertension that is often seen in patients with ARDS.

Some patients with ARDS fail to demonstrate neutrophil aggregation histologically. Maunder and colleagues[35] report the occurrence of ARDS in neutropenic patients. Although the neutrophil is important in the development of ALI, clearly it does not explain the entire story. DIC and platelet aggregation often are found in patients with ARDS and may have important roles in ALI.

The reason for the intense fibrotic response seen in some patients with ARDS is uncertain. Endotoxemia may stimulate connective tissue synthesis and alveolar macrophages, and activated lymphocytes may stimulate fibroblast proliferation.[36–38]

Whatever the reasons for the capillary leak syndrome and pulmonary fibrosis, discovery of specific therapy for their prevention or modulation is mandatory if survival is to improve in this disorder.[39]

ALTERATION IN GAS EXCHANGE

Abnormalities in gas exchange are primarily the result, at least initially, of the increased EVLW. The severe hypoxemia results from intrapulmonary shunting that occurs with alveolar flooding. Dantzker and coworkers[40] define two primary types of lung units in patients with ARDS: those that were well perfused and ventilated and those that were perfused but not ventilated. In addition, they found small areas of low but finite ventilation/perfusion ratios in 40% of their study patients.

LUNG MECHANICS

A reduction in FRC and lung compliance are hallmarks of ARDS. Alveolar flooding leads to surfactant abnormalities and widespread atelectasis. Reduced compliance is primarily the result of interstitial and alveolar edema, fibrosis, and surfactant abnormalities.

CLINICAL PRESENTATION ■

PHYSICAL EXAMINATION

After the inciting event, several hours to a day may pass before clinically apparent respiratory failure ensues. Based on work by Gomez,[41] the clinical findings in ARDS may be roughly grouped into four phases (Table 123-5). Tachypnea and tachycardia usually develop during the first 12 to 24 hours. The skin may appear moist and cyanotic. Intercostal and accessory respiratory muscles become actively involved in supporting ventilation. A dramatic increase in work of breathing can be appreciated at a glance from the bedside. High-pitched end-expiratory crackles are heard throughout all lung fields. Increasing agitation, lethargy, then obtunda-

TABLE 123-5. Progression of Clinical Findings in ARDS

PHASE 1: ACUTE INJURY

Normal physical examination and chest radiograph
Tachycardia, tachypnea, and respiratory alkalosis develop

PHASE 2: LATENT PERIOD

Lasts approximately 6–48 h after injury
Patient appears clinically stable
Hyperventilation and hypocapnia persist
Mild increase in work of breathing
Widening of the alveolar–arterial oxygen gradient
Minor abnormalities on physical examination and chest radiograph

PHASE 3: ACUTE RESPIRATORY FAILURE

Marked tachypnea and dyspnea
Decreased lung compliance
Diffuse infiltrates on chest radiograph
High-pitched crackles heard throughout all lung fields

PHASE 4: SEVERE ABNORMALITIES

Severe hypoxemia unresponsive to therapy
Increased intrapulmonary shunting
Metabolic and respiratory acidosis

ARDS, acute respiratory distress syndrome.

Taylor RW: The adult respiratory distress syndrome. In: Kirby RR, Taylor RW (eds). *Respiratory Failure*. Chicago, Year Book Medical Publishers, 1986:208.

tion may occur as the syndrome progresses. Because these clinical findings may become apparent long after hypoxemia develops, careful attention to blood gas analysis is warranted in patients at risk for ARDS.

LUNG IMAGING

The changes seen in the chest radiograph in ARDS are characteristic but nonspecific and rarely reveal the etiology of the syndrome. Acutely, pulmonary edema is seen. Interstitial infiltrates progress to a diffuse, fluffy, panacinar pattern (Fig. 123-3). Although it may be difficult to differentiate from cardiogenic pulmonary edema, there is generally an absence of pulmonary vascular redistribution, pleural effusion, or cardiomegaly. The panacinar infiltrates may consolidate and, with time, take on a patchy or nodular pattern. If the patient improves, radiographic results may revert to normal. If the disorder progresses, a pattern of diffuse interstitial fibrosis may ensue (Fig. 123-4).

Therapeutic interventions may alter the radiographic findings. Pulmonary infiltrates may increase with injudicious fluid administration. Positive-pressure ventilation and PEEP may lead to hyperinflation; subcutaneous, mediastinal, retroperitoneal, and intraperitoneal emphysema; or pneumothorax. Main stem bronchus intubation may lead to ipsilateral pneumothorax or contralateral lung collapse (Fig. 123-5).

Whereas the two-dimensional chest radiograph may suggest diffuse homogeneous infiltrates, the chest computed tomography (CT) scan usually demonstrates remarkably inhomogeneous lung involvement. Dependent regions of the lung appear to be much more involved than nondependent regions. Although chest CT scanning is not practical in the day-to-day management of patients with ARDS, in investigational trials it has provided a vivid image of dramatically reduced lung volumes in patients with this syndrome. The

chest CT also may be useful in demonstrating the presence and magnitude of pneumothoraces and pleural effusions not well seen on the standard chest radiograph. It is also useful for the positioning of thoracostomy tubes in patients with loculated pneumothoraces.

TREATMENT ■

STANDARD MANAGEMENT

Mechanical Ventilation

The clinical situation dictates when mechanical ventilation should be instituted because no specific criteria are appropriate for all situations. In general, respiratory failure is seen with the following: progressive hypoxemia with PaO_2 less than 55 mm Hg with an FIO_2 over 0.6 and a respiratory rate greater than 30 breaths/minute. The $PaCO_2$ is often low initially. If it begins to rise, even to normal levels, it is an indicator of imminent respiratory failure.[42]

The primary goal of mechanical ventilation is to provide adequate oxygenation and carbon dioxide excretion with minimal complications. To reduce the risk of oxygen toxicity, PEEP is used to increase FRC and to keep alveoli from collapsing. PEEP has no prophylactic effect in decreasing the development of ARDS in patients at risk, but low levels are not deleterious and minimize atelectasis. Despite the fact that PEEP has been used for over 25 years, disagreement exists concerning the "best PEEP." In general, PEEP should be titrated in increments of 2 to 3 cm H_2O with periodic pauses to assess its effects on oxygenation. In our experience, PEEP levels above 15 cm H_2O are rarely needed. Indiscriminate use of PEEP is associated with complications such as hemodynamic compromise, pulmonary

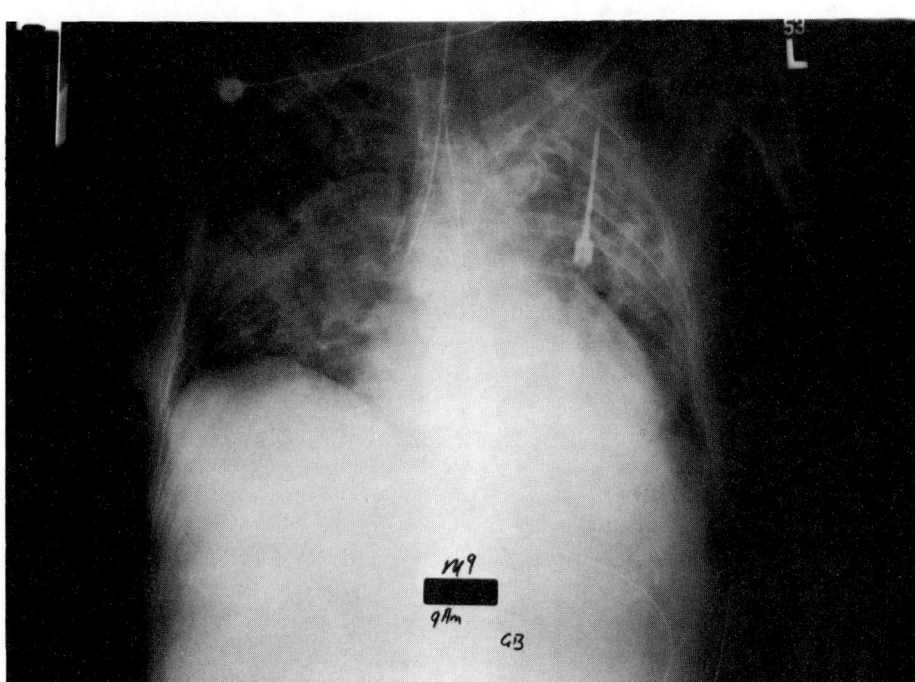

FIGURE 123-3. Diffuse interstitial and panacinar infiltrates are seen in a 36-year-old patient with acute respiratory distress syndrome. Also notice one of the complications of the respiratory support—a right mainstem intubation.

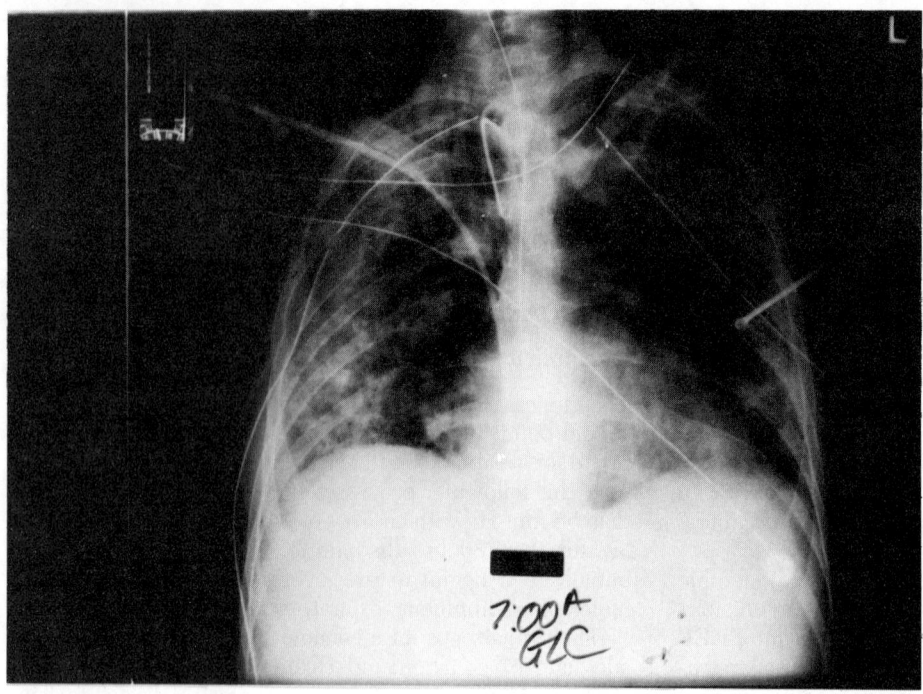

FIGURE 123-4. A pattern of diffuse interstitial fibrosis has developed in this 52-year-old patient with adult respiratory distress syndrome.

barotrauma, and volutrauma.[43] Recommended initial ventilator settings are as follows: FIO$_2$, 1.0 (titrated down as tolerated); tidal volume, 6 to 10 mL/kg ideal body weight; PEEP, 5 cm H$_2$O or less (titrated up slowly as tolerated); and flow rate, 60 L/minute.

The relatively normal areas of lung are at greatest risk of overdistension during mechanical ventilation. Alveolar overdistension has been associated with iatrogenic lung injury (volutrauma) and should be avoided. We recommend that inspiratory plateau pressures be kept under 35 cm H$_2$O if possible.[44] Strategies to avoid oxygen toxicity and ventilator-

induced complications should be considered. No single method of mechanical ventilation is optimal for all patients or even for the same patient over time.

Edema and alveolar collapse are prominent during the early phases of ALI and ARDS. Initially, higher airway pressures may be beneficial to recruit atelectatic alveolar units. As days go by, edema resolves and the lung enters the proliferative phase. Atelectasis becomes less pronounced, and increases in mean airway pressure do not lead to improvement in oxygenation as before. Inflammatory processes weaken the supporting tissues. Alveolar rupture is most likely

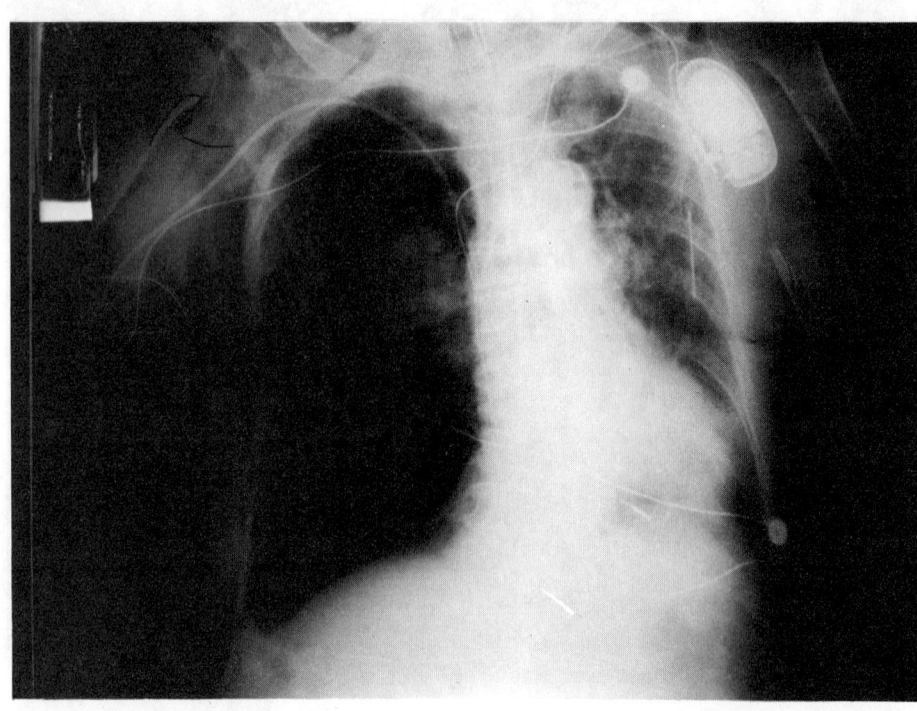

FIGURE 123-5. This 70-year-old patient with adult respiratory distress syndrome has a right tension pneumothorax and right mainstem intubation.

to occur at this point in time. Frequent patient evaluation is necessary. Adjustments in ventilatory support must keep pace with the patient's changing condition to avoid ventilator-induced lung injury.

BRONCHODILATORS

Multiple factors may lead to airflow obstruction in patients with ARDS including mucosal and interstitial edema, airway secretions, and atelectasis. Airway hyperreactivity also is a contributing factor to increased airflow resistance in many patients with ARDS in both the acute and chronic phases. Aerosolized beta-agonists can decrease airway resistance, even in patients without underlying chronic obstructive pulmonary disease or asthma. By reducing airway resistance, the work of breathing can be decreased. We recommend a therapeutic trial of inhaled bronchodilators in patients with wheezing, in those with increased resistance as measured directly, or in patients who have high peak airway pressures.[45]

ANTIBIOTICS

Because ARDS is frequently associated with sepsis, empiric antibiotics often are initiated during clinical deterioration while cultures are collected and results are pending. However, the clinician should be mindful of the fact that widespread use of broad-spectrum antibiotics may be associated with emergence of more virulent and resistant organisms.

GENERAL THERAPEUTIC MEASURES

Nutritional Support

The gut serves a critical function beyond the absorption and transport of nutrients. Enteral nutrition seems to have an advantage over parenteral nutrition in preventing gastrointestinal atrophy, in maintaining normal gut flora, and in preserving immune function in surgical patients.[46] Preliminary clinical data in the postoperative patient recovering from surgery for gastrointestinal malignancy point to the utility of enteral products containing arginine, RNA, and omega-3 fatty acids as a means of boosting immune function.[47] However, in the critically ill medical patient, no prospective randomized controlled trial has demonstrated the efficacy of routine early nutritional support. Iatrogenic complications associated with parenteral nutrition include technical problems with venous catheter insertion and catheter-related infections. We recommend institution of enteral feeding in the critically ill patient as soon as possible.

Nosocomial Infections

Nosocomial infections are covered in detail in Chapter 105. They are a leading cause of morbidity, mortality, cost, and controversy. Nosocomial pneumonia is mentioned briefly here because of its importance and prevalence in patients with ARDS. Nosocomial pneumonia is the second most frequent cause of hospital-acquired infection in the United States but is the leading cause of mortality among hospital-

acquired infections. The incidence is higher in ICU patients, especially in those requiring mechanical ventilation. Other risk factors for nosocomial pneumonia include prior antibiotic therapy, frequent changes in the ventilator circuit, iatrogenic elevation of gastric pH, use of total parenteral nutrition, chronic underlying illness, prior chest surgery, decreased mental status, intracranial pressure monitoring, and hospitalization during the fall/winter season.[48–52] Of these, the first five factors are, in part, controllable. Clinical diagnosis of ventilator-associated pneumonia is unreliable leading to overdiagnosis in greater than 60% of patients in whom pneumonia is suspected. Invasive procedures such as the bronchoscopic protected specimen brush and bronchoalveolar lavage are often necessary to confirm the diagnosis, but are less reliable if the patient has received antibiotics. Elevation of the head of the bed prevents microaspiration of enteric organisms and may minimize the effect of macroaspiration of gastric contents in the event of vomiting.[53]

Fluid Management

Fluid management in ARDS is highly controversial. As the permeability of the alveolar capillary membrane increases, pulmonary edema develops at lower pulmonary capillary pressures. The Starling equation predicts mathematically what is seen clinically. When a strategy of fluid restriction and diuresis is undertaken, EVLW is decreased, as is the duration of mechanical ventilation. Mortality in ARDS seems to be associated with net fluid gain. Adequate intravascular volume must be maintained to avoid tissue hypoperfusion. Given this, however, we recommend that the minimal amount of fluid be given and that judicious attempts at diuresis be undertaken in the hemodynamically stable patient.[54]

EXPERIMENTAL TECHNIQUES

Nitric Oxide

Acute respiratory distress syndrome is characterized by intrapulmonary shunting that leads to arterial hypoxemia. Pulmonary artery hypertension resulting from hypoxic vasoconstriction and diffuse occlusion of the pulmonary microvasculature also is common. Reducing pulmonary vascular resistance should decrease pulmonary artery pressure and improve right ventricular performance. Use of pulmonary artery vasodilators in patients with ARDS has, however, been largely unsuccessful because of unwanted systemic vasodilation and hypotension. Further, diffuse pulmonary vasodilation may increase blood flow to poorly ventilated alveolar units, thereby worsening ventilation/perfusion relationships.

In 1987, nitric oxide (NO) was reported to be a potent endothelium-derived relaxing factor.[55] It is produced by the vascular endothelium from the terminal guanidino nitrogen of L-arginine. NO activates guanylate cyclase leading to increased levels of intracellular cyclic GMP, which subsequently causes relaxation of smooth muscle in arteries and veins. NO has been given by the inhaled route to patients with ARDS. When administered in this manner, NO is distributed only to pulmonary vasculature subserving ventilated alveoli. Inhaled NO does not reach pulmonary vasculature subserving collapsed or fluid filled alveoli. While it diffuses to the surrounding vasculature of ventilated alveoli, it produces vasodilation, thereby selectively increasing blood flow to areas of good ventilation and diverting blood flow from areas of poor ventilation. The improvement in ventilation/perfusion matching is clinically seen as improved oxygenation. When NO combines with hemoglobin, it is immediately inactivated. Systemic vasodilation therefore is not seen with the inhaled administration of NO.

Important potential toxicities of inhaled NO are the development of NO_2 and the development of methemoglobinemia. The rate of formation of NO_2 from oxygen and NO depends on the concentration of oxygen and the square of the NO concentrations. The Occupational Safety and Health Association has set safety limits of 5 ppm for NO_2. NO_2 can cause pathologic changes to the lungs at doses of 25 ppm; at extremely high doses, pulmonary edema, hemorrhage, and death have been seen in animal models. NO_2 levels should be monitored as closely as possible to the endotracheal tube.[56] In clinical trials using NO at 5 to 40 ppm, NO_2 has not been a significant problem.

Methemoglobinemia is another potential but rare complication of the administration of NO. About 80% to 90% of inhaled NO is absorbed within the bloodstream, where it reacts with hemoglobin within the red blood cell to form nitrosyl-hemoglobin and methemoglobin. The primary factor determining the development of methemoglobinemia is the dose of NO given to the patient, although the hemoglobin level, oxygen saturation, and methemoglobin reductase also play a role. Native Americans more frequently have methemoglobin reductase deficiency, either partial or complete, and therefore are more susceptible to methemoglobinemia. More frequent monitoring of these patients is warranted. In clinical trials using NO at 5 to 40 ppm, methemoglobinemia has not been a significant problem.

Clinical trials using NO are ongoing. Because of improved gas exchange with inhaled NO, it is postulated that the associated reduction in FIO_2 and airway pressures necessary to support patients will lead to reduced iatrogenic lung injury and improved outcomes. When used at 5 to 40 ppm, NO has proven to be a safe therapeutic intervention. Preliminary data are encouraging. Results of ongoing clinical trials are anxiously awaited.

SURFACTANT

Surfactant dysfunction exists in ARDS. It is seen most notably in trauma victims and seems to be proportional to the severity of injury. Surfactant dysfunction also is seen in some patients at risk of developing ARDS. The greatest degree of surfactant dysfunction is seen in patients at highest risk of developing ARDS.

Administration of surfactant to patients with ARDS has received great attention recently. Surfactant decreases alveolar surface tension and alveolar edema and also has anticytokine effects. Surfactant leads to a dose-dependent inhibition in release of interleukin (IL)-1, IL-6, and tumor necrosis factor from macrophages in laboratory studies.[57] Results of clinical trials are equivocal. Early studies show that aerosolized surfactant is safe and that a trend toward improvement in mortality existed. Use of surfactant in neonates with lung inflammation demonstrates clear-cut reduction in both morbidity and mortality. Later, an international randomized placebo-controlled trial was discontinued because of a lack of efficacy.[58] Specific patients with ARDS may benefit from surfactant treatment; however, more studies are needed.

STEROIDS

Routine use of corticosteroids is not advocated, especially in the acute phase of ARDS. During the late phase, fibroproliferation often occurs in response to tissue injury. This response is damaging to the lung and is associated with persistent inflammation, which is cytokine mediated.[59] Lung injury is characterized by endothelial and epithelial damage as well as augmented fibroblast proliferation. In this setting, fever and the systemic inflammatory response syndrome are present in the absence of infection. Uncontrolled trials suggest that improvement in the fibroproliferative phase of ARDS may be seen with judicious timing of corticosteroid treatment in selected patients.[59] Proponents of this therapy recommend that a trial of corticosteroids be instituted in patients with severe ARDS after infection has been excluded. The recommended dose is 2 to 4 mg/kg/day of prednisone or its equivalent instituted on day 7 to 14. Therapy is continued for 1 to 2 weeks.

KETOCONAZOLE

Ketoconazole inhibits thromboxane synthesis, halting the production of leukotrienes. Preliminary studies demonstrate a preventive effect of ketoconazole in septic and multiple trauma patients who are at high risk of developing ARDS.[60]

PENTOXYPHYLLINE

Cytokines activate neutrophils, increasing their adhesiveness, increasing the release of proteolytic enzymes, and promoting the production of hydrogen peroxide and superoxide. Pentoxyfylline is a phosphodiesterase inhibitor that decreases chemotaxis and activation of neutrophils, especially those preexposed to inflammatory cytokines. Pentoxyphylline has been administered to a small number of patients with ARDS without detrimental effect. Beneficial effects, however, have yet to be demonstrated in humans. Ongoing studies may provide more information about the use of pentoxyfylline.[61]

ANTIOXIDANT TREATMENT

Oxygen free radicals contribute to lung injury in ARDS. Leukocytes in the pulmonary microvasculature release oxygen free radicals that attack fatty acid chains of membrane lipids, leading to peroxidation. This destroys cell membrane integrity and leads to an increase in alveolar-capillary permeability. N-acetylcysteine acts as a free radical scavenger and an anticoagulant and possibly decreases fibrin uptake in

ARDS. *N*-acetylcysteine has no beneficial effects on oxygenation.[62] As with other investigational substances, more studies are needed to determine the proper role, if any, of this agent.

NONSTEROIDAL ANTIINFLAMMATORY AGENTS

Ibuprofen acts by inhibiting prostaglandin pathways and has a demonstrated beneficial effect in experimentally induced sepsis. Healthy subjects given ibuprofen had inhibition of endotoxin-induced increases in tumor necrosis factor and reduced symptoms after the administration of *Escherichia coli* endotoxin. Clinical trials have documented a reasonable safety record for ibuprofen; however, improved outcome has not been documented.[63] Gastrointestinal and renal side effects are those most commonly seen. Routine administration of ibuprofen to patients with ARDS is not currently recommended.

PROSTAGLANDIN E₁

Prostaglandin E₁ (PGE₁) decreases the inflammatory response. Use of this agent was hoped to diminish lung damage in patients with ARDS. Early clinical studies were promising; however, a randomized, double-blind, placebo-controlled, multicenter trial failed to show a decrease in mortality.[64] The use of PGE₁ in 50 patients with ARDS resulted in reduced systemic vascular resistance that caused decreased systemic arterial blood pressure, increased stroke volume, increased heart rate, and increased cardiac output. PGE₁ may prove to be useful in high-risk patients before the development of ARDS but currently is not recommended for treating ARDS.

ANTIENDOTOXINS

Recently it was hoped that agents that inhibited or masked the effect of endotoxin would improve outcome in patients with gram-negative sepsis (Chap. 28). Perhaps a reduced incidence of ARDS or a less severe course might be seen. Unfortunately, clinical data fail to support benefit from these agents.[66-68]

PATIENT POSITIONING

Improvement in oxygenation by use of the prone position in patients with ARDS recently has been demonstrated.[69] The beneficial effect of this position is thought to primarily result from improvement in the matching of ventilation and perfusion. However, the prone position also is associated with an increased FRC and changes in hydrostatic pressure that may decrease lung edema formation.

Most centers treat patients in the supine position. Should the prone position be selected as a treatment option, great care should be exercised during the turning of the patient. Dislodgement of the endotracheal tube during the repositioning process is of concern. Care should be taken to ensure proper placement of pillows to prevent pressure-induced

injury. Problems seen with prone positioning include ocular damage, facial decubitus, and brachial plexus injuries.

NOVEL FORMS OF MECHANICAL VENTILATION

INVERSE RATIO VENTILATION

Pressure control–inverse ratio ventilation has received a fair amount of attention recently. Support for this form of mechanical ventilation stems from concern about potential ventilator-induced lung injury associated with excessive alveolar pressures and volumes. With this technique, peak inflationary pressure can be limited as inspiratory time is progressively increased. The lung is held in inflation for a longer portion of the respiratory cycle; therefore, mean airway pressure can be maintained at a lower peak inflationary pressure. Because lung involvement in patients with ARDS is a patchy process, it has been theorized that the lengthened inspiratory time may be associated with better distribution of gas to areas of lung with slow time constants, thus recruiting previously nonfunctioning alveoli. Progressive lengthening of inspiratory time is associated with development of gas trapping and auto PEEP because of incomplete lung emptying during the shortened expiratory phase. Some believe that auto PEEP is the primary reason for the observed improvement in oxygenation. If auto PEEP is excessive, the risk of barotrauma escalates. Carbon dioxide elimination is decreased with this mode of mechanical ventilation (see "Permission Hypercapnia"). Inverse ratio ventilation is not tolerated by the conscious patient and is frankly dangerous in the noncooperative patient. Heavy sedation is required and neuromuscular blockade often is indicated. This form of mechanical ventilation should be used only with great caution, with expert consultation, and in patients who do not respond to more conventional forms of mechanical ventilation. No survival advantage has been documented with this form of mechanical ventilation compared with other techniques.[70]

PERMISSIVE HYPERCAPNIA

Traditionally, the tidal volume and respiratory rate were set to avoid hypercapnia and respiratory acidosis. Dead space is increased for a variety of reasons in patients with ARDS, impairing carbon dioxide elimination. As previously mentioned, lung volume is typically reduced in this condition. Achieving a normal pH and Paco₂ may be difficult and unnecessary. Increasing minute ventilation to facilitate carbon dioxide excretion by increasing respiratory rate may be associated with unwanted auto PEEP. Further, increases in tidal volume may further predispose the patient to volutrauma and barotrauma. Given these real concerns, allowing the Paco₂ to rise seems a small price to pay, is generally well tolerated, and is termed *permissive hypercapnia*.[71] Administration of basic solutions has been advocated to treat excessive respiratory acidosis. Carbicarb is an equimolar mixture of sodium bicarbonate and sodium carbonate combined with a buffering agent. When given intravenously, it does not generate carbon dioxide and has been used to treat the depressed pH seen in this circumstance. Sodium bicarbonate infusion should be avoided because it is associated with production of carbon dioxide. Extracorporeal carbon dioxide removal also may be considered in extreme circumstances.

HIGH-FREQUENCY VENTILATION

High-frequency ventilation involves delivery of tidal volumes less than anatomic dead space at rapid rates.[72] Typical tidal volumes vary from 1 to 3 mL/kg at rates between 100 to 3000 breaths/minute. Because tidal volumes are small, peak inflationary pressures may be reduced when compared with conventional-rate mechanical ventilation. Because of this, a reduction in barotrauma has been theorized. High-frequency ventilation has been shown to improve survival in infant respiratory distress.[73] Preliminary data from a multicenter trial in adults suggest benefit in the prevention of ARDS.[74] In this study, peak airway pressures were reduced, oxygenation was improved, and no adverse hemodynamic effect was demonstrated. The near-constant airway pressure may have beneficial effects on gas distribution within the lung. It has been suggested that high-frequency ventilation allows maintenance of mean airway pressure at a lower peak pressure. Further, advocates of this technique suggest that it may be associated with less barotrauma than conventional mechanical ventilation and PEEP. Barotrauma occurred in this study[74] in patients who had previously sustained barotrauma and in those who had undergone open-lung biopsy. Greater than half of the pneumothoraces were associated with prior barotrauma.

The complications of high-frequency ventilation include tracheitis and desiccation of secretions secondary to inadequate humidification of inspired gas. Mucous desiccation is seen in about 25% of patients treated with this form of high-frequency ventilation and can be treated by aerosolization of water by the jet stream. Periodic injection of 2 mL of saline into the endotracheal tube followed by suctioning helps to ensure tube patency.

LIQUID VENTILATION

Liquid ventilation was described as long ago as 1929 by Neergaard, who showed that interfacial surface forces could be eliminated in the lung by the instillation liquid that allowed the expansion of the lung at lower pressures. Perfluorocarbon liquid has a low surface tension, allowing it to spread across the alveolar surface in various pathologic states. This liquid has a high affinity for oxygen and carbon dioxide, making it a satisfactory medium for bulk gas transport. Studies have been conducted in infant respiratory distress in patients with barotrauma and cardiovascular compromise.[75] Improvements in oxygenation and compliance are seen especially in neonates.[76,77]

EXTRACORPOREAL RESPIRATORY SUPPORT

The term *extracorporeal respiratory support* encompasses a variety of techniques. The basic model includes an artificial membrane permeable to both oxygen and carbon dioxide that acts as an artificial alveolar-capillary unit. Use of this technique theoretically protects the damaged lung from further injury by high oxygen concentrations and positive-pressure mechanical ventilation. While the extracorporeal device supports oxygenation and carbon dioxide removal, the injured lung is allowed to recover. Early studies showed worsened mortality in adults treated with extracorporeal support, and enthusiasm for the technique declined. Recent data are more promising, particularly in the infant respiratory distress syndrome. A survival benefit has not been demonstrated in adults, and the complication rate is significant. Extracorporeal support remains promising but remains experimental.

MONITORING

Monitoring the patient with ARDS is similar to monitoring other critically ill patients. Detailed descriptions of monitoring techniques can be found in Section V of this book. Common methods of monitoring used in patients with ARDS are presented in Table 123-6. Continuous monitoring of the patient's status is essential to reduce or prevent the occurrence of disastrous complications. Careful titration of therapy is best guided by attention to clinical, laboratory, and cardiorespiratory variables (see Table 123-6). The practical usefulness of some of these modalities is controversial (e.g., capnography).

COMPLICATIONS

Significant morbidity or mortality may occur during supportive therapy for ARDS. The clinician should be aware of these potential complications, many of which are outlined by Pingleton[78] (Table 123-7). Attention to detail decreases complications and may improve outcome in ARDS.

OUTCOME

In general, patients with ARDS who die within the first several days do so because of the underlying condition and because of respiratory failure. Many of those who survive the original insult succumb to sepsis or to the MODS. Of those who survive ARDS, most return to their premorbid state of respiratory function by about 6 months after extubation.[79]

Since the initial description of ARDS, the reported mortality rate has been fairly stable, about 50% to 70%. Recently, a cohort study of 918 patients from 1983 to 1993 showed a slight decline in mortality from 1989 through the end of the period.[80] The improvement in mortality was most marked in those younger than 60 years of age and in patients whose precipitating cause for ARDS was sepsis. Acute Physiology Assessment and Chronic Health Evaluation (APACHE) II scores at the onset of ARDS were higher in patients with sepsis in 1993 than in 1983, whereas the mean age at ARDS onset in 1993 (50 years) was lower than during the 1983 to 1985 period (57 years). Patients enrolled in trials of limited

TABLE 123-6. Monitoring the Patient with ARDS°

LEVEL I

Vital signs
  Temperature, heart rate, respiratory rate, arterial blood
    pressure
Weight
Intake and output
Caloric intake
Physical examination, with special emphasis on:
  Skin (texture, turgor, perspiration, emphysema)
  Respiratory (breathing pattern, lung examination)
  Cardiovascular (heart examination, peripheral pulses)
  Abdominal
  Neurologic (mental status)

LEVEL II

Continuous ECG monitoring
Chest radiography
Laboratory (CBC, electrolytes)
Gastric pH
Arterial blood gases
Vital capacity
Negative inspiratory pressure
Dead space/tidal volume ratio (V_D/V_T)
Tracheal tube cuff pressures
Ventilator settings
Pressure–volume relationship
  Lung and chest wall compliance and airways resistance
Capnography
Transcutaneous oximetry

LEVEL III

Pulmonary artery catheter
  Pulmonary artery pressures, pulmonary artery occlusion
    pressure, waveforms, cardiac index, mixed venous blood
    gases, stroke volume index, ventricular stroke work indices,
    systemic and pulmonary vascular resistance, arterial and
    mixed venous oxygen content, oxygen transport,
    arteriovenous content difference, oxygen consumption,
    oxygen extraction, venous admixture
Arterial pressure monitoring
  Beat-to-beat systolic, diastolic, and mean pressure,
    waveforms, blood sampling

ARDS, acute respiratory distress syndrome; ECG,
electrocardiographic; CBC, complete blood cell count.
°Various monitoring techniques have been divided into three
arbitrary levels. The levels are roughly ordered in terms of
increasing invasiveness and sophistication. The exact monitoring
modalities selected and the frequency with which measurements
are made must be individualized.

Taylor RW: The adult respiratory distress syndrome. In: Kirby RR,
Taylor RW (eds). *Respiratory Failure.* Chicago, Year Book Medical
Publishers, 1986:208.

TABLE 123-7. Complications Associated With ARDS

PULMONARY
  Pulmonary emboli
  Pulmonary barotrauma
  Pulmonary fibrosis
  Oxygen toxicity

GASTROINTESTINAL
  Gastrointestinal hemorrhage
  Ileus
  Gastric distention
  Pneumoperitoneum

RENAL
  Renal failure
  Fluid retention

CARDIOVASCULAR
  Invasive catheters
  Arrhythmia
  Hypotension
  Low cardiac output

INFECTION
  Sepsis
  Nosocomial pneumonia

HEMATOLOGIC
  Anemia
  Thrombocytopenia
  DIC

OTHER
  Hepatic
  Endocrine
  Neurologic
  Psychiatric
  Malnutrition

**COMPLICATIONS ATTRIBUTABLE TO INTUBATION
AND EXTUBATION**
  Prolonged attempt at intubation
  Intubation of a main stem bronchus
  Premature extubation
  Self-extubation

**COMPLICATIONS ASSOCIATED WITH ENDOTRACHEAL/
TRACHEOSTOMY TUBES**
  Tube malfunction
  Nasal necrosis
  Paranasal sinus infection
  Tracheal stenosis
  Tracheomalacia
  Polyps
  Erosion
  Fistulas
  Airway obstruction
  Hoarseness

(continued)

TABLE 113-7. *(continued)*

COMPLICATIONS ATTRIBUTABLE TO OPERATION
OF THE VENTILATOR
  Machine failure
  Alarm failure
  Alarms silenced
  Inadequate nebulization or humidification

COMPLICATIONS OCCURRING DURING POSITIVE AIRWAY
PRESSURE THERAPY
  Alveolar hypoventilation
  Alveolar hyperventilation
  Massive gastric distention
  Barotrauma
  Atelectasis
  Pneumonia
  Hypotension

ARDS, acute respiratory distress syndrome; DIC, disseminated intravascular coagulation.

Taylor RW: The adult respiratory distress syndrome. In: Kirby RR, Taylor RW (eds). *Respiratory Failure.* Chicago, Year Book Medical Publishers, 1986:208.

clinical utility were excluded from the analysis. These data indicate that supportive care of severely ill patients with ARDS has improved.

A recent prospective study of 123 patients with ALI identified on admission to an ICU found that the three major predictors of mortality were nonpulmonary organ system dysfunction before admission to the ICU, chronic liver disease, and sepsis.[81] Another negative prognostic factor was the presence of persistent metabolic acidosis on the first day of ARDS. At this point, low pH is the only reliable biochemical marker of mortality in ARDS, although many other substances such as cytokines, leukotrienes, complement components, endotoxin, and coagulation factors have been seen in abnormal concentrations. None of the other factors has been found to be specific for ARDS.[82]

REFERENCES ■

1. Kollef MH, Schuster D: The acute respiratory distress syndrome. *N Engl J Med* 1995;332:27
2. Ashbaugh DG, Bigelow DB, Petty TL, et al: Acute respiratory distress in adults. *Lancet* 1967;ii:319
3. Petty TL, Ashbaugh DG: The adult respiratory distress syndrome: clinical features, factors influencing prognosis and principles of management. *Chest* 1971;60:233
4. Petty TL: Adult respiratory distress syndrome: definition and historical perspective. *Clin Chest Med* 1982;3:3
5. Taylor RW, Duncan CA: The adult respiratory distress syndrome. *Res Medica* 1983;1:17
6. American College of Chest Physicians/Society of Critical Care Medicine Consensus Conference: Definitions for sepsis and organ failure and guidelines for the use of innovative therapies in sepsis. *Crit Care Med* 1992;20:864
7. Fowler AA, Hamman RF, Good JT, et al: Adult respiratory distress syndrome: risk with common predispositions. *Ann Intern Med* 1983;98:593
8. Pepe PE, Potkin RT, Reus DH, et al: Clinical predictors of the adult respiratory distress syndrome. *Am J Surg* 1982;144:124
9. The American–European Consensus Conference on ARDS. *Am J Respir Crit Care Med* 1994;149:818
10. Bynum LJ, Pierce AK: Pulmonary aspiration of gastric contents. *Am Rev Respir Dis* 1976;114:1129
11. Mendelson CL: The aspiration of stomach contents into the lungs during obstetric anesthesia. *Am J Obstet Gynecol* 1946;52:191
12. Wynne JW, Modell JH: Respiratory aspiration of stomach contents. *Ann Intern Med* 1977;87:466
13. Horovitz JH, Carrico CJ, Shires GT: Pulmonary response to major injury. *Arch Surg* 1974;108:349
14. Petty TL: Adult respiratory distress syndrome: historical perspective and definition. *Respir Med* 1981;2:99
15. Fulton RL, Jones CE: The cause of post-traumatic pulmonary insufficiency in man. *Surg Gynecol Obstet* 1975;140:179
16. Modell JH: Biology of drowning. *Annu Rev Med* 1978;29:1
17. Everett ED, Overholt EL: Phosgene poisoning. *JAMA* 1968;205:243
18. Close LG, Catlin FI, Cohn AM: Acute and chronic effects of ammonia burns of the respiratory tract. *Arch Otolaryngol* 1980;106:151
19. Caplin M: Ammonia-gas poisoning: 47 cases in a London shelter. *Lancet* 1941;i:95
20. Charan NB, Myers CG, Lakshminarayan S, et al: Pulmonary injuries associated with acute sulfur dioxide inhalation. *Am Rev Respir Dis* 1979;119:555
21. Ward HN: Pulmonary infiltrates associated with leukoagglutinin transfusion reactions. *Ann Intern Med* 1970;73:689
22. Kernoff PBA, Durrant IJ, Rizza CR, et al: Severe allergic pulmonary edema after plasma transfusion. *Br J Haematol* 1972;23:777
23. Bone RC, Francis PB, Pierce AK: Intravascular coagulation associated with the adult respiratory distress syndrome. *Am J Med* 1976;61:585
24. Adamson IYR, Bowden DH: Derivation of type I epithelium from type II cells in developing rat lung. *Lab Invest* 1975;32:735
25. Mason RJ: Alveolar type II cells. *Fed Proc* 1977;36:2697
26. Connors AF, McCaffree DR, Rogers RM: The adult respiratory distress syndrome. *Dis Mon* 1981;27:1
27. Lakshminarayan S, Stanford RL, Petty TL: Prognosis after recovery from adult respiratory distress syndrome. *Am Rev Respir Dis* 1976;113:7
28. Staub NC: State of the art review: pathogenesis of pulmonary edema. *Am Rev Respir Dis* 1974;109:358
29. Horn JK, Lewis FR: Acute lung injury: pathophysiology and diagnosis. In: Taylor RW, Shoemaker WC (eds). *Critical Care: State of the Art.* Fullerton, CA, Society of Critical Care Medicine, 1991:1
30. Mizamoto K, Schultz E, Health T, et al: Pulmonary intravascular macrophages and hemodynamic effects of liposomes in sheep. *J Appl Physiol* 1988;64:1143
31. Kaplan LS, Goffinet JA: Profound neutropenia during the early phase of hemodialysis. *JAMA* 1968;203:1135
32. Craddock PR, Fehr J, Dalmasso AP, et al: Hemodialysis leukopenia: pulmonary vascular leukostasis resulting from complement activation by dialyzer cellophane membrane. *J Clin Invest* 59;879:1977
33. Becker EL, Ward PA: Chemotaxis. In: Parker CW (ed). *Clinical Immunology.* Philadelphia, WB Saunders, 1980:272
34. Tate RM, Repine JE: Neutrophils and the adult respiratory distress syndrome. *Am Rev Respir Dis* 1983;128:552

35. Maunder RJ, Hackman RC, Riff E, et al: Occurrence of the adult respiratory distress syndrome in neutropenic patients. *Am Rev Respir Dis* 1986;133:313

36. Buckingham RB, Castor CW: The effect of bacterial products on synovial fibroblast function: hypermetabolic changes induced by endotoxin. *J Clin Invest* 1972;51:1186

37. Brigham LK, Meyrick B: Endotoxin and lung injury. *Am Rev Respir Dis* 1986;133:913

38. Bitterman PB, Crystal RG: Pulmonary alveolar macrophages release a factor that stimulates human lung fibroblasts to replicate [abstract]. *Am Rev Respir Dis* 1980;121(Suppl):58

39. Rinaldo JE, Rogers RM: Adult respiratory distress syndrome: changing concepts of lung injury and repair. *N Engl J Med* 1982;306:900

40. Dantzker DR, Brook CH, DeHart P, et al: Gas exchange in adult respiratory distress syndrome and the effects of positive end-expiratory pressure. *Am Rev Respir Dis* 1979;120:1039

41. Gomez AC: Pulmonary insufficiency in non-thoracic trauma [discussion]. *J Trauma* 1968;8:666

42. Slutsky AS: ACCP Consensus Conference: mechanical ventilation. *Chest* 1993;104:1833

43. Gattinoni L, Pelosi P, Crotti S, et al: Effects of positive end-expiratory pressure on regional distribution of tidal volume and recruitment in adult respiratory distress syndrome. *Am J Respir Crit Care Med* 1995;151:1807

44. Marini J: New options for the ventilatory management of acute lung injury. *New Horizons* 1993;4:489

45. Wright P, Carmichael L, Bernard G: Effect of bronchodilators on lung mechanics in the acute respiratory distress syndrome (ARDS). *Chest* 1994;106:157

46. Moore FA, Feliciano DV, Andrassy RJ, et al: Early enteral feeding, compared with parenteral, reduces postoperative septic complications. *Ann Surg* 1992;216:172

47. Koretz R: Nutritional supplemantation in the ICU. *Am J Respir Crit Care Med* 1995;151:570

48. Celis R, Torres A, Gatell JM, et al: Nosocomial pneumonia: a multivariate analysis of risk and prognosis. *Chest* 1988;93:318

49. Torres A, Aznar R, Gatell JM, et al: Incidence, risk and prognostic factors of nosocomial pneumonia in mechanically ventilated patients. *Am J Respir Crit Care Med* 1990;142:523

50. Craven DE, Kunches LM, Kilinsky V, et al: Risk factors for pneumonia and fatality in patients receiving continuous mechanical ventilation. *Am J Respir Crit Care Med* 1986;133:792

51. Kollef MH: Ventilator-associated pneumonia. *JAMA* 1993;270:1965

52. Moore FA, Moore EE, Jones TN, et al: TEN versus TPN following mafor abdominal trauma: reduced septic morbidity. *J Trauma* 1989;29:916

53. Torres A, Serra-Batlles J, Ros E, et al: Pulmonary aspiration of gastric contents in patients receiving mechanical ventilation: the effect of body position. *Ann Intern Med* 1992;116:540

54. Schuster D: Fluid management in ARDS: "keep them dry" or does it matter? *Intensive Care Med* 1995;21:101

55. Cobb JP: Nitric oxide as a target for therapy in septic shock. *Crit Care Med* 1993;21:1261

56. Puybasset L, Rouby J, Mourgeon E, et al: Factors influencing cardiopulmonary effects of inhaled nitric oxide in acute respiratory failure. *Am J Respir Crit Care Med* 1995;152:318

57. Repine JE: Scientific perspectives on adult respiratory distress syndrome. *Lancet* 1992;339:466

58. Weg JG, Balk RA, Tharratt S, et al: Safety and potential efficacy of an aerosolized surfactant in human sepsis-induced adult respiratory distress syndrome. *JAMA* 1994;272:1433

59. Meduri GU, Headley S, Tolley E, et al: Plasma and BAL cytokine response to corticosteroid rescue treatment in late ARDS. *Chest* 1995;103:1315

60. Yu M, Tomasa G: A double-blind, prospective, randomized trial of ketoconazole, a thrombaxane synthetase inhibitor, in the prophylaxis of the adult resporatory distress syndrome. *Crit Care Med* 1993;21:1635

61. Montravers P, Fagon JY, Gilbert C, et al: Pilot study of cardiopulmonary risk from pentoxifylline in adult respiratory distress syndrome. *Chest* 1993;103:1017

62. Jepsen S, Herlevsen P, Knudsen P, et al: Antioxidant treatment with N-acetylcysteine during adult respiratory distress syndrome: a prospective, randomized, placebo-controlled study. *Crit Care Med* 1992;20:918

63. Haupt MT, Jastremski MS, Clemmer TP, et al: The Ibuprofen Study Group: effect of ibuprofen in patients with severe sepsis. A randomized, double-blind, multicenter study. *Crit Care Med* 1991;19:1339

64. Bone R, Slotman G, Maunder R, et al: Randomized double-blind, multicenter study of prostaglandin E₁ in patients with the adult respiratory distress syndrome. *Chest* 1989;96:114

65. Ziegler EJ, McCutchan JA, Fierer J, et al: Treatment of gram-negative bacteremia and septic shock with human antiserum to a mutant E. coli. *N Engl J Med* 1982;307:1225

66. Ziegler EJ, Fisher CJ, Sprung CL, et al: Tratment of gram-negative bacteremia and septic shock with HA-1A human monoclonal antibody against endotoxin. *N Engl J Med* 1991;324:429

67. Bigatello LM, Green RE, Sprung Cl, et al: HA-1A in septic patiets with ARDS: results from the pivotal trial. *Intensive Care Med* 1994;20:328

68. Luce J: Introduction of new technology into critical care practice: a history of HA-1A human monoclonal antibody against endotoxin. *Crit Care Med* 1993;21:1233

69. Langer M, Mascheroni D, Marcolin R, et al: The prone position in ARDS patients: a clinical study. *Chest* 1988;94:103

70. Marini J: Inverse ratio ventilation: simply an alternative or something else? *Crit Care Med* 1995;23:224

71. Bidani A, Tzouanakis A, Cardenas V, et al: Permissive hypercapnea in acute respiratory failure. *JAMA* 1994;272:957

72. Gallager T, Boysen P, Davidson D, et al: High frequency percussive ventilation compared with conventional mechanical ventilation. *Crit Care Med* 1989;17:364

73. Arnold JH, Hanson JH, Toro-Figuero LO, et al: Prospective, randomized comparison of high-frequency oscillatory ventilation and conventional mechanical ventilation in pediatric respiratory failure. *Crit Care Med* 1994;22:1530

74. Gluck E, Heard S, Patel C, et al: Use of ultra high frequency ventilation in patients with ARDS: a preliminary report. *Chest* 1993;103:1413

75. Hirschl RB, Merz SI, Montoya JP, et al: Development and aplication of a simplified liquid ventilator. *Crit Care Med* 1995;23:157

76. Hirschl R, Parent A, Tooley R, et al: Liquid ventilation improves pulmonary function, gas exchange, and lung injury in a model of respiratory failure. *Ann Surg* 1995;221:79

77. Hirschl RB, Overbeck M, Parent A, et al: Liquid ventilation provides uniform distribution of perfluorocarbon in the setting of respiratory failure. *Surgery* 1994;116:159

78. Pingleton SK: Complications associated with the adult respiratory distress syndrome. *Clin Chest Med* 1982;5:143

79. McHugh L, Milberg J, Whitcomb M, et al: Recovery of function in survivors of the acute respiratory distress syndrome. *Am J Respir Crit Care Med* 1994;150:90

80. Doyle RL, Szaflarski N, Modin GW, et al: Identification of patients with acute lung injury: predictors of mortality. *Am J Respir Crit Care Med* 1995;152:1818

81. Bone RC, Balk R, Slotman G, et al: Adult respiratory distress syndrome: sequence and importance of development of multiple organ failure. *Chest* 1992;101:320

82. Hyers T: Prediction of survival and mortality in patients with adult respiratory distress syndrome. *New Horizons* 1993;1:466

Critical Care, Third Edition, edited by Joseph M. Civetta,
Robert W. Taylor, and Robert R. Kirby.
Lippincott-Raven Publishers, Philadelphia, PA © 1997.

CHAPTER 124

■

Community Acquired Pneumonia

Dennis P. Lawlor
Mimi Emig

IMMEDIATE CONCERNS ■

MAJOR PROBLEMS

Community acquired pneumonia (CAP) remains a common and serious illness, despite the availability of potent antimicrobials and effective vaccines. In the United States, pneumonia is the sixth leading cause of death and the number one cause of death from infectious disease.[1,2] Unlike bronchitis or tracheitis, pneumonia is frequently accompanied by fever, toxicity, pleurisy, and an infiltrate on chest radiograph. Estimates of the incidence of CAP range from 5 to 10 million cases per year, with approximately one fifth of these cases requiring hospital admission.[3–5] In the outpatient setting, mortality is 1% to 5%. However, among patients requiring hospitalization, mortality is as high as 25%, particularly in those requiring admission to the intensive care unit.[6]

Key Points

1. An assessment of the patient's age, coexisting illnesses, and severity of pneumonia is of great value in predicting likely pathogens in CAP.
2. A review of epidemiologic information, combined with laboratory and radiographic studies, can yield important clues to the cause of CAP.
3. Specific risk factors for mortality or a complicated course of CAP have been identified. Hospitalization should be strongly considered for patients with multiple risk factors for adverse outcome.

Essential Diagnostic Tests and Procedures

1. Chest radiograph, sputum Gram stain and culture, and blood cultures should be obtained in all patients hospitalized for CAP.
2. Further diagnostic testing should be directed toward the identification of likely pathogens in the individual. Extensive diagnostic testing is not indicated in uncomplicated CAP.
3. Bronchoscopy is indicated in individuals failing empiric therapy and in immunocompromised hosts.
4. Open lung biopsy (OLB) may identify unusual pathogens in immunocompromised hosts. OLB is of marginal value in immunocompetent hosts with CAP.
5. Diagnostic thoracentesis should be done on any significant parapneumonic effusion to rule out empyema. The presence of an empyema usually requires chest tube drainage plus antibiotics.
6. Repeat chest radiograph should be obtained 8 weeks after pneumonia to document clearing of the infiltrate. Persistent infiltrate at 8 weeks warrants further evaluation.

Initial Therapy

1. Empiric antibiotic therapy should be directed at the pathogens likely to cause CAP in the individual patient. Broad-spectrum therapy may initially be indicated in severely ill patients.
2. The antibiotic spectrum should be narrowed after the responsible pathogen has been identified.

1841

3. Modification of the initial therapy and invasive diagnostic testing may be indicated in patients who are worsening after 72 hours on empiric antibiotics.

CHARACTERIZATION OF PNEUMONIA ■

The characterization of CAP has become more complex as the general population has aged. Older patients have a higher prevalence of chronic obstructive lung disease (COLD), diabetes mellitus, renal insufficiency, congestive heart failure, chronic liver disease, and other comorbid conditions. Patients with comorbid diseases develop pneumonia with a broader range of pathogens. Nearly 15% of the general population of the United States is greater than 65 years of age; a minority of this age group resides in nursing homes. Institutionalized patients, however, may act as reservoirs for the development of antibiotic resistance and for the transmission of organisms capable of causing pneumonia. Penicillin-resistant pneumococcus, methicillin-resistant staphylococcal species, and vancomycin-resistant enterococcal species are increasingly being reported in institutions throughout the United States.

This chapter will focus on pneumonia acquired outside the acute care hospital; nosocomial infections are discussed in Chapter 106. With medical care increasingly coming under fiscal pressure to be performed in the outpatient setting, many conditions previously requiring hospitalization are now being taken care of in the outpatient setting or in institutions with lower acuity (i.e., nursing homes and rehabilitation facilities). Thus, patients with CAP may present with more severe illness or with unusual or resistant pathogens. The spreading epidemic of human immunodeficiency virus (HIV) into patient populations previously thought to be low-risk necessitates viewing each patient as potentially HIV-infected. A thoughtful evaluation of a patient's circumstances can narrow the spectrum of potential pathogens to reduce the use of excessively broad empiric antibiotics and avoid contributing to the development of antibiotic resistance. With the recognition of different, broader groups of pathogens with different types of chronic disease and immunosuppression, the role of invasive diagnostic testing in identifying pathogens and guiding therapy is being actively investigated. This chapter will provide a rational approach to the evaluation and treatment of the patient with CAP.

PATHOGENS IN COMMUNITY ACQUIRED PNEUMONIA ■

Community-acquired pathogens cause a spectrum of pulmonary symptoms ranging from a mild nonspecific respiratory illness to an overwhelming rapidly fatal pneumonia. A myriad of potential pathogens may cause CAP. Broad-spectrum, multidrug therapy would be required to cover all potential organisms. Epidemiologic information, combined with laboratory and radiographic studies, can yield important clues to the cause of an overwhelming pneumonia. Tables 124-1 and 124-2 list some of the more commonly recognized pathogens in CAP.

Precise determination of the frequencies of the various potential pathogens in CAP is difficult. The available methods of clinical testing are helpful but suffer from a variety of deficiencies. Adequate sputum Gram stain specimens may be discordant with culture results, and neither test detects atypical organisms (e.g., *Mycoplasma pneumoniae, Chlamydia pneumoniae,* and respiratory viruses). Acute and convalescent viral titers and serologic tests, although helpful in epidemiologic surveys, usually do not provide timely information and are not helpful in individual patient treatment decision-making. A responsible pathogen can be identified in only one half to two thirds of cases.[7] The use of antibiotics

TABLE 124-1.   Etiology of CAP in Patients not Requiring Hospitalization°

WITHOUT COMORBIDITY, AGE <60 YEARS	WITH COMORBIDITY[†] OR AGE >60 YEARS
S pneumoniae	*S pneumoniae*
M pneumoniae	Respiratory Viruses
Respiratory Viruses	*H influenzae*
C pneumoniae	Aerobic gram-negative bacilli
H influenzae	*S aureus*
Miscellaneous	Miscellaneous
Legionella spp.	*Moraxella catarrhalis*
S aureus	*Legionella* spp
M tuberculosis	*M tuberculosis*
Endemic fungi (*Coccidioides,*	Endemic fungi (*Coccidioides,*
Histoplasma, Blastomyces)	*Histoplasma, Blastomyces*)
Aerobic gram-negative bacilli	

°Identified pathogens are only found in 50–75% of cases. This grouping assumes patients are not at risk for HIV.
†Comorbidity is defined as chronic obstructive lung disease, cystic fibrosis, bronchiectasis, diabetes mellitus, chronic renal failure, congestive heart failure, chronic alcohol abuse, malnutrition, postsplenectomy.

TABLE 124-2. Etiology of CAP in Patients Requiring Hospitalization°

MILD–MODERATE HOSPITALIZED CAP	SEVERE HOSPITALIZED CAP†
S pneumoniae	*S pneumoniae*
H influenzae	*Legionella* spp.
Polymicrobial (including anaerobic bacteria)	*S aureus*
Aerobic gram-negative bacilli	Aerobic gram-negative bacilli
Legionella spp.	*M pneumoniae*
C pneumoniae	Respiratory viruses (especially Influenza)
S aureus	Miscellaneous
Respiratory Viruses (especially Influenza)	*H influenzae*
Miscellaneous	*M tuberculosis*
M pneumoniae	Endemic fungi (*Coccidioides,*
Moraxella catarrhalis	*Histoplasma, Blastomyces*)
M tuberculosis	
Endemic fungi (*Coccidioides,*	
Histoplasma, Blastomyces)	

°Identified pathogens are only found in 50–75% of cases. This grouping assumes patients are not at risk for HIV.

†Severe pneumonia is defined as respiratory rate >30 BPM, PaO_2/FiO_2 <250, requiring mechanical ventilation, multiple lobe involvement by chest radiograph, 50% or greater increase in radiographic infiltrates within 48 hours, shock (systolic blood pressure <90 mm Hg), vasopressors required for >4 hours, oliguria (<20 mL/h, or <80 mL for 4 h), or dialysis.

prior to hospitalization may contribute to the inability to identify a pathogen in some patients.

Streptococcus pneumoniae is the most common pathogen in most series of CAP. Studies done on hospitalized patients tend to overrepresent pathogens that cause a more severe clinical syndrome (e.g., gram-negative aerobes) and underrepresent pathogens with a milder clinical presentation (e.g., *Mycoplasma, Chlamydia,* and viruses). Serologic diagnosis of atypical pathogens may result in misleading epidemiologic data. For example, *C pneumoniae* is believed to cause 6% to 10% of CAP based on serologic evidence (IgM ≥ 1:16 or IgG ≥ 1:512). However, 10% to 15% of a normal healthy working population without recent symptoms of upper respiratory tract infection will also have this same serologic evidence.[8] In addition to overestimating the frequency of a pathogen using serologic methods, underestimates can occur. Again, referring to *C pneumoniae,* only 10% to 20% of older adults with pneumonia who develop immunofluorescent antibodies to *C pneumoniae* develop a positive complement fixation test.[9] Older persons are thought to be reinfected with the organism and may not develop an IgM antibody.

NEW PATHOGENS ■

Pneumocystis carinii is the most common opportunistic pathogen in HIV infection. Prior to the AIDS epidemic, *P carinii* was uncommon and only occasionally seen in immunocompromised individuals. Autopsy surveys have shown subclinical *P carinii* infection in about 5% of patients with lymphoreticular neoplasms. Two series have recently reported *P carinii* in HIV-negative individuals. The first series described five individuals without clear immune defect,

mean age 40 years, with moderate to severe pneumonia.[10] In the second series, all but one was older than 70 years of age, and these patients had a decreased lymphocyte response to T cell mitogens.[11]

Hantavirus pulmonary syndrome (HPS) is an illness recently recognized in the Four Corners area of the United States. The deer mouse, *Peromyscus maniculatus,* is the principal rodent reservoir and has a habitat throughout the United States except for the Southeast. The condition presents with a prodrome of fever, myalgias, headache, abdominal pain, nausea, and cough. Respiratory failure is abrupt with rapid development of severe hypoxia from noncardiogenic pulmonary edema, profound hypotension, and death in nearly 60% to 70% of patients.[12] Hemoconcentration and thrombocytopenia are present on admission in the majority of patients. The Centers for Disease Control and Prevention (CDC) has adopted screening criteria for HPS in patients with an unexplained respiratory illness.[13] Supportive measures are the mainstay of therapy for HPS.

Group B *Streptococcus* is now being recognized as a cause of pneumonia in debilitated elderly patients,[14] not just neonates or pregnant women. Group B streptococcal pneumonia is usually polymicrobial and mortality is high. High-dose penicillin G is the recommended treatment.

OLD PATHOGENS, NEW PROBLEMS ■

There are now several distinct syndromes of bacteremic pneumococcal pneumonia. These presentations include overwhelming bacteremia in functionally asplenic patients[15,16] and leukopenia in alcoholic patients with pneumococcal bacteremia.[17] A growing concern in treating pneumococcal pneumonia is increasing penicillin resistance. Currently, 4%

to 5% of isolates of *S pneumoniae* in the United States have intermediate to high penicillin-resistance.[18] Many penicillin-resistant strains are also resistant to multiple antibiotics including tetracycline, erythromycin, clindamycin, sulfamethoxazole and trimethoprim, and chloramphenicol.[19] Risk factors in adults for colonization with penicillin-resistant pneumococci are age greater than 70 years, prior hospitalization, and previous beta-lactam antibiotic therapy.[20]

A resurgence of increasingly virulent group A streptococcal infections recently has been recognized among young adults with competent immune systems. Group A *Streptococcus* can cause acute pharyngitis, skin and wound infection, scarlet fever, puerperal sepsis, necrotizing fasciitis, or myositis. The streptococcal toxic shock syndrome[21] can occur with infection of the skin, soft tissues, or lung, resulting in acute respiratory distress syndrome (ARDS), shock, and multiple organ failure. Group A streptococcal pneumonia[22] usually occurs after a viral illness, is well-described in military trainees, and can cause outbreaks in nursing home patients.[23] An abrupt onset is characteristic and bacteremia is present in 10% to 15% of patients. Radiographic findings are more suggestive of an atypical organism. Pleuritis is common, and empyema formation occurs in up to 40% of patients. Penicillin remains the drug of choice.

In years with no pandemics of influenza, *Staphylococcus aureus* pneumonia is a less common cause of CAP. In a recent series of hospitalized patients with CAP, most with *S aureus* were elderly or had comorbid disease; 16% were bacteremic, 30% died, and 52% tested had serologic evidence of influenza infection.[24] Cavitation is relatively common, but pneumatoceles rarely form in adults.[25] Toxic shock may occasionally complicate *S aureus* pneumonia. Methicillin-resistant *S aureus* (MRSA) initially was seen only in nosocomial infections; MRSA is now endemic in long-term care facilities.[26,27] It appears that there is no difference in virulence of MRSA compared with methicillin-sensitive *S aureus*.[28]

The major change in *Mycobacterium tuberculosis* has been the emergence of multidrug-resistant strains. Atypical presentations of tuberculosis can be seen in immunocompromised hosts (particularly in HIV infection) or in elderly nursing home residents. Epidemics of tuberculosis have been reported in nursing home residents and nursing home workers.[29]

HOST DEFENSE AND SUSCEPTIBILITY ■

Throughout the breath-to-breath process of gas exchange, the lungs are in constant interaction with an environment filled with aerosolized particulate matter and potentially pathogenic microbes. The lungs have a complex defense system to preserve gas exchange and to protect the host from infection. This defense system involves upper and lower airway mechanisms that remove debris and microbes entering the respiratory tract. These defenses include anatomic barriers, mechanical structures, mucosal secretions, and both cellular and humoral immunity (Table 124-3).

Most organisms responsible for bacterial pneumonias are found in human hosts without disease. Pulmonary infection usually results from the aspiration of a sufficient inoculum of bacteria colonizing the upper airway resulting in proliferation of the bacteria in the lung. Most organisms that cause bacterial pneumonia are acquired by direct contact and not by air droplets. Relatively few agents that cause bacterial pneumonia are transmitted by aerosol transmission (e.g., *M tuberculosis*, *Mycoplasma*, and possibly *Legionella pneumophila*). Epidemics of respiratory infection are relatively common with nonbacterial pneumonias, particularly viruses such as influenza. Legionnaire disease, *M pneumoniae*,[30] and group A streptococci[31] are examples of the uncommon epidemic bacterial pneumonia. Pneumonia from hematogenous seeding of the lungs is uncommon but can occur with organisms such as *S aureus*.

Any condition that causes obtundation, impairment of laryngeal function, or suppression of the gag reflex and cough will compromise mechanical defense of the upper airway; subsequent aspiration of nasal and oropharyngeal secretions can occur. Healthy persons normally have nonvirulent resident bacterial flora in the oropharynx, including *Neisseria* species, *Moraxella catarrhalis*, *Streptococcus* species, corynebacteria, and *Staphylococcus* species. In patients with chronic airways disease (and occasionally in normal adults), *S pneumoniae* and *Haemophilus influenzae* colonize the upper airway.[32] Factors that alter the normal flora are treatment with antibiotics, residence in a chronic care facility, and underlying diseases such as surgery, starvation, and old age. Gram-negative bacilli are uncommon flora in normal individuals[33] but are relatively common in nursing home patients[34] and patients recently hospitalized.[35] Safe and effective strategies to prevent colonization do not currently exist but are under investigation.

Beyond the conducting airways the cough reflex contributes little to removing debris. The alveolar host defense is made up of a combination of phagocytic cells (alveolar macrophages and polymorphonuclear neutrophils), opsonins, lymphocytes (some of which secrete antibody, cytokines, or function as killer cells), and enhancing mechanisms that provide cell-mediated immunity or create inflammation.[36] Several kinds of injury or illness can impair one or more of the interactions that occur in the normal alveolar space when microbes invade. Uremia may affect the motility of polymorphonuclear neutrophils and diminish the inflammatory response. Alcohol-abuse undermines host defenses by profoundly disturbing cytokine production and activity[37] and by suppressing upper airway protection in those who binge-drink. In patients with cirrhosis (from alcohol or other causes), pneumonia is nearly as frequent as subacute bacterial peritonitis (SBP), carries a higher mortality than SBP (40%), and is usually due to gram-negative bacilli.[38] The clearance of encapsulated bacteria (*S pneumoniae*, *Haemophilus*, and *Klebsiella*) requires functional opsonins. The supply of non-immune opsonins is usually sufficient in the patient without chronic illness. Patients with immunoglobulin deficiencies (see Table 124-3) can have recurrent sinopulmonary infections with encapsulated organisms. For certain microbes like mycobacteria and *L pneumophila* the macrophage must be activated to perform optimally. A number of cytokines can cause this heightened activity and are presumed to come from lymphocytes in the alveoli and

TABLE 124-3. Respiratory Host Defenses

HOST MECHANISMS	POTENTIAL DEFECT	IMPACT AND POTENTIAL INFECTION
Conducting Airways		
Mechanical barriers (larynx, etc.)	Bypassing barriers with an endotracheal tube or tracheostomy	Aspiration, direct aerosol entry of microorganisms into airway
Mucociliary clearance (cough)	Intrinsic structural defect in cilia, ciliotoxic infections	Stagnant secretions, coughing, bronchiectasis, sinusitis
Bronchoconstriction	Hyperactive airways, intrinsic asthma	Poor removal of secretions, excessive secretions
Local immunoglobulin coating-secretory IgA	IgA deficiency, functional deficiency from breakdown by bacterial IgA, proteases	Sinopulmonary infections, abnormal colonization with certain bacteria
Iron-containing proteins (transferrin, lactoferrin)	Iron deficiency	May not inhibit certain bacteria (*Pseudomonas, Escherichia coli, Legionella*)
Alveolar Milieu		
Other immunoglobulin classes (opsonic IgG)	Acquired hypogammaglobulinemia, selective IgG_4 and IgG_2 deficiency	Sinopulmonary infections, pneumonia with encapsulated bacteria
Alternative complement pathway activation	C3 and C5 deficiency	Trouble with recurrent infections
Surfactant	Decreased synthesis, acute lung injury	Loss of opsonization activity, alveolar collapse (atelectasis)
Alveolar macrophages	Subtle effects from immunosuppression, cannot kill intracellular microbes	Propensity for *Pneumocystis carinii* and *Legionella* infections, poor containment of mycobacterium
Polymorphonuclear granulocytes	Absent because of immunosuppression, intrinsic defects of motility, lack of chemotactic stimulus	Poor inflammatory response associated with gram-negative bacillary infection and fungi (*Aspergillus*)
Augmenting Mechanisms		
Initiation of immune responses (humoral antibody and cellular immunity)	Immunosuppression	Inadequate S-IgA or IgG antibody available (more susceptible to viral, mycoplasmal, and bacterial infections)
Generation of an inflammatory response (influx of polymorphonuclear granulocytes, eosinophils, lymphocytes, and fluid components)	Generally reflects supply of polymorphonuclear granulocytes, impaired adherence of polymorphonuclear neutrophils	Infection—nosocomial and opportunistic organisms

Adapted from Reynolds HY: Respiratory infections may reflect deficiencies in host defense mechanisms. *Dis Mon* 1985;31:1.

adjacent tissues. Exogenous cytokine replacement therapy or blocking of excessive levels of cytokines is not yet a reality in clinical practice.

INITIAL DIAGNOSTIC EVALUATION ■

The initial evaluation should, first, narrow the spectrum of possible pathogens, simplifying empiric therapy, and second, identify risk factors that predict complications or higher mortality. Certain infectious pathogens have clinical characteristics that help suggest their role in individual patients. Important historical features that can suggest specific pathogens are outlined in Table 124-4. A "typical" pneumonia causes fever, rigors, productive cough, and occasional pleuritic chest pain. *S pneumoniae*[39] is a pathogen that classically produces typical pneumonia. Figure 124-1 demonstrates a dense, homogeneous infiltrate caused by *S pneumoniae*. In contrast, an "atypical" pneumonia causes low-grade fever and nonproductive cough. Infection with *M pneumoniae*[40] is the characteristic cause of an atypical pneumonia. Other organisms can produce a illness indistinguishable from that caused by *Mycoplasma* (Table 124-5). Of these, *Legionella* species and influenza can cause a more fulminant pneumonia. Figure 124-2 shows radiographic changes of an atypical pneumonia, with inhomogeneous, bilateral, multilobe interstitial infiltrates.

Pneumonia caused by atypical organisms frequently has extrapulmonary features.[41] Chlamydial pneumonia often starts with hoarseness and fever, and respiratory tract symp-

TABLE 124-4. Important Historical Factors in CAP

RISK FACTORS

  HIV infection or HIV risk factors
  Aspiration risk
  Antecedent viral infection (especially influenza)
  Recent antibiotic therapy
  Underlying cardiac or pulmonary disease
  Immunosuppression from disease or medications

EXPOSURES

  Special recreational or occupational exposures
  Contact with children or ill individuals
  Recent travel

toms may not appear for days. Patients with *Mycoplasma* pneumonia may have ear pain due to bullous myringitis. *Legionella* often causes multisystem complaints, including high fevers, headaches, confusion, and gastrointestinal complaints. Although helpful, this distinction of atypical and typical oversimplifies the reality of a great deal of overlap in how these pathogens present. In a patient who has signs of pneumonia, an initial chest radiograph can demonstrate findings suggestive of specific pathogens. Cavitation is more common with *M tuberculosis*, anaerobes, *S aureus*, and *Klebsiella-Enterobacter-Serratia* species. A thorough discussion of pathogen specific radiographic changes in pneumonia is given by Fraser and and colleagues.[42] Other radiographic findings such as pleural effusions may require further evalua-

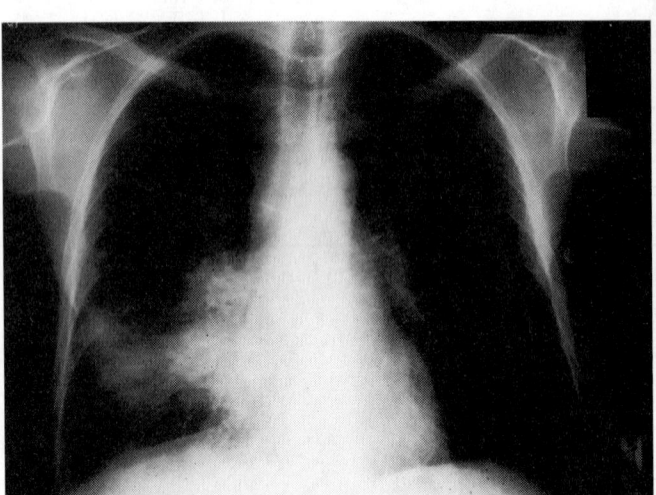
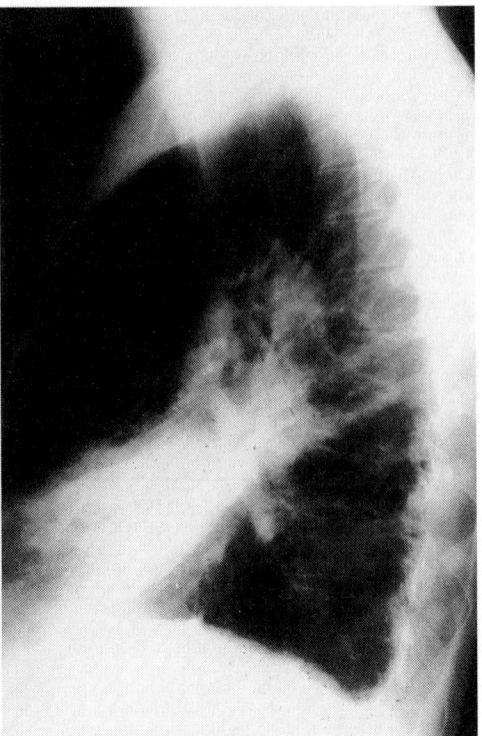

FIGURE 124-1. Typical pneumonia. A posterioranterior (**A**) and lateral (**B**) roentgenogram reveal a dense, homogeneous right middle lobe infiltrate caused by *Streptococcus pneumoniae*.

TABLE 124-5. Pathogens in Typical and Atypical Pneumonia

TYPICAL PNEUMONIA	ATYPICAL PNEUMONIA
Streptococcus pneumoniae	*Legionella pneumophila*
Hemophilus influenzae	*Chlamydia pneumoniae*
Aerobic gram-negative	*Mycoplasma pneumoniae*
Staphylococcus aureus	Viruses (influenza, respiratory
Streptococcus species	synctial virus, adenovirus)

tion (i.e., thoracentesis). The pattern of chest radiographic abnormalities may help differentiate pneumonia from conditions that mimic it. Also, certain radiographic features have prognostic implications, such as multilobar involvement at presentation, which correlate with severity of disease.

The value of examination of expectorated sputum is controversial. Some authorities have found that a Gram stain of expectorated sputum is useful in the initial evaluation if strict criteria are adhered to in accepting adequate specimens. Sensitivity of sputum Gram stains is approximately 50%. Using stringent quality criteria (>25 leukocytes, <10 squamous cells per high power field), as many as 75% of obtained specimens are judged inadequate.[43] Direct staining of sputum is diagnostic when it identifies pathogens such as *Mycobacterium* species, endemic fungi, *Legionella* species, and *P carinii*.

Bacterial cultures of sputum may demonstrate pathogenic organisms, but sensitivity and specificity is poor. In certain circumstances, sputum culture is helpful in management. The identification of pathogens not normally found in the respiratory flora such as endemic fungi, *Mycobacterium* species, and *Legionella* species is diagnostic of infection. The identification of penicillin-resistant pneumococcus or other organisms resistant to the original empiric therapy affects therapy decisions.

The impact of further laboratory testing on decision-making for hospitalization and therapy is being closely scrutinized mainly because of cost considerations. To give effective medical care and also use medical resources wisely, a knowl-

edge of what historical, physical, and laboratory findings are predictive of higher mortality or complications is necessary (Table 124-6). There are no rigid guidelines for when hospitalization is required in CAP, yet it is perhaps the single most important decision in the care of a patient with pneumonia. If multiple risk factors are clustered in a single patient, then hospitalization should be strongly considered. Social factors may play a role in the decision to hospitalize, for example, when there is no responsible caregiver or when an unstable home situation exists.

Laboratory parameters need not be checked in all patients before deciding to hospitalize or not. If a patient has few historical or physical findings suggesting a higher risk of an adverse outcome, it is unlikely that laboratory testing will affect the decision to treat as an outpatient. In the elderly, however, the expression of common clinical features of pneumonia or their severity may be atypical, obscured, or even absent.[44] In situations of clinical uncertainty, additional laboratory information may be decisive. The final decision to hospitalize a patient with CAP rests with the physician and is influenced by clinical factors and an estimate of a patient's ability to comply with therapy and subsequent followup. In the face of uncertainty, a brief hospitalization to demonstrate improvement on initial therapy is wise.

Patients who require hospitalization should have a more thorough characterization of their risk for complications. In addition to a chest radiograph, a complete blood count with differential, an arterial blood gas sample, and serum for hepatic enzymes, renal function, and electrolytes should be collected. In patients unlikely to have hypercapnia, an estimate of oxygenation from a pulse oximeter may suffice. If thrombocytopenia is present, a more complete assessment of the coagulation cascade with a prothrombin time, partial thromboplastin time, and either D-dimer or fibrin split products is warranted to look for disseminated intravascular coagulation. In addition to prognostic information, abnormal renal or hepatic function may affect the dosing antibiotics.

A more aggressive search for the etiologic agent in the hospitalized patient with CAP needs to be attempted. Two sets of blood cultures may identify the pathogen. Pneumococcal pneumonia has demonstrable bacteremia in 10% to

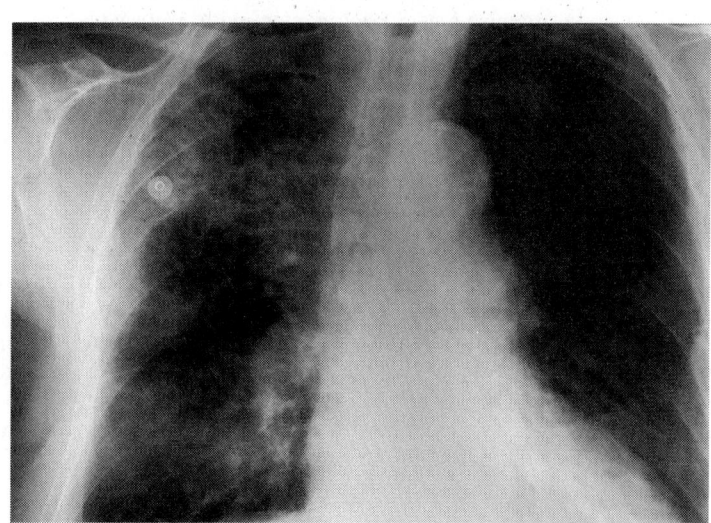

FIGURE 124-2. Atypical pneumonia. An anteriorposterior roentgenogram reveals an inhomogeneous, multilobar interstitial infiltrate predominantly involving the right lung. *Legionella pneumophilia* was identified in the sputum by direct fluorescent antibody.

TABLE 124-6. Risk Factors for Adverse Outcome in CAP

HISTORICAL INFORMATION	LABORATORY FINDINGS
Age >65 years	Leukopenia (white blood cell count <4 × 10^9/L or an absolute neutrophil count below $1 × 10^9$/L)
Previous hospitalization within 1 year	
Suspicion of aspiration	
Chronically abnormal mental status	Leukocytosis (white blood cell count >30 × 10^9/L)
Postsplenectomy state	
Underlying Diseases	Hypoxemia or hypercapnia (PaO_2 < 60 mm Hg or $PaCO_2$ > 50 mm Hg on room air)
Chronic lung disease (chronic obstructive pulmonary disease, cystic fibrosis, bronchiectasis)	Renal insufficiency (serum creatinine > 1.2 mg/dL or blood urea nitrogen > 20 mg/dL)
Diabetes mellitus	Anemia (hematocrit < 30% or hemoglobin < 9g/dL)
Chronic renal failure	Unfavorable chest radiographic findings
Congestive heart failure	More than 1 lobe involvement
Chronic liver disease	Presence of a cavity or a pleural effusion
Malnutrition	Rapid radiographic spreading
Chronic alcohol abuse	Need for mechanical ventilation
PHYSICAL FINDINGS	Other organ dysfunction to include metabolic acidosis, increased prothrombin time or partial thromboplastin time, decreased platelets, or the presence of fibrin split products > 1:40
Respiratory rate >30 breaths/min	
Hypotension (diastolic blood pressure ≤60 mm Hg or systolic ≤ 90 mm Hg)	
Fever (temperature >38.3°C, 101°F)	
Extrapulmonary site of infection (septic arthritis, meningitis, etc.)	
Confusion or decreased level of consciousness	

Modified from Niederman MS, et al. Guidelines for the initial management of adults with community-acquired pneumonia: diagnosis, assessment of severity, and initial antimicrobial therapy. *Am Rev Respir Dis* 1993;148:1418.

30% of cases and mortality with pneumococcal bacteremia is as high as 27%.[45] Overall, 60% of the cases of bacteremic pneumonia are due to *S pneumoniae*.[46] Estimates of the frequency of bacteremia for less common pathogens are difficult to find. In a retrospective series of patients with CAP with demonstrable bacteremia, nearly as many had gram-negative organisms as *S pneumoniae*, with *Klebsiella pneumoniae* predominating. Gram-negative bacteremia has a mortality rate of greater than 50%.[47] When compared with *S pneumoniae*, gram-negative pathogens result in hospitalization more frequently, are associated with bacteremia more often, and result in a higher mortality rate. Thus, in addition to identifying a pathogen, a positive blood culture can provide important prognostic information.

Tests that measure specific microbial antigens, DNA probes, acute and convalescent titers of antibodies, polymerase chain reaction amplification of DNA of microbes, etc, are not yet routinely useful in the evaluation of CAP. Even with extensive diagnostic testing the specific etiology of CAP frequently cannot be identified. More extensive testing should be reserved for patients with either identifiable risk factors for particular pathogens or severe pneumonia-failing empiric therapy directed at likely pathogens.

EVALUATION AND TREATMENT OF PLEURAL EFFUSIONS ■

Pleural effusion occurs in approximately 40% of patients who are hospitalized with pneumonia.[48] If a significant pleural effusion is identified on the initial chest radiograph in CAP, a diagnostic thoracentesis should be performed. A significant pleural effusion is one that layers greater than 1 centimeter on a lateral decubitus chest radiograph. If the effusion is difficult to identify by percussion, ultrasound guidance is helpful in localizing pleural fluid. Infection of pleural fluid (empyema) is usually a complication of a pulmonary bacterial process. The presence of an empyema warrants early closed chest tube drainage in addition to antibiotic therapy.[49] Delay in drainage results in loculation of fluid and pleural peel formation and necessitates a prolonged hospitalization and complex surgical decortication with concomitant higher morbidity and mortality.[50,51] Thus, the pleural fluid evaluation is directed at identifying the infecting pathogen and determining the need for pleural space drainage. Table 124-7 details pleural fluid characteristics suggestive of an empyema.

The identification of pathogenic bacteria is made by Gram stain of pleural fluid and both aerobic and anaerobic culture

TABLE 124-7. Characteristics of Empyema

DIAGNOSTIC OF EMPYEMA	CONSISTENT WITH EMPYEMA	NON-INFECTED FLUID
Positive Gram stain	pH < 7.1	pH > 7.25
Positive fluid culture	Glucose < 40	Glucose > 60
Frank pus	LDH > 1000	
Foul odor		

of pleural fluid. Anaerobes are commonly part of the mixed flora of an empyema. Extrapolating from data on the yield of bacterial cultures in peritonitis,[52,53] pleural fluid should be directly inoculated into blood culture bottles. As anaerobes are commonly part of the mixed flora of an empyema, both an aerobic and anaerobic bottle should be used.

Pleural fluid characteristics that are pathognomonic of an empyema are frank pus and foul odor. Forty percent of anaerobic infections lack the characteristic odor.[54] Early chest tube drainage, in addition to antibiotic therapy, is indicated for grossly purulent fluid.[55] For parapneumonic effusions with parameters worrisome for (but not diagnostic of) an empyema, repeat thoracentesis in 12 to 24 hours should be performed to see if fluid parameters have worsened.

Nonpurulent fluid that fits criteria for a complicated parapneumonic effusion recently has been managed successfully and more conservatively. One retrospective review found hospital stay shorter with systemic antibiotics plus a regimen of daily thoracentesis and instillation of local antibiotics or saline, compared to early chest tube drainage and systemic antibiotics with comparable mortality.[56] Although more conservative for the patient, this regimen is fairly labor intensive. An approach utilizing systemic antibiotics alone in non-purulent complicated parapneumonic effusions found no differences in duration of hospitalization or mortality. A trend towards cost saving in the conservative therapy group compared to immediate chest tube drainage and systemic antibiotics was noted.[57] Prolonged duration of symptoms before hospitalization, larger size of pleural effusion, presence of loculations, or demonstration of a gram-negative organism in the pleural space predict a complicated course.[50,58,59] Figure 124-3 illustrates a complex, loculated parapneumonic effusion. Failure of a conservative approach appears to be more likely if these conditions are present. If a conservative approach is elected, close follow up to monitor resolution is essential.

LUNG ABSCESS ▪

Cavitary lung disease can be due to a myriad of infectious agents, including routine bacterial pathogens, tuberculosis, and endemic mycoses. Bacterial infection with anaerobes, gram-negative rods (especially *Klebsiella* species) or *S aureus* is particularly prone to cavitation.[60] Figure 124-4 shows a large right lower lobe intraparenchymal abscess which evolved during treatment of a *S aureus* pneumonia. A radio-

graphic feature noted in this figure which helps differentiate a lung abscess from a pyopneumothorax is similar dimensions of the cavity in the frontal and lateral projections. Pyopneumothoraces tend to be much wider in one view compared to the other. It is necessary to differentiate these two processes to avoid unnecessary chest tube placement. Occasionally computed tomography (CT) is necessary to make this distinction.

Anaerobic lung abscess tends to develop more slowly than do aerobic bacterial abscesses.[61] Spontaneous rupture of a bacterial lung abscess can occur, with formation of a pyopneumothorax and rapid development of sepsis. The diagnosis of reactivation *M tuberculosis* must always be entertained in patients presenting with cavitary lung disease, since these patients require negative flow respiratory isolation and will not respond to routine antimicrobial agents. *Nocardia* or *Actinomyces* infection can produce cavitation and empyema formation (occasionally with formation of a sinus tract to the skin surface). These infections tend to be more insidious in onset than routine bacterial infections.

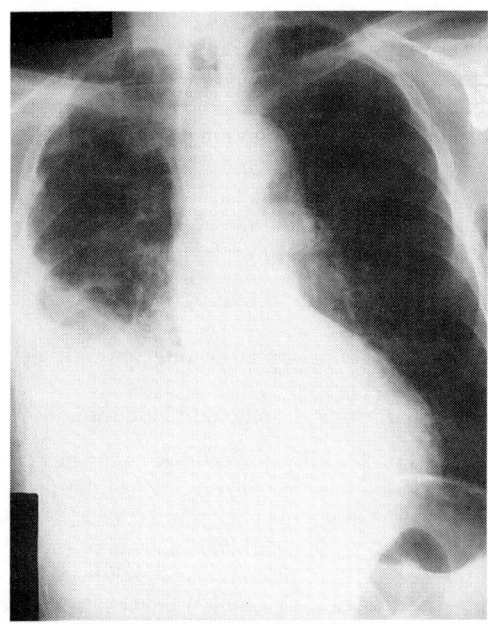

FIGURE 124-3. Complicated parapneumonic effusion. A posteroanterior roentgenogram demonstrates a moderate sized right-sided pleural effusion complicating a right lower lobe pneumonia. Note the irregular fluid meniscus along the lateral border of the mid-lung field. The haziness adjacent to this irregular meniscus suggests a posterior extension of the loculated fluid collection.

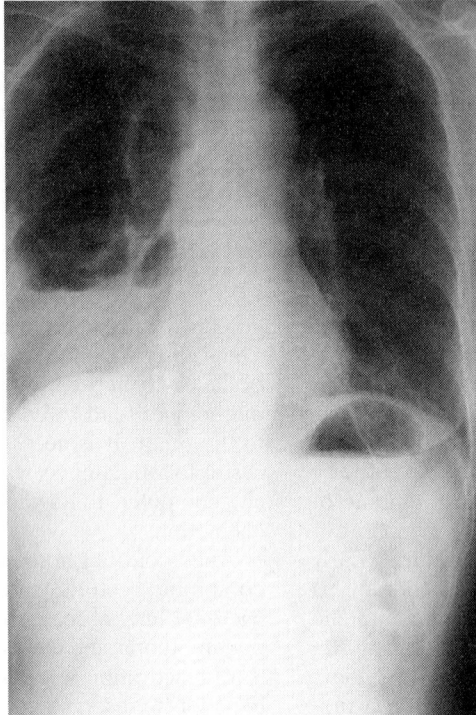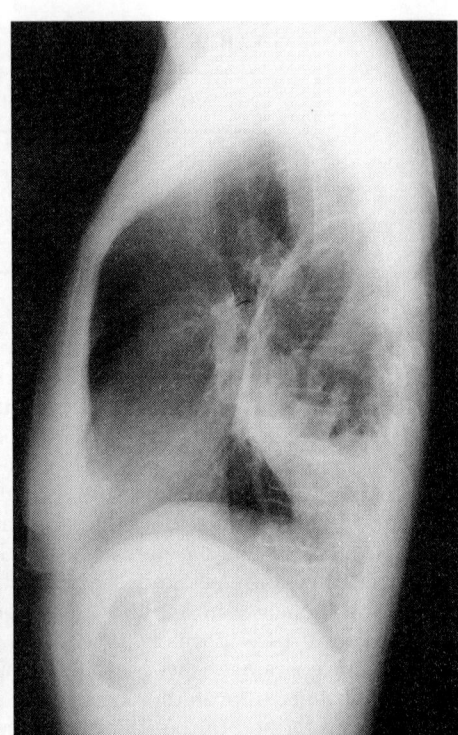

FIGURE 124-4. Large intraparenchymal lung abscess. This abscess developed during the hospital course of a patient with a *Staph aureus* pneumonia. The diameter of the abscess cavity is similar on the posteroanterior (**A**) and lateral (**B**) views, consistent with an intraparenchymal abscess rather than a pyopneumothorax.

The initial management of a bacterial lung abscess should be medical, with antibiotics directed at the responsible pathogens. Aspiration pneumonia with resultant cavitation is frequently polymicrobial, and culture of sputum may yield only "normal oral flora". Aspiration pneumonia can be effectively treated with clindamycin or with the combination of penicillin plus metronidazole.[62]

Occasionally, a bacterial lung abscess will require drainage for cure. Indications for drainage include

1. Failure to decrease in size by sequential radiographs over 2 weeks
2. Signs of ongoing sepsis despite appropriate antibiotic therapy
3. Continued fevers despite antibiotic therapy.[63]

Cavity size has prognostic implications, as cavities >6 cm in diameter are unlikely to resolve on medical therapy alone.[63] Drainage of an intraparenchymal abscess can be done with CT- or ultrasound-guided catheter placement or with open surgical resection. Blind placement of an intraparenchymal chest tube is discouraged, for it may result in excessive bleeding or creation of a pyopneumothorax. Bronchoscopic drainage has been attempted without substantial success. The suction port on flexible fiberoptic bronchoscopes is generally too small to adequately drain the collection of pus, and spillage of infected fluids into uninvolved lung parenchyma can produce new areas of pneumonia.[64]

EMPIRIC ANTIBIOTICS ■

No single antibiotic is effective against all potential pathogens in CAP. A review of the patient's clinical presentation and host defenses, combined with sputum Gram stain and knowledge of local sensitivity patterns, often narrows the list of potential pathogens. This permits the selection of narrow-spectrum antibiotics likely to be effective against the responsible organism. A useful approach to grouping pathogens to help in decision-making for empiric treatment in CAP is to combine severity of illness, age, and comorbid disease. This classification helps predict the likely microbial etiology and the patient's prognosis. An adaptation of this approach was put forth in the American Thoracic Society's guidelines for management of community acquired pneumonia.[65] Tables 124-1 and 124-2 are modifications of this grouping of pathogens in CAP.

Modification of an empiric antibiotic regimen should occur once a pathogenic organism and its sensitivities are available. Table 105-3 details the antibiotic agents of choice for human pathogens. The use of empiric therapy should never negate the need for a search for a specific pathogen. Initial therapy is often more broad-spectrum than will be required to definitively treat the cause of a pneumonia; broad-spectrum agents are more expensive and may have more side effects than directed therapy. Certain pathogens (e.g., endemic mycoses) will not be treated by even broad-spectrum antibacterial agents, and their identification has obvious impact on therapy.

OUTPATIENT THERAPY OF PATIENTS LESS THAN 60-YEARS-OLD WITHOUT COMORBID ILLNESS

Pneumonia in young patients without comorbid disease is most often caused by *S pneumoniae, Mycoplasma*, or viruses. Treatment with a macrolide (erythromycin, azithromycin, or clarithromycin) is often effective. Both azithromycin and clarithromycin are substantially more expensive than erythromycin. However, the incidence of gastrointestinal side effects is less with these agents than with erythromycin, and compliance may be better than with erythromycin due to less frequent dosing. Of note, the activity of fluoroquinolones against *S pneumoniae* is unreliable;[66,67] their use as empiric therapy in CAP is not advocated. In otherwise healthy young patients, empiric therapy with the macrolides may fail if *H influenzae* or *Chlamydia* species are responsible. If a young person is failing therapy with macrolides, tetracycline or doxycycline should be substituted to treat the above-mentioned pathogens.

OUTPATIENT THERAPY OF PATIENTS MORE THAN 60-YEARS-OLD AND THOSE WITH COMORBID ILLNESS

In older adults and those with comorbid illness, gram-negative pneumonia is possible. A review of the sputum Gram stain can be very helpful in directing antibiotic therapy (Table 124-8). If gram-positive organisms predominate, oral penicillin is a good therapeutic option; macrolides are a good

TABLE 124-8. Initial Therapy for CAP in Hospitalized Patients Based on Sputum Gram Stain*

GRAM STAIN	INITIAL THERAPY
Gram positive cocci in chains	1st generation cephalosporin or erythromycin
Gram positive cocci in clusters	Nafcillin or oxacillin[†]
Large Gram negative cocci	Trimethoprim-sulfamethoxazole or doxycycline
Pleomorphic Gram negative coccobacilli	Amoxicillin or trimethoprim-sulfamethoxazole or doxycycline
Gram-rods	Ceftazidime or cefepime plus aminoglycoside
Mixed flora or no bacteria seen or inadequate sputum specimen	Nondiagnostic, use empiric therapy given in Table 124-14

*Initial therapy should be modified based on clinical response of patient and laboratory sensitivity testing of the organism (see text).
†If the patient was recently hospitalized or institutionalized, vancomycin should be used until methicillin susceptibility testing of isolated *S aureus* is performed.

alternative for the penicillin-allergic patient. However, if gram-negatives or a mixture of gram-negatives and positives are seen, oral amoxicillin or sulfamethoxazole trimethoprim can be used. If the patient is allergic to sulfamethoxazole trimethoprim, treatment with a second-generation therapy (e.g., cefuroxime or cefamandole) is usually effective.

COMMUNITY ACQUIRED PNEUMONIA REQUIRING INPATIENT THERAPY

The clinician should aggressively seek the cause of pneumonia in patients requiring hospitalization. Sputum Gram stain should be done in these patients, as it can narrow the etiologic possibilities. Prior antimicrobial therapy should be reviewed, since the responsible pathogen may be resistant to similar agents. Institutionalized patients requiring admission for pneumonia have frequently already failed empiric oral therapy. *S aureus* and gram-negative rods must be considered if this is the case.

INPATIENT THERAPY OF MILD-TO-MODERATE COMMUNITY ACQUIRED PNEUMONIA

Patients with mild-to-moderate CAP who require hospital admission should initially be treated with a second or third generation cephalosporin or with a beta lactam-beta lactamase inhibitor combination (Table 124-9). If *Legionella* is clinically suspected, a macrolide should be added. Consideration should be given to changing to the regimen described for severe CAP if the patient is worsening despite this empiric regimen.

INPATIENT THERAPY OF SEVERE COMMUNITY ACQUIRED PNEUMONIA

Patients who are severely ill due to CAP should be treated empirically for *Legionella, S aureus*, pneumococcus, and gram-negative pathogens. An effective regimen against these pathogens is the combination of a macrolide *plus* one of the following: ceftazidime, cefepime, an antipseudomonal

TABLE 124-9. Empiric Antibiotic Therapy for Pneumonia Requiring Hospitalization

MILD TO MODERATE ILLNESS	SEVERE ILLNESS
2nd or 3rd generation cephalosporin *or* beta lactam/beta lactamase inhibitor ± erythromycin 1 g q 6 hr*	Erythromycin 1 g q 6 hr[†] *and* ceftazidime or cefepime[‡]

*Erythromycin should be used if *Legionella* is suspected; rifampin should be added if *Legionella* is documented.
†Rifampin should be added if *Legionella* is documented.
‡In penicillin-allergic patients, quinolones may be substituted. If *Pseudomonas* pneumonia, add aminoglycoside for first 3–5 days of therapy.

penicillin, or cilastatin-imipenem. Because of the broad-spectrum nature of this combination, it is particularly important to narrow the antibiotic coverage after an etiologic pathogen has been identified.

DURATION OF THERAPY ■

The duration of therapy is influenced by the responsible pathogen and the severity of the patient's illness. In critically ill patients, initial antibiotic therapy is almost always given intravenously. Absorption from the oral or intramuscular route may be unpredictable in critically ill patients, with a resultant potential for subtherapeutic levels of antibiotics. Once a patient is clinically improving and is no longer critically ill, consideration should be given to changing to an oral antibiotic regimen. Oral antibiotics are usually less expensive than their intravenous counterparts. Changing to oral therapy may also decrease the duration of intravenous (IV) access, thus reducing the risk of IV catheter-related infection. Intravenous therapy is generally continued for longer in patients with documented pneumonia-related bacteremia, especially prolonged bacteremia. This is because of the concern for endocarditis or metastatic focus of infection, though the benefit of this over oral agents has not been clearly demonstrated.

Table 124-10 lists the recommended duration of therapy for specific causes of CAP. Of note, pneumonia complicated by abscess formation, empyema, endocarditis, or metastatic foci of infection may require a more prolonged course of antibiotics. The overall condition of the patient and the patient's response to therapy should influence the duration of therapy.

TABLE 124-10. Suggested Duration of Antibiotic Therapy°

ORGANISM	DURATION OF THERAPY
Anaerobes	At least 3 weeks and until cavity resolves
Chlamydia pneumoniae	10–14 days
Chlamydia psittaci	At least 14 days
Gram negative rods-coliforms	21 days
Haemophilus influenzae	14 days
Legionella	21 days
Moraxella catarrhalis	10–14 days
Mycoplasma pneumoniae	7–14 days
Nocardia	3–6 months
S aureus	21 days
S pneumoniae	10–14 days

°Therapy may need to be extended beyond the duration listed based upon clinical response to therapy and the presence of complications of infection (e.g., for lung abscess, metastatic foci of infection, etc.).

ADJUNCTIVE TREATMENT ■

In addition to antimicrobial therapy, attention to supportive therapy needs to be maintained, particularly in the hospitalized patient. Aerosolized bronchodilator therapy is appropriate in those with concomitant chronic airway disease. Upper and lower airway infection frequently exacerbates obstructive lung diseases, and intensification of the bronchodilator regimen is often required. Short courses of corticosteroids are appropriate for patients with reactive airways disease who manifest acute bronchospasm. The clinical effects of glucocorticoids in bacterial pneumonia have not been well studied. Although glucocorticoids are useful in moderate to severe *P carinii* pneumonia in HIV infection, there are no studies to support an analogous approach in CAP.

Other important adjuncts are supplemental oxygen and respiratory therapy to manage excessive bronchial secretions. If hospitalization lasts more than several days, nutritional support becomes essential. Lastly, vigilance for complications of therapy (e.g., drug fever, allergy, renal toxicity, or fluid overload from high salt or fluid loads of certain antibiotic regimens) needs to be maintained.

CLINICAL RESPONSE TO THERAPY ■

Effective antibiotic therapy often improves the clinical manifestations of pneumonia in 48 to 72 hours. Host or pathogen factors can delay clinical improvement. The initial empiric therapy should not be changed during this time unless there is a marked clinical deterioration or a pathogen resistant to the chosen regimen is isolated.

Radiographic resolution does not follow the same time course as clinical resolution. Despite improving clinical symptoms the chest radiograph may worsen with progression of the infiltrate or the development of a pleural effusion. Evaluation of the delayed pleural effusion is similar to that previously described for the initially recognized pleural effusion.

INVASIVE TESTING ■

Not all patients respond to initial empiric therapy. Table 105-6 lists reasons for failure of an initial empiric antibiotic regimen. Failure to improve after 72 hours or clinical deterioration in severely ill patients without an etiologic diagnosis are indications for a more aggressive diagnostic evaluation. Radiographic worsening in the setting of severe CAP carries a poor prognosis, predictive of higher mortality.[68]

Prior to invasive testing, a careful repeat of the history is essential. Table 124-11 lists animal exposures and travel which may predispose to uncommon pathogens. These pathogens can be detected with special serologic tests or cultures, and specific therapy is available for many of these unusual pathogens. Clues to host immune defects may be present. An inquiry into a patient's sexual practices or history

TABLE 124-11. Unusual Pathogens in
Non-resolving Pneumonia

PATHOGEN	EXPOSURE
Q Fever (*Coxiella burnetii*)	Parturient cats, cattle, sheep, or goats
Hantavirus pulmonary syndrome	Rodents, ticks
Rickettsia	Ticks
Tularemia (*Francisella tularensis*)	Infected rabbits and ticks
Psittacosis (*Chlamydia psittaci*)	Birds, including chickens
Plague (*Yersinia pestis*)	Rodents (rats, mice, occ squirrels)
Leptospirosis	Rodents (seen in sewer/sanitation workers, animal handlers, veterinarians, farm workers)
Melioidosis (*Pseudomonas pseudomallei*)	Travel to South East Asia (remote or recent)
Paragonimiasis	Travel to Asia, Africa, or Central and South America
Anthrax (*Bacillus anthracis*)	Industrial exposure to animal hair, wool, skins, or bones originating in Africa or Asia

of injection drug use may suggest that HIV testing is important. A review of the patient's recent past and current medications may identify a lengthy period of treatment with immunosuppressive therapy such as corticosteroids or recently completed chemotherapy. These abnormal host factors may prompt an earlier invasive diagnostic approach due to the broader spectrum of possible pathogens.

Careful physical examination may reveal extrapulmonary complications of pneumonia. Metastatic sites of infection can occur in up to 10% of bacteremic pneumococcal pneumonia[69] with resultant meningitis, arthritis, endocarditis, pericarditis, or peritonitis. Repeat blood cultures and chest radiographs should be performed to look for the cause of the clinical deterioration. Repeat blood cultures may detect intermittent bacteremia and identify the original pathogen or an additional pathogen. The chest radiograph may demonstrate an empyema that requires drainage, a pneumothorax from necrotizing pneumonia that requires evacuation, or the development of significant atelectasis that will respond to better pulmonary toilet.

BRONCHOSCOPY

Greater than 90%[70] of patients with CAP, including those requiring hospitalization, will respond to empiric antibiotic therapy. Bronchoscopy will not add anything other than cost to the care of those who respond to empiric therapy. Invasive testing has been used in CAP for severely ill patients requiring ICU admission[70,71] and for those who fail to improve or worsen on empiric antibiotics.[72,73] Bronchoscopy has been used in CAP using both bronchoalveolar lavage (BAL) and telescoping-plugged catheter (TPC) cultures. TPC and BAL

quantitative cultures have the highest yield when performed prior to antibiotic therapy but still achieve a bacteriologic diagnosis in nearly half of the patients on antibiotic therapy.[74] In approximately 40% of cases of nonresolving CAP, a nonbacteriologic diagnosis can be made by BAL and transbronchial biopsy (TBB). There will still be a significant minority of patients with nonresolving pneumonia on antibiotic therapy who do not receive a diagnosis despite TPC, BAL, and TBB with bronchoscopy. In the studies to date, it appears most of these patients will slowly improve on antibiotic therapy suggesting that they have undiagnosed infectious pneumonia with delayed improvement. Applying a pneumococcal antigen test (either latex agglutination or countercurrent immunoelectrophoresis) to BAL fluid, 50% of patients with no etiology established by BAL cultures had positive antigen tests.[75] This would suggest that in a body fluid unlikely to be contaminated with oral secretions (BAL fluid with < 2% squamous epithelial cells), half of the undiagnosed cases of CAP may be due to *S pneumoniae* and can be identified with pneumococcal antigen testing. Antigen testing is particularly helpful in patients currently or previously on antibiotic therapy.

TRANSTHORACIC NEEDLE ASPIRATION

If an infiltrate is in an area not easily accessible to bronchoscopy, percutaneous fine needle aspiration (FNA) with either fluoroscopy or CT guidance can help determine the cause of life-threatening pneumonia. It is usually not the procedure of choice in critically ill patients. Pneumothorax may develop in up to 25% of patients who undergo FNA.[76] Mechanical ventilation is usually considered a contraindication to FNA due to its particularly high risk of pneumothorax. Other contraindications include the inability to tolerate a significant pneumothorax, bullous emphysema, and an untreatable bleeding diathesis. The diagnostic yield of FNA ranges from 26%[77] to 73%[78] for infectious etiologies in pneumonia in both immunocompetent and immunocompromised individuals. A recent series reported an initial bacteriologic diagnostic yield of 50% which rose to 78% with the addition of pneumococcal antigen testing by latex agglutination on the aspirate from the FNA.[79]

OPEN LUNG BIOPSY

Open lung biopsy (OLB) has traditionally been used in immunocompromised patients with undiagnosed diffuse pulmonary infiltrates; its role in these patients is somewhat controversial. In some series a specific diagnosis is frequently made,[80] but others have found it infrequently finds a treatable cause or results in a change of therapy or outcome.[81] In a series of 1 118 patients with severe CAP, 26 underwent OLB.[82] Of the 26 undergoing OLB, all but 8 were newly diagnosed as immunocompromised. Of the remaining 8 nonimmunocompromised patients with progressive deterioration and negative conventional cultures, a 25% yield on OLB was obtained, similar to previous reports.[83] The majority of patients had non-specific histologic findings. Mortality was nearly 40%, though not specifically attributed to the OLB. In patients who required mechanical ventilation or met traditional intubation criteria, mortality was 60% to 75% post-operatively.[84]

To summarize, OLB is rarely necessary in CAP. In those patients being considered for OLB without a diagnosed etiology for their severe CAP, a majority may be immunocompromised. Mortality is high in this subset of patients, and OLB is of limited use in identifying the cause of their pneumonia.

CHRONIC LUNG INFECTIONS ■

Slow resolution of pneumonia may reflect derangement in host defenses, inadequate or inappropriate antimicrobial therapy, unusual pathogens, or a noninfectious pneumonic process. Delayed clinical resolution has historically been due more commonly to host factors than to an unusual pathogen.[85,86] The factors most commonly associated with delayed clinical resolution are age greater than 50 years, alcoholism, and chronic illness. The most common chronic illnesses are those listed at the bottom of Table 124-1.

Chronic pneumonia is an illness that lasts at least 6 weeks and is caused by a microorganism. A protracted course over several weeks to months suggests either a more indolent pathogen (e.g., fungi, mycobacteria, etc) or a noninfectious cause.[87,88] Chest radiographs are non-specific but are rarely normal, with either diffuse or focal shadows. Tuberculosis in the elderly may present in an atypical fashion. The majority of cases of unsuspected tuberculosis in community hospitals occur in elderly patients.[89] Between 35%[90] and 50%[91] of elderly patients with active tuberculosis will have atypical radiographic findings, with nonspecific mid- or lower-lobe inflammatory changes and pleural reaction. Tuberculin testing may be negative in 10% to 20% of elderly patients with active disease.[92] A two-step tuberculin test may be useful because of waning delayed hypersensitivity. When the diagnosis is sought, positive acid-fast stains of sputum can be obtained in a majority of patients.[93]

Atypical mycobacteria causing chronic pulmonary disease usually mimic tuberculosis in presentation.[94] Exclusive of patients with AIDS, disease from the atypical mycobacteria is predominantly seen in middle-aged or elderly patients with pre-existing chronic lung disease. *Mycobacterium kansasii* and *Mycobacterium avium* complex are the common species affecting the lungs. The diagnosis of lung disease caused by non-tuberculous mycobacteria usually is not difficult and often can be made without a lung biopsy. Colonization with atypical mycobacteria is not uncommon and must be distinguished by demonstrating acid-fast bacillus (AFB) on two or more sputum samples. The American Thoracic Society has published guidelines for diagnostic criteria and treatment of atypical mycobacteria causing lung disease.[95]

Aspergillus has several distinct forms of pulmonary disease that are indistinguishable from CAP. Chronic necrotizing aspergillosis is a semi-invasive form of infection,[96] with features of mycetoma formation and tissue invasion. It is most commonly seen in elderly patients with chronic lung disease. Invasive aspergillosis typically is seen in patients with prolonged severe neutropenia. Additionally, invasive *Aspergillus* can cause non-resolving pneumonia in patients

with COLD treated with long courses of corticosteroids.[97] Diagnosis is made by culture of TBB or FNA specimens in the appropriate clinical setting. Serologic tests are not definitively diagnostic.

Exposure to endemic fungi occurs in specific geographic areas (Table 124-12). These fungi have similar acute clinical characteristics and can cause a nonspecific illness with fever, chills, and cough. Characteristic radiographic findings include mass-like pulmonary infiltrates in blastomycosis, and thin-walled cavities in *Coccidiomycosis*. However, in general, these fungi can not be distinguished radiographically. Diagnosis can be made by Giemsa smear or potassium hydroxide smears of sputum, and may occasionally require lung biopsy. Serologic testing can be helpful. IgM antibodies become positive in the first few weeks of infection and disappear after about a month. Skin testing is positive in more than 90% of the population in endemic areas and is not usually helpful.

Chronic bacterial pneumonia has been described.[98] Cough, fatigue, dyspnea, and weight loss were the predominant symptoms. Symptoms were present on average for 6 months before diagnosis. The majority of patients had underlying lung disease or systemic disease predisposing to infection. Bronchoscopy with an unprotected cytology brush was used to collect specimens for bacterial culture, and growth greater than 4000 colony forming units (CFU) was defined as significant. Predominant organisms identified were *H influenzae*, α-hemolytic streptococci, *Pseudomonas aeruginosa*, and *S aureus*. The use of an unprotected brush to culture lung secretions and the pathogens identified raise the question of saprophytic colonization in patients with chronic disease. However, the authors noted resolution of symptoms and chest radiograph findings in 93% of patients when treated with prolonged courses of antibiotics, usually 4 weeks or greater.

A wide spectrum of noninfectious diseases and clinical syndromes can mimic CAP (Table 124-13). Distinguishing noninfectious causes of lung infiltrates from infection may be difficult. Noninfectious etiologies tend to present with a more indolent course, similar to a chronic infection. The presence of multiorgan involvement should raise the possibility of a noninfectious, inflammatory cause. Radiographic findings do not separate infectious from noninfectious causes. Peripheral blood eosinophilia is unusual in CAP, but may be seen in mycobacterial or fungal infections.[99] Eosinophilia should raise the possibility of an immune-mediated lung disease (e.g., drug reaction, chronic eosinophilic pneumonia, allergic bronchopulmonary aspergillosis, vasculitis, or rheumatologic disorder). The clinical description and evaluation of this complex category of diseases is comprehensively reviewed by Lynch and Sitrin.[100]

TABLE 124-12. Geographic Distribution of Endemic Fungi

Histoplasma capsulatum	Mississippi and Ohio river valley
Coccidioides immitis	San Joaquin Valley in California, Southwest US
Blastomyces dermatitidis	Southeast and Midwest US

TABLE 124-13. Noninfectious Conditions That May Mimic CAP

IMMUNE-MEDIATED OR IDIOPATHIC DISORDERS	NEOPLASTIC DISORDERS

IMMUNE-MEDIATED OR IDIOPATHIC
  DISORDERS

Hypersensitivity pneumonitis
Chronic eosinophilic pneumonia
Bronchiolitis obliterans organizing
  pneumonia (BOOP)
Drug-induced lung disease

Systemic Necrotizing Vasculitis (SNV)

Wegener Granulomatosis
Churg-Strauss angiitis
Polyarteritis nodosa (PAN) group

Alveolar Hemorrhage Syndromes

Antiglomerular basement membrane
  antibody disease
Microscopic SNV
Connective tissue disorders
Idiopathic rapidly progressive
  glomerulonephritis
Drug-induced hemorrhage (crack, cocaine,
  D-penicillamine, trimellitic anhydride,
  isocyanates, lymphangiographic dye)
Idiopathic pulmonary hemosiderosis
Pulmonary alveolar proteinosis
Collagen vascular disease
Sarcoidosis

NEOPLASTIC DISORDERS

Bronchoalveolar carcinoma
Pulmonary lymphangitic
  carcinomatosis
Primary pulmonary lymphoma
Lymphomatoid granulomatosis
Primary lymphoproliferative disorders
Multiple myeloma/plasmacytoma

MISCELLANEOUS

Pulmonary emboli
Lipoid pneumonia

Adapted from Lynch JP, Sitrin RG. Noninfectious mimics of community-acquired pneumonia. *Semin Respir Infect* 1993;8:14.

RADIOGRAPHIC RESOLUTION ■

Delayed radiographic resolution of an infiltrate in the setting of clinical improvement suggests the need for further evaluation. For many clinicians, "slow radiographic resolution" raises the possibility of an underlying neoplasm. In reality, host factors or common pathogens (e.g., *S pneumoniae* or *Legionella*) are more often responsible for delayed radiographic resolution. Mittl and colleagues[101] performed sequential chest radiographs every 2 weeks until resolution in patients with CAP. The chest radiograph remained abnormal at 4 weeks in 33% of patients, at 8 weeks in 15%, and at 16 weeks in 10%. Radiographic consolidation had not resolved in only 5% at 8 weeks. Factors associated with delayed resolution were older age and multilobe involvement. In a retrospective series of 1011 hospitalized patients with CAP, 13 (1.3%) were found to have an undiagnosed pulmonary carcinoma.[102] Most of these malignancies (62%) were suspected from chest radiographs taken while the patient was still hospitalized. This low prevalence of bronchogenic carcinoma agrees well with other series.[103] If the patient is clinically improving, convalescent chest radiography need not be repeated before 6 to 8 weeks unless a mass lesion or hilar adenopathy is suspected from the initial films. Further evaluation for bronchogenic carcinoma with CT of the chest and fiberoptic bronchoscopy should be limited to those with persistent consolidative changes on their convalescent chest radiographs. Additionally, if only those patients greater than 50 years of age and with significant smoking histories are evaluated, a lung malignancy is rarely missed.[104]

PROPHYLAXIS ■

IMMUNIZATIONS

The pneumococcal vaccine is an intramuscular polyvalent vaccine against the 23 most common serotypes of *S pneumoniae*. The vaccine is both safe and effective against preventing serious infections with these strains.[105] Local reactions can occur in patients with recent pneumococcal pneumonia. Repeat immunization can be given every 6 years for those at highest risk of declining antibody levels, including patients with HIV infection and patients over 65 years of age.[106]

The influenza vaccine should be given to those at risk of acquiring or spreading influenza infection. Due to antigenic shifts in the virus, vaccination must be given annually. The vaccine is contraindicated in those with severe allergic reactions to eggs. Post-exposure prophylaxis for influenza is covered in the section on prophylaxis in Chapter 105.

Table 124-14 lists indications for influenza and pneumococcal vaccination.[107] Consideration should be given to immunizing adults who have pneumonia, since these patients are at increased risk for recurrent pneumonia. The exact timing of immunization of vaccination in a patient with pneu-

TABLE 124-14. Indications for Immunization

PATIENT CHARACTERISTIC	PNEUMOCOCCAL VACCINE	ANNUAL INFLUENZA VACCINE
Age ≥ 65	Y	Y
Splenectomy	Y	N
HIV (+)	Y	Y
Renal failure or diabetes	Y	Y
Homeless or alcoholic	Y	Y
Nursing home resident	Y	Y
Organ transplant or immunosuppressed	Y	Y
Health care worker, daycare personnel, college students, military recruits	N	Y

monia remains controversial. The pneumococcal vaccine theoretically may be less effective if given during an episode of pneumonia. Patients who are likely to follow up should receive their vaccine 8 weeks after their pneumonia;[108] this coincides with the time for a follow up chest radiograph. For patients who may not follow up, vaccination can be done while the patient is hospitalized for their pneumonia.[109]

INTRAVENOUS IMMUNOGLOBULIN

Intravenous immunoglobulin (IVIG) is obtained from pooled human serum. Replacement therapy is indicated in those with an immunoglobulin deficiency.[110] IVIG is effective in preventing pneumonia and sepsis in multiple myeloma.[111] Due to the high cost of IVIG, its use in multiple myeloma and other hematologic malignancies remains controversial.

EVALUATION OF RECURRENCE ■

Recurrent pneumonia is generally defined as two or (usually) more separate episodes of lower respiratory tract infection accompanied by fever, leukocytosis, and purulent sputum production.[112] Clinical and radiographic improvement results after appropriate antimicrobial treatment. These episodes are usually separated by an asymptomatic period and the chest radiograph should clear during the asymptomatic period. Possible etiologies are structural abnormalities, underlying medical conditions, and immunologic abnormalities.

A pneumonia recurring in the same radiographic location after interval clearing suggests an anatomic abnormality of the bronchial tree (Table 124-15). An unrecognized foreign body aspiration can occasionally result in a focal obstruction with resultant recurrent pneumonia in the same lung region. This cause is more common in children and in adults with poor protection of their upper airway. Structural abnormalities like bronchiectasis are best visualized with high resolution CT. Foreign bodies and endobronchial masses are best evaluated with bronchoscopy.

Recurrent pneumonia affecting varying regions of the lung may be due to recurrent aspiration, multifocal bronchial abnormalities, or a host immune defect. Videofluoroscopy has high sensitivity and specificity for swallowing dysfunction and can identify patients at risk for aspiration pneumonia.[113]

Aspiration as demonstrated by videofluoroscopy occurs in nearly 30% of elderly patients with Alzheimer's disease.[114] Esophageal manometry and 24-hour pH monitoring are effective at identifying recurrent aspiration from gastroesophageal reflux.[115] Which method of testing is better is not clear, and institutional experience may dictate which testing modalities are used. Multifocal bronchial abnormalities such as diffuse bronchiectasis are unusual and best identified with an anatomic study such as high resolution CT. Rayner and coworkers[116] has outlined a comprehensive approach to the evaluation and treatment of bronchiectasis. Specific types of bronchiectasis, notably cystic fibrosis, have unusual pathogens causing recurrent pulmonary infection. Antibiotic and other medical strategies to prevent the progressive decline in lung function in these unique patients is rapidly evolving.[117,118]

Host immune defects can take many different forms. Chronic alcohol abuse, uremia, diabetes mellitus, and cirrhosis are common chronic illnesses that affect immune function. Immunosuppressive therapy also should be relatively obvious as a potential cause of immune suppression. Evaluation for less obvious causes of immune dysfunction is indicated if no cause for recurrent pneumonia is apparent. In a review of patients with 3 or more episodes of pneumonia, nearly 30% were found to have underlying immunoglobulin deficiencies.[119] Recurrence of pneumococcal pneumonia occurs in 8% to 25% of patients with HIV infection compared with 7% in control subjects.[120] In addition to a careful clinical history to look for chronic illnesses or treatments which could contribute to immune deficiency, total gammaglobulin and selective IgG_2 and IgG_4 levels should be checked. If not previously tested, HIV status should be evaluated. Specific tests of functional abnormalities of alveolar macrophages or polymorphonuclear leukocytes are rarely clinically useful.

FUTURE DIRECTIONS ■

Despite the introduction of a cornucopia of antibiotic agents, the mortality rate for moderate-to-severe pneumonia remains high. Rapid diagnostic tests with improved sensitivity and specificity for atypical pathogens (e.g., *Chlamydia*, *Mycoplasma*, *M tuberculosis*) are needed. Polymerase chain reaction for detection of *M tuberculosis* is currently a re-

TABLE 124-15. Etiology of Recurrent Pneumonia

SAME LOCATION	VARYING LOCATION
Endobronchial mass	Host immune defect
Primary lung malignancy	HIV infection
Metastatic malignancy to lung	Hypogammaglobulinemia
(e.g., breast, colon, sarcoma, melanoma)	Diffuse bronchiectasis
Benign tumor (e.g., carcinoid, hamartoma)	Cystic fibrosis
Broncholith	Primary ciliary dyskinesia
Foreign body aspiration	Allergic bronchopulmonary aspergillosis
Extrinsic compression	Panhypogammaglobulinemia
Lymphadenopathy	Recurrent aspiration
Benign (Sarcoid, mediastinal TB)	
Malignant (lung cancer, lymphoma)	
Localized bronchiectasis	
Pulmonary sequestration	

search tool and may facilitate more rapid detection of this organism. DNA probes to detect antimicrobial resistance may also prove useful, particularly in the case of multidrug-resistant tuberculosis.

Due to the high morbidity and mortality of severe CAP, active investigation into new effective interventions is ongoing. In addition to the continuing search for more effective antimicrobial therapy, non-antibiotic therapies are being tested. Areas of active research include

1. Augmenting the immune response to infection (e.g., G-CSF in nonneutropenic hosts, τ-interferon, pentoxifylline)
2. Blocking exuberant inflammatory cytokine responses (e.g., TNF-α, IL-1, PAF)
3. Alternative ventilatory strategies (e.g., permissive hypercapnia, inverse-ratio ventilation, high-frequency ventilation)
4. Improving ventilation-perfusion matching (e.g., indomethacin, inhaled prostacyclin, inhaled nitrous oxide)

REFERENCES ■

1. Garibaldi RA: Epidemiology of community-acquired respiratory tract infections in adults: incidence, etiology, and impact. *Am J Med* 1985;78:32S
2. U. S. Department of Commerce, Bureau of the Census: Statistical Abstract of the United States, 104th ed. Washington DC: USGPO, 1984
3. Marrie TJ, Durant H, Yates L: Community-acquired pneumonia requiring hospitalization: a 5 year prospective study. *Rev Infect Dis* 1989;11:586
4. Woodhead MA, MacFarlane JT, McCracken JS, et al: Prospective study of the aetiology and outcome of pneumonia in the community. *Lancet* 1987;1:671
5. Ortqvist A, Sterner G, Nilsson JA: Severe community-acquired pneumonia: factors influencing need of intensive care treatment and prognosis. *Scand J Infect Dis* 1985;17:377
6. Detailed diagnoses and procedures, national hospital discharge survey, 1990: National Center for Health Statistics. Hyattsville, MD, 1992
7. Fang GD, Fine M, Orloff J, et al: New and emerging etiologies for community-acquired pneumonia with implications for

therapy: a prospective multicenter study of 359 cases. *Medicine* 1990;69:307
8. Kern DG, Neill MA, Schachter J: A seroepidemiologic study of *Chlamydia pneumoniae* in Rhode Island. *Chest* 1993; 104:208
9. Grayston JT: Pneumonia due to *Chlamydia pneumoniae* strain TWAR (correspondence). *Clin Infect Dis* 1993;17:926
10. Cano S, Apote F, Pereira A, et al: *Pneumocystis carinii* pneumonia in patients without predisposing illnesses: acute episode and follow-up of five cases. *Chest* 1993;104:376
11. Jacobs JL, Libby DM, Winters RA, et al: A cluster of *Pneumocystis carinii* pneumonia in adults without predisposing illnesses. *N Engl J Med* 1991;324:246
12. Hughes JM, Peters CJ, Cohen ML, et al: Hantavirus pulmonary syndrome: an emerging infectious disease. *Science* 1993; 262:850
13. Centers for Disease Control: Update: hantavirus pulmonary syndrome: United States. *MMWR* 1993;42:816
14. Farley MM, Harvey RC, Stull T, et al: A population-based assessment of invasive disease due to group B streptococcus in nonpregnant adults. *N Engl J Med* 1993;328:1807
15. Gopal V, Bisno AL: Fulminant pneumococcal infections in normal asplenic hosts. *Arch Intern Med* 1977;137:1526
16. Huatekeete ML, Berneman ZN, Bieger R, et al: Purpura fulminans in pneumococcal sepsis. *Arch Intern Med* 1986; 146:497
17. Perlino CA, Rimland DL: Alcoholism, leukopenia and pneumococcal sepsis. *Am Rev Respir Dis* 1985;132:757
18. Caputo GM, Appelbaum PC, Liu HH: Infections due to penicillin-resistant pneumococci: clinical, epidemiologic and microbiologic features. *Arch Intern Med* 1993;153:1301
19. Jacobs MR, Koornhof HJ, Robins-Browne RM, et al: Emergence of multiply-resistant pneumococci. *N Engl J Med* 1978;299:735
20. Pallares R, Gudiol F, Linares J, et al: Risk factors and response to antibiotic therapy in adults with bacteremic pneumonia caused by penicillin-resistant pneumococci. *N Engl J Med* 1987;317:18
21. Stevens DL, Tanner MH, Winship J, et al: Severe group A streptococcal infections associated with a toxic shock-like syndrome and scarlet fever toxin A. *N Engl J Med* 1989;321:1
22. Basiliere JL, Bistrong HW, Spence WF: Streptococcal pneumonia: recent outbreaks in military recruit populations. *Am J Med* 1968;44:580
23. Hansen JL, Paulissen JP, Larson AL, et al: Nursing home outbreaks of invasive group A streptococcal infections: Illinois, Kansas, North Carolina, Texas. *MMWR* 1990;39:577

24. Woodhead MA, Radvan J, MacFarlane JT: Adult community-acquired staphylococcal pneumonia in the antibiotic era: a review of 61 cases. *Quart J Med* 1987;64:783

25. Davidson AC, Creach M, Cameron IR: Staphylococcal pneumonia, pneumatoceles, and the toxic shock syndrome. *Thorax* 1990;45:639

26. Bradley SF, Ramsay MA, Terpenning MS, et al: Methicillin-resistant Staphylococcus aureus: colonization and infection in a long-term care facility. *Ann Intern Med* 1991;115:417

27. Muder RR, Brennan C, Wagener MM, et al: Methicillin-resistant staphylococcal colonization and infection in a long term care facility. *Ann Intern Med* 1991;114:107

28. Bradley SF: Methicillin-resistant *Staphylococcus aureus* infection. *Clin Geriatr Med* 1992;8:853

29. Esposito AL: Pulmonary infections acquired in the workplace: a review of occupation-associated pneumonia. *Clinics in Chest Medicine* 1992;13:355

30. Couch RB: Mycoplasma pneumonia. In: Mandell GL, Douglas RG, Bennett JE (eds). Principles and Practices of Infectious Diseases, 3rd ed. New York, Churchill Livingstone, Inc, 1990:1446

31. Basiliere JL, Bistrong HW, Spence WF: Streptococcal pneumonia: recent outbreaks in military recruit populations. *Am J Med* 1968;44:580

32. Mackowiak PA: The normal microbial flora. *N Engl J Med* 1982;307:83

33. Rosenthal S, Tager I: Prevalence of Gram-negative rods in the normal pharyngeal flora. *Ann Intern Med* 1975;83:355

34. Valenti WM, Trudell RG, Bentley BWL: Factors predisposing to oropharyngeal colonization with Gram-negative bacilli in the aged. *N Engl J Med* 1978;298:1108

35. Johanson WG, Peirce AK, Sanford JP: Changing pharyngeal bacterial flora of hospitalized patients: emergence of Gram-negative bacilli. *N Engl J Med* 1969;281:1137

36. Reynolds HY: Respiratory infections may reflect deficiencies in host defense mechanisms. *Dis Mon* 1985;31:1

37. Spitzer JJ, Bautista AP: Alcohol, cytokines and immunodeficiency. *Advances in Experimental Medicine & Biology* 1993; 335:159

38. Caly WR, Strauss E: A prospective study of bacterial infections in patients with cirrhosis. *J Hepatology* 1993;18:353

39. Levin DC, Schwartz MI, Matthay RA, et al: Bacteremic *Hemophilus influenzae* pneumonia in adults: a report of 24 cases and a review of the literature. *Am J Med* 1977;62:219

40. Reimann HA: An acute infection of the respiratory tract with atypical pneumonia. *JAMA* 1938;11:2377

41. Johnson DH, Cunha BA: Atypical pneumonias: clinical and extrapulmonary features of chlamydia, mycoplasma, and legionella infections. *Postgraduate Medicine* 1993;93:69

42. Fraser RG, Pare JA, Pare PD, et al: Diagnosis of Diseases of the Chest. Philadelphia, WB Saunders, 1988:3032

43. Leach RP, Coonrod JD: Detection of pneumococcal antigens in the sputum in pneumococcal pneumonia. *Am Rev Respir Dis* 1977;116:847

44. Venkatesan P, Gladman J, MacFarlane JT, et al: A hospital study of community-acquired pneumonia in the elderly. *Thorax* 1990;45:254

45. Ostergaard L, Andersen PL: Etiology of community-acquired pneumonia: evaluation by transtracheal aspiration, blood culture, or serology. *Chest* 1993;104:1400

46. Marrie TJ, Durant H, Yates L: Community-acquired pneumonia requiring hospitalization: a 5 year prospective study. *Rev Infect Dis* 1989;11:586

47. Chen CW, Jong GM, Shiau JJ, et al: Adult bacteremic pneumonia: bacteriology and prognostic factors. *J Formosan Med Assoc* 1992;91:754

48. Light RW, Girard WM, Jenkinson SG, et al: Parapneumonic effusions. *Am J Med* 1980;69:507

49. Light RW: Management of Empyema. *Seminars Resp Med* 1992;13:167

50. Light RW, MacGregor MI, Ball WC Jr, et al: Diagnostic significance of pleural fluid pH and PCO_2. *Chest* 1973;64:591

51. Light RW: Management of parapneumonic effusions. *Arch Intern Med* 1981;141:1339

52. Kammerer J, Dupeyron C, Vuillemin N, et al: Apport des examens cytologiques et bacteriologiques du liquide d'ascite cirrhotique au diagnostic de peritonite bacterienne. *Med Chir Dig* 1982;11:243

53. Runyon BA, Umland ET, Merlin T: Inoculation of blood culture bottles with ascitic fluid: improved detection of spontaneous bacterial peritonitis. *Arch Intern Med* 1987;147:73

54. Bartlett JG: Respiratory tract and other thoracic infections. In: Finegold SM and George WL (eds). *Anaerobic infections in humans*. San Diego, CA, Academic Press, 1989:318

55. Lemmer JH, Botham MJ, Orringer MB: Modern management of adult thoracic empyema. *J Thorac Cardiovasc Surg* 1985;90:849

56. Storm HK, Krasnik M, Bang K, et al: Treatment of pleural empyema secondary to pneumonia: thoracentesis versus chest tube drainage. *Thorax* 1992;47(10):821

57. Berger HA, Morganroth ML: Immediate drainage is not required for all patients with complicated parapneumonic effusions. *Chest* 1990;97:731

58. Light RW, Girard WM, Jenkinson SG, et al: Parapneumonic effusions. *Am J Med* 1980;69:507

59. Potts DE, Levin DC, Sahn SA: Pleural fluid pH in parapneumonic effusions. *Chest* 1976;70:328

60. Bartlett JG: Anaerobic bacterial infections of the lung. *Chest* 1987;91:901

61. Bartlett JG: Lung Abscess. *Johns Hopkins Med J* 1982;150:141

62. Levison ME, Mangura CT, Lorber B, et al: Clindamycin compared with penicillin for the treatment of anaerobic lung abscess. *Ann Intern Med* 1983;98:466

63. Bartlett JG: Anaerobic bacterial infections of the lung. *Chest* 1987;91:901

64. Räsänen J, Bools JC, Downs JB, et al: Endobronchial drainage of undiagnosed lung abscess during chest physical therapy: a case report. *Phys Ther* 1988;68:371

65. Niederman MS, Bass JB, Campbell GD, et al: Guidelines for the initial management of adults with community-acquired pneumonia: diagnosis, assessment of severity, and initial antimicrobial therapy. *Am Rev Respir Dis*, 1993;148:1418

66. Eliopoulos GM, Eliopoulos CT: Activity in vitro of the quinolones. In: Hooper DC, Wolfson JD (eds). Quinolone Antimicrobial Agents, 2nd ed. Washington DC, American Society of Microbiology, 1993:161

67. Wolfson JS, Hooper DC: Fluoroquinolone antimicrobial agents. *Clin Microbiol Rev* 1989;2:378

68. Torres A, Serra-Batlles J, Ferrer A, et al: Severe community-acquired pneumonia: epidemiology and prognostic factors. *Am Rev Respir Dis* 1991;144:312

69. Marrie TJ: Bacteremic pneumococcal pneumonia: a continuously evolving disease. *J Infect* 1992;24:247

70. Levy M, Dromer F, Brion N, et al: Community-acquired pneumonia: importance of initial noninvasive bacteriologic and radiographic investigations. *Chest* 1988;92:43

71. Sorensen J, Forsberg P, Hakanson E, et al: A new diagnostic approach to the patient with severe pneumonia. *Scand J Infect Dis* 1989;21:33

72. Ortqvist A, Kalin M, Lejdeborn L, et al: Diagnostic fiberoptic bronchoscopy and protected bush culture in patients with community-acquired pneumonia. *Chest* 1990;97:576

73. Feinsilver SH, Fein AM, Niederman MS, et al: Utility of fiberoptic bronchoscopy in nonresolving pneumonia. *Chest* 1990;98:1322

74. Jiminez P, Saldias F, Meneses M, et al: Diagnostic fiberoptic bronchoscopy in patients with community-acquired pneumonia: comparison between bronchoalveolar lavage and telescoping plugged catheter cultures. *Chest* 1993;103:1023

75. Jimenez P, Meneses M, Saldias F, et al: Pneumococcal antigen detection in bronchoalveolar lavage fluid from patients with pneumonia. *Thorax* 1994;49:872

76. Salazar AM, Westcott JL: The role of transthoracic needle biopsy for the diagnosis and staging of lung cancer. *Clin Chest Med* 1993;14:99

77. Greenman R, Goodall P, King D: Lung biopsy in immunocompromised hosts. *Am J Med* 1975;59:488

78. Bandt P, Blank N, Castellino R: Needle diagnosis of pneumonitis: value in high risk patients. *JAMA* 1972;220:1578

79. Bella F, Tort J, Morera MA, et al: Value of bacterial antigen detection in the diagnostic yield of transthoracic needle aspiration in severe community-acquired pneumonia. *Thorax* 1993;48:1227

80. Wilson WR, Coerill FR, Rosenow EC: Pulmonary disease in the immunocompromised host. *Mayo Clin Proc* 1985;60:610

81. Donowitz GR, Mandell GL: Acute pneumonia. In: Mandell GL, Douglas RG, Bennett JE (eds). Principles and Practice of Infectious Diseases, 3rd ed. New York, Churchill Livingstone Inc, 1990;69:307

82. Dunn IJ, Marrie TJ, MacKeen AD, et al: The value of open lung biopsy in immunocompetent patients with community-acquired pneumonia requiring hospitalization. *Chest* 1994;106:23

83. Matthay RA, Moritz ED: Invasive procedures for diagnosing pulmonary infections: a critical review. *Clin Chest Med* 1981;2:3

84. LoCicero J: Does every patient with enigmatic lung disease deserve a lung biopsy? The continuing dilemma. *Chest* 1994;106:706

85. Gleichman TK, Leder M, Zahn DW: Major etiological factors producing delayed resolution in pneumonia. *Am J Med Sci* 1949;218:309

86. Israiel HL, Wiss W, Eisenberg GM, et al: Delayed resolution of pneumonias. *Med Clin North Am* 1956;40:1291

87. Luby JP: Pneumonia caused by mycoplasma pneumoniae infection. *Clin Chest Med* 1991;12:237

88. Ruben FL, Nguyen MLT: Viral pneumonitis. *Clin Chest Med* 1991;12:257

89. Counsell SR, Tan JS, Dittus RS: Unsuspected pulmonary tuberculosis in a community teaching hospital. *Arch Int Med* 1989;149:1274

90. Kahn MA, Kovnat DN, Bachus B, et al: Clinical and roentgenographic spectrum of pulmonary tuberculosis in the adult. *Am J Med* 1977;62:31

91. Morris CDW: The radiology, hematology and biochemistry of tuberculosis in the aged. *Q J Med* 1989;71:529

92. Kent DC, Schwartz R: Active pulmonary tuberculosis with negative tuberculin skin reactions. *Am Rev Resp Dis* 1967;95:411

93. Katz PR, Reichman W, Dube D, et al: Clinical features of pulmonary tuberculosis in young and old veterans. *J Am Geriatr Soc* 1987;35:512

94. Wolinsky E, Rynearson TK: Mycobacteria in soil and their relation to disease-associated strains. *Am Rev Respir Dis* 1968;97:1032

95. Wallace RJ, O'Brien R, Glassroth J, et al: Diagnosis and treatment of disease caused by nontuberculous mycobacteria. *Am Rev Respir Dis* 1990;142:940

96. Binder RE, Faling LJ, Pugatch RD, et al: Chronic necrotizing pulmonary aspergillosis: a discrete clinical entity. *Medicine* 1982;61:109

97. Rodrighes J, Niederman MS, Fein AM, et al: Nonresolving pneumonia in steroid-treated patients with obstructive lung disease. *Amer J Med* 1992;93:29

98. Kirtland SH, Winterbauer RH, Drets DF, et al: A clinical profile of chronic bacterial pneumonia: report of 115 cases. *Chest* 1994;106:15

99. Marcy TW: Eosinophilia in patients presents with pulmonary infiltrates and fever. *Semin Respir Infect* 1988;3:247

100. Lynch JP, Sitrin RG: Noninfectious mimics of community-acquired pneumonia. *Seminars in Respiratory Infections* 1993;8:14

101. Mihl RL, Schwab RJ, Duchinn JS, et al. Radiographic resolution of community acquired pneumonia. *Am J Respir Crit Care Med* 1994;149:630-5

102. Holmberg H, Kragsbjerg P: Association of pneumonia and lung cancer: the value of convalescent chest radiography and follow-up. *Scandanavian J of Inf Dis* 1993;25:93

103. Marrie TJ: Pneumonia and carcinoma of the lung. *J Infection.* 1994;29:45

104. Gibson SP, Weir DC, Burge PS: A prospective audit of the value of fiberoptic bronchoscopy in adults admitted with community acquired pneumonia. *Respiratory Medicine* 1993;87:105

105. Shapiro ED, Berg AT, Austrian R, et al. The protective efficacy of polyvalent pneumococcal vaccine. *NEJM* 1991;325:1453

106. Stein BE: Adult vaccinations: protecting your patients from avoidable illness. *Geriatrics* 1993;48:46

107. ACP Guide for Adult Immunization, 2nd Ed. Philadelphia: American College of Physicians, 1990

108. Hedlund JU, Kalin ME, Ortquist AB, et al: Antibody response to pneumococcal vaccine in middle-aged and elderly patients recently treated for pneumonia. *Arch Intern Med* 1994;154:1961

109. Hedlund JU, Ortquist AB, Kalin M, et al: Risk of pneumonia in patients previously treated in hospital for pneumonia. *Lancet* 1992;340:396

110. Sweinberg SK, Wodell RA, Grodofsky MP, et al: Retrospective analysis of the incidence of pulmonary disease in hypogammaglobulinemia. *J Allergy Clin Immunology* 1991;88:96

111. Chapel HM, Lee M, Hargreaves R, et al: Randomised trial of intravenous immunoglobulin as prophylaxis against infection in plateau-phase multiple myeloma. *Lancet* 1994;343:1059

112. Geppert EF: Chronic and recurrent pneumonia: seminars in respiratory infections. 1992;7:282

113. Martin BJ, Corlew MM, Wood H, et al: The association of swallowing dysfunction and aspiration pneumonia. *Dysphagia* 1994;9:1

114. Horner J, Alberts MJ, Dawson DV, et al: Swallowing in Alzheimer's disease. *Alzheimer Disease & Associated Disorders* 1994;8:177

115. Patt MG, Debas HT, Pellegrini CA: Esophageal manometry and 24-hour pH monitoring in the diagnosis of pulmonary aspiration secondary to gastroesophageal reflux. *American Journal of Surgery* 1992;163(4):401

116. Rayner CFJ, Cole PJ, Wilson R: Management of chronic bronchial sepsis due to bronchiectasis. *Clin Pulm Med* 1994;1:348

117. Neijens HJ: Strategies and perspectives in treatment of respiratory infections. *Acta Paediatr Scand Suppl* 1989;363:66

118. Knowles MR: New therapies for cystic fibrosis. (supplement) *Chest* 1995;107:52S

119. Ekdahl K, Braconier JH, Rollof J: Recurrent pneumonia: a review of 90 adult patients. *Scandinavian Journal of Infectious Diseases* 1992;24:71

120. Janoff EN, Freiman RD, Daley CL, et al: Pneumococcal disease during HIV infection: epidemiologic, clinical and immunologic perspectives. *Ann Intern Med* 1992;117:314

Critical Care, Third Edition, edited by Joseph M. Civetta,
Robert W. Taylor, and Robert R. Kirby.
Lippincott-Raven Publishers, Philadelphia, PA © 1997.

CHAPTER 125

■

Aspiration Syndromes

Salvatore R. Goodwin

IMMEDIATE CONCERNS ■

MAJOR PROBLEMS

Aspiration pneumonia was known as a clinical problem as
early as 400 BC when Hippocrates recognized "Dangers
of Aspiration."[1] In 1946, Mendelson presented a series of
parturients suspected of having aspirated stomach contents
during labor or anesthesia induction.[2] Subsequently, his laboratory investigations led him to the conclusion that two
entirely separate clinical entities existed. One followed the
aspiration of solid food and produced the picture of laryngeal
or bronchial obstruction, whereas the other resulted from
direct acid injury to the lung and produced the "asthma-
like" syndrome that carries his name.

Signs and symptoms depend on the quality and quantity
of the aspirate. Because most aspirations involve gastric contents, be aware of those situations in which patients are at
higher risk for this problem (Table 125-1). The pathophysiologic changes that occur are dependent on the type of aspiration. In general, particulate obstructive aspiration results in
significant hypoxemia, which rapidly progresses to cardiovascular collapse if the obstruction is unrelieved. As in any
anoxic-ischemic event, the resultant sequelae are dependent
on the degree and duration of the hypoxemia. Acid aspiration
injury can be thought of as potentially producing four stages.[3]
The major problem depends on the stage in which the patient presents (Table 125-2).

Particulate nonobstructive and the various forms of liquid
aspiration result in a broad spectrum of pathophysiologic
changes, depending on the degree of lung injury. The major
problem initially may be bronchospasm, which can be mild
to severe regardless of the type of aspiration. Aspiration of
irritating particulate matter, acid gastric contents, or both
is likely to bring the added dimension of local lung injury

with an associated inflammatory response. Mild hypoxemia
and tachypnea often progress to the acute respiratory distress
syndrome (ARDS) and respiratory failure.

STRESS POINTS

1. Food articles large enough to cause complete obstruction usually have not yet passed into the stomach. The
   "cafe coronary" is caused by an obstructed airway from
   partially masticated food that is aspirated during
   swallowing.
2. Particulate gastric aspiration of neutral materials not
   sufficiently large to cause airway obstruction often
   causes a prolonged inflammatory process similar in
   many respects to acid aspiration.
3. Inhalation of any amount of fluid with a pH less than
   2.5 is likely to damage lung tissue extensively.
4. The pulmonary lesion in near-drowning depends on
   the amount of water aspirated.[4] Because of laryngospasm and breath-holding, 12% of patients do not
   aspirate.[5]
5. Blood in the lungs may occur as a consequence of
   hematemesis, intrapulmonary hemorrhage, and surgical procedures involving the upper airway, pharynx, or
   maxillofacial areas. Immediately after blood aspiration,
   patients have an increased pulse and respiratory rate
   and may become cyanotic if the amount inhaled is
   sufficient to cause intrapulmonary shunting.
6. Ingestion of hydrocarbons such as kerosene, furniture
   polish, lighter fluid, gasoline, and other petroleum solvents accounts for 18% of accidental poisoning in children. Pulmonary toxicity occurs only if the hydrocarbon is aspirated either during ingestion or after it
   is regurgitated.[6]

TABLE 125-1.   Risk Factors in Gastric Aspiration

PERIOPERATIVE

   Parturition
   Emergencies
   Obesity
   Outpatients
   Gastrointestinal dysfunction
   Hiatal hernia
   Scleroderma
   Intestinal obstruction
   Esophageal diverticulae
   Gastroesophageal reflux

DEPRESSED LEVEL OF CONSCIOUSNESS

   Head injury
   Drug overdose
   Metabolic coma
   CNS infections
   Seizures
   Hypothermia
   Sepsis

LARYNGEAL INCOMPETENCE

   CNS disease causing bulbar dysfunction
   Guillain-Barré syndrome
   Multiple sclerosis
   Brain stem cerebrovascular accidents
   Posterior fossa tumors
   Muscular dystrophy
   Myasthenia gravis
   Amyotrophic lateral sclerosis
   Traumatic vocal cord paralysis
   Extensive surgery of the pharynx and hypopharynx

NASOGASTRIC FEEDING

ARTIFICIAL AIRWAYS

   Tracheostomy tube
   Endotracheal tube

GASTROINTESTINAL HEMORRHAGE

ESSENTIAL DIAGNOSTIC TESTS AND PROCEDURES

1. Success in diagnosing pulmonary aspiration depends on maintaining a high index of suspicion for its occurrence in at-risk patients. In 63% of cases, regurgitation is witnessed.
2. Frequently, the diagnosis is confirmed by the visualization of gastric contents in the airway or hypopharynx during tracheal intubation or by tracheal suction retrieval of gastric contents. However, 37% of patients have either silent or unwitnessed aspirations.
3. When clinical findings suggest pulmonary aspiration, further evaluation is essential. Arterial blood gas and pH analysis affords the most useful initial laboratory test. Oxygen partial pressure (PaO_2) ranging from 30 to 70 mm Hg when the patient breathes room air is a ubiquitous finding with significant aspiration.

4. Approximately 88% to 94% of people who aspirate gastric contents eventually demonstrate pulmonary infiltrates on chest radiographs.[7] Thus, a normal finding on chest radiograph does not exclude the possibility of aspiration.
5. Because the initial physical findings and blood gas values may be identical in acid and nonacid aspiration, determination of the pH of any remaining gastric or pharyngeal fluid can be helpful. If the fluid is highly acidic, anticipate a worsening course.
6. A finding of nonacidic fluid may be factitious because of dilution with secretions and is not of much help. The clinical course and response to therapy provide important information regarding the extent and type of aspiration.

INITIAL THERAPY

1. Initial management depends on whether aspiration is imminent, occurring, or completed. When regurgitation occurs in an obtunded patient, clear the airway and tilt the patient's head down and to the side.
2. Be sure to have suction equipment available and ready to use in areas where this problem is likely to occur (operating, delivery, and emergency rooms, postanesthesia care unit, and the ICU).
3. Oxygen should be administered immediately to all patients suspected of pulmonary aspiration.
4. Secure the airway by intubating the trachea, then suction any particulate aspirate. Suctioning has no beneficial effect with acid aspiration because the injury is immediate.
5. No benefit is derived from alkaline tracheal lavage; the practice actually is detrimental.
6. Removal of large particulate matter requires rigid bronchoscopy. Fiberoptic techniques permit the removal of only extremely small particles.

CLASSIFICATION   ■

PARTICULATE OBSTRUCTIVE

Patients are unable to breathe or speak and rapidly become cyanotic with particulate obstruction. If the obstruction continues, they become comatose and die of hypoxemia. Five of Mendelson's 66 patients had this type of aspiration, and two died.[2] Partial tracheal or bronchial obstruction may result from gastric aspiration of intermediate-sized particles and lead to the symptoms common to any foreign body aspiration. Stridor, tachypnea, coughing, and wheezing frequently are present with radiographic findings of atelectasis, expiratory emphysema, and pneumonia. Occasionally, a history of recurrent pneumonia is elicited with an associated choking spell preceding the symptoms. Foreign bodies such as food, bones, or coins also can lodge in the esophagus, resulting in respiratory distress with stridor, wheezing, and tachypnea, and can be fatal.[8]

TABLE 125-2. Stages of Acid Aspiration Lung Injury

Stage 1	Mechanical airways obstruction (leading to) obstructive atelectasis	Hypoventilation, hypercarbia, increased shunt, hypoxemia
Stage 2	Chemical burn of airway (early onset) Bronchoconstriction Bronchorrhea Bronchial edema Alveolar edema (only in extreme cases) Impaired mucociliary action	Decreased lung compliance and FRC, increased work of breathing, increasing V̇/Q̇ mismatch, further increase in shunt
Stage 3	Lung inflammatory response (delayed 1–2 d) Neutrophil, platelet sequestration Release of chemoattractants, prostanoids, leukotrienes, proteases, oxygen radicals Increased pulmonary vascular permeability Vascular thrombosis Surfactant denaturation, patchy atelectasis	Increasing pulmonary hypertension, low-pressure high-protein edema, increasing shunt, hypoxemia, marked decrease in compliance and FRC, atelectasis may be bilateral, increasing deadspace, hypercaphia, decreased oxygen delivery, hypovolemia
Stage 4	Secondary lung infection (3–5 d) Bacterial pneumonia—most common form Lung abscess	Hyperdynamic state with onset of sepsis, lactic acidosis, evolving to MSOF (if uncontrolled)

FRC, functional residual capacity; V̇/Q̇, ventilation/perfusion ratio; MSOF, multiple system organ failure.

From Britto J, Demling RH: Aspiration lung injury. *New Horizons* 1993;1:436.

PARTICULATE NONOBSTRUCTIVE

Patients manifest tachypnea, cyanosis, wheezing, cough, sputum production, and occasionally shock with particulate nonobstructive aspiration. Although 96% of the patients become symptomatic within the first hour after aspiration, 4% have a delayed onset of up to 2 hours.[7] The initial presentation may be mild with gradual worsening as the inflammatory response develops.

ACIDIC LIQUID: pH LESS THAN 2.5

Although the critical liquid acidic volume for injury is commonly held to be 25 mL (0.4 mL/kg), lower volumes can also result in lung injury.[4,9] Larger quantities produce more severe sequelae, sometimes causing pulmonary edema within minutes. Tachypnea, dyspnea, cyanosis, wheezing, and hypotension may be the presenting signs. Smaller volumes cause more subtle changes initially but ultimately produce a similar picture. Arterial blood gas analysis reveals hypoxemia and increasing alveolar-to-arterial oxygen gradient. Hypoxemia occurs within seconds of acid aspiration, and decreasing pulmonary compliance follows shortly thereafter. Patients may hyperventilate initially until the work of breathing increases enough to result in hypoventilation.

WATER: NEAR-DROWNING

In near-drowning aspiration, tachypnea, wheezing, cyanosis, and pulmonary edema depend on the amount aspirated. Pulmonary compliance is decreased. These changes are seen with either fresh or salt water. However, the pulmonary findings usually are short lived, and those who survive the initial insult generally have no long-term alteration in pulmonary function. Gastric dilation often leads to vomiting and aspiration of gastric contents during resuscitation.

BLOOD

The acute phase of blood aspiration often mimics acid aspiration, but the symptoms usually disappear rapidly, and patients suffer sequelae only if large quantities are aspirated. Animal experiments document the benign lesion produced by blood aspiration.

HYDROCARBON

Rapid onset of severe hypoxemia and intrapulmonary shunting are induced by hydrocarbon aspiration.[10] The clinical presentation seems to be independent of the type of hydrocarbon ingested. An initial burning sensation of the mouth and oropharynx is accompanied by choking, coughing, and gagging. The characteristic hydrocarbon odor is usually detected on the patient's breath. Respirations become rapid and labored, and cyanosis follows.

Central nervous system (CNS) irritability is manifested by dizziness, weakness, lethargy, twitching, and, rarely, convulsions. This last problem may be caused or enhanced by hypoxemia. When present, respiratory symptoms usually worsen over the first 24 hours. Patients who aspirate substantial quantities may develop pulmonary edema, hemoptysis, and respiratory failure. Those who aspirate small to moderate amounts usually improve over the next 2 to 5 days. In the first 24 to 48 hours, most patients have fever, which is not infectious in origin.

FURTHER DIAGNOSTIC CONCERNS ■

ACUTE ASPIRATION

As mentioned previously, 63% of aspirations are witnessed. In others, the acute onset of wheezing, tachypnea, tachycardia, and cyanosis in patients at risk for acute aspiration makes the diagnosis relatively simple. The differential diagnosis is limited primarily to cardiogenic pulmonary edema, ARDS from any other cause (Table 125-3), and negative-pressure pulmonary edema.

CHRONIC ASPIRATION

Chronic aspiration of gastric or oropharyngeal secretions is different from the full-blown acute syndrome. Patients often present with recurrent pneumonia or interstitial lung disease of undetermined etiology. Most frequently involved are patients with neurologic disease or injury affecting either glottic closure, the level of consciousness, or both.

Chronic aspiration also results from gastroesophageal reflux associated with the presence of a feeding tube. The incidence rate of pneumonia in patients receiving nasoenteral feeding whose tracheas are not intubated is 13%. In adult ICU patients intubated with low-pressure/high-volume cuffed endotracheal tubes, the incidence rate is 20%, and 15% to 17% with low-pressure/high-volume cuffed tracheotomy tubes. It increases to 77% in infants and children with uncuffed endotracheal tubes and to 80% in neonates. The incidence rate decreased to 16% in one study of infants, but the endotracheal tubes used were large enough to prevent

TABLE 125-3. Causes of Adult Respiratory Distress Syndrome

Aspiration	Pancreatitis
Chemical lung injury	Prolonged cardiopulmonary
Disseminated intravascular	bypass
coagulation	Radiation injury
Drug ingestion	Sepsis
Fat or air emboli	Shock
Massive transfusion	Trauma, thoracic uremia
Trauma	Oxygen toxicity

an audible air leak, and hence predisposed to potential airway complications.

Severe gastroesophageal reflux is diagnosed by a barium swallow, whereas more subtle problems are documented with esophageal pH probe studies (Tuttle test) and isotope scans. Lipid-laden alveolar macrophages may serve as markers for chronic aspiration pneumonia, as can milk antibody concentrations in small children. A suggested approach to suspected chronic aspiration is provided in Figure 125-1. In difficult cases, 24-hour tracheal pH monitoring has been advocated.[11]

CHEST RADIOGRAPHS

Radiographic findings often lag behind the clinical symptoms for 12 to 24 hours. In severe aspiration, diffuse bilateral infiltrates and pulmonary edema may be present (Fig. 125-2). Lack of cardiac enlargement and congested pulmonary veins distinguish this condition from heart failure. Less severe lesions initially cause atelectasis followed by alveolar infiltrates. Because the right main stem bronchus offers the most direct accessible path for aspirated material, the right lower lobe is the most frequently and severely affected when

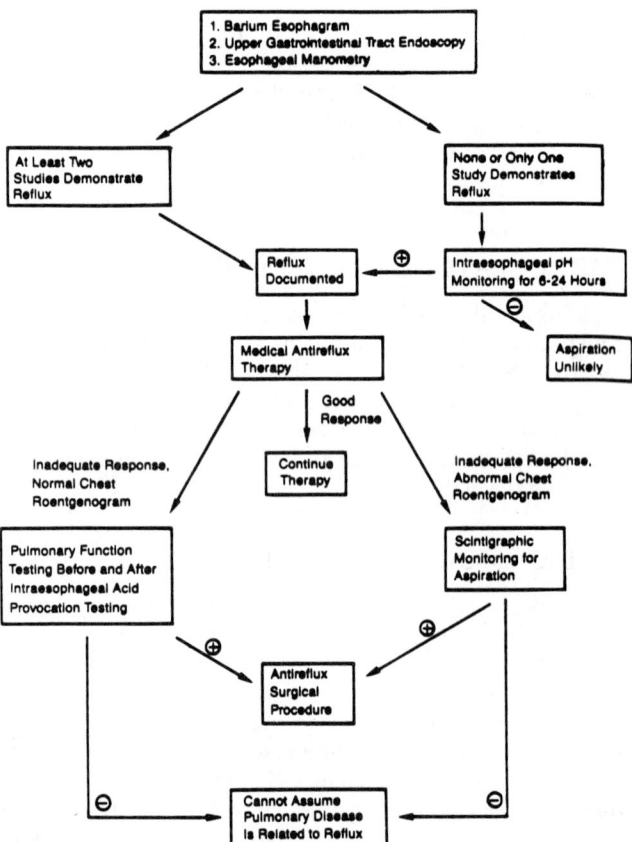

FIGURE 125-1. Suggested approach to patients with suspected reflux-induced respiratory disease. (Barish CF, Wu WC, Castell DO: Respiratory complications of gastroesophageal reflux. *Arch Intern Med* 1985;145:1882.)

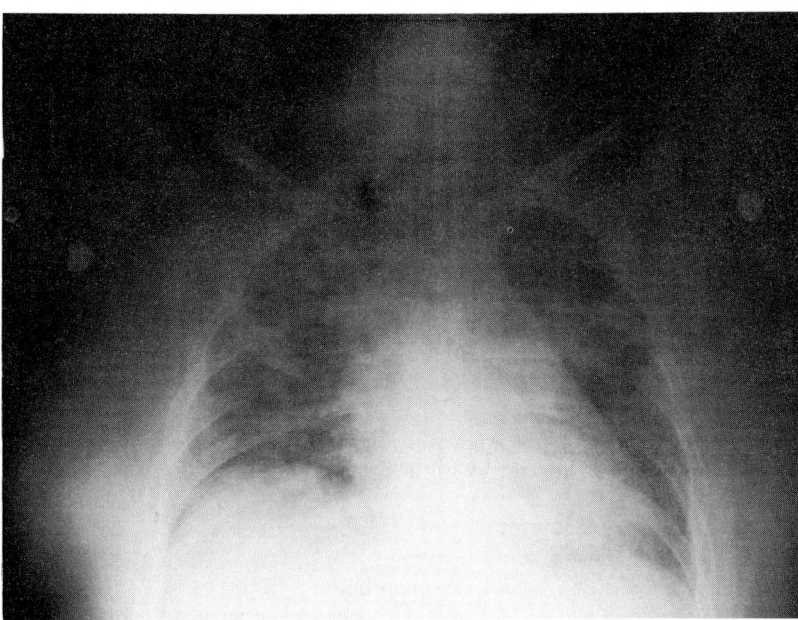

FIGURE 125-2. Diffuse, bilateral pulmonary infiltrates in a pediatric patient with pulmonary aspiration of gastric contents.

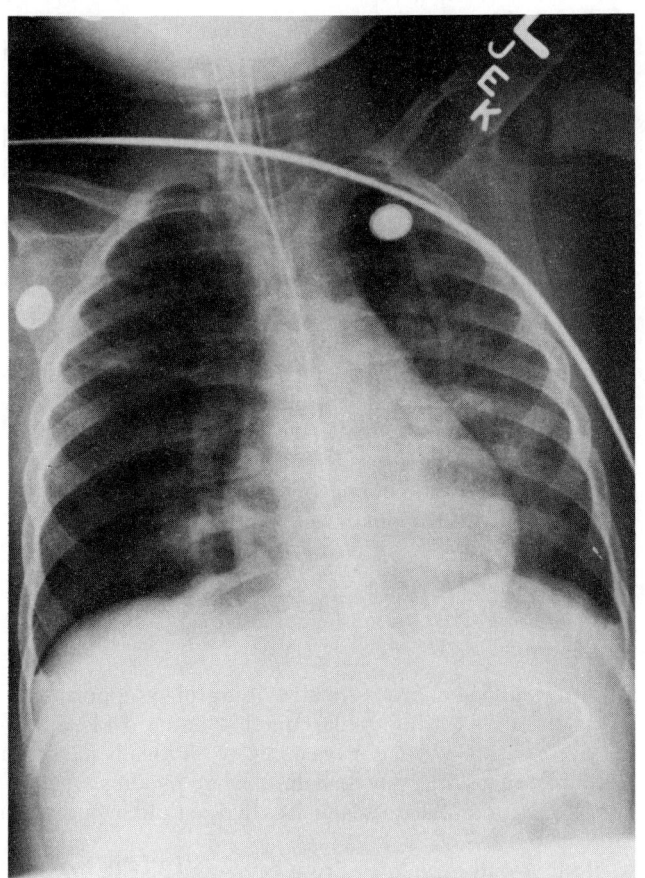

FIGURE 125-3. Delayed radiographic manifestations of hydrocarbon ingestion.

only one lobe is involved (60%); the left lower lobe is next (42%), followed by the right middle lobe (32%). Aspiration of particulate material may cause bronchial obstruction.

Initially, the chest radiograph sometimes appears normal, but expiratory emphysema may be present. Subsequently, the blocked segment loses volume. Aspiration of water occurs in 88% of near-drowning patients. In one series, 20 of 90 near-drowning victims (22%) had normal findings on chest radiograph at hospital admission.[9] The other 70 victims had lesions ranging from lobar infiltrates to extensive bilateral pulmonary edema.

Chest radiographic abnormalities may be seen within 30 minutes of direct hydrocarbon aspiration. If aspiration occurs after ingestion, patients develop infiltrates within 12 hours (Fig. 125-3). Hypoxemia and respiratory acidosis occur rapidly.

SUBSEQUENT MANAGEMENT

Further therapy is designed to support the patient during the injury and healing phases and to prevent further damage. Face mask oxygen increases PaO_2 and may be all that is necessary in mild cases. However, if symptoms worsen, the patient becomes obtunded, or hypoxemia persists despite supplemental oxygen, tracheal intubation and mechanical ventilation are often indicated.

The value of early intervention is debated. Some experts believe that as long as the patient is not hypoxemic (PaO_2 of 60 mm Hg or more when the inspired oxygen concentration is 0.50 or less) and is alert, tracheal intubation is unnecessary. Others believe that intubation and continuous positive airway pressure (CPAP) shorten the course of the disease.[12] I strongly support the early use of CPAP in pulmonary aspiration syndrome. Aspiration causing severe intrapulmonary shunting and hypoxemia must be treated aggressively. Positive-pressure ventilation with and without CPAP improves arterial blood gas values and may improve survival.

If the patient is alert, cooperative, and not at risk for further aspiration, face mask CPAP to a maximum of 14 mm Hg is sometimes useful. Higher levels exceed the lower esophageal sphincter tone and can promote gastric distention and further emesis.

CORTICOSTEROIDS

Corticosteroids are of no benefit in any of the aspiration syndromes and may interfere with healing.[13,14]

BRONCHODILATORS

Wheezing and air trapping are common findings in the various aspiration syndromes. Aerosolized bronchodilators may be beneficial, followed by intravenous bronchodilators if a therapeutic response is observed. Inhaled β_2-selective sympathomimetics are effective bronchodilators. These can be administered as often as every 20 minutes if needed to treat bronchospasm (Table 125-4). Inhaled ipratroprium bromide, 0.25 to 0.5 mg, may be added to the β_2-agents for additional bronchodilation. This quaternary ammonium anticholinergic does not cause the CNS symptoms that frequently accompany administration of its analog, atropine sulfate.

FLUIDS

Fluid management is difficult in severe aspiration. Intravascular volume is depleted because of diffusely increased pulmonary capillary permeability (except possibly in early freshwater aspiration).[8] Therapy may be further complicated by high levels of CPAP with the attendant compromise in cardiac filling. Careful monitoring of urinary output and vital signs is adequate to guide therapy in mild to moderate cases; invasive hemodynamic monitoring with central venous or pulmonary artery catheters is sometimes indicated for more severe lesions. The controversy over which type of fluid is best for volume repletion exists with this condition, as in many others. Some investigators believe colloid administra-

tion is beneficial; others show a detrimental effect of such therapy. My view is that no convincing evidence supports the use of colloids or indicates improvement in outcome when they are used.

EMESIS OR LAVAGE

Gastric lavage or induced emesis after ingestion of large amounts of hydrocarbon may well lead to subsequent aspiration. I believe this is a dangerous practice. The major life-threatening lesion is caused by pulmonary aspiration, not gastrointestinal absorption. Such therapy should be used only if a cuffed endotracheal tube is in place.

RESPIRATORY SUPPORT

Patients with aspiration of nonacidic fluid usually respond to the initial therapeutic measures. They can be weaned rapidly from ventilatory support in most instances. Those patients who aspirate acid or particulate material usually develop clinical and pathologic findings associated with any form of ARDS. The pathophysiologic process has been studied extensively in acid aspiration. Rapid injury to the trachea and alveoli is associated with early intraalveolar hemorrhage and interstitial edema.[11]

After several hours, loss of cilia and desquamation of the trachea and bronchi occurs, and bronchiolitis develops. At this time, the alveoli demonstrate edema, hemorrhage, and leukocyte infiltration, with destruction of type I and II pneumocytes. Hyaline membrane formation occurs after approximately 48 hours. Within 72 hours, evidence of healing and regeneration can occur with appearance of fibroblasts and decrease in inflammatory cells.

Factors such as volume, pH, the particulate content of the aspirate, secondary infection, and host response determine the degree to which injury occurs and whether the process leads to healing with preservation of function or the development of ARDS or fibrosis. Common denominators with other types of ARDS are type II pneumatocyte dysfunction, decreased surfactant production, and leaky pulmonary capillaries, which ultimately lead to hypoxemia and increased work of breathing[15] (Fig. 125-4). Decreased compliance and bronchospasm result not only in hypoxemia but also in hypoventilation. These patients benefit from ventilatory assistance and therapy to improve oxygenation.

Conventional Mechanical Ventilation, PEEP, and CPAP

Intermittent mandatory ventilation is useful to support ventilation, preserve cardiovascular function, and provide a rational approach to ventilator weaning. Occasionally, sedation or muscle relaxation may be helpful when patients are combative once potential causes such as hypoxia and hypercapnia are ruled out.

Positive end-expiratory airway pressure (PEEP) or CPAP is the mainstay of treatment for hypoxemia in aspiration pneumonia. Such therapy allows the inspired oxygen concentration to be lowered to safer (nontoxic) levels. Arbitrary upper limits originally were placed on CPAP, but levels

TABLE 125-4. Dosages of Inhaled Beta-2 Agents°

	ADULTS (mg)	CHILDREN (mg/kg)
Albuterol (Salbutamol)	2.5–5	0.15 (5 mg maximum)
Terbutaline	1–5	0.1 (2 mg maximum)
Metaproterenol	10–15	
Fenoterol	0.5–2.5	

°Initial dosages. Subsequent doses can be adjusted if side effects occur.

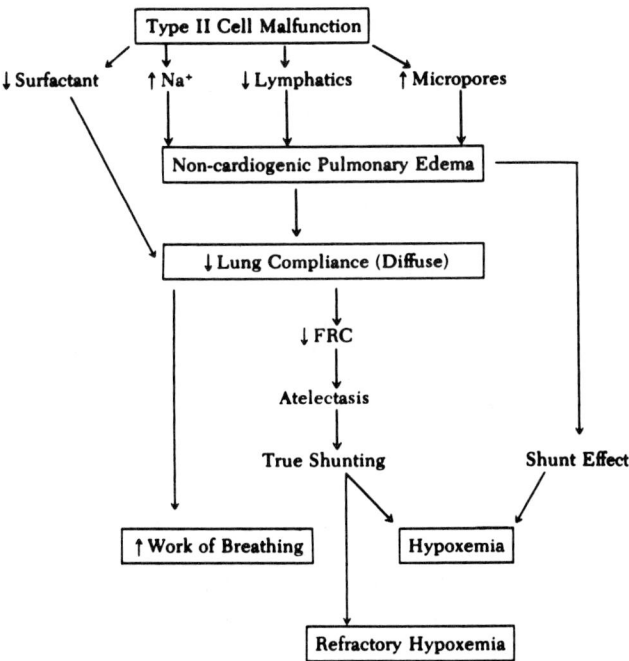

FIGURE 125-4. A proposed pathophysiologic course leading to the acute respiratory distress syndrome. FRC, functional residual capacity. (Shapiro BA, Harrison RA, Trout CA: *Clinical Application of Respiratory Care.* Chicago, Year Book Medical Publishers, 1979.)

as high as 40 mm Hg are believed to be useful in some circumstances. Several techniques are used to attain the most benefit with the least harm. Oxygen delivery is dependent not only on hemoglobin concentration and oxygen content but also on cardiac output.

If CPAP compromises cardiac output so that improved oxygenation does not improve oxygen delivery, the therapy is counterproductive. Furthermore, if excessive pressure overdistends normal alveoli, barotrauma can occur. A pulmonary artery catheter can be used to ascertain changes in cardiac output and intrapulmonary shunt. I use such monitoring in the rare patients who require more than 12 to 15 mm Hg PEEP/CPAP or in those who show evidence of impaired cardiovascular function at lower levels.

Permissive Hypercapnia

Many strategies of mechanical ventilation have been advocated for the treatment of ARDS. My current practice is to use the technique that provides adequate oxygenation with the lowest inspiratory pressures and oxygen concentrations possible. I allow $PaCO_2$ to rise to 50 to 60 mm Hg or more if a pH of 7.2 or above is maintained, in deference to using high peak airway pressures. Such *"gentilation,"* also known as *controlled hypoventilation* or *permissive hypercapnia,* may decrease overdistension of alveoli and barotrauma in patients with a variety of types of respiratory failure.[16-18] This important concept was discussed in the 1993 report of the American College of Chest Physicians' Consensus Conference on Mechanical Ventilation, cosponsored by the Society

of Critical Care Medicine and the European Society of Intensive Care Medicine (Table 125-5).

Pressure Support and Pressure Control–Inverse Ratio Ventilation

For spontaneously breathing patients, I use *pressure support ventilation* to help decrease the work of breathing imposed by decreased lung compliance, the breathing circuit, and endotracheal tube. In selected cases, *pressure control–inverse ratio ventilation* is helpful to reduce shunt and peak airway pressure.[20-23] This technique allows collapsed or fluid-filled alveoli to participate in gas exchange with less chance of overdistending the more normal alveoli. Familiarity with this approach and the potential complications are essential before its use.

Surfactant Replacement

Because aspiration and ARDS lung injury include loss of pulmonary surfactant function, considerable interest exists in surfactant replacement therapy. Although case reports and animal studies support the use of artificial surfactant such as dipalmitylphosphotidalcholine (DPPC; Exosurf) in ARDS,[24-29] the international multicenter company–sponsored study showed no improvement in mortality or oxygenation.[30] The study had enrolled 498 patients when it was

TABLE 125-5. Clinical Recommendations From the ACCP Consensus Conference on Mechanical Ventilation: Mechanical Ventilation for ARDS°

---

1. Select a ventilator mode that has been shown to be capable of supporting oxygenation and ventilation in ARDS patients and that the clinician has experience in using.

2. An acceptable SaO_2 (usually ≥90%) should be targeted.

3. When plateau pressure equals or exceeds 35 cm H_2O, the tidal volume can be decreased (to as low as 5 mL/kg or lower, if necessary) unless decreases in chest wall compliance mandate pressures somewhat exceeding this value.

4. $PaCO_2$ can be permitted to slowly rise (permissive hypercapnia) unless contraindicated, such as in situations of elevated intracranial pressure.

5. PEEP is useful in supporting oxygenation but may also be associated with deleterious effects and thus should be minimized to the level required and reevaluated on a regular basis.

6. FIO_2 should be minimized. The relative risk of pressure and FIO_2 are of significant concern; consideration for accepting a SaO_2 slightly less than 90% is reasonable.

7. When oxygenation is inadequate, sedation, paralysis, and position change are possible therapeutic measures. Hemoglobin and cardiac output should also be considered as other factors of oxygen delivery.

°Abstracted guidelines.

ACCP, American College of Chest Physicians; ARDS, acute respiratory distress syndrome; SaO_2, saturation with oxygen (arterial blood); PEEP, positive end-expiratory pressure; FIO_2, fraction of inspired oxygen.

discontinued after analysis revealed a 41% mortality rate in both groups. Many hypotheses have been proposed as to why this product was ineffective. The dose was 5 mL/kg (13.5 mg dipalmitylphosphotidalcholine [DPPC]) per milliliter and was administered by aerosol. This product contains no surfactant proteins (SP-A, SP-B, SP-BC, or SP-BD), which are responsible for adsorption and spreading of the surface active DPPC.

Gregory and others[31] recently reported success using Survanta in ARDS resulting from multiple causes in a pilot study of 59 patients. This substance is a natural minced bovine product that contains SP-B and SP-C with added DPPC. In hydrocarbon aspiration, I have found that artificial surfactant improves survival in an animal model.[32] This approach requires clinical investigation for verification.

ANTIBIOTICS

Secondary infection rates may be as high as 50%. Severe and prolonged pulmonary insufficiency is likely to be associated with secondary infection. In general, antibiotics should be withheld until clinical evidence of infection is present and appropriate cultures are obtained. If empirical therapy is chosen, remember that patients with abscesses, empyema, and pneumonia after aspiration may harbor oropharyngeal anaerobic infection[33] as well as colonization with *Staphylococcus* and *Pseudomonas* species.

Lung abscesses associated with aspiration involve anaerobic bacteria 90% of the time. The predominant organisms are peptostreptococci, *Bacteroides*, and *Fusobacterium*. Clues to infectious complications include new or enlarging infiltrates, progressive leukocytosis, persistent fever, cavitation or abscess formation with or without empyema, foul-smelling sputum, and the culture of distinctive organisms. Culture specimens should be obtained from blood, pleural fluid, or sputum collected during fiberoptic bronchoscopy or from transtracheal collections. Bronchoalveolar lavage and protected bronchial brush specimens produce the most reliable culture results. Expectorated sputum is of no value because of upper tract contamination.

Although penicillin G historically has been considered the drug of choice for anaerobic chest infections, the emergence of penicillinase-producing strains of *Bacteroides* requires the substitution of clindamycin in treating these infections. Dosages of 1200 to 2700 mg/day in three or four divided administrations are recommended for mild to moderate infections. Higher dosages are needed for life-threatening infections. Children should receive 40 mg/kg/day in three or four divided doses. Alternatives to clindamycin are erythromycin and metronidazole, which are likely less effective when staphylococcal infection is suspected.

Vancomycin, 2 g/day, should be divided into two or four doses. Pediatric patients older than 1 month of age should receive 40 mg/kg/day in three or four doses. Vancomycin must be administered over 1 hour to avoid many of the infusion-related reactions, including hypotension. Antibiotic therapy should be coupled with adequate drainage of infected fluid collections.

PREVENTION

Many techniques are useful to decrease pulmonary aspiration of gastric contents (Table 125-6). The extremes to which one must go to prevent aspiration depend on the likelihood of aspiration and the potential sequelae, should it occur. Therefore, identify at-risk groups (see Table 125-1).

AT-RISK FACTORS

The various risk factors for aspiration share one or more of the following variables: (1) increased gastric acidity (pH <2.5); (2) increased gastric volume (>0.4 mL/kg); (3) gastroesophageal reflux; and (4) laryngeal reflex dysfunction.

Pregnancy

Pregnant patients undergo physiologic changes that predispose them to gastric aspiration. Hormonal alterations decrease gastric motility and lower esophageal sphincter tone. The growing uterus exerts mechanical forces that increase intragastric pressure. Laboring patients frequently have a full stomach and are nauseated. Pulmonary aspiration of stomach contents is responsible for 30% to 50% of anesthesia-related maternal mortality.[34]

TABLE 125-6. Methods to Reduce the Risk of Pulmonary Aspiration Syndrome

REGURGITATION

    Decrease gastric volume
        Stop intake (NPO)
        Facilitate emptying (metoclopramide)
    Sellick's maneuver (cricoid pressure)
    Head-up positioning
    Surgical approach
        Nissen fundoplication
        Gastric division

ASPIRATION

    Maintain consciousness
    Lateral and head-down positioning
    Endotracheal tubes
    Surgical approaches
        Tracheostomy
        Laryngotracheal closure
        Laryngeal stent
        Total laryngectomy
        Epiglottoaryepiglottopexy

GASTRIC ACIDITY

    Antacids
        Particulate
        Clear
    Histamine (H₂)-antagonists
        Cimetidine
        Ranitidine

NPO, nothing by mouth.

Aspiration of smaller volumes of a lower pH can be fatal. Fifty-five percent of patients presenting for cesarean section are at risk by the previously mentioned criteria.[35] Although mechanical changes are alleviated after delivery, hormonal factors persist. Seventy-three percent of postpartum patients are at risk within the first 8 hours after delivery, and 40% are at risk in the next 16 hours. This fact is important to consider for patients who are scheduled to undergo postpartum tubal ligation.

Surgery

Surgical patients requiring emergency procedures and those who are obese are at increased risk of aspiration pneumonitis. Both groups have high gastric acidity, and the former often have a full stomach. Tracheal intubation frequently is more difficult in obesity. Outpatients have a higher gastric volume and similar pH compared with inpatients[36] (Fig. 125-5). This observation is important considering that 40% to 50% of all surgery currently is performed on outpatients. The risk of aspiration in patients scheduled for elective surgery is inversely related to age[37] (Table 125-7).

Neurologic and Neuromuscular Disease

Obtunded patients are at increasingly higher risk of aspiration as their level of consciousness decreases. They are less able to protect the airway because of diminished to absent gag and swallowing reflexes. In addition, their primary problem may also cause nausea and emesis.

Patients with muscular dystrophies or polymyositis are predisposed to dysphagia and, potentially, aspiration. Infants with muscular dystrophies have severe swallowing difficulty that frequently leads to aspiration. Adult-onset variant muscular dystrophy is also associated with swallowing difficulty and aspiration. Approximately half of patients with polymyositis experience dysphagia, and as many at 62% of this subgroup have evidence of aspiration.[38]

Progressive bulbar dysfunction frequently occurs with poliomyelitis, botulism, and the Guillain-Barré and Eaton-Lambert syndromes. This cranial nerve dysfunction results in swallowing difficulty and, frequently, aspiration. Cranial nerve dysfunction and altered consciousness can result from cerebrovascular accidents, placing these patients at particular risk for aspiration.

Laryngeal Dysfunction

Laryngeal dysfunction from any cause predisposes to the aspiration of secretions, medications, food, and regurgitated material. Patients with a progressive neuropathy need frequent assessment of their ability to protect their airway.

Enteral Feeding

Enteral alimentation through a nasogastric feeding tube is associated with a 5.7% incidence rate of aspiration[39] (range, 1% to 38%). Transpyloric feeding tubes may decrease the risk of feeding aspiration, but gastric secretions can accumulate, thereby increasing the risk of acid aspiration.

Artificial Airways

Aspiration around tracheotomy and endotracheal tubes was discussed previously. To minimize the danger of this problem, use a tube with a low-pressure/high-volume, thin-walled cuff inflated to between 18 and 25 mm Hg whenever possible. Leakage around the tube between the tracheal folds is decreased while adequate capillary flow is maintained.

PREVENTIVE MEASURES

Because aspiration pneumonia is associated with substantial morbidity and mortality, aggressive preventive measures should be taken in high-risk patients. This goal can be achieved by using a regional anesthetic technique, when appropriate, in surgical or obstetric patients. Mechanical, medical, and surgical methods can also be used.

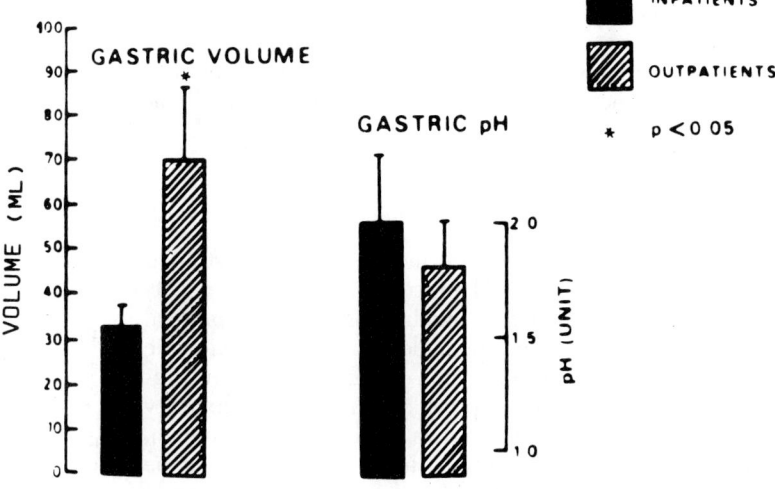

FIGURE 125-5. Mean gastric volume and pH of hospitalized inpatients (*solid*) and outpatients (*shaded*). (Ong BY, Palahniuk RJ, Cumming M: Gastric volume and pH in out-patients. *Can Anaesth Soc J* 1978;25:36.)

TABLE 125-7.   Frequency of Aspiration Risk Factors in Children, Adults, and Elderly Patients

ASPIRATION RISK FACTORS	NO. (AND PERCENTAGE) OF PATIENTS HAVING THE RISK FACTOR			DIRECTIONS AND SIGNIFICANCE OF DIFFERENCE
	Children ≤12 y (N = 25)	Adults ≥18–<65 y (N = 50)	Elderly >65 y (N = 25)	
pH <2.5	23 (92)	38 (76)	15 (60)	C = A; A = E; C > E
Volume ≥0.3 mL/kg	21 (84)	24 (48)	5 (20)	C > A > E
pH ≤2.5 plus volume ≥0.3 mL/kg	20 (80)	22 (44)	5 (20)	C > A > E
Volume ≥0.4 mL/kg	15 (60)	16 (32)	3 (12)	C > A > E
pH ≤2.5 plus volume ≥0.4 mL/kg	15 (60)	14 (28)	3 (12)	C > A = E

C, children; A, adults; E, elderly patients.

Modified from Manchikanti L, Colliver JA, Marrero TC, et al: Assessment of age-related acid aspiration risk factors in pediatric, adult, and geriatric patients. *Anesth Analg* 1985;64:11.

Mechanical

Several steps may be taken in selected patients. Stop oral intake and intubate the trachea while the patient is awake or after rapid-sequence induction of anesthesia while using Sellick's maneuver.[40] Evacuation of the stomach (emesis or large-bore tubes) and mechanical blockage of the esophagus with balloon tube devices have been used but are poorly tolerated by conscious patients. The latter technique is associated with potentially lethal complications.

When using Sellick's maneuver, apply pressure with the thumb, index, and middle fingers over the *cricoid* cartilage. Maintain pressure until intubation is accomplished and the cuff is inflated. Properly applied cricoid pressure prevents regurgitation in most cases because it "seals" the esophagus against pressures of up to approximately 75 mm Hg.[41] However, esophageal perforation can occur if active vomiting ensues. The clinical significance of this potential problem is unclear. Positive airway pressure may reduce the incidence of aspiration around endotracheal tubes,[38] but this possibility is not substantiated.

Some evidence suggests that the simple maneuver of elevating the head of the bed decreases regurgitation and aspiration in intubated, mechanically ventilated patients. The semirecumbent (45-degree angle) position is associated with a lower incidence of regurgitation and aspiration in at least one report.[42]

Medical

Medical prophylactic measures include the administration of antacids, histamine-2 (H_2) receptor antagonists, agents that hasten gastric emptying and increase lower esophageal sphincter tone (metoclopramide), and anticholinergic agents. Continuous alkalinization of the stomach can promote bacterial growth and provide a source for pulmonary infection.[43] Thus, the relative risks of gastric acid aspiration, gastric ulceration, and gastric bacterial overgrowth must be weighed when deciding to alter the pH of the stomach.

Sucralfate protects against gastric ulceration but does not protect against gastric aspiration. In fact, aspiration of sucralfate has been shown to cause acute lung injury in animals.[44] Because acidity is not altered, bacterial growth is not promoted.

ANTACIDS.   Antacids commonly are administered to high-risk patients. However, some investigations report no difference in mortality after such therapy.[45] Further evaluation reveals an injurious effect of particulate antacids on lung tissue[46] (Fig. 125-6). Clear antacids such as Bicitra[47] and

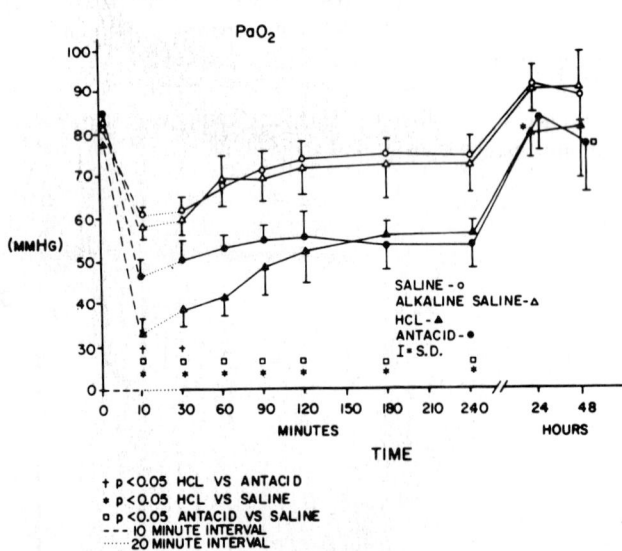

FIGURE 125-6. Measured values of PaO_2 of animals receiving antacid aspirate differ only slightly from those of animals receiving acid aspirate. Saline and alkaline saline aspirates produce smaller changes, which revert to control values by 4 hours. °*p* <0.05, HCl and antacid versus saline; †*p* <0.05, HCl versus antacid. (Gibbs CP, Schwartz DJ, Wynne JW, et al: Antacid pulmonary aspiration in the dog. *Anesthesiology* 1979;51:380.)

Alka-Seltzer[48] elevate gastric pH without the danger of particulate injury.

Concern over the additional volume imposed by antacids placed within the stomach prompted investigations into the relative importance of volume versus pH. Buffered gastric fluid can be tolerated at volumes higher than those previously reported, whereas low volumes of acidic fluid, as observed earlier, are associated with a high mortality rate. Despite literature in support of routine administration of clear antacid to high-risk patients, a recent report shows that nearly one fifth of obstetric patients in the United Kingdom receive no prophylaxis and that one half are given a particulate antacid.[49] For maximal benefits, antacids should be given within 60 minutes of a surgical procedure.[50]

H₂ ANTAGONISTS. Acid is secreted from the gastric parietal cells in response to one of three secretagogues: histamine, acetylcholine, and gastrin. H₂ antagonists competitively inhibit acid secretion stimulated by histamine, and noncompetitively inhibit acid secretion stimulated by acetylcholine and gastrin, thereby reducing the volume and hydrogen ion concentration of gastric fluid.

Cimetidine. Cimetidine initially was used for the treatment of peptic ulcer disease but soon thereafter was suggested to be useful as a preoperative medication to reduce the risk of acid aspiration.[51] For elective surgery, an oral dose of 300 mg the preceding night plus an intramuscular dose 1 hour before surgery are most effective (Table 125-8). The dose in children is 7.5 mg/kg. Cimetidine does not reduce the pH of gastric fluid already present within the stomach, but decreases the volume and increases the pH of fluid produced thereafter. Oral antacids are superior for acute therapy.

Cimetidine is associated with numerous side effects during short-term and long-term use. Short-term side effects include cardiovascular depression with rapid intravenous injection, headache, fatigue, dizziness, muscle pain, and fever. Side effects associated with longer use are gynecomastia in men and galactorrhea in women; mental status changes; bone marrow suppression (rarely); and microsomal enzyme inhibition, which causes a delayed clearance of many drugs used in the ICU, including theophylline, diazepam, propranolol, phenytoin, and warfarin.[52]

Ranitidine. Ranitidine also effectively decreases gastric hydrogen ion concentration and volume. It seems to have several advantages over cimetidine, including a longer duration of action (8 hours compared with 4 hours), less interference with hepatic drug metabolism, and fewer adverse reactions. The dose most often recommended is 150 mg orally and 50 mg parenterally.

Both drugs are more effective for perioperative prophylaxis when administered in a two-dose regimen, with one dose given the evening before and one on the morning of surgery. When given intravenously, they should be administered at least 45 minutes before anesthetic induction to assure effectiveness. Some effectiveness has been observed in as little as 30 minutes.[53]

Famotidine. This H₂ receptor antagonist has a potency 20 times that of cimetidine and 7.5 times that of ranitidine. It offers the potential advantages of longer duration, fewer side effects, fewer drug interactions, and greater decrease of gastric volume. Initial studies demonstrate a reduced volume of gastric secretion compared with ranitidine, which has little effect on volume.[54] With a duration of action of 12 hours, a single dose on the night before surgery effectively increases gastric pH to low-risk levels.[55]

Nizatidine and Roxatidine. Nizatidine and roxatidine, which are H₂ receptor antagonists, are being evaluated for potentially unique properties. The former may provide reduction in gastric volume and is commercially available; the latter may offer a longer duration of action.

OMEPRAZOLE. Omeprazole is a substituted benzimidazole "prodrug" that decreases gastric acid secretion by inhibiting the proton pump H^+-K^+-ATPase. This pump exchanges luminal potassium for cellular hydrogen ions. Acting on the final step in the acid secretion process, it is believed to be more potent than H₂ receptor antagonists. Perhaps it binds the enzyme irreversibly, requiring new ATPase to be synthesized before acid secretion can resume. A single oral dose of 40 mg effectively increases gastric pH to above 3.5 in elective surgery patients without an effect on gastric volume.[56]

The drug is inactivated by gastric acidity and is formulated in an enteric-coated tablet that permits duodenal absorption.

TABLE 125-8. Dosages of Antisecretory Agents

DRUG	ORAL (mg)	IV DOSE (mg)	PEDIATRIC IV DOSE (mg/kg)
Cimetidine	800	300°	5–10 per dose 4 times daily
Famotidine	40		
Nizatidine	300		
Omeprazole	20–80	40	
Ranitidine	150, twice daily	50°	0.5 per dose 4 times daily
Roxatidine	150		

°Administer over 15–20 min.

IV, intravenous.

Intravenous omeprazole administered 1 hour before surgery is effective in increasing gastric pH to greater than 2.5. When metoclopramide is added to enhance gastric motility, the efficacy of omeprazole in reducing aspiration risk in obstetric patients is enhanced.[57]

PROKINETIC DRUGS

Metoclopramide.   Metoclopramide acts peripherally by stimulating acetylcholine release, resulting in increased gastrointestinal motility, increased lower esophageal sphincter tone, and decreased pyloric tone. It also acts centrally, exerting antidopaminergic activity. Its *gastroprokinetic* effects hasten gastric emptying, potentially decreasing the risk of regurgitation and aspiration. Some investigators show a decrease of gastric volume in at-risk patients. This drug can cause extrapyramidal side effects including tardive dyskinesia.

Cisapride.   Cisapride is a prokinetic drug that works similarly to metoclopramide. Extrapyramidal side effects seem not to be a problem. At a dosage of 10 mg orally four times daily it has been shown to accelerate gastric emptying in critically ill patients during enteral feeding.[58]

COMBINATION THERAPY

H₂ Receptor Antagonists and Antacids. An effervescent cimetidine–sodium citrate mixture seems to be more effective than sodium citrate alone. In one study, a combination of 400 mg of cimetidine and 0.9 g of sodium citrate was compared with sodium citrate alone when administered to cesarean section parturients entering the operating room. The combination was more effective and resulted in fewer patients with a gastric pH greater than 2.5.[59]

ANTICHOLINERGIC AGENTS. Atropine and glycopyrrolate are antimuscarinic agents, inhibiting only the acetylcholine stimulus for gastric acid secretion. They decrease lower esophageal sphincter tone, thereby decreasing the barrier to regurgitation. No evidence supports their use in the prevention of aspiration. Some evidence shows that they increase the risk of aspiration.[60]

Surgical

Aggressive surgical methods to prevent the continued passage of secretions, food, or regurgitated material into the larynx are used primarily when other measures fail.[61] They are useful mostly in patients with disabling CNS disease or primary laryngeal disorders (see Table 125-6).

Patients with gastroesophageal reflux and life-threatening complications such as aspiration, apnea (infants), or choking are candidates for antireflux procedures. Nissen fundoplication is 95% successful in preventing reflux in children. Children with impaired oral intake who require gastrostomy placement may benefit from a protective antireflux procedure, even if reflux cannot be documented preoperatively.[62] Isolated gastrostomy does not protect against gastroesopha-

geal reflux. In fact, gastrostomy tube placement may worsen reflux in some patients when an antireflux procedure is not performed. A small percentage continue to reflux even after the combined procedure.[63]

REFERENCES   ■

1. Chadwick J, Mann WN: *Medical Works of Hippocrates.* Oxford, C & J Adlard, 1950
2. Mendelson CL: The aspiration of stomach contents into the lungs during obstetric anesthesia. *Am J Obstet Gynecol* 1946;52:191
3. Britto J, Demling RH: Aspiration lung injury. *New Horizons* 1993;1:435
4. Modell JH, Moya F: Effects of volume of aspirated fluid during chlorinated fresh water drowning. *Anesthesiology* 1966;27:662
5. Modell JH, Graves SA, Ketover A: Clinical course of 91 consecutive near-drowning victims. *Chest* 1976;70:231
6. Dice WH, Ward B, Kelly J, et al: Pulmonary toxicity following gastrointestinal absorption of kerosene. *Ann Emerg Med* 1982;11:138
7. Bynum K, Pierce AK: Pulmonary aspiration of gastric contents. *Am Rev Respir Dis* 1976;114:1129
8. Mittleman M, Perik J, Kolkov Z, et al: Fatal aspiration pneumonia caused by an esophageal foreign body. *Ann Emerg Med* 1985;14:365
9. James CR, Modell JH, Gibbs CP, et al: Pulmonary aspiration: Effects of volume and pH in the rat. *Anesth Analg* 1984;63:665
10. Goodwin SR, Berman LS, Tabling BB, et al: Kerosene aspiration: immediate and early pulmonary and cardiovascular effects. *Vet Hum Toxicol* 1988;30:521
11. Jack CI, Walshaw MJ, Tran J, et al: Twenty-four–hour tracheal pH monitoring: a simple and non-hazardous investigation. *Respir Med* 1994;88:441
12. Wynne JW, Modell JH: Respiratory aspiration of stomach contents. *Ann Intern Med* 1977;87:466
13. Downs JB, Chapman RL, Modell JH, et al: An evaluation of steroid therapy in aspiration pneumonitis. *Anesthesiology* 1974;40:129
14. Wynne JW, Reynolds JC, Hood CI, et al: Steroid therapy for pneumonitis induced in rabbits by aspiration of foodstuff. *Anesthesiology* 1979;51:11
15. Shapiro BA, Harrison RA, Trout CA: *Clinical Application of Respiratory Care,* 2nd ed. Chicago, Year Book Medical Publishers, 1979:491
16. Kolobow T, Moretti MP, Fumagalli R, et al: Severe impairment in lung function induced by high peak airway pressure during mechanical ventilation. *Am Rev Respir Dis* 1987;135:312
17. Darioli R, Perret C: Mechanical controlled hypoventilation in status asthmaticus. *Am Rev Respir Dis* 1984;129:385
18. Hickling KG, Henderson SJ, Jackson R: Low mortality associated with permissive hypocapnia in severe adult respiratory distress syndrome. *Intensive Care Med* 1990;16:372
19. Slutsky AS: AACP consensus conference: mechanical ventilation. *Chest* 1993;104:1833
20. Lain DC, DiBenedetto R, Morris SL, et al: Pressure control inverse ratio ventilation as a method to reduce peak inspiratory pressure and provide adequate ventilation and oxygenation. *Chest* 1989;95:1081
21. Anderson JB: Ventilatory strategy in catastrophic lung disease. Inverse ratio ventilation (IRV) and combined high frequency ventilation (CHFV). *Acta Anaesth Scand* 1989;33:145

22. Abraham E, Yoshihara G: Cardiorespiratory effects of pressure controlled inverse ratio ventilation in severe respiratory failure. *Chest* 1989;96:1356
23. Tharatt RS, Allen RP, Albertson TE: Pressure controlled inverse ratio ventilation in severe adult respiratory failure. *Chest* 1988;94:755
24. Lewis JF, Jobe AH: Surfactant and the adult respiratory distress syndrome. *Am Rev Respir Dis* 1993;147:218
25. Lachmann B: The role of pulmonary surfactant in the pathogenesis and therapy of ARDS. In: Vincent JL (ed). *Update in Intensive Care and Emergency Medicine*. Berlin, Springer-Verlag, 1987:123
26. Richman PS, Spragg RG, Robertson B, et al: The adult respiratory distress syndrome: first trials with surfactant replacement. *Eur Respir J* 1989;2:109s
27. Nosaka S, Sakai T, Yonekura et al: Surfactant for adults with respiratory failure. *Lancet* 1990;336:947
28. Wiedemann H, Baughmann R, Deboisblanc B, et al: A multicenter trial in human sepsis-induced ARDS of an aerosolized synthetic surfactant (Exosurf). *Am Rev Resp Dis* 1992; 45:A184
29. Reines HD, Silverman H, Hurst J, et al: Effects of two concentrations of nebulized surfactant (Exosurf) in sepsis-induced adult respiratory distress syndrome (ARDS). *Crit Care Med* 1992;20:S61
30. Anzueto A, Baughman R, Guntupalli K, et al: An international, randomized, placebo-controlled trial evaluating the efficacy of aerosolized surfactant in patients with sepsis-induced ARDS. *Am J Resp Crit Care* 1994;149:A567
31. Gregory FJ, Gadek JE, Weiland JE, et al: Survanta supplementation in patients with acute respiratory distress syndrome (ARDS). *Am J Resp Crit Care* 1994;149:A567
32. Widner L, Goodwin, SR, Berman LS, et al: Artificial surfactant administration as rescue therapy in hydrocarbon induces lung injury in a sheep model. *Crit Care Med* 1993;21:S289
33. Bartlett JF, Gorbach SL, Finegold SL: The bacteriology of aspiration pneumonia. *Am J Med* 1974;56:202
34. James CF, Gibbs CP, Banner T: Postpartum perioperative risk of aspiration pneumonia. *Anesthesiology* 1984;61:756
35. Roberts RB, Shirley MA: Reducing the risk of acid aspiration during cesarean section. *Anesth Analg* 1974;53:859
36. Ong BY, Palahniuk RJ, Cumming M: Gastric volume and *p*H in out-patients. *Can Anaesth Soc J* 1978;25:36
37. Manchikanti L, Colliver JA, Marrero TC, et al: Assessment of age-related risk factors in pediatric, adult, and geriatric patients. *Anesth Analg* 1985;64:11
38. Brin MF, Younger D: Neurologic disorders and aspiration. *Otolaryngol Clin North America* 1988;21:691
39. Matheny NA, Eisenberg P, Speis M: Aspiration pneumonia in patients fed through nasoenteral tubes. *Heart Lung* 1986; 15:256
40. Sellick BA: Cricoid pressure to control regurgitation of stomach contents during induction of anesthesia. *Lancet* 1961;2:404
41. Janson BA, Poulton TJ: Does PEEP reduce the incidence of aspiration around endotracheal tubes? *Can Anaesth Soc J* 1986;33:157
42. Torres A, Serra-Battles J, Ros E, et al: Pulmonary aspiration of gastric contents in patients receiving mechanical ventilation: the effect of body position. *Ann Intern Med* 1992;116:540
43. Atherton ST, White DJ: Stomach as source of bacteria colonising respiratory tract during artificial ventilation. *Lancet* 1978;ii:968
44. Shepherd KE, Faulkner CS, Leiter JC: Acute effects of sucralfate aspiration: clinical and laboratory observations. *J Clin Anesth* 1994;6:119
45. Tomkins J, Turnbull A, Robson G, et al: *Report on Confidential Inquiries into Maternal Deaths in England and Wales, 1976–1978*. London, Her Majesty's Stationery Office, 1982
46. Gibbs CP, Schwartz DJ, Wynne JW, et al: Antacid pulmonary aspiration in the dog. *Anesthesiology* 1979;51:380
47. Gibbs CP, Banner TC: Effectiveness of Bicitra as a preoperative antacid. *Anesthesiology* 1984;61:97
48. Chen CT, Toung TJK, Haupt HM, et al: Evaluation of the efficacy of Alka-Seltzer effervescent in gastric acid neutralization. *Anesth Analg* 1984;63:325
49. Sweeney B, Wright I: The use of antacids as a prophylaxis against Mendelson's syndrome in the United Kingdom: a survey. *Anaesthesia* 1986;41:419
50. Dewan DM, Floyd HM, Thistlewood JM, et al: Sodium citrate pretreatment in elective cesarean section patients. *Anesth Analg* 1985;64:34
51. Toung T, Cameron JL: Cimetidine as a preoperative medication to reduce the complications of aspiration of gastric contents. *Surgery* 1980;87:205
52. Manchikanti L, Kraus JW, Edds SP: Cimetidine and related drugs in anesthesia. *Anesth Analg* 1982;61:595
53. Rout CC, Rocke DA, Gousw E: Intravenous ranitidine reduces the risk of acid aspiration of gastric contents at emergency cesarean section. *Anesth Analg* 1993;76:156
54. Escolono F, Castano J, Pares N, et al: Comparison of the effects of famotidine and ranitidine on gastric secretion in patients undergoing elective surgery. *Anaesthesia* 1989;44:212
55. Gallagher EG, White M, Ward S, et al: Prophylaxis against acid aspiration syndrome. *Anesthesia* 1988;43:1011
56. Wingtin LNG, Glomaud D, Hardy F, et al: Omeprazole for prophylaxis of acid aspiration in elective surgery. *Anaesthesia* 1990;45:436
57. Orr DA, Bill KM, Gillon KR, et al: Effects of omeprazole, with and without metoclopramide, in elective obstetric anaesthesia. *Anaesthesia* 1993;48:114
58. Spapen HD, Duinslaeger L, Diltoer M, et al: Gastric emptying in critically ill patients is accelerated by adding cisapride to a standard enteral feeding protocol: results of a prospective, randomized, controlled trial. *Crit Care Med* 1995;23:481
59. Ormezzano X, Francois TP, Viaud JY, et al: Aspiration pneumonitis prophylaxis in obstetric anaesthesia: comparison of effervescent cimetidine-sodium citrate mixture and sodium citrate. *Br J Anaesth* 1990;64:503
60. Randell T, Saarnivaara L, Oikkonen M, et al: Oral atropine enhances the risk for acid aspiration in children. *Acta Anaesth Scand* 1991;35:651
61. Laurian N, Shvilli Y, Zohar UY: Epiglotto-aryepiglottopexy: a surgical procedure for severe aspiration. *Laryngoscope* 1986; 96:78
62. Jolley SG, Smith EI, Tunell WP: Protective antireflux operation with feeding gastrostomy. *Ann Surg* 1985;201:736
63. Bui HD, Dang CV, Chaney RH, et al: Does gastrostomy and fundoplication prevent aspiration pneumonia in mentally retarded persons? *Am J Ment Retard* 1989;94:16

Critical Care, Third Edition, edited by Joseph M. Civetta,
Robert W. Taylor, and Robert R. Kirby.
Lippincott-Raven Publishers, Philadelphia, PA © 1997.

CHAPTER 126

◼

Drowning and Near-Drowning

Eric T. Kunichika
Lawrence S. Berman

IMMEDIATE CONCERNS ◼

MAJOR PROBLEMS

Approximately 4700 cases of death attributable to drowning occurred in the United States in 1990,[1] and 140,000 cases per year occur worldwide.[2] Near-drowning events occur daily. In the United States, drowning is the second most common cause of accidental deaths among young children. In pediatric cases, the incidence of drowning peaks at two different ages[3] (Fig. 126-1). The first peak is in toddlers aged 2 to 4 years. This fact explains why 50% of all drownings occur in swimming pools, and 98% of all drownings take place in fresh water.

The second peak occurs in the adolescent to young adult age group. Alcohol plays a major role in many of these deaths.[4] One third of adults who drown have positive results on blood alcohol testing.[5] Drug use and peer group pressure are important factors contributing to this peak. Many boys attempt to impress their friends and themselves by hyperventilating before swimming under water. There are potentially fatal dangers inherent to this practice.

Drowning in adults frequently occurs around boating activities. Alcohol also plays a part here. Of 924 boating fatalities reported by the U.S. Coast Guard for 1991, 60% of the fatalities had elevated blood alcohol levels.[6] Because only 18% of the deaths involved collisions with other vessels or objects, many involved falling overboard.

STRESS POINTS

1. Physiologic changes are of great interest. Experimentally, occlusion of an endotracheal tube, which is analogous to breath-holding, causes only a 6 mm Hg/minute rise in $PaCO_2$ in 1 minute,[7] whereas PaO_2 falls from about 92 mm Hg before occlusion to 40 mm Hg after 1 minute and 10 mm Hg 3 minutes after obstruction[2] (Table 126-1).

2. A similar change has been found in volunteers who could breath-hold for an average of 87 seconds at resting conditions,[8] resulting in a $PaCO_2$ of 51 mm Hg and a PaO_2 of 73 mm Hg. After hyperventilation, breath-holding could be maintained for 146 seconds. The $PaCO_2$ rose only to 46 mm Hg, whereas the PaO_2 dropped to 58 mm Hg.

3. Hyperventilation preceded by exercise, as would occur during swimming, resulted in breath-holding for 85 seconds. Although the $PaCO_2$ was only 49 mm Hg, the PaO_2 decreased to 43 mm Hg.

4. After hyperventilation and artificial depression of $PaCO_2$, victims can become hypoxic and lose consciousness before their central respiratory drive "reminds" them to ascend to the surface for a breath. Physical exertion further hastens the fall of PaO_2 and the rise of $PaCO_2$. In addition, hyperventilation may also lower the seizure threshold and can precipitate seizures in victims who are prone to epilepsy.

1875

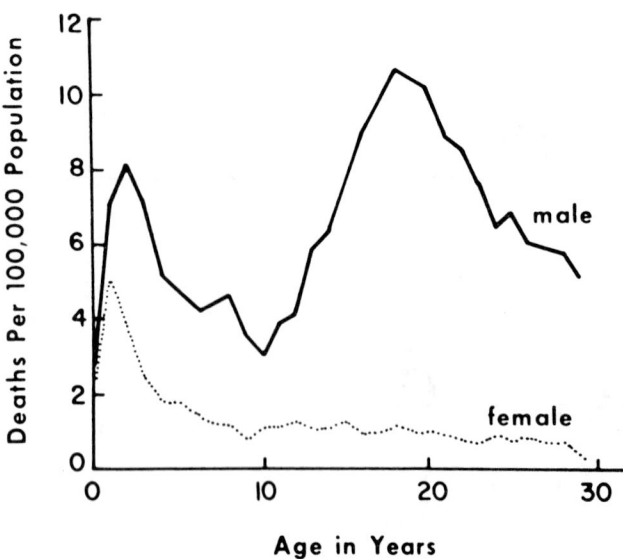

FIGURE 126-1. Male and female death rates from drowning. Male drowning rates peak at 2 years of age, decline until age 10, and then sharply rise to a maximum of age 18 years. Female drownings are highest in number at 1 year of age and then sharply decline and do not rise again. (Orlowski JP: Drowning, near-drowning, and ice-water submersions. *Pediatr Clin North Am* 1987;34:75.)

5. In the United States, male drownings outnumber female drownings by a ratio of 3.3 to 1. The drowning rate for black children (4.5 per 100,000) is nearly twice the rate for white children (2.6 per 100,000).[9]

6. Even more alarming is the incidence of nonfatal immersion events. An estimated 31,000 children are brought each year to emergency departments for near-drowning.[10] The largest emergency department study demonstrated a near-drowning visit to admission ratio of 4 to 1.

ESSENTIAL DIAGNOSTIC TESTS, PROCEDURES, AND THERAPY

1. Restoration of oxygenation begins with the establishment of a patent airway. Foreign bodies must be cleared from the mouth. The tongue and oropharyngeal soft tissues must not obstruct airflow through the trachea. However, until the cervical spine has been evaluated thoroughly, the head and neck should be manipulated cautiously using in-line cervical traction and immobilization.

2. Most victims of submersion injury fail to aspirate large quantities of water. In fact, approximately 10% of all drowning victims aspirate no water at all.[11] Fresh water, even if aspirated, is rapidly absorbed into the lungs. Therefore, except in the rare circumstance when a solid foreign body is obstructing the trachea,[12] the Heimlich maneuver is not indicated.[13-15] Indeed, performance of the Heimlich maneuver may induce vomiting and increase the propensity for aspiration of gastric contents.[15]

3. After the upper airway is adequately assessed and stabilized, the next function that must be addressed is breathing. In a near-drowning patient with altered mental sensorium, inefficient ventilation or profound hypoxia, the need for tracheal intubation and manual or mechanical ventilation is unquestioned.

4. Treatment alternatives for an awake, alert, but marginally oxygenated patient are more perplexing. Does the patient's clinical condition mandate insertion of an artificial airway? The answer to this question can be ascertained by determining the severity of alveolar damage as reflected by oxygen saturation less than 95% with an inspired fraction of oxygen (FIO_2) more than 0.4, PaO_2 less than 90 mm Hg with a FIO_2 more than 0.5, or PaO_2/FIO_2 ratio less than 300 mm Hg.

5. These values should be correlated with respiratory rate, the degree of neurologic insult as evaluated by the Glasgow Coma Score (GCS) (Tables 126-2 and 126-3), or focal changes.

6. Face mask continuous positive airway pressure (CPAP) may be a consideration in a spontaneously breathing patient who remains alert but has compromised oxygenation despite increasing concentrations of supplemental oxygen.[7] A patient should have a $PaCO_2$ less than 45 mm Hg to be considered a candidate for mask CPAP.[16]

7. A rise in $PaCO_2$ above 50 mm Hg, intolerance of the CPAP mask, diminution of mental status, gastric distention, vomiting, or persistent hypoxemia are indications for tracheal intubation and ventilation.[17]

8. The subset of patients who appear normal in the emergency department and who have normal chest radiograph findings but present with a history of submersion

TABLE 126-1. Arterial Blood Gas and pH Values Before and After Acute Tracheal Obstruction°

TIME (min)	pH	$PaCO_2$ (mm Hg)	PaO_2 (mm Hg)	BASE EXCESS (mEq/L)
0	7.45 ± 0.06	30 ± 5	92 ± 22	−1 ± 3
1	7.37 ± 0.06	36 ± 5	40 ± 6	−3 ± 2
3	7.32 ± 0.06	42 ± 5	10 ± 2	−4 ± 2
5	7.21 ± 0.06	48 ± 6	4 ± 1	−9 ± 2
10	7.15 ± 0.10	53 ± 9	1 ± 1	−12 ± 3

°Each value represents the mean and standard deviation of studies in 5 dogs.

TABLE 126-2. Glasgow Coma Scale (Recommended for Ages 4 Through Adult

	SCORE
EYES	
Open	
Spontaneously	4
To verbal command	3
To pain	2
No response	1
BEST MOTOR RESPONSE	
To verbal command	
Obeys	6
To painful stimulus	
Localizes pain	5
Flexion-withdrawal	4
Flexion-abnormal	3
Extension	2
No response	1
BEST VERBAL RESPONSE	
Oriented and converses	5
Disoriented and converses	4
Inappropriate words	3
Incomprehensible sounds	2
No response	1
GCS TOTAL	3–15

GCS, Glasgow Coma Scale.

TABLE 126-3. Children's Coma Scale (Modified Glasgow Coma Scale; Recommended for Age 3 y and Younger)

	SCORE
EYE OPENING	
Spontaneous	4
Reactions to speech	3
Reaction to pain	2
No response	1
BEST MOTOR RESPONSE	
Spontaneous (obeys verbal command)	6
Localizes pain	5
Withdraws in response to pain	4
Abnormal flexion in response to pain (decorticate posture)	3
No response	1
BEST VERBAL RESPONSE	
Smiles, oriented to sound, follows objects, interacts	5

Crying	*Interacts*	
Consolable	Inappropriate	4
Inconsistently consolable	Moaning, irritable	3
Inconsolable	Restless	2
No response	No response	1

CCS TOTAL	3–15

CCS, Children's Coma Scale.

for more than 1 minute, cyanosis during initial resuscitation, or requirement for mouth-to-mouth resuscitation should be observed and serially evaluated for at least 12 to 24 hours.[8]

9. Late-onset fulminant pulmonary edema occurring as long as 12 hours after the initial near-drowning event has been reported.[18] Delayed cerebral edema with late-onset neurologic deterioration also has been documented.[19]

PRESENTATION ■

That a person surfaces three times before drowning *is* a myth. Of 34 cases for which this information is available, 30 persons did not surface at all, three surfaced once, and one victim surfaced twice.[20] Although no data in humans are available, the sequence of events after immersion in water in animals is as outlined in Table 126-4.[21]

The clinical presentation and medical sequelae of drowning are consequences of varying degrees of hypoxia. Initial concerns should accordingly be directed toward the primary elements of advanced cardiac life support: management of *airway*, *breathing*, and *circulation*. Other injuries must not be overlooked simply because the victim is found in water.

Cervical spine injuries secondary to diving, air embolism secondary to rapid ascent during scuba diving, inebriation,[22] drug use, myocardial infarction, seizure disorder, cerebral vascular accidents, and attempted murder are just a few entities that can precipitate a drowning incident. Patient manipulation and steps at initial management should be undertaken with the assumption that some of these injuries have occurred. Do not forget the potential for cervical spine injury. Radiographs of the cervical spine are indicated if this injury is possible.

PATHOPHYSIOLOGY ■

SEAWATER

Seawater is hypertonic. When aspirated into the alveoli, it acts like a physiologic sponge and draws fluid into the alveoli from the plasma. In animals, tracheal instillation of 22 mL/kg of seawater results in gravity drainage of 33 mL/kg of

TABLE 126-4. Sequence of Events After Experimental Immersion

1. An immediate struggle for freedom, with or without an inspiratory effort
2. Suspension of movement with exhalation of air and frequent swallowing
3. A violent struggle for freedom
4. Seizure activity; exhalation of air; spasmodic inspiratory efforts with disappearance of reflexes
5. Death

fluid after 5 minutes.[23] Alveoli that are fluid filled cannot participate in gas exchange. Ventilation is impeded, and functional residual capacity is reduced. Perfusion, however, remains fairly constant, and intrapulmonary shunting results. Although surfactant quantity is decreased, surfactant function remains largely unchanged.[24]

FRESH WATER

Aspiration of fresh water results in rapid absorption of fluid from the alveoli into the circulation.[25] Experimentally, significant amounts of fluid cannot be drained from the lungs after freshwater aspiration.[23] The hypotonic nature of fresh water destroys surfactant function, and alveolar stability is lost. Alveolar surface tension increases, atelectasis results, and the loss of ventilation with preservation of perfusion produces intrapulmonary shunting and hypoxemia. Thus, intrapulmonary shunting is more likely caused by alveolar collapse in freshwater near-drowning and pulmonary edema in seawater near-drowning.[26,27]

Although the underlying pathophysiologic mechanisms in freshwater versus saltwater drownings differ, the clinical manifestations of severe near-drowning are the same.

TREATMENT ■

CARDIOPULMONARY

The primary goal during resuscitation of the near-drowned patient is the maintenance of tissue oxygenation. Supplemental oxygen must be administered to all patients until a complete evaluation is performed and the degree of neurologic and cardiopulmonary compromise can be ascertained. A rescuer should administer mouth-to-mouth ventilation as soon as a victim is reached in the water.

If indicated, cardiac compressions should be instituted as soon as feasible. Aquatic (in the water) chest compressions are usually ineffective. Mean carotid blood flow of only 3% to 6% of control values can be achieved, even by specially trained rescuers.[28,29] Chest compressions are probably ineffective until the victim is on a firm surface. As previously discussed, the airway should be assessed and intubation performed when indicated.

Many near-drowning victims are unidentified and arrive at a hospital unaccompanied. No medical history or even weight is available. A useful formula approximating a young pediatric victim's weight for resuscitation can be derived by estimating the patient's age:

$$\text{Weight (kg)} = (\text{age [years]} \times 2) + 8$$

PEEP/CPAP

CPAP is the mainstay of therapy in near-drowning. By increasing functional residual capacity and counteracting the effects of pulmonary edema and atelectasis, CPAP, with or without positive-pressure ventilation, increases PaO_2 and decreases the associated intrapulmonary shunt. Titrating the optimal amount of CPAP to maximize arterial oxygen content, while minimizing FIO_2 and the potential for pulmonary oxygen toxicity, are the primary objectives of therapy.[30,31]

Because tissue oxygen delivery is dependent on cardiac output and arterial oxygen content, cardiac output must be maintained during ventilator therapy. Necessary increases in CPAP or positive end-expiratory pressure (PEEP) may be associated with decreases in cardiac output,[32,33] causing oxygen delivery to fall despite increases in PaO_2. Invasive monitoring of central venous pressure, cardiac output, blood pressure, mixed venous oxyhemoglobin saturation, blood gas partial pressures, and pH may be extremely helpful in optimizing tissue oxygen delivery in cases of severe near-drowning.

Prophylactic use of inotropes when higher levels of CPAP are required does not necessarily improve tissue oxygen delivery. More important is to assure adequate intravascular resuscitation and to administer fluids when needed rather than to administer inotropes to victims who are volume depleted.[34]

OPTIMAL PEEP. What is "optimal PEEP?"[35] Unfortunately, no preset formula defines this value, nor is there a "maximum PEEP." Downs and Modell[36] define optimal PEEP as the level of PEEP required to minimize intrapulmonary shunting with minimal negative effects on cardiac output. Clinically, however, PEEP is often adjusted without measurement of cardiac output by selecting the level that produces the maximum PaO_2 without affecting blood pressure or heart rate. Clearly, a point exists beyond which further increases in PEEP will decrease cardiac output or increase alveolar dead space.[32] This point may not be apparent by simply calculating intrapulmonary shunt.

Intrapulmonary Shunting

The severity and trend of intrapulmonary shunting can be monitored clinically by the alveolar-to-arterial oxygen gradient, $P(A - a)O_2$.[37] The alveolar partial pressure of oxygen (PAO_2) is calculated by the following equation:

$$PAO_2 = (PB - PH_2O) \times FIO_2 - \frac{PaCO_2}{0.8}$$

where 0.8 represents the respiratory quotient; PB represents barometric pressure; and PH_2O denotes partial pressure of water vapor (47 mm Hg at 37°C). In a normal subject breathing a FIO_2 of 1.0, the $P(A - a)O_2$ is 35 mm Hg. The gradient can rise as high as 600 mm Hg as the degree of intrapulmonary shunting increases.

The validity of this formula is predicated on a normal cardiac output and oxygen consumption. Accuracy is also dependent on a linear relationship between dissolved oxygen content and alveolar and arterial oxygen partial pressures. This relationship is lost when arterial hemoglobin is not completely saturated, and PaO_2 values must be greater than 150 mm Hg to assure that small changes in oxygen partial pressure are not associated with large changes in oxygen content related to desaturation of hemoglobin.

Because the $P(A - a)O_2$ gradient frequently is calculated while the patient breathes a FIO_2 of 1.0 and changes if the FIO_2 is varied, the arterial-to-alveolar ratio may be more useful clinically. This ratio normally should be greater than 0.75.

Dead Space

The arterial to end-tidal carbon dioxide gradient $[P(a - ET)CO_2]$ may be valuable[38] (Fig. 126-2). This value, obtained by measuring $PaCO_2$ from the arterial blood gas and $PETCO_2$ from a capnograph, should be smallest with maximal recruitment of perfused alveoli that are not overdistended. It can be a useful tool when PEEP is titrated without a pulmonary artery catheter. Remember that decreases in $PETCO_2$ and increases in the gradient can occur in situations other than PEEP-induced alveolar overdistention and increases in dead space ventilation. Pulmonary emboli, sudden decreases in cardiac output, and tension pneumothorax, all of which can occur in a critically ill, bedridden patient on high PEEP, also cause increased dead space, reduced $PETCO_2$, and widening of the gradient.

Acceptable Oxygenation

In patients who require a high FIO_2 despite high levels of PEEP, PaO_2 values as low as 55 mm Hg, oxygen saturations of 90%, or both can be acceptable. Oxygen toxicity compounds the alveolar damage secondary to near-drowning. To facilitate suctioning with minimal loss of airway pressure, patients treated with significant levels of PEEP should have an endotracheal suction adapter at the junction of the endotracheal tube–ventilator connection.

Mechanical Ventilation

The type of ventilatory support should be determined by the needs of the patient, coupled with equipment availability and physician experience. If a concomitant neurologic injury is present, intermittent mandatory ventilation has some theoretical advantages over controlled mechanical ventilation or assist-control ventilation.[39-41] This factor may be important when intracranial pressure (ICP) is a concern, because positive-pressure ventilation impedes venous blood return from the head and can reduce mean arterial pressure. Pressure support ventilation can reduce work of breathing significantly, and pressure-controlled inverse ratio ventilation may limit pulmonary hyperinflation and high peak airway pressure.

High-frequency jet ventilation and oscillation have not proven to be advantageous. For patients who have mild pulmonary injury or require ventilator support mainly for neurologic therapy, airway pressure release ventilation may be an attractive choice. Because this method of mechanical support allows ventilation with peak inspiratory pressures that never exceed the level of CPAP, it minimizes the risk of barotrauma and reduces mean airway pressure.[42] Reductions in mean airway pressure allow optimal cerebral venous return and cardiac output, an obvious advantage if ICP control is a concern. Controlled studies must be done to assess its definitive role, and the question may be moot, because airway pressure release ventilation is unavailable in commercially available mechanical ventilators.

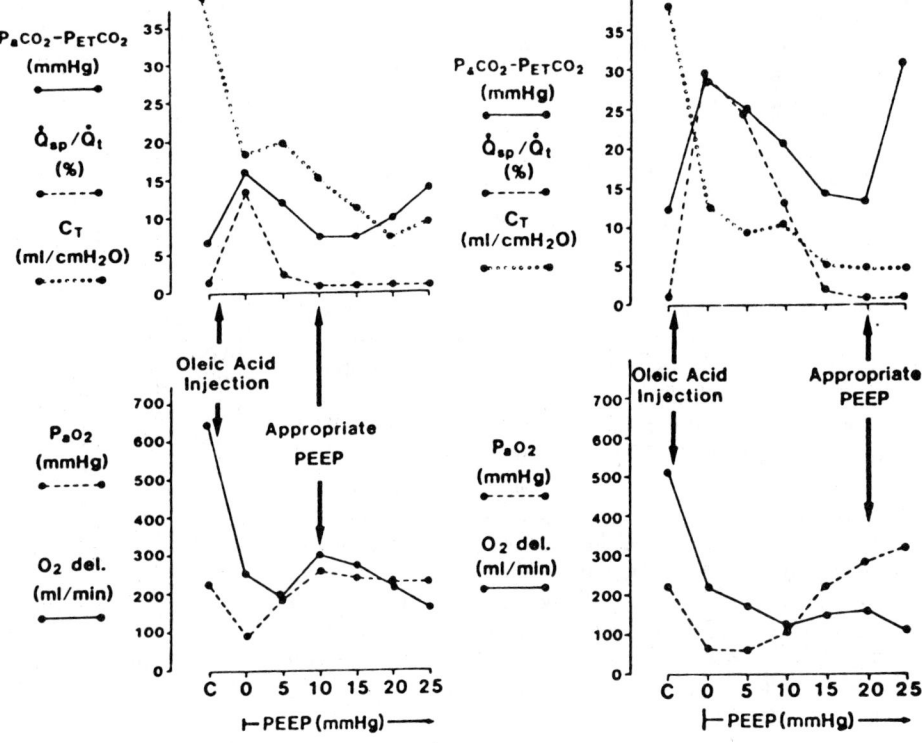

FIGURE 126-2. The arterial minus end tidal carbon dioxide tension gradient ($PaCO_2$ − $PETCO_2$), intrapulmonary physiologic shunt ($\dot{Q}sp/\dot{Q}t$), arterial oxygen tension (PaO_2), total compliance (CT), and oxygen delivery (O_2 del) for two animals from series are plotted before (*left*) and after (*right*) an intravenacaval injection of oleic acid. Positive end-expiratory pressure (PEEP) was added in 5 mm Hg increments from 0 to a total of 25 mm Hg. The "appropriate level of PEEP" is indicated by the arrow. (Murray IP, Modell JH, Gallagher TJ, et al: Titration of PEEP by the arterial minus end-tidal carbon dioxide gradient. *Chest* 1984;85:100.)

Adjunctive Measures

Steroids[43] and prophylactic antibiotics are not indicated.[44,45] The value of extracorporeal membrane oxygenation and administration of artificial surfactant has yet to be established.

NEUROLOGIC SEQUELAE ■

GENERAL CONSIDERATIONS

The most important complication of near-drowning, anoxic/ischemic encephalopathy is a consequence of hypoxia, either from the initial insult or from intrapulmonary shunting. The ultimate goal of resuscitation is directed at rapid restoration of cerebral oxygen delivery. Although the cardiovascular system can be revived after even 40 minutes of warm-water submersion, permanent neurologic deficit can result after just 1 to 3 minutes of hypoxia. Adequate blood flow to the brain may be maintained but with inadequate cerebral oxygenation. In severe cases, the result is survival in a persistent vegetative state.[46]

VENTILATORY SUPPORT AND CEREBRAL PERFUSION

The combination of pulmonary and neurologic injury in near-drowning victims presents a dilemma to the clinician who is attempting to maximize tissue oxygenation with CPAP/PEEP, while concurrently minimizing ventilator and CPAP-induced reductions in cerebral perfusion pressure (CPP). The CPAP necessary to assure adequate oxygenation can decrease mean arterial pressure. Concomitantly, CPAP may increase ICP by impeding venous blood return from the brain; intracranial blood volume increases, hence ICP rises.[20] The magnitude of this effect depends on the severity of the reduction in lung compliance and how much pressure is transmitted to the vascular bed.

ASSESSMENT OF INTRACRANIAL PRESSURE

Global cerebral ischemia is common after a significant immersion injury. ICP rises as cellular swelling progresses and cerebral perfusion is compromised. Progressive clinical deterioration and permanent neurologic damage may result. Computed tomography (CT) of the head can help determine the presence of cerebral edema and may be repeated if delayed neurologic findings develop.

Monitoring of ICP may be fruitless: maintenance of ICP below 20 mm Hg and CPP greater than 50 mm Hg improves survival but not residual brain function.[52] Osmotic agents and hyperventilation improve cerebral blood flow, but the areas of the brain that have the greatest cellular injury and edema are least likely to reap the benefit. Studies have shown that elevations in ICP frequently occur, not at the onset of hypoxic injury but on the second or third hospital day. Elevated ICP may be a reflection of irreversible cerebral injury rather than its cause.[53] The current trend is away from such monitoring.

GLASGOW COMA SCORE

The GCS (see Tables 126-2 and 126-3) is useful in following the neurologic trend of the patient. Most patients who are awake or who have blunted consciousness with a GCS of 7 or greater need not be hyperventilated. Comatose patients can be divided into three categories: decorticate, decerebrate, and flaccid. These patients (GCS <7), victims with CT-documented cerebral edema, or patients with rapidly declining neurologic status should be assumed to have elevated ICP.

HYPOTHERMIA

Because hypothermia reduces cerebral metabolic rate and barbiturates decrease ICP, could a combination of these treatment regimens improve neurologic outcome in drowning? Conn and associates[47] in 1978 suggested that cerebral salvage may be improved if the victim is hydrated, hyperventilated, paralyzed, rendered hypothermic, placed in barbiturate coma, and given corticosteroids. Such HYPER therapy (*H*yperhydration, h*Y*perventilation, hyper*P*yrexia, hyper*E*xcitability, hyper*R*igidity), however, has demonstrated no improvement in outcome.[48] Hypothermia, instead, was found to increase the risk of septicemia and multiple organ failure.[49] In addition, barbiturate coma does not improve outcome and is associated with significant side effects.[50,51] Cardiac output is depressed by slower heart rates and lower stroke volume.

FLUIDS AND ELECTROLYTES ■

Clinically significant alterations in serum sodium, potassium, or chloride do not occur in usual seawater or freshwater drownings. A review of 91 human drowning cases showed that all electrolyte values fell within a range compatible with life[45] (Fig. 126-3). No patient in this series required corrective electrolyte therapy.

Electrolytes, including calcium, should be evaluated during therapy for severe near-drowning because of the potential for associated secondary abnormalities. Freshwater drowning of young infants may result in the swallowing of a great amount of water and consequent hyponatremia. Central diabetes insipidus, renal compromise with secondary hyperkalemia, and a primary electrolyte disturbance induced by seizures are just a few potential associated anomalies. Glucose-containing intravenous fluids should be avoided during the initial stages of resuscitation. Neurologic outcome allegedly is worse when glucose is administered in a nonhypoglycemic patient.

RENAL FAILURE ■

Renal failure may be associated with both seawater and freshwater drowning. Acute tubular necrosis, secondary to hypoxia and decreased renal blood flow, is the likely etiology.

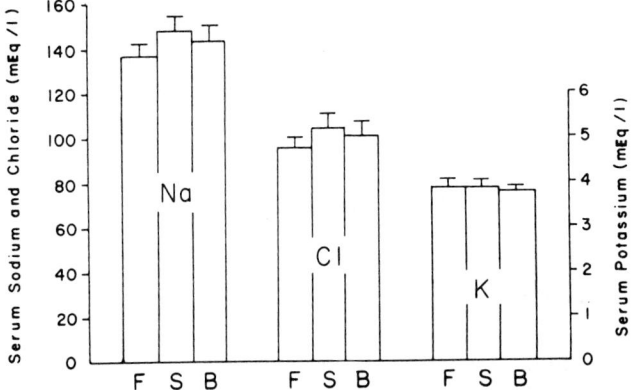

FIGURE 126-3. Serum concentrations (mean ± SD) of sodium, chloride, and potassium in patients who experienced near-drowning in fresh (F), sea (S), or brackish (B) water. (Modell JH, Graves SA, Ketover A: Clinical course of 91 consecutive near-drowning victims. *Chest* 1976;70:231.)

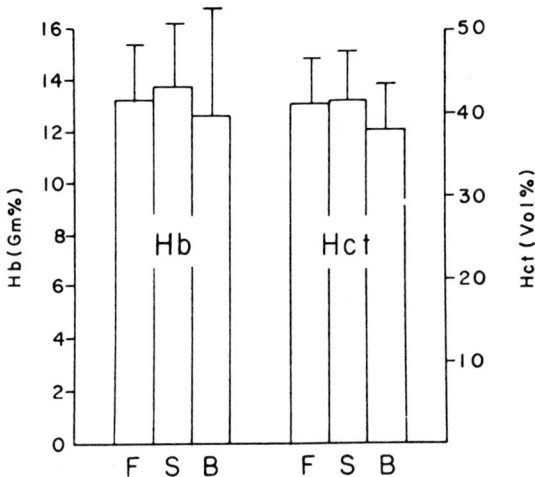

FIGURE 126-4. Hemoglobin (Hb) levels and hematocrit (Hct) readings (mean ± SD) in patients who experienced near-drowning in fresh (F), sea (S), or brackish (B) water. (Modell JH, Graves SA, Ketover A: Clinical course of 91 consecutive near-drowning victims. *Chest* 1976;70:230.)

Myoglobinuria and hemolysis with hemoglobin deposition in the renal tubules are other postulated mechanisms of renal injury.

Restoration of circulating volume with maintenance of renal oxygenation and perfusion are important factors in preventing renal insufficiency. Initial urinalysis, blood urea nitrogen, creatinine, and electrolytes should be documented. Urine output should be meticulously followed. If myoglobinuria is present, serum free hemoglobin should be checked, and mannitol may be used to maintain patency of renal tubules. Should renal compromise be suspected, normal saline rather than potassium-containing lactated Ringer's solution may be the crystalloid of choice. Low-dose dopamine (3 μg/kg/minute) may possibly improve renal blood flow and urine output. Peritoneal dialysis, hemodialysis, and hemofiltration are considerations in patients with significantly altered renal function.[20]

HEMATOLOGIC CHANGES ■

Although experimental aspiration of large quantities of fresh water (hypotonic) can result in hemolysis, and aspiration of seawater (hypertonic) can result in hemoconcentration, these changes seldom occur in the clinical setting[45] (Fig. 126-4). However, disseminated intravascular coagulation secondary to hypoxia, hypoperfusion, acidosis, and sepsis and thrombocytopenia secondary to cold water exposure have been reported.[20,54]

Patients with significant submersion injury should have screening studies that include prothrombin time, partial thromboplastin time, and platelet count. If these are abnormal, fibrinogen levels, d-diamers, and thrombin time should be measured. Supplementation of deficient coagulation fac-

tors with fresh frozen plasma and administration of platelets may be necessary to prevent bleeding.

SEQUELAE ■

Major problems that arise in near-drowning are cerebral edema with herniation and barotrauma associated with rapid ascent from depth or treatment of pulmonary insufficiency. Clinicians must be extremely vigilant to minimize these problems; however, much of this damage may have occurred before resuscitation. Continuous monitoring using pulse oximetry, the electrocardiogram, arterial blood pressure, and heart rate are mandatory in patients with major injury.

Subcutaneous emphysema can be a prelude to more significant barotrauma. Sudden arterial desaturation, with or without hypotension and tachycardia, is the hallmark of a tension pneumothorax. The patient's clinical status is ever changing, and dynamic medical support must likewise be modulated to reflect therapeutic needs. Improvement in pulmonary compliance without a concomitant decrease in the level of ventilator support can be disastrous. All alveoli are not uniformly affected in drowning. Alveoli with normal compliance are at greatest risk for barotrauma.

Patients treated with greater than 15 to 18 cm H_2O CPAP and mechanical ventilation may sustain barotrauma by coughing during suctioning, exhaling against a high-resistance ventilator expiratory valve, or both. Until intrapulmonary shunting is improved, prophylactic muscle relaxation should be considered in these patients. A tension pneumothorax not only compromises oxygenation, ventilation, and cardiac output, but also profoundly increases ICP.

ICE WATER SUBMERSION ■

NEUROLOGIC OUTCOME

Numerous reports of good neurologic outcome after ice water submersion have been published, mostly in children,[55] but also in adults.[56] Such instances usually occur in water less than 10°C. Bolte and colleagues[55] in Salt Lake City, Utah, report intact neurologic outcome in a 2-year-old child who was submerged for at least 66 minutes in 5°C water, the longest documented submersion with intact cerebral function. The case illustrates many of the factors that potentiate a favorable outcome:

1. Children have larger body surface–to–weight ratios to facilitate surface cooling.
2. Ice water submersion may induce rapid cooling and muscular paralysis without panic or struggle.
3. Swallowing of ice water may speed the rapidity of cooling. Contrary to widespread belief, the diving reflex is probably not involved in cerebral protection in human ice water near-drowning.[57,58]

Moderate hypothermia (35° to 32°C) is associated with increased sympathetic output and oxygen consumption. More profound hypothermia (<32°C) causes decreased oxygen consumption, decreased cerebral blood flow, and increased propensity for ventricular fibrillation and asystole.

CARDIOPULMONARY RESUSCITATION

Should rescuers commence with cardiopulmonary resuscitation (CPR) in victims found in extreme cold water? Several cases of ventricular fibrillation have occurred during rescue or resuscitation of the profoundly hypothermic patient. Defibrillation at body temperatures less than 30°C is often unsuccessful.[59] The exact risk of converting bradycardia to ventricular fibrillation is unknown. Current recommendations are to check pulses for at least 1 minute, withhold vigorous resuscitation in profoundly hypothermic victims who have any heartbeat and are breathing, and administer CPR to any asystolic patients.[54]

REWARMING

Once the victim is hospitalized, rewarming should take place with constant monitoring and preparation for further resuscitation. Patients with core temperatures below 29.5°C should be rapidly rewarmed. Thermal blankets, gastric and bladder lavage with warmed fluids, warmed intravenous solutions, and heated humidified oxygen may be used. Peritoneal lavage and even extracorporeal blood rewarming may be helpful.[59]

Patients with core temperatures between 29.5° and 32°C can be rewarmed slowly with blankets and warmed solutions. Victims with temperatures above 32°C are usually hemodynamically stable. However, shivering at this temperature can increase oxygen consumption and carbon dioxide production by up to 500%,[60] a critical finding in patients who are only marginally oxygenated.

Any patients who are found in extremely cold water should not be assumed to be dead until they are warmed or are found to be unresponsive to CPR. Hyperkalemia greater than 6.5 mMol/L may differentiate terminal hypothermic patients from potential survivors.[61] Blood gas partial pressures and pH should be measured without temperature correction.[62] The ideal treatment and management of the hypothermic nearly-drowned patient is still unresolved.

PROGNOSIS AND OUTCOME ■

The ultimate outcome in near-drowning is usually determined within the first few minutes of immersion. Once cerebral anoxia has occurred, irreversible neurologic damage results and attempts at resuscitation to full recovery are futile.[63] Survival in a persistent vegetative state has been described as "a fate worse than death."[46] Numerous attempts have been made to predict the ultimate neurologic outcome in near-drowning.[64,65]

INDICATORS

The length of time from onset of immersion to initiation of rescue efforts has been used as a prognostic tool. This time is difficult to determine accurately. A report of successful resuscitation after submersion in warm water for as long as 40 minutes[66] negates the use of this variable as the sole determining factor for initiating and pursuing aggressive resuscitative efforts. Core temperature, initial arterial pH, absence of spontaneous respiration, lack of response to pain, and pupillary nonreactivity have been found to be unreliable predictors of outcome.[67]

Glasgow Coma Score

The GCS (see Tables 126-2 and 126-3) alone cannot be used as the sole outcome prognosticator. Dean and McComb[53] and Nussbaum and Galant[68] found that despite the minimum GCS of 3, 15% to 29% of patients recovered; 2% to 12% were normal neurologically. Lavelle and Shaw[69] found that unreactive pupils in the emergency room and a GCS score of 5 or less on arrival to the ICU were the best independent predictors of poor neurologic outcome. The GCS alone has an unacceptably large error of false pessimism[70]; however, improvement during the first few hours after immersion may indicate a better outcome.[71]

Orlowski Score

The Orlowski Score[3] contains five variables that attempt to predict poor prognosis:

1. Age 3 years or older
2. Estimated submersion time greater than 5 minutes
3. No attempts at resuscitation for at least 10 minutes after rescue
4. Patient coma on admission to the emergency department
5. Arterial blood pH greater than or equal to 7.10

Patients with two or less of these variables have a 90% chance of good recovery after standard therapy. Patients with three or more variables have only a 5% chance of normal recovery. An error of false pessimism of 1 in 20 patients may still be too high.[72]

ICP, CPP, and Evoked Potentials

Mean ICP and mean CPP are reliable in predicting survival but not neurologic outcome.[64,72,73] They should not be used to guide the intensity of resuscitative therapy. Multimodality-evoked potential recordings may be useful in predicting poor neurologic recovery. Cumulative results in about 1000 comatose patients show that evoked potentials have a low error of false pessimism.[74–76] Normal results, however, do not necessarily portend favorable outcome.[77]

CARDIOPULMONARY RESUSCITATION

The need for cardiotonic medications to reestablish perfusing cardiac rhythm[78,79] and flaccid coma with a GCS of 3 are also associated with poor prognosis.[64] A retrospective review of 72 pediatric near-drownings presenting to the emergency department found that all 14 patients who required CPR on arrival either died or had permanent anoxic encephalopathy.[80] False optimism is tragic when CPR is successful in the absence of central nervous system recovery. Yet, false pessimism is unacceptable. In the normothermic patient, use of all prognostic indices may help to determine which patients should receive aggressive therapy. Emphasis must be placed on neuroresuscitation and prevention.

OTHER CONCERNS ■

CHILD ABUSE

In the pediatric population, clinicians should be especially alert to signals that point toward nonaccidental injury. In 1986, an estimated 1.6 million children were abused or neglected.[9] Near-drownings that occur in bathtubs, especially in infants and preschool-aged children, may be secondary to child abuse.[81] Foreign material in the lungs, injuries to the face, retinal hemorrhages, and burns to the soles of the feet and buttocks are associated with abuse.

WATER INTOXICATION

Another unusual presentation occurs in infants receiving swimming instruction who present with water intoxication and hyponatremia.[82] These children may be restless, weak, nauseated, and have vomiting, muscle twitching, and seizures. Treatment of the hyponatremia results in resolution of the symptoms.

THERAPEUTIC GOALS

In near-drowning, the focus of therapy should be directed at immediate restoration of circulation and oxygenation. The first 5 to 10 minutes after submersion are critical in de-

termining the outcome of resuscitation. Supplemental oxygen and positive airway pressure therapy are the mainstays of pulmonary resuscitation. Unfortunately, neurologic outcome may be largely determined before institution of hospital therapy.[69] Hyperventilation in patients with cerebral edema is indicated, but maintenance of adequate CPP may affect mainly survival, not function.

PREVENTION AND EDUCATION

The focus in drowning must shift toward prevention and medical education.[6] Adequate enclosures surrounding swimming pools decrease the mortality and morbidity rates secondary to drowning by up to 45%.[83,84] An enclosure that stands 150 cm (5 ft) high and surrounds all four sides of the pool is recommended.[85] The gate should have a self-latch as high as possible. The 95th percentile of vertical grip reach for boys 3 to 4.5 years of age is 129 cm (4.3 ft).

Children should be taught water safety and should learn how to swim. However, forced submersion is not recommended, and children younger than 2 years of age should have limited in-water class time of 30 minutes.[82,85] Parents must not get a false sense of security from toddlers who "can swim." No preschooler should be considered "water safe." Parents must be reminded that children are fantastic imitators. The bathtub is often full of water toys; bathing is usually a pleasurable and playful experience. Therefore, toys in the pool can be irresistible. Almost half of childhood swimming pool drownings occur with toys in the pool.[86] Even the pool cleaner, disguised to look like an alligator or sea creature, can lure a child into the pool.

A free-floating pool cover may be a casket for a small child who attempts to walk on it. Education of children and adults to the dangers of drugs, alcohol, and hyperventilation while swimming will prevent a few drownings. Community-wide basic CPR training will facilitate restoration of perfusion and oxygenation during the crucial initial stages of resuscitation.

Drownings and near-drownings are sudden and unexpected events. The victim's family and loved ones are devastated. Whether or not our therapeutic measures are successful, the true art of medicine begins, perhaps, after all of the technologic marvels available to us are exhausted.[87]

REFERENCES ■

1. Itasca IL: *Accident Facts*. Chicago: National Safety Council, 1993:6
2. Clarke EB, Niggemann EH: Near-drowning. *Heart Lung* 1975;4:946
3. Orlowski JP: Drowning, near-drowning, and ice-water submersions. *Pediatr Clin North Am* 1987;34:75
4. Wintemute GJ, Kraus JF, Teret SP, et al: The epidemiology of drowning in adulthood: implications for prevention. *Am J Prev Med* 1988;4:343
5. Dietz PE, Baker SP: Drowning epidemiology and prevention. *Am J Public Health* 1974;64:303
6. Howland J, Smith GS, Mangione T, et al: Missing the boat on drinking and boating. *JAMA* 1993;270:91

7. Modell JH: *The Pathophysiology and Treatment of Drowning and Near-Drowning.* Springfield, IL, Charles C Thomas, 1971

8. Craig AB Jr: Causes of loss of consciousness during underwater swimming. *J Appl Physiol* 1961;16:583

9. MMWR: Fatal injuries to children—United States, 1986. *JAMA* 1990;264:952

10. Wintemute GJ: Childhood drowning and near-drowning in the United States. *Am J Dis Child* 1990;144:663

11. Giammona ST: Drowning: pathophysiology and management. *Curr Probl Pediatr* 1971;1:3

12. Heimlich HJ, Patrick EA: Using the Heimlich maneuver to save near-drowning victims. *Postgrad Med* 1988;84:62

13. Heimlich HJ: Subdiaphragmatic pressure to expel water from the lungs of drowning persons. *Ann Emerg Med* 1981;10:476

14. Orlowski JP: Heimlich maneuver for near-drowning questioned. *Ann Emerg Med* 1982;11:111

15. Ornato JP: The resuscitation of near-drowning victims. *JAMA* 1986;256:75

16. Greenbaum DM, Millen JE, Eross B, et al: Continuous positive airway pressure without tracheal intubation in spontaneously breathing patients. *Chest* 1976;69:615

17. Hoff BH: Multisystem failure: a review with special reference to drowning. *Crit Care Med* 1979;7:310

18. Pearn JH: Secondary drowning in children. *Br Med J* 1980; 281:1103

19. Oakes DD, Scherck JP, Maloney JR, et al: Prognosis and management of victims of near-drowning. *J Trauma* 1982;22: 544

20. Press E, Walker J, Crawford I: An interstate drowning study. *Am J Public Health* 1968;58:2275

21. Karpovich PV: Water in the lungs of drowned animals. *Arch Pathol* 1933;15:828

22. Howland J, Hingson R: Alcohol as a risk factor for drownings: a review of the literature (1950–1985). *Accident Anal Prev* 1988;20:19

23. Modell JH, Gaub M, Moya F, et al: Physiologic effects of near-drowning with chlorinated fresh water, distilled water, and isotonic saline. *Anesthesiology* 1966;27:33

24. Modell JH, Moya F, Newby EJ, et al: The effects of fluid volume in seawater drowning. *Ann Intern Med* 1967;67:68

25. Swan HG, Brucer M, Moore C, et al: Freshwater and seawater drowning: a study of the terminal cardiac and biochemical events. *Tex Rep Biol Med* 1947;4:423

26. Modell JH: The pathophysiology and treatment of drowning. *Acta Anaesthesiol Scand* 1967–1968:27;263

27. Giommona ST, Modell JH: Drowning by total immersion. *Am J Dis Child* 1967;114:662

28. Kizer KW: Aquatic rescue and in-water CPR. *Ann Emerg Med* 1982;11:166

29. March NF, Matthews RC: New techniques in external cardiac compressions: aquatic cardiopulmonary resuscitation. *JAMA* 1980;244:1229

30. Modell JH, Calderwood HW, Ruiz BC, et al: Effects of ventilatory patterns on arterial oxygenation after near-drowning in seawater. *Anesthesiology* 1974;40:376

31. Glasser KL, Civetta JM, Flor RJ: The use of spontaneous ventilation with constant-pressure in the treatment of saltwater near-drowning. *Chest* 1975;67:355

32. Downs JB, Douglas ME: Assessment of cardiac filling pressure during continuous positive pressure ventilation. *Crit Care Med* 1980;8:285

33. Downs JB, Klein EF Jr, Modell JH: The effect of incremental PEEP on PaO_2 in patients with respiratory failure. *Anesth Analg* 1973;53:210

34. Tabeling BB, Modell JH: Fluid administration increases oxygen delivery during continuous positive pressure ventilation after freshwater near-drowning. *Crit Care Med* 1983;11:693

35. Gallagher TJ, Civetta JM, Kirby RR: Terminology update: optimal CEEP. *Crit Care Med* 1978;6:323

36. Downs JB, Modell JH: Patterns of respiratory support aimed at pathophysiologic conditions. *ASA Refresh Courses Anesthesiol* 1977;7:71

37. Modell JH, Moya F, Williams HD, et al: Changes in blood gases and $AaDO_2$ during near-drowning. *Anesthesiology* 1968;29:456

38. Murray IP, Modell JH, Gallagher TJ, et al: Titration of PEEP by the arterial minus end-tidal carbon dioxide gradient. *Chest* 1984;85:100

39. Kirby RR, Downs JB, Civetta JM, et al: High level positive end expiratory pressure (PEEP) in acute respiratory insufficiency. *Chest* 1975;67:156

40. Downs JB, Douglas ME, Sanfelippo PM, et al: Ventilatory pattern, intrapleural pressure, and cardiac output. *Anesth Analg* 1977;56:88

41. Kirby RR, Perry JC, Calderwood HW, et al: Cardiorespiratory effects of high positive end-expiratory pressure. *Anesthesiology* 1975;43:533

42. Florete OG, Banner MJ, Rodriguez JC, et al: Airway pressure release ventilation in a patient with acute pulmonary injury. *Chest* 1989;96:679

43. Anderson DD, Cranford RE: Corticosteroids in ischemic stroke. *Stroke* 1979;10:68

44. Gonzalez R, Rothi RJ: Near-drowning: consensus and controversies in pulmonary and cerebral resuscitation. *Heart Lung* 1987;16:474

45. Modell JH, Graves SA, Ketover A: Clinical course of 91 consecutive near-drowning victims. *Chest* 1976;70:231

46. Feinberg WM, Ferry PC: A fate worse than death: the persistent vegetative state in childhood. *Am J Dis Child* 1984;138:128

47. Conn AW, Edmonds JF, Barker GA: Near-drowning in cold fresh water: current treatment regimen. *Can Anaesth Soc J* 1978;25:259

48. Modell JH: Treatment of near-drowning: is there a role for H.Y.P.E.R. therapy? *Crit Care Med* 1986;14:593

49. Bohn DJ, Biggar WD, Smith CR, et al: Influence of hypothermia, barbiturate therapy, and intracranial pressure monitoring on morbidity and mortality after near-drowning. *Crit Care Med* 1986;14:529

50. Nussbaum E, Magge JC: Pentobarbital therapy does not improve neurologic outcome in nearly drowned, flaccid-comatose children. *Pediatrics* 1988;81:630

51. Lyrene RK, Truog WE: Adult respiratory distress syndrome in a pediatric intensive care unit: predisposing conditions, clinical course, outcome. *Pediatrics* 1981;67:790

52. Nussbaum E, Galant SP: Intracranial pressure monitoring as a guide to prognosis in the nearly-drowned, severely comatose child. *J Pediatr* 1983;102:215

53. Dean JM, McComb JG: Intracranial pressure monitoring in severe pediatric near-drowning. *Neurosurgery* 1981;9:627

54. Cohen IJ, Amir J, Gedaliah A, et al: Thrombocytopenia of neonatal cold injury. *J Pediatr* 1984;104:620

55. Bolte RG, Black PG, Bowers RS, et al: The use of extracorporeal rewarming in a child submerged for 66 minutes. *JAMA* 1988;260:377

56. Edwards ND, Timmins AC, Randalls B et al.: Survival in adults after cardiac arrest due to drowning. *Intensive Care Med* 1990;16:336

57. Hayward JS, Hay C, Mathews BR, et al: Temperature effect on the human dive response in relation to cold water near-drowning. *J Appl Physiol* 1984;56:202

58. Ramey CA, Ramey DN, Hayward JS: Dive response of children in relation to cold water near-drowning. *J Appl Physiol* 1987;63:665

59. Ornato JP: Special resuscitation situations: Near-drowning, traumatic injury, electric shock, and hypothermia. *Circulation* 1986;74(Suppl):IV-23

60. Sessler DI, Israel D, Pozos RS, et al: Spontaneous post-anesthetic tremor does not resemble thermoregulatory shivering. *Anesthesiology* 1988;68:843

61. Schaller MD, Fischer AP, Perrett CH: Hyperkalemia is a prognostic factor during acute severe hypothermia. *JAMA* 1990; 264:1842

62. Orlowski JP: Drowning, near-drowning and ice-water drowning. *JAMA* 1988;260:390

63. Bell TS, Ellenberg L, McComb JG: Neuropsychological outcome after severe pediatric near-drowning. *Neurosurgery* 1985;17:604

64. Allman FD, Nelson WB, Pacentine GA, et al: Outcome following cardiopulmonary resuscitation in severe pediatric near-drowning. *Am J Dis Child* 1986;140:571

65. O'Rourke PP: Outcome of children who are apneic and pulseless in the emergency room. *Crit Care Med* 1986;14:466

66. Siebke H, Breivik H: Survival after 40 minutes submersion without cerebral sequelae. *Lancet* 1975;1:1275

67. Kruss S, Bergstrom L, Suutarinen T, et al: The prognosis of near-drowned children. *Acta Paediatr Scand* 1979;68:315

68. Nussbaum E, Galant SP: Intracranial pressure monitoring as a guide to prognosis in the nearly drowned severely comatose child. *J Pediatr* 1983;102:215

69. Lavelle JM, Shaw KN: Near-drowning: is emergency department cardiopulmonary resuscitation or intensive care unit cerebral resuscitation indicated? *Crit Care Med* 1993;21:368

70. Dean JM, Kaufman ND: Prognostic indicators in pediatric near-drowning: the Glasgow coma scale. *Crit Care Med* 1981; 9:536

71. Bratton SL, Jardine DS, Morray, JP: Serial neurologic examinations after near-drowning and outcome. *Arch Pediatr Adoles Med* 1994;148:167

72. Nussbaum E: Prognostic variables in nearly drowned, comatose children. *Am J Dis Child* 1985;139:1058

73. Sarnaik AP, Preston G, Lieh-Lai M, et al: Intracranial pressure and cerebral perfusion pressure in near-drowning. *Crit Care Med* 1985;13:224

74. Rosenberg C, Wogensen KSA: Auditory brainstem and middle- and long-latency evoked potentials in coma. *Arch Neurol* 1984;41:835

75. Orlowski JP, Abulleil MM, Phillips JM: The hemodynamic and cardiovascular effects of near-drowning in hypotonic, isotonic, and hypertonic solutions. *Ann Emerg Med* 1989;18:1044

76. Goodwin SR, Friedman WA, Bellefleur M: Is it time to use evoked potentials to predict outcome in comatose children and adults? *CCM* 1991;19:518

77. Tsao CY, Ellingson RJ: Normal somatosensory evoked potentials in a child in persistent coma. *Pediatr Neurol* 1989;5: 257

78. Nichter MA, Everett PB: Childhood near-drowning: is cardiopulmonary resuscitation always indicated? *Crit Care Med* 1989;17:993

79. Weinberg HD: Prognostic variables in nearly drowned, comatose children. *Am J Dis Child* 1986;140:329

80. Peterson B: Morbidity of childhood near-drowning. *Pediatrics* 1977;59:364

81. Griest KJ, Zumwait RE: Child abuse by drowning. *Pediatrics* 1989;83:41

82. Kropp RM, Schwartz JF: Water intoxication from swimming. *J Pediatr* 1982;101:947

83. Orlowski JP: It's time for pediatricians to 'rally' round the pool fence. *Pediatrics* 1980;83:1065

84. Winemute GJ, Wright MA: Swimming pool owners' opinions of strategies for prevention of drowning. *Pediatrics* 1990;85: 63

85. Spyker DA: Submersion injury: epidemiology, prevention, and management. *Pediatr Clin North Am* 1985;32:113

86. Present P: *Child Drowning Study: A Report on the Epidemiology of Drownings in Residential Pools to Children Under Age Five.* Washington, DC, US Consumer Product Safety Commission, 1987

87. Robinson MD, Seward PN: Submersion injury in children. *Pediatr Emerg Care* 1987;3:44

Critical Care, Third Edition, edited by Joseph M. Civetta,
Robert W. Taylor, and Robert R. Kirby.
Lippincott-Raven Publishers, Philadelphia, PA © 1997.

CHAPTER 127

■

Venous Thrombosis and Pulmonary Embolism

Mandeep R. Mehra
Frederick R. Bode

IMMEDIATE CONCERNS ■

MAJOR PROBLEMS

Prevention is better than cure. Every patient entering the intensive care unit (ICU) should be considered at risk of thromboembolism and immediately assessed for prophylaxis and choice of prophylaxis. Some patients unsuitable for pharmacologic or other conventional prophylaxis, such as multiple trauma patients, may be candidates for vena caval interruption. Do not forget prophylaxis.

STRESS POINTS

1. If acute pulmonary embolism (PE) is suspected, administer a bolus dose of heparin, unless contraindicated, then concentrate on establishing a precise diagnosis.
2. The test selected for diagnosis should be one that enables continuation of adequate therapy.

ESSENTIAL DIAGNOSTIC TESTS AND PROCEDURES

1. Figure 127-1 depicts an overview of an algorithm for the diagnosis of venous thromboembolism.
2. In very ill patients, it may be appropriate to diagnose a lower extremity deep venous thrombus (DVT) using duplex ultrasound, even if hemodynamically stable PE is suspected, since it provides the armamentarium for definitive therapy.

3. When the potential hazards of planned therapy are preeminent in your mind, you may proceed to definitive diagnosis using pulmonary angiography. In most cases, a perfusion lung scan that can be performed at the bedside is the best first step.
4. Once the diagnosis of thromboembolism is suspected, pursue it until a definitive answer is achieved.
5. A normal or nearly normal perfusion lung scan finding essentially rules out significant PE.
6. A low-probability scan finding, in conjunction with a normal lower extremity duplex examination, allows most clinicians to temporarily stop the diagnostic pursuit, initiate prophylaxis, and repeat a lower extremity ultrasound study in 3 to 5 days.
7. A high-probability scan finding should lead to therapeutic intervention. Any other scan result should be deemed nondiagnostic, and a decision to proceed with pulmonary angiography should be considered.

INITIAL THERAPY

1. Therapy should not be conservative. The goal is to initiate therapy rapidly and achieve effective levels of anticoagulation promptly.
2. Patients who demonstrate evidence of any hemodynamic compromise should be quickly evaluated for thrombolytic therapy.
3. Vena caval interruption should be considered when indicated or in situations where other options are unsuitable and the patient must be protected from recurrent embolism.

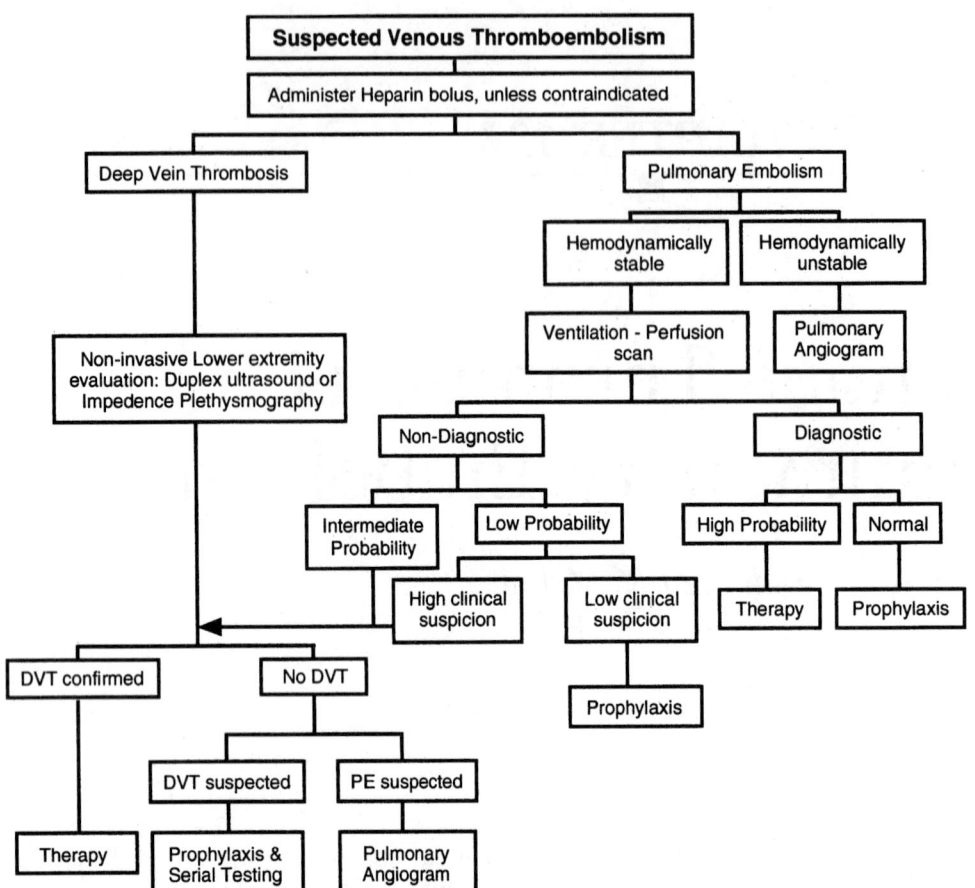

FIGURE 127-1. An overview of the algorithmic approach to the clinical diagnosis of pulmonary embolism and deep venous thrombosis (DVT). PE, pulmonary embolism.

4. Remember that surgical embolectomy can be considered as a last choice.
5. Iatrogenic thromboembolism is an evil that looms large in the ICU. Avoid prolonged intravascular access that predisposes to thrombosis and assess the appropriateness of prophylactic measures daily.
6. When treating the patient diagnosed with thromboembolism, remember that recurrent events can occur.
7. To avoid confusion, it is a good idea to assess the new "normal" baseline diagnostic test profile that can be used for future comparisons.
8. Thus, a repeat perfusion scan after therapy establishes the presence of any defects that might cause future conflicts in interpretation.
9. Similarly, a lower extremity ultrasound after successful therapy of DVT clarifies any residual venous abnormalities.

VENOUS THROMBOEMBOLISM: UBIQUITOUS YET UNDIAGNOSED ■

An autopsy study of the frequency of pulmonary thromboembolism in humans by Freiman and others[1] in the 1960s found evidence of subclinical pulmonary emboli in 64% of consecutive autopsies in patients with various causes of

death. This important information underscores the elusive nature of venous thromboembolism and emphasizes that most events escape clinical recognition. A population-based survey conducted in 16 hospitals found that the annual incidence of DVT was 48 per 100,000, whereas the incidence of PE with or without DVT was 23 per 100,000.[2] Extrapolation from these data suggests that approximately 170,000 new cases of venous thromboembolism occur in hospitalized patients, with as many as 100,000 cases resulting from recurrent disease; yet, these are conservative estimates, and the exact incidence and prevalence remains a mystery. More importantly, 50,000 deaths annually in the United States are attributable to fatal PE.[3] Indeed, the mortality rate of untreated venous thromboembolism approaches 30%, but prompt recognition and treatment can reduce this to under 10%.[4] Most cases of PE arise as a result of thrombosis in the deep veins of the legs; thus, amelioration of this devastating complication lies in religious surveillance and prophylaxis for DVT.

Data regarding use of venous thromboembolism prophylaxis in the medical ICU are sparse. A prospective investigation in 152 medical ICU patients by Keane and coworkers[5] demonstrates that prophylaxis was used in only 33% of patients at risk of DVT, and, moreover, was initiated at least 48 hours late. Furthermore, it was found that 87% of the patients had at least one thromboembolic risk factor whereas 52% had multiple indications for prophylaxis. This remarkable underutilization of prophylaxis for an easily preventable disease underscores the need to remember this simple yet indispensable adjunct to the therapeutic regimen of every medical ICU patient.

THE MEDICAL ICU AND DEEP VENOUS THROMBOSIS: THE CASE FOR ROUTINE PROPHYLAXIS

Rudolph Virchow recognized DVT in 1856 and described the classic triad of vessel wall inflammation, hypercoagulability, and venostasis that underlie all risk factors for venous thrombosis. Patients who enter the medical ICU have at least one and often many well-recognized factors predisposing them to the initiation and propagation of DVT. The most common factors are recent surgery, trauma, serious systemic illness, immobility, congestive heart failure, stroke, and malignancy. The postoperative patient is particularly at high risk of DVT, not only because of the ubiquitous presence of early venous stasis from immobility and elevated central venous pressures, but also because of the presence of several derangements in blood coagulability. This cascade in surgical patients begins with anesthesia, which causes a fall in vascular tone with at least a 50% reduction in blood flow through the popliteal and iliac veins. Antithrombin III levels fall intraoperatively and remain depressed for 3 to 5 days. Additionally, plasma viscosity progressively increases because of elevation in fibrinogen, which peaks by postoperative day 5. Thus, it is not surprising that this thrombogenic milieu—along with prolonged immobility, local venous trauma through compression (as in femoral fractures), and endovas-

cular trauma (as with catheter insertions)—places the postoperative patient at a particularly higher risk of developing DVT. Table 127-1 lists some of the commonly encountered risk factors for DVT in the medical ICU.

One important fact is the notorious unreliability of clinical features to suggest acute DVT. Moreover, it is easy to miss the development of venous thromboembolism in critically ill patients because of the multiplicity of ongoing problems. Therefore, efforts targeted to the prevention of this silent but deadly force not only decrease the morbidity of patients entering the ICU, but also prove to be cost efficient in the long term. The method of prophylaxis used depends on the assessment of the patient's risk for venous thromboembolism in the context of the individual clinical scenario. Table 127-2 outlines a scheme for dividing patients into risk categories, along with the expected incidence of venous thromboembolism. This enables selection of the preventive modality most likely to benefit the patient. Thus, appropriate prophylaxis for each patient (1) involves facets of considering prophylaxis for all patients entering the ICU, and (2) entails proper selection of preventive modalities: pharmacologic, nonpharmacologic, or a combination thereof.

NONPHARMACOLOGIC PROPHYLAXIS

General Measures

In the awake and cooperative patient, several general measures help to avoid venous stasis. All such patients should be encouraged to exercise their legs by repeatedly flexing their ankles, thus allowing adequate emptying of the lower extremity veins. Additionally, the knees should be frequently flexed and extended. If possible, these simple yet effective

TABLE 127-1. Risk Factors for Acute DVT

FACTOR	SPECIAL CONSIDERATIONS
Older age	Incremental increase beyond age 40 y
Previous thromboembolism	Established past diagnosis increases future risk by threefold
Pregnancy	Highest risk is during parturition
Surgical procedures	Orthopedic, neurosurgical, and abdominal procedures impart the greatest risk
Anesthesia	General anesthesia has a higher risk than regional anesthesia
Multiple trauma	Particularly high risk if reparative surgical procedures are performed
Immobilization	Obesity, critical care settings, orthopedic events (hip fracture), and paralytic strokes associated with highest rate of DVT
Malignancy	Occult cancers increase the risk by twofold to 19-fold, particularly in the young; overt cancers have an increased risk during chemotherapy
Hypercoagulable states	Antithrombin III, proteins C & S deficiency; Activated protein C resistance; polycythemia; antiphospholipid syndromes
Drug therapy	Estrogens
Cardiovascular conditions	Myocardial infarction; heart failure

DVT, deep venous thrombosis.

TABLE 127-2. Risk Stratification for Prophylaxis

RISK STRATA	THROMBOEMBOLIC EVENTS	CLINICAL PROFILE
Low risk	0.2–0.4%	No clinical risk factors; age <40 y
Moderate risk	1–4%	No clinical risk factors; age >40 y; major surgery with general anesthesia
High risk	2–8%	Clinical risk factors; age >40 y
Very high risk	10–20%	Multiple clinical risk factors; age >40 y; high-risk surgery (orthopedic, neurosurgical, gynecologic, trauma)

adjunctive measures should be explained to patients before an anticipated period of prolonged immobility.

Specific Measures

There are three main measures of nonpharmacologic prophylaxis: (1) graduated compression stockings (GCSs), (2) intermittent pneumatic compression (IPC) boots, and (3) inferior vena caval (IVC) interruption.

GRADUATED COMPRESSION FLOW STOCKINGS. Using GCSs achieves higher femoral vein flow than uniform compression, with a 35% increase in femoral blood flow velocities.[6] A metaanalysis of 12 studies assessing the efficacy of GCSs in postoperative prophylaxis after moderate-risk surgery (abdominal, gynecologic, and neurologic) suggests a 68% overall risk reduction rate for DVT.[7] Thus, GCSs should be considered as first-line prophylaxis against venous thromboembolism for all low- to moderate-risk hospitalized patients who do not have peripheral vascular disease.

INTERMITTENT PNEUMATIC COMPRESSION BOOTS. Use of IPC boots involves placing air-filled sleeves around the limb, providing intermittent inflation, which can increase femoral vein blood flow velocity by as much as 180% for a single-chamber IPC boot and 240% when used in a sequentially graded manner.[8] Thus, this prophylactic technique is more effective than GCSs; however, it has the disadvantage of being cumbersome and uncomfortable with prolonged use.

The mechanism by which the IPC boot is effective involves more than the amelioration of venous stasis; effectiveness may accrue from activation of the endogenous fibrinolytic system. Indeed, a study by Knight and Dawson[9] that randomly placed patients into either "arm" of IPC boots or no prophylaxis demonstrates a significant reduction of "leg" DVT in the prophylaxis group, which suggests the presence of a systemically beneficial influence of IPC boots. Also, IPC boots should be shunned when treating a patient with acute DVT.

Also of significance is the fact that GCSs and IPC boots are not supplementary but may be complementary to each other because they work by several different mechanisms. GCSs prevent venous stasis and dilatation by continuous increase in venous flow velocity, whereas IPC boots do so only briefly. Scurr and others[10] found that the combination was more effective than either alone in preventing venous thromboembolism.

INFERIOR VENA CAVAL INTERRUPTION. IVC interruption is accomplished by placing a filter device that acts as a mechanical barrier to embolism. Therefore, such devices do not have any effect on the thrombotic process itself. However, situations may arise that require using this modality as an embolism prophylaxis in certain high-risk clinical settings. Thus, IVC interruption may be preferred when a contraindication for pharmacologic agents (active bleeding) coexists with the inability to use IPC boots (e.g., recent acute DVT). This approach should be used only in high-risk situations (such as orthopedic surgeries) and applied only after careful consideration of other modes of prophylaxis. A more detailed discussion of IVC interruption follows later in this chapter.

PHARMACOLOGIC PROPHYLAXIS

Methods for pharmacologic prophylaxis include use of fixed low-dose unfractionated heparin, adjusted-dose heparin, low molecular weight heparin (LMWH), dextran, and warfarin either as a low dose or as an adjusted dose. The advantages, disadvantages, and limitations of each of these modalities must be recognized to select them appropriately.

FIXED-DOSE UNFRACTIONATED HEPARIN. The standard method of low-dose heparin (LDH) administered subcutaneously (5000 U every 8 to 12 hours) is highly effective as prophylaxis in medical patients immobilized for 48 hours or in patients undergoing elective abdominal or gynecologic surgery. Collins and associates[11] performed a metaanalysis of more than 70 randomized studies that evaluated the role of LDH versus placebo and demonstrated that this approach can decrease the incidence of DVT by two thirds and of PE by one half. More significantly, the rate of fatal PE was reduced by 64% with heparin prophylaxis administered until the patient was ambulatory. Optimally, heparin prophylaxis must begin 2 hours before any planned surgery or medical event requiring immobilization.

ADJUSTED-DOSE UNFRACTIONATED HEPARIN. Heparin in adjusted doses was developed to provide effective prophylaxis beyond fixed-dose heparin in patients undergoing orthopedic procedures. A dose of 3500 U injected subcutaneously every 8 hours is begun 2 days before surgery and then adjusted to maintain the activated partial thromboplastin time (aPTT) in the high-normal range. This approach seems to be more effective than fixed LDH but with a slightly increased risk of bleeding complications.

LOW MOLECULAR WEIGHT HEPARIN. LMWHs are fragments of heparin with greater anti–factor Xa affinity. The advantages of LMWHs lie in their longer half-life (not affected by heparin binding proteins), more predictable anticoagulant response, and, possibly, a reduced risk of heparin-induced thrombocytopenia. In a metaanalysis that assessed the usefulness of LMWH in venous thrombosis, Rosendaal and coworkers[12] examined 62 studies with up to 20,000 subjects and found that LMWH was not only effective when compared with placebo, but also significantly reduced the rates of venous thrombosis when compared with unfractionated heparin by 20% to 30%. LMWH also has been found to be better than warfarin in patients undergoing major hip or knee surgery.[13]

DEXTRAN. Dextran occupies a niche in prophylaxis of patients who are at grave risk of bleeding from continuous heparin therapy but who possess a high risk for venous thrombosis requiring more than just subcutaneous heparin. Further use can be found in treating patients with heparin-associated thrombocytopenia.[14] However, effective dextran prophylaxis is not without risk: anaphylaxis, renal failure, and congestive heart failure have been reported. The usual dose is 500 mL intravenously over 6 hours as a once daily dose. The prophylactic effect of dextran accrues from its effect on platelet aggregation and adhesion, as well as by altering the structure of the thrombus.

WARFARIN. Warfarin has been found to be effective as prophylaxis in most situations when adjusted to achieve an International Normalized Ratio (INR) of approximately 2.0. Indeed, if using warfarin prophylaxis, the drug must be started preoperatively and continued postoperatively, particularly for orthopedic procedures.[15] Notice that adequate anticoagulation by this technique is not achieved until at least 3 days after starting warfarin, despite a prolongation in the prothrombin time. This results from the rapid inhibition of factor VII, which has a short half-life and causes a prolongation in the prothrombin time even in the presence of circulating factor II, which is not depleted for at least 3 days, and thereby provides a procoagulant milieu. One other prophylactic use in the ICU merits discussion. Very low dose warfarin (1 mg/day) has been advocated for thrombosis prophylaxis in the presence of indwelling subclavian venous catheters by the demonstration of its efficacy in a randomized study conducted by Bern and colleagues,[16] who found

that untreated patients were three to four times more likely to develop thrombosis than those treated with low-dose warfarin.

Prophylaxis is the most important way of decreasing the mortality associated with PE and the morbidity that accompanies DVT. Using well-defined clinical criteria, patients should be sorted into low- or high-risk groups (see Table 127-2). Thereafter, the appropriate choice of prophylaxis can be chosen for each patient under consideration. This schema is outlined in Table 127-3.

NATURAL HISTORY OF VENOUS THROMBOEMBOLISM

The natural history of untreated DVT is associated with a frightening rate of complications. First, up to 30% of isolated calf vein thrombi propagate into the proximal popliteal vein. Second, almost 50% of proximal vein thrombi result in PE.[17] Furthermore, partial treatment of proximal vein thrombi is associated with a 40% recurrence rate.[18] Indeed, even symptomatic calf vein thrombi, if treated with short-term heparin without continuation of long-term warfarin, are associated with a 20% recurrence rate.[19]

The most dreaded morbid complication of DVT, the postphlebitic syndrome, results from destruction of the venous architecture, with consequent ambulatory venous hypertension that causes edema and pain in the lower extremity. Indeed, in patients with iliofemoral thrombosis, the pain and swelling may never disappear. However, in most patients, the symptoms resolve in a few weeks to months. Chronic venous stasis can develop into venous ulcers and recurrent cellulitis.

More importantly, in patients with more than one episode of venous thromboembolism, the recurrence rate, even after 3 months of anticoagulation, approaches 25% in the first year alone with a mortality rate of 5%.[20] These data emphasize the utmost importance not only of prophylaxis, but also of prompt and early diagnosis and treatment of this syndrome of venous thromboembolism.

CLINICAL FEATURES AND DIAGNOSIS OF VENOUS THROMBOEMBOLISM

DEEP VENOUS THROMBOSIS

Clinical Features

The clinical diagnosis of DVT most often is inaccurate. Indeed, the sensitivity of the clinical diagnosis is low because of the clinically silent nature of most thrombi. Sevitt[21] reports that up to 60% of autopsy-proven fatal pulmonary emboli resulting from DVT were clinically silent. Conversely, almost 70% of ambulatory patients who are thought to have venous thrombosis on clinical grounds are found to have another explanation for their symptoms.[22] Thus, nonthrombotic disorders such as cellulitis, lymphangitis, myositis, vasculitis, tendinitis, muscle tears, and spontaneous muscle hematomas may mimic venous thrombosis with alarming frequency. The

TABLE 127-3.   Recommendations for DVT Prophylaxis

SURGICAL SITUATIONS

1. In low-risk patients, no specific prophylaxis other than early ambulation is recommended.
2. ES, LDUH (given 2 h before and every 12 h after operations), or IPC should be used in moderate-risk patients.
3. LDUH (every 8 h) or LMWH should be used in higher risk patients.
4. In high-risk general surgery patients who are prone to wound complications such as hematomas and infections, IPC is a good alternative prophylaxis.
5. In very high-risk surgery patients with multiple risk factors, pharmacologic methods (LDUH, LMWH, or dextran) combined with IPC are most effective. LDUH and LMWH therapy should be started preoperatively and dextran given intraoperatively. IPC should be applied intraoperatively, if possible. Alternatively, perioperative warfarin (INR, 2.0–3.0) therapy may be used.
6. In patients undergoing total hip replacement surgery, postoperative, subcutaneous twice-daily fixed-dose unmonitored LMWH, low-intensity (INR, 2.0–3.0) oral anticoagulation (started preoperatively or immediately after operation), or adjusted-dose unfractionated heparin (started preoperatively) are the most effective anticoagulant-based prophylaxis regimens. Adjuvant prophylaxis with ES or IPC may provide additional efficacy.
7. In patients undergoing total knee replacement surgery, postoperative subcutaneous twice-daily fixed-dose unmonitored LMWH is the most effective anticoagulate-based prophylaxis regimen. IPC is the most effective nonpharmacologic prophylaxis regimen and provides a reduction in relative risk comparable to LMWH.
8. In patients undergoing hip fracture surgery, either preoperative subcutaneous fixed-dose unmonitored LMWH or oral anticoagulation (INR, 2.0–3.0) is effective.
9. Prophylactic inferior vena cava filter replacement should be limited to high-risk patients in whom other forms of anticoagulant-based prophylaxis are not feasible because of contraindications.
10. IPC with or without ES should be used in patients undergoing neurosurgery. LDUH therapy may be an acceptable alternative. IPC and LDUH may be more effective in combination than individually.
11. Aspirin is ineffective prophylaxis and should not be used.

MEDICAL SITUATIONS

1. In multiple trauma patients, IPC, warfarin, or LMWH should be used when feasible. Because of the high risk of venous thromboembolism and the inability to apply standard methods of prophylaxis, serial surveillance with duplex ultrasonography may be a successful strategy. In selected very high-risk patients, prophylactic inferior vena caval filter placement may be employed.
2. LDUH should be used in patients with myocardial infarction. Full-dose anticoagulation is also effective. IPC and possibly ES may be useful when heparin is contraindicated.
3. In patients with ischemic stroke and lower extremity paralysis, LDUH and LMWH are effective. IPC and ES are also probably effective.
4. In patients with acute spinal cord injury with paralysis, treatment with adjusted-dose heparin or LMWH is recommended for prophylaxis. Warfarin prophylaxis also may be effective. LDUH, ES, and IPC when used alone are ineffective.
5. In general medical patients with clinical risk factors for venous thromboembolism, particularly those with heart failure or chest infections, LDUH and LMWH are effective.
6. In patients with long-term indwelling central vein catheters, warfarin, 1 mg daily, should be used to prevent axillary-subclavian venous thrombosis.

DVT, deep vein thrombosis; ES, elastic stockings; INR, international normalized ratio; IPC, intermittent pneumatic compression; LDUH, low-dose unfractionated heparin; LMWH, low molecular weight heparin.

Adapted from Clagett GP, Anderson FA Jr, Heit J, et al. Prevention of venous thromboembolism. *Chest* 1995;108:312S.

clinical suspicion of venous thrombosis therefore must always provoke objective testing.

Homan's sign, a time-honored diagnostic clue to venous thrombosis is, in fact, insensitive and nonspecific. This sign, elicited by discomfort in the calf as a result of forced dorsiflexion of the foot, can be present in up to 50% of symptomatic patients who do not have thrombosis and is found in fewer than one third of patients with established thrombosis.[22] Therefore, this sign should no longer be used clinically in establishing the diagnosis of venous thrombosis.

Diagnostic Testing

Various techniques for the objective diagnosis of DVT have been introduced in clinical practice: venography, plethysmography, and ultrasonography have been substantially validated in diagnosing DVT, yet the choice of test depends on the clinical circumstances of the particular patient. In this regard, the intensive care patient poses a special problem. Because these patients are sometimes not even temporarily movable, the test must be performed at the bedside. Furthermore, it should not be physiologically challenging and must be accurate enough to allow therapeutic decisions based on a high sensitivity and specificity.

ASCENDING CONTRAST VENOGRAPHY. Although contrast venography has been termed the "gold standard" for the diagnosis of venous thrombosis, it is often imperfect. Venography requires the patient to be mobile, involves use of contrast agents, is painful, and has been associated with induction of DVT in as many as 3% to 4% of patients.[23]

When properly performed, venography can detect a clot in the calf as well as the thigh up to the common iliac vein; however, it often misses thrombosis in the internal iliac vein and other pelvic veins. In addition, venography can produce negative results in up to a third of patients with proven PE.[24] This is thought to result from embolization in toto. Inadequate venography is encountered 5% of the time, and visualization of the external and common iliac veins is inadequate in as many as 18% of cases.[22,23] More importantly, studies of interobserver variability have revealed variations in 10% of reports regarding the presence or absence of a thrombus.[25] Venography requires services that might not be easily available on an urgent basis at most hospitals and requires moving the patient to the radiology department for its performance. Thus, we believe that venography, although imperfect by most standards, has become the gold standard merely by default of its usefulness as an arbitrator of confusing results of noninvasive testing.

NONINVASIVE TESTS. In 1981, the search for a noninvasive diagnostic modality led investigators to advocate the use of impedance plethysmography (IPG) in combination with radiolabeled fibrinogen leg scanning in lieu of venography in patients thought to have DVT.[26] This modality gained respect only because of the demonstration that it was safe to withhold anticoagulation from patients having negative results from noninvasive studies. Thereafter, it was reported that IPG used alone was able to allow treatment decisions to be made in a safe manner.[27] These studies ushered in the era of noninvasive testing as a clinically feasible entity for the diagnosis of DVT. Duplex ultrasonography has evolved to supplant the other two modalities, which are largely archaic, in the diagnostic evaluation of venous thrombosis. A brief discussion of the merits and disadvantages of various noninvasive tests follows.

Impedance Plethysmography. IPG depends on the demonstration of volume changes and impaired venous emptying to make a diagnosis of DVT. Currently available data suggest that IPG can detect proximal vein thrombi with a great sensitivity (95%), but that it is insensitive to calf thrombi (less than 30%).[28]

This method is based on the observation that blood volume changes in the lower limb produced by maximum respiratory effort or inflation and deflation of a pneumatic cuff

on the thigh produce alterations in electrical resistance ("impedance"; Fig. 127-2). Thus, the diagnosis of DVT using IPG is based on a decrease in capacitance with thigh cuff compression and the decrease in venous outflow observed within 3 seconds after release.[29]

IPG cannot distinguish between thrombotic and nonthrombotic obstructions, such as those resulting from extraneous compression or when venous emptying is retarded by elevated central venous pressures, as in the presence of congestive heart failure or in mechanically ventilated patients. Furthermore, reduced arterial inflow leads to decreased outflow and causes a false-positive IPG finding. Conversely, false-negative test results also occur in the presence of nonocclusive thrombi, low ambient temperatures, and obesity.[30,31]

Bilaterally abnormal IPG findings should not always be assumed to be false-positive. Indeed, Curley and colleagues[32] have found evidence of DVT in 26% of patients with bilaterally abnormal IPG results who were subsequently discovered to have venous thrombosis. This also can result from thrombosis in the vena cava itself.

Ultrasonography. Real time ultrasound evaluation of the deep veins has been a welcome addition to diagnostic capabilities. Not only does this modality provide anatomic visualization and localization of the thrombus, it is also movable to the patients bedside, quick to perform, and thereby suitable for most patients in an ICU or those restrained by orthopedic devices.[33] When Doppler measurement of blood flow is added to the two-dimensional image of ultrasound, the combination is called a duplex scan. In addition, color-coded flow velocity data can be superimposed on the ultrasound image to create color-flow imaging. Thus, areas of

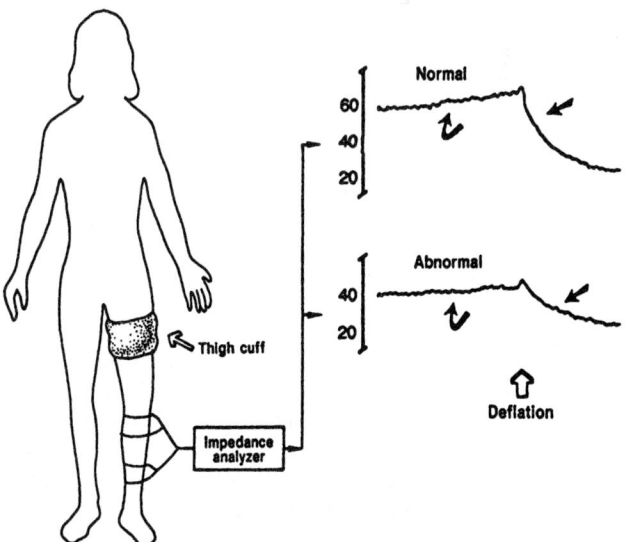

FIGURE 127-2. The technique of impedance plethysmography involves positioning an occlusive cuff on the mid-thigh, which is inflated to 40 mm Hg and then deflated. The venous pooling is recorded by estimation of electrical impedance. Abnormal pooling is characterized by a "dampened" initial rise and reduced rate of fall compared with normals.

minor alterations in venous flow can be detected by this modality, even if a thrombus is nonocclusive or if collateral veins carry enough venous drainage to bypass local venous congestion.

The accuracy of Doppler ultrasonography has been compared with contrast venography in patients with symptoms of acute DVT. At the outset, notice that the clinical value of this procedure is operator-dependent and varies with the expertise of the technician. Lensing and others[34] report a sensitivity rate of 100% and a specificity rate of 99% in the detection of proximal, symptomatic deep venous thrombi, yet others report less dramatic sensitivity (65% to 100%) and specificity rates (72% to 98%) in the diagnosis of DVT, likely resulting from differences in technical experiences.[35] However, once strict objective criteria are applied, the overall predictive value can be expected to be in excess of 90%.[36]

Compressive duplex ultrasound images veins as nonechogenic structures, either longitudinally or transversely. Objective criteria for demonstrating DVT include visualization of thrombi, absence of spontaneous flow by Doppler, absence of phasicity of flow with respiration, and lack of compressibility of the vein with probe pressure. A combination of these criteria must be used for a diagnosis, and no single factor can confirm the diagnosis in isolation. Additionally, the criterion of vein compressibility has been heavily emphasized by some investigators. Caution must be used because sensitivity of this criterion is low, as it is often not possible to compress the superficial femoral vein as it enters the adductor canal in normal controls.[35]

In an investigation by Kellewich and associates,[37] the most reliable criteria obtainable by ultrasound were demonstrated to be the absence of spontaneous flow and phasicity of flow with respiration. Thus, the most effective use of duplex scanning may lie in using the ultrasound for anatomic visualization and location of the vein and then using the Doppler to define the presence of thrombosis.

A distinct advantage of duplex ultrasound examination lies in sorting out the differential diagnosis of symptomatic DVT. For instance, spontaneous calf hematomas and ruptured Baker's cyst can be easily diagnosed by this modality. In addition, false-positive test results are unusual above the knee. However, duplex scanning is relatively insensitive for common iliac thrombi, but they are extremely rare.[38] Thus, we believe that if available, duplex ultrasound should be the preferred method for detecting DVT in the ICU setting.

Scintigraphy and Other Techniques. Other techniques for diagnosis of DVT are of substantially limited value and include iodine 125 fibrinogen leg scanning and radionuclide venography using several labeling agents such as indium 111 or technetium 99m in conjunction with macroaggregated albumin, human albumin microspheres, red blood cells, streptokinase, urokinase (UK), plasmin, or sulfur colloid.[39,40] Plethysmography, thermography, and blood tests that reflect vascular fibrin formation and fibrin proteolysis also have been studied.[41–43] Although radiofibrinogen leg scanning is an extraordinarily potent diagnostic test for detecting calf vein thrombosis, it requires a 24- to 48-hour waiting period after injection, before making a definitive diagnosis. Furthermore, it cannot be used in pregnant or lactating women.

Blood Tests. Plasma measurements of D-dimer as a diagnostic aid in suspected venous thromboembolism has been suggested as a simple noninvasive marker for evaluating DVT.[44] A pooled analysis of 11 studies disclosed a sensitivity rate of 97% and a specificity rate of 35% for DVT when using an enzyme-linked immunosorbent assay method.[45] Notice that figures obtained for latex assays were definitely lower, precluding their successful use in the diagnostic approach for DVT. Thus, D-dimer may be of potential clinical value in the exclusion of DVT; however, its use cannot be recommended until management studies are completed and the fast D-dimer tests are validated.

PULMONARY EMBOLISM

Clinical Features

The most common clinical presentation of PE consists of sudden-onset dyspnea, tachycardia, tachypnea, or low-grade fever. Indeed, Leeper and coworkers[46] found that dyspnea or tachypnea were seen in 96% of subjects with PE in their series and suggest that the absence of either of these symptoms argues strongly against a diagnosis of PE. Apprehension, cough, fatigue, and oppressive chest discomfort are other common complaints. The lung examination is usually unremarkable, but focal wheezing may be observed.[47] Furthermore, pleuritic chest pain is also commonly seen in patients with acute PE.[48] Although these clinical appearances are useful, keep in mind that ICU patients may display subtle complexes of symptoms and signs that do not meet with classic conformity and often are masked by symptoms of other primary pathologic states.

Benotti and Dalen[49] describe subtle manifestations of PE in ICU patients that should heighten suspicion for the diagnosis:

1. Worsening arterial hypoxemia and respiratory alkalosis in a spontaneously ventilating patient
2. Persistent dyspnea and hypoxemia unresponsive to bronchodilators despite a reduction in $PaCO_2$ in a patient with chronic lung disease and history of carbon dioxide retention
3. Unexplained fever, atelectasis, or pleural-based infiltrates
4. Sudden development of pulmonary hypertension in a hemodynamically monitored patient
5. Unexplained elevation in the central venous pressure
6. Unexplained tachycardia or tachypnea
7. Worsening hypoxemia, hypercapnia, and respiratory acidosis in a sedated patient on controlled mechanical ventilation

Differentiating worsening chronic lung disease from acute PE in the medical ICU can be a daunting dilemma. Clinical examination and radioisotope scans are often not helpful. Lippman and Fein[50] recommend that the diagnosis be suspected in a patient whose worsening dyspnea is unresponsive to bronchodilators. Furthermore, the diagnosis is supported by a reduction in the arterial $PaCO_2$ in previously hypercapnic patients. In this situation, pulmonary angiography must often be performed to diagnose PE.

Diagnostic Testing

The usefulness and limitations of routinely available laboratory tests also must be recognized in the diagnostic scrutiny of PE.

ARTERIAL BLOOD GASES. Arterial hypoxemia in conjunction with respiratory alkalosis is the general rule, and the size of the embolic process relates to the degree of oxygen reduction.[51] However, a normal PaO_2 by no means excludes the diagnosis of PE. Indeed, in the Urokinase Pulmonary Embolism Trial (UPET), 12% of the patients with angiographic disease had PaO_2 values exceeding 80 mm Hg and 6% were well above 90 mm Hg. In this regard, the arterial oxygen gradient $[P(A - a)O_2]$ may be elevated. Even the use of the $P(A - a)O_2$ can be fallible because it has been demonstrated that up to 8% to 10% of patients with PE have a normal $P(A - a)O_2$.[52]

CHEST RADIOGRAPHY. The principal value lies in excluding competing diagnoses such as pneumothorax and in the interpretation of ventilation/perfusion scintigraphy. Moreover, a normal chest radiograph finding in an otherwise dyspneic patient should invite suspicion for the diagnosis of acute PE,[53] yet almost 60% of patients have some abnormality on the radiograph such as atelectasis, pleural effusion, infiltrates, or an elevated hemidiaphragm.[54] Data from the UPET study indicate that the two most common abnormalities on the affected side were an infiltrate or consolidation (40%) and elevation of the hemidiaphragm (40%).[52] Indeed, the combined presence of these two abnormalities helps to exclude pneumonia because the hemidiaphragm on the affected side is not elevated in a purely pneumonic process.

Certain radiographic signs that were once thought to be specific for PE have been reevaluated and found to be insensitive and nonspecific. In a study by Greenspan and colleagues,[55] the finding of a Hampton's hump (a pleural-based rounded density with hilar convexity) and Westermark's sign (regional oligemia with proximal vascular fullness) were not accurate markers for the presence of PE (Fig. 127-3).

ELECTROCARDIOGRAPHY. Unless the patient has had a massive PE that results in acute right ventricular overload, the electrocardiogram (ECG) is unlikely to be diagnostic. In such cases, the ECG reveals sinus tachycardia, right axis shifts, incomplete or complete right bundle branch block, and a deep S wave in limb lead I with a prominent Q wave in lead III, along with inversion of the T wave in lead III (S_1, QIII, TIII pattern). These findings signal embolic obstruction of at least 35% of the vasculature.[56] Notice that normal ECGs were found in only 6% of patients with massive embolism and 23% of cases with submassive embolism in the UPET trial.[52] Thus, the principal utility of ECG lies in excluding other etiologic explanations for the patient's symptomatology such as acute pericarditis and myocardial ischemia (Fig. 127-4).

VENTILATION/PERFUSION LUNG SCANNING. In the 1960s, Taplin and others[57] developed the principles and tech-

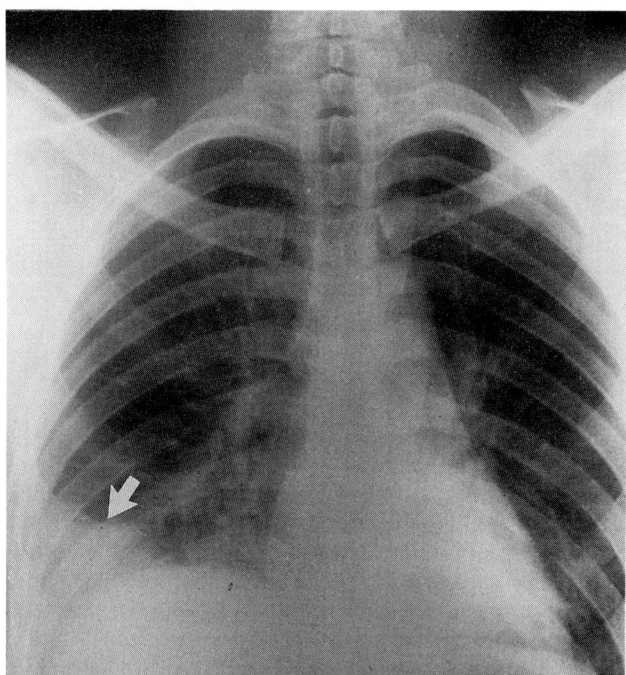

FIGURE 127-3. Chest radiograph demonstrating Hampton's hump (*arrow*) secondary to pulmonary infarction.

niques of pulmonary scanning, a noninvasive test that has entrenched itself as one of the best initial evaluation techniques in the clinical assessment of PE. The basic principles that underlie interpretation of the test involve characterization of the regional distribution of pulmonary arterial blood flow in relation to changes in ventilation. The technique of perfusion scanning involves intravenous (IV) injection of small aggregate particles of albumin or microspheres labeled with a suitable radionuclide (e.g., technetium 99m) that are detected radiographically as they traverse the pulmonary bed, such that their relative distribution reflects pulmonary blood flow. The pivotal nature of this test accrues from its ability to exclude a PE when it is normal.

Ventilation scanning, often performed with xenon, is usually added to the perfusion scan to increase test specificity. Therefore, it is preferable to perform the perfusion scan first and proceed with a ventilation scan only if the initial perfusion scan result is abnormal. Combining the ventilation scan and the perfusion scan is based on the assumption that an embolic vascular obstruction causes a perfusion abnormality without affecting ventilation, the classic appearance of a $\dot{V}/\dot{Q}$ mismatch. Most other processes, such as lung consolidation, bronchial obstructive disease, and restrictive disease that cause perfusion defects, also likely result in ventilatory defects.

The scintigraphic hallmark of acute PE are large, wedge-shaped, pleural-based perfusion defects in areas that ventilate normally and are not associated with any roentgenic abnormality. Criteria for the interpretation of ventilation/perfusion scans vary among different investigators, and this has led to considerable confusion. The most widely used set of clinical guidelines that we recommend has been devel-

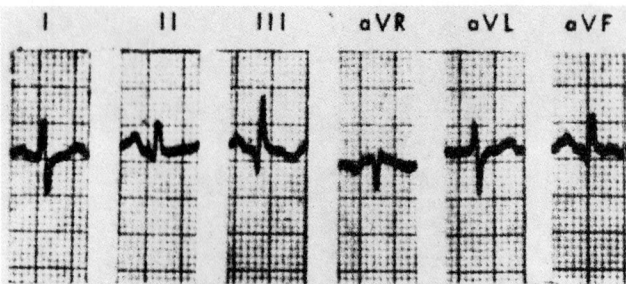

FIGURE 127-4. An echocardiogram shows the classic right ventricular strain pattern. If these findings are new, consider acute pulmonary embolus as a likely diagnosis.

oped for the Prospective Investigation of Pulmonary Embolism Diagnosis (PIOPED).[58] The major significance of the PIOPED diagnostic criteria lies in the fact that these criteria were defined in a prospective manner and are therefore subject to clinical generalization. However, the strengths and limitations of such information must be recognized. A high-probability scan result was associated with angiographic PE in 87% of cases; however, fewer than half of all cases with PE had such a diagnostic scan (sensitivity, 41%; specificity, 97%). Conversely, a low-probability scan finding excluded the diagnosis of PE in 86% of cases; however, this was a finding in only 34% of the study population. Thus, nearly 40% of the study population had indeterminate scan results, a finding of dubious and uninformative clinical value. A normal or nearly normal scan result was seen in only 14% of the study cohort. Therefore, although the use of scanning is important, application of scan criteria alone provides definitive or nearly definitive clinical information in only half of all patients suspected of having acute PE (Fig. 127-5).

The PIOPED investigators further investigated the combined utility of clinical impression of the event probability in conjunction with radiographic criteria and found that this enhanced the predictive value of noninvasive scanning considerably and with greater clinical relevance.[58] Thus, if both clinical impression and scan indicated a high probability for event, the diagnosis was likely in 96% of the cases. Similarly, a low clinical likelihood in combination with a low probability scan result excluded the diagnosis with greater than 90% certainty.

Whereas this information might sound daunting and somewhat confusing, we recommend that the results of scanning be simplified and interpreted into two major classes consisting of either a diagnostic scan (low clinical probability in conjunction with a scan result of normal, nearly normal, or low probability; high clinical probability with a high-probability scan result), or a nondiagnostic scan (all other clinical and radiographic probabilities). Thus, a therapeutic decision to either discard the diagnosis or to initiate therapy can be safely made in situations where the scan is diagnostic. Conversely, most patients in the nondiagnostic class should have a continued search for thromboembolism using other diagnostic techniques. This clinical schema is delineated in Figure 127-1.

PULMONARY ANGIOGRAPHY. Pulmonary angiography is the current gold standard for the diagnosis of PE, yet is clinically feared for its invasive nature and antecedent risk. The decision to perform angiography should be carefully weighed against the magnitude of clinical yield, and in situations where it is deemed essential, the patient must be suitably prepared. Safeguards for a proper study include a detailed precatheterization evaluation, optimal oxygen administration, minimization of the amount of contrast medium (preferably using nonionic media), and the immediate

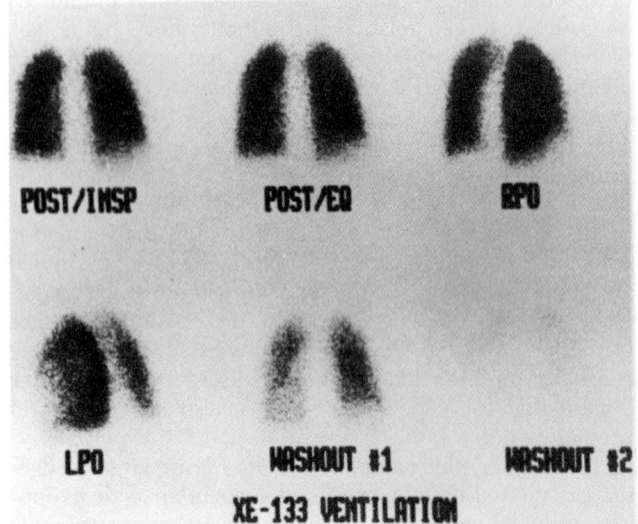
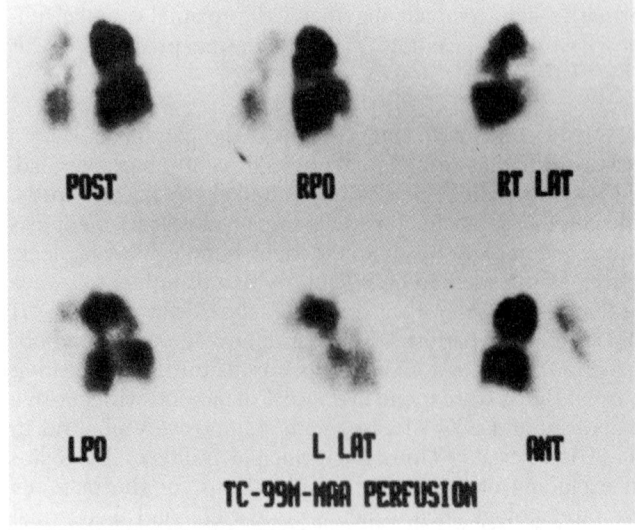

FIGURE 127-5. High-probability ventilation/perfusion lung scan. (**A**) Normal ventilation is demonstrated. (**B**) Multiple segmental and subsegmental perfusion defects are seen on the perfusion scan. (Dellinger RP, Taylor RW. *Self-Assessment in Multidisciplinary Critical Care: A Comprehensive Review.* Fullerton, CA, Society of Critical Care Medicine, 1987:340.

availability of complete resuscitative capabilities. The mortality risk in experienced hands approaches 0.3% with a morbidity rate of 1% to 4%.[59] The most serious complications of pulmonary angiography are ventricular arrhythmias, acute right-sided heart failure, and right ventricular perforation.

The clinician should recognize that angiography is definitive only when properly performed. Angiography that is performed simply by the injection of contrast agent into the main pulmonary artery with filming in the anteroposterior position is inadequate and merely excludes large central emboli. Peripheral emboli, which are more common, are detected with angiography performed in multiple projections with selective regional contrast injections. The specific findings for a PE include filling defects and abrupt vascular cutoff. Other findings that suggest PE include oligemia, delayed filling in the lower zones, asymmetric filling, and a prolonged arterial phase.[59,60] Furthermore, the findings should be interpreted in the context of perfusion scan findings because cutoff of a vessel to a lung zone that is normal on perfusion imaging should heighten the suspicion for an artifact. One issue that is often raised is the case of distal peripheral microemboli that can be picked up by perfusion scanning in a more sensitive manner than angiography.[61] The clinical ramifications of this lie in the obvious question, "What is the clinical outcome of patients who have negative angiograms but high clinical suspicion? Should these patients be treated anyway?" Novelline and others[62] provided answers to these questions by examining the course of 167 patients with normal angiogram findings in the presence of a strong clinical event probability, following them for a minimum of 6 months. During the study period, none of the patients died of thromboembolism. These data underscore the strong negative predictive value of a pulmonary angiogram.

Patients who are in a high-risk category for PE include those with a recent myocardial infarction, history of troublesome ventricular arrhythmias, and those with pulmonary hypertension, particularly with a right ventricular end-diastolic pressure in excess of 20 mm Hg.[63] In such patients, the safety of the angiographic procedure can be further enhanced by using perfusion scan guided selective lobar or segmental injections and by using nonionic contrast media.[64]

When should a clinician obtain a pulmonary angiogram? The following situations warrant obtaining one:

1. Nondiagnostic noninvasive studies for thromboembolism, especially in patients with preexisting cardiopulmonary disease
2. Patients deemed at high risk of bleeding complications from anticoagulation
3. Before embolectomy
4. Before thrombolytic therapy, particularly in the setting of right ventricular hemodynamic compromise where lung scanning gives equivocal results
5. Recurrent PE preceding vena caval interruption

TRANSESOPHAGEAL ECHOCARDIOGRAPHY. Transesophageal echocardiography (TEE) allows high-resolution images of the main pulmonary artery and the proximal portions of the left and right pulmonary arteries. Numerous reports describe visualization of pulmonary emboli by this technique. In fact, this modality may be able to segregate thrombi into fresh and mobile ones with echolucent centers from chronic thrombi that are immobile and fixed to the vessel wall. Patel and colleagues[65] describe a group of 14 critically ill patients wherein TEE was performed for other reasons but picked up the presence of unsuspected pulmonary emboli. Notice that the principal utility of this technique lies in patients with nondiagnostic radionuclide scans in whom logistic reasons preclude pulmonary angiography. Furthermore, TEE is sensitive only to proximal emboli and does not define distal embolism.

OTHER DIAGNOSTIC TESTS. A brief discussion of available diagnostic modalities that are either experimental or of limited diagnostic use is provided here. Digital substraction angiography allows lesser contrast volume use while allowing more peripheral injections.[66] However, this technique lacks accuracy in diagnosing embolism in subsegmental pulmonary arteries. Pulmonary angioscopy has been used in the setting of chronic pulmonary emboli where endarterectomy is contemplated.[67] In this situation, the angiogram is often difficult to interpret and lung scanning lacks sensitivity. Development of radiolabeled monoclonal antibodies to thrombi and vascular imaging using magnetic resonance may hold promise for the future.

THERAPY OF VENOUS THROMBOEMBOLISM

DEEP VENOUS THROMBOSIS

General Principles and Anticoagulation

The principal therapeutic objectives in treating acute DVT are threefold: (1) to achieve rapid and effective initiation of anticoagulant therapy (discussed later); (2) to use adjunctive measures for symptomatic relief; and (3) to prevent long-term sequelae, particularly the development of postphlebitic syndrome. The role of anticoagulant drugs not only relates to preventing further thrombus development, but also to minimizing the potential for PE. Adjuvant measures to reduce edema and pain include bedrest, extremity elevation, and use of analgesics. Ambulation may begin once the symptoms have abated.

Thrombolytic Therapy

The use of thrombolytic therapy in acute DVT has been demonstrated to restore early venous patency. A compilation of comparative data between streptokinase and heparin for the indication of DVT reveals that thrombolytic therapy resulted in a long-term patency of 49% versus 4% for heparin-treated patients. Furthermore, venous valvular function was maintained in a greater number of thrombolytic-treated subjects (41% versus 15%).[68] Although these data allude to the potentially beneficial role of thrombolytic therapy in reducing postphlebitic syndrome, this remains to be proven definitively. Also, no evidence supports that thrombolytic agents afford a greater protection against embolic potential than heparin alone. Analysis of patient subsets most likely to benefit from thrombolytic therapy include those having symptoms having less than 5 days and those with extensive lower extremity involvement (Fig. 127-6).

Surgical Therapy

Surgical thrombectomy has been mainly advocated for use in relieving the morbid state of phlegmasia cerulea dolens, a condition of extensive venous occlusion with a compromised adjacent arterial circulation.[69] In this grave situation, even a minimal improvement in venous return results in limb salvage. The major limitation of surgical thrombectomy is the creation of venous endothelial damage that often results in reocclusion. If surgical thrombectomy facilities are not available, then a justification can be made for the use of thrombolytic agents as a limb salvage therapy in patients with concomitant arterial circulation compromise.

PULMONARY EMBOLISM

General Principles

The primary goal of therapy is to prevent recurrent thromboembolism in a stable patient who is thought to have a pulmonary embolus. In unstable patients, however, the goals are different and include not only prevention of second events, but also stabilization of cardiopulmonary parameters by relief of hypoxemia and reversal of acute cor pulmonale. Therefore, therapy must be tailored to the patient's clinical circumstances.

Anticoagulation

INITIAL THERAPY.   The time-honored treatment of venous thromboembolism is the rapid and optimal initiation of heparin followed by 3 to 6 months of oral warfarin therapy.[70] This approach has been shown to reduce the mortality rate to under 10% from venous thromboembolism. The principal benefit of rapid heparin therapy lies in the prevention of recurrent embolism by interfering with development of new thrombus. Therefore it is rarely appropriate to delay heparin therapy while awaiting a firm diagnosis. Furthermore, the risk of recurrence of PE is greatest in the first 48 hours postoperatively, and thus every effort must be made to attain therapeutic levels of anticoagulation during this critical period.[71]

The efficacy of heparin anticoagulation is a linear function of the dose used. Conventional heparin therapy with a standard bolus dose followed by a fixed infusion rate has been shown to grossly underestimate the anticoagulation needs in the first 48 hours of therapy.[72] To obviate this problem, investigators have developed weight-based nomograms to better guide therapy. Raschke and coworkers[73] established the efficacy of a weight-based nomogram in a randomized controlled trial of 115 patients. Starting with a 80-U/kg IV bolus dose followed by a 18-U/kg/hour infusion, the investigators demonstrated a reduced rate of recurrent thromboembolism (relative risk, 0.2) at a less than 1% incidence rate of bleeding. The heparin nomogram currently in use at the University of Missouri-Columbia hospitals is illustrated in Table 127-4.

The aPTT is the most widely used heparin monitoring test. Retrospective analyses of anticoagulant therapy indicate that the risk of recurrent embolism is infrequent when the aPTT is more than 1.5 times the control value.[74,75] To that end, it has been shown that failure to maintain this minimal threshold of anticoagulation is associated with a 20% to 25% rate of recurrence risk. Clinicians have long wondered about the inability of high-dose heparin in some patients to achieve therapeutic anticoagulation, and such patients are often labeled as having "heparin resistance." It has been shown that the anticoagulant effect of heparin can be suppressed by the presence of heparin-binding proteins in plasma, and in other instances by increased levels of factor VIII activity as a manifestation of acute-phase reaction.[76]

One newer therapeutic approach to initial anticoagulation relates to the development of LMWH. Currently available data suggest that subcutaneously administered LMWH is as effective as IV heparin in the initial anticoagulation of patients with venous thrombosis. This approach has been pre-

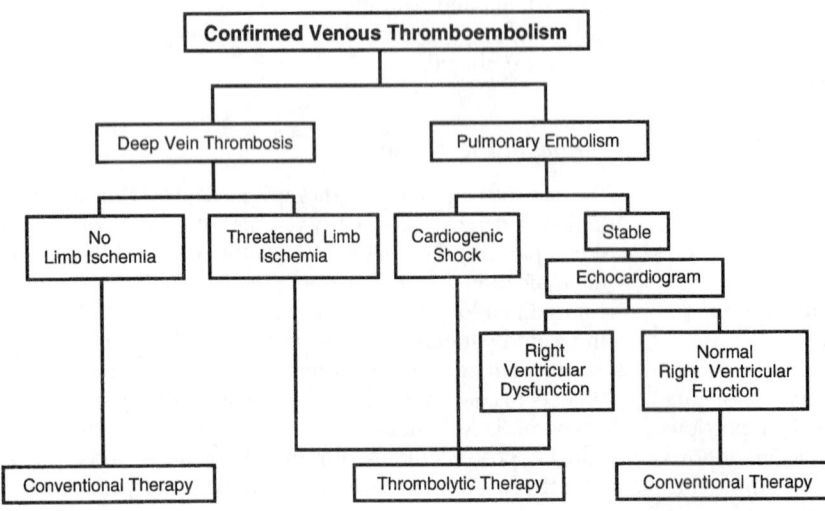

FIGURE 127-6. A suggested strategy for consideration of thrombolytic therapy in venous thromboembolism.

TABLE 127-4. Heparin Dosing Nomogram–Based Protocol

1. Bolus with 80 U/kg
2. Begin continuous infusion (25,000 U in 250 mL 0.45% NaCl = 100 U/mL) at 18 U/kg/h
3. Adjust to aPTT as follows:

aPTT	INFUSION CHANGES
<35	Re-bolus, 80 U/kg
	Increase rate by 4 U/kg/h
35–45	Re-bolus, 40 U/kg
	Increase rate by 2 U/kg/h
46–70	No change
71–90	Reduce rate by 2 U/kg/h
>90	Hold heparin for 1 h
	Reduce rate by 3 U/kg/h

Round off to nearest mL/h
Repeat aPTT every 4–6 h after a dose change
4. When 2 consecutive aPTTs are therapeutic, order aPTT every 24 h
5. Begin warfarin on d 2 of heparin infusion

NaCl, sodium chloride; aPTT, activated partial thromboplastin time.

dominantly tested in the setting of lower extremity DVT and not in PE.[77] The pooled results of current studies suggest that LMWH is soon to replace IV heparin as the initial anticoagulant of choice, and allude to the ambulatory use of LMWH in the treatment of venous thrombosis.

CHRONIC ORAL ANTICOAGULATION. Oral therapy with warfarin can be started within 24 hours of IV heparin, provided that therapeutic levels of anticoagulation are being maintained. This point must be emphasized because early institution of warfarin therapy can be associated with a procoagulant milieu as a result of depletion of proteins C and S, which are vitamin K–dependent anticoagulant proteins that have a short half-life. Therefore, a large bolus dose of warfarin may seem to prolong the prothrombin time as a result of rapid factor VII depletion, yet the overall anticoagulant effect may be marred by the depletion of anticoagulant proteins C and S.[78,79] This is why most studies suggest the necessity of a few days of overlap between warfarin and heparin therapy.

It has been demonstrated that monitoring the effectiveness of oral warfarin requires standardization of prothrombin time measurement. A calibration system has been developed to account for the marked variabilities in the sensitivities of commonly used thromboplastin reagents for performance of the prothrombin time assay. This system requires that all prothrombin time values be reported as an INR, which denotes the prothrombin time ratio raised to the power value that represents the sensitivity of the thromboplastin used[80,81]:

$$INR = \left(\frac{\text{patient prothrombin time}}{\text{control prothrombin time}}\right)^{ISI}$$

where ISI is the International Sensitivity Index. Succinctly stated, the INR represents the prothrombin time ratio that would have been obtained by using the reference thromboplastin from the World Health Organization.

The intensity of oral anticoagulation necessary to achieve long-term efficacy in venous thromboembolism seems to be a target INR of 2.0 to 3.0. Trials comparing high-intensity regimens with low-intensity regimens demonstrate that low-level anticoagulation at an INR of 2.0 to 3.0 achieves equivalent therapeutic protection at a lower bleeding risk.[82]

IVC Filters

Inferior vena cava filters prevent PE in carefully selected patients at risk for lethal embolism who have failed anticoagulation therapy or who have developed absolute contraindications to the use of these agents. Widespread use of IVC filters, particularly the Greenfield filter, has instilled faith in the long-term patency of IVC flow that can be maintained by these devices, along with high clinical efficacy. At least five filters are available for use in the United States.[83]

APPLICATIONS. Filter insertion is an irreversible therapeutic action. Therefore, the clinical decision for its necessity should rest on sound evidence. Besides clear indications, which include the inability to use anticoagulant therapy, IVC filters are a recommended consideration in patients with a tenuous cardiopulmonary status, particularly in the presence of massive acute DVT and documented PE where a second embolic event is highly likely. Prophylactic insertion of these filters is becoming more common. Such use has been reported before pulmonary embolectomy, in the presence of freely mobile proximal DVT, or for prophylaxis in clinical conditions of high perioperative DVT risk such as hip fractures and head trauma.

FILTER CHOICE. The optimal filter has not been created. Nevertheless, all of the currently available filters seem to be effective in preventing major PE. Whereas most filters are limited to use in vessels with a diameter of 30 mm or less, the Bird's nest filter can be used in the vena cava, even up to 40 mm. The Simon-Nitinol filter is advantageous in two situations. First, since it is narrow, it can be inserted through vessels of narrow caliber, such as the internal jugular veins, when bilateral femoral access is limited. Second, because this filter is short, it is particularly suitable for implantation in situations where the distance between the renal veins and the iliac bifurcation is limited.

NEED FOR ANTICOAGULATION. The placement of an IVC filter does not obviate the necessity for anticoagulation. These patients remain at risk for thrombosis above the filter insertion site as well as below the filter because of impaired venous flow. Therefore, whenever possible, anticoagulation should be continued to maintain an INR of 2.0 to 3.0.

COMPLICATIONS OF IVC FILTERS. In experienced hands, the incidence of technical complications is infrequent, with a magnitude of approximately 5%. These include air embolism, filter misplacement, retroperitoneal pain, and insertion site DVT. This last complication has been reported in 2% of filter insertions. Anchoring the filter hooks to the wall is associated with IVC wall perforation, but only rarely does this lead to clinical consequences. Indeed, radiographic evidence of IVC perforation can be found in 20% of Greenfield filter placements without significant clinical sequelae.[84]

Thrombolytic Therapy for Pulmonary Embolism

GENERAL PRINCIPLES.   The use of thrombolytic therapy in acute PE has been proposed to improve abnormalities seen on lung scan as well as provide rapid resolution of hemodynamic compromise. In addition, use of thrombolytic agents results in better pulmonary gas exchange, vascular flow dynamics, and restoration of pulmonary microcirculation to its premorbid state. These benefits translate into improved short- and long-term exercise capacity; however, whether thrombolytic therapy provides a survival benefit over and above that of routine anticoagulation remains unproven. This is so mainly because of the high survival characteristics of patients treated with heparin and warfarin therapy (mortality rate, less than 10%), and proof of a survival benefit requires comparisons of these agents in extremely large patient populations to achieve a statistically significant difference in mortality.[85–89]

We believe that thrombolytic therapy should be used in patients who present with acute massive PE with acute cor pulmonale. In such patients, if the diagnosis of PE has been made with reasonable certainty along with proven evidence of right ventricular compromise, thrombolytic therapy should be the preferred approach. The effectiveness of thrombolytic agents in such a situation most certainly outweighs any potential risks of therapy. Traditionally, it has been recommended that before thrombolytic therapy, the diagnosis of PE must be established by angiography. Current thinking has shifted to earlier use of thrombolysis even with noninvasive diagnostic confirmation, such as in the setting of a high-probability lung scan along with echocardiographic evidence of right ventricular dysfunction where the clinical suspicion for thromboembolism is also high. In summary, contemporary PE thrombolysis can be applied without mandatory angiography, with a brief infusion through a peripheral vein, and with no special additional tests.[90]

A significant difference exists between thrombolytic therapy for myocardial infarction and PE. For one, the window of therapeutic use is wider and can be used for up to 2 weeks after the index PE. Second, partial dissolution of the clot is usually the norm, largely because of the older age of the clots. These factors have led to the development of treatment strategies that require shorter and less intense thrombolytic regimens.

Clinical Trials of Thrombolysis

INITIAL STUDIES.   The first evidence of a potentially beneficial effect of thrombolytic therapy came from the randomized, open-label UPET, which compares a 24-hour infusion of UK and heparin with heparin alone.[52] This study of 160 patients reveals a trend toward a survival benefit in the thrombolytic therapy group and alludes to a lesser incidence of recurrent embolism. A later study by Sharma and colleagues[87] demonstrates that patients treated with thrombolytic therapy had a more complete resolution of PE with evidence of preserved exercise pulmonary dynamics and less functional disability at 7 years of follow-up.[87,91]

RECENT TRIALS.   The development of recombinant tissue plasminogen activator (rTPA) ushered in the era of target clot-specific thrombolysis with less systemic hematologic aberrations. Whereas earlier thrombolytic regimens focused on 24- to 48-hour drug infusions, the potency of rTPA allowed consideration of shorter duration of bolus therapy. Meyer and others,[92] on behalf of the European Cooperative Study Group Investigators, compared 100 mg of rTPA over 2 hours to a regimen of weight-adjusted UK administered as a 4400-U/kg bolus followed by 4400 U/kg/hour for 12 hours and followed hemodynamic parameters with a view to assessing pulmonary vascular resistance. This study demonstrates an early advantage of rTPA in reducing pulmonary resistance compared with UK, but these initial differences failed to persist at 6 hours. Other studies by Goldhaber and others[93,94] demonstrate that rTPA provides better clot dissolution with greater rapidity and safety than UK. In this 1988 study, rTPA caused thrombolysis in 82% at 2 hours compared with 48% of UK-treated patients. More striking was the finding that 39% (9 of 23) of the UK-treated patients could not complete their infusion as a result of allergy or bleeding-related side effects.

Goldhaber and colleagues[95] compare right ventricular function and pulmonary perfusion in a randomized study of rTPA thrombolysis (100 mg over 2 hours followed by heparin) versus heparin therapy. All patients in this trial were hemodynamically stable, and only 20% underwent a pulmonary angiogram for definitive diagnosis. This trial concluded that twice as many rTPA-treated patients demonstrated improvement in right ventricular function compared with heparin alone. More important, however, was the finding that no patients in the rTPA-treated group had recurrent embolism, whereas 9% of heparin-treated patients had fatal and nonfatal recurrent events. Notice that all of these patients presented with echocardiographic evidence of right ventricular hypokinesis, which suggests that the presence of echocardiographic right ventricular involvement, even when hemodynamically stable, might signal a high-risk patient who should be considered for thrombolytic therapy. In such a situation, thrombolytic therapy may prevent the precipitation of clinical right ventricular failure resulting from secondary embolic events. Table 127-5 lists current Food and Drug Administration–approved thrombolytic regimens. Figure 127-6 outlines a suggested algorithm for the use of thrombolytic therapy.

Surgical Pulmonary Artery Embolectomy

Consideration for surgical pulmonary artery embolectomy should not be undertaken casually. Candidates for acute embolectomy should demonstrate evidence of massive PE with cardiopulmonary shock along with an established contraindication to thrombolytic therapy. Furthermore, the availability of an experienced surgical team is essential be-

TABLE 127-5. Thrombolytic Therapy for Venous Thromboembolism

AGENT	DOSAGE SCHEDULE°
Recombinant tissue plasminogen activator (rTPA)	100-mg total dose administered as a continuous infusion over 2 h
Streptokinase	250,000 IU loading dose over 30 min followed by 100,000 IU/h infusion for 24 h
Urokinase	4400 IU/kg loading dose, followed by 4400 IU/kg/h maintenance for 12–24 h

°Food and Drug Administration–approved dosing schedules.

cause even in such hands, the postoperative outcome is commonly associated with adult respiratory distress syndrome, renal failure, and infectious sequelae, particularly mediastinitis.[96]

Transvenous Percutaneous Embolectomy

An alternative approach to embolus extraction is the use of a balloon-tipped steerable catheter device that can be used to extract pulmonary emboli by suction technique. This technique is not without morbidity, and controlled series report a mortality rate of up to 28%.[97] Therefore, this approach should be used only in the setting where thrombolysis is unsuccessful or contraindicated and an experienced interventional team and laboratory is available.

Cardiopulmonary Bypass

Cardiopulmonary bypass can often be lifesaving in hemodynamic collapse caused by PE because its application provides a hiatus until definitive therapy becomes available. This approach requires the placement of large-bore femoral cannulas that can be emergently placed even in an emergency room setting.

FUTURE DIRECTIONS

The future will bring even more challenges in this everchanging area of medicine. Venous thromboembolism too often is left undiagnosed with a consequence of unacceptable morbidity and mortality. In the ICU, a greater exploitation of the diagnostic capabilities of noninvasive ultrasound imaging will evolve. In the therapeutic arena, the use of low molecular weight heparin will increase and may even replace unfractionated heparin as the initial therapy of choice. Furthermore, criteria for the use of thrombolytic therapy will become less stringent and will allow its use in a less restricted manner. Finally, the greatest challenge of the future will lie in perfecting the diagnosis of venous thromboembolism, with emphasis on early, accurate, and noninvasive detection. However, we must not forget the seminal importance of prevention of venous thromboembolism as the cardinal challenge of not only the future, but also the present.

ACKNOWLEDGMENTS

The authors appreciate the editorial assistance provided by Jeanette Cothren.

REFERENCES

1. Freiman DG, Suyemoto J, Wessler S: Frequency of pulmonary thromboembolism in man. *N Engl J Med* 1965;272:1278
2. Anderson FA, Wheeler B, Goldberg RJ, et al: A population based perspective of the hospital incidence and case-fatality rates of deep venous thrombosis and pulmonary embolism: the Worcester DVT study. *Arch Intern Med* 1991;151:933
3. Dalen JE, Alpert JS: Natural history of pulmonary embolism. *Prog Cardiovasc Dis* 1975;17:257
4. Alpert JS, Smith R, Carlson J, et al: Mortality in patients treated for pulmonary embolism. *JAMA* 1976;236:1477
5. Keane MG, Ingenito EP, Goldhaber SZ: Utilization of venous thromboembolism prophylaxis in the medical intensive care unit. *Chest* 1994;106:13
6. Sigel B, Edelstein AL, Savitch L, et al: Type of compression for reducing venous stasis: a study of lower extremities during active recumbency. *Arch Surg* 1975;110:171
7. Wells PS, Lensing AW, Hirsh J: Graduated compression stockings in the prevention of postoperative venous thromboembolism: a meta analysis. *Arch Intern Med* 1994;154:67
8. Nicolaides AN, Fernandes JF, Pollack AV: Intermittent sequential pneumatic compression of the legs in the prevention of venous stasis and postoperative deep venous thrombosis. *Surgery* 1980;87:69
9. Knight MTN, Dawson R: Effect of intermittent compression of the arms on deep venous thrombosis in the legs. *Lancet* 1976;ii:1265
10. Scurr JH, Coleridge-Smith PD, Hasty JH: Regimen for improved effectiveness of intermittent pneumatic compression in deep venous thrombosis prophylaxis. *Surgery* 1987;102:816
11. Collins R, Scrimgeour A, Yusuf S, et al: Reduction in fatal pulmonary embolism and venous thrombosis by perioperative administration of subcutaneous heparin: overview of results of randomized trials in general, orthopedic, and urologic surgery. *N Engl J Med* 1988;318:1162
12. Rosendaal FR, Nurmohamed MT, Buller HR, et al: Low molecular weight heparin in the prophylaxis of venous thrombosis: a meta analysis. *Thromb Haemost* 1991;65:927
13. Hull R, Raskob G, Pineo G, et al: A comparison of subcutaneous low molecular weight heparin with warfarin sodium for

prophylaxis against deep venous thrombosis after hip or knee implantation. *N Engl J Med* 1993;329:1370

14. Ljungstrom KG: The antithrombotic efficacy of dextran. *Acta Chir Scand* 1988;543:26

15. Powers PJ, Gent M, Jay RM, et al: A randomized trial of less intense postoperative warfarin or aspirin therapy in the prevention of venous thromboembolism after surgery for fractured hip. *Arch Intern Med* 1989;149:771

16. Bern MM, Lokich JJ, Wallach SR, et al: Very low doses of warfarin can prevent thrombosis in central venous catheters: a randomized prospective trial. *Ann Intern Med* 1990;112:423

17. Kakkar VV, Planc C, Howe CT, et al: Natural history of postoperative deep-vein thrombosis. *Lancet* 1969;ii:230

18. Hull R, Delmore T, Genton E, et al: Warfarin sodium versus low dose heparin in the long term treatment of venous thrombosis. *N Engl J Med* 1979;301:855

19. Lagerstedt CI, Olsson CG, Fagher BO, et al: Need for long term anticoagulant treatment in symptomatic calf-vein thrombosis. *Lancet* 1985;ii:515

20. Hull RD, Carter CJ, Jay RM, et al: The diagnosis of acute, recurrent, deep venous thrombosis: a diagnostic challenge. *Circulation* 1983;67:901

21. Sevitt S: Venous thrombosis and pulmonary embolism. In: Clark R, Badger FG, Scott S (eds). *Modern Trends in Accident Medicine and Surgery*. London, Butterworth, 1959

22. Hull RD, Raskob GE, Hirsh J: The diagnosis of clinically suspected venous thrombosis. *Arch Surg* 1962;85:738

23. Redman HC: Deep venous thrombosis: is contrast venography the "gold standard"? *Radiology* 1988;163:277

24. Hull RD, Hirsh J, et al: Pulmonary angiography, ventilation lung scanning, and venography for clinically suspected pulmonary embolism with abnormal perfusion lung scan. *Ann Intern Med* 1983;98:891

25. McLachlan MSF, Thomson JG, Taylor DW, et al: Observer variation in the interpretation of lower limb venograms. *Am J Radiol* 1979;132:227

26. Hull RD, Hirsh J, Sackett D, et al: Replacement of venography in suspected venous thrombosis by impedance plethysmography and ^{125}I-fibrinogen leg scanning. *Ann Intern Med* 1981;94:12

27. Hull RD, Hirsh J, Carter CJ, et al: Diagnostic efficacy of impedance plethysmography for clinically suspected deep-vein thrombosis. *Ann Intern Med* 1985;102:21

28. Huisman MV, Buller HR, Tencate JW, et al: Serial impedance plethysmography for suspected deep venous thrombosis in outpatients. *N Engl J Med* 1986;314:823

29. Wheeler HB, Mullick SC: Detection of venous destruction in the leg by measurement of electrical impedance. *Ann NY Acad Sci* 1970;170:804

30. Ramchandani P, Soulen RL, Fedullo LM, et al: Deep vein thrombosis: significant limitations of non invasive tests. *Radiology* 1985;156:47

31. Patterson RB, Fowl RJ, Keller JD, et al: The limitations of impedance plethysmography in the diagnosis of acute deep venous thrombosis. *J Vasc Surg* 1989;9:725

32. Curley FJ, Pratter MR, Irwin RS, et al: The clinical implications of bilaterally abnormal impedance plethysmography. *Arch Intern Med* 1987;147:125

33. White RH, McGahan JP, Daschbach MM, et al: Diagnosis of deep venous thrombosis using duplex ultrasound. *Ann Intern Med* 1989;111:297

34. Lensing AW, Pradoni P, Brandjes D, et al: Detection of deep vein thrombosis by real time B-mode ultrasonography. *N Engl J Med* 1989;320:342

35. Wright DJ, Shepard AD, McPharlin, et al: Pitfalls in lower extremity venous duplex scanning. *J Vasc Surg* 1990;11:675

36. Lensing AW, Levi MM, Buller HR, et al: An objective Doppler method for the diagnosis of deep vein thrombosis. *Ann Intern Med* 1990;113:9

37. Kellewich LA, Bedford GR, et al: Diagnosis of deep venous thrombosis: a prospective study comparing duplex scanning to contrast venography. *Circulation* 1989;79:810

38. Cronan JJ, Dorfman GS, Grusmark J: Lower-extremity deep venous thrombosis: further experience with and refinements of ultrasound assessment. *Radiology* 1988;168:101

39. Jonckheer MH, Abramovici J, Jeghers O, et al: The interpretation of phlebograms using fibrinogen labeled with ^{99m}Tc. *Eur J Nucl Med* 1978;3:233

40. Davis HH, Siegel BNM, Sherman LA, et al: Scintigraphy with 111-indium labeled autologous platelets in venous thromboembolism. *Radiology* 1980;136:203

41. Cranley JJ, Gay AY, Grass AM, et al: A plethysmographic technique for the diagnosis of deep venous thrombosis of the lower extremities. *Surg Gynecol Obstet* 1973;136:385

42. Cooke ED, Pilcher MF: Deep vein thrombosis: a preclinical diagnosis by thermography. *Br J Surg* 1974;61:971

43. Yudelman IM, Nossel HL, et al: Plasma fibrinopeptide A levels in symptomatic venous thromboembolism. *Blood* 1978;51:1189

44. Bounameaux H, Cirafici P, de Moerloose P, et al: Measurement of D-dimer in plasma as diagnostic aid in suspected pulmonary embolism. *Lancet* 1991;337:196

45. Bounameaux H, DeMoerloose P, Perrier A, et al: Plasma measurement of D-dimer as diagnostic aid in suspected venous thromboembolism: an overview. *Thromb Haemost* 1994;71:1

46. Leeper KV, Popovich J, et al: Clinical manifestations of acute PE: Henry Ford Hospital experience. A five year review. *Henry Ford Hosp Med J* 1988;36:29

47. Webster JR, et al: Wheezing due to pulmonary embolism-treatment with heparin. *N Engl J Med* 1966;274:931

48. Bell WR, Simon TL: Current status of pulmonary thromboembolic disease: pathophysiology, diagnosis, prevention, and treatment. *Am Heart J* 1982;103:239

49. Benotti JR, Dalen JE: Pulmonary embolism. In: Rippe JM, et al (eds). *Intensive Care Medicine*. Boston, Little, Brown, 1985:129

50. Lippman M, Fein A: Pulmonary embolism in the patient with COPD. *Chest* 1981;79:39

51. McIntyre KM, Sasahara AA: The hemodynamic response to pulmonary embolism without prior cardiopulmonary disease. *Am J Cardiol* 1971;28:288

52. The Urokinase Pulmonary Embolism Trial: a national cooperative study. *Circulation* 1973;47:1

53. Stein PD, Willis PW: Diagnosis, prophylaxis, and treatment of acute pulmonary embolism. *Arch Intern Med* 1971;143:991

54. Kelly MJ, Elliott LP: The radiologic evaluation of the patient with suspected pulmonary thromboembolic disease. *Med Clin North Am* 1975;59:3

55. Greenspan RH, Ravin CE, Polansky SM, et al: Accuracy of the chest radiograph in diagnosis of pulmonary embolism. *Invest Radiol* 1982;17:539

56. Stein PD, Dalen JE, McIntyre KM, et al: The electrocardiogram in acute pulmonary embolism. *Prog Cardiovasc Dis* 1975;17:247

57. Taplin GV, Johnson DE, Dore EK, et al: Suspensions of radioalbumin aggregates for photoscanning of liver, spleen, lung, and other organs. *J Nucl Med* 1964;5:259

58. The PIOPED Investigators: Value of ventilation/perfusion scan in acute pulmonary embolism: results of the PIOPED study. *JAMA* 1990;263:2753

59. Sasahara AA, Stein M, Simon M, et al: Pulmonary angiography in the diagnosis of thromboembolic disease. *N Engl J Med* 1964;279:1075

60. Bettman MA: Pulmonary angiography. In: Hirsch J (ed). *Venous Thrombosis and Pulmonary Embolism: Diagnostic Methods*. New York, Churchill Livingstone, 1987:150

61. McIntyre KM, Sasahara AA, Sharma GVRK: Pulmonary thromboembolism: current concepts. *Ann Intern Med* 1972; 18:199

62. Novelline RA, Baltarowich OH, Athanavsoulis MD, et al: The clinical course of patients with suspected pulmonary embolism and a negative angiogram. *Radiology* 1978;126:561

63. Nicod P, Peterson KL: Pulmonary angiography in chronic severe pulmonary hypertension. *Ann Intern Med* 1987;107:565

64. Granger RA: The clinical and financial implications of low-osmolar radiologic contrast media. *Clin Radiol* 1984;35:251

65. Patel JJ, Chandrasekaran K, Maniet AR, et al: Impact of the incidental diagnosis of clinically unsuspected central pulmonary artery embolism in treatment of critically ill patients. *Chest* 1994;105:986

66. Pond GT, Ovitt TW, Capp PM: Comparison of conventional angiography with intravenous digital substraction angiography for pulmonary embolic disease. *Radiology* 1983;147:345

67. Shure D: Pulmonary angioscopy. In: Goldhaber SZ (ed). *Pulmonary Embolism and Deep Venous Thrombosis*. Philadelphia, WB Saunders, 1985:269

68. Rogers LQ, Lutcher CL: Streptokinase therapy for deep vein thrombosis: a comprehensive review of the English literature. *Am J Med* 1990;88:389

69. Mavor GE, Galloway JMD: Iliofemoral venous thrombosis: pathological considerations and surgical management. *Br J Surg* 1969;56:45

70. Baritt DW, Jordan SC: Anticoagulant drugs in the treatment of pulmonary embolism: a controlled clinical trial. *Lancet* 1960;i:1309

71. Lilienfeld DE, Chan E, Ehland J, et al: Mortality from pulmonary embolism in the United States: 1962–1984. *Chest* 1990;98:1067

72. Cruikshank MK, Levine MN, Hirsch J, et al: A standard heparin nomogram for the management of heparin therapy. *Arch Intern Med* 1991;151:333

73. Raschke RA, Reilly BM, Guidry JR, et al: The weight-based heparin dosing nomogram compared with a "standard care" nomogram. *Ann Intern Med* 1993;119:874

74. Basu D, Ballus A, Hirsch J, et al: A prospective study of the value of monitoring heparin treatment with the activated partial thromboplastin time. *N Engl J Med* 1972;287:325

75. Hull RD, Raskob GE, Hirsch J, et al: Continuous intravenous heparin compared with intermittent subcutaneous heparin in the initial treatment of proximal-vein thrombosis. *N Engl J Med* 1986;315:1109

76. Young E, Pruis M, Levine MN, et al: Heparin binding to plasma proteins: an important mechanism for heparin resistance. *Thromb Haemost* 1992;67:639

77. Lensing AWA, Prins MH, Davidson BL, et al: Treatment of deep venous thrombosis with low-molecular-weight heparins: a meta analysis. *Arch Intern Med* 1994;155:601

78. Weitz JI, Hudoba M, Massel D, et al: Clot bound thrombin is protected from inhibition by heparin-antithrombin III but is susceptible to inactivation by antithrombin III-independent inhibitors. *J Clin Invest* 1990;86:385

79. Furie B, Diuguid CF, Jacobs M, et al: Randomized prospective trial comparing the native prothrombin antigen with the prothrombin time for monitoring anticoagulant therapy. *Blood* 1990;75:344

80. Kirkwood TBL: Calibration of reference thromboplastins and standardization of the prothrombin time ratio. *Thromb Haemost* 1983;49:238

81. Hirsch J: Is the dose of warfarin prescribed by American physicians unnecessarily high? *Arch Intern Med* 1987;147:769

82. Hull R, Hirsch J, Jay R, et al: Different intensities of oral anticoagulant therapy in the treatment of proximal-vein thrombosis. *N Engl J Med* 1982;307:1676

83. Grassi CJ, Goldhaber SZ: Interruption of the inferior vena cava for prevention of pulmonary embolism: transvenous filter devices. *Herz* 1989;14:182

84. Greenfield LJ, Peyton R, Crate S, et al: Greenfield vena caval filter experience: late results in 156 patients. *Arch Surg* 1981; 16:1451

85. National Heart, Lung, and Blood Institute: Urokinase Pulmonary Embolism Trial: Phase I results. *JAMA* 1970;214: 2163

86. National Heart, Lung, and Blood Institute: Urokinase Pulmonary Embolism Trial: Phase II results. *JAMA* 1974;229: 1606

87. Sharma GVRK, Burleson VA, Sasahara AA, et al: Effect of thrombolytic therapy on pulmonary capillary blood volume in patients with pulmonary embolism. *N Engl J Med* 1980;303:842

88. Marder VK, Sherry S: Thrombolytic therapy. II. Current status. *N Engl J Med* 1988;348:1585

89. Sasahara AA, Sharma GVRK, McIntyre KM, et al: Does thrombolytic therapy alter the prognosis of pulmonary embolism? *Haemostasis* 1986;16(Suppl 3):51

90. Goldhaber SZ: Contemporary pulmonary embolism thrombolysis. *Chest* 1995;107:45S

91. Sharma GVRK, Folland ED, McIntyre KM, et al: Long term hemodynamic benefit of thrombolytic therapy in pulmonary embolic disease [abstract]. *J Am Coll Cardiol* 1990;15:65A

92. Meyer G, Sors H, Charbonnier B, et al: Effects of intravenous urokinase versus alteplase on total pulmonary resistance in acute massive pulmonary embolism. *J Am Coll Cardiol* 1992; 19:239

93. Goldhaber SZ, Vaughan DE, Markis JE, et al: Acute pulmonary embolism treated with tissue plasminogen activator. *Lancet* 1986;ii:886

94. Goldhaber SZ, Kessler CM, Heit JA, et al: A randomized controlled trial of recombinant tissue plasminogen activator versus urokinase in the treatment of acute pulmonary embolism. *Lancet* 1988;ii:293

95. Goldhaber SZ, Haire WD, Feldstein ML, et al: Alteplase versus heparin in acute pulmonary embolism:randomized trial assesing right ventricular function and pulmonary perfusion. *Lancet* 1993;341:507

96. Meyer G, Tamisier D, Sors H, et al: Pulmonary embolectomy: a 20-year experience at one center. *Ann Thorac Surg* 1991; 51:232

97. Timsit J-F, Reynaud P, Meyer G, et al: Pulmonary embolectomy by catheter device in massive pulmonary embolism. *Chest* 1991;100:655

Critical Care, Third Edition, edited by Joseph M. Civetta,
Robert W. Taylor, and Robert R. Kirby.
Lippincott-Raven Publishers, Philadelphia, PA © 1997.

CHAPTER 128

■

Other Embolic Syndromes

Scott A. Deppe
Dan R. Thompson
Roger R. Barrette

IMMEDIATE CONCERNS ■

MAJOR PROBLEMS

1. Other chapters in this section deal with venous thromboembolic disease and pulmonary thromboembolism,
including their diagnosis, treatment, and complications.
2. Other embolic syndromes are seen in the critically ill
patient, necessitating rapid diagnosis and treatment to
avoid life-threatening sequelae.

STRESS POINTS

The other embolic syndromes include the following and
emphasis is placed on their causes, clinical diagnoses, and
treatments:

1. Arterial air embolism
2. Cholesterol embolism
3. Fat embolism
4. Venous air embolism
5. Traumatic fat embolism
6. Amniotic fluid embolism.

ARTERIAL EMBOLISM OF GAS, CHOLESTEROL, OR FAT ■

An arterial embolus can result from the acute expansion of
air (decompression) with subsequent embolization; from the
embolization of venous air, fat, or foreign body embolus

occurring with right-to-left shunts, for example, patent foramen ovale, or noncardiac shunts; from the release of cholesterol into the arterial supply; or from the direct administration of air or fat into the arterial system.

Arterial air embolus is a reported complication seen with
percutaneous thin-needle biopsy of the lung,[1-3] laser bronchoscopy,[4] transbronchial biopsy,[5] mechanical ventilation
during adult respiratory distress syndrome (ARDS),[6] penetrating chest injuries,[7] other pulmonary barotrauma syndromes (emphysematous bulla in scuba divers),[8] indwelling
arterial catheters,[9] coronary balloon angioplasty,[10] cardiopulmonary bypass, and dysbaric arterial gas embolism (neurologic decompression sickness).[11-14] Symptoms and signs of
arterial air emboli are specific for the body region embolized.
The most common, potentially damaging, areas affected are
the cerebral and coronary circulation.

Dysbarism is a term related to problems that result from
either increases or decreases in ambient atmospheric pressure.[15] Dysbaric air embolism (DAE) is caused by rapid or
uncontrolled surface ascent with sudden onset of symptoms
from a compressed air device, usually with signs of an acute
brain injury. Neurologic decompression sickness, the most
serious form of DAE, can also occur while flying at high
altitudes without a pressurized environment. *Decompression
sickness* manifests itself either as type I, or simple decompression sickness, a mild illness characterized by pain in the
joints (particularly shoulders and elbows), pruritus, rash,
cutis marmorata (purple-hued skin mottling), or as type II
decompression sickness (also known as neurologic decompression sickness, arterial gas embolism [AGE], or DAE);
manifested by severe neurologic illness with ataxia, vertigo,
altered mental status, weakness, disturbances of vision and

1905

consciousness, loss of sensation, loss of bladder or bowel control, and pelvic pain. The clinical findings for these diagnoses are summarized in Table 128-1. Although exact occurrence and morbidity rates are unknown for many types of arterial gas embolism, there is an increasing store of data available regarding incidence and complications for known DAE. Studies done by Kizer[11] from 1976 through 1979 in Hawaiian scuba divers and reports from the Diver's Alert Network in 1989,[12] have recorded information on the scope, morbidity, and mortality of decompression sickness. There are between 500 to 600 injuries (50% are < 35 age) and 75 to 100 deaths reported yearly from undersea diving accidents.[12] Kizer[11] identified cases of DAE in which 18% of patients required recompression for diving related disorders. Patients with presumed DAE but who died before recompression treatment were not included due to incomplete data. Of the 42 patients studied, 52% had clinically apparent cerebral arterial air embolism, but with inadequate or omitted recompression (hyperbaric oxygen or return to depth) or confounding neurologic decompression sickness, and 48% had classic cerebral air embolism. The most common presenting signs were asymmetric multiplegia—asymmetric diplegia in lower extremities in 21%, hemiplegia in 19%, monoplegia in 12%, quadriplegia–triplegia in 12%, and unilateral facial nerve palsy with a combination of extremity motor deficits in 10%. Other common findings were sensory disturbances in 62%, vertigo in 43%, visual disturbances in 43% (two initially blind), headaches in 19%, loss of consciousness in 17%, slurred speech in 10%, apnea in 5%, hemoptysis in 5%, and pneumomediastinum in 1 patient. In patients who presented with these complaints, 36% had partial resolution and 20% had complete resolution before recompression therapy. Two patients who arrived at the recompression chamber alive subsequently died (5%), and a total of 78% had complete

or substantial recovery. Most commonly the cause was running out of air at significant depth necessitating an emergency free ascent. Inexperienced divers (20 dives or less) constituted 60% of mortalities.[12] Osteonecrosis is a known, late complication.

The pathophysiology of decompression sickness is based on a disequilibrium arising from changes in atmospheric pressure, particularly when breathing compressed air. At higher atmospheric pressures, large amounts of nitrogen and oxygen become dissolved in tissues and the blood stream. In fatty tissues (neural tissues) the solubility of the gases is high. Nitrogen is not metabolized like oxygen and tends to accumulate. If decompression occurs too rapidly, nitrogen bubbles form in the blood stream and the tissues. Since central nervous system (CNS) tissue has a high fat content, the presence of gas in myelin sheaths is common, as are CNS symptoms and complications. Pulmonary barotrauma occurs with rapid decompression, causing air trapped in the lungs to expand, exceeding the distention limits of the alveoli, resulting in lung parenchymal tears, allowing respired gas into the pulmonary veins and thus into the arterial circulation, which leads to arterial gas embolization distributed in a flow dependent fashion. Additionally, mediastinal emphysema and pneumothorax are both reported complications due to air entry into the mediastinal and pleural spaces.

Onset of symptoms in type II decompression sickness is usually acute, whereas type I decompression sickness symptoms may be delayed for up to 12 hours. Symptoms can progress over several hours. Symptoms are related to the specific tissues involved (see descriptions of types I and II illness earlier and Table 128-1), and manifestations of both type I and type II decompression sickness may present simultaneously. There are significantly less serious cases of decompression sickness in divers who inspire a mixture of oxygen and helium (heliox) as compared to compressed air.[15] It is suggested that all unexplained deaths in diving mishaps should be investigated beginning with plain chest radiographs and subsequent CT scans of the head, neck, and chest.[16] Recompression therapy (hyperbaric oxygen with at least 3 atmospheres absolute [ATA] and 100% oxygen) is recommended for all individuals historically at risk and for all symptomatic individuals.

Arterial air emboli may also occur with venous air in the presence of a right-to-left intracardiac shunt, the most common being a patent foramen ovale (PFO). This problem is well reported in the neuroanesthesiology literature, the entity known as paradoxic air embolism. Venous air embolism is documented to occur in 30% to 45% of patients who undergo intracranial surgery in the sitting position. A PFO is estimated to be present post mortem in 20% to 35% of individuals without a history of cardiac disease.[17] Techniques of transthoracic or transesophageal contrast echocardiography, Doppler, and color flow mapping are valuable in the search for the etiology of all unexplained arterial gas embolism events.[18–20]

Common acute physical findings of arterial gas embolism are focal livedo reticularis, signs of cerebral involvement (including focal defects and seizures), signs of myocardial injury (including arrhythmia, hypotension, and infarction), and facial angioedema.[6,21] Identification of gas in the systemic

TABLE 128-1. Clinical Findings of Decompression Sickness

TYPE I: MILD, SIMPLE DECOMPRESSION SICKNESS

No neurologic symptoms or signs
Joint pain characteristically in the knees, elbows, and shoulders ("the bends")
Itching ("the niggles") of the skin, sometimes associated rashes or cutis marmorata
Fatigue

TYPE II: SERIOUS, NEUROLOGIC DECOMPRESSION SICKNESS

Neurologic signs:
  Coma, convulsions, hemiplegia
  Auditory and visual disturbances (cortical blindness)
  Dysesthesias and sensory deficits
  Coordination deficits, vertigo
  Memory loss, disturbances in mentation
  Dysarthria or aphasia
  Bladder dysfunction (urinary retention)
  Paraplegia or quadriplegia (lower spinal segments more at risk)
  Back, girdle, pelvic pain
Mixture of type I symptoms

Adapted from Greer and Massey 1992,[12] Lowenherz 1992,[14] and James, 1993.[15]

circulation may be difficult because (1) only small quantities of air are necessary to cause significant sympto—[6,21] (2) Intravascular gas clears rapidly (especially when oxygen-rich);[6,21,22] and (3) direct demonstration of air usually requires ultrasonography, CT scanning, or surgery.[6,16,23] Patient positioning significantly dictates the subsequent areas embolized when air is present in the left ventricle. Specifically, the upright position favors embolization of the right carotid, right coronary, and right internal mammary arteries, and the Trendelenburg position favors embolization of the coronary circulation.[6,21]

Arterial air embolism produces vasospasm followed by vasodilation.[21,22,24] Platelet-fibrin occlusion sometimes occurs. Depending on the amount of air and location of embolization, the spectrum of complications can be either transient and reversible or irreversible and fatal. Diagnostic techniques commonly employed include ultrasonography, and immediate computed tomography (CT) of the head and other involved areas.[23,25,26] To prevent air embolism, ultrasonic probes may be used during cardiopulmonary bypass and during neurosurgical procedures.[6,26,27]

The treatment of arterial gas embolism not related to decompression sickness includes institution of 100% oxygen (preferably by mechanical ventilation) to promote more rapid absorption of air bubbles, aggressive institution of anticonvulsants for control or prophylaxis of seizures, and proper positioning of the patient.[2] Proper positioning is probably the prone position with head elevation of 30 degrees to prevent ongoing embolization to the cerebral and coronary circulation.[6,7] Occasionally, depending on logistic considerations and patient stability, hyperbaric oxygen therapy has been successfully used.[2,11] There is little efficacy for previously advocated therapies of intravenous steroids and antiplatelet agents.[2,11] A high index of suspicion, given the right clinical scenario, is needed to diagnose arterial air embolization and thus allow proper therapy and institution of subsequent, protective modalities.

Arterial embolization of cholesterol, also known as the *cholesterol emboli syndrome,* is a known complication of atherosclerotic disease. These events may occur spontaneously, or as the result of an invasive vascular procedure. The multiple cholesterol emboli syndromes are usually the result of invasive procedures.[28–30] Manifestations reported include lower extremity ischemia, renal failure, bowel infarction—hemorrhage or pseudopolyp formation, hemorrhagic gastric ulcers, ischemic cholecystitis, and cerebral vascular accident.[31–33] Early diagnosis and removal of the cholesterol source, when feasible, in conjunction with aggressive supportive care are the mainstays of therapy. However, avoidance of invasive techniques, particularly in the at risk patient, whenever prudent, represents the best solution for this potentially lethal complication.

Finally, arterial embolization of fat has been demonstrated in rare clinical cases.[34,35] This syndrome is reported with a lethal, posttraumatic fat embolism syndrome (FES) (see later) in a patient with a patent foramen ovale, which may suggest a cause for the systemic manifestations of severe FES. It is also reported after autologous glabellar fat injection for treatment of frown lines, manifesting as a middle cerebral artery infarction with unilateral vision loss. Al-

though uncommon, the proper clinical scenario should make the clinician consider this possibility.

VENOUS AIR EMBOLISM

Venous air embolism occurs either as an iatrogenic complication from invasive procedures or as the result of accidental trauma.[36,37] There are multiple known causes of entry of air into the venous system in which systemic complications have resulted, including surgical procedures (total hip arthroplasty, arthroscopy, hysteroscopy, laparoscopy, cesarean section, head–neck or neurologic surgery, liver transplantation, misuse of closed-wound suction units, venous reconstruction, peritoneovenous shunt, cryosurgery); traumatic injury (neck–craniofacial, open thoracic, blunt abdominal trauma); cardiovascular procedures (cardiopulmonary bypass, pulmonary artery catheters, central venous catheters); and other diffuse medical causes such as injection of contrast media, epidural analgesia, hemodialysis, gastrointestinal endoscopy, laser induced hyperthermia, hydrogen peroxide ingestion, and orogenital sex during pregnancy.[36–69]

Small amounts of air transported to the right ventricle and lungs may be completely asymptomatic due to rapid removal. Repeated small injections have experimentally and clinically produced pulmonary hypertension and noncardiogenic pulmonary edema.[68–73] A large bolus of air into the right ventricle can completely obstruct pulmonary blood flow causing cardiac arrest.[74] In addition, both experimentally and clinically, venous air embolism is shown to cause arterial embolization via shunts from passage of air through the pulmonary circulation.[75,76]

Although the exact incidence is unknown, venous air embolus is likely a common phenomenon. Since most episodes are asymptomatic, precise clinical data are lacking. For example, the incidence of venous air embolism during upright neurosurgical procedures is recorded between 40% and 100% versus approximately 25% for all craniotomies.[74–78] Other studies estimate the incidence of venous air embolism in central venous catheter insertions to range from between 1:47 and 1:3000.[36–37,79–80]

Symptoms and signs are dependent on the severity of the insult. Venous air embolism to the lung mimics pulmonary thromboembolism. Presentation includes agitation, confusion, cough, dyspnea, chest pain, wheezing, tachycardia, and hypotension. On immediate auscultation, a mill wheel murmur may be heard.[78] Arterial hypoxemia, hypercapnia, and acidosis are present in severe cases, and the chest radiograph may reveal pulmonary edema, air–fluid levels, or both in the main pulmonary arterial system.[81,82] Representative electrocardiographic findings are sinus tachycardia, P-wave depressions, ST-segment depression, and evidence of acute right ventricular strain.[83] When a pulmonary arterial catheter is present, acute elevation of the central venous and pulmonary artery pressures without elevation of pulmonary artery occlusion pressure usually occurs; however, pulmonary artery pressure may remain normal.[37] The use of capnography shows a widened arterial minus end-tidal carbon dioxide pressure (PCO_2) gradient compatible with increased dead space ventilation.[84]

The emphasis in venous air embolism should be on prevention. Because venous air embolism is a potential surgical complication whenever the operative site is more than 5 cm above the right atrium,[85] if this situation is anticipated, computer-assisted precordial or esophageal audio Doppler should be used.[77,86] Either capnography or mass spectrometry is also advisable.[85] Continuous precordial auscultation alerts the anesthesiologist to this potentially fatal complication.[87] Recently, transesophageal echocardiographic probes demonstrated more sensitivity than precordial Doppler sensors.[88] Surgical procedures with high risk for air embolus (cesarean section, craniotomy, etc) also must be monitored closely, as outlined earlier. Care in following prescribed techniques for catheter placement, including assurance that jugular and subclavian central venous cannulation occurs with the patient in a Trendelenburg position and that the catheter is securely sutured, significantly lessens the risk. Luer-Lok connectors help to prevent detachment. Attention to detail during catheter removal, preferably with the patient performing a Valsalva maneuver in the Trendelenburg position, followed by placement of an airtight dressing, also prevents this complication.

The treatment of venous air embolism consists of immediate placement of the patient in Trendelenburg position with a left lateral decubitus tilt. One hundred percent oxygen should be instituted as rapidly as possible. If a central venous catheter is in position near the right atrium, air aspiration should be attempted and has been effective experimentally.[36,37,89,90] Closed cardiac massage may be as effective as placement of the patient in the left lateral decubitus position. Occasionally, resuscitative drugs with cardiorespiratory support may be necessary. In surgical procedures, as the patient's condition improves, the heart should be elevated above the surgical site if feasible to minimize further air entrainment.[91] In severe cases, mortality may be as high as 50%, emphasizing the need to rapidly diagnose and treat the problem.[92] If immediately available, hyperbaric oxygen therapy has a place in the treatment of severe cases. Hyperbaric oxygen not only decreases bubble size, but also potentiates high oxygen delivery to ischemic tissues.[36,68] Even if delayed, hyperbaric oxygen therapy may have beneficial effects on morbidity and mortality.[93]

FAT EMBOLISM SYNDROME ■

The classic presentation of FES is associated with the clinical triad of dyspnea, mental confusion, and petechiae. A more rigorous criteria for diagnosis is respiratory distress that meets the definition for adult respiratory distress syndrome (ARDS), associated with petechial rash and global neurologic deficits.[36] Although most commonly noted following long-bone–pelvic fractures, its association with a variety of other traumatic and nontraumatic entities is suggested, as summarized in Table 128-2. All age groups, including the pediatric population, may develop FES.[94–96]

A distinction is made between the phenomenon of fat embolism and the clinical entity known as fat embolism syndrome. In virtually all long-bone fractures the phenome-

TABLE 128-2. Possible Causes of the Fat Embolism Syndrome*

Long-bone fractures*
Pelvic fractures*
Total hip or knee replacement*
Lymphangiography*
Other fractures
Median sternotomy
External cardiac massage
Blood transfusions
Bone marrow transplantation
Acute decompression sickness
Septic shock
Acute pancreatitis
Cardiopulmonary bypass
Corticosteroids
Burns
Renal transplantation

---

*Etiologies most commonly associated with fat embolism syndrome.

non of fat embolism occurs.[97,98] The incidence of FES is generally thought to range from 0.5% to 2% in isolated long-bone fractures, to 5% to 10% in multiple, long-bone–pelvic fractures.[99,100] Ganong studied young healthy skiers who sustained isolated fractures to the tibia or femur and suggests FES incidence at 23%, 19% with fractured tibia and 75% with fractured femur.[101] In his study, it is noteworthy that the mortality was 0%. One major problem in determining the incidence is the lack of a standard definition.[36] A spectrum of pathophysiologic changes occurs with the phenomenon of fat embolism. At one end of this spectrum, only subclinical changes occur; while at the extreme, major pathophysiologic changes result in what is diagnosed as fat embolism syndrome.

Absence of immobilization, improper fracture immobilization, closed long-bone fractures, multiple long-bone fractures, delayed operative stabilization, conditions that increase marrow fat content, and shock are all suggested as risk factors that increase the likelihood of developing FES.[102–106] Experimentally, pulmonary fat embolism is demonstrated in rabbits by forced immobilization.[107] FES has been reported in the absence of trauma in a child with muscular dystrophy.[108] FES characteristically presents within the first 72 hours after a traumatic injury. Twenty-five percent of cases are noted within 12 hours, 60% within 24 hours, and 85% within 48 hours.[109] All cases probably develop in the first 72 hours after the insult.[101]

Pulmonary sequelae associated with fat embolism represent the most significant clinical and pathophysiologic changes. In the vast majority of cases, arterial hypoxemia is the earliest indicator of significant fat embolism and remains the cornerstone to the early recognition of FES. Although dyspnea is established as one of the symptoms of the FES triad, arterial hypoxemia is most commonly present before dyspnea.

Three pulmonary patterns of presentation are identified with fat embolism. The first, a hyperacute or fulminant pattern, is characterized by massive embolization and obstruction of the pulmonary capillary bed.[110] Marked elevations in pulmonary artery pressures, drastic reductions in cardiac output, and severe arterial hypoxemia are all usually present. Electrocardiographic abnormalities suggestive of right heart strain may be noted. Death is typically the result of acute cor pulmonale. The second presentation, the subacute pattern, is the classically described presentation of FES. ARDS is the characteristic, pathologic feature.[111] Dyspnea and tachypnea are prominent clinical features associated with hypocapnia and hypoxemia. Thrombocytopenia is a common laboratory finding with this pattern. A temporal delay of 12 to 24 hours in the radiographic appearance in comparison with the onset of clinical symptoms is usually noted. Chest radiographs often demonstrate bilateral, interstitial, or alveolar edema. The third presentation, the subclinical pattern, manifests by mild arterial desaturation (90% to 97%) without associated clinical signs and symptoms.[112] Chest radiographs are usually normal.

Numerous systemic sequelae also may be observed, yet with lesser frequency than pulmonary sequelae. The CNS, retina, skin, and coagulation cascade have significant end-organ responses to systemic fat embolism. Mechanisms proposed to explain entry into the systemic circulation include (1) patent foramen ovale; (2) presence of pulmonary arteriovenous communications; and (3) existence of bronchopulmonary venous shunts. The significance of quantitative fat present in the pulmonary vasculature as sampled from pulmonary capillary blood as a diagnostic tool to assist in quantitation of cardiopulmonary dysfunction is controversial as an etiologic factor.[113–115] The presence of other systemic sequelae, in addition to tachycardia (120 to 140 beats per minute) and unexplained fever (38° to 40°C), are important to establishing the diagnosis of FES and to differentiating fat embolism sequelae from other abnormalities.[116]

CNS manifestations of fat embolism are diverse and nonspecific, ranging from irritability and confusion (common) to focal deficits, seizures, and coma (infrequent).[117] Rare cases of isolated cerebral fat embolism without synchronous pulmonary involvement have been reported. However, arterial hypoxemia before the onset of CNS dysfunction is most typically encountered.[118] Neurologic abnormalities are present in as many as 85% of those who succumb to FES.[36,119]

Retinal lesions develop in 50% to 60% of patients with FES.[119] The presence of retinal lesions remains the only access to in vivo visualization of fat embolism. Initial ophthalmologic examination may demonstrate migrating solitary retinal light reflections within central or choroidal vessels.[120] Later "cotton-wool" exudates and streaky hemorrhages appear along the course of retinal vessels. With time, cotton-wool exudates evolve into a drusen type of fibrotic pigmentation.[121] Transient and occasionally permanent visual disturbances, for example, scotoma, have been reported.

Skin petechiae are present in 50% of patients who develop FES. Petechiae characteristically distribute over the anterior chest, base of the neck, conjunctiva, and axilla.[122] Emergence of petechiae typically occurs 24 to 48 hours from the initial trauma after the appearance of hypoxemia, and other times in association with cerebral fat embolism.[123]

With FES, coagulation abnormalities such as a low-grade consumptive coagulopathy are common.[124] This subclinical form of disseminated intravascular coagulation (DIC) influences platelet activities, coagulation factors V and VIII, and the fibrinolytic system.[125] Despite these changes, clinically observed bleeding disorders are rare. Thrombocytopenia is a frequently observed phenomenon in association with the subacute pulmonary pattern of presentation. The degree of platelet consumption–sequestration appears to be a reliable marker for the severity of pulmonary dysfunction seen in FES.[126–128] Osteonecrosis is another complication associated with the intravascular coagulation manifest in FES.[129]

The diagnosis of FES has as its cornerstone the presence of arterial hypoxemia with associated systemic sequelae confirming this clinical syndrome. Associated sequelae may include fever, petechial rash, and neurologic dysfunction. Although a number of objective scoring indices and criteria for the diagnosis of FES have been suggested,[130,131] lack of specificity and validation makes them of questionable value.[132,133] Other laboratory markers, such as lipuria, sputum fat content, CSF fat, and lipase levels have been unreliable or nonspecific in identifying patients with FES.[116,127,134–136] Study of fat-laden pulmonary macrophages obtained by bronchoalveolar lavage, although originally promising,[137,138] has been shown to be nonspecific.[139,140] Reports on the use of lung perfusion scans utilizing Tc 99m MAA have demonstrated characteristic diffuse subsegmental, mottled perfusion defects in patients with FES that can be helpful in differentiation from fibrin clot type of pulmonary emboli.[141–143] Cerebral fat emboli may be diagnosed by magnetic resonance imaging (MRI) and single photon emission computed tomography (SPECT) scanning.[144]

Aggressive supportive care remains the mainstay of therapy. Effective fracture immobilization, immediate definitive treatment of long-bone fractures, and aggressive resuscitation from hypoperfusion states are important elements in minimizing the risk of developing FES.[103–106,145] Early continuous monitoring of patients at high risk for pulmonary sequelae with pulse oximetry is essential. In the 1960s and early 1970s, mortality from FES ranged from 12% to 50%. More recently, it has been suggested that the mortality from FES approaches zero, with the mortality observed in this traumatized population reflecting the severity of associated injuries.[146] Aggressive supportive pulmonary care, improvements in ventilator technology, and use of ventilatory techniques that minimize both toxic oxygen concentration and ventilator-associated complications may in part explain this decrease in mortality. Historically, hypertonic glucose, intravenous ethanol, aspirin, heparin, and low-molecular-weight dextran had been used in the treatment of FES based on their lipolytic action, inhibition of lipase production, or ability to decrease platelet aggregation. Lack of efficacy and associated side effects have led to abandonment of these forms of therapy.[147–151] The use of corticosteroids in the treatment and prophylaxis of FES has been advocated.[131,151–153] Definitive evidence demonstrating a beneficial effect from corticosteroids in overall survival is lacking. However, adverse effects of corticosteroids appear to play a significant role in the morbidity of other steroid-treated trauma victims.[154,155] To date, no study has examined the benefit-to-risk ratio of corticosteroids in the treatment of FES. Likewise, at least experimentally, prophylaxis with nonsteroidal antiinflammatory agents has been disappointing.[156]

AMNIOTIC FLUID EMBOLISM ▪

Pulmonary embolism in obstetric cases includes two frequent causes—obstetric thromboembolism and amniotic fluid embolism (AFE).[157] The most frequent causes of peripartum maternal death are pulmonary thromboembolism (21%), hypertensive disorders (19%), ectopic pregnancies (12%), AFE (7%), and hemorrhage (7%).[158] AFE is "one of the most catastrophic events possible in the gravid female."[159] Although infrequent by total numbers of cases, AFE remains one of the leading causes of maternal death in the United States.[160] The estimated incidence of AFE as a peripartum complication is between 1:8000 to 1:80,000 (see later), with a mortality of at least 80%.[161] Since most patients die within 1 hour without diagnosis and treatment,[162] the emphasis on early diagnosis and treatment is obvious. Generally, the patient with AFE presents in the peripartum or postabortion period with the sudden onset of life-threatening hypoxemia, shock, and DIC. Since the occurrence of the disorder is uncommon, few physicians have extensive experience in its treatment.[163]

Meyer wrote the first description of AFE in 1926.[164] Recognition of the disorder came with the landmark publication by Steiner and Luschbaugh in 1941.[165] They described eight women with unexpected shock and death following hard or violent labor. Restlessness, dyspnea, cyanosis, and sometimes chills, delirium or vomiting characterized the onset of their illnesses. Rales were consistently heard and each woman died after the onset of shock. On autopsy, evidence of pulmonary edema with widespread pulmonary emboli composed of epithelial squamae, amorphous debris, or mucin were consistently found. None of 14 control patients, who died during labor or immediately postpartum, demonstrated any of the analogous pathologic findings mentioned in the 8 index patients at autopsy. Liban and Raz reported similar observations for 14 cases in 1969,[166] and likewise Morgan reviewed 272 similar cases in 1979.[167] The incidence of AFE is apparently dependent on specific health care regions of the world and methods of reporting the complication. Incidence ranges from 1:8000 for births in the original report of Steiner and Luschbaugh,[165] to 1:27,000,[168] 1:47,300 to 1:63,500,[169] and 1:80,000[170] for live births in Southeast Asia, the United States, and Great Britain, respectively. Within the first hour after the onset of symptoms, up to 50% of these patients died,[167] and in the next 5 hours, an additional 25% died, largely from cardiovascular causes with DIC contributing in other cases.[171–173] In Steiner and Luschbaugh's original study, the average patient was 32 years old, multiparous, and generally had very strong contractions (frequently described as tetanic). Uterine rupture was rare.[165,174] In forty-five percent of patients, AFE is associated with premature placental separation (abruptio placentae or placenta previa).[175] Some data support the contention of higher rates in the later childbearing ages, with higher parity, but the relationship between violent contractions and hard labor is less apparent.[170] Other papers correlate relationships between AFE and cesarean deliveries, or rapid, uncontrolled and violent labor (including the use of uterine stimulants).[176–181] Although the diagnosis

of AFE was originally held in doubt if the patient survived, difficulties with definitions, diagnosis, and underreporting were probably the cause. There are multiple case reports and other literature documenting AFE with survival of both mothers and infants without significant clinical sequelae.[182–185]

AFE causes 12% of the deaths related to legal abortion in the United States.[186] There is a greater associated abortion mortality with the use of the saline instillation method compared with the dilatation and evacuation method.[187] Additionally, AFE is occasionally seen with first-trimester curettage abortion; second-trimester abortion with saline, prostaglandin, urea and hysterectomy; uncomplicated second-trimester pregnancy; abdominal trauma; amniocentesis; and saline amnioinfusion.[188] The onset of symptoms is usually prompt, but rarely, delays up to 48 hours after the event is recorded.[189]

Lung pathology involves alveolar hemorrhage, rupture of alveolar walls, emboli, and polymorphonuclear infiltration. Squamae, amorphous debris, and mucin compose the emboli. The mucin emboli probably originate from meconium mucus or from the mucus producing uterine glands, while the amorphous emboli consist of material resembling the caseous ground substance of vernix caseosa. Polymorphonuclear leukocytes are noted within or on emboli. Emboli are usually found lodged in pulmonary vessels less than 1 mm in diameter. Experimentally, an analogous pathologic picture can be produced in rabbits following injection of amniotic materials.[165] Characteristic lung findings may persist for as long as 5 weeks after delivery.[190] Common pathologic findings in nonsurviving patients are pulmonary edema, pulmonary hemorrhage, and subendocardial hemorrhage. Histologic features include squamous epithelial emboli, fibrin microthrombi, alveolar–interstitial inflammation, and focal myocardial and hepatocellular necrosis.[191]

Clinical features of AFE are biphasic; the initial phase involves profound alterations in cardiac and pulmonary dynamics and a consumptive coagulopathy. The classic presentation consists of the sudden onset of dyspnea and hypotension followed by cardiorespiratory arrest. Presenting signs include respiratory failure and cyanosis in 51%, cardiovascular collapse in 27%, convulsions in 10%, and hemorrhage in 12%.[167] Metabolic acidosis is usually extreme. If the patient survives the initial events, a second phase of respiratory failure characterized by ARDS occurs in up to 70%.[189–192]

Historically, definitive diagnosis occured at autopsy, yet attempts to demonstrate debris and cells in the maternal central circulation have met with some success. Withdrawal of blood from central venous or pulmonary artery catheters shows the presence of squamous and trophoblastic cells. Unless special care is taken in handling the specimen, contamination by adult squames from the mother or the technician may render the use of this finding unreliable.[193] In addition, asymptomatic normal patients also may have squamous and trophoblastic cells in their central circulation during the peripartum period.[194] Still, there is a quantitative difference in the number of cells between patients with and without AFE. The exact limits that allow differentiation between AFE and non-AFE patients remain to be established. Yet, the quantitative and qualitative differences may explain the wide variation in the clinical severity of the disorder.[195] For example, investigators have not noted mucus threads or fat droplets in normal postpartum patients, and more careful characterization may allow differentiation using this finding. Clinical presentation and supportive laboratory findings usually suffice in making the diagnosis. Extensive sampling of cervical debris may be important in suspected cases.[196] Maternal blood sampling for fetal squamous cells and mucin, a new monoclonal antibody that recognizes a structure for a component of meconium and amniotic fluid, and zinc coproporphyrin (present in meconium) all hold promise as noninvasive and sensitive tests for future early diagnosis.[197–199]

At the onset, the differential diagnosis may include aspiration pneumonia, bilateral pneumothoraces, pulmonary embolism, eclampsia, abruptio placentae, ruptured uterus, inverted uterus, septic and hemorrhagic shock, venous air embolism, acute myocardial infarction with other causes of acute left ventricular failure, and cerebrovascular accident.[163] Hemorrhagic shock and pulmonary thromboembolism are usually the most important diagnoses to consider in the clinical setting compatible with AFE.

The postulated sites of entry of amniotic fluid into the right side of the central circulation are 1) through endocervical veins (lacerated even during normal labor); 2) from placental sites (especially when associated with placenta previa, uterine rupture, premature separation of placenta, or cesarean section); and 3) the uterine veins at sites of uterine trauma.[200] Early efforts at developing an animal model confirmed the lethality of an intravenous injection of human amniotic fluid and meconium. Highly conflicting data have come from subsequent animal models. Results have varied depending on species, the source of amniotic fluid (human or animal), the concentration of amniotic fluid particulate matter in the injectate, and the presence or absence of pregnancy. It appears that the pathophysiology, particularly the finding of right ventricular failure, may be secondary to the concentration of the amniotic fluid injected. Two studies in primates have demonstrated that the injection is entirely innocuous, even when the volume of amniotic fluid injected is equivalent to 80% of the total present in the normal woman.[201,202] The conclusion of these studies suggests that pathophysiology in women who died of AFE involved only severe pulmonary artery hypertension secondary to obstruction of the pulmonary bed by emboli or vasospastic changes leading to acute cor pulmonale. These assumptions provided the early basis for therapy.

Animal models fail to explain the noncardiogenic pulmonary edema that is present in up to 70% of patients.[203] Courtney[204] has proposed a two-phase model. The primary phase involves a response of the pulmonary vasculature to amniotic fluid and debris characterized by intense vasospasm leading to severe pulmonary hypertension, profound hypoxemia, and systemic hypotension. An anaphylactoid reaction, direct mechanical obstruction of the microvasculature by particulate material, or pulmonary vasoconstriction induced by vasoactive substances such as complement, prostaglandins, or leukotrienes could trigger these events. In the animal mod-

els, this phase resolves within 30 minutes and could account for the deaths of the nearly 50% of patients who die within the first hour. A correlation between amniotic fluid surfactant and leukotriene production has also been established.[205]

The second phase includes left ventricular failure and decrease in left ventricular contractility. The left ventricular dysfunction may be the result of hypoxia and acidosis, a direct depressant activity of amniotic fluid on the myocardium, or both. The finding of decreased myometrial contractility due to amniotic fluid in vitro, and the frequent finding of uterine atony in AFE, support the theory of direct myocardial depressant activity of amniotic fluid.[206] Several authors have reported patients with evidence of left as well as right ventricular failure.[206–209] Echocardiographic evidence does not support pulmonary hypertension with a right-to-left shift of the interventricular septum to explain the left ventricular dysfunction.[210] One report describes a patient with echocardiographic evidence of elevated end-systolic volume and decreased fiber shortening. This patient had a normal endocardial biopsy, a rapid return to normal cardiac function, and survived.[206] The frequent finding of pulmonary edema out of proportion to the measured pulmonary capillary wedge pressure supports increased permeability (noncardiogenic) pulmonary edema. Still, ARDS and increased hydrostatic pressure both may be implicated in the pulmonary edema of AFE.

Between 40% to 50% of patients with AFE develop DIC.[211,212] Laboratory evidence of coagulopathy may present before the onset of clinical symptoms. Amniotic fluid contains an activator of factor X and a plasmin proactivator; thus activations are independent of particulate matter. Associated fibrinolysis appears to be on a secondary basis.[211–213] Amniotic fluid can activate complement directly through the alternative pathway. Complement activation and leukotriene production may initiate coagulation and eicosanoid cascades leading to DIC and ARDS. The circumstance is probably due to a potentially activating fluid combining with potentially activatable plasma.[212]

After suspecting the diagnosis of AFE, immediate attention to life-sustaining support and treatment is mandatory. Because of initial profound hypoxemia, clinicians should direct their initial efforts at maintaining the highest possible level of tissue oxygenation. The use of moderate levels of positive end-expiratory pressure (PEEP) in the early portion of the disorder is controversial, because of potential concern about overloading an already failing right ventricle. The rapidly changing nature of AFE hemodynamics over the first 30 to 90 minutes, with cardiogenic shock replacing obstructive shock as the underlying pathophysiology, makes prompt placement of a pulmonary artery catheter to guide optimization of oxygen delivery to tissues essential. Support of a failing myocardium with fluid loading, diuresis, or infusion of inotropic agents to improve myocardial contractility must be carefully titrated. In severe cases, successful treatment has been reported with institution of cardiopulmonary bypass and performance of pulmonary artery thromboembolectomy.[214]

The high incidence of DIC mandates monitoring for the impending development of a coagulopathy.[189,190] For treatment of impending or actual DIC, some advocate the administration of cryoprecipitate.[215,216] The rationale proposed for the use of cryoprecipitate is based on the theoretic relationship between the fibronectin level and the functional integrity of the reticuloendothelial system, rather than on the replacement of the fibrinogen consumed.[216] Low fibronectin levels are associated with early signs of fibrinolysis.[213] Theoretically, low fibronectin levels impair the ability of the reticuloendothelial system to phagocytize blood-borne particulate matter leading to pulmonary dysfunctions associated with lodging of the particulate material in the microvasculature. In a patient described by Rodgers and Heymach, 25 units (400 mL) of cryoprecipitate therapy was followed by rapid improvement in hematologic status with a decrease in intrapulmonary shunt fraction. The patient subsequently was extubated and survived.[215] Others have rejected the significance of cryoprecipitate use in this situation, suggesting that improvement may be merely consistent with the natural course of ARDS associated with an isolated thrombocytopenia.[216]

The rationale for heparin use in this setting is based on several factors including in vitro and animal studies.[217] There are several regimens for heparinization. Uszynski[218] described 4 patients that were heparinized rapidly with an initial intravenous bolus of 5000 units of heparin repeated as necessary to reach a therapeutic level. Effectiveness of therapy was monitored by a variety of coagulation tests (activated clotting time, activated partial thromboplastin time (aPTT), or thrombin time). This study recommended maintenance of the aPTT time at 1.5 to 2.5 times normal and continuous heparin infusion for 2 to 3 days followed by subcutaneous heparin. Masson also suggests routine heparinization as a part of the active treatment.[216] Weiner[211] recommends administration of a single intravenous dose of 3000 to 5000 units after making the diagnosis. If this regimen fails to prevent the onset of DIC, therapy should shift instead to replacement of factors with component therapy. Weiner further recommends the use of the antifibrinolytic agents (ε-aminocaproic acid 4 to 6 g every 4 to 6 hours). Premedication with aspirin is not considered helpful.[217] Therapy with nonsteroidal antiinflammatory agents has not been studied.

The literature lists increasing numbers of survivors, particularly when the therapeutic approach is consistent with the present understanding of the pathophysiology of AFE. Most papers that describe the care of the AFE patient mention either the hemodynamic or hematologic problems, rarely with emphasis on both or the total patient. Permanent disability from the effects of the profound cerebral hypoxemia and systemic deposition of embolic material characterize the long-term adverse effects of AFE. Bilateral retinal arteriolar occlusions and permanent pulmonary damage from ARDS secondary to AFE have been described in survivors of AFE.[212,219]

In treating the patient with AFE, one cannot forget the fetus. The onset of AFE may be heralded by fetal distress and Clark[203] recommends monitoring of fetal heart rate, and with sufficient gestational age, intervention for fetal distress. As previously stated, successful outcome for both mother

and infants is a current clinical possibility.[182–185]

REFERENCES

1. Omenaas E, Moerkve O, Thomassen L, et al: Cerebral air embolism after transthoracic aspiration with a 0.6 mm (23 gauge) needle. *Eur Respir J* 1989;2:908
2. Aberle DR, Gamsu G, Golden JA: Fatal systemic arterial air embolism following lung needle aspiration. *Radiology* 1987;165:351
3. Cianci P, Posin JP, Shimshak RR, et al: Air embolism complicating percutaneous thin needle biopsy of the lung. *Chest* 1987;92:749
4. Peachy T, Eason J, Moxham J, et al: Systemic air embolism during laser bronchoscopy. *Anaesthesia* 1988;43:872
5. Strange C, Heffner JE, Collins BS, et al: Pulmonary hemorrhage and air embolism complicating transbronchial biopsy in pulmonary amyloidosis. *Chest* 1987;92:367
6. Marini JJ, Culver BH: Systemic gas embolism complicating mechanical ventilation in the adult respiratory distress syndrome. *Ann Intern Med* 1989;110:699
7. Thomas AN: Air embolism following penetrating chest injuries. *J Thorac Cardiovasc Surg* 1973;66:533
8. Mellem H, Emhjellen S, Horgen O: Pulmonary barotrauma and arterial gas embolism caused by an emphysematous bulla in a scuba diver. *Aviat Space Environ Med* 1986;57:931
9. Chang C, Dughi J, Shitabata P, et al: Air embolism and the radial arterial line. *Crit Care Med* 1988;16:141
10. Kahn JK, Hartzler GO: The spectrum of symptomatic coronary air embolism during balloon angioplasty: causes, consequences, and management. *Am Heart J* 1990;119:1374
11. Kizer KW: Dysbaric cerebral air embolism in Hawaii. *Ann Emerg Med* 1987;16:535
12. Greer HD, Massey EW: Neurological injury from undersea diving. *Neurol Trauma* 1992;10:1031
13. Jerrad DA: Diving medicine. *Emerg Med Clin North Am* 1992;10:329
14. Loewenherz JW: Pathophysiology and treatment of decompression sickness and gas embolism. *J Fla Med Assoc* 1992;79:620
15. James PB: Dysbarism: the medical problems from high and low atmospheric pressure. *J R Coll Physicians Lond* 1993;27:367
16. Williamson JA, King GK, Callanan VI, et al: Fatal arterial gas embolism: detection by chest radiography and imaging before autopsy. *Med J Aust* 1990;153:97
17. Petrozza PH: Preoperative echocardiography and the sitting position [Editorial]. *J Neurosurg Anesthesiol* 1994;6:71
18. Schwarz G, Fuchs G, Weihs W, et al: Sitting position for neurosurgery: experience with preoperative contrast echocardiography in 301 patients. *J Neurosurg Anesthesiol* 1994;6:83
19. Konstadt SN, Louie EK, Black S, et al: Intraoperative detection of patent foramen ovale by transesophageal echocardiography. *Anesthesiology* 1991;74:212
20. Nemec JJ, Marwick TH, Lorig RJ, et al: Comparison of transcranial doppler ultrasound and transesophageal contrast echocardiography in the detection of right-to-left interatrial shunts. *Am J Cardiol* 1991;68:1498
21. Durant TM, Oppenheimer MJ, Webster MR, et al: Arterial air embolism. *Am Heart J* 1949;38:481
22. Goldfarb D, Bahnson HT: Early and late effects on the heart of small amounts of air in the coronary circulation. *J Thorac Cardiovasc Surg* 1963;46:368

23. Hwang TL, Fremaux R, Sears ES, et al: Confirmation of cerebral air embolism with computerized tomography. [Letter]. *Ann Neurol* 1983;13:214

24. Menkin M, Schwartzman RJ: Cerebral air embolism. *Arch Neurol* 1977;34:168

25. Jensen ME, Lipper MH: CT in iatrogenic cerebral air embolism. *AJNR* 1986;7:823

26. Maroon JC, Albin MS: Air embolism diagnosed by Doppler ultrasonography. *Anesth Analg* 1974;53:399

27. Albin MS: The sights and sounds of air. *Anesthesiology* 1983; 58:113

28. Hendel RC, Cuenoud HF, Giansiracusa DF, et al: Multiple cholesterol emboli syndrome: bowel infarction after retrograde angiography. *Arch Intern Med* 1989;149:2371

29. Henderson MJ, Manhire AR: Cholesterol embolization following angiography. *Clin Radiol* 1990;42:281

30. Kawakami Y, Hirose K, Watanabe Y, et al: Management of multiple cholesterol embolization syndrome—a case report. *Angiology* 1990;41:248

31. Fuks DF, Griguoli RE, Borracci RA, et al: Cholesterol embolization following coronary angioplasty. *Rev Port Cardiol* 1992;11:1089

32. Grant DJ, Sanders DSA, Marion ET, et al: Recurrent anaemia due to ischaemic colonic ulceration caused by cholesterol embolism. *Postgrad Med J* 1993;69:320

33. Cheville JC, Mitros FA, Vanderzalm G, et al: Atheroemboli-associated polyps of the sigmoid colon. *Am J Surg Pathol* 1993;17:1054

34. Pell ACH, Hughes D, Keating J, et al: Brief report: fulminating fat embolism syndrome caused by paradoxical embolism through a patent foramen ovale. *N Engl J Med* 1993;329:926

35. Egido JA, Arroyo R, Marcos A, et al: Middle cerebral artery embolism and unilateral visual loss after autologous fat injection into the glabellar area. *Stroke* 1993;24:615

36. King MB, Harmon KR: Unusual forms of pulmonary embolism. *Clin Chest Med* 1994;15:561

37. Orebaugh SL: Venous air embolism: clinical and experimental considerations. *Crit Care Med* 1992;20:1169

38. Spress BD, Sloan MS, McCarthy RJ, et al: The incidence of venous air embolism during total hip arthroplasty. *J Clin Anesth* 1988;1:25

39. Habegger R, Siebenmann R, Kieser CH: Lethal air embolism during arthroscopy. *J Bone Joint Surg Br* 1989;314

40. Brundin J, Thomasson K: Cardiac gas embolism during carbon dioxide hysteroscopy: risk and management. *J Obstet Gynecol Reprod Biol* 1989;33:241

41. Lantz PE, Smith JD: Fatal carbon dioxide embolism complication in attempted laparoscopic cholecystectomy—case report and literature review. *J Forensic Sci* 1994;39:1468

42. DePlates RMH, Jones ISC: Non-fatal carbon dioxide embolism during laparoscopy. *Anaesth Intens Care* 1989;359

43. Lowenwirt IP, Chi DS, Handwerker SM: Nonfatal venous air embolism during cesarean section: a case report and review of the literature. *Obstet Gynecol Sur* 1994;49:72

44. Meyer RM: Venous embolism during cesarean section. [Letter] *Anesth Analg* 1990;70:668

45. Younker D, Rodriguez V, Kavanagh J: Massive air embolism during cesarean section. *Anesthesiology* 1986;65:77

46. Phillips RJL, Mulliken JB: Venous air embolism during a craniofacial procedure (case report). *Plast Reconstr Surg* 1988;82:155

47. Losasso TJ, Martino JD, Muzzi DA: Venous air embolism in the recovery room producing unexplained cardiac dysrhythmias: a case report. *Anesthesiology* 1990;72:203

48. Prager MC, Gregory GA, Ascher N, et al: Massive venous embolism during orthotopic liver transplantation. *Anesthesiology* 1990;72:198

49. King S, Shuckett B: Sonographic diagnosis of portal venous gas in two pediatric liver transplant patients with benign pneumatosis intestinalis: a case report and literature review. *Pediatr Radiol* 1992;22:577

50. Ramsay MA, Klintmalm G, Brajtbord D, et al: Air embolism during liver transplantation. [Letter]. *Anesthesiology* 1988; 68:829

51. Fatal air embolism from misuse of closed-wound suction units. *ECRI Problem Reporting System* 1990;19:200

52. Smelt WLH, DeLange JJ: Delayed air embolism during vascular surgery. *Mt Sinai J Med* 1990;57:112

53. Ahmat KP, Riley RH, Sims C: Fatal air embolism following anesthesia for insertion of peritoneovenous shunt. *Anesthesiology* 1989;70:702

54. Dwyer DM, Thorne AC, Healey JH, et al: Liquid nitrogen instillation can cause venous gas embolism. *Anesthesiology* 1990;73:179

55. Adams VI, Hirsch CS: Venous air embolism from head and neck wounds. *Arch Pathol Lab Med* 1989;113:498

56. Vaulhey JN, Matthews CC: Portal vein air embolization after blunt abdominal trauma. *Am Surg* 1988;54:586

57. Kimura BJ, Chaux GE, Maisel AS: Delayed air embolism simulating pulmonary thromboembolism in the intensive care unit: role of echocardiography. *Crit Care Med* 1994;22: 1884

58. Jastremski MS, Chelluri L: Air embolism and cardiac arrest in a patient with a pulmonary artery catheter: a possible association. *Resuscitation* 1986;14:113

59. Kuhn M, Fitting JW, Leuemberger PH: Acute pulmonary edema caused by venous air embolism after removal of a subclavian catheter. *Chest* 1987;92:364

60. Kane G, Hewins B, Grannis FW: Massive air embolism in an adult following positive pressure ventilation. *Chest* 1988; 93:874

61. Price DB, Nardi D, Teitcher J: Venous air embolization as a complication of pressure injection of contrast media: CT findings. *J Comput Assist Tomogr* 1987;11:294

62. Sleigh JW, Saddler JM: Air embolus and epidural anaesthesia [Letter]. *Anaesthesia* 1986;41:878

63. Air embolism associated with hemodialysis. *ECRI Problem Reporting System* 1989;18:406

64. Lowdon JD, Tidmore TL: Fatal air embolism after gastrointestinal endoscopy. *Anesthesiology* 1988;69:622

65. Schroeder TM, Puolakkainen PA, Hahl J, et al: Fatal air embolism as a complicating factor of laser-induced hyperthermia. *Lasers Surg Med* 1989;9:183

66. Rackoff WR, Merton DF: Gas embolism after ingestion of hydrogen peroxide. *Pediatrics* 1990;85:593

67. Cina SJ, Downs CU, Conradi SE: Hydrogen peroxide: a source of lethal oxygen embolism. A case report and review of the literature. *Am J Forensic Med Pathol* 1994;15:44

68. Bernhardt TL, Goldmann RW, Thombs PA, et al: Hyperbaric oxygen treatment of cerebral air embolism from orogenital sex during pregnancy. *Crit Care Med* 1988;16:729

69. Kaufman BS, Kaminsky SJ, Rackow EC, et al: Adult respiratory distress syndrome following orogenital sex during pregnancy. *Crit Care Med* 1987;15:703

70. Matthay RA, Matthay MA: Pulmonary thromboembolism and other pulmonary vascular diseases. In: George RB, Light RW, Matthay RA (eds). *Chest Medicine*, New York, Churchill Livingstone, 1983:323

71. Ohkuda K, Nakahara K, Binder A, et al: Venous air emboli in sheep: reversible increase in lung microvascular permeability. *J Appl Physiol* 1981;51:887

72. Santoro IH, Lang RM: Iatrogenic air embolism causing the adult respiratory distress syndrome. *Cathet Cardiovasc Diagn* 1989;17:84

73. Lam KK, Hutchinson RC, Gin T: Severe pulmonary oedema after venous air embolism. *Can J Anaesth* 1993;40:964

74. Flanigan J, Gradishar I, Gross R, et al: Air embolism: a lethal complication of subclavian venipuncture. *N Engl J Med* 1969; 281:488

75. Gottdiener JS, Papademetriou V, Notargiacomo A, et al: Incidence and cardiac effects of systemic venous air embolism. *Arch Intern Med* 1988;148:795

76. Marquez J, Sladen A, Gendell H, et al: Paradoxical cerebral air embolism without an intracardiac septal defect. *J Neurosurg* 1981;55:997

77. Hybels C: Venous air embolism in head and neck surgery. *Laryngoscope* 1980;90:946

78. O'Quin RJ, Lakshminarayan S: Venous air embolism. *Arch Intern Med* 1982;142:2173

79. Doblar DD, Hinkle JC, Fay ML, et al: Air embolism associated with pulmonary artery catheter introducer kit. *Anesthesiology* 1982;56:307

80. Feliciano DV, Mattox KL, Graham JM, et al: Major complications of percutaneous subclavian vein catheters. *Am J Surg* 1979;138:869

81. Kinard RE, Williams JE, Orrison WW: Venous air embolism. *South Med J* 1987;80:96

82. Peters SG: Mediastinal air-fluid level and respiratory failure. *Chest* 1988;94:1063

83. Dasher WA, Weiss W, Bogen E: The electrocardiographic pattern in venous air embolism. *Dis Chest* 1955;27:542

84. Nunn JF: Pulmonary embolism. In: Nunn JF (ed). *Applied Respiratory Physiology,* 3rd ed, Boston, Butterworth, 1987: 447

85. Temple AP, Katz J: Air embolization: a potentially lethal surgical complication. *AORN J* 1987;45:387

86. Gibby GL, Ghani GA: Computer-assisted doppler monitoring to enhance detection of air emboli. *J Clin Monit* 1988;4:64

87. Matthews RL: Fatal air embolism. [Editorial]. *Can J Anaesth* 1990;37:12

88. Muzzi DA, Losasso TJ, Black S, et al: Comparison of a tranesophageal and precordial ultrasonic Doppler sensor in the detection of venous air embolism. *Anesth Analg* 1990;70:103

89. Stallworth JM, Martin JB, Postlethwait RW: Aspiration of the heart in air embolism. *JAMA* 1956;143:1250

90. Alvaran SB, Toung JK, Graff TE, et al: Venous air embolism: comparative merits of external cardiac massage, intracardiac aspiration, and the lateral decubitus position. *Anesth Analg* 1978;57:166

91. Fong J, Gadalla F, Gimbel AA: Precordial Doppler diagnosis of haemodynamically compromising air embolism during Caesarean section. *Can J Anaesth* 1990;37:262

92. Kaskuk JL, Penn I: Air embolism after central venous catheterization. *Surg Gynecol Obstet* 1984;159:249

93. Dunbar EM, Fox R, Watson B, et al: Successful late treatment of venous air embolism with hyperbaric oxygen. *Postgrad Med* 1990;66:469

94. Weisz GM, Rang M, Salter RB: Posttraumatic fat embolism in children. *J Trauma* 1973;13:529

95. Limbird TJ, Ruderman RJ: Fat embolism in children. *Clin Orthop* 1978;136:267

96. Dines DE, Lindsheid RL: Fat embolism in elderly patients. *Geriatrics* 1971;26:60

97. Gossling HR, Pellegrini VD: Fat embolism syndrome. *Clin Orthop* 1982;165:68

98. Szabo G, Sereny P, Kocsar L: Fat embolism: fat absorption from the site of injury. *Surgery* 1963;756

99. Peltier LF, Collins JA, Evarts CM, et al: Fat embolism. *Arch Surg* 1974;109:12

100. Fabian TC, Hoots AV, Stanford DS, et al: Fat embolism syndrome: prospective evaluation in 92 fracture patients. *Crit Care Med* 1990;18:42

101. Ganong RB: Fat emboli syndrome in isolated fractures of the tibia and femur. *Clin Orthop* 1993;291:208

102. Aach R, Kissane J: Fat embolism. *Am J Med* 1971;51:258

103. Derks CM, Peters RM: The role of shock and fat embolus in leakage from pulmonary capillaries. *Surg Gynecol Obstet* 1973;137:945

104. Cloutier CT, Lowery BD, Strickland TG, et al: Fat embolism in Vietnam battle casualties in hemorrhagic shock. *Milit Med* 1970;135:369

105. Riska EB, von Bonsdorff H, Hakkinen S, et al: Prevention of fat embolism by early internal fixation of fractures in patients with multiple injuries. *Injury* 1976;8:110

106. Riska EB, von Bonsdorff H, Hakkinen S, et al: Primary operative fixation of long bone fractures in patients with multiple injuries. *J Trauma* 1977;17:111

107. Xue H, Zhang YF: Pulmonary fat embolism in rabbits induced by forced immobilization. *J Trauma* 1992;32:415

108. Pender ES, Pollack CV, Evans OB: Fat embolism syndrome in a child with muscular dystrophy. *J Emerg Med* 1992;10:705

109. Sevitt S: *Fat Embolism.* London, Butterworth, 1962

110. Curtis AM, Knowles GD, Putnam CE, et al: The three syndromes of fat embolism: pulmonary manifestations. *Yale J Biol Med* 1979;52:149

111. Wertzberger JJ, Peltier LF: Fat embolism: the importance of arterial hypoxia. *Surgery* 1968;63:626

112. Pazell JA, Peltier LF: Experience with sixty-three patients with fat embolism. *Surg Gynecol Obstet* 1972;135:77

113. Castella X, Valles J, Cabezuelo MA, et al: Fat embolism syndrome and pulmonary microvascular syndrome. *Chest* 1992; 101:1710

114. Gatlin TA, Seidel T, Cera PJ, et al: Pulmonary microvascular fat: the significance? *Crit Care Med* 1993;21:673

115. Bone RC: Pulmonary microvascular fat in lung injury: an epiphenomenon? [Editorial] *Crit Care Med* 1993;21:644

116. Tachakra SS, Sevitt S: Hypoxaemia after fractures. *J Bone Joint Surg* 1975;57B:197

117. Chan KM, Tham KT, Chow YN, et al: Post-traumatic fat embolism: Its clinical and subclinical presentations. *J Trauma* 1984;24:45

118. Knowles GD, Putnam CE, Smith W, et al: Fat embolism associated with an atrial septal defect. *J Trauma* 1976;16:71

119. Jacobson DM, Terrence CF, Reinmuth OM: The neurologic manifestations of fat embolism. *Neurology* 1986;36:847

120. Findlay JM, DeMajo W: Cerebral fat embolism. *Canad Med Assoc J* 1984;131:755

121. Pollak R, Myers RAM: Early diagnosis of the fat embolism syndrome. *J Trauma* 1978;18:121

122. Roden D, Fitzpatrick G, O'Donoghue H, et al: Purtscher's retinopathy and fat embolism. *Br J Opthalmol* 1989;73:677

123. Arbus L, Fabre J, Bechac G, et al: Clinical, ophthalmoscopic and biological findings in systemic fat embolism. *Acta Neurochir* 1973;29:89

124. Adams CBT: The retinal manifestations of fat embolism. *Injury* 1971;2:221

125. Kearns TP: Fat embolism to the retina. *Am J Opthalmol* 1956;4:1

126. Tachakra SS: Distribution of skin petechiae in fat embolism rash. *Lancet* 1976;1:284
127. Shier MR, Wilson RF: Fat embolism syndrome: traumatic coagulopathy with respiratory distress. *Surg Annu* 1980; 12:139
128. Bergentz SE, Nilsson IM: Effect of trauma on coagulation and fibrinolysis in dogs. *Acta Chir Scand* 1961;122:21
129. Jones JP Jr: Fat embolism, intravascular coagulation, and osteonecrosis. *Clin Orthop* 1993;292:294
130. Gurd AR: Fat embolism: an aid to diagnosis. *J Bone Joint Surg* 1970;52B:732
131. Schonfeld SA, Ploysongsang Y, DiLisio R, et al: Fat embolism prophylaxis with corticosteroids. *Ann Intern Med* 1983;99: 438
132. Nolte WJ, Olofsson T, Schersten T, et al: Evaluation of the Gurd test for fat embolism. *J Bone Joint Surg* 1974;56B:417
133. Lindeque BGP, Schoeman HS, Dommisse GF, et al: Fat embolism and the fat embolism syndrome: a double-blind therapeutic study. *J Bone Joint Surg* 1987;69B:128
134. Cole WG: Urinary fat and fat embolism. *Med J Aust* 1973; 1:1187
135. Peltier LF: Fat embolism: a perspective. *Clin Orthop* 1988; 232:263
136. Cross HE: Examination of CSF in fat embolism. *Arch Intern Med* 1965;115:470
137. Benzer A, Ofner D, Totsch M, et al: Early diagnosis of fat embolism syndrome by automated image analysis of alveolar macrophages. *J Clin Monit* 1994;10:213
138. Chastre J, Fagon JY, Soler P, et al: Bronchoalveolar lavage for rapid diagnosis of the fat embolism syndrome in trauma patients. *Ann Intern Med* 1990;113:583
139. Stanley JD, Hanson RR, Hicklin GA, et al: Specificity of bronchoalveolar lavage for the diagnosis of fat embolism syndrome. *Am Surg* 1994;60:537
140. Vedrinne JM, Guillame C, Gagnieu MC, et al: Bronchoalveolar lavage in trauma patients for the diagnosis of fat embolism syndrome. *Chest* 1992;102:1323
141. Skarzynski JJ, Slavin JD, Spencer RP, et al: "Matching" ventilation/perfusion images in fat embolization. *Clin Nucl Med* 1986;11:40
142. Williams AG, Mettler FA, Christie JH, et al: Fat embolism syndrome. *Clin Nucl Med* 1986;11:495
143. Park HM, Ducret RP, Brindley DC: Pulmonary imaging in fat embolism syndrome. *Clin Nucl Med* 1986;11:521
144. Erdem E, Namer IJ, Saribas O, et al: Cerebral fat embolism studied with MRI and SPECT. *Neuroradiology* 1993;35:199
145. Riska EB, Myllynen P: Fat embolism in patients with multiple injuries. *J Trauma* 1982;22:891
146. Guenter CA, Braun TE: Fat embolism syndrome: changing prognosis. *Chest* 1981;79:143
147. Adler F, Lai SP, Peltier LF: Fat embolism: prophylactic treatment with lipase inhibitors. *Surg Forum* 1961;12:453
148. Gardiner AM, Harrison MH: Report of the treatment of experimental fat embolism with heparin. *J Bone Joint Surg* 1957;39B:538
149. Lewis A, Pappas AM: Experimental fat embolism: evaluation and treatment with low molecular weight dextran. *J Trauma* 1969;9:49
150. Morton KS, Kendall MJ: Failure of intravenous alcohol in the treatment of experimental pulmonary fat embolism. *Can J Surg* 1966;9:286
151. Chintz JL, Kim KE, Onesti G, et al: Pathophysiology and prevention of dextran 40 induced anuria. *J Lab Clin Med* 1971;77:76
152. Kallenbach J, Lewis M, Zaltzman M, et al: "Low-dose" corticosteroid prophylaxis against fat embolism. *J Trauma* 1987; 27:1173
153. Fischer JE, Turner RH, Herndon JH: Massive steroid therapy in severe fat embolism. *Surg Gynecol Obstet* 1971;132:667
154. Deutschman CS, Konstantinides FN, Raup S, et al: Steroids potentiate the metabolic abnormalities and malnutrition of isolated closed-head injury. *Surg Forum* 1985;36:46
155. Huang JC, Gay R, Khella SL: Sickling crisis, fat embolism, and coma after steroid use. *Lancet* 1994;344:951
156. Byrick RJ, Wong PY, Mullen JB, et al: Ibuprofen pretreatment does not prevent hemodynamic instability after cemented arthroplasty in dogs. *Anesth Anal* 1992;75:515
157. Ravindran J: Sudden maternal deaths probably due to obstetrical pulmonary embolism in Malaysia in 1991. *Med J Malaysia* 1994;49:53
158. Davies MG, Harrison JC: Amniotic fluid embolism: maternal mortality revisited. *Br J Hosp Med* 1992;47:775
159. Price TM, Baker VV, Cefalo RC: Amniotic fluid embolism: Three case reports with a review of the literature. *Obstet Gynecol Survey* 1985;40:462
160. Kaunitz AM, Hughes JM, Grimes DA: Causes of maternal mortality in the United States. *Obstet Gynecol* 1985;65:605
161. Olefsky JM: Obesity. In: Wilson JD, Braunwald E, Isselbacher KJ, et al (eds). *Harrison's Principles of Internal Medicine.* New York, McGraw-Hill, 1991:411
162. Lau G: Amniotic fluid embolism as a cause of sudden maternal death. *Med Sci Law* 1994;34:213
163. Cruikshank DP: Amniotic fluid embolism. In: Berkowitz RL (ed). *Critical Care of the Obstetric Patient,* New York, Churchill Livingstone, 1983:431
164. Meyer JR: Embolis pulmonar-caseosa. *Brasil-medico* 1926; 2:301
165. Steiner PE, Luschbaugh CC: Maternal pulmonary embolism by amniotic fluid. *JAMA* 1941;117:1245, 1340
166. Liban E, Raz S: A clinicopathologic study of fourteen cases of amniotic fluid embolism. *Am J Clin Pathol* 1969;51:477
167. Morgan M: Amniotic fluid embolism. *Anesthesia* 1979;34:20
168. Watamamili R, Benjawongkulchai S, Boosiri B: Amniotic fluid embolism: report of five cases. *Southeast Asian J Trop Med Public Health* 1979;10:424
169. Resnik R, Swartz WH, Plumver MH, et al: Amniotic fluid embolism with survival. *Obstet Gynecol* 1976;47:295
170. Department of Health and Social Security: Report on health and social subjects No. 26. In: *Report on confidential enquiries into maternal deaths in England and Wales, 1976–1978.* London: Her Majesty's Stationery Office, 1982
171. Moore PG, James OF, Saltos N: Severe amniotic fluid embolism: case report with haemodynamic findings. *Anaesth Intens Care* 1982;10:40
172. Clark SL, Montz FJ, Phelan JP: Hemodynamic alterations associated with amniotic fluid embolism: a reappraisal. *Am J Obstet Gynecol* 1985;151:617
173. Dudney TM, Elliott CG: Pulmonary embolism from amniotic fluid, fat, and air. *Prog Cardiovasc Dis* 1994;36:447
174. Sperry K: Amniotic fluid embolism: to understand an enigma. *JAMA* 1986;255:2183
175. Peterson M, Taylor H: Amniotic fluid embolism: an analysis of 40 cases. *Obstet Gynecol* 1970;35:787
176. Roungsipragarn R, Herabutya Y: Amniotic fluid embolism: a case report. *J Med Assoc Thai* 1993;76(Suppl 1):105
177. Sisson MC: Amniotic fluid embolism. *Crit Care Nurs Clin North Am* 1992;4:667
178. Sprung J, Cheng EY, Patel S, et al: Understanding and management of amniotic fluid embolism. *J Clin Anesth* 1992;4:235

179. Sisson MC: Amniotic fluid embolism. *NAACOG's Clinical Issues* 1992;3:469
180. Noble WH, St-Armand J: Amniotic fluid embolus. *Can J Anaesth* 1993;40:971
181. Martindale E, Oates S: Amniotic fluid embolism and pregnancy. [Letter] *Br J Hosp Med* 1992;48:135
182. Clark SL: Successful pregnancy outcomes after amniotic fluid embolism. *Am J Obstet Gynecol* 1992;167:511
183. Brown MD: Nonfatal amniotic fluid embolism: three possible cases and a new clinical definition. *Arch Fam Med* 1993;2:989
184. Hwang JJ, Chuang HI, Wei TT, et al: Successful resuscitation of amniotic fluid embolism during cesarean section: a case report. *Acta Anaesthesiol Sin* 1993;31:191
185. Masson RG: Amniotic fluid embolism. *Clin Chest Med* 1992;13:657
186. Guidotti R, Grimes D, Cates W: Fatal amniotic fluid embolism during legally induced abortion in the United States, 1971–1978. *Am J Obstet Gynecol* 1981;141:257
187. Grimes DA, Schulz KF: Morbidity and mortality from second-trimester abortions. *J Reprod Med* 1985;30:505
188. Maher JE, Wenstrom KD, Hauth JC, et al: Amniotic fluid embolism after saline amnioinfusion: two cases and review of the literature. *Obstet Gynecol* 1994;83:851
189. Clark SL: New concepts of amniotic fluid embolism: a review. *Obstet Gynecol Surv* 1990;45:360
190. Attwood HD, Delprado WJ: Amniotic fluid embolism: fatal case confirmed at autopsy five weeks after delivery. *Pathology* 1988;20:381
191. Lau G, Chui PPS: Amniotic fluid embolism: a review of 10 fatal cases. *Singapore Med J* 1994;35:180
192. Koegler A, Sauder P, Jaeger A: Amniotic fluid embolism: a case of non-cardiogenic pulmonary edema. *Intensive Care Med* 1994;20:45
193. Grampaolo C, Schneider V, Kowalski BH, et al: The cytologic diagnosis of amniotic fluid embolism: a critical reappraisal. *Diagn Cytopathol* 1987;3:126
194. Lee W, Ginsburg KA, Cotton DB, et al: Squamous and trophoblastic cells in the maternal pulmonary circulation identified by invasive hemodynamic monitoring during the peripartum period. *Am J Obstet Gynecol* 1986;155:999
195. Kuhlman K, Hidegi D, Tamura RK, et al: Is amniotic fluid material in the central circulation of peripartum patients pathologic? *Am J Perinatol* 1985;2:295
196. Cheung ANY, Luk SC: The importance of extensive sampling and examination of cervix in suspected cases of amniotic fluid embolism. *Arch Gynecol Obstet* 1994;255:101
197. Kobayashi H, Hidekazu O, Terao T: A simple, noninvasive, sensitive method for diagnosis of amniotic fluid embolism by monoclonal antibody TKH-2 that recognizes NeuAcalpha$_2$-6GalNAc. *Am J Obstet Gynecol* 1993;168:848
198. Kanayama N, Yamazaki T, Naruse H, et al: Determining zinc coproporphyrin in maternal plasma—a new method for diagnosing amniotic fluid embolism. *Clin Chem* 1992;38:529
199. Sprung J: Understanding and management of amniotic fluid emboli. [Letter]. *J Clin Anesth* 1992;4:504
200. Weinberger SE, Weiss ST, Cohen WR, et al: Pregnancy and the lung. *Am Rev Respir Dis* 1980;121:559
201. Adamson K, Mueller-Heubach E, Myer RE: The innocuousness of amniotic fluid infusion in the pregnant rhesus monkey. *Am J Obstet Gynecol* 1971;109:977
202. Stolte L, Van Kessel H, Seelen J, et al: Failure to produce the syndrome of amniotic fluid embolism by infusion of amniotic fluid and meconium into monkeys. *Am J Obstet Gynecol* 1967;98:694
203. Clark SL: Amniotic fluid embolism. *Clin Perinatol* 1986;13:801
204. Courtney LD: Coagulation failure in pregnancy. *BMJ* 1970;1:691
205. Lee HC, Yamaguchi M, Ikenoue T, et al: Amniotic fluid embolism and leukotrienes—the role of amniotic fluid surfactant in leukotriene production. *Prostaglandins Leukot Essent Fatty Acids* 1992;47:117
206. Girard P, Mal H, Laine JF, et al: Left heart failure in amniotic fluid embolism. *Anesthesiology* 1986;64:262
207. Peterson EP, Taylor HB: Amniotic fluid embolism: an analysis of 40 cases. *Obstet Gynecol* 1970;35:787
208. Clark SL, Cotton DB, Gonik B, et al: Central hemodynamic alterations in amniotic fluid embolism. *Am J Obstet Gynecol* 1988;158:1124
209. Vanmaele L, Noppen M, Vincken W, et al: Transient left heart failure in amniotic fluid embolism. *Intensive Care Med* 1990;16:269
210. Anderson DG: Amniotic fluid embolism: a re-evaluation. *Am J Obstet Gynecol* 1967;98:336
211. Weiner CP: The obstetric patient and disseminated intravascular coagulation. *Clin Perinatol* 1986;13:705
212. Hammerschmidt DE, Ogburn PL, Williams JE: Amniotic fluid activates complement. *J Lab Clin Med* 104:901
213. Rodgers GP, Heymach GJ: Amniotic fluid embolism. [Letter]. *JAMA* 1986;256:1892
214. Esposito RA, Grossi EA, Coppa G, et al: Successful treatment of postpartum shock caused by amniotic fluid embolism with cardiopulmonary bypass and pulmonary artery thromboembolectomy. *Am J Obstet Gynecol* 1990;163:572
215. Rodgers GP, Heymach GJ: Cryoprecipitate therapy in amniotic fluid embolization. *Am J Med* 1984;76:916
216. Masson RG: Cryoprecipitate therapy in amniotic fluid embolization. *Am J Med* 1985;79:A45
217. Strickland MA, Bates GW, Whitworth NS: Amniotic fluid embolism: Prophylaxis with heparin and aspirin. *South Med J* 1985;78:377
218. Uszynski M: Heparin therapy in the primary phase of amniotic fluid embolism. *Thromb Haemost* 1984;52:362
219. Chang M, Herbert WN: Retinal arteriolar occlusions following amniotic fluid embolism. *Ophthalmology* 1984;91:1634

CHAPTER 129

■

Acute Respiratory Failure in Chronic Obstructive Lung Disease

Michael J. Cicale
Frederick L. Trent

IMMEDIATE CONCERNS ■

MAJOR PROBLEMS

Acute respiratory failure occurs when the respiratory system is unable to maintain alveolar ventilation sufficient to eliminate carbon dioxide produced by the body. Therefore, acute respiratory failure is associated with alveolar hypoventilation and elevation of the arterial partial pressure of carbon dioxide ($PaCO_2$). At the level of the alveolar capillary membrane, the amount of oxygen added and carbon dioxide eliminated is reduced, resulting in the development of hypoxemia and hypercapnia.[1]

STRESS POINTS

1. Patients with acute respiratory failure superimposed on chronic obstructive lung disease (COLD) generally have dyspnea and worsening of their chronic cough, productive of thick mucoid or purulent sputum, for several days.
2. These symptoms are associated with a deterioration in the arterial oxygen partial pressure (PaO_2), often with elevation of the $PaCO_2$.
3. Acute respiratory failure with alveolar hypoventilation and elevated $PaCO_2$ in a patient with previously normal blood gas partial pressures is associated with a proportionately decreased pH but only a slightly higher than normal serum bicarbonate level.
4. This situation is in contrast to patients with chronic respiratory failure and alveolar hypoventilation with an elevated $PaCO_2$. The kidneys retain bicarbonate to compensate for the elevated $PaCO_2$, resulting in a low-normal arterial pH, an increased serum bicarbonate concentration, and a proportionately decreased serum chloride level.
5. Patients with acute respiratory failure superimposed on COLD usually can be distinguished from patients with chronic respiratory failure by arterial blood gas analysis.[1]
6. The first step in the acute setting is to establish a prior diagnosis of chronic bronchitis or emphysema by history, physical examination, chest radiograph, electrocardiogram (ECG), arterial blood gas analysis, and previously performed pulmonary function tests.
7. Patients with COLD generally have a long history of regular tobacco use. Those with chronic bronchitis typically manifest a chronic productive cough, progressive dyspnea on exertion, and, occasionally, wheezing.
8. The predominant symptom in patients with emphysema is chronic and progressive exertional dyspnea; a productive cough and wheezing are usually absent.

ESSENTIAL DIAGNOSTIC TESTS AND PROCEDURES

1. Physical examination of patients with COLD reveals prolonged expiration and diffusely reduced breath sounds. Chronic bronchitis patients may appear cyanotic, with rhonchi and wheezing; emphysematous patients are characterized by asthenia and a barrel-shaped chest and may have dry crackles.
2. Patients with moderate to severe COLD often have associated hypoxemia. Chronic hypoxemia, either intermittent or continuous, results in secondary erythrocytosis, pulmonary hypertension, and cor pulmonale.
3. Physical and laboratory manifestations of cor pulmonale include a loud pulmonary component of the second heart sound, a right ventricular heave, jugular venous distention, lower extremity edema, and ECG evidence of right ventricular hypertrophy and P-pulmonale.
4. The chest radiograph usually shows evidence of hyperinflation. Characteristically, in a posteroanterior radiograph, the dome of the diaphragm is below the tenth interspace posteriorly. In addition, specifically in patients with chronic bronchitis, increased peribronchial and bronchial markings may be noticed. Patchy areas of hyperlucency and fibrosis, flat hemidiaphragms, and attenuated pulmonary vasculature are frequently seen in emphysematous patients.
5. Routine pulmonary function testing is useful in diagnosing and characterizing patients with COLD. The pathophysiologic hallmark is a decrease in the ratio of the forced expiratory volume in 1 second (FEV_1) to forced vital capacity.
6. In addition to decreased expiratory flow rates, patients with chronic bronchitis often manifest an elevated residual volume, hypoxemia, and, in moderately severe disease, hypercapnia. Significant improvement in spirometric testing often occurs after they inhale bronchodilators.
7. Patients with emphysema have an increase in residual volume and total lung capacity, a decrease in the diffusing capacity for carbon monoxide, and relatively well-preserved PaO_2 and $PaCO_2$ until late stages of disease. They have minimal improvement in spirometry after inhaling bronchodilators.
8. These historical, physical, and laboratory features are useful in identifying patients with COLD. The clinical distinction between chronic bronchitis and emphysema is largely artificial, however, because most patients have features of both disease processes.
9. When acute respiratory failure complicates underlying COLD, cough and dyspnea are exacerbated. Clinical signs of acute hypoxemia and hypercapnia, although often present, are nonspecific.
10. Disturbances of consciousness, headache, and abnormal muscle movements may be observed. A bounding pulse, tachycardia, and initial hypertension are followed in severe cases by hypotension with associated vasodilatation and diaphoresis. Definitive assessment of the adequacy of oxygenation and ventilation depends on arterial blood gas analysis.[1]

INITIAL THERAPY

1. Therapeutic approaches are divided conveniently into conservative and nonconservative (aggressive).
2. Conservative therapy includes the following:
   A. Controlled oxygen therapy applied with nasal cannula or face mask
   B. Bronchodilators (β_2-agonists, anticholinergics, and methylxanthines)
   C. Corticosteroids
   D. Antibiotics when a bacterial infection is suspected (or confirmed)
   E. Hydration, tracheal toilet, and occasionally acetylcysteine when tenacious mucus is problematic
   F. Physical stimulation
   G. Heparin
   H. ICU admission
   I. Noninvasive positive-pressure ventilation (PPV) (i.e., continuous positive airway pressure [CPAP] or bilevel positive airway pressure [BIPAP]), mechanical ventilation, or both
3. Aggressive therapy includes the following:
   A. Tracheal intubation or tracheotomy
   B. Mechanical ventilation, with or without positive end-expiratory pressure (PEEP) or CPAP
   C. Carefully controlled weaning and extubation
4. Ancillary measures include nutritional support
5. Complications of the disease and therapy must be considered at all times, including alkalosis syndrome, cardiac arrhythmias, barotrauma, endotracheal tube misplacement and cuff-induced damage, and ventilator malfunction.

DEFINITIONS ■

Chronic obstructive lung disease is a generic term that encompasses a variety of disease processes, the most common of which are chronic bronchitis, emphysema, asthma, bronchiectasis, and cystic fibrosis. This chapter emphasizes the diagnosis and management of adult patients with exacerbation of chronic bronchitis or emphysema; however, many of the principles also apply to patients with other types of obstructive lung disease.

Chronic bronchitis is defined clinically by a chronic productive cough, present on most days for at least 3 months of the year, for at least 2 consecutive years. Pathophysiologically, it is defined as excessive mucus secretion and mucous gland hypertrophy within the tracheobronchial tree. Emphysema is defined as the anatomic alteration of the lung characterized by an abnormal enlargement of the airspaces distal to the terminal and respiratory bronchioles. Additionally, this anatomic alteration is associated with destructive changes of the alveolar walls and alveolar capillary membranes.[2] Although we emphasize a distinction between chronic bronchitis and emphysema, most patients with COLD have features of both disease processes.

ETIOLOGY ▪

Respiratory infection, including acute tracheobronchitis and pneumonia, is the most common cause of an acute exacerbation of underlying obstructive lung disease. *Mycoplasma* infection or viral infection with respiratory syncytial virus, adenovirus, and influenza A$_2$ virus is reported in more than half of these cases. Acute bacterial pneumonia precipitated by infection with *Streptococcus pneumoniae* or *Hemophilus influenzae* also is a common infectious cause of acute respiratory failure in this group.

Congestive heart failure (CHF) causes interstitial and alveolar edema, abnormal alveolar ventilation/perfusion ($\dot{V}A/\dot{Q}$) ratios, and the subsequent development of hypoxemia, hypercapnia, and acidosis. Chronic hypoxemia results in pulmonary hypertension and subsequent right ventricular strain and hypertrophy. Right ventricular muscle fiber bundles cross the interventricular septum and interdigitate with those from the left ventricle. Thus, right ventricular dysfunction in patients with COLD may be associated with simultaneous left ventricular dysfunction.[3]

Oxygen is of major importance in the treatment of hypoxemia during acute exacerbations of COLD. Some patients with chronic bronchitis and emphysema are stimulated to breathe by a hypoxic drive mechanism. If oxygen is administered injudiciously, the PaO$_2$ may rise to a level at which the hypoxic drive is blunted, resulting in alveolar hypoventilation. Medications with sedative properties also are hazardous in patients with carbon dioxide retention. They lead to further alveolar hypoventilation and acute respiratory failure. The most common offending agents are hypnotics and minor tranquilizers.

Acute pulmonary thromboembolism can precipitate acute respiratory failure. A high index of suspicion for this problem is necessary. Because patients with acute exacerbations of obstructive airways disease have $\dot{V}A/\dot{Q}$ ratio inequalities, a routine $\dot{V}A/\dot{Q}$ lung scan is not likely to be helpful in confirming or excluding a diagnosis of pulmonary embolus. Pulmonary angiography is necessary in most instances. A final precipitating cause is the development of a pneumothorax, which usually can be diagnosed without difficulty.[3]

PATHOPHYSIOLOGY ▪

Chronic obstructive lung disease is characterized by alterations in the mechanical properties of the lung that result in an increased workload for the respiratory muscles. Changes in the geometric configuration of the respiratory muscles from hyperinflation and thoracic cage abnormalities and impaired gas exchange resulting primarily from $\dot{V}A/\dot{Q}$ ratio inequalities occur in patients with COLD. To overcome these abnormalities and to achieve a requisite level of alveo-

lar ventilation, patients with COLD must increase their minute ventilation. However, their response to acutely imposed respiratory failure may be insufficient to prevent alveolar hypoventilation and carbon dioxide retention.[4]

MANAGEMENT ▪

Arterial PaCO$_2$ is related to carbon dioxide production ($\dot{V}CO_2$) and to the amount of carbon dioxide eliminated by alveolar ventilation ($\dot{V}A$):

$$PaCO_2 = \frac{\dot{V}CO_2}{\dot{V}A} \times 0.863$$

Treatment of an acute exacerbation of COLD is designed to provide adequate oxygenation, to decrease carbon dioxide production by decreasing the work of breathing, and to increase alveolar ventilation, thus decreasing PaCO$_2$.[2] Management should be directed toward identifying and treating the specific factors that precipitate acute respiratory failure. If acute bacterial infection is suspected, sputum Gram stain tests and cultures of sputum and blood should be obtained, and the patient should be placed on appropriate antibiotic coverage. In similar fashion, CHF must be treated with digitalis and diuretics; inappropriate oxygen therapy corrected by careful and controlled oxygen administration; the injudicious use of sedatives eliminated; a pulmonary thromboembolus treated by heparin or thrombolytic infusion; and a pneumothorax relieved by tube thoracostomy.

CONSERVATIVE THERAPY

In most patients, a specific precipitating cause may not be identified, although an acute viral upper respiratory tract infection often is responsible. Most of these patients respond favorably to conservative treatment, including continuous supplemental oxygen administration, inhaled and intravenous bronchodilators, intravenous steroids and antibiotics, vigorous hydration, aggressive chest physical therapy and tracheal suctioning, avoidance of sedatives, physical stimulation to keep them awake, and diuretics as needed to control pulmonary congestion.[3,5] In one study of 91 consecutive hospitalized patients, 81 were managed successfully on this regimen. Acute mortality for this group was 13%.[5]

Oxygen

The low PaO$_2$ often seen with acute exacerbations of COLD responds well to administered oxygen in terms of increased arterial oxygen saturation, arterial oxygen content (CaO$_2$), and tissue oxygenation[6] (Fig. 129-1). Overall improvement is effected without raising the PaO$_2$ to normal levels that may, in this subgroup of patients, depress respiratory drive.[3] The rise in PaCO$_2$ seen after administering supplemental oxygen often has been ascribed to elimination of the hypoxic stimulus to breathe. Other causes, such as the effect of oxygen on the carbon dioxide dissociation curve of blood (Haldane effect), are also implicated.

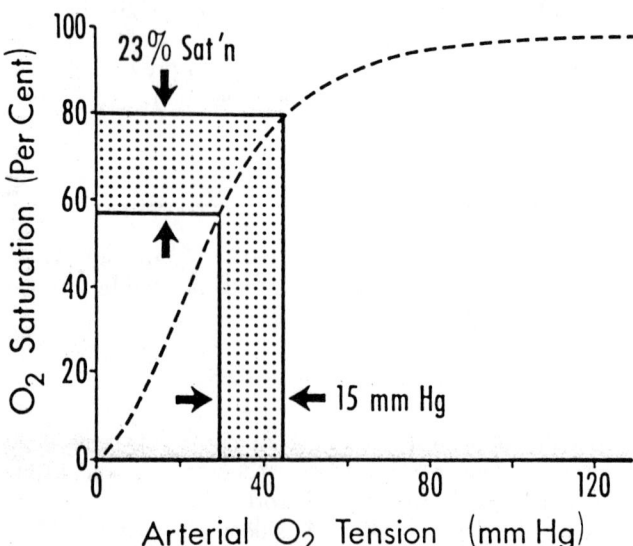

FIGURE 129-1. Oxyhemoglobin dissociation curve illustrates the effect of a 15 mm Hg increase in Pao$_2$ occurring on the steep portion of the curve on percent oxygen saturation. (Block AJ: Practical management of pulmonary insufficiency. In: Eliot RS [ed]. *The Acute Cardiac Emergency: Diagnosis and Management.* Mount Kisco, NY, Futura Publishing, 1972:194.)

The problem was evaluated by Aubier and colleagues[7] in 22 patients with COLD and acute airway infection. After 15 minutes of oxygen administration, minute ventilation decreased slightly to 93% of the control value, and Paco$_2$ increased by an average of 23 mm Hg. Presumably, if no other changes occurred, the decrease in minute ventilation should have resulted in only a 5 mm Hg increase in Paco$_2$. An additional 7 mm Hg increase in Paco$_2$ might be explained by the Haldane effect, leaving almost half of the increase in Paco$_2$ from increased carbon dioxide production or dead space ventilation (i.e., an inhomogeneity of $\dot{V}A/\dot{Q}$ throughout the lungs).

APPLIANCES.   Oxygen can be safely administered by a Venturi mask or nasal cannula. We believe that the safest technique for hypoxemic and hypercapnic COLD patients uses a 28% Venturi mask. A 5 L/minute oxygen flow through the jet entrains 50 L of air to produce an accurate 28% inspired oxygen concentration (FIO$_2$) at a total 55 L/minute flow, which exceeds the patient's minute ventilation.[3]

Although we prefer the Venturi mask, a low-flow nasal cannula system also works well. Bone and coworkers[8] compared oxygen therapy with either a 24% or 28% Venturi mask and low-flow nasal cannula oxygen adjusted to maintain Pao$_2$ between 50 and 60 mm Hg. Twenty-six percent of patients treated with Venturi masks subsequently developed worse carbon dioxide retention, became stuporous, and required tracheal intubation and mechanical ventilation. Patients with more severe hypoxemia and acidosis failed conservative therapy. Sixteen of the 73 patients (22%) treated with nasal cannulae subsequently required tracheal intubation and mechanical ventilation. In this group, initial admission arterial blood gas values predicted the success of conservative medical therapy. Apparently, Venturi mask and low-flow nasal cannula oxygen therapy result in a similar incidence of carbon dioxide narcosis.

Bronchodilators

β_2-AGONISTS.   The relief of bronchial obstruction is desirable to decrease the work of breathing, carbon dioxide production, and alveolar hypoventilation. Various inhaled β_2-selective sympathomimetics are available (Table 129-1). Most have an onset of action between 5 and 15 minutes and a duration between 3 and 6 hours.

Metaproterenol is administered by either a metered-dose inhaler or a gas-powered nebulizer. The usual dose is 0.3 mL of a 5% solution diluted with 2.5 mL of normal saline. Albuterol has a slightly longer duration of action than metaproterenol and is administered by a metered-dose inhaler or nebulizer. The dosage for nebulization is 2.5 to 5 mg administered every 4 hours. Like metaproterenol, terbutaline can be administered by either a metered-dose inhaler or nebulizer. The dosage for nebulization is 5 mL of a 0.1% solution administered every 4 hours.

TABLE 129-1.   MDI Bronchodilators

DRUG	CONCENTRATION/PUFF
Terbutaline Brethaire	200 μg

Albuterol
  Proventil
  Ventolin
	90 μg

Metaproterenol
  Alupent
  Metaprel
	650 μg

Isoetharine Bronkometer	340 μg
Bitolterol Tornalate	370 μg

Isoproterenol
  Isuprel Mistometer
  Medihaler-Iso
	
	130 μg
	75 μg

Isoproterenol and
  phenylephrine
  Duo–Medihaler
	160 μg Iso
	
	240 μg Phenyl

Epinephrine
  Asthmahler
  Bronitin Mist
  Bronkaid Mist
  Medihaler-Epi
  Primatene Mist
	160 μg

Ipratropium Atrovent	18 μg

MDI, metered dose inhaler; Iso, Isoproterenol; Phenyl, phenylephrine.

Modified from: Gold MI, Marcial E: An anesthetic adaptor for all metered dose inhalers [letter]. *Anesthesiology* 1988;68:965.

In general, we prefer to administer these agents by metered-dose inhaler; however, when faced with uncooperative patients or those who are unable to use a metered-dose inhaler correctly, we use a gas-powered nebulizer. Our dosage schedule is every 2 to 4 hours, regardless of the variable half-lives of the different drugs. Oral preparations of all the β_2-sympathomimetics are available; however, we strongly believe that the inhalation route is the preferred delivery method and is better tolerated with fewer side effects by most patients.

ANTICHOLINERGICS.   Additional bronchodilation may be achieved by administering an inhaled anticholinergic agent. Ipratropium bromide, a quaternary ammonium compound related to atropine, may be given by metered dose inhaler or nebulizer (see Table 129-1). It is associated with few side effects because it is not systemically absorbed. The recommended dosage of ipratropium is two inhalations every 4 hours and it can be doubled or tripled without notable side effects.[9] The recommended dosage for a nebulized treatment is 0.5 mg in 2.5 mL of normal saline solution every 4 hours. In addition to its bronchodilating properties, ipratropium reduces the volume of sputum without altering its viscosity or dry weight.[10]

When comparing the efficacy of inhaled anticholinergics versus β_2-agonists, the results of controlled trials in COLD are controversial, mostly because it has been difficult to establish equipotent doses of two agents. In comparison with β_2-agonists, ipratropium bromide has a slower onset of action but a longer duration of action. However, most trials suggest that ipratropium bromide is equally efficacious to β_2-agonists,[11,12] and neither medication potentiates the action of the other. Braun and colleagues[13] in a short-term study compared the effect of ipratropium bromide (two inhalations or 36 μg) versus albuterol (two inhalations or 200 μg) in patients with moderate to severe COLD. They reported that 15 of 25 patients who did not have a significant bronchodilator response to albuterol did respond to ipratropium bromide, which was effective significantly longer than albuterol.

Our practice is to use a combination of both medications in a staggered fashion to avoid using higher doses of β_2-agonists, which may be associated with an increase in side effects including hypokalemia, tremors, and tachycardia. Because ipratropium bromide has become widely available, we rarely use atropine in a nebulized solution but it can be administered at a dosage of 0.05 mg/kg every 4 hours.

METHYLXANTHINES.   The role of theophylline is controversial but remains useful in the therapeutic armamentarium for COLD. In addition to its pharmacologic relaxation of bronchial and vascular smooth muscle, it augments cardiac rate and contractility and acts as a respiratory stimulant.[14] Theophylline also possesses other actions typical of the methylxanthines: coronary vasodilation, diuresis, and cerebral and skeletal muscle stimulation. Other physiologic effects of theophylline that might benefit patients with COLD include enhancement of mucociliary clearance and reduction of pulmonary vascular resistance.

Murciano and colleagues[15] believe diaphragm strength is improved and fatigue decreased in patients with stable COLD treated with theophylline. An increase in forced vital capacity, FEV_1, and maximum transdiaphragmatic pressure can be demonstrated, thus indicating an increase in the maximal inspiratory diaphragmatic force. These effects are observed 7 days after therapy is initiated and persist for 30 days, suggesting that theophylline has a potent and long-lasting effect of diaphragmatic strength in patients with fixed airway obstruction. In a subsequent, randomized, controlled trial of theophylline in patients with severe COLD, Murciano and coworkers[16] also found that theophylline significantly improved the arterial partial pressure of oxygen and carbon dioxide by increasing tidal volumes and minute ventilation.

Oral and intravenous theophylline preparations are available. Many intravenous theophylline products are supplied as aminophylline in which ethylenediamine is added to solubilize theophylline. Each milligram of aminophylline dihydrate contains approximately 0.8 milligrams of theophylline anhydrous. In acutely ill patients, we prefer to administer intravenous theophylline. In patients who have not taken methylxanthines regularly, theophylline should be given as a 5 mg/kg loading dose over approximately 30 minutes followed by a continuous intravenous maintenance dosage of 0.4 mg/kg/hour (equivalent dosage for aminophylline is 6 mg/kg loading dose followed by 0.5 mg/kg maintenance). When patients have taken theophylline preparations chronically but do not have evidence of toxicity, one half of the loading dose should be administered. Patients who routinely take theophylline preparations and have symptoms or signs of toxicity on hospital admission should not receive any methylxanthines until the serum theophylline level is known.

Although the standard maintenance infusion dosage is 0.4 mg/kg/hour, actual dosages may vary between 0.25 and 0.9 mg/kg/hour. Regular cigarette smokers have a markedly increased theophylline clearance and often require much higher doses of methylxanthines. Decreased clearance occurs in patients who are critically ill with COLD, pulmonary edema, CHF, cirrhosis, or pneumonia and in patients receiving cimetidine or erythromycin. Because of the wide individual variation in theophylline metabolism, serum level determinations are extremely useful in patient management.

When patients demonstrate subjective and objective evidence of improvement and no longer require intravenous medications, the correct oral theophylline dose can be calculated from the previously required theophylline infusion rate. Simply multiply the theophylline infusion rate (milligrams per hour) by the desired dosage interval in hours. For example, if a patient requires 37.5 mg/hour of theophylline to maintain a serum theophylline level in the therapeutic range, and you want to administer a slow-release theophylline preparation twice daily, multiply 37.5 mg/hour by 12 hours to compute the dose. Slow-release, sustained-action theophylline preparations are popular because they require dosing usually only once or twice daily. Theophylline should not be administered as a rectal suppository because of its unpredictable absorption.[14]

The usual therapeutic theophylline range is between 10 and 20 μg/mL. For patients receiving oral theophylline preparations, measurement should be performed at the time of peak absorption to avoid toxicity. Measurement just before administration of a slow-release, sustained-action preparation indicates a trough level that may be useful in maximizing theophylline effectiveness.

Because of theophylline's narrow therapeutic window, symptoms and signs of toxicity are common. Manifestations include nausea, vomiting, diarrhea, central nervous system stimulation, and cardiac stimulation (usually sinus tachycardia). Potentially serious manifestations include cardiac arrhythmias, specifically sinus tachycardia at a rate greater than 120 beats per minute with associated premature ventricular beats. Severe intoxication is associated with frequent premature ventricular beats, runs of premature ventricular beats, ventricular tachycardia, and grand mal seizures.[10]

Corticosteroids

Corticosteroids are an important component of conservative treatment. They should be reserved for patients with acute exacerbations that do not seem to be caused by bacterial infections and commonly are used in cases of acute, probably viral, tracheobronchitis. Their mechanisms of action in this population is to decrease inflammation, thereby relieving bronchospasm.

Albert and coworkers[17] studied the effects of methylprednisolone in patients with acute exacerbation of chronic bronchitis. Asthmatic patients were excluded from the study population because it was anticipated that they would have dramatic improvement with corticosteroid therapy. Patients received intravenous aminophylline, nebulized isoproterenol, ampicillin or tetracycline, and oxygen by nasal cannula to maintain an oxygen saturation equal to or above 85%. They were then randomly assigned to receive either methylprednisolone, 0.5 mg/kg, or placebo every 6 hours for a total of 72 hours. Although both prebronchodilator and postbronchodilator FEV_1 were greater for the steroid-treated group than the placebo group, no difference was observed with respect to $PaCO_2$ or pH. One patient developed presumed steroid-induced psychosis, and one patient in each group developed gastrointestinal bleeding.

We routinely use similar doses of intravenous corticosteroids in this type of patient, but we generally administer them for more than 3 days. After patients demonstrate subjective and objective evidence of improvement in air flow obstruction, we switch to a tapering course of prednisone over several weeks. Inhaled corticosteroids do not have any role in the management of acute respiratory failure complicating COLD.

Antibiotics

The routine use of antibiotics in patients with COLD exacerbation in whom pneumonia is not identified is controversial. Although the most common inciting infectious agents are viral, the complication of bacterial invasion is also well established.[18] The most commonly encountered bacterial pathogens in patients with acute exacerbation of COLD include *Streptococcus pneumoniae, Hemophilus influenzae,* and *Moraxella (Branhamela) catarrhalis.* Other important pathogens that can cause an acute exacerbation of COLD include *Legionella, Chlamydia pneumoniae,* and *Mycoplasma.*

Acute bacterial pneumonia should be suspected in patients who present with fever, a cough productive of purulent sputum, localized crackles or consolidation, leukocytosis, and radiographically demonstrated pulmonary infiltrates. Initial antibiotic therapy should be guided by the findings on sputum Gram stain and modified according to sputum, pleural fluid, or blood culture results. Antibiotics are also indicated in patients with a change in their sputum production but without clear evidence of bacterial infection.

We recommend initial parenteral therapy with a broad-spectrum antibiotic such as ampicillin, erythromycin, or a second-generation cephalosporin. In toxic patients, antibiotic coverage should be extended to cover gram-negative infections until the results of sputum, pleural fluid, and blood cultures are available. In less ill patients, antibiotic therapy can be initiated orally with either ampicillin, tetracycline, cephalexin, or trimethoprim/sulfamethoxazole.

Erythromycin is an attractive choice because it is an alternative to penicillin in pneumococcal infections, and it covers infections with *Legionella, Mycoplasma,* and *C. pneumoniae.* The newer macrolide antibiotics such as clarithromycin are also effective in treating the most common pathogens found in patients with acute exacerbations of COLD. When anaerobic infections are suspected, a penicillin, second-generation cephalosporin, or clindamycin are appropriate choices.

Miscellaneous Adjuncts

HYDRATION. Most patients have thick mucoid or purulent tracheobronchial secretions. Vigorous intravenous hydration is indicated to facilitate expectoration. Aggressive chest physical therapy should be performed every 4 hours after inhalation of bronchodilators to mobilize secretions. Nasotracheal suctioning should be performed as needed to remove secretions in weak and debilitated patients or in those with an ineffective cough. When secretions are extremely tenacious and cannot be mobilized, the mucolytic agent, acetylcysteine, may be beneficial. The dose is 5 mL of a 20% solution administered four times daily with a gas-powered nebulizer. This drug should be administered in combination with an inhaled β_2-selective sympathomimetic to counteract bronchospasm.

Pulmonary hypertension and acute cor pulmonale are known complications of acute respiratory failure. Cor pulmonale results in fluid retention and subsequent pulmonary congestion. A low-sodium diet and diuretics should be used to ameliorate intravascular volume overload. The use of digitalis for cor pulmonale is controversial and probably should be reserved for patients with cardiomegaly and a clinical diagnosis of CHF.

PHYSICAL STIMULATION. Many patients become severely hypoxemic, hypercapnic, and acidotic when they fall asleep. Therefore, when they are initially admitted to the hospital, they should receive continuous physical stimulation so that they do not sleep. The goal is to improve their condition sufficiently during the first 24 to 48 hours of hospitalization so that they can then take short naps. Hypnotics, minor tranquilizers, or other drugs with sedative properties should not be administered.

HEPARIN. Most patients with acute exacerbations of COLD initially are placed at bed rest. During this period, heparin should be administered in a subcutaneous dosage of 5000 U twice daily to prevent deep venous thrombosis and subsequent pulmonary thromboembolism. Few studies actually document the effectiveness of this regimen. However, because few side effects occur, and because several studies confirm the effectiveness of low-dose subcutaneous heparin in other bedridden patients, its use in COLD patients seems indicated.

RESPIRATORY STIMULANTS. Various respiratory stimulants have been used, but little evidence supports their efficacy. Doxapram acts through the peripheral carotid chemoreceptors, and at higher dosages it is a respiratory center stimulant. Medroxyprogesterone acetate is used in the treatment of certain types of respiratory failure. Aubier and associates[4] measured the mouth occlusion pressure ($P_{0.1}$, pressure generated 100 milliseconds after the onset of an inspiratory effort performed against a closed glottis at functional residual capacity) in 20 patients with acute exacerbations of COLD and in 11 normal control subjects. All of the patients with acute respiratory failure had hypoxemia, hypercapnia, an increased respiratory rate, decreased tidal volume, and a $P_{0.1}$ that averaged five times the control level, indicating a markedly increased respiratory drive. Treatment with supplemental oxygen resulted in an increased PaO_2 and $PaCO_2$ and a decreased respiratory rate. Although $P_{0.1}$ also decreased, it still remained greater than in control subjects, again indicating an increased respiratory drive.

This evidence suggests that alveolar hypoventilation associated with acute exacerbations of COLD probably is not caused by a decrease in respiratory drive and minute ventilation, but perhaps by an increase in either carbon dioxide production or dead space ventilation. Therefore, treatment with pharmacologically active respiratory stimulants has little physiologic basis in this group of patients.

ICU ADMISSION. Patients with severe hypoxemia and acute respiratory acidemia should be admitted to the ICU. Serious cardiac arrhythmias warrant continuous monitoring of heart rate and rhythm. Frequent recording of vital signs, regular and effective chest physical therapy and tracheal suctioning, and assessment of arterial blood gases and pH are more easily performed in this environment.

Noninvasive Positive-Pressure Ventilation

Noninvasive PPV refers to techniques of improving alveolar ventilation and oxygenation without the use of an endotracheal tube. The theoretical advantages of this approach are avoidance of tracheal intubation and its attendant risks and complications, improved patient comfort, preservation of speech, and swallowing. The goals of noninvasive ventilation include the correction of hypoxemia, hypoventilation, and respiratory acidosis. Different techniques can be used with face and nasal masks including volume-cycled flow generators (VCFGs), CPAP, and BIPAP.

CPAP. By reducing the inspiratory mechanical load, CPAP decreases the inspiratory work of breathing in patients with COLD and acute respiratory failure who are mechanically ventilated.[19] CPAP can also be administered by a facial or nasal tight-fitting mask in selected patients. A major advantage of CPAP flow generators is that they are substantially cheaper than both the BIPAP and VCFGs. High levels of CPAP are poorly tolerated, however, because of the difficulty in exhaling.

BIPAP. Compared with CPAP, BIPAP does seem to provide a theoretical advantage in that pressure support ventilation can be added to decrease the work of breathing. The BIPAP ventilator system is a pressure support ventilator for the application of intermittent positive-pressure ventilation. A pressure-controlling valve maintains pressure at one of two different levels: the expiratory positive airway pressure level, which is equivalent to PEEP on conventional mechanical ventilators; or the inspiratory positive airway pressure level, which is equivalent to pressure support. With BIPAP, the patient cycles between different levels of positive airway pressure and spontaneous ventilation.

The clinician may set the BIPAP system to deliver a certain expiratory positive airway pressure, inspiratory positive airway pressure, and respiratory rate. In addition, it offers three options for providing pressure support ventilation: spontaneous, spontaneous/timed, and timed modes. Another characteristic of BIPAP is that the inhalation-to-exhalation ratio can be adjusted, usually at less than 1, to facilitate expiration. The device lacks alarms or monitors, however, and patients who are ventilator dependent or who have limited ventilatory reserve are not candidates for this form of ventilation. Frequent monitoring of symptoms and arterial blood gas analysis therefore is required.

In a study of 31 consecutive patients with respiratory failure in whom treatment with intubation and mechanical ventilation was being strongly considered, alternative ventilatory support by a BIPAP ventilatory system was used.[20] BIPAP improved patient comfort, slowed the respiratory rate, and improved oxygenation. Twenty-two of 29 patients (76%) recovered from their episode of respiratory failure and were successfully treated with BIPAP and nasal mask, avoiding tracheal intubation. Most of these patients were postsurgical patients, however, with only 5 patients having COLD.

POSITIVE-PRESSURE VENTILATION BY FACE MASK. Brochard and others[21] studied 13 patients with acute exacerbation of COLD treated with inspiratory positive airway pressure delivered by a tight fitting face mask. Of these patients, only one required tracheal intubation and mechanical ventilation. By contrast, in the control group with similar acute exacerbation of COLD, 11 of 13 patients required tracheal intubation and mechanical ventilation.

Marino[22] studied 13 patients admitted for exacerbation of chronic respiratory failure, 10 of whom had COLD. These patients, only 1 of whom had an acute exacerbation before admission, were treated with volume-cycled positive-pressure intermittent mechanical ventilation with a close-fitting nasal CPAP mask. Nine of 13 patients responded to PPV by nasal mask with improvement in blood gas values and clinical status. The 4 remaining patients failed to improve their ventilation, blood gas levels, or clinical status.

CRITIQUE. To our knowledge, no study has directly compared one technique to another in patients with acute respiratory failure; however, Elliott and associates[23] compared different modes of noninvasive ventilatory support and evaluated the effects on ventilation and inspiratory muscle effort and oxygen saturation in stable, awake outpatients with COLD or neuromusculoskeletal disease. Compared with spontaneous ventilation, oxygen saturation and tidal volume increased and inspiratory muscle effort and respiratory rate decreased, the largest changes occurring with BIPAP. No clinically significant differences were observed between VCFG and BIPAP techniques, but CPAP was less effective.

The investigators point out that in acutely ill patients with erratic breathing, small differences between the different modes may assume greater significance. Although these studies show that noninvasive ventilation may be useful in the treatment of acute respiratory failure from COLD, no trials have compared success rates and outcomes to standard therapy with tracheal intubation. In addition, no study has discussed criteria for the discontinuation of noninvasive positive pressure ventilation; thus it remains a clinical judgment. Further comparative studies are required to evaluate the benefit of these devices in acute respiratory failure.

Some of the problems with this alternative mode of noninvasive ventilation include carbon dioxide retention and inability to correct the respiratory acidosis, aspiration, aerophagia, and abrasions on the nasal bridge. Because of the risk of aspiration, face mask ventilation should not be instituted in lethargic or uncooperative patients. Patients who are unable to protect their upper airway are therefore not candidates for noninvasive PPV. Those with copious sputum production are at risk for mucus plugging and atelectasis, and pulmonary toilet may be best achieved by placing an endotracheal tube.

Patients who are hemodynamically unstable or with acute cardiac problems, including ischemia or arrhythmias, also are not ideal candidates for noninvasive PPV. When weaning a patient from face mask ventilation, we recommend increasing periods off the mask while the patient receives supplemental oxygen with a Venturi mask or nasal cannula.

We emphasize the importance of strict selection criteria in determining which patient population can be successfully treated with one of the noninvasive ventilatory techniques. Finally, noninvasive PPV places greater demands on nurses and therapists to closely monitor patients using it.[24] We do not recommend its use in units that are understaffed.

AGGRESSIVE, NONCONSERVATIVE THERAPY

When conservative medical therapy is unsuccessful, tracheal intubation and mechanical PPV are indicated. The timing of intubation and assisted ventilation cannot be predicted on specific arterial blood gas values or tests of lung function. However, stupor and coma caused by carbon dioxide retention or severe respiratory acidemia are indications for intubation. Other indications include the necessity to protect the airway in comatose patients, to aid in the control of profuse and viscous secretions in debilitated patients who are unable to cough effectively, and to prevent intolerable respiratory muscle workloads and fatigue.

Tracheal Intubation

We prefer nasotracheal intubation because of patient comfort and because of the ease in securing the endotracheal tube to prevent migration within the trachea. Large-bore, cuffed endotracheal tubes should be inserted. Our choices are 7.5- to 8.0-mm internal diameter endotracheal tubes for nasotracheal intubation and 8.0- to 8.5-mm internal diameter tubes for orotracheal insertion.

Currently available endotracheal tubes have large-volume, low-pressure cuffs to decrease the incidence of pressure necrosis of the trachea. Immediately after intubation, the endotracheal tube cuff should be inflated to allow a minimal leak around the tube. Tube location within the tracheobronchial tree should be confirmed by physical examination and a portable chest radiograph.

Tracheotomy

Patients may require prolonged tracheal intubation and mechanical ventilation. In such cases, a tracheotomy should be considered. Stauffer and coworkers[25] reviewed the complications and consequences of tracheal intubation and tracheotomy in 150 acutely ill patients. Ninety-seven patients underwent only tracheal intubation; the other 53 underwent tracheotomy, most after a period of tracheal intubation. After 2 days of intubation, patients were randomized to continue tracheal intubation (not to exceed 21 days) or to undergo tracheotomy. Two hundred sixty-eight early clinical problems of tracheal intubation were identified, the most common including excessive cuff pressure, self-extubation, and inability to seal the airway (Table 129-2). Of the 226 total tracheal intubations, 140 (62%) were complicated by one or more early clinical problems.

Eighty-seven early clinical problems of tracheotomy were identified, including stomal infection, stomal hemorrhage, and excessive cuff pressure (Table 129-3). Overall, 34 of the 53 patients who underwent tracheotomy (66%) developed one or more early clinical problems of tracheotomy. The percentage of patients who developed any signs of early clinical problems, therefore, was not different between the two groups.

Laryngotracheal injury was detected at the time of autopsy in 39 of 41 patients (95%) who were treated with tracheal intubation alone. In these patients, the location of the laryngotracheal injury was either supraglottic or at the level of the glottis. Similarly, 20 of 22 patients (91%) who had undergone tracheotomy had laryngotracheal injuries documented at autopsy. However, injuries in this group were infraglottic. The abnormalities included mucosal ulcers, inflammation, edema, and submucosal hemorrhage.

TABLE 129-2. Early Clinical Problems of Tracheal Intubation°

CLINICAL PROBLEM	NO.	PERCENTAGE OF ALL ET
Excessive cuff pressure to achieve seal by minimal occluding pressure technique	42	19
Self-exubation	29	13
Inability to seal airway	24	11
Right main stem bronchus intubation	21	9
Aspiration	17	8
Lip ulceration, cellulitis	16	7
Pharyngeal injury, bleeding	15	7
Mechanical problems with endotracheal tube	14	6
Difficulty suctioning via endotracheal tube	12	5
Pain in nose, mouth, pharynx, or chest related to endotracheal tube	8	4
Glottic edema	5	2
Oral mucous membrane injury	5	2
Tooth avulsion	4	2
Laryngospasm at time of extubation	3	1
Pneumothorax	2	1
Esophageal intubation	2	1
Miscellaneous	49	22
Total	268	

°226 intubations.

Stauffer JL, Olson DE, Petty TL: Complications and consequences of endotracheal intubation and tracheotomy. *Am J Med* 1981;70:65.

Laryngotracheal tomograms were performed in some patients during follow-up evaluation. Evidence of tracheal stenosis was detected in 5 of 27 patients (19%) who had undergone tracheal intubation and in 11 of 17 patients (65%) who underwent tracheotomy. Thus, patients with tracheotomy were more likely to develop tomographic evidence of tracheal stenosis. The study did not confirm an association between the duration of tracheal intubation and the degree of laryngotracheal injury. The mortality associated with tracheotomy was 3%, whereas that with tracheal intubation was negligible.

Both tracheal intubation and tracheotomy are commonly associated with early clinical problems and with evidence of laryngotracheal injury at autopsy. However, the incidence of tracheal stenosis and mortality is much greater after tracheotomy.[25] We recommend tracheotomy only when a major complication of tracheal intubation occurs or after intubation of 3 to 4 weeks' duration.

Mechanical Ventilation

When it is used, mechanical ventilation should incorporate a time-cycled, volume-limited, positive-pressure ventilator. The techniques most commonly used are intermittent mandatory ventilation/synchronized intermittent mandatory ventilation (IMV/SIMV) and assist-control mechanical ventilation (AMV).

IMV/SIMV. IMV delivers a preset tidal volume at preselected intervals but allows spontaneous breathing between ventilator-delivered breaths. Initially, the ventilator can be set to provide most of the patient's minute ventilation. As subjective and objective evidence of improvement occurs, the IMV/SIMV rate is decreased, maintaining constant tidal volume, and the patient's spontaneous ventilation increases.

Many advantages and potential disadvantages are claimed for IMV/SIMV (Table 129-4). Asynchronous breathing between patient and ventilator is decreased, thus improving patient tolerance. Respiratory alkalemia is decreased, and patients "set" their own level of alveolar ventilation. Respiratory muscle function is supported, and the cardiovascular side effects of mechanical ventilation with PEEP are reduced. IMV was initially introduced as a weaning technique and is claimed to shorten weaning time. Potential disadvantages include increased oxygen consumption caused by increased ventilatory work with spontaneous breathing. In addition, IMV/SIMV cannot respond to changes in the patient's respiratory status and, therefore, may require more intensive cardiopulmonary monitoring.[26]

TABLE 129-3. Early Clinical Problems of Tracheotomy°

CLINICAL PROBLEM	NO.	PERCENTAGE OF ALL T
Stomal infection	19	36
Stomal hemorrhage, moderate or greater	19	36
Excessive cuff pressure	12	23
Subcutaneous emphysema	5	9
Stomal erosion or breakdown	5	9
Excessively long skin incision	4	8
Aspiration	4	8
Cardiorespiratory arrest	2	4
Pneumomediastinum	2	4
Mediastinitis	2	4
Septicemia	2	4
Difficulty suctioning by T tube	2	4
Dislodgement of tube resulting in airway obstruction	2	4
Inability to seal airway	2	4
Pneumothorax	2	4
Massive arterial hemorrhage	2	4
Miscellaneous	1	2
Total	87	

T, tracheotomies.

°51 standard tracheotomies

Stauffer JL, Olson DE, Petty TL: Complications and consequences of endotracheal intubation and tracheotomy. *Am J Med* 1981:70:65.

TABLE 129-4. Claimed Advantages and Disadvantages of IMV

ADVANTAGES

1. Prevents asynchronous breathing ("fighting the ventilator")
2. Prevents respiratory alkalemia and allows patients to set their own $PaCO_2$
3. Decreases oxygen consumption because of decreased respiratory alkalemia
4. Shortens weaning time
5. Benefits some patients psychologically and allows weaning of otherwise unweanable patients
6. Maintains respiratory muscle function
7. Improves ventilatory responsiveness to CO_2
8. Reduces cardiovascular effects of mechanical ventilation with PEEP
9. Decreases ventilator-related complications and the amount of equipment needed for ventilatory support
10. Lessens necessity for frequent ventilatory measurements and close monitorinig

DISADVANTAGES

1. Cannot respond to changes in patient status and therefore requires more monitoring
2. Increases oxygen consumption resulting from increased ventilatory work during spontaneous breathing
3. Prolongs weaning, especially if improperly used
4. Increases cost to patient if not built into ventilator or used properly
5. Increases risk of barotrauma by "stacking" breaths

IMV, intermittent mandatory ventilation; PEEP, positive end-expiratory pressure.

Luce JM, Pierson DJ, Hudson LD: Intermittent mandatory ventilation. *Chest* 1981;79:678. Used with permission of American College of Chest Physicians.

AMV. AMV guarantees a minimal level of ventilation with a preselected tidal volume and respiratory rate and provides an assist mechanism so that spontaneous inspiratory effort triggers the ventilator to deliver the same preselected tidal volume. Whenever the spontaneous (assist) rate falls below the preselected control rate, the ventilator "takes over," acting as a backup system to provide the minimum number of breaths per minute.[27]

A potential disadvantage of AMV is respiratory alkalemia,[28,29] which causes cerebral vasoconstriction and induces a leftward shift of the oxyhemoglobin dissociation curve, impairing tissue oxygen delivery. Cardiac arrhythmias and lowering of the seizure threshold may result. Prolonged respiratory alkalemia is associated with the renal excretion of bicarbonate. Subsequently, when spontaneous ventilation resumes, patients with COLD may not be able to maintain the same $PaCO_2$ and acidemia ensues. Respiratory alkalemia usually can be corrected with sedative medication, additional dead space in the ventilator circuit, or adjustment of the ventilator-triggering sensitivity.

Much controversy centers on IMV/SIMV and AMV as the preferred ventilatory modes. Hudson and colleagues[28]

studied 26 patients with acute respiratory failure treated with AMV who developed a respiratory alkalemia. Patients were then switched to IMV at a respiratory rate one half that of the AMV rate. Ten subjects also were treated with IMV at one fourth the AMV rate. The mean arterial pH decreased by 0.03 pH units when IMV was used. The difference was statistically but not clinically significant. Carbon dioxide production significantly increased with IMV, but no change in alveolar ventilation occurred. The decrease in pH with IMV was thought to result from increased carbon dioxide production associated with the increased work of spontaneous breathing. A later publication reported similar findings.[29]

CRITIQUE. We believe that too much controversy has been generated to define the superiority of one ventilatory mode over the other. Extensive clinical experience proves that both techniques are capable of achieving adequate oxygenation and ventilation in patients with acute respiratory failure. We prefer IMV/SIMV because of our familiarity, extensive experience, and successful application.

Initial tidal volume should be adjusted between 10 and 15 mL/kg. Inspired oxygen should be adjusted to maintain a PaO_2 between 75 and 90 mm Hg. When IMV is used, the initial ventilator rate should be set between four and eight breaths per minute and adjusted to maintain a normal pH. With AMV, the initial control ventilator rate also should be set between eight and ten breaths per minute. Adequate humidification is essential in intubated COLD patients.

CPAP. CPAP can be combined with both IMV/SIMV and AMV in treating refractory hypoxemia associated with diffuse alveolar infiltrative diseases. Functional residual capacity is increased, and more normal $\dot{V}A/\dot{Q}$ ratios and oxygenation often result. Hypoxemia in patients with acute exacerbations of COLD usually responds to relatively low concentrations of supplemental oxygen. However, in patients with cardiogenic and noncardiogenic pulmonary edema and hypoxemia that are poorly responsive to the administration of an FIO_2 of 0.5, CPAP may be beneficial.

Major complications associated with CPAP are pulmonary barotrauma and hypotension with resultant decreased tissue oxygenation. Because of these potentially serious complications, and because most patients do not have refractory hypoxemia, CPAP plays a minor role in this patient population.

WEANING. Weaning from mechanical ventilation should be initiated when acute respiratory failure resolves and the patient is clinically stable with no arrhythmias, normal body temperature, adequate oxygenation with a FIO_2 less than 0.5, an improving or "stable" chest radiograph, and a hematocrit above 30%. The major techniques are IMV/SIMV or spontaneous T-tube breathing.

Before IMV/SIMV weaning is started, the FIO_2 should be adjusted to maintain the PaO_2 between 55 and 65 mm Hg to ensure that carbon dioxide retention does not result from removal of the hypoxic stimulus to breathe. The IMV/SIMV rate is then decreased by one or two breaths per minute, as long as the pH remains above 7.35. Arterial blood gas measurements should be obtained after each ventilator adjustment. If the patient remains clinically stable at a rate of zero to one breath per minute, discontinuation of mechanical support and tracheal extubation follow. Oxygen at a slightly higher concentration than was used with mechanical ventilation should be delivered by face mask as soon as the patient is extubated.

When a T tube is used, a variety of ventilatory function measurements are obtained during weaning. If the results of these tests indicate adequate respiratory function, the patient is connected to a T tube, and supplemental oxygen at a concentration slightly higher than that used during mechanical ventilation is delivered. After a brief period of observation, if the patient remains clinically stable and arterial blood gas analysis results are acceptable, extubation can be performed.

Sahn and Lakshiminarayan[30] evaluated 100 ICU patients to identify the factors predictive of successful T-tube weaning. When the patients' clinical condition was stable and PaO_2 was greater than 55 mm Hg while they breathed a FIO_2 less than 0.4, minute ventilation, maximal voluntary ventilation (MVV), and inspiratory peak negative pressure (PNP) were ascertained. Subsequently, they were allowed to breathe spontaneously through a T tube, and arterial blood gas analysis was performed. Patients were separated into three groups.

Seventy-six patients with a minute ventilation less than 10 L were able to double their ventilation with MVV. The patients in this group had a mean inspiratory PNP of 31.5 cm H_2O and were weaned successfully. Seventeen patients in group 2 had a minute ventilation greater than 10 L or could not double their minute ventilation with MVV. They could not be weaned, and their mean PNP was only 17.2 cm H_2O. Seven patients in group 3 had minute ventilation and MVV similar to those in the second group. However, group 3 patients were weaned successfully, and their mean PNP was 28.4 cm H_2O.

NUTRITIONAL THERAPY

Much attention is focused on the nutritional assessment and supplementation of patients in the ICU. Driver and coworkers[31] studied 18 control patients with COLD and 9 subjects treated with tracheal intubation and mechanical ventilation because of acute respiratory failure complicating COLD. Body weight, triceps skin-fold thickness, and arm muscle circumference were all decreased in the latter subjects compared with the control group, indicating a significant depletion of body fat and protein stores.

Because of protein and calorie malnutrition in this subgroup of patients, nutritional supplementation seems reasonable. However, no data support the contention that parenteral nutrition helps in the resolution of respiratory failure, decreases ventilator dependence, or decreases time spent in the ICU and hospital. We recommend nutritional supplementation in patients who appear to be malnourished. Those who are not intubated should be fed orally. Nutritional substrates can be administered enterally or parenterally. We prefer enteral nutrition through a transnasal pediatric feeding tube placed into the duodenum when the gastrointestinal tract is intact and functional. Feeding should not be commenced until the tube is in the duodenum; otherwise, gastric distention, regurgitation, and subsequent pulmonary aspiration can result.

If the gastrointestinal tract is nonfunctional, we use total parenteral nutrition administered through a central venous catheter or a lipid solution infused through a peripheral cannula. Large infusions with high concentrations of glucose increase carbon dioxide production. Patients with COLD often cannot increase their minute ventilation to compensate for the increased $PaCO_2$, and respiratory acidemia is exacerbated.

Herve and associates studied hypercapnic acidemia induced by parenteral nutrition in mechanically ventilated patients. Patients received three different 48-hour nutritional regimens, each of which provided a constant daily nitrogen intake. The *control* regimen used 5% glucose; the *glucose* regimen added 50% glucose; and the *lipid* regimen added 20% fat emulsion. Low and high minute ventilation was used. The respiratory quotient increased in patients receiving the glucose nutritional regimen compared with the control nutritional regimen. Both carbon dioxide production and oxygen consumption increased proportionally in patients treated with the lipid nutritional regimen so that the respiratory quotient was unchanged. Increased $PaCO_2$ and decreased pH occurred at both high and low minute ventilation; however, at low levels, respiratory acidemia improved when the patients were switched from glucose to lipid.

COMPLICATIONS ■

Asmundsson and Kilburn[32] report complications in 146 men during 239 exacerbations of COLD. Seventy-seven patients died during hospitalization. Although this study may be outdated in terms of the number of patients who died, the types of complications observed still occur. They subdivided their complications into ventilatory, infectious, and circulatory categories (Table 129-5).

The most common ventilatory complication was the alkalosis syndrome, which was manifested by tachypnea, confusion, tremors, asterixis, myoclonic jerking, seizures, and cardiac arrhythmias. This syndrome is precipitated by attempts to "normalize" the $PaCO_2$ rather than the pH. Other fatal complications included errors in airway and ventilator management, oxygen toxicity, and severe hypercapnia. Infectious complications included pneumonia, with or without superimposed pulmonary edema. Fatal circulatory complications included acute myocardial infarction, cardiac arrhythmias, hypotension, and pulmonary embolus.

CARDIAC ARRHYTHMIAS

Hudson and associates[33] report that the most common major cardiac arrhythmias in their study were multifocal atrial tachycardia, occurring in 17% of patients, and atrial tachycardia, occurring in 16%. Major supraventricular tachyarrhythmias and ventricular arrhythmias occurred in 47%. Mortality rate with the combination of major supraventricular tachyar-

TABLE 129-5. Fatal Complications During Hospitalization Based on 77 Deaths (53 Autopsies)

VENTILATORY

Alkalosis syndrome	12
Errors of airway management	8
Severe hypercapnia	3
Expanding lung cyst	1
Oxygen toxicity	3
Total	27

INFECTIOUS

Necrotizing pneumonia	18
(with pneumothorax caused by abscesses)	(6)
Pneumonia with pulmonary edema	4
Total	22

CIRCULATORY

Acute myocardial infarction	12
Arrhythmias (ventricular)	11
Intractable low cardiac output	3
Pulmonary emboli	2
Bleeding aortic aneurysm	1
Intracranial bleeding	1
Total	30

OTHERS

Gastrointestinal bleeding	5
Jaundice	3
Renal failure	3
Spinal cord compression	1
Total	12

Asmundsson T, Kilburn KH: Complications of acute respiratory failure. *Ann Intern Med* 1969;70:487. Used with permission of American College of Physicians.

rythmias and ventricular arrhythmias, or with ventricular arrhythmias alone, was 100%, compared with a mortality of 31% to 46% in patients with minor or major supraventricular tachyarrhythmias. Because of the frequency of cardiac arrhythmias and the high associated mortality rate, continuous ECG monitoring is indicated.

MECHANICAL VENTILATION

Complications of mechanical ventilation are common. Zwillich and coworkers[34] prospectively studied 304 medical and surgical patients during 354 episodes of acute respiratory failure (Table 129-6). Complications were subdivided into four classes: those attributable to intubation and extubation, those associated with artificial airways, those attributable to ventilator operation, and those occurring during assisted ventilation. Their findings are as follows.

Intubation/Extubation

The most common complication associated with intubation or extubation was a prolonged intubation attempt, occurring in 30% of patients. Right mainstem bronchial intubation occurred approximately 10% of the time and was associated with increased mortality, hyperventilation, pneumothorax, and atelectasis. Premature extubation occurred in 7% of patients, and self-extubation occurred in 8.5% of patients.

Endotracheal Tubes

Complications associated with endotracheal tubes included cuff air leak in 6% of patients and nasal necrosis in 2% of patients, with one instance of airway obstruction caused by herniation of the cuff over the distal lumen of the endotracheal tube.

Ventilator Function

Complications attributable to ventilator operation were uncommon. Mechanical ventilatory failure occurred in 1.7% of patients. The ventilatory alarms were noted to be turned off in 9% of patients, and ventilatory alarm failure occurred in 4% of patients. The most common complication was inadequate nebulization, occurring 13% of the time. Several medical complications occurred. The two most common were the development of alveolar hyperventilation in 11% of patients and alveolar hypoventilation in 10%. The latter problem was associated with increased mortality.

TABLE 129-6. Complications Observed Prospectively

COMPLICATIONS ATTRIBUTABLE TO INTUBATION AND EXTUBATION

Prolonged intubation attempt
Intubation of right main stem bronchus
Premature extubation
Self-extubation

COMPLICATIONIS ASSOCIATED WITH ENDOTRACHEAL–TRACHEOSTOMY TUBES

Tube malfunction
Nasal necrosis

COMPLICATIONS ATTRIBUTABLE TO OPERATION OF THE VENTILATOR

Machine failure
Alarm failure
Alarm found off
Inadequate nebulization or humidification
Overloading of inspired air

MEDICAL COMPLICATIONS OCCURRING DURING ASSISTED VENTILATION

Alveolar hypoventilation
Alveolar hyperventilation
Massive gastric distention
Pneumothorax
Atelectasis
Pneumonia
Hypotension

Zwillich CW, Pierson DJ, Creagh CE, et al: Complications of assisted ventilation. *Am J Med* 1974;57:161.

Miscellaneous

Atelectasis, pneumonia, and hypotension occurred in about 4% of patients. Pneumothorax occurred in about 4% of patients overall; however, it was observed in 23% of patients treated with PEEP compared with 3.5% of patients treated with mechanical ventilation alone.

PROGNOSIS ■

Although many patients with acute exacerbations of COLD are critically ill and likely to develop several serious and potentially life-threatening complications, the short- and long-term prognosis is actually good. Martin and associates[35] studied patients with COLD and acute respiratory failure secondary to bronchitis. Most were treated conservatively with supplemental oxygen administered by a nasal cannula; intravenous aminophylline, tetracycline, or penicillin; inhaled isoproterenol; chest physical therapy; and, in half of the cases, intravenous methylprednisolone.

Of the 36 patients studied, 34 (94%) survived the acute episode. Only 2 patients died, 1 because of seizures resulting from alcohol withdrawal and aminophylline administration, and 1 from respiratory failure. Only 1 patient failed conservative therapy, necessitating tracheal intubation with mechanical ventilation. This patient subsequently improved and survived. Twenty-six of 36 patients (72%) survived for more than 2 years after hospitalization. Only three required additional hospitalizations during the follow-up period. Eight patients who initially survived the acute episode of respiratory failure died after hospital discharge, but none as a result of respiratory failure.

The onset of right heart failure in 7 patients during the follow-up period was a poor prognostic sign. All eventually required therapy with supplemental home oxygen administration, and only 3 of the 7 patients (43%) survived for 2 years.

This study supports the contention that patients with acute exacerbation of COLD have a better prognosis than is commonly recognized. With appropriate therapy, they have a low hospital mortality rate, and tracheal intubation with mechanical ventilation is rarely required. The 2-year survival rate is similar to that observed in stable outpatients with a similar degree of COLD.[35]

REFERENCES ■

1. Cherniack RM: The management of acute respiratory failure. *Chest* 1970;58:427
2. American Thoracic Society: A statement by the Committee on Diagnostic Standards for Nontuberculous Respiratory Diseases: definitions and classifications of chronic bronchitis, asthma, and pulmonary emphysema. *Am Rev Respir Dis* 1962;85:762
3. Block AJ: Practical management of pulmonary insufficiency. In: Eliot RS (ed). *The Acute Cardiac Emergency: Diagnosis and Management.* Mount Kisco, NY, Futura Publishing, 1972:189
4. Aubier M, Murciano D, Fournier M, et al: Central respiratory drive in acute respiratory failure of patients with chronic obstructive pulmonary disease. *Am Rev Respir Dis* 1980;122:191
5. Smith JP, Stone RW, Muschenheim C: Acute respiratory failure in chronic lung disease. *Am Rev Respir Dis* 1968;97:791
6. Campbell EJM: The J. Burns Lecture: The management of acute respiratory failure in chronic bronchitis and emphysema. *Am Rev Respir Dis* 1967;96:626
7. Aubier M, Murciano D, Milic-Emili J, et al: Effects of the administration of O₂ on ventilation and blood gases in patients with chronic obstructive pulmonary disease during acute respiratory failure. *Am Rev Respir Dis* 1980;122:747
8. Bone RC, Pierce AK, Johnson RL: Controlled oxygen administration in acute respiratory failure in chronic obstructive pulmonary disease. *Am J Med* 1978;65:896
9. Ferguson GT, Cherniack RM: Management of chronic obstructive pulmonary disease. *N Engl J Med* 1993;328:1017
10. Ghafouri MA, Patil KD, Kass I: Sputum changes associated with the use of ipratropium bromide. *Chest* 1984;86:387
11. LeDoux EJ, Morris JF, Temple WP, et al: Standard and double dose ipratropium bromide and combined ipratropium bromide and inhaled metaproterenol in COPD. *Chest* 1989;95:1013
12. Karpel JP: Bronchodilator response to anticholinergic and beta-adrenergic agents in acute and stable COPD. *Chest* 1991;99:871
13. Braun SR, McKenzie WN, Copeland C, et al: A comparison of the effect of ipratropium and albuterol in the treatment of chronic obstructive airway disease. *Arch Intern Med* 1989;149:544
14. Matthay RA, Depew CC: Obstructive airway disease: rational therapy with theophylline agents. *Geriatrics* 1980;35:65
15. Murciano D, Aubier M, Lecocguic Y, et al: Effects of theophylline on diaphragmatic strength and fatigue in patients with chronic obstructive pulmonary disease. *N Engl J Med* 1984;311:349
16. Murciano D, Auclair MH, Pariente R, et al: A randomized, controlled trial of theophylline in patients with severe chronic obstructive pulmonary disease. *N Engl J Med* 1989;320:1521
17. Albert RK, Martin TR, Lewis SW: Controlled clinical trial of methylprednisolone in patients with chronic bronchitis and acute respiratory insufficiency. *Ann Intern Med* 1980;92:753
18. Tager I, Speizer FE: Role of infection in chronic bronchitis. *N Engl J Med* 1975;292:563
19. Petrof BJ, Legare M, Goldberg P, et al: Continuous positive airway pressure reduces work of breathing and dyspnea during weaning from mechanical ventilation in severe chronic obstructive pulmonary disease. *Am Rev Respir Dis* 1990;141:281
20. Pennock BE, Kaplan PD, Carlin BW, et al: Pressure support ventilation with a simplified ventilatory support system administered with a nasal mask in patients with respiratory failure. *Chest* 1991;100:1371
21. Brochard L, Isabey D, Piquet J, et al: Reversal of acute exacerbation of chronic obstructive lung disease by inspiratory assistance with a face mask. *N Engl J Med* 1990;323:1523
22. Marino W: Intermittent volume cycled mechanical ventilation via nasal mask in patients with respiratory failure due to COPD. *Chest* 1991;99:681
23. Elliott MW, Aquilina R, Green M, et al: A comparison of different modes of noninvasive ventilatory support: effects on ventilation and inspiratory muscle effort. *Anesthesia* 1994;49:279
24. Chevrolet JC, Jolliet P, Abajo B, et al: Nasal positive pressure ventilation in patients with acute respiratory failure. *Chest* 1991;100:775
25. Stauffer JL, Olson DE, Petty TL: Complications and conse-

quences of endotracheal intubation and tracheostomy. *Am J Med* 1981;70:65

26. Luce JM, Person DJ, Hudson LD: Intermittent mandatory ventilation. *Chest* 1981;79:678

27. Spearman CB, Sanders HG: Physical principles and functional designs of ventilators. In: Kirby RR, Smith RA, Desautels DA (eds). *Mechanical Ventilation.* New York, Churchill Livingstone, 1985:69

28. Hudson LD, Hurlow RS, Craig KC, et al: Does intermittent mandatory ventilation correct respiratory alkalosis in patients receiving assisted mechanical ventilation? *Am Rev Respir Dis* 1985;132:1071

29. Groeger JS, Levinson MR, Carlon GC: Assist control versus synchronized intermittent mandatory ventilation during acute respiratory failure. *Crit Care Med* 1989;17:607

30. Sahn SA, Lakshiminarayan S: Bedside criteria for discontinuation of mechanical ventilation. *Chest* 1973;63:1002

31. Driver AG, McAlvevy MT, Smith JL: Nutritional assessment of patients with chronic obstructive pulmonary disease and acute respiratory failure. *Chest* 1982;82:568

32. Asmundsson T, Kilburn KH: Complications of acute respiratory failure. *Ann Intern Med* 1969;70:487

33. Hudson LD, Kurt TL, Petty TL, et al: Arrhythmias associated with acute respiratory failure in patients with chronic airway obstruction. *Chest* 1973;63:661

34. Zwillich CW, Pierson DJ, Creagh CE, et al: Complications of assisted ventilation. *Am J Med* 1974;57:161

35. Martin TR, Lewis SW, Albert RK: The prognosis of patients with chronic obstructive pulmonary disease after hospitalization for acute respiratory failure. *Chest* 1982;82:310

Critical Care, Third Edition, edited by Joseph M. Civetta,
Robert W. Taylor, and Robert R. Kirby.
Lippincott-Raven Publishers, Philadelphia, PA © 1997.

CHAPTER 130

∎

Life-Threatening Bronchospasm in the Asthmatic

R. Phillip Dellinger

IMMEDIATE CONCERNS ∎

MAJOR PROBLEMS

Critically ill asthmatic patients are often encountered in the emergency department and the ICU. The term *status asthmaticus* is used to imply that the patient is refractory to traditional beta-agonist and theophylline therapy. This condition is usually associated with a prolonged asthma attack and implies that inflammatory changes have occurred that are not easily reversed by standard bronchodilator therapy.

STRESS POINTS

1. Antiinflammatory therapy, although not immediately effective, is essential.
2. The *initial* management of severe, life-threatening bronchospasm centers around aggressive use of bronchodilator therapy.
3. The primary cause of respiratory demise in the patient with severe asthma is acute respiratory acidosis and ventilatory insufficiency. This is related to the increased work of breathing due to a combination of decreased lung compliance and increased minute ventilation requirements. Acute respiratory acidosis may lead to depressed level of consciousness and loss of airway protection.
4. Patients with status asthmaticus may be unresponsive to initial therapeutic intervention and may require prolonged and aggressive therapy.[1,2]
5. This disease process, at its severest, offers great challenge to the intensivist, both from a medical therapy and ventilatory strategy standpoint.

ESSENTIAL DIAGNOSTIC TESTS AND PROCEDURES

1. History and physical examination
2. Arterial blood gases
3. Chest radiograph
4. Complete blood count (CBC), serum chemistries
5. Peak expiratory flow measurements

INITIAL THERAPY

1. Initial concerns in the asthmatic patient with severe bronchospasm should be directed toward early, aggressive medical therapy; decisions for intubation and mechanical ventilation; and recognition of disease complications and their treatment.
2. Although supplemental oxygen is administered to the severely ill asthmatic patient, severe hypoxemia is not usually a problem. Although a significant increase in alveolar-arterial oxygen gradient $P(A - a)O_2$ is present due to low ventilation-perfusion $(\dot{V}/\dot{Q})$ areas, it can

usually be adequately compensated for by increasing inspired oxygen concentration (FIO_2).

3. Criteria for intubation before aggressive therapy include depressed level of consciousness, altered mental status, central cyanosis, or extreme distress.[3]

4. In severely ill asthmatic patients who are hypotensive prior to intubation, the primary consideration should be tension pneumothorax (diagnosis by physical examination and empiric therapy), arrhythmias (monitoring is important), and severe respiratory acidosis.

5. In addition, the possibility of decreased cardiac filling secondary to converting normally negative intrathoracic pressure to a positive value after institution of mechanical ventilation as well as intrinsic PEEP needs to be considered as a cause of hypotension.[4] Treatment of the former is volume therapy. Suspect intrinsic PEEP in patients who are receiving a high number of ventilatory breaths/minute (this may be a problem with assist-control ventilation) and treat by decreasing inspiratory time (best done by converting to synchronized intermittent mandatory ventilation or controlled ventilation [heavy sedation or sedation–paralysis] at a lower ventilator rate).

6. Aggressive inhaled beta-agonist therapy is the treatment of choice. The addition of subcutaneous beta-agonist therapy should be considered in the most severe cases. The threshold for subcutaneous use of a beta-agonist should be lower in patients with little risk for coronary artery disease.

7. In the patient with acute, life-threatening bronchospasm, the addition of inhaled anticholinergics is recommended.

8. Intravenous (IV) aminophylline is controversial. If IV aminophylline is selected, it should be used cautiously in patients at risk for hypokalemia or arrhythmias.

9. Although IV steroids may not have an immediate benefit, they are indicated in all patients with life-threatening bronchospasm or when hospital admission is anticipated.

Case Report: A 30-year-old patient with a 15-year history of asthma was seen in the emergency department (ED) three times over a 2-week period. After the first visit, he was discharged, significantly improved, with a peak expiratory flow rate (PEFR) of 260 L/minute. He gave a history of previous tracheal intubation during an acute asthmatic attack. He was again discharged following the second ED visit with significant improvement and a PEFR of 240 L/minute. Discharge medications included adequate oral theophylline, inhaled β_2-selective agonist, and high-dose oral steroids. On the third ED visit, he had a cardiorespiratory arrest shortly after arrival and could not be resuscitated. Gross examination of the lungs at autopsy revealed marked mucus plugging (Fig. 130-1). Microscopic examination of the lungs revealed mucosal edema (Fig. 130-2), proliferation of bronchial smooth muscle (Fig. 130-3), and a marked inflammatory infiltrate (Fig. 130-4). Charcot-Leyden crystals (Fig. 130-5) thought to be secondary to excretions from large numbers of eosinophils were also present.

This unfortunate case emphasizes the need for a clear understanding of the pathophysiology and treatment of acute asthma.

PATHOPHYSIOLOGY AND PULMONARY FUNCTION IN SEVERE ASTHMA ■

Like chronic obstructive lung disease (COLD), asthma is characterized by obstruction to expiratory gas flow. Smooth muscle contraction produces varying degrees of obstruction that may be largely reversible with therapy. In contrast, patients with COLD have a large-component fixed airway

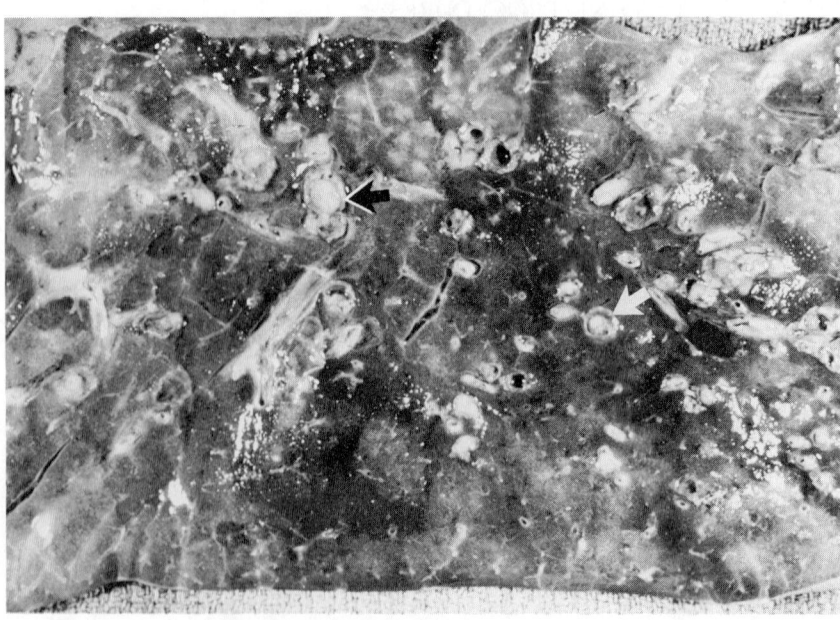

FIGURE 130-1. Gross necropsy material from a patient dying of asthma. The patient had been seen three times over 8 days and was on maximum outpatient medication with unknown compliance. On the third visit to the hospital the patient arrested and could not be resuscitated. Profound mucous plugging of segmental and subsegmental bronchi is seen (*arrows*).

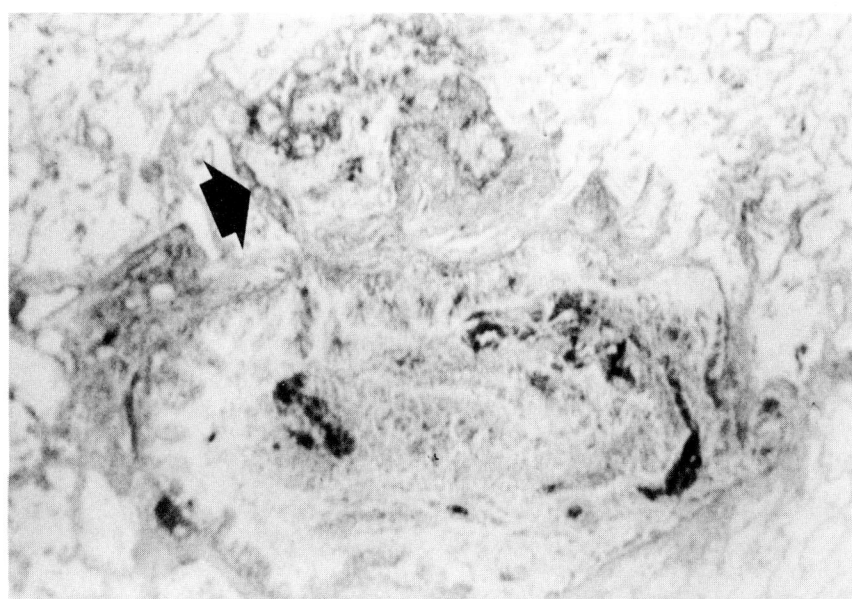

FIGURE 130-2. Same patient as in Figure 130-1. This scanning low-power photomicrograph demonstrates two bronchioles. The smaller of the two bronchioles (*arrow*) is depicted at the top. Both are occluded with mucus and debris.

obstruction that is not as amenable to bronchodilator therapy.[5] Severe asthma is characterized not only by bronchial smooth muscle contraction but also bronchial inflammation causing mucosal edema and mucus plugging.

In severe asthma, obstruction to airflow leads to $(\dot{V}/\dot{Q})$ mismatching. An increased $P(A - a)O_2$ develops and hypoxemia follows if hyperventilation does not compensate for the increased $P(A - a)O_2$. Expiratory obstruction decreases forced expiratory volume in the first second (FEV_1). In mild asthma the forced vital capacity (FVC) is normal, but in severe asthma with associated air trapping it is reduced. The hallmark of asthma is a decreased FEV_1/FVC. As bronchospasm worsens, the patient is unable to complete expiration due to expiratory airway resistance and limited expiratory time. This leads to air trapping and an increasing functional residual capacity as well as a decreased FVC. Air trapping also leads to hyperinflation and increased work of breathing. Edema and airway secretions further compromise inspiratory flow and, in the mechanically ventilated patient, often lead to high peak inspiratory pressures. The cardinal feature of bronchospasm is expiratory obstruction. The cause of respiratory arrest in asthmatics, however, is usually failure of the *inspiratory* muscles. Respiratory acidosis may be preceded by an anion-gap metabolic acidosis due to increased lactate production by the failing inspiratory muscles.[6] Decreased liver perfusion related to increased intrathoracic pressure and aggressive use of beta-agonist therapy may also contribute to elevated serum lactate,[7] as well as blood flow diverted away from the liver to muscles of respiration. A nonanion-gap acidosis may also be observed in patients with

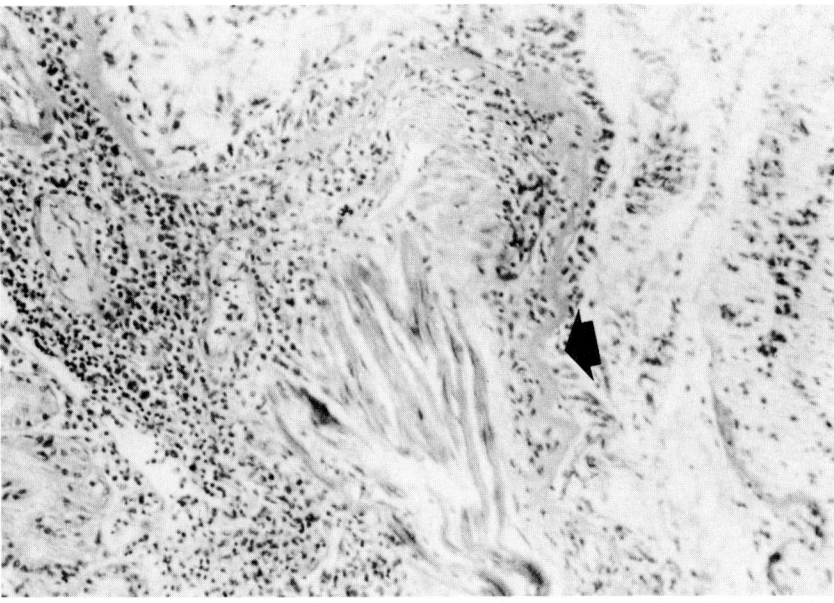

FIGURE 130-3. Same patient as in Figure 130-1. This higher magnification view depicts, on the right side, mucus and debris within an airway lumen. The wall of the lumen, depicted on the left (*arrow*), demonstrates hyperplasia of the smooth muscle and eosinophilic infiltration.

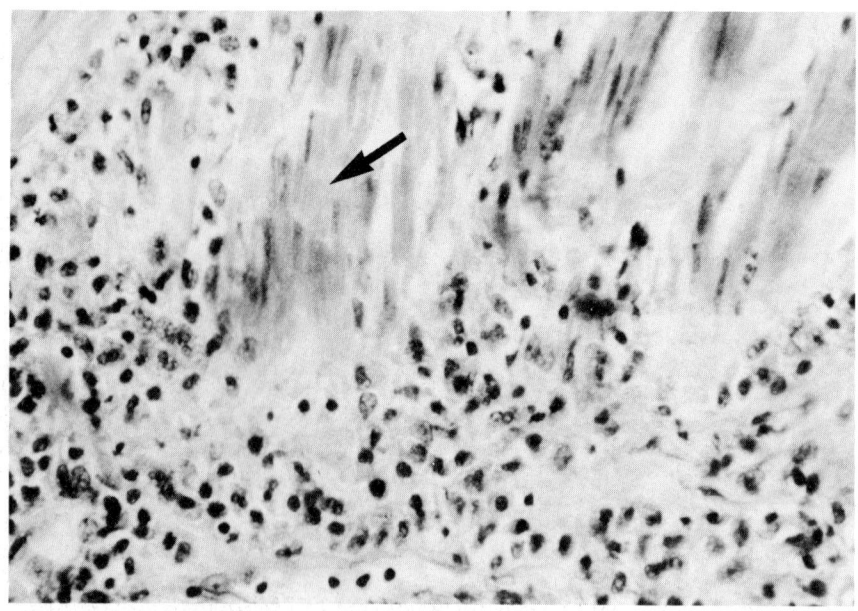

FIGURE 130-4. Same patient as in Figure 130-1. An even higher magnification demonstrates smooth muscle proliferation (*arrow*) and massive pulmonary infiltration of eosinophils.

severe asthma if several days of hyperventilation leading to renal compensation for a chronic respiratory alkalosis have preceded presentation at the hospital.

DIAGNOSIS ■

DIFFERENTIAL DIAGNOSIS

The differential diagnosis of patients with wheezing includes asthma, COLD, "cardiac asthma" (acute congestive heart failure), upper airway obstruction, endobronchial obstruction, pulmonary embolism, anaphylaxis, and toxic fume exposure (Table 130-1). A wheezing patient with a long smoking

history and no history of childhood asthma is more likely to have COLD. Treatment for COLD is similar to that for acute asthma, but response to bronchodilator therapy is less satisfactory.

Upper airway obstruction is characterized by stridor (inspiratory wheezing) heard loudest over the upper airway. Risk factors are usually evident and include foreign body aspiration, previous tracheal intubation, upper respiratory tract infection, or neck mass. Endobronchial obstruction does not usually produce acute respiratory distress in adults unless it is of acute onset (e.g., foreign body aspiration superimposed on poor respiratory reserve).

Rarely, patients with acute congestive heart failure (CHF) present with wheezing. This is probably caused by accumula-

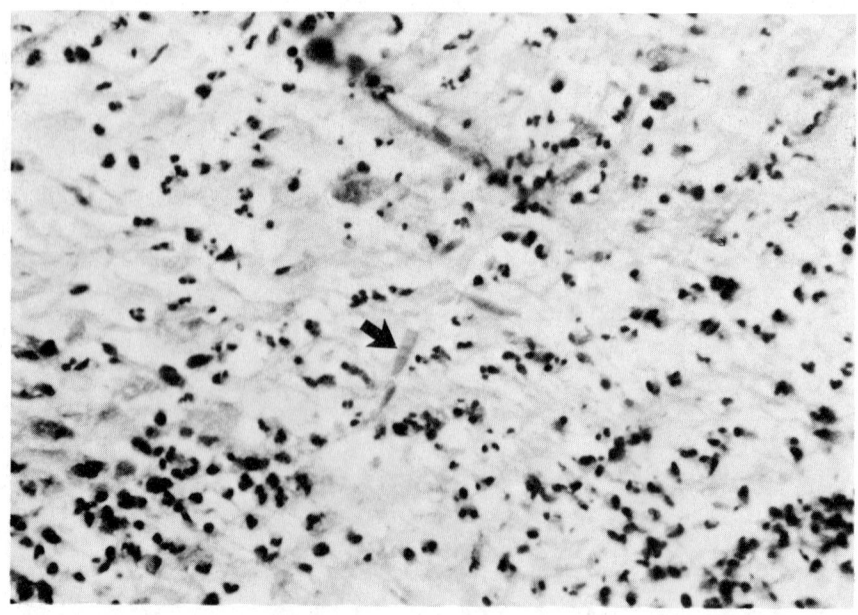

FIGURE 130-5. Same patient as in Figure 130-1. This high magnification view vividly shows mucosal debris with an admixture of exfoliated respiratory epithelium and eosinophils. A Charcot-Leyden crystal is noted in the center of the field (*arrow*). These elongated amorphous structures are thought to be produced from excretions of eosinophils.

TABLE 130-1. Differential Diagnosis of Asthma

ENTITY	CLUE
COLD	Smoking history, less responsive to bronchodilators
CHF	History, cardiomegaly, rales, wheezes
Upper airway obstruction	History, wheezing heard loudest over neck and upper chest
Endobronchial obstruction	History, localized wheezing
Pulmonary embolism	Rare, risk factors, chest pain
Anaphylaxis	Insect sting, recent medication history, urticaria
Toxic fume exposure	History, poorly responsive to bronchodilators

tion of lung water in the bronchovascular bundle and extrinsic compression of the bronchiole. Wheezing patients who have risk factors for both CHF and bronchospasm present a management dilemma. This problem is compounded in patients with COLD who may also have right ventricular failure. Jugular venous distention and peripheral edema are unreliable markers in this setting. The chest radiograph is particularly helpful in establishing the primary cause of respiratory distress in this circumstance.

Pulmonary embolism rarely presents with wheezing and, unless other signs are prominent, does not enter the differential diagnosis. Asthma produces significant perfusion defects on the lung scan in the absence of pulmonary embolism, making interpretation difficult.

SYMPTOMS AND SIGNS

Wheezing may be both expiratory and inspiratory and correlates with the degree of obstruction if adequate air movement is present[8]; however, an objective measurement of expiratory flow is still necessary.[9] The absence of wheezing is an ominous finding in the severely distressed asthmatic patient because it implies minimal air movement and is a harbinger of respiratory arrest. With air trapping comes progressive flattening of the diaphragm. This leads to a mechanical disadvantage and decreased force of diaphragmatic contraction. Contraction of the sternocleidomastoid muscles and other accessory muscles is indicative of severe obstruction ($FEV_1 < 1$).[10] With severe asthma, the patient may be unable to speak or may have an altered level of consciousness or central cyanosis.

Intense inspiratory effort leads to large swings in intrathoracic pressure and to an accentuated pulsus paradoxus (representing a decreased stroke volume during inspiration). The paradoxic pulse is often appreciated during routine blood pressure measurement as the systolic blood pressure falls dramatically during inspiration. Normally this fall is not greater than 10 mm Hg. A value greater than 15 mm Hg in an acute asthmatic patient is usually associated with an FEV_1 of less than 0.9 L.[11] The cause of increased pulsus paradoxus in severe asthma is related to the large swings in pleural pressure and likely multifactorial. Significant positive

pressure generated in the thorax during forced expiration diminishes blood return to the right ventricle, while vigorous inspiratory effort during inspiration augments blood return to the right ventricle. The increased filling of the right ventricle in early inspiration may shift the intraventricular septum toward the left ventricle reducing compliance and leading to a decrease in stroke volume index. Other potential contributing causes include the increased negative pleural pressure produced as an increase in left ventricular afterload with associated reduction in stroke volume, as well as the direct effect of lung hyperinflation on increasing right ventricular afterload and deterring movement of blood from right to left ventricle. Pulsus paradoxus is nonspecific and occurs in other disease states such as pericardial tamponade, cardiomyopathy, severe COLD, and acute hemorrhage.

Ominous signs and findings in the acute severe asthmatic, if not quickly reversed, include diaphoresis, inability to recline, increased $PaCO_2$, PEFR less than 100, and use of accessory muscles.

OBJECTIVE MEASUREMENT OF OBSTRUCTION

History and physical examination alone do not reliably predict the severity of airway obstruction in patients with acute asthma.[12] Therefore, more objective measures are desirable.[15] Although spirometry is the best objective measure of airway obstruction, the severely ill asthmatic patient is rarely able to perform a full FVC maneuver.[13]

An objective assessment of airway obstruction in the severe asthmatic can usually be made by measuring the PEFR.[14-16] This test requires patient cooperation only in the early part of the FVC maneuver. Because the greatest expiratory flow rates exist in early expiration, most patients with severe asthma are able to produce a reliable PEFR value. Normal expiratory flow rates vary considerably with age, sex, and height. In adults, a PEFR less than 100 to 125 L/minute implies severe obstruction to airflow.[17] The response of PEFR to initial aggressive bronchodilator therapy is the best predictor of morbidity in the severe acute asthmatic patient.[18-20]

LABORATORY AND RADIOGRAPHIC DATA

Asymmetric breath sounds or chest pain should alert the physician to the possibility of pneumothorax and mandate an early chest radiograph. Auscultatory findings suggesting pneumonia or the presence of fever also indicate a need for chest radiography. A history of sputum production is a poor predictor of pneumonia in the asthmatic patient who, in the absence of infection, may produce large amounts of clear, white, green, or gray sputum. Yellow, brown, blood-tinged, or foul-smelling sputum is uncommonly due to asthma alone and should point the physician to the possibility of pneumonia. An elevated white blood cell count (WBC) may be difficult to interpret because it may be elevated by asthma alone in the absence of infection and may be further elevated with subcutaneous epinephrine. Elderly patients and those receiving diuretics or steroids are often hypokalemic. Both beta-adrenergic receptor agonists and theophylline shift potassium intracellularly. Hypokalemia-induced arrhythmias may be more common following intensive bronchodilator therapy in these groups. CK (non-MB fraction) may also be elevated due to strenuous activity of ventilatory muscles.[21]

Severe asthma may show right ventricular strain on ECG that resolves with clinical improvement.[22] Although arterial blood gases (ABGs) are useful for decisions regarding hospital admission or tracheal intubation, they add little in the early management of acute asthma. Most asthmatic patients respond dramatically to initial therapy so that ABGs obtained on presentation are rarely predictive of outcome. Often the patient dramatically improves with aggressive therapy before the ABG result is available. Therefore, early attention in the asthmatic patient should center around aggressive therapeutic intervention.

ABGs may also be used to stage asthma. Stage I is characterized by normal blood gases. Patients in stage II have a decreased $PaCO_2$ and a normal PaO_2 (hyperventilation has led to normalization of PaO_2). Stage III is associated with a decrease in both $PaCO_2$ and PaO_2 (hyperventilation is now unable to compensate totally for a widened $P(A - a)O_2$. Stage IV is characterized by a normal $PaCO_2$ and a further decrease in PaO_2 (inspiratory fatigue is now prominent). Patients in stage V have respiratory failure with an increased $PaCO_2$ and a marked decrease in PaO_2. These findings indicate an impending respiratory arrest. A normal $PaCO_2$ in a distressed asthmatic should alert the physician to respiratory fatigue and the danger of respiratory arrest. This classification system is best applied after initial aggressive treatment of asthmatic patients and may be inappropriate if applied before initial therapy. In contrast to asthma, this classification has little usefulness in patients with COLD.

ADMISSION DECISIONS ■

Identifying the acute asthmatic patient who will probably deteriorate with outpatient treatment and who is at risk for developing status asthmaticus is more difficult.[23] Reasons favoring the need for hospitalization in the asthmatic patient with continued significant dyspnea include an increased $PaCO_2$ in any other than the initial pretreatment or early treatment ABGs, pneumonia, pneumothorax, history of tracheal intubation due to asthma (unless the event is a rare occurrence in a patient frequently discharged with success), initial PEFR less than 60 L/minute (assumes that the patient adequately cooperated), posttreatment PEFR less than 200 L/minute, inability to improve the medical regimen, noncompliance, and frequent emergency department visits (Table 130-2).

The physician should be extremely concerned if a patient has returned to the emergency department for a second or third visit for treatment of the same asthma attack without returning to baseline. This implies failure of the medications to reverse bronchospasm or patient noncompliance—either factor is a major concern.[24]

TABLE 130-2. Hospitalization Criteria and Guidelines for Asthma

Pneumonia
Pneumothorax
Previous intubation for asthma
Initial PEFR < 60 L/min (assumes cooperation)
Inability to increase PEFR to ≥200 L/min
Multiple emergency department visits for the same attack
Inability to improve the medical regimen
Increased $PaCO_2$ other than at the time of presentation
Noncompliance

THERAPY ■

BETA-ADRENERGIC THERAPY

Inhaled β_2-selective agonists are the cornerstone of treatment for patients with asthma and COLD.[25] Fears that frequent use of beta-agonist inhalation therapy before emergency department presentation might make subsequent use of these agents less effective are unfounded.[26]

Albuterol and metaproterenol are β_2-selective agents and should be delivered by inhalation as the preferred agents in treating acutely ill asthmatic patients. Albuterol probably offers some increased β_2 selectivity, but the clinical impact of this may be negligible in most patients.[27,28] Larger doses and more frequent dosing intervals for inhaled beta-agonist therapy are needed in acute severe asthma due to decreased deposition at site of action (low tidal volumes and narrowed airways), alteration in dose-response curve, and altered duration of activity. I begin initial therapy in the acutely ill asthmatic with 2.5 to 5.0 mg of albuterol (0.5–1.0 mL of 0.5% solution in 5 mL normal saline) by nebulization every 15 minutes for three to four doses followed by treatments hourly during the initial hours of therapy. Fewer doses can be administered in patients with less severe airflow obstruction and patients who demonstrate a quick response to therapy. However, inhaled treatments can be given continuously to severely obstructed patients until either an adequate clinical response is achieved or adverse side effects limit further administration (excessive tachycardia thought to be related to the inhaled beta-agonist or arrhythmias). The NIH Expert Panel report recommends 2.5 mg of albuterol delivered by nebulizer in three doses over 60 to 90 minutes for acute asthma.[29] The Canadian Association of Emergency Physicians, Lung Association, and Thoracic Society recommends for the initial management of the severely ill adult asthma patient (FEV_1 or peak expiratory flow rate less than 40% of predicted) in the emergency department, 5 mg albuterol by nebulizer every 15 to 20 minutes three times.[30] Continuous nebulization of albuterol using a large reservoir system to deliver up to 15 mg/hour for 2 hours may also be appropriate in some circumstances of severe life-threatening asthma.[31,32] In these circumstances, tachycardia and hypokalemia may occur.[33]

When β_2-selective agents are delivered parenterally or orally, they lose much of their β_2 selectivity. When subcutaneous terbutaline is compared with subcutaneous epinephrine, equal cardiac side effects are seen.[34] Terbutaline is, however, the parenteral agent of choice in pregnancy.[35] Oral β_2-selective agents should not be used as primary treatment for patients with acute asthma because the therapeutic-to-toxicity ratio is less than with inhaled agents.[36] Subcutaneous beta-agonist therapy (epinephrine, terbutaline) also has a disadvantageous therapeutic-to-toxicity ratio when compared with inhaled β_2-selective agonists. Subcutaneous epinephrine or terbutaline might, however, be useful in several situations. Inhaled agents are often difficult to administer to children. In addition, the pediatric population has a reduced susceptibility to β_1 toxicity making subcutaneous administration a useful route of drug delivery. Rapid delivery of beta-agonists to the airway is desirable in seriously ill asthmatic patients with impending respiratory arrest. The combination of inhaled and subcutaneously administered beta-agonists in this circumstance has been useful in my experience. It has been argued that bronchodilation is enhanced when drug is delivered by the airway and by the circulation. No clear data support this concept; however, the subcutaneous administration of beta-agonists induces greater peripheral airway bronchodilation than an equal amount of inhaled agent.[37,38] This has not been shown to be clinically significant. There is also a concern, again not documented, that subcutaneous adrenergic therapy is indicated in patients with severe bronchospasm because inhaled agents may not be adequately delivered to the peripheral sites of action. The fact that many patients with severe asthma present in extreme distress with a PEFR less than 60 L/minute and respond very briskly to inhaled beta-agonist therapy seems to refute this contention. If patients do not respond to initial inhaled therapy, particularly if the attack has lasted several days and mucus plugging is a possibility, I administer subcutaneous therapy. I use a subcutaneous beta-agonist initially in combination with an inhaled β_2-selective agonist in all patients presenting with life-threatening asthma. If subcutaneous adrenergic therapy is chosen, the epinephrine dose for adults is 0.3 to 0.5 mL of a 1:1000 dilution, depending on age and weight. This may be repeated in the initial management every 15 minutes as many as three times. An alternative agent is subcutaneous terbutaline, 0.25 mg.

β_1-adrenergic stimulators are given subcutaneously with caution to the elderly and to those with documented or suspected coronary artery disease. This group of patients is at risk for toxicity associated with β_1 stimulation. It is best to avoid parenteral adrenergic therapy in these patients if possible. However, when faced with the situation of severe life-threatening asthmatic bronchospasm in the cardiac patient with impending respiratory failure, subcutaneous adrenergic therapy in addition to inhaled therapy is probably indicated. No clinical studies document the benefit of subcutaneous terbutaline over subcutaneous epinephrine. Patients in the ICU who have persistent severe bronchospasm and who are unresponsive to inhaled bronchodilator therapy may be placed on intermittent subcutaneous adrenergic therapy. In this circumstance I do give terbutaline subcutaneously as frequently as every 2 hours.

Larger doses of aerosol bronchodilators must be administered to patients with intense bronchospasm because peripheral airway distribution of these drugs is decreased due to high inspiratory frequencies and flow rates, low tidal volumes, and narrowed airways.[39] Adequate delivery of beta-agonists can be accomplished by a metered-dose inhaler with spacer during acute bronchospasm if proper technique is used and doses are increased.[39–41] The argument is that use of such devices would be quicker and cheaper. Four puffs of albuterol (0.36 mg) delivered with a spacer should be expected to be equipotent to 2.5 mg of albuterol by nebulization in patients with severe disease.[42] This method is usually undesirable in the severe asthmatic due to poor patient cooperation. Even when stable asthmatic patients receive proper instructions for handling a metered-dose inhaler with spacer, studies reveal that improper technique is used by a majority of patients.[43] It is advisable, therefore, to deliver the beta-agonist by nebulization in most acutely ill asthmatic patients because this delivery technique requires minimal coordination and cooperation of the patient and less bedside instruction and supervision by the health care professional.

Two types of nebulizer systems are available for inhalation therapy: the face mask and the hand-held nebulizer with a mouthpiece. The mouthpiece is preferred because it delivers more drug. However, more patient cooperation is required with the hand-held system because a good seal must be maintained around the mouthpiece. In the severely ill asthmatic patient, the face mask system may be necessary.

Aggressive inhaled beta-agonist therapy is preferred to intravenous albuterol as the risk-benefit ratio of the preponderance of literature favors inhaled therapy and the same endpoint can usually be achieved with less toxicity.[44–48] Intravenous albuterol may be considered as an alternative when patients with life-threatening asthma have failed to respond to inhaled therapy.

INHALED ANTICHOLINERGIC THERAPY

Although ipratropium produces less bronchodilatation at peak effect than beta-agonist and is associated with a less predictable clinical response, literature in general supports the use of ipratropium as adjunctive therapy in patients with acute severe asthma.[49,50] Ipratropium bromide appears to reliably augment the bronchodilating effect of beta-agonists in acute asthma.[49,51,52] It is particularly useful in the presence of beta-blockade.[53] Recommended dose is 0.25 to 0.5 mg by nebulizer. This can be combined with an albuterol dose. Contrary to patients with chronic stable disease, ipratropium may produce a clinical significant response within minutes of administration. A paradoxic bronchoconstrictive response to ipratropium, although much rarer than initially reported, may occur and is due to the preservative in the solution.[54] If ipratropium is to be delivered by metered-dose inhaler, ten puffs (.018 mg/puff) are recommended. If ipratropium bromide is delivered by metered-dose inhaler, a spacer is indicated. I initially dose ipratropium every 2 hours until the patient improves and then go to an every-4-hour dosing interval. Nebulized glycopyrrolate, although not extensively studied in acute asthma, is also an effective anticholinergic agent.[55] The hand-held mouthpiece nebulizer system should be used if anticholinergic medication is being administered. Contamination of the ocular area with precipitation of narrow-angle glaucoma may occur in susceptible individuals if a face mask is used for delivery of an anticholinergic agent. Inhaled atropine is an inferior anticholinergic agent when compared to ipratropium. It is systemically absorbed and has a narrow therapeutic window causing tachycardia. Systemic effects include precipitation of glaucoma and bladder neck obstruction and inhaled atropine should be not be used in patients with these disorders.

THEOPHYLLINE

Theophylline, when compared with a placebo, is clearly an effective bronchodilator in the patient with acute bronchospasm. An inhaled beta-agonist is accepted to be a much better single therapeutic agent than theophylline.[56] The question, however, is whether theophylline plus adequate dosing of an inhaled beta-agonist produces greater bronchodilatation than adequate dosing of beta-agonist alone in the patient with acute asthma. The addition of theophylline to a full course of an inhaled beta-agonist remains debatable. The majority of studies have demonstrated no significant additional improvement in physiologic or outcome variables when theophylline is added to full doses of inhaled beta-agonist therapy.[57] In addition, theophylline toxicity is a concern.[58–60] Extrapolating data from short-term studies showing no additional benefit of theophylline may be problematic since other studies have shown benefits evident at 24 or 48 hours. Several studies do offer evidence for the use of theophylline as adjunctive therapy, demonstrating (1) improvement in ventilatory function at 1 and 24 hours; (2) improvement in FEV_1 during the first 3 hours and at 48 hours; and (3) improvement in FEV_1 at 4 hours.[61–63] Therefore, there are no data to definitively support or reject the use of theophylline in this setting. I use theophylline added to a full dose of inhaled beta-agonist and ipratropium bronchodilator regimen in patients with an initial clinical impression of life-threatening bronchospasm, as well as patients admitted to the ICU. Theophylline might also be considered in any patient who fails to respond to initial therapy with inhaled beta-agonists. The following should be used as guidelines for administration of IV theophylline in the severe asthmatic if the decision is made to use theophylline. If the patient has not been receiving a theophylline preparation, I give a loading dose of aminophylline, 5 mg/kg, over 15 to 30 minutes. After the loading dose is given, I administer aminophylline by continuous infusion with an infusion pump at a rate of 0.6 mg/kg/hour. Higher doses may be used in children. The rate of metabolism is highly variable and may be affected by many factors. Suggestions for modification of the IV aminophylline maintenance doses are shown in Table 130-3. Other factors that decrease aminophylline clearance and necessitate a lowering of continuous infusion rates include cimetidine use, erythromycin use, upper respiratory tract infections, pneumonia, and COLD.[64,65] A therapeutic drug level should be obtained in 6 hours and the rate adjusted accordingly.

TABLE 130-3. Maintenance Doses of Aminophylline in Acute Asthma

CONDITION	INITIAL CONTINUOUS INFUSION DOSE° (mg/kg/h)
Otherwise healthy adult	0.5
Teenager	0.7
Older than age 50	0.4
History of cardiac or liver dysfunction	0.2
Smoking adult	0.7

°Adjust up or down using serum theophylline levels.

All patients evaluated for acute bronchospasm who have been receiving a theophylline preparation should have a theophylline level determined, the results of which are useful in later dosing decisions. Theophylline levels correlate only roughly with toxicity. Patient symptoms are unreliable in predicting the theophylline level.[66,67] The longer acting the oral theophylline compound, the more likely it is to be associated with a higher initial level. If aminophyline is to be used, a decreased loading dose (2 mg/kg) is recommended in the severely bronchospastic asthmatic patient who admits to poor or partial compliance in taking medications. I target a therapeutic range of serum theophylline at 8 to 12 µg/mL to minimize risk for toxicity.

A 1 mg/kg IV aminophylline dose increases the serum level roughly 2 µg/mL with considerable scatter.[68] A 5 mg/kg dose is, therefore, estimated to give a level of 10 µg/mL. This relationship of loading dose to incremental increase in blood level can also be used for additional dosing considerations after the theophylline level is known.

Theophylline has been demonstrated in vitro and in vivo to have nonbronchodilator effects of potential clinical benefit. It lowers the threshold of diaphragmatic fatigue[69] and is an inotrope and a nonspecific respiratory stimulant. It is doubtful, however, that any of these effects exert a significant clinical impact. Theophylline is a nonselective phosphodiesterase inhibitor and would be expected to produce an increase in intracellular cyclic adenosine monophosphate levels, in turn causing bronchial smooth muscle relaxation. Although this is an attractive mechanism to explain its beneficial effect in the asthmatic patient, it is probably incorrect because other phosphodiesterase inhibitors have not demonstrated significant bronchodilation.[70]

STEROIDS

Corticosteroids are an essential part of in-hospital asthma therapy.[71] Minimal or no side effects occur with a single large dose of IV steroid. Some enhancement of beta-agonist effect may be seen as early as 1 hour; however, 4 to 6 hours are required for antiinflammatory activity. Methylprednisolone given in a dose of 60 to 125 mg every 4 to 6 hours has become accepted therapy in the early management of the hospitalized asthmatic patient.[72] The benefit derived by the asthmatic is probably due to a combination of enhancement of β_2-receptor responsiveness, interruption of arachidonic acid inflammatory pathways, decrease in capillary basement membrane permeability, decreased leukocyte attachment, modulation of calcium migration intracellularly, reduction in airway mucus production, and suppression of IgE receptor binding.

Although use of steroids in the hospitalized asthmatic is well supported by medical literature, the use of a single dose of IV steroids at the time of presentation independent of decisions to admit or discharge the patient from the emergency department is controversial. One study indicates that 125 mg of methylprednisolone given intravenously at the onset of management of acute asthma has a significant beneficial effect on the patient's course.[73] A follow-up study using a similar experimental design failed to show similar benefit.[74] A possible reason for the difference may be more aggressive inhaled beta-agonist therapy in the latter study. In patients presenting to the emergency department who are judged to have life-threatening asthma and in whom admission will follow, the decision to initiate steroid therapy immediately is appropriate and I recommend its use.

MAGNESIUM SULFATE

Magnesium's potential to reverse bronchoconstriction is multifactorial and is based on characteristics of inhibition of the calcium channel and decreased acetylcholine release. As with theophylline, considerable controversy exists as to the potential benefit of magnesium sulfate as adjunctive therapy in acute asthma. Following initial reports of benefit in acute asthma refractory to treatment with inhaled beta-agonists (the majority being case series),[75-79] subsequent, better controlled studies have cast doubt on its role.[80,81] A recent study suggests that magnesium sulfate is of benefit in severe acute asthma.[82] Originally described benefits of magnesium sulfate were reported in patients with both normal magnesium levels as well as hypomagnesemia. Subsequent larger prospective studies have failed to confirm a benefit of magnesium in acute asthma. These randomized double-blinded placebo controlled studies included patients with initial PEFR less than 200 L/minute who failed to double peak inspiratory flow rate after two albuterol treatments, as well as emergency department patients with acute asthma poorly responsive to inhaled albuterol. Dosing of magnesium sulfate has varied from a single 2-g dose to a 2-g dose followed by continuous infusion. The large amount of anecdotal case report literature of response coupled with the safety profile of the drug should still lead to consideration of the drug in dire circumstances in which patients have failed treatment with other agents. In that circumstance I would administer 2 g over 20 minutes. It is not recommended for routine use, however.

HELIUM–OXYGEN MIXTURES

A blended mixture of helium and oxygen (Heliox) is available in mixtures of 60:40, 70:30, and 80:20. Heliox is less dense than air and can be delivered through a tight-fitting nonrebreathing mask or, in the intubated patient, through the ventilatory circuit. This less dense gas mixture results in

decreased airway resistance. Studies have shown the ability of Heliox to decrease both physical examination findings of pulsus paradoxus as well as physiologic improvement measured by both inspiratory and expiratory flow.[83-86] Heliox may have potential benefit in delaying need for intubation while bronchodilators exert their effect as well as decreasing peak airway pressures in the mechanically ventilated patient. In the latter case its potential to decrease auto PEEP may be particularly useful. A mixture of 60:40 blend of Heliox is recommended as initial therapy carefully monitoring oxygenation status. Recalibration of gas blenders and flowmeters are required to obtain accurate measures of oxygen concentration and tidal volumes when this mixture is used in the mechanically ventilated patient. It must be remembered that despite reported anecdotal success, no controlled trials have demonstrated alteration of outcome variables.

OTHER TREATMENT ISSUES

Antibiotic therapy in the asthma patient is indicated only if bacterial infection is present. Typically, the diagnosis is bacterial pneumonia. Patients with severe bronchospasm should have an IV catheter placed simultaneously with or immediately after inhaled beta-agonist therapy is initiated. A theophylline level should be determined if the patient is taking an oral theophylline preparation. If the patient is volume-depleted, normal saline is used. In elderly patients or those with cardiac disease, dextrose 5% in water is routinely used. There is no evidence that excess volume replacement liquefies or facilitates loosening of secretions.

PRECIPITATING FACTORS

β-Adrenergic receptor blockers, aspirin, nonsteroidal antiinflammatory drugs, inhaled irritants, reflux esophagitis, sinusitis, cold, exercise, and emotional stress may all precipitate acute asthma in selected patients. These factors should certainly be eliminated or treated.

INDICATIONS FOR TRACHEAL INTUBATION ∎

Indications for early tracheal intubation include apnea or near apnea, central cyanosis, mental status changes, or depressed level of consciousness. Inability to adequately oxygenate or ventilate an asthmatic patient mandates tracheal intubation. A sustained respiratory rate in excess of 40 breaths/minute may imply impending respiratory fatigue and mandates consideration of tracheal intubation. Intubation should be accomplished using the technique in which the operator feels most proficient (see subsequent section, Sedation for Intubation and Mechanical Ventilation).

MECHANICAL VENTILATION IN THE ASTHMATIC

Mechanical ventilation in the asthmatic patient is often feared by the clinician because of published reports of a significant increase in morbidity and mortality with its use.

It is more likely that the morbidity and mortality is related to the severity of the disease that necessitated intubation and not due to the intervention itself. Significant complications do occur in the mechanically ventilated asthmatic patient, including barotrauma, machine failure, endotracheal tube malfunction, and pneumonia (Fig. 130-6).[87]

Westerman and coworkers mechanically ventilated 39 patients with severe asthma.[88] Four patients died during the hospitalization. Thirty-two of the 35 patients discharged were followed up at 4 to 5 years. There were nine deaths among this group. Deaths occurred in those patients who had either labile airway obstruction or increasing airway obstruction and not among those who had stable obstruction or who were well controlled. Zimmerman and colleagues reviewed a large series of intubated and mechanically ventilated patients at a county hospital.[89] Only 1 patient died among those who reached the emergency department with

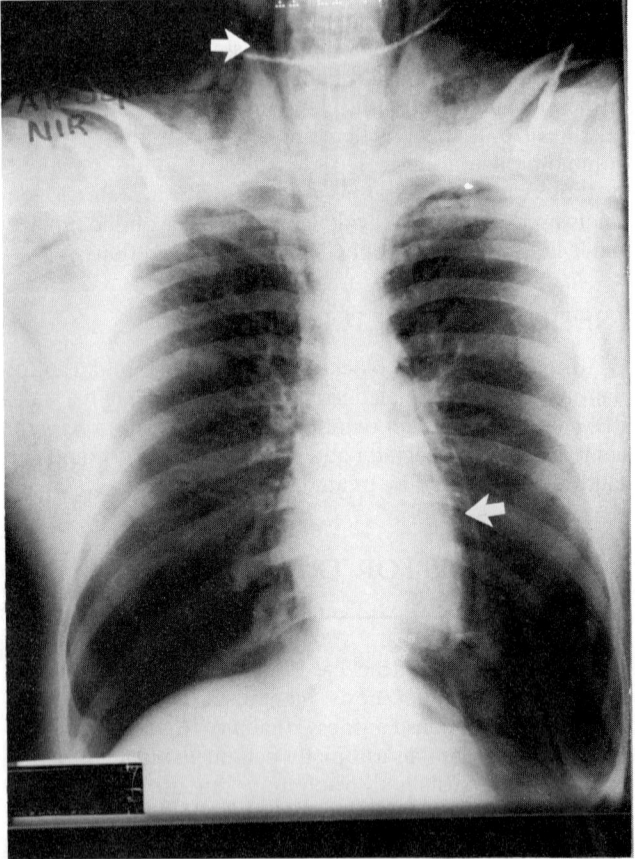

FIGURE 130-6. This anteroposterior supine portable chest radiograph was obtained in a patient with status asthmaticus following tracheal intubation and mechanical ventilation. The radiograph demonstrates evidence of severe barotrauma. Marked subcutaneous and mediastinal emphysema is present (*arrows*). This patient developed bilateral subpulmonic tension pneumothoraces. The crisp outline of the hemidiaphragm and the hyperlucent area over the left upper quadrant (deep sulcus sign) are indicative of pneumothorax. These findings all resolved after bilateral thoracostomy tubes were inserted.

a pulse. These data suggest that the prognosis for most mechanically ventilated asthmatic patients is good.

AEROSOL DELIVERY

Aerosol delivery in the intubated, mechanically ventilated patient poses a significant problem. Only a small percentage of nebulized agent reaches the lung parenchyma in the mechanically ventilated patient.[90] Most is deposited in the endotracheal tube, probably because of its 90-degree curve. An altered breathing pattern and regional lung pathology may decrease the effectiveness of the delivered drug. It is important to connect the ventilator circuit nebulizer system as close to the patient as possible and to consider increasing the amount of active agent in each treatment. I routinely double the dose I would use in the nonintubated patient. Metered-dose inhaler with spacer has been advocated to be effective in delivering bronchodilator medication in mechanically ventilated patients. Some data, however, have questioned its efficacy compared with wet nebulization.[91] More importantly, either method may give varying delivery based on technique and ventilator as well as patient variables.[92]

SEDATION FOR INTUBATION AND MECHANICAL VENTILATION

Sedation and analgesia is almost always required in preparation for intubation in the severe asthmatic patient. Choices include benzodiazepines, narcotics, ketamine, and propofol. Midazolam and lorazepam are the most frequently chosen benzodiazepines, with initial low doses titrated to higher doses to achieve desired effects. Bolus morphine is typically avoided because of the possibility of histamine release and systemic hypotension. Ketamine may offer an advantage due to its bronchodilating effect as well as its minimal respiratory depression potential.[93,94] It may, however, increase heart rate and blood pressure related to sympathomimetic release. A significant percentage of adults also have dramatic mood alterations associated with ketamine administration.

Propofol has a similar onset of action when compared with midazolam and a similar effect on hemodynamic parameters.[95] It can also be used to titrate for depth of sedation. Once the patient is intubated successfully and mechanical ventilation has been instituted, a combination of benzodiazepines and opioids offer optimal sedation. I recommend initially a combination of lorazepam and morphine delivered by continuous infusions. Although adequate control of ventilation may be reached in some patients with a combination of benzodiazepine and morphine, many patients require paralyzing agents, especially early in their ventilatory course. Neuromuscular blockade may also be required in some patients to facilitate intubation.

INITIATING MECHANICAL VENTILATION

Initial ventilator settings recommended are a tidal volume of 8 to 10 mL/kg and a frequency of 10 to 12 breaths/minute.[96,97] If volume ventilation is used, peak inspiratory flow rates should be set at 80 to 100 L/minute with a square waveform. The use of noncompressible tubing facilitates lowering of inspiratory time. Controlled mechanical ventilation is ideal and requires heavy sedation and analgesia or more typically sedation, analgesia, and muscle paralysis. Assist-control ventilation predisposes the patient to hyperinflation.[98]

Heavy sedation or sedation–paralysis reduces carbon dioxide production, facilitates measurement of end-inspiratory and expiratory pressures, and facilitates mechanical ventilation of the severe asthmatic patient.[99,100] Prolonged neuromuscular blockade is, however, ideally avoided. Attempts to withdraw neuromuscular blockade over the 24- to 48-hour period after intubation are appropriate. If the patient is to be continuously paralyzed, a peripheral nerve stimulator should be used to limit paralysis to a recording of one or two twitches in response to a train of four stimuli as opposed to higher degrees of paralysis.[101,102] Prolonged neuromuscular blockade may lead to persistent neuromuscular weakness after withdrawal of neuromuscular blockade. This is particularly likely to occur in patients with renal impairment, females, the presence of hypophosphatemia, higher degrees of paralysis, and when concomitant steroids are given. The latter is particularly problematic since steroids are a critical component of medical therapy for life-threatening asthma.

AUTO PEEP

Auto PEEP occurs when ventilator settings dictate an inspiration-to-expiration ratio that does not allow adequate expiratory time for total exhalation of the delivered ventilator breath. After the first breath delivered in a setting conducive to auto PEEP, the next breath is delivered before complete emptying of the first breath. Thereafter, with each subsequent breath failing to completely empty, end-expiratory lung volume rises as does flow and pressure at end-expiration. End-inspiratory lung volume also rises (risk for barotrauma) and intrathoracic pressure rises (risk for decreased cardiac output). With continued delivery of previous tidal volume (volume-cycled ventilation with peak pressures not exceeding alarm limit or pressure-limited, time-cycled ventilation in which equilibration of pressures between ventilator system and patient does not occur), end-inspiratory lung volume and peak alveolar pressure rise until barotrauma occurs or equilibrium is reached. Equilibrium is established due to the distention-induced larger caliber of airways (reduced resistance to expiratory flow) and the increased lung recoil (due to increased end-inspiratory lung volume) eventually allowing complete emptying of the delivered tidal volume. Equilibrium is reached, however, with significant end-expiratory flow still occurring when the next ventilator breath is delivered. The continued expiratory flow at end-expiration represents positive pressure relative to atmospheric pressure. Positive end-expiratory pressure therefore exists even though it is not set on the ventilator (auto PEEP). This is associated with significant increases in mean intrathoracic pressure. This condition may be accompanied by a marked elevation in intrathoracic pressure with associated hypotension (decreased venous return to heart) and barotrauma (pneumothorax).

It should also be noted that with pressure-limited time cycled ventilation, the rise in lung volumes with increasing auto-PEEP will produce a progressive drop in tidal volume due to decreased lung elastance. This will favor an eventual equilibrium with increased end-inspiratory/end-expiratory lung volumes and decreased tidal volume delivered at the same pressure settings.

Because obstructive airways disease increases expiratory time, mechanically ventilated patients with asthma are at increased risk for auto PEEP.

When there is no other obvious cause (e.g., tension pneumothorax), auto PEEP should be suspected clinically in asthmatic patients who are hypotensive after institution of mechanical ventilation. Higher minute ventilation likely to occur in assist-control ventilation in the awake asthmatic patient in distress predisposes the patient to auto PEEP. Auto PEEP is treated by decreasing total inspiratory time. This is best accomplished by decreasing inspiratory rate. Decreasing tidal volume is also effective. Increasing inspiratory flow rate with volume ventilation is less effective. If hypotension resolves, this is both a diagnostic and a therapeutic maneuver. Shortening the total inspiratory time by increasing flow rate is a less effective way of decreasing auto PEEP and may actually hyperinflate areas of lung with short time constants for filling.

Auto PEEP frequently manifests itself when the water manometer dial of the ventilator fails to return to set PEEP at end-expiration. Severe auto PEEP may, however, be present in the absence of this finding. Auto PEEP can be detected easily with graphic flow displays showing expiratory gas flow still present at the onset of the next inspiration. Measurement of auto PEEP can be accomplished with either the end-expiratory occlusion pressure technique or esophageal balloon technique. Occlusion of the expiratory and inspiratory circuit of the ventilator just before the onset of the next breath causes the pressure in the lungs and ventilator circuit to equilibrate and the displayed pressure represents the level of auto PEEP. With the esophageal balloon technique, the negative deflection in esophageal pressure (representing pleural pressure) from the onset of inspiratory effort to the onset of inspiratory flow represents the inspiratory muscle pressure necessary to counterbalance the end-expiratory elastic recoil of the respiratory system, and therefore represents the amount of auto PEEP. In the absence of an esophageal balloon, the ability to accurately reflect the auto PEEP–related pressure at the alveolar level in the intubated asthmatic patient ideally depends on a prolonged end-expiratory hold (3 to 4 seconds) and the absence of patient inspiratory or expiratory effort during measurement. Measurement is unlikely to be accurate unless the patient is heavily sedated or sedated–paralyzed. Unless full equilibration to a no-flow state is allowed at end-inspiration with the system closed to the ventilator, the auto PEEP level exerted at the alveolar level is typically underestimated. The typical end-expiratory hold used in clinical practice of 0.4 to 1 second is less likely to provide a reliable auto PEEP measurement.

Auto PEEP in the presence of assisted ventilation modes (assist-control and synchronized intermittent mandatory ventilation [SIMV]) implies that the patient must initiate gas flow by producing inspiratory effort equal to not only the sensitivity setting of the demand valve, but the level of auto PEEP as well. In the presence of auto PEEP, this implies significant increase in inspiratory work of breathing. If it is not advantageous or possible to eliminate auto PEEP, applying or raising ventilator-set PEEP to a level slightly below total PEEP decreases patient effort necessary to trigger a ventilator breath. One must be careful, however, as inappropriately set ventilator PEEP offers additional risks to the patient. I recommend this approach only by health care professionals well-schooled in the intricacies of mechanical ventilation.

BAROTRAUMA

The risk for barotrauma in the intubated asthmatic patient correlates best with inspiratory plateau pressure. Auto PEEP and peak inspiratory pressures are less reliable predictors of barotrauma.[98,103] Peak inspiratory pressure, although correlating to some degree with inspiratory plateau and end-inspiratory lung volume, also reflects resistance in the endotracheal tube and tracheobronchial tree that may be considerable in the presence of a small endotracheal tube, airway secretions, mucosal thickening, and bronchoconstriction.[103] In the heavily sedated or the sedated–paralyzed patient, inspiratory plateau measurement is the best indicator of hyperinflation and risk for barotrauma. In the presence of normal chest wall and abdominal compliance factors, an inspiratory plateau pressure greater than 35 cm H_2O puts the patient at risk for exceeding alveolar size at total lung capacity. Literature supports a decrease in barotrauma when inspiratory plateau pressure is maintained below this value.[104] This can usually be accomplished by using low tidal volumes and minimizing auto PEEP. The degree of auto PEEP is not itself a risk factor for barotrauma, but defines the end-expiratory lung volume on which the next tidal volume is delivered. This influences barotrauma by its effect on inspiratory plateau pressure. In addition, auto PEEP estimated by measuring end-expiratory pressure following an end-expiratory pause (occlusion of inspiratory and expiratory ventilator limbs), may underestimate the degree of auto PEEP. This is because airway collapse before end-expiration may prevent equilibration with acinar units at the highest levels of auto PEEP. These airways are then, however, open during inspiration and exert an effect on end-inspiratory lung volumes. The ability to decrease inspiratory plateau pressure while holding tidal volume constant may be a better reflection of diminution of auto PEEP than actual measurement of the end-expiratory pressure. Since the primary determinant of barotrauma is a high inspiratory plateau pressure and this value is reduced by lowering tidal volume, reduction in the tidal volume should be the primary strategy in decreasing the risk of barotrauma in the presence of hyperinflation and auto PEEP. If after heavy sedation or sedation–paralysis, inspiratory plateau pressure remains greater than 35 cm H_2O despite decreases in tidal volume to the lowest value that allows an acceptable pH, typically 7.25 or greater, the use of bicarbonate infusion to allow acceptable pH with further lowering of tidal volume should be considered.[105] Bicarbonate should be infused slowly by continuous infusion

to avoid possible acute worsening of intracellular pH. The concept of lowering the tidal volume to decrease alveolar inflation and accepting a higher $PaCO_2$ and lower pH is called permissive hypercapnia and should be considered in the mechanically ventilated asthmatic patient with life-threatening asthma, severe hyperinflation, and inability to achieve a satisfactory inspiratory plateau pressure without producing an unacceptable acidemia.[106,107] Permissive hypercapnia is well tolerated in most patients even with $PaCO_2$ up to 90 mm Hg as long as pH remains at or greater than 7.20.[108] It should, however, be avoided in the presence of increased intracranial pressure and clinically significant myocardial dysfunction.[109]

NONINVASIVE POSITIVE-PRESSURE VENTILATION

Noninvasive positive-pressure ventilation (NPPV) by face or nasal mask, although more frequently used and more beneficial in treating acute respiratory acidosis in severe COLD, may offer utility in patients with acute asthma. A word of caution, however, should start any discussion of NPPV in asthma. Distinct disadvantages include increased risk of aspiration of gastric content secondary to gastric insufflation and a technique that is significantly inferior to invasive mechanical ventilation for controlling a patient's ventilatory status. If noninvasive ventilation is successful as a bridge to allow the effect of medical therapy to negate the need for intubation and its associated complications, it is a worthwhile endeavor. The primary potential benefit of noninvasive ventilation is the ability of inspiratory positive pressure to decrease the patient's work of breathing. The potential for NPPV-applied positive end-expiratory pressure to benefit the severely ill asthmatic patient is a more controversial and sophisticated concept with less established clinical relevance. If NPPV is used in the acute asthmatic patient, I recommend an initial inspiratory pressure of 8 cm H_2O and an expiratory pressure of 0 to 2 cm H_2O. Inspiratory pressure can then be titrated upward for effect.

SUMMARY OF TREATMENT PRIORITIES ∎

Initial beta-agonist inhaled therapy at the time of presentation in the patient with severe asthma is recommended every 15 minutes three or four times followed by a dose every hour until the patient improves. After improvement, the interval between β_2-selective agonist treatments is slowly increased to every 2, 3, and 4 hours. Steroids should be instituted in all admitted asthmatic patients. Initial therapy at the time of presentation to the emergency department seems appropriate in life-threatening asthma. IV aminophylline therapy and inhaled anticholinergic therapy as an adjunct to inhaled beta-agonists and steroids are controversial. Until further studies are available, I recommend use of inhaled ipratropium initially in all severe acutely ill asthmatic patients (PEFR < 100) and in all asthmatic patients in whom hospital admission is anticipated or known, and use of theophylline in all patients with life-threatening presentations of asthma as well as asthmatic patients admitted to the ICU.

Careful patient monitoring is extremely important. In a patient with severe life-threatening asthma, inhaled β_2-selective agonist therapy does not typically produce any sympathomimetic toxic effects above those due to the distress of the asthma. It seems reasonable in this patient group to rely primarily on aggressive use of the single best therapy (β_2-selective agonists) until improvement is observed or toxicity is produced. I believe that patients in the ICU with life-threatening asthma, and especially those who are intubated, should have frequent inhaled β_2-selective agonists. In some circumstances, initial continuous administration is appropriate. After stabilization, the frequency should be reduced as noted earlier. Therapy should always be decreased or stopped at the first sign of toxicity.

My recommendation for initial anticholinergic therapy is hourly ipratropium. Following improvement, anticholinergic therapy may be delivered every 4 to 6 hours and given 15 minutes after β_2-selective agonist treatments. This may facilitate deposition of the anticholinergic drug. IV aminophylline may be given by continuous infusion to maintain a serum level of 8 to 12 μg/mL. Methylprednisolone is initially given intravenously in a dose of 125 mg. I then reduce the dose to 60 to 125 mg given every 4 hours for six times, then every 6 hours for four times. If the patient is improving, oral steroids are started on day 2 or 3, and IV steroids are tapered rapidly as long as the patient continues to improve. My recommendation is to continue oral steroids for at least 7 to 10 days, and if the patient has previously received steroids (continuous or intermittent), steroids may be tapered slowly over weeks. Inhaled steroids may be added at the time of hospital discharge. If mechanical ventilation is needed, goals should be acceptable oxygenation, maintenance of pH at or greater than 7.20, and limiting inspiratory plateau pressure to less than or equal to 35 cm H_2O.

NONTRADITIONAL THERAPY OF SEVERE BRONCHOSPASM ■

Asthmatic patients who fail to respond to traditional therapy for life-threatening bronchospasm should be considered for nontraditional therapy. I consider nontraditional therapy after 12 hours of standard therapy in the presence of either refractory hypercapnia (difficulty in maintaining pH $\geq$ 7.20), persistent severe hyperinflation (inspiratory plateau pressure > 35 cm H_2O), or FIO_2 requirements greater than 0.6 after 48 hours (oxygenation of the mechanically ventilated asthmatic patient is usually not a major problem).

Nontraditional treatment alternatives include intensification of beta-agonist therapy beyond routinely recognized standards, heliox therapy (see earlier discussion), general anesthetic agents, and bronchial lavage. Intensive beta-agonist therapy has been used successfully in patients who have not responded to traditional therapy and who are at risk for morbidity secondary to bronchospastic disease.[110] Under these circumstances the risk of β_1-adrenergic toxic side effects may be outweighed by the benefits of the medication.

Treatment alternatives include continuous β_2-selective agonist nebulized therapy, frequent subcutaneous β_2-agonist therapy, and IV β_2-agonist therapy. Continuous IV albuterol has been used successfully in Europe but is not available in the United States.[111] Intravenous isoproterenol and terbutaline have been used in children but is not recommended in adults. Controlled studies would also indicate that the same or similar effect can usually be achieved with more aggressive use of inhaled beta-agonists.

Anecdotal success with isoflurane or halothane anesthesia[112,113] and rectally administered ether[114] has been reported. Intravenous thiopental has also been used.[115]

Success has been reported with bronchial lavage in patients with obstructive airways disease who could not be weaned from ventilatory support.[116,117] Mucus plugs impacted in airways may be expelled using the fiberoptic bronchoscope for lavage, thus improving ventilation and oxygenation.[118,119] Critically ill mechanically ventilated asthmatic patients are, however, poor candidates for bronchial lavage. The procedure is likely to produce a significant increase in auto PEEP and worsening of hypoxemia.

Controlled trials demonstrating efficacy of nonstandard therapy with aggressive beta-agonist therapy, anesthetic agents, or bronchial lavage do not exist.

ACKNOWLEDGMENT ■

The author thanks Dr. S. Donald Greenburg for help in preparation and interpretation of the photomicrographs.

REFERENCES ■

1. Corbridge TC, Hall JB: The assessment and management of adults with status asthmaticus. *Am J Respir Crit Care Med* 1995;151:1296
2. Henderson A, Wright M: Status asthmatiucs: experience of 100 consecutive admissions to an intensive care unit. *Clin Intensive Care* 1992;3:148
3. Bishop GF, Hillman KM: Acute severe asthma. *Intensive Care World* 1993;10:166
4. Franklin C, Samuel J, Hu TC: Life-threatening hypotension associated with emergency intubation and the initiation of mechanical ventilation. *Am J Emerg Med* 1994;12:425
5. Bone RC: Treatment of respiratory failure due to advanced chronic obstructive lung disease. *Arch Intern Med* 1980;140:1018
6. Appel D, Rubenstein R, Schrager K, Williams MH: Lactic acidosis in severe asthma. *Am J Med* 1983;75:580
7. O'Connell MB, Iber C: Continuous intravenous terbutaline infusions for adult patients with status asthmaticus. *Ann Allergy* 1990;64:213
8. Smith CS, Williams MH: Relationship of wheezing to the severity of obstruction in asthma. *Arch Intern Med* 1983;143:890
9. Centor RM, Yarbrough B, Wood JP: Inability to predict relapse in acute asthma. *N Engl J Med* 1984;310:577
10. McFadden ER Jr, Kiser R, DeGroot WJ: Acute bronchial asthma: Relations between clinical and physiologic manifestations. *N Engl J Med* 1973;288:221
11. Gerschke GL, Baker FJ, Rosen P: Pulsus paradoxus as a

parameter in treatment of the asthmatic. *J Am Coll Emerg Physicians* 1977;6:191

12. Shim CS, Williams MH: Evaluation of the severity of asthma: patients versus physicians. *Am J Med* 1980;68:11

13. Fanta CH, Rossing TH, McFadden ER: Emergency room treatment of asthma. *Am J Med* 1982;72:416

14. Nowak RM, Pensler MI, Sarkar DD, et al: Comparison of peak expiratory flow and FEV_1 admission criteria for acute bronchial asthma. *Ann Emerg Med* 1982;11:64

15. Brandstetter RD, Gotz VP, Mar DD: Identifying the acutely ill patient with asthma. *South Med J* 1981;74:713

16. Martin TG, Elenbaas RM, Pingleton SH: Use of peak expiratory flow rates to eliminate unnecessary arterial blood gases in acute asthma. *Ann Emerg Med* 1982;11:70

17. National Heart, Lung, and Blood Institute. National Asthma Education Program: Expert Panel Report: guidelines for the diagnosis and management of asthma. *J Allergy Clin Immunol* 1991;88:425

18. Rodrigo G, Rodrigo C: Assessment of the patient with acute asthma in the emergency department: a factor analytic study. *Chest* 1993;104:1325

19. Banner AS, Shah RS, Addington WW: Rapid prediction of need for hospitalization in acute asthma. *JAMA* 1976;235:1337

20. Fanta CH, Rossing TH, McFadden ER: Emergency room treatment of asthma: relationships among therapeutic combinations, severity of obstruction and time course of response. *Am J Med* 1982;72:416

21. Burki NK, Diamond L: Serum creatine phosphokinase activity in asthma. *Am Rev Respir Dis* 1977;116:327

22. Grossman J: The occurrence of arrhythmias in hospitalized asthma patients. *J Allergy Clin Immunol* 1976;57:310

23. Brenner BE: The acute asthmatic in the emergency department. *Am J Emerg Med* 1985;3:74

24. Hopewell PC, Miller RT: Pathophysiology and management of severe asthma. *Clin Chest Med* 1984;5:623

25. Shim CS, Williams MH: Bronchodilator response to oral aminophylline and terbutaline versus aerosol albuterol in patients with chronic obstructive pulmonary disease. *Am J Med* 1983;75:697

26. Rossing TH, Fanta CH, McFadden ER: Effect of outpatient treatment of asthma with beta agonists on the response to sympathomimetics in an emergency room. *Am J Med* 1983; 75:781

27. Kennedy MCS, Simpson WT: Human pharmacological and clinical studies on salbutamol: a specific beta-adrenergic bronchodilator. *Br J Dis Chest* 1969;63:165

28. Paterson JW, Evans RJC, Prime FJ: Selectivity of bronchodilator action of salbutamol in asthmatic patients. *Br J Dis Chest* 1971;65:21

29. National Heart, Lung, and Blood Institute, National Institutes of Health: International Consensus Report on Diagnosis and Management of Asthma. NIH Pub No. 92-3091. Bethesda, MD, US Department of Health and Human Services, Offices of Prevention, Education, and Control, 1992

30. Beveridge R, Grunfeld A, Hodder R, Verbeek R, and members of the CAEMP/CTS Consensus Panel: Guidelines for the emergency management of adult asthma (poster). Ottawa, Canada: Canadian Association of Emergency Medicine Physicians and the Canadian Thoracic Society, 1994

31. Rudnitsky GS, Eberlein RS, Schoffstall JM, et al: Comparison of intermittent and continuously nebulized albuterol for treatment of asthma in an urban emergency department. *Ann Emerg Med* 1993;22:1842

32. Lin RY, Sauter D, Newman T, et al: Continuous versus intermittent albuterol nebulization in the treatment of acute asthma. *Ann Emerg Med* 1993;22:1847

33. Lin RY, Smith AJ, Hergenroeder P: High serum albuterol levels and tachycardia in adult asthmatics treated with high-dose continuously aerosolized albuterol. *Chest* 1993;103:221

34. Amory DW, Burnham SC, Cheney FW: Comparison of the cardiopulmonary effects of subcutaneously administered epinephrine and terbutaline in patients with reversible airway obstruction. *Chest* 1975;67:279

35. Rosenfeld CR, Barton MD, Meschia G: Effects of epinephrine on distribution of blood flow in the pregnant ewe. *Am J Obstet Gynecol* 1972;124:156

36. Shim C, Williams J: Bronchial response to oral versus aerosol metaproterenol in asthma. *Ann Intern Med* 1980;93:428

37. Tashkin DP, Trevor E, Chopra SK, et al: Sites of airway dilatation in asthma following inhaled versus subcutaneous terbutaline. *Am J Med* 1980;68:14

38. Appel D, Karpel P, Sherman M: Epinephrine improves expiratory airflow rates in patients with asthma who do not respond to inhaled metaproterenol sulfate. *J Allergy Clin Immunol* 1989;84:90

39. Newhouse MT, Dolovich MB: Control of asthma by aerosols. *N Engl J Med* 1986;315:870

40. Idris AH, McDermott MF, Raucci JC, et al: Emergency department treatment of severe asthma: metered-dose inhaler plus holding chamber is equivalent in effectiveness to nebulizer. *Chest* 1993;103:665

41. Jasper AC, Mohsenifar Z, Kahan S, et al: Cost-benefit comparison of aerosol bronchodilator delivery methods in hospitalized patients. *Chest* 1987;91:614

42. Busse WW: Mechanisms of inflammation in the asthmatic patient. *Allergy Proc* 1993;14:5

43. Eptstein SW, Manning CPR, Ashley MJ, et al: Survey of the clinical use of pressurized aerosol inhalers. *Can Med Assoc J* 1979;120:813

44. Williams S, Seaton A: Intravenous or inhaled salbutamol in severe acute asthma. *Thorax* 1977;32:555

45. Lawford P, Jones BMJ, Milledge JS: Comparison of intravenous and nebulised salbutamol in initial treatment of severe asthma. *BMJ* 1978;1:84

46. Williams SJ, Winner SJ, Clark TJH: Comparison of inhaled and intravenous terbutaline in acute severe asthma. *Thorax* 1981;36:629

47. Bloomfield P, Carmichael J, Petrie GR, et al: Comparison of salbutamol given intravenously and by intermittent positive-pressure breathing in life-threatening asthma. *BMJ* 1979; 1:848

48. Salmeron S, Brochard L, Mal H, et al: Nebulized versus intravenous albuterol in hypercapnic acute asthma: a multicenter, double-blind, randomized study. *Am J Respir Crit Care Med* 1994;149:1466

49. Rebuck AS, Chapman KR, Abboud P: Nebulized anticholinergic and sympathomimetic treatment of asthma and chronic airways disease in the emergency room. *Am J Med* 1987;82:59

50. Ward MJ, Fentem PH, Smith WHR, et al: Ipratropium bromide in acute asthma. *BMJ* 1981;282:598

51. Kelly HW, Murphy S: Should anticholinergics be used in acute severe asthma? *Ann Pharmacother* 1990;24:409

52. Bryant DH, Rogers P: Effects of ipratropium bromide nebulizer solution with and without preservatives in the treatment of acute and stable asthma. *Chest* 1992;102:742

53. Gross N: The use of anticholinergic agents in the treatment of airways disease. *Clin Chest Med* 1988;9:591

54. Rafferty P, Beasley R, Howarth PH: Bronchoconstriction induced by ipratropium bromide in asthma; relation to bromide ion. *BMJ* 1986;293:1538

55. Gilman MJ, Meyer L, Carter J, et al: Comparison of aerosolized glycopyrrolate and metaproterenol in acute asthma. *Chest* 1990;98:1095

56. Rossing TH, Fanta CH, Goldstein DH, et al: Emergency therapy of asthma: comparison of acute effects of parenteral and inhaled sympathomimetics and infused aminophylline. *Am Rev Respir Dis* 1980;122:365

57. Littenberg B: Aminophylline in severe, acute asthma: a meta-analysis. *JAMA* 1988;259:1678

58. Siegel D, Sheppard D, Gelb A, et al: Aminophylline increases the toxicity but not the efficacy of an inhaled beta-adrenergic agonist in the treatment of acute exacerbations of asthma. *Am Rev Respir Dis* 1985;132:283

59. Murphy DG, McDermott MF, Rydman RJ, et al: Aminophylline in the treatment of acute asthma when beta-two adrenergics and steroids are provided. *Arch Intern Med* 1993;153:1784

60. Josephson GW, Kennedy HL, MacKenzie EJ, et al: Cardiac dysrhythmias during the treatment of acute asthma: a comparison of two treatment regimens by double blind protocol. *Chest* 1980;78:429

61. Huang D, O'Brien RG, Harman E, et al: Does aminophylline benefit adults admitted to the hospital for an acute exacerbation of asthma? *Ann Intern Med* 1993;119:1155

62. Lalla S, Saleh A, Faroog J, et al: Intravenous aminophylline in acute, severe bronchial asthma. *Chest* 1991;100(Suppl):60S

63. Kelly HW, Murphy S: Should we stop using theophylline for the treatment of the hospitalized patient with status asthmaticus. *DICP* 1989;23:995

64. Bukowskyj M, Nakatsu K, Munt PW: Theophylline reassessed. *Ann Intern Med* 1984;101:63

65. Bauman JH, Lalonde RL, Self TH: Factors modifying serum theophylline concentrations: an update. *Immunol Allergy Pract* 1985;7:259

66. Emerman CL, Nowak RM, Tomlanovich MC, et al: Theophylline concentrations in the emergency treatment of acute bronchial asthma. *Am J Emerg Med* 1983;1:12

67. Jenne JW: Theophylline use in asthma: some current issues. *Clin Chest Med* 1984;5:645

68. Rothstein RJ: Intravenous theophylline therapy in asthma: a clinical update. *Ann Emerg Med* 1980;9:327

69. Aubier M, Troyer AD, Sampson M, et al: Aminophylline improves diaphragmatic contractility. *N Engl J Med* 1981;305:249

70. Miech RP, Stein M: Methylxanthines. *Clin Chest Med* 1986;7:331

71. Dunlap NE, Fulmer JD: Corticosteroid therapy in asthma. *Clin Chest Med* 1984;5:669

72. Haskell RJ, Wong BM, Hansen JE: A double-blind, randomized clinical trial of methylprednisolone in status asthmaticus. *Arch Intern Med* 1983;143:1324

73. Littenberg B, Gluck EH: A controlled trial of methylprednisolone in the emergency treatment of acute asthma. *N Engl J Med* 1986;314:150

74. Stein LM, Cole RP: Early administration of corticosteroids in emergency room treatment of acute asthma. *Ann Intern Med* 1990;112:822

75. Skobeloff EM, Spivey WH, McNamara RM, et al: Intravenous magnesium sulfate for the treatment of acute asthma in the emergency department. *JAMA* 1989;262:1210

76. Noppen M, Vanmaele L, Impens N, et al: Bronchodilating effect of intravenous magnesium sulfate in acute severe asthma. *Chest* 1990;97:373

77. Rolla G, Bucca C, Caria E, et al: Acute effect of intravenous magnesium sulfate on airway obstruction of asthmatic patients. *Ann Allergy* 1986;61:388

78. Okayama H, Okayama M, Aikawa T, et al: Treatment of status asthmaticus with intravenous magnesium sulfate. *J Asthma* 1991;28:11

79. Bloch H, Silverman R, Mancherje N, et al: Magnesium sulfate is a useful adjunct to standard therapy for acute severe asthma. *Chest* 1992;102(Suppl):83S

80. Green SM, Rothrock SG: Intravenous magnesium for acute asthma: failure to decrease emergency treatment duration or need for hospitalization. *Ann Emerg Med* 1992;21:260

81. Tiffany BR, Berk W, Todd IK, et al: Magnesium bolus or infusion fails to improve expiratory flow in acute asthma exacerbations. *Chest* 1993;104:831

82. Bloch H, Silverman R, Mancherje N, et al: Intravenous magnesium sulfate as an adjunct in the treatment of acute asthma. *Chest* 1995;107:1576

83. Gluck EH, Onorato DJ, Castriotta R: Helium-oxygen mixtures in intubated patients with status asthmaticus and respiratory acidosis. *Chest* 1990;98:693

84. Kass JE, Castriotta RJ: Heliox therapy in acute severe asthma. *Chest* 1995;107:757

85. Madison JM, Irwin RS: Heliox for asthma: a trial balloon. [Letter]. *Chest* 1995;107:597

86. Manthous CA, Hall JB, Melmed A, et al: Heliox improves pulsus paradoxus and peak expiratory flow in nonintubated patients with severe asthma. *Am J Respir Crit Care Med* 1995;151:310

87. Scoggin CH, Sahn SA, Petty TL: Status asthmaticus: a nine-year experience. *JAMA* 1977;238:1158

88. Westerman DE, Benatar SR, Potgierter PD, et al: Identification of the high-risk asthmatic patient. *Am J Med* 1979;66:565

89. Zimmerman JL, Dellinger RP, Shah, AN, et al: Endotracheal intubation and mechanical ventilation in severe asthma. *Crit Care Med* 1993;21:1727

90. MacIntyre NR, Silver RM, Miller CW, et al: Aerosol delivery in intubated, mechanically ventilated patients. *Crit Care Med* 1985;13:81

91. Manthous CA, Hall JB, Schmidt GA, et al: Metered-dose inhaler versus nebulized albuterol in mechanically ventilated patients. *Am Rev Respir Dis* 1993;148:1567

92. Diot P, Morra L, Smaldone GC: Albuterol delivery in a model of mechanical ventilation. *Am J Respir Crit Care Med* 1995;152:1391

93. Corssen G, Gutierrez J, Reves JG, Huber FC: Ketamine in the anaesthetic management of asthmatic patients. *Anesth Analg* 1972;51:588

94. Huber FC, Gutierrez J, Corssen G: Ketamine: its effect on airways resistance in man. *South Med J* 1972;65:1176

95. Clarkson K, Power CK, O'Connell F, et al: A comparative evaluation of propofol and midazolam as sedative agents in fiberoptic bronchoscopy. *Chest* 1993;104:1029

96. Williams TJ, Tuxen DV, Scheinkestel CD, et al: Risk factors for morbidity in mechanically ventilated patients with acute severe asthma. *Am Rev Respir Dis* 1992;146:607

97. Tuxen DV, Williams TJ, Scheinkestel CD, et al: Use of a measurement of pulmonary hyperinflation to control the level of mechanical ventilation in patients with acute severe asthma. *Am Rev Respir Dis* 1992;146:1136

98. Leatherman JW, Ravenscraft SA, Iber C, et al: Does measured auto-PEEP accurately reflect the degree of dynamic hyperinflation during mechanical ventilation of status asthma? *Am Rev Respir Dis* 1993;147:877A

99. Hall JB, Wood LDH: Management of the critically ill asthmatic patient. *Med Clin North Am* 1990;74:779

100. Tuxen DV, Lane S: The effects of ventilatory pattern on hyperinflation, airway pressures, and circulation in mechanical ventilation of patients with severe air-flow obstruction. *Am Rev Respir Dis* 1987;136:872

101. Isenstein D, Venner DS, Duggan J: Neuromuscular blockade in the intensive care unit. *Chest* 1992;102:P1258

102. Wheeler AP: Sedation, analgesia, and paralysis in the intensive care unit. *Chest* 1993;104:566

103. Williams TJ, Tuxen DV, Scheinkestel CD, et al: Risk factors for morbidity in mechanically ventilated patients with acute severe asthma. *Am Rev Respir Dis* 1992;146:607

104. Leatherman J: Life-threatening asthma. *Clin Chest Med* 1994;15:453

105. Menitove SM, Goldring RM: Combined ventilator and bicarbonate strategy in the management of status asthmaticus. *Am J Med* 1983;74:898

106. Bidani A, Tzouanakis AE, Cardenas VJ, et al: Permissive hypercapnia in acute respiratory failure. *JAMA* 1994;272:957

107. Feihl F, Perret C: Permissive hypercapnia: how permissive should we be? *Am J Respir Crit Care Med* 1994;150:1722

108. Darioli R, Perret C: Mechanical controlled hypoventilation in status asthmaticus. *Am Rev Respir Dis* 1984;129:385

109. Tuxen DV: Permissive hypercapnic ventilation. *Am J Respir Crit Care Med* 1994;150:870

110. Clark SW, Newman SP: Therapeutic aerosols. 2. Drugs available by the inhaled route. *Thorax* 1984;39:1

111. Bloomfield P, Carmichael J, Petrie GR, et al: Comparison of salbutamol given intravenously and by intermittent positive-pressure breathing in life-threatening asthma. *Br Med J* 1979;1:848

112. Rosseel P, Lauwers LF, Baute L: Halothane treatment in life-threatening asthma. *Intensive Care Med* 1985;11:241

113. Schwartz SH: Treatment of status asthmaticus with halothane. *JAMA* 1984;251:2688

114. Robertson CE, Sinclair CJ, Steedman D, et al: Use of ether in life-threatening acute severe asthma. *Lancet* 1985;1:187

115. Grunberg G, Cohen JD, Keslin J, et al: Facilitation of mechanical ventilation in status asthmaticus with continuous intravenous thiopental. *Chest* 1991;99:1216

116. Lang, DM, Simon RA, Mathison DA, Timms RM, Stevenson DD: Safety and possible efficacy of fiberoptic bronchoscopy with lavage in the management of refractory asthma with mucous impaction. *Ann Allergy* 1991;67:324

117. Henke CA, Hertz M, Gustafson P: Combined bronchoscopy and mucolytic therapy for patients with severe refractory status asthmaticus on mechanical ventilation: a case report and review of the literature. *Crit Care Med* 1994;22:1880

118. Millman M, Goodman AH, Goldstein IM, et al: Status asthmaticus: use of acetylcysteine during bronchoscopy and lavage to remove mucous plugs. *Ann Allergy* 1983;50:85

119. Weinstein HJ, Bone RC, Ruth WE: Pulmonary lavage in patients treated with mechanical ventilation. *Chest* 1977;72:583

Critical Care, Third Edition, edited by Joseph M. Civetta,
Robert W. Taylor, and Robert R. Kirby.
Lippincott-Raven Publishers, Philadelphia, PA © 1997.

CHAPTER 131

■

Inhalation Injury

David A. Striker
Robert W. Taylor

IMMEDIATE CONCERNS ■

MAJOR PROBLEMS

1. Acute injury to the respiratory system may develop
   after exposure to a variety of toxic chemical inhalants
   and smoke.
2. Following exposure, a wide spectrum of clinical conditions can develop ranging from mild irritation of the
   upper airways to pulmonary edema and death (Fig.
   131-1).

STRESS POINTS

1. The pattern and severity of injury depends on the
   type and concentration of material inhaled, duration
   of exposure, rate and depth of respiration, and the
   presence of other injuries or preexisting conditions.
2. Toxic inhalants can be subdivided into categories on
   the basis of their mechanism of injury.
   a. Simple asphyxiants
   b. Tissue asphyxiants
   c. Chemical irritants
   d. Systemic toxins
   e. Volatilized hydrocarbons
   f. Metal fume fever
   g. Bronchospasm inducers (Table 131-1)
3. Despite the many types of toxins and various exposure
   environments there are only two basic mechanisms of
   pathogenesis: direct pulmonary injury and systemic
   absorption of inhaled poisons.
4. A typical environment for exposure to toxic inhalants
   includes industrial workplaces, areas in which cleaning
   supplies are used, and fires.

5. Fire smoke is a complex mixture of ingredients that
   varies from fire to fire, during the time course of a
   single fire, and between victims of the same fire.
6. A wide mixture of chemical toxins are produced during
   fires by combustion or pyrolysis (Table 131-2).
7. Thermal decomposition in the presence of oxygen results in combustion and in its absence, pyrolysis and
   asphyxia.

ESSENTIAL DIAGNOSTIC TESTS
AND PROCEDURES

1. There are no absolute diagnostic criteria for inhalation
   injury; therefore the diagnosis requires that the clinician has a high index of suspicion and is conscious of
   the subtle signs and symptoms that may be present in
   an exposed patient.
2. Some patients may present without any symptoms initially but can develop life-threatening complications
   hours to days after the exposure. All unconscious fire
   victims, patients with thermal skin burns, and those
   with a history of exposure in an enclosed space are at
   risk to develop inhalation lung injury.
3. Spirometric testing, fiberoptic bronchoscopy, and xenon lung scans can be useful adjunctive tests to determine the patient population that has sustained significant pulmonary injury.
4. Carboxyhemoglobin levels, while useful as an indirect
   marker of exposure, have no utility in determining the
   degree of pulmonary involvement or prognosis.

1947

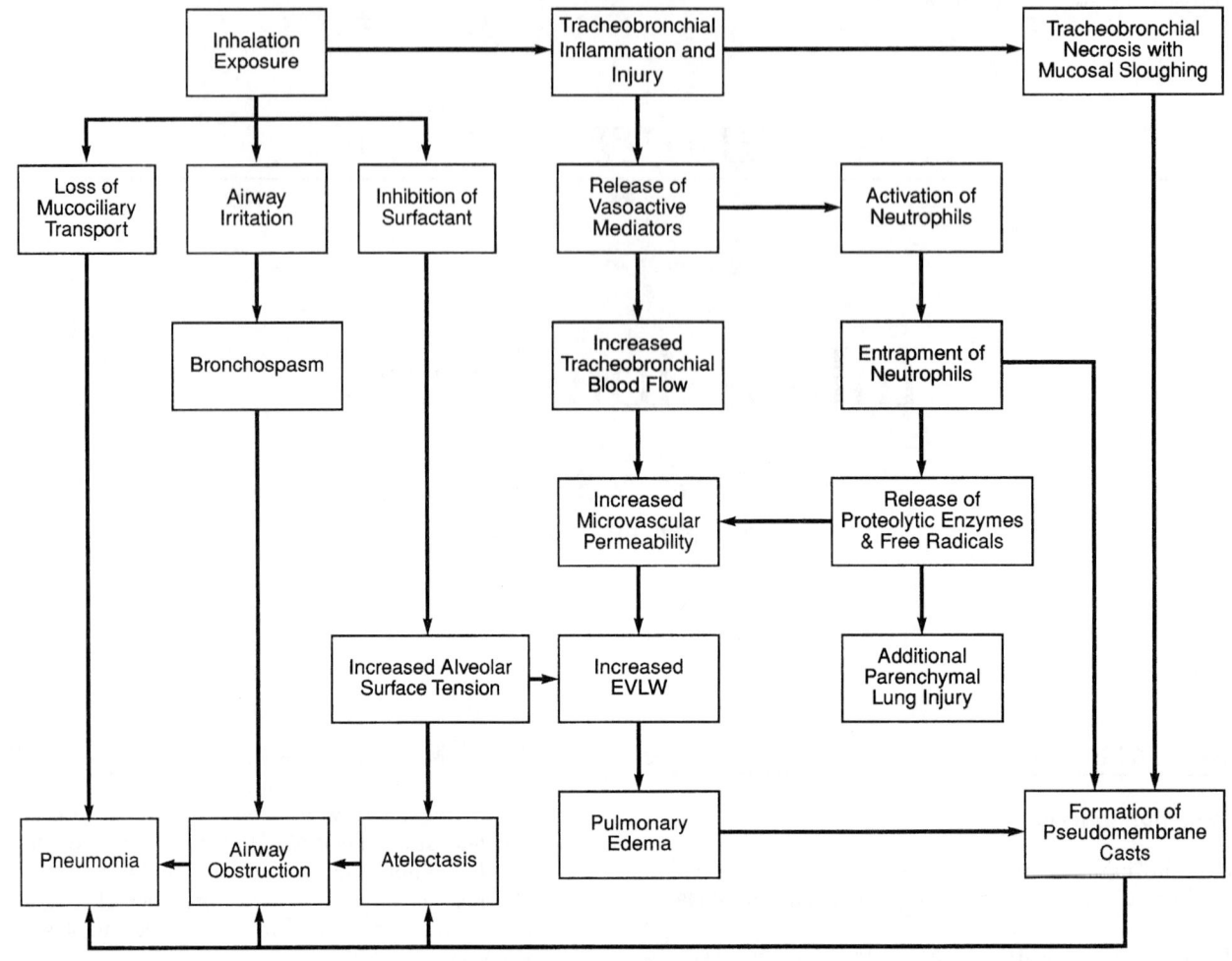

FIGURE 131-1. Pathophysiology of inhalation injury. EVLW, extravascular lung water.

INITIAL THERAPY

1. Initial treatment is supportive and follows basic resuscitation guidelines because it is often difficult or impossible to determine the type or concentration of toxins inhaled.
2. Maintenance of airway patency is extremely important and early intubation may be necessary to prevent airway obstruction and to aid in the clearance of secretions and debris.
3. Application of 100% oxygen should occur immediately, since this hastens the elimination of carboxyhemoglobin.
4. After the patient has been stabilized and removed from the exposure environment, a secondary assessment for associated injuries should be performed.
5. Further treatments are guided by the severity of the pulmonary injury. Aggressive bronchopulmonary hygiene with addition of beta-agonists or theophylline to treat bronchospasm is beneficial.
6. Prophylactic antibiotics and steroids have no role in the treatment of inhalation injury and can increase mortality.
7. Patients with significant inhalation exposure should be monitored for at least 24 hours to observe for delayed effects that may develop and cause a rapid deterioration.

FIRE AND SMOKE

Smoke inhalation is the most common cause of death in fires and results from inhalation of gaseous or particulate matter of incomplete combustion. Inhalation injury should be suspected in all unconscious fire victims and in those fires that produce a heavy smoke or occur in an enclosed area. The incidence of inhalation injury in all hospitalized burn patients varies between 5 and 35 percent.[1] Inhalation injury has been shown to increase mortality in all thermally injured patients regardless of age and total body surface area involved and is associated with a threefold prolongation of hospital stay.[2] Smoke is defined as the airborne products released by thermal decomposition of matter and is composed of gases, volatized organic molecules, free radicals, systemic toxins, respiratory irritants, and particulate matter.

TABLE 131-1. Classification of Toxic Inhalants

PHYSICAL ASPHYXIANTS	*Volatile Hydrocarbons*
Argon	Acetone
Carbon dioxide	Aniline
Ethane	Benzene
Hydrogen	Butane
Methane	Chloroform
Nitrogen	Cyclohexane
	Freon
RESPIRATORY IRRITANTS	Hexane
	Methylene chloride
Acetic acid	Phenol
Acrolein	Toluene
Ammonia	Xylene
Chlorine	
Diborane	*Miscellaneous*
Formaldehyde	Arsine
Hydrogen chloride	Butyl nitrate
Hydrogen fluoride	Mercury vapor
Nitrogen dioxide	Metallic oxide
Ozone	Methyl chloride
Phosgene	Organophosphates
Silicon tetrachloride	Phosphine
Sulfur dioxide	
Zinc chloride	PULMONARY SENSITIZERS
	Acid anhydrides
SYSTEMIC TOXINS	Amines
	Isocyantes
CHEMICAL ASPHYXIANTS	Metals
	Organic dusts
Carbon monoxide	
Hydrogen cyanide	
Hydrogen sulfide	
Acrylonitrile	

TABLE 131-2. Toxic Substances Produced in Fires

SOURCE	SUBSTANCE
Wood	Acrolein, aldehydes, carbon monoxide, HCL
Cotton	Acrolein, aldehydes, HCL acid
Paper	Sulfur oxides, HCL, aldehydes, acrolein
Polyvinyl chloride	HCL acid
Nylon, silk	Ammonia, cyanide, isocyanates
Fuel	Oxides of nitrogen, carbon monoxide
Batteries, paint	Cadmium, zinc, manganese, cobalt

HCL, Hydrogen chloride.

TABLE 131-3. Clinical Presentation

Chest tightness	Alteration of sensorium
Wheezing	Conjunctival irritation
Stridor	Singed nasal hairs
Hoarseness	Facial burns
Dyspnea	Uvular edema
Tachypnea	Carbonaceous sputum

The type of products liberated during a fire depends on the amount and composition of material burned, the amount of water present, the degree of heat, and the partial pressure of oxygen. As the water content of a fire increases, the amount of aerosolized solid and liquid particles increases as does its heat carrying capacity.[3] The principal gases found in smoke include oxygen, carbon dioxide, carbon monoxide, and hydrogen cyanide. Most of the toxic compounds liberated during a fire are not produced in concentrations that are lethal but contribute to mortality by potentiating the asphyxiant effects of carbon monoxide and hydrogen cyanide.

Particulate matter can cause pulmonary injury by several mechanisms. The particles can act as a direct airway irritant, they may be coated with chemical irritants and transport these toxins into the airways, or they may be hot and act as a vehicle for thermal injury to the lower airways.[4] The distance that chemicals travel into the respiratory system depends on the size of the particles on which they are carried. Particles 5 to 30 μm in diameter become lodged in the upper respiratory tract and those less than 0.5 μm are usually exhaled. Particles 1 to 5 μm in diameter are deposited in the trachea and major bronchi and those less than 1 μm enter the alveolar zone.[5] In fires, tissue anoxia can develop both directly and indirectly. Initially, the hypoxic atmosphere of the fire leads to a fall in blood oxygen content. Second, incomplete combustion results in the formation of carbon monoxide, which preferentially binds to hemoglobin and reduces its oxygen carrying capacity. Third, carbon monoxide and hydrogen cyanide interfere with oxygen utilization in the mitochondria. Lastly, inhalation of toxic materials from the fire can have a depressant effect on the cardiovascular system with a decrease in oxygen delivery.

THERMAL INJURY ■

Thermal injury is usually confined to the nasopharynx and upper airways. The extent of thermal damage that occurs depends not only on the temperature of the inhaled substance but also on the water content, or heat carrying capacity of the inhaled gas. The nasopharynx and upper airways provide an extremely efficient cooling system that filters out heated inhaled particles.[6] An inhaled substance of 260°C can be cooled to 50°C before reaching the major airways. The glottis and vocal cords function as an additive protective mechanism by reflexly closing after exposure to heat.[7] As a result of these protective mechanisms, thermal injury below the vocal cords occurs in less than 5% of patients with cutaneous burns.[8] The lower airways may be subjected to thermal injury after contact with hot particulate matter or partially oxidized gases that continue to burn after entering the airway. In addition, steam, which has a specific heat carrying capacity 4000 times that of air, can overcome the protective mechanisms of the upper airways.

Heat damage to the upper airways occurs by direct contact with the respiratory mucosa leading to swelling, ulceration, congestion, and hemorrhage. The most important complication of thermal injury is obstructive asphyxia from upper airway and laryngeal edema. Thermal injury is best managed by preventing airway obstruction with early insertion of an endotracheal tube before the airway becomes compromised.

PATHOGENESIS   ■

Inhaled toxins produce damage to both the tracheobronchial and parenchymal regions of the lung. The resultant injury is due to direct local cell damage by components of the inhalant and the activation of systemic vasoactive mediators generated during the inflammatory cascade. Almost immediately following exposure the cilia of the tracheobronchial mucosa are inactivated with subsequent loss of the mucociliary transport mechanism and bacterial clearance. Surfactant is also inactivated soon after exposure leading to development of atelectasis and an increase in extravascular lung water (EVLW). Bronchospasm is induced by stimulation of irritant receptors in the airways, which worsens atelectasis and ventilation–perfusion relationships in the lung.[9]

Intense tracheobronchial inflammation develops within hours of exposure and blood flow to the tracheobronchial region increases 10- to 20-fold.[10] The vasoactive mediators produced during inflammation and the increased blood flow result in an increased concentration of activated neutrophils in the pulmonary microcirculation and interstitium. These neutrophils become trapped by hypoxic vasoconstriction and damaged or obstructed blood vessels. The sequestered neutrophils degranulate releasing oxygen free radicals and proteolytic enzymes such as trypsin, elastase, and beta-glucuronidase.[11] Under normal conditions enzymatic degradation of the lung is prevented by soluble antiproteases that bind to and inactivate these enzymes. However, following exposure to the inhalants, the antiproteases become depleted and parenchymal injury can develop. The proteolytic enzymes are then allowed to destroy fibronectin and other glycoproteins, which weakens the intercellular bonds of the epithelial and endothelial cells creating gaps. These gaps allow leakage of protein and fluid into the interstitial space.[12] As the volume of fluid increases in the interstitial space the integrity of the alveolar epithelium may be compromised and rupture, and the interstitial fluid enters the alveolar space. The production of free radicals by neutrophils or present as constituents of the inhaled toxin can intensify the pulmonary damage. Free radicals can oxidize and inactivate antiproteases and stimu-

late production of chemotactic factors. In addition, they can stimulate contractile elements of epithelial and endothelial cells that change the cell's shape and create gaps in the tight junctions allowing additional protein and fluid leakage and an increase in EVLW.[13]

The lining epithelium of the trachea and bronchi die as a result of the inhaled toxins and products released during inflammation. The necrotic cells slough into the airway and mix with the protein-rich exudate, neutrophils, and mucus to form pseudomembrane casts.[11] These casts fill the airway resulting in obstruction, atelectasis, and worsening air exchange. Areas of hyperinflation secondary to partial obstruction and air trapping may be seen. Tracheobronchitis and pneumonia may subsequently develop.

HISTOPATHOLOGY   ■

Specimen examination with light and electron microscopy reveals many changes in the lung after inhalation of smoke and other toxins. Within 1 hour of exposure to toxic inhalants or smoke the tracheobronchial epithelium undergoes major changes including loss of cilia. Clumping and swelling of the epithelial cells is also seen, which can progress to cell necrosis and surface erosion. These changes are not seen uniformly throughout the lung but there is patchy involvement with areas of normal mucosa mixed with areas of minor and severe damage.[14–16]

The alveolar epithelium may also become involved, with findings of intracellular edema of type I pneumocytes that may eventually die. The exposed alveolar surface can then become covered by hyaline membranes. The alveolar septum and perivascular space become thickened as a result of interstitial edema. Type II pneumocytes develop changes in the membrane-bound vacuoles but are otherwise spared of damage and play an important role during the reparative phase. Capillary endothelial cells are usually well preserved with only mild intracellular edema formation and development of intercellular gaps, as previously described.

CLINICAL PRESENTATION AND DIAGNOSIS   ■

Signs of pulmonary injury may occur from the 1st to the 15th day after exposure, with a peak incidence at day 2.[17,18] There are no absolute criteria to make the diagnosis of inhalation injury but a clinical picture is suggestive (Table 131-3). The presence of these clinical findings after an episode of exposure suggests inhalation injury and the need for further observation after initial evaluation. Carbonaceous sputum serves only as an indicator of exposure and has no prognostic importance. Stridor, hoarseness, and abnormal phonation is suggestive of an upper airway injury and the upper airway should be evaluated by direct visualization to assess the degree of mucosal involvement and to remove necrotic debris.

Several tests are available to aid in the diagnosis of inhalational lung injury. The chest radiograph is readily available and easily performed but is insensitive in detecting even severe inhalation injury. Clark and coworkers found the chest radiograph to have a false-negative rate of 92% when obtained on the day of presentation.[19] Radiographic evidence of inhalation injury does not usually appear until 24 hours after the initial event and may be difficult to distinguish from pulmonary edema and volume overload.

Spirometric testing can be useful in excluding inhalation injury. Patients with inhalation injury have normal lung volumes on spirometric testing but have a decrease in the maximum expiratory flow volume, FEV_1, forced vital capacity (FVC), and an increase in the work of breathing secondary to an increase in pulmonary resistance. Normally spirometry can exclude the diagnosis of inhalation lung injury and has a negative predictive value of 94% to 100%.[9]

Fiberoptic bronchoscopy is a safe and accurate method to evaluate the supra- and infraglottic regions for mucosal damage. A false-positive result may be seen in heavy smokers and FOB may fail to detect injury of the distal airways resulting from particles less than 1 μm in diameter. Bronchoscopic findings confirm exposure to smoke but do not correlate with severity of illness or mortality. FOB may also be usefull as a treatment modality to improve clearance of secretions and debris.[20,21]

[133]Xe ventilation lung scans should be performed in patients with suspected inhalation injury and a negative result on FOB. An unequal lung field radiation density or retention of the radiolabeled gas in a lung region 90 seconds after inhalation of xenon is a positive scan. Hyperventilation can produce a false-negative scan, and conditions that cause air trapping such as asthma, chronic bronchitis, or bronchiectasis can result in a false-positive study. Scans performed early (3 to 4 hours after exposure) or late (>72 hours after exposure) can produce false-negative results. Xenon scanning is inaccurate in diagnosing upper airway injury but is more sensitive in identifying parenchymal and lower airway injury.[22]

Elevated carboxyhemoglobin levels are responsible for profound hypoxemia but do not cause direct pulmonary damage. Carboxyhemoglobin levels can only be used as an indirect marker of exposure and do not correlate with the degree of respiratory failure, mortality, or prognosis. Normal carboxyhemoglobin levels do not rule out exposure because levels are dependent on the interval between exposure and blood sampling, and whether supplemental oxygen has been administered prior to sampling.

TREATMENT ■

At the present time there is no specific therapy for patients with inhalational lung injury that prevents tissue damage and reduces the increased risk of pulmonary infections. In addition, it is virtually impossible to predict which poisons

a patient has inhaled. Any fire victim who arrives with a skin burn should be considered a patient with potential airway injury. A history of exposure in an enclosed space, even in the absence of immediate clinical signs, warrants a high index of suspicion for occult pulmonary injury, as does an episode of loss of consciousness during an exposure.

A basic treatment protocol should include stabilization of the patient with attention to airway management and circulatory support. Subsequent decontamination and supportive care are also needed. Control of the upper airway is extremely important and early intubation should be performed if signs of impending airway obstruction are seen, the patient is comatose or has depressed respirations, or in patients who exhibit posterior pharyngeal swelling, nasolabial full-thickness burns, or circumferential neck burns.[23] Any patient with a history of significant exposure should be monitored for at least 24 hours because several agents have delayed effects and despite presenting without symptoms, some patients subsequently develop complications.

The treatment of inhalation injury is guided by the severity of the resulting pulmonary insufficiency. Supportive therapy is designed to prevent complications such as laryngeal edema, airway obstruction, excessive secretions, pneumonia, pulmonary edema, bronchospasm, adult respiratory distress syndrome (ARDS), and delayed neurologic sequelae. Each patient with suspected inhalation injury should receive high flow oxygen as early as possible to shorten the half-life of carboxyhemoglobin, since carbon monoxide is a major causative agent of mortality in fires. The use of humidified oxygen may allow more efficient mobilization of secretions and debris, and inhaled beta-agonists may be needed to treat bronchospasm. An aggressive pulmonary toilet with frequent suctioning aids in the clearance of secretions, debris, and bronchial casts. Prophylactic antibiotics have no benefit in preventing bronchopneumonia and can increase the incidence of resistant organisms.[24]

In general, the use of steroids in inhalation lung injury should be avoided. There are no clinical human studies that demonstrate a beneficial effect from steroids, and several studies have shown no improvement in arterial blood gases, pulmonary dynamics, or pathologic changes. Several studies have demonstrated that patients receiving parenteral steroids for as short as 48 hours had an increased incidence of infectious complications and a significantly higher mortality when compared with patients of similar burn size and inhalation injury not receiving steroids.[9,24] Steroids may, however, be useful in treating severe bronchospasm not responsive to beta-agonists and theophylline. In addition, after nitrogen dioxide exposure, cortocosteroids are indicated for up to 8 weeks to prevent the development of bronchiolitis obliterans.[25]

The use of hyperbaric oxygen in the treatment of inhalation lung injury remains controversial. Hyperbaric oxygen can be used to further shorten the half-life of carboxyhemoglobin and may be beneficial in preventing the development of delayed neurologic sequelae after exposures.[26] In addition, there are reports of clinical benefit of hyperbaric oxygen therapy with hydrogen cyanide poisoning.[27]

CLASSIFICATION ■

ASPHYXIANTS

A significant exposure to physical or chemical asphyxiants can occur without a person's knowledge and without direct pulmonary damage. Simple or physical asphyxiants are biologically inert agents that displace or remove oxygen from the inspired air resulting in asphyxiation from hypoxemia. These exposures usually occur in enclosed spaces such as wells, silos, sewers, and mines. After breathing in an oxygen-deficient environment, the partial pressure of oxygen delivered to the tissues falls and cellular hypoxia ensues. Symptoms of asphyxia including headache, sweating, and hyperventilation occur when the oxygen concentration falls to 15%. Stupor, memory loss, and incoordination are seen with levels of 10 percent, and loss of consciousness and death can occur when the ambient oxygen concentration falls below 6% to 8%.[28]

Tissue or chemical asphyxiants interfere with oxygen delivery and use at the cellular level resulting in anaerobic metabolism. These agents can be further subclassified into those that inhibit the binding of oxygen to hemoglobin (carbon monoxide and nitrogen dioxide) and those that block oxidative phosphorylation at the cellular level (hydrogen cyanide, carbon monoxide, hydrogen sulfide, and acrylonitrile).

CARBON DIOXIDE. Carbon dioxide is a physical asphyxiant that is a byproduct of carbohydrate fermentation and is a derivative of dry ice. It is odorless and colorless and is heavier than air. It collects in areas that are poorly ventilated such as caves, mine shafts, and on ships. Treatment is supportive and removal from the area of exposure with application of 100% oxygen.

METHANE. Methane is an odorless and colorless gas that is less dense than air and is produced by decaying organic matter. Typical exposure sites include coal mines and natural gas pockets (it is a constituent of natural gas). Like other simple asphyxiants, 85 percent of the inspired air must be replaced before adverse effects develop. Treatment is removal from the toxic environment and supplemental oxygen.[29]

CARBON MONOXIDE. Incomplete combustion of natural and synthetic organic matter (wood, coal, gasoline, and tobacco) results in the formation of carbon monoxide. Carbon monoxide is present in almost all fires, is colorless, odorless, nonirritating to mucous membranes, and is the most common cause of poisoning deaths in the United States.[30] Morbidity and mortality are greater in patients with preexisting cardiovascular disease, age greater than 60, and in those patients who have suffered an episode of loss of consciousness during the exposure period. Acute mortality from carbon monoxide may be mediated through cerebral hypoxia secondary to respiratory depression or from direct pulmonary shunting and ventilation-perfusion imbalance.

Carbon monoxide does not injure the lung directly but produces its toxic effects by binding to hemoglobin and other cellular proteins including myoglobin. Inhaled carbon monoxide rapidly diffuses across the alveoli and binds to hemoglobin with a relative affinity 200 times greater than that of oxygen.[31] Carboxyhemoglobin decreases the oxygen carrying capacity of hemoglobin and increases the affinity of unbound hemoglobin for oxygen creating a leftward shift of the oxyhemoglobin dissociation curve. The shift in the curve results in a further decrease in oxygen carrying capacity and inhibition of oxygen unloading at the tissue level. When carbon monoxide binds to myoglobin it interferes with oxygen use in the muscle cells. Carbon monoxide also weakly binds to cytochrome oxidase in the mitochondria and partially interferes with oxidative phosphorylation.[32] The net result of the hypoxemia is anaerobic metabolism and lactic acidosis.

The symptoms of carbon monoxide poisoning are due primarily to decreased oxygen delivery and use. Tissues with an active oxygen metabolism such as the brain, kidney, and heart are more sensitive to carbon monoxide poisoning than those with lower oxygen requirements. Individuals with low levels of exposure (CO–Hgb levels <20%) may experience headache, tinnitus, and nausea. Those with moderate exposure (CO–Hgb 20% to 40%) demonstrate weakness and a depressed mental state. Levels greater than 40% are associated with arrhythmias and obtundation. Neurologic deterioration may occur after acute exposure from hypoxemia and an ischemic CNS insult. Delayed neurologic sequelae such as mental deterioration, mutism, gait abnormalities, peripheral neuropathies, cortical blindness, urinary incontinence, and choreoathetosis can occur from 2 to 40 days after the event.[33]

Carbon monoxide is primarily eliminated by the lungs and its elimination depends on the level of inspired oxygen concentration. The goal of treatment of carbon monoxide poisoning is to increase the amount of physically dissolved oxygen in the plasma, which accelerates dissociation of carbon monoxide from hemoglobin. When breathing room air the elimination half-life is 3 to 4 hours and decreases to 30 to 40 minutes with 100% oxygen. Under hyperbaric conditions the half-life can fall to 15 to 20 minutes.[34] Supplemental oxygen in the highest available concentration should be administered as early as possible in all patients with suspected inhalation injury. Oxygen administration should continue until carboxyhemoglobin levels return to normal, although there is no direct correlation between the carboxyhemoglobin levels and the severity of symptoms. The use of hyperbaric oxygen to treat carbon monoxide poisoning is controversial, but anecdotal reports and uncontrolled studies have demonstrated some benefit in preventing the development of the delayed neurologic symptoms.[35,36]

HYDROGEN CYANIDE. Hydrogen cyanide is a chemical asphyxiant and should be suspected in fires in which plastics or chemicals are fuels. Hydrogen cyanide is produced by combustion of natural and synthetic household materials such as paper, nylon, polyurethane, wool, silk, and synthetic polymers. Occupational exposure may occur during electroplating, photographic development, and with use of certain jewelry cleaners. Cyanide is normally present in the body at low concentrations and is metabolized to thiocyanate by the liver. Hydrogen cyanide vapor has a characteristic bitter almond odor; however, 20% to 40% of the population is genetically incapable of detecting it. Hydrogen cyanide is rapidly fatal following inhalation or ingestion. When combined with carbon monoxide, hydrogen cyanide can have a synergistic effect and increase mortality.[37]

Hydrogen cyanide binds to the ferric iron in cytochrome-C oxidase preventing oxygen from reoxidizing the reduced enzyme, thus inhibiting electron transport, and blocking cellular respiration and production of adenosine triphosphate.[38] Cellular anoxia, anaerobic metabolism, and lactic acidosis develop. Hydrogen cyanide also has a weak affinity for hemoglobin and may interfere with oxygen binding. Early symptoms after exposure include headache, palpitations, and dyspnea. Late signs such as bradycardia, vomiting, hypotension, convulsions, coma, and apnea follow.

Cyanide levels can be measured but results usually take hours or days to obtain and are not clinically useful. In addition, blood cyanide levels may not correlate with intracellular levels.[39] Suspicion of cyanide poisoning should be considered if severe hypoxemia is seen without cyanosis, there is a difference of greater than 5 percentage points between the measured (SpO_2) and calculated arterial oxygen saturation (SaO_2), or the patient has a significant anion-gap metabolic acidosis without another explainable etiology.

Treatment of cyanide poisoning can be purely supportive or may require use of specific antidotes. Use of antidotes should be considered in unconscious patients with a history of exposure in an enclosed space and a metabolic acidosis. The primary mechanism of detoxification is to prevent hydrogen cyanide from entering the mitochondria and assisting the body's natural elimination mechanisms. Inhaled amyl nitrite and intravenous sodium nitrite are admistered initially to oxidize hemoglobin to methemoglobin. Methemoglobin competes with cytochrome oxidase for hydrogen cyanide and cyanomethemoglobin is formed. As cyanomethemoglobin dissociates, free cyanide is released and can be converted to thiocyanate by rhodanase, a mitochondrial enzyme found in the liver.[40] Thiocyanate is then excreted in the urine. Methemoglobin forming agents should not be used in patients who cannot have levels followed closely. Second, cobalt edetate or hydroxycobalamin is given as a chelating agent that binds to free cyanide and is excreted in the urine. Thiosulfate can also be administered intravenously to enhance conversion of cyanide to thiocyanate by rhodanase.[41] Hyperbaric oxygen has been reported to be beneficial in the treatment of cyanide poisoning but other studies dispute these findings.[37]

HYDROGEN SULFIDE. Hydrogen sulfide is a byproduct of decay that can be found in oil refineries, natural gas processing plants, fishing industries, and industries that manufacture fertilizers, chemicals, and rubber. Exposures can also occur in sewers and mines. Hydrogen sulfide is more dense than air and has an odor similar to rotten eggs.[42] Its mechanism of action, similar to hydrogen cyanide, is by inhibition of cellular respiration and disruption of several intracellular enzyme systems. High concentrations may depress the central respiratory drive. Hydrogen sulfide is also a respiratory irritant and can cause cough, chest pain, and pulmonary edema. Treatment is similar to cyanide intoxication.[43]

RESPIRATORY IRRITANTS

Respiratory irritants are responsible for the majority of toxic inhalations and produce irritation and inflammation of the respiratory system following dissolution in the fluids of the respiratory mucosa. A wide spectrum of clinical illnesses can develop including tracheobronchitis, pulmonary edema, airway hyperreactivity, obstruction, and pneumonia, all of which can cause hypoxemia. The location and type of injury resulting after an exposure depends on the chemical involved, its particle size, concentration, pH, water solubility, and duration of exposure.

Irritant gases that are highly water soluble such as ammonia, sulfur dioxide, and hydrogen chloride have a rapid onset of injury and usually affect the mucosa of the eyes, nose, mouth, and upper respiratory tract. The lower airways may become involved after prolonged exposure or with high concentrations. Agents with low water solubilities such as oxides of nitrogen, ozone, and phosgene have a delay between exposure and clinical manifestations of injury and preferentially damage the distal airways and alveoli. The cytotoxic tissue effects seen after exposure also vary depending on the type of product generated. Acids (chlorine, hydrogen chloride, phosgene, sulfur dioxide, and oxides of nitrogen) cause tissue coagulation. Alkalis (ammonia) cause a liquefaction necrosis and may penetrate deeper into the mucosal layers. Free radicals formed from chlorine, ozone, and oxides of nitrogen cause lipid peroxidation and inhibit antiproteases in the lung.

NITROGEN DIOXIDE AND OXIDES OF NITROGEN. Nitrogen dioxide is a red-brown pungent gas that is poorly water soluble and is derived by the fermentation of grain nitrates into nitrites and oxygen. Under dry, hot conditions nitrites combine with organic acids to form nitrous acid that decomposes to nitrogen dioxide and nitrogen tetroxide. These agents are the primary mediators of pulmonary toxicity. Sources of exposure include welding, electroplating, metal cleaning, coal mining, as a component of jet engine fuels, as a byproduct of diesel combustion, and in the manufacturing of dyes and lacquers. Farmers may be exposed when entering silos with fresh hay and can develop silo filler's disease when exposed to concentrated grain silage.[28]

Nitrogen dioxide causes damage to the distal airways because of its low water solubility. The nitrogen oxides react with water in the airways and produce nitric acid causing free radical production and lipid peroxidation. The target cells affected are the ciliated secretory cells of the membranous bronchioles and type I alveolar cells. Respiratory symptoms develop within hours after exposure and include wheezing, cough, chest pain, fever, diaphoresis, and tachypnea. Pulmonary edema and ARDS may develop. The pulmonary injury may resolve in some patients but others have progression of the disease and develop bronchiolitis obliterans. Many recover from this stage while others have persistent symptoms or may die.[3] In addition to the local pulmonary damage produced, nitrogen dioxide can be dissolved in body fluids and contributes to hypoxemia, acidosis, and cardiovascular depression. Nitrate ions react with hemoglobin to form methemoglobin, and nitrite ions induce systemic hypotension by their direct actions on vascular smooth muscle.

Treatment is mainly supportive but if significant methemoglobinemia is present, intravenous methylene blue (2 mg/kg) should be administered. The use of steroids is somewhat controversial but most experts believe that 40 to 80 mg/day should be administered for 8 weeks after exposure to prevent the development of bronchiolitis obliterans.[45]

ACROLEIN.   Acrolein is a three-carbon aldehyde with a pungent odor that is released during combustion of wood, cotton, and several man-made products. It is used in the manufacturing of plastics, pharmaceuticals, synthetic fibers, resins, textiles, and herbicides. It is an irritant of the upper rspiratory tract and can cause lacrimation, pulmonary edema, and mucosal sloughing at concentrations as low as 10 ppm. Aldehydes can also impair the chemotactic and phagocytic properties of alveolar macrophages leading to an increased risk of infection. Direct skin contact can cause irritation, erythema, and burns. Treatment is supportive.[28]

CHLORINE.   Chlorine is a dense, heavy, green-yellow gas that has an intermediate water solubility and can cause damage throughout the respiratory tract. Chlorine reacts with water in the mucous membranes to form hydrochloric acid and potent oxygen free radicals. Increased pulmonary vascularity and pulmonary edema may develop. Treatment is supportive.[46,47]

HYDROGEN CHLORIDE.   Hydrogen chloride is highly water soluble and can be inhaled as a gas or as an aerosol. It is used in the manufacturing of dyes, fertilizers, textiles, and rubber. It is formed during the combustion of polyvinyl chloride and during metal ore refining.[48] Exposure to low concentrations causes irritation of the conjunctivae, mucous membranes, and upper airways. Dyspnea, cough, wheezing, and airflow obstruction may be seen. Pulmonary edema may develop after prolonged exposures or with high concentrations. Treatment is supportive.[49]

HYDROGEN FLUORIDE.   Hydrogen fluoride is produced in metal refining, welding, and etching and is similar to hydrogen chloride. The site of injury is usually limited to the upper airways and exposed mucous membranes. Treatment is supportive.

SULFUR DIOXIDE AND SULFURIC ACID.   Sulfur dioxide is used in the manufacturing of paper products, refrigeration, fumigation, metal smelting of sulfide containing ores (copper, lead, and zinc), oil refining, combustion of coal and fuel oils, mining, and wine and food processing. Sulfur dioxide is a highly water soluble, colorless gas that is heavier than air. It is rapidly hydrated on contact with mucosal surfaces and is oxidized to sulfurous acid. Exposures with concentrations of 5 to 10 ppm causes irritation of the conjunctivae and nasal mucosa. Exposures to greater than 50 ppm can cause damage throughout the entire respiratory tract extending to the alveoli. Mucoal sloughing, bronchoconstriction, pulmonary edema, and ARDS have been reported. Treatment is supportive.[50]

PHOSGENE.   Phosgene is a colorless, sweet smelling gas that is poorly water soluble and heavier than air. Workers exposed to heated chlorinated hydrocarbons are at risk of exposure, as are firemen, welders, and paint strippers. It is also used in the manufacturing of pesticides and dyes. Phosgene enters distal airways and alveoli and is slowly hydrolyzed to hydrochloric acid and carbon dioxide with resultant mucosal damage, pulmonary edema, and hemorrhage. Treatment is supportive.[51,52]

FORMALDEHYDE.   Formaldehyde is a colorless gas with a pungent odor that is used in the production of agricultural products, pharmaceuticals, fumigants, and disinfectants. Formaldehyde based resins are used in the manufacturing of plywood, particle board insulation, paper, plastics, textiles, and rubber products. Formaldehyde is liberated when these products are burned and can cause irritations of the skin, eyes, and respiratory system. Airway irritation and bronchospasm may also develop. Treatment is supportive.[53,54]

OZONE.   Ozone is a sweet smelling gas with a moderate water solubility that is produced in the upper atmosphere and is also used in paper bleaching. Exposure from 0.8 to 2 ppm can cause chest pain, cough, and dyspnea. Levels greater than 2 ppm can lead to respiratory failure and noncardiogenic pulmonary edema. Death has been reported with exposures in excess of 5 ppm. Treatment is supportive.[55]

SILICON TETRACHLORIDE.   Silicon is used in the manufacturing of microchips for electronic and computer use and as an agent of chemical warfare. On contact with the moisture of the respiratory system silicon is hydrolyzed to hyrochloric acid in a manner similar to phosgene, but its effects are primarily limited to irritation of the upper airways, eyes, nose, and mucous membranes. Treatment is supportive and should also include a careful ophthalmologic examination.[56]

AMMONIA.   Ammonia is a strongly alkaline, highly water soluble, colorless gas with a very pungent odor used in the production of fertilizers, nitric acid, dyes, plastics, explosives, and synthetic fibers. Ammonium hydroxide is formed after the gas combines with water of the respiratory mucosa and liquefaction necrosis develops. Symptoms of exposure are usually confined to the upper respiratory tract because of ammonia's high water solubility. Symptoms include lacrimation, laryngeal irritation, and cough following mild exposures (50 to 150 ppm) and laryngeal edema, tracheitis, and airway obstruction with higher levels of exposure (>150 ppm). Treatment is supportive.[57-59]

SYSTEMIC TOXINS

Systemic toxins are chemicals that are absorbed from the alveoli into the blood stream after inhalation. They can cause acute and chronic symptoms of the lung and other organ systems. The lung parenchyma may be damaged or may be spared of any injury. Chemical or tissue asphyxiants can also be classified as systemic toxins because they are absorbed from the lung and have widespread tissue effects.

VOLATILE HYDROCARBONS. Volatile hydrocarbons are a group of organic toxicants that are used in the production of solvents, cleaning products, paints, dyes, lacquers, glues, and cements. Gasoline, lighter fluid, and kerosene are created by mixing volatile hydrocarbons. Exposure is usually through intentional inhalation because these products can produce mind altering effects. After inhalation they are absorbed systemically and can have generalized effects because they are highly lipophilic and reach high concentrations in the CNS.[60] Their mechanism of action is unclear but they produce an anesthetic state in the CNS and can cause peripheral neuropathies, hyperreflexia or areflexia, muscle irritability, and coma. They can cause injury in the liver and kidney and can produce cardiac arrhythmias. Bone marrow involvement can develop with resultant blood dyscrasias. Leukemia has been seen after exposure to benzene. When inhaled in high concentrations they can produce severe pulmonary irritation. Sudden death has been reported acutely after inhalation and is believed to be the result of cardiac arrhythmias.[61,62] Treatment is removal from the exposure environment and supportive care.

ARSENIC. Arsine gas is produced when acids are combined with metals and ores containing arsenic. Arsenic is used in the manufacturing of microelectronics and semiconductors and in soldering, galvinizing, and the refinement of metals such as tin, zinc, and lead. Exposures usually cause headache, nausea, vomiting, malaise, and dizziness after systemic absorption with sparing of the respiratory system. The triad of hemoglobinuria, abdominal pain, and jaundice should raise suspicion of arsenic exposure. Treatment is supportive.

ORGANOPHOSPATES. These agents are commonly used as insecticides and in chemical warfare. Their mechanism of action after absorption is to inhibit cholinesterase with a resultant rise in acetylcholine levels. Muscarinic signs of intoxication include lacrimation, salivation, pupillary miosis, vomiting, diarrhea, and bradycardia. The nicotinic effects include muscle fasciculations, CNS depression, and respiratory paralysis.[64] Treatment is twofold: Intravenous atropine acts as a competitive inhibitor of acetylcholine at the receptor sites and reverses the muscarinic effects. Pralidoxime is also administered intravenously to regenerate plasma and red blood cell cholinesterase.[65]

CADMIUM. Cadmium can be inhaled as a dry powder or mist and becomes a gas at high temperatures. Occupational exposures occur during welding, electroplating, smelting, and during the manufacturing of paints, batteries, pesticides, plastics, and semiconductors. In the air, cadmium fumes react with oxygen to form cadmium oxide. Inhalation causes diffuse alveolar and airway damage. The site of injury in the lung depends on particle size. Systemic absorption can occur following inhalation, and deposition of cadmium may occur in the liver, pancreas, and thyroid; in the kidney tubular necrosis can develop. Treatment is supportive.[66,67]

METAL AND POLYMER FUME FEVER. Metal fume fevers are a syndrome of flulike illnesses occurring after exposure to metal oxides.[68] Zinc and copper are the most common

causes but the syndrome may be seen after exposure to mercury, cadmium, magnesium, antimony, nickel, chromium, beryllium, manganese, vanadium, cobalt, tin, and platinum salts. These metal particles enter the alveoli and cause a chemical pneumonitis. The exact mechanism of the systemic symptoms is unclear but tumor necrosis factor and interleukins may play a role. Symptoms include throat irritation, cough, dyspnea, altered taste, weakness, myalgias, and arthralgias. Fever, rigors, leukocytosis, pneumonitis and tracheobronchitis may also develop. The symptoms appear several hours after exposure and last 1 to 2 days. Treatment is supportive and the patient should avoid other exposures.[69]

A similar syndrome called polymer fume fever may be seen after exposure to the fumes of polytetrafluoroethylene (PTFE, Teflon). Exposures may occur in textile and electronic manufacturing plants while smoking cigarettes contaminated with soluble PTFE. The symptoms and time course are similar to metal fume fever. Severe cases have been associated with the development of noncardiogenic pulmonary edema. Treatment is supportive.[70]

PULMONARY SENSITIZERS

Repeated inhalation of these agents produce a hypersensitivity pneumonitis (extrinsic allergic alveolitis). This is an immune-mediated inflammation of the pulmonary parenchyma involving the alveoli and terminal airways. Nonimmunologic processes may also play a role. Approximately 150 low-molecular-weight chemicals have been associated with this condition.[71] The clinical presentation varies and can be acute, subacute, or chronic depending on the duration of exposure. Symptoms include cough, fever, chills, and dyspnea from acute bronchoconstriction. The preferred treatment is avoidance, with bronchodilators and corticosteroids administered as needed.

ORGANIC DUSTS. Examples include moldy hay, grain (oats, wheat, barley, corn), and silage. Inhalation of these organic dusts causes a syndrome referred to as farmer's lung. Pet birds (bird fancier's lung), heating, cooling, and humidification systems (humidifier's lung), and other less commonly encountered materials are known to cause hypersensitivity pneumonitis. Treatment is supportive with avoidance of further exposures.[72,73]

ISOCYANATES. Toluene diisocyanate[74] and trimellitic anhydride[75] are liquids used to manufacture foams, rubber, plastics, adhesives, alkyl resins, and insulation materials. Their vapors induce symptoms of cough, fever, chills, and wheezing, along with irritation of the skin and mucous membranes. Repeated exposures may lead to chronic airway obstruction.

SUMMARY

Toxic inhalants cause pulmonary injury by several different modes of action leading to the development of a combined local and systemic inflammatory response. The degree of injury and the location within the respiratory tree may vary after exposure to different agents depending on their chemical characteristics. A typical exposure, especially with fire smoke, involves inhalation of several different toxic compounds that can cause injury to multiple sites, and certain toxins can potentiate the harmful effects of other inhalants.

The majority of patients with simple asphyxiant and chemical irritant exposures have a good prognosis. Long-term and chronic pulmonary changes may develop such as emphysema, fibrosis, airflow obstruction, and bronchiolitis obliterans. An awareness of patients at risk for inhalation injury and supportive therapy to maintain airway patency and adequate ventilation can improve prognosis.

REFERENCES ■

1. Clark WR: Smoke inhalation: diagnosis and treatment. *World J Surg* 1992;16:24
2. Tridget EE, Shankowsky HA, Taerum TV, et al: The role of inhalation injury in burn trauma: a Canadian experience. *Ann Surg* 1990;212:720
3. Ainslie G: Inhalation injuries produced by smoke and nitrogen dioxide. *Respir Med* 1993;87:169
4. Clark WR, Bonaventura M, Myers W: Smoke inhalation and airway management at a regional burn unit: 1974–1983. Part I: Diagnosis and consensus of smoke inhalation. *J Burn Care Rehabil* 1989;10:52
5. Klaussen CD: Nonmetallic environmental toxicants: air pollutants, solvents, vapors, and pesticides. In: Goodman LS, Gilman A, Rall TW, et al (eds). *The Pharmacological Basis of Therapeutics*, p 1628. New York, Macmillan, 1990
6. Chu C: New concepts of pulmonary burn injury. *J Trauma* 1981;21:958
7. Moylan JA: Smoke inhalation and burn injury. *Surg Clin North Am* 1980;60:1533
8. Fein A, Lefe A, Hopewell PC: Pathophysiology and management of the complications resulting from fire and the inhaled products of combustion: review of the literature. *Crit Care Med* 1980;8:94
9. Mosely S: Inhalation injury: a review of the literature. *Heart Lung* 1988;17:3
10. Herndon DN, Traber DL, Niehaus GD, et al: The pathophysiology of smoke inhalation injury in a sheep model. *J Trauma* 1984;24:1044
11. Herndon DN, Thompson PB, Linares HA, et al: Postgraduate course: respiratory injury. Part I: Incidence, mortality, pathogenesis, and treatment of pulmonary injury. *J Burn Care Rehabil* 1986;7:184
12. Neihaus GD, Kimura R, Traber LD, et al: Administration of a synthetic antiprotease reduces smoke induced drug injury. *J Applied Physiol* 1990;69:694
13. Traber DL, Linares HA, Herndon DN, et al: The pathophysiology of inhalation injury—a review. *Burns Incl Therm Inj* 1988;14:357
14. Linares HA, Herndon DN, Traber DL: Sequence of morphologic events in experimental smoke inhalation. *J Burn Care Rehabil* 1984;10:52
15. Young CJ, Moss J: Smoke inhalation: diagnosis and treatment. *J Clin Anesth* 1989;1:377
16. Hubbard GB, Longlinais PC, Shimozu T, et al: The morphology of smoke inhalation injury in sheep. *J Trauma* 1991;31:1477
17. Birky MM, Clark FB: Inhalation of toxic products from fires: *Bull N Y Acad Med* 1981;57:997
18. Anderson RA, Willetts P, Cheng KN: Fire deaths in the United Kingdom, 1976–1982. *Fire Materials* 1983;7:67
19. Clark WR, Bonaventura M, Myers W: Smoke inhalation and airway management at a regional burn unit: 1974–1983; diagnosis and consequences of smoke inhalation. *J Burn Care Rehabil* 1989;10:52
20. Harvey JS, Watkins CS, Sherman RT: Emergent burn care. *South Med J* 1984;77:204
21. Moylan JA, Alexander G Jr: Diagnosis and treatment of inhalation injury: *World J Surg* 1978;2:185
22. Di Vincenti FC, Pruitt BA Jr, Reckler JM: Inhalation injuries. *J Trauma* 1971;11:109
23. Bartlett RH, Nicole M, Travis MJ, et al: Acute management of the upper airway in facial burns. *Arch Surg* 1976;111:744
24. Haponik EF, Ciapo RO, Herndon DN, et al: Smoke inhalation. *Am Rev Respir Dis* 1988;138:1060
25. Ramirez JR, Dowell AR: Silo filler's disease: nitrogen dioxide induced lung injury. *Ann Intern Med* 1971;74:569
26. Thorn SR: Smoke inhalation. *Emerg Med Clin North Am* 1989;7:371
27. Litovitz TL, Larkin RF, Myers RA: Cyanide poisoning treated with hyperbaric oxygen. *Am J Emerg Med* 1983;1:94
28. Rorison DG, McPherson SJ: Acute toxic inhalations. *Emerg Med Clin North Am* 1992;10:409
29. Weiss SM, Lakshminarayan S: Acute inhalation injury. *Clin Chest Med* 1994;15:103
30. Thorn SR, Klein LW: Carbon monoxide poisoning: a review—epidemiology, pathophysiology, clinical findings, and treatment options including hyperbaric oxygen therapy. *J Toxicol Clin Toxicol* 1989;27:141
31. Rodkey FL, O'Neal JD, Collison HA, et al: Relative affinity of hemoglobin S and hemoglobin A for carbon monoxide and oxygen. *Clin Chem* 1974;20:83
32. Goldbaum LR, Orellano T, Dergal E: Mechanism of the toxic actions of carbon monoxide. *Ann Clin Lab Sci* 1976;6:372
33. Choi IS: Delayed neurologic sequelae in carbon monoxide intoxication. *Arch Neurol* 1983;40:433
34. Winter PM, Miller JN: Carbon monoxide poisoning. *JAMA* 1976;236:1502
35. Mathieu D, Nolf M, Durocher A, et al: Acute carbon monoxide poisoning; risk of late sequelae and treatment by hyperbaric oxygen. *Clin Toxicol* 1985;23:315
36. Norkool DM, Kirpatrick JN: Treatment of acute carbon monoxide poisoning with hyperbaric oxygen: a review of 115 cases. *Ann Emerg Med* 1985;14:1168
37. Barillo DJ, Goode R, Esch V: Cyanide poisoning in victims of fires: analysis of 364 cases and review of the literature. *J Burn Care Rehabil* 1994;15:46
38. Hall AH, Rumak BH: Clinical toxicology of cyanide. *Ann Emerg Med* 1986;15:1067
39. Vogel SN, Sultan TR, Treneyck RP: Cyanide poisoning. *Clin Toxicol* 1981;18:367
40. Levine MS, Radford EP: Occupational exposures to cyanide in Baltimore fire fighters. *J Occup Med* 1978;20:53
41. Saunders JP, Himwich WA: Properties of the transulfurase responsible for conversion of cyanide to thiocyanate. *Am J Physiol* 1950;163:404
42. Smith RP, Gosselin RE: Hydrogen sulfide poisoning. *J Occup Med* 1979;21:93
43. Stine RJ, Slosberg B, Beacham BE: Hydrogen sulfide intoxication. *Ann Intern Med* 1976;85:756
44. Prien T, Traber DL: Toxic smoke compounds and inhalation injury—a review. *Burns* 1988;14:451
45. Horvath EP, Do Pico GA, Barbee RA, et al: Nitrogen dioxide induced pulmonary disease. *J Occup Med* 1978;20:103

46. Adelson L, Kaufman J: Fatal chlorine poisoning. report of 2 cases with clinicopathologic correlation. *Am J Clin Pathol* 1971;56:430

47. Beach RXM, Jones ES, Scarrow GD: Respiratory effects of chlorine gas. *Br J Industr Med* 1969;26:231

48. Dyer RF, Esch VH: Polyvinyl chloride toxicity in fires. *JAMA* 1976;235:393

49. Higgins EA, Fioca V, Thomas AA, et al: Acute toxicity of brief exposures to HF, HCL, NO_2, and HCN with and without CO. *Fire Tech* 1972;8:120

50. Rabinovitch S, Greyson ND, Weiser W, et al: Clinical and laboratory features of acute sulfur dioxide inhalation poisoning: two year follow-up. *Am Rev Respir Dis* 1989;139:556

51. Everett ED, Overhold EL: Phosgene poisoning. *JAMA* 1968; 205:103

52. Bardley BL, Unger KM: Phosgene inhalation: a case report. *Tex Med* 1982;78:51

53. Harris JC, Rumak BH, Aldrich FD: Toxicology of urea formaldehyde and polyurethane foam insulation. *JAMA* 1981;245:243

54. Loomis TA: Formaldehyde toxicity. *Arch Pathol Lab* 1979; 103:321

55. Kerr HD, Kulle TJ, McIlhany MC, et al: Effects of ozone on pulmonary function in normal subjects. *Am Rev Respir Dis* 1975;111:763

56. Kizer GW, Garb LJ, Hine CH: Health effects of silicon tetrachloride: report of an urban accident. *J Occup Med* 1984;26:33

57. Leduc D, Gris P, Lheureux P, et al: Acute and long term respiratory damage following inhalation of ammonia. *Thorax* 1992;47:755

58. Close LG, Catlin FI, Cohn AM: Acute and chronic effects of ammonia burns of the respiratory tract. *Arch Otolaryngol* 1980; 106:151

59. Montague TJ, MacNeil AR: Mass ammonia inhalation. *Chest* 1980;77:496

60. Sourindhrin I: Solvent abuse. *BMJ* 1985;290:94

61. Bass M: Sudden sniffing death. *JAMA* 1970;212:2075

62. Anderson HR, MacNair RS, Ramsey JD: Deaths from abuse of volatile substances: a national epidemiologic survey. *BMJ* 1985;290:304

63. Fowler BA, Weissberg JB: Arsine poisoning. *New Engl J Med* 1974;291:1171

64. Sidell FR: Clinical manifestations and treatment of accidental poisoning by organophosphates. *Clin Toxicol* 1974;7:1

65. Dunn MA, Sidell FR: Progress in medical defense against nerve agents. *JAMA* 1989;262:649

66. Barnhart S, Rosenstock L: Cadmium chemical pneumonitis. *Chest* 1984;86:789

67. Benton DC, Andrews GS, Davies HJ, et al: Acute cadmium fume poisoning. *Br J Med* 1966;23:292

68. McCord CP: Metal fume fever as an immunological disease. *Industr Med Surg* 1960;29:101

69. Mueller EJ, Segere DL: Metal fume fever: a review. *J Emerg Med* 1985;2:271

70. Silver MJ, Young DK: Acute noncardiogenic pulmonary edema due to polymer fume fever. *Clev Clin J Med* 1993;60:479

71. O'Neil CE. Review: mechanisms of occupational airways diseases induced by exposure to organic and inorganic chemicals. *Am J Med Sci* 1990;299:265

72. Dyer EL: Farmer's lung: industrial hazard for rural inhabitants. *South Med J* 1980;73:353

73. Fraser RG, Pare JAP: Extrinsic allergic alveolitis. *Semin Roentgenol* 1975;10:31

74. Brugsch HG, Elkins HB: Toluene di-isocyanate (TDI) toxicity. *N Engl J Med* 1963;268:353

75. Zeiss CR, Patterson R, Pruzansky JJ, et al: Trimellitic anhydride airway syndromes: clinical and immunologic studies. *J Allergy Clin Immunol* 1977;60:96

Critical Care, Third Edition, edited by Joseph M. Civetta,
Robert W. Taylor, and Robert R. Kirby.
Lippincott-Raven Publishers, Philadelphia, PA © 1997.

CHAPTER 132

■

Pulmonary Barotrauma

David L. Brown
Robert R. Kirby

IMMEDIATE CONCERNS ■

MAJOR PROBLEMS

Pulmonary barotrauma (PBT) is a complication of traumatic thoracic injury and therapeutic interventions. Included in the general category of barotrauma are pneumothorax, pulmonary interstitial emphysema (PIE), subcutaneous emphysema, pneumomediastinum, pneumopericardium, pneumoperitoneum and pneumoretroperitoneum, and venous or arterial air embolization.

Because PBT is usually a complication of some other major problem, the outcome of therapy directed specifically at the barotrauma is difficult to assess. Obviously, relief of a tension pneumothorax in a patient with a major crushing injury to the chest can be immediately lifesaving. However, the eventual outcome is more likely related to the magnitude of the associated injuries to the heart and great vessels, and the success in their treatment.

Outside of the ICU, scuba diving–related pulmonary overpressurization accidents are an increasingly common problem because of the popularity and growth of sport diving. Although physicians uncommonly see many patients with barotrauma occurring while diving, they must understand the basic pathophysiology to treat the affected patients properly. In like fashion, we hope that early recognition and treatment (i.e., tube thoracostomy) will decrease the morbidity and mortality associated with traumatic injuries and resultant barotrauma.

The prospects for reducing in-hospital, mechanical ventilator–induced barotrauma seem brighter. Most available evidence suggests that large tidal volume and high peak inflation pressure (PIP) are responsible for lung injuries. An interesting observation is that pneumothorax frequently occurs during the resolution phase, when lung volume and compliance are improving. The level of support in such cases may not be decreased as rapidly as lung function improves. Thus, higher than necessary pressure and volume are delivered. Adjustment of ventilator pressure and volume to the lowest levels consistent with satisfactory ventilation and oxygenation is indicated.

Selected ventilatory techniques may reduce the overall incidence of barotrauma. Intermittent mandatory ventilation (IMV) and synchronized intermittent mandatory ventilation generally provide fewer mechanical breaths per minute than control or assist-control modes and are reported to decrease the incidence of pneumothoraces. Airway pressure release ventilation (APRV) has the lowest peak and mean airway pressure of any conventional method currently used. APRV is indicated for minimal-to-moderate respiratory insufficiency, particularly during the recuperative phase.

STRESS POINTS

1. Providing the required ventilatory assistance without superimposing additional morbidity or mortality is a central problem in managing patients with PBT.
2. Maintain oxygenation with positive airway pressure and as much spontaneous breathing as can be tolerated. Simultaneously reduce the number of positive-pressure mechanical breaths.
3. Limit the peak and mean airway pressures and decrease mechanical tidal volumes. Pressure-controlled mechanical ventilation may be an option, but when used with reversed inspiratory-to-expiratory ratios, it often requires paralysis.

1959

4. Consider pressure support ventilation (PSV) and APRV to achieve the above goals.
5. Sepsis, acute respiratory distress syndrome (ARDS), and pneumonia increase by the risk of PBT.
6. Hypovolemia predisposes patients to PBT, although this relationship is seldom recognized. The same factors that increase the incidence of PBT (high pressures, large tidal volumes) also potentially compromise the circulation.
7. PBT can be associated with venous (and occasionally arterial) air embolism. Sudden cardiovascular collapse should cause one to look for this complication. It can be instantaneously lethal.
8. Other forms of PBT also can be problematic (pneumopericardium, pneumomediastinum, and pneumoperitoneum). They often are difficult to treat.

ESSENTIAL DIAGNOSTIC TESTS AND PROCEDURES

1. Maintain constant vigilance for the injuries that predispose to PBT.
2. Sudden deterioration in a previously stable patient is tension pneumothorax or air embolism until proven otherwise. Cardiovascular insufficiency may appear before clear-cut evidence of PBT.
3. A chest radiograph usually provides diagnostic results for subcutaneous emphysema, pneumomediastinum, pneumopericardium, and tension pneumothorax. Small pneumothoraces can be missed with standard anteroposterior views. In rare cases, a chest computed tomography (CT) scan may be necessary.
4. Arterial blood gas partial pressures and pH can help but are not diagnostic. Decreased pH may reflect cardiac and pulmonary compromise.
5. Physical signs (altered breath sounds, unequal chest expansion) are frequently overlooked in the flurry of activity when a patient deteriorates or collapses.

INITIAL THERAPY

1. For tension pneumothorax, a 16-gauge catheter with a three-way stopcock and attached syringe should be inserted in the second anterior intercostal space on the suspected (or documented) side if immediate decompression is essential.
2. Follow with tube thoracostomy. Adequate decompression occasionally requires CT guidance.
3. Don't delay. Morbidity and mortality increase significantly if treatment is delayed more than 30 minutes.
4. Don't rule out PBT because a chest tube is already in place. It may be plugged, kinked, or outside of the chest cavity.
5. Be judicious with ventilator therapy. Reduce volume and pressure to the lowest levels compatible with adequate oxygenation and ventilation.

PNEUMOTHORAX ■

PATHOPHYSIOLOGY

Thoracic injuries customarily are referred to as penetrating and nonpenetrating. However, elements of both may be present in a given patient. Penetrating injuries commonly result from bullets, knives, and ice picks but also follow attempts at vascular cannulation. Subclavian venipuncture is associated with an incidence rate of pneumothorax ranging from 1% to 2%. Nonpenetrating thoracic injuries may be categorized as blunt or deceleration (most commonly in motor vehicle accidents) and blast (explosions).

Pneumothorax also results from internal forces associated with mechanical ventilation.[1] In such instances, high airway pressure and large tidal volumes overdistend relatively normal alveoli, predisposing to rupture of these air sacs into the contiguous perivascular sheathes. The extra-alveolar air then dissects medially, over the pleural reflections of the great vessels and into the mediastinum.[2] From this point, it may then rupture into the pleural space. Characterization of pneumothorax by the portal of pleural entry is useful for classification (Table 132-1).

Whatever the cause of a pneumothorax may be, the basic result is the same. Normally, "negative" (subambient) pleural pressure equilibrates with atmospheric pressure or may become positive (tension pneumothorax). The latter circumstance is usually associated with manual or mechanical positive-pressure ventilation. Ventilation is significantly impaired and intrapulmonary shunting is often profound. Of even greater concern, however, is the effect on the cardiovascular system. The increase of pleural pressure impairs venous return, and the mediastinum becomes shifted to the contralateral side, twisting the great vessels and further decreasing stroke volume and cardiac output. Cardiovascular collapse may occur within minutes.

TABLE 132-1.   Source of Pulmonary Barotrauma

Alveolar rupture
  Deceleration/blast injury
  Hypovolemia
  Cough
  Necrotizing pneumonia
  Positive airway pressure (mechanical ventilation/PEEP/CPAP)
Parietal pleura
  Penetrating injury (bullets/knives)
  Tracheal/esophageal perforation
  Tracheostomy, nephrectomy, rib resection
  Spinal fusion
Visceral pleura
  Nerve blocks
  Vascular cannulation
  Emphysematous blebs/bullae
  Liver, lung, kidney biopsies

PEEP, positive end-expiratory pressure; CPAP, continuous positive airway pressure.

A central problem in the management of PBT is to provide the required ventilatory assistance without additional compromise. The mortality rate from acute respiratory failure ranges from 7% to 80%, whereas barotrauma-related mortality during mechanical ventilation is less than 1%.[1] Thus, effort should be made to maintain oxygenation through increased positive end-expiratory pressure (PEEP), continuous positive airway pressure, and the fraction of inspired oxygen (FIO_2) while the number of mechanically administered positive-pressure breaths is reduced. Such alterations of ventilator therapy (Table 132-2) may decrease the incidence and progression of PBT, although the major factor appears primarily related to the underlying pulmonary disease.[1]

MECHANICAL VENTILATION

Frequency of Mechanical Breaths

Mechanical ventilation of the neonate with respiratory distress syndrome provides much of our understanding of PBT. In 1976, Mannino and colleagues[3] reported that lowering the number of mechanically delivered breaths with IMV compared with controlled ventilation decreased the incidence rate of neonatal PBT from 69% to 18%. Similar findings were reported by Mathru and associates[4] in adults. They found the incidence rate of PBT was 22% in patients treated with controlled ventilation and PEEP versus 7% in a similar IMV and PEEP group (Table 132-3).

Peak Inspiratory Pressure and Volume

In addition to decreasing the number of mechanically delivered breaths, the PIP also should be reduced whenever possible. Early data supporting this concept also came from neonatal studies. Moylan and colleagues[5] noticed a change in the incidence of PBT after an alteration in ventilatory management technique in neonates with respiratory distress syndrome at the Massachusetts General Hospital (Boston). From 1971 until 1974, ventilatory pressures were maintained while the FIO_2 was decreased during the weaning of mechanically ventilated neonates. From 1974 to 1975, the FIO_2 was maintained while the ventilatory pressures were decreased. This study showed significant differences in the two periods and clarified the relationship of PIP to PBT (Table 132-4).

TABLE 132-2. Decreasing the Incidence of Pulmonary Barotrauma

Minimize the number of mechanically delivered breaths
Minimize peak inspiratory pressures (flow rates, sedation, relaxants)
Maintain intravascular volume
Use selective (independent) lung ventilation if indicated
(Do not allow respiratory death to occur by avoiding high
  PEEP/CPAP)

PEEP, positive end-expiratory pressure; CPAP, continuous positive airway pressure.

TABLE 132-3. Incidence of Pulmonary Barotrauma in Adults with Alteration of Ventilation Mode

	CMV	IMV
MV rate	12/min	6/min (initially)
PIP (cm H_2O)	34 ± 9	51 ± 14
PEEP/CPAP (cm H_2O)	15 ± 4	27 ± 5
PBT	22%	7%
PA catheterization	5%	48%

CMV, controlled mechanical ventilation; IMV, intermittent mandatory ventilation, MV, mechanical ventilation; PIP, peak inspiratory pressure; CPAP, continuous positive airway pressure; PBT, pulmonary barotrauma; PA, pulmonary artery.

Mathru M, Rao TLK, Venus B: Ventilator-induced barotrauma in controlled mechanical ventilation versus intermittent mandatory ventilation. *Crit Care Med* 1983;11:359.

This association also has been found in adults. Petersen and Baier[6] observed stratification of the PBT incidence in patients requiring increased PIP (Table 132-5). Because of the relationship of high PIP to PBT in many reports, high-frequency ventilation (HFV) is suggested as a method to decrease the incidence. Carlon and coworkers[7] report on 309 patients with acute respiratory failure at Memorial Sloan-Kettering Cancer Institute (New York) who were selected randomly to receive either conventional volume-controlled IMV or HFV. Mechanical ventilation in all cases lasted more than 12 hours. PBT occurred in 3.8% of HFV patients and in 2.6% of conventionally ventilated patients. These differences were clinically and statistically nonsignificant. Mean airway pressures were 12 cm H_2O in the HFV patients and 37 cm H_2O in the conventionally ventilated patients, suggesting that the relationship between PIP and PBT may not be causal and may instead reflect only the noncompliance of the patient's lungs. Occult PEEP associated with HFV may be a contributing factor.

Parker and associates[8] showed that ventilation with large tidal volumes produced stress fractures of capillary endothelium, basement membranes, and epithelium. The mechanical damage led to extravasation of fluid, blood, and protein into air and tissue spaces and the leakage of air into tissue spaces. Damage can be minimized by preventing overdistention of functional lung units, perhaps by adjustment of the ventilator technique chosen.

Intravascular Volume

The aforementioned recommendations for reducing the incidence of PBT are reasonably well supported. Less clear is the connection between hypovolemia and PBT. In 1969, Lenaghan and associates[9] reported a study of expansion rupture of the lung in normovolemic and hypovolemic dogs. Normovolemic dogs did not experience PBT until airway pressures of 62 ± 9 cm H_2O were reached, whereas dogs rendered hypovolemic by hemorrhage sustained PBT at 33

TABLE 132-4.   Incidence of Alveolar Rupture in Infants With RDS

VENTILATORY PRESSURES MAINTAINED UNTIL FIO$_2$ REDUCED TO LESS THAN 0.4		VENTILATORY PRESSURES MINIMIZED ONCE FIO$_2$ REDUCED TO LESS THAN 0.6
60 ± 18 hr	PIP > 40 cm H$_2$O	8 ± 2 hr
17 ± 7 hr	PIP > 50 cm H$_2$O	1 ± 0.7 hr
90 ± 14 hr	PEEP > 5 cm H$_2$O	71 ± 7 hr
51%	Alveolar rupture	24%

From Moylan FMB, Walker AAA, Kramer SS, et al: The relationship of bronchopulmonary dysplasia to the occurrence of alveolar rupture during positive pressure ventilation. *Crit Care Med* 1978;6:140.

± 7 cm H$_2$O. Thus, prevention of hypovolemia may be important in decreasing the risk of PBT.

Mathru and colleagues[4] documented a difference in the incidence of PBT in two groups of patients receiving different ventilatory management. Hypovolemia as a contributing factor to PBT was not directly addressed. However, only 5% of the patients in the group with a 22% incidence rate of PBT underwent pulmonary artery catheterization, whereas in the group with a 7% incidence rate of PBT, almost 50% had pulmonary artery catheters inserted, perhaps with more attention to maintenance of intravascular volume. Because the question of hypovolemia was not central to this study, no definitive statements can be made in this regard. Nevertheless, hypovolemia is a likely contributor to an increased incidence of PBT.

Selective Ventilation

Asynchronous independent lung ventilation also is an option for patients with unilateral lung disease as a cause of PBT or for those with primarily unilateral PBT.[10] If the air leak lateralizes, ventilation to that lung can be altered to provide decreased frequency and PIP of mechanical breaths. Such therapy, although attractive in principle, is difficult to achieve clinically because of problems with placement and maintenance of double-lumen endotracheal tubes in the appropriate location.

TABLE 132-5.   Peak Inspiratory Pressures During Positive-Pressure Ventilation and Incidence of Pulmonary Barotrauma

PIP (cm H$_2$O)	INCIDENCE OF PBT
>70	43% (10/23)
50–70	8% (4/53)
<50	0% (0/157)

PIP, peak inspiratory pressure; PBT, pulmonary barotrauma.

From Peterson GW, Baier H: Incidence of pulmonary barotrauma in a medical ICU. *Crit Care Med* 1983;11:67.

DIAGNOSIS

Physical Findings

PBT usually can be readily ascertained if one has a high index of suspicion for its presence. A knowledge of the types of injuries predisposing to barotrauma is of paramount importance in this regard (see Table 132-1). Physical findings may be obvious (subcutaneous emphysema extending into the neck) or subtle (decrease in breath sounds over the ipsilateral hemithorax). Sudden cardiopulmonary deterioration in a patient who has sustained chest trauma or is treated with mechanical ventilation, or both, should suggest the possibility of a tension pneumothorax (Table 132-6).

Abrasions and ecchymoses over the thorax indicate that underlying pulmonary injury may be present. Often, however, a significant impact or deceleration injury occurs with little or no external physical evidence. Rib fractures may be evident after palpation and are usually anterolateral in position. Paradoxical chest wall motion (flail chest) with spontaneous ventilation usually is present. It can be masked, however, if the underlying rib fractures are posterior and the patient is lying supine. Such fractures are evidence of a severe thoracic injury and indicate the need to evaluate carefully for the presence of a pulmonary contusion and barotrauma.

Radiographic Signs

A chest radiograph usually is diagnostic for the presence of subcutaneous emphysema, pneumomediastinum, and pneumopericardium. On occasion, however, the patient's condition or position when the radiograph is obtained may preclude an adequate examination. In addition, the radiographic manifestations of pneumothorax are sometimes delayed; hence, repeated examinations are indicated. In supine patients, two radiographic changes associated with an otherwise obscure pneumothorax are (1) the lateral sulcus sign (intrapleural air ascending into the anterior costophrenic sulcus producing a "deep" lateral costophrenic angle), and (2) the presence of a dark, lucent band between the medial lung and mediastinum.[11]

TABLE 132-6. Signs and Symptoms of Tension Pneumothorax

Tachypnea/dyspnea
Cyanosis
Decreased blood pressure/cardiac output
Increased or decreased pulse
Hyperresonance to percussion ipsilateral side
Asymmetric chest movement with ventilation

Oxygenation and Ventilation

The effects of pneumothorax on oxygenation and ventilation are often profound. Hypoxemia resulting from increased intrapulmonary shunting can be exacerbated by the reduction of cardiac output with tension pneumothorax. Hypercapnia as a result of decreased ventilation leads to respiratory acidemia. Cyanosis, when present, reflects both pulmonary and cardiovascular impairment.

TREATMENT

Catheter Aspiration

The development of pneumothorax during positive-pressure ventilation demands efficient evaluation and decompression if barotrauma morbidity is to be minimized. If the patient is experiencing pulmonary or cardiovascular compromise, an intravenous cannula (16-gauge, 6.4-cm [2.5-inch] long) with attached syringe can be placed in the second anterior intercostal space on the side of the suspected pneumothorax. In the presence of a tension pneumothorax, the plunger will be forced out of the syringe barrel if the pressure is sufficiently high, and the pneumothorax will be temporarily relieved.

Tube Thoracostomy

When a pneumothorax is present or suspicion of pneumothorax is sufficiently high, a chest tube should be placed. If the patient is not severely compromised and time is available for evaluation, a chest radiograph should be obtained before placement. Tube thoracostomy should be performed using a 30-French or larger tube placed in the midaxillary line through the fifth intercostal space. This location avoids the pectoralis major and latissimus dorsi muscles, and the catheter may be easily directed to the superior aspect of the pleural space, allowing efficient drainage of the pleural air.[12]

Although radiographic-assisted chest tube placement is seldom used in patients requiring long-term ventilatory therapy, radiographic guidance, including computerized tomography, may be necessary to decompress the air collection adequately (Fig. 132-1). Patients who require tube thoracostomy for pneumothorax during a period of positive-pressure ventilation often require pleural drainage for a longer period than the usual 2 to 4 days when they are breathing spontaneously.

The importance of timely treatment is supported by data from Steier and coworkers,[13] who showed that a delay of

longer than 30 minutes in chest tube insertion of patients with a ventilator-related pneumothorax was associated with 31% mortality rate (nine deaths in 29 patients). When immediate decompression was carried out (less than 30 minutes after recognition of pneumothorax), mortality rate was only 7% (3 of 45 patients). Zwillich and associates[14] prospectively analyzed the complications of assisted ventilation and found no correlation between the occurrence of pneumothorax and ventilator-related mortality.

PITFALLS. The presence of an ipsilateral chest tube should not lull one into thinking a tension pneumothorax cannot also be present. Gobein and colleagues[15] determined that tension pneumothorax occurs in mechanically ventilated ARDS patients with a functioning ipsilateral chest tube in place. In 15 of the 16 patients reviewed, a loculated tension pneumothorax was present in the subpulmonic or paracar-

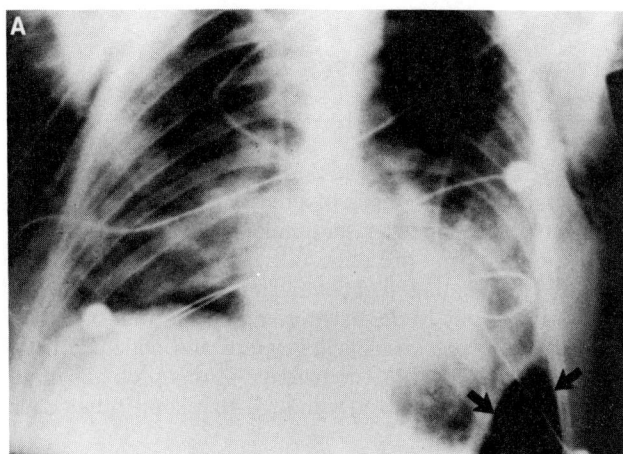

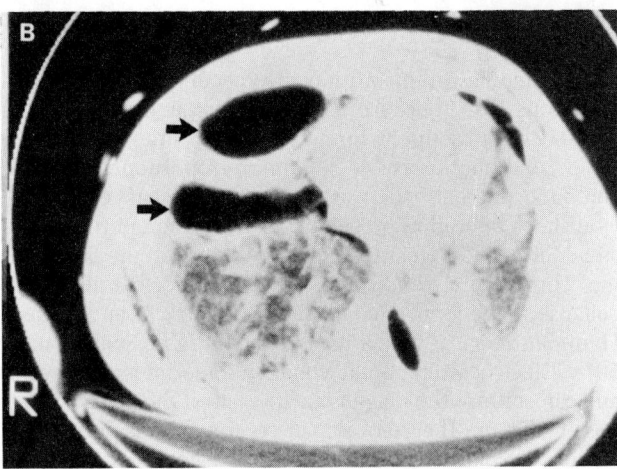

FIGURE 132-1. Radiographs from a 22-year-old with acute respiratory distress syndrome after 30 days of mechanical ventilation. (**A**) Anteroposterior radiograph illustrates only one pleural air collection (*arrows*), at the left costophrenic angle. (**B**) A CT scan demonstrates two unrecognized right lung extraparenchymal air collections (*arrows*), which necessitated CT scan–guided decompressions.

diac region, although no shift of the mediastinum was clinically detectable. Reines[16] reported a second pneumothorax in 11 of 16 patients (78%) with acute respiratory failure who were treated with more than 15 cm H_2O PEEP despite a functioning ipsilateral chest tube. Six of 11 (54%) were loculated and under tension. Pollack and associates[17] described similar findings in six infants with pneumothorax after cardiac surgical procedures. Five of the six infants (83%) had a second pneumothorax while an ipsilateral chest tube was in place.

ALTERNATIVE THERAPY. As an alternative to conventional tube thoracostomy, Bell[18] and others recommend the McSwain dart for temporary prehospital care and transport. This device consists of a 16-French trochar with a polyethylene catheter and Heimlich valve that can be used instead of the previously described 16-gauge intravenous catheter.

OTHER EXTRA-ALVEOLAR AIR CONDITIONS ■

Other extra-alveolar air conditions that may require immediate therapy include pneumomediastinum, pneumopericardium, and, occasionally, intravascular air. Bricker and associates[19] verified the presence of venous air embolism in mechanically ventilated patients. They used transesophageal echocardiography to demonstrate embolism that otherwise was not suspected on clinical grounds and concluded that there is a relatively high occurrence of this problem in patients with PBT associated with high ventilator-induced airway pressure.

PNEUMOMEDIASTINUM

Pneumomediastinum infrequently occurs as the only sign of serious PBT, because mediastinal air is usually decompressed by subsequent formation of subcutaneous emphysema, pneumothorax, or pneumoretroperitoneum. If an anatomic anomaly such as prior pleural scarring or previous neck operation prevents decompression of the mediastinal air, the excessive pressure (tension mediastinum) may compromise venous return and produce cardiovascular collapse. Patients may complain of chest pain, and a classic Hamman's sign ("mediastinal crunch") is present in up to 50%. Electrocardiographic changes sometimes are present and can confuse the diagnosis, especially if the patient develops chest pain. If cardiovascular compromise is present and tension mediastinum is diagnosed, decompression is required.[20] In infants, relief can be provided by insertion of a small catheter into the anterior mediastinum. In adults, the most efficient method of mediastinal decompression is by incision 2 to 3 cm cephalad to the suprasternal notch, followed by opening of the deep fascia beneath the sternum. The infrequency of this complication makes this a rarely needed technique.

PNEUMOPERICARDIUM

Pneumopericardium can also require immediate therapy.[21,22] Isolated signs of cardiac tamponade may be present if the mediastinal air selectively decompresses into the pericardium. Therapy may include pericardiocentesis using a technique similar to that for decompressing a pericardial effusion.

AIR EMBOLISM

If entrainment of intravascular air appears to have occurred, a head down–left lateral decubitus position (Durant's) is often recommended. Barotrauma-induced intravascular air may also be found in the left side of the heart, making the choice of the decubitus position problematic. If air entrainment is nonlethal and the patient is stabilized, hyperbaric oxygen therapy may be indicated; this is an unusual clinical problem.

Several reports of carbon dioxide embolization during laparoscopic surgery have been published.[23-25] This complication results from direct insufflation through the Verres needle or trochar into a systemic vein. Alternatively, it may follow from gas trapping in the portal circulation with delayed release into the hepatic veins.[26]

We see air embolism in divers whose ascent from depth is too rapid.[27] It may be associated with other forms of barotrauma, such as pneumomediastinum and pneumothorax, and has a high morbidity and mortality. Treatment in such cases includes recompression in a hyperbaric facility. Frequently, these victims sustain near-drowning, pulmonary aspiration of gastric contents, or both. Their care is particularly difficult. Special ventilators and techniques are necessary during hyperbaric treatments. Neurologic sequelae, often severe, are common.

PREVENTION OF BAROTRAUMA AND RELATED COMPLICATIONS ■

LIMITATION OF PRESSURE AND VOLUME

Patients at risk for PBT range from infants receiving "physiologic" continuous positive airway pressure (5 cm H_2O)[22] to adults requiring controlled mechanical ventilation and high levels of PEEP.[4,28] Certain features help to stratify a patient's risk of developing PBT (Table 132-7), and some are amena-

TABLE 132-7. Factors Predisposing to Pulmonary Barotrauma

High airway pressures
Frequent positive pressure breaths
Pulmonary infection
Systemic infection
Diffuse pulmonary injury (ARDS)
Hypovolemia

ARDS, adult respiratory distress syndrome.

ble to corrective action (see Table 132-2). PIP requirements remain the single best predictor of PBT because of the higher pressures necessary to deliver an adequate minute volume when the lungs sustain a severe injury that decreases pulmonary compliance.[24]

Peterson and Baier[6] studied 171 patients who required mechanical ventilation. PBT occurred in 14 (8%) of their patients, and PIP seemed to be related to the development of PBT (see Table 132-5). Patients in this series and in that of Zwillich and associates[14] who sustained barotrauma were younger (often less than 30 years of age) than those without barotrauma.

Zwillich and colleagues[14] hypothesized that younger patients more often "fought the ventilator," thus exposing their lungs to higher airway pressures. Another interpretation of these data is that the younger patients more commonly experienced respiratory failure as a result of ARDS, whereas older patients developed respiratory failure as a result of exacerbations of chronic obstructive lung disease (COLD). Patients with COLD most often have increased pulmonary compliance compared with those with ARDS; thus, young patients with ARDS are exposed to an increased risk of PBT because of requirements for higher PIP during mechanical ventilation.

LIMITATION OF RATE

Patients ventilated at higher frequencies also seem to be at increased risk of PBT.[3,5] This association is related to the decrease in pulmonary compliance, which increases the work of breathing. A point may be reached when the entire minute ventilation must be delivered mechanically. The problem likely is more frequent when PEEP is withheld for fear of inducing PBT, thereby causing further deterioration of pulmonary compliance.

INFECTION CONTROL

Another risk factor for PBT is infection. Fleming and Bowen[29] detected pneumothorax in 19 of 128 patients in a Vietnamese evacuation hospital who received postoperative controlled mechanical ventilation for more than 24 hours. These investigators were the first to suggest that concurrent pulmonary infection played an important role in the incidence of PBT. Necrotizing pulmonary infections were present in 17 of the 19 pneumothorax patients (80%).

This relationship of infection, pulmonary and systemic, to PBT and mortality is strengthened by two reports from the University of South Carolina (Columbia, SC). Gobein and colleagues[15] documented that of 16 patients with ARDS who developed a pneumothorax, 11 (69%) died, and 10 of the 11 (91%) had superimposed infection. In the 5 pneumothorax patients who survived, only 1 had an infectious process (viral pneumonia). In the second report, Reines[16] noted that 11 of 16 (69%) patients who were treated with PEEP above 15 cm H_2O died during mechanical ventilation for respiratory failure. Nine of the 11 (82%) had pulmonary infections or were septic, whereas no documented infections were present in the five survivors.

Investigators studying patients who were treated with mechanical ventilation or extracorporeal membrane oxygenation concluded that "the combination of ARDS, sepsis, intrapulmonary infection, and increasing levels of PEEP is the setting in which PBT occurs."[30]

SURVEILLANCE FOR PULMONARY BAROTRAUMA ∎

Can any type of monitoring warn of impending PBT and thus provide the opportunity to prevent or reduce its incidence? The initial manifestation (and its unifying mechanism) is development of PIE. This problem occurs when air ruptures from alveoli into the perivascular (interstitial) space surrounding the pulmonary vessels, perhaps when PIP exceeds 40 cm H_2O. Woodring[31] found that 13 of 15 patients with ARDS (87%) demonstrated PIE. In 12 of the 13, PIE occurred after PIP exceeded 40 cm H_2O.

The identification of PIE on a standard anteroposterior chest radiograph in the ICU may be difficult. Interstitial air is manifested by small parenchymal cysts, air patterns that fail to taper toward the peripheral lung margins, and halos or crescents of air that are observed surrounding the pulmonary vessels. In addition, subpleural air dissection, producing either linear collections of air or frank air cysts, is possible.[31,32] The most common early manifestation of PBT recognized radiographically by nonradiologists probably is mediastinal emphysema, because PIE initially tracks to the mediastinum. Subcutaneous emphysema, pneumothorax, and pneumopericardium follow. Reines[16] demonstrated pneumomediastinum in 12 of 16 patients with ARDS; pneumothorax later developed in 10 of these 12. Woodring's data indicate that the peak incidence of pneumothorax occurs within 12 hours of the appearance of PIE. In his patients, no pneumothorax occurred before PIE developed.[31]

Another potential early warning sign of PIE may be increased pulmonary artery pressure. Patients studied by McLoud and colleagues[33] had abrupt elevations of pulmonary artery diastolic pressure (8 to 12 mm Hg) before developing pneumothoraces. Perhaps air tracking along the perivascular sheaths toward the hilum of the lung causes obliteration of a portion of the vascular bed, either peripherally or at a central hilar location. This sequence may result in higher pulmonary artery pressures.

SPECIAL CONSIDERATIONS

Ventilator-related PBT probably occurs in 3% to 7% of all patients requiring mechanical ventilation, although the reported range is from 0.5%[34] to 41%[5] (Tables 132-8 through 132-10). All patients treated with mechanical ventilation are at risk. Several factors seem to be associated with the development of PBT, which raises the question of the common mechanism that causes inspired air to become extra-alveolar in location and to produce a pneumothorax.

The unifying mechanism of PBT was unknowingly detailed in 1888 by the German physician, Mueller,[35] who

TABLE 132-8.   Incidence of Pulmonary Barotrauma in Retrospective Clinical Studies

| | PBT | | |
STUDY	No.	Incidence (%)	PATIENT POPULATION
Fleming (1970)	19/128	15	Adult
Steier (1965–72)	74/4800	1.5	Adult
Kirkpatrick (1972–73)	15/37	41	Pediatric
Leonidas (1971–72)	48/222	22	Pediatric
Kirby (1973–74)	4/28	14	Adult
Rohlfing (1972–75)	38/1545	2.5	Adult
Moylan (1971–75)	41/99	41	Pediatric
Pollack (1975–78)	10/179	5.6	Pediatric
Cullen (1974–76)	1/200	0.5	Adult
Mathru (1971–76)	44/292	15	Adult

Brown DL: Pulmonary barotrauma. In: Kirby RR, Taylor RW (eds). *Respiratory Failure.* Chicago, Year Book Medical Publishers, 1986:602.

TABLE 132-9.   Incidence of Pulmonary Barotrauma in Prospective Clinical Studies

| | PBT | | |
STUDY	No.	Incidence (%)	PATIENT POPULATION
Zwillich (1974)	15/354	4.5	Adult
Petersen (1983)	14/171	8	Adult
Carlon (1983)	10/309	3.2	>20 kg
Pepe (1984)	22/92	23	Adul

Brown DL: Pulmonary barotrauma. In: Kirby RR, Taylor RW (eds). *Respiratory Failure.* Chicago, Year Book Medical Publishers, 1986:602.

TABLE 132-10.   Incidence of Pulmonary Barotrauma in Combined Retrospective and Prospective Studies

VARIABLE	RETROSPECTIVE	PROSPECTIVE
Time interval	1965–78	1972–82
Age	Neonates to adult	>20 kg to adult
Total number patients	8055	926
Number experiencing PBT	303	61
Incidence of PBT	3.8%	6.6%

PBT, pulmonary barotrauma.

Brown DL: Pulmonary barotrauma. In: Kirby RR, Taylor RW (eds). *Respiratory Failure.* Chicago, Year Book Medical Publishers, 1986:602.

reported that air from the lungs appeared in the mediastinum. The Macklins,[2] Canadian investigators, clearly outlined the mechanism of PBT during the 1930s and 1940s. Evaluation of rabbits and cats that were subjected to alveolar overinflation with intermittent positive-pressure ventilation showed that extra-alveolar air resulting from alveolar rupture tracked from the alveoli along pulmonary vascular sheaths, principally the arterioles, and then into the mediastinum. From this location, it could rupture by way of the more delicate mediastinal pleura into the pleural space to cause a pneumothorax.

Mediastinal air also may decompress into other areas to produce subcutaneous emphysema, pneumopericardium, and pneumoretroperitoneum[36] (Fig. 132-2). This experimental work was extended to human postmortem studies by Tucker and Langsten,[37] and the mechanism was documented to be similar. Once PIE and vascular sheath air dissection begin, they continue even at lower airway pressures than those needed initially to produce the lesions.[12]

PBT also occurs as a result of thoracic trauma, attempts at central venous catheter placement, cardiopulmonary resuscitation, prior thoracotomy, surgical procedures, and many other less common factors. Nevertheless, the percentage of PBT related to mechanical ventilation varies from 5% to 35% of extra-alveolar air found in ICU patients (Table 132-11).

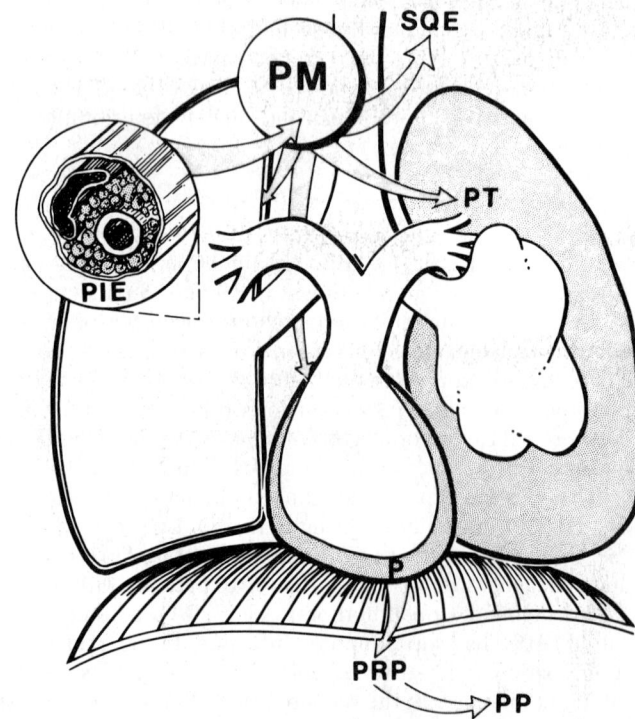

FIGURE 132-2. Mechanisms of pulmonary barotrauma. Alveolar air dissects along the pulmonary vascular sheaths to the mediastinum. After the pneumomediastinum (PM) develops, subcutaneous emphysema (SQE), pneumothorax (PT), pneumoretroperitoneum (PRP), pneumoperitoneum (PP), and pneumopericardium (P) are all possible. P/E, pulmonary interstitial emphysema.

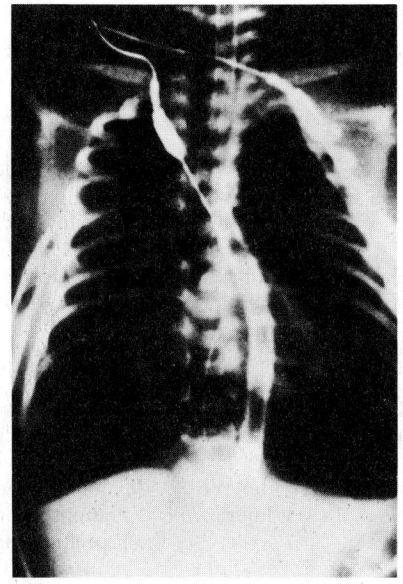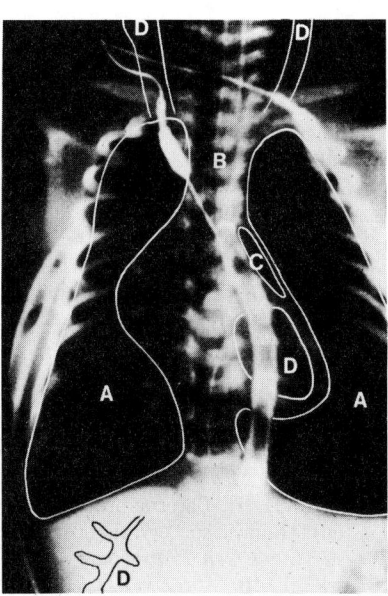

FIGURE 132-3. Postmortem chest radiograph of a mechanically ventilated infant who sustained lethal barotrauma, including bilateral tension pneumothoraces (*A*), pneumomediastinum (*B*), pneumopericardium (*C*), and intravascular air in heart, great vessels, and hepatic veins (*D*).

UNUSUAL AND RARE PRESENTATIONS

PBT may cause cardiovascular embarrassment through the development of tension pneumothorax, tension pneumomediastinum, tension pneumopericardium, and even tension subcutaneous emphysema.[38] Pneumothorax, pneumomediastinum, pneumoperitoneum, and subcutaneous emphysema have been reported to compromise ventilation. In addition, subcutaneous emphysema may cause ventilatory compromise by producing tracheal obstruction.[11,37] Intracranial pressure increases are reported to be associated with massive subcutaneous emphysema.[39]

The diagnosis of air embolism secondary to mechanical ventilation is difficult to make with certainty. It requires timely pathologic examination, coupled with the clinical suspicion of intravascular air in the differential diagnosis of death. This combination is not often achieved in clinical practice. The radiograph in Figure 132-3 is an extreme example of PBT-related intravascular air that makes a postmortem examination unnecessary. If a patient experiences abrupt cardiovascular collapse during mechanical ventilatory therapy, and more common causes such as tension pneumothorax and pericardial tamponade are ruled out, the diagnosis of air embolism should be considered.

REFERENCES

1. Brown DL: Pulmonary barotrauma. In: Kirby RR, Taylor RW (eds). *Respiratory Failure*. Chicago, Year Book Medical Publishers, 1986:602
2. Macklin MT, Macklin CC: Malignant interstitial emphysema of the lungs and mediastinum as an important occult complication in many respiratory diseases and other conditions: an interpretation of the clinical deterioration in light of the laboratory experiment. *Medicine* 1984;23:281
3. Mannino FL, Feldman BH, Heldt GP, et al: Early mechanical ventilation in RDS with prolonged inspiration. *Pediatr Res* 1976;10:464
4. Mathru M, Rao TLK, Venus B: Ventilator-induced barotrauma in controlled mechanical ventilation versus intermittent mandatory ventilation. *Crit Care Med* 1983;11:359
5. Moylan FMB, Walker AM, Kramer S, et al: The relationship of bronchopulmonary dysplasia to the occurrence of alveolar rupture during positive pressure ventilation. *Crit Care Med* 1978;6:140
6. Petersen GW, Baier H: Incidence of pulmonary barotrauma in a medical ICU. *Crit Care Med* 1983;11:67
7. Carlon GC, Howland WS, Ray C, et al: High frequency jet ventilation: a prospective randomized evaluation. *Chest* 1983;84:551
8. Parker JC, Hernandez LA, Peevy KJ: Mechanisms of ventilator-induced lung injury. *Crit Care Med* 1993;21:131
9. Lenaghan R, Silva YJ, Walt AJ: Hemodynamic alterations associated with expansion rupture of the lung. *Arch Surg* 1969;99:339
10. Hillman KM, Barber JD: Asynchronous independent lung ventilation (AILV). *Crit Care Med* 1980;8:390
11. Bryan CL: Radiology in the ICU. In: Kirby RR, Taylor RW

TABLE 132-11. Proportion of Pulmonary Barotrauma Related to Mechanical Ventilation in Critically Ill Patients

STUDY	TOTAL	PBT RELATED TO MV
Steier (1965–72)	544	74 (14%)
Kumar (1966–71)	53	17 (30%)
Rohlfing (1972–75)	108	38 (35%)
Cullen (1974–76)	22	1 (5%)
Total	727	130 (18%)

PBT, pulmonary barotrauma; MV, mechanical ventilation.

(eds). *Respiratory Failure*. Chicago, Year Book Medical Publishers, 1986:414

12. Hillman KM: Pulmonary barotrauma. *Clin Anaesthesiol* 1985; 3:877
13. Steier M, Ching N, Roberts EB, et al: Pneumothorax complicating continuous ventilatory support. *J Thorac Cardiovasc Surg* 1974;67:17
14. Zwillich W, Pierson DJ, Creagh CE, et al: Complications of assisted ventilation: a prospective study of 354 consecutive episodes. *Am J Med* 1974;57:161
15. Gobein RP, Reines HD, Schabel SI: Localized tension pneumothorax: unrecognized form of barotrauma in adult respiratory distress syndrome. *Radiology* 1982;142:15
16. Reines HD: Manifestations of barotrauma in acute respiratory failure. *Am Surg* 1981;47:421
17. Pollack MM, Fields AL, Holbrook PR: Pneumothorax and pneumomediastinum during pediatric mechanical ventilation. *Crit Care Med* 1979;7:536
18. Bell WH III: Barotrauma: invited comment. In: Webb WR (ed). Thoracic surgery: surgical management of chest injuries. *Int Trends Gen Thorac Surg* 1991;70
19. Bricker MB, Morris WP, Allen SJ, et al: Venous air embolism in patients with pulmonary barotrauma. *Crit Care Med* 1994;22:1692
20. Van Stiegmann G, Brantigan CO, Hopeman AR: Tension pneumomediastinum. *Arch Surg* 1977;112:1212
21. Hurd TE, Novak R, Gallagher TJ: Tension pneumopericardium: a complication of mechanical ventilation. *Crit Care Med* 1984;12:200
22. Alpan G, Goder K, Glick B, et al: Pneumopericardium during continuous positive airway pressure in respiratory distress syndrome. *Crit Care Med* 1984;12:1080
23. Yacoub OF, Cardona I Jr, Coveler LA, et al: Carbon dioxide embolism during laparoscopy. *Anesthesiology* 1982;57:533
24. Diakun TA: Carbon dioxide embolism: successful resuscitation with cardiopulmonary bypass. *Anesthesiology* 1991;74:1151
25. Joris JL: Anesthetic management of laparoscopy. In: Miller RD (ed). *Anesthesia*, 4th ed. New York, Churchill Livingstone, 1994:2015
26. Root B, Leby MN, Pollack S, et al: Gas embolism death after laparoscopy delayed by "trapping" in portal circulation. *Anesth Analg* 1978;57:232
27. Bradley ME: Pulmonary barotrauma. In: Bove AA, Davis JC (eds). *Diving Medicine*, 2nd ed. Philadelphia, WB Saunders Co, 1990:188
28. Kohn S, Bellamy P: Pulmonary barotrauma in patients with adult respiratory distress syndrome (ARDS) during continuous positive pressure ventilation (CPPV). *Am Rev Respir Dis* 1982;125:129A
29. Fleming WH, Bowen JC: Early complications of long-term respiratory support. *J Thorac Cardiovasc Surg* 1972; 64:729
30. Browdie DA, Deane R, Shinozaki T, et al: Adult respiratory distress syndrome (ARDS), sepsis and extracorporeal membrane oxygenation (ECMO). *J Trauma* 1977;17:579
31. Woodring JH: Pulmonary interstitial emphysema in the adult respiratory distress syndrome. *Crit Care Med* 1985;13:786
32. Johnson TH, Altman AR, McCaffree RD: Radiologic considerations in the adult respiratory distress syndrome treated with positive end-expiratory pressure (PEEP). *Clin Chest Med* 1982;3:89
33. McLoud TC, Barash PG, Ravin CE, et al: Elevation of pulmonary artery pressure as a sign of pulmonary barotrauma (pneumothorax). *Crit Care Med* 1978;6:81
34. Cullen DJ, Caldera DL: The incidence of ventilator-induced pulmonary barotrauma in critically ill patients. *Anesthesiology* 1979;50:185
35. Mueller F: Uber emphysema des mediastinum. *Klin Wochenschr* 1888;25:205
36. Marchand P: The anatomy and applied anatomy of the mediastinal fascia. *Thorax* 1951;6:359
37. Tucker AM, Langsten HT: The perivascular space of the pulmonary vessels. *Thorac Surg* 1952;23:539
38. Tonnesen AS, Wagner W, Mackey-Hargadine J: Tension subcutaneous emphysema. *Anesthesiology* 1985;62:90
39. Cotelho JC, Tonnesen AS, Allen SJ, et al: Intracranial hypertension secondary to tension subcutaneous emphysema. *Crit Care Med* 1985;13:512

Neurologic Disease and Dysfunction

Critical Care, Third Edition, edited by Joseph M. Civetta,
Robert W. Taylor, and Robert R. Kirby.
Lippincott-Raven Publishers, Philadelphia, PA © 1997.

CHAPTER 133

■

Altered Mental Status and Coma

Warren J. Strittmatter

IMMEDIATE CONCERNS ■

A rapid, effective, and orderly evaluation of the patient in coma is critical in the first minutes after arrival in the emergency department. After this initial evaluation is completed and the patient is stabilized, a more comprehensive evaluation is necessary to determine the anatomy of the lesion producing coma and then to establish the etiology of the coma. The outcome may rest on therapy initiated within minutes of the patient's arrival. This chapter outlines the necessary initial steps to be taken in the emergency evaluation of coma. A more detailed evaluation of the comatose patient is then described, to help define the anatomy of the lesion and guide subsequent evaluation. The three processes that cause coma—bilateral hemispheric lesions, brain stem lesions, and diffuse metabolic–toxic lesions—are discussed. Finally, the assessment and treatment of the deteriorating comatose patient, including patterns of brain herniation, are described.

EMERGENCY EVALUATION ■

When the comatose patient is brought into the emergency department, a rapid, simple, and methodic evaluation must be conducted.[1,2] This 5-minute evaluation is designed to reveal any problems that may lead to death or prolonged morbidity if left untreated.

AIRWAY–BREATHING

Check respirations. First, check the airway and respiratory excursions. If in doubt, tracheally intubate. Elective intubation in an unrushed, controlled setting is far preferable to emergency intubation after the patient develops acute respiratory distress. Check arterial blood gases to ensure adequate ventilation. If the patient is suspected to have a neck injury, radiographic assessment must be done first to prevent injury to the spinal cord. If time does not permit radiographic assessment, a cricothyroidotomy or emergency tracheostomy is indicated.

The patient may require mechanical ventilation, based on the arterial blood gas values and the physician's clinical judgment. Keep in mind that a comatose patient who initially presents with adequate ventilation may subsequently deteriorate, particularly if the coma is caused by acute intoxication or trauma.

CIRCULATION

Check the blood pressure and pulse. Remember that cardiac dysfunction (myocardial infarction or arrhythmia) or hypotension (due to blood loss or septic shock) may cause coma. As described later, acute brain dysfunction during herniation may secondarily alter cardiac rate, rhythm, and blood pressure. Whatever the cause, maintenance of adequate cardiac output and blood pressure is essential to survival. Cardiac rate and rhythm must be continuously monitored, and abnormalities treated aggressively.

1971

METABOLIC

Draw blood for laboratory studies and give glucose. The laboratory evaluation is sometimes critical in diagnosing the cause of coma. Blood should be drawn for determination of serum electrolytes, glucose, urea nitrogen, complete blood count, Chemscreen-20, and prothrombin and partial thromboplastin times. Additional blood is drawn in serum tubes for studies indicated from the later evaluation (e.g., drug screen, liver function tests, and serum ammonia). Glucose should be administered intravenously as early as possible to *all* patients in coma, without waiting for laboratory results. Hypoglycemia is often neglected as a cause of coma, or is recognized too late. Hypoglycemia can produce all degrees of alteration of consciousness, from lethargy to coma, and can cause focal neurologic signs.

Stop seizures. Seizures may cause additional brain damage, primarily due to anoxia, as discussed in Chapter 134. The most widely recommended treatment is intravenous (IV) diazepam (approximately 10 mg) to stop the seizure, followed by IV phenytoin (500 mg to 1 g at a rate less than 50 mg/minute). These drugs are not benign in this setting. Diazepam may cause respiratory depression or arrest, and phenytoin may cause hypotension or bradycardia. Adequate respiratory support, including artificial ventilation, if necessary, and frequent monitoring of vital signs are critical. A more detailed discussion of treating status epilepticus is found in Chapter 134.

Treat metabolic disturbances. Metabolic acidosis or alkalosis may cause or worsen coma. Abnormalities of acid–base balance and blood chemistry should be corrected. Similarly, hypo- or hyperthermia can contribute to the patient's altered mental state and must be treated.

Administer thiamine, and consider other drugs as a cause of coma. Wernicke's encephalopathy is a rare but potentially treatable cause of coma. The administration of glucose may precipitate Wernicke's encephalopathy in a patient who is alcoholic or malnourished. Thiamine, 50 mg to 100 mg, should be administered.

A common cause of coma is abuse of legal or illegal drugs. The primary treatment of drug overdose is supportive, particularly in maintaining ventilation. More specific therapy is available for narcotic overdose and for anticholinergic sedative overdose. Narcotic overdose is treated with naloxone hydrochloride, 0.4 mg IV every 5 minutes until the patient is conscious. The duration of action is 2 to 3 hours. Because many narcotic agents, including methadone, have a longer half-life, the patient may relapse and need to be treated again. Sedatives with anticholinergic effects, such as the tricyclic antidepressants, can produce coma.

Lower intracranial pressure. Increased intracranial pressure (ICP) may result from some causes of coma and can cause morbidity or death if not aggressively treated.

Treat infection. Infection of the CNS may produce an altered mental state. Infection elsewhere in the body may also alter the level of consciousness. Blood cultures and lumbar puncture may need to be obtained quickly.

All points previously outlined must be evaluated in every patient in coma, and evaluation must be initiated within minutes after the patient's arrival in the emergency room. A patient who is brought in comatose after an automobile accident, for example, may have had the accident because of hypoglycemia.

BEDSIDE EVALUATION OF COMA ■

After the initial evaluation is completed and the patient has been stabilized, a comprehensive evaluation is conducted to determine the anatomic lesion causing coma. The simple, brief bedside evaluation of the comatose patient outlined usually reveals the level of the neuraxis responsible for the altered mental state.

The descriptions of acutely altered mental state are easier to label than to define. The spectrum of states between "alert" and "comatose" is difficult to quantitate. Decreasing levels of consciousness are commonly described by the following terms: clouding of consciousness, delirium, obtundation, stupor, and coma. A stuporous patient is unresponsive except to vigorous stimuli, whereas a comatose patient is unresponsive to all external stimuli.

Lesions in either of two anatomic sites can impair consciousness. Stupor or coma is produced by bilateral hemispheric lesions affecting the ascending reticular activating system, or by a brain stem lesion affecting the reticular core. The bedside neurologic examination helps to determine the site of the lesion.

The reticular activating system occupies the central core of the brain stem. This dense population of neurons receives collaterals from every major somatic and spinal sensory pathway.[3] Experimental lesions in animals and neuropathologic studies in humans demonstrate that a lesion in the brain stem reticular core can cause coma. Specifically, lesions in the midbrain and pons, extending anywhere from the posterior hypothalamus to the lower third of the pons, produce coma.[4,5] Brain stem lesions causing coma are paramedian and ventral to the ventricular system, involving both sides of the midline and most of the dorsal-ventral axis of the tegmentum. Brain stem lesions exclusively localized to the medulla do not impair consciousness.

The brain stem reticular core communicates with the cerebral hemispheres through a diffuse fiber pathway, the ascending reticular activating system, which ascends primarily through the central tegmental fasciculus.[3] Three major ascending pathways arise from the reticular formation. One pathway ascends to the thalamic reticular nucleus and then to the cortex. The second ascends through the hypothalamus to the basal forebrain. The third pathway originates in the midbrain raphe and locus ceruleus and projects to the neocortex. Lesions in the cerebral hemispheres that produce coma must be large and bilateral.[6] A lesion involving exclusively one hemisphere does not produce coma unless it secondarily affects the function of the other hemisphere.

The bedside neurologic examination of the comatose patient determines whether the lesion is in the brain stem, involving the reticular core, or in both hemispheres, involving the ascending reticular activating system. This evaluation consists of examining spontaneous and induced movements, the pattern of respiration, pupils, and ocular movements.

SPONTANEOUS AND INDUCED MOVEMENTS

Simple observation of the patient at bedside reveals much about the depth of stupor or coma and about the anatomic lesion. The patient may have semipurposeful movements (e.g., arm flailing) or may have no movements. More spontaneous or evoked movement may be present on one side, indicating a lesion involving one corticospinal tract more than the other. The patient may have tonic or clonic movements that can be either massive or subtle and focal (indicating seizure activity). Movement evoked by a mildly painful stimulus is examined next. Noxious stimuli include rubbing the sternum with a closed fist or pressing the nasal bridge. The pattern of motor response elicited by pain may reveal the anatomic level producing the altered mental state. Purposeful movement (e.g., withdrawing the examiner's hand) indicates a higher level of function than no movement. Painful stimuli may also produce posturing, which has great localizing value. Decerebrate rigidity is induced by painful stimuli, and involves extension, adduction, and pronation of the arms, and extension of the legs with plantar flexion of the feet. Decerebrate posturing almost always signifies a brain stem lesion, from the mesencephalon to the vestibular nuclei.[7] Decorticate posturing produces flexion of the arms with extension of the legs. Lesions of the cerebral hemispheres produce decorticate posturing.[8]

RESPIRATION

Examination of the respiratory pattern may facilitate anatomic localization.[1,2] Figure 133-1 diagrams the various respiratory patterns commonly encountered in the comatose patient and their anatomic localization. Cheyne-Stokes respiration is a regular crescendo–decrescendo pattern in the depth of respiration; there may be a brief apneic spell between cycles. Cheyne-Stokes respirations are seen commonly in patients with deep bilateral subcortical lesions. Hyperventilation—a sustained hyperpnea—can result from lesions in the brain stem, but most frequently is a compensatory mechanism for primary pulmonary dysfunction. True central neurogenic hyperventilation is present when the patient is breathing room air and arterial blood gases reveal an elevated PO_2, lowered PCO_2, and an elevated pH. Patients meeting these strict criteria are rare, and usually have lesions in the low midbrain and middle third of the pons. Most frequently, comatose patients who are hyperventilating are attempting to compensate for pulmonary dysfunction and are mildly hypoxic. Apneustic breathing is characterized by a long inspiratory pause at full inspiration. This respiratory pattern indicates a lesion at the midpontine level, involving the dorsolateral tegmentum. Ataxic breathing is characterized by chaotic respiration of random depth and rate. Lesions of the dorsomedial medulla, compromising the primary respiratory centers, produce this respiratory pattern. Cluster breathing consists of clusters of breaths with irregular

pauses, and is produced by lesions in the lower pons or upper medulla.

OCULAR MOVEMENTS

Examination of eye movements elicited by stimulation of the vestibular mechanism often reveals important localizing information. Two tests of ocular function are easily conducted at the bedside, and are important components of the initial neurologic assessment. Both the oculocephalic maneuver and the ice water caloric test rely on the same anatomic pathways to produce eye movements.

To perform the oculocephalic test, the patient's head is rapidly rotated from side to side, which stimulates both the vestibular apparatus and proprioceptors in the neck. A normal response in the comatose patient is conjugate deviation of the eyes in the direction opposite the head turning. Conjugate deviation of the eyes implies that the pathways between the vestibular nuclei, the abducens nuclei, and the oculomotor nuclei are all intact, and therefore indicates that the brain stem is functional. A patient with an intact oculocephalic response usually has a bilateral hemispheric lesion causing coma. If no eye deviation is produced by the oculocephalic maneuver, no anatomic conclusions can be drawn, and the ice water caloric test, which uses a more effective stimulus, must be employed. An oculocephalic test producing disconjugate eye movements suggests a brain stem lesion preventing effective communication between the vestibular and ocular nuclei, as shown in Figure 133-1.

To conduct the ice water caloric test, the ears are first examined to determine whether the tympanic membrane is intact, and the patient's head is elevated 30 degrees above the horizontal plane, thereby placing the lateral semicircular canal in the vertical plane. Up to 120 mL of ice water is instilled into the external canal by a catheter attached to a syringe. The eye movements are then observed. In the conscious patient, cold water stimulation of the semicircular canal produces tonic conjugate deviation of the eyes toward the side of the stimulus with superimposed nystagmus, the fast component away from the side of the stimulus. The tonic eye movements are mediated by information arising in the vestibular nuclei, traveling to the paramedian pontine reticular formation, then to the abducens and oculomotor nuclei.[9] The fast saccadic nystagmus is mediated by impulses traveling from the posterior portion of the frontal lobes, descending through the genu of the internal capsule. In the comatose patient with bilateral hemispheric lesions, ice water vestibular stimulation therefore produces tonic conjugate eye deviation and no nystagmus, because the tonic deviation is mediated by the brain stem and the nystagmus results from fibers originating in the frontal lobes.

The comatose patient with a brain stem lesion usually demonstrates either of two abnormalities. The lesion may be in the middle or upper brain stem, involving the medial longitudinal fasciculus, which transmits information from the abducens nuclei to the oculomotor nucleus. In this case, the eye opposite the side of stimulation does not adduct across the midline (due to failure of the oculomotor nucleus), whereas the eye on the side of stimulation fully abducts (due

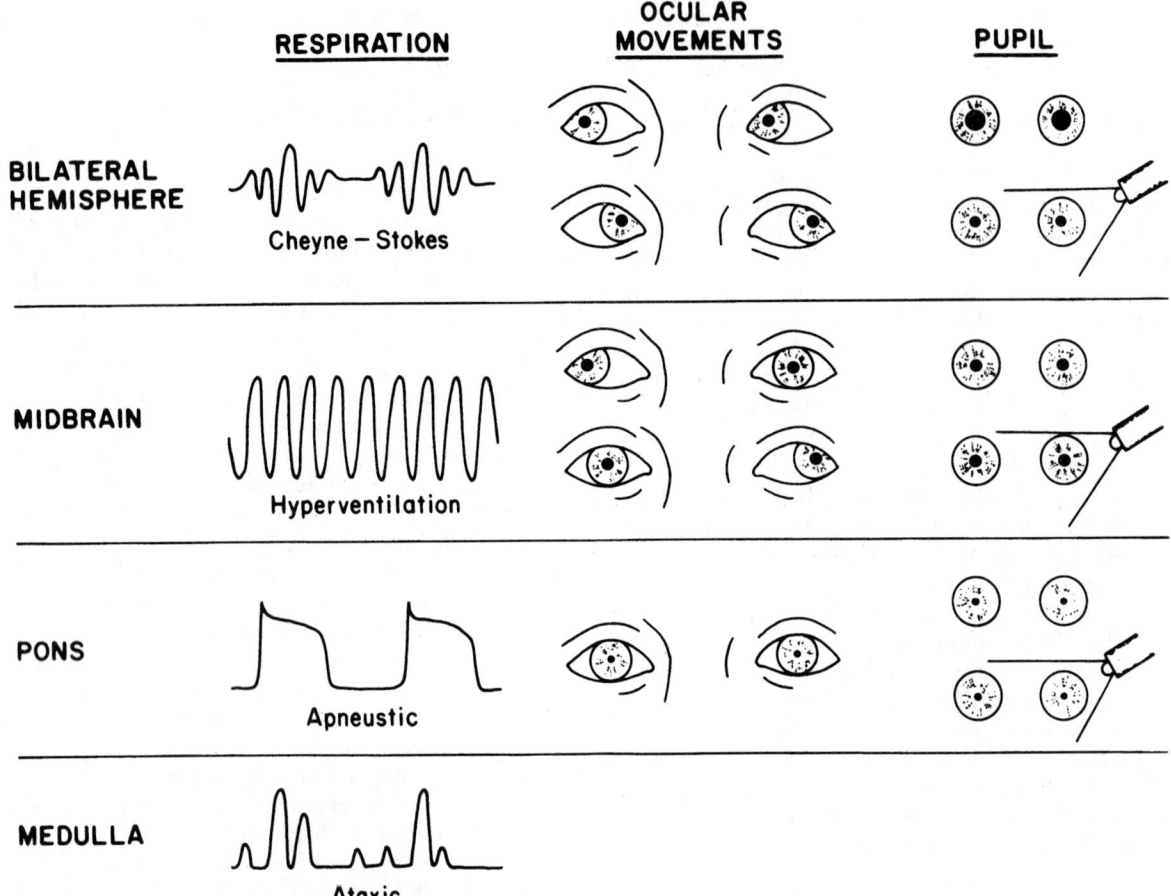

FIGURE 133-1. Respiratory patterns, extraocular movements, and pupillary findings in comatose patients with lesions in different locations of the central nervous system. (Adapted from figures in Plum F, Posner JB: *The Diagnosis of Stupor and Coma.* Philadelphia, FA Davis, 1980.)

to the normal function of the abducens nucleus). If the lesion is in the lower brain stem, the patient may have no response to ice water stimulation due to destruction of the vestibular nuclei or of the paramedian pontine reticular formation ("lateral gaze centers") near the abducens nuclei.

PUPILS

The size of the pupil represents a balance between parasympathetic input, which constricts the pupil, and sympathetic input, which dilates the pupil. The pupillary examination is critical because it often reveals important anatomic information and can be quantitatively assessed to help evaluate the patient over time. Therefore, a careful measure of the pupils, recorded in the hospital chart, is essential. A table displaying pupillary diameters recorded in millimeters in ambient light and with direct and consensual stimuli must be a part of the initial and follow-up evaluations. A "large pupil" recorded by a physician in the emergency room may or may not be the same "large pupil" seen later by the ICU physician.

The pupils in a comatose patient with bilateral cortical lesions are usually small and reactive. There are three drugs that may produce coma by depressing bilateral cortical function and can also produce pupillary disturbances directly. Atropine and scopolamine are muscarinic receptor antagonists that directly inhibit the parasympathetic input to the eye and therefore produce fixed and dilated pupils. Glutethimide overdose can produce coma and frequently produces unequal pupils that are 4 to 8 mm. Opiates (such as heroin and morphine) can also produce coma by depressing cortical function and produce pinpoint pupils.[1,2]

Brain stem lesions causing coma may produce pupillary abnormalities with localizing value. Lesions in the midbrain, involving the tectum, interrupt the pupillary light reflex and produce midposition pupils that do not respond to light. Lesions of the midbrain tegmentum interrupt both parasympathetic and sympathetic pathways to produce midposition, fixed, and nonreactive pupils. A lesion involving the third cranial nerve, or oculomotor nucleus in the midbrain, may produce a dilated pupil that is sluggishly reactive to light, and may also produce ocular motor paresis.

A pontine lesion producing coma destroys the descending sympathetic fibers and stimulates the parasympathetic input, producing pinpoint pupils. The light reflex is still intact, although it is often difficult to see without a magnifying glass.

Lesions of the medulla, by themselves, do not produce coma, as noted previously. However, if a lesion producing coma extends to the lateral medulla, Horner syndrome may result from interruption of the sympathetic pathway, producing pupillary constriction and ptosis (see Fig. 133-1).[1,2]

The orderly bedside examination of the comatose patient for spontaneous and evoked motor movement, respirations, ocular movements, and pupillary size and response is an invaluable aid in assessing whether the patient is comatose from a bilateral hemispheric lesion or a brain stem lesion. These observations, in addition to the routine history and physical examination, help direct the subsequent evaluation.

ADDITIONAL STUDIES ■

Four studies are commonly used in the emergency evaluation of the comatose patient: (1) computed tomographic (CT) scanning, (2) lumbar puncture, (3) electroencephalography (EEG), and (4) laboratory studies.

The CT scan has revolutionized the evaluation of the comatose patient. Virtually every patient who presents with acute onset of stupor or coma needs an emergency CT scan to detect mass lesions, destructive lesions, or blood in either the supratentorial or infratentorial compartments. Evaluation with CT often helps determine the anatomy, etiology, and size of the lesion.[10] This information is critical in determining therapy and is prerequisite to decisions about surgery. Unfortunately, movement of the stuporous patient may preclude adequate studies. Intravenous doses of diazepam (3 to 10 mg) are therefore sometimes indicated. For all comatose patients, the physician must be in attendance during the CT scan to detect and treat failing respirations, cardiovascular changes, seizures, or deteriorating mental state.

Lumbar puncture is often vital in evaluating the comatose patient. It must be performed, on an emergency basis, whenever acute bacterial meningitis is suspected. If acute bacterial meningitis is suspected in a febrile comatose patient, the lumbar puncture should be performed and therapy instituted before the CT scan is performed. For most other patients, the lumbar puncture is best deferred until after the CT scan.

The EEG sometimes helps in the emergency evaluation of the comatose patient.[11] First, the EEG helps to differentiate true coma from psychogenic unresponsiveness. Second, the EEG may help in uncovering the etiology of the coma. Status epilepticus, which may manifest as "electrical status" with no motor movement, produces unresponsiveness and requires recognition and aggressive anticonvulsant therapy (see Chap. 134). Patients with metabolic disease, such as hepatic failure, may have characteristic triphasic waves that alert the physician to the etiology and help direct therapy. The EEG is also helpful in the nonemergency evaluation of the comatose patient, because it is more sensitive than the clinical examination in detecting improvement or worsening of the clinical condition.

Laboratory tests are vital in the emergency evaluation of the comatose patient. At the time of presentation, all patients need to have determination of electrolytes and glucose and arterial blood gases. Additional tests may also be obtained after a more thorough clinical evaluation, including a screen for sedative and toxic drugs, liver function tests, coagulation tests, thyroid and adrenal evaluation, blood cultures, and viral titers.

As stressed previously, two basic lesions may cause coma: brain stem lesions affecting the reticular core and bilateral hemispheric lesions affecting the ascending reticular activating system. Lesions causing coma may therefore be confined to the brain stem or the cerebral hemispheres, or may be diffuse, affecting the entire brain, as seen in intoxication and other metabolic insults. The following sections describe the diagnosis and management of the comatose patient who presents with a bilateral hemispheric lesion, a brain stem lesion, or a toxic, metabolic, or diffuse lesion.

BILATERAL HEMISPHERIC LESIONS ■

Bilateral hemispheric lesions causing coma should be suspected in any patient with a history of headache or trauma. The examination may show the signs of hemispheric dysfunction mentioned in the previous section: Cheyne-Stokes respiration, equal and reactive pupils, ice water caloric testing producing tonic conjugate eye deviation (with no nystagmus), and either semipurposeful movement or decorticate posturing. The major exception to these generalizations is the hemispheric mass lesion causing coma, which compresses the third cranial nerve directly to produce a dilated, and eventually fixed, pupil. (This condition is described in a later section.) Patients demonstrating marked focal neurologic signs, such as tonic eye deviation or hemiparesis, and patients deteriorating rapidly should be suspected of harboring bilateral hemispheric lesions.

Key considerations in the evaluation of a comatose patient with bilateral hemispheric lesions are the depth, progression, and duration of coma. Clearly, a patient brought to the emergency room comatose after an automobile accident, whose level of function continues to deteriorate, must be treated with utmost urgency. Once the patient is stabilized and assessed, an emergency CT scan must be performed. If CT is unavailable, cerebral angiography should be considered. These studies usually provide definitive information revealing the site, size, and etiology of the lesion. In patients who are deteriorating rapidly or undergoing herniation, treatment of increased ICP usually takes precedence over radiographic studies. If the CT scan does not reveal a mass lesion, the patient may have a metabolic or toxic encephalopathy.

Lesions in only one hemisphere produce coma by one of two processes: secondarily compromising the function of the other hemisphere (to produce bilateral hemispheric dysfunction) or compromising the function of the brain stem. A lesion affecting one hemisphere exclusively, without affecting the other hemisphere or the brain stem, does not cause coma.

Hemispheric lesions producing coma may occur in the extracerebral spaces or in the intracerebral space. Lesions found in the extracerebral space include neoplasm, infection, and hematoma. Lesions found in the intracerebral space include neoplasm, hemorrhage, infarction, and abscess. Early recognition and treatment of these hemispheric lesions are important; by the time they produce coma, their effects have extended beyond simply compromising function of one hemisphere.

EXTRACEREBRAL LESIONS

Neoplasms rarely present for the first time by producing coma. In general, the course of extracerebral neoplasm is insidious, with headache, focal neurologic signs, and seizures occurring over weeks, months, or even years before the patient's level of consciousness is altered.

Hematomas in the extracerebral compartment often develop precipitously. Their prompt recognition and surgical treatment are often critical. A patient with a clear history of head trauma, a car accident, or a fall who lapses into coma must be quickly evaluated for an expanding hematoma. Unfortunately, the level of suspicion is often not high if the patient fails to give such a history. Keep in mind that the patient may be confused or demented and simply may not recall the trauma. Also remember that patients with blood dyscrasias (e.g., thrombocytopenia or leukemia) and those receiving anticoagulants may develop a "spontaneous" hematoma.[12]

Blood in the extracerebral spaces may be extradural. Extradural hemorrhage most commonly arises in the temporal fossa, from laceration of the middle meningeal artery, and may rapidly expand and cause death if not recognized and treated surgically. Extradural hemorrhage commonly follows head injury, sometimes of a trivial nature, and often produces only headache. The patient's mental state may then progressively deteriorate to coma and death. Focal neurologic signs of hemiparesis and third cranial nerve dysfunction are often seen. Emergency CT scanning or angiography is necessary. In a patient who is deteriorating too rapidly for these studies, emergency trephine of the skull may be performed for both diagnosis and therapy.

Blood may accumulate in the subdural space and produce coma. Subdural hematoma can be acute, subacute, or chronic. A unilateral subdural hematoma commonly produces coma by producing direct effects on one cerebral hemisphere, with secondary displacement downward to affect the brain stem. Commonly, no history of trauma is elicited and the diagnosis is not suspected. A CT scan with contrast enhancement usually reveals the diagnosis. Chronic subdural hematoma may produce a lesion that is isodense with cortex and may be difficult to visualize. In such cases, cerebral angiography is helpful.

Extracerebral infection may cause coma by producing a subdural empyema. This infection is most frequently seen with acute bacterial sinusitis, but may also be seen after trauma, surgery, or a ruptured cerebral abscess. The usual clinical setting is a patient with a history of nose or ear infection who develops headache, fever, and focal neurologic signs. Angiography or CT scanning, followed by a lumbar puncture, is necessary to make the diagnosis and to initiate the appropriate therapy.

INTRACEREBRAL LESIONS PRODUCING COMA

Intracerebral neoplasm, hemorrhage, infarction, and abscess may produce coma.[12] Cerebral hemorrhage is the most common vascular cause of coma, producing unconsciousness in 25% of cases. Cerebral hemorrhage severe enough to produce coma has a dismal prognosis; most patients die. The diagnosis of intracerebral hemorrhage is made by CT scan. If blood pressure is severely elevated, it should be lowered in an attempt to limit further damage. Surgical intervention should be considered. Blood in the ventricular space usually results from dissection of an intracerebral hemorrhage and can produce acute obstructive hydrocephalus. In this situation, surgical placement of a ventricular drain may partially alleviate symptoms and improve recovery.

Coma is rare with simple hemispheric infarction. Patients with hemispheric infarction who are comatose at the time of admission often have some common underlying disease process, such as hypotension due to myocardial infarction or cardiac arrhythmia. Coma can result from hemispheric infarction due to brain swelling, which is maximal 2 to 4 days after infarction.

Venous thrombosis is often overlooked as a cause of coma. Venous thrombosis may occur during bacterial infection, may result from direct venous occlusion by tumor, or may be produced by a hypercoagulable state. Patients presenting with headache, focal signs, and seizures should be suspected of harboring venous thrombosis.[13] Lumbar puncture commonly reveals increased intracranial pressure (ICP) and both red and white blood cells. The definitive diagnosis is made by examining the venous phase of cerebral angiograms, which reveals occluded venous sinus or draining veins.

Intracranial tumors may cause coma, but their usually insidious course prompts aggressive workup long before the tumor alters consciousness.

BRAIN STEM LESIONS   ■

Brain stem lesions causing coma are either intrinsic to the brain stem or are extrinsic and compress the brain stem. Before lapsing into coma, the patient may have occipital headache or symptoms of vertigo, diplopia, or ataxia. Nausea and vomiting frequently occur. On neurologic examination, these patients commonly have brain stem signs, with respiratory pattern abnormalities, abnormalities of extraocular movements elicited by ice water caloric testing, and other cranial nerve abnormalities described previously. A CT scan may prove helpful by revealing an etiology, such as a cerebellar hemorrhage compromising the brain stem. If the CT scan is normal, particular attention must be paid to the metabolic tests outlined previously, as well as lumbar puncture. Comatose patients with brain stem lesions may be undergoing herniation and may need aggressive therapy for increased ICP.

Lesions within the brain stem cause coma by directly destroying the reticular activating system or by impairing the blood supply to this region. By far the most common intrinsic brain stem lesion causing coma is cerebrovascular disease. Mass lesions caused by neoplasms, abscesses, and granulomas may also compromise brain stem function.

Lesions outside the brain stem can cause coma by directly pressing against the pons or midbrain, secondarily affecting the reticular activating system; by pushing the cerebellar vermis up through the tentorial notch, compromising midbrain function; or by pushing the cerebellar tonsils down through the foramen magnum, affecting lower brain stem function.

Basilar artery thrombosis is a common cause of coma. Typically, patients develop transient signs and symptoms for days before becoming comatose. These symptoms may wax and wane, and may affect different areas of the brain stem causing a multitude of symptoms. Intermittent dysarthria, dysphagia, diplopia, ataxia, and weakness are common. If the ischemia progresses to produce coma, a number of previously described clinical signs may be observed, which localize the deficit to the brain stem level. In these comatose patients, a CT scan should be performed to rule out hemorrhage, and anticoagulation should be considered.

Pontine hemorrhage commonly presents precipitously with coma, and usually occurs in patients with hypertension. The diagnosis of pontine hemorrhage is usually simple because of the typical history and neurologic findings. The onset of coma is rapid, the ice water caloric tests produce no ocular movements, the patient is quadriplegic, and the pupils are pinpoint. Hemorrhages large enough to produce coma are usually revealed on CT scan.

Cerebellar hemorrhage is an uncommon cause of coma, but overlooking this possibility is unfortunate because surgical evacuation of the hemorrhage can often effectively improve the patient's outcome.[14] Most patients with cerebellar hemorrhage have a history of hypertension, and the remainder harbor an angioma. Commonly, the patient presents with a history of occipital headache, nausea and vomiting, vertigo, and difficulty in walking. On examination, the patient may have ipsilateral ataxia, nystagmus, and a gaze paresis toward the site of the hematoma. The patient may be alert, but any subtle change in mental state is ominous and indicates impending decompensation. A physician examining such a patient must have a high index of suspicion and must move quickly. Suboccipital craniotomy with evacuation is a potentially lifesaving procedure in cerebellar hemorrhage. Emergency CT scanning makes the diagnosis. In the patient who is deteriorating rapidly, an emergency craniotomy may be necessary without delaying the CT scan study.

Cerebellar infarction may produce clinical findings similar to cerebellar hemorrhage. The symptoms and signs of cerebellar infarction usually evolve over a longer period. These findings often remain the same for 1 to 3 days before renewed progression to coma. The diagnosis is made by CT scanning. Surgery is warranted for two complications: (1) herniation of the swollen cerebellum with continuing clinical decompensation and (2) appearance of obstructive hydrocephalus on CT scan.

Nonvascular destructive lesions in the brain stem may cause coma, but usually present with a relentlessly progressive picture of focal brain stem dysfunction before altering consciousness. Granulomas, metastatic tumors, and abscesses are the most common of these causes of coma.

METABOLIC–TOXIC ETIOLOGIES ■

Coma of diffuse, metabolic, or toxic etiology is frequently seen in the ICU, and is often the most difficult to diagnose. Unlike the causes of coma discussed in the previous two sections, no mass lesions are visualized on CT scan that pinpoint the anatomic site of dysfunction or the etiology. The differential diagnosis is further complicated by the wide range of mechanisms by which coma can be produced.

The usual metabolic–toxic coma is preceded by hours, days, or weeks of progressive confusion and disorientation. The examination usually reveals no focal signs, and the level of dysfunction reveals a lesion anywhere from bilateral hemispheric to the low brain stem. Tremor, asterixis, or myoclonus should alert the physician to a metabolic etiology. A patient who has recently ingested large quantities of sedative medication may be found with adequate respiration but may deteriorate rapidly as the level of brain stem function is further depressed. Vigilance regarding respiratory and cardiovascular function is essential in the emergency evaluation of a patient with metabolic–toxic coma. The metabolic and toxic etiologies of coma that are treatable and that may otherwise lead to death include drug overdose, hypoglycemia, metabolic acidosis, hyperosmolar states, bacterial meningitis, endocarditis, hypoxia, and electrolyte imbalance.

DEPRIVATION OF OXYGEN, SUBSTRATE, OR METABOLIC COFACTORS

Cerebral hypoxia causes coma. Immediate evaluations of the airway, respirations, pulse, and blood pressure, followed by arterial blood gas analysis and electrocardiogram, are mandatory. Deprivation of oxygen to the brain for 1 to 2 minutes may lead to longstanding or even permanent encephalopathy or stupor. Deprivation longer than 4 minutes results in neural death, particularly in the hippocampus and cerebellum.[15]

Hypoglycemia must be rapidly treated to prevent long-term sequelae or death. Most commonly, hypoglycemia severe enough to produce coma results from insulin overdose, either accidental or intentional. Hypoglycemia may cause seizures and may produce focal neurologic signs that wax and wane. Because of the potential for reversal, as well as the necessity for rapid treatment, all stuporous and comatose patients should have blood drawn for serum glucose determination, followed immediately by intravenous administration of glucose.

Thiamine deficiency may produce coma or may alter the mental status of the malnourished patient who has been given glucose.

ORGAN DYSFUNCTION

Dysfunction of virtually any organ can result in coma. Liver failure is a common cause of encephalopathy that may progress to coma. The typical history is a delirium that usually progresses over days. Hyperventilation is invariably seen and the patient may have either a metabolic or a respiratory alkalosis. The patient usually has a history of chronic liver disease with the associated stigmata. Measurement of serum ammonia and liver function makes the diagnosis.

Renal failure resulting in uremia may cause confusion, stupor, and coma. The biochemical mechanism by which renal failure causes coma is not known. Blood urea nitrogen is elevated but correlates poorly with the degree of cerebral depression, and is not the cause. In treating patients with severe renal failure, particular attention must be paid to associated electrolyte abnormalities, which may by themselves depress consciousness or cause seizures.

Pancreatitis rarely causes stupor or coma. The patient may present with days of abdominal pain followed by delirium, hallucinations, and seizures.

Diabetes can cause coma by at least three mechanisms: a hyperosmolar state, diabetic ketoacidosis, or diabetic lactic acidosis. Never forget that diabetic patients can become comatose from hypoglycemia.

Abnormal adrenal function resulting in either hypoadrenal or hyperadrenal dysfunction can lead to stupor or coma, but more commonly presents with more protean symptoms. Likewise, both hyperthyroidism and hypothyroidism can alter the mental state. Hypothyroidism commonly presents with hypothermia and hypoventilation. The definitive diagnosis is made by thyroid function testing, but occasionally therapy with triiodothyronine must be initiated before laboratory confirmation. Hyperthyroidism commonly causes tremor, anxiety, sweating, tachycardia, pulmonary edema, and congestive heart failure.

EXOGENOUS POISONS

The list of drugs (licit or illicit), toxins, and poisons that may cause coma is extensive. Intoxication with drugs and toxins is an extremely common cause of coma. The level of mental state depression may be subtle (mild confusion) or profound (deep coma with no respirations and absent caloric response). The physician must be vigilant in determining whether the patient is deteriorating. The potential for complete neurologic recovery is excellent in most cases, unless other complications such as hypoxia develop. Emergency care is primarily supportive; however, clinical suspicion or specific toxicologic assays may indicate more specific therapies.

INFECTIONS AND INFLAMMATION

Acute bacterial meningitis must always be suspected in the patient presenting with coma, because early diagnosis and treatment is essential for a favorable outcome (see Chap. 110). *Haemophilus influenzae*, *Streptococcus pneumoniae*, *Neisseria meningitidis*, and *Listeria monocytogenes* are most frequently encountered.[16] A high level of suspicion for meningitis must be maintained and a lumbar puncture should be performed early in the evaluation. Keep in mind that signs of meningeal irritation, such as stiff neck, are frequently absent in the stuporous or comatose patient.

Encephalitis can also be caused by viruses, rickettsiae, protozoa, and nematodes. Only two groups of viruses are encountered in the United States that cause coma: the arboviruses (Eastern equine, Western equine, and St. Louis encephalitis) and herpes simplex.[1] The cerebrospinal fluid (CSF) usually contains increased white cells, mostly mononuclear, and an elevated protein; CSF glucose may be normal or slightly depressed.

Cerebral vasculitis is a rare cause of coma. Granulomatous angiitis is a small vessel vasculitis limited to the brain.[17] Systemic lupus erythematosus produces neurologic dysfunction in the majority of cases, presenting with focal waxing and waning symptoms, psychiatric symptoms, seizures, and, less commonly, altered sensorium. Lupus should be considered in any patient, particularly a young female, who presents in coma with focal signs and seizures. The diagnosis is supported by a history of arthralgia, skin rash, and renal failure.

Subarachnoid hemorrhage commonly arises from rupture of a berry aneurysm in the circle of Willis. Subarachnoid hemorrhage may cause coma by acutely increasing ICP, and later by causing vasospasm. Hydrocephalus may develop weeks after the acute bleed. Patients may present with a history of subacute or acute headache with signs of increased ICP (papilledema and subhyaloid hemorrhages). The diagnosis of subarachnoid hemorrhage in the comatose patient is best made by CT scan.

THE DETERIORATING COMATOSE PATIENT

The physician must be alert to changes in the comatose patient. Deterioration of the clinical condition can occur abruptly, in minutes, or may evolve slowly over days. Recognition of deterioration is vital. Additional supportive measures may need to be initiated rapidly. In some cases, the patient may require reevaluation for different causes of coma. For example, a patient treated for bacterial meningitis may suddenly become less responsive because of hypoxia due to pulmonary emboli. Additional therapy may be required to treat the lesion producing the coma, or measures may be needed to reduce ICP. The key to recognizing deterioration is documentation in the chart of specific findings. The statement that the patient "responds to pain" is not helpful to the physician called in later to see the patient. *How* does the patient respond—by decerebrate posturing, decorticate posturing, semipurposeful movements, or by withdrawing the examiner's hand? Similarly, the notation of pupils being equal and reactive to light is of no use to the physician who later documents 4-mm pupils. Be specific, and wherever possible, quantitate. The level of stimulation necessary to evoke reaction in the stuporous or comatose patient and the extent and pattern of motor response are good indicators of function and should be specifically noted. Pupillary size and response should be quantitated. Respiratory pattern and rate must be noted. Ocular movements in response to oculocephalic or ice water stimulation should be regularly checked.

Two patterns of changes in these neurologic functions indicate deterioration and should alert the physician that additional diagnostic and therapeutic efforts are necessary. Decompensating cerebral lesions may produce either the uncal syndrome, which causes signs of third cranial nerve and midbrain compression, or the central syndrome, which produces bilateral diencephalic signs.[1] After these two distinctive early phases, deterioration proceeds similarly in both syndromes, compromising brain stem function continuously from the midbrain down.

The uncal syndrome is most commonly encountered with expanding unilateral hemispheric lesions. With expansion of the hemisphere, the medial edge of the hippocampus is pushed toward the midline and over the edge of the tentorium, pressing against the third cranial nerve. Dilation of the pupil on the side of the lesion is the earliest sign. As the lesion continues to expand, third cranial nerve function is further compromised and the dilated pupil becomes unresponsive to light. In addition, medial rectus function may be destroyed, producing disconjugate gaze on ice water caloric testing. Motor signs of decorticate or even decerebrate posturing may be seen.

The central syndrome is seen commonly with increasing pressure exerted more or less evenly by both hemispheres. In this syndrome, the earliest signs are changes in respiration, with the development of Cheyne-Stokes respiration and small, minimally reactive pupils. In the earliest stages, motor responses to painful stimuli may be appropriate, but with further deterioration, bilateral decorticate posturing may develop.

After these two distinctive early stages, both central and uncal herniation produce similar patterns of brain stem function. At the point of midbrain function, the patient is hyperventilating. Pupils are midposition and nonreactive, and oculocephalic testing may show medial rectus weakness. With further deterioration to the pontine or medullary level, the respiratory pattern may be ataxic, and ice water caloric testing elicits no response. The pupils are midposition and fixed.

With the appearance of either uncal or central herniation, the physician is forced to reevaluate therapy. Emergency surgery may be indicated if a lesion producing the herniation can be surgically treated (e.g., subdural hematoma). Specific measures to treat increased ICP need to be initiated while additional diagnostic and therapeutic measures are considered. Hyperventilation is the most rapid technique to reduce ICP. The $PaCO_2$ should be between 20 and 25 mm Hg. Since the reduction in pressure is only transient, additional therapy must also be started. Hyperosmotic agents reduce increased ICP by pulling water from the intracranial to the vascular compartments. Mannitol (20%) given by bolus injection at 1.5 to 2.0 g/kg reduces ICP for several hours.

Steroids may reduce edema only in certain lesions, but nevertheless are widely used. The effective dose is not established, but 16 mg of dexamethasone daily in divided doses is widely used.

After these measures are initiated, a CT scan is indicated, even in patients who have been recently scanned. A neurosurgical evaluation should be done as soon as possible because the neurosurgeon may elect to place bur holes even before the scan is obtained. Pulmonary and cardiovascular status should be carefully evaluated and metabolic status reevaluated. After these emergency measures are instituted, more definitive therapy is started.

REFERENCES ■

1. Plum F, Posner JB: *The Diagnosis of Stupor and Coma.* Philadelphia, FA Davis, 1980
2. Bates D: The management of medical coma. *J Neurol Neurosurg Psychiatry* 1993;56:589
3. Peele TL: *The Neuroanatomic Basis for Clinical Neurology.* 3rd ed. New York, McGraw-Hill, 1977:248
4. Von Economo C: *Encephalitis Lethargica: Sequelae and Treatment.* London, Oxford University Press, 1931
5. Brian R: The physiologic basis of consciousness. *Brain* 1958; 81:426
6. Magoun HW: *The Waking Brain.* 2nd ed. Springfield, IL, Charles C Thomas, 1963
7. Purpura DP: Operations and processes in thalamic and synaptically related neural subsystems. In: *The Neurosciences Second Study Program.* New York, Rockefeller University Press, 1970: 458
8. Feldman MH: The decerebrate state in the primate. I. Studies in monkeys. *Arch Neurol* 1971;25:501
9. Glaser J: *Neuroopthalmology.* Hagerstown, MD, Harper & Row, 1978:247
10. Kinkel W: Computerized tomography in clinical neurology. In: Baker AB, Joynt RJ (eds): *Clinical Neurology.* Philadelphia, Harper & Row, 1986
11. Prensky AL, Coben LA: Electroencephalography. In: Baker AB, Joynt RJ (eds): *Clinical Neurology* Philadelphia, Harper & Row, 1986
12. Edwards RH, Simon RP: Coma. In: Baker AB, Joynt RJ (eds): *Clinical Neurology.* Philadelphia, Harper & Row, 1986
13. Smith BH: Infections of the dura and its venous sinus. In: Baker AB, Joynt RJ (eds): *Clinical Neurology* Philadelphia, Harper & Row, 1986
14. McKissock W, Richardson A, Walsh L: Spontaneous cerebellar hemorrhage: a study of 34 consecutive cases treated surgically. *Brain* 1960;83:1
15. Weinberger LM, Gibbon MH, Gibbon JH Jr: Temporary arrest of the circulation to the central nervous system: II. Pathologic effects. *Arch Neurol Psychiatry* 1940;43:961
16. Romer FK: Bacterial meningitis: a 15 year review of bacterial meningitis from departments of internal medicine. *Dan Med Bull* 1977;24:35
17. Jellinger K: Giant cell granulomatous angitis of the central nervous system. *J Neurol* 1977;215:175

Critical Care, Third Edition, edited by Joseph M. Civetta,
Robert W. Taylor, and Robert R. Kirby.
Lippincott-Raven Publishers, Philadelphia, PA © 1997.

CHAPTER 134

■

Status Epilepticus

Paul A. Rutecki

IMMEDIATE CONCERNS ■

MAJOR PROBLEMS

In the most general terms, status epilepticus is defined as
"epileptic seizures that are so frequently repeated or so
prolonged as to create a fixed and lasting epileptic condition."[1] In most cases status epilepticus consists of recurrent
seizures without an intervening return to normal consciousness.

STRESS POINTS

1. Any of the classified seizures can develop into status
   epilepticus; however, generalized tonic–clonic (convulsive) status epilepticus is a medical emergency and
   is the focus of most of this chapter.
2. Mortality and morbidity of generalized tonic–clonic
   status increase with duration of the status.[2,3,4] It is
   critical that convulsive status be stopped within 60
   minutes to prevent both systemic[5,6] and neurologic[7,8]
   complications.

ESSENTIAL DIAGNOSTIC TESTS
AND PROCEDURES

1. History and physical examination
2. Blood work including a stat blood glucose (see later)
3. Arterial blood gases
4. Anticonvulsant blood levels and toxicology screen
5. Electrocardiogram (ECG), pulse oximetry monitoring,
   and, optimally, electroencephalogram (EEG)

INITIAL THERAPY

1. A protocol for treating generalized tonic–clonic status
   epilepticus is presented in Table 134-1. As with most
   medical emergencies, initial treatment should be directed toward maintaining cardiorespiratory function
   and correcting any precipitating causes. An airway
   should be inserted and oxygen administered; if necessary, the patient should be intubated and artificially
   ventilated. A large-gauge intravenous catheter should
   be inserted and blood obtained for laboratory studies.
   Intravenous infusion of normal saline should be
   started, and 50 mL of 50% glucose should be administered along with thiamine. The ECG and blood pressure should be monitored.
2. The next step in treatment is to stop the seizures
   and prevent their recurrence. In 80% of cases, the
   intravenous administration of lorazepam or diazepam
   and phenytoin is effective.[9,10] If status continues following adequate dosages of these medications, intravenous phenobarbital is administered. At this point,
   intubation should be performed, laboratory results assessed, and metabolic abnormalities treated. Convulsive status that lasts longer than 60 minutes requires
   drug or inhalation anesthesia and continuous EEG
   monitoring.
3. Frequent monitoring of vital signs is essential during
   treatment to detect the consequences of convulsive
   status and the side effects of pharmacologic therapy.

TABLE 134-1. Protocol for Treatment of Generalized Tonic–Clonic Status

1. Provide for maintenance of vital signs. Maintain airway; give oxygen. Observe and examine patient. Obtain any pertinent history (0–10 m).
2. Obtain 50 mL of blood for determination of glucose, calcium, magnesium, electrolytes, BUN, liver functions, anticonvulsant levels, CBC, and toxicology screen. Assess oxygenation with pulse oximetry or arterial blood gases. Begin normal saline IV. If hypoglycemia is established or glucose determination is unavailable, give 50 mL of 50% glucose and 100 mg of thiamine. Monitor ECG, blood pressure, and, if possible, EEG (6–10 m).
3. If patient is having clinical seizures, use IV lorazepam 0.1 mg/kg given 1–2 mg/m. Alternatively, may use IV diazepam 0.2 mg/kg at 5 mg/m repeating dose in 5 m for recurrent or continuous seizures (10–30 m).
4. If using diazepam or if seizures persist after lorazepam, then load with phenytoin (18 mg/kg) IV at a rate of 50 mg/m or less. If cardiac arrhythmia or hypotension occurs, then stop until resolution and resume at a slower rate (10–30 m).
5. If seizures persist 10–20 m after phenytoin infusion is completed, may give additional 5–10 mg/kg of phenytoin. Alternatively, or if seizures persist after additional phenytoin, intubate patient and give phenobarbital IV 20 mg/kg at a rate of 50–100 mg/m (30–60 m).
6. If seizures continue after 60 m, review laboratory results and correct any abnormalities. Arrange for anesthesia, neuromuscular blockade, and EEG monitoring. For refractory status epilepticus, options include sodium pentobarbital (5–15 mg/kg loading dose, followed by 0.5–5 mg/kg/h), midazolam (0.15–0.20 mg/kg loading dose, followed by 0.06–1.1 mg/kg/h), or isoflurane anesthesia.

Systemic complications of convulsive status (hypoxia, acidosis, rhabdomyolysis, hyperthermia, dehydration, cardiac arrhythmia) should be prevented or corrected. Further evaluation of the cause of the convulsive status should be undertaken after the patient has been stabilized.

DEFINITIONS AND CLASSIFICATION ■

Seizures are classified as *generalized* or *partial*. *Generalized seizures* are accompanied by synchronous epileptiform activity in both cerebral hemispheres. In *primary* generalized seizures, bilaterally synchronous epileptiform activity occurs in both cerebral hemispheres from onset; *secondary* generalized seizures begin as partial seizures that spread and result in epileptiform activity in both cerebral hemispheres. Primary generalized seizures include *tonic–clonic* (grand mal), tonic, clonic, myoclonic, atonic, and absence (petit mal) seizures. *Partial seizures,* those that begin with epileptiform activity in one brain region, are defined as *simple partial* if consciousness is not impaired during the seizure and as *complex partial* if consciousness is impaired. The initial clinical manifestation of partial seizures depends on the function of the brain region involved in the seizure onset. For example, if the motor strip is the site of origin, the initial manifes-

tation is abnormal motor activity, usually clonic, of the contralateral limbs.

Although this classification scheme is helpful in addressing the clinical and EEG characteristics of seizures, a more useful classification with regard to the management and treatment of status epilepticus divides the status into convulsive, nonconvulsive, and simple partial (Table 134-2). Convulsive status includes generalized tonic–clonic seizures with either a partial or generalized onset. Tonic, clonic, or myoclonic seizures may also occur with sufficient frequency to constitute a convulsive status; however, these seizure types (discussed later) rarely develop into status in adults.[1] Subtle convulsive status refers to patients who are comatose with minimal motor signs but with EEG-defined generalized seizure activity (see Special Cases).[3,4] Nonconvulsive status includes absence and complex partial seizures; it is not accompanied by major motor signs but is associated with various degrees of impaired consciousness and automatic behavior. Simple partial status is usually characterized by unilateral, restricted motor seizures that are continuous and do not impair consciousness (epilepsia partialis continua). Because generalized tonic–clonic status (also referred to as convulsive status) is the most common form of status epilepticus in adults,[1] it is the main focus of this chapter. The diagnosis and treatment of nonconvulsive status and simple partial status are addressed at the end of the chapter.

ETIOLOGY ■

Each year between 50,000 to 60,000 people in the United States develop convulsive status epilepticus.[2] About 50% of adult patients with convulsive status epilepticus have a preexisting diagnosis of epilepsy.[11-13] Convulsive status is rarely the presenting symptom of primary generalized epilepsy.[11] About 25% of patients have cryptogenic or idiopathic seizures[13] (i.e., seizures without a definite etiology). The other 75% have symptomatic seizures (i.e., caused by a brain lesion or metabolic abnormality). Only about 1% to 2% of patients with cryptogenic seizures develop status, whereas about 9% of those with symptomatic epilepsy develop convulsive status.[13]

In two series of adult patients presenting with convulsive status to a metropolitan public hospital emergency room, the most common cause of status epilepticus is anticonvulsant drug noncompliance (about 30% of all patients; 50% of patients with preexisting epilepsy).[11,12] Other causes include association with alcohol withdrawal (15% to 25%), cerebrovascular lesions (5% to 10%), drug intoxication (10%), and

TABLE 134-2. Classification of Status Epilepticus

I. Convulsive	II. Non-convulsive
Generalized tonic–clonic	Absence
Tonic	Complex partial
Clonic	III. Simple partial
Myoclonic	Epilepsia partialis continua
Subtle	

acute metabolic derangement (8%). In other series, 5% to 25% of patients with convulsive status had brain tumors (usually in the frontal lobes), 10% to 25% had an acute or chronic traumatic lesion, 10% to 25% had an acute or old cerebrovascular lesion, and 5% to 10% had a central nervous system (CNS) infection.[2,4,13]

Seizures may occur in association with acute or chronic cerebrovascular lesions (infarction, intracerebral hemorrhage, subarachnoid hemorrhage). Metabolic etiologies include hyponatremia, hypoglycemia, hypocalcemia, uremia, hepatic encephalopathy, anoxic-hypoxic encephalopathy, and hyperosmolar states.[11,12] Commonly used or abused drugs that may produce seizures and status are theophylline and its derivatives, isoniazid, lidocaine, tricyclic antidepressants, phenothiazines, antibiotics (imipenem/cilastatin, penicillins, ciprofloxacin), cocaine, and amphetamines.[14]

In most series, the seizures of more than 50% of patients had focal features.[1,11] These included asymmetric tonic or clonic motor activity and eye deviation. The presence of focal central nervous system (CNS) lesions was not a prerequisite for the seizures to have focal features.[11] Even metabolic etiologies can be accompanied by seizures with focal features, and in such situations the focus of seizure origin may shift or alternate between sides.

In summation, convulsive status manifested by generalized tonic–clonic seizures is associated with a precipitating etiology in at least 75% to 85% of patients.[11–13] In patients with previously diagnosed epilepsy, the most common precipitating causes are anticonvulsant medication, noncompliance, or alcohol withdrawal. Other considerations include systemic infections, sleep deprivation, metabolic alterations, or drug intoxication. In patients without a previous seizure history, convulsive status is usually associated with a CNS lesion or acute metabolic derangement. In this group of patients, neoplasm, trauma, and cerebrovascular insults must be considered, as well as any acute metabolic insult. During the course of treatment, these considerations must be kept in mind and appropriate laboratory studies ordered.

PATHOPHYSIOLOGY ■

Convulsive status produces a number of physiologic changes. During the first 20 to 30 minutes of convulsive status, compensatory mechanisms appear to prevent CNS damage. If status lasts longer than 30 to 60 minutes, the compensatory mechanisms begin to fail, and, after 60 minutes of status, CNS damage may result. Furthermore, the systemic complications of status epilepticus predispose the heart to arrhythmia. Initially, there is an increase in systemic and pulmonary blood pressure[5,6,15] and a 200% to 600% increase in cerebral blood flow (CBF).[15] The increase in blood pressure is secondary to elevations in circulating norepinephrine and epinephrine and to muscular contractions.[5,6,15] The CNS venous pressure increases in part because of muscular contractions. Initially, there is a decrease in the cerebral arterial-venous oxygen difference; however, with prolonged status (25 to 30 minutes), blood pressure and CBF decrease, and the arterial-venous oxygen difference increases.[5] After 20 minutes

of status in experimental animals, the partial pressure of oxygen and the oxidized state of cytochrome oxidase in brain tissue fall below baseline levels.[16] Initially, hyperglycemia is present, but as status continues, hypoglycemia is produced.[5] These changes result in a mismatch between CNS metabolic demand and supply, leading to tissue damage.[7] Excessive and prolonged exposure to excitatory amino acid neurotransmitters may also contribute to neuronal death.[17]

In convulsive status, severe acidosis results from the muscular activity and associated lactate production.[5,6,8] There is often accompanying respiratory acidosis. In one third of patients, arterial pH falls below 7.0.[11] There may be associated hyperkalemia from the acidosis, or muscle necrosis, and hyperkalemia may potentiate the acidosis in producing cardiac arrhythmia. In addition to a systemic acidosis, the brain also has increased lactate production, which leads to vasodilatation and increased intracranial pressure (ICP). After a single seizure, the resulting metabolic acidosis usually corrects itself within 60 minutes and is not associated with hyperkalemia.[18] Paralysis and bicarbonate administration help to prevent these changes in experimental animals,[6,8] but even in ventilated and paralyzed animals, CNS damage can occur when electrical status lasts more than 60 minutes.[8] The use of bicarbonate in status in humans has been recommended by some authors,[19] but there is little support for rapid correction, and rebound alkalosis can occur.[15]

The marked hyperactivity of the autonomic nervous system associated with convulsive status produces hyperpyrexia, increased pulmonary secretions, excessive sweating, dehydration, and tachycardia, and may predispose to cardiac dysrhythmia.[6,15] Neurogenic pulmonary edema may occur,[15] and can further compromise respiratory function. Hyperpyrexia and the duration of status were the main predictors of CNS damage in an experimental model of status.[7] About one third of the patients have a temperature above 100°F (38°C), more than half have a peripheral leukocytosis, and 18% have a CSF pleocytosis.[11] Dehydration from hyperpyrexia and sweating, coupled with any rhabdomyolysis that might occur, can lead to renal failure.

In summation, convulsive status produces a number of physiologic consequences. Status lasting more than 60 minutes may lead to irreversible CNS damage and can occur even when experimental animals are paralyzed and artificially ventilated. The morbidity and mortality associated with status increase with its duration. The acidosis, hypoxia, and autonomic hyperactivity can produce fatal cardiac arrhythmia. Prolonged status may also be associated with cardiovascular collapse.[5,6] For these reasons, it is essential to treat convulsive status as soon as possible. General anesthesia must be used to terminate status that persists beyond 60 minutes.

INITIAL THERAPY AND MANAGEMENT ■

The first step in management is to determine whether the patient is in status epilepticus. Convulsive status can be defined as successive generalized tonic–clonic seizures without an intervening return to normal consciousness. If a patient presents with a single convulsion, it is not considered status unless he or she has a second convulsion before regaining consciousness. Most patients with generalized convulsive status do not have continuous generalized seizures but have four or five generalized tonic–clonic seizures per hour.[1] Between seizures, the patient is comatose or markedly obtunded. In rare cases, a comatose patient may have minimal motor activity associated with an EEG that demonstrates generalized electric seizure activity, a condition termed subtle generalized status epilepticus (see Special Cases).[3,4] A continuous seizure that lasts more than 30 minutes is also considered to be status epilepticus; however, a tonic–clonic seizure that lasts more than 10 minutes requires pharmacologic therapy.[3]

The initial therapy for a patient who has a history of a recent seizure and has not regained consciousness consists of maintaining adequate ventilation and circulation. An airway should be inserted and oxygen given by mask. If the patient is having a tonic–clonic seizure, no attempt should be made to open the mouth with a tongue depressor or other device; doing so might damage the gums or tongue or could dislodge teeth that the patient might then aspirate. Instead, oxygen should be administered, and the patient's head should be turned to one side to prevent aspiration. The seizure usually terminates within a few minutes, and an airway can then be inserted. Airways aid in suctioning secretions that accompany tonic–clonic seizures. The tonic component of generalized seizures is associated with cyanosis and hypoxia; however, intubation is usually not necessary unless there is evidence of respiratory depression following the seizure. If neuromuscular blockade is required for intubation, a short-acting agent should be used unless EEG monitoring is available.

An intravenous catheter should be inserted, and at least 50 mL of blood should be obtained for laboratory studies. Studies should include determinations of serum electrolytes, blood urea nitrogen (BUN), liver function, calcium, magnesium, glucose, anticonvulsant drug levels, a complete blood count, alcohol level, and toxicology screen. Arterial blood gas and pulse oximetry determinations may be useful but must be interpreted in light of the consequences of a generalized convulsion (see earlier). After the blood is drawn, an infusion of normal saline should be started. If hypoglycemia is confirmed or results cannot be obtained immediately, then 50 mL of 50% glucose is given. Because a carbohydrate load in a patient deficient in thiamine may precipitate Wernicke's encephalopathy, 100 mg of thiamine should also be administered. Normal saline should be used because phenytoin precipitates in glucose-containing solutions.[20]

During this initial period, the physician should observe and be able to describe the patient's seizure activity. A brief physical examination is done for signs of systemic disease, trauma, and any focal neurologic signs. If the patient presents without a history, look for an identification tag stating that he or she has epilepsy or for medications he or she may be carrying. If the patient is already hospitalized, the diagnosis and the medications that the patient is receiving should be reviewed. The next step in treatment depends on whether the patient is in convulsive status epilepticus or

is merely in a postictal state. If the patient has a second generalized seizure before regaining consciousness, appropriate pharmacologic therapy should be instituted, as outlined later. Intravenous diazepam or derivatives should not be given to a patient who has had a single seizure and is postictal. This initial pharmacologic therapy should be given only when the patient is in convulsive status (i.e., successive generalized tonic–clonic seizures without an intervening return to full consciousness or a continuous seizure lasting more than 10 minutes).

PHARMACOLOGIC THERAPY   ■

Patients in convulsive status epilepticus should be treated with parenteral anticonvulsants so that the actual dose given is known. This avoids variables associated with intramuscular, nasogastric, and rectal administration that are dependent on the patient's vascular perfusion, which may be compromised by status. I also favor direct administration of medications into the intravenous line so that the actual dose given is known. Administration from a reservoir may lead to precipitation or to binding of drugs to plastic; thus, the actual dose received may not be the dose administered. When status is treated with intravenous medication, it is necessary to monitor the ECG and to make frequent blood pressure determinations to assess whether the therapy is causing cardiac arrhythmia or hypotension. After a loading dose of a drug is given, the serum level should be determined to confirm a therapeutic level. Ideally, the EEG should also be monitored to determine whether the desired effect of therapy on the electrical seizure is being achieved.

The drugs of choice for initially stopping convulsions are diazepam or lorazepam, a diazepam derivative.[3,21,22] Both drugs can produce respiratory depression when given in dosages required to stop seizures.[22] An airway should be in place, and the physician must be prepared to intubate patients when these drugs are used. I am most comfortable with giving 0.1 mg/kg lorazepam intravenously (IV) at a rate of 1 to 2 mg/minute. Alternatively diazepam 0.2 mg/kg IV at rate of 5 mg given over 1 to 2 minutes may be used. If the seizure persists following the initial dose of diazepam, the treatment may be repeated after 5 minutes. Diazepam stops the seizures in 33% of patients within 3 minutes and in 80% within 5 minutes.[10] Although diazepam is used to stop seizures, it is not an effective medication for preventing seizure recurrence because of its short effective anticonvulsant half-life (due to tissue redistribution).[21] Because effective anticonvulsant doses are associated with some sedation, in cases in which the level of consciousness must be monitored (as in acute head trauma), diazepam or lorazepam should be avoided and phenytoin used instead.

Recent studies have supported the use of lorazepam rather than diazepam in the initial management of convulsive status.[21,22] Lorazepam is less lipid soluble than diazepam and has a longer effective anticonvulsant half-life.[21] In a double-blind study, lorazepam was effective in stopping status in

89% of patients, compared with 76% of those given diazepam.[22] With both drugs, respiratory depression, hypotension, or excessive sedation occurred in 12% to 13% of the patients. Because of its longer effective half-life, lorazepam alone may successfully stop status epilepticus alone, whereas diazepam must be accompanied by another treatment to ensure effective antiepileptic coverage for the next 8 to 12 hours.

As already mentioned, diazepam is effective in stopping most generalized tonic–clonic seizures; to prevent the recurrence of convulsive seizures, phenytoin is the drug of choice.[9,10] Phenytoin is available for parenteral administration; however, the pH of this preparation is about 12, and propylene glycol is used as a solvent.[20] For this reason, phenytoin may crystallize if given intramuscularly, and it precipitates in glucose-containing solutions.[9,20] Phenytoin should be administered as a slow IV push or diluted in normal saline (10 to 20 mg/mL)[20] and infused at rates of 50 mg/minute or less. Intravenous administration can cause a chemical phlebitis, and IV patency should be confirmed after every 50 to 100 mg if being given by slow IV push. Care must also be taken to prevent extravasation from an intravenous site, because tissue necrosis may occur. In the near future, a new phenytoin preparation, fosphenytoin, that is more water-soluble should make parenteral administration easier.

The main side effects of intravenous phenytoin are hypotension and cardiac arrhythmia; these effects may be related to the propylene glycol used as a solvent.[9] These side effects are usually seen in older patients or patients with underlying cardiac disease or sepsis. The ECG and blood pressure should be monitored when phenytoin is given intravenously. If hypotension or cardiac arrhythmia develop, the infusion should be stopped and then resumed at a slower rate when the blood pressure returns to normal or the arrhythmia ceases.

A total dose of 18 mg/kg should be given. At this dose, a therapeutic level is obtained within 10 to 20 minutes after the onset of infusion and, in most patients, is sustained for 24 hours.[9] An extra 5 to 10 mg/kg of phenytoin may be given after the initial loading dose if seizures persist.[3] Diazepam and phenytoin therapy is effective in 80% to 90% of patients who do not have an acute metabolic or anoxic encephalopathy.[9,10]

If the patient continues to have seizures 10 to 20 minutes after a loading dose of phenytoin, intravenous phenobarbital should be used. If phenobarbital is used, I usually intubate the patient at this stage because phenobarbital given after diazepam or lorazepam is likely to depress respiration. Phenobarbital can be given intravenously at a rate of 50 to 100 mg/minute. I administer 250 to 500 mg intravenously and repeat this dose if the seizures continue, up to a total dose of 20 mg/kg.[3,23] The main side effects are respiratory depression or arrest and circulatory collapse. The latter occurs in less than 1% of patients.[23]

By this stage in the treatment process, laboratory results should be available, and any metabolic cause for the status should be corrected. If the seizures continue despite the therapy described above, anesthesia should be used to stop them. Antiepileptic drug levels should be checked and addi-

tional medication should be given to achieve a phenytoin level of 20 to 30 μg/mL and phenobarbital of >40 μg/mL.

Paraldehyde, valproate, and lidocaine have been used to control status.[3,24] Paraldehyde is no longer available for intravenous administration. Paraldehyde and valproate can be given rectally but the absorption is slow compared with that in intravenous administration. The doses of lidocaine used for status (1.5 to 2.0 mg/kg loading dose followed by an infusion of 2 to 4 mg/kg/hour) can produce seizures.[3,24]

If the patient continues to have seizures, anesthesia with neuromuscular blockade must be used. The patient must have EEG monitoring during these procedures to determine whether the seizure activity is controlled. Continued electrical status epilepticus results in CNS damage.[8] Three basic types of anesthetics can be used: barbiturate, inhalation, or benzodiazepines.

Pentobarbital can be used, with an initial intravenous dose of 5 to 15 mg/kg. Anesthesia is then maintained with an infusion of 0.5 to 5.0 mg/kg/hour to obtain a suppression-burst EEG pattern.[25] Barbiturate administration is stopped every 8 to 12 hours to assess whether the electrical seizure activity is still present. Because barbiturates may protect the brain from ischemic and other types of injury as well as decrease intracranial pressure (ICP), their use is favored by some. Others believe that the withdrawal of barbiturate therapy may produce rebound or withdrawal seizures and argue that barbiturates may lead to circulatory collapse.[26] If barbiturates are used, hemodynamic monitoring is necessary so that fluid replacement and the use of inotropic agents can be appropriately managed. Fifty percent of the patients receiving barbiturate anesthesia require dopamine for blood pressure maintenance.[25] An alternative is inhalation anesthesia and neuromuscular blockade. Either halothane or isoflurane may be used. Halothane may increase ICP and may have more detrimental hemodynamic effects than isoflurane;[26] thus, isoflurane may be the better choice.

Pentobarbital has adverse cardiovascular effects that complicate its use, and isoflurane has technical limitations regarding its administration. Newer agents are being considered for refractory status epilepticus. Bleck advocates the use of midazolam after lorazepam and phenytoin failure.[27] A 0.15 to 2.0 mg/kg loading dose of midazolam is given and followed by a 0.06 to 1.1 mg/kg/hour infusion titrated to seizure suppression defined by EEG monitoring. The midazolam dosage can be decreased and tapered when the serum phenytoin level is 20 to 30 μg/mL and phenobarbital level is greater than 40 μg/mL. If midazolam does not stop seizure activity within an hour, then pentobarbital should be used.[27] Recent reports have also documented successful treatment of refractory status epilepticus using high-dose IV lorazepam (1 to 9 mg/hour)[28] or the IV anesthetic propofol (1 to 3 mg/kg loading dose followed by 5 to 10 mg/kg/hour).[29]

The most common reasons for treatment failure are inadequate dosages, failure to maintain respiratory function, incorrect route of medication administration, failure to continue therapy, and misdiagnosis. Some patients with nonepileptic or pseudoseizures may appear to be in status epilepticus and may not respond to initial drug therapies. Most patients who are refractory to nonanesthetic therapy have either metabolic abnormalities or major structural lesions that are inherently associated with high morbidity and mortality. When convulsive status lasts longer than 60 minutes, the systemic consequences must be prevented or treated effectively. This may require correction of acidosis and insertion of a pulmonary artery catheter to ensure proper volume correction. The patient's temperature should also be kept near normal to help prevent irreversible CNS damage.

LABORATORY EVALUATION ▪

Laboratory data obtained during the initial management of a patient in status epilepticus often reveal the etiology. Further evaluation depends on the clinical setting and whether the patient has been diagnosed previously as having epilepsy. An EEG is helpful in determining whether the patient has a generalized epileptiform abnormality, a focal epileptiform abnormality, or an underlying metabolic abnormality. If a patient presents with convulsive status as a first seizure and without an obvious metabolic etiology, a complete evaluation should be performed to determine whether there is an underlying lesion. Unenhanced computed tomography (CT) of the brain should be performed to detect the presence of acute hemorrhage, and an enhanced CT should be done to detect neoplasms, abscesses, or vascular malformations. Magnetic resonance imaging (MRI) may detect lesions (especially low-grade neoplasms) not seen with CT scan and is an appropriate alternative in some cases.

Lumbar puncture is indicated whenever an infectious etiology or a subarachnoid hemorrhage not seen on CT scan is suspected. When focal features or papilledema are detected on examination or there is a clinical picture of transtentorial herniation, a CT or MRI scan should be performed before the lumbar puncture. Antibiotic treatment should not be delayed by waiting for a scan and lumbar puncture. Patients with convulsive status epilepticus may have elevated temperatures and increased white blood cell (WBC) counts that are not accompanied by underlying infection. Nonetheless, these findings require that a CNS infection be ruled out by lumbar puncture. As many as 18% of patients with recent convulsive status may have a pleocytosis without CNS infection.[11] Usually, the total WBC count is below 100 and may consist of either polymorphonuclear or mononuclear cells. The protein is often elevated, but the glucose is usually normal or higher than normal. These abnormalities are believed to be a consequence of a blood–brain barrier breakdown during status. Patients with pleocytosis and fever should be treated as if they had meningitis until cultures are negative.

PROGNOSIS ▪

The prognosis for patients with convulsive status epilepticus depends on the duration of the status and on the underlying etiology. Mortality has decreased recently but is still approximately 10%.[2–4] In most cases, death results from the underlying pathology responsible for the patient's seizures.[2,3] In adults, the neurologic sequelae of status have not been well studied. Intellectual impairment may occur as a consequence of the patient's status rather than the underlying pathology. The morbidity of status epilepticus is higher in children than in adults. Most studies have found that the longer that convulsive status remains uncontrolled, the greater the associated morbidity and mortality.[2–4,11]

SPECIAL CASES ▪

SUBTLE CONVULSIVE STATUS EPILEPTICUS

There are some patients who have EEG features consistent with generalized tonic–clonic status but are comatose and display only subtle movements.[4,30] These patients cannot be diagnosed without an accompanying EEG and may represent the end stage of prolonged status[4] or the sequelae of metabolic derangements, infection, or cardiac arrest.[30] The mortality associated with this condition is high (>50%); however, treatment should be undertaken to suppress well-defined EEG seizure activity.

CONVULSIVE STATUS EPILEPTICUS OTHER THAN GENERALIZED TONIC–CLONIC

Tonic, clonic, and myoclonic seizures may occur with sufficient frequency to be termed status epilepticus. Tonic seizures are brief episodes of generalized muscle stiffening, often accompanied by opisthotonos. They are most often seen in children with mental retardation, as slow spike-and-wave abnormalities in the EEG, and a variety of seizure manifestations (Lennox-Gastaut syndrome).[1] In these patients, intravenous diazepam may actually precipitate tonic seizures. Tonic status may be difficult to treat and may last several days. The consequences of tonic status are not as severe as those of generalized tonic–clonic status; hence, general anesthesia is not used, and the side effects of therapy must be weighed against the effects of the seizures. There have been reports of adult patients with an anoxic or hypoxic encephalopathy who have developed tonic status.[11] These patients are refractory to most forms of therapy, and the "seizures" may be a consequence of a brain stem release phenomenon.

Clonic status is usually seen only in infants or very young children, and the reader is referred to other sources for reviews of this topic.[1] Myoclonic status occurs mainly in children epilepticus.[1] Children and adolescents with myoclonic epilepsy may have continuous myoclonus with relatively preserved consciousness. These patients with relatively benign forms of primary generalized epilepsy respond well to lorazepam and divalproex sodium therapy.

Adult patients may develop myoclonic status. Recurrent abrupt, brief, uncontrollable, jerklike contractions of one or more muscles may be associated with EEG discharges and represent myoclonic status epilepticus.[31,32] These patients usually have an acute metabolic encephalopathy (especially postanoxic encephalopathy, but also hepatic encephalopathy or renal failure) or end-stage degenerative neurologic disease (neurolipidosis, Jakob-Creutzfeldt disease, or other rare disorders). Myoclonic status in patients with anoxic encephalopathy, metabolic abnormalities, or degenerative neurologic disease is associated with a 90% mortality.[31] The treatment depends on the etiology and consequences of the myoclonus. When myoclonus is a sign of irreversible anoxic encephalopathy, treatment may include neuromuscular paralysis.[32]

NONCONVULSIVE STATUS EPILEPTICUS

There are basically two types of nonconvulsive status epilepticus: *absence* (petit mal) and *complex partial.* In both situations, the patient has impaired consciousness, ranging from inattention to a fuguelike state, and may display a variety of automatisms and semipurposeful motor behaviors. It is often difficult to distinguish between absence and complex partial status on clinical grounds alone, and past history can be extremely helpful. The EEG can distinguish between absence and complex partial seizures and should be used to confirm the diagnosis and to evaluate therapy.[33,34]

Absence status epilepticus is associated with lethargy, slowness, and decreased higher cortical function.[1,33] Although eye blinking, brief myoclonic jerks, and automatisms may occur, frank tonic–clonic or unilateral clonic activity is not present. The EEG demonstrates almost continuous generalized spike-and-slow-wave or polyspike-and-slow-wave activity.[1,33] Absence status epilepticus is most often a manifestation of primary generalized epilepsy. It may occur at any age over 3 years and may be the presenting sign of epilepsy.[33] Intravenous diazepam given at dosages used for convulsive status usually terminates the attack, and patients may return to normal almost instantly; this is in contrast to complex partial status, which is followed by postictal confusion. Ethosuximide (15 to 20 mg/kg/day in divided doses) is the drug of choice for maintenance therapy of absence seizures.[33] If ethosuximide is ineffective or if the patient also has generalized tonic–clonic seizures, valproic acid or divalproex sodium (15 to 60 mg/kg/day) should be used.

Complex partial status epilepticus is manifested by repeated complex partial seizures without an intervening return to normal consciousness. Prolonged complex partial status may be associated with persistent impairment of memory and should be treated aggressively when recognized.[34] Patients with complex partial status appear to be in a twilight state, and there are fluctuations in their responsiveness. EEG monitoring is usually necessary to confirm the diagnosis and is helpful in assessing therapy.[34] Once the diagnosis is made, therapy consists of intravenous diazepam or lorazepam and maintenance with either phenytoin or carbamazepine.

SIMPLE PARTIAL STATUS EPILEPTICUS

The most common form of simple partial status epilepticus consists of continuous small jerks or twitches of a group of muscles confined to one side of the body (often involving just one limb or the face); they do not spread or develop into a secondarily generalized tonic–clonic seizure. Consciousness is not impaired, but there may be weakness of the involved side. This form of simple partial status has been termed *epilepsia partialis continua* (EPC). The EEG

sometimes shows focal spikes or sharp waves that may be continuous or periodic; however, it may not demonstrate well-delineated epileptiform activity.[35] The most common causes of EPC are cerebral infarction, hemorrhage, neoplasm, encephalitis, and metabolic abnormality.[35] Nonketotic hyperglycemia is the most common metabolic abnormality associated with this disorder, and often an underlying structural lesion is also present.[36]

Phenytoin, phenobarbital, and carbamazepine can all be effective therapies, either alone or in combination. Intravenously administered diazepam is usually effective in suppressing the seizures; however, because of the potential hazards of intravenous diazepam, EPC rarely justifies its repeated use. Despite appropriate pharmacologic therapy, EPC may last for years.[35] Appropriate therapy depends on the cause, the severity of the movement, and the side effects of the serum levels of anticonvulsants needed to stop the movements.

ACKNOWLEDGEMENTS ■

The author thanks Michael Collins, John C. Jones, Nancy Spencer, and Thomas Sutula for helpful comments.

REFERENCES ■

1. Gastaut H: Classification of status epilepticus. In: Delgado-Escueta AV, Wasterlain CG, Treiman DM, Porter RJ (eds): *Advances in Neurology, vol 34. Status Epilepticus.* New York, Raven Press, 1983:15
2. Hauser WA: Status epilepticus: Epidemiologic considerations, sequelae. *Neurology* 1990;40(Suppl 2):9
3. Epilepsy Foundation of America: Treatment of convulsive status epilepticus: Recommendations of the Epilepsy Foundation of America's Working Group on Status Epilepticus. *JAMA* 1993;270:854
4. Treiman DM: Generalized convulsive status epilepticus in the adult. *Epilepsia* 1993;34(Suppl 1):S2
5. Meldrum BS, Horton RW: Physiology of status epilepticus in primates. *Arch Neurol* 1973;28:1
6. Wasterlain CG: Mortality and morbidity from serial seizures: an experimental study. *Epilepsia* 1974;15:155
7. Meldrum BS, Brierley JB: Prolonged epileptic seizures in primates: ischaemic cell change and its relationship to ictal physiological events. *Arch Neurol* 1973;28:10
8. Meldrum BS, Vigouroux RA, Brierley JB: Systemic factors and epileptic brain damage. Prolonged seizures in paralyzed, artificially ventilated baboons. *Arch Neurol* 1973;29:82
9. Cranford RE, Leppik IE, Patrick B, et al: Intravenous phenytoin: clinical and pharmacokinetic aspects. *Neurology* 1978;28:874
10. Delgado-Escueta AV, Enrile-Bacsal F: Combination therapy for status epilepticus: Intravenous diazepam and phenytoin. In: Delgado-Escueta AV, Wasterlain CG, Treiman DM, et al (eds). *Advances in Neurology, vol 34. Status Epilepticus.* New York, Raven Press, 1983;477
11. Aminoff MJ, Simon RP: Status epilepticus: causes, clinical features and consequences in 98 patients. *Am J Med* 1980;69:657
12. Lowenstein DH, Alldredge BK: Status epilepticus at an urban public hospital in the 1980s. *Neurology* 1993;43:483

13. Janz D: Etiology of convulsive status epilepticus. In: Delgado-Escueta AV, Wasterlain CG, Treiman DM, et al (eds). *Advances in Neurology, vol 34. Status Epilepticus.* New York, Raven Press, 1983:47

14. Kuniask TA, Augenstein WL: Drug- and toxin-induced seizures. *Emerg Med Clin North Am* 1994;12:1027

15. Simon RP: Physiologic consequences of status epilepticus. *Epilepsia* 1985;26:S58

16. Kreisman NR, Rosenthal M, LaManna JC, et al: Cerebral oxygenation during recurrent seizures. In: Delgado-Escueta AV, Wasterlain CG, Treiman DM, et al (eds). *Advances in Neurology, vol 34. Status Epilepticus.* New York, Raven Press, 1983:231

17. Rothman SM, Olney JW: Glutamate and the pathophysiology of hypoxic-ischemic brain damage. *Ann Neurol* 1986;19:105

18. Orringer CE, Eustace JC, Wunsch CD, et al: Natural history of lactic acidosis after grand-mal seizures: a model for the study of an anion-gap acidosis not associated with hyperkalemia. *N Engl J Med* 1977;297:696

19. Treiman DM: General principles of treatment: responsive and intractable status epilepticus in adults. In: Delgado-Escueta AV, Wasterlain CG, Treiman DM, et al (eds). *Advances in Neurology, vol 34. Status Epilepticus.* New York, Raven Press, 1983:377

20. Cloyd JC, Bosch DE, Sawchuk RJ: Concentration-time profile of phenytoin after admixture with small volumes of intravenous fluids. *Am J Hosp Pharm* 1978;35:45

21. Greenblatt DJ, Divoll M: Diazepam versus lorazepam: relationship of drug distribution to duration of clinical action. In: Delgado-Escueta AV, Wasterlain CG, Treiman DM, et al (eds). *Advances in Neurology, vol 34. Status Epilepticus.* New York, Raven Press, 1983:487

22. Leppik IE, Derivan AT, Homan RW, et al: Double-blind study of lorazepam and diazepam in status epilepticus. *JAMA* 1983;249:1452

23. Goldberg MA, McIntyre HB: Barbiturates in the treatment of status epilepticus. In: Delgado-Escueta AV, Wasterlain CG, Treiman DM, et al (eds). *Advances in Neurology, vol 34. Status Epilepticus.* New York, Raven Press, 1983:499

24. Browne TR: Paraldehyde, chlormethiazole, and lidocaine for treatment of status epilepticus. In: Delgado-Escueta AV, Wasterlain CG, Treiman DM, et al (eds). *Advances in Neurology, vol 34. Status Epilepticus.* New York, Raven Press, 1983;509

25. Lowenstein DH, Aminoff MJ, Simon RP: Barbiturate anesthesia in the treatment of status epilepticus: clinical experience with 14 patients. *Neurology* 1988;38:395

26. Kofke WA, Snider MT, Young RSK, et al: Prolonged low flow isoflurane anesthesia for status epilepticus. *Anesthesiology* 1985;62:653

27. Bleck TP: Advances in the management of refractory status epilepticus. *Crit Care Med* 1993;21:955

28. Labar DR, Auslim A, Root J: High-dose intravenous lorazepam for the treatment of refractory status epilepticus. *Neurology* 1994;44:1400

29. Borgeat A, Wilder-Smith OHG, Jallon P, et al: Propofol in the management of refractory status epilepticus. *Intensive Care Med* 1994;20:148

30. Lowenstein DH, Aminoff MJ: Clinical and EEG features of status epilepticus in comatose patients. *Neurology* 1992;42:100

31. Jumao-as A, Brenner RP: Myoclonic status epilepticus: a clinical and electroencephalographic study. *Neurology* 1990;40:1199

32. Wijdicks EFM, Parisi JE, Sharbrough FM: Prognostic value of myoclonus status in comatose surviors of cardiac arrest. *Ann Neurol* 1994;35:239

33. Porter RJ, Penry JK: Petit mal status. In: Delgado-Escueta AV, Wasterlain CG, Treiman DM, et al (eds). *Advances in Neurology, vol 34. Status Epilepticus.* New York, Raven Press, 1983:61

34. Treiman DM, Delgado-Escueta AV: Complex partial status epilepticus. In: Delgado-Escueta AV, Wasterlain CG, Treiman DM, et al (eds). *Advances in Neurology, vol 34. Status Epilepticus.* New York, Raven Press, 1983:69

35. Thomas JE, Reagan TJ, Klass DW: Epilepsia partialis continua: a review of 32 cases. *Arch Neurol* 1977;34:266

36. Singh BM, Stobos RJ: Epilepsia partialis continua associated with nonketotic hyperglycemia: clinical and biochemical profile of 21 patients. *Ann Neurol* 1980;8:155

Critical Care, Third Edition, edited by Joseph M. Civetta,
Robert W. Taylor, and Robert R. Kirby.
Lippincott-Raven Publishers, Philadelphia, PA © 1997.

CHAPTER 135

∎

Cerebrovascular Disease

Ken P. Madden
Loren A. Rolak ·

IMMEDIATE CONCERNS ∎

MAJOR PROBLEMS

The first concern is to verify that the diagnosis of stroke
is correct.

STRESS POINTS

1. Abrupt neurologic deficit is the hallmark of stroke,
   with symptoms of unilateral weakness or sensory loss,
   visual disturbance, speech–language disorder, or impaired coordination.
2. Nonfocal symptoms, such as confusion or lethargy,
   appear much less frequently and a diagnosis of stroke
   should be made with caution in patients who have a
   significantly altered mental status.
3. Strokes may be thrombotic (from atherosclerotic stenosis or occlusion of a large vessel), embolic (especially
   from cardiac or carotid sources), lacunar (from deep
   intraparenchymal small vessel disease), or hemorrhagic (from the rupture of a conducting artery or an
   intraparenchymal arteriole).
4. Besides determining the etiology, the other major goal
   of stroke assessment is localizing its anatomy to either
   the anterior circulation (carotid artery and its
   branches) or the posterior circulation (vertebral basilar
   system and its branches). Although the immediate
   management of the stroke may be similar in these
   two different distributions, definitive therapy (such as
   carotid endarterectomy, anticoagulation, etc.) often
   varies depending on the anatomic pathology.

ESSENTIAL DIAGNOSTIC TESTS
AND PROCEDURES

1. A computed tomography (CT) scan of the brain is
   almost always indicated to guide the initial evaluation
   and critical care management of the stroke patient.
2. Magnetic resonance imaging (MRI) is more sensitive
   than CT but it is usually less available urgently and
   patients must remain still and calm for a much longer
   period of time.
3. Carotid duplex Doppler testing, sometimes coupled
   to transcranial Doppler, allows rapid bedside assessment of abnormal flow within the major intracranial
   and extracranial arteries, and can provide valuable immediate information about the vascular physiology to
   supplement the anatomic information provided by the
   CT scan.
4. An echocardiogram, transthoracic or transesophageal,
   may identify potential sources of cerebral emboli.
5. An electrocardiogram (ECG) and routine laboratory
   studies, with attention paid to coagulation parameters,
   generally completes the initial evaluation.
6. Lumbar puncture may be necessary for diagnosis in
   patients with subarachnoid hemorrhage.

INITIAL THERAPY

1. The care of the ischemic stroke patient is largely supportive, with special attention paid to aspiration pneumonia, pulmonary emboli, and cardiac disease. Patients should be monitored, by telemetry if necessary,
   in the acute period after a stroke.
2. A common practice in the acute setting of thrombotic
   stroke is to begin heparin, without an initial loading

bolus, to maintain the partial thromboplastin time (PTT) at 1.5 times normal. Patients may then be maintained on more chronic therapy if their subsequent evaluation indicates this would be beneficial, as in the setting of a cardiac source of embolus.

3. An intracerebral hemorrhage causes abrupt focal neurologic deficits resembling those of an ischemic stroke, but the mass of blood usually also produces an altered mental status and decreased level of consciousness. A CT scan is extremely sensitive for detecting such intraparenchymal hemorrhages. Therapy focuses on reducing the increased intracranial pressure, especially by lowering the systemic blood pressure, and maintaining supportive measures similar to those previously mentioned for patients with ischemic stroke.

4. Subarachnoid hemorrhages differ from other types of cerebrovascular disease in that they only rarely cause focal findings, and instead usually present as a sudden severe headache accompanying a collapse and decreased or lost consciousness. Although a CT scan is sensitive for showing the blood around the brain, lumbar puncture may be necessary to confirm the diagnosis. Most spontaneous subarachnoid hemorrhages arise from ruptured berry aneurysms, and cerebral angiography is often performed acutely to identify the site of the bleeding. In patients with a relatively preserved mental status and only mild neurologic deficit, urgent surgery to clip the aneurysm is the preferred treatment. For patients who are stuporous or suffer severe neurologic deficits, the complication rate of acute surgery is unacceptably high, and medical management must support the patient for 2 or 3 weeks, until surgery can be safely performed. In all patients with subarachnoid hemorrhage, key management issues include careful attention to electrolytes, maintenance of normovolemia, and treatment with calcium channel blockers to prevent vasospasm. After surgical clipping of the aneurysm, aggressive measures to prevent vasospasm can include hypertensive–hypervolemic treatment.

STROKE

DIFFERENTIAL DIAGNOSIS

Most patients who suddenly develop a localized neurologic problem have, in fact, had a stroke. It is by far the most common acute, focal, nontraumatic brain disease. The differential diagnosis of stroke thus is not extensive, but there is nevertheless an unfortunate tendency to assume that any neurologic symptom that appears abruptly must be due to vascular disease.

As shown in Table 135-1, there are a number of stroke symptoms that may occur alone, unaccompanied by other evidence of neurologic damage, that are not an expression of vascular disease. Thus, an elderly patient with a sudden attack of isolated vertigo is unlikely to be experiencing a stroke, and is more likely to have labyrinthitis or benign

TABLE 135-1. Symptoms Seldom Resulting From Cerebrovascular Disease

Vertigo alone	Confusion
Dysarthria alone	Memory loss
Dysphagia alone	Delirium
Diplopia alone	Coma
Headache	Syncope
Tremor	Incontinence
Tonic–clonic motor activity	Tinnitus

positional vertigo. Similarly, dysarthria, headache, and double vision have multiple etiologies, in which vascular disease appears far down the list. It is particularly important that changes in mental status not be attributed to cerebrovascular disease until other, more likely, metabolic, toxic, and infectious etiologies have been excluded. Confusion, delirium, memory loss, and coma are rarely caused by stroke. Most of the errors in the diagnosis of stroke occur in patients with altered mental status. Beware of attributing such nonfocal symptoms to strokes. Stroke causes focal deficits, either of strength, sensation, vision, speech–language, or coordination. Hemiparesis, ranging from mild weakness to complete paralysis of the limbs on one side of the body and involving the face, arm, or leg in any combination, is the hallmark of stroke. There is often some degree of numbness or sensory loss in a distribution similar to the weakness. Most patients with this deficit have had a stroke.

Table 135-2 lists the diseases most commonly mistaken for stroke. Epilepsy mimics stroke more often than any other condition. In one study of 821 consecutive patients admitted to a stroke unit, only 13% had a disease other than stroke, but almost 40% of these misdiagnosed patients had seizures.[1] The next largest group of mistaken diagnoses occur in patients suffering confusion and neurologic deficits from drug intoxication, alcohol, or metabolic abnormalities. Focal mass lesions such as cerebral tumors, abscesses, and subdural hematomas may present suddenly, simulating a stroke. In young patients, multiple sclerosis and migraine are common causes of rapidly developing focal neurologic deficits. Occasionally, labyrinthitis, encephalitis, hypoglycemia, and hysterical or psychogenic symptoms can also be confused with stroke. Establishing a correct diagnosis of these conditions usually depends heavily on the patient's history, and the physician must specifically probe for these diseases in every patient presenting with the clinical picture of a stroke. A

TABLE 135-2. Conditions Most Frequently Mistaken for Stroke

Seizures	Peripheral neuropathy and
Metabolic encephalopathy	Bell's palsy
Cerebral tumor	Multiple sclerosis
Subdural hematoma	Hypoglycemia
Cerebral abscess	Encephalitis
Vertigo, Ménière's disease	Migraine
	Psychogenic illness

thorough history and physical examination, combined with appropriate laboratory testing and brain imaging such as MRI or CT scan, can usually exclude conditions that mimic a stroke.

ANATOMY

Crucial to evaluating a patient with cerebrovascular disease is determining whether the symptoms arise from the anterior circulation (carotid artery and its main branches, the anterior and middle cerebral arteries) or the posterior circulation (vertebral, basilar, and posterior cerebral arteries). The pathogenesis, diagnostic evaluation, therapy, and prognosis of stroke in these two vascular regions are usually different.

The two symptoms that most accurately reflect carotid circulation disease are aphasia and monocular blindness (Table 135-3). The capacity for language resides in the dominant (usually left) hemispheric cortex, within the territory of the carotid artery. A stroke causing aphasia must therefore involve the carotid distribution. Similarly, the blood supply of the eye arises largely from the ophthalmic artery, a direct branch from the carotid artery, and monocular ischemia therefore implicates the carotid circulation.

Because the brain stem, with its numerous neurologic structures, is a more tightly compacted region than the cerebral hemispheres, clinical syndromes in the posterior circulation are usually more complex than those in the cerebral hemispheres. In brain stem stroke, bilateral neurologic signs are frequently present and cranial nerve and cerebellar abnormalities are usually prominent (Table 135-4). Cranial nerve dysfunction (dysarthria, dysphagia, diplopia, dizziness), when seen in conjunction with hemiparesis or hemisensory loss—especially in a bilateral or crossed fashion—is the most reliable indication of brain stem disease.

Although only a few clues absolutely differentiate carotid from vertebro basilar ischemia, doubt is usually resolved in favor of a carotid localization since vascular pathology in this territory accounts for 80% of all strokes. This anatomic distinction has practical importance because of the difference in the pathogenesis and prognosis of strokes in these different vascular beds. The internal carotid and middle cerebral arteries are the major points of attack for atherosclerosis in the cerebrovascular system, and most strokes in the

TABLE 135-3. Most Common Symptoms of Carotid Circulation Ischemia

SYMPTOM	INCIDENCE (%)
Hemiparesis	65
Hemisensory loss	60
Monocular blindness	35
Facial numbness	30
Lower facial weakness	25
Aphasia	20
Headache	20
Dysarthria	15
Visual field loss	15

TABLE 135-4. Most Common Symptoms of Vertebrobasilar Circulation Ischemia

SYMPTOM	INCIDENCE (%)
Ataxia	50
Crossed or hemisensory loss	30
Vertigo	30
Crossed or hemiparesis	25
Dysarthria–dysphagia	25
Syncope or lightheadedness	25
Headache	20
Deafness or tinnitus	10
Diplopia	10

carotid distribution are due to atherosclerotic stenosis and thrombosis of these vessels. Most emboli from the carotid artery or the heart travel to the middle cerebral artery. By contrast, atherosclerosis is less prominent in the posterior circulation, and emboli less commonly travel the tortuous route through the vertebral arteries. Brain stem strokes are more often due to occlusion of small penetrating arterioles emerging directly from the vertebro basilar arteries. Evaluation of a patient with carotid ischemia therefore usually focuses on atherosclerotic disease of the neck, with a view ultimately toward carotid endarterectomy, and on cardiac sources of emboli. Therapeutic options are more limited for disease of the posterior circulation, since surgical repair usually is less feasible. However, the prognosis may well be better for posterior circulation strokes since they are more often due to small vessel disease.

PATHOGENESIS

Vascular disease of the brain takes four major forms: thrombotic, embolic, lacunar, and hemorrhagic.[2] Each has a different etiology, a different emphasis in its diagnostic evaluation, a different therapy, and a different prognosis (Table 135-5).

Thrombotic strokes are the most common, accounting for about 40% of all ischemic cerebrovascular disease. Thrombotic strokes are usually due to atherosclerotic stenosis or occlusion of a large blood vessel, especially the carotid or middle cerebral artery. Because thrombotic occlusion of a vessel commonly occurs as a gradual process, the damage it produces often has a slower onset than the deficits of other kinds of strokes and may present in an evolving fashion (i.e., a stuttering or stepwise progression of symptoms over hours or even days). Very similar symptoms may briefly appear and then disappear as warning signs preceding a stroke, and as many as 50% of all patients with thrombotic strokes report such previous transient ischemic attacks (TIAs). Thrombosis also commonly occurs at night, and the patient who awakens in the morning with a new deficit has probably had a thrombotic stroke. Because atherosclerosis generally involves large vessels, the ischemia produced by thrombotic strokes often leads to severe impairment.

Emboli cause 30% of all strokes, and their relative importance may be increasing as antihypertensive drugs and better

TABLE 135-5. Characteristics of Different Types of Strokes

TYPE OF STROKE	PERCENTAGE OF ALL STROKES	ONSET	PRECEDING TIAs (%)	SEIZURE AT ONSET (%)	COMA (%)	ATRIAL FIBRIL-LATION (%)	KNOWN CORONARY ARTERY DISEASE (%)	MRI OR CT SCAN	OTHER FEATURES
Thrombotic	40	Stuttering, gradual	50	1	5	10	50	Ischemic infarction	Carotid bruit; stroke during sleep
Embolic	30	Sudden	10	10	1	35	35	Superficial (cortical) infarction	Underlying heart disease; peripheral emboli or strokes in different vascular territories
Lacunar	20	Gradual or sudden	30	0	0	5	35	Normal, or small, deep infarction	Pure motor or pure sensory stroke
Hemorrhagic	10	Sudden	5	10	25	5	10	Hyperdense mass	Nausea and vomiting; decreased mental status

control of atherosclerotic risk factors begin to lower the incidence of thrombotic stroke.[3,4] Embolic strokes arise from platelets, cholesterol, fibrin, or other bits of hematogenous material breaking off from an arterial wall or from the heart. Most strokes occurring in the setting of cardiac disease, such as atrial fibrillation or myocardial infarction, are embolic in origin, and the emboli often travel peripherally, causing renal infarcts or splinter hemorrhages in the conjunctiva and fingers. Embolic strokes have a very abrupt onset, as the embolic material travels up the arterial tree to lodge suddenly in a smaller-caliber blood vessel. Because emboli float in the circulation until encountering a vessel with a sufficiently small diameter to stop them, they usually occlude distal small cortical vessels. For this reason, cortical deficits are the hallmark of embolic strokes; these include seizures, aphasia (in the dominant hemisphere), and denial and neglect (in the nondominant hemisphere). Emboli may be showered or sprayed to multiple vessels, but they occasionally cause repeated strokes in the same vascular territory, and are most common in the carotid distribution.

Lacunar strokes represent approximately 20% of all strokes.[5] These are very small infarctions (by most definitions, <1 cm^3) that occur only where small perforating arterioles branch directly off large vessels. This distinctive vascular anatomy occurs in two areas of the brain: in the deep structures of the basal ganglia, thalamus, and internal capsule and in the brain stem. These are the regions in which lacunae develop. Because these very small perforating arterioles are exposed to the same constant high pressures and flows of the large arteries from which they branch, they become damaged over the years, particularly if they are also buffeted by hypertension. The vessels become thickened and hyalinized; they then thrombose, resulting in small infarcts in the

discrete territory supplied by the arteriole. This chronic process may produce symptoms resembling large vessel thrombosis, including a gradual onset and preceding TIAs. Because they occur in the deep subcortical regions of the brain, lacunae do not cause aphasia, neglect, seizures, or other cortical symptoms.

Lacunae are best diagnosed by the discrete and specific clinical deficits they produce, by far the most common being a pure motor stroke, or hemiparesis without any sensory loss. Similarly, a pure sensory stroke, causing numbness but not motor deficits, may also be seen. Although these deficits may be severe, infarctions are small and the prognosis is generally excellent, with about 85% of patients making a very satisfactory recovery.[6]

Intracerebral hemorrhage, which accounts for only 10% of all strokes, is the most rare but most catastrophic type of cerebrovascular accident.[7] The onset is typically very sudden, although continued bleeding may progress over minutes or hours. The clinical key to recognition of hemorrhagic strokes is the presence of increased intracranial pressure (ICP) from the sudden outpouring of blood into the brain, resulting in headaches, nausea, vomiting, and a decreased level of consciousness. The stroke patient who is lethargic or comatose has probably had a bleed. Hemorrhages tend to occur in the same location as lacunae, namely, deep within the brain in the region of the basal ganglia and internal capsule, and in the brain stem. Here, hypertension can rupture the penetrating arterioles, causing hemorrhage. Occasionally, intracerebral hematomas may appear after rupture of a cavernous angioma or arteriovenous malformation, but hypertension is by far the more common cause. In addition to altered mental status, hemiplegia, hemisensory loss, and visual field defects occur frequently. The prognosis for recovery from hemorrhage is very poor, with an initial mortality of 50% to 70%. However, if the patient does recover, the blood may be reabsorbed, leaving only mild deficits and thus a potentially satisfactory outcome.

CLINICAL EVALUATION

The history, focusing on the characteristic features of each type of stroke previously discussed, is the most reliable, reproducible, and cost-effective way of evaluating cerebrovascular disease. The neurologic examination complements the history, but examination of the vascular system itself is usually surprisingly unrewarding. Atherosclerosis may present few outward signs.

Carotid bruits are vexatious physical findings. No characteristic feature, including the volume, pitch, or duration of the bruit, reliably indicates the degree or the nature of constriction of the vascular lumen. Many bruits reflect benign conditions. The clinical significance of carotid bruits is minimized because they are audible in many asymptomatic persons without atherosclerosis who never suffer from cerebrovascular disease, but may be absent in severely diseased vessels. Therefore, even if a carotid bruit is detected, it may be difficult to decide whether it is relevant to the patient's symptoms, and it should not be given undue emphasis in the overall evaluation.[8,9]

Examination of the heart should focus on detecting thrombogenic diseases, including myocardial infarction, arrhythmias, prosthetic valves, and bacterial endocarditis. The presence of heart disease is important because of the high morbidity and mortality from coronary artery disease after stroke and because the determination that a stroke is embolic may rest on finding a cardiac source of embolus. As many as 9% of patients with stroke have had a concomitant myocardial infarction, which is often silent.[10] The history must therefore address chest pain, diaphoresis, nausea, dyspnea, and other symptoms of cardiac ischemia. Palpitations, dizziness, and lightheadedness are clues to dysrhythmias.

The physician should inquire about intravenous drug use and search for needle tracks, especially in younger patients. A fourth heart sound may indicate a recent myocardial infarction, whereas murmurs may reflect underlying valvular heart disease.

LABORATORY INVESTIGATION

A major goal in the care of patients with stroke is determining the underlying etiology of the ischemic event. Both acute management and prophylactic strategies may vary by causative mechanism. Much of the initial evaluation can be done noninvasively, and the cost of such a directed workup is outweighed by its benefits. With invasive procedures such as angiography, the value of knowledge gained should be weighed against the procedural risk. Unfortunately, the relevance of discovered pathology to the ischemic event almost always requires clinical judgment and educated hypotheses. A direct causal link can rarely be proved.

CT scan of the brain is the standard initial evaluation of stroke. CT is very sensitive to the presence of hemorrhage, which is the primary reason for its use in the acute setting.

CT may also be useful for detection of the presence and type of prior infarctions, as well as for exclusion of other pathologies that may mimic ischemia (tumor, abscess, etc.). CT is not sensitive for detection of an acute cerebral infarction (Fig. 135-1), and the lack of abnormality on CT within the first 24 hours should not dissuade physicians from this diagnosis. The timing of CT for suspected infarction is therefore a matter of judgment. As a rule, CT should be obtained urgently for patients presenting with acute focal neurologic signs, and is mandatory if anticoagulation is considered. For the rare patient who presents with mild nonprogressive deficit, with no headache and no disturbance of consciousness, and for whom anticoagulation is not intended, a single delayed (24 to 48 hours) CT may be most appropriate.

MRI is more sensitive for cerebral infarction, particularly the lacunar type (Fig. 135-2), but may still be falsely negative within the first 12 hours. MRI is of special value in brain stem and posterior circulation strokes, since infarcts are so often obscured by bony artifacts with CT scanning (Fig. 135-3). In addition, many imaging units have the capacity to display flow-related enhancement of the vasculature, resulting in a magnetic resonance (MR) "angiogram" displayable in 360-degree projection.[11] Disadvantages of MRI include increased cost and less availability. The patient must also be more cooperative and remain motionless for a longer period than for a CT scan. MRA requires a skilled interpreter and often overestimates the degree of arterial stenoses.

Carotid duplex scanning provides a rapid noninvasive assessment of carotid artery disease, based on abnormalities of either flow (Doppler) or morphology (B-mode). Sensitivity is quite operator dependent, but with experienced technicians and interpreters, duplex provides a reproducible, accurate screening examination for this common underlying etiology of stroke. Disadvantages include poor discrimination of high-grade carotid stenosis (highly treatable) from complete occlusion (untreatable).

Transcranial Doppler (TCD) allows rapid bedside assessment of abnormal flow within the major intracranial arteries.[12] The 2-MHz ultrasonic signal can penetrate various bony "windows" and its gated character allows identification of arteries by "depth" of the reflected signal. In the majority of patients, TCD can examine proximal portions of all arteries of the circle of Willis, but is insensitive for pathology of smaller distal vessels. Newer applications include detection of microemboli and on-line monitoring of arterial flow during invasive or therapeutic procedures (Figure 135-4). Multiple disadvantages include major dependency on operator skill, a high prevalence of acoustically inadequate bony windows, and multiple explanations for recorded abnormalities.

Though relatively insensitive, echocardiography is a useful tool to assess the potential for arterial embolization of cardiac origin. Physicians must be attentive not only to visualized thrombus but also to other pathologic states associated with systemic embolization. These include left ventricular (particularly anterior) wall motion abnormalities, chamber dilatation, valvular disease, and septal defects. Transthoracic echocardiography can be routinely performed and is a superior study for the detection of ventricular apex pathology,

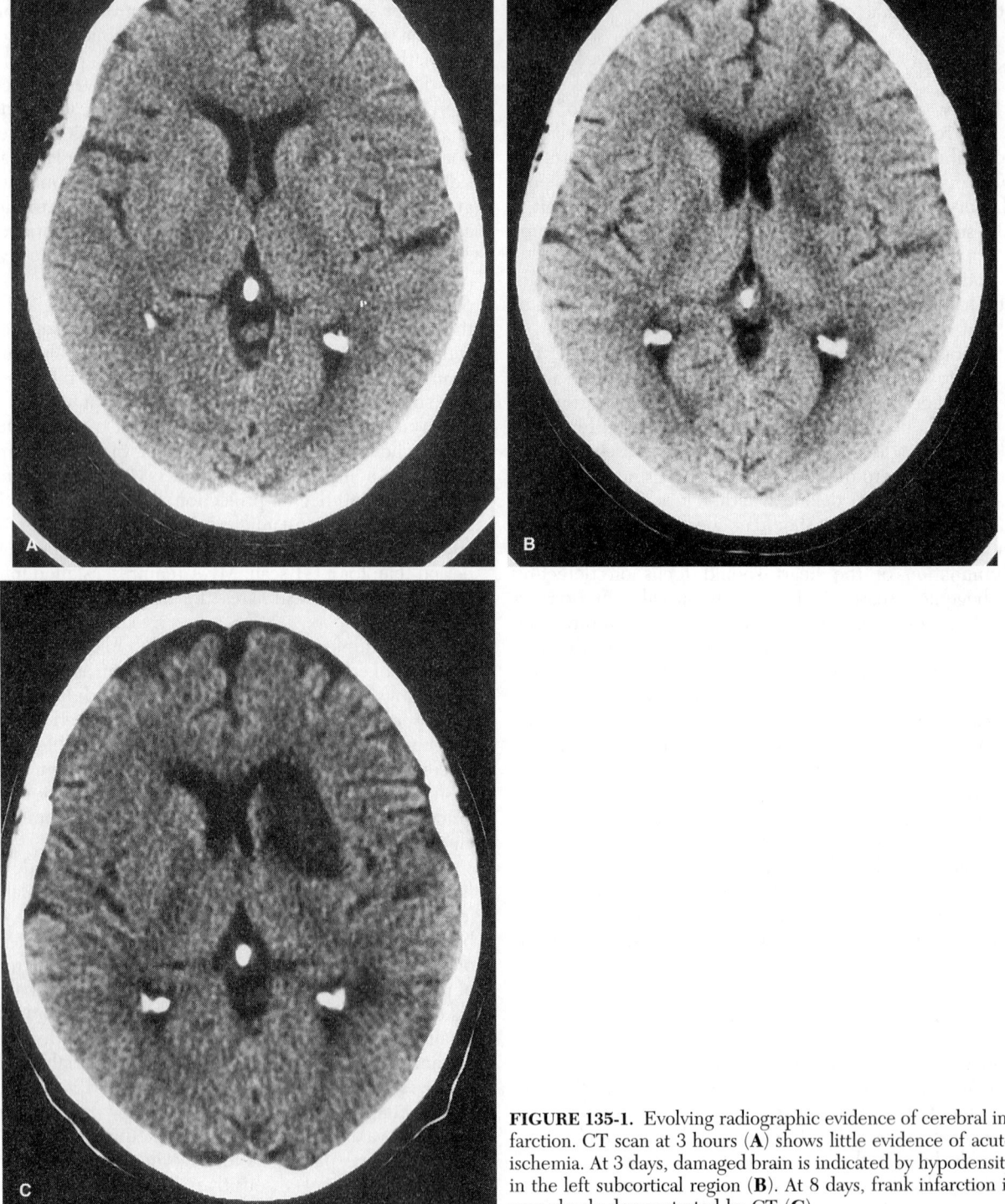

FIGURE 135-1. Evolving radiographic evidence of cerebral infarction. CT scan at 3 hours (**A**) shows little evidence of acute ischemia. At 3 days, damaged brain is indicated by hypodensity in the left subcortical region (**B**). At 8 days, frank infarction is now clearly demonstrated by CT (**C**).

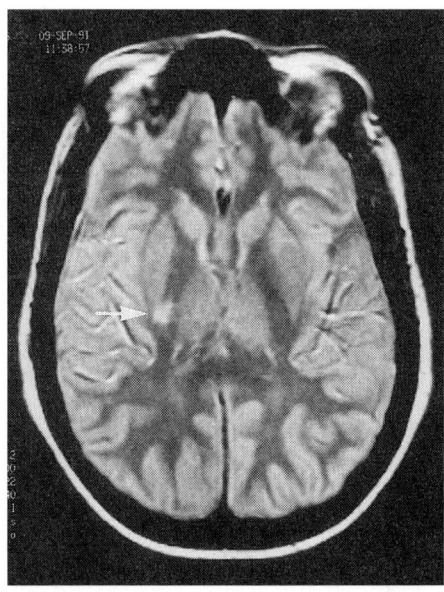

FIGURE 135-2. Lacunar infarction of the right internal capsule demonstrated by MRI.

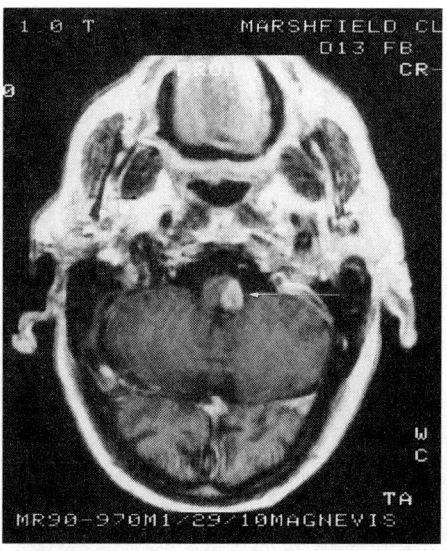

FIGURE 135-3. MRI demonstrates enhancing left lateral medullary infarction in a patient with Wallenberg's syndrome.

left ventricle thrombus, and views of prosthetic valves. Transesophageal echocardiography is an invasive but safe[13] procedure that provides much improved ultrasonic resolution of the left atrial appendage, intraatrial septum, atrial aspect of mitral–tricuspid valves, and the ascending aorta. Sensitivity for pathology is estimated to be several times that of standard transthoracic echocardiography.[14] Sedation is required, however, and it is more physician-intensive than the standard study.

Cerebral angiography is an invasive procedure with associated morbidity of aproximately 1%.[15] Its indications include suspicion of severe intracranial atherosclerosis, cerebral vasculitis, arterial dissection, arteriovenous malformation, or aneurysm. Angiography is commonly performed to define the degree of extracranial carotid stenosis and associated vascular anatomy in anticipation of endarterectomy.

Hematologic evaluation of patients with stroke should include a complete blood count (erythrocytosis or marked leukocytosis may limit perfusion through "sludging") and chemistry profile. A fasting lipid profile should be obtained for potential vascular risk factor modification. In patients for whom an unusual cause of stroke is suspected (young patient or minimal vascular risk factors), laboratory investigation of prothrombotic states should be initiated. Analysis should include levels of anticardiolipin antibody, test for the lupus anticoagulant, antinuclear antibody, erythrocyte sedimentation rate, proteins C and S, antithrombin III, and homocysteine. Toxicology screening should be performed on hospital admission, with attention directed to amphetamines, phencyclidine, ephedrine, and cocaine.[16]

Recommended initial investigations for various patient presentations are listed in Table 135-6. Laboratory evaluation in a patient with stroke, however, requires individualized assessment. Known clinical profiles and pathologies of patients may allow a more directed evaluation. More extensive testing may be required to evaluate detected pathology (e.g.,

cerebral angiography for carotid disease suggested by duplex) or if the etiology remains uncertain.

MANAGEMENT OF THE PATIENT WITH STROKE

Basics of Care

Following a completed stroke, basic care of the patient should emphasize supportive measures. The patient should be admitted to the hospital and a diagnostic workup initiated, as already outlined. The airway, breathing, and circulation should be supported if the patient is comatose or unstable. It is usually preferable to err on the side of hypertension in patients with ischemic stroke; lowering the blood pressure too quickly may further enlarge the area of ischemia. Most patients have a transient blood pressure elevation after a stroke, and this can usually be monitored without intervention. Other support includes maintenance of hydration and normal blood glucose, as well as proper electrolyte balance.

While most patients eventually improve substantially after a stroke, early clinical deterioration is not uncommon (Table 135-7). The leading causes of death after a stroke are not neurologic; critical care of the stroke patient usually centers around management of medical problems. Pneumonia is the leading cause of morbidity and mortality after a stroke. Aspiration is the usual cause, since stroke often causes weakness of facial and pharyngeal muscles and disturbance of the swallowing reflexes. Patients should have their oral intake restricted until it is clear that they can swallow well. Fever after a stroke is almost always due to an infection and should prompt a search for pneumonia or urinary tract infection.[17] Stroke patients who are either bedridden or have lost mobility in their limbs are at high risk for deep venous thrombosis, and pulmonary embolism is another common cause of complications following stroke. For those patients who are not

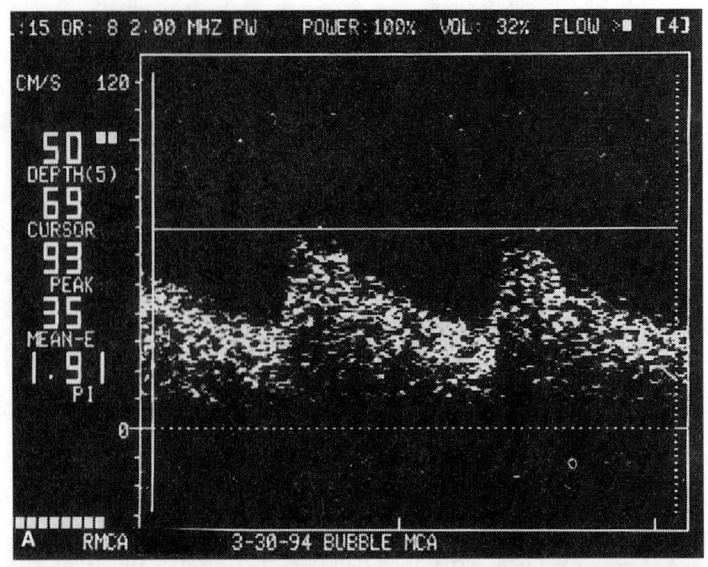

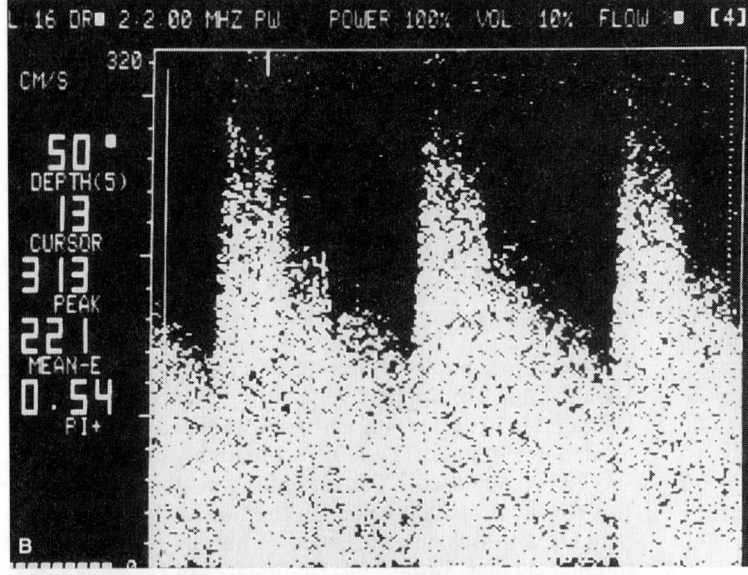

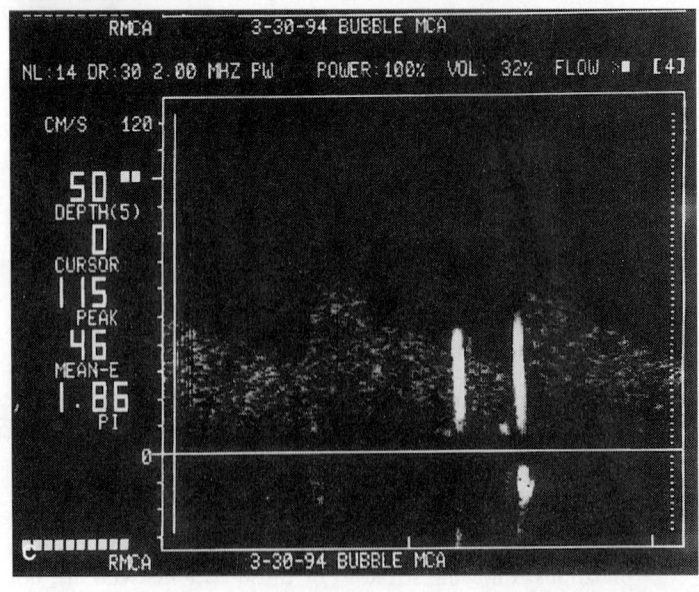

FIGURE 135-4. Transcranial Doppler. The normal flow-velocity profile through the middle cerebral artery (velocity plotted over time during three cardiac cycles) is demonstrated in (**A**). Elevated flow velocities as a result of the arterial spasm associated with subarachnoid hemorrhage is demonstrated in (**B**). In (**C**), two microemboli are detected through the middle cerebral artery as transient high-intensity signals.

TABLE 135-6. Typical Laboratory Investigation of Stroke

Anterior circulation ischemia	Carotid duplex, echocardiography, CT scan (MRI if lacunar)
Posterior circulation ischemia	Echocardiography, MRI (CT if unavailable), TCD or MRA
The "unexpected stroke" (minimal risk factors or stroke in the young)	MRA (including cervical views) or conventional angiography, echocardiography (TEE preferred), toxicology screen, prothrombotic workup

MRA, Magnetic resonance angiography; TCD, transcranial Doppler; TEE, transesophageal echocardiography.

being treated with intravenous heparin, sequential pressure stockings or low-dose subcutaneous heparin therapy (e.g., 5000 units bid)[18] should be initiated.

There is a definite correlation between atherosclerosis in the coronary and cerebral arteries, and most patients admitted with a stroke have underlying coronary artery disease.[19] Many patients with a stroke have had a concomitant myocardial infarction or will suffer one within a few days. The myocardial ischemia is often "silent" or unrecognized, and the patient must be questioned and examined diligently for any symptoms that could indicate cardiac ischemia. Because patients are often aphasic, confused, or unresponsive after a stroke, their ECG (and possibly serum creatine kinase level) should always be examined so that a myocardial infarction is not overlooked.[20] Preexisting heart disease, combined with the catecholamine release that often accompanies a stroke, accounts for a high incidence of cardiac arrhythmias in stroke patients. At least 24 hours of telemetry or Holter monitoring is therefore indicated, and an event recorder may be required to capture intermittent arrhythmias.

Neurologic causes of clinical deterioration include progressive or recurrent stroke, hemorrhagic transformation of the infarct, and local cerebral edema. The latter is the most common cause of deterioration and may well cause fatal herniation in large infarctions. Ischemia-related edema is maximal on about the third day after stroke and resolves slowly thereafter. This type of "cytotoxic" cerebral edema is unfortunately not very responsive to treatments useful for vasogenic edema. Corticosteroids, in particular, do not appear helpful, and hyperglycemia associated with their use may worsen clinical outcome.[21] Mannitol (1 g/kg bolus, then 0.3 g/kg every 6 hours), mechanical hyperventilation (to arterial PCO_2 of 25 to 30 mm Hg), or use of albumin and furosemide to raise colloid oncotic pressure[22] (to 25 to 30 mm Hg) may all provide mild benefit. Hemorrhagic transformation of a stroke occurs commonly in larger cerebral infarctions and usually represents petechial transudation of blood products into the ischemic tissue bed. Generally, this phenomenon occurs in a delayed fashion with no associated clinical deterioration—not uncommonly surprising the treat-

TABLE 135-7. Deterioration in a Patient With Stroke

COMPLICATION	CLINICAL FEATURES	DIAGNOSTIC TESTS	THERAPY
Progressive thrombosis	Worsening or new neurologic deficits	Clinical exam (delayed CT scan may confirm)	Similar to primary stroke
Recurrent embolism	New neurologic deficits	Clinical exam (delayed CT scan may confirm)	Similar to primary stroke
Hemorrhage (major)	Lethargy, headache, worsening or new neurologic deficits	CT scan	Hold ongoing anticoagulation, consider protamine or fresh frozen plasma
Increased ICP (edema-related mass effect)	Decreased alertness, worsened headache, herniation syndrome	CT scan	Mannitol, hyperventilation
Hydrocephalus	Decreased alertness, worsened headache, herniation syndrome	CT scan	Ventriculostomy drainage or shunt, surgical excision of hematoma
Infection	Confusion, lethargy	Panculture, chest X-ray, urinalysis	Appropriate antibiotic
Deep venous thrombosis; pulmonary embolism	Leg pain–swelling; dyspnea, hypoxia	Venous Doppler or venogram; V̇/Q̇ scan or pulmonary arteriogram	Anticoagulation, venous filter; embolectomy

ing physician who has watched the patient steadily improve following the stroke. Specific therapy is not usually required, although any ongoing anticoagulation should be held for 1 to 2 weeks. If the hemorrhage is associated with clinical deterioration, pharmacologic reversal of anticoagulation should be initiated.

Early initiation of physical, occupational, and speech therapy services hastens functional recovery from stroke. Each patient requires individualized assessment for potential benefit from these services. Speech therapists are also commonly involved in formal assessment of aspiration risk. A videofluoroscopy swallowing study is the most sensitive measure and should be a consideration for most patients with a stroke. At the least, bedside swallowing function should be observed by a trained technician, nurse, or physician before oral intake is resumed.

Acute Therapy

Clinically, cerebral ischemia is most commonly related to arterial pathology, usually abrupt occlusion from a variety of causes. The ensuing oligemic neuronal environment leads to local tissue dysfunction. Clearly, there is likely to be a population of neurons that cannot be salvaged no matter how aggressively treated. These are the neurons exposed to the extreme deprivation of nutrients that results in cell death within minutes. The treating physician, however, must presume that the observed loss of function does not represent irreversibly infarcted tissue. In any stroke, there is likely a large portion of tissue that is not receiving sufficient nutrient delivery to function properly, but that is not yet irreparably damaged. This zone of hypoperfused, *but salvageable,* brain has been termed the ischemic penumbra. If maintained, hypoperfusion can and often does ultimately result in infarction. Animal studies have shown the "tolerance" of the neurons to be related to the severity of oligemia,[23] and clinically the latter commonly exceeds the former. This oligemic tolerance, however, provides the basis for a "therapeutic window" for CNS ischemia.

Three primary treatment strategies are now evolving for therapy of cerebral ischemia. The first strategy attends to the arterial occlusive process itself: remove the occlusion and thereby shorten the duration of tissue ischemia. A second goal is to pharmacologically increase cerebral tolerance to the existing ischemic conditions, maintaining viability until spontaneous or induced thrombolysis occurs. The final goal is use of pharmacologic or other means to protect the ischemic tissue from potentially toxic mechanisms associated with reperfusion.

Thrombolytic and antithrombotic therapy has now been clearly demonstrated as efficacious for other arterial occlusive diseases in coronary, pulmonary, and aortofemoral vascular beds and therefore has obvious potential for similar benefit in cerebral artery occlusions. Although undoubtedly beneficial in selected patients, use of these drugs carries an elevated risk of brain hemorrhage. Acute major hemorrhage in a region of brain compromised by ischemia occurs spontaneously in approximately 5% of stroke patients,[24] an underappreciated incidence until demonstration by placebo-controlled acute stroke therapy trials. Thrombolytic therapy with tissue plasminogen activator, urokinase, or streptokinase, given via the intravenous or intraarterial route, increases this incidence significantly. Risk-benefit profiles for the varying temporal and vascular characteristics of stroke patients await definition by clinical trial; until then, their use is not recommended.

Antithrombotic drugs such as heparin or its low-molecular-weight derivatives may be beneficial for acute stroke by prevention of progressive thrombosis or recurrent embolization, though this still awaits verification by clinical trial. A common current practice is to use anticoagulation, barring contraindications (see later), until the underlying etiology of stroke is defined. A CT scan must first be obtained to exclude any intracerebral hemorrhage. If the scan result is negative, the patient is then begun on intravenous heparin, administered at the rate of approximately 1000 units/hour, with close monitoring of the prothrombin time (PT) and partial thromboplastin time (PTT). Many authorities advocate that the patient not be given a bolus or loading dose of heparin, since this may increase the likelihood of intracerebral hemorrhage. The PTT should be maintained at approximately 1.5 times normal, and over the next few days the patient can usually be switched to warfarin to maintain the PT at the same level. Indications for long-term anticoagulation in patients who recover from stroke are based on presumed stroke etiology (likely most effective for cardioembolic, variable for thrombotic, and least effective for lacunar disease), risk of recurrence (higher risk favors more "aggressive" prophylaxis), and perceived risk from bleeding. The contraindications to anticoagulation include very advanced age or pronounced medical frailty, a large cerebral infarction (which would contain a great deal of necrotic brain tissue), uncontrolled hypertension, or the presence of active bleeding (either within the head or at another site, such as a gastrointestinal hemorrhage).

Many drugs are currently under investigation for potential benefit as "neuroprotectants." Drugs in this category are likely to be useful in combination with maneuvers to directly treat the occlusive process, or may be solely used when such treatment is contraindicated. Types of drugs under investigation include calcium channel blockers, intracellular calcium chelators, free radical scavengers, and neurotransmitter modulators (e.g., glutamate antagonists, glycine antagonists, GABA agonists). Preliminary benefit has been demonstrated, but use of these agents also awaits verification of efficacy by clinical trial.

A number of biochemical mechanisms occur with reperfusion into an ischemic vascular bed that may be harmful to the compromised tissue. Drugs with the potential to limit this secondary injury are also in clinical trial. They will likely be most useful in "cocktail" form with thrombolytics or antithrombotics, or both.

OTHER CEREBROVASCULAR DISEASES ■

TRANSIENT ISCHEMIC ATTACK

Transient ischemic attacks (TIAs) are episodes of temporary neurologic dysfunction of ischemic origin with rapid onset followed by swift and complete resolution. By arbitrary definition, signs and symptoms must last less than 24 hours, but most TIAs resolve within 30 minutes. Actual death of cerebral tissue thus does not occur. Patients with TIAs are seldom critically ill. The importance of TIAs is that they may be harbingers of more devastating strokes in the future. The diagnosis of TIA depends almost entirely on the skill with which the history is taken and interpreted, since the deficit is transient and seldom witnessed by the physician. Since TIAs are actually reversible strokes, evaluation and long-term management mirrors that outlined earlier for stroke. The major objectives of the physician are to identify the cause of the ischemic event and determine the optimal strategy for prevention of recurrent cerebral ischemia.

INTRACEREBRAL HEMORRHAGE

Primary intracerebral hemorrhage (ICH) frequently causes profound neurologic impairment that mandates intensive care management. Primary ICH should be distinguished from hemorrhagic transformation of an initially ischemic stroke (see earlier). In contrast to the latter, primary ICH involves bleeding, usually of arterial origin, into normally perfused brain. The resultant confluent mass causes direct injury to local brain tissue and compressive toxicity to neighboring regions by the expanding hematoma. The former generally results in permanent deficits, but the compressive effects are potentially reversible.

Diagnosis of ICH is usually not difficult. Like ischemic stroke, patients present with focal neurologic deficits related to the site of the injury. Unlike a primary ischemic event, level of consciousness is commonly altered early in the clinical course as mass effect impairs bilateral hemispheric or brain stem function. CT scanning is extremely sensitive for this disorder (Fig. 135-5) and should be obtained emergently when suspected.

Once confirmed, other laboratory evaluation may be required to define the underlying etiology. Chronic hypertension is considered the most common cause of ICH, with hemorrhage usually occurring in deep basal ganglia, thalamic, or pontine sites. Patients with the appropriate clinical history and a typical site of hemorrhage probably do not require extensive etiologic investigation. Other causes of ICH include medical illnesses that predispose to bleeding in other bodily tissues, and complete investigation of coagulation parameters should therefore be performed. Metastases from certain malignancies such as melanoma or renal cell carcinoma may cause arterial necrosis resulting in ICH. If suspicion exists for this pathology and initial CT does not reveal other intracranial lesions, repeat neuroimaging may be required after spontaneous resorption of the hematoma (3 to 4 weeks). Primary CNS vasculopathies such as arteriovenous malformation or cavernous angioma may require diagnostic cerebral angiography but this can be delayed until the patient has stabilized and the hematoma has resorbed. Cerebral sinus thrombosis is a rare cause of ICH that may require urgent angiography, though MRI and particularly dedicated MR angiography are sensitive noninvasive tests. Amyloid angiopathy is a primary CNS vasculopathy that is more prevalent with advancing age and is one of the few

disorders that cause recurrent ICH. This should be suspected in the elderly patient with one or more cortically based hemorrhages, particularly if a coexistent dementia is suspected. Diagnostic brain biopsy is impractical, however, and the diagnosis is usually based on clinical findings. Iatrogenic causes of ICH include use of anticoagulants, most often in supratherapeutic degree, and thrombolytics. The associated hemorrhage may be multifocal in such cases, possibly implying an underlying vasculopathy such as amyloid.

Management of the patient with ICH (Table 135-8) is similar to the management of ischemic stroke, with two notable exceptions. Intracranial hemorrhage is occasionally progressive and blood pressure should therefore be aggressively controlled to target the normotensive range. Second, more aggressive neurosurgical management may also be required. The neurologic deficit related to compressive effects of the hematoma may be only transiently reversible. With persistent compression, local vascular insufficiency and metabolic derangement eventually lead to neuronal death. In addition, life-threatening herniation syndromes can be aborted with surgical extraction of the hematoma and nonviable brain, often with only modest residual deficit. This is particularly relevant with ICH of the posterior fossa (brain stem or cerebellum). Hemorrhage at these sites should be considered neurosurgical emergencies and prompt urgent consultation. Surgical excision of the hematoma may also be considered in hemispheric ICH, though this is controversial. Most neurosurgeons consider extraction of peripherally based (cortical) hematomas, but not hematomas of deep basal ganglia or thalamic bleeds. If there is intraventricular extension of the hemorrhage or compression of cerebrospinal fluid (CSF) channels, ventriculostomy drainage may be necessary to treat hydrocephalus. Neurosurgical opinions should be sought for these patients.

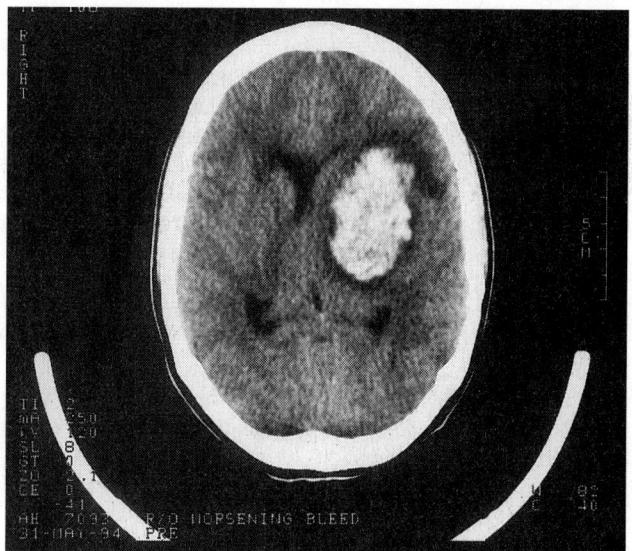

FIGURE 135-5. Intracerebral hemorrhage of the left basal ganglia. Hyperdense appearance of blood on the CT scan easily defines the extent of hemorrhage.

TABLE 135-8. Complications of Intracerebral Hemorrhage

COMPLICATION	CLINICAL FEATURES	DIAGNOSTIC TESTS	THERAPY
Increased ICP	Decreased alertness, worsened headache, herniation syndrome	ICP monitor	Mannitol, hyperventilation, surgical excision of hematoma
Hydrocephalus	Decreased alertness, worsened headache, herniation syndrome	CT scan	Ventriculostomy drainage or shunt, surgical excision of hematoma
Cerebral infarction (arterial compression)	Worsening or new neurologic deficits	Neurologic exam, CT scan	Primary stroke therapy, surgical excision of hematoma
Seizure	Sudden behavioral change or uncontrolled motor activity	EEG	Anticonvulsants
Expanding hematoma	Worsening or new neurologic deficits	CT scan	Treat existing coagulopathy, maintain normotension
Infection	Confusion, lethargy	Panculture, chest X-ray, urinalysis	Appropriate antibiotic

SUBARACHNOID HEMORRHAGE

Subarachnoid hemorrhage (SAH) is a relatively uncommon, but often devastating type of stroke. Incidence is estimated at 30,000 patients per year in the United States, with a mortality that exceeds 50%. While head trauma is the most frequent cause of subarachnoid hemorrhage, aneurysmal rupture results in the greatest morbidity and mortality. Clinically, this is an apoplectic disorder. Most commonly, patients perceive a sudden severe headache with rapid impairment of consciousness, both symptoms related to the sudden release of irritating blood products into the meningeal spaces surrounding the brain. Focal neurologic symptoms such as hemiparesis, sensory loss, or diplopia may occur if loculation of subarachnoid blood or intraparenchymal extension of the hemorrhage develops. The most important features of the neurologic examination are the assessment of level of consciousness, cranial nerve function, and motor function. Clinical severity of SAH is graded on these findings[25] (grades I to V, Table 135-9), and can be rough prognostic indicators.

Diagnosis of SAH is based on neuroimaging or CSF analysis. Brain CT scan is a very sensitive indicator of the presence of subarachnoid blood, although close examination must be paid to subarachnoid spaces surrounding the brain stem and over the cerebral convexities (Fig. 135-6). Brain parenchyma itself most commonly displays no acute abnormalities. Erythrocyte concentration in CSF below approximately 30,000 cells/mm^3 may not result in the diagnostic increased density within CSF on CT scans. In approximately 10% of patients, diagnosis therefore requires CSF analysis through lumbar puncture. In addition to elevated erythrocyte count, CSF xanthochromia and elevation of CSF D-dimer can often be detected in true subarachnoid hemorrhage. The latter two findings may help distinguish bloody CSF from a "traumatic tap," as these serve as markers of the breakdown of thrombosis or blood products. Serial cell counts should always be obtained, however, whenever SAH is suspected. Cell counts in SAH should be roughly equivalent in all tubes, while a declining count is usual in traumatic punctures. It should be stressed that lumbar puncture should be avoided in any patient with depressed level of consciousness until CT scan excludes a focal mass (such as intraparenchymal or subdural hemorrhage). If bacterial meningitis is a concern, blood cultures should be obtained and antibiotics started while awaiting results of the CT scan.

Management

Patients with acute SAH are at high risk for a multitude of complications[26] (Table 135-10) that usually mandate admission to an intensive care facility. All patients should be placed on strict bed rest with appropriate precautions for deep venous thrombosis and aspiration. Patients with progressive lethargy may require intubation for airway protection and mechanical ventilation. Until the aneurysm has been ablated, blood pressure should be kept in the normotensive range and isotonic intravenous fluids should be used to maintain normovolemia. All patients should be started on nimodipine at 60 mg every 4 hours (duration 21 days), either orally or through a nasogastric tube, for prevention of vasospasm (see later). Since seizures occur in 25% of patients and may complicate the morbidity of subarachnoid hemorrhage, prophylactic use of anticonvulsants is recommended (e.g., phenytoin, 15 mg/kg loading dose, followed by 300 mg/day,

TABLE 135-9. Severity Grade of Subarachnoid Hemorrhage

Grade 1: Fully conscious, no neurologic deficit, headache only
Grade 2: Mild drowsiness, no neurologic deficits other than cranial nerve dysfunction
Grade 3: Drowsy, mild neurologic deficit
Grade 4: Stuporous, moderate to severe neurologic deficits
Grade 5: Coma

From Hunt WE, Hess RM: Surgical risk as related to the time of intervention in the repair of intracranial aneurysms. *J Neurosurg* 1968;28:14.

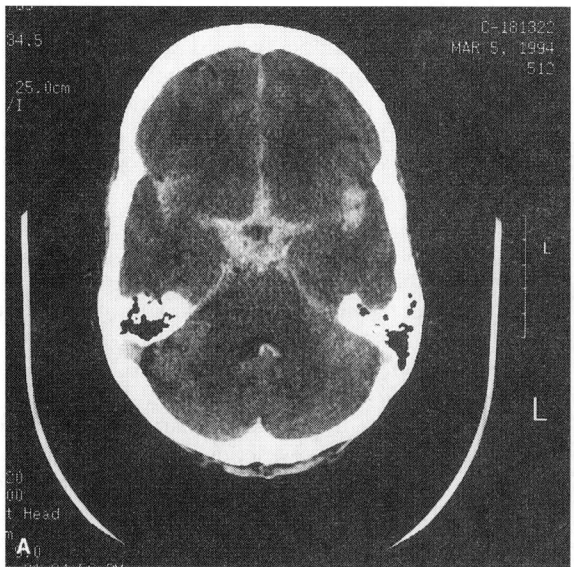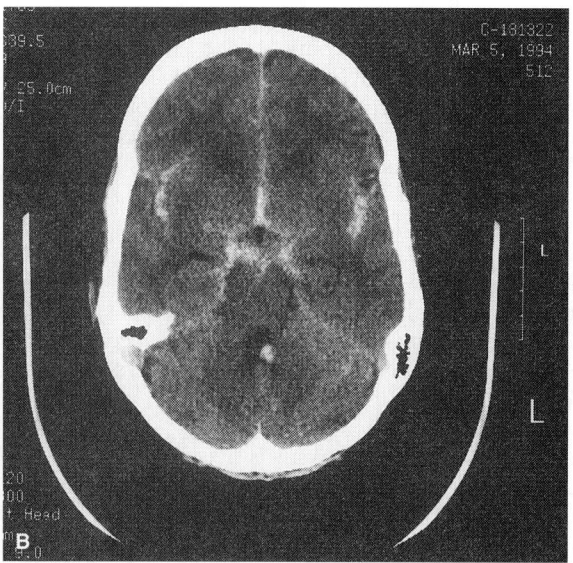

FIGURE 135-6. Subarachnoid hemorrhage. Blood is imaged as hyperdense fluid within the cisterns surrounding the brain stem and within bilateral sylvian fissures.

adjusted by levels). In nondiabetic patients, dexamethasone (10 mg loading dose, then 4 to 6 mg every 6 hours) may be of value in reducing cerebral edema. An ECG with rhythm strip is mandatory because the catecholamine surge and hypertension after SAH often precipitate cardiac arrhythmias. Bleeding parameters should also be measured, including prothrombin time (PT), PTT, and platelet count. Serum electrolytes should be followed at least daily.

In those patients surviving the initial hemorrhage, the two most feared complications are cerebral artery vasospasm and rebleeding from an aneurysm. Unfortunately, therapy directed at lowering the risk of one may well increase the risk of the other. Further management of patients therefore depends in large degree on their neurologic condition. In those patients with Hunt and Hess grades I to III, a directed

investigation for the presence of cerebral aneurysm should be initiated as soon as possible. If a surgically accessible cerebral aneurysm is detected with cerebral angiography (Fig. 135-7) or other means, prompt clipping of the aneurysm minimizes the risk of a second, often fatal, hemorrhage. Unclipped aneurysms rebleed at a rate of 4% on day 1, then 1% to 2% a day for the next 4 weeks. Early surgery also allows aggressive management of vasospasm, manipulations that would increase the risk of rebleeding from an unclipped aneurysm. Patients with a higher initial Hunt and Hess grade are less likely to survive and more likely to suffer surgical morbidity during the acute phase of hemorrhage. In these patients, angiography and surgery are believed best delayed for at least 14 days.

The exact cause of arterial vasospasm following SAH is

TABLE 135-10. Complications of Subarachnoid Hemorrhage

COMPLICATION	CLINICAL FEATURES	DIAGNOSTIC TESTS	THERAPY
Increased ICP	Decreased alertness, worsened headache, herniation syndrome	ICP monitor	Mannitol, steroids, hyperventilation
Hydrocephalus	Decreased alertness, worsened headache, herniation syndrome	CT scan	Ventriculostomy drainage or shunt
Vasospasm	Delayed focal neurologic deficit	TCD, angiography	Nimodipine, hypervolemia, hypertension, angioplasty
Rebleed	Worsened neurologic condition, especially level of consciousness	CT scan, lumbar puncture	Ablation of aneurysm
Seizure	Sudden behavioral change or uncontrolled motor activity	EEG	Anticonvulsants
Hyponatremia	Confusion, seizure	Serum electrolytes	Isotonic fluids to achieve euvolemia or hypervolemia
Infection	Confusion, lethargy	Panculture, chest X-ray, urinalysis	Appropriate antibiotic

TCD, Transcranial Doppler.

unknown, but its incidence does appear to be correlated with the density of blood products. The site of greatest vasospasm is not necessarily related to the location of the aneurysm, however. Severe vasospasm may result in cerebral infarction within the vascular distribution of the involved artery. Vasospasm begins about 3 days after the bleed and may persist for 3 weeks. Transcranial Doppler is a sensitive, noninvasive indicator of the presence and degree of vasospasm within proximal arteries, although it may not detect vasospasm restricted to smaller peripheral vessels. This technique may be used daily to guide and monitor management strategies. Angiography may occasionally be necessary to confirm vasospasm. The calcium channel blockers nimodipine and nicardipine can reduce the incidence of vasospasm, as well as associated cerebral infarction.

Once ablation of the aneurysm is accomplished, vasospasm can be managed aggressively. During the operative procedure, neurosurgeons attempt to flush as much blood from the subarachnoid space as possible. Following surgery, IV fluids should be pushed to the tolerance of the patient (up to 400 mL/hour). Since congestive heart failure is a potential complication, central pressure monitoring should be used in patients at risk. Optimal central venous pressure is 8 to 12 mm Hg. If hypervolemic therapy is not adequate to control vasospasm, hypertension can be initiated by cessation of antihypertensives or use of vasopressors (e.g., phenylephrine 10 to 40 μg/minute; dopamine 5 to 15 μg/kg/minute), targeting mean arterial pressures of 120 to 140 mm Hg. For symptomatic vasospasm refractory to these therapies, selective transluminal angioplasty can be considered at experienced medical centers. Even using the most aggressive management strategies, vasospasm remains a leading cause of morbidity and mortality after subarachnoid hemorrhage.

Acute hydrocephalus occurs in approximately 20% of survivors of SAH, either as a result of direct obstruction of CSF channels or by impeding CSF absorption at arachnoid granulations. Likelihood of hydrocephalus increases with worsening grade of hemorrhage. Ventriculostomy drainage is recommended for patients with acute hydrocephalus and decreased level of consciousness. Improvement can be expected in over 50% of patients.

Hyponatremia occurs in approximately 30% of patients with subarachnoid hemorrhage. The occurrence seems to parallel that of vasospasm, and is worse in those patients with higher grades of hemorrhage. The hyponatremia was initially thought secondary to the syndrome of inappropriate ADH secretion, but in actuality the ADH release in this disorder may be entirely appropriate. The sodium disturbance is now thought to be secondary to an elevated natriuretic peptide. Fluid restriction for this disorder should definitely be avoided, particularly since this may precipitate vasospasm. The administration of large volumes of isotonic fluid is recommended, with volume status monitored by central pressure catheters in severe cases.

REFERENCES

1. Norris JW, Hachinski VC: Misdiagnosis of stroke. *Lancet* 1982;1:328
2. Mohr JP, Caplan LR, Melski JW, et al: The Harvard cooperative stroke registry. *Neurology* 1978;28:754
3. Cerebral Embolism Task Force: Cardiogenic brain embolism. *Arch Neurol* 1986;43:71
4. Kittner SJ, Sharkness CM, Price TR, et al: Infarcts with a cardiac source of embolism in the Nincos Stroke data bank. *Neurology* 1990;40:281
5. Mohr JP: Lacunes. *Stroke* 1982;13:3
6. Arboix A, Marti-Vilalta JL, Garcia JH: Clinical study of 227 patients with lacunar infarcts. *Stroke* 1990;21:842
7. Hier DB, Davis KR, Richardson EP, et al: Hypertensive putaminal hemorrhage. *Ann Neurol* 1977;1:152
8. Hart RG, Easton JD: Management of cervical bruits and carotid stenosis in preoperative patients. *Stroke* 1983;14:290
9. Wiebers DO, Whisnant JR, Sandok BA, et al: Prospective comparison of a cohort with asymptomatic carotid bruit and a population-based cohort without carotid bruit. *Stroke* 1990;21:989
10. Dimant J, Grob D: Electrocardiographic changes and myocardial damage in patients with acute cerebrovascular accidents. *Stroke* 1977;8:448
11. Anderson CM, Edelman RR, Turski PA: *Clinical Magnetic Resonance Angiography.* New York, Raven Press, 1993
12. Newell DW, Auslid R: *Transcranial Doppler.* New York, Raven Press, 1992
13. Daniel WG, Erbel R, Kasper W, et al: Safety of transesophageal echocardiography: a multicenter survey of 10,419 examinations. *Circulation* 1991;83:817
14. DeRook FA, Comess KA, Albers GW, et al: Transesophageal echocardiography in the evaluation of stroke. *Ann Intern Med* 1992;117:922
15. Hankey GJ, Warlow CP, Sellar RJ: Cerebral angiographic risk in mild cerebrovascular disease. *Stroke* 1990;21:209
16. Sloan MA, Kittner SJ, Rigamonti D, Price TR: Occurrence of stroke associated with use/abuse of drugs. *Neurology* 1991; 41:1358

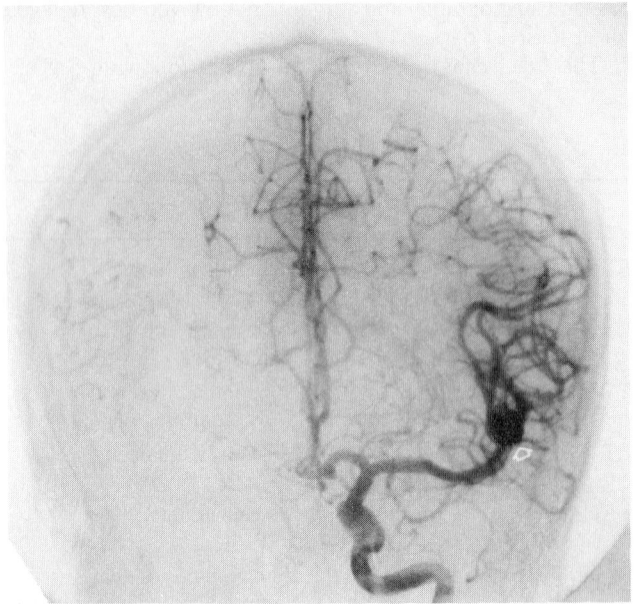

FIGURE 135-7. Aneurysm at the bifurcation of the left middle cerebral artery demonstrated by angiography. (Courtesy of R. Nick Bryan, MD, Baylor College of Medicine, Houston, TX.)

17. Przelomski MM, Roth RM, Gleckman RA, et al: Fever in the wake of a stroke. *Neurology* 1986;36:427

18. McCarthy ST: Low dose heparin as a prophylaxis against deep-vein thrombosis after acute stroke. *Lancet* 1977;2:800

19. Rokey R, Rolak LA, Harati Y, et al: Coronary artery disease in patients with cerebrovascular disease: a prospective study. *Ann Neurol* 1984;16:50

20. Rolak LA, Rokey R: *Coronary and Cerebral Vascular Disease.* New York, Futura, 1990

21. Lees KR: Therapeutic interventions in acute stroke. *Br J Clin Pharmacol* 1992;34:486

22. Tone O, Ito U, Tomita H, et al: High colloid oncotic therapy for brain edema with cerebral hemorrhage. *Acta Neurochir Suppl Wien* 1994;60:568

23. Jones TH, Morawetz RB, Crowell RM, et al: Thresholds of focal cerebral ischemia in awake monkeys. *J Neurosurg* 1981;54:773

24. Wardlaw JM, Warlow CP: Thrombolysis in acute ischemic stroke: does it work? *Stroke* 1992;23:1826

25. Hunt WE, Hess RM: Surgical risk as related to the time of intervention in the repair of intracranial aneurysms. *J Neurosurg* 1968;28:14

26. Mayberg MR, Batjer HH, Dacey R, et al: Guidelines for the management of aneurysmal subarachnoid hemorrhage. *Circulation* 1994;90:2592

Critical Care, Third Edition, edited by Joseph M. Civetta,
Robert W. Taylor, and Robert R. Kirby.
Lippincott-Raven Publishers, Philadelphia, PA © 1997.

CHAPTER 136

■

Neuromuscular Disorders

Stephen Derdak

IMMEDIATE CONCERNS ■

MAJOR PROBLEMS

Neuromuscular disorders are a relatively common cause
of admissions to ICUs in large university medical centers.
Diseases leading to respiratory failure include Guillain-Barré
syndrome, myasthenia gravis, amyotrophic lateral sclerosis,
and polymyositis (Table 136-1). Patients with neuromuscular
diseases usually come under the care of the intensivist because of acute respiratory decompensation necessitating
close monitoring or mechanical ventilation. Precipitating factors include exacerbation of the underlying disease (e.g.,
rapidly progressive ascending motor paralysis in Guillain-
Barré syndrome), pulmonary infection (e.g., muscular dystrophy), and myasthenic crisis (e.g., precipitated by infection
or surgery) in patients with myasthenia gravis. A common
pathogenic factor in all these disorders is the rapid development of profound respiratory muscle and diaphragm weakness leading to ineffective cough, inability to clear secretions,
atelectasis, and hypercapneic respiratory failure.

STRESS POINTS

1. The development of respiratory failure in patients with
   neuromuscular disorders often occurs abruptly in the
   face of recent "normal" arterial blood gases. Frequently these patients were said to have "looked good"
   before a catastrophic respiratory arrest, because of the
   relative absence of facial clues of distress or use of
   accessory muscles of respiration that are normally seen
   in other patients before frank respiratory failure (as
   in severe asthmatic patients).
2. Patients with neuromuscular diseases who have evidence of increasing muscle weakness should undergo
   serial monitoring with tests of respiratory muscle

strength (e.g., negative inspiratory pressure and forced
vital capacity [FVC] maneuvers) in order to anticipate
the need for elective intubation.
3. The principles of management of neuromuscular disorders include careful attention to pulmonary toilet
   (frequent suctioning and turning), thrombosis prophylaxis, prompt treatment of infections, nutritional
   support, and specific therapies depending on the underlying disease (e.g., plasmapheresis for patients with
   Guillain-Barré syndrome).
4. Providing emotional support to the patient (who frequently is in a "locked-in" state, aware of his or her
   surroundings but unable to communicate because of
   muscle paralysis and intubation) and family is essential
   in helping them cope with these catastrophic diseases.
5. The remainder of this chapter focuses on Guillain-
   Barré syndrome and myasthenia gravis because specific treatments are available for these two diseases
   and because the general management principles are
   applicable to other neuromuscular disorders resulting
   in respiratory failure.

GUILLAIN-BARRÉ SYNDROME (ACUTE AUTOIMMUNE INFLAMMATORY DEMYELINATING POLYNEUROPATHY) ■

ESSENTIAL DIAGNOSTIC TESTS AND PROCEDURES

1. Lumbar puncture (cells <10, elevated protein), spinal
   magnetic resonance imaging (MRI) with gadolinium
   enhancement (characteristic lumbosacral root enhancement with Guillain-Barré syndrome) and nerve
   conduction studies are warranted.

TABLE 136-1. Neuromuscular Disorders Affecting
Respiratory Function

MOTOR NEURON

Poliomyelitis
Tetanus
Amyotrophic lateral sclerosis

PERIPHERAL NEUROPATHIES

Acute ascending sensorimotor paralysis
　Guillain-Barré syndrome
　Mononucleosis, diphtheria, prophyria, drugs (thallium,
　　FK506)
　Human immunodeficiency virus
　Cytomegalovirus
　Critical illness polyneuropathy
Chronic sensorimotor polyneuropathy
　Charcot-Marie-Tooth disease
　Lyme polyradiculitis
Critical illness polyneuropathy

NEUROMUSCULAR JUNCTION

Myasthenia gravis
Botulism

MYOPATHIES

Muscular dystrophy
Myotonic disorders
Polymyositis
Glycogen storage disorders

2. Exclude infectious etiologies for which specific treatment may exist: cytomegalovirus (AIDS patients, solid
organ and bone marrow transplantation), Epstein-Barr
virus (EBV), herpes simplex, herpes zoster virus, human immunodeficiency virus (HIV), *Borrelia burgdorferi, Mycoplasma pneumoniae,* and *Campylobacter
jejuni* (Penner serotype 19).
3. Monitor inspiratory pressure and FVC. If FVC is less
than 20 mL/kg and progressive weakness is demonstrated, the patient should be monitored in a critical
care setting. Consider elective intubation for FVC less
than 15 mL/kg—***before*** arterial blood gases deteriorate. Succinylcholine to facilitate intubation is ***contraindicated*** because of the risk of inducing severe hyperkalemia and cardiac arrythmias.

INITIAL THERAPY

1. For Guillain-Barré patients with progressive weakness, plasma exchange and intravenous immunoglobulin (IVIg) appear equally effective. Both therapies may
result in relapse of weakness within days of completing
therapy and may respond to a second course of treatment. Corticosteroids are not considered useful.
2. Careful attention to general supportive measures for
paralyzed patients on ventilators includes frequent
turning or kinetic beds (reduced risk of pressure ulcers, nosocomial pneumonia), thrombosis prophylaxis

(low-dose heparin, low-molecular-weight heparin, low-
dose warfarin sodium [Coumadin]), nutrition (early
enteral feeding), water restriction for hyponatremia
associated with syndrome of inappropriate antidiuretic
hormone (SIADH), and vigilance for nosocomial infections (pneumonias, urinary tract infections).
3. Autonomic manifestations may require specific treatment (e.g., beta-blockers for persistent sinus tachycardia associated with hypertension).

CAPSULE

Guillain-Barré syndrome (GBS) remains one of the most
common neurologic disorders that may cause a previously
healthy person to develop, over a course of several days to
weeks, complete muscle paralysis and respiratory failure.
The syndrome became a household word following the National Influenza Immunization Program of 1976 when over
1000 cases of GBS were reported. Persons who received the
A/New Jersey/76 (swine) influenza vaccine had an increased
incidence of GBS of approximately five to six times that of
unvaccinated persons. An estimated 10 cases of GBS for
every 1 million persons vaccinated occurred in the 10 to 12
weeks after vaccination. Younger persons (<25 years old)
appeared to have a lower relative risk of GBS and a lower
case-fatality rate. Subsequent national influenza vaccination
programs have not demonstrated an increased risk of developing GBS.

Typically, patients present with initial complaints of paresthesias and pain in the distal extremities—most commonly
beginning in the feet and legs. The discrepancy between
the subjective complaints of tingling, numbness, and pain
often mislead the unwary clinician into suspecting functional
illness. An ascending motor paralysis associated with areflexia rapidly dominates the clinical picture over the subsequent days to weeks. Involvement of respiratory muscles
may result in precipitous respiratory failure that must be
anticipated and properly managed. Paralysis of bulbar and
facial muscles results in difficulty handling secretions and
dsyphagia. Severe cases may manifest autonomic nervous
system involvement marked by wide swings in blood pressure, cardiac arrythmias, facial flushing, and urinary retention. The diagnosis depends on recognition of the typical
clinical pattern of acute onset of ascending motor weakness,
areflexia, and minimal sensory deficit in the absence of other
recognized causes (Table 136-2). The clinical impression is
supported by finding an increased cerebrospinal fluid (CSF)
protein (sometimes as high as 1300 mg/dL) with minimal
to absent pleocytosis—so-called albuminocytologic dissociation. Nerve conduction testing indicating demyelination is
the most sensitive and specific laboratory finding in GBS.
Occasionally, otherwise typical cases may reveal nearly normal findings on electromyography and nerve conduction
testing.

Plasmapheresis or IVIg are the accepted treatments of
choice for patients with GBS. Early institution of either
therapy has been shown to shorten the duration of mechanical ventilation and the time to achieve independent walking
as well as to reduce the incidence of chronic neurologic

TABLE 136-2. Criteria for Diagnosis of Guillain-Barré Syndrome

I. Features Required for Diagnosis
   A. Progressive motor weakness of more than one limb. The degree ranges from minimal weakness of the legs, with or without mild ataxia, to total paralysis of the muscles of all four extremities and the trunk, bulbar and facial paralysis, and external ophthalmoplegia.
   B. Areflexia (loss of tendon jerks). Universal areflexia is the rule, though distal areflexia with definite hyporeflexia of the biceps and knee jerks will suffice if other features are consistent.
II. Features Strongly Supportive of the Diagnosis
   A. Clinical features (ranked in order of importance)
      1. Progression. Symptoms and signs of motor weakness develop rapidly but cease to progress by 4 weeks into the illness. Approximately 50% will reach the nadir by 2 weeks, 80% by 3 weeks, and more than 90% by 4 weeks.
      2. Relative symmetry. Symmetry is seldom absolute, but usually, if one limb is affected, the opposite is as well.
      3. Mild sensory symptoms or signs.
      4. Cranial nerve involvement. Facial weakness occurs in approximately 50% and is frequently bilateral. Other cranial nerves may be involved, particularly those innervating the tongue and muscles of deglutition, and sometimes the extraocular motor nerves. On occasion (less than 5%) the neuropathy may begin in the nerves to the extraocular muscles or other cranial nerves.
      5. Recovery. It usually begins two to four weeks after progression stops. Recovery may be delayed for months. Most patients recover functionally.
      6. Autonomic dysfunction. Tachycardia and other dysrhythmias, postural hypotension, hypertension, and vasomotor symptoms, when present, support the diagnosis. These findings may fluctuate. Care must be exercised to exclude other bases for these symptoms, such as pulmonary embolism.
      7. Absence of fever at the onset of neuritic symptoms.
      Variants (not ranked)
      1. Fever at the onset of neuritic symptoms.
      2. Severe sensory loss with pain
      3. Progression beyond 4 weeks. Occasionally, a patient's disease will continue to progress for many weeks longer or the patient will have a minor relapse.
      4. Cessation of progression without recovery or with major permanent residual deficit remaining.
      5. Sphincter function. Usually the sphincters are not affected, but transient bladder paralysis may occur during the evolution of symptoms.
      6. Central nervous system involvement. Ordinarily, Guillain-Barré syndrome is thought of as a disease of the peripheral nervous system. Evidence of central nervous system involvement is controversial. In occasional patients, such findings as severe ataxia interpretable as cerebellar in origin, dysarthria, extensor plantar responses, and ill-defined sensory levels are demonstrable, and these need not exclude the diagnosis if other features are typical.
   B. Cerebrospinal fluid features strongly supportive of the diagnosis
      1. CSF protein. After the first week of symptoms, CSF protein is elevated or has been shown to rise on serial lumbar punctures.
      2. CSF cells. Counts of 10 or fewer mononuclear leukocytes/mm^3 in CSF.
      Variants
      1. No CSF protein rise in the period of 1 to 10 weeks after the onset of symptoms (rare).
      2. Counts of 11 to 50 mononuclear leukocytes/mm^3 of CSF.
   C. Electrodiagnostic features strongly supportive of the diagnosis
      Approximately 80% will have evidence of nerve conduction slowing or block at some point during the illness. Conduction velocity is usually less than 60% of normal, but the process is patchy and not all nerves are affected. Distal latencies may be increased to as much as three times normal. Use of F-wave responses often gives good indication of slowing over proximal portions of nerve trunks and roots. Up to 20% of patients will have normal conduction studies. Conduction studies may not become abnormal until several weeks into the illness.
III. Features Casting Doubt on the Diagnosis
   1. Marked, persistent asymmetry of weakness.
   2. Persistent bladder or bowel dysfunction.
   3. Bladder or bowel dysfunction at onset.
   4. More than 50 mononuclear leukocytes/mm^3 in CSF.
   5. Presence of polymorphonuclear leukocytes in CSF.
   6. Sharp sensory level.
IV. Features That Rule Out the Diagnosis
   1. A current history of hexacarbon abuse (volatile solvents; N-hexane and methyl N-butyl ketone. This includes huffing of paint lacquer vapors or addictive glue sniffing.
   2. Abnormal porphyrin metabolism indicating a diagnosis of acute intermittent porphyria. This would manifest as increased excretion of porphobilinogen and δ-aminolevulinic acid in the urine.
   3. A history or finding of recent diphtheritic infection, either faucial or wound, with or without myocarditis.
   4. Features clinically consistent with lead neuropathy (upper limb weakness with prominent wrist drop; may be asymmetric) and evidence of lead intoxication.
   5. The occurrence of a purely sensory syndrome.
   6. A definite diagnosis of a condition such as poliomyelitis, botulism, paralysis, or toxic neuropathy (e.g., from nitrofurantoin, dapsone, or organophosphorus compounds), which occasionally may be confused with Guillaim-Barré syndrome.

(Criteria for diagnosis of Guillain-Barré syndrome. *Ann Neurol* 1978;3:565)

deficit. Vigilant monitoring for incipient respiratory failure, in addition to intensive nursing care after generalized paralysis has supervened, is essential. Recognition and appropriate management of associated autonomic dysfunction (e.g., ileus, obstipation, bradycardia) are important. Prevention of complications common to all bedridden paralyzed patients such as pressure ulcers, compression neuropathies, tendon contractures, malnutrition, nosocomial pneumonias, urinary tract infections, and thromboembolism is essential to a good outcome. With the advent of modern intensive and respiratory care, the mortality for patients with GBS is now less than 5% in most centers.

PATHOGENESIS

The cause of GBS is unknown, although a growing body of evidence has implicated both humoral and cellular immune factors. In 50% to 75% of patients an infectious illness precedes onset of neurologic symptoms by several weeks; previous diarrheal illness occurs in 10% to 30% of patients (Table 136-3). Interestingly, a frequent association between preceding *C jejuni* (especially serotype Penner 019) infection and GBS has been reported.[1-3] Stool cultures at the onset of neurologic symptoms have yielded *C jejuni* in greater than 25% of cases and serology studies indicate recent *C jejuni* infection in 20% to 40% of patients. Sera from GBS patients following *C jejuni* infection have autoantibody to GM_1 ganglioside, an inhibitor of motoneuron excitability. Molecular mimicry between infectious agents and nerve tissue components may trigger an autoimmune attack on peripheral nerve myelin. In support of this hypothesis are anecdotal reports of GBS developing after administration of parenteral gangliosides. Examination of biopsied and postmortem neural tissue typically shows inflammatory lesions throughout the peripheral nervous system consisting of lymphocyte and macrophage invasion of the myelin sheaths with segmental demyelination. Although cranial nerve lesions are common, central nervous system demyelination has not been noted. Severe cases of GBS are associated with axonal disruption and wallerian degeneration. Electrodiagnostic studies that disclose evidence of primarily axonal destruction (e.g., fibrillations, positive sharp waves) predict a prolonged course with residual neurologic impairment.[4,5] Similar pathologic lesions have been noted in the autonomic nervous system and seem to correlate with the autonomic derangements that may complicate the clinical course.[6]

EPIDEMIOLOGY

Since the epidemic of GBS following the National Influenza Immunization Program of 1976, the annual reported incidence of GBS in the United States and Europe has been 0.4 to 1.7 per 100,000 population. The reported incidence is influenced by the diagnostic criteria adopted as well as by the thoroughness of case-finding. The disorder may occur at any age, with no discernible geographic or seasonal distributions. Most cases are sporadic, although infrequent clusters have been identified. A minor respiratory or gastrointestinal infection within the previous 8 weeks is typically present in approximately 65% of affected patients (Table 136-4). Approximately 30% of patients ultimately require mechanical ventilation for periods ranging from several weeks to over 1 year.[1] With meticulous intensive supportive care, the case-fatality rate has been reduced to approximately 5%. Over the last decade, new patient groups have been identified that may be predisposed to developing Guillain-Barré–like syndromes. These include patients with AIDS, in whom cytomegalovirus (CMV) may cause a polyradiculomyelitis

TABLE 136-3.   Factors Associated With Onset of Guillain-Barré Syndrome

---

Immunizations (e.g., swine flu vaccine 1976, *Haemophilus influenza* conjugate vaccine)
Infections
   Viruses (e.g., EBV, HIV-1, HSV-1, HSV-6, CMV, hepatitis A virus, rubella)
   Mycoplasma pneumoniae
   Camplylobacter jejuni (Penner serotype 019)
   Coxiella burnetii
Allogeneic bone marrow transplant
Solid-organ transplant
Pregnancy
Preexisting illnesses
   Hodgkin disease
   Lymphoma
   Systemic lupus erythematosus
Drugs
   Streptokinase
   Tacrolimus (FK506)

TABLE 136-4.   Experience With Guillain-Barré Syndrome at Massachusetts General Hospital (1962–1979)

VARIABLE	FINDING
Number of cases	157
Average age	39 years
Age range	8–81 years
Prior illness	Upper respiratory infection (approximately 70%)
Onset to maximal deficit and plateau	Average = 17 days 40% by first week 77% by second week 89% by third week
Mortality	1.25%
Respiratory failure requiring endotracheal intubation	29%
Average hospitalization	61 days
Average intubation	51 days
Residual deficit at 1 year	23% (severe in 8%)

Ropper AH: Management of Guillain-Barré syndrome. In Ropper AH, Kennedy SK, Zervas NT (eds): *Neurological and Neurosurgical Intensive Care*, pp 163–174. Baltimore, University Park Press, 1983

with characteristic findings on contrast MRI.[7-9] Additionally, patients with solid organ and bone marrow transplants may be at risk for CMV polyradiculomyelitis.

CLINICAL FEATURES

The clinical presentation of patients with GBS may be variable and may not always fit the typical case description (see Table 136-2). Initial symptoms are often sensory and consist of paresthesias, dysesthesias, and neuritic-type pain. Patients may initially be misdiagnosed as having conversion symptoms, somatization disorder, or hysteria. The onset of objective weakness and areflexia within hours to days should alert the clinician that one is not dealing with functional weakness. Symmetric weakness usually begins in the lower extremities and progresses to muscles of the trunk, diaphragm, arms, and facial muscles. Bilateral facial paresis eventually develops in more than 50% of patients. Proximal muscle weakness is typically more prominent than distal weakness. Involvement of bulbar muscles may impair swallowing and the ability to handle secretions. Autonomic demyelination results in marked lability of the blood pressure with rapid and unpredictable swings between hypertension and hypotension.[6]

Other autonomic manifestations of GBS are persistent facial flushing, urinary retention, tachyarrythmias, and bradyarrythmias. Neuropathic lesions in the afferent limb of the baroreceptor system may lead to SIADH and resultant hyponatremia. Extreme elevations in CSF protein (>1500 mg/dL) have been associated with symptoms of increased intracranial pressure and clinical papilledema. Occasionally patients have evidence of mild glomerulonephritis manifested as transient proteinuria, sometimes in the nephrotic range. In the typical case, maximum neurologic deficit is reached within 2 to 3 weeks followed by stabilization and gradual recovery over weeks to months.

Several clinical variants of GBS have been identified including ophthalmoplegia, ataxia, and areflexia (Miller-Fisher syndrome); "descending paralysis" with ocular, facial, and pharyngeal paresis occurring before limb paresis; almost pure respiratory muscle failure; and pure dysautonomic syndromes.

Occasionally patients seemingly recover from the acute paralysis and then suffer a relapse of paresis with a subsequent protracted course. Other patients may have a progressive course following the initial attack of GBS. These syndromes are referred to as chronic relapsing polyneuropathy and differ from acute demyelinating polyneuropathy in that the chronic form appears to be more responsive to corticosteroid therapy. The chronic relapsing syndrome has been associated with neurofibromatosis and HLA-Aw30 and HLA-Aw31.

DIAGNOSIS

Criteria to assist in the diagnosis of GBS are illustrated in Table 136-2. Recognition of a typical case is usually not difficult; however, patients may present with unusual features (e.g., focal weakness) that may confuse the initial diagnosis. The initial CSF protein may be normal for the first 7 to 10 days after onset of symptoms. Typical electrodiagnostic

abnormalities may likewise not be apparent shortly after onset of symptoms. In atypical cases, repeated lumbar puncture and electrodiagnostics should be combined with continued clinical observation before the diagnosis of GBS is accepted. Contrast-enhanced MRI shows lumbosacral roots and cauda equina and may have diagnostic utility, particularly in ruling out other disorders (e.g., transverse myelitis, cord compression).[8] In HIV-seropositive patients with demyelinating neuropathy, the mean CSF cell count was 23 cells/mm on average compared with fewer than 3 cells/mm of CSF in HIV-seronegative patients with GBS. Thus, in HIV-seropositive patients the variant has become the norm for CSF pleocytosis.[7] The clinical presentation of urinary retention, flaccid paraparesis, back or leg pain, and "saddle anesthesia" in a patient with AIDS should suggest the diagnosis of CMV polyradiculomyelitis. Diffuse enhancement of the cauda equina on postcontrast MRI is strongly supportive of this diagnosis.[9]

A number of diseases may superficially resemble GBS but can usually be excluded based on clinical criteria, CSF examination, electrodiagnostics, gadolinium-enhanced MRI, and laboratory evaluation (Table 136-5).

Laboratory tests that should be considered include an antinuclear antibody, serum cold agglutinins, serum protein electrophoresis, and serology for *M pneumoniae*, HIV, CMV, and *B burgdorferi*. Stool cultures for *C jejuni* should be obtained.

TREATMENT

The most immediate threat to life of the patient with GBS is respiratory failure from intercostal and diaphragmatic muscle paralysis. Patients often "look good" only to suffer precipitous respiratory arrest because of lack of appreciation of the extent of weakness. Arterial blood gas monitoring is worthwhile but it should be emphasized that hypoxemia and hypercapnea are late findings and indicate that respiratory arrest is imminent. Intubation should not be delayed until there is evidence of deteriorating blood gases. Respiratory

TABLE 136-5. Conditions That Resemble Guillain-Barré Syndrome

Lyme meningoradiculitis (*Borrelia burgdorferi*)
Cytomegalovirus polyradiculopathy (AIDS, posttransplant)
Critical illness polyneuropathy
Poliomyelitis
Botulism
Tick paralysis
Diphtheria
Myasthenia gravis
Spinal cord disease or compression (tumor, acute transverse myelitis)
Pontine infarction
Central pontine myelinolysis (severe hyponatremia)
Hyperkalemia or hypokalemia
Vasculitic neuropathy
Polymyositis
Toxic neuropathy (lead, dapsone, organophosphates)

reserve is best monitored by serial determinations of forced inspiratory vital capacity and negative inspiratory force at least every 2 hours until stabilization. Patients with rapidly declining vital capacity (or values less than 18 to 19 mL/kg) or cardiovascular manifestations should be observed in the CCU. Elective intubation should be performed when the vital capacity approaches 15 mL/kg (approximately 1 L in the average adult) or sooner if there is associated pharyngeal paresis and difficulty handling secretions. As the vital capacity drops farther, the ability to effectively cough and clear secretions is impaired; this results in atelectasis and ventilation-perfusion mismatch with resultant hypoxemia. Hypercapnea usually occurs after the appearance of hypoxemia when the bellows function of the diaphragm and intercostal muscles is lost. The use of succinylcholine to facilitate intubation is *contraindicated* because of the risk of hyperkalemia and cardiac arrest.[10,11]

The most common error in caring for GBS patients is failure to intubate a patient with marginally compensated ventilatory mechanics. Failure to intubate early in the course may result in the need for emergent intubation under suboptimal conditions, thereby causing unnecessary risk to the patient. After the patient is intubated, it is unnecessary to proceed to immediate tracheostomy. Some patients may experience recovery within several days to 2 weeks, thereby obviating the need for tracheostomy. If, after a period of 10 to 14 days, the patient shows no signs of imminent recovery, tracheostomy should be considered. On the other hand, if the patient has been steadily gaining strength, one might choose to wait an additional several days before proceeding with tracheostomy.

Meticulous attention to monitoring the patient and the ventilator is essential to prevent mechanical mishaps that may result in death of the patient. Ventilator alarms should be checked daily to ensure that they are working. Remember that a paralyzed patient with a tube through the vocal cords cannot call for help!

Frequent chest physiotherapy, tracheal suction, and kinetic beds may help reduce the risk of nosocomial pneumonia; however, the incidence of acquired pneumonia in GBS patients remains high and should be anticipated. Prophylactic antibiotics are not advised; when pulmonary infiltrates and fever develop, empiric antibiotic therapy should be started pending the results of Gram stains, cultures, and sensitivities. The initial choice of antibiotics should be based on the likely pathogens and sensitivity patterns unique to the particular hospital.

Frequent turning (every 2 hours) or use of a kinetic bed decreases the risk of skin breakdown and decubitus ulcer formation. Attention should be paid to limb positioning to avoid compressive neuropathies, particularly around the ulnar and peroneal nerves. Physical therapy should be initiated to prevent contractures, footdrop, and muscle atrophy.

Autonomic dysfunction usually responds to the appropriate pharmacologic agents (e.g., use of beta-blockers for persistent tachycardia associated with hypertension). The development of asystole or advanced degrees of heart block may require emergent insertion of a temporary transvenous pacemaker.

Hyponatremia from SIADH is usually manageable by free water restriction.

Neuritic pain in the limbs and back is common and may respond to quinine or tricyclic antidepressants. Narcotics may occasionally be required to obtain adequate analgesia.

Adequate nutrition must be maintained to avoid a catabolic state and help reduce the risk of infection. Sufficient calories can usually be given by the enteral route using a small nasogastric feeding tube. Occasionally, autonomic derangements are of sufficient severity to result in ileus and inability to effectively use the gastrointestinal tract for feeding. Parenteral nutrition may initially be started through a peripheral vein; if gastrointestinal dysfunction is persistent, long-term central hyperalimentation should be used.

Lower extremity thromboembolism and pulmonary embolism are significant risks in the bedridden, paralyzed patient. Additionally, anticardiolipin antibody has been reported in patients with GBS, which may further increase the risk of thrombosis. Compressive pneumatic boots have been advocated but may result in pressure neuropathy of the peroneal nerve as it crosses the fibula head. Since pulmonary emboli have occurred in some patients treated with fixed-dose subcutaneous heparin, it may be preferable to use adjusted-dose subcutaneous heparin (i.e., adjusting the dose to maintain a 6-hour postdose partial thromboplastin time [PTT] in the upper 5 seconds of control). Although FDA-approved only for prevention of deep vein thrombosis after hip replacement surgery, low-molecular-weight heparin (e.g., enoxaparin 30 mg twice daily) is less likely to cause heparin-induced thrombocytopenia and associated thrombotic complications compared with unfractionated heparins.[12] Additional advantages include the absence of a requirement for daily anticoagulant monitoring and a greater therapeutic index (less risk of bleeding for a given antithrombotic effect). Alternatively, warfarin sodium may be used to maintain an international normalized ratio (INR) 1.25 to 1.5. Since the above regimens may still not be sufficient to prevent deep vein thrombosis from occurring, it is my practice to obtain periodic (every 7 to 10 days) bilateral lower extremity compression–Doppler ultrasound studies to monitor for deep vein thrombosis in these high-risk immobilized patients.[13]

Plasmapheresis or IVIg are the specific treatments of choice for GBS. Controlled studies have clearly demonstrated that both modalities reduce the time it takes to achieve independent walking, ventilator days, and long-term neurologic deficit.[14-16] The type of replacement fluid (e.g., fresh frozen plasma versus albumin) used during plasmapheresis does not appear to make a difference in outcome.[17] In hospitals in which plasmapheresis machines are not available, similar improvement of patients has been observed using exchange transfusions. With this technique, a unit of whole blood is removed and centrifuged to remove the plasma. Fresh pooled plasma is then added back to the patient's cells, and the reconstituted blood is returned to the patient.

Corticosteroid therapy (e.g., prednisone) has not been convincingly shown to alter the course of GBS. A controlled study on the use of high-dose intravenous methylprednisolone with or without plasmapheresis given early in the course of GBS showed no significant benefit from steroid treatment.[18]

IVIg therapy appears at least as effective as plasmapheresis and may be superior.[19] A recent multicenter randomized trial comparing IVIg (0.4 g/kg/day for five doses) with plasma exchange (200 to 250 mL/kg in five sessions over 7 to 14 days) showed more significant strength improvement (34% with plasma exchange versus 53% with IVIg) and shorter time to improvement (41 days with plasma exchange versus 27 days with IVIg). IVIg may have important practical advantages over plasmapheresis, since it is available in more hospitals and can be administered without delay. Ten percent to 20% of patients demonstrate treatment-related fluctuations in strength or late relapse after either plasmapheresis or IVIg. If symptoms are mild, watchful waiting may be appropriate. Significant losses of strength may respond to additional courses of IVIg or plasmapheresis.[20]

A careful search for infectious diseases that can mimic idiopathic GBS is important since a specific treatment may be available. CMV polyradiculoneuropathy in transplant or HIV-infected patients may respond to specific therapy with ganciclovir and CMV immune globulin (CytoGam). Polyradiculitis associated with Epstein-Barr virus, herpes simplex, and herpes zoster virus may respond to specific therapy with acyclovir. Lyme meningoradiculitis has been treated successfully with ceftriaxone and IVIg. Depression and psychological aberrations related to the "locked-in syndrome" are common and should be anticipated. Speaking tracheostomy tubes (Portex "talk" tube) may be an excellent adjunct to the ventilator-dependent patient's emotional well-being.[21]

Althought the outlook for recovery is generally favorable, mortality from GBS is 3% to 8% occurring primarily from sepsis, pulmonary embolism, adult respiratory distress syndrome, or rare cases of cardiac arrest. Permanent disabling weakness or sensory loss occurs in 7% to 10% of survivors with 50% to 65% having persistent mild neurologic deficits (e.g., footdrop, distal sensory loss, mild weakness). An optimistic and empathic attitude on the part of the physician, nursing, and rehabilitation staff is essential.

MYASTHENIA GRAVIS

ESSENTIAL DIAGNOSTIC TESTS AND PROCEDURES

1. Patients who have or are suspected of having myasthenia gravis and are experiencing increasing weakness should have inspiratory pressures and FVC measured. An FVC less than 20 mL/kg in a patient with progressive weakness warrants admission to the CCU for close monitoring.
2. An edrophonium (Tensilon) test may demonstrate objective improvement in strength, confirming a myasthenic crisis. Lack of improvement suggests an alternative diagnosis (or possible cholinergic crisis if the patient is already on anticholinesterase medication).
3. Electromyography (EMG) using repetitive low-frequency nerve stimulation (3 Hz/second) demonstrates characteristic progressive decrement (more than 15%) in muscle action potential amplitude.

4. Anti-acetycholine receptor antibodies (anti-AChRabs) are measurable in 85% of generalized myasthenia and 65% of limited myasthenia patients.
5. Infection (e.g., pneumonia) and drugs are common precipitants of myasthenic crisis.
6. Patients with newly diagnosed myasthenia gravis should have a chest computed tomography (CT) scan to evaluate for thymoma.
7. Associated thyroid disease (hypo- or hyperthyroidism) is present in up to 8% of myasthenics.

INITIAL THERAPY

1. Intubation and mechanical ventilation is required if the patient shows decreasing FVC or inspiratory pressure (FVC <15 mL/kg).
2. If myasthenic crisis requiring intubation occurs, an anticholinesterase drug "holiday" for 48 to 72 hours is recommended, followed by oral retitration of pyridostigmine. Neostigmine may be given parenterally at an approximate ratio of 1 mg for every 60 mg of pyridostigmine.
3. Plasma exchange is indicated for myasthenic crisis and as preoperative therapy for thymectomy (or other major surgery). IVIg and pulse methylprednisolone therapy may also be effective for severe cases.
4. Chronic therapy includes thymectomy and chronic immunosuppressive therapy (e.g., corticosteroids, azathioprine, cyclosporine), which may predispose to opportunistic infections.

CAPSULE

Myasthenia gravis (MG) is an autoimmune neuromuscular disorder characterized by fatigability and weakness of skeletal muscles resulting from decreased availability of acetylcholine receptors in the postsynaptic membrane. The disorder most frequently presents with involvement of the extraocular muscles leading to complaints of diplopia and ptosis. Severe cases may have generalized progression with involvement of the muscles of respiration and swallowing—the *myasthenic crisis*, which requires rapid diagnosis and intensive respiratory and supportive care. Excessive dosage of anticholinesterase medications may also lead to exacerbation of generalized weakness, which can result in respiratory compromise. Differentiation between myasthenic crisis and cholinergic crisis can usually be made from a carefully taken history and physical examination, although performance of a low-dose edrophonium (Tensilon) test may be needed to confirm the clinical suspicion. Diagnosis of the typical case is based on a history of fatigability of skeletal muscles with repetitive use, particularly if the extraocular muscles are involved. Physical examination demonstrates muscle fatigue with prolonged repetitive effort. The clinical impression of MG is confirmed by results of an edrophonium test, repetitive nerve stimulation, and assay for anti-AChRab. Treatment of mild cases of MG consists of anticholinesterase medications (e.g., pyridostigmine) and prednisone. Severe cases with generalized involvement are treated with thymectomy, immunosuppressives (e.g., azothioprine, cyclosporine), plasmapheresis, and

IVIg. With improved management of the disorder, the incidence of myasthenic crisis requiring intensive care and mechanical ventilation has decreased in recent years. Of particular importance to the intensivist is the perioperative management of the myasthenic patient undergoing thymectomy or other surgical procedures.

EPIDEMIOLOGY

MG is an uncommon disease with a prevalence of 50 to 125 cases per million population. Age of peak onset differs markedly between the sexes with women mostly afflicted in young adulthood (third to fourth decades) and men afflicted later in life, during the sixth and seventh decades. Undetermined genetic factors may play a role in the pathogenesis of MG. There is an increased incidence of HLA-B8 and DRw3 in young females with MG and thymic hyperplasia. In contrast to nonaffected infants born to mothers with GBS, transient neonatal weakness has been noted in 10% to 20% of infants born to mothers with MG. The occurrence of neonatal weakness does not correlate with the severity of the mother's illness or the titer of anti-AChRab.

Pathogenesis

The essential feature that leads to the skeletal muscle weakness of patients with MG is decreased transmission across the neuromuscular junction because of a decreased number of acetylcholine receptors on the postsynaptic membrane.[22] The normal acetylcholine receptor of skeletal muscle is composed of four subunits arranged in a rosette around a cation channel. Acetylcholine released from the presynaptic terminal into the neuromuscular junction attaches to subunits of the acetylcholine receptor rosette resulting in opening of the cation channel. A flux of cations enters the open channel resulting in depolarization of the muscle cell membrane and subsequent muscle contraction. Patients with MG appear to develop one or more antibodies to subunits of the acetylcholine receptor (anti-AChRab). Anti-AChRabs have been found in approximately 85% of patients with generalized MG and in 65% of those with myasthenia confined to the extraocular muscles alone. Although the precise mechanisms remain uncertain, it appears as though these antibodies decrease the number of functional acetylcholine receptors. The serum level of anti-AChRab does not correspond with the severity of the clinical illness. However, the functional ability of anti-AChRab to accelerate degradation or block acetylcholine receptors closely correlates with clinical severity.[23,24]

Seventy-five percent of myasthenic patients have abnormalities of the thymus gland. Of these, approximately 85% have germinal cell hyperplasia (typically young females), whereas the remaining 15% have gross or microscopic thymomas (typically elderly males). Although the relationship of thymic abnormalities to the etiology of the disease is uncertain, thymectomy has become an accepted form of therapy for adolescents past the age of puberty and adults up to 60 years old with generalized disease. Patients with limited ocular MG, children, and elderly patients represent more controversial treatment groups. Thymectomy may be

expected to produce clinical remission or significant improvement in up to 70% of patients, although benefit may not be apparent for 1 year or more. Initiating factors that trigger B lymphocytes to produce anti-AChRabs and the precise role that the thymus gland plays in the pathogenesis of the disease remain to be elucidated.

A number of other autoimmune diseases have been associated with MG, particularly thyroid disease, which may be present in up to 10% of myasthenic patients. The incidence of rheumatoid arthritis, systemic lupus erythematosus, and pernicious anemia also appears to be increased in myasthenic patients. Numerous autoantibodies including antinuclear antibodies, antiparietal cell antibodies, and antithyroglobulin antibodies may be found in myasthenic serum. Antibodies to striated muscle have been particularly associated with thymoma.

The autoimmune nature of chronic graft-versus-host disease, which develops in up to 30% of long-term survivors following allogeneic bone marrow transplant, may predispose to the formation of antibodies to acetylcholine receptors and the subsequent development of clinical MG in this patient population.[25]

Penicillamine, a drug commonly used to treat rheumatoid arthritis and Wilson disease, has been associated with the development of clinical myasthenia and formation of anti-AChRabs. Withdrawal of the drug results in clinical improvement of weakness and decreased titers of anti-AChRab.

CLINICAL FEATURES

The dominant feature of MG is progressive weakness of muscles when used repetitively, and partial recovery following a period of rest. The disease usually develops insidiously over a period of weeks to months, although explosive onset with rapid generalized weakness is sometimes seen. Initial bouts of weakness are transient and may resolve with a good night's rest. Unilateral or bilateral ptosis with diplopia are common complaints, reflecting predominant involvement of the extraocular muscles. Up to 20% of patients have disease confined to the eye muscles and are said to have "ocular myasthenia" (Table 136-6).

Any weakness of muscle groups in addition to the extraocular muscles is referred to as *generalized myasthenia*. If generalized progression does not occur within several years, it is unlikely to occur at all.

Involvement of bulbar muscles may manifest as weakness of the jaw muscles while chewing food with inability to retract the corners of the mouth leading to a peculiar transverse, snarling smile ("myasthenic facies"). Weakness of the pharyngeal and laryngeal muscles may cause a nasal, garbled-sounding voice with reduced volume on prolonged talking. Regurgitation of swallowed liquids through the nose may be reported by the patient. Involvement of the arm, leg, and trunk muscles may occur asymmetrically in any combination. Typically, proximal muscle weakness is more prevalent than distal weakness. Weakness may not be apparent in the well-rested patient, but can usually be elicited with repetitive exercise (ptosis developing with sustained upward gaze). Patients with extensive involvement may be weak even at

TABLE 136-6. Clinical Stages of Myasthenia Gravis

Stage 1	Eyelid or ocular muscle involvement only (15%–20% of patients); patients rarely have crises requiring intensive care.
Stage 2A	Mild generalized myasthenia in addition to ocular and bulbar involvement (25% of patients); usually managed with anticholinesterase medications; patients may occasionally experience acute worsening.
Stage 2B	Moderately severe disease involving ocular, bulbar, and limb muscles (30% of patients); crisis not uncommon; thymectomy often performed if patient is between 15 and 50 years old.
Stage 3	Acute, fulminating myasthenia evolving over days to weeks (10% of patients); patients require early respiratory support; thymoma is commonly associated.
Stage 4	Chronic, severe weakness of long duration; treatment measures are unsuccessful or response is partial.

Note: Patients in stages 2B, 3, and 4 often require intensive care during the course of their illness.

rest. Muscle atrophy is rare but can occasionally be seen in older myasthenic patients.

The remainder of the physical examination is usually normal. A number of factors may lead to an exacerbation of weakness and precipitation of myasthenic crisis (Tables 136-7 and 136-8).

DIAGNOSIS

Confirmation of the clinical diagnosis of MG is aided by performance of the edrophonium (Tensilon) test and by repetitive nerve stimulation. Edrophonium is a short-acting acetylcholinesterase inhibitor that allows a buildup of acetylcholine in the neuromuscular junction, thereby improving motor strength in the myasthenic patient. Before administration of edrophonium, baseline testing of muscle strength is performed. Edrophonium (10 mg/1 mL ampule) is withdrawn into a syringe and 2 mg is administered through a previously established intravenous catheter. Muscle strength is retested after approximately 30 seconds with particular attention to respiratory function (measuring vital capacity or negative inspiratory force), swallowing, extremity strength (dynamometry), and oculomotor function. If no improvement in strength occurs, the remaining 8 mg is injected. A definite improvement in strength that occurs within 1 minute and lasts several minutes strongly supports a diagnosis of MG. If functional weakness is a possibility, the test should also be performed using an injectable saline control. Pretreatment with atropine (0.5 to 1.0 mg) may help block distressing muscarinic side effects. Occasionally patients with myasthenia may show an ambiguous response to edrophonium, particularly patients with limited ocular myasthenia.

EMG using repetitive low-frequency nerve stimulation (3 Hz/second) demonstrates characteristic progressive decrement (more than 15%) in muscle action potential amplitude. Diagnosis is enhanced if weak muscles or several proxi-

TABLE 136-7. Factors That May Precipitate Crisis in Myasthenia Gravis

Infection (especially respiratory)
Drugs (procainamide, aminoglycosides)
Excessive anticholinesterase dosage ("cholinergic crisis")
Hyperthyroidism
Initiation of steroid therapy
Iodinated contrast agents
Pulmonary embolism
Environmental heat stress
Surgery
Menstruation
Immunizations
Emotional distress

mal muscles are tested. Single-fiber EMG may increase sensitivity in making the diagnosis in difficult cases.

Anti-AChRab testing is specific for MG but detectable in only 85% of patients with generalized MG.

Routine chest radiographs may disclose evidence of macroscopic thymoma. Chest CT scan or MRI improves the detection rate of thymoma and should be done in all newly diagnosed patients. Radioisotope scanning with gallium 67 (^{67}Ga) has been reported to give good imaging of thymomas and may be particularly valuable in detecting recurrences of malignant thymoma following surgery.

Thyroid function tests should be obtained because up to 8% of MG patients may have associated hyperthyroidism. A tuberculin test should be obtained in all patients in anticipation of the need for chronic immunosuppressive therapy.

In patients with generalized MG, careful assessment of respiratory muscle strength and fatigue (e.g., maximum expiratory and inspiratory pressures, maximum voluntary ventilation and FVC) should be obtained as a baseline for comparison if subsequent exacerbations occur.

TREATMENT

Persons affected with myasthenia gravis who complain of dyspnea or difficulty in swallowing should be admitted to the hospital immediately. Rapid assessment of respiratory function should be carried out. If vital capacity is less than 15 to 18 mL/kg (or negative inspiratory pressure is <40 cm H_2O), the patient should be admitted to an ICU for close observation and possible elective intubation (Table 136-9).

TABLE 136-8. Drugs That May Worsen Myasthenia Gravis

Aminoglycoside antibiotics
Tetracyclines
Colistin
Morphine
Procainamide
Quinidine
Quinine
Lithium carbonate
D-Tubocurarine

TABLE 136-9.   Indications for Intubation in Myasthenia Gravis

---

Respiratory rate > 30/min
Vital capacity < 15 mL/kg
Negative inspiratory pressure ≤ 30 cm H_2O
Inability to handle oral secretions
Progressive dyspnea despite anticholinesterase medications
Increasing $PaCO_2$ (indicates respiratory arrest is imminent)

Weakened facial muscles may make using the Wright spirometer difficult, in which case a negative inspiratory force is a better parameter to follow. One should not delay intubation if the patient has marginal respiratory compensation. It is better to perform a timely elective intubation because patients can abruptly fatigue and suffer respiratory arrest or mucus plugging from voluminous secretions.[26]

A careful search for infection (especially pneumonia) is mandatory because these patients are frequently on immunosuppressive therapy. However, even myasthenic patients not on immunosuppressives appear to be at increased risk of infection because of difficulty handling secretions and poor pulmonary toilet from weakened respiratory muscles. A common mistake is to delay initiation of antibiotics too long or to miss a seemingly trivial infection that may have precipitated the crisis. Although aminoglycosides may produce mild neuromuscular blockade and weakness, if required because of the source of infection (or sensitivity reports), they may be used.

Patients with respiratory failure should have a clear airway maintained with repeated gentle suction, postural drainage, and periodic inflations with intermittent positive-pressure breathing to prevent segmental atelectasis and hypostatic pneumonia. Repeated incentive spirometry may cause respiratory muscle fatigue and should be avoided. If intubaton and mechanical ventilation is required, anticholinesterase drugs should be withdrawn for 48 to 72 hours. The ventilator should be set up with the goal of minimizing the patient's work of breathing and allowing "rest" of the neuromuscular junction (e.g., assist-control mode, flow triggering during inspiratory phase, adequate inspiratory flow rate and tidal volume; see Chapter 48 for a full discussion on the application of mechanical ventilation). Anticholinesterase therapy can be reintroduced in small doses by nasogastric tube, starting with 30 to 60 mg of pyridostigmine every 8 hours (maximum dose, 120 mg by mouth every 4 hours), until bowel function is restored.

Plasmapheresis is indicated for myasthenic patients in crisis, especially in conjunction with the initiation of immunosuppressive therapy with corticosteroids or azothioprine.[22] Plasmapheresis is also useful in preparing patients for thymectomy or other elective surgery (especially if the vital capacity is less than 2 L), and as an adjunct to initiating immunosuppressive therapy to effect more rapid improvement. A typical approach is to perform five exchanges of 3 to 4 L each over 14 days. Typically the response to plasmapheresis occurs within days; however, the improvement wanes within a few weeks. Refractory cases have also been treated with IVIg (400 mg/kg daily for 5 days) with favorable outcome.[27] The use of pulse therapy with high-dose methylprednisolone (2 g infused intravenously over 12 hours repeated at 5-day intervals for a total of two or three doses) may also be of benefit for severe myasthenic patients in crisis.[28] Pulse therapy appears to produce less initial worsening and more rapid improvement in severe myasthenic patients than conventional doses of prednisone.

If elective surgery is required in a myasthenic patient, oral anticholinesterase medication may be stopped and the equivalent dose given by intravenous (IV) infusion (1 mg IV neostigmine equivalent to 60 mg of oral pyridostigmine). The amount of neostigmine required should be infused over the time interval that approximates the oral dosing interval (pyridostigmine 60 mg by mouth every 4 hours may be given as neostigmine 1 mg IV infusion over each 4 hours). The immediate postoperative requirement for anticholinesterase medication may be reduced for several days (especially following thymectomy); therefore, a dose reduction to approximately 75% of the preoperative dose should be considered. Intravenous methylprednisolone may be substituted for oral prednisone in a dose equivalent to the "on" day if the patient has been on alternate-day steroids. A preoperative course of plasmapheresis using the above regimen should be considered in patients with residual weakness or reduced vital capacity. Nondepolarizing muscle relaxants should be avoided if possible during anesthesia. If it is necessary to use nondepolarizing muscle relaxants intraoperatively, small amounts (one third of the normal dose) of a short-acting drug (e.g., atracurium or vecuronium) should be used.[29,30] Patients in apparent clinical remission can have prolonged paralysis after administration of nondepolarizing agents.

Neonatal myasthenia occurs in up to 20% of infants born to myasthenic mothers. The incidence is unrelated to the severity of the mother's illness or the titer of anti-AChRabs. Neonatal MG is usually manifested by weakness of sucking and crying, impaired swallowing, and impaired respiration. Occasionally, generalized weakness is noted. Neostigmine, 0.05 to 0.1 mg every 3 to 4 hours by constant infusion pump usually results in clinical improvement and should be continued until strength improves. Pyridostigmine syrup can be substituted when oral medications can be taken.

SUMMARY ■

Patients with respiratory failure resulting from neuromuscular disorders can be effectively managed by serial monitoring of respiratory muscle strength and timely provision of mechanical ventilation when indicated. The goal of ventilator support in these patients is to provide respiratory muscle rest while supportive and specific treatment (if available) is given for the underlying disease (e.g., plasmapheresis for GBS). For diseases in which no specific therapy is available (muscular dystrophies) or in which residual respiratory muscle weakness prevents complete weaning from mechanical ventilation, the use of home mechanical ventilation may be a viable option in carefully selected patients. The use of intermittent positive-pressure ventilation with a nasal mask has recently offered selected patients with chronic neuromuscular failure an option for home ventilation without the requirement for tracheostomy.[31]

REFERENCES ■

1. Ropper AH: The Guillain-Barré syndrome. *N Engl J Med* 1992;326:1130
2. Mishu B, Ilyas A, Koski C, et al: Serologic evidence of previous *Camplylobacter jejuni* infection in patients with Guillain-Barré syndrome. *Ann Intern Med* 1993;118:947
3. von Wulffen H, Hartard C, Scharein E: Seroreactivity to *Camplylobacter jejuni* and gangliosides in patients with Guillain-Barré syndrome. *J Infect Dis* 1994;170:828
4. Ropper AH, Wijdicks EFM, Shahani BT: Electrodiagnostic abnormalities in 113 patients with Guillain-Barré syndrome. *Arch Neurol* 1990;47:881
5. Ropper AH: Severe acute Guillain-Barré syndrome. *Neurology* 1986;36:429
6. Zochodne DW: Autonomic involvement in Guillain-Barré syndrome: a review. *Muscle Nerve* 1994;17:1145
7. Simpson DM, Tagliati M: Neurologic manifestations of HIV infection. *Ann Intern Med* 1994;121:769
8. Bertorini T, Halford H, Lawrence J, Wassef M: Contrast-enhanced magnetic resonance imaging of the lumbosacral roots in the dysimmune inflammatory polyneuropathies. *J Neuroimaging* 1995;5:9
9. Whiteman ML, Dandapani BK, Shebert RT, Post MJ: MRI of AIDS-related polyradiculomyelitis. *J Comput Assist Tomog* 1994;18:7
10. Reilly M, Hutchinson M: Suxamethonium is contraindicated in the Guillain-Barré syndrome. [Letter]. *J Neurol Neurosurg Psychiatry* 1991;54:1018
11. Dalman JE, Verhagen WI: Cardiac arrest in Guillain-Barré syndrome and the use of suxamethonium. *Acta Neurol Belg* 1994;94:259
12. Warkentin TE, Levine MN, Hirsh J, et al: Heparin-induced thrombocytopenia in patients treated with low-molecular-weight heparin or unfractionated heparin. *N Engl J Med* 1995;332:1330
13. Rosenow EC: Venous and pulmonary thromboembolism: an algorithmic approach to diagnosis and management. *Mayo Clin Proc* 1995;70:45
14. The Guillain-Barré Syndrome Study Group: Plasmapheresis and acute Guillain-Barré syndrome. *Neurology* 1985;35:1096
15. Osterman PO, Lundemo G, Pirskanen R, et al: Beneficial effects of plasma exchange in acute inflammatory polyradiculopathy. *Lancet* 1984;2:1296
16. Dyck PJ, Kurtzke JF: Plasmapheresis in Guillain-Barré syndrome. *Neurology* 1985;35:1105
17. French Cooperative Group on Plasma Exchange in Guillain-Barré syndrome: efficiency of plasma exchange in Guillain-Barré syndrome: role of replacement fluids. *Ann Neurol* 1987;22:753
18. Guillain-Barré Syndrome Steroid Trial Group: Double-blind trial of intravenous methylprednisolone in Guillain-Barré syndrome. *Lancet* 1993;341:586
19. van der Meche FGA, Schmitz PIM: A randomized trial comparing intravenous immune globulin and plasma exchange in Guillain-Barré syndrome. *N Engl J Med* 1992;326:1123
20. Kleyweg RP, Van der Meche FGA: Treatment related fluctuations in Guillain-Barré syndrome after high-dose immunoglobulins or plasma exchange. *J Neurol Neurosurg Psychiatry* 1991;54:957
21. Leder SB: Importance of verbal communication for the ventilator-dependent patient. *Chest* 1990;98:792
22. Drachman DB: Myasthenia gravis. *N Engl J Med* 1994;330:1797
23. Drachman DB, Adams RN, Josifek LF, et al: Functional activities of autoantibodies to acetylcholine receptors and the clinical severity of myasthenia gravis. *N Engl J Med* 1982;307:769
24. Linton DM, Philcox D: Myasthenia gravis. *Dis Mon* 1990;36:559
25. Bolger GB, Sullivan KM, Spence AM, et al: Myasthenia gravis after allogeneic bone marrow transplantation: relationship to chronic graft-versus-host disease. *Neurology* 1986;36:1087
26. Bennet DA, Bleck TP: Recognizing impending respiratory failure from neuromuscular causes. *J Crit Illness* 1988;3:46
27. Arsura EL, Bick A, Brunner NG, et al: High-dose intravenous immunoglobulin in the management of myasthenia gravis. *Arch Intern Med* 1986;146:1365
28. Arsura EL, Brunner NG, Namba T, et al: High-dose intravenous methylprednisolone in myasthenia gravis. *Arch Neurol* 1985;42:1149
29. Macdonald AM, Keen RI, Pugh ND: Myasthenia gravis and atracurium. *Br J Anaesth* 1984;56:651
30. Redfern N, McQuillan PJ, Conacher ID, et al: Anaesthesia for trans-sternal thymectomy in myasthenia gravis. *Ann R Coll Surg Engl* 1987;69:289.
31. Meyer TJ, Hill NS: Noninvasive positive pressure ventilation to treat respiratory failure. *Ann Intern Med* 1994;120:760

Critical Care, Third Edition, edited by Joseph M. Civetta,
Robert W. Taylor, and Robert R. Kirby.
Lippincott-Raven Publishers, Philadelphia, PA © 1997.

CHAPTER 137

■

Behavioral Disturbances

Michael G. Wise
Ned H. Cassem

IMMEDIATE CONCERNS ■

MAJOR PROBLEMS

This chapter provides a road map to the evaluation and treatment of behavioral disturbances in the intensive care unit (ICU). If the guidelines are followed (Fig. 137-1), the reasons for many, if not most, behavioral disturbances in hospitalized patients are identifiable and specific treatment is possible. However, behavioral disturbances (e.g., agitation, confusion) are not specific diagnoses; rather, these are behavioral manifestations of an underlying problem, and a thoughtful evaluation is necessary to define their cause.

Behavioral disturbances occur commonly in individuals who are seriously ill. For example, the prevalence of delirium on acute medical and surgical wards ranges from 11% to 16%, and the incidence of delirium (i.e., new cases that develop during hospitalization) ranges from 4% to 31%.[1] The prevalence of delirium increases in elderly patients, patients with central nervous system disorders (e.g., Alzheimer's dementia, Parkinson's disease, human immunodeficiency virus infection), patients who have undergone surgery (e.g., cardiotomy), patients with severe burns, and patients who are in drug withdrawal, especially from alcohol or sedative-hypnotics.[2] Other behavioral disorders result from a critically ill patient's fear, anxiety, denial, anger, depression, dependency, and personality and are encountered daily by physicians and critical care nurses (see Fig. 137-1).

Regardless of the clinician's expertise, psychiatric consultation is often needed for patients who are critically ill. Physicians should look for a psychiatrist with sound medical skills; that is, he or she should use a mental status examination and a physical, especially a basic neurologic, examination. Most good medical training programs give graduates these basic skills. From the medical graduates who choose

psychiatry, those who love medicine and relish the challenge of diagnosis and treatment make the best consultants.[3] They are able to integrate the current physiologic state of the patient with the psychosocial aspects of the situation.

The consulting psychiatrist must also be able to communicate information in a clear, concise fashion to the requesting physician. Psychiatric jargon is not appropriate in this process. In addition, the psychiatrist must follow the patient until the problem is under control or resolved and, if necessary, arrange psychiatric care for the patient after discharge.

STRESS POINTS

1. If faced with a patient who has a behavioral disturbance, the first question is whether the patient has evidence of cognitive dysfunction. In other words, does the patient have evidence of delirium (acute brain dysfunction), dementia (chronic brain dysfunction), or both? This determination is a crucial point in the evaluation (see Fig. 137-1).
2. If a delirium or acute confusional state is present, the focus of the differential diagnosis becomes the medical disorder or substance that is causing the problem.
3. The importance of discovering and correcting the underlying cause of delirium cannot be overemphasized.
4. If cognitive impairment (delirium) is not present, the clinician can take an alternative approach to the patient's behavioral difficulties (see Fig. 137-1).
5. Two lines of investigation are likely to illuminate the cause of the behavioral problem. These are examination of the patient's underlying areas of concern (most often unrealistic expectations about the illness) and thorough review of the patient's medications to ensure that the behavioral disturbances are not drug-induced side effects.

2017

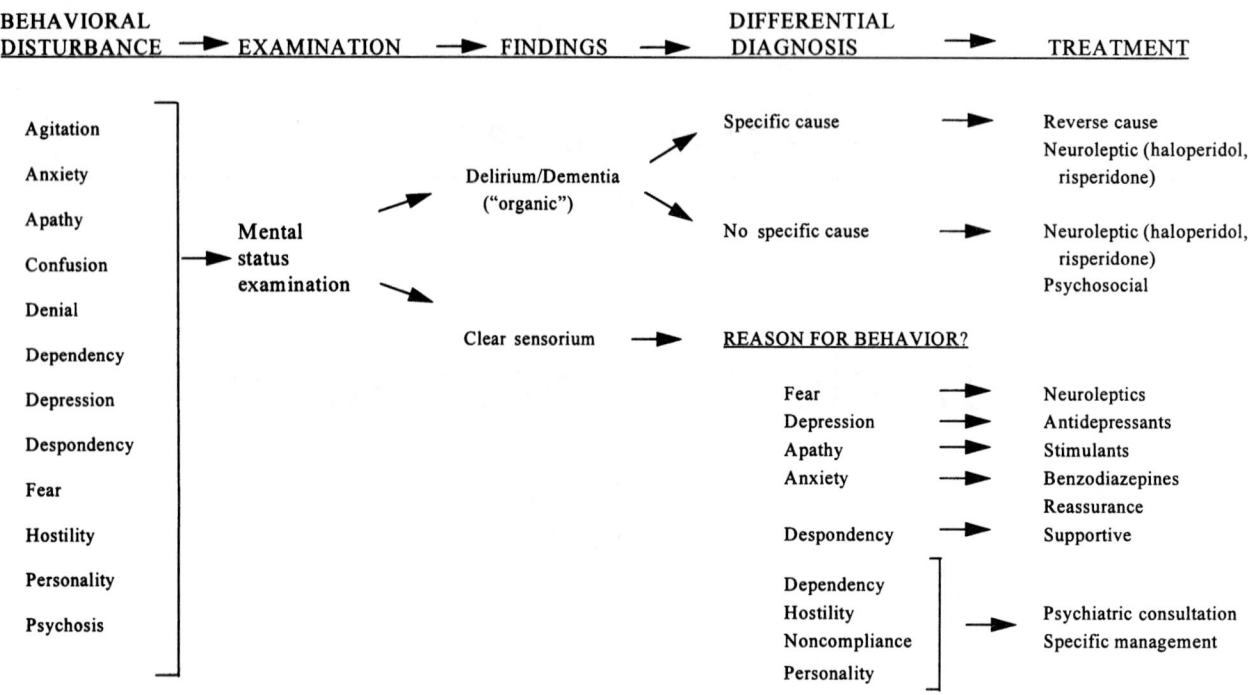

FIGURE 137-1. Overview of the evaluation and treatment of behavioral disturbances in the ICU.

INITIAL DIAGNOSIS, TESTING, AND THERAPY

1. Testing mental status for cognitive dysfunction is not difficult. Folstein's Mini-Mental State (MMS) examination[4] (Fig. 137-2) provides a good, rapid screening tool for organicity and is also used to follow the patient's clinical course serially. The disadvantage of the MMS is that it is insensitive and cannot detect patients who have mild but significant brain dysfunction or individuals who have nondominant brain disease.

2. The MMS examination tests for orientation, memory, attention, dysgraphia, and constructional apraxia. Out of a total score of 30, a score of 0 to 10 indicates severe cognitive impairment, 11 to 20 moderate impairment, 21 to 25 mild impairment, and 26 to 30 questionable impairment or intact function.

3. Delirium and dementia are not the only possible reasons for a low score on the MMS examination. Other causes include deafness, blindness, mutism, inability to understand English, aphasia, mental retardation, an educational level less than eighth grade, and deliberate lack of cooperation.

4. The clinical history helps to separate patients who have delirium from those who have dementia (Table 137-1). A clinical history of chronicity, found in the demented patient, should be distinguished from the acute presentation found in the delirious patient.

5. Demented patients have a lower threshold for developing delirium; therefore, both disorders can appear in the same patient. If they occur simultaneously, treatment of delirium improves the patient's behavior.

6. The electroencephalogram (EEG) is diagnostically helpful in difficult cases. Delirium is a clinical manifestation of global cerebral dysfunction. The EEG char-

acteristically, but not always, shows global cerebral slowing. A low-voltage, fast-activity pattern, as in delirium tremens, also can be present.[5] Pro and Wells reported that EEG changes virtually always accompany delirium.[6]

7. In the delirious patient, the EEG findings appear worse than those of the mental status examination; conversely, the mental status examination of the demented patient is usually much worse than predicted from simple review of the EEG.

8. Haloperidol is the drug of choice for treatment of delirium. Other potentially useful drugs include thiothixine, droperidol, thioridazine, and chlorpromazine. Close observation and orientation to time and place are important adjunctive measures.

DIAGNOSIS AND CLINICAL FEATURES OF A DELIRIUM ■

Numerous terms are used by clinicians to label a patient who has a delirium. These include acute brain failure, acute confusion state, acute organic brain syndrome, acute encephalopathy, and so on. The pseudodiagnostic term "ICU psychosis" is sometimes used. This label implies a cause-and-effect relation between the ICU setting and delirium, hinting that the problem naturally follows or is expected if a patient is critically ill and therefore can be ignored.

The evidence for such an relation is flimsy. There is no such diagnosis as ICU fever or ICU arrhythmia. The brain's highly complex, multifactorial reaction to metabolic, anoxic, toxic, and infectious insults is delirium. Delirium is the tangible sign of cerebral insufficiency, just as angina is the ordi-

Patient_____

Examiner_____

Date_____

"MINI-MENTAL STATE"

Maxi-mum score	Score	
		Orientation
5	( )	What is the (year) (day) (month)?
5	( )	Where are we: (state) (county) (town) (hospital) (floor).
		Registration
3	( )	Name 3 objects;1 second to say each. Then ask the patient all 3 after you have said them. Give 1 point for each correct answer. Then repeat them until he learns all 3. Count trials and record.
		Trials _____
		Attention and Calculation
5	( )	Serial 7's. 1 point for each correct. Stop after 5 answers. Alternatively spell "world" backwards.
		Recall
3	( )	Ask for the 3 objects repeated above. Give 1 point for each correct.
		Language
9	( )	Name a pencil, and watch (2 points) Repeat the following "no ifs ands or buts." (1 point) Follow a 3-stage command: "Take a paper in your right hand, fold it in half, and put it on the floor" (3 points) Read and obey the following:

Close YOUR eyes (1 point)

Write a sentence (1 point)
Copy design (1 point)
Total Score
ASSESS level of consciousness
along a continuum ___ Alert   Drowsy   Stupor   Coma

INSTRUCTIONS FOR ADMINISTRATION OF MINI- MENTAL STATE EXAMINATION

Orientation

(1) Ask for the date. Then ask specifically for parts omitted, e.g., "Can you also tell me what season it is?" One point for each correct.
(2) Ask in turn "Can you tell me the name of this hospital?" (town, county, etc.). One point for each correct.

Registration

Ask the patient if you may test his memory. Then say the names of 3 unrelated objects, clearly and slowly, about one second for each. After you have said all 3, ask him to repeat them. This first repetition determines his score (0-3) but keep saying them until he can repeat all 3, up to 6 trials. If he does not eventually learn all 3, recall cannot be meaningfully tested.

Attention and Calculation

Ask the patient to begin with 100 and count backwards by 7. Stop after 5 subtractions (93,86,79,72,65). Score the total number of correct answers.

If the patient cannot or will not perform this task, ask him to spell the word 'World' backwards. The score is the number of letters in correct order. E.g., dlrow = 5, dlorw = 3.

Recall

Ask the patient if he can recall the 3 words you previously asked him to remember. Score 0-3.

Language

Naming: Show the patient a wristwatch and ask him what it is. Repeat for pencil. Score 0-2.
Repetition: Ask the patient to repeat the sentence after you. Allow only one trial. Score 0 or 1.
3-Stage command: Give the patient a piece of plain blank paper and repeat the command. Score 1 point for each part correctly executed.
Reading: On a blank piece of paper print the sentence "Close your eyes", in letters large enough for the patient to see clearly. Ask him to read it and do what it says. Score 1 point only if he actually closes his eyes.
Writing: Give the patient a blank piece of paper and ask him to write a sentence for you. Do not dictate a sentence, it is to be written spontaneously. It must contain a subject and verb and be sensible. Correct grammar and punctuation are not necessary.
Copying: On a clean piece of paper, draw intersecting pentagons, each side about 1 in., and ask him to copy it exactly as it is. All 10 angles must be present and 2 must intersect to score 1 point. Tremor and rotation are ignored.

Estimate the patient's level of sensorium along a continuum, from alert on the left to coma on the right.

FIGURE 137-2. (**A**) The Mini-Mental State examination. (**B**) Instructions for administration of the Mini-Mental State examination. (Folstein MF, Folstein SE, McHugh PR: "Mini-mental state": A practical method for grading the cognitive state of patients for the clinician. *J Psychiatr Res* 1975;12:189)

nary warning sign of heart ischemia. The appearance of a delirium, which is often referred to as acute brain failure, should promote marshaling of the same medical forces as failure of any other vital organ.

Mortality rates associated with delirium further emphasize the need for action. From 20% to 76% of acutely ill patients diagnosed with delirium die within a few months.[7,8] Far from being a natural phenomenon or a "disease of medi-

cal progress," brain failure is ominous and signals a need for renewed concern and prompt attention.[9]

CHARACTERISTICS

Three sources of information are used to determine whether a patient is delirious. They are the medical record, particularly the nurses' notes; past and present observations of the

TABLE 137-1. Clinical Comparison of Delirium and Dementia

	DELIRIUM	DEMENTIA
COGNITIVE DYSFUNCTION	Acute or sudden onset	Insidious onset, longstanding problems
MENTAL STATUS	Marked fluctuation that can occur rapidly during the day	Chronically impaired cognitive function that is stable
	Occasionally completely lucid; may "sundown" (i.e., show increased confusion during the night)	Is never completely lucid; may "sundown"
ELECTROENCEPHALOGRAPHY FINDINGS	Diffuse, bilateral slowing	Normal until late in course with Alzheimer's dementia; focal abnormalities with vascular dementias

family; and examination of the patient. A delirium has certain clinical characteristics (Table 137-2). The patient often manifests prodromal symptoms such as restlessness, anxiety, irritability, or sleep disruption before onset.

Confusion and Attention Deficits

One of the hallmarks of delirium is rapid fluctuation in the degree of confusion. Patients may be grossly confused and hallucinate during the night and have brief, lucid intervals interspersed with confusional periods during the day. They also have difficulty sustaining attention. During the interview, they typically are distracted by environmental events, such as a loud noise or a nurse checking the intravenous infusion, and forget the question asked. An inability to sustain attention and a preoccupation with internal events undoubtedly play key roles in the severe memory impairment and orientation difficulties found in delirium.

Disorientation and Amnesia

Delirious patients, except during lucid intervals, are usually disoriented to time, and often disoriented to place, but very rarely disoriented to their identity. After recovery from a delirium, some patients are amnesic regarding the entire episode, others have islands of memory, and a few recall the entire period. Those patients who experience paranoid delusions with a relatively clear sensorium usually recall the ICU experience.

Apathy, Somnolence, and Hyperactivity

Another clinical feature of delirium deserves particular emphasis. Although usually aroused, the reticular activating system of the brain stem may be hypoactive in delirium, in which case a patient appears apathetic, somnolent, and quietly confused. The medical staff often diagnose this patient as depressed. Such a diagnosis in an apathetic, quietly confused patient sometimes leads to inappropriate treatment with antidepressant medications and worsening confusion.

In many patients, reticular activating system hyperactivity occurs, inducing agitation, hypervigilance, and psychomotor hyperactivity. Some patients vacillate back and forth between hypoactive and hyperactive states; this condition is usually referred to as a mixed delirium. The sleep-wake cycle of delirious patients is often reversed. They may be somnolent during the day and active during the night when the nursing staff is sparse. Restoration of the normal diurnal sleep cycle is an important part of treatment.

Thought Patterns

Thought patterns of delirious patients are disorganized, and their reasoning is defective. They often experience misconceptions involving illusions, delusions, and hallucinations. These misperceptions often are woven into a loosely-knit, delusional, paranoid system. Visual hallucinations are common and can involve simple visual distortions or complex scenes. During a delirium, they occur more frequently than auditory hallucinations. Tactile hallucinations are the least

TABLE 137-2. Clinical Features of Delirium

Prodrome
Rapidly fluctuating course; reversible, lucid intervals
Altered arousal and psychomotor abnormality
Decreased attention
Sleep-wake disturbance
Impaired memory
Disorganized thinking and speech
Altered perceptions
Disorientation
Emotional lability
Dysgraphia/constructional apraxia/dysomic aphasia
Motor abnormalities

frequent. As the severity of the delirium increases, spontaneous speech becomes incoherent and rambling.

Neuropsychiatric Signs

A number of neuropsychiatric signs accompany delirium, including dysgraphia, constructional apraxia, and motor system abnormalities. Dysgraphia is one of the most sensitive indicators of a delirium. In the study of Chedru and Geschwind, 33 of 34 acutely confused patients had writing problems that ranged from motor limitations (tremor to illegible scribble) and spatial impairments (letter malalignment and line disorientation) to misspelling and linguistic errors.[10] Constructional apraxia also is a sensitive indicator of a confusional state and can be evaluated at the bedside by asking the patient to draw a clock showing a particular time, or to draw a three-dimensional cube.

Motor Abnormalities

Motor system abnormalities such as tremor, myoclonus, asterixis ("liver flap"), and reflex and muscle tone changes can also be present. The tremor associated with delirium, particularly if toxic-metabolic in origin, is absent at rest but apparent during movement. Myoclonus and asterixis occur in many toxic and metabolic conditions. Symmetric reflex and muscle tone changes also are seen.

DIFFERENTIAL DIAGNOSIS

The differential diagnosis of delirium is extensive. Confusional states, particularly in the elderly, can have multiple contributory causes. An elderly, delirious patient may have a low hematocrit and multiorgan system disease (e.g., pulmonary insufficiency, cardiac failure, preexisting brain damage) and may be taking multiple medications. Each potential contribution to the delirium needs to be pursued and, to whatever degree possible, reversed. A method for organizing the differential diagnosis of a delirious patient is helpful. The diagnostic system found in Table 137-3 is represented by the mnemonic WHHHHIMP. The diagnoses contained in the WHHHHIMP mnemonic can also help the clinician recall these critical items.

Among hospital and emergency room patients, prescribed medications are common causes of delirium (Table 137-4). A thorough medication history and a review of the patient's medication records are essential. The doctor's order sheets can be misleading because drugs may have been ordered but not given. Correlation of changes in behavior with medication administration or discontinuation can be helpful in sorting through a difficult case.

A more comprehensive list of conditions and agents that can cause delirium is summarized in Table 137-5. The mne-

TABLE 137-3. Differential Diagnosis of Delirium

Wernicke's encephalopathy/withdrawal
Hypertensive encephalopathy
Hypoglycemia
Hypoperfusion of central nervous system
Hypoxemia
Intracranial bleeding/Infection
Meningitis/Encephalitis
Poisons/Medications

TABLE 137-4. Drugs Causing Delirium (Reversible Dementia)

ANALGESICS

  Meperidine
  Opiates
  Pentazocine
  Salicylates

ANTIBIOTICS

  Acyclovir, gangciclovir
  Aminoglycosides
  Amodiaquine
  Amphotericin B
  Cephalexin
  Cephalosporins
  Chloramphenicol
  Chloroquine
  Ethambutol
  Gentamicin
  Interferon
  Sulfonamides
  Tetracycline
  Ticarcillin
  Vancomycin

ANTICHOLINERGIC DRUGS

  Antihistamines
    (chlorpheniramine)
  Antispasmodics
  Atropine/homatropine
  Belladonna alkaloids
  Benztropine
  Biperidin
  Diphenhydramine
  Phenothazines (especially
    thioridazine)
  Promethazine
  Scopolamine
  Tricyclic antidepressants
    (especially amitriptyline)
  Trihexyphenidyl

ANTICONVULSANTS

  Phenobarbital
  Phenytoin
  Valproic acid

ANTIINFLAMMATORY DRUGS

  Corticosteroids
  Ibuprofen
  Indomethacin
  Naproxen
  Phenylbutazone
  Steroids

ANTINEOPLASTIC DRUGS

  Aminoglutethimide
  Asparaginase
  Dacarbazine
  5-fluorouracil
  Hexamethylenamine
  Methotrexate (high dose)
  Tamoxifen
  Vinblastine
  Vincristine

ANTIPARKINSON DRUGS

  Amantadine
  Bromocriptine
  Carbidopa
  Levodopa

ANTITUBERCULOUS DRUGS

  Isoniazid
  Rifampin

CARDIAC DRUGS

  β-Blockers (propranolol)
  Captopril
  Clonidine
  Digitalis
  Disopyramide
  Lidocaine
  Mexiletine
  Methyldopa
  Procainamide
  Quinidine
  Tocainamide

DRUG WITHDRAWAL

  Alcohol
  Barbiturates
  Benzodiazepines

SEDATIVE-HYPNOTICS

  Barbiturates
  Benzodiazepines
  Glutethimide

SYMPATHOMIMETICS

  Aminophylline
  Amphetamines
  Cocaine
  Ephedrine
  Epinephrine
  Phenylephrine
  Phenylpropanolamine
  Theophylline

MISCELLANEOUS DRUGS

  Baclofen
  Bromides
  Chlorpropamide
  Cimetidine
  Disulfiram
  Ergotamines
  Lithium
  Metrizamide
  Metronidazole
  Phenelzine
  Podophylline (by
    absorption)
  Procarbazine
  Propylthiouracil
  Quinacrine
  Ranitidine
  Timolol ophthalmic

Wise MG, Brandt GT: Delirium. In: Hales RE, Yudofsky SC (eds). *Textbook of Neuropsychiatry*, 2nd ed. Washington DC, American Psychiatric Press, 1992.

TABLE 137-5.   Causes of Delirium

Infectious	Encephalitis, meningitis, and syphilis
Withdrawal	Alcohol, barbiturates, sedative-hypnotics, benzodiazepine
Acute metabolic	Acidosis, alkalosis, electrolyte disturbance, hepatic failure, renal failure
Trauma	Heat stroke, postoperative severe burns, closed-head injury
Central nervous system pathology	Abscesses, hemorrhage, normal-pressure hydrocephalus, seizures, stroke, tumors, vasculitis
Hypoxia	Anemia, carbon monoxide poisoning, hypotension, pulmonary/cardiac failure
Deficiencies	B_{12}/niacin/thiamine; hypovitaminosis
Endocrinopathies	Hyper- or hypo-adrenalcorticism, hyperglycemia, hypoglycemia, parathyroid
Acute vascular	Hypertensive encephalopathy, shock
Toxins/drugs	Medications, pesticides, solvents
Heavy metals	Lead, manganese, mercury

monic used, I WATCH DEATH, may seem melodramatic, but the mortality rate within the first 3 months after the diagnosis of delirium is approximately 30%. Tesar and Stern[11] and Wise[12] include complete discussions of the differential diagnosis of delirium.

In virtually every delirious patient, the evaluative process includes review of historical information as well as basic and advanced laboratory tests (Table 137-6). If information concerning the patient's mental and physical status is com-

bined with the basic laboratory battery, the specific cause or causes are usually apparent. If not, the case should be reviewed and further diagnostic studies considered.

TREATMENT

The goal of evaluation is to discover specific reversible causes for delirium. Therefore, locating the precise time of the abnormal change in mental status is most helpful. A delirious

TABLE 137-6.   Evaluation of the Behaviorally Disturbed Patient

MENTAL STATUS

Interview (assess level of consciousness, psychomotor activity, appearance, affect, mood, intellect, thought processes)

Performance tests (for memory, concentration, reasoning, motor and constructional apraxia, dysgraphia, dysnomia, dysphasia)

PHYSICAL STATUS

Brief neurologic examination (reflexes, limb strength, Babinski's sign, cranial nerves, meningeal signs, gait)

Review past and present vital signs (pulse, temperature, blood pressure, respiration rate)

Review chart (laboratory work, any abnormal behavior noted, onset of behavior)

Review medication records (correlate abnormal behavior with starting or stopping of medications)

LABORATORY EXAMINATION—BASIC

Blood chemistries (electrolytes, glucose, Ca^{2+}-albumin, BUN, NH_4^+, liver functions, Mg^{2+}, PO_4^{2-}, thyroid function tests)

Blood count (hematocrit, leukocyte count, differential, mean corpuscular volume, sedimentation rate)

Drug levels (need toxic screen or medication blood levels?)

Arterial blood gases

Urinalysis

Electrocardiogram

Chest radiograph

LABORATORY TESTS—AS APPROPRIATE

Electroencephalogram (seizures? local lesion? Confirm delirium)

Computed tomography (normal pressure hydrocephalus, stroke, space-occupying lesion)

Additional blood chemistries (heavy metals, thiamine and folate levels, lupus erythematosus, antinuclear antibodies, urinary porpholbilinogen)

Lumbar puncture (if indication of infection or intracranial bleed)

patient with a blood pressure of 260/150 mm Hg and papilledema must immediately receive antihypertensive medications. The alcoholic patient who is having withdrawal symptoms must immediately receive appropriate pharmacologic intervention with drugs such as thiamine and a benzodiazepine. If a specific cause for the confusional state cannot be found, a number of interventions are helpful in controlling unacceptable behavior.

Haloperidol

Haloperidol is the drug of choice to treat a delirium of unknown cause.[13,14] It is a potent antipsychotic, with virtually no anticholinergic or hypotensive properties; it is not a respiratory depressant; and it can be given parenterally. Intravenous haloperidol has been used in high doses for many years in seriously ill patients without harmful side effects.[14,15] In 60% of ICUs surveyed, physicians used haloperidol for sedation,[16] usually by intermittent intravenous infusion or intramuscular administration or, least frequently, by continuous infusion.[17]

Despite haloperidol's frequent use in ICU settings, it is not approved by the Food and Drug Administration for intravenous use. If such use is desired, we recommend that the hospital's pharmacy and therapeutics committee authorize use of the drug with careful monitoring of results. Because haloperidol is the safest drug for control of agitation in the critically ill patient, it is certainly justifiable as an innovative therapy. After monitoring of the results is complete, the committee can authorize use of the intravenous haloperidol, if necessary to care for the medically ill patient.

The only potentially dangerous adverse effect associated with intravenous haloperidol is torsade de pointes. Wilt and colleagues[18] reported four cases over a 3-year period during which about 1100 patients were treated with a combination of haloperidol and lorazepam. Other case reports also have appeared.[19,20]

Although extrapyramidal side effects are more likely with the higher-potency antipsychotic drugs such as haloperidol, the actual occurrence rate in medically ill patients, particularly with intravenous administration, is low. This observation may be related to the fact that medically ill patients frequently receive concomitant benzodiazepines or β-blockers, which ameliorate extrapyramidal syndromes, or that psychiatric patients have a lower threshold for extrapyramidal syndromes.[21]

Recommended dosages of haloperidol for the agitated patient are summarized in Table 137-7. The initial dosage for the elderly patient is at the lower end of the dosage schedule. It is repeated every 30 minutes until the patient is sedated or calm. (The oral dose is twice the parenteral dose.)

The calming effects of an antipsychotic drug are not immediate. The therapeutic delay may cause the physician and nursing staff to believe the medication is not effective. After calm is achieved, agitation then becomes the sign for a repeat dose. After confusion has cleared, it is important to continue the medications for 3 to 5 days. Abrupt discontinuation immediately after improvement is usually followed by recurrence of the delirium within 24 hours. A more rational approach is to taper the medication over a 3- to 5-day period, administering the largest dose before bedtime to help nor-

TABLE 137-7. Guidelines for Intravenous Use of Haloperidol

LEVEL OF AGITATION	STARTING DOSE
Mild	0.5–2.0 mg
Moderate	2.0–5.0 mg
Severe	5.0–10.0 mg

1. Clear intravenous tubing with normal saline
2. For elderly patients, use starting doses in the low range
3. Allow at least 30 min between doses
4. For continued agitation, double previous use
5. After 3 doses, give 0.5–1.0 mg of intravenous lorazepam concurrently, or alternate lorazepam with haloperidol every 30 min
6. If patient's agitation is poorly controlled with intermittent doses of haloperidol, consider a constant intravenous infusion
7. After patient is calm, determine the total number of milligrams of haloperidol given and administer same number of milligrams over the next 24 h. Can divide total into two doses with largest part at bedtime.
8. Assuming the patient remains calm, reduce dose by 50% every 24 hrs.
9. Oral dose is twice the intravenous dose.

malize the sleep-wake cycle. Small doses of intravenous lorazepam, particularly in patients who have not responded to high doses of haloperidol alone, are a useful adjunct.[22]

Other Antipsychotic Medications

Other useful antipsychotic medications include thiothixene (Navane) and droperidol (Inapsine). Droperidol is used as a preanesthetic agent and for control of nausea and vomiting. It is a butyrophenone, like haloperidol, and has comparable antipsychotic potency. Droperidol is approved for intravenous use but has the disadvantage of having a higher potential than haloperidol for causing hypotension. Continuous infusion of droperidol is sometimes used in ICUs to control an agitated delirium.[23]

Less potent antipsychotic medications are thioridazine (Mellaril) and chlorpromazine (Thorazine). Because higher milligram doses are required, they are more likely to cause hypotension and they have more anticholinergic side effects; they should be used with caution in the unstable patient with cardiovascular disease. We recommend that psychiatric consultation be obtained before thioridazine or chlorpromazine is used in critically ill patients.

Ancillary Measures

Other interventions are also necessary. All nonessential medications should be discontinued. The patient should be placed in a room near the nursing station so that vital signs can be obtained frequently. Increased observation by the nursing staff ensures closer evaluation of medical deterioration and frequent monitoring for dangerous behavior (e.g., crawling over bedrails, pulling out central venous or arterial catheters). Fluid input and output are monitored, and good oxygenation is ensured.

TABLE 137-8. Distribution of Consultation Requests According to Type of Intensive Care Unit (ICU)

CORONARY CARE UNIT	SURGICAL ICU	RESPIRATORY ICU	MEDICAL ICU
Anxiety	Delirium	Depression	Delirium
Depression	Depression	Anxiety on weaning from	Management (suicide attempt)
Management (sign-out against	Anxiety on weaning from	ventilator	Depression
medical orders, dependency)	ventilator	Management (drug	Anxiety
Hostility		dependency, dependency)	
Delirium			

Having a calm family member remain with a paranoid, agitated patient is reassuring and can prevent mishaps. In lieu of a family member, close supervision by reassuring staff is important. Both nurses and family members can frequently reorient the disoriented patient to date and surroundings. Placing a clock, calendar, and familiar objects in the room may be helpful. Adequate light in the room decreases frightening illusions at night. Despite recommendations to the contrary, a private room for the delirious patient is appropriate only if adequate supervision can be ensured. A room with a window is helpful to orient the patient to normal diurnal cues.[24]

If the patient normally wears eyeglasses or a hearing aid, improving the quality of sensory input by returning these devices is useful. A common error on medical and surgical wards is to group delirious patients in the same room. This process slows recovery and makes reorientation of confused patients virtually impossible.

BEHAVIORAL DISORDERS WITHOUT COGNITIVE DYSFUNCTION ■

CHARACTERISTICS

If the patient has a behavioral disorder but the MMS examination and recent clinical history indicate that no cognitive dysfunction is present, the next concern is whether a change in medical status prompted the behavior. For example, shortness of breath may prompt agitation and anxiety. The physician's concern about the patient's medical condition not only rules out problems but also helps to establish rapport. After medical problems are discounted and rapport is established, the interviewer can ask open-ended questions about the current situation. A direct approach is used to uncover and correct the critically ill patient's unrealistic or distorted expectations. The interviewer may ask, for example, "What is worrying you most right now?" Some patients can easily identify fears, anxiety, and depressive ideas concerning their medical condition, but this task is not always easy. Certain characteristic emotional responses are encountered in different intensive care settings (Table 137-8). If sufficient rapport cannot be established or the patient is unable or unwilling to talk, a psychiatric consultation should be requested.

Although little research concerning the sequence of emotional and behavioral reactions in critically ill patients has been published, Cassem and Hackett have developed a useful hypothetical sequence of patient reactions to a coronary care unit (CCU) based on the timing of psychiatric consultations[25] (Fig. 137-3). The majority of behavioral problems during the first 2 days in the CCU are caused by *fear and anxiety*, probably resulting from the threat to life posed by a heart attack. In many patients' experience, they were healthy one moment and bedridden in an ICU the next. By the second or third day, patients frequently convince

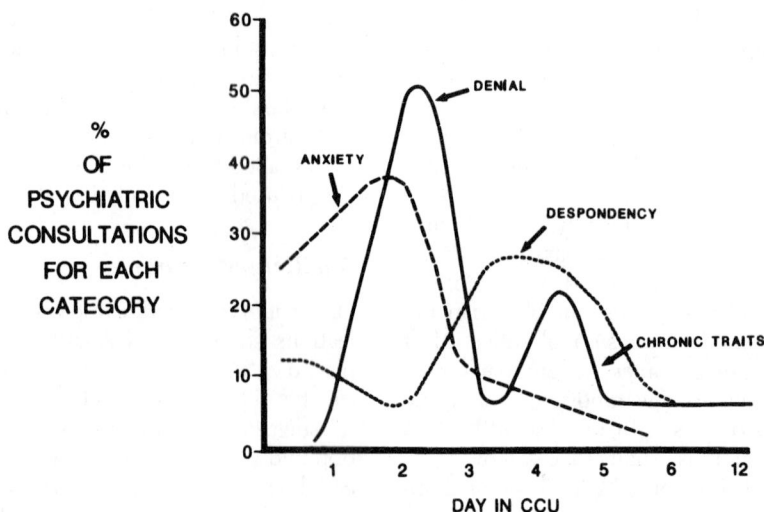

FIGURE 137-3. Hypothetical sequence of emotional and behavioral reactions in a critical care unit.

themselves that nothing serious has occurred and that the physicians' and nurses' concerns are misplaced. During this period of *denial*, noncompliance with medical advice occurs and sign-out against medical advice is threatened.

As evidence mounts that something did injure the myocardium, patients become depressed or appear demoralized and express pessimism about the future. Behavioral problems that occur later in the course of illness often result from chronic personality traits. Patients with these problems are difficult to get along with and are often disliked by the staff.

Several behavioral disturbances deserve individual discussion.

AGITATION AND ANXIETY

Causes

Agitation is excessive motor activity that results from a patient's internal discomfort. This discomfort may result from physical pain, anxiety, fear, or akathisia (an internal sense of discomfort, often with motor restlessness, that occurs as a side effect of antipsychotics and other medications that block dopamine, such as metoclopramide). As Tesar and Stern point out, "Agitation is usually a manifestation of a delirium."[11] If a delirium is not present, other sources for the agitation should be explored.

PAIN. Physical pain is common in the critically ill patient and can result in agitation. If pain is the cause of restlessness, the patient usually makes it known. The critical care nurse commonly asks about pain and administers a previously ordered narcotic. Dasta and colleagues[26] found that parenteral morphine was prescribed for agitation and pain 76% of the time. Agitated patients may not be able to communicate pain severity if they are intubated. Before an analgesic trial, a brief mental status evaluation is recommended, because an underlying delirium, and therefore underlying medical problems, can be masked by narcotic analgesics. Sometimes, however, a trial of morphine is required.

FEAR OF DEATH. For many critically ill patients, the cause of their anxiety and fear is the threat of death. In conversations with a patient who looks afraid, the health care worker may ask, "You look scared. How are you doing?" or ask directly, "Are you worried that you may die?" If the patient answers in the affirmative, the response depends on the reality of those fears. If dying is an unrealistic possibility, reassurance and realistic explanations about the current situation will markedly decrease the level of anxiety and fear. If dying is a likely or definite outcome of the illness, the patient may be asked, "What frightens you most about dying?" The patient may reply, "I'm afraid of the pain I will have" or "I have never been religious and don't know what to expect." In the former instance, the patient can be reassured that he or she will be kept comfortable and free from moderate or severe pain. In the latter case, the health care worker can offer to arrange a consultation visit from a chaplain who can offer reassurance and advice.

Some critically ill patients inquire spontaneously about dying. This direct question, especially if asked without much

anxiety, means that the patient wants to be told the truth. The patient usually suspects that he or she is dying when the question is posed. The quick reply, "You'll be just fine," is usually frustrating and decreases chances of meaningful communication about the patient's predicament. Patients sometimes ask about dying in a near-panic. They really are asking for reassurance. Such patients often ask the nurse and usually avoid asking the physician.

If the patient's outcome is in doubt, the health care worker may say, "My focus is more on getting people well than on predicting death. You sound scared. What is it?" Another approach may be, "No one gets in this unit without being seriously ill. Why do you ask a question about dying now?" The patient can then clarify why the inquiry was made. Whenever anxiety seems to threaten overall stability, judicious use of medication or consultation with the psychiatrist is appropriate.

Treatment

BENZODIAZEPINES. Medications are helpful in treating anxiety and fear. Benzodiazepines reduce acute anxiety in most patients (Table 137-9). For critically ill patients, the half-life of the drug, onset of action, drug interactions, and routes of metabolism and elimination should be considered.[27] Diazepam is very lipophilic and rapidly enters the central nervous system; therefore, it is clinically useful if rapid tranquilization is desired.

Drug interactions can result in behavioral changes. For example, cimetidine increases the half-life of longer-acting benzodiazepines, resulting sometimes in confusion or lethargy.[28] Short-acting benzodiazepines, such as oxazepam or lorazepam, are recommended in patients with liver damage to prevent buildup of sedating drugs and their active metabolites.

MAJOR TRANQUILIZERS. If anxiety is severe and is manifested as fear, major tranquilizers (neuroleptics) are usually more efficacious than benzodiazepines. The following example is illustrative.

A young man is admitted to the CCU to rule out a myocardial infarction. He is extremely anxious with agitation. Oxazepam, 15 mg orally four times a day, is ordered. Despite the medication, agitation and hypervigilance continue and he resists sleep. MMS examination is unremarkable (30 correct out of 30 possible). Inquiry into the patient's concerns reveals a strong family history of deaths associated with heart attacks. The patient is afraid to sleep "because I might not wake up," and he is "watching the monitors in case the alarms don't work." On a 0-to-10 scale of anxiety (0, "no anxiety"; 10, "terror"), the patient reports a 9.5 (*with* benzodiazepine treatment). He is then prescribed perphenazine (Trilafon), 2 mg orally three times each day. His anxiety promptly drops to a self-rating of 3 out of 10, and all objective signs of emotional discomfort disappear.

If panic emerges, as it did in this patient, low-dose major tranquilizers such as haloperidol, 1 or 2 mg twice per day; perphenazine, 2 mg orally three times per day; thiothixene, 1 or 2 mg three times per day; or trifluoperazine (Stelazine), 2 mg three times per day, can markedly reduce the level of anxiety. The newest available agent is risperidone (Risper-

TABLE 137-9. Profile for Use of Benzodiazepines

	EQUIVALENT ORAL DOSE (mg)	ONSET OF ACTION	ACTIVE METABOLITE	HALF-LIFE OF PARENT COMPOUND (h)	DEGREE OF SEDATION
Midazolam (Versed)	—°	Fast	Yes	2–5	+++
Diazepam (Valium)	5.0	Fast	Yes	20–70	+++
Clorazepate (Tranxene)	7.5	Fast	Yes	P	++
Flurazepam (Dalmane)	15.0	Fast	Yes	P	+++
Triazolam (Halcion)	0.25	Intermediate	No	1.5–5	++
Lorazepam (Ativan)†	1.0	Intermediate	No	10–20	+++
Alprazolam (Xanax)	0.5	Intermediate	Yes	12–15	+
Halazepam (Paxipam)	20.0	Intermediate	Yes	12–15	++
Chlordiazepoxide (Librium)	10.0	Intermediate	Yes	5–30	++
Oxazepam (Serax)†	15.0	Slow	No	5–15	+
Temazepam (Restoril)†	15.0	Slow	No	9–12	++
Clonazepam (Klonopin)	0.5	Slow	No	18–50	++
Prazepam (Centrax)	10.0	Slow	Yes	P	+

°Available only in parenteral form in the United States
†Direct hepatic glucuronide conjugation
P, Prodrugs–metabolites are the active agents and have long half-lives (30–200 h); +, mild; ++, moderate; +++, strong.

dal), 1 mg twice a day, which is also effective but quite expensive.

DOPAMINE BLOCKERS. Medications that block dopamine, including droperidol, prochlorperazine (Compazine), and metoclopramide (Reglan), are associated with extrapyramidal side effects such as akathisia. Patients usually report a sense of inner restlessness and sometimes manifest agitation. Akathisia is difficult to treat and may or may not be improved by giving the patient diphenhydramine (Benadryl), benzodiazepines (usually diazepam), or anticholinergic drugs such as trihexyphenidyl (Artane) or benztropine mesylate (Cogentin). Propranolol may also reduce akathisia.[21] If symptoms do not clear, the medication may have to be discontinued.

DEPRESSION

If a medically ill patient lacks energy and appears to have no interest in his or her medical condition, is the patient apathetic or depressed? The question of depression versus apathy is important because the differential diagnosis and treatment are different.

Characteristics

Clinical depression consists of a depressed mood with a symptom constellation that includes sleep disturbance, decreased interests, increased sense of guilt, decreased energy, decreased ability to concentrate, decreased (or, more rarely, increased) appetite, altered psychomotor state (either agitation or retardation), and suicidal ideation or preoccupation with death.

The mnemonic in Table 137-10, SIG: E CAPS (prescribe energy capsules), may help the clinician recall the eight clinical features, in addition to depressed mood, of a major depression. If five out of eight symptoms are present and the patient's mood is depressed, he or she meets diagnostic criteria for depression set out in the Diagnostic and Statistical Manual of Mental Disorders, fourth edition.[29] Many of these symptoms are quite difficult to interpret in a patient who is seriously medically ill, because almost all such patients have difficulties with sleep, energy, appetite, and, to some degree, concentration.

The following characteristics help to identify critically ill patients who are also clinically depressed: sustained depressed mood; either increased (agitation) or decreased psychomotor movements; suicidal ideation; and, most important, a sense of helplessness, hopelessness, or worthlessness about the current situation.[30] If these symptoms are present, the patient requires treatment for depression. One approach is to make a strict criterion for both depressed mood (almost all the time) and loss of interest (in almost everything), then count the other seven symptoms without regard for the "cause." This method is valid.

TABLE 137-10. Clinical Features of Depression

Sleep disturbance
Interests decrease
Guilt increases
Energy decreases
Concentration difficulties
Appetite alteration
Psychomotor alteration
Suicidal ideation

Treatment

Failure to treat depression increases the mortality, morbidity, and cost of all medical illness.[31,32] Most moderate to severe depressive syndromes require antidepressant medication or electroconvulsive therapy. The selection of a particular antidepressant for a given patient is based on matching the medical status of the patient with the side effect profile of the medication (Table 137-11).

APATHY

Apathy and depression can coexist in certain patients. For example, depressed patients often are apathetic about the future. Apathy, however, also exists as a separate entity.

Characteristics

Apathetic patients are indifferent about their current medical condition but do not feel sad, hopeless, or worthless. They are not clinically depressed, although they may be misdiagnosed as such. One could say they are pseudodepressed (personal communication, G. B. Murray, MD, Massachusetts General Hospital). Apathy in this group of patients is a product of brain dysfunction, probably as a result of injury to or dysfunction of the frontal lobe. Apathy occurs in hypoaroused delirious patients, in demented patients, and in some patients with stroke or brain damage.

Treatment

Nondepressed apathetic patients are not likely to respond to antidepressant medications. In fact, their mental status may worsen because of the anticholinergic side effects of these drugs. A subgroup respond to stimulants. Methylphenidate (Ritalin) in doses of 10 mg twice per day, or dextroamphetamine 10 mg once per day, may energize the patient and improve rehabilitation.[33,34] The afternoon dose of stimulants should be given before 3:00 P.M. so that the patient's ability to fall asleep is not impaired.

TABLE 137-11. Side Effect Profile of Antidepressant Drugs

	SEDATIVE EFFECTS	ORTHOSTATIC EFFECTS	ANTICHOLINERGIC EFFECTS	CARDIAC CONDUCTION/ARRHYTHMIAS
TRICYCLIC AGENTS				
Amitriptyline (Elavil)	High	Moderate	Highest	Yes
Clomipramine (Anafranil)	Moderate	Moderate	Moderate	Yes
Desipramine (Norpramin)	Low	Low	Moderate	Yes
Doxepin (Sinequan)	High	Moderate	Moderate	Yes
Imipramine (Tofranil)	Moderate	High	Moderate	Yes
Nortriptyline (Pamelor)	Moderate	Low	Moderate	Yes
Protriptyline (Vivactil)	Low	Low	High	Yes
Trimipramine (Surmontil)	High	?Moderate	Moderate	Yes
OTHER AGENTS				
Amoxapine	Moderate	Low	Moderate	Rare
Bupropion	None	None	Very low	Very rare
Fluoxetine	Low	None	Very low	Very rare
Maprotiline	Moderate	Low	Moderate	Rare
Nefazodone (Serzone)°	Moderate	Low	Very low	None
Paroxetine (Paxil)°	Low	None	Moderate	None
Sertraline (Zoloft)°	Low	None	Very low	None
Trazodone	High	Moderate	Very low	Rare
Venlafaxine (Effexor)°	Low	None	Very low	None
MONOAMINE OXIDASE INHIBITORS				
Phenelzine	Low	High	None	Very rare
Tranylcypromine	Low	High	None	Very rare
Isocarboxazid	Low	Moderate	None	Very rare
PSYCHOSTIMULANTS†				
Dextroamphetamine	None	None	None	Rare
Methylphenidate	None	None	None	Rare

°Paroxetine (Paxil), sertraline (Zoloft), venlafaxine (Effexor), and nefazodone (Serzone) are new antidepressants, and their profiles may change with additional clinical experience.
†Psychostimulants are not approved by the FDA for treating depression.

Because certain medications are depressogenic, a review of the depressed patient's medication regimen is necessary. Frequent offenders are reserpine, methyldopa, guanethidine, hydralazine, steroids, and clonidine.

REFUSAL TO COOPERATE

Characteristics

A patient's refusal to cooperate can manifest as denial of serious illness, such as a threatening to sign out against medical advice, or as refusal to follow a treatment plan, such as sneaking cigarettes or failing to remain in bed while ordered on strict bed rest. As Hackett and Cassem suggest, "Although the threat to sign out can mean that the individual does not take the illness seriously (e.g., is not frightened enough), the threat to sign out issued by an acutely ill patient should be assumed to be a reaction to panic unless proven otherwise."[25] Basically, if faced with fight-or-flight response to the severe stress of acute illness, the patient opts for flight.

Treatment

If the patient is incompetent (i.e., does not understand the situation because of mental dysfunction), a psychiatric consultation can be requested to document the mental status. If the patient is competent and is demanding to leave against medical advice, the following approach is recommended.

Remain calm. Anger is a tempting response to this situation, but an adversarial stance rarely changes the patient's decision. In a calm, direct way, inform the patient about the medical difficulties, stressing the fact that the illness is manageable. Mobilize the patient's family. If certain members of the family can help to calm the patient, they are invaluable resources in this situation. If the family is as panicky as the patient, which is very rarely the case, keep the family and the patient separated. As soon as possible, medicate the patient with a low-dose antipsychotic medication such as haloperidol, 1 or 2 mg, or perphenazine, 2 to 5 mg orally. Medication is important; however, "If calm is achieved it should not be expected to last."[25]

Patients who do not comply with a medical regimen are sometimes frightened. The previously described young male in the CCU did not remain in bed. The usual translation of this behavior is something like, "My heart is not so damaged that I can't walk to the bathroom!" If the staff demand that the patient return to bed and do not understand the unspoken message, the behavior is then repeated to the increasing frustration of all parties involved. Instead of an adversarial statement, a better approach would be, "Your heart is damaged and needs time to heal. The damaged part is like cement that is setting; right now it is soft and can be damaged more. If you allow the cement (scar) to harden, your heart will be as strong or stronger than before."

Many patients who refuse to comply with medical treatment are rebelling against dependency. The natural response of the staff to this rebellious behavior is to demand complete compliance (i.e., complete dependency). To do so is to fight a losing battle in which the staff attempt to function as the police and the patient feels like a misunderstood criminal.

If patients believe that their bodies have forsaken them by becoming ill, and that now the medical staff is demanding total surrender, it is certainly a fertile setting for rebellion! The staff in this situation should review the treatment plan and decide where flexibility is possible and where it is contraindicated. Choices should be offered, such as, "Would you like your sponge bath this morning or in the evening?" or "Your digitalis should be taken on schedule to keep your heart rhythm regular, but you can refuse your Valium. If you want the Valium later, just let us know." This approach gives patients some sense of control in a situation in which they are feeling totally powerless.

HOSTILITY

Anger in the critically ill person springs from many roots. Patients may be frightened or feel threatened. They commonly ask, "What did I do to deserve this?" The nursing and physician staff may be the recipients of the resultant anger. If patients have complaints, the staff should hear them out and correct the problem if appropriate. They can express empathy with the patient's situation: "I know you are having a difficult time." For most patients, anger is a temporary state of affairs and passes as they and the staff become adjusted to each other and to the situation. However, a few patients who exhibit chronic hostility have lifelong difficulties with interpersonal relationships. A psychiatric consultation is indicated. These individuals are difficult even for the psychiatrist to treat, and marginal management of the anger is often as much as can be achieved.

DEPENDENCY

Critically ill patients who regress to an infantile state during hospitalization (helpless behavior and unrealistic demands) usually irritate the medical staff. The staff may become so intent on controlling their own anger that they overcompensate and give in to the patient's demands. Unfortunately, acquiescence to unreasonable demands results in further regression and more demands. If dealing with a regressed patient, the staff must enforce reasonable limits and guide the patient toward rehabilitation. Firm demands for self-care and increased independence are recommended.

Transfer from the ICU environment, in which the staff is constantly vigilant and attentive, has both good and bad aspects. The patient is improving, but the level of medical observation and monitoring is significantly reduced. The patient should be told in advance about the transfer and provided reassurance that less monitoring is appropriate because medical improvement has occurred. In some cases, a transitional status, such as a step-down unit, offers reassurance before transfer to a general medical ward.

SUMMARY ■

The first task in the evaluation of a behaviorally disturbed, critically ill patient is to determine whether cognitive dysfunction is present. A brief mental status examination, such as the MMS examination, should be used. If acute brain failure (delirium) is present, an immediate search for the cause of the brain dysfunction is indicated. If a delirium is present and no clear cause is found, haloperidol is the drug of choice to control confused behavior.

If the behaviorally disturbed patient is not delirious or demented, the underlying emotional reason for the disturbance should be sought. Fear and anxiety are the most common causes. When dealing with behavioral problems in critically ill patients, there is no substitute for the ability to give calm reassurance and prescribe medications wisely. A good psychiatric consultant for difficult cases is essential.

REFERENCES ■

1. Wise MG: Delirium due to a general medical condition, delirium due to multiple etiologies, and delirium not otherwise specified. In: Gabbard GO (ed). *Treatments of Psychiatric Disorders: The DSM-IV Edition*. Washington, DC, American Psychiatric Press, 1995
2. Wise MG, Trzepacz P: Delirium (confusional states). In: Rundell JR, Wise MG (ed). *The American Psychiatric Press Textbook of Consultation-Liaison Psychiatry*. Washington, DC, 1996:258
3. Glickman L: *Psychiatric Consultation in the General Hospital*. New York, Marcel Dekker, 1980:x (preface)
4. Folstein MF, Folstein SE, McHugh PR: "Mini-mental state:" a practical method for grading the cognitive state of patients for the clinician. *J Psychiat Res* 1975;12:189
5. Kennard MA, Bueding E, Wortis WB: Some biochemical and electroencephalographic changes in delirium tremens. *Q J Stud Alcohol* 1945;6:4
6. Pro JD, Wells CE: The use of the electroencephalogram in the diagnosis of delirium. *Dis Nerv Syst* 1977;38:804
7. Epstein LJ, Simon A: Organic brain syndromes in the elderly. *Geriatrics* 1967;22:145
8. Flint FJ, Richards SM: Organic basis of confusional states in the elderly. *BMJ* 1956;2:1537
9. McKegney FB: Intensive care syndrome: Definition, treatment and prevention of new "disease of medical progress." *Conn Med* 1966;30:633
10. Chedru F, Geschwind N: Writing disturbances in acute confusional states. *Neuropsychologia* 1972;10:343
11. Tesar GE, Stern TA: Evaluation and treatment of agitation in the intensive care unit. *J Intensive Care Med* 1986;1:137
12. Wise MG: Delirium. In: Hales RE, Yudofsky SC (eds). *The American Psychiatric Press Textbook of Neuropsychiatry*. Washington DC, American Psychiatric Press, 1987:89
13. Lipowski ZJ: Delirium updated. *Compr Psychiatry* 1980;21:190
14. Cassem NH: Acute and subacute psychiatric disorders. In: Parrillo JE, Bone RC (eds). *Critical Care Medicine: Principles of Diagnosis and Management*. Philadelphia, Mosby–Year Book, 1994:2013
15. Tesar GE, Murray GB, Cassem NH: Use of high-dose intravenous haloperidol in the treatment of agitated cardiac patients. *J Clin Psychopharmacol* 1985;5:344
16. Adams F: Neuropsychiatric evaluation and treatment of delirium in the critically ill cancer patient. *Cancer Bull* 1984;36:156
17. Wilson LM: Intensive care delirium. *Arch Intern Med* 1972;130:225
18. Wilt JL, Minnema AM, Johnson RF, et al: Torsade de pointes associated with the use of intravenous haloperidol. *Ann Intern Med* 1993;119:391
19. Metzger E, Friedman R: Prolongation of the corrected QT and torsade de pointes cardiac arrhythmia associated with intravenous haloperidol in the medically ill. *J Clin Psychopharmacol* 1993;13:128
20. Zeifman CWE: Torsade de pointes: Potential consequence of intravenous haloperidol in the intensive care unit. *Intensive Care World* 1994;11:109
21. Lipinski JF, Zubenko GS, Cohen BM, et al: Propranolol in the treatment of neuroleptic-induced akathisia. *Am J Psychiatry* 1984;141:412
22. Adams F: Neuropsychiatric evaluation and treatment of delirium in the critically ill cancer patient. *Cancer Bull* 1984;36:156
23. Frye MA, Coudreault MF, Hakeman SM, et al: Continuous droperidol infusion for management of agitated delirium in an intensive care unit. *Psychosomatics* 1995;36:301
24. Wilson LM: Intensive care delirium. *Arch Intern Med* 1972;130:225
25. Cassem NH, Hackett TP: The setting of intensive care. In: Hackett TP, Cassem NH (eds). *Massachusetts General Hospital Handbook of General Hospital Psychiatry*. St Louis, CV Mosby, 1978:319
26. Dasta JF, Fuhrman TM, McCandles C: Patterns of prescribing and administering drugs for agitation and pain in patients in a surgical intensive care unit. *Crit Care Med* 1994;22:974
27. Wise MG, Taylor SE: Anxiety and mood disorders in medically ill patients. *J Clin Psychiatry* 1990;51:27
28. Desmond PV, Patwardhan RV, Schenker S, et al: Cimetidine impairs elimination of chlordiazepoxide (Librium) in man. *Ann Intern Med* 1980;93:266
29. American Psychiatric Association: *Diagnostic and Statistical Manual of Mental Disorders*, 4th ed. Washington, DC, American Psychiatric Association, 1994
30. Chochinov HM, Wilson KG, Enns M, et al: Prevalence of depression in the terminally ill: Effects of diagnostic criteria and symptom threshold judgements. *Am J Psychiatry* 1994;151:537
31. Avery D, Winokur G: Mortality in depressed patients with electroconvulsive therapy and antidepressants. *Arch Gen Psychiatry* 1976;33:1029, 1976
32. Hall, Wise MG: The clinical and financial burden of mood disorders: Cost and outcome. *Psychosomatics* 1995;36:S11
33. Katon W, Raskind M: Treatment of depression in the medically ill with methylphenidate. *Am J Psychiatry* 1980;137:963
34. Kaufmann MW, Murray GB, Cassem NH: Use of psychostimulants in medically ill depressed patients. *Psychosomatics* 1982;23:817

Gastrointestinal Disease and Dysfunction

Critical Care, Third Edition, edited by Joseph M. Civetta,
Robert W. Taylor, and Robert R. Kirby.
Lippincott-Raven Publishers, Philadelphia, PA © 1997.

CHAPTER 138

■

Gastrointestinal Bleeding

Jack A. DiPalma

IMMEDIATE CONCERNS ■

MAJOR PROBLEMS

The initial approach to patients with gastrointestinal (GI) hemorrhage is an exercise in resuscitation. The following questions should be addressed and acted on immediately. Is the airway adequate? Is the intravenous (IV) access adequate? Is the circulating blood volume adequate? In reality diagnostic and therapeutic modalities are initiated simultaneously. Eighty percent of all GI bleeding stops spontaneously regardless of treatment. The clinician's responsibility in managing GI hemorrhage is to prevent or treat the consequences of GI blood loss. The general approach to patients admitted to the ICU with upper GI hemorrhage is presented in Table 138-1.

STRESS POINTS

1. Is there GI bleeding?
2. What is the magnitude of the blood loss (Table 138-2)?
3. What is the specific lesion?

ESSENTIAL DIAGNOSTIC TESTS
AND PROCEDURES

1. History and physical examination
2. Vital signs
3. Gastric lavage
4. Stool guaiac
5. Upper or lower GI endoscopy (as indicated)
6. Contrast radiography (barium studies) (as indicated)
7. Nuclear medicine tagged red blood cells (RBC) studies (as indicated)
8. Angiography (as indicated)

INITIAL THERAPY

1. Prevention of stress gastritis should be undertaken in patients at risk with H_2 receptor antagonists or sucralfate. Risk factors for stress gastritis include respiratory failure requiring mechanical ventilation, coagulopathy, major trauma, sepsis, and shock.
2. H_2 receptor antagonists are commonly used in the management of upper GI hemorrhage although there is no convincing evidence that these agents alter the course of acute bleeding or improve patient outcome.
3. Drugs that induce vasoconstriction, such as vasopressin, are frequently used in the management of GI hemorrhage; however, clinical trials have failed to show improvement in patient outcome.
4. Endoscopic hemostatic modalities such as electrocoagulation, heater probe, laser, and injection may be highly effective depending on the specific lesion.
5. Surgical consultation is warranted in cases of severe GI hemorrhage.

OVERVIEW ■

The management of gastrointestinal hemorrhage presents to critical care practitioners a diagnostic, therapeutic, and economic challenge. Unfortunately, the rationale for making clinical decisions concerning these patients is not firmly based on well-designed clinical trials. In the United States, there are 250,000 admissions (50 to 100 per 100,000 population) with GI bleeding each year.[1] Despite advances in technology and changes in therapy and treatment, mortality from GI hemorrhage has remained at 8% to 10% over the past 25 years.[1-6]

TABLE 138-1. Approach to Gastrointestinal Bleeding

DIAGNOSIS	TREATMENT
1. Is there GI bleeding?	
2. What is the magnitude of the blood loss?	Resuscitation: fluids, blood products
3. Is the bleeding upper GI?	Gastric lavage
4. What is the specific lesion?	
Varices	Vasopressin; sclerotherapy; balloon tamponade
Mallory-Weiss tear	Observation; vasopressin
Acute mucosal lesion	Gastric neutralization; drugs
Gastric ulcer	Endoscopic techniques
Duodenal ulcer	Angiographic techniques
Tumor	Surgery

TABLE 138-2. Indicators of Major Blood Loss

1. Resting tachycardia (> 100 beats/min)
2. Orthostasis (pulse increase > 20 beats/min, systolic BP decrease > 20 mm Hg, diastolic BP decrease > 10 mm Hg)
3. Acidosis
4. Azotemia (BUN ≥ 40 mg/dL without prior renal disease)
5. Transfusion requirements > 1 U q 8 h (or 6 U total)
6. Hematochezia from upper GI source
7. Failure to clear bright red blood from gastric lavage
8. Continued bleeding or rebleeding during endoscopy

Some patients are admitted to the CCU for gastrointestinal hemorrhage; however, critically ill patients often suffer initially from a single well-defined problem, then develop additional complications such as GI bleeding. The critical care environment is characterized by invasive monitoring and vasoactive and other drugs that affect mesenteric oxygen delivery. Additionally, complications such as heart failure and sepsis can have profound effects on GI function. In the critically ill, endoscopically evident gastritis or ulceration has been documented in 75% to 100% of patients, and clinically evident bleeding occurs in 20%.[7,8] GI bleeding has also been recognized as part of the syndrome of multiple organ failure along with renal, hematologic, respiratory, neurologic, and cardiovascular complications.[9,10] Increasing the awareness and understanding of GI bleeding in the critically ill leads to better detection and therapy.

APPROACH TO DIAGNOSIS AND MANAGEMENT OF UPPER GASTROINTESTINAL BLEEDING ■

IS GASTROINTESTINAL BLEEDING PRESENT?

The first question the clinician must ask when evaluating gastrointestinal hemorrhage is, "Is there GI bleeding?"[11] Historically, information about color and quantity of stool is helpful.[3] Melena suggests a minimum blood loss of 200 mL. Hematemesis, hematochezia, and vomiting of "coffee ground" material is evidence of hemorrhage. A positive nasogastric aspirate for red blood or coffee ground material confirms the presence of upper GI bleeding, whereas a negative nasogastric aspirate does not rule out an upper GI source of bleeding. Testing stool or emesis during an acute episode of bleeding is not usually helpful.[3] Using material designed to detect occult hematochezia in colon cancer screening programs can confirm a clinical impression of the presence of blood in the stool. Testing of gastric contents can frequently be misleading because of nasogastric tube trauma. In addition, the low pH of gastric contents interferes

with the guaiac test's design for occult blood testing in stool, giving false results. Laboratory evaluation noting anemia may also be evidence for existence of GI bleeding.

HOW MUCH BLEEDING?

Estimation and replacement of blood loss is the single most important aspect of care in patients with gastrointestinal hemorrhage. Most complications occur secondary to the effects of hypovolemia on organs and are compounded by the presence of preexisting atherosclerosis or previous organ damage. Blood loss is usually underestimated. Estimation requires an accurate assessment of vital signs, central pressure, hemoglobin and hematocrit, and a degree of clinical experience. Indicators of major blood loss are outlined in Table 138-2. Severe hemorrhage is usually defined as a greater than 1000-mL blood loss. Hematocrit determination after rapid blood loss is particularly unreliable, requiring as long as 72 hours for total equilibration from the initial hematocrit.

Physiologic responses to blood loss are acute and chronic. The acute responses include orthostatic changes with acute fluid shifts, vascular insufficiency from peripheral vasoconstriction, and acute impairment of central organ function. Chronic blood loss usually is associated with stable hemodynamic responses, retention of hypotonic fluid, and an absence of impaired organ function. Other factors may impair or mask normal responses to blood loss. Those factors include drugs, preexisting dehydration, oxygen desaturation from pulmonary disease, the state of the cardiovascular system (particularly atherosclerotic cerebrovascular disease), abnormal concentration of plasma proteins, and miscellaneous conditions such as spinal cord disease, neuropathy, renal dysfunction, toxic shock, and congestive heart failure.

SOURCE OF BLEEDING

Historic clues such as hematemesis or melena can help to determine whether bleeding is from the upper or the lower GI tract. Hematemesis and melena suggest an upper GI source, whereas hematochezia usually suggests bleeding that originates in the lower GI tract. It must be remembered that a significant percentage of patients with ascending colon sources of bleeding may present with melena. Nasogastric aspirate should be used to confirm upper GI hemorrhage. Melena is most often caused by upper GI blood loss. Thus, patients who present with GI hemorrhage, even if it appears to be of a lower GI etiology, need a diagnostic gastric lavage. In patients with persistent melena of unclear etiology, an upper endoscopy should be performed to exclude upper GI bleeding even if the nasogastric lavage is negative.

Clinical and laboratory data may also indicate whether GI bleeding is from an upper or a lower source. Hyperactive bowel sounds imply an upper GI source of bleeding. An elevated blood urea nitrogen (BUN)–creatinine ratio usually indicates an upper GI source as well as major blood loss.[5,12] Patients without intrinsic renal disease who have a BUN greater than 25 mg/dL have lost a minimum of 1 L of blood. Persistent azotemia (>24 hours) is an indication of hypovolemia because volume loss contributes quantitatively more than the digestion of blood in raising BUN and is the sole determinant of azotemia 24 hours after cessation of bleeding.[5,13]

IS THERE A SPECIFIC LESION?

Generally pain implies a mucosal lesion such as peptic ulcer disease; vomiting before the onset of bleeding suggests a Mallory-Weiss tear.[14] When previous bleeding occurred from a known lesion, there is a 70% probability that the repeat bleeding is from that lesion. When there has been previous bleeding from an unknown source despite an earlier diagnostic evaluation, arteriovenous malformations should be considered. Careful drug history with specific attention to proprietary medicines is important because of the relationship of major upper GI hemorrhage to the use of aspirin and other nonsteroidal analgesics.[15,16] Physical examination may reveal evidence of trauma, a hemorrhagic diathesis, or stigmata of chronic liver disease. A national survey of upper GI hemorrhage in 1981 revealed that ulcer disease or inflammation accounts for approximately 85% of patients admitted to CCUs.[17] Varices or Mallory-Weiss tears accounts for the remainder.

The most expeditious and accurate method of diagnosing a specific cause for upper GI hemorrhage is upper endoscopy. An adequate endoscopic examination requires a stable patient and removal of blood and clots from the stomach, and is hindered by recent use of barium contrast radiography and antacids. Emergency examinations are more difficult and less accurate, and therefore should be avoided. No study exists with conclusive findings that endoscopy has significantly altered overall outcome of GI hemorrhage.[11,18] However, endoscopic complications are higher during emergency examinations. Morbidity (0.2%) and mortality (0.006%) are low but measurable.[19] Continued development of endoscopic techniques to control GI hemorrhage is likely to change our approach to the timing of diagnostic procedures in the future.

TREATMENT FOR GASTROINTESTINAL BLEEDING ■

CAPSULE

The importance of resuscitation in patients with GI bleeding cannot be overemphasized. The initial emergency assessment should note vital signs. The patient should be "tilted" for orthostatic change unless there is shock or resting tachycardia with pulse greater than 120 beats/minute. Intravenous access should rapidly be obtained and fluids and blood replaced as necessary. There should be an assessment for impaired organ function or underlying disease.

ICU ADMISSION CRITERIA

Not all patients need ICU admission. Criteria such as greater than 500-mL blood loss, hypotension, or hypovolemic shock have been used as indications for CCU admission,[1] but there are no universally accepted guidelines. Bordley and coworkers[20] define clinical predictors of good outcome: (1) age less than 75 years; (2) no unstable comorbid illness; (3) no ascites on initial examination; (4) normal prothrombin time; (5) systolic blood pressure greater than or equal to 100 mm Hg within 1 hour after presentation; and (6) a nasogastric aspirate free from fresh (red) blood within 1 hour after presentation. Others are evaluating admission criteria and demographics to predict poor outcome and risk of further bleeding.[6,11,21,22] Endoscopy can also be used to assess the risk of rebleeding.[23,24] Peptic ulcers with active bleeding or a nonbleeding visible vessel has a high risk of rebleeding and patients should be watched in the ICU for 24 hours and observed in the hospital ward for 48 to 72 hours. Patients with clean based ulcers or Mallory-Weiss tears can be discharged when otherwise clinically stable or within 1 day.[24] A review of hospital care and duration of stay in acute nonvariceal bleeding has shown that despite dramatic reductions in length of stay from 1981 to 1991, patient outcome remains excellent with short hospitalizations.[25] The fact that the mortality of patients with GI bleeding has not changed in the last 25 years despite technologic and therapeutic advances leads to a conservative approach when deciding whether a patient would benefit from critical care monitoring. After an initial assessment and diagnostic lavage have been completed, specific therapy can be considered.

EMPIRIC THERAPY FOR UPPER GASTROINTESTINAL HEMORRHAGE

Empiric treatment should stop upper GI hemorrhage and prevent its recurrence. Since this form of treatment must be administered without a diagnosis, it must be relatively safe and easily administered by physicians without special skills.[5]

GASTRIC LAVAGE

The use of iced saline lavage came into vogue in 1959 after Wangensteen produced evidence that hepatic and gastric blood flow was reduced with gastric cooling produced by an indwelling balloon containing circulating cold fluid.[26] These data were extrapolated to the use of iced saline lavage in patients with upper GI hemorrhage. Since that time, several studies have examined the usefulness of this technique in a model of canine gastric ulcer. Iced saline appears to offer no advantage over room temperature saline in arresting upper GI hemorrhage and may, in fact, produce hypothermia and prolong hemorrhage.[27,28] Although iced saline may reduce gastric blood flow by 50%, bleeding time is increased threefold, offering a possible explanation for prolongation of hemorrhage.[29] Saline has been compared with water in a similar animal model and no difference was found in duration of hemorrhage, serum sodium, potassium, or osmolality.[30] The addition of levarterenol to the lavage solution appears to do little to control bleeding and does not appear to be warranted.[31]

There is no controlled clinical trial evaluating the efficacy of gastric lavage in the treatment of upper GI hemorrhage. Animal data reveal no benefit in its use and actually suggest that lavage may ultimately prolong hemorrhage. At present, the use of gastric lavage should be limited to the localization and estimation of severity of upper GI hemorrhage and to the preparation of the upper GI tract for endoscopy. Existing data suggest that room temperature tap water is the lavage fluid of choice.

PHARMACOLOGIC INTERVENTION

Medical therapy in upper GI hemorrhage, outlined in Table 138-3, has been directed toward one of three entities: (1) raising gastric pH; (2) inducing vasoconstriction and therefore reducing blood flow to the "feeder vessel" disrupted by the disease process; or (3) inhibiting clot dissolution. All modalities could potentially be used as empiric therapy.

DRUGS THAT RAISE GASTRIC PH

Drugs that raise gastric pH, such as H_2 antagonists, antacids, secretin and somatostatin, should be of value in the treatment of patients with upper GI hemorrhage. These drugs accelerate ulcer healing and inactivate pepsin. Pepsin has been shown to promote platelet disaggregation and is inactivated at a pH greater than 4.5. It has been shown in vitro that prothrombin time (PT) and partial thromboplastin time

(PTT) are prolonged in the presence of pH less than 7.3. Acid pH also decreases platelet aggregation and promotes disaggregation.[32]

Although H_2 antagonists are commonly used in the management of upper GI hemorrhage, there is no convincing evidence that these agents improve outcome. Approximately 30 clinical trials have evaluated the various H_2 antagonists. Pooled data from over 2500 patients enrolled in these various trials have been analyzed to achieve a large enough sample size to reveal a statistically significant difference in outcome between the drug- and placebo-treated groups.[33] The use of H_2 antagonists resulted in a 10% decrease in rebleeding rate or cessation of ongoing hemorrhage compared with that found with use of a placebo—a difference that was not statistically significant. The need for emergent surgery in the H_2 antagonist group was reduced by approximately 20% ($p = 0.02$). This analysis suggests that H_2 antagonists probably have a therapeutic influence, albeit small, on patients with upper GI hemorrhage. Interestingly, patients with gastric ulcers appeared to benefit from H_2 antagonist therapy to a greater degree than those with duodenal ulcers.

Somatostatin has a theoretic use in the empiric treatment of upper GI hemorrhage. Somatostatin lowers splanchnic blood flow, decreases portal pressure and hepatic blood flow, inhibits gastric acid, gastrin and pepsin secretion, and increases gastric mucus production. One large controlled, clinical trial of more than 500 patients showed no statistically significant reduction in rebleeding rate in somatostatin-treated patients.[34] Also, there was no reduction in mortality or need for surgical intervention. Additionally, a smaller study involving 95 patients failed to show a significant reduction in rebleeding rates or transfusions, but a significant reduction in the number of patients undergoing surgery was seen in the somatostatin-treated group.[35] Somatostatin presently is available in the United States but not approved by the Food and Drug Administration for use in upper GI hemorrhage.

Administration of pharmacologic doses of secretin have been shown to result in a reduction in serum gastrin levels and in gastric acid secretion, although these findings have been challenged. No double-blind trial using secretin in patients with upper GI hemorrhage has been performed, but some uncontrolled studies have suggested a slight benefit.[36-38]

DRUGS THAT INDUCE VASOCONSTRICTION

Lysine vasopressin has been used for the treatment of GI hemorrhage for more than 20 years. Clinical trials have failed to show an improvement in patient outcome even in patients with documented bleeding esophageal varices, the entity in which vasopressin is thought to be most effective.[5] The gastrointestinal effects of vasopressin center around its ability to contract vascular smooth muscle, resulting in a decrease in splanchnic blood flow. As a result, portal venous flow, portal venous pressure, and total hepatic flow are reduced, presumably leading to a decrease in esophageal variceal flow and a reduction in variceal hemorrhage. The systemic side effects of vasopressin are considerable, including an increase in heart rate, a reduction in coronary blood flow,

TABLE 138-3. Medications Used in the Empiric Treatment of Upper GI Hemorrhage

Drugs that raise gastric pH
    H_2 receptor antagonists
    Antacids
    Somatostatin
    Secretin
Drugs that induce splanchnic vasoconstriction
    Lysine vasopressin
    Glycine vasopressin
    Somatostatin
Drugs that inhibit fibrinolysis
    Tranexamic acid

a reduction in cardiac output, peripheral vasoconstriction, arterial hypertension, increased GI peristalsis, increased fibrinolysis, and a decrease in free water excretion with resulting hyponatremia and its attendant complications. Studies comparing selective intraarterial infusion with peripheral venous infusion have found no advantage to the arterial route.[39,40] The use of nitroglycerin in combination with vasopression has been shown to reverse the detrimental hemodynamic effects of vasopressin and decrease cardiovascular complications without altering efficacy.[24]

Glycine vasopressin (Glypressin), a long-acting congener of lysine vasopressin, has recently been approved for use in patients with variceal bleeding in the United Kingdom and in several other European countries. Besides the increase in half-life over that of lysine vasopressin, Glypressin has the theoretic advantage of not increasing fibrinolysis. The clinical relevance of this feature is not known. No controlled clinical trials showing an improvement in outcome with Glypressin therapy exist.

Somatostatin, in addition to its antisecretory effects, lowers azygous vein (and presumably esophageal variceal) blood flow in portal hypertension. One study comparing somatostatin with vasopressin showed it to be equally effective for control of esophageal variceal hemorrhage with fewer side effects.[41] In other studies somatostatin achieved hemostasis more effectively than vasopressin[42] or a placebo.[43]

DRUGS THAT INHIBIT FIBRINOLYSIS

The antifibrinolytic agent tranexamic acid (Cyklokapron, Kabi Vitrum AB, Sweden) has been investigated in several trials. The largest of these placebo-controlled trials involved over 400 patients and revealed a statistically significant reduction in mortality in upper GI hemorrhage from 10.5% in the placebo group to 3.6% in the treatment group (p = .0072).[44] Virtually all of the studies involving this drug have shown some improvement in the need for transfusion, in surgery, or in mortality; however, many differences were not statistically significant. A metaanalysis of earlier work with tranexamic acid suggests that its use could result in a 20% reduction in bleeding, a 30% reduction in the need for surgery, and a 40% reduction in mortality.[45] These results should be viewed with caution because of the many objections to this type of analysis on pooled data.[10] Superficial thrombophlebitis and deep venous thrombosis are common complications of this therapy. However, most complications are not serious. Overall, tranexamic acid is considered to be relatively safe and inexpensive.[10] It is not available in the United States.

CRITICAL ASSESSMENT OF AVAILABLE INTERVENTIONS ∎

No form of available empiric medical therapy has been conclusively shown to improve outcome in upper GI hemorrhage. The inability of current trials to prove drug efficacy in upper GI hemorrhage is probably related to the large number of patients who stop bleeding spontaneously, the mixture of patients and bleeding etiologies included in these trials, the relatively small number of patients included, and the lack of a truly potent drug to use in upper GI bleeding. A study of 10,000 patients with upper GI hemorrhage is required to show the statistically significant reduction in mortality of 20%.[5,33] Because of their attendant safety, ease of administration, and a suggestion of efficacy when patients from multiple trials are pooled, intravenous administration of an H_2 antagonist at the time of admission in patients with upper GI hemorrhage is frequently recommended. The oral route should be used whenever possible to reduce the cost of therapy. Currently, Somatostatin, secretin, vasopressin, and tranexamic acid cannot be recommended for the empiric therapy of upper GI hemorrhage due to their side effects, lack of efficacy, or lack of availability. Both somatostatin and tranexamic acid show some promise in treatment for upper GI hemorrhage but must be considered investigational therapy at the present time.

ENDOSCOPY

Many endoscopic techniques have been introduced in an attempt to avoid surgery in high-risk patients. Those likely to benefit from early endoscopic intervention are patients who have acute GI bleeding and (1) present with shock or hemodynamic instability; (2) present with hemoglobin less than 8; (3) have a coexistent catabolic state, coagulopathy, advanced age, or serious concomitant disease; (4) have bright red nasogastric aspirate after 4 hours of initial resuscitation; and (5) have onset of bleeding while in the hospital.[46-48] Hemostatic mechanisms include topical, injectable, mechanical, and thermal techniques.[49-51] Table 138-4 outlines a comparison of hemostatic modalities. Surgery remains the standard of care in most cases of severe, uncontrolled GI hemorrhage. The current trend is for more conservative procedures, optimally timed and of limited extent.[10,52] Such management requires a team approach, incorporating members of the departments of medicine, surgery, and radiology. A skilled nursing staff is required for consistent outcome.

STRESS ULCERATION ∎

Stress ulceration is a topic of clinical and economic importance in the CCU. Without prophylaxis, more than 75% of patients admitted to a critical care facility develop active mucosal disease.[1,7,8] Fifty percent of these patients show evidence of recent bleeding,[53] and as many as 20% have clinically evident hemorrhage.[7,53] If surgery is required to control hemorrhage, mortality may exceed 70%.[8] Various pharmacologic agents have been recommended for prophylaxis but not all have been subjected to randomized clinical trials.

HISTORIC PERSPECTIVE

Gastroduodenal mucosal lesions associated with stress, trauma, and burns have been recognized for more than a century.[1,7] Rokitansky's "gastric mucosal decubiti" were

TABLE 138-4. Comparison of Hemostatic Modalities

	MONOPOLAR ELECTROCOAGULATION	BIPOLAR COAGULATION	HEATER PROBE	LASER	INJECTION*
Efficacy for control of bleeding	++	++	+++	++	++
Tissue erosion	++++	+	+	++++	+
Ease of use	++	++	++	++	++
Portability	++	++	++	Not	++
Cost	++	++	++	++++	+

*Nonvariceal injection sclerotherapy.

Adapted from Hartfelder RC: Endoscopic control of gastrointestinal bleeding. In: Di Palma JA (ed). *Problems in Critical Care—Gastrointestinal Complications.* Philadelphia, JB Lippincott, 1989:351

considered a result of postmortem autolysis for decades before it was recognized as an antemortem event. Cushing's gastroduodenal lesions related to head trauma were described in 1933.[53] Acute duodenal ulcerations associated with burns were reported in 1923 by London surgeon, Joseph Swan, and termed *Curling's ulcers* after Curling's 1842 report. Stress-related mucosal injury refers to these lesions and the mucosal erosions noted in most untreated critically ill patients.

ETIOLOGY

The pathogenesis of stress ulceration remains poorly understood. Various factors and mechanisms, alone or in combination, are probably responsible for these lesions. One can think of stress lesions as a result of an imbalance between protective and aggressive factors.[8] The aggressive factors include acid, pepsin, and bile salts. Some patients who develop stress ulceration demonstrate hypersecretion of acid.[1,7] Pepsin and bile salts can damage gastric mucosa in the absence of acid; however, it does not seem that ulcerations or erosions occur in patients with achlorhydria.[1] Therefore, hypersecretion of acid and pepsin seems to be a prerequisite for stress mucosal injury. Protective factors are those that prevent gastric epithelium autodigestion. Mucosal blood flow, the gastric mucus layer, bicarbonate secretion, prostaglandins, and epithelial cell renewal are factors that protect overall mucosal integrity from the aggressive factors.

The concept of a mucosal barrier has been developed to describe the constellation of defense mechanisms that permits a high hydrogen ion gradient between lumen and tissue without damage to the tissue.[8] This thin layer of mucus gel is a matrix of glycoprotein moieties joined by physical noncovalent molecular interactions.[8] In addition to providing mechanical protection and trapping bicarbonate, mucus delays the diffusion of the hydrogen ion and pepsin, leading to a near neutral environment of the mucosal cell surface.[8] Endogenous prostaglandins in the stomach, prostaglandin E_2 and I_2, may help to maintain the integrity of the mucus–bicarbonate barrier. In its most simplistic description, compromise of this "barrier" leads to back diffusion of hydrogen ions. These hydrogen ions lead to permeability changes and

development of edema. Pepsin is activated, which leads to local tissue destruction.[1]

Several "barrier breakers" have been described.[1] Aspirin, nonsteroidal antiinflammatory drugs, and alcohol are unionized at low pH and may break the mucosal barrier. Nonsteroidal antiinflammatory drugs block the formation of these protective prostaglandins, potentially leading to changes in the mucus layer and its polysaccharides. Free radicals may also compromise the barrier. Alcohol by itself does not produce free radicals, but it decreases glutathione, a free radical scavenger.[1] Urea in chronic renal failure also compromises the barrier. Steroid drugs potentiate other barrier breakers. Steroids also decrease mucus production and lead to changes in the polysaccharide portion of the mucus.[1]

Ischemia promotes epithelial damage by a variety of mechanisms.[8] Inadequate tissue oxygenization and nutrition lead to a compromise of aerobic metabolism resulting in a decrease of high-energy phosphate compounds and subsequently leading to cell death. This deficit of high-energy phosphate compounds seems to be greater in the fundus than in the antrum of the stomach; this may be one of the explanations for the distribution of stress mucosal lesions.[7,8] Ischemia also disrupts the acid–base balance at the luminal–mucosal interface. Blood flow is required to dispose of the hydrogen ions that back diffuse to the gastric epithelial surface and supply bicarbonate for buffering the acid. Ischemia additionally promotes the development of oxygen derived radicals, or superoxides, which damage cell organelles and membranes.[8] Shock or hypoperfusion does not directly cause gastric mucosal erosions. The breaks in the mucosa occur with reperfusion. These events support a superoxide, oxygen-derived free radical injury theory.

The rate of gastric epithelial turnover is decreased during stress. Because agents that stimulate the growth of mucosa appear to be effective in reducing stress injury, it has been proposed that the rate of epithelial turnover may be an important factor in the development of stress ulceration.

PATIENTS AT RISK

Critically ill patients who have a predisposition for developing stress-related mucosal injury include those with burns, sepsis, major trauma, and respiratory, renal, or hepatic insuf-

TABLE 138-5. Risk Factors for Stress Hemorrhage

RISK FACTOR I (SEVERE)	RISK FACTOR II (MODERATE)	RISK FACTOR III (ONLY IN COMBINATION WITH I, II)
History of ulcer	Transplantation	Repeat laparotomy
Acute renal insufficiency	Coagulopathy	Ileus
Burn > 25% body	Neurogenic shock	Anaphylactic shock
surface area	Intracranial bleeding	Septic shock
Sole cerebral trauma with	Transfusion (> 4 U)	Cerebral trauma with neurologic
neurologic deficit	Age > 65 y	defect (in combination with
Severe infection	Heparin use	polytrauma)
Severe polytrauma	Hemoglobin < 10 g/dL	Corticosteroid use
Cardiogenic shock	for > 24 h	
Pancreatitis	Systolic BP < 100 mm Hg	
Kidney disease	for > 2 h (single	
Gastroenterologic disease	episode or cumulative)	
Respiratory insufficiency	Systolic BP > 200 mm Hg	
Septic shock	for > 4 d (single	
	episode or cumulative)	

Adapted from Tryba M: Risk of acute stress bleeding and nosocomial pneumonia in ventilated intensive care unit patients: sucralfate versus antacids. *Am J Med* 1987;83(Suppl 38):117

ficiency. Patients with burns over more than 35% of their body surface are at risk to develop Curling's ulcers. Patients with head trauma may develop Cushing's ulcers. Table 138-5 outlines factors used to score the severity of the patient's risk for developing hemorrhage in randomized clinical trials of prophylactic therapy.[54] Such a system may be used to objectively quantify the risk of stress injury in individual patients. Sepsis may be an independent risk factor. In various studies of agents used for stress ulcer prophylaxis, those patients who had bleeding and were refractory to control of gastric pH were usually septic.

Not all patients admitted to the CCU require prophylactic therapy. Monitoring of gastric pH may predict those patients who need therapy. Stothert and coworkers, in a study using gastric pH monitoring as a prognostic indicator for the prophylaxis of stress ulceration, found that the indication for prophylaxis was identified when gastric pH was less than 4.[55] Patients who had gastric pH greater than 4 did not develop stress ulceration or bleeding. In an attempt to identify patients who would be at low risk of bleeding and not need stress prophylaxis, Cook and collaborators found that prophylaxis can safely be withheld from critically ill patients unless they have coagulopathy or require mechanical ventilation.[56] This study, however, excluded those with burns, transplants, head injury, recent peptic ulcer, or GI bleeding underscoring the need for prophylaxis in these patients.

TREATMENT

The initial therapy for stress ulceration and its prevention should be directed toward the underlying disease.[8] The intensivists must pay attention to hemodynamic metabolic and physiologic factors to provide adequate mucosal blood flow. Special attention should be focused on the possibilities of

sepsis, hypovolemia, acidosis, respiratory failure, and nutritional deficiencies.

PROPHYLAXIS

Various agents have been used in an attempt to prevent acute mucosal stress injury in the critically ill. Only recently have many of these agents been subjected to carefully performed randomized clinical trials to document efficacy. Antacids, histamine receptor antagonists, and sucralfate (a cytoprotective agent) have been studied.[1,7,8,53,54,57–60] These reports document that prophylactic therapy significantly reduces the risk of upper gastrointestinal hemorrhage. Efficacy is similar for each studied agent. There seems to be no difference in the ability of antacids, cimetidine, ranitidine, famotidine, or sucralfate to prevent stress injury and bleeding. It is important to emphasize that acid-modulating therapy with antacids or H₂ receptor antagonists requires control of gastric pH. When gastric acidity is titrated to a desired pH goal, the overall bleeding rate is low. Inability to control pH is associated with stress ulceration and bleeding. It is, therefore, important to monitor gastric pH during therapy with these agents. Relatively inexpensive, simple systems to directly measure pH using electrodes located at the tip of nasogastric tubes are available.[61] These devices have been shown to be accurate when compared with laboratory techniques to titrate pH and superior to litmus paper measurements.[61] Litmus paper is a particularly inaccurate method for measuring pH in the ICU.[62] Sucralfate is a mucosal cytoprotective agent that has efficacy in stress ulceration[58,59] by means of a mechanism that is independent of gastric pH. It is not necessary to monitor gastric pH while using sucralfate.

Other agents have been used for stress injury prophylaxis. Most of these have not been subjected to clinical trials. Conflicting data exist concerning prostaglandin E$_2$ preparations for prevention of stress bleeding.[7,63] Other agents such as omeprazole, glucagon, and lithium seem promising but have not been carefully studied. Another promising therapy would be the use of oxygen radical scavengers and xanthine oxidase inhibitors such as allopurinol.[8] Agents such as pentagastrin, carbenoxolone, vitamin A, and growth hormone may protect or stimulate mucosal growth and may be effective in stress ulceration therapy.[7] Gastrin, isoproterenol, and anticholinergic agents also seem promising but have not been studied. Enteral alimentation has been advocated by many authors but conclusive data are forthcoming. Stress ulceration may be a manifestation of the systemic inflammatory response syndrome with the gut playing a central role in the metabolic disturbances of the syndrome.[64] It has been proposed that translocation of luminal GI bacteria to extraintestinal sites triggers organ dysfunction. Early enteral feedings help preserve gut mucosal integrity and should be favored over parenteral feeding. Small amounts of enteral feeding can be protective even when ileus or other medical conditions would usually not allow enteral nutrition.[64]

CHOICE OF AGENT

The choice of an agent for stress prophylaxis can be difficult; however, an agent with proved efficacy in randomized clinical trials should be used. Since efficacy of various agents may be similar, ease of administration and cost become important considerations. Parenteral agents are more expensive than oral agents but require less nursing time. Titrated antacids are expensive and provide a significant volume load to the stomach. Sucralfate and antacids require a functioning gut.

Sucralfate (1 g every 6 hours) may be used when the gut can tolerate an oral agent. It is relatively inexpensive when compared with parenteral agents and does not require monitoring of gastric pH. In addition, stress ulcer prophylaxis with sucralfate reduces the risk for late-onset pneumonia in ventilated patients compared with antacids or ranitidine.[65] Antacids are not acceptable since they provide a large volume load and require gastric pH monitoring. When a parenteral agent is necessary, infusion is recommended rather than bolus therapy. With use of a primed infusion, a continuous infusion of the parenteral agent is begun after a bolus IV dose.[60,66] This allows rapid attainment of a therapeutic serum level of the medication and, it is hoped, provides continuous hypochlorhydria. Gastric pH is monitored to use the lowest necessary dose. Cimetidine, ranitidine, and famotidine are acceptable, efficacious agents for stress ulcer prophylaxis. With cimetidine, one needs to be attentive to adverse experiences in elderly patients and avoid predictable drug interactions.[67]

THERAPY FOR STRESS HEMORRHAGE

Surgical mortality in stress bleeding has been reported to be greater than 75%.[1,8] Fortunately, patients who develop stress ulceration are no more likely to bleed or require surgery than those with typical acid peptic disease. The poor outcome from surgery underscores the importance of prevention of stress bleeding. In an attempt to avoid surgery in this condition, various endoscopic therapies have been used. Endoscopic techniques to control gastrointestinal hemorrhage include nonvariceal injection sclerotherapy, heater probe or laser thermal coagulation, and electrocoagulation.[50,51] Other nonsurgical measures include arteriography with embolization or intraarterial vasopressin.[8] If surgery is unavoidable, preoperative endoscopy is helpful in guiding the limits of resection. Various surgical procedures have been tried including vagotomy and pyloroplasty, vagotomy and gastric resection, total gastric resection, and gastric devascularization. The results have been dismal for all operative procedures designed to treat stress ulcerations.[7]

APPROACH TO LOWER GASTROINTESTINAL BLEEDING

There are many possible causes of gastrointestinal hemorrhage from the lower GI tract. Table 138-6 lists many of these lesions.[5] In patients presenting to the CCU with acute lower GI bleeding, diverticular disease and angiodysplasias are the most common causes. However, in patients who develop lower GI bleeding while in the CCU, nonocclusive mesenteric ischemia deserves particular attention. In this disorder, hemodynamic and systemic abnormalities may predispose the patient to functional intestinal ischemia with or without preexisting anatomic vascular obstruction.[7] Causes include shock, low cardiac output, congestive failure, injudicious use of diuretics, hemoconcentration, and arrhythmias. Management is based on correcting underlying abnormalities with restoration of circulating blood volume. Harmful drugs such as vasoconstrictors and digitalis preparations must be avoided.

EVALUATION OF LOWER GASTROINTESTINAL HEMORRHAGE

The initial approach in evaluating lower GI bleeding should be similar to that discussed for upper GI hemorrhage. Anoscopy or sigmoidoscopy is recommended during the initial evaluation. If it is clear that hemorrhage has stopped spontaneously, elective barium enema radiographic examinations or colonoscopy can be used.[68,69] If the radiographic approach is preferred, a wait of 48 to 72 hours is suggested. Performing barium studies early interferes with angiographic studies if bleeding recurs. If bleeding continues, recurs, or is massive, it should be localized with a nuclear medicine RBC study or angiography as indicated. When angiography is performed, the inferior mesenteric artery, superior mesenteric artery, and celiac axis all should be studied. If a bleeding site is identified, the use of intraarterial vasopressin may arrest bleeding and prevent surgery. Selective intraarterial digital subtraction angiography (DSA) has received recent attention for localization and embolization of bleeding lesions.[70] "Urgent" colonoscopy may be used as an initial diag-

TABLE 138-6. Summary of Lesions Causing Moderate to Severe Bleeding

SOURCE OF LESION	INCIDENCE (%)	
	Range	*Estimate*
Upper GI tract	0–15	10
Varices		
Acid peptic disease		
Small intestine	0–10	5
Children		
Intussusception, Mechel diverticulum		
Adults		
Neoplasm		
Crohn disease		
Arterial–enteric fistulas		
Colonic	75–100	85
Diverticulosis	1–72	25
Vascular dysplasia	0–11	10
Neoplasm	4–36	15
Cancer		10
Polyp		5
Inflammatory bowel disease	0–16	5
Ischemic colitis	0–3	2
Miscellaneous	0–21	8
Undiagnosed	0–57	20

nostic procedure. In the hemodynamically stable patient, bowel preparation with a polyethylene glycol–electrolyte lavage solution (PEG-ELS, GoLytely, Colyte, NuLytely) can be undertaken early in the course of management.[71-73] This not only prepares the bowel for colonoscopy or surgery but allows monitoring for new bleeding because old blood is purged from the GI tract.[5] Any further blood passed through the rectum indicates recurrent or ongoing hemorrhage. Many of the previously discussed endoscopic methods to control GI hemorrhage can be used during colonoscopy.

CONCLUSIONS ■

The successful management of the patient with GI hemorrhage demands an organized, multidisciplinary approach. Resuscitation takes precedence over all other measures of intervention. The physician must confirm that GI bleeding is present, determine the magnitude of bleeding to guide resuscitation, and then localize the bleeding to the upper or lower GI tract.[5] Following localization, the choice of empiric therapy, diagnostic evaluation, and therapeutic intervention must be made. The urgency of diagnostic and therapeutic intervention depends on the patient's condition, the etiology and severity of the hemorrhage, and the resources available. New therapies must continue to be evaluated in controlled settings to reduce the morbidity and mortality of gastrointestinal bleeding.

REFERENCES ■

1. Hurst JM: Gastrointestinal bleeding. In: Civetta JM, Taylor RW, Kirby RR (eds). *Critical Care Medicine.* Philadelphia, JB Lippincott, 1988:1271
2. Gostout CJ: Acute gastrointestinal bleeding—a common problem revisited. *Mayo Clin Proc* 1988;63:596
3. Schaffner J: Acute gastrointestinal bleeding. *Med Clin North Am* 1986;70:1055
4. Kinard HB III, Powell DW, Sandler RS, et al: A current approach to acute upper gastrointestinal bleeding. *J Clin Gastroenterol* 1981;3:231
5. Rowell WG, DiPalma JA: Critical care approach to gastrointestinal hemorrhage. In: DiPalma JA (ed). *Problems in Critical Care—Gastrointestinal Complications.* Philadelphia, JB Lippincott, 1989:341
6. Morgan AG, Clamp SE: OMGE International Upper Gastrointestinal Bleeding Survey, 1978–1986. *Scand J Gastroenterol* 1988;23(Suppl 144):51
7. Gottlieb JE, Menashe PI, Cruz E: Gastrointestinal complications in critically ill patients: the intensivist's overview. *Am J Gastroenterol* 1986;81:227
8. Chamberlain CE, Peura DA: Stress ulceration and prevention. In: DiPalma JA (ed). *Problems in Critical Care—Gastrointestinal Complications.* Philadelphia, JB Lippincott, 1989:371
9. Bumaschny E, Doglio G, Pusajo J, et al: Postoperative acute gastrointestinal tract hemorrhage and multiple-organ failure. *Arch Surg* 1988;123:722
10. Dykes PW, Walt RP: Acute gastrointestinal hemorrhage. *Curr Opin Gastroenterol* 1989;5:852
11. Peterson WL: Gastrointestinal bleeding. In: Sleisenger MH, Fordtran JS (eds). *Gastrointestinal Disease.* Philadelphia, WB Saunders, 1989:397
12. Felber S, Rosenthal P, Henton D: The BUN/creatinine ratio in localizing gastrointestinal bleeding in pediatric patients. *J Pediatr Gastroenterol Nutr* 1988;7:685
13. Stellato T, Rhodes RS, McDougal WS: Azotemia in upper gastrointestinal hemorrhage: a review. *Am J Gastroenterol* 1980;73:486
14. Harris JM, DiPalma JA: Clinical significance of Mallory-Weiss tears. *Am J Gastroenterol* 1993;88:2056
15. Levy M, Miller DR, Kaufman DW, et al: Major upper gastrointestinal tract bleeding—relation to use of aspirin and other non-narcotic analgesics. *Arch Intern Med* 1988;148:281
16. Kurata JG, Abbey DE: The effect of chronic aspirin use on duodenal and gastric ulcer hospitalizations. *J Clin Gastroenterol* 1990;12:260
17. Silverstein FE, Gilbert DA, Tedesco FJ, et al: International A/S/G/E survey on upper gastrointestinal bleeding. *Gastrointest Endosc* 1981;27:73
18. Eastwood GL: Does the patient with upper gastrointestinal bleeding benefit from endoscopy? Reflections and discussion of recent literature. *Dig Dis Sci* 1981;26:22s
19. Beck DE, DiPalma JA: Complication of gastrointestinal procedures. In: DiPalma JA (ed). *Problems in Critical Care—Gastrointestinal Complications.* Philadelphia, JB Lippincott, 1989:361
20. Bordley DR, Mushlin AI, Dolan JG, et al: Early clinical signs identify low-risk patients with acute upper gastrointestinal hemorrhage. *JAMA* 1985;253:3282
21. Clamp SE, Morgan AG, Kotwal MR, et al: Use of a multinational survey to provide clinical guidelines for upper gastrointestinal bleeding in developing countries. *Scand J Gastroenterol* 1988;23(Suppl 144):63
22. Garrigues-Gil V, Clamp SE, Morgan AG, et al: Do the stigmata

of recent hemorrhage have additional prognostic value in patients with bleeding duodenal ulcer? *Scand J Gastroenterol* 1988;23(Suppl 144):59

23. Laine L, Peterson WL: Bleeding peptic ulcer. *N Engl J Med* 1994;331:717

24. Laine L: Rolling review: upper gastrointestinal bleeding. *Aliment Pharmacol Ther* 1993;7:207

25. Longstreth GF, Feitelberg SP: Hospital care of acute nonvariceal upper gastrointestinal bleeding: 1991 versus 1981. *J Clin Gastroenterol* 1994;19:189

26. Wangensteen OH, Salmon PA, Griffen WO Jr, et al: Studies of local gastric cooling as related to peptic ulcer. *Ann Surg* 1959;150:346

27. Gilbert DA, Saunders DR, Peoples J, et al: Failure of iced saline lavage to suppress hemorrhage from experimental bleeding ulcers. *Gastroenterology* 1979;76:1138

28. Ponsky JL, Hoffman M, Swayngim DS: Saline irrigation in gastric hemorrhage: the effect of temperature. *J Surg Res* 1980; 28:204

29. Waterman NG, Walker JL: The effect of gastric cooling on hemostasis. *Surg Gynecol Obstet* 1973;137:80

30. Bryant LR, Mobin-Uddin K, Dillon ML, et al: Comparison of ice water with iced saline solution for gastric lavage in gastroduodenal hemorrhage. *Am J Surg* 1972;124:570

31. Waterman NG, Walker JL: Effect of a topical adrenergic agent on gastric blood flow. *Am J Surg* 1974;127:241

32. Green FW, Kaplan MM, Curtis LE, et al: Effect of acid and pepsin on blood coagulation and platelet aggregation: a possible contributor to prolonged gastroduodenal mucosal hemorrhage. *Gastroenterology* 1978;74:38

33. Collins R, Langman M: Treatment with histamine H₂ antagonists in acute upper gastrointestinal hemorrhage: implications of randomized trials. *N Engl J Med* 1985;313:660

34. Somerville KW, Henry DA, Davies JG, et al: Somatostatin in treatment of haematemesis and melaena. *Lancet* 1985;1:130

35. Magnusson I, Ihre T, Johansson C, et al: Randomized double blind trial of somatostatin in the treatment of massive upper gastrointestinal haemorrhage. *Gut* 1985;26:221

36. Becker HD, Schafmayer A, Borger HW, et al: Die Behandlung der Blutung aus akuten Schleimhaut lasionen des Magens und Duodenums durch secretin. *Chirurg* 1979;50:87

37. Berg P, Bar U, Hausamen TU, et al: Vergleichende Behandlung gastroduodenaler Blutungen mit Sekretin und Cimetidin. Eine multizentrische studie. *Dtsch Med Wochenschr* 1982;107:1831

38. Wagner PK, Rothmund M, Gronniger J: Sekretin versus somatostatin bei akuter Blutung aus gastroduodenalen ulcera und erosionen, eine randomisiete studie. *Klin Wochenschr* 1983;61:285

39. Johnson WC, Widrich WC, Ansell JE, et al: Control of bleeding varices by vasopressin: a prospective randomized study. *Ann Surg* 1977;186:369

40. Chojkier M, Groszmann RJ, Atterbury CE, et al: A controlled comparison of continuous intraarterial and intravenous infusions of vasopressin in hemorrhage from esophageal varices. *Gastroenterology* 1979;77:540

41. Kravetz D, Bosch J, Teres J, et al: Comparison of intravenous somatostatin and vasopressin infusions in treatment of acute variceal hemorrhage. *Hepatology* 1984;4:442

42. Saari A, Klvilaakso E, Iaberg M, et al: Comparison of somatostatin and vasopressin in bleeding esophageal varices. *Am J Gastroenterol* 1990;85:804

43. Burroughs AK, McCormick PA, Hughes MD, et al: Randomized, double-blind placebo-controlled trial of somatostatin for variceal bleeding. *Gastroenterology* 1990;99:1388

44. Barer D, Ogilvie A, Henry D, et al: Cimetidine and tranexamic acid in the treatment of acute upper-gastrointestinal-tract bleeding. *N Engl J Med* 1983;308:1571

45. Henry DA, O'Connell DL: Effects of fibrinolytic inhibitors on mortality from upper gastrointestinal haemorrhage. *Br Med J* 1989;29:1142

46. Gilbert DA: Epidemiology of gastrointestinal bleeding. *Gastrointest Endosc* 1990;36:58

47. Johnson JH: Endoscopic risk factors for bleeding peptic ulcer. *Gastrointest Endosc* 1990;36:516

48. Castell DO, Blankenbaker RG, Bozymski EM, et al (Consensus development panel): Consensus statement on therapeutic endoscopy and bleeding ulcers. *Gastrointest Endosc* 1990;36:562

49. Steele RJ: Endoscopic haemostasis for non-variceal upper gastrointestinal hemorrhage. *Br J Surg* 1989;76:219

50. Fleischer D: Endoscopic therapy of upper gastrointestinal bleeding in humans. *Gastroenterology* 1986;90:217

51. Hartfelder RC: Endoscopic control of gastrointestinal bleeding. In: DiPalma JA (ed). *Problems in Critical Care—Gastrointestinal Complications*. Philadelphia, JB Lippincott, 1989: 351

52. Hoak BA, Tiley E, Kudminsky R, et al: Parietal cell vagotomy for bleeding duodenal ulcers. *Am Surg* 1988;54:249

53. Shuman RB, Schuster DP, Zuckerman GR: Prophylactic therapy for stress ulcer bleeding: a reappraisal. *Ann Intern Med* 1987;106:562

54. Tryba M: Risk of acute stress bleeding and nosocomial pneumonia in ventilated intensive care unit patients: sucralfate versus antacids. *Am J Med* 1987;83(Suppl 3B):117

55. Stothert JC Jr, Dellinger EP, Simonowitz DA, et al: Gastric pH monitoring as a prognostic indicator for the prophylaxis of stress ulceration in the critically ill. *Am J Surg* 1980;140:761

56. Cook DJ, Fuller HD, Guyatt GH, et al: Risk factors for gastrointestinal bleeding in critically ill patients. *N Engl J Med* 1994;330:377

57. Peura DA, Johnson LF: Cimetidine for prevention and treatment of gastroduodenal mucosal lesions in patients in an intensive care unit. *Ann Intern Med* 1985;103:173

58. Bresalier RS, Grendell JG, Cello JP, et al: Sucralfate suspension vs titrated antacid for the prevention of acute stress-related gastrointestinal hemorrhage in critically ill patients. *Am J Med* 1987;83(Suppl 3B):110

59. Driks MR, Craven DE, Celli BR, et al: Nosocomial pneumonia in intubated patients given sucralfate as compared with antacids or histamine type 2 blockers: the role of gastric colonization. *N Engl J Med* 1987;317:1376

60. Aoki T: Clinical benefits of intravenously administered famotidine in the treatment of upper gastrointestinal hemorrhage caused by peptic ulcer and stress ulcer disease. *Scand J Gastroenterol* 1987;22(Suppl 134):41

61. Durham RM, Weigelt JA: Monitoring gastric pH levels. *Surg Gynecol Obstet* 1989;169:14

62. Caballero GA, Ausman RK, Quebbeman EJ, et al: Gastric secretion pH measurement: what you see is not what you get! *Crit Care Med* 1990;18:396

63. Zinner MJ, Rypins EB, Martin LR, et al: Misoprostil versus antacid titration for preventing stress ulcers in postoperative surgical ICU patients. *Ann Surg* 1989;210:590

64. DiPalma JA: Editorial overview: gastrointestinal complications in the critically ill and the role of the gut in multiple organ dysfunction syndrome. In: DiPalma JA (ed). *Current Opinion in Critical Care*. Philadelphia, Current Science 1995;1:121

65. Prod'hon G, Levenberger P, Roerfer J, et al: Nosocomial pneumonia in mechanically ventilated patients receiving antacid, ranitidine, or sucralfate as prophylaxis for stress ulcer: a randomized controlled trial. *Ann Intern Med* 1994;120:653

66. Morris DL, Markham SJ, Beechey A, et al: Ranitidine—bolus

or infusion prophylaxis for stress ulcer. *Crit Care Med* 1988;16:229

67. McGuigan JE: A consideration of the adverse effects of cimetidine. *Gastroenterology* 1981;80:181
68. Levinson SE, Powell DW, Callahan WT, et al: A current approach to rectal bleeding. *J Clin Gastroenterol* 1981;3(Suppl 1):9
69. Tedesco FJ, Gottfried EB, Corless JK, et al: Prospective evaluation of hospitalized patients with nonactive lower intestinal bleeding—timing and role of barium enema and colonoscopy. *Gastrointest Endosc* 1984;30:281

70. Rees CR, Palmaz JC, Alvarado R, et al: DSA in acute gastrointestinal hemorrhage: clinical and in vitro studies. *Radiology* 1988;169:499
71. Jensen DM, Machicado GA: Diagnosis and treatment of severe hematochezia: the role of urgent colonoscopy after purge. *Gastroenterology* 1988;95:1569
72. DiPalma JA, Brady CE: Colon cleansing for diagnostic and surgical procedures: polyethylene glycol–electrolyte lavage solution. *Am J Gastroenterol* 1989;84:1008
73. Berry MA, DiPalma JA (Review article): Orthograde lavage for colonoscopy. *Aliment Pharmacol Ther* 1994;8:391

Critical Care, Third Edition, edited by Joseph M. Civetta,
Robert W. Taylor, and Robert R. Kirby.
Lippincott-Raven Publishers, Philadelphia, PA © 1997.

CHAPTER 139

■

Fulminant Hepatic Failure

Marc G. Webb
Andreas G. Tzakis

IMMEDIATE CONCERNS ■

MAJOR PROBLEMS

Encephalopathy, cerebral edema leading to brain stem
herniation, severe coagulopathy, renal failure with volume
overload, hemodynamic instability, and a high incidence of
infectious complications makes management of fulminant
hepatic failure (FHF) especially challenging. Patients who
survive with medical management alone must be distinguished from those who require liver transplantation, and
management of both groups of patients requires a keen
understanding and aggressive management of the complications of liver failure.

STRESS POINTS

1. Medical therapy is supportive, should be given in the
   ICU, and is directed toward the treatment and prevention of complications while awaiting regeneration in
   good-prognosis patients, or transplantation in poor-
   prognosis patients. Medical therapy alone in patients
   with grade III or IV hepatic encephalopathy is associated with a survival rate of less than 20% in most series.
2. Encephalopathy is a major complication of FHF, predisposes to other complications, and confuses assessment and treatment of cerebral edema. Clinical signs
   usually associated with increased intracerebral pressure—myoclonus, focal seizures, decerebrate posturing, and loss of brain stem reflexes—may result from
   metabolic encephalopathy. After initial assessment,
   the focus should be on identification and treatment
   of reversible causes of encephalopathy.

3. Cerebral edema is the leading cause of death. The
   usual signs of elevated intracranial pressure (ICP) are
   usually absent. Major issues include the early diagnosis
   and management of intracranial hypertension, and the
   identification of patients with irreversible neurologic
   injury, in whom transplantation is contraindicated.
4. Coagulopathy is a common problem in FHF. Complete correction of coagulopathy in the absence of
   bleeding is controversial and may not be indicated.
   When epidural monitors are in place or when other
   invasive procedures are being performed, it is prudent
   to keep the platelet count above 50,000 to 75,000 and
   to correct the prothrombin time to within 3 seconds
   of normal.
5. Loss of vasomotor tone may make it difficult to differentiate the high-output/low systemic resistance state
   of advanced liver failure from that of sepsis. Management of the FHF patient's hemodynamic status should
   be guided by early placement of a pulmonary artery
   catheter. Pressor support may be necessary.
6. Acute renal dysfunction is frequently present in cases
   of FHF, and oliguric renal failure is associated with
   decreased survival. Conventional hemodialysis has not
   been shown to improve patient survival and has been
   supplanted largely by continuous venovenous hemofiltration (CVVH).
7. Sepsis and impaired immune response are common
   in liver failure. Up to 80% of patients have been found
   to have bacterial infections in the first week of ICU
   stay. Infection should be strongly suspected whenever
   a patient's clinical status deteriorates.
8. Many other methods of artificial liver support have
   been tried. None have found widespread acceptance

or clinical applicability, and none are available outside the few centers where they are undergoing experimental trials.

9. Liver transplantation has changed the prognosis of FHF. Survival rates of 55% to 75% in early series have improved to 90% to 100% in selected centers. Patients with a poor prognosis for survival with medical management alone should be listed for transplantation if no contraindications exist.

ESSENTIAL DIAGNOSTIC TESTS AND PROCEDURES

1. Baseline neurologic examination and ongoing monitoring
2. Baseline laboratory and imaging studies
3. Placement of hemodynamic and volume status monitoring devices, including central venous or pulmonary artery catheters, an arterial catheter, and a Foley catheter
4. Placement of a nasogastric (NG) tube and aspiration for diagnosis of possible upper gastrointestinal (GI) tract bleeding
5. Neurologic consultation and ICP monitoring for grade III-IV encephalopathy.
6. Exclusion or diagnosis and treatment of infectious processes by review of chest radiographs, urinalyses, cell counts in body cavity fluid samples, and surveillance cultures

INITIAL THERAPY

1. Admit the patient to an ICU where appropriate care is available.
2. Use a dextrose drip titrated to keep the patient normoglycemic.
3. Give H-2 blockers to reduce risk of GI bleeding.
4. Supply pulmonary care directed against atelectasis, hypoxia, hypercapnia, and the risk of aspiration.
5. Support blood pressure as needed with judicious volume replacement and vasopressors.
6. Use early antibiotic treatment based on clinical suspicion and surveillance cultures.
7. Control volume overload with volume restriction, diuresis, or ultrafiltration.

FHF is a syndrome characterized by a rapid onset of hepatic dysfunction in an individual previously free of liver disease. It has been further delimited as the development of encephalopathy with or without cerebral edema in less than 8 weeks of the onset of illness,[1] although some authorities use a 2-week period to distinguish fulminant from subfulminant failure.[2] Approximately 2000 cases of FHF in the United States annually.

Mortality with medical management has historically been high, although modest improvements recently can be attributed to improved understanding and treatment of the complications of this disorder. Improved survival is seen in selected patients with liver transplantation.

ETIOLOGY AND PROGNOSIS   ■

Etiology is not always possible to establish and can be identified in only 60% to 80% of cases. Viral infections are the most common cause, followed by hepatotoxic drug reactions and a score of other etiologies (Table 139-1). Establishing an etiology may allow an early tentative assessment of risk, with hepatitis A having historically a 67% survival rate with medical management, acetaminophen poisoning 53%, fulminant hepatitis B 40%, and all others having a less than 20% survival rate. In the case of acetaminophen poisoning, early knowledge may lead to an effective therapeutic intervention (intravenous acetylcysteine). More often, this information is important from an epidemiologic point of view but will not influence early therapy.

Prognosis also depends on nonetiologic factors, such as age older than 40 years or younger than 11 years, markedly prolonged prothrombin time, markedly elevated bilirubin, metabolic acidosis, degree of encephalopathy, time greater than 1 week to the development of encephalopathy, uncorrectable cerebral hypertension, prolonged decreased cerebral perfusion pressure, evidence of cerebral herniation, presence of sepsis, and the presence of extrahepatic organ dysfunction such as renal failure[3] (Table 139-2).

TABLE 139-1.   Possible Etiologies in Fulminant Hepatic Failure

Acetaminophen poisoning
Acute fatty liver of pregnancy
Bactrim
Budd-Chiari syndrome
Chemotherapy
Designer drugs (i.e., Ecstasy)
Dilantin
Ebstein-Barr virus
Fipexide
Halothane
Heat stroke
Heaptitis A, B, C, D, E
Hydroxychloroquine
Isoniazid
Ketoconazole
Lepiota Helveola poisoning
Leukemia/lymphoma
Minocycline
Mushroom poisoning
Nicotinic acid
Octrieatide
Reyes syndrome
Rifampin
Sea anemone stings
Sulfasalazine
Tetracycline
Tricyclics
Valproic acid
Varicella
Vicodin
Wilson's disease

TABLE 139-2. Prognosis–Kings College Criteria

Age younger than 11 or older than 40
Poor prognosis etiology
Greater than 1 week to development to encephalopathy
Markedly elevated prothrombin time (INR >6.5)
Markedly elevated total bilirubin
One + criterion: 80% mortality with medical treatment
Three + criteria: 95% mortality

INR, international normalized ratio; +, positive.

COMPLICATIONS AND TREATMENT ■

OVERVIEW

Medical therapy is supportive, should be given in the ICU, and is directed toward the treatment and prevention of complications while awaiting regeneration in good-prognosis patients or transplantation in poor-prognosis patients (Tables 139-3 and 139-4). Medical therapy alone in patients with grade III or IV hepatic encephalopathy is associated with a survival rate of less than 20% in most series, and cerebral edema is the most common cause of death. No artificial hepatic support system has be shown to be reliably successful in patients with FHF.

A recent trend to better outcomes may be related to improved care in specialized units or may represent the efficacy of advanced methods for treatment of intracranial hypertension in the treatment of these patients.[4-7] A prearranged team for managing these patients is desirable. Early recognition of patients with FHF who are unlikely to survive with medical management alone has focused efforts toward preparation for possible liver transplantation, since the formerly overall dismal prognosis in this condition has been transformed by the availability of liver transplantation.

ENCEPHALOPATHY

Encephalopathy is a major complication of FHF. It predisposes to other complications and confuses assessment and treatment of cerebral edema. The clinical signs usually associated with increased intracerebral pressure (myoclonus, focal seizures, decerebrate posturing, and loss of brainstem reflex) may be caused by metabolic encephalopathy, whereas other signs of cerebral edema may not be apparent, although the ICP is elevated.[7] Determination of the grade of encephalopathy (Table 139-5) allows immediate assessment of prognosis and of the risk of other complications such as respiratory failure, aspiration, and cerebral edema, and also establishes the need for advanced monitoring and treatment modalities such as cerebral blood flow (CBF) studies, ICP monitoring, and prophylactic intubation. After initial assessment of encephalopathy, further abrupt deterioration of the patient's mental status may occur, and serial neurologic examinations should be performed every 2 to 3 hours to monitor possible progressive neurologic deterioration in grade I and II patients. Prognosis for recovery without neurologic

deficit and without need for transplantation is excellent for patients who do not progress beyond grade II.

After initial assessment, identification and treatment of reversible causes of encephalopathy should be the next focus. The causes of encephalopathy include the following:

Drugs (sedatives or pain medication)
Electrolyte imbalances and dehydration
Azotemia
Infection
GI bleeding
Protein load
Constipation
Hypoxia
Hypoglycemia

Electrolyte imbalances should be corrected carefully to avoid fluid overload, because nonhydrostatic pulmonary edema may occur even with moderate filling pressures. Treatment of GI bleeding, with mechanical lavage or enemas to eliminate the resulting protein load, may be necessary. Dietary protein is avoided. Lactulose may be given by NG tube every 6 hours initially, and adjusted to give two to three loose stools per day.

Overtreatment with lactulose may lead to diarrhea and result in dehydration or hypernatremia.

Neomycin orally may be contraindicated in cases of borderline renal function because it is variably absorbed and is nephrotoxic. Hypoxia should be ruled out or treated. Serum glucose may be low, and a continuous drip should be provided. Infection is common in this population and can precipitate encephalopathy.[8,9] Midozalam can be used in low doses in agitated patients, but in general, sedatives should be used with caution because they complicate clinical assessment and precipitate progression of encephalopathy. Opiates should be avoided.

Flumazenil treatment may be helpful in reversing the trend into deeper levels of encephalopathy.[10,11]

CEREBRAL EDEMA

Cerebral edema is the leading cause of death, accounting for roughly 50% of all preoperative deaths and approximately 40% of deaths after transplantation.[12-14] The usual signs of

TABLE 139-3. Philosophical Goals in the Management of FHF

1. Recognition of the nature and severity of the condition
2. Admission or transfer to an appropriate care facility
3. Establishment of etiology and assessment of prognosis
4. Treatment of potentially reversible causes of FHF
5. Institution of optimal supportive care
6. Treatment and prevention of further complications
7. Sustain liver function long enough to allow regeneration in good-prognosis patients
8. Investigate and exclude indicators of unacceptably poor outcome
9. Prepare for transplantation

FHF, fulminant hepatic failure.

TABLE 139-4.   Practical Treatment of Fulminant Failure

1. Admit to the ICU
2. Baseline neurologic examination and follow-up exam q 2 to 3 h
3. Baseline laboratory studies: CBC, chemistry profile, ABGs, PT, ammonia, blood type and crossmatch, serologies, blood cultures, an acetaminophen level and other diagnostic tests as indicated, urinalysis, urine electrolytes, and creatinine clearance
4. CBC and electrolytes q 6 h; serum osmolality q 6 h if receiving mannitol therapy; ABGs q 6 h if intubated; prothrombin time q 6–8 h if coagulopathic; serum glucose levels q 2–3 h if encephalopathic
5. Placement of nasogastric tube if encephalopathy is grade II or greater, monitor gastric pH
6. Routine H-2 blocker therapy
7. Vitamin K 10 mg qd IV (not SQ or IM)
8. Lactulose to promote 2–3 soft bowel movements daily
9. Dextrose drip to maintain normal glucose levels
10. Mannitol infusions q 4 h as needed for elevated ICP
11. Correct electrolyte abnormalities
12. Treat fever and agitation
13. CT of the head and EEG for encephalopathy grade II or greater
14. ICP monitor for grade III–IV encephalopathy
15. Screening chest radiograph
16. Pulmonary care and supplemental oxygen
17. Correct hypoxia and hypercapnia
18. Intubation and ventilatory support as necessary
19. Foley catheter
20. Placement of arterial line
21. Treat hypertension and hypotension—avoid vasodilators
22. Place CVP line or pulmonary artery catheter
23. Optimize fluid status and transfuse if indicated
24. Support MAP with dopamine or norepinephrine
25. Initiate diuretic treatment or continuous venovenous hemofiltration if needed
26. Fresh frozen plasma drip as needed to keep PT <25–30
27. Correct coagulopathy for procedures
28. Aggressive surveillance cultures: blood, urine, sputum and ascites if present—bronchoscopy if indicated
29. Consider prophylactic antibiotics
30. Consult transplant team, nephrology, gastroenterology or hepatology, social work, and neurosurgery regarding the patient's anticipated needs
31. Doppler ultrasound to determine portal vein patency and to screen for masses in the liver
32. Consider transjugular biopsy exam, examination

CBC, complete blood cell count; ABGs, arterial blood gases; q, every; IV, intravenously; SQ, subcutaneously; IM, intramuscularly; ICP, intracranial pressure; CT, computed tomography; EEG, electroencephalogram; qd, daily; CVP, central venous pressure; PT, prothrombin time; MAP, mean arterial pressure.

elevated ICP—headache, papilledema, and bradycardia—are usually absent. The risk of death in patients with grade III–IV encephalopathy is high enough to justify placement of a ICP monitor. Causes are not fully known but include hypoproteinemia, a hyperdynamic circulation, disrupted cerebral vasoregulation with altered permeability of the blood-brain barrier, and uncoupling of CBF to demand (luxury perfusion[15]). There is also a probable direct cytotoxic effect on astroglial cells in the brain.[16] Cerebral edema rarely occurs in patients with encephalopathy from chronic liver disease. Major issues include the early diagnosis and management of intracranial hypertension and the identification of patients with irreversible neurologic injury secondary to intracranial hypertension in whom liver transplantation is contraindicated.

Assessment is difficult but is essential for successful management. Unfortunately, clinical assessment is confounded

by encephalopathy, and computed tomographic (CT) scanning is not sensitive enough to reliably detect early stages of cerebral edema. Swelling detected on CT scanning is a late sign. In one series, 8 of 12 patients found to have elevated ICP had no CT evidence of edema.[17] In another, 3 of 3 patients with "severe swelling" died.[4] The main use of CT scanning of the head may be to exclude subdural hematomas and other mass lesions. Modern therapy is directed by determinations of CBF, ICP monitoring, and monitoring of cerebral arterial—venous oxygen content differences $[C(a - v)O_2]$ differences after placement of a jugular bulb catheter.[5] CBF is normally coupled to the demands of cerebral metabolism: both are usually reduced in coma. Cerebral metabolic rates generally reduced in FHF to an average of less than 50% of normal, but in one series of patients with FHF and grade III–IV encephalopathy, CBFs were reduced in 50% of patients, were within normal range

TABLE 139-5. Clinical Grade of Hepatic Encephalopathy

I. Confused state with altered mood, sleep habits or behavior, loss of spatial orientation, slowed mentation, asterixis
II. Sleepiness with slow arousability but responsive, inappropriate behavior, incontinence, marked asterixis
III. Stuporous with marked confusion, or coma responsive to painful stimuli
IV. Coma unresponsive to painful stimuli

in 26% and were above normal in 24%.[5] Higher CBFs were correlated with elevations in ICP, swelling on CT scan, greater depths of coma, and ultimately a higher risk of mortality.[5,18] CBF can be determined by xenon-CT,[18] or by xenon-clearance nuclear scan at the bedside[19]; the results of these tests are highly correlated with one another.[5] A correction is performed for variations in $PaCO_2$ within and between patients. Adjusted CBF (aCBF), expressed in milliliters per 100 grams tissue per minute, can be calculated as follows:

$$aCBF = \frac{CBF}{1 - 0.028(32 - PaCO_2)}$$

Although constant CBF monitoring is not practical, these measurements can predict risk for elevated ICP, can provide an indication for ICP monitor placement, and can be used to monitor therapy.

The gold standard is direct measurement of ICP with epidural, subarachnoid, or ventricular monitors, allowing minute-to-minute assessment of intracranial hypertension and results of therapy. Clinical reviews have demonstrated that survival is associated with ICP levels maintained at less than 20 mm Hg.[5] Prolonged elevation of the ICP to greater than 40 mm Hg is strongly correlated with neurologic death.[20] Measurement of ICP also allows one to calculate the cerebral perfusion pressure (CPP), defined as the difference between mean arterial pressure (MAP) and ICP. Reviews of FHF patients have shown that a sustained CCP less than 40 mm Hg for 2 hours was associated with neurologic death or significant neurologic handicap.[7,20,21] The CCP should be kept greater than 50 mm Hg.

A third advanced modality in monitoring the effects of treatment is the calculation of cerebral $C(a - v)O_2$ after placement of a catheter in the internal jugular vein directed cephalad into the jugular bulb. Correct position is confirmed by a lateral skull radiograph. After placement is confirmed, arterial and jugular bulb oxygen concentrations are compared every 4 hours, or more often as indicated. Like CBF, corrections for variability in $PaCO_2$ within and between patients are performed. Adjusted $C(a - v)O_2$, expressed as volume percent (vol%), can be calculated as follows:

$$\text{Adjusted } C(a - v)O_2 = C(a - v)O_2 \times [1 - 0.028(32 - PaCO_2)]$$

Oxygen extraction is usually low in FHF (normal range, 5 to 9 vol%). A narrow $C(a - v)O_2$ indicates supply in excess of demand (luxury perfusion) secondary to loss of cerebral vasoregulation, and may indicate a need for hyperventilation. A wide $C(a - v)O_2$ is characteristic of ischemia secondary to overextraction and may indicate a need for measures to increase CPP, or to reduce hyperventilation.[5]

Treatment of Cerebral Edema

In general, the treatment of cerebral edema demands a balance between measures that reduce ICP with those that reduce CPP. The simplest form of treatment—augmenting venous return and lowering ICP by seeking an optimal position of the head--may be helpful, but it is limited in its effect. It may be helpful to raise the head to 20 degrees; further elevation did not improve ICP and was shown to decrease CCP in one study.[22] A midline posture also probably reduces impedance to venous drainage.[20] Numerous factors are known to exacerbate elevated ICPs, and these should be avoided or treated:

> Valsalva maneuvers (sneezing, coughing, straining, vomiting)
> Positive end-expiratory pressure
> Head turning (i.e., Doll's eyes maneuver) or body rolling
> Trendelenburg positioning
> Painful stimuli, agitation
> Hypertension or hypotension
> Hypoxia or hypercapnia
> Fevers or shivering
> Seizures

Doll's eyes maneuvers in the neurologic examination may transiently raise ICP and are discouraged. Vasodilators, such as nitroprusside, are avoided in treating hypertension because they may worsen cerebral hyperemia. Esmolol or labetalol have been shown to be reasonable alternatives. Tracheal suctioning should be limited to 15 seconds at a time, and preoxygenation should be performed. Control of painful stimuli helps to prevent intermittent rises in ICP.

Reduction of cerebral metabolic demand allows a wider margin of safety between reducing hyperemia and inducing ischemia. Control of seizures is mandatory, because cerebral metabolic demand and ICP are elevated during seizures. Control of fevers is also important, with use of ketorolac 60 mg IM, hypothermia blankets, or both. If these simple maneuvers are not sufficient to keep the ICP below 20 to 25 mm Hg, pharmacologic coma can be induced. Pharmacologic coma reduces cerebral metabolic activity and cerebral oxygen demand. Agents employed include pentobarbital (3 to 5 mg/kg followed by a 0.5 to 3 mg/kg/hour infusion), thiopentone (250 mg over 15 minutes, followed by a 50 to 250 mg/hour drip titrated to maintain satisfactory MAP, CPP, and ICP[23]), and propofol. Hypotension is common, and inotropes or vasopressors may be needed.

Because of the inability to conduct continuous clinical assessments, direct arterial and ICP monitoring are recommended in cases of induced coma treatment. The infusion is stopped twice or thrice a day to allow for assessment of brain stem reflexes and possible return of consciousness. Brain stem reflexes can be lost in induced states of coma, and under no circumstances should a patient be pronounced dead during induced pharmacologic coma.

Manipulation of arterial carbon dioxide levels by hyperventilation has long been known to reduce CBF and hence lower ICP. FHF patients have been shown to retain this responsiveness to changes in PaCO₂. This strategy may be harmful if CBF is reduced below that needed to supply cerebral metabolism, inducing ischemia. General goals are to keep PaCO₂ in the 25 to 35 range with frequent monitoring of the arterial blood gases. $C(a - v)O_2$ should be monitored and maintained in the normal range to protect against excessive hyperventilation. In one series, PaCO₂ was lowered by increasing ventilation when the $C(a - v)O_2$ was less than 5.5 vol%, or the ICP was greater than 20 mm Hg. Ventilation was reduced when $C(a - v)O_2$ was greater than 9 vol%, as an inference of overventilation and induction of cerebral ischemia.[5] Caution should be exercised regarding the interpretation of a narrow $C(a - v)O_2$ because this may result from other causes, such as malposition of the jugular catheter or end-stage neurologic disease with failing cerebral metabolism.

Reduction of ICP may also be accomplished by measures aimed at correcting fluid overload such as diuresis, dialysis, and CVVH, but MAP and CPP must be maintained. Mannitol infusion (0.5 to 1 g/kg every 4 hours, not to exceed a total dose of 100 g every 4 hours) may reduce cerebral tissue water, but serum osmolality must be determined and should not be allowed to exceed 310 mOsm. Mannitol infusions may be contraindicated in renal failure because they may exacerbate hyperemia unless hemodialysis or CVVH are used concomitantly to remove excess fluids. Steroids, although frequently used, have not been shown to benefit this population.[24] Prostacycline infusions should be avoided because they have been shown to increase ICP and decrease CPP. An uncontrolled trial of prostaglandin E infusions in FHF is encouraging but needs further validation.

The decision to initiate ICP monitoring should be gauged by the inferred risk of elevated ICP and subsequent herniation. Patients in grade III-IV coma—particularly those shown to have evidence of hyperemia by increased CBF studies, edema on CT scanning, or high mixed venous O₂ saturation by pulmonary artery catheter—should be considered. Goals include the reduction of ICP to less than 20 mm Hg and maintaining CPP greater than 50 mm Hg. Maintaining an adequate MAP may be essential in preserving an adequate CPP. Frequent calculation of CPP may guide changes in other aspects of patient management as well. A prolonged ICP greater than 40 mm Hg has been associated with eventual herniation, poor neurologic function even if herniation is avoided, and postoperative neurologic death in patients who have undergone transplantation.[20] The patient with refractory intracranial hypertension will develop irreversible neurologic damage and should not undergo transplantation. ICP monitoring is discontinued when the patient regains consciousness or when the ICP is consistently less than 12 mm Hg.

Complications of ICP monitoring include infection and hemorrhage. A national survey revealed a substantially lower rate of infection (0.6% versus 3%) and hemorrhage (3.1% versus 18%) with epidural rather than subdural or parenchymal monitors.[7,25,26] These complications are best avoided by limiting the procedure to patients who would benefit from it, having an experienced team place the monitor, using epidural rather than subdural or intraventricular devices,

and having the equipment checked once or twice daily by the neurosurgical team. Before placement of an ICP monitor it is prudent to correct an existing coagulopathy with factor replacement until the prothrombin time is within 3 seconds of normal, and to administer antibiotics with gram positive coverage at the time of the procedure. Uncorrectable coagulopathy may preclude placement of an ICP monitoring device. A dramatic rise in ICP should prompt an emergent CT scan of the head to rule out intracranial hemorrhage.

COAGULOPATHY

Coagulopathy is a common problem in FHF. All coagulation factors except factor VIII are made in the liver; because the basic deficit is hepatocellular injury, this coagulopathy is generally resistant to vitamin K administration. In addition to factor deficiencies, circulating fibrinolytic factors are not well cleared by the failing liver. Disseminated intravascular coagulation may be seen secondary to sepsis or multiorgan system failure. Thrombocytopenia secondary to alcoholism or hypersplenism may be an additional contributing factor.

Complete correction of coagulopathy in the absence of bleeding is controversial and may not be indicated. Nonetheless, in many centers patients receive round-the-clock fresh frozen plasma to keep the prothrombin time less than 25 to 30 seconds. Thromboelastograms, factor V levels, and coagulation profiles may be useful in guiding replacement therapy. In the absence of bleeding, platelet transfusions may be held until the count falls below 20,000 per mm³. When epidural monitors are in place or when other invasive procedures are being performed, it is more prudent to keep the platelet count above 50,000 to 75,000 per mm³ and to aggressively correct the prothrombin time to within 3 seconds of normal by fresh frozen plasma and cryoprecipitate administration. CVVH or plasmapheresis may be necessary to avoid fluid overload.

GASTROINTESTINAL BLEEDING

GI bleeding is not as common in this population as in end-stage liver disease (ESLD), in which portal hypertension is more common. Esophageal varices are rarely observed.

Nevertheless, significant GI bleeding can occur because of the combination of a severe coagulopathy and stress ulceration or gastritis, and can complicate management. Significant GI bleeding deepens the levels of encephalopathy, complicates correction of coagulopathy and fluid status, and compromises tissue and cerebral perfusion secondary to hypovolemia and anemia. For these reasons, stress ulcer prophylaxis with intravenous H-2 blockers or omeprazole, monitoring of gastric pH, correction of coagulopathy in bleeding patients, and transfusion to maintain tissue perfusion and hemodynamic stability are essential early management principles. Because portal hypertension and esophageal varices are rare, there is no reason not to place a NG tube, whereas esophagogastroduodenoscopy and Sengstaken-Blakemore tubes are rarely indicated.

Transjugular intrahepatic portosystemic shunt procedures, useful in temporizing the bleeding patient in ESLD with portal hypertension, are rarely needed in FHF. Nasogastric lavage or repeated enemas may be necessary to remove the protein load produced by blood in the GI tract and avoid worsening the level of encephalopathy.

LOSS OF VASOMOTOR TONE AND HIGH-OUTPUT FAILURE

Loss of vasomotor tone is a central phenomenon in liver failure and complicates many phases of patient management. The etiology is poorly understood and is probably multifactorial. Factors thought to be contributory include impaired vasoconstriction resulting from norepinephrine depletion, arteriovenous shunting, and increased concentrations of vasodilatory substances normally cleared by the liver: endotoxins, prostaglandins, bradykinins, substance P, vasoactive intestinal polypeptide, histamine, γ-aminobutyric acid, glucagon, and others.[27] Vasodilation and a hyperdynamic state—with an elevated cardiac output, low systemic vascular resistance (SVR), and relative arterial hypotension—are common.

It may be difficult to differentiate the high-output/low systemic resistance state of advanced liver failure from that of sepsis, particularly because liver failure renders patients vulnerable to infection.

Unfortunately, this is an important distinction to make, because the presence of sepsis or an extrahepatic source of infection is a contraindication to transplantation.

Management of the FHF patient's hemodynamic status should be guided by early placement of a pulmonary artery catheter. Ideally, pulmonary artery occlusion pressures should be maintained in the range of 8 to 12 mm Hg. Overcorrection of postulated fluid deficiencies may lead to nonhydrostatic pulmonary edema, or worse yet, to exacerbate cerebral hyperemia. Pressor support with low-to-moderate dose dopamine, or with renal dose dopamine and norepinephrine, may be necessary to maintain a MAP greater than 80 mm Hg, the CPP greater than 40 mm Hg, and to redistribute blood away from the nonvital organs.[27] Hemodynamic status has been seen to improve in acetaminophen poisoning patients after infusion of acetylcysteine, but these anecdotal observations require further validation. Clearance of circulating vasoactive substances may be responsible for the frequently observed improvement of renal function and hemodynamic status in ESLD and FHF patients undergoing CVVH, presumably resulting from correction of the nonphysiologic shunting. Whatever the underlying causes, this phenomenon is one of the contributors to cerebral hyperemia.

OLIGURIC RENAL FAILURE AND FLUID OVERLOAD

Acute renal dysfunction is present in 75% of acetaminophen poisoning patients and 30% of all other cases of FHF. Oliguric renal failure is associated with decreased survival, especially in the patient with acetaminophen toxicity.[3] Renal dysfunction may fall under the categories of prerenal azotemia, acute tubular necrosis, or hepatorenal syndrome. Interactive etiologies include diminished intravascular volume from third-space losses and hypoalbuminemia, the effects of sepsis, injudicious diuretic management, diarrhea from lactulose administration, and decreased oral intake. Another important contributing factor is loss of vasomotor regulation with inappropriate shunting of blood flow to skeletal muscle and skin. Endotoxemia, with reduced renal perfusion, may be a factor. In this setting, urea production may be a poor measure of renal function. A 24-hour creatinine clearance should be checked as well as urine electrolytes to distinguish acute tubular necrosis from hepatorenal syndrome.

Treatment should include measures to monitor filling pressures, cardiac output, and systemic vascular resistance accurately. Dopamine or norepinephrine may be useful in counteracting loss of vasomotor tone and inappropriate shunting. Cautious fluid administration may be required, or diuretics with or without salt-poor albumin may be given. Deteriorating renal function may be an indication for early ultrafiltration or dialysis to control azotemia and fluid overload, or to allow for administration of needed blood products. Conventional hemodialysis has not been shown to improve patient survival, possibly because of adverse effects on CPP and MAP, leading to increases in ICP. CVVH can control volume status without the adverse effects on cardiac output, ICP, or CPP seen in conventional dialysis. The clearance of poorly characterized vasodilatory mediators may improve hemodynamics and renal output.

Complications of fluid overload are frequently seen, caused by loss of vasomotor regulation, hypoproteinemia, hyperdynamic circulation, and possible superimposed effects of sepsis. Lower extremity and pulmonary edema are more common than ascites and pleural effusions. A significant association between pulmonary and cerebral edema has been noted.[28]

SEPSIS AND IMPAIRED IMMUNE RESPONSE

Sepsis and impaired immune response are common in liver failure, whether ESLD or FHF, possibly caused in part by failure of the hepatic reticuloendothelial system to clear enteric organisms in the portal venous drainage. The numbers of invasive procedures may be a factor, as well as the loss of phagocytic function associated with decreased levels of complement and fibronectin made in the liver. Bacteremia is found in 20% to 25% of patients, and up to 80% of patients will be found to have bacterial infections in the first week in the ICU.[8] Fungal infections have been observed in up to 35% of patients, pneumonia in 50% of patients, and urinary tract infections in 24%.

Infection was the principal cause of death in 11% of autopsy-studied fatal cases in one series.[29]

Fever and leukocytosis may be absent and appropriate cultures should be obtained if infection is suspected. Empiric antibiotic coverage may be indicated. Occult infections may be suspected by the appearance of acidosis, disseminated intravascular coagulation, increased encephalopathy, a drop in the SVR, urine output, or blood pressure. Prophylactic antibiotic coverage may be appropriate in high-risk patients.

The hyperdynamic state may mimic sepsis. Fever and leukocytosis may be present secondary to hepatocellular necrosis. It may be impossible to diagnose or exclude infection in a given patient.

Failure to make an accurate diagnosis may allow an infected patient to undergo transplantation and immunosuppression, which portends a poor prognosis. Failure to settle the issue may result in the patient being denied a life-saving procedure.

RESPIRATORY CARE

Because of progressive encephalopathy, loss of protective reflexes, inanition, loss of immunologic defenses, and prolonged hospital stays, these patients are at extremely high risk for aspiration and nosocomial pneumonia. Hypoxia may be caused by pleural effusions, nonhydrostatic pulmonary edema, intrapulmonary shunting, or simple hypoventilation and atelectasis. For this reason, aggressive pulmonary care or protective intubation may be appropriate. Early intubation and judicious use of positive end-expiratory pressure permits adequate oxygenation with minimal oxygen toxicity. Hyperventilation may be instituted to compensate for a metabolic acidosis, or to control ICP, and should be adjusted to $PaCO_2$ or $C(a - v)O_2$ if available.

METABOLIC DISORDERS

Metabolic acidosis may be a result of renal failure, failure of adequate tissue perfusion despite elevated cardiac outputs, or inability of the failing liver to clear circulating lactic acid.

Intervention should be guided by data obtained by pulmonary artery catheterization, including filling pressures, cardiac output, oxygen delivery, and SVR. Cardiac performance and oxygen delivery should be optimized, and elevating inappropriately low SVRs resulting from peripheral shunting should improve oxygen delivery to the vital tissues.

Bicarbonate infusions and CVVH or dialysis may be necessary. Uncorrected acidosis may worsen cardiac performance and is a possible indicator of ongoing dysfunctional shunting in the periphery.

Although FHF patients are generally well nourished because of the absence of chronic disease, they tend to be intensely catabolic. Hypoglycemia is seem in almost 50% of patients and may result from impaired gluconeogenesis, lack of glycogen stores, or failure of insulin clearance. A dextrose infusion should be started and its rate adjusted to normalizing blood sugars as assessed by frequent measurements. Amino acid and protein feedings are avoided until encephalopathy is resolved. Hypokalemia or hyperkalemia are common and should be managed with supplementation or dialysis as necessary. Serum osmolality and phosphate, magnesium, and calcium levels should be monitored and corrected.

TRANSPLANTATION

The availability of liver transplantation has changed the prognosis of FHF. Survival rates of 55% to 75% after transplantation in early series have improved to 86% to 100% in recent series, as exclusion criteria were developed and medical management improved.[5,6,30,31] According to Unified Network

TABLE 139-6.   Contraindications to Transplantation

Sustained cerebral hypertension >50 mm Hg
Prolonged decreased cerebral perfusion pressure (<40 mm Hg for 2 h)
Evidence of cerebral herniation
Preexisting neurodegenerative disease
Unresectable malignant disease
Uncontrollable sepsis
Active infection outside of the liver or biliary tract
HIV infection
Severe cardiopulmonary disease
Hemorrhagic pancreatitis

HIV, human immunodeficiency virus.

for Organ Sharing (UNOS) sources, approximately 5% to 9% of orthotopic liver transplantations (OLTxs) are done for FHF. Serious problems remain: historically, 30% to 50% of FHF patients have died awaiting OLTx, either because donors organs are not available, or because complications of FHF preclude transplantation.[30] Postoperative neurologic problems have marred otherwise successful transplants, with up to 40% of postoperative deaths resulting from neurologic causes, and infections in 20%.[32]

The first task is determining whether a given patient is a candidate for transplantation. As observed earlier, good- and poor-prognosis patients for medical management can be determined on the the basis of etiologic, clinical, and biochemical grounds. Patients with a poor prognosis for survival with medical management alone should be listed for transplantation if no contraindications to OLTx exist (Table 139-6). It has been suggested that because of the average 2-day delay in obtaining a suitable transplant donor, the FHF patient in grade III-IV coma should be listed promptly, and reevaluated when a donor is identified.[6,32]

In one series, a liver biopsy was used to determined whether patients were likely to require transplantation. If greater than 30% viable hepatocytes remained, the patients were managed medically: 10 of 11 recovered and 1 underwent OLTx after clinical deterioration. The patients with less than 30% viable hepatocytes were listed for transplantation.[5] Because of the coagulopathy found in these patients, transjugular biopsy has been the main route to obtain a specimen for histologic analysis. Unfortunately, the tissue cores obtainable may be so small as to make confident interpretation difficult.

Preparation for OLTx should include obtaining a blood type and cross-matching of blood components, sending blood for viral serologies and for tissue cross-matching. A human immunodeficiency virus test should be performed. A Doppler ultrasound should be obtained to rule out portal vein thrombosis and hepatic masses, an echocardiogram should be obtained to estimate cardiac risk and aid anesthesia management, and if time and the patient's condition allows, a CT scan for liver size may be done. A CT scan of the head may reveal evidence of irreversible neurologic injury, tumor, or conditions demanding immediate neurologic management. An estimation of neurologic prognosis in comatose patients is important so that successful transplantation is not followed by an unacceptable neurologic outcome. Active infections should be excluded, or if present, should be treated with intention to clear before transplantation. Medical management for treatable contraindications and prevention of further complications should be continued to provide the best possible status at the time of transplantation.

OTHER TREATMENT MODALITIES

In desperate attempts to treat these sick patients, many modalities have been offered for the "cleansing of blood" and the provision of artificial support. Charcoal hemofiltration initially showed some promise of efficacy but was ineffective in a randomized prospective trial.[33] High-volume plasma exchange transfusions have also been tried, as well as plasmapheresis. Many other methods of artificial liver support have been tried, including extracorporeal liver perfusion, injection of encapsulated liver cells into the peritoneum, and filtering blood through extracorporeal circuits.[34,35] The common goals of all of these methods have been the support of the patient until regeneration of the liver can take place, improvement of patient status so that transplantation can be considered, or prevention of further complications while a patient is waiting for transplantation. None have found widespread acceptance or clinical applicability, and none are available outside of the few centers where they are undergoing experimental trials.

Hepatectomy has been performed in critically ill FHF patients with the intent of removing the agent of injury: if the patient's condition stabilizes, urgent transplantation is performed; otherwise, death supervenes. This step is taken only when it is apparent that all other forms of treatment are ineffective and the patient is at imminent risk of fatal decompensation.

REFERENCES

1. Trey C, Davidson CS: The management of fulminant hepatic failure. *Prog Liver Dis* 1970;3:282
2. Bernuau J, Rueff B, Bebganou JP: Fulminant and subfulminant liver failure: definitions and causes. *Semin Liver Dis* 1986; 6:97
3. O'Grady JG, Alexander JM, Hayllar KM, et al: Early indicators of prognosis in fulminant hepatic failure. *Gastroenterology* 1989;97:439
4. Aggarwal S, Yonas H, Kang Y, et al: Relationship of cerebral blood flow and cerebral swelling to outcome in patients with acute fulminant hepatic failure. *Transplant Proc* 1991;23:1978
5. Aggarwal S, Kramer D, Yonas H, et al: Cerebral hemodynamic and metabolic changes in fulminant failure: a retrospective study. *Hepatology* 1994;19:80
6. Ascher N, Lake J, Emond J, et al: Liver transplantation for fulminant hepatic failure. *Arch Surg* 1993;128:677
7. Lidofsky LD, Bass MN, Prager MC, et al: Intracranial pressure monitoring and liver transplantation for fulminant hepatic failure. *Hepatology* 1992;16:1
8. Rolando N, Harvey F, Javier B, et al: Prospective study of

9. Rolando N, Harvey F, Brahm J, et al: Fungal infection: a common, recognized complication of acute liver failure. *J Hepatol* 1991;12:1
10. Grimm G, Ferenchi P, Katzenschlager R, et al: Improvement of hepatic encephalopathy treated with flumazenil. *Lancet* 1988:1392
11. Howard CD: Flumazenil in the treatment of hepatic encephalopathy. *Ann Pharmacother* 1993;27:46
12. Bismuth H, Samuel D, Gugenheim J, et al: Emergency liver transplantation for fulminant hepatitis. *Ann Intern Med* 1987;107:337
13. Edmond J, Peter P, Aran P, et al: Liver transplantation in the management of fulminant hepatic failure. *Gastroenterology* 1989;96:1583
14. Sherlock S: Hepatic encephalopathy. In: *Disease of the Liver and Biliary System,* 8th ed. London: Blackwell Scientific Publications, 1989:85
15. Lassen NA: The luxury-perfusion syndrome and its possible relation to acute metabolic acidosis localised within the brain. *Lancet* 1966:1113
16. Kato M, Hughes RD, Keays RT, et al: Electron microscopic study of brain capillaries from fulminant hepatic failure. *Hepatology* 1992;15:1060
17. Munoz SJ, Robinson M, Northrup B, et al: Elevated intracranial pressure and computed tomography of the brain in fulminant hepatocellular failure. *Hepatology* 1991;13:209
18. Obrist WD, Langfeet TW, Jaggi JL, et al: Cerebral blood flow and metabolism in comatose patients with acute head injury. *J Neourosurg* 1984;61:241
19. Yonas H, Darby JM, Marks EC, et al: CBF measured by Xe-CT: approach to analysis and normal values. *J Cereb Blood Flow Metab* 1991;11:716
20. Schafer DF, Shaw BW: Fulminant hepatic failure and orthotopic liver transplantation. *Semin Liver Dis* 1989;9:189
21. Jenkins JG, Gasglow JFT, Black GW, et al: Reye's syndrome: assessment of intracranial monitoring. *Br Med J* 1987;294:337
22. Davenport A, Will E, Davison A: Effect of posture on intracranial pressure and cerebral perfusion in patients with fulminant hepatic and renal failure after acetaminophen self-poisoning. *Crit Care Med* 1990;18:286
23. Forbes A, Alexader JM, O'Grady JG, et al: Thiopental infusion in the treatment of intracranial hypertension complicating fulminant hepatic failure. *Hepatology* 1989;10:306
24. Canalese J, Gimson AE, Davis C, et al: Controlled trial of dexamethasone and mannitol for the cerebral oedema of fulminant hepatic failure. *Gut* 1982;23:625
25. Blei A, Olafsson S, Webster S, et al: Complications of intracranial pressure monitoring in fulminant hepatic failure. *Lancet* 1993;341:157
26. Kanazi G, Plekela D, Marin E, et al: How helpful is intracranial pressure monitoring in patients with acute hepatic failure? *Transplant Proc* 1993;25:1819
27. Sherlock S: Vasodilatation associated with hepatocellular disease: relation to functional organ failure. *Gut* 1990;31:365
28. Trewby PN, Warren R, Contini S, et al: Incidence and pathophysiology of pulmonary edema in fulminant hepatic failure. *Gastroenterology* 1978;74859
29. Gazzard BG, Portmann B, Murray-Lyon IM, Williams R. Causes of death in fulminant hepatic failure and relationship to quantitative histological assessment of parenchymal damage.

bacterial infection in acute liver failure: an analysis of fifty patients. *Hepatology* 1990;11:49

Q J Med 1975;44:615

30. Campbell D, Ham J, McCurry K et al: Liver transplant for fulminant hepatic failure. *Am Surg* 1991;57:546

31. Friedman AL, Maller E, Piccoli D, Plona L, Hoffman MA, Lau HT. Encouraging experience with aggressive liver transplantation for children with fulminant failure at a single transplant center. *Transplant Proc* 1994;26:65

32. Lidofsky SD: Liver transplantation for fulminant hepatic failure. *Gastroenterol Clin North Am* 1993;22:257

33. O'Grady JG, Gimson AES, O'Brien CJ, et al: Controlled trials of charcoal hemoperfusion and prognostic factors in fulminant hepatic failure. *Gastroenterology* 1988;94:1186

34. Fox IJ, Langnas AN, Fristoe LW, et al: Successful application of extracorporeal liver perfusion: a technology whose time has come. *Am J Gastroenterol* 1993;88:1876

35. Sussman NL, Gislason GT, Kelly JG: Extracorporeal liver support: application to fulminant hepatic failure. *J Clin Gastroenterol* 1994;18:320

Critical Care, Third Edition, edited by Joseph M. Civetta,
Robert W. Taylor, and Robert R. Kirby.
Lippincott-Raven Publishers, Philadelphia, PA © 1997.

CHAPTER 140

■

Pancreatic Disease

Danny Sleeman
Joe U. Levi

IMMEDIATE CONCERNS ■

MAJOR PROBLEMS

Pancreatitis is an unpredictable disease that forms a spectrum from mild to progressively lethal. The intensive care specialist usually sees patients who present with the most severe initial forms or those with multiple complications that last for a protracted time. The complications can be both systemic (hypovolemia, respiratory failure, sepsis), similar to those associated with any serious disease, and local (related to the pancreas and surrounding structures).

STRESS POINTS

1. Pancreatitis has many causes. Determination of cause is important to direct initial therapy (e.g., if the cause is biliary) or to prevent future attacks (e.g., if the cause is related to alcohol, drugs, hyperparathyroidism, or toxins).
2. The International Symposium in Atlanta in 1992 produced a new classification system that divides pancreatitis into seven clinical conditions: acute pancreatitis, severe acute pancreatitis, mild acute pancreatitis, acute fluid collections, pancreatic necrosis, pseudocyst, and pancreatic abscess.
3. The Ranson criteria remain a reliable predictor of the clinical course. The admission criteria are as follows: age older than 55 years, blood glucose level greater than 200 mg/dL, leukocyte count greater than 16,000/mm^3, serum lactate dehydrogenase (LDH) level greater than 350 IU/L, and SGOT greater than 250 Sigma Frankel units (aspartate aminotransferase [AST] greater than 20 U/L). The criteria to be deter-

mined within 48 hours are as follows: serum calcium level less than 8 mg/dL, arterial partial pressure of oxygen (PaO$_2$) less than 60 mm Hg, base deficit greater than 4 mEq/L, increase in blood urea nitrogen (BUN) of more than 5 mg/dL, decrease in hematocrit of more than 10 percentage points, and more than 6 L fluid sequestration.

4. The nonsurgical treatment of pancreatitis includes general resuscitative and supportive measures (especially volume replacement and ventilatory support), suppression of exocrine function, and nutritional support.
5. Surgical treatment of pancreatitis includes removal of the offending cause (e.g., common bile duct stones) and the treatment of pseudocysts, pancreatic abscess, infected necrosis, bleeding, and bowel complications.
6. Pseudocysts are more often treated by percutaneous drainage than by a direct surgical approach. Percutaneous drainage is also helpful for the diagnosis of infection in fluid collections and as a temporizing measure to stabilize critically ill patients before an operation.
7. Vascular complications may be diagnosed and treated by angiography and embolization.
8. Necrotizing pancreatitis has a better outcome if treated by an open technique. Percutaneous drainage of collections that form away from the open area is beneficial.

ESSENTIAL DIAGNOSTIC TESTS

1. The history must be determined, including previous episodes, medications, substance abuse, hyperlipidemia, recent endoscopic retrograde cholangiopancreatography (ERCP), and specific associated diseases.

2. Amylase, lipase, calcium, hematocrit, leukocyte count, liver function tests, and lipid profile help establish diagnosis, cause, and severity.
3. Sequential computed tomography (CT) scanning with intravenous contrast is now the test of choice for diagnosis, follow-up, and management (CT-guided drainage).
4. Ultrasound is used to diagnose associated biliary tract disease and in follow-up of pseudocysts.
5. Angiography plays a role in the diagnosis and treatment (embolization) of arterial vascular complications, especially bleeding and pseudoaneurysms, and in the diagnosis of venous complications such as splenic vein or portal vein thrombosis.
6. ERCP is used as both a diagnostic and a therapeutic modality.

INITIAL THERAPY

1. Establish the diagnosis. Rule out disease necessitating urgent surgery and determine causes amenable to direct treatment, such as common bile duct stones.
2. Cardiovascular, pulmonary, and renal support are the cornerstones of initial therapy in severe pancreatitis.
3. If a patient's condition deteriorates after initial therapy, local complications must be suspected and, if present, treated.

OVERVIEW ◼

No other entity presents with such varied origins, clinical manifestations with multisystem involvement, and diagnostic difficulties as does pancreatitis; no other demands more days in the intensive care unit (ICU) or more hours of multidisciplinary care, and no other carries such an indeterminate prognosis for such long periods. Although numerous causes of pancreatitis are known—including alcohol, biliary disease, trauma, postoperative states, drugs, hyperlipidemia, hyperparathyroidism, collagen vascular disease, viruses, and toxins—these suggest only a possible initiation or association of the inflammatory process and do little to explain the exact pathophysiology or course of the disease. The pancreatic digestive enzymes have the capacity to digest protein, carbohydrates, lipids, and even nucleic acids, and when released and activated, these enzymes have the capability of autodigesting the gland itself and the body around it. The clinical course of pancreatitis may be self-limited, requiring no surgical intervention and resulting in little, if any, structural anatomic alteration of the gland. All complications of this disease, however, are potentially lethal and may require surgical intervention along with aggressive intensive care management to control or abort the process and to support the patient during the period of resolution.

DIAGNOSIS OF THE DISEASE PROCESS ◼

At times, diagnosing acute pancreatitis may be as difficult as predicting the course or defining the treatment. Even with history, physical examination, and laboratory, radio-

graphic, and special procedures, a conclusive diagnosis of acute pancreatitis and its complications is often elusive.

The best approach is to elucidate the history of a similar attack or hospitalization, along with associated etiologic factors such as alcohol or biliary tract disease. After the patient develops peritoneal signs, pancreatitis can mimic all other acute abdominal crises, especially those necessitating immediate surgery.

The recurrence rate of acute pancreatitis has been reported to be as high as 33%[1] and even higher in the alcoholic population.[2] Isolated disease of the pancreatic head or tail may localize the pain of pancreatitis to the right or left upper quadrant with diaphragmatic irritation and referred pain to the subcapsular areas, but the classic epigastric pain with radiation to the back may be present in only 50% of the patients evaluated.

LABORATORY TESTING

Of the biochemical diagnostic criteria, the most commonly used is the serum amylase level.[3] Although the serum amylase concentration begins to rise shortly after onset of the disease, it may return to normal levels in 2 to 4 days. A single normal level may not exclude the disease, and the peak value may have no relation to the severity. Some of the highest serum amylase values are associated with a biliary tract origin of pancreatitis. Because pancreatitis mimics many other abdominal processes, the physician must always be aware of the differential diagnosis of hyperamylasemia, which includes perforated or penetrating peptic ulcer, ruptured ectopic pregnancy, and intestinal obstruction or infarction. Determinations of urinary amylase, amylase-to-creatinine clearance ratios,[4] and amylase isoenzymes[5] have shown little advantage clinically, except possibly to rule out macroamylasemias.

Serum lipase levels, although thought to be more specific for pancreatic destruction, play little role in today's ICU therapy. An elevated concentration of serum lipase, however, is quite sensitive for diagnosis of acute pancreatitis secondary to alcohol.[6] Lipase levels tend to remain elevated longer than amylase concentrations. Therefore, an elevated lipase level can be useful information for patients who present later in the course of disease and who may have a normal amylase concentration. Methemoglobinemia[7] does not differentiate the milder forms from acute hemorrhagic pancreatitis, and neither lipase nor methemoglobinemia is useful in the ICU.

Except for differentiation of other bacterial sources of peritonitis or diagnosis of complications of pancreatitis that would necessitate surgery, diagnostic peritoneal lavage has had little role in our institution in making the definitive diagnosis or assessing the prognosis of a given episode of pancreatitis.

RADIOLOGIC AND DIAGNOSTIC STUDIES

There are numerous findings suggestive of, but not specific for, pancreatitis. These include dilatation of the first portion of the duodenum (duodenal ileus), dilatation of the first loop of the jejunum (jejunal ileus or "sentinel loop"), dilatation of the transverse colon or "colon cut-off" sign (secondary to a transverse colonic ileus), and elevated hemidiaphragm and pleural effusion, especially on the left side (secondary to diaphragmatic irritation and sympathetic pleural effusions).

Pancreatic ultrasonography is not sensitive in the diagnosis of acute pancreatitis, often because of gas in the bowel. It can be helpful in detection of early complications of pancreatitis and identification of associated biliary tract disease.[8] Ultrasonography frequently provides an incomplete view of the pancreas and the peripancreatic area, especially in patients who are obese with severe disease and excessive bowel gas secondary to ileus. In addition, if imaging of the tail of the pancreas is necessary, an incomplete view may occur because of a poor sonic window.

The current modality of choice to diagnose and follow pancreatitis is sequential contrast-enhanced CT. Changes in gland size, attenuation, abnormalities of the pancreatic ducts, and thickening of the renal and perirenal fascia, as well as peripancreatic fluid collections, small gas and fluid collections, and pancreatic phlegmon can be detected and differentiated from abscess and pancreatic necrosis.[9,10] A means for using percutaneous aspiration to confirm diagnosis and possibly even convert to an external catheter drainage is also provided.

Although angiography does not play a role among the usual diagnostic techniques for pancreatitis, it has become essential for localizing hemorrhagic complications of the disease and extremely useful for nonoperative or preoperative control of bleeding vessels before surgery.

ENDOSCOPIC RETROGRADE CHOLANGIOPANCREATOGRAPHY

ERCP can demonstrate ductal disruptions in traumatic pancreatitis. It is also helpful in establishing biliary tract disease as the cause of pancreatitis and in demonstrating stones. It can also demonstrate pancreatic divisum, thought to be one of the rare causes of this disease.

CLASSIFICATION ■

The Marseilles classification of pancreatitis into four types—acute pancreatitis, recurrent acute pancreatitis, relapsing chronic pancreatitis, and chronic pancreatitis—has been useful to characterize the pathology of the gland and clinical episodes.[11] A recent advance is the clinical classification by Bradley,[12] the result of an International Symposium in 1992. Seven entities were defined: (1) acute pancreatitis, (2) severe acute pancreatitis, (3) mild acute pancreatitis, (4) acute fluid collection, (5) pancreatic necrosis, (6) pseudocysts, and (7) pancreatic abscess.

The most relevant classification to the intensivist determines the degree of severity and progress of an individual episode of pancreatitis. Ranson and colleagues[13,14] established 11 clinical criteria, 5 of which were assessed on admission and 6 within 48 hours. They are well correlated with morbidity, number of days' stay in the ICU, and eventual mortality. The admission criteria are as follows: age

older than 55 years, blood glucose level greater than 200 mg/dL, leukocyte count greater than 16,000/mm³, serum LDH level greater than 350 IU/L, and SGOT greater than 250 Sigma Frankel units. The criteria to be determined within 48 hours are as follows: serum calcium level less than 8 mg/dL, PaO_2 less than 60 mm Hg, base deficit greater than 4 mEq/L, increase in BUN of more than 5 mg/dL, decrease in hematocrit of more than 10 percentage points, and more than 6 L fluid sequestration. The presence of fewer than 3 of these 11 criteria within 48 hours of admission usually correlates with a more benign form and course of disease, with an eventual mortality rate of 3%. The presence of three or more of these parameters on admission or within 48 hours usually implies a more severe form of pancreatitis and is associated with high risk of death and major complications.

ICU admission is indicated for patients with acute pancreatitis if they meet three or more of Ranson's criteria (because of the predicted severity) or if there is need for monitoring and managing large-volume resuscitation, respiratory insufficiency requiring ventilatory support, metabolic imbalances and impending renal insufficiency, cardiovascular collapse, or sepsis with multiple organ system failure.

TREATMENT OF ACUTE PANCREATITIS ■

It is difficult to discuss the treatment of an entity that is so hard to diagnose, with such obscure and varied causes, and whose pathogenesis and course are poorly understood. Our goal is to discuss the various presentations and complications of this disease, along with an approach to the diagnostic and therapeutic measures used to define, control, and abort them.

An overall approach to the therapy for acute pancreatitis would include placing the pancreas "at rest," supporting the patient's nutritional and metabolic needs, correcting the acute causes of mortality (i.e., cardiovascular collapse, respiratory insufficiency, and renal failure), detecting those complications of disease that require surgical intervention, and preventing and treating delayed causes of mortality (i.e., septic complications).

GLAND SUPPRESSION

Suppression of the secretory function of the pancreatic gland has been attempted by elimination of oral fluids,[15,16] suppression of acid secretion with various H_2-blockers[17,18] and antacids, and use of anticholinergics[11,19] and proteolytic enzyme inhibitors.[20] Calcitonin[21] and somatostatin,[22] which are potent inhibitors of pancreatic enzyme secretion, have also been subjected to clinical trials. Although there may be a good physiologic rationale, controlled randomized studies have not shown significant improvement. However, early feeding may increase the severity of the disease and reexacerbate the inflammatory process. Most patients admitted to the ICU have pancreatitis of sufficient severity and associated ileus that justifies NPO (nothing by mouth) orders, nasogastric tube decompression, and some form of acid suppression or neutralization, even if the goal is just to prevent bleeding from erosive gastritis.

METABOLIC AND NUTRITIONAL SUPPORT

Nutritional support is not an option but an essential requirement for long-term management of these patients. Solutions may be either lipid- or glucose-based as long as triglyceridemia and glucose levels are monitored.[23] Lipid emulsions have been questioned with respect to exacerbation of pancreatitis. The issue is unresolved, but the current recommendation is to use only an amount sufficient to prevent essential fatty acid deficiency. Glucose intolerance is common during the acute phase. It may recur during the chronic phase as one of the more subtle manifestations of a septic complication. Insulin drips, sliding scales, and insulin added to total parenteral nutrition solutions are all options that may be used. Enteral feedings should be low in fat and should be delivered distal to the ligament of Treitz, based on the theory (not data) of keeping the pancreas at rest.

Hypocalcemia in acute pancreatitis has many possible causes, including hypoalbuminemia[24] with decreased protein binding, formation of calcium soaps in the presence of fat necrosis,[25] stimulation of calcitonin secretion[26] by increased serum glucagon,[27] and decreased parathormone secretion by various mechanisms,[28] but rarely is there a clinically significant decrease in ionized calcium. If deficits are found, however, calcium and magnesium are easily replaced.

CARDIOVASCULAR COLLAPSE, RENAL FAILURE, AND RESPIRATORY INSUFFICIENCY

Other supportive therapies include vigorous rehydration and correction of electrolyte abnormalities, as well as maintenance of adequate renal urinary output, circulatory perfusion, and ventilatory assistance to avoid tissue hypoxia and damage. All of these are attempts to abort the acute-phase determinants of early mortality: cardiovascular collapse, renal failure, and pulmonary insufficiency.

Hypovolemia is easy to explain as a result of the chemical peritonitis that develops in these patients; the associated increased capillary permeability, relative lymphatic obstruction, and partial splanchnic venous obstruction can account for sequestration of up to 40% of the patient's circulatory plasma volume in just a few hours. Renal insufficiency may be a result of this massive fluid loss. If it is present, the association of renal failure in acute pancreatitis markedly increases the mortality in these patients.[29]

Whether or not there is a myocardial depressant factor associated with severe pancreatitis,[30] inotropic agents may be required to improve cardiac function if cardiac output remains low despite adequate left atrial filling pressures.

The respiratory insufficiency associated with severe pancreatitis is much more complex and is probably a combination of a decrease in functional residual capacity and shunting, which may be related to elevated paralyzed hemidiaphragms, basilar atelectasis, pleural effusion, empyema, pneumonia, micropulmonary emboli, or alveolar collapse secondary to the decrease in pulmonary surfactant, which is degraded by circulating pancreatic enzymes. Respiratory

assistance with positive end-expiratory pressure is required until the process resolves and the patient can maintain minute ventilation and oxygenation.

THERAPEUTIC PERITONEAL LAVAGE

Short-term (48- to 96-hour) therapeutic peritoneal lavage has clearly been demonstrated by Ranson and Spencer to improve the early clinical condition of patients with acute pancreatitis.[31] In their randomized, prospective studies, the mortality rate during the first 10 days decreased from 45% in control subjects to 0% in patients treated with peritoneal lavage. Cardiovascular instability and respiratory insufficiency improved and did not result in early mortality. The overall survival rate, however, was not significantly improved; the cause of death only shifted from cardiovascular and respiratory insufficiency to late infection of devitalized pancreatic and peripancreatic tissue.

Controlled clinical trials of long-term (7-day) peritoneal lavage in severe acute pancreatitis showed a reduction in both the incidence of pancreatic sepsis and its associated mortality rate.[32] This therapy is a major undertaking, because it involves hourly lavage for at least 7 days. The fluid used was Dianeal (Baxter Health Care), an approximately isotonic, balanced electrolyte solution containing 15 g/L of dextrose; 8 mEq potassium, 1000 USP units of heparin, and 250 mg of ampicillin were added to each 2 L of fluid. An alternative antibiotic was used if the patient had a history of penicillin allergy.

Peritoneal lavage should be considered as adjuvant therapy in the unstable patient with severe pancreatitis (i.e., if more than 5 of Ranson's criteria are present at 48 hours).

ANTIBIOTICS

The late complications of severe pancreatitis are related to sepsis and account for up to 80% of deaths from this disease. Although it seems logical to administer antibiotics to patients with severe pancreatitis, *prophylactic* administration has never been shown to prevent the septic complications of this disease and usually only hastens colonization by resistant bacterial and fungal organisms. There are no randomized clinical studies showing effective antibiotic prophylaxis.[33] Prophylactic ampicillin did not show any benefit in preventing septic complications in a randomized study.[34] Although newer agents have not been studied, prophylaxis is not recommended. If therapy is deemed necessary after sepsis has developed, antibiotics should be selected that can exceed the in vitro concentration (MIC-90) in pancreatic secretion and tissue. The enteric pathogens that invade the pancreas include *Escherichia coli*, *Klebsiella pneumoniae*, enterococcus, *Staphylococcus aureus*, *Pseudomonas aeruginosa*, *Proteus mirabilis*, *Streptococcus* species, *Enterobacter aerogenes*, and *Bacteroides fragilis*.[35]

Antibiotics are used in pancreatic necrosis, infected necrosis, and infected pseudocysts, based on the susceptibility data of the cultured bacteria. Gram-negative bacteria are the most common pathogens. Secondary fungal infections are not uncommon in patients with complications. A continued septic course despite adequate drainage and antibacterial antibiotics should alert the clinician to the possibility of a fungal infection.

SURGICAL MANAGEMENT ■

Surgery may be indicated for confirmation of the diagnosis of pancreatitis, for treatment of an underlying biliary tract problem, or for treatment of complications.

CONFIRMATION OF THE DIAGNOSIS

Many surgical emergencies can mimic acute pancreatitis, with diffuse peritoneal signs and even amylasemia. Exploratory laparotomy may be required to diagnose and treat the condition definitively. No patient should be allowed to die from progression of pancreatitis without an exploratory laparotomy to confirm the diagnosis, to eliminate other treatable entities that can mimic pancreatitis, and to attempt to correct the complications of pancreatitis that otherwise may lead to death. Diagnostic laparoscopy may be helpful to identify a process that needs surgical treatment and avoid laparotomy; we have used bedside laparoscopy in the ICU in critically ill patients to avoid the hazards associated with transport.

TREATMENT OF THE BILIARY CAUSE

Biliary pancreatitis is usually associated with the passage of a small common bile duct stone. Typically, the highest serum amylase levels may be present initially but they return to normal, as do the patient's clinical signs. Occasionally, a stone may become impacted at the ampulla; rapid progressive deterioration in the patient's clinical course may soon follow. The therapeutic procedure of choice to relieve the obstruction is endoscopic papillotomy and stone extraction. Operative intervention may carry higher risks. If common bile duct exploration can not retrieve the impacted stone, the duodenum must be opened to attempt a sphincteroplasty. The duodenal suture line then necessary is in jeopardy in the face of pancreatitis, and dehiscence is a disastrous complication. If an impacted stone can not be removed through the common bile duct at the operation, an interoperative ERCP should be considered. ERCP can also be performed postoperatively. Little evidence supports emergency surgery for these patients if they have passed their common bile duct stones, because any alteration of their clinical course cannot be confirmed after such an emergency surgical procedure.[36,37] Later, definitive biliary surgery can be justified during that same admission to prevent recurrence of biliary pancreatitis (>50% probability) in a patient who is waiting for elective readmission.[38]

TREATMENT OF DISEASE COMPLICATIONS

Most complications of pancreatitis require surgical and radiologic consultations and procedures. The complications of pancreatitis may be outlined as vascular complications, pancreatic pseudocyst formation, and complications related to pseudocysts, biliary obstruction, and pancreatic abscess and necrosis.

Vascular Complications

Vascular complications of pancreatitis may be divided into systemic and local. The *systemic vascular effects* of acute pancreatitis are probably related to the release of pancreatic proteases, such as trypsin, which locally and distally may activate complement C5a and precipitate the coagulation cascade.[39] This causes microscopic and physiologic changes in granulocytes that induce a cell-to-cell interaction and clumping. The clumps may then embolize and set the stage for further fibrin deposition and thrombosis. This phenomenon explains the leukoembolic damage of the posterior fundus of the eye in the syndrome of sudden blindness associated with severe trauma and pancreatitis (Purtscher's retinopathy).[40] Other systemic effects of C5a may be granulocyte aggregation and leukoembolization of other vital tissues, such as the lung, kidney, and splanchnic and systemic vascular beds, which may explain some of the respiratory distress syndromes, renal insufficiency, splanchnic venous thrombosis, and incidence of pulmonary emboli in these patients.[39]

There are both arterial and venous *local vascular effects* and complications of pancreatitis. Bleeding from pancreatic pseudocysts and ruptured pseudoaneurysms is the most often fatal complication of pancreatitis, carrying a mortality rate of 25% to 40%.[41-43] Bleeding may present as melena from erosion into the proximal gastrointestinal tract or as hypovolemia and abdominal pain if there is rupture into the peritoneal cavity. Diagnosis is usually made late in the patient's clinical course or only at postmortem examination. Most patients with gastrointestinal tract bleeding secondary to acute or chronic pancreatitis are alcoholics, and the cause of the bleeding is usually missed because of more common causes of serious bleeding in this patient population (e.g., peptic ulcer disease, gastritis, varices, Mallory-Weiss tears). The development of aneurysms is probably related to the severe inflammation and enzymatic autodigestion of the pancreatic and peripancreatic arteries with eventual formation of a pseudoaneurysm. With growth and expansion, the pseudoaneurysms may rupture into pseudocysts, adjacent viscera, the peritoneal cavity, or the pancreatic duct.

The most common vessel involved in splanchnic pseudoaneurysms related to pancreatitis is the splenic artery, followed by the gastroduodenal and the inferior pancreaticoduodenal, but such involvement may occur with any of the adjacent splanchnic vessels.[44] Patients with chronic pancreatitis may have as high as a 10% incidence of pseudoaneurysms demonstrated on angiographic studies, but bleeding from these rarely occurs unless they are associated with pseudocysts.[45] The treatment of ruptured pseudoaneurysms requires that the diagnosis be recognized; therefore, the clinician must know of it, must have a high index of suspicion, and must have a well-defined diagnostic and therapeutic plan, including emergency upper endoscopy, selective visceral angiography, ultrasonography, and CT scanning. Temporary control can be rendered by selective arterial infusion of vasopressin,[45] Gelfoam and autogenous clot embolization,[46] transcatheter electrocoagulation,[47] detachable intravascular balloons,[48] Gianturco coils,[49] or polymerizing adhesives.[49] These procedures should be considered as temporizing measures until the patient's clinical condition improves sufficiently for definitive operative control. At surgery, the initial approach should be that of proximal vascular control, which can be performed preoperatively with inflatable balloon catheters, local manual tamponade or packing, digital compression, or intraluminal Fogarty balloon catheters.

Intracystic suture ligation alone is attended by a higher incidence of recurrent bleeding, and therefore both intracystic suture ligation and proximal and distal ligation with either resection or internal drainage of the pseudocyst may be necessary for complete control of the problem.[51]

Hemoductal pancreatitis or hemosuccus pancreatitis is the complication of pseudoaneurysm rupture into the pancreatic duct and usually encompasses the triad of gastrointestinal bleeding, pancreatitis with epigastric pain, and partial common bile duct obstruction.[52] The diagnosis can be confirmed by selective visceral angiography or ERCP. The treatment of this rare complication requires ligation of the pseudoaneurysm and possible pancreatic resection.

Venous complications of acute pancreatitis, although not as dramatic, may be just as lethal as their arterial counterparts. Venous thrombosis of the portal vein is a potential complication of acute or chronic pancreatitis. The patient's course is complicated by acute decompensation, hypotension with sequestration in the splanchnic vascular bed, acidosis, hepatic enzyme elevation, alteration in clotting studies, and venous infarction of the bowel. Patients who survive this insult all develop portal hypertension, and some present months to years later with bleeding esophageal varices. Selective splenic venous thrombosis occurs more frequently, and patients usually present with an increased spleen size, unexplained blood loss, pain in the left upper quadrant and subscapular area, and, possibly, hypotension and cardiovascular collapse because the subcapsular hematoma ruptured into the free peritoneal cavity. The treatment is splenectomy with preoperative vascular control by angiographic techniques and balloons. The intensivist must simultaneously manage resuscitation, coordination of the surgeons and interventional radiologists, and transportation of the patient. Selective pancreatic surgery, such as external drainage of pancreatic abscess or resection or internal drainage of a pseudocyst, is desirable.

During drainage procedures for pancreatic pseudocysts in the presence of associated splenic venous thrombosis, the transgastric approach should be avoided in order to decrease postoperative bleeding from the rich submucosal plexus of high-pressure veins. In the absence of bleeding gastric varices, one may elect to leave the spleen in situ even with splenic vein thrombosis, because not all patients develop bleeding from the gastric varices.

Pseudocyst Formation

Pseudocyst formation is not an uncommon complication of acute pancreatitis; it is seen more frequently in alcoholic than nonalcoholic patients.[53,54] Most pseudocysts are benign, varying from lesser sac fluid collections to true pseudocysts, and may spontaneously resolve during the first 6 weeks.

Pseudocysts that persist longer than 6 weeks rarely resolve; furthermore, because there is an increase in incidence of complications, definitive treatment is justified.[55] Complications include infection; visceral or biliary tract obstruction; free rupture into the peritoneal cavity or pleural space, or transenterically; and hemorrhagic complications.

The diagnosis of a pseudocyst is easily made with CT scanning and can be followed by ultrasonography. The complication of secondary infection of a pseudocyst can be confirmed by percutaneous needle aspiration with Gram stain and culture. The infected pseudocyst can be drained percutaneously and continuously by a catheter placed in the cavity. This fluid is not as viscous as that seen in a pancreatic abscess, and infected pseudocysts are well handled with this approach.

Pseudocysts may cause gastrointestinal tract obstruction by their direct compression on adjacent viscera, most commonly the duodenum, but they can also cause gastric, jejunal, or even colonic obstruction. The therapy here, too, may initially be percutaneous drainage; if this fails or the pseudocyst recurs, operative internal decompression may be required. Small or large pseudocysts may rupture freely into the peritoneal cavity, causing acute chemical peritonitis[56] and chronic pancreatic ascites, or they may track retroperitoneally into the pleural space, causing chronic pleural effusions.[57] The initial therapy for this complication is peritoneal lavage and drainage or pleural space closed-tube drainage with the placing of the pancreas "at rest." If this fails, more aggressive attempts at sealing the leak, either with anterior and posterior port radiation to transiently stop the secretory process[58] or with the combination of ERCP and definitive internal surgical drainage, may be necessary.[59] Transenteric perforation of a pseudocyst may resolve the problem with spontaneous internal drainage but more commonly heralds further complications: contamination of the pseudocyst or bleeding from the submucosal plexus of the adjacent bowel structure. The hemorrhagic complications and their management have already been discussed.

A preoperative percutaneous aspirate of the pseudocyst should be sent for cytologic examination to rule out neoplasm, for culture and Gram stain, and for examination for blood to determine whether a pseudoaneurysm has formed, requiring angiographic identification and control of the proximal vessel before surgery. About 20% of these pseudocysts do not recur after complete aspiration,[60] and those that do can be treated with either percutaneous transgastric drainage[61] or definitive surgical resection or internal drainage. Bleeding after a cystogastrostomy is most commonly related to the suture line and can be prevented by avoiding running sutures[62] or controlled with aggressive endoscopic cauterization techniques.

Obstruction Due to Pancreatic Inflammation

Biliary obstruction may be found in as many as 25% of cases presenting with acute pancreatitis,[63] and this obstruction, caused by pancreatic swelling, can be confused with a stone lodged at the ampulla. The intrapancreatic portion of the common bile duct becomes involved in the inflammatory process, but this usually resolves over the course of the disease.[64] If the biliary obstruction does not resolve, a work-up including ultrasonography, ERCP, or transhepatic cholangiography, may be necessary to define the problem and the anatomy so that an appropriate decompressive procedure can be performed. If the patient develops cholangitis and becomes septic from infected bile in the obstructed duct, transhepatic cholangiography and drainage may be lifesaving to provide decompression without subjecting the patient in septic shock to an emergency operation.

Pancreatic Necrosis and Abscess

Little is known of what triggers the release of activated pancreatic enzymes that autodigest the gland and surrounding retroperitoneal tissue and convert acute interstitial or edematous pancreatitis to pancreatic necrosis.[1] If venous thrombosis and erosion to the small peripancreatic vessels occur, the combination is hemorrhagic necrotizing pancreatitis. Enteric bacterial contamination results in combined abscess and infected necrosis, which carries the highest mortality rate.[65] The timing of this sequence of presentations is important. It is rare to see septic complications in the first week of presentation but not unusual after the second week, and they are almost universally present if the patient's course requires therapy for more than 3 weeks. Clinical signs of abdominal pain, fever, and leukocytosis; associated severe systemic manifestations of hypotension, cardiovascular collapse, pulmonary insufficiency, and renal failure; and associated mental disorientation all strongly suggest the onset of this complication.

Of significance has been the ability to predict abscess formation in patients with an increasing number of Ranson's early objective signs. Thirty-four percent of patients presenting with three or more positive prognostic signs developed pancreatic or peripancreatic sepsis.[66] The problem is rarely that of making the diagnosis of sepsis but that of differentiating pancreatic necrosis and abscess formation from other sources of sepsis such as pneumonia, urinary tract infection, and intravascular catheter-related infection.

Sequential CT scanning is the best tool available for diagnosing and following this disease process. The study is diagnostic of abscess formation if air is seen in the phlegmon. Percutaneous needle aspiration of the intrapancreatic or peripancreatic fluid collections can be used to confirm bacterial contamination.

If necrosis is demonstrated on CT scan, aspirates are sterile, and the patient is not toxic, a conservative approach may be attempted. If the patient shows signs of increasing toxicity and sepsis, then exploration, debridement, sequestrectomy, and drainage are recommended. In the unstable patient, aspiration and catheter drainage under CT guidance and drainage of an abscess as a temporizing measure before surgery may improve the patient's overall condition. Recently, multiple, large percutaneous catheters have provided better drainage for the thick material in abscesses and have increased utility of nonoperative treatment (see Chap. 38). Surgical techniques are still necessary for debridement and drainage if percutaneous drainage does not improve the septic course. Operative intervention must not be delayed too long. Both open and closed drainage techniques have been proposed. Degidio and Schein,[67] in a collaborative review of 920 patients, compared three strategies: (1) resection followed by drainage and reoperation as needed, (2) necrosectomy plus local lavage, and (3) necrosectomy and open management. The latter two methods were associated with improved survival.

We use the open technique of marsupialization[68,69] of the lesser sac along with packing that can be changed daily in the ICU. The marsupialization essentially compartmentalizes the abdomen to contain the infected area. Even with this technique, other collections can form, usually in the pericolic gutters. If present, these can be drained through flank incisions, although we have begun to rely increasingly on the placement of large percutaneous drainage tubes under CT guidance for this purpose. Pancreatic necrosis and abscess formation, whether treated in an open or closed fashion, have been associated with arterial hemorrhage (which is treated by packing and embolization of the offending artery) and with necrosis of the transverse colon (which requires resection and a proximal colostomy).

Early operation directed toward debridement of devitalized tissue to prevent septic complications has only led to increased morbidity and incidence of sepsis.[70] Therefore, it is extremely important to differentiate the phlegmon or necrotic pancreatic process from abscess formation and infected necrosis.

Intestinal fistulization from the colon and duodenum usually results from prolonged tube drainage with erosion into the adjacent viscera. The management of the controlled fistula probably carries with it less morbidity than does reexploration because of premature removal of lesser sac drains.

REFERENCES ■

1. Satiani B, Stone HH: Predictability of present outcome and future recurrence in acute pancreatitis. *Arch Surg* 1979; 114:711
2. Trapnell JE, Duncan EHL: Patterns of incidence in acute pancreatitis. *Br Med J* 1975;1:179
3. Salt WB II, Schenker S: Amylase—its clinical significance: A review of the literature. *Medicine* 1976;55:269
4. Warshaw AL, Fuller FF Jr: Specificity of increased renal clearance of amylase in diagnosis of acute pancreatitis. *N Engl J Med* 1975;292:325
5. Levitt MD: Clinical use of amylase clearance and isoamylase measurements. *Mayo Clin Proc* 1979;54:428
6. Gumaste V,. Diagnostic tests for acute pancreatitis. *The Gastroenterologist* 1994;2:119
7. Northam BE, Rowe DS, Winstone NE: Methemalbumin in the differential diagnosis of acute hemorrhagic and aedematous pancreatitis. *Lancet* 1963;1:348
8. Lawson TL: Acute pancreatitis and its complications: Computed tomography and sonography. *Radiol Clin North Am* 1983;21:495
9. Block S, Maier W, Bittner R, et al: Identification of pancreas necrosis in severe acute pancreatitis: Imaging procedures versus clinical staging. *Gut* 1986;27:1035
10. White EM, Wittenberg J, Mueller PR: Pancreatic necrosis: CT manifestations. *Radiology* 1986;158:343
11. Sarles H: Pancreatitis: Symposium of Marseilles, 1963. Basel, Skarger, 1965.

12. Bradley E. A clinically based classification system for acute pancreatitis. *Arch Surg* 1993;128:586

13. Ranson JHC, Rifkind KM, Turner JW: Prognostic signs and nonoperative peritoneal lavage in acute pancreatitis. *Surg Gynecol Obstet* 1976;143:209

14. Ranson JHC, Spencer FC: The role of peritoneal lavage in severe acute pancreatitis. *Ann Surg* 1978;187:565

15. Levant JA, Secrist DLM, Resin H, et al: Nasogastric suction in the treatment of alcoholic pancreatitis: A controlled study. *JAMA* 1974;229:51

16. Sarr MG, Sanfey H, Cameron JL: Prospective randomized trial of nasogastric suction in patients with acute pancreatitis. *Surgery* 1986;100:500

17. Meshkinpour H, Molinari MD, Gardner L, et al: Cimetidine in the treatment of acute alcoholic pancreatitis. *Gastroenterology* 1979;77:687

18. Broe PJ, Zinner MJ, Cameron JL: A clinical trial of cimetidine in acute pancreatitis. *Surg Gynec Obstet* 1982;154:13

19. Switz DM, Vlahcevic JR, Ferrar JT: The effect of anticholinergic and/or nasogastric suction on the outcome of acute alcoholic pancreatitis: A controlled trial. *Gastroenterology* 1975;68:994

20. Trapnell JE, Rigby CC, Talbot CH, Duncan EHL: A controlled trial of Trasylol in the treatment of acute pancreatitis. *Br J Surg* 1974;61:177

21. Goebell H, Ammann R, Herfarth CH, et al: A double-blind trial of synthetic salmon calcitonin in the treatment of acute pancreatitis. *Scand J Gastroenterol* 1979;14:881

22. Usadel KH, Leuschner U, Uberla KK: Treatment of acute pancreatitis with somatostatin: A multicenter double-blind trial. *N Engl J Med* 1980;303:999

23. Sitzmann JV, Steinborn PA, Zinner MJ, Cameron JL: Total parenteral nutrition and alternate energy substrates in treatment of severe acute pancreatitis. *Surg Gynecol Obstet* 1989;168:311

24. Imrie CW, Allam BF, Ferguson JC: Hypocalcaemia of acute pancreatitis: The effect of hypoalbuminaemia. *Curr Med Res Opin* 1976;4:101

25. Storck G, Bjorntorp P: Chemical composition of fat necrosis in experimental pancreatitis in the rat. *Scand J Gastroenterol* 1971;6:225

26. Canale DD, Donabedian RK: Hypercalcitoninemia in acute pancreatitis. *J Clin Endocrinol Metab* 1975;40:738

27. Donowitz M, et al: Glucagon secretion in acute and chronic pancreatitis. *Ann Intern Med* 1975;83:778

28. Robertson GM, et al: Inadequate parathyroid response in acute pancreatitis. *N Engl J Med* 1976;294:512

29. Balslov JT, Jorgensen HE, Nielsen R: Acute renal failure complicating severe pancreatitis. *Acta Chir Scand* 1962;124:348

30. Ito K, Ramirez-Schon G, Shah PM, et al: The myocardial depressant factor in acute hemorrhagic pancreatitis. *Trans Am Soc Artif Intern Organ* 1980;26:149

31. Ranson JHC, Spencer FC: The role of peritoneal lavage in severe acute pancreatitis. *Ann Surg* 1978;187:565

32. Ranson JHC, Berman RS: Long peritoneal lavage decreases pancreatic sepsis in acute pancreatitis. *Ann Surg* 1990;211:708

33. Bradley EL III: Antibiotics in acute pancreatitis: Current status and future directions. *Am J Surg* 1989;158:472

34. Finch WT, Sawyers JL, Schender S. A prospective study to determine the efficiency of antibiotics in acute pancreatitis. *Ann Surg* 1976;183:667

35. Lumsden A, Bradley EL III: Secondary pancreatic infections: Abscess, infected necrosis, and infected pseudocyst. *Surg Gynecol Obstet* 1990;170:459

36. Stone HH, Fabian TC, Dunlop WE: Gallstone pancreatitis: Biliary tract pathology in relation to time of operation. *Ann Surg* 1981;194:305

37. Acosta JM, Rossi R, Galli OMR, et al: Early surgery for acute gallstone pancreatitis: Evaluation of a systemic approach. *Surgery* 1978;83:367

38. Mayer AD, McMahon MJ, Benson EA, et al: Operations upon the biliary tract in patients with acute pancreatitis: Aims, indications, and timing. *Ann R Coll Surg Engl* 1984;66:179

39. Jacob HS, Craddock PR, Hammerschmidt DE, et al: Complement-induced granulocyte aggregation: An unsuspected mechanism of disease. *N Engl J Med* 1980;302:789

40. Jones WL: Purtscher's retinopathy associated with acute pancreatitis. *Am J Optom Physiol Opt* 1981;58:855

41. Frey CF: Pancreatic pseudocyst: Operative strategy. *Ann Surg* 1978;188:652

42. Gadacz TR, Trunkey D, Kieffer RF Jr: Visceral vessel erosion associated with pancreatitis. *Arch Surg* 1978;113:1438

43. Stanley JC, Frey CF, Miller TA, et al: Major arterial hemorrhage: A complication of pancreatic pseudocysts and chronic pancreatitis. *Arch Surg* 1976;111:435

44. Stabile BE, Wilson SE, Debas HT: Reduced mortality from bleeding pseudocysts and pseudoaneurysms caused by pancreatitis. *Arch Surg* 1983;118:45

45. White AF, Baum S, Buranasiri S: Aneurysms secondary to pancreatitis. *AJR Am J Roentgenol* 1976;127:393

46. Vujic I, Anderson MC, Meredith HC, et al: Successful embolization of the dorsal pancreatic artery to control massive upper gastrointestinal hemorrhage. *Ann Surg* 1980;46:184

47. Prasad JK, Chatterjee KS, Johnston DWB: Unusual case of massive gastrointestinal bleeding: Pseudoaneurysm of the head of the pancreas. *Can J Surg* 1975;18:490

48. Kaufman SL, Strandberg JD, Barth KH, et al: Therapeutic embolization with detachable silastic balloons: long-term effects in swine. *Invest Radiol* 1979;14:156

49. Wallace S, Gianturco C, Anderson JH, et al: Therapeutic vascular occlusion utilizing steel coil technique: Clinical application. *AJR Am J Roentgenol* 1976;127:381

50. Goldman ML, Freeny PC, Tallman JM, et al: Transcatheter vascular occlusion therapy with isobutyl 2-cyanoacrylate (bucylate) for control of massive upper-gastrointestinal bleeding. *Radiology* 1978;129:41

51. Greenstein A, Demaio EF, Nabseth DC: Acute hemorrhage associated with pancreatic pseudocysts. *Surgery* 1971;69:56

52. Harper PC, Gamelli RL, Kaye MD: Recurrent hemorrhage into the pancreatic duct from a splenic artery aneurysm. *Gastroenterology* 1984;87:417

53. Sankaran S, Walt AJ: The natural and unnatural history of pancreatic pseudocysts. *Br J Surg* 1975;62:377

54. Bradley EL III, Salam AA: Hyperbilirubinemia in inflammatory pancreatic disease: Natural history and management. *Ann Surg* 1978;188:626

55. Bradley EL III, Clements JL Jr, Gonzalez AC: The natural history of pancreatic pseudocysts: A unified concept of management. *Am J Surg* 1979;137:135

56. Hanna WA: Rupture of pancreatic cysts: Report of a case and review of the literature. *Br J Surg* 1960;47:495

57. Cameron JL, Kieffer RS, Anderson WJ, et al: Internal pancreatic fistulas: Pancreatic ascites and pleural effusions. *Ann Surg* 1976;183:587

58. Morris SJ, Barkin JS, Kalser MH, et al: Radiation therapy of a pancreatic fistula. *Am J Gastroenterol* 1979;72:431

59. Cameron JL, Kieffer RS, Anderson WJ, et al: Internal pancreatic fistulas: Pancreatic ascites and pleural effusions. *Ann Surg* 1976;184:587

60. Barkin JS, Smith FR, Pereira R Jr, et al: Therapeutic percutaneous aspiration of pancreatic pseudocysts. *Dig Dis Sci* 1981; 26:585

61. Nunez D Jr, Yrizarry JM, Russell E, et al: Transgastric drainage of pancreatic fluid collections. *AJR Am J Roentgenol* 1985; 145:815

62. Hutson DG, Zeppa R, Warren WD: Prevention of postoperative hemorrhage after pancreatic cystogastrostomy. *Ann Surg* 1973;177:689

63. Frieden JH: The significance of jaundice in acute pancreatitis. *Arch Surg* 1965;90:422

64. Bradley EL III, Salam AA: Hyperbilirubinemia in inflammatory pancreatic disease: Natural history and management. *Ann Surg* 1978;188:626

65. Bolooki H, Jaffe B, Gliedman ML: Pancreatic abscesses and lesser omental sac collections. *Surg Gynecol Obstet* 1968; 128:1301

66. Ranson JHC: Acute pancreatitis. *Curr Probl Surg* 1979;16:1

67. Degidio A, Schein M: Surgical strategies in the treatment of pancreatic necrosis and infection. *Br J Surg* 1991;78:133

68. Davidson ED, Bradley EL III: "Marsupialization" in the treatment of pancreatic abscess. *Surgery* 1981;89:252

69. Gliedman ML, Bolooki H, Rosen RG: Acute pancreatitis. *Curr Probl Surg* 69(70), 1970:1

70. Ranson JHC, Rifkind KM, Roses DF, et al: Prognostic signs and the role of operative management in acute pancreatitis. *Surg Gynecol Obstet* 1974;139:69

Critical Care, Third Edition, edited by Joseph M. Civetta,
Robert W. Taylor, and Robert R. Kirby.
Lippincott-Raven Publishers, Philadelphia, PA © 1997.

CHAPTER 141

Inflammatory Bowel Disease

Charles E. Brady
Oscar A. Alvarez

IMMEDIATE CONCERNS

MAJOR PROBLEMS

Inflammatory bowel disease produces several complications that may require admission to an intensive care unit. Fulminant colitis, toxic megacolon, perforation, and massive hemorrhage are the most serious of these complications from an acute life-threatening standpoint and may occur in ulcerative colitis, Crohn's disease, and various infections.[1-11] Toxic megacolon is a well known and serious clinical entity usually identified as a complication of inflammatory bowel disease; because of its fulminant nature, the frequent need for surgery, and the potentially life-threatening complications associated with a high mortality, there has been great debate regarding medical management and the appropriate time for surgical intervention.

STRESS POINTS

1. Toxic megacolon is defined as a severe attack of colitis seen in several inflammatory conditions involving the large bowel and accompanied by total or segmental dilation of the colon.
2. Two components must be present: toxicity and dilation of the colon.
3. Although this entity is uncommon, morbidity and mortality can be high.
4. Fulminant colitis and toxic megacolon have multiple etiologies.
5. Exact cause is unknown, but several triggering factors seem to predispose to the development of fulminant colitis or toxic megacolon.
6. Frequent clinical assessment and abdominal radio-

graphs are crucial in diagnosing and managing such patients.
7. Immediate surgery is indicated for perforation and massive hemorrhage, whereas an initial attempt at medical management is indicated in most patients.

ESSENTIAL DIAGNOSTIC TESTS AND PROCEDURES

1. Frequent physical examination with vital signs
2. Stool studies: stool culture, tests for ova and parasites and for *Clostridium difficile* enterotoxin
3. Blood studies every 24 to 48 hours: complete blood count, serum electrolytes, serum albumin, and sedimentation rate
4. Daily obstructive radiographic series
5. Flexible sigmoidoscopy to 20 cm, if indicated

INITIAL THERAPY

1. Hospitalization, consultation with a surgeon
2. Aggressive fluid and electrolyte replacement, transfusion as necessary
3. Avoidance of oral intake, use of intravenous nutritional support
4. Intestinal decompression using nonendoscopic methods
5. Appropriate antibiotics and intravenous corticosteroids
6. In selected patients, cyclosporine, 4 mg/kg per day[12,13]
7. Surgery for perforation, massive bleeding, deterioration despite intensive therapy, or failure to respond after an appropriate period of medical management.

FULMINANT COLITIS AND TOXIC MEGACOLON

The terms *severe* or *fulminant colitis* and *toxic megacolon* are often used interchangeably, but *such use is not correct.* The syndrome of toxic megacolon more appropriately refers specifically to colonic dilation superimposed on a toxic state of acute fulminant colitis. Although most frequently seen with ulcerative colitis, fulminant colitis and toxic megacolon may occur in patients with Crohn's disease, amebic colitis, *Shigella* or *Salmonella* infection, pseudomembranous colitis, ischemic bowel disease, mucosal ulcerative colitis,[8] cytomegalovirus infection,[9] Chagas' disease,[10] and anti-cancer chemotherapy.[11]

Regardless of the cause, fulminant colitis implies an acutely ill patient with a diseased colon and toxic megacolon signifies that the colonic diameter has progressed to the point of imminent perforation and death. This is a medical-surgical emergency that requires hospitalization and integrated multidisciplinary care. When strictly defined, toxic megacolon is a relatively rare complication, but perforation can occur without megacolon.[14]

CLINICAL FEATURES

Patients with severe or fulminant colitis are usually extremely ill with frequent, often bloody diarrheal stools, fever, anemia, hypoalbuminemia, weakness, and severe general debility. Fulminant ulcerative colitis may occur as a complication in a patient with a short- or long-standing history of inflammatory bowel disease and commonly occurs as the initial presentation of the illness.[1,4,5,15] Toxic megacolon is defined as a severe attack of colitis accompanied by total or segmental dilation of the colon and can be regarded as a phase of toxic colitis. Use of the term *toxic* conjures up images of desperately ill patient with fever, tachycardia, and shock. However, an exact definition of *toxicity* is difficult to find. Some investigators consider toxicity to be present when at least three of the following four conditions exist: fever over 38.6°C (101.5°F), tachycardia greater than 120 beats per minute (bpm), white blood cell count greater than 10,500/mm^3, and anemia with a hemoglobin concentration less than 60% of normal. In addition, as the disease progresses, one of the following has to be present: dehydration, mental changes, electrolyte disturbance, or hypotension. Clinical or radiographic evidence of colonic distention combined with this degree of toxicity constitutes the entity of toxic megacolon.

At the Cleveland Clinic,[1] a patient is considered toxic if, in addition to a chart notation to that effect, there is evidence of a least two of the following: tachycardia greater than 100 bpm, fever over 38.6°8C (101.5°8F), white blood cell count greater than 10,000/mm^3, and hypoalbuminemia with a serum albumin less than 3.0 g/dL. The presence of abdominal distention is also documented, and megacolon is defined as being present if the colon diameter measures 5 cm or more and the haustral pattern is disturbed or absent. Other features commonly present, but not necessary for the diagnosis, are abdominal tenderness, hypotension, electrolyte imbalance, and anemia.

The features observed in toxic megacolon represent a spectrum of illnesses, presence of underlying malnutrition, and fulminant nature of the attack.[1,16] Although the patient usually complains of abdominal pain, this is not always present because delirium, steroids, or analgesics may modify this symptom. Symptoms and signs of acute colitis with severe, frequently bloody diarrhea usually have been present for at least 1 week before megacolon supervenes.

On physical examination, vital signs show fever and tachycardia. Toxicity may be further manifested by lethargy, pallor, hypotension, mental change, and signs of dehydration. Abdominal distention may be present, and frequently the contour of the dilated transverse colon can be seen or felt during examination. Bowel sounds are usually diminished, and the abdomen is often tympanitic on percussion. Localized tenderness, especially in the left upper quadrant, implies local peritonitis and impending perforation. Generalized tenderness, rebound tenderness, guarding, and complaints of shoulder tip pain indicate free perforation, but surprisingly few clinical signs of frank peritonitis may be present in some patients. Some of these findings may be modified or masked by concurrent steroid therapy or disturbances of the patient's sensorium, and, in this particular situation, the abdominal radiographic examination assists the clinician in the diagnosis of toxic megacolon.[17,18] Toxic psychosis and delirium should be regarded as sinister signs and are a reflection of toxemia. Gram-negative septicemia may be present but unrecognized.

Laboratory studies usually show anemia, leukocytosis, electrolyte disturbances, hypoalbuminemia, and elevated sedimentation rate.[7] Hypokalemia secondary to gastrointestinal loss is common and may contribute to the development of colonic dilation,[19] whereas other investigators believe that a clear-cut relationship has not been shown.[14] Hypoalbuminemia is usually evidence for chronicity or severity of illness, but a rapid drop implies increasing toxicity.

DIAGNOSIS

In all patients thought to have severe or fulminant colitis or toxic megacolon of any etiology, plain abdominal radiographs are essential. Anteroposterior recumbent and upright or left lateral decubitus radiographs should be obtained in all patients. Such radiographs not only provide some information on distribution and extent of involvement, but also are particularly important for diagnosing perforation and toxic megacolon.[1] The plain recumbent radiograph is usually diagnostic in patients with toxic megacolon.[1,4,14,16–18] Colonic dilation may affect the entire colon but is usually segmental, with the transverse colon being the most prominently dilated segment. The descending and sigmoid colon also are often distended; the rectum is rarely distended. Although dilatation of the transverse colon on a plain supine abdominal radiograph is a most conspicuous finding, it does not have specific pathophysiologic significance. Distention of the transverse colon in toxic megacolon is the result of its anterior position, and repositioning the patient redistributes gas to other segments, depending on the position used.[20] Dilation beyond 5.5 cm generally is considered abnormal,[1] and attempts have been made to fix the definition of toxic mega-colon on the basis of the diameter of the transverse colon. However, strict criteria cannot be applied because the caliber of the distended segments varies greatly. It is best not to rely on a single measurement of this type but to consider the radiographic appearance as only one factor, with the clinical manifestations being of equal importance.

Haustra may be absent but may be thickened early and subsequently disappear. The mucosal surface may display multiple broad-based nodular intraluminal protrusions caused by pseudopolyps. Occasionally, a radiolucent line paralleling the bowel lumen can be seen and is believed to represent intramuscular air dissection, suggesting that perforation may be imminent.[1] Although perforation is rare in the absence of toxic dilatation, for unclear reasons it is more likely to occur during the initial severe attack of ulcerative colitis.[1,4] Perforation is most common in patients with pancolitis and is most frequent in the sigmoid colon. In most cases, free intraperitoneal air is easily demonstrated on the upright or lateral decubitus radiographs.

When the classic features of toxicity and colonic dilation occur in a patient with known idiopathic inflammatory bowel disease, a diagnosis of fulminant colitis or toxic megacolon can be confidently made. In other patients, the diagnosis may be less clear, and sigmoidoscopy should be performed to exclude the other much less frequent causes that can present in the same fashion.[1,4,5,8-11,16,17,21] Most patients with inflammatory bowel disease should undergo sigmoidoscopy to exclude a superimposed infectious colitis (e.g., amebiasis) because steroid therapy could have devastating results. Sigmoidoscopy should be done with gentle, minimal manipulation and without preparation or air insufflation, the scope should not be passed above 20 cm, and, if necessary, it can be done in the left lateral position in bed. Occasionally, features are observed that are highly suggestive of a specific entity (amebiasis, pseudomembranous colitis, Crohn's disease), but this is certainly the exception rather than the rule. More commonly, a fierce, nonspecific rectal inflammation with pus and blood is seen, and a clear distinction cannot be made. Biopsy should not be done; instead, mucosal scrapings should be collected for culture (*Salmonella*, *Shigella*, *Campylobacter*, *Clostridium*, *Yersinia*) and to look for amebas. These samples should not be obtained with a cotton swab, but rather a metal spoon or suction trap because amebas adhere to the cotton. To enhance recovery of infectious agents, fresh stool samples also should be sent to the laboratory for culture and to check for ova and parasites, particularly if sigmoidoscopy is not performed. In the appropriate clinical setting, amebic serologic studies should be done and stool assayed for *C difficile* toxin. These steps should not be overlooked because a specific underlying disorder could mandate more specific therapy. However, keep in mind that most cases of fulminant colitis or toxic megacolon result from inflammatory bowel disease.

There are few indications for performing a barium enema in patients with fulminant colitis, and it is not required for routine management. The role of a barium enema in precipitating toxic megacolon is unclear, but it is generally believed to be contraindicated in toxic megacolon because of the risk of colonic perforation.[17] There is little need for ultrasonography or computed tomography in the diagnosis and management of toxic megacolon.

MANAGEMENT

Fulminant colitis and toxic megacolon are medical-surgical emergencies requiring hospitalization, usually in an intensive care unit, and integrated multidisciplinary care. Regardless of the etiology, if the initial assessment reveals perforation, immediate surgical intervention is mandatory. If perforation is not present, a trial of medical management is indicated. The goals of therapy are the following:

1. Replace fluid, blood, and electrolyte losses rapidly.
2. Institute aggressive medical therapy.
3. Avoid precipitating toxic megacolon.
4. Monitor closely to avoid perforation.
5. Use surgery early if prompt and sustained improvement is not achieved.

The goals of therapy for megacolon are similar to those for fulminant colitis, with the addition goal of bowel decompression. Nursing care is crucial in managing these severely ill patients, and a sophisticated knowledge of nutrition, wound healing, and fluid and electrolyte balance helps to ensure an optimal outcome.

Several triggering factors have been implicated as contributing to toxic dilation in patients with a severe attack of colitis. Various medications that interfere with gut motility such as opiates (codeine, diphenoxylate), anticholinergic agents, and the synthetic antidiarrheal agent loperamide have been accused of inducing toxic megacolon. Although controversial, it is recommended that these medications be avoided or discontinued.[1,4,7,14-16] In one author's experience, early discontinuation or marked decrease in dosages of therapeutic medications has been a common contributing factor.[7] The possible relation of toxic megacolon to electrolyte abnormalities, particularly hypokalemia, and barium enema already has been mentioned. Although colonoscopy may be safe in acute colitis, there are anecdotal reports of precipitating toxic megacolon, and total colonoscopy is generally believed to be contraindicated in toxic megacolon.[7]

Treatment consists of general supportive measures and efforts to arrest the necrotic process in the colon. Oral intake is discontinued and a nasogastric tube (16 French) is placed and connected to intermittent suction to aspirate swallowed air to minimize bowel distention. Proper positioning of the nasogastric tube is necessary for effective decompression: the tip should point to or cross the spine when checked by fluoroscopy or abdominal plain radiograph. Long intestinal tubes have been found useful by some[7] but not advocated by others because of placement difficulty and lack of clear benefit. Rectal tubes should not be used because the risk of perforation.

Air does tend to accumulate preferentially in the transverse colon because the patient is usually supine in bed. Great success in preventing further air accumulation and actual decompression can be achieved by a rolling technique.[7] The patient rolls prone for 10 to 15 minutes every 2 to 3 hours and is encouraged to pass flatus in this position. A knee-to-chest position also may be helpful.

Restoring plasma volume is essential, along with correcting the deficits that result from severe diarrhea, protein loss, bleeding, and often inanition. Fluid and electrolytes deficits may be profound (water deficit may be as great as 10% of body weight), and special attention to potassium, magnesium, and calcium levels is important. Commonly, 80 to 120 mEq of potassium chloride is needed during the first 24 hours to correct hypokalemia. Orthostatic changes in vital signs usually indicate inadequate fluid or blood replacement. Blood transfusions should be given when indicated (anemia, volume depletion from blood loss, significant colonic bleeding). Persistent tachycardia may indicate inadequate volume replacement or continued disease activity. Prolonged prothrombin time is treated with vitamin K. Parenteral alimentation (central or peripheral) is usually indicated to improve nutrition but is not a successful temporizing measure in patients with fulminant colitis or toxic megacolon.[7] Some believe preoperative total parenteral nutrition to be contraindicated in the presence of free perforation or in patients needing emergency surgery because of the potential for preoperative complication.

Because extensive ulceration may facilitate bacterial invasion with resultant bacteremia and because frank perforation is a constant danger, broad-spectrum antibiotics are recommended.[1,4,15,16,19] Mortality resulting from toxic megacolon increases in the presence of sepsis and malnutrition, and the appropriate use of antibiotics can be lifesaving. Because most intraabdominal infections are caused by a mixture of aerobic and anaerobic bacteria, treatment should incorporate antibiotic coverage against both. An aminoglycoside (gentamicin) is an appropriate agent for aerobic gram-negative bacilli; a second agent (clindamycin, cefoxitin, metronidazole) directed against anaerobes is a reasonable combination. The addition of ampicillin provides more complete coverage against enterococci. Acceptable regimens are ampicillin-gentamicin-clindamycin or metronidazole and cefoxitin-gentamicin. Using metronidazole can be an additional advantage because it is also effective in Crohn's disease, amebiasis, and in cases of *C difficile*–superimposed colitis. When amebiasis is suspected, intravenous metronidazole should be used. In patients in whom diarrhea is persistent despite resolution of toxicity and colonic dilation, stools should be rechecked for the *C difficile* toxin.

Most authors agree on the use of corticosteroids in treating fulminant colitis or toxic megacolon from ulcerative colitis or Crohn's disease.[1–4,7,14–15,19] There is concern that steroids might mask signs of perforation and peritonitis; therefore, careful monitoring is important. Obviously, corticosteroids should not be used in cases caused by infectious agents. Because this complication most frequently is caused by idiopathic inflammatory bowel, this rarely presents a problem. There is no evidence that corticosteroids precipitate or adversely influence the outcome of fulminant colitis or toxic megacolon. Steroids should be continued for two main reasons: (1) most patients seen in the hospital develop their toxic dilatation while receiving steroids; (2) if steroids are discontinued when this complication arises, the patient will be at risk for adrenal insufficiency. For patients with fulminant colitis or toxic megacolon, parenteral steroids should

be used for 48 to 72 hours, and many consider surgery to be indicated if there is no improvement within this time. Few data support a specific timing for surgical intervention because only a few well-defined clinical trials use standardized therapeutic regimens. Patients who do not respond promptly or those who develop colonic perforation or even suspected perforation require prompt surgical attention. Although many of these patients ultimately come to surgery, it is reasonable to try steroids in all patients because remissions can be long lasting. Surgery can often be performed later under safer elective conditions. However, therapy should not be prolonged in the patient who fails to respond or deteriorates, in which case emergency surgery is indicated. We usually give intravenous prednisolone, 60 mg/day in divided doses. Doses of 100 to 200 mg have been used, but whether this is more beneficial is unknown. Equivalent doses of hydrocortisone (100 to 400 mg/day) have the same efficacy. Evidence suggests that corticotropin (80 to 120 U/day) may be more effective in patients who have not previously received oral steroids. We are not supporters of this approach because we believe that corticosteroids may be more precisely regulated, do not depend on adrenal responsiveness, cause fewer and less serious side effects, and are less expensive. Sulfasalazine, 5-aminosalicylic acid, metronidazole, and the immunosuppressants with slow onset of action, such as 6-mercaptopurine and azathioprine, have no role in the acute management of fulminant colitis or toxic megacolon. Intravenous cyclosporine, 4 mg/kg per day, has been shown to be effective in severe active ulcerative colitis refractory to steroid therapy.[12,13] Although cyclosporine has not been used in toxic megacolon, once the megacolon has been decompressed, cyclosporine therapy should be considered.

MONITORING THE PATIENT

Thus far, the patient has been diagnosed and resuscitated, and medical therapy instituted. Because surgical intervention is required in many patients, a team approach is required; considering that such patients can deteriorate rapidly, monitoring by both medical and surgical teams should be done once, twice, or more times daily. Vital signs are monitored frequently and physical examination should include evaluation for abdominal and rebound tenderness as well as percussion for distention and loss of hepatic dullness. Hypotension or postural changes in pulse or blood pressure and persistent tachycardia may indicate hypovolemia or continued toxicity.

The frequency, volume, and nature of diarrhea should be recorded. Improvement in the patient's diarrhea to the point of absolute constipation is a sinister feature and reflects diminished colonic evacuation rather than improvement. Misinterpretation of this change may be avoided by examining the patient's abdomen, which reveals distention, diminished bowel sounds, and tenderness. A plain abdominal radiograph may confirm continued colonic dilatation, and upright or left decubitus radiographs can indicate perforation. The corollary is also true that recurrence of diarrhea during medical treatment of toxic megacolon implies improvement in the patient's condition. Serial abdominal girth measurements may be an additional useful objective parameter in assessing overall abdominal distention. A daily obstructive radiographic series should be done.

Laboratory studies are important and should be done on presentation and every 24 to 48 hours; they should to include a complete blood count with differential, serum electrolytes, chemistries with albumin levels, and possibly a sedimentation rate. Electrolyte abnormalities should be aggressively treated and the patient transfused if anemia is significant. A poor prognosis has been associated with alkalosis using arterial pH samples. No single parameter, however, is ideal to follow. For example, dramatic response to medical treatment may occur in the absence of radiographic improvement. A synthesis of the overall clinical picture is essential for determining whether the patient is responding.

SIGNS OF IMPENDING PERFORATION

Signs of impending perforation include spiking fever, leukocytosis, tachycardia, hypotension, worsening abdominal pain or tenderness, abdominal distention, and a decrease in diarrhea as an ileus occurs. Steroids may mask signs and symptoms, causing the so-called silent perforation. The physician or nurse examining the patient may notice increasing toxicity, restlessness, or lethargy.

PATTERNS OF RESPONSE TO MEDICAL TREATMENT

Medical treatment can result in three types of response: improvement, illusory improvement, or deterioration. Few patients experience a dramatic decrease in distention with return of bowel sounds and resolution of the other signs and symptoms of toxicity. Abdominal radiographs in such patients demonstrate progressive diminution of colonic dilatation. High-dose corticosteroids should be continued for 10 to 14 days, then gradually tapered and the patient changed to oral corticosteroids when oral intake is resumed. Antibiotics should be continued for 2 weeks because intraabdominal abscess may still complicate recovery in this time period. Deterioration at any point is an absolute indication for surgery. Patients with illusory improvement with fluctuating degrees of toxicity should be operated on if their attacks have not remitted during 5 to 7 days of intensive medical treatment.

SURGERY

Views differ regarding the necessity of surgical treatment of toxic megacolon. Most authorities agree that the current surgical option is total abdominal colectomy with end ileostomy.[7,8] The rectal segment is left in place, minimizing morbidity from a pelvic dissection in the acute setting and leaving the ileoproctostomy as an available option. The diverting ileostomy and decompressive colostomy (blowhole procedure) is not widely used, and we do not recommend this procedure.

SPECIAL CONSIDERATIONS

Fulminant Colitis and Toxic Megacolon During Pregnancy

Treating fulminant colitis and toxic megacolon during pregnancy is much the same as for nonpregnant patients. In the second and third trimester, gentle proctoscopy may be performed; in the first trimester, the procedure should be avoided unless sufficiently warranted by the situation. In the second and third trimester, radiographs can be performed with minimal risk using current technology and safeguards. When absolutely necessary, radiographs can be obtained in the first trimester, preferably with informed consent. Strict attention should be paid to detail while using modern technology, equipment, and safeguards. Severe colitis is not regarded as an indication for therapeutic abortion because there is no evidence that it improves the clinical course. The indications for colectomy in the severely ill patient are the same as for the nonpregnant patient.

Toxic Megacolon From Infectious Causes

Infectious agents (amebas, *Salmonella*, *Shigella*, *Clostridium*, cytomegalovirus, Chagas' disease) occasionally may cause toxic megacolon. Management should follow exactly the same general principles already outlined. This implies a trial of medical therapy with emergency colectomy if there is not a swift response. If an infective agent is known or suspected, even in an accessory role, appropriate antibiotic therapy should be used to cover surgery.

COLONIC PERFORATION AND MASSIVE HEMORRHAGE ■

Patients who present with colonic perforation or who develop this complication during medical treatment require surgery after adequate resuscitation. Massive hemorrhage is rare in inflammatory bowel disease, usually subsides spontaneously, and only rarely requires colectomy to control bleeding. The same general principles that pertain to the management of any gastrointestinal bleeding apply to these patients and have been discussed in a previous chapter.

REFERENCES ■

1. Farmer RG, Hamilton SR, Morson BC, et al: Ulcerative colitis. In: Berk JE (ed). *Bockus Gastroenterology*, ed 5. Philadelphia, WB Saunders, 1995:1326
2. Meyers S, Hamilton SR, Morson BC, et al: Crohn's disease. In: Berk JE (ed). *Bockus Gastroenterology*, ed 5. Philadelphia, WB Saunders, 1995:1398
3. Kornbluth A, Salomon P, Sachar DB: Crohn's disease. In: Sleisinger MH, Fordtran JS (eds). *Gastrointestinal Disease: Pathophysiology, Diagnosis, Management*, ed 5. Philadelphia, WB Saunders, 1993:1270
4. Jewell DP: Ulcerative colitis. In: Sleisinger MH, Fordtran JS

(eds). *Gastrointestinal Disease: Pathophysiology, Diagnosis, Management*, ed 5. Philadelphia, WB Saunders, 1993:1305

5. Targan SR, Shanahan F (eds): *Inflammatory Bowel Disease: From Bench to Bedside*. Baltimore, Williams & Wilkins, 1994

6. Smith JN, Winship DH: Complications and extraintestinal problems in inflammatory bowel disease. *Med Clin North Am* 1980;64:1161

7. Present DH: Gastrointestinal emergencies: toxic megacolon. *Med Clin North Am* 1993;77:1129

8. Binderow SR, Wexner SD: Current surgical therapy for mucosal ulcerative colitis. *Dis Colon Rectum* 1994;37:610

9. Beaugerie L, Ngo Y, Goujard F, et al: Etiology and management of toxic megacolon in patients with human immunodeficiency virus infection. *Gastroenterology* 1994;107:858

10. Kobayasi S, Mendes EF, Rodriguez MA, et al: Toxic dilatation of the colon in Chagas' disease. *Br J Surg* 1992;79:1202

11. de Gara CJ, Gagic N, Arnold A, et al: Toxic megacolon associated with anticancer chemotherapy. *Can J Surg* 1991;34:339

12. Lichtiger S, Present DH: Preliminary report: cyclosporine in treatment of severe active ulcerative colitis. *Lancet* 1990;336:16

13. Lichtiger S, Present DH, Kornbluth A, et al: Cyclosporine in severe ulcerative colitis refractory to steroid therapy. *N Engl J Med* 1994;330:1841

14. Truelove SC, Marks SG: Toxic megacolon. *Clin Gastroenterol* 1981;10:107

15. Present DH: Ulcerative colitis. In: Bayless TM (ed). *Current Therapy in Gastroenterology and Liver Disease*, ed 4. St Louis, CV Mosby, 1994:387

16. Danovitch SH: Fulminant colitis and toxic megacolon. *Gastroenterol Clin North Am* 1989;18:73

17. Ott DJ, Chen MY: Specific acute colonic disorders. *Radiol Clin North Am* 1994;32:871

18. Caroline DF, Friedman AC: The radiology of inflammatory bowel disease. *Med Clin North Am* 1994;78:1353

19. Cassidy D, Boyd WP Jr: Toxic megacolon. In: Nord HJ, Brady PG (eds). *Critical Care Gastroenterology*. New York, Churchill Livingstone, 1982:317

20. Kramer P, Wittenburg J: Colonic gas distribution in toxic megacolon. *Gastroenterology* 1981;80:433

21. Perkel MS: Acute inflammatory bowel disease. *Crit Care Q* 1982;5:21

Critical Care, Third Edition, edited by Joseph M. Civetta,
Robert W. Taylor, and Robert R. Kirby.
Lippincott-Raven Publishers, Philadelphia, PA © 1997.

CHAPTER 142

■

Esophageal Disorders

Jack A. DiPalma

IMMEDIATE CONCERNS ■

A variety of esophageal disorders may require intensive care
or may develop in the critically ill. This chapter briefly reviews some of these disorders with attention to those that
require emergency evaluation and treatment. As a rule,
esophageal disorders become emergent when the airway is
compromised either by the initial insult or by a high risk of
aspiration. Protection of the airway is of major importance.
Disorders of the esophagus that require emergency evaluation and treatment include obstruction, foreign bodies, corrosive injury, perforation, trauma, esophagitis in the immunocompromised host, medication injury, and bleeding.
Esophageal bleeding, reviewed in Chapter 138, is usually
dramatic; however, the other disorders may have subtle presentations and the patient, at first glance, may not appear
very ill.

STRESS POINTS

1. Protection of the airway from aspiration
2. Consideration of aspiration and secondary pulmonary
   insult occurring *before* presentation
3. Elimination of ongoing damage (as in the case of
   corrosives)
4. Avoidance of long-term complications by careful initial management

ESOPHAGEAL OBSTRUCTION ■

CAPSULE

It is not unusual for patients to present with sudden onset
of the inability to swallow food, liquids, or saliva. Most are not
critically ill, but life-threatening complications may develop.
Occasionally, they may be orthostatic or dehydrated or may
have aspirated gastrointestinal (GI) contents. The goal of
management is to relieve the obstruction and to prevent
potential complications such as aspiration, bleeding, or
esophageal perforation. Most authors recommend immediate esophagoscopy to confirm the suspicion of obstruction
and the use of endoscopic techniques to remove the impacted bolus or foreign body. Several nonendoscopic removal techniques and pharmacologic interventions are used
as alternative approaches, particularly when endoscopy is not
available or is considered risky. After obstruction is relieved,
subsequent management is directed at evaluation of underlying esophageal pathology.

PRESENTATION

Most patients with food impaction and esophageal obstruction present with acute onset of dysphagia and complete
inability to swallow food or liquids, even their own saliva.
It is not unusual for these persons to delay presentation for
24 to 96 hours and have resultant dehydration or orthostasis.
Pulmonary aspiration of esophageal contents may occur before they seek treatment. Some may have experienced minor, transient episodes in the past and expected this prolonged event to resolve similarly. Typically, symptoms are
temporarily related to swallowing a poorly chewed food bolus, usually meat. The descriptive names "steakhouse syndrome" or "backyard barbecue syndrome," therefore, have
been applied.[1] Many patients admit concurrent alcohol use
or inebriation. Steakhouse syndrome is more common in
older persons who may be edentulous or have poorly fitting
dentures. Chest pain, odynophagia, hypersalivation, retching, and vomiting are associated complaints.

Physical examination should determine the consequences
of fluid or electrolyte depletion or pulmonary aspiration.

2071

DIAGNOSTIC APPROACH

Immediate esophagoscopy is the current approach recommended for diagnostic evaluation and treatment. It may be necessary to lavage the obstructed esophagus before the procedure, particularly if long delays occurred before the patient appeared for care. Esophagoscopy with flexible fiberoptic instruments is safe and rapid in the hands of experienced endoscopists. Most patients tolerate endoscopy well. It is probably the most acceptable approach to food impaction, allowing rapid confirmation of the esophageal obstruction, treatment and, in most cases, evaluation for underlying esophageal pathology. Barium contrast radiographs can also be used to confirm obstruction and define the nature or location of the impaction. Figure 142-1 shows an esophagram with esophageal obstruction and impacted food bolus in the distal esophagus seen as a large filling defect. Contrast studies are neither necessary or desirable because the presence of barium in the esophagus complicates removal of the bolus by compromising endoscopic visualization.[2] Meglumine diatrizoate (Gastrografin) is avoided because it is hypertonic and results in severe pneumonitis if aspirated. If contrast radiographs are performed, an attempt should be made to carefully aspirate residual loose food, fluids, and barium before endoscopy. In cases where perforation is a concern, water-soluble contrast media may be used.

MANAGEMENT

Therapeutic options are endoscopic bolus retrieval, pharmacologic interventions to relieve obstruction, and nonendoscopic retrieval techniques. We prefer endoscopic management.

Endoscopy allows relief of bolus impaction to be attempted under direct visual guidance. The bolus can be retrieved and extracted using endoscopy forceps, graspers, or polyp retrieval devices. The bolus can also be desiccated by visually guided catheter lavage or broken up with enzyme-containing lavage solutions. The bezoar should not, however, be forced into the stomach until the nature of any underlying esophageal lesion is known.

Several alternatives to the endoscopic approach can be tried when a competent endoscopist is not available or when the planned endoscopic procedure and necessary sedation pose an unacceptable risk to the patient. The traditional approach has been to confirm impaction and obstruction with a barium sulfate contrast radiograph. Occasionally, the weight of the barium column above the impaction may relieve the obstruction. If the impaction is persistent, hormonal relaxation using 1 mg glucagon or 0.4 mg atropine intravenously given slowly may be tried.[3] Sublingual nitroglycerin and oral hydralazine have been used as smooth muscle relaxants. The calcium channel blocker, nifedipine, has been suggested for esophageal spasm and obstruction. Nifedipine in doses of 20 mg given orally or buccally dramatically decreases distal esophageal and lower sphincter pressures in normal volunteers. In patients with achalasia, sphincter pressures after 20 mg nifedipine may be reduced more than 60%. These reductions are similar to those seen in patients

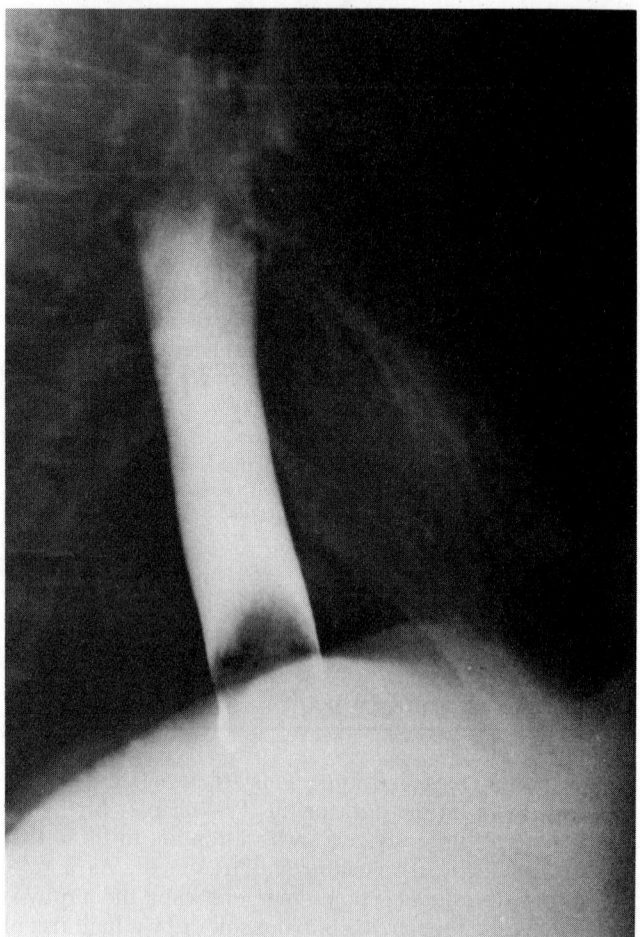

FIGURE 142-1. Barium esophagram shows food bolus impaction obstructing the distal esophagus.

who undergo surgical cardiomyotomy. We have had varying success using nifedipine for the food-obstructed esophagus. Doses of 20 mg of nifedipine are necessary because in the distal esophagus the pharmacologic effect of the commonly used 10-mg dose is minimal. Caution is advised when nifedipine doses of 20 mg or more are used, because blood pressure may be reduced and should be monitored carefully. Experience with other calcium blockers is limited.

Enzymatic therapy using papain or meat tenderizers has long been used in attempts to dissolve the food bolus.[4] Such approaches are time-consuming and specifically not advised in patients who have had obstruction for more than 24 hours. Patients with prolonged obstruction have some element of esophageal ischemia, and dissolution enzymes pose a risk in this situation.

Nonendoscopic procedures for food bolus removal have involved tubes for suction or retrieval with radiographically guided graspers or balloons to pull out the bolus. We have removed a food bolus using a 34F large-bore tube modified by cutting off the distal 8 to 9 cm with the side holes and making sure that the cut end is smooth.[5] The patient's hypopharynx is anesthetized with lidocaine spray or gargle. We then put the patient in a left lateral decubitus position and pass the tube through the mouth to the level of the bolus. The procedure is guided by fluoroscopy, if available. Suction is applied using the 120-mL lavage syringe supplied in the tube kit. The food bolus is partially aspirated into the end of the large-bore tube and carefully extracted. Special caution is advised because the bolus could potentially be dropped while passing through the hypopharynx, posing a risk of tracheal aspiration and obstruction. This suction technique should be attempted only by personnel experienced in gastrointestinal tube placement and airway management.

SPECIAL CONSIDERATIONS FOR SUBSEQUENT MANAGEMENT AND "STEAKHOUSE SPASM"

Most authors have approached steakhouse syndrome and esophageal obstruction as disorders in which a food bolus impacts in or above a preexisting esophageal lesion. Reported lesions include neoplastic, peptic, or caustic strictures, webs, distal rings, and vascular anomalies. However, we reported data on several patients with food impaction and complete obstruction for 72 to 96 hours who had no underlying anatomic lesions.[6] Subsequent endoscopy and barium radiographs were normal, but esophageal motility disorders were defined by esophageal manometry. A careful review of previous literature revealed that the majority of reported cases of steakhouse syndrome had no anatomic explanation for obstruction, and we call this variant "steakhouse spasm" to emphasize the spastic nature of the obstruction. Before endoscopic bolus retrieval is attempted in these patients, we recommend correcting the fluid and electrolyte imbalance and using 20 mg buccal or sublingual nifedipine.

FOREIGN BODIES ▪

CAPSULE

Foreign bodies other than meat bolus are a common cause of esophageal injury. Endoscopic removal is the preferred management. Special attention should be made to protect the airway.

PRESENTATION

It has been reported that over 1500 people die yearly because of foreign body ingestions.[2,7] In this condition, the flexible fiberoptic endoscope has had a significant impact on management. Commonly ingested items include coins, batteries, sharp and pointed objects, and cocaine packets. As previously discussed, food impaction is probably the most common upper GI foreign body that requires medical management. Over 75% of foreign body obstructions occurs in pediatric patients.[7] Children more often ingest coins and toys, whereas adults have problems with meat and bones. Prisoners and psychiatric patients have been known to ingest multiple and unusual objects.[2]

MANAGEMENT

Most objects pass spontaneously, but approximately 10% to 20% need to be removed endoscopically, and about 1% may require surgery.[7]

The preferred management for most foreign body obstructions of the upper GI tract is removal with a flexible endoscope. As a rule, pushing agents into the stomach is not recommended. An overtube or some other protective device is recommended to protect the upper GI mucosa from damage or perforation from sharp or pointed foreign bodies, particularly razor blades.[8] Although less than 1% of foreign bodies may perforate the gut, all sharp and pointed objects should be removed before they pass the stomach in an attempt to avoid distal intestinal perforation. Batteries, particularly the new small button battery type, may cause caustic mucosal injury. In the esophagus, esophagoaortic fistula has been reported. Batteries that reach the stomach do not pose as serious a risk to mucosal damage because of the acid milieu. Batteries in the stomach may be followed radiographically with endoscopic removal if symptoms develop or if the battery remains in the stomach for more than 36 to 48 hours. After the object is beyond the reach of the upper endoscope, it usually passes without difficulty. If it fails to progress or if the patient becomes symptomatic, surgical intervention may be necessary. In recent years, drugs (most commonly cocaine) have been swallowed in packet form for transport or other reasons for concealment. Endoscopy is not recommended in these conditions because of the risk of packet rupture. Surgery is the safest way to remove these agents.

Foreign bodies lodged in the hypopharynx or proximal esophagus may require rigid esophagoscopy. Most other objects are amenable to removal with a flexible endoscope. It must be emphasized that the airway should be protected because of the risk of dropping and aspirating the object as it passes the hypopharynx. When there is any doubt or risk, tracheal intubation or rigid esophagoscopy with general anesthesia can be used.

CORROSIVE INJURY ▪

CAPSULE

When presented with a patient who has ingested a caustic substance, immediate attention is focused on the overall condition, presence of systemic complications, status of oropharynx and airway, nature of the offending agent, and extent of injury.[9,10] If the victim is seen within 1 hour of ingestion, neutralization of alkali with water or dilute vinegar, and neutralization of acids with milk or antacids can be tried. Emetics are contraindicated. If 1 hour has lapsed from ingestion of the substance, the patient should be kept NPO (nothing by mouth) and vigorously hydrated intravenously. The oropharynx should be examined carefully and radiographs of the chest and abdomen obtained. The extent and severity of damage should be assessed early using fiberoptic endoscopy. The value of antibiotics or steroid therapy is controversial, but antibiotics should be used for suspected aspiration or perforation and steroids for laryngeal edema. After initial stabilization, the goals of management are to observe the patient for complications such as infection or perforation and to prevent late sequelae of stricture formation.

PRESENTATION

The clinical presentation of a patient with corrosive injury is dependent on the type (alkali or acid) and nature (solid or liquid) of the caustic substance.[11] Liquid alkali is swallowed rapidly, causing less oropharyngeal injury but extensive damage to the esophagus and stomach. Solid alkali causes severe burns to the oropharynx and induces severe pain and expectoration such that little corrosive is actually swallowed. Acid ingestion injury is more localized to the gastric antrum, but systemic acidosis and toxicity have been reported. Thus, mouth pain, hoarseness, dysphagia, odynophagia, or abdominal pain can occur as determined by the agent ingested and location of the injury. Stridor, aphonia, dyspnea, and hoarseness suggest laryngeal edema. Substernal, abdominal, or back pain raises concern for mediastinitis or peritonitis.

Physical examination of the lips, mouth, and pharynx can reveal a spectrum of injuries from mild erythema to erosions, ulcers, and obvious severe burns. Some authors have graded the injury by the presence and severity of oropharyngeal findings at the time of admission. It is often possible to estimate the degree of esophageal injury from the state of the oropharynx and type of agent ingested, but esophageal damage has been seen in patients without oropharyngeal burns.

DIAGNOSTIC APPROACH

After the history and physical examination have been obtained, with particular attention devoted to the oropharyngeal and airway status, laboratory evaluation is directed at determining complications of the ingestion such as renal or hepatic insufficiency or anemia. Chest and abdominal radiographs should be performed to look for evidence of aspiration, visceral perforation, or mediastinal air. After the patient has been stabilized, the extent and severity of disease can be evaluated by fiberoptic endoscopy. When endoscopy was initially introduced as a diagnostic procedure for evaluating caustic ingestions, concern was raised about the risk of perforation. Authors opposed using early endoscopy or recommended not passing the endoscope beyond the first burned area. Recent work suggests that endoscopy can be safely performed early in the course and provides information about severity and extent of damage that may influence management.[10] When possible, a complete endoscopic examination evaluating the esophagus, stomach, and duodenum should be accomplished.

Radiographic examination can be helpful, particularly when endoscopy is not available or is dangerous because of suspected perforation. In these situations, water-soluble contrast agents should be used.

COMPLICATIONS

Chemical injury to the gastrointestinal tract and resultant complications depend on the nature of the agent, the quantity and concentration of the agent, and the contact time duration. Liquid alkali such as Liquid Plumbr was a 20% sodium hydroxide solution when introduced in the late 1960s and was subsequently reduced to a 5% solution after being implicated in 20% of reported caustic ingestions. Liquid alkalis have a high specific gravity and pass rapidly through the esophagus to the stomach. In dogs, violent regurgitation of gastric contents and pyloric and cricopharyngeal spasm cause a "seesaw" action that prolongs contact time. Solid alkali is usually in crystal form and causes severe pain that limits further ingestion. Crystals adhere to mucous membranes of mouth, pharynx, and upper esophagus, causing predominantly proximal burns. Alkali produces injury by liquefaction necrosis. This type of injury enhances alkali penetration and prevents surface neutralization that results in full-thickness burns.

Concentrated acids produce a coagulative necrosis that forms eschar, which, with the coagulum, limits penetration to deeper muscular coats. Surface sloughing and perforation are therefore common problems. Late complications relate to location and extent of injury. Gastric injury may result in pyloric obstruction, antral stenosis, or "hourglass" deformity. Esophageal stricture may be proximal or distal and despite careful management develops in 10% to 20% of patients with caustic ingestion. In these patients, esophageal cancer has an estimated incidence of 2% to 4%, with a 1000-fold increase over normal persons more than 20 years after the caustic burn.

In attempts to avoid cicatricial esophageal stenosis, several interventions have been tried with controversial results. Traditional approaches have used antibiotics, steroids, and early "prophylactic" dilations, but these cannot be supported by any well-controlled studies. Corticosteroids, in particular, have been shown not to be of benefit in treating children who have ingested caustic substances.[12] Total parenteral nutrition, agents that impair collagen synthesis, penicillamine, and intraluminal splinting with large-bore Silastic tubes or nasogastric tubes have also been used, but the role of these techniques in stricture prevention remains unclear.

MANAGEMENT

Initial efforts are directed toward stabilizing the patient and replacing fluids and blood as appropriate.[13] The need for careful assessment of the airway cannot be overemphasized. Translaryngeal intubation or tracheostomy may be necessary. Evidence of esophageal perforation requires early surgical intervention. The corrosive should be neutralized only when the patient is seen within 1 hour of ingestion. Milk or antacids are used for acid ingestions and water or vinegar for alkali ingestions. Nasogastric intubation should be avoided unless the tube is placed under direct vision.

Early endoscopy is used when feasible. Complete examination of the esophagus, stomach, and duodenum should be attempted. If no significant injury is found, the patient can be discharged. In patients with significant injury, hospitalization and careful management are necessary. The use of steroids or antibiotics is not routinely advocated. Broad-spectrum antibiotic coverage is used for signs of aspiration, infection, or suspected perforation, or it may be used when deep ulcers are present and perforation seems imminent. Laryngeal edema is treated with short courses of high-dose steroids. Early bougienage using mercury-weighted rubber (Maloney) or polyvinyl dilators can be used in an attempt to prevent strictures and is usually started 2 to 3 weeks after the ingestion. Patients are kept NPO until they can swallow their saliva. Then clear liquids are allowed, advancing the diet thereafter as tolerated. Parenteral nutrition should be started early after stabilization.

It must be remembered that corrosive injuries are often severe, causing full-thickness mucosal destruction and perforation. The patients must be carefully observed for the need of surgical intervention.[14]

ESOPHAGEAL PERFORATION ■

CAPSULE

Esophageal perforation is a catastrophic event that is uniformly fatal if left untreated. Despite improved understanding, potent antibiotics, and advances in surgical technique, the mortality remains at 15% to 20%. Identified poor prognostic factors are delayed treatment, severe underlying esophageal disease, the need for major extirpative procedures, and thoracic location of perforation. Early recognition and prompt diagnosis are essential because treatment delays greater than 12 hours are associated with increased mortality. Plain radiographs are valuable and suggestive of perforation in 90% of cases. Contrast radiographs using barium sulfate or water-soluble contrast agents provide pertinent information about the site and extent of perforation. Management includes broad-spectrum antibiotics, NPO status, intravenous hydration, nasogastric suction, and parenteral nutrition. Definitive treatment is usually surgical, but there is a place for conservative, nonoperative management of small, contained, instrumental injuries or pharyngeal perforations.

PRESENTATION

Esophageal perforations may be iatrogenic or noniatrogenic. Iatrogenic causes occur as complications of instrumentation such as esophagoscopy, attempts at endotracheal intubation or obturator airway placement, or esophageal tubes or stents. Dilatation procedures and surgical misadventures or leaks also lead to perforation of the esophagus. Noniatrogenic etiologies are usually barogenic ruptures. The most well-known "spontaneous" rupture occurred in the gluttonous Dutch admiral Baron Van Wassanaer. The admiral gorged himself and induced forceful vomiting for relief. His autopsy by Hermann Boerhaave was published in 1724 and described the pathologic findings of barogenic esophageal rupture. Resultant signs and symptoms are similar for Boerhaave syndrome and iatrogenic perforations. Pain is a near-universal experience, and 30% of patients develop acute pain. Fever and leukocytosis are also common.

Other presentations are influenced by the site of perforation. Patients with abdominal esophageal segment tears have had retroperitoneal air and vague epigastric pain. Patients with thoracic perforations often complain of abdominal and back pain. Cervical perforations are associated with subcutaneous emphysema and chest pain. Symptoms that occur during or shortly after an esophageal procedure should raise concern for iatrogenic perforations. Other clinical findings in patients with esophageal tears include pleural effusion, pneumothorax, dysphagia, cervical crepitus, hematemesis, and shock. However, asymptomatic perforations have been demonstrated radiographically, which emphasizes the importance of an accurate history and a high index of suspicion.

DIAGNOSTIC APPROACH

The diagnosis of esophageal perforation may be fairly obvious, particularly in the iatrogenic group. Plain chest radiographs may suggest perforation in over 90% of patients (Fig. 142-2).[15] Findings include mediastinal air, pneumothorax, pleural effusion, infiltrate, or subcutaneous emphysema. Hyperextended neck films can reveal widened spaces, air, or esophageal displacement. Fears of barium mediastinitis have

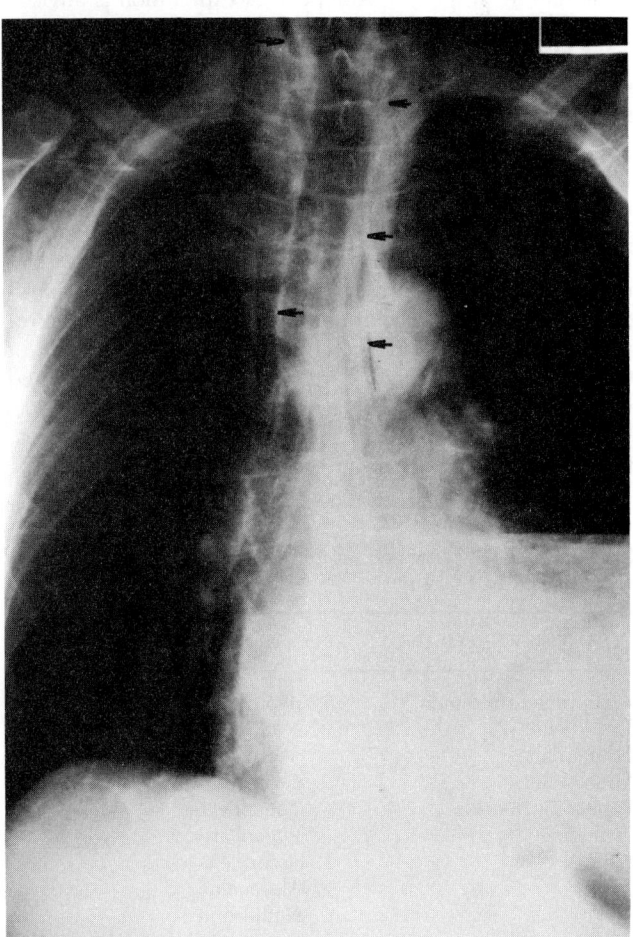

FIGURE 142-2. Chest radiograph in Boerhaave's syndrome. Note left pleural effusion, esophageal deviation, and presence of mediastinal and subcutaneous air (*arrows*).

traditionally led to the use of water-soluble contrast media.[16] Recent reports indicate that iodinated water-soluble contrast radiographs may be normal in 20% to 25% of thoracic and 50% of cervical perforations.[15] Therefore, negative or equivocal findings on water-soluble studies should be immediately reexamined with barium sulfate contrast radiographs. Other authors believe that barium does not potentiate mediastinal inflammation. Because it is more palatable than water-soluble agents and less dangerous if aspirated into the bronchial tree, many use dilute barium in the initial examination to take advantage of its better coating and definition. Regardless of the agent used, it is important to examine the entire esophagus in multiple positions.

MANAGEMENT

Early diagnosis of esophageal perforation is essential for successful management. Intravenous access should be obtained and intravenous hydration initiated. The patient is placed NPO, and high-dose, broad-spectrum antibiotic therapy is started. Nasogastric suction and parenteral nutrition are used. Some authors recommend treating small instrumental tears or pharyngeal perforations nonoperatively, but most large instrument tears, trauma, or spontaneous perforations require surgery.[17] Prompt neck exploration is advised for large cervical perforations. Absolute indications for operative intervention are sepsis, shock, respiratory failure, pneumothorax, pneumoperitoneum, and mediastinal emphysema. Most thoracic surgeons advise exploration with primary repair and drainage as the procedure of choice.[18]

SPECIAL CONSIDERATIONS

The development of small-bore fiberoptic endoscopy techniques has dramatically decreased the incidence of iatrogenic instrumental perforation from esophagoscopy.[17] Previously used rigid esophagoscopy had a perforation rate of 0.2% to 1.9%. Perforation during esophagoscopy performed with modern flexible fiberscopes is approximately .01%. However, current palliative therapy for esophageal and gastric cardia neoplasms may have perforation rates above 10%.

TABLE 142-1.   Drugs Implicated in Drug-Induced Esophageal Mucosal Injury

COMMONLY REPORTED	MISCELLANEOUS DRUGS
Emepronium bromide	Aspirin
Doxycycline	Nonsteroidal antiinflammatory
Tetracycline	drugs
Minocycline	Cromolyn
Potassium chloride	Theophylline
Quinidine	Phenobarbital
	Ascorbic acid
	Alprenolol
	Naftidrofury
	Ferrous sulfate
	Clindamycin
	Lincomycin

Aggressive therapeutic endoscopy techniques use laser photocoagulation and bipolar electrocoagulation, dilatation, or intubation with prosthetic stents. One report of 34 perforations occurring after palliative intubation notes favorable experience with nonsurgical management, particularly for pharyngeal tears, and advocates conservative management.[19]

Before World War II, traumatic external injury to the esophagus was uncommonly reported.[20] In an approach similar to that for spontaneous or instrumental perforations to the esophagus, early detection and prompt surgical exploration is emphasized. It must be remembered that with esophageal injury both esophagoscopy and the radiographic esophagram can give false-negative results.[20] Both studies have been recommended as a preoperative evaluation for ideal management in a patient in stable condition.

MEDICATION INJURY ■

CAPSULE

In the critical care unit, we cannot ignore esophageal injury from prescribed medications.

PRESENTATION

Accidental or suicidal injury with caustic agents has been previously discussed, but typical therapeutic doses of commonly used medications can cause significant esophageal injury. Patients predisposed to injury are those who are supine and who do not receive concurrent ingestion of adequate amounts of fluids. Such patients are frequent residents of the critical care unit. The American College of Gastroenterology (ACG) Committee on Food and Drug Administration (FDA)-related matters published a review of 127 cases of drug induced esophagitis in 1987.[21] Eighty-nine percent of the cases were related to quinidine, potassium chloride, emepronium bromide, and tetracycline and its derivatives. The remaining 11% were caused by 14 other medications. Serious sequelae, including death, were linked to esophageal injury from medications, particularly those that may be potassium induced.

In the ACG report, the most common presenting symptoms of medication injury were retrosternal pain, odynophagia, and dysphagia. Retrosternal pain was seen in 61%, odynophagia in 50%, and dysphagia in 40%. Hematemesis and low-grade fever occurred, and complete aphagia with the inability to swallow oral secretions was not uncommon. Medication injury should be suspected in critically ill patients with unexplained esophageal symptoms. The diagnosis can be offered and made by clinical history alone, but radiographic or endoscopic diagnostic studies can add additional information concerning the nature of the injury.

Drugs implicated in medication esophageal injury are outlined in Table 142-1. Emepronium bromide is a quaternary ammonium anticholinergic agent with a peripheral effect similar to that of atropine. It is used predominantly in Great Britain for women with urinary frequency and urgency in an attempt to reduce muscular tone of the urinary bladder. Tetracycline, doxycycline, and minocycline are also frequent offenders. Sustained-release potassium chloride preparations were involved in 18 of the 127 cases of drug induced esophagitis reported by the ACG. Potassium chloride solution and nonenteric preparations of potassium chloride are also reported to cause esophageal injury. A common area for esophageal stricture from these agents is at the level of the compression of the esophagus by the aortic arch or left antrum. In the group of patients reported, six deaths were related to potassium esophageal injury. Two patients developed fistulas from the esophagus to the aorta or left antrum. One patient had perforation to the mediastinum and died from sepsis. Another patient died from a bleeding esophageal ulcer. Quinidine is also a commonly reported agent of esophageal mucosal injury. In some of the reported cases, the patients were also taking medications that may have contributed to the injury, and some patients had underlying esophageal obstruction disease.

MANAGEMENT

Most cases of medication esophageal injury resolve without sequelae when the medication is discontinued. Liquid preparations may be substituted when it is not possible to discontinue the offending medication. Antacids, H_2 receptor antagonists, and cytoprotective agents can be given. Severe odynophagia may be treated with a topical anesthetic agent. Esophageal stricture may be treated with bougienage.

In the critical care unit, prevention of esophageal injury is the best approach to the problem. If possible, patients should have the head of the bed elevated during oral medication administration with sufficient quantities of water given afterward. Certain medicines should be used with caution in patients with cardiomegaly or in those who are elderly or have known or suspected underlying esophageal obstruction. Oral potassium should be avoided in critically ill patients.

REFERENCES ■

1. Palmer ED: Backyard barbecue syndrome: steak impaction in the esophagus. *JAMA* 1976;125:277
2. Brady PG: Management of esophageal and gastric foreign bodies. A/S/G/E Clinical Update 1994;2:1
3. Ferrucci JT, Long JA: Radiologic treatment of foreign food impaction using intravenous glucagon. *Radiology* 1977;135:25
4. Goldner F, Danley D: Enzymatic digestion of esophageal meat impaction—a study of Adolph's Meat Tenderizer. *Dig Dis Sci* 1985;30:456
5. Kozarek RA, Sanowski RA: Esophageal food impaction: description of a new method for bolus removal. *Dig Dis Sci* 1980;25:100
6. DiPalma JA, Brady CE III: Steakhouse spasm. *J Clin Gastroenterol* 1987;9:274
7. Webb WA: Management of foreign bodies in the upper gastrointestinal tract. *Gastroenterology* 1988;94:204
8. Marcon NE: Overtubes and foreign bodies. *Can J Gastroenterol* 1990;4:599
9. Goldman LP, Weigert JM: Corrosive substance ingestion: a review. *Am J Gastroenterol* 1984;79:85
10. Zargar SA, Kochhar R, Nagi B, et al: Ingestion of strong corrosive alkalis: spectrum of injury to upper gastrointestinal tract and natural history. *Am J Gastroenterol* 1992;87:337
11. Oakes DD, Sherck JP, Mark JBD: Lye ingestion—clinical patterns and therapeutic implications. *J Thorac Cardiovasc Surg* 1982;83:194
12. Anderson KD, Rouse TM, Randolph JG: A controlled trial of corticosteroids in children with corrosive injury of the esophagus. *N Engl J Med* 1990;323:637
13. Tucker JA, Yarington CT: The treatment of caustic ingestion. *Otolaryngol Clin North Am* 1979;12:343
14. DiCostanzo J, Noirclerc M, Jouglard J, et al: New therapeutic approach to corrosive burns of the upper gastrointestinal tract. *Gut* 1980;21:370
15. Phillips LG, Cunningham J: Esophageal perforation. *Radiol Clin North Am* 1984;22:607
16. Foley MJ, Ghahremani GG, Rogers LF: Reappraisal of contrast media used to detect upper gastrointestinal perforations—comparison of Jonic water-soluble media with barium sulfate. *Radiology* 1982;144:231
17. Beck DE, DiPalma JA: Complications of gastrointestinal procedures. In: DiPalma JA (ed). *Problems in Critical Care: Gastrointestinal Complications*. Philadelphia, JB Lippincott 1989: 361
18. Richardson JD, Martin LF, Borzotta AP, et al: Unifying concepts in treatment of esophageal leaks. *Am J Surg* 1985;149: 157
19. Hine KR, Atkinson M: The diagnosis and management of perforations of esophagus and pharynx sustained during intubation of neoplastic esophageal strictures. *Dig Dis Sci* 1986; 31:571
20. Cheadle W, Richardson JD: Options in management of trauma of the esophagus. *Surg Gynecol Obstet* 1982;155:380
21. Bott S, Prakasah C, McCallum RW, et al: Medication-esophageal injury: survey of the literature. *Am J Gastroenterol* 1987; 82:758

Renal and Endocrine Disease and Dysfunction

Critical Care, Third Edition, edited by Joseph M. Civetta,
Robert W. Taylor, and Robert R. Kirby.
Lippincott-Raven Publishers, Philadelphia, PA © 1997.

CHAPTER 143

■

Acute Renal Failure

Richard S. Muther

IMMEDIATE CONCERNS ■

MAJOR PROBLEMS

1. Acute renal failure (ARF) is usually defined as an abrupt decrease in glomerular filtration rate (GFR) caused by intrinsic renal parenchymal disease or alterations in intrarenal hemodynamics resulting in the accumulation of waste products (e.g., urea, creatinine, potassium) in the blood.
2. Decreased renal perfusion (prerenal azotemia) or obstruction of urine flow (postrenal azotemia) are reversible causes of acute azotemia, and excluding each is a prerequisite to the diagnosis of ARF.

STRESS POINTS

1. Although oliguria may have prognostic implications in ARF,[1] it is not a requirement for diagnosis. In fact, urine output may range from total anuria to polyuria in patients with ARF.
2. Several factors help distinguish acute from chronic azotemia (Table 143-1). These include patient symptoms and history, renal size, hematocrit, serum albumin, and the daily change of serum creatinine.

ESSENTIAL DIAGNOSTIC TESTS AND PROCEDURES

1. The immediate diagnostic and therapeutic steps in patients with acute azotemia are outlined in Table 143-2. Details of this evaluation follow in the section Differential Diagnosis.

2. Once prerenal, postrenal, and pseudorenal causes of acute azotemia are excluded, the clinician can approach the possibility of ARF using the diagnostic and therapeutic outline presented in Table 143-3.

DIFFERENTIAL DIAGNOSIS OF ACUTE AZOTEMIA ■

In addition to ARF, various factors may cause acute azotemia. *Pseudorenal failure* refers to azotemia not related to a decrease in GFR (Table 143-4). For example, corticosteroids, gastrointestinal (GI) bleeding, or high protein intake may all increase blood urea nitrogen (BUN) by increasing the substrate for urea production. Serum creatinine can increase when muscle breakdown (rhabdomyolysis) causes creatine release, when drugs (cimetidine, trimethoprim) block renal tubular creatinine secretion, or when substances (cefoxitin, acetone, alpha-methyldopa) interfere with the creatinine assay.[2] Excepting rhabdomyolysis, which may easily double or triple serum creatinine, the rise in serum creatinine due to these artifacts approximates 20%. Spillage of urine into the peritoneal cavity (e.g., urinoma following trauma or surgery) may spuriously elevate both BUN and serum creatinine. The diagnosis of pseudorenal failure is primarily based on the history.

Prerenal azotemia (Table 143-5) results when renal perfusion is compromised by an absolute decrease in intravascular volume (hemorrhage, GI fluid losses, burns), a decrease in the effective circulating volume (heart failure, cirrhosis with ascites), or the sequestration of fluid in the third space (i.e., one not readily accessible to the vascular space). This latter phenomenon commonly complicates severe burns or abdominal catastrophes such as pancreatitis, bowel surgery,

TABLE 143-1. Acute Versus Chronic Azotemia

	ACUTE	CHRONIC
Renal size	Normal–large	Usually small°
Hematocrit	Usually normal	Decreased
Serum albumin	Usually normal	Decreased
Rate of creatinine rise	0.5–2.0 mg/dL/d	0–0.5 mg/dL/d
Previous history of renal disease	Negative	Positive

°Exceptions are diabetic nephropathy and infiltrative diseases (myeloma, lymphoma, amyloidosis.)

perforation, or ischemia. Rhabdomyolysis or localized soft tissue trauma may also cause third spacing.

In most series, prerenal azotemia is associated with a less than 10% in-hospital mortality. However, if unrecognized and untreated the hemodynamic compromise underlying prerenal azotemia can produce ARF, increasing mortality to 50% or greater. An aggressive approach to the diagnosis and correction of prerenal azotemia is therefore mandatory.

Prerenal azotemia is best diagnosed by physical examination of the patient and chemical analysis of the urine. Resting tachycardia, orthostatic hypotension, flat neck veins in the supine position, and dry mucous membranes suggest an absolute decrease in extracellular fluid volume (ECV). Alternatively, pulmonary rales, S_3 heart gallop, jugular venous distention, and edema suggest cardiac failure as a cause of prerenal azotemia. In other less obvious cases, determining the pulmonary artery occlusion pressure (PAOP) may be necessary.

The urinary diagnostic indices that differentiate ARF from prerenal azotemia are listed in Table 143-6. Because renal tubular cell integrity is maintained in patients with prerenal azotemia, the urine is very concentrated (specific gravity >1.020; Uosm >400 mOsm/L) and relatively devoid of sodium (U_{NA} <20 mEq/L) due to the appropriate reab-

sorption of water and sodium respectively. Patients with ARF lack the ability to conserve water or sodium and demonstrate isosthenuria (specific gravity = 1.012; Uosm = 300 mOsm/L) and urinary sodium wasting (U_{NA} >30 mEq/L).

In some circumstances, these parameters may fail to differentiate the patient with prerenal azotemia. A more specific test is the fractional excretion of sodium (FENA), which is the fraction of filtered sodium that is ultimately excreted by the nephron. The FENA measures the ratio of the sodium excreted (urinary NA × volume) to the sodium filtered (plasma NA × GFR) by the following formula:

$$FE_{NA} = \frac{U_{NA} \times V}{P_{NA} \times \dfrac{U_{Cr} \times V}{P_{Cr}}} \times 100\%$$

where U = urine, P = plasma, Cr = creatinine, and V = volume. Because the volumes cancel, the test can be done with spot sample of urine and blood.

Patients with a potent stimulus for sodium reabsorption (as in prerenal azotemia) should have low urinary sodium (<10 mEq/L) and FENA (<1%). In other words, the fractional reabsorption is greater than 99% of all filtered sodium. However, in patients with ARF, poor tubular function prevents sodium reabsorption, and the FENA is elevated (>1%). If used properly, this test can differentiate acute tubular necrosis from prerenal azotemia in more than 90% of cases.[3]

There are several exceptions to the reliability of the FENA. Any condition decreasing sodium reabsorption (e.g., chronic renal insufficiency, diuretics, glucosuria) can spuriously increase the FENA in patients with prerenal azotemia. Conditions enhancing tubular sodium reabsorption (e.g., severe congestive failure, cirrhosis with ascites) can spuriously lower the FENA in patients with established ARF.[4] Acute glomerulonephritis, intravenous contrast, rhabdomyolysis, and severe sepsis are also causes of ARF that can be associated with a low FENA, particularly early in the clinical course.[5] The clinician must be alert to these exceptions, prudent with fluid therapy, and frequently reevaluate the patient's ECV.

TABLE 143-2. Immediate Diagnostic and Therapeutic Steps for Patients With Acute Azotemia

STEP	DIAGNOSTIC TESTS	THERAPEUTIC OPTIONS
1. Exclude pseudorenal	History of GI bleed, hyperalimentation, certain drugs, ketosis? CK to exclude rhabdomyolysis	Treat bleed Stop offending agent, treat ketosis Expand ECV
2. Exclude postrenal	Foley catheterization Ultrasound (or CT) Retrograde pyelogram?	Foley catheterization Ureteral stent? Percutaneous nephrostomy?
3. Exclude prerenal:	FE_{NA} BUN:Cr ratio Urine NA, Urine Osm	
a. ECV depletion?	Physical exam (PEx)	Isotonic fluids
b. Heart failure?	PEx, chest radiograph, PAOP?	Inotropes, diuretics; dopamine?
c. Third space?	Soft tissue injury or trauma?	Isotonic fluids; colloid?

CK, Creatine kinase.

TABLE 143-3.   Approach to Diagnosis and Therapy for Acute Renal Failure

ETIOLOGY	DIAGNOSTIC TESTS	THERAPEUTIC OPTIONS
Step 1. Glomerular disease:	UA, sediment	Treat hypertension
Hemodynamic	Nitroprusside, nifedipine, NSAIDs, ACEI, sepsis, hepatorenal?	Stop drug; Dopamine?
Glomerulonephritis	ANA, C_3, C_4, ANCA, Anti-GBM antibody Biopsy	Specific therapy
Step 2. Interstitial disease	UA, sediment, Biopsy	
Allergic	Eosinophilia/uria?	Stop drug, Steroids
Infectious	Urine, blood cultures	Antibiotics?
Myeloma	Urine protein electrophoresis	Specific therapy.
Step 3. Vascular disease	UA, sediment	Treat hypertension.
Thrombosis–embolus	Atrial fib? WBC, LDH Renal scan. Angiogram	Anticoagulation. Surgery/angioplasty?
Atheroemboli	Eosinophilia? Livedo?	Stop angicoagulants.
Microangiopathy	Periph smear, bili, LDH, platelets	Plasmapheresis?
Vasculitis	?Systemic disease. ANCA. Biopsy	Specific therapy.
Step 4. Acute tubular necrosis		
Toxic	Aminoglycosides, contrast, Rhabdo, Platinum, Cyclosporine?	Stop offending agent.
Ischemic	Trauma, surgery, sepsis, shock?	Specific therapy. Volume expand. Vasopressors.

Prerenal azotemia is confirmed if the urinary output improves and the azotemia resolves with the administration of isotonic fluids or improvement in the underlying condition (e.g., heart failure).

Postrenal azotemia (Table 143-7) is also reversible as long as the obstruction is relatively recent (days to weeks) and the serum creatinine relatively low (<5 mg/dL). As in prerenal azotemia, failure to recognize and correct urinary obstruction early significantly worsens renal prognosis and patient mortality. Lower urinary tract obstruction can be effectively excluded and treated by placement of a Foley catheter. Renal ultrasonography can usually exclude hydronephrosis (Fig. 143-1), but computed tomography (CT) scanning should be performed if retroperitoneal disease is suspected. Retrograde pyelography is occasionally necessary, usually in patients with a solitary kidney. Chemical analysis of the urine cannot reliably exclude obstruction. Any obstruction must be promptly treated by mechanical drainage.

The causes of obstructive uropathy include disorders of the urethra (stricture, calculus, foreign body), prostate (hy-

TABLE 143-4.   Pseudorenal Failure: Nonrenal Factors Affecting Serum Urea and Creatinine

SUBSTANCE	INCREASED	DECREASED
Urea	Prerenal azotemia, upper GI bleeding, catabolic state, corticosteroids, hyperalimentation	Heaptocellular failure, low protein intake, water excess

Creatinine	Rhabdomyolysis
	Blocked secretion
	  Trimethoprim, cimetidine
	Chemical interference
	  Cefoxitin, ascorbic acid, acetone, alpha-methyldopa, 5-flucytosine
		Decreased muscle mass, hepatocellular failure

TABLE 143-5. Causes of Prerenal Azotemia

Decreased Extracellular Volume (ECV)
  Gastrointestinal losses
    Diarrhea
    Vomiting
    Fistula
  Renal losses
    Diuretics
    "Salt losing" nephropathy
    Hypoaldosteronism
  Burns
  Hemorrhage
Decreased Effective Circulating Volume
  Cardiac failure
  Cirrhosis–ascites
  Nephrotic syndrome
  Positive-pressure ventilation
Third-Spaced Volume
  Acute or postoperative abdomen
  Soft tissue trauma
  Hypoalbuminemia

TABLE 143-7. Causes of Postrenal Azotemia

Urethral
  Clot
  Stricture
  Stone
  Foreign Body
Prostatic
  Hypertrophy
  Carcinoma
  Clot
Bladder
  Tumor
  Neurogenic bladder
Ureter
  Tumor
  Clot
  Stone
  Stricture
  Retroperitoneal fibrosis
  Ligation

pertrophy, tumor), bladder (neurogenic, tumor) and ureter (calculus, tumor, sloughed papillae, ligation, or retroperitoneal disease).

Taken together, pseudorenal, prerenal, and postrenal factors account for 20% to 50% of hospital-acquired acute azotemia.[6] Once these are excluded, the clinician can focus attention on the possible intrarenal hemodynamic and parenchymal diseases that produce ARF.

DIFFERENTIAL DIAGNOSIS OF ACUTE RENAL FAILURE ■

Because there are four primary histologic structures in the kidney, ARF can conveniently be classified into disorders of the glomerulus (e.g., glomerulonephritis, alterations of intraglomerular hemodynamics), blood vessels (e.g., vasculitis), interstitium (e.g., interstitial nephritis), and tubules (e.g., acute tubular necrosis) (Table 143-8).

Fulminant *glomerulonephritis* (GN) due to bacterial endocarditis, systemic lupus erythematosus, foreign body asso-ciated staphylococcal septicemia, visceral abscesses, hepatitis B antigenemia, Goodpasture syndrome, or idiopathic rapidly progressive (crescentic) GN are not uncommon in a major ICU. Once considered, these diagnoses are not difficult to make. The urinalysis shows dysmorphic red cells with multiple surface irregularities (Fig. 143-2), red blood cell casts, and moderate to heavy proteinuria. Hypertension may or may not be present. Blood cultures; serologic testing including antineutrophilic cytoplasmic antibodies (ANCA), antinuclear autoantibodies (ANA), C3, C4, HBsAg, anti-GBM antibody; and a search for visceral abscess may be rewarding but an *early* renal biopsy is usually necessary when acute GN causes ARF.

TABLE 143-6. Diagnostic Indices Distinguishing Prerenal Azotemia From Acute Renal Failure

	PRERENAL	ARF
BUN:serum Cr ratio	20	10
Urine specific gravity	>1.020	1.010–1.015
Urine osmolarity (mOsm/L)	>350	300
Urine–plasma osmolarity	>1.5	1.0
Urine Na (mEq/L)	<20	>30
FE_{NA}	<1%	>1%

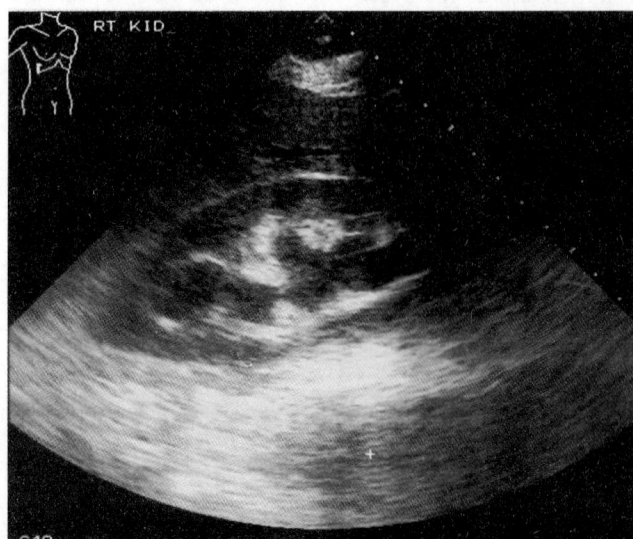

FIGURE 143-1. Renal ultrasound demonstrates acute obstructive uropathy in a patient with acute renal failure.

TABLE 143-8. Causes of Acute Renal Failure

GLOMERULAR DISEASE
  Glomerulonephritis
    Infectious (bacterial endocarditis, shunt nephritis, visceral
      abscess)
    Vasculitis (polyarteritis, Wegener granulomatosis,
      hypersensitivity)
    Systemic lupus erythematosis
    Goodpasture syndrome
    Idiopathic, rapidly progressive
  Hemodynamic changes
    Hepatorenal syndrome
    NSAIDs
    ACE inhibitors
    Nifedipine
    Nitroprusside
    Cytokines

INTERSTITIAL NEPHRITIS
  Allergic interstitial nephritis
    Antibiotics (penicillins, sulfonamides, cephalosporins)
    NSAIDs
    Diuretics
  Infections (bacterial, *Legionella*, viral)
  Immune (lupus, transplant rejection)
  Infiltrative (sarcoidosis, lymphoma)
  Tubular obstruction (uric acid, oxalate, myeloma)

VASCULAR DISEASE
  Hypertensive
  Atherosclerotic
    Thrombosis–thromboembolism
    Diffuse cholesterol microemboli
  Traumatic (avulsion, intimal flap)
  Renal vein (thrombosis, ligation)
  Microangiography (hemolytic uremic syndrome, thrombotic
    thrombocytopenia purpura)
  Vasculitis (polyarteritis, Wegener granulomatosis,
    hypersensitivity)

ACUTE TUBULAR NECROSIS (ATN)
  Toxic
    Drugs (aminoglycosides, cisplatin)
    Radiographic contrast agents
    Rhabdomyolysis–myoglobinuria (trauma, seizures, cocaine,
      lovastatin)
    Metals (Pb, Cd, Hg)
    Solvents (CCl$_4$, ethylene glycol, hydrocarbons)
  Ischemic
    Hemorrhage
    Hypotension–shock
    Sepsis
    Progressive prerenal azotemia

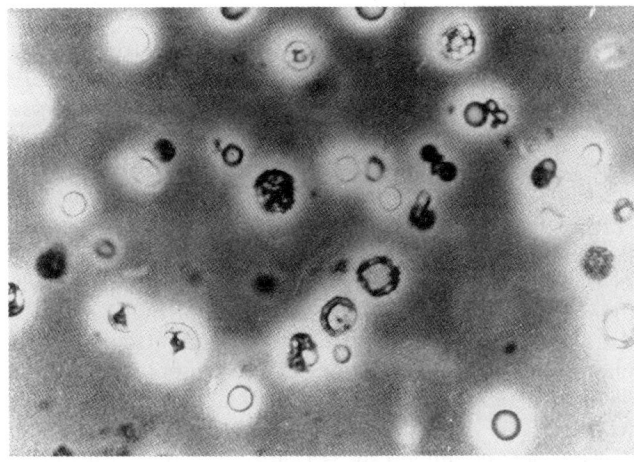

FIGURE 143-2. Dysmorphic changes of urinary erythrocytes indicate glomerular disease.

Alterations in *glomerular hemodynamics* are an increasingly recognized cause of ARF. These include the afferent arteriolar vasoconstriction due to the hepatorenal syndrome[7] or efferent arteriolar vasodilatation from angiotensin converting enzyme (ACE) inhibitors.[8] The latter is usually seen when renal blood flow is already compromised by severe cardiac failure[8] or renal artery stenosis.[9] In addition, less well defined derangements in intrarenal hemodynamics are likely responsible for the ARF of sepsis,[10] potent vasodilators such as nitroprusside[11] and nifedipine[12] and the nonsteroidal antiinflammatory drugs (NSAIDs).[13] In most of these cases, the ARF is functional. The urine sediment is usually bland and the renal biopsy (if performed) is normal. Recovery of renal function is expected provided the offending drug is removed or the underlying condition is corrected.

Acute *interstitial nephritis* is usually due to a drug allergy: penicillins, cephalosporins, sulfonamides, diuretics, and NSAIDs being the most common. Patients usually have fever, rash, arthralgias, and eosinophilia–eosinophiluria[14] (excepting NSAIDs). Other causes of ARF due to interstitial nephritis are rare but include bacterial pyelonephritis, myeloma kidney, acute uric acid nephropathy, tumor lysis syndrome, and occasionally infiltrative disorders such as lymphoma, leukemia, and sarcoidosis. Oxalate nephropathy may complicate ethylene glycol ingestion or methoxyflurane anesthesia. The urine sediment in these cases is usually bland, but crystalluria, pyuria, and white blood cell (WBC) casts can be seen, even in the absence of infection. Urine protein electrophoresis and immunoelectrophoresis usually demonstrates a monoclonal paraprotein if myeloma is responsible for ARF.

Vascular disease is frequently overlooked as a cause of ARF.[15] Nevertheless, malignant hypertension remains a common problem.[16] Retinopathy, thrombocytopenia, and microangiopathy of the peripheral blood smear usually accompany this syndrome. Microangiopathy and thrombocytopenia also occur when ARF is caused by hemolytic uremic syndrome or thrombotic thrombocytopenic purpura.[17] Renal infarction due to trauma (with intimal flap), arterial embolus, or thrombosis of a previously atherosclerotic vessel can cause ARF. Renal artery embolism is usually associated with intermittent atrial fibrillation. These patients usually have fever, hematuria, acute flank pain, ileus, leukocytosis and an elevated lactic dehydrogenase (LDH).[18] The syndrome sometimes mimics an acute abdomen and may persist for several days. Renal atherosclerotic or cholesterol microemboli com-

monly occur following aortic manipulation (surgery or catheterization) or systemic anticoagulation. Besides ARF, gastrointestinal bleeding (due to microinfarcts), livido reticularis
of the lower extremities, patchy areas of ischemic necrosis
in the toes, hypocomplementemia, and eosinophilia are common with atheromatous–cholesterol emboli.[19] Finally, renal
vasculitis (Wegener granulomatosis, polyarteritis nodosa
[PAN], hypersensitivity vasculitis, and Henoch-Schönlein
purpura) often causes ARF. These syndromes are identified
by their multisystem manifestations, very active urine sediment (hematuria, pyuria, red blood cell [RBC] and WBC
casts, proteinuria) and the presence of antineutrophilic cytoplasmic antibodies (ANCA), which are present in the serum
of most patients with Wegener granulomatosis and many
with PAN.[20]

The most common cause of hospital and ICU acquired
ARF remains *acute tubular necrosis* (ATN).[6] The diagnosis
of ATN is often made by default if glomerular, interstitial,
or vascular disease are not found. Nevertheless, renal tubular
epithelial cells and granular casts are typical features of the
urine sediment. Urine chemistries demonstrate inappropriate salt wasting (U$_{Na}$ >30 mEq/L; FE$_{Na}$ >1%) and isosthenuria (specific gravity = 1.012 ±; U$_{osm}$ = 300 mOsm/
L). The patient may be oliguric or nonoliguric.

ATN is broadly divided into toxic and ischemic etiologies.
The *aminoglycoside antibiotics* continue to be one of the
more common toxins causing ATN. Risk factors for aminoglycoside nephrotoxicity include volume contraction, age,
hypokalemia, concomitant use of other nephrotoxins, and a
short dosing interval.[21] After an initial loading dose (2 to 3
mg/kg), the maintenance dose (1 mg/kg) should be adjusted
based on the patient's creatinine clearance, estimated by
the formula: C$_{Cr}$ = body weight (kg) ÷ serum creatinine.
The routine use of peak and trough serum levels does not
decrease the likelihood of ATN.[22]

Radiographic contrast agents commonly cause ARF, particularly in patients with preexisting renal insufficiency, diabetes mellitus and poor left ventricular function or when
multiple studies are done in a 24-hour period.[23] The volume
of contrast used (>1.5 mL/kg) also appears directly related
to nephrotoxicity. In the subgroup patients at very high risk
for contrast nephropathy, nonionic contrast is less nephrotoxic.[24] However, volume expanding these high-risk patients
with intravenous crystalloid (500 to 1000 mL over previous
6 to 12 hours) appears the best prevention.[25] Theophylline
(5 mg/kg over 20 minutes) given 90 minutes before contrast
infusion may abrogate ARF in patients with chronic azotemia.[26] Intravenous mannitol and furosemide have not proved
beneficial separate from crystalloid loading. Calcium channel
blockers may be of adjunctive value although properly controlled studies are not available. Most cases of contrast nephrotoxicity are nonoliguric and resolve within a few days.
Rarely, a patient requires acute dialysis. Permanent loss of
renal function may rarely occur in diabetics with severe
preexisting azotemia (serum creatinine >3 mg/dL).

Rhabdomyolysis produces ARF in our CCUs at an increasing rate. Drugs (e.g., heroin, cocaine, lovastatin) and
major crush injuries have joined alcohol, seizures, and muscle compression as common etiologies. All have the potential
of producing myoglobinuria and ARF, particularly if ECV

depletion or shock exist simultaneously. Hyperkalemia, hyperuricemia, hyperphosphatemia, and hypercreatinemia (low
BUN:Cr ratio) are commonly seen with rhabdomyolysis.
Hypocalcemia occurs early but hypercalcemia (often as high
as 12 to 14 mg/dL) may appear during recovery.[27] Dark
heme-positive urine without RBCs in the urinary sediment
is a major diagnostic clue. Prophylaxis against ATN in patients with rhabdomyolysis depends on aggressive IV crystalloid (one half normal saline or normal saline at 250 to
500 mL/hour).[28] Mannitol (12.5 g/L) and sodium bicarbonate
(50 mEq/L) may be added initially to increase urine flow
and alkalinize the urine, measures that may decrease myoglobin nephrotoxicity.

Ischemic insults to the kidney occur with prolonged hypotension, suprarenal aortic or renal artery occlusion (either
with clot or clamp), and sepsis. The renal tubular cells at
the corticomedullary junction are particularly susceptible
to ischemic insult because their baseline balance between
oxygen supply and demand is tenuous.[29] Thus, whenever
systemic or intrarenal blood flow decreases slightly, ischemic
insult to the tubular cells can occur (see Pathophysiology
below). This may help to explain the beneficial affects attributed to loop diuretics shown in some studies. By inhibiting
active chloride and sodium transport in the ascending limb
of the loop of Henle, these agents decrease metabolic work
and therefore oxygen requirements, rendering the cells less
susceptible to ischemic injury.[30]

More than 50% of all cases of oliguric ARF in the ICU
are due to *sepsis*.[31] This condition appears related to a simultaneous decrease in systemic vascular resistance and increase
in renal vascular resistance, reducing renal plasma flow and
GFR.[32] In these patients, ARF can occur independently of
systemic hypotension. Fever, leukocytosis, and other overt
signs of sepsis may also be absent. A mild alteration in mental
status or respiratory akalosis may be the only clinical clue.
Oliguria or azotemia, or both in this setting should be considered occult septicemia unless disproved.

PATHOPHYSIOLOGY ■

For many years, the mechanisms responsible for the initiation and maintenance of ARF have remained elusive. This
is due to several factors including (1) the relatively poor
clinical applicability of animal models, (2) the heterogeneity
of etiologies of ARF, (3) the multiple causes of ARF often
seen in any particular patient, (4) the "ischemic" nature of
certain "toxins," and (5) the regenerative and repair processes that occur simultaneous to the clinical syndrome of
ARF, notably decreased GFR.

While recent evidence has begun to clarify this pathophysiology, ARF is best thought of as a spectrum of clinical
conditions, caused by multiple potential factors, manifested
commonly as a decrease in GFR (Fig. 143-3). For example,
a given etiology may cause a direct toxic or ischemic insult
to renal tubular cells. Injury to these cells results in a fall
in GFR by a process termed tubuloglomerular feedback
(TGF).[33] Local production of angiotensin II, endothelin, interleukin 2, adenosine, or vasoconstrictor prostaglandins may

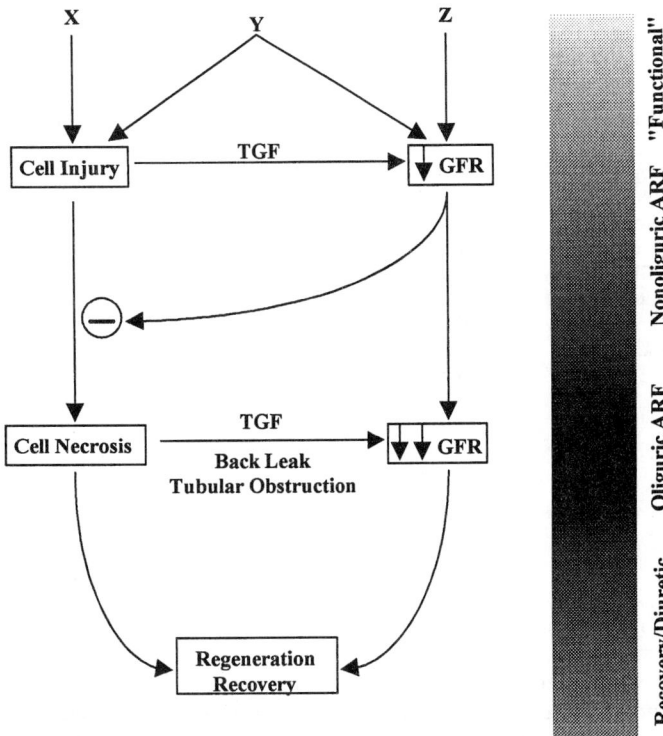

FIGURE 143-3. Pathophysiology of acute renal failure with clinical correlation. GFR may fall after a cellular insult (X) stimulates tubuloglomerular feedback (TGF) or because of a direct hemodynamic alteration (Z). Some etiologies (Y) may directly affect tubular injury and GFR. In its mildest form, functional renal failure results and resolves without oliguria or histologic evidence of cell necrosis. More severe or prolonged insults may cause cell necrosis with tubular obstruction and backleak of ultrafiltrate contributing to oliguria. Tubular cell regeneration and recovery of GFR usually correspond to a diuretic phase clinically.

mediate this phenomenon. Alternatively, a variety of etiologies may directly decrease GFR by effecting a fall in renal blood flow (severe hypotension), altering glomerular hemodynamics (e.g., hepatorenal syndrome, ACE-I, sepsis), or changing glomerular permeability (e.g., hypercalcemia). Sepsis appears to simultaneously cause both tubular cell injury and a decrease in GFR.[10,32] In its mildest form, these events may produce a functional and quickly reversible decrease in GFR not associated with morphologic or structural changes. More severe or prolonged insults can produce nonoliguric or oliguric ARF clinically with or without actual tubular necrosis histologically. The more severe the insult, the more likely is frank tubular necrosis as well as backleak of ultrafiltrate across damaged basement membranes and tubular obstruction from necrotic tubular cells that contributes to prolonged decrements in GFR and protracted oliguria.

When histologic evidence of tubular necrosis is found in patients with ARF, it usually involves cells of the S_3 segment of the proximal tubule and thick ascending limb of the loop of Henle.[34] These renal tubular cells are uniquely susceptible to toxic or ischemic insult because under normal conditions, oxygen supply is limited (due to arteriovenous shunting in the vasa recta) and oxygen demand is high because these metabolically active cells reabsorb significant amounts of sodium and chloride.[29] Because basal oxygen balance is marginal, the presence of a nephrotoxin, any decrease in oxygen supply or increase in oxygen demand can produce significant cellular injury. This appears to be important not only to the initiation but also the maintenance and recovery of ARF. In any given patient with ARF, a balance between several exogenous and endogenous substances appears to

control medullary oxygen supply, the extent of tubular cell injury, and thus the clinical course. Some of these factors affecting medullary oxygenation are outlined in Figure 143-4.

The actual mechanisms involved in cellular injury are not clearly defined and may vary depending on the etiology. Nevertheless, the proximate derangement appears to be decreased production and increased degradation of adenosine triphosphate (ATP) that activates phospholipases and increases cellular hypoxanthine and adenosine.[35] Activated phospholipases destabilize cellular membranes. Calcium influx may cause additional membrane changes and contribute to the production of xanthine oxidase. When catalyzed by xanthine oxidase, hypoxanthine produces oxygen free radicals (superoxide, hydrogen peroxide, hydroxyl radical), particularly after the initial ischemic event resolves and reperfusion occurs. Free radicals further contribute to cell injury by altering protein structure and forming lipid peroxides in cell membranes.[36] Adenosine dilates the glomerular efferent arteriolar sphincter, lowering intraglomerular hydrostatic pressure that, in the face of compromised renal blood flow, decreases GFR.[36] Local production of platelet activating factor, angiotensin II, vasoconstrictive prostaglandins, and endothelin are other factors that may affect intraglomerular hemodynamics or glomerular capillary permeability in such a way as to decrease GFR (e.g., TGF).[33]

TGF moderates tubular injury by preventing massive sodium diuresis and hypovolemia, improving medullary blood flow (due to adenosine) and limiting tubular cell work (and thus oxygen demand) by limiting sodium delivery to and reabsorption by the ascending limb of the loop of Henle. This homeostatic phenomenon therefore protects the organism

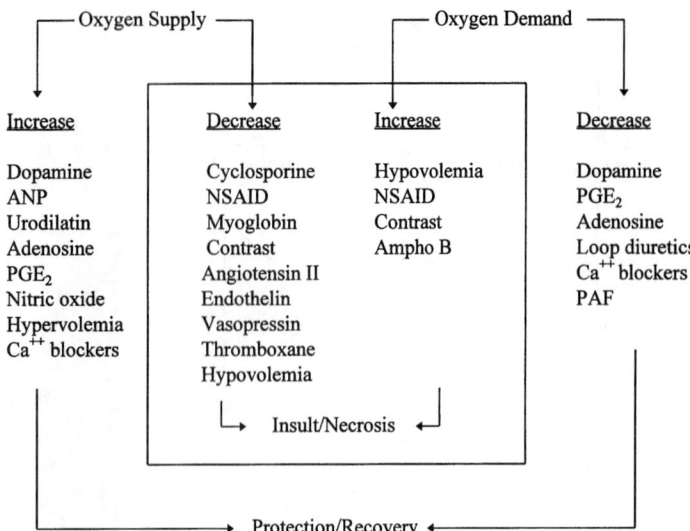

FIGURE 143-4. Factors affecting oxygen supply and demand in the medullary thick ascending limb, the cells most susceptible to ischemic injury. A decrease in oxygen supply or increase in oxygen demand tends to cause cellular injury and necrosis. Factors increasing oxygen supply or decreasing oxygen demand tend to protect the cell from injury and aid in recovery.

while tending to limit further tubular cell injury ("acute renal success").[37]

Simultaneous with these events causing cellular injury and renal functional decline, other factors appear to begin the regenerative or repair process. Release of various cytokines from injured cells recruit and activate macrophages that synthesize growth factors, such as epidermal growth factor (EGF), insulinlike growth factor (IGF), and transforming growth factor (TGF), stimulating renal tubular regeneration.[38] Local production of vasodilatory prostaglandins and nitric oxide may aid this recovery.[39] Clinically, the recovery phase is marked by increasing urinary volume in oliguric patients and a gradual return of GFR provided that subsequent insults (e.g., hypotension, sepsis, toxins) are minimal. The kidney is unique in this ability to evolve from near total failure to essentially complete recovery.

The pathophysiology described offers hope of specific therapy to improve intrarenal hemodynamics (ANP, antiendothelin antibodies, endothelin receptor antagonists, adenosine inhibitors), restore cellular ATP ($MgCl_2$ infusions, 5' nucleotidase inhibitors), limit cell injury (diuretics, free radical scavengers), and stimulate growth (EGF, IGF, TGF). See Treatment and Supportive Care later in chapter.

PREVENTION OF ARF ∎

Because the mortality from ARF is high and the treatment largely supportive, prevention in those patients at high risk is extremely important. The strongest risk factor for ARF is renal hypoperfusion.[6,40] This includes ECV depletion, heart failure, active liver disease, and third spacing of fluids (e.g., with pancreatitis or burns).[41] Preexisting azotemia and chronic hypertension are less important, whereas age and diabetes mellitus are not consistently identified as risk factors. Most patients who develop ARF in the hospital have more than one risk factor and most suffer more than one specific insult.[40] The common insults include severe infections, sepsis, nephrotoxins, and metabolic derangements.

Insults may occur simultaneously or sequentially and because each represents a spectrum of severity, they may be thought of as risk factors as well.

Several factors appear to predict not only the incidence but also the severity of ARF.[41–43] These include extreme hypotension (shock), sepsis, multiple antibiotics used concurrently, pancreatitis, peritonitis, active liver disease, and respiratory failure with mechanical ventilation. Such patients are more likely to be oliguric, suffer a prolonged course, require more dialysis, endure more complications, and have greater mortality.

Table 143-9 lists several of the most common renal risk factors and strategies for their prevention. ECV expansion with crystalloid is indicated in patients with a diminished intravascular volume (absolute volume contraction, third spacing of fluids, positive pressure ventilation) and for most receiving nephrotoxins. Intravenous colloids may be of value in patients with shock, severe hypoalbuminemia, and those with third spacing of fluids. Inotropic agents are indicated in patients with poor myocardial contractility.[44] "Renal dose" dopamine (1.5 to 3.0 μg/kg/minute) is more controversial but appears to "protect" patients when renal perfusion is compromised by heart failure, liver disease, and perhaps sepsis.[45] Dopamine does not appear to improve risk in patients receiving nephrotoxins. ACE inhibitors and NSAIDs should be avoided or used cautiously until renal hypoperfusion of any cause is corrected.

TREATMENT AND SUPPORTIVE CARE ∎

Unfortunately, specific therapy does not exist for most causes of ARF. Table 143-10 categorizes some of the causes of ARF that may respond to specific treatments. For example, steroids and cyclophosphamide are indicated for patients with systemic vasculitis[46] (e.g., polyarteritis, Wegener granulomatosis) or the diffuse proliferative glomerulonephritis of lupus erythematosus.[47] Plasmapheresis is indicated for the hemolytic uremic syndrome[48] and Goodpasture syndrome[49]

TABLE 143-9. Prevention of ARF in Patients at High Risk

RISK FACTOR	STRATEGY FOR PREVENTION
Renal hypoperfusion	Avoid nephrotoxins
ECV depletion	Isotonic crystalloid
Hypotension	Crystalloid, colloid, vasopressors
Congestive failure	Inotropic agents; cautious use of ACE inhibitors
Cirrhosis–ascites	Dopamine? Peritoneovenous shunt? Avoid NSAIDs
Third space	Colloid, isotonic crystalloid
PEEP	Isotonic crystalloid
Renal artery stenosis	Avoid ACE inhibitors with diuretics
Preexisting azotemia	Avoid ECV depletion; cautious use of nephrotoxins
Sepsis	Avoid ECV depletion; cautious use of nephrotoxins; dopamine?
Nephrotoxins	Avoid ECV depletion and other nephrotoxins
Aminoglycosides	Use alternative agent if possible; lengthen dosing interval; correct hypokalemia
Chemotherapy	Expand ECV; mannitol
Radiocontrast	Expand ECV; theophylline; limit dose; nonionic contrast with diabetes and preexisting azotemia
Cyclosporine	Calcium blockers
NSAIDs	Cautious use in CHF, cirrhosis, ECV depletion; avoid triamterene
Rhabdomyolysis	Expand ECV; mannitol; HCO_3
Hyperuricemia	Expand ECV; alkalinize urine; allopurinol
Electrolyte disorders	
Hypokalemia	Correct
Hypophosphatemia	Correct
Hyperphosphatemia	Avoid calcium therapy; expand ECV
Hypercalcemia	Avoid phosphorus therapy; expand ECV; furosemide

TABLE 143-10. Causes of Acute Renal Failure in Which Specific Treatment Is Indicated

CAUSE	TREATMENT
VASCULAR DISEASE	
Malignant hypertension	Antihypertensives
Thrombosis–embolism	Anticoagulants
Cholesterol emboli	Support; avoid anticoagulants
HUS–TTP	Plasma exchange–pheresis
Vasculitis°	Steroids; cyclophosphamide
GLOMERULAR DISEASE	
Hemodynamic (ACE inhibitor, nifedipine, nitroprusside)	Stop offending agent, ? low-dose dopamine
Infectious glomerulonephritis (BE, shunt nephritis)	Antibiotics
Lupus nephritis (DPGN)	Steroids, cyclophosphamide
Goodpasture syndrome	Steroids, plasmapheresis, cyclophosphamide
Idiopathic RPGN°	Steroids, cyclophosphamide, plasmapheresis
Allergic interstitial nephritis	Discontinue agent, steroids
Infection (pyelonephritis)	Antibiotics
Uric acid	Dialysis
Multiple myeloma	Plasmapheresis and chemotherapy
ACUTE TUBULAR NECROSIS	Supportive

°Serology and immunofluorescence microscopy define specific syndromes and therapy.
HUS, Hemolytic uremic syndrome; TTP, thrombotic thrombocytopenic purpura; BE, bacterial endocarditis; DPGN, diffuse proliferative glomerulonephritis; RPGN, rapidly progressive glomerulonephritis.

and as adjunctive therapy for multiple myeloma.[50] Corticosteroids may also be indicated in allergic interstitial nephritis, particularly if the renal failure does not improve after discontinuation of the offending drug. For pyelonephritis and infectious glomerulonephritis (e.g., bacterial endocarditis, shunt nephritis), antibiotics should be administered.

The pathophysiologic concepts previously discussed offer the hope of specific therapy for ATN. Restoration of ATP (ATP–MgCl$_2$; inhibition of 5′ nucleotidase),[51,52] free radical scavengers, and adenosine inhibitors (e.g., theophylline) have shown promise in experimental trials.[52] So too have antagonists to platelet activating factor[53] and endothelin (antiendothelin antibodies; endothelin receptor antagonists).[52,54] However, for most patients with ARF, treatment is largely supportive and expectant management is the rule. Stimulating urinary output, avoiding subsequent renal insults and systemic complications, supporting nutrition, and performing dialysis are important strategies.

Whether converting a patient from oliguric to nonoliguric ARF influences mortality is unknown, but it does appear to limit morbidity and simplify management. Therefore, our practice is to stimulate urine output by high-dose loop diuretics (e.g., furosemide 200 mg q 12 hours or 10 to 20 mg/hour continuously). Occasionally, the addition of proximal (acetazolamide 250 mg IV q 12 hours) and distal (chlorothiazide 500 mg IV q 12 hours) diuretics may also improve urine output. Renal-dose dopamine (1.5 to 3.0 μg/kg/minute) may increase urinary volume in some patients with ARF.[45] Atrial natriuretic factor not only improves urine output but also creatinine clearance when given to oliguric patients with established ATN.[55]

Subsequent renal insults may delay recovery and increase the mortality of ATN. These include nephrotoxins, sepsis and hypotension, which may cause ischemic damage.[56] Biocompatible dialysis membranes can limit hemodialysis-induced hypotensive episodes and improve survival in ARF patients requiring dialysis.[57] The use of these synthetic membranes (polysulfone, PMA, PMNA) has replaced cellulose acetate and cupraphane as standard dialysis procedure in critically ill patients.

If hypotension or shock do not respond to volume expansion, inotropic agents or vasopressor doses of dopamine or norepinepherine should be started. Norepinepherine is a more effective pressor agent and improves renal perfusion in intractable septic shock.[58]

Care must be taken to avoid extracellular volume excess and to limit occult sources of potentially toxic electrolytes such as potassium (K penicillin, salt substitutes, oral tobacco products, drugs), phosphorus, and magnesium (laxatives, antacids). Drug dosage often requires adjustment as outlined by several practical guides.[59]

Bleeding is a common and potentially serious complication of ARF. Cryoprecipitate,[60] desmopressin,[61] and conjugated estrogens[62] effectively shorten the prolonged bleeding time and favorably influence clinical bleeding. Hemodialysis can easily be performed without heparin if necessary (see Chap. 42).

Several studies suggest that hyperalimentation improves tubular cell recovery and regeneration[63] and improves survival in patients with ARF.[64] Compared to total parenteral nutrition (TPN), enteral nutrition appears to be more efficient, less expensive, and with fewer complications. In animal models of peritonitis with sepsis and hemorrhagic shock, enteral nutrition significantly reduced mortality compared with TPN.[65] This reduction in mortality is probably related to the integrity of the gut as a mucosal barrier to infection and its protection by enteral feedings.[66] Without enteral feedings, the gut mucosa atrophies, predisposing to the overgrowth of bacterial and fungal organisms and their translocation to the lymphatics and blood. This may contribute to the central role of sepsis in the multiple organ failure syndrome. However, not every patient is an acceptable candidate for enteral nutrition. Pulmonary aspiration may occur in as many as 30% of patients receiving gastric feedings. This can be markedly reduced (to a rate similar to TPN) by placing the feeding tube past the pylorus to a duodenal or jejunal site. This may require fluoroscopy, endoscopy, or surgery. Diarrhea may also occur, but this is usually related to a drug reaction or infection (*Clostridium difficile*) and not the feeding solutions. Certain problems contraindicate enteral nutrition, including small bowel obstruction or ileus, bowel ischemia or infarction, severe bowel dilatation, severe pancreatitis, diarrhea, or fistula.

Whether administered enterally or parenterally, the formulation of hyperalimentation starts with protein requirements. Generally, 1.0 to 1.5 g/kg/day is sufficient, but this may range from 0.6 to 0.8 g/kg/day in unstressed patients and 2.5 g/kg/day in the very critically ill. To effectively use protein or anabolism, enough nonprotein calories (i.e., glucose, fat) must be provided to satisfy energy requirements. The optimal nonprotein caloric nitrogen ratio is approximately 90 to 110:1 (i.e., 100 nonprotein calories per gram of nitrogen) divided roughly evenly between carbohydrate and fat. If carbon dioxide retention occurs, a greater percentage of fat can be used. The clinician must determine the total fluid, electrolyte, and mineral needs for each patient with ARF. Regardless of the route of administration, the hyperalimentation formula must be individualized and reevaluated daily in patients with ARF.

Dialysis is often necessary especially when hypervolemia, hyperkalemia, metabolic acidosis, or uremic symptoms occur. Although intermittent hemodialysis has been the standard dialysis treatment for years, several potential hazards exist such as hypotension, dysequilibrium syndrome, bleeding, hypoxemia, and bioincompatibility. Several other dialysis techniques (peritoneal dialysis and continuous renal replacement therapies) are available to critically ill patients. A detailed discussion of these therapies is presented in Chapter 42.

PROGNOSIS AND RECOVERY

In most clinical series, mortality from ARF continues to average 50%. Mortality in nonoliguric patients may be as low as 25%; with oliguric ARF, it approaches 70%.[1,43] The major determinants of outcome are the precipitating event and preexisting disease. ARF associated with sepsis, trauma, abdominal catastrophe, and burns carries a mortality of 70%

to 80%, but the mortality is 25% to 30% for patients with ARF due to aminoglycosides, radiographic contrast, or other drug reactions.[42,43,64]

Mortality is highest in the very young and very old.[64,67] The number of complications also influences prognosis. Mortality from ARF approaches 100% if three or more major organ systems have failed simultaneously.[40,64] The severity of azotemia, number of dialysis treatments, "aggressive" dialysis, or the dialysis modality do not seem to influence survival.[68]

Infection is the most common cause of death and is usually due to overwhelming sepsis from resistant gram-negative bacteria or yeast. One report related this to the number of antibiotics administered to the patient before renal failure.[67] Other common causes of death are cardiovascular compromise (e.g., strokes, myocardial infarction), respiratory failure (often with nosocomial pneumonia), and gastrointestinal bleeding.

If the patient with ARF survives, recovery is usually prompt and clinically complete.[67,69] The period of oliguria averages 10 to 14 days. Urinary volume recovers gradually over the next 3 to 7 days. Fluid therapy is needed to support this obligatory diuretic phase. Although the BUN and creatinine continue to rise during this phase, dialysis can usually be discontinued. Most survivors regain essentially complete renal function within 30 days; rarely, a patient requires 60 to 90 days. In one large series, 97% of survivors regained renal function, almost all within 30 days.[69] Those patients who have delayed or no recovery are usually older, with preexisting renal insufficiency who suffer acute ischemic insults to the kidney.

Although renal recovery is usually clinically complete, as many as 50% of patients have minor decrements in GFR, decreased concentrating ability, or defects in maximal urinary acidification.

REFERENCES ■

1. Anderson RJ, Linas SL, Berns AS, et al: Nonoliguric acute renal failure. *N Engl J Med* 1977;296:1134
2. Muther RS: Drug interference with renal function tests. *Am J Kidney Dis* 1983;3:118
3. Espinel CH, Gregory AW: Differential diagnosis of acute renal failure. *Clin Nephrol* 1980;2:73
4. Diamond JR, Yoburn DC: Nonoliguric acute renal failure associated with a low fractional excretion of sodium. *Ann Intern Med* 1982;96:597
5. Brosins FL, Lau K: Low fractional excretion of sodium in acute renal failure: role of timing of the test and ischemia. *Am J Nephrol* 1986;6:450
6. Hou SH, Bushinsky DA, Wish JB, et al: Hospital-acquired renal insufficiency: a prospective study. *Am J Med* 1983;74:243
7. Moore K, Wendon J, Frazer M, et al: Plasma endothelin immunoreactivity in liver disease and the hepatorenal syndrome. *N Engl J Med* 1992;327:1774
8. Schwartz D, Averbuch M, Pines A, et al: Renal toxicity of enalapril in very elderly patients with progressive, severe congestive heart failure. *Chest* 1991;100:1558
9. Hricik DE: Captopril induced renal insufficiency and the role of sodium balance. *Ann Intern Med* 1989;108:222
10. Parillo JE (moderator): Septic shock in humans: advances in the understanding of pathogenesis, cardiovascular dysfunction, and therapy. *Ann Intern Med* 1990;113:227
11. Reid GM, Muther RS: Nitroprusside-induced acute azotemia. *Am J Nephrol* 1987;7:313
12. Diamond JR, Cheung JY, Fang LST: Nifedipine-induced renal dysfunction. *Am J Med* 1984;77:905
13. Clive DM, Stoff JS: Renal syndromes associated with nonsteroidal antiinflammatory drugs. *N Engl J Med* 1984;310:563
14. Nolan CR, Anger MS, Kelleher SP: Eosinophiluria—a new method of detection and definition of the clinical spectrum. *N Engl J Med* 1986;315:1516
15. Abuelo JG: Diagnosing vascular causes of renal failure. *Ann Intern Med* 1995;123:601
16. Nolan CR 3d, Linas S: Malignant hypertension and other hypertensive crises. In: Schrier RW, Gottschalk CW (eds). *Disease of the Kidney*, vol 2. Boston, Little, Brown; 1993:1555
17. Eknoyan G, Riggs SA: Renal involvement in patients with thrombotic thrombocytopenic purpura. *Am J Nephrol* 1986;6:117
18. Lessman RK, Johnson SF, Coburn JW, Kaufman JJ: Renal artery embolism: clinical features and long term follow-up of 17 cases. *Ann Intern Med* 1978;89:477
19. Meyrier A, Bucket P, Simon P, et al: Atheromatous renal disease. *Am J Med* 1988;85:139
20. Lesavre P: Antineutrophil cytoplasmic autoantibodies antigen specificity. *Am J Kidney Dis* 1991;18:159
21. Kapusnik JE, Sande MA: Challenging conventional aminoglycoside dosing regimens: the value of experimental models. *Am J Med* 1986;80(suppl 6B):179
22. Schentag JJ, Cerra FB, Plaut ME: Clinical and pharmacokinetic characteristics of aminoglycoside nephrotoxicity in 201 critically ill patients. *Antimicrob Agents Chemother* 1982;21:721
23. Taliercio CP, Vlietstra RE, Fisher LD, Burnett JL: Risks for renal dysfunction with cardiac angiography. *Ann Intern Med* 1986;104:501
24. Rudnick MR, Goldfarb S, Wexler L, et al: Nephrotoxicity of ionic and nonionic contrast media in 1196 patients: a randomized trial. *Kidney Int* 1995;47:254
25. Solomon R, Werner C, Mann DO, et al: Effects of saline, mannitol and furosemide on acute decreases in renal function induced by radiocontrast agents. *N Engl J Med* 1994;331:1416
26. Erley CM, Duda SH, Schlepckow S, et al: Adenosine antagonist theophylline prevents the reduction of glomerular filtration rate after contrast media application. *Kidney Int* 1994;45:1425
27. Akmal MD, Bishop JE, Telfer N, et al: Hypocalcemia and hypercalcemia in patients with rhabdomyolysis with and without acute renal failure. *J Clin Endocrinol Metab* 1986;63:137
28. Better OS, Stein JH: Early management of shock and prophylaxis of acute renal failure in traumatic rhabdomyolysis. *N Engl J Med* 1990;322:825
29. Brezis MD, Rosen S: Hypoxemia of the renal medulla—its implications for disease. *N Engl J Med* 1995;332:647
30. Heyman SN, Brezis MD, Greenfeld Z, et al: Protective role of furosemide and saline in radiocontrast-induced acute renal failure in the rat. *Am J Kidney Dis* 1989;14:377
31. Muther RS, Murray M, Bennett WM: Assessing university nephrology training as preparation for community consultative practice. *Acad Med* 1989;64:677
32. Cumming AD, Driedger AA, McDonald JWD, et al: Vasoactive hormones in the renal response to systemic sepsis. *Am J Kidney Dis* 1988;11:23
33. Briggs JP, Schnermann J: The tubuloglomerular feedback mechanism: functional and biochemical aspects. *Annu Rev Physiol* 1987;49:251
34. Brezis M, Dinour D, Greenfield Z, et al: Susceptibility of

Henle's loop to hypoxic and toxic insults. *Adv Nephrol Necker Hosp* 1991;2041:56

35. Bonventre J: Mechanism of ischemic acute renal failure. *Kidney Int* 1993;43:1160

36. Dinour D, Brezis M: Effects of adenosine on intrarenal oxygenation. *Am J Physiol* 1991;261:F787

37. Thurau K, Boylan JW: Acute renal success. *Am J Med* 1976; 61:308

38. Toback FG: Regeneration after acute tubular necrosis. *Kidney Int* 1992;42:226

39. Agmon Y, Peleg H, Greenfield Z, et al: Nitric oxide and prostanoids protect the renal outer medulla from radiocontrast toxicity in the rat. *J Clin Invest* 1994;94:1069

40. Rasmussen HH, Ibels LS: Acute renal failure: multivariate analysis of causes and risk factors. *Am J Med* 1982;73:211

41. Groeneveld ARJ, Tran DD, Van der Meulen, Nauta JJP, Thijs LG: Acute renal failure in the medical intensive care unit: predisposing, complicating factors and outcome. *Nephron* 1991;59:602

42. Jochimsen F, Schafer JH, Mauerer A, Distler A: Impairment of renal function in medical intensive care: predictability of acute renal failure. *Crit Care Med* 1990;18:480

43. Spiegel DM, Ullian ME, Zerbe GO, Berl T: Determinants of survival and recovery in acute renal failure patients dialyzed in intensive-care untis. *Am J Nephrol* 1991;11:44

44. Duke GJ, Briedis J, Weaver RA: Renal support in critically ill patients: low dose dopamine or low dose dobutamine? *Crit Care Med* 1994;22:1919

45. Parker S, Carlon GC, Isaacs MD, et al: Dopamine administration in oliguria and oliguric renal failure. *Crit Care Med* 1981;9:630

46. Fauci AS, Haynes BF, Katz P, et al: Wegener's granulomatosis: prospective clinical and therapeutic experience with 85 patients for 21 years. *Am Intern Med* 1983;98:76

47. Austin HA, Klippel JH, Balow JE, et al: Therapy of lupus nephritis: a controlled trial of prednisone and cytotoxic drugs. *N Engl J Med* 1986;314:614

48. Rock GA, Shumak KH, Buskard NA, et al: Comparison of plasma exchange with plasma infusion in the treatment of thrombotic thrombocytopenic purpura. The Canadian Apheresis Study Group. *N Engl J Med* 1991;325:393

49. Pusey CD, Lockwood CM, Peters DK: Plasma exchange and immunosuppresive drugs in the treatment of glomerulonephritis due to antibodies in the basement membrane. *Int J Artif Organs* 1983;6(Suppl);15

50. Johnson WJ, Kyle RA, Pineda AA, et al: Treatment of renal failure associated with multiple myeloma. *Arch Intern Med* 1990;150:863

51. VanWaarde A, Stromski ME, Thuliri G, et al: Protection of the kidney against ischemic injury by inhibition of 5′ nucleotidase. *Am J Physiol* 1989;256:F298

52. Fischereder MD, Trick W, Nath KA: Therapeutic strategies in the prevention of acute renal failure. *Semin Nephrol* 1994;14:41

53. Lopez-Farre A, Bernabeou F, Gomez-Garre DO, et al: Platelet activating factor antagonist treatment protects against postischemic acute renal failure in rats. *J Pharm Exp Ther* 1990;253:328

54. Luscher TF, Bock HA, Yang Z, et al: Endothelium derived relaxing and contracting factors: perspectives in nephrology. *Kidney Int* 1991;39:575

55. Rahman SN, Kim GE, Mathew AS, et al: Effects of atrial natriuretic peptide in clinical acute renal failure. *Kidney Int* 1994;45:1731

56. Kelleher SP, Robinette JB, Miller F, Conger JD: Effect of hemorrhagic reduction in blood pressure on recovery from acute renal failure. *Kidney Int* 1987;31:725

57. Hakim RM, Wingard R, Parker RA: Effect of the dialysis membrane in the treatment of patients with acute renal failure. *N Engl J Med* 1994;331:1338

58. Meadows DO, Edwards DO, Wilkins RG, et al: Reversal of intractable septic shock with norepinephrine therapy. *Crit Care Med* 1988;16:663

59. Bennett WM, Aronoff G, Golper TA, et al: *Drug Prescribing in Renal Failure: Dosing Guidelines for Adults*, 3rd ed. Philadelphia, Am College Physicians, 1994

60. Jason PA, Jubelirer SJ, Weinstein MJ, Deykin DO: Treatment of the bleeding tendency in uremia with cryoprecipitate. *N Engl J Med* 1980;303:1318

61. Mannucci PM, Remuzzi G, Pusinori F, et al: Deamino-8-D-arginine vasopressin shortens the bleeding time in uremia. *N Engl J Med* 1983;308:8

62. Livio MD, Mannucci PM, Vigano G: Conjugated estrogen for the management of bleeding associated with renal failure. *N Eng J Med* 1986;315:731

63. Toback FG, Dodd RC, Mayer ER, et al: Amino acid administration enhances renal protein metabolism after acute tubular necrosis. *Nephron* 1983;33:238

64. McMurray SD, Luft FC, Maxwell DR, et al: Prevailing patterns and predictor variables in patients with acute tubular necrosis. *Arch Intern Med* 1978;139:950

65. Peterson VM, Moore EE, Jones TN, et al: Total enteral nutrition versus total parenteral nutrition after major torso injury: attenuation of hepatic protein reprioritization. *Surgery* 1988; 104:199

66. Alverdy JC, Aoys E, Moss GS: Total parenteral nutrition promotes bacterial translocation from the gut. *Surgery* 1988; 104:185

67. Spurney RF, Fulkerson WJ, Schwab SJ: Acute renal failure in critically ill patients: prognosis for recovery of kidney function after dialysis support. *Crit Care Med* 1991;19:8

68. Gillum DM, Dixon BS, Nanover MJ, et al: The role of intensive dialysis in acute renal failure. *Clin Nephrol* 1986;25:249

69. Kjellstrand CM, Gormick C, Davin T: Recovery from acute renal failure. *Clin Exp Dial Apheresis* 1981;5:143

Critical Care, Third Edition, edited by Joseph M. Civetta,
Robert W. Taylor, and Robert R. Kirby.
Lippincott-Raven Publishers, Philadelphia, PA © 1997.

CHAPTER 144

■

Impact of Chronic
Renal Failure

Gerald M. Reid
Richard S. Muther

IMMEDIATE CONCERNS ■

MAJOR PROBLEMS

1. Patients with chronic renal failure present for intensive
   care with clinical problems similar to patients with
   normal renal function.
2. Common presentations include hypotension, chest
   pain, cardiac arrhythmias, respiratory distress, and altered consciousness.
3. In each of these cases, special considerations apply in
   the advanced renal failure patient. Disordered volume
   control, solute and acid-base homeostasis, and pharmacokinetics present unique challenges in the acute
   intensive care setting in this population.
4. Physiologic characteristics common to chronic renal
   patients must be taken into account.

STRESS POINTS

1. In the renal failure patient with hypotension, the primary considerations are hypovolemia, reduced cardiac
   performance, and sepsis. Hypovolemia often results
   from overaggressive ultrafiltration dialysis and is aggravated by myocardial dysfunction, systolic or diastolic.
   Gastrointestinal bleeding is common as well. In the
   presence of abdominal pain (patient not on peritoneal
   dialysis), intestinal ischemia and pancreatitis are more
   common than in the general population.
2. Reduced cardiac performance is typically due to coronary artery disease. Myocardial ischemia without chest

pain is not infrequent, especially in diabetics. Pericarditis with possible tamponade or constrictive pericarditis must be considered in this patient population.
3. Sepsis with peripheral vasodilatation causing hypotension is contributed to by altered immune function with
   azotemia and dialysis. In hemodialysis patients, the
   vascular access is the most likely source. With peritoneal dialysis, peritonitis must be excluded.
4. Chest pain in patients with chronic renal failure is
   usually due to angina or pericarditis. Increased arteriosclerosis and coronary artery disease are more common than in the general population. Chest pain is
   typical for angina in most patients, as are electrocardiographic (ECG) changes. Nonspecific ECG changes
   are also more common in dialysis patients, probably
   due to chemical alterations.
5. Patients with cardiac arrythmias are more likely to
   have electrolyte or acid-base disturbances. Abnormal
   magnesium and potassium levels are particularly common. Antiarrhythmic drug dosing must be carefully
   considered.
6. When a patient with chronic renal failure has respiratory distress, circulatory overload must be excluded.
   The chest radiograph is often atypical. Frequently, a
   trial of volume reduction with dialysis or potent diuretics yields excellent relief. Pulmonary emboli may be
   less frequent than with other chronic diseases, but
   certainly do occur. Pneumonias are due to usual organisms, with opportunistic infections less commonly seen.
7. Altered consciousness may be due to the uremic state

2093

before dialysis or it may occur with overly aggressive dialysis (dialysis dysequilibrium syndrome). Technical complications of dialysis (air embolism, dialysate contamination) are rare but should be considered. The incidence of cerebrovascular accident is very high in the dialysis population.

HYPOTENSION ■

HYPOVOLEMIA

Hypovolemic hypotension in patients with chronic renal failure is frequently due to overaggressive ultrafiltration dialysis. Careful physical examination aids in recognition. Treatment is isotonic volume replacement. This problem can be avoided by carefully following pre- and postdialysis body weight.

Hypovolemic hypotension is accentuated by frequently present myocardial dysfunction. Ischemic coronary artery disease often accompanied by decreased left ventricular ejection fraction, accounts for most of the serious cardiac morbidity in the chronic renal failure population.[1-3] Even in patients without coronary disease or preexisting cardiac abnormalities, characteristic changes in myocardial performance occur with time on maintenance dialysis. Dilatation of the left ventricle (LV) is common[4,5] and is associated with three factors: the presence of an arteriovenous shunt; chronic sodium overload with extracellular fluid (ECF) expansion; and anemia. Permanent correction of anemia with erythropoietin is accompanied by diminution in size of the left ventricle.[6] Rarely, patients without other demonstrable cardiac disease suffer from progressive global cardiomyopathy; these patients may respond dramatically to renal transplantation.[7]

Left ventricular hypertrophy (LVH) is seen even more frequently. It is found in over 50% of chronic hemodialysis patients.[8] LVH is an independent risk factor for mortality in end-stage renal disease.[9] An essential feature of LVH in these patients is its asymmetry.[10] Diastolic dysfunction with poor LV compliance is characteristic.[11] Because of the increased filling pressures required with both systolic and diastolic dysfunction, volume depletion can lead to rapid and severe drops in blood pressure, requiring urgent volume restoration. In patients presenting with hypotension, even without volume depletion or chest pain, acute myocardial ischemia or pericardial tamponade must be considered (see later).

Possible gastrointestinal bleeding is a common concern in the hypotensive renal failure patient. Gastritis is often present.[12] Angiodysplasia of the upper gastrointestinal tract and erosive esophagitis are more common causes of bleeding in chronic renal failure patients than in those without renal failure. Duodenal or gastric ulcers may occur as frequently as in the general population, but clinically significant bleeding is more common.[13,14] This is partially due to anticoagulants administered during the hemodialysis procedure, as well as to chronic aspirin or even warfarin therapy used to prevent vascular access clotting. Uremic bleeding tendency due to platelet dysfunction is another important contributing factor.

The uremic platelet disorder has been well characterized. Mild thrombocytopenia is not infrequent, but the platelet count does not fall below 70,000 from uremia alone. Multiple defects in platelets and platelet–vessel wall interaction have been described.[15,16] The cutaneous bleeding time is used clinically to assess the degree of uremic platelet dysfunction. Anemia affects the bleeding time independently. Transfusions of red blood cells to raise the hematocrit above 30%[17] or correction of anemia with erythropoietin can shorten the bleeding time.[18]

The therapeutic approach to the chronic renal failure patient with active gastrointestinal (or other) bleeding is multifaceted. Platelet transfusions are not effective, since normal platelets exposed to uremic plasma quickly acquire functional abnormalities. Initiating or increasing dialysis shortens the bleeding time, but not always into the normal range.[15] Transfusions to raise the hematocrit above 30% should be routine. If bleeding continues and the bleeding time remains prolonged, several other measures have been shown to be of value (Table 144-1). Concentrated cryoprecipitate shortens the bleeding time, usually into the normal range.[19] The amount of precipitate obtained from 10 units of plasma is infused over 30 minutes into a peripheral vein. The beneficial effects wear off within 24 hours. Intravenous deamino-D-arginine-vasopressin (dDAVP) infusions also shorten the bleeding time in uremic patients,[20] with temporary effects lasting 6 to 8 hours. Successive infusions produce a reduced response. Conjugated estrogens are also beneficial when given as daily intravenous infusions for 5 consecutive days.[21]

CARDIOGENIC

The preponderance of ischemic coronary artery disease leads to the strong consideration of cardiogenic shock in the hypotensive renal failure patient. In diabetic patients, chest pain is absent more frequently. Angiographic cardiac evaluation and the consideration of cardiac bypass surgery or angioplasty requires special concerns (see section on Chest Pain).

PERICARDIAL DISEASE

Pericardial disease is common in renal failure patients and may result in hypotension. Pericarditis may occur before or during the first several weeks after initiating chronic dialysis therapy. This is termed *uremic pericarditis*.[22] Alternatively,

TABLE 144-1. Treatment of Uremic Bleeding Defects

Initiate or intensify dialysis treatments.
Administer red blood cells to Hct >30%.
Administer cryoprecipitate, 10 units IV over 30 min. May repeat every 24 h.
Administer dDAVP, 0.3 μg/kg. Give in 50 mL NS over 30 min. May repeat the following day.
Conjugated estrogens, 0.6 mg/kg IV daily for 5 d.

---

patients well-established on dialysis may develop pericarditis, termed *dialysis-associated pericarditis*.[23] In either case, two serious complications may lead to hypotension: cardiac tamponade or constrictive pericarditis.

Most patients with uremic pericarditis respond well to the initiation or intensification of chronic dialysis therapy. Although blood urea nitrogen and creatinine concentrations are not significantly different from chronic renal failure patients without pericarditis, the predictable response to dialysis strongly implicates retained uremic toxins as causative factors.[24] These patients are not likely to present with chest pain or develop serious complications.

On the other hand, patients with dialysis-associated pericarditis are more prone to complications. Heparin therapy, viral infections,[25] accumulation of "middle molecules,"[26] and immunologic mechanisms[27] all have been implicated in pathogenesis. Chest pain, fever, and a scratchy or grating pericardial friction rub are usually present. Cardiomegaly with clear lung fields is seen on chest radiographs, sometimes accompanied by pleural effusion from concomitant pleuritis. Echocardiography reveals the presence and size of any pericardial effusion. Daily dialysis is instituted, without systemic heparinization. Pericardiocentesis with local steroid instillation can be performed if no improvement occurs after 10 to 14 days of dialysis.[28] If pericarditis fails to resolve or recurs after these measures, surgical pericardiectomy is indicated. Indomethacin may relieve chest pain, but does not affect the overall course.[29]

Acute *cardiac tamponade* must be quickly recognized and treated. Hypotension with a narrow pulse pressure, distended neck veins, dyspnea, tachypnea, and apprehension are typically seen. Pulsus paradoxus is often present but may be absent with severe LV failure[30] or extreme hypotension. Prompt right ventricular catheterization demonstrates the characteristic equilibration of atrial, ventricular, and pulmonary artery diastolic pressures.

Pericardiocentesis should be performed acutely, with catheter drainage and the local instillation of corticosteroids. Some sources advocate moving invariably to open surgical procedures such as pericardiotomy or pericardiectomy. Others take a more conservative approach. Recurrent tamponade certainly requires definitive surgery.

Chronic *constrictive pericarditis* may develop consequent to acute pericarditis. The course is more subacute, with evidence of right ventricular failure and hypotension during hemodialysis. The diagnosis may be subtle and typically requires echocardiography, cardiac angiography, or both.

SEPSIS

Patients with chronic renal failure may present with hypotension due to peripheral vasodilatation from septic shock. Defects in immune function have been repeatedly demonstrated in these persons. The precise nature and causes of these defects continue to be the subject of lively debate and investigation.[31] Defects in various lymphocyte and neutrophil functions have been documented. These defects are often not improved and may even be exacerbated by hemodialysis therapy. This is particularly true when complement activating dialysis membranes are used. Nutritional factors are also likely to play a role in diminished immune competence.

In spite of these demonstrated immune deficits, clinical sepsis is likely to be related to bacterial entry through the dialysis access. Opportunistic infections are rare. When they do occur, they are most often related to additional immunosuppressive therapy.[32]

In hemodialysis patients, vascular access is the most likely source of bacterial sepsis. *Staphylococcus aureus* and *Staphylococcus epidermidis* are both common pathogens entering from skin.[33] A local site of infection involving the access itself can usually be found. Synthetic arteriovenous grafts are more likely to become infected than native vein fistulas.[34] Temporary large-bore double-lumen intravenous (IV) dialysis catheters carry a particularly high risk of staphylococcal colonization and subsequent sepsis. Another common bacterial pathogen in hemodialysis patients is *Escherichia coli,* entering through the urinary tract.[32,33] In addition, entry through cutaneous ulcers or sores is common, particularly in patients with severe peripheral vascular disease and neuropathy such as diabetics.

Infection in the peritoneal dialysis patient is likely to originate in the peritoneal cavity. The typical sources of entry are contamination of the sterile exchange procedure and migration through the peritoneal catheter tunnel from an infected exit site. The development of cloudy dialysate and dialysate leukocytosis (>100 white blood cells per mm^3) are characteristic. In bacterial peritonitis, greater than 50% of leukocytes are neutrophils. Abdominal pain and tenderness almost always occur, but fever is often absent in milder cases.

The ability to obtain a positive culture result in bacterial peritonitis is largely dependent on culture technique. Proper technique may increase the yield of positive cultures from 50% to more than 90%. Currently recommended are the use of standard blood culture media for initial incubation, the concentration of the specimen by centrifugation or membrane filtration, and minimum observation periods of 7 days for aerobic cultures and 2 to 3 weeks for fastidious organisms.

The most common peritoneal infecting organism, *S epidermidis*, tends to produce milder infections that are easily treated. Severe infections, which might require intensive care and produce systemic manifestations, should raise the suspicion of *S aureus* or gram-negative bacteria, including *Pseudomonas aeruginosa*. Fecal peritonitis, arising from a bowel source such as diverticulitis, appendicitis, ischemic bowel, or perforation, may be particularly virulent. Occasionally, fecal material is apparent in the peritoneal drainage. This diagnosis must also be suspected when multiple organisms are cultured from the peritoneal fluid, including gram-negative organisms and sometimes anaerobes.

As in any infected patient, recovery of the offending organism and identification of its source are of primary importance. If no likely source is discovered, the dialysis access must be strongly considered. Antibiotic dosage and timing must be adjusted for the lack of renal metabolism and clearance. If at all possible, hemodialysis with cellulosic membranes should be avoided and membranes with greater biocompatibility substituted. Cellulosic membranes appear to have deleterious effects on neutrophil function. The dialysis procedure may also significantly lower antibiotic concentration, requiring supplemental dosages after treatment.

As already mentioned, careful culture techniques enable the recovery of the offending organism in most cases of peritonitis. Two initial rapid exchanges through the peritoneal catheter help relieve pain. Loading doses of antibiotics may be given intravenously or intraperitoneally. Antibiotic levels are then maintained through continuous addition to the peritoneal dialysate. Empiric broad-spectrum coverage appropriate for both gram-positive and gram-negative organisms is begun until culture results are known. Coverage is then narrowed, guided by in vitro susceptibilities. Dialysate leukocyte counts are followed to ensure resolution of the infection.

CHEST PAIN ■

The increased prevalence of ischemic coronary artery disease in this patient population is well documented.[2] Hypertension is probably the most important risk factor for atherogenesis.[35,36] Other contributing factors are dyslipidemia, abnormal calcium and phosphorus metabolism, and abnormal glucose tolerance. The renal failure patient presenting with chest pain must therefore be suspected of having myocardial ischemia or infarction. As previously discussed, pericardial disease must also be kept in mind.

The evaluation of the acutely ill renal patient with suspected coronary disease requires the consideration of coronary angiography. In the patient who is already dialysis-dependent, the risk of radiocontrast agents is small. However, the hyperosmolar nature of these agents may cause pulmonary congestion from circulatory overload. If volume overload is a potential problem, arrangements should be made for acute dialysis following the angiographic procedure. The patient with preexisting renal insufficiency, not yet requiring dialysis, is clearly at increased risk for contrast-induced acute renal failure.[37,38] The simultaneous presence of diabetes, volume depletion, and LV dysfunction increase the risk.[39–41] Although results in different studies are variable, roughly 25% of patients with at least moderate renal insufficiency develop significant renal dysfunction after cardiac angiography. The risk doubles when diabetic nephropathy

TABLE 144-2. Minimizing the Risk of Contrast Nephropathy

Ensure adequate hydration[43]:
  Diabetics—0.5 NS at 1 mL/kg/h. Starting 12 h before procedure, continuing for 24 h postprocedure
  Nondiabetics—Add mannitol 25 g to run 3 h before and 3 h postprocedure
If LV function is compromised:
  Inotropic agents
  Dopamine at 2 µg/kg/min (nondiabetics only)
Limit dye load to less than 125 mL of contrast agent[40]
Nonionic contrast agent[42]
Theophylline[65]

is present. Five to 10 percent of patients require dialysis, rarely permanently. Careful preparation can reduce the risk of contrast nephropathy (Table 144-2). Recent studies have shown that nonionic contrast agents lessen the risk of nephrotoxicity in patients with preexisting azotemia (creatinine >1.8).[42] The prophylactic use of furosemide can no longer be recommended.[43] The most effective prophylaxis appears to be simple intravascular volume expansion with crystalloids.[43] Theophylline may be of adjunctive value.[44]

The indications for and usage of heparin or thrombolytic agents for acute myocardial infarction are unchanged in the patient with chronic renal failure.[45,46] However, dosages should be carefully titrated to achieve therapeutic effect because uremic bleeding may be potentiated. Recent puncture sites in a hemodialysis access can lead to troublesome hemorrhage when thrombolytics are given. Recent studies have looked at coronary artery bypass surgery and coronary angioplasty in the dialysis patient. For bypass surgery, perioperative mortality is variable, usually in the range of 5% to 10%.[47–50] Longer-term postoperative survival is similar to the dialysis population at large and relief of symptoms is excellent.[49–51] For these reasons, indications for bypass surgery are the same in the dialysis population as in patients without renal disease. Extra care must be taken in assessing the possibility of bleeding. Template bleeding time should be checked. Normalizing bleeding defect (see Table 144-1) decreases the risk of significant hemorrhage. Several disappointing studies have appeared with regard to coronary angioplasty,[50,52,53] documenting a very high restenosis and failure rate. There is therefore less enthusiasm for this procedure in the end-stage renal disease population than in patients without renal disease.

CARDIAC ARRHYTHMIAS ■

When patients with renal failure present with cardiac arrhythmias, disorders of electrolytes or acid-base abnormalities must be identified and corrected. In addition, coronary artery disease should be strongly suspected.

Ventricular arrhythmias may frequently occur during, and for several hours after, hemodialysis. Patients prone to ventricular arrhythmias include those with impaired cardiac performance and high calcium–phosphorus concentration products.[54] Nonsustained ventricular tachycardia is frequently seen before sudden death in these patients.

The search for abnormalities of acid-base, electrolytes, calcium, and magnesium must be complete. Severe acidemia (serum pH <7.10 or alkalemia pH >7.60) clearly predisposes to ventricular arrhythmias especially in patients with underlying cardiac disorders. Hypokalemia is associated with variable cardiac rhythm disturbances, especially in the presence of digitalis. Progressive rhythm disturbances leading to ventricular standstill due to hyperkalemia are not uncommonly seen. Hypocalcemia, hyponatremia, and acidemia all enhance the cardiac toxicity of hyperkalemia. Heart block has rarely been reported with hypocalcemia alone.

Recent literature has emphasized the role of hypomagnesemia in ventricular and supraventricular arrhythmias.[55,56]

TABLE 144-3. Antiarrhythmic Drug Dosing in Renal Failure

DRUG	ELIMINATION AND METABOLISM	DOSAGE	ADJUSTMENT–MAINTENANCE DOSE (GFR mL/min)		REMARKS
			10–50	*<10*	
Amiodarone	Hepatic	Load 800–1600 mg/d for 1–3 wk. Then 400–600 mg/d	No change	No change	Frequent toxicity; pulmonary hepatic thyroid; no supplement postdialysis
Bretylium	Renal	5–10 mg/kg q 6 h or constant infusion 1–2 mg/mL after load	25–50% of dose	25% of dose	Hypotension common; supplement 50% of dose postdialysis
Disopyramide	Renal, hepatic	100–150 mg q 6 h	50% of dose	25–50% of dose	Postdialysis supplement probably necessary
Lidocaine	Hepatic, renal	0.7–1.4 mg/kg IV load; 1–4 mg/min infusion	No change	No change	No supplement postdialysis
Flecainide	Hepatic, renal	100 mg bid to start; titrate up to 200–300 mg bid	No change	50% of dose	
Mexiletine	Hepatic, renal	200–300 mg q 8 h	No change	No change	
Procainamide	Renal, hepatic	2–4 g/d in divided doses or IV load up to 600 mg; infuse 2–6 mg/min	50%	25% of dose; avoid, if metabolites accumulate	Must closely follow drug and NAPA (metabolite) levels; excess may provoke torsades des pointes
Propafenone	Hepatic, renal	150–300 mg q 8 h	No change	No change	Decrease dose with hepatic dysfunction
Quinidine	Hepatic, renal	200–500 mg q 8 h	No change	No change	No supplemental dose postdialysis
Sotalol	Renal	80–160 mg bid	25–50% of dose	25% of dose	May need to individualize dosage with very low GFR. Avoid hypokalemia

GFR, Glomerular filtration rate; NAPA, *N*-acetylprocainamide.

Hypomagnesemia is surprisingly common in dialysis patients, especially immediately after dialysis and in those on diuretics. Magnesium infusions are increasingly recommended in the setting of acute arrhythmias. Of course, in patients with renal failure, hypermagnesemia may occur. However, toxic effects are rarely severe and tend to occur only at very high magnesium levels. Measurements of serum magnesium concentration are readily available and should be carefully followed.

The overall approach to antiarrhythmic therapy is not altered by the presence of renal failure, except as it affects the pharmacokinetics of therapeutic agents (Table 144-3).

RESPIRATORY FAILURE ■

Respiratory failure in patients with chronic azotemia is usually caused by circulatory overload. Several factors may contribute including dietary noncompliance, arterial hypertension, and systolic or diastolic myocardial dysfunction, as outlined earlier. Acute myocardial infarction must also be excluded. In addition, there is evidence that some uremic patients have increased pulmonary capillary membrane permeability and so-called uremic pulmonary edema.[57] The chest radiograph typically reveals cardiomegaly, evidence of pulmonary vascular congestion, or frank pulmonary edema with pleural effusion. However, uremic patients may also present with atypical chest radiograph findings (including unilateral or segmental infiltrates) but still respond well to therapy aimed at ECF contraction alone.

Therapy is initially targeted to reducing volume overload. If residual renal function is present, diuretics may be useful. Loop diuretics have the greatest efficacy, but large doses are needed due to limited delivery into the urine in patients with marked renal insufficiency. Furosemide, 80 mg IV (160 mg PO), or bumetanide, 4 mg IV or PO, are recommended starting doses. If the response is inadequate, a "ceiling" dose of furosemide (200 mg IV or 400 mg PO) or bumetanide (10 mg IV or PO) may be tried.[58,59] (Intravenous infusions should run over 15 to 20 minutes to avoid ototoxicity.) Higher doses are unlikely to produce added benefit. The addition of a thiazide or metolazone may produce a diuresis when combined with the loop diuretic in the unresponsive patient.

Torsemide is a recently released loop diuretic that may have greater efficiency in patients with renal failure or heart failure.[60] The intravenous and oral dosage regimens feature a direct milligram-for-milligram conversion. With renal insufficiency, a 50-mg or 100-mg dose should be tried. The recommended ceiling dosage is 200 mg. Doses can be repeated every 8 to 12 hours.

The use of continuous furosemide infusions has gained increasing clinical acceptance.[61] Increased diuretic efficiency, especially in difficult patients, is seen. An initial bolus of 40 mg IV is followed by a continuous infusion of 10 to 20 mg/hour, usually in a 1:1 solution mixed in dextrose 5% in water.

Ultrafiltration dialysis is the mainstay of therapy in the fluid-overloaded CRF patient. With the use of "dry" ultrafiltration (with no dialysate but simply a negative pressure applied across the dialyzer membrane), fluid removal is rapid, measured, and complicated by less hypotension than standard hemodialysis. In the peritoneal dialysis patient, hypertonic dialysate exchanges with dwell times shortened to 60 to 90 minutes optimize fluid removal.

When volume overload is accompanied by hypertension, the increased afterload contributes to pulmonary congestion. Volume reduction alone may lower blood pressure effectively. Sometimes, antihypertensive agents are needed. With severe hypertension, sodium nitroprusside is a highly reliable vasodilator. Unfortunately, the toxic metabolite thiocyanate may accumulate in renal failure, producing metabolic acidosis and neurologic changes. Infusions should be limited to 48 hours or less unless thiocyanate levels can be carefully monitored in a timely fashion. Minoxidil is also a potent and effective vasodilator but must be given orally. Metabolism is unchanged in renal failure. Of the calcium channel blockers, dihydropyrolidines are the most potent antihypertensives and require no special considerations in the renal failure patient. Due to their negative inotropic effects, beta-blockers are usually avoided in this circumstance. Angiotensin converting enzyme (ACE) inhibitors may be used, but half-lives are markedly prolonged; for this reason once or twice daily captopril is favored rather than the longer-acting agents. Enalapril is available intravenously, but initial doses should be very low (0.625 mg IV q 6 to 12 hours).

In the intensive care setting, many patients cannot be treated by the enteral route. Intravenous nitroprusside and enalapril have already been mentioned. Other good choices include intravenous labetalol (intermittent or continuous infusion), intravenous diltiazem (continuous infusion), or transcutaneus clonidine patches.

Other causes of respiratory compromise must also be considered. Chronic renal failure patients with central neurologic abnormalities or frequent hypotensive episodes on dialysis are predisposed to pneumonia. Impaired neutrophil function, as discussed previously, may slow the response to treatment. Although opportunistic infections are rare, outbreaks of tuberculosis have been reported in some dialysis populations.[32] The incidence of clinically significant pulmonary emboli is certainly lower in this population than in other groups with chronic diseases.[62] However, pulmonary embolism can occur and must be considered in the appropriate setting.[63] The issue of prophylaxis with low-dose intermittent heparin is unsettled.

When the patient with preexisting renal failure presents with unusual pulmonary manifestations, the so-called pulmonary-renal syndromes should be considered. Anti–glomerular basement membrane (GBM) antibody-induced renal disease, which presents initially without pulmonary involvement, almost never produces pulmonary hemorrhage in a delayed fashion. On the other hand, renal involvement may precede pulmonary manifestations in Wegener granulomatous vasculitis, occasionally by several years. Antineutrophilic cytoplasmic antibodies are helpful in diagnosis of these patients.

DISORDERED CONSCIOUSNESS ■

The patient with chronic renal failure may present with disordered consciousness severe enough to require intensive care. Special diagnostic considerations related to the uremic state or the dialysis procedure should be entertained.

The predialysis uremic patient may present with delirium, seizures, or even coma. There is typically a history of progressive symptoms of increasing severity. The initiation of dialysis leads to resolution of these symptoms within several days. Toxic concentrations of medications metabolized or excreted by the kidneys also must be considered.

The patient newly initiated on hemodialysis may develop *dialysis dysequilibrium syndrome*.[64] New dialysis patients may have very high levels of urea and other retained solutes in the extracellular fluid. Rapid removal quickly lowers ECF osmolarity causing water to shift into the relatively hypertonic intracellular space. Brain cell swelling can produce manifestations of cerebral edema, including headache, nausea, vomiting, and even seizures, coma, or death. The syndrome is prevented by initiating dialysis with short, low-flow sessions using dialyzers with small surface area. Intravenous mannitol is also used in the first few sessions to maintain the tonicity of the ECF.

Widespread hypertension and atherosclerosis predispose to cerebrovascular accident, with typical presentation. Subarachnoid bleeding occurs with greater frequency in hemodialysis patients, partly related to anticoagulant excess. Subdural hematoma is also surprisingly common in this patient population. The manifestations may be acute or chronic. Wernicke encephalopathy is also occasionally seen in chronic dialysis patients. Thiamine is a water-soluble vitamin that is lost into the dialysate. If this vitamin is not adequately replaced, deficiency can develop. As in other cases, intravenous thiamine is indicated for treatment.

Technical complications of the dialysis procedure can result in severe, acute neurologic disorders. Errors in proportioning of dialysate can lead to hypo- or hyperosmolar syndromes, resulting in seizures, coma, or death. Acute copper intoxication may occur when acidic water comes into contact with copper tubing. The dialysate changes from colorless to blue-green in this circumstance. Symptoms include headache, nausea, emesis, and confusion.

Finally, patients may develop a progressive neurologic syndrome known as *dialysis dementia*. This is a rapidly progressive myoclonic dementia, occasionally accompanied by seizures. It is most closely associated with exposure to aluminum especially through contaminated dialysate water.[65] Some cases occur in patients with a history of substantial intake of aluminum-containing phosphate binders. Treatment consists of deferoxamine chelation therapy, with some reports of improvement. Generally, the disorder is irreversible.

REFERENCES ■

1. Lazarus JM, Lowrie EG, Hampers CL, et al: Cardiovascular disease in uremic patients on hemodialysis. *Kidney Int* 1975;7(Suppl 2):167
2. Lindner A, Charra B, Sherrard DJ, et al: Accelerated atherosclerosis in prolonged maintenance hemodialysis. *N Engl J Med* 1974;290:697
3. Johnson WJ, Kurtz SB, Mitchell JC, et al: Results of treatment of center hemodialysis patients. *Mayo Clin Proc* 1984;59:669
4. Lai KN, Ng J, Whitford J, et al: Left ventricular function in uremia: echocardiographic and radionuclide assessment in patients on maintenance hemodialysis. *Clin Nephrol* 1985;23:125
5. London GM, Marchais SJ, Guerin AP, et al: Cardiovascular function in hemodialysis patients. *Adv Nephrol* 1991;20:249
6. Low I, Grutzmacher P, Bergmann M, et al: Echocardiographic findings in patients on maintenance hemodialysis substituted with recombiant human erythropoietin. *Clin Nephrol* 1989;31:26
7. Burt RK, Gupta-Burt S, Suki WN, et al: Reversal of left ventricular dysfunction after renal transplantation. *Ann Intern Med* 1989;111:635
8. Ikram H, Lynn KL, Bailey RR, et al: Cardiovascular changes in chronic hemodialysis patients. *Kidney Int* 1983;24:371
9. Silberberg JS, Barre PE, Prichard SS, et al: Impact of left ventricular hypertrophy on survival in end-stage renal disease. *Kidney Int* 1989;36:286
10. Huting J, Kramer W, Charra B, et al: Asymmetric septal hypertrophy and left atrial dilatation in patients with end stage renal disease on long-term hemodialysis. *Clin Nephrol* 1989;32:276
11. Kramer W, Wisemann V, Lammlein G, et al: Systolic and diastolic properties of the left ventricle assessed by invasive methods. *Contrib Nephrol* 1986;52:97
12. Boyle JM, Johnston B: Acute upper gastrointestinal hemorrhage in patients with chronic renal disease. *Am J Med* 1983;75:409
13. Zuckerman GR, Cornette GL, Clouse RE, et al: Upper gastrointestinal bleeding in patients with chronic renal failure. *Ann Intern Med* 1985;102:588
14. Rosenblah SG/lm, Drake S, Fadem S, et al: Gastrointestinal blood loss in patients with chronic renal failure. *Am J Kidney Dis* 1987;1:232
15. DiMinno G, Martinez J, McLean ML, et al: Platelet dysfunction in uremia. *Am J Med* 1985;79:552
16. Jubelirer SJ: Hemostatic abnormalities in renal disease. *Am J Kidney Dis* 1985;5:219
17. Liuio M, Marchese D, Remuzzi G, et al: Uraemic bleeding: role of anaemia and beneficial effect of red cell transfusions. *Lancet* 1982;2:1013
18. Moia M, Vizzotto L, Cattaneo M, et al: Improvement in the hemostatic defect in uremia after treatment with human erythropoietin. *Lancet* 1987;2:1227
19. Janson PA, Jubelirer SJ, Weinstein MJ, et al; Treatment of the bleeding tendency in uremia with cryoprecipitate. *N Engl J Med* 1980;303:1318
20. Mannucci PM, Remuzzi G, Dusineri F, et al: Deamino-8-

21. arginine vasopressin shortens the bleeding time in uremia. *N Engl J Med* 1983;308:8
22. Liuio M, Manucci PM, Vigano G, et al: Conjugated estrogens for the management of bleeding associated with renal failure. *N Engl J Med* 1986;315:731
23. Luft FC, Gilman JK, Weyman AE: Pericarditis in the patient with uremia: clinical and echo-cardiographic evaluation. *Nephron* 1980;25:160
24. Silverberg S, Oreopoulas DG, Wise DJ, et al: Pericarditis in patients undergoing long-term hemodialysis and peritoneal dialysis. *Am J Med* 1977;63:874
25. Drueke T, lePuilleur C, Zingraff J, et al: Uremic cardiomyopathy and pericarditis. *Adv Nephrol* 1980;9:33
26. Osanloo E, Shalhoub RJ, Cioffi RF, et al: Viral pericarditis in patients receiving hemodialysis. *Arch Intern Med* 1979;139:301
27. Asaba H, Alvestrand A, Bergstrom J, et al: Uremic middle molecules in non-dialysis azotemic patients: relation to symptoms and clinical biochemistries. *Clin Nephrol* 1982;17:90
28. Twardowski ZJ, Alpert MA, Gupta RC, et al: Circulating immune complexes: possible toxins responsible for serositis in renal failure. *Nephron* 1983;35:190
29. Buselmeier TJ, Davin TD, Simmons RC, et al: Treatment of intractable uremic pericardial effusion. *JAMA* 1978;240:1358
30. Spector D, Alfred H, Siedlecki M, et al: A controlled study of the effect of indomethacin in uremic pericarditis. *Kidney Int* 1983;24:663
31. Reddy PS, Curtis EI, O'Toole JD, et al: Cardiac tamponade: hemodynamic observations in man. *Circulation* 1978;58:265
32. Nelson J, Ormrod DJ, Miller TE: Host immune status in uremia: leukocyte response to bacterial infection in chronic renal failure. *Nephron* 1985;39:21
33. Goldman M, Vanderwegham JL: Bacterial infections in chronic hemodialysis patients. *Adv Nephrol* 1990;19:315
34. Keane WF, Shapiro FL, Raij CR: Incidence and type of infections occurring in 445 chronic hemodialysis patients. *Trans Am Soc Artif Intern Organs* 1977;23:41
35. Nsouli KA, Lazarus JM, Schoenbaum SC, et al: Bacteremic infection in hemodialysis. *Arch Intern Med* 1979;139:1255
36. Rostand SG, Kirk KA, Rutsky EA: Relationship of coronary risk factors to hemodialysis-associated ischemic heart disease. *Kidney Int* 1982;22:304
37. Charra B, Calemard E, Cuche M, et al: Control of hypertension and prolonged survival on maintenance hemodialysis. *Nephron* 1983;33:96
38. D'Elia JA, Gleason RE, Alday M, et al: Nephrotoxicity from angiographic contrast material. *Am J Med* 1982;72:719
39. Cochran ST, Wong WS, Roe DJ: Predicting angiography induced acute renal function impairment. *AJR* 1983;141:1027
40. Manske CL, Sprafka JM, Strong JT, et al: Contrast nephropathy in azotemic diabetic patients undergoing coronary angiography. *Am J Med* 1990;89:615
41. Taliercio CP, Vlietstra RE, Fisher LD, et al: Risks for renal dysfunction with cardiac angiography. *Ann Intern Med* 1986;109:501
42. Paredero UM, Dixon SM, Baker JD, et al: Risk of renal failure after major angiography. *Arch Surg* 1983;118:1417
43. Rudnick MR, Goldfarb S, Wexler L, et al: Nephrotoxicity of ionic and non-ionic contrast media in 1196 patients: a randomized trial. *Kidney Int* 1995;47:254
44. Solomon R, Werner C, Mann D, et al: Effects of saline, mannitol and furosemide on acute declines in renal function induced by radiocontrast agents. *N Engl J Med* 1994;331:1416
45. Erlive CM, Duda SH, Schlepekow S, et al: Adenosine antagonist theophylline prevents the reduction of glomerular filtration rate after contrast media application. *Kidney Int* 1994;45:1425

45. Bell WR, Meek AG: Guidelines for the use of thrombolytic therapy. *N Engl J Med* 1979;301:1266

46. Teien AN, Bjornson J: Heparin elimination in uremic patients on hemodialysis. *Scand J Hematol* 1977;17:29

47. Kaul TE, Fields BL, Reddy MA, et al: Cardiac operations in end stage renal disease. *Ann Thorac Surg* 1994;57:691

48. Deutsch E, Bernstein RC, Addomzio VP, et al: Coronary artery bypass surgery in patients on chronic hemodialysis: a case-control study. *Ann Intern Med* 1989;110:369

49. Owen CH, Cummings RG, Sell TL, et al: Coronary artery bypass grafting in patients with dialysis-dependent renal failure. *Ann Thorac Surg* 1994;58:1729

50. Rinehart AL, Herzog CA, Collins AJ, et al: A comparison of coronary angioplasty and coronary artery bypass grafting outcomes in chronic dialysis patients. *Am J Kidney Dis* 1995;25:281

51. Zamora JL, Burdine JT, Karlberg HK, et al: Cardiac surgery in patients with end stage renal disease. *Ann Thorac Surg* 1986;42:113

52. Ahmed WH, Shubrooks SJ, Gibson CM, et al: Complications and long term outcome after percutaneus coronary angioplasty in chronic hemodialysis patients. *Am Heart J* 1994, 128:252

53. Reusser LM, Osborn LA, White HJ, et al: Increased morbidity after coronary angioplasty in patients on chronic hemodialysis. *Am J Cardiol* 1994;73:965

54. Kimura K, Tabei K, Asano Y, et al: Cardiac arrhythmias in hemodialysis patients. *Nephron* 1989;53:201

55. Iseri LT: Role of magnesium in cardiac tachyarrhythmias. *Am J Cardiol* 1990;65:47K

56. Tzivoni D, Keren A: Suppression of ventricular arrythmias by magnesium. *Am J Cardiol* 1990;65:1397

57. Rackow EC, Fein IA, Sprung G, et al: Uremic pulmonary edema. *Am J Med* 1978;64:1084

58. Brater DC: Use of diuretics in chronic renal insufficiency and nephrotic syndrome. *Semin Nephrol* 1988;8:333

59. Brater DC, Anderson SA, Cartwright DB: Response to furosemide in chronic renal insufficiency: rationale for limited doses. *Clin Pharmacol Ther* 1986;40:134

60. Gehr TW, Rudy DW, Matzke GR, et al: The pharmacokinetics of intravenous and oral torsemide in patients with chronic renal insufficiency. *Clin Pharmacol Ther* 1994;56:31

61. Martin SJ, Danziger LH: Continuous infusion of loop diuretics in the critically ill: a review of the literature. *Crit Care Med* 1994;22:1323

62. Mossey RT, Kasabian AA, Wilkes BM, et al: Pulmonary embolism: low incidence in chronic renal failure. *Arch Intern Med* 1982;142:1986

63. Guntupalli K, Soffer O, Baciewicz P: Pulmonary embolism in end stage renal disease. *Intensive Care Med* 1990;16:405

64. Rose SM, O'Connor K, Shaldon S: Hemodialysis dysequilibrium. *BMJ* 1964;2:672

65. Flending JA, Kruis H, Das HA: Aluminum and dialysis dementia. *Lancet* 1976;1:1235

Critical Care, Third Edition, edited by Joseph M. Civetta,
Robert W. Taylor, and Robert R. Kirby.
Lippincott-Raven Publishers, Philadelphia, PA © 1997.

CHAPTER 145

■

Disordered Glucose Metabolism

Dan R. Thompson

IMMEDIATE CONCERNS ■

MAJOR PROBLEMS

1. Diabetes is a common illness that all physicians see in one form or another. Diabetic ketoacidosis (DKA) and hyperglycemic hyperosmolar nonketotic state (HHNK) represent opposite ends of the spectrum of the same disease.
2. Patients may present with diabetes mellitus (DM) alone or in association with other diseases.
3. Familiarity with the basic concepts of diabetic pathophysiology and treatment including the use of insulin permits the physician to rapidly control the situation.
4. This chapter reviews the more urgent and emergent aspects of treatment of the diabetic patient and focuses particularly on DKA and HHNK.

STRESS POINTS

1. DKA develops in patients with relative or absolute insulin lack.
2. Hydrolysis of triglycerides causes release of free fatty acids (FFA) into the blood stream.
3. FFA are converted to ketone bodies causing metabolic acidosis.
4. The patient with HHNK has low but residual insulin secretion. This balances counterregulatory hormone activity and suppresses ketone body formation.
5. In the absence of insulin, glucose cannot enter cells and the extracellular space becomes profoundly hyperosmolar.

6. An osmotic diuresis ensues. Patients with DKA and HHNK are often profoundly volume depleted.
7. Total body potassium depletion may be dramatic.

ESSENTIAL DIAGNOSTIC TESTS AND PROCEDURES

1. A careful history and physical examination is important.
2. A search for the cause of DKA or HHNK is warranted.
3. Frequent determinations of blood glucose, ketones, and electrolytes should be performed initially. Hourly blood glucose determinations should be performed until the blood glucose reaches 200 to 250 mg/dL.

INITIAL THERAPY

1. Institute volume expansion with intravenous (IV) normal saline. Give 1 L within the first hour.
2. Treat any underlying cause of DKA or HHNK (infection, etc.).
3. Institute intravenous regular insulin treatment (0.1 unit/kg bolus, followed by 0.1 unit/kg/hour continuous infusion). Adjust the insulin infusion according to the patient's response. The patient with HHNK may be very responsive to insulin.
4. Begin potassium replacement when serum potassium falls into normal range.
5. Switch to dextrose-containing solutions (D5 0.9 saline, D5 0.45 saline) when the blood glucose reaches 200 to 250 mg/dL.

DISORDERED GLUCOSE METABOLISM ■

EPIDEMIOLOGY

The National Institutes of Health reports that 3.6% of the US population has diabetes mellitus (DM) and between 90% and 95% of the population has non–insulin dependent diabetes mellitus (NIDDM). About 3.2% of the population meets the criteria for diagnosis, but they have not been diagnosed and 11.2% has impaired glucose tolerance.[1] Lebovitz reports that in 1987, 1.25% of hospital admissions were for DKA and in these patients the mortality was 2%, or 0.25 per 1000 admissions.[2] DKA was an admitting diagnosis for 8.6% of insulin dependent diabetes mellitus (IDDM) patients in the preceding 12 years.

Mortality is primarily related to sepsis, or cardiopulmonary complications. Age has a profound influence on mortality. Patients greater than 65 years of age experience a 20% mortality compared with 2% in younger adults. It is rare for children to die of DKA. The capacity to withstand the stresses of DM diminishes with age and the ravages of the disease, and when coexisting medical illnesses occur these factors become more crucial in determining outcome. In our ICU rarely is death secondary to DKA. Yet one must constantly be prepared for the other medical problems that coexist in these patients. Patients may present with diabetes or the episode may mark the beginning of their disease.

DIABETIC KETOACIDOSIS ■

CLINICAL DESCRIPTION

The diagnosis of DKA is usually not difficult (Table 145-1). About 20% of DKA patients represent newly diagnosed IDDM. Seventy-five percent of patients have an identifiable cause (Table 145-2). Of these patients, 50% have infection as the underlying basis, 20% have DKA secondary to noncompliance with their treatment regimen, and 30% represent inadequate insulin use by patient or physician. Taking a careful history may provide the answers. DKA most often occurs in the patient with IDDM but may occur in NIDDM. The physician must remember that the two diseases are ends of a spectrum.

PATHOGENESIS[3–6]

DKA develops in a condition of relative or absolute insulin deficiency and relative excess of three counterregulatory hormones: epinephrine, cortisol, and glucagon. Metabolism

TABLE 145-1. Diagnosis of Diabetic Ketoacidosis

1. Hyperglycemia >250 mg/dL
2. Low bicarbonate <15 mEq/L
3. Low pH <7.3
4. Ketonemia >1:2 dilution
5. Moderate ketonuria

TABLE 145-2. Precipitating Factors in DKA–Hyperosmolar Coma

1. Insulin insufficiency
   Relative
   Absolute
2. Infection
   Urinary tract infection
   Other
   May be trivial
3. Insufficient water intake
   Suppressed thirst
   Lack of access to water
4. Stress
   Cortisol release
   Epinephrine release
5. Hypokalemia
   Inhibits insulin secretion
   Decreases insulin sensitivity
6. Drugs
   Alcohol
   Glucocorticoids
   Beta-blockers
   Thiazides and other diuretics
   Phenytoin
   Calcium channel blockers

in the liver, adipose tissue, and muscle converts to a state of profound catabolism. Catabolism in the liver results in the breakdown of glycogen stores to glucose; in adipose tissue catabolism results in the hydrolysis of fat to triglyceride, and in the muscle catabolism results in breakdown of muscle protein to amino acids and conversion to glucose.

In adipose tissue hormone-sensitive lipase causes hydrolysis of triglycerides and release of FFA. The excess of glucagon and lack of insulin reset the metabolism of the liver. FFA are converted to ketones in contrast to the usual conversion to carbon dioxide or storage as triglyceride. Abnormal tissue metabolism does not allow for ketone use and as a result ketone levels accumulate. Ketones are composed of the strong acids beta-hydroxybutyric acid and acetoacetate. The third component is acetone, which contributes little other than the odor characteristic of patients in DKA. These strong acids (pK 3.8 at body pH) are buffered by bicarbonate and by the proteins of the body's buffering system, resulting in a net loss of bicarbonate. Excretion of the buffered acids and the loss of total buffering capacity result in acidosis. The appearance of acidemia depends on failure of the buffering capacity and failure of the urinary acidification systems. Ketones are excreted as sodium and potassium salts. Loss of ketones represents loss of potential bicarbonate on treatment with insulin and recovery.[7]

Gluconeogenesis results in the production of tremendous amounts of glucose. Amino acids are rapidly converted to glucose, but because of the relative lack of insulin, glucose cannot be transported into the cells nor metabolized. There is a combination of overproduction and decreased peripheral use. The result is hyperglycemia.

The balance of the two processes determines whether DKA or HHNK is the result. The relative activity of insulin determines whether ketoacidosis is present. Ketoacidosis is primarily a consequence of a profound lack of insulin.

The tremendous amount of glucose presented to the intravascular space results in profound diuresis from the osmolar load. Saturation of the reabsorption transport system allows massive amounts of glucose to remain in the tubules, and production of an osmotic gradient incompatible with water concentration. The resulting losses include not only water, bicarbonate and glucose, but also ketones, nitrogen, sodium, potassium, bicarbonate, phosphate, and magnesium.

LABORATORY FEATURES

The glucose concentrations can exceed 800 mg% but usually average between 500 mg% and 700 mg/dL. In 15% of patients, blood glucose levels at presentation may be less than 350 mg/dL. Alcoholics and pregnant patients, in particular, may present with lower blood glucose levels. Actively drinking alcoholics may have low levels because ethanol inhibits gluconeogenesis. In pregnancy, the fetus does not depend on insulin secretion by the mother for absorption and acts as a glucose sink for the mother's blood.

By definition, these patients usually present with significant metabolic acidosis. We have seen patients with a pH of less than 6.8 on admission who have survived. The acidosis is usually of the anion gap type. We can calculate the anion gap with the following formula:

$$\text{Anion gap} = Na^+ \text{ mEq} + (Cl^- \text{ mEq} + HCO_3 \text{ mEq})$$

$$= 8 \text{ to } 12 \text{ mEq}$$

Some newer chemistry instruments for analyzing electrolytes produce higher levels of chloride resulting in reduction of the calculated anion gap.[8] By not recognizing that the normal anion gap is actually lower, the patient with a high anion gap may be missed. Decreases in the anion gap secondary to instrumentation may obscure ketones when they are in fact present. We need to know what a normal anion gap is in a particular hospital. The anion gap represents the anions that are not part of the routine measurement with chloride and bicarbonate.

Albumin is the predominant anion not normally measured. In DKA, increased ketones add to the anion gap. Patients may also present with an existing hyperchloremic metabolic acidosis and have a low anion gap. The patient with ketones has retained these molecules because of a lower urinary clearance secondary to dehydration. Patients who present with low ketones and high chlorides most likely represent a state of better preservation of volume. Ketones are excreted as sodium and potassium salts.

Water losses are about 10% of body weight or 100 mL/kg. Because of the derangements in sodium, creatinine and glucose, the usual laboratory features of dehydration may not be obvious. The patient may actually appear to be vasodilated with dehydration and abdominal pain secondary to excess prostaglandin production.[3]

Sodium levels are usually low. The patient with severe dehydration, however, may have a serum sodium of greater than 150 mEq/L. Total body deficits are about 7 to 10 mEq/

kg. Serum hyperosmolarity causes redistribution of fluid into the intravascular space and results in low sodium concentration. The sodium level without the effects of fluid shift by glucose may be calculated by the following formula:

$$Na^+ \text{ mEq} = \frac{(\text{glucose} - 100)}{100} \times 1.6 \text{ mEq} + Na^+ \text{ mEq}$$

The actual level is not factitious but is an artifact caused by the inward movement of water. Sodium levels may be factitiously low if the patient has hyperlipidemia. Lipid increases the measured volume, but the sodium is contained only in the water. The result is hyponatremia. Lactescent serum may be a clue to those performing the analysis.

Potassium levels may be low (4%), normal (74%), or elevated (22%).[3] Normally the serum level represents only 2% of total body stores. High potassium level is secondary to several factors. The acidemia causes exchange of hydrogen ion for potassium ion in the intracellular space, potassium shifts out of the cells secondary to the hyperosmolarity of the intravascular space, and potassium production is increased during breakdown of proteins to amino acids. Potassium is not carried into the cell as usual with transport of glucose.[3] Urinary losses are high in combination with ketones and then both potassium and ketones are excreted. Hyperaldosteronism, secondary to dehydration, causes urinary excretion of potassium rather than sodium.

Patients with low potassium levels may have major preexisting total body depletion of potassium secondary to diuretic therapy or protracted vomiting. These patients may be at great risk of developing malignant arrhythmias and other manifestations of low potassium. Treatment with insulin moves glucose into the cells, corrects acidemia, and reverses the hydrogen–potassium exchange. These factors may aggravate critically low intravascular potassium levels. Some have advocated careful treatment with potassium and volume replacement before giving insulin to prevent further hypokalemia. Total body potassium losses represent 3 to 5 mEq/kg and may total up to 300 to 600 mEq.

Magnesium deficiency is seldom important and losses are very modest. Total body loss ranges from 0.2 to 1.0 mM/kg. Phosphate therapy causing calcium precipitation may unmask low magnesium levels that may occur in treating hypokalemia. Hypomagnesemia may manifest itself by carpal tunnel syndrome, muscle spasms, and tetany.[9]

Phosphate levels are normally elevated in DKA. The phosphate deficit is about 1 mM/kg or 60 mM to 70 mM of a total body phosphate of 6000 to 8000 mM. Increased levels in the face of decreased total body stores are secondary to dehydration and the decrease in renal clearance associated with profound diuresis or diarrhea.

Thirty percent of patients with DKA have abdominal pain, particularly those with bicarbonate levels of less than 10 mEq/L.[3] The older diabetic patient with abdominal pain usually represents a major concern because of the propensity for abdominal pathology. Patients with DKA frequently also have elevated amylase levels. Some patients have abdominal pain and elevated amylase levels and some have one or the other. Critically ill patients frequently have elevations of amylase, the source of which has been found to be from the pancreas in only 40% of cases. In the other 60%, the source has been clearly identified as the salivary glands. Investigations of patients with DKA have found that hyperamylasemia is secondary to salivary gland pathology. These findings are confirmed by fractionation of the enzyme and lack of inflammation of the pancreas on abdominal computed tomography (CT) scan.[10] Hyperamylasemia has been found to be a feature of acidosis and not necessarily indicative of pancreatis in DKA.[11]

Cross-reaction of the reagents involved in the creatinine determination may falsely elevate the results of this test. Renal function may be better assessed by blood urea nitrogen level (BUN).

TREATMENT

The treatment of DKA involves restoration of volume, correction of abnormal electrolytes, and resolution of serum glucose and ketone levels with appropriate doses of insulin. The details are summarized in Table 145-3.[12]

Fluid

Treatment of the volume deficit before the institution of insulin therapy is now accepted as routine therapy. While the early administration of fluid does not affect the acidosis, it does decrease the levels of counterregulatory hormones.

TABLE 145-3. Protocol for Management of Diabetic Ketoacidosis

---

Rapid but careful history and physical examination with special attention to: patency of airway, mental status, cardiovascular and renal status, source of infection, and state of hydration.

Initial biochemical evaluation should consist of immediate emergency room assessment of blood "ketones" and blood glucose (finger stick) and urine "ketones" by Keto-Diastix, including immediate order for plasma glucose, blood gases and pH, serum electrolytes, BUN, amylase, complete blood count, and urinalysis; chest film, ECG, and appropriate bacterial cultures are also to be obtained if indicated.

As soon as the initial chemistries are drawn, give 1 L of 0.9% sodium chloride solution in the first hour, with subsequent infusion of 0.45% sodium chloride 200–1000 mL/h. Do not exceed total fluid of 5 L in 8 hours.

With the confirmation of diagnosis of diabetic ketoacidosis, give 0.4 U of regular insulin/kg body weight (half as IV push and half as subcutaneous [SC] in deltoid area). (In comatose patients or intensive care unit admissions, give 7–10 U of insulin per hour as continuous infusion)

Determine plasma glucose hourly and electrolytes and blood gases every 2–4 hours as needed. If plasma glucose does not fall by 10% in the first hour, repeat initial priming dose of insulin or double the rate of insulin infusion.

After satisfactory glucose decrement, give 7 U regular insulin per hour as either IM or SC intermittent injection or IV infusion until plasma glucose reaches 200 mg/dL.

As soon as plasma glucose reaches 200 mg/dL, switch to D5% in 0.45% saline if sodium is > 140 mEq/L or D5% in 0.9% saline if sodium is < 140 mEq/L. Use rate of 100–300 mL/h depending on state of hydration. Give insulin 10 U/2h SC until diabetic ketoacidosis is controlled (defined as PG < 200 mg/dL, HCO_3 > 15 mEq/L, and pH > 7.3, and serum ketone negative at 1:2 dilution).

If initial potassium is < 3.5 mEq/L, potassium supplements should be provided at the rate of 40 mEq/L with the initial insulin therapy (1/3 as KPO_4 and 2/3 as KCl). Give 20–30 mEq of potassium/L after the first liter of solution if potassium > 3.5 but < 5.5 mEq/L, and urinary output is adequate. Give no potassium if potassium > 5.5 mEq/L. With abnormal potassium, repeat serum potassium every 1–2 hours.

No bicarbonate is given for pH > 7.0; for pH < 7.0, but > 6.9, give 1 ampule (44–50 mEq) of $NaHCO_3$; for pH < 6.9, give 2 ampules (88–100 mEq) of $NaHCO_3$. Each ampule of $NaHCO_3$ to run in 30 min with 15 mEq of KCL.

Repeat above every 2 hours until pH > 7.0.

Ancillary measures: stomach aspiration in unconscious patient; O_2 therapy for PO_2 < 80 mm Hg; plasma expander for consistent hypotension and antibiotic therapy, as needed.

Continue to look for precipitating factor; monitor patient's clinical condition and assess management frequently.

Based on University of Tennessee, Memphis, protocol, revised March 1994. Kitabchi AE, Wall BM: Diabetic ketoacidosis. *Med Clin North Am* 1995;79:9

Most advocate administration of 1 L of fluid in the first hour. Normal saline is usually the fluid of choice, but half-normal saline may be used in severe hypernatremia (sodium >150 mEq/dL.) Normal saline usually stays in the extracellular space and represents primarily the fluid that is lost to osmotic diuresis.[2] Undertreatment and overzealous treatment have been described. Undertreatment is a common source of treatment failure. Overzealous treatment with volume can cause congestive heart failure (CHF), adult respiratory distress syndrome (ARDS), and delay correction of the acidosis. The resulting fluid produces an increase in diuresis and may result in the loss of ketones that are potential bicarbonate ions. Insulin induces the metabolism of ketones, but ketone losses in the urine result in less substrate with which to produce bicarbonate by the action of insulin. Excessive fluid administration is associated with a prolongation in correction of ketosis.[6]

Careful monitoring and assessment of the patient's fluid state before treatment can minimize both over and under treatment. Should there be doubt about the ability of the patient to tolerate fluid, more intensive monitoring with a pulmonary artery catheter it indicated. The hypotensive patient should initially be treated with albumin-containing solutions to expand the intravascular space before proceeding with crystalloids. Adrogue and coworkers have reported that in patients without extreme volume deficits a less aggressive approach may be used. Of note, there were no patients with shock, severe renal insufficiency, or persistent oliguria included in the study. They suggest an infusion rate of 750 mL/hour for 4 hours, then dropping the rate to 375 mL/hour. This approach may be associated with less hyperchloremia and more rapid correction of the bicarbonate decrement.[13]

Insulin

In the ICU we use the intravenous route of insulin administration rather than the intramuscular or subcutaneous routes. While it once was almost mandatory to admit a patient with DKA to the ICU, it is now more important to admit them to a floor or nursing unit where they can be monitored carefully. The availability of bedside glucose monitoring (BGM) has made therapy easier on the floor. BGM costs slightly more in our institution but the results are immediately available. While the cost is slightly more, the time for adjustment in therapy is considerably shortened resulting in less time to correction of blood glucose levels.

The amount of insulin administered has changed from the megadoses given historically. Today therapy with lower doses of insulin tends to give insulin blood levels of 100 to 200 mU/mL. Higher insulin levels do not result in more rapid correction of blood glucose levels. There is some controversy whether to give a bolus of insulin before starting an infusion. Some advocate a 0.1 U/kg loading dose followed by a continual infusion of the same dose. Others recommend no loading dose.

Large doses of insulin have been associated with hypokalemia and hypoglycemia later during treatment. Larger doses also result in longer insulin effect, since it requires more time for the blood concentration to fall to a level that is

necessary to produce resolution of the hyperglycemia and ketosis. Insulin given during the first few hours of treatment promotes fuel storage rather than glucose oxidation. Glucose oxidation occurs when other preferred fuel competitors are removed.[14] About 50% of glucose reduction in the early part of treatment of DKA is the result of urinary losses.

Intravenous insulin has a half-life of 4 to 5 minutes with a biologic half-life of less than 20 minutes. If glucose concentration does not fall by 100 mg/dL in the first 2 hours of treatment, then the dose should be doubled. If the level does not fall in the next 2 hours by 100 mg/dL, then the dose should again be doubled.

Some patients are either slow responders or require high doses of insulin. This may not be apparent before initiation of treatment unless the patient is known to require large doses of insulin in chronic treatment. All patients in DKA have some resistance to insulin. Peripheral dispersal of glucose is one factor in insulin resistance.[15] Additionally, acidemia, phosphorus deficiency, and high levels of counterregulatory hormones contribute. Use of large doses of insulin should be expected to give prolonged biologic action that needs to be carefully monitored as blood glucose levels decrease.

Plasma glucose levels should be measured every hour until the blood glucose levels reach 200 to 250 mg/dL. In a comatose patient the goal is to maintain blood glucose levels at 300 mg/dL until the patient wakes up. Once either level is reached, then intravenous solutions should be changed to 5% dextrose solutions. If the sodium is less than 140 mEq/L, then use 0.9% normal saline. If the sodium is greater than 140/L mEq, then use 0.45% normal saline.

It is important to anticipate the fall in blood glucose and add dextrose before the blood glucose actually reaches target levels. While individual patients vary somewhat in blood glucose reduction, generally this is between 75 to 100 mg/dL/hour. Therapeutic levels are achieved in 6 to 8 hours. It is important not to lower the rate of insulin administration until the ketoacidosis is controlled, that is, bicarbonate concentrations of 15 to 18 mEq/L or a pH of greater than 7.3. Failure to follow this rule results in a delay in correction of, or a worsening of, the ketosis. The combination of insulin and glucose ensures continued metabolism of ketones. If the starting glucose is less than 350 mg/dL, then dextrose solutions should be used initially. Glucose use is severely compromised to about 10 to 15% of normal. Administration of between 5 and 10 g/hour of glucose is sufficient. Once DKA is corrected, a combination of 10 g of glucose, 2 units of insulin, and 2 mEq/hour of potassium is a good starting point (Table 145-4).

Electrolytes

Sodium losses are corrected along with correction of the water deficit. Selection of normal saline or half-normal saline depends on the sodium serum level. The decision point is a serum sodium of 150 mEq/L early-on in treatment and 140 mEq/L during treatment.

Potassium depletion requires prompt attention. Although only some patients are admitted with hypokalemia (less than

TABLE 145-4.   Deficits in Diabetic Ketoacidosis Based on Body Weight

Water	70–120 mL/kg
Sodium	7–10 mEq/kg
Potassium	2–5 mEq/kg
Chloride	5 mEq/kg
Magnesium	0.2–1.0 mEq/kg
Phosphate	1 mM/kg
Bicarbonate	4–5 mEq/kg

Modified from Martin HE, Smith K, Wilson ML: The fluid and electrolyte therapy of severe diabetic acidosis and ketosis. *Am J Med* 1958;24:376

3.5 mEq/L), these patients are the ones at risk for hypokalemia secondary to treatment. It is important to begin potassium repletion early with these patients, before administering insulin, or even in the first liter of fluid. Loss of total body potassium has been discussed previously. Most patients are admitted with normal potassium and can receive a more modest amount of potassium supplementation after the first liter of fluid. Elevated potassium levels (greater than 5.5 mEq/L) require no insulin to start. Once urine output has increased, potassium administration should be cautious. Potassium determinations should be every 1 to 2 hours at least, if the levels are abnormal. Administration of potassium should be as one third potassium phosphate and two thirds potassium chloride. The electrocardiogram can be used as an adjunct to monitor potassium levels. About 50% to 80% of the administered potassium is lost in the urine.[6]

Phosphorus losses are small. Physiologic problems secondary to low levels seem to occur rarely, presumably because of the relatively short duration.[16] Serum phosphate levels tend to mirror potassium levels. Theoretically phosphate is important for 2,3 diphosphoglycerate (2,3-DPG) levels, and diaphragmatic contraction,[17] but there is no evidence to suggest that supplementation with phosphate alters the outcome in DKA.[18] Rapid correction has hazards. Phosphate supplementation with potassium is appropriate therapy for this problem.

Magnesium deficiency exists, but rarely requires supplementation unless potassium replacement fails and requires replacement of magnesium to conserve potassium ion. Magnesium levels may fall with phosphate repletion.

Bicarbonate has no place in the *routine* treatment of DKA (Table 145-5).[19] Only at very low pH levels is any treatment necessary. Recent literature has suggested a reduction of myocardial contractility associated with the administration of bicarbonate[20] and fall in serum ketones.[21] Change in acidosis does not change the outcome in DKA. Appropriate therapy involves the use of small doses of bicarbonate at a pH

TABLE 145-5.   Potential Disadvantages of Bicarbonate Therapy

Worsening of hypokalemia
Paradoxical CNS acidemia
Intracellular acidosis from CO_2 production
Prolongation of ketone metabolism

of less than 7.0 (50 mEq) and less than 6.9 (100 mEq). Potassium should be administered simultaneously with bicarbonate over 30 to 60 minutes.

COMPLICATIONS

ARDS has been described during the treatment of DKA.[11] Reduction in colloid oncotic pressures correlate with increases in hypoxemia. Production of pulmonary edema[16] is not related to increased hydrostatic pressures but probably to reduction in colloid osmotic pressure.[22] Large doses of crystalloid may be related or causal and there also may be an association with an increased incidence of cerebral edema secondary to reduction of colloid osmotic pressure.

Brain swelling may occur particularly in children with treatment of DKA. Children have less room to allow swelling of the brain in the cranial vault. Some have thought brain swelling is related to the rapidity of lowering the blood sugar producing edema or vasodilatation.[23] They suggest caution not to let the blood glucose level fall below 300 to 350 mg/dL before dextrose is added to the fluids. Others have suggested that the brain produces idiogenetic osmoles to protect itself from the osmolar effects of hyperglycemia and that correction time is needed to allow dissolution of these compounds. Occurrence of brain edema may be as high as 1 in 200 with mortality as high as 90%.[24] Mannitol and steroid administration, while unproved, have been suggested.

Other complications related to underlying medical problems may occur. Pulmonary aspiration may occur secondary to decreased levels of consciousness and inability to protect the airway. Acute myocardial infarction, either as result of the stress of DKA or as a precipitating factor, may be present. Hyperchloremic metabolic acidosis may occur as previously mentioned because of loss of ketones before insulin therapy. On rare occasions persistence of the hyperchloremia may require treatment with bicarbonate, although usually this condition is benign. Hypoglycemia, poor glucose control, or electrolyte abnormalities can occur with less than adequate attention to the disease process.

HYPEROSMOLAR HYPERGLYCEMIC NONKETOTIC DIABETES[25,26]   ■

HHNK often occurs in older obese diabetic patients particularly those with NIDDM. HHNK may occur in those who are not known to have DM. The lack of ketosis and acidosis results in a delay in seeking medical attention. The average delay is 12 days for HHNK in contrast to 3 days for DKA. The postponement results in more profound water losses and higher accumulation of glucose. Impaired thirst and impaired renal conservation of water because of advanced age also may contribute to the water imbalance.

A negative nitroprusside test result indicates that acetoacetate is not a component of the syndrome and the mild acidosis has been attributed to lactic acid or beta-hydroxybutyric acid. Altered mental status may be secondary to hyperosmolarity or focal neurologic changes of local microthrombosis.

Usually a coexisting illness precipitates the syndrome. These may include burns, infection, pancreatitis, or the stress of dialysis. Generally these patients are easier to control once they are over the acute episode. One must remember, however, that they represent part of the spectrum of DKA and HHNK.

PATHOGENESIS

Ketoacidosis is lacking in these patients. Marked hyperglycemia is present without FFA elevations. There are two hypotheses for this paradox. It has been suggested that there is enough insulin present to inhibit lipolysis, but not enough insulin to promote glucose uptake by the tissues. There is increased production but not increased uptake.[4] Alternatively, there are not enough counterregulatory hormones present or there is an adipose tissue unresponsiveness to these hormones so that there is not enough substrate to form FFA and ketones. Portal insulin concentrations are lower in DKA patients than with HHNK and may explain the difference. The syndrome may be perpetuated by the hyperosmolarity. Hyperosmolarity decreases the response of adipose tissue to insulin.

Hyperglycemia causes a shift in water from the extravascular to the intravascular space causing a dilution in the serum sodium. The increased intravascular volume promotes hydrostatic as well as hyperosmolar diuresis. Osmolar diuresis persists causing intravascular dehydration. The dehydration process involves both extracellular and intracellular space. Urine losses are equivalent to half-normal saline with equal amounts of potassium as well as sodium. The severe water loss causes an increase in serum sodium, and elevation of BUN and creatinine.

LABORATORY FEATURES

HHNK differs from DKA in the degree of ketoacidosis. Blood glucose levels tend to run higher but may overlap (600 to 2700 mg/dL, average 1200 mg/dL). Acidosis, if present, is generally milder but can have a wide range (pH 6.81 to 7.49, average 7.26.) The etiology of the acidosis is discussed earlier. Underlying medical conditions and pharmacologic therapy may alter acid-base status. Metabolic alkalosis secondary to diuretic use before the onset of the syndrome may further confuse the situation.

Osmolarity is a component but not a distinguishing feature of HHNK; however, comatose patients tend to have higher osmolarities (373 ± 6.4 mOsm/L) compared to the patient who has DKA without coma (331 ± 5.5 mOsm/L). Coma seems related to osmolarity greater than 340 mOsm/L. Siperstein suggests that calculation of "effective osmolarity" is a better reflection of the level critical for coma.[4] Effective osmolarity may be calculated as follows:

$$\text{Effective osmolarity} = 2\,(Na^+\,mEq + K^+\,mEq) + \text{glucose}/20$$

BUN is eliminated because of the fact that it readily crosses into the intracellular space. Although the level is high it does not contribute to the effective osmolar gradient.

Glucose by comparison does not cross into the cell and therefore is a major component of the osmolarity. Normal levels are 280 to 295 mOsm/L. The patient who is comatose and has an effective osmolarity of less than 340 mOsm/L does not have coma secondary to HHNK. Other studies are needed to determine the etiology of the coma.

TREATMENT

Many treatment principles discussed in DKA apply to HHNK. The water and potassium deficits are often greater. There is a greater tendency for these patients to be hypotensive and therefore initial fluid should be normal saline whether the patient is hypotensive or not. Because of the high osmolarity, the normal saline is hypotonic to the level of the blood, and until intravascular volume is repleted this should be the fluid of choice. Half-normal saline may be substituted after reaching this point. Frequent measurement of sodium guides the selection of resuscitation fluid.

It is mandatory to treat volume loss before the institution of insulin therapy. HHNK patients may be very sensitive to the actions of insulin and resultant precipitous falls in blood glucose levels. Additionally, restoration of effective circulating volume and also of urine output may dilute blood glucose levels. Effective circulating volume restarts urine output with excretion of glucose by the kidneys, rapidly lowering the blood glucose. The principles of insulin therapy for DKA may be applied, but require extremely close monitoring.

Potassium repletion must be monitored closely because of existing large deficits and continued loss in the urine. Again DKA guidelines can apply.

COMPLICATIONS

Mortality in HHNK patients, particularly those with coma, may be high. These patients have a high incidence of coexisting medical problems that may be the prime cause for the increased mortality. HHNK coma is only a contributing factor. Hyperosmolarity carries with it an increased incidence for intravascular thrombosis, acute tubular necrosis, cerebral vascular accident, and myocardial infarction.

DECOMPENSATED DIABETES MELLITUS IN PATIENTS WITH COEXISTENT MEDICAL OR SURGICAL PROBLEMS ■

The stress of medical illness or surgery can cause a loss of control of DM secondary to release of counterregulatory hormones. Hyperglycemia, HHNK, and even DKA may result. Economics no longer permit the admission of a patient days before surgery to establish control of the DM. Preparation of a plan before the situation arises is important. The regimen described in Table 145-6 is such a plan. The goal of therapy is a blood sugar level of 90 to 180 mg/dL. Separation of the insulin infusion from the glucose–potassium infusion enhances uptake of both solutions and minimizes wasting.

TABLE 145-6. Management of Diabetes Complicated by Medical Illness or Surgery

1. Prepare an infusion of dextrose 10% in 0.9% saline with KCl 20 mEq.
2. Infuse at a rate of glucose 10 g and KCl 2 mEq/h (100 mL).
3. Prepare insulin infusion of 500 mL NS and 50 U regular insulin (0.1 U/mL). Prime tubing with 50 mL of infusion.
4. Infuse insulin at 3 U/h (30 mL/h).
5. Measure blood sugar every hour and regulate insulin—goal 90–180 mg/dL.
   a. Blood sugar 90–180 mg/dL keep on same rate.
   b. Blood sugar > 180 mg/dL increase insulin by 0.5 U/h.
   c. Blood sugar < 90 mg/dL decrease insulin by 0.5 U/h.
6. Measure potassium every 1 to 2 h—goal 3.5 to 5.5 mEq/L.
   a. If K 3.5–5.5 mEq/L keep same rate.
   b. If K >5.5 mEq/L stop the potassium in infusion.
   c. If K <3.5 mEq/L double the potassium concentration.

Modified from Alberti KG: *Insulin Therapy in Diabetic Ketoacidosis and Surgery. Insulin Update.* Amsterdam, Excerpta Medica, 1982:260

The insulin–glucose ratio can be used to initiate the insulin component of the treatment plan. Normally this ratio is 0.1 with steps for pregnancy and obesity to 0.15 to 0.2, liver disease to 0.5, infection or administration of glucocorticoids to 0.7, and the stress of surgery or DKA to 1.0.[27] Understanding these ratios permit better control of blood glucose levels and correction of the dose of administered insulin.

Alternatively, control of hyperglycemia can be more conventional without administration of glucose-containing solutions and blood glucose levels controlled with variable insulin by constant infusion. A second treatment plan is outlined in Table 145-7 for use without glucose administration.[28] Modification for the individual patient is necessary. Once obtaining hyperglycemic control, the patient may be maintained on an infusion of glucose 10 g/hour and the insulin adjusted to a goal of a blood glucose level of 90 to 180 mg/dL. Both techniques can be used in the same patient at

TABLE 145-7. Algorithm for Control of Hyperglycemia in Poorly Controlled Diabetes

GLUCOSE CONCENTRATION (mg/dL)	INTRAVENOUS INFUSION RATE (mL/h)	INSULIN INFUSION RATE (U/h)
>250	50	5.0
201–250	40	4.0
171–200	30	3.0
141–170	20	2.0
121–140	15	1.5
101–120	10	1.0
81–100	8	0.8
61–80	5	0.5
<60	0	0

Based on insulin concentration of 0.1 U/mL. Bedside glucose determinations every hour.

White NH, Skor D, Santiago JV: Practical closed-loop insulin delivery. *Ann Intern Med* 1982;97:210

different times. Control of hyperglycemia in the ICU allows the close observation of the patient limiting the risk of close regulation of blood glucose. Good control of blood glucose levels ensures fewer complications in the long term.[29]

REFERENCES ∎

1. Harris MI, Hadden WC, Knowler WC, Bennett PH: Prevalence of diabetes and impaired glucose tolerance and plasma glucose levels in U.S. population aged 20–74. *Diabetes* 1987; 36:523
2. Lebovitz HE: Diabetic ketoacidosis. *Lancet* 1995;345:767
3. Cefalu WT: Diabetic ketoacidosis. *Crit Care Clin* 1991;7:89
4. Siperstein MD: Diabetic ketoacidosis and hyperosmolar coma. *Endocrinol Metab Clin North Am* 1992;21:415
5. Foster DW: Insulin deficiency and hyperosmolar coma. *Adv Intern Med* 1974;19:159
6. Fleckman AM: Diabetic ketoacidosis. *Endocrinol Metab Clin North Am* 1993;22:181
7. Adrogue HJ, Wilson H, Boyd AE, et al: Plasma acid-base patterns in diabetic ketoacidosis. *N Engl J Med* 1982;307:1603
8. Winter SD, Pearson R, Gabow PA, et al: The fall of the serum anion gap. *Arch Intern Med* 1990;150:311
9. Zipf WB, Bacon GE, Spencer ML, et al: Hypocalcemia, hypomagnesemia, and transient hypoparathyroidism during therapy with potassium phosphate in diabetic ketoacidosis. *Diabetes Care* 1979;2:265
10. Warshaw AL, Feller ER, Lee KH: On the cause of raised serum-amylase in diabetic ketoacidosis. *Lancet* 1977;1:1619
11. Eckfeldt JH, Leatherman JW, Levitt MD: High prevalence of hyperamylasemia in patients with acidemia. *Ann Intern Med* 1986;104:362
12. Kitabchi EA, Wall BM: Diabetic ketoacidosis. *Med Clin North Am* 1995;79:9
13. Adrogue HJ, Barbiero J, Eknoyan G: Salutary effects of modest fluid replacement in the treatment of adults with diabetic ketoacidosis. *JAMA* 1989;262:2108
14. Owen OE, Trapp VE, Reichard GA, et al: Effects of therapy on the nature and quantity of fuels oxidized during diabetic ketoacidosis. *Diabetes* 1980;29:365
15. Barrett EJ, DeFronzo RA, Bevilacqua S, et al: Insulin resistance in diabetic ketoacidosis. *Diabetes* 1982;31:923
16. Fisher JN, Kitabchi AE: A randomized study of phosphate therapy in the treatment of diabetic ketoacidosis. *J Clin Endocrinol Metab* 1983;57:177
17. Aubier M, Murciano D, Lecocguic Y, et al: Effect of hypophosphatemia on diaphragmatic contractility in patients with acute respiratory failure. *N Engl J Med* 1985;313:420
18. Kebler R, McDonald FD, Cadnapaphornchai P: Dynamic changes in serum phosphorus levels in diabetic ketoacidosis. *Am J Med* 1985;79:571
19. Stacpoole PW: Lactic acidosis: the case against bicarbonate therapy. *Ann Intern Med* 1986;105:276
20. Weil MH, Rackow EC, Trevino R, et al: Difference in acid-base state between venous and arterial blood during cardiopulmonary resuscitation. *N Engl J Med* 1986;315:153
21. Hale PJ, Crase J, Nattrass M: Metabolic effects of bicarbonate in the treatment of diabetic ketoacidosis. *BMJ (Clin Res Ed)* 1984;289:1035
22. Fein IA, Rackow EC, Sprung CL, et al: Relation of colloid osmotic pressure to arterial hypoxemia and cerebral edema during crystalloid volume loading of patients with diabetic ketoacidosis. *Ann Intern Med* 1982;96:570

23. Krane EJ, Rockoff MA, Wallman JK, Wolfsdorf JI: Subclinical brain swelling in children during treatment of diabetic ketoacidosis. *N Engl J Med* 1985;312:1147
24. Fish LH: Diabetic ketoacidosis: treatment strategies to avoid complications. *Postgrad Med* 1994;96:75
25. Kitabchi AE, Matteri R, Murphy MB: Optimal insulin delivery in diabetic ketoacidosis (DKA) and hyperglycemic hyperosmolar nonketotic coma (HHNC). *Diabetes Care* 1982;5:78
26. Gerich JE, Martin MM, Recant L: Clinical and metabolic characteristics of hyperosmolar nonketotic coma. *Diabetes* 1971;20:228
27. Alberti KG: *Insulin Therapy in Diabetic Ketoacidosis and Surgery. Insulin Update*. Amsterdam, Excerpta Medica, 1982:260
28. White NH, Skor D, Santiago JV: Practical closed-loop insulin delivery: a system for maintenance of overnight euglycemia and the calculation of basal insulin requirements in insulin-dependent diabetics. *Ann Intern Med* 1982;97:210
29. DCCT Research Group: The effect of intensive treatment of diabetes on the development and progression of long term complications in insulin-dependent diabetes mellitus. *N Engl J Med* 1993;329:977

Critical Care, Third Edition, edited by Joseph M. Civetta,
Robert W. Taylor, and Robert R. Kirby.
Lippincott-Raven Publishers, Philadelphia, PA © 1997.

CHAPTER 146

■

Hypothalamic and Pituitary Disease

Charles A. Reasner II
Gary L. Mueller

IMMEDIATE CONCERNS　　　■

MAJOR PROBLEMS

In the critically ill patient, lack of thyroid hormone, cortisol, and antidiuretic hormone (ADH) may lead to life-threatening complications. Loss of pituitary function may become manifest only when the patient is stressed by a severe underlying disorder such as sepsis, myocardial infarction, or trauma. Clues to loss of pituitary function include the following: obtundation with hypothermia and bradycardia (lack of thyroid hormone), hypotension unresponsive to fluids (cortisol deficiency), and polyuria with hypernatremia and a decreased urine osmolality (lack of vasopressin).

STRESS POINTS

1. The manifestation of pituitary dysfunctions depends on the extent of hormone loss, rapidity of onset, and the underlying stress.
2. Replacement therapy should not await laboratory confirmation of thyroid hormone deficiency or vasopressin deficiency if panhypopituitarism is suspected in a critically ill patient.
3. Evaluation of the hypothalamic–pituitary–gonadal axis should be done when the patient has recovered from the acute illness.

ESSENTIAL DIAGNOSTIC TESTS AND PROCEDURES

1. If thyroid hormone lack is suspected, free thyroxine (T_4) and thyrotropin (TSH) levels should be measured.
2. A cosyntropin (Cortrosyn) stimulation test is the procedure of choice to diagnosis adrenal insufficiency. A cortisol level above 20 μg/dL is normal.
3. A serum sodium, osmolality, and urine volume and osmolality should be used to diagnosis diabetes insipidus (DI) in conjunction with an assessment of volume status. Patients with DI should have a serum sodium greater than 145 mg/dL and an inappropriately dilute urine.

INITIAL THERAPY

1. If the patient is believed to be in myxedema coma, 0.2 to 0.5 mg of levothyroxine may be given by intravenous push. If central nervous system (CNS) symptoms are not present, the patient should be treated with low doses of levothyroxine (0.025 mg orally daily) and the dose gradually titrated up over 2 to 3 months until full replacement doses are reached.
2. A stress dose of steroids is 75 mg of hydrocortisone given intravenously every 6 hours. This dose may be tapered over 2 to 3 days if the underlying stress has resolved.

3. 1-Desamino-8-D-arginine vasopressin (DDAVP) should be given as a 1- to 2-μg dose intravenously (IV) in the patient believed to have DI. The patient should be allowed to "break through" once each day to prevent iatrogenic hyponatremia.

OVERVIEW ■

This chapter considers the derangements of the hypothalamic–pituitary axis that affect the critically ill patient. Functionally, the hypothalamic–pituitary axis is divided into a hypothalamic–anterior pituitary unit (adenohypophysis) and a hypothalamic–posterior pituitary unit (neurohypophysis). Although hypofunction of both units may occur simultaneously, only one unit is commonly affected. Therefore, this chapter has been divided into aspects of hypothalamic–anterior pituitary hypofunction and of neurohypophyseal hypofunction. Hyperfunction of the hypothalamic–anterior pituitary unit is not discussed because it is rarely of concern in the seriously ill patient. Hyperfunction of the neurohypophysis (syndrome of inappropriate secretion of ADH) is discussed in Chapter 29.

HYPOTHALAMIC–ANTERIOR PITUITARY UNIT ■

The clinical manifestation of anterior pituitary failure ranges from asymptomatic patients who require sophisticated testing procedures to make the diagnosis of pituitary insufficiency to patients with acute life-threatening illness. The presentation depends largely on the underlying destructive process as well as the extent and rapidity of hormone loss.

The hypothalamus communicates with the anterior pituitary through a vascular network that extends down the pituitary stalk (Fig. 146-1). Arterial blood from the internal carotid arteries drains into a unique portal plexus that transports regulating hormones produced in the hypothalamus to the anterior pituitary. The predominant effect of the hypothalamic hormones on the secretion of growth hormone (GH), the gonadotropins (follicle-stimulating hormone [FSH] and luteinizing hormone [LH]), TSH, and corticotropin (ACTH) is stimulatory, whereas the hypothalamic influence on prolactin (PRL) secretion is inhibitory.

In the critically ill patient, common symptoms of anterior pituitary insufficiency include fatigue, weakness, postural hypotension, and hypoglycemia (ACTH deficiency); and cold intolerance, dry skin, and mental dullness (TSH deficiency). If anterior pituitary dysfunction is suspected, a careful history, physical examination, routine laboratory screening tests, and basal level of all six anterior pituitary hormones are required. In addition, a free T_4 level, cosyntropin stimulation test, and a computed tomography (CT) scan of the pituitary gland is usually necessary to determine the cause and extent of anterior pituitary failure.

Therapy should not be withheld pending study results in a seriously ill patient. To restore intravascular volume, 5% dextrose in normal saline should be given initially. Hydrocortisone, 75 mg, should be administered IV every 6 hours. Separate mineralocorticoid replacement is usually not required. Replacement T_4 should be initiated at low doses (0.025 mg orally or intravenously per day) only after the patient is given glucocorticoid replacement, or the pituitary–adrenal axis is shown to be intact.

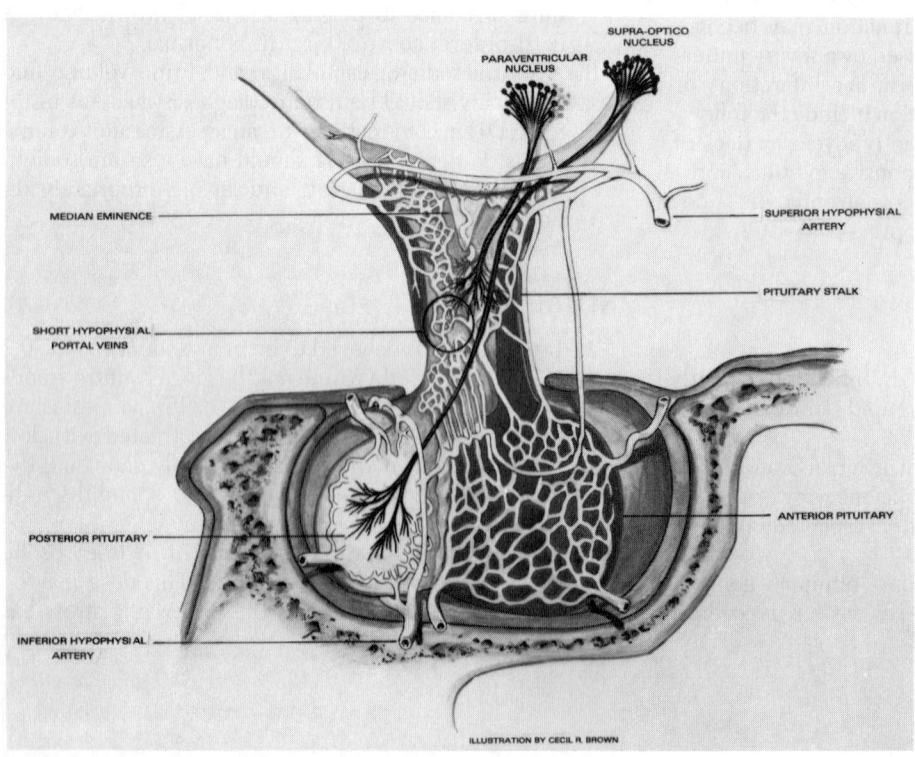

FIGURE 146-1. Functional anatomy of the hypothalamus and anterior and posterior pituitary.

EXAMINATION OF THE PATIENT

The endocrine manifestations of anterior pituitary failure depend on the patient's age, the extent and severity of the specific hormonal deficiencies, and the rapidity of onset. Disturbances of the hypothalamic–anterior pituitary unit may result in insufficient amounts of one, more than one, or all of the six hormones normally produced by the anterior pituitary. Although hormone loss may occur in any order, the following sequence is often observed: GH and PRL, FSH and LH, TSH, and ACTH.

In an adult, inadequate amounts of GH, PRL, FSH, and LH may cause few, if any, symptoms, whereas loss of TSH and ACTH may be life-threatening. The slowly progressive loss of anterior pituitary function commonly seen with tumors generally results in vague complaints, causing the diagnosis to be delayed for months or years. Sudden loss of anterior pituitary function such as occurs after surgical hypophysectomy or pituitary apoplexy may require lifesaving measures within hours. This spectrum of clinical presentation can be best understood by reviewing the effects of individual hormone deficiencies and the common etiologies of anterior pituitary failure.

Individual Hormone Deficiencies

GROWTH HORMONE. GH stimulates somatomedin production primarily by the liver. Somatomedin seems to play a key role in the control of growth in children. Although GH plays a role in intermediary metabolism, GH deficiency in the critically ill adult is not clinically significant.

PROLACTIN. PRL plays a role in breast development and the initiation and maintenance of lactation. Prolactin deficiency leads to failure of postpartum lactation.

GONADOTROPINS. Both FSH and LH stimulate ovulation in women and spermatogenesis in men. They also initiate and maintain sex hormone production in both sexes. Women with FSH and LH deficiency complain of breast atrophy, vaginal dryness, and amenorrhea. Men notice softening of the testes and loss of testicular volume, diminished libido, and loss of muscular development. In the prepubertal child, gonadotropin deficiency leads to pubertal failure and a eunuchoid appearance because of delayed long bone epiphyseal closure.

THYROTROPIN. TSH causes thyroid hormone production and release. Deficiency results in nongoitrous hypothyroidism with clinical features including bradycardia, dry skin, cold intolerance, and mental slowing. In children, hypothyroidism causes growth retardation unresponsive to GH.

CORTICOTROPIN. ACTH is synthesized as part of the larger prohormone pro-opiomelanocortin (POMC). In addition to ACTH, POMC contains beta-lipotropin and the opioid-like peptides beta-endorphin and the enkephalins. ACTH stimulates cortisol secretion primarily and has a secondary role in aldosterone production, which is primarily controlled by the renin–angiotensin system. Adrenal sex steroids also are stimulated by ACTH. Patients who are ACTH deficient manifest weakness and postural hypotension. Hypoglycemia may be present, particularly after ethanol ingestion. Because gonadal function is not ACTH dependent, decreased libido and loss of sexual hair is unusual in isolated ACTH deficiency.

ACTH AND GH INTERACTION WITH INSULIN. A dramatic reduction in the insulin requirements of an insulin-treated diabetic may signal the development of hypopituitarism. This reduction is caused by the loss of GH and cortisol, which are antagonistic to insulin's actions.

Common Etiologies of Anterior Pituitary Failure

HEMORRHAGE. Panhypopituitarism caused by hemorrhage into the pituitary is termed *pituitary apoplexy*. It is the most dramatic cause of pituitary function loss. The patient presents with severe headache, visual loss, ophthalmoplegia, and signs of meningeal irritation. The signs result from lateral and superior expansion of the sellar contents. Although this degree of hemorrhage is unusual, bleeding may occur in as many as 17% of pituitary adenomas.[1] Pituitary radiation may lead to hemorrhage from weakening of the vascular endothelium. Bleeding generally occurs during the first 3 weeks of radiation therapy.[2] Rupture of an intrasellar aneurysm can mimic hemorrhage into a pituitary tumor. Intrasellar aneurysms account for 2% of all intracranial aneurysms and may be mistaken for pituitary tumors.[3]

Up to one third of pregnant women with hypotension from severe uterine bleeding during delivery develop some degree of pituitary failure (Sheehan's syndrome), which may not manifest itself clinically for months or years after delivery.[4] The susceptibility of the pituitary gland to damage at delivery results from the 50% increase in size from lactotroph hyperplasia during pregnancy. Ischemia compresses the already hyperplastic pituitary, causing increased intrasellar pressure and diminishing tissue perfusion in the unyielding sella turcica. Sheehan's syndrome classically presents with failure to lactate and resume menses. Postpartum pituitary damage may occur in the absence of circulatory collapse, but an underlying disease that decreases tissue perfusion, such as diabetes mellitus, hypertension, arteritis, or sickle cell anemia, is usually present.[5]

A uniformly fatal syndrome characterized by central diabetes mellitus and insipidus, brain edema, cerebral herniation, and infarction of the hypothalamic pituitary unit has been described in young women. The patients all presented with symptomatic hyponatremia after elective surgery. It is postulated that a hormonal abnormality predisposed these premenopausal women to develop brain edema secondary to hyponatremia.[6]

PITUITARY TUMORS. Pituitary tumors are usually benign lesions that become evident in approximately 70% of cases because of hypersecretion of a single hormone. In contrast, large, nonfunctioning pituitary adenomas become manifest because of pituitary hypofunction, which develops insidiously from the impaired secretory capacity of nontumorous pituitary tissue. Occasionally, hypopituitarism is sudden in onset because of pituitary apoplexy. Finally, the tumors may present with neurologic deficits, such as the classic bitemporal hemianopsia caused by suprasellar extension and optic chiasm compression by the tumor.

TRAUMA AND RADIATION.   Radiation treatments for malignant disease of the head and neck may cause hypopituitarism in adults if doses of more than 8000 to 9000 rad are administered. Pituitary tumors are usually treated with approximately 5000 rad, a dose that usually does not cause complete pituitary insufficiency. Obviously, surgical hypophysectomy for whatever reason produces hypopituitarism or exacerbates partial hypopituitarism.

IMMUNOLOGIC.   Women are at particular risk for lymphocytic destruction of the pituitary, especially in the postpartum period.[7] Patients generally present with headache or symptoms of hypopituitarism and CT scan findings that suggesti a pituitary tumor. If suspected, the diagnosis may be made by biopsy; however, in the past, the diagnosis had been made only at autopsy.

INFECTION OR INFILTRATION.   Infections rarely cause panhypopituitarism, but bacteremia may cause a pituitary abscess that mimics pituitary apoplexy. Over one third of pituitary abscesses are associated with pituitary tumors.[8] Granulomatous involvement of the pituitary or hypothalamus may occur with histiocytosis or sarcoidosis. In hemochromatosis, excessive iron deposition in the pituitary causes hypogonadism in more than 50% of patients. Adrenal and thyroid hypofunction also are rarely observed in patients with hemochromatosis. Postmortem examination of patients with acquired immunodeficiency syndrome has documented direct infectious involvement in 12% of pituitary glands.[9] Anterior pituitary involvement is most common with cytomegalovirus infection; however, clinical pituitary failure has not been reported to be caused by cytomegalovirus infiltration. In contrast, *Toxoplasma gondii* infection may cause massive pituitary necrosis and panhypopituitarism.[10]

SECONDARY HYPOPITUITARISM.   Secondary hypopituitarism may result from damage to the pituitary stalk or hypothalamus. Destruction of the stalk is most commonly caused by surgery or trauma, but tumors and vascular lesions may cause it as well. Because the dominant hypothalamic influence on pituitary PRL secretion is inhibitory, stalk section results in elevated PRL levels if the blood supply to the pituitary is intact. In addition to anterior pituitary dysfunction, DI suggests hypothalamic involvement.[11] Vascular lesions, tumors, trauma, immunologic diseases, infections, and infiltrative diseases may destroy the hypothalamus.

DIAGNOSIS

Patients with nonendocrine disorders such as chronic malnutrition, hepatic failure, and depression may present with weakness, lethargy, cold intolerance, and decreased libido, suggesting hypopituitarism. In these patients, basal anterior pituitary and target hormone levels are normal. In all critically ill patients, pituitary imaging and endocrine function testing is necessary to define the etiology and extent of hormone loss.

Scanning

A CT scan or magnetic resonance imaging (MRI) is mandatory in patients with suspected anterior pituitary failure. Solid pituitary adenomas characteristically are enhanced with contrast media. Tumors that have undergone central hemorrhagic necrosis frequently have a rim of tissue enhancement. MRI is the preferred imaging method if an infectious or infiltrating disorder of the hypothalamus is suspected. Pituitary aneurysms sometimes can be diagnosed with CT scanning or MRI alone, but angiography may be required as well.

Endocrine Testing

ACTH STIMULATION.   The 1-hour cosyntropin stimulation test is the procedure of choice in the initial assessment of patients with suspected adrenocortical insufficiency.[12] In this test, 250 μg of synthetic 1-24, alpha-ACTH is administered intravenously. Blood samples for cortisol determination are obtained immediately before injection, and 30 and 60 minutes after injection. A rise in the cortisol value to 20 μg/dL or greater rules out primary adrenal insufficiency with 95% certainty. Most patients with secondary adrenal insufficiency also are unable to respond normally to the cosyntropin challenge because chronic ACTH deficiency causes adrenal cortical atrophy. Primary adrenal failure may be differentiated from secondary adrenal failure by measuring ACTH levels. Patients with primary failure have ACTH values greater than 250 pg/mL; patients with secondary failure have ACTH levels less than 50 pg/mL.

Rarely, patients with partial pituitary insufficiency may have a normal cosyntropin test result. These patients produce enough ACTH to prevent adrenal cortical atrophy, but they cannot increase ACTH production in response to stress.

Thyroid Function Testing

A normal free T_4 index (FT_4I) or a normal level of directly measured free T_4 excludes clinically significant dysfunction of the hypothalamic–pituitary–thyroid axis. Low levels of T_4 and TSH combined with evidence of other pituitary hormone deficiencies indicate secondary thyroid failure. Differentiation of hypothalamic from pituitary failure has no therapeutic implications. Because isolated TSH deficiency is rare, low TSH and low T_4 values in the absence of other pituitary hormone deficiencies suggest the euthyroid sick syndrome. Glucocorticoids and dopamine infusions also lower the basal level of TSH. The euthyroid sick syndrome was found in 69% of patients admitted to the intensive care unit (ICU) in one study and may be seen in any critically ill patient.[13] Initially, peripheral 5'-deiodinase activity is depressed, leading to decreased levels of total triiodothyronine (T_3) and elevated levels of reverse T_3 (rT_3) (Fig. 146-2). As the patient becomes more ill, the T_4 level also decreases because of decreased T_4-binding globulin affinity, which leads to increased T_4 clearance.[14] The magnitude of the decrease in serum T_4 concentration may be used to predict clinical outcome. In one study, ICU patients with total T_4 values less than 3.0 µg/dL had an 84% mortality rate; total T_4 values between 3.0 and 5.0 µg/dL were associated with a 50% mortality rate.[15] The free T_4 measured by equilibrium dialysis is usually normal in these patients. Therefore, an elevated rT_3 and near normal free T_4 equilibrium dialysis reliably distinguishes the euthyroid sick patient from the patient with secondary hypothyroidism.

MANAGEMENT

In the critically ill adult, GH, PRL, FSH, and LH deficiencies have minimal clinical importance, and sophisticated testing and definitive treatment should be delayed until the patient has recovered. Deficiencies in TSH and ACTH cause thyroid and adrenal failure and require replacement therapy without delay. In addition to hormone replacement, surgical decompression is required for patients with pituitary apoplexy.

TSH Deficiency

Because isolated TSH deficiency is extremely rare, the physician must ensure that glucocorticoid deficiency does not exist before thyroid hormone replacement is initiated. Increasing the metabolic rate in a patient with untreated adrenal insufficiency may precipitate an adrenal crisis. Replacement L-T_4 therapy should be initiated cautiously. Elderly patients or those with ischemic heart disease should be started on 0.025 mg/day. This dosage may be increased by 0.025 mg every 3 to 4 weeks as long as the patient does not develop angina or signs of hyperthyroidism. The final maintenance dosage should be determined by assessing the patient and the FT_4I. Obviously, TSH measurement is not useful in patients with secondary hypothyroidism. Most adults require 0.1 to 0.2 mg L-T_4 daily and feel best with a FT_4I near the upper end of the normal range. Thyroid USP and T_3 are not recommended for chronic replacement therapy.

Currently, replacement therapy is not recommended for patients with euthyroid sick syndrome. In a randomized, prospective study of 23 hypothyroxinemic patients admitted to a medical ICU, T_4 therapy did not improve survival.[16] Similarly, no improvement in survival was observed in critically ill patients receiving T_3 replacement.[17]

ACTH Deficiency

ACUTE.   Replacement glucocorticoid therapy should not be withheld pending study results in a seriously ill patient with suspected adrenal insufficiency. Intravascular volume repletion with 5% dextrose in normal saline is initially administered to replace sodium losses and prevent hypoglycemia. Hydrocortisone (75 mg) every 6 hours should be given until the precipitating cause is identified and corrected, and the patient is clearly responding to therapy. The glucocorticoid dose may then be reduced by 50% every day until maintenance levels are reached. Mineralocorticoid replacement is seldom necessary in the acute setting, but electrolyte and fluid status should be carefully monitored. If glucocorticoid replacement must be initiated before the completion of the cosyntropin stimulation test, dexamethasone should be given in place of hydrocortisone because dexamethasone is not measured in the cortisol assay. The patient may be switched to hydrocortisone replacement when the cosyntropin stimulation test is completed.

PERIOPERATIVE PERIOD.   Patients believed to have adrenal insufficiency of any cause should receive glucocorticoid coverage until the physician is certain that the pituitary–adrenal axis is intact postoperatively. A commonly used ste-

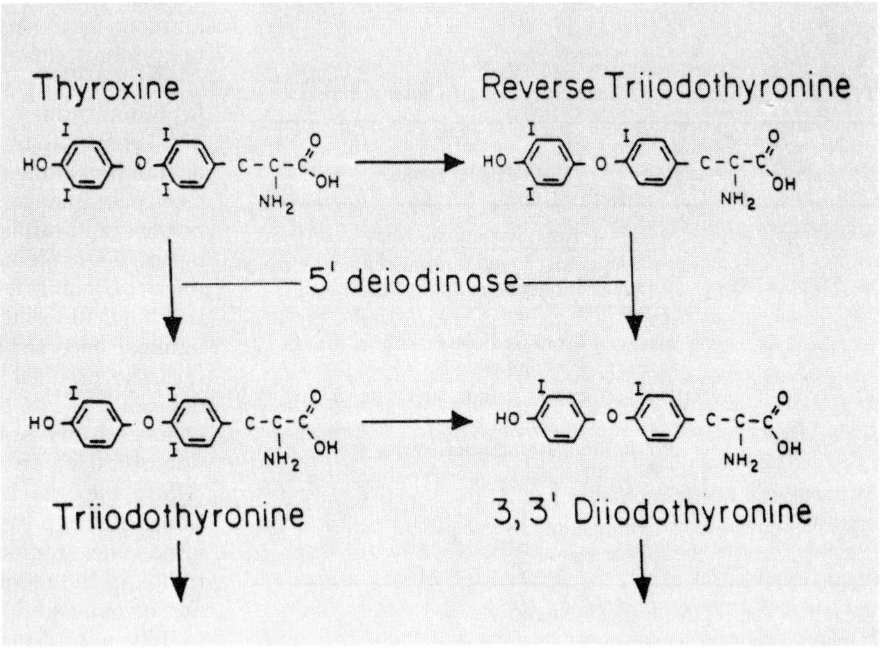

FIGURE 146-2. Conversion of thyroxine to triiodothyronine, reverse triiodothyronine, and diiodothyronine.

roid schedule is outlined in Table 146-1.[18] If the patient's cortisol value on day 5 is low, replacement therapy (i.e., 5 mg of prednisone in the morning) should be given. Thyroid function testing should be performed 4 to 6 weeks after surgery to ensure thyroid sufficiency. Gonadal function can be assessed 2 months postoperatively.

CHRONIC STEROID THERAPY.   When glucocorticoids are administered for more than 5 days, the pituitary–adrenal axis may be suppressed. The degree of suppression depends on the medication used, the dosage, and the time of administration. Long-acting steroids (dexamethasone) cause greater suppression than the short-acting agents. Pharmacologic doses of glucocorticoirds, especially if given in the evening, cause maximal ACTH suppression. A dosage of 50 mg of prednisone givenor 5 days causes decreased ACTH responsiveness for up to 1 week.[19] When large doses have been given chronically, recovery of the pituitary–adrenal axis may require 9 to 12 months. Because of the trophic influence of ACTH on the adrenal cortex, the hypothalamic–pituitary axis must first recover. Eventually, supranormal levels of ACTH stimulate the atrophied adrenal cortices, cortisol production rises to normal, and ACTH levels return to normal as a result of negative feedback inhibition.[20]

Steroid withdrawal in patients who have been receiving suppressive doses of glucocorticoids should be done slowly because rapid reductions may precipitate adrenal insufficiency. Signs and symptoms of adrenal insufficiency may occur even at supraphysiologic dose levels of steroids.[21] If the symptoms persist, the steroid dosage should be increased to its previous level with the taper reinstituted at a slower rate. It is usually safe to taper prednisone by 2.5 mg a week until a dosage of 5 mg each morning is tolerated. When the morning cortisol level (determined before the morning steroid dose is given) is greater than 10 μg/dL, the normal early morning endogenous ACTH surge has returned and replacement therapy may be discontinued. A normal response to cosyntropin indicates a normally functioning axis

TABLE 146-1.   Perioperative Steroid Replacement Schedule

POSTOPERATIVE DAY	STEROID DOSE
0	Hydrocortisone sodium succinate, 100 mg preoperatively and 50 mg added to each liter of intravenous fluid given during surgery
1	Hydrocortisone sodium succinate, 50 mg IV or IM every 8 h
2	Hydrocortisone sodium succinate, 50 mg IV or IM every 12 h
3°	Prednisone, 10 mg orally, twice a day
4°	Observe patient on no steroid replacement
5°	If 8 AM cortisol greater than 10 μg/dL, continue to observe patient on no steroid replacement

IV, intravenously; IM, intramuscularly.
°Only if patient is nonstressed.

in most cases. If major surgery is anticipated and partial pituitary insufficiency is suspected, an insulin tolerance test may be used to assess the pituitary's ability to mount a stress response.

The daily maintenance dose of steroid should be doubled in patients on chronic maintenance therapy who develop intercurrent febrile illnesses. The maintenance dose can be resumed when the patient has been afebrile for 24 to 48 hours. Major illnesses that require hospitalization need stress coverage in the range of 300 mg of hydrocortisone daily or a pharmacologically equivalent amount of another glucocorticoid.

NEUROHYPOPHYSIS   ■

Central DI is caused by inadequate secretion of ADH by the neurohypophysis (Chap. 29). Lack of ADH leads to the dramatic onset of polyuria because the patient is unable to produce a concentrated urine. If the intake of water is insufficient, this condition leads to hypertonic encephalopathy from hypernatremia, circulatory collapse from volume depletion, or both.

The neurohypophysis extends from the hypothalamus to the posterior pituitary (see Fig. 146-1). ADH is produced by the neurosecretory cells concentrated in the supraoptic and paraventricular nuclei of the hypothalamus, transported in neurosecretory granules down the cell's axon, and stored in terminal dilatations of the axon. On its release into the bloodstream, ADH functions as a true hormone. Although most axons terminate in the posterior pituitary, a large minority terminate high in the pituitary stalk and release ADH into the portal venous system that drains into the anterior pituitary.[22] Destruction of the hypothalamic neurosecretory cells or high transection of the stalk is associated with permanent DI. Distal stalk transection or removal of the posterior pituitary produces only transient polyuria because sufficient hormone can be released from axons terminating higher in the pituitary stalk to prevent permanent DI.[23]

The cardinal effect of ADH is to allow the formation of hypertonic urine by increasing the water permeability of the distal convoluted tubule and collecting duct. The collecting duct passes through the renal medullary interstitium, whose osmolality increases to 1200 to 1400 mOsm/kg. In normal persons, approximately 20 L of fluid daily reach the collecting system hypotonic to plasma, having been diluted in the thick ascending limb of the loop of Henle. When ADH is absent, the water permeability of the collecting duct is minimal, and most of the hypotonic fluid is excreted. Therefore, the maximal degree of polyuria resulting from ADH deficiency is less than 20 L/24 hours. Patients with urine volumes in excess of 20 L should be suspected of psychogenic water drinking. In the presence of ADH, water can passively diffuse into the hypertonic renal medullary interstitium. Thus, in the presence of maximal ADH stimulation, the urine concentration equals, but never exceeds, the concentration of the medullary interstitium. Urine concentrations in the young adult with normal renal function vary from 50 to 100 mOsm/kg when ADH is lacking to 1200 to 1400 mOsm/kg when maximal concentrations of ADH are present and renal function is intact. The elderly are unable to concentrate the urine to this degree because of decreased secretion of ADH and because of a decreased capacity of the kidney tubule to respond to ADH. Consequently, the elderly must increase their fluid intake to excrete the obligatory solute load.[24]

Both osmotic and nonosmotic factors may regulate ADH release. Osmoreceptors lie near the neurosecretory cells in the hypothalamus. A 1% to 2% increase in plasma osmolality shrinks the osmoreceptors and triggers the release of ADH. The osmoreceptors are not equally sensitive to all solutes. Sodium that is restricted to the extracellular compartment causes maximal cell shrinkage and is a potent stimulus for ADH release. Urea that can freely pass through the cellular membranes causes little change in cell size, and no increase in ADH secretion is observed. Glucose is intermediate in its ability to stimulate ADH release.[25]

Nonosmotic factors capable of stimulating ADH release include volume depletion and hypotension. Stretch receptors located in the left atrium increase ADH release when exposed to decreased pressure. Thus, volume depletion, positive pressure ventilation, and upright posture all reduce intrathoracic blood volume and produce maximal antidiuresis.[26] Conversely, volume expansion, balloon distention of the left atrium, and paroxysmal atrial tachycardia all increase left atrial pressure and result in suppression of ADH release. Baroreceptors located in the carotid bifurcations and aortic arch modulate ADH release by parasympathetic pathways in the vagus and glossopharyngeal nerves.[27] Hypotension causes maximal ADH release to maintain arterial blood pressure. Under normal physiologic conditions, only osmotic changes affect ADH release because a fall in blood volume of 7% to 10% is necessary to stimulate left atrial stretch receptors or baroreceptors. Once stimulated, however, these relatively insensitive receptors are able to override the less potent osmotic stimuli.

A wide variety of drugs may affect ADH levels. Cyclophosphamide, vincristine, nicotine, and clofibrate increase ADH production, whereas alcohol and phenytoin inhibit its release. Chlorpropamide potentiates the action of ADH on the renal tubules; lithium and tetracycline block ADH effects.

Input from the sympathetic nervous system and CNS also influences ADH release. The alpha-adrenergic system suppresses and the beta-adrenergic system stimulates ADH release. Pain, nausea, and stress are associated with transient antidiuresis.

Central DI may result from any condition that damages the neurohypophyseal system. Accidental or neurosurgical head trauma may cause DI if the injury is high on the pituitary stalk. Because only 15% of the neurohypophyseal secretory capacity is required to maximally concentrate the urine, DI after trauma is most often transient. Idiopathic DI occurs at any age and affects either sex. It is second only to trauma as a cause of central DI.[28] Intracranial neoplasms are the third most common cause of central DI. In children, craniopharyngiomas predominate as causes of DI; metastatic lung or breast carcinomas are the common offenders in adults. Granulomatous diseases infiltrating the hypothala-

mus, CNS infections, vascular lesions, and an inherited form of central DI also should be considered in the differential diagnosis of DI. Herpes simplex encephalitis complicating the acquired immunodeficiency syndrome has been reported to cause central DI.[29] Pituitary tumors rarely cause central DI because they seldom reach sufficient size to disrupt the neurosecretory function of axons terminating high in the stalk. Therefore, if a patient with DI also has an abnormal sella, the tumor is more likely to be of suprasellar origin with extension downward into the sella rather than a primary pituitary neoplasm.

Clinically significant central DI has traditionally been treated with DDAVP. DDAVP is a structural analogue of ADH, which has potent antidiuretic properties and negligible pressor effects, making it safe for patients with cardiovascular disease. Its twice-daily dosage is well tolerated, and water intoxication is rare.

EXAMINATION OF THE PATIENT

Because central DI is rare, osmotic diuresis and volume overload must be considered before treating the patient for lack of vasopressin. Hyperglycemia, myoglobinuria, and intravenous contrast infusions all are examples of osmotic insults that mimic DI. The medical history and a urine osmolality that is not maximally dilute should suggest the correct diagnosis. Overhydration with isotonic fluid often occurs during an operative procedure or resuscitation efforts. This volume overload produces a physiologic free water diuresis. If intravenous fluids are given to match urinary losses, sustained polyuria may be mistaken for DI. In these cases, the serum sodium should not be elevated. As the amount of administered fluid is decreased, the patient decreases the urine output and begins to concentrate their urine. If the urine does not become concentrated and the serum sodium becomes elevated with fluid restriction, the possibility of DI should be entertained. A plasma sample should be obtained for a vasopressin measurement, and 2 μg DDAVP should be administered IV. Urine osmolality increases by 50% if the patient has central DI.

Patients with central DI generally describe the abrupt onset of polyuria and polydipsia. Urine volumes of 10 to 12 L/day are common. Nocturia is present; the patient may complain of fatigue resulting from disturbed sleep. If the underlying disease that destroyed the neurohypophysis causes no symptoms, the patient may appear surprisingly well. With an intact thirst mechanism and free access to water, the patient matches fluid intake to output and maintains a normal serum sodium and osmolality.[30] The inability to obtain water, which frequently occurs after head trauma or anesthesia, may lead to life-threatening hypernatremia. A careful record of urine volumes and serum osmolalities in patients with CNS trauma prevents this complication. Rarely, the patient with central DI also may have destruction of the thirst receptors in the hypothalamus. These patients must be taught to take fluids at regular intervals to prevent the development of hypernatremia.

Patients who eventually develop permanent DI after surgical destruction of the neurohypophysis may undergo a characteristic response consisting of an initial 4- to 5-day period of polyuria immediately after the surgery followed by a 5- to 6-day period of oliguria before the polyuria and polydipsia of permanent central DI supervene.[31] This triphasic response parallels the neurosecretory cell's response to injury. The initial trauma causes a shock paralysis of neurosecretory function, and ADH is not released. During the oliguric phase, cellular degeneration causes release of preformed hormone into the circulation. Finally, neurosecretory cell death causes permanent DI to appear. Failure to appreciate this sequence of events may lead to the following two common management errors: (1) water intoxication may develop during the oliguric phase if hypotonic fluids routinely given postoperatively are not appropriately restricted; and (2) the patient's ability to concentrate urine 6 to 10 days postoperatively may be mistakenly interpreted as a sign of permanent recovery of neurohypophyseal function. Fortunately, most patients have lesser damage to the neurohypophysis and recover fully. The physician managing an early case of postsurgical DI should avoid premature judgments regarding the permanence of the condition.

MANAGEMENT

The preferred medication for treating central DI is DDAVP. This structural analogue of arginine vasopressin has a deaminated hemicysteine at position 1, which produces a prolonged duration of action and enhances the antidiuretic effect.[32] Substitution of the D-isomer for the L-isomer at position 8 markedly decreases the molecule's pressor activity. The final result is a potent analogue of ADH with a 6- to 24-hour duration of action and extremely low pressor:antidiuretic activity ratio.

DDAVP is administered by a metered-dose nasal spray dispenser. Patients who have "colds" need only blow their noses before DDAVP administration because absorption is usually satisfactory. The initial dose of DDAVP should be small, about 5 μg. The urine output and osmolality should be monitored. When polyuria returns, the dose may be increased to 10 μg and the duration of action determined. Most patients require a dose before bedtime to prevent nocturia and a dose in the morning to allow normal daily activity without frequent interruptions. Excessive amounts of DDAVP may produce water retention, hyponatremia, and natriuresis. If nasal packing prevents intranasal administration, DDAVP may be given subcutaneously, intramuscularly, or IV.[33] When administered by one of these latter three methods, similar antidiuretic effects are seen at less than 10% of the intranasal dose. Therefore, 0.5 μg to 1.0 μg should be tried initially. This produces antidiuresis for 8 to 12 hours.

Arginine vasopressin has significant pressor activity in addition to its antidiuretic effects. When given as an intravenous bolus, it may induce angina or hypertension.

Vasopressin tannate in oil is a long-acting preparation that should not ordinarily be used in critically ill patients. Water intoxication is common because of its long duration of action (up to 72 hours). Its relatively potent vasoconstrictive properties are of concern in the patient with cardiovascular disease.

Transient DI is common after neurosurgical procedures. Once osmotic loads and overhydration has been excluded (see earlier), the flow rate of intravenous fluids should be decreased and the serum Na^+ concentration and urine output and osmolality should be measured hourly. The combination of polyuria (more than 4 mL/minute) with an osmolality of less than 150 mOsm/kg and a serum Na^+ greater than 145 mMol/L is consistent with DI. Intravenous DDAVP can be started at a 1-μg dose. The return of a dilute urine signals the need for subsequent doses. Excess hypotonic fluid may lead to severe hyponatremia when given with DDAVP.

Patients with unrecognized DI may develop hypertonic encephalopathy that requires emergency treatment. Rapid infusion of hypotonic solutions may produce cerebral edema and generalized seizure activity in up to 40% of these patients.[34] Normal saline should be administered if there are signs of circulatory collapse until the patient is no longer orthostatic. Hypotonic saline solutions may then be used cautiously. Generally speaking, the serum sodium level should be normalized over 36 to 48 hours.

REFERENCES ■

1. Wakai S, Fukushima T, Teramoto A, Sano K: Pituitary apoplexy: its incidence and clinical significance. *J Neurosurg* 1981;55:187
2. Weisberg LA: Pituitary apoplexy. *Am J Med* 1977;63:109
3. White JC, Ballantin HJ: Intrasellar aneurysms simulating hypophyseal tumors. *J Neurosurg* 1972;36:640
4. Barkan AL: Pituitary atrophy in patients with Sheehan's syndrome. *Am J Med Sci* 1989;298:38
5. Schlak DS, Burday SZ: Antepartum pituitary insufficiency in diabetes mellitus. *Ann Intern Med* 1971;74:357
6. Fraser CL, Arieff AI: Fatal central diabetes mellitus and insipidus resulting from untreated hyponatremia: a new syndrome. *Ann Intern Med* 1990;112:113.
7. Asa SC, Bilboa JM, Kovacs K, et al: Lymphocytic hypophysitis of pregnancy resulting in hypopituitarism. *Ann Intern Med* 1981;95:166
8. Lindholm J, Rasmussen P, Korsgaard B: Intrasellar tumor or pituitary abscess. *J Neurosurg* 1973;38:616
9. Sano T, Kovacs K, Scheithauer BW, et al: Pituitary pathology in acquired immunodeficiency syndrome. *Arch Pathol Lab Med* 1989;113:1066.
10. Milligan SA, Katz MS, Craven PC, et al: Toxoplasmosis presenting as panhypopituita rism in a patient with the acquired immune deficiency syndrome. *Am J Med* 1984;77:760.
11. Stuart CA, Neelon FA, Lebovitz HE: Hypothalamic insufficiency: the cause of hypopituitarism in sarcoidosis. *Ann Intern Med* 1978;88:589
12. May ME, carey RM: Rapid adrenocorticotropic hormone test in practice: retrospective review. *Am J Med* 1985;79:679
13. Kaptein EM, Weiner JM, Robinson WJ, et al: Relationship of altered thyroid hormone indices to survival in nonthyroidal illnesses. *Clin Endocrinol (Oxf)* 1982;16:565
14. Chopra IS, Solomon DH, Chua Teco GN, et al: An inhibitor of the binding of thyroid hormones to serum proteins is present in extrathyroid tissue. *Science* 1982;215:407
15. Slay MF, Morley JE, Elson MK, et al: Hypothroxinemia in critically ill patients as a predictor of high mortality. *JAMA* 1981;245:43

16. Brent GA, Hershman JM: Thyroxine therapy in patients with severe nonthyroidal illnesses and low serum thyroxine concentrations. *J Clin Endocrinol Metab* 1986;63:1
17. Becker RA, Vaughn GM, Zeigler MG, et al: Hypermetabolic low triiodothyronine syndrome of burn injury. *Crit Care Med* 1982;10:870
18. Daughaday WH: The anterior pituitary. In: Wilson JD, Foster DW (eds). *Textbook of Endocrinology*, ed 7. Philadelphia, WB Saunders, 1985:593
19. Streck WF, Lockwood DH: Pituitary adrenal recovery following short term suppression with corticosteroids. *Am J Med* 1979;66:910
20. Graber AL, Ney RL, Nicholson WE, et al: Natural history of pituitary–adrenal recovery following long-term suppression with corticosteroids. *J Clin Endocrinol Metab* 1965;25:11
21. Amatruda TT, Hurst MM, D'Esopo ND: Certain endocrine and metabolic facets of the steroid withdrawal syndrome. *J Clin Endocrinol Metab* 1965;25:1207
22. Zimmerman EA, Robinson AG: Hypothalamic neurons secreting vasopressin and neurophysin. *Kidney Int* 1976;10:12
23. Coggins CH, Leaf AL: Diabetes insipidus. *Am J Med* 1967;42:807
24. Brown WW, Davis BB, Spry LA, et al: Aging and the kidney. *Arch Intern Med* 1986;146:1790
25. Robertson GL, Athar S, Shelton RL: Osmotic control of vasopressin function. In: Andreoli TE, et al (eds). *Disturbances in Body Fluid Osmolality*. Bethesda, American Physiological Society, 1977:215
26. Annat G, Viak JP, Bui Xuan B, et al: Effect of PEEP ventilation on renal function, plasma renin, aldosterone, neurophysins and urinary ADH, and prostaglandins. *Anesthesiology* 1983;58:136
27. Buonocorc CM, Robinson AG: The diagnosis and management of diabetes insipidus during medical emergencies. *Endocrinol Metab Clin North Am* 1993;22:411
28. Blotner H: Primary or idiopathic diabetes insipidus: a system disease. *Metabolism* 1958;7:191
29. Madhoun ZT, Dubois DB, Rosenthal J, et al: Central diabetes insipidus: a complication of herpes simplex type 2 encephalitis in a patient with AIDS. *Am J Med* 1991;90:658
30. Barlow ED, DeWardener HE: Compulsive water drinking. *Q J Med* 1959;28:235
31. Randall RV, Clark EC, Dodge HW, et al: Polyuria after operation for tumors in the region of the hypophysis and hypothalamus. *J Clin Endocrinol* 1960;20:1614
32. Sawyer WH, Acosta M, Balaspiri L, et al: Structural changes in the arginine vasopressin molecule that enhance antidiuretic activity and specificity. *Endocrinology* 1974;95:140
33. Rado JP, Marosi J, Fischer J: Comparison of the antidiuretic effects of single intravenous and intranasal doses of DDAVP in diabetes insipidus. *Pharmacology* 1977;15:40
34. Morris-Jones PH, Houston IB, Evans RC: Prognosis of neurological complications of acute hyponatremia. *Lancet* 1967;ii:1385

Critical Care, Third Edition, edited by Joseph M. Civetta,
Robert W. Taylor, and Robert R. Kirby.
Lippincott-Raven Publishers, Philadelphia, PA © 1997.

CHAPTER 147

Adrenal Disease

Robert B. Constant
Richard J. Barth

IMMEDIATE CONCERNS

MAJOR PROBLEMS

Adrenal diseases are infrequent admitting diagnoses to
ICUs. However, patients with unrecognized or previously
diagnosed and stable underlying disease of the hypothalamic-
pituitary-adrenal (HPA) axis can sometimes demonstrate
severe decompensation in the setting of other critical illnesses. In addition, steroid medications (derived from adrenal glucocorticoid hormones) are commonly used in the care
of the critically ill. For these reasons, the clinical problems
associated with the HPA axis and the use of glucocorticoid
hormones must be understood by the intensive care provider.

STRESS POINTS

1. The adrenal gland makes numerous hormones, including the glucocorticoid hormones. The principal glucocorticoid hormone secreted by the adrenal gland is
   cortisol, which is regulated closely by the pituitary
   through its production of adrenocorticotropin hormone (ACTH).
2. Glucocorticoid insufficiency (hypoadrenalism) is the
   most important clinical problem involving the adrenal
   gland in the ICU setting. It can occur as the result
   of diseases affecting the adrenal gland itself (primary
   adrenal insufficiency) or because of a lack of ACTH
   stimulation of the adrenal gland (secondary adrenal
   insufficiency). In its extreme form (adrenal crisis), glucocorticoid insufficiency can result in severe systemic
   symptoms, numerous electrolyte abnormalities, and
   cardiovascular decompensation with shock. Unrecognized, these problems commonly result in death. The

clinical findings associated with adrenal insufficiency
and the management of acute adrenal crisis are found
in Tables 147-1 and 147-2.
3. There are a number of glucocorticoid steroid medications available for use in the ICU setting. The type
   and dose of the steroid medication chosen depends
   largely on the indications for its use. In general, to
   reduce the incidence of serious side effects, the physician should prescibe the lowest dose of medication for
   the shortest period of time that produces the desired
   therapeutic endpoint. In many instances, steroid medications cannot be abruptly stopped, but need to be
   tapered slowly. The principles of steroid withdrawl are
   included in this chapter.

ESSENTIAL DIAGNOSTIC TESTS
AND PROCEDURES

1. The various symptoms, physical signs, and general laboratory findings that suggest hypoadrenalism are
   shown in Table 147-1.
2. A listing and description of the procedures for performing various adrenal function tests are shown at the
   end of this chapter. It is essential to perform hormonal
   testing to confirm the diagnosis of adrenal insufficiency. In emergent situations, the short adrenocorticotropic hormone (ACTH) stimulation test is adequate
   to verify hypoadrenalism.

INITIAL THERAPY

The principles of management of hypoadrenalism depend on
the severity of clinical findings. The stepwise management of
acute adrenal crisis is shown in detail in Table 147-2. The

TABLE 147-1.   Clinical Findings in Adrenal Insufficiency

Symptoms
    Weakness/fatigue
    Anorexia
    Gastrointestinal symptoms
    Orthostatic symptoms
    Myalgias/arthralgias
Signs
    Weight loss
    Orthostatic hypotension
    Hyperpigmentation
    Vitiligo
General laboratory findings
    Hyponatremia
    Hyperkalemia
    Acidosis
    Prerenal azotemia
    Lymphocytosis/eosinophilia
    Hypoglycemia

principles for the use and withdrawl of steroid medications are included in a separate section of this chapter.

PHYSIOLOGY OF THE ADRENAL GLAND   ■

The adrenal glands are two pyramid-shaped glands, each weighing about 5 to 10 g, located just superior to the kidneys. Each adrenal gland is divided into two distinct areas, the cortex and the medulla. The adrenal cortex is responsible for the secretion of multiple steroid hormones. Centrally located within each gland, the adrenal medulla is responsible for the secretion of catecholamines. Adrenocortical insufficiency and the use of some of these steroid hormones in critically ill patients are discussed in this chapter; the major disease of the adrenal medulla, pheochromocytoma, is discussed in Chapter 148.

REGULATION OF ADRENAL HORMONE SYNTHESIS

Adrenal hormone production is closely regulated by the hypothalamus and the pituitary gland. Corticotropin-releasing hormone (CRH) is produced in the hypothalamus and acts on specialized cells in the pituitary, stimulating production of ACTH, which serves, in turn, to stimulate adrenal cortical cells to produce numerous steroid hormones. Finally, in completing the classic negative feedback loop typical of many endocrine systems, the adrenal hormones have a negative influence at the level of the hypothalamus and pituitary, inhibiting CRH and ACTH release. Therefore, abnormalities in circulating levels of adrenal steroid hormones can be due to either adrenal or hypothalamic–pituitary disease.

TABLE 147-2.   Management of Acute Adrenal Crisis

I. Initial management—*all patients*
    1. Obtain baseline blood samples for cortisol, electrolytes, glucose, BUN, and creatinine while establishing IV lines for therapy.
II. Glucocorticoid therapy
    A. For patients with *diagnosis well established*
        1. Administer hydrocortisone hemisuccinate 100-mg IV bolus.
        2. Establish hydrocortisone hemisuccinate IV infusion at 75–100 mg every 6 h.
        3. After resuscitation, taper to standard replacement doses (hydrocortisone 30 mg/24 h) as rapidly as patient's condition allows.
    B. For patients with *diagnosis not established*
        1. Administer dexamethasone phosphate 4-mg IV bolus.
        2. Establish dexamethasone phosphate IV infusion at 4 mg every 8 h.
        3. Switch to hydrocortisone hemisuccinate after diagnostic procedures are completed.
III. Fluid management—*all patients*
    1. Administer isotonic saline IV in volumes sufficient to support blood pressure.
    2. If patient is hypoglycemic, use 5% dextrose in isotonic saline.
    3. Assume patient has at least 20% of extracellular fluid depleted.
    4. Hemodynamic monitoring is advised.
IV. Diagnostic procedures
    A. For patients with *diagnosis well established*
        1. No special diagnostic procedures are necessary.
    B. For patients with *diagnosis not established*
        1. Perform short ACTH stimulation test after therapy is initiated.
        2. If the short ACTH test is abnormal, perform long ACTH stimulation test after stabilization.
V. Other supportive measures—*all patients*
    1. Mineralocorticoid replacement is not usually necessary as long as isotonic saline is administered as required.
    2. Treat underlying problem that precipitated the episode of adrenal crisis.
    3. Prophylactic antibiotic use is not indicated.

TYPES OF ADRENAL HORMONES

The adrenal cortex produces more than 50 different steroids. All of these hormones are derived from cholesterol and can be grouped into three major classes: glucocorticoids, named for their effects on carbohydrate metabolism; mineralocorticoids, involved in the maintenance of normal electrolyte balance; and sex hormones.

Glucocorticoid production is regulated closely by ACTH. The principal glucocorticoid secreted from the adrenal gland is cortisol. The principal mineralocorticoid is aldosterone, which is regulated not only by ACTH but also by serum sodium and potassium levels and by the renin–angiotensin system. Mineralocorticoids exert their primary effect on distal renal tubule cells, resulting in renal sodium retention at the expense of potassium loss in the urine. A third major class of adrenal steroids are the sex hormones: dehydroepiandrosterone (DHEA), DHEA-sulfate, and androstenedione. Like the glucocorticoids, these steroid hormones are regulated primarily by ACTH. They function mainly as precursors for the primary circulating androgen, testosterone, and also may undergo separate conversion to estrogen hormones. In ICU patients, glucocorticoids are the steroid hormones of greatest concern, and so they are the focus of the remainder of this discussion.

GLUCOCORTICOID ACTION

Current thinking suggests that the actions of glucocorticoids, like those of all steroid hormones, result from the ability of glucocorticoids to regulate protein synthesis. Since glucocorticoid receptors have been found on nearly every nucleated cell in the body, and since each cell type has its own expression of glucocorticoid effect, it follows that glucocorticoids have many effects in the body.[1] This is equally true of endogenously produced glucocorticoid hormones or exogenously administered glucocorticoid medications.

Metabolic Effects

Glucocorticoid hormones have a profound influence on carbohydrate metabolism. They increase hepatic production of glucose and glycogen and decrease peripheral use of glucose. These steroids also affect fat and protein metabolism. They increase lipolysis both directly and indirectly through their actions on other hormones. They elevate free fatty acid (FFA) levels in the plasma and enhance any tendency to ketosis. Glucocorticoids stimulate peripheral protein metabolism, using the amino acid products as gluconeogenic precursors. In the liver, they stimulate protein synthesis.

Immunologic Effects

Perhaps of more immediate importance to the ICU physician are the immunologic effects of glucocorticoids.[2] They increase the number of circulating neutrophils by 2000 to 5000 cells/mm^3, usually demonstrating a peak effect in this regard by 4 to 6 hours after administration of a single dose. At the same time, they cause a decrease in the numbers of lymphocytes, monocytes, eosinophils, and basophils. The decrease in circulating lymphocytes is due primarily to a redistribution of T lymphocytes from the circulating pool into lymphoid tissue. The most important immunosuppressive effect of glucocorticoids, however, is their ability to impair recruitment of neutrophils, monocytes, and macrophages into an area of inflammation. They also affect humoral immunity by impairing release of effector substances, antigen processing, and antibody formation by B lymphocytes.

Other Effects

Glucocorticoids have many other effects, including their ability to produce significant mood changes and even psychosis in some patients. Also well known is the association of cataract formation and increased intraocular pressure with use of glucocorticoid medications. These hormones tend to lower serum calcium levels also. This occurs by several mechanisms, including their ability to block calcium absorption from the gut, decrease renal calcium reabsorption (resulting in hypercalciuria), and promote a shift of calcium from extracellular to intracellular compartments. Glucocorticoids can also affect the production and action of a number of other hormones, including insulin, thyroxine (T$_4$), and gonadal hormones.

ADRENAL HORMONE INSUFFICIENCY ■

Hypoadrenalism can occur on the basis of diseases that involve the adrenal gland directly (primary adrenal insufficiency), or because of the lack of stimulation by ACTH of an otherwise normal adrenal gland secondary to hypothalamic–pituitary disease (secondary adrenal insufficiency). Although the treatment of these two problems is similar, they have widely divergent causes and some differences in clinical presentation.

DIFFERENTIAL DIAGNOSIS

The most common cause of primary hypoadrenalism in the United States is autoimmune adrenalitis, which is responsible for almost 70% of cases described in this country. This disorder is associated with numerous other autoimmune-mediated endocrinopathies. In adults, these include thyroiditis and diabetes mellitus (Schmidt's syndrome). Occasionally, these patients may demonstrate other autoimmune disorders such as hypogonadism, vitiligo, and pernicious anemia.[3]

The second most common cause of primary adrenal insufficiency is destruction of the gland secondary to *Mycobacterium tuberculosis*. This rarely occurs except in the presence of other extrapulmonary tuberculosis, especially with involvement of the genitourinary system. In contrast to autoimmune adrenalitis, tuberculosis adrenal disease is not associated with other endocrine diseases. In addition, the adrenal glands are frequently enlarged and may be calcified in this disorder compared with the atrophied, noncalcified glands seen with autoimmune involvement.

Other much less common etiologies of primary hypoadrenalism are acquired immunodeficiency syndrome, bilateral hemorrhage of the glands secondary to bacterial infection with sepsis and shock, other granulomatous diseases such as sarcoidosis and systemic fungal infections, metastatic malignancies, and amyloidosis.

The differential diagnosis of secondary hypoadrenalism involves disorders of the hypothalamus or the pituitary. The most common disorders involving these organs are pituitary adenomas and hypothalamic neoplasms such as craniopharyngiomas. Metastatic carcinomas, most commonly from the lung or breast, or lymphoproliferative malignancies with involvement of the pituitary or hypothalamus can also produce adrenal insufficiency. Pituitary infarction in the immediate postpartum state (Sheehan's syndrome), traumatic lesions such as basilar skull fractures, infections such as tuberculosis, nocardiosis, actinomycosis, and other infiltrative diseases such as sarcoidosis, hemochromatosis, and amyloidosis have also been known to produce a similar condition. Overall, however, the most common cause of secondary adrenal insufficiency in this country is iatrogenic. The common use of high-dose glucocorticoid medications sufficient to suppress the HPA axis and increasing use of pituitary surgery and irradiation frequently result in adrenal insufficiency.

CLINICAL PRESENTATION

Although the symptoms, signs, and general laboratory results seen in adrenal insufficiency are nonspecific, taken together they form a pattern of findings that should suggest the possibility of hypoadrenalism. These findings are listed in Table 147-1. Virtually all patients describe significant weakness, fatigue, and loss of appetite. Most also complain of nausea and diarrhea, with occasional vomiting and abdominal pain. Less frequently, they note symptoms of myalgias, arthralgias, and orthostatic dizziness.

On physical examination, patients with adrenal insufficiency usually demonstrate weight loss and orthostatic hypotension. The blood pressure abnormalities are the result of decreased inotropic changes on the heart and decreased systemic vascular resistance, which can lead to severe hypotension even with a normal circulating blood volume. Patients with primary adrenal insufficiency may also show hyperpigmentation, especially of the tongue, buccal mucosa, palmar creases, and scar tissue. This occurs as the result of increased production of ACTH from the pituitary. Of course, hyperpigmentation is notably absent in secondary hypoadrenalism. If the underlying problem is autoimmune adrenalitis, the patient may show evidence of vitiligo, pernicious anemia, or one of the endocrinopathies commonly associated with this disorder.[4]

Laboratory evaluation of patients with suspected adrenal insufficiency is essential. The electrolyte abnormalities that occur depend on whether the patient has a combined glucocorticoid and mineralocorticoid deficiency (typical of primary adrenal disease) or an isolated glucocorticoid deficit (characteristic of secondary adrenal insufficiency). Those with a combined deficit of adrenal hormones commonly show evidence of hyponatremia, hyperkalemia, decreased serum bicarbonate levels, and elevated blood urea nitrogen (BUN), primarily due to mineralocorticoid deficiency, which leads to renal sodium loss, potassium retention, and dehydration with acidosis and prerenal azotemia.

Patients with secondary adrenal insufficiency usually have milder electrolyte abnormalities. Their normal adrenal glands are able to produce sufficient amounts of mineralocorticoid even in the absence of normal ACTH stimulus. These patients commonly demonstrate mild hyponatremia with normokalemia, presumably on the basis of decreased free water clearance. They often show little evidence of dehydration, and may actually gain weight secondary to water retention.

Other abnormal laboratory findings include anemia and a relative lymphocytosis with eosinophilia. These patients may also demonstrate hypoglycemia, which occurs as the result of increased utilization of glucose and decreased gluconeogenesis in the face of glucocorticoid deficiency.

Hormonal testing is necessary to confirm the diagnosis of adrenal insufficiency. Serum cortisol levels increase significantly in patients with normal adrenal function who are in shock. The finding of a cortisol level less than 20 μg/dL in the setting of shock is highly suggestive of compromised adrenal function.[5] As a rule, however, baseline serum and urine hormonal measurements are inadequate to confirm the diagnosis. Adrenal insufficiency can be determined effectively by ACTH stimulation tests. The short ACTH stimulation test (described in detail at the end of this chapter) is an excellent screening examination for adrenal insufficiency and may be performed without difficulty in an ICU patient.[6] If results are abnormal, the test should be followed at a later date by the long ACTH stimulation test which requires a prolonged ACTH infusion but can differentiate between primary and secondary adrenal insufficiency.

MANAGEMENT

The management of patients with adrenal insufficiency depends on whether the patient complains of mild symptoms suggestive of chronic hypoadrenalism and is felt to have normal cardiovascular hemodynamics or whether he or she presents in shock with symptoms of acute adrenal insufficiency (adrenal crisis).

Acute Adrenal Insufficiency

In the patient with suspected adrenal crisis, proper management requires immediate glucocorticoid therapy and intravenous (IV) administration of fluids, if necessary. Steps in the therapeutic and diagnostic management of acute adrenal insufficiency are outlined in Table 147-2.

It is essential to obtain baseline blood samples for cortisol levels, electrolytes, glucose, and renal function tests before the initiation of any therapy. The blood can be drawn for later use when intravenous lines are being placed to prevent any undue delay in starting therapy. Immediately after this, glucocorticoid therapy should begin. An excellent glucocorticoid medication to use is hydrocortisone hemisuccinate, which should be delivered initially as a 100-mg IV bolus, followed by a continuous IV infusion set to deliver approximately 75 to 100 mg of the medication every 6 hours. After resuscitation, as rapidly as their clinical condition allows, patients should receive tapered standard replacement doses of glucocorticoid, such as hydrocortisone 30 mg/24 hours or its equivalent (Table 147-3). Typically, mineralocorticoid therapy is not required in adrenal crisis as long as the patient is receiving isotonic saline.

For the patient with suspected adrenal crisis in whom no previous diagnosis of adrenal disease has been made, a short ACTH stimulation test is required to fully evaluate the patient for hypoadrenalism; this can easily be performed after resuscitative therapy has begun. Administration of hydrocortisone hemisuccinate results in increased serum cortisol levels, however, and interferes with the tests to establish the diagnosis of hypoadrenalism. In this instance, dexamethasone phosphate, which does not alter serum cortisol levels,

TABLE 147-3. Daily Replacement Doses for Several Common Glucocorticoid Medications

MEDICATION	DAILY DOSE (mg)
Hydrocortisone	30
Cortisone acetate	38
Prednisone	5
Prednisolone	5
Methylprednisolone	4
Dexamethasone	1

can be used to initiate glucocorticoid therapy while diagnostic tests are performed. The patient can be safely maintained on dexamethasone phosphate until the ACTH stimulation tests have been completed, at which time changing to appropriate doses of hydrocortisone hemisuccinate is suggested.

Fluid therapy should be administered in the form of isotonic saline to replace urinary salt losses. Occasionally the patient may be hypoglycemic, in which case 5% dextrose should be added to the isotonic saline infusion. It is important to treat patients for the underlying problem that precipitated the adrenal crisis. Prophylactic use of antibiotics is not beneficial in this regard, but specific infections should be treated aggressively with appropriate antibiotic therapy.

Chronic Adrenal Insufficiency

In patients who have slowly developed hypoadrenalism over the years, replacement therapy can be safely initiated after a full diagnostic evaluation is completed. Glucocorticoid replacement can be administered in the form of oral hydrocortisone at a dose of 30 mg/24 hours.[7] Although this can be given as a single dose, many patients prefer receiving 20 mg in the morning and 10 mg in the afternoon. An advantage of hydrocortisone is that it possesses some mineralocorticoid activity. As such, many patients with primary adrenal insufficiency can be treated with hydrocortisone alone as long as they receive adequate salt content in their diet. If the patient is unable to maintain normal salt balance while taking hydrocortisone alone (as evidenced by weight loss, hypotension, hyponatremia, and hyperkalemia), mineralocorticoids can be administered in the form of fludrocortisone acetate, 25 to 200 μg/24 hours.

Equally important to replacement hormone therapy is adequate patient instruction. Patients with adrenal insufficiency should be instructed to wear a medical alert bracelet. They should be supplied with a parenteral form of glucocorticoid and taught to self-administer the medication in the event of an emergency in which medication cannot be given orally. Finally, they should be instructed concerning those clinical situations in which increased amounts of glucocorticoid are required. For a minor degree of stress (an uncomplicated febrile illness), doubling or tripling the usual maintenance dose for a few days is probably adequate.[8] For severe stress (major accident, injury, illness, or surgery), patients should be instructed to notify their physicians of their clinical condition, because intravenous administration of a dose of glucocorticoid medication equivalent to hydrocortisone, 300 mg/24 hours, may be required.

ADRENAL HORMONE EXCESS (CUSHING'S SYNDROME) ∎

The constellation of characteristic signs and symptoms in the patient who has been chronically exposed to elevated levels of corticosteroids is termed *Cushing's syndrome* after Harvey Cushing, who first described the syndrome in 1912.[9]

Many different clinical situations can result in Cushing syndrome. The various etiologies can be divided into ACTH-mediated and non–ACTH-mediated categories. The ACTH-mediated causes include excessive production of ACTH by the pituitary, either from primary pituitary tumors or from excessive stimulation of the pituitary by CRH, and ectopic production of ACTH by nonpituitary tumors. The non–ACTH-mediated causes include iatrogenic Cushing's syndrome due to use of glucocorticoid drugs, and benign or malignant adrenal neoplasms with autonomous secretion of glucocorticoids.

The diagnosis and management of Cushing's syndrome is usually accomplished outside the critical care setting and therefore is beyond the scope of this discussion. Screening tests for this disorder (urine free-cortisol excretion and the overnight dexamethasone suppression test) are included with the adrenal function tests at the end of this chapter. Also included is a discussion of the long dexamethasone suppression test, which distinguishes many of the causes of Cushing's syndrome.

CLINICAL USE OF GLUCOCORTICOID MEDICATIONS ∎

There is a bewildering array of adrenal hormones available for use; it is up to the clinician to decide which one, at what dosage, and under what conditions it should be used. The most commonly used glucocorticoids are hydrocortisone, cortisone acetate, prednisone, prednisolone, methylprednisolone, and dexamethasone. A rough estimate of the relative glucocorticoid potency for each of these medications is provided by the doses of the medications suggested for normal daily glucocorticoid replacement (see Table 147-3). Cortisone acetate and prednisone must be converted in the liver to active metabolites before they have appreciable glucocorticoid activity. This may influence the choice of therapy in a patient with severe hepatic dysfunction. Hydrocortisone and cortisone acetate possess some mineralocorticoid activity, although at normal replacement doses of these medications, specific mineralocorticoid supplementation (fludrocortisone acetate 25 to 200 μg/24 hour) may be required.

GLUCOCORTICOID DOSAGE

The proper dose for a particular glucocorticoid medication is determined largely by the indications for its use. The choice of a particular steroid and its dose becomes a matter of reported clinical experience, pharmacologic (versus physiologic) effects, and prescribing habits. For example, glucocorticoids are commonly used for acute trauma to the central nervous system (CNS) in doses that are orders of magnitude beyond those that produce maximum glucocorticoid effects.[10] Despite this, a dose–response relationship exists between the dose of a glucocorticoid and the clinical outcome. The pharmacology of glucocorticoids in these massive doses is not well understood, and their use is guided by clinical experience and experimental data from animal models in which they have been beneficial.

A principal guideline in using steroid hormone medications is to accomplish the therapeutic endpoint while using the least amount of glucocorticoid for the shortest length of time. This is done to minimize the side effects and complications of glucocorticoid therapy, as well as to prevent suppression of the HPA axis. In addition to their well-known metabolic and immunologic effects, glucocorticoids have been associated with various complications, such as glaucoma, posterior subcapsular cataracts, benign intracranial hypertension, psychiatric symptoms, pancreatitis, edema, aseptic necrosis of bone, and poor wound healing, among others.[11]

A major concern in the use of large doses of glucocorticoids is suppression of the HPA axis, placing the patient at risk for adrenal insufficiency in times of stress. In general, doses of glucocorticoids equivalent to 20 to 30 mg of prednisone daily for 1 week probably do not cause clinically important adrenal suppression.[12] For larger doses or more prolonged usage, the physician can assume some degree of adrenal suppression has occurred. This is supported by abnormal findings on ACTH stimulation testing (discussed at the end of this chapter). Realizing that these laboratory findings may not correlate with clinically significant adrenal suppression, common practice is to treat patients as if they have adrenal insufficiency in times of stress for at least 1 year after cessation of prolonged or high-dose glucocorticoid therapy, unless the HPA axis had been shown to be functioning properly.[13]

PRINCIPLES OF TAPERING GLUCOCORTICOIDS

The decision to stop glucocorticoid therapy can be a major clinical problem. If there is any doubt as to the functional capability of the HPA axis, the medications should be tapered rather than abruptly discontinued. The rate at which the taper occurs should vary in different clinical situations. The choice of a particular tapering schedule must take into account the duration and magnitude of therapy to estimate to what degree the HPA axis had been suppressed: the more the suppression, the slower the taper. In addition, the underlying disease process must be considered; a self-limited acute allergic reaction might require only 3 days of large doses with no taper, whereas an aggressive inflammatory arthritis might require a taper lasting months to prevent a disease flareup.

Typically, a steroid taper follows these general guidelines. First, drug administration should be switched from an intravenous to an oral route. Next, a change should be made from divided doses of glucocorticoids to a single morning dose using a short-acting medication. Of the commonly used glucocorticoids, dexamethasone has the longest duration of action whereas hydrocortisone and cortisone acetate have the shortest durations of action. Use of short-acting agents allows some escape from the ACTH-suppressive effects of the drug in the early morning hours, allowing the HPA axis to be stimulated. The absolute amount of glucocorticoid that can be withdrawn depends in some measure on the total amount of steroid that the patient is taking. In general, for glucocorticoid doses greater than 40 mg of prednisone or its equivalent, individual decrements of 10 mg can be used; when the prednisone dose is 20 to 40 mg, decrements should be limited to 5 mg; when the prednisone dose falls below 20 mg, individual decrements of no more than 2.5 mg should be attempted. Finally, the timing of each decrement may vary from 1 day to several weeks, depending on the clinical situation. The glucocorticoid dose is tapered only as rapidly as the patient's clinical condition permits to prevent relapse of the underlying disease state.

Specific guidelines for managing withdrawal from steroid therapy have been previously published.[14] In general, medication should be tapered to a single 20-mg morning dose of hydrocortisone. When the basal serum cortisol level measured at 7:00 to 8:00 AM (and obtained before the usual morning hydrocortisone dose) is greater than 10 μg/dL, glucocorticoid supplementation can be discontinued, although the patient should still be considered to have a suppressed HPA axis in times of stress. Full recovery of the HPA axis is determined by normalization of the serum cortisol response to ACTH as noted in the short ACTH stimulation test.

For anticipated prolonged use of glucocorticoids, alternative-day therapy should be considered. The rationale for this approach is that the antiinflammatory effects of the medications last longer than the glucocorticoid effects. Thus, by using a short-acting glucocorticoid once every other morning, the underlying disease process may be controlled, yet HPA suppression can be prevented and the development of drug side effects minimized. Despite careful tapering of the glucocorticoid dosage, the patient may still experience symptoms of glucocorticoid withdrawal, including fever, anorexia, nausea, lethargy, arthralgias, desquamation of the skin, weakness, and weight loss.

ADRENAL FUNCTION TESTS ■

The following section lists important common biochemical tests for evaluating patients with adrenal disease.

SERUM CORTISOL

PROCEDURE. Serum is collected for a standard radioimmunoassay. It is important to note the time of collection, because cortisol levels vary throughout the day.

NORMAL VALUES. 7:00 to 8:00 AM, 5 to 25 μg/dL; 10:00 to 11:00 PM, 5 to 10 μg/dL.

COMMENTS. Serum cortisol levels vary in a circadian pattern, with peak levels in the early morning and nadirs late at night. Basal cortisol levels alone are not very useful in the evaluation of adrenal disease, but are important in conjunction with maneuvers that stimulate or suppress the adrenal gland.

High-normal cortisol levels with loss of the normal circadian pattern is suggestive of Cushing's syndrome. In untreated hypotensive patients with suspected acute adrenal insufficiency, a cortisol level less than 20 μg/dL strongly suggests the diagnosis.[5]

URINE FREE-CORTISOL EXCRETION

PROCEDURE. A quantitated 24-hour urine specimen is collected and measured for free-cortisol levels. The 24-hour urine free-cortisol excretion is calculated based on the measured urine volume. Measurement of urine creatinine is suggested to assess for the adequacy of the collection.

NORMAL VALUES. 20 to 90 μg/24 hours.

COMMENTS. The urine free-cortisol excretion correlates well with cortisol production integrated over 24 hours. The test is extremely useful in screening for patients with Cushing syndrome, who excrete elevated amounts of the hormone.[15]

ACTH LEVELS

PROCEDURE. Serum is collected for a standard radioimmunoassay. Since ACTH levels vary throughout the day, it is important to obtain the sample between 7:00 and 8:00 AM.

NORMAL VALUES. Less than 70 pg/mL.

COMMENTS. ACTH levels vary in a circadian pattern, with peak levels in the early morning and nadirs late at night. These levels are most useful in differentiating between those patients who have ectopic ACTH syndrome and those with adrenal adenomas as the etiology of Cushing syndrome.[9] Patients in both of these groups have elevated glucocorticoid levels unresponsive to high-dose dexamethasone suppression. Patients with ectopic ACTH syndrome have high ACTH levels, however, whereas the ACTH levels are suppressed in patients with adrenal adenomas. ACTH levels are rather poor in differentiating patients with Cushing disease from normals[16] and should not be used regularly for that purpose.

SHORT ACTH STIMULATION TEST

PROCEDURE. Serum samples are obtained just before and 30 and 60 minutes after an IV injection of 250 μg of cosyntropin (synthetic 1,24-ACTH).

NORMAL VALUES. A normal response is defined as an increase in the cortisol level of at least 7 μg/dL over the basal level *and* a rise in serum cortisol to an absolute level of at least 20 μg/dL. Note that *both* conditions must be met for a normal response.

COMMENTS. The short ACTH stimulation test is a simple, effective test for evaluating adrenal insufficiency,[6] and can be performed in an ICU. It does not differentiate between primary and secondary hypoadrenalism.

LONG ACTH STIMULATION TEST

PROCEDURE. Urine 17-hydroxycorticosteroid (17-OHCS) excretion is measured daily on quantitated 24-hour urine collections while the patient is receiving an IV infusion of ACTH in the following manner: 250 μg of cosyntropin is placed in 500 mL of normal saline, and the solution is infused over 8 hours during each 24-hour period for 2 to 5 consecutive days.

NORMAL VALUES. A normal response is defined as 17-OHCS excretion of at least 10 mg/24 hours.

COMMENTS. This stimulation test is required to differentiate primary from secondary adrenal insufficiency in those patients with abnormal responses to the short ACTH stimulation test.[17] It can be performed after a patient has been fully stabilized.

Patients with primary hypoadrenalism do not respond in a normal fashion. Patients with secondary hypoadrenalism have a delayed response, normalizing 17-OHCS excretion as early as the second day of collection, but at times requiring up to 5 days of ACTH infusion to produce a normal response.

OVERNIGHT DEXAMETHASONE SUPPRESSION TEST

PROCEDURE. Dexamethasone, 1.0 mg, is administered orally at 11:00 PM on day 1. Serum is collected for measurement of a cortisol level at 7:00 to 8:00 AM on day 2.

NORMAL VALUES. A normal response is for the morning serum cortisol level to be suppressed to less than 5 μg/dL following administration of dexamethasone the night before.

COMMENTS. The overnight dexamethasone suppression test is an excellent screening test for the evaluation of Cushing syndrome.[18] If abnormal, it should be followed by the long dexamethasone suppression test.

LONG DEXAMETHASONE SUPPRESSION TEST

PROCEDURE. Urine 17-OHCS excretion is measured daily for 6 days with quantitated 24-hour urine collections. Measurement of urine creatinine is suggested to assess for the adequacy of the collections.

On days 1 and 2 the patient receives no glucocorticoid medication. These collections represent the baseline 17-OHCS excretion levels. On days 3 and 4 the patient receives 0.5 mg dexamethasone every 6 hours (a total of eight 0.5-mg doses is given during this 48-hour period). This is defined as the low-dose dexamethasone suppression test. On days 5 and 6 the patient receives 2.0 mg dexamethasone every 6 hours (a total of eight 2.0-mg doses is given during this 48-

hour period). This is defined as the high-dose dexamethasone suppression test.

In place of the 17-OHCS excretion, measurement of 24-hour urine free-cortisol excretion or serum cortisol levels may be made to quantitate cortisol production, but the normal responses of these tests to low- and high-dose dexamethasone suppression are less well standardized.

NORMAL VALUES.   A normal response to low-dose dexamethasone administration is to suppress 17-OHCS excretion on day 4 to less than or equal to 3 mg/24 hours. An evaluation of the response to high-dose dexamethasone administration is valid only in those patients who are thought to have Cushing syndrome.

COMMENTS.   An inability to suppress 17-OHCS excretion on day 4 to less than or equal to 3 mg/24 hours strongly suggests Cushing syndrome. The high-dose dexamethasone response can then be evaluated to help determine the etiology of this disorder. If the patient suppresses the 24-hour 17-OHCS secretion on day 6 to less than 50% of the average 24-hour 17-OHCS excretion on days 1 and 2, an ACTH-producing pituitary adenoma is strongly suggested as the cause of Cushing syndrome. On the other hand, if the 24-hour 17-OHCS excretion on day 6 is not suppressed to less than 50% of the average 24-hour 17-OHCS excretion on days 1 and 2, the cause of Cushing syndrome is most likely an adrenal adenoma or ectopic ACTH syndrome.[19] These two etiologies of Cushing syndrome can usually be differentiated by measuring basal ACTH levels.

REFERENCES ■

1. Baxter JD, Forsham PH: Tissue effects of glucocorticoids. *Am J Med* 1972;53:573
2. Meuleman J, Katz P: The immunologic effects, kinetics, and use of glucocorticosteroids. *Med Clin North Am* 1985;69: 805
3. Loriaux DL: The polyendocrine deficiency syndromes. *N Engl J Med* 1985;312:1568
4. Nerup J. Addison's disease—clinical studies: a report of 108 cases. *Acta Endocrinol* 1974;76:127
5. Mattingly D, Tyler C: Plasma 11-hydroxycorticoid levels in surgical stress. *Proc R Soc Med* 1965;58:1010
6. Kehlet H, Lindholm J, Bjerre P: Value of the 30-min ACTH test in assessing hypothalamic-pituitary-adrenocortical function after pituitary surgery in Cushing's disease. *Clin Endocrinol* 1984;20:349
7. Kehlet H, Binder C, Blichert-Toft M: Glucocorticoid maintenance therapy following adrenalectomy: assessment of dosage and preparation. *Clin Endocrinol* 1976;5:37
8. Beisel WR, Bruton J, Anderson KD, et al: Adrenocortical responses during tularemia in human subjects. *J Clin Endocrinol Metab* 1967;27:61
9. Besser GM, Edwards CRW: Cushing's syndrome. *Clin Endocrinol Metab* 1972;1:451
10. Braughler JM, Hall ED: Current application of "high dose" steroid therapy for CNS injury: a pharmacologic perspective. *J Neurosurg* 1985;62:806
11. Axeirod L: Glucocorticoid therapy. *Medicine* 1976;55:39
12. Spiegel RJ, Vigersky RA, Oliff AL, et al: Adrenal suppression after short term corticosteroid therapy. *Lancet* 1979;1:630
13. Graber AL, Ney RL, Nicholson WE, et al: Natural history of pituitary-adrenal recovery following long-term suppression with corticosteroids. *J Clin Endocrinol* 1965;25:11
14. Byyny RL: Withdrawal from glucocorticoid therapy. *N Engl J Med* 1976;295:30
15. Dunlap NE, Grizzle WE, Siegel AL: Cushing's syndrome: screening methods in hospitalized patients. *Arch Pathol Lab Med* 1985;109:222
16. Croughs RJM, Tops CF, Dejong FH: Radioimmunoassay of plasma adrenocorticotropin in Cushing's syndrome. *J Endocrinol* 1973;59:439
17. Rose LI, Williams GH, Jagger PI, et al: The 48-hour adrenocorticotropin infusion test for adrenocortical insufficiency. *Ann Intern Med* 1970;73:49
18. Nugent CA, Nichols T, Tyler FH: Diagnosis of Cushing's syndrome. *Arch Intern Med* 1965;116:172
19. Liddle GW: Tests of pituitary-adrenal suppressibility in the diagnosis of Cushing's syndrome. *J Clin Endocrinol Metab* 1960;20:1539

Critical Care, Third Edition, edited by Joseph M. Civetta,
Robert W. Taylor, and Robert R. Kirby.
Lippincott-Raven Publishers, Philadelphia, PA © 1997.

CHAPTER 148

Pheochromocytoma

Gary L. Mueller
Charles A. Reasner

IMMEDIATE CONCERNS ■

MAJOR PROBLEMS

*It is important to reemphasize the seriousness of diagnosing
and treating pheochromocytoma with the aphorism of Esper-
son and Dahl-Iversen that although a pheochromocytoma
may be morphologically benign it is physiologically malignant and with Ararow's characterization of this tumor as a
"veritable pharmacological bomb." If managed appropriately by a highly skilled and professional "bomb squad," this
tumor can be removed and the patient cured in at least 90%
of cases. The secret lies in first suspecting and recognizing
the patient who has pheochromocytoma and then offering
the expert management such a patient requires.*
W.M. Manger and R.W. Gifford, Jr.[1(xiii)]

STRESS POINTS

1. Pheochromocytomas are rare tumors that arise from
   the enterochromaffin system.
2. The majority of these tumors are endocrinologically
   active, producing norepinephrine, epinephrine, and
   other secretory products.

ESSENTIAL DIAGNOSTIC TESTS
AND PROCEDURES

1. Patients may present with a wide variety of symptoms
   and signs as a result of the catecholamine excess. Chief
   among the signs is hypertension, which may be paroxysmal or sustained. Headaches, sweating, palpitations,
   tachycardia, mental status changes or "spells," and a
   plethora of other signs and symptoms may accompany
   the hypertension.
2. When the diagnosis is clinically suspected, the patient
   should be screened biochemically with a 24-hour urine
   collection for metanephrine, vanillylmandelic acid
   (VMA), and free catecholamines. The urine should be
   acidified and refrigerated during collection.
3. The patient's plasma catecholamines should be measured under standardized conditions in a nonstressed
   environment. Borderline catecholamine elevations,
   which can be seen in hypertensive patients who do
   not harbor pheochromocytomas can be investigated
   using the clonidine suppression test or the glucagon
   stimulation test.
4. After the biochemical diagnosis of pheochromocytoma is made, the tumor is localized using magnetic
   resonance imaging (MRI), computed tomography (CT),
   131-I-metaiodobenzylguanidine scanning (^{131}I-MIBG),
   or a combination of these techniques. Invasive imaging is avoided to prevent precipitation of a hypertensive "pheo crisis."

INITIAL THERAPY

1. After the tumor is localized, surgical removal is performed.
2. Preoperative preparation of the patient may involve
   the use of alpha-adrenergic blockade followed by beta-
   adrenergic blockade.
3. Anesthetic management by skilled personnel involves
   the judicious use of fluids and blood for volume expansion, adrenergic blocking agents, or pressors, combined with sophisticated intravascular pressure
   monitoring.

4. With careful attention to detail and an appropriate team approach, operative mortality should be near zero, and the patient's symptoms and signs, including the hypertension, should be relieved.

5. Patients with pheochromocytoma who present with acute medical emergencies, such as hypertensive crises, acute myocardial infarctions, cerebrovascular accidents, or other life-threatening conditions, require admission to the critical care unit. Invasive blood pressure monitoring may be necessary. Acute reduction of blood pressure can be accomplished by administering standard dilutions of drugs such as sodium nitroprusside or phentolamine in carefully titrated increments.

6. Pheochromocytomas occur sporadically or as a component of inherited syndromes, the most common of which is multiple endocrine neoplasia (MEN) type II. They are also seen in patients with neurofibromatosis, von Hippel–Lindau disease, and several more unusual syndromes. Special attention is required to exclude the diagnosis of pheochromocytoma when dealing with these conditions.

7. Pregnant women who harbor pheochromocytomas require particular care to prevent an extraordinarily high maternal and fetal morbidity and mortality rate.

8. In the rare patient with symptomatic metastatic disease, judicious catecholamine blockade can significantly improve the quality of life.

PRESENTING SYMPTOMS AND SIGNS ■

The symptoms and signs caused by pheochromocytomas are so diverse that the tumor has been called "the great imitator." Rabin and McKenna[2] devised a useful system in which these symptoms and signs are categorized as hypertension and its complications, catecholamine excess, hypermetabolism, and associated features.

HYPERTENSION AND ITS COMPLICATIONS

Pheochromocytomas are a rare cause of hypertension, accounting for approximately 0.05% to 0.1% of cases. Accurate diagnosis is important, however, because tumor resection leads to cure of the hypertension in up to 80% of patients, whereas failure to make the diagnosis and treat the patient appropriately can be fatal. Hypertension is present in 95% of pheochromocytoma patients; 50% have sustained hypertension, and 45% have paroxysmal blood pressure elevations that may be life-threatening. Five percent are relatively normotensive.[3] The hemodynamic features seen in patients with sustained hypertension are similar to those seen in patients with essential hypertension (increased peripheral resistance), whereas the hypertensive crisis is a hyperkinetic, vasoconstrictive, hypovolemic form of hypertension that combines increased cardiac rate, systemic vascular resistance, and myocardial contractility with decreased venous compliance.[4] Hypertensive crises that occur during micturition suggest a pheochromocytoma located in the bladder

wall. Possible complications caused by pheochromocytoma-induced hypertension are congestive heart failure, myocardial infarction, and cerebrovascular events. Headache is common; it is typically pounding and bitemporal. It has a rapid onset, but lasts less than 1 hour. It often occurs in the early morning and may awaken the patient from sleep. Nausea and vomiting can be present as well.

CATECHOLAMINE EXCESS

Pheochromocytomas usually release norepinephrine as their primary secretory product. (Rarely, epinephrine is the primary secretory product; these epinephrine-secreting pheochromocytomas arise almost exclusively from the adrenal medulla.) The norepinephrine released may cause sweating, cutaneous flushing, extreme anxiety or panic reactions, peripheral vasoconstriction, tachycardia with palpitations or other cardiac arrhythmias, angina pectoris, and acute abdominal pain. Some patients experience peripheral vasospasm and Raynaud's phenomenon. Livido reticularis can occur. The rare subset of patients with epinephrine, dopa, or dopamine-producing tumors may present with orthostatic hypotension (a drop of 10 mm Hg or more) or alternating hypertension–hypotension.[5]

HYPERMETABOLISM

Catecholamines are part of the "flight or fight" system. As a result, pheochromocytoma patients may exhibit signs or symptoms of hypermetabolism that resemble those seen in hyperthyroidism. Fever and profound weight loss are not uncommon. Glucose intolerance or even frank diabetes mellitus can be present. This is caused by catecholamine-induced glycolysis, lipolysis, and increased gluconeogenesis from enhanced muscle lactate production. Lactic acidosis can occur in the absence of shock. In addition, catecholamines exert a direct antiinsulin effect on the liver and other peripheral insulin-sensitive tissues. Free fatty acid levels may rise above 2000 μEq/L.

ASSOCIATED FEATURES

Associated features are primarily found as part of the diseases discussed later under Unusual Presentations. They include goiter, cholelithiasis, neurofibromas, retinal angiomatosis, and ectopic hormone production.

PATHOLOGY ■

Pheochromocytomas occur in 1 to 2 adults per 100,000 per year. The autopsy incidence in one large referral center is 0.3%.[6] Pheochromocytomas arise from cells derived from the neural crest. They are considered derivatives of the amine precursor uptake and decarboxylation (APUD) cell line. While the genetic predisposition to the development of this tumor is heterogeneous, loss of heterozygosity (LOH) involves the short arm of chromosome 1 (1p) most frequently. LOH may also occur on chromosomes 3p, 11p,

17p, or the long arm of chromosome 22 (22q).[7] Their size ranges from microscopic foci to over 2 kg. Most are 5 to 6 cm in diameter and weigh approximately 90 g. They have a fibrous capsule. The cut surface is red or gray, spongy, and obviously vascular. Focal areas of hemorrhage or cystic degeneration[8] may be present. A central white scar is often seen. Classically, tumors that contain epinephrine stain a dark mahogany brown with potassium dichromate and are "chromaffin-positive." Norepinephrine-secreting tumors do not stain and are "chromaffin-negative", or nonchromaffin tumors. Staining characteristics, however, do not correlate uniformly with tumor function.

Because of the frequent appearance of 10% in pheochromocytoma statistics, the tumor has been called a "10% disease." Ten percent of pheochromocytomas arise outside the adrenal medullae. Ten percent are bilateral, except in the MEN type II syndrome and in children, where the incidence of bilaterality is in excess of 50%. Approximately 10% of all pheochromocytomas are malignant.[9] These tumors occur in extraadrenal loci 10% of the time. Extraadrenal tumors are multicentric in 15% to 20% of patients. They have been found anywhere from the carotid bodies to the bladder. A pheochromocytoma occasionally arises below the bifurcation of the abdominal aorta in the organ of Zuckerkandl. Zuckerkandl tumors are rarely palpable and may be silent until a life-threatening pheo crisis occurs.[10]

Gross and microscopic features do not reliably differentiate benign from malignant tumors. A diagnosis of malignancy depends on the demonstration of metastases in sites where chromaffin tissue is not usually found. Common sites for metastases include bone, liver, lung, lymph nodes, bone marrow, brain, and omentum. Attempts to correlate the hypersecretion of multiple peptides or neuropeptides with malignant behavior in these tumors have been less than uniformly successful.[11] DNA ploidy patterns can be an indicator of potential aggressive behavior. DNA diploidy is more indicative of benignity while DNA aneuploidy and tetraploidy are more indicative of aggressive behavior.[12]

DIANOSIS

BIOCHEMICAL CONFIRMATION

When the possibility of a pheochromocytoma is seriously considered, biochemical confirmation must be obtained. Biochemical tests can be divided into screening tests and more sophisticated confirmatory testing. Classically, the diagnosis depended on 24-hour urine collections for VMA, metanephrine–normetanephrine metabolites, and urinary free catecholamines. When specimens are properly collected in 15 mL of 6N hydrochloric acid (pH maintained at less than 3.0) and refrigerated during collection, representative upper limits of normal in normotensive subjects are 8.0 mg, 1.3 mg, 135 μg (norepinephrine), and 37 μg (epinephrine) per 24 hours, respectively. The total urine creatinine should be determined to assess the adequacy of the collection. Whenever possible, the urine collection should be performed after any potentially interfering medications have been withdrawn. Among the many drugs that commonly

interfere with the urinary determination of catecholamine metabolites are methyldopa, L-dopa, tetracycline, erythromycin, isoproterenol, metaproterenol, terbutaline, clofibrate, nalidixic acid, labetalol, monoamine oxidase inhibitors, phenothiazines, and tricyclic antidepressants. Since urinary assays can have significant false-positive and false-negative rates, many diagnostic centers also measure plasma catecholamines for the diagnosis of pheochromocytoma.

Blood for plasma catecholamine determination should be drawn from an indwelling line placed at least 30 minutes before sampling. The patient should be supine in a quiet room and nonstressed. The sample must be processed rapidly in accordance with the laboratory's instructions. Catecholamines in whole blood deteriorate at a rate of about 30% per hour at room temperature, so prompt processing is essential. Upper limits of normal are provided by the reference laboratory performing the assays. Normotensive controls usually have norepinephrine levels below 620 ng/ L and epinephrine levels below 129 ng/L. Epinephrine constitutes 10% to 20% of the total plasma catecholamine content. Levels may rise with age, physical and mental stress, acute and chronic illness, and essential hypertension. A wide variety of drugs (indirect-acting sympathomimetics, vasodilators, alpha-adrenergic antagonists, diuretics, tobacco, marijuana, and caffeine) can also cause spurious results.[13,14] Elevated plasma metanephrines (normetanephrine, metanephrine, or both) correctly identified 52 of 52 pheochromocytoma patients (sensitivity 100%). The negative predictive value in 162 nonpheochromocytoma patients was 100%. Cardiac disease, chronic renal failure, and other types of secondary hypertension can cause plasma metanephrine elevations; so, assay results must be interpreted with caution in these groups.[14a]

Dynamic testing is usually unnecessary in patients who have unequivocal elevation of plasma or urinary catecholamines (plasma norepinephrine >1200 pg/mL, plasma epinephrine >276 pg/mL, dihydroxyphenylalanine >7000 pg/ mL, norepinephrine:dihydroxyphenylethylglycol ratio >1.09).[15] In borderline cases, such as patients with essential hypertension (160/100 mm Hg or less), suggestive symptoms, or moderate increases in catecholamine levels (plasma catecholamines 500 to 1000 pg/mL), dynamic testing may be useful.[16] In these patients, consultation with an endocrinologist is suggested. Older dynamic tests (e.g., histamine, tyramine, glucagon, and phentolamine) have fallen into disuse because of their potential to produce profound hypertensive or hypotensive crises. They have been replaced by the clonidine suppression test and the glucagon stimulation test. The clonidine suppression test takes advantage of clonidine's ability to suppress central nervous system sympathetic outflow, reducing neurogenically induced hypercatecholaminemia in normal subjects. This mechanism is not involved in the control of catecholamine production or release from pheochromocytomas. Oral administration of 0.3 mg of clonidine causes a statistically significant fall in plasma norepinephrine and epinephrine levels by 3 hours after administration in normal persons and in patients with essential hypertension. In contrast, levels in pheochromocytoma patients usually decrease insignificantly, remain the same, or even increase. Patients normally experience the minor side effects of drowsiness and dry mouth during the test, but symptomatic orthostatic hypotension and rebound signs and symptoms are not seen.[17] When plasma catecholamines are not readily available, a variation of this protocol may be useful. The patient receives 0.3 mg of clonidine orally at 9:00 PM. A timed urine specimen is collected between 9:00 PM and 7:00 AM. Normal subjects and essential hypertension patients suppress their norepinephrine and epinephrine levels to less than 60 and 20 nmol/mmol of creatinine, respectively; pheochromocytoma patients remain above these threshold values.[18]

The glucagon stimulation test is performed after an overnight fast. A cold pressor test provides a baseline reference for stress-induced blood pressure elevations. After the insertion of an indwelling intravenous (IV) line and a 30- to 60-minute reequilibration period, 1.0 mg of glucagon is injected as an IV bolus. Blood pressure and pulse are measured for 10 consecutive minutes. Blood for catecholamine measurements are drawn before glucagon injection and at 2 minutes after injection. Excessive increases in blood pressure (>200/120 mm Hg) may occur and should be managed with phentolamine, 5 to 10 mg IV, or with sodium nitroprusside by IV drip. Although generally well tolerated, glucagon can cause nausea and vomiting. An increase in plasma catecholamines to over 2000 pg/mL or a threefold increase over baseline levels constitutes a positive test. An increase in blood pressure of at least 20/15 mm Hg above the cold pressor response is also suggestive. Pretreatment with nifedipine, 10 mg orally, 30 minutes before glucagon administration, prevents the blood pressure increase, but does not interfere with the rise in catecholamines.[19] When both the clonidine suppression test and the glucagon stimulation test were negative, the diagnosis of pheochromocytoma was ruled out.[15]

Some centers measure chromogranin A in suspected pheochromocytoma patients. It is an acidic, monomeric protein that is costored and coreleased with catecholamines by exocytosis from adrenal medullary storage vesicles. In one series, plasma levels were elevated (>112 ng/mL) in 83% of their patients with proved pheochromocytomas. The specificity of the test was 96%. Overlap with normal subjects and patients with essential and secondary hypertension was minimal. Since chromogranin A is excreted by the kidneys, levels can be increased in patients with renal insufficiency.[20]

ANATOMIC LOCALIZATION

After biochemical confirmation has been obtained, anatomic localization of the tumor becomes the goal. Older diagnostic imaging techniques, such as intravenous pyelography with or without tomography, selective arteriography, adrenal venography, and diagnostic ultrasonography, as well as venous sampling for catecholamine levels, often fail to localize the lesion and subject the patient to potentially life-threatening hypertensive crises. In an attempt to improve the yield and safety of localization procedures, noninvasive imaging procedures using MRI, CT, and ^{131}I-MIBG scanning have become primary imaging modalities. CT scanning is the most widely available, noninvasive method for locating pheochromocyto-

mas. Ninety-five percent of tumors 1 cm or larger within the adrenal medullae are visualized with this technique. Extraadrenal lesions 2 cm or larger are routinely imaged. Oral or IV contrast may be necessary to reliably visualize abdominal and chest lesions.[21]

MRI also readily demonstrates both primary and metastatic pheochromocytomas. More than 95% of tumors are identified. Tumors are distinguished from adjacent structures without the use of contrast agents. Adrenal masses that are hyperintense on T2-weighted spin echo images are pathognomonic for pheochromocytomas, but T1-weighted sequences may be necessary for complete visualization of small or ectopic lesions in which tumor–fat interfaces are critical. MRI does not produce artifacts from surgical clips as CT does. It is also superior to CT for imaging extraadrenal pheochromocytomas.[22]

Although it is available at only a small number of centers, radionuclide imaging with ^{131}I-MIBG is a useful tool for anatomic localization. It has been used to image adrenal lesions, adrenal medullary hyperplasia, small tumors in patients with MEN, residual or recurrent tumors at prior operative sites, and metastases from malignant pheochromocytomas. This ^{131}I-radiolabeled guanethidine analog is actively taken up by pheochromocytoma cells. It provides a safe, specific, noninvasive technique for tumor localization. After thyroidal iodine uptake is blocked with potassium iodide, 0.5 mCi of ^{131}I-MIBG per 1.73 m^2 of body surface area (maximum dose 0.5 mCi) is administered. When obesity or known or suspected metastatic disease is present, the dose may be increased to 1.0 mCi of ^{131}I-MIBG per 1.73 m^2 of body surface area (maximum dose 1.0 mCi). Images are obtained with a large field-of-view gamma-camera with a high-energy, parallel-hole collimator at 24, 48, and 72 hours. Normal patients may have uptake in the salivary glands, left ventricle, lung bases, liver, spleen, colon, and urinary bladder. Intraadrenal pheochromocytomas usually image as intense focal uptake by 24 hours. Extraadrenal lesions or metastases are seen as focal areas of uptake in sites not seen in normal patients. All areas of uptake in pheochromocytomas become increasingly well defined between 24 and 72 hours. In 927 cases studied at the University of Michigan, the specificity of the test was 97%, with 99% sensitivity. There were 174 true-positive, 727 true-negative, four false-positive, and 22 false-negative results.[23] Medications such as labetalol, reserpine, calcium channel blockers, tricyclic antidepressants, sympathomimetics, and adrenergic blockers can decrease the uptake of ^{131}I-MIBG. They should be discontinued 1 week before radionuclide administration.[24] Single photon emission computed tomography (SPECT) using ^{123}I-MIBG, a further refinement of MIBG imaging that provides clearer visualization of both normal structures and pheochromocytomas, has been used on a limited investigational basis.

Newer methodologies for pheochromocytoma imaging include carbon-11 hydroxyephedrine (^{11}C-HED) positron emission tomography (PET) and iodine-123 or indium-111 octreotide scanning. Carbon-11 hydroxyephedrine, which structurally resembles norepinephrine, is selectively taken up by organs with rich sympathetic innervation. Within 20 minutes of IV administration, its distribution can be mapped using PET scanning. The technique yields images of superior quality over ^{131}I-MIBG techniques. In an initial study, pheochromocytomas were localized in 9 of 10 patients imaged. The tumor that did not visualize secreted predominantly dopamine.[25] The long-acting somatostatin analog octreotide can be labeled with iodine-123 or indium-111. Using this labeled hormone, paragangliomas as small as 1 cm have been demonstrated. For imaging to take place, the tumor must possess somatostatin receptors.[26]

MANAGEMENT ■

Treatment for pheochromocytoma is surgical excision of the tumor or tumors whenever possible. If excision is not possible, pharmacologic blockade is indicated to prevent the complications associated with excessive catecholamine secretion. Pharmacologic blockade may also be indicated in the preoperative period to prevent the hypertensive or hypotensive crises associated with these tumors.

Classically, phenoxybenzamine, 10 to 20 mg tid, or qid for 7 to 11 days, has been used to produce preoperative alpha-adrenergic blockade. Prazosin, 2 to 5 mg bid, has been used with good results.[27] Alpha-adrenergic blockade controls the hypertension, allows gradual reexpansion of diminished intravascular volume, and smooths anesthesia induction. Complete blockade is undesirable because it may mask the presence of a second tumor after operative removal of the first tumor. Intravascular volume expansion is necessary and reduces the incidence of postoperative hypotension. Calcium channel blockers such as nifedipine[28] attenuate the catecholamine-induced increase in blood pressure, thus neutralizing the pressor effects of catecholamines on vascular smooth muscle. These drugs may be used in combination with alpha- and beta-blockade to control blood pressure elevations in these patients. In several cases calcium channel blockers have been the sole effective therapy prescribed.[29,30] Beta-adrenergic blockade with propranolol or another agent may be necessary in some patients with cardiac arrhythmias, but it should not be given without first providing adequate alpha-adrenergic blockade to prevent severe hypertensive crises. Additional therapeutic alternatives are shown in Table 148-1.

Newer short-acting beta-adrenergic agents such as esmolol have been used successfully to manage the arrhythmias and blood pressure lability present in these patients. Esmolol's short half-life allows rapid titration of the drug to maximal therapeutic effect on blood pressure and heart rate.[31] Anesthesia and surgery should be performed by physicians experienced in the treatment of pheochromocytoma. An experienced postanesthesia care unit staff is essential.

Acute management of hypertensive crises may be accomplished with phentolamine, a short-acting alpha-adrenergic blocker, or sodium nitroprusside, a vasodilator. The physician should carefully select the lowest effective dose of either drug to prevent severe hypotension. Phentolamine, 10 μg/mL (5 mg in 500 mL of D_5W), or sodium nitroprusside, 4

μg/mL (1 mg in 250 mL of D_5W) can be infused to titrate blood pressure to acceptable levels. Volume expansion is preferred to pressors for the treatment of hypotension, if it occurs.

Unresectable metastatic pheochromocytomas may be managed with pharmacologic blockade using phenoxybenzamine, phentolamine, prazosin, calcium channel blockers, and beta-blockade (if arrhythmias are present). Metyrosine (α-methyl-L-tyrosine) has been used successfully to inhibit catecholamine biosynthesis in some of these patients; the dosage ranges from 250 mg to 1 g qid.[32] In selected patients with metastatic disease, tumor volume or hormonal activity has been reduced by therapy with 100 to 200 mCi of ^{131}I-MIBG infused over 90 minutes after thyroidal uptake of iodine-131 is blocked with iodide for 1 month. Tumor response to therapy has permitted reduction in alpha-adrenergic blockade with improvement or disappearance of symptoms in some patients. Side effects of the therapy were mild nausea and leukopenia.[33]

PREVENTION OF COMPLICATIONS ■

Pheochromocytomas arise de novo; therefore, they are not preventable. However, the complications they cause are largely preventable if the tumor is suspected in the appropriate clinical setting and proper management measures are instituted. Care should be taken not to palpate masses too vigorously when examining patients who may harbor pheochromocytomas, because this may cause catecholamine release precipitating a crisis. Similarly, older dynamic tests should be avoided. Radiologic studies that involve catheterization and administration of contrast agents should not be performed unless absolutely necessary, and then only by experienced radiologists under carefully controlled conditions. Proper preoperative, intraoperative, and postoperative management can significantly reduce morbidity and mortality. Missing the diagnosis can be fatal. Making the diagnosis early and treating the patient appropriately are life-saving or significantly ameliorate the complications that can result from these tumors.

SPECIAL CONSIDERATIONS ■

PHEOCHROMOCYTOMA IN PREGNANCY

Pheochromocytomas are particularly lethal tumors in pregnant women. Mortality is high for both mothers (17%) and fetuses (26%) if the diagnosis is missed and adequate alpha-adrenergic blockade is not instituted. When the diagnosis is made during the first trimester, therapeutic abortion followed by tumor resection may be recommended. For tumors diagnosed during the second or third trimester, alpha-adrenergic blockade followed by tumor resection has been advised. Because this may induce spontaneous abortion, alpha-adrenergic blockade may be continued until the fetus has matured

TABLE 148-1. Drugs Used in the Management of Hypertension Due to Pheochromocytoma

DRUGS	ROUTE OF ADMINISTRATION	DOSE RANGE	COMMENTS AND PRECAUTIONS
Alpha-adrenergic blockers			
Nonselective			
Phentolamine	IV	5–15 mg bolus, or 0.5–1.0 mg/min as continuous infusion	Bolus injections often used to control hypertensive paroxysms during operation.
Phenoxybenzamine	PO	10–40 mg bid or tid	Side effects include nasal congestion, headache, tachycardia, palpitations, and orthostatic hypotension.
Selective			
Prazosin	PO	1–10 mg bid	Give test dose of smallest amount and observe for orthostatic hypotension.
Terazosin	PO	1–20 mg q d	
Doxazosin	PO	1–16 mg q d	
Alpha–beta blocker			
Labetalol	PO	50–200 mg bid	Can cause paradoxic hypertension.
	IV	20–80 mg bolus prn, 2 mg/min by infusion	
Calcium antagonists			
Nifedipine	PO	10–20 mg tid	Controls tachycardia better than α_1-blockers.
Nifedipine GITS	PO	30–60 mg q d	
Nicardipine	PO	20–40 mg tid	Can be used alone or with α_1-adrenergic blocker drugs. Controls tachycardia better than α_1-blockers.
Verapamil SR	PO	120–240 mg/d	Controls tachycardia better than α_1-blockers.
Direct vasodilators			
Sodium nitroprusside	IV	0.3–10 μg/kg/min, maximal dose for no more than 10 min	Used to control hypertensive paroxysms during operation.
Nitroglycerin	IV	5–100 μg/min	
Inhibitor of catecholamine synthesis (tyrosine hydroxylase inhibitor)			
Metyrosine	PO	250–1000 mg qid	Used mostly to manage hypertension and control symptoms for patients with metastatic or inoperable pheochromocytoma. Side effects include drowsiness, crystalluria, parkinsonlike symptoms, diarrhea.

GITS, gastrointestinal treatment system.
Gifford RW Jr, Manger WM, Bravo EL: Pheochromocytoma. *Endocrinol Metab Clin North Am* 1994;23:400. Used with permission WB Saunders Company.

sufficiently to survive delivery by cesarean section. The tumor is then resected. If adequate alpha-adrenergic blockade cannot be achieved, or if the woman's condition deteriorates, early intervention may be necessary. The slight risk of teratogenesis with alpha-adrenergic receptor blockers is more than overshadowed by the reduced maternal and fetal mortality.[34]

Any pregnant patient who has severe hypertension or hypertension with paroxysmal symptoms that appears in the first 18 weeks of gestation and is accompanied by abnormal glucose tolerance or diabetes mellitus must be screened for pheochromocytoma. In addition, any pregnant patient with

suspected thyrotoxicosis or sudden cardiovascular collapse should be screened.[35]

UNUSUAL PRESENTATIONS

Although patients with pheochromocytomas usually present with headache, palpitations, diaphoresis, anxiety, and hypertension, numerous unusual presentations have been described. Some of the more common rare presentations are the type IIa and type IIb MEN syndromes, neurofibromatosis (von Recklinghausen's disease), von Hippel–Lindau disease, leiomyosarcoma with multiple pheochromocytomas (Carney's syndrome), a syndrome of neural crest tumors with massive proteinuria, renovascular hypertension due to renal artery stenosis from extrinsic pheochromocytoma compression, cardiac dysfunction, and shock.

The MEN syndromes are a heterogeneous group of familial disorders that are inherited in a mendelian dominant fashion. The gene, identified through genetic linkage analysis near the centromeric region of chromosome 10, exhibits a high degree of penetrance with variable expressivity.[36] Patients with MEN type IIa have medullary carcinoma of the thyroid (MCT), bilateral pheochromocytomas, and hyperparathyroidism caused by parathyroid chief cell hyperplasia. In MEN type IIb (formerly called type III), the patients also have multiple mucosal neuromas, ganglioneuromatosis of the gastrointestinal tract, and a marfanoid body habitus. All patients with MEN type IIa have MCT, but bilateral pheochromocytomas occur in less than 50% of these patients, and parathyroid hyperplasia occurs in only about one third of cases. In the MEN type IIb syndrome, MCT is present in all patients, and the incidence of multiple pheochromocytomas rises to greater than 90%, but parathyroid disease is rare. DNA analysis of mutations in exon 10 or 11 of the *RET* protooncogene as well as specific *RET* mutations now allow identification of family members at risk for development of MEN type II syndromes and obviates the need for yearly biochemical screening.[37] When working with patients with MEN type II, one must always consider the possibility that a pheochromocytoma may be present and remove it before attacking the other endocrinopathies. This prevents the excessively high surgical morbidity and mortality associated with procedures performed in patients with unsuspected pheochromocytomas.[38,39]

Neurofibromatosis, or von Recklinghausen's disease, is one of the more common phakomatoses. It is inherited in an autosomal dominant fashion and occurs in about 1 person in 3000. The gene locus (*NF-1*) maps to chromosome 17q.[7] Patients with von Recklinghausen's disease commonly manifest cutaneous café-au-lait spots and neurofibromas. They may also develop melanocytic hamartomas of the iris (Lisch nodules), macrocephaly, short stature, idiopathic hypertension, seizures, gliomas, meningiomas, acoustic neuromas, peripheral nerve neurofibrosarcomas, and leukemias, as well as pheochromocytomas. Five percent of all pheochromocytomas are found in these patients.[40]

Von Hippel–Lindau disease is another autosomal dominant disorder with variable penetrance. The gene locus (*VHL*) maps to chromosome 3p.[7] These patients have retinal and cerebellar hemangioblastomas; renal, hepatic, and pancreatic cysts; renal cell carcinomas; and pheochromocytomas. A small number of these patients also have pancreatic islet cell tumors that may produce insulin, glucagon, pancreatic polypeptide, calcitonin, or vasoactive intestinal polypeptide (VIP).[41] Pheochromocytoma may be the only manifestation of von Hippel–Lindau disease in up to 38% of genetic carriers.[42]

Pheochromocytoma has been reported in patients with Carney's syndrome. This rare syndrome, first reported in 1979, consists of gastric epithelioid leiomyosarcoma (a tumor that represents 0.5% of all gastric malignancies), pulmonary chondroma, and functioning extraadrenal paraganglioma (pheochromocytoma). The syndrome occurs predominantly in females (90%), with an average age at diagnosis of 16.5 years. As the condition is potentially lethal, early diagnosis and definitive surgical treatment are essential.[43]

A small number of patients have been reported in whom pheochromocytomas produced nephrotic syndrome–range proteinuria. In 1 patient, a renal biopsy revealed a glomerulopathy that resolved after the pheochromocytoma was resected. Hormonal analysis of this patient's tumor revealed the presence of adrenocorticotropic hormone, VIP, somatostatin, and leucine and methionine enkephalins. The patient also had Cushing's syndrome and diarrhea with steatorrhea.[44]

Pheochromocytomas can cause renal artery stenosis by extrinsic compression or stretching. On angiography, the pattern may be one of either stenosis or vessel interruption. In up to 30% of cases, the pheochromocytoma may be hypovascular. This rare clinical association should be considered before surgical intervention is undertaken in apparent renovascular hypertension.[45]

Cardiac dysfunction can be a clue to the presence of a pheochromocytoma. Both anatomic and functional derangements can occur. Fifty percent of patients who die with surgically uncorrected pheochromocytomas have histologic evidence of an active catecholamine-induced myocarditis on postmortem examination. Pheochromocytoma patients can present with acute myocardial infarction, congestive heart failure, life-threatening tachyarrhythmias, or sudden cardiac death. Reflex bradycardia and sick sinus syndrome have also been described. In rare cases, pheochromocytomas cause obstructive or hypertrophic cardiomyopathy. Treatment by surgical excision of the tumor and calcium channel blockade has been used effectively in these patients.[46] In extremely rare cases, pheochromocytomas can involve the heart itself. The diagnosis is often difficult with coronary angiography or ^{131}I-MIBG scanning, or both, required to localize the lesion. Cardiopulmonary bypass is usually required for curative resection.[47]

Although exceedingly rare, pheochromocytomas can present as unexplained shock at initial evaluation (12 of 540 patients). Common features in these cases included abdominal pain, pulmonary edema, intense mydriasis, profound weakness, diaphoresis, cyanosis, hyperglycemia, and leukocytosis. Patients who present with shock harboring these signs and symptoms should be managed aggressively with the possible diagnosis of pheochromocytoma firmly in mind.[48]

REFERENCES ■

1. Manger WM, Gifford RW Jr: *Pheochromocytoma.* New York, Springer-Verlag, 1977:xiii
2. Rabin D, McKenna TJ: *Clinical Endocrinology and Metabolism: Principles and Practice.* New York, Grune & Stratton, 1982:501
3. Gifford RW Jr, Manger WM, Bravo EL: Pheochromocytoma. *Endocrinol Metab Clin North Am* 1994;23:387
4. Bravo E, Fouad-Tarazi F, Rossi G, et al: A reevaluation of the hemodynamics of pheochromocytoma. *Hypertension* 1990;

15(Supp I):1128

5. Stein PP, Black HR: A simplified diagnostic approach to pheochromocytoma. *Medicine* 1990;70:46

6. Sheps SG, Jiang N, Klee GG, et al: Recent developments in the diagnosis and treatment of pheochromocytoma. *Mayo Clin Proc* 1990;65:88

7. Brodeur GM, Moley JF: Biology of tumors of the peripheral nervous system. *Cancer Metastasis Rev* 1991;10:321

8. Munden R, Adams DB, Curry NS: Cystic pheochromocytoma: radiologic diagnosis. *South Med J* 1993;86:1302

9. Gould VE, Sommers SC: Adrenal medulla and paraganglia. In: Bloodworth JMB Jr (ed). *Endocrine Pathology: General and Surgical*, 2nd ed. Baltimore, Williams & Wilkins, 1982:473

10. Whalen RK, Althausen AF, Daniels GH: Extra-adrenal pheochromocytoma. *J Urol* 1992;147:1

11. Helman LF, Cohen PS, Averbuch SD, et al: Neuropeptide Y expression distinguishes malignant from benign pheochromocytoma. *J Clin Oncol* 1989;7:1720

12. Nativ O, Grant CS, Sheps SG, et al: The clinical significance of nuclear DNA ploidy pattern in 184 patients with pheochromocytoma. *Cancer* 1992;69:2683

13. Cryer PE: Pheochromocytoma. *Clin Endocrinol Metab* 1985; 14:203

14. Rosano TG, Swift TA, Hayes LW: Advances in catecholamine and metabolite measurements for diagnosis of pheochromocytoma. *Clin Chem* 1991;37:1854

14a. Lenders JWM, Keiser HR, Goldstein DS, et al: Plasma metanephrines in the diagnosis of pheochromocytoma. *Ann Int Med* 1995;123:101

15. Grossman E, Goldstein DS, Hoffman A, et al: Glucagon and clonidine testing in the diagnosis of pheochromocytoma. *Hypertension* 1991;17:733

16. Bravo EL: Diagnosis of pheochromocytoma. *Hypertension* 1991;17:742

17. Bravo EL, Tarazi RC, Fouad FM, et al: Clonidine-suppression test: a useful aid in the diagnosis of pheochromocytoma. *N Engl J Med* 1981;305:623

18. MacDougall IC, Isles CG, Stewart H, et al: Overnight clonidine suppression test in the diagnosis and exclusion of pheochromocytoma. *Am J Med* 1988;84:993

19. Bravo EL: Evolving concepts in the pathophysiology, diagnosis, and treatment of pheochromocytoma. *Endoc Rev* 1994;15:356

20. Hsiao RJ, Parmer RJ, Takiyyuddin MA, et al: Chromogranin A storage and secretion: sensitivity and specificity for the diagnosis of pheochromocytoma. *Medicine* 1991;70:33

21. Manger WM, Gifford RW Jr: Pheochromocytoma: current diagnosis and management. *Cleve Clin J Med* 1993;60:365

22. Fink IJ, Reinig JW, Dwyer AJ, et al: MR imaging of pheochromocytomas. *J Comput Assist Tomogr* 1985;9:454

23. Shapiro B, Fig LM, Gross MD, et al: Radiochemical diagnosis of adrenal disease. *Crit Rev Clin Lab Sci* 1989;27:265

24. Khafagi FA, Shapiro B, Fig LM, et al: Labetalol reduces iodine-131 MIBG uptake by pheochromocytoma and normal tissues. *J Nucl Med* 1989;30:481

25. Shulkin BL, Wieland DM, Schwaiger M, et al: PET scanning with hydroxyephedrine: an approach to the localization of pheochromocytoma. *J Nucl Med* 1992;33:1125

26. Lamberts SWJ, Bakker WH, Reubi J et al: Somatostatin-receptor imaging in the localization of endocrine tumors. *N Engl J Med* 1990;323:1246

27. Nicholson JP Jr, Vaughn ED Jr, Pickering TG, et al: Pheochromocytoma and prazosin. *Ann Intern Med* 1983;99:477

28. Favre L, Forster A, Fathi M, et al: Calcium-channel inhibition in pheochromocytoma. *Acta Endocrinol (Copenh)* 1986; 113:385

29. Takahashi S, Nakai T, Fujiwara R, et al: Effectiveness of long-acting nifedipine in pheochromocytoma. *Jpn Heart J* 1989; 30:751

30. Proye C, Thevenin D, Cecat P, et al: Exclusive use of calcium channel blockers in preoperative and intraoperative control of pheochromocytomas: hemodynamics and free catecholamine assays in ten consecutive patients. *Surgery* 1989;106:1149

31. Mihm FG, Sandhu JS, Brown MD, et al: Short-acting beta-adrenergic blockade as initial drug therapy in pheochromocytoma. *Crit Care Med* 1990;18:673

32. Bravo EL, Gifford RW Jr: Pheochromocytoma: diagnosis, localization, and management. *N Engl J Med* 1984;311:1298

33. Shapiro B, Sisson JC, Eyre P, et al: 131-I-MIBG: a new agent in diagnosis and treatment of pheochromocytoma. *Cardiology* 1985;72(Suppl 1):137

34. Stenstrom G, Swolin K: Pheochromocytoma in pregnancy. *Acta Obstet Gynecol Scand* 1985;64:357

35. Harper MA, Murnaghan GA, Kennedy L, et al: Pheochromocytoma in pregnancy: five cases and a review of the literature. *Br J Obstet Gynaecol* 1989;96:594

36. Wells SA Jr, Donis-Keller H: Current perspectives on the diagnosis and management of patients with multiple endocrine neoplasia type 2 syndromes. *Endocrinol Metab Clin North Am* 1994;23:215

37. Lips CJM, Landsvater RM, Hoppener JWM, et al: Clinical screening as compared with DNA analysis in families with multiple endocrine neoplasia type 2A. *N Engl J Med* 1994; 331:828

38. Brunt LM, Wells SA Jr: The multiple endocrine neoplasia syndromes. *Invest Radiol* 1985;20:916

39. Raue F, Frank-Raue K, Grauer A: Multiple endocrine neoplasia type 2. *Endocrinol Metab Clin North Am* 1994;23:137

40. Ducatman DS, Scheitbauer BW, Doblin DC: Malignant bone tumors associated with neuro-fibromatosis. *Mayo Clin Proc* 1983;58:578

41. Cornish D, Pont A, Minor D, et al: Metastatic islet cell tumor in von Hippel-Lindau disease. *Am J Med* 1984;77:147

42. Neumann HPH, Berger DP, Sigmund G, et al: Pheochromocytomas, multiple endocrine neoplasia type 2, and von Hippel-Lindau disease. *N Engl J Med* 1993;329:1531

43. Carney JA: The triad of gastric epithelioid leiomyosarcoma, pulmonary chondroma, and functioning extra-adrenal paraganglioma: a five year review. *Medicine* 1983;62:159

44. Interlandi JW, Hundley RF, Kasselberg AG: Hypercortisolism, diarrhea with steatorrhea, and massive proteinuria due to pheochromocytoma. *South Med J* 1985;78:879

45. del Gaudio A: Pheochromocytoma and renal artery stenosis. *Int Surg* 1985;70:153

46. Grossman E, Knecht A, Holtzman E, et al: Uncommon presentation of pheochromocytoma: case studies. *Angiology* 1985; 36:759

47. Jebara VA, Uva MS, Farge A, et al: Cardiac pheochromocytomas. *Ann Thorac Surg* 1992;53:356

48. Bergland BE: Pheochromocytoma presenting as shock. *Am J Emerg Med* 1989;7:44

Critical Care, Third Edition, edited by Joseph M. Civetta,
Robert W. Taylor, and Robert R. Kirby.
Lippincott-Raven Publishers, Philadelphia, PA © 1997.

CHAPTER 149

■

Thyroid Disease

William L. Isley

While laboratory testing for thyroid disease has become very
sophisticated, the physician's clinical judgment is still vital
in patient management decisions. This chapter discusses
relevant information for the diagnosis and treatment of thyroid disease seen in critical care medicine, reviews the relationship of thyroid disease to applied pharmacology, considers the effects of drugs, nonthyroidal illness, and aging on
thyroid function tests, and addresses the management of
airway obstruction by goiter.

IMMEDIATE CONCERNS ■

INTERPRETATION OF THYROID FUNCTION TESTS

The American Thyroid Association recommends that measurement of serum thyroid-stimulating hormone (TSH) by
a sensitive assay and some estimate of free thyroxine (FT_4)
(by direct measurement, an analog assay, or determination
of the "free thyroxine index" [FT_4I]) be used in the diagnosis
of thyroid disease.[1] The FT_4I is derived by multiplying the
serum thyroxine (T_4) concentration by the resin triiodothyronine (T_3) uptake or similar estimation of thyroid hormone
binding capacity. (The term FT_4 in this chapter refers to
any of these measurements unless otherwise indicated). The
expected thyroid function test results in common conditions
are listed in Table 149-1. For more detailed discussion of
various disorders, the reader should see the sections later
in the chapter.

THYROTOXICOSIS ■

IMMEDIATE CONCERNS

Severe cardiac (tachyarrhythmias or heart failure) or central
nervous system (CNS) dysfunction are the likely presentations for thyrotoxicosis in the ICU. Do not expect the "classic" presentation that is described in otherwise healthy young
patients. Do not rule out thyrotoxicosis just because you
cannot appreciate a goiter.

After ordering thyroid function tests, consider using beta-
blockers to antagonize the peripheral effects of excess thyroid hormone and antithyroid drugs to inhibit thyroid hormone synthesis. If rapid restoration to the euthyroid state
is needed, use cold iodine and dexamethasone as well. Intercurrent illness in the thyrotoxic patient may result in
metabolic crisis. If you suspect thyroid storm, see later section for specific details of treatment. Do not send an unprepared patient with thyrotoxicosis for surgery.

PRESENTATION

The presentation of an anxious, perspiring, thin young
woman with proptosis and goiter is an easy diagnostic challenge for most clinicians. Table 149-2 lists the common
symptoms and signs of thyrotoxicosis.[2] However, intensive
care physicians may confront patients with "nonclassic" presentations of thyrotoxicosis or thyrotoxicosis due to processes
other than Graves disease.[3,4] Frequently small goiters are
not appreciated by the nonendocrinologist. The absence of
a recognized goiter should not deter the physician from

TABLE 149-1. Thyroid Function Test Interpretation in Common Conditions

	T$_4$	FT$_4$	TSH
Thyrotoxicosis	↑	↑	↓
Primary hypothyroidism	↓	↓	↑
Secondary hypothyroidism	↓	↓	↓, ↔
Mild nonthyroidal illness	↔, ↑	↔, ↑	↔
Severe nonthyroidal illness	↓	↓, ↔, ↑°	↓, ↔, ↑†

° Results may be assay dependent.

† ↑ Transiently and usually (though not always) <20 μU/mL during recovery of nonthyroidal illness.

considering thyroid disease in the differential diagnosis. Graves disease can occur in some patients (particularly the elderly) without palpable goiter.[5]

Toxic multinodular goiter is sometimes seen in elderly patients. The goiter should be appreciated by the careful examiner unless it is substernal. The displaced thyroid tissue is usually apparent on chest radiograph. Patients who have recently received iodinated contrast material for radiographic procedures[6] or iodine-containing medications such as amiodarone[7] may present with iodine induced thyrotoxicosis. (In this author's experience, contrast material may also temporarily ameliorate thyrotoxicosis and make diagnosis more difficult.) Rarely, a patient presents with exogenous thyroid hormone ingestion as the etiology of thyrotoxicosis. Other causes of thyrotoxicosis are so rarely seen by the intensivist that they are not discussed.

Thyrotoxic patients likely to be seen in the ICU frequently have one aspect of their disease so predominating the clinical picture that disease in a nonendocrine organ system is suspected.[3] Specifically, the patient with congestive heart failure

TABLE 149-2. Common Symptoms and Signs of Thyrotoxicosis

SYMPTOMS	SIGNS
Dyspnea	Dermopathy (if Graves disease)
Heat intolerance	Goiter
Hyperdefecation (rarely diarrhea)	Gynecomastia
Increased appetite	Hyperkinesis
Nervousness	Hyperreflexia
Palpitations	Fine hair
Scant or absent menses	Lid retraction
Sweating	Lid lag
Weakness	Onycholysis
Weight loss	Ophthalmopathy (if Graves disease)
	Proximal muscle weakness
	Smooth skin
	Tachycardia
	Thyroid bruit (if Graves disease)
	Tremor
	Warm, moist palms

or arrhythmias may be felt to have primary cardiac disease, while the patient with weight loss may be felt to have a malignancy or primary gastrointestinal disease.

Thyrotoxicosis may present in the elderly with only alterations in mental status, cardiac tachyarrhythmias, congestive heart failure, or weight loss (so called "apathetic thyrotoxicosis").[4] The physician must have a low threshold for suspicion of thyroid disease in elderly patients. Patients treated with beta-blockers may have masking of some of the classic signs and symptoms of thyrotoxicosis.[8] Diagnostic and therapeutic maneuvers may place the ill patient with unrecognized thyrotoxicosis at risk for thyroid storm, a situation with catastrophic potential.

Cardiovascular manifestations of thyrotoxicosis are particularly worthy of mention.[9–12] Findings on physical examination include a hyperdynamic precordium, tachycardia, widened pulse pressure, and a systolic murmur. The alterations in cardiovascular physiology produced by thyrotoxicosis (increased heart rate, ejection fraction, and cardiac output, and decreased systemic vascular resistance) are of particular concern in patients with preexisting heart disease and in the elderly. The increased cardiac output seen in thyrotoxic patients appears to be the result of direct effects of thyroid hormone on the heart as well as decreased systemic vascular resistance related to increased thermogenesis and peripheral vasodilatation. The stress of thyrotoxicosis may cause cardiac decompensation in the patient with intrinsic cardiac disease. Atrial fibrillation is a not uncommon presentation of thyrotoxicosis. Embolic phenomenon may occur in these patients resulting in a potentially catastrophic outcome. Some patients (usually those with intrinsic heart disease) develop frank cardiac failure. A (usually) reversible thyrotoxic cardiomyopathy may exist in some patients. Recent work suggests that diastolic dysfunction (left ventricular filling abnormalities) may be severe and take several months to resolve after resolution of the thyrotoxic state.[13] While mitral valve prolapse has been reported to be more common in thyrotoxic patients, significant mitral or tricuspid valve insufficiency is a rare finding. Occasionally thyrotoxic patients may have myocardial ischemia despite normal coronary arteries. Sick sinus syndrome has rarely been associated with thyrotoxicosis. In patients with a preexisting right-to-left shunt, the shunt is augmented by the development of thyrotoxicosis.[14]

Respiratory muscle strength is significantly reduced in thyrotoxicosis.[15] While dyspnea is a prominent symptom in some patients, respiratory failure is uncommon in thyrotoxicosis in the absence of intrinsic lung disease.

When extreme manifestations of thyrotoxicosis coexist with fever, tachycardia out of proportion to the fever, and CNS dysfunction, a diagnosis of thyroid storm is made.[3,16] Metabolic crisis occurs when the aggregate of thyroid dysfunction and nonthyroidal illness exceeds the body's usual homeostatic mechanisms. Since thyroid storm is a life-threatening disorder, therapy should be begun immediately without awaiting the results of thyroid function tests. Fever greater than 37.8°C (100°F) is necessary to make the diagnosis of thyroid storm. The patient may be comatose, highly agitated, seizing, or have some other CNS disturbance. Gastrointestinal system signs and symptoms (hyperdefecation, diarrhea, or liver function test abnormalities) may also play a prominent role in the presentation of thyroid storm. As noted previously, elderly patients present a special problem since they can have few suggestive signs and symptoms of thyrotoxicosis other than weight loss, tachyarrhythmias, congestive heart failure, or mental status changes. Precipitants of thyroid storm are listed in Table 149-3.

DIAGNOSIS

The typical patient with thyrotoxicosis has thyroid function tests as shown in Table 149-1.[1] Occasionally FT_4 values are normal, but the diagnostic suspicion for thyrotoxicosis is so high that measurement of serum T_3 or free T_3 (FT_3) is indicated to consider the possibility of T_3 toxicosis.[2] An elevation of the serum FT_3 or free T_3 index ($FT_3I = T_3$ multiplied by the resin triiodothyronine uptake [RT_3U]) is then indicative of thyrotoxicosis in these cases. However, T_4 toxicosis[11] (FT_4 elevated while FT_3 is normal) is much more common than T_3 toxicosis in severely ill patients. In the rare case when FT_4 is elevated and serum TSH is detectable, consideration should be given to the effects of nonthyroidal illness or drugs on thyroid function tests (see later), recent ingestion of l-thyroxine by a previously hypothyroid patient, or the rare possibilites of a TSH-secreting pituitary tumor or thyroid hormone resistance.[1] However, in some TSH assays, TSH may be detectable (usually low) due to nonspecific antibody binding even in the setting of thyrotoxicosis from Graves disease or other etiologies.[17] Very rarely thyrotoxic patients may have normalization of serum T_4, T_3, and FT_4 values in the face of severe nonthyroidal illness.[18] The undetectable serum TSH concentration in such cases cannot be readily distinguished from TSH suppression in nonthyroidal illness. The finding of a markedly elevated radioiodine uptake (in the absence of renal failure) supports the diagnosis of thyrotoxicosis. However, serial measurement of thyroid function is the only sure means of definitively making this diagnosis. Clearly, consultation with an endocrinologist is vital in determining the patient's thyroid status and etiology of presumed thyrotoxicosis in situations in which the thyroid function tests show "unusual" results.

Since the diagnosis of thyroid storm is a clinical one, laboratory tests do not classify a patient as having thyroid crisis. Nonetheless, FT_4 values have been reported to be higher in thyroid storm than in patients with uncomplicated thyrotoxicosis.[19]

Other laboratory findings are nonspecific in thyrotoxicosis.[2] Serum concentrations of liver enzymes and bilirubin may be eleveated. Serum cholesterol levels are low. Mild anemia and granulocytopenia can occur. Impaired glucose tolerance is occasionally seen. Mild hypercalcemia is common.

Technically the term *hyperthyroidism* refers only to thyrotoxicosis in patients with increased thyroid hormone production by the thyroid, as opposed to thyrotoxicosis caused by a destructive thyroid process (such as various forms of thyroiditis) or nonthyroidal sources (exogenous thyroid hormone ingestion or ectopic thyroid tissue).[20] The laboratory hallmark of true hyperthyroidism is an elevated radioactive iodine uptake (RAIU). Practically speaking, however, the terms *hyperthyroidism* and *thyrotoxicosis* are often used interchangeably.

In patients who do not have nodular goiters, Graves disease can usually be differentiated from other forms of thyroid disease by measuring the RAIU at 24 hours.[2] Occasional patients have such rapid turnover of iodine that the 24-hour RAIU is normal. When Graves disease is still strongly suspected, the RAIU should be measured at a shorter time interval (4 to 6 hours). The patient with a diffuse goiter or no goiter and an elevated RAIU most likely has Graves disease as the etiology of thyrotoxicosis. Patients with very low RAIU values usually have a form of thyroiditis, iodine induced thyrotoxicosis, or exogenous thyroid hormone ingestion.[2,5] However, the RAIU result is variable in patients with iodine induced thyrotoxicosis. The RAIU may not be elevated in patients with toxic nodular goiter. Patients should be off antithyroid drugs 48 to 72 hours before obtaining the RAIU. Thyroid scintiscanning is usually necessary only in certain patients with nodular thyroid disease. In severely ill patients, RAIU tests may need to be deferred so that adequate treatment with antithyroid drugs and iodides can be given without interruption until the patient's condition is stabilized.

TABLE 149-3. Precipitants of Thyroid Storm

A. Infection
B. Thyroid manipulations
   1. Surgery
   2. Radioactive therapy
   3. Vigorous palpation
   4. Withdrawal of iodine therapy
   5. Institution of iodine therapy
   6. Withdrawal of antithyroid drug therapy
C. Metabolic
   1. Diabetic ketoacidosis
   2. Hypoglycemia
D. Medical emergencies
   1. Myocardial infarction
   2. Pulmonary embolus
E. Surgical emergencies
   1. Trauma
   2. Abdominal catastrophe
F. Medication
   1. Thyroxine
   2. Haloperidol
   3. Digitalis
   4. Pseudoephedrine
G. Other
   1. Labor and delivery
   2. Diagnostic procedures
   3. ? Stress

TREATMENT

General Principles

General principles for treating thyrotoxic patients have recently been published by the American Thyroid Association.[21] Of utmost importance in dealing with the thyrotoxic patient is the determination of the rapidity with which the patient needs achievement of the euthyroid state.[3] Patients with thyrotoxic crisis, major organ system dysfunction induced by excessive thyroid hormone, or the thyrotoxic patient needing acute surgical intervention may require achievement of the euthyroid state urgently, either to prevent thyroid crisis from developing or worsening, or to enable effective treatment for the condition that is presently causing troublesome signs and symptoms and may result in significant morbidity or mortality if not promptly addressed. Antagonism of the effects of excessive thyroid hormone and inhibition of further thyroid hormone synthesis and release must be pursued immediately, although the biologic effects of thyroid hormone last for weeks. Decisions regarding definitive treatment of thyrotoxicosis can be dealt with once the patient's condition is stable.[22]

Pharmacologic Agents

Drugs for the treatment of thyrotoxic urgencies and emergencies (see Table 149-3) can generally be divided into three classes: (1) agents that inhibit thyroid hormone biosynthesis, (2) drugs that inhibit thyroid hormone release, and (3) agents that antagonize the effects of excess thyroid hormone.[3] The thionamides (antithyroid drugs) constitute the first class of drugs. The second group of drugs include cold iodine, lithium, and corticosteroids. The last group of agents includes beta-blockers, catecholamine depleting agents, and calcium antagonists.

Antithyroid drugs inhibit thyroid hormone synthesis and may suppress thyroid autoimmunity in patients with Graves disease.[23] Thionamides available in the United States are propylthiouracil (PTU) and methimazole. PTU is generally used in the critically ill patient since it has the additional effect of inhibiting the conversion of T_4 to the more active hormone T_3. Antithyroid drugs are not available in a parenteral form. Rectal administration of higher than customary doses of PTU has rarely been used in critically ill patients.[3]

Agranulocytosis is a rare but potentially lethal reaction to antithyroid drug therapy. Fear of agranulocytosis should not be a deterrent to treating severely ill patients with high-dose antithyroid drug therapy acutely unless the patient has had a previous severe reaction to thionamides. Hypersensitivity reactions can occur early in therapy (the first 3 weeks) and can include rash, pruritus, fever, arthralgias, and serum sickness. These reactions are less serious and may be handled by switching to another antithyroid drug.

Cold iodine acutely blocks the release of thyroid hormone, allowing a rapid lowering of serum T_4 levels. Iodine can be administered orally as saturated solution of potassium iodide, Lugol's solution, or oral cholecystographic dyes (which also block the conversion of T_4 to T_3), or intravenously as sodium iodide. Rarely, a patient given intravenous (IV) iodine can develop an acute hypersensitivity reaction. The administration of iodine prevents the physician from obtaining an RAIU or treating the patient with iodine 131 for several weeks.

Glucocorticoids inhibit the release of thyroid hormone in patients with Graves disease. Dexamethasone also inhibits the conversion of T_4 to T_3.

Lithium blocks the release of thyroid hormone and may block its synthesis as well. The toxic effects of lithium in the treatment of thyrotoxicosis are identical to those seen in the treatment of other disorders. Lithium is generally a second-line agent, but may be useful in patients with iodine induced thyrotoxicosis.

Beta-adrenergic blockers have revolutionized the treatment of severely ill thyrotoxic patients.[8] These agents can markedly ameliorate the signs and symptoms of thyrotoxicosis, which resemble a hyperadrenergic state, even though they have no direct effect on the thyroid. Many of the beta-blocking agents inhibit the peripheral conversion of T_4 to T_3. The risk-benefit ratio of therapy with beta-blockers in patients with reactive airway disease or congestive heart failure is a significant concern. The former problem may be alleviated by using cardioselective agents, although these drugs may not retain their cardioselectivity at higher doses. The use of beta-blockers in patients with congestive heart failure is controversial. If the heart failure is rate-dependent, the patient notes improvement with slowing of the heart rate induced by beta-blockade.

Propranolol is the time-honored beta-blocking agent af choice in the treatment of thyrotoxicosis.[3,8] The dose of propranolol necessary to achieve some degree of beta-blockade (pulse <80 to 100 beats/minute) is highly variable (40 mg to 2 g per day in the author's experience). This wide dosage range is due to the marked variability in hepatic metabolism of propranolol among thyrotoxic individuals.[24] It is mandatory that therapy be guided by the patient's response (pulse and tremor). The reported failings of propranolol to prevent or inadequately treat thyroid storm may well have been due to inadequate dosing of the medication. The ultrashort-acting cardioselective beta-blocker esmolol may be useful in patients seemingly unresponsive to propranolol or in patients requiring rapid titration to effect and rapid reversiblity of beta-blockade.[3]

Reserpine (a depleter of catecholamines) and guanethidine (which inhibits catecholamine release) have been used as treatment modalities in patients with thyrotoxicosis. These agents are rarely used in patients with severe thyrotoxicosis and reactive airway disease or seeming unresponsiveness to beta-blockers. Clonidine, a central-acting α_2-agonist that suppresses catecholamine output, has been shown to reduce thyrotoxic signs and symptoms.[25] Its role in the treatment of thyrotoxicosis in the critically ill remains to be determined.

Verapamil may be useful therapy for tachyarrhythmias in thyrotoxic patients who do not respond to beta-blockers or have a contraindication to their use.[26] Verapamil has significant negative inotropic effects and should be used with caution in patients with congestive heart failure. Diltiazem has been used in outpatients with thyrotoxicosis to ameliorate symptoms,[27] but its use in the critical care setting is unknown.

Plasmapheresis has been used as a therapeutic modality in rare cases of severe thyrotoxicosis. Plasmapheresis would appear to be most useful in the setting of thyroid hormone overdose since drugs that affect thyroid hormone synthesis and release would be of no benefit.

Thyroid Storm

All drug classes (Table 149-4) are used in the patient with thyroid storm.[3,16] A loading dose of propylthiouracil is given before the administration of iodides so that the iodine load does not become organified by the thyroid. Intensive antithyroid drug therapy is used in this life-threatening situation despite a slightly increased risk of side effects. Iodides are used to block hormone release and synthesis. Glucocorticoids have been administered due to concern over "relative adrenal insufficiency," though proof that such a condition exists is lacking. Dexamethasone inhibits T_4 to T_3 conversion and thyroid hormone release. The effects of excess thyroid hormone on body tissues are best acutely ameliorated by beta-adrenergic blocking agents. The importance of individualized dosing of beta-blockers to achieve beta-blockade cannot be overemphasized.

Supportive care in these patients includes close monitoring, intravenous dextrose-containing fluids, external cooling, acetaminophen as an antipyretic (aspirin may displace thyroid hormone from binding proteins and increase free hormone levels), and intensive therapy of the precipitating cause.[21]

Iodine Induced Thyrotoxicosis

The usual therapy for iodine induced thyrotoxicosis is to discontinue the exogenous iodine source and symptomatic therapy with beta-blockers, if needed.[28] In the setting of severe thyrotoxicosis induced by amiodarone, traditional antithyroid therapy may not be efficacious due to the very large amounts of thyroid hormone that may be already formed in the thyroid gland and the long retention of amiodarone in the body. Therapy with potassium perchlorate (to inhibit iodine uptake) combined with antithyroid drugs has been used in some patients.[29] In unresponsive cases, thyroidectomy has been used.[30]

Tachyarrhythmias

Any patient who presents with a supraventricular tachyarrhythmia (particularly atrial fibrillation) or unexplained sinus tachycardia should have thyroid function tests performed. Beta-blockers are generally used for treating tachyarrhythmias in patients known to be thyrotoxic.[3,8,12] The addition of digoxin may be necessary in the setting of atrial fibrillation. Recent studies suggest that verapamil may also be useful in this situation. There is some suggestion that thyrotoxic patients in atrial fibrillation may have a higher incidence of peripheral embolization on conversion to sinus rhythm, suggesting the need for anticoagulation before cardioversion, even if induced by treatment of the patient's thyrotoxic state.[31] The need for intensive antithyroid therapy (high-dose antithyroid drugs and iodine) in such patients depends on their general medical condition and the ease with which the tachyarrhythmias are treated with standard therapy. A patient whose heart rate and rhythm is easily controlled with beta-blockers may be treated with conventional definitive therapy. Unstable patients need rapid reversal of the thyrotoxic state and should receive intensive antithyroid therapy.

Congestive Heart Failure

A thyrotoxic patient with significant congestive heart failure may need intensive antithyroid therapy since the usual treatment for heart failure may not be efficacious and beta-blockers may not improve the patient's condition.[32] Many of the patients presumably have "high output" failure that is rate-dependent. I initiate therapy with beta-blockers acutely. The appropriate beta-blocker dose is empirically derived.

TABLE 149-4. Major Drugs Used in the Treatment of Severely Ill Patients With Thyrotoxicosis

CONVENTIONAL ANTITHYROID THERAPY	INTENSIVE ANTITHYROID THERAPY
INHIBIT THYROID HORMONE SYNTHESIS Propylthiouracil 100–200 mg tid	INHIBIT THYROID HORMONE SYNTHESIS Propylthiouracil 800–1200 mg PO, then 200–300 mg q 6 h
	INHIBIT THYROID HORMONE RELEASE Oral: Lugol's solution 3–5 drops tid, or SSKI° ≥1 drop tid Dexamethasone 2 mg q 6 h Intravenous: Sodium iodide 0.5 g q 12 h Dexamethasone 2 mg q 6 h
ANTAGONIZE EFFECTS OF EXCESS THYROID HORMONE Oral: Propranolol 20 mg q 6 h and adjust dose by response	ANTAGONIZE EFFECTS OF EXCESS THYROID HORMONE Oral: Propranolol 40 mg q 6 h and adjust dose by response Intravenous: Propranolol 1 mg over 5 min and adjust dose by response

°Saturated solution of potassium iodide.

The ultrashort-acting intravenous agent esmolol may be tried if a need for rapid reversal of beta-blockade and ease of dosage titration is desired.[3] If signs and symptoms of congestive heart failure worsen, beta-blockers should be discontinued. Intensive antithyroid therapy should clearly be used unless the patient responds promptly to initial therapy.

Severe Concomitant Medical Illness

Patients with thyrotoxicosis and severe concomitant medical illness are presumably at risk for the development of thyroid storm. The literature does not give clear guidelines for treatment of such patients. I treat such patients with intensive antithyroid therapy and beta-blockers to minimize the perceived risk of thyroid storm or the possible deleterious effect of thyrotoxicosis on the patient's other medical problems.[3]

Concomitant Surgical Emergencies

The stress of anesthesia or surgery may precipitate thyroid storm in uncontrolled thyrotoxic patients. While there are some reports of thyrotoxic patients undergoing thyroidectomy with minimal or no pretreatment, I recommend treatment to antagonize the peripheral effects of excess thyroid hormone and prevent further release of thyroid hormone.[3] Intravenous beta-blockers are used with the dose titrated to the patient's pulse rate response. Esmolol may prove to be especially useful in this setting. Inhibition of thyroid hormone synthesis and release can be accomplished with propylthiouracil, iodine, and dexamethasone.

Special Situations

The critically ill pregnant patient presents a special challenge to the physician.[3,33] Antithyroid drugs should be used in the smallest dose possible since these agents cross the placenta and may affect fetal thyroid function. Thyroid hormone does not cross the placenta in sufficient quantities to prevent fetal hypothyroidism and goiter development. PTU is the antithyroid drug of choice in the pregnant woman since it is highly protein bound and does not cross the placenta as readily as methimazole. A fetal scalp defect has been reported with methimazole. Iodine administered to the mother can be a fetal goitrogen. The safety of beta-blockers in pregnancy is controversial. In life-threatening cases I administer high-dose antithyroid drugs, dexamethasone, and beta-blockers acutely. The doses of these drugs should be decreased as soon as the patient's condition has stabilized. The goal in most non–life-threatening situations is to give antithyroid drugs in a dose that keeps the serum FT_4 at the upper limit of the normal range or mildly elevated.[33]

Thyroid hormone overdose may be accompanied by few thyrotoxic signs and symptoms, or be associated with florid thyrotoxicosis.[3] The serum half-life of thyroxine is approximately 1 week, while the biologic half-life is considerably longer. Therefore the toxic effects may not be seen until a considerable time after the ingestion. (Triiodothyronine ingestions are associated with a much shorter time course.) Antagonism of the biologic effects of thyroid hormone is the primary drug therapy. Agents that accelerate thyroxine metabolism such as phenytoin and rifampin theoretically may be of benefit. Cholestyramine has been used to induce intestinal loss of thyroid hormone in patients with iatrogenic thyrotoxicosis.[34] Plasmapheresis has been rarely used in settings of thyroid hormone overdose.

Thyrotoxic patients with renal failure can be treated similarly to those patients with normal renal function.[35] Rare patients with thyrotoxicosis present with extreme cachexia (usually the elderly or the mentally retarded in my experience). These patients may be candidates for intensive antithyroid therapy so that their nutritional status can be improved as quickly as possible.

HYPOTHYROIDISM   ■

IMMEDIATE CONCERNS

Congestive heart failure, respiratory failure, CNS dysfunction, or hyponatremia are likely to be the manifestations of hypothyroidism encountered in the intensive care unit. Elderly patients are of particular concern. Intercurrent illness, diagnostic and therapeutic interventions, and exposure may lead to metabolic decompensation in previously undiagnosed hypothyroid patients. Profoundly hypothyroid patients with infectious processes may lack fever and leukocytosis. If you suspect myxedema coma, see later section specifically related to the therapy of that disorder. General supportive care, treatment of the specific manifestations of disease, and treatment of concomitant illness are as important as thyroid hormone replacement in seriously ill hypothyroid patients. Do not forget that hypothyroidism slows the metabolism of many drugs, placing the patient at increased risk for untoward side effects.

PRESENTATION

While many patients with hypothyroidism have mild symptoms, critically ill patients are rarely encountered who have significant hypothyroidism. Such patients often have significant cardiovascular compromise, respiratory failure, altered sensorium, or hyponatremia. In this author's experience, the failure to obtain a history of previous radioactive iodine therapy in a seriously ill patient with multisystem dysfunction may delay the diagnosis of hypothyroidism and ultimately be associated with a poor outcome.

Common symptoms and signs of hypothyroidism are listed in Table 149-5.[2] The symptoms are nonspecific and the degree of severity of these symptoms and signs is varied from patient to patient. Goiter may or may not be present depending on the cause of the hypothyroidism. Of particular note to intensive care physicians is the fact that hypothyroid patients, like patients with other endocrine deficiency states, may not display a fever when an infectious process is present.

Cardiovascular manifestations of hypothyroidism are particularly germane to critical care medicine.[10] Cardiac output is reduced secondary to diminished inotropic and chronotropic activity of the heart. Peripheral vascular resistance is increased while intravascular volume is decreased. The patient may be hypertensive. Enlargement of the cardiac

TABLE 149-5. Common Symptoms and Signs of Hypothyroidism

SYMPTOMS	SIGNS
Cold intolerance	Bradycardia
Constipation	Bradykinesia
Dry skin	Coarse hair
Hoarseness	Delayed relaxation phase of deep
Lethargy	tendon reflexes
Paresthesias	Dry and coarse skin
Peripheral edema	Periorbital edema
Weakness	
Weight gain	

silhouette may be seen on chest radiography, often due to pericardial effusion. Rarely, these effusions produce hemodynamic compromise. Occasionally frank cardiac failure develops, usually in patients with intrinsic heart disease. Low voltage and nonspecific changes may be present on the electrocardiogram. Patients with hypothyroid heart disease may be more sensitive to the toxic effects of digitalis preparations since drug metabolism is slowed. There may be confusion in the diagnosis of acute myocardial infarction in hypothyroid patients since creatine kinase (CK) and CK-MB levels may be elevated due to the hypothyroid state.

Patients with hypothyroidism have decreased hypoxic and hypercapnic ventilatory drives.[36] There may be obstruction of the airway by an enlarged tongue. Sleep apnea is more common in hypothyroid patients.[37] Respiratory muscles are weak in hypothyroidism. Rarely, goiters can produce significant airway obstruction irrespective of the patient's thyroid status. Fortunately, only rarely do patients with hypothyroidism develop major respiratory difficulties. However, in my experience, failure to make such a diagnosis in a timely fashion in the patient with respiratory compromise may have catastrophic results.

Less common manifestations of hypothyroidism[2,38] include bowel obstruction and liver function test abnormalities. Occasionally frank ascites or pleural effusions can occur, though pleural effusions should be considered etiologic of another disease process until proved otherwise.[39] Many hypothyroid patients have achlorhydria. Urinary amylase levels can be elevated. Patients may complain of joint and muscle aches. Peripheral neuropathies can be related to hypothyroidism. Deafness occasionally occurs. Profoundly hypothyroid patients may appear dull mentally and desire to sleep more.

Hypothyroidism may cause hyponatremia due to a decrease in free water excretion. Rarely hypercalcemia may be present. Hypercholesterolemia is common, and hypertriglyceridemia may occur. Interestingly, lipids may be normal in patients with secondary hypothyroidism. Hematologic manifestations of hypothyroidism include mild anemia and prolongation of the partial thromboplastin time (PTT).

The most likely causes of hypothyroidism include previous thyroid ablative procedures (^{131}I therapy, radiation therapy for Hodgkin disease, and thyroidectomy,) chronic thyroiditis, thyroid dysfunction induced by immune-modulating agents (interferon, interleukin-2, and granulocyte colony stimulating factor [GCSF]), iron deposition in transfusion-dependent states (thalassemia and sickle cell disease) residual hypothyroidism after subacute, silent, or postpartum thyroiditis, iodine excess (from radiographic contrast agents and certain drugs such as amiodarone), drugs (antithyroid drugs or lithium), loss of thyroid hormone in the urine in nephrotic states, and rarely, secondary hypothyroidism (pituitary tumors or hypothalamic disorders such as sarcoidosis).[2] Transient hypothyroidism can occur after withdrawal of prolonged l-thyroxine treatment; during the course of chronic, subacute, silent and postpartum thyroiditis; and after radioactive iodine administration. (Most patients with chronic thyroiditis have permanent hypothyroidism.)

Myxedema coma is fortunately a rare manifestation of hypothyroidism.[40] Metabolic crisis is apparently due to nonthyroidal illness, resulting in CNS and cardiovascular decompensation. Recognized precipitants of myxedema coma are listed in Table 149-6.

The hallmarks of myxedema coma are severe depression of the sensorium and hypothermia, though some reported patients have normal temperatures. It is usually seen in elderly patients during the winter months and in hospitalized elderly patients with undiagnosed hypothyroidism who receive CNS depressant medications, undergo diagnostic procedures, or develop intercurrent medical or surgical illnesses leading to metabolic decompensation. A normal temperature in such a patient may indicate bacterial infection. Most comatose, hypothermic patients do not have myxedema coma. However, the risk of untreated myxedema coma far outweighs the risk of empiric thyroxine treatment. Thus the intensive care physician should have a low threshold to treat patients for presumptive myxedema coma.

If information from the patient's family is available, the physician should inquire carefully about a previous history of radioiodine treatment, neck surgery, or l-thyroxine therapy. I have found that questioning family members about past signs and symptoms of thyrotoxicosis (and then learning that the patient had an "iodine treatment") is useful in determining the likelihood of hypothyroidism in severely ill patients.

The typical patient has dry, scaly skin; periorbital puffiness; thinning hair and eyebrows (lateral third); yellowish

TABLE 149-6. Precipitating Factors for Myxedema Coma

Cerebrovascular accident
Congestive heart failure
Drugs (phenothiazines, barbiturates, narcotics, anesthetics, diuretics)
Exposure to cold
Gastrointestinal hemorrhage
Infection
Metabolic disturbances (hypoglycemia, hyponatremia, hypoadrenalism)
Respiratory failure
Seizures
Surgery
Trauma

skin; and bradycardia. Many patients are comatose. Temperatures below 26.7°C (80°F) have been reported, so temperature measurements should be made with a thermometer that registers below 34.4°C (94°F). Myxedema coma patients do not shiver. Survival is inversely proportional to body temperature.

Patients may present in cardiovascular collapse or be hypertensive. If respiratory failure has not yet occurred, it may be impending due to the combined effects of airway obstruction, decreased sensitivity of central respiratory centers to hypoxic and hypercapnic drives, and respiratory muscle weakness. The examiner should look closely for a thyroidectomy scar. Goiters are rarely seen in patients with myxedema coma. Pleural and pericardial effusions and ascites may be present. The patient may appear to have bowel obstruction due to decreased gastrointestinal motility. Localizing neurologic signs may be seen.

None of the usual laboratory tests are pathognomonic for myxedema coma. Leukocytosis may not occur despite overwhelming infection. Hyponatremia is common and hypoglycemia may be present. Hypercalcemia is rarely seen. The patient may have respiratory acidosis due to respiratory failure or metabolic acidosis if hypoperfusion is present. The cerebrospinal fluid protein may be elevated. Changes in cardiac enzymes and the electrocardiogram induced by hypothyroidism may complicate the diagnosis of myocardial infarction in these patients.

The examiner should be especially alert to possible precipitating factors for myxedema coma. Pulmonary infection is the most common such factor.

DIAGNOSIS

Typical thyroid function test results in hypothyroid patients are shown in Table 149-1[1] Measuring serum T_3 has no place in the evaluation of hypothyroidism. The metabolic status of otherwise well patients with normal FT_4 but minimal elevation in TSH is debatable (through I frequently err on the side of calling such patients hypothyroid). Severely ill patients may have transient elevation of the serum TSH concentration during recovery from nonthyroidal illness as the patient's serum T_4 concentration returns to normal. Serum TSH may also be mildly elevated in primary adrenal insufficiency. Dopamine and pharmacologic doses of glucocorticoids can lower serum TSH concentrations in hypothyroid patients.[2]

Most critical care physicians are aware of the diagnostic dilemma presented by the finding of a low serum T_4 concentration and normal or low serum TSH concentration in severely ill patients. The measured FT_4 concentration may be low, normal, or high. The overwhelming majority of these patients have the "euthyroid sick syndrome"[1] and should have repeat thyroid function testing during and after recovery from the acute illness. However, secondary hypothyroidism is a diagnostic possibility. If other signs and symptoms point to possible pituitary or hypothalamic disease in such patients, secondary hypothyroidism should be considered. Complete testing of the pituitary (if indicated) should be carried out when the patient is not gravely ill. The simplest tests to do in the acute situation are assessments of adrenal and gonadal function. The administration of α-1-24-corticotropin (see Chap. 147) provides useful information if inadequate adrenal reserve is shown (though it is not a formal test of the entire hypothalamic-pituitary-adrenal axis). Presumptive evidence of secondary hypogonadism (amenorrhea in premenopausal women, inappropriately low serum concentrations of gonadotropins in postmenopausal women, or low serum testosterone and gonadotropin concentrations in men) give support to the diagnosis of secondary hypothyroidism, though severe illness may induce a degree of secondary hypogonadism. Some patients with secondary hypothyroidism have mild elevations of the serum TSH concentration.[41] The TSH in such cases is presumed to be immunoreactive but relatively bioinactive. If the endocrine status of a severely ill patient with known hypothalamic or pituitary disease is in doubt, the patient should be assumed to have endocrine insufficiency, be it hypothyroidism or adrenal insufficiency, until recovery from nonthyroidal illness takes place.

TREATMENT

General Principles

General principles for treating hypothyroid patients have recently been published by the American Thyroid Association.[23] L-Thyroxine is the appropriate treatment for hypothyroidism.[42] With the possible exception of treating myxedema coma, there is generally no indication for the use of combination thyroxine–triiodothyronine preparations or for using triiodothyronine alone in treating hypothyroidism since most T_3 is formed in peripheral tissues from T_4. Presumably the body can more appropriately regulate serum and tissue T_3 levels than can the physician. The usual oral replacement dose of l-thyroxine is approximately 1.6 μg/kg/day (75 to 100 μg/day for women, 100 to 150 μg/day for men).[47] The replacement dose decreases with age, and increases with pregnancy, malabsorption syndromes, and the concomitant administration of certain drugs (see later section on drugs and thyroid function). Patients with normal FT_4 and mildly elevated TSH levels can probably be treated with full replacement doses with impunity. Patients with established or possible coexistent coronary artery disease (virtually any man ≥ 55 years of age and any woman ≥ 65 years of age, though younger age cutoffs seem appropriate if a patient has other cardiac risk factors) should receive replacement more cautiously (25 μg l-thyroxine daily, with a 25-μg increase in the dose every 8 weeks). Any patient with severe long-standing hypothyroidism deserves cautious thyroid replacement (due to possible secondary adrenal insufficiency). Normalization of the serum TSH concentration is the desired hormonal endpoint for patients with primary hypothyroidism. The serum TSH is checked approximately 8 weeks after instituting what is presumed to be a replacement dose of l-thyroxine. The dose may be titrated as needed. In patients with secondary hypothyroidism, the FT_4 should be at least midnormal range, though higher doses of l-thyroxine should be administered if symptoms of hypothyroidism have not abated.

Myxedema Coma

The diagnosis of myxedema coma is a clinical one. Since there are no proved deleterious effects of thyroxine treatment in euthyroid comatose patients, it is better to treat patients suspected to have myxedema coma and be proved wrong than to delay treatment pending laboratory test results. Most comatose, hypothermic patients do not have myxedema coma, but suffer from exposure, the effects of depressant drugs, other major organ failure, or hypoglycemia.

Before beginning treatment, blood should be obtained for the measurement of serum TSH and FT_4. The adrenal reserve of these patients should be evaluated (see Chap. 147) with the onset of therapy even though steroids are typically given concomitantly with thyroid hormone for the first few days.

Treatment of myxedema coma is outlined in Table 149-7.[40] Patients should be passively warmed with blankets. Active warming may cause peripheral vasodilatation and hypotension. Since the intravascular volume is decreased in hypothyroid patients, the use of diuretics may lead to hypotension. If the patient is hypotensive, vigorous fluid replacement (isotonic solutions) must be given. If necessary, vasopressor agents can be administered, though hypothyroid patients have a diminished response to such agents and are at increased risk for development of arrhythmias. Continuous cardiac monitoring is vital in these patients. Glucose-containing solutions should be given. The airway should be secured by endotracheal intubation in most cases. Mechanical ventilation may be necessary. Glucocorticoids should be administered empirically due to the risk of coexistent adrenal insufficiency. A diligent search for a precipitant should be undertaken, and vigorous treatment of any recognized precipitant initiated. In myxedema coma patients who have severe hyponatremia, a free water diuresis can be induced by the administration of furosemide while monitoring carefully for signs of volume depletion and hypotension. Patients with severe hyponatremia and seizures may be treated with hypertonic saline, furosemide, and vigorous replacement of sodium and potassium losses. Patients with protracted hypotension may benefit from central monitoring. The effects of hypothyroidism on drug metabolism should be considered before prescribing any therapeutic agent for these patients.

TABLE 149-7. Treatment of Myxedema Coma

Treat underlying cause.
Passively warm patient.
Treat hypotension with isotonic fluids.
Use pressors if needed cautiously.
Secure the airway and mechanically ventilate if necessary.
Administer hydrocortisone 100 mg IV q 8 h.
Administer l-thyroxine 500 μg IV followed by:
   100 μg l-thyroxine IV qd, or
   25 μg triiodothyronine IV q 6 h.

There are two different approaches to thyroid hormone administration in patients with myxedema coma.[40] The administration of 300 to 500 μg l-thyroxine intravenously saturates protein binding sites and establishes a relatively normal serum T_4 concentration.[43] Such therapy should result in an improvement in the patient's cardiovascular status within a few hours and mental status within a day, virtually clinching the diagnosis of myxedema coma even before the results of thyroid function tests are available. Subsequent replacement therapy can either take the form of intravenous l-thyroxine 100 μg daily, or IV triiodothyronine 25 μg every 6 hours. Advocates of triiodothyronine administration use this form of thyroid hormone since triiodothyronine therapy of the hypothyroid patient normalizes some parameters more rapidly than l-thyroxine treatment and severely ill patients have impaired conversion of T_4 to T_3.[40]

Respiratory Failure

Occasional patients present with respiratory failure and hypothyroidism. It is frequently difficult to determine if the patient's respiratory problems constitute primary lung disease or the combined effects of hypothyroidism on muscle function and central respiratory drive and primary lung disease. No clear guidelines can be drawn from the literature regarding the rapidity with which these patients should receive thyroid replacement. Recent research suggests that normalization of ventilatory drive occurs far earlier than return of normal muscle function.[44] The desire to reverse the deleterious effects of hypothyroidism on normal respiratory physiology must be weighed against the risk of induction of myocardial ischemia if rapid thyroid replacement is pursued. I generally recommend slow replacement to patients who are otherwise stable, but rapid replacement in patients who are deteriorating.

Concomitant Coronary Artery Disease

Thyroid replacement of patients with significant hypothyroidism and concomitant coronary artery disease (or a significant possibility for concomitant coronary disease) is a lengthy process, possibly requiring several months.[45] The increase in myocardial oxygen demand induced by thyroid replacement in these patients may precipitate significant myocardial ischemia. Since the biologic half-life of thyroxine is several weeks, angina developing in the setting of thyroid hormone replacement should be considered to be unstable angina. Such patients need vigorous antianginal therapy and possibly coronary angioplasty or coronary artery bypass grafting (in addition to the temporary discontinuation of thyroxine therapy). Rarely hypothyroid patients are unable to receive full thyroid replacement due to recurring ischemia when normal or near-normal serum thyroid hormone concentrations are achieved. L-Thyroxine therapy is initiated at low doses (25 to 50 μg daily), and the dose is increased incrementally (12.5 to 25.0 μg) every month. I err on the side of slower thyroid replacement since, in my experience, thyroid replacement–induced ischemia may be difficult to treat medically.

Concomitant Adrenal Insufficiency

While slow thyroid replacement is not acutely a risk in patients with adrenal insufficiency, rapid thyroid replacement can precipitate Addisonian crisis. Addison disease is increased in frequency in patients (though still not very common) with chronic thyroiditis. In the outpatient setting, screening for concomitant adrenal insufficiency is usually unnecessary in the absence of suggestive signs and symptoms. However, critically ill patients should be tested for adrenal insufficiency (see Chap. 147) and empirically treated with glucocorticoids while awaiting test results if there is any significant possibility of coexistent adrenal and thyroid failure.

Patients with long-standing hypothyroidism often have pituitary enlargement due to thyrotroph hyperplasia. These patients may have partial hypopituitarism.[46] Pituitary function normalizes with thyroid hormone replacement over time, but administration of full replacement doses of thyroxine initially may precipitate adrenal crisis. If rapid thyroxine repletion is deemed necessary, steroid treatment is indicated in the short term.

Patients with known secondary hypothyroidism are likely to have coexistent deficiency of other pituitary hormones. Weakness and cachexia may predominate in these patients. The examiner should be alert to symptoms and signs suggesting hypogonadism (decreased libido, amenorrhea in females, diminished sex hormone–dependent hair, or small testes in males) as a clue that the hypothyroidism is secondary. Patients with secondary hypothyroidism should have empiric corticosteroid therapy pending test results of the hypothalamic-pituitary-adrenal axis (see Chap. 147).

Concomitant Surgical Emergency

Surgery can be carried out in hypothyroid patients, though minor complications may be increased.[47] The anesthesiologist must pay careful attention to altered drug metabolism in these patients.

DRUGS, THYROID DISEASE, AND THYROID FUNCTION ∎

A number of pharmacologic agents affect thyroid function tests. A list of agents likely to be encountered in intensive care patients is given in Table 149-8.[48,49] The metabolism of drugs is generally accelerated in thyrotoxicosis and slowed in hypothyroidism.[50] Oral anticoagulants are less potent in hypothyroid patients and more potent in patients with thyrotoxicosis due to alterations in clearance of vitamin K–dependent clotting factors in these disease states. When available, serum drug levels may greatly aid treatment of patients with thyroid disease.

THYROID FUNCTION IN NONTHYROIDAL ILLNESS AND AGING ∎

Multiple studies have shown a very high frequency of abnormal thyroid function tests in patients with severe medical or surgical illness.[51,52] Rather than representing an endocrine disease process, abnormalities of thyroid function tests seen in nonthyroidal illness appear to represent an adaptive process by the body to maintain tissue metabolism at an optimum level. It is often difficult to ascertain the metabolic status of severely ill patients by history and physical examination. The clinician must know about the effects of nonthyroidal illness on thyroid function tests and be able to identify patients who may actually have primary alterations in thyroid function.

Older patients may have a low serum TSH concentration with normal FT_4. Many of these patients do not go on to develop frank thyrotoxicosis. However, over the course of time, a suppressed TSH value appears to be a risk factor for the ultimate development of atrial fibrillation.[53]

Patients with *high T_4* syndrome have high serum T_4 concentrations.[54] This abnormality may occur due to increases in thyroxine-binding globulin (TBG). However, the FT_4 will be normal. Serum T_4 may be transiently elevated in other ill patients, particularly those with acute psychosis. Serum T_3 concentrations are normal or low while other thyroid test results are usually normal. Serum T_4 may also be increased in patients taking certain drugs (see Table 149-8). If the serum FT_4 concentraion is elevated, the patient should be assumed to have thyrotoxicosis. Occasionally, only time and further observation will delineate the thyroid status of the individual patient.

Patients with *low T_3* syndrome have normal serum T_4, FT_4, and TSH levels, but low serum T_3 concentrations.[54] Low T_3 syndrome is of no known clinical significance and is not ascertained if T_3 measurements are not routinely done.

The biggest dilemma is caused by patients who have low serum T_4 concentrations (low T_4 syndrome) and normal or low serum TSH levels.[54] FT_4 values are often normal, but may be low or high depending on the assay used.[55] Mortality is significantly increased in intensive care patients with low serum T_4 values, and is inversely proportional to the serum T_4 concentration.[56] If patients recover, their thyroid function tests return to normal. Interestingly, TSH values may be transiently elevated in the recovery phase from nonthyroidal illness.[57] Studies have failed to show an improvement in survival in patients with low T_4 syndrome when treated with l-thyroxine.[58]

How does one decide whether a specific patient with a low serum T_4 is euthyroid or hypothyroid? Patients with a significant elevation of the serum TSH concentration (>20 mU/mL) usually have primary hypothyroidism. Patients with a low or normal serum TSH concentration and low FT_4 usually have the *euthyroid sick syndrome*. If a patient has any suggestion of hypothalamic or pituitary disease, consideration should be given to secondary hypothyroidism.

In human immunodeficiency virus (HIV) infection, thyroxine-binding globulin is increased compared with nonin-

TABLE 149-8. Common Drugs and Illnesses That Affect Thyroid Function Tests

ANTITHYROID ACTION

Decrease FT_4, increase TSH
 Lithium
 Interferon
 Interleukins
 6-Mercaptopurine
 Iodine-containing medications
 Nitroprusside

INTERFERE WITH L-THYROXINE ABSORPTION

Decrease FT_4, increase TSH in treated
  primary hypothyroid patients
 Ferrous sulfate
 Bile acid sequestrants
 Sodium polystyrene sulfonate
 Aluminum hydroxide
 Sucralfate

INHIBIT T_4 TO T_3 CONVERSION

Increase T_4, decrease T3
 Propranolol
 Radiographic contrast agents
 Amiodarone
 Severe medical illness
 Surgery

INCREASE THYROID HORMONE
DEGRADATION

Decrease T_4; decrease FT_4, increase TSH in
  treated primary hypothyroid patients
 Anticonvulsants
 Rifampin

DECREASE TSH

Dopamine
Glucocorticoids
Octreotide
Severe medical illness

INCREASE TBG

Decrease RT_3U, increase T_4, normal FT_4,
  TSH; increase thyroid hormone
  requirement in hypothyroid patients
 Estrogens
 Methadone
 5-Fluorouracil
 Perphenazine
 Niacin
 Inflammatory liver disease
 Pregnancy
 HIV

DECREASE TBG

Increase RT_3U, decrease T_4, normal FT_4, TSH;
  decrease thyroid hormone requirement in
  hypothyroid patients
 Androgens
 Tamoxifen
 Glucocorticoids
 L-Asparaginase

INTERFERE WITH THYROID HORMONE
BINDING

May increase RT_3U, decrease T_4, normal or
  decreased FT_4, normal TSH
 NSAIDs
 Phenytoin
 Heparin
 Penicillin
 Furosemide
 Severe medical illness

---

fected subjects, leading to a decrease in the RT_3U and similar tests.[59] Serum T_4 and T_3 remain relatively normal (though the T_4 and T_3 values may be in the high normal range) until severe intercurrent illness strikes, when serum T_3 and T_4 concentrations decline.

Serum TSH concentrations may be suppressed in elderly patients without other laboratory or clinical evidence of thyrotoxicosis.[60,61] While the long-term risk for atrial fibrillation or clinical thyrotoxicosis of these patients is increased, many of these patients never develop clinical thyrotoxicosis and may have spontaneous normalization of the abnormal thyroid function tests. While isolated FT_3 toxicosis has recently been reported[62] and should be considered as a diagnostic possibility in patients with a low serum TSH concentration, most patients with an isolated low TSH have normal concentrations of other thyroid parameters and should be considered to be euthyroid. Follow-up of abnormal thyroid function tests must be done.

Isolated elevations in the FT_4I have been observed in elderly chronically ill nursing home residents.[63] With a normal serum TSH and T_3 concentration, it seems likely that these patients are euthyroid.

Increases in the serum TSH concentration, often mild, with a normal FT_4 are common in older patients. Most of these patients continue to have elevation of the TSH and some ultimately develop hypothyroxinemia as well.[64]

AIRWAY OBSTRUCTION ∎

Although airflow compromise is common in patients with goiters, rarely the enlarged (usually benign) thyroid can cause significant airway obstruction.[65] The performance of a flow-volume loop is helpful in identifying these patients.[66] In the author's experience, prophylactic intubation while awaiting thyroidectomy seems prudent in patients with evidence of carbon dioxide retention.

REFERENCES ■

1. Surks MI, Chopra IJ, Mariash CN, et al: American Thyroid Association guidelines for use of laboratory test in thyroid disorders. *JAMA* 1990;263:1529
2. Utiger RD: The thyroid: physiology, thyrotoxicosis, hypothyroidism, and the painful thyroid. In: Felig P, Baxter JD, Frohman LA (eds). *Endocrinology and Metabolism*, 3rd ed. St Louis, McGraw-Hill, 1995:435
3. Reasner CA II, Isley WL: Thyrotoxicosis in the critically ill. *Crit Care Clin* 1991;7:57
4. Hamilton CR, Maloof F: Unusual types of hyperthyroidism. *Medicine* 1973;52:195
5. Davis P, Davis F: Hyperthyroidism in patients over the age of 60 years. *Medicine* 1974;53:161
6. Martin FIR, Tress BW, Colman PG, Deam DR: Iodine-induced hyperthyroidism due to nonionic contrast radiography in the elderly. *Am J Med* 1993;95:78
7. Sanmarti A, Permanyer-Miralda G, Castellanos JM, et al: Chronic administration of amiodarone and thyroid function: a follow-up study. *Am Heart J* 1984;108:1262
8. Feely J, Peden N. Use of β-adrenoceptor blocking drugs in hyperthyroism. *Drugs* 1984;27:425
9. Klein I: Thyroid hormone and the heart. *Am J Med* 1990;88:631
10. Ladenson PW: Recognition and management of cardiovascular disease related to thyroid dysfunction. *Am J Med* 1990;88:638
11. Levey GS: Catecholamine–thyroid hormone interactions and the cardiovascular manifestations of hyperthyroidism. *Am J Med* 1990;88:642
12. Woeber KA: Thyrotoxicosis and the heart. *N Engl J Med* 1992;327:94
13. Thomas MR, McGregor AM, Jewitt DE: Left ventricle filling abnormalites prior to and following treatment of thyrotoxicosis—is diastolic dysfunction implicated in thyrotoxic cardiomyopathy? *Eur Heart J* 1993;14:662
14. Orme SM, Sebastian JP, Page MD, et al: Thyrotoxicosis increases right to left shunt in congenital cyanotic heart disease. *Clin Endocrinol* 1993;39:253
15. Siafakas NM, Milona I, Salesiotou V, et al: Respiratory muscle strength in hyperthyroidism before and after treatment. *Am Rev Respir Dis* 1992;146:1025
16. Burch HB, Wartofsky L: Life-threatening thyrotoxicosis. *Clin Endocrinol Metab* 1993;22:263
17. Laurberg P: Persistent problems with the specificity of immunometric TSH assays. *Thyroid* 1993;4:279
18. Lum SMC, Kaptein EM, Nicoloff JT: Influence of nonthyroidal illnesses on serum thyroid hormone in hyperthyroidism. *West J Med* 1983;138:670
19. Brooks MH, Waldstein SS: Free thyroxine concentrations in thyroid storm. *Ann Intern Med* 1980;93:694
20. Braverman LE, Utiger RD: Introduction to thyrotoxicosis. In: Braverman LE, Utiger RD (eds). *The Thyroid*, 6th ed. Philadelphia, JB Lippincott, 1991:645
21. Singer PA, Cooper DS, Levy EG, et al: Treatment guidelines for patients with hyperthyroidisim and hypothyroidism. *JAMA* 1995;273:808
22. Klein I, Becker DV, Levey GS: Treatment of hyperthyroid disease. *Ann Intern Med* 1994;121:281
23. Cooper DS: Antithyroid drugs. *N Engl J Med* 1984;311:1353
24. Feely J, Stevenson IH, Crooks J: Increased clearance of propranolol in thyrotoxicosis. *Ann Intern Med* 1981;94:472
25. Herman VS, Joffe BI, Kalk WJ, et al: Clinical and biochemical responses to nadolol and clonidine in hyperthyroidism. *J Clin Pharmacol* 1989;29:1117
26. Dahlstrom CG, Ladefoged SD: Verapamil in atrial fibrillation in hyperthyroidism. *BMJ* 1987;294:1384
27. Roti E, Montermini M, Roti S, et al: The effect of diltiazem, a calcium channel-blocking drug, on cardiac rate and rhythm in hyperthyroid patients. *Arch Intern Med* 1988;148:1919
28. Fradkin JE, Wolff J: Iodide-induced thyrotoxicosis. *Medicine* 1983;62:1
29. Newnham HH, Topliss DJ, Le Grand BA, et al: Amiodarone-induced hyperthyroidism: assessment of the predictive value of biochemical testing and response to combined therapy using propylthiouracil and potassium perchlorate. *Aust N Z J Med* 1987;18:37
30. Farwell AP, Abend SL, Huang SKS, et al: Thyroidectomy for amiodarone-induced thyrotoxicosis. *JAMA* 1990;263:1526
31. Bar-Sela S, Ehrenfeld M, Eliakim M: Arterial embolism in thyrotoxicosis with atrial fibrillation. *Arch Intern Med* 1981;141:1191
32. Forfar JC, Muir AL, Sawers SA, et al: Hyperthyroid heart disease. *Clin Endocrinol Metab* 1985;14:491
33. Burrow BN: The management of thyrotoxicosis in pregnancy. *N Engl J Med* 1983;313:562
34. Shakir KM, Michaels RD, Jays JH, Potter BB: The use of bile acid sequestrants to lower serum thyroid hormones in iatrogenic hyperthyroidism. *Ann Intern Med* 1993;118:112
35. Cooper DS, Steigerwalt S, Migdal S: Pharmacology of propylthiouracil in thyrotoxicosis and chronic renal failure. *Arch Intern Med* 1987;147:785
36. Zwillich CW, Pierson DJ, Hofeldt F, et al: Ventilatory control in myxedema and hypothyroidism. *N Engl J Med* 1975;292:662
37. Rajagopal KR, Abbrecht PH, Derderian SS, et al: Obstructive sleep apnea in hypothyroidism. *Ann Intern Med* 1984;101:491
38. Klein I, Levey GS: Unusual manifestations of hypothyroidism. *Ann Intern Med* 1984;144:123
39. Gottehrer A, Roa J, Stanford GG, et al: Hypothyroidism and pleural effusions. *Chest* 1990;98:1120
40. Nicoloff JT, LoPresti JS: Myxedema coma: a form of decompensated hypothyroidism. *Clin Endocrinol Metab* 1993;22:279
41. Faglia G, Bitensky L, Pinchera A, et al: Thyrotropin secretion in patients with central hypothyroidism: evidence for reduced biological activity of immunoreactive thyrotropin. *J Clin Endocrinol Metab* 1979;48:989
42. Mandel SJ, Brent GB, Larsen PR: Levothyroxine therapy in patients with thyroid disease. *Ann Intern Med* 1993;119:492
43. Ladenson PW, Goldenheim PD, Ridgway EC: Rapid pituitary and peripheral tissue responses to intravenous L-triiodothyronine in hypothyroidism. *J Clin Endocrinol Metab* 1983;56:1252
44. Duranti R, Gheri RG, Gorini M, et al: Control of breathing in patients with severe hypothyroidism. *Am J Med* 1993;95:29
45. Becker C: Hypothyroidism and atherosclerotic heart disease: pathogenesis, medical management, and the role of coronary artery bypass surgery. *Endocr Rev* 1985;6:432
46. Bigos ST, Ridgway EC, Kourides IA, et al: Spectrum of pituitary alterations with mild and severe thyroid impairment. *J Clin Endocrinol Metab* 1978;46:317
47. Litt L, Roizen F: Anesthetic and surgical risk in hypothyroidism. *Arch Intern Med* 1984;144:657
48. Burger AG: Effects of pharmacologic agents on thyroid hormone metabolism. In: Braverman LE, Utiger RD (eds). *The Thyroid*, 6th ed. Philadelphia, JB Lippincott, 1991:335
49. Kaplan MM: Interactions between drugs and thyroid hormones. *Thyroid Today* 1981;4(5):1
50. Shenfield GM: Influence of thyroid dysfunction on drug pharmacokinetics. *Clin Pharm* 1981;6:275

51. DeGroot LJ, Mayor G: Admission screening by thyroid function tests in an acute general care teaching hospital. *Am J Med* 1992;93:558

52. Simons FJ, Simon JM, Demers LM, Santen RJ: Thyroid dysfunction in elderly hospitalized patients. *Arch Intern Med* 1990;150:1249

53. Sawin CT, Geller A, Wolf PA, et al: Low serum thyrotropin concentrations as a risk factor for atrial fibrillation in older persons. *N Engl J Med* 1994;331:1249

54. Chopra IJ, Hershman JM, Pardridge WM, et al: Thyroid function in nonthyroidal illnesses. *Ann Intern Med* 1983;98:946

55. Wong TK, Pekary AE, Hoo GS, et al: Comparison of methods for measuring free thyroxin in nonthyroidal illness. *Clin Chem* 1992;38:720

56. Slag MR, Morley JE, Elson MK, et al: Hypothyroxinemia in critically ill patients as a predictor of high mortality. *JAMA* 1981;245:43

57. Hamblin PS, Dyer SA, Mohr VS, et al: Relationship between thyrotropin and thyroxine changes during recovery from severe hypothyroxinemia of critical illness. *J Clin Endocrinol Metab* 1986;67:717

58. Brent GA, Hershman JM: Thyroxine therapy in patients with severe nonthyroidal illnesses and low serum thyroxine concentration. *J Clin Endocrinol Metab* 1986;63:1

59. LoPresti JS, Fried JC, Spencer CA, Nicoloff JT: Unique alterations of thyroid hormone indices in the acquired immunodeficiency syndrome (AIDS). *Ann Intern Med* 1989;110:970

60. Sawin CT, Geller A, Kaplan MM, et al: Low serum thyrotropin (thyroid-stimulating hormone) in older persons without hyperthyroidism. *Arch Intern Med* 1991;151:165

61. Bagchi N, Brown TR, Parish RF: Thyroid dysfunction in adults over age 65 years. *Arch Intern Med* 1990;150:785

62. Bitton RN, Wexler C: Free triiodothyronine toxicosis: a distinct entity. *Am J Med* 1990;88:531

63. Drinka PJ, Nolten WE, Voeks S, et al: Misleading elevation of the free thyroxine index in nursing home residents. *Arch Pathol Lab Med* 1991;115:1208

64. Parle JV, Franklyn JA, Cross KW, et al: Prevalence and follow-up of abnormal thyrotrophin (TSH) concentrations in the elderly in the United Kingdom. *Clin Endocrinol* 1991;34:77

65. Miller MR, Pincock AC, Oates GD, et al: Upper airway obstruction due to goitre: detection, prevalence and results of surgical management. *Q J Med* 1990;274:177

66. Geraghty JG, Coveney EC, Kiernan M, O'Higgins NJ: Flow volume loops in patients with goiters. *Ann Surg* 1992;215:83

Skin and Muscle Disease and Dysfunction

Critical Care, Third Edition, edited by Joseph M. Civetta,
Robert W. Taylor, and Robert R. Kirby.
Lippincott-Raven Publishers, Philadelphia, PA © 1997.

CHAPTER 150

Critical Care of Rheumatic Disease

Jay B. Higgs
Ramon A. Arroyo
Kenneth F. Des Rosier
Matthew T. Carpenter

IMMEDIATE CONCERNS

MAJOR PROBLEMS

The rheumatic diseases arise from disorders of the immune system and other poorly defined pathophysiologic processes and present with a wide variety of manifestations, depending on which organ systems are targeted for destruction. The central pathophysiologic process is dysregulation of the immune system, a complex array of many cellular and humoral components. In most rheumatic diseases, however, the precise cause has not been discovered, and treatment is empirical. Direct threats to life and limb include vascular compromise with ischemia of multiple possible organ sites, acute and chronic renal disease, cerebritis, pulmonary disease, cardiac disease, and cervical spine instability. Secondary threats are infection and complications of antirheumatic therapy.

The opinions expressed herein are those of the authors and do not reflect policy of the United States Air Force or the Department of Defense.

STRESS POINTS

General

1. Patients with known rheumatic disease may present to the critical care setting with new manifestations of their illness, antirheumatic medication complications, or medically altered presentations of common illnesses.
2. Joints compromised by inflammatory diseases are more prone to infection, and the expected local manifestations of joint sepsis in these patients may be mild or absent.
3. Inflammatory joint disease can render the cervical spine unstable. Extra caution must be exercised in patients with potentially unstable necks during transportation and intubation.
4. Abdominal pain in the patient with rheumatic disease may be a harbinger of catastrophe. The initial examination may appear disarmingly benign, especially in the face of corticosteroid therapy. Careful, thorough evaluation and serial observation are required.

Vasculitis

1. The vasculitides all are characterized by inflammation within or through a vessel wall, with resultant compromise of blood flow and vessel wall integrity. The vari-

ous clinical syndromes result from tissue ischemia and systemic features of inflammation (fever, malaise, weight loss).

2. Involvement may include one or many organ systems and vessels of predominately one or multiple sizes. Determining both predominant vessel size involvement and pattern of organ involvement is useful in working through the differential diagnosis.

Systemic Lupus Erythematosus

1. Indicators of life-threatening systemic lupus erythematosus (SLE) include renal disease, central nervous system (CNS) involvement, severe hemolysis or thrombocytopenia, pulmonary parenchymal disease, and, less commonly, vasculitis or myocarditis.
2. Fever in a patient with SLE should always trigger a search for infection. Shaking chills, leukocytosis, increased complement components, and absence of multisystem lupus activity favor an infectious etiology.
3. Fever, disproportionate tachycardia, and cardiomegaly with or without pericarditis or congestive heart failure (CHF) are features of lupus myocarditis. Creatine kinase (CK) levels and echocardiography are useful in making this diagnosis.

Systemic Sclerosis

1. Life-threatening complications of systemic sclerosis (SSc) include pulmonary fibrosis, pulmonary hypertension, myocardial fibrosis, and scleroderma renal crisis.
2. Optimal management of SSc in the critical care setting includes attention to problems of esophageal dysmotility, Raynaud's phenomenon, skin fragility, and poor gut motility.

ESSENTIAL DIAGNOSTIC TESTS AND PROCEDURES

General

1. The diagnosis of suspected rheumatic disease hinges first on an adequate history and physical examination, then on laboratory tests aimed at defining organ damage, and finally on appropriate serologic testing.
2. Accurate diagnosis is critical in the management of pulmonary failure in the face of rheumatic disease, especially when treatment includes immunosuppressive medications. In more severe presentations, efforts should be more invasive, even to the point of open-lung biopsy.

Vasculitis

1. Once vasculitis is suspected, the diagnosis usually relies on biopsy of involved tissue or arteriography.
2. The histopathologic hallmarks of medium-sized muscular artery vasculitis are inflammation, vessel wall necrosis, and disruption of the internal elastic lamina. Small vessel vasculitis is evidenced by perivascular

inflammation and is termed *leukocytoclastic* when nuclear debris is seen.

Systemic Lupus Erythematosus

1. Aside from history and physical, basic laboratory testing is more important than serologic studies in determining the seriousness of the presentation. Hypocomplementemia and elevated anti–double-stranded DNA titers are associated with more severe disease, but this is not universally reliable.
2. Any patient with new anemia should have careful examination of the peripheral smear for evidence of intravascular or extravascular hemolysis; thrombotic thrombocytopenic purpura should be suspected if there is microangiopathic hemolysis, particularly when simultaneous CNS or renal disease is present.

Systemic Sclerosis

1. Laboratory features of SSc renal crisis include elevated serum creatinine, which may rise as rapidly as 1 mg/dL per day, microangiopathic hemolytic anemia, reticulocytosis, and mild thrombocytopenia. If renal crisis is suspected, examination of a peripheral blood smear by a physician for schistocytes is mandatory.
2. Rheumatologic serologies are of little diagnostic utility in the critical care of SSc.
3. High-resolution computed tomography (CT) of the lungs and bronchoalveolar lavage (BAL) are important in guiding therapy of interstitial lung disease.

INITIAL THERAPY

General

1. For life- or organ-threatening inflammatory diseases, glucocorticoids are usually the first line of treatment and have the most rapid onset of action. Other immunosuppressive agents tend to have a delayed effect and are used in conjunction with steroids, either to decrease steroid requirement or improve disease prognosis.
2. The toxicity profile of all antirheumatic medications mandates informed consent and close monitoring.
3. Disease modifying antirheumatic drugs such as gold compounds, penicillamine, hydroxychloroquine, and sulfasalazine can usually be discontinued in the face of acute severe intercurrent illness with little adverse effect.
4. In patients already under treatment with immunosuppressive (cytotoxic) agents for known rheumatic illness, the decision whether to withhold these medications in the face of acute nonrheumatic illness hinges on balancing the risk of immunocompromise or other-drug side effects versus the severity of the rheumatic disease.
5. When possible, nonsteroidal antiinflammatory drugs (NSAIDs) should be withheld in the critical care setting.

Vasculitis

1. In life- or organ-threatening vasculitis, treatment may need to begin before the diagnosis is firmly established.
2. Cytotoxic agents are added to steroids in specific situations of steroid failure, unacceptable steroid morbidity, and in the vasculidites for which the prognosis is improved with cytotoxic agents over steroids alone.

Systemic Lupus Erythematosus

1. Rapidly progressive decline in renal function may be salvageable with aggressive immunosuppressive therapy. Renal biopsy is helpful in estimating prognosis and predicting treatment response.
2. Although many neuropsychiatric manifestations of lupus are self-limiting, acute and progressive mental status changes or seizures associated with either abnormal cerebral spinal fluid (CSF) findings or multifocal ischemic findings on magnetic resonance imaging (MRI) warrant aggressive immunosuppressive therapy.
3. Focal thrombotic CNS ischemia associated with antiphospholipid antibodies (aPLs) should be treated initially with anticoagulation.

Systemic Sclerosis

1. Recognition of SSc renal crisis is critical, because early management with angiotensin converting enzyme (ACE) inhibitors preserves renal function and decreases mortality.
2. Narcotics and anticholinergic agents may precipitate severe ileus. Glucocorticoid therapy may precipitate normotensive renal crisis. Beta-blockers may exacerbate Raynaud's phenomenon.
3. Pulmonary hypertension in SSc patients with limited skin disease (CREST) is an important cause of mortality. Patients may respond to continuous intravenous iloprost.
4. Pseudo-obstruction of the small intestine or colon is best managed conservatively, even when air appears in the bowel wall.

OVERVIEW

This chapter is divided into four sections: general concepts, vasculitis, SLE, and SSc. This material offers important concepts in the initial management of rheumatic disease in the critical care setting. Further literature research may be necessary for the many specific questions that arise in the care of these patients. Many of the references cited are review articles or book chapters; this is intentional to facilitate research from text to review article and then specific topics as necessary. When no clear solution to a given problem can be found in the literature, we offer a consensus of personal preference, and have so noted in the text.

PRINCIPLES AND PITFALLS IN THE CRITICAL CARE OF RHEUMATIC DISEASE

Caring for patients with rheumatic disease in the critical care setting can be intimidating. In some cases, the rheumatic disease is the primary, yet undiagnosed threat to life. In others, complications of a preexisting rheumatic disease or its treatment may be in the differential diagnosis of a confusing clinical presentation. Given the rarity of many rheumatic diseases, their protean and often overlapping manifestations, and the complexity of laboratory tests available, it is not surprising that diagnostic and therapeutic dilemmas often result.

EARLY MANAGEMENT

The initial evaluation and management of the critically ill patient with known or suspected rheumatic disease follows the same principles of airway, breathing, and circulation as for other patients. However, a few pitfalls (outlined later) must be kept in mind from the outset. Once the patient is stabilized, further diagnostic efforts can be made. Early involvement of a rheumatologist with experience in the diagnosis and management of these disorders improves patient care and saves the time, expense, and morbidity of unnecessary tests or treatments.

DIAGNOSTIC STRATEGY

The diagnosis of suspected rheumatic disease hinges first on an adequate history and physical examination. Often, when a rheumatic disease is suspected, the first reflex is to order a large panel of "serologies." When some of these results are positive, a diagnosis is then attempted, primarily from laboratory findings. Experienced rheumatologists first go to the bedside and collect all of the history and physical examination data possible. The next most valuable data come from laboratory tests which look for evidence of organ damage. For example, the simple complete blood cell count (CBC) and urinalysis provide crucial information about possible nephritis, hemolysis, leukopenia, and thrombocytopenia in patients with vasculitis or SLE. Finally, the results of serologic testing can be incorporated into the diagnostic picture. The results of all available noninvasive data are then compiled and used to determine appropriate therapy or invasive testing. When key questions remain, consultation of primary literature sources is a must.

PREEXISTING RHEUMATIC DISEASE IN THE CRITICAL CARE SETTING

There are several important considerations in critical care patients admitted with preexisting rheumatic disease. The first is that the critical health problem may, in fact, be a new manifestation of the disease. Second, possible complications of all of the patient's current and previous treatments must be considered as contributors to the current clinical picture. Third, even when the rheumatic disease appears uninvolved with the current illness, special precautions are

TABLE 150-1.   Selected Noninfectious Antirheumatic Drug Complications Most Likely to Be Encountered in the Critical Care Setting°

ANTIRHEUMATIC DRUG	SKIN	GASTROINTESTINAL/ HEPATIC	PULMONARY
Sulfasalazine	Toxic epidermal necrolysis, Stevens-Johnson syndrome	Pancreatitis, acute hepatitis	Fibrosing alveolitis, pneumonitis, brochospasm, bronchiolitis obliterans
Hydroxychloroquine, chloroquine			Cardiorespiratory failure with overdose
Penicillamine	Pemphigus		Pneumonitis, bronchiolitis obliterans, Goodpasture's syndrome
Gold compounds	Exfoliative dermatitis	Severe enterocolitis, intrahepatic cholestasis	Pneumonitis, bronchiolitis obliterans
Methotrexate		Hepatic cirrhosis, enterocolitis	Acute pneumonitis, chronic fibrosis, noncardiogenic pulmonary edema
Azathioprine		Enterocolitis, cholestatic jaundice, hepatic vein thrombosis, transaminitis	Pneumonitis, fibrosis
Cyclophosphamide			Acute pneumonitis, chronic fibrosis, noncardiogenic pulmonary edema
Cyclosporine		Transaminitis, elevated bilirubin	
NSAIDs	Toxic epidermal necrolysis	Gastritis or ulcers with bleeding, enterocolitis, exacerbation of inflammatory bowel, cholestatic jaundice, transaminitis	Bronchospasm, adult respiratory distress syndrome, pulmonary infiltrate with eosinophilia
Corticosteroids		Peptic ucler disease in association with NSAIDs, fatty liver, pancreatitis	
Allopurinol	Stevens-Johnson syndrome	Hepatic necrosis, granulomatous hepatitis	
Colchicine		Diarrhea/dehydration, gastritis/hemorrhage, hepatic necrosis	Noncardiogenic pulmonary edema

NSAIDs, nonsteroidal antiinflammatory drugs; G6PD, glucose-6 phosphate dehydrogenase.
°Not all complications of these drugs are listed; specific literature or the package insert should be consulted when potential complications not listed in the table are being considered.

needed to ensure an optimal outcome for the patient once the crisis passes.

When a patient with known rheumatic disease is admitted with an acute problem, consider whether the problem could be a manifestation of that illness. For instance, a patient with a history of Wegener's granulomatosis (WG) is admitted with an acute myocardial infarction. With only a few minutes of effort, a specific computer-assisted literature search looking for any connection between the two reveals that coronary vasculitis should be considered.[1]

ANTIRHEUMATIC MEDICATION CONSIDERATIONS

The patient with a history of rheumatic disease may present to the critical care setting with complications of therapy or with a common illness that presents atypically because of the effects of treatment.[2] Some of the complications of antirheumatic treatment that are likely to be encountered in the critical care setting are listed in Table 150-1, which is not all-inclusive. The first class of medications considered

RENAL	HEMATOLOGIC	MISCELLANEOUS
Rare proteinuria	Aplastic anemia, agranulocytosis, hemolysis (especially with G6PD deficiency), methemoglobinemia	Serum sickness, pyrexia
	Hemolysis (especially with G6PD deficiency)	Arrythmia, cardiomyopathy, seizures
Proteinuria, Goodpasture's syndrome	Thrombocytopenia, granulocytopenia, aplastic anemia, hemolysis	Myasthenia gravis, polymyositis, systemic lupus erythematosus
Proteinuria	Thrombocytopenia, granulocytopenia, aplastic anemia	Gullian-Barré syndrome, encephalopathy
	Thrombocytopenia, granulocytopenia	
	Thrombocytopenia, granulocytopenia	
Syndrome of inappropriate secretion of antidiuretic hormone	Thrombocytopenia, granulocytopenia	Hemorrhagic cystitis, cardiomyopathy
Renal insufficiency, hypertension, hyperkalemia	Leukopenia	Seizures
Renal insufficiency, interstitial nephritis, hyponatremia, hyperkalemia, analgesic nephropathy	Platelet dysfunction, hemolysis, neutropenia, red cell aplasia	Metabolic acidosis in salicylate toxicity, anaphylaxis, aseptic meningitis, Reye's syndrome
Hypokalemia, hypertension		Adrenal axis suppression, hyperglycemia, impaired wound healing
Interstitial nephritis, oxypurinal stones		Hypersensitivity vasculitis
	Bone marrow suppression	Severe multisystem failure in overdose

here is the immunosuppressive agents, which include corticosteroids, cyclosporine, and cytotoxic agents such as cyclophosphamide, azathioprine, and methotrexate.[2,3] Infectious complications must be be considered in the acutely ill immunocompromised host and are addressed elsewhere in this text. Even if complications from immunosuppressive agents are uninvolved in the current illness, these therapies may need to be altered in the setting of acute illness. A key question that often arises in caring for critically ill and possibly infected patients taking these medications is whether the immunosuppressive agent should be continued. The answer lies in weighing the risk of continued immunosuppression against exacerbation of the underlying rheumatic disease; that is, well-controlled rheumatoid arthritis (RA)

tolerates cessation of therapy much better than active CNS vasculitis.

In corticosteroid-treated patients, this last question may be moot when there is a need for stress-dose corticosteroids, which if given as hydrocortisone, 100 mg intravenously (IV) every 8 hours, works out to approximately the equivalent of 60 mg/day of prednisone in divided doses (the principles of stress dose corticosteroids and adrenal insufficiency are discussed in Chap. 147). In cases where stress dosing is not needed and the patient has a fever that could be either from the rheumatic disease or infection, our approach is to continue the medication at its current dosing (if less than 0.5 mg/kg/day of prednisone or the equivalent) while the patient is being further evaluated. In cases of higher corticosteroid dosing where there seems to be no immediate threat to life from the rheumatic disease, we lower the corticosteroid dose to at least 0.5 mg/kg of prednisone or the equivalent while the fever is being evaluated. In cases of life- or organ-threatening rheumatic disease complicated by fever, we are occasionally forced into continuation of high-dose corticosteroids with careful monitoring. In the patient treated with corticosteroids or other immunosuppressive agents in whom there is a reasonable suspicion of infection or impending sepsis, we empirically add broad-spectrum antibiotic coverage after initial cultures are obtained. Other steroid therapeutic and toxicity issues in rheumatic disease have been recently reviewed.[4] It cannot be emphasized too strongly that steroid therapy, even in moderate doses, can mask abdominal or other catastrophes, and a high index of suspicion is needed to avoid a delay in diagnosis.

Some antirheumatic medications such as gold, penicillamine, hydroxychloroquine, and sulfasalazine have little adverse effect on host defenses against infection unless they are complicated by idiosyncratic bone marrow suppression. However, these medications also may cause severe and unusual side effects that would complicate matters for acutely ill patients.[2,5] Because these medications are seldom used to treat life-threatening manifestations of rheumatic disease, our practice is to temporarily discontinue them during severe acute illness.

The side effects of NSAIDs have been well described.[2,6,7] Several special precautions in the critical care setting should be mentioned. Because these patients are already under significant stress and are often corticosteroid treated as well, the potential for NSAID-induced gastrointestinal (GI) bleeding is magnified. The use of injectable NSAIDs does not obviate this risk. Second, when administering oral NSAIDs to a recumbent ill patient, the physician must recognize the risk of pharyngeal or esophageal erosion when the medication is incompletely swallowed. Third, the risk of a fall in the glomerular filtration rate as a result of prostaglandin inhibition and the consequences of decreased renal clearance for other medications being administered must be considered. Conditions in which the intrarenal blood flow is particularly prostaglandin dependent include CHF, cirrhosis with ascites, and intravascular volume depletion (e.g. dehydration or GI bleeding). Unless clearly needed we withhold NSAIDs in the acute care setting and use acetaminophen or narcotics for pain relief.

Preexisting Joint Disease

Several pitfalls in caring for patients with rheumatic disease should be considered when these patients enter the critical care setting. The first of these relates to preexisting joint disease. Joints compromised by inflammatory diseases such as RA are more prone to infection, perhaps related both to local mechanical factors and systemic compromise of the immune system. In addition, the expected local manifestations of joint sepsis (severe pain, erythema, heat) may be absent or mild in these patients. Patients with prosthetic joints may harbor indolent infection, either introduced at the time of surgery or from hematogenous seeding. Therefore, a high index of suspicion for joint infection is needed in patients with preexisting joint disease who present with mainly systemic manifestations of sepsis.

Preexisting joint disease also is important to consider in managing the patient's cervical spine. Most autoimmune diseases that cause peripheral joint destruction also compromise the stability and mobility of the cervical spine. Cervical subluxation in RA from ligamentous laxity and bone destruction is a classic example of this principle.[8] Ankylosing spondylitis causes fusion in the neck, but paradoxically, the structure is weak and also should be respected. The most important point to remember is that any patient with inflammatory peripheral joint destruction should be considered to have a potentially unstable neck until proven otherwise, and that minor trauma or forced neck flexion (as in endotracheal intubation) can result in destruction of the spinal cord at a high cervical level. Protective measures, such as elective nasotracheal (rather than endotracheal) intubation in the appropriate setting and extra care in transferring the unconscious patient, should be employed until lateral cervical spine radiographs in flexion and extension can be obtained to rule out instability. We recommend that inflammatory arthritis patients with potentially unstable necks who require transportation, such as to the operating room, wear at least a soft cervical collar. This does not directly protect the neck, but it signals all handlers to use extra care. When a detailed examination of the spinal cord and canal is required, MRI is the best test.

The last point to make about preexisting joint disease relates to rehabilitation. Patients with compromised joints who become bedridden for even a short period of time may lose significant function. Flexion contractures develop quickly in unused arthritic joints and are difficult to overcome once the critical illness passes. This is particularly true for the knees, which contract quickly in the bedridden patient. Loss of periarticular motor strength also rapidly develops and is just as disabling. Bedside physical therapy with twice-daily full range of motion of the joints and, if possible, muscle strengthening exercises minimizes these complications.

Pulmonary Failure

One of the most difficult critical care presentations in patients with rheumatic disease is that of pulmonary failure. The differential diagnosis of this presentation includes infection, complications of the rheumatic disease (pulmonary fibrosis, hemorrhage, thrombosis, vasculitis, pleuritis, hypertension, diaphragmatic dysfunction, restriction, or acute pneumonitis),[9,10] and pulmonary compromise secondary to immunomodulatory medications.[5] Given that the correct diagnosis leads down much different treatment pathways (e.g., antibiotics, corticosteroids, institution or withdrawal of immunomodulatory agents), it is critical to make the correct diagnosis early. With increasing seriousness of pulmonary parenchymal disease, our practice is to move quickly from empirical therapy to bronchoscopy or open-lung biopsy.

Raynaud's Phenomenon

Raynaud's phenomenon also is an important pitfall in the critical care of patients with rheumatic disease.[11] Patients with this problem typically experience intermittent pain and color changes of the hands, precipitated most often by body cooling and stress. The initial phase of Raynaud's phenomenon is ischemia from vasospasm of the digital arteries. This results in cyanotic or blanched and painful digits, followed by erythema on rewarming. Critical care patients with this problem are at risk for severe digital ischemia, which can cause complete necrosis of the digits. In addition, vasospasm of internal organs may occur. One precipitating event is body cooling; hence, maintaining appropriate body core and extremity temperatures are both important in preventing this complication. Although the use of beta-adrenergic blocking agents in patients with Raynaud's phenomenon has been thought to pose a risk for increased vasospasm, this concept has been recently challenged. Until further data accumulate on the safety of beta-blockers in Raynaud's phenomenon, we urge that this drug class be used with great caution and only when a reasonable alternative agent does not exist. Severe ischemia with digital necrosis may be seen after complicated treatment courses in the critical care setting; two potential causes are vasopressors and hypotension. Treatment may include body warming, calcium channel blockers, topical nitroglycerin paste, or surgical sympathectomy (cervical or digital), depending on the severity of ischemia and on the patient's ability to tolerate these interventions. Acute pain may be relieved with narcotic agents, both for patient comfort and theoretically to reduce sympathetic vascular tone. Caution is needed, however, because of the negative effect of narcotics on gut motility, especially in patients with SSc (see later). Iloprost, a prostaglandin analogue, is a potent vasodilator that has been used IV on an experimental basis for severe Raynaud's phenomenon. Success has been reported in a placebo-controlled trial, but iloprost has not yet received approval by the Food and Drug Administration for this use. When, despite our best efforts, severe ischemia results in digital infarction, we most often let the necrotic digits autoamputate.

Sicca Syndrome

A final pitfall in the care of patients with rheumatic disease is sicca syndrome. Patients with Sjogren's syndrome or other causes of sicca have severe mucosal dryness for which they must compensate with frequent sips of water, artificial tears, and ocular ointment at bedtime. In the conscious state, symptoms clearly direct the patient to appropriate mucosal care, but this may not be possible in the critical care situation. Mucosal dryness impairs first-line host defenses against infection; hence, attention to appropriate humidification of inspired air and to local mucosal moisturization is important. Topical hydration with ocular ointment and taping the eyelids closed becomes important in the unconscious state.

VASCULITIS ∎

The recognition and treatment of systemic vasculitis is challenging. First, a reasonable working classification of the different vasculitides and of the diseases that may produce a similar picture is needed. The diagnosis of vasculitis must be as precise and definitive as possible because the treatment and prognosis vary in different vasculitic syndromes. The clinician's most valuable tools in this process are the history and physical examination. Recognition of the clinical patterns is more valuable than sophisticated serologic studies. Ultimately, the definitive diagnosis often is dependent on biopsy or angiography of involved or symptomatic sites. With this in mind, we approach this difficult clinical problem by discussing a general description of the systemic vasculitides, how to recognize them in the acutely ill patient, the differential diagnosis, and treatment.

Vasculitis is a clinical and pathologic process caused by inflammation of blood vessels. It may arise de novo or it may be associated with other systemic conditions, such as RA. All vasculidites share features of vascular inflammation, vascular necrosis, and varying degrees of target-organ ischemia. In each patient, the clinical picture depends on the nature and intensity of the inflammatory response, distribution of vessel involvement, and degree of target-organ damage. The vasculitic process is believed to be immunologically mediated, and only rarely is a causative agent found. Classification is particularly important in dealing with vasculitis. The classification of vasculitis has been confusing mainly because of overlap in both clinical and pathologic features in the various syndromes.[12] Table 150-2 lists the major vasculitic syndromes according to the primary blood vessel size involved. We find it most clinically useful to describe the vasculitis by following this classification.[13] However, some vasculitides span more than one vessel size.

TABLE 150-2. Classification of Vasculitis

LARGE BLOOD VESSEL PREDOMINANT
    Takayasu's arteritis
    Temporal arteritis

MEDIUM-SIZED BLOOD VESSEL PREDOMINANT
    Polyarteritis nodosa
    Wegener's granulomatosis
    Churg-Strauss syndrome
    Vasculitis associated with collagen vascular diseases
        SLE
        Systemic sclerosis
        Behcet's syndrome
        Other

SMALL VESSEL (HYPERSENSITIVITY OR LEUKOCYTOCLASTIC) VASCULITIS
    Secondary to exogenous antigen
        Drugs
        Infections
        Henoch-Schönlein purpura
    Secondary to endogenous antigen
        Autoimmune disorders (e.g., SLE, RA, Sjogren's)
        Malignancy (leukemia, myeloma, solid tumors)
        Essential mixed cryoglobulinemia
        Urticarial vasculitis

SLE, systemic lupus erythematosus; RA, rheumatoid arthritis.

CLASSIFICATION

Large Vessel Vasculitis

The two vasculidites of major blood vessels are Takayasu's arteritis and temporal arteritis (TA). Takayasu's arteritis is a chronic inflammatory disorder of unknown etiology primarily affecting the aorta and its major branches, occurring most commonly in female patients younger than 40 years of age.[14] The clinical picture includes an early systemic phase characterized by malaise, fever, night sweats, and fatigue. This is followed by an occlusive phase with symptoms of upper limb claudication, headaches, postural dizziness, and visual disturbances. These symptoms require careful examination of pulses and blood pressure in all four extremities. Asymmetry of findings suggests the diagnosis. Arteriography is the critical diagnostic procedure. Findings include bilateral, asymmetric, smooth stenosis and tapered occlusions of the aorta or its major branches. Presentations to the critical care setting may include stroke, myocardial ischemia, pericarditis, CHF, and severe hypertension, particularly in young persons. The mainstay of therapy during inflammatory disease is oral glucocorticoids, with cytotoxic agents reserved for refractory cases. In late disease, the vascular insufficiency may be a result of permanent vascular damage rather than active inflammation. In this situation, angioplasty or vascular surgery may be the only remedy.

TA is a vasculitis of unknown etiology occurring primarily in the elderly.[15] There is a wide range of symptoms, but most patients have clinical findings related to the involved arteries. Frequent features include fatigue, headaches (most common symptom), jaw claudication, loss of vision, scalp tenderness, polymyalgia rheumatica (stiffness, fatigue, low-grade fever, weight loss), and a highly elevated erythrocyte sedimentation rate (ESR). Unlike other forms of vasculitis, TA rarely involves the skin, kidney, or lungs. Once suspected,

the diagnosis may be made by biopsy of the temporal artery. Because vascular involvement may be only segmental, negative biopsy findings may occur even in the most typical cases. The temporal artery biopsy specimen must be substantial (larger than 5 cm), and multiple sections must be processed if the initial results are negative. The diagnostic yield may be further enhanced by biopsy of the opposite temporal artery when the result from the first side is negative. Diagnosis should lead to immediate initiation of steroid therapy at 1 mg/kg/day of prednisone or equivalent. Unless there is a contraindication to corticosteroids, treatment must be initiated while diagnostic procedures are being planned because visual loss in untreated patients may be sudden, total, and irreversible.

Medium-Size Vessel Vasculitis

The prototype of this class is polyarteritis. Polyarteritis, also called polyarteritis nodosa (PAN) is a condition characterized by inflammation of small and medium-sized arteries.[16] It most commonly involves the vessels of the skin, kidney, peripheral nerves, muscle, and gut. Involvement of other organs (e.g., lungs) is rare. The disease presents in a variety of ways. Typically, the patient experiences constitutional features of fever, malaise, and weight loss, along with manifestations of multisystem involvement (Table 150-3). Presentations to the critical care setting may include catastrophic ischemia of one or multiple organ systems, hypertension, renal failure, myocardial infarction, CHF, seizure, or cerebrovascular accident. Laboratory abnormalities are nonspecific. Elevated ESR, normocytic normochromic anemia, thrombocytosis, and diminished levels of albumin are usually present. Once PAN is suspected, the diagnosis should be determined by biopsy of the most accessible clinically involved tissue (e.g., sural nerve biopsy in mononeuritis multi-

TABLE 150-3. Clinical Manifestations of Polyarteritis Nodosa

ORGAN	MANIFESTATION	ESTIMATED PREVALENCE RATE (%)
Peripheral nerves	Mononeuritis multiplex	50–70
Kidney	Focal necrotizing glomerulonephritis	70
Skin	Palpable purpura, infarction, livedo	50
Joint	Arthralgia, arthritis	50
		20
Muscle	Myalgia	50
Gut	Abdominal pain, liver function abnormalities	30
Heart	Congestive heart failure, myocardial infarction	Low
Central nervous system	Seizure, CVA	Low
Lung	Interstitial pneumonitis	Low
Temporal artery	Jaw claudication	Low
Testis	Pain	Low
Eye	Retinal hemorrhage	Low

CVA, cerebrovascular accident.

plex). Biopsy of uninvolved sites such as muscle also may yield a positive result. When this is not possible, the diagnostic procedure of choice is an arteriogram, usually of abdominal viscera. The major arteriographic findings are microaneurysms, occlusion, and stenoses of the small and medium-sized vessels of the viscera (Fig. 150-1). Treatment of PAN depends on the extent of the disease, the rate of progression, and the organs involved. For example, cutaneous PAN without internal organ involvement is a benign recurrent condition requiring only intermittent corticosteroid therapy, whereas serious internal organ involvement requires corticosteroids and cytotoxic agents (treatment is further discussed later).

Another major form of medium- and small-vessel vasculitis is WG.[17] WG is a necrotizing granulomatous vasculitis that affects the small and medium-sized arteries and veins, usually sparing large vessels. This vasculitis has a predilection for the upper and lower respiratory tract. Common presenting signs and symptoms include the following: sinusitis, pulmonary infiltrates or nodules, fever, arthralgia, otitis, hearing loss, hemoptysis, and ocular problems. Nasal and sinus disease tend to be destructive. Permanent damage to nasal and sinus structures in WG often leads to impaired mucosal immunity and recurrent upper airway infections. WG renal involvement is usually in the form of focal segmental glomerulonephritis, tends to follow respiratory disease within weeks to months, and may progress rapidly. Ocular abnormalities occur in 52% of patients and include conjunctivitis, episcleritis, scleritis, uveitis, retinal vasculitis, corneoscleral ulcerations, dacryocystitis, and proptosis. Although this condition usually presents insidiously, challenging presentations to the critical care setting such as renal failure, pulmonary failure, or major organ ischemia are well described. Most of the laboratory abnormalities are nonspecific (elevated ESR, anemia, thrombocytosis, leukocytosis), except for the antineutrophil cytoplasmic antibody (c-ANCA).

When properly performed, c-ANCA testing has been reported to be highly specific for this disease, and titers correlate with disease activity. However, in most presentations, there are serious differential diagnostic considerations, and we believe that a positive c-ANCA result should not replace the vigorous pursuit of a histologic diagnosis. Nasal biopsy is less invasive but often nonspecific. Renal biopsy may reveal a glomerulonephritis but does not make a definitive diagnosis. In cases with lung involvement, transbronchial biopsy may be useful to exclude some infections; however, open-lung biopsy best shows the granulomatous inflammation and necrotizing arteritis. Immunosuppressive therapy with corticosteroids and cyclophosphamide is the cornerstone therapy for this condition.

A more rare condition in the small or medium-sized arteritis group is Churg-Strauss Syndrome (CSS).[18] CSS is a granulomatous inflammation of small and medium-sized vessels associated with peripheral eosinophilia. Three phases occur in this condition. The first phase is a prodromal phase. This phase may persist for years and consists of allergic manifestations of rhinitis, nasal polyposis, and asthma. The second phase includes peripheral blood and tissue eosinophilia, frequently causing a picture resembling Loeffler's syndrome (shifting pulmonary infiltrates), chronic eosinophilic pneumonia, or eosinophilic gastroenteritis. This second phase may remit or recur over years before the third phase. The third phase is a life-threatening systemic vasculitis. These three phases may appear simultaneously, and they do not have to follow in sequence. The characteristic laboratory abnormality in CSS is eosinophilia. Anemia, elevated ESR, and elevated IgE levels also may be found. The diagnosis is corroborated by biopsy of involved tissue. The characteristic findings are small necrotizing granulomas and necrotizing vasculitis. The presence of rhinitis, sinusitis, and pulmonary involvement can lead to confusion with WG. Table 150-4 gives some hints on differentiating between

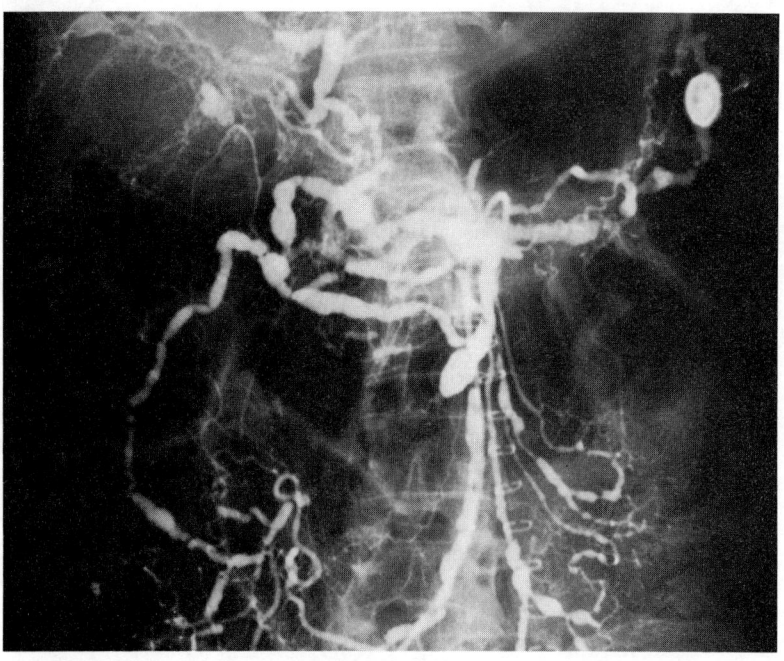

FIGURE 150-1. A visceral angiogram in polyarteritis nodosa (PAN) demonstrates aneurysms in the hepatic, splenic, celiac, and mesenteric circulations.

TABLE 150-4. Differentiation Between Churg-Strauss Syndrome and Wegener's Granulomatosis

	CHURG-STRAUSS SYNDROME	WEGENER'S GRANULOMATOSIS
ENT	Rhinitis, polyposis	Necrotizing lesions
Allergy, bronchial asthma	Frequent	Not more frequent than in general population
Renal involvement	Uncommon	Common
Eosinophilia	>10% of peripheral leukocytes	Minimally elevated
Histologic features	Eosinophilic necrotizing granulomas	Necrotizing epitheloid granulomas
Prognosis	Major cause of death: cardiac	Major cause of death: pulmonary and renal
cANCA	Negative	Positive

ENT, ear–nose–throat; ANCA, antineutrophil cytoplasmic antibody.

these two entities. The treatment of choice for CSS is glucocorticoids.

Small and medium-sized vessel vasculitis also is a common complication of most connective tissue disorders.[19] Here we mention a few clinical clues that pertain to vasculitis in the setting of SLE and RA. Markers of systemic vasculitis in SLE include a variety of skin lesions and a PAN-like picture with multisystem organ involvement. The skin lesions can present as palpable purpura, nail fold or digital ulcerations, splinter hemorrhages, urticarial lesions, livedo reticularis, or palmar vasculitic lesions simulating Osler's nodes and Janeway lesions. Vasculitic lesions of the digits may result in gangrene. The histopatholgic picture of involved tissue is similar to PAN. Rheumatoid vasculitis usually presents in male patients with longstanding high-titer seropositive RA. Mononeuritis multiplex and infarction of the skin are the two most characteristic presentations. Angiography or tissue biopsy corroborate the diagnosis. The histopathologic features of rheumatoid and SLE vasculitis resemble those of PAN.

Small Vessel Vasculitis

Small vessel vasculitis[20,21] includes a variety of conditions that are grouped together because of involvement of small blood vessels of the skin, especially arterioles and venules. *Leukocytoclastic vasculitis* (LCV) or *necrotizing vasculitis* are terms used to describe the usual histopathologic picture, in which leukocytoclasis (nuclear debris) from neutrophils is seen in and around acute vascular lesions. The two main etiologic categories of small vessel vasculitis include that which is secondary to (1) an exogenous antigen (drugs, infectious agents, vaccination), and (2) an endogenous antigen (autoimmune disorders, malignancy, essential mixed cryoglobulinemia, urticarial vasculitis). Palpable purpura is the most common primary lesion in LCV (Fig. 150-2). Urticarial lesions are the second most common cutaneous presentation. Other less common skin lesions include ulcers, papules, vesicles, urticaria, livedo reticularis, nodules, or erythema multiforme. Constitutional symptoms (fever, arthralgia, myalgia) frequently accompany the skin lesions. Occasionally, renal failure or GI manifestations (particularly GI bleeding)

require critical care support, but other organ involvement is less common. Laboratory abnormalities are usually nonspecific. These patients require a full medical evaluation and appropriate laboratory testing, depending on the clinical situation. It is important to look for those patients in whom LCV is part of a more severe process such as PAN, WG,

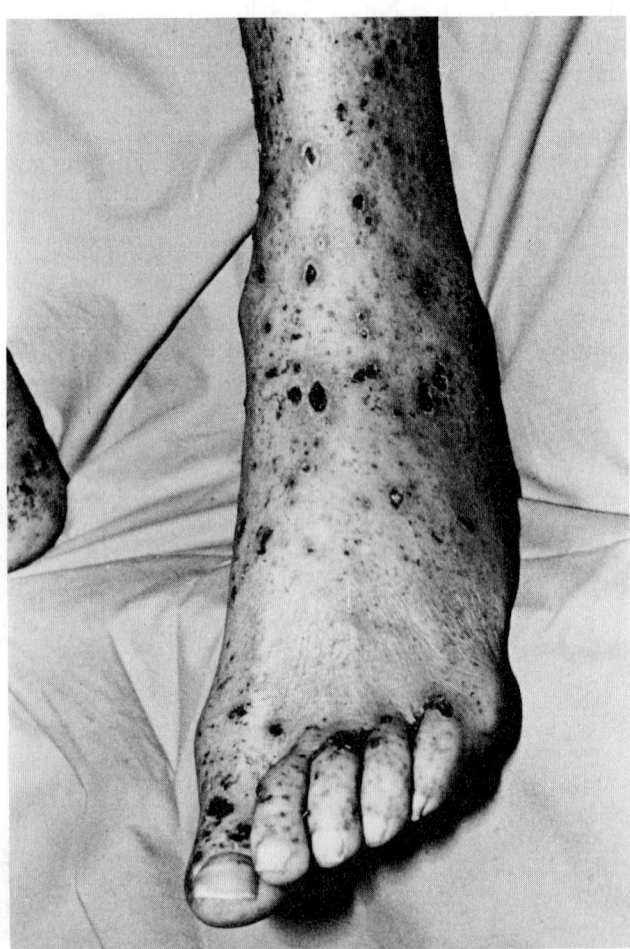

FIGURE 150-2. Leukocytoclastic vasculitis secondary to quinidine that resolved without specific therapy after the drug was removed.

CSS, or SLE, emphasizing again the importance of a detailed history and physical examination. Diagnosis is made by skin biopsy. The treatment has to be determined individually. If the associated disorder can be identified, then treatment of the underlying condition may result in resolution of the vasculitis. Any potential drug or antigen should be discontinued or removed. In mild cases without internal organ involvement, no specific treatment is needed. If systemic symptoms or internal organ involvement are present, glucocorticoids are usually the treatment of choice.

DIFFERENTIAL DIAGNOSIS

The nonspecific multisystem critical care presentations of possible vasculitis are challenging from the standpoint of differential diagnosis[22,23] (Table 150-5). Systemic vasculitis should be considered in any patient in whom multisystem disease cannot be readily explained. Important differential diagnoses include infection (sepsis, endocarditis), endocrinopathy, drug toxicity, coagulopathy, malignancy, left atrial myxoma, and multiple emboli (e.g., cholesterol or mycotic). There are some important clues regarding these vasculitis simulators. Cardiac myxoma is a neoplasm that presents with obstructive, embolic, or systemic manifestations simulating vasculitis. Confusing symptoms include Raynaud's phenomenon, arthralgia, petechiae, and erythematous rashes. This is the only tumor known to produce arterial aneurysm with embolization simulating PAN. Echocardiogram is the key to this diagnosis. Cholesterol emboli syndrome is another vasculitis simulator that usually presents in the sixth to eighth decades in patients with severe atherosclerosis. It most typically occurs after a procedure (arterial catheterization, car-

TABLE 150-5. Diseases Simulating Vasculitis

SMALL VESSEL

Infectious endocarditis
Septicemia
Platelet disorders (ITP, TTP)
Drug reactions
Causes of purpura (amyloid, scurvy, senility, steroid)

MEDIUM VESSELS

Atrial myxoma
Cholesterol emboli
Vasculopathy of antiphospholipid antibody syndrome
Ergotism
Arsenic poisoning
Hypertensive crisis
Malignancies (lymphoma, leukemia, myeloma)

LARGE VESSELS

Congenital coarctation
Fibromuscular dysplasia
Thoracic outlet syndrome
Radiation fibrosis
Neurofibromatosis

ITP, idiopathic thrombocytopenic purpura; TTP, thrombotic thrombocytopenic purpura.

diopulmonary resuscitation), after trauma, with anticoagulation, or spontaneously. Multisystem involvement simulates vasculitis including the presence of petechiae, purpura, livedo reticularis, proteinuria, stroke, ischemic bowel, and constitutional symptoms. Important clues include history of a recent vascular procedure, normal peripheral pulses, and Hollenhorst plaques on funduscopic examination. Diagnosis is by lesional skin biopsy with demonstration of cholesterol clefts. aPLs are associated with venous and arterial thrombosis, recurrent spontaneous abortion, thrombocytopenia, and a variety of skin manifestations that can simulate systemic vasculitis. Clues to the presence of aPLs include false-positive VDRL, anticardiolipin antibodies, the lupus anticoagulant (LAC), and histologic features showing primarily thrombosis with minimal inflammation. Chronic ergotism mimics vasculitis by presenting with symptoms of claudication, commonly of lower extremities and less frequently of the hands. On angiography, vessels may show narrowing and occlusion. Radiation arteriopathy is manifested by intimal and mural thrombosis, aneurysm formation, or progressive fibrosis. A history of irradiation to a vascular bed, atypical areas of vessel involvement, and absence of a systemic inflammatory process suggest this diagnosis. Neurofibromatosis is an autosomal dominant disorder of neural crest tissue. Approximately 10% of patients have vascular involvement of small and large arteries. Vascular involvement presents as aneurysm and renovascular hypertension. Histologic examination shows small arteries with diffuse intimal thickening by spindle cells. Large vessels usually have aberrant nervous system tissue circumferentially compressing the vessel.

APPROACH TO THE DIAGNOSIS OF VASCULITIS

Certain features enhance the suspicion for vasculitis: persistent fever, palpable purpura, peripheral neuropathy, preexisting connective tissue disorders, and ischemic symptoms, especially in young patients.[24] Making the diagnosis as early as possible is important because the disease may progress to involve vital organs. Evidence of vascular involvement should be established by biopsy or angiography. The likelihood of finding vasculitis is greatest when early lesions of clinically abnormal tissues are examined. The most accessible tissues are skin, sural nerve, skeletal muscle, liver, rectum, and testicle. Renal biopsy may be of help if no other tissue is involved or available for diagnosis. It usually reveals a focal necrotizing glomerulonephritis.[25] Focal necrotizing glomerulonephritis can be seen in most medium-vessel vasculitides, so it is impossible to differentiate between them based on renal biopsy alone. Together with the clinical picture, however, even nonspecific histopathologic findings can be helpful. When clinically involved tissue is not available for biopsy, the diagnostic procedure of choice is an angiogram. The best plan is to study the kidney, liver, spleen, stomach, and small bowel. In rare cases, hand and foot arteriography is necessary. The major angiographic findings are microaneurysm, occlusion, and stenoses of small and medium-sized vessels of the viscera. Although the overall angiographic findings of vasculitis are relatively specific, other diseases must be excluded. The diagnoses to be considered in the angiographic differential are arteriosclerosis, thoracic outlet syndrome, Buerger's disease, and ergotism. Useful clues to this differential are as follows:

1. Patient age: The younger age of patients with Takayasu's arteritis, WG, CSS, and PAN makes atherosclerosis less of a consideration.
2. Location: Arteriosclerotic changes are predominantly found in the legs, whereas most medium-sized vasculitides are visceral. Large-vessel vasculitides are in the aorta and its proximal branches.
3. Pattern of stenosis: The pattern in atherosclerosis is one of short, eccentric narrowing by irregular atheromatous plaques, whereas stenoses are smooth and tapered in vasculitis.

MANAGEMENT

Before discussing the management of systemic vasculitis, some basic therapeutic principles should be reviewed[26,27]:

1. Accurate diagnosis is essential for successful therapy.
2. Early diagnosis is essential. Acute and possibly irreversible renal failure, respiratory failure, bowel infarction, stroke, and other tissue ischemia all may be consequences of delayed diagnosis. Sometimes it may be necessary to simultaneously initiate therapy for acute life-threatening vasculitis and other confounding conditions (e.g., infection) before all clinical data are available.
3. Successful treatment of vasculitis requires determination of when disease activity has been controlled. Certain disorders are associated with reliable markers of disease activity (e.g., the ESR in TA). In others, we depend on clinical findings or follow-up angiography. Clinical parameters are the most often used indicators of disease activity, but certain organs demonstrate little improvement even after disease activity has been suppressed (e.g., brain and peripheral nerves).
4. Vasculitides are rare and, with few exceptions, therapy has not been subjected to rigorous controlled therapeutic trials.

Except for a few conditions, the first line of therapy in life- or organ-threatening vasculitis is corticosteroids. Corticosteroids usually are given in high doses (1 mg/kg/day of prednisone or equivalent) and tapered slowly according to clinical response. Some patients with fulminant disease progression such as respiratory failure, catastrophic ischemic event, or renal failure might be salvageable if treated aggressively with high-dose "pulse" intravenous methylprednisolone (e.g., 1 g/day IV for 3 days). If corticosteroid treatment seems to be ineffective, certain issues should first be addressed before considering additional therapy: (1) Is the diagnosis correct? (2) Does the patient have an intercurrent illness (e.g., infection) that gives a false impression of progressive disease? (3) Has the steroid been tapered too rapidly? and (4) Is this deterioration a result of drug toxicity? Once it has been determined that life- or organ-threatening disease continues to be active despite adequate corticoste-

roid therapy, additional measures to include cytotoxic agents should be considered.

Cytotoxic agents should be strongly considered in the following situations: (1) when, on the initial evaluation, a rapidly progressive vasculitis with significant visceral involvement (i.e., progressive renal insufficiency, bowel infarction, CNS disease, cardiac disease, or life-threatening limb involvement) is present; (2) when prednisone in high daily doses fails to control the activity and progression of the vasculitis; (3) when prednisone cannot be tapered to tolerable levels because of continued disease activity; and (4) in patients with WG where the combination of cyclophosphamide and corticosteroids has been shown to reduce mortality. Of the cytotoxic drugs available, cyclophosphamide seems to be the most efficacious, but azathioprine also has been used in some cases with the benefit of a less severe toxicity profile. Consultation with a rheumatologist is important in the initial therapeutic choice and follow-up monitoring of these medications.

CRITICAL CARE OF SYSTEMIC LUPUS ERYTHEMATOSUS ■

GENERAL PRINCIPLES

Systemic lupus erythematosus is a disease entity that is characterized and diagnosed by the recognition of its clinical manifestations. Eleven clinical features are considered specific enough to define SLE (Table 150-6) in addition to a multitude of less specific features. Diagnosis is often challenging because most patients manifest only a few of these features at any time, and many varied combinations are observed. In the ICU setting, two situations may arise: (1) a patient with known SLE may present with a life-threatening complication of the disease or its therapy; or (2) a patient may present with life-threatening undiagnosed SLE, direly needing that disease to be recognized in the ICU. The detailed approach to the diagnosis of SLE is thus important but beyond the scope of this text. The reader is referred to general rheumatologic textbooks for a discussion of this subject.[28–30] The remainder of this chapter discusses specific manifestations of SLE that may occur in critical care situations and may confound the evaluation or management process.

FEVER

Fever is a nonspecific but common expression of disease activity in SLE. The most important diagnostic alternative to consider, however, is the possibility of an infectious etiology. This is particularly important in the SLE patient being treated with immunosuppressive drugs, which significantly increase infection risk. Almost one third of deaths in lupus patients are attributable to infection, and fever may be the sole initial manifestation. Patients with SLE have been shown to have increased susceptibility to infection, even in the absence of corticosteroid or immunosuppressive therapy. The most common outpatient infections involve the respira-

TABLE 150-6. 1982 Classification Criteria for Systemic Lupus Erythematosus°

1. Malar rash
2. Discoid rash
3. Photosensitivity
4. Oral ulcers
5. Arthritis
6. Serositis
   Pleuritis *or*
   Pericarditis
7. Renal disorder
   Proteinuria >0.5 g/d *or*
   Cellular casts
8. Neurologic disorder
   Seizures *or*
   Psychosis
9. Hematologic disorder
   Hemolytic anemia *or*
   Leukopenia *or*
   Lymphopenia *or*
   Thrombocytopenia *or*
10. Immunologic disorder
    Positive LE cell preparation *or*
    anti-DNA *or*
    Anti-Smith *or*
    False-positive serologic test for syphilis
11. Antinuclear antibody

LE, lupus erythematosis.
°Four of 11 criteria must be present, serially *or* simultaneously, in any interval of observation.

Tan EM, Cohen AS, Fries JF, et al: The 1982 revised criteria for the classification of systemic lupus erythematosus (SLE). *Arthritis Rheum* 1982;25:1271.

tory or urinary tract with *Staphylococcus aureus, Proteus mirabilis,* and *Escherichia coli.* Septic arthritis caused by infection with *Neisseria gonorrhoeae, Staphylococcus, Mycobacterium tuberculosis,* or *Salmonella* also is typical. Corticosteroid use increases the incidence of infection as much as fourfold. When immunosuppressive treatment is present, opportunistic infection also must be considered. *Salmonella* cellulitis leading to gangrene and infection with *Candida, Nocardia, Cryptococcus, Toxoplasmosis,* and *Pneumocystis* are common. Mortality rate in hospitalized lupus patients with opportunistic infection is approximately 10% when lupus is inactive. In contrast, mortality rate exceeds 60% if active lupus is complicated by opportunistic infection.[31] Life-threatening pneumococcal sepsis may occur, particularly in those with a history of lupus thrombocytopenia treated with splenectomy or who are functionally asplenic. Hospitalized patients with lupus are approximately ten times as likely to develop a hospital-acquired infection compared with non-SLE patients.

The dilemma of the febrile patient with SLE in the ICU is that presentations of SLE may be difficult to distinguish from infection. The presence of shaking chills, leukocytosis in the absence of steroid therapy (rather than leukopenia typical of SLE), increased levels of complement components

(C3, C4), and an absence of manifestations of lupus activity in other organ systems favor an infectious etiology. The ESR and C-reactive protein lack consistent correlation with activity in either SLE or SLE complicated by infection. The approach to an ill, febrile lupus patient thus requires: (1) culture of all potential sites of infection, including blood, urine, sputum, and any abnormal fluid collections; (2) early empirical broad-spectrum antibiotic coverage; (3) consideration of treatment with stress-dose corticosteroids (see previous section); and (4) early aggressive diagnostic measures such as bronchoscopy, bone marrow evaluation, arthroscopic synovial biopsy, pericardiocentesis, or open-lung biopsy, directed at the most likely area of clinical involvement.

PULMONARY PROBLEMS

General Issues

Pulmonary manifestations of SLE include asymptomatic restrictive pulmonary defects and decreased diffusion capacity, pleural inflammation with or without effusion, neuromuscular dysfunction (including the diaphragm), chronic interstitial lung disease, acute pneumonitis, pulmonary hemorrhage, pulmonary hypertension, and pulmonary embolism. In addition, bronchiolitis obliterans (BO) and bronchiolitis obliterans organizing pneumonia (BOOP) have been reported, and may be underrecognized.

Pleuritis and Pleural Effusion

Because pleural involvement rarely results in massive effusion, pleuritis often is not a serious threat in lupus. In fact, asymptomatic small effusions are common. A sick or febrile lupus patient with a new pleural effusion should undergo diagnostic thoracentesis to characterize the effusion and rule out infection. The pleural fluid in lupus is exudative. Leukocyte counts vary and rarely exceed $50,000/mm^3$. Polymorphonuclear leukocytes predominate in acute lupus pleural effusions, being replaced by lymphocytes within 1 or 2 weeks. Pleural fluid glucose is reduced but not as severely as in rheumatoid effusions. A pleural fluid glucose of 50 mg/dL is typical in SLE. Lupus erythematosus cells can be observed by experienced examiners and are specific for SLE. Pleural fluid anti-nuclear antibody (ANA) titers greater than 1:160 are suggestive of a lupus pleural effusion.

Lupus pleural effusions do not ordinarily present a management problem, being responsive to NSAIDs or low-dose corticosteroids in patients for whom treatment is desired because of symptoms. The major problem is the broad differential diagnosis, especially if bilateral, which includes infection, CHF, uremia, and pulmonary embolism.

Acute Lupus Pneumonitis

This potentially life-threatening manifestation of SLE occurs in less than 5% of lupus patients, although it can be the initial presenting manifestation.[32] The mortality rate in cases complicated by respiratory failure exceeds 50%. Initial symptoms include dyspnea, nonproductive cough, fever, and pleuritic chest pain. Tachypnea, tachycardia, and hypoxemia are frequently observed. Infiltrates, typically in the lower lobes, may be unilateral or bilateral. Concomitant atelectasis and pleural effusion also may be observed. The symptoms and signs of acute lupus pneumonitis are indistinguishable from infection, which is a critical differential diagnosis. Alveolar hemorrhage and pulmonary embolism, also manifestations of SLE, must be considered as well.

The approach to a lupus patient with this presentation must include aggressive measures to uncover an infectious process. Empiric treatment for presumed acute lupus pneumonitis should be avoided, except for those so desperately ill that diagnostic studies cannot be performed nor treatment delayed. In the latter instance, it would be necessary to presumptively treat both possible infectious and autoimmune processes simultaneously.

Initial evaluation should include sputum, blood, and urine cultures. However, an early decision to perform BAL or fiberoptic bronchoscopy with transbronchial biopsy is the approach most likely to permit timely intervention with specific therapy. If BAL or transbronchial biopsy reveal no evidence of infection, immunosuppressive therapy may be initiated. The histologic appearance in acute lupus pneumonitis includes alveolar damage, necrosis, inflammatory infiltrates, hemorrhage, and hyaline membranes. All of these are nonspecific. Open-lung biopsy may be needed, especially in immunosuppressed SLE patients in whom *Pneumocystis*, *Aspergillus*, or *Candida* infection is possible, because bronchoscopy with brushings and BAL are less sensitive in detecting these infections.[33]

There are no prospective or controlled trials of therapy in acute lupus pneumonitis. Our approach is to initiate therapy with high-dose corticosteroids. In cases without respiratory failure, 1 mg/kg/day of prednisone is usually sufficient, initially in three or four divided doses. If the patient cannot take oral medication, equivalent doses of methylprednisolone are administered IV. In more severe cases, methylprednisolone, 1 g IV each day is administered for the first 3 days. If no improvement in respiratory function occurs within 48 hours and no evidence of infection has been discovered, then cytotoxic agents should be considered. Daily oral (or parenteral) cyclophosphamide, 2 mg/kg/day, is an effective immunosuppressive regimen. Alternatively, monthly pulse intravenous cyclophosphamide may be used. Azathioprine also has been used successfully in some cases.[34] The role of plasmapheresis in refractory cases has not been established.

Pulmonary Hemorrhage

A rare but lethal pulmonary manifestation of SLE, pulmonary hemorrhage, may be difficult to distinguish from acute lupus pneumonitis when hemoptysis is lacking. Both may present with fever, dyspnea, hypoxemia, and diffuse alveolar infiltrates. The infiltrates are usually symmetric but are occasionally unilateral. If the hemorrhage stops, infiltrates resolve in 2 to 4 days. Mortality of lupus pulmonary hemorrhage exceeds 50%.[35] Differential diagnosis also should include CHF, pneumonia, uremia, and multiple pulmonary emboli. A decreasing hematocrit may be the only clue to the etiology.

This manifestation usually occurs in patients with known SLE in the setting of active extrapulmonary illness. The occurrence of pulmonary hemorrhage in the absence of active lupus elsewhere should trigger a search for alternative etiologies such as infection, primary pulmonary hemosiderosis, or Goodpasture's syndrome. Fiberoptic bronchoscopy may reveal gross blood in the tracheobronchial tree, and hemosiderin-laden macrophages may be observed in BAL samples. Histopathologic study generally is not diagnostic; vasculitis or necrosis is rarely seen, immune complex deposition is variable, and septal inflammatory infiltrates are minimal.

Once suspected, treatment of this condition must begin immediately to maximize the chances for the patient's recovery.[36] No prospective or randomized treatment trials evaluate the role of corticosteroids or other treatment options for this syndrome. Hence, all treatment regimens are empirically based on case reports and clinical experience. We begin patients on methylprednisolone, 1 g IV daily for 3 days, followed by prednisone, 1 mg/kg/day. Symptoms, CBC, and serial chest radiographs are followed as a measure of response. If the patient is critically ill or does not respond to corticosteroids within 24 to 48 hours, then either oral daily or pulse monthly intravenous cyclophosphamide is our next choice. Other options might include azathioprine, plasmapheresis, or lymphoplasmapheresis. Additional treatments that may be required include red blood cell transfusion and mechanical ventilation with a small amount of positive end-expiratory pressure.

Pulmonary Emboli

Pulmonary emboli, often multiple, can occur in patients with SLE. Presentation may be similar to acute lupus pneumonitis or pulmonary hemorrhage, with fever, dyspnea, cough, and transient pulmonary infiltrates. An association with aPLs has been described.[37] Subclinical emboli may occur more frequently than is recognized.

Diagnosis may be suggested by findings of dyspnea and hypoxemia with no or minor radiographic abnormalities, although infiltrates also may be observed. Ventilation/perfusion ($\dot{V}/\dot{Q}$) radionuclide scans are helpful in patients stable enough to undergo this evaluation. Problems with interpretation of $\dot{V}/\dot{Q}$ scans, addressed elsewhere, apply to SLE patients as well. Pulmonary angiography remains the definitive diagnostic tool and may be the only one available to patients in respiratory distress. Diagnosis of pulmonary embolism in an SLE patient should trigger a search for aPLs. A prolonged partial thromboplastin time with or without a false-positive serologic test result for syphilis are suggestive of the presence of aPLs. This may be confirmed by specific enzyme-linked immunosorbent assays for detecting IgG and IgM anticardiolipin antibodies, or detection of aPLs on a LAC battery.

Treatment of aPL-associated pulmonary emboli acutely should include anticoagulation with intravenous heparin followed by warfarin. Because patients with aPL-associated thrombotic or embolic complications appear subject to recurrent events, prolonged prophylaxis with warfarin is advised. Cases which recur despite adequate anticoagulation have been treated with corticosteroid or immunosuppressive therapy aimed at reducing circulating aPLs,[38] but the response has been variable.

Chronic Interstitial Lung Disease

SLE may be complicated during its course by slowly progressive dyspnea from interstitial lung disease. The course, histologic features, and prognosis of chronic interstitial lung disease in lupus is similar to idiopathic interstitial pneumonia. Treatment, once fibrosis is established, is seldom beneficial.

Bronchiolitis Obliterans and Bronchiolitis Obliterans Organizing Pneumonia

Both BO and BOOP are rare inflammatory and fibrotic processes affecting the small airways and may occur in SLE and other collagen vascular diseases, as well as with infection, toxic gas exposure, transplantation, and as a complication of certain medications.[30] In both conditions, an inflammatory exudate occludes or obliterates bronchiolar lumina resulting in airway obstruction. When the inflammation extends into the alveolar space, resulting in alveolar consolidation, the term "organizing pneumonia" is added to the description.

Both syndromes present with acute or subacute fever and cough. Noninvasive evaluation includes pulmonary spirometry, which may show a restrictive or mixed restrictive-obstructive pattern. Diffusing capacity may be decreased in BOOP. Chest radiographs may help differentiate BO and BOOP, although definitive diagnosis of either condition requires transbronchial or open-lung biopsy. BOOP may spontaneously remit, and most patients remit on high-dose corticosteroid regimens (1 mg/kg/day of prednisone or the equivalent)[39] within 4 to 6 weeks. BO, however, usually progresses relentlessly despite such treatment. No data report the efficacy of cyclophosphamide or azathioprine. Table 150-7 contrasts features of these conditions.

Miscellaneous Pulmonary Conditions

Pulmonary hypertension occurs in SLE patients but is not well studied. Patients tend to be young women with dyspnea, fatigue, and chest pain. An increased pulmonary component of the second heart sound, right ventricular heave, and systolic murmur suggest the diagnosis. Evaluation includes electrocardiogram, chest radiograph, and echocardiogram. Occasionally, multiple pulmonary emboli are detected by V̇/Q̇ scan or angiography. Histologically, medial hyperplasia with intimal fibrosis is usually advanced by the time symptoms bring the problem to medical attention. Treatment responses have been reported with intravenous prostacyclin infusion and with calcium channel blockers. Warfarin may decrease mortality (in primary pulmonary hypertension). Corticosteroids or immunosuppressive treatment responses are anecdotal.

CARDIOVASCULAR MANIFESTATIONS

Pericardial Disease

Inflammatory manifestations of SLE may involve the pericardium, myocardium, or endocardial structures such as valves.[40] Cardiac lesions usually do not result in significant dysfunction and may not cause overt symptoms at all. Pericarditis, for example, occurs in up to 30% of SLE patients, yet may be asymptomatic. Rarely does pericarditis in lupus result in massive pericardial effusion. The major concern in this instance is the possibility of infection. Evidence of extracardiac disease activity is usually present during episodes of lupus pericarditis. Atrial arrhythmias may occur during episodes. Pericardiocentesis or a pericardial window with culture of effusion may be necessary if infection is deemed likely. Fever, leukocytosis, increased complement components, and the absence of active lupus in other sites indicate that infection should be considered. However, leukopenia, lymphopenia, decreased complement components, and active lupus elsewhere can be treated as SLE, and invasive studies can be deferred. Pericardial tamponade oc-

TABLE 150-7. Clinical Features of BO and BOOP

	BO	BOOP
Organizing inflammatory bronchiolar exudate	Yes	Yes
Alveolar consolidation	No	Yes
Clinical course	Subacute, chronic, progressive	Acute, subacute, spontaneous remission, fever, cough, constitutional symptoms
Chest radiographs	Normal or hyperinflation Reticulonodular	Alveolar, interstitial, or reticulonodular infiltrates
Pulmonary function tests	Restrictive or mixed DLCO may be normal or mildly decreased	Restrictive Diminished DLCO
Prognosis	Treatment response poor	Corticosteroid responsive
Diagnostic procedure	Open-lung biopsy	Open-lung biopsy

BO, bronchiolitis obliterans; BOOP, bronchiolitis obliterans organizing pneumonia; DLCO, diffusing capacity for carbon monoxide.

curs in less than 1% of patients. Case reports of constrictive pericarditis also have been described. Mild pericarditis generally responds to therapy with NSAIDs. Corticosteroids can be used for moderate or refractory pericarditis. Prednisone, 20 to 40 mg/day is usually effective. In severe pericarditis associated with constriction or tamponade, high-dose intravenous corticosteroids may decrease the effusion and improve symptoms promptly.

Myocardial Disease

Although myocarditis is seen histologically in 50% of autopsy cases, the most common cause of CHF in SLE is a combination of hypertension, renal insufficiency, and volume overload from corticosteroids. Fever, disproportionate tachycardia, cardiomegaly, and pericarditis in a patient with active lupus raise the suspicion of lupus myocarditis. CK levels may be elevated, specifically the muscle–brain fraction (CK-MB). Endomyocardial biopsy has been used to establish the diagnosis in selected patients.[41] Treatment includes high-dose corticosteroids and occasionally immunosuppressive therapy.

Valvular Heart Disease

The classic cardiac manifestation of SLE is described by Libman and Sacks:[41a] 1- to 4-mm verrucous vegetations, sometimes occurring in clusters, found on valve edges, valve rings, commissures, and occasionally on chordae tendinea. Physical findings and echocardiography are nondiagnostic. These valve lesions usually do not cause significant valvular dysfunction. They do predispose to bacterial endocarditis; and ruptured chordae tendineae, thromboemboli, and cerebral emboli have occurred. Treatment of Libman-Sacks vegetations includes endocarditis prophylaxis and valve replacement for hemodynamically significant lesions. In the absence of vegetations, significant aortic or mitral insufficiency requiring valve replacement also occurs in SLE patients. Surgery in these patients can be successful with acceptable mortality rates.[42]

ABDOMINAL EMERGENCIES IN SLE

Abdominal pain is common in SLE, and although usually trivial and self-limited, may be the initial manifestation of catastrophe.[43] Fever often accompanies abdominal pain, and peritoneal signs are present in about 10% of patients, although both may be masked by concomitant corticosteroid treatment. Etiologies are diverse and include duodenal or gastric ulceration, gastritis, acute pancreatitis, serositis, bowel inflammation, infarction, and mesenteric vasculitis. An apparently benign abdominal examination in a lupus patient with abdominal pain, especially when corticosteroids are in use, should never cause the clinician to feel secure. A serious life-threatening process may be evolving. Aggressive and complete evaluation should begin with CBC, amylase, and blood chemistry to detect acidosis. Abdominal flat and upright radiographs should be observed for free air, pseudo-

obstruction, and bowel wall thickening. Free air, or acidosis with free peritoneal fluid and hyperamylasemia, warrant immediate surgical consultation. In other cases, additional studies are individualized and may include upper and lower GI radiocontrast studies, CT, MRI, gallium or indium radionuclide scans, or angiography.

Inflammatory Bowel in SLE

Colitis may be diffuse or local and is indistinguishable from idiopathic ulcerative colitis.[44] Inflammatory ileitis, however, is extremely rare. Inflammation can lead to ileus, hemorrhage, intussusception, and perforation and may be associated with mesenteric vasculitis. Radiocontrast studies can reveal bowel wall edema and loss of rugal folds. The problem usually responds to treatment with high-dose corticosteroids, such as 1 to 2 mg/kg/day of parenteral prednisolone or the equivalent. Massive ascites suggests bowel perforation, pancreatitis, or peritonitis caused by either lupus or bacterial infection.

Acute Pancreatitis in SLE

Severe epigastric pain, nausea, vomiting, dehydration, and hyperamylasemia suggest acute pancreatitis. This may be serious, with mortality rates as high as 75% in some series. Confusion may exist concerning the cause of pancreatitis because many lupus patients are receiving corticosteroids, azathioprine, thiazide diuretics, or other medications known to cause pancreatitis. Lupus pancreatitis tends to occur concurrently with active multisystem SLE and responds to an increase in steroid dose.[45] In contrast, drug-induced pancreatitis lacks evidence of SLE activity in other organs and does not respond to increasing corticosteroids.

Mesenteric Vasculitis

Constant or cramping abdominal pain associated with fever, vomiting, and diffuse rebound tenderness suggest mesenteric vasculitis. Fever and peritoneal signs may be masked by concomitant corticosteroid treatment, and symptoms may be insidiously progressive, with perforation occurring before the patient begins to appear significantly ill. Cases are usually associated with concomitant active SLE involving other organs, particularly CNS disease, ischemic bone necrosis, and peripheral vasculitis.[46] Diagnosis is challenging and requires an aggressive approach. A declining hematocrit suggests internal hemorrhage. Hematochezia may be present. Paracentesis may reveal hemoperitoneum or increased leukocyte counts and amylase. Thumbprinting, a sign revealed in radiocontrast study resulting from focal bowel wall edema, is believed to strongly suggest ischemic bowel. CT with contrast also may be helpful. Mesenteric angiogram may be normal. If the colon is involved, endoscopy may reveal ischemic injury. If surgical resection becomes necessary, histologic study reveals vasculitis similar to that seen in PAN. Treatment with high-dose parenteral corticosteroids and complete bowel rest is often effective, although mortality in these patients is significant.

RENAL DISEASE AND SLE

Renal disease is usually insidious in onset, with asymptomatic urinary sediment abnormalities or proteinuria being the most common initial presentation. Be aware that some patients can develop a rapidly progressive nephritis, and treatment must be started in these patients as soon as the diagnosis of lupus nephritis is confirmed.

Rapidly progressive glomerulonephritis is a renal syndrome defined by a 50% or greater loss of renal function within three months. In lupus, this presentation most often results from diffuse proliferative glomerulonephritis. The rate of decline in glomerular function is important, although data such as prior serum creatinine or 24-hour creatinine clearances often are not available. When the rate of progression is unknown, assess the patient for causes of acute renal failure, such as medication use (NSAIDs, aminoglycosides, cisplatin), infection (pyelonephritis), or obstruction. Appropriate early studies include direct examination of urinary sediment and ultrasonic assessment of renal size and ureteral dilatation. Although each case is determined on an individual basis, we recommend renal biopsy in most cases for prognostic information and to detect lesions other than those resulting from SLE, such as poststreptococcal glomerulonephritis, IgA nephropathy, membranoproliferative glomerulonephritis, Goodpasture's syndrome, and pauciimmune crescentic glomerulonephritis, including WG.[47]

Diffuse proliferative glomerulonephritis may respond to corticosteroid treatment alone, but most often requires concomitant treatment with monthly intravenous cyclophosphamide pulses. This decision must be individualized, and the renal biopsy result may be pertinent to formulating a treatment plan. Biopsy and treatment of lupus nephritis is a highly controversial area, and here we offer our consensus opinion. Milder renal insufficiency with predominantly focal proliferative lesions on biopsy may be treated initially with corticosteroids alone. A 4- to 6-week course of prednisone, 1 mg/kg/day, initially in three-times-daily divided doses consolidated to single daily doses in 1 to 2 weeks, should result in improved renal function and clearing of urinary sediment. Prednisone is then tapered slowly over the next 6 to 12 months. If no response occurs after the initial 4 weeks of prednisone, or for diffuse proliferative glomerulonephritis, monthly intravenous cyclophosphamide may be added. If the patient has severe renal failure or histopathologic examination shows both active proliferation and chronicity, then a more aggressive approach with cyclophosphamide in addition to high-dose corticosteroids at the initiation of therapy should be considered. If minimal activity, high chronicity, and many senescent glomeruli are present, then, in all likelihood, the patient will not respond to aggressive therapy. A trial of therapy may be worth undertaking in hopes of delaying progression to end-stage renal disease, but the potential medication toxicity should be weighed against allowing dialysis or transplantation sooner. If urinary sediment or proteinuria persist or renal function continues to deteriorate

despite therapy, then immunosuppressive agents can be discontinued and preparations made for dialysis. Additional measures include sodium restriction if hypertension is present, aggressive management of hypertension, and avoidance of NSAIDs and other nephrotoxic medications. In active cases refractory to high-dose corticosteroids and immunosuppressive agents, we have obtained anecdotal success with the addition of lymphoplasmapheresis. This experience is not universal, however.[48] In the acute ICU setting, serum creatinine and blood pressure should be followed closely. Other parameters such as urine sediment, creatinine clearance, 24-hour urine protein, serum albumin, and C3 should be checked every 2 weeks until improved and stable.

CNS DISEASE AND SLE

The subject of CNS manifestations in SLE often is a confusing one. Multiple small observational series span the decades, observations frequently are contradictory, and difficulties in comparison arise from a lack of clearly defined criteria for this group of lupus-associated disorders. Most agree that the overall category of CNS involvement is common, perhaps as high as 50% sometime during the course of SLE. However, the serious manifestations that are likely to result in hospitalization, and which may be life threatening, are much less common. These are the conditions that are discussed in the sections that follow.

Acute Cerebritis (Vasculitis)

Acute cerebritis also is referred to as *cerebral vasculitis* by some authors who acknowledge that this entity rarely has been found to involve a true vasculitis. Here we use the term *acute cerebritis*. Presentation of this syndrome is dramatic, with the acute onset of fever, headache, and confusion followed within hours or a few days by progressive mental dysfunction, seizures, encephalomyelitis, or coma. Acute cerebritis is distinguished from more benign presentations of isolated psychosis, affective disorders, and seizures (described later). Acute cerebritis often is lethal and usually occurs with active multisystem SLE. Pathologic study of brain sections reveals microinfarcts with hemorrhage, thrombosis, and perivascular inflammation without disruption of vessel walls or fibrinoid necrosis typical of vasculitis. Lesions are usually widely scattered and of varied age, implying an additive rather than simultaneous onset.

Evaluation should proceed promptly. Brain CT or MRI may reveal multiple intracerebral infarcts, although initial scan findings may be normal. CSF sampling is important to rule out infection as well as to document typical findings of pleocytosis and increased levels of CSF protein, IgG, oligoclonal bands, IgG synthesis, or IgG:albumin ratios. These tests are usually normal in seizures secondary to thromboembolism, drugs, alcohol, or scar foci from prior cerebritis. If infection is excluded, even when the MRI does not reveal significant abnormality, the above CSF findings in association with the clinical syndrome warrant early and aggressive therapy.

Specific therapy for lupus cerebritis includes high-dose corticosteroids, which are associated with recovery in a greater proportion of patients in studies done during the modern era. Parenteral prednisolone, 1 mg/kg/day, or the equivalent may be sufficient in early or less severe cerebritis. In the presence of status epilepticus, encephalomyelitis, or coma, we prefer to give 1 g of methylprednisolone per day IV for the first 3 days. In refractory cases, cyclophosphamide may be considered. Consultation with a rheumatologist experienced in the treatment of this disorder is critical. Anticonvulsant therapy should be used concomitantly in patients affected by seizures.

When seizures occur without fever, confusion, or progressive mental dysfunction, it is equally important to investigate for the presence of infection, thromboembolic disease, hypertension, uremia, and other non-SLE causes. If no other etiology is found and the CSF is normal, then treatment with anticonvulsant therapy is usually all that is required. If the CSF is abnormal, as described earlier, then treatment with moderate- to high-dose oral corticosteroids and anticonvulsants is appropriate.

More frequently than the acute cerebritis described earlier, SLE patients may present with isolated seizures, acute psychoses, or affective disorders. The key to differentiating SLE patients from those with acute cerebritis is the presentation: SLE without cerebritis has only a single manifestation in a patient with an otherwise clear sensorium. In these cases, the CSF is usually normal and MRI or CT scan reveal no generalized or focal abnormalities. The clinical course is more benign, and anticonvulsant or psychotropic medication is the treatment of choice. We add corticosteroids to patients with severe psychosis, but avoid cytotoxic drugs, which have not been shown to benefit this group of patients.

Thromboembolic Disease

Presenting as transient ischemic attacks, cerebral infarction or hemorrhage, or subarachnoid hemorrhage, the occurrence of thromboembolic disease in SLE seems to be strongly associated with the LAC or other aPLs. Cerebral infarction or hemorrhage is usually focal, and seizures may occur secondarily. Occasional cases of multifocal infarcts are observed. Except in the case of subarachnoid hemorrhage, CSF is usually normal. CT or MRI may reveal infarction or hemorrhage. Evaluation also should include partial thromboplastin time, rapid plasma reagin (RPR), anticardiolipin antibody, and LAC profile. Selected cases may require other hypercoagulability testing, including plasma viscosity, cryoglobulin, protein C, and protein S. Echocardiogram to identify a cardiac embolic source should be performed in most hemorrhagic or multiple infarct cases. If aPLs are detected, treatment may require long-term anticoagulation to minimize the risk of recurrence. Corticosteroids do not seem to be beneficial.

Transverse Myelitis

Inflammation of the spinal cord presenting as paresis or paralysis in one or more limbs is an uncommon manifestation of SLE, and thus may be underrecognized. Paralysis is flaccid

or spastic, and spontaneous resolution is the exception. Some patients develop a syndrome identical clinically to Guillain-Barré syndrome. CSF pleocytosis and elevated protein are usually present. CSF glucose is normal or decreased. Serum LAC or anticardiolipin antibodies are frequently detected. In pathologic specimens, inflammatory infiltrates and occasional extensive necrotizing myelitis have been described. Rarely, vasculitis has been observed. MRI findings may be normal or show an increased signal intensity, although this is often transient.[49] Other etiologies must be excluded, including compression fracture, spondylolisthesis, herniated disc, spinal stenosis, and *M tuberculosis* infection. Response to treatment with high-dose corticosteroids is variable. Early treatment seems to improve the chance of recovery, although full recovery is not assured. Corticosteroids can be started while awaiting cultures and modified if infection is confirmed. If aPLs are present, some authors recommend anticoagulation. Cyclophosphamide has been studied in small uncontrolled trials.[50] Deaths in these patients usually result from respiratory compromise or sepsis.

HEMATOLOGIC EMERGENCIES IN SLE

Autoimmune Hemolytic anemia

Autoimmune hemolytic anemia occurs in 7% to 15% of SLE patients.[51] Autoimmune hemolytic anemia also may be the initial manifestation of SLE. "Warm" IgG antierythrocyte antibodies are the most common type, and "cold" IgM antibodies occasionally coexist. The anemia may develop acutely, and patients usually exhibit symptoms of fever, weakness, and dizziness. Jaundice occasionally is present, with dark urine resulting from increased urinary bilirubin. The spleen is the major site of sequestration and phagocytosis of antibody-coated erythrocytes, and may be enlarged. Peripheral smears usually reveal spherocytes and polychromatophilia; however, red blood cell fragments seen with intravascular hemolysis are lacking. The hemolysis usually responds to high-dose corticosteroid administration. Prednisone, 1 to 1.5 mg/kg/day, is commonly used. If the patient is severely symptomatic or the anemia is rapidly progressive, then daily methylprednisolone IV for the first 3 days is preferred. Failure to respond within 1 week indicates a need for additional therapeutic options. Immunosuppressive therapy with azathioprine, 2 mg/kg/day, in addition to high-dose corticosteroids is effective in many of these patients. Other options include danazol, intravenous immune globulin (IVIG), and plasmapheresis. IVIG may be useful only temporarily. Splenectomy may be helpful in some patients but rarely results in remission that enables discontinuation of medical treatment. We have found splenectomy to be useful in decreasing the steroid requirement in patients who cannot be maintained on low-dose corticosteroids. Before splenectomy, it is critical to administer pneumococcal vaccination.

Acute Hemophagocytic Syndrome

Acute hemophagocytic syndrome is a rare disorder that also is observed in certain infectious or neoplastic conditions and results in fever associated with severe pancytopenia. The bone marrow contains histiocytes that have phagocytosed erythrocytes, erythroblasts, platelets, and granulocytes.[52] Prompt treatment with 1 to 2 mg/kg/day of prednisone is usually effective.

Acute Immune Thrombocytopenia

Occasional patients with SLE develop an acute thrombocytopenia, often associated with purpura, which clinically cannot be distinguished from idiopathic immune thrombocytopenic purpura. Thrombocytopenia may be the initial manifestation of SLE, or it may occur any time during the course of SLE. aPLs often are detected in the serum. Occasional patients present with profound thrombocytopenia, epistaxis, bleeding gums, or heavy menstrual flow. Cerebral hemorrhage is the dire complication of unrecognized or untreated thrombocytopenia. Acutely, patients respond to IVIG, which may be helpful if life-threatening bleeding is present or urgent surgery is anticipated. Prednisone, 1 to 1.5 mg/kg/day, or its equivalent, is also effective and should be started if the platelet count acutely drops below 50,000. Severe cases may require intravenous pulse methylprednisolone, cyclophosphamide, danazol, azathioprine, or dapsone. Splenectomy does not prevent recurrence in most patients but may decrease the corticosteroid requirement. Stable moderate thrombocytopenia associated with aPLs does not require treatment.

Thrombotic Thrombocytopenic Purpura

Thrombotic thrombocytopenic purpura or related hemolytic-uremic syndrome also may occur in SLE patients,[53,54] although the incidence is rare. Patients present with headache, confusion, and sometimes paresis, so lupus cerebritis, myelitis, or both should be considered in the differential diagnosis, just as thrombotic thrombocytopenic purpura needs to be considered in any lupus patient presenting with neurologic symptoms or thrombocytopenia. Fever also is common, and thrombocytopenic purpura, microangiopathic hemolytic anemia, and renal dysfunction complete the picture. Examination of the peripheral smear should be performed in all SLE patients presenting with thrombocytopenia or neurologic or renal dysfunction, and may reveal fragmented and nucleated erythrocytes. Lactate dehydrogenase is increased, and indirect hyperbilirubinemia is often present. Histologic specimens, including renal biopsy, may reveal microthrombi. Mortality is high despite high-dose corticosteroids, antiplatelet agents, splenectomy, plasma exchange, and plasmapheresis. In most patients, therapy should be guided by joint collaboration with the hematologist, nephrologist, and rheumatologist. Early plasmapheresis with plasma exchange and high-dose corticosteroids offer the best chance of recovery.

SYSTEMIC SCLEROSIS ■

GENERAL CONSIDERATIONS

Although the special problems of SSc (previously termed *scleroderma*) are most often addressed in the outpatient setting, there are several general considerations and organ-specific problems of great importance in the critical care management of these patients. For the SSc patient in the critical care setting, rheumatologic serologies such as complement components, ESR, C-reactive protein, rheumatoid factor (RF), ANA, or even the SSc-specific autoantibodies Scl-70 and anticentromere antibody are of little diagnostic utility. Vascular access may be difficult because of skin thickening in the distal extremities, including the antecubital fossae. Central venous catheters may be necessary. Intravenous fluids and ambient room temperature should be relatively warm to avoid precipitating vasospasm, although fluid warmers are not usually necessary. Beta-blockers may precipitate severe Raynaud's phenomenon (see the earlier discussion on Raynaud's phenomenon), as may ergot alkaloids. Decreased oral aperture complicates oral hygiene and intubations, which may need to be nasotracheal.

Scleroderma skin ulcerates easily. Caution should be exerted to avoid abrading affected areas. Even minor skin ulcerations may become infected because of poor blood flow and require prompt attention. Occupational therapists may be able to furnish protective padding. Distinguishing whether an area of cutaneous calcinosis is infected or just inflamed is difficult. The safest approach is to assume infection. Similarly, distinguishing osteomyelitis and osteonecrosis in SSc may be difficult without bone biopsy.

Reflux and esophageal dysmotility are universal problems in SSc patients. The head of the bed should be elevated to avoid reflux and aspiration. Pills should be administered with the patient upright for at least 30 minutes after swallowing. We recommend treatment with H_2 receptor antagonists or omeprazole for all SSc patients in the ICU. NSAIDs should be used judiciously, with the effect on reflux symptoms kept in mind.

Gut motility in the SSc patient is precarious at best. The effect on gut motility needs to be considered in all drugs administered to SSc patients. Narcotics should be used cautiously to avoid precipitating ileus.

SYSTEMIC SCLEROSIS RENAL CRISIS

Renal crisis is typically seen early (less than 4 years) into the course of diffuse SSc. Features that predict increased risk of renal crisis include rapidly progressive skin thickening, new-onset asymptomatic pericardial effusion, and new-onset anemia (not a typical laboratory feature of early SSc). Treatment with high-dose glucocorticoids, for example, in SSc associated myositis, may precipitate normotensive renal crisis manifested by rising creatinine in a patient with normal blood pressure. The presence of urinalysis abnormalities or previous mild hypertension do not predict increased risk for renal crisis.[55]

Onset of renal crisis is heralded by hypertension. Usually diastolic blood pressure is greater than 90 mm Hg and frequently is greater than 120 mm Hg. However, persons who have low to normal blood pressures at baseline may initially show only increased blood pressures in the normal range. Symptoms are related to malignant hypertension and include headache, visual disturbance, encephalopathy, seizure, oliguria or anuria, edema, CHF, or arrhythmia. Physical examination reveals hypertension and the typical skin changes of SSc, as well as retinal hemorrhages or papilledema, jugulo-venous distention, rales, tachycardia with S_3 or S_4 gallop and edema. Laboratory features include elevated serum creatinine, which may rise as rapidly as 1 mg/dL/day, microangiopathic hemolytic anemia, reticulocytosis, and mild thrombocytopenia. If renal crisis is suspected, examination of a peripheral blood smear by a physician for schistocytes is mandatory. Microangiopathic hemolytic anemia is a constant feature of normotensive renal crisis. An elevated serum renin level is typical, but prolonged turnaround time by the laboratory makes this impractical as a diagnostic aid.

The pathophysiologic course of renal crisis is based on a state of hyperreninemia. Small arteries of the kidneys are affected by a bland vasculopathy that causes progressive vessel narrowing. The kidneys are subject to the same vasospastic tendencies that cause Raynaud's phenomenon in the extremities. Vasospasm in the setting of arteriolar narrowing induces relative ischemia, which stimulates the juxtaglomerular apparatus to secrete renin. Angiotensin II produced in response to renin exacerbates the vasoconstriction, leading to malignant hypertension.

Understanding the pathophysiologic mechanism of renal crisis has lead to a revolution in treatment with ACE inhibitors. With the use of ACE inhibitors, mortality from renal crisis has dropped dramatically. The goal of therapy is normalization of blood pressure. Treatment begins with an oral dose of captopril, 12.5 mg, followed by 25 mg 6 hours later. The dose is increased by 25 mg every 8 hours as needed, up to 100 mg.[56] The maximum dose of captopril is 200 mg in 24 hours. The dose may need to be adjusted for renal insufficiency. If a patient is unable to take oral medications, intravenous enalapril may be substituted. An adverse reaction to captopril may require changing to a different ACE inhibitor. If maximum-dose ACE inhibitors fail to control blood pressure within 48 hours, ACE inhibitors are continued and additional antihypertensives are added. We begin with nifedipine, 10 to 30 mg every 8 hours. Other antihypertensive agents that have been used include prazosin, hydralazine, and minoxidil.[55,56]

Severe diastolic hypertension with seizures, encephalopathy, or cardiac symptoms requires immediate control of blood pressure with intravenous nitroprusside. When skin changes or severe Raynaud's phenomenon preclude the use of radial or brachial sites for arterial blood pressure monitoring, a femoral site may be required. Control of blood pressure with nitroprusside does not remove the need for therapy with ACE inhibitors. Basic ICU management of scleroderma renal crisis includes chest radiograph and electrocardiogram, with monitoring of daily weights and fluid balance. CHF usually responds promptly to control of blood pressure. If diuretics are necessary, care must be exerted to avoid hypovolemia and hypotension. An echocardiogram may be performed if pericardial effusion is suspected.

Even if blood pressure control is achieved, serum creatinine may continue to rise for a week or more. Older men with serum creatinine of 3 mg/dL or more and preexisting SSc cardiac disease are more likely to have fatal outcomes, particularly if the blood pressure cannot be controlled within 72 hours.[55] If renal failure develops and dialysis is required,

ACE inhibitor therapy should be maintained because renal function may improve gradually in this setting. Initially, dialysis may be accomplished using temporary catheters or the peritoneal route. In the era of ACE inhibitors, there is no role for nephrectomy to control hyperreninemia. For patients with normotensive renal crisis, treatment with low doses of ACE inhibitors may be attempted.

CARDIOPULMONARY DISEASE

Ischemic cardiomyopathy

Progressive vasculopathy of small arteries in the heart may lead to ischemic cardiomyopathy with CHF, arrhythmias, and sudden death. Management is the same as for CHF from other causes. Nifedipine should also be administered if the patient is stable because it reduces microvascular spasm and may improve myocardial perfusion.[56]

Myocarditis

If CHF accompanies myositis with a high serum CK, it is presumed to be secondary to myocarditis. Management is with prednisone, 1 mg/kg daily.[56]

Pulmonary Hypertension

The limited skin disease variant of SSc (or CREST) is complicated by pulmonary hypertension in 10% of cases. Pathophysiology and manifestations are the same as for primary pulmonary hypertension. Clinical manifestations include dyspnea and chest pain with clear lung fields on radiographs, and normal spirometry with an isolated reduction in diffusion capacity. Supportive measures for pulmonary hypertension include oxygen, warfarin anticoagulation, and diuretics. To optimize dosage of nifedipine or other vasodilators in pulmonary hypertension, a right heart catheterization may be necessary to monitor pulmonary artery pressures. Continuous intravenous administration of iloprost holds great promise in improving the quality of life for these patients.[57] If the patient is otherwise systemically well, heart and lung transplantation may be considered.

Interstitial Lung Disease

Interstitial lung disease is the leading cause of death directly attributable to SSc.[56,58,59] In rapidly progressive cases, the diagnosis may be in doubt and ICU care warranted. If there is any question whether the patient's symptoms are a toxic effect of penicillamine, such as in BOOP, penicillamine should be withheld. Pulmonary fibrosis caused by SSc presents similarly to other forms of interstitial lung disease. Patients complain of nonproductive cough and breathlessness. Severe cases are accompanied by cor pulmonale and right-sided CHF. Physical examination reveals dry rales on auscultation. Spirometry has a restrictive pattern, and diffusion capacity is decreased. High-resolution CT may demonstrate a ground glass appearance suggestive of acute alveolitis. BAL is useful to exclude atypical infections in rapidly progressing cases. In a nonsmoker SSc patient, BAL fluid with a high percentage of neutrophils indicates active alveolitis, which may respond to cyclophosphamide.[56,58,59] High-dose glucocorticoids may contribute to the development of normotensive renal crisis[56] or avascular necrosis of bone, and should be avoided.

GASTROINTESTINAL DISEASE

Management of problems related to bowel dysmotility often is the dominant concern for SSc patients in the clinic.[56–59] Small bowel dysmotility is caused by diminished peristalsis, loss of smooth muscle, and ultimately fibrosis. Early in the course abdominal pain, bloating and diarrhea reflect small bowel dysmotility with or without bacterial overgrowth. Patients are treated with prokinetic agents and cycles of antibiotics. Colonic dysmotility causes constipation. Later, the gut may be atonic, resulting in serious malnutrition requiring long-term total parenteral nutrition. We prefer to avoid barium studies because impaction of barium with perforation has catastrophic consequences. As the gut becomes less motile, patients may be admitted to the ICU with severe abdominal pain and small bowel or colonic distention on radiographs. Such pseudo-obstruction should be managed conservatively with bowel rest, nasogastric suction, intravenous fluids, and intravenous antibiotics. Electrolyte abnormalities are aggressively corrected. The appearance of air in the bowel wall signals the presence of pneumatosis cystoides intestinalis or coli. This is a benign condition, and management remains conservative. Laparotomy should be avoided because the result may be prolonged postoperative ileus and poor outcome.

REFERENCES ■

1. Grant SCD, Venning MC, Brooks NH: Wegener's granulomatosis and the heart. *Br Heart J* 1994;71:82
2. Boyce E, Mandell BF: Pharmacology and acute toxicity of antirheumatic and immunological therapy. In: Mandell BF (ed). *Acute Rheumatic and Immunological Diseases*. New York, Marcel Dekker, 1994:57
3. Furst DE, Clements PJ: SAARDs. Part II. In: Klippel JH, Dieppe PA (eds). *Rheumatology*. St Louis, CV Mosby, 1994:8.13.1
4. Boumpas DT, Chrousos GP, Wilder RL, et al: Glucocorticoid therapy for immune-mediated diseases: basic and clinical correlates. *Ann Intern Med* 1993;119:1198
5. Cannon GW: Pulmonary complications of antirheumatic drug therapy. *Semin Arthritis Rheum* 1990;19:353
6. Brooks PM: NSAIDs. In: Klippel JH, Dieppe PA (eds). *Rheumatology*. St Louis, CV Mosby, 1994:8.10.1
7. Simon LS: Nonsteroidal anti-inflammatory drug toxicity. *Curr Opinion Rheumatol* 1993;5:265
8. Kramer J, Jolesz F, Kleefield J: Rheumatoid arthritis of the cervical spine. *Rheum Dis Clin North Am* 1991;17:757
9. Owens G: Respiratory insufficiency in patients with connective tissue disease. In: Mandell BF (ed). *Acute Rheumatic and Immunological Diseases*. New York, Marcel Dekker, 1994:443
10. Byrd SL, Case BA, Boulware DW: Pulmonary manifestations of rheumatic disease. *Postgrad Med* 1993;93:149
11. Wigley FM : Raynaud's phenomenon. *Curr Opinion Rheumatol* 1993;5:773
12. Lie JT: Diagnostic histopathology of major systemic and pulmonary vasculitic syndromes. *Rheum Dis Clin North Am* 1990;16:269
13. Fauci AS, Haynes BF, Katz P: The spectrum of vasculitis: clinical, pathologic, immunologic and therapeutic considerations. *Ann Intern Med* 1978;89:660
14. Kerr GS, Hallahan CW, Girodano J, et al: Takayasu arteritis. *Ann Intern Med* 1994;120:919
15. Hunder GG: Giant cell (temporal) arteritis. *Rheum Dis Clin North Am* 1990;16:399
16. Conn DL: Polyarteritis. In: Klippel JH, Dieppe PA (eds). *Rheumatology*. St Louis, CV Mosby, 1994:6.17.1.
17. Hoffman GS, Fauci AS: Wegener's granulomatosis. In: Klippel JH, Dieppe PA (eds). *Rheumatology*. St Louis, CV Mosby, 1994:6.19.1
18. Lanham JG, Elkon KB, Pusey CD, et al: Systemic vasculitis with asthma and eosinophilia: a clinical approach to the Churg-Strauss syndrome. *Medicine* 1984;63:65
19. Fauci AS, Leavitt RY: Vasculitis. In: McCarty DJ (ed). *Arthritis and Allied Condititions*. Philadelphia, Lea & Febinger, 1993:1301
20. Conn DL, Hunder GG, O'Duffy, et al: Vasculitis and related disorders. In: Kelley WN, Harris ED, Ruddy S, et al (eds). *Texbook of Rheumatology*. Philadelphia, WB Saunders, 1993:1077
21. Gibson LE, Su DWP: Cutaneous vasculitis. *Rheum Dis Clin North Am* 1990;16:309
22. Hoffman GS, Kerr GS: Recognition of systemic vasculitis in the acutely ill patient. In: Mandell BF (ed). *Acute Rheumatic and Immunological Diseases*, New York, Marcel Dekker, 1994:279
23. Lie JT: Vasculitis simulators and vasculitis look-alikes. *Curr Opin Rheumatol* 1992;4:47
24. Lightfoot RW: Overview of the inflammatory vascular diseases. In: Klipple JH, Dieppe PA (eds). *Rheumatology*. St Louis, CV Mosby, 1994:6.16.1
25. Couser WG: Rapidly progressive glomerulonephritis: classification, pathogenic mechanism, and therapy. *Am J Kidney Dis* 1988;11:449
26. Calabrese LH, Hoffman GS, Guillevin L, et al: Therapy of resistant systemic necrotizing vasculitis: polyarteritis, Churg-Strauss syndrome, Wegener's granulomatosis, and hypersensitivity vasculitis group disorders. *Rheum Dis Clin North Am* 1995;21:1
27. Gross WL: New developments in the treatment of systemic vasculitis. *Curr Opinion Rheumatol* 1994;6:11
28. Schur PH: Clinical features of SLE. In: Kelley WN, Harris ED, Ruddy S, et al (eds). *Textbook of Rheumatology*. Philadelphia, WB Saunders, 1993:1017
29. Gladman DD, Urowitz MB: Systemic lupus erythematosus: clinical features. In: Klippel JH, Dieppe PA (eds). *Rheumatology*. St Louis, Mosby–Year Book Europe Limited, 1994:6.2.1.
30. Wallace DJ: The clinical presentation of systemic lupus erythematosus. In: Wallace DJ, Hahn BH (eds). *Dubois' Lupus Erythematosus*. Philadelphia, Lea & Febiger, 1993:317
31. Wallace DJ: Infections in systemic lupus erythematosus. In: Wallace DJ, Hahn BH (eds). *Dubois' Lupus Erythematosus*. Philadelphia, Lea & Febiger, 1993:454
32. Orens JB, Martinez FJ, Lynch JP III: Pleuropulmonary manifestations of systemic lupus erythematosus. *Rheum Dis Clin North Am* 1994;20:159
33. McCabe RE: Diagnosis of pulmonary infections in immunocompromised patients. *Med Clin North Am* 1988;72:1067
34. Matthay RA, Schwarz MI, Petty TL, et al: Pulmonary manifes-

tations of systemic lupus erythematosus: review of 12 cases of acute lupus pneumonitis. *Medicine* 1974;54:397

35. Abud-Mendoza C, Diaz-Jouanen E, Alarcon-Segovia D: Fatal pulmonary hemorrhage in systemic lupus erythematosus; occurrence without hemoptysis. *J Rheumatol* 1985;12:558

36. Eagen JW, Memoli VA, Roberts JL, et al: Pulmonary hemorrhage in systemic lupus erythematosus. *Medicine* 1978;57:545

37. Asherson RA, Cervera R: Review: antiphospholipid antibodies and the lung. *J Rheumatol* 1995;22:62

38. Pines A, Kaplinsky N, Olchovsky D, et al: Pleuro-pulmonary manifestations of systemic lupus erythematosus: clinical features of its subgroups. *Chest* 1985;88:129

39. Gammon RB, Bridges TA, Al-Nezir H, et al: Bronchiolitis obliterans organizing pneumonia associated with systemic lupus erythematosus. *Chest* 1992;102:1171

40. Carrete S: Cardiopulmonary manifestations of systemic lupus erythematosus. *Rheum Dis Clin North Am* 1988;14:135

41. Quismorio FP Jr: Cardiac abnormalities in systemic lupus erythematosus. In: Wallace DJ, Hahn BH (eds). *Dubois' Lupus Erythematosus*. Philadelphia, Lea & Febiger, 1993:332

41a. Libman E, Sacks B: A hitherto undescribed form of valvular and mural endocarditis. *Arch Intern Med* 1924;33:701

42. Galve E, Candell-Riera J, Pigrau C, et al: Prevalence, morphologic types, and evolution of cardiac valvular disease in systemic lupus erythematosus. *N Engl J Med* 1988;319:817

43. Zizic TM, Classen JN, Stevens MB: Acute abdominal complications of systemic lupus erythematosus and polyarteritis nodosa. *Am J Med* 1982;73:525

44. Hoffman BI, Katz WA: The gastrointestinal manifestations of systemic lupus erythematosus: a review of the literature. *Semin Arthritis Rheum* 1980;9:237

45. Reynolds JC, Inman RD, Kimberly RP, et al: Acute pancreatitis in systemic lupus erythematosus: report of 20 cases and a review of the literature. *Medicine* 1982;61:25

46. Wallace DJ: Gastrointestinal manifestations and related liver and biliary disorders. In: Wallace DJ, Hahn BH (eds). *Dubois' Lupus Erythematosus*. Philadelphia, Lea & Febiger, 1993:410

47. Jennette JC, Falk RJ: Diagnosis and management of glomerulo-nephritis and vasculitis presenting as acute renal failure. *Med Clin North Am* 1990;74:893

48. Lewis EJ, Hunsicker LG, Lan SP, et al: A controlled trial of plasmapheresis therapy in severe lupus nephritis. *N Engl J Med* 1992;326:1373

49. Salmaggi A, Lamperti E, Eoli M, et al: Spinal cord involvement and systemic lupus erythematosus: clinical and magnetic resonance findings in five patients. *Clin Exp Rheumatol* 1994;12:389

50. Barile L, LaValle C: Transverse myelitis in systemic lupus erythematosus: the effect of IV pulse methylprednisolone and cyclophosphamide. *J Rheumatol* 1992;19:370

51. Quisimoro FP: Hemic and lymphatic abnormalities in SLE. In: Wallace DJ, Hahn BH (eds). *Dubois' Lupus Erythematosus*. Philadelphia, Lea & Febiger, 1993:418

52. Wong K, Hui P, Chan JKC, et al: The acute lupus hemophagocytic syndrome. *Ann Intern Med* 1991;114:387

53. Hess DC, Sethi K, Awad E: Thrombotic thrombocytopenic purpura in systemic lupus erythematosus and antiphospholipid antibodies; effective treatment with plasma exchange and immunosuppression. *J Rheumatol* 1992;19:1474

54. Bray VJ, West SG, Kristo DA: Simultaneous presentation of thrombotic thrombocytopenic purpura and systemic lupus erythematosus. *South Med J* 1994;87:827

55. Steen VD, Medsger TA: Scleroderma renal crisis. In: Mandell BF (ed). *Acute Rheumatic and Immunological Disease*. New York, Marcel Dekker, 1994:353

56. Legerton CW, Smith EA, Silver RM: Systemic sclerosis: clinical management of its major complications. *Rheum Dis Clin North Am* 1995;21:203

57. De la Mata J, Gomez-Sanchez MA, Aranzana M, et al: Long term iloprost infusion for severe pulmonary hypertension in patients with connective tissue diseases. *Arthrits Rheum* 1994;37:1528

58. Torres MA, Furst DE: Treatment of generalized systemic sclerosis. *Rheum Dis Clin North Am* 1990;16:217

59. Van den Hoogen FHJ, van de Putte LBA: Treatment of systemic sclerosis. *Curr Opinion Rheumatol* 1994;6:637

Critical Care, Third Edition, edited by Joseph M. Civetta,
Robert W. Taylor, and Robert R. Kirby.
Lippincott-Raven Publishers, Philadelphia, PA © 1997.

CHAPTER 151

■

Dermatologic Conditions

Richard L. Spielvogel

IMMEDIATE CONCERNS ■

The dermatologic diseases discussed in this chapter provide
a serious challenge to the clinician. They require astute
attention to clinical and historical data, as well as prompt
diagnosis and institution of appropriate therapy. The final
outcome depends on the clinician's ability to recognize or
suspect the clinical entity and on a thorough and dynamic
approach to treatment. These diseases often are best managed in an inpatient setting with a multispecialty approach.
The dermatologist often plays a unifying role.

Dermatologic conditions are often viewed as annoying
accompaniments of systemic disease and at one time were
handled by the overly simplified approach, "If it's wet, dry
it up, and if it's dry, make it wet." A few dermatologic conditions, however, are serious, with potentially high morbidity
and mortality and should be recognized and aggressively
treated.

ERYTHEMA MULTIFORME ■

A heterogeneous clinical syndrome, erythema multiforme
(EM) is a cutaneous or multisystem hypersensitivity reaction
pattern to one of many etiologic factors.[1] The reaction is
self-limited and benign in most patients; it usually resolves
spontaneously within a 2-week period. Patients with severe
forms may require intensive inpatient care, and death from
septicemia or pneumonia is possible.[1] Stevens-Johnson syndrome is a severe form of EM with marked oral mucosal and
ocular involvement. These patients may develop extensive
epidermal necrosis with large denuded areas simulating toxic
epidermal necrolysis.

ETIOLOGY

Medications and infections are the most common causes
of EM (Table 151-1). Immunizations, multisystem disease,
sunlight, and radiotherapy of tumors have been reported as
rare causes.[1]

PRESENTATION

The natural course of the disease depends on its severity
and the organs affected. Some patients are free of lesions
within 2 weeks, but many patients with bullous and mucosal
involvement may have persistent lesions for up to 6 weeks.[1]

EM erupts with a sudden onset of erythematous macules
and papules. The center may progress to a vesiculobullous
lesion with a dusky hue. These "target" lesions are considered the pathognomonic skin lesions of EM, and some dermatologists are unwilling to make a firm diagnosis if they
are not present. There are patients who are best classified
in the EM spectrum but who do not exhibit target lesions
during the course of their disease. Target lesions are composed of a central erythematous papule, elevated plaque,
or small grayish vesicle surrounded by concentric rings or
normal-appearing skin and erythema (Fig. 151-1). The eruption is symmetric, with a predilection for the dorsal aspect
of the hands and feet, palms and soles, and extensor extremities. Nonspecific prodromal symptoms may precede the
eruption. Successive crops of lesions persist for 1 to 2 weeks.
Complete resolution usually occurs in 4 to 6 weeks. Oral
lesions may be seen in as many as 25% of patients. Recurrences are common. In one study, recurrences ranged from
2 to 24 attacks per year, most patients had oral mucosal
involvement, 71% of attacks were preceded by herpes simplex infection, and acyclovir was helpful when initiated early
in the disease course.[2]

TABLE 151-1. Causative Agents of Erythema Multiforme

Medications
  Sulfa preparations
  Phenytoin
  Phenylbutazone
  Penicillin
  Barbiturates
  Tetracycline
Infections
  Herpes simplex labialis (up to one third of cases)
  Hepatitis B
  HIV (often with drugs)
  Mycoplasma pneumonia
  Influenza
  Streptococcal pharyngitis
  Histoplasmosis
Vaccinations/immunizations
Multisystem diseases
  Collagen-vascular
Physical agents
  Sunlight
  Radiotherapy of tumors

HIV, human immunodeficiency virus.

In the severe form (EM major), a prodromal phase with fever, malaise, and focal or confluent cutaneous erythema may be seen. This is followed by the development of macules, papules, vesicles, bullae, or target (iris) lesions.

Stevens-Johnson syndrome is distinguished by the severity of oral mucosal (Fig. 151-2) and ocular (Fig. 151-3) involvement and may have a variable, but almost always less severe, cutaneous component.

DIAGNOSIS

Erythema multiforme is diagnosed clinically because the histologic picture may not be as helpful in the early stages. A superficial dermal perivascular mononuclear infiltrate, combined with an interface dermatitis and necrotic epidermal cells, strongly suggests the diagnosis. Immunofluorescence study results are negative, but they may help to differentiate EM from other dermatoses. Laboratory tests are not diagnostic. Viral cultures of bullae should be performed to rule out a generalized herpes simplex infection. Cold agglutinins, a chest radiograph, and an otoscopic examination help to determine a mycoplasmic etiology. The etiology often is not determined despite extensive laboratory testing.

MANAGEMENT

When EM is suspected, a thorough history must be obtained with emphasis on medications and illness. If an infectious source is clinically evident, it should be treated appropriately. Removal of an offending drug usually brings about recovery. Only supportive therapy is required for the mild forms. Rarely has progression from EM minor to EM major (the Stevens-Johnson syndrome) occurred. High-potency corticosteroid creams applied two to three times daily may be beneficial. Aluminum acetate soaks (Burow's solution) help to control exudation from eroded sites and dry the blisters. Antihistamines may be helpful for pruritus. An ophthalmology consultation is important for patients with ocular involvement (Stevens-Johnson syndrome). Keratitis leading to leukoma formation and visual loss from bulbar perforation have been reported.[1] Many patients need supportive topical therapy to reduce pain and assist food and fluid intake. Glycerin-coated sticks, lozenges, and lidocaine-containing preparations are helpful. If the patient is unable to eat or swallow, the intravenous route should be used for hydration.

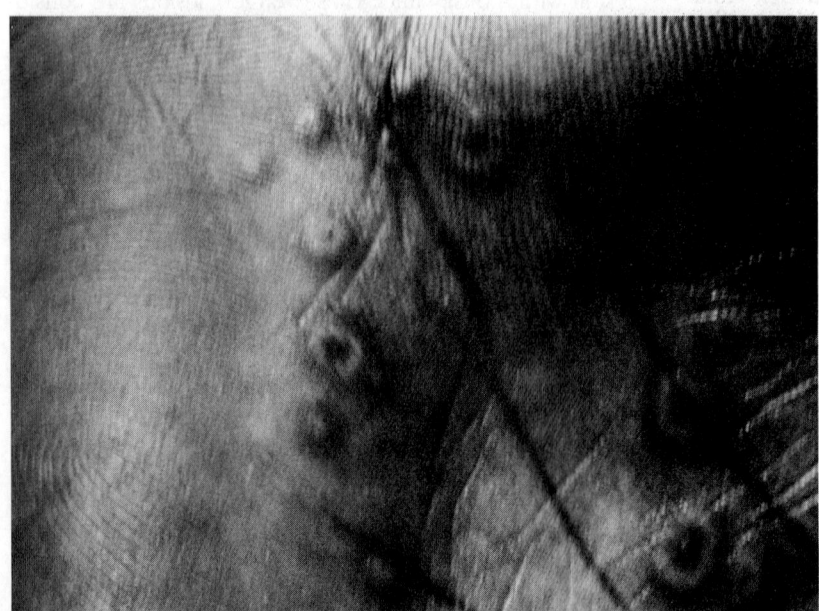

FIGURE 151-1. Typical target lesion of erythema multiforme on palm.

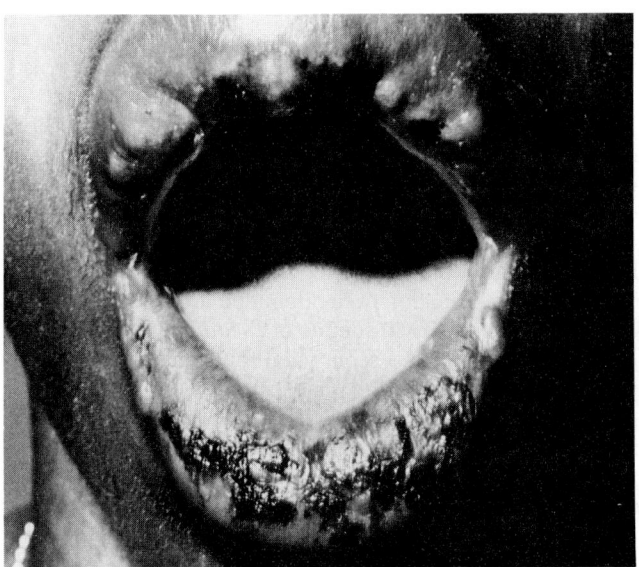

FIGURE 151-2. Vesiculobullous and crusted lip lesions are common features of the Stevens-Johnson syndrome.

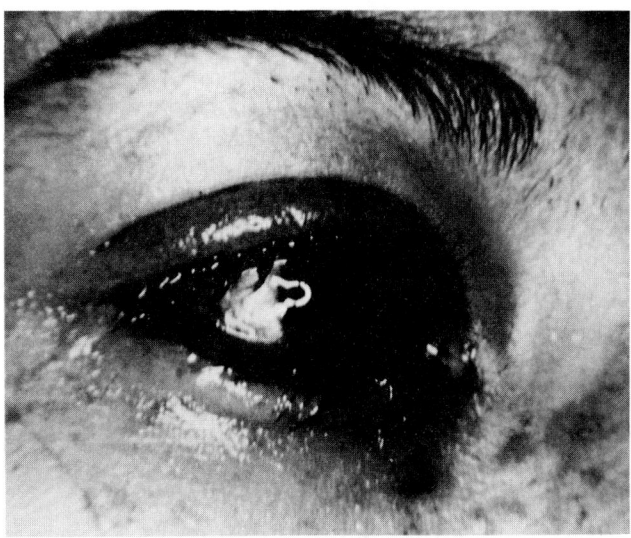

FIGURE 151-3. Ocular conjunctival involvement is a serious clinical manifestation of the Stevens-Johnson syndrome.

The use of systemic corticosteroid therapy in this disease is controversial. In selected patient groups, corticosteroid use has been associated with a higher complication rate and prolongation of disease. Other practitioners favor the use of this therapy in symptomatic patients with rapidly evolving severe disease.[3–5] If systemic corticosteroids are used, they should be administered in appropriate early morning dosages (oral prednisone, 60 to 100 mg/day in adults; 30 to 60 mg/day orally in children) until symptoms and skin lesions begin to involute. Dosages should be tapered gradually over 2 to 3 weeks. This regimen minimizes the possibility of disease exacerbation if corticosteroids are discontinued too early. Levamisole alone at 150 mg per day for 3 days or in combination with prednisone,[6] and thalidomide have been helpful.

For patients with mucosal involvement (Stevens-Johnson syndrome) who progress to widespread epidermal necrosis, the prognosis is worse. They should be managed in the same manner as patients with extensive burns. Bacterial septicemia, fluid-electrolyte abnormalities, and organ failure are responsible for fatalities. Fortunately, most patients with EM have a self-limited course. Recurrences are common, especially if drugs, hormonal changes, or herpetic infections are the triggering factors.

TOXIC EPIDERMAL NECROLYSIS ■

Toxic epidermal necrolysis is manifested by a severe vesiculobullous cutaneous reaction to an etiologic agent, most commonly a drug, followed by infection and multisystem complications. The prodrome is sudden with fever, malaise, skin tenderness, and prostration. This is followed by focal or confluent erythema, urticarial plaques, papules, or vesiculobullous lesions. The skin findings rapidly evolve toward extensive epidermal necrosis. Septicemia from bacterial colo-

nization of the denuded skin is common, and death occurs in over 20% of cases.[7] Some believe that the early administration of corticosteroids may be lifesaving, but once epidermal necrosis is extensive, their use seems to be associated with increased morbidity and mortality.[3]

ETIOLOGY

Toxic epidermal necrolysis is caused by a drug in most instances. Patients with graft-versus-host disease may develop toxic epidermal necrolysis as a severe manifestation of the clinical syndrome.[8] Other causes are listed in Table 151-2.

TABLE 151-2. Toxic Epidermal Necrolysis—Etiology

Drugs
   Sulfonamides
   Phenylbutazone barbiturates
   Phenytoin
   Carbamazepine
   Penicillin derivatives
   NSAIDs
Infections
   Viral (including HIV, often with drugs)
Immunizations
   Polio
   Diphtheria
   Tetanus
Preexisting diseases
   Collagen-vascular
   Graft-versus-host disease
   Stevens-Johnson syndrome
   Neoplasia (lymphoma)
Physical agents
   Radiotherapy of tumors

NSAIDs, nonsteroidal antiinflammatory drugs; HIV, human immunodeficiency virus.

PRESENTATION

There is a sudden onset of fever, malaise, skin tenderness, and focal or confluent skin erythema, papules, or urticarial lesions. This picture rapidly evolves toward a vesiculobullous state as the patient becomes more toxic (Fig. 151-4). Lateral shearing pressure on normal-appearing skin adjacent to a vesiculobullous lesion results in the rubbing off of the epidermis, leaving a moist erosion (positive Nikolsky's sign). Oral mucosal involvement resulting in painful erosions and conjunctivitis may be prominent. The patient has severe pain because of the erosions and may become dehydrated and mentally confused as the disease progresses. Despite intensive supportive therapy with antibiotics or corticosteroids, patients with extensive epidermal necrosis have a high mortality rate. Septicemia and fluid-electrolyte disturbances with subsequent internal organ failure contribute to death.

DIAGNOSIS

The sudden development of epidermal necrosis in a toxic, febrile patient should alert the clinician to the diagnosis. A biopsy of the skin adjacent to a bulla or erosion should be performed and histologic sections examined. The examination of the roof of a bulla by frozen section technique is also recommended. If performed early, the section may demonstrate a suprabasilar separation. At a later stage, a biopsy may show full-thickness epidermal necrosis and eventually the formation of a subepidermal bulla. The skin biopsy is an important diagnostic tool in this disease, but the clinician's initial diagnosis is based primarily on a thorough dermatologic examination.

MANAGEMENT

These patients should be managed in an ICU or a burn unit by a multispecialty team. A rotating bed frame is helpful in providing access to all affected skin areas. Topical wet dressings with Burow's solution or weak silver nitrate preparations (0.25% to 0.5%) reduce the accumulation of crusts and also act as a local antiseptic.

Silver sulfadiazine (Silvadene) cream provides a soothing cover that counteracts the colonization of bacteria on the open skin. If a sulfa drug is suspected as the etiologic factor, do not use silver sulfadiazine or silver nitrate because either one may cross-react with the offending agent and prolong the clinical reaction.

Periodic examination of the denuded areas with a Wood's lamp may detect early evidence of *Pseudomonas* infections, because fluorescence is seen when the local bacteria count reaches a critical level.

Careful monitoring of fluid intake and output and electrolyte status is mandatory. Because these patients usually cannot ingest fluid, intravenous replacement is necessary.

Corticosteroid therapy has a place in the management of these patients if given at an early stage before extensive epidermal necrosis occurs. At an advanced stage, such therapy seems to be associated with increased morbidity and mortality primarily from septic complications.[9] The drugs are usually administered intravenously. I use a prednisone equivalency level of 80 to 160 mg/day, depending on severity. Plasmapheresis has been used successfully in a limited number of patients. It may remove the antigenic stimulus (drug), decrease the circulating antibody response, or remove a circulating cytotoxic agent that may be responsible for the pathologic changes.[10] Cyclosporine has been reported to be effective.[11]

STAPHYLOCOCCAL SCALDED SKIN SYNDROME ■

The staphylococcal scalded skin syndrome is a self-limited disease. The disease affects infants and children of preschool age; however, a few adults also have developed a similar

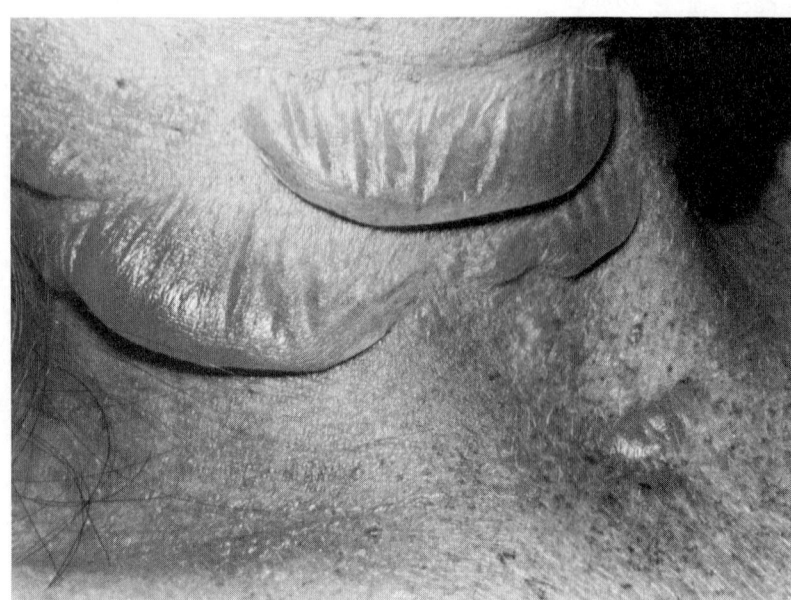

FIGURE 151-4. Flaccid bullae may be present in the early stage of toxic epidermal necrolysis.

condition. Adults may have a severe course with kidney failure, and the condition has been reported in human immunodeficiency virus (HIV)–positive patients. Treatment with penicillin derivatives is recommended to eradicate a staphylococcal focus and to reduce the possibility of septicemia. Staphylococcal toxic shock syndrome may clinically mimic staphylococcal scalded skin syndrome.

ETIOLOGY

The disease process is caused by the action of epidermolytic exotoxins (A and B) produced by *Staphylococcus aureus* groups I, II, and III with multiple and varied phage types.[12]

PRESENTATION

The onset of the disease may follow an upper respiratory infection or infection of the umbilical stump. It evolves rapidly with periorificial and intertriginous bullae and extensive exfoliation. The patient may be febrile and irritable.

DIAGNOSIS

The clinical diagnosis is based on the presence of periorificial and intertriginous crusting and a scalded skin appearance in this particular age group (Fig. 151-5). A skin biopsy for permanent and frozen section examination of a blister roof confirms the diagnosis by showing superficial epidermal necrosis and cleavage within or near the granular cell layer. Tzanck preparations of lesions show acantholytic keratinocytes. Although a definite source of the *S. aureus* organisms cannot be determined in many cases, bacterial cultures of affected skin, nasopharynx, circumcision area, and umbilical stump are recommended.

MANAGEMENT

The disease runs a self-limited course of 10 to 14 days. The epidermal necrosis is superficial and, therefore, usually no serious problems occur with fluid-electrolyte losses or superimposed bacterial infections. Most patients are treated as outpatients with supportive measures such as topical astringent soaks (Burow's solution). They should be treated with penicillin derivatives or other appropriate antibiotics to eliminate an occult staphylococcal focus and to prevent the spread of the disease. Corticosteroids are not indicated for this condition. Resolution comes rapidly, and most patients recover without complications.

GENERALIZED PUSTULAR PSORIASIS (VON ZUMBUSCH) ■

Generalized pustular psoriasis is characterized by the abrupt onset of fever and prostration preceding or accompanying a peculiar generalized eruption. The primary skin lesions are pustules, which arise on erythematous skin or psoriasiform plaques. Chills and leukocytosis may be the initial symptom and sign, respectively, leading the physician to search for an infection. An unpredictable clinical course with variable response to therapy magnifies the clinical challenge. Superimposed bacterial infections, fluid-electrolyte disturbances, and organ failure may lead to death.

ETIOLOGY

Generalized pustular psoriasis can be precipitated by the administration of systemic corticosteroids and other medications to patients with preexisting classical plaque-type psoria-

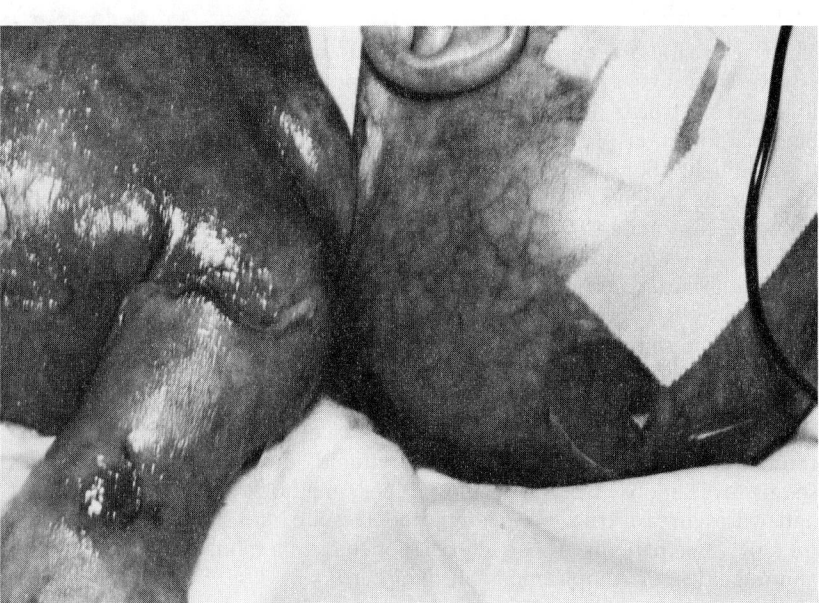

FIGURE 151-5. Scalded skin appearance in infant with staphylococcal scalded skin syndrome.

sis.[13] This clinical conversion most frequently occurs after corticosteroids are withdrawn. Respiratory, urinary tract, and periodontal infections, as well as postsurgical hypoparathyroidism, have been implicated as triggering factors.[14] Most cases are classified as idiopathic (Table 151-3). The underlying cause of psoriasis remains an enigma, although a strong genetic component exists.

PRESENTATION

The disease usually runs a prolonged course with acute exacerbations and periods of remission. During the acute episodes, patients may develop fever and chills, appear irritable, and sometimes become delirious, suggesting an acute infectious process. The initial febrile episode lasts a few days and is accompanied or followed by the onset of generalized erythroderma or psoriasiform plaques with multiple sterile pustules (Fig. 151-6). The pustulation occurs in waves and may persist for days or weeks.

DIAGNOSIS

Generalized pustular psoriasis is diagnosed by careful assessment of the patient's clinical picture. Biopsy of involved skin reveals the presence of intraepidermal spongiform pustules (Kogoj). A few reports in the dermatologic literature have described women in their last trimester of pregnancy who develop an acute febrile episode with a skin eruption that is sometimes identical to generalized pustular psoriasis. Hypocalcemia has been a prominent feature in these cases, as well as a significant cause of maternal and fetal mortality. This clinical syndrome has been named impetigo herpetiformis and histologically is indistinguishable from generalized pustular psoriasis. Many dermatologists believe that it represents a clinical variant of pustular psoriasis.

MANAGEMENT

The therapy for generalized pustular psoriasis includes supportive measures as well as specific measures to correct fluid and electrolyte disturbances and to treat superimposed bacterial infections. Long-term psoralen and long-wave ultraviolet light photochemotherapy (PUVA) have been effective in some patients.[15] The oral administration of synthetic retinoids, etretinate (0.5 to 1.0 mg/kg/day) and isotretinoin (1.5 to 2.0 mg/kg/day), has provided an alternative to methotrexate or systemic corticosteroids in the management of severe cases.[16] They successfully control acute pustulation and systemic symptoms but usually must be used for prolonged periods, and the patient's liver functions and cholesterol and triglyceride levels must be monitored carefully. As with other therapies, the disease may exacerbate once retinoids are discontinued. Of these two retinoids, etretinate seems to be more effective. Cyclosporine,[17] methotrexate, and hydroxyurea also have been employed. Despite intensive therapy, some patients die of bacterial septicemia, metabolic abnormalities, or complications of therapy.

TABLE 151-3.   Causes of Generalized Pustular Psoriasis

Systemic corticosteroid therapy and its subsequent withdrawal
Other medications
    Sulfa drugs
    Penicillin
    Cough medicine
    Salicylates
    Potassium iodide
Infections
    Bacterial—skin infections, dental abscesses
    Viral—upper respiratory infections
Pregnancy
    Impetigo herpetiformis?
Postsurgical hypoparathyroidism
Idiopathic
    No preexisting psoriasis or identifiable extraneous
      precipitating factor

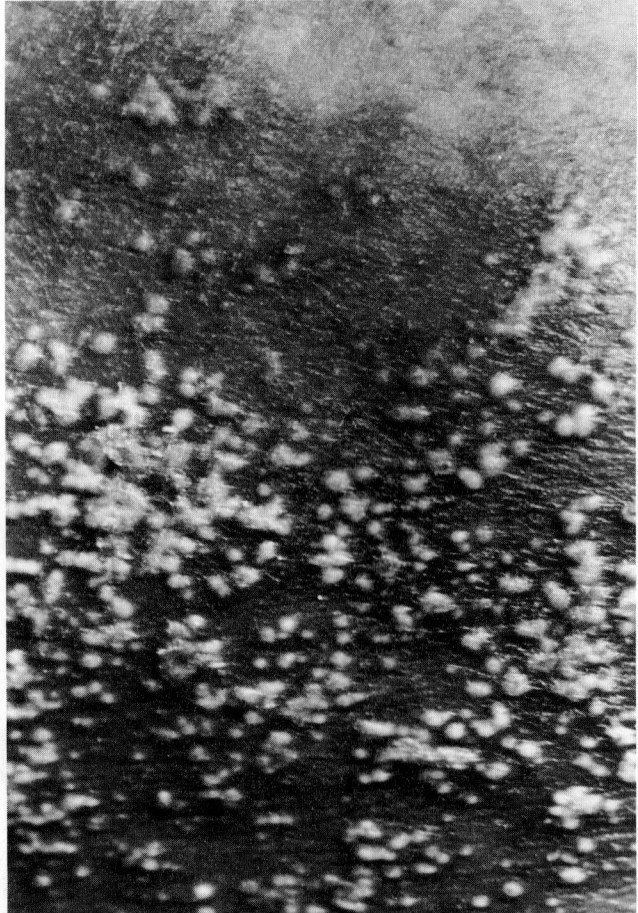

FIGURE 151-6. Multiple pustules arising on inflamed skin are a common presentation for generalized pustular psoriasis.

ERYTHRODERMA AND EXFOLIATIVE DERMATITIS ∎

Erythroderma is characterized by either a rapid or insidious onset of extensive cutaneous erythema. Edema or exfoliation of scales (exfoliative erythroderma) may occur simultaneously (Fig. 151-7). Life-threatening metabolic, cardiovascular, or thermoregulatory complications may occur in elderly, debilitated patients with preexisting cardiovascular disease. These include high-output heart failure, iron deficiency anemia, hypoalbuminemia, and excess heat or fluid loss through inflamed skin.[18] The condition follows a chronic course with exacerbations and remissions. The prognosis is generally better when a drug is the causative agent because its discontinuation usually promotes resolution of the inflammatory process. Management is directed toward hydrating and moisturizing the patient's skin and improving the overall physiologic status. Administering corticosteroids may temporarily suppress the erythroderma. Because of potential complications, they should be reserved as a last measure for patients who are not doing well.

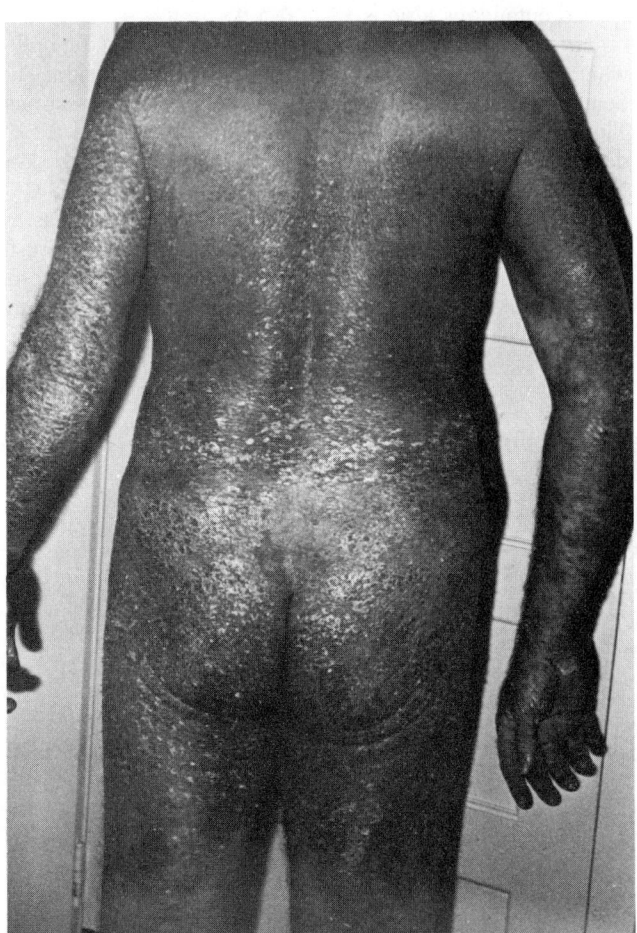

FIGURE 151-7. Extensive skin involvement with erythema, exfoliation, and lichenification in patient with erythroderma.

ETIOLOGY

The most common cause of erythroderma is the exacerbation of a preexisting dermatologic disease such as psoriasis vulgaris or eczema. Other causes are listed in Table 151-4.

PRESENTATION

The onset of erythroderma may be sudden or insidious. The patient may have fever, skin tenderness, and paroxysmal shivering. Patches of erythema become confluent, and cutaneous edema becomes a prominent clinical feature. The edema may restrict limb motion and may be a sign of hypoalbuminemia or impending heart failure. Exfoliation of scales of more than 9 g/m²/day has been documented.[19] Pruritus may be intense, especially if the underlying process is an eczematous or lymphoproliferative disorder. Excoriations may lead to erosions with secondary impetiginization, lichenification, and hyperpigmentation. A "leathery" skin appearance, generalized hair loss, and loss of nails are commonly seen in the patient with chronic erythroderma.

Reactive lymphadenopathy is common in patients with underlying benign dermatoses. In patients with indurated lymph nodes, a lymph node biopsy for diagnosis should be considered.

DIAGNOSIS

The diagnosis is made by clinical observation because these patients exhibit a unique appearance and clinical course. Skin biopsy is not diagnostic but may show features of the underlying dermatosis. The presence of atypical mononuclear cells in the dermal infiltrate may provide the earliest sign of an evolving cutaneous lymphoma. Periodic skin biop-

TABLE 151-4. Causes of Erythroderma and Exfoliative Dermatitis

---

Exacerbation of preexisting dermatologic disease
    Dermatophyte infections
    Eczema
    Lichen planus
    Pemphigus foliaceous
    Pityriasis rubra pilaris
    Psoriasis
    Scabies
Malignancies
    Leukemia
    Lymphoma
Contact dermatitis
Drugs
    Barbiturates
    Gold
    Penicillin
    Sulfonamides
Idiopathic
    No preexisting disease or identifiable precipitating factor

---

Shuster S: The metabolic and hemodynamic effects of skin disease. *Am Clin Res* 1971; 3:135.

sies and evaluations of the peripheral blood smear for atypical circulating mononuclear cells (Sézary syndrome) are mandatory.

MANAGEMENT

There is no universally effective therapy for erythroderma. PUVA and tar-ultraviolet light therapy have been helpful in patients with underlying psoriasis or eczema. Systemic corticosteroids are reserved for patients with a rapidly deteriorating physiologic status. Once corticosteroids are discontinued, erythroderma usually recurs. Wet compresses with saline or tap water are a value in the acute phase of erythroderma. They promote vasoconstriction of superficial cutaneous vessels. This response may be important in limiting the development of dermal edema produced by the extravasation of intravascular fluid.

In patients with severe exfoliation, emollient creams and ointments (Eucerin, Aquaphor, petrolatum) are beneficial. The clinician should monitor the patient's cardiovascular and metabolic status. Early detection of an evolving lymphoproliferative process is important. Increased activity and hyperthermia may precipitate congestive heart failure in patients with erythroderma, particularly in the elderly. Close monitoring of fluid intake and output with frequent weight checks is mandatory.

PEMPHIGUS ■

Pemphigus is an autoimmune blistering disorder affecting the skin and mucous membranes. It is more prevalent in Jewish people and most commonly affects persons in their fourth or fifth decade of life. The two main types are pemphigus vulgaris and pemphigus foliaceus. The former is a more common and more severe disease. The presenting sign may be painful oral mucosal lesions, usually followed by widespread skin involvement. The primary lesions in pemphigus are vesicles and bullae that break, leaving a painful denuded area (Fig. 151-8).

ETIOLOGY

Pemphigus is an autoimmune disease. Serum autoantibodies (mainly IgG) react with cell surface or intercellular antigens located between keratinocytes or mucosal cells. This reaction results in decreased cellular cohesiveness and eventual acantholysis.[20]

PRESENTATION

Pemphigus vulgaris is the most common and severe condition within this rare group of blistering disorders. It is the most likely disease in this group to present with a degree of severity requiring urgent care. The typical patient is in the fourth or fifth decade of life, and the most common initial complaint is a history of recent painful oral erosions. These may precede by weeks or months the onset of widespread cutaneous lesions.

The primary lesion in this disease is a vesicle or bulla, which arises on normal-appearing or erythematous skin. The head, upper trunk, and periorificial areas are likely locations. The clear fluid in the bullae becomes turbid within 2 to 4 days, and the lesions rupture, leaving painful denuded skin. Nikolsky's sign is positive.

The fluid content of the vesiculobullous lesions has an offensive odor, and the development of extensive crusts creates an unattractive cosmetic effect. As the disease progresses, the patient becomes debilitated and remains uncomfortable.

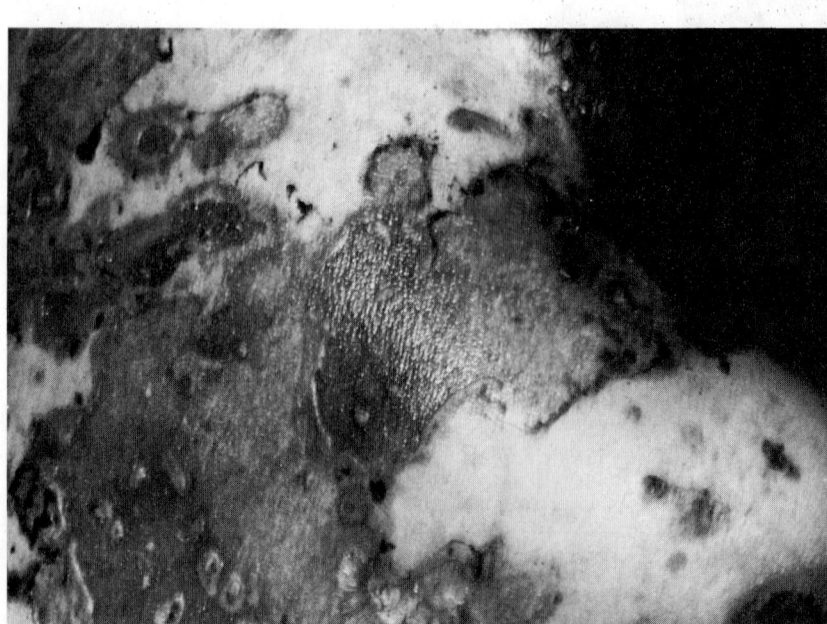

FIGURE 151-8. Large eroded areas with local crusting in patient with pemphigus vulgaris.

DIAGNOSIS

Pemphigus must be suspected in any patient who presents with recurrent painful oral erosions. During periods of exacerbation, the presence of flaccid bullae, painful denuded skin, and a positive Nikolsky's sign should alert the clinician to this diagnosis. A definitive diagnosis is supported by a biopsy of normal-appearing skin adjacent to a bulla or denuded area. Acantholysis of keratinocytes, combined with a "tombstone" appearance of a basal cell layer, are characteristic of pemphigus vulgaris. Direct immunofluorescence studies show deposition of IgG and complement (mainly C3) in intercellular areas of the epidermis. Circulating IgG antibodies are found in patients with pemphigus vulgaris as detected by indirect immunofluorescence.

MANAGEMENT

Without corticosteroid therapy, pemphigus vulgaris is invariably fatal. The painful oral lesions result in inadequate fluid intake and nutrition. Debility, combined with superimposed infections and epidermal fluid and electrolyte losses, contribute to the patient's death.

A high corticosteroid dose (200 to 400 mg/day of prednisone orally) is used for several weeks until the disease activity decreases significantly (no new blisters or few blisters).[21] Prednisone dosage may then be reduced to about 40 mg/day, and an immunosuppressant is usually added (azathioprine, 100 mg/day) to reduce total steroid dosage.

Three weeks later, the corticosteroid dose is changed to an alternate-day schedule of 40 mg for 1 year. Attempts to decrease the prednisone dose are made at that time. If the condition flares, high-dose treatment is reinstituted. With this regimen, many patients have cleared and remained free of disease for years.

The mortality rate with this therapeutic approach has been reduced to about 10%. Methotrexate, cyclophosphamide, pulse cyclophosphamide, sulfones, gold salts, cyclosporine, and plasma pheresis have been used as alternative therapies with variable results. Antibiotics should be restricted to the management of proven infections and not be used prophylactically.[21]

Patients undergoing penicillamine therapy for rheumatologic diseases may develop vesiculobullous lesions that on biopsy exhibit superficial epidermal acantholysis in a pattern indistinguishable from pemphigus foliaceus.[20] Direct immunofluorescence testing demonstrates deposition of immunoglobulins in intercellular areas of the epidermis as in pemphigus foliaceus. In most cases, the disease begins 6 to 12 months after the initiation of penicillamine therapy and runs a relatively mild course. Once medication is discontinued, the patient may continue to develop vesiculobullous lesions for several months. The selection of therapy for this special form of pemphigus depends on the severity of the disease. Astringent soaks, topical corticosteroids, sulfapyridine, sulfones, and systemic corticosteroids may be used. If systemic corticosteroids are required, the effective dosage is generally much lower than that used in pemphigus vulgaris. In the rare instances of severe life-threatening disease, initial high corticosteroid dosages are indicated. Paraneoplastic pemphigus is a newly recognized disease that mimics, but can be distinguished, from pemphigus vulgaris in some patients with lymphoproliferative neoplasms and solid tumors.[22]

BULLOUS PEMPHIGOID ■

An uncommon blistering disease, bullous pemphigoid is more prevalent in elderly patients. It runs a self-limited course of approximately 5 to 6 years with periods of exacerbation and remission. Initially, the patient may manifest either localized or extensive skin involvement. Some patients with the localized form never develop generalized disease. Oral mucosal lesions are present in about one third of cases.[20]

The pathognomonic change is a subepidermal bulla that occurs as a result of damage to the lamina lucida of the basement membrane zone.

ETIOLOGY

Bullous pemphigoid is an autoimmune disease. A bullous pemphigoid antigen resides in the basal cell layer or superficial basement membrane zone. This antigen stimulates the development of circulating antibodies with subsequent complement activation. Degranulation of inflammatory cells may release proteolytic enzymes near the lamina lucida, producing the blister.

PRESENTATION

The cutaneous eruption is characterized by vesicles and tense bullae that arise on normal or inflamed skin (Fig. 151-9). Itching associated with the lesions is common, but once ruptured, the exposed skin is not as painful to the patient as in pemphigus vulgaris. Nikolsky's sign is negative in most cases. There is no proven association between internal malignancy and this disease.

DIAGNOSIS

A perilesional skin biopsy shows a subepidermal vesicle or bulla with a variable number of eosinophils in the inflammatory infiltrate and blister fluid. Direct immunofluorescence studies show the linear deposition of immunoglobulin and complement (mainly C3) at the basement membrane zone in a tubular pattern.

MANAGEMENT

The selection of therapy for bullous pemphigoid depends on its severity. Localized forms may be controlled with astringent soaks and high-potency topical corticosteroids. The combination of nicotinamide, 500 mg three times daily, and tetracycline, 500 mg four times daily, is a useful alternative therapy to steroids in mild to moderately severe cases.[23] In severe life-threatening cases, sulfones (dapsone, 50 to 150 mg/day), sulfapyridine (2 to 4 g/day), or systemic corticosteroids (prednisone, 80 to 100 mg/day or higher) may be needed.

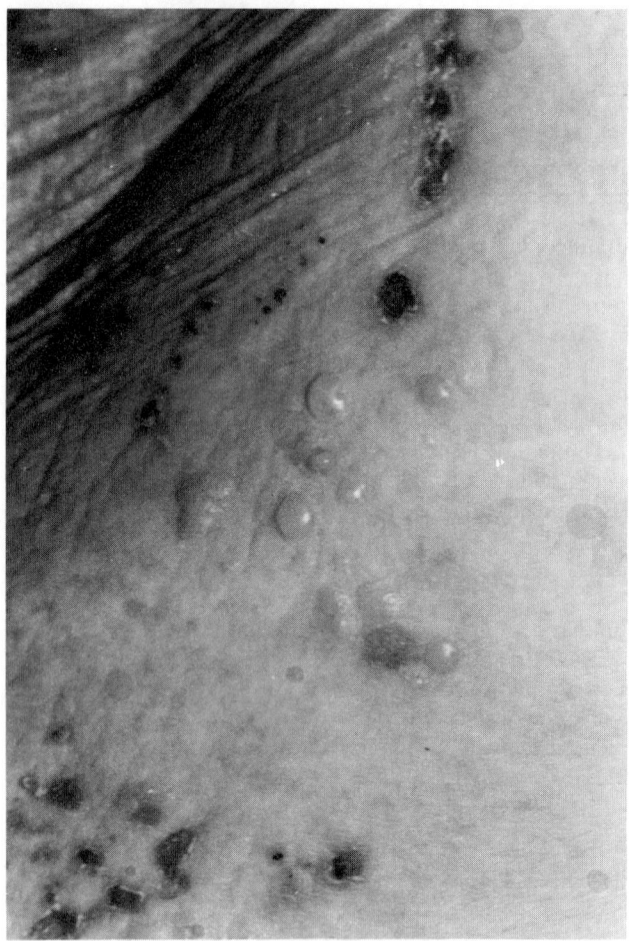

FIGURE 151-9. Vesicles, tense bullae, and crusted sites are seen in patients with bullous pemphigoid.

If high-dose systemic corticosteroids are used, as soon as the disease is under control, alternate-day therapy at a reduced dose (40 mg) is initiated, and an immunosuppressant (azathioprine, 100 mg/day) may be added.[20] Because the disease is self-limited with long periods of remission, attempts to discontinue the corticosteroid therapy are successful in most instances when new blisters have ceased to form. The immunosuppressant alone may control the disease activity in patients requiring long-term management. Eventually, the immunosuppressant also can be discontinued.

ECZEMA HERPETICUM (KAPOSI'S VARICELLIFORM ERUPTION) ■

Herpes simplex and varicella-zoster viruses are DNA-containing agents capable of producing life-threatening clinical manifestations. The outcome of the infection depends on early clinical diagnosis, the patient's age and immunologic status, and coexistence of neoplasia. Severely affected patients may require multispecialty management in an ICU. Data obtained from recent randomized clinical studies demonstrate that acyclovir is the most effective therapeutic agent

available for disseminated herpes simplex and varicella-zoster infections.[24]

A condition first described by Kaposi in 1894, eczema herpeticum results from the inoculation of inflamed skin by herpes simplex virus. A similar pathophysiologic process was responsible for the dissemination of vaccinia virus in atopic patients (eczema vaccinatum) when smallpox vaccination was a common practice in this country. Acyclovir is an effective treatment for eczema herpeticum and can be administered orally or intravenously. Astringent soaks and systemic antibiotics, when indicated, also are valuable therapeutic agents.

PRESENTATION

The infection is usually seen in patients with severe, eczematous atopic dermatitis and is characterized by the presence of multiple superficial crusted lesions that evolve from small umbilicated vesicles or pustules (Fig. 151-10). The patient may remain asymptomatic or demonstrate fever and malaise. Superimposed bacterial infection may lead to septicemia with subsequent internal organ failure. This has been responsible for most fatalities.

ETIOLOGY

Eczema herpeticum is caused by herpes simplex virus. A cellular immunity defect on the part of the host facilitates the development of the clinical syndrome.

DIAGNOSIS

The clinical presentation of multiple crusted erosions, umbilicated vesicles, or pustules in a patient with preexisting atopic eczema is usually diagnostic. Appropriate supportive diagnostic studies include a positive Tzanck preparation and herpes simplex cultures. The Tzanck test is helpful and can be performed rapidly. The base of a vesicular lesion is scraped using a no. 15 surgical blade, the blade is rubbed against a glass slide, the slide is air-dried, and undiluted Giemsa stain (or Wright's stain) is applied. After 30 seconds, the excess stain is removed with gently flowing tap water. The slide is blotted dry with filter paper or a paper towel, and a cover slip is applied. The slide is examined under low and high power to locate multinuclear epidermal squamous cells (epithelial giant cells), which demonstrate abundant basophilic nuclear material (Fig. 151-11). If multinucleated giant cells are seen in the presence of multiple superficial crusted lesions, vesicles, or pustules in a patient with known atopic eczema, a diagnosis of eczema herpeticum is most likely, and appropriate therapy may be initiated without delay. The Tzanck test also is positive in varicella-zoster infections.

MANAGEMENT

Acyclovir has been an effective therapy, shortening the natural course and preventing serious complications. The drug should be given orally or intravenously in a weight-adjusted dosage[25,26] (Table 151-5). Antibiotic therapy should be insti-

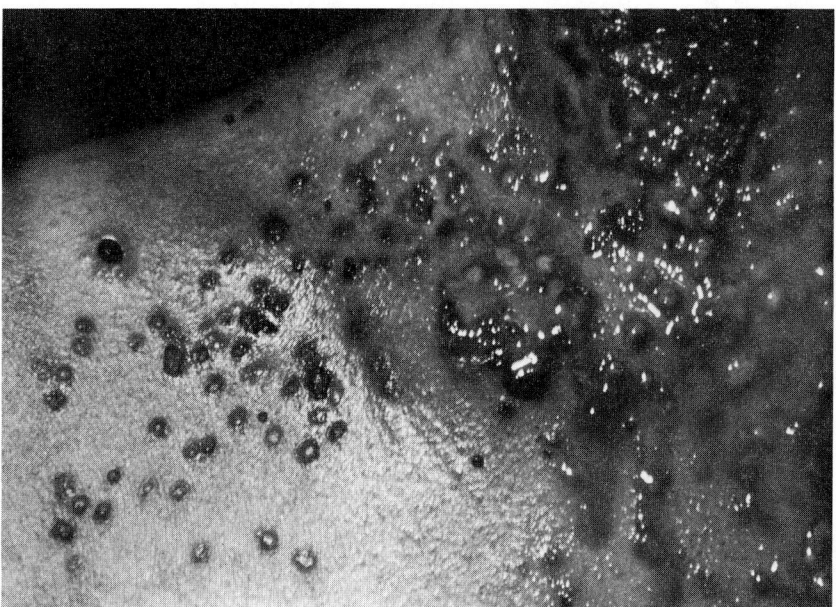

FIGURE 151-10. Multiple vesicles, erosions, and crusted sites are prominent features of eczema herpeticum.

tuted for patients with superimposed bacterial infections. Astringent soaks (Burow's) are helpful in decreasing exudation and crust formation from ruptured vesicles or pustules.

VARICELLA-ZOSTER INFECTIONS ■

Disseminated varicella-zoster infection with visceral involvement occurs in about 2% of the patients with "shingles" but in a much higher percentage of immunosuppressed patients with underlying Hodgkin's disease or other conditions, including HIV infection.

ETIOLOGY

The varicella-zoster virus is responsible for life-threatening infections like encephalitis and pneumonitis in susceptible individuals. They occur as a sequela to primary (varicella) or recurrent (herpes zoster) infections.

PRESENTATION

Viral pneumonitis and encephalitis are ominous clinical developments in these patients. Cough, respiratory difficulty, chest pain, or neurologic abnormalities may be clinical signs

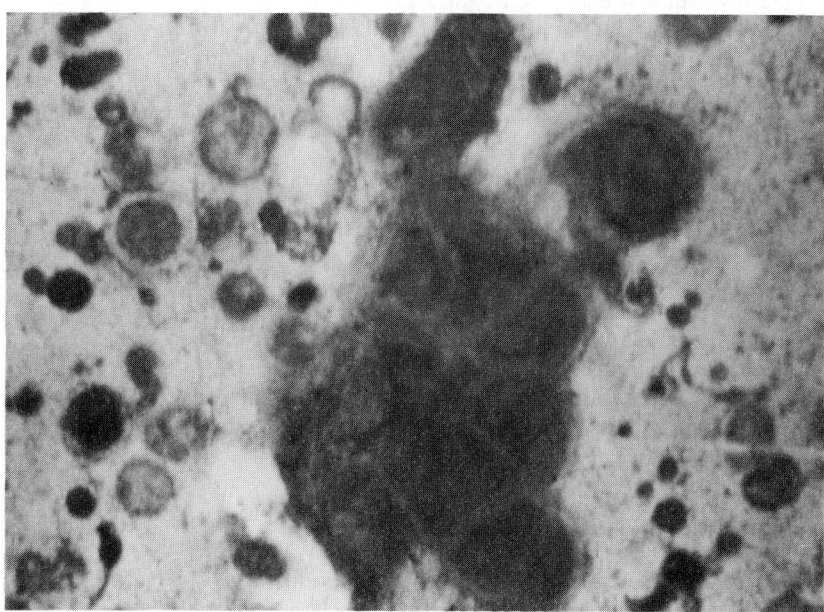

FIGURE 151-11. Tzanck smear demonstrates multinucleated epidermal giant cells (originial magnification ×400).

TABLE 151-5. Therapy for Life-Threatening Viral Infections

Eczema herpeticum
　Acylovir
　　25 mg/kg/d orally for 5 d; give individual doses every 4 h, 5
　　　times/d
　　5 mg/kg/8 h IV for 5 d
Antibiotics
　IV or orally for treatment of superimposed bacterial infections
Disseminated varicella-zoster infections with organ involvement
　(encephalitis or pneumonitis)
Acyclovir
　10 mg/kg/d IV for 10d°
Vidarabine
　10 mg/kg/d IV for 5d

IV, intravenously.
°Infuse over at least 1 h to prevent crystallization in renal tubules.
Monitor creatinine clearance during therapeutic course.

of varicella-zoster virus dissemination in a patient with ante-cedent dermatomal herpes zoster or chicken pox. Multiple vesicular lesions occurring away from the original derma-tome of involvement are the dermatologic sign of dissemina-tion in patients with herpes zoster (Fig. 151-12). In most instances, it represents increased viral activity resulting from the host's immunocompromised status.

DIAGNOSIS

The correlation between the clinical picture and a positive Tzanck smear from an active lesion is usually diagnostic. Viral cultures provide confirmation of the initial clinical impressions.

MANAGEMENT

These patients should be managed in an ICU once internal organ involvement is apparent. Intravenous administration of acyclovir or vidarabine has been helpful (see Table 151-5). Acyclovir is the most effective preventive and therapeutic agent.[27] The outcome is usually dictated by the primary illness and associated host immune status.

DRUG ERUPTIONS ■

Drug eruptions affect at least 2% to 3% of all medical inpa-tients and many are not reported.[28,29] In my experience, they are the most common reason a dermatologist is consulted in an ICU. Eruptions vary in morphologic appearance and severity and are classified as morbilliform, urticarial, and bullous. EM, Stevens-Johnson syndrome, and toxic epider-mal necrolysis also are included.

MORBILLIFORM

Typical morbilliform eruptions occur within the first 7 days of initiation of therapy. However, with ampicillin the rash may occur after 1 to 28 days of administration. It may also

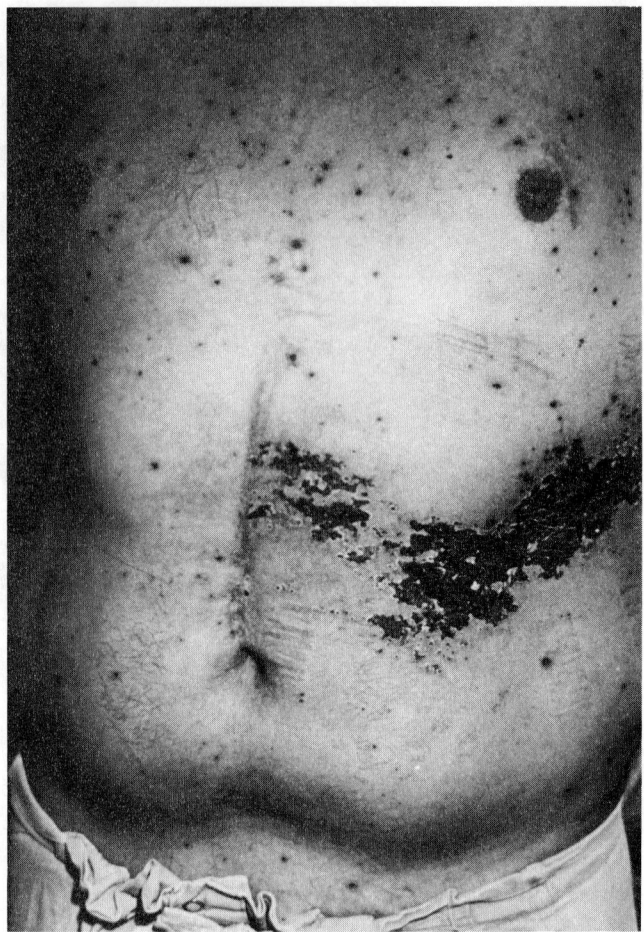

FIGURE 151-12. Herpes zoster with dermatomal involvement and disseminated lesions.

appear up to 2 weeks after termination of therapy and persist for 1 to 2 weeks.

The eruptions are maculopapular, and initially they occur on the trunk or in dependent areas, especially in ICU pa-tients. The erythematous macules and papules are usually symmetric and tend to become confluent (Fig. 151-13). Involvement of mucous membranes, palms, and soles is variable.

When the physician sees a red morbilliform eruption, several questions should be asked. What is the etiology of this rash? If it is a drug eruption, which drug? Will therapy need altering? Finally, will the eruption be treated? Viral exanthems cause the most confusion in differentiation from a drug eruption. The clinical setting is sometimes helpful, but occasionally they are impossible to differentiate, even with biopsy.

First, make a list of the patient's medications and tempo-rally relate them to the onset of the rash. When this is complete, decide if the patient has just taken any medica-tions with a high incidence of drug eruptions. Most eruptions are caused by relatively few medications. The greatest inci-dence occurs with the penicillins, sulfonamides, phenytoin, and barbiturates. Blood products also produce a high inci-

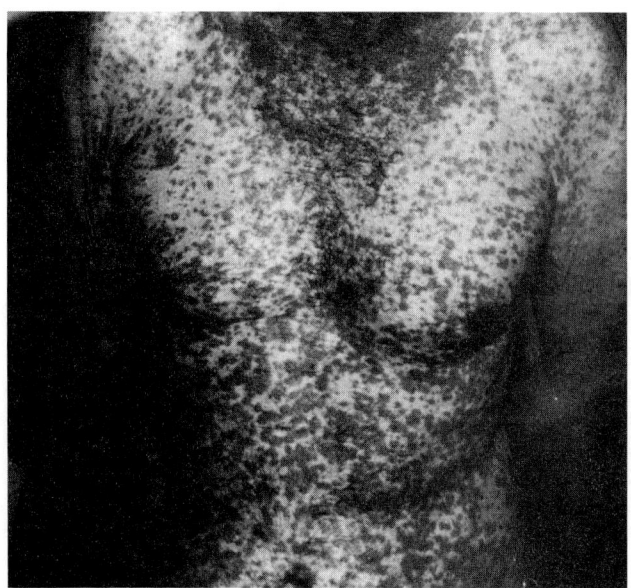

FIGURE 151-13. Diffuse morbilliform drug eruption.

dence of eruptions. Interestingly, aspirin, hydrochlorothiazide, and tetracycline caused no reactions in one study.[28]

Although I recommend switching to another medication when feasible, if necessary, continue a drug in the face of a morbilliform eruption without fear of precipitating an anaphylactic episode. In some instances, the eruption fades with continued therapy. Pruritus, usually the only complication, is treated with topical antipruritics. A hydrocortisone 1% cream or ointment or Sarna lotion containing menthol and phenol is useful. Oral antihistamines, alone or in combination, are titrated to relieve the itching.

Progression of the rash to an exfoliative erythroderma demands close monitoring. High-output cardiac states occur secondary to cutaneous vasodilation. Anemia, eosinophilia, and hypoalbuminemia are common. Intake and output should be monitored because of an excess of extrarenal water loss. For cutaneous therapy, use open wet dressings, total body if applicable, followed by a mild steroid ointment, either hydrocortisone or a nonfluorinated steroid. The key to this therapy is evaporation. Wet dressings are applied by placing a thin cotton material (e.g., bed linen) in lukewarm water, wringing it out, and laying it over the red skin for 15 to 20 minutes. This procedure is repeated every 3 to 4 hours while the patient is awake. The cooling, vasoconstrictive effect of evaporation is desired. Soaks and wet compresses are not as effective. Plain water is as beneficial as astringent tablets.

The pathogenesis of a morbilliform eruption remains unknown; however, it does not seem to be allergic in origin. Some investigators believe, especially with antibiotic reactions, that the rash may be secondary to the release of bacterial endotoxins. Others think it may be a manifestation of an underlying systemic disease.

URTICARIAL

The term *urticaria* encompasses a broad spectrum of disease. The diagnosis of urticaria is relatively easy, but determining its etiology may be difficult. Acute urticaria and chronic urticaria (present for more than 6 weeks) can be associated with neoplasia, collagen vascular disease, infections, and other chronic diseases. For this discussion, assume the urticaria is acute and secondary to a medication.

Urticarial eruptions may occur within minutes of administration of the drug as part of an anaphylactic reaction. Those occurring within 12 to 36 hours may be part of an IgE-dependent accelerated reaction. Urticaria arising 7 to 10 days after administration of a medication may signify a serum sickness syndrome or the nonimmunologic activation of effector pathways.

Clinically, the dermis is infiltrated with fluid that gives an indurated orange peel appearance to the skin (Fig. 151-14). The lesions can attain great size and may appear arcuate.

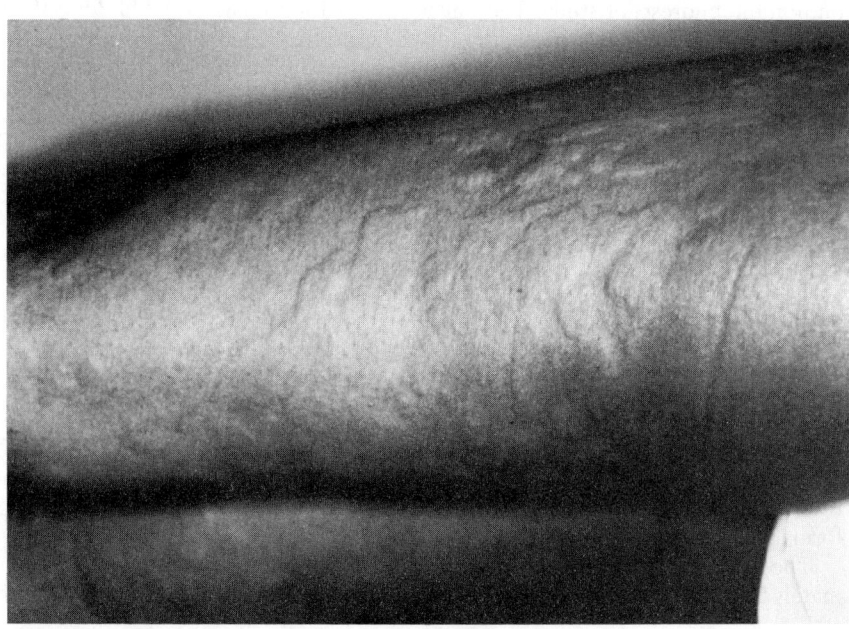

FIGURE 151-14. Large plaque of urticaria.

Purpura may accompany the lesions, especially in dependent areas, secondary to hydrostatic pressure. The plaques resolve in 12 to 24 hours without residua. If the lesions persist more than 48 hours and are associated with pain and purpura, a biopsy should be obtained to rule out urticarial vasculitis.

No specific laboratory tests yield abnormal results, and a skin biopsy is usually unnecessary. History often suffices in disclosing a temporal relationship between the urticaria and initiation of therapy.

Treatment consists of identifying and discontinuing the offending medication. Dietary restrictions also may be helpful. For example, patients with a penicillin allergy should avoid dairy products because they may contain traces of penicillin. In about 25% of patients with drug-induced urticaria, the pathogenesis involves an IgE-mediated type 1 immunologic reaction. Patients should be advised to never again take that medication for fear of an anaphylactic episode. They may also be referred to an allergist for more intensive skin testing.

Oral antihistamines of the H_1 type are the mainstay of therapy. Combinations consisting of two or three H_1 antihistamines can be used in the more difficult cases. Doxepin hydrochloride (Sinequan), which has potent H_1-blocking effects and some evidence of H_2-blocking effects, is being used in difficult cases with good results. Severe urticarial reactions associated with wheezing, laryngeal edema, and circulatory collapse may require subcutaneous epinephrine, tracheal intubation, and systemic corticosteroids.

BULLOUS

Bullous drug reactions have been documented secondary to the drug itself, the drug plus light, and in drug overdoses—the so-called coma blisters. Bromides, iodides, mercury, arsenic, salicylates, phenolphthalein, minoxidil, and penicillamine have been associated with generalized bullous reactions.[30] These bullae may be hemorrhagic. The mechanism of blister formation is unknown. The diagnosis is made by combining the history with a skin biopsy and negative results on immunofluorescent study. The bullae recur with rechallenge. Therapy consists of discontinuing the causative agent and using supportive skin care. Large bullae may require aspiration and topical antibiotic coverage. Phototoxic bullous drug eruptions can be caused by furosemide, tetracycline, psoralen, and nalidixic acid.

Patients in coma secondary to a narcotic overdose, carbon monoxide poisoning, accident, or illness may develop bullae. Classically, erythema followed by cyanosis and blister formation appears over pressure points, usually within the first 24 hours. Bullae may be solitary or multiple, of varying size, usually with clear fluid. They resolve spontaneously, without scarring, in 10 to 14 days.

The diagnosis is made by history, and the skin biopsy is diagnostic. Extensive sweat gland necrosis is found with occasional similar involvement of the pilosebaceous glands. Supportive therapy is similar to that for bullous drug reactions. Constant attention to pressure points inhibits blister formation.

The incidence rate of blisters in drug overdoses is approximately 5%.[30] The exact mechanism of formation is unknown.

Speculation on causative factors includes hypoxia, trauma, or a direct toxic effect of the drug. Bullae have been reported with central nervous system disease, and this should be kept in mind. Furthermore, it does not seem that coma is essential for blister formation. Duration of pressure seems to play a major role.

PURPURA ■

Purpura is a condition characterized by hemorrhage into the skin. Petechiae are hemorrhagic macules less than 3 mm in size, whereas ecchymoses are hemorrhagic macules greater than 3 mm. If purpura is suspected, diascopy should be done first. The failure of a lesion to completely blanch on pressure from a glass slide is a reliable indication that extravasated red blood cells may be present. Next, determine if the lesions are palpable. Palpable purpura implies vasculitis until proven otherwise. Flat purpura is an extremely uncommon manifestation of vasculitis. Finally, determine whether the purpuric pattern is vasculitic (round or oval) or infarctive (sharply angulated).

SENILE

Perhaps the most common type of purpura is senile purpura. Occurring predominantly in elderly patients, senile purpura is diagnosed clinically. Large, flat, violaceous ecchymoses are observed principally on the dorsal aspects of the arms and hands. These lesions fade over 1 to 2 weeks without scarring. The typical color changes of a resolving bruise become evident. The underlying mechanism seems to be trauma to cutaneous vessels in skin with minimal supporting stroma. All clotting parameters are normal. There is no specific therapy. However, if the skin becomes too fragile and tears, an antibiotic ointment should be applied to prevent secondary infection. Corticosteroids, either topical or oral, compound the situation.

MECHANICAL

Mechanical purpura is a phenomenon caused by either decreased outside capillary pressure or increased intracapillary pressure. Petechiae near the eyes or soft palate can be caused by coughing or vomiting. Externally applied suction cups, such as those used during an electrocardiographic examination, may result in round flat ecchymoses. This type of purpura resolves spontaneously without sequelae. All clotting parameters are normal.

DRUG-INDUCED

Other important causes of purpura are medications. Some medications (e.g., aspirin) impair platelet function, whereas others cause vasculitis. Up to 20% of thrombocytopenic purpura may be drug induced. Diagnosis is made by history and laboratory findings. Any new medication should be dis-

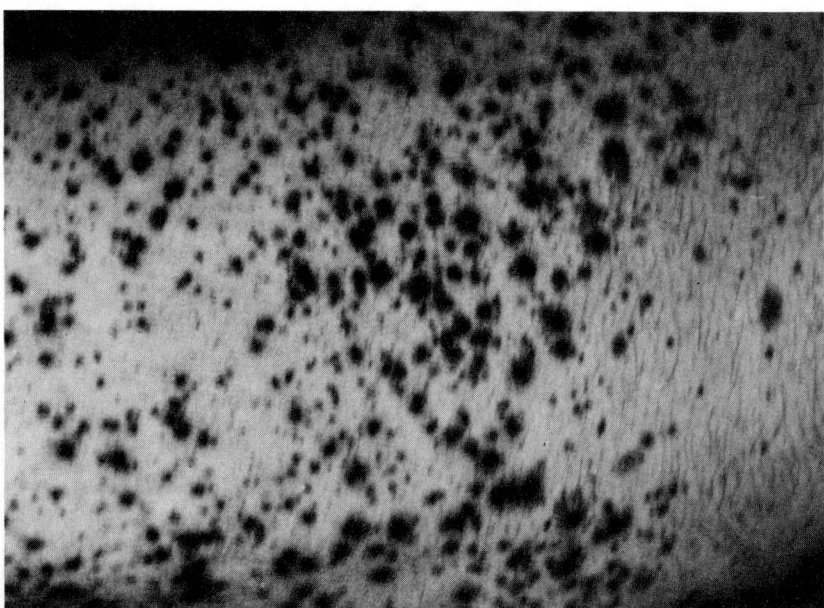

FIGURE 151-15. Multiple round to oval purpuric papules of leukocytoclastic vasculitis.

continued, and a comparable medication of different chemical structure administered. Platelets, bleeding time, clotting parameters, and bone marrow biopsy may be indicated. If the thrombocytopenia persists 2 weeks after cessation of the medication, then an etiology other than that of medication should be sought.

VASCULITIC

The term *vasculitis* means inflammation of blood vessel walls. There are many different types of vasculitis, but this section concentrates on an immune complex disease of the postcapillary venules called leukocytoclastic vasculitis (LCV), which is an allergic or hypersensitivity vasculitis. Its clinical presentation, diagnosis, etiology, and treatment are discussed.

Clinically, LCV generally presents as palpable purpura of the lower extremities, occasionally with edema (Fig. 151-15), often accompanied by abdominal pain, arthralgia, and renal involvement. Because the postcapillary venules are inflamed, the vessels leak. Extravasated red blood cells then percolate to the surface and form round or oval areas of palpable purpura, which may coalesce to become polycyclic. The morphologically round purpuric papules form the so-called vasculitic pattern of purpura. This is an extremely important clinical finding. Opposed to this is the infarctive pattern described later.

The finding of palpable purpura implies a vasculitis until proven otherwise. The workup consists of a detailed history for a possible etiology and a complete physical examination to determine the presence and extent of systemic involvement. A skin biopsy confirms the diagnosis, and the laboratory tests listed in Table 151-6 should be considered. A urinalysis should be performed during the initial examination to look for proteinuria and microscopic hematuria; this should be repeated in 3 to 4 days, and again, after the vasculitis has resolved. If abnormalities persist, further renal workup is indicated. The remainder of laboratory results direct future investigations.

There are many etiologies of LCV, including streptococcal infections and viral influenza, medications, foreign proteins, and systemic disease (e.g., collagen vascular diseases and malignancies). An in-depth analysis is found in many reviews.[31]

Treatment consists of first identifying the offending agent and removing it, if possible. Further therapy is determined by the extent and severity of renal disease. Other possible considerations for therapeutic intervention are involvement of joints and the gastrointestinal tract. If the patient is asymptomatic and the blood test results are normal, no therapy is indicated. Antihistamines to decrease vascular permeability and aspirin for its antiinflammatory and antichemotactic activity may be used. If the kidneys are involved, oral corticosteroids are indicated. If the patient's condition deteriorates,

TABLE 151-6. Laboratory Workup for Leukocytoclastic Vasculitis

Skin Biopsy
Urinalysis
Antistreptolysin O titer
Antinuclear antibody, rheumatoid factor
Sedimentation rate
Complete blood count
Chest radiograph
Hematest stool
Hepatitis panel
Cryoglobulins
Total complement
Throat culture, if indicated

cytotoxic agents should be used. Fauci and coworkers[32] found cyclophosphamide (2 mg/kg/day) to be effective.

INFARCTIVE

Fortunately, the infarctive pattern of hemorrhage into the skin is not common. There are two major differences in the pathogenesis of the vasculitic versus the infarctive pattern. Leakage of the superficial postcapillary venule forming round, purpuric papules is the hallmark of the vasculitic pattern. Blockage of distal blood flow of the deeper dermal and subcutaneous arterioles results in the infarctive pattern. The end result of this blockage is irregularly outlined areas of purpura with sharp, angulated borders. Four basic pathophysiologic mechanisms are involved in infarctive lesions:

1. Hypoperfusion—cardiac failure
2. Vasospasm—medications, Raynaud's disease, cold injury, livedo vasculitis
3. Embolic—septic, cholesterol, cryoglobulin, disseminated intravascular coagulation, hemoglobinopathies
4. Inflammation surrounding the vessel—polyarteritis nodosa, Wegener's granulomatosis, allergic granulomatosis

The underlying mechanism is cessation of blood flow through the deep dermal plexus.

Infarctive patterns of purpura are much more serious and important skin findings and demand prompt intervention. Acute meningococcemia is an excellent example of infarctive purpura (Fig. 151-16). Diagnosis and workups are individualized to the clinical setting. Blood work, cultures, and skin biopsy are usually required immediately. Treatment varies with the underlying disease.

ANTICOAGULANT NECROSIS

Anticoagulant therapy has been associated with purpuric skin findings. Although rare, a higher incidence is expected in an emergency setting where these medications are frequently required.

Coumarin

Coumarin necrosis is a well-defined entity. Classically, between day 3 and 10 of coumarin loading, the symptoms begin. A sudden onset of pain is followed by purpura, bulla formation, and necrosis. More than 90% of affected patients are women, obese, and middle-aged.[33] The usual sites are those with significant areas of subcutaneous adipose tissue, such as the breasts, buttocks, abdomen, and thighs. Interestingly, the lesions do not progress with continued use of the medication. Furthermore, coumarin necrosis does not necessarily recur with subsequent courses of therapy.

The diagnosis is made according to the clinical setting and morphologic appearance of the lesions. A skin biopsy is helpful in ruling out vasculitis. Coagulation studies eliminate excessive anticoagulant therapy as an etiology. A relationship with protein C deficiency, and occasionally protein S deficiency, often can be documented.

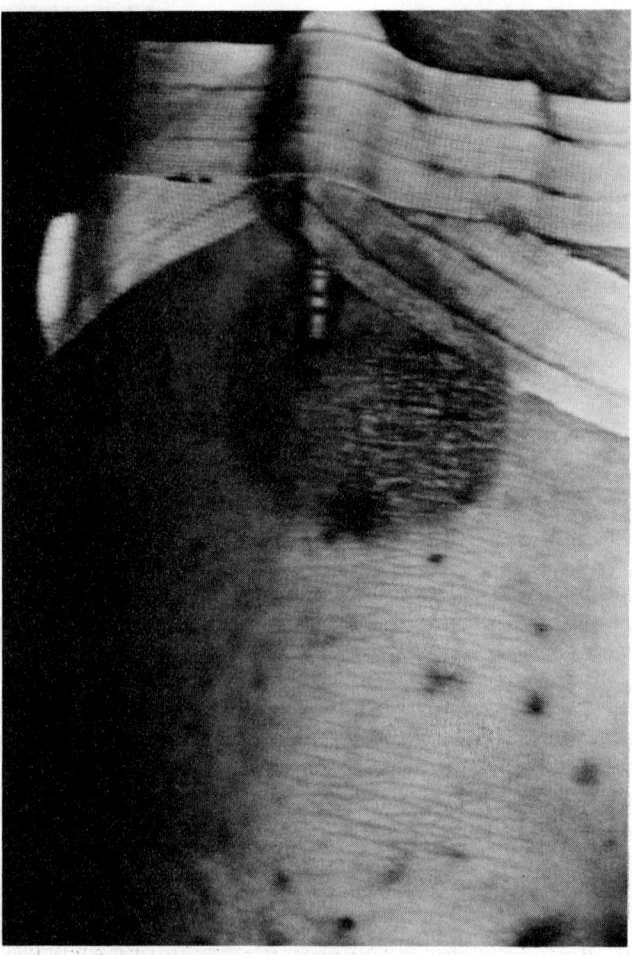

FIGURE 151-16. Infarctive pattern of hemorrhage in patient with acute meningococcemia.

Therapy is supportive. Management of the necrotic areas varies with the depth of involvement. In some instances, grafting may be necessary.

Other cutaneous manifestations of coumarin therapy consist of hemorrhage, vesicular and morbilliform eruptions, alopecia, and the "purple toe" syndrome. Purple toes appear 3 to 8 weeks after initiation of coumarin; they can be tender and blanch with pressure or elevation.

Heparin

Cutaneous ecchymoses, usually at the site of injection, are the most common adverse reaction to heparin therapy. Other reported areas of bleeding are the adrenal glands, urinary tract, and gastrointestinal tract. Heparin necrosis is a far less common occurrence but of much more clinical importance. Skin necrosis usually occurs at the injection site but has been documented at distant locations. Obese, middle-aged, diabetic women are particularly vulnerable. Treatment with broad-spectrum antibiotics has been shown to increase the risk.[34]

Heparin necrosis seems to follow a typical course. A burning pain appears 6 to 13 days after start of therapy. Localized erythema quickly develops into a bulla followed by frank necrosis. This evolution occurs in 12 to 24 hours.

The diagnosis is made based on the clinical setting and is suggested by skin biopsy. A platelet count is extremely important. Evidence suggests that heparin induces the development of a platelet-aggregating factor.[34] The end result of this process is intravascular thrombosis. Skin necrosis can then be a harbinger of a dangerous triad consisting of skin necrosis, thrombocytopenia, and myocardial infarction.

Cutaneous ecchymoses are a common clinical finding requiring no therapy. Skin necrosis with thrombocytopenia is much more ominous. Heparin therapy should be discontinued and coumarin considered. Localized supportive skin care as described for coumarin necrosis is appropriate.

ACQUIRED IMMUNODEFICIENCY SYNDROME ■

An extensive and ever-expanding variety of skin findings have been reported in acquired immunodeficiency syndrome (AIDS)[35] (Table 151-7). In a 2.8-year study of 684 HIV-infected subjects, each individual averaged 3.7 separate skin diagnoses.[36] The most important clinical consideration is that the skin eruptions in these immunocompromised patients may appear atypical. Clinical suspicion must be high, especially for infectious disorders such as candidiasis, herpes simplex, cryptococcosis, and bacillary angiomatosis. Severe infections with *Candida*, fungi, herpes simplex, or herpes zoster may be the first sign of AIDS and should be investigated with a thorough history, physical examination, and HIV serologic studies. Oral hairy leukoplakia presents as distinct white, verrucous "hairy" plaques on the sides of the tongue and is a combined infection with *Candida*, Epstein-Barr virus, and papilloma virus.[37]

Kaposi's sarcoma is classically described as violaceous nodules on the lower extremities of elderly men. In AIDS patients, these patches, plaques, or firm nodules may resemble ecchymoses, nevi, dermatofibromas, or even eczema (Fig. 151-17). Biopsy is necessary to discriminate the recently described entity of bacillary epithelioid angiomatosis.[38] In this condition, multiple violaceous nodules that simulate Kaposi's sarcoma and pyogenic granulomas appear rapidly. The etiologic agent is similar to the cat scratch bacillus and responds rapidly to oral antibiotic therapy.

CONTACT DERMATITIS ■

Between 5% to 10% of a dermatologist's practice consists of patients with contact dermatitis. It can be caused by either an allergy or an irritant, with the latter being the most common. First, obtain a history for any substance applied to the skin and any activities, especially outdoors, that may have exposed the patient to an allergen. These include topical medications, cleansing agents, and all type of plants, foods, and chemicals. Then examine the patient.

Clinically, vesicles on an erythematous base, in a linear arrangement, are the hallmark of contact dermatitis. The physician should look for sharply angulated arrangements and right angles in an eruption. These signal an "outside contact" as opposed to a systemic finding. The eruption is localized to the area of the contact. Irritant reactions occur in numerous patients immediately after exposure to the irritant, do not require a previous exposure or sensitization, and are not immunologic reactions. Allergic contact reactions are type IV delayed hypersensitivity reactions, occur 24 to 72 hours after exposure, and require previous sensitization.

A typical history of an allergic contact dermatitis reaction to a topical medication consists of an eruption initially re-

TABLE 151-7. Cutaneous Skin Findings Associated with AIDS

Kaposi's sarcoma
Thrombocytopenic purpura
Seborrheic dermatitis, severe
Infections: molluscum contagiosum, herpes simplex, herpes zoster, verruca vulgaris, condyloma acuminatum, syphilis, cytomegalic virus, cryptococcosis, histoplasmosis, *Mycobacterium*, scabies, cutaneous *Pneumocystis carinii*
Bacillary epithelioid angiomatosis
Oral candidiasis
White, hairy oral leukoplakia
Evanescent maculopapular eruption
Eosinophilic pustular folliculitis
Chronic acne-like follicular inflammation (often in the axilla)
Impetigo in neck and beard area
Dermatophyte infections
Acquired keratoderma of soles
Acquired ichthyosis
Alopecia
Morbilliform drug eruptions
Reiter's syndrome and psoriasis

AIDS, acquired immunodeficiency syndrome.

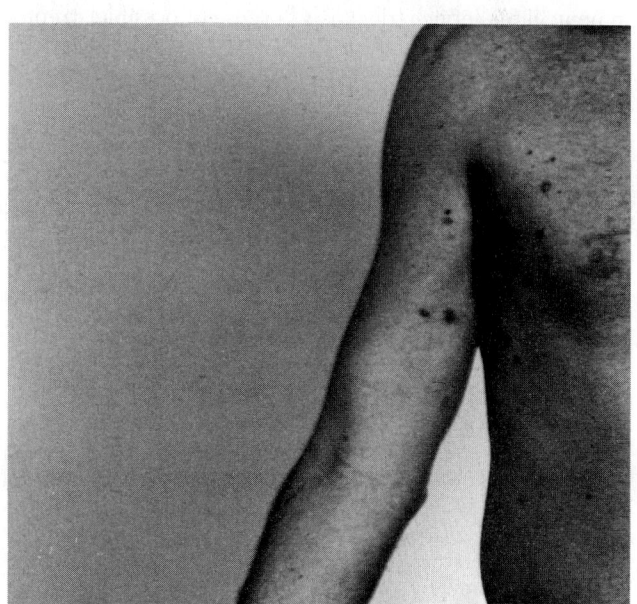

FIGURE 151-17. Multiple violaceous papules of Kaposi's sarcoma in an AIDS patient.

sponding to an applied cream, but then becoming much worse. Remember that even topical steroids may contain sensitizing chemicals. Patients also may be sensitized to topical medications by cross-reacting oral medication.

Treatment consists of discontinuing the topical medication or irritant and finding an alternative. Open wet dressings followed by a topical steroid ointment are indicated. Antihistamines titrated to eliminate pruritus also may be necessary, especially at night. Oral corticosteroids are indicated in acute contact dermatitis if the reaction is widespread. I prefer a 3-week tapering course of prednisone and prescribe 60 mg orally for 1 week, then 40 mg orally the second week, followed by 20 mg daily the final week in an average-sized individual.

NECROTIZING FASCIITIS ■

Necrotizing fasciitis is a relatively rare, severe, and life-threatening, infectious process that involves the sheaths around skeletal muscles. It presents as a deep cellulitis with a warm, tender, indurated, erythematous plaque. The key to suspecting the deeper and more serious involvement is the rapid extension, of both depth and induration, and overall progression in size.

A recent publication[39] documents a marked increase in incidence in several countries including the United States, the United Kingdom, and the Netherlands. Group A streptococci of various subtypes are the etiologic agents. Case fatality rates range from 20% to 50% with rapid, widespread necrosis of muscle.

Most isolates have been sensitive to penicillin. Immediate treatment of all clinically suspected cases with 2.4 g of benzylpenicillin every 4 hours is recommended.[39] Additionally, clindamycin, 0.6 to 1.2 g every 6 hours, should be considered in more severe cases. Erythromycin is not a good substitute in penicillin-allergic individuals because of possible streptococcal antibiotic resistance.

REFERENCES ■

1. Huff JC, Weston WL, Tonnesen MG: Erythema multiforme: a critical review of characteristics, diagnostic criteria, and causes. *J Am Acad Dermatol* 1983;8:763
2. Schofield JK, Tatnell FM, Leigh FM: Recurrent erythema multiforme: clinical features and treatment in a large series of patients. *Br J Dermatol* 1993;128:542
3. Prendiville JS, Herbert AA, Greenwald MJ, et al: Management of Stevens-Johnson syndrome and toxic epidermal necrolysis in children. *J Pediatr* 1989;115:881
4. Renfrol L, Grant-Kels JM, Feder HM Jr, et al: Controversy: are systemic steroids indicated in the treatment of erythema multiforme? *Pediatr Dermatol* 1989;6:43
5. Patterson R, Dykewicz MS, Gonzales A, et al: Erythema multiforme and Stevens-Johnsons syndrome: descriptive and therapeutic controversy. *Chest* 1990;98:331
6. Lozada-Nur F, Cram D, Gorsky M: Clinical response to levamisole in 39 patients with erythema multiforme: an open prospective stydy. *Oral Surg Oral Med Oral Pathol* 1992;74:294
7. Lyell A: A review of toxic epidermal necrolysis in Britain. *Br J Dermatol* 1967;79:662
8. Peck G, Gerzig GP, Elias PM: Toxic epidermal necrolysis in a patient with graft-vs-host reaction. *Arch Dermatol* 1972; 105:561
9. Ward DJ, Krzeminska EC, Tanner NS: Treatment of toxic epidermal necrolysis and review of six cases. *Burns* 1990;16:97
10. Kamanabros D, Schnmitz-Laudgraf W, Czarnelski BM: Plasmapheresis in severe drug-induced toxic epidermal necrolysis. *Arch Dermatol* 1985;121:1548
11. Hewitt J, Ormerod AD: Toxic epidermal necrolysis treated with cyclosporin. *Clin Exp Dermatol* 1992;17:264
12. Murono K, Fujita K, Yoshioka H: Microbiologic characteristics of exfoliative toxin-producing staphylococcus. *Pediatr Infect Dis J* 1988;7:313
13. Baker H, Ryan TJ: Generalized pustular psoriasis: a clinical and epidemiological study of 104 cases. *Br J Dermatol* 1968;80:771
14. Ryan TJ, Baker H: The prognosis of generalized pustular psoriasis. *Br J Dermatol* 1971;85:407
15. Honigsmann H, Gschnait F, Konrad K, et al: Photochemotherapy for pustular psoriasis (von Zumbusch). *Br J Dermatol* 1977;97:119
16. Fristsch PO: Retinoids in psoriasis and disorders of keratinization. *J Am Acad Dermatol* 1992;27:58
17. Meinardi MM, deRie MA, Bos JD: Oral cyclosporin A in the treatment of psoriasis. *Br J Dermatol* 1990;122(7
18. Shuster S: The metabolic and haemodynamic effects of skin disease. *Ann Clin Res* 1971;3:135
19. Freedberg I, Baden H: The metabolic response to exfoliation. *J Invest Dermatol* 1962;38:277
20. Lever WF: Pemphigus and pemphigoid: a review of the advances made since 1964. *J Am Acad Dermatol* 1979;1:2
21. Lever WF, Schaumburg-Lever G: Treatment of pemphigus vulgaris: results obtained in 84 patients between 1961 and 1982. *Arch Dermatol* 1984;120:44
22. Mutasin DF, Pelc NJ, Anhalt GJ: Paraneoplastic pemphigus. *Dermatol Clin* 1993;11:473
23. Fivenson DP, Breneman DL, Rosen GB, et al: Nicotinamide and tetracycline therpay of bullous pemphigoid. *Arch Dermatol* 1994;130:753
24. Bork K, Brauninger W: Increasing incidence of eczema herpeticum: analysis of 75 cases. *J Am Acad Dermatol* 1988;19:1024
25. Woolfson H: Oral acyclovir in eczema herpeticum. *Br Med J* 1984;288:531
26. David TJ, Longson M: Herpes simplex infections in atopic eczema. *Arch Dis Child* 1985;60:338
27. Shepp DH, Dandliker PS, Meyers JD: Treatment of varicella-zoster virus infection in severely immunocompromised patients: a randomized comparison of acyclovir and vidarabine. *N Engl J Med* 1986;314:208
28. Arndt KA, Jick H: Rates of cutaneous reactions to drugs. *JAMA* 1976;235:918
29. Roujeau JC, Stern RS: Severe adverse cutaneous reactions to drugs. *N Engl J Med* 1994;331:1272
30. Murray JC: Miscellaneous blistering diseases. *Dermatol Clin* 1983;1:318
31. Jeanette CJ, Milling DM, Falk RJ: Vasculitis affecting the skin. *Arch Dermatol* 1994;130:899
32. Fauci A, Katz S, Haynes P, et al: Cyclophosphamide therapy of severe systemic necrotizing vasculitis. *N Engl J Med* 1979; 301:235
33. Anderson DR, Brill-Edwards P, Walker I: Warfarin induced skin necrosis in two patients with protein S deficiency: successful reinstatement of warfarin therapy. *Haemostasis* 1992;22:124
34. Gross AS, Thompson FL, Arzubiag MC, et al: Heparin associated thrombocytopenia and thrombosis presenting with livedo reticularis. *Int J Dermatol* 1993;32:276

35. Cockerall CJ: Cutaneous manifestations of HIV infection other than Kaposi's sarcoma: clinical histologic aspects. *J Am Acad Dermatol* 1990;22:1260
36. Stern RS: Epidemiology of skin diseases in HIV infection: a cohort study of health maintenance organization members. *J Invest Dermatol* 1994;102:345
37. Resnick L, Herbst JS, Raab-Traub N: Oral hairy leukoplakia. *J Am Acad Dermatol* 1990;22:1278
38. Leboit PE, Egbert B, Stolen MH, et al: Epithelioid haemangioma-like vascular proliferations in AIDS: manifestation of cat scratch disease bacillus infection? *Lancet* 1988;i:960
39. Necrotizing fasciitis. *Wkly Epidemiol Rec* 1994;69:165

Critical Care, Third Edition, edited by Joseph M. Civetta,
Robert W. Taylor, and Robert R. Kirby.
Lippincott-Raven Publishers, Philadelphia, PA © 1997.

CHAPTER 152

Rhabdomyolysis

J. Christopher Farmer

IMMEDIATE CONCERNS ■

MAJOR PROBLEMS

Rhabdomyolysis is a clinical and laboratory syndrome resulting from skeletal muscle injury with release of cell contents into the plasma.[1] Clinical sequelae result from local injury (e.g., muscle injury, edema formation, and regional neurovascular compression) and from the systemic effects of the many biochemical toxins released (e.g., effects of myoglobin on the kidney).

STRESS POINTS

1. The causes of rhabdomyolysis are listed in Table 152-1.
2. Generally, these conditions lead to rhabdomyolysis when demand for oxygen and metabolic substrate exceeds available supply or when an inability to use the available supply develops.
3. Primary muscle injury, infection, and various toxins also may cause rhabdomyolysis.
4. Alcohol, drugs of abuse, overexertion, seizures, viral infections, and compression or crush syndromes are most frequently cited as etiologies.[2-5]
5. In particular, human immunodeficiency virus (HIV) infection and cocaine-associated rhabdomyolysis are increasingly common entities in urban populations.[6-12]
6. A complete list of toxins associated with rhabdomyolysis is provided in Table 152-2.

ESSENTIAL DIAGNOSTIC TESTS AND PROCEDURES

1. A diagnosis of rhabdomyolysis often cannot be determined by physical examination. Myoedema, myalgia,

and "doughy"-feeling muscles are classically described but are inconsistent findings at best.
2. Diagnosis usually depends on a high index of clinical suspicion in the appropriate clinical setting, followed by confirmatory laboratory findings.[13]
3. The presence of myoglobin in the urine and elevated muscle enzyme activity in the serum (skeletal muscle creatine kinase [MM-CK], aldolase, carbonic anhydrase III) are diagnostic. However, clinically significant rhabdomyolysis may occur without grossly visible myoglobin pigment in the urine.
4. Other important admission laboratory findings are hyperkalemia, hypocalcemia, hyperphosphatemia, and hyperuricemia. The blood urea nitrogen (BUN):creatinine ratio is decreased. Ratios as low a 2 to 3 have been reported, strongly suggesting the diagnosis of rhabdomyolysis.[14]
5. Hypomagnesemia also may be seen in alcoholic patients with this disorder and may contribute to its development.[15,16]
6. The calculated anion gap in patients with pigment-induced acute renal failure is markedly elevated in patients with rhabdomyolysis compared with that found from other causes of renal failure.[1]
7. Disseminated intravascular coagulation (DIC) is invariably present to a greater or lesser degree. Thrombocytopenia also is common (with or without DIC).
8. Electrocardiographic changes (ST segment depression, T wave inversion) have been reported in a young adult patient without underlying cardiac disease, and were presumed to represent involvement of cardiac muscle by the same process that incited rhabdomyolysis.[17] These changes were self-limited and without sequelae.

TABLE 152-1.   Etiologic Factors in Rhabdomyolysis

TRAUMATIC	Hypothyroidism/hyperthyroidism
Cold salt water near-drowning	Sickle cell trait
Crush syndrome	Electrolyte deficiencies
Prolonged compression	Hypokalemia
Ischemia (embolization)	Hypophosphatemia
Postexertional	Hypomagnesemia
Seizures	Severe hyponatremia
Heat stroke	Inflammatory muscle disease
Malignant hyperthermia	Polymyositis
Electric shock/burns	Dermatomyositis
Prolonged CPR/repeated defibrillation	Arteritis/vasculitis
Decerebrate posturing	Idiopathic paroxysmal myoglobinuria
	Infection
NONTRAUMATIC	CMV
	EBV
Medical Disorders	Adenovirus
Peripheral blood stem cell transplantation	Streptococcus pneumoniae bacteremia
Status asthmaticus	Hepatitis
Addisonian crisis	Influenza/coxsackie viruses
Becker's muscular dystrophy	Shigellosis
Duchenne's muscular dystrophy	Salmonellosis
Pancreatitis	Gram-negative septic shock
Metabolic disorders	Legionella
Myophosphorylase deficiency	Leptospirosis
Phosphofructokinase deficiency	Rocky Mountain spotted fever
Carnitine palmityltransferase deficiency	Trichinosis
Phosphoglycerate mustase deficiency	Tetanus
Myoadenylate deaminase deficiency	Gag gangrene
Diabetic ketoacidosis	Human immunodeficiency virus
Nonketotic hyperosmolar coma	

CPR, cardiopulmonary resuscitation; CMV, cytomegalovirus; EBV, Epstein-Barr virus.

INITIAL THERAPY

1. Mannitol and loop diuretics (furosemide) have been suggested as prophylactic therapy against the development of pigment-induced acute renal failure.
2. Intravenous administration of bicarbonate-containing solution to alkalinize the urine also is espoused to prevent the development of acute renal failure, especially in patients with posttraumatic rhabdomyolysis. In theory, these solution have potential benefit, but no absolute, conclusive evidence exists to support their universal administration.[18–20]
3. In most patients, little morbidity results from an infusion of mannitol (1 g/kg), and it is recommended because it is potentially beneficial. However, loop diuretics can theoretically worsen renal tubular acidosis and may potentiate pigment-induced nephropathy.[20] Likewise, elderly patients with nontraumatic rhabdomyolysis and other debilitating chronic diseases may not tolerate the large volumes of salt and water required to alkalinize the urine to a salutary pH endpoint.
4. Patients who are even marginally intravascularly volume depleted, and who have myoglobinuria, are at greater risk to develop renal failure. Early, aggressive volume repletion is mandatory, especially when osmotic diuretics are given.[21–23]

5. Therapy for hyperkalemia may be required because it can be fulminant. Hydration and forced diuresis are usually adequate therapy; however, more specific measures, such as intravenous glucose and insulin administration or even emergency dialysis, may be required.
6. Hypocalcemia occurs commonly in patients with rhabdomyolysis but is rarely associated with adverse sequelae so that calcium administration is rarely required.
7. Hyperphosphatemia generally responds to phosphate-binding antacid administration (generally reserved for patients with acute renal failure). Hyperuricemia often is present, independent of underlying renal function. Therapy beyond hydration (to facilitate its excretion) is not required.

COMPLICATIONS

Prevention of acute renal failure is the preeminent concern for all patients presenting with rhabdomyolysis. In a 1988 retrospective study, several predictive factors were identified (using multiple regression analysis) for the development of acute renal failure.[24] These included the following: peak CK elevation, degree of serum potassium elevation on admis-

TABLE 152-2.   Drugs and Toxins Associated with Rhabdomyolysis

Alcohol	Doxapin	Pemoline
Alteplas	Emetine	Pentamidine
p-Aminosalicylate	Enflurane	Perphenazine
Amitriptyline	Epsilon aminocaproic acid	Phenazone
Amoxapine	Ethanol	Phenazopyridine
Amphetamines	Ethchlorvynol	Phencyclidine
Amphotericin-B	Ethylene glycol	Phenelzine
Anticholinergics	Etretinate	Phenformin
Antihistamines	Ecstasy	Phenmetrazine
Antimalarials	Fendluramine	Phenothiazines
Antipyrine	Fluoxetine	Phenylopropanolamine
5-Azacytidine	Fluphenazine	Phenytoin
Barbiturates	Gasoline fumes	Phosphorus
Benzodiazepines	Glutethimide	Phosphine
Betamethasone bezafibrate	Glycyrrhizate (licorice)	Plasmocid
Butyrophenones	Halothane	Potassium-wasting diuretics
Caffeine	Heroin	Potassium-wasting laxatives
Carbenoxolone	5HT uptake inhibitors	Potassium-wasting emetics
Carbon monoxide	HMG-CoA reductase inhibitors	Procainamide
Carbromal	Hymenoptera sting venom	Promethazine
Cathine	Hydrocarbons	Protriptyline
Centipede sting	Hydrogen sulfide	Quinidine
Chlorazepate	Imipramine	Retinoids
Chlorpromazine	Iodoacetate	Salicylate
Chlordiazepoxide	Isoflurane	Sedatives (prolonged compression)
Chlorinated hydrocarbon	Isoniazid	Selenium
Insecticides	Isopropyl alcohol	Snake venom
Chlormethiazole base	Isotretinoin	Spider venom
Chlorphenoxyl herbicides	Lindane	Streptokinase
Chlorpromazine	Lithium	Strychnine
Chlorthalidone	Lovostatin/gemfibrozil	Succinylcholine
Clofibrate	Lovostatin/Erythromycin	Suxamethonium bromide
Cimetidine	Loxapine	Tetraethyl lead
Codeine	LSD	Terbutaline
Colchicine	Marijuana	Theophylline
Copper sulfate	MAO inhibitors	Thiopental
Corticosteroids	Mercuric chloride	Thioridazine
Cotrimazole	Mescaline	Thiothixine
Cocaine	Methadone	Toxaphene
Cyamemazine	Methanol	2,4,5-Trichlorophenoxyacetic acid
Cyanide	Mineralocorticoids	Tricyclic antidepressants
Cyclosporin-A	Molindone	Triethylene tetramine dihydrochloride
Dextromoramide	Morphine	Trifluoroperazine
Diaminobenzene	Moxalactam	Trimethoprim sulfamethoxazole
2,4 Dichlorophenoxyacetic acid	Opioids	Toluene
Didanosine	Oxyprenolol	Triazolam
Diphenhydramine	Palfium	Vasopressin
Diquat	Paraquat	Valproic acid
Doxylamine	Peanut oil	Zidovudine

MAO, monoamine oxidase; 5HT, 5-hydroxtrypophan; HMG-CoA, 3-hydroxy-3-methylglutaryl CoA reductase; LSD, lysergic acid diethylamide.

sion, degree of serum phosphate elevation on admission, decrease in serum albumin, and clinical evidence of dehydration at presentation. However, these criteria have not been prospectively applied to patient populations at risk for the development of rhabdomyolysis-associated acute renal failure and so their utility remains unproven. More recently, two studies have dealt with the incidence and the prediction of acute renal failure in patients with rhabdomyolysis. Sinert and others[25] report a 0% incidence rate of acute renal failure in 35 patients with exercise-induced rhabdomyolysis who presented with a mean CK of 40,471 U/L, unless other comorbid nephrotoxic factors supervened (e.g., significant hypovolemia). Again, early, aggressive volume repletion is essential. Feinfeld and coworkers[26] correlated quantitative urinary myoglobin concentrations with acute renal failure. All 4 patients whose urinary myoglobin concentrations exceeded 1000 ng/mL developed acute renal failure. Finally, venous bicarbonate concentrations may correlate with the development of acute renal failure in some patients with traumatic rhabdomyolysis.[27] In patients with values less than 17 mmol/L, 4 of 5 patients subsequently developed acute renal failure, irrespective of their CK values. Unfortunately, all of these studies target different patient populations, are narrow in scope, and do not involve many patients with rhabdomyolysis. Therefore, these observations should be interpreted and applied to individual patients with discretion.

When acute renal failure develops, the outlook generally is good. Morbidity is most directly associated with incomplete management of associated metabolic perturbations (e.g., hyperkalemia). Most patients recover baseline renal function in 3 to 4 weeks. Dialysis during this interval is not associated with a significant increase in clinical complications. Early institution of continuous arteriovenous hemofiltration with or without dialysis in patients with acute renal failure may speed recovery of renal function. Continuous arteriovenous hemofiltration with dialysis is an efficient and effective method of dialyzing myoglobin from the plasma.[28] Thus, a shorter duration of ongoing dialysis may be required.[29,30]

Muscular swelling leading to compression of intracompartmental muscles within a narrow fascial sheath poses a substantial risk in rhabdomyolysis. This swelling may ultimately threaten additional muscle viability, along with other local vascular and nerve structures. Complaints of worsening pain, development of paresthesia, or tense muscular compartments on physical examination should prompt direct measurement of intracompartmental pressures, followed serially, so that pressure can be relieved before the development of permanent muscle or nerve damage. Emergency fasciotomy may be required to relieve high intracompartmental pressures when vascular compromise is already evident. Remember, too, that as volume repletion is maintained, muscle swelling and a "compartment syndrome" may develop as a later finding. Volume repletion remains paramount, however.

Life-threatening ventricular arrhythmias can result with severe hyperkalemia seen in rhabdomyolysis. In this setting, calcium administration may help limit the arrhythmogenic effects of hyperkalemia. The otherwise indiscriminate use of calcium may further complicate the clinical picture by potentiating muscle cell injury and worsening rhabdomyolysis (the mechanism is described later). Rhabdomyolysis also can lead to severe DIC with clinical bleeding. The role of heparin therapy in this setting is not defined.

THE CLINICAL SYNDROME OF RHABDOMYOLYSIS ▄

ETIOLOGIES

Causes of rhabdomyolysis can be arbitrarily divided into traumatic and nontraumatic. Traumatic causes are best exemplified by the so-called "crush syndrome," which was originally described in battle-related injuries but also is occasionally seen in civilian trauma patients. The syndrome is characterized by an effective reduction in circulating plasma volume, hypotension, and hemoconcentration.[13,31] On release

of the compressing objects from the area of injured muscle, circulation is temporarily restored and is followed by a massive loss of both fluid and electrolytes into the injured tissues. This results in myoedema and decreased circulating plasma volume. Together with myoglobinuria, acute renal failure is the inevitable result if specific therapy is not rapidly undertaken. Rhabdomyolysis also is seen in patients unaccustomed to sustained exercise who exceed their normal tolerance limits (e.g., postexertional rhabdomyolysis in military recruits).[32] They, too, have skeletal muscle necrosis, although usually to a lesser extent. Ongoing generalized seizure activity also may result in traumatic rhabdomyolysis, as can heat stroke syndrome.[33] Notably, many patients with heat stroke syndrome also are hypokalemic, further increasing their risk of rhabdomyolysis.

Nontraumatic causes of rhabdomyolysis are diverse, and diagnosis is often difficult to establish clinically. Myositis and myoedema are not evident at physical examination in as many as 60% of patients. Another study reports a history of muscle pain in only 25 of 50 documented episodes of rhabdomyolysis, and findings of muscle swelling in just 4 of 87 episodes, and then only after intravenous fluid administration. Alcohol and muscle compression were cited as the most common nontraumatic causes of rhabdomyolysis, which is consistent with the findings of others.[1]

Alcohol seems to have a direct toxic effect on skeletal muscle in some patients, both chronically and acutely. Binge drinking may precipitate myoglobinuria, with the extent of muscle breakdown correlating roughly with the total amount of alcohol consumed.[13] Fifty percent of these patients develop acute renal failure as part of their clinical presentation. In addition, these patients often are malnourished, with concomitant metabolic abnormalities such as hypokalemia, hypophosphatemia, and hypomagnesemia-/all of which may contribute independently to the development of skeletal muscle injury.[15] Finally, when alcohol abusers (or drug abusers) become comatose, they directly injure skeletal muscle from the prolonged, unrelieved compression of their body weight, thus leading to ischemia or muscle necrosis.[34] Other operative mechanisms in drug overdose–related rhabdomyolysis include hypotension, hypothermia, hypoxia from respiratory depression, and metabolic acidosis. Certain other drugs, such as epsilon-aminocaproic acid and clofibrate, are direct mycotoxins, whereas succinylcholine alters the cellular metabolism of muscle cells. Phencyclidine increases myotonic activity but does not have a known direct toxic effect.

Some authors suggest checking a screening CK value in all patients presenting with hyperosmolar nonketotic diabetic coma.[35,36] Furthermore, they point out that significant rhabdomyolysis may occur in this patient population without routinely detectable myoglobinuria.

Anesthetic agents must be administered with caution in patients with primary muscle disorders. In particular, patients with muscular dystrophy of a variety of types are susceptible to rhabdomyolysis and life-threatening metabolic abnormalities. Inhalational agents (e.g., halothane) and muscle relaxants (e.g., succinylcholine) pose a significant risk to muscular dystrophy patients.[37]

Psychotropic and neuroleptic drugs are commonly administered in critical care units. These have the potential to induce the neuroleptic malignant syndrome, which is characterized by fever, muscular rigidity, and neurologic changes (usually catatonia). Prompt recognition and discontinuation of the offending medication is important. Rhabdomyolysis with end-organ failure is well described.[38,39]

Infections are uncommon causes of rhabdomyolysis. They are typically viral and usually are seen almost exclusively in elderly patients as a cause of rhabdomyolysis. Of these, influenza A is most frequently reported. Other associated infections include Legionnaire's disease, tetanus, leptospirosis, Rocky Mountain spotted fever, hepatitis (types A, non-A, and non-B), shigellosis, and HIV.[11,40] In the last 3 years, HIV-associated rhabdomyolysis has become an increasingly recognized entity.[40] In the largest of these studies (11 patients), immune-mediated myositis, the use of psychotropic drugs (e.g., haloperidol) and other medications (e.g., pentamidine, zidovudine-induced mitochondrial myopathy), tumoral infiltration of muscle, HIV wasting syndrome, and other vasculidities were most commonly associated with the development of clinically significant rhabdomyolysis.

LABORATORY FEATURES

Skeletal muscle contains about 110 mMol of potassium per kilogram of muscle. After massive muscle injury, release of potassium into the free circulation can cause overwhelming hyperkalemia, and lethal arrhythmias may ensue, especially during the first 1 to 3 days after injury. Additionally, metabolic acidosis and oliguria with decreased renal clearance of potassium often are present, both of which may exacerbate serum hyperkalemia. Of these, renal function seems to be the most important predictor for the development of significant hyperkalemia.[41]

Hypocalcemia occurs frequently in rhabdomyolysis. This is usually seen early in the clinical course when measured serum proteins such as albumin are normal or elevated. Two mechanisms are hypothesized to explain these observations. Calcium carbonate and calcium phosphate salts are diffusely deposited in injured or necrotic skeletal muscle. Furthermore, several authors suggest that hyperphosphatemia, the resultant decrease in 1,25-$(OH)_2$-D_3 levels, and skeletal resistance to vitamin D all contribute to the development of hypocalcemia.[32,32] Others have been unable to correlate high serum phosphate with low serum calcium levels in their patient cohorts.[44] The fact that calcium is deposited in injured muscle is well established, however.

Hypercalcemia may be seen in patients with myoglobinuria who develop acute renal failure and who are in the diuretic phase of their illness. Almost all of these patients have hypocalcemia during the early clinical stages of their rhabdomyolysis. This is thought to represent the release of calcium from injured muscle or perhaps inappropriate 1,25-$(OH)_2$-D_3 levels.[42]

Hyperuricemia is usually present and is marked in patients who have postexertional rhabdomyolysis. The rate of rise of serum urate levels generally exceeds the rate of renal excretion and is thought to represent overproduction as purines are released from injured muscle and are metabolized to uric acid. Additionally, urate excretion may be impaired, because both lactate and urate are actively excreted by the same distal tubular mechanism and because strenuous exer-

tion often causes anaerobic metabolism and lactate generation. The degree of uric acid elevation does not correlate with the degree of azotemia, however.[45]

Patients with rhabdomyolysis and acute renal failure have anion gap metabolic acidosis. When compared with a group of patients with acute renal failure from other causes, the calculated anion gap in patients rhabdomyolysis-induced renal failure is greater.[1]

Phosphorus content of skeletal muscle is 2.25 g/kg of muscle. Like potassium, it leaks from injured muscle cells whose membrane integrity is disrupted, resulting in serum hyperphosphatemia. Additionally, some phosphate present may result from hydrolization of phosphate bonds in adenosine triphosphate (ATP). Phosphate may, in turn, precipitate with calcium and deposit in blood vessel walls, soft tissues (including muscle), and the cornea.[46]

Skeletal muscle breakdown results in creatine release, a storage compound of high-energy phosphate (in the form of phosphocreatine). Creatinine, in turn, is the metabolic waste product of creatine degeneration and is filtered by glomeruli, but not reabsorbed. About 2% of body creatine stores are metabolized to creatinine each 24 hours. Creatinine formation is proportional to body muscle mass. In rhabdomyolysis, conventional teaching is that creatinine formation exceeds its filtration rate, such that measured serum creatinine levels increase out of proportion to BUN levels. As a result, the calculated BUN:creatinine ratio is typically low. Recently, these tenets have been questioned by some investigators, who instead suggest that the rate of rise is lower in other forms of renal failure because of the lower muscle mass of these patients, and that rhabdomyolysis represents a more typical expected rate of rise of serum creatinine values.[47]

Measured serum CK is invariably elevated in rhabdomyolysis. Its concentration in skeletal muscle and myocardium is high. Appreciable amounts also are present in brain tissue. Release of CK from injured muscle or myocardium is a fairly specific marker of their injury, particularly when elevations are profound. Lesser degrees of elevation also are seen in patients with pulmonary edema or pulmonary infarction. Generally, CK levels peak during the first 24 hours after injury. Thereafter, levels should decrease at a rate of 50% each 48 hours. If a second rise in serial CK values is observed, recurrent or ongoing muscle injury and necrosis should be considered, and a compartment syndrome should be investigated. Aldolase, another muscle enzyme, is released when skeletal muscle injury occurs, resulting in an elevation of measured serum aldolase levels. In most hospitals, these values are less readily obtained so that following aldolase levels becomes less practical. Similarly, carbonic anhydrase III is a highly specific biochemical marker of skeletal muscle injury.[48] This enzyme is not present in cardiac muscle and may be useful to differentiate myocardial from skeletal muscle injury. Unfortunately, it, too, is not widely available as a routine screening tool.

Myoglobin is an oxygen-binding respiratory protein found in muscle in an amount of 2.5 g per 100 g of skeletal muscle. It binds molecular oxygen and transports it across muscle cell membranes to the mitochondrial apparatus, where oxidative phosphorylation occurs. Myoglobin is normally present in serum at concentrations less than 85 ng/mL, of which 50%

is bound to an α_2-globulin. It is released from injured skeletal muscle and normally appears in the urine when serum levels exceed 1500 to 3000 ng/mL. Myoglobin may be measured quantitatively in urine and serum, or it may be detected with an orthotolidine dipstick or stool guaiac card, both of which are readily available. The presence of detectable myoglobin in the urine suggests that at least 100 to 200 g of muscle are injured. Grossly visible myoglobinuria is a function of the plasma concentration of myoglobin, the extent of myoglobin binding in the plasma, the glomerular filtration rate, and the rate of urine flow.[33] In other words, the presence or absence of visible myoglobinuria does not correlate with the underlying extent of muscle injury.

Hepatic dysfunction is common in patients with nontraumatic rhabdomyolysis. In one study, 25% of patients had reversible liver function abnormalities.[49] These abnormalities included elevated levels of lactate dehydrogenase, hepatic transaminases (aspartate aminotransferase, alanine aminotransferase), and total bilirubin as well as prolonged prothrombin times, not related to DIC. With the exception of the lactate dehydrogenase, all of these laboratory findings were significantly more common in patients who developed acute renal failure.

The use of ^{99m}Tc-diphosphonate highlights areas of muscle injury. One should be able to establish a diagnosis of rhabdomyolysis by other means. However, scanning gives a rough quantitation of the extent of muscle injury and can detect previously unsuspected areas of damage that may be susceptible to such complications as a compartment syndrome. The findings are particularly striking in patients who develop renal failure. Reversion to a normal scan may take months.[34]

THERAPEUTIC APPROACH

Adequate maintenance of the circulating plasma volume is the most important aspect of treating a patient with rhabdomyolysis. Additional therapy aimed at any contributing or underlying cause of this disorder (e.g., carbon monoxide poisoning, infection) also is important. Adjunctive measures to control such problems as hyperkalemia and others (mentioned earlier) also should be accomplished.

The prevention of acute renal failure remains a priority in the early treatment of rhabdomyolysis. Acute tubular necrosis is said to be mediated by several factors, including decreased circulating plasma volume and renal hypoperfusion, acid urine pH (which facilitates the dissociation of myoglobin into ferrihemate and its globin moiety), tubular obstruction caused by precipitation of heme proteins (and possibly urate), and, finally, possibly tubular cell anoxia related to an inadequate supply of oxygen and metabolic substrate during times of increased tubular cell metabolic demands.[50]

Traditionally, it is thought that myoglobin dissociates into ferrihemate (hematin) and its globin moiety at or below a pH of 5.6. Furthermore, a widely held opinion is that ferrihemate has a direct toxic effect on tubular cells, whereas myoglobin does not. Early in vitro research suggested that alkalinization of the urine may inhibit this process and therefore aid in the prevention of renal failure.[18,19] However, recent work indicates this may not be accurate. In Zager's

experiments,[51] aciduria was not a prerequisite for renal injury to develop after exposure of renal tubular cells to myoglobin. In addition, electrophoretic experiments demonstrated that myoglobin did not dissociate to hematin in an acid pH but did become less soluble and was subsequently retained to a greater extent by renal tubular cells. Finally, any protective effects of bicarbonate seem to result from solute loading and not from the effects of alkalinization per se.

Well-controlled clinical trials in patients with traumatic or nontraumatic rhabdomyolysis that conclusively demonstrate benefit from urinary alkalinization using bicarbonate containing intravenous solutions do not exist. Despite this lack of conclusive results, most clinicians favor their use when possible.[31,52] However, this use must be weighed against the potential risks of salt and water overload, which may occur in the amounts needed to raise the urinary pH above 5.6. In my opinion, measurable clinical benefits from the early administration of bicarbonate-containing solutions to a volume-depleted patient with traumatic rhabdomyolysis are just as likely related to prompt restoration of plasma volume, renal blood flow, and urine flow, and are probably unrelated to specific effects on pH.

Loop diuretics (e.g., furosemide) or osmotic agents (e.g., mannitol) are traditionally thought to prevent renal failure associated with rhabdomyolysis by maintaining urine flow, thereby decreasing tubular concentrations of myoglobin and hematin. Additionally, as these agents increase tubular urine flow, they also decrease active sodium reabsorption, an energy-requiring process. This may decrease the overall need for oxygen and metabolic substrate, potentially limiting the development of anoxic tubular cell damage.[19] In more recent work, Zager and coworkers[53,54] have additionally studied the effects of mannitol and deferoxamine on pigment-induced acute renal failure. Catalytic iron concentrations increase dramatically after respiratory pigment injury, and may contribute to the tubular anoxic damage through oxidant mechanisms (hydroxyl radical formation). Deferoxamine may therefore be of value. Clinical trails have not been published, and this remains an "of interest only" item. Finally, mannitol is an osmotic diuretic that dilutes toxic concentrations of catalytic iron at the tubular cell level. However, it does not confer any cytoprotection against oxidant injury. Given all of these points, I recommend considering mannitol administration (rather than a loop diuretic) because it is not associated with a potential risk of exacerbating renal tubular cell acidosis and may lessen the risk of oxidant-related renal injury.

It is tempting to treat the often profound hypocalcemia seen during the early stages of rhabdomyolysis. As mentioned earlier, however, hypocalcemia associated with rhabdomyolysis is rarely of clinical consequence, whereas exogenous administration of calcium may exacerbate muscle injury. Under normal physiologic circumstances, a cell membrane protein carrier regulates intracellular calcium ion concentration through a sodium–calcium exchange mechanism, combined with the activity of the sodium–potassium ATPase enzyme. When muscle cell membrane integrity is disrupted, intracellular calcium ion concentrations increase, leading to stimulation of intracellular neutral proteases and causing further cell destruction.[55] Administration of exogenous calcium may lead to even greater intracellular calcium ion concentrations and thus even greater protease enzyme activity. Conversely, drugs such as verapamil may ultimately prove to be beneficial in modulating muscle cell injury. Therapy for hypocalcemia, therefore, is recommended only in the setting of life-threatening ventricular arrhythmias from uncontrolled hyperkalemia.

Lack of recognition of progressive elevation in intrafascial muscle compartment pressures (as myoedema worsens) can be devastating and can cause permanent disability. Close attention should be paid to findings at physical examination, especially that of a progressive increase in palpable muscle tension and tenderness. A patient who presents with pain and paresthesia should receive immediate attention. Renewed elevation of CK levels should also alert the clinician to the possibility of a developing compartment syndrome. Measurement of intracompartmental pressure can be performed using a probe and transducer. Intracompartmental pressures greater than 30 mm Hg generally require fasciotomy to prevent neurovascular damage. The tibialis anterior, in particular, is susceptible to this complication because it is normally a tight compartment with little room for expansion.[56] An incision down to the muscle to check the contractile response to pinching may be required to assess the need for fasciotomy.

DIC can be severe, sometimes to the point of clinical bleeding. Therapy should be primarily supportive; the use of blood products, including repletion of coagulation proteins with fresh frozen plasma, is indicated. Heparin therapy for DIC associated with rhabdomyolysis is not recommended. Therapy for hyperuricemia is not needed. Hyperphosphatemia, particularly in acute renal failure patients, usually responds to orally administered phosphate-binding antacids.

UNUSUAL PRESENTATIONS

Rhabdomyolysis is said to be an uncommon disorder of uncommon causes. Several categories are discussed here. McArdle's disease is hereditary, characterized by the absence of the phosphorylase enzyme, which enables glycogen utilization during anaerobic exercise. Continued exertion by these affected patients may result in muscle ischemia and necrosis, despite a seemingly adequate supply of metabolic substrate. Other enzyme deficiency states such as carnitine palmityl transferase and phosphofructokinase also have been associated with rhabdomyolysis.[57]

Primary muscle inflammatory diseases such as polymyositis and dermatomyositis also are associated with muscle weakness and destruction. Additionally, vasculitic processes may mimic their clinical presentations. Muscle biopsy may be required for diagnosis. Besides the therapy for rhabdomyolysis outlined earlier, corticosteroids often are necessary.

Salmonellosis, shigellosis, trichinosis, Rocky Mountain spotted fever, Legionnaire's disease, leptospirosis, and infectious hepatitis have been associated with rhabdomyolysis.[58,59] Their clinical courses are widely variable.

Both hypothyroidism and hyperthyroidism have been described as causal in rhabdomyolysis.[60] Hypothyroidism may induce a reversible defect in glycogenolysis, thus precipitat-

ing rhabdomyolysis when physical exertion ensues.[61] More frequently, elevated CK values are observed with clinical hypothyroidism, but typically these patients are without evidence of significant muscle destruction. Rhabdomyolysis associated with hyperthyroidism is rare.

REFERENCES ∎

1. Gabow PA, Kaehny WD, Kelleher SP: The spectrum of rhabdomyolysis. *Medicine* 1982;61:141
2. Koffler A, Friedler RM, Massry SG: Acute renal failure due to nontraumatic rhabdomyolysis. *Ann Intern Med* 1976;85:23
3. Poels PJ, Gabreels FJ: Rhabdomyolysis: a review of the literature. *Clin Neurol Neurosurg* 1993;95:175
4. Collins AJ, Burzstein S: Renal failure in disasters. *Crit Care Clin* 1991;7:421
5. Knochel JP: Mechanisms of rhabdomyolysis. *Curr Opin Rheumatol* 1993;5:725
6. Ahijado F, Garcia de Vinuesa S, Luno J: Acute renal failure and rhabdomyolysis following cocaine abuse. *Nephron* 1990;54:268
7. Curry SC, Chang D, Connor D: Drug- and toxin-induced rhabdomyolysis. *Ann Emerg Med* 1989;18:1068
8. Parks JM, Reed G, Knochel JP: Cocaine-associated rhabdomyolysis. *Am J Med Sci* 1989;297:334
9. Steingrub JS, Sweet S, Teres D: Crack-induced rhabdomyolysis. *Crit Care Med* 1989;17:1073
10. Welch RD, Todd K, Krause GS: Incidence of cocaine-associated rhabdomyolysis. *Ann Emerg Med* 1991;20:154
11. Chariot P, Ruet E, Authier FJ, et al: Acute rhabdomyolysis in patients infected by human immunodeficiency virus. *Neurology* 1994;44:1692
12. Prendergast BD, George CF: Drug-induced rhabdomyolysis: mechanisms and management. *Postgrad Med J* 1993;69:333
13. Flamenbaum W, Dubrow A: Acute renal failure associated with myoglobinuria and hemoglobinuria. In: Brenner BM, Lazurus JM (eds). *Acute Renal Failure*, ed 2. New York, Churchill Livingstone, 1988:279
14. Grossman RA, Hamilton RW, Morse BM, et al: Nontraumatic rhabdomyolysis and acute renal failure. *N Engl J Med* 1974;291:807
15. Haller RG, Knochel JP: Skeletal muscle disease in alcoholism. *Med Clin North Am* 1984;68:91
16. Hellman RN, O'Neill MJ: The clinical spectrum of alcohol-related nontraumatic rhabdomyolysis. *Minnesota Med* 1988;71:769
17. Subramaniam PN, Garcia CA, Hill MK: ECG abnormalities in myoglobinuria: review of the literature. *Am J Med Sci* 1987;293:45
18. Ron D, Taitelman U, Michaelson M, et al: Prevention of acute renal failure in traumatic renal failure. *Arch Intern Med* 1984;144:277
19. Eneas JF, Schoenfeld PY, Humphreys MH: The effect of infusion of mannitol-sodium bicarbonate on the clinical course of myoglobinuria. *Arch Intern Med* 1979;139:801
20. Better OS, Stein JH: Early management of shock and prophylaxis of acute renal failure in traumatic rhabdomyolysis. *N Engl J Med* 1990;322:825
21. Veenstra J, Smit WM, Krediet RT, Arisz L: Relationship between elevated creatine phosphokinase and the clinical spectrum of rhabdomyolysis. *Nephrol Dial Transpl* 1994;9:637
22. Knochel JP: Rhabdomyolysis and myoglobinuria. *Ann Rev Med* 1982;33:435
23. Hamilton RW, Hopkins MB, Shihabi ZK: Myoglobinuria, he-

moglobinuria, and acute renal failure. *Clin Chem* 1989;35: 1713

24. Ward MM: Factors predictive of acute renal failure in rhabdomyolysis. *Arch Intern Med* 1988;148:1553
25. Sinert R, Kohl L, Rainone T, et al: Exercise-induced rhabdomyolysis. *Ann Emerg Med* 1994;23:1301
26. Feinfeld DA, Cheng JT, Beysolow TD, et al: A prosepective study of urine and serum myoglobin levels in patients with acute rhabdomyolysis. *Clin Nephrol* 1992;38:193
27. Muckart DJ, Moodley M, Maidu AG, et al: Prediction of acute renal failure following soft-tissue injury using the venous bicarbonate concentration. *J Trauma* 1992;33:813
28. Berns JS, Cohen RM, Rudnick MR: Removal of myoglobin by CAVH-D in traumatic rhabdomyolysis. *Am J Nephrol* 1991;11:73
29. Winterberg B, Ramme K, Tenschert W, et al: Hemofiltration in myoglobinuric acute renal failure. *Int J Artif Organs* 1990;13:113
30. Winterberg B, Tenschert W, Rolf N, et al: CAVH in myorenal syndrome. *Adv Exp Med Biol* 1989;252:385
31. Better OS: Traumatic rhabdomyolysis ("crush syndrome"): updated 1989. *Isr J Med Sci* 1989;25:69
32. Soni SN, McDonald E, Marino C: Rhabdomyolysis after exercise. *Postgrad Med* 1993;94:128
33. Knochel JP: Rhabdomyolysis and myoglobinuria. *Semin Nephrol* 1981;1:75
34. Chaikin HL: Rhabdomyolysis secondary to drug overdose and prolonged coma. *South Med J* 1980;73:990
35. Trump D, O'Hanlon S, Rinsler M, et al: Hyperosmolar nonketotic diabetic coma and rhabdomyolysis. *Postgrad Med J* 1994;70:44
36. Leung CB, Li PK, Lui SF, et al: Acute renal failure (ARF) caused by rhabomyolysis due to diabetic hyperosmolar nonketotic coma: a case report and literature review. *Ren Fail* 1992;14:81
37. Farrell PT: Anesthesia-induced rhabdomyolysis causing cardiac arrest: case report and review of anaesthesia and the dystrophinopathies. *Anaesth Intensive Care* 1994;22:597
38. Becker BN, Ismail N: The neuroleptic malignant syndrome and acute renal failure. *J Am Soc Nephrol* 1994;4:1406
39. Jermain DM, Crismon ML: Psychotropic drug-related rhabdomyolysis. *Ann Pharmacother* 1992;26:948
40. del Rio C, Soffer O, Widell JL, et al: Acute human immunodeficiency virus infection temporally associated with rhabdomyolysis, acute renal failure, and nephrosis. *Rev Infect Dis* 1990;12:282
41. Cadnapaphornchai P, Taher S, McDonald FD: Acute drug-associated rhabdomyolysis: an examination of its diverse renal manifestations and complications. *Am J Med Sci* 1980;280:66
42. Akmal M, Bishop JE, Telfer N, et al: Hypocalcemia and hypercalcemia in patients with rhabdomyolysis with and without renal failure. *J Clin Endocrinol Metab* 1986;63:137
43. Llach F, Felsenfeld AJ, Haussler MR: The pathophysiology of altered calcium metabolism in rhabdomyolysis-induced acute renal failure: interactions of parathyroid hormone, 25-hydroxycholecalciferol, and 1,25-dihydroxycholecalciferol. *N Engl J Med* 1981;305:117
44. Massry SG, Arieff AI, Coburn JW, et al: Divalent ion metabolism in patients with acute renal failure: studies of the mechanism of hypocalcemia. *Kidney Int* 1974;5:437
45. Schiff HB, MacSearraigh ETM, Kallmeyer JC: Myoglobinuria, rhabdomyolysis, and marathon running. *Q J Med* 1978;47:463
46. Akmal M, Goldstein DA, Tefler N, et al: Resolution of muscle calcification in rhabdomyolysis and acute renal failure. *Ann Intern Med* 1978;89:928
47. Oh MS: Does serum creatinine rise faster in rhabdomyolysis? *Nephron* 1993;63:255
48. Syrjala H, Vuori J, Huttunen K, et al: Carbonic anhydrase III as a serum marker for diagnosis of rhabdomyolysis. *Clin Chem* 1990;36:696
49. Akmal M, Massry SG: Reversible hepatic dysfunction associated with rhabdomyolysis. *Am J Nephrol* 1990;10:49
50. Braun SR, Weiss FR, Keller AI, et al: Evaluation of the renal toxicity of heme proteins and their derivatives: a role in the genesis of acute tubular necrosis. *J Exp Med* 1970;131:443
51. Zager RA: Studies of mechanisms and protective maneuvers in myoglobinuric acute renal injury. *Lab Invest* 1989;60:619
52. Koppel C: Clinical features, pathogenesis and management of drug-induced rhabdomyolysis. *Med Toxicol* 1989;4:108
53. Zager RA: Combined mannitol and deferoxamine therapy for myohemaglobinuric renal injury and oxidant tubular stress: mechanistic and therapeutic implications. *J Clin Invest* 1992;90:711
54. Zager RA, Foerder C, Bredl C: The influence of mannitol on myoglobinuric acute renal failure: functional, biochemical, and morphological assessments. *J Am Soc Nephrol* 1991;2:848
55. Reddy MK, Etlinger JD, Rabinowitz M, et al: Removal of z-lines and alpha-actinin from isolated myofibrils by a calcium activated neutral protease. *J Biol Chem* 1975;250:4278
56. Whiteside TE, Haney TC, Morimoto K, et al: Tissue pressure measurements as a determinant for the need of fasciotomy. *Clin Orthop* 1975;113:43
57. Tonin P, Lewis P, Servidei S, et al: Metabolic causes of myoglobinuria. *Ann Neurol* 1990;27:181
58. Spataro V, Marone C: Rhabdomyolysis associated with bacteremia due to streptococcus pneumoniae: case report and review. *Clin Infect Dis* 1993;17:1063
59. Bando T, Fujimura M, Noda Y, et al: Rhabdomyolysis associated with bacteremic pneumonia due to Staphlococcus aureus. *Intern Med* 1994;33:454
60. Bennett WR, Huston DP: Rhabdomyolysis in thyroid storm. *Am J Med* 1984;77:733
61. Sekine N, Yamamoto M, Michikawa M, et al: Rhabdomyolysis and acute renal failure in a patient with hypothyroidism. *Int Med* 1993;32:269

Critical Care, Third Edition, edited by Joseph M. Civetta,
Robert W. Taylor, and Robert R. Kirby.
Lippincott-Raven Publishers, Philadelphia, PA © 1997.

CHAPTER 153

∎

Preventive Care

Deborah Weppler
Joseph M. Civetta

The term *intensive care* usually creates an initial image of
dramatic crises, minute-to-minute interventions, and the
highest technology. Although crises certainly exist and require emergency interventions, these patients eventually stabilize and often receive prolonged care. In such cases, many
less-spectacular and uninteresting details assume an increasingly important role in determining the success or failure
of treatment, as well as creating a major demand for the
increasingly scarce resource of patient care.

Fundamental nursing care plays an important role in
improving the patient's sense of well-being, avoiding lingering complications such as decubitus ulcers, which may markedly prolong hospitalization, and in lessening the patient's
sense of loss of control and overwhelming feelings of dependency. The team concept of intensive care fosters the practice of individual specialties monitoring themselves (i.e.,
nurses monitoring nursing care and physicians monitoring
medical care); however, care is most efficient when all components are truly understood and highly valued by all members of the team.

This chapter discusses common bedside problems and
activities along with useful corrective measures to provide
the physician with the knowledge necessary to create a harmonious care plan. The effects of these problems on the
functioning of the unit and the well-being of patients and
families are markedly underestimated. "An ounce of prevention is worth a pound of cure": at today's prices for intensive
care, we cannot afford to be ignorant of these fundamental
aspects of intensive care.

SKIN AND SUBCUTANEOUS TISSUES ∎

Simple protocols are necessary for managing wounds; the
skin surrounding drains, stomas, or open wounds; stomas
and drains; decubitus ulcers; and superficial yeast infections. Each unit develops its own preferences, but the following recommendations are based on reasonably general principles.

WOUNDS

Wounds are closed in most clean cases and in some clean-
contaminated cases. The skin is approximated with sutures
or staples. It is usually covered with a dry sterile dressing
for the first 24 to 48 hours—the time necessary for the
wound to seal. Thereafter, the dressing may be changed or
the wound may be left open to the air if no drainage is
present. A light dressing may be used to promote comfort
and convenience and to prevent bedclothes from catching
on the sutures or staples. Routine nursing actions include
observing and characterizing any drainage (color, odor,
amount, and consistency). The wound is observed for erythema around the sutures or staples and collections of fluid
or pus around individual sutures or under the line of incision
(which may indicate a loculated infection).

Contaminated wounds are usually managed in an "open"
fashion. Typically, the fascia is closed, but the subcutaneous
tissues and skin are not approximated to avoid superficial

wound infections. Occasionally, particularly after multiple dehiscences, the fascia itself is left open and abdominal contents are visible in the base of the wound. Other wounds may be left entirely open; the fascia, subcutaneous tissue, and skin are left open if the wound is grossly infected, and daily irrigations and debridement are necessary. Occasionally, because of massive fluid resuscitation intraoperatively, it is impossible to close the fascia. In either of these cases, an artificial covering may be need to be used over the open peritoneal cavity. Several types of temporary coverings can be used: Marlex, Goretex, and reinforced Silastic (Fig. 153-1). If edematous bowels are the problem, the mesh is tightened at the bedside on a daily basis as the edema resolves. When the surgeon believes that the fascia can be closed, the patient is returned to the operating suite for formal closure.

If the wound is infected, daily bedside irrigations are performed by the surgeon. A zipper (large toothed, nylon, 48 cm [18 inch], gas sterilized) is sewn into the mesh to allow easy access to the wound (Fig. 153-2). Many types of dressings are used. The only solutions demonstrated to be nontoxic to tissues are 0.9% saline and Pleuronic F-68.[1,2] Several solutions should not be placed in a wound. Providine-iodine scrub and soaps containing hexachlorophene are especially damaging to normal tissue.[3] Dakin's (0.05% sodium hypochlorite) and 0.25% acetic acid are toxic to fibroblasts, impair neutrophil function, and slow epithelialization. Hydrogen peroxide kills fibroblasts in culture and causes histologic damage to tissues.

The dictum, "Don't put in a wound what you wouldn't put in your eye," is a valid guideline.

WOUND DRESSINGS

For centuries, wounds have been dressed to protect them from the harmful external environment. Clearly the principal

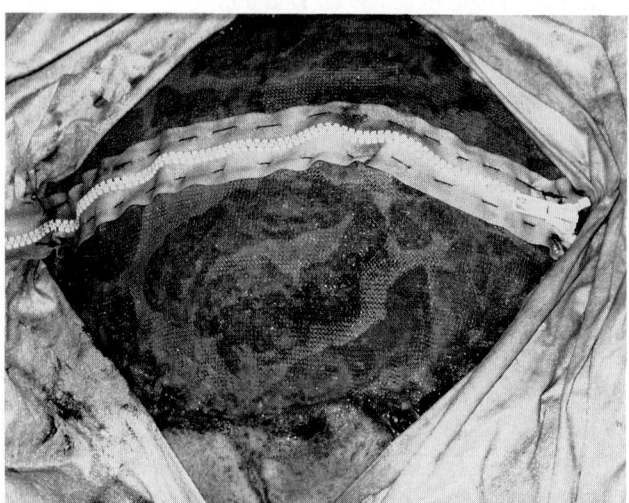

FIGURE 153-2. A nylon zipper is used in this Prolene mesh to provide easy access to the wound. This allows bedside exploration and irrigation of the peritoneal cavity.

function of a wound dressing is to provide an optimal healing environment.

The materials designed to dress wounds are designed to control local hydration and oxygen tension. *Occlusion* is the ability of a dressing to transmit moisture vapor from a wound to the external atmosphere. It also describes the relative permeability of that dressing to gases. Occlusion influences both epidermal resurfacing and dermal repair.

The advantages of moist healing include the following:

Reduced pain—resulting from insulation and protection of sensitive nerve endings
Rapid healing
Rapid debridement—enhanced autolysis
Ease of use
Waterproof quality
Fewer dressing changes
Cost-effectiveness: although the cost of the occlusive dressing is greater, the time saved from fewer dressing changes and time of healing reduces the total cost of care
Bacterial barrier

Several new types of dressings are available on the market that provide a moist environment for healing.

Films—transparent adherent dressings that can be used on stage I breakdown (see later) as a secondary dressing. Their backing is either polyurethane or copolyester, they are microporous, which allows for the escape of moisture vapor from the skin and the permeation of gases from the external environment, and the size of the pores is small enough to impede the entrance of bacteria. (Examples: OpSite, Bioclusive, Tegaderm, Blisterfilm)
Hydrocolloids—dressings that contain hydrophilic colloid particles; they interact with the fluid at the wound site and hydrate to form a soft protective gel; they are direct descendants of materials used historically as

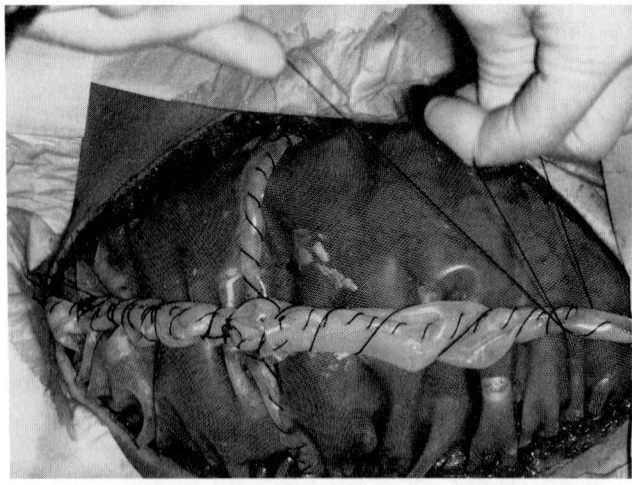

FIGURE 153-1. After exploratory laparotomy for traumatic diaphragmatic hernia, the abdominal wall fascia could not be closed because of massive bowel edema. Reinforced Silastic mesh was sewn in place as a temporary measure. Two days later, as the edema began to subside, the mesh was tightened with suture material to begin approximating the wound edges.

ostomy barriers (Examples: Duoderm, Intrasite, Tegasorb)

Hydrogels—complex lattices in which a dispersion medium, such as a cross-linked polymer as polyethyleneoxide, is trapped. Gels can be used for safe autolytic debridement and desloughing while a moist wound environment is maintained (Fig. 153-3). (Examples: Vigilon, Geliperm, Elastogel, IntraSite gel.) Hydrogels do not adhere well and contain large amounts of water; careful attention should be paid to the selection of an appropriate secondary dressing that holds the gel in place (Fig. 153-4).

Impregnated dressing—designed not to adhere to the wound; therefore, close attention must be paid to the type of secondary dressing used (Examples: Vaseline gauze, Biobrane, Scarlet Red)

Absorption powders—used in heavily draining, chronic wounds. These powders usually consist of starch copolymers or colloidal, hydrophilic particles; these "super slurpers" absorb up to 100 times their weight in fluid and extend the life of the dressing. (Examples: Bard Absorption Dressing, Hollister Exudate Absorber, Debrisan Beads, Duoderm Granules)

Foams—combine the benefits of a moist environment and absorbency. They can be hydrophilic or hydrophobic. Because foams may reinjure tissue if allowed to dry, selection of an appropriate secondary cover is important. (Examples: Synthaderm, Lyofoam, Allevin)

The role of wound dressings in wound management has changed from a passive role to an interactive role, because an environment is created to optimize the healing process. Correct selection of dressings is essential for optimal healing and improved cost-effectiveness.[4] The choice of the dressing is based on several variables such as wound type (acute or chronic), depth of injury, amount of eschar or slough, likelihood of drainage, wound location, and infections. During the healing process, attention should be given to the wound at its different stages because the suitability of dressings may vary along the way.[5]

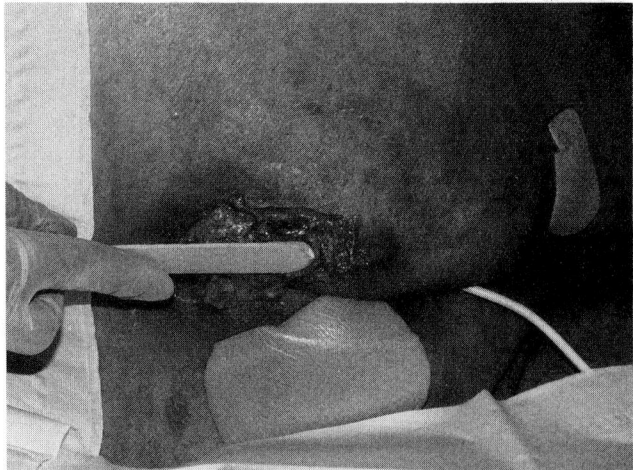

FIGURE 153-3. A grade II sacral decubitus is treated with hydrogel to maintain a moist wound environment and facilitate debridement.

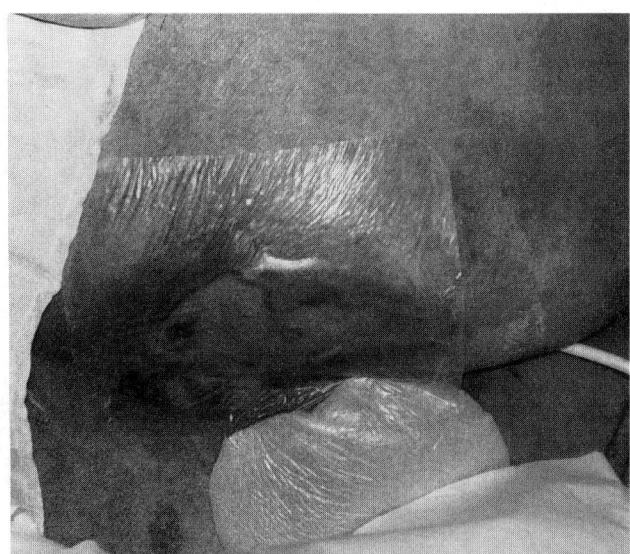

FIGURE 153-4. Adherent transparent film dressing is used as a secondary dressing over hydrogel to maintain a moist environment.

Wound dressings are changed every 4 to 12 hours, depending on the amount of secretions and the degree of inflammation. Nurses generally select the specific hours for dressing changes. The physician should arrange to be called or should find a convenient time so that physician and nurse can examine the wound together. The wound is examined for pockets or loculated collections. All tracts are packed open to ensure drainage and debridement. Again, the characteristics of the drainage are observed. In addition, the characteristics of the tissue or organs are observed (e.g., pink, pale, dusky, necrotic, shaggy).

SKIN SURROUNDING WOUNDS, DRAINS, OR STOMAS

The skin surrounding open wounds, drains, and fistulas must be kept intact. This can be accomplished by using Skin Prep on the skin or by placing a hydrocolloid dressing or skin barrier around the edge of the wound on the intact skin.

Bodily secretions and some of the solutions used to dress wounds may be caustic and may damage the surrounding skin. Dry dressings are used for protection. If wounds require frequent changing, removal of the tape may cause excoriations. In these situations, Montgomery straps are applied; when the dressing is changed, the straps are tied together, thus eliminating frequent removal of the adhesive tape.

STOMAS

The stoma itself is observed for viability. Instead of a pink and healthy color, edema, dusky mucosa, and even frank necrosis may be observed. The temperature of the mucosa can be estimated by touching with the finger. In the presence of an adequate blood supply, the mucosa is usually warm to the touch. Dusky mucosa that is cold probably has insuffi-

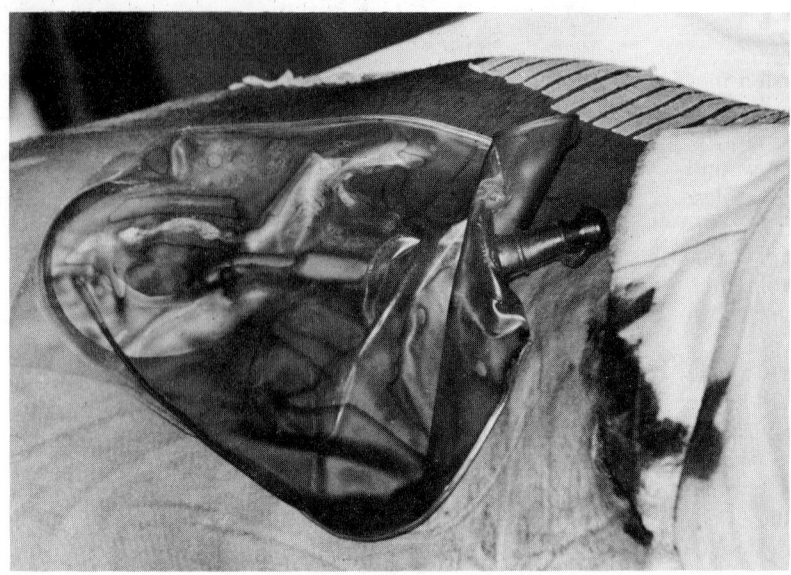

FIGURE 153-5. Catheter-Penrose drain, placed above a liver laceration, is enclosed in an ostomy bag. The opening has been tailored to leave little exposed skin, for protection; by capturing the drainage, the number of dressing changes may be reduced and the amount of drainage measured.

cient blood supply and will become necrotic. The skin surrounding the stoma is susceptible to breakdown. Duodenostomies or jejunostomies secrete fluids that are more irritating than those secreted by ileostomies or colostomies.

All stomas must be framed with a karaya ring, which should be approximately 0.6 cm (0.25 inch) larger than the stoma. The ring is covered with a protective collection device (ostomy bag). This appliance should be changed only if leakage develops rather than on a routine basis. Skin breakdown occurs from frequent removal of adhesives as well as from the direct effects of the drainage. Characteristics of the drainage are usually observed as well. Excoriation can be severe, and simple measures may not permit application of a tight seal. Karaya gum powder can be "dusted" on the excoriated skin to provide a base for the karaya ring. An enterostomal therapist (if available) may be able to provide helpful strategies if difficult problems arise.

DRAINS AND FISTULAS

Both open and closed drainage systems are currently used. Closed drainage systems are used to prevent external contaminants from traveling into the drainage tract, resulting in internal contamination. These drains are usually connected to a suction apparatus and the amount of drainage is recorded daily. Other characteristics are observed as well. If open drains are used, the use of dry dressings and frequent changes may be sufficient if the amount of drainage is small. However, an ostomy bag can be used if an opening is tailored to surround the exit wound (Fig. 153-5). This helps to prevent skin excoriation and provides a method of quantitating the amount of drainage. Patients may have many drains or fistulas (Fig. 153-6). Whenever possible, individual ostomy bags should be used for each, with both characteristics and amounts of drainage observed individually, and a labeled

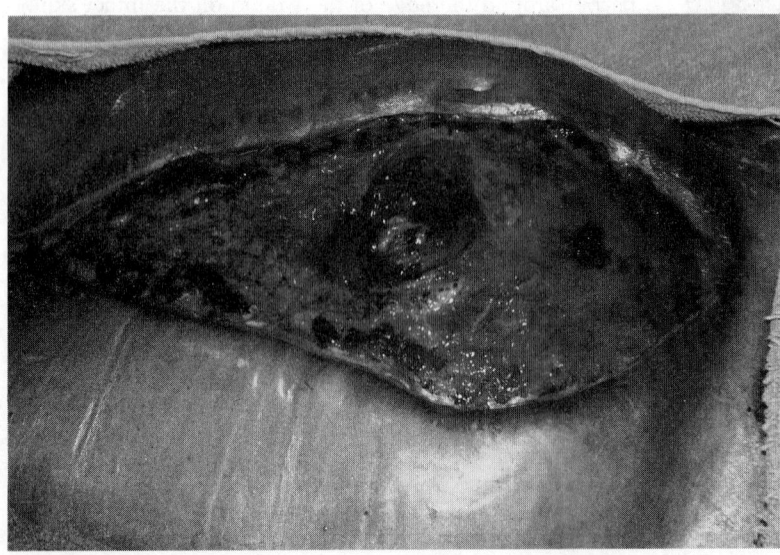

FIGURE 153-6. Complex abdominal wound with several small and large bowel fistulas.

diagram should be placed in the chart and the nursing care plan.

Fistulas, particularly enteric fistulas, may pose perplexing management problems. The drainage may be irritating, and if the tract or site is irregular, it may be difficult to secure any appliance to protect the skin and to quantitate the drainage.

DECUBITUS ULCERS

Decubitus ulcers tend to be associated with long-term patients in nursing homes who do not receive ideal nursing care. However, decubitus ulcers may develop in the intensive care unit (ICU). They are caused by pressure exerted on the subcutaneous tissue and skin when compressed between the weight of the body and a mattress or chair. The pressure affects capillary perfusion and interrupts the blood supply, producing ischemia and preventing the removal of cellular waste. When this pressure is unrelieved, cell necrosis may occur. The patient in shock or with cardiovascular instability has a marked decrease in cutaneous blood flow, initiated by primary compensatory mechanisms. Although events seem to occur on a minute-to-minute basis, many hours may elapse while monitoring devices are inserted and interventions are initiated in sequence. If the patient is not turned and the pressure is not relieved because of "instability" or because there are "too many other things to do," pressure necrosis may occur, despite the fact that the patient was surrounded by numerous physicians and nurses delivering the "best" type of care.

Decubitus ulcers can be classified as superficial or deep. Superficial ulcers may be subdivided into four stages that are useful in planning effective treatment.

Stage I—skin intact with redness or shallow breakdown, no further than the dermis
Stage II—skin breakdown limited to the junction between the dermis and subcutaneous tissue; irregular edges, shallow ulcer with subcutaneous fat at the base
Stage III—skin breakdown that extends to the deep fascia; extensive undermining; possible infection
Stage IV—skin breakdown that extends beyond the fascia to involve muscle, bone, and joints; possible infection

Deep pressure ulcers develop in tissues under the skin and tend to occur in response to shearing forces. Necrosis begins beneath the skin rather than in the epidermis, as described in the development of superficial decubitus ulcers. Deep ulcers may present initially as blisters that change into eschars. The lesion itself may be well developed before any signs are visible. Classic signs include a hard mass under the skin and purplish discoloration of the skin area subjected to pressure. The amount of tissue damage is usually much more extensive than indicated by the amount of skin area involved.

Patients susceptible to decubitus ulcers include those who are bedridden, elderly, or immobile. Other potentially predisposing characteristics are hyperactivity, obesity, cachexia, poor nutritional status, neurologic disease, conditions that impair sensation (e.g., peripheral vascular disease or diabetes mellitus), and orthopedic problems.

In addition to sites in the sacral area, decubitus ulcers may develop on the back of the head, behind the ear, and over the scapular spines, on the iliac crest, heels, and elbows. Preventive measures start with the recognition of susceptible patients. Then, it is necessary to ensure that change of position, good body alignment, and proper skin care are part of the initial *medical* care plan, even in patients with cardiovascular instability. The "egg crate" mattress, "bunny boots," and elbow protectors should be used, especially in patients with peripheral vascular disease or diminished sensation.

Treatment

Prevention of decubitus ulcers is clearly the best treatment. Improving nutritional status and ensuring frequent position changes are fundamental. Susceptible areas should be observed frequently to detect any signs of pressure, especially during their earliest stages. For stage I lesions, use of the egg crate mattress for comfort and good skin care should suffice, because the redness disappears when the pressure is eliminated. In stage II lesions, karaya gum may be placed over the affected area, and an absorbable gelatin sponge can provide an artificial layer to absorb pressure over a bony prominence. The involved area itself can be surrounded by support so that there is no direct pressure. Stage III is a deeper ulcer. In cases of thick, shaggy, necrotic tissue, surgical debridement also may be necessary. Local wound measures as described earlier may then be used.

Stage IV lesions usually require extensive surgical debridement with local measures used to provide a clean granulating base. Often, formal operations, including resection of bony prominences and creation of a skin flap, are necessary.

TOPICAL YEAST INFECTIONS

Patients who receive long-term broad-spectrum antibiotics and those who are immunocompromised comprise the two groups at risk for topical yeast infections. The lesions are characterized by erythema, scale formation, peripheral papules, and pustules and are often pruritic. They commonly occur under skin folds in the neck, abdomen, thigh, axillae, and under the breasts. Therapeutic measures include keeping the area cool and dry and applying topical nystatin (Mycostatin) powder every 12 hours or clotrimazole cream every 6 to 12 hours. *Thrush* is the term used to describe a candidal infection in the oral cavity. A thick, white, scaly coating is observed over the tongue and in other areas of the mouth. Nystatin liquid, 5 to 10 mL, is used as an oral rinse ("swish and swallow") four to six times a day. Patients who develop superficial yeast infections should be evaluated for more serious yeast infections in the wound, urine, or blood.

MUSCULOSKELETAL SYSTEM CONSIDERATIONS ■

COMPARTMENT SYNDROMES

Patients who have had crush injuries or have conditions producing vascular interruption may develop compartment syndromes, commonly in the lower leg. The injury itself or the ischemia induced by vascular interruption results in increasing tissue edema. The pressure within the compartment, limited by bone and fascia, rises first above venous and then arterial pressure. At this point, necrosis of the entire compartment contents occurs. Early signs and symptoms may be difficult to elicit in patients with multiple injuries, who may not be fully responsive because of a closed-head injury or the continued effects of sedatives or anesthesia. Pain, numbness, and loss of sensation are common findings. Swelling of the compartment may be observed, as well as limb paralysis and sensory deficits.

Any extremity subjected to trauma or ischemia should be monitored for all of these signs and symptoms; the diagnosis must be made early enough so that when the pressure is relieved surgically (by fasciotomy), function can return (Fig. 153-7). This cannot be the case if ischemic necrosis has occurred.

LOCALIZED ISCHEMIA

Three clinical settings can lead to the development of patchy or localized ischemia. First, the edges of a wound, particularly in flap reconstructions, may have insufficient vascularity, and circumscribed areas of ischemia and necrosis may occur. Second, in association with generalized septicemia, emboli may lodge in end arterioles of the skin. These septic emboli may progress to produce an infected necrotic area. The third cause, ischemia secondary to vascular cannulation, is probably the most common. The frequency of this complication depends on several factors, including size and type of catheter, site selected, coexisting vascular disease, duration of catheterization, and the external pressure monitoring system. Color, sensation, muscle function, and temperature must be evaluated during each nursing shift. This problem must be recognized promptly so that the catheter may be removed before tissue necrosis occurs. Small emboli may break off from an indwelling arterial catheter and produce a localized patchy area of necrosis in one or more digits. If the artery itself has become thrombosed and there is insufficient collateral circulation (no matter how carefully the circulation was evaluated at the time of insertion), the

viability of the hand, foot, or even the entire extremity (depending on the site of insertion) may be in jeopardy.

Most ICUs adhere to a protocol for the types of catheters inserted and the conditions of insertion. The best method to prevent ischemia is to use the smallest catheter, made of the least reactive substance, in the largest artery, and for the shortest period of time. If there are any signs of ischemia or changes in color, temperature, or sensation, the line must be removed as quickly as possible. If the artery is not fully thrombosed, this may provide a small increase in flow that is sufficient to reverse the ischemia. If ischemia persists, a sympathetic block should be performed, monitoring temperature in the digits before and after injection to document efficacy. Repeated sympathetic blocks with long-acting agents may provide a sufficient increment in blood flow through collateral circulation to maintain viability. Direct surgical repair also has been effective. Thrombectomy and reconstruction should be considered before the damage becomes irreversible. Thrombolysis also may be considered. Unfortunately, frank necrosis is a recognized complication. In these situations, amputation is delayed as long as necessary to allow the most distal demarcation possible.

CONTRACTURES

Elderly patients who remain immobilized for long periods of time and patients with neurologic impairment may develop contractures while in the ICU. Our attention, again, is usually focused on "life-threatening" and "attention-grabbing" pathophysiologic changes, such as acute hypotension or hypoxia. These long-term patients, who seem to make little or no discernible improvement, may actually be slipping away from a potentially functional life if contractures develop. Mobilization of such patients, with their many monitoring lines, tubes, and ventilators, is a difficult task that is sometimes easier left undone. However, early and repeated mobilization is an important method to forestall the development of contractures. Usually, the physicians in the unit must provide physical assistance in the process of mobilizing these

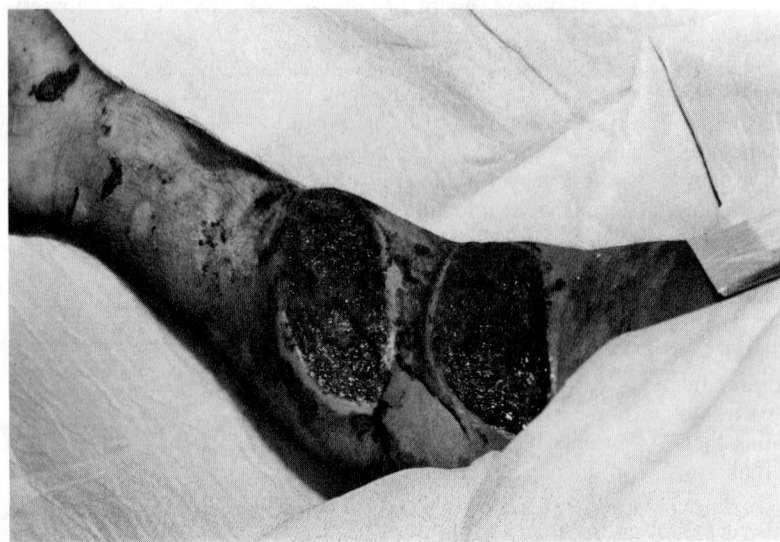

FIGURE 153-7. A compartment syndrome in the forearm after fractures of radius and ulna, treated by fasciotomies. The wound edges separated and the bases are granulating. Split-thickness skin grafts may be necessary to close large defects.

patients. Bunny boots provide relief of pressure points; there is also an external device that can be adjusted to provide dorsiflexion in an attempt to prevent footdrop. Range-of-motion exercises should be performed by a nurse or technician on each shift to avoid contractures. This is usually done with the hygienic care.

If a patient is considered to be at high risk for developing musculoskeletal problems, the physical therapist should be consulted early, before problems occur. In addition to supervising exercises to prevent contractures, the physical therapist may be of inestimable value in helping to motivate these long-term patients, who often seem to prefer to "slip away." The experience gained in motivating difficult patients during long-term rehabilitation makes the physical therapist an invaluable asset to the ICU team.

SUBTLE INFECTIOUS PROCESSES

Typical sources of postoperative fever or sepsis in the ICU patient are well known. Sepsis can be related to the primary problem, such as peritonitis, and a relatively short list of other sources, such as urinary tract or wound infection and nosocomial pneumonia. Some sources are less obvious and may be overlooked, especially in the long-term patient.

PHLEBITIS

Phlebitis, especially in a previous intravenous site, is common. It may be merely sterile inflammation caused by irritating substances in the intravenous solution. If the inflammation is septic, it can produce both local and systemic problems. Local infection, including purulence, is the most common manifestation; septicemia may be persistent and septic emboli may also occur. The incidence of phlebitis increases markedly after 48 to 72 hours of peripheral intravenous infusion. Lines that were placed under adverse circumstances (e.g., during emergency resuscitation or in a crowded emergency room) may be associated with a higher incidence of phlebitis. To prevent phlebitis, these lines should be removed as soon as replacement sites can be cannulated. The dressings over existing peripheral intravenous catheters are usually done according to hospital standards. Most protocols prescribe daily care and limit duration of infusion to 72 hours.

If the site becomes reddened or painful, the intravenous line should be removed and warm compresses applied. Elevation of the extremity helps to resolve edema. If the patient shows signs of systemic infection or if pus can be expressed from the needle entry site, surgical exploration is indicated. Proper therapy consists of opening the skin and removing the entire section of involved vein. Antibiotic therapy may be necessary if septicemia has developed.

SINUSITIS

Inflammation and infection of one or more paranasal sinuses are often related to tubes passed through the nares. Although nasotracheal intubation may often be the easier route in patients with head injury, the incidence of sinusitis is high and there is a general preference to avoid prolonged nasal intubation. Feeding tubes, nasogastric tubes, or other enteric tubes may be a sufficient stimulus to induce the edema that occludes the ostium of the sinus and thus creates the conditions for sinusitis. Generally, the most common symptom of sinusitis is pain; however, this is difficult to evaluate in an intubated or unconscious ICU patient. The diagnosis may be made if purulent drainage is observed around the indwelling tube. More frequently, however, sinusitis is diagnosed after specific tests have been ordered because the diagnosis was entertained. Sinus radiographs are difficult to obtain in the ICU and are of questionable value. Many cases of sinusitis occur in association with head injury, and the sinuses should be evaluated on the patient's computed tomography scans.

Indwelling nasotracheal tubes should be removed in all patients as soon as possible. In a patient with sinusitis, prompt removal is mandatory. An orotracheal tube or tracheostomy should be substituted for the nasotracheal tube. The nasogastric tube should be removed and replaced through the mouth, although tubes in this position are often more difficult to maintain and may be less comfortable for the patient. Systemic and local vasoconstrictive agents may re-open the ostia, and antibiotic therapy may be used. When spiking temperatures persist, if air-fluid levels are seen by radiograph, the sinus can be aspirated to obtain a culture specimen. An antral window may be necessary to promote better drainage.

PERINEAL INFECTIONS

Although they are more commonly associated with the emergency room, perirectal abscesses may occur in ICU patients, particularly those at prolonged bed rest. Incision and drainage with subsequent packing are necessary after the abscess has matured.

Epididymitis is an infrequent and often unsuspected cause of sepsis in male patients with long-term indwelling Foley catheters. Physicians in the ICU tend to examine the heart and lungs and surgeons examine the abdomen, but perineal examinations are "deferred"; hence, perirectal abscesses and epididymitis are easily overlooked because physicians are not looking for them.

COMPLICATIONS ASSOCIATED WITH ICU DEVICES

Whenever we violate the patient's physical integrity during monitoring and therapy, specific complications may result in disfiguring cosmetic problems that persist long after the "lifesaving" ICU care is but a dim memory. Pressure from indwelling tubes may produce local ischemia that may progress to necrosis if this possibility is not considered and preventive and therapeutic measures are not part of the daily care plan.

Endotracheal Tubes

It is often difficult to secure an endotracheal tube so that its distal tip remains in a constant position in the trachea,

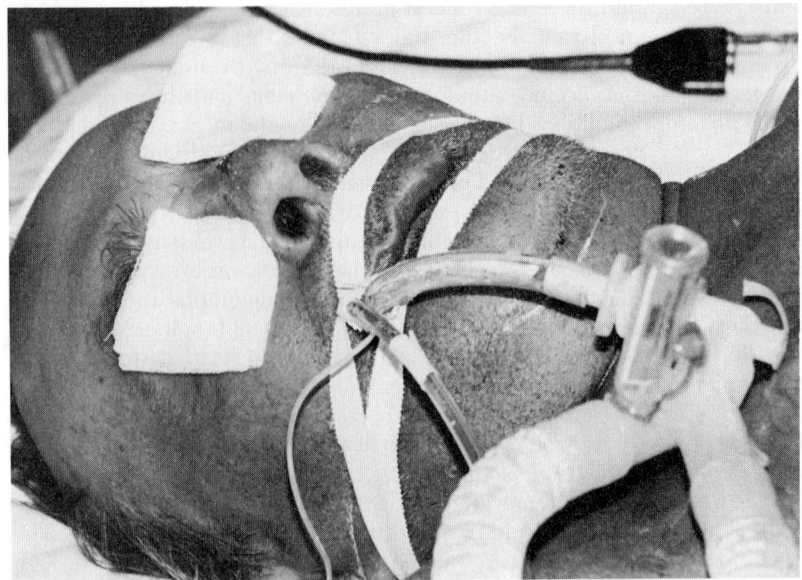

FIGURE 153-8. The oral endotracheal tube has been secured with tape passing around the patient's neck and across the upper and lower lips. This patient with a closed head injury had undergone emergency nasotracheal intubation but developed fever; maxillary sinutis was diagnosed by CT scan. Notice that both the endotracheal tube and the tube for gastric decompression exit through the mouth.

neither too close to the vocal chords nor progressing into the mainstem bronchi. These tubes must be taped securely around the head (Fig. 153-8). It is essential to avoid local pressure induced by the method of taping or angulation or by excessive weight when the tube is attached to the ventilator circuit. The tip of the nose, the alar cartilage, and the corner of the mouth are particularly vulnerable. We prefer to alternate sides of the mouth every 24 to 48 hours to avoid prolonged pressure. If nasal tubes are employed, it is extremely important to avoid angulation and pressure at the tip of the nose. Again, nasotracheal intubation, often preferred on the basis of the increased patient comfort and ease of fixation, has a significant complication rate in terms of pressure necrosis and sinusitis.

Nasogastric and Feeding Tubes

Nasogastric and feeding tubes should be taped so that neither angulation nor pressure can occur. Often, the tubes may be taped in a position that does not cause pressure, but then the tube is angulated after suction apparatus or feedings are attached, resulting in unwanted and unexpected pressure (Fig. 153-9).

Tracheostomy Tapes

Umbilical tapes are often used to secure tracheostomy tubes in place. These should be tied snugly, but there should be space for one finger to fit between the patient's neck and the tape itself. If excoriation occurs under the tape or near the stoma, the neck should be padded with plain gauze pads before the ties are secured.

Traction Helmet

Bleeding esophageal varices are life-threatening and difficult to control. Inflation of the gastric and esophageal balloons

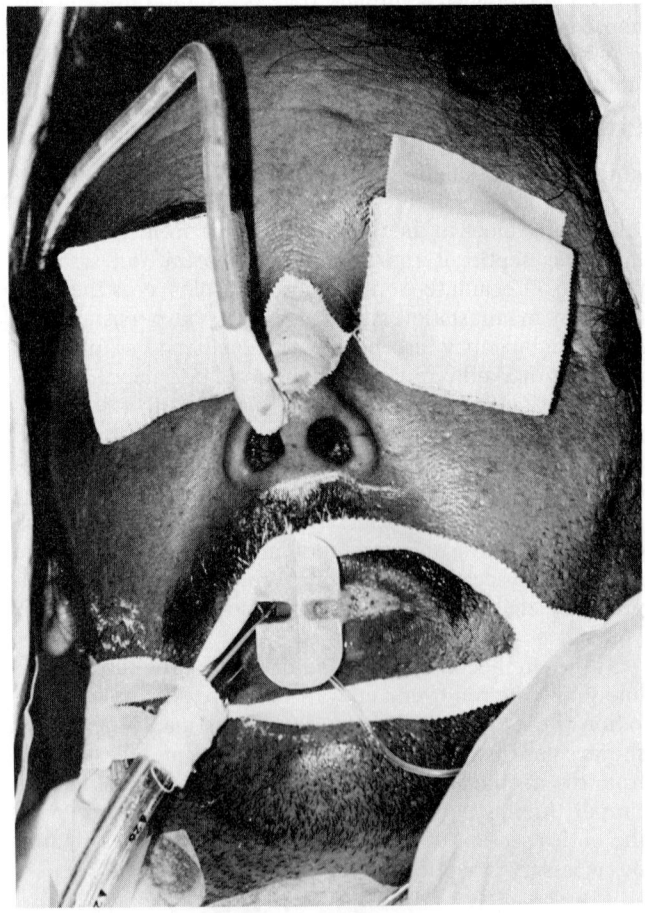

FIGURE 153-9. This nasogastric tube was placed and taped with the tubing in line with the arc entering the nose. For illustrative purposes, the tube was angulated when connected to the suction apparatus. If the tube was left in this position, pressure would be placed on the tip of the nose at the angle formed by the septum and alar surface. Ultimately, necrosis would result.

of the various tubes used often is insufficient to control bleeding unless traction is added. Pulley systems and weights at the end of the bed are extremely difficult to use for protracted periods of time. The traction helmet permits constant traction to be maintained relatively easily. However, if this traction is applied too forcefully, necrosis of the forehead and cheeks can occur. Large areas of full-thickness skin necrosis on the face are too common. After the patient survives hospitalization, disfiguring scars remain. This complication may be prevented if the helmet is secured with all three of the straps so that no shearing pressure occurs. Abdominal combined dressings may be used to provide additional padding between the helmet and the patient's face. Despite the need to maintain traction, the affected areas of the skin must be examined to preclude ischemia and necrosis.

Arterial Catheter Armboard

To facilitate the placement of a radial artery catheter, the hand is usually fixed with the wrist extended, the fingers are secured, and padding is placed beneath the dorsum of the hand. Excoriations, ischemia, and breakdown may occur. The tapes may need to be loosened, especially if edema develops. The armband position can usually be adjusted so that the character of the arterial tracing is unchanged but pressure is avoided (Fig. 153-10).

Military Antishock Trousers

Military antishock trousers (MAST) were originally designed for prehospital use in patients with profound hypotension presumed secondary to acute blood loss. The anticipated duration of such use included only the time to move the patient from the scene of the accident to the emergency room and, subsequently, to the operating room. However, external compression also has been used to control bleeding from pelvic fractures and in association with dilutional or hypothermic coagulopathies in patients who have received multiple blood transfusions. Patients treated in this manner may remain in the MAST for 24 to 48 hours. Pressure is usually maintained at approximately 30 to 40 mm Hg, which is sufficient to create two potential complications. The first complication, more serious but fortunately rarer, is a compartment syndrome similar to that described earlier in this chapter. Patients maintained in the MAST must, therefore, have frequent assessments of color, temperature, motion, and sensation in the feet to detect changes before rising compartment pressures produce ischemic and irreversible changes. The second complication, which is almost universal in patients who are in the MAST for 24 to 48 hours, consists of blistering of the skin that was covered by the garment. Management is similar to that of blisters induced by thermal injury. We generally pad the inside of the MAST with towels and pillowcases to distribute the pressure as evenly as possible, to pad protuberances, and to minimize blister formation.[6]

MISCELLANEOUS CONDITIONS ■

MISSED EXTREMITY FRACTURES

In the initial assessment of the multitrauma patient, life-threatening injuries must be the primary focus. Emergency operative intervention often may be necessary, and evaluation can be completed only after admission to the ICU. The symptoms that would be of use in evaluating an alert patient in the emergency room include pain, limited range of motion, or actual deformity. Postoperative or unconscious patients cannot be assessed in this manner. In addition, complications of extremity fracture, such as compartment syndrome or vascular compromise, must be detected by repetitive examinations of color, temperature, muscular function, sensation, and pulses. An area that is deemed suspicious should be further evaluated by a radiograph.

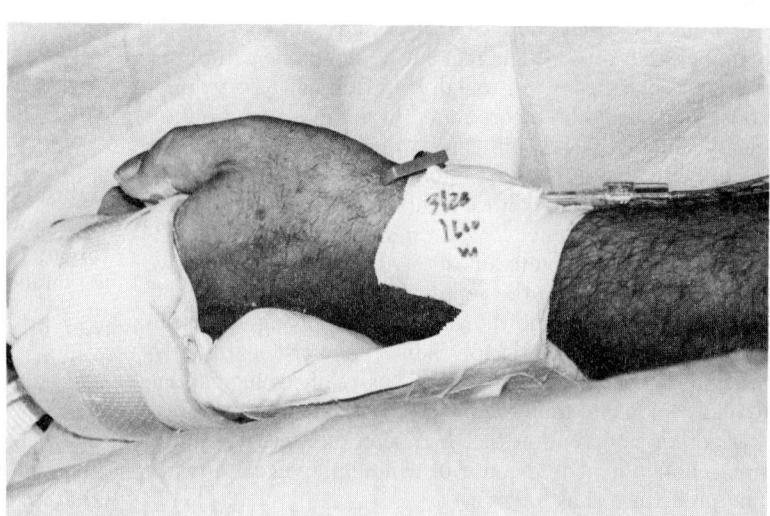

FIGURE 153-10. The hand containing a radial artery catheter is padded, fixed to an armboard, and restrained. Angulation and pressure have been minimized while maintaining function of the catheter and fixation.

ALTERATIONS IN BOWEL FUNCTION

Constipation per se is not a common ICU problem. Ileus secondary to retroperitoneal hemorrhage (after emergency aortic aneurysmectomy or fracture of the lumbosacral spine), peritonitis, or gastrointestinal surgery may be expected to be protracted. Many "nostrums" are used to stimulate "bowel function," but none has proved useful in the ICU setting.

The most common problem in the ICU is diarrhea, which can be particularly distressing for the patient and the entire staff; it may be difficult to control, creates unpleasant chores for the caregivers, and increases the patient's dependency and discomfort. It is commonly associated with the administration of antacids to prevent stress gastrointestinal bleeding and the use of enteral feedings. Diarrhea also may be a side effect of many antibiotics and medications, such as lactulose. It can also occur during resolution of protracted ileus.

Treatment is most successful if the cause can be eliminated. Antacids containing aluminum seem to be less diarrheagenic than those containing magnesium. Enteral feedings should not be advanced too rapidly in either rate or concentration. Patients seem to differ in their tolerance of different formulas; therefore, a process of trial and error may be necessary. The addition of sodium chloride often decreases diarrhea. Antidiarrheal medications seem to be more effective if given at normal doses at specified intervals rather than by adding a similar total quantity to the enteral feeding mixture. Medications that may be of some value include diphenoxylate, 10 mL every 6 hours as necessary, or loperamide, 2 mg every 6 hours. Lactobacillus can be used to reestablish normal bowel flora and is given in doses of about one package every 8 hours.

Persistent diarrhea is certainly psychologically demeaning to the patient and frustrating to the nursing staff. In some instances, we resort to the use of a rectal tube to ameliorate the situation temporarily while other measures are "juggled" to achieve more permanent control. A 30-French Foley catheter with a 30-mL balloon is inflated in the rectal ampulla and attached to gravity drainage. The balloon should be deflated and the tube repositioned during each shift to prevent pressure necrosis. Strong feelings often accompany the use of rectal tubes. Especially in cases of lower pelvic surgery, this approach should be discussed with the surgical team before it is used. The rectal tube should be withdrawn as soon as diarrhea is controlled. If the amounts are voluminous, they should be incorporated in the intake and output measurements. Good skin care with the use of ointments may be of value in preventing or treating excoriation.

Other measures to control fecal incontinence are the use of a fecal incontinence bag or perineal pouch, which is similar in construction to an ostomy bag. It has an adhesive backing with a hole in the center. Before applying this bag, prepare the skin around the anus when applying any appliance, shave the area, and apply Skin Prep to protect underlying skin. The incontinence bag also has a self-sealing passage to allow for rectal temperatures.

Another intervention that has been effective for liquid stool containment is the use of a nasopharyngeal airway.[7] The procedure is as follows:

1. Explain the procedure to the patient.
2. Position the patient on his or her side.
3. Lubricate the trumpet portion (the part designed to stick out of the nose) of the airway with a water-soluble lubricant.
4. Insert the airway into the rectum, past the external and internal sphincters.
5. Connect the airway tubing to a straight drainage system.
6. Stabilize drainage tubing on the bed surface.
7. For patients able to get out of bed, a disposable diaper can help maintain the tube's position; create an opening in the diaper's perineal section.
8. Change the airway every 2 days; wait approximately 1 hour before reinsertion.
9. Use the barrier system to protect the surrounding skin.

This intervention and the rectal tube should be used only as a short-term management methods.

ALTERATIONS IN BLADDER FUNCTION

The duration of Foley catheterization has been clearly demonstrated to correlate with the incidence of urinary tract infection. If a closed system is used and maintained, the incidence of nosocomial urinary tract infection is no higher in the ICU than in the general wards. However, Foley catheters, the almost ubiquitous monitoring device, are often left in place in ICU patients far longer than is necessary for monitoring purposes or even hygienic reasons. Elimination of constant bladder drainage is a high priority because urinary tract infections are the most frequent iatrogenic infectious complications in this country. A highly dramatic resuscitation and operation may "save" a patient with a ruptured liver, but the same patient may later die of septic shock after nosocomial urinary tract infection. An external "Texas" catheter is an option for male patients. However, after the catheter is removed, the patient must be evaluated for overflow incontinence or inability to void. A recommendation for long-term management of paraplegics and quadriplegics is intermittent straight catheterization rather than continuous drainage by a Foley catheter.

Yeast may often be identified in urinalysis or in urine cultures in long-term ICU patients. Most often, there is no systemic evidence of pyelonephritis. If catheterization must be continued, we often use continuous bladder irrigation (50 mg of amphotericin B in 1000 mL sterile water per day) through a three-way Foley catheter. An alternative is an infusion of one-quarter strength acetic acid at approximately the same rate (40 mL/hour). This is usually continued for about 1 week; after it is stopped, urinalysis and culture are obtained to check again for the presence of yeast.

TYPES OF ICU BEDS ■

The typical ICU bed is of low-leakage construction so that the patient is protected from external sources of electricity that might be transmitted by the invasive monitoring catheters. It is usually adjustable for the comfort of the patient and to accommodate commonly used treatment positions, such as the Trendelenburg position. As mentioned previously, however, pressure sores can develop in ICU patients who may be difficult to move about or position because of their size, requirements for immobility, or the paraphernalia used in treatment. Other types of beds have been introduced to counteract these problems.[8]

In providing effective pressure relief, pressure and time must be considered. Necrosis may occur with high pressure over a short period of time or with low pressure over a long period of time. Devices for pressure relief are specialty beds such as those with air-fluidized therapy or low air loss therapy. Pressure-reduction devices are defined as mattresses that reduce pressure compared with the standard hospital mattress surface, yet do not keep interface pressure consistently below capillary closing pressure. Capillary closing pressure is 25 to 30 mm Hg; however, this pressure may be significantly lower in the elderly and those with compromised tissue perfusion.[9]

AIR FLUIDIZED

The air fluidized bed, also called the static high air loss bed, is recommended for patients with severe skin disorders. The patient lies on a loose-fitting sheet that yields to the contours of the body without shearing or friction. Under the sheet is a tub-shaped vessel filled with thousands of tiny ceramic beads, creating a fluid-like movement as if the patient is floating on sand.

ADVANTAGES

It places minimal pressure on bony prominences.
Drying effect decreases skin maceration.
Alkaline substance in beads decreases the risk of infection.
Fluidization makes turning easier.

DISADVANTAGES

Weight of bed makes transport difficult.
Bed cannot be elevated.
Foam backrest provides limited head elevation.
Patient cannot be placed in upright position.
Drying effect of beads may overdry open wounds.
Difficult to get patients out of bed with the aid of an automatic lift device.
Beads leak from the bed.
Drainage difficulty with catheters so that a longer length of tubing is required to place drains to dependent drainage.

EXAMPLES

Clintron (Support Systems International, Columbia, SC)
FluidAir (Kinetic Concepts, San Antonio, TX)

STATIC, LOW AIR LOSS

Static, low air loss beds are used for patients at high risk for skin breakdown. The mattress is made of many air-filled cushions divided into four or five sections from the head of the bed to the foot. Separate controls permit each section to be inflated to a different degree of firmness, to give necessary support yet minimize pressure on bony prominences.

ADVANTAGES

Bed adjusts to a variety of positions.
Filter reduces risk of airborne contamination.
Cushions provide pressure relief.
Heavy-duty cushions are available for obese patients.

DISADVANTAGES

Bed does not absorb fluid.
Separate unit is required to keep bed inflated during transport.

EXAMPLES

KinAir (Kinetic Concepts)
Flexicair (Support Systems International)
Mediscus (The Mediscus Group, Buena Park, CA)

ACTIVE, LOW AIR LOSS

The active low air loss bed looks exactly like the static low air loss bed except for one additional feature: it gently pulsates or rotates from side to side. This feature may stimulate capillary blood flow and may help loosen pulmonary secretions.

ADVANTAGES

It has the same advantages as static air loss bed.
Bed protects skin integrity and may promote removal of pulmonary secretions.

DISADVANTAGES

It has the same disadvantages as the static air loss bed.

EXAMPLES

BioDyne (Kinetic Concepts)
TheraPulse (Kinetic Concepts)
Restcue (Support Systems International)
Pulmonair 40 (The Mediscus Group)

STATIC, STEEP FOWLER'S POSITION

This bed adjusts to a more upright position than a standard hospital bed. It is also called a *cardiopulmonary bed*. It moves easily into a variety of positions.

ADVANTAGES

Bed relieves pressure on sternum, heart, and lungs.
Bed frame can move up and down while in the reclining chair position.

BEDS FOR OBESITY

Beds for obese patients are designed to give extra support to patients weighing 135 kg (300 lb) or more. This bed is sturdier and wider than the average bed. It comes with a set of foam blocks and wedges that keep patients in a semireclining position.

ADVANTAGES

Added support is given to morbidly obese patients.
Hand supports help patients move to standing position.

DISADVANTAGES

There is still not enough width for ease of repositioning.
Short patients may have difficulty reaching hand grasps.

EXAMPLES

Burke Bariatric (Kinetic Concepts)
Magnum 800 (The Mediscus Group)

ROTATIONAL THERAPY

Rotational therapy beds are indicated for patients with spinal cord injuries. This bed may also be used for patients with unilateral or severe pulmonary problems. Consisting of a flat surface with adjustable foam support packs that serve as a mattress and to maintain body alignment, this type of bed turns either intermittently or continuously from side to side. Hatches underneath the bed give access for skin care to the head and shoulder region, as well as to the back and buttocks area.

ADVANTAGES

It is said to increase gastrointestinal motility and help remove pulmonary secretions.
Fabric-covered cushions help protect skin integrity.
Spinal column alignment is maintained.

DISADVANTAGES

Waterproof cushions may cause sweating.
Movement increases risk of friction and shearing.
Motion sickness may result.
Patient needs to be fitted in bed properly to ensure alignment.

EXAMPLES

Keane Mobility (The Mediscus Group)
RotoRest (Kinetic Concepts)

CONCLUSION ■

The prominent and often exclusive focus on profound physiologic abnormalities and lifesaving interventions that forms the initial concept of intensive care must be discarded. Attention to the details of daily bedside care makes a tremendous difference in the comfort and mental state of the patient, in the easing of unglamorous but overwhelming nursing tasks, in the cost and outcome of the entire care process, and thus on the overall ICU milieu. Knowledge of these problems and of their prevention and treatment undoubtedly enhances the physician's ability to improve the care that is given and the result that is obtained.

REFERENCES ■

1. Rodeheaver G, Bellamy W, Kody M, et al: Bacterial activity and toxicity of iodine-containing solutions in wounds. *Arch Surg* 1982;117:181
2. Rodeheaver G, Turnbull V, Edgerton MT, et al: Pharmacokinetics of a new skin cleanser. *Am J Surg* 1976;132:67
3. Lineaweaver W, Howard R, Soucy D, et al: Topical antimicrobial toxicity. *Arch Surg* 1985;120:267
4. Rodeheaver G: Controversies in wound management. *Wound* 1989;1:19
5. Alverez O: Moist environment for healing: matching the dressing to the wound. *Ostomy Wound Management* 1988;21:64
6. *Jackson Memorial Hospital Nursing Policy and Procedure Manual*, 1990:806A
7. Watterworth B, Ryzewski J: Managing fecal incontinence. *J Enterostomal Ther* 1990;17:180
8. Lovell H, Anderson C: Put your patient on the right bed. *RN* 1990;67
9. Petrie L, Hummel R: A study of interface pressure for pressure reduction and relief mattresses. *J Enterostomal Ther* 1990;17:212

Hematologic and Oncologic Disease and Dysfunction

Critical Care, Third Edition, edited by Joseph M. Civetta,
Robert W. Taylor, and Robert R. Kirby.
Lippincott-Raven Publishers, Philadelphia, PA © 1997.

CHAPTER 154

∎

Coagulation Disorders

Robert I. Parker

IMMEDIATE CONCERNS ∎

MAJOR PROBLEMS

The critical care physician needs to accurately assess the potential causes of bleeding in a critically ill patient and begin an appropriate workup to confirm the diagnosis. In situations such as the postsurgical patient, bleeding may be caused by an anatomic lesion, although a systemic coagulopathy needs to be investigated and ruled out to initiate the most appropriate therapy (e.g., return to the operating room), whereas in other clinical situations, potential causes may be related but require different therapy (e.g., liver disease versus vitamin K deficiency). This assessment requires the clinician to understand the most likely clinical presentation for the bleeding resulting from platelet defects, systemic coagulopathies, or anatomic lesions. Furthermore, the clinician needs to have a working understanding of the appropriateness and limitations of coagulation testing.

STRESS POINTS

1. Inhibitors or deficiencies of soluble clotting factors (e.g., factor VIII) present with deep bleeding (e.g., muscle hematoma, hemarthrosis), whereas platelet defects and von Willebrand disease present with mucosal-type bleeding. A thorough family history often points the clinician in the direction of an inherited coagulopathy; multiple males on the mother's side of the family with clinically significant bleeding may point toward an X-linked disorder such as factor VIII or IX deficiency.
2. Always consider "surgical bleeding" in a postoperative patient who presents with localized bleeding in the region of a recent surgery. Clinically significant con-

sumptive coagulopathy rarely presents with localized bleeding in a critically ill patient.
3. A consumptive coagulopathy (e.g., disseminated intravascular coagulation [DIC]) is frequently sought but relatively infrequently found in intensive care unit (ICU) patients. Fibrin(ogen) split products (FSPs) usually are mildly elevated (above 10 and less than 40 μg/dL) in postoperative patients and in liver disease. To convincingly make a diagnosis of DIC, one should have thrombocytopenia, hypofibrinogenemia, and elevations of FSPs above 80 μg/dL along with a microangiopathic picture on peripheral blood smear.
4. Bleeding is rarely caused by thrombocytopenia alone with platelet counts over 40,000 to 60,000/μL in a nonpostoperative patient, or with platelets above 80,000/μL in a postoperative patient. Minor prolongations of the prothrombin time (PT; less than 2 seconds) or activated partial thromboplastin time (aPTT; less than 4 seconds) rarely result in clinically significant bleeding in and of themselves.
5. The inappropriate use of blood products may make a clinical situation worse (e.g., platelet transfusions in heparin-induced thrombocytopenia, fresh frozen plasma fresh frozen plasma (FFP) infusions for hypofibrinogenemia in patients with volume overload).
6. Significant hypofibrinogenemia (less than 100 mg/dL) or hyperfibrinogenemia (over 800 mg/dL) may result in prolongation of PT, aPTT, and thrombin time (TT); only hypofibrinogenemia results in a hemorrhagic risk.

ESSENTIAL DIAGNOSTIC TESTS AND PROCEDURES

1. All studies and physical findings must be interpreted in the context of the patient's immediate past medical

history including drug exposure: aspirin and related compounds inhibit platelet function and may result in significant postoperative bleeding; cardiopulmonary bypass surgery may result in a quantitative and qualitative platelet defect; and aggressive transfusion or fluid resuscitation may result in a "washout" coagulopathy.

2. The PT measures the "extrinsic" cascade and is most sensitive to abnormalities in factor VII; the aPTT or PTT measures the "intrinsic" cascade and is most sensitive to abnormalities in factors VIII but also is prolonged with abnormalities of factors XII, XI, and IX. Both tests (aPTT and PTT) should be prolonged with abnormalities of factors V, X, II (prothrombin), or fibrinogen. The TT measures the conversion of fibrinogen to fibrin and is sensitive to abnormalities in fibrinogen or to inhibitors of thrombin (e.g., heparin) or to fibrin polymerization (e.g., FSPs).

3. Initial studies to be obtained on a bleeding patient include a complete blood cell count with platelet count and peripheral smear, PT, aPTT, and fibrinogen. Assays for FSPs or fibrin(ogen) degradation products (FDPs) are unlikely to be informative if the platelet count and fibrinogen level are normal, and can be omitted from the initial laboratory workup unless platelets, fibrinogen, or both have recently fallen to less than 50% of baseline levels.

INITIAL THERAPY

1. FFP is the treatment of choice for a coagulopathy of unknown origin (prolonged PT, aPTT, or both with normal fibrinogen).

2. If significant hypofibrinogenemia is present (less than 75 mg/dL), cryoprecipitate may be given to raise the fibrinogen level. Cryoprecipitate is not a standardized product; a usual dose is 1 bag/10 kg body weight (or significant fraction thereof).

3. Platelet transfusions should be given for significant thrombocytopenia (less than 40,000 to 80,000/μL) unless immune destruction of platelets is believed to be present. In general, 1 unit of random platelets (or its equivalent) can be expected to increase the circulating platelet count by a minimum of 5000 to 10,000/μL in a 70-kg adult unless significant platelet destruction is occurring. Platelet transfusions are contraindicated in the presence of heparin if heparin-induced thrombocytopenia is suspected.

4. All anticoagulants should be stopped. If the bleeding is thought to result from vitamin K deficiency, this should be administered subcutaneously or by slow intravenous infusion (longer than 5 minutes because of a small risk of anaphylaxis), and not by intramuscular injection because of the risk of muscle hematoma formation. Response to vitamin K is often blunted in the critically ill patient; 10 mg subcutaneously three times each day is an appropriate therapeutic trial. Protamine sulfate may be given to neutralize excess heparin (1 mg protamine sulfate neutralizes approximately 100 USP units of heparin; no single dose of protamine should exceed 50 mg).

TABLE 154-1. Overview of Coagulation Disorders Seen in the ICU

CONDITIONS ASSOCIATED WITH SERIOUS BLEEDING OR A HIGH PROBABILITY OF BLEEDING

Disseminated intravascular coagulation (DIC)
Liver disease/hepatic insufficiency
Vitamin K deficiency/depletion
Massive transfusion syndrome
Anticoagulant overdose (heparin, warfarin)
Thrombocytopenia (drug induced, immunologic)
Acquired platelet defects (drug induced, uremia)

THROMBOTIC CLINICAL SYNDROMES

Thombotic thrombocytopenia purpura/hemolytic uremic syndrome
Deep venous thrombosis
Pulmonary embolism
Coronary thrombosis/acute myocardial infarction

LABORATORY ABNORMALITIES NOT ASSOCIATED WITH CLINICAL BLEEDING

Lupus anticoagulant
Reactive hyperfibrinogenemia

OTHER SELECTED CLINICAL SYNDROMES

Hemophilia (A and B)
Specific factor deficiencies associated with specific diseases
    Amyloidosis–factor X, Gaucher's–factor IX, nephrotic syndrome–factor IX, antithrombin III
Cyanotic congenital heart disease (polycythemia, qualitative platelet defect)
Depressed clotting factor levels (newborns)

OVERVIEW ■

This chapter focuses on a variety of pathophysiologic conditions associated with abnormal hemostasis or abnormal laboratory measurements of hemostasis. These conditions are arbitrarily divided into four categories: conditions associated with serious bleeding or a high probability of bleeding; thrombotic syndromes; laboratory abnormalities that do not result in bleeding; and selected other syndromes. Most of the hematologic problems encountered in an ICU fall within the first category; therefore, most of the chapter is devoted to this area. A topical listing of these conditions is included for review in Table 154-1. The order in which these categories are listed suggests their relative importance to the critical care practitioner.

AN APPROACH TO THE PATIENT WITH AN ACTUAL OR SUSPECTED COAGULATION DISORDER ■

CLINICAL HISTORY

Diagnostic assessment begins at the bedside. The medical history, both past and present, may lend some insight into the risk for significant bleeding.[1] A prior history of prolonged or excessive bleeding or of recurrent thrombosis is important. Specific questions regarding bleeding should investigate the occurrence of any of the following: spontaneous, easy, or disproportionately severe bruising; intramuscular hematoma formation (either spontaneous or related to trauma); spontaneous or trauma-induced hemarthrosis; spontaneous mucous membrane bleeding; prior problems with bleeding related to surgery (including dental extractions, tonsillectomy, and circumcision); the need for transfusions in the past; menstrual history; and, finally, current medications. There are innumerable aspirin-containing medications available to the consumer, all of which can potentially interfere with platelet-mediated primary hemostasis. Many other drugs used in the ICU also are associated with bleeding abnormalities and are discussed later in this chapter. In situations involving trauma (either surgical or accidental), it is important to determine the severity of injury relative to the magnitude of bleeding that followed. A prior history of significant thrombosis (e.g., deep venous thrombosis, pulmonary embolus, stroke) also suggests the possibility that a hypercoagulable condition may be present. These include antithrombin III deficiency, protein C or S deficiency, factor V Leiden, vasculitis associated with an "autoimmune" disorder such as systemic lupus erythematosus (SLE). In addition, the family history also may separate congenital from acquired disorders.

In a general sense, one can separate defects in primary or secondary hemostasis according to the nature of the bleeding. Patients with primary hemostatic defects tend to manifest "capillary type bleeding"—oozing from cuts or incisions, mucous membrane bleeding, or excessive bruising. This type of bleeding is seen in patients with quantitative or qualitative platelet defects and von Willebrand's disease. In contrast, patients with dysfunction of secondary hemostasis have "large vessel bleeding" characterized by hemarthroses, intramuscular hematomas, and the like. This type of bleeding is most often associated with specific coagulation factor deficiencies or inhibitors.

PHYSICAL EXAMINATION

Development of generalized bleeding in critically ill ICU patients presents a special problem. Such bleeding is often a marker of severe underlying multiple organ system dysfunction. Thus, correction of the coagulopathy usually requires improvement in the patient's overall clinical status.[2,3] Supportive evidence or physical findings of other concurrent organ system dysfunction (e.g., oliguria or anuria, respiratory failure, hypotension) often are readily apparent. With the exception of massive transfusion syndrome (discussed later), such bleeding is usually caused by DIC or severe liver dysfunction.[2–6]

The physical examination of the patient with a bleeding disorder should answer several basic questions. Is the process localized or diffuse? Is it related to an anatomic or surgical lesion? Is there mucosal bleeding? And finally, when appropriate, Are there signs of thrombosis (either arterial or venous)? These answers may give clues to the cause of the problem (primary versus secondary hemostatic dysfunction).

During the course of the general examination, particular attention should be paid to the presence of several specific physical findings that may be helpful in determining the etiology of a measured hemostatic abnormality. For example, the presence of an enlarged spleen coupled with thrombocytopenia suggests that splenic sequestration may be responsible for a suspected primary hemostatic abnormality. Further, evidence of liver disease (e.g., portal hypertension, ascites), points to decreased factor synthesis as the etiology of a prolonged PT or aPTT. When lymphadenopathy or other findings of disseminated malignancy are detected, acute or chronic DIC should be suspected as the cause of prolonged coagulation times, hypofibrinogenemia, and thrombocytopenia. Purpura that are palpable suggest capillary leak from vasculitis, whereas purpura associated with thrombocytopenia or qualitative platelet defects are not elevated and cannot be distinguished by touch. Finally, venous and arterial telangiectasias may be seen in von Willebrand's disease and liver disease, respectively. When selective pressure is centrally applied to an arterial telangiectasia, the whole lesion fades, whereas a venous telangiectasia requires confluent pressure across the entire lesion (as with a glass slide) for blanching to occur.

LABORATORY EVALUATION

Chapter 18 discusses the laboratory evaluation of hemostasis. This chapter focuses on selecting appropriate tests that enable the clinician to sort out information from the history, physical examination, or previously obtained (and often confusing) laboratory data. Before we proceed, however, the importance of correct specimen collection for hemostatic evaluation must be emphasized. In the ICU, it is common for laboratory samples to be drawn through an indwelling arterial or central venous cannula, often because other access is no longer available. Heparin is, therefore, invariably present, either in solutions used to flush the cannula, to transduce a waveform, or as a component of the intravenous infusion. Depending on the concentration of heparin in the infusing fluid and the volume of blood withdrawn, several tests can be influenced. FDPs can be falsely elevated and fibrinogen can be falsely low. Likewise, the PT, aPTT, and TT can be spuriously prolonged. A minimum of 20 mL of blood should therefore be withdrawn through the cannula and either discarded or used for other purposes before obtaining a specimen for laboratory hemostasis analysis.[7] This should minimize any influence of heparin on the results. Because the aPTT is sensitive to the presence of small remnants of heparin, the presence of an unexpected significantly prolonged aPTT obtained through a heparinized catheter should raise the suspicion of sample contamination. In this setting, the TT also will be prolonged but will be normal if the contaminating heparin is neutralized (e.g., with toluidine blue or Hepasorb).

The presence of most suspected bleeding disorders can be confirmed using readily available tests. These include evaluation of the peripheral blood smear (including an estimate of the platelet count and platelet and red blood cell morphologic features); measurement of the template bleeding time, PT, aPTT, and the TT; and, finally, assays for

TABLE 154-2.   Hemorrhagic Syndromes and Associated Laboratory Findings

CLINICAL SYNDROME	SCREENING TESTS	SUPPORTIVE TESTS
DIC	Prolonged PT, aPTT, TT; decreased fibrinogen, platelets	(+) FDPs, D-dimer; decreased factors V, VIII, and II (late)
Massive transfusion	Prolonged PT, aPTT; decreased fibrinogen, platelets ± Prolonged TT	All factors decreased; (−) FDPs, D-dimer (unless DIC develops); (+) transfusion history
Anticoagulant overdose		
Heparin	Prolonged aPTT, TT; ± prolonged PT	Toluidine blue/protamine corrects TT; reptilase time normal
Warfarin (same as vitamin K deficiency)	Prolonged PT; ± prolonged aPTT (severe); normal TT, fibrinogen, platelets	Vitamin K–dependent factors decreased; factors V, VIII normal
Liver disease		
Early	Prolonged PT	Decreased factor VII
Late	Prolonged PT, aPTT; decreased fibrinogen (terminal liver failure); normal platelet count (if splenomegaly absent)	Decreased factors II, V, VII, IX, and X; decreased plasminogen; ± FDPs unless DIC develops
Primary fibrinolysis	Prolonged PT, aPTT, TT; decreased fibrinogen ± platelets decreased	(+) FDPs, (−) D-dimer; short euglobulin clot lysis time

PT, prothrombin time; aPTT, activated partial thromboplastin time; TT, thrombin time; DIC, disseminated intravascular coagulation; FDPs, fibrin degredation products.

fibrinogen or the presence of FDPs or FSPs. Discretion should be used in determining which of these tests are most appropriate for assessment; they need not be ordered as a blanket panel on all patients with known or suspected bleeding disorders. Table 154-2 summarizes several major categories of hemorrhagic disorders and the tests that are characteristically abnormal in each. In most instances, measurement of the platelet count, fibrinogen level, PT, aPTT, and TT should provide sufficient information for determining the correct diagnosis—or at least making an educated guess. By using these five screening tests and assessing other more specific tests only when an absolute diagnosis is necessary, inappropriate use of laboratory resources may be avoided.

CONDITIONS ASSOCIATED WITH SERIOUS BLEEDING OR A HIGH PROBABILITY OF BLEEDING ■

DISSEMINATED INTRAVASCULAR COAGULATION

Pathogenesis

Because it often occurs in conjunction with more serious, life-threatening disorders, DIC is one of the more ominous hemostatic defects seen in the ICU. The clinical syndrome itself results from the activation of blood coagulation, which then leads to excessive thrombin generation. The final result of this process is the widespread formation of fibrin thrombi in the microcirculation, with resultant consumption of certain clotting factors and platelets. Ultimately, this consumption is largely responsible for the development of significant bleeding.[2,3] Table 154-3 reviews several specific conditions in which DIC occurs secondarily. These include a wide variety of disorders that share as their common feature the ability to initiate coagulation to varying degrees. The mechanisms involved generally can be considered in two categories: (1) those intrinsic processes that enzymatically activate procoagulant proteins; and (2) those that cause the release of tissue factor, which then triggers coagulation. These are complex events that can lead to significant bleeding and often complicate the management of an already critically ill patient.

Fibrinolysis invariably accompanies thrombin formation in DIC.[2,3,8,9] The intrinsic pathway of coagulation (i.e., thrombin generation) or release of tissue plasminogen activator usually initiates this process. Plasmin is generated and then digests fibrinogen and fibrin clots as they form. Plasmin also inactivates several activated coagulation factors and impairs platelet aggregation. As such, DIC represents an imbalance between the activity of thrombin, which leads to microvascular thrombi with coagulation factor and platelet consumption, and plasmin, which degrades these fibrin-based clots as they form. Therefore, thrombin-induced coagulation, factor

TABLE 154-3.   Underlying Diseases Associated With Disseminated Intravascular Coagulation

Sepsis	Retained placenta
Liver disease	Hypertonic saline abortion
Shock	Amniotic fluid embolus
Penetrating brain injury	Retention of a dead fetus
Necrotizing pneumonitis	Eclampsia
Tissue necrosis/crush injury	Localized endothelial injury
Intravascular hemolysis	(aortic aneurysm, giant
Acute promyelocytic leukemia	hemangiomata, angio-
Thermal injury	graphy)
Freshwater drowning	Disseminated malignancy
Fat embolism syndrome	(prostate, pancreatic)

consumption, thrombocytopenia, and plasmin generation contribute to the presence of bleeding.

In addition to bleeding complications, the presence of fibrin thrombi in the microcirculation also can lead to ischemic tissue injury. Pathologic data indicate that renal failure, acrocyanosis, multifocal pulmonary emboli, and transient ischemic attacks may be related clinically to the presence of such thrombi.[2,3] The liberation of fibrinopeptides A and B (resulting from enzymatic cleavage of fibrinogen) can lead to pulmonary and systemic vasoconstriction, which can potentiate an existing ischemic injury. This appears to be an inherent property of these peptides. In a given patient with DIC, either bleeding or thrombotic tendencies may predominate; in most patients, bleeding is usually the predominant problem. In up to 10% of patients with DIC, the presentation is exclusively thrombotic (e.g., pulmonary emboli with pulmonary hypertension) without hemorrhage.

Presentation and Diagnosis

The suspicion that DIC is present usually stems from one of two situations: (1) unexplained, generalized oozing or bleeding; or (2) unexplained abnormal laboratory parameters of hemostasis. This usually occurs in the context of a likely clinical scenario or associated disease (see Table 154-3). As discussed earlier, thrombotic sequelae occasionally may dominate the clinical presentation. Certain other organ system dysfunctions predispose to DIC, namely, hepatic insufficiency or splenectomy.[3–5] Both of these conditions are associated with impaired reticuloendothelial system function; therefore, clearance of activated coagulation proteins and FDP and FSPs may be significantly reduced.

The clinical severity of DIC often is judged in part by the severity of evident bleeding, although clinical severity and prognosis also correlate roughly with the extent of aberration in the measured laboratory tests. Although this general rule cannot be applied at the outset of the disorder, once the diagnosis of DIC has been established, a progressive deterioration in laboratory tests of hemostasis does seem to correlate with an increased severity of the clinical disorder and portends a worse outcome.[2,3]

The combination of a prolonged PT, hypofibrinogenemia, and thrombocytopenia in the appropriate clinical setting is sufficient to establish the diagnosis of DIC in most instances. Severe hepatic insufficiency (with splenomegaly and splenic sequestration of platelets) also can yield a similar laboratory profile. It remains to be seen whether the laboratory findings measured in severe liver disease result exclusively from the liver disease itself or at least in part from concomitant DIC, which often occurs in cases of severe hepatic insufficiency.[5,6]

In addition to liver disease, several other conditions have presentations similar to DIC and must be considered in the differential diagnosis:

Liver disease
Massive transfusion
Fibrinolysis
Thrombotic thrombocytopenic purpura
Heparin therapy
Dysfibrinogenemia

With the exception of massive transfusion syndrome, these disorders generally have only two of the three characteristic laboratory findings of DIC; other confirmatory tests may be required to establish the proper diagnosis. Measurement of FDPs in the serum is helpful in confirming the presence of DIC, particularly when they are present in concentrations greater than 40 μg/mL (for most of the commonly used assay methods). The TT is a less sensitive test for DIC, but may be useful in cases of suspected heparin overdose because it corrects in the test tube with the addition of protamine sulfate or toluidine blue. Similarly, the euglobulin clot lysis time may not be sensitive to fibrinolysis associated with DIC but is significantly shortened in most cases of primary fibrinolysis. The D-dimer assay, which measures a degradation fragment of polymerized fibrin, also may be used as a more specific measure of a FDP. Its presence essentially excludes primary fibrinogenolysis as the sole cause of measurable FDPs in the serum. Interpretation of D-dimer assay results must be undertaken with some degree of skepticism (Chap. 18). Other tests of purported value either have problems with sensitivity or are impractical for widespread use outside of research settings.

Management

The primary treatment for DIC is correction of the underlying problem that led to its development. Specific therapy for DIC should not be undertaken unless the patient has significant bleeding or organ dysfunction secondary to DIC, significant thrombosis has occurred, or treatment of the underlying disorder (i.e., acute promyelocytic leukemia) is likely to increase the severity of DIC.

Supportive therapy for DIC includes the use of several component blood products. Packed red blood cells are given according to accepted guidelines in the face of active bleeding. Fresh whole blood (i.e., less than 24 to 48 hours old) also may be given to replete both volume and oxygen-carrying capacity, with the additional potential benefit of providing coagulation proteins, including fibrinogen and platelets. Cryoprecipitate contains a much higher concentration of fibrinogen than whole blood or FFP and therefore is more likely to provide the quantity of fibrinogen needed to replete that which is consumed by DIC. In this regard, FFP is of limited value for the treatment of significant hypofibrinogenemia because of the inordinate volumes required to make any meaningful contribution to plasma fibrinogen concentration. FFP does effectively replete other coagulation factors consumed with DIC. The use of cryoprecipitate or FFP is open to debate, however, because of concern that these products merely provide further substrate for ongoing DIC and thus increase the amount of fibrin thrombi formed. Currently, clinical (autopsy) studies have failed to confirm this concern.[2,3]

If the serum fibrinogen level is less than 50 mg/dL or the patient cannot receive or is unresponsive to heparin therapy, repletion with cryoprecipitate to raise plasma levels to 100 mg/dL or higher is reasonable.[9] For a 70-kg patient, this equates to roughly 10 bags every 8 to 12 hours. Platelet packs also may be used when thrombocytopenia is thought to contribute to ongoing bleeding. Many of the FDPs impair qualitative platelet function. This may be clinically significant at the concentration of FDPs achieved with DIC. In the absence of bleeding, platelet transfusions are given in many conditions when the platelet count falls below 20,000/μL. Platelet transfusions in patients with DIC should be considered at platelet counts higher than this level (e.g., up to 60,000 to 80,000/mL), although transfused platelets also may acquire an FDP-associated qualitative defect.

Pharmacologic therapy for DIC has two primary aims: to "turn off" ongoing coagulation so that repletion of coagulation factors may begin, and to impede thrombus formation and ensuing ischemic injury. The most widely used drug is heparin, although this is still the center of much controversy.[2,3,9,10] My practice is to consider heparin therapy in DIC if treatment of the underlying disorders is likely to worsen the DIC (e.g., acute promyelocytic leukemia), in "thrombotic" DIC, or if one is unable to control the DIC with blood product support. Objective data from randomized, disease-matched, prospective studies documenting its efficacy do not exist, however.

The goal of heparin therapy in these patients differs from that in patients requiring aggressive anticoagulation (e.g., thromboembolic disease). The amount of heparin typically given should not influence the aPTT unless the patient's condition causes impaired heparin elimination (i.e., significant renal and hepatic insufficiency). A bolus dose of 25 U/kg is given, followed by a continuous infusion of 5 to 10 U/kg/hour. The use of a continuous infusion is less likely to cause bleeding complications than intermittent bolus dosing.[9] Clinical signs of improvement include decreased bleeding and improved organ function in systems previously impaired by the effects of fibrin thrombi and ischemia. Platelet counts, plasma fibrinogen levels, and specific coagulation factor levels (e.g., factor V) should improve when heparin therapy is successful. The ongoing dose of heparin should be titrated according to these clinical and laboratory parameters and *not* to a target aPTT value.

In the more acute forms of DIC, duration of therapy is most closely linked to improvement in the underlying disease. Chronic DIC, particularly in association with disseminated malignancy, may require heparin therapy for the duration of the patient's life. Specific contraindications to heparin therapy parallel other situations of heparin use. Heparin should be avoided in patients with intracranial disease or recent intracranial surgery. Further, heparin-induced thrombocytopenia may develop idiosyncratically and should be considered in patients with persistently low platelet counts who are receiving heparin.[11]

Epsilon aminocaproic acid (EACA) was originally administered to patients with DIC to control the unremitting bleeding attributed to fibrinolysis. When used as a single agent, however, EACA may precipitate catastrophic thrombosis in patients with DIC.[2,3] Inhibition of fibrinolysis without control of coagulation is the apparent cause of thrombosis. Therefore, any patient with DIC who receives EACA also should receive heparin. The actions of thrombin usually have greater consequences than those of plasmin. Laboratory measurement of α₂-antiplasmin can be used to identify patients in whom the effects of plasmin predominate. Most clinical experience in this regard is limited to patients with acute promyelocytic leukemia.[10,12] If the assayed level of α₂-antiplasmin is less than 40% of normal, the use of EACA is reasonable. A loading dose of 3 to 4 g of EACA is given, followed by a continuous infusion at 1 g/hour until the α₂-antiplasmin level rises above 40% of normal. Because EACA is teratogenic, it is contraindicated in pregnant women.

LIVER DISEASE AND HEPATIC INSUFFICIENCY

Abnormal Hemostasis in Liver Disease

Liver disease is a common cause of abnormal hemostasis in ICU patients, with abnormal coagulation studies or overt bleeding occurring in approximately 15% of patients with either clinical or laboratory evidence of hepatic dysfunction.[5,6] It is a common cause of a prolonged PT or aPTT, often without any clinical sequelae. The hemostatic defect associated with liver disease is multifactorial, that is, multiple aspects of hemostasis are affected.

In liver disease, synthesis of several plasma coagulation proteins is impaired. These include factors II, V, VII, IX, and X. Fibrinogen synthesis by the liver usually can be maintained at levels that prevent bleeding until terminal liver failure supervenes.[5,6] The physiologic action of this fibrinogen is suspect, however, because it has been shown to have an increased carbohydrate content in its structure (sialic acid) and may be dysfunctional. Factor XIII activity also is often decreased in the setting of hepatocellular disease. However, the clinical significance of this decrease in factor XIII is uncertain because levels as low as 3% provide for normal fibrin clot stabilization. Although it is apparently synthesized by the liver, factor VIII (i.e., factor VIII:C, AHF) synthesis seems to be independent of the state of hepatic function. In fact, factor VIII levels may be increased in some types of liver disease. Plasma protein C and antithrombin III levels are low in many conditions of hepatic insufficiency, with variable effects.[13]

In addition to these deficiencies in plasma coagulation protein synthesis, many patients with liver disease have increased fibrinolytic activity. The mechanism for this heightened fibrinolytic state is not clear, although increased amounts of plasminogen activator often can be demonstrated. It may be difficult to discern whether fibrinolysis occurs solely because of underlying severe liver disease or as a result of concurrent DIC. The clinical distinction can be virtually impossible if active bleeding is present. In liver disease, levels of FDPs can be increased by both increased fibrinolysis and by decreased hepatic clearance.[5,6] Finally, clinically significant fibrinolysis is a frequent occurrence in patients who undergo portacaval shunt procedures.

Thrombocytopenia may be present to a variable degree in patients with hepatic dysfunction. This is usually ascribed to splenic sequestration. It is rarely profound and should not interfere with hemostasis as a quantitative defect. In vitro platelet aggregation is often affected, however. Increased plasma concentrations of FDPs are a possible cause of these abnormalities. The further addition of the hemostatic defects described earlier may result in bleeding that is difficult to manage clinically, particularly if all aspects of the problem are not addressed.

Presentation

The hemostatic defect in liver disease is multifactorial, and each patient should be approached accordingly. The most common scenario is a patient with liver disease and a prolonged PT in whom the potential for bleeding is a concern.[5,6] Factor VII has a half-life of only 4 to 6 hours. In patients with liver disease and impaired synthetic capabilities, particularly those who are critically ill, factor VII activity levels are usually the first to decrease. This results in a prolonged PT, whereas hepatic insufficiency remains relatively mild. As the severity of liver disease increases, the aPTT also may be affected, reflecting more severely impaired synthetic function. In this setting, plasma concentrations of the vitamin K–dependent coagulation proteins decrease, as do those of factor V (which is not vitamin K dependent). Although fibrinogen synthesis occurs in the liver, its plasma level is maintained until the disease approaches end-stage. When the fibrinogen levels begin to drop, liver failure has typically reached the terminal phase.

In more severe forms of liver disease, fibrinolysis may complicate clinical management.[14] The differentiation between concomitant DIC and fibrinolysis attributable to liver disease alone may be difficult. The D-dimer assay result should be negative in the patient who has liver disease and elevated FDPs but no active bleeding. Further clinical distinction usually is not possible.

Management

If the patient is not actively bleeding, no specific therapy is required, with certain provisos. In patients with a prolonged PT who are in a postoperative state or are scheduled for an invasive procedure, correction of the PT should be attempted. FFP provides the most immediate source of specific coagulation factors (i.e., factor VII) and usually corrects an isolated mild PT prolongation. Cryoprecipitate is rarely required because fibrinogen levels are maintained. Vitamin K deficiency also is relatively common in this patient population, and replacement may be needed. Correction of the PT in vitamin K–responsive critically ill patients typically requires longer than 12 to 24 hours. Patients with significant hepatic impairment may not respond at all. The immediate use of FFP is therefore appropriate when rapid correction is necessary.

When the synthetic capability of the liver becomes more profoundly impaired, and the aPTT is also prolonged, greater volumes of FFP or more specific therapy may be needed. The use of factor IX concentrates (prothrombin complex concentrates) has been advocated, particularly if bleeding is present. However, their use remains controversial. These pooled concentrates from multiple donors carry a significant risk of hepatitis (both B and C). In addition, they may provoke DIC and actually worsen hemostasis. The use of prothrombin complex concentrates should be reserved for patients with poorly controlled bleeding that is unresponsive to other more established therapeutic modalities.

A comprehensive therapeutic approach is needed in the patient with active bleeding. FFP, 2 to 4 units, should be given every 6 to 8 hours until bleeding slows significantly, and should then be continued at maintenance levels as dictated by clinical status and coagulation studies. Platelet transfusions also may be required, depending on the clinical situation. Vitamin K should be empirically administered on the presumption that part of the synthetic defect may result from a lack of this cofactor. Transfusions of packed cells are given as deemed appropriate by the clinician. If DIC is present, heparin therapy may be considered, using the guidelines previously discussed, although its use in this setting is even less well defined.

VITAMIN K DEFICIENCY

The most common cause of a prolonged PT in the ICU is vitamin K deficiency. Vitamin K is necessary for the gamma-carboxylation of factors II, VII, IX, and X, without which these factors cannot function normally. Factor VII has the shortest half-life of these coagulation proteins; accordingly, the PT is the most sensitive early indicator of vitamin K deficiency.

Vitamin K deficiency is relatively common in critically ill patients for several reasons. Many of the second- and third-generation cephalosporins directly interfere with vitamin K absorption from the gut lumen. The metabolites of these antibiotics may even act as competitive inhibitors of vitamin K. In addition, these and other antibiotics may kill or inhibit the growth of gut bacterial flora and thus limit the amounts of vitamin K they normally produce and excrete into the gut lumen. Malnutrition also may contribute to the development of vitamin K deficiency, although this usually requires 2 weeks to develop in the complete absence of vitamin K intake. The use of parenteral alimentation without vitamin K supplementation is one example of this pattern. When this is coupled with antibiotic use, however, significant vitamin K depletion, with prolongation of the PT, can occur within only 2 to 3 days. Finally, fat malabsorption states are associated with vitamin K deficiency. Vitamin K is fat soluble and is not absorbed well in some conditions of biliary tract and intrinsic small bowel disease. In the ICU, vitamin K deficiency usually results from the interaction of several of these factors and is rarely limited to one of the conditions mentioned. It is the responsibility of the clinician to maintain an awareness of the potential for vitamin K deficiency and to treat accordingly.

The differential diagnosis of an isolated prolongation of the PT without bleeding, other than vitamin K deficiency, is primarily limited to liver disease. These patients may present in much the same fashion as those with vitamin K deficiency. In fact, the distinction sometimes can be made only on the basis of the response (or lack thereof) to empirical vitamin K therapy. Warfarin administration (either overt or covert) also should be excluded as a cause of a prolonged PT, as should the presence of a specific inhibitor or congenital deficiency of factor VII. The clinician also must be aware of the existence of newer, long-acting vitamin K antagonists (so-called "superwarfarin"), which, when ingested, produce a profound, prolonged, vitamin K–resistant reduction in vitamin K–dependent clotting factors. Treatment of poisoning with these agents requires aggressive prolonged use of vitamin K, and, in the bleeding patient, FFP infusions.[15] Methods to detect these drugs in plasma and tissues are available.

The laboratory findings of an isolated vitamin K deficiency, in addition to a prolonged PT, include a normal fibrinogen level, platelet count, and factor V level. Factor V is not a vitamin K–dependent protein and should therefore be normal except in cases of DIC (consumption) or severe liver disease (decreased production). Prolongation of the aPTT from vitamin K deficiency is a relatively late event and occurs initially as a result of factor IX depletion.

The management of vitamin K deficiency consists primarily of its repletion, usually by intravenous or subcutaneous routes in critically ill patients. Therapy should not await the development of bleeding or oozing but should be administered when the PT abnormality is detected and vitamin K deficiency is thought to be responsible. As with other drugs administered subcutaneously (e.g., insulin), a near-normal blood pressure is needed to ensure reliable absorption from the soft tissues. Concern about the possibility of anaphylactoid reactions with the intravenous use of vitamin K exists. This risk is almost completely negated when the drug is given as a piggyback infusion over 30 to 45 minutes in a small volume of fluid rather than as a bolus or "slow-push" dose. This is the preferred method of drug administration in hemodynamically unstable patients. The usual dose of vitamin K is 5 to 10 mg intravenously or subcutaneously. In an otherwise healthy person, the PT should correct within 12 to 24 hours after this dose. Serial dosing of critically ill patients is often needed, however, and the PT may require up to 72 hours to normalize. If the PT does not correct within 72 hours after three daily doses of vitamin K, intrinsic liver disease should be suspected. Further administration of vitamin K is of no additional benefit in this setting.

When the patient is actively bleeding, it is not sufficient to give vitamin K alone. A more immediate restoration of coagulation is required. FFP usually contains sufficient amounts of vitamin K–dependent coagulation proteins to stem further bleeding. Fresh whole blood may be used when hemoglobin is also required. To restore hemostasis to an acceptable level (30% to 50%) of normal enzyme activity, 4 to 6 units of plasma or fresh whole blood is typically required. A similar approach is used in patients previously given warfarin.

MASSIVE TRANSFUSION SYNDROME

Transfusion of large quantities of blood can result in a multifactorial hemostatic defect. The genesis of this problem is related to the "washout" of plasma coagulation proteins and platelets, and it may be exacerbated by the development of DIC with consequent factor consumption or, rarely, by citrate toxicity or hypocalcemia. These variables often act in combination to cause the coagulopathy.[16]

A washout syndrome can result from the transfusion of large amounts of stored blood products devoid of clotting factors and platelets. This develops most commonly in patients who require vigorous resuscitation with blood products (e.g., trauma victims, patients with massive gastrointestinal hemorrhage or hepatectomy, or those undergoing cardiopulmonary bypass). Factors V and VII have short shelf half-lives and are often deficient in blood that has been banked longer than 48 hours. More importantly, qualitative hemostatic platelet activity in whole blood is typically lost within hours of its storage, especially if an acid–citrate–dextrose solution is used. These platelets lose essentially all functional activity. The subsequent development of a washout coagulopathy is directly dependent on the volume of blood transfused relative to the blood volume of the patient. As a general rule, residual plasma clotting activity after one blood volume exchange falls to 18% to 37% of normal; whereas after a two blood volume exchange, residual activity is only 3% to 14%; and after a three-blood-volume exchange, less than 5% of normal clotting function remains.[16]

As previously discussed, DIC may develop in many clinical settings, including some associated with major hemorrhage or massive transfusion. In the presence of hypotension associated with hypovolemia or hemorrhagic shock, DIC is a common sequela. Major trauma itself, especially with the release of tissue factors into the plasma, also can result in the development of DIC. Exsanguinating hemorrhage sometimes requires blood replacement faster than a type and crossmatch of each unit can be performed, and unmatched blood is given as a lifesaving measure. Donor–recipient incompatibility—even when the mismatch is only of the minor blood group systems—can lead to DIC. Human error resulting in major incompatibility can produce lethal hemorrhage. Finally, microaggregates that form within stored blood products also can cause DIC. The advent of smaller pore, more effective filtering systems for blood product administration, however, has essentially eliminated this as a source of problems.

Citrate toxicity in adults as a result of massive transfusion does not seem to be as significant a problem as was once thought. In patients who receive massive transfusions, the development of citrate toxicity seems more closely related to the rate of blood administration than to the absolute amount transfused. There are several other predisposing and virtually prerequisite factors for its development. These include hypovolemia or hypotension, liver disease, hypothermia, preexisting hyperkalemia, and severe metabolic alkalosis. Significant citrate toxicity rarely develops in the absence of these factors unless blood is given at rates exceeding 1 unit every 5 minutes in an average 70-kg man.

Calcium depletion, in addition to the effects of citrate on platelets, has been suggested as a cause of the observed coagulopathy because calcium is a requisite cofactor for the vitamin K–dependent coagulation proteins. Electrocardiographic QT interval prolongation seems to be the only measurable clinical sequela of such calcium depletion and is insignificant in almost all instances. Finally, metabolic abnormalities previously seen with citrate-containing solutions are almost nonexistent with the current use of phosphate-buffered mixtures.

The patient who is bleeding as a consequence of massive transfusion or washout presents with diffuse oozing and bleeding from all surgical wounds and puncture sites. Laboratory abnormalities include prolonged PT, aPTT, and TT. Fibrinogen levels and platelet counts are typically decreased; FDPs are not usually increased unless concurrent DIC is present. The magnitude of the problem can be estimated from the amount of bleeding that has occurred and the blood volume administered relative to the patient's blood volume (i.e., the number of blood volume exchanges that have been given).

The therapeutic approach to patients who develop a coagulopathy from massive transfusion is supportive. Platelets and FFP are given to replete the components of coagulation that are typically lacking. Platelet administration may help stem bleeding from anatomic wounds. Bleeding associated with thrombocytopenia alone is uncommon unless counts fall below 20,000 to 30,000/μL of blood. The complex nature of bleeding seen with massive transfusion, however, may benefit from platelet transfusion at counts even as high as 80,000 to 100,000/μL. FFP is preferred over cryoprecipitate because it has a more complete coagulation protein composition. Cryoprecipitate may be specifically given when fibrinogen depletion is thought to be a major contributor to abnormal hemostasis.

Prospective identification of those at risk to develop a coagulopathy from massive transfusion is important. When the magnitude of the insult and the anticipated need for blood are large, both platelets and FFP should be given before a coagulopathy develops. Four units of platelets and 1 unit of FFP should be given for each 5 units of whole blood or packed cells transfused. This should prevent washout and its attendant bleeding.

When the patient continues to bleed despite what should be adequate therapy for massive transfusion syndrome, other causes should be considered. Specifically, the possibility of DIC should be investigated, particularly if the patient is at risk. Therapy for DIC should then follow guidelines previously mentioned.

ANTICOAGULANT OVERDOSE

Anticoagulant therapy is commonplace in the ICU, and the possibility of errors in administration exists. Methods of prophylactic anticoagulant use, systemic anticoagulation, and thrombolytic therapy are sometimes poorly standardized and can lead to overdose.

Heparin

Heparin is a repeating polymer of two disaccharide glycosaminoglycans and is commercially prepared from either porcine intestinal mucosa or bovine lung. Heparin has an immediate effect on coagulation that is exerted primarily through its influence on antithrombin III. The resulting heparin–antithrombin III complex then inactivates thrombin, as well as factors VII, IX, X, and XI. The extent of heparin's effects seems to be dose related, that is, at low plasma concentrations the heparin–antithrombin III complex primarily inhibits factors X and thrombin, whereas

higher concentrations of heparin inactivate factor VII. Therefore, the TT is most sensitive to the early effects of heparin, followed by the aPTT, and finally the PT. The results of these laboratory tests then may be used to gauge the dose effects of heparin in a given patient, including situations of overdose.

Heparin is metabolized in the liver by the "heparinase" enzyme in a dose-dependent fashion. As the rate of heparin administration is increased, the half-life of the drug is prolonged. For example, when a 100-U/kg bolus of heparin is infused parenterally, the average half-life of the drug is 1 hour. If the bolus is increased to 400 or 800 U/kg, however, the half-life is prolonged to 2.5 and 5 hours, respectively.[17] Therefore, when the dose of heparin is increased, so are its effects. This is an area of potential misunderstanding that can lead to heparin overdose. The nonlinear response results in greater drug effects on coagulation with smaller dosage increments. When one "reboluses" or increases a heparin infusion rate in response to insufficient anticoagulation (i.e., inadequate prolongation of the aPTT), a point will be reached when further small increments in the heparin infusion rate result in a substantially greater prolongation of the aPTT. Although this is usually of little consequence, it has been shown that pathologic bleeding associated with heparin usually occurs during overzealous anticoagulation or inadvertent over-anticoagulation, producing prolongation of the aPTT beyond the therapeutic window.[18] As a corollary, administration of heparin as a continuous parenteral infusion rather than in an intermittent bolus dose regimen is less likely to be associated with pathologic bleeding.

Serious bleeding associated with heparin overdose can be rapidly reversed by protamine sulfate. Protamine binds ionically with heparin to form a complex that lacks any anticoagulant activity. As a general rule, 1 mg of protamine neutralizes approximately 100 U of heparin (specifically, 90 USP units of bovine heparin or 115 USP units of porcine heparin). The dose of protamine needed is calculated from the number of units of active heparin remaining in the patient's system. This, in turn, is estimated from the original heparin dose and the typical half-life for that infusion rate. The aPTT is used to gauge the residual effects of heparin. Protamine itself potentially has anticoagulant effects, and precautions are necessary during its administration. The drug should be given by slow intravenous push over 8 to 10 minutes. A single dose should not exceed 50 mg. This dose may be repeated, but no more than 100 mg should be given as a cumulative dose without rechecking coagulation parameters. The dose of protamine should always be monitored by coagulation studies. Significant side effects are most commonly seen in situations of overly rapid drug administration and include hypotension and anaphylactoid-like reactions.

Warfarin

Warfarin and vitamin K share a similar chemical structure in their respective 4-hydroxycoumarin nucleus and naphthoquinone ring. In fact, evidence suggests that the mechanism of action of warfarin is through competitive binding at the vitamin K receptor site, where postribosomal modification of the vitamin K–dependent coagulation proteins (factors

II, VII, IX, and X) occurs. When warfarin is present in sufficient plasma concentrations, there is depletion of the active forms of vitamin K–dependent factors.

The PT is a reasonable indicator of the effects of warfarin when its use has continued beyond 2 or 3 days. Factor VII has a half-life of only 4 to 6 hours and is rapidly depleted after one or two doses of warfarin. The remainder of the vitamin K–dependent factors may take up to a week to become depleted. The PT becomes prolonged with factor VII depletion alone but does not reflect an overall state of anticoagulation until an equilibrium period of several days has passed. Over this time, the other vitamin K–dependent factors are depleted and PT prolongation can then be used to assess the anticoagulant effects of warfarin. In severe cases of warfarin overdose, the aPTT also becomes prolonged.

Several drugs and pathophysiologic conditions are associated with potentiation of warfarin's effects on coagulation. Table 154-4 lists many of the drugs known to prolong the effects of warfarin.[17] These drugs have a variety of mechanisms, which generally include either inhibition of function or competitive binding of the enzymes responsible for active warfarin metabolism. Aspirin does not seem to have any direct influence on warfarin metabolism but can so profoundly influence qualitative platelet function that it must be considered as a potentiator of warfarin's anticoagulant effects. The same is true for clofibrate. Large ingestion of aspirin may also impair prothrombin (factor II) synthesis, further increasing the effects of warfarin administration. Warfarin is metabolized by the liver. Conditions of acute and chronic hepatic dysfunction can alter warfarin metabolism and vitamin K–mediated Gamma-carboxylation of the vitamin K–dependent coagulation proteins. Broad-spectrum antibiotics also may limit vitamin K availability through their alteration of the gut flora (in addition to their direct effects on vitamin K metabolism). All of these factors may ultimately influence a patient's response to warfarin.

When over-anticoagulation with warfarin presents with bleeding, immediate reversal is usually mandated. The treatment of choice is FFP, which provides prompt restoration of the deficient vitamin K–dependent coagulation proteins, along with restoration of hemostatic function. Four to 6 units of FFP are usually sufficient. Vitamin K also may be administered, particularly in situations that are less acute (see section "Vitamin K Deficiency").

Warfarin necrosis is characterized pathologically by the thrombosis of small blood vessels in the fat and subcutaneous tissues, with consequent necrosis. Protein C also is a vitamin K–dependent anticoagulant protein and is subject to the effects of warfarin as well. In some situations (particularly when an initial dose of warfarin greater than 10 to 15 mg is given), levels of protein C may fall before those of the vitamin K–dependent coagulation proteins reach "anticoagulant" levels. Under these conditions, thrombosis may be precipitated. This generally can be avoided if heparin and warfarin therapy are overlapped until "coumadinization" is complete and if large loading doses of warfarin are avoided.

PLATELET DISORDERS

Platelet disorders are a common cause of clinical bleeding in the ICU. They can be grouped into quantitative and qualitative defects. Table 154-5 presents an overview of platelet disorders based on this classification scheme.

Quantitative Disorders

A decrease in the number of circulating platelets reflects either increased peripheral destruction–sequestration, decreased marrow production, or a combination of these factors. Examples of increased peripheral destruction include immune-mediated processes (both autoimmune and drug induced), abnormal consumption (as in DIC), and mechanical destruction (e.g., cardiopulmonary bypass, hyperthermia). Autoimmune processes such as idiopathic thrombocytopenic purpura (ITP), SLE, or acquired immunodeficiency syndrome can result in increased peripheral destruction and increased splenic sequestration of platelets. Autoimmune destruction also may occur in conjunction with lymphocytic leukemia or lymphoma. The prototypic example of these processes is ITP, in which IgG directed against specific platelet antigens is thought to be responsible for platelet destruction. Acute ITP is usually self-limited, with life-threatening bleeding occurring only rarely. In contrast, chronic ITP generally requires therapy. Steroids may be given (1 to 2 mg/kg day of prednisone or its equivalent). Splenectomy also may be required to avert serious bleeding complications in patients who do not respond to steroids. Agents such as vincristine/vinblastine and cyclophosphamide also have been used as immunosuppressants, with variable success. More recently, high doses of intravenous gamma globulin (1 to 2 g/kg given over 2 to 5 days) have been useful in producing at least transient elevations in platelet counts. In many clinical conditions, intravenous IgG has been shown to be as efficacious as corticosteroids in improving the platelet count.

Drug-induced immune-mediated platelet destruction is a common cause of thrombocytopenia seen in the ICU. Fortunately, it is usually reversible; withdrawal of the offending drug prevents further immune-mediated platelet destruction. The exact mechanism of platelet destruction seems to be related to the binding (coating) of a drug to

TABLE 154-4. Drugs That Potentiate the Anticoagulant Effects of Warfarin

ANTIBIOTICS	Phenylbutazone (oxy-phenbutazone)
Broad-spectrum antibiotics (especially cephalosporins)	Sulfinpyrazone
Griseofulvin (oral)	
Metronidazole	OTHER DRUGS
Sulfonamides	Cimetidine
Trimethoprim-sulfamethoxazole	Clofibrate
	Disulfiram
ANTIINFLAMMATORY DRUGS	Phenytoin
	Thyroxine (both D- and L-isomers)
Steroids (anabolic, in particular)	Tolbutamide
Acetylated salicylates	

TABLE 154-5. Platelet Disorders Seen in the ICU

QUANTITATIVE	QUALITATIVE

INCREASED DESTRUCTION
    Immune
        Idiopathic thrombocytopenic purpura
        Systemic lupus erythematosus
        Acquired immunodeficiency syndrome
        Drugs (gold salts, heparin, sulfonamides,
            quinidine, quinine)
        Sepsis
    Nonimmune
        Thrombotic thrombocytopenic purpura/
            hemolytic uremic syndrome
        Mechanical destruction (e.g., cardiopulmonary
            bypass, hyperthemia)
        Consumption (i.e., DIC)
 	
DECREASED PRODUCTION
    Marrow suppression
        Chemotherapy
        Viral illness (e.g., cytomegalovirus, Epstein-Barr
            virus, herpes simplex, parvovirus)
        Drugs (thiazides, ethanol, cimetidine)
    Marrow replacement
        Tumor
        Myelofibrosis
    Other conditions
        Splenic sequestration
        Dilution (see massive transfusion syndrome)
	DRUGS
	    Antiinflammatory agents
	        Aspirin (irreversible)
	        Nonsteroidal anti-inflammatory agents
	        Corticosteroids
	    Antibiotics
	        Penicillins (e.g., ampicillin,
	            carbenicillin, ticarcillin, penicillin-G)
	        Cephalosporins (e.g., cephalothin)
	        Nitrofurantoin
	        Chloroquine, hydroxychloroquine
	    Phosphodiesterase inhibitors
	        Dipyridamole
	        Methylxanthines (e.g., theophylline)
	    Other drugs
	        Antihistamines
	        Alpha-blockers (e.g., phentolamine)
	        Beta-blockers (e.g., propranolol)
	        Dextran
	        Ethanol
	        Furosemide
	        Heparin
	        Local anesthetics (e.g., lidocaine)
	        Phenothiazines
	        Tricyclic antidepressants
	        Nitrates (e.g., sodium nitroprusside,
	            nitroglycerin)
	
	METABOLIC CAUSES
	    Uremia
	    Stored whole blood
	    Disseminated intravascular coagulation
	        (i.e., FDPs)
	    Hypothyroidism

the platelet membrane surface, with subsequent binding to the platelet, platelet–drug complex, or both, of a specific antibody. The resulting platelet–drug–antibody complexes then are cleared by the reticuloendothelial system and thrombocytopenia develops. Drugs used in the ICU that are most commonly associated with this clinical picture include quinidine, quinine, heparin, gold salts, various penicillin and cephalosporin antibiotics, and the sulfonamides. In all of these immune-mediated conditions, thrombopoiesis is usually preserved unless the disorder is multifactorial.

A variety of drugs are associated with the nonimmune development of thrombocytopenia by bone marrow suppression. Several of the cancer chemotherapeutic agents currently used may adversely influence thrombopoiesis. The thiazide diuretics, cimetidine, ethanol, and several of the cephalosporin and penicillin antibiotics may suppress platelet production. Generalized infection, such as bacterial sepsis, and many viral illnesses also are associated with bone marrow suppression and thrombocytopenia. The extent of thrombocytopenia alone is infrequently sufficient to cause

significant clinical bleeding, however. Bone marrow replacement with tumor cells and myelofibrosis are uncommon causes of thrombocytopenia in the ICU.

Consumption of platelets also can cause thrombocytopenia. Mechanical destruction invariably occurs during the use of cardiopulmonary bypass machines. Platelets also are destroyed by the high body temperatures seen in severe hyperthermic syndromes and consumed during active coagulation in DIC. In many of these circumstances, the development of thrombocytopenia is associated with significant clinical bleeding, primarily caused by the coexistence of other abnormalities of hemostasis.

Heparin-Induced Thrombocytopenia

The special problems associated with heparin merit emphasis. Heparin use is ubiquitous in the ICU. Heparin-induced thrombocytopenia may develop in one of two ways.[11] Acute nonidiosyncratic heparin-induced thrombocytopenia is seen in approximately 10% to 15% of patients receiving heparin.

It usually remits despite continued use of the drug. The thrombocytopenia that develops is mild and is usually of little or no clinical significance. Heparin need not be stopped in these patients. Idiosyncratic heparin-induced thrombocytopenia is of much greater clinical consequence. Although it is a less frequent occurrence (typically seen in fewer than 5% of patients receiving heparin), it has a much greater potential for clinical morbidity. Arterial thrombosis is the usual problem and may be life threatening in that it may cause myocardial infarction, cerebrovascular accident, or pulmonary embolism. The mechanism of thrombosis is thought to be a consequence of the deposition of platelet aggregates in the microcirculation. Thrombocytopenia, like other immune-mediated drug reactions, seems to involve the formation of platelet aggregates mediated by the binding of specific antibody to platelets in the presence of heparin. This process seems to require minuscule amounts of heparin. Clinical bleeding is an infrequent problem in these patients.

From a practical perspective, the diagnosis of heparin-induced thrombocytopenia is usually one of exclusion. Diagnostic markers do exist (e.g., heparin-dependent platelet serotonin release), but these tests are best considered confirmatory and not exclusive. The diagnosis may be difficult to confirm because coexisting clinical illnesses with the potential to cause thrombocytopenia also may be present. Heparin-induced thrombocytopenia is more likely to be associated with the use of bovine lung heparin, although it may occur after exposure to porcine heparin as well. The clinician must balance the relative importance of the primary thrombosis for which heparin is being given against the risk that a new secondary focus of arterial thrombosis will develop from its continued use. Unless thrombocytopenia becomes severe, it is rarely necessary to discontinue heparin on the basis of platelet count alone.[7]

Qualitative Disorders

These disorders are particularly important in the ICU, where virtually all drugs used can be potential causes of qualitative platelet dysfunction. Many drugs associated with qualitative platelet dysfunction often are used in the sickest patients. These individuals often have other underlying pathophysiologic conditions that can predispose to bleeding. Table 154-5 provides an abbreviated list of the drugs that can affect at least in vitro platelet function.

All unnecessary drugs should be viewed as suspect and discontinued in patients with evidence of qualitative platelet dysfunction. Terminating the offending drugs usually results in a restoration of normal platelet functional activity.

Aspirin is the notable exception. It irreversibly inhibits platelet cyclooxygenase, resulting in a defect that lasts for the duration of the platelet life span (8 to 9 days). The effect is profound: a single 325-mg aspirin tablet results in a qualitative platelet hemostatic defect that remains in 50% of the circulating platelets 5 days after its ingestion.

Nonsteroidal antiinflammatory agents similarly affect the platelet cyclooxygenase enzyme. However, their effects are reversible, and normal platelet function is usually restored within 24 hours of the last dose. The β-lactam antibiotics stearically hinder the binding of a platelet aggregation agonist (e.g., ADP) to its specific platelet receptor, thus resulting in impaired platelet aggregation under circumstances of normal physiologic stimulation. This, too, is reversed on removal of the drug. Many of these same antibiotics can also influence the vitamin K–dependent coagulation proteins, resulting in an additional impediment to normal hemostatic function.

Management

Because many of the adverse drug-related platelet effects are reversible, all unnecessary medications should be discontinued promptly when primary hemostasis seems affected. The more controversial issue is deciding whether platelet transfusions are warranted in a particular patient.

The relationship of thrombocytopenia to clinical bleeding is relative, that is, it is difficult to identify a specific, arbitrary platelet count (threshold) beyond which bleeding is likely to occur. Several conditions, such as massive transfusion syndrome and DIC, may respond to empirical platelet transfusion at counts as high as 80,000 or even 100,000 platelets/μL. With other causes, such as thrombocytopenia seen with cancer chemotherapy and bone marrow aplasia, therapy may not be required until counts fall below 20,000/μL. Thrombocytopenia related to peripheral destruction is less likely to respond to platelet transfusion.

The morbidity and mortality related to bleeding increase markedly in patients undergoing induction chemotherapy for acute leukemia when the platelet count falls below 10,000 to 20,000/μL. Empirical administration of platelets to these patients significantly limits both morbidity and mortality. This finding, however, has been generalized to virtually all patients with platelet counts in this range. The efficacy of this approach is doubtful. A major concern that should temper the empirical use of platelet transfusion is the development of alloimmunization to transfused platelets, potentially negating any future benefit from platelet transfusion in a time of need. Patients with acute leukemia typically have self-limited marrow aplasia resulting from chemotherapy. Therefore, the need for platelet transfusion is also limited and the chances for development of antiplatelet antibodies are greatly decreased. Patients with aplastic anemia, however, have an ongoing need for platelet transfusion, so their risk of alloimmunization is high. Autoimmune disorders associated with increased peripheral platelet destruction, disorders of splenic sequestration, and drug-related thrombocytopenia are unlikely to benefit from platelet transfusion. An exception is related to planned invasive procedures with an increased risk of bleeding. In this situation, empirical platelet transfusion immediately before the procedure may be reasonable.

Empiric platelet transfusion should be reserved for significant thrombocytopenia related to transient marrow aplasia secondary to cancer chemotherapy, massive transfusion syndrome, the situations in DIC outlined previously, conditions in which active bleeding already is present, and invasive procedures that are potentially associated with bleeding.

Uremia

Uremia can cause reversible impairment of qualitative platelet function and is commonly seen in the ICU. The "toxin" responsible for this defect is not well defined, although its effect seems to be related to impaired platelet–von Willebrand factor interactions. The degree of impairment seems to be related to the severity of uremia for a given patient.

Several approaches may modulate the qualitative platelet defect associated with uremia. The primary therapy in this setting is dialysis. Cryoprecipitate, 1-deamino-8-D-arginine vasopressin (DDAVP), and conjugated estrogens have been given to patients with severe uremia and an isolated primary hemostatic defect with good results.[19–21] The mechanism of action of both cryoprecipitate and DDAVP is related to the consequent increase in the plasma concentration of the large multimeric forms of von Willebrand factor, thus greatly improving platelet adhesion. The durations of action of these agents, however, are limited, reaching their zenith between 2 and 6 hours. Additional doses of DDAVP during the same 24-hour period can result in a diminished response to the drug (tachyphylaxis). Patients may ultimately become refractory to DDAVP for 48 to 72 hours when the drug is given this frequently. The mechanism of action of the conjugated estrogens is not known. In contrast to the first two therapies described, the effect of estrogen is more protracted and does not diminish with repeat dosing.

THROMBOTIC SYNDROMES

The following thrombotic disorders occur commonly in the ICU:

Thrombotic thrombocytopenic purpura/hemolytic-uremic syndrome
Deep venous thrombosis
Pulmonary embolism sydrome
Heparin-induced thrombocytopenia
Thrombotic DIC
Coronary thrombosis/acute myocardial infarction
Stroke
Peripheral vascular disease/arterial thrombosis

Many of these, particularly venous thromboembolic diseases, often develop while the patient is in the ICU and may be preventable. Most of these disorders are discussed in detail throughout the text.

LABORATORY ABNORMALITIES NOT ASSOCIATED WITH BLEEDING

LUPUS ANTICOAGULANT

The lupus anticoagulant has received much attention as a potential cause of bleeding by virtue of its name and its associated laboratory abnormalities. As an isolated hemostatic defect, thrombosis is the more likely problem (25%

incidence rate), with bleeding in one series occurring in only 1 of 219 patients with the lupus anticoagulant.[22,23]

The PT and aPTT assays depend on the interaction of various coagulation factors with either a lipoprotein or phospholipid to activate coagulation efficiently. The lupus anticoagulant seems to be an antiphospholipid antibody directed against these phospholipids or lipoproteins and produces prolongation of the PT, aPTT, or the measured recalcification time of platelet-rich plasma. Prolongation of the aPTT is much more common than prolongation of the PT. Twenty-five percent of patients with active SLE and the lupus anticoagulant also have associated thrombocytopenia or hypoprothrombinemia and are therefore at risk for bleeding (unlike those with the lupus anticoagulant alone). Although the lupus anticoagulant was originally described in patients with SLE, it is not limited to this class of diseases. Indeed, lupus anticoagulants or anticardiolipin antibodies, or both, have been demonstrated in large percentages of patients with human immunodeficiency virus infection, hemophilia A, or both. Lupus anticoagulants also are observed in disorders accompanied by chronic inflammation.

Thrombotic events may occur independently of the underlying disorder and seem to be directly related to the lupus anticoagulant itself. The relationship of these immunoglobulins to thrombosis is not understood. Some forms of the disorder, such as that associated with pregnancy, do respond to antiinflammatory drugs such as aspirin or prednisone. Thrombosis, when it occurs, is equally likely to be venous or arterial. Venous thrombosis is more common in the extremities while arterial thrombosis is more common in the central nervous system. Placental infarcts are frequently seen in placental specimens in those patients with repeated fetal wastage. Stroke, myocardial infarction, and pulmonary embolization are also well described in patients with the lupus anticoagulant.

REACTIVE HYPERFIBRINOGENEMIA

Hyperfibrinogenemia is defined as a plasma fibrinogen concentration greater than 800 mg/dL. Usually the plasma fibrinogen concentration is measured with the Clauss method. Plasma from the patient is allowed to clot in the presence of excess thrombin. The time to clotting in this setting is proportional to the amount of fibrinogen present in the sample. When excessive amounts of fibrinogen are present, clotting is incomplete and fibrin fragments that inhibit further fibrin clot formation are formed. Other hematologic parameters, such as the aPTT, PT, and the TT, are consequently prolonged, suggesting a potential (artefactual) for bleeding despite a high fibrinogen level. This is evaluated by diluting the plasma to a normal fibrinogen concentration using saline or defibrinated plasma. These same clotting studies will now be normal. Bleeding is not seen unless the fibrinogen also is a dysfibrinogen, although even in these patients, bleeding remains an uncommon problem. In patients with dysfibrinogenemia, clotting studies fail to correct when either saline or defibrinated plasma dilutions are undertaken, thus distinguishing them from patients with reactive hyperfibrinogenemia.

SELECTED DISORDERS ■

SYSTEMIC DISEASES ASSOCIATED WITH FACTOR DEFICIENCIES

Amyloidosis, Gaucher's disease, and the nephrotic syndrome are occasionally seen in the ICU. Each may have one or more associated factor deficiencies that may complicate patient management and cause bleeding. Patients with either amyloidosis or Gaucher's disease may develop factor IX deficiency. Factor X deficiency also has been associated with amyloidosis. These deficiencies generally result from the absorption of the specific clotting factor onto the abnormal proteins present with each disorder. In the nephrotic syndrome, factor IX deficiency also may develop. Although it was originally thought that proteinuria was responsible for the development of factor IX deficiency, this does not appear to be the case. The deficiency typically remits with corticosteroid therapy. Finally, antithrombin III deficiency can be seen along with the nephrotic syndrome and may lead to thrombosis. The loss of antithrombin III does appear to be related to proteinuria.

REFERENCES ■

1. Messmore HL Jr, Godwin J: Medical assessment of the bleeding surgical patient. *Med Clin North Am* 1994;78:625
2. Feinstin DI: Treatment of disseminated intravascular coagulation. *Semin Thromb Hemost* 1988;14:351
3. Bick RL: Disseminated intravascular coagulation: objective criteria for diagnosis and management. *Med Clin North Am* 1994;78:545
4. Bick RL: Coagulation abnormalities in malignancy: a review. *Semin Thromb Hemost* 1992;19:184
5. Parmo JA, Rocha E: Hemostasis in advanced liver disease. *Semin Thromb Hemost* 1993;19:184
6. Mammen EF: Coagulation abnormalities in liver disease. *Hematol Oncol Clin North Am* 1992;6:1247
7. Barton JC, Poon MC: Coagulation testing of the Hickmann catheter blood in patients with acute leukemia. *Arch Intern Med* 1986;146:2165
8. Fareed J, Hoppenstedt D, Bick RL, et al: Drug-induced alterations of hemostasis and fibrinolysis. *Hematol Oncol Clin North Am* 1992;6:1229
9. Phillips LL: Transfusion support in acquired coagulation disorders. *Clin Hematol* 1984;13:137
10. Gralnick HR, Bagley J, Abrell E: Heparin treatment for the hemorrhagic diathesis of acute promyelocytic leukemia. *Am J Med* 1972;52:167
11. Warkentin TE, Kelton JG: Heparin-induced thrombocytopenia. *Ann Rev Med* 1990;41:1
12. Schwartz BS, Williams EC, Conlon MG, et al: Epsilon-aminocaproic acid in the treatment of patients with acute promyelocytic leukemia and acquired alpha-2-plasmin inhibitor deficiency. *Ann Intern Med* 1986;105:873
13. Clouse LH, Comp PC: The regulation of hemostasis: the protein C system. *N Engl J Med* 1986;314:1298
14. Stump DC, Taylor FB, Nesheim ME, et al: Pathologic fibrinolysis as a cause of clinical bleeding. *Semin Thromb Hemost* 1990;16:260
15. Routh CR, Triplett DA, Murphy MJ, et al: Superwarfarin ingestion and detection. *Am J Hematol* 1991;36:50
16. Gralnick HR: Massive transfusion. In: Colman RW, Hirsh J, Marder VJ, et al (eds): *Hemostasis and Thrombosis: Basic Principles and Clinical Practice.* Philadelphia, JB Lippincott, 1982
17. Majerus PW, Broze GJ Jr, Miletich JP, et al: Anticoagulant, thrombolytic and antiplatelet drugs. In: Gilman AG, Rall TW, Nies AS, et al (eds). *Goodman and Gilman's The Pharmacologic Basis of Therapeutics*, ed 8. New York, Pergamon Press, 1990
18. Penner JA: Managing the hemorrhagic complications of heparin therapy. *Hematol Oncol Clin North Am* 1993;7:1281
19. Janson PA, Jubelirer SJ, Weinstein MJ, et al: Treatment of the bleeding tendency in uremia with cryoprecipitate. *N Engl J Med* 1980;303:1318
20. Livio M, Mannucci PM, Vigano G, et al: Conjugated estrogens for the management of bleeding associated with renal failure. *N Engl J Med* 1986;315:731
21. Mannucci PM, Remuzzi G, Pusineri F, et al: Deamino-8-D-arginine vasopressin shortens the bleeding time in uremia. *N Engl J Med* 1983;308:8
22. Asherson RA, Khamashta MA, Ordi-Ros J, et al: The "primary" anti-phosopholipid syndrome: major clinical and serologic features. *Medicine* 1989;68:366
23. Bick RL, Ancypa D: The antiphospholipid and thrombosis (APL-T) syndromes: clinical and laboratory correlates. *Clin Lab Med* 1995;15:63

Critical Care, Third Edition, edited by Joseph M. Civetta,
Robert W. Taylor, and Robert R. Kirby.
Lippincott-Raven Publishers, Philadelphia, PA © 1997.

CHAPTER 155

■

Hematologic Diseases

David A. Sears

REDUCED BLOOD COUNTS ■

ANEMIA

The most immediate concern for the physician confronted by a patient with severe anemia is to decide whether the patient requires transfusion with red blood cells. The answer to this important question does not depend simply on the laboratory values for hematocrit or hemoglobin concentration, but on the physiologic state of the patient with regard to intravascular volume and tissue oxygen delivery.[1,2] Table 155-1 shows the basic indications for transfusion of red blood cells, the guidelines to be used in arriving at a decision to transfuse, and alternatives or adjuncts to transfusion. The hematocrit level associated with findings that dictate transfusion varies widely among patients depending on oxygen demand, cardiac output, distribution of blood flow, and affinity of hemoglobin for oxygen. Volume expansion with colloid or electrolyte solutions often improves the physiologic state of the hypovolemic patient, even if it results in a marked drop in hematocrit. Administering oxygen to the patient whose saturation is already 100% only increases blood oxygen content by the small volume of oxygen that can be dissolved in plasma. However, in the severely anemic patient, that small increment may mean a 20% to 25% increase in blood oxygen-carrying capacity. Patients with severe aplastic anemia, who may be candidates for bone marrow transplantation in the future, warrant special consideration. Transfusion should be avoided, if possible, because it diminishes the success rate of the procedure.[3] Principles of transfusion therapy in critical care are covered in more detail in Chapter 43.

If a patient requires transfusion, the question must be asked: What diagnostic studies may be altered by transfusion and should, therefore, be obtained before blood is administered? A complete blood count should be obtained, including at least hematocrit or hemoglobin concentration and mean cell volume, a reticulocyte count, and a stained blood smear in all cases. If a hemoglobinopathy is suspected, hemoglobin electrophoresis should be obtained before transfusion. If folic acid deficiency is suspected, it may be appropriate to order the red blood cell folic acid level before transfusion. If immune hemolytic disease is suspected, antiglobulin (Coombs') tests should be ordered. The sample sent to the blood bank for typing and crossmatching usually suffices for necessary immediate immunologic diagnostic studies. Other pretransfusion tests are necessary only in certain circumstances. For example, it is not necessary to obtain serum iron or vitamin B_{12} levels routinely, because these deficiencies can be diagnosed even after red blood cell transfusion. The reticulocyte count, converted to "reticulocyte index" by correction for (1) the degree of the anemia and (2) early release of erythroid cells from the marrow, provides an estimate of the rate of red cell production and, therefore, destruction.[4] Immediate determination of serum bilirubin, haptoglobin, or lactic acid dehydrogenase is not required to identify hemolytic disease. Table 155-2 summarizes these principles.

Autoimmune Hemolytic Anemia

When a patient is critically ill from autoimmune hemolytic anemia (AIHA), the presenting signs and symptoms are those of normovolemic anemia.[5] Mild jaundice also may be present. Initial laboratory data show an elevated reticulocyte index (greater than 2) identifying the mechanism of the anemia as hemolytic, and the blood smear shows increased numbers of diffusely basophilic (polychromatophilic) red cells (reflecting the increased reticulocytes) and variable numbers of microspherocytes and fragmented cells. In rare instances, the urine may be discolored (red, brown, or black) if there has been sufficient intravascular hemolysis to produce hemoglobinuria. A positive result on direct antiglobulin

TABLE 155-1. Transfusion of Red Blood Cells

INDICATIONS	GUIDELINES	ALTERNATIVES
Reduced blood volume (acute blood loss)	Tachycardia Hypotension Instability of heart rate and blood pressure on sitting up or standing	Non-red cell–containing volume-expanding fluids
Reduced oxygen-carrying capacity	Tachypnea Evidence of hypoxia of specific organs (e.g., confusion, angina, lactic acidosis)	Oxygen therapy

(Coombs') test, indicating that immunoglobulin or complement is on the surface of the circulating red cells, identifies the immune etiology of the hemolysis. In the absence of recent transfusion, the diagnosis of AIHA is confirmed. This information may first become available when the blood bank attempts to crossmatch the patient's blood for transfusion.

It is important to determine, by history and appropriate laboratory studies, whether the hemolysis could be related to a drug the patient is taking and whether it is caused by warm-reacting (usually IgG) or cold-reacting (usually IgM) antibodies. The mechanisms whereby drugs produce immune hemolysis are not absolutely clear, but evidence suggests an alteration of red cell surface antigens by the drug and production of antibodies that lead to hemolysis.[6] In some instances, the drug must be present for hemolysis to occur (e.g., quinidine, penicillin); in others, hemolysis occurs even in the absence of the drug (e.g., methyldopa). Underlying diseases that may be associated with AIHA include infections, such as infectious mononucleosis and pneumonia caused by *Mycoplasma pneumoniae*, collagen vascular diseases (especially systemic lupus erythematosus), and lymphoproliferative disorders such as chronic lymphocytic leuke-

TABLE 155-2. Effects of Transfusions on Diagnostic Laboratory Tests

STUDIES THAT SHOULD BE OBTAINED *BEFORE* TRANSFUSION OF RED BLOOD CELLS

In all anemic patients
    Complete blood count
    Reticulocyte count
    Stained blood smear
In certain anemic patients
    Hemoglobin electrophoresis
    Red blood cell folic acid
    Antiglobulin (Coombs') tests°

STUDIES THAT ARE USUALLY VALID *AFTER* TRANSFUSION OF RED BLOOD CELLS

    Serum iron
    Serum B_{12}
    Serum folic acid

°The blood sent for "type and crossmatch" usually suffices for necessary immunologic studies.

mia.[7] In some instances, the AIHA may be the presenting manifestation of the underlying disease.

The mainstay of treatment of AIHA caused by warm-reacting antibodies is corticosteroids, usually given in dosages equivalent to 60 to 80 mg/day of prednisone. In patients who do not respond to steroids, splenectomy, high-dose intravenous gamma globulin, or treatment with immunosuppressive drugs may be useful. Steroids are usually ineffective in AIHA that is caused by cold-reactive antibodies (cold agglutinin disease), but responses have been observed using larger doses.[8] Patients with cold agglutinins may have symptoms related to impaired blood flow in acral parts where the blood temperature is low enough to permit agglutination of red blood cells by antibodies. Warming usually prevents or alleviates such symptoms; but, in a small percentage of cases, plasmapheresis to reduce the concentration of the offending IgM antibodies may be required. In drug-induced immune hemolysis, discontinuing the drug is usually the only treatment needed.

In the patient with AIHA who has a critical degree of anemia, transfusion must be considered.[9] It may be impossible to find "compatible" red blood cells by the usual crossmatching procedures, and transfused cells may be subject to rapid antibody-mediated destruction. On the other hand, the patient must not be allowed to die because of undue caution regarding the transfusion of "incompatible" red cells. The key to optimal care in this critical situation is close communication between the clinician and the blood bank physician. In some cases, identification of the specificity of the offending antibody may permit selection of more compatible units. In other cases, the blood bank must simply resort to selection of the "least incompatible" donor units that can be identified by in vitro testing. Regardless of test results, when an AIHA patient is transfused, the patient must be observed closely for signs of accelerated hemolysis, such as visible hemoglobin in the plasma or urine.

Certain special considerations pertain to transfusion of patients with cold-reacting antibodies. Administered blood should be warmed to body temperature. Transfusion of plasma, which contains complement, should be avoided because hemolysis is complement mediated and may be limited by depletion of complement in vivo.

If hemolysis is massive and associated with hypotension and significant hemoglobinuria, acute renal failure may occur. Therapeutic efforts should be directed at maintenance of blood pressure, renal blood flow, and urinary output. Intravenous fluids and diuretics such as furosemide should be used to maintain a urine flow of 100 mL/hour.

Hemolytic Anemia From G6PD Deficiency

Red blood cell glucose-6-phosphate dehydrogenase (G6PD) deficiency is inherited as an X-linked recessive disorder and affects various population groups around the world.[10] In the United States, African-Americans are the group most often affected, with a gene frequency of about 11%. They have the G6PD A–variant of the enzyme and a mild to moderate deficiency. The red cell G6PD levels in affected men are 8% to 20% of normal. Clinically significant hemolysis occurs when red cells are subjected to an oxidative metabolic challenge, as may occur with exposure to certain drugs or with certain illnesses. Among drugs producing hemolysis are some sulfonamides, nitrofurantoins, and antimalarials such as primaquine. Illnesses most likely to trigger hemolysis are acute infections. Infectious hepatitis, in particular, has been associated with severe hemolytic episodes in G6PD-deficient patients.[11]

Hemolysis in the G6PD-deficient patient may be sudden and massive, usually becoming apparent 1 to 3 days after the inciting stress, such as administration of an oxidant drug. Hemoglobinemia and hemoglobinuria may occur. The blood smear shows polychromatophilia within a few days, reflecting the developing reticulocytosis. Microspherocytes and red cells with eccentrically distributed hemoglobin may be present. Early in the course of the hemolytic episode, Heinz bodies may be identified in red cells by special staining methods. These precipitates of oxidatively denatured hemoglobin provide a useful diagnostic clue and should be sought if G6PD deficiency is suspected as a cause of acute hemolysis. However, the absence of Heinz bodies does not exclude this diagnosis. The red cell enzyme deficiency may be readily detected by laboratory assay when the patient is in a stable state, but may be more difficult to demonstrate during a hemolytic episode. This is because the enzyme deficiency is greatest in the oldest red cells. These cells are the first destroyed in a hemolytic episode, and as they are replaced by newly produced young cells, the overall red cell enzyme level may rise to the normal range. This replacement of susceptible erythrocytes by more resistant cells also tends to produce amelioration of the hemolysis with time.

If the diagnosis is suspected, any potentially offending drugs should be stopped. Otherwise, supportive care is usually all that is necessary. Although the deficiency is an X-linked trait, female heterozygotes may have hemolytic episodes.

Hemolytic Anemia From Red Cell Injury in the Circulation

Fragmentation and destruction of red cells in the circulation may result from increased shear stresses caused by turbulent blood flow.[12] The two major categories of disease in which this kind of hemolysis occurs are malfunctioning intravascular prosthetic devices (e.g., heart valves, vascular grafts, and shunts) and disorders affecting blood vessels to produce so-

called microangiopathic hemolytic disease (e.g., disseminated intravascular coagulation, thrombotic thrombocytopenic purpura [TTP], hemolytic uremic syndrome, and various vasculitides). These forms of hemolytic disease are rarely of sufficient severity to require critical care.

Because hemolysis is intravascular, hemoglobinemia and hemoglobinuria may be present. Characteristically, the blood smear shows red cell fragmentation producing micropoikilocytes (schistocytes). Specific treatment is directed at the underlying disorder. Supportive measures may be required for the effects of hemolysis itself and to minimize any adverse renal consequences of hypotension and hemoglobinuria. These may include blood transfusion and hydration to ensure good urine flow. Occasionally, a badly malfunctioning prosthesis, such as an artificial heart valve, may require replacement, but this is more often necessary to correct a life-threatening hemodynamic abnormality than to alleviate severe hemolysis. Even severe degrees of hemolysis may be well tolerated, and the hemoglobinemia and hemoglobinuria are, in themselves, not usually harmful.

Sickle Cell Anemia

Many of the complicating syndromes occurring in the sickle cell disorders are labeled "crises" and present as problems requiring critical care.[13] Table 155-3 presents a partial list. "Hemolytic crisis" is not mentioned; moderate to severe worsening of anemia resulting from accelerated hemolysis is not characteristic of sickle cell diseases. If hemolysis does increase significantly, a second disorder, such as G6PD deficiency or AIHA, should be sought.

The discussion here is directed primarily toward homozygous sickle cell disease. Patients with related, commonly occurring, doubly heterozygous conditions, such as sickle cell-hemoglobin C disease and sickle cell-β-thalassemia, may have similar complications. It is important to recognize that sickle cell trait, the heterozygous sickle cell state, rarely causes symptoms, signs, or laboratory abnormalities.[14]

PAINFUL CRISIS.   The painful or vasoocclusive crisis is the most common symptomatic event in sickle cell disease.[15] Its onset is unpredictable and usually without known precipitants. It is manifested by severe deep pain, which occurs most often in musculoskeletal areas of the extremities and back but also may affect the chest and abdomen. There are

TABLE 155-3.   Complications of Sickle Cell Disorders

Painful (vasoocclusive) crisis
Chest syndrome
Hepatic crisis
Cholelithiasis
Aseptic necrosis of bone
Bone marrow necrosis and fat embolism
Cerebral vascular occlusion
Hematuria
Priapism
Splenic infarction and sequestration
Asplenic sepsis syndrome

no pathognomonic signs, and laboratory test and radiograph results are inconclusive. The diagnosis thus is made by the patient's history and exclusion of other possible diagnoses by appropriate physical examination and laboratory testing. The frequency of painful crises is variable in different patients and in a given patient over time. The crisis is self-limited and may last only minutes or as long as 2 to 3 weeks.

Treatment of the painful crisis is supportive. Dehydration, acidosis, and hypoxemia all promote red cell sickling and should be prevented or corrected. Adequate relief of pain in the hospitalized patient usually requires parenteral administration of opioid analgesics. Physicians are sometimes concerned about drug dependence, but the addiction potential of narcotics administered for pain in the hospital is low. Physicians also worry about dangerous side effects of opiates, such as respiratory depression, but these are rare in the sickle cell patient with painful crisis. Sufficient analgesics should be used to relieve pain. Oxygen is often administered in sickle cell crisis, but its benefits are uncertain. If the arterial oxygen saturation is normal, it need not be given. As is discussed later, red cell transfusion or exchange transfusion is recommended for some severe complications of sickle cell disease. However, because there is no clear evidence that transfusion therapy shortens simple painful crises and because the crisis is unpredictable and self-limited, transfusion is not a treatment for the uncomplicated painful crisis.

LUNGS.   The term *acute chest syndrome* is used to describe the clinical situation in which painful crisis is accompanied by pleuritic chest pain, fever, and a pulmonary infiltrate on chest radiograph.[16] The usual etiology is probably in situ vasoocclusion, but infection and thromboembolism are difficult to exclude. The major concern is that a vicious cycle may be initiated of pulmonary vasoocclusion, poor oxygenation of the blood, increased red cell sickling, and more vasoocclusion. Arterial blood gases must be followed closely in this situation, and if the Po_2 cannot be maintained above 75 mm Hg, transfusion or exchange transfusion must be considered. Transfusion in this circumstance is not to increase oxygen-carrying capacity but to "dilute out" hemoglobin S–containing red cells capable of sickling in the circulation and thus to prevent the "logjams" of sickle cells that produce vascular occlusions. There are no proven guidelines for the extent of transfusion therapy required, but a hematocrit of 25% with 50% non–hemoglobin S-containing red cells is an acceptable goal. Fever and leukocytosis are common in the chest syndrome, as in other types of painful crisis; pneumonia is usually in the differential diagnosis and is difficult to rule out. Prescription of antibiotics on an empirical basis is frequently justifiable. Chest radiographic changes in the chest syndrome caused by vasoocclusion may be evanescent, disappearing rapidly with or without exchange transfusion.

LIVER.   A modest increase in conjugated serum bilirubin may be seen in sickle cell crises, presumably as a result of intrahepatic sickling and cholestasis. A small percentage of patients may manifest a much more striking cholestatic syndrome with extreme elevations of serum bilirubin.[17] In many of these patients (usually adolescents), severe illness does not ensue, and the syndrome resolves spontaneously. On the other hand, rare patients may go on to hepatic failure and death. Anecdotal experience suggests that these patients may benefit from timely exchange transfusion. Like other patients with chronic hemolytic disease, patients with sickle cell disease have a high incidence of bile pigment gallstones. Thus, if abdominal symptoms are present, the possibilities of cholecystitis and complications of cholelithiasis must be considered. Posttransfusion hepatitis is a threat in sickle cell patients who have received blood products.

BONES, BONE MARROW, AND JOINTS.   Bone pain is a common manifestation of painful crisis and is probably caused by microinfarctions of bone or bone marrow.[18] Rarely, bone marrow infarction may be extensive and may produce the syndrome of fat embolism.[19] This syndrome is manifested by severe bone pain, fever, neurologic abnormalities, and respiratory distress. It may be fatal. In the past, it was rarely diagnosed in life. It can be identified by observing refractile (fat) bodies in the retinal circulation, lipiduria, or fat in the sputum or bronchial washings. Treatment by exchange transfusion may be lifesaving. Fat embolism may be a cause of some cases of acute chest syndrome.[20] Other skeletal or joint manifestations of sickle cell disease include avascular necrosis of bone, osteomyelitis (often caused by salmonella organisms), joint effusion secondary to adjacent bone necrosis, gout caused by the increased nucleic acid catabolism associated with accelerated red cell production, and dactylitis (the hand-foot syndrome), which is a self-limited acute painful swelling of one or more extremities that occurs primarily in young children.

CENTRAL NERVOUS SYSTEM.   Strokes occur in a significant percentage of sickle cell patients.[21] Except for the rare case of fat embolism resulting from bone marrow necrosis, the pathogenesis is usually in situ vasoocclusion. Treatment should be by exchange transfusion. Such patients are at increased risk for recurrent strokes, and there is evidence that the frequency of these events can be reduced by a maintenance transfusion program.[22] Radiographic contrast media may cause sickling in vitro. The risks of angiographic procedures to sickle cell patients are, however, uncertain. If patients require exchange transfusion, it seems prudent to perform the transfusion before angiography if possible.

GENITOURINARY SYSTEM.   Hematuria occurs as a complication of the sickle cell diseases, including sickle cell trait, and may be severe.[14] It is thought usually to result from sickling and vasoocclusion in the renal medulla, but other causes unrelated to sickle disease must be excluded. Supportive treatment with hydration, and perhaps urinary alkalinization, is often sufficient for this self-limited complication. Transfusion or exchange transfusion is rarely required. Nephrectomy must be avoided because recurrence on the other side is the rule. Priapism, a frequent and painful complication of sickle cell disease, arises from vasoocclusion that produces congestion and sickling in the corpora cavernosa.[23,24] It may resolve spontaneously, and initial conservative treatment with analgesics, hydration, and alkalinization is appropriate. Exchange transfusion and various surgical procedures have been successful in terminating priapism, but controlled studies of these forms of therapy have not been reported. Recurrent or prolonged attacks frequently result in impotence.

SPLEEN.   Acute splenic sequestration is an important cause of morbidity and mortality in the first few years of life in patients with sickle cell anemia. In this syndrome, the spleen, for unknown reasons, suddenly traps a large proportion of the red cell mass, causing left upper quadrant pain, a rapid fall in hematocrit, shock, and occasionally death. Transfusion reverses the process rapidly and should be administered immediately. By adulthood, most patients with sickle cell disease have undergone "autosplenectomy" because of repeated splenic infarctions and, therefore, are not susceptible to this syndrome. However, in other sickle cell diseases, like hemoglobin SC disease, in which splenomegaly often persists, splenic infarction and sequestration may occur in adults.[25] The functional asplenia of most sickle cell patients renders them susceptible to fulminant septicemia caused by encapsulated organisms, such as *Streptococcus pneumoniae* and *Haemophilus influenzae.*[26] Preventive strategies include prophylactic penicillin in children and administration of pneumococcal vaccine to children and adults. In addition, early and vigorous treatment of any possible pneumococcal infection is mandatory.

TRANSFUSION.   There are certain caveats about transfusion in sickle cell disease.[27] First, there is an inverse relationship between hematocrit and frequency of vasoocclusion. Thus, if transfusion planned to dilute out sicklable cells will elevate the hematocrit significantly above its usual level, exchange transfusion must be considered. Secondly, alloimmunization is common in sickle cell patients.[28] Therefore, many authorities recommend extended typing of the recipient's blood and of donor units to avoid administration of red cells bearing foreign antigens, which commonly elicit antibody formation. Finally, because of frequent prior transfusion and alloimmunization, sickle cell patients are at risk for delayed hemolytic transfusion reactions[29] (Chap. 43).

Aplastic Crisis in Hemolytic Anemia

Sudden intensification of anemia in hemolytic disease resulting from precipitous reduction in the rate of red cell production is known as aplastic crisis.[30] It may occur in the course of any hemolytic disease but has been most commonly reported in congenital hemolytic disorders such as hereditary spherocytosis and sickle cell anemia. It is most common in children but also occurs in adults. Patients characteristically have fever, anorexia, nausea, and vomiting; abdominal pain and headache are common. Their anemia is usually severe and may be life threatening. Mild leukopenia and thrombocytopenia are often present. The "aplastic" nature of the anemia is demonstrated by extremely low reticulocyte counts and marked reduction in erythroid precursors in the bone marrow. The episode is self-limited, and recovery usually begins by 2 weeks. In the recovery phase, there is a return of vigorous erythropoiesis and often an outpouring of nucleated red cells and reticulocytes into the blood, fre-

quently accompanied by leukocytosis and immature white blood cells. Simultaneous or sequential aplastic crises may occur in other family members with hemolytic anemia. There is convincing evidence that parvovirus B19 is the cause of most aplastic crises.[31]

Prompt recognition of this syndrome is important because of the suddenness and severity of the anemia. A reticulocyte count, which should be done in every patient with hemolytic disease admitted to the hospital, is the major clue to the diagnosis. Treatment is transfusion with red blood cells. The volume given should be sufficient to alleviate signs or symptoms of inadequate tissue oxygenation; that amount need not be exceeded because episodes are self-limited, and the patient's hematocrit will return rapidly to its baseline level.

LEUKOPENIA

The term *leukopenia,* as used in this chapter, refers to granulocytopenia or neutropenia, that is, a circulating granulocyte count below 1500/mm[3]. Agranulocytosis implies severe neutropenia or complete absence of granulocytes. The clinical importance of granulocytopenia is in the associated increased risk of bacterial infection. This risk is slightly increased if the absolute neutrophil count is 500 to 1000/mm[3]. If neutrophil counts below 500/mm[3] persist, bacterial infection becomes the rule. Three patient groups are discussed as most pertinent to critical care situations: patients with neutropenia from malignant diseases or cytotoxic treatment, patients in whom neutropenia exists alone or in combination with other cytopenias as an aplastic process, and patients with neutropenia or agranulocytosis caused by immunologic mechanisms.

Malignant Disease and Cytotoxic Treatment

Malignant diseases involving the bone marrow, particularly those of hematopoietic origin, commonly produce neutropenia, and the cytotoxic therapy currently used to treat these diseases almost invariably does so. A vast literature exists in this area dealing with such issues as prophylactic antibiotic therapy and empirical antibiotic therapy for fever. These issues are addressed in the following sections, but remember that the long-term prognosis is heavily dependent on the success achieved in treating the underlying neoplastic disease.

Various regimens, many of them containing trimethoprim-sulfamethoxazole, have been investigated for their efficacy in preventing infection in the neutropenic patient. The results have been too variable to justify blanket recommendations.[32,33]

When the patient with severe neutropenia (absolute granulocyte count less than 500/mm[3]) develops fever above 38.3°C (101°F) in the absence of other possible pyrogenic influences (e.g., transfusion of blood products), infection must be assumed to be the cause. A full physical examination must be carried out, with particular attention to the mouth, groin, and perianal areas. The findings may be minimal because local manifestations of infection may depend on white blood cells. Thus, the common effects of bacterial infections—purulent sputum in pneumonia, pyuria in urinary tract infection, or abscess formation—may be absent. It has even been suggested that radiographic findings of pulmonary infiltrates in pneumonia appear later in the severely neutropenic patient. Cultures of blood, sputum, and urine should be obtained in all patients, and other sites should be cultured as indicated in individual patients. Because infections that may be rapidly fatal occur in these patients, antibiotics must be given promptly on an empirical basis before the results of the cultures are available. Many regimens have been tested, and guidelines for a rational approach to therapy have been formulated.[34] The choice of antibiotic regimen should take into account any findings in the individual patient that suggest a specific site of infection and any knowledge of patterns of infection in a given institution.

If cultures are positive, antibiotic treatment should be adjusted accordingly. If cultures are negative, as is frequently the case, empirical therapy should be continued if the patient remains febrile and neutropenic. Even if the patient becomes afebrile, it is advisable to continue antibiotics for a minimum course of 7 to 10 days.[35] When fever continues and the patient's general condition deteriorates, it is appropriate in selected patients to prescribe empirical treatment with an antifungal agent, such as amphotericin B, because of the frequency of fungal infections in neutropenic patients.

Recombinant hematopoietic growth factors, such as granulocyte colony stimulating factor, which stimulates the proliferation and maturation of neutrophil progenitor cells and enhances the function of mature cells, may be useful in certain neutropenic patients.[36] Indications for treatment and its timing are the subject of clinical trials, but some guidelines are available.[37] Granulocyte colony stimulating factor may be used as a standard part of chemotherapeutic regimens in which there is a high incidence of febrile neutropenia and in conjunction with bone marrow or peripheral blood stem cell transplantation. It should not be used routinely in patients presenting with fever and neutropenia.

Bone Marrow Aplasia

Neutropenia is part of the pancytopenia commonly present in aplastic anemia.[38] Some cases of aplastic anemia seem to have an autoimmune basis; in others, a drug or chemical exposure may be suspected as a cause.[39] No tests are available to prove an association in individual cases. Benzene and its derivatives are potentially toxic to the bone marrow, and many other chemicals, such as dichlorodiphenyltrichloroethane (DDT) and other insecticides, are suspect. Toluene exposure in glue sniffers may be associated with aplastic anemia. Many medications have been associated with aplastic anemia, which occurs as an idiosyncratic reaction in a small percentage of patients exposed to a given drug. Drugs for which an etiologic role seems likely include chloramphenicol, phenylbutazone, indomethacin, diphenylhydantoin, sulfonamides, and gold preparations. In at least half the cases of aplastic anemia, no etiology is found or suspected.

Isolated neutropenia from bone marrow hypoplasia also may be an idiosyncratic reaction to drug ingestion. Drugs prominently involved include those associated with aplastic anemia and also the phenothiazines and antithyroid drugs.

Many drugs have been implicated, and for practical purposes, virtually any drug must be considered a possible culprit.

The principles of treating infectious complications resulting from neutropenia in aplastic states are the same as those outlined earlier for neutropenia in malignant diseases. Treatment of aplastic anemia is not discussed except to point out that bone marrow transplantation may be used in suitable severely affected patients, and immunosuppressive therapy, particularly with antithymocyte globulin, has been successful in a significant percentage of idiopathic cases.

Immune Granulocytopenia

Certain drugs are associated with sudden, severe granulocytopenia that occurs by immune mechanisms involving the drug and serum antibodies and leads to granulocyte destruction.[40] The onset may be a few days after the drug is taken for the first time or immediately after a repeated exposure. Phenylbutazone, sulfonamides, antipsychotic drugs, and antithyroid drugs may produce granulocytopenia in this way or by the slower marrow-suppressive mechanism discussed earlier. The characteristic clinical syndrome, usually called agranulocytosis, includes high fever, chills, and severe sore throat ("agranulocytic angina") caused by bacterial infection. Oral and pharyngeal ulcers, necrotizing tonsillitis, pharyngeal abscesses, and bacteremia may occur. The blood shows virtual absence of granulocytes. The bone marrow may show absence of all granulocyte precursors or only the mature cells. The picture may superficially resemble acute leukemia or a state of "maturation arrest." After discontinuation of the drug, recovery occurs over a period of about 1 week. The return of granulocytes to the blood may be heralded by the appearance of monocytes and marked by an outpouring of immature neutrophils. Because this disease can be fatal, early recognition and appropriate antibiotic and supportive therapy are important. Obviously, the suspected offending drug must be discontinued and its future use avoided.

Neutropenia may occur in rheumatoid, collagen vascular, or lymphoproliferative diseases on an autoimmune basis.[41] Treatment of the neutropenia itself is rarely necessary or warranted and is usually alleviated by successful treatment of the underlying disease. Felty's syndrome is a triad of rheumatoid arthritis, splenomegaly, and neutropenia that rarely occurs in advanced rheumatoid arthritis. If it is associated with frequent infections, treatment with immunosuppressive drugs or splenectomy may be advisable.[42]

THROMBOCYTOPENIA

The types of bleeding characteristically seen with thrombocytopenia differ from those resulting from abnormalities of coagulation or fibrinolysis. Hemarthroses, large hematomas in soft tissues, and hemorrhages into body cavities are characteristic of plasma coagulation abnormalities. The earliest hemorrhagic lesions caused by thrombocytopenia are typically petechiae in dependent body parts. Larger skin lesions (purpura or ecchymoses) and mucosal hemorrhages (petechiae and hemorrhagic bullae) also may occur. When thrombocytopenia is severe, epistaxis, menometrorrhagia, hematuria, and gastrointestinal and intracranial bleeding may be seen. Blood vessel defects and qualitative platelet disorders may present with bleeding similar to that seen in thrombocytopenia. If small hemorrhagic skin lesions are raised or produce itching or pain, they are more likely to be caused by vasculitis than thrombocytopenia. Bleeding caused by disturbed platelet function, as seen in uremia, myeloproliferative diseases, dysproteinemias, and with many drugs (notably aspirin) is discussed in Chapter 154.

Confirmation of suspected thrombocytopenia or the diagnosis of asymptomatic thrombocytopenia requires a platelet count. Although a count less than 150,000/mm^3 is abnormally low, bleeding with ordinary trauma ("easy bruising") rarely occurs unless the count is less than 50,000/mm^3, and severe spontaneous bleeding is seen only at counts less than 10,000/mm^3 unless other defects are present. The mechanism by which the thrombocytopenia arises may influence the severity of bleeding at a given platelet count. If platelet destruction is the mechanism, the young platelets present have increased hemostatic effectiveness.

When a low platelet count is reported by the laboratory, there are at least two important reasons to examine the platelets on a stained peripheral blood smear. First, the presence of large platelets, which are young newly released cells, provides a clue that the thrombocytopenia results from increased platelet destruction rather than decreased bone marrow production. Second, if the number of platelets seen on the blood smear appears greater than would be expected for the reported platelet count or if platelet clumps are seen, pseudothrombocytopenia must be suspected.[43] Spuriously low platelet counts, whether done by automated counter or in a counting chamber, may arise by several mechanisms, including clumping induced by the commonly used anticoagulant ethylenediaminetetraacetic acid, platelet cold agglutinins, partial clotting of the blood sample, and platelet satellitosis, a disorder in which platelets cluster around white blood cells. When pseudothrombocytopenia is suspected, close communication and cooperation with the laboratory is necessary to confirm the diagnosis.

The first step in the diagnosis of true thrombocytopenia is to consider the mechanism.[44] Is the thrombocytopenia caused by increased destruction, decreased production, or sequestration of platelets? As noted earlier, the presence of large platelets on the blood smear suggests active thrombopoiesis, but this finding may be equivocal. Therefore, examination of the bone marrow for the presence of megakaryocytes often is necessary to distinguish between increased destruction (megakaryocytes present) and decreased production (megakaryocytes absent). The presence of splenomegaly raises the possibility of sequestration. Other laboratory tests are not necessary to evaluate the thrombocytopenia itself. The bleeding time is usually prolonged in patients with platelet counts less than 100,000/mm^3 and is not useful in assessing thrombocytopenia.

Treatment of thrombocytopenia depends on the cause and is discussed under specific diseases in the following sections. First, general principles of platelet transfusion are outlined.[45] When thrombocytopenia is caused by destruction or sequestration of the patient's own platelets, transfused platelets are subject to the same fate. Thus, platelet transfusions usually are of little benefit and are reserved for treatment of severe bleeding. When thrombocytopenia is caused by decreased platelet production, as in hematologic malignancies, serious hemorrhage can be prevented by regular transfusion of platelets. Some authorities advise "prophylactic" transfusion at a certain platelet count, usually 10,000/mm^3 to 20,000/mm^3; others recommend transfusion only when a low platelet count is accompanied by bleeding manifestations. In the stable patient, transfusion of 6 to 8 units of platelets two to three times weekly prevents serious hemorrhage. The effectiveness of platelet transfusions is diminished in febrile, infected patients, who may require larger and more frequent transfusions. Chronically transfused patients may become refractory to platelet transfusions from random donors because of alloimmunization. Single-donor platelets limit exposure to foreign platelet antigens and may delay immunization. Platelets obtained from family members by platelet pheresis may be effective in patients refractory to random-donor platelets.

Idiopathic (Autoimmune) Thrombocytopenic Purpura

In idiopathic thrombocytopenic purpura (ITP), an IgG autoantibody with broad reactivity is produced, and severe thrombocytopenia results from the accelerated destruction of platelets in the reticuloendothelial system.[46] In children, the disease often follows a viral infection and is self-limited. In adults, the thrombocytopenia usually persists unless treatment is applied, although spontaneous remissions and relapses may occur. Patients present with bleeding and thrombocytopenia. Splenomegaly is rarely present. The mechanism of the thrombocytopenia is established by the presence of ample megakaryocytes on bone marrow examination, and the presumptive diagnosis of ITP is made by excluding other possible causes of accelerated platelet destruction. Reliable clinical laboratory methods to identify antiplatelet antibodies are not generally available.

Many forms of treatment have demonstrated effectiveness in ITP. Because of the numerous therapeutic options, individualization of therapy is possible. For the reasons cited earlier, platelet transfusions are used only in the case of severe (life-threatening) hemorrhage. The initial therapy is usually with corticosteroids in a dosage equivalent to 1 mg/kg/day of prednisone. If the platelet count does not rise substantially within 2 to 3 weeks, splenectomy is usually the next step. The spleen is a site of autoantibody production and of destruction of sensitized platelets, and splenectomy produces prolonged remissions in most cases. Splenectomy also may be necessary in patients who have responded to steroids but cannot be weaned from the drug without the recurrence of thrombocytopenia. The 10% to 20% of patients who fail to respond to splenectomy may benefit from treatment with vincristine or immunosuppressive agents like cyclophosphamide. The anabolic steroid danazol, when given for periods of several months, also has been effective in some cases of ITP. Large doses of intravenous gamma globulin also may increase platelet counts in ITP, perhaps through blockage of reticuloendothelial sites of platelet destruction. The high cost of this therapy and the short duration of responses limit its use to certain specific circumstances.

Because ITP is common in young women, it is often seen in conjunction with pregnancy. The IgG autoantibody may cross the placenta and produce thrombocytopenia in the fetus. Management of the disease during pregnancy and delivery presents special challenges.[47]

Thrombocytopenic purpura also may occur as one of the autoimmune complications of collagen vascular diseases (e.g., systemic lupus erythematosus) or lymphoproliferative diseases (e.g., chronic lymphocytic leukemia) and may even be the presenting manifestation of these disorders. It occurs frequently in individuals infected with the human immunodeficiency virus.[48] Treatment of thrombocytopenic purpura may be complicated by treatment required for these underlying diseases but generally follows the principles outlined earlier. Thrombocytopenia from immune mechanisms may be induced by drugs, and the disorder resembles ITP in most respects.[49] The drug and antidrug antibody attach to the platelet membrane and mediate its destruction. Among the many drugs that have been incriminated are quinine, quinidine, and various sulfonamides. Differentiation between drug-induced thrombocytopenia and ITP may be impossible in an individual case. Any potentially responsible drug must be discontinued; if the thrombocytopenia is severe, it is prudent to initiate steroid therapy as well.

Heparin-associated thrombocytopenia is an important drug-related problem.[50] The incidence rate varies in reported series but may exceed 1%. The mechanism is probably immunologic with heparin, platelet constituents, and antibody reacting on the surface of platelets, endothelial cells, or both. The disorder differs in several ways from the more typical immune drug-induced thrombocytopenias, such as that associated with quinidine. Thrombocytopenia occurs 6 to 12 days after the initiation of heparin therapy or immediately after a repeated exposure to the drug. The exposure to the drug may be minimal (e.g., flushes of indwelling venous lines with dilute heparin or even heparin-coated intravenous catheters). The thrombocytopenia may be accompanied by major arterial thromboses; thrombosis is responsible for the major morbidity and mortality of the syndrome. Platelet counts should be done regularly in all patients receiving heparin and the drug discontinued if the count falls significantly.

Thrombotic Thrombocytopenic Purpura

Thrombotic thrombocytopenic purpura and its closely related disorders, hemolytic-uremic syndrome and postpartum renal failure, may be catastrophic and rapidly fatal.[51–53] Thus, prompt recognition and therapy are important. The causes of TTP remain unknown, but some pathogenetic features have been elucidated. Factors in the plasma of some patients with TTP enhance platelet aggregation, and this effect may be inhibited by factors in normal plasma. In patients with chronic relapsing TTP, there is evidence that unusually large multimers of von Willebrand's factor, perhaps arising from endothelial cells and persisting abnormally in the plasma, contribute to platelet aggregation.[54] Other factors and mechanisms have been postulated. Whatever the underlying and

initiating factors, platelet aggregation and occlusion of arterioles and capillaries by hyaline thrombi are important features of the disease. The thrombi contain platelets and fibrin-like material, but disseminated intravascular coagulation is not characteristically present.

Because TTP is a syndrome without pathognomonic features, diagnosis remains a matter of clinical judgment and depends on the presence of the major triad or pentad of features (Table 155-4): thrombocytopenia from increased platelet destruction, microangiopathic hemolytic anemia caused by mechanical damage to red cells as a result of the vascular lesions, and neurologic abnormalities (the triad), plus renal abnormalities and fever (the pentad). Clinical presentation is variable, but the thrombocytopenia and hemolytic anemia are often severe. A wide variety of fluctuating neurologic abnormalities may be present, including seizures, altered consciousness, delirium, and paresis. Renal abnormalities may include uremia, hematuria, and proteinuria. The reasons for fever are unclear. The laboratory findings in TTP are basically those related to the above features: thrombocytopenia, hemolytic anemia with red cell fragmentation, and renal dysfunction. Elevation of serum lactic acid dehydrogenase from intravascular hemolysis, and perhaps also damage to other tissues, is an index of activity of the disease. Coagulation tests are usually normal.

The characteristic hyaline thrombi may be present in the small arterioles and capillaries of any tissue. Biopsies of bone marrow or gingival tissue have a fairly high yield, but their usefulness as regular diagnostic studies is limited by the fact that negative findings do not exclude the diagnosis.

Because the cause of TTP is unknown, treatment has evolved largely on empirical grounds. This fact, plus the remitting, relapsing nature of the disease in patients who survive, has led to claims of efficacy for many therapies. The infrequency, variability, and severity of the disease have militated against controlled studies of treatment. Therapies considered to be beneficial include plasmapheresis, transfusions of plasma or the plasma supernatant fluid remaining after removal of cryoprecipitate, corticosteroids, vincristine, immunosuppressive agents, and splenectomy. Because platelets contribute to the hyaline thrombi, which are responsible for most of the adverse effects of TTP, platelet transfusions should be avoided except as a last-ditch measure in the presence of life-threatening hemorrhage.

The following approach to treatment of TTP may be recommended, with the warning that our understanding of TTP is rapidly evolving and new approaches may be

TABLE 155-4. Diagnostic Pentad of Thrombotic Thrombocytopenic Purpura

1. Thrombocytopenia°
2. Microangiopathic hemolytic anemia°
3. Neurologic abnormalities°
4. Renal abnormalities
5. Fever

°Nos. 1 through 3 comprise the diagnostic "triad" of thrombotic thrombocytopenic purpura.

anticipated. When the diagnosis is made, corticosteroid therapy is begun with prednisone at a dosage of 1 mg/kg/day or the equivalent dosage of another steroid. Arrangements are made for plasmapheresis to be started as soon as possible. If it will be more than 2 to 4 hours before the procedure—as is often the case because of delays in assembling personnel, setting up the equipment, and obtaining the necessary venous access—transfusion with fresh frozen plasma should be started. Several units may be administered, depending on the patient's tolerance of the volume load. When plasmapheresis is begun, the removed plasma should be replaced with fresh frozen plasma or cryoprecipitate-free plasma. The patient's response to therapy is monitored by clinical symptoms and signs, platelet count, and serum level of lactic acid dehydrogenase. Daily plasma exchange procedures should be carried out until there is definite improvement, or failure of response is apparent. Intermittent plasma exchange for long periods may be necessary in some patients. Empirical use of the other forms of therapy indicated earlier is appropriate in refractory patients.

The hemolytic-uremic syndrome resembles TTP except that neurologic manifestations are absent, thrombocytopenia is often less marked, renal impairment is often more severe, and it is less likely to be recurrent. It is a disease primarily of early childhood and often follows a febrile respiratory illness or gastroenteritis caused by a verotoxin-producing serotype of *Escherichia coli* or *Shigella*. In adults, it may follow administration of certain chemotherapeutic agents. With dialysis and other supportive care, most children survive and regain normal renal function. The prognosis is less favorable in the rare adult cases. The syndrome of postpartum renal failure closely resembles the hemolytic-uremic syndrome.

Other Thrombocytopenias

DISSEMINATED INTRAVASCULAR COAGULATION.   Thrombocytopenia is a hallmark of this syndrome, along with coagulation abnormalities and thrombotic complications (Chap. 154).

BACTERIAL SEPSIS.   Thrombocytopenia, occasionally of marked degree, commonly accompanies septicemia.[55] The mechanism in most instances is uncertain. It is usually present without overt disseminated intravascular coagulation and consumption of plasma coagulation factors, although these may occur. An immunologic mechanism has been implicated by studies showing increased amounts of IgG associated with platelets in septic patients.[56] Successful treatment of the septicemia cures the thrombocytopenia. Platelet transfusions may be necessary if the thrombocytopenia is severe and there is significant bleeding.

ALCOHOLISM.   Platelet counts less than 100,000/mm^3 are present in over one fourth of acutely ill alcoholic patients.[57] There are many possible etiologies for thrombocytopenia in such patients, including hypersplenism and folic acid deficiency, but it is important to recognize that reversible severe thrombocytopenia may occur as a direct effect of alcohol ingestion in some patients. Studies of the mechanism have

demonstrated elements of both decreased effective platelet production and shortened platelet survival. Abnormalities of platelet function have been noted as well. Recovery begins 2 to 3 days after cessation of alcohol ingestion, and maximum platelet counts are reached in 1 to 3 weeks. There is often an "overshoot" to abnormally high platelet counts, which then return to baseline levels. Therapy consists of discontinuing alcohol ingestion and providing appropriate supportive measures.

BONE MARROW DISORDERS.   Severe thrombocytopenia from impaired platelet production is a frequent concomitant of bone marrow disorders, such as aplastic anemia and the leukemias or other malignancies metastatic to the bone marrow, and also may result from cytotoxic chemotherapy of such disorders. Treatment is directed at the underlying disease. Transfusion of platelets, according to the principles outlined earlier, is important supportive therapy.

INCREASED BLOOD COUNTS ■

ERYTHROCYTOSIS

Erythrocytosis (i.e., an abnormally increased red cell mass) may require critical care because of the complications of hyperviscosity of the blood or because of hemorrhagic or thromboembolic complications that threaten some of these patients. The initial clue to the presence of erythrocytosis is usually a high value for the hematocrit or hemoglobin concentration. Such values may be present without true erythrocytosis if the plasma volume is contracted. This circumstance is usually apparent, but it is often advisable to quantify the red cell mass by direct measurement using radioisotopic red cell labels. The red cell mass is usually increased when the hematocrit is above 60% in a man or 57% in a woman.[58]

True erythrocytosis results from one of two general mechanisms. Polycythemia vera (PV) is a clonal abnormality of bone marrow stem cells resulting in autonomous overproduction of red cells and often of granulocytes and platelets. Secondary erythrocytosis results from excess erythropoietin production in response to hypoxemia, abnormalities of oxygen release from hemoglobin, or autonomous hormone production (e.g., by renal or other tumors). When the red cell mass is expanded and the hematocrit increased, blood viscosity is increased, and diminished blood flow, stasis, thrombosis, and tissue hypoxia may ensue. On the other hand, blood volume is increased, resulting in vascular distention and a tendency toward increased blood flow. The latter effect may lead to a hemorrhagic tendency, particularly in PV, where elevated platelet counts and abnormalities of platelet function also may be present.

Polycythemia Vera

Criteria for the diagnosis of PV are shown in Table 155-5.[59]

Risks in uncontrolled PV are primarily hyperviscosity and thromboembolic or hemorrhagic events. Patients at highest risk are those whose disease has shown particularly active

TABLE 155-5.   Criteria for the Diagnosis of Polycythemia Vera

Increased red cell mass
Arterial O$_2$ saturation >92%
+
Splenomegaly or 2 of the following
    Platelet count >400,000/mm^3
    White blood cell count >12,000/mm^3 without infection or fever
    Leukocyte alkaline phosphatase score >100
    Serum B$_{12}$ >900 pg/mL or Serum unbound B$_{12}$ binding capacity
        >2200 pg/mL

cell proliferation requiring extensive therapy, those with a prior history of complications, and the elderly. The height of the hematocrit or platelet count is not a reliable predictor. Symptoms resulting from decreased cerebral flow, such as headache, dizziness, and changes in vision, are the most common manifestations of hyperviscosity. Hemorrhage or thrombosis can affect almost any body part. Peptic ulcer disease with bleeding is common. Thromboses may be arterial or venous. Surgery poses an enormous risk in the patient with uncontrolled PV because of a high incidence of thrombotic or hemorrhagic complications.[60]

Patients with PV whose disease is uncontrolled, as manifested by a significantly increased hematocrit and red cell mass, may require urgent therapy of the PV itself in the event of one of the complications described earlier, a serious concurrent illness, or a requirement for surgery. The mainstay of such therapy is phlebotomy to reduce the red cell mass. This may be done as rapidly as 1 unit of blood every other day. Electrolyte solutions or plasma expanders should be administered with phlebotomy, as necessary, to avoid circulatory instability from sudden changes in blood volume. Elderly patients may tolerate phlebotomy less well, so that removal of volumes of 200 to 300 mL at less frequent intervals may be necessary. Simultaneous use of cytotoxic chemotherapy may be needed in some patients, although the effects on blood counts will be delayed for at least several days. Hydroxyurea is often used for this purpose, in an initial dose of 15 to 30 mg/kg/day. In rare cases, thrombocytosis may be of sufficient magnitude that plateletpheresis is advisable as emergency therapy (see discussion of thrombocytosis). Because of the risks of bleeding, anticoagulants or inhibitors of platelet aggregation, such as aspirin, generally should be avoided in patients with PV.

Secondary Erythrocytosis

The diagnosis of secondary erythrocytosis is made in a patient with an increased red cell mass in whom the criteria for PV are not met. Identification of an etiology, such as hypoxemic state, is confirmatory. Indications for phlebotomy in secondary erythrocytosis are less clear than in PV. In this instance, the increase in red cell mass is a physiologic response that may improve oxygen delivery by increasing the oxygen-carrying capacity of the blood. This response also may be deleterious, however, if blood viscosity is increased

to a level that significantly impairs blood flow and therefore tissue oxygenation. Despite considerable experimentation and theoretical calculation, an optimal hematocrit for all hypoxemic patients cannot be stipulated. It has been shown in some instances that phlebotomy improves cerebral blood flow,[61] and some authorities advise maintaining a hematocrit below 60%. The best current advice is to individualize therapy so as to maximize the patient's exercise tolerance and overall sense of well-being.

THROMBOCYTOSIS

Thrombocytosis, which may be defined as a platelet count greater than 600,000/mm^3, occurs as a clonal bone marrow proliferative disorder or as a secondary phenomenon in several disorders, including infection, the postoperative state, solid tumors, bleeding, iron deficiency, the postsplenectomy state, and others. As a marrow disorder, thrombocytosis may occur as part of myeloproliferative diseases like PV, myelofibrosis with myeloid metaplasia, or chronic myelocytic leukemia, or it may present as "essential thrombocythemia," in which other cell lines are not included in the proliferative process.

The diagnosis of essential thrombocythemia is basically one of exclusion of diseases associated with secondary or reactive thrombocytosis and of the other myeloproliferative diseases listed earlier.[62,63] Patients with essential thrombocythemia or thrombocytosis in association with other myeloproliferative disorders are at increased risk for both hemorrhagic and thromboembolic events. Thrombotic complications may be arterial or venous. The risk probably increases with increasing platelet counts, but there are no reliable guidelines based on controlled clinical studies or tests of platelet function to dictate when treatment is indicated. It is generally agreed, however, that reducing the platelet count reduces the risks of complications. Thus, it is reasonable to recommend that the platelet count be lowered if it exceeds 1,000,000/mm^3 in a patient who is experiencing hemorrhagic or thrombotic complications or 1,500,000/mm^3 in an asymptomatic patient. Platelet-lowering treatment also should be given if the patient is elderly or has other risk factors for vascular disease. In patients with complications, the platelet count can be reduced most rapidly by platelet pheresis. More gradual reduction in the count can be achieved by myelosuppressive agents, such as hydroxyurea, administered at an initial dose of 15 to 30 mg/kg/day. Some patients with thrombocythemia develop erythromelalgia, a syndrome of redness and burning pain in the distal parts of the extremities caused by disturbances of neurovascular circulation.[64] Treatment with aspirin or indomethacin provides relief. Except in this circumstance, one should use inhibitors of platelet aggregation with caution in essential thrombocythemia because of the risk of bleeding.

Secondary or reactive thrombocytosis is reversed by successful treatment of the underlying disease. The thrombocytosis itself does not require therapy. If thrombosis occurs, it should be treated as in a patient with a normal platelet count.

LEUKOCYTOSIS

When leukocytosis is extreme and immature cells are present, certain symptoms and signs may occur that constitute what has been called "hyperleukocytosis syndrome." This occurs in leukemic states when the white blood cell count is high. Signs and symptoms are most commonly related to the central nervous system, eyes, and lungs. They include stupor, altered mentation, dizziness, visual blurring, retinal abnormalities (venous dilation, hemorrhages, exudates, papilledema), dyspnea, tachypnea, and hypoxia. Intracranial and pulmonary infarction or hemorrhage and sudden death may occur. Priapism and peripheral vascular insufficiency have also been associated with the syndrome. Although the pathogenesis is incompletely understood, autopsies have shown white cell aggregates, microthrombi, and microvascular invasion (leukostatic tumors).[65] Immature white blood cells are poorly deformable, increase blood viscosity when present in large numbers, and may consume oxygen to produce local tissue hypoxia.[66] The syndrome occurs more commonly in acute and chronic myelocytic leukemia than in acute lymphocytic leukemia and occurs rarely, if ever, in chronic lymphocytic leukemia. The level of white blood cell count at which the syndrome appears is variable, depending perhaps on the maturity and size of the white blood cells present and the degree of coexisting anemia. Leukemic blast cell counts exceeding 50,000/mm^3 in acute myelocytic leukemia or the accelerated phase of chronic myelocytic leukemia are an indication for prompt treatment, and signs or symptoms attributable to the hyperleukocytosis syndrome are an indication for urgent reduction of the white blood cell count.

The safest method for reducing the white blood cell count rapidly is leukapheresis. It avoids the hazards of rapid leukemic cell destruction that may be associated with large doses of cytotoxic chemotherapy (see discussion on tumor lysis syndrome, Chap. 156). At the same time, chemotherapy should be initiated, and treatment with allopurinol started in anticipation of the hyperuricemia that will occur with cell death. Hydroxyurea is frequently used initially to produce rapid leukemic cell kill.

ALTERED BLOOD RHEOLOGY

The relationship between blood viscosity measured in vitro and blood flow in vivo is complex and unpredictable. Nevertheless, clinical syndromes are recognizable in which rheologic characteristics of the blood are altered, with symptoms that appear to result from sluggish blood flow. The viscosity of blood, or resistance to flow, largely results from its formed elements, particularly the red cells.[67] Thus, impaired blood flow may result from increased concentration of red cells, as in PV and secondary erythrocytosis, or from qualitative abnormalities of the cells, as in sickle cell diseases. Antibody-induced agglutination of red cells, as in cold agglutinin disease, also may produce hyperviscosity. These disorders have been discussed previously. Abnormalities of serum proteins may result in increased serum viscosity, but the clinically important effects of high serum protein levels on blood flow probably also result from effects on red cells through enhancement of aggregation or rouleaux formation.

SERUM PROTEIN ABNORMALITIES

The disease most commonly associated with increased serum viscosity is Waldenström's macroglobulinemia, in which a malignant proliferation of plasmacytoid lymphocytes results in overproduction of monoclonal macroglobulin.[68] These IgM molecules, because of their molecular size and shape, frequently produce increased serum viscosity and the clinical picture of the "hyperviscosity syndrome." A lower incidence of the hyperviscosity syndrome is seen in multiple myeloma, the malignant plasma cell dyscrasia in which monoclonal IgA or IgG is overproduced. Because of its greater tendency to aggregate, IgA is more often associated with hyperviscosity than is IgG. Hyperviscosity may occur in cryoglobulinemia, in which cold-precipitable immunoglobulins or immune complexes are responsible for the abnormalities.

The most common manifestations of the hyperviscosity syndrome are neurologic and include headache, visual disturbances, hearing loss, vertigo, altered consciousness (ranging from stupor to coma), paresis, seizures, and peripheral neuropathy. These symptoms, presumably caused by sluggish or occluded blood flow, may be fluctuating. Plasma volume is frequently expanded in states of increased viscosity, which, along with the hyperviscosity and frequently associated anemia, predisposes these patients to congestive heart failure. A bleeding tendency may exist because of associated thrombocytopenia or interference by the abnormal protein with the function of platelets or plasma coagulation factors.

Specific physical findings are often lacking. However, careful examination of the optic fundi is important because the presence of alternating bulges and constrictions in the column of blood in retinal veins (so-called "boxcar" or "sausage-link" abnormalities) is highly suggestive of hyperviscosity. Direct measurement of serum viscosity can be carried out in the laboratory. A simple rapid screening test also is available.[69]

The most rapidly effective form of therapy for hyperviscosity from serum protein abnormalities is plasmapheresis. It is particularly efficient in macroglobulinemic disorders because most of the IgM is in the plasma. Extravascular pools are larger for IgA and IgG. Therapy may be followed with serum viscosity measurements as well as protein electrophoresis. Plasmapheresis is then repeated as necessary to control viscosity and symptoms. The only effective means to prevent recurrence of the syndrome over the long term is to treat the underlying disease.

REFERENCES

1. Welch HG, Meehan KR, Goodnough LT: Prudent strategies for elective red blood cell transfusion. *Ann Intern Med* 1992;116:393
2. American College of Physicians: Practice strategies for elective red blood cell transfusion. *Ann Intern Med* 1992;116:403

3. Armitage JO: Bone marrow transplantation. *N Engl J Med* 1994;330:827

4. Hillman RS, Finch CA: The misused reticulocyte. *Br J Haematol* 1969;17:313

5. Pirofsky B: Clinical aspects of autoimmune hemolytic anemia. *Semin Hematol* 1976;13:251

6. Salama A, Mueller-Eckhardt C: On the mechanisms of sensitization and attachment of antibodies to RBC in drug-induced immune hemolytic anemia. *Blood* 1987;69:1006

7. Petz LD, Garratty G: *Acquired Immune Hemolytic Anemias.* New York, Churchill Livingstone, 1980:26

8. Rosse WF: *Clinical Immunohematology: Basic Concepts and Clinical Applications.* Boston, Blackwell Scientific Publications, 1990:555

9. Rosenfield RE, Jagathambal: Transfusion therapy for autoimmune hemolytic anemia. *Semin Hematol* 1976;13:311

10. Beutler E: G6PD deficiency. *Blood* 1994;84:3613

11. Chan TK, Todd D: Haemolysis complicating viral hepatitis in patients with glucose-6-phosphate dehydrogenase deficiency. *Br Med J* 1975;1:131

12. Young TW, Keeney GL, Bull BS: Red cell fragmentation in human disease: a light and scanning electron microscope study. *Blood Cells* 1984;10:493

13. Mills ML: Life-threatening complications of sickle cell disease in children. *JAMA* 1985;254:1487

14. Sears DA: Sickle cell trait. In: Embury SH, Hebbel RP, Mohandas N, et al (eds). *Sickle Cell Disease: Basic Principles and Clinical Practice.* New York, Raven Press, 1994:381

15. Shapiro BS, Ballas SK: The acute painful episode. In: Embury SH, Hebbel RP, Mohandas N, et al (eds). *Sickle Cell Disease: Basic Principles and Clinical Practice.* New York, Raven Press, 1994:531

16. Castro O, Brambilla DJ, Thorington B, et al: The acute chest syndrome in sickle cell disease: incidence and risk factors. *Blood* 1994;84:643

17. Johnson CS, Omata M, Tong MJ, et al: Liver involvement in sickle cell disease. *Medicine* 1985;64:349

18. Milner PF, Joe C, Burke GJ: Bone and joint disease. In: Embury SH, Hebbel RP, Mohandas N, et al (eds). *Sickle Cell Disease: Basic Principles and Clinical Practice.* New York, Raven Press, 1994:645

19. Shapiro MP, Hayes JA: Fat embolism in sickle cell disease: report of a case with brief review of the literature. *Arch Intern Med* 1984;144:181

20. Vichinsky E, Williams R, Das M, et al: Pulmonary fat embolism: a distinct cause of severe acute chest syndrome in sickle cell anemia. *Blood* 1994;83:3107

21. Powars D, Wilson B, Imbus C, et al: The natural history of stroke in sickle cell disease. *Am J Med* 1978;65:461

22. Russell MO, Goldberg HI, Hodson A, et al: Effect of transfusion therapy on arteriographic abnormalities and on recurrence of stroke in sickle cell disease. *Blood* 1984;63:162

23. Hamre MR, Harmon EP, Kirkpatrick DV, et al: Priapism as a complication of sickle cell disease. *J Urol* 1991;145:1

24. Sharpsteen JR Jr, Powars D, Johnson C: Multisystem damage associated with tricorporal priapism in sickle cell disease. *Am J Med* 1993;94:289

25. Sears DA, Udden MM: Splenic infarction, splenic sequestration, and functional hyposplenism in hemoglobin S-C disease. *Am J Hematol* 1985;18:261

26. Serjeant GR: *Sickle Cell Disease.* New York, Oxford University Press, 1985:124

27. Wayne AS, Kevy SV, Nathan DG: Transfusion management of sickle cell disease. *Blood* 1993;81:1109

28. Vichinsky EP, Earles A, Johnson RA: Alloimmunization in sickle cell anemia and transfusion of racially unmatched blood. *N Engl J Med* 1990;322:1617

29. Cox JV, Steane E, Cunningham G, et al: Risk of alloimmunization and delayed hemolytic transfusion reactions in patients with sickle cell disease. *Arch Intern Med* 1988;148:2485

30. Conklin GT, George JN, Sears DA: Transient erythroid aplasia in hemolytic anemia: a review of the literature with two case reports. *Tex Rep Biol Med* 1974;32:2

31. Lefrere JJ, Courouce AM, Bertrand Y, et al: Human parvovirus and aplastic crisis in chronic hemolytic anemias: a study of 24 observations. *Am J Hematol* 1986;23:271

32. Estey E, Maksymiuk A, Smith T, et al: Infection prophylaxis in acute leukemia: comparative effectiveness of sulfamethoxazole and trimethoprim, and ketoconazole, and a combination of the two. *Arch Intern Med* 1984;144:1562

33. Karp JE, Merz WG, Hendrickson C, et al: Oral norfloxacin for prevention of gram-negative bacterial infections in patients with acute leukemia and granulocytopenia. *Ann Intern Med* 1987;106:1

34. Pizzo PA: Management of fever in patients with cancer and treatment-induced neutropenia. *N Engl J Med* 1993;328:1323

35. Joshi JH, Schimpff SC, Tenney JH, et al: Can antibacterial therapy be discontinued in persistently febrile granulocytopenic cancer patients? *Am J Med* 1984;76:450

36. Fleischman RA: Clinical use of hematopoietic growth factors. *Am J Med Sci* 1993;305:248

37. American Society of Clinical Oncology recommendations for the use of hematopoietic colony-stimulating factors: evidence-based clinical practice guidelines. *J Clin Oncol* 1994;12:2471

38. Camitta BM, Storb R, Thomas ED: Aplastic anemia: pathogenesis, diagnosis, treatment, and prognosis. *N Engl J Med* 1982;306:645

39. International Agranulocytosis and Aplastic Anemia Study: Risks of agranulocytosis and aplastic anemia: a first report of their relation to drug use with special reference to analgesics. *JAMA* 1986;256:1749

40. Pisciotta AV: Drug induced agranulocytosis: peripheral destruction of polymorphonuclear leukocytes and their marrow precursors. *Blood Rev* 1990;4:226

41. Bux J, Mueller-Eckhardt C: Autoimmune neutropenia. *Semin Hematol* 1992;29:45

42. Logue G: Felty's syndrome: granulocyte-bound immunoglobulin G and splenectomy. *Ann Intern Med* 1976;85:437

43. Payne BA, Pierre RV: Pseudothrombocytopenia: a laboratory artifact with potentially serious consequences. *Mayo Clin Proc* 1984;59:123

44. Sheehan RG: Thrombopoiesis and thrombokinetics: an approach to the evaluation of thrombocytopenia. *Am J Med Sci* 1985;289:168

45. Kelton JG, Ali AM: Platelet transfusions: a critical appraisal. *Clin Oncol* 1983;2:549

46. George JN, El-Haraka MA, Raskob GE: Chronic idiopathic thrombocytopenic purpura. *N Engl J Med* 1994;331:1207

47. McCrae KR, Samuels P, Schreiber AD: Pregnancy-associated thrombocytopenia: pathogenesis and management. *Blood* 1992;80:2697

48. Walsh C, Krigel R, Lennette E, et al: Thrombocytopenia in homosexual patients: prognosis, response to therapy, and prevalence of antibody to the retrovirus associated with the acquired immunodeficiency syndrome. *Ann Intern Med* 1985;103:542

49. Salama A, Mueller-Eckhardt C: Immune-mediated blood cell dyscrasias related to drugs. *Semin Hematol* 1992;29:54

50. Schmitt BP, Adelman B: Heparin-associated thrombocytopenia: a critical review and pooled analysis. *Am J Med Sci* 1993;305:208

51. Bell WR, Braine HG, Ness PM, et al: Improved survival in thrombotic thrombocytopenic purpura–hemolytic uremic syndrome: clinical experience in 108 patients. *N Engl J Med* 1991;325:398

52. Neild GH: Haemolytic uraemic syndrome in practice. *Lancet* 1994;343:398

53. Hayslett JP: Postpartum renal failure. *N Engl J Med* 1985; 312:1556

54. Moake JL, McPherson PD: Abnormalities of von Willebrand factor multimers in thrombotic thrombocytopenic purpura and the hemolytic-uremic syndrome. *Am J Med* 1989;87:3-9N

55. Wilson JJ, Neame PB, Kelton JG: Infection-induced thrombocytopenia. *Semin Thromb Hemost* 1982;8:217

56. Poskitt TR, Poskitt PKF: Thrombocytopenia of sepsis: the role of circulating IgG-containing immune complexes. *Arch Intern Med* 1985;145:891

57. Cowan DH: Effect of alcoholism on hemostasis. *Semin Hematol* 1980;17:137

58. Adamson JW: The polycythemias: diagnosis and treatment. *Hosp Pract* 1983;December:49

59. Berk PD, Goldberg JD, Donovan PB, et al: Therapeutic recommendations in polycythemia vera based on polycythemia vera study group protocols. *Semin Hematol* 1986;23:132

60. Wasserman LR, Gilbert HS: Surgery in polycythemia vera. *N Engl J Med* 1963;269:1226

61. York EL, Jones RL, Menon D, et al: Effects of secondary polycythemia on cerebral blood flow in chronic obstructive pulmonary disease. *Am Rev Respir Dis* 1980;121:813

62. Murphy S, Iland H, Rosenthal D, et al: Essential thrombocythemia: an interim report from the Polycythemia Vera Study Group. *Semin Hematol* 1986;23:177

63. Mitus AJ, Schafer AI: Thrombocytosis and thrombocythemia. *Hematol Oncol Clin North America* 1990;4:157

64. Michiels JJ, Abels J, Steketee J, et al: Erythromelalgia caused by platelet-mediated arteriolar inflammation and thrombosis in thrombocythemia. *Ann Intern Med* 1985;102:466

65. McKee C Jr, Collins RD: Intravascular leukocyte thrombi and aggregates as a cause of morbidity and mortality in leukemia. *Medicine* 1974;53-463

66. Lichtman MA: The relationship of excessive white cell accumulation to vascular insufficiency in patients with leukemia. In: Meiselman HJ, Lichtman MA, LaCelle PL (eds). *White Cell Mechanics: Basic Science and Clinical Aspects*. New York, Alan R Liss, 1984:295

67. LaCelle PL, Weed RI: The contribution of normal and pathologic erythrocytes to blood rheology. *Prog Hematol* 1971; 7:1

68. Dimopoulos MA, Alexanian R: Waldenström's macroglobulinemia. *Blood* 1994;83:1452

69. Wright DJ, Jenkins DE Jr: Simplified method for estimation of serum and plasma viscosity in multiple myeloma and related disorders. *Blood* 1970;36:516

Critical Care, Third Edition, edited by Joseph M. Civetta,
Robert W. Taylor, and Robert R. Kirby.
Lippincott-Raven Publishers, Philadelphia, PA © 1997.

CHAPTER 156

Oncologic Emergencies

Robert J. Downey
Jeffrey S. Groeger

Approximately 500,000 Americans, or 4 of 10 patients who get cancer this year, will be alive 5 years after diagnosis. When adjusted for normal life expectancy, a "relative" 5-year survival rate of 54% is seen for all cancers.[1] New chemotherapeutic agents, interstitial radiation, autologous and allogeneic bone marrow transplantation,[2] the expansion of biologic therapy with monoclonal antibodies,[3] and new cytokines[4] offer hope, but may lead to complications rarely seen in the nononcologic patient. It is beyond the scope of this chapter to discuss all aspects of cancer that warrant admission to an intensive care unit, and such topics as infection in the immunocompromised host, shock, coagulation abnormalities, and multisystem organ failure are discussed elsewhere in this book. This chapter focuses on clinical conditions that arise either as a direct result of a neoplasm or of antineoplastic therapies.

CANCER HYPERCALCEMIA ■

Hypercalcemia develops in 10% to 20% of all patients with malignancy.[5] Serum calcium levels above 13 mg/dL—when corrected for changes in plasma proteins or a clinical picture consistent with hypercalcemia, regardless of the serum calcium concentration—warrant urgent intervention.

CLINICAL PRESENTATION

No symptom or sign is pathognomonic of hypercalcemia. Clinical manifestations of hypercalcemia are frequently related to the rapidity of onset rather than the absolute concentration of serum calcium. Patients may present with full-blown hypercalcemic crisis, presenting with somnolence, lethargy, general weakness, and nausea and vomiting—a

clinical pattern easily confused with terminal features of the underlying malignancy or with side effects of chemotherapy or radiation therapy—or they may be asymptomatic. In hypercalcemic crisis, nausea, vomiting, abdominal pain, lethargy, dehydration, and renal failure are present. Elevation of serum calcium levels impairs the kidney's ability to concentrate urine, causing polyuria and polydipsia. Contraction alkalosis with progressive dehydration leads to further renal impairment, and frank renal failure may ensue, especially in the patient with underlying multiple myeloma. Infrequently, hypercalcemia may present as acute abdominal pain, peptic ulcer disease, or pancreatitis. Hypertension also has been reported.[6] Psychotic behavior, visual abnormalities, hyporeflexia, stupor and coma, and occasional localizing signs on neurologic examination (often thought to be secondary to metastatic disease) may disappear with therapy that lowers the patient's serum calcium.[7] In contradistinction to primary hyperparathyroidism, hypercalcemia of malignancy is rarely associated with nephrocalcinosis and nephrolithiasis; hypercalciuria must be chronic for these renal manifestations to develop.

Electrocardiographic (ECG) changes associated with hypercalcemia,[8] such as shortening of the QT interval, bradycardia, T wave changes, changes in atrioventricular conduction, and increased automaticity and arrhythmias, are not usually associated with clinically significant hemodynamic alterations, even with extreme elevations of the serum calcium.

Calcium is normally present in plasma in two forms: 50% an ionized free fraction, and 50% protein bound, primarily to albumin. Either hypoalbuminemia or the presence of abnormal binding proteins, as seen in multiple myeloma, may lead to inaccurate estimates of the ionized fraction. As a rule, for every 1-g/dL decrease in the serum albumin, there is a 0.8-mg/dL decrease in the serum calcium. In the critically ill or cancer patient with hypoalbuminemia, ionized calcium becomes a larger fraction of the total serum calcium, and therefore, total calcium levels may understate the severity of hypercalcemia. Measurement of ionized calcium, the clinically relevant fraction that correlates best with signs and symptoms of hypercalcemia, is essential. Although ionized calcium levels increase with acidosis and decrease with alkalosis, these changes are relatively small and lead to no clinically significant events.[9]

DIFFERENTIAL DIAGNOSES

Malignancies and primary hyperparathyroidism account for approximately 90% of all cases of hypercalcemia and may coexist in the critically ill cancer patient. Among hospitalized patients, neoplastic disease is the more common cause. Solid tumors (predominantly breast and lung carcinoma) account for 80% of malignancy-associated hypercalcemia; hematologic malignancies such as multiple myeloma and lymphoma account for most of the remaining 20%.[7,10] Renal failure, sarcoidosis, thyrotoxicosis, vitamin D or A intoxication, immobilization, milk alkali syndrome, adrenal insufficiency, familial hypocalciuric hypercalcemia, and medications such as thiazide, lithium, estrogens, and tamoxifen are also included in the differential diagnoses.

PATHOPHYSIOLOGY

Tumors associated with hypercalcemia of malignancy are not a homogeneous group, and there is no single unifying mechanism.[7,11] Increased bone resorption is widely accepted as the major cause of hypercalcemia of malignancy.[12–15] In the hematologic malignancies, local bone-resorbing factors may be responsible, whereas with solid tumors associated with advanced osteolytic metastasis, there is extensive local bone destruction. In other solid tumors, the mechanism of increased bone resorption is tumor secretion of parathyroid hormone–like proteins.[16–18] Osteoclast activating factor, transforming growth factors, interleukin-1, tumor necrosis factor, interferon-gamma, and lymphotoxin (tumor necrosis factor-beta) may act independently or synergistically in the pathophysiologic mechanism of hypercalcemia.[19] Because the kidneys are major regulatory organs for calcium homeostasis, any alteration in renal function can lead to hypercalcemia in a patient with increased bone resorption by effecting a decrease in the filtered calcium load.

LABORATORY INVESTIGATION

Immunoreactive parathyroid hormone (PTH) levels, as measured by immunoradiometric assays, are suppressed in hypercalcemia of malignancy and remain among the best tests for differentiating causes of hypercalcemia.[20] Combining measurements of parathormone with total or ionized serum calcium identifies primary hyperparathyroidism in a large percentage of cases.[21] Approximately 25% of cancer patients with hypercalcemia also have elevations of PTH. In addition to raising the serum calcium concentration, PTH lowers

serum phosphate and increases the serum chloride concentration.[22] Hypophosphatemia results from reduced renal tubular reabsorption of phosphate, whereas the elevation of serum chloride is caused by hyperchloremic acidosis resulting from PTH-induced renal bicarbonate loss. The chloride-to-phosphorus ratio is expected to rise with increases of PTH. Ninety-six percent of patients with hyperparathyroidism have ratios above 33, whereas ratios less than 30 are found in 92% of patients with hypercalcemia from other causes.[22] Hypophosphatemia usually is not seen in breast carcinoma, and its occurrence should lead to suspicion of coexisting hyperparathyroidism.

More sophisticated tests are available to assist in the evaluation of the hypercalcemic patient, but most tend to be expensive and few offer much assistance in the differential diagnosis. Urinary calcium measurements may not be helpful because tubular reabsorption of calcium may be elevated with cancer hypercalcemia. Plasma cyclic adenosine monophosphate (cAMP) and urinary cAMP offer little assistance in separating primary from secondary hypercalcemia.[23] Clinically significant hypokalemia predisposing to cardiac arrhythmias may be seen when the calcium level is greater than 14 mg/dL.[24] Forced diuresis, especially with furosemide, may exacerbate this problem. The hypokalemia may be secondary to decreased oral intake, gastrointestinal loss from diarrhea, chemotherapy, emesis, or anorexia.

THERAPY OF HYPERCALCEMIA

Several reviews of the therapy of cancer hypercalcemia are available.[13,25,26] This section focuses on measures used for immediate reduction of calcium levels to non–life-threatening values. The only effective long-term means of reversing malignancy-associated hypercalcemia is reduction in the tumor burden. The aggressiveness of the therapeutic approach depends on the potential for significant palliation or cure.

Restoration of intravascular volume in patients who are dehydrated usually increases urinary calcium secretion by 100 to 300 mg/day.[27] A urine output of 1.5 to 2 mL/kg/minute is desirable. Calciuresis is enhanced by a provoked natriuresis, which can be facilitated by administering furosemide, a loop diuretic. Careful attention is given to volume and electrolyte repletion, especially potassium. All agents capable of precipitating hypercalcemic crisis should be discontinued, including vitamins A and D, thiazide diuretics, and, especially, estrogens or antiestrogens used as therapy for breast carcinoma.

Rehydration with calciuresis may offer transient reduction in ionized calcium, and therapy must be instituted to correct the underlying process of excessive bone resorption. Plicamycin,[27] calcitonin,[28] gallium nitrate,[29] and biphosphonates[19,30,31] all are administered parenterally and are effective in treating acute hypercalcemia.

Calcitonin, a synthetic polypeptide of 32 amino acids in the same sequence as naturally occurring salmon calcitonin, decreases plasma calcium levels by inhibiting bone resorption.[28] A dosage of 8 to 16 International Units/kg intravenously or intramuscularly every 12 hours usually produces a partial and mild response in lowering calcium level. This agent is nontoxic, well tolerated, and particularly useful in patients with congestive heart failure or renal failure who cannot tolerate saline and diuresis. The effect is rapid but, unfortunately, transient. Tachyphylaxis may occur with continued use.

Plicamycin, if given in dosages of 25 μg/kg IV over 4 to 12 hours lowers, lowers serum calcium levels by 48 hours,[28] and the effect usually lasts 4 to 6 days. The mechanism of action seems to be direct action on osteoclasts with retardation of bone resorption rather than promotion of calciuresis. Reduction of bone resorption occurs without affecting the rate of bone accretion. Thrombocytopenia, mild reversible hepatic dysfunction,[32] hemorrhagic diathesis, and nephrotoxicity may all follow the administration of plicamycin, although usually at higher doses than mentioned and with repeated administration. Plicamycin should be used with calcitonin for life-threatening hypercalcemia because calcitonin, although less effective, has a much more rapid onset of action.

Intravenous phosphates uniformly and promptly lower calcium levels in a dose-dependent manner. This route of administration is extremely toxic and is associated with extraskeletal calcification of the lung, kidney, or both.[26] Minor myocardial calcification also has been seen. Deaths have been ascribed to the use of intravenous phosphate, and it should be used to lower calcium only when all other therapies have either failed or are contraindicated.

Gallium nitrate inhibits bone resorption and increases calcium content of bone.[29,33] Administered at a daily dose of 200 mg/m² for 5 days, gallium nitrate lowers serum calcium levels to normal levels in approximately 85% of cancer patients. It is well tolerated and is associated with a decrease in serum concentration of inorganic phosphorus. Significant decreases of serum calcium levels occur, whereas symptoms of hypocalcemia are avoided. Because gallium nitrate is a heavy metal, it may be associated with renal impairment in patient with preexisting renal disease.

Etidronate disodium and pamidronate disodium, structural analogues of pyrophosphate, are inhibitors of osteoclastic bone resorption. Unlike pyrophosphate, both agents are resistant to enzymatic hydrolysis. The principal action of diphosphonate in the treatment of hypercalcemia associated with malignant neoplasms is the reduction of abnormal bone resorption with no direct antineoplastic activity. Etidronate is administered as an infusion of 7.5 mg/kg slowly over 4 to 6 hours for 3 consecutive days. With this regimen, 50% to 73% of patients obtain normalization of serum calcium levels. Pamidronate is administered as a single 60-mg dose over 4 to 6 hours. When the corrected calcium exceeds 13.5 mg/dL, the dose is increased to 90 mg. A minimum of 7 days should elapse before retreatment is considered to fully evaluate the effect of pamidronate. Biphosphonates are generally well tolerated when administered for short periods.[34]

Although unpredictable, glucocorticoids may be of some benefit in steroid-responsive tumors such as multiple myeloma and non-Hodgkin's lymphoma. Responses may take 7 to 14 days; therefore, one cannot count on their being useful in acute situations.[26]

ACUTE TUMOR LYSIS SYNDROME

DEFINITION AND PATHOPHYSIOLOGY

Renal and metabolic complications may result from acute dissolution of bulky tumors highly sensitive to radiation or chemotherapeutic drugs. Intracellular products, when rapidly released into the circulation, can produce life-threatening hyperkalemia, hyperuricemia (defined as a uric acid value above 18 mg/dL), hyperphosphatemia, and hypocalcemia, with or without acute renal failure (ARF).[35-40] The degree of biochemical disarray is related to baseline renal function and to tumor mass. Classically, the syndrome is seen with Burkitt's lymphoma, among other lymphomas, and acute and chronic leukemia.[38-40] ARF can result from intratubular precipitation of uric acid or calcium phosphate crystals.[36,37] If the release of uric acid occurs more slowly, uric acid stones forming in the renal pelvis may lead to ureteral obstruction.

CLINICAL MANAGEMENT

Patients with bulky abdominal disease, markedly elevated plasma lactate dehydrogenase levels, evidence of renal dysfunction, or metabolic alterations require careful monitoring and renal protection during the induction of antineoplastic therapy. If the metabolic burden proves great or ARF ensues, dialysis is initiated.

The mainstay in prophylaxis against ARF in this setting is vigorous hydration and maintenance of a urine output of at least 2 mL/kg/hour. If diuresis cannot be achieved by saline hydration alone, an infusion of dopamine, 1.5 μg/kg/minute, is useful in initiating and maintaining urine flow.[41] If this is unsuccessful, patients may be given either an intravenous bolus of furosemide, 80 to 120 mg, or mannitol, 12.5 g of a 25% solution. Mannitol is preferred when intravascular volume is decreased, whereas furosemide is used in patients with normal or elevated intravascular volume. Diuresis can be maintained by continuous infusion of furosemide, 3 to 5 mg/kg/day, or mannitol, 5 g/hour. Urine losses in excess of total volume infused hourly are replaced with dextrose 2.5% with 0.45% saline, allowing for insensible fluid losses. Careful attention to fluid retention, as evidenced by progressive weight gain and accumulation of edema, is mandatory. As with the management of any severe fluid and electrolyte disorder, the clinician may consider the insertion of a flow-directed pulmonary artery catheter to help direct fluid management to maintain the diuresis.

Allopurinol, 10 mg/kg orally or IV, is given to control hyperuricemia. While the patient remains hyperuricemic, the urine pH can be maintained at or above 7 with intravenous sodium bicarbonate to provide maximal solubility of urate without intratubular calcium phosphate precipitation. Bicarbonate administration can be discontinued when serum uric acid is normalized or when the arterial pH is above 7.5. Acetazolamide, 250 mg to 500 mg IV, alkalinizes the urine without bicarbonate administration. Hydration remains important in preventing xanthine crystallization and stone formation; xanthine excretion is increased with allopurinol use.[37]

At times, when tumor lysis may be predicted to occur, potassium, phosphorus, calcium, uric acid, magnesium, arterial pH, creatinine, and blood urea nitrogen levels should be measured at least once daily. Rapid release of intracellular phosphorus results in reciprocal depression of serum calcium. Bicarbonate infusion is beneficial for hyperkalemia because alkalosis causes intracellular shift of this cation. However, alkalosis may further lower ionized calcium. Calcium is not administered unless there is a positive Chvostek's or Trousseau's sign, other signs of impending tetany, or significant ECG abnormalities. Administration of calcium in the presence of a calcium-phosphorus product above 60 may produce metastatic calcifications. Hyperphosphatemia should be anticipated and phosphate-binding antacids started before therapy. Hypertonic glucose and insulin administered intravenously or the initiation of total parenteral nutrition may help control hyperphosphatemia and hyperkalemia. Dialysis should be initiated if oliguria develops or there is significant hyperkalemia or other electrolyte imbalance.

OBSTRUCTIVE SYNDROMES ■

SUPERIOR VENA CAVA OBSTRUCTION

Clinical Presentation

Superior vena cava (SVC) obstruction may be the first presentation of lung carcinoma or lymphoma or may develop in the patient with previously documented neoplastic disease. Patients with SVC obstruction usually exhibit marked plethora or cyanosis of the head, neck, upper thorax, and upper extremities. Edematous conjunctiva, jugular venous distension, and subcutaneous venous collaterals all may be evident above the level of the obstruction. This clinical presentation is often dramatic and leads to the conclusion that SVC obstruction is an oncologic emergency; however, it is our experience and that of others that this is not a life-threatening event unless there is coexisting airway compromise and respiratory failure.[42] Depending on the location of the tumor mass, one may see an associated Horner's syndrome, recurrent nerve palsy, or airway obstruction. Respiratory insufficiency may be worse in the supine position as the weight of the mediastinal structures impinges on the tracheobronchial tree. Vague symptoms of pain, headache, cough, dysphagia, nausea, vomiting, drowsiness, and vertigo also may occur.[43]

Diagnostic Investigations

Once the clinical diagnosis of SVC obstruction is suspected, confirmation can be obtained using both nuclide and radiologic techniques. Posteroanterior and lateral chest radiographs reveal a superior mediastinal mass in most patients with clinical SVC compression. Computed tomograms (CT) with contrast enhancement have largely replaced SVC venography, which involves the simultaneous injection of intravenous contrast into both upper extremities. In addition to confirming the diagnosis, CT delineates the extent of mediastinal and hilar disease and may help in differentiating

neoplasm from inflammatory conditions such as mediastinal fibrosis. In the critically ill patient who cannot be transported, a short-lived isotope such as ^{99m}Tc-phosphate can be injected into a peripheral vein and the upper thorax scanned with a portable nuclear camera to reveal obstruction.

Therapy

Venous access should be established from below the diaphragm. The patient's head should be elevated above 45 degrees to minimize pressure on posterior mediastinal masses and to favor hydrostatic drainage of venous blood from the head. Although intracaval clot may be present, we have found no role for systemic heparinization. Therapy for the tumor is based on knowledge of the tissue type and relative sensitivity to radiation or chemotherapy. A careful search for evidence of extrathoracic disease, which sometimes can be readily apparent on biopsy, may help delineate therapy. The mainstay of treatment has been radiation therapy; recently, angiographically placed intracaval stents have proven effective. There is little role for surgical intervention in malignant caval obstruction. Before initiating radiation therapy, high-dose corticosteroids may be started to decrease edema and inflammation of the tumor during therapy.

OROPHARYNGEAL AND TRACHEAL OBSTRUCTION

Acute Airway Obstruction

Sudden upper airway obstruction is uncommon with cancer of the head and neck. Life-threatening intrathoracic airway obstruction occurs with some frequency with carcinoma of the lung and mediastinal tumors such as Hodgkin's and non-Hodgkin's lymphoma. Upper airway obstruction may result from direct invasion of the trachea, as seen with thyroid carcinoma, bulky supraglottic or glottic lesions of the trachea, oropharyngeal tumors, or from external compression of the trachea by lymphoma. Tumors of the larynx, pharynx, thyroid, and base of the tongue usually are slow growing, and obvious symptoms of airway compromise are evident before an emergency situation develops. During performance of a thorough head and neck examination, care should be taken minimize trauma to large friable tumors because bleeding may lead to complete airway obstruction. Obstruction from a bulky oropharyngeal or thyroid carcinoma may be best managed by elective tracheostomy, but if the obstruction is caused by an external compression of the trachea by lymphoma or other tissue highly sensitive to radiation or chemotherapy, then nasal or orotracheal intubation alone may be used to maintain airway patency in anticipation of a rapid reduction in tumor mass.[44]

Intrathoracic Obstruction

Lymphoma may present with bulky intrathoracic adenopathy causing airway compression. Because these tumors are extremely sensitive to radiation and chemotherapy, and may regress rapidly regardless of initial size, every attempt to maintain ventilation in these patients is warranted. Intrathoracic airway obstruction should be suspected when a patient complains of dyspnea, wheezing, or chest discomfort. Examination may reveal tachycardia, tachypnea, and occasionally a significant pulsus paradox. There may be evidence of extrathoracic adenopathy and other signs consistent with the diagnosis of lymphoma. Chest examination may reveal a prolonged expiratory time and wheezing. Respiratory symptoms occasionally may be unilateral, and chest radiographs may reveal asymmetric lung fields, particularly at end expiration. Stable patients should have a flow–volume loop performed and may need bronchoscopy or mediastinal exploration for diagnosis if no tissue specimen is more easily accessible. When mechanical ventilation is necessary, the clinician should be alert to hemodynamic compromise resulting from asymmetric obstruction and significant increases in airway pressure distal to the obstruction.

Metastatic and primary tumors of the lung also may present with intrathoracic obstruction; therapy is based on tissue type. Radiation (either external beam or endobronchial), surgical resection, bronchoscopy with debridement or stent placement, or chemotherapy all may play a role.

NEUROLOGIC SYNDROMES ■

SPINAL CORD COMPRESSION

Etiology and Pathophysiology

Spinal cord compression is a profoundly debilitating but usually nonfatal manifestation of neoplastic disease, and occurs in 5% of patients with malignant disease. Any tumor capable of metastasizing may give rise to this problem, but lung cancer, myeloma, prostate cancer, melanoma, lymphomas, carcinomas of unknown primary, and breast cancer each account for 10% to 15% of cases. In 85% of cases, cord compression is caused by epidural metastasis[45–49]; the tumor usually involves the vertebral body and compresses the anterior surface of the cord. Approximately 10% of cases are caused by direct extension into the intravertebral space of lymphomatous lymph nodes arising within the retroperitoneal space. Intramedullary metastases account for fewer than 4% of all cases.[48] Other causes of cord compression in the cancer patient include vertebral subluxation or spinal subdural hematomas.[50]

Clinical Presentation

Pressure on the cord results in decreased blood supply to the area of compression, edema of the spinal cord, occlusion and stasis of the epidural venous plexus, and distortion of the neural tissue. Pain, muscle weakness or paralysis, sensory loss, bowel or bladder dysfunction, or ataxia all may be associated with epidural spinal cord compression. Symptoms may be present from 5 days to 2 years before the diagnosis is confirmed by myelogram.[46]

Pain, usually close to the site of the lesion, is usually present. Complaints of localized pain occasionally can be misleading if there is cancerous involvement of other vertebral bodies producing pain without cord compression. Pain

is usually constant but may be exacerbated by movement, coughing, or Valsalva maneuvers. The discomfort is usually worse when the patient is recumbent, and affected individuals often elect to sleep sitting up. Direct tenderness of the involved vertebral body is evident in one third of the patients. Neck flexion often reproduces symptoms, particularly if the lesion is in the thoracic region. Straight leg raising identifies lumbosacral disease. Radicular pain, unilateral or bilateral, is most common with lumbosacral disease but can be seen with all spinal lesions. Bilateral involvement is common with thoracic disease. The mechanism of the pain may involve stretching or compression of pain-conducting nerve fibers situated in the anterior and posterior spinal ligaments, in the annulus of the intervertebral disc, and in the dura and the apophyseal joints.[46,48]

Three quarters of patients complain of weakness, and more than 85% have demonstrable weakness. Half complain of numbness and paresthesia, and more than 75% have objective sensory deficits. Autonomic dysfunction usually is not a complaint, but most patients have bowel or bladder deficits on examination.[46] Herpes zoster, clinically apparent at the site of extradural compression, is an unusual presentation; this is thought to result from activation of latent virus by tumor involvement of the posterior ganglia.[46]

Radiologic Investigation of Spinal Cord Compression

The onset of new back pain with associated radiographic evidence of vertebral involvement in any cancer patient warrants myelography, even with normal findings on neurologic examination,[45] because radiologic studies of the vertebral bodies demonstrate abnormalities in two thirds of patients with new pain. If the results from neurologic examination and the radiographs are normal, or if the patient has a plexopathy with normal radiographic findings, the clinician may choose careful observation.[48] An extradural block of greater than 80% on myelography confirms the diagnosis of cord compression. Complete blocks warrant cisternal myelography to delineate the upper margin of the tumor. Magnetic resonance imaging with surface coils affords excellent delineation of bone, soft tissue, cord, and tumor, and is especially useful when surgery is planned.

Therapy

Diagnosis of epidural compression mandates immediate therapy, even before completion of radiologic examinations, and particularly in the patient with rapidly evolving neurologic signs. Dexamethasone, 100 mg IV followed by 24 mg IV every 6 hours for 72 hours and then tapered over 2 weeks, offers substantial amelioration of pain for most patients, often within hours.[46,48] Consultation for external-beam radiation therapy to the involved area should be obtained immediately. There seems to be no difference in outcome between radiation therapy alone or combined surgery–radiotherapy. Surgery should not be considered in the patient who presents with paraplegia because the outlook for neurologic recovery is dismal. When diagnosis is in doubt, the nature of the tumor is unknown, or a bone protrusion causes the block, surgery is indicated. Relapse after radiation therapy when no further radiation can be administered and progression of symptoms despite ongoing radiation also are indications for surgery, preferably by an anterior approach.[49]

CARDIAC TAMPONADE

Primary neoplasms of the myocardium and pericardium are uncommon, but metastatic disease to the pericardial space is frequently seen.[51-55] Pericardial metastasis is possible with most malignancies and is common in patients with lung or breast carcinomas, leukemia, and Hodgkin's or non-Hodgkin's lymphoma. Malignancy is the cause of approximately 50% of all cases of cardiac tamponade in medical patients; therefore, idiopathic pericarditis, radiation-related pericarditis or constriction (subacute effusive constrictive pericarditis), hemorrhagic or purulent pericarditis, and restrictive myopathies all must be considered in the differential diagnosis,[56,57] even if a history of malignancy is elicited. Clinical syndromes observed include arrhythmias (especially supraventricular), pericarditis, and diastolic cardiac failure. The clinical, diagnostic, and therapeutic aspects of diastolic cardiac disease and arrhythmias are discussed elsewhere in this text.

Pericardial effusions may become large and remain relatively hemodynamically asymptomatic; however, eventually the enlarged pericardial sac compresses surrounding structures such as the airway, leading to symptoms like coughing. Symptoms of incipient hemodynamic compromise include a sense of fullness in the head and neck, and vague gastrointestinal distress as a result of visceral engorgement. Eventually, signs of more significant hemodynamic impairment ensue: tachycardia, narrow pulse pressure, pulsus paradoxus, and, eventually, systolic hypotension. Chest radiographs are helpful if an enlarged cardiac silhouette without pulmonary congestion is seen. As small amounts of pericardial fluid can be hemodynamically significant, a normal chest radiograph finding does not rule out the presence of a significant effusion. Electrocardiographic changes are nonspecific; sinus tachycardia, ST segment elevation, or electrical alternans may be seen. Echocardiography can document effusions as small as 20 mL; tamponade is suggested by the findings of right ventricular and atrial compression, as well as plethora of the inferior vena cava without fluctuation in size during the respiratory cycle. Right heart catheterization may reveal elevation and equalization of central pressures.

Treatment consists of drainage of the pericardial fluid, with the possible addition of either sclerotherapy or the creation of a permanent "window" to allow free drainage of recurrent fluid into another body space. There are multiple ways to drain the pericardial fluid,[58] including creation of a window, either through a subxiphoid incision, a limited left anterior thoracotomy,[59] or thoracoscopically[60]; catheter drainage under echocardiographic guidance[61]; or, less commonly, percutaneous balloon pericardiostomy[62,63] or placement of a pericardial–peritoneal shunt or window.[64,65] Complications, recurrence rates, and cost of all methods are probably equivalent, and the choice of a particular method should be based on the circumstances of any individual patient's illness. If tamponade is present, pericardial fluid should be drained slowly and accompanied by an immediate attempt at diuresis; otherwise, the increased intravascular volume retained as compensation for the obstruction to venous return may lead to pulmonary edema once the increased intrapericardial pressure is relieved.[66] Pericardial fluid and tissue should be sent for pathologic examination and culture. In a review of our experience of 25 patients seen over 2 years who had known malignancies and then developed pericardial effusions, malignancy was detected in the pericardial fluid alone in 8, in the pericardial tissue alone in 4, in both the fluid and the pericardium in 3, and in neither in 10.[67]

GASTROINTESTINAL EMERGENCIES: NEUTROPENIC ENTEROCOLITIS

Neutropenic enterocolitis (also known as necrotizing enteropathy, typhlitis, or ileocecal syndrome,[68,69]) is a pathologic syndrome of fever, diarrhea, and abdominal pain and distension in the oncologic patient with treatment-related neutropenia. The most common malignancy associated with this syndrome is leukemia, although it may be seen in patients with other hematologic malignancies, and rarely, solid tumors.

Histopathologic findings consist of mucosal inflammation of the ileum, cecum, or ascending colon. The mechanism of bowel injury is probably multifactorial. Involvement of the bowel mucosa by lymphomatous or leukemic cells may lead to mucosal ulceration.[70] Cytotoxic drugs may induce mucosal injury.[71] The prior administration of antibiotics may lead to the selection and overgrowth of virulent organisms. Ileus may either precede and predispose to the syndrome (e.g., if induced by antispasmodics) or arise as a response to inflammation; in either case, ileus, by leading to bowel distension, increased transmural pressure, and mucosal ischemia, probably increases the susceptibility of the bowel to secondary invasion by pathologic organisms. If present, thrombocytopenia predisposes to the formation of intramural hematomas, which increase the risk of necrosis in the distended bowel.

The chief differential diagnoses are appendicitis,[72] *Clostridium difficile*–associated pseudomembranous enterocolitis, and ischemic colitis.[73] Pathologic conditions seen in the oncologic patient that should be kept in mind are the pseudoacute abdomen associated with leukemia,[74] and the abdominal pain and diarrhea associated with the administration of chemotherapeutic agents.[75,76]

As mentioned earlier, the clinical features that suggest neutropenic enterocolitis are fever, loose bowel movements, and abdominal pain, distension, and tenderness. Unfortunately, the diagnosis of neutropenic colitis must be considered a diagnosis of exclusion. Fever is so common in hospitalized neutropenic patients as to be nonspecific.[77] The abdominal pain is diffuse, whereas the tenderness is elicited primarily in the right lower quadrant.[78] Blood work usually is not helpful in establishing the diagnosis of neutropenic enterocolitis, but blood tests may help to rule out other causes of abdominal pain such as hepatobiliary disorders or pancreatitis, and to establish the severity of sepsis, for example, by the degree of acidemia.

Plain abdominal radiographs also are relatively nonspecific and may show distended loops of bowel, "thumb-printing," and pneumatosis intestinalis, or may suggest a mass.[79,80] Such radiographs are most helpful if they suggest a clear indication for surgical intervention such as free air. CT scans of the abdomen may demonstrate findings such as thickening of the right colon wall with edema of the adjacent tissues, but also are most helpful in either suggesting alternative etiologies such as pancreatitis, or providing clear-cut indications for intervention such as free air or abscess cavities.[81] Both barium enemas and colonoscopy generally should be avoided because of the risk of bowel perforation.

Medical therapy consists of bowel rest by parenteral nutrition and possibly, nasogastric suction, and the administration of broad-spectrum antimicrobial agents effective against bowel flora. The need for surgical intervention may be clear-cut if a perforation is present; but, more commonly, the decision is difficult, and exploration is performed in an attempt to salvage a patient who is failing to improve.[82] Improvement and eventual survival is closely related to recovery of the white blood cell count[83]; therefore, granulocyte transfusions have been advocated,[84] although the effectiveness is unproven.

Patients who recover but required further chemotherapy are at risk of recurrent bouts of enterocolitis,[81] and 40% of these patients will require surgery.[82] Therefore, if further chemotherapy is performed, bowel rest and avoidance of bowel antispasmodics is indicated. The role for prophylactic colectomy or diverting ileostomy is as unproven.

TOXICITY OF CHEMOTHERAPY

PULMONARY TOXICITY

Pulmonary toxicity, both acute and chronic, is seen increasingly with numerous antineoplastic agents.[85] Respiratory failure may present as an acute hypersensitivity reaction, chronic insidious pulmonary fibrosis, and rarely, as noncardiogenic pulmonary edema.[86] Symptoms can appear immediately or months after termination of therapy, as seen with acute radiation-induced pneumonitis. Synergistic toxicity also occurs (e.g., radiation and bleomycin). Patients with a history of bleomycin therapy and respiratory failure should ideally be managed with as low a fraction of inspired oxygen as is clinically possible, with a goal of less than 0.3, because oxygen causes synergistic toxicity.[87]

Mitomycin in combination with *Vinca* alkaloids have come into wide use in the treatment of ovarian, breast, and small cell lung cancer. Acute dyspnea associated with hypoxemia has been reported 1 to 2 hours after administration of the *Vinca* alkaloids. Bilateral rales and wheezing is common. The chest radiograph most commonly reveals interstitial infiltrates. Symptoms usually resolve within 12 hours and are treated with supplemental oxygen, bronchodilators, and occasionally steroids. Severe symptomatology has

required intubation. The etiology of this acute dyspnea syndrome is unknown.[88]

CARDIAC TOXICITY

Cardiac toxicity is seen with anthracycline antibiotics such as doxorubicin (Adriamycin). Chronic administration may be associated with subclinical ventricular dysfunction or overt congestive heart failure. Acute toxicities of anthracyclines are infrequent but can present with ECG abnormalities, myocarditis–pericarditis, or transient deterioration of left ventricular function. Chest pain mimicking myocardial infarction or pulmonary emboli is reported, although rarely with infusions of bleomycin,[89] whereas chest pain with coronary spasm and ischemic changes on ECG progressing to myocardial infarction is seen with continuous infusion of 5-fluorouracil.[90]

Cyclophosphamide is ordinarily lethal at doses above 50 to 100 mg/kg, although this amount is routinely administered as preparation for bone marrow transplantation. A potential side effect is a severe hemorrhagic myocarditis.[91] The ventricular dysfunction is significantly worse in patients who have received prior anthracyclines or mediastinal radiation. Invasive monitoring to optimize hemodynamic function is usually required. Serial echocardiograms may reveal progressive pericardial effusion in the setting of deteriorating cardiac function. Separating critical cardiac tamponade from profound myocardial dysfunction, even with a pulmonary artery catheter in place, is commonly impossible. Pericardiocentesis should not be performed in these thrombocytopenic patients unless absolutely indicated. When able to support vital functions through the acute decompensation, cardiac function usually returns to baseline.

Subacute effusive constrictive pericarditis may be seen after mediastinal radiation.[92,93] Patients present with signs and symptoms of critical pericardial tamponade; however, on removal of pericardial fluid, intracardiac filling pressures remain elevated because of restrictive pericarditis. Pericardiectomy often is necessary to relieve the embarrassed diastolic ventricular filling associated with the restrictive state.

Most cancer therapy is associated with some toxicity. The reader is referred to other general references for a detailed discussion of the toxicities of cancer therapy.[94–98]

REFERENCES

1. *Cancer Facts & Figures 1995.* New York, American Cancer Society, 1995
2. O'Reilly RJ: New promises for autologous marrow transplants in leukemia. *N Engl J Med* 1986;3:186
3. Rabin RS: Monoclonal antibodies: use in the detection and treatment of cancer. *Postgrad Med* 986;79:293
4. Rosenberg SA, Lotze MT, Muul LM, et al: Observations on the systemic administration of autologous lymphokine-activated killer cells and recombinant interleukin-2 to patients with metastatic cancer. *N Engl J Med* 1985;313:1485
5. Myers WPL: Differential diagnosis of hypercalcemia and cancer. *CA* 1977;27:258

6. Nainby-Luxmoore JC, Langford HG, Nelson NC, et al: A case-comparison study of hypertension and hyperparathyroidism. *J Clin Endocrinol Metab* 1982;55:303

7. Cogan MG, Covey GM, Arieff AL, et al: Central nervous system manifestations of hyperparathyroidism. *Am J Med* 1978; 65:963

8. Hoff HE, Smith PK, Winkler W: Electrocardiographic changes and concentrations of calcium in serum following intravenous injection of calcium chloride. *Am J Physiol* 1938;125:162

9. Mundy GR, Martin TJ: The hypercalcemia of malignancy: pathogenesis and management. *Metabolism* 1982;31:1247

10. Fisken RA, Health DA, Somers S, et al: Hypercalcemia in hospital patients: clinical and diagnostic aspects. *Lancet* 1981; i:202

11. Steward Af, Horst R, Deftos L, et al: Biochemical evaluation of patients with malignancy-associated hypercalcemia: evidence for humoral and non-humoral groups. *N Engl J Med* 1980;330:1377

12. McDonnell GD, Dunstan CR, Evans RA, et al: Quantitative bone histology in the hypercalcemia of malignant disease. *J Clin Endocrinol Metab* 1982;55:1066

13. Mundy GR: Hypercalcemia of malignancy revisited. *J Clin Invest* 1988;82:1

14. Orloff JJ, Wu TL, Stewart AF: Parathyroid hormone-like proteins: biochemical responses and receptor interactions. *Endocr Rev* 19989;10:476

15. Broadus A, Mangin M, Ikeda K, et al: Humoral hypercalcemia of cancer: identification of a novel parathyroid hormone-like peptide. *N Engl J Med* 1988;319:556

16. Leung SC, Rosenblatt M, Nissensoon RA: Parathyroid hormone-like protein from human renal carcinoma cella: structural and functional homology with parathyroid hormone. *J Clin Invest* 1987;80:1803

17. Mosely JM, Kubota M, Diefenbach-Jagger H, et al: Parathyroid hormone-related protein purified from a human lung cancer cell line. *Proc Natl Acad Sci* 1987;84:5048

18. Stewart AF, We T, Goumas D, et al: N-terminal amino acid sequence of two novel tumor-derived adenylate cyclase-stimulating proteins: identification of parathyroid hormone-like and parathyroid hormone-unlike domains. *Biochem Biophys Res Commun* 1987;146:672

19. Mundy GR, Ibbotson KJ, D'Souza SM: Tumor products and the hypercalcemia of malignancy. *J Clin Invest* 1985;76:391

20. Nussbaum S, Zahradnik R, LaVigne J, et al: Highly sensitive two-site immunoradiometric assay parathyroid hormone and its clinical utility in evaluating patients with hypercalcemia. *Clin Chem* 1987;33:1364

21. Boyd JC, Ladenson JH: Value of laboratory tests in the differential diagnosis of hypercalcemia. *Am J Med* 1984;77:863

22. Palmer FJ, Nelson JC, Bacchus H: The chloride–phosphate ratio in hypercalcemia. *Ann Intern Med* 1974;80:200

23. Rude RK, Sharp CF, Fredericks RS, et al: Urinary and nephrogenous adenosine 3′,5′-monophosphate in the hypercalcemia of malignancy. *J Clin Endocrinol Metab* 1981;52:765

24. Saldinger KA, Samaan NA: Hypokalemia with hypercalcemia: prevalence with significance in treatment. *Ann Intern Med* 1977;87:571

25. Warrell RP Jr, Bockman RS: Metabolic emergencies. In: DeVita VTY, Hellman S, Rosenberg SA (eds). *Cancer: Principles and Practice of Oncology*. Philadelphia, JB Lippincott, 1989: 1986

26. Attie MF: Treatment of hypercalcemia. *Endocrinol Metab Clin North Am* 1989;18:807

27. Kiang DT, Loken MK, Kennedy BJ: Mechanism of the hypocalcemic effect of mithramycin. *J Clinc Endocrinol Metab* 1979;48:341

28. Silva OL, Becker KL: Salmon calcitonin in the treatment of hypercalcemia. *Arch Intern Med* 1973;132:337

29. Warrell RP, Skelos A, Alcock N, et al: Gallium nitrate for acute treatment of cancer related hypercalcemia: clinicopharmacological and dose response analysis. *Cancer Res* 1986;46:4208

30. White DA, Schwartzberg LS, Kris MG, et al: Acute chest pain syndrome during bleomycin infusions. *Cancer* 1987;59:1582

31. Jacobs TP, Gordon AC, Silberberg SJ, et al: Neoplastic hypercalcemia: physiologic response to intravenous etiidronate disodium. *Am J Med* 1987;82:42

32. Green L, Donehower RC: Hepatic toxicity of low doses of mithramycin in hypercalcemia. *Cancer Treat Rep* 1984;68:1379

33. Warrell RP, Israel R, Fisone Me, et al: Gallium nitrate for acute treatment of cancer related hypercalcemia: a randomized double-blind comparison to calcitonin. *Ann Intern Med* 1988;108:669

34. Ralston SH, Patel U, Fraser WD, et al: Comparison of three intravenous biphosphonates in cancer-associated hypercalcemia. *Lancet* 1989;ii:1180

35. Flombaum CD: Electrolyte and renal abnormalities. In: Groeger JS (ed). *Critical Care of the Cancer Patient*. St Louis, Mosby–Year Book 1991:140

36. Simpson DP, Wen SF, Chesney RW: Fluid and electrolyte abnormalities due to tumors: their products or metabolites. In: Rieselbach RE, Garnick MB (eds). *Cancer and the Kidney*. Philadelphia, Lea & Febiger, 1982:534

37. Banck PR, Silverberg DS, Henderson JF: Xanthine nephropathy in patients with lymphosarcoma treated with allopurinol. *N Engl J Med* 1970;283:354

38. Arseneau JC, Bagley CM, Anderson T, et al: Hyperkalemia: a sequel to chemotherapy of Burkitt's lymphoma. *Lancet* 1973; i:10

39. Zusman J, Brown DM, Nesbit ME: Hyperphosphatemia, hyperphosphaturia, and hypocalcemia in acute lymphoblastic leukemia. *N Engl J Med* 1973;289:1333

40. Lynch Re, Kjellstrand CM, Coccia PF: Renal and metabolic complications of childhood non-Hodgkin's lymphoma. *Semin Oncol* 1977;4(3):325

41. Parker S, Carlon GC, Isaacs M, et al: Dopamine administration in oliguria and oliguric renal failure. *Crit Care Med* 1981;9:630

42. Ahman F: A reassessment of the clinical implications of the superior vena caval syndrome. *J Clin Oncol* 1984;2:8

43. Simpson JR Perez CA, Presant BJ, et al: Superior vena cava syndrome. In: Yabro JW, Bornstein RS (eds). *Oncologic Emergencies*. New York, Grune & Stratton, 1981:43

44. Strong EW: Head and neck emergencies: life threatening emergencies in the cancer patient. Part II. *Curr Probl Cancer* 1979;4:36

45. Barr LR, Nealon N: Neurologic complications. In: Groeger JS (ed). *Critical Care of the Cancer Patient*. St Louis, Mosby–Year Book 1991:226

46. Gilbert RW, Kim JH, Psoner JB: Epidural spinal cord compression from metastatic tumor: diagnosis and treatment. *Ann Neurol* 1978;3:40

47. Greenberg HS, Kin JH, Posner JB: Epidural spinal cord compression from metastatic tumor: results with a new treatment protocol. *Ann Neurol* 1980;8:361

48. Rodichok L, Harper Gr, Ruckdeschell JC, et al: Early diagnosis of spinal epidural metastasis. *Am J Med* 1981;70:1181

49. Siegel T, Siegal T, Robin G, et al: Anterior decompression of the spine for metastatic epidural compression: a promising avenue of therapy? *Ann Neurol* 1982;11:28

50. Edelson RN, Chernik NL, Posner JB: Spinal subdural hematomas complicating lumbar puncture. *Arch Neurol* 1974;31:134

51. Pierri MK: Heart disease. In: Groeger JS (ed). *Critical Care of the Cancer Patient*. St Louis, Mosby–Year Book 1991:64

52. Griffiths GC: A review of primary tumors of the heart. *Prog Cardiovasc Dis* 1965;7:465

53. Berge T, Sievers J: Myocardial metastases: a pathological and electrocardiographic study. *Br Heart J* 1986;30:383

54. Goodwin JF: Symposium on cardiac tumors: the spectrum of cardiac tumors. *Am J Cardiol* 1968;21:307

55. Theologides A: Neoplastic cardiac tamponade. *Semin Oncol* 1958;5:181

56. Hancock EW: Subacute effusive-constrictive pericarditis. *Circulation* 1971;43:183

57. Brosius FC, Waller Bf, Roberts WC: Radiation heart disease: analysis of 16 young (aged 15–32 years) necropsy patients who received over 3,500 rads to the heart. *Am J Med* 1981;70:519

58. Vaitkus PT, Herrman HC, Le Winter MM: Treatment of malignant pericardial effusion. *JAMA* 1994;272:59

59. Moores DW, Allen KB, Faber LP, et al: Subxiphoid pericardial drainage for pericardial tamponade. *J Thorac Cardiovasc Surg* 1995;109:546

60. Liu HP, Chang CH, Lin PJ, et al: Thorascopic management of effusive pericardial disease: indications and technique. *Ann Thorac Surg* 1994;58:1695

61. Hingorani AD, Bloomberg TJ: Ultrasound-guided pigtail catheter drainage of malignant pericardial effusions. *Clin Radiol* 1995;50:15

62. DiSegni E, Lavee J, Kaplinsky E, et al: Percutaneous balloon pericardiostomy for treatment of cardiac tamponade. *Eur Heart J* 1995;16:184

63. Ziskind AA, Pearce AC, Lemmon CC, et al: Percutaneous balloon pericardiotomy for the treatment of cardiac tamponade and large pericardial effusions: description of technique and report of the first 50 cases. *J Am Coll Cardiol* 1993;21:1

64. Wang N, Feikes JR, Mogansen T, et al: Pericardioperitoneal shunt: alternative treatment for malignant pericardial effusion. *Ann Thorac Surg* 1994;57:289

65. Olson JE, Ryan MB, Blumenstock DA: Eleven years' experience with pericardial-peritoneal window in the management of malignant and benign pericardial effusions. *Ann Surg Oncol* 1995;2:165

66. Downey RJ, Bessler M, Weissman C: Acute pulmonary edema following pericardiocentesis for chronic cardiac tamponade secondary to trauma. *Crit Care Med* 1991;19:1323

67. Downey RJ, Keefe D, Groeger J, et al: Correlation of echocardiographic, cytologic, and histologic findings of pericardial effusions in patients with malignancy. *Chest* 1995;108:150S

68. Amromin GD, Solomon RD: Necrotizing enteropathy: a complication of treated leukemia or lymphoma patients. *JAMA* 182:23;1962

69. Sherman NJ, Woolley MM: The ileocecal syndrome in acute childhood leukemia. *Arch Surg* 1973;107:39

70. Newbold KM: Neutropenic enterocolitis: clinical and pathological review. *Dig Dis* 1989;7:281

71. Vlasveld LT, Zwaan, FE, Fibbe WE, et al: Neutropenic enterocolitis following treatment with cytosine araginoside-containing regiments for hematological malignancies: a potentiating role for amsacrine. *Ann Hematol* 1991;62:129

72. Angel CA, Rao BN, Wrenn E Jr, et al: Acute appendicitis in children with leukemia and other malignancies: still a diagnostic dilemma. *J Pediatr Surg* 1992;27:476

73. Dosik GM, Luna M, Valdivieso M, et al: Necrotizing colitis in patients with cancer. *Am J Med* 1979;67:646

74. Prolla JC, Kirsner JB: The gastrointestinal lesions and complications of the leukemias. *Ann Intern Med* 1964;61:1084

75. Rosenthal S, Kaufman S: Vincristine neurotoxicity. *Ann Intern Med* 1974;80:733

76. Slavin RE, Dias MA, Saral R: Cytosine arabinoside induced gastrointestinal toxic alterations in sequential chemotherapeutic protocols. *Cancer* 1978;42:1747

77. Gurwith MJ, Brunton JL, Land BA, et al: Granulocytopenia in hospitalized patients: prognostic factors and etiology of fever. *Am J Med* 1978;64:121

78. Archibald RB, Nelson JA: Necrotizing enterocolitis in acute leukemia: radiographic findings. *Gastrointest Radiol* 1978;3:63

79. Mower WJ, Hawkins JA, Nelson EW: Neutropenic enterocolitis in adults with acute leukemia. *Arch Surg* 1986;121:571

80. Adams GW, Rauch RF, Kelvin FM, et al: CT detection of typhlitis: a case report. *J Comput Assist Tomogr* 1985;9:363

81. Stellato TA, Shenk RR: Gastrointestinal emergencies in the oncology patient. *Semin Oncol* 1989;16:521

82. Glenn J, Funkhouser WK, Schneider PS: Acute illness necessitating urgent abdominal surgery in neutropenic cancer patients: description of 14 cases and review of the literature. *Surgery* 1989;105:778

83. Gandy W, Greenberg BR: Successful medical management of neutropenic enterocolitis. *Cancer* 1983;51:1551

84. Moir Cr, Scudamore CH, Bennyt WB: Typhilitis: selective surgical management. *Am J Surg* 1986;151:563

85. White DA, Orenstein M, Godwin TA, et al: Chemotherapy-associated pulmonary toxic reactions during treatment of breast cancer. *Arch Intern Med* 1984;144:953

86. Cooper JA Jr, White DA, Matthay RA: Drug-induced pulmonary disease: state of art. *Am Rev Respir Dis* 1986;133:321

87. Goldiner PL, Carlon GC, Cvitkovic E, et al: Factors influencing post-operative morbidity and mortality in patients treated with bleomycin. *Br Med J* 1978;1:664

88. Pisters K, Rivera P, Kris M: Acute toxicities of cancer therapy. In: Groeger JS (ed). *Critical Care of the Cancer Patient*. St Louis, Mosby–Year Book, 1991

89. White DA, Schwartzberg LS, Kris MG, et al: Acute chest pain syndrome during bleomycin infusions. *Cancer* 1987;59:1582

90. LaBianca R, Beretta G, Clerici M, et al: Cardiac toxicity of 5-FU: a study on 1083 patients. *Tumori* 1982;68:505

91. Mills BA, Roberts RW: Cyclophosphamide-induced cardiomyopathy. *Cancer* 1979;43:2223

92. Gottdiener JS, Aplebaum FR, Ferrans J, et al: Delayed pericardial disease after radiotherapy. *Am J Cardiol* 1981;47:210

93. Applefeld MM, Slawson RG, Hall-Craigs M, et al: Delayed pericardial disease after radiotherapy. *Am J Cardiol* 1981;47:210

94. Groeger JS (ed): *Critical Care of the Cancer Patient*. St Louis, Mosby–Year Book Publishers, 1991

95. Yarbro Jw, Bornstein RS (eds): *Oncologic Emergencies*. New York, Grune & Stratton, 1981

96. Perry MC (ed): Toxicity of chemotherapy. *Semin Oncol* 1982;9(1):1

97. DeVita VT Jr, Hellman S, Rosenberg SA (eds): *Cancer: Principles and Practice of Oncology*. Philadelphia, JB Lippincott, 1993

98. Turnbull A (ed): *Surgical Emergencies in Oncology*. Chicago, Year Book Medical Publishers, 1987

APPENDIX

Critical Care Catalog

Stephen M. Koch

APPENDIX A: PREFIXES AND CONVERSIONS

TABLE A-1. METRIC PREFIXES

MULTIPLE	PREFIX	ABBREVIATION
10^{12}	tera-	T
10^{9}	giga-	G
10^{6}	mega-	M
10^{3}	kilo-	k
10	deca-	da
10^{-1}	deci-	d
10^{-2}	centi-	c
10^{-3}	milli-	m
10^{-6}	micro-	μ
10^{-9}	nano-	n
10^{-12}	pico-	p
10^{-15}	femto-	f
10^{-18}	atto-	a

TABLE A-2. FAHRENHEIT AND CELSIUS TEMPERATURE CONVERSIONS

Celsius scale (°C): Degree of Celsius (or centigrade) equals 1/100th of the difference in temperature of melting ice and boiling water at the atmospheric pressure of 760 mm Hg.

Fahrenheit scale (°F): The interval between freezing and boiling is divided into 180 degrees.

$$°C = (5/9°F) - 32$$
$$°F = (9/5°C) + 32$$

°C	°F	°C	°F
45	113.0	32	89.6
44	111.2	31	87.8
43	109.4	30	86.0
42	107.6	29	84.2
41	105.8	28	82.4
40	104.0	27	80.6
39	102.2	26	78.8
38	100.4	25	77.0
37	98.6	24	75.2
36	96.8	23	73.4
35	95.0	22	71.6
34	93.2	21	69.8
33	91.4	20	68.0

APPENDIX B: DUBOIS BODY SURFACE AREA NOMOGRAM AND FORMULA ∎

Body Surface Area = ([height in cm]$^{0.718}$) ([weight in kg]$^{0.427}$) (74.49)

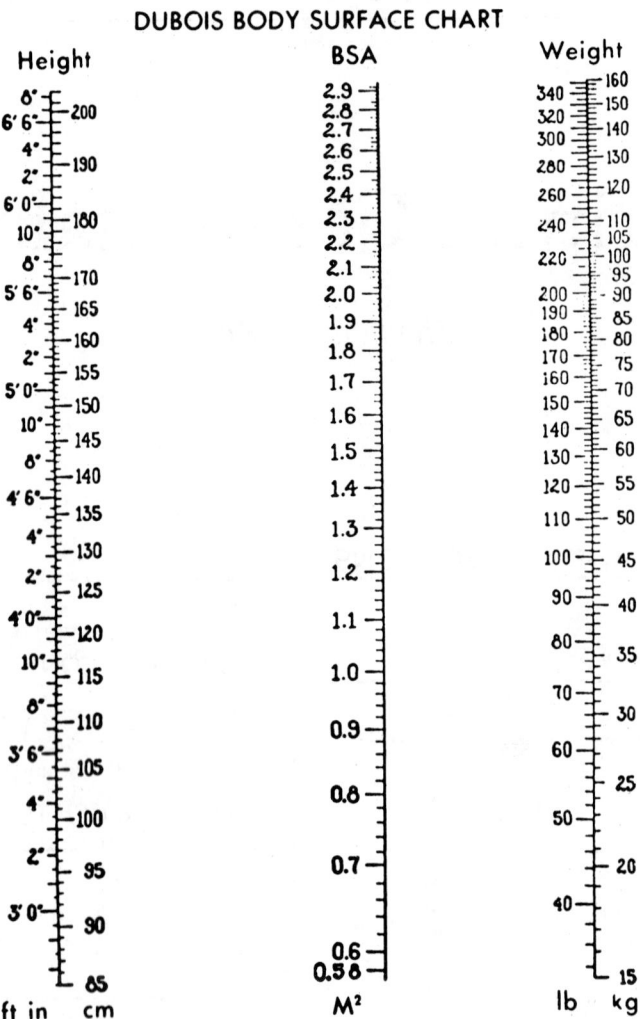

DUBOIS BODY SURFACE CHART

FIGURE B-1. Nomogram for determination of body surface area in adults. A straight edge is placed so that it connects the patient's height (*left column*) with his weight (*right column*) crossing the center column at the point indicating the body surface area. (From DuBois D, DuBois EF. *Arch Intern Med* 1916;17:863. Used by permission.)

From reference 1 with permission.

APPENDIX C: FLUIDS AND ELECTROLYTES

TABLE C-1. INTRAVENOUS FLUIDS

SOLUTION		pH	Na	Cl	K	Ca	Mg	ACETATE	GLUCONATE	ALBUMIN	LACTATE	DEXTROSE
Units	*mOsm/L*		*mMol/L*			*mg/dL*				*g/L*		
5% Dextrose (D₅W)	250–253	5	—	—	—	—	—	—	—	—	—	50
0.45% NaCl (½ NS)	155	5–5.6	77	77	—	—	—	—	—	—	—	—
0.9% NaCl (NS)	308	5.7	154	154	—	—	—	—	—	—	—	—
0.45% NaCl + D₅W (D₅½NS)	406	4–4.4	77	77	—	—	—	—	—	—	—	50
0.9% NaCl + D₅W (D₅NS)	561	4–4.4	154	154	—	—	—	—	—	—	—	50
Ringer's solution	309	6	147	156	4	4–4.5	—	—	—	—	—	—
Lactated Ringer's (LR)	275	6.7	130	109	4	3	—	—	—	—	28	—
5% Dextrose + lactated Ringer's (D₅LR)	525–530	4.7–5	130	109	4	3	—	—	—	—	28	50
Plasma protein fractions 5%	294	6.7–7.3	130–160	90	0–5	—	0–3	0–27	0–23	0–12.5	—	—
3% NaCl	1026	5.8	513	513	—	—	—	—	—	—	—	—
5% NaCl	1710	5–6	855	855	—	—	—	—	—	—	—	—
Mannitol 5%	275	6										
Mannitol 10%	550	6										
Mannitol 15%	825	6										
Mannitol 20%	1100	6										
Mannitol 25%	1375	6										
Fresh frozen plasma	310–330		168	76	3.2	8.2	—	—	—	—	—	—
Dextran-40 in NS	310	5–5.5	154	154	—	—	—	—	—	—	—	—
Dextran-70 in D₅W	287	3.5–7										50
5% Albumin	300	6.9	145	145						50		
25% Albumin		6.9	145	145						250		
Hydroxyethyl starch 6% (Hetastarch)	310	5.5	154	154								

Na, sodium; Cl, chloride; K, potassium; Ca, calcium; Mg, magnesium; D₅W, 5% dextrose in water; NaCl, sodium chloride; NS, normal saline.

TABLE C-2. ELECTROLYTE COMPOSITION OF VARIOUS BODY FLUIDS

FLUID (IN mMoL/L)	Na$^+$	K$^+$	Cl$^-$	HCO$_3^-$	VOLUME (L/d)
Saliva	30	20	35	15	1–1.5
Gastric fluid (pH <4)	60	10	90	—	2.5
Gastric fluid (pH >4)	100	10	100	—	2
Bile	145	5	110	40	1.5
Duodenum	140	5	80	50	—
Pancreas	140	5	75	90	0.7–1.0
Ileum	130	10	110	30	3.5
Cecum	80	20	50	20	—
Colon	60	30	40	20	—
Sweat	50	5	55	—	0–3
New ileostomy	130	20	110	30	0.5–2.0
Adapted ileostomy	50	5	30	25	0.4
Colostomy	50	10	40	20	0.3

Modified from reference 2 with permission.

OSMOLALITY

Calculated serum osmolality

$$= 2[\text{Na}^+] + \frac{[\text{glucose}]}{18} + \frac{[\text{BUN}]}{2.8} + \frac{[\text{mannitol}]}{18} + \frac{[\text{EtOH}]}{4.6} + \frac{[\text{ethylene glycol}]}{6.2} + \frac{[\text{methanol}]}{3.2}$$

[275–290 mMol/kg]

Osmolar gap

= Measured serum osmolality − Calculated serum osmolality
[0–5 mOsm/kg]

Sodium (Na$^+$)

Pseudohyponatremia with hyperglycemia
Each 100-mg/dL increase in serum glucose (above 100 mg/dL) decreases Na$^+$ by 1.6 mMol/L

Free water deficit in hypernatremia

$$= (0.6)\,(\text{body weight in kg}) \left(\frac{[\text{Na}^+]}{140} - 1\right)$$

Free water excess in hyponatremia

$$= (0.6)\,(\text{body weight in kg}) \left(1 - \frac{[\text{Na}^+]}{140}\right)$$

POTASSIUM (K$^+$)

[K$^+$] increases 0.6 mMol/L for each 0.1 unit decrease in pH
[K$^+$] decreases 0.6 mMol/L for each 0.1 unit increase in pH

APPENDIX D: ACID-BASE

OVERVIEW

Acidosis: process that tends to decrease pH
Alkalosis: process that tends to increase pH
Normal pH range: 7.36–7.44
Acidemia/alkalemia: refers to the actual pH, not the etiologic process
Changes affecting [HCO_3^-] are metabolic disturbances
Changes affecting $PaCO_2$ are respiratory disturbances
Henderson-Hasselbach equation:

$$pH = pK + \log \frac{[HCO_3^-]}{[H_2CO_3]}$$

Simple acid-base disturbance: a single primary process *and* its expected compensations
Mixed acid-base disturbance: two or more primary processes *and* their expected compensation
Buffer: a substance that can absorb or donate H^+ ions and thereby mitigate, *but not entirely prevent*, a change in pH
Carbonic acid (H_2CO_3) and bicarbonate (HCO_3^-) buffer system:

$$H^+ + HCO_3^- \rightleftharpoons H_2CO_3 \rightleftharpoons CO_2 + H_2O$$

Anion gap = difference between measured cations and anions

$$= [Na^+] - ([Cl^-] + [HCO_3^-])$$

TABLE D-1. ACID-BASE DISTURBANCES AND COMPENSATION

DISTURBANCE	PRIMARY CHANGE	SECONDARY CHANGE
Metabolic acidosis	Decrease HCO_3^- (retention of fixed acid or loss of alkali)	Decrease $PaCO_2$ (increase ventilation)
Respiratory acidosis	Increase $PaCO_2$ (hypoventilation)	Increase HCO_3^- (increased renal regeneration of HCO_3^-)
Metabolic alkalosis	Increase HCO_3^- (loss of fixed acid or increased HCO_3^-)	Increase $PaCO_2$ (hypoventilation)
Respiratory alkalosis	Decrease $PaCO_2$ (hyperventilation)	Decrease HCO_3^- (decreased renal acid excretion and HCO_3^- regeneration)

TABLE D-2. ANTICIPATED CHANGES IN SIMPLE DISTURBANCES

PRIMARY DISORDER	PRIMARY	SECONDARY	COMPENSATION	LIMIT	NET EFFECT
Metabolic acidosis	↓ [HCO_3]	↓ $PaCO_2$	$\delta\ PaCO_2 = 1.0–1.4 \times \delta\ [HCO_3]$	10 mm Hg	↑ [H^+](↓ pH)
Metabolic alkalosis	↑ [HCO_3]	↑ $PaCO_2$	$\delta\ PaCO_2 = 0.5–1.0 \times \delta\ [HCO_3]$	55 mm Hg No hypoxia	↓ [H^+](↑ pH)
Respiratory acidosis	↑ $PaCO_2$	↑ [HCO_3]	Acute: $\delta\ [H^+]\ 0.75\ \delta\ PaCO_2$ $\delta\ [HCO_3] = 1$ mMol/L ↑/10 mm Hg ↑ $PaCO_2$ $\delta\ [HCO_3] = 0.1 \times \delta\ PaCO_2$ Chronic: $\delta\ [HCO_3] = 0.35 \times PaCO_2$ $\delta\ [HCO_3]$ = mMol/L ↑/10 mm Hg ↑ $PaCO_2$	30 mMol/L HCO_3 45 mMol/L HCO_3	↑ [H^+](↓ pH)
Respiratory alkalosis	↓ $PaCO_2$	↓ [HCO_3]	Acute: $\delta\ [HCO_3] = 0.2 \times \delta\ PaCO_2$ $\delta\ [HCO_3] = 1$ mMol/L ↓/10 mm Hg ↓ $PaCO_2$ $\delta\ [H^+]\ 0.75\ \delta\ PaCO_2$ Chronic: $\delta\ [HCO_3] = 0.5 \times \delta\ PaCO_2$ $\delta\ [HCO_3] = 2–5$ mMol/L ↓/10 mm Hg ↓ $PaCO_2$	18 mMol/L 12–15 mMol/L	↓ [H^+](↑ pH)

CAUSES OF SIMPLE
ACID-BASE DISTURBANCES

A. Metabolic acidosis
  1. Increased anion gap (usually decreased chloride)
    a. Acidosis
      1. Alcoholic ketoacidosis
      2. Diabetic ketoacidosis
      3. Starvation ketoacidosis
      4. Ethylene glycol ingestion
      5. Paraldehyde
      6. Methanol ingestion
      7. Lactic acidosis
      8. Uremic acidosis
      9. Hyperosmolar nonketotic coma
    b. Nonacidosis
      1. Hypokalemia
      2. Hypocalcemia
      3. Hypomagnesemia
      4. Hyperalbuminemia
      5. Nitrate usage
      6. Penicillin/carbenicillin
      7. Pseudohypernatremia
      8. Pseudohypochloremia
      9. False decrease in serum HCO_3^-
  2. Normal anion gap (usually increased chloride)
    a. Acidosis
      1. Carbonic anhydrase inhibitors
      2. Ureterosigmoidostomy
      3. Ileostomy
      4. Diarrhea
      5. Pancreatic fistula
      6. Parenteral nutrition
      7. Ingestion of NH_4Cl
      8. Ingestion of HCl or other acid
      9. Renal tubular acidosis
      10. Dilutional acidosis
      11. Following respiratory alkalosis
      12. Cholestyramine
      13. Normal saline infusions
    b. Nonacidosis
      1. Hyperkalemia
      2. Hypocalcemia
      3. Hypomagnesim
      4. Hypoalbuminemia
      5. IgG
      6. Lithium
      7. Pseudohyponatremia

  8. Pseudohyperchloremia
  9. False increase in serum HCO_3^-
B. Metabolic alkalosis
  1. Loss of H^+
    a. Gastrointestinal loss
      1. Vomiting, nasogastric suction
      2. Antacids
      3. Chloride-losing diarrhea
    b. Renal loss
      1. Diuretics
      2. Excess mineralocortiocoid
      3. Postchronic hypercapnia
      4. Decreased chloride intake
      5. High-dose penicillins
      6. Hypercalcemia
    c. Intracellular H^+ Shift
      1. Hypokalemia
      2. Refeeding
  2. HCO_3^- retention
    a. Massive transfusions
    b. $NaHCO_3$ therapy
    c. Milk-alkali syndrome
  3. Volume contraction
    a. Diuretics
    b. Gastrointestinal losses in patients with achlorhydria
    c. Sweat losses in cystic fibrosis
C. Respiratory acidosis
  1. CNS depression
  2. Chronic obstructive lung disease
  3. Severe asthma
  4. Pneumothorax
  5. Abdominal distention
  6. Pulmonary edema
  7. Mechanical underventilation
  8. Idiopathic hypoventilation
  9. Neuromuscular disease
D. Respiratory alkalosis
  1. Salicylate toxicity
  2. Hepatic failure
  3. Psychogenic hyperventilation
  4. Pulmonary edema
  5. Asthma
  6. Systemic inflammatory response syndrome
  7. Restrictive lung disease
  8. Primary CNS disease
  9. Mechanical overventilation
  10. Hypoxemia

ACID-BASE NOMOGRAM

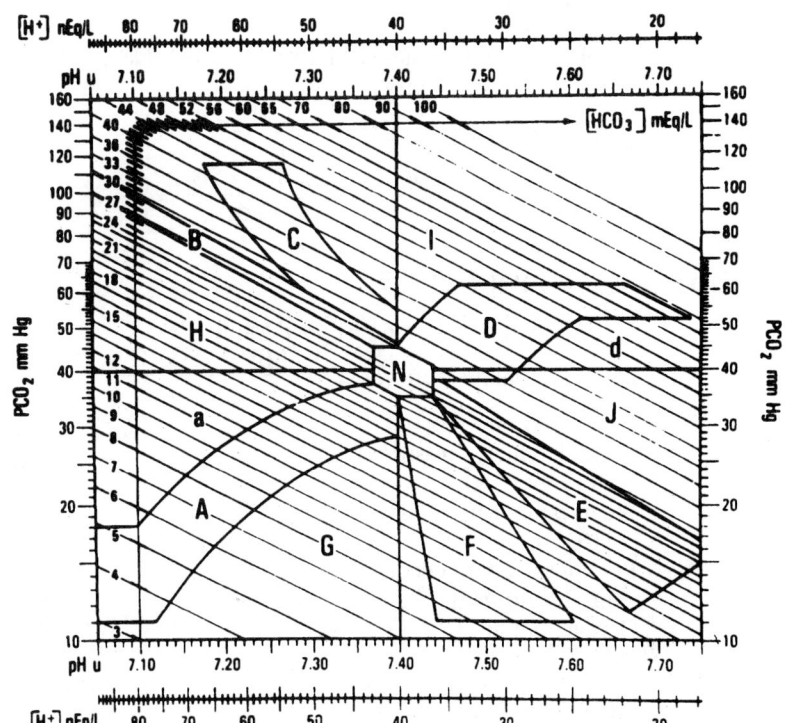

FIGURE D-1. Areas of the acid base map

A-compensated metabolic acidosis

a-metabolic acidosis without respiratory compensation

B-compensated acute respiratory acidosis

C-compensated chronic respiratory acidosis

D-compensated metabolic alkalosis

d-metabolic alkalosis without respiratory compensation

E-compensated acure respiratory alkalosis

F-compensated chronic respiratory alkalosis

G-mixed metabolic acidosis and respiratory alkalosis

H-mixed metabolic acidosis and respiratory acidosis

I-mixed metabolic alkalosis and respiratory acidosis

J-mixed metabolic alkalosis and respiratory alkalosis

°-The areas labeled A, B, C, D, E, and F may represent either a pure primary disturbance or a complex mixed disturbance. (From Meerott JC: An easy-to-read acid-base nomogram. *Hosp Prac* 1987:187; with permission.)

APPENDIX E: FORMULAS (NORMAL RANGES IN BRACKETS) ■

CEREBRAL/NEUROLOGIC FORMULAS

Glasgow coma scale (GCS) = eyes + motor + verbal [Normal: 15]

Eye opening:

Spontaneous	4
To speech	3
To pain	2
Negative	1

Motor Response:

Obeys commands	6
Localizes pain	5
Withdraws	4
Abnormal flexion	3
Abnormal extension	2
Negative	1

Verbal response:

Oriented	5
Confused, conversant	4
Inappropriate words	3
Incomprehensible sounds	2
Negative	1

Intracranial pressure (ICP)

[<20 cm H_2O, <15 mm Hg]

Cerebral perfusion pressure (CPP) = MAP − ICP

[70–100 mm Hg]

Cerebral vascular resistance (CVR)

[1.5–2.1 mm Hg/100 g/min/mL]

Cerebral blood flow (CBF) = CPP/CVR

[75 mL/100 g gray matter/min]
[45 mL/100 g white matter/min]
Jugular bulb saturation $(S_{jv}O_2)$
[55–70%]
Cerebral metabolic rate $(CMRo_2) = (CBF) (CaO_2 - C_{jv}O_2)$
[3–3.5 mL/100 g/min]

$$\text{Cerebral oxygen extraction} = \frac{CMRo_2}{(CBF)(CaO_2)}$$
$$= \frac{CaO_2 - C_{jv}O_2}{CaO_2}$$

HEMODYNAMIC FORMULAS

Pulse pressure = systolic BP − diastolic BP

$$\text{Mean arterial pressure (MAP)} = \frac{SBP + 2(DBP)}{3}$$

[70–105 mm Hg]
Central venous pressure (CVP)
[0–8 mm Hg]
Mean pulmonary artery pressure $(\overline{PA})$
[10–20 mm Hg]
Pulmonary artery occlusion pressure (PAOP)
[4–12 mm Hg]
Cardiac output (CO) = stroke volume (SV) × heart rate (HR)
[4–8 L/min]

$$\text{Cardiac index (CI)} = \frac{CO}{BSA}$$

[2.5–4.0 L/min/m²]

$$\text{Pulmonary vascular resistance (PVR)} = \frac{(\overline{PA} - PAOP)\,80}{CO}$$

[150–250 dyne/s/cm⁻⁵/m²]

$$\text{Pulmonary vascular resistance index (PVRI)} = \frac{(\overline{PA} - PAOP)\,80}{CI}$$

[100–240 dyne/s/cm⁻⁵/m²]

$$\text{Systemic vascular resistance (SVR)} = \frac{(MAP - CVP)\,80}{CO}$$

[800–1200 dyne/s/cm⁻⁵/m²]

$$\text{Systemic vascular resistance index (SVRI)} = \frac{(MAP - CVP)\,80}{CI}$$

[1300–2900 dyne/s/cm⁻⁵/m²]

$$\text{Stroke volume index (SVI)} = \frac{CI}{HR}$$

[40 ± 7 mL/beat/m²]
Right ventricular stroke work index (RVSWI)
  = SVI $(\overline{PA} - CVP)$ (0.0136)
  [6–10 g/beat/m²]
Left ventricular stroke work index (LVSWI)
  = SVI(MAP − PAOP) (0.0136)
  [43–56 g/beat/m²]
Arterial O_2 content $(CaO_2) = O_2$ combined with hemoglobin + O_2 dissolved in the plasma
  [1 g Hb binds 1.36 mL O_2]
  = (1.36) (Hb) (SaO_2) + 0.003 (PaO_2)
  [20 mL O_2/dL]
Mixed venous O_2 saturation $(S\overline{v}O_2)$
  [75%]
Mixed venous O_2 content $(C\overline{v}O_2) = (1.36)$ (Hb) $(S\overline{v}O_2)$ + 0.0003 (PaO_2)
  [15 mL O_2/dL]
O_2 delivery $(\dot{D}O_2) = CO \times CaO_2 \times 10$
  [600–1000 mL O_2/min]

O_2 availability (O_2AVI) = $CI \times CaO_2 \times 10$
[500–600 mL/min/m^2]

O_2 consumption ($\dot{V}O_2$) = $CI (CaO_2 - C\bar{v}O_2)$
[110–150 mL/min/m^2]

O_2 extraction ratio = $\dfrac{(CaO_2 - C\bar{v}O_2)}{CaO_2}$
[25%]

RESPIRATORY FORMULAS

OXYGENATION

Fraction of inspired O_2 (FIO_2)
[0.21–1.0]

Respiratory quotient (R) = CO_2 inspired/O_2 expired
[Normal: 0.8]

Barometric pressure (PB)
[760 mm Hg at sea level]

Partial pressure of H_2O (PH_2O)
[47 mm Hg at 37°C]

Partial pressure of inspired O_2 (PIO_2) = $FIO_2(PB - PH_2O)$
[150 mm Hg at sea level]

Partial pressure of alveolar O_2 (PAO_2) (alveolar gas equation)

$$PAO_2 = FIO_2(PB - PH_2O) - \frac{PaCO_2}{R}$$
$$= (FIO_2 \times 713) - (PaCO_2/0.8) \text{ (at sea level)}$$
$$= 150 - (PaCO_2/0.8) \text{ (at sea level on room air)}$$

[Range: 100 mm Hg on room air; 673 mm Hg on 100% O_2]

Partial pressure of arterial O_2 (PaO_2)
[70–100 mm Hg]
Increased: hyperventilation, increased FIO_2, contaminated sample
Decreased: hypoventilation, decreased FIO_2, $\dot{V}/\dot{Q}$ mismatch, intrapulmonary or anatomic
R → L shunt, diffusion abnormalities

Alveolar–arterial O_2 gradient ($P(A\text{-}a)O_2$) = $PAO_2 - PaO_2$
[3–16 mm Hg on room air; 25–65 mm Hg on 100% O_2]

VENTILATION

Partial pressure of arterial CO_2 ($PaCO_2$)
[46 mm Hg]

Partial pressure of alveolar (expired) CO_2 ($PECO_2$)

Dead space ventilation (VD): portion of VT that does not participate in gas exchange
VD = anatomic dead space + physiologic dead space
[150 mL]

Engelhoff modification of the Bohr formula for dead space
$$\frac{VD}{VT} = \frac{PaCO_2 - PECO_2}{PaCO_2}$$

Minute ventilation (VE) = respiratory rate $\times$ VT

Pulmonary capillary blood O_2 content (CcO_2)
$$= 1.36 \, (Hb) \, (SaO_2) \, (FIO_2) + 0.003 \, (PBH_2O - PaCO_2) \, (FIO_2)$$

Shunt fraction ($\dot{Q}s/\dot{Q}t$) = $\dfrac{CcO_2 - CaO_2}{CcO_2 - CvO_2}$

LUNG VOLUMES

Tidal volume (VT): volume inspired/expired with each breath
[500 mL (6–7 mL/kg lean body weight]

Inspiratory reserve volume (IRV): maximal inspired volume end-tidal inspiration
[25% of vital capacity (VC)]

Inspiratory capacity (IC): maximal volume inspired from resting expiratory level
IC = IRV + VT

[1–2.4 L]
Expiratory reserve volume (ERV: maximal expired volume from end-tidal inspiration
    [25% of vital capacity (VC)]
Residual volume (RV): volume remaining in lungs after maximal expiration
    [1–2.4 L]
Functional residual capacity (FRC): volume remaining in lungs at end-tidal expiration
    FRC = ERV + RV
    [1.8–3.4 L]
Vital capacity (VC): maximal volume expelled by forceful effort after maximal inspiration
    VC = IRV + ERV + VT
    [3–5 L; 50–60 mL/kg lean body weight in females; 70 mL/kg lean body weight in males]
Total lung capacity (TLC): volume in lungs at end of maximal inspiration
    TLC = VC + RV
    [4–6 L]

LUNG MECHANICS

Plateau pressure (Pplat)
Peak inspiratory pressure (PIP)
Positive end-expiratory pressure (PEEP)
Compliance = change in volume/change in pressure

$$\text{Static compliance (Cst)} = \frac{V_T}{\text{Pplat} - \text{PEEP}}$$

[70–160 mL/cm H_2O (paralyzed/anesthesized and supine)]

$$\text{Dynamic compliance (Cdyn)} = \frac{V_T}{\text{PIP} - \text{PEEP}}$$

[50–80 mL/cm H_2O (paralyzed/anesthesized and supine)]

RENAL FORMULAS

$$\text{Creatinine clearance (Cl}_{\text{Creat}}) = \frac{(U_{\text{Creat}})\,(\text{urine volume})}{P_{\text{creat}}}$$

Fractional excretion of sodium (FeNa$^+$)

$$= \frac{\text{urine [Na}^+]}{\text{plasma [Na}^+]} \times \frac{\text{plasma [creatinine]}}{\text{urine [creatinine]}} \times 100$$

Free water clearance

$$= \text{urine vol} - \frac{\text{urine osmolality}}{\text{plasma osmolality}} \times \text{urine vol}$$

TABLE E-1. DAILY RENAL EXCRETION OF CATIONS AND ANIONS IN NORMALS

ELECTROLYTE	URINARY EXCRETION (mMol/d)
CATIONS	
Na	127 ± 6
K	49 ± 2
Ca	4 ± 1
Mg	11 ± 1
NH_4	28 ± 2
Total	$\mathbf{219 \pm 3}$
ANIONS	
Cl	135 ± 5
SO_4	34 ± 1
PO_4	20 ± 1
Organic anions	29 ± 1
Total	$\mathbf{221 \pm 6}$

Na, sodium; K, potassium; Ca, calcium; Mg, magnesium; NH_4, ammonia; Cl, chloride; SO_4, sulfate; H_2PO_4, phosphate.

From reference 4 with permission.

TABLE E-2. USE OF URINE ELECTROLYTES

DIAGNOSTIC PROBLEM	URINARY VALUE	PRIMARY DIAGNOSTIC POSSIBILITIES
Volume depletion	Na = 0–10 mMol/L	Extrarenal sodium loss
	Na >10 mMol/L	Renal salt wasting or adrenal insufficiency
Acute oliguria	Na = 0–10 mMol/L	Prerenal azotemia
	Na >30 mMol/L	Acute tubular necrosis
Hyponatremia	Na = 0–10 mMol/L	Severe volume depletion, edematous
	Na >dietary intake	Inappropriate antidiuretic hormone ADH secretion; adrenal insufficiency
Hypokalemia	K = 0–10 mMol/L	Extrarenal K loss
	K >10 mMol/L	Renal K loss
Metabolic alkalosis	Cl = 0–10 mMol/L	Cl-responsive alkalosis
	Cl = dietary intake	Cl-resistant alkalosis

Na, sodium; K, potassium; Cl, chloride; ADH, antidiuretic hormone.

From reference 6 with permission.

TABLE E-3. INTERPRETATION OF URINE ELECTROLYTES

ELECTROLYTE	NORMAL RESPONSE	PATIENT RESPONSE	POTENTIAL PITFALLS
Na^+	Reflects diet and ECF volume <10 mMol if ECF vol contracted	>20 mMol in ECF vol contraction suggests renal tubular damage	Diuretic use Nonreabsorbed anions Recent vomiting, drugs
Cl^-	Reflects diet and ECF volume <10 mM if ECF vol contracted	>20 mM with ECF vol contraction suggests renal damage	Diuretic Diarrhea
K^+	Reflects diet, plasma [K], aldosterone action	If hypokalemia and urine [K] >20 mM or rate of K excretion >30 mmol/d. then K excretion too high	K-sparing diuretics Low urine [Na] Water diuresis

(continued)

TABLE E-3. (*continued*)

ELECTROLYTE	NORMAL RESPONSE	PATIENT RESPONSE	POTENTIAL PITFALLS
pH	Depends on acid-base status Useful for bicarbonaturia	Useful once low NH_4^+ excretion confirmed to define cause of low NH_4^+	Unreliable for urine NH_4^+ Urinary tract infection
HCO_3^-	Depends on diet and acid-base status >10 mM indicates HCO_3^- load 0 in acidemia	High urine HCO_3^- with chronic metabolic alkalosis indicates vomiting or HCO_3^- input High urine HCO_3^- with acidemia in pRTA	Urinary tract infection Carbonic anhydrase inhibitors
(Na^+, K^+, Cl^-)	Depends on diet and acid-base status	$Na + K > Cl$ = low urine NH_4^+ $Cl > Na + K$ = high urine NH_4^+	Ketonuria Drug anions Alkaline urine

Na^+, sodium; Cl, chloride; K^+, potassium; HCO_3^-, carbonate; NH_4^+, ammonia; ECF, extracellular fluid; pRTA, partial renal tubular acidosis. From reference 5 with permission.

TOXICOLOGY FORMULAS

Serum methanol concentration [MeOH] in mg/dL = 3.2 (Osm_s − (2 × [Na^+]) − ([BUN]/2.8) − ([glucose]/18) − ([ETOH]/4.6) − 10)

Ethylene glycol concentration = 6.2 (Osm_s − (2 × [Na^+]) − ([BUN]/2.8) − ([glucose]/18) − ([EtOH]/4.6) − 10)

APPENDIX F: PHARMACOLOGY ■

DRUG FORMULAS

Drug clearance = V_d × K_{el}

Drug half-life ($T_{1/2}$) = $0.693/K_{el}$

Drug elimination constant (K_{el}) = $\dfrac{\ln([\text{peak}]/[\text{trough}])}{t_{peak} - t_{trough}}$

Drug loading dose = V_d × [target peak]

Drug dosing interval
= $(-1/K_{el})$ × ln ([desired trough]/[desired peak]) + infusion time (h)

TABLE F-1. DRUG DOSAGE ADJUSTMENTS IN RENAL FAILURE

	DOSE ADJUSTMENT	GFR (mL/min)			REMOVED BY	
		>50	*10–50*	*<10*	*Hemodialysis*	*Peritoneal Dialysis*
Aminoglycosides						
Gentamicin	D	60–90	30–70	20–30	Yes	Yes
	I	8–12	12	24		
Tobramycin	D	60–90	30–70	20–30	Yes	Yes
	I	8–12	12	24		
Antifungals						
Amphotericin B	I	24	24	24–36	No	No
Flucytosine	I	6	12–24	24–48	Yes	Yes
Antituberculous						
Ethambutol	I	24	24–36	48	Yes	Yes
Isoniazid	D	100	100	66–75	Yes	Yes
Rifampin	I	None	None	None	No	No

Antivirals						
Acyclovir	I	8	24	48	Yes	—
Amantadine	I	12–24	48–72	168	No	No
Cephalosporins						
Cefamandole	I	6	6–8	8	Yes	—
Cefazolin	I	6	12	24–48	Yes	—
Cefotaxime	I	6–8	8–12	12–24	Yes	—
Cefoxitin	I	8	8–12	24–48	Yes	—
Cephalothin	I	6	6	8–12	Yes	Yes
Chloramphenicol	D	None	None	None	Yes	No
Clindamycin	D	None	None	None	No	No
Erythromycin	D	None	None	None	No	No
Metronidazole	I	8	8–12	12–24	Yes	No
Nitrofurantoin	D	100	Avoid	Avoid	Yes	—
Penicillins						
Amoxicillin	I	6	6–12	12–16	Yes	No
Ampicillin	I	6	6–12	12–16	Yes	No
Carbenicillin	I	8–12	12–24	24–48	Yes	Yes
Dicloxacillin	D	None	None	None	No	—
Nafcillin	D	None	None	None	No	—
PCN G	I	6–8	8–12	12–16	Yes	No
Piperacillin	I	4–6	6–8	8	Yes	—
Ticarcillin	I	8–12	12–24	24–28	Yes	Yes
Sulfas/trimethoprim						
Sulfamethoxazole	I	12	18	24	Yes	No
Trimethoprim	I	12	18	24	Yes	No
Tetracyclines						
Doxycycline	I	12	12–18	18–24	No	No
Minocycline	D	None	None	None	No	No
Vancomycin	I	24–72	72–240	240	No	No
Antihypertensives						
Atenolol	D	None	50	25	Yes	—
Captopril	D	None	None	50	Yes	—
Clonidine	D	None	None	50–75	No	—
Hydralazine	D	8	8	12–24	No	No
Methyldopa	I	6	9–18	12–24	Yes	Yes
Metroprolol	D	None	None	None	Yes	—
Minoxidil	D	None	None	None	Yes	—
Nadolol	D	None	50	25	Yes	—
Nitroprusside	D	None	None	None	Yes	—
Prazosin	D	None	None	None	No	No
Propranolol	D	None	None	None	No	—
Antiarrhythmics						
Bretylium	D	None	25–50	Avoid	?	—
Disopyramide	I	None	12–24	24–40	Yes	—
Lidocaine	D	None	None	None	No	—
Procainamide	I	4	6–12	8–24	Yes	—
Quinidine	I	None	None	None	Yes	Yes
Calcium Blockers						
Diltiazem	D	None	None	None	—	—
Nifedipine	D	None	None	None	—	—
Verapamil	D	None	None	None	No	—
Digoxin	D	100	25–75	10–25	No	No
	I	24	36	48		
H$_2$ Blockers						
Cimetidine	D	800/d	600/d	400/d	No	No
Ranitidine	D	None	150/d	150/d	No	—
Nizatidine	D	None	150/d	150 qod	—	—
Famotidine	D	None	None	20/d or (40 qod)	—	—

GFR, glomerular filtration rate; PCN G, penicillin G; D, dosage reduction method of dosage adjustment; I, interval extension method of dosage adjustment; qod, every other day; H$_2$, histamine.

From reference 7 with permission.

DRUGS COMMONLY USED IN THE INTENSIVE CARE UNIT (EXCLUDING ANTIBIOTICS)

Adenosine
  a. Action: slows atrioventricular (AV) nodal conduction; produces short-term (seconds) high-degree AV blockade
  b. Indications: antiarrhythmic; useful for diagnosing supraventricular tachycardias and effective for terminating reentrant AV tachyarrhythmias
  c. Loading dose: 6- or 12-mg intravenous (IV) bolus followed with a rapid saline flush
  d. Dose interval/infusion: wait 1–2 min between doses; no continuous infusion
  e. Comments: give through central venous catheter; contraindicated in heart block; sick sinus syndrome (except if pacemaker present), venticular arrhythmias

Alfentanyl
  a. Action: potent opiate receptor ligand; produces decreases in heart rate; respiratory depressant; may produce skeletal muscle rigidity
  b. Indications: opioid analgesia
  c. Loading dose: 5–150 µg/kg used, depending on additional anesthetic agents used; lower dose required in the elderly
  d. Dose interval/infusion: maintenance of anesthesia usually with 0.5–3.0 µg/kg/min
  e. Comments: $\frac{1}{5}$ to $\frac{1}{3}$ as potent as fentanyl; more rapid onset of action with shorter duration than other opioids

Aminophylline
  a. Action: bronchodilator, improves diaphragm contractility; positive inotrope and chronotrope; natriuretic and diuretic
  b. Indications: bronchoconstriction
  c. Loading dose: 5–6 mg/kg lean body weight over 20 min (if patient already taking aminophylline/theophylline then check level, begin infusion and then adjust dose based on baseline value)
  d. Dose interval/infusion: 0.2–0.8 mg/kg/min (use increased dosage with smokers; decreased dosage with elderly, patients with heart or liver disease)
  e. Comments: produces increased irritability, agitation, tachycardia, arrhythmias, nausea, and vomiting

Amrinone/Milrinone
  a. Action: inhibit cellular phosphodiesterase producing extracellular to intracellular calcium shift; increased contractility but with arterial and venous dilatation
  b. Indications: positive inotrope
  c. Loading dose: amrinone 0.75–3.0 mg/kg over 2–3 min; milrinone 50 µg/kg over 10 min
  d. Dose interval/infusion: amrinone 5–10 µg/kg/min continuous infusion; milrinone 0.375–0.75 µg/kg/min
  e. Comments: synergistic with dobutamine (because of receptor downregulation in congestive heart failure); hepatic metabolism; renal excretion; rapid onset of action; dose-related thrombocytopenia with prolonged use of amrinone

Atracurium
  a. Action: nondepolarizing neuromuscular blocker; minimal dose-dependent histamine (H_2) release; no vagal activity
  b. Indications: intermediate acting neuromuscular blockade
  c. Loading dose: 0.4–0.5 mg/kg intubating dose
  d. Dose interval/infusion: 4–12 µg/kg/min continuous infusion
  e. Comments: titrate to effect in ICU patients (monitor with train-of-four testing); onset within 3–5 min; 25–35 min duration; 40–60 min recovery; no dose adjustment in hepatorenal dysfunction

Bretylium
  a. Action: initial norepinephrine (NE) release followed by blockade of NE reuptake; prolongs refractory period; increases ventricular fibrillation threshold
  b. Indications: treatment of sustained ventricular tachycardia, ventricular fibrillation, or both (refractory to lidocaine and defibrillation)
  c. Loading dose: 5–10 mg/kg bolus
  d. Dose interval/infusion: rebolus of 5–10 mg/kg every 6–8 h or continuous infusion of 1–5 mg/min
  e. Comments: produces an initial increase in blood pressure and heart rate with subsequent hypotension; may produce nausea and vomiting

Bumetanide
  a. Action: acts at loop of Henle to prevent chloride and sodium uptake; diuretic
  b. Indications: decreased urine output, mobilize edema fluid, pulmonary edema, treat hypercalcemia
  c. Loading dose: 0.5–1.0 mg over 1–2 min
  d. Dose interval/infusion: repeat dose every 2–3 h; up to 10 mg/d
  e. Comments: observe for secondary electrolyte disturbances (hyponatremia, hypokalemia)

Calcium Chloride/Gluconate
  a. Action: required for wide variety of cellular functions
  b. Indications: ionized hypocalcemia; vasopressor; hypermagnesemia/hyperkalemia (stabilizes cell membrane); calcium channel blocker overdose
  c. Loading dose: 90 mg Ca IV bolus (chloride: 1 g = 272 mg [13.6 mMol] Ca) (gluconate: 1 g = 90 mg [4.65 mMol] Ca)
  d. Dose interval/infusion: 0.5–2.0 mg/h adjust to ionized calcium value
  e. Comments: monitor for hypercalcemia, hypophosphatemia, and decreased sensorium

Clonidine
  a. Action: central α_2-receptor agonist
  b. Indications: hypertension; withdrawal syndromes (opiates, nicotine); modulate sympathetic hyperactivity of closed head injury
  c. Loading dose: 0.1 mg transdermal weekly (may require 2–3 d for response); for hypertensive urgencies use 0.2 mg orally hourly until pressure controlled
  d. Dose interval/infusion: usually twice daily when taken orally, no intravenous formulation
  e. Comments: usual maximum dose 2.4 mg/d; rebound hypertension with acute withdrawal

dDAVP
  a. Action: synthetic vasopressin; decreased excretion of free water; increases factor VIII levels

b. Indications: central (neurogenic) diabetes insipidus (DI); bleeding in patients with decreased factor VIII levels

c. Loading dose: 2–4 μg IV or subcutaneously (SQ) for DI; 0.3 μg/kg IV over 15–30 min for bleeding

d. Dose interval/infusion: twice daily

e. Comments: dose for central DI by following urine output/osmolarity and serum sodium/osmolarity

Diazepam

a. Action: benzodiazepine

b. Indications: sedation, anxiety, agitation; ethanol withdrawal; seizures

c. Loading dose: 5 mg

d. Dose interval/infusion: begin at 5 mg/h and titrate to effect

e. Comments: CNS depression

Diltiazem

a. Action: calcium channel blockade; negative inotrope and peripheral vasodilator; depresses sinoatrial (SA) and AV node

b. Indications: hypertension, angina; rate control in atrial fibrillation/flutter

c. Loading dose: 0.25 mg/kg IV over 2 min

d. Dose interval/infusion: 5–15 mg/h

e. Comments: maximum dose 360 mg/d

Dobutamine

a. Action: positive inotrope, peripheral vasodilator, increases automaticity of SA node and enhances conduction through AV node and ventricles

b. Indications: low cardiac output states, especially with increased systemic vascular resistance

c. Loading dose: 2.5–20.0 μg/kg/min

d. Dose interval/infusion: titrate to effect

e. Comments: no dopaminergic effects on renal vessels; tachycardia may be a problem; contraindicated in idiopathic hypertrophic subaortic stenosis; tolerance may develop

Dopamine

a. Action: dose-dependent vasopressor acting at multiple receptor sites

b. Indications: hypotension; increase renal blood flow and subsequently urine output

c. Loading dose: none

d. Dose interval/infusion: dopaminergic 0.5–2.0 μg/kg/min; beta plus dopaminergic 2–10 μg/kg/min; alpha, beta, and dopaminergic at >10 μg/kg/min

e. Comments: tachycardia may be significant; necrosis at injection site with extravasation (treat with phentolamine)

Epinephrine

a. Action: alpha- and beta-receptor agonist; vasopressor, positive inotrope and chronotrope; bronchodilatation; increased glycogenolysis

b. Indications: bronchoconstriction; allergic reactions; advanced cardiac life support; refractory hypotension

c. Loading dose: 1-mg bolus IV

d. Dose interval/infusion: 1–4 μg/min titrated to effect

e. Comments: increased myocardial oxygen consumption with arrhythmias and ischemia; hypertension; hyperglycemia; poor renal perfusion

Esmolol

a. Action: short-acting beta-blockade ($\beta_1 > \beta_2$)

b. Indications: supraventricular tachyarrhythmias; hypertension

c. Loading dose: 0.5–1.0 mg/kg over 1 min

d. Dose interval/infusion: 10–300 μg/kg/min

e. Comments: hypotension; bradycardia; bronchospasm; may prolong neuromuscular blockade effects of succinylcholine; contraindicated in bradycardia, heart block, cardiogenic shock

Fentanyl

a. Action: potent opiate receptor ligand; produces decreases in heart rate, blood pressure, and cardiac index; respiratory depressant; may produce skeletal muscle rigidity

b. Indications: opioid analgesia

c. Loading dose: 1–3 μg/kg, depending on additional anesthetic agents used

d. Dose interval/infusion: 0.01–0.3 μg/kg/h

e. Comments: approximately 100 times as potent as morphine; no histamine release

Flumazenil

a. Action: benzodiazepine antagonist; acts centrally at benzodiazepine receptors

b. Indications: complete or partial reversal of sedative effects of benzodiazepines; reversal effects occur within 1 min of intravenous dose

c. Loading dose: 0.2 mg IV over 15–30 s

d. Dose interval/infusion: can repeat 0.2 mg every 60 s up to total dose of 1 mg; may use up to 3 mg in suspected benzodiazepine overdose; no continuous infusion

e. Comments: effective reversal of benzodiazepine effects lasts 20 min, so repeated dosing with flumazenil may be necessary; liver metabolism

Furosemide

a. Action: inhibits chloride and sodium reabsorption in ascending loop of Henle producing a diuretic effect

b. Indications: decreased urine output, acute oliguric renal failure, mobilize edema fluid, pulmonary edema, hypercalcemia

c. Loading dose: 10–200 mg, depending on the clinical situation

d. Dose interval/infusion: begin at 5 mg/h and titrate to effect

e. Comments: hepatic metabolism, renal excretion; up to 6 g/d has been given by continuous infusion; observe for electrolyte disturbances (hyponatremia, hypomagnesemia, hypokalemia)

Glucagon

a. Action: increases glycogenolysis and gluconeogenesis producing hyperglycemia; increases lipolysis; positive inotrope; decreases gastrointestinal (GI) motility and secretions

b. Indications: hypoglycemia; beta-blocker and calcium channel blocker overdoses; hypotension

c. Loading dose: 0.5–1.0 mg SQ/IV/intramuscularly (IM)

d. Dose interval/infusion: repeat loading dose every 15 min; 1–20 mg/h as continuous infusion

e. Comments: hyperglycemia; tachycardia; hypokalemia

Haloperidol

a. Action: dopaminergic blockade acting as an antipsychotic

b. Indications: agitation; acute psychosis

c. Loading dose: 0.5–5.0 mg IV/IM

d. Dose interval/infusion: can be given hourly; 1–20 mg/h as continuous infusion

e. Comments: decrease dose in hepatic dysfunction; observe closely for dystonic reactions and sedative effects; alpha-blockade

Heparin

a. Action: anticoagulant acting through antithrombin III complexes

b. Indications: deep venous thrombosis (acute and prophylaxis); pulmonary embolism; acute myocardial infarction; hemodialysis; catheter patency

c. Loading dose: wide variety, depending on clinical situation

d. Dose interval/infusion: adjusted to desired anticoagulant effect, usually based on following serial activated partial thromboplastin time (aPTT)

e. Comments: side effects include hemorrhage, thrombocytopenia, fever

H$_2$ Blockers (cimetidine, famotidine, ranitidine)

a. Action: H$_2$ receptor competitive antagonist decreasing gastric acid secretion

b. Indications: prophylaxis for stress ulcer GI bleeding, acute/chronic peptic ulcer disease, acid hypersecretory diseases, reflux disease

c. Loading dose for stress ulcer prophylaxis: cimetidine 300 mg IV every 6 h; famotidine 20 mg IV every 12 h; ranitidine 50 mg IV every 8 h

d. Dose interval/infusion: total daily dose divided into continuous infusion, may be placed in parenteral nutritional formulas

e. Comments: adjust dose based on creatinine clearance

Isoproterenol

a. Action: nonspecific beta-agonist; positive inotrope and chronotrope; bronchodilator

b. Indications: bronchoconstriction; symptomatic bradycardia; beta-blocker overdose

c. Loading dose: 0.02–0.06 mg IV

d. Dose interval/infusion: 2–20 μg/min

e. Comments: tachycardia; arrhythmias (torsade de pointes); myocardial ischemia; anxiety

Labetalol

a. Action: α$_1$- and nonspecific beta-blocker

b. Indications: hypertension

c. Loading dose: 5–20 mg IV

d. Dose interval/infusion: boluses can be repeated every 5 min; continuous infusion of 1–2 mg/min titrated to effect

e. Comments: observe for bronchospasm, bradycardia

Lidocaine

a. Action: antiarrhythmic and local anesthetic

b. Indications: local anesthesia; ventricular arrhythmias; prophylaxis in acute myocardial infarction

c. Loading dose: 1.0–1.5 mg/kg bolus IV (maximum load, 3 mg/kg)

d. Dose interval/infusion: bolus repeated in 20 min; 1–4 mg/min continuous infusion

e. Comments: observe for metabolic acidosis, altered mental status (including seizures), and myocardial depression; (hepatic metabolism; methemoglobinemia

Lorazepam

a. Action: benzodiazepine

b. Indications: agitation; seizures; supplemental sedation with neuromuscular blockade

c. Loading dose: 2-mg bolus IV

d. Dose interval/infusion: begin at 1 mg/h and titrate to effect

e. Comments: CNS depression

Magnesium

a. Action: coenzyme; muscular contractility; nerve conduction; membrane stabilization; antiseizure; inhibits uterine contractility

b. Indications: hypomagnesemia; arrhythmias; preeclampsia and eclampsia

c. Loading dose: 1–4 g over 15 min (infuse over 4 h for treatment of asymptomatic hypomagnesemia)

d. Dose interval/infusion: subsequent dosing based on desired clinical effect and serum levels

e. Comments: observe for hypotension and heart block; respiratory and CNS depressant (primarily in patients with renal dysfunction)

Metocurine

a. Action: nondepolarizing neuromuscular blocker; moderate H$_2$ release; some bradycardia

b. Indications: long-acting neuromuscular blockade

c. Loading dose: 0.2–0.4 mg/kg for intubation

d. Dose interval/infusion: 5–10 mg/h

e. Comments: titrate to effect in ICU patients (monitor with train-of-four testing); onset within 1.5–10 min; 70–90 min duration of action; 90–180 min recovery; partial renal excretion

Midazolam

a. Action: short-acting benzodiazepine

b. Indications: sedation, anxiety, agitation; ETOH withdrawal; seizures

c. Loading dose: 1–4 mg

d. Dose interval/infusion: 1–20 mg/h titrated to effect

e. Comments: CNS depression; active metabolites; respiratory depression when used in combination with narcotics; 3–4 times the potency of diazepam

Mivacurium

a. Action: nondepolarizing neuromuscular blocker; minimal to moderate H$_2$ release; minimal tachycardia

b. Indications: short-acting neuromuscular blockade

c. Loading dose: 0.1–0.25 mg/kg intubating dose

d. Dose interval/infusion: 5–15 μg/kg/min continuous infusion; onset in 2–4 min; 13–40 min duration of action; 6–14 min recovery

e. Comments: titrate to effect in ICU patients (monitor with train-of-four testing)

Morphine

a. Action: opioid analgesia; venodilatation

b. Indications: analgesia, sedation; pulmonary edema

c. Loading dose: 1–5 mg IV

d. Dose interval/infusion: rebolus every 2–3 h; 1–10 mg/

h continuous infusion titrated to effect

e. Comments: CNS disturbances; hypotension (especially if intravascular volume depletion is present); respiratory depression; histamine release

Nicardipine

a. Action: noncardiosuppressive calcium channel antagonist

b. Indications: postoperative hypertension, prevention of vasospasm from subarachnoid hemorrhage; angina

c. Loading dose: 5 mg/h and increase by 2.5 mg/h every 15 min

d. Dose interval/infusion: 1–15 mg/h; 20–40 mg orally three times daily

e. Comments: hypotension; reflex tachycardia

Nifedipine

a. Action: calcium channel blocker; minimal myocardial depression with slowing of conduction; smooth muscle relaxation

b. Indications: angina, hypertension

c. Loading dose: 10–20 mg orally or sublingual

d. Dose interval/infusion; hourly as needed, no intravenous preparation; maximum dose 180 mg/d

e. Comments: hypotension and reflex tachycardia

Nimodipine

a. Action: calcium channel antagonist; minimal cardiovascular effect

b. Indications: prevention of vasospasm due to subarachnoid hemorrhage

c. Loading dose: none, no IV formulation available

d. Dose interval/infusion: 60 mg orally or sublingually every 4 h for 21 d

e. Comments: hypotension may occur

Nitroglycerin

a. Action: smooth muscle relaxation through nitric oxide pathway; pulmonary vasculature and venous vasodilator; decreased preload; improved coronary blood flow

b. Indications: myocardial ischemia; hypertension; congestive heart failure; esophageal spasm

c. Loading dose: none necessary in intravenous dosing

d. Dose interval/infusion: 10–400 μg/min titrated to effect

e. Comments: liver metabolism; renal excretion; tolerance; rare methemoglobinemia; increased cerebral blood flow (CBF); hypotension

Nitroprusside

a. Action: arterial and venous vasodilatation through nitric oxide pathway; coronary vasodilatation; increased CBF and volume with subsequent increased intracranial pressure

b. Indications: hypertension; acute left ventricular failure

c. Loading dose: not indicated

d. Dose interval/infusion: 0.5–10 μg/kg/min and titrate to effect

e. Comments: coronary steal (angina) possible with coronary vasodilatation; metabolic acidosis; follow thiocyanate levels if toxicity suspected (toxicity: amyl nitrate and sodium nitrite converts hemoglobin to methemoglobin; methemoglobin binds cyanide; sodium thiosulfate converts cyanide to thiocyanate)

Norepinephrine

a. Action: alpha and β₁-agonist; arterial and venous vaso-

constriction; minimal chronotropic effect

b. Indications: hypotension

c. Loading dose: not indicated

d. Dose interval/infusion: 2–40 μg/min titrated to effect

e. Comments: decreased renal perfusion; peripheral vasoconstriction; arrhythmias; tissue necrosis with extravasation

Octreotide

a. Action: mimics effects of somatostatin; increases GI motility while decreasing GI and pancreatic secretions; decreases splanchnic blood flow

b. Indications: gut neuroendocrine tumors, diarrhea, excess GI/pancreatic secretions; variceal hemorrhage

c. Loading dose: 250-μg bolus

d. Dose interval/infusion: 25–100 μg three times daily or 50–250 μg/h infusion

e. Comments: total dose, 50–1500 μg/d; both hypoglycemia and hyperglycemia

Pancuronium

a. Action: nondepolarizing neuromuscular blocker; no histamine release, modest to marked vagal block with tachycardia

b. Indications: long-acting neuromuscular blockade

c. Loading dose: 0.1-mg/kg intubating dose

d. Dose interval/infusion: 1–2 μg/kg/min continuous infusion

e. Comments: titrate to effect in ICU patient (monitor with train-of-four testing); onset within 2–4 min and duration of action of 60–100 min; recovery within 120–180 min; primarily renal excretion

Phentolamine

a. Action: alpha-blocker; vasodilatation

b. Indications: hypertension; pheochromochytoma

c. Loading dose: 5 mg IV/IM to effect

d. Dose interval/infusion: no continuous infusion

e. Comments: monitor for hypotension

Phenylephrine

a. Action: alpha-agonist; arterial and venous vasoconstriction; vasopressor with reflex decrease in heart rate

b. Indications: hypotension

c. Loading dose: not indicated

d. Dose interval/infusion: 10–40 μg/min titrated to effect

e. Comments: hypertension, bradycardia, myocardial ischemia, decreased renal perfusion

Procainamide

a. Action: antiarrhythmic; vasodilatation

b. Indications: supraventricular and ventricular arrhythmias; recurrent atrial fibrillation/flutter

c. Loading dose: 50 mg/min to effect or total dose of 17 mg/kg

d. Dose interval/infusion: 2–6 mg/min continuous infusion

e. Comments: observe for conduction disturbances (including torsade) and myocardial depression

Propofol

a. Action: alkylphenol

b. Indications: short acting sedative

c. Loading dose: 1.5–3 mg/kg

d. Dose interval/infusion: titrate to effect; usual dose is 10–50 μg/kg/min

e. Comments: no analgesic properties; very short duration of action (2–3 min); reduce dosage in the elderly; monitor triglyceride values

Propranolol

a. Action: nonspecific beta-blockade; decreased heart rate and contractility; antiarrhythmic

b. Indications: supraventricular tachyarrhythmias, angina, hypertension, acute myocardial infarct

c. Loading dose: 0.5–1.0 mg bolus IV

d. Dose interval/infusion: repeat bolus every 5 min to effect

e. Comments: bradycardia, hypotension, bronchospasm

Protamine

a. Action: heparin antagonist (complexes with heparin)

b. Indications: reverse the effects of heparin

c. Loading dose: 1 mg/90 IU bovine heparin; 1 mg/115 IU porcine heparin over 1–3 min

d. Dose interval/infusion: titrate to aPTT

e. Comments: maximum dose of 50 mg in any 10-min period; observe for bleeding after large dosages; hypotension

Rocuronium

a. Action: nondepolarizing neuromuscular blocker; minimal H_2 release; minimal to moderate vagal blockade

b. Indications: intermediate-acting neuromuscular blockade

c. Loading dose: 0.4–1.2 mg/kg intubating dose

c. Dose interval/infusion: 10–12 μg/kg/min continuous infusion

e. Comments: titrate to effect in ICU patients (monitor with train-of-four testing); 1–3 min onset of action; 22–67 min duration of action; recovery in 10–20 min

Succinylcholine

a. Action: depolarizing neuromuscular blocker; no H_2 release, some vagal stimulation

b. Indications: rapid onset of paralysis; short-acting neuromuscular blockade

c. Loading dose: 0.3–1.5 mg/kg

d. Dose interval/infusion: continuous infusion of 7.1–142 μg/kg/min

e. Comments: onset in 0.5–5 min with duration of action of 2–3 min and recovery within 10 min; hyperkalemia; prolonged blockade in patients with atypical pseudocholinesterase; increased intracranial pressure (ICP)

Sufentanil

a. Action: potent opiate receptor ligand; produces decreases in heart rate, blood pressure, and cardiac index; respiratory depressant; may increase ICP in patients with compromised intracranial compliance; may produce skeletal muscle rigidity

b. Indications: opioid analgesia

c. Loading dose: 1–30 μg/kg, depending on other anesthetic agents used

d. Dose interval/infusion: as needed, no infusion

e. Comments: 5–10 times as potent as fentanyl with a shorter duration of action; muscle rigidity

Thiopental

a. Action: barbiturate with hypnotic and anesthetic properties

b. Indications: general anesthesia, seizures, increased ICP

c. Loading dose: 3–5 mg/kg for induction of anesthesia; 75–125 mg for treatment of seizures

d. Dose interval/infusion: additional doses as clinically indicated; no continuous infusion

e. Comments: observe clinically and use blood levels as necessary; respiratory depression

Thrombolytics (Streptokinase, Urokinase, Tissue Plasminogen Activator)

a. Action: plasminogen activators; plasmin produced; plasmin degrades fibrinogen and fibrin, dissolving preexisting thrombi

b. Indications: pulmonary embolism, acute myocardial infarction, venous thrombosis, graft thrombosis, catheter occlusion

c. Loading dose: varies, depending on agent used and clinical condition

d. Dose interval/infusion: variable

e. Comments: bleeding (about 5% of patients); absolute contraindications include active hemorrhage, recent (2 mo) neurologic injury/surgery/tumor

Vasopressin

a. Action: decreases hepatic blood flow and portal pressure; increased clotting; decreased free water excretion; increases gut motility

b. Indications: central (neurogenic) DI; bleeding esophageal varices

c. Loading dose: central DI—aqueous vasopressin 5–10 IU IM/SQ

d. Dose interval/infusion: central DI—two to four times daily dosing (follow polyuria and serum sodium); GI bleeding—aqueous vasopressin 0.2–1.0 U/min IV

e. Comments: CNS disturbances, hypertension, angina, hyponatremia; metabolic acidosis

Vecuronium

a. Action: nondepolarizing neuromuscular blocker; no H_2 release; no vagal activity or tachycardia

b. Indications: intermediate-acting neuromuscular blockade

c. Loading dose: 0.08 mg/kg intubating dose

d. Dose interval/infusion: 1–2 μg/kg/min continuous infusion

e. Comments: titrate to effect in ICU patients (monitor with train-of-four testing); onset within 2.5–4.5 minutes; 35–45 min duration; recovery within 45–60 minutes; renal and hepatic excretion

Verapamil

a. Action: antiarrhythmic; calcium channel blockade

b. Indications: treatment of angina, hypertension, hypertrophic cardiomyopathy, and supraventricular tachyarrhythmias (SVT) (slows ventricular response in atrial fibrillation or flutter and may convert SVT to sinus rhythm)

c. Loading dose: 0.075–0.15 mg/kg (5–10 mg) IV over 2–3 min; may repeat bolus in 10 min

d. Dose interval/infusion: continuous infusion of 5 mg/h titrated to effect

e. Comments: may produce hypotension: bradycardia and AV block in patients treated with concomitant beta-blockers

APPENDIX G: DERMATOMES ■

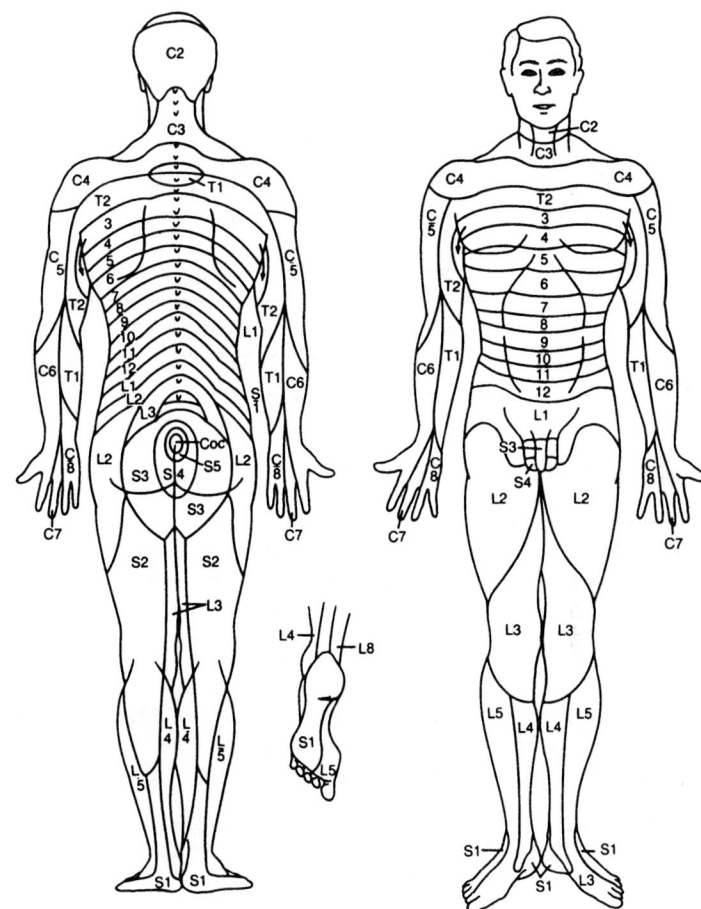

FIGURE G-1.

APPENDIX H: ORGAN INJURY SCALING ■

The Organ Injury Scaling Committee of the American Association for the Surgery of Trauma devised injury severity scores for individual organs to facilitate clinical research. The classification scheme is an anatomic description scaled from 1 (least severe injury) to 5 (most severe injury).

TABLE H-1. SPLENIC INJURY SCALE

GRADE°	INJURY DESCRIPTION†	ICD-9	AIS-85	AIS-90
I. Hematoma:	Subcapsular, nonexpanding <10% surface area	865.01 865.11	2	2
Laceration:	Capsular tear, nonbleeding, <1 cm parenchymal depth	865.02 865.12		
II. Hematoma:	Subcapsular, nonexpanding, 10–50% surface area; Intraparenchymal, nonexpanding, <2 cm in diameter	865.01 865.11	2	2
Laceration:	Capsular tear, active bleeding; 1–3 cm parenchymal depth that does not involve a trabecular vessel	865.02 865.12	2	2
III. Hematoma:	Subcapsular, >50% surface area or expanding; Ruptured subcapsular hematoma with active bleeding; Intraparenchymal hematoma >2 cm or expanding		3	3

(continued)

TABLE H-1. (*continued*)

GRADE°	INJURY DESCRIPTION[†]	ICD-9	AIS-85	AIS-90
Laceration:	>3 cm parenchymal depth or involving trabecular vessels	865.03 865.13	3	3
IV. Hematoma:	Ruptured intraparenchymal hematoma with active bleeding		3	4
Laceration:	Laceration involving segmental or hilar vessels producing major devascularization (>25% of spleen)	865.04 865.14	3	4
V. Laceration:	Completely shattered spleen	865.04 865.14	5	5
Vascular:	Hilar vascular injury which devascularizes spleen		5	5

°Advance one grade for multiple injuries to the same organ.
[†]Based on most accurate assessment at autopsy, laparotomy, or radiologic study.

From reference 8 with permission.

TABLE H-2. LIVER INJURY SCALE

GRADE°	INJURY DESCRIPTION[†]	ICD-9	AIS-85	AIS-90
I. Hematoma:	Subcapsular, nonexpanding, <10% surface area	864.01 864.11	2	2
Laceration:	Capsular tear, nonbleeding, <1 cm parenchymal depth	864.02 864.12	2	2
II. Hematoma:	Subcapsular, nonexpanding, 10–50% surface area; Intraparenchymal, nonexpanding, <2 cm in diameter	864.01 864.11	2	2
Laceration:	Capsular tear, active bleeding; 1–3 cm parenchymal depth, <10 cm in length	864.03 864.13	2	2
III. Hematoma:	Subcapsular, >50% surface area or expanding; Ruptured subcapsular hematoma with active bleeding; Intraparenchymal hematoma >2 cm or expanding		3	3
Laceration:	>3 cm parenchymal depth	864.04 864.14	3	3
IV. Hematoma:	Ruptured intraparenchymal hematoma with active bleeding		3	4
Laceration:	Parenchymal disruption involving 25–50% of hepatic lobe	864.04 864.14	4	4
V. Laceration:	Parenchymal disruption involving >50% of hepatic lobe		5	5
Vascular:	Juxtahepatic venous injuries; i.e., retrohepatic vena cava/major hepatic veins		5	5
VI. Vascular:	Hepatic avulsion			6

°Advance one grade for multiple injuries to the same organ.
[†]Based on most accurate assessment at autopsy, laparotomy, or radiologic study.

From reference 8 with permission.

TABLE H-3. RENAL INJURY SCALE

GRADE°	INJURY DESCRIPTION[†]	ICD-9	AIS-85	AIS-90
I. Contusion:	Microscopic or gross hematuria; urologic studies normal		2	2
Hematoma:	Subcapsular, nonexpanding without parenchymal laceration	866.01 866.11	2	2
II. Hematoma:	Nonexpanding perirenal hematoma confined to renal retroperitoneum	866.01 866.11	2	2
Laceration:	<1.0 cm parenchymal depth of renal cortex without urinary extravasation	866.02 866.12	2	2
III. Laceration:	>1.0 cm parenchymal depth of renal cortex without collecting system rupture or urinary extravasation	866.02 866.12	3	3

IV. Laceration:	Parenchymal laceration extending through the renal cortex, medulla and collecting system		3	4
Vascular:	Main renal artery or vein injury with contained hemorrhage		3	4
V. Laceration:	Completely shattered kidney	866.03	5	5
Vascular:	Avulsion of renal hilum which devascularizes kidney	866.13	5	5

°Advance one grade for multiple injuries to the same organ.
†Based on most accurate assessment at autopsy, laparotomy, or radiologic study.

From reference 8 with permission.

TABLE H-4. PANCREATIC INJURY SCALE

GRADE°		INJURY DESCRIPTION†	ICD-9	AIS-85	AIS-90
I	Hematoma	Minor contusion without duct injury	863.81–863.84	2	2
	Laceration	Superficial laceration without duct injury		2	2
II	Hematoma	Major contusion without duct injury or tissue loss	863.81–863.84	3	2
	Laceration	Major laceration without duct injury or tissue loss		3	3
III	Laceration	Distal transection or parenchymal injury with duct injury	863.92–863.94	3	3
IV	Laceration	Proximal† transection or parenchymal injury involving ampulla	863.91	3	4
V	Laceration	Massive disruption of pancreatic head	863.91	5	5

.81, .91 = Head; .82, .92 = Body; .83, .93 = Tail

°Advance one grade for multiple injuries to the same organ.
†Based on most accurate assessment at autopsy, laparotomy, or radiologic study.
‡Proximal pancreas is to the patient's right of the superior mesenteric vein.

From reference 9 with permission.

TABLE H-5. DUODENUM INJURY SCALE

GRADE°		INJURY DESCRIPTION†	ICD-9	AIS-85	AIS-90
I	Hematoma	Involving single portion of duodenum	863.21	2	2
	Laceration	Partial thickness, no perforation	863.21	2	3
II	Hematoma	Involving more than one portion	863.21	2	2
	Laceration	Disruption <50% of circumference	863.31	3	4
III	Laceration	Disruption 50–75% circumference of D2	863.31	4	4
		Disruption 50–100% circumference of D1, D3, D4		4	4
IV	Laceration	Disruption >75% circumference of D2	863.31	4	5
		Involving ampulla or distal common bile duct		4	5
V	Laceration	Massive disruption of duodenopancreatic complex	863.31	5	5
	Vascular	Devascularization of duodenum	863.31	5	5

D1, 1st portion duodenum; D2, 2nd portion duodenum; D3, 3rd portion duodenum; D4, 4th portion duodenum.
°Advance one grade for multiple injuries to the same organ.
†Based on most accurate assessment at autopsy, laparotomy, or radiologic study.

From reference 9 with permission.

TABLE H-6. SMALL BOWEL INJURY SCALE

GRADE°		INJURY DESCRIPTION†	ICD-9	AIS-85	AIS-90
I	Hematoma	Contusion or hematoma without devascularization	863.20	2	2
	Laceration	Partial thickness, no perforation	863.20	2	2
II	Laceration	Laceration <50% of circumference	863.30	3	3

(continued)

TABLE H-6. (*continued*)

GRADE°		INJURY DESCRIPTION†	ICD-9	AIS-85	AIS-90
III	Laceration	Laceration ≥50% of circumference without transection	863.30	3	3
IV	Laceration	Transection of the small bowel	863.30	4	4
V	Laceration	Transection of the small bowel with segmental tissue loss	863.30	4	4
	Vascular	Devascularized segment	863.30	4	4

°Advance one grade for multiple injuries to the same organ.
†Based on the most accurate assessment at autopsy, laparotomy, or radiologic study.

From reference 9 with permission.

TABLE H-7. COLON INJURY SCALE

GRADE°		INJURY DESCRIPTION†	ICD-9	AIS-85	AIS-90
I	Hematoma	Contusion or hematoma without devascularization	863.40–863.44	2	2
	Laceration	Partial thickness, no perforation	863.40–863.44	3	2
II	Laceration	Laceration <50% of circumference	863.50–863.54	4	3
III	Laceration	Laceration ≥50% of circumference without transection	863.50–863.54	4	3
IV	Laceration	Transection of the colon	863.50–863.54	5	4
V	Laceration	Transection of the colon with segmental tissue loss	863.50–863.54	5	4
	Vascular	Devascularized segment	863.50–863.54	5	4

.41, .51 = Ascending; .42, .52 = Transverse; .43, .53 = Descending; .44, .54 = Rectum

°Advance one grade for multiple injuries to the same organ.
†Based on the most accurate assessment at autopsy, laparotomy, or radiologic study.

From reference 9 with permission.

TABLE H-8. RECTAL INJURY SCALE

GRADE°		INJURY DESCRIPTION†	ICD-9	AIS-85	AIS-90
I	Hematoma	Contusion or hematoma without devascularization	863.45	2	2
	Laceration	Partial thickness laceration	863.45	3	2
II	Laceration	Laceration <50% of circumference	863.55	4	3
III	Laceration	Laceration ≥50% of circumference	863.55	4	4
IV	Laceration	Full-thickness laceration with extension into the perineum	863.55	5	5
V	Vascular	Devascularized segment	863.55	5	5

°Advance one grade for multiple injuries to the same organ.
†Based on most accurate assessment at autopsy, laparotomy, or radiologic study.

From reference 9 with permission.

TABLE H-9. CHEST WALL INJURY SCALE*

GRADE[†]	INJURY TYPE	DESCRIPTION OF INJURY	ICD-9	AIS-85	AIS-90
I	Contusion	Any size	911.0/922.1	1	1
	Laceration	Skin and subcutaneous	875.0	1	1
	Fracture	<3 ribs, closed;	807.01/807.02	1	1–2
		nondisplaced clavicle, closed	810.00–810.03	2	2
II	Laceration	Skin, subcutaneous and muscle;	875.1	1	1
	Fracture	≥3 adjacent ribs, closed;	807.03–807.09	2	2–3
		open or displaced clavicle;	810.10–810.13	2	2
		nondisplaced sternum, closed;	807.02	2	2
		scapular body, open or closed	811.00–811.19	2	2
III	Laceration	Full thickness including pleural penetration	862.29	2	2
	Fracture	Open or displaced sternum; flail sternum	807.2/807.3	3	2
		Unilateral flail segment (<3 ribs);	807.4	4	3–4
IV	Laceration	Avulsion of chest wall tissues with underlying rib fractures	807.10–807.19	4	4
	Fracture	Unilateral flail chest (≥3 ribs);	807.4	4	3–4
V	Fracture	Bilateral flail chest (≥3 ribs on both sides)	807.4	4	5

*This scale is confined to the chest wall alone and does not reflect associated internal thoracic or abdominal injuries. Therefore, further delineation of upper versus lower or anterior versus posterior chest wall was not considered, and a grade VI was not warranted. Specifically, *thoracic crush* was not used as a descriptive term; instead, the geography and extent of fractures and soft tissue injury were used to define the grade.
†Upgrade by one grade for bilateral injuries.

From reference 10 with permission.

TABLE H-10. ABDOMINAL VISCERAL ORGAN INJURY SCALE*

	OIS GRADE	ICD-9	AIS-85	AIS-90
Grade I[†]				
Nonnamed superior mesenteric or superior mesenteric vein branches	I	902.20/902.39	NS	NS
Nonnamed inferior mesenteric artery or inferior mesenteric vein branches	I	902.27/902.32	NS	NS
Phrenic artery/vein	I	902.89	NS	NS
Lumbar artery/vein	I	902.89	NS	NS
Gonadal artery/vein	I	902.89	NS	NS
Ovarian artery/vein	I	902.81/902.82	NS	NS
Other nonnamed small arterial or venous structures requiring ligation	I	902.90	NS	NS
Grade II[†]				
Right, left or common hepatic artery	II	902.22	3	3
Splenic artery/vein	II	902.23/902.34	3	3
Right or left gastric arteries	II	902.21	3	3
Gastroduodenal artery	II	902.24	3	3
Inferior mesenteric artery, trunk or inferior mesenteric vein, trunk	II	902.27/902.32	3	3
Primary named branches of mesenteric artery (e.g., ileocolic artery) or mesenteric vein	II	902.26/902.31	3	3
Other named abdominal vessels requiring ligation/repair	II	902.89	3	3
Grade III[†]				
Superior mesenteric vein, trunk	III	902.31	3	3
Renal artery/vein	III	902.41/902.42	3	3

(continued)

TABLE H-10. (*continued*)*

	OIS GRADE	ICD-9	AIS-85	AIS-90
Iliac artery/vein	III	902.53/902.54	3	3
Hypogastric artery/vein	III	902.51/902.52	3	3
Vena cava, infrarenal	III	902.10		3
Grade IV†				
Superior mesenteric artery, trunk	IV	902.25	3	3
Celiac axis proper	IV	902.24	3	3
Vena cava, suprarenal and infrahepatic	IV	902.10	3	3
Aorta, infrarenal	IV	902.00	4	4
Grade V†				
Portal vein	V	902.33	3	3
Extraparenchymal hepatic vein	V	902.11	3 (hepatic vein)	3 (hepatic vein)
			5 (liver vein)	5 (liver + veins)
Vena cava, retrohepatic or suprahepatic	V	902.19	5	5
Aorta, suprarenal, subdiaphragmatic	V	902.00	4	4

NS, not significant.
*This classification system is applicable for extraparenchymal vascular injuries. If the vessel injury is within 2 cm of the organ parenchyma, refer to specific organ injury scale.
†Increase one grade for multiple grade III or IV injuries involving >50% vessel circumference. Downgrade one grade if <25% vessel circumference laceration for grades IV or V.

From reference 10 with permission.

TABLE H-11. URETER INJURY SCALE

GRADE°	INJURY TYPE	DESCRIPTION OF INJURY	ICD-9	AIS-85	AIS-90
I	Hematoma	Contusion of hematoma without devascularization	867.2/867.3	2	2
II	Laceration	<50% transection	867.2/867.3	2	2
III	Laceration	>50% transection	867.2/867.3	3	3
IV	Laceration	Complete transection with 2-cm devascularization	867.2/867.3	3	3
V	Laceration	Avulsion with >2 cm of devascularization	867.2/867.3	3	3

°Advance one grade if multiple lesions exist.
From reference 10 with permission.

TABLE H-12. BLADDER INJURY SCALE

GRADE°	INJURY TYPE	DESCRIPTION OF INJURY	ICD-9	AIS-89	AIS-90
I	Hematoma	Contusion, intramural hematoma	867.0/867.1	2	2
	Laceration	Partial thickness		3	3
II	Laceration	Extraperitoneal bladder wall laceration <2 cm	867.0/867.1	4	4
III	Laceration	Extraperitoneal (>2 cm) or intraperitoneal (<2 cm) bladder wall lacerations	867.0/867.1	4	4
IV	Laceration	Intraperitoneal bladder wall laceration >2 cm	867.0/867.1	4	4
V	Laceration	Intra or extraperitoneal bladder wall laceration extending into the bladder neck or ureteral orifice (trigone)	867.0/867.1	4	4

°Advance one grade if multiple lesions exist.
From reference 10 with permission.

TABLE H-13. URETHRA INJURY SCALE

GRADE°	INJURY TYPE	DESCRIPTION OF INJURY	ICD-9	AIS-85	AIS-90
I	Contusion	Blood at urethral meatus; urethrography normal	867.0/867.1	2	2
II	Stretch injury	Elongation of urethra without extravasation on urethrography	867.0/867.1	2	2
III	Partial disruption	Extravasation of urethrography contrast at injury site with contrast visualized in the bladder	867.0/867.1	2	2
IV	Complete disruption	Extravasation of urethrography contrast at injury site without visualization in the bladder; <2 cm of urethral separation	867.0/867.1	3	3
V	Complete disruption	Complete transection with >2 cm urethral separation, or extension into the prostate or vagina	867.0/867.1	4	4

°Advance one grade if multiple injuries exist.

From reference 10 with permission.

TABLE H-14. THORACIC VASCULAR INJURY SCALE

GRADE°	INJURY DESCRIPTION[†]	ICD-9	AIS-90	GRADE°	INJURY DESCRIPTION[†]	ICD-9	AIS-90
I	Intercostal artery/vein	901.81	2–3		Inferior vena cava (intrathoracic)	902.10	3–4
	Internal mammary artery/vein	901.82	2–3		Pulmonary artery, primary intraparenchymal branch	901.41	3
	Bronchial artery/vein	901.89	2–3				
	Esophageal artery/vein	901.9	2–3		Pulmonary vein, primary intraparenchymal branch	901.42	3
	Hemiazygous vein	901.89	2–3				
	Unnamed artery/vein	901.9	2–3	V	Thoracic aorta, ascending and arch	901.0	5
II	Azygous vein	901.89	2–3				
	Internal jugular vein	900.1	2–3		Superior vena cava	901.2	3–4
	Subclavian vein	901.3	3–4		Pulmonary artery, main trunk	901.41	4
	Innominate vein	901.3	3–4		Pulmonary vein, main trunk	901.42	4
III	Carotid artery	900.01	3–5	VI	Uncontained total transection	901.0	5
	Innominate artery	901.1	3–4		of thoracic aorta or	901.41	4
	Subclavian artery	901.1	3–4		pulmonary hilum	901.42	
IV	Thoracic aorta, descending	901.0	4–5				

°Increase one grade for multiple grade III or IV injuries if >50% circumference, decrease one grade for grade IV and V injuries if <25% circumference.
[†]Based on most accurate assessment at autopsy, operation, or radiologic study.

From reference 11 with permission.

TABLE H-15. LUNG INJURY SCALE

GRADE°	INJURY TYPE	INJURY DESCRIPTION[†]	ICD-9	AIS-90
I	Contusion	Unilateral, <1 lobe	861.12/861.31	3
II	Contusion	Unilateral, single lobe	861.20/861.30	3
	Laceration	Simple pneumothorax	860.0/1 860.4/5	3
III	Contusion	Unilateral, >1 lobe	861.20/861.30	3
	Laceration	Persistent (>72 h), airleak from distal airway	860.0/1 860.4/5 862.0/861.30	3–4
	Hematoma	Nonexpanding intraparenchymal		

(*continued*)

TABLE H-15. (*continued*)

GRADE°	INJURY TYPE	INJURY DESCRIPTION[†]	ICD-9	AIS-90
IV	Laceration	Major (segmental or lobar) airway leak	862.21/861.31	4–5
	Hematoma	Expanding intraparenchymal		
	Vascular	Primary branch intrapulmonary vessel disruption	901.40	3–5
V	Vascular	Hilar vessel disruption	901.41/901.42	4
VI	Vascular	Total, uncontained transection of pulmonary hilum	901.41/901.42	4

°Advance one grade for bilateral injuries; hemothorax is graded according to the thoracic vascular OIS.
[†]Based on most accurate assessment at autopsy, operation, or radiologic study.

From reference 11 with permission.

TABLE H-16. CARDIAC INJURY SCALE

GRADE°	INJURY DESCRIPTION	ICD-9	AIS-90
I	Blunt cardiac injury with minor ECG abnormality (nonspecific ST or T wave changes, premature atrial, ventricular contraction or persistent sinus tachycardia)	861.01	3
	Blunt or penetrating pericardial wound without cardiac injury, cardiac tamponade, or cardiac herniation		
II	Blunt cardiac injury with heart block (right or left bundle branch, left anterior fasicular, or atrioventricular) or ischemic changes (ST depression or T wave inversion) without cardiac failure	861.01	3
	Penetrating tangential myocardial wound up to, but not extending through endocardium, without tamponade	861.12	3
III	Blunt cardiac injury with sustained (≥5 beats/min) or multifocal ventricular contractions	861.01	3–4
	Blunt or penetrating cardiac injury with septal rupture, pulmonary or tricuspid valvular incompetence, papillary muscle dysfunction, or distal coronary arterial occlusion without cardiac failure	861.01	3–4
	Blunt pericardial laceration with cardiac herniation		
	Blunt cardiac injury with cardiac failure	861.01	3–4
	Penetrating tangential myocardial wound up to, but not extending through endocardium, with tamponade	861.12	3
IV	Blunt or penetrating cardiac injury with septal rupture, pulmonary or tricuspid valvular incompetence, papillary muscle dysfunction or distal coronary arterial occlusion producing cardiac failure	861.12	3
	Blunt or penetrating cardiac injury with aortic or mitral valve incompetence		
	Blunt or penetrating cardiac injury of the right ventricle, right atrium, or left atrium	861.03 861.13	5
V	Blunt or penetrating cardiac injury with proximal coronary arterial occlusion		
	Blunt or penetrating left ventricular perforation	861.03 861.13	5
	Stellate injuries <50% tissue loss of the right ventricle, right atrium or left atrium	861.03 861.13	5
VI	Blunt avulsion of the heart; penetrating wound producing >50% tissue loss of a chamber		6

ECG, electrocardiographic.
°Advance one grade for multiple penetrating wounds to a single chamber or multiple chamber involvement.

From reference 11 with permission.

TABLE H-17. DIAPHRAGM INJURY SCALE

GRADE°	INJURY DESCRIPTION	ICD-9	AIS-90
I	Contusion	862.0	2
II	Laceration $\leq$2 cm	862.1	3
III	Laceration 2–10 cm	862.1	3
IV	Laceration >10 cm with tissue loss $\leq$25 cm^2	862.1	3
V	Laceration with tissue loss >25 cm^2	862.1	3

°Advance one grade for bilateral injuries.

From reference 11 with permission.

REFERENCES ■

1. DuBois D, DuBois EF: *Arch Intern Med* 1916;17:863
2. Lyerly HK: The renal system. In: *Handbook of Surgical Intensive Care: Practices of the Surgery Residents at the Duke University Medical Center*, ed 2. Chicago, Year Book Medical Publishers, 1989:171
3. Meerott JC: An easy-to-read acid-base nomogram. *Hosp Pract* 1987;187
4. Goldstein MB, Bear R, Richardson RMA, et al: The urine anion gap: a clinically useful index of ammonium excretion. *Am J Med Sci* 1986;292:198
5. Halperin ML, Goldstein MB: *Fluid, Electrolyte and Acid-Base Emergencies*. Philadelphia, WB Saunders, 1988
6. Harrington JT, Cohen JJ: Measurement of urinary electrolytes: indications and limitations. *N Engl J Med* 1975;293:1241
7. Bennett WM, Aronoff GR, Golper TA, et al: *Drug Prescribing in Renal Failure*. Philadelphia, American College of Physicians, 1987
8. Moore EE, Shackford SR, Pachter HL, et al: Organ injury scaling: Spleen, liver, and kidney. *J Trauma* 1989;29:1664
9. Moore EE, Cogbill TH, Malangoni MA, et al: Organ injury scaling. II. Pancreas, duodenum, small bowel, colon, and rectum. *J Trauma* 1990;30:1427
10. Moore EE, Cogbill TH, Jurkovich GJ, et al: Organ injury scaling. III. Chest wall, abdominal vascular, ureter, bladder, and urethra. *J Trauma* 1992;33:337
11. Moore EE, Malangoni MA, Cogbill TH, et al: Organ injury scaling. IV. Thoracic vascular, lung, cardiac, and diaphragm. *J Trauma* 1994;36:229

Index

Abdomen. *See also* Intraabdominal *entries; specific organs and disorders*
  acute. *See* Acute abdomen
  anterior, 1077
  computed tomography of, 974, 976, 977f, 978f
  intrathoracic, 1077
  open. *See* Postoperative abdomen, open
  in poisonings and toxic exposures, 1471
  postoperative. *See* Postoperative abdomen
Abdominal abscesses
  acute abdomen and, 1105
  postoperative, drainage of, 592, 593f
Abdominal distention, abdominal radiography in, 970–971, 972f, 973f
Abdominal drains, postoperative abdomen and, 1118f, 1119, 1119f
Abdominal infections, anaerobic, 1678
Abdominal injuries, 1075–1096. *See also specific injuries*
  anatomy and, 1077
  blunt, 1080–1082
    diagnostic laparotomy for, 1081–1082
    organ injury and, incidence of, 1082, 1082t
  delayed diagnosis of, 1055
  detection of, peritoneal lavage for, 563
  diagnostic evaluation and management of, 1078–1079
  diagnostic tests and procedures for, 1076
  initial therapy for, 1076–1077
  major problems with, 1075
  mechanism of injury and, 1077–1078
  mortality and morbidity in, 1082
  in obstetric patients. *See* Trauma, in obstetric patients
  penetrating, 1079–1080
  shearing, 1085

  stress points with, 1075–1076
Abdominal ischemia, abdominal radiography in, 971
Abdominal pain
  in acute abdomen, 1100–1101, 1101t
  in diabetic ketoacidosis, 2103
  in HIV-infected patients, 1629–1630
  in systemic lupus erythematosus, 2168
Abdominal radiography, 969–971
  in abdominal distention, 970–971, 972f, 973f
  in acute abdomen, 1103, 1103f
  free intraperitoneal air and, 970, 971f, 972f
  in fulminant colitis, 2066–2067
  infections and, 1596
  in ischemic disease, 971
  in neutropenic enterocolitis, 2251
  in toxic megacolon, 2066–2067
Abdominal surgery. *See also specific procedures*
  to lower abdomen, postoperative management and, 1255t, 1255–1256
  pulmonary assessment for, 992–994
    clinical application of, 992–994, 993t
  pulmonary consultation for, 989
  to upper abdomen, postoperative management and, 1254–1255
Abdominal thrusts, subdiaphragmatic, 493
Abdominal visceral organ injury scale, 2277t–2278t
Abdominal wall injuries, 1083–1085
ABO incompatibility, 1370, 1370t
Abortion, as stress response, 320
Abruptio placentae, 1403–1404, 1404f, 1404t
  diagnosis of, 1403
  trauma and, 1423
  treatment of, 1404

Abscesses
  abdominal
    acute abdomen and, 1105
    postoperative, drainage of, 592, 593f
  of brain
    anaerobic, 1678
    clinical presentation and initial diagnostic measures for, 1638–1639
  epidural, 818
    cranial, clinical presentation and initial diagnostic measures for, 1638
    spinal, clinical presentation and initial diagnostic measures for, 1637–1638
  of lung
    in aspiration syndromes, treatment of, 1868
    in pneumonia, 1849–1850, 1850f
  in pancreatitis, surgical treatment of, 2061
  percutaneous catheter drainage of. *See* Catheter drainage, percutaneous
  perinephric, in pyelonephritis, 1653
  renal, in pyelonephritis, 1653
Absence seizures, 1987
Absence status epilepticus, 1987
Absolute refractory period, 229
Absorption, of drugs, in renal disease, 478
Absorption atelectasis
  denitrogenation, 930
  oxygen therapy and, 707
Absorption powders, 2205
Accelerated idioventricular rhythm, 1784
Acceleration, of aircraft, 806–807
Acetaminophen
  for heart transplantation, 1335
  poisoning by, 1483–1486
    antidote for, 1465t
    clinical manifestations of, 1484

Acetaminophen, poisoning by (*continued*)
  toxicology and, 1483–1484
  treatment of, 1484–1486, 1485f
Acetazolamide
  for acute renal failure, 2090
  for acute tumor lysis syndrome, 2247
  for intracranial hypertension, 284
N-Acetylcysteine (Mucomyst), for acetaminophen
    poisoning, 1465t, 1483, 1484–1486,
    1485f
N-Acetyl procainamide, therapeutic serum level
    of, 479t
Acid(s). *See also* pH
  administration of, for metabolic alkalosis,
    262–263
  chemistry of, 255–256
  ingestion of. *See* Corrosive injuries, esophageal
  loss of, metabolic alkalosis and, 262
Acid-base balance, 255–263
  definitions and, 255–256, 256t
    actual concentrations and pH and,
      255–256, 256t
  metabolic disturbances of, 257t, 257–258,
      260–263, 2259t–2261t. *See also*
      specific disturbances
  respiratory compensation for, 259, 259t
  physiology of, 926–927
    anion gap and, 927
    base excess/deficit and, 926–927
    bicarbonate deficiency estimation and, 927,
      927t
    renal buffers and, 926
  problem solving and, 259–260
  respiratory disturbances of, 257, 263, 263t,
      2259t–2261t. *See also specific*
      disturbances
    metabolic compensation for, 258t, 258–259
  temperature correction and, 936–937
  tourniquets and, 1246, 1246f
Acidemia, 256
  acetaminophen poisoning and, 1486
  metabolic, 927–928
Acidosis, 256, 921
  diabetic ketoacidosis. *See* Diabetic
      ketoacidosis (DKA)
  of gastric mucosa, in surgical patients,
      448–450, 449f
  metabolic. *See* Metabolic acidosis
  prevention of, in cyclic antidepressant
      poisoning, 1492
  respiratory, 263, 922t
    venous, during cardiopulmonary
      resuscitation, 935
Acid-pepsin problems, renal transplantation
    and, 1306
Acinetobacter infections, 1669
Acquired immunodeficiency syndrome (AIDS),
    1439–1444. *See also* Human
    immunodeficiency virus (HIV)
    infections
  acute abdomen in, 1104
  epidemiology of, 1440
  historical background of, 1439–1440
  neurologic infections in, 1645, 1645t
  skin disorders in, 2191, 2191f, 2191t
  transfusion therapy and, 648, 655

Acrolein, inhalation injury due to, 1954
Acrylamide poisoning, antidote for, 1465t
Actin filaments, 229, 230, 230f, 231
Actinomycosis, 1675–1676
Action potentials, cardiac electrical activity and,
      227–229
  automaticity and, 228
  depolarization and repolarization and,
      227–228, 228f
  refractoriness and excitability and, 228–229
Activated charcoal
  for acetaminophen poisoning, 1484
  for cyclic antidepressant poisoning, 1491
  for poisonings and toxic exposures,
      1473–1474, 1474t
  for salicylate poisoning, 1489
  for theophylline poisoning, 1500
Activated partial thromboplastin time (aPTT), 270
Active, low air loss beds, 2213
Active electrodes, 832
Active external rewarming, for hypothermia,
      1453–1454
Actuators, for microprocessor-controlled
      mechanical ventilators, 719
Acute abdomen, 1099–1107
  acute mesenteric ischemia and, 1107
  anatomy and, 1100–1101, 1101t
  biliary tract disease and, 1104–1105
  definition of, 1100
  diagnostic peritoneal lavage and, 1102
  diagnostic tests and procedures for, 1099–1100
  in immune compromised patients, 1104
  initial therapy for, 1100
  laboratory evaluation of, 1102
  in neutropenic cancer patients, 1104
  in obstetric patients, 1424
  patient history and, 1101
  physical examination and, 1102
  pneumoperitoneum and, 1105–1106, 1106f
  pseudo-obstruction of colon and, 1106, 1106f
  radiographic studies of, 1103, 1103f
  stress points with, 1099
  therapy of, 1103–1104
Acute Infarction Ramipril Efficacy Study
      (AIRE), 1756
Acute lung injury (ALI)
  acute, respiratory distress syndrome and, 1828
  mechanisms of, 1829–1830
  structural response to, 1828f, 1828–1829,
      1829f, 1829t
Acute myocardial infarction (AMI), 1727–1744
  angiotensin-converting enzyme inhibitors for,
      1736–1737
  aspirin in, 1727–1728, 1728f
  beta-blocking agents for, 1734t, 1734–1735
  calcium channel blockers for, 1735–1736
  cardiogenic shock and, 1737, 1738
  cocaine abuse and, 1516
  heart failure and, 1737
    approach to, 1739–1740
    differentiation from, 1737, 1737t
    mechanical complications of, 1737–1738
  hemodynamic monitoring guidelines for,
      1738–1739, 1739t
  heparin in, 1733–1734
  immediate concerns with, 1727

left ventricular, 390–392, 391t
  lidocaine for, 1736
  nitroglycerin for, intravenous, 1735
  noninvasive imaging techniques for,
      1740–1742
    echocardiography, 1741–1742, 1742t
    gated radionuclide angiography, 1741
    technetium 99m isonitriles, 1740–1741
    technetium 99m scanning, 1741
    thallium-201 scintigraphy, 1740
  percutaneous transluminal coronary
      angioplasty for, 1733, 1733f
  Q wave and non-Q wave, 1742–1744
    diagnosis of, 1742
    noninvasive predischarge assessment of,
      1743–1744
    prognosis of, 1742–1743
  right ventricular, 392–393
    diagnosis and therapy of, 1738
  thrombolytic therapy for. *See* Thrombolytic
      therapy, for acute myocardial infarction
Acute Physiology and Chronic Health Evaluation
      (APACHE), 42, 57, 57t
  APACHE II, 43, 57, 57t
    outcome prediction and, 138, 139, 139t, 141,
      141t, 143f, 143–145, 144f, 144t, 145t
  APACHE III, 57, 57t
    outcome prediction and, 138–139, 140f, 141,
      142, 145
    outcome prediction and, 135, 136, 138, 141t,
      141–145, 142f–144f, 144t, 145t
Acute renal failure (ARF), 2081–2091. *See also*
      Renal failure
  in autoimmune hemolytic anemia, 2232–2233
  in burn patients, 1270
  in cancer, prophylaxis of, 2247
  contrast-induced, 2086
  diagnostic tests and procedures for, 2081,
      2082t, 2083t
  differential diagnosis of, 2084–2086, 2085f,
      2085t
  differential diagnosis of acute azotemia and,
      2081–2084, 2083t, 2084f, 2084t
  major problems with, 2081
  pathophysiology of, 2086–2088, 2087f, 2088f
  prevention of, 2088, 2089t
  prognosis and recovery from, 2090–2091
  in rhabdomyolysis, prevention of, 2196–2198,
      2200
  stress points with, 2081, 2082t
  treatment and supportive care for, 2083t, 2088,
      2089t, 2090
Acute respiratory distress syndrome (ARDS),
      1825–1838
  following cardiac surgery, 1156
  chest radiography in, 962–963
  clinical presentation of, 1830–1831
    lung imaging and, 1831, 1831f, 1832f
    physical examination and, 1830t, 1830–1831
  complications of, 1836, 1837t–1838t
  in diabetic ketoacidosis, 2106
  diagnostic tests and procedures for, 1825–1826
  etiology of, 1826–1828, 1827t
  major problems with, 1825
  monitoring in, 1836, 1837t
  outcome of, 1836, 1838

pathophysiology of, 1828–1830
  alteration in gas exchange and, 1830
  lung mechanics and, 1830
  mechanisms of acute lung injury and,
    1829–1830
  noncardiogenic pulmonary edema and, 1829
  structural response to injury and, 1828f,
    1828–1829, 1829f, 1829t
shock and, 371
stress points with, 1825
synonyms of, 1826t
treatment of, 1831–1835
  antibiotics in, 1833
  antiendotoxins for, 1835
  antioxidants for, 1834–1835
  bronchodilators in, 1833
  fluid management in, 1833
  initial therapy for, 1826
  ketoconazole for, 1834
  mechanical ventilation for. *See* Mechanical
    ventilation, for acute respiratory
    distress syndrome
  nitric oxide for, 1833–1834
  nonsteroidal anti-inflammatory drugs for,
    1835
  for nosocomial infections, 1833
  nutritional support in, 1833
  patient positioning for, 1835
  phentoxyphylline for, 1834
  prostaglandin E_1 for, 1835
  steroids for, 1834
  surfactant for, 1834
Acute stress disorder, 89–90
Acute tubular necrosis (ATN), acute renal failure
  due to, 2086
Acyclovir, 1570–1571, 1696, 1699–1700, 1700t
  for eczema herpeticum, 2184, 2186t
  for heart-lung transplantation, 1319t
  for herpes simplex virus infections
    in bone marrow transplant recipients, 1613
    in HIV-infected patients, 1619t
  for lung transplantation, 1319t
  prophylactic
    heart transplantation and, 1339
    for varicella-zoster virus infections, 1566
  for varicella-zoster virus infections, 2186t
    in bone marrow transplant recipients, 1614
Address buses, of microprocessor-controlled
  ventilators, 718
Adenitis, mesenteric, *Yersinia*, 1672
Adenohypophyseal disorders. *See*
    Hypopituitarism
Adenosine
  actions, indications, and dosing of, 2268
  for arrhythmias, 1785, 1786
  for cardiopulmonary resuscitation, 504–505
    complications of, 504–505
    dosage of, 504
    indications for, 504
Adhesive arachnoiditis, 818
Adjusted-dose unfractionated heparin, for deep
  venous thrombosis prophylaxis, 1891
Admission(s). *See also under specific disorders*
  clinical decision-making at time of, 56
  source of, clinical decision-making and,
    55–56, 56t

Admission criteria, as continuous quality
    improvement indicator, 166, 168, 168t
Adolescents
  bone marrow transplantation in, growth and
    development following, 1379
  terminal, levels of care for, 122
Adrenalectomy, postoperative management and,
  1254–1255
Adrenal function tests, 2126–2128
Adrenal gland
  glucocorticoid action and, 2123
  hyperfunction of, coma and, 1978
  physiology of, 2122–2123
    regulation of adrenal hormone synthesis
      and, 2122
    types of adrenal hormones and, 2122–2123
Adrenal hormone excess, 2125
Adrenal insufficiency, 2113, 2115–2116,
    2121–2122, 2123–2125
  chronic steroid therapy and, 2116
  clinical presentation of, 2124
  coma and, 1978
  diagnostic tests and procedures for, 2121
  differential diagnosis of, 2123–2124
  in HIV-infected patients, 1628–1629
  hypothyroidism with, treatment of, 2146
  major problems with, 2121
  management of, 2124–2125
    in acute insufficiency, 2124–2125, 2125t
    following adrenalectomy, 1255
    in chronic insufficiency, 2125
    initial therapy for, 2121–2122
  during perioperative period, 2115–2116, 2116t
  stress points with, 2121, 2122t
Adrenalitis, autoimmune, 2123
Adrenal shock, 368
Adrenal suppression, in surgical patients, 1008
Adrenergic agonists. *See also specific drugs*
  alpha, for ethanol withdrawal, 1514
  beta, for acute respiratory failure, 1920t,
    1920–1921
  intracranial pressure and, 281
  for opiate withdrawal, 1518–1519
Adrenergic blocking agents
  alpha, for pheochromocytomas, 2133, 2134t
  beta
    for cardiopulmonary resuscitation, 504
    complications of, 504
    dosage of, 504
    indications for, 504
Adrenocortical insufficiency, fever and,
    1600–1601
Adrenocorticotropic hormone (ACTH)
  Cushing's syndrome and, 2125
  deficiency of. *See* Adrenal insufficiency
  for fulminant colitis, 2068
  interaction with insulin, 2113
  serum level of, 2127
  for toxic megacolon, 2068
Adrenocorticotropic hormone (ACTH)
    stimulation
  in hypopituitarism, 2114
  long ACTH stimulation test and, 2127
  short ACTH stimulation test and, 2127
Adult(s)
  airway management in, anatomical

    considerations and, 759–760, 760f, 761f
  antibiotic selection for neurologic infections
    in, 1641t
  cardiac surgery in, postoperative management
    of. *See* Cardiac surgery, postoperative
    management of adult patients and
  closed chest cardiac compression in, 496
  extracorporeal membrane oxygenation in. *See*
    Extracorporeal membrane oxygenation
    (ECMO), in adults
Adult respiratory distress syndrome. *See* Acute
    respiratory distress syndrome (ARDS)
Advance directives, 29–31. *See also* Do-not-
    resuscitate (DNR) orders
  termination of cardiopulmonary resuscitation
    and, 161
Advanced life support (ALS), 492
Adverse drug reactions (ADRs), 482–486, 483t.
    See also specific drugs, drug types,
    and reactions
  drug interactions and, 485–486
    pharmacodynamic, 486
    pharmacokinetic, 485–486, 486t
  management of, 486
Aeromonas infections, 1675
Affective capacity, informed consent and, 86
Affidavits, 33–34
Afterload. *See* Respiratory muscles; Ventricular
    afterload
Afternoon rounds, 38
Age. *See also specific age groups*
  antibiotic selection for neurologic infections
    and, 1641, 1641t
  outcome of cardiopulmonary resuscitation
    and, 157
  termination of cardiopulmonary resuscitation
    and, 159
Agitation, 2025–2026
  causes of, 2025
  in head injury, 1204
  postanesthetic, 1030
    evaluation of, 1030, 1030t
    treatment of, 1030
  treatment of, 2025–2026
    benzodiazepines for, 2025, 2026t
    dopamine blockers for, 2026
    major tranquilizers for, 2025–2026
    sedation for, 823
Agranulocytosis, antithyroid agents as cause of,
    2140
Air, blending with oxygen, 704
  jet entrainment for, 704
  mechanical, 704, 704f
Aircraft. *See* Interhospital transport, aircraft for
Air embolism, 783, 1964
  arterial, 1905, 1906–1907
  clinical manifestations of, 783
  dysbaric, 1905–1906, 1906t
  invasive pressure monitoring and, 844
  presentation of, 783, 783t
  systemic, in trauma patients, 1051
  treatment of, 783
  venous, 1907–1908
    in obstetric patients, 1413
    in trauma patients, 1051
Air entrainment masks, 705–706, 706f

Air exchange. *See* Gas exchange
Air fluidized beds, 2213
Airway
  in comatose patients, emergency evaluation
    of, 1971
  difficult, 761
  initial triage of trauma patients and, 1040–1041
  following lung and heart-lung transplantation,
    1320–1321, 1323f, 1324f
  lung and heart-lung transplantation and,
    management of, 1329, 1329f
  in rheumatoid arthritis, 1244
  secondary triage of trauma patients and,
    1047–1048
  tracheal intubation causing injuries to, 767–768
Airway adjuncts. *See also* Artificial airways;
    specific artificial airways
  in cardiopulmonary resuscitation, 493–494,
    494f, 495f
Airway management, 492–495, 757–772
  airways for. *See* Artificial airways; *specific*
    artificial airways
  anatomic considerations and, 759–761
    in adults, 759–760, 760f, 761f
    assessment of, 760–761, 761f
    pediatric, 760
  cuff inflation for. *See* Cuff inflation
  diagnostic tests and procedures for, 758
  drugs for, 762t, 762–763
    barbiturates, 762
    benzodiazepines, 762
    ketamine, 763
    local anesthetics, 762
    muscle relaxants, 762
    narcotics, 762
    propofol, 763
  in dysoxia, 340–341
  fiberoptic bronchoscopy in. *See*
    Bronchoscopy, fiberoptic
  foreign body removal for, 493
  general principles of, 758–759, 759f, 759t
  in head injury, 1204
  initial therapy and, 758
  intubation for. *See* Intubation; *specific types*
    of intubation
  major problems with, 757
  in poisonings and toxic exposures, 468
    cyclic antidepressants and, 1491
  positioning for, 492–493, 493f
  in rheumatoid arthritis, 1245
  in shock, 374
  in spinal cord injury, 1209–1210
  stress points with, 757–758
  surgical techniques for, 495
    cricothyroidotomy, 770, 1210
    tracheostomy. *See* Tracheostomy
    tracheotomy. *See* Tracheotomy
Airway obstruction, 869
  in anaphylaxis, 1548
  in asthma, measurement of, 1935
  in cancer, 2248
  by goiters, 2147–2148
  in head injury, 1201, 1201f
  tracheal intubation causing, 768
  of upper airway
    asthma versus, 1934

fiberoptic bronchoscopy in, 697–698
Airway pressure
  decreased, mechanical ventilation and, 741
  measurement of, 735f, 735–736, 736f
    cardinal pressure and, 735–736
    rationale for, 735–736
Airway pressure release ventilation (APRV),
    732–734, 749–750
  advantages of, 750
  cardiorespiratory effects of, 734
  continuous positive airway pressure selection
    for, 734
  disadvantages of, 750
  equipment for, 733, 733f
  initial settings for, 750
  operational principles of, 732–733
  patient selection for, 734
  pressure-controlled inverse ratio ventilation
    compared with, 734
  setup parameters for, 750, 750f
  tidal volume control for, 733–734, 734f
  work of breathing and, 750
Airway resistance, 196–198
  anatomic considerations and, 196–197
  changes in, 197–198
    airway pressure changes and, 197
    clinical correlates of, 198
    complicating factors and, 197–198
    gas trapping and auto positive end-expiratory
     pressure and, 197
    mechanics of, 197
    peptides and, 197
  distribution of ventilation and, 201–202
  laminar and turbulent flow and, 196
  lung and heart-lung transplantation and, 1326
  pressure support ventilation titration and,
    220–221, 222f
Alanine, metabolism of, in critical illness, 328–329
Alarm(s), on mechanical ventilators, 719
Alarm capabilities, of cardiopulmonary
    assessment, 868
Albumin
  for depressed gastrointestinal pH, 452
  in diabetic ketoacidosis, 2103
  hemostasis and, 436
  following hepatic resection, 1126
Albuterol
  for acute respiratory failure, 1921
  for asthma, 1936, 1937
  preoperative, 994t
Alcoholism. *See* Ethanol, abuse of
Aldosterone, osmolality and, 439
Alfentanil
  actions, indications, and dosing of, 2268
  cost of, 827t
Alkalemia, 256
  metabolic, 928
  specific therapy for, 928
Alkali. *See also* Bases
  administration of, metabolic alkalosis and, 262
  ingestion of. *See* Corrosive injuries, esophageal
Alkalosis, 256, 921. *See also* Metabolic alkalosis
  respiratory, 263, 263t, 922t
    with hypoxemia, blood gas analysis in, 926
    with metabolic acidosis, 261
    without hypoxemia, blood gas analysis in, 926

Allergic bronchopulmonary aspergillosis, 1688
Allergy. *See* Hypersensitivity reactions; Immune
    system function
Allopurinol
  for acute tumor lysis syndrome, 2247
  adverse effects of, 2156t–2157t
Alpha-adrenergic agonists, for ethanol
    withdrawal, 1514
Alpha-adrenergic blocking agents, for
    pheochromocytomas, 2133, 2134t
Alpha coma, electroencephalography in, 943, 944f
Alprazolam, 825t
Alprostadil
  for heart-lung transplantation, 1319t
  for lung transplantation, 1319t
Althesin, during pregnancy, 320
Alveolar ventilation
  inhalational anesthetic delivery and, 1015
  in obstetric patients, 1411, 1411t
  $PaCO_2$ and, 924
Alveoli, gas composition in, 198–199
Amantadine, 1571, 1700t, 1700–1701
  prophylactic, for influenza, 1566
Ambulances
  air. *See* Interhospital transport, aircraft for
  ground, 805
American Medical Association (AMA), treatment
    withdrawal policy of, 73
Americans with Disabilities Act (ADA), 114
Amikacin, 1568, 1568t
  cost and initial dosage of, 1562t
  for *Mycobacterium avium* complex infections,
    in HIV-infected patients, 1619t
  for *Nocardia* infections, 1608
  therapeutic serum level of, 479t
Amino acids, metabolism of, in critical illness,
    328–329
ε-Aminocaproic acid (EACA)
  for amniotic fluid embolism, 1912
  for disseminated intravascular coagulation,
    2222
  transfusion therapy and, 662
Aminoglycoside antibiotics, 1567–1568. *See also*
    specific drugs
  acute renal failure due to, 2086
  dosing of, 1568, 1568t
  for infective endocarditis, 1793
  for urinary tract infections, 1652
Aminophylline
  actions, indications, and dosing of, 2268
  for anaphylaxis, 1547t
Amiodarone, dosing of, in chronic renal failure,
    2097t
Amitriptyline (Elavil), side effects of, 2027t
Ammonia, inhalation injury due to, 1954
Amnesia, in delirium, 2020
Amniotic fluid embolism (AFE), 1406, 1413,
    1910–1912
  disseminated intravascular coagulation and,
    1911–1912
Amoxapine (Asendin)
  poisoning by, 1493
  side effects of, 2027t
Amoxicillin, prophylactic
  for infective endocarditis, 1798t, 1799t
  for surgical patients, 1010t

Amphotericin B (AMB), 1570, 1690t, 1690–1691
  for *Aspergillus* infections, in bone marrow transplant recipients, 1614
  for *Candida* infections, in HIV-infected patients, 1619t
  for coccidioidomycosis, in HIV-infected patients, 1619t
  for cryptococcosis, in HIV-infected patients, 1619t
  for heart-lung transplantation, 1329
  for histoplasmosis, in HIV-infected patients, 1619t
  for infections in granulocytopenic patients, 1606
  for infective endocarditis, 1793
  for intestinal transplantation, 1361
  for lung transplantation, 1329
  for meningitis, in renal transplant recipients, 1612
  for multivisceral transplantation, 1361
  for urinary tract infections, 1655, 2212
Ampicillin
  cost and initial dosage of, 1562t
  for infective endocarditis, 1794t
  for *Listeria monocytogenes* infections, 1608
  prophylactic
    for infective endocarditis, 1799t
    for surgical patients, 1010t
  for urinary tract infections, 1652
Ampicillin/sulbactam, cost and initial dosage of, 1562t
Amplifier systems, for invasive pressure monitoring, 840
Amrinone
  actions, indications, and dosing of, 2268
  for cardiac contractility augmentation, following cardiac surgery, 1153
  following cardiac surgery in pediatric patients, 1166, 1166f, 1167t
  for cardiomyopathy, peripartum, 1396
  for shock, 363t
Amylase, in diabetic ketoacidosis, 2103–2104
Amyl nitrate, for cyanide poisoning, 1466t
Amyloidosis, coagulation disorder associated with, 2230
Anacrotic limb, 850
Anaerobic cocci, 1675
Analgesia. *See* Pain control
Analgesia service function, 819
Analog signals, 718–719, 719t
Analog-to-digital converters, 719
Analysis bias, 7
Analysis of variance (ANOVA), 16
Anaphylactic and anaphylactoid reactions, 483, 1543–1550
  clinical manifestations of, 1544–1546, 1545t–1547t
  to drugs, 1598, 1599t
  implications and outcome of, 1550
  major problems with, 1543
  management of, 1546–1549, 1547t, 1549f
    initial therapy for, 1544
  pathogenesis of, 1550
  prevention of, 1549–1550
  shock, 368

  adjunctive and experimental management techniques for, 380–381
  stress points with, 1543–1544
Anemia, 2231–2235, 2232t
  aplastic, 2236
  chronic, transfusion therapy for, 644, 644t
  hemolytic. *See* Hemolytic anemia
  in rheumatoid arthritis, 1244
  sickle cell, 2233t, 2233–2235
    painful crisis in, 2233–2234
Anencephaly, 1292
Anesthesia, 1013–1033. *See also specific anesthetics*
  combined, 1028
    advantages of, 1028
    applications for, 1028
  for deep venous thrombosis prevention, 1241
  for fiberoptic bronchoscopy, 687–689, 689t
  general, stress response and, 1027–1028
  inhalational. *See* Inhalational anesthetics; *specific anesthetics*
  local. *See* Local anesthetic(s); Local anesthetic blocks; *specific drugs*
  major problems with, 1013, 1014f
  postanesthetic problems and, 1026–1033
    agitation and sedation, 1030, 1030t
    hypoxemia, 1026–1027
    malignant hyperthermia, 483, 483t, 1032t, 1032–1033, 1033t
    pain, 1027–1030
    residual neuromuscular blockade, 1031t, 1031–1032, 1032t
  during pregnancy, 320
  for pulmonary thromboembolism prevention, 1241
  regional, stress response and, 1028
  rhabdomyolysis due to, 2198
  stress points with, 1013, 1015
  techniques for critically ill patients and, 1026
Aneurysms
  aortic. *See* Aortic dissection
  false, management of, 1188
  falsein pancreatitis, surgical treatment of, 2059–2060
  left ventricular
    cardiogenic shock and, 395
    surgical intervention for, 402
  thoracic, dissecting, echocardiography in, 884, 885t
Angina pectoris, chest pain and, 1723
Angiographic embolization, for pelvic fractures, 1061
Angiography
  in abdominal injuries, 1081
  cerebral, in stroke patients, 1995
  of kidney, penetrating trauma and, 1259–1260, 1261f
  in pancreatitis, 2057
  pulmonary, in pulmonary embolism, 1720–1721, 1896–1897
  radionuclide
    in acute myocardial infarction, 1743–1744
    gated, in acute myocardial infarction, 1741
  in thoracic trauma, 1138
Angiotensin-converting enzyme inhibitors. *See also specific drugs*

  for acute myocardial infarction, 1736–1737
    for limitation of infarct size, 397
  for heart failure, 1755–1756, 1757
    clinical use of, 1756
    pooled studies of, 1756
  for hypertension
    in hypertensive emergencies, 1819
    vascular surgery and, 1179
  for renal crisis, in systemic sclerosis, 2172
Angiotensin II receptor antagonists, for dilated cardiomyopathy, 1763
Anion(s), daily renal excretion of, 2265t
Anion gap, 927
Anisoylated plasminogen-streptokinase activator complex (APSAC), 623, 623t, 1729–1732, 1730t, 1731t, 1732f
Ankle, venous cutdown at, 569, 573f
Anorectal injuries, 1093–1094
  with pelvic fractures, 1059
  rectal injury scale and, 2276t
Anorexia, in refractory advanced heart failure, 1758
Antacids, for aspiration prophylaxis, 1870f, 1870–1871, 1872
Antecubital fossa, venous cutdown in, 570–571, 574d
Anthozoa envenomations, 1533t, 1533–1534
  clinical manifestations of, 1533–1534
  treatment of, 1534
Anthracycline antibiotics, cardiac toxicity of, 2251
Anthrax, 1668
Antiarrhythmic agents. *See also specific drugs*
  adverse reactions to, 484
  dosing of, in chronic renal failure, 2097t
  during pregnancy, 1397
Antibiotics, 1555–1571. *See also specific drugs*
  for acute abdomen, 1104, 1105
  for acute respiratory distress syndrome, 1833
  for acute respiratory failure, 1922
  adverse effects of, 1652
  aminoglycoside. *See* Aminoglycoside antibiotics
  anthracycline, cardiac toxicity of, 2251
  antibacterial, effectiveness of, 1558t–1560t
  antifungal, 1570. *See also specific drugs*
    effectiveness of, 1560t
  antiviral, 1570–1571, 1696, 1699–1700, 1700t. *See also specific drugs*
    effectiveness of, 1560t
  for aspiration syndromes, 1868
  bactericidal, 1561
    for neurologic infections, 1641–1642
  bacteriostatic, 1561
  following cardiac surgery in adults, 1159–1160
  following cardiac surgery in pediatric patients
    prophylactic, 1171–1172
    therapeutic, 1172
  combination therapy using
    monotherapy versus, 1562–1564
    for neurologic infections, 1642
  cost and initial dosage of, 1562t
  diagnostic tests and procedures and, 1555
  dosage and administration routes for, 1561, 1562t
  for fractures, 1228
  for fulminant colitis, 2068
  for heart-lung transplantation, 1319t

Antibiotics (*continued*)
  initial therapy and, 1555, 1562t
  β-lactam, 1567
    penicillins combined with, 1566
  for leukopenia, 2236
  for liver transplantation, 1348–1350
    antiviral, prophylactic, 1348–1349
    empiric, 1348
  for lung transplantation, 1319t
  major problems with, 1555
  metabolism of, antibiotic selection and,
      1557t, 1557–1558
  minimum inhibitory concentrations of, 1793
  monotherapy versus combination therapy
      using, 1562–1564
    in specific clinical settings, 1563–1564
  for neurologic infections, empiric selection of,
      1641t, 1641–1642
  for nosocomial pneumonia, 1577
  for pancreatitis, 2058–2059
  for pneumonia, 1850–1852, 1851t
    clinical response to, 1852
    duration of therapy with, 1852, 1852t
    empiric, 1594
  in pregnancy, 1425, 1557t, 1557–1558
  prophylactic, 1565–1566
    for bacterial meningitis, 1642t, 1643
    heart transplantation and, 1339
    for infective endocarditis, 1796–1797, 1798t,
        1799t, 1800
    for liver transplantation, 1348–1349
  reassessment of therapy using, 1564t,
      1564–1565
  resistance to, 1652
    pneumonia due to, 1844
    of *Staphylococcus aureus*, 1661
    of *Streptococcus pneumoniae*, 1665
  selection of, 1556–1561
    diagnosis of infection and, 1558,
        1558t–1560t, 1560–1561
    host factors and, 1556–1558
  spectrum of activity of, 1561, 1652
  stress points with, 1555
  surgical patients and, 1009, 1009t–1010t
    following thoracic surgery, 1136
  toxicity of, 1561–1562, 1563t
  for toxic megacolon, 2068
  for varicella-zoster virus infections, 2186t
Antibodies. *See* Immunoglobulins; Intravenous
    immunoglobulin (IVIg)
Antibody-dependent cellular cytotoxicity
    (ADCC) cells, inhalational anesthetics
    and, 1019–1020
Anticholinergic agents. *See also specific drugs*
  for acute respiratory failure, 1921
  for aspiration prophylaxis, 1872
  inhaled, for asthma, 1937–1938
  for neuromuscular blocking agent reversal,
      1032t
  poisoning by, antidote for, 1465t
Anticholinergic toxidrome, 1468, 1469t
Anticholinesterases. *See also specific drugs*
  for neuromuscular blocking agent reversal,
      1032t
  for reversal of neuromuscular blockade,
      834–835, 835t

Anticoagulant agents. *See also specific drugs*
  for deep venous thrombosis, 1897
  extracorporeal membrane oxygenation and, 674
  with extracorporeal renal replacement
      therapies, 635–636
  necrosis due to, purpura and, 2190–2191
  during pregnancy, 1425
  prophylactic
    for deep venous thrombosis, 1239–1241
    for pulmonary thromboembolism,
        1239–1241
  for pulmonary embolism, 1898–1899
    chronic, 1899
    with inferior vena caval filters, 1899
    initial therapy, 1898–1899, 1899t
  surgical patients and, 1009
Anticonvulsant agents. *See also specific drugs*
  for preeclampsia/eclampsia, 1392
  prophylactic, in brain injury, 286
Antidepressant agents. *See also specific drugs*
  tricyclic
    poisoning by, antidote for, 1465t
    side effects of, 2027t
    tricyclic antidepressant toxidrome and,
        1468, 1469t
Antidiarrheal agents, 2212
Anti-digoxin Fab therapy, 311, 312t, 1466t, 1499
Antidiuretic hormone (ADH)
  diabetes insipidus and, 2116–2118
    management of, 2118
    patient examination in, 2117–2118
  osmolality and, 439
  secretion of, in head injury, 1207
  sodium regulation and, 415
  syndrome of inappropriate antidiuretic
      hormone and, hyponatremia and, 417,
      418
Anti-dumping law, 114–115
Antiendotoxins, for acute respiratory distress
    syndrome, 1835
Antifungal agents, 1570. *See also specific drugs*
  effectiveness of, 1560t
Antigen clearance, 306–307, 306–308
  effector cell function and, 306–307, 307t
  immunoglobulin and complement and, 306
  inflammation and, 308
Antigen presenting cells (APCs), 303, 304, 305,
    306
Antihistamines. *See also specific drugs*
  with amphotericin B, 1570
Antihypertensive agents. *See also specific drugs*
  for preeclampsia/eclampsia, 1392
  during pregnancy, 1425
  surgical patients and, 1008
  withdrawal of, hypertensive emergencies and,
      1818
Antiinflammatory agents. *See also* Nonsteroidal
    anti-inflammatory drugs (NSAIDs);
    specific drugs
  surgical patients and, 1009
Antilymphocyte agents
  for heart-lung transplantation, 1320
  for lung transplantation, 1320
  for renal transplantation, 1304–1305
Antioxidants
  for acute respiratory distress syndrome,

1834–1835
  for head injury, 1206
  pulmonary oxygen toxicity and, 708
Antiplatelet agents, 613–615. *See also specific
    drugs*
  aspirin as, 613–614, 614t, 615f, 2228
  carotid/subclavian reconstructions and, 1182
  dextran as, 615
  for infrainguinal reconstructions, 1186
  monoclonal antibody to platelet glycoprotein
      IIb/IIIa as, 615
  ticlopidine as, 614
Antiplatelet integrin receptor, 312t
Antipsychotic agents. *See also specific drugs*
  neuroleptic malignant syndrome and. *See*
      Neuroleptic malignant syndrome
      (NMS)
  poisoning by, 1494–1495
    toxicology and clinical manifestations of,
        1494–1495
    treatment of, 1495
  rhabdomyolysis due to, 2198–2199
Antireflux surgery, for aspiration prophylaxis,
    1872
Antirheumatic agents, 2156–2159
  adverse effects of, 2156t–2157t
Antithrombin-3, prophylactic
  for deep venous thrombosis, 1239
  for pulmonary thromboembolism, 1239
Antithrombotic therapy, 613, 615–622
  heparin for, 615–619
    for cardiovascular disorders, 617–618
    for central nervous system disorders,
        618–619
    low-molecular-weight, 619f, 619–620
    for venous thromboembolism prophylaxis,
        616, 616t, 617t
    for venous thromboembolism treatment,
        616–617, 617t, 618t
  hirudin for, 620
  for stroke, 1998–1999
  warfarin for, 620–622, 621t
    for atrial fibrillation, 621–622, 622f
    for hypercoagulable states, 622, 622t
    for myocardial infarction, 622
    for prosthetic heart valves, 622
    for venous thromboembolism prophylaxis,
        620–621, 1891, 1892t
    for venous thromboembolism treatment, 621
Antithymocyte globulin (ATG)
  for heart transplantation, 1335
  for simultaneous pancreas/kidney
      transplantation, 1314
Antithyroid agents, 2140
Antivenins
  for black widow spider bites, 1529, 1530t
  for snake bites, 1466t, 1527t, 1527–1528
Antiviral agents, 1570–1571, 1696, 1699–1700,
    1700t. *See also specific drugs*
  effectiveness of, 1560t
Ant stings, anaphylaxis and, 1545, 1546t, 1548
Anxiety, 2025–2026. *See also* Fear; Stress
    (emotional)
  causes of, 2025
  treatment of, 2025–2026
    benzodiazepines for, 2025, 2026t

dopamine blockers for, 2026
major tranquilizers for, 2025–2026
sedation for, 822, 823t
Any laboratory test available syndrome, 100
Aorta
coarctation of, during pregnancy, 1395
injury of
of abdominal aorta, management of, 1188
of thoracic aorta, management of, 1188
in trauma patients, 1055, 1057t
rupture of, 1141–1142
Aortic dissection, 1191
chest pain and, 1721–1722
diagnosis of, 1191
hypertensive emergencies and, 1817
management of, 1191
Aortic impedance, 235–236, 236f
Aortic insufficiency, during pregnancy, 1394
Aortic reconstruction, 1184–1186
acute cholecystitis and, 1185
acute pancreatitis and, 1185
aortoenteric fistulas and, 1185
distal embolization and, 1184
hemodynamics and, 1184
intestinal ischemia and, 1184–1185
mortality and, 1185–1186
sigmoid ischemia following, 1111
Aortic regurgitation, 1774–1776
acute, 1775–1776
clinical presentation of, 1775
diagnostic studies for, 1776
etiology of, 1775
pathophysiology of, 1775
therapy of, 1776
chronic, 1774–1775
clinical presentation of, 1774–1775
diagnostic studies for, 1775
etiology of, 1774
pathophysiology of, 1774
therapy of, 1775
with mitral regurgitation, 1778
with mitral stenosis, 1778
Aortic stenosis, 1773–1774
chest pain and, 1723
clinical presentation of, 1772
diagnostic studies for, 1773–1774
etiology of, 1772
with mitral regurgitation, 1778
with mitral stenosis, 1778
pathophysiology of, 1772
during pregnancy, 1394
therapy of, 1774
Aortocaval compression, during labor, 1431
Aortoenteric fistulas (AEFs), aortic
reconstructions and, 1185
diagnosis of, 1185
etiology of, 1185
incidence of, 1185
therapy of, 1185
Apathy, 2027–2028
characteristics of, 2027
in delirium, 2020
treatment of, 2027–2028
Aphasia, stroke and, 1991
Aplastic anemia, 2236
Aplastic crisis, in hemolytic anemia, 2235

Apnea
cardiopulmonary resuscitation and, 495
pressure support ventilation for, 725
Apoplexy, pituitary, 2113
Appendicitis, in HIV-infected patients,
1629–1630
Arbovirus infections
encephalitis due to, 1694
meningoencephalitis due to, 1647, 1647t
Arginine vasopressin
actions, indications, and dosing of, 2272
for diabetes insipidus, 421t, 2118
Arm examination, for femorofemoral and
axillofemoral bypass procedures, 1186
Arrhythmias, 227, 1781–1786. *See also specific
arrhythmias*
following cardiac surgery in adults, 1150
therapy of, 1150
following cardiac surgery in pediatric
patients, 1170–1171
in chronic renal failure, 2096–2097, 2097t
in cyclic antidepressant poisoning, 1490
diagnostic methods for
pacing techniques, 1783
physical examination, 1781
recording techniques and, 1783
vagal maneuvers, 1781, 1782t
ethanol intoxication and, 1513
immediate concerns with, 1781, 1782t
insecticide poisoning and, 1507
junctional, 1783
management of, 1785
lightning injuries and, 1541
management of, 1784–1786
following cardiac surgery, 1150
general principles for, 1784
in spinal cord injury, 1213–1214
in thyrotoxicosis, 2141
in organ donors, 1294
outcome after out-of-hospital cardiac arrest
and, 151, 151f, 152, 152f, 152t, 153f
during pregnancy, 1397
respiratory failure and, 1927–1928
in rhabdomyolysis, 2198
in spinal cord injury, treatment of, 1213–1214
thermodilution and, 894
following thoracic surgery, 1145
in thyrotoxicosis, treatment of, 2141
tracheal intubation causing, 768
waveform analysis in, central venous catheters
for, 852–853
Arsenic
inhalation injury due to, 1955
poisoning by, antidote for, 1465t
Arterial air embolism, 1906–1907
Arterial blood gases (ABGs). *See also* Blood gas
analysis
arterial catheters for measurement of, 852
in asthma, 1936
in pulmonary embolism, 1895
Arterial cannulation, 538–542
peripheral, 539–542, 540t
complications of, 541t, 541–542
insertion techniques for, 540–541
of pulmonary artery, 538–539
complications of, 539

indications for, 538, 538t
insertion technique for, 538–539, 539f
Arterial catheter(s), 850–852
arterial blood sampling and, 852
in dysoxia, 339
indications for, 850
infection related to, 1581
insertion of. *See* Arterial cannulation
peripheral, following thoracic surgery, 1134
positive end-expiratory pressure effects and,
851f, 851–852
physiologic significance of, 851–852
for preoperative assessment, 1005, 1005t
pressure measurements using, 850
waveform analysis and, 850–851
contour changes and, 850f, 850–851
stroke volume analysis and, 851
Arterial catheter armboards, infections associated
with, 2211, 2211f
Arterial cholesterol embolism, 1907
Arterial disorders. *See also specific disorders*
in pancreatitis, surgical treatment of,
2059–2060
Arterial embolism, 1905–1907
air, 1905
cholesterol, 1907
fat, 1907
Arterial injuries, with fractures, management
of, 1188
Arterial oxygenation. *See* Blood gas analysis,
arterial oxygenation and
Arterial pH
during cardiopulmonary resuscitation, 935
evaluation of, 921, 922t
Arterial thrombosis, tourniquets and, 1246
Arterial venous cannulation, 537
Arterial venous oxygen content difference, 916
Arterial volume clamp method, for blood pressure
measurement, 873
Arteriography
pulmonary, for pulmonary embolism, 587–588
in vascular trauma, 1187
with extremity injuries, 1187
with thoracic and neck injuries, 1187
Arteriovenous block, 1784
Arteriovenous fistulas, management of, 1188
Arteritis
Takayasu's, 2160
temporal, 2160
Arthritis
rheumatoid. *See* Rheumatoid arthritis (RA)
septic, staphylococcal, 1660–1661
Arthroplasty
hip, complications of, 1234–1235
knee, complications of, 1235
shoulder, complications of, 1235
Artificial airways
aspiration pneumonitis and, 1869
esophageal obturator, 493, 494f, 763, 763f
laryngeal mask, 493, 494, 495f, 764, 764f, 765f
nasal, 763
in cardiopulmonary resuscitation, 493
nasopharyngeal, for diarrhea, 2212
oropharyngeal, 763
in cardiopulmonary resuscitation, 493
pharyngeal tracheal lumen, 763

Artificial hearts, 611–612
  following cardiac surgery, 1159
Ascites
  in cirrhosis. *See* Cirrhosis
  following hepatic resection, 1126
  paracentesis in, 561–562
Aseptic meningitis, clinical presentation and
      initial diagnostic measures for, 1637
A Severity Characterization of Trauma
      (ASCOT), 55
Aspartate, for head injury, 1206
Aspergillomas, 1688
Aspergillus infections, 1688
  Aspergillus fumigatus, in renal transplant
      recipients, 1612
  in bone marrow transplant recipients, 1614
  following lung and heart-lung transplantation,
      1323
Asphyxiants. *See also specific substances*
  inhalation injury due to, 1952–1953
Aspiration (diagnostic and therapeutic)
  fine-needle, in pneumonia, 1853
  for pneumothorax, 1963
  transthoracic
    for diagnosis of pneumonia, 1577
    in pneumonia, 1853
  transtracheal, 580–581
    complications of, 581
    procedure for, 580, 580f, 581f
Aspiration (pathologic), 1861–1872
  acidic liquid volume and, 1863
  acute, 1864, 1864t
  of blood, 1863
  chest radiography in, 1864–1865, 1865f
  chronic, 1864, 1864f
  diagnostic tests and procedures for, 1862
  of foreign bodies, fiberoptic bronchoscopy in,
      696–697
  of gastric contents
    enteral nutrition and, 469
    in obstetric patients, 1414, 1414t, 1868–1869
    perioperative, 1007
    prevention of, 1009
    following thoracic surgery, 1137
    tracheal intubation causing, 768
  of hydrocarbons, 1863–1864
  infections in, treatment of, 1868
  major problems with, 1861
  management of, 1865–1868
    antibiotics for, 1868
    bronchodilators for, 1866, 1866t
    corticosteroids for, 1866
    emesis or lavage for, 1866
    fluids for, 1866
    initial therapy for, 1862
    respiratory support for, 1866–1868, 1867f,
      1867t
  particulate
    nonobstructive, 1863
    obstructive, 1862
  pneumonia due to, 1678
  prevention of, 1868t, 1868–1872
    at-risk factors and, 1868–1869, 1869f, 1870t
    mechanical measures for, 1870
    medical methods for, 1870f, 1870–1872,
      1871t

surgical methods for, 1872
  pulmonary, acute respiratory distress syndrome
      and, 1826–1827
  stress points with, 1861
  of water, in near-drowning, 1863
Aspiration pneumonia, 1861. *See also*
      Aspiration (pathologic)
  anaerobic, 1678
Aspirin. *See also* Salicylates
  in acute myocardial infarction, 1727–1728,
      1728f
  for antiplatelet therapy, 613–614, 614t, 615f
  for intestinal transplantation, 1361
  for multivisceral transplantation, 1361
  platelet defects due to, 2228
Asplenia
  pathogens associated with, 1556t
  prevention of bacterial meningitis in, 1643
Assist control ventilation (ACV), 750–751
  advantages of, 751
  disadvantages of, 751
  initial settings for, 751
  for respiratory failure, 1926
  setup parameters for, 750–751, 751f
  work of breathing and, 751
Assisted suicide, 113–114
Assisted ventilation. *See* Patient-triggered
      ventilation
Asthma, 1931–1943
  admission decisions with, 1936, 1936t
  chest pain and, 1724
  diagnosis of, 1934–1936
    differential diagnosis and, 1934–1935, 1935t
    laboratory and radiographic data for,
      1935–1936
    objective measurement of obstruction and,
      1935
    signs and symptoms and, 1935
    tests and procedures for, 1931
  fiberoptic bronchoscopy in, 698
  major problems with, 1931
  mechanical ventilation for. *See* Mechanical
      ventilation, for asthma
  noninvasive positive-pressure ventilation for,
      1942
  nontraditional, 1943
  in obstetric patients, 1415
  pathophysiology and pulmonary function in,
      1932–1934
  status asthmaticus in, fiberoptic bronchoscopy
      in, 698
  stress points with, 1931
  therapy of, 1936–1939
    beta-adrenergic agents for, 1936–1937
    helium-oxygen mixtures for, 1939
    inhaled anticholinergics for, 1937–1938
    initial, 1931–1932, 1932f–1934f
    magnesium sulfate for, 1939
    precipitating factors and, 1939
    steroids for, 1938–1939
    theophylline for, 1938, 1938t
    treatment priorities for, 1942–1943
  tracheal intubation in, 1939–1942
    for aerosol delivery, 1940
    mechanical ventilation and, 1939–1942,
      1940f

sedation for, 1940
Asystole, 1784
Atelectasis
  absorption
    denitrogenation, 930
    oxygen therapy and, 707
  fiberoptic bronchoscopy in, 689, 690f, 691, 691f
  tube thoracostomy as cause of, 560
Atherosclerotic disease, clinical features of, 1178
Atlantoaxial subluxation, in rheumatoid arthritis,
      1244f, 1244–1245
Atmosphere, in aircraft, 806, 806f, 806t
Atovaquone, for *Pneumocystis carinii* infections,
      in HIV-infected patients, 1620t
Atracurium, 829, 830t
  actions, indications, and dosing of, 2268
Atrial arrhythmias. *See also specific arrhythmias*
  in advanced heart failure, as prognostic
      factor, 1755
Atrial fibrillation, 1783
  following cardiac surgery in pediatric
      patients, 1171
  cardioversion for, 575, 576f
  ethanol intoxication and, 1513
  management of, 1785
  during pregnancy, 1397
  warfarin for, 621–622, 622f
Atrial flutter, 1783
  following cardiac surgery in pediatric
      patients, 1171
  cardioversion for, 575, 576f
Atrial mitral insufficiency, cardiogenic shock
      and, 393–394
Atrial natriuretic peptide, neurohormonal
      activation in advanced heart failure
      and, 1753
Atrial septal defect (ASD), during pregnancy,
      1395
Atrial tachycardia
  ectopic, 1783
    diagnosis of, 1783
    management of, 1785
  multifocal (chaotic), 1783
    management of, 1785
  paroxysmal, 1783
    cardioversion for, 575, 575f
    diagnosis of, 1783
Atropine
  for arrhythmias, 1785
  for cardiopulmonary resuscitation, 502
    complications of, 502
    dosage of, 502
    indications for, 502
  for esophageal obstruction, 2072
  for fiberoptic bronchoscopy, 688–689
  for neuromuscular blocking agent reversal, 835,
      835t, 1032t
  poisoning by, antidote for, 1465t
  for poisonings, 1467t
    beta-blockers and, 1497
    insecticides and, 1506
  for scorpion stings, 1533t
Attending physicians, 36
Attention deficits, in delirium, 2020
Auscultation
  of acute abdomen, 1102

in cardiac assessment, 870
in pulmonary assessment, 869
Austin-Flint murmurs, 1775
Autoimmune adrenalitis, 2123
Autoimmune hemolytic anemia (AIHA),
    2231–2233
  in systemic lupus erythematosus, 2170
Automaticity, 228
Autonomic dysfunction
  in Guillain-Barré syndrome, 2009
    treatment of, 2010
  lightning injuries and, 1541
Autonomic innervation, cardiovascular, in
    children, 1163
Autonomy, 23, 25
  informed consent and, 85–86
  as medicomoral principle, 67
Auto positive end-expiratory pressure (auto
    PEEP)
  airway resistance and, 197–198
  in asthma, 1941–1942
  fiberoptic bronchoscopy for, 684
  treatment of, in dysoxia, 341
Autopsy correlation, as continuous quality
    improvement indicator, 173, 175, 175t
Autotransfusion, 648, 663–665
  normovolemic hemodilution and, 664
  predonation for, 664
    advantages of, 664
    complications of, 664
    recommendations for, 664
    risk and cost-benefit ratios for, 664
  salvage of shed blood for, 664–665
    complications of, 665
    indications for, 664–665
    methodology for, 665
Axillary catheters
  insertion of, 540t, 541
  for peripheral nerve blocks, 813
Axillofemoral bypass, 1186
  arm examination for, 1186
  brachial plexus injury and, 1186
  graft tunnels for, 1186
  mortality and, 1186
  positioning for, 1186
Azathioprine (Imuran), 312t
  adverse effects of, 2156t–2157t
  for autoimmune hemolytic anemia, in systemic
    lupus erythematosus, 2170
  for bullous pemphigoid, 2184
  for heart-lung transplantation, 1317, 1319t,
    1320
  for heart transplantation, 1335, 1336
  for liver transplantation, 1345
  long-term, problems with, 1308
  for lung transplantation, 1317, 1319t, 1320
  for renal transplantation, 1304, 1306
  for simultaneous pancreas/kidney
    transplantation, 1314
Azoles, 1570. *See also specific drugs*
Azotemia
  acute, differential diagnosis of, 2081–2084,
    2083t, 2084f, 2084t
  acute renal failure differentiated from, 2082,
    2084t
  following bone marrow transplantation, 1374

hemolytic uremic syndrome and, 2239
platelet disorders due to, 2094, 2094t, 2229
postrenal, 2083–2084, 2084f, 2084t
prerenal, 2081–2083, 2084t
Aztreonam, 1567
  cost and initial dosage of, 1562t
  for infective endocarditis, 1796t
Azygous vein, in congestive heart failure, chest
    radiography and, 962, 963f

Baby K decision, 114, 115
Baby L decision, 114
Bacillus infections, 1668
Back, definition of, 1077
Backyard barbecue syndrome. *See* Esophageal
    obstruction
Baclofen poisoning, antidote for, 1465t
Bacteremia
  anaerobic, 1678
  definition of, 406t
  in HIV-infected patients, 1627
  in pyelonephritis, 1651
  staphylococcal, 1657–1658
    Staphylococcus aureus endocarditis
      differentiated from, 1792, 1792t
Bacterial infections, 1657–1682, 1658t. *See also*
    specific infections
  endocarditis. *See* Infective endocarditis
  endotoxins and, 407, 407t
  meningitis. *See* Meningitis, bacterial
  transfusion therapy and, 655
Bag-valve-mask ventilation, 495–496, 758–759,
    759f
  contraindications to, 759
Bainbridge reflex, 243f, 243–244
Balanced electrolyte solutions, 262
Barber decision, 71, 72–73, 112, 113, 115
Barbiturate(s). *See also specific drugs*
  for airway management, 762
  as anesthetics, 1022–1023, 1023t
  cardiorespiratory effects of, 1023
  neurologic effects of, 1023
  pharmacokinetics and pharmacodynamics of,
    1022–1023, 1023t
  for sedation, 825, 825t
Barbiturate coma
  for brain injury, 285–286, 1206
  for cerebral edema, in fulminant hepatic
    failure, 2049
Barium enema, in fulminant colitis and toxic
    megacolon, 2067
Barotrauma. *See* Pneumothorax; Pulmonary
    barotrauma (PBT)
Barrier protection, 1631
Bartling v Superior Court, 68, 70–71
Bartonella (Rochalimaea) infections, 1679
Bases. *See also* Acid-base balance; pH
  chemistry of, 255–256
  excess/deficit of, 926–927
    estimating excess and, 927, 927t
  ingestion of. *See* Corrosive injuries, esophageal
Basic disinfection, 510
Basic life support, 492
Basilar artery thrombosis, coma and, 1977
Basilic vein, cutdown of, 570, 574f

Baxter formula, 1267–1268, 1268f
Beds, 2212–2214
  active, low air loss, 2213
  air fluidized, 2213
  for obesity, 2214
  rotational therapy, 2214
  static
    low air loss, 2213
    steep Fowler's position, 2213–2214
  transport, 793
Bedside care, 29
Bee stings, anaphylaxis and, 1545, 1546t, 1548
Behavioral disturbances, 2017–2029
  consultations for, 2024, 2024t
  delirium. *See* Delirium
  initial diagnosis, testing, and therapy of, 2018,
    2019f, 2019t
  major problems with, 2017, 2018f
  psychosis
    intensive care, 93
    sedation for, 823
  sedation for, 822–823, 823t
  stress points with, 2017
  without cognitive dysfunction, 2024–2028
    agitation, 2025–2026
    anxiety, 2025t, 2025–2026
    apathy, 2027–2028
    characteristics of, 2024f, 2024–2025
    dependency, 2028
    depression, 2026t, 2026–2027
    hostility, 2028
    refusal to cooperate, 2028
Belief systems, treatment decisions and, 75
Bellows, of mechanical ventilators, 714t, 715f
Beneficence, 22, 24–25
  informed consent and, 85
  physician aid-in-dying and, 77–78
Bentley autotransfusion system, 665
Benzodiazepines, 823–825. *See also specific drugs*
  for agitation and anxiety, 2025, 2026t
  for airway management, 762
  as anesthetics, 1025
  cardiorespiratory effects of, 1025
  efficacy of, 824, 824t, 825t
  for ethanol withdrawal, 1514
  for fiberoptic bronchoscopy, 688
  neurologic effects of, 1025
  parenteral, 824–825
  pharmacokinetics and pharmacodynamics of,
    1025
  poisoning by, 1495–1496
    antidote for, 1465t
    toxicology and clinical manifestations of,
      1495
    treatment of, 1495–1496
  reversal with flumazenil, 825
  safety of, 824
  for sedation, 823–825
  for seizures
    in brain injury, 286
    in hyperthermia, 1457
  site of action of, 823–824
  tolerance and dependence on, 484
Benztropine mesylate (Cogentin)
  for agitation and anxiety, 2026
  for neuroleptic malignant syndrome, 828

Benzylisoquinolines, 829, 830t. *See also specific drugs*

Benzylpenicillin, for necrotizing fasciitis, 2192

Best interest standard, 121

Beta-adrenergic agents, for asthma, 1936–1937

Beta-adrenergic agonists. *See also specific drugs*
    for acute respiratory failure, 1920t, 1920–1921

Beta-blocking agents. *See also specific drugs*
    for acute myocardial infarction, 1734t, 1734–1735
    for arrhythmias, 1784
    for cardiopulmonary resuscitation, 504
        complications of, 504
        dosage of, 504
        indications for, 504
    for dilated cardiomyopathy, 1763
    for limitation of infarct size, 396–397
    poisoning by, 1496–1497
        antidote for, 1465t
        clinical manifestations of, 1497
        toxicology and, 1496–1497
        treatment of, 1497
    for Raynaud's phenomenon, 2159
    for theophylline poisoning, 1500–1501
    for thyrotoxicosis, 2140

Beta-lactam antibiotics, 1567
    penicillins combined with, 1566

Bezold-Janish reflex, 243

Bias, in research studies, 7

Bicarbonate. *See also* Sodium bicarbonate
    deficiency of, estimating, 927, 927t
    excess of, 928

Bile, postoperative drainage of, 1111
    following cholecystectomy, 1127

Bilevel positive airway pressure (BIPAP), 747
    advantages of, 747
    disadvantages of, 747
    initial settings for, 747
    for respiratory failure, 1923
    setup parameters for, 747
    work of breathing and, 747

Biliary fistulas, postoperative, 1114, 1114t
    after cholecystectomy, 1128
    hepatic injuries and, 1087
    following hepatic resection, 1126

Biliary obstruction
    in pancreatitis, surgical treatment of, 2060–2061
    ultrasonography in, 977–978, 981f

Biliary surgery, postoperative ICU care for, 1111

Biliary tract. *See also* Hepatobiliary disease; *specific disorders*
    injuries to, extrahepatic, 1090–1091

Biliary tubes, postoperative abdomen and, 1116f, 1117

Bilirubin, hepatic graft function assessment and optimization and, 1346, 1346f

Bilomas, drainage of, 594

Binasal pharyngeal airway (BNPA), 763

Binding-insensitive drugs, 482

Binding-sensitive drugs, 482

Bioavailability, of drugs, 478
    in renal disease, 478

Bioimpedence, for cardiac output determination, 883–884, 884f

Biopsy. *See specific types of biopsies*

Biostatistics. *See* Statistics

Biotin, requirement for, 464, 464t

Bitolterol, preoperative, 994t

Black widow spider bites, 1528f, 1528t, 1528–1530, 1530t

Bladder function, alterations in, 2212

Bladder injuries
    blunt, 1258–1259, 1259f
    with pelvic fractures, 1059
    penetrating, 1261

Bladder injury scale, 2278t

Blastomyces dermatitidis infections, 1688–1689

Bleeding. *See* Gastrointestinal bleeding; Hemorrhage

Blinding, in research studies, 5

Blindness, monocular, stroke and, 1991

Blisters, fracture, 1227

Blood. *See also* Hematologic disorders; *specific blood cells; specific disorders*
    aspiration of, 1863
    autologous donation of. *See* Autotransfusion
    coagulation of. *See* Anticoagulant agents; Coagulation; Coagulation factors; Coagulopathy; Fibrinolysis; Hemostasis
    crossmatched, incomplete, 652
    drug-induced disorders of, 484
    in extracerebral spaces, coma and, 1976
    hemoglobin and. *See* Carboxyhemoglobin; Hemoglobin; Methemoglobin; Oxyhemoglobin
    loss of. *See also* Gastrointestinal bleeding; Hemorrhage
        passive, 665–666
        scoliosis correction and, 1233
        total hip arthroplasty and, 1235
    rheological alterations of, 2241
        serum protein abnormalities and, 2241
    Rh-negative, hyperimmune anti-D globulin for, 1425
    shed, salvage of, 664–665
        complications of, 665
        indications for, 664–665
        methodology for, 665
    shock and, 372
    transfused, age of, 652
    in urine
        in sickle cell anemia, 2234
        following simultaneous pancreas/kidney transplantation, 1313
    viscosity of, maneuvers to increase cerebral blood flow and, 285
    volume of
        deficit of. *See* Hypovolemia
        excess of. *See* Hypervolemia
        hemoglobin concentration and, 645–646

Blood cultures, in infective endocarditis, 1791

Blood flow. *See also* Circulation
    cerebral. *See* Cerebral blood flow (CBF)
    endocardial, reduction of, spontaneous breathing and, 740
    peripheral, neural control of, 244–245
    pulmonary. *See* Pulmonary blood flow
    to spinal cord, interruption of, 818
    splanchnic. *See* Gastrointestinal system

Blood gas(es). *See also specific gases*
    arterial

arterial catheters for measurement of, 852
    in asthma, 1936
    in pulmonary embolism, 1895
    composition of, 199
    in dysoxia, 339
    mixed venous blood sampling for, 859–860

Blood gas analysis, 921–938
    in aberrant intracellular metabolism, 934
    in acute respiratory failure, 926
        respiratory alkalosis with hypoxemia and, 926
        respiratory alkalosis without hypoxemia and, 926
    arterial oxygenation and, 923–924
        hemoglobin-oxygen affinity and, 923, 924f
        hypoxemia assessment and, 923–924
        oxygen content calculation and, 923, 923t
        oxyhemoglobin measurement and, 923
    for assessment of oxygenation, 928–929
        alternatives to shunt calculation for, 929, 929t
        interpretive guidelines for, 929
        lungs as oxygenators and, 928–929
        shunt calculation and, 929
    capnography and, 931–932
        end-tidal and arterial $PaCO_2$ and, 931
        trending dead space ventilation and, 931–932, 932f
    carbon dioxide stores and, 932–933
        in acute alveolar hyperventilation-on-chronic ventilatory failure, 933
        in acute-on-chronic ventilatory failure, 933
        central, 932
        peripheral, 932t, 932–933
    in carbon monoxide poisoning, 933–934
    cardiopulmonary resuscitation and low flow states and, 934–936
        acid-base balance and, 935
        arterial blood gases and, 935
        bicarbonate administration and, 935–936
        venous blood gases and, 935
    in hypoxemia and oxygen therapy, 929–930
        denitrogenation absorption atelectasis and, 930
        hypoxic pulmonary vasoconstriction and, 930
    interpretive guidelines for, 921–922
        evaluation of arterial PaO_2 and, 921–922, 922t, 923t
        evaluation of arterial pH and $PaCO_2$ and, 921, 922t
    in metabolic acid-base imbalances, 926–928
        acid-base physiology and, 926–927
        acidemia, 927–928
        alkalemia, 928
        electrolyte abnormalities and, 928
        lactic acidosis, 934
        specific therapy and, 928
    parameters derived from, 849t, 851
    parenteral hyperalimentation and, 934
    preoperative, 1003
    pulse oximetry and, 931
    in sepsis, 934
    temperature correction and, 936t, 936–938
        clinical relevance of, 937
        definition of, 936
        physiologic considerations and, 936–937
        point of care analyzers and blood gas monitors and, 938

recommendations for, 937–938
tissue oxygenation and, 930–931
  mixed venous oxygen saturation and, 930
  oxygen delivery and, 930
  oxygen demand and, 931
  oxygen extraction and, 930, 930t
transcutaneous carbon dioxide electrode and, 932
transcutaneous oxygen electrode and, 932
ventilation and, 924–926
  acute ventilatory failure and, 925–926
  impending ventilatory failure and, 926
  physiology of, 924–925
  work of breathing and, 925
Blood pressure. *See also* Hypertension; Hypotension
arterial, following cardiac surgery, 1150
carotid/subclavian reconstructions and, 1182
in head injury, 1201
mean. *See* Mean arterial pressure (MAP); Mean pressure (MP)
proportional, in refractory advanced heart failure, 1758–1759
systolic, variation of, 851f, 851–852
Blood pressure measurement, 870–873
automated-continuous method for, 873
conventional manual technique for, 870–872
  cuff deflation and, 871
  cuff size and, 870–871
  Korotkoff sounds and, 871f, 871–872
  manometer calibration for, 871
  mean arterial pressure and, 872
Doppler techniques for, 872
invasive. *See* Arterial catheter(s); Central venous catheters; Invasive pressure monitoring; Pulmonary artery (PA) catheters
oscillometry for, 872f, 872–873, 873f
palpation for, 872
photoplethysmography for, 872
Blood product(s). *See also* Transfusion therapy; *specific blood products*
conservation of, as continuous quality improvement indicator, 170, 172, 175f
for sepsis, 410
Blood substitutes, 666
Blood transfusions. *See* Transfusion therapy
Blood urea nitrogen (BUN)
in hyperosmolar hyperglycemic nonketotic diabetes, 2107
in rhabdomyolysis, 2199
Blood vessels. *See also* Cardiovascular *entries*; Vascular *entries*; *specific vessels*
coagulation and, 266
Body fluids. *See also specific body fluids*
electrolyte composition of, 2258t
Body surface area (BSA), 861
Dubois nomogram and formula for, 2256t
Body temperature
following cardiac surgery in pediatric patients, 1171
extremes of. *See also* Fever; Hyperpyrexia; Hyperthermia; Hypothermia; Malignant hyperthermia (MH); Neuroleptic malignant syndrome
  major problems with, 1451

stress points with, 1451
maintenance of, during intrahospital transport, 794
in poisonings and toxic exposures, 1470
regulation of. *See* Thermoregulation
following thoracic surgery, 1136
Boerhaave's syndrome. *See* Esophageal perforation
Bone. *See also* Fracture(s); Musculoskeletal *entries*; Orthopedic complications; *specific disorders*
cryptococcal infections of, 1689
injuries to. *See also* Fracture(s); *specific sites*
  delayed diagnosis of, 1054, 2211
Bone marrow
aplastic anemia and, 2236
bacterial infections of, 2239
in sickle cell anemia, 2234
suppression of, thrombocytopenia due to, 2227
venous cannulation into, 537
Bone marrow transplantation (BMT), 1367–1380
acute graft versus host disease following, 1375–1377, 1376t
blood products for, 1369–1370, 1370t
cataracts following, 1379–1380
conditioning regimens for, 1367, 1368t
diarrhea following, 1371–1372
electrolytes and, 1369
engraftment and, 1374–1375, 1375t
fertility following, 1379
fever following, 1371
fluids and hypotension and, 1369
graft versus host disease following, chronic, 1377–1378, 1378t
growth and development following, 1379
heart failure following, 1373–1374
hypothyroidism following, 1379
infection prophylaxis for, 1370–1371
  for cytomegalovirus, 1377
infections following, 1613t, 1613–1614
  Epstein-Barr virus lymphoproliferative disease, 1377
  hemorrhagic cystitis, 1372
  herpes zoster, 1378
  late, 1614
  post-engraftment, 1613–1614
  pretransplant to engraftment, 1613
mucositis following, 1371
neutropenia following, 1371
pulmonary function following, 1380
relapse following, 1378–1379
renal function following, 1374, 1380
respiratory failure following, 1373
secondary malignancy following, 1378
stem cell harvest for, 1368–1369
stem cell infusion in, 1369
venoocclusive disease of liver following, 1372t, 1372–1373
Bone pain, in sickle cell anemia, 2234
Borrelia burgdorferi infections, 1682, 1708, 1709
Borreliosis, 1708–1709
Botulism, 1676
Bowel. *See* Intestinal *entries*; *specific intestinal disorders*
Box-jellyfish envenomations, 1533

Brachial artery cannulation, 540t, 541
Brachial plexus injuries, femorofemoral and axillofemoral bypass procedures and, 1186
diagnosis of, 1186
etiology of, 1186
incidence of, 1186
therapy of, 1186
Bradyarrhythmias, in cyclic antidepressant poisoning, 1491
Bradycardia
calcium channel blocker poisoning and, 1498
cardiac pacing for, 545
following cardiac surgery in pediatric patients, 1171
fetal, 1434
management of, 1784–1785
in poisonings and toxic exposures, 1471
during pregnancy, 1397
sinus, 1783
in spinal cord injury, treatment of, 1213–1214
Brain
abscesses of
  anaerobic, 1678
  clinical presentation and initial diagnostic measures for, 1638–1639
cerebrovascular disease and. *See* Cerebrovascular disease; Stroke; Transient ischemic attacks (TIAs)
edema of
  cerebral. *See* Cerebral edema
  in diabetic ketoacidosis, 2106
  insecticide poisoning and, 1507
  shock and, 359, 371
Brain death, 1291–1292
anencephaly and, 1292
cardiac arrest during evaluation for, 1298
consent for organ donation and, 1292, 1296
legal issues related to, 122–123
maternal, 1425–1426
persistent vegetative state and, 1292
Brain injuries, 273–287, 1198–1208
cardiovascular concerns during resuscitation and, 282–283
  hypertension, 282–283
  hypotension and fluid resuscitation, 282
coagulation disorders and, 1207
coma and. *See* Coma
computed tomography and diagnosis of emergent surgical lesions and, 279–280
cytoprotection for, 286–287
diagnosis of, 1200
  tests and procedures for, 273–274, 1196, 1196t
fluid and electrolyte problems and, 1206–1207
guidelines for intensive care and ICU admission for, 1200–1201
initial stabilization and, 278–279, 279t, 280t
intracranial pressure and. *See* Intracranial hypertension; Intracranial pressure (ICP)
intrahospital transport and, 789, 789t, 797, 800
long-term management problems with, 1207
major problems with, 273, 1195
maneuvers to increase cerebral blood flow and, 285

Brain injuries, maneuvers to increase cerebral blood flow and (*continued*)
  blood viscosity and intravascular volume and, 285
  iatrogenic hypotension and, 285
  maneuvers to increase metabolic demand and, 285–286
    barbiturate coma, 285–286
    seizures and, 286
    temperature regulation, 285
  maternal death due to, 1423
  mechanisms of, 274t, 274–278, 275f, 279t
    brain edema and, 278
    cerebral blood flow and, 276f, 276–277
    cerebral metabolism and, 277–278, 278t
    intracranial pressure and, 275f, 275–276
  metabolic concerns during resuscitation and, 283
  outcome after, 1207–1208, 1208t
  pathophysiology of, 1198–1200
    of herniation syndromes, 1199–1200
    of intracranial injuries, 1199
    intracranial pressure, volume, and blood flow and, 1198–1199
    of penetrating injuries, 1200
    of scalp lacerations, 1200
    of skull fractures, 1200
  penetrating
    antibiotic selection for neurologic infections in, 1641t
    pathophysiology of, 1200
  pharmacologic agents and intracranial pressure and, 280–281
  pulmonary concerns during resuscitation and, 281–282
    hypoxemia and abnormal ventilation, 281
    intubation and mechanical ventilation, 281–282
  stress points with, 273, 1195–1196
  treatment of, 1201–1206
    airway and, 1201, 1201f
    barbiturate coma for, 285–286, 1206
    blood pressure and, 1201
    central nervous system function monitoring and, 1203–1204
    general measures in, 1204–1205
    initial therapy for, 274, 1196–1197
    for intracranial hypertension, 1205
    intracranial pressure monitoring and, 1202–1203
    neurologic monitoring and, 1201–1202, 1202f
Brain stem evoked responses (BAERs), for monitoring cerebral function, 945f, 945–946
Brain stem lesions, coma and, 1976–1977
Breast feeding, following cardiac surgery in pediatric patients, 1174
Breath, in poisonings and toxic exposures, 1471
Breathing. *See also* Gas exchange; Respiratory *entries;* Ventilation; Ventilatory *entries*
  cardiopulmonary resuscitation and, 495–496
    apnea and, 495
    techniques for, 495–496
  in comatose patients, emergency evaluation of, 1971

discoordinate, 869
initial triage of trauma patients and, 1041–1042
pattern of, respiratory muscle loading and, 217t, 217–218, 218f
in poisonings and toxic exposures, 468
secondary triage of trauma patients and, 1048
spontaneous
  assisted, 218
  continuous positive airway pressure. *See* Continuous positive airway pressure (CPAP)
  positive end-expiratory pressure. *See* Positive end-expiratory pressure (PEEP), spontaneous
  side effects and complications of, 739–740
    hemodynamic, 739–740
work of. *See* Respiratory muscles, decreasing afterload of; Respiratory muscles, loading; Work of breathing (WOB)
Bretylium
  actions, indications, and dosing of, 2268
  for cardiopulmonary resuscitation, 503–504
    dosage of, 504
    indications for, 503
  dosing of
    for cardiopulmonary resuscitation, 504
    in chronic renal failure, 2097t
Bronchiectasis, in obstetric patients, 1415
Bronchiolitis obliterans (BO)
  following lung and heart-lung transplantation, 1323, 1325f
  lung and heart-lung transplantation and, management of, 1330
  in systemic lupus erythematosus, 2167, 2167t
Bronchiolitis obliterans organizing pneumonia (BOOP), in systemic lupus erythematosus, 2167, 2167t
Bronchitis, chronic
  definition of, 1918–1919
  in obstetric patients, 1415–1416
Bronchoalveolar lavage (BAL)
  for diagnosis of pneumonia, 693t, 693–694, 1576–1577, 1594
  lung and heart-lung transplantation and, 1327
Bronchodilators. *See also specific drugs*
  for acute respiratory distress syndrome, 1833
  for acute respiratory failure, 1920t, 1920–1922
  for aspiration syndromes, 1866, 1866t
  for asthma, 1937
  preoperative, 994, 994t
  response to, preoperative assessment of, 990
  surgical patients and, 1008
Bronchopleural fistulas
  fiberoptic bronchoscopy in, 696
  tube thoracostomy as cause of, 559–560
Bronchoscopy
  fiberoptic, 683–699, 687t, 688f, 689f, 698t
    in acute upper airway obstruction, 697–698
    anesthesia for, 687–689, 689t
    in atelectasis, 689, 690f, 691, 691f
    complications of, 684t, 684–686, 685t
    in foreign-body aspiration, 696–697
    in hemoptysis, 691–692, 692t
    immediate concerns with, 683–684
    in inhalation injury, 697, 1951
    in pneumonia, 692–695, 693t, 695t

    in status asthmaticus, 698
    in tracheobronchial trauma, 695t, 695–696
    in tuberculosis, 698–699
    lung and heart-lung transplantation and, 1326–1327
    in pneumonia, 692–695, 693t, 695t, 1853
Bronchospasm, in asthma. *See* Asthma
Bronchospirometry
  in inhalation injury, 1951
  lung and heart-lung transplantation and, 1327
  preoperative, 991, 1003
Brophy decision, 112, 115
Brown recluse spider bites, 1530–1532, 1531f, 1531t
Brucellosis, 1706–1707
Brudzinski sign, 1635
Bubonic plague, 1671–1672, 1708
Budd-Chiari syndrome, 1127
Buffers
  acid-base disorders and, 257–258
    metabolic acidosis, 261
  renal, 926
Bullet embolism, management of, 1188
Bullet wounds. *See* Trauma; *specific sites and injuries*
Bullous drug eruptions, 2188
Bullous pemphigoid, 2183–2184
  diagnosis of, 2183
  etiology of, 2183
  management of, 2183–2184
  presentation of, 2183, 2184f
Bumetanide
  actions, indications, and dosing of, 2268
  for respiratory failure, in chronic renal failure, 2097
Buprenorphine, for opiate withdrawal, 1518
Bupropion, side effects of, 2027t
Burns, 1265–1274
  bleeding disorders and, 1270–1271
    coagulopathies, 1270
    gastrointestinal hemorrhage and, 1270–1271
  cardiovascular problems with, 1267–1268
    hypertonic salt solutions for, 1268
    loss of intravascular volume and, 1267
    postresuscitation diuresis and, 1268
    resuscitation of burn shock and, 1267–1268, 1268f
  complications of resuscitation and, 1268–1269
    escharotomies and, 1269
    fluids and electrolytes and, 1269
    septic shock and, 1269
  diagnostic tests and procedures for, 1266
  electrolyte and acid-base problems and, 1269–1270
    serum potassium concentration disturbances and, 1270
    serum sodium concentration disturbances and, 1269–1270
  hypertensive emergencies and, 1819
  infections and, 1272–1273
    diagnosis of, 1272
    herpes simplex, 1695
    immunosuppression of burn injury and, 1272
    infection control and, 1272
    Pseudomonas aeruginosa, 1674
    treatment of, 1273

inhalation injury and, 1949–1950
initial therapy for, 1266
major problems with, 1265
nutritional support for, 1271–1272
  enteral, 1271
  estimation of caloric needs for, 1271, 1272t
  hypermetabolism of burns and, 1271
  parenteral, 1271
  protein repletion and, 1271–1272
  transition to oral feeding and, 1272
physiotherapy for, 1274
  heterotopic ossification and, 1274
  prevention of contractors and, 1274
psychosocial needs of patient and family and, 1274
  consciousness level and, 1274
  counseling and, 1274
  pain management and, 1274
renal failure and, 1270
  acute, 1270
  burn wound as "third kidney" and, 1270
respiratory problems with, 1266–1267
  carbon monoxide poisoning and, 1266
  indications for extubation and, 1266–1267
  indications for tracheostomy and, 1267
  maintenance of adequate air exchange and, 1266
  smoke inhalation and, 1266
  ventilation-perfusion problems and, 1267
stress points with, 1265–1266
team approach to, 1274
wound care for, 1273–1274
  depth of injury and, 1273
  excision of wound and, 1273
  topical treatment in, 1273–1274
Burn shock, resuscitation of, 1267–1268, 1268f
Busulfan, for bone marrow transplantation, 1368t

Cadmium, inhalation injury due to, 1955
Calcitonin, for hypercalcemia, 429t
  in cancer, 2246–2247
Calcium, 426–429
  deficiency of. *See* Hypocalcemia
  excess of. *See* Hypercalcemia
  functions of, 426
  metabolism of, disorders of, in spinal cord injury, 1215
  myocardial handling of, abnormalities of, 1750–1751
  regulation of, 426–428
    chelating agents and, 427
    parathyroid hormone and, 427
    vitamin D and, 427–428
  requirement for, 461t, 462
  for scorpion stings, 1533t
  serum level of, following cardiac surgery, 1154
Calcium administration
  for acute tumor lysis syndrome, 2248
  for hyperkalemia, 427t
  for hypocalcemia, 428t
  for salicylate poisoning, 1488
Calcium channel blocking agents. *See also specific drugs*
  for acute myocardial infarction, 1735–1736
  for brain injury, 286–287

for cardiopulmonary resuscitation, 504
  complications of, 504
  dosage of, 504
  indications for, 504
  for hypertension, following liver transplantation, 1345
  for limitation of infarct size, 396
  for pheochromocytomas, 2133, 2134t
  poisoning by, 1497–1498
    clinical manifestations of, 1497
    toxicology and, 1497
    treatment of, 1497–1498
Calcium chloride
  actions, indications, and dosing of, 2268
  actions and indications for, 2268
  for calcium channel blocker poisoning, 1498
  following cardiac surgery in pediatric patients, 1167t
  for cardiopulmonary resuscitation, 505
    complications of, 505
    dosage of, 505
    indications for, 505
  dosing of, 2268
    for cardiopulmonary resuscitation, 505
Calcium edetate, for lead poisoning, 1465t
Calcium gluconate
  actions, indications, and dosing of, 2268
  for black widow spider bites, 1530t
  following cardiac surgery in pediatric patients, 1167t
  poisoning by, antidote for, 1466t
Calibration, for invasive pressure monitoring, 841
Caloric needs, of burn patients, estimation of, 1271, 1272t
Campbell diagram, 213, 214f
Campylobacter fetus species *fetus* infections, 1669
Campylobacter jejuni infections, 1669
Cancer. *See* Malignancies; Oncologic emergencies; *specific malignancies*
Cancer chemotherapy
  for leukemia, bleeding caused by, 2228
  leukopenia due to, 2235–2236
  toxicity of, 2251
    cardiac, 2251
    pulmonary, 2251
Candida infections, 1685–1688
  clinical disease in, 1686–1688, 1687t
  disseminated, 1686
    diagnosis of, 1583
    nosocomial, 1583
    treatment of, 1583
  in HIV-infected patients, 1629
    treatment of, 1619t
  microbiology and pathogenesis of, 1685–1686
  oropharyngeal, 1686
    in HIV-infected patients, treatment of, 1619t
    treatment of, 2207
Capillaries
  permeability of, colloid fluid therapy and, 434
  pulmonary
    gas exchange in, 198, 198f
    integrity of, pulmonary fluid and protein homeostasis and, 204
Capnocytophaga infections, 1679–1680
Capnography, 931–932
  end-tidal and arterial Pco₂ and, 931

trending dead space ventilation and, 931–932, 932f
Capnometry, 877–883
  capnometric phases and, 878–879
  clinical applications of, 880–882
    for assessment of ventilatory adequacy, 880
    during cardiopulmonary resuscitation, 882, 882f
    causes of PaCO₂-PETCO₂ difference and, 880f, 880–881
    during transport, 881–882
  principles of, 877–880, 878f, 878t
    chemical indicators and, 878
    electronic monitoring and, 878–879
    Mapleson D breathing system and, 879, 879f
    in nonintubated patients, 879–880
Capreomycin, for *Mycobacterium tuberculosis* infections, in HIV-infected patients, 1620t
Captopril
  for acute myocardial infarction, 1737
  for heart failure, 1756
  for hypertension
    in hypertensive emergencies, 1819
    in hypertensive urgencies, 1820, 1820t
    for renal crisis, in systemic sclerosis, 2172
Carbamate poisoning
  antidote for, 1467t
  cholinergic syndrome and, 1504–1505
  clinical manifestations of, 1505
  treatment of, 1506–1507
Carbamazepine
  for diabetes insipidus, 421t
  therapeutic serum level of, 479t
Carbapenem, for infections in granulocytopenic patients, 1606
Carbohydrates. *See also specific arbohydrates*
  intolerance of, nutritional support and, 468
  metabolism of, in critical illness, 329t, 329–330, 330t
Carbon dioxide
  acid-base disorders and, 257
  arterial pressure of
    during cardiopulmonary resuscitation, 935
    in dysoxia, 340
    evaluation of, 921, 922t
    temperature correction and, 937
  central control of ventilation and, 204
  decreased arterial level of, during brain resuscitation, 281
  end-tidal concentration of, termination of cardiopulmonary resuscitation and, 159
  excess of. *See* Hypercapnia
  extracorporeal removal of, with venovenous bypass, 753
  inhalation injury due to, 1952
  measurement of. *See* Capnometry
  stores of, 932–933
    central, 932
    peripheral, 932t, 932–933
Carbon-11 hydroxyephedrine, for pheochromocytoma localization, 2132–2133
Carbon monoxide
  inhalation injury due to, 1952
  poisoning by, 784

Carbon monoxide, poisoning by (*continued*)
   blood gas analysis in, 933–934
   with burns, 1266
   severity of, 784
   treatment of, 784
Carboplatin, for bone marrow transplantation,
      1368t
Carboxyhemoglobin
   in inhalation injury, 1951
   pulse oximetry and, 875
Cardiac arrest
   cardiopulmonary resuscitation for. *See*
      Cardiopulmonary resuscitation
   as continuous quality improvement indicator,
      168t, 170
   in-hospital, 155f, 155–157
      age as predictive factor for outcome of
         cardiopulmonary resuscitation and, 157
      factors during resuscitation predicting
         increased mortality and, 156, 156t
      factors predicting mortality after successful
         resuscitation and, 156–157
      influence on in-hospital location of cardiac
         arrest on survival and, 157
      prearrest medical conditions predicting
         increased mortality and, 156
      survival and functional status after hospital
         discharge and, 157
   in organ donors, 1294, 1298
      during evaluation for brain death, 1298
      sudden, in previously relatively healthy
         patients, 1298
   out-of-hospital, 150–155
      bystander cardiopulmonary resuscitation
         and, 152–154, 153t
      cardiac rhythm and, 151, 151f, 152t
      community emergency medical services
         system and, 150–151, 151f
      hospital course and, 154, 154t
      location of, 154
      survival after hospital discharge and,
         154–155
      time to definitive care and resuscitation and,
         154, 154f
      ventricular fibrillatory waveform amplitude
         and postcountershock rhythm and, 152,
         152f, 153f
      witnessed versus unwitnessed, 152
Cardiac arrhythmias. *See* Arrhythmias; *specific
      arrhythmias*
Cardiac assist devices. *See also* Intraaortic balloon
      pump (IABP); Ventricular assist
      devices (VADs)
   synchronized coronary venous retroperfusion
      and, 611
Cardiac compliance
   following cardiac surgery, 1148–1149
      cardiovascular changes and, 1149
      time course of changes in, 1148–1149
   left ventricular, reduced, waveform analysis
      in, 858
Cardiac compression, closed chest, 496–497
   in adults, 496
   in children, 496
   complications of, 497
   compression rate for, 496–497

   with single rescuer, 497
   with two rescuers, 496–497
   effectiveness of, 496, 497
      compression-relaxation cycle and, 496
      G-suits and, 496
Cardiac contractility
   following cardiac surgery, 1152–1153
      drug therapy to augment, 1152–1153, 1153f
   contractile reserve and, in advanced heart
      failure, as prognostic factor, 1754
   determination of, 862
   inhalational anesthetics and, 1017
   intrinsic regulation of, 233–234
   myocardial, inhalational anesthetics and, 1017
Cardiac contraction, 231–233, 236–241
   in intact heart, 233
   in isolated muscle preparations, 231f–233f,
      231–233
   pressure-flow relations and, 240f, 240–241
   pressure-volume relations and, 236–240,
      237f–240f
Cardiac contusions, 1140f, 1140–1141
Cardiac disorders. *See also specific disorders*
   chemotherapy toxicity as cause of, 2251
   congenital heart disease, during pregnancy,
      1394–1395
      left-to-right shunt and, 1395
      right-to-left shunt and, 1395
   pheochromocytomas and, 2135
   right-sided, following cardiac surgery in
      pediatric patients, 1168–1169
      pulmonary hypertension and, 1168, 1169t
      therapy of, 1168–1169
   scoliosis correction and, 1233
   shock and, 359–360
Cardiac electrical activity, 227–231
   action potentials and, 227–229
      automaticity and, 228
      depolarization and repolarization and,
         227–228, 228f
      refractoriness and excitability and, 228–229
   excitation-contraction coupling and, 229t,
      229–231
      ultrastructural changes and, 229–231, 230f,
         231f
   impulse conduction and, 229
Cardiac function
   assessment of, 869–870
      auscultation in, 870
      inspection in, 869–870
      palpation in, 870
   in hypokalemia, 423–424
   intrinsic regulation of. *See* Cardiovascular
      physiology, intrinsic regulation of
      cardiac function and
   in obese surgical patients, 1278
   postoperative ICU care and, 1110
Cardiac index, 861, 1153
Cardiac injuries, blunt, 1052
Cardiac injury scale, 2280t
Cardiac ischemia
   chest pain and, 1722–1723
   myocardial
      following cardiac surgery, 1149
      hypertensive emergencies and, 1817–1818
      myocardial metabolism and, 251, 252f

Cardiac monitoring, vascular surgery and, 1178,
      1179t
Cardiac output (CO), 861
   anesthetic uptake from lungs and, 1016
   bioimpedance-determined, 883–884, 884f
   capnometry for determination of, 882
   following cardiac surgery, 1153–1154
   continuous thermodilution for measurement
      of, 895
   Doppler-determined, 883
   dye dilution for measurement of, 895
   Fick technique for measurement of, 895
   illness and, inhalational anesthetic uptake and
      distribution and, 1017
   pulmonary artery catheters for measurement
      of, 860
   right ventricular ejection fraction for
      measurement of, 895
   in shock, 377t
   stress response and, 1028
   thermodilution for determination of. *See*
      Thermodilution
Cardiac pacing
   for arrhythmias, 1783, 1785
   following cardiac surgery
      in adult patients, 1150–1151
      in pediatric patients, 1170
   external pacemakers for, 547–548, 548f, 549f
   permanent pacemakers for, following cardiac
      surgery in pediatric patients, 1171
   pulmonary artery catheters for, 861
   temporary, 545–552
      electrode catheters and external pacemaker
         units for, 546–549, 547f–549f
      external noninvasive approach for, 552, 552f
      for heart transplantation, 1337
      indications for, 545–546, 546t
      initial therapy for, 545
      major problems with, 545
      prophylactic, 546
      stress points with, 545
      transthoracic, 551f, 551–552
      transvenous, 548–551
   transvenous. *See* Transvenous cardiac pacing
Cardiac rhythm. *See also* Arrhythmias
   following cardiac surgery, 1150–1151
      in adult patients, 1150–1151
      in pediatric patients, 1165, 1165f, 1166f
   inhalational anesthetics and, 1017–1018
   outcome after out-of-hospital cardiac arrest
      and, 151, 151f, 152t
Cardiac surgery. *See also specific procedures*
   for cardiogenic shock, 401–402
   for infective endocarditis, 1793, 1796, 1798t
   postoperative management of adult patients
      and, 1147–1160
      antibiotic therapy in, 1159–1160
      arterial blood pressure and, 1150
      bleeding and, 1155–1156
      cardiac output and, 1153–1154
      catheter sepsis and, 1159
      central nervous system sequelae and, 1157
      contractility and, 1152–1153, 1153f
      diagnostic tests and procedures for, 1148
      diuretic therapy for, 1156

during first 8 postcardiopulmonary bypass hours, 1148
heart rate and rhythm and, 1150–1151
initial therapy for, 1148
major problems with, 1147
mechanical cardiac assistance and, 1158–1159
mixed venous saturation and, 1154
during next 16 postcardiopulmonary bypass hours, 1148–1149
nitroprusside toxicity and, 1158, 1158f, 1159f
pancreatitis and, 1159
renal failure and, 1156–1157
during second 24 postcardiopulmonary bypass hours, 1149
sedation and paralysis and, 1157–1158
serum ionized calcium and potassium and, 1154–1155
serum lactic acid/lactate and, 1154
stress points with, 1147–1148
during third 24 postcardiopulmonary bypass hours, 1149–1150
urine output and, 1155
ventilatory, 1156
ventricular afterload and, 1152
ventricular preload and, 1151f, 1151–1152
postoperative management of pediatric patients and, 1161–1175
bleeding and, 1173
cardiac rhythm and pacing and, 1170–1171
cardiac rhythm and rate and, 1165, 1165f, 1166f
cardiac tamponade and, 1173
chylous collections and, 1173
complete repair and, 1163, 1163t
diagnostic tests, procedures, and therapy for, 1162
diastolic function and, 1165
echocardiography and Doppler studies and, 1174–1175
fluid replacement and, 1164–1165
infections and, 1171–1172
inotropes for, 1166, 1166f, 1167t–1168t, 1168
laboratory values and, 1170
limb ischemia and, 1172–1173
major problems with, 1161
nutritional, 1173–1174
palliative procedures and, 1163–1164
physiologic differences in children and, 1162–1163
renal failure and, 1172
respiratory, 1169–1170
right-sided heart dysfunction and, 1168–1169, 1169t
sedation and paralysis and, 1171
stress points with, 1162
temperature and, 1171
tissue oxygen delivery and, 1164
transplantation and, 1175
vasodilators and, 1166
ventilator weaning and extubation and, 1174
during pregnancy, 1397–1398
pregnancy after, 1398
Cardiac tamponade, 1805–1808
in cancer, 2250

following cardiac surgery in pediatric patients, 1173
cardiogenic shock and, 395
in chronic renal failure, 2095
clinical features of, 1806–1807, 1807f, 1808f
echocardiography in, 885
pericardial, waveform analysis in, central venous catheters for, 853
pericardiocentesis for, 577
in trauma patients, 1051
thoracic trauma and, 1142
treatment of, 1807–1808
Cardiac transplantation, 1333–1339. *See also* Heart-lung transplantation (HLT)
current status of, 1290
hemodynamic assessment for, 1333–1334
heterotopic, for heart failure, 1762
initial ICU management for, 1336–1339
acute rejection and, 1338
diagnostic tests and procedures for, 1339
drug toxicity and, 1338
hypertension and, 1338
infection and, 1338–1339
inotropic support in, 1336
primary graft dysfunction and, 1336–1337
right ventricular failure and, 1337
stress points with, 1339
temporary pacing and, 1337
initial postoperative management and, 1334–1335
immunosuppression and, 1334–1335
intracerebral, 1333
major problems with, 1335–1336
organ allocation for, 1297
in pediatric patients, 1175
Cardiac valves, prosthetic
endocarditis of, 1661–1662
staphylococcal, 1659
placement of, warfarin for, 622
Cardiogenic shock, 366, 389–403, 391f
acute myocardial infarction and, 1737, 1738
adjunctive and experimental management techniques for, 380
clinical manifestations of, 395
diagnostic tests and procedures for, 389
etiology of, 390–395, 391t
left ventricular acute myocardial infarction and, 390–392, 391t
mechanical defects and, 393t, 393–395
right ventricular infarction and, 392–393
major problems with, 389
right ventricular infarct and, 366
adjunctive and experimental management techniques for, 380
stress points with, 389
therapy of, 395–403
adjunctive and experimental management techniques for, 380
assist devices for, 402–403
initial, 389–390
inotropic agents in, 398f, 398–401
pharmacologic limitation of infarct size and, 395–397
surgical, 401–402
thrombolytic, 397–398
Cardiomyopathy

dilated, beta-blocking agents for, 1763
ischemic, in systemic sclerosis, 2172
peripartum, 1395–1396
clinical considerations in, 1396
Cardiomyoplasty, for heart failure, 1762
Cardiopulmonary assessment, 867–895
alarm capabilities and, 868
blood pressure measurement. *See* Blood pressure measurement
capnometry in. *See* Capnometry
of cardiac output. *See* Cardiac output (CO)
clinical, 868–870, 870t
cardiac, 869–870
pulmonary, 868–869
costs of, 868
data acquisition for, 868
echocardiography in. *See* Echocardiography
electrocardiography in. *See* Electrocardiography (ECG)
pulse oximetry in. *See* Pulse oximetry
risks of, 868
thermodilution in. *See* Thermodilution
user involvement in, 867–868
Cardiopulmonary bypass (CPB). *See also* Cardiac surgery
postoperative bleeding due to, 1072–1073, 1073f
for pulmonary embolism, 1901
weaning time following, as continuous quality improvement indicator, 172
Cardiopulmonary disorders. *See also specific disorders*
electrical injuries and, 1539
in systemic sclerosis, 2172–2173
Cardiopulmonary function
assessment of. *See* Cardiopulmonary assessment
during pregnancy, at term, 316–317
scoliosis correction and, 1232–1233
blood loss and, 1233
cardiac impairment and, 1233
lung mechanics and, 1232–1233, 1233t
Cardiopulmonary parameters, 849t, 861–863
based on analysis of blood gas partial pressure, 863
clinical applications of, 862–863
hemodynamic, 861–862
Cardiopulmonary resuscitation (CPR), 149–161, 491–505
airway patency and. *See* Airway management
blood gas analysis during. *See* Blood gas analysis, cardiopulmonary resuscitation and low flow states and
breathing and, 495–496
apnea and, 495
techniques for, 495–496
capnometry during, 882, 882f
circulation and, 496–497
closed chest cardiac compression and, 496–497
precordial thump and, 497
clinical decision-making regarding, 50f–52f, 50–52
electrical cardioversion and, 498–499, 499f, 500f
for ice water submersion, 1882

Cardiopulmonary resuscitation (CPR)
(*continued*)
immediate concerns with, 149–150, 491–492
diagnostic tests and procedures, 492
initial therapy, 492
major problems, 491
stress points, 491–492
initial considerations with, 492
advanced life support, 492
basic life support, 492
intermediate life support, 492
for near-drowning, 1878, 1883
outcomes of, 150–1157
after in-hospital cardiac arrest, 155–157
neurologic, 157
after out-of-hospital cardiac arrest, 150–155
pharmacotherapy for, 499–505
adenosine in, 504–505
β-adrenergic blockers in, 504
atropine in, 502
bretylium in, 503–504
calcium channel blocking agents in, 504
calcium chloride in, 505
epinephrine in, 499–501
lidocaine in, 502–503
nitroglycerin in, 505
procainamide in, 503
sodium bicarbonate in, 501–502
during pregnancy, 1398
as prognostic indicator in near-drowning,
1883
pulseless activity, bradycardia, and asystole and,
499, 501f, 502f
termination of, 157–161
advance directives and, 161
age as factor in, 159
bases for decision to terminate and, 158t,
158–159
coronary perfusion pressure and, 159
cost of patient care and, 159
end-tidal carbon dioxide concentration
and, 159
family interests and, 161
legal implications of, 160
in normothermic adults, 149–150
out-of-hospital, 160
quality of life and, 159
responsibility for decision to terminate
and, 159
ventricular defibrillation and, 497–498, 498f
Cardiovascular, function, monitoring of, following
cardiac surgery. *See specific parameters*
Cardiovascular collapse, in pancreatitis, treatment
of, 2058
Cardiovascular disorders. *See also specific*
disorders
in acute respiratory distress syndrome, 1837t
anaphylaxis and, 1544, 1545t
antibiotics and, 1563t
black widow spider bites and, 1529
with burns. *See* Burns, cardiovascular
problems with
chest pain in, 1718t
life-threatening, 1721–1723
in cyclic antidepressant poisoning, 1491–1492
digitalis poisoning and, 1498–1499

extracorporeal membrane oxygenation and, in
neonates, 677–678
in fat embolism syndrome, 1238
heparin for, 617–618
in hypothyroidism, 2142–2143
lithium toxicity and, 1494
in obese surgical patients, 1278–1279
cardiac function and, 1278
clinical implications of, 1278–1279
hypertension, 1278
pulmonary vascular changes and, 1278
opiate abuse and, 1518
postoperative, prevention of, 1006–1007
preoperative evaluation of, 1001–1002
history and physical examination in,
1001–1002
laboratory examination in, 1002
renal transplantation and, 1305
in rheumatoid arthritis, 1243
in spinal cord injury, treatment of, 1213–1214
in systemic lupus erythematosus, 2167–2168
thyrotoxicosis and, 2138
Cardiovascular function. *See also* Vascular *entries*
barbiturates and, 1023
benzodiazepines and, 1025
during brain resuscitation, 282–283
hypertension and, 282–283
hypotension and fluid resuscitation and, 282
following cardiac surgery, 1149
in hyperkalemia, 426t
in hyperosmolar states, 441t
in hypokalemia, 424t
in hypomagnesemia, 432t
during intrahospital transport, 789, 791t
ketamine and, 1025–1026
monitoring of, following cardiac surgery. *See*
Cardiac surgery
during pregnancy, 316
propofol and, 1024
in sepsis, 407–408
spinal cord injury and, 1210
Cardiovascular physiology, 227–251
cardiac contraction and, 231–233
in intact heart, 233
in isolated muscle preparations, 231f–233f,
231–233
coronary autoregulation and myocardial oxygen
balance and, 250–251, 251f
electrical activity and. *See* Cardiac electrical
activity
heart as pump and, 236–241
pressure-flow relations and, 240f, 240–241
pressure-volume relations and, 236–240,
237f–240f
intrinsic regulation of cardiac function and,
233–236
afterload and, 235–236, 236f
contractility and, 233–234
preload and, 234f–236f, 234–235
ischemic effects on myocardial metabolism
and, 251, 252f
metabolic demand of heart and, 248f, 248–249
extrinsic requirements and, 248–249, 249f
intrinsic requirements and, 249, 249f
supply-demand ratio and, 250, 250f
metabolic supply of heart and, 249–250, 250f

supply-demand ratio and, 250, 250f
neurogenic control and, 242–245
of heartbeat, 242–244, 243f, 244f
of peripheral blood flow, 244–245, 245f
pediatric, 1162–1163
autonomic innervation and, 1163
ischemia and, 1163
pulmonary vascular resistance and, 1163
ventricular independence and, 1163
systemic and coronary artery size and
vasomotion and, 246–247
active control of, 246f, 246–247, 247f
passive control of, 246
ventricular interaction and, 241
ventricular vascular coupling and, 241–242,
242f
Cardioversion, 1785
electrical, 498–499, 499f, 500f, 575f–577f,
575–577
complications of, 576–577
energy level for, 499
procedure for, 576
technique for, 498–499
Carmustine (BCNU), for bone marrow
transplantation, 1368t
Carney syndrome, pheochromocytomas and, 2135
Carotid bruits, in stroke patients, 1993
Carotid reconstruction, 1182–1183
antiplatelet therapy and, 1182
blood pressure and, 1182
chest radiography and, 1182
mortality and, 1183
neurologic assessment and, 1182
postoperative complications of, 1182–1183
Casts
complications of, 1247
for fractures, 1221
Cataracts, following bone marrow
transplantation, 1379–1380
Catecholamines. *See also specific catecholamines*
excess of, pheochromocytoma and, 2130
regulation of metabolic responses to critical
illness and, 331–332
Categorical data, 9
Cathartics, for cyclic antidepressant poisoning,
1491
Catheter(s)
Heimlich, insertion of, 560–561
procedure for, 561, 561f
for oxygen delivery, 705
transtracheal, 705
for parenteral nutrition
care of, 467
complications of, 470
urinary
in dysoxia, 340
urinary tract infections associated with,
1655, 2212
vascular. *See* Arterial catheter(s); Central
venous catheters; Interventional
radiology, vascular procedures;
Pulmonary artery (PA) catheter(s);
Vascular catheters
Catheter drainage, percutaneous, 591–594
catheter maintenance for, 592
complications of, 592

imaging and, 591–594
locations and types of collections and, 592–594
technique for, 592
Catheter electrodes, for cardiac pacing, 546–547, 547f
Catheter-related infections, 844, 1577–1581
with arterial catheters, 1581
following cardiac surgery, 1159
clinical significance of, 1577
colonization and, 1578t
contamination and, 1578t
definition of, 1577–1578, 1578t
diagnostic techniques for, 1580
fever associated with, 1594–1595
with multilumen central venous catheters, 1581
pathogenesis of, 1578–1579
prevention of, 1579–1580. *See also* Vascular cannulation
dressing change regimens for, 1579
duration of insertion and, 1579–1580
guidewire exchange and, 1580
site care for, 1579
with pulmonary artery catheters, 1580–1581
rate of, as continuous quality improvement indicator, 169
risk factors for, 1579
septicemia, 1578t
staphylococcal, 1662
through the catheter cultures of, 1577–1578, 1580
Cations, daily renal excretion of, 2265t
Caustic ingestions. *See* Corrosive injuries, esophageal
Caval interruption, for pulmonary embolism, 588
CD markers, 304–306, 305f
Cecostomy tubes, 1118
Cefazolin
for bacterial endocarditis, 1658
for cellulitis, staphylococcal, 1661
cost and initial dosage of, 1562t
for infective endocarditis, 1794t, 1796t
for orbital cellulitis, staphylococcal, 1660
Cefoperazone, dosage adjustment for, in hepatic disease, 482t
Cefotaxime
cost and initial dosage of, 1562t
for Lyme disease, 1709
Cefotetan, cost and initial dosage of, 1562t
Cefoxitin, cost and initial dosage of, 1562t
Ceftazidime
cost and initial dosage of, 1562t
for heart-lung transplantation, 1319t
for infections in granulocytopenic patients, 1606
for lung transplantation, 1319t
Ceftizoxime, cost and initial dosage of, 1562t
Ceftriaxone
for *Hemophilus influenzae* infections, 1710
for infective endocarditis, 1794t
for Lyme disease, 1709
prophylactic, for meningococcal disease, 1565
Cefuroxime, cost and initial dosage of, 1562t
Cell-mediated immunity, disorders of, 310
Cellular injury, shock and, 369
Cellulitis, staphylococcal, 1661
orbital, 1660

Celsius temperature conversions, 2255t
Centers for Disease Control, handwashing guidelines of, 509
Central Limit Theorem, 11
Central nervous system disorders. *See also* Neurologic disorders; *specific disorders*
following cardiac surgery, 1157
heparin for, 618–619
infectious. *See also* Neurologic infections; *specific disorders and infections*
in renal transplant recipients, 1611
methanol poisoning and, 1502
opiate abuse and, 1518
Central nervous system function. *See also* Brain *entries*; Spinal cord *entries*
antidiuretic hormone release and, 2117
in hypernatremia, 420, 420t
in hyperosmolar states, 441
in hyperthermia, 1456
in hyponatremia, 417, 417t, 419
monitoring of, in head injury, 1203–1204
during pregnancy
direct hormonal effects on, 319
at term, 317
Central processing units, of microprocessor-controlled ventilators, 715–716
Central syndrome, in comatose patients, 1979
Central venous catheters, 852–853
bacteremia associated with, in HIV-infected patients, 1627
chest radiography and, 968–969, 970f
indications for, 852
insertion of. *See* Venous cannulation, central
multilumen, infection related to, 1581
position of, following thoracic surgery, 1135
pressure measurements using, 852
in shock, 376
following thoracic surgery, 1134
thrombolytic therapy for, 626
waveform analysis and, 852–853, 853f
Centruroides exilicauda stings, 1532–1533, 1533t
Centruroides suffusus stings, 1532–1533, 1533t
Cephalic vein, cutdown of, 570–571, 574f
Cephalosporins, 1567. *See also specific drugs*
first-generation, 1567
for infections in granulocytopenic patients, 1606
second-generation, 1567
third-generation, 1567
Cephalothin, for infective endocarditis, 1794t, 1796t
Cerebellar hemorrhage, coma and, 1977
Cerebellar infarction, coma and, 1977
Cerebral angiography, in stroke patients, 1995
Cerebral blood flow (CBF)
cerebral oxygen consumption and, 277–278, 278t
maneuvers to increase, in brain injury, 285
blood viscosity and intravascular volume and, 285
iatrogenic hypotension and, 285
monitoring of, 946–947
in head injury, 1203
nitrous oxide saturation and, 946–947
single-photon emission computed tomography for, 947

stable xenon-enhanced computed tomography for, 947
xenon 133 clearance for, 947
pathological alterations of, 277
hyperemia and vasospasm and, 277
hypoperfusion after brain injury and, 277
regulation of, 276f, 276–277
Cerebral edema
cytotoxic, 278
in fulminant hepatic failure, 2047–2050
treatment of, 2049–2050
ischemic, 278
near-drowning and, 1881
peritumor, treatment of, 280t
treatment of, 280t
Cerebral embolism, with infective endocarditis, 1789
Cerebral function, monitoring of. *See* Neurologic monitoring, of cerebral function
Cerebral hemorrhage, coma and, 1976
Cerebral hypoxia
coma and, 1977
electroencephalography in, 945
Cerebral infarction, with intracerebral hemorrhage, 2000t
Cerebral ischemia
electroencephalography in, 944
treatment of, 280t
Cerebral malaria, 1711
Cerebral metabolism, 277–278, 278t
maneuvers to increase demand and, 285–286
monitoring of, 951–952
jugular venous saturation for, 951–952
near-infrared spectroscopy for, 952
Cerebral/neurologic formulas, 2261t–2262t
Cerebral oxygen consumption, 277–278, 278t
Cerebral perfusion, monitoring of. *See* Neurologic monitoring, of cerebral perfusion
Cerebral perfusion pressure (CPP)
cerebral blood flow regulation and, 276
near-drowning and, as prognostic indicator, 1883
Cerebral survival, as goal of cardiopulmonary resuscitation, 491
Cerebral vasculitis
coma and, 1978
in systemic lupus erythematosus, 2169–2170
Cerebral vasospasm
cerebral blood flow and, 277
with subarachnoid hemorrhage, 2001t
treatment of, 2002
treatment of, 280t
Cerebritis, acute, in systemic lupus erythematosus, 2169–2170
Cerebrospinal fluid (CSF)
drainage of, for intracranial hypertension, 284, 1205
examination of, 1639–1640, 1640t
Cerebrospinal fluid (CSF) rhinorrhea, antibiotic selection for neurologic infections in, 1641t
Cerebrospinal fluid (CSF) shunts, staphylococcal infections of, 1662
Cerebrovascular disease, 1989–2002. *See also* Stroke; Transient ischemic attacks (TIAs)

Cerebrovascular disease (*continued*)
  diagnostic tests and procedures for, 1989
  dialysis and, 2098
  initial therapy for, 1989–1990
  intracerebral hemorrhage, 1999–2000, 2000t
  major problems with, 1989
  stress points with, 1989
  subarachnoid hemorrhage, 2000t, 2000–2002, 2001f
    management of, 2001t, 2001–2002, 2002f
Cervical canal, alignment of, in spinal cord injury, 1211
Cervical spine
  control of, initial triage of trauma patients and, 1040–1041
  immobilization of, for spinal cord injury, 1209
  in rheumatoid arthritis, 1244–1245
    atlantoaxial subluxation and, 1244f, 1244–1245
  surgery of, complications of, 1234
Cervical spine collars, complications of, 1247, 1247f
Chaotic atrial tachycardia, 1783
  management of, 1785
Charcoal. *See* Activated charcoal
Chediak-Higashi syndrome, 309t
Chelating agents, calcium regulation and, 427
Chemical injuries. *See* Corrosive injuries, esophageal; Poisonings and toxic exposures
Chemokines, host response and, 294
Chemotherapy. *See* Cancer chemotherapy; Medications; *specific drugs and drug types*
Chest. *See also* Thoracic *entries; specific organs*
  flail, 1138–1139
    conservative management of, 1138
    internal stabilization with ventilator support for, 1138
Chest pain, 1717–1724
  atypical, 1719–1720
  in chronic renal failure, 2096, 2096t
  classic, 1719
  cocaine abuse and, 1516
  diagnostic tests and procedures for, 1717–1718
  differential diagnosis of life-threatening causes of, 1720–1724
    cardiovascular, 1721–1723
    gastrointestinal, 1723–1724
    pulmonary, 1720–1721
  differential diagnosis of non-life-threatening causes of, 1724
  major problems with, 1717, 1718t, 1719f
  pathophysiology and differentiation of, 1719–1720
  psychosomatic, 1724
  in sickle cell anemia, 2234
  stress points with, 1717
Chest radiography, 957–965
  in acute respiratory distress syndrome, 962–963, 1831, 1831f, 1832f
  in aspiration syndromes, 1864–1865, 1865f
  carotid/subclavian reconstructions and, 1182
  in chest pain, 1718
  in congestive heart failure, 960–962
    azygous vein and, 962, 963f

pulmonary edema and, 961–962, 963f
  pulmonary vasculature and, 960–961, 962f
  in esophageal perforation, 2075f, 2075–2076
  in hydropneumothorax, 959, 961f
  in lobar collapse, 964f–965f, 965
  in myasthenia gravis, 2013
  pleural effusions and, 958–959, 961f
  in pneumomediastinum, 963, 964f
  in pneumonia, 963, 965
  in pneumothorax, 1962
  in pulmonary embolism, 1895, 1895f
  in simple pneumothorax, 957–958, 958f–960f
  in tension pneumothorax, 959, 962f
  following thoracic surgery, 1135–1136
  in thoracic trauma, 1137–1138
  in valvular heart disease, 1770, 1771, 1772, 1773, 1775, 1776, 1777, 1778
Chest syndrome, acute, in sickle cell anemia, 2234
Chest tube(s). *See also* Tube thoracostomy
  clamping of, 1136–1137
  output of, following thoracic surgery, 1135–1136
Chest tube bottles, 561, 561f, 562f
Chest wall
  injuries of, of lower wall, 1083–1085
  lung interaction with, pulmonary compliance and, 195–196, 196f
Chest wall injury scale, 2277t
Chickenpox, in immunocompromised patients, 1695
Child abuse, near-drowning and, 1883
Child Abuse Amendment of 1984, 122
Children. *See* Adolescents; Infants; Neonates; Pediatric patients
Chironex fleckeri envenomations, 1533
Chi-square test, 13
Chlamydia infections, 1680
  antibiotics effective against, 1559t
  Chlamydia pneumoniae, pneumonia due to, 1843
  endocarditis due to, treatment of, 1793
Chloramphenicol
  for bubonic plague, 1671–1672, 1708
  dosage adjustment for, in hepatic disease, 482t
  for *Hemophilus influenzae* infections, 1710
  for Q fever, 1706
  for tularemia, 1708
Chlordiazepoxide (Librium), 825t
  for agitation and anxiety, 2026t
Chloride, loss of, 928
Chloride-wasting nephropathy, 262
Chlorine, inhalation injury due to, 1954
Chloroquine, adverse effects of, 2156t–2157t
Chlorothiazide, for acute renal failure, 2090
Chlorpromazine (Thorazine)
  for delirium, 2023
  for hyperthermia, 1457
Chlorpropamide, for diabetes insipidus, 421t
Cholangiopancreatography, retrograde, endoscopic
  for biliary pancreatitis, 2059
  diagnostic, in pancreatitis, 2057
Cholangitis, 1128
Cholecystectomy, biliary fistulas following, 1128
Cholecystitis
  acalculous

fever associated with, 1596
    postoperative, 1115
    in spinal cord injury, treatment of, 1214
  acute
    acute abdomen and, 1105
    in obstetric patients, 1424
  aortic reconstructions and, 1185
    diagnosis of, 1185
    etiology of, 1185
    incidence of, 1185
    therapy of, 1185
  postoperative, 1127–1128
Cholecystostomy, percutaneous, 594
Cholesterol embolism, arterial, 1907
Cholinergic toxidrome, 1468, 1469t, 1504–1505. *See also* Insecticides, poisoning by
Choriomeningitis, lymphocytic, 1694
Chromium, requirement for, 462t, 463
Chromogranin A, in pheochromocytomas, 2132
Chronic obstructive lung disease (COLD)
  acute respiratory failure in. *See* Respiratory failure, acute
  asthma versus, 1934, 1935t
  chest pain and, 1724
  definition of, 1918
  oxygen therapy in, 707
  pulmonary function testing and, 989
  waveform analysis in, 859, 859f
Chronic renal failure (CRF), 2093–2099. *See also* Renal failure
  arrhythmias in, 2096–2097, 2097t
  chest pain in, 2096, 2096t
  disordered consciousness in, 2098–2099
  hypotension in, 2094–2096
    cardiogenic, 2094
    hypovolemic, 2094, 2094t
    pericardial disease and, 2094–2095
    sepsis and, 2095–2096
  major problems with, 2093
  respiratory failure in, 2097–2098
  stress points with, 2093–2094
Churg-Strauss syndrome (CSS), 2161–2162, 2162t
Chylothorax, tube thoracostomy for, 557
Chylous collections, following cardiac surgery in pediatric patients, 1173
Cigarette smoking
  cessation of, preoperative, 995
  pulmonary function testing and, 989
Cilastin-imipenem, for *Nocardia* infections, 1608
Cimetidine
  actions, indications, and dosing of, 2270
  for aspiration prophylaxis, 1871, 1871t
  dosage adjustment for, in hepatic disease, 482t
C1 inhibitor deficiency, 309t
Ciprofloxacin, 1569
  cost and initial dosage of, 1562t
  for infective endocarditis, 1795t
  for *Mycobacterium avium* complex infections, in HIV-infected patients, 1619t
  prophylactic, for meningococcal disease, 1565
  for *Rhodococcus equi* infections, in HIV-infected patients, 1620t
Circulation. *See also* Blood flow
  assessment of, vascular surgery and, 1178
  cardiopulmonary resuscitation and, 496–497

closed chest cardiac compression and, 496–497
  precordial thump and, 497
central nervous system, monitoring of, in head injury, 1203
in comatose patients, emergency evaluation of, 1971
compromise of, in cyclic antidepressant poisoning, 1491
extracorporeal. *See* Extracorporeal membrane oxygenation (ECMO)
fetal, persistent, extracorporeal membrane oxygenation for, 671
inhalational anesthetics and, 1017–1018, 1018t
initial triage of trauma patients and, 1042
intrinsic, return of, determination of, 882
in poisonings and toxic exposures, 468
red cell injury in, hemolytic anemia due to, 2233
secondary triage of trauma patients and, 1048–1049
Cirrhosis, 1122–1125
  avoidance of ascites in, 1122–1123
  chylous ascites and, 1123
  early postshunt complications of, 1123–1125
    bleeding, 1123–1124
    encephalopathy, 1124
    hepatorenal syndrome, 1124–1125
    infected ascites, 1124
    leaking ascites, 1124
    pancreatitis, 1125
  shunt procedures for ascites in, 1125
    options for, 1125
    prevention and treatment of complications and, 1125
Cisapride, for aspiration prophylaxis, 1872
Cisplatin, for bone marrow transplantation, 1368t
Citrate
  in banked blood, 1058
  with extracorporeal renal replacement therapies, 636
  toxicity of, massive transfusion and, 2224
Clarithromycin, for *Mycobacterium avium* complex infections, in HIV-infected patients, 1619t
Clavicular venous cannulation, 532–536
  anatomy and, 532f, 532–533, 533f
  techniques for, 533–534
    infraclavicular, 529t, 536
    supraclavicular, 529t, 533–536, 534f, 535f
Clearance, of drugs, 477
Clear and convincing evidence standard, 121
Clindamycin, 1569
  cost and initial dosage of, 1562t
  dosage adjustment for, in hepatic disease, 482t
  for heart-lung transplantation, 1319t
  for lung transplantation, 1319t
  for *Pneumocystis carinii* infections, in HIV-infected patients, 1620t
  prophylactic
    for infective endocarditis, 1798t, 1799t
    for surgical patients, 1010t
  for *Toxoplasma* infections, in HIV-infected patients, 1620t
Clinical care, elements of, 52–55
Clinical data, as scientific variables, 50
Clinical decision-making, 49–50

on admission, 56
assessment of likely effects of therapy and, 53
cardiopulmonary resuscitation and do-not-resuscitate orders and, 50f–52f, 50–52
clinical data as scientific variables and, 50
clinical decisions and, 53–54
continued ICU care and, 57–58
discharge from ICU and, 59
health care status of patient and, 53
judicial involvement in, 105–115
  beginnings of, 106–107
  consensus in, 107–114
  lack of consensus in, 114–115
long-term ICU patients and, 58t, 58–59
new information and, 54
newly acquired diseases and complications and, 53
outcome definition and, 54f, 54–55
selection and sequencing of diagnostic evaluation and, 53
short- and long-term objectives and, 54
short-term ICU outcome and, 56–57, 57t
source of admissions and, 55–56, 56t
termination of cardiopulmonary resuscitation and. *See* Cardiopulmonary resuscitation, termination of
time and, 55, 55f
Clinical status, antibiotic selection for neurologic infections and, 1641, 1641t
Clitocybe poisoning, antidote for, 1467t
Clofazimine, for *Mycobacterium avium* complex infections, in HIV-infected patients, 1619t
Clofibrate, for diabetes insipidus, 421t
Clomipramine (Anafranil), side effects of, 2027t
Clonazepam (Klonopin), 825t
  for agitation and anxiety, 2026t
Clonic status epilepticus, 1986
Clonidine
  actions, indications, and dosing of, 2268
  for hypertension
    in hypertensive emergencies, 1815
    in hypertensive urgencies, 1819–1820, 1820t
  for opiate withdrawal, 1518–1519
Clonidine suppression test, in pheochromocytomas, 2131–2132
Clorazepate (Tranxene), for agitation and anxiety, 2026t
Closed chest cardiac compression. *See* Cardiac compression, closed chest
Closed-tube thoracostomy. *See* Tube thoracostomy
Clostridium botulinum infections, 1676
Clostridium difficile infections, 1583–1584, 1676–1677
Clostridium perfringens infections, 1677
Clostridium tetani infections, 1677–1678
Clot removal, mechanical, for pulmonary embolism, 588
Clotrimazole (Mycelex), 1690t
  for *Candida* infections, 2207
    in HIV-infected patients, 1619t
  prophylactic
    for heart transplantation, 1339
    for renal transplantion, 1305

Clotting, of blood. *See* Anticoagulant agents; Coagulation; Coagulation factors; Coagulopathy; Fibrinolysis; Hemostasis
CMV-specific immunoglobulin (CytoGan), for lung transplantation, 1330
Coagulase-negative staphylococci. *See* Staphylococci, coagulase-negative
Coagulation, 265–272. *See also* Anticoagulant agents; Hemostasis
  extrinsic pathway of, 270
  fibrinolysis and. *See* Fibrinolysis
  final common pathway to, 270
  host response and, 299
  insurgical patients, cardiac surgery in pediatric patients and, 1173
  as integrated system, 272
  intrinsic pathway of, 269–270
  during pregnancy, 1403
  stress points with, 265
  in surgical patients, 1008
  following transfusion therapy, 643
Coagulation factors
  contact, 268, 268t
  decreased production of, postoperative bleeding due to, 1069
  depletion of, by massive transfusion, 1057
  impaired function of, postoperative bleeding due to, 1069
  increased destruction of, postoperative bleeding due to, 1069–1071, 1070t
  replacement of, fresh frozen plasma for, 649
  thrombin-sensitive, 269, 269t
  vitamin K-dependent, 268–269
Coagulopathy, 2217–2230, 2218t
  anticoagulant overdose and, 2225–2226
    of heparin, 2220t, 2225
    of warfarin, 2220t, 2225–2226, 2226t
  in burn patients, 1270
  clinical history in, 2218–2219
  consumptive, postoperative bleeding due to, 1069–1071, 1070t
  diagnosis of, 1067
    tests and procedures for, 2217–2218
  disseminated intravascular coagulation. *See* Disseminated intravascular coagulation (DIC)
  in fat embolism syndrome, 1909
  fresh frozen plasma for, 648–649, 2221, 2225
  in fulminant hepatic failure, 2050
  in head injury, 1207
  heparin for, 619
  following hepatic resection, 1126
  in hyperthermia, 1457
  initial therapy for, 2218
  following intestinal transplantation, 1360
  intestinal transplantation and, 1357, 1357t
  laboratory evaluation for, 2219–2220, 2220t
  in liver disease, 2220t, 2222–2223
    hemostatic abnormalities and, 2222–2223
    management of, 2223
    presentation of, 2223
  following liver transplantation, 1343, 1343f
    assessment of, 1343, 1343f
    treatment of, 1343
  lupus anticoagulant and, 2229
  major, 265, 266t

Coagulopathy (*continued*)
  major problems with, 2217
  massive transfusion syndrome and, 2220t, 2224–2225
  following multivisceral transplantation, 1360
  multivisceral transplantation and, 1356
  in obstetric patients, 1406
  physical examination for, 2219
  platelets and. *See* Platelet disorders
  postoperative bleeding due to, 1068–1071
    primary hemostatic failure and, 1068–1069
    secondary hemostatic failure and, 1069–1071, 1070t
  prevention of, fresh frozen plasma for, 649
  reactive hyperfibrinogenemia, 2229
  in salicylate poisoning, 1488
  stress points with, 2217
  systemic diseases associated with, 2230
  vitamin K deficiency and, 2220t, 2223–2224
  warfarin for, 622, 622t
Cocaine
  abuse of, 1514–1517
    diagnosis of, 1516
    toxicity and, 1515t, 1515–1516
    treatment of, 1516–1517
    withdrawal and, 1517
  for airway management, 762
Coccidiomycosis infections
  Coccidioides immitis, 1688
    in HIV-infected patients, 1624–1625
  in HIV-infected patients, 1624–1625
    treatment of, 1619t
  pneumonia due to, 1854
Coelenterata envenomations, 1533t, 1533–1534
  clinical manifestations of, 1533–1534
  treatment of, 1534
Cognitive function. *See also* Dementia
  incompetent patients and
    informed consent and, 118–119
    informed consent in care of, 83
    right to refuse treatment, 108–111
  informed consent and, 86
Colchicine, adverse effects of, 2156t–2157t
Colectomy, abdominal, total, for toxic megacolon, 2069
Colitis
  in HIV-infected patients, treatment of, 1619t
  neutropenic enterocolitis, in cancer, 2250–2251
  pseudomembranous, 1583–1584, 1676–1677
  ulcerative. *See* Fulminant colitis; Inflammatory bowel disease; Toxic megacolon
Collaborative care. *See* Team care
Collateral ventilation, 721
Colloids. *See also* Fluid therapy
  as blood substitute, 666
Colon. *See also specific colonic disorders*
  pseudo-obstruction of, acute abdomen and, 1106, 1106f
Colonic fistulas, postoperative, 1114
Colonic injuries, 1093
Colonic injury scale, 2276t
Colonic perforation, massive hemorrhage and, 2069
Colonization, 510
  of catheters, 1578t

Colonoscopy, in pseudo-obstruction of colon, 1106, 1106f
Colony stimulating factors
  for leukopenia, 2236
  regulation of metabolic responses to critical illness and, 332t
Colyer decision, 120
Coma, 1971–1979
  barbiturate
    for brain injury, 285–286, 1206
    for cerebral edema, in fulminant hepatic failure, 2049
  bedside evaluation of, 1972–1975
    ocular movements in, 1973–1974
    pupils in, 1974–1975
    respiration in, 1973, 1974f
    spontaneous and induced movements in, 1973
  bilateral hemispheric lesions causing, 1975–1976
    extracerebral, 1976
    intracerebral, 1976
  brain stem lesions causing, 1976–1977
  computed tomography in, 1975
  in cyclic antidepressant poisoning, 1490
    management of, 1492
  electroencephalography in, 943, 943f, 944f, 1975
  emergency evaluation of, 1971–1972
    airway and breathing in, 1971
    circulation in, 1971
    metabolic, 1972
  etiology of, differentiation of, 1471–1472
  Glasgow Coma Scale and. *See* Glasgow Coma Scale (GCS)
  immediate concerns with, 1971
  laboratory tests in, 1975
  lumbar puncture in, 1975
  metabolic-toxic etiologies of, 1977–1979
    deprivation of oxygen, substrate, or metabolic cofactors and, 1977
    deterioration and, 1978–1979
    exogenous poisons and, 1978
    infections and inflammation and, 1978
    organ dysfunction and, 1978
  myxedema
    presentation of, 2143t, 2143–2144
    treatment of, 2145, 2145t
  in poisonings and toxic exposures, 1471–1472
  poisonings and toxic exposures and, 468
  in salicylate poisoning, 1489
Communication
  for intrahospital transport, 792
  with patients, problems in, 93
  among team members, 36–37
Community acquired pneumonia (CAP), 1841–1857
  adjunctive treatment for, 1852
  antibiotics for, 1850–1852, 1851t
    clinical response to, 1852
    duration of therapy with, 1852, 1852t
  characterization of, 1842
  chronic, 1854, 1854t, 1855t
  future directions for, 1856–1857
  host defense and susceptibility to, 1844, 1845t, 1846

initial diagnostic evaluation for, 1846f, 1846t–1848t, 1846–1848, 1847f
  initial therapy for, 1841–1842
  invasive testing in, 1852–1854, 1853t
    bronchoscopy, 1853
    open lung biopsy, 1853–1854
    transthoracic needle aspiration, 1853
  lung abscess in, 1849–1850, 1850f
  major problems with, 1841–1842
  pathogens in, 1842t, 1842–1844, 1843t
    new, 1843
    new problems associated with, 1843–1844
  pleural effusions in, evaluation and treatment of, 1848–1849, 1849f, 1849t
  pneumococcal, bacteremic, 1843–1844
  prophylaxis of, 1855–1856
    immunizations for, 1855–1856, 1856t
    intravenous immunoglobulin for, 1856
  radiographic resolution of infiltrates in, 1855
  recurrence of, 1856, 1857t
Compartment syndromes, 1235–1237, 2207–2208
  bullet, 1188–1189
  clinical presentation of, 1236, 1236f
  diagnosis of, 1236, 1236t
  fasciotomy for, 1236–1237, 1237f
  with fractures, 1227–1228
  intraabdominal, in trauma patients, 1053–1054
  military antishock trousers for, 1235–1236
  postoperative care for, 1237
  sequelae of, 1237
  in trauma patients, 1052f, 1052–1053, 1052–1054
  treatment of, 2208, 2208f
Compensatory renal metabolic alkalosis, 256
Complement
  activation of, 306
  defects of, critical illness and, 308–309, 309t
  host response and, 296–297, 297f
Complex partial seizures, 1982, 1987
Complex partial status epilepticus, 1987
Compression stockings, for deep venous thrombosis prophylaxis, 1890
Computed tomography (CT), 972–976
  abdominal, 974, 976, 977f, 978f
    in abdominal injuries, 1081
    in acute abdomen, 1103
    in hepatic injuries, 1087
    infections and, 1597–1598
    sepsis and, 1113
  in comatose patients, 1975
  of head, 973f–976f, 973–974
    in brain injury, 279–280
    in stroke patients, 1993, 1994f
    xenon-enhanced, for cerebral blood flow monitoring, 947
  in hypopituitarism, 2114
  limitations of, 976
  for neurologic infections, 1640
  in pancreatitis, 2057
  of percutaneous catheter drainage, 591, 592
  single-photon emission computed tomography
    in acute myocardial infarction, 1740
    for cerebral blood flow monitoring, 947
  in thoracic trauma, 1138

Concentration effect, inhalational anesthetic
    delivery and, 1015
Conditioning regimens, for bone marrow
    transplantation, 1367, 1368t
Confidence intervals (limits), 18–19, 19f
Confounding, in research studies, 7
Confusion
    causes of, 484
    in delirium, 2020
Congenital heart disease, during pregnancy,
    1394–1395
    left-to-right shunt and, 1395
    right-to-left shunt and, 1395
Congestive heart failure (CHF)
    approach to, 1739–1740
    asthma versus, 1934–1935
    chest radiography in, 960–962
        azygous vein and, 962, 963f
        pulmonary edema and, 961–962, 963f
        pulmonary vasculature and, 960–961, 962f
    postoperative, prevention of, 1006
    respiratory failure and, 1919
    in thyrotoxicosis, treatment of, 2141–2142
Congo-Crimean hemorrhagic fever, 1696
Conjugated estrogens, for uremic bleeding
    defects, 2094t
Connective tissue, during pregnancy, at term,
    317–318
Conroy decision, 112
Consciousness, 1198
    disordered, in chronic renal failure, 2098–2099
    level of. *See also* Coma
        burns and, 1274
Consent
    implied, 118
    informed. *See* Informed consent
    for organ donation, 1292, 1296
Constant physician care, 24
Constipation, 2212
    renal transplantation and, 1306
Consultants, 36
Consultations
    in dysoxia, 340
    elective, evaluation of, 39
Consumptive coagulopathy, postoperative
    bleeding due to, 1069–1071, 1070t
Contact activation proteins, host response and,
    297–299, 298f
Contact dermatitis, 2191–2192
Contact factors, 268, 268t
Contamination, of catheters, 1578t
Continuous arteriovenous hemodiafiltration
    (CAVHD), 635f, 637
Continuous arteriovenous hemofiltration
    (CAVH), 634–636, 635f
    following cardiac surgery, 1157
Continuous data, 9
Continuous hemodiafiltration, 634–636, 635f
Continuous positive airway pressure (CPAP),
    729f, 729–734, 730f
    airway pressure release ventilation and. *See*
        Airway pressure release ventilation
        (APRV)
    for aspiration syndromes, 1866–1867
    complications of, neurologic, 1880
    demand-flow valves for, 731–732, 732t

equipment for, 730, 730f
expiratory pressure valves for, 730–731, 731f
face mask, 745–746
    advantages of, 745
    disadvantages of, 745
    initial settings for, 745
    setup parameters for, 745
    work of breathing and, 745–746
nasal, 746
    advantages of, 746
    disadvantages of, 746
    initial settings for, 746
    setup parameters for, 746, 746f
    work of breathing and, 746
for near-drowning, 1878–1880
    adjunctive measures and, 1880
    intrapulmonary shunting and, 1878–1879
    mechanical ventilation and, 1879
for pulmonary manifestations in HIV-infected
    patients, 1622
for respiratory failure, 1923, 1926
side effects and complications of, 740, 741
work of breathing and, 731, 732f
Continuous positive-pressure ventilation
    (CPPV), 719
Continuous quality improvement (CQI), 95,
    163–185
    critical paths and, 175–176
        benefits of, 176
        concept of, 175
        documentation of, 176
        implementation of, 176, 177f–184f
        physician participation and, 176
    establishing programs for, 164–165
        indicator selection for, 164, 165t
        scope of practice and, 164, 165t
        start-up of, 164
        steering committee for, 164
        thresholds for, 164–165
    JCAHO surveys and, 176, 185
        personnel involvement in, 185
        specific analyses and, 185
    risk management and, 175
    for surgical critical care, 165–175
        admission and discharge criteria and, 166,
            168, 168t
        autopsy correlation and, 173, 175, 175t
        blood product conservation and, 170, 172,
            175f
        cardiac arrest and, 168t, 170
        catheter infection rate and, 169
        cerebrovascular accidents and, 168t, 170
        data collection for, 166, 166f, 167f
        decubitus ulcers and, 168t, 169, 174f
        mortality and, 173, 175f
        organizational framework for, 165–166
        pneumothorax rate and, 168t, 169, 170f–173f
        readmission rate and, 168, 168t
        reintubation rate and, 168t, 169
        self-extubation and, 168–169
        setting and, 165
        weaning time following cardiopulmonary
            bypass procedures and, 172
Contraction, cardiac. *See* Cardiac contractility;
    Cardiac contraction
Contractures, prevention of

with burns, 1274
in elderly patients, 2208–2209
Contrast venography, for deep venous thrombosis
    diagnosis, 1242
Control, loss of, 90–91
Control buses, of microprocessor-controlled
    ventilators, 718
Control groups, 5
Controlled mechanical ventilation (CMV). *See*
    Mechanical ventilation, controlled
Conversions
    Fahrenheit and Celsius, 2255t
    metric, 2255t
Convulsions. *See* Seizure(s); Status epilepticus
Cooperative North Scandinavian Enalapril
    Survival Study (CONSENSUS), 1755
Copper, requirement for, 462t, 462–463
Copperhead bites, 1525f, 1525–1528, 1526t
    antidote for, 1466t, 1527t, 1527–1528
Coral envenomations, 1533t, 1533–1534
    clinical manifestations of, 1533–1534
    treatment of, 1534
Coral snake bites, 1525, 1525f, 1526t,
    1526–1527, 1528
    antidote for, 1527t, 1528
Core-rewarming, invasive, for hypothermia, 1454
Coronary arteries, size and vasomotion of
    active control of, 246f, 246–247
    passive control of, 246
Coronary artery disease (CAD)
    hemoglobin concentration in, optimal, 646
    hypothyroidism with, treatment of, 2145–2146
    ischemia, in chronic renal failure, 2096
Coronary autoregulation, myocardial oxygen
    balance and, 250–251, 251f
Coronary perfusion pressure (CPP), 863
    termination of cardiopulmonary resuscitation
        and, 159
Corpus callosum, venous cannulation into,
    537–538
Correlation, 7–8, 8f
Corrosive injuries, esophageal, 2073–2075
    complications of, 2074
    diagnostic approach to, 2074
    management of, 2074–2075
    presentation of, 2074
Corticosteroids. *See also specific corticosteroids*
    for acute respiratory distress syndrome, 1834
    for acute respiratory failure, 1922
    adverse effects of, 2156t–2157t
    for aspiration syndromes, 1866
    for asthma, 1938–1939
    for fulminant colitis, 2068
    for Guillain-Barré syndrome, 2010
    as immunosuppressive drugs, 312t
        for heart-lung transplantation, 1318, 1319t,
            1319–1320
        for lung transplantation, 1318, 1319t,
            1319–1320
        for simultaneous pancreas/kidney
            transplantation, 1314
    infections in patients treated with, 1606–1609
        Legionella, 1609
        Listeria monocytogenes, 1608–1609
        Nocardia, 1607–1608
        Pneumocystis carinii, 1607

Corticosteroids (*continued*)
 for inhalation injury, 1951
 for intracranial hypertension, 284–285
 for sepsis, 410
 for shock, 381
 surgical patients and, 1008
 tapering, 2116
 for toxic megacolon, 2068
 for vasculitis, 2164
Corticotropin. *See* Adrenocorticotropic
  hormone (ACTH)
Cortisol
 regulation of metabolic responses to critical
  illness and, 331–332
 serum level of, 2126–2127
 urine free-cortisol excretion and, 2127
Cortisone acetate, for adrenal insufficiency, 2125t
Corynebacteria, 1668
Cost(s). *See also* Third-party reimbursement
 of analgesics, 827t, 828
 of antibiotics, 1562t
 of cardiopulmonary assessment, 868
 of colloid therapy, 436, 436t
 of extracorporeal membrane oxygenation, in
  neonates, 678
 of intrahospital transport, 792
 outcome prediction and, 127–128
  cost and cost effectiveness and, 129, 129f
  cost-containment and, 130–131
 of sedatives, 827t, 828
 termination of cardiopulmonary resuscitation
  and, 159
 treatment decisions and, 76
 treatment objectives and, 22
 of venous saturation monitoring, 915–916, 916t
Cost-containment, outcome prediction and,
  130–131
Cost effectiveness, outcome prediction and,
  129, 129f
Costochondritis, chest pain and, 1724
Cosyntropin stimulation test, in
  hypopituitarism, 2114
Cottonmouth bites, 1525f, 1525–1528, 1526t
 antidote for, 1466t, 1527t, 1527–1528
Coumadin, prophylactic
 for deep venous thrombosis, 1239, 1240–1241
 for pulmonary thromboembolism, 1239,
  1240–1241
Coumarin, necrosis due to, purpura and, 2190
Coumarin derivative poisoning, antidote for,
  1465t
Counseling, for burn patients and their
  families, 1274
Countersinks, for leaking ascites, 1124
Court proceedings, to secure approval of decision
  to withhold or withdraw treatment,
  110–111
Coxiella burnetii infections, 1703, 1705–1706
Cranial abscesses, epidural, clinical presentation
  and initial diagnostic measures for, 1638
Creatine kinase (CK), in rhabdomyolysis, 2199
Creatinine
 clearance of, 479–480
 in rhabdomyolysis, 2199
CREST syndrome, 2172

Cricothyroidotomy, 770
 in spinal cord injury, 1210
Cricothyroid ventilation, needle-catheter, for
  anaphylaxis, 1548, 1549f
Critical care team. *See* Team care
Critical paths. *See* Continuous quality
  improvement, critical paths and
Crohn's disease. *See* Fulminant colitis;
  Inflammatory bowel disease; Toxic
  megacolon
Crotalidae bites, 1525f, 1525–1528, 1526t
 antidote for, 1466t, 1527t, 1527–1528
Crush injury syndrome, 1595
 rhabdomyolysis due to, 2198
Cruzan decision, 70, 107, 109–110, 113
Cryoprecipitate, 649
 for disseminated intravascular coagulation,
  2221
 for uremic bleeding defects, 2094t
Cryopreservation, of red blood cells, 647
Cryotherapy, for snake bites, 1526
Cryptococcus neoformans infections, 1689
 in HIV-infected patients, 1624, 1626
  treatment of, 1619t
 in renal transplant recipients, 1612
Crystalloids. *See also* Fluid therapy
 prophylactic, for acute tubular necrosis, 2086
Cuff inflation, 770–772
 with high-pressure, low-volume cuffs, 770, 770f
 with low-pressure, high-volume cuffs, 771f,
  771–772
  cuff size for, 771, 771f
  inflation volume and pressure for, 771
  intermittent inflation and, 772
  minimal leak inflation and, 772
  no leak inflation and, 772
  pressure and volume measurement and,
   771–772
Cushing's syndrome, 2121–2122, 2125
 diagnostic tests and procedures for, 2121
 initial therapy for, 2121–2122
 major problems with, 2121
 stress points with, 2121, 2122t
Cutaneous disorders. *See* Skin disorders;
  specific disorders
Cyanide poisoning
 antidote for, 1466t
 methemoglobin and, 1953
 with sodium nitroprusside, 1158, 1158f, 1159f
Cyclic antidepressants. *See also specific drugs*
 poisoning by, 1489–1493
  antidote for, 1465t
  initial treatment of, 1490–1491
  with second-generation agents, 1493
  toxicology and, 1490
  treatment of complications of, 1491–1492
  triage of, 1492–1493
 side effects of, 2027t
 tricyclic antidepressant toxidrome and, 1468,
  1469t
Cyclophosphamide
 for acute lupus pneumonitis, 2166
 adverse effects of, 2156t–2157t
 for bone marrow transplantation, 1368t
 cardiac toxicity of, 2251

 for heart-lung transplantation, 1320
 for heart transplantation, 1336
 for lung transplantation, 1320
Cycloserine, for *Mycobacterium tuberculosis*
  infections, in HIV-infected patients,
  1620t
Cyclosporine (cyclosporin A), 312t
 administration of, 1344
 adverse effects of, 2156t–2157t
 elimination of, hepatic graft function
  assessment and optimization and, 1347
 for fulminant colitis, 2068
 for heart-lung transplantation, 1317–1319,
  1319t
 for heart transplantation, 1334–1335
 for liver transplantation, 1344
 for lung transplantation, 1317–1319, 1319t
 metabolism of, drugs affecting, 1350
 nephrotoxicity of, 1338
 renal effects of, 1344
 for renal transplantation, 1303–1304, 1304t,
  1306
 for simultaneous pancreas/kidney
  transplantation, 1314
 therapeutic serum level of, 479t
 for toxic megacolon, 2068
Cystectomy, radical, postoperative management
  and, 1255–1256
Cystic fibrosis, in obstetric patients, 1416
Cystitis, 1650
 hemorrhagic, following bone marrow
  transplantation, 1372
Cytarabine, for bone marrow transplantation,
  1368t
Cytokines. *See also specific cytokines*
 host response and, 292, 294
 as immunosuppressive agents, 312t
 inflammation and, 308
 multiple organ system failure and, 352, 352f
 regulation of metabolic responses to critical
  illness and, 332t, 332–333
 sepsis and, 407, 407t
Cytomegalovirus (CMV) infections
 following bone marrow transplantation, 1614
  prophylaxis of, 1377
 encephalitis due to, 1694
 following heart transplantation, 1339
 in HIV-infected patients, 1625–1626, 1629
  treatment of, 1619t
 in immunocompromised patients, 1696
 intestinal transplantation and, 1361–1362
  prophylaxis of, 1361
 liver transplantation and, 1348
  prophylaxis of, 1348–1349
 following lung and heart-lung transplantation,
  1322–1323
  management of, 1329–1330
 following multivisceral transplantation,
  1361–1362
  prophylaxis of, 1361
 following renal transplantation, 1306–1307,
  1611–1612
  diagnosis of, 1611
  presentation of, 1611
  therapy of, 1611–1612

transfusion therapy and, 656
Cytomegalovirus-specific immunoglobulin
(CytoGan), for heart-lung
transplantation, 1330
Cytomegalovirus syndrome, following lung and
heart-lung transplantation, 1322–1323
Cytoprotection, in brain injury, 286–287
Cytotoxic agents, 312t. *See also specific drugs*
for vasculitis, 2164
Cytotoxic edema, cerebral, 278

Dactylometra quinquecirrha envenomations,
1533
Dantrolene
for black widow spider bites, 1530t
for malignant hyperthermia, 483, 1033, 1033t,
1460–1461, 1600
for neuroleptic malignant syndrome, 827
Dapsone
for bullous pemphigoid, 2183
for *Pneumocystis carinii* infections
prophylactic, 1566
treatment of, in HIV-infected patients, 1620t
Data
accumulating, repeat analyses of, 15
acquisition of, for cardiopulmonary
assessment, 868
clinical, as scientific variables, 50
quantal, fourfold table for, 9–10, 10t
statistical analysis of. *See* Statistics
types of, 9
Data buses, of microprocessor-controlled
ventilators, 718
D-dimer fibrin degradation product, assays for,
271–272
Dead space, 199
near-drowning and, 1879, 1879f
Dead space ventilation, 924–925
trending, capnography and, 931–932, 932f
Death. *See also* Brain death; Terminal patients
abdominal injuries as cause of, 1082
acute respiratory distress syndrome as cause of,
1836, 1838
aortic reconstructions and, 1185–1186
following cardiac arrest. *See* Cardiac arrest
carotid endarterectomy and, 1183
certification of, 1293
confirmatory tests for, 1293
documentation of, 1293
as continuous quality improvement indicator,
173, 175f
drowning as cause of, 1875, 1876f
femorofemoral and axillofemoral bypass
procedures and, 1186
heart failure as cause of, 1751–1752
imminent, families' reactions to, 93–94
infrainguinal reconstructions and, 1187
intraabdominal sepsis as cause of, 1105
mesenteric and renal artery reconstructions
and, 1184
multiple organ system failure as cause of, 1598
nosocomial infections and, 1575
physician aid-in-dying and, 77–79, 113–114
pulmonary oxygen toxicity as cause of, 708

Débridement
in obese surgical patients, 1281
for snake bites, 1528
Deciding to Forego Life-Sustaining Treatments,
107
Decision-making. *See* Clinical decision-making;
Ethical considerations
Decision trees, for test selection, 132–134,
133t, 134t
Decompression sickness, 783–784, 1905–1906,
1906t
diagnosis of, 784
presentation of, 784
treatment of, 784
Decubitus ulcers, 100–101, 2207
as continuous quality improvement indicator,
168t, 169, 174f
prevention of, 2207
treatment of, 2207
Deep venous thrombosis (DVT), 1239–1243. *See
also* Venous thromboembolism
clinical features of, 1891–1892
diagnosis of, 1241–1242, 1242t, 1892–1894
ascending contrast venography for, 1893
contrast venography for, 1242
duplex ultrasonography for, 1242
impedance plethysmography for, 1242,
1893, 1893f
scintigraphy for, 1894
ultrasonography for, 1893–1894
infrainguinal reconstructions and, 1186–1187
therapy of, 1186–1187
prevention of, 1239–1241, 1241t, 1889t,
1889–1891, 1890t
anesthetic choices for, 1241
anticoagulation for, 1239–1241
external compression devices for, 1241
nonpharmacologic, 1889–1890
pharmacologic, 1890–1891
risk factors for, 1239
therapy of, 1242–1243, 1243t, 1897–1898
anticoagulation in, 1897
general principles of, 1897
surgical, 1898
thrombolytic therapy for, 1191
thrombolytic therapy in, 1897–1898, 1898f
Defense mechanisms, 89–90
Deferoxamine (Desferal), for iron poisoning,
1466t
Defibrillation, ventricular. *See* Ventricular
defibrillation
Dehydration
following intestinal transplantation, 1362–1363
following multivisceral transplantation, 1363
Delio decision, 115
Delirium, 2018–2024
following cardiac surgery, 1157
characteristics of, 2019–2020, 2020t
dementia compared with, 2018, 2019t
differential diagnosis of, 2020–2022, 2021t,
2022t
sedation for, 823
treatment of, 2022–2024, 2023t
Delirium tremens (DTs), 1514
Delivery, following maternal trauma, 1425

Demand-flow valves, for continuous positive
airway pressure and spontaneous
positive end-expiratory pressure,
731–732, 732t
Demeclocycline, for syndrome of inappropriate
antidiuretic hormone secretion, 418
Dementia
delirium compared with, 2018, 2019t
dialysis, 2098–2099
Demyelinating polyneuropathy, inflammatory,
autoimmune, acute. *See* Guillain-Barré
syndrome (GBS)
Denial, 90
Denitrogenation absorption atelectasis, 930
Deontology, 64
Deoxyspergualin, for simultaneous pancreas/
kidney transplantation, 1314
Dependency, 2028
Depolarization, 227–228, 228f
Depression, 2026–2027
characteristics of, 2026, 2026t
treatment of, 2027, 2027t
Dermatitis
contact, 2191–2192
exfoliative. *See* Exfoliative dermatitis
Dermatologic disorders. *See* Skin disorders;
specific disorders
Dermatomes, 2273
1-Desamino-8-D-arginine-vasopressin. *See*
Desmopressin (DDAVP)
Descriptive statistics. *See* Statistics, descriptive
Desipramine (Norpramin), side effects of, 2027t
Desmopressin (DDAVP)
actions, indications, and dosing of, 2268–2269
for bleeding time correction, 686
for diabetes insipidus, 420, 421t, 2118
in head injury, 1207
transfusion therapy and, 651, 662
for uremic bleeding defects, 2094t
Development, following bone marrow
transplantation, 1379
Dexamethasone
for adrenal insufficiency, 2124–2125, 2125t
for intracranial hypertension, 285
long dexamethasone suppression test and,
2127–2128
overnight dexamethasone suppression test
and, 2127
for seizures, with subarachnoid hemorrhage,
2001
for spinal cord compression, 2249
for thyrotoxicosis, 2141
Dextran
for antiplatelet therapy, 615
for deep venous thrombosis prophylaxis, 1891
hemostasis and, 436
low-molecular-weight
for intestinal transplantation, 1361
for multivisceral transplantation, 1361
Dextroamphetamine, side effects of, 2027t
Dextrose
for coma, in poisonings and toxic exposures, 468
in surgical patients, 437–438
hyponatremia and renal function and,
437–438, 438t

Dextrose, in surgical patients (*continued*)
  lack of solute for urine formation and, 438, 438t
Diabetes insipidus (DI), 419–420
  central, 419–420, 2116–2118
    initial therapy for, 2111–2112
    management of, 2118
    patient examination in, 2117–2118
    stress points with, 2111
    treatment of, 420, 421t
  diagnostic tests and procedures for, 2111
  in head injury, 1207
  major problems with, 2111
  nephrogenic, 419
    treatment of, 420
  following neurosurgical procedures, 2118
  partial, treatment of, 420
Diabetes mellitus (DM), 2101–2108
  coma and, 1978
  decompensated, in patients with coexistent medical or surgical problems, 2107–2108, 2108t
  diagnostic tests and procedures for, 2101
  epidemiology of, 2102
  hyperosmolar hyperglycemic nonketotic. *See* Hyperosmolar hyperglycemia nonketotic diabetes (HHNK)
  initial therapy for, 2101
  insulin-dependent, 2102
  ketoacidosis and. *See* Diabetic ketoacidosis (DKA)
  major problems with, 2101
  non-insulin-dependent, 2102
  renal transplantation and, 1305–1306
  sepsis and, in obese surgical patients, 1281
  silent disease and, 1313
  simultaneous pancreas/kidney transplantation for, 1312–1313
  stress points with, 2101
Diabetes of injury, 329, 329t
Diabetic ketoacidosis (DKA), 2102–2106
  clinical description of, 2102, 2102t
  complications of, 2106
  laboratory features of, 2103–2104
  pathogenesis of, 2102–2103
  treatment of, 2104t, 2104–2106
    electrolytes in, 2105–2106
    fluid management in, 2104–2105
    insulin in, 2105, 2106t
Diagnostic evaluation. *See also under specific disorders*
  delayed diagnosis of bone injuries and, 1054, 2211
  misdiagnosis and, 96
  selection and sequencing of, 53
  tests for. *See also* Laboratory tests; *specific tests*
    statistical analysis of, 18, 18f
Diagnostic peritoneal lavage, 563–568
  for abdominal injuries, 1079–1081
  for acute abdomen, 1102
  closed technique for, 564, 566
    dialysis catheter and trocar method of, 564, 566, 566f
    prepackaged kit for, 566, 567f
  complications of, 566
  open technique for, 564, 564f, 565f

results with, 566–568, 568t
Dialysis
  for acute renal failure, 2090
  following cardiac surgery, 1156–1157
    goal of, 1157
    indications for, 1157
    techniques for, 1157
  disordered consciousness associated with, 2098–2099
  hemodialysis. *See* Hemodialysis
  periotneal. *See* Peritoneal dialysis
  in sepsis, 411
  ultrafiltration
    for heart failure, 1762
    for respiratory failure, 2098
Dialysis dementia, 2098–2099
Dialysis disequilibrium syndrome, 2098
Dialysis membranes, for intermittent hemodialysis, 633
Dialyzers, for intermittent hemodialysis, 632–633
Diaphragm, 210–212
  actions of, 211–212
  dysfunction of
    following lung and heart-lung transplantation, 1323
    lung and heart-lung transplantation and, management of, 1330
  injuries to, 1085
    delayed diagnosis of, 1055, 1056f
    diaphragmatic injury scale and, 2281t
    rupture due to, 1142
  muscle fiber types of, 211, 211t
    endurance and strength and, 211
    force generation and fatigue and, 211
    oxidative properties and, 211
    recruitment and, 211
Diaphragmatic injury scale, 2281t
Diarrhea, 2212. *See also specific disorders*
  following bone marrow transplantation, 1371–1372
  enteral nutrition and, 469
  in fulminant colitis. *See* Fulminant colitis
  in HIV-infected patients, 1629
  following intestinal transplantation, 1362–1363
  following multivisceral transplantation, 1363
  in toxic megacolon. *See* Toxic megacolon
Diastolic dysfunction, 1764–1765
  following cardiac surgery in pediatric patients, 1165
  in heart failure. *See* Heart failure, diastolic dysfunction in
Diazepam (Valium), 824, 824t, 825t
  actions, indications, and dosing of, 2269
  for agitation and anxiety, 2026t
  for black widow spider bites, 1530, 1530t
  for cocaine intoxication, 1516
  cost of, 827t
  dosage adjustment for, in hepatic disease, 482t
  pharmacokinetics and pharmacodynamics of, 1023t, 1025
  for seizures
    in brain injury, 286
    in cyclic antidepressant poisoning, 1492
    in hyperthermia, 1457
    in status epilepticus, 1982t, 1984

Diazoxide (Hyperstat), for hypertension, in hypertensive emergencies, 1813, 1814t
Dicloxacillin, for infective endocarditis, 1796t
Dicrotic notch, 850
Dideoxyinosine (ddI), 1571
Diffusing capacity (DLCO)
  decreased, following bone marrow transplantation, 1380
  placental, 1433, 1433t
  preoperative assessment of, 990
Diffusion hypoxia, 1016
Digital displays, for invasive pressure monitoring, 840–841
Digitalis
  for cardiogenic shock, 400
  for heart failure, 1757
  poisoning by, 1498–1499
    antidote for, 1466t
    toxicology and clinical manifestations of, 1498–1499
    treatment of, 1499
Digitalis Investigators Group Trial (DIG), 1757
Digital signals, 718–719, 719t
Digital-to-analog converters, 719
Digitoxin, therapeutic serum level of, 479t
Digoxin
  following cardiac surgery in pediatric patients, 1167t
  for heart failure, 1757
  therapeutic serum level of, 479t
Digoxin immune fab (Digibind), 311, 312t, 1466t, 1499
Diltiazem
  actions, indications, and dosing of, 2269
  for arrhythmias, 1785
  for hypertension, following liver transplantation, 1345
Dimercaprol, for metal poisoning, 1465t
Dipalmitylphosphotidalcholine (DPPC), for aspiration syndromes, 1868
Diphenhydramine
  for anaphylaxis
    prevention of, 1549
    treatment of, 1547t, 1548
  for antipsychotic poisoning, 1495
  for black widow spider bites, 1529
  for heart transplantation, 1335
  for neuroleptic malignant syndrome, 827
  for sedation, 826
Diphenoxylate, for diarrhea, 2212
2,3-Diphosphoglycerate, red blood cells enriched with, 646
Diphtheroids, 1668
  endocarditis due to, treatment of, 1796t–1797t
Disability
  initial triage of trauma patients and, 1043
  secondary triage of trauma patients and, 1049
Discharge, from ICU, clinical decision-making and, 59
Discharge criteria, as continuous quality improvement indicator, 166, 168, 168t
Disclosure, degrees of, 81–82, 118
Disconnect alarms, on mechanical ventilators, 719
Discoordinate breathing, 869
Discrete data, 9

Disinfection
  basic, 510
  hygienic, 509
    with residual action, 509
  recommendations for, 1631
  surgical, 509–510
Dislocations, diagnosis of, 1220–1221
Disopyramide
  dosing of, in chronic renal failure, 2097t
  therapeutic serum level of, 479t
Disorientation, in delirium, 2020
Display, for invasive pressure monitoring,
    844–845
Dissecting thoracic aneurysms, echocardiography
    in, 884, 885t
Disseminated gonococcal infection (DGI), 1667
Disseminated intravascular coagulation (DIC),
    2220t, 2220–2222
  amniotic fluid embolism and, 1911–1912
  autotransfusion and, 665
  diagnosis of, 2221
  in hyperthermia, 1456–1457
  management of, 2221–2222
  massive transfusion and, 2224
  pathogenesis of, 2220t, 2220–2221
  presentation of, 2221
  in rhabdomyolysis, 2200
Distribution, volume of, 476–477
Distributive justice, 22–23, 24–25
Distributive shock, 367–368, 390. *See also*
    Septic shock
  adrenal, 368
  anaphylactic, 368
    adjunctive and experimental management
      techniques for, 380–381
  neurogenic, 368
  septic, 367–368
Diuresis
  forced
    for poisonings and toxic exposures, 1474
    for salicylate poisoning, 1489
  postresuscitation, for burns, 1268
Diuretics. *See also specific drugs*
  following cardiac surgery
    in adult patients, 1156
    in pediatric patients, 1172
  for heart failure, 1761–1762
  for hypertension, in hypertensive
      emergencies, 1815–1816
  for intracranial hypertension, 284, 1205
  loop
    for acute renal failure, 2090
    for renal dysfunction, in sepsis, 411
    for rhabdomyolysis, 2200
  during pregnancy, 1425
  surgical patients and, 1008
  thiazide, for diabetes insipidus, 421t
Divalproex sodium, for status epilepticus, 1987
Dobutamine
  actions, indications, and dosing of, 2269
  following cardiac surgery
    for cardiac contractility augmentation, 1153
    in pediatric patients, 1167t
  for heart failure, 1760–1761, 1761t
    administration mode for, 1761
    congestive, 1740

  in shock, 379
  for heart transplantation, 1336
  for hypotension
    in cyclic antidepressant poisoning, 1492
    in shock, 379
  for shock, 363t, 379
    cardiogenic, 399, 399t
Documentation
  of critical paths, 176
  of date and time of death, 1293
Donors
  of blood, 648
  of organs. *See* Organ donors
Do-not-resuscitate (DNR) orders, 26. *See also*
    Treatment, refusal of
  clinical decision-making regarding, 50f–52f,
      50–52
  lack of requirement of judicial approval for,
      111–112
  for surgical patients, 1009
  termination of cardiopulmonary resuscitation
      and, 161
Dopamine
  actions, indications, and dosing of, 2269
  for acute renal failure, 2090
  for acute tumor lysis syndrome, 2247
  following cardiac surgery
    for cardiac contractility augmentation,
      1152–1153, 1153f
    in pediatric patients, 1166, 1167t, 1168, 1172
  for cyclosporine nephrotoxicity, 1338
  for heart-lung transplantation, 1319t
  for heart transplantation, 1336
  for hypotension
    in cyclic antidepressant poisoning, 1492
    in shock, 379
  for lung transplantation, 1319t
  prophylactic, for contrast nephropathy, 2096t
  for renal dysfunction, in sepsis, 411
  for shock, 363, 363t, 379
    cardiogenic, 398–399
Dopamine blockers, for agitation and anxiety,
    2026
Doppler techniques
  in acute myocardial infarction, 1741, 1742t
  for blood pressure measurement, 872
  for cardiac output determination, 883
  following cardiac surgery in pediatric
      patients, 1174–1175
  for deep venous thrombosis diagnosis, 1242t
  for fetal assessment, following maternal
      trauma, 1422
  laser Doppler flowmetry, 950–951
  in stroke patients, 1995, 1996f
  transcranial, 949f–951f, 949–950
  in valvular heart disease, 1776
Dorsalis pedis artery cannulation, 540t, 541
Double-burst suppression (DBS), for evaluation
    of neuromuscular blockade, 831
Double-lung transplantation (DLT), 1317–1330
  indications for, 1317, 1318f, 1318t
  initial management for, 1317–1320
    immunosuppression and, 1318–1320
    preoperative, 1317–1318, 1318t–1319t
  postoperative management for, 1320–1330
    acute rejection and, 1321–1322, 1324f

  airway complications and, 1320–1321,
      1323f, 1324f
  bleeding and, 1320, 1321f
  bronchiolitis obliterans and, 1323, 1325f
  diagnostic tests and procedures for,
      1325–1327, 1326f
  diaphragmatic dysfunction and, 1323
  infection and, 1322–1323
  initial therapy and, 1327–1330, 1328f, 1329f
  reimplantation response and, 1320, 1322f
  stress points with, 1323, 1325
Doxacurium, 829, 830t
Doxapram, for acute respiratory failure, 1923
Doxazosin, for pheochromocytomas, 2134t
Doxepin (Sinequan), side effects of, 2027t
Doxorubicin (Adriamycin), cardiac toxicity of,
    2251
Doxycycline, for bubonic plague, 1671
Drain(s)
  abdominal, postoperative abdomen and, 1118f,
      1119, 1119f
  care of, 2206, 2206f
  for major liver injuries, 1086
  percutaneous, postoperative abdomen and,
      1118
  skin care around, 2205
Drainage
  for acute abdomen, 1104
  of bile, postoperative, 1111
    following cholecystectomy, 1127
  of brain abscesses, 1639
  for cardiac tamponade, 1807–1808
  of cerebrospinal fluid, for intracranial
      hypertension, 284, 1205
  chest tube. *See* Chest tube(s); Tube
      thoracostomy
  nasogastric, following cardiac surgery in
      pediatric patients, 1173–1174
  of pancreatic pseudocysts, 2060
  percutaneous. *See* Catheter drainage,
      percutaneous
  of pericardial fluid, for cardiac tamponade,
      2250
  of perinephric abscesses, 1653
  of renal abscesses, 1653
Dressings, 2204–2205, 2205f
  catheter-related infection prevention and, 1579
  for vascular catheter insertion, 512
  changing, 514
Droperidol (Inapsine)
  for agitation and anxiety, 2026
  for delirium, 2023
  for vascular cannulation, 522
Drowning. *See also* Near-drowning
  incidence of, 1875, 1876f
  pathophysiology of, 1877–1878
    fresh water and, 1878
    seawater and, 1877–1878
  presentation of, 1877, 1877t
Drug(s). *See* Medications; Substance abuse and
    withdrawal; *specific drugs and drug
    types*
Drug allergies, 1598–1599, 1599t
Drug eruptions, 2186–2188
  bullous, 2188
  morbilliform, 2186–2187, 2187f

Drug eruptions (*continued*)
  urticarial, 2187f, 2187–2188
Drug formulas, 2266t
Drug interactions, 485–486
  in liver transplant patients, 1350
  pharmacodynamic, 486
  pharmacokinetic, 485–486, 486t
  in renal transplant recipients, 1307t, 1308
  of warfarin, 2226, 2226t
Drug overdoses. *See* Poisoning and toxic
    exposures
Ductal closure, extracorporeal membrane
    oxygenation and, 674
Duodenal fistulas, 1090
  postoperative, 1114, 1114t
Duodenal injuries, 1089–1090
Duodenal injury scale, 2275t
Duodenostomy tubes, 1117
Durable Power of Attorney for Health Care, 70
  form for, 32–33
Dural puncture, headache and, 817
Dusts, inhalation injury due to, 1955
Dye dilution, for cardiac output determination,
    895
Dysbaric air embolism (DAE), 1905–1906, 1906t
Dysgammaglobulinemia, pathogens associated
    with, 1556t
Dysoxia, 337–341
  diagnostic tests and procedures for, 339–340
  initial therapy for, 340–341
  major problems with, 337–338, 338f
  stress points with, 338f, 338–339
Dysphagia, in HIV-infected patients, 1629
Dyspnea, in refractory advanced heart failure,
    1758
Dysrhythmias. *See* Arrhythmias

Ear(s), aminoglycoside toxicity and, 1568
Earle Spring decision, 106
Ebola virus infections, 1696, 1709, 1710
Echocardiography, 884–886
  following cardiac surgery in pediatric
      patients, 1174–1175
  in cardiac tamponade, 885
  in chest pain, 1718
  choice of method for, 884
  in dissecting thoracic aneurysms, 884, 885t
  Doppler
      in acute myocardial infarction, 1741, 1742t
      in valvular heart disease, 1776
  heart transplantation and, 1339
  in infective endocarditis, 885, 886f, 886t, 1791
  in pericardial effusion, 885
  pericardiocentesis and, 578–579
  principles of, 884
  in stroke patients, 1995
  transesophageal. *See* Transesophageal
      echocardiography (TEE)
  transthoracic, 884–886
      in thoracic trauma, 1138
  two-dimensional, in acute myocardial
      infarction, 1741–1742, 1742t
  in valvular heart disease, 885, 1770, 1771–1772,
      1773–1774, 1775, 1776, 1777, 1778
  in ventricular function assessment, 885–886,
      887f

Eclampsia. *See* Preeclampsia/eclampsia
Economics. *See* Cost(s); Third-party
    reimbursement
Ectopic atrial tachycardia (EAT), 1783
  diagnosis of, 1783
  management of, 1785
Eczema herpeticum, 2184–2185
  diagnosis of, 2184, 2185f
  etiology of, 2184
  management of, 2184–2185, 2186t
  presentation of, 2184, 2185f
Edema
  cerebral. *See* Cerebral edema
  of legs. *See* Legs, edema of
  peripheral, following hepatic resection, 1126
  pulmonary. *See* Pulmonary edema
Edrophonium
  for neuromuscular blocking agent reversal,
      1032t
  for reversal of neuromuscular blockade,
      834–835, 835t
Education, for prevention of drowning, 1883
Edwin Smith Surgical papyrus, 21
Effective refractory period, 229
Ehrlichiosis, 1703, 1706
Elapidae bites, 1525, 1525f, 1526t, 1526–1527,
    1528
  antidote for, 1527t, 1528
Elastance, pressure support ventilation titration
    and, 220–221, 222f
Elastic forces, pulmonary compliance and,
    193–194, 194f
Elastic pressure, ventilation and, 191
Elderly patients
  contracture prevention in, 2208–2209
  postoperative ICU care for, 1110
  preoperative evaluation of, 1004, 1004t
      pulmonary function testing in, 989
  thyroid function in, 2146, 2147
Electrical activity, cardiac. *See* Cardiac
    electrical activity
Electrical cardioversion. *See* Cardioversion,
    electrical
Electrical injuries, 1537–1542
  classification of, 1538
  clinical manifestations and treatment of,
      1539–1541
      for cardiopulmonary manifestations, 1539
      for musculoskeletal and cutaneous injuries,
          1540
      for neurologic manifestations, 1540
      for renal manifestations, 1539–1540
  diagnostic tests and procedures for, 1538
  initial therapy for, 1538
  lightning and, 1541t, 1541–1542
  major problems with, 1537, 1538t
  mechanisms in, 1538–1539
  prevention of, 1541
  stress points with, 1537
Electrocardiography (ECG), 873–875, 942–944,
    943f, 944f
  in acute pericarditis, 1722, 1804–1805, 1806f
  in angina pectoris, 1723
  in chest pain, 1719
  fetal monitoring and, 1430
  heart transplantation and, 1339
  in hyperthermia, 1456

  ischemia detection using, 874–875
      lead V_4 and, 874, 874f
      modified V_5 lead and, 874, 874f
      trouble-shooting and, 874–875
  in myocardial infarction, 1723
  principles of, 873–874
  in pulmonary embolism, 1895, 1896f
  in thoracic trauma, 1138
Electrodes, placement of, for evaluation of
    neuromuscular blockade, 832
Electroencephalography (EEG). *See also* ST
    segment monitoring
  brain death and, 123
  in comatose patients, 1975
  in dysoxia, 339
  frequency domain analysis and, 944f, 944–945
Electrolyte(s). *See also* Fluid and electrolyte
    disorders; *specific electrolytes and
    electrolyte disorders*
  in body fluids, 2258t
  following bone marrow transplantation, 1369
  requirements for, 461t, 461–462
  urinary, 2265t–2266t
Electrolyte management
  for diabetic ketoacidosis, 2105–2106
  near-drowning and, 1880
  for organ donors, 1295
Electrolyte solutions, balanced, 262
Electromyography (EMG)
  for evaluation of neuromuscular blockade, 831
  in myasthenia gravis, 2013
Electrophysiologic monitoring, in head injury,
    1204
Embolectomy
  percutaneous, transvenous, for pulmonary
      embolism, 1901
  pulmonary, for pulmonary embolism,
      1900–1901
Embolic stroke, 1991–1992, 1992t
Embolic syndromes, pulmonary artery catheters
    for, 860–861
Embolism. *See also* Thromboembolism; Venous
    thromboembolism; *specific disorders*
  air (gas). *See* Air embolism
  of amniotic fluid, 1406, 1413, 1910–1912
      disseminated intravascular coagulation and,
          1911–1912
  antithrombotic therapy for. *See*
      Antithrombotic therapy
  bullet, management of, 1188
  cerebral, with infective endocarditis, 1789
  fat. *See* Fat embolism; Fat embolism
      syndrome (FES)
  with infective endocarditis, 1789
  microemboli
      fat, autotransfusion and, 665
      platelet, autotransfusion and, 665
  pulmonary. *See* Pulmonary embolism
Embolization
  angiographic, for pelvic fractures, 1061
  aortic reconstructions and, 1184
      diagnosis of, 1184
      etiology of, 1184
      incidence of, 1184
      therapy of, 1184
  distal, thrombolytic therapy and, 1190
  venous, tourniquets and, 1246

Emepromium bromide, esophageal injury caused by, 2076

Emergencies, exception to informed consent and, 118

Emergency medical services (EMS) system, outcome after out-of-hospital cardiac arrest and, 150–151, 151f

Emergency medical technicians (EMT-As), 804

Emergency Medical Treatment and Active Labor Act, 114–115

Emesis, for aspiration syndromes, 1866

Emphysema, in obstetric patients, 1415–1416

Empyema
    subdural, clinical presentation and initial diagnostic measures for, 1638
    following thoracic trauma, 1143, 1145

Enalapril
    for acute myocardial infarction, 1737
    for heart failure, 1755–1756
    for respiratory failure, 2098

Enalaprilat, for hypertension, in hypertensive emergencies, 1814t, 1816

Encephalitis
    aseptic, 1693–1694
    coma and, 1978
    herpes, clinical presentation and initial diagnostic measures for, 1639
    in HIV-infected patients, treatment of, 1620t
    parainfectious, 1647
    Toxoplasma gondii, in HIV-infected patients, 1626–1627
    viral, 1694
        parainfectious, 1647, 1647t

Encephalopathy
    electroencephalography in, 944
    in fulminant hepatic failure, 2047, 2049t
    intestinal transplantation and, 1357, 1357t
    multivisceral transplantation and, 1356
    postshunt, 1124
    shock and, 371
    Wernicke's, prevention of, in comatose patients, 1972

End-diastolic pressure
    left ventricular, 856, 861, 863
        following cardiac surgery, 1149, 1151
    in pulmonary artery, 857, 857f

End-inspiratory pause (plateau), 720–721
    clinical applications of, 720–721
    operational principles of, 720, 721f, 721t

Endocardial blood flow, reduction of, spontaneous breathing and, 740

Endocarditis
    antibiotic combination therapy for, 1564
    in aspergillosis, 1688
    bacterial. *See* Infective endocarditis
    candidal, 1687
    prosthetic valve, staphylococcal, 1659, 1661–1662

Endocrine system. *See also* Hormones; *specific endocrine glands and hormones*
    disorders of. *See also specific disorders*
        lithium toxicity and, 1494
        during pregnancy, direct hormonal effects on, 319–320
    regulation of metabolic responses to critical illness and, 331–332

Endogenous pyrogens, 1591

Endogenous transmission, 510–511

Endoscopic retrograde cholangiopancreatography (ERCP)
    for biliary pancreatitis, 2059
    diagnostic, in pancreatitis, 2057

Endoscopy
    for esophageal corrosive injury, 2074–2075
    for esophageal foreign bodies, 2073
    for esophageal obstruction, 2072
    for gastrointestinal bleeding, 2037, 2038t

Endothelial cells
    activation of, host response and, 294–296, 295f
    interactions with leukocytes, host response and, 296

Endothelial permeability, pulmonary fluid and protein homeostasis and, 202

Endothelin, 246

Endothelium-derived relaxing factors (EDRFs), 246f, 246–247

Endotoxins, sepsis and, 407, 407t

Endotracheal intubation
    complications of, 1837t
    fiberoptic bronchoscopy for, 686–687, 689f, 697t

Endotracheal tubes
    complications of, 1928
    infections associated with, 2209–2210, 2210f
    position of, following thoracic surgery, 1135
    work of breathing and, 215–216, 216f, 734–735

Endotracheal venous cannulation, 537

Endurance, of diaphragm, 211

Energy
    expenditure of, protein-sparing modified fast and, in obese surgical patients, 1283–1284, 1284f
    metabolism of
        cellular, gastrointestinal, 444–445
        hepatic graft function assessment and optimization and, 1347
    requirement for, 460–461
    supply and demand of, respiratory muscle loading and, 216–217

Enteral nutrition. *See* Feeding tube placement; Nutritional support, enteral

Enteral perforations. *See also specific organs*
    renal transplantation and, 1306

Enteric abscesses, drainage of, 593

Enteric fever, 1670

Enterobacteriaceae infections, 1669
    endocarditis due to, treatment of, 1796t–1797t

Enterococci, 1666
    endocarditis due to, treatment of, 1793, 1796t–1797t

Enterocolitis
    neutropenic, in cancer, 2250–2251
    Yersinia, 1672

Enteropathy, necrotizing, in cancer, 2250–2251

Entropy, intrahospital transport and, 793

Envenomations, 1523–1534
    initial therapy for, 1524
    major problems with, 1523
    marine animals and, 1533f, 1533–1534
        clinical manifestations of, 1533–1534
        treatment of, 1534
    scorpion stings and, 1532–1533, 1533t
    snake bites and, 1524–1528, 1525f, 1526t, 1527t

antidote for, 1466t, 1527t, 1527–1528
    spider bites and, 1528–1532
        black widow spiders and, 1528f, 1528t, 1528–1530, 1530t
        brown recluse spiders and, 1530–1532, 1531f, 1531t
    stress points with, 1523–1524

Enzymatic therapy
    antioxidant
        for acute respiratory distress syndrome, 1834–1835
        for head injury, 1206
        pulmonary oxygen toxicity and, 708
    for esophageal obstruction, 2072

Enzyme-inducing agents, 486, 486t

Epididymitis, 2209

Epidural abscesses, 818, 1199
    cranial, clinical presentation and initial diagnostic measures for, 1638
    spinal, clinical presentation and initial diagnostic measures for, 1637–1638

Epidural analgesia, 815–816
    postoperative, 995–996, 1029–1030
    following thoracic surgery, 1134

Epidural catheters
    for anesthesia, 815–816
    complications of, 1247–1249
        catheter removal and, 1249
        clinical studies and recommended guidelines for, 1248t, 1248–1249

Epidural hematomas (EDHs), 818, 1199

Epidural local anesthetic blocks, 812
    complications of, 818

Epidural puncture, 814–815, 815t, 816f
    midline approach for, 814–815, 816f
    paramedian approach for, 815, 816f
    thoracic approach for, 815

Epiglottitis, 1710

Epilepsia partialis continua (EPC), 1987

Epilepsy. *See* Seizure(s); Status epilepticus

Epinephrine
    actions, indications, and dosing of, 2269
    for anaphylaxis, 1547t, 1547–1548
    following cardiac surgery
        for cardiac contractility augmentation, 1153
        in pediatric patients, 1166, 1167t
    for cardiomyopathy, peripartum, 1396
    for cardiopulmonary resuscitation, 499–501
        administration route for, 501
        dosage of, 500–501
        indications for, 500
    pheochromocytoma and, 2130
    preoperative, 994t
    regulation of metabolic responses to critical illness and, 331–332
    for shock, 363t

Epsilon aminocaproic acid (EACA)
    for amniotic fluid embolism, 1912
    for disseminated intravascular coagulation, 2222
    transfusion therapy and, 662

Epstein-Barr virus infections
    encephalitis due to, 1694
    in immunocompromised patients, 1695
        following bone marrow transplantation, lymphoproliferative disease due to, 1377

Epstein-Barr virus infections, in immunocompromised patients (*continued*)
  following lung and heart-lung transplantation, 1330
  following renal transplantation, 1307
Error
  in diagnosis, 96
  laboratory, 99t, 99–100, 100t
  type I and type II (α and β), 16–17
Erythema chronicum migrans (ECM), 1682
Erythema multiforme, 2175–2177
  diagnosis of, 2176
  etiology of, 2175, 2176t
  management of, 2176–2177
  presentation of, 2175–2176, 2176f, 2177f
Erythrocytosis, 2239–2240
  in polycythemia vera, 2239–2240, 2240t
  secondary, 2240
Erythroderma, 2181f, 2181–2182
  diagnosis of, 2181–2182
  etiology of, 2181, 2181t
  management of, 2182
  presentation of, 2181
Erythromycin, 1569
  cost and initial dosage of, 1562t
  dosage adjustment for, in hepatic disease, 482t
  for *Legionella* infections, 1609, 1673
  for pneumonia, 1851t
  prophylactic
    for infective endocarditis, 1798t
    for surgical patients, 1010t
  for *Rhodococcus equi* infections, in HIV-infected patients, 1620t
Erythropoietin, red blood cell production and, 663
Escharotomy, 1269
Escherichia coli infections, 1670
E-selectin, host response and, 294–295
Esmolol
  actions, indications, and dosing of, 2269
  for arrhythmias, 1785
  for cardiac contractility augmentation, following cardiac surgery, 1153
  for hypertension, in hypertensive emergencies, 1814t, 1816
Esophageal disorders, 2071–2077. *See also specific disorders*
  corrosive. *See* Corrosive injuries
  foreign bodies, 2073
    management of, 2073
    presentation of, 2073
  immediate concerns with, 2071
  medication-induced, 2076–2077
    management of, 2077
    presentation of, 2076t, 2076–2077
  stress points with, 2071
Esophageal gastric tube airway, 493, 494f
Esophageal injuries, 1091
  chest pain and, 1723–1724
Esophageal obstruction, 2071–2073
  diagnostic approach to, 2072, 2072f
  by foreign bodies, 2073
    management of, 2073
    presentation of, 2073
  management of, 2072–2073

presentation of, 2071
  special considerations for, 2073
Esophageal obturator airway (EOA), 493, 494f, 763, 763f
Esophageal perforation, 1142, 2075–2076
  diagnostic approach to, 2075f, 2075–2076
  management of, 2076
  presentation of, 2075
  special considerations with, 2076
Esophageal rupture, chest pain and, 1723–1724
Esophageal spasm, chest pain and, 1724
Esophageal stenosis, in corrosive injury, prevention of, 2074
Esophageal tracheal comitube (ETC), 763
Esophageal ulcers, in HIV-infected patients, 1629
Esophagitis
  herpes simplex virus, 1695
  in HIV-infected patients, 1629
  treatment of, 1619t
Esophagoscopy
  in esophageal obstruction, 2072, 2072f
  rigid
    for esophageal foreign bodies, 2073
    esophageal perforation during, 2076
Estrogens
  conjugated, for uremic bleeding defects, 2094t
  during pregnancy, direct effects of, 318t, 318–320
Ethambutol
  for *Mycobacterium avium* complex infections, in HIV-infected patients, 1619t
  for *Mycobacterium tuberculosis* infections, in HIV-infected patients, 1619t
Ethanol
  abuse of, 1512–1514
    acute toxicity and, 1512t, 1512–1513, 1513t
    bacterial, 2239
    chronic disease and, 1514
    rhabdomyolysis due to, 2198
    treatment of acute intoxication and, 1513
    withdrawal and, 1513–1514
  for ethylene glycol poisoning, 1446t, 1503
  for methanol poisoning, 1466t, 1502
Ethical considerations, 63–79
  deontology and utilitarianism and, 64
  factors compelling treatment even in likelihood of negative outcome and, 74–77
  futility debate and, 73–74
  in informed consent, 83–84, 85–86
  law and, 64, 72–73
  medicomoral principles and, 64f, 64–73, 65f, 69t–70t
    autonomy and, 67
    critical care team and, 71–73
    family's role and, 71
    justice and, 67
    limitation or refusal of treatment and, 68, 70–71, 72
    nonmaleficence and, 66–67
    potential for salvageability and, 66
    preservation of life and, 66
    society's impact on, 73
  morality and, 63–64
  parties to decision-making process and, 68, 69t–70t, 70–73
  physician aid-in-dying and, 77–79

Ethionamide, for *Mycobacterium tuberculosis* infections, in HIV-infected patients, 1620t
Ethosuximide
  for status epilepticus, 1987
  therapeutic serum level of, 479t
Ethylene glycol poisoning, 1501, 1502–1503
  antidote for, 1466t
Etidomate, 825t, 825–826
  during pregnancy, 320
Etidronate disodium, for hypercalcemia, in cancer, 2247
Etoposide, for bone marrow transplantation, 1368t
Etretinate, for generalized pustular psoriasis, 2180
Euglobulin clot lysis time, 271
Euthyroid sick syndrome, 2114–2115, 2115f, 2146
Euvolemia, hyponatremia and
  causes of, 417
  treatment of, 418
Evisceration, 1085
Evoked potentials
  for monitoring cerebral function, 945f, 945–946
  near-drowning and, as prognostic indicator, 1883
Excitability, cardiac, 228–229
Excitation-contraction coupling, 229t, 229–231
  ultrastructural changes and, 229–231, 230f, 231f
Excitatory amino acid (EAA) neurotransmitters, for brain injury, 286
Exercise testing
  preoperative, 990–991
  submaximal, in acute myocardial infarction, 1743
Exercise tolerance, in advanced heart failure, as prognostic factor, 1754
Exfoliative dermatitis, 2181f, 2181–2182
  diagnosis of, 2181–2182
  etiology of, 2181, 2181t
  management of, 2182
  presentation of, 2181
Exogenous transmission, 510
Expiratory plateau, capnometry and, 879
Expiratory pressure valves, for continuous positive airway pressure and spontaneous positive end-expiratory pressure, 730–731, 731f
Expiratory reserve volume (ERV), in obese surgical patients, 1279
Expiratory upstroke, capnometry and, 879
Exposure
  for initial triage of trauma patients, 1043
  for secondary triage of trauma patients, 1050
Extensive nursing requirement, 24
External compression devices
  for deep venous thrombosis prevention, 1241
  for pulmonary thromboembolism prevention, 1241
External fixation, for fractures, 1223–1225, 1224f
  pelvic, 1060, 1061
External rewarming, for hypothermia, 1453–1454
External transcutaneous cardiac pacing, 552, 552f

Extracardiac obstructive shock, 367
Extracorporeal membrane oxygenation (ECMO), 669–680
  in adults
    complications of, 678
    historical background of, 670
    pathophysiology and, 671
    patient selection for, 672
    results of, 678–679
    techniques and management of, 675
  cardiac support using, 679–680
    complications of, 680
    outcome of, 679
    techniques for, 679–680
  in children
    following cardiac surgery, 1174
    historical background of, 670–671
    results of, 678
  complications of, 677–678
  ECMO team and, 676f, 676–677
  historical background of, 670–671
    in trauma, 671
  laboratory investigations for, 679
  major problems with, 669
  in neonates
    complications of, 677–678
    historical background of, 670
    pathophysiology and, 671
    patient selection for, 671–672
    results of, 678
    techniques and management of, 672–674
  pathophysiology and, 671
  patient selection for, 671–672
  results of, 678–679
  stress points with, 669–670
  techniques and management of, 672–675
  techniques and management with
    anticoagulation, transfusion, and fluid therapy and, 674
    circuit preparation and, 672, 672f
    circulation and, 673, 673f
    ductal closure and, 674
    mechanical ventilation and, 673
    surgical preparation and, 672, 673f
    therapeutic endpoints and, 674, 674f
    weaning and, 674
  in trauma, historical background of, 671
  venovenous, 675–676
    advantages of, 675, 676f
    outcome with, 675–676
    rationale for, 675
Extracorporeal respiratory support, for acute respiratory distress syndrome, 1836
Extradural hematomas, 818, 1199
Extrapyramidal toxidrome, 1468, 1469t
Extra-renal fluid removal. See also Hemofiltration; Peritoneal dialysis
  ultrafiltration for
    for heart failure, 1762
    for respiratory failure, 2098
Extravascular lung water, in shock, 377t
Extremities. See also Legs
  ankle, venous cutdown at, 569, 573f
  arm examination for femorofemoral and axillofemoral bypass procedures and, 1186

ischemia of, following cardiac surgery in pediatric patients, 1172–1173
  in poisonings and toxic exposures, 1471
  vascular injuries of
    arteriography in, 1187
    management of, 1188–1189
Extrinsic coagulation pathway, 270
Extubation
  complications of, 1837t, 1928
  inadvertent, 768
  indications for, with burns, 1266–1267
Eyes. See also Ocular disorders; specific disorders
  decontamination of, 1473
    for insecticide poisoning, 1506
  movements of, in comatose patients, evaluation of, 1973–1974
  pupils of
    in comatose patients, evaluation of, 1974–1975
    local anesthetics and, 819
    in poisonings and toxic exposures, 1471–1472

Face masks, 705–706
  air entrainment, 705–706, 706f
  nonrebreathing, 705
  partial rebreathing, 705, 705f
  simple, 705
Factor assays, 270
Fahrenheit temperature conversions, 2255t
Failure-to-cycle alarms, on mechanical ventilators, 719
Falls, 101
False aneurysms, management of, 1188
Families
  of burn patients, counseling for, 1274
  consent for organ donation and, 1292, 1296
  in decision-making process, 69t, 71
  futile care insisted on by, 114–115
  of incompetent patients, informed consent and, 83
  as presumptively appropriate surrogate, 110
  psychological reactions of. See Psychological factors
  reaction to imminent death, 93–94
  staff involvement with, 91–92
    methods for involving families and, 91–92
  termination of cardiopulmonary resuscitation and, 161
  treatment objectives and, 26–27
  withdrawal of treatment and, 113
Famotidine
  actions, indications, and dosing of, 2270
  for aspiration prophylaxis, 1871, 1871t
Fascia, abdominal, postoperative dehiscence of, 1115–1116
Fasciitis, necrotizing, 2192
Fasciotomy
  for compartment syndromes, 1236–1237, 1237f
  for snake bites, 1528
Fat, mobilization and oxidation of, in obese surgical patients, protein-sparing modified fast for, 1283, 1284f
Fat embolism
  arterial, 1907

in obstetric patients, 1413
Fat embolism syndrome (FES), 1237–1239, 1908t, 1908–1909
  diagnosis of, 1237–1238
    cardiovascular manifestations and, 1238
    neurologic manifestations and, 1237–1238
  pathogenesis of, 1237, 1238f
  treatment of, 1238–1239
    fracture stabilization and, 1238–1239, 1240t
Fatigue, of respiratory muscles, 193, 193t
  diaphragm, 211
  loading and, 216, 217f
Fat microemboli, autotransfusion and, 665
Fatty acids
  deficiency of, prevention of, in obese surgical patients, 1284
  free, metabolism in critical illness, 330–331, 331f
Fear, 90. See also Anxiety; Stress (emotional)
Fecal fistulas, postoperative, 1114t
Fecal incontinence bags, for diarrhea, 2212
Feeding tube(s), infections associated with, 2210
Feeding tube placement, 599–606
  diagnostic tests and procedures for, 600
  initial therapy for, 600
  major problems with, 599
  placement technique options for, 602–605
    nasoduodenal and nasojejunal, 602–603, 603f
    nasogastric, 602
    novel, 605
    percutaneous gastrostomy, 603–604
    percutaneous jejunostomy, 604
    surgical gastrostomy, 604–605
    surgical jejunostomy, 605, 605f, 606f
  stress points with, 599–600
  tube options for, 601–602
  type, site, and placement technique determination for, 600–601, 602f
Femoral artery cannulation, 540t, 541
Femoral vein cannulation, 526–527
Femorofemoral bypass, 1186
  arm examination for, 1186
  brachial plexus injury and, 1186
  graft tunnels for, 1186
  mortality and, 1186
  positioning for, 1186
Fenoldopam mesylate, for hypertension, in hypertensive emergencies, 1816
Fentanyl
  actions, indications, and dosing of, 2269
  following cardiac surgery, 1157–1158
  cost of, 827t
Fertility, following bone marrow transplantation, 1379
Fetal assessment, following maternal trauma, 1422–1423, 1423f
Fetal circulation, persistent, extracorporeal membrane oxygenation for, 671
Fetal demise, intrauterine, 1406
Fetal heart rate
  assessment of, following maternal trauma, 1422, 1423f
  monitoring of, 1432
    limitations of, 1432
    modifications of, 1432

Fetal monitoring, 1429–1435
  acute adaptations and, 1434t, 1434–1435
    bradycardia and, 1434
    of lactate metabolism, 1434
    of metabolic rate, 1434
    spontaneous movement and, 1435
  background of, 1430–1431
    electrocardiographic monitoring and, 1430
    maternal-fetal interactions and, 1430–1431
    oxygen deprivation and hypoglycemia and, 1430
  chronic adaptations and, 1433t, 1433–1434
    compensatory, 1433–1434
    of placental diffusion capacity, 1433, 1433t
  diagnostic tests and procedures for, 1429–1430
  of heart rate, 1432
    limitations of, 1432
    modifications of, 1432
  initial therapy for, 1430
  major problems with, 1429
  of oxygenation, 1431–1432
    oxygen consumption and, 1431
    oxygen supply and availability and, 1431
    stress of labor and, 1431
  of scalp pH, 1432–1433
  stress points with, 1429
  of transition changes, 1433
Fever, 1589–1601. *See also* Hyperpyrexia; Hyperthermia
  in adrenocortical insufficiency, 1600–1601
  antibiotics and, 1562
  following bone marrow transplantation, 1371
  causes of, 1592, 1592t
    blood transfusions, 1599–1600
    drugs, 484, 1598–1599, 1599t
  definition of, 1591
  diagnostic tests and procedures for, 1590
  in head injury, 1205
  in HIV-infected patients, 1630
  infectious sources of, 1593–1598
    catheter-related, 1594–1595
    in granulocytopenic patients, 1605
    intraabdominal, 1596–1598
    neurologic, 1595–1596
    respiratory, 1593–1594
    surgical and traumatic wounds, 1595
    urinary tract, 1594
  initial therapy for, 1590–1591, 1591f
  major problems with, 1589, 1590f
  in malignant hyperthermia. *See* Malignant hyperthermia (MH)
  in neuroleptic malignant syndrome. *See* Neuroleptic malignant syndrome (NMS)
  pathophysiology of, 1591
  as predictor of infection, 1592–1593
  with pulmonary embolism, 1601
  purpose of, 1591
  stress points with, 1589
  in systemic lupus erythematosus, 2164–2165
Fiberoptic bronchoscopy. *See* Bronchoscopy, fiberoptic
Fibrinogen
  evaluation of, in coagulation disorders, 1067
  reactive hyperfibrinogenemia and, 2229
Fibrinolysis, 270–272

chemical, for pulmonary embolism, 588
  components of, 270t, 270–271
  drugs inhibiting, for gastrointestinal bleeding, 2037
  function in normal coagulation, 271
  host response and, 299
  laboratory assessment of, 271–272
  primary, hemorrhage and, 2220t
Fick technique, for cardiac output determination, 895
Film dressings, 2204
Filters
  high-efficiency particulate air filtration, for infection prophylaxis following bone marrow transplantation, 1371
  inferior vena caval. *See* Inferior vena caval (IVC) filters
  for pulmonary embolism, 588
Fine-needle aspiration (FNA), in pneumonia, 1853
Firearm wounds. *See* Trauma; *specific sites and injuries*
Fire coral envenomations, 1533t, 1533–1534
  clinical manifestations of, 1533–1534
  treatment of, 1534
Fistulas
  aortoenteric. *See* Aortoenteric fistulas (AEFs)
  arteriovenous, management of, 1188
  biliary. *See* Biliary fistulas
  bronchopleural
    fiberoptic bronchoscopy in, 696
    tube thoracostomy as cause of, 559–560
  care of, 2206–2207, 2247
  colonic, 1114
  duodenal, 1090, 1114, 1114t
  fecal, 1114t
  gastric, 1114, 1114t
  ileal, 1114, 1114t
  intestinal, 1090, 1114t, 1114–1115
  jejunal, 1114
  open abdomen and, 1115
  pancreatic, 1114, 1114t
    in pancreatitis, 2061
  postoperative, 1113–1115
  tracheoesophageal, following thoracic surgery, 1143
  tracheoinnominate, following thoracic surgery, 1143
  treatment of, 1114–1115
Fixation
  external, for fractures, 1223–1225, 1224f
    pelvic, 1060, 1061
  internal, for fractures, 1225f, 1225–1226
FK-506, *See* Tacrolimus (FK–506; Prograf)
Flail chest, 1138–1139
  conservative management of, 1138
  internal stabilization with ventilator support for, 1138
  surgical management of, 1138
Flanks, definition of, 1077
Flaps, compromised, hyperbaric oxygen therapy for, 781
Flavobacterium infections, 1672
Flecainide, dosing of, in chronic renal failure, 2097t
Flora, resident and transient, 509

Flosequinan, for heart failure, 1757
Flow-cycled ventilators, 713
Flow valves, microprocessor-controlled, of mechanical ventilators, 714t
Flucloxacillin, for infective endocarditis, 1794t
Fluconazole, 1570, 1690t, 1691
  for *Candida* infections, in HIV-infected patients, 1619t
  for coccidioidomycosis, in HIV-infected patients, 1619t
  for cryptococcosis, in HIV-infected patients, 1619t
  for meningitis, in renal transplant recipients, 1612
  for urinary tract infections, 1655
5-Flucytosine (5-FC)
  for meningitis, in renal transplant recipients, 1612
  therapeutic serum level of, 479t
  for urinary tract infections, 1655
Fludrocortisone, for hyperkalemia, 426
Fluid and electrolyte disorders, 413–443. *See also* Electrolyte management; Fluid therapy; Hyperosmolar states; Hypoosmolar states; *specific disorders; specific electrolytes*
  antibiotics and, 1563t
  diagnostic tests for
    for composition disorders, 414
    for volume disorders, 414
  electrolyte imbalances
    in advanced heart failure, as prognostic factor, 1754–1755
    digitalis poisoning and, 1498
    nutritional support and, 469
    in theophylline poisoning, 1501
  fluid compartments and, 414–415
    distribution and, 414, 414t
    effects of fluid administration and, 414–415, 415t
  in head injury, 1206–1207
  hypervolemic. *See* Hypervolemia
  hypovolemic. *See* Hypovolemia; Hypovolemic shock
  initial therapy for
    for composition disorders, 414
    for volume disorders, 414
  major problems with, 413
  stress points and, 413–414
Fluid collections
  infected. *See* Abscess(es); *specific sites*
  noninfected, drainage of, 593–594
  percutaneous catheter drainage of. *See* Catheter drainage, percutaneous
  pericardial
    in cancer, 2250
    echocardiography in, 885
    pericardiocentesis and, 577
  pleural. *See* Pleural effusions
  thoracic, drainage of, 593
Fluid homeostasis
  following intestinal transplantation, 1360
  following multivisceral transplantation, 1360
  pulmonary, 202–204
    anatomic considerations and, 202–203
    fluid flux and, 203

pulmonary edema and, 203–204
shifts in, hyperkalemia due to, 425
Fluid therapy, 433–437
 for acute respiratory distress syndrome, 1833
 for acute respiratory failure, 1922
 for acute tumor lysis syndrome, 2247
 for aspiration syndromes, 1866
 for bone marrow transplantation, 1369
 during brain resuscitation, 282
 for burn patients, 1269
 following cardiac surgery in adult patients,
  1151f, 1151–1152
 following cardiac surgery in pediatric
  patients, 1164–1165
  preload and afterload adjustment and, 1164
  specific indications for, 1164–1165
 colloids for, 434–435
  capillary permeability changes and, 434
  following cardiac surgery, 1152
  complications of, 437
  crystalloids versus, 435f, 435–437
  distribution of, 434, 437
  hemostasis and, 436–437
  oncotic pressure gradients and, 434–435
  role of, 435–436
 crystalloids for, 433–434, 434t
  following cardiac surgery, 1152
  colloids versus, 435f, 435–437
  complications of, 437
  distribution of, 433–434, 437
 for diabetic ketoacidosis, 2104–2105
 for dysoxia, 341
 effects of fluid administration and, 414–415,
  415t
 extracorporeal membrane oxygenation and, 674
 for hypercalcemia, in cancer, 2246
 for hyperosmolar hyperglycemic nonketotic
  diabetes, 2107
 for hyperthermia, 1457
 hypertonic solutions for, 437
  complications of, 437
  distribution of, 437
 initial triage of trauma patients and, 1043
 intravenous fluids for, 2257t
 following liver transplantation, 1343–1344,
  1344f
 mesenteric and renal artery reconstructions
  and, 1183
 for multiple organ system failure, 353–354
 near-drowning and, 1880, 1881f
 for organ donors, 1294, 1295
 for sepsis, 410
 for shock, 378
 in trauma patients, 1049
Flumazenil (Romazicon)
 actions, indications, and dosing of, 2269
 for antipsychotic poisoning, 1495–1496
 for benzodiazepine poisoning, 1465t
 benzodiazepine reversal with, 825
5-Fluorocytosine, 1690t
Fluoxetine, side effects of, 2027t
Flurazepam (Dalmane), 825t
 for agitation and anxiety, 2026t
Flush devices, for invasive pressure monitoring,
  840
Foams, for wounds, 2205

Folate, red blood cell production and, 663
Folic acid
 for methanol poisoning, 1502
 requirement for, 464, 464t
Folinic acid, for *Toxoplasma* infections, in HIV-
  infected patients, 1620t
Follicle-stimulating hormone (FSH), deficiency
  of, 2113
Food bolus, esophageal obstruction by. *See*
  Esophageal obstruction
Food poisoning, *Clostridium perfringens*, 1677
Forced expiratory volume in 1 second,
  preoperative assessment of, 990
Forced vital capacity (FVC), preoperative
  assessment of, 989, 989t
Force-velocity curve, for cardiac contraction,
  232f, 232–233, 233f
Foreign bodies
 aspiration of
  fiberoptic bronchoscopy for, 696–697
  removal from airway, in cardiopulmonary
   resuscitation, 493
 esophageal, 2073
  management of, 2073
  presentation of, 2073
 radiologic interventions for, 590
 wound management and, 782
Formaldehyde, inhalation injury due to, 1954
Foscarnet (Foscavir), 1571
 cost and initial dosage of, 1562t
 for cytomegalovirus infections, in HIV-infected
  patients, 1619t
 for heart-lung transplantation, 1330
 for herpes simplex virus infections, in HIV-
  infected patients, 1619t
 for lung transplantation, 1330
Fracture(s), 1219–1229. *See also* Orthopedic
  complications; *specific sites*
 casts and splints for, 1221
 complications of, 1227–1229
  compartment syndrome. *See* Compartment
   syndromes
  infection, 1228–1229
  limitation of joint motion, 1228
  neurovascular compromise, 1227
  swelling, 1227
 diagnosis of, 1220–1221
  delayed, 1054, 2211
  tests and procedures for, 1219–1220
 external fixation of, 1223–1225, 1224f
 initial therapy for, 1220
 internal fixation of, 1225f, 1225–1226
 major problems with, 1219
 multiple trauma and, 1226–1227
 open, 1226
  infection and, 1228–1229
 stabilization of, in fat embolism syndrome,
  1238–1239, 1240t
 stress points with, 1219
 traction for, 1221–1223
  cervical, 1223
  skeletal, 1221–1223, 1222f
  skin, 1221, 1221f
 vascular injuries with, management of, 1188
Fracture blisters, 1227
Francisella tularensis infections, 1672

Frank-Starling principle, 234f–236f, 234–235,
  238, 238f
Free radicals
 pulmonary oxygen toxicity and, 707
 reperfusion injury and, 445–446, 446f
 scavengers for
  for brain injury, 286
  for head injury, 1206
Free wall rupture
 cardiogenic shock and, 394–395
 surgical intervention for, 402
Frequency domain analysis, 944f, 944–945
Fresh frozen plasma (FFP), 648–649
 for coagulopathy, 648–649
  due to massive transfusion, 2225
 for disseminated intravascular coagulation,
  2221
 for hemolytic abnormalities in liver disease,
  2223
 indications for, 648–649
Fresh water, aspiration of, 1878. *See also*
  Drowning; Near-drowning
Fulminant colitis, 2066–2069
 clinical features of, 2066
 diagnosis of, 2066–2067
 from infectious causes, 2069
 management of, 2067–2068
 patient monitoring in, 2068–2069
 patterns of response to medical treatment of,
  2069
 during pregnancy, 2069
 signs of impending perforation in, 2069
 surgical treatment of, 2069
Fulminant glomerulonephritis, acute renal failure
  due to, 2084, 2085f, 2085t
Fulminant hepatic failure (FHF), 2045–2053
 complications and treatment of, 2047t,
  2047–2053, 2048t
  cerebral edema and, 2047–2050
  coagulopathy and, 2050
  encephalopathy and, 2047, 2049t
  gastrointestinal bleeding and, 2050–2051
  initial therapy for, 2046
  loss of vasomotor tone and high-output
   failure and, 2051
  metabolic disorders and, 2052
  oliguric renal failure and fluid overload
   and, 2051
  respiratory care and, 2052
  sepsis and impaired immune response and,
   2051–2052
  transplantation for, 2052t, 2052–2053
 diagnostic tests and procedures for, 2046
 etiology and prognosis of, 2046, 2046t, 2047t
 major problems with, 2045
 stress points with, 2045–2046
Functional residual capacity (FRC), 189–190,
  190f, 191t
 in obese surgical patients, 1279, 1279f
 maintenance of, 1279–1280, 1280f
Fundoplication, Nissen, for aspiration
  prophylaxis, 1872
Fungal infections, 1685–1691. *See also specific*
  infections
 antibiotics effective against, 1560t
 endocarditis due to, 1792

Fungal infections, endocarditis due to
  (*continued*)
    treatment of, 1793
  nosocomial, 1583
  pneumonia due to, 1688–1689
    in HIV-infected patients, 1624–1625
  topical, 2207
  treatment of. *See* Antifungal agents; *specific drugs*
  of urinary tract, 1655
Furosemide
  actions, indications, and dosing of, 2269
  for acute renal failure, 2090
  following cardiac surgery in pediatric patients, 1172
  for hypercalcemia, 429t
  for intracranial hypertension, 284
  for respiratory failure, in chronic renal failure, 2097, 2098
Fusidic acid, for infective endocarditis, 1794t
Futile care
  cardiopulmonary resuscitation as, 158t, 158–159
  family insistence on, 114–115

Galambos cocktail, for hepatorenal syndrome, 1124
Gallbladder necrosis, fever associated with, 1596
Gallium nitrate, for hypercalcemia, in cancer, 2247
Gallium scans, abdominal, sepsis and, 1113
Gallstones, ultrasonographic detection of, 977, 980f
Gamma globulin, intravenous. *See* Intravenous immunoglobulin (IVIg)
Ganciclovir (Cytovene), 1571, 1700, 1700t
  cost and initial dosage of, 1562t
  for cytomegalovirus infections
    in HIV-infected patients, 1619t
    in renal transplant recipients, 1611–1612
  for heart-lung transplantation, 1319t, 1330
  for interstitial pneumonitis, in bone marrow transplant recipients, 1614
  for intestinal transplantation, 1361
  for lung and heart-lung transplantation, 1330
  for lung transplantation, 1319t, 1330
  for multivisceral transplantation, 1361
  prophylactic, heart transplantation and, 1339
Gangrene
  gas, hyperbaric oxygen therapy for, 780
  synergistic, abdominal, postoperative, 1115
Gas(es)
  blood. *See* Arterial blood gases (ABGs); Blood gas(es); Blood gas analysis; *specific gases*
  toxic, inhalation of. *See* Inhalation injuries
Gas embolism. *See* Air embolism
Gas exchange, 198–199
  alterations in, acute respiratory distress syndrome and, 1830
  alveolar gas composition and, 198–199
  blood gas composition and, 199
  gas transfer and, 199
  lung and heart-lung transplantation and, 1325–1326, 1326f
  maintenance of, with burns, 1266

in obese surgical patients, support of, 1280
  in pulmonary capillaries, 198, 198f
Gas flow, for intermittent mandatory ventilation, 723
Gas gangrene, hyperbaric oxygen therapy for, 780
Gas trapping, airway resistance and, 197–198
Gastric atony, in spinal cord injury, treatment of, 1214
Gastric contents, aspiration of. *See* Aspiration, of gastric contents
Gastric distension, enteral nutrition and, 469
Gastric emptying
  delayed, postoperative, 1111
  in poisonings and toxic exposures, 1473–1474, 1474t
Gastric fistulas, postoperative, 1114, 1114t
Gastric hypersecretion, in spinal cord injury, treatment of, 1214
Gastric injuries, 1091–1092
Gastric lavage
  for acetaminophen poisoning, 1484
  for aspiration syndromes, 1866
  for cyclic antidepressant poisoning, 1491
  for gastrointestinal bleeding, 2035–2036
  for insecticide poisoning, 1506
  for poisonings and toxic exposures, 1473–1474, 1474t
Gastric mucosa, cytoprotection of, for sepsis, 410
Gastroenteritis, bacteremia associated with, in HIV-infected patients, 1627
Gastrointestinal access, for enteral nutrition, 465–466. *See also* Feeding tube(s); Feeding tube placement
  complications of, 469
Gastrointestinal bleeding, 2033–2041
  in burn patients, 1270–1271
  in chronic renal failure, 2094, 2094t
  colonic perforation and, 2069
  diagnostic tests and procedures for, 2033
  in fulminant hepatic failure, 2050–2051
  hemobilia and, 1127
  intestinal transplantation and, 1356
  liver transplantation and, 1348
  lower, 2040–2041, 2041t
    evaluation of, 2040–2041
    radiologic interventions for, 589–590
  major problems with, 2033, 2034t
  multivisceral transplantation and, 1356
  postshunt, 1123–1124
  stress points with, 2033
  stress ulceration as cause of. *See* Stress ulceration
  treatment of, 2035–2037
    critical assessment of, 2037
    empiric, for upper gastrointestinal bleeding, 2035
    endoscopy in, 2037
    gastric lavage in, 2035–2036
    ICU admission criteria and, 2035
    initial therapy for, 2033
    pharmacologic, 2036t, 2036–2037
    radiologic interventions for, 589–590
  upper
    amount of, 2034, 2034t
    diagnostic and management approach for, 2034–2035

empiric therapy for, 2035
    lesions causing, 2035
    radiologic interventions for, 589
    source of, 2034–2035
Gastrointestinal disorders. *See also specific disorders*
  in acute respiratory distress syndrome, 1837t
  anaphylaxis and, 1545t
  antibiotics and, 1563t
  antirheumatic agents as cause of, 2156t
  in cancer, 2250–2251
  candidal, 1686
  chest pain in, 1718t
    life-threatening, 1723–1724
  enteral nutrition and, 469
  in HIV-infected patients, 1629–1630
    abdominal pain and, 1629–1630
    diarrhea, 1629
    dysphagia and odynophagia, 1629
  lithium toxicity and, 1494
  in obstetric patients, 1424
  parenteral nutrition and, 470
  in poisonings and toxic exposures, 1471–1472
  in refractory advanced heart failure, 1758
  renal transplantation and, 1306
  shock and, 372
  in systemic sclerosis, 2173
Gastrointestinal function. *See also* Intestinal function
  in hypokalemia, 424t
  in hypomagnesemia, 432t
  intravenous narcotics and, 1022
Gastrointestinal obstruction
  esophageal. *See* Esophageal obstruction
  intestinal, colonic pseudo-obstruction and, acute abdomen and, 1106, 1106f
  pancreatic pseudocysts and, surgical treatment of, 2060
Gastrointestinal surgery, postoperative ICU care for, 1111
Gastrointestinal system. *See also specific organs*
  cellular energy metabolism of, 444–445
  dysoxic versus normoxic state and, 446
  eliminating poisons from, 1473–1474, 1474t
  global parameters of oxygen delivery and utilization in, 446–447
  microcirculation of, 443–444, 444t
  multiple organ system failure and, 447f, 447–448, 448f
  pH of
    acidosis of gastric mucosa in surgical patients and, 448–450, 449f
    depressed, therapy of, 452
    future research directions for, 452–453
    gastric, drugs raising, 2036
    tonometric monitoring of, 443, 450–452
  reperfusion injury of, 445–446, 446f
Gastrostomy
  percutaneous, 595
    for feeding tube placement, 603–604
  surgical, for feeding tube placement, 604–605
Gastrostomy tubes, 1116f, 1117
Gated radionuclide angiography, in acute myocardial infarction, 1741
Gaucher's disease, coagulation disorder associated with, 2230

Generalizability, 5–6
Generalized myasthenia, 2012
Generalized pustular psoriasis, 2179–2180
  diagnosis of, 2180
  etiology of, 2179–2180, 2180t
  management of, 2180
  presentation of, 2180, 2180f
Generalized seizures, 1982
Genitalia, external
  penile venous cannulation and, 537–538
  priapism and, 2234–2235
  trauma to, 1261–1262
    penile, 1262
    of skin and scrotum, 1261–1262
Genitourinary disorders. *See also specific disorders*
  candidal, 1687–1688
  in sickle cell anemia, 2234–2235
  in spinal cord injury, management of, 1215
Genitourinary injury scales, 2278t–2279t
Gentamicin, 1568, 1568t
  following cardiac surgery in pediatric patients, 1172
  cost and initial dosage of, 1562t
  for infective endocarditis
    prophylactic, 1799t
    treatment of, 1793, 1794t, 1795t, 1796
  in renal disease, 480–481
    volume of distribution of, 480–481, 481t
  therapeutic serum level of, 479t
  for tularemia, 1707–1708
Geriatric patients. *See* Elderly patients
Glands. *See also* Hormones; *specific glands and hormones*
  during pregnancy, direct hormonal effects on, 319–320
Glasgow Coma Scale (GCS), 941–942, 942f, 942t
  in head injury, 1195, 1196, 1196t, 1197, 1202
    intracranial pressure and, 1203
  near-drowning and, 1880
    as prognostic indicator, 1882
  outcome prediction and, 138
Glasgow Outcome Scale, 1207–1208
Glomerular filtration rate (GFR), acute renal failure and, 2086–2087, 2087f
Glomerular hemodynamics, alterations in, acute renal failure due to, 2085
Glomerulonephritis (GN)
  fulminant, acute renal failure due to, 2084, 2085f, 2085t
  in systemic lupus erythematosus, 2169
Glucagon
  actions, indications, and dosing of, 2269–2270
  for cardiogenic shock, 401
  for esophageal obstruction, 2072
  for poisonings, 1465t
    beta-blockers and, 1497
    calcium channel blockers and, 1498
  regulation of metabolic responses to critical illness and, 331–332
Glucagon stimulation test, in pheochromocytomas, 2132
Glucocorticoids. *See also specific glucocorticoids*
  actions of, 2123
  production of, 2122
  therapeutic, 2125–2126. *See also specific drugs*

dosage of, 2125–2126
  for hypercalcemia, in cancer, 2247
  for shock, 381
  tapering of, 2126
  for thyrotoxicosis, 2140
Glucose
  deficit of
    coma and, 1977
    fetal, oxygen deprivation and, 1430
  excess of. *See* Hyperglycemia
  levels following cardiac surgery in pediatric patients, 1170
  metabolism of. *See also* Diabetes mellitus (DM)
    in critical illness, 329t, 329–330, 330t
  requirement for, in salicylate poisoning, 1488
  therapeutic use of
    for diabetes mellitus, complicated by medical illness or surgery, 2108t
    for ethanol intoxication, 1513
    for hyperkalemia, 427t
    for status epilepticus, 1984
Glucose insulin potassium infusions, for limitation of infarct size, 397
Glucose-6-phosphate dehydrogenase (G6PD) deficiency, hemolytic anemia due to, 2233
Glutamate, for head injury, 1206
Glutamine
  for depressed gastrointestinal pH, 452
  metabolism of, in critical illness, 328–329
Glycerol, metabolism in critical illness, 331
Glycine vasopressin (Glyopressin), for gastrointestinal bleeding, 2037
Glycopyrrolate
  for fiberoptic bronchoscopy, 688–689
  for neuromuscular blocking agent reversal, 1032t
  for reversal of neuromuscular blockade, 835, 835t
Goiters
  airway obstruction by, 2147–2148
  multinodular, toxic, 2138
Gold compounds, adverse effects of, 2156t–2157t
Gonorrhea, 1667
  endocarditis due to, treatment of, 1793
Graduated compression stockings (GCSs), for deep venous thrombosis prophylaxis, 1890
Graft function
  compromised, hyperbaric oxygen therapy for, 781
  disorders of
    following bone marrow transplantation, 1374–1375, 1375t
    early, following liver transplantation, 1342
    primary, heart transplantation and, 1336–1337
  liver transplantation and, assessment and optimization of. *See* Hepatic transplantation, graft function assessment and optimization and
Graft infections
  of prosthetic heart valves, staphylococcal, 1662
  vascular surgery and, 1111, 1181–1182
    diagnosis of, 1181
    etiology of, 1181

  incidence of, 1181
  therapy of, 1181–1182
Graft rejection
  acute
    following heart transplantation, 1338
    following intestinal transplantation, 1362
    following lung and heart-lung transplantation, 1321–1322, 1324f, 1329
    following multivisceral transplantation, 1362
  hyperacute, following heart transplantation, 1335–1336
Graft stenosis, mesenteric and renal artery reconstructions and, 1183
  diagnosis of, 1183
  etiology of, 1183
  incidence of, 1183
  therapy of, 1183
Graft thrombosis
  intestinal transplantation and, prophylaxis of, 1361
  multivisceral transplantation and, prophylaxis of, 1361
  following vascular surgery, 1111, 1180–1181
    diagnosis of, 1180, 1183
    etiology of, 1180, 1183
    incidence of, 1180, 1183
    mesenteric and renal artery reconstructions, 1183
    therapy of, 1181, 1183
Graft tunnels, for femorofemoral and axillofemoral bypass procedures, 1186
Graft-versus-host disease (GVHD), 653–654
  following bone marrow transplantation, 1368, 1613–1614
    acute, 1375–1377, 1376t
    chronic, 1377–1378, 1378t
    clinical grading of, 1376t, 1376–1377
    diarrhea due to, 1372
    prevention of, 1376
  clinical presentation of, 653
  following intestinal transplantation, 1362
  morbidity and mortality due to, 654
  following multivisceral transplantation, 1362
Gram-negative bacilli infections
  anaerobic, 1678–1679
    aspiration pneumonia due to, 1679
    bacteremia due to, 1678
    brain abscess due to, 1679
    head and neck infections due to, 1678
    intraabdominal infections due to, 1678
  antibiotics effective against, 1559t
  in critical care settings, 1658t
Gram-negative cocci infections
  antibiotics effective against, 1558t
  in critical care settings, 1658t
Gram-negative rod infections
  ICP monitoring devices and, 1643
  meningitis due to, 1643, 1646
  neurologic, epidemiologic and clinical clues to, 1637
Gram-positive bacilli infections
  antibiotics effective against, 1558t
  in critical care settings, 1658t
Gram-positive cocci infections
  antibiotics effective against, 1558t

Gram-positive cocci infections (*continued*)
in critical care settings, 1658t
Gram staining, for diagnosis of infections, 1561
Granulocyte colony stimulating factor, for
leukopenia, 2236
Granulocytic ehrlichiosis (HGE), 1706
Granulocytopenia. *See also* Leukopenia
immune, 2236
infections and, 1605–1606
diagnosis of, 1606
presentation of, 1605
therapy of, 1606
pathogens associated with, 1556t
Granulomatous disease
chronic, 309t
following extubation, 769
Wegener's granulomatosis, 2156, 2161, 2162t
Greater omentum injuries, 1092–1093
Great vessels, injuries of, management of,
1187–1188
Groin, venous cutdown in, 569–570, 574f
Ground ambulances, 805
Growth, following bone marrow transplantation,
1379
Growth factors
hematopoietic
for infections in granulocytopenic patients,
1606
for leukopenia, 2236
as immunosuppressive agents, 312t
regulation of metabolic responses to critical
illness and, 332t
Growth hormone (GH)
deficiency of, 2113
interaction with insulin, 2113
G-suits, 496
Guidewire exchange (GWX), 1580
semiquantitative culture specimens using,
515f–517f, 515–517
guidelines for, 517–518
Guillain-Barré syndrome (GBS), 2005–2011
clinical features of, 2009
diagnosis of, 2006, 2007t, 2009, 2009t
tests and procedures for, 2005–2006
epidemiology of, 2008t, 2008–2009
pathogenesis of, 2008, 2008t
treatment of, 2006, 2008, 2009–2011
initial therapy for, 2006
Gunshot wounds. *See* Trauma; *specific sites and
injuries*
Gut-liver axis, multiple organ system failure
and, 351
Gut motor hypothesis, of multiple organ system
failure, 447, 448, 448f
Gut starter hypothesis, of multiple organ system
failure, 447f, 447–448
Gyromitra poisoning, antidote for, 1466t

HACEK organisms, 1673
endocarditis due to, treatment of, 1794t–1795t
Haemonetics Cell Saver, 665
Hageman factor, 297–298
Halazepam (Paxipam), for agitation and anxiety,
2026t
Half-lives, of drugs, 477f, 477–478

Hallucinogenic toxidrome, 1468, 1469t
Haloperidol, 826–828, 827t
actions and indications for, 2270
complications of, 827–828
cost of, 827t
for delirium, 2023, 2023t
dosage of, 826–827, 2270
side effects of, 827
Handwashing, 507–510
CDC recommendations for, 509
compliance with guidelines for, 509
efficacy of, 509–510
encouraging, 508–509
factors influencing, 508
linkage with nosocomial infection, 508
scope of nosocomial infection problem and,
507–508
H₂ antagonists. *See also specific drugs*
actions, indications, and dosing of, 2270
for aspiration prophylaxis, 1871, 1871t, 1872
for gastrointestinal bleeding, 2036
Hantavirus infections, 1696
pulmonary, 1709, 1843
Hantavirus pulmonary syndrome (HPS), 1709,
1843
Harris-Benedict equation, 20
Head
computed tomography of, 973f–976f, 973–974
in brain injury, 279–280
in comatose patients, 1975
xenon-enhanced, for cerebral blood flow
monitoring, 947
injury of. *See* Brain injuries
Headache, dural puncture and, 817
Head and neck infections, 1710–1711
anaerobic, 1678
deep-space, of neck, 1710–1711
epiglottitis, 1710
Health care proxy designation and acceptance
form, 31–32
Health care status, clinical decision-making
and, 53
Health care surrogate designation form, 32–33
Health care workers. *See also* Physicians; Team
care
emergency medical technicians, 804
HIV transmission and. *See* Human
immunodeficiency virus (HIV)
infections
immunization against hepatitis and, 1447
for intrahospital transport, 792
involvement in JCAHO surveys, 185
involvement with families. *See* Families
Heart. *See also* Cardiac *entries;* Cardiopulmonary
entries; Cardiovascular *entries;* Left
ventricular *entries;* Myocardial *entries;*
Right ventricular *entries*
artificial, 611–612
following cardiac surgery, 1159
electrical activity of. *See* Cardiac electrical
activity
in poisonings and toxic exposures, 1471
shock and, 359, 370
size of, in advanced heart failure, as prognostic
factor, 1754
in stroke patients, 1993

ventricular interaction of, 241
ventricular vascular coupling and, 241–242,
242f
Heartbeat, neurogenic regulation of, 242–244
parasympathetic, 242
reflex control and, 243f, 243–244, 244f
sympathetic, 242–243
Heart block, 1784
in cyclic antidepressant poisoning, 1491
Heart failure, 1749–1765
acute myocardial infarction and, 1737
approach to, 1739–1740
differentiation of, 1737, 1737t
mechanical complications of, 1737–1738
angiotensin-enzyme inhibitors in
clinical use of, 1756
pooled studies of, 1756
following bone marrow transplantation,
1373–1374
clinical trials in medical management of,
1755–1758, 1758t
congestive. *See* Congestive heart failure (CHF)
diagnostic tests and procedures for, 1749
diastolic dysfunction in, 1764–1765
definition of, 1764
diagnostic pitfalls with, 1764–1765
etiology of, 1764, 1764t
prevalence of, 1764
prognosis of, 1764
therapeutic goals for, 1765
emerging therapies for, 1763
epidemiology of, 1751–1752
etiology of, 1752, 1752f
extracorporeal membrane oxygenation for. *See*
Extracorporeal membrane oxygenation
(ECMO)
initial therapy for, 1749–1750
inotropic agents for, 1756–1757, 1760–1761
mechanism of action of, 1760, 1760f
left ventricular, acute, hypertensive
emergencies and, 1818
major problems with, 1749
myocardial cellular abnormalities and,
1750–1751
of calcium handling, 1750–1751
myocardial remodeling and, 1751
ventricular hypertrophy and, 1751
neurohormonal activation in, 1752–1753
adaptiveness versus maladaptiveness of,
1753, 1753f
atrial natriuretic peptide and, 1753
as prognostic factor, 1755
renin-angiotensin-aldosterone, 1752–1753
sympathetic, 1752
non-pharmacological cardiac assistance for,
1762–1763
biologic systems for, 1762
implantable, selection criteria for, 1763
mechanical systems for, 1762–1763
prognostic factors in, 1753–1755, 1754t
atrial and ventricular dysrhythmias, 1755
cardiac size, 1754
contractile reserve, 1754
electrolyte abnormalities, 1754–1755
etiology, 1755
exercise tolerance, 1754

hemodynamic abnormalities, 1754
    left ventricular function, 1753–1754
    neurohumoral activation, 1755
    refractory. *See* Refractory heart failure
    right ventricular
        heart transplantation and, 1337
        waveform analysis in, 858, 858f
    in shock, treatment of, 379
    stress points with, 1749
    tailored medical therapy for, 1759–1760
        cardiac output and, 1760
        hemodynamic goals of, 1759
        hemodynamic responses to therapy and
            survival and, 1759–1760, 1760t
        systemic vascular resistance and, 1760
Heart-lung transplantation (HLT), 1317–1330
    indications for, 1317, 1318f, 1318t
    initial management for, 1317–1320
        immunosuppression and, 1318–1320
        preoperative, 1317–1318, 1318t–1319t
    postoperative management for, 1320–1330
        acute rejection and, 1321–1322, 1324f
        airway complications and, 1320–1321,
            1323f, 1324f
        bleeding and, 1320, 1321f
        bronchiolitis obliterans and, 1323, 1325f
        diagnostic tests and procedures for,
            1325–1327, 1326f
        diaphragmatic dysfunction and, 1323
        infection and, 1322–1323
        initial therapy and, 1327–1330, 1328f,
            1329f
        reimplantation response and, 1320, 1322f
        stress points with, 1323, 1325
Heart rate
    following cardiac surgery, 1150
        in pediatric patients, 1165
    fetal. *See* Fetal heart rate
Heatstroke syndrome, 1454–1455, 1455t
Heilicobacter pylori infections, 1669
Heimlich catheters, insertion of, 560–561
    procedure for, 561, 561f
Heimlich maneuver, 493
Helga Wanglie decision, 114
Helium-oxygen mixture (Heliox), for asthma,
    1939
HELLP syndrome, 1393
Hematocrit, following cardiac surgery in pediatric
    patients, 1170
Hematologic disorders, 2231–2241. *See also*
    specific disorders
    in acute respiratory distress syndrome, 1837t
    anaphylaxis and, 1545t
    antibiotics and, 1563t
    antirheumatic agents as cause of, 2157t
    with increased blood counts, 2239–2241
    near-drowning and, 1881, 1881f
    with reduced blood counts, 2231–2239
    in systemic lupus erythematosus, 2170–2171
Hematologic evaluation, in stroke patients, 1995
Hematomas
    drainage of, 593–594
    epidural (extradural), 818, 1199
    expanding, with intracerebral hemorrhage,
        2000t

extracerebral, coma and, 1976
    retroperitoneal. *See* Retroperitoneal injuries,
        hematomas due to
    subdural, 1199
Hematopoietic growth factors
    for infections in granulocytopenic patients,
        1606
    for leukopenia, 2236
Hematuria
    in sickle cell anemia, 2234
    following simultaneous pancreas/kidney
        transplantation, 1313
Hemispheric infarction, coma and, 1976
Hemobilia, 1127
    postoperative, hepatic injuries and, 1087
Hemodiafiltration. *See also* Hemofiltration
    continuous, 634–636, 635f
Hemodialysis
    intermittent, 632–634, 634t
    for methanol poisoning, 1502
    pericarditis and, 2095
    for poisonings and toxic exposures, 1475, 1475t
    for salicylate poisoning, 1489
Hemodilution, normovolemic, 664
Hemodynamic disorders. *See also specific*
        disorders
    in advanced heart failure, as prognostic
        factor, 1754
Hemodynamic formulas, 2262t–2263t
Hemodynamic function
    aortic reconstructions and, 1184
    assessment of, heart transplantation and,
        1333–1334, 1339
    following cardiac surgery. *See* Cardiac surgery
    in cardiac tamponade, 1807
    glomerular, alterations in, acute renal failure
        due to, 2085
    inhalational anesthetics and, 1018, 1018t
    following intestinal transplantation, 1357,
        1357t, 1360
    intravenous narcotics and, 1021
    following liver transplantation, 1343–1344
    following multivisceral transplantation, 1356,
        1360
    during pregnancy, 1389–1390, 1390t
    in refractory advanced heart failure, 1759–1760
        cardiac output and, 1760
        goals for, 1759
        responses to therapy and survival and,
            1759–1760, 1760t
        systemic vascular resistance and, 1760
Hemodynamic monitoring
    in acute myocardial infarction, 1738–1739,
        1739t
    invasive, 847–863. *See also* Arterial catheters;
        Central venous catheters; Pulmonary
        artery catheters
        cardiopulmonary parameters and, 849t,
            861–863
        diagnostic tests, procedures, and therapy
            and, 848, 849t
        major problems with, 847
        stress points with, 847–848, 848t
    in multiple organ system failure, 344–345
    in shock, 376t–377t, 376–378

Hemodynamic support
    lung and heart-lung transplantation and,
        1327–1328
    for organ donors, 1293–1294
    for sepsis, 409–410
Hemofiltration
    continuous, 634–636, 635f, 637
        following cardiac surgery, 1157
    for fulminant hepatic failure, 2053
    for heart failure, 1762
Hemoglobin. *See also* Carboxyhemoglobin;
        Methemoglobin; Oxyhemoglobin
    concentration of
        blood volume and, 645–646
        in dysoxia, 339
        minimally acceptable, 645–646
        optimal, 646
    oxygen affinity of, 923, 924f
    plasma-free, increased, autotransfusion and,
        665
    solutions of, 666
Hemolysis, intravascular, brown recluse spider
        bites and, 1531
Hemolytic anemia, 2231–2233
    aplastic crisis in, 2235
    autoimmune, 2231–2233
        in systemic lupus erythematosus, 2170
    drugs causing, 1599t
    from glucose-6-phosphate dehydrogenase
        deficiency, 2233
    from red cell injury in circulation, 2233
Hemolytic transfusion reactions, 1599–1600
    acute, 652–653
        management of, 653
        renal failure and, 653
Hemolytic uremic syndrome (HUS), 2239
Hemoperfusion
    for poisonings and toxic exposures, 1475
    for salicylate poisoning, 1489
    for theophylline poisoning, 1500
Hemophagocytic syndrome, acute, in systemic
        lupus erythematosus, 2170
Hemophilus influenzae infections, 1672–1673
    antibiotic prophylaxis for, 1565
    epiglottitis due to, 1710
    neurologic, epidemiologic and clinical clues to,
        1636, 1636t
Hemoptysis
    fiberoptic bronchoscopy in, 691–692, 692t
    following thoracic trauma, 1145
Hemorrhage
    anterior pituitary failure and, 2113
    anticoagulant overdose and, 2220t,
        2225–2226, 2226t
    into biliary passages, 1127
        postoperative, hepatic injuries and, 1087
    following cardiac surgery in adult patients,
        1155–1156
        cardiac tamponade and, 1155–1156
        causes of, 1155
        treatment of, 1155
    following cardiac surgery in pediatric
        patients, 1173
    central nervous system
        coma and, 1976, 1977, 1978
        hypertensive emergencies and, 1816

Hemorrhage, central nervous system
(*continued*)
intracerebral, 1976, 1977, 1993, 1999f,
1999–2000, 2000t
stroke and, 1992t, 1993
coagulation disorders and. *See* Coagulopathy
continued, following transfusion therapy, 643
in disseminated intravascular coagulation. *See*
Disseminated intravascular
coagulation (DIC)
extracorporeal membrane oxygenation and, in
neonates, 677
gastrointestinal. *See* Gastrointestinal bleeding
following heart transplantation, 1335
hepatic, traumatic, 1086
following hepatic resection, 1126
intracerebral, 1999f, 1999–2000, 2000t,
2000–2002, 2001f
coma and, 1976, 1977
stroke and, 1992t, 1993
following lung and heart-lung transplantation,
1320, 1321f
management of, 1328–1329
massive
colonic perforation and, 2069
transfusion therapy for. *See* Transfusion
therapy, for acute massive hemorrhage
in obstetric patients, 1401–1406
amniotic fluid embolism and, 1406
cardiovascular changes with obstetric drugs
and, 1402–1403
coagulation changes and, 1403
diagnostic tests and procedures for, 1402
intrauterine fetal demise and, 1406
placental abruption and, 1403–1404,
1404f, 1404t
placenta previa and, 1404–1405, 1405f
postpartum, 1406
sepsis and, 1406
stress points with, 1401–1402, 1402f
uterine rupture and, 1405t, 1405–1406
in platelet disorders. *See* Platelet disorders
pontine, coma and, 1977
postoperative, 1008, 1065–1073
cardiopulmonary bypass as cause of,
1072–1073, 1073f
coagulation disorders as cause of,
1068–1071, 1070t
diagnostic tests and procedures for, 1066
evaluation of, 1067
hepatic injuries and, 1087
hepatobiliary disease as cause of, 1071
initial therapy for, 1066
liver trauma as cause of, 1072
local hemostatic failure as cause of,
1067–1068
major issues with, 1065
stress points with, 1065–1066
transfusion-induced, 1071–1072
vascular surgery and, 1180
preoperative evaluation of, 1005, 1005t
pulmonary, in systemic lupus erythematosus,
2166
stress, treatment of, 2040
subarachnoid, 2000t, 2000–2002, 2001f
coma and, 1978

in surgical patients, 1008
thrombolytic therapy and, 626, 1190
through prosthetic grafts, thrombolytic therapy
and, 1190
in trauma patients
with pelvic fractures, 1059–1061
persistent shock and, 1050
tube thoracostomy as cause of, 558–559
vascular surgery and, 1180
diagnosis of, 1180
etiology of, 1180
therapy of, 1180
Hemorrhagic fever, 1709–1710
Hemorrhagic fever with renal syndrome
(HFRS), 1709
Hemorrhagic shock, 1457
acute respiratory distress syndrome and, 1827
emergency transfusion in, 651–652
Hemorrhagic shock and encephalopathy
syndrome (HSE), 1457
Hemorrhagic stress-induced serum factor,
inhalational anesthetics and, 1020
Hemorrhagic stroke, 1992t, 1993
Hemostasis
colloids and, 436–437
local failure of, postoperative bleeding due
to, 1067–1068
primary, 265–267
components of, 265–266
function in normal coagulation, 266
laboratory assessment of, 266–267
primary failure of, postoperative bleeding due
to, 1068–1069
secondary, 267–270
components of, 267f, 267–269
function in normal coagulation, 269–270
laboratory assessment of, 270
secondary failure of, postoperative bleeding
due to, 1069–1071, 1070t
Hemothorax
in trauma patients, 1050–1051
retained, following thoracic trauma, 1143
tube thoracostomy for, 557
Heparin
actions, indications, and dosing of, 2270
for acute myocardial infarction, 1733–1734
for acute respiratory failure, 1923
for amniotic fluid embolism, 1912
for antithrombotic therapy. *See* Antithrombotic
therapy, heparin for
for deep venous thrombosis prophylaxis,
1890–1891
for disseminated intravascular coagulation,
2222
with extracorporeal renal replacement
therapies, 635
idiopathic thrombocytopenic purpura induced
by, 2238
for intestinal transplantation, 1361
for multivisceral transplantation, 1361
necrosis due to, purpura and, 2190–2191
overdose of, hemorrhage and, 2220t, 2225
poisoning by, antidote for, 1466t
for pulmonary embolism, 1898–1899
for simultaneous pancreas/kidney
transplantation, 1313

for stroke, 1997
thrombocytopenia due to, 484
thrombocytopenia induced by, 2227–2228
Hepatectomy, for fulminant hepatic failure, 2053
Hepatic disorders. *See also specific disorders*
antirheumatic agents as cause of, 2156t
hemorrhage and, 2220t
hemostatic abnormalities in, 2222–2223
management of, 2223
presentation of, 2223
intestinal transplantation and, 1356–1357
multivisceral transplantation and, 1356
pharmacotherapy for, 481t, 481–482
in rhabdomyolysis, 2200
in rheumatoid arthritis, 1244
in sickle cell anemia, 2234
venoocclusive, following bone marrow
transplantation, 1372t, 1372–1373
Hepatic failure
acetaminophen poisoning and, 1486
coma and, 1978
fulminant. *See* Fulminant hepatic failure
(FHF)
following hepatic resection, 1127
high-output, 2051
Hepatic function
in hyperthermia, 1456
inhalational anesthetics and, 1018
following intestinal transplantation, 1360
following multivisceral transplantation, 1360
during pregnancy, 316
Hepatic injuries, 1085–1087
liver injury scale and, 2274t
major, 1086
minor, 1085
nonoperative management of, 1087
postoperative complications with, 1086–1087
bleeding, 1072
scale for, 1083t
vascular, 1086
Hepatic insufficiency
hemostatic abnormalities in, 2222–2223
management of, 2223
presentation of, 2223
nutritional support in, 468
Hepatic resection, 1126–1127
albumin administration following, 1126
bile fistulas following, 1126
jaundice following, 1126
liver failure following, 1127
nutritional support following, 1126
postoperative coagulopathy and bleeding and,
1126
postoperative ICU care for, 1110
sepsis following, 1127
Hepatic transplantation, 1341–1350
for acetaminophen poisoning, 1486
coagulation abnormalities following, 1343
assessment of, 1343, 1343f
treatment of, 1343
consultations for, 1350
current status of, 1290
diagnostic tests and procedures for, 1342
early graft function and primary nonfunction
following, 1342
for fulminant hepatic failure, 2052t, 2052–2053

gastrointestinal complications of, 1348
graft function assessment and optimization
    and, 1346–1347
    bilirubin secretion and, 1346, 1346f
    elimination of drugs and metabolic waste
      and, 1346–1347
    energy metabolism and, 1347
    protein synthesis and, 1347
    radiologic assessment and, 1347
hemodynamic function and fluid therapy
    following, 1343–1344, 1344f
hypertension following, 1345
hypoxemia following, 1346
immunosuppression for, 1344–1345
    cyclosporin A and FK506 for, 1344
    mycophenolate mofetil for, 1345
    poly- and monoclonal antibodies for,
      1344–1345
    steroids and azathioprine for, 1345
infections following, 1348–1350
    early, 1348–1349
    late, 1349–1350
initial therapy for, 1342
late readmissions to ICU following, 1349t, 1350
major problems with, 1341
organ allocation for, 1297
pulmonary complications of, 1347
renal complications of, 1347–1348
right pleural effusion following, 1345
seizures following, 1345
stress points with, 1341–1342
Hepatitis, 1444–1448
  epidemiology of, 1444
  hepatitis A, 1444–1445
    clinical ans serologic features of, 1445
    prevention of, 1445
    transmission of, 1445
  hepatitis B, 1445–1446
    antibody formation and, 1445–1446
    chronic carriers of, 1446
    clinical and serologic features of, 1445
    composition of, 1445
    risk of infection with, 1445
    transmission of, 1446
  hepatitis D, 1447
  hepatitis E, 1447
  herpes simplex virus, 1695
  immunization against, 1447
  non-A, non-B, 1446–1447
    clinical features of, 1446
    serologic features of, 1447
    therapy of, 1447
    transmission of, 1446
  secondary, 1448
  transfusion therapy and, 648, 656
Hepatobiliary disorders, 1121–1128. *See also*
    Biliary *entries; specific disorders*
  acute abdomen and, 1104–1105
  diagnostic tests and procedures for, 1121–1122
  in HIV-infected patients, 1630
  initial therapy for, 1122
  major problems with, 1121
  postoperative bleeding due to, 1071
  stress points with, 1121
Hepatorenal syndrome, postshunt, 1124–1125
Herniation syndromes, 1199–1200

in comatose patients, 1979
Heroin abuse. *See* Opiates, abuse of
Herpes simplex virus (HSV) infections
  in bone marrow transplant recipients, 1613
  eczematous. *See* Eczema herpeticum
  in HIV-infected patients, 1629
    treatment of, 1619t
  in immunocompromised patients, 1695
  meningitis due to, 1694
Herpesvirus hominis (HVH), encephalitis due
    to, 1639
Herpes zoster infections
  following bone marrow transplantation, 1378
  chest pain and, 1724
  encephalitis due to, 1694
Heterotopic ossification, with burns, 1274
High-efficiency particulate air (HEPA) filtration,
    for infection prophylaxis, following bone
    marrow transplantation, 1371
High-frequency ventilation (HFV), 737–738,
    738f, 752–753
  for acute respiratory distress syndrome, 1836
  advantages of, 752
  disadvantages of, 753
  initial settings for, 752
  jet ventilators and, 737–738
    controls for, 737, 737t
    potential problems with, 737t, 737–738, 738t
  for near-drowning, 1879
  setup parameters for, 752
  for tracheobronchial injuries, 1142
  work of breathing and, 753
High T$_4$ syndrome, 2146
Hip replacement, complications of, 1234–1235
  blood loss, 1235
  pulmonary embolization, 1234–1235
Hirudin, for antithrombotic therapy, 620
Histoplasma capsulatum infections, 1688
  in HIV-infected patients, 1625, 1628
    disseminated, 1628
    treatment of, 1619t
"Holiday heart" syndrome, 1513
Hormonal activation, in heart failure. *See* Heart
    failure, neurohormonal activation in
Hormonal therapy, red blood cell production
    and, 663
Hormones. *See also specific hormones and glands*
  hyperkalemia due to, 425
  during pregnancy
    direct effects of, 318t, 318–320
    interactions of, 320
  regulation of metabolic responses to critical
    illness and, 331–332
  sex, production of, 2123
Hornet stings, anaphylaxis and, 1545, 1546t, 1548
Hospital
  in decision-making process, 70
  iatrogenesis related to, 97. *See also* Catheter-
    related infections; Nosocomial
    infections
  patient transport between. *See* Interhospital
    transport
  patient transport within. *See* Intrahospital
    transport
Host defense, susceptibility to pneumonia and,
    1844, 1845t, 1846t

Hostility, 2028
Host response, 291–300, 292f, 293f
  immunity and, 291, 299–300
  plasma protein defenses and, 296–299
    coagulation and, 299
    complement and, 296–297, 297f
    contact activation proteins and, 297–299,
      298f
    fibrinolysis and, 299
  reticuloendothelial system and, 291, 292,
    294–296
    endothelial cell activation and, 294–296,
      295f
    leukocyte effector functions and, 296
    leukocyte-endothelial cell interactions and,
      296
    mononuclear phagocytes and, 292, 294
H$_2$ receptor antagonists. *See* H$_2$ antagonists
Human immunodeficiency virus (HIV) infections,
    1617–1632. *See also* Acquired
    immunodeficiency syndrome (AIDS)
  adrenal insufficiency in, 1628–1629
  antibiotic prophylaxis in, 1565–1566
  bacteremia in, 1627
  Bartonella (Rochalimaea) infections associated
    with, 1679
  bias against people with, 1440
  diagnosis of pneumonia in, 694–695, 695t
  diagnostic tests and procedures for, 1618
  disseminated histoplasmosis in, 1628
  fever in, 1630
  gastrointestinal manifestations of, 1629–1630
    abdominal pain and, 1629–1630
    diarrhea, 1629
    dysphagia and odynophagia, 1629
  ICU control of, 1630–1632
    infection control guidelines for, 1631
    management of exposures to HIV and,
      1631–1632, 1632t
    transmission from health care workers to
      patients and, 1631
  ICU utilization in, 1630
  initial therapy for, 1618, 1618t–1621t
  major problems with, 1617
  neurologic manifestations of, 1626–1627, 1628f
    focal lesions of central nervous system,
      1626–1627
    meningitis, 1626
  prevention of, 1442–1444
    invasive precautions for, 1443, 1443t
    laboratory precautions for, 1443, 1443t
    needle punctures and, 1443
    responsibility to health care workers and,
      1444
    responsibility to patients and, 1444
    sharp injuries and, 1443
    universal precautions for, 1442–1443, 1443t
  pulmonary manifestations of, 1618, 1620–1626,
    1622t, 1623f
    bacterial pneumonia, 1623–1624
    fungal pneumonia, 1624–1625
    mucobacterial pneumonia, 1625
    noninfectious, 1626
    Pneumocystis carinii pneumonia, 1622–1623
    viral infections, 1625–1626
  stress points with, 1617, 1618t

Human immunodeficiency virus (HIV) infections (*continued*)
testing health care workers for, 1441–1442
thyroid function in, 2146–2147
transmission of, 1440–1441
from health care workers to patients, 1440, 1631
implications of, 1441
incidence of, 1440–1441
from patients to health care workers, 1441
seroconversion and, 1441
Humanitarianism, critical care team's decision-making and, 72
Human tetanus immunoglobulin, 1677
Humeral depression, spontaneous breathing and, 740
Humidification
for intermittent mandatory ventilation, 723
for oxygen therapy, 405, 707f
Hyaluronidase, for limitation of infarct size, 397
Hydralazine
for esophageal obstruction, 2072
for heart failure, 1755–1756
for hypertension, in hypertensive emergencies, 1814t, 1815
Hydration. *See also* Fluid therapy
withdrawal of, rules regarding, 112–113
Hydrocarbons
aspiration of, 1863–1864
inhalation injury due to, 1955
Hydrocephalus
with intracerebral hemorrhage, 2000t
with subarachnoid hemorrhage, 2001t
treatment of, 2002
Hydrocolloid dressings, 2204–2205
Hydrocortisone
for adrenal insufficiency, 1601, 2115, 2124, 2125, 2125t
following adrenalectomy, 1255
with amphotericin B, 1570
for anaphylaxis, 1547t, 1548
for depressed gastrointestinal pH, 452
for dysoxia, 341
for fulminant colitis, 2068
for hypercalcemia, 429t
for rheumatic disorders, 2157
for shock, 381
for toxic megacolon, 2068
Hydrofluoric acid, for calcium gluconate poisoning, 1466t
Hydrogel wound dressings, 2205, 2205f
Hydrogen chloride, inhalation injury due to, 1954
Hydrogen cyanide, inhalation injury due to, 1952–1953
Hydrogen fluoride, inhalation injury due to, 1954
Hydrogen ions
acid-base disorders and, 257t, 257–258
potassium regulation by, 422
Hydrogen sulfide, inhalation injury due to, 1953
Hydropneumothorax, chest radiography in, 959, 961f
Hydrostatic forces, pulmonary fluid and protein homeostasis and, 203
Hydroxychloroquine, adverse effects of, 2156t–2157t
Hydroxyethyl starch, hemostasis and, 436–437

Hydroxyurea, for polycythemia vera, 2240
Hydrozoa envenomations, 1533t, 1533–1534
clinical manifestations of, 1533–1534
treatment of, 1534
Hygiene, for obese surgical patients, 1281
Hygienic hand disinfection, 509
with residual action, 509
Hymenoptera stings, anaphylaxis and, 1545, 1546t, 1548
Hyperactivity
in delirium, 2020
motor, in cyclic antidepressant poisoning, 1490
Hyperadrenalism, 2125
Hyperalimentation. *See* Nutritional support
Hyperamylasemia, in diabetic ketoacidosis, 2103–2104
Hyperbaric oxygen (HBO) therapy, 777–784
care before, 781–784
for air embolism, 783, 783t
for carbon monoxide poisoning, 784
for decompression sickness, 783–784
techniques for, 781–782
wound management and, 782–783
diagnostic tests, procedures, and therapy and, 778–779
indications for, 780–781
for inhalation injury, 1951
major problems with, 777, 778t
mechanism of action of, 779, 779t
stress points with, 777–778, 778t
transcutaneous oximetry and, 779
Hypercalcemia, 428–429
in cancer, 2245–2247
clinical presentation of, 2245–2246
differential diagnosis of, 2246
laboratory investigation of, 2246
pathophysiology of, 2246
therapy of, 2246–2247
causes and clinical effects of, 428–429, 429t, 430t
in rhabdomyolysis, 2199
treatment of, 430
Hypercapnia
oxygen therapy and, 707
permissive, 753
for acute respiratory distress syndrome, 1835–1836
for aspiration syndromes, 1867, 1867t
Hypercoagulable states, warfarin for, 622, 622t
Hyperdynamic sepsis, blood gas analysis in, 934
Hyperemia, cerebral blood flow and, 277
Hyperfibrinogenemia, reactive, 2229
Hyperglycemia
in diabetes complicated by surgery or medical illness, control of, 2108
in head injury, 1207
in hyperosmolar hyperglycemic nonketotic diabetes, 2107
nutritional support and, 469
in obese surgical patients, prevention of, 1283
Hyperimmune anti-D globulin, during pregnancy, 1425
Hyperkalemia, 425–426
in burn patients, 1270
causes of, 425–426
fluid shifts, hormones, and drugs as, 425

renal dysfunction as, 425, 425f
sodium reabsorption as, 425–426
clinical effects of, 426, 426t
following transfusion therapy, 655, 1057
treatment of, 426, 427t
"Hyperleukocytosis syndrome," 2241
Hypermagnesemia, 433
causes of, 433
clinical effects of, 433
treatment of, 433
Hypermetabolism
of burns, 1271
pheochromocytoma and, 2130
Hypernatremia, 419–420
causes of, 419f, 419–420
central nervous system dysfunction and, 420, 420t
hypertonicity with, 443
hypovolemic, 419, 419f
treatment of, 420, 420t, 421t
Hyperosmolar hyperglycemia nonketotic diabetes (HHNK), 2106–2107
complications of, 2107
laboratory features of, 2107
pathogenesis of, 2107
treatment of, 2107
Hyperosmolar states, 439–443
clinical features of, 440–441
fluid shifts and central nervous system changes, 441, 441t
onset and, 440
signs and symptoms, 440–441
evaluation of, 439–440, 440f
normal regulation of osmolality and, 439
aldosterone and, 439
renal function and, 439
thirst and antidiuretic hormone and, 439
treatment of, 441–443, 442f
in hypernatremia, 443
in hyponatremia, 452
in sodium overload, 443
Hyperphosphatemia, 430
in diabetic ketoacidosis, 2103
in rhabdomyolysis, 2199
Hyperpyrexia. *See also* Fever; Hyperthermia
cocaine abuse and, 1516
postoperative, hepatic injuries and, 1087
salicylate poisoning and, 1488
Hypersensitivity reactions. *See also* Anaphylactic and anaphylactoid reactions; Immune system function
to *Aspergillus* antigens, 1688
to drugs, 483–484, 1598–1599, 1599t
antibiotics, 1561–1562
thrombolytic, 626, 1190
to transfusion therapy, 653
Hypertension. *See also* Hypertensive emergencies
arterial, in head injury, 1204
during brain resuscitation, 282–283
cocaine abuse and, 1516, 1517
heart transplantation and, 1337, 1338
intraabdominal, in trauma patients, 1053–1054
intracranial. *See* Intracranial hypertension
following liver transplantation, 1345
management of

maneuvers to increase cerebral blood flow and, 285
mesenteric and renal artery reconstructions and, 1183
vascular surgery and, 1178–1179
in obese surgical patients, 1278
perioperative, 1819
persistent, of newborn, extracorporeal membrane oxygenation for, 671
pheochromocytoma and, 2130
in poisonings and toxic exposures, 1470–1471
during pregnancy, 1392–1393, 1818
pulmonary
following cardiac surgery in pediatric patients, 1168, 1169t
heart transplantation and, 1337
waveform analysis in, 858
Hypertensive emergencies, 1811–1819
acute left ventricular failure and, 1818
antihypertensive withdrawal and, 1818
burns and, 1819
central nervous system damage and, 1816–1817
diagnostic tests and procedures for, 1811–1812
dissecting aortic aneurysm and, 1817
drugs used in, 1813, 1814–1815t, 1815–1816
initial therapy for, 1812–1813, 1813f, 1814t–1815t
major problems with, 1811, 1812t
myocardial ischemia and, 1817–1818
pediatric, 1818–1819
perioperative, 1819
pheochromocytoma and, 1818
preeclampsia/eclampsia and, 1818
renal insufficiency and, 1817
stress points with, 1811
Hypertensive urgencies, 1819–1820
drugs used in, 1819–1820, 1820t
Hyperthermia, 1454–1457. *See also* Fever; Hyperpyrexia
clinical syndrome of, 1455–1456
cocaine abuse and, 1517
complications of, 1456–1457
heatstroke syndrome and, 1454–1455, 1455t
malignant. *See* Malignant hyperthermia (MH)
temperature correction and, 936
temperature regulation and, 1455
therapeutic approach to, 1457
Hyperthyroidism, 2139. *See also* Thyrotoxicosis
Hypertonic solutions, 437
for burns, 1268
complications of therapy using, 437
distribution of, 437
Hyperuricemia, in rhabdomyolysis, 2199
Hyperventilation
for cerebral edema, in fulminant hepatic failure, 2049–2050
for intracranial hypertension, 284, 1205
for salicylate poisoning, 1488
Hyperviscosity syndrome, 2241
Hypervolemia
in fulminant hepatic failure, 2051
hyponatremia and
causes of, 417
treatment of, 418–419
nutritional support in, 468

Hypoadrenalism. *See* Adrenal insufficiency
Hypocalcemia, 428
causes of, 428, 428t, 429t
clinical effects of, 428
in pancreatitis, treatment of, 2058
in rhabdomyolysis, 2199
treatment of, 2200–2201
following transfusion therapy, 654–655, 2224
treatment of, 428, 2200–2201
Hypocapnia, during brain resuscitation, 281
Hypogammaglobulinemia, pathogens associated with, 1556t
Hypoglycemia
coma and, 1977
fetal, oxygen deprivation and, 1430
Hypoglycemic agents
poisoning by, antidote for, 1465t
surgical patients and, 1008
Hypokalemia, 422–425
in burn patients, 1270
causes of, 422–423, 423f
loss of potassium as, 422–423
potassium shifts as, 423
clinical effects of, 423–424, 424t
cardiac, 423–424
in diabetic ketoacidosis, 2103
treatment of, 2105–2106
in salicylate poisoning, 1488
following transfusion therapy, 655
treatment of, 424t, 424–425
in diabetic ketoacidosis, 2105–2106
replacement in, 424–425
Hypomagnesemia, 431–433
causes of, 431–432
clinical effects of, 432, 432t
magnesium shifts as, 432
obligate loss as, 432
renal, 432
in chronic renal failure, 2097
in diabetic ketoacidosis, 2103
treatment of, 2106
treatment of, 432–433, 433t
for acute symptomatic depletion, 432
for chronic depletion, 432–433
in diabetic ketoacidosis, 2106
Hyponatremia, 416–419
in burn patients, 1269–1270
causes of, 416f, 416–417
central nervous system effects of, 417, 417t, 419
in diabetic ketoacidosis, 2103
treatment of, 2105
euvolemic
causes of, 417
hypovolemic, 418
hypertonicity with, 442
hypervolemic
causes of, 417
hypovolemic, 418–419
in hypothyroidism, 2143
hypovolemic
causes of, 416–417
treatment of, 417–418
with subarachnoid hemorrhage, 2001t
treatment of, 2002
in surgical patients, 437–438, 438t
treatment of, 417–419, 418t

in diabetic ketoacidosis, 2105
with subarachnoid hemorrhage, 2002
Hypoosmolar states, 437–438
dextrose and water in surgical patients and, 437–438
hyponatremia and renal function and, 437–438, 438t
lack of solute for urine formation and, 438, 438t
Hypoperfusion
after brain injury, cerebral blood flow and, 277
in sepsis, treatment of, 410
in shock, treatment of, 373t
Hypophosphatemia, 429–430, 431t
causes of, 429–430
treatment of, 430
in diabetic ketoacidosis, 2106
Hypopituitarism
adrenal insufficiency due to, 2123–2124
diagnosis of, 2114–2115
endocrine testing in, 2114
scanning in, 2114
thyroid function testing in, 2114–2115, 2115f
etiology of, 2113–2114
individual hormone deficiencies in, 2113
management of, 2115–2116
for adrenocorticotropic hormone deficiency, 2115–2116
for thyroid-stimulating hormone deficiency, 2115
secondary, 2114
Hypotension
antidiuretic hormone release and, 2117
arterial, in shock, 359
following bone marrow transplantation, 1369
during brain resuscitation, 282
cardiogenic, in chronic renal failure, 2094
definition of, 406t
in dysoxia, 340
epidural anesthetics and, 819
hypovolemic, in chronic renal failure, 2094, 2094t
intermittent hemodialysis and, 633–634, 634f
in poisonings and toxic exposures, 1470
calcium channel blockers and, 1498
cyclic antidepressants and, 1491–1492
insecticides and, 1507
salicylates and, 1489
theophylline and, 1501
in sepsis, management of, 410
in shock
arterial, 359
treatment of, 373t, 374–375, 378–379, 381
in trauma patients, 1048–1049, 1050t
spinal cord injury and, 1210
Hypothalamic-anterior pituitary unit disorders, 2111–2116, 2112f
diagnostic tests and procedures for, 2111
initial therapy for, 2111–2112
major problems with, 2111
stress points with, 2111
Hypothalamic disorders, adrenal insufficiency due to, 2123–2124
Hypothermia, 1451–1454, 1452t
clinical syndrome of, 1452–1453, 1453f
ice water submersion and, 1882

Hypothermia (*continued*)
near-drowning and, 1880
platelet function and, 650–651
in poisonings and toxic exposures, 1470
salicylates and, 1488
temperature correction and, 936
temperature regulation and, 1452
therapeutic approach to, 1453f, 1453–1454
therapeutic use of
for brain injury, 285
for organ donors, 1295, 1296
thermodilution and, 894
transfusion therapy and, 643, 655, 1057–1058
Hypotheses, 4
null, 11
implying or stating, 14
proving, 14–15
Hypothyroidism, 2142–2146
following bone marrow transplantation, 1379
diagnosis of, 2144
immediate concerns with, 2142
presentation of, 2142–2144, 2143t
in rhabdomyolysis, 2200
treatment of, 2144–2146
for concomitant adrenal insufficiency, 2146
for concomitant coronary artery disease, 2145–2146
for concomitant surgical emergencies, 2146
general principles of, 2144
for myxedema coma, 2145, 2145t
for respiratory failure, 2145
Hypovolemia
antidiuretic hormone release and, 2117
with burns, 1267
in head injury, 1206
hypernatremia and, 419, 419f
in hyperosmolar states, 441, 441t
hyponatremia and
causes of, 416–417
treatment of, 417–418
in pancreatitis, treatment of, 2058
response to, shock and, 369, 369f
transfusion therapy for. See Transfusion therapy
in trauma patients, 1048–1049
Hypovolemic shock, 365–366, 390
in trauma patients, 1048–1049
waveform analysis in, 858, 859f
Hypoxemia, 921
assessment of, 923–924
blood gas analysis and, 929–930
denitrogenation absorption atelectasis and, 930
pulmonary vasoconstriction and, 930
during brain resuscitation, 281
intermittent hemodialysis and, 634
following liver transplantation, 1346
postanesthetic, 1026–1027
respiratory alkalosis with, blood gas analysis in, 926
Hypoxia
cerebral
coma and, 1977
electroencephalography in, 945
diffusion, 1016
intestinal, 445

pulmonary vasoconstriction and, 201
wound management and, 782
Hypoxic pulmonary vasoconstriction (HPV), inhalational anesthetics and, 1018

Iatrogenesis, 95–102
decubitus ulcers and, 100–101
falls and, 101
incorrectly diagnosed disorders and, 96
infectious. See Nosocomial infections
laboratory error and, 99t, 99–100, 100t
legal aspects of, 101–102
procedure-related, 97–99, 98t, 99t
therapy-related, 96–97
IBM blood cell processor, 665
Ice water caloric test, in comatose patients, 1973
Ice-water submersion, 1882
cardiopulmonary resuscitation for, 1882
neurologic disorders and, 1882
rewarming following, 1882
ICU attending physicians, 36
ICU fellows, 35
functions and interrelationships of, 37–39
ICU junior residents, 36
ICU utilization, for HIV-infected patients, 1630
Idiogenic osmoles, 441
Idiopathic thrombocytopenic purpura (ITP), 2226, 2237–2238
heparin-associated, 2238
Idiosyncratic reactions, to drugs, 483–484
Ifosfamide, for bone marrow transplantation, 1368t
Ileal fistulas, postoperative, 1114, 1114t
Ileal loop urostomy, postoperative management and, 1256, 1256f
Ileocecal syndrome, in cancer, 2250–2251
Ileus, 2212
in spinal cord injury, treatment of, 1214
Illness. See Medical illness; *specific disorders*
Iloprost, for Raynaud's phenomenon, 2159
Imaging, 957–982. See also *specific sites and modalities*
abdominal, 969–971
abdominal distention and, 970–971, 972f, 973f
free intraperitoneal air and, 970, 971f, 972f
in ischemic disease, 971
contrast agents for. See Radiographic contrast agents
for evaluation of life-support and monitoring devices, 965–969
central venous catheters, 968–969, 970f
intraaortic counterpulsation balloons, 969, 970f
pulmonary artery catheters, 967–968, 968f, 969f
ventilatory support tubes, 966–967, 967f
graft function assessment and optimization and, 1347
neurologic, 952
in neurologic infections, 1640
in percutaneous catheter drainage, 591–592
during pregnancy, traumatic injuries and, 1421–1422, 1422t
in spinal cord injury, 1210–1211

compression and, 2249
^{131}I-MIBG, for pheochromocytomas, 2133, 2134t
^{131}I-MIBG scintigraphy, for pheochromocytoma localization, 2132
Imipenem, 1567
cost and initial dosage of, 1562t
for *Nocardia* infections, in HIV-infected patients, 1620t
for *Rhodococcus equi* infections, in HIV-infected patients, 1620t
Imipenem-cilastin, for infections in granulocytopenic patients, 1606
Imipramine (Tofranil), side effects of, 2027t
Immune complex reaction, to drugs, 1598–1599, 1599t
Immune granulocytopenia, 2236
Immune system function, 303–313
adverse drug reactions and, 483–484
alteration in critically ill patients, 1575
antigen clearance and, 306–308
effector cell function and, 306–307, 307t
immunoglobulin and complement and, 306
inflammation and, 308
antigen recognition and processing and, 304–306, 305f
critical illness and, 308–311, 309t
cell-mediated immunity disorders and, 310
complement defects and, 308–309
immunoglobulin abnormalities and, 309–310
phagocytic cell abnormalities and, 310–311
diagnostic tests and procedures for, 303–304
drug-induced immune-mediated platelet destruction and, 2226–2227
glucocorticoids and, 2123
host responses and, 291, 299–300
hypopituitarism and, 2114
impairment of. See also Acquired immunodeficiency syndrome (AIDS); Human immunodeficiency virus (HIV) infections; Immunocompromised patients; *specific organ transplantations*
in fulminant hepatic failure, 2051–2052
pathogens associated with, 1556, 1556t
inhalational anesthetics and, 1019t, 1019–1020
initial therapy and, 304
intravenous anesthetics and, 1026
intravenous narcotics and, 1022
major problems in, 303
stress points for, 303
Immune thrombocytopenia, acute, in systemic lupus erythematosus, 2171
Immunity
cell-mediated, disorders of, 310
mediators of, 306–307, 307t
Immunizations. See Vaccines
Immunocompromised patients. See also Acquired immunodeficiency syndrome (AIDS); Human immunodeficiency virus (HIV) infections
acute abdomen in, 1104
infections in, 1603–1614
antibiotic selection for, 1641t
Bartonella (Rochalimaea), 1679
in bone marrow transplant recipients, 1613t, 1613–1614

in corticosteroid-treated patients, 1606–1609
diagnostic approach to, 1604–1605
diagnostic tests and procedures for, 1604
in granulocytopenic patients, 1605–1606
initial therapy for, 1604
major problems with, 1603
minimizing, 1305
neurologic, 1641t, 1644–1646, 1645t
pneumonia, diagnosis of, 694–695, 695t
in renal transplant recipients, 1609–1612, 1610f
stress points with, 1603–1604
viral, 1694–1696
organ transplantation and. *See specific organ transplantations*
Immunoglobulins
antilymphocyte
for heart-lung transplantation, 1320
for lung transplantation, 1320
for renal transplantation, 1304–1305
cytomegalovirus-specific
for heart-lung transplantation, 1330
for lung transplantation, 1330
deficiencies of, 309t, 309–310
to hepatitis B, formation of, 1445–1446
host response and, 295
therapeutic administration of
intravenous. *See Intravenous immunoglobulin (IVIg)*
therapeutic administration of, 311, 312t
Immunologic transfusion reactions, 652–654
allergic, 653
delayed, 653
graft-versus-host disease, 653–654
clinical presentation of, 653
morbidity and mortality due to, 654
hemolytic, acute, 652–653
management of, 653
renal failure and, 653
in immunosuppressed patients, 654
nonhemolytic/noninfectious, 653
Immunomodulatory drugs, 312t
Immunosuppression, 312t. *See also specific drugs*
burn injury and, 1272
cell-mediated, pathogens associated with, 1556t
for heart-lung transplantation, 1318–1320
for heart transplantation, 1334–1335
for intestinal transplantation, 1360–1361
for liver transplantation, 1344–1345
for lung transplantation, 1318–1320
for multivisceral transplantation, 1360–1361
for renal transplantation. *See Renal transplantation, immunosuppressants for*
for simultaneous pancreas/kidney transplantation, 1314–1315
transfusion reactions and
organ transplantation and, 654
septic complications of, 654
tumor recurrence and, 654
wound management and, 782
Immunotherapy, 303, 311, 312t, 313. *See also Immunosuppression*
complications of, 313

for sepsis, 411
Impedance plethysmography
for deep venous thrombosis diagnosis, 1242, 1242t, 1893, 1893f
for pulmonary thromboembolism diagnosis, 1242
Implied consent, 118
Impregnated dressings, 2205
Impulse conduction, cardiac, 229
Inactive electrodes, 832
Incision and suction, for snake bites, 1526–1527
Incisura, 850–851
Incompetent patients
informed consent and, 83, 118–119
right to refuse treatment, 108–111
Indanedione derivative poisoning, antidote for, 1465t
Independent samples, 12
Indicators, for continuous quality improvement programs. *See also Continuous quality improvement*
selection of, 164, 165t
Indomethacin
for acute pericarditis, 1805
for heart transplantation, 1335
Infants
breast feeding of, following cardiac surgery in pediatric patients, 1174
closed chest cardiac compression in, 496
newborn. *See Neonates*
Infarction
cerebellar, coma and, 1977
cerebral, with intracerebral hemorrhage, 2000t
hemispheric, coma and, 1976
intestinal. *See Intestinal infarction*
myocardial. *See Acute myocardial infarction (AMI); Myocardial infarction*
Infarctive purpura, 2190, 2190f
Infection(s). *See also Sepsis; specific infections*
abscesses. *See Abscesses*
acquisition of, antibiotic selection and, 1556t, 1556–1557
in acute respiratory distress syndrome, 1837t
acute respiratory distress syndrome and, 1827
of ascites, 1124
in aspiration syndromes, treatment of, 1868
bacterial, 1657–1682, 1658t. *See also specific infections*
transfusion therapy and, 655
following bone marrow transplantation, prophylaxis of, 1370–1371
in burn patients. *See Burns, infections and*
following cardiac surgery in pediatric patients, 1171–1172
prophylaxis of, 1171–1172
treatment of, 1172
catheter-related. *See Catheter-related infections*
clinical epidemiology of, 1685, 1686t
coma and, 1978
definition of, 406t
diagnosis of, antibiotic selection and, 1558, 1558t–1560t, 1560–1561
endogenous transmission of, 510–511
exogenous transmission of, 510
extracerebral, coma and, 1976

fever as predictor of, 1592–1593
fever associated with. *See Fever, infectious sources of*
with fractures, 1228–1229
fungal. *See Fungal infections; specific infections*
of grafts. *See Graft infections*
heart transplantation and, 1329–1330, 1338–1339
host response to. *See Host response*
hypopituitarism and, 2114
iatrogenic, 97–99, 98t, 99t
immune defects and. *See Immune system function*
in immunocompromised patients. *See Immunocompromised patients, infections in*
inflammatory response to. *See Sepsis*
infrainguinal reconstructions and, 1186
intestinal transplantation and, 1356, 1361–1362
prophylaxis of, 1361
with intracerebral hemorrhage, 2000t
liver transplantation and, 1348–1350
early, 1348–1349
late, 1349–1350
following lung and heart-lung transplantation, 1322–1323
lung and heart-lung transplantation and, management of, 1329–1330
in multiple organ system failure, evaluation for, 345
multivisceral transplantation and, 1356, 1361–1362
prophylaxis of, 1361
necrotic, hyperbaric oxygen therapy for, 780
neurologic. *See Neurologic infections; specific disorders and infections*
nosocomial. *See Nosocomial infections*
nutritional support and, 468–469
in obese surgical patients, 1281–1282
peritoneal dialysis and, 2095
postoperative, subtle, 2209–2211
pulmonary
acute respiratory distress syndrome and, 1827
transtracheal aspiration in, 580
in renal transplant recipients, 1306–1308
respiratory. *See also Pneumonia*
fever associated with, 1593–1594
respiratory failure and, 1919
rhabdomyolysis due to, 2199
scoliosis correction and, 1234
secondary, 1562
in shock, treatment of, 373t
of shunts
for ascites, 1125
cerebrospinal fluid, staphylococcal, 1662
soft tissue
streptococcal, 1663
wound management and, 782
with subarachnoid hemorrhage, 2001t
superinfections, 1562
toxic megacolon due to, 2069
transfusion therapy and, 648, 655–656
tube thoracostomy as cause of, 560
of vascular grafts. *See Graft infection*
viral. *See Viral infections; specific infections*

Infection control
for bacterial meningitis, 1643
for barotrauma prevention, 1965
burns and, 1272
for exotic viral infections, 1698t–1699t
for human immunodeficiency virus. *See*
Acquired immunodeficiency syndrome
(AIDS); Human immunodeficiency
virus (HIV) infections
invasive precautions for, 1443, 1443t
laboratory precautions for, 1443, 1443t
preoperative, 995
universal precautions for, 1442–1443, 1443t
Infectious mononucleosis, in
immunocompromised patients, 1695
Infective endocarditis, 1787–1800
acute, 1788
clinical manifestations of, 1790, 1790t
culture-negative, 1792t, 1792–1793
diagnostic criteria for, 1789, 1789t
diagnostic tests and procedures for, 1787,
1790t, 1790–1791
echocardiography in, 885, 886f, 886t
epidemiology of, 1788
major problems with, 1787
microbiology of, 1791t, 1791–1793, 1792t
pathology and pathogenesis of, 1788–1789
prophylaxis of, 1565, 1796–1797, 1798t,
1799t, 1800
pseudomonal, 1674
staphylococcal, 1658–1659, 1661–1662
stress points with, 1787
subacute, 1788
therapy of, 1793, 1794t–1799t, 1796–1797,
1800
initial, 1787
Inferential statistics. *See* Statistics, inferential
Inferior vena caval (IVC) filters, for pulmonary
embolism, 1899–1900
anticoagulation with, 1899
applications of, 1899
choice of, 1899
complications of, 1899–1900
Inferior vena caval (IVC) interruption, for deep
venous thrombosis prophylaxis, 1890
Infiltration, hypopituitarism and, 2114
Inflammation. *See also* Sepsis
antigen clearance and, 308
coma and, 1978
mediators of, 306–307, 307t
Inflammatory bowel disease, 2065–2069. *See also*
Fulminant colitis; Toxic megacolon
colonic perforation and massive hemorrhage
in, 2069
diagnostic tests and procedures for, 2065
initial therapy for, 2065
major problems with, 2065
stress points with, 2065
in systemic lupus erythematosus, 2168
Inflammatory response
in shock, treatment of, 373t
in systemic inflammatory response syndrome,
367
definition and, 406t
multiple organ system failure and, 345,
348, 351
nosocomial infections and, 1576

Influenza vaccine
Guillain-Barré syndrome and, 2008
for pneumonia, 1855–1856, 1856t
Influenza virus infections, 1691–1693
antibiotic prophylaxis for, 1566
Informational overload, iatrogenesis related to,
100
Informed consent, 81–87, 117–119
degrees of disclosure and, 81–82, 118
elements of, 81
ethical foundations of, 85–86
exceptions to, 118
implied consent and, 118
incompetent patients and, 83, 118–119
level of information and, 118
for pediatric patients, 118–119
preventive ethics and, 83–84
refusal of treatment and, 84–85
special considerations regarding, 86
strategies for obtaining, 82
for vascular cannulation, 521
Infraclavicular cannulation, 529t, 536
Infrainguinal reconstruction, 1186–1187
antiplatelet agents for, 1186
infection and, 1186
leg edema and, 1186–1187
leg elevation for, 1186
mortality and, 1187
Inhalational anesthetics, 1015–1020. *See also*
specific anesthetics
distribution of, 1015, 1016–1017
effects of illness on, 1016–1017
organ system function and, 1017t–1019t,
1017–1020
uptake of, 1015t, 1015–1017
delivery and, 1015
effects of illness on, 1016–1017
from lungs, 1015–1016, 1016t
production and, 1015
Inhalation injuries, 1266, 1947–1956
acute respiratory distress syndrome and,
1827–1828
asphyxiants and, 1952–1953
clinical presentation and diagnosis of, 1949t,
1950–1951
diagnostic tests and procedures for, 1947
fiberoptic bronchoscopy in, 697
fire and smoke and, 1266, 1948–1949
fiberoptic bronchoscopy in, 697
histopathology of, 1950
major problems with, 1947, 1948f
pathogenesis of, 1950
pulmonary sensitizers and, 1955
respiratory irritants and, 1953–1954
stress points with, 1947, 1949t
systemic toxins and, 1954–1955
thermal, 1949–1950
treatment of, 1951
initial therapy for, 1948
Injectors, of mechanical ventilators, 714t
Injuries. *See also* Trauma; *specific sites and
injuries*
diabetes of, 329, 329t
host response to. *See* Host response
metabolic response to. *See* Metabolic response
to injury and illness
Inocybe poisoning, antidote for, 1467t

Inotropic agents. *See also specific drugs*
following cardiac surgery
in pediatric patients, 1166, 1166f,
1167t–1168t, 1168
weaning of, 1149
for cardiogenic shock, 398f, 398–401
for dysoxia, 341
for heart failure, 1756–1757, 1760–1761
congestive heart, 1740
mechanism of action of, 1760, 1760f
for heart transplantation, 1336
In re Hamlin, 120
Insecticides
inhalation injury due to, 1955
poisoning by, 1504–1507
antidote for, 1467t
cholinergic syndrome and, 1504–1505
clinical manifestations of, 1505
treatment of, 1506–1507
Inspection
in cardiac assessment, 869–870
in pulmonary assessment, 868–869
Inspiratory baseline, for capnometry, 878–879,
879f
Inspiratory downstroke, capnometry and, 879
Inspiratory flow, triggering of. *See* Work of
breathing (WOB), triggering inspiratory
flow and
Inspiratory flow waveforms, 713, 714t, 715, 715f
Insulin
for diabetes mellitus, complicated by medical
illness or surgery, 2108t
for diabetic ketoacidosis, 2104t, 2105, 2106t
for hyperkalemia, 427t
interaction with adrenocorticotropic hormone
and growth hormone, 2113
surgical patients and, 1008
Insulin resistance, 332
Insurance, organ transplantation and, 124–125
Intensive care psychosis, 93
Intercostal nerve blocks, 813
Interferons
regulation of metabolic responses to critical
illness and, 332t
for viral infections, 1700t, 1701
Interhospital transport, 803–807
aircraft for, 805–807
acceleration of, 806–807
atmosphere in, 806, 806f, 806t
isolation and cabin constraints in, 807
noise in, 807
temperature in, 806
vibration of, 807
approach to, 807
ground ambulances for, 805
major problems with, 803
prehospital practitioners and, 804–805
basic emergency medical technicians, 804
paramedics, 804–805
procedures essential for, 803
stress points with, 803
Interleukin-1 (IL-1)
host response and, 292, 294
multiple organ system failure and, 347,
348–349, 349f, 350
regulation of metabolic responses to critical
illness and, 332t, 332–333

Interleukin-2 (IL-2)
  host response and, 292, 294
  regulation of metabolic responses to critical
      illness and, 333
Interleukin-6 (IL-6)
  multiple organ system failure and, 347, 348,
      349f
  regulation of metabolic responses to critical
      illness and, 333
Interleukin-8 (IL-8), multiple organ system
      failure and, 347, 348, 349f
Intermediate life support, 492
Intermittent mandatory ventilation (IMV),
      722–723, 747–748
  advantages of, 748
  following cardiac surgery, 1156
  clinical applications of, 722, 723f
  disadvantages of, 748
  equipment for, 723
  initial settings for, 747
  for near-drowning, 1879
  operational principles of, 722
  for respiratory failure, 1925, 1926t
  setup parameters for, 747, 748f
  side effects and complications of, 741
  synchronized. *See* Synchronized intermittent
      mandatory ventilation (SIMV)
  work of breathing and, 748
Intermittent pneumatic compression (IPC) boots,
      for deep venous thrombosis
      prophylaxis, 1890
Internal fixation, for fractures, 1225f, 1225–1226
Interrater reliability, 6
Interstitial edema, cerebral, treatment of, 280t
Interstitial lung disease
  pneumonitis, in bone marrow transplant
      recipients, 1613–1614
  in systemic lupus erythematosus, 2167
  in systemic sclerosis, 2172–2173
Interstitial nephritis, acute, acute renal failure due
      to, 2085
Interventional radiology, 587–596. *See also*
      specific procedures
  nonvascular procedures, 590–596
    catheter drainage. *See* Catheter drainage,
        percutaneous
    cholecystostomy, 594
    gastrostomy, 595
    nephrostomy, 595–596
    transgastric jejunostomy, 595
  vascular procedures, 587–590
    for acute ischemia, 588–589
    for foreign body manipulation, 590
    for gastrointestinal bleeding, 589–590
    for pulmonary embolism, 587–588
    for vascular trauma, 590, 591f
Intestinal anastomosis, postoperative
      management and, 1256
Intestinal fistulas
  in pancreatitis, 2061
  postoperative, 1114, 1114t
Intestinal function
  alterations in, 2212. *See also* Diarrhea
    dysmotility in systemic sclerosis, 2173
  following intestinal transplantation, 1362–1363
  following multivisceral transplantation,
      1362–1363

Intestinal infarction, following revascularization,
      1183–1184
  diagnosis of, 1183
  etiology of, 1183
  incidence of, 1183
  therapy of, 1183–1184
Intestinal injuries
  colonic, 1093
    colonic injury scale and, 2276t
  duodenal, 1089–1090
    duodenal injury scale and, 2275t
  rectal, 1093–1094
    with pelvic fractures, 1059
    rectal injury scale and, 2276t
  to small intestine, 1092–1093
Intestinal injury scales, 2275t–2276t
Intestinal ischemia, 445
  aortic reconstructions and, 1184–1185
  diagnosis of, 1184
  etiology of, 1184
  incidence of, 1184
  therapy of, 1184–1185
Intestinal necrosis, postoperative, 1111
Intestinal obstruction
  colonic pseudo-obstruction and, acute
      abdomen and, 1106, 1106f
  in obstetric patients, 1424
Intestinal perforation
  colonic, massive hemorrhage and, 2069
  impending, signs of, 2069
Intestinal transplantation, 1353–1364
  candidate evaluation and treatment for, 1355t,
      1355–1357, 1357t
  diagnostic tests and procedures for, 1354
  initial therapy for, 1354
  major problems with, 1353, 1354
  operative procedure for, 1358, 1358f, 1359f,
      1360
  outcome with, 1364
  postoperative care and, 1354, 1360–1364
    early problems and, 1360–1361, 1361t
    graft rejection and, 1362, 1363t
    infection and, 1361–1362
    late problems and, 1361
    lymphoproliferative disease and, 1363–1364
    nutrition and intestinal function and,
        1362–1363
  preparation for, 1357–1358
  stress points with, 1353, 1354
Intestinal tubes, long, postoperative abdomen
      and, 1117
Intoxications. *See* Poisonings and toxic exposures;
      Substance abuse and withdrawal;
      specific substances
Intraabdominal hypertension, in trauma
      patients, 1053–1054
Intraabdominal infections, fever associated
      with, 1596
Intraabdominal pressure measurement, 568–569
  procedure for, 568f, 569
Intraaortic balloon pump (IABP)
  following cardiac surgery, 1159
  for cardiogenic shock, 402
  complications with, 611
  contraindications to, 610–611
  for heart failure, 1762
  indications for, 610

purpose of, 609–610, 610f
Intraaortic counterpulsation balloons, chest
      radiography and, 969, 970f
Intracardiac shunts
  left-to-right
    arterial emboli with, 1906
    during pregnancy, 1395
  right-to-left, during pregnancy, 1395
  thermodilution and, 894
Intracerebral hemorrhage (ICH), 1999f,
      1999–2000, 2000t
  stroke and, 1993
Intraconazole, for *Candida* infections, in HIV-
      infected patients, 1619t
Intracranial hypertension, 275–276
  with intracerebral hemorrhage, 2000t
  management of, 1205
  with subarachnoid hemorrhage, 2001t
  treatment of, 280t, 283–285
    corticosteroids for, 284–285
    in fulminant hepatic failure, 2049–2050
    hyperventilation for, 284
    nonosmotic diuresis and cerebrospinal fluid
        drainage for, 284
    osmotic agents for, 284
Intracranial injuries, 1199
Intracranial pressure (ICP)
  elevated. *See* Intracranial hypertension
  head injury and, 1198–1199
  monitoring of, 947f, 947–949, 948f, 949t
    bacterial meningitis due to, 1643
    complications of, 2050
    in head injury, 1202–1203
  near-drowning and, 1880
    as prognostic indicator, 1883
  pharmacologic agents and, 280–281
Intrahospital transport, 787–800
  basic issues in, 788
  cardiovascular system and, 789
  central nervous system and, 789, 789t
  cost and benefit of, 792
  between critical care areas, 790–792
  from critical care areas, 789, 790, 791t
    contributing factors and, 790
    manual versus mechanical techniques for,
        790
    physiological impact of, 790
  to critical care areas, 789
  critical monitors for, 795, 796f, 796t
  diagnostic tests and procedures for, 788
  of hemodynamically unstable patients, 797
  individualizing approaches to, 795f, 795–800
  magnetic resonance imaging and, 800
  major problems with, 787
  of neurotrauma patients, 789, 789t, 797, 800
  oxygenation and, 788–789
  posttransport stabilization and, 794–795
  preparatory phase of, 792–794
    body temperature maintenance and, 794
    communication and, 792
    entropy and, 793
    equipment and supplies and, 793
    general considerations for, 792
    integrated approaches and, 793–794, 794f
    personnel and, 792
    TRAM system and, 793
    transport beds and, 793

Intrahospital transport (*continued*)
  stress points with, 787–788
  transport phase of, 794
  of ventilator-dependent patients, 795–797,
    797t
    manual versus mechanical techniques for,
      790
    ventilators and, 796–797, 798t–799t, 800f
Intraperitoneal air, free, abdominal radiography
    and, 970, 971f, 972f
Intraperitoneal infections, antibiotic combination
    therapy for, 1564
Intrapleural pressure, 189, 190f
  during spontaneous breathing, changes in, 739
Intrapulmonary shunts
  for near-drowning, 1878–1879
  venous saturation monitoring and, 916–917
Intrarater reliability, 6
Intrathoracic abdomen, 1077
Intravascular catheters. *See* Arterial cannulation;
    Central venous catheters; Pulmonary
    artery (PA) catheters; Vascular
    catheters; Venous cannulation
Intravascular hemolysis, brown recluse spider
    bites and, 1531
Intravascular oxygenators (IVOXs), 753–754
Intravascular volume
  deficit of. *See* Hypovolemia
  excess. *See* Hypervolemia
  maneuvers to increase cerebral blood flow
    and, 285
  mechanical ventilation and, 1961–1962
Intravenous access, for parenteral nutrition, 467
Intravenous anesthetics, 1021–1026. *See also*
    specific anesthetics
  barbiturate, 1022–1023, 1023t
  immune system function and, 1026
  narcotic, 1021t, 1021–1022
Intravenous immunoglobulin (IVIg)
  for cytomegalovirus infections, 1612
  for Guillain-Barré syndrome, 2006, 2008,
    2010, 2011
  for idiopathic thrombocytopenic purpura,
    2226, 2237–2238
  for myasthenia gravis, 2014
  for pneumonia, 1856
Intrinsic coagulation pathway, 269–270
Intubation
  during brain resuscitation, 281
  bronchial, chest radiography and, 966–967,
    967f
  complications of, 1837t
  endotracheal
    complications of, 1837t
    fiberoptic bronchoscopy for, 686–687,
      689f, 697t
  for enteral nutrition. *See* Feeding tube
    placement; Feeding tube(s)
  esophageal, chest radiography and, 967, 967f
  extubation and
    complications of, 1837t, 1928
    inadvertent, 768
    indications for, with burns, 1266–1267
  in Guillain-Barré syndrome, 2010
  for mechanical ventilation, complications of,
    1928

  for myasthenia gravis, 2014
  nasal, in spinal cord injury, 1209–1210
  nasoduodenal, for enteral nutrition, 602–603,
    603f
  nasogastric
    following cardiac surgery in pediatric
      patients, 1173–1174
    for enteral nutrition, 602
  nasojejunal, for enteral nutrition, 602–603,
    603f
  nasotracheal. *See* Nasotracheal intubation
  orotracheal, techniques for, 766
    with curved blades, 766
    with straight blades, 766
  for salicylate poisoning, 1489
  for sepsis, 410
  in spinal cord injury, 1212
  tracheal. *See* Tracheal intubation
Invasive core-rewarming, for hypothermia, 1454
Invasive precautions, 1443, 1443t
Invasive pressure monitoring, 839–845. *See also*
    specific catheters and cannulations
  complications of, 844
  equipment for, 839–841, 840f
    amplifier system, 840
    catheters, 839
    continuous flush devices, 840
    oscilloscope display, 840
    pressure transducers, 840
    pressure tubing, 839
    processor/digital display, 840–841
    recorder, 841
    stopcocks, 839, 840
  equipment setup for, 841–844
    calibration and, 841
    checking and optimizing dynamic response
      characteristics and, 841–842, 842f, 843f
    clinical versus laboratory measurement of
      dynamic response and, 842–844, 843f
    transducer selection and, 844
    zeroing transducers and, 841, 841f
  signal amplification, processing, and display
    for, 844–845
Inverse ratio ventilation (IRV), 751–752
  for acute respiratory distress syndrome, 1835
  advantages of, 752
  for aspiration syndromes, 1867
  disadvantages of, 752
  initial settings for, 752
  pressure-controlled. *See* Pressure-controlled
    inverse ratio ventilation (PC-IRV)
  setup parameters for, 752, 753f
  work of breathing and, 752
Iodine
  radioactive, uptake of, in thyrotoxicosis, 2139
  for thyrotoxicosis, 2140, 2141
  thyrotoxicosis induced by, treatment of, 2141
Ipecac, for salicylate poisoning, 1488
Ipratropium bromide
  for acute respiratory failure, 1921
  for asthma, 1937–1938
  preoperative, 994t
Iron
  deposition of, transfusion therapy and, 655
  poisoning by, antidote for, 1466t
  red blood cell production and, 663

  requirement for, 462, 462t
Ischemia
  abdominal, abdominal radiography in, 971
  acute, radiologic interventions for, 588–589
  acute renal failure due to, 2086
  cardiac, chest pain and, 1722–1723
  cerebral
    electroencephalography in, 944
    treatment of, 280t
  in children, 1163
  cocaine abuse and, 1516
  electrocardiographic detection of, 874–875
    modified V_5 lead and, 874, 874f
    trouble-shooting and, 874–875
    V_4 lead and, 874, 874f
  intestinal. *See* Intestinal ischemia
  of limbs, following cardiac surgery in pediatric
    patients, 1172–1173
  localized, prevention of, 2208
  mesenteric, acute
    acute abdomen and, 1107
    radiologic interventions for, 588–589
  of muscles, tourniquets and, 1246
  myocardial
    following cardiac surgery, 1149
    hypertensive emergencies and, 1817–1818
    myocardial metabolism and, 251, 252f
  preoperative, significance of, 900–901
  sigmoid, following vascular surgery, 1111
  silent, prevalence of, 899–900, 900t
  stress ulceration and, 2038
  ST segment monitoring for. *See* ST segment
    monitoring
  wound management and, 782
Ischemic cardiomyopathy, in systemic sclerosis,
    2172
Ischemic edema, cerebral, 278
  treatment of, 280t
Isocarboxazid, side effects of, 2027t
Isocyanates, inhalation injury due to, 1955
Isoetharine, preoperative, 994t
Isoflurane, for status epilepticus, 1982t
Isolation
  in aircraft, 807
  of HIV-infected patients, 1631
  for prevention of bacterial meningitis, 1643
  for viral infections, 1691, 1692t
Isometric contraction, 231
Isoniazid
  for *Mycobacterium tuberculosis* infections, in
    HIV-infected patients, 1619t, 1620t
  poisoning by, antidote for, 1466t
  prophylactic, for tuberculosis, 1565
Isopropanol poisoning, 1501, 1503–1504
Isoproterenol
  actions, indications, and dosing of, 2270
  following cardiac surgery in pediatric
    patients, 1167t
  for heart-lung transplantation, 1319t
  for heart transplantation, 1336
  for lung transplantation, 1319t
  preoperative, 994t
  for shock, 363t
    cardiogenic, 400
Isosorbide dinitrate, for heart failure, 1755–1756

Isotretinoin, for generalized pustular psoriasis, 2180
Isovolemic contraction, 231
Isradipine (DynaCirc), for hypertension, following liver transplantation, 1345
Itraconazole, 1570, 1690t, 1691
  for coccidioidomycosis, in HIV-infected patients, 1619t
  for heart-lung transplantation, 1329
  for histoplasmosis, in HIV-infected patients, 1619t
  for lung transplantation, 1329

Jaundice, following hepatic resection, 1126
Jaw-thrust method, modified, for airway management, 1209
Jehovah's Witnesses, refusal of transfusion therapy by, 656
Jejunal fistulas, postoperative, 1114
Jejunostomy
  percutaneous, for feeding tube placement, 604
  surgical, for feeding tube placement, 605, 605f, 606f
  transgastric, 595
Jejunostomy tubes, 1117f, 1117–1118
Jellyfish envenomations, 1533t, 1533–1534
  clinical manifestations of, 1533–1534
  treatment of, 1534
Jet entrainment, 704
Jet ventilators, 737–738
  controls for, 737, 737t
  potential problems with, 737t, 737–738, 738t
J.F.K. Memorial Hospital v. Bludworth, 120
Job's syndrome, 309t
Joint(s)
  disorders of. *See specific disorders*
  motion of, limitation of, fractures and, 1228
  in sickle cell anemia, 2234
Joint Commission on Accreditation of Healthcare Organizations (JCAHO)
  iatrogenesis and, 95
  surveys by, 176, 185
    personnel involvement in, 185
    specific analyses in, 185
Joint replacement, 2158
  complications of, 1234–1235
    with total hip arthroplasty, 1234–1235
    with total knee arthroplasty, 1235
    with total shoulder arthroplasty, 1235
Judicial involvement, in treatment decisions. *See* Clinical decision-making, judicial involvement in
Jugular vein cannulation
  of external jugular vein, 529t, 530–531, 531f
  of internal jugular vein, 527–530, 528t, 529t
    anatomy and, 527
    approaches for, 527
    complications of, 530, 531t
    technique for, 527–530, 530f
    tip position and, 530
Jugular venous distension, in refractory advanced heart failure, 1758, 1759t
Jugular venous saturation, cerebral metabolism and, 951–962
Junctional arrhythmias, 1783

management of, 1785
Junior residents, 36
Justice
  distributive, 22–23, 24–25
  as medicomoral principle, 67

Kallikrein, 298
Kaposi's sarcoma (KS), in HIV-infected patients, 1626
Kaposi's varicelliform eruption. *See* Eczema herpeticum
Karya rings, 2206
Kayexalate (sodium polystyrene sulfonate), for hyperkalemia, 427t
Kernig sign, 1635
Kernohan's notch, 1200
Ketamine, 825t, 826, 1025–1026
  for airway management, 763
  cardiovascular effects of, 1025–1026
  cost of, 827t
  neurologic effects of, 1025
  pharmacodynamics of, 1025
  pharmacokinetics of, 1023t, 1025
  respiratory effects of, 1026
  for vascular cannulation, 522
Ketoacidosis. *See* Diabetic ketoacidosis (DKA)
Ketoconazole, 1570, 1690t, 1691
  for acute respiratory distress syndrome, 1834
  for *Candida* infections, in HIV-infected patients, 1619t
Ketorolac, for cerebral edema, in fulminant hepatic failure, 2049
Kidney(s). *See also* Renal *entries*
  potassium regulation by, 421–422
  shock and, 371–372
  ultrasonography of, 976–977, 979f
Kinins, 298
Klebsiella infections, 1670
Knee replacement, complications of, 1235
Knife wounds. *See* Trauma; *specific sites and injuries*
Korotkoff sounds, 871f, 871–872
Kussmaul's sign, in constrictive pericarditis, 853
Kyphoscoliosis, in obstetric patients, 1416

Labetalol
  actions and indications for, 2270
  dosage of, 2270
    in hepatic disease, 482t
  for hypertension
    cocaine abuse and, 1517
    in hypertensive emergencies, 1813, 1814t, 1815, 1819
    following liver transplantation, 1345
    vascular surgery and, 1179
  for pheochromocytomas, 2134t
Labor
  amniotic fluid embolism and, 1910
  drugs used to arrest, cardiovascular changes with, 1402–1403
  preterm, 320
  postoperative, 1424–1425
  stress of, 1431
    aortocaval compression and, 1431

Laboratory error, 99t, 99–100, 100t
Laboratory error syndromes, 100
Laboratory precautions, 1443, 1443t
Laboratory tests. *See also specific tests*
  for acute abdomen, 1102
  following cardiac surgery in pediatric patients, 1170
  in comatose patients, 1975
  criteria and judgment for choosing, 131–134, 132t
    deletion of standing orders for testing and, 132
    management principles and, 132, 133t
    no orders for repeated testing and, 134, 134t
    structured decision trees, 132–134, 133t, 134t
  overuse of, 96
  in poisonings and toxic exposures, 1472–1473
  in shock, 375
β-Lactam antibiotics, 1567
  penicillins combined with, 1566
Lactate
  in dysoxia, 339
  fetal metabolism of, 1434
  serum level of
    following cardiac surgery in adult patients, 1154
    following cardiac surgery in pediatric patients, 1170
Lactic acid, serum level of, following cardiac surgery, 1154
Lactic acidosis. *See* Metabolic acidosis, lactic
Lactulose, for postshunt encephalopathy, 1124
Lacunar stroke, 1992t, 1992–1993
Laminar flow, 196
Laparoscopy
  for abdominal injuries, 1081
  for acute abdomen, 1103, 1105
  pneumoperitoneum due to, 1105–1106, 1106f
Laparotomy
  for abdominal injuries, 1080, 1081–1082
  infections and, 1598
  pneumoperitoneum due to, 1105–1106, 1106f
Laryngeal disorders. *See also specific disorders*
  aspiration pneumonitis and, 1869
  in rheumatoid arthritis, 1245, 1245f
Laryngeal edema, following extubation, 769
Laryngeal injuries, tracheal intubation causing, 768, 1924
Laryngeal mask airway (LMA), 493, 494, 495f, 764, 764f, 765f
Laryngoscopes, 764–765
  blades of, 765
Laser Doppler flowmetry (LDF), 950–951
Lassa virus infections, 1696, 1710
Lateral position test, preoperative, 991
Latrodectus bites, 1528f, 1528t, 1528–1530, 1530t
Leach v. Akron General Medical Center, 111
Lead poisoning, antidote for, 1465t
Left atrial pressure (LAP), 856
Left-to-right intracardiac shunts
  arterial emboli with, 1906
  during pregnancy, 1395
Left ventricle, free wall rupture of
  cardiogenic shock and, 394–395
  surgical intervention for, 402

Left ventricular afterload, spontaneous breathing and, 739

Left ventricular aneurysms
cardiogenic shock and, 395
surgical intervention for, 402

Left ventricular assist devices (LVADs)
following cardiac surgery in pediatric patients, 1174
for cardiogenic shock, 402–403

Left ventricular compliance, reduced, waveform analysis in, 858

Left ventricular end-diastolic pressure (LVEDP), 856, 861, 863
following cardiac surgery, 1149, 1151

Left ventricular failure, acute, hypertensive emergencies and, 1818

Left ventricular function
in advanced heart failure, as prognostic factor, 1753–1754
assessment of, in acute myocardial infarction, 1743
decreased, spontaneous breathing and, 740

Left ventricular hypertrophy (LVH), in chronic renal failure, 2094

Left ventricular infarction, 390–392, 391t

Legal issues, 117–125
brain death, 122–123
critical care team's decision-making and, 72–73
ethics and, 64
iatrogenesis and, 101–102
informed consent. *See* Informed consent
organ transplantation, 124–125
refusal of treatment. *See* Treatment, refusal of
regarding clinical decision-making. *See* Clinical decision-making, judicial involvement in
terminal patients and. *See* Terminal patients
termination of cardiopulmonary resuscitation and, 160
threat of litigation and, 76–77
withdrawal of treatment and, 27–29, 28f, 110–111, 112–114

Legionella infections, 1673
in immunocompromised patients, 1609
diagnosis of, 1609
presentation of, 1609
therapy of, 1609
pneumonia due to, *Mycoplasma pneumoniae* pneumonia distinguished from, 1846, 1847f, 1847t

Legs
edema of, infrainguinal reconstructions and, 1186–1187
diagnosis of, 1186
etiology of, 1186
incidence of, 1186
therapy of, 1186–1187
elevation of, for infrainguinal reconstructions, 1186
venous cutdown at ankle and, 569, 573f

Leiurus quinquestriatus stings, 1532–1533, 1533t

Lennox-Gastaut syndrome, 1986

Leptospirosis, 1682

Leucovorin
for methotrexate poisoning, 1467t
for *Pneumocystis carinii* infections, 1607

Leukapheresis, for leukocytosis, 2241

Leukemia
aspergillosis associated with, 1688
chemotherapy for, bleeding caused by, 2228

Leukocyte(s)
effector functions of, host response and, 296
host response and, 296
interactions with endothelial cells, host response and, 296

Leukocyte adhesion deficiency (LAD), 291, 296, 309t

Leukocytoclastic vasculitis (LCV), 2162f, 2162–2163, 2189f, 2189t, 2189–2190

Leukocytosis, 2241

Leukopenia, 2235–2236. *See also* Granulocytopenia; Neutropenia
bone marrow aplasia and, 2236
immune granulocytopenia and, 2236
malignant disease and cytotoxic treatment as cause of, 2235–2236

Levamisole, 312t

Libman-Sacks vegetations, in systemic lupus erythematosus, 2168

Lidocaine
actions and indications for, 2270
for acute myocardial infarction, 1736
for airway management, 762
for arrhythmias, 1786
for cardiopulmonary resuscitation, 502–503
complications of, 503
dosage of, 503
indications for, 503
toxicity of, 503
for depressed gastrointestinal pH, 452
dosing of, 2270
in chronic renal failure, 2097t
in hepatic disease, 482t
for fiberoptic bronchoscopy, 689, 689t
for status epilepticus, 1984
therapeutic serum level of, 479t
for vascular cannulation, 531–533

Life
preservation of, as medicomoral principle, 66
quality of, termination of cardiopulmonary resuscitation and, 159

Life-support systems, treatment decisions and, 75–76

Light, ambient, pulse oximetry and, 875

Lightning injuries, 1541t, 1541–1542

Lightning psychorecidivism, 1542

Limbs. *See* Extremities; Legs

Lipid emulsions, for parenteral nutrition, complications of, 470

Lipid metabolism, in critical illness, 330t, 330–331, 331f

Lipopolysaccharide (LPS)
host response and, 292, 294
sepsis and, 407, 407t

Liquid ventilation, for acute respiratory distress syndrome, 1836

Lisinopril, for acute myocardial infarction, 1737

Listeria monocytogenes infections, 1668
in immunocompromised patients, 1608–1609
diagnosis of, 1608
presentation of, 1608
renal transplant recipients, 1612

therapy of, 1608–1609

Lithium
poisoning by, 1493–1494
clinical manifestations of, 1493–1494
toxicology and, 1493
treatment of, 1494
for syndrome of inappropriate antidiuretic hormone secretion, 418
therapeutic serum level of, 479t
for thyrotoxicosis, 2140

Litigation. *See also* Clinical decision-making, judicial involvement in; Legal issues
threat of, 76–77

Liver. *See also* Hepatic *entries;* Hepatobiliary disease; *specific disorders*
assessment of
for intestinal transplantation, 1356
for multivisceral transplantation, 1356
interactions with lungs, multiple organ system failure and, 351–352, 352f
potassium regulation by, 422
shock and, 372

Liver injury scale, 2274t

Living wills, 29–31

Lobar collapse
chest radiography in, 964f–966f, 965
in spinal cord injury, 1212–1213

Local anesthetic(s). *See also specific drugs*
for airway management, 762
hypotension and, 819
pupillary effects of, 819
subdural catheter placement for delivery of, 819
total spinal block and, 818–819
toxicity of, 818

Local anesthetic blocks, 812
epidural, 812
neuraxial, 813–816
anatomy and, 813, 813f–815f
epidural catheter technique for, 815–816
epidural puncture for, 814–815, 815t, 816f
equipment for, 813, 815t
spinal puncture for, 816
peripheral, 812
axillary catheter for, 813
intercostal, 813
technique for, 813

Logical operations, of microprocessor-controlled ventilators, 716–717, 717f

Lomustine (CCNU), for bone marrow transplantation, 1368t

Long ACTH stimulation test, 2127

Long dexamethasone suppression test, 2127–2128

Longeway decision, 113

Loop diuretics. *See also specific drugs*
for intracranial hypertension, 1205
for renal dysfunction, in sepsis, 411
for rhabdomyolysis, 2200

Loperamide, for diarrhea, 2212

Lorazepam (Ativan), 824, 824t, 825, 825t
actions and indications for, 2270
for agitation and anxiety, 2026t
cost of, 827t
dosage of, 2270
in hepatic disease, 482t

for heart-lung transplantation, 1319t
for lung transplantation, 1319t
pharmacokinetics and pharmacodynamics of, 1023t, 1025
for seizures
in brain injury, 286
in status epilepticus, 1982t, 1984
Low-dose heparin (LDH), for deep venous thrombosis prophylaxis, 1890–1891
Low flow states, blood gas analysis during. *See* Blood gas analysis, cardiopulmonary resuscitation and low flow states and
Low-molecular-weight dextran
for intestinal transplantation, 1361
for multivisceral transplantation, 1361
Low-molecular-weight heparin (LMWH)
for antithrombotic therapy, 619f, 619–620
for deep venous thrombosis prophylaxis, 1891
prophylactic
for deep venous thrombosis, 1239–1241
for pulmonary thromboembolism, 1239–1241
for pulmonary embolism, 1898–1899
Low T$_3$ syndrome, 2146
Loxosceles bites, 1530, 1530t
Ludwig's angina, 1710–1711
Lugol's solution, for thyrotoxicosis, 2140, 2141
Lumbar puncture
in comatose patients, 1975
in status epilepticus, 1986
Lung(s). *See also* Cardiopulmonary *entries;* Pulmonary *entries;* Respiratory *entries; specific disorders*
acute lung injury and
acute, respiratory distress syndrome and, 1828
mechanisms of, 1829–1830
structural response to, 1828f, 1828–1829, 1829f, 1829t
anesthetic uptake from, 1015–1016
alveolar-mixed venous anesthetic partial pressure gradient and, 1016
cardiac output and, 1016
solubility and, 1015–1016, 1016t
cavitary lesions of, surgical management of, 1144f, 1145
collapse of, in spinal cord injury, 1213
interactions with liver, multiple organ system failure and, 351–352, 352f
lobar collapse of
chest radiography in, 964f–966f, 965
in spinal cord injury, 1212–1213
mechanics of. *See* Pulmonary mechanics
as oxygenators, 928–929
oxygen toxicity and. *See* Oxygen, pulmonary toxicity of
physiology of. *See* Airway resistance; Lung volumes; Pulmonary compliance; Pulmonary physiology; Ventilation
in poisonings and toxic exposures, 1471
shock and, 371
zones of, pulmonary blood flow and, 200
Lung biopsy
for diagnosis of pneumonia, 695
open-lung, in pneumonia, 695, 1853–1854
Lung capacity, preoperative assessment of, 990

Lung injury scale, 2279t–2280t
Lung perfusion scans. *See also* Ventilation/perfusion (V/Q) scans
in chest pain, 1718
in pulmonary embolism, 1720
Lung transplantation. *See also* Double-lung transplantation (DLT); Heart-lung transplantation (HLT); Single-lung transplantation (SLT)
current status of, 1290
organ allocation for, 1297
Lung volumes
formulas for, 2263t–2264t
mechanical ventilation and, 1961
in obstetric patients, 1411, 1411t
postoperative maintenance of, 995
preoperative assessment of, 990
static, 189–193
functional residual capacity and, 189–190, 190f, 191t
mechanics of ventilation and, 190–191, 192f
pleural pressure and, 189, 190f
respiratory muscles and, 191–193
Lupus. *See* Systemic lupus erythematosus (SLE)
Lupus anticoagulant, 2229
Lupus pneumonitis, acute, 2165–2166
Luteinizing hormone (LH), deficiency of, 2113
Lyme disease, 1682, 1708, 1709
Lymphadenectomy, retroperitoneal, postoperative management and, 1255
Lymphoceles, drainage of, 594
Lymphocytes, inhalational anesthetics and, 1020
Lymphomas
aspergillosis associated with, 1688
central nervous system, in HIV-infected patients, 1627
tracheal obstruction due to, 2248–2249
Lymphoproliferative disease
Epstein-Barr virus infections and, following bone marrow transplantation, 1377
following intestinal transplantation, 1362–1363
following multivisceral transplantation, 1363–1364
Lysine vasopressin, for gastrointestinal bleeding, 2036–2037

McArdle's disease, 2200
McMemar test, 13
Macrolides, 1569. *See also specific drugs*
Mafenide acetate cream, for burn wounds, 1273
Magnesium, 430–433
actions, indications, and dosing of, 2270
deficiency of. *See* Hypomagnesemia
distribution of, 430–431
excess of, 433
causes of, 433
clinical effects of, 433
treatment of, 433
function of, 430
obligate loss of, hypomagnesemia due to, 432
regulation of, 431
requirement for, 461t, 462
shifts in, hypomagnesemia due to, 432
supplementation of, for hypomagnesemia, 432–433, 433t

Magnesium sulfate
for asthma, 1939
during pregnancy
cardiovascular changes with, 1402–1403
for preeclampsia/eclampsia, 1392
for torsade de points, in antipsychotic poisoning, 1495
Magnetic resonance imaging (MRI), 978–981
abdominal, infections and, 1598
in hypopituitarism, 2114
intrahospital transport and, 800
in musculoskeletal injuries, 980
for neurologic infections, 1640
for pheochromocytoma localization, 2132
of spinal cord, 980, 983f
in stroke patients, 1993, 1995, 1995f
of vascular abnormalities, 980–981
Magnetic resonance venography, for deep venous thrombosis diagnosis, 1242t
Major histocompatibility complex (MHC), 304–306, 305f
Major tranquilizers, for agitation and anxiety, 2025–2026
Malaria, cerebral, 1711
Malignancies. *See also* Oncologic emergencies; *specific malignancies*
chemotherapy for. *See* Cancer chemotherapy
leukopenia due to, 2235–2236
neutropenia and, acute abdomen in, 1104
radiation therapy for
anterior pituitary failure caused by, 2114
constrictive pericarditis due to, 2251
secondary, following bone marrow transplantation, 1378
Malignant hyperthermia (MH), 483, 483t, 1032t, 1032–1033, 1457–1461, 1600
clinical syndrome of, 1458–1460, 1459t–1460t
complications of, 1460
diagnosis of, 1033
historical background of, 1032–1033
temperature regulation and, 1458, 1458t
treatment of, 1033, 1033t, 1460–1461
Mallampati signs and classifications, 760–761, 761f
Management principles, outcome prediction and, 132, 133t
Mandatory minute ventilation (MMV), 729
clinical applications of, 729
operational principles of, 729
Mannitol
for acute tumor lysis syndrome, 2247
following cardiac surgery in pediatric patients, 1172
for head injury, 1206–1207
for intracranial hypertension, 284, 1205
in fulminant hepatic failure, 2050
prophylactic
for acute tubular necrosis, 2086
for compartment syndromes, 1237
Manometer calibration, for blood pressure measurement, 871
Mapleson D breathing system, capnometry and, 879, 879f
Maprotiline (Ludiomil)
poisoning by, 1493
side effects of, 2027t

Marburg virus infections, 1696, 1710
Marfan's syndrome, 1775
    during pregnancy, 1395
Marine envenomations, 1533t, 1533–1534
    clinical manifestations of, 1533–1534
    treatment of, 1534
Marsupialization, for pancreatic necrosis and
        abscesses, 2061
Massive transfusion syndrome, 2220t, 2224–2225
Maternal-fetal interactions, fetal monitoring
        and, 1430–1431
Matter of Strorar, 106
Maximal voluntary ventilation (MVV),
        preoperative assessment of, 990
Mean(s), sampling variance of, 11
Mean arterial pressure (MAP)
    cerebral blood flow regulation and, 276
    measurement of, 872
Mean pressure (MP), 861
Measure 16 (Oregon), 78
Meat tenderizer, for esophageal obstruction, 2072
Mechanical cardiac assist devices. *See also*
        Intraaortic balloon pump (IABP);
        Ventricular assist devices (VADs)
    synchronized coronary venous retroperfusion
        and, 611
Mechanical purpura, 2188
Mechanical ventilation, 711–741. *See also*
        Microprocessor-controlled ventilators;
        Ventilators
    for acute respiratory distress syndrome,
        1831–1833, 1835–1836
        extracorporeal respiratory support and,
            1836
        high-frequency, 1836
        inverse ratio, 1835
        liquid ventilation and, 1836
        permissive hypercapnia and, 1835–1836
    airway pressure release. *See* Airway pressure
        release ventilation (APRV)
    for aspiration syndromes, 1866–1867
        control-inverse, 1867
        conventional, positive end-expiratory
            pressure, and continuous positive
            airway pressure, 1866–1867
        permissive hypercapnia and, 1867, 1867t
        pressure-support, 1867
    assist control. *See* Assist control ventilation
        (ACV)
    for asthma, 1939–1942, 1940f
        aerosol delivery and, 1940
        auto positive end-expiratory pressure and,
            1941–1942
        barotrauma and, 1942
        initiating, 1940–1941
        sedation for, 1940
    during brain resuscitation, 281–282
    following cardiac surgery
        in adult patients, 1156
        in pediatric patients, 1168–1169
    complications of, 1832, 1928t, 1928–1930
        endotracheal tubes and, 1928
        intubation and extubation and, 1928
        neurologic, 1880
        ventilator function and, 1928
    controlled, 719

    as backup for patient-triggered ventilation,
        720
        clinical applications of, 719
        operational principles of, 719, 720f
    end-inspiratory pause and, 720–721
        clinical applications of, 720–721
        operational principles of, 720, 721f, 721t
    extracorporeal membrane oxygenation and, 673
    failure to wean from, sepsis and, 1112
    for flail chest, 1138
    for Guillain-Barré syndrome, 2010
    high-frequency. *See* High-frequency
        ventilation (HFV)
    intermittent mandatory. *See* Intermittent
        mandatory ventilation (IMV);
        Synchronized intermittent mandatory
        ventilation (SIMV)
    inverse ratio. *See* Inverse ratio ventilation
        (IRV); Pressure-controlled inverse ratio
        ventilation (PC-IRV)
    low-volume, augmented, spontaneous, 754
    lung and heart-lung transplantation and,
        1327, 1328f
    major problems with, 711
    mandatory minute volume, 729
        clinical applications of, 729
        operational principles of, 729
    minimal excursionary, 753–754
        extracorporeal carbon dioxide removal with
            venovenous bypass and, 753
        intravascular oxygenator and, 753–754
        permissive hypercapnia and, 753
    for myasthenia gravis, 2014
    for near-drowning, 1879
    patient-triggered (assisted). *See* Patient-
        triggered ventilation
    peak inflation pressure and, 711, 712
    pneumothorax and, 1961–1962
        frequency of mechanical breaths and,
            1961, 1961t
        intravascular volume and, 1961–1962
        peak inspiratory pressure and volume and,
            1961, 1962t
        selective ventilation and, 1962
    postoperative, 996, 996t, 997t
        avoidance of, 1007, 1007t
    pressure augmentation and, 727
        operational principles of, 727, 728f
    pressure-controlled inverse ratio. *See* Pressure-
        controlled inverse ratio ventilation
        (PC-IRV)
    pressure support. *See* Pressure support
        ventilation (PSV)
    proportional assist, 727–729
        clinical applications of, 728
        operational principles of, 728
        potential problems with, 728–729
    for respiratory failure, 1925–1927
        assist-control, 1926
        continuous positive airway pressure and,
            1926
        intermittent mandatory ventilation and
            synchronized intermittent mandatory
            ventilation, 1925, 1926t
        weaning from, 1926–1927
    for salicylate poisoning, 1489

    for sepsis, 410
    in shock, 374
    side effects and complications of, 741
        hemodynamic, 741
        pneumothorax. *See* Mechanical ventilation,
            pneumothorax and
        pulmonary barotrauma, 741
    spontaneous breathing and. *See* Continuous
        positive airway pressure (CPAP);
        Positive end-expiratory pressure
        (PEEP), spontaneous; Spontaneous
        breathing
    stress points with, 711–712
    following thoracic surgery, 1135
    during transport, 738–739, 739f, 739t,
        795–797, 797t
        manual versus mechanical techniques for,
            790
        ventilators and, 796–797, 798t–799t, 800f
    weaning from. *See* Ventilator weaning
Mediastinum
    injuries of, delayed diagnosis of, 1055, 1057t
    shift of, following thoracic surgery, 1135
Medicaid, organ transplantation and, 125
Medical ethics. *See* Ethical considerations
Medical illness. *See also specific disorders*
    chronic, ethanol abuse and, 1514
    critical
        antibiotic monotherapy for, 1563–1564
        metabolic response to. *See* Metabolic
            response to injury and illness
        prolonged neuromuscular blockade and, 834
    decompensated diabetes mellitus and, 708,
        2108t
    metabolic response to. *See* Metabolic response
        to injury and illness
    thyroid function in, 2146–2147
    in thyrotoxicosis, treatment of, 2142
Medical literature, 3–20
    critical reading of, 4t, 4–9
        abstract or summary and, 9
        data analysis and, 6–8, 8f
        discussion and conclusions and, 8–9
        methodology and observations and, 6
        negative studies and, 8–9
        objective and hypothesis and, 4
        presentation of findings or results and, 6
        study design and, 4–6
    interpretation of study results and, 14–20
        analysis of diagnostic tests and, 18, 18f
        cautions regarding, 14–16
        confidence intervals and, 18–19, 19f
        regression analyses and, 19–20
        sample size and, 17–18
        type I and type II errors and, 16–17
    statistics and. *See* Statistics
Medicare, organ transplantation and, 125
Medications. *See also* Drug *entries; specific drugs
    and drug types*
    absorption of, in renal disease, 478
    actions, indications, and dosing of, 2268–2272
    adverse reactions to. *See* Adverse drug reactions
    antidiuretic hormone release and, 2117
    for arrest of labor, cardiovascular changes
        with, 1402–1403
    binding-insensitive, 482

binding-sensitive (restrictive), 482
bioavailability of, in renal disease, 478
clearance of, 477
　in hepatic disease, 481–482, 482t
delirium due to, 2021, 2021t
dosing of
　adjustment for hepatic disease, 482t
　adjustments for renal failure, 2266t–2267t
　for obese surgical patients, 1282
elimination of, hepatic graft function
　　assessment and optimization and,
　　1346–1347
emotional immobilization by, 93
enhancing neuromuscular blocking agent
　　effects, 831t
esophageal injury caused by, 2076–2077
　management of, 2077
　presentation of, 2076t, 2076–2077
half-life of, 477f, 477–478
hypercalcemia due to, 428, 430t
hyperkalemia due to, 425
hypocalcemia due to, 428, 429t
iatrogenesis related to, 96–97
immune-mediated platelet destruction induced
　　by, 2226–2227
for increase of uterine tone, cardiovascular
　　changes with, 1403
intracranial pressure and, 280–281
pharmacodynamics and, 475
　relationship to pharmacokinetics, 475, 476f
pharmacokinetics and, 475–478
　one-compartment model of, 476
　relationship to pharmacodynamics, 475, 476f
　two-compartment model of, 476–478, 477f
platelet disorders due to, 2226–2228
　heparin and, 2227–2228
　immune mediated, 2226–2227
during pregnancy, 320t, 320–321, 1425
purpura caused by, 2188–2189
for renal diseases, 478–481, 479t
　creatinine clearance and, 479–480
　gentamicin in, 480–481, 481t
rhabdomyolysis due to, 2197t, 2198–2199
for rheumatoid arthritis, side effects of, 1243t
surgical patients and, 1008–1009
thyroid function tests and, 2146, 2147t
tissue binding of, in renal disease, 478
Medroxyprogesterone, for acute respiratory
　　failure, 1923
Melphalan, for bone marrow transplantation,
　　1368t
Membrane oxygenators. *See also* Extracorporeal
　　membrane oxygenation (ECMO)
　extracorporeal carbon dioxide removal using,
　　with venovenous bypass, 753
Memory, in delirium, 2020
Memory (computer), of microprocessor-
　　controlled ventilators, 718, 718f
Meningitis
　aseptic, clinical presentation and initial
　　diagnostic measures for, 1637
　bacterial, 1595–1596
　　acute, coma and, 1978
　　clinical presentation and initial diagnostic
　　　measures for, 1635–1637, 1636t
　　complications of, 1643–1644, 1644t

gram-negative rod, 1643, 1646
　listerial, 1668
　meningococcal, 1666–1667
　partially treated, 1646
　prevention of, 1642t, 1642–1643
　staphylococcal, 1660
　streptococcal, 1664–1665
chronic, 1647, 1647t
fever associated with, 1595–1596
in HIV-infected patients, 1626
　treatment of, 1619t
nosocomial, 1584
pseudomonal, 1674
in renal transplant recipients, 1611
tuberculous, 1681
　in HIV-infected patients, 1626
viral, 1693t, 1693–1694, 1694t
Meningococcus infections
　acute meningococcemia, purpura and, 2190,
　　2190f
　antibiotic prophylaxis for, 1565
　neurologic, epidemiologic and clinical clues
　　to, 1636t
Meningoencephalitis, viral, 1647, 1647t
Mental confusion. *See* Confusion
Meperidine
　with amphotericin B, 1570
　cost of, 827t
　dosage adjustment for, in hepatic disease, 482t
Mercury poisoning, antidote for, 1465t
Mesenteric injuries, 1092–1093
Mesenteric ischemia, acute
　acute abdomen and, 1107
　radiologic interventions for, 588–589
Mesenteric reconstruction, 1183–1184
　fluid management and, 1183
　hypertension management and, 1183
　intestinal infarction and, 1183–1184
　mortality and, 1184
　renal artery graft stenosis/thrombosis and, 1183
Mesenteric vasculitis, in systemic lupus
　　erythematosus, 2168
Metabolic acidemia, 927–928
Metabolic acidosis, 259, 259t, 260–261, 922t
　during cardiopulmonary resuscitation, 935
　causes of, 260
　in diabetic ketoacidosis, 2103
　lactic
　　blood gas analysis in, 934
　　during brain resuscitation, 283
　　idiopathic, 261
　　in shock, 359, 379
　　in trauma patients, 1051–1052
　　in neonates, 261
　in poisonings and toxic exposures, 1472–1473
　　methanol and, 1502
　with respiratory alkalosis, 261
　in rhabdomyolysis, 2199
　tourniquets and, 1246
　treatment of, 260–261
Metabolic alkalemia, 928
Metabolic alkalosis, 259, 261–263, 922t
　causes of, 261–262, 262t
　drug-induced, 484
　renal, compensatory, 256
　treatment of, 262–263

Metabolic disorders. *See also specific disorders*
　coma and. *See* Coma, metabolic-toxic
　　etiologies of
　ethanol intoxication and, 1513
　in fulminant hepatic failure, 2052
　lithium toxicity and, 1494
　nutritional support and, 468–469
　following transfusion therapy, 654–655
Metabolic monitoring, in multiple organ system
　　failure, 344–345
Metabolic rate, fetal, 1434
Metabolic response to injury and illness, 325–334
　clinical care and, 333–334
　ebb phase of, 326, 326t
　flow phase of, 326
　intermediary metabolism and, 327–331
　　of amino acids, 328–329
　　of carbohydrates, 329t, 329–330, 330t
　　of lipids, 330t, 330–331, 331t
　　of protein, 327–328, 328f
　major problems with, 325
　regulation of, 331–333
　　cytokines and, 332t, 332–333
　　endocrine mediators and, 331–332
　shock and, 370
　starvation and, 326–327
　stress points with, 325–326
Metabolic support, for pancreatitis, 2058
Metabolic waste, elimination of, hepatic graft
　　function assessment and optimization
　　and, 1346–1347
Metabolism
　of antibiotics, antibiotic selection and, 1557t,
　　1557–1558
　during brain resuscitation, 283
　cardiac. *See* Cardiovascular physiology
　cerebral. *See* Cerebral metabolism
　of comatose patients, emergency evaluation
　　of, 1972
　of energy
　　cellular, gastrointestinal, 444–445
　　hepatic graft function assessment and
　　　optimization and, 1347
　glucocorticoids and, 2123
　hypermetabolism
　　of burns, 1271
　　pheochromocytoma and, 2130
　in hypokalemia, 424t
　in hypomagnesemia, 432t
　of lactate, fetal, 1434
　pheochromocytoma and, 2130
　pulmonary, 205–206
Metal fume fever, 1955
Metaproterenol
　for acute respiratory failure, 1920
　preoperative, 994t
Methane, inhalation injury due to, 1952
Methanol poisoning, 1501–1502
　antidote for, 1466t
Methemoglobin, cyanide poisoning and, 1953
Methemoglobinemia, nitric oxide and, 1834
Methemoglobin inducer poisoning, antidote for,
　　1467t
Methicillin-resistant *Staphylococcus aureus*
　　(MRSA), 1661
　pneumonia due to, 1844

Methimazole, 2140
Methocarbamol, for black widow spider bites, 1530t
Methohexital, 825t
  pharmacokinetics of, 1023
Methotrexate
  adverse effects of, 2156t–2157t
  for heart-lung transplantation, 1320
  for lung transplantation, 1320
  poisoning by, antidote for, 1467t
Methylene blue, for methemoglobin inducer poisoning, 1467t
Methylergonovine, during pregnancy, cardiovascular changes with, 1403
Methylphenidate (Ritalin)
  for apathy, 2027
  side effects of, 2027t
Methylprednisolone
  for acute cerebritis, in systemic lupus erythematosus, 2170
  for acute respiratory failure, 1922
  for adrenal insufficiency, 2125t
  for asthma, 1938, 1939
  for heart-lung transplantation, 1318, 1319t, 1320
  for heart transplantation, 1335, 1338
  for intracranial hypertension, 285
  for lung transplantation, 1318, 1319t, 1320
  for myasthenia gravis, 2014
  for pulmonary hemorrhage, in systemic lupus erythematosus, 2166
  for spinal shock, 1212
  for vasculitis, 2164
4-Methylpyrazole, for methanol poisoning, 1502
Methylxanthines. *See also specific drugs*
  for acute respiratory failure, 1921–1922
Metoclopramide (Reglan)
  for agitation and anxiety, 2026
  for aspiration prophylaxis, 1872
Metocurine, 829, 830t
  actions, indications, and dosing of, 2270
Metoprolol
  for dilated cardiomyopathy, 1763
  for limitation of infarct size, 396–397
Metric system, 2255t
Metronidazole, 1569
  for *Clostridium difficile* infections, 1677
  cost and initial dosage of, 1562t
Metyrosine, for pheochromocytomas, 2133, 2134t
Mexiletine, dosing of, in chronic renal failure, 2097t
Miconazole (Monistat), 1690t, 1691
  prophylactic, for renal transplant recipients, 1305
Microemboli
  fat, autotransfusion and, 665
  platelet, autotransfusion and, 665
Microprocessor-controlled ventilators, 715–719
  basic operation of, 715f, 715–716, 716f, 716t
    central processing unit and, 715–716
  data manipulation and logic and, 716–717
    logical operations and, 716–717
    microprocessor control and, 717
    relational operations and, 716
  digital and analog signals and, 718–719, 719t
    analog-to-digital converters and, 719

digital-to-analog converters and, 719
flow valves of, 714t
microprocessor systems of, 718
  data transfer, access and control and, 718
  random-access and read-only memory and, 718, 718f
Micrurus fulvius antivenin, 1527t, 1528
Midazolam (Versed), 824t, 824–825
  actions, indications, and dosing of, 2270
  for agitation and anxiety, 2026t
  for continuous sedation, 1030
  cost of, 827t
  pharmacokinetics and pharmacodynamics of, 1023t, 1025
  for status epilepticus, 1982t, 1984
  for vascular cannulation, 522
Midflow measurements, preoperative, 990
Military antishock trousers (MAST)
  for compartment syndromes, 1235–1236
  infections associated with, 2211
  for pelvic fractures, 1060, 1061
Milrinone
  actions, indications, and dosing of, 2268
  following cardiac surgery in pediatric patients, 1168t
  for heart failure, 1757, 1761, 1761t
  for heart transplantation, 1336
  for shock, 363t
Mineralocorticoids, production of, 2122
Mini-Mental State (MMS) examination, 2018, 2019f
Minimum inhibitory concentrations (MICs), 1793
Minocycline
  for methicillin-resistant *Staphylococcus aureus* infections, 1661
  for *Nocardia* infections, 1608
  prophylactic, for bacterial meningitis, 1642t
Minoxidil, for hypertensive urgencies, 1820, 1820t
Minute ventilation, 214
Miosis, in poisonings and toxic exposures, 1472
Misdiagnosis, 96
Misoprostol, for cyclosporine nephrotoxicity, 1338
Missile wounds. *See* Trauma; *specific sites and injuries*
Mithramycin, for hypercalcemia, 429t
Mitoxantrone, for bone marrow transplantation, 1368t
Mitral insufficiency
  acute, waveform analysis in, 857–858, 858f
  atrial, cardiogenic shock and, 393–394
  during pregnancy, 1394
    clinical considerations in, 1394
Mitral regurgitation, 1771–1773
  acute, 1772–1773
    clinical presentation of, 1772
    diagnostic studies for, 1772–1773
    etiology of, 1772
    pathophysiology of, 1772
    therapy of, 1773
  with aortic regurgitation, 1778
  with aortic stenosis, 1778
  chronic, 1771–1772
    clinical presentation of, 1771
    diagnostic studies for, 1771–1782
    etiology of, 1771

pathophysiology of, 1771
  therapy of, 1772
Mitral stenosis, 1770–1771
  with aortic regurgitation, 1778
  with aortic stenosis, 1778
  clinical presentation of, 1770
  diagnostic studies for, 1770
  etiology of, 1770
  pathophysiology of, 1770
  during pregnancy, 1393–1394
    clinical considerations in, 1393–1394
  therapy of, 1770–1771
Mitral valve prolapse, during pregnancy, 1396
  clinical considerations in, 1396
Mivacurium, 829, 830t
  actions, indications, and dosing of, 2270
Mixed lymphocyte reaction, inhalational anesthetics and, 1020
Mizoribin, for simultaneous pancreas/kidney transplantation, 1314
Mobitz block, 1784
Monitoring. *See also specific disorders; specific types of monitoring*
  equipment for. *See also specific devices*
    insertion of, during secondary triage of trauma patients, 1050
    for intrahospital transport, 793, 795, 796f, 796t
  orders for, 43–44, 44f, 44t, 45f
  of organ donors, 1293, 1294t
  outcome prediction and, 131
  as treatment objective, 23–24
Monoamine oxidase inhibitors. *See also specific drugs*
  side effects of, 2027t
Monoclonal antibodies. *See also specific monoclonal antibodies*
  for liver transplantation, 1344–1345
  to platelet glycoprotein IIb/IIIa, for antiplatelet therapy, 615
  for renal transplantation, 1305
Monocytic ehrlichiosis (HME), 1706
Monomethyl-hydrazine-containing mushroom poisoning, antidote for, 1466t
Mononuclear phagocytes, host response and, 292, 294
Mononucleosis, infectious, in immunocompromised patients, 1695
Monroe-Kellie doctrine, 275, 1195, 1198
Moral principles, 63–64. *See also* Ethical considerations
  governing treatment objectives, 22–23
Moraxella (Branhamella) catarrhalis infections, 1666
Morbilliform drug eruptions, 2186–2187, 2187f
Morphine
  actions, indications, and dosing of, 2270–2271
  for black widow spider bites, 1530, 1530t
  cost of, 827t
  dosage adjustment for, in hepatic disease, 482t
  for hypertension, in hypertensive emergencies, 1818
Morphine sulfate
  for heart-lung transplantation, 1319t
  for lung transplantation, 1319t
  following thoracic surgery, 1133

Mortality. *See* Death

Motion. *See* Movements

Motor abnormalities
in delirium, 2020
hyperactivity, in cyclic antidepressant
poisoning, 1490

Mouth-to-mask breathing, 495

Mouth-to-mouth breathing, 495

Movements
fetal, spontaneous, 1435
ocular, in comatose patients, evaluation of,
1973–1974
pulse oximetry and, 875
spontaneous and induced, in comatose
patients, 1973

Mucociliary transport, central control of
ventilation and, 205

Mucormycosis, 1689–1690

Mucosal barrier, stress ulceration and, 2039

Mucositis, following bone marrow
transplantation, 1371

Muerto Canyon virus infections, 1696

Multifocal atrial tachycardia (MAT), 1783
management of, 1785

Multiple comparisons procedures, 15–16

Multiple endocrine neoplasia (MEN) syndromes,
pheochromocytomas and, 2134–2135

Multiple organ dysfunction syndrome (MODS),
346, 372–373
treatment of, 373t

Multiple organ system failure (MOSF), 343–355
acute abdomen and, 1104
clinical features of, 352–353
definitions for, 345–346, 346t, 406t
diagnostic tests and procedures for, 344–345
epidemiology of, 346–347
gastrointestinal tract and, 447–448
gut motor hypothesis of, 447, 448, 448f
gut starter hypothesis of, 447f, 447–448
major problems with, 343
mortality due to, 1598
organ system interactions and, 351–352, 352f
outcome prediction and, 144
pathogenesis of, 347t, 347–351, 348f–351f,
348t
prevention of, 353–355, 354t
in sepsis, 408
shock and, 362t
stress points with, 343–344
treatment of, 353–355, 354t
initial therapy for, 345

Multiple organ transplantation. *See also*
Multivisceral transplantation; *specific
procedures*
current status of, 1290–1291

Multiple trauma, fractures and, 1226–1227

Multivisceral transplantation, 1353–1364
candidate evaluation and treatment for, 1355t,
1355–1357, 1357t
diagnostic tests and procedures for, 1354
initial therapy for, 1354
major problems with, 1353, 1354
operative procedure for, 1358, 1358f, 1359f,
1360
outcome with, 1364
postoperative care and, 1354, 1360–1364

early problems and, 1360–1361, 1361t
graft rejection and, 1362, 1363t
infection and, 1361–1362
late problems and, 1361
lymphoproliferative disease and, 1363–1364
nutrition and intestinal function and,
1362–1363
preparation for, 1357–1358
stress points with, 1353, 1354

Mupirocin, for methicillin-resistant
Staphylococcus aureus infections, 1661

Murine typhus, 1703, 1705

Muscarine-containing mushroom poisoning,
antidote for, 1466t, 1467t

Muscle(s). *See also* Neuromuscular *entries;*
Orthopedic complications; *specific
muscles*
function of, in hypokalemia, 424t
ischemia of, tourniquets and, 1246
myopathy due to prolonged neuromuscular
blockade and, 834
respiratory. *See* Diaphragm; Respiratory
muscles
rhabdomyolysis and. *See* Rhabdomyolysis
smooth
during pregnancy, direct hormonal effects
on, 319
at term, 317, 317t
spasms of, black widow spider bites and, 1529
strength of, in poisonings and toxic
exposures, 1471–1472
swelling of, in rhabdomyolysis, 2198
therapeutic paralysis of. *See* Neuromuscular
blocking agents (NMBAs); *specific
drugs*

Muscle relaxants. *See* Neuromuscular blocking
agents (NMBAs); *specific drugs*

Musculoskeletal disorders. *See also*
Neuromuscular disorders; Orthopedic
complications; *specific disorders*
chest pain in, 1718t
electrical injuries and, 1540

Musculoskeletal injuries. *See also* Bone, injuries
to; Fracture(s); Orthopedic
complications; *specific sites*
magnetic resonance imaging of, 980

Mushroom poisoning, antidote for, 1466t, 1467t

Myasthenia gravis (MG), 2011–2014
clinical features of, 2012–2013, 2013t
diagnosis of, 2013
tests and procedures for, 2011
epidemiology of, 2012
generalized myasthenia and, 2012
in neonates, 2014
pathogenesis of, 2012
treatment of, 2013–2014, 2014t
initial therapy for, 2011

Myasthenic crisis, precipitation of, 2013, 2013t

Mycobacterium avium complex (MAC)
infections, 1680
in HIV-infected patients, 1625
prophylaxis of, 1619t
treatment of, 1619t
pneumonia due to, 1854

Mycobacterium kansasii infections, 1680
pneumonia due to, 1854

Mycobacterium tuberculosis infections,
1680–1681
adrenal insufficiency due to, 2123
central nervous system manifestations of, 1646
meningitis, 1681
fiberoptic bronchoscopy in, 698–699
in HIV-infected patients, 1625, 1626
prophylaxis of, 1620t
treatment of, 1619t–1620t
miliary, 1681
in obstetric patients, 1415
pericarditis associated with, 1681
pneumonia due to, 1844
prophylaxis of
antibiotics for, 1565
in HIV-infected patients, 1620t
pulmonary, 1680–1681
treatment of, 1681
antibiotic combination therapy for, 1564
in HIV-infected patients, 1619t–1620t

Mycophenolate mofetil (Cellcept; RS-61443)
for heart-lung transplantation, 1320
for liver transplantation, 1345
for lung transplantation, 1320
for renal transplantation, 1304
for simultaneous pancreas/kidney
transplantation, 1314

Mycoplasma infections, 1681
antibiotics effective against, 1559t
Mycoplasma pneumoniae, pneumonia due to,
Legionella pneumonia distinguished
from, 1846, 1847f, 1847t

Mydriasis, in poisonings and toxic exposures,
1472

Myelitis, transverse, in systemic lupus
erythematosus, 2170

Myocardial cell abnormalities. *See* Heart failure,
myocardial cellular abnormalities and

Myocardial contractility, inhalational anesthetics
and, 1017

Myocardial disease, acute, hypoxemia with, 926

Myocardial infarction
acute. *See* Acute myocardial infarction (AMI)
chest pain and, 1723
left ventricular, 390–392, 391t
perioperative, prevention of, 1006f, 1006t,
1006–1007, 1007t
pharmacologic limitation of infarct size in,
395–397
during pregnancy, 1396–1397
clinical considerations in, 1396–1397
right ventricular, 392–393
adjunctive and experimental management
techniques for, 380
diagnosis of, 1738
therapy of, 1738
warfarin for, 622

Myocardial ischemia
following cardiac surgery, 1149
hypertensive emergencies and, 1817–1818
myocardial metabolism and, 251, 252f

Myocardial oxygen balance. *See* Cardiovascular
physiology

Myocardial oxygen consumption, following
cardiac surgery, 1149

Myocardial remodeling, heart failure and, 1751

Myocarditis
  in systemic lupus erythematosus, 2168
  in systemic sclerosis, 2172
Myoclonic status epilepticus, 1986–1987
Myoclonus, in cyclic antidepressant poisoning, 1490
Myofibrils, 229
Myoglobin, in rhabdomyolysis, 2199–2200
Myopathy, prolonged neuromuscular blockade and, 834
Myosin filaments, 229–230, 230f, 231
Myxedema coma
  presentation of, 2143t, 2143–2144
  treatment of, 2145, 2145t

Nafcillin
  for bacterial endocarditis, 1658
  for cellulitis
    orbital, staphylococcal, 1660
    staphylococcal, 1661
  cost and initial dosage of, 1562t
  for infective endocarditis, 1793, 1794t, 1795t, 1796t
  for meningitis, staphylococcal, 1660
  for osteomyelitis, staphylococcal, 1660
Nail polish, pulse oximetry and, 875
Naloxone (Narcan)
  for ethanol intoxication, 1513
  for opiate intoxication, 468, 1467t, 1518
  for respiratory depression, 817, 817t
Nanoequivalents, 256
Narcotics. See Opiates; *specific opiates*
Nasal airways, in cardiopulmonary resuscitation, 493
Nasal cannulae, 705
  for acute respiratory failure, 1920
Nasal disorders, anaphylaxis and, 1545t
Nasal intubation, in spinal cord injury, 1209–1210
Nasoduodenal intubation, for enteral nutrition, 602–603, 603f
Nasogastric drainage, following cardiac surgery in pediatric patients, 1173–1174
Nasogastric intubation
  following cardiac surgery in pediatric patients, 1173–1174
  for enteral nutrition, 602
Nasogastric tubes
  infections associated with, 2210, 2210f
  postoperative abdomen and, 1117
Nasojejunal intubation, for enteral nutrition, 602–603, 603f
Nasopharyngeal airway, for diarrhea, 2212
Nasotracheal intubation
  for respiratory failure, 1924
  techniques for, 766–767
    blind, 766
    with direct vision, 766–767
Nasotracheal tubes, sinusitis and, 2209
National Organ and Transplantation System, 1296
National Organ Transplant Act of 1984, 124, 1296–1297
Natural Death Act, 68, 70
Natural killer (NK) cells, inhalational anesthetics and, 1019

Near-drowning, 1863, 1875–1883
  acute respiratory distress syndrome and, 1827
  child abuse and, 1883
  clinical presentation of, 1877, 1877t
  diagnostic tests and procedures for, 1876–1877, 1877t
  fluids and electrolytes and, 1880, 1881f
  hematologic changes and, 1881, 1881f
  major problems with, 1875–1965, 1876f
  neurologic disorders and, 1880
  pathophysiology of, 1877–1878
    fresh water and, 1878
    seawater and, 1877–1878
  prevention and education for, 1883
  prognosis and outcome of, 1882–1883
    cardiopulmonary resuscitation and, 1883
    indicators for, 1882–1883
  renal failure and, 1880–1881
  sequelae of, 1881
  stress points with, 1875–1876, 1876t
  treatment of, 1878–1880
    cardiopulmonary, 1878, 1883
    positive end-expiratory pressure and continuous positive airway pressure in, 1878–1880, 1879f
    therapeutic goals for, 1883
  water intoxication and, 1883
Nebulization, for oxygen therapy, 706, 706f
Neck
  infections of. See Head and neck infections
  vascular trauma to, arteriography in, 1187
Necrosis
  of deep tissues, lightning injuries and, 1541
  of gallbladder, fever associated with, 1596
  hyperbaric oxygen therapy for, 780
  intestinal, postoperative, 1111
  in pancreatitis, surgical treatment of, 2061
  warfarin, 2226
Necrotizing enteropathy, in cancer, 2250–2251
Necrotizing fasciitis, 2192
  hyperbaric oxygen therapy for, 780
Necrotizing vasculitis, 2162f, 2162–2163
Needle-catheter cricothyroid ventilation, for anaphylaxis, 1548, 1549f
Needle punctures, 1443
Nefazodone (Serzone), side effects of, 2027t
Neisseria gonorrheae infections, 1667
  endocarditis due to, treatment of, 1793
Neisseria meningitidis infections, 1666–1667
  neurologic, epidemiologic and clinical clues to, 1636
Neonates
  antibiotic selection for neurologic infections in, 1641t
  breast feeding of, following cardiac surgery, 1174
  extracorporeal membrane oxygenation in. See Extracorporeal membrane oxygenation (ECMO), in neonates
  hypertrophic pyloric stenosis in, following cardiac surgery, 1174
  metabolic acidosis in, 261
  myasthenia gravis in, 2014
  persistent hypertension of newborn in, extracorporeal membrane oxygenation for, 671

Neostigmine
  for myasthenia gravis
    before elective surgery, 2014
    in neonates, 2014
  for neuromuscular blocking agent reversal, 835t, 1032t
Nephrectomy, radical, postoperative management and, 1255
Nephritis. See also Glomerulonephritis (GN); Pyelonephritis
  bacterial, focal, acute, in pyelonephritis, 1653
  interstitial, acute, acute renal failure due to, 2085
Nephronia, focal, acute, in pyelonephritis, 1653
Nephropathy, chloride-wasting, 262
Nephrosis, in pyelonephritis, 1653–1654
Nephrostomy, percutaneous, 595–596
  for pyonephrosis, 1654
Nephrotic syndrome, coagulation disorder associated with, 2230
Nephrotoxicity
  of aminoglycosides, 1568
  of immunosuppressants, 1338
Nerve blocks. See Local anesthetic blocks
Nerve injuries. See also Neurologic disorders; *specific disorders*
  carotid/subclavian reconstructions and, 1182–1183
    diagnosis of, 1182–1183
    etiology of, 1182
    incidence of, 1182
    therapy of, 1183
  with fractures, 1227
Netilmicin, therapeutic serum level of, 479t
Neural depression, spontaneous breathing and, 740
Neural receptors, central control of ventilation and, 204
Neurofibromatosis, pheochromocytomas and, 2135
Neurogenic control, of cardiovascular system, 242–245
  of heartbeat, 242–244
  of peripheral blood flow, 244–245
Neurogenic shock, 368
Neurohormonal activation, in heart failure. See Heart failure, neurohormonal activation in
Neurohumoral responses, shock and, 369f, 369–370
Neurohypophyseal disorders, 2116–2118
  management of, 2118
  patient examination in, 2117–2118
Neuroleptic agents. See Antipsychotic agents; *specific drugs*
Neuroleptic malignant syndrome (NMS), 827–828
  clinical syndrome of, 1458–1460
  complications of, 1460
  fever and, 1600
  temperature regulation and, 1458, 1458t
  therapeutic approach to, 1460–1461
Neurologic disorders. See also *specific disorders*
  anaphylaxis and, 1545t
  antibiotics and, 1563t
  aspiration pneumonitis and, 1869

autonomic
 in Guillain-Barré syndrome, 2009, 2010
 lightning injuries and, 1541
 following cardiopulmonary resuscitation, 157
 electrical injuries and, 1540
 epidural blocks and, 818
 in fat embolism syndrome, 1237–1238, 1909
 ice water submersion and, 1882
 lithium toxicity and, 1493–1494
 near-drowning and, 1880
 preoperative evaluation of, 1003–1004
  history and physical examination in, 1003t, 1003–1004
  laboratory examination in, 1004
 spinal cord compression. *See* Spinal cord, compression of
 in systemic lupus erythematosus, 2169–2170
Neurologic function
 assessment of
  carotid/subclavian reconstructions and, 1182
  in dysoxia, 340
  in spinal cord injury, 1210, 1211f
 barbiturates and, 1023
 benzodiazepines and, 1025
 in hyperosmolar states, 441t
 in hypokalemia, 424t
 during intrahospital transport, 789, 789t, 791t
 intravenous narcotics and, 1022
 ketamine and, 1025
 in poisonings and toxic exposures, 1471–1472
 propofol and, 1024
Neurologic infections, 1635–1647. *See also specific disorders and infections*
 antibiotic selection for, 1641t, 1641–1642
 clinical presentation and initial diagnostic measures for, 1635–1639
  with suspected infection with focal neurologic signs, 1637–1649
  with suspected infection with no focal neurologic signs, 1635–1637
 cryptococcal, 1689
 establishing diagnoses for, 1639–1641
  cerebrospinal fluid examination for, 1639–1640, 1640t
  radiologic tests for, 1640
  serologic tests for, 1640–1641, 1641t
 focal lesions and, in HIV-infected patients, 1626–1627
 immediate concerns with, 1635
 in immunocompromised patients, 1644–1646, 1645t
 tuberculous, 1646
Neurologic injuries. *See also* Brain injury; Nerve injuries; Spinal cord injuries; *specific nerves*
 intrahospital transport of patients and, 789, 789t, 797, 800
Neurologic monitoring, 941–953
 of cerebral function, 941–946
  electrocardiographic, 942–945, 943f, 944f
  evoked potentials for, 945f, 945–946
  frequency domain analysis for, 944f, 944–945
  neurologic examination for, 941–942, 942f, 942t
 of cerebral metabolism, 951–952

jugular venous saturation for, 951–952
 near-infrared spectroscopy for, 952
of cerebral perfusion, 946–951
 cerebral blood flow and, 946–947
 intracranial pressure and, 947f, 947–949, 948f, 949t
 laser Doppler flowmetry for, 950–951
 transcranial Doppler for, 949f–951f, 949–950
in head injury, 1201–1202, 1202f
imaging in, 952
Neuromuscular blocking agents (NMBAs), 828–835. *See also specific drugs*
 antagonism or residual blockade with, 834–835, 835t
 following cardiac surgery in pediatric patients, 1171
 depolarizing, 828–829
  for airway management, 762
 drugs enhancing effects of, 831t
 indications for, 828
 monitoring and, 830–833, 832t
  clinical applications of, 832–833, 833f, 834t
  double-burst suppression and, 831
  electrode placement for, 832
  posttetanic count and, 831
  titration of paralysis and, 833
  train-of-four, 831, 832f
  twitch response and, 831
 nondepolarizing, 829
  for airway management, 762
 physiology and pharmacology of neuromuscular transmission and, 828–829
 prolonged paralysis with, 833–834, 834t
  critical illness and, 834
  myopathy and, 834
  overdose and, 833–834
  postanesthesia, 1031t, 1031–1032, 1032t
 reversal of, 1031–1032, 1032t
Neuromuscular disorders, 2005–2015. *See also* Guillain-Barré syndrome (GBS); Myasthenia gravis (MG)
 aspiration pneumonitis and, 1869
 major problems with, 2005, 2006t
  stress points with, 2005
Neuromuscular function
 in hyperkalemia, 426t
 in hypomagnesemia, 432t
"Neuroprotectants," for stroke, 1999
Neuropsychiatric signs, in delirium, 2020
Neurosurgery, diabetes insipidus following, 2118
Neurotransmitters, excitatory, for head injury, 1206
Neurotrauma. *See* Brain injuries; Nerve injuries; Neurologic injuries; Spinal cord injuries; *specific nerves*
Neutropenia, 309t. *See also* Leukopenia
 acute abdomen in, 1104
 antibiotic monotherapy for, 1564
 antibiotic prophylaxis for, 1565
 in aplastic anemia, 2236
 following bone marrow transplantation, 1371
 enterocolitis and, in cancer, 2250–2251
 in immune granulocytopenia, 2236

Neutrophils
 acute lung injury and, 1829–1830
 inhalational anesthetics and, 1020
 polymorphonuclear
  fibrinolysis and, 271
  multiple organ system failure and, 347, 349–350, 350f
Newborn infants. *See* Neonates
Niacin, requirement for, 463–464, 464t
Nicardipine
 actions, indications, and dosing of, 2271
 for hypertension, in hypertensive emergencies, 1815t, 1816
 for pheochromocytomas, 2134t
Nicotinamide, for bullous pemphigoid, 2183
Nifedipine (Procardia)
 actions, indications, and dosing of, 2271
 for esophageal obstruction, 2072, 2073
 for hypertension
  in hypertensive emergencies, 1815
  in hypertensive urgencies, 1820, 1820t
  following liver transplantation, 1345
 for pheochromocytomas, 2134t
 for renal crisis, in systemic sclerosis, 2172
Nikolsky's sign, in pemphigus, 2182
Nimbus hemopump, for cardiogenic shock, 402–403
Nimodipine
 actions, indications, and dosing of, 2271
 for brain injury, 286–287
Nissen fundoplication, for aspiration prophylaxis, 1872
Nitrates, for limitation of infarct size, 396
Nitric oxide (NO)
 for acute respiratory distress syndrome, 1833–1834
 following cardiac surgery in pediatric patients, 1169
 toxicity of, 1834
Nitrite poisoning, antidote for, 1467t
Nitrogen oxides, inhalation injury due to, 1953–1954
Nitroglycerin (NTG)
 actions, indications, and dosing of, 2271
 for acute myocardial infarction, 1735
 following cardiac surgery in pediatric patients, 1168t
 for cardiopulmonary resuscitation, 505
  complications of, 505
  dosage of, 505
  indications for, 505
 for hypertension, vascular surgery and, 1179
 for limitation of infarct size, 396
 for pheochromocytomas, 2134t
 for reduction of ventricular afterload, following cardiac surgery, 1152
Nitroprusside. *See* Sodium nitroprusside (Nipride; SNP)
Nitrous oxide saturation, cerebral blood flow and, 946–947
Nizatidine, for aspiration prophylaxis, 1871, 1871t
Nocardia infections, 1668–1669
 in HIV-infected patients, 1624
  treatment of, 1620t
 in immunocompromised patients, 1607–1608
  diagnosis of, 1608

Nocardia infections, in immunocompromised
patients (*continued*)
presentation of, 1607–1608
therapy of, 1608
Nocardia asteroides, in renal transplant
recipients, 1612
Noise, in aircraft, 807
Nominal variables, 9
Non-A, non-B hepatitis. *See* Hepatitis, non-A,
non-B
Noninvasive positive-pressure ventilation (NPPV)
for asthma, 1942
for respiratory failure, 1923–1924
Nonmaleficence, 22, 24–25
as medicomoral principle, 66–67
Nonparoxysmal junctional tachycardia, 1783
management of, 1785
Non-Q wave myocardial infarction, 1742–1744
diagnosis of, 1742
noninvasive predischarge assessment of,
1743–1744
prognosis of, 1742–1743
Nonrebreathing masks, 705
Nonsteroidal anti-inflammatory drugs (NSAIDs).
See also specific drugs
for acute respiratory distress syndrome, 1835
adverse effects of, 2156t–2157t, 2158
platelet defects due to, 2228
Norepinephrine
actions, indications, and dosing of, 2271
for anaphylaxis, 1548
following cardiac surgery in pediatric
patients, 1167t
for hypotension, in cyclic antidepressant
poisoning, 1492
pheochromocytoma and, 2130
regulation of metabolic responses to critical
illness and, 331
for shock, 363t
cardiogenic, 399–400
Nortriptyline (Pamelor)
side effects of, 2027t
therapeutic serum level of, 479t
Nosocomial infections, 1573–1584
in acute respiratory distress syndrome
treatment of, 1833
antibiotic-associated pseudomembranous
colitis, 1583–1584
of blood stream, 510
catheter-related. *See* Arterial cannulation;
Catheter-related infections; Vascular
cannulation; Venous cannulation
device-associated, 2209–2211
diagnostic tests and procedures for, 1574
fungal, 1583
in immunocompromised patients,
minimizing, 1305
initial therapy for, 1574–1575
linkage with handwashing, 508
major problems with, 1573
meningitis, 1584
respiratory, 1575–1577, 1576t
risk factors for, 1575
scope of problem, 507–508, 1575
sinusitis, 1583
stress points with, 1573–1574

of surgical wounds, 1581–1582
tracheal intubation causing, 768
of urinary tract, 1582–1583, 1654–1655
ventriculitis, 1584
Nuchal rigidity, 1635
Nuclear medicine. *See* Interventional radiology;
specific procedures
Nucleoside analogues, 1571. *See also specific
drugs*
Null hypothesis, 11
implying or stating, 14
proving, 14–15
Nurse(s), as team members, 39, 40
Nursing care
allocation of, 40–41, 41t
allocation of resources and, 41–47, 42t, 43t
extensive requirement for, 24
orders for, 44–46
outcome prediction and, 131
functions of, 41
Nutrition
intestinal transplantation and, 1356
multivisceral transplantation and, 1356
red blood cell production and, 663
Nutritional support, 457–470
for acute renal failure, 2090
for acute respiratory distress syndrome, 1833
for burn patients. *See* Burns, nutritional
support for
carbohydrate intolerance and, 468
following cardiac surgery in pediatric
patients, 1173–1174
complications of, 468–470
general and metabolic, 468–469
diagnostic tests and procedures for, 457–458
emteral
gastrointestinal access for. *See also* Feeding
tube(s); Feeding tube placement
enteral, 464–467
for acute renal failure, 2090
aspiration pneumonitis and, 1869
for burn patients, 1271
following cardiac surgery in pediatric
patients, 1173
complications of, 469
feeding mixtures for, 466f, 466–467
gastrointestinal access for, 465–466, 469
infections associated with tubes for, 2210
nutrient delivery for, 467
for obese surgical patients, 1282
parenteral nutrition compared with,
464–465
tube placement for. *See* Feeding tube
placement
in Guillain-Barré syndrome, 2010
hepatic insufficiency and, 468
following hepatic resection, 1126
initial therapy for, 458
for intestinal transplantation, 1361
major problems with, 457
for multivisceral transplantation, 1361
nutritional assessment and patient selection for,
459f, 459–460
nutritional requirements and, 460–464
for electrolytes, 461t, 461–462
for energy, 460–461

for protein, 460, 460t
for trace elements, 462t, 462–463
for vitamins, 463–464, 464t
nutritional support service and, 459
for obese surgical patients, 1282–1284
enteral, 1282
parenteral, 1282
protein-sparing modified fast and, 1282f,
1282–1284
for pancreatitis, 2058
parenteral, 467–468. *See also* Total parenteral
nutrition (TPN)
adverse effects of, 1282
blood gas analysis in, 934
for burn patients, 1271
catheter and tubing care for, 467
catheters for, 513
complications of, 470
enteral nutrition compared with, 464–465
formulations for, 467
intravenous access for, 467
nutrient delivery for, 468
for obese surgical patients, 1282
renal insufficiency and, 468
for respiratory failure, 1927
for sepsis, 410
stress points with, 457
volume restriction and, 468
withdrawal of, rules regarding, 112–113
wound management and, 782
Nystagmus, in poisonings and toxic exposures,
1472
Nystatin (Mycostatin)
for *Candida* infections, in HIV-infected
patients, 1619t
for heart-lung transplantation, 1319t
for intestinal transplantation, 1361
for lung transplantation, 1319t
for multivisceral transplantation, 1361
prophylactic, heart transplantation and, 1339
for yeast infections, 2207

Obesity
beds for, 2214
definition of, 1278
postoperative ICU care and, 1110
pulmonary function testing and, 989
in surgical patients. *See* Surgical patients, obese
weight loss and, preoperative, 995
Objective(s), of research study, 4
Objective standard, 121
Observation
orders for, 43–44, 44f, 44t, 45f
outcome prediction and, 131
in poisonings and toxic exposures, 1474–1475
as treatment objective, 23–24
Observational research, 5
Observation bias, 7
Obstetric patients. *See* Hemorrhage, in obstetric
patients; Pregnancy; Trauma, in
obstetric patients
Obstructive shock, 390
Octreotide, actions, indications, and dosing of,
2271

Ocular disorders. *See also specific disorders*
　anaphylaxis and, 1545t
　in aspergillosis, 1688
　cataracts, following bone marrow
　　　transplantation, 1379–1380
　in poisonings and toxic exposures, 1471–1472
　　methanol and, 1502
　retinal
　　in fat embolism syndrome, 1909
　　retinitis, in HIV-infected patients, treatment
　　　of, 1619t
　stroke and, 1991
Ocular movements, in comatose patients,
　　evaluation of, 1973–1974
Odynophagia, in HIV-infected patients, 1629
Ofloxacin, 1569
　cost and initial dosage of, 1562t
OKT3, 312t
　for heart-lung transplantation, 1320
　for heart transplantation, 1335, 1336, 1338
　for lung transplantation, 1320
　for renal transplantation, 1305
　for simultaneous pancreas/kidney
　　transplantation, 1314
Older patients. *See* Elderly patients
Oligemic shock, 365–366, 390
　in trauma patients, 1048–1049
　waveform analysis in, 858, 859f
Oliguria
　salicylate poisoning and, 1488
　shock and, 371–372
Omeprazole, for aspiration prophylaxis,
　　1871–1872
Oncologic emergencies, 2245–2251
　acute tumor lysis syndrome, 2247–2248
　　clinical management of, 2247–2248
　cardiac tamponade, 2250
　chemotherapy toxicity, 2251
　　cardiac, 2251
　　pulmonary, 2251
　hypercalcemic. *See* Hypercalcemia, in cancer
　neutropenic enterocolitis, 2250–2251
　obstructive, 2248–2249
　　oropharyngeal, 2248
　　superior vena cava obstruction, 2248
　　tracheal, 2248–2249
　spinal cord compression. *See* Spinal cord,
　　compression of
Oncotic pressure
　colloid fluid therapy and, 434–435
　pulmonary fluid and protein homeostasis
　　and, 203
Open-lung biopsy (OLB), in pneumonia, 695,
　　1853–1854
Opiates. *See also specific drugs; specific opiates*
　abuse of, 1517t, 1517–1519
　　heroin body packers and, 1519
　　toxicity and, 1517–1518, 1518t
　　treatment for acute intoxication and, 1518
　　treatment for withdrawal and, 1518–1519,
　　　1519t
　for airway management, 762
　as anesthetics, 1021t, 1021–1022, 1022t
　classification of, 1517t
　gastrointestinal effects of, 1022
　general properties of, 1021

hemodynamic effects of, 1021
immune function and, 1022
neuraxial, 817
　side effects of, 817
neurologic effects of, 1022
for pain control. *See* Pain control, narcotics for
pharmacokinetics and pharmacodynamics of,
　　1021, 1021t
poisoning by, antidote for, 468, 1467t
renal effects of, 1022
respiratory effects of, 1021–1022
surgical stress and, 1022, 1022t
following thoracic surgery, 1133–1134
tolerance and dependence on, 484
Opiate toxidrome, 1468, 1469t
Opsonization, 306
Oral feeding, transition to, in burn patients,
　　1272
Ordinal variables, 9
Organ donors
　assessment of, 1292
　certification of death of, 1293
　　confirmatory tests for, 1293
　　documentation of, 1293
　living, 1297–1298
　management of, 1293–1295
　　fluid and electrolyte management in, 1295
　　general considerations in, 1293
　　hemodynamic support in, 1293–1294
　　hypothermia in, 1295, 1296
　　monitoring and, 1293, 1294t
　　problems in, 1295
　　ventilatory support in, 1294–1295
　non-heart-beating, 1298
　　cardiac arrest during evaluation for brain
　　　death and, 1298
　　sudden cardiac arrest in previously relatively
　　　healthy patients and, 1298
　　withdrawal of life-sustaining therapy and,
　　　1298
　potential, 1291
　　brain death and, 1291. *See also* Brain death
　　categories of, 1291
　recognition of, 1292
　xenotransplantation and, 1298
Organic brain syndrome, 93
Organic dusts, inhalation injury due to, 1955
Organ injury scaling, 2273t–2281t
Organizing, by ICU fellows, 37
Organophosphates
　inhalation injury due to, 1955
　poisoning by, 1504–1507
　　antidote for, 1467t
　　cholinergic syndrome and, 1504–1505
　　clinical manifestations of, 1505
　　treatment of, 1506–1507
Organ procurement organizations (OPOs),
　　1295–1296
　consent and, 1296
　responsibilities of, 1295
　transplant coordinators and, 1295–1296
Organ transplantation, 1289–1298. *See also*
　　specific organs
　brain death concept and. *See* Brain death
　current status of, 1290–1291
　cytomegalovirus infection following, 1696

donors for. *See* Organ donors
immunosuppression and, transfusion reactions
　　and, 654
legal issues related to, 124–125
major problems with, 1289, 1290t
　stress points with, 1289–1290
need versus supply and, 1291
　potential donors and, 1291
organ allocation for, 1296–1298
　living donors and, 1297–1298
　non-heart-beating donors and, 1298
　United Network for Organ Sharing and,
　　1296–1297
　xenotransplantation and, 1298
organ recovery and preservation for, 1296
posttransplant lymphoproliferative disease and
　following intestinal transplantation,
　　1362–1363
　following multivisceral transplantation,
　　1363–1364
procedural considerations in, 1292–1295
　certification of death, 1293
　donor management. *See* Organ donors
　organ procurement, recovery, and
　　preservation, 1295–1296
Orientation, by ICU fellows, 38–39
Orlowski score, near-drowning and, as prognostic
　　indicator, 1882–1883
Oropharyngeal airways, in cardiopulmonary
　　resuscitation, 493
Orotracheal intubation, techniques for, 766
　with curved blades, 766
　with straight blades, 766
Orthodeoxia, following liver transplantation, 1346
Orthopedic complications, 1231–1249
　cervical spine collars and, 1247, 1247f
　compartment syndromes. *See* Compartment
　　syndromes
　diagnostic tests and procedures for, 1232
　epidural catheters and, 1247–1249
　　catheter removal and, 1249
　　clinical studies and recommended guidelines
　　　for, 1248t, 1248–1249
　fat embolism. *See* Fat embolism
　of joint replacement, 1234–1235
　　of hip, 1234–1235
　　of knee, 1235
　　of shoulder, 1235
　major problems with, 1231
　rheumatoid arthritis. *See* Rheumatoid
　　arthritis (RA)
　of spinal surgery, 1232–1234
　　cervical, 1234
　　scoliosis correction, 1232–1234, 1233t
　stress points with, 1231–1232
　thromboembolic. *See* Deep venous thrombosis
　　(DVT); Pulmonary embolism;
　　Thromboembolism; Venous thrombosis
　tourniquets and. *See* Tourniquets
Orthopnea, in refractory advanced heart failure,
　　1758
Orthotopic liver transplantation (OLTx). *See*
　　Hepatic transplantation
Oscillometry, 872f, 872–873m 873f
Oscilloscope displays, for invasive pressure
　　monitoring, 840

Osmolality, 2258t. *See also* Hyperosmolar states; Hypoosmolar states
Osmolarity, in hyperosmolar hyperglycemic nonketotic diabetes, 2107
Osmoreceptors, antidiuretic hormone release and, 2117
Osmotic agents, for intracranial hypertension, 284
Osmotic demyelination syndrome, 418
Osmotic pressure, pulmonary fluid and protein homeostasis and, 203
Osteomyelitis, staphylococcal, 1660
Ostomy bags, for drainage, 2206, 2206f
Ototoxicity, of aminoglycosides, 1568
Outcome(s)
  definition of, clinical decision-making and, 54f, 54–55
  prediction of. *See* Outcome predictions
  short-term, clinical decision-making and, 56–57, 57t
Outcome predictions, 127–146
  cost considerations and, 127–128
  definition of outcome and, 128–131
    cost and cost effectiveness and, 129, 129f
    cost-containment efforts and, 130–131
    resource utilization and, 130
    severity of illness and, 129, 130t
  quantitative indices for, 134–136, 136t–139t, 138–139, 140f, 141–145. *See also* Acute Physiology and Chronic Health Evaluation (APACHE); Therapeutic Intervention Scoring System (TISS)
    values and limitations of, 141t, 141–145, 142f–144f, 144t, 145t
  treatment goals and, 131–134, 132t
    deletion of standing orders for testing and, 132
    management principles and, 132, 133t
    nor orders for repeated testing and, 134, 134t
    structured decision trees to select tests and, 132–134, 133t, 134t
Outcome research, 128
Outcomes management, 128
Outflow valves, for intermittent mandatory ventilation, 723
Over-diagnosis, 96
Overdoses. *See* Poisonings and toxic exposures
Over-interpretation of physical finding syndrome, 96
Overnight dexamethasone suppression test, 2127
Overwhelming postsplenectomy infection (OPSI), 1088
Oxacillin
  for bacterial endocarditis, 1658
  following cardiac surgery in pediatric patients, 1172
  for cellulitis, staphylococcal, 1661
  for infective endocarditis, 1793, 1794t, 1796t
  for meningitis, staphylococcal, 1660
  for osteomyelitis, staphylococcal, 1660
Oxazepam (Serax), 825t
  for agitation and anxiety, 2026t
Oximetry
  dual, pulmonary artery catheters for, 860
  pulse. *See* Pulse oximetry
  transcutaneous, 779
  venous. *See* Venous saturation monitoring

Oxygen
  blending with air, 704
    jet entrainment for, 704
    mechanical, 704, 704f
  central control of ventilation and, 204
  gastrointestinal metabolism of
    dysoxic versus normoxic state and, 446
    global parameters of, 446–447
  hemoglobin affinity for, 923, 924f
  pulmonary toxicity of, 707–708
    antioxidants and, 708
    death due to, 708
    early manifestations of, 708
    granular pneumocytes and, 708
    oxygen free radicals and, 707
    pulmonary effects of, 708
Oxygenation. *See also* Hypoxemia; Hypoxia; Mechanical ventilation; Oxygen therapy; Ventilation
  clinical assessment of, blood gas analysis for. *See* Blood gas analysis
  fetal, monitoring of, 1431–1432
    oxygen consumption and, 1431
    oxygen supply and availability and, 1431
    stress of labor and, 1431
  during intrahospital transport, 788–789
  in pneumothorax, 1963
  temperature correction and, 936, 937
Oxygenation formulas, 2263t
Oxygenators
  intravascular, 753–754
  membrane. *See also* Extracorporeal membrane oxygenation (ECMO)
    extracorporeal carbon dioxide removal using, with venovenous bypass, 753
Oxygen carriers, 666
Oxygen consumption, 910
  cerebral, 277–278, 278t
  fetal, 1431
Oxygen delivery, 911
  following cardiac surgery
    in adult patients, 1154
    in pediatric patients, 1164
  deficient. *See* Dysoxia
  stress response and, 1028
  tissue oxygenation and, 930
Oxygen demand, 910
  reduction of, in dysoxia, 341
  tissue oxygenation and, 931
Oxygen deprivation, fetal, hypoglycemia and, 1430
Oxygen extraction, tissue oxygenation and, 930, 930t
Oxygen free radicals. *See* Free radicals
Oxygen metabolism, cardiac. *See* Cardiovascular physiology
Oxygen pressure tension
  alveolar
    evaluation of, 921–922, 922t, 923t
    inhalational anesthetic delivery and, 1015
  arterial, values for, 921–922, 922t, 923t
Oxygen supply, fetal, 1431
Oxygen therapy, 703–708
  for acute respiratory failure, 1919–1920, 1920f
    appliances for, 1920
  air-oxygen blending techniques for, 704

  jet entrainment for, 704
  mechanical, 704, 704f
  blood gas analysis and, 929–930
  complications of, 707–708
    absorption atelectasis, 707
    hypercapnia, 707
    oxygen toxicity, 707–708
  diagnostic tests and procedures for, 703–704
  humidification for, 706–707, 707f
  hyperbaric. *See* Hyperbaric oxygen (HBO) therapy
  initial therapy and, 704
  nebulization for, 706, 706f
  oxygen delivery systems for, 704–706, 705f, 706f
  stress points with, 703
Oxygen transport
  definition of, 911
  venous saturation monitoring and. *See* Venous saturation monitoring
Oxygen uptake, 911
Oxygen utilization, following cardiac surgery, 1154
Oxygen utilization coefficient, 911
Oxyhemoglobin
  massive transfusion and, 1058
  measurement of, 923
Oxytocin, during pregnancy, cardiovascular changes with, 1403
Ozone, inhalation injury due to, 1954

Pacing, cardiac. *See* Cardiac pacing; Transvenous cardiac pacing
Paclitaxel, for bone marrow transplantation, 1368t
Pain
  abdominal. *See* Abdominal pain
  in chest. *See* Chest pain
  postoperative, 1027–1030
    combined anesthesia and, 1028
    management techniques for, 995–996, 1007, 1029–1030
    prevention of, 1007
    stress response and, 1027–1028
  radicular, in spinal cord compression, 2249
  in sickle cell anemia, 2233–2234
Pain control, 809–819
  analgesia service function and, 819
  for burn patients, 1274
  cost of, 827t, 828
  diagnostic tests and procedures for, 810
  inadequate analgesia and, 816–817
  initial therapy for, 810–811
  local anesthetic blocks for. *See* Local anesthetic blocks
  major problems with, 809
  narcotics for, 811–812
    epidural or intrathecal, 811–812, 812f, 812t
    intramuscular, 811
    intravenous, 811, 812–813
    postoperative, 995–996
  neuraxial narcotics for, 817
    pharmacologic advances in, 819
    side effects of, 817
  patient-controlled. *See* Patient-controlled analgesia (PCA)

patient selection for, 811, 811t
postoperative, 995–996, 1007, 1029–1030
preoperative, 1029
problems and complications of, 817–819
  adhesive arachnoiditis, 818
  epidural abscess, 818
  epidural hematoma, 818
  headache, 817
  interruption of blood supply, 818
  local anesthetic-related, 818–819
  neurologic, 818
  pneumothorax, 819
  respiratory depression, 817, 817t
in rheumatoid arthritis, 1245
stress points with, 809–810, 810f, 810t
for vascular cannulation, 531–533
vascular surgery and, 1179–1180
Paired samples, 12
Palpation
  for blood pressure measurement, 872
  in cardiac assessment, 870
  in pulmonary assessment, 869
Pamidronate disodium, for hypercalcemia, in
  cancer, 2247
Pancreas, shock and, 372
Pancreas transplantation. *See also* Simultaneous
  pancreas/kidney (SPK) transplantation
  current status of, 1290
  living donors for, 1297
  organ allocation for, 1297
Pancreatic abscesses, in pancreatitis, surgical
  treatment of, 2061
Pancreatic fistulas, postoperative, 1114, 1114t
Pancreatic gland, suppression of secretory
  function of, for pancreatitis, 2057–2058
Pancreatic injuries, 1088–1089
Pancreatic injury scale, 2275t
Pancreatic pseudocysts, drainage of, 592–593
Pancreatic surgery, postoperative ICU care for,
  1111
Pancreatitis, 2055–2061
  acute, in systemic lupus erythematosus, 2168
  aortic reconstructions and, 1185
    diagnosis of, 1185
    etiology of, 1185
    incidence of, 1185
    therapy of, 1185
  following cardiac surgery, 1159
  classification of, 2057
  coma and, 1978
  diagnosis of, 2056–2057
    endoscopic retrograde
      cholangiopancreatography for, 2057
    laboratory tests for, 2056
    radiologic and diagnostic studies for,
      2056–2057
    tests for, 2055–2056
  hemoductal (hemosuccus), surgical treatment
    of, 2060
  in HIV-infected patients, 1629
  initial therapy for, 2056
  insecticide poisoning and, 1507
  major problems with, 2055
  necrotizing, postoperative, 1116
  postshunt, 1125
  stress points with, 2055

surgical management of, 2059–2061
  confirmation of diagnosis and, 2059
  for treatment of biliary cause, 2059
  for treatment of complications, 2059–2061
treatment of, 2057–2059
  antibiotics for, 2058–2059
  for cardiovascular collapse, renal failure, and
    respiratory insufficiency, 2058
  gland suppression for, 2057–2058
  metabolic and nutritional support in, 2058
  peritoneal lavage for, 2058
  surgical. *See* Pancreatitis, surgical
    management of
Pancuronium bromide, 829, 830t
  actions, indications, and dosing of, 2271
  for cocaine intoxication, 1516
Pancytopenia, in aplastic anemia, 2236
Panhypopituitarism, hemorrhage as cause of,
  2113
Pantothenate, requirement for, 464, 464t
Papain, for esophageal obstruction, 2072
Papaverine, for acute mesenteric ischemia, 1107
Papillary muscles, cardiogenic shock and, 393t
Papillary necrosis, acute, in pyelonephritis, 1654
Papillotomy, endoscopic, for biliary pancreatitis,
  2059
Para-aminosalicylic acid (PAS), for
  Mycobacterium tuberculosis infections,
  in HIV-infected patients, 1620t
Paracentesis, 561–563
  complications of, 563
  for hepatorenal syndrome, 1124
  procedure for, 562f, 562–563, 563t
Paralysis
  diagnostic tests, procedures, and therapy and,
    821–822
  lightning injuries and, 1542
  major problems with, 821
  stress points with, 821
  therapeutic. *See* Neuromuscular blocking
    agents (NMBAs); *specific drugs*
  tourniquets as cause of, 1246
Paramedics (EMT-Ps), 804–805
Paranasal sinus infections, 2209
  prevention of, 2209
  treatment of, 1583
Parasites, transfusion therapy and, 656
Parasympathetic control, of heartbeat, 242
Parathyroid hormone (PTH)
  calcium regulation and, 427
  in hypercalcemia, in cancer, 2246
Parenteral nutrition. *See* Nutritional support,
  parenteral; Total parenteral nutrition
  (TPN)
Parkland formula, 1267–1268, 1268f
Paroxetine (Paxil), side effects of, 2027t
Paroxysmal atrial tachycardia (PAT), 1783
  cardioversion for, 575, 575f
  diagnosis of, 1783
Paroxysmal junctional tachycardia, 1783
Paroxysmal nocturnal errors, 100
Paroxysmal ventricular tachycardia, 1784
Partial rebreathing masks, 705, 705f
Partial seizures, 1982, 1987
Partial thromboplastin time (PTT), 852
  in coagulation disorders, 1067

Passive external rewarming, for hypothermia,
  1453
Pasteurella infections, 1673
Patent foramen ovale (PFO), arterial emboli
  with, 1906
Pathologic dead space, 199
Patient(s)
  autonomy of. *See* Autonomy
  in decision-making process, 69t
  dependent, 2028
  hostile, 2028
  incompetent
    informed consent and, 83, 118–119
    right to refuse treatment, 108–111
  newly admitted, 38
  psychological reactions of. *See* Psychological
    factors
  rights of, 25
  terminal. *See* Terminal patients
  transport of. *See* Interhospital transport;
    Intrahospital transport; Transport
  uncooperative, 2028
Patient-controlled analgesia (PCA)
  postoperative, 995, 1030
    lung function and, 996
    following thoracic surgery, 1134
Patient selection, 22–23
Patient Self-Determination Act, 70
Patient-triggered ventilation, 719–720
  clinical applications of, 720
  controlled backup ventilation with, 720
  operational principles of, 719
  potential problems with, 720
Peak pressures
  inflation, 711, 712
  inspiratory, mechanical ventilation and, 1961,
    1962t
  ventilation and, 192
Pediatric patients. *See also* Adolescents; Infants;
  Neonates
  abuse of, near-drowning and, 1883
  airway management in, anatomical
    considerations and, 760
  antibiotic selection for neurologic infections
    in, 1641t
  bone marrow transplantation in, growth and
    development following, 1379
  cardiac surgery in, postoperative management
    of. *See* Cardiac surgery, postoperative
    management of pediatric patients and
  cardiovascular physiology of. *See*
    Cardiovascular physiology, pediatric
  extracorporeal membrane oxygenation in,
    historical background of, 670–671
  hypertensive emergencies in, 1818–1819
  hyperthermia in, 1457
  informed consent and, 118–119
  terminal, levels of care for, 121–122
  thermodilution in, 894–895
Pelvic fractures, 1058–1061
  anatomy and, 1058–1059
  angiographic embolization for, 1061
  diagnosis of, 1059, 1060f
  initial management of, 1059–1061
  injuries associated with, 1059
  military antishock trousers for, 1061

Pelvic fractures (*continued*)
skeletal fixation for, 1061
Pelvic infections, antibiotic combination therapy for, 1564
Pemphigoid, bullous. *See* Bullous pemphigoid
Pemphigus, 2182f, 2182–2183
diagnosis of, 2183
etiology of, 2182
management of, 2183
presentation of, 2182
Penicillamine
adverse effects of, 2156t–2157t
for metal poisoning, 1465t
Penicillin(s), 1566
anaphylaxis and, 1546t
anto-pseudomonal, 1566
benzylpenicillin, for necrotizing fasciitis, 2192
extended spectrum, 1566
for infective endocarditis, 1788, 1793
β-lactams combined with, 1566
penicillinase-resistant, 1566
penicillin G, 1566
for aspiration syndromes, 1868
for *Clostridium perfringens* infections, 1677
cost and initial dosage of, 1562t
for infective endocarditis, 1794t, 1795t
for *Listeria monocytogenes* infections, 1608
for *Streptococcus agalactiae* infections, 1664
for syphilis, 1682
penicillin VK, for streptococcal pharyngitis, 1663
Penile venous cannulation, 537–538
Penis
in sickle cell anemia, 2234–2235
trauma to, 1262
Pentamidine
cost and initial dosage of, 1562t
for *Pneumocystis carinii* infections, 1607
in HIV-infected patients, 1620t
Pentastarch, hemostasis and, 437
Pentobarbital
for cerebral edema, in fulminant hepatic failure, 2049
for head injury, 1206
for status epilepticus, 1982t, 1984
Penumbra effect, pulse oximetry and, 876
Peptic ulcers
esophageal, in HIV-infected patients, 1629
renal transplantation and, 1306
stress. *See* Stress ulceration
Peptides
airway resistance and, 197–198
regulatory. *See* Cytokines; *specific cytokines*
Percentages, 9–10
Percussion, in pulmonary assessment, 869
Percutaneous drains, postoperative abdomen and, 1118
Percutaneous procedures. *See* Interventional radiology, nonvascular procedures; *specific procedures*
Percutaneous transluminal coronary angioplasty (PTCA), for acute myocardial infarction, 1733, 1733f
Perfluorocarbons, as oxygen carriers, 666
Perfusion. *See also* Lung perfusion scans; Ventilation-perfusion relationships; Ventilation/perfusion (V/Q) scans

assessment of, with pulse oximetry, 876, 877f
cerebral. *See* Cerebral perfusion pressure (CPP); Neurologic monitoring, of cerebral perfusion
coronary perfusion pressure and, 863
termination of cardiopulmonary resuscitation and, 159
hemoperfusion and
for poisonings and toxic exposures, 1475
for salicylate poisoning, 1489
for theophylline poisoning, 1500
hypoperfusion and
after brain injury, cerebral blood flow and, 277
in sepsis, treatment of, 410
in shock, treatment of, 373t
Pericardial effusions
in cancer, 2250
echocardiography in, 885
pericardiocentesis and, 577
Pericardial resection, subxiphoid, for cardiac tamponade, 1807–1808
Pericardial tamponade, waveform analysis in, central venous catheters for, 853
Pericardiocentesis, 577–580
for cardiac tamponade, 1807, 2095
complications of, 580
needle, 579
procedure for, 577f–579f, 579–580
Pericardiotomy
balloon, percutaneous, for cardiac tamponade, 1808
postpericardiotomy syndrome and, 1809
Pericarditis
acute, 1803–1805, 1805t
chest pain and, 1722, 1722t
clinical features of, 1804–1805, 1806f
treatment of, 1805
constrictive, 1808, 1809f
in chronic renal failure, 2095
radiation therapy as cause of, 2251
waveform analysis in, central venous catheters for, 853
dialysis-associated, 2095
effusive-constrictive, 1808, 1809f
staphylococcal, 1660
in systemic lupus erythematosus, 2167–2168
tuberculous, 1681
uremic, 2094–2095
Pericardium, 1803
pneumopericardium and, 1964
Perineal infections, 2209
Perineal pouches, for diarrhea, 2212
Perinephric abscesses, in pyelonephritis, 1653
Peripheral blood flow, neural control of, 244–245
vasovagal response and, 245, 245f
Peripheral nerve blocks, 812
axillary catheter for, 813
intercostal, 813
technique for, 813
Peripheral vascular disease, thrombolytic therapy for, 626, 626f
Peripheral venous access, 522–524
Peritoneal dialysis, 636
following cardiac surgery in pediatric patients, 1172

catheter infections and, staphylococcal, 1662–1663
for heart failure, 1762
infections associated with, 2095
for poisonings and toxic exposures, 1474
Peritoneal lavage
diagnostic. *See* Diagnostic peritoneal lavage
for pancreatitis, 2058
Peritoneovenous shunts, for ascites, 1125
Peritoneum
free air in, abdominal radiography and, 970, 971f, 972f
infections of, antibiotic combination therapy for, 1564
Peritonitis
diffuse, in obstetric patients, 1424
persistent, diffuse, postoperative, 1116
Peritumor edema, cerebral, treatment of, 280t
Permissive hypercapnia, 753
for acute respiratory distress syndrome, 1835–1836
for aspiration syndromes, 1867, 1867t
Perphenazine (Trilafon), for agitation and anxiety, 2025
Persistent fetal circulation (PFC), extracorporeal membrane oxygenation for, 671
Persistent vegetative state (PSV), 1292
Petechiae, in fat embolism syndrome, 1909
pH, 255–256, 256t. *See also* Acid(s); Acid-base balance; Bases
arterial
during cardiopulmonary resuscitation, 935
evaluation of, 921, 922t
of fetal scalp, monitoring of, 1432–1433
gastric, drugs raising, 2036
gastrointestinal. *See* Gastrointestinal system, pH of
potassium regulation by, 422
Phagocytic cells
abnormalities of, 310–311
mononuclear, host response and, 292, 294
Phagocytosis, inhalational anesthetics and, 1019
Pharmacodynamics, 475
relationship to pharmacokinetics, 475, 476f
Pharmacokinetics, 475–478
one-compartment model of, 476
relationship to pharmacodynamics, 475, 476f
two-compartment model of, 476–478, 477f
Pharmacotherapy. *See* Cancer chemotherapy; Medications; *specific drugs and drug types*
Pharyngeal tracheal lumen airway (PTLA), 763
Pharyngitis, streptococcal, 1663
Phenazopyridine poisoning, antidote for, 1467t
Phenelzine, side effects of, 2027t
Phenobarbital
dosage adjustment for, in hepatic disease, 482t
for scorpion stings, 1533t
for status epilepticus, 1982t, 1984
therapeutic serum level of, 479t
Phenoxybenzamine
following adrenalectomy, 1255
for pheochromocytomas, 2133, 2134t
Phentolamine
actions, indications, and dosing of, 2271
for hypertension, in hypertensive emergencies, 1814t, 1815, 1818, 1819

for pheochromocytomas, 2133, 2134t
for scorpion stings, 1533t
Phentoxyphylline, for acute respiratory distress
syndrome, 1834
Phenylephrine
actions, indications, and dosing of, 2271
for airway management, 762
following cardiac surgery in pediatric
patients, 1167t
preoperative, 994t
for shock, 363t
Phenytoin
for cyclic antidepressant poisoning, 1491
dosage adjustment for, in hepatic disease, 482t
for seizures
in brain injury, 286
in status epilepticus, 1982t, 1984
with subarachnoid hemorrhage, 2001
therapeutic serum level of, 479t
Pheochromocytomas, 2129–2135
diagnosis of, 2131–2133
anatomic localization and, 2132–2133
biochemical confirmation and, 2131–2132
tests and procedures for, 2129
hypertensive emergencies and, 1818
major problems with, 2129
management of, 2133, 2134t
initial therapy for, 2129–2130
pathology of, 2130–2131
in pregnancy, 2133–2134
presenting signs and symptoms of, 2130
prevention of complications with, 2133
stress points with, 2129
unusual presentations of, 2134–2135
Phlebitis, 2209
Phlebography, for deep venous thrombosis
diagnosis, 1242t
Phlebotomy
for polycythemia vera, 2240
for secondary erythrocytosis, 2240
Phosgene, inhalation injury due to, 1954
Phosphates, for hypercalcemia, in cancer, 2247
Phosphodiesterase inhibitors, for cardiogenic
shock, 400–401
Phosphorus, 429–430
deficiency of, 429–430, 431t
causes of, 429–430
treatment of, 430
excess of, 430
requirement for, 461t, 462
Photoplethysmography, 872
Phrenic nerve injuries, following lung and heart-
lung transplantation, 1323
Phycomycosis, 1689–1690
Physalia physalis envenomations, 1533t,
1533–1534
clinical manifestations of, 1533–1534
treatment of, 1534
Physical stimulation, for acute respiratory
failure, 1922–1923
Physicians
aid-in-dying provided by, 77–79, 113–114
attending, 36
compliance with termination orders over
ethical objections of, 115
constant care by, 24
orders for, 46–47

degrees of disclosure by, 81–82, 118
before development of ICUs, 35
ICU fellows, 35
functions and interrelationships of, 37–39
involvement with families. *See* Families
junior residents, 36
lack of assertiveness by, 76
participation in critical paths, 176
practice style of, iatrogenesis related to, 100
as team members, 35–36, 36f, 39–40
Physiotherapy, for burns, 1274
heterotopic ossification and, 1274
for prevention of contractures, 1274
Physostigmine (Antilirium), for poisonings, 1465t
cyclic antidepressants and, 1492
Phytonadione, for poisonings, 1465t
Pimobendan, for heart failure, 1757
Pimobendan Multi-Center Research Group
Study, 1757
Pipecuronium, 829, 830t
Piperacillin
cost and initial dosage of, 1562t
for urinary tract infections, 1652
Piperacillin/tazobactam
cost and initial dosage of, 1562t
for heart-lung transplantation, 1319t
for lung transplantation, 1319t
Pistons, of mechanical ventilators, 714t, 717f
Pituitary apoplexy, 2113
Pituitary disorders
anterior. *See* Hypopituitarism; Hypothalamic-
anterior pituitary unit disorders
posterior, 2116–2118
management of, 2118
patient examination in, 2117–2118
tumors, anterior pituitary failure caused by,
2113–2114
Pit viper bites, 1525f, 1525–1528, 1526t
antidote for, 1466t, 1527t, 1527–1528
Placenta, diffusing capacity of, 1433, 1433t
Placental abruption, 1403–1404, 1404f, 1404t
diagnosis of, 1403
trauma and, 1423
treatment of, 1404
Placenta previa, 1404–1405, 1405f
diagnosis of, 1404–1405
treatment of, 1405
Plague, bubonic, 1671–1672, 1708
pneumonia and, antibiotic prophylaxis for, 1565
Plasma, fresh frozen. *See* Fresh frozen plasma
(FFP)
Plasmapheresis, 311, 313
for acute renal failure, 2088, 2090
for Guillain-Barré syndrome, 2006, 2010
for myasthenia gravis, 2014
for serum protein abnormalities, 2241
for thyrotoxicosis, 2140
Plasmin, 271
Plasminogen, activation of, 271
Plasmodium falciparum infections, cerebral, 1711
Platelet(s)
concentration of, 650
consumption of, thrombocytopenia due to,
2227
function of, 650–651
future research directions for, 651

hypothermia and, 650–651
platelet mass and, 650
storage and, 650
in primary hemostasis, 265–266
transfusion of. *See* Transfusion therapy, of
platelets
Platelet disorders, 2226–2229, 2227t
drug-induced, 2226–2228
heparin and, 2227–2228
immune mediated, 2226–2227
management of, 2228
postoperative bleeding due to, 1068–1069
qualitative, 2228
quantitative, 2226–2228
heparin-induced thrombocytopenia,
2227–2228
thrombocytosis, 2240
in uremia, 2229
Platelet microemboli, autotransfusion and, 665
Platelet plug retraction, 271
Plesiomonas infections, 1675
Plethysmography
impedance
for deep venous thrombosis diagnosis,
1242, 1242t
for pulmonary thromboembolism
diagnosis, 1242
photoplethysmography, for blood pressure
measurement, 872
Pleural effusions
chest radiography and, 958–959, 961f
in pneumonia, evaluation and treatment of,
1848–1849, 1849f, 1849t
right, following liver transplantation, 1345
in systemic lupus erythematosus, 2165
thoracentesis for diagnosis of, 553–556
complications of, 556
procedure for, 553–554, 554f, 555f, 556
Pleural pressure, 189, 190f
during spontaneous breathing, changes in, 739
Pleuritis, in systemic lupus erythematosus, 2165
Plicamycin, for hypercalcemia, in cancer, 2247
Pneumatic compression boots, for deep venous
thrombosis prophylaxis, 1890
Pneumococcal vaccine, 1855–1856, 1856t
Pneumococcus infections
neurologic, epidemiologic and clinical clues
to, 1636t
pneumonia due to, bacteremic, 1843–1844
Pneumocystis carinii infections
antibiotic prophylaxis for, 1566
diagnosis of, 694–695, 695t
in HIV-infected patients, 1618, 1622–1623
prophylaxis of, 1620t
treatment of, 1620t
in immunocompromised patients, 1607
diagnosis of, 1607
lung and heart-lung transplant recipients,
1330
presentation of, 1607
renal transplant recipients, 1611
therapy of, 1607
pneumonia due to, 1843
Pneumocytes, granular, pulmonary oxygen
toxicity and, 708
Pneumomediastinum, 1964
chest radiography in, 963, 964f

Pneumonia
  aspiration, 1861. *See also* Aspiration
      (pathologic)
  bacterial
    anaerobic, 1678
    in HIV-infected patients, 1623–1624
  bronchiolitis obliterans organizing, in systemic
      lupus erythematosus, 2167, 2167t
  chest radiography in, 963, 965
  community acquired. *See* Community acquired
      pneumonia (CPE)
  diagnosis of, fiberoptic bronchoscopy in,
      692–695, 693t, 695t
  fever associated with, 1593–1594
  fungal, 1688–1689
    in HIV-infected patients, 1624–1625
  following lung and heart-lung transplantation,
      1323
  mycobacterial, in HIV-infected patients, 1625
  nosocomial, 1575–1577
    diagnosis of, 1576–1577, 1577t
  plague, antibiotic prophylaxis for, 1565
  *Pneumocystis carinii. See Pneumocystis
      carinii* infections
  pseudomonal, 1673–1674
  staphylococcal, 1659
  streptococcal, 1663, 1664
  viral, 1691–1692
Pneumonitis
  following bone marrow transplantation, 1377
  herpes simplex virus, 1695
  in HIV-infected patients
    cytomegalovirus, 1625–1626
    treatment of, 1619t
  interstitial, in bone marrow transplant
      recipients, 1613–1614
  lupus, acute, 2165–2166
Pneumopericardium, 1964
Pneumoperitoneum, acute abdomen and,
      1105–1106, 1106f
Pneumothorax, 1960–1964. *See also*
      Hydropneumothorax
  chest pain and, 1721
  diagnosis of, 1962–1963
    oxygenation and ventilation and, 1963
    physical findings and, 1962, 1963t
    radiographic signs and, 1962
  iatrogenic, tube thoracostomy for, 556
  local anesthetics and, 819
  mechanical ventilation and. *See* Mechanical
      ventilation, pneumothorax and
  pathophysiology of, 1960t, 1960–1961, 1961t
  rate of, as continuous quality improvement
      indicator, 168t, 169, 170f–173f
  recurrent, tube thoracostomy as cause of, 560
  simple, chest radiography in, 957–958,
      958f–960f
  spontaneous
    following thoracic surgery, 1137
    tube thoracostomy for, 556
  tension
    chest radiography in, 959, 962f
    in trauma patients, 1050–1051
    tube thoracostomy for, 556
    following thoracic surgery, 1135
  traumatic, tube thoracostomy for, 556

treatment of, 1963–1964
  catheter aspiration for, 1963
  tube thoracostomy for, 1963f, 1963–1964
Poikilothermia, in spinal cord injury, management
    of, 1214–1215
Point of care blood gas analyzers, 938
Point of care blood gas monitors, 938
Poisonings and toxic exposures, 1463–1481,
    1483–1507. *See also specific substances*
  accidental poisoning and, 1464
  chemotherapeutic agents and, 2251
    cardiac manifestations of, 2251
    pulmonary manifestations of, 2251
  clinical evaluation in, 1468–1473, 1469t
    gastrointestinal disturbance and, 1472
    laboratory evaluation in, 1472–1473
    medical history in, 1468–1470
    physical examination in, 1470
    seizures and, 1472
    vital signs in, 1470–1472
  coma and, 1978
  deliberate self-poisoning and, 1464
  diagnostic tests and procedures for, 1463
  elimination of poison and, 1473–1474, 1474t
    enhanced elimination of absorbed
      substances and, 1474, 1475t
  emergency management and, 1468
  historical background of, 1464, 1467
  homicidal poisoning and, 1464, 1467
  initial therapy for, 1463–1464, 1464f,
      1465t–1467t
  major problems with, 1463
  observation and disposition for, 1474–1475
  during pregnancy, 1475
  rhabdomyolysis and, 2197t
  stress points with, 1463
  therapeutic poisoning and, 1467
  toxicology information sources and, 1475–1481
  toxidromes and, 1468, 1469t
  uncooperative patients and, 1475
Polarizing solution, for limitation of infarct size,
    397
Polyarteritis nodosa (PAN), 2160t, 2160–2161
Polyclonal activators, inhalational anesthetics
    and, 1020
Polyclonal antibodies, for liver transplantation,
    1344
Polycythemia vera (PV), 2239–2240, 2240t
Polydipsia, psychogenic, 418
Polyethylene glycol (Colyte; GoLytely), for
    lithium poisoning, 1494
Polymer fume fever, 1955
Polymorphonuclear neutrophils (PMNs)
  fibrinolysis and, 271
  multiple organ system failure and, 347,
      349–350, 350f
Polymyxin B, for depressed gastrointestinal pH,
    452
Polyvalent sera, for renal transplantation,
    1305
Pontine hemorrhage, coma and, 1977
Portuguese man-of-war envenomations, 1533t,
    1533–1534
  clinical manifestations of, 1533–1534
  treatment of, 1534
Position, pulse oximetry and, 875

Positive end-expiratory pressure (PEEP),
    729–734. *See also* Auto positive end-
    expiratory pressure (auto PEEP)
  for acute respiratory distress syndrome,
      1831–1832
  arterial waveform and, 851f, 851–852
  for aspiration syndromes, 1866–1867
  during brain resuscitation, 282
  following cardiac surgery, 1156
  complications of, neurologic, 1880
  intrinsic, 214–215
  for near-drowning, 1878–1880
    acceptable oxygenation and, 1879
    adjunctive measures and, 1880
    dead space and, 1879, 1879f
    intrapulmonary shunting and, 1878–1879
    mechanical ventilation and, 1879
    optimal, 1878
    pulmonary artery occlusion pressure and,
      856–857
  spontaneous, 729f, 729–732, 730f
    demand-flow valves for, 731–732, 732t
    equipment for, 730, 730f
    expiratory pressure valves for, 730–731, 731f
    side effects and complications of, 740
    work of breathing and, 731, 732f
Positive-pressure ventilation
  for asthma, 1942
  bilevel. *See* Bilevel positive airway pressure
      (BIPAP)
  continuous. *See also* Airway pressure release
      ventilation (APRV); Continuous
      positive airway pressure (CPAP)
    continuous positive-pressure ventilation
      and, 719
  for respiratory failure, 1923–1924
Post-inflation hold, 720–721
  clinical applications of, 720–721
  operational principles of, 720, 721f, 721t
Postoperative abdomen, 1109–1119
  abdominal drains and, 1118f, 1119, 1119f
  acalculous cystitis and, 1115
  biliary tubes and, 1116f, 1117
  cecostomy tubes and, 1118
  duodenostomy tubes and, 1117
  evaluation of, 1110–1111
    following complicated gastrointestinal and
      biliary procedures, 1111
    diagnostic tests and procedures for,
      1109–1110
    following liver resection, 1110
    following major vascular procedures, 1111
    following pancreatic operations, 1111
    reasons for ICU care and, 1110
    for sepsis, 1112–1113
  fistulas and, 1113–1115, 1114t
  gastrostomy tubes and, 1116f, 1117
  initial therapy for, 1110
  jejunostomy tubes and, 1117f, 1117–1118
  long intestinal tubes and, 1117
  major problems with, 1109
  nasogastric tubes and, 1117
  normal postoperative course and, 1111–1112
  open, 1115–1116
    dehiscence of fascia and, 1115–1116
    diffuse persistent peritonitis and, 1116

fistulas and, 1115
  loss of abdominal domain and, 1116
  necrotizing pancreatitis and, 1116
percutaneous drains and, 1118
stress points with, 1109
warning signs for sepsis and, 1112
wound infection and synergistic gangrene
  and, 1115
Postpartum hemorrhage, 1406
Postpericardiotomy syndrome, 1809
Posttetanic count, for evaluation of
  neuromuscular blockade, 831
Posttourniquet syndrome, 1246–1247
Posttransplant lymphoproliferative disease
  (PTLD)
  following intestinal transplantation, 1362–1363
  following multivisceral transplantation,
    1363–1364
Potassium, 421–426
  deficiency of. *See* Hypokalemia
  excess of. *See* Hyperkalemia
  functions of, 421
  loss of, 928
    hypokalemia due to, 422–423
  regulation of, 421–422
    hydrogen ion and, 422
    renal, 421–422
    tissues involved in, 422
  requirement for, 461, 461t
  serum level of, following cardiac surgery,
    1154–1155
  shifts in, hypokalemia due to, 423
Potassium-binding resins, for hyperkalemia, 427t
Potassium chloride, sustained-release, esophageal
  injury caused by, 2077
Potassium repletion
  for diabetic ketoacidosis, 2104t
  for hyperosmolar hyperglycemic nonketotic
    diabetes, 2107
  for hypokalemia, 424–425
  for metabolic alkalosis, 262
Power, of statistical tests, 17
Pralidoxime (Protopam; 2-Pam), for insecticide
  poisoning, 1506
  organophosphates and, 1467t, 1504
Prazepam (Centrax), 825t
  for agitation and anxiety, 2026t
Prazosin, for pheochromocytomas, 2133, 2134t
Precordial thump, 497
Prednisolone
  for acute cerebritis, in systemic lupus
    erythematosus, 2169
  for adrenal insufficiency, 2125t
  for fulminant colitis, 2068
  for toxic megacolon, 2068
Prednisone
  for acute lupus pneumonitis, 2166
  for acute pericarditis, 1805
  for acute respiratory distress syndrome, 1834
  for adrenal insufficiency, 2116, 2125t
  for anaphylaxis prevention, 1549
  for autoimmune hemolytic anemia, 2232
    in systemic lupus erythematosus, 2170
  for bronchiolitis obliterans organizing
    pneumonia, in systemic lupus
    erythematosus, 2167

for bullous pemphigoid, 2183–2184
for contact dermatitis, 2192
for erythema multiforme, 2177
for glomerulonephritis, in systemic lupus
  erythematosus, 2169
for heart-lung transplantation, 1319t, 1320
for hemophagocytic syndrome, in systemic
  lupus erythematosus, 2170
for hypercalcemia, 429t
for idiopathic thrombocytopenic purpura,
  2226, 2237
for inflammatory bowel disease, in systemic
  lupus erythematosus, 2168
for interstitial lung disease, in systemic
  sclerosis, 2172–2173
for lung transplantation, 1319t, 1320
for myocarditis, in systemic sclerosis, 2172
for pemphigus, 2183
for *Pneumocystis carinii* infections, in HIV-
  infected patients, 1620t
for rheumatic disorders, 2157–2158
  tapering, 2116
for thrombotic thrombocytopenic purpura,
  2239
for toxic epidermal necrolysis, 2178
for vasculitis, 2164
  Takayasu's arteritis, 2160
Predonation, of blood. *See* Autotransfusion,
  predonation for
Preeclampsia/eclampsia, 1392–1393, 1818
  clinical considerations in, 1392–1393
  etiology of, 1392
  HELLP syndrome and, 1393
  management of, 1392
  pathophysiology of, 1392
Prefixes, metric, 2255t
Pregnancy, 315–321
  amniotic fluid embolism in, 1406, 1413,
    1910–1912
  antibiotics in, 1557t, 1557–1558
  aspiration of gastric contents during, risk of,
    1868–1869
  after cardiac surgery, 1398
  cardiopulmonary resuscitation during, 1398
  cardiovascular disease in, 1389–1399
    arrythmias, 1397
    asymmetric septal hypertrophy, 1396
    cardiomyopathy, 1395–1396
    congenital heart disease, 1394–1395
    diagnostic tests and procedures for, 1391,
      1391t
    hypertension, 1392–1393
    major problems with, 1389
    myocardial infarction, 1396–1397
    stress points with, 1389–1390, 1390f, 1390t
    surgical treatment of, 1397–1398
    valvular lesions, 1393–1394, 1396
  changes at term and, 316–318
    cardiopulmonary, 316–317
    of central nervous system, 317
    of connective tissue, 317–318
    of smooth muscle, 317, 317t
    uterine, 317
  coordination of, 318t, 318–321, 319t
    direct hormonal effects and, 318–320
    drugs and anesthesia and, 320t, 320–321

hormonal interactions and, 320
    premature labor and abortion and, 320
    stress and, 320
  dating of, 1422
  diseases of, 315–316
  eclamsia in. *See* Preeclampsia/eclampsia
  fetal heart rate during. *See* Fetal heart rate
  fulminant colitis in, 2069
  hemodynamic changes in, 1389–1390, 1390t
  hemorrhage during. *See* Hemorrhage, in
    obstetric patients
  hypertension in. *See* Preeclampsia/eclampsia
  pheochromocytomas in, 2133–2134
  poisonings and toxic exposures during, 1475
  preeclamsia in. *See* Preeclampsia/eclampsia
  Rh-negative pregnant women and,
    hyperimmune anti-D globulin for, 1425
  Sheehan's syndrome in, 2113
  stress imposed by, 315–316, 320
    characteristics of, 315
    response to, 315–316
  surgery during, 1424–1425
  thyrotoxicosis in, treatment of, 2142
  toxic megacolon in, 2069
  trauma during. *See* Trauma, in obstetric
    patients
  ultrasonography in, 978, 982f
  vomiting during, 319
Prekallikrein, 298
Preload. *See* Ventricular preload
Premature atrial contractions (PACs), 1783
  management of, 1785
Premature junctional contractions (PJCs), 1783
  management of, 1785
Premature labor, 320
  postoperative, 1424–1425
Premature ventricular contractions, following
    cardiac surgery in pediatric patients,
    1170–1171
Preoperative evaluation
  of diffusing capacity, 990
  exercise testing in, 990–991
  of high-risk patients, 999–1010, 1000t
    adrenal suppression and, 1008
    aspiration of gastric contents and, 1007
    bleeding and clotting problems and, 1008
    concurrent disease and, 1001–1004, 1002t
    diagnostic tests and procedures for, 1000
    don-not-resuscitate patients, 1009–1010
    initial therapy and, 1000
    major problems with, 999
    medications and, 1008–1009
    methods for, 1004–1006, 1005t
    prevention of complications and, 1006–1007
    stress points with, 999–1000
    timing of, 1004, 1004t
  lateral position test in, 991
  of pulmonary disorders, 1002–1003
    history and physical examination in,
      1002–1003
    laboratory examination in, 1003
  pulmonary function testing in. *See* Pulmonary
    function tests; *specific surgical
    procedures*
  of response to bronchodilators, 990
  for thoracic surgery, 1133

Preoperative evaluation (*continued*)
  ventilation/perfusion lung scans in, 991–992
Prerenal azotemia, 2081–2083, 2084t
Preservation
  of organs for transplantation, 1296
  of red blood cells, 647–648
President's Commission, brain death criteria of, 123
Pressor agents, for dysoxia, 341
Pressure-controlled inverse ratio ventilation (PC-IRV), 721–722
  advantages and disadvantages of, 722
  airway pressure release ventilation compared with, 734
  clinical applications of, 721
  operational principles of, 721, 722f
Pressure-cycled ventilators, 713
Pressure-flow relations, during cardiac contraction, 236–240, 237f–240f, 240f, 240–241
Pressure gradients
  distribution of ventilation and, 201
  pulmonary fluid and protein homeostasis and, 202–203
Pressure-support ventilation (PSV), 218, 724–727, 748–749
  advantages of, 749
  for aspiration syndromes, 1867
  clinical applications of, 724–725, 725f
    in apnea, 725
    for high-level PSV, 725
    for low-level PSV, 724
  disadvantages of, 749
  flow rate and pressure rise and, 725–726
  initial settings for, 748–749
  operational principles of, 724, 724f, 725t
  patient-ventilator interaction and, 726f, 726–727, 727f
  pressure augmentation and, 727
    operational principles of, 727, 728f
  setup parameters for, 748, 749f
  therapeutic objectives of, 219, 219f, 220f
  titration of, 219–221, 222f
  work of breathing and, 749
    assessment of, 725
Pressure transducers, for invasive pressure monitoring, 840
  selecting, 844
  zeroing, 841, 841f
Pressure ulcers, 100–101, 2207
  as continuous quality improvement indicator, 168t, 169, 174f
  prevention of, 2207
  treatment of, 2207
Preterm labor, 320
  postoperative, 1424–1425
Priapism, in sickle cell anemia, 2234–2235
Primaquine, for *Pneumocystis carinii* infections, in HIV-infected patients, 1620t
Primate organ donors, 1298
Primidone, therapeutic serum level of, 479t
Prioritization, by ICU fellows, 37
Probability, certainty versus, 74
Procainamide
  actions and indications for, 2271
  for cardiopulmonary resuscitation, 503

complications of, 503
  dosage of, 503
  indications for, 503
  dosing of, 2271
    for cardiopulmonary resuscitation, 503
    in chronic renal failure, 2097t
  therapeutic serum level of, 479t
Processors, for invasive pressure monitoring, 840–841
Prochlorperazine (Compazine), for agitation and anxiety, 2026
Procyclidine, for neuroleptic malignant syndrome, 828
Professional community standard, of disclosure, 81, 118
Progesterone, during pregnancy, direct effects of, 318t, 318–320
Prokinetic drugs, for aspiration prophylaxis, 1872
Prolactin (PRL), deficiency of, 2113
Propafenone, dosing of, in chronic renal failure, 2097t
Propionibacterium acnes infections, 1678
Propofol, 825t, 826, 1023–1024
  actions, indications, and dosing of, 2271–2272
  for airway management, 763
  cardiovascular effects of, 1024
  for continuous sedation, 1030
  cost of, 827t
  neurologic effects of, 1024
  pharmacokinetics and pharmacodynamics of, 1023t, 1023–1024
  respiratory effects of, 1024
  for status epilepticus, 1984
Proportion(s), sampling variance of, 11
Proportional assist ventilation (PAV), 727–729
  clinical applications of, 728
  operational principles of, 728
  potential problems with, 728–729
Proportional blood pressure, in refractory advanced heart failure, 1758–1759
Propranolol
  actions and indications for, 2272
  for arrhythmias, 1784
  dosing of, 2272
    in hepatic disease, 482t
  for hypertension, in hypertensive emergencies, 1817
  for scorpion stings, 1533t
  for thyrotoxicosis, 2140, 2141
Propylthiouracil (PTU), 2140
  for thyrotoxicosis, 2141
Prospective Randomized Flosequinan Longevity Evaluation (PROFILE), 1757
Prospective Randomized Milrinone Survival Evaluation (PROMISE), 1757
Prostacycline, for intracranial hypertension, in fulminant hepatic failure, 2050
Prostaglandin E_1 (PGE$_1$), for acute respiratory distress syndrome, 1835
Prostatectomy, radical, postoperative management and, 1256
Prostatitis, 1654
Prosthetic heart valves
  endocarditis of, 1661–1662
    staphylococcal, 1659
  placement of, warfarin for, 622

Prosthetic joints, 2158
  complications of, 1234–1235
    with total hip arthroplasty, 1234–1235
    with total knee arthroplasty, 1235
    with total shoulder arthroplasty, 1235
Prosthetic valve endocarditis (PVE), 1661–1662
  staphylococcal, 1659
Protamine
  actions, indications, and dosing of, 2272
  with extracorporeal renal replacement therapies, 636
  for heparin poisoning, 1466t
Protected specimen brush (PSB), for diagnosis of pneumonia, 693, 1576, 1577, 1594
Protein(s)
  contact activation, host response and, 297–299, 298f
  metabolism of, in critical illness, 327–328, 328f
  repletion of, for burn patients, 1271–1272
  requirement for, 460, 460t
    in acute renal failure, 2090
  serum, abnormalities of, 2241
  synthesis of, hepatic graft function assessment and optimization and, 1347
Protein homeostasis, pulmonary, 202–204
  anatomic considerations and, 202–203
  fluid flux and, 203
  pulmonary edema and, 203–204
Protein-sparing modified fast (PSMF), for obese surgical patients, 1282f, 1282–1284
  potential benefits of, 1283f, 1283–1284
  prevention of fatty-acid deficiency and, 1284
Proteinuria, pheochromocytomas and, 2135
Proteus infections, 1670
Prothrombin time (PT), 270
  in coagulation disorders, 1067
  following shunt procedures for ascites, 1125
Protriptyline (Vivactil), side effects of, 2027t
P-selectin, host response and, 294, 295f
Pseudoaneurysms, in pancreatitis, surgical treatment of, 2059–2060
Pseudocysts
  pancreatic and peripancreatic, drainage of, 592–593
  in pancreatitis, surgical treatment of, 2060
Pseudomembranous colitis, 1583–1584, 1676–1677
Pseudomonas infections
  endocarditis due to, 1674
    treatment of, 1793, 1794t–1795t
  Pseudomonas aeruginosa, 1673–1674
    antibiotic combination therapy for, 1564
    in burn patients, 1674
    endocarditis due to, 1674
    in HIV-infected patients, 1627
    meningitis due to, 1674
    pneumonia due to, 1673–1674
  Pseudomonas (Burkholderia) cepacia, 1674–1675
  resistant strains of, 1594
Pseudoneurysms, management of, 1188
Pseudorenal failure, 2081, 2083t
Psoriasis. *See* Generalized pustular psoriasis
Psychogenic polydipsia, 418
Psychological factors, 89–94. *See also* Behavioral disturbances; Delirium

acute stress disorder and, 89–90
chest pain and, 1724
denial and, 90
fear and, 90
imminent death and, 93–94
in informed consent, 86
with lightning injuries, 1542
loss of control and, 90–91
reactions to being in ICU and, 92–93
staff involvement with families and, 91–92
Psychosis
intensive care, 93
sedation for, 823
Psychostimulants, side effects of, 2027t
Psychotropic agents. *See also* Antipsychotic
agents; *specific drugs*
rhabdomyolysis due to, 2198–2199
Pulmonary abscesses
in aspiration syndromes, treatment of, 1868
in pneumonia, 1849–1850, 1850f
Pulmonary angiography, in pulmonary embolism,
1720–1721, 1896–1897
Pulmonary arteriography, for pulmonary
embolism, 587–588
Pulmonary artery cannulation, 538–539
complications of, 539
iatrogenesic, 97–99, 98t, 99t
indications for, 538, 538t
insertion technique for, 538–539, 539f
in valvular heart disease, 1773
Pulmonary artery (PA) catheters, 853–861
cardiac output measurements using, 860
cardiac pacing and, 861
chest radiography and, 967–968, 968f, 969f
for dual oximetry, 860
in embolic syndromes, 860–861
indications for, 853–854, 854t
infection related to, 1580–1581
mixed venous blood sampling using, 859–860
positive end-expiratory pressure artifact and,
856–857
for preoperative assessment, 1005, 1005t
pressure measurement using, 855–856
clinical applications of, 855, 855f
pulmonary artery occlusion pressure, left
atrial pressure, and left ventricular end-
diastolic pressure and, 856
West's zones and, 855–856, 856f
pulmonary artery occlusion pressure and
pulmonary capillary pressure
measurement using, 857
transmural, 856
right ventricular ejection fraction measurement
using, 860
following thoracic surgery, 1134
timing of measurement with, 857
waveform analysis using, 857f, 857–859
in acute mitral insufficiency, 857–858, 858f
in chronic obstructive lung disease, 859, 859f
in decreased left ventricular compliance, 858
in hypovolemic shock, 858, 859f
in pulmonary hypertension, 858
in right ventricular failure, 858, 858f
in tachycardia, 859, 859f
Pulmonary artery occlusion pressure (PAOP),
856, 861

clinical applications of, 862
pulmonary capillary pressure and, 857
in shock, 376t–377t, 378
transmural, 856
Pulmonary artery torsion, heart transplantation
and, 1335
Pulmonary assessment, 868–869. *See also*
Pulmonary function tests
auscultation in, 869
inspection in, 868–869
palpation in, 869
percussion in, 869
Pulmonary barotrauma (PBT), 1959–1967. *See
also* Pneumothorax
air embolism and, 1964
diagnostic tests and procedures for, 1960
initial therapy for, 1960
major problems with, 1959
mechanical ventilation and, 741, 1942
near-drowning and, 1881
prevention of, 1964–1965
infection control for, 1965
pressure and volume limitation for, 1964t,
1964–1965
rate limitation for, 1965
stress points with, 1959–1960
surveillance for, 1965–1967
special considerations in, 1965–1966, 1966f,
1966t, 1967t
unusual and rare presentations and, 1967,
1967f
Pulmonary blood flow
distribution of, 200
lung zones and, 200
modifying effects of, 200
in obstetric patients, 1411
central control of respiration and, 1411,
1412f, 1412t
position changes and, 1411
Pulmonary capillaries
gas exchange in, 198, 198f
integrity of, pulmonary fluid and protein
homeostasis and, 204
Pulmonary compliance
distribution of ventilation and, 201
elastic forces and surface tension and,
193–194, 194f
lung and chest wall interaction and, 195–196,
196f
lung and heart-lung transplantation and, 1326
time, frequency, and volume dependence and,
194–195, 195f
Pulmonary contusions, 1139–1140
Pulmonary disorders. *See also specific disorders*
acute, hypoxemia with, 926
in acute respiratory distress syndrome, 1837t
antibiotics and, 1563t
antirheumatic agents as cause of, 2156t
chemotherapy toxicity as cause of, 2251
chest pain in, 1718t
life-threatening, 1720–1721
diagnostic tests and procedures for, 1410
in fat embolism syndrome, 1908–1909
initial therapy for, 1410
interstitial

pneumonitis, in bone marrow transplant
recipients, 1613–1614
in systemic lupus erythematosus, 2167
in systemic sclerosis, 2172–2173
liver transplantation and, 1347
major problems with, 1409
in obese surgical patients, 1279–1280
changes in pulmonary function and, 1279,
1279f
clinical implications of, 1279–1280, 1280f
in obstetric patients, 1409–1417
acute respiratory failure, 1414t, 1414–1415
aspiration of gastric contents, 1414, 1414t
asthma, 1415
chronic, 1415–1416
diagnosis and treatment of, 1412–1417
lung volume and alveolar ventilation and,
1411, 1411t
physiologic considerations in, 1410t,
1410–1411
pulmonary blood flow and, 1411, 1412f,
1412t
pulmonary edema, 1416, 1416t
pulmonary embolization syndromes,
1412–1413, 1413t
shock and, 1416–1417
tuberculosis, 1415
postoperative, prevention of, 1007
preoperative evaluation of, 1002–1003
history and physical examination in,
1002–1003
laboratory examination in, 1003
preoperative therapy for, 994–995
pulmonary function testing and, 989
in rheumatoid arthritis, 1244
in sickle cell anemia, 2234
stress points with, 1409–1410
in systemic lupus erythematosus, 2165–2167
following transfusion therapy, 654
Pulmonary edema, 869
colloids for, 436
in congestive heart failure, chest radiography
and, 961–962, 963f
negative-pressure, 1026–1027
neurogenic, 201
during brain resuscitation, 281
in head injury, 1204
treatment of, 1214
noncardiogenic, acute respiratory distress
syndrome and, 1829
in obstetric patients, 1416, 1416t
in poisonings and toxic exposures, 1471
salicylates and, 1489
pulmonary fluid and protein homeostasis
and, 203–204
oncotic pressure and, 203
Pulmonary embolism (PE), 587–588, 1887–1894.
See also Pulmonary thromboembolism;
Venous thromboembolism
asthma versus, 1935
chest pain and, 1720–1721
clinical features of, 1894
diagnosis of, 587, 588, 1895–1897
arterial blood gases for, 1895
chest radiography for, 1895, 1895f
electrocardiography for, 1895, 1896f

Pulmonary embolism (PE), diagnosis of
   (*continued*)
   pulmonary angiography for, 1896–1897
   tests and procedures for, 1887, 1888f
   transesophageal echocardiography for, 1897
   ventilation/perfusion lung scans for,
      1895–1896, 1896f
   in Guillain-Barré syndrome, 2010
   major problems with, 1887
   respiratory failure and, 1919
   in spinal cord injury, therapy of, 1214
   stress points with, 1887
   in systemic lupus erythematosus, 2166–2167,
      2167
   therapy of, 1898–1901
      anticoagulation in, 1898–1899, 1899t
      general principles of, 1898
      inferior vena caval filters in, 1899–1900
      initial, 1887–1888
      radiologic interventions for, 587–588
      in spinal cord injury, 1214
      surgical, 1900–1901
      thrombolytic therapy in, 1900, 1901t
   total hip arthroplasty and, 1234–1235
      with cemented implantation, 1234
      with noncemented implantation, 1234–1235
Pulmonary failure, in rheumatic disease, 2158
Pulmonary function
   following bone marrow transplantation, 1380
   during brain resuscitation, 281–282
      hypoxemia and abnormal ventilation and,
         281
      intubation and mechanical ventilation and,
         281–282
   in obese surgical patients, 1279, 1279f
   patient-controlled analgesia and, 996
   regional, preoperative assessment of, 991–992
   in sepsis, 408
Pulmonary function tests, perioperative,
      987–997, 1003. *See also specific
      surgical procedures*
   bronchodilators and, 994, 994t
   diagnostic tests and procedures and, 988
   infection control and, 995
   initial therapy and, 988
   major problems with, 987
   mechanical ventilation and work of breathing
      and, 996, 996t, 997t
   postoperative care and, 995–996
   preoperative pulmonary consultation and,
      988–989
   smoking cessation and, 995
   stress points with, 987–988
   weight loss and, 995
Pulmonary hemorrhage, in systemic lupus
      erythematosus, 2166
Pulmonary hypertension
   following cardiac surgery in pediatric patients,
      1168, 1169t
   heart transplantation and, 1337
   in systemic lupus erythematosus, 2167
   in systemic sclerosis, 2172
   waveform analysis in, 858
Pulmonary infections. *See also specific infections*
   acute respiratory distress syndrome and, 1827
   transtracheal aspiration in, 580

Pulmonary injuries, acute
   mechanisms of, 1829–1830
   respiratory distress syndrome and, 1828
   structural response to, 1828f, 1828–1829,
      1829f, 1829t
Pulmonary mechanics
   acute respiratory distress syndrome and, 1830
   formulas for, 2264t
   lung and heart-lung transplantation and,
      1325–1326
   scoliosis correction and, 1232–1233, 1233t
Pulmonary physiology, 189–206
   airway resistance and. *See* Airway resistance
   fluid and protein homeostasis and, 202–204
      anatomic considerations and, 202–203
      fluid flux and, 203
      pulmonary edema and, 203–204
   gas exchange and. *See* Gas exchange
   lung volumes and. *See* Lung volumes
   metabolic activity and, 205–206
   pulmonary compliance and. *See* Pulmonary
      compliance
   ventilation and. *See* Ventilation
   ventilation-perfusion matching and, 199–202
      distribution of pulmonary blood flow and,
         200
      distribution of ventilation and, 201–202
      pulmonary vascular resistance and, 201
Pulmonary resection, 1143
   assessment for, 989–992
      bronchodilators and, 990
      clinical application of, 992
      diffusing capacity and, 990
      exercise and, 990–991
      forced expiratory volume in 1 second and,
         990
      forced vital capacity and, 989, 989t
      lung volumes and capacities and, 990
      maximal voluntary ventilation and, 990
      midflow measurements and, 990
      tests of regional lung function and, 991–992
Pulmonary sensitizers, inhalation injury due to,
      1955
Pulmonary thromboembolism, 1239–1243. *See
      also* Pulmonary embolism (PE)
   diagnosis of, 1241–1242, 1242t
      contrast venography for, 1242
      duplex ultrasonography for, 1242
      impedance plethysmography for, 1242
   in obstetric patients, 1412–1413, 1413t
   prevention of, 1239–1241, 1241t
      anesthetic choices for, 1241
      anticoagulation for, 1239–1241
      external compression devices for, 1241
   risk factors for, 1239
   treatment of, 1242–1243, 1243t
Pulmonary toilet, following thoracic surgery, 1136
Pulmonary transplantation. *See* Double-lung
      transplantation (DLT); Heart-lung
      transplantation (HLT); Lung
      transplantation; Single-lung
      transplantation (SLT)
Pulmonary vascular pressure, microvascular,
      pulmonary fluid and protein
      homeostasis and, 203–204
Pulmonary vascular resistance (PVR), 201

   in children, 1163
   of heart transplantation patients, 1334
   hypoxic pulmonary vasoconstriction and, 201
   pathologic factors and, 201
Pulmonary vasculature. *See also specific vessels*
   changes in, spontaneous breathing and,
      739–740
   chest radiography and, in congestive heart
      failure, 960–961, 962f
   disorders of, in obese surgical patients, 1278
Pulmonary vasoconstriction, hypoxic, 201, 930
   inhalational anesthetics and, 1018
Pulmonic insufficiency, 1777–1778
   clinical presentation of, 1778
   diagnostic studies for, 1778
   etiology of, 1777
   pathophysiology of, 1778
   therapy of, 1778
Pulmonic stenosis, 1777
   clinical presentation of, 1777
   diagnostic studies for, 1777
   etiology of, 1777
   pathophysiology of, 1777
   therapy of, 1777
Pulsatile perfusion preservation, 1296
Pulse
   absence of, extremity injuries and, 1187
   in poisonings and toxic exposures, 1470
Pulse oximetry, 875–877, 931
   accuracy of, 876, 876f
   artifactual readings and, 875–876
   clinical applications of, 877
   in dysoxia, 339
   lung and heart-lung transplantation and, 1327
   perfusion assessment using, 876, 877f
   principles of, 875, 875f
   venous oximetry combined with, 916
Pulsus paradoxus
   in asthma, 1935
   pericardiocentesis and, 577–578
Pupils
   in comatose patients, evaluation of, 1974–1975
   local anesthetics and, 819
   in poisonings and toxic exposures, 1471–1472
Purified protein derivative (PPD) skin test, 1681
Purpura, 2188–2191
   in anticoagulant necrosis, 2190–2191
   drug-induced, 2188–2189
   infarctive, 2190, 2190f
   mechanical, 2188
   senile, 2188
   thrombocytopenic
      idiopathic, 2226, 2237–2238
      thrombotic, 2171, 2238t, 2238–2239
   following transfusion therapy, 654
   vasculitic, 2162f, 2162–2163, 2189f, 2189t,
      2189–2190
Pustular psoriasis. *See* Generalized pustular
      psoriasis
p values, 7
Pyelonephritis, 1650–1654
   complications of, 1653–1654
   diagnosis of, 1651
      approach to, 1654
   microbiology of, 1651
   pathophysiology of, 1650–1651

treatment of, 1651–1653
uncomplicated, 1653
urosepsis and, 1651
Pyloric stenosis, hypertrophic, following cardiac
surgery in pediatric patients, 1174
Pyonephrosis, in pyelonephritis, 1653–1654
Pyrazinamide, for *Mycobacterium tuberculosis*
infections, in HIV-infected patients,
1619t
Pyridostigmine
for myasthenia gravis, 2014
before elective surgery, 2014
for neuromuscular blocking agent reversal,
835t, 1032t
Pyridoxal. *See* Vitamin(s), vitamin B$_6$
Pyridoxamine. *See* Vitamin(s), vitamin B$_6$
Pyridoxine. *See* Vitamin(s), vitamin B$_6$
Pyrimethamine, for *Toxoplasma* infections, in
HIV-infected patients, 1620t
Pyrogens, 1591

Q fever, 1703, 1705–1706
endocarditis in, treatment of, 1793
Quality assurance (QA). *See* Continuous quality
improvement (CQI)
Quality council, 164
Quality of life, termination of cardiopulmonary
resuscitation and, 159
Quantal data, fourfold table for, 9–10, 10t
Quantitative data, 9
descriptive measures for, 10
Quazepam, 825t
Quinidine
dosing of
in chronic renal failure, 2097t
in hepatic disease, 482t
esophageal injury caused by, 2077
therapeutic serum level of, 479t
Quinlan decision, 105, 106, 108, 111, 114
Quinolones, 1569–1570. *See also specific drugs*
Q wave myocardial infarction, 1742–1744
diagnosis of, 1742
noninvasive predischarge assessment of,
1743–1744
prognosis of, 1742–1743

Rabies, 1694, 1694t
Radial artery cannulation, 540t, 541
Radiation injuries
anterior pituitary failure caused by, 2114
constrictive pericarditis due to, 2251
hyperbaric oxygen therapy for, 781
wound management and, 782
Radioactive iodine uptake (RAIU), in
thyrotoxicosis, 2139
Radiographic contrast agents
anaphylaxis and, 1546t
renal failure due to
acute, 2086
chronic, 2096
thrombolytic therapy and, 1190
Radiographic over-interpretation syndromes, 96
Radiology

diagnostic. *See* Imaging; *specific sites and
modalities*
interventional. *See* Interventional radiology;
specific procedures
Radionuclide angiography
in acute myocardial infarction, 1743–1744
gated, in acute myocardial infarction, 1741
Radionuclide scanning. *See* Scintigraphy (SCINT)
Ramipril, for acute myocardial infarction, 1737,
1756
Ramsay Scale, 822
Random-access memory (RAM), of
microprocessor-controlled ventilators,
718, 718f
Randomized Assessment of Digoxin on Inhibitors
of the Angiotensin-Converting Enzyme
(RADIANCE), 1757
Randomized studies, 5
Ranitidine
actions and indications for, 2270
for anaphylaxis, 1547t, 1548
for aspiration prophylaxis, 1871, 1871t
dosing of, 2270
in hepatic disease, 482t
for heart-lung transplantation, 1319t
for lung transplantation, 1319t
Rapamycin (siolimus), for simultaneous pancreas/
kidney transplantation, 1314
Rashes. *See* Skin disorders
Rattlesnake bites, 1525f, 1525–1528, 1526t
antidote for, 1466t, 1527t, 1527–1528
Raynaud's phenomenon, 2158–2159
Readmission rate, as continuous quality
improvement indicator, 168, 168t
Read-only memory (ROM), of microprocessor-
controlled ventilators, 718, 718f
Reasonable person standard, of disclosure, 81, 118
Rebleeding, with subarachnoid hemorrhage,
2001t, 2002
Rebound tenderness, acute abdomen and, 1102
Recorders, for invasive pressure monitoring, 841
Recording techniques, for arrhythmias, 1783
Recovery position, 493
Recruitment, by diaphragm muscle fibers, 211
Rectal injuries, 1093–1094
with pelvic fractures, 1059
Rectal injury scale, 2276t
Rectal tubes, for diarrhea, 2212
Recuronium, 829, 830t
actions, indications, and dosing of, 2272
Red blood cells
erythrocytosis and, 2239–2240
in polycythemia vera, 2239–2240, 2240t
secondary, 2240
glucose-6-phosphate dehydrogenase deficiency
of, hemolytic anemia due to, 2233
injury of, in circulation, hemolytic anemia due
to, 2233
leukocyte-depleted, 647–648
optimization of production of, 663
packed, washed, 648
transfusion of. *See* Transfusion therapy, of red
blood cells
Reflex(es), central control of ventilation and, 205
Reflex control, of heartbeat, 243f, 243–244, 244f
Refractoriness, cardiac, 228–229

Refractory heart failure
advanced systolic failure, 1758–1759
clinical features of, 1758–1759
definition of, 1758
therapeutic goals for, 1759, 1759f
diuretics for, 1761–1762
extra-renal, 1762
fluid removal in, 1761–1762
Refusal of treatment. *See* Do-not-resuscitate
(DNR) orders; Treatment, refusal of
Refusal to cooperate, 2028
characteristics of, 2028
treatment of, 2028
Regional anesthesia, stress response and, 1028
Regression, 8, 8f
Regression analyses, 19–20
Rehabilitation Act of 1973, 114
Reimplantation response, lung and heart-lung
transplantation and, management of,
1329
Reintubation rate, as continuous quality
improvement indicator, 168t, 169
Relational operations, of microprocessor-
controlled ventilators, 716
Relative refractory period, 229
Reliability, 6
Renal abscesses, in pyelonephritis, 1653
Renal artery reconstruction, 1183–1184
fluid management and, 1183
hypertension management and, 1183
intestinal infarction and, 1183–1184
mortality and, 1184
renal artery graft stenosis/thrombosis and, 1183
Renal artery stenosis, pheochromocytomas and,
2135
Renal buffers, 926
Renal crisis, in systemic sclerosis, 2171–2172
Renal disorders. *See also specific disorders*
in acute respiratory distress syndrome, 1837t
antirheumatic agents as cause of, 2157t
candidal, 1688
drug-induced, 484
antibiotics and, 1563t
lithium and, 1494
electrical injuries and, 1539–1540
hyperkalemia due to, 425, 425f
liver transplantation and, 1347–1348
pharmacotherapy for, 478–481, 479t
creatinine clearance and, 479–480
gentamicin in, 480–481, 481t
following renal transplantation, 1308
in rheumatoid arthritis, 1244
in sepsis, 411
in systemic lupus erythematosus, 2169
Renal failure
acute. *See* Acute renal failure (ARF)
azotemia and. *See* Azotemia
following bone marrow transplantation, 1374
in burn patients, 1270
acute, 1270
burn wound as "third kidney" and, 1270
following cardiac surgery in adult patients,
1156–1157
continuous arterial venous hemofiltration
for, 1157
dialysis for, 1156–1157

Renal failure, following cardiac surgery in adult patients (*continued*)
  diuretics for, 1156
  following cardiac surgery in pediatric patients, 1172
  chronic. *See* Chronic renal failure (CRF)
  coma and, 1978
  contrast-induced
    acute, 2086
    thrombolytic therapy and, 1190
  drug dosage adjustments in, 2266t–2267t
  in hyperthermia, 1457
  near-drowning and, 1880–1881
  oliguric, in fulminant hepatic failure, 2051
  in pancreatitis, treatment of, 2058
  postshunt, 1124–1125
  in thyrotoxicosis, treatment of, 2142
Renal formulas, 2264t–2266t
Renal function
  following bone marrow transplantation, 1380
  colloid therapy and, 436
  in hyperosmolar states, 441t
  in hyperthermia, 1456
  in hypokalemia, 424t
  hypomagnesemia and, 432
  inhalational anesthetics and, 1018–1019
  following intestinal transplantation, 1360
  intestinal transplantation and, 1356, 1357
  intravenous narcotics and, 1022
  following multivisceral transplantation, 1360
  multivisceral transplantation and, 1356, 1357
  osmolality and, 439
  during pregnancy, 316
  shock and, 360, 371–372
  in surgical patients, 437–438, 438t
Renal injuries
  blunt, 1257f, 1257–1258, 1258f
  penetrating, 1259–1260, 1261f, 1262f
Renal injury scale, 2274t–2275t
Renal insufficiency
  following bone marrow transplantation, 1374
  digitalis poisoning and, 1498
  hypertensive emergencies and, 1817
  nutritional support in, 468
Renal replacement therapies
  choice of, 636–637
  essential procedures for, 631–632
  extracorporeal, 632–636, 634t, 635f. *See also* Dialysis; Hemodialysis; Hemofiltration; Peritoneal dialysis
    continuous, 634–636, 635f
    intermittent hemodialysis, 632–634, 634t
  initial therapy for, 632
  major problems with, 631
  renal physiology and, 632
  stress points with, 631
Renal transplantation (KT), 1301–1308. *See also* Simultaneous pancreas/kidney (SPK) transplantation
  cardiovascular disease and, 1305
  chronic problems associated with, 1308
  current status of, 1290
  diabetes mellitus and, 1305–1306
  diagnostic tests and procedures for, 1302–1303, 1303t, 1312
  gastrointestinal disorders and, 1306

  immunosuppressants for, 1303–1305, 1314–1315
    antilymphocyte antibodies, 1304–1305
    azathioprine, 1304
    converting oral drugs to intravenous form and, 1306
    cyclosporine, 1303–1304, 1304t
    mycophenolate mofetil, 1304
    steroids, 1304
    tacrolimus, 1304
  infections following, 1306–1308, 1609–1612, 1610f
    during first month, 1610–1611
    1 to 6 months after transplant, 1611–1612
  initial therapy for, 1303, 1303t, 1312
  living donors for, 1297–1298
  major problems with, 1301–1302, 1311
  medication interactions and, 1307t, 1308, 1308t
  minimization of infection in immunocompromised patients and, 1305
  organ allocation for, 1297
  stress points with, 1302, 1311–1312
  success rate of, 1312
Renin-angiotensin-aldosterone system, neurohormonal activation in advanced heart failure and, 1752–1753
Reperfusion injury
  intestinal, 445–446, 446f
  following lung and heart-lung transplantation, 1320, 1322f
Repolarization, 227–228, 228f
Research
  as ICU fellow's role, 39
  outcome, 128
Research literature. *See* Medical literature; Statistics
Reserpine, for thyrotoxicosis, 2140
Resident(s), junior, 36
Resident flora, 509
Resistive pressure, ventilation and, 190–191
Resource utilization, outcome prediction and, 130
Respiration. *See also* Breathing; Gas exchange; Ventilation
  in comatose patients, evaluation of, 1973, 1974f
Respiratory acidosis, 263, 922t
  venous, during cardiopulmonary resuscitation, 935
Respiratory alkalosis, 263, 263t, 922t
  with hypoxemia, blood gas analysis in, 926
  with metabolic acidosis, 261
  without hypoxemia, blood gas analysis in, 926
Respiratory depression, narcotic analgesia and, 817, 817t
Respiratory disorders. *See also* Pulmonary disorders; *specific disorders*
  anaphylaxis and, 1544, 1545t
  with burns. *See* Burns, respiratory problems with
  digitalis poisoning and, 1498
  infectious. *See also* Pneumonia
    fever associated with, 1593–1594
  lightning injuries and, 1541
  postoperative, sepsis and, 1112
  in spinal cord injury, management of, 1212–1213

Respiratory failure
  acute, 1917–1929
    antibiotics for, 1922
    bronchodilators for, 1920t, 1920–1922
    complications of, 1927–1929, 1928t
    corticosteroids for, 1922
    definitions and, 1918–1919
    diagnostic tests and procedures for, 1918
    etiology of, 1919
    heparin for, 1923
    hydration for, 1922
    ICU admission for, 1923
    initial therapy for, 1918
    major problems with, 1917
    mechanical ventilation for, 1925–1927, 1926t
    noninvasive positive-pressure ventilation for, 1923–1924
    nutritional support for, 1927
    in obstetric patients, 1414t, 1414–1415
    oxygen administration for, 1919–1920, 1920f
    pathophysiology of, 1919
    physical stimulation for, 1922–1923
    prognosis of, 1929
    respiratory stimulants for, 1923
    stress points with, 1917
    tracheal intubation for, 1924
    tracheotomy for, 1924–1925, 1925t
  following bone marrow transplantation, 1373
  in chronic renal failure, 2097–2098
  extracorporeal membrane oxygenation for. *See* Extracorporeal membrane oxygenation (ECMO)
  in Guillain-Barré syndrome, treatment of, 2009–2010
  in head injury, 1204
  hypothyroidism with, treatment of, 2145
  in myasthenia gravis, treatment of, 2014
  shock and, 371
Respiratory formulas, 2263t
Respiratory function
  barbiturates and, 1023
  benzodiazepines and, 1025
  inhalational anesthetics and, 1018
  during intrahospital transport, 791t
  intravenous narcotics and, 1021–1022
  ketamine and, 1026
  postoperative ICU care and, 1110
  during pregnancy, 316
  propofol and, 1024
Respiratory infections. *See also specific infections*
  infectious, fever associated with, 1593–1594
  respiratory failure and, 1919
Respiratory insufficiency, in pancreatitis, treatment of, 2058
Respiratory irritants, inhalation injury due to, 1953–1954
Respiratory management. *See also* Mechanical ventilation; Ventilatory support
  following cardiac surgery in pediatric patients, 1169–1170
  for fulminant hepatic failure, 2052
  intestinal transplantation and, 1357, 1357t
  multivisceral transplantation and, 1356
  vascular surgery and, 1179

Respiratory muscles, 191–193, 209–223, 210f.
   See also Diaphragm
  decreasing afterload of, 219–223
    following cardiac surgery in pediatric
      patients, 1169
    partial and total unloading and, 219–221,
      221f
    therapeutic objectives of, 219, 219f, 220f
    work of breathing components and, 221,
      222f, 223, 223f, 223t
  diagnostic tests and procedures for, 210
  fatigue of, 193, 193t
    central component of, 193
    impulse generation and contractile response
      and, 193
  loading of, 213–218, 215f
    breathing apparatus and, 215–216, 216f
    breathing pattern and, 217t, 217–218,
      218f
    energy supply and demand and, 216–217
    fatigue and, 216, 217f
    intrinsic positive end-expiratory pressure
      and, 214–215
    loading factors and, 213–216, 215f
    minute ventilation and, 214
    ventilator response time and, 216
  measurement of work of breathing and, 212t,
    212–213, 213f, 214f
    Campbell diagram and, 213, 214f
  stress points and, 209–210
  therapy for, 210
  thyrotoxicosis and, 2138
  tidal ventilation and, 191–192
Respiratory stimulants. *See also specific drugs*
  for acute respiratory failure, 1923
Restrictive drugs, 482
Resuscitation
  of burn patients
    of burn shock, 1267–1268, 1268f
    complications of, 1268–1269
    diuresis following, 1268
  cardiopulmonary. *See* Cardiopulmonary
    resuscitation (CPR)
  initial, 38
  initial triage of trauma patients and, 1042–1043
  for shock, endpoints for, 375–379
Reticuloendothelial system (RES), host responses
    and. *See* Host response,
    reticuloendothelial system and
Retinal lesions, in fat embolism syndrome, 1909
Retinitis, in HIV-infected patients, treatment
    of, 1619t
Retroperitoneal injuries
  delayed diagnosis of, 1054
  hematomas due to, 1094–1095
    central-medial, 1094–1095
    lateral, 1094, 1095
    management of, 1094–1095
    pelvic, 1094, 1095
Retroperitoneal lymphadenectomy, postoperative
    management and, 1255
Retroperitoneum
  definition of, 1077
  zones of, 1077
Revised Trauma Score (RTS), 55
Rewarming

core, invasive, 1454
  external, 1453–1454
  following ice water submersion, 1882
Rhabdomyolysis, 2195–2201
  acute renal failure due to, 2086
  cocaine abuse and, 1516
  complications of, 2196–2198
  diagnostic tests and procedures for, 2195
  drugs and toxins associated with, 2197t
  etiology of, 2198–2199
  in hyperthermia, 1456
  laboratory features of, 2199–2200
  major problems with, 2195
  stress points with, 2195, 2196t, 2197t
  therapeutic approach for, 2200–2201
    initial therapy and, 2196
  unusual presentations of, 2201
Rheumatic disease, 2153–2173. *See also specific*
    disorders
  antirheumatic agents for, 2156t–2157t,
    2156–2159
    for preexisting joint disease, 2158
    with pulmonary failure, 2158
    Raynaud's phenomenon and, 2158–2159
    sicca syndrome and, 2159
  cardiac, during pregnancy, 1393
  diagnostic strategy for, 2155
  diagnostic tests and procedures for, 2154
  early management of, 2155
  initial therapy for, 2154–2155
  major problems with, 2153
  preexisting, 2155–2156
  stress points with, 2153–2154
Rheumatoid arthritis (RA), 1243t, 1243–1245
  airway abnormalities and, 1244
  airway management in, 1245
  anemia and, 1244
  cardiovascular effects of, 1243
  cervical spine abnormalities and, 1244f,
    1244–1245
  hepatic effects of, 1244
  laryngeal abnormalities and, 1245, 1245f
  pain control in, 1245
  preexisting, 2158
  pulmonary effects of, 1244
  renal effects of, 1244
  side effects of medications used to treat,
    1243t
  vasculitis in, 2162
Rh-negative pregnant women, hyperimmune
    anti-D globulin for, 1425
Rhodococcus equi infections, in HIV-infected
    patients, 1624
  treatment of, 1620t
Ribavirin, 1571, 1700t, 1701
Rib fractures, 1138
Riboflavin, requirement for, 463, 464t
Rickettsial infections, 1682, 1703–1706
  antibiotics effective against, 1559t
  endemic typhus, 1703, 1705
  epidemic typhus, 1703, 1705
  Q fever, 1703, 1705–1706
    endocarditis in, 1793
  Rocky Mountain spotted fever, 1703,
    1704–1705
  transfusion therapy and, 656

Rifabutin, for *Mycobacterium avium* complex
    infections, in HIV-infected patients,
    1619t
Rifampin
  for infective endocarditis, 1795t, 1796, 1796t
  for *Legionella* infections, 1609, 1673
  for methicillin-resistant *Staphylococcus aureus*
    infections, 1661
  for *Mycobacterium avium* complex infections,
    in HIV-infected patients, 1619t
  for *Mycobacterium tuberculosis* infections, in
    HIV-infected patients, 1619t, 1620t
  prophylactic
    for bacterial meningitis, 1642t
    for *Hemophilus influenzae* infections, 1565
    for meningococcal disease, 1565
    for tularemia, 1708
Right atrial venous cannulation, 537
Right-sided heart dysfunction, following cardiac
    surgery in pediatric patients, 1168–1169
  pulmonary hypertension and, 1168, 1169t
  therapy of, 1168–1169
Right-to-left shunt, during pregnancy, 1395
Right ventricular ejection fraction (RVEF)
  for cardiac output determination, 895
  pulmonary artery catheters for measurement
    of, 860
Right ventricular failure
  heart transplantation and, 1337
  waveform analysis in, 858, 858f
Right ventricular function, decreased,
    spontaneous breathing and, 740
Right ventricular infarction, 392–393
  adjunctive and experimental management
    techniques for, 380
  diagnosis of, 1738
  therapy of, 1738
Rimantadine, 1571, 1700t, 1700–1701
  prophylactic, for influenza, 1566
Risk management, 175
Risperidone (Risperdal), for agitation and
    anxiety, 2025–2026
Rocky Mountain spotted fever, 1703, 1704–1705
Rotational therapy beds, 2214
Roxatidine, for aspiration prophylaxis, 1871, 1871t
RS-61443. *See* Mycophenolate mofetil (Cellcept;
    RS-61443)
Rubbing alcohol poisoning, 1503–1504
Rule-utilitarianism, 64

Saikewicz decision, 106, 108, 111, 120
Salgo v. Leland Stanford Jr. University Board of
    Trustees, 117
Salicylates. *See also specific drugs*
  for acute pericarditis, 1805
  poisoning by, 1486–1489
    clinical manifestations and diagnosis of, 1487
    toxicology and, 1486–1487
    treatment of, 1487–1489
Salicylate toxidrome, 1468, 1469t
Salicylic acid, therapeutic serum level of, 479t
Salmonella infections, 1670–1671
Salvageability, potential for, as medicomoral
    principle, 66

Samples
  paired versus independent, 12
  size of, 17–18
Sampling variations, 11
Saphenous vein, cutdown of, 569–570, 573f, 574f
Sarcomas, Kaposi's, in HIV-infected patients,
      1626
Satz v. Perlmutter, 108
Scalp
  lacerations of, 1200
  pH of, fetal, monitoring of, 1432–1433
Schloendorff v. Society of New York Hospitals,
      117
Scintigraphy (SCINT)
  abdominal
    gallium, 1597
    infections and, 1597
    leukocyte, 1597
  in deep venous thrombosis, 1894
  ^{131}I-MIBG, for pheochromocytoma
      localization, 2132
  lung perfusion, in chest pain, 1718
  thallium-201, in acute myocardial infarction,
      1740, 1743
Scleroderma. *See* Systemic sclerosis (SSc)
Sclerotherapy, for cardiac tamponade, 2250
Scoliosis, correction of, 1232–1233
  cardiopulmonary effects of, 1232–1233
    blood loss and, 1233
    cardiac impairment and, 1233
    lung mechanics and, 1232–1233, 1233t
  neurologic damage due to, 1233
  postoperative care for, 1233–1234
    infection and, 1234
    neurologic, 1233
    pulmonary, 1233
    vascular, 1233
  types of scoliosis and, 1232
Scorpion stings, 1532–1533, 1533t
Scrotal injuries, 1261–1262
Scyphozoa envenomations, 1533t, 1533–1534
  clinical manifestations of, 1533–1534
  treatment of, 1534
Sea anemone envenomations, 1533t, 1533–1534
  clinical manifestations of, 1533–1534
  treatment of, 1534
Sea hydroid envenomations, 1533t, 1533–1534
  clinical manifestations of, 1533–1534
  treatment of, 1534
Sea nettle envenomations, 1533
Seat belt sign, 1085
Seawater, aspiration of, 1877–1878. *See also*
      Drowning; Near-drowning
Second gas effect, inhalational anesthetic delivery
      and, 1015
Second Veterans Administration Heart Failure
      Trial (V-HeFT-II), 1755–1756
Secretin, for gastrointestinal bleeding, 2036
Sedation, 821–828
  agents used for, 825–828. *See also specific*
      drugs
    cost of, 827t, 828
  following cardiac surgery
    in adult patients, 1157–1158
    in pediatric patients, 1171

diagnostic tests, procedures, and therapy and,
      821–822
  indications and evaluation for, 822–823, 823t
    behavioral disturbances, 822–823, 823t
    for insecticide poisoning, 1507
    for intubation and mechanical ventilation, in
        asthma, 1940
  postanesthetic, 1030
    evaluation of, 1030, 1030t
    treatment of, 1030
  therapeutic goals for, 822
Sedative-hypnotic toxidrome, 1468, 1469t
Seizure(s)
  absence, 1987
  in bacterial meningitis, 1644
  brain injury and, 286, 1204–1205
  in comatose patients, treatment of, 1972
  ethanol withdrawal and, 1514
  generalized, 1982
  in hyperosmolar states, 441t
  in hyperthermia, 1457
  instatus epilepticus. *See* Status epilepticus
  with intracerebral hemorrhage, 2000t
  following liver transplantation, 1345
  partial, 1982
  in poisonings and toxic exposures, 1471–1472
    cocaine and, 1515, 1516–1517
    cyclic antidepressants and, 1490, 1492
    salicylates and, 1489
    theophylline and, 1501
  with subarachnoid hemorrhage, 2001t
    treatment of, 2001
  tonic-clonic, 1982
Seizuregenic toxidrome, 1468, 1469t
Selection bias, 7
Selective ventilation, pneumothorax and, 1962
Selenium, requirement for, 462t, 463
Self-extubation rate, as continuous quality
      improvement indicator, 168–169
Sellick's maneuver, 1870
Senile purpura, 2188
Sepsis, 405–411. *See also* Abscess(es); Infections;
      specific infections
  acute renal failure due to, 2086
  bacterial, thrombocytopenia due to, 2239
  catheters and. *See* Catheter-related infections
  clinical manifestations of, 408t, 408–409
  definition of, 406t
  diagnosis of, 409
  diagnostic tests and procedures for, 405
  epidemiology and etiology of, 406, 406t
  in fulminant hepatic failure, 2051–2052
  following hepatic resection, 1127
  in HIV-infected patients, 1628
  hyperdynamic, blood gas analysis in, 934
  intraabdominal, fever associated with, 1596
  major problems in, 405
  management of, 409–411
    hemodynamic, 409–410
    immunotherapy in, 411
    for infection, 409
    initial therapy for, 406
  mediators of, 407, 407t
  in obese surgical patients, 1281–1282
    predisposing factors for, 1281–1282

prevention and treatment of, 1282
  in obstetrical patients, 1406
  organ system dysfunction in, 407–408
    cardiovascular, 407–408
    multiple organ system dysfunction, 408
    pulmonary, 408
  pathophysiology of, 407
    cytokines and, 407
    initiating toxins and, 407, 407t
  postoperative
    evaluation for, 1112–1113
    warning signs of, 1112
  septic shock and, 367–368
    adjunctive and experimental management
        techniques for, 380
    in burn patients, 1269
    definition of, 406t
    severe, definition of, 406t
    stress points and, 405
    following transfusion therapy,
        immunosuppression and, 654
Sepsis syndrome, 141
Septal hypertrophy, asymmetric, during
      pregnancy, 1396
Septic arthritis, staphylococcal, 1660–1661
Septicemia
  catheter-related, 1578t
  listerial, 1668
Septic shock, 367–368
  adjunctive and experimental management
      techniques for, 380
  in burn patients, 1269
  definition of, 406t
Serendipitomania, 100
Serologic tests
  in infective endocarditis, 1791
  for neurologic infections, 1640–1641, 1641t
Serotonin toxidrome, 1468, 1469t
Serratia infections, 1671
Sertraline (Zoloft), side effects of, 2027t
Serum protein abnormalities, 2241
Serum sickness, drugs and, 1598–1599, 1599t
Severe sepsis, definition of, 406t
Severity of illness, outcome prediction and,
      129, 130t
Sex hormones, production of, 2123
Sharp injuries, 1443
Shearing injuries, to abdominal wall, 1085
Sheehan's syndrome, 2113
Shigella infections, 1671
Shingles. *See* Varicella-zoster virus (VZV)
      infections
Shock, 359–382
  acute respiratory distress syndrome and, 1827
  anaphylactic, 368
    adjunctive and experimental management
        techniques for, 380–381
  burn, resuscitation of, 1267–1268, 1268f
  cardiogenic. *See* Cardiogenic shock
  classification and clinical recognition of, 360,
      360t, 361t, 362f, 365–368, 390
  definition of, 365
  diagnostic tests and procedures for, 362
  distributive. *See* Distributive shock
  hemorrhagic, 1457

acute respiratory distress syndrome and, 1827

emergency transfusion in, 651–652

hypovolemic (oligemic), 365–366, 390

in trauma patients, 1048–1049

waveform analysis in, 858, 859f

major problems with, 359–360, 360t, 361t, 362f

management of, 373t, 373–381

adjunctive and experimental techniques in, 379–381

airway management and mechanical ventilation in, 374

endpoints for resuscitation and, 375–379

initial therapy for, 362–364, 363t, 364f

initial therapy for hypotension in, 374–375

laboratory and basic studies in, 375

in obstetric patients, 1416–1417

obstructive, 390

extracardiac, 367

pathophysiology of, 368–373

cellular injury and, 369

effects on specific organs and, 370–373

metabolic responses and, 370

neurohumoral responses and, 369f, 369–370

persistent, in trauma patients, 1050t, 1050–1052

pheochromocytomas and, 2135

prognosis of, 381–382

septic, 367–368

adjunctive and experimental management techniques for, 380

in burn patients, 1269

definition of, 406t

spinal, management of, 1211–1212

stress points with, 360, 360t

toxic shock syndrome and, 1659

"warm," blood gas analysis in, 934

Short ACTH stimulation test, 2127

Shoulder(s), epaulet area of, pain referred to, 1101

Shoulder replacement, complications of, 1235

Shunt(s)

for ascites, infections of, 1125

cerebrospinal fluid, staphylococcal infections of, 1662

for cirrhosis. *See* Cirrhosis

intracardiac. *See* Intracardiac shunts

intrapulmonary

for near-drowning, 1878–1879

venous saturation monitoring and, 916–917

"Shunt gas" analysis, following cardiac surgery in pediatric patients, 1170

Sicca syndrome, 2159

Sickle cell anemia, 2233t, 2233–2235

painful crisis in, 2233–2234

Sigmoid ischemia, following vascular surgery, 1111

Signal amplification, for invasive pressure monitoring, 844–845

Signal processing, for invasive pressure monitoring, 844–845

Significance, statistical. *See* Statistics

Signing out, 38

Silent disease, 1313

Silent ischemia, prevalence of, 899–900, 900t

Silicon tetrachloride, inhalation injury due to, 1954

Silver sulfadiazine (Silvadene) cream

for burn wounds, 1273, 1274

for toxic epidermal necrolysis, 2178

Simple partial seizures, 1982

Simplified Acute Physiology Score (SAPS), outcome prediction and, 144, 144t

Simultaneous pancreas/kidney (SPK) transplantation, 1311–1315

diagnostic tests and procedures for, 1312

immunosuppressants for, 1314–1315

initial ICU admission for, 1312–1313

initial therapy for, 1312

major problems with, 1311

secondary ICU admissions for, 1315

stress points with, 1311–1312

Single-lung transplantation (SLT), 1317–1330

indications for, 1317, 1318f, 1318t

initial management for, 1317–1320

immunosuppression and, 1318–1320

preoperative, 1317–1318, 1318t–1319t

postoperative management for, 1320–1330

acute rejection and, 1321–1322, 1324f

airway complications and, 1320–1321, 1323f, 1324f

bleeding and, 1320, 1321f

bronchiolitis obliterans and, 1323, 1325f

diagnostic tests and procedures for, 1325–1327, 1326f

diaphragmatic dysfunction and, 1323

infection and, 1322–1323

initial therapy and, 1327–1330, 1328f, 1329f

reimplantation response and, 1320, 1322f

stress points with, 1323, 1325

Single-photon emission computed tomography (SPECT)

in acute myocardial infarction, 1740

for cerebral blood flow monitoring, 947

Sinus bradycardia, 1783

Sinusitis, 2209

prevention of, 2209

treatment of, 1583

Sinus tachycardia, 1783

management of, 1784

sepsis and, 1112

Siolimus (rapamycin), for simultaneous pancreas/kidney transplantation, 1314

Skeletal muscle, potassium regulation by, 422

Skin

care of

around wounds, drains, and stomas, 2205

for obese surgical patients, 1281

damage to, tourniquets and, 1246

decontamination of, for insecticide poisoning, 1506

eliminating poisons from, 1473

in poisonings and toxic exposures, 1471

preparation for vascular cannulation, 511–514, 512f–514f, 522

Skin disorders, 2175–2192. *See also specific disorders*

in acquired immunodeficiency syndrome, 2191, 2191f, 2191t

anaphylaxis and, 1545t

antibiotics and, 1563t

antirheumatic agents as cause of, 2156t

brown recluse spider bites and, 1531

decubitus ulcers, 100–101, 2207

as continuous quality improvement indicator, 168t, 169, 174f

prevention of, 2207

treatment of, 2207

drug reactions, 484–485

electrical injuries and, 1540

immediate concerns with, 2175

infectious. *See also specific infections*

cryptococcal, 1689

streptococcal, 1663

petechiae, in fat embolism syndrome, 1909

wounds. *See* Wound(s); Wound infections; Wound management

yeast infections, 2207

Skull fractures, 1200

Sleep deprivation, 92–93

Small bowel injury scale, 2275t–2276t

Small intestinal injuries, 1092–1093

Smoke inhalation, 1266, 1948–1949

fiberoptic bronchoscopy in, 697

Smoking

cessation of, preoperative, 995

pulmonary function testing and, 989

Smooth muscle, during pregnancy

direct hormonal effects on, 319

at term, 317, 317t

Snake bites, 1524–1528, 1525f, 1526t

antidote for, 1466t, 1527t, 1527–1528

Social Security Amendments of 1972, organ transplantation and, 125

Society

bias against people with HIV/AIDS and, 1440

in decision-making process, 70, 73

societal values and treatment objectives and, 27–29, 28f

Sodium, 415–420

deficiency of. *See* Hyponatremia

excess of. *See* Hypernatremia

fractional excretion of, in prerenal azotemia, 2082

overload of, hypertonicity and, 443

reabsorption of, hyperkalemia due to, 425–426

requirement for, 461, 461t

Sodium bicarbonate

for cardiopulmonary resuscitation, 501–502

blood gas analysis and, 935–936

complications of, 502

dosage of, 502

indications for, 501–502

for diabetic ketoacidosis, 2104t, 2106, 2106t

for hyperkalemia, 427t

for hypotension, in cyclic antidepressant poisoning, 1491

for malignant hyperthermia, 1033t, 1600

prophylactic, for acute tubular necrosis, 2086

for sepsis, 410

Sodium iodide, for thyrotoxicosis, 2141

Sodium nitrate, for cyanide poisoning, 1466t

Sodium nitroprusside (Nipride; SNP)

actions, indications, and dosing of, 2271

following cardiac surgery

Sodium nitroprusside (Nipride; SNP), following cardiac surgery (*continued*)
  for reduction of ventricular afterload, 1152
  ventilation and, 1156
  following cardiac surgery in pediatric patients, 1168t
  for hypertension
    cocaine abuse and, 1517
    in hypertensive emergencies, 1813, 1814t, 1816, 1817, 1818, 1819
    following liver transplantation, 1345
    vascular surgery and, 1178–1179
  for pheochromocytomas, 2133, 2134t
  toxicity of, 1158, 1158f, 1159f
Sodium polystyrene sulfonate, for hyperkalemia, 427t
Sodium thiopental. *See* Thiopental
Sodium thiosulfate, for cyanide poisoning, 1466t
Soft tissue disorders
  infectious
    streptococcal, 1663
    wound management and, 782
  in obese surgical patients, 1281
Solenoids, of mechanical ventilators, 714t
Solvent toxidrome, 1468, 1469t
Somatosensory evoked potentials (SSEPs), for monitoring cerebral function, 946
Somatostatin, for gastrointestinal bleeding, 2036, 2037
Somnolence, in delirium, 2020
Sorbitol, for hyperkalemia, 427t
Sorenson autotransfusion system, 665
Sotalol, dosing of, in chronic renal failure, 2097t
Spasms
  bronchial, in asthma. *See* Asthma
  esophageal, chest pain and, 1724
  muscular, black widow spider bites and, 1529
  vascular. *See* Cerebral vasospasm
Spectroscopy, near-infrared, cerebral metabolism monitoring using, 952
Spinal abscesses, epidural, clinical presentation and initial diagnostic measures for, 1637–1638
Spinal block, total (high), 818–819
Spinal cord
  compression of, in cancer, 2249–2250
    clinical presentation of, 2249
    etiology and pathophysiology of, 2249
    radiologic investigation of, 2249
    therapy of, 2249–2250
  interruption of blood supply to, 818
  magnetic resonance imaging of, 980, 983f
Spinal cord injuries, 789, 789t, 1051, 1208–1215
  airway control in, 1209–1210
  cardiovascular effects of, 1210
  cervical canal alignment for, 1211
  cervical immobilization for, 1209
  delivery and, 1425
  diagnostic procedures for, 1197–1198
    initial, 1210–1211
  ICU management of, 1211–1215
    of cardiovascular disorders, 1213–1214
    of gastrointestinal effects, 1214
    of genitourinary problems, 1215
    initial, 1198, 1209
    of poikilothermia, 1214–1215

  of problems associated with immobilization, 1215
  of respiratory involvement, 1212–1213
  of spinal shock, 1211–1212
  tracheostomy in, 1213
  of vasomotor tone, 1213
  of venous thrombosis and pulmonary embolism, 1214
  intrahospital transport and, 800
  major problems with, 1197
  neurologic examination in, 1210, 1211f
  scoliosis correction and, 1233
  stress points with, 1197
Spinal puncture, 816
Spinal shock, management of, 1211–1212
Spinal surgery, complications of, 1232–1234
  cervical, 1234
  scoliosis correction and, 1232–1234
Spine, cervical. *See* Cervical spine
Spirochetes, antibiotics effective against, 1559t–1560t
Spirometry
  in inhalation injury, 1951
  lung and heart-lung transplantation and, 1327
  preoperative, 1003
Splanchnic flow. *See* Gastrointestinal system
Spleen
  asplenia and
    pathogens associated with, 1556t
    prevention of bacterial meningitis in, 1643
  injuries of, 1087–1088
    nonoperative management of, 1088
    scale for, 1084t
  sequestration of, acute, in sickle cell anemia, 2235
Splenectomy
  for idiopathic thrombocytopenic purpura, 2237
  overwhelming infection following, 1088
  for splenic injuries, 1088
  for splenic venous thrombosis, in pancreatitis, 2060
Splenic injury scale, 2273t–2274t
Splints, for fractures, 1221
Split-lung function studies, preoperative, 1003
Spontaneous augmented low-volume ventilation, 754
Spontaneous breathing. *See* Breathing, spontaneous
Spontaneous fetal movement, 1435
Spring decision, 120
Sputum cultures, for diagnosis of pneumonia, 1576
Stab wounds. *See* Trauma; *specific sites and injuries*
Staff. *See* Health care workers; Physicians; Team care
Standard deviation, for sampling variations, 11
Standing orders, for testing, deletion of, outcome prediction and, 132
Staphylococcal scalded skin syndrome (SSSS), 2178–2179
  diagnosis of, 2179, 2179f
  etiology of, 2179
  management of, 2179
  presentation of, 2179
Staphylococci, coagulase-negative, 1661–1663

  cerebrospinal fluid shunt infections due to, 1662
  endocarditis due to, 1661–1662
  peritoneal dialysis catheter infections due to, 1662–1663
  prosthetic valvular graft infections due to, 1662
  vascular catheter infections due to, 1662
Staphylococcus aureus infections, 1657–1661
  bacteremia due to, 1657–1658
  cellulitis due to, 1661
    orbital, 1660
  endocarditis due to, 1658–1659, 1792
    bacteremia differentiated from, 1792, 1792t
    treatment of, 1793, 1794t–1797t
  meningitis due to, 1660
  methicillin-resistant, 1661
  osteomyelitis due to, 1660
  pericarditis due to, 1660
  pneumonia due to, 1659, 1844
  septic arthritis due to, 1660–1661
  toxic shock syndrome due to, 1659
  of wounds, 1661
Staphylococcus epidermidis infections, endocarditis due to, treatment of, 1796, 1796t–1797t
Starvation, as adaptive response, 326–327
Static, low air loss beds, 2213
Static, steep Fowler's position beds, 2213–2214
Statistics, 6–8, 8f, 9–14
  descriptive, 9–10
    data types and, 9
    descriptive measures for quantitative data and, 10
    fourfold table for quantal data and, 9–10, 10t
    normal or Gaussian distribution and, 10
  inferential, 10–14
    background and objectives of, 10–11
    paired versus independent samples for comparison of groups and, 12
    sampling variations and SE and, 11
    tests of significance and. *See* Statistics, tests of significance and
  interpretation of study results and. *See* Medical literature, interpretation of study results and
  power of statistical tests and, 17
  significance and, 7–8, 8f, 14, 15t
    interpreting tests of, 15
    multiple tests of, 15–16
    reporting of, 16
    significance level and, 11–12, 14
    significance levels and, 6–7
    specific versus general use of, 15
  tests of significance and, 11–12
    data types and study designs for comparison of groups and, 13t, 13–14, 14t
    null hypothesis and, 11–12
    one- versus two-sided tests and, 12
    rationale for, 12
Status asthmaticus, fiberoptic bronchoscopy in, 698
Status epilepticus, 1981–1987
  absence, 1987
  complex partial, 1987
  convulsive

other than generalized tonic-clonic, 1986–1987
subtle, 1986
definitions and classification of, 1982, 1982t
diagnostic tests and procedures for, 1981
etiology of, 1982–1983
initial therapy for, 1981–1982, 1982t, 1983–1984
laboratory evaluation in, 1986
major problems with, 1981
myoclonic, 1986–1987
nonconvulsive, 1987
pathophysiology of, 1983
pharmacologic therapy for, 1984–1986
refractory, therapy of, 1982t
simple partial, 1987
stress points with, 1981
Steakhouse syndrome. *See* Esophageal obstruction
Steering committees, for continuous quality improvement programs, 164
Stem cell infusion, for bone marrow transplantation, 1369
Stenotrophomonas (xanthomonas) maltophilia infections, 1675
Stepper motor flow valve, of mechanical ventilators, 714t, 716f
Sterile preparation, for vascular cannulation, 522
Sterilization, recommendations for, 1631
Steroids. *See also specific drugs*
for heart transplantation, 1335, 1336
for intestinal transplantation, 1360–1361
for liver transplantation, 1345
long-term, problems with, 1308
for multivisceral transplantation, 1360–1361
for renal transplantation, 1304
Stevens-Johnson syndrome, 2176, 2177f
Stimulant toxidrome, 1468, 1469t
Stimulation, physical, for acute respiratory failure, 1922–1923
Stoma(s), 2205–2206
framing of, 2206
skin care around, 2205
Stomach. *See Gastric entries*
Stopcocks, for invasive pressure monitoring, 839, 840
Storage
of blood products, platelets, 650
of red blood cells, 646–648
Strength, of diaphragm, 211
Streptococcal infections
enterococcal, 1666
endocarditis due to, treatment of, 1793, 1796t–1797t
Group A, pneumonia due to, 1844
Group B, pneumonia due to, 1843
Pneumococcus
neurologic, epidemiologic and clinical clues to, 1636t
pneumonia due to, bacteremic, 1843–1844
Streptococcus agalactiae, 1664
Streptococcus milleri/intermedius group, 1665–1666
Streptococcus pneumoniae, 1664–1665
endocarditis due to, treatment of, 1793

neurologic, epidemiologic and clinical clues to, 1637
pneumonia due to, 1843, 1844
Streptococcus pyogenes, 1663–1664
Streptococcus viridans, endocarditis due to, 1791–1792, 1793, 1794t–1797t
Streptokinase (SK), 623, 623t, 1189, 1191, 1191t, 1729–1732, 1730t, 1731t, 1732f
actions, indications, and dosing of, 2272
for deep venous thrombosis, 1243t
fibrinolysis and, 271
Streptomycin
for bubonic plague, 1671, 1708
for *Mycobacterium tuberculosis* infections, in HIV-infected patients, 1619t, 1620t
for tularemia, 1707
Stress (emotional). *See also* Anxiety; Fear
of families, 89–90
of patients, 93
Stress (surgical), 1027–1029
cardiac output and oxygen delivery and, 1028
combined anesthesia and, 1028
general anesthesia and, 1027–1028
goal-oriented therapy for, 1028
intravenous narcotics and, 1022, 1022t
regional anesthesia and, 1028
Stress hemorrhage, treatment of, 2040
Stress ulceration, 2037–2040
etiology of, 2038
historical background of, 2037–2038
patients at risk for, 2038–2039, 2039t
prophylaxis of, 2039–2040
treatment of, 2039
choice of agent for, 2040
Stridor, 869
Stroke, 1990–1999. *See also* Cerebrovascular disease
anatomy and, 1991, 1991t
following carotid/subclavian reconstructions, 1182
diagnosis of, 1182
etiology of, 1182
incidence of, 1182
therapy of, 1182
clinical deterioration following, 1997t, 1997–1998
clinical evaluation of, 1993
as continuous quality improvement indicator, 168t, 170
differential diagnosis of, 1990t, 1990–1991
embolic, 1991–1992, 1992t
hemorrhagic, 1992t, 1993
hypertensive emergencies and, 1816–1817
laboratory investigation of, 1993, 1994f–1996f, 1995, 1997t
lacunar, 1992t, 1992–1993
management of, 1997–1999
acute therapy for, 1998–1999
basic principles of, 1997t, 1997–1998
pathogenesis of, 1991–1993, 1992t
in sickle cell anemia, 2234
thrombotic, 1991, 1992t
Stroke volume (SV), 861
analysis of, 851
Structured decision trees, for test selection, 132–134, 133t, 134t

ST segment monitoring, 899–907
advantages of, 901–902
definition of ischemic events and, 906
indications for, 902
lead placement for, 902–903, 903t
limitations of, 902
monitor setup for, 903–905
alarm units and, 904–905, 905f
measuring points and, 903–904, 904f, 905f
pathophysiologic basis of electrocardiographic changes and, 901, 901f
preoperative ischemia and, significance of, 900–901
silent ischemia and, prevalence of, 899–900, 900t
therapeutic options and, 906
troubleshooting alarm conditions and, 905, 905f
Studies of Left Ventricular Dysfunction (SOLVD), 1755
Studies of Left Ventricular Dysfunction Prevention Arm (SOLVD-Prevention), 1756
Study groups, selection of, 5
Stupor, in salicylate poisoning, 1489
Subarachnoid hemorrhage (SAH), 2000tm 2000–2002, 2001f
coma and, 1978
Subclavian catheters, chest radiography and, 969
Subclavian reconstruction, 1182–1183
antiplatelet therapy and, 1182
blood pressure and, 1182
chest radiography and, 1182
mortality and, 1183
neurologic assessment and, 1182
postoperative complications of, 1182–1183
Subdiaphragmatic abdominal thrusts, 493
Subdural catheters, placement of, 819
Subdural empyema, clinical presentation and initial diagnostic measures for, 1638
Subdural hematomas (SDHs), 1199
Subfalcine herniations, 1200
Subjective standard, 121
of disclosure, 81–82
Subluxation, atlantoaxial, in rheumatoid arthritis, 1244f, 1244–1245
Submersion injuries. *See* Drowning; Ice-water submersion; Near-drowning
Substance abuse and withdrawal, 1511–1519. *See also* Cocaine, abuse of; Ethanol, abuse of; Opiates, abuse of
diagnostic tests and procedures for, 1511
initial therapy for, 1511–1512
major problems with, 1511
smoking and
cessation of, preoperative, 995
pulmonary function testing and, 989
stress points with, 1511
Substituted judgment standard, 121
Succimer (Chemet), for metal poisoning, 1465t
Succinylcholine, 828–829, 830t
actions, indications, and dosing of, 2272
for airway management, 762
intracranial pressure and, 281
malignant hyperthermia and, 483
Sucralfate, for stress ulceration prophylactic, 2039

Sucralfate, for stress ulceration (*continued*)
  treatment of, 2040
Suction
  for snake bites, 1526–1527
  tracheal, following thoracic surgery, 1136
Sufentanil
  actions, indications, and dosing of, 2272
  cost of, 827t
Suffering, alleviation of, as medicomoral
    principle, 67
Suicide, assisted, 113–114
Sulfadiazine
  for *Nocardia* infections, 1608
    in HIV-infected patients, 1620t
  prophylactic, for bacterial meningitis, 1642t
  for *Toxoplasma* infections, in HIV-infected
      patients, 1620t
Sulfapyridine, for bullous pemphigoid, 2183
Sulfasalazine (5-acetylsalicylic acid)
  adverse effects of, 2156t–2157t
  for fulminant colitis, 2068
  for toxic megacolon, 2068
Sulfisoxazole, for *Nocardia* infections, 1608
Sulfur dioxide, inhalation injury due to, 1954
Sulfuric acid, inhalation injury due to, 1954
Superinfection, 1562
Superior mesenteric artery (SMA) syndrome,
    scoliosis correction and, 1233
Superior vena cava (SVC) obstruction, in
    cancer, 2248
  clinical presentation of, 2248
  diagnostic investigations in, 2248
  therapy of, 2248
Supervision, by ICU fellows, 39
Supraclavicular cannulation, 529t, 533–534,
    534f, 535f
  anterior scalene/first rib approach for, 534–535
  clavicular notch approach for, 536
  junctional technique for, 533–534
Supraventricular arrhythmias, 1783
  rate abnormalities and, 1783
  rhythm abnormalities and, 1783
Supraventricular tachycardia (SVT)
  following cardiac surgery in pediatric
      patients, 1171
  cardioversion for, 575
  diagnosis of, 1783
  during pregnancy, 1397
Surface tension, pulmonary compliance and,
    193–194, 194f
Surfactant replacement
  for acute respiratory distress syndrome, 1834
  for aspiration syndromes, 1867–1868
Surgeons, before development of ICUs, 35
Surgery. *See also specific procedures and
      disorders*
  abdomen following. *See* Postoperative
      abdomen
  antibiotic prophylaxis for, 1565
  aspiration pneumonitis and, 1869, 1869f, 1870t
  in cardiopulmonary resuscitation, 495
  elective, im myasthenia gravis, 2014
  evaluation for. *See* Preoperative evaluation
  hypertension during, 1819
  pain following. *See* Pain, postoperative
  stress due to. *See* Stress (surgical)

surgical critical care quality improvement
    model for. *See* Continuous quality
    improvement, for surgical critical care
Surgery team seniors, 36
Surgical attending physicians, 36
Surgical emergencies
  in hypothyroidism, treatment of, 2146
  in thyrotoxicosis, treatment of, 2142
Surgical hand disinfection, 509–510
Surgical patients. *See also specific disorders and
      procedures*
  acidosis of gastric mucosa in, 448–450, 449f
  anesthesia and. *See* Anesthesia; Inhalational
      anesthetics; Intravenous anesthetics
  decompensated diabetes mellitus in, 708, 2108t
  dextrose and water in, 437–438
    hyponatremia and renal function and,
        437–438, 438t
    lack of solute for urine formation and, 438,
        438t
  high-risk. *See* Preoperative evaluation, of high-
      risk patients
  obese, 1277–1284
    cardiovascular disease in, 1278–1279
    diagnostic tests and procedures for, 1277
    drug dosing for, 1282
    initial therapy for, 1277–1278
    major problems with, 1277
    nutritional support for, 1282–1284
    pulmonary disease in, 1279–1280
    sepsis in, 1281–1282
    soft tissue problems in, 1281
    stress points with, 1277
    thromboembolic disease in, 1280–1281
  postoperative bleeding in. *See* Hemorrhage,
      postoperative
  preoperative evaluation of. *See* Preoperative
      evaluation
  pulmonary function testing in. *See* Pulmonary
      function tests, perioperative
  stress response in. *See* Stress (surgical)
Surgical wound infections, 1581–1582
  abdominal, 1115
  fever associated with, 1595
  in renal transplant recipients, 1610
  vascular surgery and, 1181
    diagnosis of, 1181
    etiology of, 1181
    incidence of, 1181
    therapy of, 1181
Surrogates
  family as, 110
  health care surrogate designation form and,
      32–33
  refusal of treatment and, 108–111
Survival and Ventricular Enlargement Trial
    (SAVE), 1756
Suxamethonium, sensitivity to, 483t
Swelling. *See also* Edema
  with fractures, 1227
Sympathectomy, in spinal cord injury, 1213
Sympathetic nervous system
  antidiuretic hormone release and, 2117
  control of heartbeat and, 242–243
  neurohormonal activation in advanced heart
      failure and, 1752

Sympathomimetic agents. *See also specific drugs*
  during pregnancy, cardiovascular changes
      with, 1402
  for shock, 363, 363t
Synchronized coronary venous retroperfusion,
    611
Synchronized intermittent mandatory ventilation
    (SIMV), 723–724
  following cardiac surgery, 1156
  operational principles of, 723–724
  for respiratory failure, 1925, 1926t
  side effects and complications of, 741
Syndrome of inappropriate antidiuretic hormone
    secretion (SIADH), hyponatremia and,
    417, 418
Synergistic gangrene, abdominal, postoperative,
    1115
Syphilis, 1682
  transfusion therapy and, 656
Systemic inflammatory response syndrome
    (SIRS), 367
  multiple organ system failure and, 345, 348, 351
  nosocomial infections and, 1576
Systemic inflammatory response syndrome,
    definition of, 406t
Systemic lupus erythematosus (SLE), 2164–2171
  abdominal emergencies in, 2168
  cardiovascular disorders in, 2167–2168
  central nervous system disease in, 2169–2170
  classification criteria for, 2165t
  diagnostic tests and procedures for, 2154
  fever in, 2164–2165
  hematologic emergencies in, 2170–2171
  initial therapy for, 2155
  pulmonary disorders in, 2165–2167
  renal disease in, 2169
  stress points with, 2154
  vasculitis in, 2162
Systemic sclerosis (SSc), 2171–2173
  cardiopulmonary disease in, 2172–2173
  diagnostic tests and procedures for, 2154
  gastrointestinal disease in, 2173
  initial therapy for, 2155
  renal crisis in, 2171–2172
  stress points with, 2154
Systemic vascular resistance
  in heart failure, 1760
  in shock, 377t

Tachyarrhythmias, in thyrotoxicosis, treatment
    of, 2141
Tachycardia
  atrial. *See* Atrial tachycardia
  cardiac pacing for, 546, 547f
  junctional
    nonparoxysmal, 1783
    paroxysmal, 1783
  sinus, 1783
    management of, 1784
    sepsis and, 1112
  supraventricular. *See* Supraventricular
      tachycardia (SVT)
  waveform analysis in, 859, 859f
  wide complex, 1784
    management of, 1786

Tachypnea, 868–869
Tacrolimus (FK-506; Prograf)
  administration of, 1344
  elimination of, hepatic graft function
      assessment and optimization and, 1347
  for heart-lung transplantation, 1320
  for intestinal transplantation, 1360–1361
  for liver transplantation, 1344
  for lung transplantation, 1320
  for multivisceral transplantation, 1360–1361
  renal effects of, 1344
  for renal transplantation, 1304
  for simultaneous pancreas/kidney
      transplantation, 1314
Takayasu's arteritis, 2160
T cells
  defects of, 309t
  function of, 306–307, 307t
T-connectors, 513–514
Teaching, by ICU fellows, 38
Teaching rounds, 37
Team care, 35–47
  for burns, 1274
  communications and, 36–37
  decision-making process in, 69t, 71–73
  extracorporeal membrane oxygenation and,
      676f, 676–677
  factors contributing to collaboration and, 40
  fellows' functions and interrelationships in,
      37–39
  nursing care allocation and, 40–41, 41t
  nursing care functions and, 41
  nursing resource allocation and, 41–47, 42t,
      43t
  in special situations, 37
  team functioning and, 39–40
  team members and, 35–36, 36f
Technetium 99m isonitriles, in acute myocardial
      infarction, 1740–1741
Technetium 99m scanning, in acute myocardial
      infarction, 1741
Technology, treatment decisions and, 75
Teichoic acid antibodies, in infective
      endocarditis, 1791
Temazepam (Restoril), 825t
  for agitation and anxiety, 2026t
Temperature
  in aircraft, 806
  body. *See* Body temperature;
      Thermoregulation; *specific disorders
      of thermoregulation*
  Fahrenheit and Celsius conversions for, 2255t
Temperature correction, blood gas analysis and.
      See Blood gas analysis, temperature
      correction and
Temporal arteritis (TA), 2160
Temporal artery cannulation, 540t, 541
Temporary pacing. *See* Cardiac pacing
Tenderness, rebound, acute abdomen and, 1102
Terazosin, for pheochromocytomas, 2134t
Terbutaline
  for acute respiratory failure, 1920
  for asthma, 1937
  preoperative, 994t
Terminal patients
  futile care for

cardiopulmonary resuscitation as, 158t,
    158–159
  family insistence on, 114–115
  levels of care for, 119–122
    for competent adult patients, 120
    for no longer competent adult patients,
        120–121
    for pediatric patients, 121–122
  pediatric, levels of care for, 121–122
Tetanus, 1595, 1677–1678
Tetracyclines, 1568–1569. *See also specific drugs*
  for brucellosis, 1707
  for bubonic plague, 1671, 1708
  for bullous pemphigoid, 2183
  prophylactic, for plague pneumonia, 1565
  for Q fever, 1706
  for Rocky Mountain spotted fever, 1705
Thallium-201 scintigraphy, in acute myocardial
    infarction, 1740, 1743
Theophylline
  for acute respiratory failure, 1921–1922
  for asthma, 1938, 1938t
  dosage adjustment for, in hepatic disease, 482t
  poisoning by, 1499–1501
    toxicology and clinical manifestations of,
        1499–1500
    treatment of, 1500–1501
  prophylactic, for acute renal failure due to
      contrast agents, 2086
  therapeutic serum level of, 479t
  toxicity of, 1922
Therapeutic Intervention Scoring System (TISS),
    43, 57, 57t
  outcome prediction and, 135, 136, 137t, 138t
Therapeutic privilege standard, to informed
    consent, 118
Thermal injuries. *See* Burns
Thermodilution, 886–895
  in children, 894–895
  computation constant errors in, 893
  continuous, 895
  injectate systems for, 891–892
    closed, 891–892, 892f
    open, 891
    prefilled syringes, 891
  injection technique for, 891
  monitoring of, in head injury, 1203
  patient-related factors in, 893–894
    pulmonary artery blood temperature and,
        893
    rapid-volume infusions and, 894
    timing of injection and, 893–894
  preparation for, 888–889
    catheter position and, 889
    computation constant and, 888–889
    computer check and, 889
    patient positioning and, 889
  principle of, 886–888, 887f, 888f
  procedure for, 889–890
    computation constant and, 890
    injectate solution and volume and, 890
    injectate temperature and, 889f, 889–890
    thermodilution curve and, 890, 891f
  technique-related errors in, 892–893
    injectate temperature and, 892–893
    injectate volume and, 893

Thermoregulation
  brain injury and, 285
  disorders of. *See also specific disorders*
    in spinal cord injury, management of,
        1214–1215
  hyperthermia and, 1455
  hypothermia and, 1452
  mechanisms of, 1591
Thiamine
  for comatose patients, 1972
  deficiency of, coma and, 1977
  for ethanol intoxication, 1513
  for poisonings and toxic exposures, 468
    ethylene glycol and, 1503
  requirement for, 463, 464t
  for status epilepticus, 1982t, 1984
Thiazide diuretics, for diabetes insipidus, 421t
Thiopental, 825t
  actions, indications, and dosing of, 2272
  for airway management, 762
  pharmacokinetics of, 1022–1023, 1023t
Thiopentone, for cerebral edema, in fulminant
    hepatic failure, 2049
Thioridazine (Mellaril), for delirium, 2023
Thiotepa, for bone marrow transplantation, 1368t
Thiothixene (Navane)
  for agitation and anxiety, 2025
  for delirium, 2023
Third-party reimbursement, for organ
    transplantation, 124–125
Thirst
  osmolality and, 439
  sodium regulation and, 415
Thoracentesis, 553–556
  complications of, 556
  procedure for, 553–554, 554f, 555f, 556
Thoracic aneurysms, dissecting,
    echocardiography in, 884, 885t
Thoracic collections, drainage of, 593
Thoracic duct injuries, carotid/subclavian
    reconstructions and, 1183
  diagnosis of, 1183
  etiology of, 1183
  incidence of, 1183
  therapy of, 1183
Thoracic injuries, 1137–1143
  aortic rupture due to, 1141–1142
  cardiac contusions due to, 1140f, 1140–1141
  cardiac tamponade due to, 1142
  diagnosis of, 1137–1138
  diaphragmatic rupture due to, 1142
  empyema due to, 1143, 1145
  esophageal perforation due to, 1142
  flail chest due to, 1138–1139
  hemoptysis due to, 1145
  penetrating, 1141
  pulmonary contusions due to, 1139–1140
  retained hemothorax due to, 1143
  rib injuries due to, 1138
  tracheobronchial injuries due to, 1142–1143
  vascular, arteriography in, 1187
Thoracic surgery, 1131–1145. *See also specific
    procedures*
  cardiac arrhythmias following, 1145
  diagnostic tests and procedures for, 1132
  for flail chest, 1138

Thoracic surgery (*continued*)
  initial therapy for, 1132–1133
  major problems with, 1131
  preoperative considerations for, 1133
  for pulmonary cavitary lesions, 1144f, 1145
  pulmonary consultation for, 989
  pulmonary resections, 1143
  stress points with, 1131–1132
  tracheoesophageal fistulas and, 1143
  tracheoinnominate fistulas and, 1143
  for traumatic injuries. *See* Thoracic injuries;
      specific injuries
Thoracic vascular injury scale, 2279t
Thoracoabdominal region, 1077
Thoracoscopy, in thoracic trauma, 1138
Thoracostomy, closed-tube. *See* Tube
      thoracostomy
Thoracotomy, postoperative management of,
      1133–1137
  during immediate postoperative period,
      1134–1136
  routine care in, 1133–1134
  in unusual circumstances, 1136–1137
Thought patterns, in delirium, 2020
Thresholds, for continuous quality improvement
      programs, establishing, 164–165
Thrombectomy, surgical, for deep venous
      thrombosis, 1898
Thrombin, 271, 272, 696
Thrombin-sensitive factors, 269, 269t
Thrombin time, 270
Thrombocytopenia, 2226–2228, 2236–2239
  alcoholism as cause of, 2239
  autotransfusion and, 665
  bacterial sepsis as cause of, 2239
  bleeding in, 2236–2237
  bone marrow disorders as cause of, 2227, 2239
  in disseminated intravascular coagulation. *See*
      Disseminated intravascular
      coagulation (DIC)
  drug-induced, 1599t
    heparin and, 484, 2227–2228
    immune-mediated, 2226–2227
  immune, acute, in systemic lupus
      erythematosus, 2171
  in liver disease, 2222–2223
  platelet consumption and, 2227
  postoperative bleeding due to, 1069
Thrombocytopenic purpura
  idiopathic, 2226, 2237–2238
  thrombotic, 2238t, 2238–2239
    in systemic lupus erythematosus, 2171
Thrombocytosis, 2240
Thromboelastography (TEG), 1073, 1073f
Thromboembolism
  in Guillain-Barré syndrome, 2010
  in obese surgical patients, 1280–1281
    diagnosis, prevention, and treatment of, 1281
  with pelvic fractures, 1059
  pulmonary. *See* Pulmonary embolism (PE);
      Pulmonary thromboembolism
  in systemic lupus erythematosus, 2170
  venous. *See* Deep venous thrombosis (DVT);
      Pulmonary embolism (PE); Venous
      thrombosis

Thrombolytic therapy, 613, 622–626, 623t,
      1189–1191
  for acute myocardial infarction, 624t, 624–625,
      625t, 1728–1732
    choice of agent for, 1729–1732, 1730t,
      1731t, 1732f
    contraindications to, 1729
    heparin with, 1734
    indications for, 1728–1729
  administration of, 1189–1190
  for cardiogenic shock, 397–398
  complications of, 626, 627t, 1190
  indications and contraindications to, 1189,
      1189t
  with indwelling central venous catheters, 626
  intraoperative, 1190
  new trends in, 1190–1191, 1191t
  for peripheral vascular disease, 626, 626f
  for stroke, 1998
  for venous thromboembolic disease, 625, 626t
    deep venous thrombosis, 1243, 1243t,
      1897–1898, 1898f
    pulmonary embolism, 1900, 1901t
Thrombosis, 2229. *See also specific disorders*
  antithrombotic therapy for. *See*
      Antithrombotic therapy
  arterial, tourniquets and, 1246
  basilar artery, coma and, 1977
  at catheter site, thrombolytic therapy and, 1190
  invasive pressure monitoring and, 844
  of vascular grafts. *See* Graft thrombosis
  venous, in spinal cord injury, treatment of, 1214
Thrombotic stroke, 1991, 1992t
Thrombotic thrombocytopenic purpura (TTP),
      2238t, 2238–2239
  in systemic lupus erythematosus, 2171
Through the catheter (TTC) cultures,
      1577–1578, 1580
Thrush, 1686
  in HIV-infected patients, treatment of, 1619t
  treatment of, 2207
Thyroid disease, 2137–2148. *See also*
      Hypothyroidism; Thyrotoxicosis
  airway obstruction with, 2147–2148
  digitalis poisoning and, 1498
Thyroid function, in nonthyroidal illness and
      aging, 2146–2147
Thyroid function tests
  drugs affecting, 2146, 2147t
  in hypopituitarism, 2114–2115, 2115f
  in hypothyroidism, 2144
  interpretation of, 2137, 2138t
  in myasthenia gravis, 2013
  in thyrotoxicosis, 2139
Thyroid hormones. *See also specific hormones*
  for organ donors, 1294
  overdose of, treatment of, 2142
Thyroid-stimulating hormone (TSH), deficiency
      of, 2113, 2115
Thyroid storm
  diagnosis of, 2139
  presentation of, 2138–2139
  treatment of, 2141, 2141t
Thyrotoxicosis, 2137–2142
  diagnosis of, 2139
  immediate concerns with, 2137

  presentation of, 2137–2139, 2138t, 2139t
  treatment of, 2139–2142
    for concomitant surgical emergencies, 2142
    for congestive heart failure, 2141–2142
    general principles of, 2139–2140
    for iodine induced thyrotoxicosis, 2141
    pharmacologic, 2140
    in pregnancy, 2142
    in renal failure, 2142
    for severe concomitant medical illness, 2142
    for tachyarrhythmias, 2141
    for thyroid hormone overdose, 2142
    for thyroid storm, 2141, 2141t
Thyrotropin (TSH), deficiency of, 2113
L-Thyroxine, for hypothyroidism, 2144
  with coronary artery disease, 2145–2146
  in myxedema coma, 2145
Ticarcillin/clavulanate, cost and initial dosage
      of, 1562t
Ticlopidine
  in acute myocardial infarction, 1728
  for antiplatelet therapy, 614
Tidal ventilation, 191–192
Tidal volume control, for airway pressure release
      ventilation, 733–734, 734f
Time, clinical decision-making and, 55, 55f
Time-cycled ventilators, 712–713, 713f
Tissue binding, of drugs, in renal disease, 478
Tissue-type plasminogen activator (tPA), 623,
      623t, 1189, 1190, 1191, 1191t,
      1729–1732, 1730t, 1731t, 1732f
  actions, indications, and dosing of, 2272
Tityus serrulatus stings, 1532–1533, 1533t
T lymphocytes
  defects of, 309t
  function of, 306–307, 307t
Tobramycin, 1568, 1568t
  cost and initial dosage of, 1562t
  for infective endocarditis, 1793, 1795t
  therapeutic serum level of, 479t
Toluene diisocyante, inhalation injury due to,
      1955
Tonic-clonic seizures, 1982
Tonometry, gastrointestinal, 443, 450–452
  indications for, 451–452
  trouble shooting and, 451
Tonsillar herniations, 1200
Torsade de points, in antipsychotic poisoning,
      1495
Torsemide, for respiratory failure, in chronic renal
      failure, 2097–2098
Torulopsis (Candida) glabrata infections, 1689
Total artificial heart (TAH), 611–612
  following cardiac surgery, 1159
Total hip arthroplasty (THA), complications of,
      1234–1235
  blood loss, 1235
  pulmonary embolization, 1234–1235
Total knee arthroplasty (TKA), complications
      of, 1235
Total parenteral nutrition (TPN)
  for acute renal failure, 2090
  blood gas analysis in, 934
  following cardiac surgery in pediatric
      patients, 1174
  for intestinal transplantation, 1361

for multivisceral transplantation, 1361
during pregnancy, 1425
Total shoulder arthroplasty, complications of, 1235
Tourniquets, 1245–1247
acid-base changes and, 1246, 1246f
muscle ischemia and, 1246
paralysis due to, 1246
posttourniquet syndrome and, 1246–1247
skin damage and, 1246
for snake bites, 1526
venous embolization and arterial thrombosis and, 1246
Toxic epidermal necrolysis, 2177–2178
diagnosis of, 2178
etiology of, 2177, 2177t
management of, 2178
presentation of, 2178, 2178f
Toxic inhalations. *See* Inhalation injuries
Toxic megacolon, 2066–2069
clinical features of, 2066
diagnosis of, 2066–2067
management of, 2067–2068
patient monitoring in, 2068–2069
patterns of response to medical treatment of, 2069
during pregnancy, 2069
signs of impending perforation in, 2069
surgical treatment of, 2069
Toxic multinodular goiter, 2138
Toxicology. *See* Poisonings and toxic exposures; Substance abuse and withdrawal
Toxicology formulas, 2266t
Toxic shock syndrome (TSS), 1659
Toxidromes, 1468, 1469t
Toxoplasma gondii infections
in HIV-infected patients, 1626–1627
in renal transplant recipients, 1612
Trace elements, requirements for, 462t, 462–463
Tracheal injuries. *See also* Tracheobronchial injuries
tracheal intubation causing, 768, 1924
Tracheal intubation, 759, 759t, 764–769, 869
for asthma, 1939–1942
for mechanical ventilation. *See* Mechanical ventilation, for asthma
in cardiopulmonary resuscitation, 493
complications of, 767t, 767–769
after extubation, 769, 769t
during extubation, 769
after intubation, 768–769
during intubation, 767–768
contraindications to, 759
cuff inflation and, 869
endotracheal
complications of, 1837t
fiberoptic bronchoscopy for, 686–687, 689f, 697t
equipment for, 764–766
laryngoscopes, 764–765
tracheal tubes, 765–766
nasotracheal. *See* Nasotracheal intubation
orotracheal, techniques for, 766
with curved blades, 766
with straight blades, 766
techniques for, 766–767

nasotracheal, 766–767
orotracheal, 766
Tracheal obstruction, in cancer, 2248–2249
Tracheal suctioning, following thoracic surgery, 1136
Tracheal tubes, 765–766
Tracheobronchial injuries, 1142–1143
fiberoptic bronchoscopy in, 695t, 695–696
Tracheobronchoscopy, in thoracic trauma, 1138
Tracheoesophageal fistulas, following thoracic surgery, 1143
Tracheoinnominate fistulas, following thoracic surgery, 1143
Tracheostomy
complications of, 1837t
indications for, with burns, 1267
in spinal cord injury, 1210, 1213
Tracheostomy tapes, infections associated with, 2210
Tracheotomy, 769–770
in obese surgical patients, 1280
for respiratory failure, 1924–1925, 1925t
Traction, 1221–1223
cervical, 1223
skeletal, 1221–1223, 1222f
field, 1222, 1223
roller, 1222–1223
skin, 1221, 1221f
Traction helmets, infections associated with, 2210–2211
Train-of-four monitoring, of neuromuscular blockade, 831, 832f
Tranexamic acid (Cyklokapron), for gastrointestinal bleeding, 2037
Tranquilizers. *See also specific drugs*
major, for agitation and anxiety, 2025–2026
Transbronchial biopsy (TBB)
lung and heart-lung transplantation and, 1327
in pneumonia, 1853
Transcranial Doppler (TCD), 949f–951f, 949–950
in stroke patients, 1995, 1996f
Transcricothyroid ventilation, needle-catheter, for anaphylaxis, 1548, 1549f
Transesophageal echocardiography (TEE), 884–886
in aortic dissection, 1191
in dysoxia, 340
in pulmonary embolism, 1897
in thoracic trauma, 1138
Transfusion therapy, 639–656, 661–666
ABO incompatibility and, 1370, 1370t
for acute massive hemorrhage, 640–643
bleeding and clotting and, 643
estimation of acute deficit and, 641–643, 642t
initial therapy and, 641–643
mechanics of treatment and, 640, 641t
for autoimmune hemolytic anemia, 2232
autologous donation for. *See* Autotransfusion
following bone marrow transplantation, 1369–1370, 1370t
for chronic anemia, 644, 644t
complications of, 652–656
age of transfused blood and, 652, 1058
febrile, 1599–1600

hemolytic, 1599–1600
immunologic, 652–654
infectious, 655–656
massive transfusion and, 652
metabolic, 654–655
postoperative bleeding, 1071–1072
posttransfusion purpura, 654
pulmonary, 654
component therapies for, 647, 647t
of cryoprecipitate, 649
decreasing need for, 663–666
autotransfusion and, 663–665
blood substitutes and, 666
optimization of red cell production and, 663
passive blood loss and, 665–666
designated donation for, 648
desmopressin and, 651
diagnostic tests and procedures for, 662
for disseminated intravascular coagulation, 2221–2222
donor-directed, following cardiac surgery in pediatric patients, 1173
extracorporeal membrane oxygenation and, 674
of fresh frozen plasma, 648–649
indications for, 648–649
historical background of, 644–645
initial therapy and, 662–663
following liver transplantation, 1343
major problems with, 639, 661, 662t
massive transfusion and
coagulopathy due to, 2225
hemorrhage and, 2220t, 2224–2225
in trauma patients, 1057t, 1057–1058
of platelets, 649–651
for coagulopathy due to massive transfusion, 2225
collection for, 649–650
concentration and, 650
for disseminated intravascular coagulation, 2222
for platelet disorders, 2228
platelet function and, 650–651
of red blood cells, 645–648
dilution of packed cells and, 651
2,3-diphosphoglycerate and, 646
hemoglobin concentration and blood volume and, 645–646
rationale for, 645
storage and preservation for, 646–648, 647t
refusal of, 656
in sickle cell anemia, 2235
stress points and, 639–640, 661–662
for subacute blood volume deficiency, 643–644
causes of deficiency and, 643t, 643–644
diagnosis and, 644
transfusion and, 644
technical aspects of, 651–652
dilution of packed red blood cells, 651
for emergency transfusion in hemorrhagic shock, 651–652
incomplete crossmatched blood, 652
rate of administration, 651
for trauma patients, 1049, 1060–1061
Transient flora, 509
Transient ischemic attacks (TIAs), 1999. *See also* Cerebrovascular disease

Transient ischemic attacks (TIAs) (*continued*)
  following carotid/subclavian reconstruction,
      1182
    diagnosis of, 1182
    etiology of, 1182
    incidence of, 1182
    therapy of, 1182
Transjugular intrahepatic portasystemic shunts,
      for ascites, 1125
Transplantation. *See* Organ donors; Organ
      transplantation; *specific organs*
Transplant coordinators, 1295–1296
Transport
  capnometry during, 881–882
  exotic viral infections and, 1699t
  interhospital. *See* Interhospital transport
  intrahospital. *See* Intrahospital transport
  mechanical ventilation during, 738–739,
      739f, 739t
Transport beds, 793
Transport remote acquisition monitor (TRAM)
      system, 793, 794f
Transpulmonary gradient (TPG), of heart
      transplantation patients, 1334
Transthoracic cardiac pacing, 551f, 551–552
Transthoracic echocardiography (TTE), 884–886
  clinical applications of, 884–886
  in thoracic trauma, 1138
Transthoracic needle aspiration
  for diagnosis of pneumonia, 1577
  in pneumonia, 1853
Transtracheal aspiration, 580–581
  complications of, 581
  procedure for, 580, 580f, 581f
Transtracheal catheters, 705
Transvenous cardiac pacing, 548–551
  cannulation for, 549
  catheter position for, 549, 550f, 551
  pacing and sensing threshold determinations
      for, 551
  postinsertion care and, 551
  preparation for, 549
Transverse myelitis, in systemic lupus
      erythematosus, 2170
Tranylcypromine, side effects of, 2027t
Trauma. *See also specific injuries and sites*
  anterior pituitary failure caused by, 2114
  electrical. *See* Electrical injuries
  extracorporeal membrane oxygenation for,
      historical background of, 671
  host response to. *See* Host response
  hyperbaric oxygen therapy for, 780–781
  initial triage of, 1037–1043
    airway and cervical spine control in,
        1040–1041
    breathing assessment in, 1041–1042
    circulation assessment in, 1042
    diagnostic tests and procedures for, 1038
    disability assessment in, 1043
    exposure for, 1043
    fluid resuscitation and, 1043
    during in-hospital phase, 1039–1040
    initial therapy and, 1038–1039
    major problems in, 1037
    patient history and, 1040
    during prehospital phase, 1039, 1039t
    resuscitation and, 1042–1043

  stress points in, 1037–1038
  metabolic response to. *See* Metabolic response
      to injury and illness
  multiple, fractures and, 1226–1227
  in obstetric patients, 1419–1426
    acute abdomen and, 1424
    blunt, management of, 1423–1424
    delivery concerns and, 1425
    diagnostic tests and procedures for, 1420
    fetal diagnostic studies in, 1422–1423, 1423f
    initial assessment and management of,
        1420–1421, 1421t
    initial therapy for, 1420
    major problems with, 1419
    maternal brain death and, 1425–1426
    maternal diagnostic studies in, 1421–1422,
        1422t
    medications and, 1425
    penetrating, management of, 1424
    postoperative period following, 1424–1425
    stress points with, 1419–1420
    total parenteral nutrition and, 1425
  rhabdomyolysis due to, 2198
  secondary triage of, 1045–1061
    airway assessment in, 1047–1048
    blunt cardiac injury and, 1052
    bony injuries and, 1054
    breathing assessment in, 1048
    circulation assessment in, 1048–1049
    compartment syndromes and, 1052f,
        1052–1054
    completion of, 1050
    delayed diagnoses and, 1054–1058
    diagnostic tests and procedures for, 1046
    diaphragmatic injuries and, 1055, 1056f
    disability assessment in, 1049
    exposure for, 1050
    initial therapy and, 1046–1047
    intraabdominal hypertension and,
        1053–1054
    intraabdominal injuries and, 1055
    major problems with, 1045
    massive transfusion and, 1057t, 1057–1058
    mediastinal injuries and, 1055, 1057t
    monitor insertion and, 1050
    patient history and, 1047
    pelvic fractures and, 1058–1061
    persistent shock and, 1050t, 1050–1052
    retroperitoneal injuries and, 1054
    stress points with, 1045–1046
    vascular injuries and, 1055–1057
  submersion. *See* Drowning; Near-drowning
  thermal. *See* Burns
  tracheal intubation causing, 767–768
Trauma and Injury Severity Score (TRISS), 55
Trazodone, side effects of, 2027t
Treatment. *See also specific treatments*
  assessment of likely effects of, 53
  continued, clinical decision-making and, 57–58
  decisions regarding. *See* Clinical decision-
      making
  limitation of, critical care team's role in, 72
  long-term, clinical decision-making and, 58t,
      58–59
  refusal of, 68, 70–71. *See also* Do-not-
      resuscitate (DNR) orders
    courts cases involving, 107–110, 111–112

  informed consent and, 84–85
  legal issues related to, 119
  for poisonings and toxic exposures, 1475
  right of, 25
  of transfusion therapy, 656
  right to choose and refuse, 25
  short-term, clinical decision-making and,
      56–57, 57t
  termination of, acquiescence to family's wishes
      regarding, 113
  withdrawal of
    AMA policy on, 73
    court cases involving, 110–111, 112–114
    societal values and, 27–29, 28f
  withholding, 105
Treatment objectives, 21–34
  in absence of vital signs, 25–26
  advance directives and, 29–31
  affidavit and, 33–34
  bedside care and, 29
  beneficence, nonmaleficence, and distributive
      justice and, 24–25
  Durable Power of Attorney for Health Care
      and health care surrogate designation
      form and, 32–33
  economic issues and, 22
  family and, 26–27
  generic, 23–24
  health care proxy designation and acceptance
      form and, 31–32
  outcome prediction and, 131–134, 132t
  patient autonomy as, 25
  patient selection and, 22–23
  short- and long-term, clinical decision-making
      and, 54
  societal values and, 27–29, 28f
Treatment teams. *See* Team care
Treponema pallidum infections, 1682
Triage
  of cyclic antidepressant poisoning, 1492–1493
  of trauma patients. *See* Trauma
Triazolam (Halcion), 825t
  for agitation and anxiety, 2026t
Trichosporonosis, 1689
Tricuspid insufficiency, waveform analysis in,
      central venous catheters for, 853
Tricuspid regurgitation, 1776
  clinical presentation of, 1776
  diagnostic studies for, 1776
  etiology of, 1776
  pathophysiology of, 1776
  therapy of, 1776
Tricuspid stenosis, 1776–1777
  clinical presentation of, 1777
  diagnostic studies for, 1777
  etiology of, 1777
  pathophysiology of, 1777
  therapy of, 1777
Tricyclic antidepressants (TCAs). *See also*
      specific drugs
  poisoning by, antidote for, 1465t
  side effects of, 2027t
Tricyclic antidepressant (TCA) toxidrome, 1468,
      1469t
Trifluoperazine (Stelazine), for agitation and
      anxiety, 2025
Trihexyphenidyl (Artane)

for agitation and anxiety, 2026
for neuroleptic malignant syndrome, 828
Trimetallic anhydride, inhalation injury due to, 1955
Trimethaphan camsylate, for hypertension, in hypertensive emergencies, 1814t, 1815
Trimethoprim-sulfamethoxazole (Septra; TMP-SMX), 1569
for bubonic plague, 1708
cost and initial dosage of, 1562t
for heart-lung transplantation, 1319t
for infective endocarditis, 1795t
for *Listeria monocytogenes* infections, 1608
for lung transplantation, 1319t
for *Nocardia* infections, 1608, 1668
in HIV-infected patients, 1620t
for *Pneumocystis carinii* infections, 1607
in HIV-infected patients, 1620t, 1622
prophylactic
heart transplantation and, 1339
for *Pneumocystis carinii* infections, 1566
for renal transplant recipients, 1305
for urinary tract infections, 1652
Trimetrexate, for *Pneumocystis carinii* infections, 1607
Trimipramine (Surmontil), side effects of, 2027t
Trivalent equine antitoxin, for botulism, 1676
T tubes, following cholecystectomy, 1127
Tuberculosis. *See Mycobacterium tuberculosis* infections
Tube thoracostomy, 556–560
chest tube care and, 558
complications of, 558–560
indications for, 556–557
for pneumothorax, 1963f, 1963–1964
procedure for, 557f–560f, 557–558
suggestions for, 558
Tubing
for invasive pressure monitoring, 839
for parenteral nutrition, care of, 467
D-Tubocurarine, 829, 830t
Tubular necrosis, acute, acute renal failure due to, 2086
Tularemia, 1707–1708
Tumor(s). *See also* Cancer chemotherapy; Malignancies; Oncologic emergencies; *specific tumors*
pituitary, anterior pituitary failure caused by, 2113–2114
recurrence of, immunosuppression and, 654
Tumor lysis syndrome, acute, 2247–2248
clinical management of, 2247–2248
Tumor necrosis factor (TNF)
host response and, 292, 294
multiple organ system failure and, 347–350, 348t, 349f
regulation of metabolic responses to critical illness and, 332t, 333
Turbulent flow, 196
Twitch response, for evaluation of neuromuscular blockade, 831
Two-dimensional echocardiography, in acute myocardial infarction, 1741–1742, 1742t
2 X 2 tables, 9–10, 10t
Type I error, 16
Type II error, 16–17

Typhlitis, in cancer, 2250–2251
Typhus
endemic (murine), 1703, 1705
epidemic, 1703, 1705

Ulcer(s)
decubitus, 100–101, 2207
as continuous quality improvement indicator, 168t, 169, 174f
prevention of, 2207
treatment of, 2207
peptic
esophageal, in HIV-infected patients, 1629
renal transplantation and, 1306
stress. *See* Stress ulceration
Ulcerative colitis. *See* Fulminant colitis; Inflammatory bowel disease; Toxic megacolon
Ultrafiltration
for heart failure, 1762
for respiratory failure, 2098
Ultrasonography, 976–978
abdominal
for abdominal and pelvic fluid collections, 1597
for abdominal injuries, 1081
in acute abdomen, 1103
in biliary duct obstruction, 977–978, 981f
for dating pregnancies, 1422
for fetal assessment, 1423
gallstone detection using, 977, 980f
of kidneys, 976–977, 979f
pancreatic, 2057
in pregnancy, 978, 982f, 1422
sepsis and, 1113
in deep venous thrombosis, 1893–1894
Doppler. *See* Doppler techniques
duplex
in chest pain, 1718
for deep venous thrombosis diagnosis, 1242, 1242t
in percutaneous catheter drainage, 591–592
real time, for cannulation of central veins, 536–537
Uncal herniations, 1200
in comatose patients, 1979
Uncooperativeness, 2028
characteristics of, 2028
treatment of, 2028
Uniform Anatomical Gift Act, 124
Uniform Brain Death Act, 122
Uniform Determination of Death Act, 123, 1291
United Network for Organ Sharing (UNOS), 124, 1296–1297, 1358
Universal precautions, 1442–1443, 1443t
Upper/lower limit syndromes, 100
Urea, for intracranial hypertension, 1205
Uremia. *See* Azotemia
Ureteral injuries, penetrating, 1260–1261
Ureteral injury scale, 2278t
Urethral injuries
blunt, 1259, 1260f
with pelvic fractures, 1059
Urethral injury scale, 2279t
Urinalysis, for urinary tract infection diagnosis, 1582

Urinary catheters
in dysoxia, 340
urinary tract infections associated with, 1655, 2212
Urinary diversion, postoperative management and, 1256, 1256f
Urinary tract infections (UTIs), 1649–1655. *See also* Pyelonephritis
antibiotic prophylaxis for, 1565
cystitis, 1650
hemorrhagic, following bone marrow transplantation, 1372
diagnostic tests and procedures for, 1649
fever associated with, 1594
fungal, 1655
initial therapy for, 1650
major problems with, 1649
nosocomial, 1582–1583, 1654–1655, 2212
prostatitis, 1654
in renal transplant recipients, 1610
in spinal cord injury, management of, 1215
stress points with, 1649
Urine
acidification of, 1474
alkalinization of
for poisonings and toxic exposures, 1474
for rhabdomyolysis, 2200
for salicylate poisoning, 1489
blood in
in sickle cell anemia, 2234
following simultaneous pancreas/kidney transplantation, 1313
electrolytes in, 2265t–2266t
formation of, lack of solute for, in surgical patients, 438, 438t
intraperitoneal extravasation of, 1259, 1259f
output of
following cardiac surgery, 1155
by organ donors, 1294
proteins in, pheochromocytomas and, 2135
in shock, 372
volume of, in diabetes insipidus, 2117–2118
Urine culture, for urinary tract infection diagnosis, 1582
Urine free-cortisol excretion test, 2127
Urinomas, drainage of, 594
Urogenital injuries, 1256–1262
blunt, 1257–1259
to bladder, 1258–1259, 1259f
to kidney, 1257f, 1257–1258, 1258f
to urethra, 1259, 1260f
to external genitalia, 1261–1262
to penis, 1262
to skin and scrotum, 1261–1262
penetrating, 1259–1261
to bladder, 1261
to kidney, 1259–1260, 1261f, 1262f
to ureter, 1260–1261
Urokinase (UK), 623, 623t, 1189, 1190–1191, 1191t
actions, indications, and dosing of, 2272
for deep venous thrombosis, 1243t
fibrinolysis and, 271
Urologic surgery, 1253–1256
diagnostic tests and procedures for, 1254
initial therapy for, 1253–1254
major problems with, 1253

Urologic surgery (*continued*)
    postoperative management and, 1254–1256
        for lower abdominal procedures, 1255t, 1255–1256
        for upper abdominal procedures, 1254–1255
    stress points with, 1253
Urosepsis, 1651
Urostomy, ileal loop, postoperative management and, 1256, 1256f
Urticarial drug eruptions, 2187f, 2187–2188
Uterus
    drugs used to increase tone of, cardiovascular changes with, 1403
    during pregnancy, at term, 317
    rupture of, 1405t, 1405–1406
        diagnosis of, 1405–1406
        trauma and, 1423–1424
        treatment of, 1406
Utilitarianism, 64
Uvulopalatopharyngoplasty, in obese surgical patients, 1280

Vaccines
    for bacterial meningitis, 1642t, 1643
    for hepatitis, 1447
    influenza, for pneumonia, 1855–1856, 1856t
    pneumococcal, for pneumonia, 1855–1856, 1856t
    polyvalent, for renal transplantation, 1305
    for tetanus, 1677
    trivalent equine antitoxin, for botulism, 1676
Vagal maneuvers, arrhythmias and, 1781, 1782t
Validity, 5
Valproic acid
    for status epilepticus, 1987
    therapeutic serum level of, 479t
Values, societal, treatment objectives and, 27–29, 28f
Valvular heart disease, 1769–1778. *See also specific disorders*
    complicating, in critically ill patients, 1770
    critical illness caused by, 1769–1770
    echocardiography in, 885
    immediate concerns with, 1769
    multivalvular, 1778
    during pregnancy, 1393–1394, 1396. *See also specific valvular disorders*
    of prosthetic heart valves
        endocarditis, 1659, 1661–1662
    of right heart, thermodilution and, 894
    in systemic lupus erythematosus, 2168
Vancomycin, 1569
    for aspiration syndromes, 1868
    for bacterial endocarditis, 1658–1659
    following cardiac surgery in pediatric patients, 1172
    for *Clostridium difficile* infections, 1677
    cost and initial dosage of, 1562t
    for infective endocarditis, 1793, 1794t, 1796, 1796t
    for meningitis, staphylococcal, 1660
    for osteomyelitis, staphylococcal, 1660
    prophylactic
        for infective endocarditis, 1799t
        for surgical patients, 1010t

for *Rhodococcus equi* infections, in HIV-infected patients, 1620t
    therapeutic serum level of, 479t
Varicella-zoster virus (VZV) infections
    antibiotic prophylaxis for, 1566
    in bone marrow transplant recipients, 1614
    dermatologic, 2185–2187
        diagnosis of, 2186
        eczematous. *See* Eczema herpeticum
        etiology of, 2185
        management of, 2186
        presentation of, 2185–2186, 2186f
    encephalitis due to, 1694
    in immunocompromised patients, 1695
Varicelliform eruption, Kaposi's. *See* Eczema herpeticum
Vascular cannulation, 521–542
    analgesics for, 521–522
    arterial. *See* Arterial cannulation
    dressings for, 512
    essential techniques for, 522, 523f–524f, 525t, 526t
    informed consent for, 521
    patient preparation for, 521
    practical bedside approach for, 511
    protocols for, 511
    skin preparation for, 511–512, 522
    technique for, 512f–514f, 512–514
    sources of bacteria and, 510–511
    sterile preparation of operator and cannulation site for, 522
    venous. *See* Venous cannulation
Vascular catheters, 510–518. *See also* Arterial catheter(s); Central venous catheters; Pulmonary artery (PA) catheters
    following cardiac surgery, 1150
    dressing changes and, 514
    insertion of. *See* Arterial cannulation; Vascular cannulation; Venous cannulation
    for invasive pressure monitoring, 839
    maintenance of, 514
    semiquantitative culture specimens using guidewire exchange and, 515f–517f, 515–517
        guidelines for, 517–518
    subclavian, chest radiography and, 969
    T-connectors for, 513–514
    for transvenous cardiac pacing, 549, 550f, 551
    Vietnam, 570
Vascular disorders. *See also specific disorders*
    acute renal failure due to, 2085–2086
    magnetic resonance imaging of, 980–981
    in pancreatitis, surgical treatment of, 2059–2060
    peripheral, thrombolytic therapy for, 626, 626f
Vascular endothelial cells, in primary hemostasis, 266
Vascular function, in hypokalemia, 424t
Vascular injuries, 1187–1189. *See also specific injuries*
    arteriography in, 1187
        with extremity injuries, 1187
        with thoracic and neck injuries, 1187
    delayed diagnosis of, 1055–1057
    with fractures, 1227
    hepatic, 1086

    management of, 1187–1189
    radiologic interventions for, 590, 591f
    surgical complications and, 1187, 1187t
Vascular injury scale, thoracic, 2279t
Vascular resistance, systemic
    in heart failure, 1760
    in shock, 377t
Vascular surgery, 1177–1187. *See also specific procedures*
    abdominal, postoperative ICU care for, 1111
    cardiac monitoring and, 1178, 1179t
    circulation assessment and, 1178
    clinical features of atherosclerotic vascular disease and, 1178
    diagnostic tests and procedures for, 1178
    hypertension management and, 1178–1179
    initial therapy for, 1177–1178
    pain management and, 1179–1180
    problems related to, 1180–1182
        bleeding, 1180
        graft infection, 1181–1182
        graft thrombosis, 1180–1181
        major, 1177
        wound infection, 1181
    respiratory management and, 1179
    stress points with, 1177
Vasculitis, 2159–2164
    cerebral
        coma and, 1978
        in systemic lupus erythematosus, 2169–2170
    classification of, 2159, 2159t
    diagnostic approach for, 2163–2164
    diagnostic tests and procedures for, 2154
    differential diagnosis of, 2163, 2163t
    initial therapy for, 2155
    large vessel, 2159t, 2160
    leukocytoclastic, 2162f, 2162–2163, 2189f, 2189t, 2189–2190
    management of, 2164
    medium-size vessel, 2159t, 2160t, 2160–2162, 2162f, 2162t
    mesenteric, in systemic lupus erythematosus, 2168
    purpura due to, 2162f, 2162–2163, 2189f, 2189t, 2189–2190
    in rheumatoid arthritis, 2162
    small-vessel, 2159t, 2162f, 2162–2163
    stress points with, 2153–2154
    in systemic lupus erythematosus, 2162
Vasoconstriction
    drugs inducing, for gastrointestinal bleeding, 2036–2037
    mesenteric, 444, 444t
    pulmonary, hypoxic, 201
        inhalational anesthetics and, 1018
Vasoconstrictor tone, loss of, in spinal cord injury, 1213
Vasodilators. *See also specific drugs*
    following cardiac surgery in pediatric patients, 1166
    for dysoxia, 341
    for pheochromocytomas, 2134t
Vasogenic edema, cerebral, 278
Vasomotor tone, loss of
    in fulminant hepatic failure, 2051
    in spinal cord injury, 1213

Vasopressin
actions, indications, and dosing of, 2272
for diabetes insipidus, 421t, 2118
glycine, for gastrointestinal bleeding, 2037
Vasopressors. *See also specific drugs*
for hypotension, in shock, 379
for organ donors, 1294
Vasospasm, cerebral. *See* Cerebral vasospasm
Vasovagal response, 245, 245f
Vecuronium, 829, 830t
actions, indications, and dosing of, 2272
Vegetations
in infective endocarditis, 1791
Libman-Sacks, in systemic lupus
erythematosus, 2168
Venlafaxine (Effexor), side effects of, 2027t
Venography
contrast
ascending, in deep venous thrombosis, 1893
for deep venous thrombosis diagnosis, 1242
magnetic resonance, for deep venous
thrombosis diagnosis, 1242t
Venoms. *See* Envenomations
Venoocclusive disease, of liver, following bone
marrow transplantation, 1372t,
1372–1373
Venous access, in dysoxia, 341
Venous air embolism, 1907–1908
in obstetric patients, 1413
Venous cannulation, 522–538. *See also* Central
venous catheters
arterial route for, 537
bone marrow route for, 537
central, 524–536
clavicular approaches for, 529t, 532f–535f,
532–536
of external jugular vein, 529t, 530–531, 531f
of femoral vein, 526–527
of internal jugular vein, 527–530, 528t,
529t, 530f
peripherally inserted central venous
catheters and, 524–526, 526t, 527t
real time ultrasound for, 536–537
converting single to multiple lumina and, 538
endotracheal routes for, 537
penile route for, 537–538
peripheral, 522–524, 529t
right atrial, 537
for transvenous cardiac pacing, 549
Venous cutdown, 569t, 569–572
complications of, 571–572
procedure for, 569–571, 570f–573f
at ankle, 569, 573f
at antecubital fossa, 570–571, 574f
in groin, 569–570, 574f
Venous disorders, in pancreatitis, surgical
treatment of, 2060
Venous injuries, with fractures, management of,
1188
Venous oximetry. *See* Venous saturation
monitoring
Venous oxygen saturation (SVO_2)
derivation from Fick equation, 911, 911t
in dysoxia, 339–340
monitoring of. *See* Venous saturation
monitoring

in shock, 377t, 378
tissue oxygenation and, 930
Venous return, decreased, spontaneous breathing
and, 740
Venous saturation monitoring, 909–920
applicability of, 917
arterial venous oxygen content difference
and, 916
assessment of oxygen transport balance and,
911t, 911–912
following cardiac surgery
in adults, 1154
in children, 1164
clinical examples of, 918–920
clinical usefulness of, 912f, 912–916
cost effectiveness and, 915–916, 916t
interpretation and, 913–915, 914f, 914t,
915f, 915t
pitfalls and, 915
diagnostic tests and procedures for, 910
goals of, 909
initial therapy and, 910
intrapulmonary shunt and, 916–917
jugular
cerebral metabolism and, 951–962
in head injury, 1203–1204
normal range, units, and derivation for oxygen
transport terms and, 917
objectives of, 912
patient selection for, 909
physiology of oxygen transport and, 910–911
pulse oximetry combined with, 916
stress points with, 909–910
Venous thromboembolism, 1887–1901. *See also*
Deep venous thrombosis (DVT);
Pulmonary embolism; Pulmonary
thromboembolism
clinical features and diagnosis of, 1891–1897
future directions for, 1901
natural history of, 1881
prophylaxis of
heparin for, 616, 616t, 617t
warfarin for, 620–621
subclinical, 1888–1889
tourniquets and, 1246
treatment of
heparin for, 616–617, 617t, 618t
thrombolytic therapy for, 625, 626t
warfarin for, 621
Venous thrombosis, 1887–1894. *See also* Deep
venous thrombosis (DVT); Venous
thromboembolism
coma and, 1976
diagnostic tests and procedures for, 1887, 1888f
initial therapy for, 1887–1888
major problems with, 1887
of portal vein, surgical treatment of, 2060
in spinal cord injury, treatment of, 1214
splenic, surgical treatment of, 2060
stress points with, 1887
in surgical patients, prevention of, 1009
Venovenous extracorporeal membrane
oxygenation, 675–676
advantages of, 675, 676f
outcome with, 675–676
rationale for, 675

Ventilation, 924–926. *See also* Hyperventilation
alveolar
inhalational anesthetic delivery and, 1015
in obstetric patients, 1411, 1411t
$PaCO_2$ and, 924
assessing adequacy of, capnometry for, 880
bag-valve-mask, 495–496, 758–759, 759f
contraindications to, 759
during brain resuscitation, 281
central control of, 204–205
carbon dioxide and, 204
mucociliary transport and, 205
neural receptors and, 204
oxygen and, 204
reflex activity and, 205
collateral, 721
cricothyroid, for anaphylaxis, 1548, 1549f
dead space, 924–925
trending, capnography and, 931–932, 932f
distribution of, 201–202
airway resistance and, 201–202
pressure gradients and compliance and, 201
extremes of, respiratory muscles and, 192
illness and, inhalational anesthetic uptake and
distribution and, 1016–1017
maximal voluntary, preoperative assessment
of, 990
mechanical. *See* Mechanical ventilation;
Ventilators; Ventilator weaning
mechanics of, 190–191, 192f
minute, 214
clinical applications of, 729
mandatory, 729
operational principles of, 729
in pneumothorax, 1963
during pregnancy, 316
selective, pneumothorax and, 1962
tidal, 191–192
work of breathing and. *See* Work of
breathing (WOB)
Ventilation formulas, 2263t
Ventilation lung scans, in inhalation injury, 1951
Ventilation/perfusion (V/Q) lung scans
in chest pain, 1718
preoperative, 991–992
in pulmonary embolism, 1720, 1895–1896,
1896f
Ventilation-perfusion relationships, 199–202
distribution of pulmonary blood flow and, 200
lung zones and, 200
modifying effects of, 200
distribution of ventilation and, 201–202
airway resistance and, 201–202
pressure gradients and compliance and, 201
illness and, inhalational anesthetic uptake and
distribution and, 1017
problems with, with burns, 1267
pulmonary vascular resistance and, 201
hypoxic pulmonary vasoconstriction and, 201
pathologic factors and, 201
Ventilators, 712–719
complications due to function of, 1928
cycling mechanisms of, 712–713, 713t
flow and, 713
pressure and, 713
time and, 712–713, 713f

Ventilators, cycling mechanisms of (*continued*)
  volume and, 713, 714f
  inspiratory flow waveforms and, 713, 714t,
    715, 715f
  for intrahospital transport, 796–797,
    798t–799t, 800f
  microprocessor-controlled. *See*
    Microprocessor-controlled ventilators
  patient interaction with, pressure support
    ventilation and, 726f, 726–727, 727f
  in pressure support ventilation mode, 218
    therapeutic objectives of, 219, 219f, 220f
    titration of, 219–221, 222f
  response time of, 216
Ventilator weaning
  following cardiac surgery in pediatric
    patients, 1174
    circulatory support and, 1174
    delayed, 1174
    immediate, 1174
  failure of, sepsis and, 1112
  in respiratory failure, 1926–1927
Ventilatory failure
  acute, blood gas analysis in, 925–926
  acute-on-chronic, blood gas analysis in, 933
  chronic, acute alveolar hyperventilation on,
    blood gas analysis in, 933
  impending, blood gas analysis in, 926
Ventilatory support, 745–754. *See also*
    Mechanical ventilation; Ventilators;
    Ventilator weaning
  for aspiration syndromes, 1866–1868, 1867f,
    1867t
  in head injury, 1204
  noninvasive, 745–747. *See also* Bilevel positive
    airway pressure; Continuous positive
    airway pressure (CPAP)
  for organ donors, 1294–1295
  in spinal cord injury, 1212
  to unload respiratory muscles, 209, 210
Ventilatory support tubes, chest radiography
    and, 966–967
  esophageal intubation and, 967, 967f
  inadvertent bronchial intubation and,
    966–967, 967f
Ventricles. *See also* Left Ventricular *entries;* Right
    Ventricular *entries*
  vascular coupling of, 241–242, 242f
Ventricular afterload, 235–236, 236f, 861–862
  following cardiac surgery, 1152
    reduction of, 1152
  following cardiac surgery in pediatric patients,
    fluid therapy and, 1164
  left, spontaneous breathing and, 739
  spontaneous breathing and, 739
Ventricular arrhythmias, 1783–1784
  in advanced heart failure, as prognostic
    factor, 1755
  in chronic renal failure, 2096
  management of, 1785
  during pregnancy, 1397
  in rhabdomyolysis, 2198
Ventricular assist devices (VADs), 609, 611–612
  following cardiac surgery, 1159
  for heart failure

left ventricular, 1762–1763
  selection criteria for, 1763
Ventricular catheters, for intracranial
    hypertension, 1205
Ventricular couplets, 1784
  management of, 1785–1786
Ventricular defibrillation, 497–498, 498f,
    572–575
  complications of, 574–575
  energy level for, 498
  paddle placement for, 497–498
  precautions regarding, 497
  procedure for, 573, 575f
  technique for, 497
Ventricular fibrillation, 1784
  management of, 1786
    defibrillation for. *See* Ventricular
      defibrillation
Ventricular flutter, 1784
Ventricular function. *See also* Left Ventricular
    entries; Right Ventricular *entries*
  following cardiac surgery in pediatric
    patients, 1164
  echocardiography for assessment of,
    885–886, 887f
  mechanical ventilation and, 741, 741t
Ventricular hypertrophy, 1751
  neurohumoral determinants of, 1751
Ventricular independence, in children, 1163
Ventricular interdependence, 241
  spontaneous breathing and, 739
Ventricular preload, 234f–236f, 234–235, 861
  following cardiac surgery, 1151–1152
    fluid administration and, 1151f, 1151–1152
  following cardiac surgery in pediatric patients,
    fluid therapy and, 1164
Ventricular premature beats (VPBs), 1783–1784
  management of, 1785–1786
Ventricular septal defects (VSDs)
  cardiogenic shock and, 393t, 394
  during pregnancy, 1395
  surgical intervention for, 401–402
Ventricular tachycardia
  in cyclic antidepressant poisoning, 1491
  management of, 1786
    cardioversion for, 575–576, 577f
Ventriculitis, nosocomial, 1584
Venturi mask, for acute respiratory failure, 1920
Verapamil
  actions and indications for, 2272
  for arrhythmias, 1785
  dosing of, 2272
    in hepatic disease, 482t
  for pheochromocytomas, 2134t
  for thyrotoxicosis, 2140
Vesnarinone, for heart failure, 1757
Veterans Administration Heart Failure Trial (V-
    HeFT), 1755
Vibration, of aircraft, 807
Vibrio infections, 1675
Vidarabine (adenine arabinoside), 1700, 1700t
  for varicella-zoster virus infections, 2186t
Vietnam catheter, 570
Vinca alkaloids, pulmonary toxicity of, 2251

Viral infections, 1691–1701. *See also specific*
    infections
  antibiotics effective against, 1560t
  clinical epidemiology of, 1691, 1692t
  exotic, 1696, 1697t–1699t
  in HIV-infected patients, 1625–1626
  in immunocompromised patients. *See*
    Immunocompromised patients
  meningoencephalitis due to, 1647, 1647t
  pneumonia due to, 1691–1692
  transfusion therapy and, 655–656
  treatment of. *See* Antiviral agents; *specific drugs*
Viridans streptococci, 1665t, 1665–1666
Viscerocutaneous loxoscelism, 1530, 1531
Vision. *See also* Eyes; Ocular *entries*
  stroke and, 1991
Visual evoked responses, for monitoring cerebral
    function, 945
Vital capacity, 192
Vital signs. *See also specific vital signs*
  absence of, treatment objectives and, 21–22,
    25–26
  in poisonings and toxic exposures, 1470–1472
Vitamin(s)
  red blood cell production and, 663
  requirements for, 463–464, 464t
  vitamin A, requirement for, 463, 464t
  vitamin B. *See also* Thiamine
    requirement for, 464, 464t
  vitamin B_6
    for ethylene glycol poisoning, 1503
    for isoniazid and *Gyromitra* poisonings,
      1466t
    red blood cell production and, 663
    requirement for, 464, 464t
  vitamin B_{12}, red blood cell production and, 663
  vitamin C, requirement for, 463, 464t
  vitamin D
    calcium regulation and, 427–428
    requirement for, 463, 464t
  vitamin E, requirement for, 463, 464t
  vitamin K
    deficiency of, 2220t, 2223–2224
    for poisonings, 1465t
    requirement for, 463, 464t
Vitamin K-dependent factors, 268–269
Vocal cord paralysis, following extubation, 769
Volume-cycled ventilators, 713, 714f
Volume of distribution, 476–477
Vomiting, during pregnancy, 319
Von Hippel-Lindau disease, pheochromocytomas
    and, 2135
Von Recklinghausen's disease,
    pheochromocytomas and, 2135
Vulnerable period, 229

Waldenström's macroglobulinemia, 2241
Warfarin
  for antithrombotic therapy. *See* Antithrombotic
    therapy, warfarin for
  drugs potentiating action of, 2226, 2226t
  insensitivity to, 483t
  necrosis due to, 2226

overdose of, hemorrhage and, 2220t, 2225–2226, 2226t
for pulmonary embolism, 1899
"Warm shock," blood gas analysis in, 934
Washout syndrome, massive transfusion and, 2224–2225
Wasp stings, anaphylaxis and, 1545, 1546t, 1548
Water
  aspiration of, in near-drowning, 1863
  losses of
    in diabetic ketoacidosis, 2103
    hypernatremia secondary to, 443
  submersion injury and. *See* Drowning; Ice-water submersion; Near-drowning
Waterhouse-Friderichsen syndrome, 1667
Water intoxication
  in diabetes insipidus, 2118
  hyponatremia and, 417
  near-drowning and, 1883
  in surgical patients, 437–438
    hyponatremia and renal function and, 437–438, 438t
    lack of solute for urine formation and, 438, 438t
Water moccasin bites, 1525f, 1525–1528, 1526t
  antidote for, 1527t, 1527–1528
Weaning
  from extracorporeal membrane oxygenation, 674
  from ventilators. *See* Ventilator weaning
Wegener's granulomatosis (WG), 2156, 2161, 2162t
Weight loss, preoperative, 995
Weil disease, 1682
Wernicke's encephalopathy, prevention of, in comatose patients, 1972
West's zones, 855–856, 856f
Wheezing, in asthma, 1935
White blood cells
  effector functions of, host response and, 296
  host response and, 296
  interactions with endothelial cells, host response and, 296
Wide complex tachycardia, 1784
  management of, 1786
Wills, living, 29–31
Withdrawal

from cocaine, 1517
from ethanol, 1513–1514
Withdrawal of treatment
  AMA policy on, 73
  court cases involving, 110–111, 112–114
  societal values and, 27–29, 28f
Wolff-Parkinson-White (WPW) syndrome, during pregnancy, 1397
Work of breathing (WOB), 196, 734–737, 925. *See also* Respiratory muscles, decreasing afterload of; Respiratory muscles, loading of
  airway pressure release ventilation and, 750
  assist control ventilation and, 751
  bilevel positive airway pressure and, 747
  breathing apparatus factors affecting, 215–216, 216f, 734–735
  components of, 221, 222f, 223, 223f, 223t
  continuous positive airway pressure and, 731, 732f
    face mask, 745
    nasal, 746
  high-frequency ventilation and, 753
  imposed component of, 212, 212t, 213f
  inferred, 218, 218f
  intermittent mandatory ventilation and, 748
  inverse ratio ventilation and, 752
  measurement of, 212t, 212–213, 213f, 214f
    Campbell diagram and, 213, 214f
  physiologic component of, 212, 212t
  postoperative, 996
  pressure measurement and, 735f, 735–736, 736f
    cardinal pressure and, 735–736
    rationale for, 735–736
  pressure-support ventilation and, 749
  spontaneous positive end-expiratory pressure and, 731, 732f
  triggering inspiratory flow and, 736–737
    clinical applications of, 736–737, 737f
    flow and, 736
    modifications and, 736
    pressure and, 736
Wound(s)
  dressings for, 2204–2205, 2205f
    catheter-related infection prevention and, 1579

for vascular catheter insertion, 512, 514
problem, hyperbaric oxygen therapy for, 781
skin care around, 2205
Wound infections, 2204, 2204f
  fever associated with, 1595
  staphylococcal, 1661
  of surgical wounds. *See* Surgical wound infections
  tetanus, 1595
Wound management, 782–783, 2203–2204
  for burn wounds, 1273–1274
    depth of injury and, 1273
    excision of wound and, 1273
    topical treatment in, 1273–1274
  for closed wounds, 2203
  for contaminated open wounds, 102, 2204f
  foreign bodies and, 782
  hypoxia and, 782
  immunosuppression and, 782
  ischemia and, 782
  nutritional deficits and, 782
  radiation damage and, 782
  soft tissue infections and, 782
  wound care and, 782–783

Xenon-133 clearance, for cerebral blood flow monitoring, 947
Xenon-133 ventilation lung scans, in inhalation injury, 1951
Xenotransplantation, 1298
X-linked lymphoproliferative syndrome, in immunocompromised patients, 1695

Yeast infections, topical, 2207
Yellow jacket stings, anaphylaxis and, 1545, 1546t, 1548
Yersinia enterocolitica infections, 1672
Yersinia pestis infections, 1671–1672, 1708

Zidovudine (AZT), 1571
  prophylactic, for HIV infections, 1566, 1631–1632, 1632t
Zinc, requirement for, 462, 462t